source in 5 easy-to-use sections

VOLUME 2

MANUFACTURER PROFILES

Detailed company overviews.

Contact address, telephone and fax number
FDA number
E-mail and Web addresses
Medical sales and revenue
Year founded
Number of employees, salespeople, and marketing staff
Type of ownership or parent company
Stock symbol and exchange
Quality system adherence
Federal procurement eligibility
Methods of distribution
Key company executives
Product lines and medical specialty areas
Company subsidiaries

UTAH MEDICAL PRODUCTS, INC. 800-533-4984
7043 S. 300 W., Midvale, UT 84047 801-566-1200
FDA number: 0342734 *Fax:* 801-569-4195
E-mail: info@utahmed.com
Web site: www.utahmed.com
Medical Products Sales Volume: $27,200,000
Annual Revenue: $25-$50 Million
Year Founded: 1978
Total Employees: 240 *Marketing Staff:* 5 *Sales Staff:* 23
Ownership: UTAH MEDICAL PRODUCTS, INC.
Stock Symbol: UTMD
Traded On: NASDAQ
Quality System Registration information: ISO9000; ISO9001
Produces/Sells CE-marked Devices: Y
Federal Procurement Eligibility: Small Business, VA Contract
Distribution: Manufacturer Direct, Manufacturer Through Distributor, Manufacturer Through Manufacturer Reps, OEM, Importer, Exporter
Production: Marci Clawson, Mgr. Materials
John Smith/Dir. QA
Jean Teasdale/Dir. Eng.
General Admin.: Kevin L. Cornwell/President & CEO
Paul Richins/CAO
Mktg./Adv.: Kevin L. Cornwell/Dir. Mktg.
Mark Lanman/VP Sales
Ted Paulos/Mgr. Market Research
Ben Shirley/Dir. Product Dev.
Bruce WIlson/Mgr. Intl. Sales
Apryl Zapata/Dir. Natl. Accts
Research: Ben Shirley/Mgr. R&D

Amniotome	Obstetrics/Gyn
Aspirator, Infant	General
Blade, Electrosurgery, Laparoscopic	Surgery
Catheter, Continuous Irrigation	Surgery
Catheter, Intrauterine, With Introducer	Obstetrics/Gyn
Catheter, Intravascular, Percutaneous, Long-Term	General
Catheter, Umbilical Artery	General
Catheter, Urological	Gastro/Urology
Drain, Thoracic (Chest)	Anesth/Pul Med
Electrode, Other	General
Electrosurgical Equipment, General Purpose	Surgery
Electrosurgical Equipment, Special Purpose	Surgery
Endoscope And Accessories, Battery-Powered	Surgery
Extractor, Vacuum, Fetal	Obstetrics/Gyn
Hood, Oxygen, Infant	General
Injector & Accessories, Manipulator, Uterine	Obstetrics/Gyn
Kit, Labor and Delivery	Obstetrics/Gyn
Kit, Lumbar Puncture	Neurology
Kit, Urinary Drainage Collection	Gastro/Urology
Microfilter, Blood Transfusion	Anesth/Pul Med
Tube, Gastrointestinal	Gastro/Urology
Tube, Tracheal (Endotracheal)	Anesth/Pul Med

Medical Product Subsidiaries (Listed Separately)
UTAH MEDICAL PRODUCTS LTD.

GEOGRAPHICAL INDEX

Suppliers listed alphabetically by state and city.

KANSAS

Atchison
OCEANIC MEDICAL PRODUCTS, INC. 913-874-2000
8005 Shannon Industrial Park, Atchison, KS 66002

Belleville
PRECISION DYNAMICS MIDWEST 818-897-1111
814 K St., Belleville, KS 66935
SCOTT SPECIALTIES, INC. 785-527-5627
512 M St., Belleville, KS 66935-1546

Coffeyville
AMERICAN CRAFTSMEN, INC. 316-251-3340
P.O. Box 484, Coffeyville, KS 67337-0484

Council Grove
MONARCH MOLDING INC. 620-767-5115
120 Liberty St., Council Grove, KS 66846-1218

De Soto
SEALRIGHT CO., INC. 913-583-3025
9201 Packaging Dr., De Soto, KS 66018

Derby
ROTA SYSTEMS, INC. 316-788-4531
519 North Buckner, Derby, KS 67037

TRADE NAME INDEX

Trade names associated with their manufacturers.

SURGIPAK .... BARD, INC., C.R.
SURGIPATCH .... UNITED STATES SURGICAL CORP.
SURGIPEEL .... PILLING SURGICAL
SURGIPLAN .... ELEKTA ONCOLOGY SYSTEMS INC.
SURGIPORT .... UNITED STATES SURGICAL CORP.
SURGIPRO .... UNITED STATES SURGICAL CORP.
SURGIPULSE .... LUMENIS
SURGISAFE .... COLBY MANUFACTURING CORP.
SURGISEAL .... SURGICAL SEALANTS, INC.

31st Edition

Medical Device Register®

The Official Directory of Medical Manufacturers

Produced by UBM Canon

2011

Volume 1

Keyword Index

Product Directory

GREY HOUSE PUBLISHING

Medical Device Register®

DISCLAIMER: The information in this edition was obtained from medical device suppliers, the Food and Drug Administration (FDA), and other publicly available sources, including product literature, advertising material, annual reports, and financial prospectuses. While efforts have been made to ensure accuracy, the publisher makes no representation or warranty that the information is free of error, and specifically disclaims liability for any inaccuracy. Information on list prices was obtained directly from suppliers or their publicly available price lists. Users should verify product specifications and prices with the suppliers before making purchasing decisions.

The publisher does not make any representation, warranty, or guarantee concerning any of the products described herein. The publisher has not performed, and does not perform, any testing or analysis with respect to any of the products described herein. The publisher does not assume, and expressly disclaims, any obligations to obtain or include any information with respect to any product described herein.

ISBN 13: 978-1-59237-588-2 ISSN: 0278-808X

UBM
Canon

Grey House Publishing

4919 Route 22, PO Box 56, Amenia NY 12501
518-789-8700 • 800-562-2139 • FAX 845-373-6390
www.greyhouse.com • e-mail: books@greyhouse.com
Manufactured in the United States of America

Contents

Volume 1

How to Use the *Medical Device Register*
Advertiser Index

Section I—Keyword Index .... I-1 to I-256
An alphabetical cross-reference to the nearly 8,400 standard FDA/MDR product headings in the Product Directory section. Keywords include the words in the standard headings as well as synonyms and broader functional categories. Under each keyword, all associated product headings are listed in alphabetical order.

Section II—Product Directory .... II-1 to II-1 103
The most comprehensive compilation of medical products and their manufacturers. Provides sources for some 8,400 types of products and services. Gives each source's address, phone number, and, when available, product descriptions, prices, and specifications. Organized alphabetically by FDA/MDR standard product names, listed with associated codes.

Volume 2

How to Use the Medical Device Register
Advertiser Index

Section I—Manufacturer Profiles .... I-1 to I-975
Presents detailed information on approximately 13,000 North American manufacturers listed in the MDR. Gives company name, address, telephone and fax numbers, and e-mail and Web site addresses, plus method of distribution, type of ownership, and, when available, number of employees, date founded, annual revenue and medical product sales volume, quality system information, federal procurement eligibility, key executives' names, size of sales and marketing staffs, and names of subsidiaries. Also lists each company's products and the medical specialty areas with which the products are associated. Organized alphabetically by company name.

Section II—Geographical Index .... II-1 to II-143
Lists all manufacturers profiled in Section I. Organized alphabetically by city or municipality within each state. Canadian and Mexican manufacturers are listed alphabetically by company name at the end of the section.

Section III—Trade Name Index .... III-1 to III-139
An alphabetical list of more than 27,000 brand-name products and their manufacturers.

Section IV – Subsidiary Index .... IV-1 to IV-29
An alphabetical list of manufacturers and their subsidiaries..

How to Use the Medical Device Register®

The *Medical Device Register* is the most comprehensive directory resource to the North American medical device market. This brief overview of the content and organization of the *MDR* is designed to help you unlock the full potential of the vast array of data contained within these pages.

Despite its size, the *Medical Device Register* is designed for clarity and ease of use. The two-volume directory is divided into five sections.

VOLUME 1

Section I. The **Keyword Index** cross-references the medical device product names in the *MDR* by their associated attributes and applications.

Section II. The **Product Directory** is the core of the *MDR*, listing all manufacturers of each medical device, along with available product descriptions, specifications, and prices.

VOLUME 2

Section I. The **Manufacturer Profiles** section is the reverse of the Product Directory, listing all products available from each manufacturer, together with detailed information about each company.

Section II. The **Geographical Index** identifies manufacturers by geographic location.

Section III. The **Trade Name Index** identifies manufacturers of brand-name products.

These five sections are arranged in logical order of use. What follows is a more-detailed look at the features of each section.

VOLUME 1

Keyword Index

The Keyword Index lists device names under each of their component words. Thus, the user can find any FDA/*MDR* standard medical device name by looking up any of the words that appear in it. This allows you to find a device even if you don't know the exact wording of the standard name.

SAMPLE

	Keyword ↓	Device Name ↓	Medical Specialty ↓
	GALVANIC		
FDA/*MDR* Medical Specialty Code →	84GZO	Monitor, Response, Skin, Galvanic	Neurology
	89IPF	Stimulator, Muscle, Electrical-Powered (EMS)	Physical Med
Unique Device Identification Code →	**EMS**		
	89IPF	Stimulator, Muscle, Electrical-Powered (EMS)	Physical Med

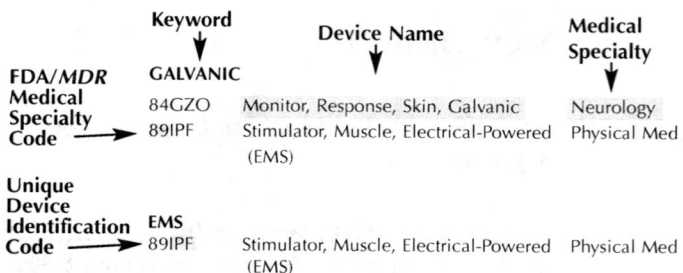

To the left of each device name in the Keyword Index is a 5-character code. This is the unique FDA/*MDR* code for each medical device and some manufacturer services. The code consists of 2 digits that identify the product's medical specialty area, and three alpha characters that identify the specific device. Together, these 5 characters supply a unique identifier for each medical device. This coding system is employed by FDA in processes for device regulation, manufacturer registration and listing, new-product approval, and product recall and risk notification. The codes are included in the *Medical Device Register* for use in inventory, filing, and ordering systems, and provide an interface compatible with current and future FDA data.

Across from the device name, the Keyword Index also shows the medical specialty area to which the device has been assigned. This information helps to confirm that you have found the correct device. It is also useful in accessing device-related FDA information, which is organized by medical specialty. However, a device's use is not necessarily limited to its officially designated specialty area. Although each device is assigned to a particular specialty's panel of experts for regulatory purposes, it may be used in other medical specialties as well. There are 19 medical specialties, corresponding to the FDA's 19 expert panels.

Due to space limitations, some medical specialty names are abbreviated in the *MDR*. The full FDA panel names, the versions used in *MDR*, and the 2-digit numeric codes, are as follows:

Medical Products

Anesth/Pul Med (73)................Anesthesiology and Pulmonary Medicine
Cardiovascular (74) ....Cardiovascular

Dental (76) ....Dental
Ear/Nose/Throat (77).............Ear, Nose, and Throat
Gastro/Urology (78) ....Gastroenterology and Urology
General (80)..........................General Hospital and Personal Use
Neurology (84).......................................Neurology
Obstetrics/Gyn (85).........................Obstetrics and Gynecology
Ophthalmic (86) ....Ophthalmic
Orthopedics (87) ....Orthopedics
Physical Med (89) ....Physical Medicine
Radiology (90) ....Radiology
Surgery (79)................General and Plastic Surgery

In Vitro Diagnostic Products

Chemistry (75) ....Chemistry
Hematology (81)..................................Hematology
Immunology (82) ....Immunology
Microbiology (83).............................Microbiology
Pathology (88)...Pathology
Toxicology (91).....................................Toxicology

Once you have found the correct FDA/*MDR* standard medical device name in the Keyword Index, you can turn to the corresponding entry in the Product Directory to identify manufacturers of the device.

Product Directory

This is the heart of the *MDR,* listing every manufacturer of each device or service. It is organized alphabetically by product or service name. If you cannot find a product in this section, it is probably because the FDA/*MDR* standard name is worded differently than the name you are looking for. Check the Keyword Index for the official FDA/*MDR* wording of the name, then turn to the corresponding entry in the Product Directory.

Alongside each device name in the Product Directory is the medical specialty area to which it's assigned, plus its unique 5-character FDA/*MDR* code. This information is followed by each of the product's manufacturers listed alphabetically, including manufacturer name, address, and telephone number.

Whenever possible, toll-free numbers are listed so that users can obtain additional product information at no cost.

SAMPLE

Device Name

Medical Specialty/Device Code — **STIMULATOR, MUSCLE, ELECTRICAL-POWERED (EMS)**
(Physical Med) 89IPF
BIODEX MEDICAL SYSTEMS, INC. — 800-224-6339 (**Toll-Free Telephone Number**)
20 Ramsay Rd.
Shirley, NY 11967-0702 — **Address**

Company Name

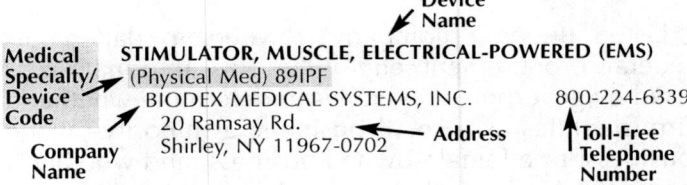

Each manufacturer's listing also includes, when available, the product's specifications and list price. The price given is based on the manufacturer's list price to hospitals for the quantity and features shown in the specs. (Actual prices vary based on quantity, special features, availability, and other factors, so you should always check with each prospective supplier before making a purchase.)

Product specifications include a variety of information. In general, the data will help you identify those manufacturers most likely to meet your needs.

Additional information on each supplier can be found in the Manufacturer Profiles section.

VOLUME 2

Manufacturer Profiles

This section contains in-depth information on all manufacturers. Entries are in alphabetical order by company name. Each name is accompanied by the manufacturer's address, telephone number, and fax number. When available, a toll-free number is included.

Beneath the company's name and address appears a 7-digit number. This is the manufacturer's unique FDA number. Like the 5-character FDA/*MDR* product code found in the Product Directory section, this number is part of FDA's system of medical device regulation, including establishment registration, manufacturing plant inspection, product approval, and product recall notification. The numbers are included in the *Medical Device Register* to help users maintain compatibility of internal data processing and filing systems with FDA.

Under the FDA number, you'll find the company's Web-site and e-mail addresses, followed by its medical-product sales volume, annual revenue, year founded, number of employees, and size of sales and marketing staffs. If the company produces CE-marked products or has a quality system in place, this is indicated as well. For publicly traded companies, stock symbols and the exchange on which the stock is traded are also reported.

Listed under a company's ownership data is its federal procurement eligibility. This information is used by government agencies to determine whether a firm qualifies as a small business, a minority-owned business, or a female-owned business, and whether it has a GSA (General Services Administration) or VA (Veterans Administration) contract.

The next field of information concerns a manufacturer's method of distributing its products. The main alternatives and their explanations are as follows:

- "Manufacturer Direct"—These companies manufacture most of their own products, and are interested in selling directly to the end user. Their products may also be available through distributors, but they would prefer to have new customers contact them directly, to be served either by the manufacturer's own employees or by a distributor assigned by the manufacturer.

- "Manufacturer through Distributor"—These companies also manufacture most of their own products, but generally prefer not to deal directly with end users. Unless negotiating a volume discount, new end users interested in these manufacturers' products should contact a local medical products distributor.

- "Exclusive Distributor"—While these companies may manufacture some of their own products, they are primarily distributors. Furthermore, each is the exclusive distributor of the products listed in its entry. End users should contact these firms directly for information on the devices they supply.

Additional distribution options can be selected by firms serving as OEMs, by those providing primarily manufacturing services, and by importers or exporters.

Also included in each manufacturer's profile are the names of several key executives, enabling you to more easily contact the appropriate individual or department for further information or quotations.

This information is followed by an alphabetical list of all medical products supplied by the company. These are the same product names under which the manufacturer is listed in the Product Directory. Across from each name is the medical specialty area associated with the product. This summary product information gives an overview of the manufacturer—how many products it offers, which medical specialties it services, and which specific products it supplies.

At the end of the company's listing are the names of any subsidiaries also listed in the *MDR*. If you cannot locate a product under the parent company's name, you should check under those of any subsidiaries. This list of subsidiaries can also be a useful indication of the total capability of the company, and may be helpful in negotiating corporate discounts based on purchases from several divisions.

Please note that complete information on each product is not contained in this section; you must turn to the appropriate entry in the Product Directory section to obtain such information, if it has been supplied. This more-detailed information in the Product Directory may clarify what the company actually offers in a given category.

Geographical Index

This index cross-references the companies presented in the Manufacturer Profiles section by their geographic location. You can use this index to identify local manufacturers or to coordinate visits to manufacturers in a particular area. Companies are listed alphabetically by state, and then by city or municipality within the state. Canadian and Mexican manufacturers are listed alphabetically by company name at the end of the section.

Trade Name Index

If you are looking for the supplier of a specific trade-named product, and the trade name is different from the manufacturer's name, the Trade Name Index is the fastest way of identifying the company.

Trade names, with the corresponding manufacturer names, are listed alphabetically. Additional information on each supplier can be found in the Manufacturer Profiles section.

Advertiser Index

A notation of a product category and page number indicates an enhanced listing in that category or display ad near the category.

SECTION I

KEYWORD INDEX

PURPOSE OF THIS SECTION

To help you find the correct FDA/*MDR* standard medical product name by referencing terms that might appear in the name, or that might relate to the name.

FEATURES

- Each of the 7,860 FDA/*MDR* standard medical product names is listed multiple times in this section. Each name is listed under the words (keywords) that appear in its name; for example, under the keyword "ULTRASONIC," all products using that technology are listed.

- Product names are also listed under alternative common names for the same products; for example, under the keyword "TIMER" is listed "Analyzer, Coagulation." In addition, product names are grouped under functional categories. Under the keyword "ENGINEERING," for example, all biomedical engineering devices are listed. Similar groupings are made under "HOME-USE," "TEST," "IMPLANT," "CLOTHING," "FURNITURE," and other categories.

- Wherever each FDA/*MDR* standard medical product name is used, the medical specialty panel the product is assigned to is shown opposite the name. For example, opposite "Cannula, Arterial" appears the specialty panel "Cardiovascular."

- Also, preceding each medical product name is the five-character FDA/*MDR* code for that product. These codes are used in automated systems.

- In general, the format for the FDA/*MDR* standard product names is "NOUN, KEY ADJECTIVE, NEXT KEY ADJECTIVE," etc. This allows for grouping of common product names together alphabetically in this and the Product Directory section; for example, "Monitors" appear together, and within that type of product, all the "Monitors, Blood Gas" appear together.

Health Resources from Grey House Publishing

The HMO/PPO Directory

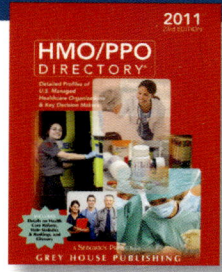

This comprehensive directory details more information about more managed health care organizations than ever before. Over 1,100 HMOs, PPOs and affiliated companies are listed, arranged alphabetically by state. Detailed listings include Key Contact Information, Drug Benefits, Enrollment, Geographical Areas served, Affiliated Physicians & Hospitals, Federal Qualifications, Status, Year Founded, Managed Care Partners, Employer References, Fees & Payment Information and more. *The HMO/PPO Directory* provides the most comprehensive information on the most companies available on the market place today.

600 pages; Softcover ISBN 978-1-59237-587-5, $325.00
Online & Directory Combo: $800.00
Online Database (Single User): $650.00

Medical Device Register

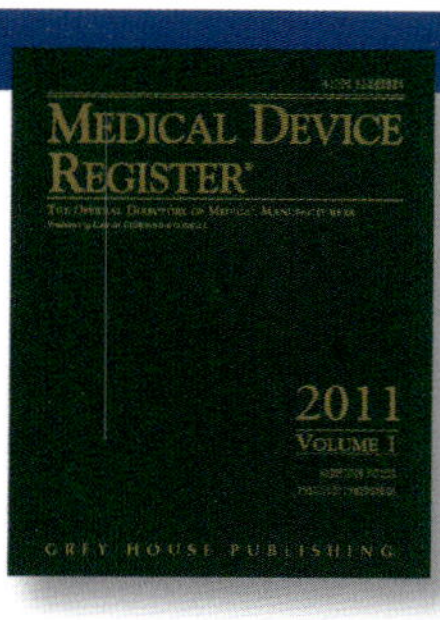

Offers fast access to over 13,000 companies - and more than 65,000 products. Volume I: Products, provides the essential information you need when purchasing or specifying medical supplies on every medical device, supply, and diagnostic available in the US. Listings provide FDA codes, Federal Procurement Eligibility, Contact information, Prices and Product Specifications. Volume 2: Suppliers, details the most complete and important data about Suppliers, Manufacturers and Distributors, with Key Executives, Contact Information along with their medical products and specialties. *Medical Device Register* is your only one-stop source for locating suppliers and products; looking for new manufacturers or hard-to-find medical devices; comparing products; know who's selling what and who to buy from cost effectively.

3,000 pages; Two Volumes; Hardcover ISBN 978-1-59237-588-2, $350.00
Online Database & Print Combo, $1,295.00

The Directory of Hospital Personnel

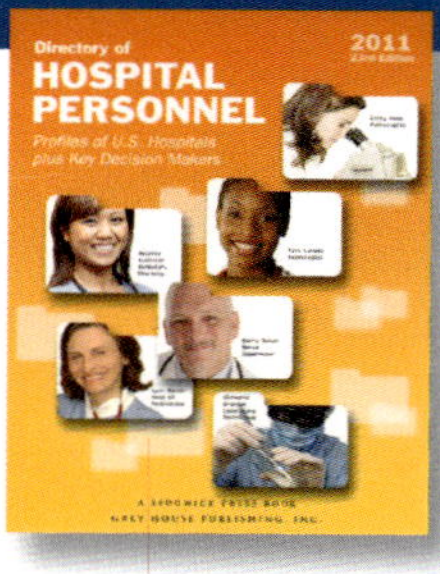

The Directory of Hospital Personnel is the best resource you can have at your fingertips when researching or marketing a product or service to the hospital market. A "Who's Who" of the hospital universe, this directory puts you in touch with over 150,000 key decision-makers. Every hospital in the U.S. is profiled, listed alphabetically by city within state. *The Directory of Hospital Personnel* is the only complete source for key hospital decision-makers by name. Whether you want to define or restructure sales territories... locate hospitals with the purchasing power to accept your proposals... or find information on which insurance plans are accepted, *The Directory of Hospital Personnel* gives you the information you need – easily, efficiently, effectively and accurately.

2,500 pages; Softcover ISBN 978-1-59237-738-1, $325.00
Online & Directory Combo: $800.00 | Online Database (Single User): $650.00

The Directory of Health Care Group Purchasing Organizations

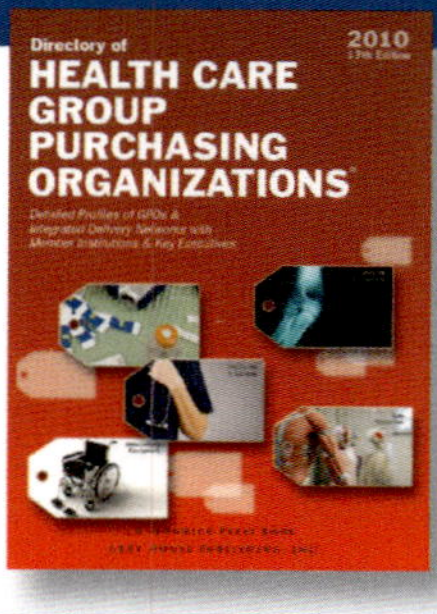

By providing in-depth information on this growing market and its members, *The Directory of Health Care Group Purchasing Organizations* fills a major need for the most accurate and comprehensive information on over 800 GPOs – Mailing Address, Phone & Fax Numbers, E-mail Addresses, Key Contacts, Purchasing Agents, Group Descriptions, Membership Categorization, Standard Vendor Proposal Requirements, Membership Fees & Terms, Expanded Services, Total Member Beds & Outpatient Visits represented and more. With its comprehensive and detailed information on each purchasing organization, *The Directory of Health Care Group Purchasing Organizations* is the go-to source for anyone looking to target this market.

1,000 pages; Softcover ISBN 978-1-59237-541-7, $325.00
Online & Directory Combo: $800.00 | Online Database (Single User): $650.00

The Comparative Guide to American Hospitals

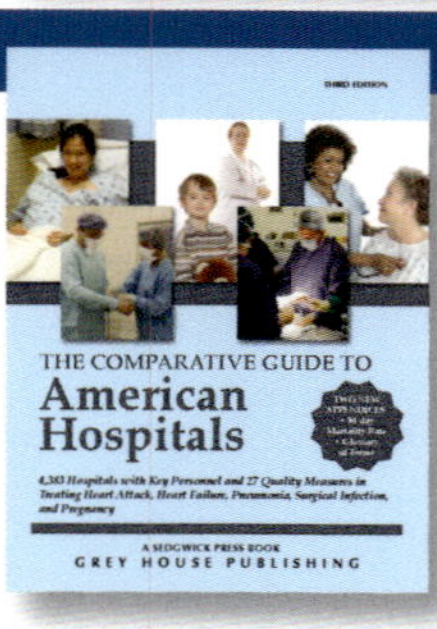

This important resource illustrates how the nation's hospitals rate when providing 24 different treatments within four broad categories: Heart Attack Care, Heart Failure Care, Surgical Infection Prevention, and Pregnancy Care. Each profile includes the raw percentage for that hospital, the state and US averages and data on the top hospital. Most importantly, *The Comparative Guide to American Hospitals* provides easy-to-use Regional State by State Statistical Summary Tables for each of the data elements to allow the user to quickly locate hospitals with the best level of service. Plus, a new 30-Day Mortality Chart, Glossary of Terms and Regional Hospital Profile Index make this a must-have source. This new, expanded edition will be a must for the reference collection at all public, medical and academic libraries.

2,000 pages; Four Volume Set; Softcover ISBN 978-1-59237-838-8, $350.00

(800) 562-2139 • www.greyhouse.com

KEYWORD INDEX

A2
81JPD Hemoglobin A2 Quantitation — Hematology

ABBEY
79RHW Holder, Needle, Other — Surgery

ABDOMEN
79MLB Device, Repeat Access (Abdomen) — Surgery

ABDOMINAL
78EXP Belt, Abdominal — Gastro/Urology
80FSD Binder, Abdominal — General
85HFR Binder, Abdominal, OB/GYN — Obstetrics/Gyn
79MDN Burr, Artificial (Velcro Fastener - Temp. Abdominal Closure) — Surgery
85HEE Chamber, Decompression, Abdominal — Obstetrics/Gyn
78SAP Elevator, Wall, Abdominal — Gastro/Urology
89KTD Orthosis, Abdominal — Physical Med
79RPM Retractor, Abdominal — Surgery
79WRZ Retractor, Abdominal, Padded, Flexible — Surgery
90RQV Scanner, Ultrasonic, Abdominal — Radiology
73MNC Stimulator, Abdominal, Electric — Anesthesiology
89RXB Support, Abdominal — Physical Med
78SCC Trocar, Abdominal — Gastro/Urology

ABDUCTION
89IOZ Splint, Abduction, Congenital Hip Dislocation — Physical Med
87WUU Splint, Abduction, Shoulder — Orthopedics

ABLATION
85MNB Device, Ablation, Thermal, Endometrial — Obstetrics/Gyn
78MIK Device, Ablation, Thermal, Ultrasonic — Gastro/Urology
74MNN Device, Ablation, Varicose Vein — Cardiovascular
74LPB Electrode, Ablation, Tissue, Conduction, Percutaneous — Cardiovascular
78MII System, Gallbladder, Thermal Ablation — Gastro/Urology

ABLATIVE
74MKI Guidewire, Peripheral, Ablative — Cardiovascular

ABNORMAL
81JCN Control, Cell Counter, Normal And Abnormal — Hematology
81JCM Control, Hemoglobin, Abnormal — Hematology
81GGC Control, Plasma, Abnormal — Hematology
81MLL Hemoglobin C (Abnormal Hemoglobin Variant) — Hematology
81GKA Quantitation, Hemoglobin, Abnormal — Hematology
81JBB Solubility, Hemoglobin, Abnormal — Hematology
81GFS Standard/Control, Hemoglobin, Normal/Abnormal — Hematology

ABO
81UJY Antiserum, ABO Blood Grouping — Hematology

ABORTION
85HGG Controller, Abortion Unit, Vacuum — Obstetrics/Gyn
85HDB Extractor, Vacuum, Fetal — Obstetrics/Gyn
85HGF Pump, Abortion Unit, Vacuum — Obstetrics/Gyn
85HHI Pump, Abortion, Vacuum, Central System — Obstetrics/Gyn
85HHQ System, Abortion, Metreurynter-Balloon — Obstetrics/Gyn

ABRASIVE
76EJR Agent, Polishing, Abrasive, Oral Cavity — Dental And Oral
76EHJ Disk, Abrasive — Dental And Oral
76EHL Point, Abrasive — Dental And Oral

ABRUPTIO
85MDH Abruptio Placentae Catheter — Obstetrics/Gyn

ABS
83GMS Anti-Human Globulin, FTA-ABS Test (Coombs) — Microbiology
83JWL Antigen, Treponema Pallidum For FTA-ABS Test — Microbiology
83GMX Antiserum, Fluorescent Antibody For FTA-ABS Test — Microbiology
83GMR Serum, Reactive And Non-Specific Control, FTA-ABS Test — Microbiology
83GMW Sorbent, FTA-ABS Test — Microbiology

ABSORBABLE
79LMF Agent, Hemostatic, Absorbable, Collagen-Based — Surgery
79LMG Agent, Hemostatic, Non-Absorbable, Collagen-Based — Surgery
85MCN Barrier, Adhesion, Absorbable — Obstetrics/Gyn
79GEM Gauze, Absorbable — Surgery
79GEL Gauze, Non-Absorbable, Medicated (Internal Sponge) — Surgery
79GEK Gauze, Non-Absorbable, Non-Medicated (Internal Sponge) — Surgery
79GDY Gauze, Non-Absorbable, X-Ray Detectable (Internal Sponge) — Surgery
86HQJ Implant, Absorbable (Scleral Buckling Method) — Ophthalmology
89MLQ Inhibitor, Peridural Fibrosis (Adhesion Barrier) — Physical Med
77ESI Polymer, Natural Absorbable Gelatin Material — Ear/Nose/Throat
77LBP Prosthesis, Ossicular (Stapes), Absorbable Gelatin Material — Ear/Nose/Throat
77LBO Prosthesis, Ossicular (Total), Absorbable Gelatin Material — Ear/Nose/Throat
79THO Sponge, Hemostatic, Absorbable Collagen — Surgery
87MNU Staple, Absorbable — Orthopedics
79GAK Suture, Absorbable — Surgery
79GAL Suture, Absorbable, Natural — Surgery
86HMO Suture, Absorbable, Ophthalmic — Ophthalmology
79GAN Suture, Absorbable, Synthetic — Surgery
79GAM Suture, Absorbable, Synthetic, Polyglycolic Acid — Surgery
79SGX Suture, Laparoscopy — Surgery
79SGW Suture, Laparoscopy, Loose — Surgery
79SGY Suture, Laparoscopy, Pre-Tied — Surgery
79GAO Suture, Non-Absorbable — Surgery
86HMN Suture, Non-Absorbable, Ophthalmic — Ophthalmology
79GAP Suture, Non-Absorbable, Silk — Surgery
79GAQ Suture, Non-Absorbable, Steel, Monofilament & Multifilament — Surgery
79GAR Suture, Non-Absorbable, Synthetic, Polyamide — Surgery
79GAS Suture, Non-Absorbable, Synthetic, Polyester — Surgery
79GAT Suture, Non-Absorbable, Synthetic, Polyethylene — Surgery
79GAW Suture, Non-Absorbable, Synthetic, Polypropylene — Surgery
87MBC Synthetic Ligaments & Tendons, Absorbable — Orthopedics

ABSORBENT
73CBL Absorbent, Carbon-Dioxide — Anesthesiology
80FOR Applicator, Tipped, Absorbent — General
80KXF Applicator, Tipped, Absorbent, Non-Sterile — General
80KXG Applicator, Tipped, Absorbent, Sterile — General
80WUM Encapsulator, Fluid — General
80FRL Fiber, Absorbent — General
82DHB Test, Radio-Allergen Absorbent (RAST) — Immunology

ABSORBER
73BSF Absorber, Carbon-Dioxide — Anesthesiology
76KHR Absorber, Saliva, Paper — Dental And Oral

ABSORPTIOMETER
90WRK Densitometer, Bone, Dual Photon — Radiology
90KGI Densitometer, Bone, Single Photon — Radiology
90WIR Densitometer, Radiography, Digital, Quantitative — Radiology

ABSORPTION
91DNE Absorption, Atomic, Antimony — Toxicology
91DNZ Absorption, Atomic, Arsenic — Toxicology

ABSORPTION *(cont'd)*

75JFN	Absorption, Atomic, Calcium	Chemistry
75JIZ	Absorption, Atomic, Iron (Non-Heme)	Chemistry
91DOF	Absorption, Atomic, Lead	Toxicology
91JII	Absorption, Atomic, Lithium	Toxicology
75JGI	Absorption, Atomic, Magnesium	Chemistry
91DPH	Absorption, Atomic, Mercury	Toxicology
79KOZ	Beads, Hydrophilic, Wound Exudate Absorption	Surgery
91JXR	Spectrophotometer, Atomic Absorption, General Use	Toxicology
81KHD	Test, Absorption, Vitamin B12	Hematology

ABUSE

91DMH	Analyzer, Alcohol	Toxicology
91DLK	Chromatograph, HPL, Drugs of Abuse (Dedicated Instrument)	Toxicology
75MPQ	Container, Specimen, Urine, Drugs Of Abuse, Over The Counter	Chemistry
91DMC	Gas Chromatograph, Drugs of Abuse (Dedicated Instruments)	Toxicology
91MVO	Kit, Test, Multiple, Drugs Of Abuse, Over The Counter	Toxicology
91MHP	Monitor, Patch, Sudromed, Drug Abuse	Toxicology
75MGX	System, Test, Drugs of Abuse	Chemistry
91JXP	Thin Layer Chromatography, Drugs of Abuse (Dedicated Instr.)	Toxicology

AC

74MPD	Auxillary Power Supply, Low Energy Defibrillator (AC or DC)	Cardiovascular

AC-POWERED

86HRG	Accessories, Engine, Trephine, AC-Powered	Ophthalmology
76EFD	Amalgamator, Dental, AC-Powered	Dental And Oral
89FNH	Bed, Water Flotation, AC-Powered	Physical Med
86HQS	Burr, Corneal, AC-Powered	Ophthalmology
86HRE	Cabinet, Instrument, AC-Powered, Ophthalmic	Ophthalmology
86HKI	Camera, Ophthalmic, AC-Powered (Fundus)	Ophthalmology
86HQR	Cautery, Radiofrequency, AC-Powered	Ophthalmology
86HQO	Cautery, Thermal, AC-Powered	Ophthalmology
86HME	Chair, Ophthalmic, AC-Powered	Ophthalmology
79GBB	Chair, Surgical, AC-Powered	Surgery
86HRN	Cryophthalmic Unit, AC-Powered	Ophthalmology
87LGH	Cutter, Cast, AC-Powered	Orthopedics
86HQE	Cutter, Vitreous Aspiration, AC-Powered	Ophthalmology
87LBB	Dynamometer, AC-Powered	Orthopedics
79GCP	Endoscope And Accessories, AC-Powered	Surgery
86HMK	Euthyscope, AC-Powered	Ophthalmology
80KZF	Examination Device, AC-Powered	General
74LIW	Fibrillator, AC-Powered	Cardiovascular
74MDO	Fibrillator, AC-Powered, Internal	Cardiovascular
86HPL	Fixation Device, AC-Powered, Ophthalmic	Ophthalmology
76EKX	Handpiece, Direct Drive, AC-Powered	Dental And Oral
86HPQ	Headlamp, Operating, AC-Powered	Ophthalmology
74QZQ	Heat Exchanger, Heart-Lung Bypass, AC-Powered	Cardiovascular
86HNO	Keratome, AC-Powered	Ophthalmology
86HLQ	Keratoscope, AC-Powered	Ophthalmology
79HJE	Lamp, Fluorescein, AC-Powered	Surgery
86HJO	Lamp, Slit, Biomicroscope, AC-Powered	Ophthalmology
80FSA	Lift, Bath, Non-AC-Powered	General
86HIX	Light, Maxwell Spot, AC-Powered	Ophthalmology
86HPO	Magnet, AC-Powered	Ophthalmology
86HLM	Measurer, Lens, AC-Powered	Ophthalmology
89IKI	Meter, Skin Resistance, AC-Powered	Physical Med
86HRM	Microscope, Operating, AC-Powered, Ophthalmic	Ophthalmology
79GEY	Motor, Surgical Instrument, AC-Powered	Surgery
86HLI	Ophthalmoscope, AC-Powered	Ophthalmology
86HOO	Perimeter, AC-Powered	Ophthalmology
86HPT	Perimeter, Automatic, AC-Powered	Ophthalmology
86HLX	Photostimulator, AC-Powered	Ophthalmology
86HLT	Preamplifier, AC-Powered, Ophthalmic	Ophthalmology
86HLG	Pupillometer, AC-Powered	Ophthalmology
86HKL	Retinoscope, AC-Powered	Ophthalmology
86HOM	Screen, Tangent, AC-Powered (Campimeter)	Ophthalmology
86HOK	Screen, Tangent, Projection, AC-Powered	Ophthalmology
77LEZ	Speech Training Aid, AC-Powered	Ear/Nose/Throat
86HMF	Stand, Instrument, AC-Powered, Ophthalmic	Ophthalmology
86HJQ	Stereoscope, AC-Powered	Ophthalmology
86HRD	Sterilizer, Soft Lens, Thermal, AC-Powered	Ophthalmology
73BXM	Stimulator, Nerve, AC-Powered	Anesthesiology
79JCX	Suction Apparatus, Ward Use, Portable, AC-Powered	Surgery
87HWE	Surgical Instrument, Orthopedic, AC-Powered Motor	Orthopedics
85HDD	Table, Obstetrical, AC-Powered	Obstetrics/Gyn
79FQO	Table, Operating Room, AC-Powered	Surgery
79JEA	Table, Surgical With Orthopedic Accessories, AC-Powered	Surgery
86HJS	Test, Spectacle Dissociation, AC-Powered (Lancaster)	Ophthalmology
86HKX	Tonometer, AC-Powered	Ophthalmology
86HJM	Transilluminator, AC-Powered, Ophthalmic	Ophthalmology
86ETJ	Transilluminator, AC-Powered, Other	Ophthalmology
85HIJ	Vibrator, Vaginal, AC-Powered	Obstetrics/Gyn

AC-POWERED *(cont'd)*

86HPF	Vision Aid, Electronic, AC-Powered	Ophthalmology
86HPI	Vision Aid, Optical, AC-Powered	Ophthalmology

ACACIA

76KOM	Acacia And Karaya With Sodium Borate	Dental And Oral
76MMU	Adhesive, Denture, Acacia & Karaya with Sodium Borate	Dental And Oral

ACCELERATION

84MHZ	Stimulator, Vestibular Acceleration, Therapeutic	Cns/Neurology

ACCELERATOR

90IYE	Accelerator, Linear, Medical	Radiology
90JAD	Therapeutic X-Ray System	Radiology

ACCELEROMETER

75TAA	Accelerometer	Chemistry

ACCESS

75QKX	Analyzer, Chemistry, Multi-Channel, Programmable	Chemistry
80LMQ	Device, Access, Peritoneal, Subcutaneous, Implantable	General
79MLB	Device, Repeat Access (Abdomen)	Surgery
78MDQ	Graft, Vascular, Biological, Hemodialysis Access	Gastro/Urology
78MCI	Graft, Vascular, Synth./Bio. Composite, Hemodialysis Access	Gastro/Urology
74THP	Port, Vascular Access	Cardiovascular
78MQS	System, Hemodialysis, Access Recirculation Monitoring	Gastro/Urology
78LTH	Vascular Access Graft	Gastro/Urology

ACCESSORIES

78KNZ	Accessories, AV Shunt	Gastro/Urology
79LYU	Accessories, Apparel, Surgical	Surgery
87VIE	Accessories, Arthroscope	Orthopedics
78MNK	Accessories, Bite Blocks (For Endoscope)	Gastro/Urology
78KOC	Accessories, Blood Circuit, Hemodialysis	Gastro/Urology
77KTI	Accessories, Bronchoscope	Ear/Nose/Throat
74KRI	Accessories, Cardiopulmonary Bypass	Cardiovascular
80WSA	Accessories, Cart, Multipurpose	General
79KGZ	Accessories, Catheter	Surgery
78KNY	Accessories, Catheter, G-U	Gastro/Urology
75JQR	Accessories, Chromatography (Gas, Gel, Liquid, Thin Layer)	Chemistry
78MNL	Accessories, Cleaning Brushes (For Endoscope)	Gastro/Urology
78FEB	Accessories, Cleaning, Endoscopic	Gastro/Urology
80VBQ	Accessories, Decorative	General
79WDY	Accessories, Electrical Power (Electrocautery)	Surgery
86HRG	Accessories, Engine, Trephine, AC-Powered	Ophthalmology
79HRF	Accessories, Engine, Trephine, Battery-Powered	Surgery
79HLD	Accessories, Engine, Trephine, Gas-Powered	Surgery
78KXM	Accessories, Extracorporeal System	Gastro/Urology
87LYT	Accessories, Fixation, Orthopedic	Orthopedics
87LYP	Accessories, Fixation, Spinal Interlaminal	Orthopedics
87LYQ	Accessories, Fixation, Spinal Intervertebral Body	Orthopedics
80WQD	Accessories, Laser	General
79SJN	Accessories, Laser, Endoscopic	Surgery
79FTA	Accessories, Light, Surgical	Surgery
88IDL	Accessories, Microtome	Pathology
79FWZ	Accessories, Operating Room, Table	Surgery
78FEM	Accessories, Photographic, Endoscopic	Gastro/Urology
84HBE	Accessories, Powered Drill	Cns/Neurology
80MRZ	Accessories, Pump, Infusion	General
90WJW	Accessories, Radiotherapy	Radiology
76EIF	Accessories, Retractor, Dental	Dental And Oral
86LYL	Accessories, Solution, Lens, Contact	Ophthalmology
79FXG	Accessories, Speculum	Surgery
79KQM	Accessories, Surgical Camera	Surgery
89ILZ	Accessories, Traction	Physical Med
87HXF	Accessories, Traction (Cart, Frame, Cord, Weight)	Orthopedics
87KRT	Accessories, Traction, Invasive	Orthopedics
80WYY	Accessories, Walker	General
89KNO	Accessories, Wheelchair	Physical Med
78LLB	Blood System, Extracorporeal (With Accessories)	Gastro/Urology
87TAU	Cannula, Drainage, Arthroscopy	Orthopedics
79WYX	Cannula, Suction/Irrigation, Laparoscopic	Surgery
78MJC	Catheter and Accessories, Urological	Gastro/Urology
85HFH	Coagulator, Hysteroscopic (With Accessories)	Obstetrics/Gyn
74WJY	Connector, Tubing, Blood	Cardiovascular
80MMP	Cover, Barrier, Protective	General
79GEH	Cryosurgical Unit	Surgery
86MMC	Dilator, Expansive Iris (Accessory)	Ophthalmology
80WSB	Dispenser, Syringe And Needle	General
84HBG	Drill, Manual (With Burr, Trephine & Accessories)	Cns/Neurology
84HBF	Drill, Powered Compound (With Burr, Trephine & Accessories)	Cns/Neurology
85HIM	Electrocautery Unit, Endoscopic	Obstetrics/Gyn
85HGI	Electrocautery Unit, Gynecologic	Obstetrics/Gyn
79BWA	Electrosurgical Unit, Anesthesiology Accessories	Surgery
78KNS	Electrosurgical, Unit, Gastroenterology	Gastro/Urology
78KOG	Endoscope	Gastro/Urology

KEYWORD INDEX

ACCESSORIES *(cont'd)*

79GCP	Endoscope And Accessories, AC-Powered	Surgery
79GCS	Endoscope And Accessories, Battery-Powered	Surgery
85HEZ	Endoscope, Transcervical (Amnioscope)	Obstetrics/Gyn
79SIV	Equipment/Accessories, Laser, Laparoscopy	Surgery
84HAP	Guide, Wire, Angiographic (And Accessories)	Cns/Neurology
80RCM	Hanger, Intravenous	General
87THC	Holder, Leg, Arthroscopy	Orthopedics
79WRY	Holder, Shoulder, Arthroscopy	Surgery
85HIH	Hysteroscope	Obstetrics/Gyn
85RCF	Injector & Accessories, Manipulator, Uterine	Obstetrics/Gyn
87HSZ	Instrument, Surgical, Powered, Pneumatic	Orthopedics
79FTN	Kit, Instruments and Accessories, Surgical	Surgery
85HET	Laparoscope, Gynecologic	Obstetrics/Gyn
86LQJ	Lens, Surgical, Laser	Ophthalmology
80WLM	Lock, Catheter	General
86HRM	Microscope, Operating, AC-Powered, Ophthalmic	Ophthalmology
85HGO	Monitor, Electroencephalographic, Fetal	Obstetrics/Gyn
79KCT	Pack, Sterilization Wrapper (Bag And Accessories)	Surgery
86HQB	Photocoagulator	Ophthalmology
76EBL	Pin, Retentive And Splinting	Dental And Oral
79GDR	Saw, Manual, And Accessories	Surgery
84HAC	Saw, Manual, Neurological (With Accessories)	Cns/Neurology
84HAB	Saw, Powered, And Accessories	Cns/Neurology
87LTO	Spacer, Cement	Orthopedics
78KOA	Surgical Instrument, G-U, Manual	Gastro/Urology
87HWE	Surgical Instrument, Orthopedic, AC-Powered Motor	Orthopedics
79KIJ	Surgical Instrument, Orthopedic, Battery-Powered	Surgery
87JDX	Surgical Instrument, Sonic	Orthopedics
78MON	System, Hemodialysis, Remote Accessories	Gastro/Urology
79JEA	Table, Surgical With Orthopedic Accessories, AC-Powered	Surgery
87JEB	Table, Surgical, Orthopedic	Orthopedics
78KNT	Tube, Gastrointestinal	Gastro/Urology
73BYX	Tubing, Flexible, Medical Gas, Low-Pressure	Anesthesiology
85MOK	Vaginoscope and Accessories	Obstetrics/Gyn

ACCESSORY

85MQG	Accessory, Assisted Reproduction	Obstetrics/Gyn
84MYU	Accessory, Barium Sulfate, Methyl Methacrylate For Cranioplasty	Cns/Neurology
73MOD	Ventilator, Continuous (Respirator), Accessory	Anesthesiology

ACCURACY

75UKH	Balance, Macro (0.1 mg Accuracy)	Chemistry
75UKF	Balance, Micro (0.001 mg Accuracy)	Chemistry
75UKG	Balance, Semimicro (0.01 mg Accuracy)	Chemistry
75UKE	Balance, Ultramicro (0.0001 mg Accuracy)	Chemistry

ACE

75KQN	Radioassay, Angiotensin Converting Enzyme	Chemistry

ACETABULAR

87JDM	Prosthesis, Hip, Acetabular Component, Metal, Non-Cemented	Orthopedics
87JDJ	Prosthesis, Hip, Acetabular Mesh	Orthopedics
87KWB	Prosthesis, Hip, Hemi-, Acetabular, Metal	Orthopedics
87JDL	Prosthesis, Hip, Semi-Constrained (Cemented Acetabular)	Orthopedics
87KWA	Prosthesis, Hip, Semi-Constrained Acetabular	Orthopedics

ACETAL

86MXY	Cannula, Ophthalmic, Posterior Capsular Polishing, Polyvinyl Acetal	Ophthalmology

ACETAMINOPHEN

91LDP	Colorimetry, Acetaminophen	Toxicology

ACETATE

75UEO	Electrophoresis Equipment, Cellulose Acetate Membrane	Chemistry
88IGB	Solution, Formalin/Sodium Acetate	Pathology
88ICG	Stain, Cresyl Violet Acetate	Pathology
75CEI	Uranyl Acetate/Zinc Acetate, Sodium	Chemistry

ACETIC

75CDA	Nitrous Acid & Nitrosonaphthol, 5-Hydroxyindole Acetic Acid	Chemistry
88IGF	Solution, Pathology, Formalin-Alcohol-Acetic Acid	Pathology

ACETONE

75UJV	Acetone	Chemistry

ACETYL

75JKW	N-Acetyl-L-Tyrosine Ethyl Ester (U.V.), Chymotrypsin	Chemistry

ACETYLACETONE

75JKK	Acetylacetone (Colorimetric), Delta-Aminolevulinic Acid	Chemistry

ACETYLCHOLINE

91JNI	Acetylcholine Iodine and DTNB, Pseudocholinesterase	Toxicology
91DLI	Reagent, Acetylcholine Chloride	Toxicology

ACETYLPROCAINAMIDE

91LAN	Enzyme Immunoassay, N-Acetylprocainamide	Toxicology

ACETYLPROCAINAMIDE *(cont'd)*

91LAZ	N-Acetylprocainamide Control Materials	Toxicology

ACID

75JKK	Acetylacetone (Colorimetric), Delta-Aminolevulinic Acid	Chemistry
81GGF	Acid Hematin	Hematology
75LFQ	Acid Reduction Of Ferric Ion, Uric Acid	Chemistry
75JMA	Acid, Ascorbic, 2, 4-dinitrophenylhydrazine (spectrophotometric)	Chemistry
88IDE	Acid, Hematein	Pathology
76LZX	Acid, Hyaluronic	Dental And Oral
89MOZ	Acid, Hyaluronic, Intraarticular	Physical Med
91DIJ	Acid, Levulinic, Amino, Delta, Lead	Toxicology
82LKL	Alpha-1-Acid-Glycoprotein, Antigen, Antiserum, Control	Immunology
75JMK	Alpha-Ketobutyric Acid And NADH (U.V.), Hydroxybutyric	Chemistry
83QAQ	Analyzer, Amino Acid	Microbiology
88ICY	Aniline Acid Fuchsin	Pathology
82MEN	Assay, Serum, Sialic Acid	Immunology
75JKL	Column, Ion Exchange With Colorimetry, Delta-Aminolevulinic	Chemistry
75JLG	Conversion Ferric Hydroxymates (Colorimetric), Fatty Acids	Chemistry
83JRZ	Culture Media, Amino Acid Assay	Microbiology
83MKZ	DNA-Probe, Nucleic Acid Amplification, Chlamydia	Microbiology
75CDF	Diazo, P-Nitroaniline/Vanillin, Vanilmandelic Acid	Chemistry
75CJX	Disodium Phenyl Phosphate, Acid Phosphatase	Chemistry
75CDK	Electrophoretic Separation, Vanilmandelic Acid	Chemistry
75JLT	Enzymatic (U.V.), Pyruvic Acid	Chemistry
75KHP	Enzymatic Method, Lactic Acid	Chemistry
91LEG	Enzyme Immunoassay, Valproic Acid	Toxicology
75CHD	Ferric Ion-Sulfuric Acid, Cholesterol	Chemistry
88LDW	Fixative, Acid Containing	Pathology
76MGG	Fluid, Hylan (For TMJ Use)	Dental And Oral
75CKH	Glycerophosphate, Beta, Phosphatase, Acid	Chemistry
75JOA	Hexane Extraction And Trifluoroacetic Acid, Vitamin A	Chemistry
75JQE	Ion Exchange Resin, Ascorbic Acid, Colorimetry, Iron Bind	Chemistry
75JQD	Ion Exchange Resin, Thioglycolic Acid, Colorimetry, Iron	Chemistry
82MEO	Kit, Antigen, RIA, Prostatic Acid Phosphatase	Immunology
75JKI	L-Leucyl B-Naphthylamide, Lactic Acid	Chemistry
76LPG	Material, Dressing, Surgical, Acid, Polylactic	Dental And Oral
79FTL	Mesh, Surgical, Polymeric	Surgery
75CKB	Naphthyl Phosphate, Acid Phosphatase	Chemistry
75CJN	Nitrophenylphosphate, Acid Phosphatase	Chemistry
75CDA	Nitrous Acid & Nitrosonaphthol, 5-Hydroxyindole Acetic Acid	Chemistry
88HZI	Osmic Acid	Pathology
75JMS	Oxalacetic Acid And NADH Oxidation (U.V.), Maleic DH	Chemistry
88KKS	Periodic Acid	Pathology
81JCI	Phosphatase, Acid	Hematology
75CHG	Phosphoric-Tungstic Acid (Spectrophotometric), Chloride	Chemistry
75CDH	Phosphotungstate Reduction, Uric Acid	Chemistry
76KOO	Polyvinyl Methylether Maleic Acid-Calcium-Sodium Dbl. Salt	Dental And Oral
76KOT	Polyvinyl Methylether Maleic Acid/Carboxymethylcellulose	Dental And Oral
75KWW	Radioimmunoassay, Cholyglycine, Bile Acids	Chemistry
75KWX	Radioimmunoassay, Conjugated Sulfalithocholic, Bile Acid	Chemistry
75CGN	Radioimmunoassay, Folic Acid	Chemistry
83UFK	Reagent, Analyzer, Amino Acid	Microbiology
88KDX	Solution, Pathology, Decalcifier, Acid Containing	Pathology
88IGF	Solution, Pathology, Formalin-Alcohol-Acetic Acid	Pathology
88IDF	Stain, Acid Fuchsin	Pathology
88HZK	Stain, Periodic Acid Schiff (PAS)	Pathology
88HZM	Stain, Phosphotungstic Acid Hematoxylin	Pathology
88GGI	Stain, Schiff, Periodic Acid	Pathology
75UIH	Standard, Amino Acid	Chemistry
79GAM	Suture, Absorbable, Synthetic, Polyglycolic Acid	Surgery
75LPT	System, Test, Acid, Methylmalonic, Urinary	Chemistry
82MVD	System, Test, Her-2/Neu, Nucleic Acid Or Serum	Immunology
75JFH	Tartrate Inhibited, Acid Phosphatase (Prostatic)	Chemistry
76KKN	Test, Acid, Ascorbic, Lingual	Dental And Oral
75JLI	Tetrahydrofolate, Enzymatic (U.V.), Formiminoglutamic Acid	Chemistry
75CJR	Thymol Blue Monophosphate, Acid Phosphatase	Chemistry
75CKE	Thymolphthalein Monophosphate, Acid Phosphatase	Chemistry
75JLH	Titrimetric, Fatty Acids	Chemistry
75KNK	Uricase (Colorimetric), Uric Acid	Chemistry
75JHB	Uricase (Coulometric), Uric Acid	Chemistry
75JHA	Uricase (Gasometric), Uric Acid	Chemistry
75JHC	Uricase (Oxygen Rate), Uric Acid	Chemistry
75CDO	Uricase (U.V.), Uric Acid	Chemistry

ACID-CALCIUM-SODIUM

76KOO	Polyvinyl Methylether Maleic Acid-Calcium-Sodium Dbl. Salt	Dental And Oral

ACIDITY

75JLK	Sodium Hydroxide/Phenol Red (Titrimetric), Gastric Acidity	Chemistry
75JLL	Tubeless Analysis, Gastric Acidity	Chemistry

ACINETOBACTER
83GSX Antisera, Acinetobacter Calcoaceticus, All Varieties — Microbiology

ACNES
83KLH Antisera, C. Acnes — Microbiology
83GOP Antiserum, C. Acnes (553, 605) — Microbiology

ACOUSTIC
77EWC Chamber, Acoustic, Testing — Ear/Nose/Throat
83UEV Microscope, Laser, Scanning, Acoustic — Microbiology
79FXD Stethoscope, Direct (Acoustic), Ultrasonic — Surgery
85MCP Stimulator, Fetal, Acoustic — Obstetrics/Gyn

ACOUSTICAL
85HHX Holograph, Fetal, Acoustical — Obstetrics/Gyn
77TAB Room, Acoustical — Ear/Nose/Throat

ACQUIRED
81VJE Test, Antibody, Acquired Immune Deficiency Syndrome (AIDS) — Hematology
82MZF Test, Hiv Detection — Immunology

ACQUISITION
80WNM Service, Publication Acquisition — General

ACRIDINE
88IDC Stain, Acridine Orange — Pathology

ACRYLIC
76VEH Curing Unit, Acrylic — Dental And Oral
76WKF Material, Acrylic, Dental — Dental And Oral

ACTH
75CKG Radioimmunoassay, ACTH — Chemistry

ACTING
75JMP Radioimmunoassay, Long-Acting Thyroid Stimulator — Chemistry

ACTIVATED
81JBP Activated Whole Blood Clotting Time — Hematology
81GFO Thromboplastin, Activated Partial — Hematology

ACTIVATOR
76EBZ Activator, Ultraviolet, Polymerization — Dental And Oral
82DAC Control, Antiserum, Antigen, Activator, C3, Complement — Immunology
82KTP Reagent, Immunoassay, Activator, C3, Complement — Immunology

ACTIVE
79FAS Electrode, Electrosurgical, Active (Blade) — Surgery
79UEB Electrode, Electrosurgical, Active, Foot Controlled — Surgery
79SJQ System, Monitoring, Electrode, Active, Electrosurgical — Surgery

ACUITY
86WQG Astigmometer — Ophthalmology
86HOX Chart, Visual Acuity — Ophthalmology
75VII Test, Taste Acuity — Chemistry
86WOO Tester, Brightness Acuity — Ophthalmology
86SFC Visometer — Ophthalmology

ACUPUNCTURE
79QJQ Chart, Acupuncture — Surgery
73QAA Kit, Acupuncture — Anesthesiology
73BWJ Locator, Acupuncture Point — Anesthesiology
73BWI Needle, Acupuncture — Anesthesiology
80MQX Needle, Acupuncture, Single Use — General
73UKR Stimulator, Acupuncture — Anesthesiology
73BWK Stimulator, Electro/Acupuncture — Anesthesiology

ACUTE
73RLA Monitor, Physiological, Acute Care — Anesthesiology
74MTE System, Pacing, Temporary, Acute, Internal Atrial Defibrillation — Cardiovascular

ADAPTER
79WDY Accessories, Electrical Power (Electrocautery) — Surgery
78KNR Adapter, AV Shunt Or Fistula — Gastro/Urology
73QAT Adapter, Anesthesia — Anesthesiology
78FFY Adapter, Bulb, Endoscope, Miscellaneous — Gastro/Urology
80WTN Adapter, Cable, Equipment — General
79GCE Adapter, Catheter — Surgery
78EYI Adapter, Catheter, Ureteral — Gastro/Urology
75QIY Adapter, Centrifuge Tube — Chemistry
78FHC Adapter, Cord, Instrument, Surgical, Transurethral — Gastro/Urology
79QTR Adapter, Electrosurgical Unit, Cable — Surgery
89IQG Adapter, Holder, Syringe — Physical Med
89ILS Adapter, Hygiene — Physical Med
77ETR Adapter, Index, Sensitivity, Increment, Short — Ear/Nose/Throat
74DRW Adapter, Lead Switching, Electrocardiograph — Cardiovascular
74DTD Adapter, Lead, Pacemaker — Cardiovascular
74WTU Adapter, Needle — Cardiovascular
78FKN Adapter, Shunt — Gastro/Urology
74DTL Adapter, Stopcock, Manifold, Cardiopulmonary Bypass — Cardiovascular
80RYL Adapter, Syringe — General

ADAPTER (cont'd)
73SBF Adapter, Tube, Tracheal — Anesthesiology
79QTS Adapter, Unit, Electrosurgical, Hand-Controlled — Surgery
78FJP Adapter, Y — Gastro/Urology
73CAI Circuit, Breathing (W Connector, Adapter, Y Piece) — Anesthesiology
78FKB Connector, Tubing, Blood, Infusion, T-Type — Gastro/Urology
73SBH Holder, Tracheostomy Tube — Anesthesiology
80SHN Vehicle/Equipment, Recreational (Handicapped) — General

ADAPTIVE
89LBE Stroller, Adaptive — Physical Med

ADAPTOMETER
86HJW Adaptometer (Biophotometer) — Ophthalmology

ADAPTOR
89ILD Adaptor, Dressing — Physical Med
78FKM Adaptor, Fistula — Gastro/Urology
89ILW Adaptor, Grooming — Physical Med
89ILT Adaptor, Recreational — Physical Med
80WSP Tubing, Connecting — General

ADDITIVE
76KLF Varnish, With Additive — Dental And Oral
76KLG Varnish, Without Additive — Dental And Oral

ADDRESS
80TDL Public Address System — General

ADENINE
81KHF Adenine Nucleotide Quantitation — Hematology

ADENOID
77KBJ Curette, Adenoid — Ear/Nose/Throat
77QZC Guillotine, Adenoid — Ear/Nose/Throat
77KBS Punch, Adenoid — Ear/Nose/Throat

ADENOSINE
81JWR ATP Release (Luminescence) — Hematology
75JLB ATP and CK (Enzymatic), Creatine — Chemistry
75CHO Radioimmunoassay, Cyclic AMP — Chemistry

ADENOTOME
77KBH Adenotome — Ear/Nose/Throat

ADENOVIRUS
83GOD Antigen, CF (Including CF Control), Adenovirus 1-33 — Microbiology
83GOB Antigen, HA (Including HA Control), Adenovirus 1-33 — Microbiology
83GOA Antiserum, CF, Adenovirus 1-33 — Microbiology
83GNY Antiserum, Fluorescent, Adenovirus 1-33 — Microbiology
83GOC Antiserum, HAI, Adenovirus 1-33 — Microbiology
83GNZ Antiserum, Neutralization, Adenovirus 1-33 — Microbiology

ADHERENT
80QQX Dressing, Non-Adherent — General

ADHESION
85MCN Barrier, Adhesion, Absorbable — Obstetrics/Gyn
81GHX Collagen, Platelet Aggregation And Adhesion — Hematology
88IFZ Gelatin For Specimen Adhesion — Pathology
89MLQ Inhibitor, Peridural Fibrosis (Adhesion Barrier) — Physical Med
89MNY Inhibitor, Post-Op Fibro., Carp. Tun. Syn.(Adhesion Barrier) — Physical Med
89MNX Inhibitor, Post-Op Fibrosis, Tenolysis (Adhesion Barrier) — Physical Med

ADHESIVE
76KOM Acacia And Karaya With Sodium Borate — Dental And Oral
80QAC Adhesive Strip, Hypoallergenic — General
80QAD Adhesive Strip, Waterproof — General
81JBZ Adhesive Study, Platelet — Hematology
80QAF Adhesive, Aerosol — General
88KEL Adhesive, Albumin Based — Pathology
76DYH Adhesive, Bracket And Conditioner, Resin — Dental And Oral
76UDQ Adhesive, Dental — Dental And Oral
76VLL Adhesive, Dental Impression — Dental And Oral
76MMU Adhesive, Denture, Acacia & Karaya with Sodium Borate — Dental And Oral
76KOP Adhesive, Denture, Karaya — Dental And Oral
76KOR Adhesive, Denture, Karaya With Sodium Borate — Dental And Oral
76EBM Adhesive, Denture, OTC — Dental And Oral
76KON Adhesive, Denture, Polymer, Polyacrylamide — Dental And Oral
80QAG Adhesive, Liquid — General
79GBJ Adhesive, Prosthesis, External — Surgery
79MPN Adhesive, Soft Tissue Approximation — Surgery
84KGF Adhesive, Tissue, Aneurysmorrhaphy — Cns/Neurology
78LNT Adhesive, Tissue, Gastroenterology/Urology — Gastro/Urology
84KGG Adhesive, Tissue, General Neurosurgery — Cns/Neurology
86LZQ Adhesive, Tissue, Ophthalmology — Ophthalmology
79MGO Adhesive, Wound Closure — Surgery
80FON Bag, Drainage, Ostomy (With Adhesive) — General
79KGX Bandage, Adhesive — Surgery
76KOS Carboxymethylcellulose Sodium & Cationic Polyacrylamide — Dental And Oral
76KOQ Carboxymethylcellulose Sodium (40-100%) — Dental And Oral

KEYWORD INDEX

ADHESIVE *(cont'd)*
76KOL Carboxymethylcellulose Sodium/Ethylene-Oxide Homopolymer — Dental And Oral
80WXA Component, Other — General
79KGT Drape, Adhesive, Aerosol — Surgery
79WVZ Drape, Incision, Surgical — Surgery
74WOV Electrode, Gel — Cardiovascular
76KXX Homopolymer, Karaya and Ethylene-Oxide — Dental And Oral
80MLX Pad, Medicated, Adhesive, Non-Electric — General
88WSX Slide, Cell Adhesive — Pathology
79KOX Solvent, Adhesive Tape — Surgery
79FPX Strip, Adhesive — Surgery
80RZE Tape, Adhesive — General
80RZF Tape, Adhesive, Hypoallergenic — General
80RZG Tape, Adhesive, Waterproof — General
80WMH Tape, Gauze, Adhesive — General

ADJUNCTIVE
90LHQ Telethermographic System (Adjunctive Use) — Radiology
90KXZ Thermographic Device, Liquid Crystal, Adjunctive — Radiology

ADJUSTABLE
80KMM Bed, Adjustable Hospital — General
89INN Chair, Adjustable, Mechanical — Physical Med
79FZM Stool, Operating Room, Adjustable — Surgery

ADMINISTRATION
80WSJ Computer Software, Hospital/Nursing Management — General
80VHN Computer, Patient Data Management — General
80QDX Kit, Administration, Blood — General
74UDD Kit, Administration, Cardioplegia Solution — Cardiovascular
78QUJ Kit, Administration, Enteral — Gastro/Urology
80WVF Kit, Administration, Intra-Arterial — General
80FPA Kit, Administration, Intravenous — General
73RJH Kit, Administration, Oxygen — Anesthesiology
78TGJ Kit, Administration, Parenteral — Gastro/Urology
78KDJ Kit, Administration, Peritoneal Dialysis, Disposable — Gastro/Urology
80RCI Kit, Intravenous, Administration, Buret — General
73BYG Mask, Oxygen, Aerosol Administration — Anesthesiology
73RGC Mask, Tracheostomy, Aerosol Administration — Anesthesiology
80LEY Oral Administration Set — General
80MQT Pump, Drug Administration, Closed Loop — General
80WZG Set, Administration, Intravenous, Needle-Free — General
80TGT System, Infusion, Administration, Drug, Implantable — General

ADMISSION
80RKC Kit, Admission (Patient Utensil) — General

ADP
75JNJ Phosphoenol Pyruvate, ADP, NADH, Pyruvate Kinase — Chemistry

ADRENOCORTICOTROPIC
75CKG Radioimmunoassay, ACTH — Chemistry

ADSON
79QTX Elevator, Adson — Surgery
79RHW Holder, Needle, Other — Surgery

ADSORBENTS
91DKO Adsorbents, Ion Exchange — Toxicology
91DMZ Adsorbents, Liquid Chromatography — Toxicology

ADSORPTION
74WTP Column, Adsorption, Lipid — Cardiovascular
80LXW Column, Adsorption, Lipoprotein, Low Density — General

ADULT
80QPL Diaper, Adult — General
80QVM Kit, Feeding, Adult (Enteral) — General
80SFJ Warmer, Radiant, Adult — General

AEBLI
86RRD Scissors, Corneal — Ophthalmology

AERATOR
80FLI Cabinet, Aerator, Ethylene-Oxide Gas — General

AEROBIC
83RBW Incubator, Aerobic — Microbiology
83JTW Transport System, Aerobic — Microbiology

AEROSOL
80QAF Adhesive, Aerosol — General
77KCK Atomizer And Tip, ENT — Ear/Nose/Throat
80VLK Cartridge, Freon — General
79KGT Drape, Adhesive, Aerosol — Surgery
80QQT Dressing, Aerosol — General
77QAH Generator, Aerosol — Ear/Nose/Throat
73BYG Mask, Oxygen, Aerosol Administration — Anesthesiology
73RGC Mask, Tracheostomy, Aerosol Administration — Anesthesiology
73CAF Nebulizer, Direct Patient Interface — Anesthesiology
73RHT Nebulizer, Heated — Anesthesiology

AEROSOL *(cont'd)*
77EPN Nebulizer, Medicinal — Ear/Nose/Throat
73CCQ Nebulizer, Medicinal, Non-Ventilatory (Atomizer) — Anesthesiology
73RHU Nebulizer, Non-Heated — Anesthesiology
73RHV Nebulizer, Ultrasonic — Anesthesiology
80RZS Tent, Mist — General
80RZT Tent, Mist, Face — General
80FNC Tent, Pediatric Aerosol — General

AERUGINOSA
83GSS Antisera, Fluorescent, Pseudomonas Aeruginosa — Microbiology

AESTHESIOMETER
86HJC Aesthesiometer — Ophthalmology

AESTHETIC
79LMI Implant, Collagen (Non-Aesthetic Use) — Surgery
79LMH Implant, Collagen, Dermal (Aesthetic Use) — Surgery
79GBI Material, Restoration, Aesthetic, External — Surgery

AFFECTIVE
80MIO Light, Therapy, Seasonal Affective Disorder (SAD) — General

AFP
82KTJ Alpha-Fetoprotein RIA Test System — Immunology
82LTQ Calibrator, AFP, Serum, Maternal, Mid-Pregnancy — Immunology
82LOJ Kit, Test, Alpha-fetoprotein For Testicular Cancer — Immunology
82LOK Test, Neural Tube Defect, Alpha-Fetoprotein (AFP) — Immunology

AFTER
86HIZ Flasher, After-Image — Ophthalmology

AFTER-IMAGE
86HIZ Flasher, After-Image — Ophthalmology

AFTERLOADER
90WIA Afterloader, Radiotherapy — Radiology

AGAR
83JTZ Culture Media, Mueller Hinton Agar Broth — Microbiology
83JSK Culture Media, Supplements — Microbiology
91KZT Disc, Diffusion, Gel, Agar, Serum Level, Gentamicin — Toxicology
91KZW Disc, Diffusion, Gel, Agar, Serum Level, Kanamycin — Toxicology
91KZX Disc, Diffusion, Gel, Agar, Serum Level, Tobramycin — Toxicology
75RBN Immunodiffusion Equipment (Agar Cutter) — Chemistry
83JTP Kit, Disc Agar Gel Diffusion, Serum Level — Microbiology
82JZP Plate, Agar, Ouchterlony — Immunology
83UJZ Test, Agar Plate — Microbiology
83UKA Test, Agar Tube — Microbiology

AGAROSE
83TDG Separation Media — Microbiology

AGENT
78LNM Agent, Bulking, Injectable (Gastro-Urology) — Gastro/Urology
88KDY Agent, Chelating, Decalcification — Pathology
79MAG Agent, Embolization/Occlusion — Surgery
79LMF Agent, Hemostatic, Absorbable, Collagen-Based — Surgery
79LMG Agent, Hemostatic, Non-Absorbable, Collagen-Based — Surgery
79MFE Agent, Injectable, Embolic — Surgery
76EJR Agent, Polishing, Abrasive, Oral Cavity — Dental And Oral
88KEM Clearing Agent — Pathology
83JSK Culture Media, Supplements — Microbiology
83MCG DNA-Probe, Agent, Listeria — Microbiology
76EHM Strip, Polishing Agent — Dental And Oral
76KLE Tooth Bonding Agent, Resin Restoration — Dental And Oral
76EJQ Wheel, Polishing Agent — Dental And Oral

AGGLUTINATING
83GPF Antigen, Agglutinating, Echinococcus SPP. — Microbiology
83GOW Antiserum, Agglutinating, B. Parapertussis — Microbiology
83GOY Antiserum, Agglutinating, B. Pertussis, All — Microbiology

AGGLUTINATION
75JHJ Agglutination Method, Human Chorionic Gonadotropin — Chemistry
83GSO Antigen, (Febrile), Agglutination, Brucella SPP. — Microbiology
83GMG Antigen, Latex Agglutination, Coccidioides Immitis — Microbiology
83GMO Antigen, Latex Agglutination, Entamoeba Histolytica & Rel. — Microbiology
83GNE Antigen, Latex Agglutination, T. Cruzi — Microbiology
83GPG Antigen, Latex Agglutination, Trichinella Spiralis — Microbiology
83GMD Antiserum, Latex Agglutination, Cryptococcus Neoformans — Microbiology
83LQN Assay, Agglutination, Latex, Rubella — Microbiology
83LLA Test, Direct Agglutination, Toxoplasma Gondii — Microbiology

AGGREGATION
81JBZ Adhesive Study, Platelet — Hematology
81RLG Analyzer, Platelet Aggregation — Hematology
81JOZ Analyzer, Platelet Aggregation, Automated — Hematology
81GHX Collagen, Platelet Aggregation And Adhesion — Hematology
81GHR Reagent, Platelet Aggregation — Hematology

AGGREGOMETER
81JBX Aggregometer, Platelet — Hematology

AGGREGOMETER *(cont'd)*

81JBY	Aggregometer, Platelet, Photo-Optical Scanning	Hematology
81GKW	Aggregometer, Platelet, Thrombokinetogram	Hematology

AGITATOR

78MEU	Agitator, Ultrasonic (Drug Dissolution)	Gastro/Urology

AID

80WYY	Accessories, Walker	General
89LFF	Aid, Control, Environmental, Controlled, Breath	Physical Med
80SHP	Aid, Living, Handicapped	General
74LIX	Aid, Resuscitation, Cardiopulmonary	Cardiovascular
77WOT	Battery, Hearing-Aid	Ear/Nose/Throat
77ETW	Calibrator, Hearing-Aid/Earphone And Analysis Systems	Ear/Nose/Throat
80UMP	Chair, Seat Lifting (Standing Aid)	General
79MBQ	Device, Peripheral Electromag. Field to Aid Wound Healing	Surgery
80QPL	Diaper, Adult	General
89WPB	Equipment, Therapy, Handicapped/Physical	Physical Med
77ESD	Hearing-Aid	Ear/Nose/Throat
77LXB	Hearing-Aid, Bone-Conduction	Ear/Nose/Throat
77MAH	Hearing-Aid, Bone-Conduction, Implanted	Ear/Nose/Throat
77MKE	Hearing-Aid, Bone-Conduction, Percutaneous	Ear/Nose/Throat
77MKP	Hearing-Aid, Cortical, Shafer	Ear/Nose/Throat
77MMB	Hearing-Aid, External, Magnet, Membrane, Tympanic	Ear/Nose/Throat
77EPF	Hearing-Aid, Group, Or Auditory Trainer	Ear/Nose/Throat
77KHL	Hearing-Aid, Master	Ear/Nose/Throat
77LRB	Hearing-Aid, Plate, Face	Ear/Nose/Throat
79LRR	Kit, First Aid	Surgery
89KNP	Orthosis, Corrective Shoe	Physical Med
73WJE	Resuscitator, Emergency, Protective, Infection	Anesthesiology
87TEO	Shoe, Orthopedic	Orthopedics
77LEZ	Speech Training Aid, AC-Powered	Ear/Nose/Throat
77LFA	Speech Training Aid, Battery-Powered	Ear/Nose/Throat
77EWM	System, Analysis, Hearing-Aid	Ear/Nose/Throat
77LRA	Tactile Hearing-Aid	Ear/Nose/Throat
79SHA	Trainer, Laparoscopy	Surgery
87UFE	Training Aid	Orthopedics
74VCZ	Training Aid, Arrhythmia Recognition	Cardiovascular
89IKX	Transfer Aid	Physical Med
89IKW	Utensil, Handicapped Aid	Physical Med
86LZP	Viscoelastic Surgical Aid	Ophthalmology
80WMV	Vision Aid, Braille	General
86HPF	Vision Aid, Electronic, AC-Powered	Ophthalmology
86HPG	Vision Aid, Electronic, Battery-Powered	Ophthalmology
86HOT	Vision Aid, Image Intensification, Battery-Powered	Ophthalmology
86HPI	Vision Aid, Optical, AC-Powered	Ophthalmology
86HPE	Vision Aid, Optical, Battery-Powered	Ophthalmology
86WOM	Vision Aid, Ultrasonic	Ophthalmology

AIDS

80WUM	Encapsulator, Fluid	General
83WKS	Equipment, Test, Western Blot	Microbiology
82MEM	Generator, Electric Field (Aids Treatment)	Immunology
80WUI	Protector, Puncture, Needle	General
80MEG	Syringe, Antistick	General
81VJE	Test, Antibody, Acquired Immune Deficiency Syndrome (AIDS)	Hematology
82MZF	Test, Hiv Detection	Immunology

AIR

79FZI	Air Handling Apparatus, Enclosure	Surgery
79FZH	Air Handling Apparatus, Room	Surgery
79FZG	Air Handling, Apparatus, Bench	Surgery
80TFU	Ambulance, Air	General
89INX	Bed, Air Fluidized	Physical Med
80WRS	Bulb, Inflation	General
86HMX	Cannula, Ophthalmic	Ophthalmology
73BTI	Compressor, Air, Portable	Anesthesiology
80VFK	Counter, Air Ion	General
78FAO	Cystometric Air Device	Gastro/Urology
78FJF	Detector, Air Bubble	Gastro/Urology
78KQR	Detector, Air Or Foam	Gastro/Urology
74QZI	Detector, Air, Heart-Lung Bypass	Cardiovascular
74KRL	Detector, Bubble, Cardiopulmonary Bypass	Cardiovascular
78QZV	Detector, Hemodialysis Unit Air Bubble-Foam	Gastro/Urology
80FRF	Equipment, Cleaning, Air	General
80WYN	Equipment, Filtering, Air, ETO	General
80QVW	Filter, Air	General
73RCO	Generator, Ionized Air	Anesthesiology
76EFB	Handpiece, Air-Powered, Dental	Dental And Oral
80RAH	Hood, Isolation, Laminar Air Flow	General
80RLY	Kit, Pressure Monitoring (Air/Gas)	General
80FLJ	Laminar Air Flow Unit	General
75RDW	Laminar Air Flow Unit, Fixed (Air Curtain)	Chemistry
75RDX	Laminar Air Flow Unit, Mobile	Chemistry
80FNM	Mattress, Air Flotation	General
73CBA	Monitor, Air Embolism, Ultrasonic	Anesthesiology
80RLZ	Pad, Pressure, Air	General
78FEQ	Pump, Air, Non-Manual, Endoscopic	Gastro/Urology

AIR *(cont'd)*

80JOI	Pump, Inflator	General
80FRA	Purifier, Air, Ultraviolet	General
80QAI	Sampler, Air	General
77KHH	Stimulator, Caloric Air	Ear/Nose/Throat
76ECB	Syringe Unit, Air And/Or Water	Dental And Oral
76DYY	Syringe, Bulb, Air Or Water	Dental And Oral
87HTA	Tourniquet, Air Pressure	Orthopedics

AIR-POWERED

76EFB	Handpiece, Air-Powered, Dental	Dental And Oral

AIRBRUSH

76KOJ	Airbrush	Dental And Oral

AIRWAY

73CBJ	Airway, Bi-Nasopharyngeal (With Connector)	Anesthesiology
73CAO	Airway, Esophageal (Obturator)	Anesthesiology
73BTQ	Airway, Nasopharyngeal (Breathing Tube)	Anesthesiology
80QAJ	Airway, Obstruction Removal (Choke Saver)	General
73CAE	Airway, Oropharyngeal, Anesthesia	Anesthesiology
80FMM	Cannula, Nasal	General
73CAT	Cannula, Nasal, Oxygen	Anesthesiology
73BZA	Connector, Airway (Extension)	Anesthesiology
73QMH	Continuous Positive Airway Pressure Unit (CPAP, CPPB)	Anesthesiology
77JOH	Cuff, Tracheostomy Tube	Ear/Nose/Throat
73SBH	Holder, Tracheostomy Tube	Anesthesiology
73CBE	Kit, Suction, Airway (Tracheal)	Anesthesiology
77RGB	Mask, Tracheostomy	Ear/Nose/Throat
73CAP	Monitor, Airway Pressure (Gauge/Alarm)	Anesthesiology
73BXR	Monitor, Airway Pressure (Inspiratory Force)	Anesthesiology
73RLV	Monitor, Airway Pressure, Continuous	Anesthesiology
73BWC	Needle, Emergency Airway	Anesthesiology
73BTR	Tube, Tracheal (Endotracheal)	Anesthesiology
73CBI	Tube, Tracheal/Bronchial, Differential Ventilation	Anesthesiology
77EQK	Tube, Tracheostomy (Breathing Tube), ENT	Ear/Nose/Throat
73BTO	Tube, Tracheostomy (W/Wo Connector)	Anesthesiology

ALANINE

75JNB	Ninhydrin And L-Leucyl-L-Alanine (Fluorimetric)	Chemistry

ALARM

74DSJ	Alarm, Blood Pressure	Cardiovascular
73QAK	Alarm, Breathing Circuit	Anesthesiology
73TAC	Alarm, Central Gas System	Anesthesiology
78FFI	Alarm, Electrosurgical	Gastro/Urology
78KPN	Alarm, Enuresis	Gastro/Urology
78THN	Alarm, Hypoglycemia	Gastro/Urology
74DSM	Alarm, Leakage Current, Portable	Cardiovascular
89IRN	Alarm, Overload, External Limb, Powered	Physical Med
73QAL	Alarm, Oxygen Depletion	Anesthesiology
78FIW	Alarm, Pillow Pressure	Gastro/Urology
90THK	Alarm, Radiation	Radiology
81QAM	Alarm, Refrigerator	Hematology
80TAD	Alarm, Voltage	General
74DSI	Detector, Arrhythmia Alarm	Cardiovascular
80WRQ	Equipment, Building Security	General
73CAP	Monitor, Airway Pressure (Gauge/Alarm)	Anesthesiology
80FLS	Monitor, Apnea	General
80QDB	Monitor, Bed Occupancy	General
80KMI	Monitor, Bed Patient	General
74DRT	Monitor, Cardiac (Cardiotachometer & Rate Alarm)	Cardiovascular
73BXC	Monitor, Oxygen (Ventilatory) W/Wo Alarm	Anesthesiology
80MLD	Monitor, ST Segment (With Alarm)	General
80RIO	Nurse Call System	General
80VAY	Security Equipment/Supplies	General
80WSZ	Sensor, Moisture	General

ALARMS

74MWI	Monitor, Physiological, Patient(without Arrhythmia Detection Or Alarms)	Cardiovascular

ALBICANS

83LHK	Antigen, ID, Candida Albicans	Microbiology

ALBUMIN

88KEL	Adhesive, Albumin Based	Pathology
82DCF	Antigen, Antiserum, Control, Albumin	Immunology
82DDZ	Antigen, Antiserum, Control, Albumin, FITC	Immunology
82DCM	Antigen, Antiserum, Control, Albumin, Fraction V	Immunology
82DFJ	Antigen, Antiserum, Control, Albumin, Rhodamine	Immunology
75CIX	Dye-Binding, Albumin, Bromcresol, Green	Chemistry
75CJW	Dye-Binding, Albumin, Bromcresol, Purple	Chemistry
75JIR	Indicator Method, Protein Or Albumin (Urinary, Non-Quant.)	Chemistry
75CJQ	Radial Immunodiffusion, Albumin	Chemistry
75CJZ	Reagent, Albumin, Colorimetric	Chemistry
75CJG	Tetrabromo-M-Cresolsulfonphthalein, Albumin	Chemistry
75CJF	Tetrabromophenolphthalein, Albumin	Chemistry
75JIQ	Turbidimetric Method, Protein Or Albumin (Urinary)	Chemistry

KEYWORD INDEX

ALCIAN
88IDA Stain, Alcian Blue — Pathology

ALCOHOL
91DJZ Alcohol Breath Trapping Device — Toxicology
91DIC Alcohol Dehydrogenase, Spec. Reagent - Ethanol Enzyme — Toxicology
91DMH Analyzer, Alcohol — Toxicology
91DNN Calibrator, Ethyl Alcohol — Toxicology
91DKC Control, Alcohol — Toxicology
91DIZ Delayed Analysis, Alcohol — Toxicology
91DMT Enzymatic Method, Alcohol Dehydrogenase, Ultraviolet — Toxicology
88LDZ Fixative, Alcohol Containing — Pathology
91DLS Gas Chromatograph, Alcohol (Dedicated Instruments) — Toxicology
91DLH Gas Chromatography, Alcohol — Toxicology
80LKB Pad, Alcohol — General
91DMI Potassium Dichromate Specific Reagent For Alcohol — Toxicology
91DOJ Potassium Dichromate, Alcohol — Toxicology
91DML Reagent, NAD-NADH, Alcohol Enzyme Method — Toxicology
91DLA Reagent, Test, Methyl Alcohol — Toxicology
88IGF Solution, Pathology, Formalin-Alcohol-Acetic Acid — Pathology
75UIB Solvent — Chemistry
80RVF Sponge, Germicidal (Alcohol) — General
80TGC Swabs, Alcohol — General
75MGX System, Test, Drugs of Abuse — Chemistry
91DMJ Test, Ethyl Alcohol — Toxicology

ALDEHYDE
88IDB Stain, Aldehyde Fuchsin — Pathology

ALDOLASE
75CJC Fructose-1, 6-Diphosphate And NADH (U.V.), Aldolase — Chemistry
75CJT Hydrazone Colorimetry, Aldolase — Chemistry

ALDOSTERONE
75CJB Chromatographic Separation/Radioimmunoassay, Aldosterone — Chemistry
75CJM Radioimmunoassay, Aldosterone — Chemistry

ALERT
80VFG Communication System, Emergency Alert, Personal — General
80UEU Identification, Alert, Medical — General
80VAY Security Equipment/Supplies — General

ALGESIMETER
73BXL Algesimeter, Manual — Anesthesiology
73BSI Algesimeter, Powered — Anesthesiology

ALGINATE
76VEF Mixer, Alginate — Dental And Oral

ALGORITHM
74MLO Electrocardiograph, Ambulatory (With Analysis Algorithm) — Cardiovascular

ALIGNER
76EHA Aligner, Beam, X-Ray (Collimator) — Dental And Oral
76ECQ Aligner, Bracket, Orthodontic — Dental And Oral

ALIGNMENT
89IQO Prosthesis Alignment Device — Physical Med
80WZF Tester, Alignment, Laser Beam — General

ALIZARIN
75CID Alizarin Sulfonate, Calcium — Chemistry
88IDD Stain, Alizarin Red — Pathology

ALKALI
81GHA Hemoglobin, Resistant, Alkali — Hematology

ALKALINE
81JCK Alkaline Hematin — Hematology
75CJO Alpha-Naphthyl Phosphate, Alkaline Phosphatase Or Isoenzyme — Chemistry
75CJL Beta Glycerophosphate, Alkaline Phosphatase Or Isoenzymes — Chemistry
75CJI Disodium Phenylphosphate, Alkaline Phosphatase Or Isoenzyme — Chemistry
75CIN Electrophoretic Separation, Alkaline Phosphatase Isoenzymes — Chemistry
75JFI Isoenzyme, Phosphatase, Alkaline (Catalytic Method) — Chemistry
81GHD Leukocyte Alkaline Phosphatase — Hematology
75CJE Nitrophenylphosphate, Alkaline Phosphatase Or Isoenzymes — Chemistry
75CJK Phenolphthalein Phosphate, Alkaline Phosphatase — Chemistry
75CKF Phenylphosphate, Alkaline Phosphatase Or Isoenzymes — Chemistry
81JCJ Phosphatase, Alkaline — Hematology
75JFG Phosphatase, Alkaline (Catalytic Method) — Chemistry
75CJH Thymol Blue Monophosphate, Alkaline Phosphatase/Isoenzymes — Chemistry
75CIO Thymolphthalein Monophosphate, Alkaline Phosphatase — Chemistry

ALKALOID
91DMO Reagent, Forming, Alkaloid, Microcrystalline — Toxicology

ALLERGEN
80LDH Delivery System, Allergen And Vaccine — General
82DHB Test, Radio-Allergen Absorbent (RAST) — Immunology

ALLERGY
80QYI Glove, Surgical, Hypoallergenic — General
80WYZ Liner, Glove — General
82WKW Syringe, Allergy — Immunology
82VKL Test, Allergy — Immunology

ALLOGENEIC
79RTO Cutter, Skin Graft — Surgery
79LCJ Expander, Skin, Inflatable — Surgery
79FZW Expander, Surgical, Skin Graft — Surgery
74WNZ Graft, Bifurcation — Cardiovascular
87QYR Graft, Bone — Orthopedics
79QYT Graft, Skin — Surgery
79RDQ Knife, Skin Grafting — Surgery

ALLOGRAFT
74MIE Allograft, Heart Valve — Cardiovascular
79LMO Allograft, Processed — Surgery
79RTO Cutter, Skin Graft — Surgery
79LCJ Expander, Skin, Inflatable — Surgery
79FZW Expander, Surgical, Skin Graft — Surgery
74WNZ Graft, Bifurcation — Cardiovascular
87QYR Graft, Bone — Orthopedics
79QYT Graft, Skin — Surgery
79RDQ Knife, Skin Grafting — Surgery

ALLOPLASTIC
78LQS Spermatocele, Alloplastic — Gastro/Urology

ALLOY
76EJJ Alloy, Amalgam — Dental And Oral
76EJT Alloy, Gold Based, For Clinical Use — Dental And Oral
76EJS Alloy, Precious Metal, For Clinical Use — Dental And Oral
76VLN Amalgam, Dental, Powder — Dental And Oral
76EHE Dispenser, Mercury And/Or Alloy — Dental And Oral
80WUL Metal, Medical — General
76VLM Well, Amalgam — Dental And Oral

ALPHA
82DBC Alpha 2, 2N-Glycoprotein, Antigen, Antiserum, Control — Immunology
82MGA Alpha-1 Microglobulin, Antigen, Antiserum, Control — Immunology
82LKL Alpha-1-Acid-Glycoprotein, Antigen, Antiserum, Control — Immunology
82DEX Alpha-1-B-Glycoprotein, Antigen, Antiserum, Control — Immunology
82DER Alpha-1-Lipoprotein, Antigen, Antiserum, Control — Immunology
82DEN Alpha-1-T-Glycoprotein, Antigen, Antiserum, Control — Immunology
82DAW Alpha-2-AP-Glycoprotein, Antigen, Antiserum, Control — Immunology
82KTJ Alpha-Fetoprotein RIA Test System — Immunology
75JMK Alpha-Ketobutyric Acid And NADH (U.V.), Hydroxybutyric — Chemistry
75CJO Alpha-Naphthyl Phosphate, Alkaline Phosphatase Or Isoenzyme — Chemistry
82DDT Antigen, Antiserum, Alpha-2-Macroglobulin, Rhodamine — Immunology
82DCO Antigen, Antiserum, Control, Alpha Globulin — Immunology
82DFF Antigen, Antiserum, Control, Alpha-1-Antichymotrypsin — Immunology
82DEM Antigen, Antiserum, Control, Alpha-1-Antitrypsin — Immunology
82DEI Antigen, Antiserum, Control, Alpha-1-Antitrypsin, FITC — Immunology
82DFB Antigen, Antiserum, Control, Alpha-1-Antitrypsin, Rhodamine — Immunology
82DEJ Antigen, Antiserum, Control, Alpha-2-Glycoproteins — Immunology
82DEF Antigen, Antiserum, Control, Alpha-2-HS-Glycoprotein — Immunology
82DEB Antigen, Antiserum, Control, Alpha-2-Macroglobulin — Immunology
82CZO Antigen, Antiserum, Control, Inter-Alpha Trypsin Inhibitor — Immunology
82DDY Antiserum, Antigen, Control, FITC, Alpha-2-Macroglobulin — Immunology
75JKH Hydrazone Derivative Of Alpha-Ketogluterate (Colorimetry) — Chemistry
82DEC Inter-Alpha Trypsin, FITC, Antigen, Antiserum, Control — Immunology
82LOJ Kit, Test, Alpha-fetoprotein For Testicular Cancer — Immunology
84GXS Monitor, Alpha — Cns/Neurology
88UMR Test, Alpha-Fetoprotein — Pathology
82LOK Test, Neural Tube Defect, Alpha-Fetoprotein (AFP) — Immunology

ALPHA-1
82MGA Alpha-1 Microglobulin, Antigen, Antiserum, Control — Immunology

ALPHA-1-ACID-GLYCOPROTEIN
82LKL Alpha-1-Acid-Glycoprotein, Antigen, Antiserum, Control — Immunology

ALPHA-1-ANTICHYMOTRYPSIN
82DFF Antigen, Antiserum, Control, Alpha-1-Antichymotrypsin — Immunology

ALPHA-1-ANTITRYPSIN
82DEM Antigen, Antiserum, Control, Alpha-1-Antitrypsin — Immunology
82DEI Antigen, Antiserum, Control, Alpha-1-Antitrypsin, FITC — Immunology
82DFB Antigen, Antiserum, Control, Alpha-1-Antitrypsin, Rhodamine — Immunology

ALPHA-1-B-GLYCOPROTEIN
82DEX Alpha-1-B-Glycoprotein, Antigen, Antiserum, Control — Immunology

ALPHA-1-LIPOPROTEIN
82DER Alpha-1-Lipoprotein, Antigen, Antiserum, Control — Immunology

ALPHA-1-T-GLYCOPROTEIN
82DEN Alpha-1-T-Glycoprotein, Antigen, Antiserum, Control — Immunology

ALPHA-2
81LGP Test, Alpha-2 Antiplasmin — Hematology

ALPHA-2-AP-GLYCOPROTEIN
82DAW Alpha-2-AP-Glycoprotein, Antigen, Antiserum, Control — Immunology

ALPHA-2-GLYCOPROTEINS
82DEJ Antigen, Antiserum, Control, Alpha-2-Glycoproteins — Immunology

ALPHA-2-HS-GLYCOPROTEIN
82DEF Antigen, Antiserum, Control, Alpha-2-HS-Glycoprotein — Immunology

ALPHA-2-MACROGLOBULIN
82DDT Antigen, Antiserum, Alpha-2-Macroglobulin, Rhodamine — Immunology
82DEB Antigen, Antiserum, Control, Alpha-2-Macroglobulin — Immunology
82DDY Antiserum, Antigen, Control, FITC, Alpha-2-Macroglobulin — Immunology

ALPHA-FETOPROTEIN
82KTJ Alpha-Fetoprotein RIA Test System — Immunology
88JCZ Analyzer, Karyotype — Pathology
82LTQ Calibrator, AFP, Serum, Maternal, Mid-Pregnancy — Immunology
82MLF Computer Software, Prenatal Risk Evaluation — Immunology
82LOJ Kit, Test, Alpha-fetoprotein For Testicular Cancer — Immunology
88UMR Test, Alpha-Fetoprotein — Pathology
82LOK Test, Neural Tube Defect, Alpha-Fetoprotein (AFP) — Immunology

ALPHA-KETOBUTYRIC
75JMK Alpha-Ketobutyric Acid And NADH (U.V.), Hydroxybutyric — Chemistry

ALPHA-KETOGLUTERATE
75JKH Hydrazone Derivative Of Alpha-Ketogluterate (Colorimetry) — Chemistry

ALPHA-NAPHTHYL
75CJO Alpha-Naphthyl Phosphate, Alkaline Phosphatase Or Isoenzyme — Chemistry

ALT
75CJJ Diazo, ALT/SGPT — Chemistry
75CKC Vanillin Pyruvate, ALT/SGPT — Chemistry

ALTERABLE
84GWO Plate, Bone, Skull, Preformed, Alterable — Cns/Neurology
84GXN Plate, Bone, Skull, Preformed, Non-Alterable — Cns/Neurology

ALTERNATING
89ILA Mattress, Alternating Pressure (Or Pads) — Physical Med
80UCU Pressure Pad, Alternating, Disposable — General
80UCV Pressure Pad, Alternating, Reusable — General
80UBG Pump, Alternating Pressure Pad — General

ALUM
88ICI Chrome Alum Hematoxylin — Pathology

ALUMINA
91DKY Alumina Fluorescent Indicator, TLC — Toxicology
91DLY Plate, Alumina, TLC — Toxicology

ALUMINUM
80QDV Blanket, Rescue — General
87RUW Splint, Molded, Aluminum — Orthopedics

ALZHEIMER'S
80RBE Bracelet, Identification — General
80UEU Identification, Alert, Medical — General
80QDB Monitor, Bed Occupancy — General
80KMI Monitor, Bed Patient — General
82MME Proteins, Amyloid And Precursor — Immunology
80VAY Security Equipment/Supplies — General
83WSI Test, Dementia, Alzheimer's — Microbiology

AMALGAM
76EJJ Alloy, Amalgam — Dental And Oral
76VLN Amalgam, Dental, Powder — Dental And Oral
76DZS Capsule, Dental, Amalgam — Dental And Oral
76EKI Carrier, Amalgam, Operative — Dental And Oral
76EKH Carver, Dental Amalgam, Operative — Dental And Oral
76EKG Condenser, Amalgam And Foil, Operative — Dental And Oral
76VLM Well, Amalgam — Dental And Oral

AMALGAMATOR
76EFD Amalgamator, Dental, AC-Powered — Dental And Oral

AMBULANCE
80QAO Ambulance — General
80TFU Ambulance, Air — General
80WMY Clothing, Protective — General
80WKO Stretcher, Collapsible — General
80FPP Stretcher, Hand-Carried — General

AMBULANCE *(cont'd)*
89INJ Stretcher, Wheeled, Mechanical — Physical Med

AMBULATION
89QAP Unit, Support, Ambulation — Physical Med

AMBULATORY
74MLO Electrocardiograph, Ambulatory (With Analysis Algorithm) — Cardiovascular
74MWJ Electrocardiograph, Ambulatory(without Analysis) — Cardiovascular
78RKM Kit, Tubing, Dialysis, Peritoneal — Gastro/Urology
74TGX Monitor, ECG, Ambulatory, Real-Time — Cardiovascular
78RKL Peritoneal Dialysis Unit (CAPD) — Gastro/Urology
80JOI Pump, Inflator — General
80VEZ Pump, Infusion, Ambulatory — General
74ROM Recorder, Long-Term, ECG, Portable (Holter Monitor) — Cardiovascular
84RON Recorder, Long-Term, EEG — Cns/Neurology
80ROP Recorder, Long-Term, Trend — General
74RQU Scanner, Long-Term, ECG, Recording — Cardiovascular
80WOI System, Delivery, Drug, Non-invasive — General
78FKX System, Peritoneal Dialysis, Automatic — Gastro/Urology

AMEBOCYTE
83VJH Test, Limulus Amebocyte Lysate (LAL) — Microbiology

AMENDMENT
84LXL Valve, Shunt, Fluid, CNS (Post-Amendment Design) — Cns/Neurology

AMIBACIN
91LGJ Fluorescence Polarization Immunoassay, Amibacin — Toxicology

AMIKACIN
91KLP Amikacin Serum Assay — Toxicology
91LDN Enzymatic Radiochemical Assay, Amikacin — Toxicology
91KLQ Radioimmunoassay, Amikacin — Toxicology

AMINO
91DIJ Acid, Levulinic, Amino, Delta, Lead — Toxicology
83QAQ Analyzer, Amino Acid — Microbiology
83JRZ Culture Media, Amino Acid Assay — Microbiology
75JMX Ninhydrin, Nitrogen (Amino-Nitrogen) — Chemistry
83UFK Reagent, Analyzer, Amino Acid — Microbiology
75UIH Standard, Amino Acid — Chemistry

AMINO-NITROGEN
75JMX Ninhydrin, Nitrogen (Amino-Nitrogen) — Chemistry

AMINOLEVULINIC
75JKK Acetylacetone (Colorimetric), Delta-Aminolevulinic Acid — Chemistry
75JKL Column, Ion Exchange With Colorimetry, Delta-Aminolevulinic — Chemistry

AMINOPEPTIDASE
75CDC L-Leucyl B-Naphthylamide, Leucine Aminopeptidase — Chemistry

AMMETER
74DSM Alarm, Leakage Current, Portable — Cardiovascular
80REQ Meter, Leakage Current (Ammeter) — General

AMMONIA
75JIG Electrode, Ion Specific, Ammonia — Chemistry
75JIF Enzymatic Method, Ammonia — Chemistry
75JIE Ion Exchange Method, Ammonia — Chemistry
75JID Photometric Method, Ammonia — Chemistry
91DPJ RIA, Amphetamine (125-I), Goat Antibody, Ammonia — Toxicology

AMMONIACAL
88ICZ Stain, Ammoniacal Silver Hydroxide Silver Nitrate — Pathology

AMMONIUM
75CEL Ammonium Molybdate And Ammonium Vanadate, Phospholipids — Chemistry
91DIQ Radioimmunoassay, Morphine (3-H), Ammonium Sulfate — Toxicology
88IGE Solution, Formalin Ammonium Bromide — Pathology

AMNIOCENTESIS
75JHG Chromatographic Separation, Lecithin-Sphingomyelin Ratio — Chemistry
75JHF Colorimetric Method, Lecithin-Sphingomyelin Ratio — Chemistry
75JHH Electrophoretic Method, Lecithin-Sphingomyelin Ratio — Chemistry
85HIO Sampler, Amniotic Fluid (Amniocentesis Tray) — Obstetrics/Gyn
85HGW Sampler, Blood, Fetal — Obstetrics/Gyn

AMNIOSCOPE
85HFA Amnioscope, Transabdominal (Fetoscope) — Obstetrics/Gyn
85HEZ Endoscope, Transcervical (Amnioscope) — Obstetrics/Gyn

AMNIOTIC
85RKH Perforator, Amniotic Membrane — Obstetrics/Gyn
85HIO Sampler, Amniotic Fluid (Amniocentesis Tray) — Obstetrics/Gyn
75WHJ Test, Maturity, Lung, Fetal — Chemistry
85SCD Trocar, Amniotic — Obstetrics/Gyn
84LID Ventriculo-Amniotic Shunt for Hydrocephalus — Cns/Neurology

AMNIOTOME
85HGE Amniotome — Obstetrics/Gyn

AMNIOTOME *(cont'd)*
85RKH Perforator, Amniotic Membrane — Obstetrics/Gyn

AMP
75CED 5-AMP-Phosphate Release (Colorimetric), 5'-Nucleotidase — Chemistry
75CHO Radioimmunoassay, Cyclic AMP — Chemistry

AMPHETAMINE
91DKZ Enzyme Immunoassay, Amphetamine — Toxicology
91DJL Free Radical Assay, Amphetamine — Toxicology
91DOD Gas Chromatography, Amphetamine — Toxicology
91DNI Liquid Chromatography, Amphetamine — Toxicology
91DPJ RIA, Amphetamine (125-I), Goat Antibody, Ammonia — Toxicology
91DJP Radioimmunoassay, Amphetamine — Toxicology
75MGX System, Test, Drugs of Abuse — Chemistry
91DIT Thin Layer Chromatography, Amphetamine — Toxicology

AMPLIFICATION
83MKZ DNA-Probe, Nucleic Acid Amplification, Chlamydia — Microbiology

AMPLIFIED
80VKO Stethoscope, Amplified — General
79FXC Stethoscope, Electronic-Amplified — Surgery

AMPLIFIER
74DRR Amplifier, Biopotential (W Signal Conditioner) — Cardiovascular
80RGO Amplifier, Microelectrode — General
84GWL Amplifier, Physiological Signal — Cns/Neurology
74DRQ Amplifier, Transducer Signal (W Signal Conditioner) — Cardiovascular
77MCK Amplifier, Voice — Ear/Nose/Throat
74KGJ Monitor, Blood Pressure, Amplifier & Associated Electronics — Cardiovascular
74RLR Monitor, Blood Pressure, Invasive (Arterial) — Cardiovascular
74RLX Monitor, Blood Pressure, Venous — Cardiovascular
74QRW Monitor, ECG — Cardiovascular
84BRR Monitor, EEG — Cns/Neurology
85TDR Monitor, Neonatal, Physiological — Obstetrics/Gyn
73RLA Monitor, Physiological, Acute Care — Anesthesiology
74RLB Monitor, Physiological, Cardiac Catheterization — Cardiovascular
74RLC Monitor, Physiological, Stress Exercise — Cardiovascular
74DQC Phonocardiograph — Cardiovascular
78FES Recorder, External, Pressure, Amplifier & Transducer — Gastro/Urology
90IZE Tube, Image Amplifier, X-Ray — Radiology

AMPULE
78QAS Ampule — Gastro/Urology
80WOF Breaker, Ampule — General
78QAR Opener, Ampule — Gastro/Urology

AMPUTATION
80WNB Amputation Protection Unit — General
79GDN Knife, Amputation — Surgery

AMSLER
86HOQ Grid, Amsler — Ophthalmology

AMYLASE
75JFJ Catalytic Method, Amylase — Chemistry
75KHM Nephelometric, Amylase — Chemistry
75CJD Nitrosalicylate Reduction, Amylase — Chemistry
75CIK Radial Diffusion, Amylase — Chemistry
75CJA Reagent, Amylase, Colorimetric — Chemistry
75CIJ Saccharogenic, Amylase — Chemistry
75CIW Starch-Dye Bound Polymer, Amylase — Chemistry

AMYLOID
82MME Proteins, Amyloid And Precursor — Immunology

ANA
82DHN Antibody, Antinuclear, Indirect Immunofluorescent, Antigen — Immunology
82LJM Antinuclear Antibody (Enzyme-Labeled), Antigen, Controls — Immunology
82LKJ Antinuclear Antibody, Antigen, Control — Immunology
82LLL Extractable Antinuclear Antibody (Rnp/Sm), Antigen/Control — Immunology

ANAEROBIC
83JTM Box, Glove — Microbiology
83VDW Chamber, Anaerobic — Microbiology
83JSL Culture Media, Anaerobic Transport — Microbiology
83RBX Incubator, Anaerobic — Microbiology
83JSP Kit, Identification, Anaerobic — Microbiology
83JTX Transport System, Anaerobic — Microbiology

ANAL
78WSS Balloon, Rectal — Gastro/Urology

ANALGESIA
73BXL Algesimeter, Manual — Anesthesiology
73BSI Algesimeter, Powered — Anesthesiology
80WRI Analgesia Unit, Cryogenic — General
84WHU Electrode, TENS — Cns/Neurology
73LEX Gas Machine, Analgesia — Anesthesiology
80THJ Gas Mixtures, Medical — General

ANALGESIA *(cont'd)*
73ELI Gas-Machine, Analgesia — Anesthesiology
73BSZ Gas-Machine, Anesthesia — Anesthesiology
76UDX Mask, Analgesia — Dental And Oral
80MEA Pump, Infusion, Patient Controlled Analgesia (PCA) — General

ANALGESIC
84UFF Stimulator, Electro-Analgesic — Cns/Neurology

ANALOG
86HMB Recorder, Analog/Digital, Ophthalmic — Ophthalmology

ANALYSIS
77ETW Calibrator, Hearing-Aid/Earphone And Analysis Systems — Ear/Nose/Throat
80WLE Computer, Image, Endoscopic — General
90UFD Computer, Radiographic Image Analysis — Radiology
91DIZ Delayed Analysis, Alcohol — Toxicology
85MNA Device, Semen Analysis — Obstetrics/Gyn
74MLO Electrocardiograph, Ambulatory (With Analysis Algorithm) — Cardiovascular
74MWJ Electrocardiograph, Ambulatory(without Analysis) — Cardiovascular
75UHG Equipment, Analysis, Photochemical — Chemistry
81JBD Hemoglobinometer, Electrophoretic Analysis System — Hematology
75MPG Kit, Urinary Carbohydrate Analysis — Chemistry
85WSC Spectroscope, Tumor Analysis, Mammary — Obstetrics/Gyn
77EWM System, Analysis, Hearing-Aid — Ear/Nose/Throat
82WUO Test, Cancer Detection, QFI — Immunology
85VIL Test, Chorionic Villi Sampling (Fetal Chromosome Analysis) — Obstetrics/Gyn
75UIS Thermogravimetric Analysis Equipment — Chemistry
75JLL Tubeless Analysis, Gastric Acidity — Chemistry

ANALYTE
75JJX Control, Analyte (Assayed And Unassayed) — Chemistry
75JJY Control, Multi Analyte, All Kinds (Assayed And Unassayed) — Chemistry
75JIX Multi Analyte Mixture, Calibrator — Chemistry
81MVU Reagents, Specific, Analyte — Hematology

ANALYTICAL
75JQO Balance, Analytical — Chemistry
80LZF Infusion Pump, Analytical Sampling — General

ANALYZER
91DMH Analyzer, Alcohol — Toxicology
83QAQ Analyzer, Amino Acid — Microbiology
83QBD Analyzer, Antibiotic Susceptibility — Microbiology
77LXV Analyzer, Apparatus, Vestibular — Ear/Nose/Throat
77RUQ Analyzer, Audio Spectrum — Ear/Nose/Throat
75QES Analyzer, BUN (Blood Urea Nitrogen) — Chemistry
80WJN Analyzer, Battery — General
73TAK Analyzer, Blood Gas pH — Anesthesiology
81TAL Analyzer, Blood Grouping — Hematology
81KSZ Analyzer, Blood Grouping/Antibody, Automated — Hematology
73VCC Analyzer, Blood Oxyhemoglobin Concentration — Anesthesiology
74MNW Analyzer, Body Composition — Cardiovascular
87MHH Analyzer, Bone, Sonic, Non-Invasive — Orthopedics
75UFO Analyzer, Carbon — Chemistry
75UFP Analyzer, Carbon Hydrogen — Chemistry
75UFQ Analyzer, Carbon Hydrogen Nitrogen — Chemistry
83TBH Analyzer, Cell Size — Microbiology
75JJG Analyzer, Chemistry, Centrifuge — Chemistry
75VIR Analyzer, Chemistry, Desk-Top — Chemistry
75UJM Analyzer, Chemistry, ELISA — Chemistry
75QTJ Analyzer, Chemistry, Electrolyte — Chemistry
75JJI Analyzer, Chemistry, Enzyme — Chemistry
75UEH Analyzer, Chemistry, Enzyme Immunoassay — Chemistry
75UEI Analyzer, Chemistry, Fluorescence Immunoassay — Chemistry
75JJF Analyzer, Chemistry, Micro — Chemistry
75QKW Analyzer, Chemistry, Multi-Channel, Fixed — Chemistry
75QKX Analyzer, Chemistry, Multi-Channel, Programmable — Chemistry
75WMG Analyzer, Chemistry, Nephelometric Immunoassay — Chemistry
75JJD Analyzer, Chemistry, Photometric, Bichromatic — Chemistry
75JJE Analyzer, Chemistry, Photometric, Discrete — Chemistry
75LCI Analyzer, Chemistry, Radioimmunoassay — Chemistry
75ROC Analyzer, Chemistry, Radioimmunoassay, Automated — Chemistry
75JJC Analyzer, Chemistry, Sequential Multiple, Continuous Flow — Chemistry
75QKY Analyzer, Chemistry, Single Channel, Programmable — Chemistry
75ULK Analyzer, Chemistry, Therapeutic Drug Monitor (TDM) — Chemistry
75KQO Analyzer, Chemistry, Urinalysis — Chemistry
75JJZ Analyzer, Chemistry, Urinalysis, Automated — Chemistry
75VEP Analyzer, Chemistry, Urine — Chemistry
75UGP Analyzer, Chromatography Infrared — Chemistry
88LNJ Analyzer, Chromosome, Automated — Pathology
81GKP Analyzer, Coagulation — Hematology
81QLM Analyzer, Coagulation, Automated — Hematology
81QLN Analyzer, Coagulation, Manual — Hematology
81JPA Analyzer, Coagulation, Multipurpose — Hematology
81KQG Analyzer, Coagulation, Semi-Automated — Hematology
81SAN Analyzer, Coagulation, Whole Blood — Hematology
75VIN Analyzer, Combination Chemistry/Hematology/Electrolyte — Chemistry
80VDN Analyzer, Composition, Weight, Patient — General

ANALYZER *(cont'd)*

74JEE	Analyzer, Concentration, Oxyhemoglobin, BP, Transcutaneous	Cardiovascular
91JFD	Analyzer, Concentration, Oxyhemoglobin, Blood Phase	Toxicology
81KSM	Analyzer, Coombs, Automated	Hematology
85HEO	Analyzer, Data, Obstetric	Obstetrics/Gyn
78MNZ	Analyzer, Diagnostic, Fiberoptic (Bladder)	Gastro/Urology
78MOA	Analyzer, Diagnostic, Fiberoptic (Colon)	Gastro/Urology
89VEM	Analyzer, Diathermy Unit, Shortwave	Physical Med
87WQP	Analyzer, Distribution, Weight, Podiatric	Orthopedics
80TEU	Analyzer, Doppler Spectrum	General
74LOS	Analyzer, ECG	Cardiovascular
80QSF	Analyzer, Electrical Safety	General
79QTT	Analyzer, Electrosurgical Unit	Surgery
80QUR	Analyzer, Ethylene-Oxide	General
87VDV	Analyzer, Gait	Orthopedics
73QZE	Analyzer, Gas, Anesthetic	Anesthesiology
73VCA	Analyzer, Gas, Argon	Anesthesiology
73JEG	Analyzer, Gas, Argon, Gaseous Phase	Anesthesiology
73CCC	Analyzer, Gas, Carbon-Dioxide, Blood Phase, Indwelling	Anesthesiology
73CCK	Analyzer, Gas, Carbon-Dioxide, Gaseous Phase (Capnograph)	Anesthesiology
73BXZ	Analyzer, Gas, Carbon-Dioxide, Partial Pressure, Blood	Anesthesiology
73CCJ	Analyzer, Gas, Carbon-Monoxide, Gaseous Phase	Anesthesiology
73VCB	Analyzer, Gas, Carbon-Monoxide, Non-Indwelling Blood Phase	Anesthesiology
91CCA	Analyzer, Gas, Carboxyhemoglobin, Blood Phase, Non-Indw.	Toxicology
73CBQ	Analyzer, Gas, Enflurane, Gaseous Phase (Anesthetic Conc.)	Anesthesiology
73CBS	Analyzer, Gas, Halothane, Gaseous Phase (Anesthetic Conc.)	Anesthesiology
73BSE	Analyzer, Gas, Helium, Gaseous Phase	Anesthesiology
73LXO	Analyzer, Gas, Hydrogen	Anesthesiology
73VCF	Analyzer, Gas, Neon	Anesthesiology
73JEF	Analyzer, Gas, Neon, Gaseous Phase	Anesthesiology
73CCI	Analyzer, Gas, Nitrogen, Gaseous Phase	Anesthesiology
73BSD	Analyzer, Gas, Nitrogen, Partial Pressure, Blood Phase (NI)	Anesthesiology
73CBR	Analyzer, Gas, Nitrous-Oxide, Gaseous Phase	Anesthesiology
73RJI	Analyzer, Gas, Oxygen, Continuous Controller	Anesthesiology
73RJJ	Analyzer, Gas, Oxygen, Continuous Monitor	Anesthesiology
73CCL	Analyzer, Gas, Oxygen, Gaseous Phase	Anesthesiology
73CCE	Analyzer, Gas, Oxygen, Partial Pr., Blood Phase, Indwelling	Anesthesiology
73CCD	Analyzer, Gas, Oxygen, Partial Pressure, Blood Phase	Anesthesiology
73RJK	Analyzer, Gas, Oxygen, Sampling	Anesthesiology
73BXA	Analyzer, Gas, Water Vapor, Gaseous Phase	Anesthesiology
75QYL	Analyzer, Glucose	Chemistry
81JOX	Analyzer, Heparin, Automated	Hematology
80VLP	Analyzer, Infusion Pump	General
73CBZ	Analyzer, Ion, Hydrogen-Ion (pH), Blood Phase, Indwelling	Anesthesiology
73CBY	Analyzer, Ion, Hydrogen-Ion pH, Blood Phase, Non-Indwelling	Anesthesiology
75RCQ	Analyzer, Iron	Chemistry
88JCZ	Analyzer, Karyotype	Pathology
80REO	Analyzer, Lead	General
75WMX	Analyzer, Mercury	Chemistry
73QCP	Analyzer, Metabolism	Anesthesiology
77RGY	Analyzer, Middle Ear	Ear/Nose/Throat
78FFX	Analyzer, Motility, Gastrointestinal, Electrical	Gastro/Urology
80WWG	Analyzer, Motion	General
83LRH	Analyzer, Overnight Microorganism I.D. System, Automated	Microbiology
83LRG	Analyzer, Overnight Suscept. System, Automated	Microbiology
73FLM	Analyzer, Oxygen, Neonatal, Invasive	Anesthesiology
73JED	Analyzer, Oxyhemoglobin Concentration, Blood Phase, Indwell.	Anesthesiology
74DTC	Analyzer, Pacemaker Generator Function	Cardiovascular
74KRE	Analyzer, Pacemaker Generator Function, Indirect	Cardiovascular
83LKS	Analyzer, Parasite Concentration	Microbiology
75UHB	Analyzer, Particle	Chemistry
79WTZ	Analyzer, Patient, Multiple Function (Surgery)	Surgery
75UHY	Analyzer, Peptide & Protein Sequence	Chemistry
86RKK	Analyzer, Peripheral Vision	Ophthalmology
83JTD	Analyzer, Petri Dish	Microbiology
81RLG	Analyzer, Platelet Aggregation	Hematology
81JOZ	Analyzer, Platelet Aggregation, Automated	Hematology
75UHL	Analyzer, Protein	Chemistry
73RNC	Analyzer, Pulmonary Function	Anesthesiology
84GZM	Analyzer, Rigidity	Cns/Neurology
81GKB	Analyzer, Sedimentation Rate, Automated	Hematology
81JPH	Analyzer, Sedimentation Rate, Erythrocyte	Hematology
74DRJ	Analyzer, Signal Isolation	Cardiovascular
84GWS	Analyzer, Spectrum, EEG Signal	Cns/Neurology
73WSV	Analyzer, Trace Gas, Breath	Anesthesiology
84RWA	Analyzer, Transcutaneous Nerve Stimulator	Cns/Neurology
80SDZ	Analyzer, Ultrasonic Unit	General
75UJB	Analyzer, Ultraviolet	Chemistry

ANALYZER *(cont'd)*

86SFB	Analyzer, Visual Function	Ophthalmology
73VCH	Analyzer, Water Vapor	Anesthesiology
75QDL	Bilirubinometer	Chemistry
73QFN	Calibrator, Anesthesia Unit	Anesthesiology
80WTI	Cart, Monitor	General
78QJW	Chloridimeter	Gastro/Urology
91MAS	Chromatography, Liquid, Performance, High	Toxicology
75JQP	Computer, Chemistry Analyzer	Chemistry
81JWS	Computer, Hematology Analyzer	Hematology
90WKA	Computer, Radiographic Data	Radiology
90VHG	Computer, Ultrasound	Radiology
83QMP	Counter, Bacteria	Microbiology
83QMQ	Counter, Cell	Microbiology
83QMR	Counter, Colony	Microbiology
91DNR	Counter, Gamma, General Use	Toxicology
91DNM	Counter, Gamma, Radioimmunoassay (Manual)	Toxicology
78QOI	Cystic Fibrosis System	Gastro/Urology
90WRK	Densitometer, Bone, Dual Photon	Radiology
90KGI	Densitometer, Bone, Single Photon	Radiology
90WIR	Densitometer, Radiography, Digital, Quantitative	Radiology
75JJJ	Detector, Beta/Gamma	Chemistry
84HCJ	Device, Measurement, Potential, Skin	Cns/Neurology
84JXE	Device, Measurement, Velocity, Conduction, Nerve	Cns/Neurology
85MNA	Device, Semen Analysis	Obstetrics/Gyn
83WKS	Equipment, Test, Western Blot	Microbiology
75JRK	Evaporator	Chemistry
75KHO	Fluorometer, Chemistry	Chemistry
81GKR	Hemoglobinometer, Automated	Hematology
81JBD	Hemoglobinometer, Electrophoretic Analysis System	Hematology
81WYW	Instrument, Coagulation, Automated	Hematology
73QEA	Monitor, Blood Gas, Carbon-Dioxide	Anesthesiology
73QEB	Monitor, Blood Gas, Oxygen	Anesthesiology
73TAJ	Monitor, Blood Gas, Transcutaneous Carbon-Dioxide	Anesthesiology
73QEC	Monitor, Blood Gas, Transcutaneous Oxygen	Anesthesiology
84QJE	Monitor, Cerebral Function	Cns/Neurology
78KLA	Monitor, Esophageal Motility, And Tube	Gastro/Urology
84GZO	Monitor, Response, Skin, Galvanic	Cns/Neurology
73ULU	Monitor, Transcutaneous, Carbon-Dioxide	Anesthesiology
73ULV	Monitor, Transcutaneous, Oxygen	Anesthesiology
75JQX	Nephelometer	Chemistry
75JJK	Oncometer, Plasma	Chemistry
75JNX	Oncometer, Plasma (Membrane Osmometry)	Chemistry
75JJM	Osmometer	Chemistry
74DPZ	Oximeter, Ear	Cardiovascular
74DQA	Oximeter, Intracardiac	Cardiovascular
80WOR	Oximeter, Pulse	General
81GLY	Oximeter, Whole Blood	Hematology
75JJO	Photometer, Flame Emission	Chemistry
91DLM	Photometer, Flame, Heavy Metals (Dedicated Instrument)	Toxicology
91DOQ	Photometer, Flame, Lithium, Toxicology	Toxicology
86SFA	Plotter, Visual Field	Ophthalmology
80WOD	Reader, Microplate	General
83WJV	Reader, Radial Immunodiffusion	Microbiology
83UFK	Reagent, Analyzer, Amino Acid	Microbiology
75JRE	Refractometer	Chemistry
74RTF	Simulator, Arrhythmia	Cardiovascular
74RTG	Simulator, Blood Pressure	Cardiovascular
74RTH	Simulator, ECG	Cardiovascular
74RTI	Simulator, Heart Sound	Cardiovascular
84LEL	Sleep Assessment Equipment	Cns/Neurology
77EWM	System, Analysis, Hearing-Aid	Ear/Nose/Throat
83QCC	System, Automated, Microbiological	Microbiology
77ETY	Tester, Auditory Impedance	Ear/Nose/Throat
74DRL	Tester, Defibrillator	Cardiovascular
74QSI	Tester, Electrocardiograph Cable	Cardiovascular
87REX	Unit, Evaluation, Height, Lift	Orthopedics
80QDG	Unit, Therapy, Behavior	General
78SEF	Urodynamic Measurement System	Gastro/Urology
90SGP	Viewer/Analyzer, 35mm Angio	Radiology
75JJL	Viscometer, Plasma	Chemistry

ANAPHYLACTIC

80UDB	Kit, Emergency, Anaphylactic	General
80RCG	Kit, Emergency, Insect Sting	General

ANASTOMOSIS

79SIW	Device, Anastomosis, Biofragmentable	Surgery
79SIY	Holder, Ring, Anastomosis	Surgery
79SIX	Sizer, Device, Anastomosis	Surgery
79GAG	Stapler, Surgical	Surgery
78LNN	Unit, Anastomosis, Gastroenterologic	Gastro/Urology

ANASTOMOTIC

74MVR	Device, Anastomotic, Microvascular	Cardiovascular

ANATOMICAL

90KXI	Anatomical Marker, Radionuclide	Radiology
80TAE	Anatomical Training Model	General

KEYWORD INDEX

ANHYDRIDE
76KQB PV Methylether Maleic Anhydride Copol./Carboxymethylcellul. — Dental And Oral
76KXY Polyvinyl Methylether Maleic Anhydride/Carboxymethylcellul. — Dental And Oral

ANILINE
88ICX Aniline — Pathology
88ICY Aniline Acid Fuchsin — Pathology
88KFD Stain, Aniline Blue — Pathology

ANIMAL
82KTS 2nd Antibody (Species Specific Anti-Animal Gamma Globulin) — Immunology
83UMA Animal, Laboratory — Microbiology
83THA Cage, Animal — Microbiology
88KIR Cultured Animal And Human Cells — Pathology
80RMA Pad, Pressure, Animal Skin — General
88KIS Serum, Animal — Pathology

ANION
91DOA Radioimmunoassay, Digoxin (125-I), Goat Anion Exchange — Toxicology

ANKLE
89ISH Ankle/Foot, External Limb Component — Physical Med
89ISW Assembly, Knee/Shank/Ankle/Foot, External — Physical Med
89KFX Assembly, Thigh/Knee/Shank/Ankle/Foot, External — Physical Med
87QDM Binder, Ankle — Orthopedics
89ITW Brace, Joint, Ankle (External) — Physical Med
89QUZ Exerciser, Leg And Ankle — Physical Med
87RBF Immobilizer, Ankle — Orthopedics
87KXC Prosthesis, Ankle, Non-Constrained — Orthopedics
87MBK Prosthesis, Ankle, Semi-, Uncemented, Porous, Metal/Polymer — Orthopedics
87KMD Prosthesis, Ankle, Semi-Constrained, Metal/Composite — Orthopedics
87HSN Prosthesis, Ankle, Semi-Constrained, Metal/Polymer — Orthopedics
87UBK Prosthesis, Ankle, Talar Component — Orthopedics
87UBL Prosthesis, Ankle, Tibial Component — Orthopedics
80RPB Restraint, Ankle/Foot — General
87RXC Support, Ankle — Orthopedics

ANKLET
89QBC Anklet — Physical Med

ANNULOPLASTY
74KRH Ring, Annuloplasty — Cardiovascular

ANOMALOSCOPE
86HIW Anomaloscope — Ophthalmology

ANOSCOPE
78FER Anoscope, Non-Powered — Gastro/Urology

ANTERIOR
86UBA Lens, Intraocular, Anterior Chamber — Ophthalmology

ANTHROPOMORPHIC
90IYP Phantom, Anthropomorphic, Nuclear — Radiology
90IXG Phantom, Anthropomorphic, Radiographic — Radiology

ANTI-ANIMAL
82KTS 2nd Antibody (Species Specific Anti-Animal Gamma Globulin) — Immunology

ANTI-CHOKE
77EWT Anti-Choke Device, Suction — Ear/Nose/Throat
77EWW Anti-Choke Device, Tongs — Ear/Nose/Throat

ANTI-DNA
82LRM Anti-DNA Antibody (Enzyme-Labeled), Antigen, Control — Immunology
82LSW Anti-DNA Antibody, Antigen and Control — Immunology
82KTL Anti-DNA Indirect Immunofluorescent Solid Phase — Immunology

ANTI-EMBOLIC
74RWI Stocking, Anti-Embolic, Pneumatic — Cardiovascular
80FQL Stocking, Elastic — General
89ILG Stocking, Elastic, Physical Medicine — Physical Med
80DWL Stocking, Support (Anti-Embolic) — General

ANTI-EMBOLISM
74QLZ Compression Unit, Intermittent (Anti-Embolism Pump) — Cardiovascular

ANTI-FOG
80WYR Solution, Instrument, Laparoscopic, Anti-Fog — General

ANTI-GASTROESOPHAGEAL
78LEI Implant, Anti-Gastroesophageal Reflux — Gastro/Urology
78UDE Prosthesis, Anti-Gastroesophageal Reflux — Gastro/Urology

ANTI-HUMAN
83GMS Anti-Human Globulin, FTA-ABS Test (Coombs) — Microbiology
81UJS Anti-Human Serum, Manual — Hematology

ANTI-PEROXIDASE
88LIJ Stain, Peroxidase Anti-Peroxidase Immunohistochemical — Pathology

ANTI-REGURGITATION
78FJK Kit, Tubing, Blood, Anti-Regurgitation — Gastro/Urology

ANTI-RIBOSOMAL
82MQA Antibodies, Anti-Ribosomal P — Immunology

ANTI-RNP-ANTIBODY
82LKO Anti-RNP-Antibody, Antigen And Control — Immunology

ANTI-SHOCK
74RLJ Suit, Pneumatic Counterpressure (Anti-Shock) — Cardiovascular
73LHX Trousers, Anti-Shock — Anesthesiology

ANTI-SM-ANTIBODY
82LKP Anti-SM-Antibody, Antigen And Control — Immunology

ANTI-SMOOTH
82DBE Antibody, Anti-Smooth Muscle, Indirect Immunofluorescent — Immunology

ANTI-SNORING
77LRK Device, Anti-Snoring — Ear/Nose/Throat

ANTI-STAMMERING
77KTH Anti-Stammering Device — Ear/Nose/Throat

ANTI-STREPTOKINASE
83GTO Anti-Streptokinase — Microbiology

ANTI-TACHYCARDIA
74LWY Dual Chamber, Anti-Tachycardia, Pulse Generator — Cardiovascular
74UMI Pacemaker, Heart, Implantable, Anti-Tachycardia — Cardiovascular
74LWW Single Chamber, Anti-Tachycardia, Pulse Generator — Cardiovascular
74LPD System, Pacing, Anti-Tachycardia — Cardiovascular

ANTI-THYROID
82WQF Antibody, Anti-Thyroid, Indirect Immunofluorescent — Immunology

ANTI-TIP
89IMR Device, Anti-Tip, Wheelchair — Physical Med

ANTIBACTERIAL
80QWM Floor Mat, Antibacterial — General
80WPU Soap — General
80TGE Solution, Antibacterial Cleaner — General
80TFM Wallpaper, Antibacterial — General

ANTIBIOTIC
83QBD Analyzer, Antibiotic Susceptibility — Microbiology
87MBB Bone Cement, Antibiotic — Orthopedics
83JSA Culture Media, Antibiotic Assay — Microbiology
83VCS Dispenser, Disc, Sensitivity, Antibiotic — Microbiology
83UJX Test, Antibiotic Susceptibility — Microbiology

ANTIBODIES
82MQA Antibodies, Anti-Ribosomal P — Immunology
82MST Antibodies, Gliadin — Immunology
82MVJ Devices, Measure, Antibodies to Glomerular Basement Membrane (gbm) — Immunology
82MSV System, Test, Antibodies, B2 - Glycoprotein I (b2 - Gpi) — Immunology

ANTIBODY
82KTS 2nd Antibody (Species Specific Anti-Animal Gamma Globulin) — Immunology
81KSZ Analyzer, Blood Grouping/Antibody, Automated — Hematology
82LRM Anti-DNA Antibody (Enzyme-Labeled), Antigen, Control — Immunology
82LSW Anti-DNA Antibody, Antigen and Control — Immunology
82LKO Anti-RNP-Antibody, Antigen And Control — Immunology
82LKP Anti-SM-Antibody, Antigen And Control — Immunology
83LJN Antibody IGM, IF, Epstein-Barr Virus — Microbiology
83LKQ Antibody Igm, If, Cytomegalovirus Virus — Microbiology
81MTP Antibody To HTLV-1, Elisa — Hematology
82DBE Antibody, Anti-Smooth Muscle, Indirect Immunofluorescent — Immunology
82WQF Antibody, Anti-Thyroid, Indirect Immunofluorescent — Immunology
82DBM Antibody, Antimitochondrial, Indirect Immunofluorescent — Immunology
82DHN Antibody, Antinuclear, Indirect Immunofluorescent, Antigen — Immunology
83WJS Antibody, Herpes Virus — Microbiology
83TFW Antibody, Monoclonal — Microbiology
81MVX Antibody, Monoclonal Blocking, Hiv-1 — Hematology
82DBL Antibody, Multiple Auto, Indirect Immunofluorescent — Immunology
83WJT Antibody, Mycoplasma SPP. — Microbiology
80WQZ Antibody, Other — General
83WJL Antibody, Polyclonal — Microbiology
83WJR Antibody, Toxoplasma Gondii — Microbiology
83WJQ Antibody, Treponema Pallidum — Microbiology
83WJU Antibody, Varicella-Zoster — Microbiology
83GPD Antigen, Fluorescent Antibody Test, Echinococcus Granulosus — Microbiology
83GNH Antigen, Fluorescent Antibody Test, Schistosoma Mansoni — Microbiology
82LJM Antinuclear Antibody (Enzyme-Labeled), Antigen, Controls — Immunology
82LKJ Antinuclear Antibody, Antigen, Control — Immunology

ANTIBODY *(cont'd)*

82DBJ	Antiparietal Antibody, Immunofluorescent, Antigen, Control	Immunology
83GMX	Antiserum, Fluorescent Antibody For FTA-ABS Test	Microbiology
83LSG	Candida Species, Antibody Detection	Microbiology
80VAN	Contract R&D, Diagnostics	General
83MKS	Device, Detection, Urinary Antibody	Microbiology
82LLL	Extractable Antinuclear Antibody (Rnp/Sm), Antigen/Control	Immunology
83LOM	Hepatitis B Test (B Core, BE Antigen & Antibody, B Core IGM)	Microbiology
88MYA	Immunohistochemistry Assay, Antibody, Estrogen Receptor	Pathology
88MXZ	Immunohistochemistry Assay, Antibody, Progesterone Receptor	Pathology
83GWD	Indirect Fluorescent Antibody Test, Entamoeba Histolytica	Microbiology
82LTM	Islet Cell Antibody (ICA) Test	Immunology
83LHL	Legionella Direct & Indirect Fluorescent Antibody Regents	Microbiology
81UJP	Potentiator, Blood Antibody	Hematology
91DPJ	RIA, Amphetamine (125-I), Goat Antibody, Ammonia	Toxicology
91DND	RIA, Digitoxin (125-I), Rabbit Antibody, Solid Phase Sep.	Toxicology
91DOW	RIA, Digitoxin (3-H), Rabbit Antibody, Coated Tube	Toxicology
91DNS	RIA, Digoxin (125-I), Rabbit Antibody, Double Label Sep.	Toxicology
91DOY	RIA, Digoxin (3-H), Goat Antibody, 2nd Antibody Sep.	Toxicology
91DNQ	RIA, Digoxin (3-H), Rabbit Antibody, Coated Tube Sep.	Toxicology
91DNA	RIA, Morphine-Barbiturate (125-I), Goat Antibody	Toxicology
75LIG	Radioassay, Intrinsic Factor Blocking Antibody	Chemistry
91DNW	Radioimmunoassay, Digitoxin (3-H), Rabbit Antibody, Char.	Toxicology
91DNJ	Radioimmunoassay, Digoxin (125-I), Goat, 2nd Antibody	Toxicology
91DNL	Radioimmunoassay, Digoxin (125-I), Rabbit, 2nd Antibody	Toxicology
91DJB	Radioimmunoassay, Gentamicin (125-I), Second Antibody	Toxicology
91DOE	Radioimmunoassay, Morphine (125-I), Goat Antibody	Toxicology
83LKT	Respiratory Syncytial Virus, Antigen, Antibody, IFA	Microbiology
88LIJ	Stain, Peroxidase Anti-Peroxidase Immunohistochemical	Pathology
82MOB	Test System, Antineutrophil Cytoplasmic Antibodies (ANCA)	Immunology
81VJE	Test, Antibody, Acquired Immune Deficiency Syndrome (AIDS)	Hematology
83LGB	Test, Antibody, Gonococcal	Microbiology
82VJD	Test, Cancer Detection, Monoclonal Antibody	Immunology
83LOL	Test, Hepatitis A (Antibody and IGM Antibody)	Microbiology
82WPH	Test, Receptor, Interleukin, Serum	Immunology

ANTICARDIOLIPIN

82MID	System, Test, Anticardiolipin, Immunological	Immunology

ANTICHYMOTRYPSIN

82DFF	Antigen, Antiserum, Control, Alpha-1-Antichymotrypsin	Immunology

ANTICOAGULANT

81GIM	Tube, Vacuum Sample, With Anticoagulant	Hematology

ANTIDEOXYRIBONUCLEASE

83GTR	Antideoxyribonuclease, Streptococcus SPP.	Microbiology

ANTIDEPRESSANT

91MLK	Chromatography, Thin Layer, Tricyclic Antidepressant Drugs	Toxicology
91LFI	High Pressure Liquid Chromatography, Tricyclic Drug	Toxicology
91LFG	Radioimmunoassay, Tricyclic Antidepressant Drugs	Toxicology
91LPX	Test, Radioreceptor, Neuroleptic Drugs	Toxicology
91LFH	U.V. Spectrometry, Tricyclic Antidepressant Drugs	Toxicology

ANTIFUNGAL

83MJE	Culture Media, Antifungal, Susceptibility Test	Microbiology

ANTIGEN

82DBC	Alpha 2, 2N-Glycoprotein, Antigen, Antiserum, Control	Immunology
82MGA	Alpha-1 Microglobulin, Antigen, Antiserum, Control	Immunology
82LKL	Alpha-1-Acid-Glycoprotein, Antigen, Antiserum, Control	Immunology
82DEX	Alpha-1-B-Glycoprotein, Antigen, Antiserum, Control	Immunology
82DER	Alpha-1-Lipoprotein, Antigen, Antiserum, Control	Immunology
82DEN	Alpha-1-T-Glycoprotein, Antigen, Antiserum, Control	Immunology
82DAW	Alpha-2-AP-Glycoprotein, Antigen, Antiserum, Control	Immunology
82LRM	Anti-DNA Antibody (Enzyme-Labeled), Antigen, Control	Immunology
82LSW	Anti-DNA Antibody, Antigen and Control	Immunology
82LKO	Anti-RNP-Antibody, Antigen And Control	Immunology
82LKP	Anti-SM-Antibody, Antigen And Control	Immunology
82DHN	Antibody, Antinuclear, Indirect Immunofluorescent, Antigen	Immunology
83GSO	Antigen, (Febrile), Agglutination, Brucella SPP.	Microbiology
83GPF	Antigen, Agglutinating, Echinococcus SPP.	Microbiology
83LIA	Antigen, All Groups, Shigella SPP.	Microbiology
83GMZ	Antigen, All Types, Escherichia Coli	Microbiology
82DDT	Antigen, Antiserum, Alpha-2-Macroglobulin, Rhodamine	Immunology
82DBA	Antigen, Antiserum, Complement C1 Inhibitor (Inactivator)	Immunology
82DCF	Antigen, Antiserum, Control, Albumin	Immunology
82DDZ	Antigen, Antiserum, Control, Albumin, FITC	Immunology
82DCM	Antigen, Antiserum, Control, Albumin, Fraction V	Immunology
82DFJ	Antigen, Antiserum, Control, Albumin, Rhodamine	Immunology
82DCO	Antigen, Antiserum, Control, Alpha Globulin	Immunology
82DFF	Antigen, Antiserum, Control, Alpha-1-Antichymotrypsin	Immunology

ANTIGEN *(cont'd)*

82DEM	Antigen, Antiserum, Control, Alpha-1-Antitrypsin	Immunology
82DEI	Antigen, Antiserum, Control, Alpha-1-Antitrypsin, FITC	Immunology
82DFB	Antigen, Antiserum, Control, Alpha-1-Antitrypsin, Rhodamine	Immunology
82DEJ	Antigen, Antiserum, Control, Alpha-2-Glycoproteins	Immunology
82DEF	Antigen, Antiserum, Control, Alpha-2-HS-Glycoprotein	Immunology
82DEB	Antigen, Antiserum, Control, Alpha-2-Macroglobulin	Immunology
82DDQ	Antigen, Antiserum, Control, Antithrombin III	Immunology
82CZQ	Antigen, Antiserum, Control, Bence-Jones Protein	Immunology
82DDN	Antigen, Antiserum, Control, Beta 2-Glycoprotein I	Immunology
82DCJ	Antigen, Antiserum, Control, Beta Globulin	Immunology
82DHX	Antigen, Antiserum, Control, Carcinoembryonic Antigen	Immunology
82DDB	Antigen, Antiserum, Control, Ceruloplasmin	Immunology
82DCY	Antigen, Antiserum, Control, Ceruloplasmin, FITC	Immunology
82DCT	Antigen, Antiserum, Control, Ceruloplasmin, Rhodamine	Immunology
82DAK	Antigen, Antiserum, Control, Complement C1q	Immunology
82DAI	Antigen, Antiserum, Control, Complement C1r	Immunology
82CZY	Antigen, Antiserum, Control, Complement C1s	Immunology
82CZW	Antigen, Antiserum, Control, Complement C3	Immunology
82DBI	Antigen, Antiserum, Control, Complement C4	Immunology
82DAY	Antigen, Antiserum, Control, Complement C5	Immunology
82DAG	Antigen, Antiserum, Control, Complement C8	Immunology
82DAE	Antigen, Antiserum, Control, Complement C9	Immunology
82DCE	Antigen, Antiserum, Control, FAB	Immunology
82DCB	Antigen, Antiserum, Control, FAB, FITC	Immunology
82DBY	Antigen, Antiserum, Control, FAB, Rhodamine	Immunology
82JZH	Antigen, Antiserum, Control, Factor B	Immunology
82DBT	Antigen, Antiserum, Control, Factor XIII A, S	Immunology
82DBF	Antigen, Antiserum, Control, Ferritin	Immunology
82DBD	Antigen, Antiserum, Control, Fibrin	Immunology
82DAZ	Antigen, Antiserum, Control, Fibrinogen And Split Products	Immunology
82DAJ	Antigen, Antiserum, Control, Free Secretory Component	Immunology
82DAH	Antigen, Antiserum, Control, Gamma Globulin	Immunology
82DAF	Antigen, Antiserum, Control, Gamma Globulin, FITC	Immunology
82DAD	Antigen, Antiserum, Control, Haptoglobin	Immunology
82DAB	Antigen, Antiserum, Control, Haptoglobin, FITC	Immunology
82CZZ	Antigen, Antiserum, Control, Haptoglobin, Rhodamine	Immunology
82CZX	Antigen, Antiserum, Control, Hemopexin	Immunology
82CZT	Antigen, Antiserum, Control, Hemopexin, FITC	Immunology
82CZR	Antigen, Antiserum, Control, Hemopexin, Rhodamine	Immunology
82CZP	Antigen, Antiserum, Control, IGA	Immunology
82CZN	Antigen, Antiserum, Control, IGA, FITC	Immunology
82CZL	Antigen, Antiserum, Control, IGA, Peroxidase	Immunology
82CZK	Antigen, Antiserum, Control, IGA, Rhodamine	Immunology
82CZJ	Antigen, Antiserum, Control, IGD	Immunology
82DGG	Antigen, Antiserum, Control, IGD, FITC	Immunology
82DGH	Antigen, Antiserum, Control, IGD, Peroxidase	Immunology
82DGE	Antigen, Antiserum, Control, IGD, Rhodamine	Immunology
82DGC	Antigen, Antiserum, Control, IGE	Immunology
82DGP	Antigen, Antiserum, Control, IGE, FITC	Immunology
82DGO	Antigen, Antiserum, Control, IGE, Peroxidase	Immunology
82DGL	Antigen, Antiserum, Control, IGE, Rhodamine	Immunology
82DEW	Antigen, Antiserum, Control, IGG	Immunology
82DFK	Antigen, Antiserum, Control, IGG (FAB Fragment Specific)	Immunology
82DAS	Antigen, Antiserum, Control, IGG (Fc Fragment Specific)	Immunology
82DFZ	Antigen, Antiserum, Control, IGG (Gamma Chain Specific)	Immunology
82DGK	Antigen, Antiserum, Control, IGG, FITC	Immunology
82DAA	Antigen, Antiserum, Control, IGG, Peroxidase	Immunology
82DFO	Antigen, Antiserum, Control, IGG, Rhodamine	Immunology
82DFT	Antigen, Antiserum, Control, IGM	Immunology
82DAO	Antigen, Antiserum, Control, IGM (Mu Chain Specific)	Immunology
82DFS	Antigen, Antiserum, Control, IGM, FITC	Immunology
82DEY	Antigen, Antiserum, Control, IGM, Peroxidase	Immunology
82DEZ	Antigen, Antiserum, Control, IGM, Rhodamine	Immunology
82CZO	Antigen, Antiserum, Control, Inter-Alpha Trypsin Inhibitor	Immunology
82DFH	Antigen, Antiserum, Control, Kappa	Immunology
82DEO	Antigen, Antiserum, Control, Kappa, FITC	Immunology
82DEK	Antigen, Antiserum, Control, Kappa, Rhodamine	Immunology
82DEG	Antigen, Antiserum, Control, Lactoferrin	Immunology
82DEH	Antigen, Antiserum, Control, Lambda	Immunology
82DES	Antigen, Antiserum, Control, Lambda, FITC	Immunology
82DFG	Antigen, Antiserum, Control, Lambda, Rhodamine	Immunology
82DFC	Antigen, Antiserum, Control, Lipoprotein, Low Density	Immunology
82DHP	Antigen, Antiserum, Control, Luteinizing Hormone	Immunology
82DGS	Antigen, Antiserum, Control, Lymphocyte Typing	Immunology
82DED	Antigen, Antiserum, Control, Lysozyme	Immunology
82DDR	Antigen, Antiserum, Control, Myoglobin	Immunology
82DGX	Antigen, Antiserum, Control, Ng1M(A)	Immunology
82WNJ	Antigen, Antiserum, Control, Other	Immunology
82DDX	Antigen, Antiserum, Control, Plasminogen	Immunology
82JZJ	Antigen, Antiserum, Control, Prealbumin	Immunology
82DDS	Antigen, Antiserum, Control, Prealbumin, FITC	Immunology
82DHL	Antigen, Antiserum, Control, Protein, Complement	Immunology
82DDF	Antigen, Antiserum, Control, Prothrombin	Immunology
81JZK	Antigen, Antiserum, Control, Red Cells	Hematology
82DFQ	Antigen, Antiserum, Control, Sperm	Immunology

ANTIGEN *(cont'd)*

82DFI	Antigen, Antiserum, Control, Spinal Fluid, Total	Immunology
82DDG	Antigen, Antiserum, Control, Transferrin	Immunology
82DDI	Antigen, Antiserum, Control, Transferrin, FITC	Immunology
82DDD	Antigen, Antiserum, Control, Transferrin, Rhodamine	Immunology
82DGR	Antigen, Antiserum, Control, Whole Human Serum	Immunology
82DAP	Antigen, Antiserum, Fibrinogen And Fibrin Split Products	Immunology
82DAX	Antigen, Antiserum, Fibrinogen And Split Products, FITC	Immunology
83GOT	Antigen, B. Parapertussis	Microbiology
83GOX	Antigen, B. Pertussis	Microbiology
83GPI	Antigen, Bentonite Flocculation, Trichinella Spiralis	Microbiology
83LSH	Antigen, Blastomyces Dermatitidis, Other	Microbiology
83MCB	Antigen, C. Difficile	Microbiology
83GOD	Antigen, CF (Including CF Control), Adenovirus 1-33	Microbiology
83GNG	Antigen, CF (Including CF Control), Coxsackievirus A 1-24	Microbiology
83GQH	Antigen, CF (Including CF Control), Cytomegalovirus	Microbiology
83GNL	Antigen, CF (Including CF Control), Echovirus 1-34	Microbiology
83GNQ	Antigen, CF (Including CF Control), Epstein-Barr Virus	Microbiology
83GQD	Antigen, CF (Including CF Control), Equine Encephalitis	Microbiology
83GNX	Antigen, CF (Including CF Control), Influenza Virus	Microbiology
83GRC	Antigen, CF (Including CF Control), Mumps Virus	Microbiology
83GQS	Antigen, CF (Including CF Control), Parainfluenza Virus	Microbiology
83GOH	Antigen, CF (Including CF Control), Poliovirus 1-3	Microbiology
83GQB	Antigen, CF (Including CF Control), Reovirus 1-3	Microbiology
83GON	Antigen, CF (Including CF Control), Rubella	Microbiology
83GQG	Antigen, CF (Including CF Controls), Respiratory Syncytial	Microbiology
83GMI	Antigen, CF And/Or ID, Coccidioides Immitis	Microbiology
83GRJ	Antigen, CF, (Including CF Control), Rubeola	Microbiology
83GQW	Antigen, CF, (Including CF Control), Varicella-Zoster	Microbiology
83JWT	Antigen, CF, Aspergillus SPP.	Microbiology
83JWW	Antigen, CF, B. Dermatitidis	Microbiology
83GQK	Antigen, CF, Lymphocytic Choriomeningitis Virus	Microbiology
83GSB	Antigen, CF, Mycoplasma SPP.	Microbiology
83GPW	Antigen, CF, Psittacosis (Chlamydia Group)	Microbiology
83GPS	Antigen, CF, Q Fever	Microbiology
83GPQ	Antigen, CF, Spotted Fever Group	Microbiology
83GNF	Antigen, CF, T. Cruzi	Microbiology
83GMN	Antigen, CF, Toxoplasma Gondii	Microbiology
83GPO	Antigen, CF, Typhus Fever Group	Microbiology
82MJB	Antigen, Cancer 549	Immunology
82LTL	Antigen, Carbohydrate (CA19-9)	Immunology
83GQN	Antigen, Cf (including Cf Control), Herpesvirus Hominis 1, 2	Microbiology
83MDU	Antigen, Enzyme Linked Immunoabsorbent Assay, Cryptococcus	Microbiology
83MCD	Antigen, Epstein-Barr Virus, Capsid	Microbiology
83GSF	Antigen, Erysipelothrix Rhusiopathiae	Microbiology
83GSZ	Antigen, Febrile	Microbiology
83GNC	Antigen, Febrile, Slide And Tube, Salmonella	Microbiology
82DAR	Antigen, Fibrinogen And Split Products, Rhodamine	Immunology
83GPD	Antigen, Fluorescent Antibody Test, Echinococcus Granulosus	Microbiology
83GNH	Antigen, Fluorescent Antibody Test, Schistosoma Mansoni	Microbiology
83GOB	Antigen, HA (Including HA Control), Adenovirus 1-33	Microbiology
83GNT	Antigen, HA (Including HA Control), Influenza Virus	Microbiology
83GQY	Antigen, HA (Including HA Control), Mumps Virus	Microbiology
83GQR	Antigen, HA (Including HA Control), Parainfluenza Virus	Microbiology
83GQA	Antigen, HA (Including HA Control), Reovirus 1-3	Microbiology
83GOL	Antigen, HA (Including HA Control), Rubella	Microbiology
83GRH	Antigen, HA (Including HA Control), Rubeola	Microbiology
83GNJ	Antigen, HA, Echovirus 1-34	Microbiology
83GMT	Antigen, HA, Treponema Pallidum	Microbiology
83GMJ	Antigen, Histoplasma Capsulatum, All	Microbiology
83LHK	Antigen, ID, Candida Albicans	Microbiology
83KHW	Antigen, ID, HA, CEP, Entamoeba Histolytica	Microbiology
83GLZ	Antigen, IF, Toxoplasma Gondii	Microbiology
83LJO	Antigen, IHA, Cytomegalovirus	Microbiology
83GND	Antigen, IHA, T. Cruzi	Microbiology
83GMM	Antigen, IHA, Toxoplasma Gondii	Microbiology
83LKC	Antigen, Indirect Hemagglutination, Herpes Simplex Virus	Microbiology
83GMG	Antigen, Latex Agglutination, Coccidioides Immitis	Microbiology
83GMO	Antigen, Latex Agglutination, Entamoeba Histolytica & Rel.	Microbiology
83GNE	Antigen, Latex Agglutination, T. Cruzi	Microbiology
83GPG	Antigen, Latex Agglutination, Trichinella Spiralis	Microbiology
83GRY	Antigen, Leptospira SPP.	Microbiology
83GMQ	Antigen, Non-Treponemal, All	Microbiology
83JWK	Antigen, Positive Control, Cryptococcus Neoformans	Microbiology
82LTJ	Antigen, Prostate-Specific (PSA), Management, Cancer	Immunology
83LSJ	Antigen, Rubella, Other	Microbiology
83GRL	Antigen, Salmonella SPP.	Microbiology
83GSL	Antigen, Slide And Tube, Francisella Tularensis	Microbiology
83GSI	Antigen, Slide And Tube, Listeria Monocytogenes	Microbiology
83LHT	Antigen, Somatic, Staphylococcus Aureus	Microbiology
83GTY	Antigen, Streptococcus SPP.	Microbiology
83JWL	Antigen, Treponema Pallidum For FTA-ABS Test	Microbiology
82MMW	Antigen, Tumor Marker, Bladder (Basement Membrane Complexes)	Immunology

ANTIGEN *(cont'd)*

82LJM	Antinuclear Antibody (Enzyme-Labeled), Antigen, Controls	Immunology
82LKJ	Antinuclear Antibody, Antigen, Control	Immunology
82DBJ	Antiparietal Antibody, Immunofluorescent, Antigen, Control	Immunology
82DDY	Antiserum, Antigen, Control, FITC, Alpha-2-Macroglobulin	Immunology
83GSN	Antiserum, Positive And Negative Febrile Antigen Control	Microbiology
82DDK	Beta-2-Glycoprotein III, Antigen, Antiserum, Control	Immunology
82DGM	Breast Milk, Antigen, Antiserum, Control	Immunology
82DGN	Breast Milk, FITC, Antigen, Antiserum, Control	Immunology
82DGI	Breast Milk, Rhodamine, Antigen, Antiserum, Control	Immunology
83LRF	Candida SPP., Direct Antigen, ID	Microbiology
82DDH	Carbonicanhydrase B, Antigen, Antiserum, Control	Immunology
82DDE	Carbonicanhydrase C, Antigen, Antiserum, Control	Immunology
91DCQ	Cholinesterase, Antigen, Antiserum, Control	Toxicology
82DGA	Cohn Fraction II, Antigen, Antiserum, Control	Immunology
82DGJ	Colostrum, Antigen, Antiserum, Control	Immunology
80VAN	Contract R&D, Diagnostics	General
82DAC	Control, Antiserum, Antigen, Activator, C3, Complement	Immunology
82DHF	D/KM-1, Antigen, Antiserum, Control	Immunology
82MLE	Enzyme, Immunoassay, Antipartietal, Antigen Control	Immunology
82LLL	Extractable Antinuclear Antibody (Rnp/Sm), Antigen/Control	Immunology
82DBN	FC, Antigen, Antiserum, Control	Immunology
82DBK	FC, FITC, Antigen, Antiserum, Control	Immunology
82DBH	FC, Rhodamine, Antigen, Antiserum, Control	Immunology
82DBB	Fibrin, FITC, Antigen, Antiserum, Control	Immunology
81DAT	Fibrin. & Split Products, Peroxidase, Antigen, Antis., Cont.	Hematology
82DAN	Fibrinopeptide A, Antigen, Antiserum, Control	Immunology
82DAL	Fraction IV-5, Antigen, Antiserum, Control	Immunology
82KHT	Fraction V, Antigen, Antiserum, Control	Immunology
82DAM	Hemoglobin, Chain Specific, Antigen, Antiserum, Control	Immunology
83LOM	Hepatitis B Test (B Core, BE Antigen & Antibody, B Core IGM)	Microbiology
82CZM	IGA, Ferritin, Antigen, Antiserum, Control	Immunology
82DFM	IGE, Ferritin, Antigen, Antiserum, Control	Immunology
82DAQ	IGG (FD Fragment Specific), Antigen, Antiserum, Control	Immunology
82DGD	IGG, Ferritin, Antigen, Antiserum, Control	Immunology
82DFL	IGM, Ferritin, Antigen, Antiserum, Control	Immunology
82DGT	INV-1, Antigen, Antiserum, Control	Immunology
82DEC	Inter-Alpha Trypsin, FITC, Antigen, Antiserum, Control	Immunology
82DFD	Kappa, Peroxidase, Antigen, Antiserum, Control	Immunology
82MEO	Kit, Antigen, RIA, Prostatic Acid Phosphatase	Immunology
83MKA	Kit, Direct Antigen, Negative Control	Microbiology
83MJZ	Kit, Direct Antigen, Positive Control	Microbiology
82DET	Lactic Dehydrogenase, Antigen, Antiserum, Control	Immunology
82DEP	Lambda, Peroxidase, Antigen, Antiserum, Control	Immunology
82DEL	Lipoprotein X, Antigen, Antiserum, Control	Immunology
82DEA	Myoglobin, FITC, Antigen, Antiserum, Control	Immunology
82DDO	Myoglobin, Rhodamine, Antigen, Antiserum, Control	Immunology
82DHI	NG3M(BO), Antigen, Antiserum, Control	Immunology
82DHQ	NG3M(G), Antigen, Antiserum, Control	Immunology
82DHY	NG4M(A), Antigen, Antiserum, Control	Immunology
82DFN	Platelets, Antigen, Antiserum, Control	Immunology
82JZI	Platelets, FITC, Antigen, Antiserum, Control	Immunology
82DFR	Platelets, Rhodamine, Antigen, Antiserum, Control	Immunology
82MGY	Radioimmunoassay, Prostate-Specific Antigen (PSA)	Immunology
82DGF	Red Cells, FITC, Antigen, Antiserum, Control	Immunology
82DFW	Red Cells, Rhodamine, Antigen, Antiserum, Control	Immunology
83LKT	Respiratory Syncytial Virus, Antigen, Antibody, IFA	Microbiology
82CZS	Retinol-Binding Protein, Antigen, Antiserum, Control	Immunology
82DGB	Seminal Fluid, Antigen, Antiserum, Control	Immunology
82DFX	Sperm, FITC, Antigen, Antiserum, Control	Immunology
88LIJ	Stain, Peroxidase Anti-Peroxidase Immunohistochemical	Pathology
81KSJ	System, Identification, Hepatitis B Antigen	Hematology
82MOI	System, Test, Immunological, Antigen, Tumor	Immunology
82LTK	Test, Antigen (CA125), Tumor-Associated, Ovarian, Epithelial	Immunology
83LLM	Test, Nuclear Antigen, Epstein-Barr Virus	Microbiology
82MTG	Test, Prostate Specific Antigen, Free, (Noncomplexed) To Distinguish Prostate Cancer from Benign Conditions	Immunology
82LTP	Test, Tissue Polypeptide Antigen (TPA)	Immunology
82DEE	Thrombin, Antigen, Antiserum, Control	Immunology
82DDC	Thyroglobulin, Antigen, Antiserum, Control	Immunology
82DDJ	Thyroglobulin, FITC, Antigen, Antiserum, Control	Immunology
82DDL	Thyroglobulin, Rhodamine, Antigen, Antiserum, Control	Immunology
82MTF	Total, Prostate Specific Antigen (noncomplexed & complexed) for Detection of Prostate Cancer	Immunology
82LTR	Tumor-Associated Antigen, Tennagen Test	Immunology
82DGQ	Whole Human Plasma, Antigen, Antiserum, Control	Immunology

ANTIMICROBIAL

83LJF	Antimicrobial Drug Removal Device	Microbiology
78MJC	Catheter and Accessories, Urological	Gastro/Urology
83JSO	Culture Media, Antimicrobial Susceptibility Test	Microbiology
83LKA	Culture Media, Antimicrobial Susceptibility Test	Microbiology
83MKR	Device, Susceptibility, Topical Antimicrobial	Microbiology
83JTN	Disc, Susceptibility, Antimicrobial	Microbiology
83JTT	Sensitivity Test Powder, Antimicrobial	Microbiology

ANTIMICROBIAL (cont'd)
80TGE Solution, Antibacterial Cleaner General
83LOP Solution, Antimicrobial Microbiology
83LTW Susceptibility Test Cards, Antimicrobial Microbiology
83LTT Susceptibility Test Panels, Antimicrobial Microbiology
83LON Test System, Antimicrobial Susceptibility, Automated Microbiology
83JWY Test, Antimicrobial Susceptibility Microbiology

ANTIMITOCHONDRIAL
82DBM Antibody, Antimitochondrial, Indirect Immunofluorescent Immunology

ANTIMONY
91DNE Absorption, Atomic, Antimony Toxicology

ANTIMYCOBACTERIA
83MJD Culture Media, Antimycobacteria, Susceptibility Test Microbiology

ANTIMYCOBACTERIAL
83MJA Powders, Antimycobacterial Susceptibility Test Microbiology

ANTINEUTROPHIL
82MOB Test System, Antineutrophil Cytoplasmic Antibodies (ANCA) Immunology

ANTINUCLEAR
82DHN Antibody, Antinuclear, Indirect Immunofluorescent, Antigen Immunology
82LJM Antinuclear Antibody (Enzyme-Labeled), Antigen, Controls Immunology
82LKJ Antinuclear Antibody, Antigen, Control Immunology
82LLL Extractable Antinuclear Antibody (Rnp/Sm), Antigen/Control Immunology

ANTIPARIETAL
82DBJ Antiparietal Antibody, Immunofluorescent, Antigen, Control Immunology

ANTIPARTIETAL
82MLE Enzyme, Immunoassay, Antipartietal, Antigen Control Immunology

ANTIPLASMIN
81LGP Test, Alpha-2 Antiplasmin Hematology

ANTIPSYCHOTIC
91LPX Test, Radioreceptor, Neuroleptic Drugs Toxicology

ANTISEPTIC
80QBE Applicator, Antiseptic General
80RYG Swabs, Antiseptic General

ANTISERA
83GSX Antisera, Acinetobacter Calcoaceticus, All Varieties Microbiology
83KLH Antisera, C. Acnes Microbiology
83LIN Antisera, Conjugated Fluorescent, Cytomegalovirus Microbiology
83GSY Antisera, Fluorescent, All Globulins, Proteus SPP. Microbiology
83GTN Antisera, Fluorescent, All Types, Staphylococcus SPP. Microbiology
83LKI Antisera, Fluorescent, Chlamydia SPP. Microbiology
83GNM Antisera, Fluorescent, Coxsackievirus A 1-24, B 1-6 Microbiology
83GRK Antisera, Fluorescent, Echovirus 1-34 Microbiology
83GOE Antisera, Fluorescent, Poliovirus 1-3 Microbiology
83GSS Antisera, Fluorescent, Pseudomonas Aeruginosa Microbiology
83LJK Antisera, IF, Toxoplasma Gondii Microbiology
83LKH Antisera, Immunoperoxidase, Chlamydia SPP. Microbiology
83GQE Antisera, Neutralization, All Types, Rhinovirus Microbiology
83GNR Antisera, Neutralization, Influenza Virus A, B, C Microbiology
83GOJ Antisera, Neutralization, Rubella Microbiology
83GPE Antisera, Positive Control, Echinococcus SPP. Microbiology

ANTISERUM
82DBC Alpha 2, 2N-Glycoprotein, Antigen, Antiserum, Control Immunology
82MGA Alpha-1 Microglobulin, Antigen, Antiserum, Control Immunology
82LKL Alpha-1-Acid-Glycoprotein, Antigen, Antiserum, Control Immunology
82DEX Alpha-1-B-Glycoprotein, Antigen, Antiserum, Control Immunology
82DER Alpha-1-Lipoprotein, Antigen, Antiserum, Control Immunology
82DEN Alpha-1-T-Glycoprotein, Antigen, Antiserum, Control Immunology
82DAW Alpha-2-AP-Glycoprotein, Antigen, Antiserum, Control Immunology
82DDT Antigen, Antiserum, Alpha-2-Macroglobulin, Rhodamine Immunology
82DBA Antigen, Antiserum, Complement C1 Inhibitor (Inactivator) Immunology
82DCF Antigen, Antiserum, Control, Albumin Immunology
82DDZ Antigen, Antiserum, Control, Albumin, FITC Immunology
82DCM Antigen, Antiserum, Control, Albumin, Fraction V Immunology
82DFJ Antigen, Antiserum, Control, Albumin, Rhodamine Immunology
82DCO Antigen, Antiserum, Control, Alpha Globulin Immunology
82DFF Antigen, Antiserum, Control, Alpha-1-Antichymotrypsin Immunology
82DEM Antigen, Antiserum, Control, Alpha-1-Antitrypsin Immunology
82DEI Antigen, Antiserum, Control, Alpha-1-Antitrypsin, FITC Immunology
82DFB Antigen, Antiserum, Control, Alpha-1-Antitrypsin, Rhodamine Immunology
82DEJ Antigen, Antiserum, Control, Alpha-2-Glycoproteins Immunology
82DEF Antigen, Antiserum, Control, Alpha-2-HS-Glycoprotein Immunology
82DEB Antigen, Antiserum, Control, Alpha-2-Macroglobulin Immunology
82DDQ Antigen, Antiserum, Control, Antithrombin III Immunology
82CZQ Antigen, Antiserum, Control, Bence-Jones Protein Immunology
82DDN Antigen, Antiserum, Control, Beta 2-Glycoprotein I Immunology
82DCJ Antigen, Antiserum, Control, Beta Globulin Immunology
82DHX Antigen, Antiserum, Control, Carcinoembryonic Antigen Immunology

ANTISERUM (cont'd)
82DDB Antigen, Antiserum, Control, Ceruloplasmin Immunology
82DCY Antigen, Antiserum, Control, Ceruloplasmin, FITC Immunology
82DCT Antigen, Antiserum, Control, Ceruloplasmin, Rhodamine Immunology
82DAK Antigen, Antiserum, Control, Complement C1q Immunology
82DAI Antigen, Antiserum, Control, Complement C1r Immunology
82CZY Antigen, Antiserum, Control, Complement C1s Immunology
82CZW Antigen, Antiserum, Control, Complement C3 Immunology
82DBI Antigen, Antiserum, Control, Complement C4 Immunology
82DAY Antigen, Antiserum, Control, Complement C5 Immunology
82DAG Antigen, Antiserum, Control, Complement C8 Immunology
82DAE Antigen, Antiserum, Control, Complement C9 Immunology
82DCE Antigen, Antiserum, Control, FAB Immunology
82DCB Antigen, Antiserum, Control, FAB, FITC Immunology
82DBY Antigen, Antiserum, Control, FAB, Rhodamine Immunology
82JZH Antigen, Antiserum, Control, Factor B Immunology
82DBT Antigen, Antiserum, Control, Factor XIII A, S Immunology
82DBF Antigen, Antiserum, Control, Ferritin Immunology
82DBD Antigen, Antiserum, Control, Fibrin Immunology
82DAZ Antigen, Antiserum, Control, Fibrinogen And Split Products Immunology
82DAJ Antigen, Antiserum, Control, Free Secretory Component Immunology
82DAH Antigen, Antiserum, Control, Gamma Globulin Immunology
82DAF Antigen, Antiserum, Control, Gamma Globulin, FITC Immunology
82DAD Antigen, Antiserum, Control, Haptoglobin Immunology
82DAB Antigen, Antiserum, Control, Haptoglobin, FITC Immunology
82CZZ Antigen, Antiserum, Control, Haptoglobin, Rhodamine Immunology
82CZX Antigen, Antiserum, Control, Hemopexin Immunology
82CZT Antigen, Antiserum, Control, Hemopexin, FITC Immunology
82CZR Antigen, Antiserum, Control, Hemopexin, Rhodamine Immunology
82CZP Antigen, Antiserum, Control, IGA Immunology
82CZN Antigen, Antiserum, Control, IGA, FITC Immunology
82CZL Antigen, Antiserum, Control, IGA, Peroxidase Immunology
82CZK Antigen, Antiserum, Control, IGA, Rhodamine Immunology
82CZJ Antigen, Antiserum, Control, IGD Immunology
82DGG Antigen, Antiserum, Control, IGD, FITC Immunology
82DGH Antigen, Antiserum, Control, IGD, Peroxidase Immunology
82DGE Antigen, Antiserum, Control, IGD, Rhodamine Immunology
82DGC Antigen, Antiserum, Control, IGE Immunology
82DGP Antigen, Antiserum, Control, IGE, FITC Immunology
82DGO Antigen, Antiserum, Control, IGE, Peroxidase Immunology
82DGL Antigen, Antiserum, Control, IGE, Rhodamine Immunology
82DEW Antigen, Antiserum, Control, IGG Immunology
82DFK Antigen, Antiserum, Control, IGG (FAB Fragment Specific) Immunology
82DAS Antigen, Antiserum, Control, IGG (Fc Fragment Specific) Immunology
82DFZ Antigen, Antiserum, Control, IGG (Gamma Chain Specific) Immunology
82DGK Antigen, Antiserum, Control, IGG, FITC Immunology
82DAA Antigen, Antiserum, Control, IGG, Peroxidase Immunology
82DFO Antigen, Antiserum, Control, IGG, Rhodamine Immunology
82DFT Antigen, Antiserum, Control, IGM Immunology
82DAO Antigen, Antiserum, Control, IGM (Mu Chain Specific) Immunology
82DFS Antigen, Antiserum, Control, IGM, FITC Immunology
82DEY Antigen, Antiserum, Control, IGM, Peroxidase Immunology
82DEZ Antigen, Antiserum, Control, IGM, Rhodamine Immunology
82CZO Antigen, Antiserum, Control, Inter-Alpha Trypsin Inhibitor Immunology
82DFH Antigen, Antiserum, Control, Kappa Immunology
82DEO Antigen, Antiserum, Control, Kappa, FITC Immunology
82DEK Antigen, Antiserum, Control, Kappa, Rhodamine Immunology
82DEG Antigen, Antiserum, Control, Lactoferrin Immunology
82DEH Antigen, Antiserum, Control, Lambda Immunology
82DES Antigen, Antiserum, Control, Lambda, FITC Immunology
82DFG Antigen, Antiserum, Control, Lambda, Rhodamine Immunology
82DFC Antigen, Antiserum, Control, Lipoprotein, Low Density Immunology
82DHP Antigen, Antiserum, Control, Luteinizing Hormone Immunology
82DGS Antigen, Antiserum, Control, Lymphocyte Typing Immunology
82DED Antigen, Antiserum, Control, Lysozyme Immunology
82DDR Antigen, Antiserum, Control, Myoglobin Immunology
82DGX Antigen, Antiserum, Control, Ng1M(A) Immunology
82WNJ Antigen, Antiserum, Control, Other Immunology
82DDX Antigen, Antiserum, Control, Plasminogen Immunology
82JZJ Antigen, Antiserum, Control, Prealbumin Immunology
82DDS Antigen, Antiserum, Control, Prealbumin, FITC Immunology
82DHL Antigen, Antiserum, Control, Protein, Complement Immunology
82DDF Antigen, Antiserum, Control, Prothrombin Immunology
81JZK Antigen, Antiserum, Control, Red Cells Hematology
82DFQ Antigen, Antiserum, Control, Sperm Immunology
82DFI Antigen, Antiserum, Control, Spinal Fluid, Total Immunology
82DDG Antigen, Antiserum, Control, Transferrin Immunology
82DDI Antigen, Antiserum, Control, Transferrin, FITC Immunology
82DDD Antigen, Antiserum, Control, Transferrin, Rhodamine Immunology
82DGR Antigen, Antiserum, Control, Whole Human Serum Immunology
82DAP Antigen, Antiserum, Fibrinogen And Fibrin Split Products Immunology
82DAX Antigen, Antiserum, Fibrinogen And Split Products, FITC Immunology
83GQO Antisera, Cf, Herpesvirus Hominis 1, 2 Microbiology
83GQL Antisera, Fluorescent, Herpesvirus Hominis 1, 2 Microbiology
81UJY Antiserum, ABO Blood Grouping Hematology
83GOW Antiserum, Agglutinating, B. Parapertussis Microbiology
83GOY Antiserum, Agglutinating, B. Pertussis, All Microbiology

ANTISERUM (cont'd)

82DDY	Antiserum, Antigen, Control, FITC, Alpha-2-Macroglobulin	Immunology
83GTE	Antiserum, Arizona SPP.	Microbiology
83GPH	Antiserum, Bentonite Flocculation, Trichinella Spiralis	Microbiology
83GTF	Antiserum, Bethesda-Ballerup Polyvalent, Citrobacter SPP.	Microbiology
83LSI	Antiserum, Blastomyces Dermatitidis, Other	Microbiology
83GOP	Antiserum, C. Acnes (553, 605)	Microbiology
83GOA	Antiserum, CF, Adenovirus 1-33	Microbiology
83GNO	Antiserum, CF, Coxsackievirus A 1-24, B 1-6	Microbiology
83GQI	Antiserum, CF, Cytomegalovirus	Microbiology
83GNK	Antiserum, CF, Echovirus 1-34	Microbiology
83GNP	Antiserum, CF, Epstein-Barr Virus	Microbiology
83GQC	Antiserum, CF, Equine Encephalitis Virus, EEE, WEE	Microbiology
83GNW	Antiserum, CF, Influenza Virus A, B, C	Microbiology
83GQJ	Antiserum, CF, Lymphocytic Choriomeningitis Virus	Microbiology
83GRB	Antiserum, CF, Mumps Virus	Microbiology
83GQT	Antiserum, CF, Parainfluenza Virus 1-4	Microbiology
83GOG	Antiserum, CF, Poliovirus 1-3	Microbiology
83GPT	Antiserum, CF, Psittacosis (Chlamydia Group)	Microbiology
83GPR	Antiserum, CF, Q Fever	Microbiology
83GPZ	Antiserum, CF, Reovirus 1-3	Microbiology
83GOM	Antiserum, CF, Rubella	Microbiology
83GRF	Antiserum, CF, Rubeola	Microbiology
83GQX	Antiserum, CF, Varicella-Zoster	Microbiology
83LIC	Antiserum, Coagglutination (Direct) Neisseria Gonorrhoeae	Microbiology
83GMP	Antiserum, Control For Non-Treponemal Test	Microbiology
91DKQ	Antiserum, Digitoxin	Toxicology
91DKA	Antiserum, Digoxin	Toxicology
83GSE	Antiserum, Erysipelothrix Rhusiopathiae	Microbiology
83GNA	Antiserum, Escherichia Coli	Microbiology
83GSW	Antiserum, Flavobacterium Meningospeticum	Microbiology
83GTH	Antiserum, Fluorescent (Direct Test), N. Gonorrhoeae	Microbiology
83GMX	Antiserum, Fluorescent Antibody For FTA-ABS Test	Microbiology
83GNY	Antiserum, Fluorescent, Adenovirus 1-33	Microbiology
83GOO	Antiserum, Fluorescent, All Globulins, Salmonella SPP.	Microbiology
83JRW	Antiserum, Fluorescent, B. Parapertussis	Microbiology
83GOZ	Antiserum, Fluorescent, B. Pertussis	Microbiology
83GSM	Antiserum, Fluorescent, Brucella SPP.	Microbiology
83GOS	Antiserum, Fluorescent, C. Diphtheriae	Microbiology
83GSP	Antiserum, Fluorescent, Campylobacter Fetus	Microbiology
83LJP	Antiserum, Fluorescent, Chlamydia Trachomatis	Microbiology
83GME	Antiserum, Fluorescent, Cryptococcus Neoformans	Microbiology
83JRY	Antiserum, Fluorescent, Epstein-Barr Virus	Microbiology
83GSD	Antiserum, Fluorescent, Erysipelothrix Rhusiopathiae	Microbiology
83GMY	Antiserum, Fluorescent, Escherichia Coli	Microbiology
83GSJ	Antiserum, Fluorescent, Francisella Tularensis	Microbiology
83GTX	Antiserum, Fluorescent, Groups, Streptococcus SPP.	Microbiology
83GRO	Antiserum, Fluorescent, Hemophilus SPP.	Microbiology
83GML	Antiserum, Fluorescent, Histoplasma Capsulatum	Microbiology
83GTB	Antiserum, Fluorescent, Klebsiella SPP.	Microbiology
83GRW	Antiserum, Fluorescent, Leptospira SPP.	Microbiology
83GSG	Antiserum, Fluorescent, Listeria Monocytogenes	Microbiology
83GRA	Antiserum, Fluorescent, Mumps Virus	Microbiology
83GRT	Antiserum, Fluorescent, Mycobacterium Tuberculosis	Microbiology
83GRZ	Antiserum, Fluorescent, Mycoplasma SPP.	Microbiology
83GTI	Antiserum, Fluorescent, N. Meningitidis	Microbiology
83GSR	Antiserum, Fluorescent, Pseudomonas Pseudomallei	Microbiology
83GPJ	Antiserum, Fluorescent, Q Fever	Microbiology
83GOI	Antiserum, Fluorescent, Rabies Virus	Microbiology
83GRE	Antiserum, Fluorescent, Rubeola	Microbiology
83GTD	Antiserum, Fluorescent, Shigella SPP., All Globulins	Microbiology
83GMA	Antiserum, Fluorescent, Sporothrix Schenekii	Microbiology
83GWB	Antiserum, Fluorescent, Streptococcus Pneumoniae	Microbiology
83GSK	Antiserum, Francisella Tularensis	Microbiology
91DJI	Antiserum, Gentamicin	Toxicology
83GRP	Antiserum, H. Influenzae	Microbiology
83GOK	Antiserum, HAI (Including HAI Control), Rubella	Microbiology
83GOC	Antiserum, HAI, Adenovirus 1-33	Microbiology
83GNS	Antiserum, HAI, Influenza Virus A, B, C	Microbiology
83GRD	Antiserum, HAI, Mumps Virus	Microbiology
83GQQ	Antiserum, HAI, Parainfluenza Virus 1-4	Microbiology
83GPY	Antiserum, HAI, Reovirus 1-3	Microbiology
83GRG	Antiserum, HAI, Rubeola	Microbiology
83GTC	Antiserum, Klebsiella SPP.	Microbiology
83GMD	Antiserum, Latex Agglutination, Cryptococcus Neoformans	Microbiology
83GRX	Antiserum, Leptospira SPP.	Microbiology
83GSH	Antiserum, Listeria Monocytogenes	Microbiology
83GPM	Antiserum, Murine Typhus Fever	Microbiology
83GSA	Antiserum, Mycoplasma SPP.	Microbiology
83GTJ	Antiserum, N. Meningitidis	Microbiology
83GNZ	Antiserum, Neutralization, Adenovirus 1-33	Microbiology
83GNN	Antiserum, Neutralization, Coxsackievirus A 1-24, B 1-6	Microbiology
83GNI	Antiserum, Neutralization, Echovirus 1-34	Microbiology
83GQM	Antiserum, Neutralization, Herpes Virus Hominis	Microbiology
83GQZ	Antiserum, Neutralization, Mumps Virus	Microbiology
83GQP	Antiserum, Neutralization, Parainfluenza Virus 1-4	Microbiology
83GOF	Antiserum, Neutralization, Poliovirus 1-3	Microbiology

ANTISERUM (cont'd)

83GQF	Antiserum, Neutralization, Respiratory Syncytial Virus	Microbiology
83GRI	Antiserum, Neutralization, Rubeola	Microbiology
83GPX	Antiserum, Neutralizing, Reovirus 1-3	Microbiology
83GSN	Antiserum, Positive And Negative Febrile Antigen Control	Microbiology
83KFG	Antiserum, Positive Control, Aspergillus SPP.	Microbiology
83KFH	Antiserum, Positive Control, Blastomyces Dermatitidis	Microbiology
83GMH	Antiserum, Positive Control, Coccidioides Immitis	Microbiology
83GMK	Antiserum, Positive Control, Histoplasma Capsulatum	Microbiology
83GST	Antiserum, Pseudomonas Pseudomallei	Microbiology
83GPK	Antiserum, Rickettsialpox	Microbiology
83GPP	Antiserum, Rocky Mountain Spotted Fever	Microbiology
83GRM	Antiserum, Salmonella SPP.	Microbiology
83GTA	Antiserum, Serratia Marcesans	Microbiology
83GNB	Antiserum, Shigella SPP.	Microbiology
83GWC	Antiserum, Streptococcus Pneumoniae	Microbiology
83GTZ	Antiserum, Streptococcus SPP.	Microbiology
83GPN	Antiserum, Typhus Fever	Microbiology
83GSQ	Antiserum, Vibrio Cholerae	Microbiology
82DDK	Beta-2-Glycoprotein III, Antigen, Antiserum, Control	Immunology
82DGM	Breast Milk, Antigen, Antiserum, Control	Immunology
82DGN	Breast Milk, FITC, Antigen, Antiserum, Control	Immunology
82DGI	Breast Milk, Rhodamine, Antigen, Antiserum, Control	Immunology
82DDH	Carbonicanhydrase B, Antigen, Antiserum, Control	Immunology
82DDE	Carbonicanhydrase C, Antigen, Antiserum, Control	Immunology
91DCQ	Cholinesterase, Antigen, Antiserum, Control	Toxicology
82DGA	Cohn Fraction II, Antigen, Antiserum, Control	Immunology
82DGJ	Colostrum, Antigen, Antiserum, Control	Immunology
82DAC	Control, Antiserum, Antigen, Activator, C3, Complement	Immunology
82DHF	D/KM-1, Antigen, Antiserum, Control	Immunology
82DBN	FC, Antigen, Antiserum, Control	Immunology
82DBK	FC, FITC, Antigen, Antiserum, Control	Immunology
82DBH	FC, Rhodamine, Antigen, Antiserum, Control	Immunology
82DBB	Fibrin, FITC, Antigen, Antiserum, Control	Immunology
81DAT	Fibrin. & Split Products, Peroxidase, Antigen, Antis., Cont.	Hematology
82DAN	Fibrinopeptide A, Antigen, Antiserum, Control	Immunology
82DAL	Fraction IV-5, Antigen, Antiserum, Control	Immunology
82KHT	Fraction V, Antigen, Antiserum, Control	Immunology
82DAM	Hemoglobin, Chain Specific, Antigen, Antiserum, Control	Immunology
82CZM	IGA, Ferritin, Antigen, Antiserum, Control	Immunology
82DFM	IGE, Ferritin, Antigen, Antiserum, Control	Immunology
82DAQ	IGG (FD Fragment Specific), Antigen, Antiserum, Control	Immunology
82DGD	IGG, Ferritin, Antigen, Antiserum, Control	Immunology
82DFL	IGM, Ferritin, Antigen, Antiserum, Control	Immunology
82DGT	INV-1, Antigen, Antiserum, Control	Immunology
82DEC	Inter-Alpha Trypsin, FITC, Antigen, Antiserum, Control	Immunology
82DFD	Kappa, Peroxidase, Antigen, Antiserum, Control	Immunology
82DET	Lactic Dehydrogenase, Antigen, Antiserum, Control	Immunology
82DEP	Lambda, Peroxidase, Antigen, Antiserum, Control	Immunology
82DEL	Lipoprotein X, Antigen, Antiserum, Control	Immunology
82DEA	Myoglobin, FITC, Antigen, Antiserum, Control	Immunology
82DDO	Myoglobin, Rhodamine, Antigen, Antiserum, Control	Immunology
82DHI	NG3M(BO), Antigen, Antiserum, Control	Immunology
82DHQ	NG3M(G), Antigen, Antiserum, Control	Immunology
82DHY	NG4M(A), Antigen, Antiserum, Control	Immunology
82DFN	Platelets, Antigen, Antiserum, Control	Immunology
82JZI	Platelets, FITC, Antigen, Antiserum, Control	Immunology
82DFR	Platelets, Rhodamine, Antigen, Antiserum, Control	Immunology
82DGF	Red Cells, FITC, Antigen, Antiserum, Control	Immunology
82DFW	Red Cells, Rhodamine, Antigen, Antiserum, Control	Immunology
82CZS	Retinol-Binding Protein, Antigen, Antiserum, Control	Immunology
82DGB	Seminal Fluid, Antigen, Antiserum, Control	Immunology
82DFX	Sperm, FITC, Antigen, Antiserum, Control	Immunology
82DEE	Thrombin, Antigen, Antiserum, Control	Immunology
82DDC	Thyroglobulin, Antigen, Antiserum, Control	Immunology
82DDJ	Thyroglobulin, FITC, Antigen, Antiserum, Control	Immunology
82DDL	Thyroglobulin, Rhodamine, Antigen, Antiserum, Control	Immunology
82DGQ	Whole Human Plasma, Antigen, Antiserum, Control	Immunology

ANTISTICK

80MEG	Syringe, Antistick	General

ANTISTREPTOLYSIN

83GTQ	Reagent, Antistreptolysin-Titer/Streptolysin O	Microbiology
83GTS	Reagent, Streptolysin O/Antistreptolysin-Titer	Microbiology

ANTISTREPTOLYSIN-TITER

83GTS	Reagent, Streptolysin O/Antistreptolysin-Titer	Microbiology

ANTITHROMBIN

82DDQ	Antigen, Antiserum, Control, Antithrombin III	Immunology
81JBQ	Quantitation, Antithrombin III	Hematology
81MMG	Response Test, Antithrombin III (ATIII)	Hematology
81JPE	Test, Antithrombin III, Two Stage Clotting Time	Hematology

ANTITRYPSIN

82DEM	Antigen, Antiserum, Control, Alpha-1-Antitrypsin	Immunology
82DEI	Antigen, Antiserum, Control, Alpha-1-Antitrypsin, FITC	Immunology

KEYWORD INDEX

APU

80WNB	Amputation Protection Unit	General

AQEOUS

76LZX	Acid, Hyaluronic	Dental And Oral

ARC

79GCT	Light Source, Endoscope, Xenon Arc	Surgery

ARCH

76KZO	Ink, Arch Tracing	Dental And Oral
87UCN	Prosthesis, Foot Arch	Orthopedics
89RXD	Support, Arch	Physical Med
87VDE	Tracing Unit, Arch	Orthopedics

ARCHITECTURAL

80VAS	Building Material	General
80VAR	Service, Architectural	General

ARCHIVING

80WQX	Camera, Video	General
80WQY	Camera, Video, Endoscopic	General
79WRX	Camera, Video, Headlight, Surgical	Surgery
79FXN	Camera, Videotape, Surgical	Surgery
80WLE	Computer, Image, Endoscopic	General
90UMF	Radiographic Picture Archiving/Communication System (PACS)	Radiology
90ROQ	Recorder, Radiographic Video Tape	Radiology
80TEF	Recorder, Videotape/Videodisc	General
78FET	Tape, Television & Video, Endoscopic	Gastro/Urology

ARDRAN-CROOKS

90IWN	Cassette, Measurement, Ardran-Crooks	Radiology

ARGININE

75JNO	N-Benzoyl-L-Arginine Ethyl Ester (U.V.), Trypsin	Chemistry
75JNN	P-Toluenesulphonyl-L-Arginine Methyl Ester (U.V.), Trypsin	Chemistry

ARGON

73VCA	Analyzer, Gas, Argon	Anesthesiology
73JEG	Analyzer, Gas, Argon, Gaseous Phase	Anesthesiology
77LMS	Laser, Argon, Microsurgical, Laryngology/Otolaryngology	Ear/Nose/Throat
77LXR	Laser, Argon, Microsurgical, Otologic	Ear/Nose/Throat
84LLF	Laser, Argon, Neurosurgical	Cns/Neurology
79ULB	Laser, Argon, Surgical	Surgery
80WQS	Laser, Combination	General
79WOH	System, Cooling, Laser	Surgery

ARIZONA

83GTE	Antiserum, Arizona SPP.	Microbiology

ARM

89QBL	Arm Rest	Physical Med
73BTX	Board, Arm	Anesthesiology
80QMX	Cover, Arm Board	General
87WLZ	Custom Prosthesis	Orthopedics
89QUV	Exerciser, Arm	Physical Med
87RBG	Immobilizer, Arm	Orthopedics
87RMN	Prosthesis, Arm	Orthopedics
90QWS	Radiographic/Fluoroscopic Unit, Mobile C-Arm	Radiology
80RPC	Restraint, Arm	General
89ILI	Sling, Arm	Physical Med
89ILE	Sling, Arm, Overhead Supported	Physical Med
89IOY	Support, Arm	Physical Med
87WUS	System, Traction, Arthroscopy	Orthopedics
80TFF	Training Manikin, Intravenous Arm	General

ARMBOARD

89IMY	Armboard, Wheelchair	Physical Med

ARMREST

89IML	Armrest, Wheelchair	Physical Med

AROUSAL

84MEI	Stimulator, Electrical, Implanted (Coma Arousal)	Cns/Neurology

ARRHYTHMIA

74QMC	Computer, ECG Interpretation (Arrhythmia)	Cardiovascular
74DSI	Detector, Arrhythmia Alarm	Cardiovascular
74QRX	Monitor, ECG, Arrhythmia	Cardiovascular
74RTF	Simulator, Arrhythmia	Cardiovascular
74VCZ	Training Aid, Arrhythmia Recognition	Cardiovascular

ARRYTHMIA

74MWI	Monitor, Physiological, Patient(without Arrhythmia Detection Or Alarms)	Cardiovascular

ARSENATE

75JMY	Citrulline, Arsenate, Nessler (Colorimetry), Ornithine CT	Chemistry

ARSENIC

91DNZ	Absorption, Atomic, Arsenic	Toxicology

ARTERIAL

74QFV	Cannula, Arterial	Cardiovascular
74QHN	Catheter, Arterial	Cardiovascular
74MUN	Device, Arterial, Temporary, For Embolization Prevention	Cardiovascular
74DTM	Filter, Blood, Cardiopulmonary Bypass, Arterial Line	Cardiovascular
74LOW	Graft, Arterial, Biological	Cardiovascular
74WTR	Guide, Catheter	Cardiovascular
80WVF	Kit, Administration, Intra-Arterial	General
73CBT	Kit, Sampling, Arterial Blood	Anesthesiology
74RLS	Monitor, Blood Pressure, Indirect (Arterial)	Cardiovascular
73BXD	Monitor, Blood Pressure, Indirect, Anesthesiology	Anesthesiology
74JOE	Monitor, Blood Pressure, Indirect, Automatic	Cardiovascular
74DXN	Monitor, Blood Pressure, Indirect, Semi-Automatic	Cardiovascular
79FYM	Monitor, Blood Pressure, Indirect, Surgery	Surgery
79FYL	Monitor, Blood Pressure, Indirect, Surgery, Powered	Surgery
73BZZ	Monitor, Blood Pressure, Indirect, Transducer	Anesthesiology
74RLR	Monitor, Blood Pressure, Invasive (Arterial)	Cardiovascular
73CAA	Monitor, Blood Pressure, Invasive (Arterial), Anesthesia	Anesthesiology
79KFO	Monitor, Cardiac Output, Dye (Central Venous & Arterial)	Surgery
79KFQ	Monitor, Cardiac Output, Trend (Arterial Pressure Pulse)	Surgery
85HEQ	Monitor, Fetal, Ultrasonic, Arterial Pressure	Obstetrics/Gyn
74FYK	Monitor, Pressure, Arterial, Internal	Cardiovascular
74RIF	Needle, Intra-Arterial	Cardiovascular
79FZC	Prosthesis, Arterial Graft, Bovine Carotid Artery	Surgery
79FZB	Prosthesis, Arterial Graft, Synthetic, Greater Than 6mm	Surgery
79JCP	Prosthesis, Arterial Graft, Synthetic, Less Than 6mm	Surgery
80FLY	Sphygmomanometer, Aneroid (Arterial Pressure)	General
80THH	Sphygmomanometer, Electronic (Arterial Pressure)	General
80UDM	Sphygmomanometer, Electronic, Automatic	General
80UDN	Sphygmomanometer, Electronic, Manual	General
80FLX	Sphygmomanometer, Mercury (Arterial Pressure)	General
87VIF	Syringe, Arterial Blood Gas	Orthopedics

ARTERIOGRAPHIC

74QBM	Arteriographic Unit, Ultrasonic	Cardiovascular

ARTERIOSCOPE

74LYK	Angioscope	Cardiovascular

ARTERIOSUS

74MAE	Occluder, Patent Ductus, Arteriosus	Cardiovascular

ARTERIOVENOUS

78KNZ	Accessories, AV Shunt	Gastro/Urology
78FIQ	Cannula, AV Shunt	Gastro/Urology
78RTB	Shunt, Arteriovenous	Gastro/Urology

ARTERY

74MFT	Band, Pulmonary Artery	Cardiovascular
74QFY	Cannula, Coronary Artery	Cardiovascular
80FOS	Catheter, Umbilical Artery	General
84HCE	Clamp, Carotid Artery	Cns/Neurology
74DXC	Clamp, Vascular	Cardiovascular
74WYD	Equipment, Ultrasound, Intravascular, 3-Dimensional	Cardiovascular
74FYS	Monitor, Pressure, Pulmonary Artery, Powered	Cardiovascular
79FZC	Prosthesis, Arterial Graft, Bovine Carotid Artery	Surgery
74WWF	Shunt, Carotid	Cardiovascular
74DWX	Stripper, Artery, Intraluminal	Cardiovascular
74WTW	Syringe, Angioplasty	Cardiovascular
74WYC	System, Infusion, Enzyme, Thrombolytic	Cardiovascular
74LPE	System, Retroperfusion, Artery, Coronary	Cardiovascular

ARTHRITIS

80WYB	Equipment, Management, Pain, Radiofrequency, Non-Invasive	General
89MKC	Stimulator, Arthritis, Non-Invasive	Physical Med
82WVP	Test, Disease, Lyme	Immunology

ARTHROGRAM

87QBO	Arthrogram Kit	Orthopedics

ARTHROMETER

87LYH	Arthrometer	Orthopedics

ARTHROPLASTY

87KQY	Prosthesis, Finger and Toe, Hemi-Arthroplasty	Orthopedics

ARTHROSCOPE

87VIE	Accessories, Arthroscope	Orthopedics
87HRX	Arthroscope	Orthopedics
87TAU	Cannula, Drainage, Arthroscopy	Orthopedics

ARTHROSCOPIC

76MGG	Fluid, Hylan (For TMJ Use)	Dental And Oral

ARTHROSCOPY

87WHX	Aspirator, Arthroscopy	Orthopedics
87TAU	Cannula, Drainage, Arthroscopy	Orthopedics
80WVY	Cart, Equipment, Video	General
87THC	Holder, Leg, Arthroscopy	Orthopedics
79WRY	Holder, Shoulder, Arthroscopy	Surgery
79RCH	Insufflator, Other	Surgery

ARTHROSCOPY *(cont'd)*
87WUR Needle, Suture, Arthroscopy — Orthopedics
87WUS System, Traction, Arthroscopy — Orthopedics

ARTICULATION
76EFK Forceps, Articulation Paper — Dental And Oral
76EFH Paper, Articulation — Dental And Oral
87JWI Prosthesis, Wrist, 2 Part Metal-Plastic Articulation — Orthopedics
87JWJ Prosthesis, Wrist, 3 Part Metal-Plastic-Metal Articulation — Orthopedics

ARTICULATORS
76EJP Articulators — Dental And Oral

ARTIFACT
74RLJ Suit, Pneumatic Counterpressure (Anti-Shock) — Cardiovascular

ARTIFICIAL
79MDN Burr, Artificial (Velcro Fastener - Temp. Abdominal Closure) — Surgery
86NCK Button, Iris, Eye, Artificial — Ophthalmology
73BYD Condenser, Heat And Moisture (Artificial Nose) — Anesthesiology
84HCG Device, Embolization, Artificial — Cns/Neurology
86HQI Eye, Artificial, Custom — Ophthalmology
86HQH Eye, Artificial, Non-Custom — Ophthalmology
74LOZ Heart, Artificial — Cardiovascular
77ESE Larynx, Artificial Battery-Powered — Ear/Nose/Throat
74RMT Prosthesis, Heart — Cardiovascular
74DSO Prosthesis, Heart, With Control System — Cardiovascular
76LFD Saliva, Artificial — Dental And Oral
76ELK Teeth, Artificial, Backing And Facing — Dental And Oral
76ELJ Teeth, Artificial, Posterior With Metal Insert — Dental And Oral

ASCORBIC
75JMA Acid, Ascorbic, 2, 4-dinitrophenylhydrazine (spectrophotometric) — Chemistry
75JQE Ion Exchange Resin, Ascorbic Acid, Colorimetry, Iron Bind — Chemistry
76KKN Test, Acid, Ascorbic, Lingual — Dental And Oral

ASH
75JIK Dry Ash Method, Protein Bound Iodine — Chemistry
75JIJ Wet Ash Method, Protein Bound Iodine — Chemistry

ASPERGILLUS
83JWT Antigen, CF, Aspergillus SPP. — Microbiology
83KFG Antiserum, Positive Control, Aspergillus SPP. — Microbiology

ASPIRATING
74QFW Cannula, Aspirating — Cardiovascular
73BSY Catheter, Suction (Tracheal Aspirating Tube) — Anesthesiology
79QCL Drain, Suction, Closed — Surgery
79ULE Tip, Suction Tube (Yankauer, Poole, Etc.) — Surgery
73BYY Tube, Aspirating, Flexible, Connecting — Anesthesiology
77KTR Tube, Aspirating, Rigid Bronchoscope Aspirating — Ear/Nose/Throat
73JEM Tube, Bronchoscope, Aspirating — Anesthesiology

ASPIRATION
73CBD Bottle, Collection, Breathing System (Calibrated) — Anesthesiology
73CBC Bottle, Collection, Breathing System (Uncalibrated) — Anesthesiology
86HMX Cannula, Ophthalmic — Ophthalmology
79WZU Cannula, Suction, Pool-Tip — Surgery
79KDH Catheter, Aspiration — Surgery
73QLT Collector, Sputum — Anesthesiology
86HQE Cutter, Vitreous Aspiration, AC-Powered — Ophthalmology
86HKP Cutter, Vitreous Aspiration, Battery-Powered — Ophthalmology
84LBK Device, Fragmentation and Aspiration, Neurosurgical — Cns/Neurology
80QDT Kit, Biopsy, Ultrasonic Aspiration — General
86RCT Kit, Irrigation, Eye — Ophthalmology
79GAA Needle, Aspiration And Injection, Disposable — Surgery
79GDM Needle, Aspiration And Injection, Reusable — Surgery
79RIJ Needle, Aspiration, Cyst, Laparoscopic — Surgery
85MHK Needle, Oocyte Aspiration — Obstetrics/Gyn
79SIS Needle, Puncture — Surgery
79SJC Probe, Electrosurgery, Endoscopy — Surgery
73BTA Pump, Aspiration, Portable — Anesthesiology
80WVE Syringe, Other — General

ASPIRATOR
87WHX Aspirator, Arthroscopy — Orthopedics
80QBQ Aspirator, Emergency Suction — General
85HFC Aspirator, Endocervical — Obstetrics/Gyn
85HFF Aspirator, Endometrial — Obstetrics/Gyn
80QBS Aspirator, Infant — General
79MFF Aspirator, Liposuction — Surgery
78QBR Aspirator, Low Volume (Gastric Suction) — Gastro/Urology
77QBT Aspirator, Nasal — Ear/Nose/Throat
86WKR Aspirator, Ophthalmic — Ophthalmology
79QBU Aspirator, Surgical — Surgery
74QBV Aspirator, Thoracic (Suction Unit) — Cardiovascular
77QBW Aspirator, Tracheal — Ear/Nose/Throat
85MGI Aspirator, Ultrasonic — Obstetrics/Gyn
80QBZ Aspirator, Wound Suction Pump — General
80KDQ Bottle, Collection, Vacuum (Aspirator) — General

ASPIRATOR *(cont'd)*
74DWM Canister, Suction — Cardiovascular
85HGG Controller, Abortion Unit, Vacuum — Obstetrics/Gyn
76QOE Cuspidor — Dental And Oral
78FFD Evacuator, Bladder, Manually Operated — Gastro/Urology
78FHF Evacuator, Fluid — Gastro/Urology
76EHZ Evacuator, Oral Cavity — Dental And Oral
85HDB Extractor, Vacuum, Fetal — Obstetrics/Gyn
79WIF Filter, Aspirator — Surgery
79QUQ Probe, Suction, Irrigator/Aspirator, Laparoscopic — Surgery
85HGF Pump, Abortion Unit, Vacuum — Obstetrics/Gyn
85HHI Pump, Abortion, Vacuum, Central System — Obstetrics/Gyn
85HGX Pump, Breast, Powered — Obstetrics/Gyn
76EBR Pump, Suction Operatory — Dental And Oral
73SEI Pump, Vacuum, Central — Anesthesiology
78ROX Regulator, Suction, Low Volume (Gastric) — Gastro/Urology
80CBB Regulator, Suction, Surgical — General
73ROZ Regulator, Suction, Thoracic — Anesthesiology
77RPA Regulator, Suction, Tracheal (Nasal, Oral) — Ear/Nose/Throat
79GCX Suction Apparatus, Operating Room, Wall Vacuum-Powered — Surgery
79GCY Suction Apparatus, Single Patient, Portable, Non-Powered — Surgery
79JCX Suction Apparatus, Ward Use, Portable, AC-Powered — Surgery
73SBZ Trap, Mucus — Anesthesiology

ASSAULT
85QXO Kit, Forensic Evidence, Sexual Assault — Obstetrics/Gyn

ASSAY
91KLP Amikacin Serum Assay — Toxicology
83MDU Antigen, Enzyme Linked Immunoabsorbent Assay, Cryptococcus — Microbiology
83LQN Assay, Agglutination, Latex, Rubella — Microbiology
75LTC Assay, Disease, Membrane, Hyaline — Chemistry
83MZO Assay, Enzyme Linked Immunosorbent, Hepatitis C Virus — Microbiology
83MYL Assay, Enzyme Linked Immunosorbent, Parvovirus B19 Igg — Microbiology
83MYM Assay, Enzyme Linked Immunosorbent, Parvovirus B19 Igm — Microbiology
91MAR Assay, Serum, Cyclosporine and Metabolites, TDX — Toxicology
82MEN Assay, Serum, Sialic Acid — Immunology
91DKD Bacillus Subtilis, Microbiological Assay, Gentamicin — Toxicology
82KTQ Complement — Immunology
83JRZ Culture Media, Amino Acid Assay — Microbiology
83JSA Culture Media, Antibiotic Assay — Microbiology
83JSB Culture Media, Vitamin Assay — Microbiology
91LDN Enzymatic Radiochemical Assay, Amikacin — Toxicology
91KLO Enzymatic Radiochemical Assay, Gentamicin — Toxicology
91LDO Enzymatic Radiochemical Assay, Tobramycin — Toxicology
83LJC Enzyme Linked Immunoabsorbent Assay, Chlamydia Group — Microbiology
83MIY Enzyme Linked Immunoabsorbent Assay, Coccidioides Immitis — Microbiology
83LFZ Enzyme Linked Immunoabsorbent Assay, Cytomegalovirus — Microbiology
83LGC Enzyme Linked Immunoabsorbent Assay, Herpes Simplex Virus — Microbiology
83MIZ Enzyme Linked Immunoabsorbent Assay, Histoplasma Capsulatum — Microbiology
83LJY Enzyme Linked Immunoabsorbent Assay, Mumps Virus — Microbiology
83LJZ Enzyme Linked Immunoabsorbent Assay, Mycoplasma SPP. — Microbiology
83LIR Enzyme Linked Immunoabsorbent Assay, Neisseria Gonorrhoeae — Microbiology
83MCE Enzyme Linked Immunoabsorbent Assay, Resp. Syncytial Virus — Microbiology
83LIQ Enzyme Linked Immunoabsorbent Assay, Rotavirus — Microbiology
83LFX Enzyme Linked Immunoabsorbent Assay, Rubella — Microbiology
83LJB Enzyme Linked Immunoabsorbent Assay, Rubeola — Microbiology
83MIU Enzyme Linked Immunoabsorbent Assay, T. Cruzi — Microbiology
83LGD Enzyme Linked Immunoabsorbent Assay, Toxoplasma Gondii — Microbiology
83LIP Enzyme Linked Immunoabsorbent Assay, Treponema Pallidum — Microbiology
83MDT Enzyme Linked Immunoabsorbent Assay, Trichinella Spiralis — Microbiology
83LFY Enzyme Linked Immunoabsorbent Assay, Varicella-Zoster — Microbiology
83MXJ Enzyme-Linked Immunosorbent Assay, Herpes Simplex Virus, HSV-1 — Microbiology
83MYF Enzyme-Linked Immunosorbent Assay, Herpes Simplex Virus, HSV-2 — Microbiology
75LPJ Estrogen Receptor Assay Kit — Chemistry
91DJL Free Radical Assay, Amphetamine — Toxicology
91DIR Free Radical Assay, Cocaine — Toxicology
91DPC Free Radical Assay, Heavy Metals — Toxicology
91DOL Free Radical Assay, LSD — Toxicology
91DPP Free Radical Assay, Methadone — Toxicology
91DOK Free Radical Assay, Morphine — Toxicology
91DKT Free Radical Assay, Opiates — Toxicology

ASSAY *(cont'd)*
83MIV Immunofluorescent Assay, T. Cruzi — Microbiology
88MYA Immunohistochemistry Assay, Antibody, Estrogen Receptor — Pathology
88MXZ Immunohistochemistry Assay, Antibody, Progesterone Receptor — Pathology
82JFR Indirect Copper Assay, Ceruloplasmin — Immunology
75LPI Kit, Assay, Receptor, Progesterone — Chemistry
75LTD Paraquat Assay — Chemistry
88MHR System, Assay, Chemoresponse — Pathology
81LCP Test, Glycosylated Hemoglobin Assay — Hematology

ASSAYED
75JJX Control, Analyte (Assayed And Unassayed) — Chemistry
75JJR Control, Electrolyte (Assayed And Unassayed) — Chemistry
75JJT Control, Enzyme (Assayed And Unassayed) — Chemistry
75JJY Control, Multi Analyte, All Kinds (Assayed And Unassayed) — Chemistry
75JJW Control, Urinalysis (Assayed And Unassayed) — Chemistry

ASSAYS
81MAN Interleukin - 2 Assays — Hematology
83LSD Rubella, Other Assays — Microbiology

ASSEMBLY
89ISW Assembly, Knee/Shank/Ankle/Foot, External — Physical Med
89KFT Assembly, Shoulder/Elbow/Forearm/Wrist/Hand, Mechanical — Physical Med
89KFW Assembly, Shoulder/Elbow/Forearm/Wrist/Hand, Powered — Physical Med
89KFX Assembly, Thigh/Knee/Shank/Ankle/Foot, External — Physical Med
76EBX Bracket, Table Assembly, N2O Delivery System — Dental And Oral
80WXA Component, Other — General
80WVW Contract Assembly — General
80VAC Contract Manufacturing — General
80VAO Contract Packaging — General

ASSESSMENT
84LEL Sleep Assessment Equipment — Cns/Neurology

ASSIST
73CCO Bed, Rocking, Breathing Assist — Anesthesiology
74QKD Circulatory Assist Unit, Cardiac — Cardiovascular
74QKE Circulatory Assist Unit, Intra-Aortic Balloon — Cardiovascular
74DSQ Circulatory Assist Unit, Left Ventricular — Cardiovascular
74QKF Circulatory Assist Unit, Venous Return — Cardiovascular
74QLZ Compression Unit, Intermittent (Anti-Embolism Pump) — Cardiovascular
73LYM Device, Assist, CPR — Anesthesiology
74QZM Heart-Lung Bypass Unit (Cardiopulmonary) — Cardiovascular
74RMT Prosthesis, Heart — Cardiovascular
74DRN Pump, Counterpulsating, External — Cardiovascular
74RNE Pump, Extracorporeal Perfusion — Cardiovascular
74RPH Resuscitator, Cardiopulmonary — Cardiovascular
74JOW Sleeve, Compressible Limb — Cardiovascular
74RWI Stocking, Anti-Embolic, Pneumatic — Cardiovascular
80DWL Stocking, Support (Anti-Embolic) — General
74RLJ Suit, Pneumatic Counterpressure (Anti-Shock) — Cardiovascular
74MFZ System, Pump & Control, Cardiac Assist, Axial Flow — Cardiovascular
74DRP Tourniquet, Automatic Rotating — Cardiovascular

ASSISTANT
87SHK Assistant, Surgical, Orthopedic, Automated — Orthopedics

ASSISTED
85MQG Accessory, Assisted Reproduction — Obstetrics/Gyn
85MQF Catheter, Assisted Reproduction — Obstetrics/Gyn
81KST Collector, Blood, Vacuum-Assisted — Hematology
85MQK Labware, Assisted Reproduction — Obstetrics/Gyn
85MQJ Micromanipulators and Microinjectors, Assisted Reproduction — Obstetrics/Gyn
85MQH Microtools, Assisted Reproduction — Obstetrics/Gyn
85MQI Microtools, Fabrication, Assisted Reproduction — Obstetrics/Gyn
85MQE Needle, Assisted Reproduction — Obstetrics/Gyn
85MGK Scanner, Breast, Thermographic, Ultrasonic, Computer-Asstd. — Obstetrics/Gyn
85MTW System, Water, Reproduction, Assisted, And Purification — Obstetrics/Gyn

ASSISTIVE
77LZI Device, Assistive Listening — Ear/Nose/Throat

ASSOCIATED
81LLG Kit, Platelet Associated IGG — Hematology
74KGJ Monitor, Blood Pressure, Amplifier & Associated Electronics — Cardiovascular
82LTK Test, Antigen (CA125), Tumor-Associated, Ovarian, Epithelial — Immunology
82LTR Tumor-Associated Antigen, Tennagen Test — Immunology

ASSURANCE
90TDZ Tester, Radiology Quality Assurance — Radiology

AST
75JFK Catalytic Method, AST/SGOT — Chemistry
75CIT NADH Oxidation/NAD Reduction, AST/SGOT — Chemistry

AST *(cont'd)*
75CIF Vanillin Pyruvate, AST/SGOT — Chemistry

ASTIGMATISM
86QVI Eyeglasses — Ophthalmology

ASTIGMOMETER
86WQG Astigmometer — Ophthalmology

ATAXIAGRAPH
84GWW Ataxiagraph — Cns/Neurology

ATHERECTOMY
74LIT Catheter, Angioplasty, Transluminal, Peripheral — Cardiovascular
74MCX Catheter, Coronary, Atherectomy — Cardiovascular
74MCW Catheter, Peripheral, Atherectomy — Cardiovascular
74LPC Laser, Angioplasty, Coronary — Cardiovascular
74LWX Laser, Angioplasty, Peripheral — Cardiovascular
74WTW Syringe, Angioplasty — Cardiovascular
74MKX System, Carotid Atherectomy — Cardiovascular
74MKH System, Renal Atherectomy, Ivt — Cardiovascular

ATIII
81MMG Response Test, Antithrombin III (ATIII) — Hematology

ATMOSPHERIC
80QUM Monitor, Gas, Atmospheric, Environmental — General

ATOMIC
91DNE Absorption, Atomic, Antimony — Toxicology
91DNZ Absorption, Atomic, Arsenic — Toxicology
75JFN Absorption, Atomic, Calcium — Chemistry
75JIZ Absorption, Atomic, Iron (Non-Heme) — Chemistry
91DOF Absorption, Atomic, Lead — Toxicology
91JII Absorption, Atomic, Lithium — Toxicology
75JGI Absorption, Atomic, Magnesium — Chemistry
91DPH Absorption, Atomic, Mercury — Toxicology
91JXR Spectrophotometer, Atomic Absorption, General Use — Toxicology

ATOMIZER
77KCK Atomizer And Tip, ENT — Ear/Nose/Throat
75JQS Atomizer, Flameless — Chemistry
91DLC Atomizer, TLC — Toxicology
77KCO Inhaler, Nasal — Ear/Nose/Throat
73CCQ Nebulizer, Medicinal, Non-Ventilatory (Atomizer) — Anesthesiology

ATP
81JWR ATP Release (Luminescence) — Hematology
75JLB ATP and CK (Enzymatic), Creatine — Chemistry
75JLZ Nadh, Phosphoglycerate Mutase, Atp (u.v.) 2, 3-diphosphoglyceric Acid — Chemistry

ATRAUMATIC
79QKT Forceps, Grasping, Atraumatic — Surgery
79QLE Forceps, Grasping, Traumatic — Surgery
79QQR Gauge, Thickness, Tissue — Surgery

ATRIAL
84UBJ Catheter, Hydrocephalic, Atrial — Cns/Neurology
74FYQ Monitor, Pressure, Cardiac, Atrial — Cardiovascular
74MTE System, Pacing, Temporary, Acute, Internal Atrial Defibrillation — Cardiovascular

ATRIOVENTRICULAR
74RAD Detector, His Bundle — Cardiovascular

ATROX
81JCO Reagent, Bothrops Atrox — Hematology

ATTACHED
73KHB Filter, Tobacco Smoke (Attached) — Anesthesiology

ATTACHMENT
89UMM Attachment, Bag (Crutch, Walker, Wheelchair) — Physical Med
78FEJ Attachment, Binocular, Endoscopic — Gastro/Urology
73BYE Attachment, Breathing, Positive End Expiratory Pressure — Anesthesiology
89INB Attachment, Commode, Wheelchair — Physical Med
73CBO Attachment, Intermittent Mandatory Ventilation (IMV) — Anesthesiology
89IMQ Attachment, Narrowing, Wheelchair — Physical Med
80TDH Attachment, Oxygen Canister/IV Pole, Wheelchair — General
76EGG Attachment, Precision — Dental And Oral
80WRS Bulb, Inflation — General
76EGS Handpiece, Contra- And Right-Angle Attachment, Dental — Dental And Oral
88IDN Microtome, Freezing Attachment — Pathology
78FEA Teaching Attachment, Endoscopic — Gastro/Urology

ATTACK
75VIQ Test, Myocardial Infarction (Heart Attack) — Chemistry

ATTENTION
84LQD Recorder, Attention Task Performance — Cns/Neurology

ATTIC
77JYX Punch, Attic — Ear/Nose/Throat

KEYWORD INDEX

AUTOPSY *(cont'd)*

88RQM	Saw, Autopsy	Pathology
88RQP	Scale, Autopsy	Pathology
88VFV	Station, Autopsy	Pathology
88RYV	Table, Autopsy	Pathology

AUTOTRANSFUSION

73CAC	Autotransfusion Unit (Blood)	Anesthesiology
74UMG	Hemoconcentrator	Cardiovascular
78RAB	Hemofiltration Unit	Gastro/Urology

AUXILLARY

74MPD	Auxillary Power Supply, Low Energy Defibrillator (AC or DC)	Cardiovascular
74MPE	Auxillary Power Supply, Pacemaker, Cardiac, External Trans.	Cardiovascular

AV

78KNZ	Accessories, AV Shunt	Gastro/Urology
78KNR	Adapter, AV Shunt Or Fistula	Gastro/Urology
78FIQ	Cannula, AV Shunt	Gastro/Urology
78RTB	Shunt, Arteriovenous	Gastro/Urology

AVERSION

84HCB	Device, Conditioning, Aversion	Cns/Neurology
84RWC	Stimulator, Aversion Conditioning (Behavior Modification)	Cns/Neurology

AWL

87HWJ	Awl	Orthopedics

AXIAL

78LBW	Kit, Dialysis, Single Needle (Co-Axial Flow)	Gastro/Urology
90VHB	Phantom, Computed Axial Tomography (CAT, CT)	Radiology
74MFZ	System, Pump & Control, Cardiac Assist, Axial Flow	Cardiovascular

AZAN

88ICT	Stain, Azan Counterstain	Pathology

AZO

75CJY	Azo-Dye, Calcium	Chemistry
75JJB	Azo-Dyes, Colorimetric, Bilirubin And Conjugates	Chemistry

AZO-DYE

75CJY	Azo-Dye, Calcium	Chemistry

AZO-DYES

75JJB	Azo-Dyes, Colorimetric, Bilirubin And Conjugates	Chemistry

AZOCARMINE

88ICR	Stain, Azocarmine B	Pathology
88ICS	Stain, Azocarmine G	Pathology

AZURE

88ICQ	Stain, Azure A	Pathology
88KJL	Stain, Azure C	Pathology

B-NAPHTHYLAMIDE

75JKI	L-Leucyl B-Naphthylamide, Lactic Acid	Chemistry
75CDC	L-Leucyl B-Naphthylamide, Leucine Aminopeptidase	Chemistry

B. DERMATITIDIS

83JWW	Antigen, CF, B. Dermatitidis	Microbiology

B. PARAPERTUSSIS

83GOT	Antigen, B. Parapertussis	Microbiology
83GOW	Antiserum, Agglutinating, B. Parapertussis	Microbiology
83JRW	Antiserum, Fluorescent, B. Parapertussis	Microbiology

B. PERTUSSIS

83GOX	Antigen, B. Pertussis	Microbiology
83GOY	Antiserum, Agglutinating, B. Pertussis, All	Microbiology
83GOZ	Antiserum, Fluorescent, B. Pertussis	Microbiology

B12

75CDD	Radioimmunoassay, Vitamin B12	Chemistry
81KHD	Test, Absorption, Vitamin B12	Hematology

B19

83MYL	Assay, Enzyme Linked Immunosorbent, Parvovirus B19 Igg	Microbiology
83MYM	Assay, Enzyme Linked Immunosorbent, Parvovirus B19 Igm	Microbiology

B2

82MSV	System, Test, Antibodies, B2 - Glycoprotein I (b2 - Gpi)	Immunology

BABY

80QCD	Care Kit, Baby	General

BACILLUS

91DKD	Bacillus Subtilis, Microbiological Assay, Gentamicin	Toxicology
91DID	Test, Bacillus Subtilis Microbiology, Tobramycin	Toxicology

BACK

80QCE	Back Rest	General

BACK *(cont'd)*

80FPS	Board, Bed	General
74QGJ	Board, Cardiac Compression	Cardiovascular
87RUV	Board, Spine	Orthopedics
89QVE	Exerciser, Other	Physical Med
73CAX	Flowmeter, Back-Pressure Compensated, Thorpe Tube	Anesthesiology
73CCN	Flowmeter, Gas, Non-Back-Pressure Compensated, Bourdon Gauge	Anesthesiology
87RXE	Support, Back	Orthopedics

BACK-PRESSURE

73CAX	Flowmeter, Back-Pressure Compensated, Thorpe Tube	Anesthesiology
73CCN	Flowmeter, Gas, Non-Back-Pressure Compensated, Bourdon Gauge	Anesthesiology

BACKING

76ELK	Teeth, Artificial, Backing And Facing	Dental And Oral

BACTERIA

83LKS	Analyzer, Parasite Concentration	Microbiology
83QMP	Counter, Bacteria	Microbiology
80WOX	Filter, Bacteria, Pump, Breast	General
88KPA	Stainer, Slide, Automated	Pathology
88KIN	Stainer, Slide, Contact Type	Pathology
80WWZ	Test, Bacteria Characterization	General

BACTERIAL

83JSQ	Chromatographic Bacterial Identification	Microbiology
73CAH	Filter, Bacterial, Breathing Circuit	Anesthesiology
83UFL	Meter, Bacterial Culture Growth	Microbiology
83VLF	Test, Bacterial Diagnostic	Microbiology

BACTERIOLOGICAL

75UHT	Enclosure, Bacteriological Safety	Chemistry
75UGC	Filter, Bacteriological, Laboratory	Chemistry

BADGE

90QQI	Dosimeter, Radiation	Radiology
80WIP	Monitor, Contamination, Environmental, Personal	General

BAG

89UMM	Attachment, Bag (Crutch, Walker, Wheelchair)	Physical Med
78EXF	Bag, Bile Collection	Gastro/Urology
81ULQ	Bag, Blood	Hematology
81KSR	Bag, Blood, Collection	Hematology
80WNA	Bag, Body	General
73QEK	Bag, Breathing	Anesthesiology
80FOC	Bag, Collection, Urine, Newborn	General
78QQK	Bag, Drainage (Incontinence)	Gastro/Urology
80WOQ	Bag, Drainage, Nasogastric	General
80FON	Bag, Drainage, Ostomy (With Adhesive)	General
80QUF	Bag, Enema	General
80QVL	Bag, Enteral Feeding	General
80VAU	Bag, Garbage	General
78FCB	Bag, Hemostatic	Gastro/Urology
80KYR	Bag, Ice	General
79KGY	Bag, Intestine	Surgery
80TCV	Bag, Laundry, Infection Control	General
80REJ	Bag, Laundry, Operating Room	General
78FAQ	Bag, Leg	Gastro/Urology
80RGJ	Bag, Medical, Physician	General
80WNK	Bag, Plastic	General
74DSW	Bag, Polymeric Mesh, Pacemaker	Cardiovascular
73BTC	Bag, Reservoir (Blood)	Anesthesiology
79WZP	Bag, Specimen, Laparoscopic	Surgery
79GDS	Bag, Stomal	Surgery
80SEB	Bag, Urinary Collection	General
80SEC	Bag, Urinary Collection, Precision Measure (Urine Meter)	General
78EXG	Bag, Urinary Collection, Ureterostomy	Gastro/Urology
78EXH	Bag, Urinary, Ileostomy	Gastro/Urology
78FGD	Catheter, Retention, Barium Enema With Bag	Gastro/Urology
80KPE	Container, IV	General
78WLL	Device, Incontinence, Fecal	Gastro/Urology
79KCT	Pack, Sterilization Wrapper (Bag And Accessories)	Surgery
80RVT	Packaging, Sterilization	General
80VLU	Pump, Urinary Collection Bag	General
90RQJ	Sand Bag	Radiology
90SGN	Sand Bag, X-Ray	Radiology

BAGOLINI

86HPD	Lens, Bagolini	Ophthalmology

BAKER

78QIB	Catheter, Jejunostomy	Gastro/Urology
78VHP	Tube, Gastrointestinal Decompression, Baker Jejunostomy	Gastro/Urology

BALANCE

77LXV	Analyzer, Apparatus, Vestibular	Ear/Nose/Throat
75DOI	Balance (General Use)	Chemistry
75JQO	Balance, Analytical	Chemistry
75QCF	Balance, Electronic	Chemistry

BALANCE *(cont'd)*

75UKH	Balance, Macro (0.1 mg Accuracy)	Chemistry
75QCG	Balance, Mechanical	Chemistry
75UKF	Balance, Micro (0.001 mg Accuracy)	Chemistry
75UKG	Balance, Semimicro (0.01 mg Accuracy)	Chemistry
75UKE	Balance, Ultramicro (0.0001 mg Accuracy)	Chemistry
88RQP	Scale, Autopsy	Pathology
75RQT	Scale, Laboratory	Chemistry
80FQA	Scale, Surgical Sponge	General

BALANCED

88KIP	Solution, Balanced Salt	Pathology

BALL

80QMO	Ball, Cotton	General
87LZY	Hip, Hemi-, Femoral, Metal Ball	Orthopedics
87JDF	Prosthesis, Hip (Metal Stem/Ceramic Self-Locking Ball)	Orthopedics

BALLISTOCARDIOGRAPH

74DXR	Ballistocardiograph	Cardiovascular

BALLOON

74MKG	Balloon, Angioplasty, Coronary, Heated	Cardiovascular
74MKF	Balloon, Angioplasty, Peripheral, Heated	Cardiovascular
77EMX	Balloon, Epistaxis (Nasal)	Ear/Nose/Throat
78WNS	Balloon, Gastric	Gastro/Urology
74DSP	Balloon, Intra-Aortic (With Control System)	Cardiovascular
79SJI	Balloon, Manipulation, Tissue	Surgery
77MGL	Balloon, Middle Ear	Ear/Nose/Throat
84LHH	Balloon, Occlusion, Cerebrovascular	Cns/Neurology
78WSS	Balloon, Rectal	Gastro/Urology
79WZS	Cannula With Inflatable Balloon (Distal Tip)	Surgery
74LOX	Catheter, Angioplasty, Coronary, Transluminal, Percut. Oper.	Cardiovascular
74LIT	Catheter, Angioplasty, Transluminal, Peripheral	Cardiovascular
79GBA	Catheter, Balloon (Foley Type)	Surgery
78QIU	Catheter, Balloon, Dilatation, Vessel	Gastro/Urology
86LOG	Catheter, Balloon, Reattachment, Retinal	Ophthalmology
74GBR	Catheter, Cardiovascular, Balloon Type	Cardiovascular
77QHU	Catheter, Esophageal Balloon	Ear/Nose/Throat
74QHY	Catheter, Intra-Aortic Balloon	Cardiovascular
74MJN	Catheter, Intravascular Occluding, Temporary	Cardiovascular
78EZL	Catheter, Retention Type, Balloon	Gastro/Urology
85MKN	Catheter, Transcervical, Balloon Tuboplasty	Obstetrics/Gyn
74QKE	Circulatory Assist Unit, Intra-Aortic Balloon	Cardiovascular
85HDN	Dilator, Cervical, Expandable	Obstetrics/Gyn
79SJJ	Dissector, Balloon, Surgical	Surgery
78EYJ	Holder, Catheter	Gastro/Urology
74DQP	Kit, Balloon Repair, Catheter	Cardiovascular
79KFN	Monitor, Cardiac Output, Thermal (Balloon Type Catheter)	Surgery
74MAV	Syringe, Balloon Inflation	Cardiovascular
85HHQ	System, Abortion, Metreurynter-Balloon	Obstetrics/Gyn
74MFB	System, Reprocessing, Catheter, Balloon Angioplasty	Cardiovascular
78FEF	Tube, Single Lumen, W Mercury Wt Balloon	Gastro/Urology
74LWT	Vena Cava Balloon Occluder	Cardiovascular

BANA

75MGT	Test, Diagnostic, Bana Hydrolase, Dental Plaque	Chemistry

BAND

76ECI	Band, Elastic, Orthodontic	Dental And Oral
76DYO	Band, Material, Orthodontic	Dental And Oral
76UDY	Band, Matrix	Dental And Oral
85HFY	Band, Occlusion, Tubal	Obstetrics/Gyn
76ECM	Band, Preformed, Orthodontic	Dental And Oral
74MFT	Band, Pulmonary Artery	Cardiovascular
89ISR	Band, Support, Pelvic	Physical Med
80WXC	Band, Sweat	General
76ECT	Driver, Band, Orthodontic	Dental And Oral
76ECS	Pusher, Band, Orthodontic	Dental And Oral
76ECR	Setter, Band, Orthodontic	Dental And Oral

BANDAGE

80QAC	Adhesive Strip, Hypoallergenic	General
80QAD	Adhesive Strip, Waterproof	General
79KGX	Bandage, Adhesive	Surgery
80QCH	Bandage, Butterfly	General
89ITG	Bandage, Cast	Physical Med
80MHW	Bandage, Compression	General
80FQM	Bandage, Elastic	General
80QCI	Bandage, Gauze	General
79KMF	Bandage, Liquid	Surgery
80QCO	Bandage, Other	General
80QCK	Bandage, Scultetus	General
80QCM	Bandage, Traction	General
80QCN	Bandage, Tubular	General
80QLD	Clip, Bandage	General
87LGF	Component, Cast	Orthopedics
80FRO	Dressing, Other	General
79MGP	Dressing, Wound and Burn, Occlusive	Surgery

BANDAGE *(cont'd)*

79NAE	Dressing, Wound, Hydrogel W/out Drug And/or Biologic	Surgery
79NAC	Dressing, Wound, Hydrophilic	Surgery
79NAD	Dressing, Wound, Occlusive	Surgery
80WMU	Pin, Safety	General
80RPJ	Retainer, Bandage (Elastic Net)	General
80RRB	Scissors, Bandage/Gauze/Plaster	General
79FPX	Strip, Adhesive	Surgery

BANK

81KSO	Centrifuge, Blood Bank, Diagnostic	Hematology
81QNO	Equipment, Bank, Blood, Cryogenic (Liquid Nitrogen)	Hematology
86TCI	Freezer, Eye Bank	Ophthalmology
81RHG	Mixer, Blood Bank, Donor Blood	Hematology
81ROT	Refrigerator, Blood Bank	Hematology
86ULM	Refrigerator, Eye Bank	Ophthalmology
80WXG	Service, Tissue Bank	General
81MMH	Software, Blood Bank (Stand-Alone Products)	Hematology
81KSS	Supplies, Blood Bank	Hematology

BANKING

81KSE	Freezer, Blood Storage	Hematology
81KSF	Kit, Quality Control, Blood Banking	Hematology

BAR

76EHO	Bar, Preformed	Dental And Oral
86HKW	Bar, Prism, Ophthalmic	Ophthalmology
80VFR	Computer, Bar Code	General
80WNL	Label, Bar Code	General
80VAH	Labeling Equipment	General
80WMT	Printer, Bar Code	General
80WMS	Reader, Bar Code	General
86HJY	Reader, Bar, Ophthalmic	Ophthalmology
80SHI	System, Drug Dispensing, Pharmacy, Automated	General

BARBITURATE

91DKX	Chromatographic Barbiturate Identification (Thin Layer)	Toxicology
91DIS	Enzyme Immunoassay, Barbiturate	Toxicology
91DMF	Gas Liquid Chromatography, Barbiturate	Toxicology
91DLX	Hemagglutination Inhibition, Barbiturate	Toxicology
91KZY	High Pressure Liquid Chromatography, Barbiturate	Toxicology
91DJN	Mercury Dithiazone, Colorimetry, Barbiturate	Toxicology
91DNA	RIA, Morphine-Barbiturate (125-I), Goat Antibody	Toxicology
91DKN	Radioimmunoassay, Barbiturate	Toxicology
75MGX	System, Test, Drugs of Abuse	Chemistry

BARIUM

84MYU	Accessory, Barium Sulfate, Methyl Methacrylate For Cranioplasty	Cns/Neurology
78FGD	Catheter, Retention, Barium Enema With Bag	Gastro/Urology
78FCD	Kit, Barium Enema, Disposable	Gastro/Urology
90UJW	Media, Gastroenterographic Contrast (Barium Sulfate)	Radiology

BARON

80WNO	Tube, Suction	General

BAROREFLEX

84LIK	Prosthesis, Baroreflex	Cns/Neurology

BARRIER

85MCN	Barrier, Adhesion, Absorbable	Obstetrics/Gyn
90IWX	Barrier, Control Panel, X-Ray, Moveable	Radiology
77MSC	Barrier, Std, Oral Sex	Ear/Nose/Throat
80MMP	Cover, Barrier, Protective	General
75UGD	Filter, Membrane	Chemistry
89MLQ	Inhibitor, Peridural Fibrosis (Adhesion Barrier)	Physical Med
89MNY	Inhibitor, Post-Op Fibro., Carp. Tun. Syn.(Adhesion Barrier)	Physical Med
89MNX	Inhibitor, Post-Op Fibrosis, Tenolysis (Adhesion Barrier)	Physical Med

BARRON

80RNF	Pump, Food (Enteral Feeding)	General

BARS

89IOE	Bars, Parallel, Exercise	Physical Med
89IRR	Bars, Parallel, Powered	Physical Med
89RJY	Bars, Parallel, Walking	Physical Med
87RVM	Bars, Spreader	Orthopedics
80TEB	Rail, Bath	General

BART'S

81LGL	Test, Hemoglobin Bart's	Hematology

BARTHOLIN

78QHO	Catheter, Bartholin Gland	Gastro/Urology

BASAL

73QCP	Analyzer, Metabolism	Anesthesiology

BASE

76EBI	Base, Denture, Relining, Repairing, Rebasing, Resin	Dental And Oral
80WVN	Base, Roller, Tank, Oxygen	General
76EJH	Metal, Base	Dental And Oral

BASE (cont'd)
76EEA Plate, Base, Shellac — Dental And Oral

BASED
88KEL Adhesive, Albumin Based — Pathology
79LMF Agent, Hemostatic, Absorbable, Collagen-Based — Surgery
79LMG Agent, Hemostatic, Non-Absorbable, Collagen-Based — Surgery
76EJT Alloy, Gold Based, For Clinical Use — Dental And Oral
75CGL Ion Electrode Based Enzymatic, Creatinine — Chemistry

BASEMENT
82MMW Antigen, Tumor Marker, Bladder (Basement Membrane Complexes) — Immunology
82MVJ Devices, Measure, Antibodies to Glomerular Basement Membrane (gbm) — Immunology

BASIC
88KKW Fuchsin, Basic — Pathology
82MEL Kit, RIA, Basic Protein, Myelin — Immunology
75RDU Labware, Basic, Disposable — Chemistry
75RDV Labware, Basic, Reusable — Chemistry
82LTN Test, Myelin, Basic Protein — Immunology

BASIN
77UEF Basin, Ear — Ear/Nose/Throat
80FNY Basin, Emesis — General
80QCR Basin, Sponge — General
80TAF Basin, Wash — General
80QCQ Stand, Basin — General

BASKET
78TEH Basket, Biliary Stone Retrieval — Gastro/Urology
78FFL Dislodger, Stone, Basket, Ureteral, Metal — Gastro/Urology
80VLO Stretcher, Basket, Portable — General
80WIG Stretcher, Emergency, Other — General

BASSINET
80QCS Bassinet (Infant Bed) — General

BATH
80VDN Analyzer, Composition, Weight, Patient — General
75ULO Bath, Dry (Constant Temperature) — Chemistry
75ULP Bath, Freezing — Chemistry
89ILJ Bath, Hydro-Massage (Whirlpool) — Physical Med
83UGO Bath, Ice — Microbiology
75UGS Bath, Kinematic Viscosity — Chemistry
80TAG Bath, Leg — General
89IMC Bath, Paraffin — Physical Med
80QCU Bath, Portable — General
89KTC Bath, Sitz, Non-Powered — Physical Med
89ILM Bath, Sitz, Physical Medicine — Physical Med
80QCW Bath, Steam — General
79LZZ Bath, Sterilizer — Surgery
83QCX Bath, Tissue Flotation — Microbiology
88IDY Bath, Tissue Flotation, Pathology — Pathology
75UJJ Bath, Viscosity — Chemistry
75QCY Bath, Water (Constant Temperature) — Chemistry
80VKA Bathtub — General
80QCT Boot, Bath — General
80QJF Chair, Bath — General
80QJN Chair, Sitz Bath — General
75SFW Circulator, Water Bath — Chemistry
75JRH Incubator/Water Bath — Chemistry
83JTQ Incubator/Water Bath, Microbiology — Microbiology
89HHC Kit, Sitz Bath — Physical Med
80FSA Lift, Bath, Non-AC-Powered — General
78VKM Lithotriptor, Electro-Hydraulic, Extracorporeal — Gastro/Urology
78LNS Lithotriptor, Extracorporeal Shock-wave, Urological — Gastro/Urology
80RLD Pillow, Bath — General
80TEB Rail, Bath — General
75WID Support, Tube, Test — Chemistry
80RZD Tank, Full Body (Bath) — General
81VLV Warmer, Blood, Water Bath — Hematology

BATHOPHENANTHROLINE
75JQF Bathophenanthroline, Iron Binding Capacity — Chemistry

BATHTUB
80VKA Bathtub — General
80QCZ Bathtub, Portable — General
80RZD Tank, Full Body (Bath) — General

BATTERY
79HRF Accessories, Engine, Trephine, Battery-Powered — Surgery
80WJN Analyzer, Battery — General
74MPD Auxillary Power Supply, Low Energy Defibrillator (AC or DC) — Cardiovascular
74MPE Auxillary Power Supply, Pacemaker, Cardiac, External Trans. — Cardiovascular
80VDY Battery — General
77WOT Battery, Hearing-Aid — Ear/Nose/Throat

BATTERY (cont'd)
90VGM Battery, Mobile Radiographic Unit — Radiology
74DSZ Battery, Pacemaker — Cardiovascular
74MOR Battery, Rechargeable, Replacement for Class III Device — Cardiovascular
79MOQ Battery, Replacement, Rechargeable — Surgery
89IQH Biofeedback Equipment, Myoelectric, Battery-Powered — Physical Med
78FCP Box, Battery, Pocket (Endoscopic) — Gastro/Urology
78FCO Box, Battery, Rechargeable (Endoscopic) — Gastro/Urology
86HOG Burr, Corneal, Battery-Powered — Ophthalmology
86HOP Campimeter, Stereo, Battery-Powered — Ophthalmology
80WRU Capacitor, Defibrillator — General
86HQQ Cautery, Radiofrequency, Battery-Powered — Ophthalmology
86HQP Cautery, Thermal, Battery-Powered — Ophthalmology
80WJM Charger, Battery — General
80WKG Component, Electrical — General
86HKP Cutter, Vitreous Aspiration, Battery-Powered — Ophthalmology
74QOR Defibrillator, Battery-Powered — Cardiovascular
74DRK Defibrillator, Battery-Powered, High Energy — Cardiovascular
74LDD Defibrillator, Battery-Powered, Low Energy — Cardiovascular
74QOO Defibrillator/Monitor, Battery-Powered — Cardiovascular
79QSK Electrocautery Unit, Battery-Powered — Surgery
86HPY Electrolysis Unit, Battery-Powered, Ophthalmic — Ophthalmology
79GCS Endoscope And Accessories, Battery-Powered — Surgery
86HML Euthyscope, Battery-Powered — Ophthalmology
86HKJ Fixation Device, Battery-Powered, Ophthalmic — Ophthalmology
86HPP Headlamp, Operating, Battery-Operated — Ophthalmology
86HMY Keratome, Battery-Powered — Ophthalmology
86HLR Keratoscope, Battery-Powered — Ophthalmology
77ESE Larynx, Artificial Battery-Powered — Ear/Nose/Throat
80KYT Light, Examination, Battery-Powered — General
89IPD Massager, Battery-Powered — Physical Med
89IKJ Meter, Skin Resistance, Battery-Powered — Physical Med
86HLJ Ophthalmoscope, Battery-Powered — Ophthalmology
86HJP Penlight, Battery-Powered — Ophthalmology
80QUD Power Supply, Endoscopic, Battery-Operated — General
86HLW Preamplifier, Battery-Powered, Ophthalmic — Ophthalmology
86HKM Retinoscope, Battery-Powered — Ophthalmology
86HMJ Screen, Tangent, Projection, Battery-Powered — Ophthalmology
86HLK Screen, Tangent, Target, Battery-Powered — Ophthalmology
77LFA Speech Training Aid, Battery-Powered — Ear/Nose/Throat
86HJR Stereoscope, Battery-Powered — Ophthalmology
86HRC Sterilizer, Soft Lens, Thermal, Battery-Powered — Ophthalmology
80FLW Stethoscope, DC-Powered — General
73BXN Stimulator, Nerve, Battery-Powered — Anesthesiology
79KIJ Surgical Instrument, Orthopedic, Battery-Powered — Surgery
86HLO Test, Spectacle Dissociation, Battery-Powered (Lancaster) — Ophthalmology
76MMD Toothbrush, Ionic, Battery-Powered — Dental And Oral
86HJN Transilluminator, Battery-Powered — Ophthalmology
89IPE Vibrator, Battery-Powered — Physical Med
85HIK Vibrator, Vaginal, Battery-Powered — Obstetrics/Gyn
86HPG Vision Aid, Electronic, Battery-Powered — Ophthalmology
86HOT Vision Aid, Image Intensification, Battery-Powered — Ophthalmology
86HPE Vision Aid, Optical, Battery-Powered — Ophthalmology

BATTERY-OPERATED
86HPP Headlamp, Operating, Battery-Operated — Ophthalmology
80QUD Power Supply, Endoscopic, Battery-Operated — General

BATTERY-POWERED
79HRF Accessories, Engine, Trephine, Battery-Powered — Surgery
89IQH Biofeedback Equipment, Myoelectric, Battery-Powered — Physical Med
86HOG Burr, Corneal, Battery-Powered — Ophthalmology
86HOP Campimeter, Stereo, Battery-Powered — Ophthalmology
86HQQ Cautery, Radiofrequency, Battery-Powered — Ophthalmology
86HQP Cautery, Thermal, Battery-Powered — Ophthalmology
86HKP Cutter, Vitreous Aspiration, Battery-Powered — Ophthalmology
74QOR Defibrillator, Battery-Powered — Cardiovascular
74DRK Defibrillator, Battery-Powered, High Energy — Cardiovascular
74LDD Defibrillator, Battery-Powered, Low Energy — Cardiovascular
74QOO Defibrillator/Monitor, Battery-Powered — Cardiovascular
79QSK Electrocautery Unit, Battery-Powered — Surgery
86HPY Electrolysis Unit, Battery-Powered, Ophthalmic — Ophthalmology
79GCS Endoscope And Accessories, Battery-Powered — Surgery
86HML Euthyscope, Battery-Powered — Ophthalmology
86HKJ Fixation Device, Battery-Powered, Ophthalmic — Ophthalmology
86HMY Keratome, Battery-Powered — Ophthalmology
86HLR Keratoscope, Battery-Powered — Ophthalmology
77ESE Larynx, Artificial Battery-Powered — Ear/Nose/Throat
80KYT Light, Examination, Battery-Powered — General
89IPD Massager, Battery-Powered — Physical Med
89IKJ Meter, Skin Resistance, Battery-Powered — Physical Med
86HLJ Ophthalmoscope, Battery-Powered — Ophthalmology
86HJP Penlight, Battery-Powered — Ophthalmology
86HLW Preamplifier, Battery-Powered, Ophthalmic — Ophthalmology
86HKM Retinoscope, Battery-Powered — Ophthalmology
86HMJ Screen, Tangent, Projection, Battery-Powered — Ophthalmology
86HLK Screen, Tangent, Target, Battery-Powered — Ophthalmology
77LFA Speech Training Aid, Battery-Powered — Ear/Nose/Throat

BENZOYLECGNONINE

91DNG	Free Radical, Benzoylecgnonine	Toxicology
91DLN	Hemagglutination, Cocaine Metabolites (Benzoylecgnonine)	Toxicology
91DOM	Thin Layer Chromatography, Benzoylecgnonine	Toxicology

BERTHELOT

75CDL	Indophenol, Berthelot, Urea Nitrogen	Chemistry

BEST'S

88ICO	Stain, Best's Carmine	Pathology

BETA

82DDN	Antigen, Antiserum, Control, Beta 2-Glycoprotein I	Immunology
82DCJ	Antigen, Antiserum, Control, Beta Globulin	Immunology
75CJL	Beta Glycerophosphate, Alkaline Phosphatase Or Isoenzymes	Chemistry
82DDK	Beta-2-Glycoprotein III, Antigen, Antiserum, Control	Immunology
75JNK	Beta-D-Fructose & NADH Oxidation (U.V.), Sorbitol DH	Chemistry
75JJJ	Detector, Beta/Gamma	Chemistry
75CKH	Glycerophosphate, Beta, Phosphatase, Acid	Chemistry
82JZG	Test, Beta 2 - Microglobulin	Immunology
86HRL	Unit, Radiation, Beta, Ophthalmic	Ophthalmology

BETA-2-GLYCOPROTEIN

82DDK	Beta-2-Glycoprotein III, Antigen, Antiserum, Control	Immunology

BETA-D-FRUCTOSE

75JNK	Beta-D-Fructose & NADH Oxidation (U.V.), Sorbitol DH	Chemistry

BETATRON

90IYG	Betatron, Medical	Radiology

BETHESDA-BALLERUP

83GTF	Antiserum, Bethesda-Ballerup Polyvalent, Citrobacter SPP.	Microbiology

BI-NASOPHARYNGEAL

73CBJ	Airway, Bi-Nasopharyngeal (With Connector)	Anesthesiology

BIB

80QDJ	Bib	General

BICHROMATIC

75JJD	Analyzer, Chemistry, Photometric, Bichromatic	Chemistry

BICYCLE

74QUN	Ergometer, Bicycle	Cardiovascular
89QUW	Exerciser, Bicycle	Physical Med

BIEBRICH

88ICN	Stain, Biebrich Scarlet	Pathology

BIFOCAL

86ULH	Lens, Contact, Bifocal	Ophthalmology

BIFURCATION

74WNZ	Graft, Bifurcation	Cardiovascular

BILE

78EXF	Bag, Bile Collection	Gastro/Urology
78WIL	Lithotriptor, Multipurpose	Gastro/Urology
75KWW	Radioimmunoassay, Cholylglycine, Bile Acids	Chemistry
75KWX	Radioimmunoassay, Conjugated Sulfalithocholic, Bile Acid	Chemistry

BILIARY

78TEH	Basket, Biliary Stone Retrieval	Gastro/Urology
78FGE	Catheter, Biliary	Gastro/Urology
79GCA	Catheter, Biliary, General & Plastic Surgery	Surgery
78LQR	Dislodger, Store, Biliary	Gastro/Urology
78QXB	Forceps, Gallbladder (Biliary Duct)	Gastro/Urology
78QTO	Introducer, T-Tube	Gastro/Urology
78LQC	Lithotriptor, Mechanical, Biliary	Gastro/Urology
78FTK	Pancreatoscope, Biliary	Gastro/Urology
85UAN	Stent, Other	Obstetrics/Gyn

BILIRUBIN

75JJB	Azo-Dyes, Colorimetric, Bilirubin And Conjugates	Chemistry
75MQM	Bilirubin (Total and Unbound) Neonate Test System	Chemistry
75JFM	Enzymatic Method, Bilirubin	Chemistry
80TCX	Light, Bilirubin (Phototherapy)	General
80RKZ	Phototherapy Unit (Bilirubin Lamp)	General
75CIG	Reagent, Bilirubin (Total Or Direct Test System)	Chemistry

BILIRUBINOMETER

75QDL	Bilirubinometer	Chemistry
80UDF	Bilirubinometer, Cutaneous (Jaundice Meter)	General
75VEO	Hematofluorimeter (Bilirubinometer)	Chemistry

BILLING

80VAX	Computer Equipment	General
80VHN	Computer, Patient Data Management	General
80WTG	Monitor, Utilization, Equipment	General

BIN

80VKB	Bin, Storage	General

BIN *(cont'd)*

90UAB	Storage Unit, X-Ray Film	Radiology

BIND

75JQE	Ion Exchange Resin, Ascorbic Acid, Colorimetry, Iron Bind	Chemistry

BINDER

80QCK	Bandage, Scultetus	General
80FSD	Binder, Abdominal	General
85HFR	Binder, Abdominal, OB/GYN	Obstetrics/Gyn
87QDM	Binder, Ankle	Orthopedics
85HEF	Binder, Breast	Obstetrics/Gyn
80QDN	Binder, Chest	General
80KMO	Binder, Elastic	General
80MDR	Binder, Medical, Therapeutic	General
80FQK	Binder, Perineal	General
80QDO	Binder, Scultetus	General
87QDP	Binder, T	Orthopedics
87QDQ	Binder, Wrist	Orthopedics

BINDING

75JQF	Bathophenanthroline, Iron Binding Capacity	Chemistry
75CIX	Dye-Binding, Albumin, Bromcresol, Green	Chemistry
75CJW	Dye-Binding, Albumin, Bromcresol, Purple	Chemistry
75JMO	Ferrozine (Colorimetric) Iron Binding Capacity	Chemistry
75CEE	Radioimmunoassay, Thyroxine Binding Globulin	Chemistry
75JQG	Radiometric, Fe59, Iron Binding Capacity	Chemistry
82CZS	Retinol-Binding Protein, Antigen, Antiserum, Control	Immunology

BINOCULAR

78FEJ	Attachment, Binocular, Endoscopic	Gastro/Urology
86HJH	Loupe, Binocular, Low Power	Ophthalmology

BIOCHEMICAL

83JSE	Culture Media, Multiple Biochemical Test	Microbiology
83JSF	Culture Media, Single Biochemical Test	Microbiology
83LTS	Test, Reagent, Biochemical, Neisseria Gonorrhoeae	Microbiology

BIODEGRADABLE

87MBJ	Fastener, Fixation, Biodegradable, Hard Tissue	Orthopedics
87MAI	Fastener, Fixation, Biodegradable, Soft Tissue	Orthopedics
87MBI	Fastener, Fixation, Non-Biodegradable, Soft Tissue	Orthopedics

BIOFEEDBACK

84HCC	Biofeedback Device	Cns/Neurology
89IQH	Biofeedback Equipment, Myoelectric, Battery-Powered	Physical Med
89IRC	Biofeedback Equipment, Myoelectric, Powered	Physical Med
84HCB	Device, Conditioning, Aversion	Cns/Neurology
89IOA	Diathermy, Microwave	Physical Med
89IKA	Electrode, Biopotential, Surface, Composite	Physical Med
89IKB	Electrode, Biopotential, Surface, Metallic	Physical Med
89IKI	Meter, Skin Resistance, AC-Powered	Physical Med
89IKJ	Meter, Skin Resistance, Battery-Powered	Physical Med
84GZO	Monitor, Response, Skin, Galvanic	Cns/Neurology
84GZJ	Stimulator, Nerve, Transcutaneous (Pain Relief, TENS)	Cns/Neurology

BIOFRAGMENTABLE

79SIW	Device, Anastomosis, Biofragmentable	Surgery

BIOLOGIC

79NAE	Dressing, Wound, Hydrogel W/out Drug And/or Biologic	Surgery

BIOLOGICAL

83UFW	Disintegrator, Biological Cell	Microbiology
75UKL	Freezer, Laboratory, Biological	Chemistry
74LOW	Graft, Arterial, Biological	Cardiovascular
74MAK	Graft, Vascular, Biological	Cardiovascular
78MDQ	Graft, Vascular, Biological, Hemodialysis Access	Gastro/Urology
78MCI	Graft, Vascular, Synth./Bio. Composite, Hemodialysis Access	Gastro/Urology
74MAL	Graft, Vascular, Synthetic/Biological Composite	Cardiovascular
80MRB	Indicator, Biological, Liquid Chemical Steril. Process	General
80QDR	Monitor, Biological (Contamination Testing)	General
74DYE	Prosthesis, Cardiac Valve, Biological	Cardiovascular
83ROS	Refrigerator, Biological	Microbiology
91UHZ	Serum, Biological, General	Toxicology
88UIG	Stain, Biological, General	Pathology
80FRC	Sterilization Process Indicator, Biological	General
80WLS	Test, Equipment, Sterilization	General

BIOMICROSCOPE

86HJO	Lamp, Slit, Biomicroscope, AC-Powered	Ophthalmology

BIOPHOTOMETER

86HJW	Adaptometer (Biophotometer)	Ophthalmology

BIOPOTENTIAL

74DRR	Amplifier, Biopotential (W Signal Conditioner)	Cardiovascular
89IKA	Electrode, Biopotential, Surface, Composite	Physical Med
89IKB	Electrode, Biopotential, Surface, Metallic	Physical Med

KEYWORD INDEX

BIOPSY
74DWZ Biopsy Device, Endomyocardial — Cardiovascular
78KNW Biopsy Instrument — Gastro/Urology
78FCF Biopsy Instrument, Mechanical, Gastrointestinal — Gastro/Urology
78FCK Biopsy Instrument, Suction — Gastro/Urology
73BTG Brush, Biopsy, Bronchoscope (Non-Rigid) — Anesthesiology
79GEE Brush, Biopsy, General & Plastic Surgery — Surgery
80WKZ Brush, Cytology — General
78FDX Brush, Cytology, Endoscopic — Gastro/Urology
73WVG Catheter, Culture, Pulmonary — Anesthesiology
74WTL Cleaner, Forceps, Biopsy — Cardiovascular
78FFF Cover, Biopsy Forceps — Gastro/Urology
73BST Curette, Biopsy, Bronchoscope (Non-Rigid) — Anesthesiology
73JEL Curette, Biopsy, Bronchoscope (Rigid) — Anesthesiology
79MJG Device, Biopsy, Percutaneous — Surgery
79QRD Drill, Biopsy — Surgery
79SIR Forceps, Biopsy — Surgery
73BWH Forceps, Biopsy, Bronchoscope (Non-Rigid) — Anesthesiology
73JEK Forceps, Biopsy, Bronchoscope (Rigid) — Anesthesiology
78KGE Forceps, Biopsy, Electric — Gastro/Urology
85HFB Forceps, Biopsy, Gynecological — Obstetrics/Gyn
78FCL Forceps, Biopsy, Non-Electric — Gastro/Urology
80WXY Guide, Device, Ultrasonic — General
79QQU Instrument, Dissecting, Laparoscopic — Surgery
79QQY Instrument, Dissecting, Myoma, Laparoscopic — Surgery
80QDS Kit, Biopsy — General
78FCG Kit, Biopsy Needle — Gastro/Urology
78FCH Kit, Biopsy, Gastro-Urology — Gastro/Urology
80QDT Kit, Biopsy, Ultrasonic Aspiration — General
74DWO Needle, Biopsy, Cardiovascular — Cardiovascular
85WJD Needle, Biopsy, Mammary — Obstetrics/Gyn
78FCI Punch, Biopsy — Gastro/Urology
76EME Punch, Biopsy, Surgical — Dental And Oral
85WWA Retractor, Mammary — Obstetrics/Gyn

BIPOLAR
85HIN Coagulator/Cutter, Endoscopic, Bipolar — Obstetrics/Gyn
79SJX Forceps, Laparoscopy, Bipolar, Electrosurgical — Surgery
79SJW Needle, Cutting, Bipolar, Electrocauterization — Surgery
87MJT Prosthesis, Shoulder, Humeral, Bipol., Hemi-, Constr., M/P — Orthopedics
79SJL Scissors, Laparoscopy, Bipolar, Electrosurgical — Surgery

BIRTHING
80QDE Bed, Birthing — General
85QJG Chair, Birthing — Obstetrics/Gyn
85HDD Table, Obstetrical, AC-Powered — Obstetrics/Gyn
85HHP Table, Obstetrical, Manual — Obstetrics/Gyn

BISMARCK
88KJM Stain, Bismarck Brown Y — Pathology

BISTOURY
77KCC Bistoury, Tracheal — Ear/Nose/Throat

BIT
87HTW Bit, Drill — Orthopedics
79GFG Bit, Surgical — Surgery

BITE
78MNK Accessories, Bite Blocks (For Endoscope) — Gastro/Urology
84JXL Block, Bite — Cns/Neurology
77JPL Block, Bite, ENT — Ear/Nose/Throat
73BTW Block, Bite, Intubation — Anesthesiology
80RTX Kit, Snake Bite — General
80KYQ Kit, Snake Bite, Chemical Cold Pack — General
80KYP Kit, Snake Bite, Suction — General

BLACK
88KJQ Stain, Chlorazol Black E — Pathology
88HZZ Stain, Sudan Black B — Pathology

BLADDER
78MNZ Analyzer, Diagnostic, Fiberoptic (Bladder) — Gastro/Urology
82MMW Antigen, Tumor Marker, Bladder (Basement Membrane Complexes) — Immunology
78FFD Evacuator, Bladder, Manually Operated — Gastro/Urology
78SIQ Extractor, Gall Bladder — Gastro/Urology
78WYI Instrument, Volume, Bladder — Gastro/Urology
78RCR Kit, Irrigation, Bladder — Gastro/Urology
78EZT Pacemaker, Bladder — Gastro/Urology
78RPN Retractor, Bladder — Gastro/Urology
78FHK Spreader, Bladder Neck — Gastro/Urology
78EZW Stimulator, Electrical, For Incontinence — Gastro/Urology
84GZD Stimulator, Spinal Cord, Implantable, Bladder Evacuator — Cns/Neurology
78UAE Stimulator, Urinary — Gastro/Urology
82NAH System, Test, Tumor Marker, For Detection Of Bladder Cancer — Immunology
78FGK Tripsor, Stone, Bladder — Gastro/Urology

BLADE
87LXT Appliance, Fix., Nail/Blade/Plate Comb., Multiple Component — Orthopedics
87QDU Blade, Bone Cutting — Orthopedics
79SIH Blade, Electrosurgery, Laparoscopic — Surgery
79QVD Blade, Knife, Laparoscopic — Surgery
87TAI Blade, Saw, Cast Cutting — Orthopedics
74DWH Blade, Saw, Surgical, Cardiovascular — Cardiovascular
79GES Blade, Scalpel — Surgery
79GFA Blade, Surgical, Saw, General & Plastic Surgery — Surgery
79FWQ Blade, Tongue — Surgery
80FMA Depressor, Tongue — General
76EJC Depressor, Tongue, Dental — Dental And Oral
77KBL Depressor, Tongue, ENT, Metal — Ear/Nose/Throat
77EWF Depressor, Tongue, ENT, Wood — Ear/Nose/Throat
79FAS Electrode, Electrosurgical, Active (Blade) — Surgery
79RDE Handle, Knife Blade — Surgery
79QWG Handle, Knife, Laparoscopic — Surgery
79RCZ Jar, Blade — Surgery
79QWI Knife, Laparoscopic — Surgery
87KWK Nail/Blade/Plate Appliance — Orthopedics
76EGR Osteotome, Roto With Blade — Dental And Oral
80WZH Remover, Blade, Scalpel — General
88RSH Sharpener, Microtome Blade — Pathology
80SFS Waste Disposal Unit, Sharps — General

BLAKEMORE
78SCV Tube, Esophageal, Blakemore — Gastro/Urology

BLANKET
80QDA Bed Cradle — General
80LDI Blanket, Fire — General
80QDW Blanket, Infant — General
80QDV Blanket, Rescue — General
80WHO Cover, Other — General
74BTE Device, Hyperthermia (Blanket, Plumbing & Heat Exchanger) — Cardiovascular
80RAZ Hypo/Hyperthermia Blanket — General
73BTF Hypothermia Unit (Blanket, Plumbing & Heat Exchanger) — Anesthesiology
80SFF Warmer, Blanket — General

BLASTOMYCES
83LSH Antigen, Blastomyces Dermatitidis, Other — Microbiology
83LSI Antiserum, Blastomyces Dermatitidis, Other — Microbiology
83KFH Antiserum, Positive Control, Blastomyces Dermatitidis — Microbiology
83MDC DNA-Probe, Blastomyces Dermatitidis — Microbiology
83MJL EIA, Blastomyces Dermatitidis — Microbiology

BLEACHING
76EEG Source, Heat, Bleaching, Teeth, Dental — Dental And Oral

BLEEDING
81JCA Bleeding Time Device — Hematology
78FFW Locator, Bleeding, Gastrointestinal, String And Tube — Gastro/Urology

BLENDER
88IHJ Blender, Sputum — Pathology
75JRO Blender/Mixer — Chemistry
73QMK Controller, Oxygen (Blender) — Anesthesiology

BLIND
89IPS Cane — Physical Med
86HQI Eye, Artificial, Custom — Ophthalmology
86HQH Eye, Artificial, Non-Custom — Ophthalmology
86QVI Eyeglasses — Ophthalmology
86QVJ Eyeglasses, Aphakic — Ophthalmology
86HQZ Frame, Spectacle (Eyeglasses) — Ophthalmology
79FWO Prosthesis, Eye, Internal (Sphere) — Surgery
86HQY Sunglasses (Including Photosensitive) — Ophthalmology
86HIT Tester, Color Vision — Ophthalmology
80WMV Vision Aid, Braille — General
86HPF Vision Aid, Electronic, AC-Powered — Ophthalmology
86HPG Vision Aid, Electronic, Battery-Powered — Ophthalmology
86HOT Vision Aid, Image Intensification, Battery-Powered — Ophthalmology
86HPI Vision Aid, Optical, AC-Powered — Ophthalmology
86HPE Vision Aid, Optical, Battery-Powered — Ophthalmology
86WOM Vision Aid, Ultrasonic — Ophthalmology

BLOCK
78MNK Accessories, Bite Blocks (For Endoscope) — Gastro/Urology
90IXI Block, Beam Shaping, Radionuclide — Radiology
84JXL Block, Bite — Cns/Neurology
77JPL Block, Bite, ENT — Ear/Nose/Throat
73BTW Block, Bite, Intubation — Anesthesiology
77JXS Block, Cutting, ENT — Ear/Nose/Throat
75JRG Block, Heating — Chemistry
90WKV Block, Therapy, Radiation — Radiology
87MBE Bone, Block, Filler, Metal, Porous, Uncemented — Orthopedics
79MIB Elastomer, Silicone Block — Surgery
75UIK Electrophoresis Equipment, Starch Block — Chemistry

BLOCK *(cont'd)*

79UAO	Reconstruction Block, Plastic Surgery	Surgery

BLOCKADE

73UFG	Stimulator, Peripheral Nerve, Blockade Monitor	Anesthesiology

BLOCKING

81MVX	Antibody, Monoclonal Blocking, Hiv-1	Hematology
75LIG	Radioassay, Intrinsic Factor Blocking Antibody	Chemistry

BLOOD

75JKP	51 Chromium, Blood Volume	Chemistry
78KOC	Accessories, Blood Circuit, Hemodialysis	Gastro/Urology
81JBP	Activated Whole Blood Clotting Time	Hematology
74WTU	Adapter, Needle	Cardiovascular
79LMF	Agent, Hemostatic, Absorbable, Collagen-Based	Surgery
79LMG	Agent, Hemostatic, Non-Absorbable, Collagen-Based	Surgery
74DSJ	Alarm, Blood Pressure	Cardiovascular
75QES	Analyzer, BUN (Blood Urea Nitrogen)	Chemistry
73TAK	Analyzer, Blood Gas pH	Anesthesiology
81TAL	Analyzer, Blood Grouping	Hematology
81KSZ	Analyzer, Blood Grouping/Antibody, Automated	Hematology
73VCC	Analyzer, Blood Oxyhemoglobin Concentration	Anesthesiology
81SAN	Analyzer, Coagulation, Whole Blood	Hematology
74JEE	Analyzer, Concentration, Oxyhemoglobin, BP, Transcutaneous	Cardiovascular
91JFD	Analyzer, Concentration, Oxyhemoglobin, Blood Phase	Toxicology
73CCC	Analyzer, Gas, Carbon-Dioxide, Blood Phase, Indwelling	Anesthesiology
73BXZ	Analyzer, Gas, Carbon-Dioxide, Partial Pressure, Blood	Anesthesiology
73VCB	Analyzer, Gas, Carbon-Monoxide, Non-Indwelling Blood Phase	Anesthesiology
91CCA	Analyzer, Gas, Carboxyhemoglobin, Blood Phase, Non-Indw.	Toxicology
73BSD	Analyzer, Gas, Nitrogen, Partial Pressure, Blood Phase (Nl)	Anesthesiology
73CCE	Analyzer, Gas, Oxygen, Partial Pr., Blood Phase, Indwelling	Anesthesiology
73CCD	Analyzer, Gas, Oxygen, Partial Pressure, Blood Phase	Anesthesiology
73CBZ	Analyzer, Ion, Hydrogen-Ion (pH), Blood Phase, Indwelling	Anesthesiology
73CBY	Analyzer, Ion, Hydrogen-Ion pH, Blood Phase, Non-Indwelling	Anesthesiology
73JED	Analyzer, Oxyhemoglobin Concentration, Blood Phase, Indwell.	Anesthesiology
79WTZ	Analyzer, Patient, Multiple Function (Surgery)	Surgery
81JPH	Analyzer, Sedimentation Rate, Erythrocyte	Hematology
90WNR	Angio-Dynograph	Radiology
81UJY	Antiserum, ABO Blood Grouping	Hematology
73CAC	Autotransfusion Unit (Blood)	Anesthesiology
81ULQ	Bag, Blood	Hematology
81KSR	Bag, Blood, Collection	Hematology
73BTC	Bag, Reservoir (Blood)	Anesthesiology
78LLB	Blood System, Extracorporeal (With Accessories)	Gastro/Urology
80WMK	Calibrator, Blood Gas	General
84HBY	Catheter, Angiographic	Cns/Neurology
81KSO	Centrifuge, Blood Bank, Diagnostic	Hematology
80FML	Chair, Blood Donor	General
80WZB	Chair, Blood Drawing	General
78UCO	Clamp, Hemodialysis Unit Blood Line	Gastro/Urology
78FIG	Clamp, Tubing, Blood, Automatic	Gastro/Urology
81KST	Collector, Blood, Vacuum-Assisted	Hematology
81JIO	Colorimetric, Occult Blood in Urine	Hematology
80WON	Column, Immunoadsorption	General
74DSK	Computer, Blood Pressure	Cardiovascular
74WJY	Connector, Tubing, Blood	Cardiovascular
78FKB	Connector, Tubing, Blood, Infusion, T-Type	Gastro/Urology
75JJS	Control, Blood Gas	Chemistry
81GJP	Control, Platelet	Hematology
80LHE	Controller, Glucose, Blood, Closed-Loop	General
80LSX	Controller, Pressure, Blood, Closed-Loop	General
74DXQ	Cuff, Blood Pressure	Cardiovascular
74ULR	Detector, Blood Flow, Ultrasonic (Doppler)	Cardiovascular
78FJD	Detector, Blood Leakage	Gastro/Urology
78FJC	Detector, Blood Level	Gastro/Urology
78MKL	Device, Measuring, Blood Loss	Gastro/Urology
81GIF	Diluent, Blood Cell	Hematology
81GKH	Diluter, Blood Cell, Automated	Hematology
74WSD	Doppler, Blood Flow, Transcranial	Cardiovascular
73QSO	Electrode, Blood Gas, Carbon-Dioxide	Anesthesiology
73QSP	Electrode, Blood Gas, Oxygen	Anesthesiology
75CHL	Electrode, Blood pH	Chemistry
80WUM	Encapsulator, Fluid	General
85HGK	Endoscope, Fetal Blood Sampling	Obstetrics/Gyn
75TGO	Enzymatic Method, Blood, Occcult, Fecal	Chemistry
75JIP	Enzymatic Method, Blood, Occult, Urinary	Chemistry
81JBE	Enzyme, Cell (Erythrocytic And Leukocytic)	Hematology
81QNO	Equipment, Bank, Blood, Cryogenic (Liquid Nitrogen)	Hematology
74DTM	Filter, Blood, Cardiopulmonary Bypass, Arterial Line	Cardiovascular
74JOD	Filter, Blood, Cardiotomy Suction Line, Cardiopulmonary	Cardiovascular
78FKJ	Filter, Blood, Dialysis	Gastro/Urology
74DPW	Flowmeter, Blood, Intravenous	Cardiovascular

BLOOD *(cont'd)*

78FIT	Flowmeter, Blood, Non-Invasive Electromagnetic	Gastro/Urology
74WSR	Flowmeter, Blood, Other	Cardiovascular
78QWP	Flowmeter, Blood, Ultrasonic	Gastro/Urology
74CAS	Flowmeter, Blood, Ultrasonic, Transcutaneous (W/WO Calibr.)	Cardiovascular
84UEW	Flowmeter, Meter, Cerebral Blood, Xenon Clearance	Cns/Neurology
81KSP	Freezer, Blood Cell	Hematology
81KSE	Freezer, Blood Storage	Hematology
81JBM	Glucose-6-Phosphate Dehydrogenase (Erythrocytic), Electro	Hematology
81JBF	Glucose-6-Phosphate Dehydrogenase (Erythrocytic), Screening	Hematology
81JBG	Glucose-6-Phosphate Dehydrogenase (Erythrocytic), Spot	Hematology
84HAP	Guide, Wire, Angiographic (And Accessories)	Cns/Neurology
74QZM	Heart-Lung Bypass Unit (Cardiopulmonary)	Cardiovascular
74WWI	Hemoglobin	Cardiovascular
81UJR	Identification Panel, Blood Cell	Hematology
80RLQ	Infuser, Pressure (Blood Pump)	General
74DXT	Injector, Angiographic (Cardiac Catheterization)	Cardiovascular
78FKL	Insert, Blood Pump	Gastro/Urology
90WIB	Irradiator	Radiology
90MOT	Irradiator, Blood to Prevent Graft Vs Host Disease	Radiology
78NAX	Irradiator, Blood, Extracorporeal	Gastro/Urology
80QDX	Kit, Administration, Blood	General
90VGB	Kit, Angiographic, Digital	Radiology
90VGC	Kit, Angiographic, Special Procedure	Radiology
74RKS	Kit, Blood Collection, Phlebotomy	Cardiovascular
81QDZ	Kit, Blood Donor	Hematology
74QIX	Kit, Blood Pressure, Central Venous	Cardiovascular
80BRZ	Kit, Blood, Transfusion	General
81KSF	Kit, Quality Control, Blood Banking	Hematology
73CBT	Kit, Sampling, Arterial Blood	Anesthesiology
80RQG	Kit, Sampling, Blood	General
80RQH	Kit, Sampling, Blood Gas	General
78FJK	Kit, Tubing, Blood, Anti-Regurgitation	Gastro/Urology
75JKA	Labware, Blood Collection	Chemistry
80FMK	Lancet, Blood	General
81JWO	Meter, Volume, Blood	Hematology
75JKO	Meter, pH, Blood	Chemistry
73CAK	Microfilter, Blood Transfusion	Anesthesiology
81RHG	Mixer, Blood Bank, Donor Blood	Hematology
81GLE	Mixer, Blood Tube	Hematology
81KSQ	Mixer/Scale, Blood	Hematology
85HEP	Monitor, Blood Flow, Ultrasonic	Obstetrics/Gyn
73QEA	Monitor, Blood Gas, Carbon-Dioxide	Anesthesiology
74DRY	Monitor, Blood Gas, On-Line, Cardiopulmonary Bypass	Cardiovascular
73QEB	Monitor, Blood Gas, Oxygen	Anesthesiology
74UMH	Monitor, Blood Gas, Real-Time	Cardiovascular
73TAJ	Monitor, Blood Gas, Transcutaneous Carbon-Dioxide	Anesthesiology
73QEC	Monitor, Blood Gas, Transcutaneous Oxygen	Anesthesiology
78TGM	Monitor, Blood Glucose (Test)	Gastro/Urology
73TAM	Monitor, Blood Potassium	Anesthesiology
74KGJ	Monitor, Blood Pressure, Amplifier & Associated Electronics	Cardiovascular
74WZC	Monitor, Blood Pressure, Finger	Cardiovascular
74RLS	Monitor, Blood Pressure, Indirect (Arterial)	Cardiovascular
73BXD	Monitor, Blood Pressure, Indirect, Anesthesiology	Anesthesiology
74JOE	Monitor, Blood Pressure, Indirect, Automatic	Cardiovascular
74DXN	Monitor, Blood Pressure, Indirect, Semi-Automatic	Cardiovascular
79FYM	Monitor, Blood Pressure, Indirect, Surgery	Surgery
79FYL	Monitor, Blood Pressure, Indirect, Surgery, Powered	Surgery
73BZZ	Monitor, Blood Pressure, Indirect, Transducer	Anesthesiology
74RLR	Monitor, Blood Pressure, Invasive (Arterial)	Cardiovascular
73CAA	Monitor, Blood Pressure, Invasive (Arterial), Anesthesia	Anesthesiology
74BXE	Monitor, Blood Pressure, Transducer, Indwelling	Cardiovascular
74RLX	Monitor, Blood Pressure, Venous	Cardiovascular
74KRK	Monitor, Blood Pressure, Venous, Cardiopulmonary Bypass	Cardiovascular
79FYO	Monitor, Blood Pressure, Venous, Central	Surgery
79FYP	Monitor, Blood Pressure, Venous, Peripheral	Surgery
84LME	Monitor, Cerebral Blood Flow, Thermal Diffusion	Cns/Neurology
75WXU	Monitor, Glucose, Blood, Non-Invasive	Chemistry
80FLP	Monitor, Neonatal, Blood Pressure, Invasive	General
80FLQ	Monitor, Neonatal, Blood Pressure, Ultrasonic/Doppler	General
84HAQ	Needle, Angiographic	Cns/Neurology
80RHY	Needle, Blood Collection	General
81GLY	Oximeter, Whole Blood	Hematology
90RKT	Phonoangiograph	Radiology
81UJP	Potentiator, Blood Antibody	Hematology
74DPT	Probe, Blood Flow, Extravascular	Cardiovascular
79RTA	Probe, Detector, Flow, Blood, Laparoscopy, Ultrasonic	Surgery
81KSW	Processor, Frozen Blood	Hematology
79FZC	Prosthesis, Arterial Graft, Bovine Carotid Artery	Surgery
79FZB	Prosthesis, Arterial Graft, Synthetic, Greater Than 6mm	Surgery
79JCP	Prosthesis, Arterial Graft, Synthetic, Less Than 6mm	Surgery
74DYF	Prosthesis, Vascular Graft, Less Than 6mm Diameter	Cardiovascular
74DSY	Prosthesis, Vascular Graft, Of 6mm And Greater Diameter	Cardiovascular
80WUI	Protector, Puncture, Needle	General

KEYWORD INDEX

BLOOD *(cont'd)*

74KFM	Pump, Blood, Cardiopulmonary Bypass, Non-Roller Type	Cardiovascular
74DWB	Pump, Blood, Cardiopulmonary Bypass, Roller Type	Cardiovascular
78FIR	Pump, Blood, Extra-Luminal	Gastro/Urology
78QZW	Pump, Blood, Hemodialysis Unit	Gastro/Urology
90VLE	Radiographic Unit, Digital Subtraction Angiographic (DSA)	Radiology
90IZI	Radiographic/Fluoroscopic Unit, Angiographic	Radiology
90VHC	Radiographic/Fluoroscopic Unit, Angiographic, Digital	Radiology
80WRG	Reagent, Blood Gas/pH	General
75UMB	Reagent, Blood Urea Nitrogen (BUN)	Chemistry
81GGG	Reagent, Guaiac	Hematology
81KHE	Reagent, Occult Blood	Hematology
74ROK	Recorder, Long-Term, Blood Pressure, Portable	Cardiovascular
81ROT	Refrigerator, Blood Bank	Hematology
74DTN	Reservoir, Blood, Cardiopulmonary Bypass	Cardiovascular
85HGW	Sampler, Blood, Fetal	Obstetrics/Gyn
81RQR	Scale, Blood	Hematology
90IYN	Scanner, Ultrasonic (Pulsed Doppler)	Radiology
90IYO	Scanner, Ultrasonic (Pulsed Echo)	Radiology
90VCV	Scanner, Ultrasonic, Vascular	Radiology
74DTY	Sensor, Blood Gas, In-Line, Cardiopulmonary Bypass	Cardiovascular
81GKT	Separator, Blood Cell, Automated	Hematology
78LKN	Separator, Blood Cell/Plasma, Therapeutic	Gastro/Urology
78MDP	Separator, Blood Cell/Plasma, Therapeutic, Membrane, Auto.	Gastro/Urology
81UJU	Serum, Screening, Blood	Hematology
74RTG	Simulator, Blood Pressure	Cardiovascular
81MMH	Software, Blood Bank (Stand-Alone Products)	Hematology
81MTQ	Software, Blood Virus Applications	Hematology
80FLY	Sphygmomanometer, Aneroid (Arterial Pressure)	General
80THH	Sphygmomanometer, Electronic (Arterial Pressure)	General
80UDM	Sphygmomanometer, Electronic, Automatic	General
80UDN	Sphygmomanometer, Electronic, Manual	General
80FLX	Sphygmomanometer, Mercury (Arterial Pressure)	General
75WTX	Strip, Test	Chemistry
81KSX	Substance, Grouping, Blood (Non-Human Origin)	Hematology
81KSS	Supplies, Blood Bank	Hematology
87VIF	Syringe, Arterial Blood Gas	Orthopedics
83MDB	System, Blood Culturing	Microbiology
75NBW	System, Test, Blood Glucose, Over-The-Counter	Chemistry
81RYW	Table, Blood Donor	Hematology
81LIM	Test, D Positive Fetal Rbc	Hematology
81KQE	Test, Erythrocytic Glucose-6-Phosphate Dehydrogenase	Hematology
83MSQ	Test, Urea (Breath or Blood)	Microbiology
75LCH	Tonometer (Calibration And Q.C. Of Blood Gas Instruments)	Chemistry
80SBD	Tourniquet	General
73BXG	Transducer, Blood Flow, Invasive	Anesthesiology
73BXF	Transducer, Blood Flow, Non-Invasive	Anesthesiology
80SBW	Transducer, Blood Pressure	General
74DXO	Transducer, Blood Pressure, Catheter Tip	Cardiovascular
74DRS	Transducer, Blood Pressure, Extravascular	Cardiovascular
81KSB	Transfer Unit, Blood	Hematology
81GJE	Tray, Blood Collection	Hematology
75SCN	Tube, Blood Collection	Chemistry
75SCM	Tube, Blood Microcollection	Chemistry
81GIO	Tube, Capillary Blood Collection	Hematology
81KSY	View Box, Blood Grouping	Hematology
81KZL	Warmer, Blood and Plasma	Hematology
81SFG	Warmer, Blood, Coil	Hematology
81SFH	Warmer, Blood, Dry Heat	Hematology
81BSA	Warmer, Blood, Electromagnetic Radiation	Hematology
81SFI	Warmer, Blood, Microwave	Hematology
73BSB	Warmer, Blood, Non-Electromagnetic Radiation	Anesthesiology
81VLV	Warmer, Blood, Water Bath	Hematology
81SFO	Washer, Cell (Frozen Blood Processor)	Hematology
81KHG	Whole Blood Hemoglobin Determination	Hematology

BLOT

83WKS	Equipment, Test, Western Blot	Microbiology
81MVW	Kit, Western Blot, Hiv-1	Hematology

BLOW

73BYO	Bottle, Blow (Exerciser)	Anesthesiology

BLOWER

77KCL	Blower, Powder, ENT	Ear/Nose/Throat

BLUE

81GHP	Brilliant Cresyl Blue	Hematology
75CIA	Methylthymol Blue, Calcium	Chemistry
75CEQ	Molybdenum Blue Method, Phospholipids	Chemistry
88IDA	Stain, Alcian Blue	Pathology
88KFD	Stain, Aniline Blue	Pathology
88KJN	Stain, Brilliant Cresyl Blue	Pathology
88ICJ	Stain, Carbol Night Blue	Pathology
88GHZ	Stain, Gugol Blue Solution	Pathology
88HYR	Stain, Leuco-Patent Blue	Pathology
88HYT	Stain, Luxol Fast Blue	Pathology

BLUE *(cont'd)*

88KFC	Stain, Methylene Blue	Pathology
88KKM	Stain, Methylene Blue Thiocyanate	Pathology
81GFR	Stain, Methylene Blue, New	Hematology
88HZE	Stain, Nile Blue	Pathology
88HZN	Stain, Picro Methyl Blue	Pathology
88IAB	Stain, Toluidine Blue	Pathology
81GIX	Stain, Toluidine Blue, Hematology	Hematology
88LGY	Stain, Trypan Blue	Pathology
75CJR	Thymol Blue Monophosphate, Acid Phosphatase	Chemistry
75CJH	Thymol Blue Monophosphate, Alkaline Phosphatase/Isoenzymes	Chemistry
75CHC	Titrimetric Permanganate And Bromophenol Blue, Calcium	Chemistry

BLUNT

79WZY	Dilator, Blunt	Surgery
80RHZ	Needle, Blunt	General

BOARD

80KMP	Board (Bed and Cardiopulmonary Resuscitation)	General
73BTX	Board, Arm	Anesthesiology
80FPS	Board, Bed	General
74QGJ	Board, Cardiac Compression	Cardiovascular
80FOA	Board, Cardiopulmonary Resuscitation	General
88WMB	Board, Dissecting	Pathology
87QWT	Board, Foot	Orthopedics
89RNR	Board, Quadriceps (Exerciser)	Physical Med
89KNL	Board, Scooter, Prone	Physical Med
87RUV	Board, Spine	Orthopedics
80QMX	Cover, Arm Board	General
87RBJ	Immobilizer, Infant (Circumcision Board)	Orthopedics
87RVB	Splint, Wire Board	Orthopedics
89IMX	Tray, Wheelchair	Physical Med

BODY

87LYQ	Accessories, Fixation, Spinal Intervertebral Body	Orthopedics
74MNW	Analyzer, Body Composition	Cardiovascular
80VDN	Analyzer, Composition, Weight, Patient	General
87KWQ	Appliance, Fixation, Spinal Intervertebral Body	Orthopedics
80WNA	Bag, Body	General
90JAN	Counter, Whole Body, Nuclear	Radiology
87MQP	Device, Spinal Vertebral Body Replacement	Orthopedics
80UDO	Exhaust System, Body	General
90LNG	Hyperthermia System, Whole-Body	Radiology
87WUW	Immobilizer, Upper Body	Orthopedics
87MAT	Orthosis, Fixation, Cervical Intervertebral Body, Spinal	Orthopedics
73CCM	Plethysmograph, Pressure (Body)	Anesthesiology
73JEI	Remover, Foreign Body, Bronchoscope (Non-Rigid)	Anesthesiology
80FMQ	Restraint, Protective (Body)	General
90THS	Scanner, Computed Tomography, X-Ray, Full Body	Radiology
81GJJ	Stain, Heinz Body	Hematology
80RZD	Tank, Full Body (Bath)	General
73BYT	Ventilator, External Body, Negative Pressure, (Cuirass)	Anesthesiology
80FLH	Washer, Receptacle, Waste, Body	General

BOILING

76ECG	Sterilizer, Boiling Water	Dental And Oral

BOLSTER

79RXQ	Bolster, Suture (Bumper)	Surgery

BOLT

87HTN	Bolt, Nut, Washer	Orthopedics

BONDING

76KLE	Tooth Bonding Agent, Resin Restoration	Dental And Oral

BONE

86HRG	Accessories, Engine, Trephine, AC-Powered	Ophthalmology
79HRF	Accessories, Engine, Trephine, Battery-Powered	Surgery
79HLD	Accessories, Engine, Trephine, Gas-Powered	Surgery
87LYT	Accessories, Fixation, Orthopedic	Orthopedics
87MHH	Analyzer, Bone, Sonic, Non-Invasive	Orthopedics
87QDU	Blade, Bone Cutting	Orthopedics
87LOD	Bone Cement	Orthopedics
87MBB	Bone Cement, Antibiotic	Orthopedics
87LYS	Bone Mill	Orthopedics
87MBE	Bone, Block, Filler, Metal, Porous, Uncemented	Orthopedics
80WVO	Brush, Other	General
87JDT	Cap, Bone	Orthopedics
77MLI	Cement, Bone, Ionomer	Ear/Nose/Throat
79MGN	Cement, Hydroxyapatite	Surgery
87QIW	Cement, Orthopedic (Bone)	Orthopedics
76EML	Chisel, Bone, Surgical	Dental And Oral
87HXD	Clamp, Bone	Orthopedics
84JXJ	Cutter, Bone, Ultrasonic	Cns/Neurology
90WRK	Densitometer, Bone, Dual Photon	Radiology
90KGI	Densitometer, Bone, Single Photon	Radiology
90WIR	Densitometer, Radiography, Digital, Quantitative	Radiology
87QRE	Drill, Bone	Orthopedics

BONE *(cont'd)*

76DZI	Drill, Bone, Powered	Dental And Oral
87QRO	Driver, Bone Staple	Orthopedics
87HXJ	Driver, Bone Staple, Powered	Orthopedics
76DZJ	Driver, Wire, And Bone Drill, Manual	Dental And Oral
87QRM	Driver/Extractor, Bone Nail/Pin	Orthopedics
87QRN	Driver/Extractor, Bone Plate	Orthopedics
87HTE	Elevator, Orthopedic	Orthopedics
87WRR	Equipment, Screening, Scoliosis	Orthopedics
76EMI	File, Bone, Surgical	Dental And Oral
89MBS	Filler, Bone Void, Non-Osteoinduction	Physical Med
89MBP	Filler, Bone Void, Osteoinduction	Physical Med
87TCH	Freezer, Bone	Orthopedics
87QYR	Graft, Bone	Orthopedics
76KMW	Handpiece, Rotary Bone Cutting	Dental And Oral
77LXB	Hearing-Aid, Bone-Conduction	Ear/Nose/Throat
77MAH	Hearing-Aid, Bone-Conduction, Implanted	Ear/Nose/Throat
77MKE	Hearing-Aid, Bone-Conduction, Percutaneous	Ear/Nose/Throat
79KIK	Hook, Bone	Surgery
87WII	Hydroxyapatite	Orthopedics
76LYC	Implant, Endosseous (Bone Filling and/or Augmentation)	Dental And Oral
87VID	Indicator, Bone Healing	Orthopedics
80LWE	Kit, Collection/Transfusion, Marrow, Bone	General
87HXL	Mallet, Bone	Orthopedics
87JDS	Nail, Fixation, Bone	Orthopedics
79SGU	Needle, Bone Marrow	Surgery
79HWM	Osteotome (Orthopedic)	Surgery
79GFI	Osteotome, Manual (Plastic Surgery)	Surgery
76JEY	Plate, Bone, Orthodontic	Dental And Oral
84RLI	Plate, Bone, Skull (Cranioplasty)	Cns/Neurology
84GWO	Plate, Bone, Skull, Preformed, Alterable	Cns/Neurology
84GXN	Plate, Bone, Skull, Preformed, Non-Alterable	Cns/Neurology
87HRS	Plate, Fixation, Bone	Orthopedics
87NDF	Plate, Fixation, Bone, Non-Spinal, Metallic	Orthopedics
87UCR	Prosthesis, Bone Cerclage	Orthopedics
79MEP	Prosthesis, Craniofacial, Bone-Anchored	Surgery
77JAZ	Prosthesis, Facial, Mandibular Implant	Ear/Nose/Throat
87MIL	Prosthesis, Hip, Semi-Const., Uncem., M/P, Bone Morph. Prot.	Orthopedics
87RNJ	Punch, Bone	Orthopedics
87HTR	Rasp, Bone	Orthopedics
87ULN	Refrigerator, Bone	Orthopedics
87HSO	Saw, Bone Cutting	Orthopedics
87VHR	Saw, Bone Cutting, Micro	Orthopedics
87RQN	Saw, Bone, Pneumatic	Orthopedics
76DZH	Saw, Electric Bone	Dental And Oral
87HWC	Screw, Fixation, Bone	Orthopedics
87NDJ	Screw, Fixation, Bone, Non-Spinal, Metallic	Orthopedics
87HWO	Skid, Bone	Orthopedics
90MUA	Sonometer, Bone	Radiology
87JDR	Staple, Fixation, Bone	Orthopedics
87HWD	Starter, Bone Screw	Orthopedics
76LYD	Stimulator, Growth, Bone, Electromagnetic, Dental	Dental And Oral
87LOE	Stimulator, Growth, Bone, Invasive	Orthopedics
87LOF	Stimulator, Growth, Bone, Non-Invasive	Orthopedics
87HTM	Stimulator, Osteogenesis, Electric, Invasive	Orthopedics
87WNT	Stimulator, Osteogenesis, Electric, Non-Invasive	Orthopedics
89MBO	Substitute, Graft, Bone	Physical Med
87HWX	Tap, Bone	Orthopedics
87SBA	Tongs, Bone	Orthopedics
87HWK	Trephine, Bone	Orthopedics
76LPK	Tricalcium Phosphate Granules for Dental Bone Repair	Dental And Oral
77TFL	Vibrator, Audiometric Bone	Ear/Nose/Throat
79MTJ	Wax, Bone	Surgery
87UBT	Wire, Bone	Orthopedics
87LMJ	Xenograft for Bone Growth/Stimulation	Orthopedics

BONE-ANCHORED

79MEP	Prosthesis, Craniofacial, Bone-Anchored	Surgery

BONE-CONDUCTION

77LXB	Hearing-Aid, Bone-Conduction	Ear/Nose/Throat
77MAH	Hearing-Aid, Bone-Conduction, Implanted	Ear/Nose/Throat
77MKE	Hearing-Aid, Bone-Conduction, Percutaneous	Ear/Nose/Throat

BOOT

80QCT	Boot, Bath	General
89IPG	Shoe, Cast	Physical Med

BOOTH

89LEJ	Booth, Sun Tan	Physical Med
77EWC	Chamber, Acoustic, Testing	Ear/Nose/Throat

BORATE

76KOM	Acacia And Karaya With Sodium Borate	Dental And Oral
76MMU	Adhesive, Denture, Acacia & Karaya with Sodium Borate	Dental And Oral
76KOR	Adhesive, Denture, Karaya With Sodium Borate	Dental And Oral
75CEJ	Tetraphenyl Borate, Colorimetry, Potassium	Chemistry

BORRELIA

83LSR	Reagent, Borrelia, Serological	Microbiology
82WVP	Test, Disease, Lyme	Immunology

BOTHROPS

81JCO	Reagent, Bothrops Atrox	Hematology

BOTTLE

73BYO	Bottle, Blow (Exerciser)	Anesthesiology
73CBD	Bottle, Collection, Breathing System (Calibrated)	Anesthesiology
73CBC	Bottle, Collection, Breathing System (Uncalibrated)	Anesthesiology
80KDQ	Bottle, Collection, Vacuum (Aspirator)	General
78QEE	Bottle, Endoscopic Wash	Gastro/Urology
80TAN	Bottle, Evacuated	General
80FPF	Bottle, Hot/Cold Water	General
80VFT	Bottle, Medicine Spray	General
85TAO	Bottle, Nursing	Obstetrics/Gyn
80QEF	Bottle, Sterile Solution	General
88KJC	Bottle, Tissue Culture, Roller	Pathology
73RJL	Canister, Oxygen	Anesthesiology
88KER	Container, Embedding	Pathology
80KPE	Container, IV	General
88KDT	Container, Specimen Mailer And Storage	Pathology
88KDW	Container, Specimen Mailer And Storage, Temperature Control	Pathology
80FMH	Container, Specimen, All Types	General
80SEE	Container, Urine Specimen	General
73QVA	Exerciser, Respiratory	Anesthesiology
80FNN	Nipple, Feeding	General
73SBZ	Trap, Mucus	Anesthesiology
83SCS	Tube, Culture	Microbiology
78LJH	Urological Irrigation System	Gastro/Urology

BOUFFANT

79FYF	Cap, Surgical	Surgery
79RXN	Cover, Head, Surgical	Surgery

BOUGIE

78FAT	Bougie, Esophageal, And Gastrointestinal, Gastro-Urology	Gastro/Urology
77KCD	Bougie, Esophageal, ENT	Ear/Nose/Throat
77KBI	Bougie, Eustachian (Ear)	Ear/Nose/Throat
78FAX	Bougie, Urological	Gastro/Urology
78EZM	Dilator, Esophageal (Metal Olive) Gastro-Urology	Gastro/Urology

BOUIN'S

88IGN	Fluid, Bouin's	Pathology

BOUND

75JIK	Dry Ash Method, Protein Bound Iodine	Chemistry
75CIW	Starch-Dye Bound Polymer, Amylase	Chemistry
75JIJ	Wet Ash Method, Protein Bound Iodine	Chemistry

BOURDON

73CCN	Flowmeter, Gas, Non-Back-Pressure Compensated, Bourdon Gauge	Anesthesiology

BOVIE

79QTV	Electrosurgical Unit, General Purpose (ESU)	Surgery

BOVINE

79QYS	Graft, Bovine	Surgery
79FZC	Prosthesis, Arterial Graft, Bovine Carotid Artery	Surgery
91DPL	Radioimmunoassay, Digitoxin (125-I), Bovine, Charcoal	Toxicology
91DOR	Radioimmunoassay, Digoxin (3-H), Bovine, Charcoal	Toxicology

BOW

76KCR	Face Bow	Dental And Oral

BOWEL

78WLL	Device, Incontinence, Fecal	Gastro/Urology
78SIB	Kit, Bowel	Gastro/Urology

BOWL

80QEG	Bowl, Solution	General
80QEH	Bowl, Sponge	General
76QOE	Cuspidor	Dental And Oral
87JDZ	Mixing Equipment, Cement	Orthopedics

BOX

78FCP	Box, Battery, Pocket (Endoscopic)	Gastro/Urology
78FCO	Box, Battery, Rechargeable (Endoscopic)	Gastro/Urology
83JTM	Box, Glove	Microbiology
80WYL	Box, Transportation, Container, Specimen	General
80WPQ	Container, Medication, Home-Use	General
90IXC	Illuminator, Radiographic Film	Radiology
90JAG	Illuminator, Radiographic Film, Explosion-Proof	Radiology
81KSY	View Box, Blood Grouping	Hematology
83WHV	View Box, Microtiter	Microbiology
81SEY	View Box, Rh Typing	Hematology

BRACE

87HXY	Brace, Drill	Orthopedics

KEYWORD INDEX

BROMOPHENOL
75CHC Titrimetric Permanganate And Bromophenol Blue, Calcium — Chemistry

BRONCHIAL
77KCE Cannula, Bronchial — Ear/Nose/Throat
77RWV Stylet, Bronchial — Ear/Nose/Throat
77ENZ Telescope, Laryngeal-Bronchial — Ear/Nose/Throat
73BTS Tube, Bronchial (W/Wo Connector) — Anesthesiology
73CBI Tube, Tracheal/Bronchial, Differential Ventilation — Anesthesiology

BRONCHOSCOPE
77KTI Accessories, Bronchoscope — Ear/Nose/Throat
77BTN Bronchoscope, Non-Rigid — Ear/Nose/Throat
77EOQ Bronchoscope, Rigid — Ear/Nose/Throat
73BTJ Bronchoscope, Rigid, Non-Ventilating — Anesthesiology
73BTH Bronchoscope, Rigid, Ventilating — Anesthesiology
73BTG Brush, Biopsy, Bronchoscope (Non-Rigid) — Anesthesiology
73BST Curette, Biopsy, Bronchoscope (Non-Rigid) — Anesthesiology
73JEL Curette, Biopsy, Bronchoscope (Rigid) — Anesthesiology
73BWH Forceps, Biopsy, Bronchoscope (Non-Rigid) — Anesthesiology
73JEK Forceps, Biopsy, Bronchoscope (Rigid) — Anesthesiology
73JEI Remover, Foreign Body, Bronchoscope (Non-Rigid) — Anesthesiology
77KTR Tube, Aspirating, Rigid Bronchoscope Aspirating — Ear/Nose/Throat
73JEJ Tube, Bronchoscope — Anesthesiology
73JEM Tube, Bronchoscope, Aspirating — Anesthesiology

BRONCHUS
77QKJ Clamp, Bronchus — Ear/Nose/Throat

BROTH
83JSC Culture Media, General Nutrient Broth — Microbiology
83JTZ Culture Media, Mueller Hinton Agar Broth — Microbiology
83JSD Culture Media, Selective Broth — Microbiology
83TDG Separation Media — Microbiology

BROWN
89ITN Splint, Denis Brown — Physical Med
88KJM Stain, Bismarck Brown Y — Pathology

BRUCELLA
83GSO Antigen, (Febrile), Agglutination, Brucella SPP. — Microbiology
83GSM Antiserum, Fluorescent, Brucella SPP. — Microbiology

BRUSH
78MNL Accessories, Cleaning Brushes (For Endoscope) — Gastro/Urology
78FEB Accessories, Cleaning, Endoscopic — Gastro/Urology
76KOJ Airbrush — Dental And Oral
73BTG Brush, Biopsy, Bronchoscope (Non-Rigid) — Anesthesiology
79GEE Brush, Biopsy, General & Plastic Surgery — Surgery
76QEO Brush, Burr Cleaning — Dental And Oral
81WIT Brush, Centrifuge — Hematology
77EPE Brush, Cleaning, Tracheal Tube — Ear/Nose/Throat
80WKZ Brush, Cytology — General
78FDX Brush, Cytology, Endoscopic — Gastro/Urology
76QEP Brush, Dental Plate (Denture) — Dental And Oral
79GFE Brush, Dermabrasion — Surgery
79GED Brush, Dermabrasion, Manual — Surgery
85HFE Brush, Endometrial — Obstetrics/Gyn
76QER Brush, Gum (Gingival) — Dental And Oral
86HIY Brush, Haidinger, With Macular Integrity — Ophthalmology
86QEQ Brush, Ophthalmic — Ophthalmology
80WVO Brush, Other — General
79GEC Brush, Scrub, Operating Room — Surgery
79QQB Dispenser, Brush — Surgery
76EFW Toothbrush, Manual — Dental And Oral
76JEQ Toothbrush, Powered — Dental And Oral

BUBBLE
78WNS Balloon, Gastric — Gastro/Urology
74VCJ Bubble Defoamer, Cardiopulmonary Bypass — Cardiovascular
80QNI Cover, Crib Top (Bubble) — General
78FJF Detector, Air Bubble — Gastro/Urology
74QZI Detector, Air, Heart-Lung Bypass — Cardiovascular
74KRL Detector, Bubble, Cardiopulmonary Bypass — Cardiovascular
78QZV Detector, Hemodialysis Unit Air Bubble-Foam — Gastro/Urology
74SBY Trap, Bubble — Cardiovascular

BUBBLE-FOAM
78QZV Detector, Hemodialysis Unit Air Bubble-Foam — Gastro/Urology

BUCKET
80RDC Liner, Kick Bucket — General
80RDD Waste Receptacle, Kick Bucket — General

BUCKLING
86HQJ Implant, Absorbable (Scleral Buckling Method) — Ophthalmology
86TEL Scleral Buckling Instrument — Ophthalmology

BUCKY
90IXJ Grid, Radiographic — Radiology
90VGT Holder, X-Ray Film Cassette, Vertical — Radiology

BUFFER
81JCC Buffer, pH — Hematology
75UHD Solution, pH Buffer — Chemistry

BUFFERED
88IFP Formalin, Neutral Buffered — Pathology

BUILDING
80VAS Building Material — General
80TBA Cabinet Casework, General Purpose — General
75TBB Cabinet Casework, Laboratory — Chemistry
80TBC Cabinet Casework, Modular — General
80TBE Cabinet Casework, Patient Room — General
80TBF Cabinet Casework, Pharmacy — General
80VBB Carpeting — General
80UMS Column, Life Support (Electrical/Gas) — General
80VBT Control System, Energy — General
80QTZ Elevator, Other — General
90VGS Entrance, X-Ray Darkrooms — Radiology
80WRQ Equipment, Building Security — General
80TCD Floor, Conductive — General
80VBC Flooring — General
80RLO Headwall System (Patient Room) — General
80TGZ Mirror, Corridor Safety — General
80VAY Security Equipment/Supplies — General
90RSV Shield, X-Ray, Brick — Radiology
90TDY Shield, X-Ray, Door — Radiology
80UMU Station, Nourishment — General
80TBD Station, Nursing — General
80TFM Wallpaper, Antibacterial — General

BUILT-IN
80WOB Meter, Patient Height — General
80WOE System, Pipeline, Gas — General

BULB
78FFY Adapter, Bulb, Endoscope, Miscellaneous — Gastro/Urology
80WRS Bulb, Inflation — General
78FCY Bulb, Inflation (Endoscope) — Gastro/Urology
80RYU Syringe, Bulb — General
76DYY Syringe, Bulb, Air Or Water — Dental And Oral
76EIB Syringe, Irrigating, Dental — Dental And Oral

BULBOUS
78MES Stent, Urethral, Bulbous, Permanent/Semi-Permanent — Gastro/Urology

BULK
80UDL Sterilizer, Bulk, Steam & Ethylene-Oxide — General
80UDJ Sterilizer, Ethylene-Oxide, Bulk — General
80UCS Sterilizer, Steam, Bulk — General

BULKING
78LNM Agent, Bulking, Injectable (Gastro-Urology) — Gastro/Urology

BULLDOG
79QKK Clamp, Bulldog — Surgery

BUMPER
79RXQ Bolster, Suture (Bumper) — Surgery
80TBM Bumper Guard, Corner — General

BUN
75QES Analyzer, BUN (Blood Urea Nitrogen) — Chemistry
75UMB Reagent, Blood Urea Nitrogen (BUN) — Chemistry

BUNDLE
74RAD Detector, His Bundle — Cardiovascular

BUNION
87RSR Shield, Bunion — Orthopedics

BURET
75QET Buret — Chemistry
80RCI Kit, Intravenous, Administration, Buret — General

BURGDORFERI
82WVP Test, Disease, Lyme — Immunology

BURN
79KGN Dressing, Burn, Porcine — Surgery
79MSA Dressing, Wound And Burn, Occlusive, Heated — Surgery
79MGQ Dressing, Wound and Burn, Hydrogel — Surgery
79MGR Dressing, Wound and Burn, Interactive — Surgery
79MGP Dressing, Wound and Burn, Occlusive — Surgery
80QEU Kit, Burn — General
80WMD Pad, Pressure, Gel, Operating Table — General
80FPY Sheet, Burn — General
89WIN Stimulator, Wound Healing — Physical Med
80WTK Support, Cover, Bed — General

BURNER
75UFM Burner — Chemistry

KEYWORD INDEX

CABLE *(cont'd)*

74WLG	Cable/Lead, ECG, Radiolucent	Cardiovascular
74DSA	Cable/Lead, ECG, With Transducer And Electrode	Cardiovascular
84VDF	Cable/Lead, EEG	Cns/Neurology
84VDG	Cable/Lead, EMG	Cns/Neurology
84VDH	Cable/Lead, TENS	Cns/Neurology
80RWO	Strap, Cable	General
74QSI	Tester, Electrocardiograph Cable	Cardiovascular

CADAVER

80WNA	Bag, Body	General
88RYV	Table, Autopsy	Pathology

CAGE

83THA	Cage, Animal	Microbiology
89ITM	Cage, Knee	Physical Med

CALCITONIN

75JKR	Radioimmunoassay, Calcitonin	Chemistry

CALCIUM

75JFN	Absorption, Atomic, Calcium	Chemistry
75CID	Alizarin Sulfonate, Calcium	Chemistry
75CJY	Azo-Dye, Calcium	Chemistry
75CIC	Complexone, Cresolphthalein, Calcium	Chemistry
75CHZ	DI (O-Hydroxyphenylimine) Ethane, Calcium	Chemistry
80LJJ	Electrode, In Vivo Calcium Ion Selective	General
75JFP	Electrode, Ion Specific, Calcium	Chemistry
87MQV	Filler, Calcium Sulfate Preformed Pellets	Orthopedics
76EJK	Liner, Cavity, Calcium Hydroxide	Dental And Oral
75CIA	Methylthymol Blue, Calcium	Chemistry
76KOO	Polyvinyl Methylether Maleic Acid-Calcium-Sodium Dbl. Salt	Dental And Oral
87MAZ	Prosthesis, Hip, Semi-Const., M/P, Por. Uncem., Calc./Phos.	Orthopedics
87MEH	Prosthesis, Hip, Semi-Const., Uncem., Non-P., M/P, Ca./Phos.	Orthopedics
75JFO	Reagent, Calcium (Test System)	Chemistry
88IGD	Solution, Pathology, Formol Calcium	Pathology
75SAY	Titrator, Calcium	Chemistry
75CHC	Titrimetric Permanganate And Bromophenol Blue, Calcium	Chemistry
75CHW	Titrimetric With EDTA And Indicator, Calcium	Chemistry

CALCOACETICUS

83GSX	Antisera, Acinetobacter Calcoaceticus, All Varieties	Microbiology

CALCULATED

81JPJ	Red Cell Indices, Calculated	Hematology

CALCULATOR

80SHP	Aid, Living, Handicapped	General
85MPT	Calculator, Contraception	Obstetrics/Gyn
90WSH	Calculator, Technique, Radiographic	Radiology
75JHZ	Programmable Calculator, Enzyme Calculator	Chemistry

CALCULI

75JNP	Infrared Spectroscopy Measurement, Urinary Calculi (Stone)	Chemistry
78UEP	Lithotriptor	Gastro/Urology
78VKM	Lithotriptor, Electro-Hydraulic, Extracorporeal	Gastro/Urology
78FFK	Lithotriptor, Electro-Hydraulic, Percutaneous	Gastro/Urology
78LNS	Lithotriptor, Extracorporeal Shock-wave, Urological	Gastro/Urology
78WSU	Lithotriptor, Laser	Gastro/Urology
78FEO	Lithotriptor, Ultrasonic	Gastro/Urology
75JNQ	Qualitative Chemical Reactions, Urinary Calculi (Stone)	Chemistry

CALCULUS

76ELA	Hand Instrument, Calculus Removal	Dental And Oral

CALIBRATED

73CBD	Bottle, Collection, Breathing System (Calibrated)	Anesthesiology
73BXY	Flowmeter, Gas (Oxygen), Calibrated	Anesthesiology
73BXK	Gas, Calibrated (Specified Concentration)	Anesthesiology

CALIBRATION

80WRA	Reagent, Calibration	General
83LIE	Reagent, Inoculator Calibration (Laboratory)	Microbiology
73WTC	Syringe, Calibration Testing, Spirometer	Anesthesiology
75LCH	Tonometer (Calibration And Q.C. Of Blood Gas Instruments)	Chemistry

CALIBRATOR

90IXD	Calibrator Source, Nuclear Sealed	Radiology
82LTQ	Calibrator, AFP, Serum, Maternal, Mid-Pregnancy	Immunology
73QFN	Calibrator, Anesthesia Unit	Anesthesiology
77EWA	Calibrator, Audiometer	Ear/Nose/Throat
90WPC	Calibrator, Beam	Radiology
80WMK	Calibrator, Blood Gas	General
81KRX	Calibrator, Cell Indices	Hematology
90KPT	Calibrator, Dose, Radionuclide	Radiology
78TAQ	Calibrator, Drop-Rate, Infusion	Gastro/Urology
91DKB	Calibrator, Drug Mixture	Toxicology

CALIBRATOR *(cont'd)*

91DLJ	Calibrator, Drug Specific	Toxicology
91DNN	Calibrator, Ethyl Alcohol	Toxicology
73BXX	Calibrator, Gas, Pressure	Anesthesiology
73BXW	Calibrator, Gas, Volume	Anesthesiology
77ETW	Calibrator, Hearing-Aid/Earphone And Analysis Systems	Ear/Nose/Throat
81KRZ	Calibrator, Hemoglobin And Hematocrit Measurement	Hematology
80WML	Calibrator, Mass Spectrometer	General
81KRY	Calibrator, Platelet Counting	Hematology
73QFO	Calibrator, Pressure Transducer	Anesthesiology
75JIS	Calibrator, Primary, Clinical Chemistry	Chemistry
90QFP	Calibrator, Radioisotope	Radiology
81KSA	Calibrator, Red Cell And White Cell Counting	Hematology
73QFQ	Calibrator, Respiratory Therapy Unit	Anesthesiology
75JIT	Calibrator, Secondary, Clinical Chemistry	Chemistry
75JIW	Calibrator, Surrogate, Clinical Chemistry	Chemistry
86HLA	Calibrator, Tonometer	Ophthalmology
74CAS	Flowmeter, Blood, Ultrasonic, Transcutaneous (W/WO Calibr.)	Cardiovascular
75JIX	Multi Analyte Mixture, Calibrator	Chemistry
74RTF	Simulator, Arrhythmia	Cardiovascular
74RTG	Simulator, Blood Pressure	Cardiovascular
74RTH	Simulator, ECG	Cardiovascular
74RTI	Simulator, Heart Sound	Cardiovascular
73RTK	Simulator, Respiration	Anesthesiology
80RTM	Simulator, Temperature	General

CALIPER

90WSH	Calculator, Technique, Radiographic	Radiology
87KTZ	Caliper	Orthopedics
74VLH	Caliper, ECG	Cardiovascular
85HEN	Caliper, Fetal Head, Ultrasonic	Obstetrics/Gyn
86HOE	Caliper, Ophthalmic	Ophthalmology
87HSY	Caliper, Orthopedic	Orthopedics
80QFR	Caliper, Skinfold	General
79FTY	Tape, Measuring, Ruler And Caliper	Surgery

CALL

80RIO	Nurse Call System	General

CALLOUS

79QVU	File, Callous	Surgery

CALORIC

77QFS	Irrigator, Caloric	Ear/Nose/Throat
77KHH	Stimulator, Caloric Air	Ear/Nose/Throat
77ETP	Stimulator, Caloric Water	Ear/Nose/Throat

CALORIMETER

75UFN	Calorimeter	Chemistry

CAMERA

79KQM	Accessories, Surgical Camera	Surgery
79FTS	Camera, Cine, Endoscopic (With Audio)	Surgery
79FWL	Camera, Cine, Endoscopic (Without Audio)	Surgery
79FWK	Camera, Cine, Microsurgical (With Audio)	Surgery
79FWJ	Camera, Cine, Microsurgical (Without Audio)	Surgery
79FWI	Camera, Cine, Surgical (With Audio)	Surgery
79FWH	Camera, Cine, Surgical (Without Audio)	Surgery
90IXH	Camera, Focal Spot, Radiographic	Radiology
90IYX	Camera, Gamma (Nuclear/Scintillation)	Radiology
80QFT	Camera, Identification	General
83TAR	Camera, Microscope	Microbiology
90LMC	Camera, Multi Format	Radiology
90TAS	Camera, Multi-Image	Radiology
86HKI	Camera, Ophthalmic, AC-Powered (Fundus)	Ophthalmology
83QFU	Camera, Oscilloscope	Microbiology
80WKP	Camera, Other	General
78EXZ	Camera, Physiological, Function Monitor	Gastro/Urology
90IZC	Camera, Positron	Radiology
90VER	Camera, Radiographic Photospot	Radiology
79FXM	Camera, Still, Endoscopic	Surgery
79FTH	Camera, Still, Microsurgical	Surgery
79FTT	Camera, Still, Surgical	Surgery
79FWG	Camera, Television, Endoscopic (With Audio)	Surgery
79FWF	Camera, Television, Endoscopic (Without Audio)	Surgery
79FWE	Camera, Television, Microsurgical (With Audio)	Surgery
79FWD	Camera, Television, Microsurgical (Without Audio)	Surgery
79FWC	Camera, Television, Surgical (With Audio)	Surgery
79FWB	Camera, Television, Surgical (Without Audio)	Surgery
80WQX	Camera, Video	General
80WQY	Camera, Video, Endoscopic	General
79WRX	Camera, Video, Headlight, Surgical	Surgery
80WZQ	Camera, Video, Multi-Image	General
79FXN	Camera, Videotape, Surgical	Surgery
90IZJ	Camera, X-Ray, Fluorographic, Cine Or Spot	Radiology
80SHM	Coupler, Optical, Laparoscopic	General
79TBN	Cover, Camera	Surgery
79FXT	Film, Camera	Surgery

KEYWORD INDEX

CAPD
78KQR Detector, Air Or Foam — Gastro/Urology
78KPP Filter, Peritoneal Dialysate — Gastro/Urology
78RKM Kit, Tubing, Dialysis, Peritoneal — Gastro/Urology
78RKL Peritoneal Dialysis Unit (CAPD) — Gastro/Urology
78KPM Shunt, Peritoneal — Gastro/Urology
78LLJ Solution, Dialysis — Gastro/Urology
80SDJ Tube, Transfer — General
78KQQ Tubing, Dialysate (And Connector) — Gastro/Urology

CAPILLARY
78FJI Dialyzer, Capillary, Hollow Fiber (Hemodialysis) — Gastro/Urology
75JNW Timed Flow in Capillary, Plasma Viscometry — Chemistry
75SCO Tube, Capillary — Chemistry
81GIO Tube, Capillary Blood Collection — Hematology

CAPNOGRAPH
73CCK Analyzer, Gas, Carbon-Dioxide, Gaseous Phase (Capnograph) — Anesthesiology

CAPSID
83MCD Antigen, Epstein-Barr Virus, Capsid — Microbiology

CAPSULAR
86MXY Cannula, Ophthalmic, Posterior Capsular Polishing, Polyvinyl Acetal — Ophthalmology

CAPSULATUM
83GMJ Antigen, Histoplasma Capsulatum, All — Microbiology
83GML Antiserum, Fluorescent, Histoplasma Capsulatum — Microbiology
83GMK Antiserum, Positive Control, Histoplasma Capsulatum — Microbiology
83MIZ Enzyme Linked Immunoabsorbent Assay, Histoplasma Capsulatum — Microbiology

CAPSULE
76DZS Capsule, Dental, Amalgam — Dental And Oral

CAPSULOTOMY
86LOI Laser, Neodymium:YAG (Excl. Post. Capstmy./Pupilloplasty) — Ophthalmology
86LXS Laser, Neodymium:YAG, Ophthalmic (Post. Capsulotomy) — Ophthalmology

CAR
80QAO Ambulance — General
89WHH Vehicle, Handicapped — Physical Med

CARBAMAZEPINE
91KLT Enzyme Immunoassay, Carbamazepine — Toxicology
91LGI Fluorescence Polarization Immunoassay, Carbamazepine — Toxicology
91LDB U.V. Spectrometry, Carbamazepine — Toxicology

CARBAZONE
75CHK Mercuric Nitrate And Diphenyl Carbazone (Titrimetric) — Chemistry

CARBOHYDRATE
82LTL Antigen, Carbohydrate (CA19-9) — Immunology
75MPG Kit, Urinary Carbohydrate Analysis — Chemistry
75UII Standard, Carbohydrate — Chemistry

CARBOL
88ICL Stain, Carbol Fuchsin — Pathology
88ICJ Stain, Carbol Night Blue — Pathology

CARBON
73CBL Absorbent, Carbon-Dioxide — Anesthesiology
73BSF Absorber, Carbon-Dioxide — Anesthesiology
75UFO Analyzer, Carbon — Chemistry
75UFP Analyzer, Carbon Hydrogen — Chemistry
75UFQ Analyzer, Carbon Hydrogen Nitrogen — Chemistry
73CCC Analyzer, Gas, Carbon-Dioxide, Blood Phase, Indwelling — Anesthesiology
73CCK Analyzer, Gas, Carbon-Dioxide, Gaseous Phase (Capnograph) — Anesthesiology
73BXZ Analyzer, Gas, Carbon-Dioxide, Partial Pressure, Blood — Anesthesiology
73CCJ Analyzer, Gas, Carbon-Monoxide, Gaseous Phase — Anesthesiology
73VCB Analyzer, Gas, Carbon-Monoxide, Non-Indwelling Blood Phase — Anesthesiology
75CIL Colorimetry, Cresol Red, Carbon-Dioxide — Chemistry
75CHS Coulometric Method, Carbon-Dioxide — Chemistry
79QUA Cylinder, Carbon-Dioxide — Surgery
78FAP Cystometric Gas (Carbon-Dioxide) Or Hydraulic Device — Gastro/Urology
80WSE Dressing, Layer, Charcoal — General
73QSO Electrode, Blood Gas, Carbon-Dioxide — Anesthesiology
73QTG Electrode, Transcutaneous, Carbon-Dioxide — Anesthesiology
75KHS Enzymatic, Carbon-Dioxide — Chemistry
91JKT Gas Chromatograph, Carbon-Monoxide — Toxicology
78FCX Insufflator, Carbon-Dioxide, Automatic (For Endoscope) — Gastro/Urology
85HES Insufflator, Carbon-Dioxide, Uterotubal — Obstetrics/Gyn
77EWG Laser, Carbon-Dioxide, Microsurgical, ENT — Ear/Nose/Throat
79UKZ Laser, Carbon-Dioxide, Surgical — Surgery
79KKY Material, PTFE/Carbon, Maxillofacial — Surgery
73QEA Monitor, Blood Gas, Carbon-Dioxide — Anesthesiology
73TAJ Monitor, Blood Gas, Transcutaneous Carbon-Dioxide — Anesthesiology

CARBON (cont'd)
73LKD Monitor, Carbon-Dioxide, Cutaneous — Anesthesiology
73ULU Monitor, Transcutaneous, Carbon-Dioxide — Anesthesiology
91JKS Oxyhemoglobin/Carboxyhemoglobin Curve, Carbon-Monoxide — Toxicology
75KMS Phenolphthalein Colorimetry, Carbon-Dioxide — Chemistry
77ESF Polymer, ENT Composite Synthetic PTFE With Carbon-Fiber — Ear/Nose/Throat
87KMB Prosthesis, Knee, Non-Const. (M/C Reinf. Polyeth.) Cemented — Orthopedics
79KDA Prosthesis, PTFE/Carbon-Fiber — Surgery
91DKM Reagent, Test, Carbon Monoxide — Toxicology
75CHR Titrimetric Phenol Red, Carbon-Dioxide — Chemistry
75CIE Volumetric/Manometric, Carbon-Dioxide — Chemistry
75JFL pH Rate Measurement, Carbon-Dioxide — Chemistry

CARBON-DIOXIDE
73CBL Absorbent, Carbon-Dioxide — Anesthesiology
73BSF Absorber, Carbon-Dioxide — Anesthesiology
73CCC Analyzer, Gas, Carbon-Dioxide, Blood Phase, Indwelling — Anesthesiology
73CCK Analyzer, Gas, Carbon-Dioxide, Gaseous Phase (Capnograph) — Anesthesiology
73BXZ Analyzer, Gas, Carbon-Dioxide, Partial Pressure, Blood — Anesthesiology
79WTZ Analyzer, Patient, Multiple Function (Surgery) — Surgery
75CIL Colorimetry, Cresol Red, Carbon-Dioxide — Chemistry
75CHS Coulometric Method, Carbon-Dioxide — Chemistry
79QUA Cylinder, Carbon-Dioxide — Surgery
78FAP Cystometric Gas (Carbon-Dioxide) Or Hydraulic Device — Gastro/Urology
73QSO Electrode, Blood Gas, Carbon-Dioxide — Anesthesiology
73QTG Electrode, Transcutaneous, Carbon-Dioxide — Anesthesiology
75KHS Enzymatic, Carbon-Dioxide — Chemistry
78FCX Insufflator, Carbon-Dioxide, Automatic (For Endoscope) — Gastro/Urology
85HES Insufflator, Carbon-Dioxide, Uterotubal — Obstetrics/Gyn
77EWG Laser, Carbon-Dioxide, Microsurgical, ENT — Ear/Nose/Throat
79UKZ Laser, Carbon-Dioxide, Surgical — Surgery
80WQS Laser, Combination — General
73QEA Monitor, Blood Gas, Carbon-Dioxide — Anesthesiology
73TAJ Monitor, Blood Gas, Transcutaneous Carbon-Dioxide — Anesthesiology
73LKD Monitor, Carbon-Dioxide, Cutaneous — Anesthesiology
73ULU Monitor, Transcutaneous, Carbon-Dioxide — Anesthesiology
79RKN Needle, Insufflation, Laparoscopic — Surgery
75KMS Phenolphthalein Colorimetry, Carbon-Dioxide — Chemistry
75CHR Titrimetric Phenol Red, Carbon-Dioxide — Chemistry
75CIE Volumetric/Manometric, Carbon-Dioxide — Chemistry
75JFL pH Rate Measurement, Carbon-Dioxide — Chemistry

CARBON-FIBER
77ESF Polymer, ENT Composite Synthetic PTFE With Carbon-Fiber — Ear/Nose/Throat
79KDA Prosthesis, PTFE/Carbon-Fiber — Surgery

CARBON-MONOXIDE
73CCJ Analyzer, Gas, Carbon-Monoxide, Gaseous Phase — Anesthesiology
73VCB Analyzer, Gas, Carbon-Monoxide, Non-Indwelling Blood Phase — Anesthesiology
91CCA Analyzer, Gas, Carboxyhemoglobin, Blood Phase, Non-Indw. — Toxicology
91JKT Gas Chromatograph, Carbon-Monoxide — Toxicology
80QUM Monitor, Gas, Atmospheric, Environmental — General
91JKS Oxyhemoglobin/Carboxyhemoglobin Curve, Carbon-Monoxide — Toxicology

CARBONATE
88KKP Solution, Silver Carbonate — Pathology

CARBONIC
82KTK Carbonic Anhydrase B And C Immunoassay Reagents — Immunology

CARBONICANHYDRASE
82DDH Carbonicanhydrase B, Antigen, Antiserum, Control — Immunology
82DDE Carbonicanhydrase C, Antigen, Antiserum, Control — Immunology

CARBOWAX
88IER Polyethylene Glycol (Carbowax) — Pathology

CARBOXYHEMOGLOBIN
91CCA Analyzer, Gas, Carboxyhemoglobin, Blood Phase, Non-Indw. — Toxicology
81GHS Carboxyhemoglobin — Hematology
91JKS Oxyhemoglobin/Carboxyhemoglobin Curve, Carbon-Monoxide — Toxicology

CARBOXYMETHYLCELLULOSE
76KXW Carboxymethylcellulose Sodium — Dental And Oral
76KOS Carboxymethylcellulose Sodium & Cationic Polyacrylamide — Dental And Oral
76KOQ Carboxymethylcellulose Sodium (40-100%) — Dental And Oral
76KOL Carboxymethylcellulose Sodium/Ethylene-Oxide Homopolymer — Dental And Oral
76KQB PV Methylether Maleic Anhydride Copol./Carboxymethylcellul. — Dental And Oral

CARE

80QCD	Care Kit, Baby	General
80FRR	Chamber, Isolation, Patient Care	General
80QHG	Kit, Catheter Care	General
73SBG	Kit, Tracheostomy Care	Anesthesiology
80VLB	Lotion, Skin Care	General
73RLA	Monitor, Physiological, Acute Care	Anesthesiology
80VLI	Swabs, Oral Care	General
73SEW	Ventilator, Volume (Critical Care)	Anesthesiology

CARIES

76LFC	Detector, Caries	Dental And Oral
76LXD	Optical Caries Detection Device	Dental And Oral
76LMW	Solution, Removal, Caries	Dental And Oral

CARINII

83LYF	Pneumocystis Carinii	Microbiology

CARMINE

88ICO	Stain, Best's Carmine	Pathology
88KJP	Stain, Carmine	Pathology

CARNOY'S

88IGM	Solution, Pathology, Carnoy's	Pathology

CAROTID

84HCE	Clamp, Carotid Artery	Cns/Neurology
79FZC	Prosthesis, Arterial Graft, Bovine Carotid Artery	Surgery
74WWF	Shunt, Carotid	Cardiovascular
74DSR	Stimulator, Carotid Sinus Nerve	Cardiovascular
74MKX	System, Carotid Atherectomy	Cardiovascular

CARPAL

89MNY	Inhibitor, Post-Op Fibro., Carp. Tun. Syn.(Adhesion Barrier)	Physical Med
87HSM	Prosthesis, Carpal	Orthopedics
87KWN	Prosthesis, Wrist, Carpal Lunate	Orthopedics
87KWO	Prosthesis, Wrist, Carpal Scaphoid	Orthopedics
87KYI	Prosthesis, Wrist, Carpal Trapezium	Orthopedics

CARPETING

80VBB	Carpeting	General

CARRIED

80FPP	Stretcher, Hand-Carried	General

CARRIER

76EKI	Carrier, Amalgam, Operative	Dental And Oral
80WUT	Carrier, Container, Oxygen, Portable	General
79GEJ	Carrier, Ligature	Surgery
78FGS	Carrier, Sponge, Endoscopic	Gastro/Urology
73QXW	Cart, Gas Cylinder (Carrier)	Anesthesiology
73VFZ	Container, Liquid Oxygen	Anesthesiology
73VFF	Cylinder, Oxygen	Anesthesiology
77EQH	Fiberoptic Light Source & Carrier	Ear/Nose/Throat
79FSZ	Light, Surgical, Carrier	Surgery
73QXX	Stand, Gas Cylinder	Anesthesiology
80SBK	Track And Carrier, Cubicle Curtain	General
80SBL	Track And Carrier, Intravenous	General

CART

80WSA	Accessories, Cart, Multipurpose	General
87HXF	Accessories, Traction (Cart, Frame, Cord, Weight)	Orthopedics
73QGO	Cart, Anesthetist's	Anesthesiology
80QGP	Cart, Dressing	General
73BZN	Cart, Emergency, Cardiopulmonary Resuscitation (Crash)	Anesthesiology
80WVY	Cart, Equipment, Video	General
80TAX	Cart, Foodservice	General
73QXW	Cart, Gas Cylinder (Carrier)	Anesthesiology
80TAY	Cart, Housekeeping	General
79QGQ	Cart, Instrument	Surgery
79QZT	Cart, Instrument/Equipment, Laparoscopy	Surgery
80QGR	Cart, Isolation	General
80TAZ	Cart, Laundry	General
80QGS	Cart, Medicine	General
80WTI	Cart, Monitor	General
80QGT	Cart, Multipurpose	General
87QGU	Cart, Orthopedic Supply (Cast)	Orthopedics
80QGW	Cart, Other	General
73BWM	Cart, Patient (Stretcher)	Anesthesiology
80TAW	Cart, Supply	General
79FSK	Cart, Supply, Operating Room	Surgery
80VFB	Cart, Tissue	General
87QGV	Cart, Traction	Orthopedics
80WVR	Cart, Waste	General
80WKB	Cover, Cart	General
73QXX	Stand, Gas Cylinder	Anesthesiology
80WVS	Unloader, Cart	General
80SFN	Washer, Cart	General

CARTILAGE

79HWM	Osteotome (Orthopedic)	Surgery

CARTILAGE *(cont'd)*

79GFI	Osteotome, Manual (Plastic Surgery)	Surgery

CARTRIDGE

80VLG	Cartridge, Ethylene-Oxide	General
80VLK	Cartridge, Freon	General
90TER	Silver Recovery Equipment	Radiology
76EJI	Syringe, Cartridge	Dental And Oral

CARVER

76EKH	Carver, Dental Amalgam, Operative	Dental And Oral
76EIK	Carver, Wax, Dental	Dental And Oral

CASE

86LYL	Accessories, Solution, Lens, Contact	Ophthalmology
86LRX	Case, Contact Lens	Ophthalmology
80WSG	Case, Protection, Equipment	General
80RVS	Container, Sterilization (Tray)	General
79VEE	Container, Surgical Instrument	Surgery

CASEWORK

80TBA	Cabinet Casework, General Purpose	General
75TBB	Cabinet Casework, Laboratory	Chemistry
80TBC	Cabinet Casework, Modular	General
80TBE	Cabinet Casework, Patient Room	General
80TBF	Cabinet Casework, Pharmacy	General
80UMU	Station, Nourishment	General
80TBD	Station, Nursing	General

CASSETTE

74MCU	Cassette, Audio Tape	Cardiovascular
90IWN	Cassette, Measurement, Ardran-Crooks	Radiology
90IXA	Cassette, Radiographic Film	Radiology
88IDZ	Cassette, Tissue	Pathology
90IZP	Changer Programmer, Radiographic Film/Cassette	Radiology
90IXT	Changer, Cassette, Radiographic	Radiology
90KPX	Changer, Radiographic Film/Cassette	Radiology
90EAL	Film, X-Ray	Radiology
90IXY	Holder, Radiographic Cassette, Wall-Mounted	Radiology
76EGZ	Holder, X-Ray Film	Dental And Oral
90VGT	Holder, X-Ray Film Cassette, Vertical	Radiology
74DSF	Recorder, Paper Chart	Cardiovascular

CAST

87LGG	Applier, Cast	Orthopedics
89ITG	Bandage, Cast	Physical Med
87TAI	Blade, Saw, Cast Cutting	Orthopedics
87QGU	Cart, Orthopedic Supply (Cast)	Orthopedics
87QHE	Cast	Orthopedics
87QHC	Cast Walking Heel	Orthopedics
87LGF	Component, Cast	Orthopedics
80KIA	Cover, Cast	General
87QGZ	Cutter, Cast	Orthopedics
87LGH	Cutter, Cast, AC-Powered	Orthopedics
80WKI	Padding, Cast/Splint	General
89IPG	Shoe, Cast	Physical Med
87RUA	Sock, Cast Toe	Orthopedics
87RVN	Spreader, Plaster (Cast)	Orthopedics
87QHB	Stockinette, Cast	Orthopedics
87QGY	Vacuum, Cast Cutter	Orthopedics

CASTERS

80WVN	Base, Roller, Tank, Oxygen	General
80UKP	Casters, Hospital Equipment	General
89INM	Chair, With Casters	Physical Med

CASTING

76QHD	Casting Unit, Dental	Dental And Oral
76UDT	Material, Casting	Dental And Oral
76QOZ	Ring, Dental (Casting)	Dental And Oral
87UES	Stand, Casting	Orthopedics

CASTROVIEJO

86RRD	Scissors, Corneal	Ophthalmology

CAT

83UMA	Animal, Laboratory	Microbiology
90VHB	Phantom, Computed Axial Tomography (CAT, CT)	Radiology
90WMF	Scanner, Computed Tomography, Cine	Radiology
84JXD	Scanner, Computed Tomography, X-Ray (CAT, CT)	Cns/Neurology
90THS	Scanner, Computed Tomography, X-Ray, Full Body	Radiology
90TEI	Scanner, Computed Tomography, X-Ray, Head	Radiology
90JAK	Scanner, Computed Tomography, X-Ray, Special Procedure	Radiology
90WJP	Stand, Cardiovascular	Radiology
90WLW	Stand, Vascular	Radiology

CATALASE

81JBI	Glucose-6-Phosphate Dehydrogenase (Erythrocytic), Catalase	Hematology

CATHETER *(cont'd)*

78QIS	Catheter, Urinary, Condom	Gastro/Urology
78QIT	Catheter, Urinary, Irrigation	Gastro/Urology
78KOD	Catheter, Urological	Gastro/Urology
74DWF	Catheter, Vascular, Cardiopulmonary Bypass	Cardiovascular
74DYD	Catheter, Vascular, Long-Term	Cardiovascular
74JAP	Catheter, Vascular, Opaque	Cardiovascular
84HCA	Catheter, Ventricular	Cns/Neurology
79GBS	Catheter, Ventricular, General & Plastic Surgery	Surgery
78FFE	Catheter, Water Jet, Renal	Gastro/Urology
79GCD	Connector, Catheter	Surgery
74WJY	Connector, Tubing, Blood	Cardiovascular
78FKB	Connector, Tubing, Blood, Infusion, T-Type	Gastro/Urology
78EYK	Connector, Ureteral Catheter	Gastro/Urology
74DXX	Control System, Catheter, Steerable	Cardiovascular
79GCC	Dilator, Catheter	Surgery
78EZN	Dilator, Catheter, Ureteral	Gastro/Urology
78QAN	Drain, Nasobiliary	Gastro/Urology
74QSQ	Electrode, Catheter Tip	Cardiovascular
85VIK	Equipment, In Vitro Fertilization/Embryo Transfer	Obstetrics/Gyn
74WTR	Guide, Catheter	Cardiovascular
74DQX	Guidewire, Catheter	Cardiovascular
90JAJ	Guidewire, Catheter, Radiological	Radiology
78EYJ	Holder, Catheter	Gastro/Urology
74DQW	Holder, Guide, Catheter	Cardiovascular
80KMK	Holder, Intravascular Catheter	General
80RCJ	Immobilizer, Intravenous Catheter-Needle	General
78FJT	Intracatheter, Dialysis	Gastro/Urology
74DYB	Introducer, Catheter	Cardiovascular
78QUJ	Kit, Administration, Enteral	Gastro/Urology
74DQP	Kit, Balloon Repair, Catheter	Cardiovascular
80QHG	Kit, Catheter Care	General
74QHK	Kit, Catheterization, Cardiac	Cardiovascular
74QHL	Kit, Catheterization, Intravenous, Winged	Cardiovascular
78QHM	Kit, Catheterization, Urinary	Gastro/Urology
74UCH	Lead, Pacemaker (Catheter)	Cardiovascular
74QIG	Lead, Pacemaker, Implantable Endocardial	Cardiovascular
80WLM	Lock, Catheter	General
80WNC	Molding, Custom	General
79KFN	Monitor, Cardiac Output, Thermal (Balloon Type Catheter)	Surgery
79GCB	Needle, Catheter	Surgery
74DQT	Occluder, Catheter Tip	Cardiovascular
74DXW	Phonocatheter System, Intracavitary	Cardiovascular
78QHJ	Plug, Catheter	Gastro/Urology
80MDX	Port & Catheter, Infusion, Implanted, Subcut., Intraperit.	General
80MDV	Port & Catheter, Infusion, Implanted, Subcutaneous, Intraspinal	General
73DQZ	Probe, pH Catheter	Anesthesiology
78FEX	Punch, Catheter	Gastro/Urology
84UCC	Reservoir, Hydrocephalic Catheter	Cns/Neurology
78RTB	Shunt, Arteriovenous	Gastro/Urology
84RTC	Shunt, Hydrocephalic	Cns/Neurology
73BZW	Stethoscope, Esophageal	Anesthesiology
74DRB	Stylet, Catheter	Cardiovascular
78EZB	Stylet, Catheter, Gastro-Urology	Gastro/Urology
80RYO	Syringe, Catheter	General
74MKX	System, Carotid Atherectomy	Cardiovascular
74WYC	System, Infusion, Enzyme, Thrombolytic	Cardiovascular
74MFB	System, Reprocessing, Catheter, Balloon Angioplasty	Cardiovascular
73BSQ	Tip, Suction	Anesthesiology
79ULE	Tip, Suction Tube (Yankauer, Poole, Etc.)	Surgery
74DXO	Transducer, Blood Pressure, Catheter Tip	Cardiovascular
74WLT	Transducer, Flow, Catheter Tip	Cardiovascular
73BTS	Tube, Bronchial (W/Wo Connector)	Anesthesiology
78MIQ	Tube, Colostomy	Gastro/Urology
78FFA	Tube, Drainage	Gastro/Urology
80WNG	Tubing, Radiopaque	General
74QHH	Valve, Catheter Flush	Cardiovascular
74QHI	Valve, Catheter Flush, Continuous	Cardiovascular

CATHETER-NEEDLE

80RCJ	Immobilizer, Intravenous Catheter-Needle	General

CATHETERIZATION

90QKB	Cineangiograph (Cardiac Catheterization)	Radiology
74QMA	Computer, Cardiac Catheterization Laboratory	Cardiovascular
74DRE	Dilator, Vessel, Percutaneous Catheterization	Cardiovascular
74DXT	Injector, Angiographic (Cardiac Catheterization)	Cardiovascular
74QHK	Kit, Catheterization, Cardiac	Cardiovascular
74QHL	Kit, Catheterization, Intravenous, Winged	Cardiovascular
78FCM	Kit, Catheterization, Sterile Urethral	Gastro/Urology
78QHM	Kit, Catheterization, Urinary	Gastro/Urology
74RLB	Monitor, Physiological, Cardiac Catheterization	Cardiovascular
90RKW	Photofluoroscope (Cardiac Catheterization)	Radiology
90THR	Radiographic/Fluoroscopic Unit, Special Procedure	Radiology

CATHODE

74DXJ	Display, Cathode-Ray Tube	Cardiovascular

CATHODE-RAY

74DXJ	Display, Cathode-Ray Tube	Cardiovascular

CATIONIC

76KOS	Carboxymethylcellulose Sodium & Cationic Polyacrylamide	Dental And Oral

CAUDAL

73QAV	Kit, Anesthesia, Caudal	Anesthesiology

CAUTERIZATION

79WWP	Cover, Tip, Probe, Cauterization	Surgery
79QYU	Laser, Nd:YAG, Laparoscopy	Surgery
79QEZ	Probe, Electrocauterization, Multi-Use	Surgery
79QHA	Probe, Electrocauterization, Single-Use	Surgery
79QIJ	Tip, Instrument, Electrocauterization, Monopolar	Surgery

CAUTERY

79SIH	Blade, Electrosurgery, Laparoscopic	Surgery
86HQR	Cautery, Radiofrequency, AC-Powered	Ophthalmology
86HQQ	Cautery, Radiofrequency, Battery-Powered	Ophthalmology
86HQO	Cautery, Thermal, AC-Powered	Ophthalmology
86HQP	Cautery, Thermal, Battery-Powered	Ophthalmology
79QSK	Electrocautery Unit, Battery-Powered	Surgery
85HIM	Electrocautery Unit, Endoscopic	Obstetrics/Gyn
85HGI	Electrocautery Unit, Gynecologic	Obstetrics/Gyn
79QSL	Electrocautery Unit, Line-Powered	Surgery
79SII	Electrode, Electrosurgery, Laparoscopic	Surgery
79SIJ	Instrument, Electrosurgery, Laparoscopic	Surgery
79SIG	Module, Control, Electrosurgery	Surgery

CAVA

74QGG	Cannula, Vena Cava	Cardiovascular
74DST	Clip, Vena Cava	Cardiovascular
74QWE	Filter, Vena Cava	Cardiovascular
74LWT	Vena Cava Balloon Occluder	Cardiovascular

CAVITY

76EJR	Agent, Polishing, Abrasive, Oral Cavity	Dental And Oral
79SJA	Dispenser, Laparoscopic	Surgery
74SIZ	Dispenser, Thorascopic	Cardiovascular
76EHZ	Evacuator, Oral Cavity	Dental And Oral
76EJK	Liner, Cavity, Calcium Hydroxide	Dental And Oral
85WSK	Meter, Cavity, Intrauterine	Obstetrics/Gyn
76EBJ	Primer, Cavity, Resin	Dental And Oral
76LBH	Varnish, Cavity	Dental And Oral

CEA

82DHX	Antigen, Antiserum, Control, Carcinoembryonic Antigen	Immunology

CEILING

80TCY	Lamp, Examination, Ceiling Mounted (Light)	General
79FSY	Light, Surgical, Ceiling Mounted	Surgery
79UMJ	Mount, Surgical Microscope	Surgery
80WRN	Rails, Equipment	General

CELL

83TBH	Analyzer, Cell Size	Microbiology
81JPH	Analyzer, Sedimentation Rate, Erythrocyte	Hematology
80WKZ	Brush, Cytology	General
78FDX	Brush, Cytology, Endoscopic	Gastro/Urology
81KRX	Calibrator, Cell Indices	Hematology
81KSA	Calibrator, Red Cell And White Cell Counting	Hematology
75UID	Cell, Spectrophotometer	Chemistry
81JQC	Centrifuge, Cell Washing	Hematology
81KSN	Centrifuge, Cell Washing, Automated, Immuno-Hematology	Hematology
88ICI	Chrome Alum Hematoxylin	Pathology
80WON	Column, Immunoadsorption	General
81JCN	Control, Cell Counter, Normal And Abnormal	Hematology
81GJR	Control, Red Cell	Hematology
81GGL	Control, White Cell	Hematology
83QMQ	Counter, Cell	Microbiology
81GKL	Counter, Cell Or Particle, Automated	Hematology
81GKZ	Counter, Cell, Differential Classifier, Automated	Hematology
81LKZ	Counter, Cell, Photometric	Hematology
88KIT	Culture Media, Synthetic Cell And Tissue	Pathology
81GIF	Diluent, Blood Cell	Hematology
81GKH	Diluter, Blood Cell, Automated	Hematology
83UFW	Disintegrator, Biological Cell	Microbiology
83VFS	Disrupter, Cell	Microbiology
81JBE	Enzyme, Cell (Erythrocytic And Leukocytic)	Hematology
88KET	Filter, Cell Collection, Tissue Processing	Pathology
81JCG	Fluid, Manual Cell Diluting	Hematology
81GJN	Fluid, Red Cell Diluting	Hematology
81GGK	Fluid, Red Cell Lysing	Hematology
81GGJ	Fluid, White Cell Diluting	Hematology
83UFR	Fractionator, Cell	Microbiology
81KSP	Freezer, Blood Cell	Hematology
81JBM	Glucose-6-Phosphate Dehydrogenase (Erythrocytic), Electro	Hematology

CELL (cont'd)

81JBF	Glucose-6-Phosphate Dehydrogenase (Erythrocytic), Screening	Hematology
81JBG	Glucose-6-Phosphate Dehydrogenase (Erythrocytic), Spot	Hematology
81GII	Glutathione, Red Cell	Hematology
83UFS	Harvester, Cell	Microbiology
81UJR	Identification Panel, Blood Cell	Hematology
82LTM	Islet Cell Antibody (ICA) Test	Immunology
74MFY	Kit, Cell Harvesting, Endothelial	Cardiovascular
81GHD	Leukocyte Alkaline Phosphatase	Hematology
81GIA	Leukocyte Peroxidase	Hematology
81JOY	Locator, Cell, Automated	Hematology
88IJS	Locators, Metaphase Cell	Pathology
81GLQ	Mixture, Control, Indices, White and Red Cell	Hematology
81KQH	Red Cell Indices	Hematology
81JPJ	Red Cell Indices, Calculated	Hematology
81JBW	Red Cell Indices, Measured	Hematology
81JWP	Red Cell Survival Test	Hematology
85RRS	Scraper, Cytology (Cervical)	Obstetrics/Gyn
81GKT	Separator, Blood Cell, Automated	Hematology
78LKN	Separator, Blood Cell/Plasma, Therapeutic	Gastro/Urology
78MDP	Separator, Blood Cell/Plasma, Therapeutic, Membrane, Auto.	Gastro/Urology
88WSX	Slide, Cell Adhesive	Pathology
88KEX	Sorter, Cell (Separator)	Pathology
85HHT	Spatula, Cervical, Cytology	Obstetrics/Gyn
88KJE	Spinner System, Cell Culture	Pathology
88KPA	Stainer, Slide, Automated	Pathology
88KIN	Stainer, Slide, Contact Type	Pathology
83RTR	Stainer, Slide, Cytology	Microbiology
88KJF	Suspension System, Cell Culture	Pathology
81MZJ	System, Concentration, Hematopoietic Stem Cell	Hematology
81LIM	Test, D Positive Fetal Rbc	Hematology
81KQE	Test, Erythrocytic Glucose-6-Phosphate Dehydrogenase	Hematology
82WPH	Test, Receptor, Interleukin, Serum	Immunology
81GHM	Test, Sickle Cell	Hematology
81MAP	Test, Squamous Cell Carcinoma	Hematology
81LJX	Test, Urine Leukocyte	Hematology
81SFO	Washer, Cell (Frozen Blood Processor)	Hematology

CELL-MEDIATED

83NCD	Test, Immunity, Cell-Mediated, Mycobacterium Tuberculosis	Microbiology

CELL-WASHING

81SFO	Washer, Cell (Frozen Blood Processor)	Hematology

CELLOIDIN

88IEZ	Celloidin	Pathology

CELLS

81JZK	Antigen, Antiserum, Control, Red Cells	Hematology
88KIR	Cultured Animal And Human Cells	Pathology
75JMQ	M. Lysodeikticus Cells (Spectrophotometric), Lysozyme	Chemistry
82DGF	Red Cells, FITC, Antigen, Antiserum, Control	Immunology
82DFW	Red Cells, Rhodamine, Antigen, Antiserum, Control	Immunology
81UJT	Reverse Grouping Cells	Hematology

CELLULOSE

91DJO	Cellulose Fluorescent Indicator, TLC	Toxicology
75UEO	Electrophoresis Equipment, Cellulose Acetate Membrane	Chemistry
91DKG	Plate, Cellulose, TLC	Toxicology
80RVI	Sponge, Rayon Cellulose	General

CEMENT

87LOD	Bone Cement	Orthopedics
87MBB	Bone Cement, Antibiotic	Orthopedics
77MLI	Cement, Bone, Ionomer	Ear/Nose/Throat
76EMA	Cement, Dental	Dental And Oral
79MGN	Cement, Hydroxyapatite	Surgery
87QIW	Cement, Orthopedic (Bone)	Orthopedics
84MLG	Cement, Silicate (Cranioplasty)	Cns/Neurology
78EZR	Cement, Stomal Appliance, Ostomy	Gastro/Urology
76MZW	Dental Cement w/out Zinc-Oxide Eugenol as an Ulcer Covering for Pain Relief	Dental And Oral
87KIH	Dispenser, Cement	Orthopedics
87JDY	Evacuator, Vapor, Cement Monomer	Orthopedics
87JDZ	Mixing Equipment, Cement	Orthopedics
87LZN	Obturator, Cement	Orthopedics
87JDK	Prosthesis, Hip, Cement Restrictor	Orthopedics
87KWR	Prosthesis, Shoulder, Constr., Metal/Metal or Polymer/Cem.	Orthopedics
87KWT	Prosthesis, Shoulder, Non-Constrained, Metal/Polymer Cem.	Orthopedics
87KWS	Prosthesis, Shoulder, Semi-Constrained, Metal/Polymer Cem.	Orthopedics
87UCF	Restrictor, Orthopedic Cement	Orthopedics
76KZP	Solution, Cement Dissolving	Dental And Oral
87LTO	Spacer, Cement	Orthopedics

CEMENT (cont'd)

76RUE	Spatula, Cement	Dental And Oral
87LZV	System, Extraction, Cement Removal	Orthopedics
87KII	Tube, Cement Ventilation	Orthopedics

CEMENTED

87LBC	Prosthesis, Finger, Constrained, Metal, Cemented	Orthopedics
87JDM	Prosthesis, Hip, Acetabular Component, Metal, Non-Cemented	Orthopedics
87JDG	Prosthesis, Hip, Femoral Component, Cemented, Metal	Orthopedics
87LPF	Prosthesis, Hip, Semi-Const., Metal/Ceramic/Ceramic, Cem.	Orthopedics
87JDL	Prosthesis, Hip, Semi-Constrained (Cemented Acetabular)	Orthopedics
87MRA	Prosthesis, Hip, Semi-constrained, Metal/ Ceramic/ Ceramic/ Metal, Cemented or Uncemented	Orthopedics
87MAY	Prosthesis, Hip, Semi-constrained, Metal/Ceramic/Polymer, Cemented or Non-porous Cemented, Osteophilic Finish	Orthopedics
87MBM	Prosthesis, Hip, Semi/Hemi-Const., M/PTFE Ctd./P, Cem./Unc.	Orthopedics
87KMB	Prosthesis, Knee, Non-Const. (M/C Reinf. Polyeth.) Cemented	Orthopedics

CENTRAL

73TAC	Alarm, Central Gas System	Anesthesiology
80WQH	Catheter, Central Venous	General
74QIA	Catheter, Intravenous, Central	Cardiovascular
78FKQ	Dialysate Delivery System, Central Multiple Patient	Gastro/Urology
80RBA	Hypo/Hyperthermia Unit, Central	General
74QIX	Kit, Blood Pressure, Central Venous	Cardiovascular
80WOB	Meter, Patient Height	General
74RLX	Monitor, Blood Pressure, Venous	Cardiovascular
79FYO	Monitor, Blood Pressure, Venous, Central	Surgery
79KFO	Monitor, Cardiac Output, Dye (Central Venous & Arterial)	Surgery
74FYN	Monitor, Pressure, Venous, Central, Powered	Cardiovascular
85HHI	Pump, Abortion, Vacuum, Central System	Obstetrics/Gyn
73SEI	Pump, Vacuum, Central	Anesthesiology
84JXG	Shunt, Central Nerve, With Component	Cns/Neurology
80WOE	System, Pipeline, Gas	General

CENTRIFUGE

75QIY	Adapter, Centrifuge Tube	Chemistry
75JJG	Analyzer, Chemistry, Centrifuge	Chemistry
81WIT	Brush, Centrifuge	Hematology
81KSO	Centrifuge, Blood Bank, Diagnostic	Hematology
81JQC	Centrifuge, Cell Washing	Hematology
81KSN	Centrifuge, Cell Washing, Automated, Immuno-Hematology	Hematology
75UKI	Centrifuge, Continuous Flow	Chemistry
75UKJ	Centrifuge, Explosion-Proof	Chemistry
88QJA	Centrifuge, Floor	Pathology
91DOT	Centrifuge, General (Over 5,000 rpm)	Toxicology
88KDR	Centrifuge, General (Up to 5,000 rpm)	Pathology
81GKG	Centrifuge, Hematocrit	Hematology
81QJB	Centrifuge, Microhematocrit	Hematology
81GHK	Centrifuge, Microsedimentation	Hematology
88QJC	Centrifuge, Refrigerated	Pathology
88QJD	Centrifuge, Tabletop	Pathology
88IFB	Cytocentrifuge	Pathology
81GKF	Hematocrit, Automated	Hematology
81JPI	Hematocrit, Manual	Hematology
75SCP	Tube, Centrifuge	Chemistry
75SDV	Ultracentrifuge	Chemistry

CENTROMERE

88IJW	Detector, Centromere	Pathology

CEP

83KHW	Antigen, ID, HA, CEP, Entamoeba Histolytica	Microbiology

CEPHALOMETER

76EAG	Cephalometer	Dental And Oral

CERAMIC

80VFE	Component, Ceramic	General
87JDF	Prosthesis, Hip (Metal Stem/Ceramic Self-Locking Ball)	Orthopedics
87LPF	Prosthesis, Hip, Semi-Const., Metal/Ceramic/Ceramic, Cem.	Orthopedics
87LZO	Prosthesis, Hip, Semi-Constr., Metal/Ceramic, Cemented/NC	Orthopedics
87MRA	Prosthesis, Hip, Semi-constrained, Metal/ Ceramic/ Ceramic/ Metal, Cemented or Uncemented	Orthopedics
87MAY	Prosthesis, Hip, Semi-constrained, Metal/Ceramic/Polymer, Cemented or Non-porous Cemented, Osteophilic Finish	Orthopedics

CERAMICS

87LMM	Ceramics, Triphos./Hydroxyapatite, Ca. (Load Bearing)	Orthopedics
87LMN	Ceramics, Triphos./Hydroxyapatite, Ca. (Non-Load Bearing)	Orthopedics

CERCLAGE

87HXN	Applier, Cerclage	Orthopedics
87JDQ	Cerclage, Fixation	Orthopedics
85HDH	Needle, Cerclage, Gynecological	Obstetrics/Gyn
78UDE	Prosthesis, Anti-Gastroesophageal Reflux	Gastro/Urology
87UCR	Prosthesis, Bone Cerclage	Orthopedics
85HHY	Prosthesis, Suture, Cerclage	Obstetrics/Gyn

CEREBELLAR

84LKR	Stimulator, Cerebellar, Full Implant	Cns/Neurology
84LGW	Stimulator, Cerebellar, Full Implant (Pain Relief)	Cns/Neurology

CEREBRAL

84UEW	Flowmeter, Meter, Cerebral Blood, Xenon Clearance	Cns/Neurology
84RFM	Kit, Lumbar Puncture	Cns/Neurology
84LME	Monitor, Cerebral Blood Flow, Thermal Diffusion	Cns/Neurology
84QJE	Monitor, Cerebral Function	Cns/Neurology
80CAQ	Monitor, Cerebral Spinal Fluid Pressure (CSF)	General
80CAR	Monitor, Cerebral Spinal Fluid Pressure, Electrical	General
84GZA	Stimulator, Cerebral, Implantable	Cns/Neurology

CEREBROSPINAL

84QHQ	Catheter, Cerebrospinal	Cns/Neurology

CEREBROVASCULAR

84LHH	Balloon, Occlusion, Cerebrovascular	Cns/Neurology
84LJA	Catheter, Cerebrovascular, Everting	Cns/Neurology

CERULOPLASMI

82JFQ	P-Phenyl-Enediamine/EDTA (Spectrophotometric), Ceruloplasmi	Immunology

CERULOPLASMIN

82DDB	Antigen, Antiserum, Control, Ceruloplasmin	Immunology
82DCY	Antigen, Antiserum, Control, Ceruloplasmin, FITC	Immunology
82DCT	Antigen, Antiserum, Control, Ceruloplasmin, Rhodamine	Immunology
82CHN	Immunochemical, Ceruloplasmin	Immunology
82JFR	Indirect Copper Assay, Ceruloplasmin	Immunology

CERVICAL

85HDR	Cap, Cervical	Obstetrics/Gyn
87QLP	Collar, Cervical Neck	Orthopedics
80WMR	Collar, Extrication	General
85LLQ	Contraceptive Cervical Cap	Obstetrics/Gyn
85HDN	Dilator, Cervical, Expandable	Obstetrics/Gyn
85HDQ	Dilator, Cervical, Fixed Size	Obstetrics/Gyn
85MCR	Dilator, Cervical, Hygroscopic, Synthetic	Obstetrics/Gyn
85HDY	Dilator, Cervical, Hygroscopic-Laminaria	Obstetrics/Gyn
85HHG	Dilator, Cervical, Vibratory	Obstetrics/Gyn
85HFL	Drain, Cervical	Obstetrics/Gyn
85TBX	Drill, Cervical	Obstetrics/Gyn
87RBH	Immobilizer, Cervical	Orthopedics
85MCO	Kit, Smear, Cervical	Obstetrics/Gyn
85HDZ	Knife, Cervical Cone	Obstetrics/Gyn
89IQK	Orthosis, Cervical	Physical Med
89IQF	Orthosis, Cervical-Thoracic, Rigid	Physical Med
87MAT	Orthosis, Fixation, Cervical Intervertebral Body, Spinal	Orthopedics
87RLE	Pillow, Cervical	Orthopedics
77MYB	Pillow, Cervical(for Mild Sleep Apnea)	Ear/Nose/Throat
88MNM	Reader, Slide, Cytology, Cervical, Automated	Pathology
85RRS	Scraper, Cytology (Cervical)	Obstetrics/Gyn
85HHT	Spatula, Cervical, Cytology	Obstetrics/Gyn
85LOB	Synthetic Osmotic Cervical Dilator	Obstetrics/Gyn
88LIY	Test, Cervical Mucous Penetration	Pathology
85LHZ	Viscometer, Mucus, Cervical	Obstetrics/Gyn

CERVICAL-THORACIC

89IQF	Orthosis, Cervical-Thoracic, Rigid	Physical Med

CF

83GOD	Antigen, CF (Including CF Control), Adenovirus 1-33	Microbiology
83GNG	Antigen, CF (Including CF Control), Coxsackievirus A 1-24	Microbiology
83GQH	Antigen, CF (Including CF Control), Cytomegalovirus	Microbiology
83GNL	Antigen, CF (Including CF Control), Echovirus 1-34	Microbiology
83GNQ	Antigen, CF (Including CF Control), Epstein-Barr Virus	Microbiology
83GQD	Antigen, CF (Including CF Control), Equine Encephalitis	Microbiology
83GNX	Antigen, CF (Including CF Control), Influenza Virus	Microbiology
83GRC	Antigen, CF (Including CF Control), Mumps Virus	Microbiology
83GQS	Antigen, CF (Including CF Control), Parainfluenza Virus	Microbiology
83GOH	Antigen, CF (Including CF Control), Poliovirus 1-3	Microbiology
83GQB	Antigen, CF (Including CF Control), Reovirus 1-3	Microbiology
83GON	Antigen, CF (Including CF Control), Rubella	Microbiology
83GQG	Antigen, CF (Including CF Controls), Respiratory Syncytial	Microbiology
83GMI	Antigen, CF And/Or ID, Coccidioides Immitis	Microbiology
83GRJ	Antigen, CF, (Including CF Control), Rubeola	Microbiology
83GQW	Antigen, CF, (Including CF Control), Varicella-Zoster	Microbiology
83JWT	Antigen, CF, Aspergillus SPP.	Microbiology
83JWW	Antigen, CF, B. Dermatitidis	Microbiology
83GQK	Antigen, CF, Lymphocytic Choriomeningitis Virus	Microbiology
83GSB	Antigen, CF, Mycoplasma SPP.	Microbiology

CF *(cont'd)*

83GPW	Antigen, CF, Psittacosis (Chlamydia Group)	Microbiology
83GPS	Antigen, CF, Q Fever	Microbiology
83GPQ	Antigen, CF, Spotted Fever Group	Microbiology
83GNF	Antigen, CF, T. Cruzi	Microbiology
83GMN	Antigen, CF, Toxoplasma Gondii	Microbiology
83GPO	Antigen, CF, Typhus Fever Group	Microbiology
83GQN	Antigen, Cf (including Cf Control), Herpesvirus Hominis 1, 2	Microbiology
83GQO	Antisera, Cf, Herpesvirus Hominis 1, 2	Microbiology
83GOA	Antiserum, CF, Adenovirus 1-33	Microbiology
83GNO	Antiserum, CF, Coxsackievirus A 1-24, B 1-6	Microbiology
83GQI	Antiserum, CF, Cytomegalovirus	Microbiology
83GNK	Antiserum, CF, Echovirus 1-34	Microbiology
83GNP	Antiserum, CF, Epstein-Barr Virus	Microbiology
83GQC	Antiserum, CF, Equine Encephalitis Virus, EEE, WEE	Microbiology
83GNW	Antiserum, CF, Influenza Virus A, B, C	Microbiology
83GQJ	Antiserum, CF, Lymphocytic Choriomeningitis Virus	Microbiology
83GRB	Antiserum, CF, Mumps Virus	Microbiology
83GQT	Antiserum, CF, Parainfluenza Virus 1-4	Microbiology
83GOG	Antiserum, CF, Poliovirus 1-3	Microbiology
83GPT	Antiserum, CF, Psittacosis (Chlamydia Group)	Microbiology
83GPR	Antiserum, CF, Q Fever	Microbiology
83GPZ	Antiserum, CF, Reovirus 1-3	Microbiology
83GOM	Antiserum, CF, Rubella	Microbiology
83GRF	Antiserum, CF, Rubeola	Microbiology
83GQX	Antiserum, CF, Varicella-Zoster	Microbiology

CHAIN

82DFZ	Antigen, Antiserum, Control, IGG (Gamma Chain Specific)	Immunology
82DAO	Antigen, Antiserum, Control, IGM (Mu Chain Specific)	Immunology
82DAM	Hemoglobin, Chain Specific, Antigen, Antiserum, Control	Immunology

CHAIR

89INN	Chair, Adjustable, Mechanical	Physical Med
80QJF	Chair, Bath	General
85QJG	Chair, Birthing	Obstetrics/Gyn
80FML	Chair, Blood Donor	General
80WZB	Chair, Blood Drawing	General
76QJH	Chair, Dental	Dental And Oral
76KLC	Chair, Dental (With Unit)	Dental And Oral
78WQV	Chair, Dialysis (With Scale)	Gastro/Urology
78FKS	Chair, Dialysis, Powered (Without Scale)	Gastro/Urology
78FIA	Chair, Dialysis, Unpowered (Without Scale)	Gastro/Urology
80FRK	Chair, Examination And Treatment	General
80QJI	Chair, Flotation Therapy	General
80FRJ	Chair, Geriatric	General
80FRM	Chair, Geriatric, Wheeled	General
80UDI	Chair, Infant Treatment	General
84HBN	Chair, Neurosurgical	Cns/Neurology
76EFG	Chair, Operative	Dental And Oral
86HME	Chair, Ophthalmic, AC-Powered	Ophthalmology
86HMD	Chair, Ophthalmic, Manual	Ophthalmology
80QJO	Chair, Other	General
80QJJ	Chair, Pediatric	General
90IZN	Chair, Pneumoencephalographic	Radiology
84HBK	Chair, Pneumoencephalographic, Neurology	Cns/Neurology
87QJK	Chair, Podiatric	Orthopedics
89INO	Chair, Position, Electric	Physical Med
73BYN	Chair, Posture, For Cardiac And Pulmonary Treatment	Anesthesiology
80QJL	Chair, Rehabilitation	General
84WHW	Chair, Rotating	Cns/Neurology
80UMP	Chair, Seat Lifting (Standing Aid)	General
80QJM	Chair, Shower	General
80QJN	Chair, Sitz Bath	General
79GBB	Chair, Surgical, AC-Powered	Surgery
79FZK	Chair, Surgical, Non-Electrical	Surgery
89INM	Chair, With Casters	Physical Med
80KMN	Chair/Table, Medical	General
80QLV	Commode (Toilet)	General
80TFX	Lift, Stair Climbing	General
80FNI	Mattress, Silicone, And Chair Cushion	General
80RQS	Scale, Chair	General
80WXD	Scale, Chair, Transfer	General
87SBP	Traction Unit, Static, Chair	Orthopedics
77ETF	Unit, Examining/Treatment, ENT	Ear/Nose/Throat

CHAMBER

83JTM	Box, Glove	Microbiology
77EWC	Chamber, Acoustic, Testing	Ear/Nose/Throat
83VDW	Chamber, Anaerobic	Microbiology
83UFT	Chamber, Constant Temperature (Environmental)	Microbiology
85HEE	Chamber, Decompression, Abdominal	Obstetrics/Gyn
81KSH	Chamber, Environmental, Platelet Storage	Hematology
75VFW	Chamber, Freezing	Chemistry
73CBF	Chamber, Hyperbaric	Anesthesiology
89IQD	Chamber, Hyperbaric Oxygen	Physical Med
80UKU	Chamber, Hypobaric	General

CHAMBER *(cont'd)*

80FRR	Chamber, Isolation, Patient Care	General
80LGN	Chamber, Isolation, Patient Transport	General
79KPJ	Chamber, Oxygen, Topical, Extremity	Surgery
88KIY	Chamber, Slide Culture	Pathology
75UHI	Chamber, Ultraviolet Polymerization	Chemistry
73VFZ	Container, Liquid Oxygen	Anesthesiology
74LWY	Dual Chamber, Anti-Tachycardia, Pulse Generator	Cardiovascular
74LWP	Dual Chamber, Implantable Pulse Generator	Cardiovascular
86UBA	Lens, Intraocular, Anterior Chamber	Ophthalmology
86UBD	Lens, Intraocular, Posterior Chamber	Ophthalmology
74ULJ	Pacemaker, Heart, Implantable, Dual Chamber	Cardiovascular
74WST	Pacemaker, Heart, Implantable, Rate Responsive	Cardiovascular
80LGM	Patient Isolation Chamber	General
77TAB	Room, Acoustical	Ear/Nose/Throat
74LWW	Single Chamber, Anti-Tachycardia, Pulse Generator	Cardiovascular
74LWO	Single Chamber, Sensor Driven, Implantable Pulse Generator	Cardiovascular

CHANGE

80FQZ	Thermometer, Chemical Color Change	General

CHANGER

90IZP	Changer Programmer, Radiographic Film/Cassette	Radiology
90IXT	Changer, Cassette, Radiographic	Radiology
90IXS	Changer, Film, Radiographic	Radiology
90KPX	Changer, Radiographic Film/Cassette	Radiology
73LNZ	Changer, Tube, Endotracheal	Anesthesiology

CHANNEL

75QKW	Analyzer, Chemistry, Multi-Channel, Fixed	Chemistry
75QKX	Analyzer, Chemistry, Multi-Channel, Programmable	Chemistry
75QKY	Analyzer, Chemistry, Single Channel, Programmable	Chemistry
74DPS	Electrocardiograph, Single Channel	Cardiovascular
80TEZ	Telemetry Unit, Physiological, Multiple Channel	General
74QRY	Transmitter/Receiver System, ECG, Telephone Multi-Channel	Cardiovascular
74QRZ	Transmitter/Receiver System, ECG, Telephone Single-Channel	Cardiovascular

CHARACTERIZATION

80WWZ	Test, Bacteria Characterization	General

CHARCOAL

80WSE	Dressing, Layer, Charcoal	General
80WXR	Media, Filter	General
75SFX	Purification Filter, Water, Charcoal	Chemistry
91DPL	Radioimmunoassay, Digitoxin (125-I), Bovine, Charcoal	Toxicology
91DNW	Radioimmunoassay, Digitoxin (3-H), Rabbit Antibody, Char.	Toxicology
91DPB	Radioimmunoassay, Digoxin (125-I), Rabbit, Charcoal	Toxicology
91DOR	Radioimmunoassay, Digoxin (3-H), Bovine, Charcoal	Toxicology
91DPD	Radioimmunoassay, Digoxin (3-H), Rabbit, Charcoal	Toxicology

CHARGED

90LHN	Radiotherapy Unit, Charged-Particle	Radiology

CHARGED-PARTICLE

90LHN	Radiotherapy Unit, Charged-Particle	Radiology

CHARGER

80WJM	Charger, Battery	General
74KRF	Charger, Pacemaker	Cardiovascular

CHART

80QGT	Cart, Multipurpose	General
79QJQ	Chart, Acupuncture	Surgery
80UKS	Chart, Anatomical Training	General
87QJR	Chart, Posture	Orthopedics
86HOX	Chart, Visual Acuity	Ophthalmology
80WSM	Component, Paper	General
80RGK	Holder, Medical Chart	General
80QJP	Paper, Chart, Record, Medical	General
80WUP	Paper, Recording, Data	General
80VLR	Paper, Recording, ECG/EEG	General
80RGL	Rack, Medical Chart	General
75UHR	Recorder, Chart, Laboratory	Chemistry
74DSF	Recorder, Paper Chart	Cardiovascular
86HIT	Tester, Color Vision	Ophthalmology

CHECK

80MJF	Check Valve, Retrograde Flow (In-Line)	General
73MJJ	Valve, CPB Check, Retrograde, In-Line	Anesthesiology

CHELATING

88KDY	Agent, Chelating, Decalcification	Pathology

CHEMICAL

90VGU	Chemical, Film Processor	Radiology
74LIS	Chemical, Heparin Coating	Cardiovascular
75RAF	Hood, Chemical	Chemistry
75JRN	Hood, Fume, Chemical	Chemistry

CHEMICAL *(cont'd)*

80MRB	Indicator, Biological, Liquid Chemical Steril. Process	General
80KYQ	Kit, Snake Bite, Chemical Cold Pack	General
90WHY	Mixer, Chemical, Film, X-Ray	Radiology
80FRS	Pack, Cold, Chemical	General
80FRY	Pack, Hot, Chemical	General
89UED	Pad, Heating, Chemical	Physical Med
75JNQ	Qualitative Chemical Reactions, Urinary Calculi (Stone)	Chemistry
88LED	Stain, Chemical Solution	Pathology
80RVU	Sterilization Process Indicator, Chemical	General
80JOJ	Sterilization Process Indicator, Physical/Chemical	General
80MLR	Sterilizer, Chemical	General
80WLS	Test, Equipment, Sterilization	General
80FQZ	Thermometer, Chemical Color Change	General

CHEMICALLY

85MHT	Tampon, Chemically Modified	Obstetrics/Gyn

CHEMICALS

80WXH	Contract Manufacturing, Pharmaceuticals/Chemicals	General

CHEMILUMINESCENT

85MPU	Source, Chemiluminescent Light	Obstetrics/Gyn

CHEMISTRY

75JJG	Analyzer, Chemistry, Centrifuge	Chemistry
75VIR	Analyzer, Chemistry, Desk-Top	Chemistry
75UJM	Analyzer, Chemistry, ELISA	Chemistry
75QTJ	Analyzer, Chemistry, Electrolyte	Chemistry
75JJI	Analyzer, Chemistry, Enzyme	Chemistry
75UEH	Analyzer, Chemistry, Enzyme Immunoassay	Chemistry
75UEI	Analyzer, Chemistry, Fluorescence Immunoassay	Chemistry
75JJF	Analyzer, Chemistry, Micro	Chemistry
75QKW	Analyzer, Chemistry, Multi-Channel, Fixed	Chemistry
75QKX	Analyzer, Chemistry, Multi-Channel, Programmable	Chemistry
75WMG	Analyzer, Chemistry, Nephelometric Immunoassay	Chemistry
75JJD	Analyzer, Chemistry, Photometric, Bichromatic	Chemistry
75JJE	Analyzer, Chemistry, Photometric, Discrete	Chemistry
75LCI	Analyzer, Chemistry, Radioimmunoassay	Chemistry
75ROC	Analyzer, Chemistry, Radioimmunoassay, Automated	Chemistry
75JJC	Analyzer, Chemistry, Sequential Multiple, Continuous Flow	Chemistry
75QKY	Analyzer, Chemistry, Single Channel, Programmable	Chemistry
75ULK	Analyzer, Chemistry, Therapeutic Drug Monitor (TDM)	Chemistry
75KQO	Analyzer, Chemistry, Urinalysis	Chemistry
75JJZ	Analyzer, Chemistry, Urinalysis, Automated	Chemistry
75VEP	Analyzer, Chemistry, Urine	Chemistry
75VIN	Analyzer, Combination Chemistry/Hematology/Electrolyte	Chemistry
75JIS	Calibrator, Primary, Clinical Chemistry	Chemistry
75JIT	Calibrator, Secondary, Clinical Chemistry	Chemistry
75JIW	Calibrator, Surrogate, Clinical Chemistry	Chemistry
80VBH	Computer Software	General
75JQP	Computer, Chemistry Analyzer	Chemistry
75KHO	Fluorometer, Chemistry	Chemistry
75WHL	Inoculator, Laboratory	Chemistry
80WOC	Microplate	General
80WOD	Reader, Microplate	General
80WRA	Reagent, Calibration	General

CHEMORESPONSE

88MHR	System, Assay, Chemoresponse	Pathology

CHEMOTHERAPY

90WJA	Container, Substance, Radioactive	Radiology
80FSB	Perfusion Unit	General
80VEZ	Pump, Infusion, Ambulatory	General
80TGT	System, Infusion, Administration, Drug, Implantable	General
82VJK	Test, Chemotherapy Sensitivity (Tumor Colony Forming)	Immunology
80SFU	Waste Receptacle, Contaminated	General
90SFV	Waste Receptacle, Radioactive	Radiology

CHEST

80QDN	Binder, Chest	General
80VDK	Chest, Dry Ice	General
73QQO	Drain, Thoracic (Chest)	Anesthesiology
89QUX	Exerciser, Chest	Physical Med
80QJS	Kit, Chest Drainage (Thoracentesis Tray)	General
90QJT	Radiographic Unit, Diagnostic, Chest	Radiology
73ROZ	Regulator, Suction, Thoracic	Anesthesiology

CHILLING

89IMF	Chilling Unit	Physical Med

CHIN

79FWP	Prosthesis, Chin, Internal	Surgery

CHISEL

79KDG	Chisel (Osteotome)	Surgery
76EML	Chisel, Bone, Surgical	Dental And Oral
77JYD	Chisel, Mastoid	Ear/Nose/Throat
77JYE	Chisel, Middle Ear	Ear/Nose/Throat
77KAN	Chisel, Nasal	Ear/Nose/Throat

CHISEL *(cont'd)*

87QJU	*Chisel, Orthopedic*	*Orthopedics*
76EMM	*Chisel, Osteotome, Surgical*	*Dental And Oral*
79QJV	*Chisel, Other*	*Surgery*
79FZO	*Chisel, Surgical, Manual*	*Surgery*

CHLAMYDIA

83GPW	*Antigen, CF, Psittacosis (Chlamydia Group)*	*Microbiology*
83LKI	*Antisera, Fluorescent, Chlamydia SPP.*	*Microbiology*
83LKH	*Antisera, Immunoperoxidase, Chlamydia SPP.*	*Microbiology*
83GPT	*Antiserum, CF, Psittacosis (Chlamydia Group)*	*Microbiology*
83LJP	*Antiserum, Fluorescent, Chlamydia Trachomatis*	*Microbiology*
83MGM	*Chlamydia Trachomatis*	*Microbiology*
83LSK	*Chlamydia, DNA Reagents*	*Microbiology*
83MKZ	*DNA-Probe, Nucleic Acid Amplification, Chlamydia*	*Microbiology*
83LJC	*Enzyme Linked Immunoabsorbent Assay,* Chlamydia Group	Microbiology

CHLORAL

91DJW	*Reagent, Test, Chloral Hydrate*	*Toxicology*

CHLORAZOL

88KJQ	*Stain, Chlorazol Black E*	*Pathology*

CHLORIDE

75QTJ	*Analyzer, Chemistry, Electrolyte*	*Chemistry*
75JFS	*Coulometric, Chloride*	*Chemistry*
78QOI	*Cystic Fibrosis System*	*Gastro/Urology*
75CGZ	*Electrode, Ion Specific, Chloride*	*Chemistry*
75JGK	*Ferric Chloride, Phenylketones (Urinary, Non-Quantitative)*	*Chemistry*
91JKQ	*Gold Chloride (Colorimetric), Bromide*	*Toxicology*
88HYQ	*Iron Chloride-Weigert*	*Pathology*
88IFQ	*Mercuric Chloride Formulations For Tissue*	*Pathology*
75CHG	*Phosphoric-Tungstic Acid (Spectrophotometric), Chloride*	*Chemistry*
91DLI	*Reagent, Acetylcholine Chloride*	*Toxicology*
75CHJ	*Reagent, Chloride (Test System)*	*Chemistry*
88HYH	*Stain, Gold Chloride*	*Pathology*
75JNS	*Stannous Chloride - Hydrazine, Phospholipids*	*Chemistry*
80SDR	*Tubing, Polyvinyl Chloride*	*General*

CHLORIDE-WEIGERT

88HYQ	*Iron Chloride-Weigert*	*Pathology*

CHLORIDIMETER

78QJW	*Chloridimeter*	*Gastro/Urology*
78QOI	*Cystic Fibrosis System*	*Gastro/Urology*
75QTF	*Electrode, Sweat Test*	*Chemistry*

CHLOROFORM

76MMT	*Resin, Filling, Root Canal (Containing Chloroform)*	*Dental And Oral*

CHOKE

80QAJ	*Airway, Obstruction Removal (Choke Saver)*	*General*
77EWT	*Anti-Choke Device, Suction*	*Ear/Nose/Throat*
77EWW	*Anti-Choke Device, Tongs*	*Ear/Nose/Throat*

CHOLANGIOGRAPHY

79GBZ	*Catheter, Cholangiography*	*Surgery*
79WZW	*Clamp, Fixation, Cholangiography*	*Surgery*
74RIB	*Needle, Cholangiography*	*Cardiovascular*

CHOLECYSTECTOMY

78QAN	*Drain, Nasobiliary*	*Gastro/Urology*
78SHX	*Kit, Cholecystectomy*	*Gastro/Urology*

CHOLEDOCHOSCOPE

78FBN	*Choledochoscope, Flexible Or Rigid*	*Gastro/Urology*
78WZV	*Choledochoscope, Mini-Diameter (5mm or Less)*	*Gastro/Urology*

CHOLERAE

83GSQ	*Antiserum, Vibrio Cholerae*	*Microbiology*

CHOLESTEROL

74WTP	*Column, Adsorption, Lipid*	*Cardiovascular*
75LBT	*Electrophoresis, Cholesterol Via Esterase-Oxidase, HDL*	*Chemistry*
75CHH	*Enzymatic Esterase-Oxidase, Cholesterol*	*Chemistry*
75CHD	*Ferric Ion-Sulfuric Acid, Cholesterol*	*Chemistry*
75LBS	*LDL & VLDL Precipitation, Cholesterol Via* Esterase-Oxidase	*Chemistry*
75NAQ	*Lipoprotein, High Density, HDL, Over-The-Counter*	*Chemistry*
78MMY	*Lipoprotein, Low Density, Removal*	*Gastro/Urology*
75CGO	*Reagent, Cholesterol (Total Test System)*	*Chemistry*

CHOLINESTERASE

91DCQ	*Cholinesterase, Antigen, Antiserum, Control*	*Toxicology*
91DIH	*Colorimetry, Cholinesterase*	*Toxicology*
91DOH	*Electrometry, Cholinesterase*	*Toxicology*
91DMR	*M-Nitrophenol Solution, Specific Reagent For* Cholinesterase	Toxicology
91DIG	*Test Paper, Cholinesterase*	*Toxicology*

CHOLYGLYCINE

75KWW	*Radioimmunoassay, Cholyglycine, Bile Acids*	*Chemistry*

CHORD

76LTG	*Paste, Injectable, Augmentation, Chord, Vocal*	*Dental And Oral*

CHORIOMENINGITIS

83GQK	*Antigen, CF, Lymphocytic Choriomeningitis Virus*	*Microbiology*
83GQJ	*Antiserum, CF, Lymphocytic Choriomeningitis Virus*	*Microbiology*

CHORIONIC

75JHJ	*Agglutination Method, Human Chorionic Gonadotropin*	*Chemistry*
85LLX	*Catheter, Sampling, Chorionic Villus*	*Obstetrics/Gyn*
75JHI	*Radioimmunoassay, Human Chorionic Gonadotropin*	*Chemistry*
75JZM	*System, Gonadotropin, Chorionic, Human (Non-RIA)*	*Chemistry*
85VIL	*Test, Chorionic Villi Sampling (Fetal Chromosome Analysis)*	*Obstetrics/Gyn*
82JZN	*Test, Human Chorionic Gonadotropin*	*Immunology*
82DHA	*Test, Human Chorionic Gonadotropin, Serum*	*Immunology*
75LFS	*Test, Radioreceptor, Human Chorionic Gonadotropin*	*Chemistry*
75JHK	*Titrimetric Method, Human Chorionic Gonadotropin*	*Chemistry*

CHROMATIN

88LNJ	*Analyzer, Chromosome, Automated*	*Pathology*
83UGH	*Genetic Engineering*	*Microbiology*
83WPR	*Micro-Injector, Transplant, Gene*	*Microbiology*
83WNY	*Test, DNA-Probe, Other*	*Microbiology*

CHROMATOGRAPH

91DLK	*Chromatograph, HPL, Drugs of Abuse (Dedicated* Instrument)	Toxicology
91DLS	*Gas Chromatograph, Alcohol (Dedicated Instruments)*	*Toxicology*
91JKT	*Gas Chromatograph, Carbon-Monoxide*	*Toxicology*
91DMC	*Gas Chromatograph, Drugs of Abuse (Dedicated* Instruments)	Toxicology

CHROMATOGRAPHIC

83JSQ	*Chromatographic Bacterial Identification*	*Microbiology*
91DKX	*Chromatographic Barbiturate Identification (Thin Layer)*	*Toxicology*
75CFB	*Chromatographic Derivative, Total Lipids*	*Chemistry*
75JHT	*Chromatographic Separation, CPK Isoenzymes*	*Chemistry*
75CEX	*Chromatographic Separation, Lactate Dehydrogenase* Isoenzyme	Chemistry
75JHG	*Chromatographic Separation, Lecithin-Sphingomyelin Ratio*	*Chemistry*
75CJB	*Chromatographic Separation/Radioimmunoassay,* Aldosterone	Chemistry
75CDG	*Chromatographic Separation/Zimmerman* 17-Ketogenic Steroids	Chemistry
75CDE	*Chromatographic Separation/Zimmerman, 17-Ketosteroids*	*Chemistry*
75JLD	*Chromatographic, Cystine*	*Chemistry*
75JLN	*Chromatographic, Glutathione*	*Chemistry*
75JMI	*Chromatographic, Histidine*	*Chemistry*
75JGL	*Chromatographic, Inorganic Phosphorus*	*Chemistry*
75JNT	*Chromatographic, Phospholipids*	*Chemistry*
75CHQ	*Chromatographic/Fluorometric Method, Catecholamines*	*Chemistry*
75CEA	*Triglyceride, Separation, Chromatographic, TLC*	*Chemistry*

CHROMATOGRAPHY

75JQR	*Accessories, Chromatography (Gas, Gel, Liquid,* Thin Layer)	Chemistry
91DMZ	*Adsorbents, Liquid Chromatography*	*Toxicology*
75UGP	*Analyzer, Chromatography Infrared*	*Chemistry*
91KIE	*Apparatus, High Pressure Liquid Chromatography*	*Toxicology*
75UJG	*Cabinet, Chromatography (U.V.) Viewing*	*Chemistry*
91KZQ	*Chromatography (Gas), Clinical Use*	*Toxicology*
91KZR	*Chromatography (Liquid, Gel), Clinical Use*	*Toxicology*
91KZS	*Chromatography (Thin Layer), Clinical Use*	*Toxicology*
75QJY	*Chromatography Equipment, Gas*	*Chemistry*
91DJY	*Chromatography Equipment, Ion Exchange*	*Toxicology*
75QJZ	*Chromatography Equipment, Liquid*	*Chemistry*
75QKA	*Chromatography Equipment, Paper*	*Chemistry*
91DPA	*Chromatography Equipment, Thin Layer*	*Toxicology*
75JLR	*Chromatography, Gas, Pregnanetriol*	*Chemistry*
91MAS	*Chromatography, Liquid, Performance, High*	*Toxicology*
75WYT	*Chromatography, Supercritical Fluid (SFC)*	*Chemistry*
91MLK	*Chromatography, Thin Layer, Tricyclic* Antidepressant Drugs	Toxicology
75JNC	*Column Or Paper Chromatography Plus Ninhydrin,* Phenylalanin	Chemistry
75QJX	*Column, Chromatography*	*Chemistry*
75JMM	*Column, Chromatography, Hydroxyproline*	*Chemistry*
91DII	*Column, GLC*	*Toxicology*
91DPM	*Column, Liquid Chromatography*	*Toxicology*
91LEQ	*Detector, Electrochemical, Chromatography, Liquid*	*Toxicology*
75JMN	*Extraction/Chromatography, Ninhydrin, Hydroxyproline*	*Chemistry*
75UIY	*Fitting, Gas Chromatography Tube*	*Chemistry*
91DLH	*Gas Chromatography, Alcohol*	*Toxicology*
91DOD	*Gas Chromatography, Amphetamine*	*Toxicology*
91KZZ	*Gas Chromatography, Benzodiazepine*	*Toxicology*
91DIN	*Gas Chromatography, Cocaine*	*Toxicology*
91LAD	*Gas Chromatography, Codeine*	*Toxicology*
91DKH	*Gas Chromatography, Diphenylhydantoin*	*Toxicology*
91DIY	*Gas Chromatography, Ethosuximide*	*Toxicology*

CLAMP (cont'd)

85HFX	Clamp, Circumcision	Obstetrics/Gyn
78FGW	Clamp, Electrical	Gastro/Urology
86HOD	Clamp, Eyelid, Ophthalmic	Ophthalmology
79WZW	Clamp, Fixation, Cholangiography	Surgery
78UCO	Clamp, Hemodialysis Unit Blood Line	Gastro/Urology
78QKL	Clamp, Hemorrhoidal	Gastro/Urology
78RBT	Clamp, Incontinence	Gastro/Urology
78QKM	Clamp, Intestinal	Gastro/Urology
79WZX	Clamp, Laparoscopy	Surgery
78FKK	Clamp, Line	Gastro/Urology
86HOB	Clamp, Muscle, Ophthalmic	Ophthalmology
78FFN	Clamp, Non-Electrical	Gastro/Urology
77JYF	Clamp, Ossicle Holding	Ear/Nose/Throat
79QKR	Clamp, Other	Surgery
79QKN	Clamp, Patent Ductus	Surgery
78FHA	Clamp, Penile	Gastro/Urology
74QKO	Clamp, Peripheral Vascular	Cardiovascular
78QKP	Clamp, Rectal	Gastro/Urology
76EEF	Clamp, Rubber Dam	Dental And Oral
84QKQ	Clamp, Skull	Cns/Neurology
79GDJ	Clamp, Surgical, General & Plastic Surgery	Surgery
80WUF	Clamp, Tubing	General
78FIG	Clamp, Tubing, Blood, Automatic	Gastro/Urology
85HFW	Clamp, Umbilical	Obstetrics/Gyn
85HGC	Clamp, Uterine	Obstetrics/Gyn
74DXC	Clamp, Vascular	Cardiovascular
76ECN	Clamp, Wire, Orthodontic	Dental And Oral
79QLI	Clip, Towel	Surgery
79TBO	Cover, Clamp	Surgery
78FFR	Device, Locking, Clamp, Instestinal	Gastro/Urology
76EJG	Forceps, Rubber Dam Clamp	Dental And Oral
84HBL	Holder, Head, Neurosurgical (Skull Clamp)	Cns/Neurology
78FHN	Ligator, Hemorrhoidal	Gastro/Urology
85REZ	Ligator, Umbilical	Obstetrics/Gyn
79WUZ	Pad, Clamp	Surgery

CLAMPS

78QXE	Forceps, Intestinal (Clamps)	Gastro/Urology

CLARKE'S

88IGK	Solution, Clarke's	Pathology

CLASP

76EHP	Clasp, Preformed	Dental And Oral
76EJW	Clasp, Wire	Dental And Oral

CLASS

74MOR	Battery, Rechargeable, Replacement for Class III Device	Cardiovascular

CLASSIFIER

81GKZ	Counter, Cell, Differential Classifier, Automated	Hematology

CLAVICLE

89IQJ	Splint, Clavicle	Physical Med
87RWP	Strap, Clavicle	Orthopedics
87RXG	Support, Clavicle	Orthopedics

CLAW

73JEI	Remover, Foreign Body, Bronchoscope (Non-Rigid)	Anesthesiology

CLEANER

80QKS	Cleaner, Bedpan (Sterilizer)	General
76EFT	Cleaner, Denture	Dental And Oral
76JER	Cleaner, Denture, Mechanical	Dental And Oral
79UMT	Cleaner, Electrosurgical Tip	Surgery
74WTL	Cleaner, Forceps, Biopsy	Cardiovascular
86LPN	Cleaner, Lens, Contact	Ophthalmology
80MDZ	Cleaner, Medical Device	General
80QKU	Cleaner, Needle	General
80QKV	Cleaner, Syringe	General
76ECA	Cleaner, Ultrasonic, Dental Laboratory	Dental And Oral
80FLG	Cleaner, Ultrasonic, Medical Instrument	General
80QPZ	Disinfector, Liquid	General
80RQL	Sanitizer	General
80TGE	Solution, Antibacterial Cleaner	General
80TGF	Solution, Instrument Cleaner	General
80THI	Sterilizer/Washer, Endoscope	General
80SFN	Washer, Cart	General
75SFP	Washer, Labware	Chemistry
75SFQ	Washer, Pipette	Chemistry
75UJA	Washer, Pipette, Ultrasonic	Chemistry
80FLH	Washer, Receptacle, Waste, Body	General
80SFR	Washer, Utensil	General
80SFM	Washer/Sterilizer	General

CLEANERS

80LRJ	Medical Disinfectants/Cleaners for Instruments	General

CLEANING

78MNL	Accessories, Cleaning Brushes (For Endoscope)	Gastro/Urology

CLEANING (cont'd)

78FEB	Accessories, Cleaning, Endoscopic	Gastro/Urology
76QEO	Brush, Burr Cleaning	Dental And Oral
77EPE	Brush, Cleaning, Tracheal Tube	Ear/Nose/Throat
80WVO	Brush, Other	General
80FRF	Equipment, Cleaning, Air	General
80VBI	Housekeeping Equipment	General
78FCE	Kit, Enema (For Cleaning Purposes)	Gastro/Urology
80LKB	Pad, Alcohol	General
80WPU	Soap	General
80WWK	Washer/Disinfector	General
80WPO	Wipe, Instrument	General

CLEANROOM

80VAA	Cleanroom Equipment	General
80WQM	Equipment/Service, Quality Control	General
83UGI	Germ-Free Apparatus	Microbiology
80RAH	Hood, Isolation, Laminar Air Flow	General
80FLJ	Laminar Air Flow Unit	General
75RDW	Laminar Air Flow Unit, Fixed (Air Curtain)	Chemistry
75RDX	Laminar Air Flow Unit, Mobile	Chemistry

CLEANSER

76KJJ	Cleanser, Root Canal	Dental And Oral

CLEARANCE

84UEW	Flowmeter, Meter, Cerebral Blood, Xenon Clearance	Cns/Neurology

CLEARING

88KEM	Clearing Agent	Pathology
88IJZ	Clearing Oil	Pathology

CLEFT

77UCZ	Obturator, Cleft Palate	Ear/Nose/Throat

CLEIDOCLAST

85HHN	Cleidoclast	Obstetrics/Gyn

CLIMBER

89IMN	Climber, Curb, Wheelchair	Physical Med

CLIMBING

80TFX	Lift, Stair Climbing	General
89IMK	Wheelchair, Stair Climbing	Physical Med

CLINICAL

76EJT	Alloy, Gold Based, For Clinical Use	Dental And Oral
76EJS	Alloy, Precious Metal, For Clinical Use	Dental And Oral
75JIS	Calibrator, Primary, Clinical Chemistry	Chemistry
75JIT	Calibrator, Secondary, Clinical Chemistry	Chemistry
75JIW	Calibrator, Surrogate, Clinical Chemistry	Chemistry
91KZQ	Chromatography (Gas), Clinical Use	Toxicology
91KZR	Chromatography (Liquid, Gel), Clinical Use	Toxicology
91KZS	Chromatography (Thin Layer), Clinical Use	Toxicology
75QMB	Computer, Clinical Laboratory	Chemistry
75JJH	Concentrator, Clinical Sample	Chemistry
91DOP	Mass Spectrometer, Clinical Use	Toxicology
75RHH	Mixer, Clinical Laboratory	Chemistry
75JRP	Monochromator, for Clinical Use	Chemistry

CLIP

80QBF	Applicator, Clip (Forceps)	General
84HCI	Applier, Aneurysm Clip	Cns/Neurology
78WZN	Applier, Clip, Repair, Hernia, Laparoscopic	Gastro/Urology
84HBT	Applier, Hemostatic Clip	Cns/Neurology
79SJF	Applier, Ligature Clip	Surgery
79GDO	Applier, Surgical, Clip	Surgery
84HCH	Clip, Aneurysm (Intracranial)	Cns/Neurology
80QLD	Clip, Bandage	General
85HEA	Clip, Drape, Lithotomy	Obstetrics/Gyn
79MCH	Clip, Hemostatic	Surgery
79FZP	Clip, Implantable	Surgery
84HBP	Clip, Implantable, Malleable	Cns/Neurology
79QLF	Clip, Instrument	Surgery
84HBS	Clip, Instrument, Forming/Cutting	Cns/Neurology
86HOC	Clip, Iris Retractor	Ophthalmology
86VEU	Clip, Lens Implantation	Ophthalmology
86HPB	Clip, Lens, Trial, Ophthalmic	Ophthalmology
79SJG	Clip, Ligature	Surgery
73BXJ	Clip, Nose	Anesthesiology
79QLK	Clip, Other	Surgery
78QLG	Clip, Penis	Gastro/Urology
79FZQ	Clip, Removable (Skin)	Surgery
84HBO	Clip, Scalp	Cns/Neurology
79QLH	Clip, Suture	Surgery
78FBF	Clip, Suture, Stomach And Intestinal	Gastro/Urology
86HQW	Clip, Tantalum, Ophthalmic	Ophthalmology
79QLI	Clip, Towel	Surgery
85HGB	Clip, Tubal Occlusion	Obstetrics/Gyn
74DSS	Clip, Vascular	Cardiovascular
74DST	Clip, Vena Cava	Cardiovascular

COATING *(cont'd)*

80SHH	Equipment, Device Coating, Protective	General
91DLG	Liquid Coating, GLC	Toxicology
80SHG	Service, Device Coating, Protective	General

COBALT

90IWH	Source, Teletherapy, Radionuclide	Radiology
90JAD	Therapeutic X-Ray System	Radiology

COCAINE

91JXO	Enzyme Immunoassay, Cocaine	Toxicology
91DIO	Enzyme Immunoassay, Cocaine And Cocaine Metabolites	Toxicology
91DIR	Free Radical Assay, Cocaine	Toxicology
91DIN	Gas Chromatography, Cocaine	Toxicology
91DKL	Hemagglutination, Cocaine	Toxicology
91DLN	Hemagglutination, Cocaine Metabolites (Benzoylecgnonine)	Toxicology
91LAC	High Pressure Liquid Chromatography, Cocaine & Metabolites	Toxicology
91KLN	Radioimmunoassay, Cocaine Metabolite	Toxicology
75MGX	System, Test, Drugs of Abuse	Chemistry
91DMN	Thin Layer Chromatography, Cocaine	Toxicology

COCCIDIOIDES

83GMI	Antigen, CF And/Or ID, Coccidioides Immitis	Microbiology
83GMG	Antigen, Latex Agglutination, Coccidioides Immitis	Microbiology
83GMH	Antiserum, Positive Control, Coccidioides Immitis	Microbiology
83MIY	Enzyme Linked Immunoabsorbent Assay, Coccidioides Immitis	Microbiology
83MDF	Reagent, DNA-Probe, Coccidioides Immitis	Microbiology

COCHLEA

77MLJ	Device, Otoacoustic	Ear/Nose/Throat

COCHLEAR

77MCM	Implant, Cochlear	Ear/Nose/Throat
77UAI	Prosthesis, Cochlear	Ear/Nose/Throat

CODE

80VFR	Computer, Bar Code	General
80WNL	Label, Bar Code	General
80VAH	Labeling Equipment	General
80WMT	Printer, Bar Code	General
80WMS	Reader, Bar Code	General
80SHI	System, Drug Dispensing, Pharmacy, Automated	General

CODEINE

91LAD	Gas Chromatography, Codeine	Toxicology
91LAE	High Pressure Liquid Chromatography, Codeine	Toxicology
91DLD	Thin Layer Chromatography, Codeine	Toxicology

CODING

76UDU	System, Coding, Color, Instrument	Dental And Oral

CODY

77ESX	Tack, Sacculotomy (Cody)	Ear/Nose/Throat

COHENT

73CBL	Absorbent, Carbon-Dioxide	Anesthesiology

COHN

82DGA	Cohn Fraction II, Antigen, Antiserum, Control	Immunology

COIL

78FKD	Canister, Coil	Gastro/Urology
90MOS	Coil, Magnetic Resonance, Specialty	Radiology
78FHS	Dialyzer, Single Coil (Hemodialysis)	Gastro/Urology
78FJJ	Dialyzer, Twin Coil	Gastro/Urology
81SFG	Warmer, Blood, Coil	Hematology

COLCHICINE

88IAY	Colchicine	Pathology

COLD

80KYR	Bag, Ice	General
80FPF	Bottle, Hot/Cold Water	General
89IMF	Chilling Unit	Physical Med
80QLR	Collar, Ice	General
80QLW	Compress, Cold	General
80RAZ	Hypo/Hyperthermia Blanket	General
80RBA	Hypo/Hyperthermia Unit, Central	General
80RBB	Hypo/Hyperthermia Unit, Mobile	General
80RBC	Hypothermia Unit	General
73BTF	Hypothermia Unit (Blanket, Plumbing & Heat Exchanger)	Anesthesiology
80KYQ	Kit, Snake Bite, Chemical Cold Pack	General
89RHK	Moist Therapy Pack	Physical Med
89RHJ	Moist Therapy Pack Conditioner	Physical Med
80QLO	Pack, Cold	General
80FRS	Pack, Cold, Chemical	General
89IMD	Pack, Hot Or Cold, Disposable	Physical Med
89IME	Pack, Hot Or Cold, Reusable	Physical Med
89ILO	Pack, Hot Or Cold, Water Circulating	Physical Med
76LFE	Solution, Sterilizing, Cold	Dental And Oral

COLD *(cont'd)*

89UEC	Support, Hot/Cold Pack	Physical Med

COLI

83GMZ	Antigen, All Types, Escherichia Coli	Microbiology
83GNA	Antiserum, Escherichia Coli	Microbiology
83GMY	Antiserum, Fluorescent, Escherichia Coli	Microbiology
80WWZ	Test, Bacteria Characterization	General

COLLAGEN

79LMF	Agent, Hemostatic, Absorbable, Collagen-Based	Surgery
79LMG	Agent, Hemostatic, Non-Absorbable, Collagen-Based	Surgery
84MFQ	Collagen, Hemostatic, Microsurgical	Cns/Neurology
77MGF	Collagen, Injectable (For Vocal Cord Augmentation)	Ear/Nose/Throat
77LMT	Collagen, Lyophilized	Ear/Nose/Throat
81GHX	Collagen, Platelet Aggregation And Adhesion	Hematology
74WYE	Device, Closure, Puncture, Hemostatic	Cardiovascular
79LMI	Implant, Collagen (Non-Aesthetic Use)	Surgery
79LMH	Implant, Collagen, Dermal (Aesthetic Use)	Surgery
79GBI	Material, Restoration, Aesthetic, External	Surgery
77KHK	Polymer, ENT Natural Collagen Material	Ear/Nose/Throat
86MOE	Shield, Corneal, Collagen	Ophthalmology
79THO	Sponge, Hemostatic, Absorbable Collagen	Surgery

COLLAGEN-BASED

79LMF	Agent, Hemostatic, Absorbable, Collagen-Based	Surgery
79LMG	Agent, Hemostatic, Non-Absorbable, Collagen-Based	Surgery

COLLAPSIBLE

80WKO	Stretcher, Collapsible	General

COLLAR

87QLP	Collar, Cervical Neck	Orthopedics
80WMR	Collar, Extrication	General
76QLQ	Collar, Gingival	Dental And Oral
80QLR	Collar, Ice	General
76EIR	Scissors, Collar And Crown	Dental And Oral

COLLECTION

74WTU	Adapter, Needle	Cardiovascular
78EXF	Bag, Bile Collection	Gastro/Urology
81KSR	Bag, Blood, Collection	Hematology
80FOC	Bag, Collection, Urine, Newborn	General
80WOQ	Bag, Drainage, Nasogastric	General
80SEB	Bag, Urinary Collection	General
80SEC	Bag, Urinary Collection, Precision Measure (Urine Meter)	General
78EXG	Bag, Urinary Collection, Ureterostomy	Gastro/Urology
73CBD	Bottle, Collection, Breathing System (Calibrated)	Anesthesiology
73CBC	Bottle, Collection, Breathing System (Uncalibrated)	Anesthesiology
80KDQ	Bottle, Collection, Vacuum (Aspirator)	General
80WZB	Chair, Blood Drawing	General
80SEE	Container, Urine Specimen	General
88KET	Filter, Cell Collection, Tissue Processing	Pathology
85LTY	Fluid, Collection, Cytological	Obstetrics/Gyn
73KGK	Gas, Collecting Vessel	Anesthesiology
74RKS	Kit, Blood Collection, Phlebotomy	Cardiovascular
80LWE	Kit, Collection/Transfusion, Marrow, Bone	General
80RGZ	Kit, Mid-Stream Collection	General
78FCN	Kit, Urinary Drainage Collection	Gastro/Urology
75JKA	Labware, Blood Collection	Chemistry
80FMK	Lancet, Blood	General
80RHY	Needle, Blood Collection	General
80VLU	Pump, Urinary Collection Bag	General
78LNL	Stimulator, Collection, Sperm, Electrical	Gastro/Urology
80RYI	Swabs, Specimen Collection	General
73BXT	System, Collection, Gas	Anesthesiology
73SBZ	Trap, Mucus	Anesthesiology
81GJE	Tray, Blood Collection	Hematology
75SCN	Tube, Blood Collection	Chemistry
81GIO	Tube, Capillary Blood Collection	Hematology

COLLECTOR

81KST	Collector, Blood, Vacuum-Assisted	Hematology
75QLS	Collector, Fraction	Chemistry
78EXB	Collector, Ostomy	Gastro/Urology
83LIO	Collector, Specimen	Microbiology
73QLT	Collector, Sputum	Anesthesiology
75VCX	Collector, Sweat	Chemistry
78KNX	Collector, Urine	Gastro/Urology
78FFH	Collector, Urine, Disposable	Gastro/Urology

COLLIMATOR

76EHA	Aligner, Beam, X-Ray (Collimator)	Dental And Oral
90IZW	Collimator, Radiographic, Automatic	Radiology
90IZX	Collimator, Radiographic, Manual	Radiology
90IYL	Collimator, Therapeutic X-Ray, Dermatological	Radiology
90IYK	Collimator, Therapeutic X-Ray, High Voltage	Radiology
90IYJ	Collimator, Therapeutic X-Ray, Low Voltage	Radiology
90IYI	Collimator, Therapeutic X-Ray, Orthovoltage	Radiology
76EHB	Collimator, X-Ray	Dental And Oral

KEYWORD INDEX

COMMUNICATION *(cont'd)*

90UMF	Radiographic Picture Archiving/Communication System (PACS)	Radiology
90LMD	System, Communication, Image, Digital	Radiology
74MSX	System, Network And Communication, Physiological Monitors	Cardiovascular
80VAT	Telephone Equipment	General
89UME	Telephone, Handicapped Use	Physical Med
77WRO	Valve, Speaking, Tracheal	Ear/Nose/Throat

COMPACTOR

80WVR	Cart, Waste	General
80TBJ	Compactor, Fixed	General
80TBK	Compactor, Portable	General
80WLA	Equipment, Control, Pollution	General
80WWY	Sterilizer/Compactor	General

COMPENSATED

73CAX	Flowmeter, Back-Pressure Compensated, Thorpe Tube	Anesthesiology
73CCN	Flowmeter, Gas, Non-Back-Pressure Compensated, Bourdon Gauge	Anesthesiology

COMPLEMENT

82DBA	Antigen, Antiserum, Complement C1 Inhibitor (Inactivator)	Immunology
82DAK	Antigen, Antiserum, Control, Complement C1q	Immunology
82DAI	Antigen, Antiserum, Control, Complement C1r	Immunology
82CZY	Antigen, Antiserum, Control, Complement C1s	Immunology
82CZW	Antigen, Antiserum, Control, Complement C3	Immunology
82DBI	Antigen, Antiserum, Control, Complement C4	Immunology
82DAY	Antigen, Antiserum, Control, Complement C5	Immunology
82DAG	Antigen, Antiserum, Control, Complement C8	Immunology
82DAE	Antigen, Antiserum, Control, Complement C9	Immunology
82DHL	Antigen, Antiserum, Control, Protein, Complement	Immunology
83GNF	Antigen, CF, T. Cruzi	Microbiology
82KTQ	Complement	Immunology
82DAC	Control, Antiserum, Antigen, Activator, C3, Complement	Immunology
82KTP	Reagent, Immunoassay, Activator, C3, Complement	Immunology

COMPLEXED

82MTF	Total, Prostate Specific Antigen (noncomplexed & complexed) for Detection of Prostate Cancer	Immunology

COMPLEXES

82MMW	Antigen, Tumor Marker, Bladder (Basement Membrane Complexes)	Immunology

COMPLEXONE

75CIC	Complexone, Cresolphthalein, Calcium	Chemistry

COMPONENT

89ISH	Ankle/Foot, External Limb Component	Physical Med
82DAJ	Antigen, Antiserum, Control, Free Secretory Component	Immunology
87LXT	Appliance, Fix., Nail/Blade/Plate Comb., Multiple Component	Orthopedics
87LGF	Component, Cast	Orthopedics
80VFE	Component, Ceramic	General
80WKG	Component, Electrical	General
80VAF	Component, Electronic	General
89IOD	Component, Exercise	Physical Med
80WOS	Component, Metal, Other	General
80SHS	Component, Optical	General
80WXA	Component, Other	General
80WSM	Component, Paper	General
80VAE	Component, Plastic	General
80VAL	Component, Rubber	General
80VAM	Component, Silicone	General
87JEC	Component, Traction, Invasive	Orthopedics
87KQZ	Component, Traction, Non-Invasive	Orthopedics
89KNN	Component, Wheelchair	Physical Med
80WVW	Contract Assembly	General
80VAC	Contract Manufacturing	General
80WLY	Contract Manufacturing, Product, Disposable	General
80WLX	Contract Manufacturing, Product, Durable	General
87KTT	Fixation Appliance, Multiple Component	Orthopedics
87KTW	Fixation Appliance, Single Component	Orthopedics
89IRA	Hand, External Limb Component, Mechanical	Physical Med
89IQZ	Hand, External Limb Component, Powered	Physical Med
89IQX	Hook, External Limb Component, Mechanical	Physical Med
89IQW	Hook, External Limb Component, Powered	Physical Med
89IRD	Joint, Elbow, External Limb Component, Mechanical	Physical Med
89IRE	Joint, Elbow, External Limb Component, Powered	Physical Med
89ISL	Joint, Hip, External Limb Component	Physical Med
89ISY	Joint, Knee, External Limb Component	Physical Med
89IQQ	Joint, Shoulder, External Limb Component	Physical Med
89ISZ	Joint, Wrist, External Limb Component, Mechanical	Physical Med
80WUL	Metal, Medical	General
79WUZ	Pad, Clamp	Surgery
80WTJ	Polymer, Synthetic, Other	General
87UBK	Prosthesis, Ankle, Talar Component	Orthopedics
87UBL	Prosthesis, Ankle, Tibial Component	Orthopedics

COMPONENT *(cont'd)*

87UBN	Prosthesis, Elbow, Humeral Component	Orthopedics
87UBO	Prosthesis, Elbow, Radial Component	Orthopedics
87UBP	Prosthesis, Elbow, Ulna Component	Orthopedics
87JDM	Prosthesis, Hip, Acetabular Component, Metal, Non-Cemented	Orthopedics
87JDG	Prosthesis, Hip, Femoral Component, Cemented, Metal	Orthopedics
89ISS	Prosthesis, Thigh Socket, External Component	Physical Med
80WSO	Pump, Industrial	General
80WWC	Resin, Other	General
80WSZ	Sensor, Moisture	General
84JXG	Shunt, Central Nerve, With Component	Cns/Neurology
89ILH	Splint, Hand, And Component	Physical Med
89ITC	Stirrup, External Brace Component	Physical Med
80WWE	Tubing, Other	General
89KGH	Wrist, External Limb Component, Powered	Physical Med

COMPONENTS

88KPB	Mycoplasma Detection Media and Components	Pathology

COMPOSITE

76VLQ	Compound, Resinous, Composite	Dental And Oral
89IKA	Electrode, Biopotential, Surface, Composite	Physical Med
78MCI	Graft, Vascular, Synth./Bio. Composite, Hemodialysis Access	Gastro/Urology
74MAL	Graft, Vascular, Synthetic/Biological Composite	Cardiovascular
77ESF	Polymer, ENT Composite Synthetic PTFE With Carbon-Fiber	Ear/Nose/Throat
87KMD	Prosthesis, Ankle, Semi-Constrained, Metal/Composite	Orthopedics
87MEJ	Prosthesis, Hip, Semi-Const., Composite/Polymer	Orthopedics
87KMC	Prosthesis, Hip, Semi-constrained, Composite/metal	Orthopedics

COMPOSITION

74MNW	Analyzer, Body Composition	Cardiovascular
80VDN	Analyzer, Composition, Weight, Patient	General

COMPOUND

76VLQ	Compound, Resinous, Composite	Dental And Oral
84HBF	Drill, Powered Compound (With Burr, Trephine & Accessories)	Cns/Neurology
75JKB	Radioimmunoassay, Compound S (11-Deoxycortisol)	Chemistry
76UDV	Resinous Compound	Dental And Oral
84UCK	Resinous Compound, Cranial	Cns/Neurology
90VHD	Scanner, Ultrasonic, Compound B	Radiology

COMPRESS

80QLW	Compress, Cold	General
80QLX	Compress, Gauze	General
89QLY	Compress, Moist Heat	Physical Med

COMPRESSED

73ECX	Cylinder, Compressed Gas, With Valve	Anesthesiology

COMPRESSIBLE

80LLK	Legging, Compression, Non-Inflatable	General
74JOW	Sleeve, Compressible Limb	Cardiovascular

COMPRESSION

80MHW	Bandage, Compression	General
74QGJ	Board, Cardiac Compression	Cardiovascular
87HWN	Compression Instrument	Orthopedics
74QLZ	Compression Unit, Intermittent (Anti-Embolism Pump)	Cardiovascular
74WTT	Legging, Compression, Inflatable, Sequential	Cardiovascular
80LLK	Legging, Compression, Non-Inflatable	General
80WVI	Sock, Non-Compression	General

COMPRESSOR

80QBQ	Aspirator, Emergency Suction	General
73BTI	Compressor, Air, Portable	Anesthesiology
74DRM	Compressor, Cardiac, External	Cardiovascular
80FQD	Compressor, External, Cardiac, Manual	General
80FQI	Compressor, External, Cardiac, Powered	General
86HOA	Compressor, Orbital	Ophthalmology
73BTZ	Resuscitator, Cardiac, Mechanical, Compressor	Anesthesiology

COMPUTED

90VHB	Phantom, Computed Axial Tomography (CAT, CT)	Radiology
90WMF	Scanner, Computed Tomography, Cine	Radiology
84JXD	Scanner, Computed Tomography, X-Ray (CAT, CT)	Cns/Neurology
90THS	Scanner, Computed Tomography, X-Ray, Full Body	Radiology
90TEI	Scanner, Computed Tomography, X-Ray, Head	Radiology
90JAK	Scanner, Computed Tomography, X-Ray, Special Procedure	Radiology
90KPS	Scanner, Emission Computed Tomography	Radiology
90THG	Scanner, Nuclear Emission Computed Tomography (ECT)	Radiology

COMPUTER

89LFF	Aid, Control, Environmental, Controlled, Breath	Physical Med
75QKX	Analyzer, Chemistry, Multi-Channel, Programmable	Chemistry
75QKY	Analyzer, Chemistry, Single Channel, Programmable	Chemistry
85HEO	Analyzer, Data, Obstetric	Obstetrics/Gyn

COMPUTER (cont'd)

87VDV Analyzer, Gait — Orthopedics
86SFB Analyzer, Visual Function — Ophthalmology
87SHK Assistant, Surgical, Orthopedic, Automated — Orthopedics
80WKP Camera, Other — General
74QGK Cardiac Output Unit, Direct Fick — Cardiovascular
74UDP Cardiac Output Unit, Dye Dilution — Cardiovascular
74QGL Cardiac Output Unit, Indicator Dilution (Thermal) — Cardiovascular
74QGM Cardiac Output Unit, Other — Cardiovascular
74TAV Cardiac Output Unit, Radioisotope Probe — Cardiovascular
80VAF Component, Electronic — General
80VAX Computer Equipment — General
80VBH Computer Software — General
80WVJ Computer Software, Home Healthcare — General
80WSJ Computer Software, Hospital/Nursing Management — General
80WSN Computer Software, Industrial — General
82MLF Computer Software, Prenatal Risk Evaluation — Immunology
80LNX Computer and Software, Medical — General
86LQB Computer and Software, Medical, Ophthalmic Use — Ophthalmology
77WQJ Computer, Audiometry — Ear/Nose/Throat
80VFR Computer, Bar Code — General
74DSK Computer, Blood Pressure — Cardiovascular
84VKG Computer, Brain Mapping — Cns/Neurology
74QMA Computer, Cardiac Catheterization Laboratory — Cardiovascular
75JQP Computer, Chemistry Analyzer — Chemistry
75QMB Computer, Clinical Laboratory — Chemistry
74DXG Computer, Diagnostic, Pre-Programmed, Single-Function — Cardiovascular
74DQK Computer, Diagnostic, Programmable — Cardiovascular
74QMC Computer, ECG Interpretation (Arrhythmia) — Cardiovascular
81JWS Computer, Hematology Analyzer — Hematology
80WLE Computer, Image, Endoscopic — General
79WIY Computer, Imaging, Presurgery — Surgery
90QMD Computer, Nuclear Medicine — Radiology
86WQK Computer, Ophthalmology — Ophthalmology
73BZL Computer, Oxygen-Uptake — Anesthesiology
80VHN Computer, Patient Data Management — General
73QME Computer, Patient Monitor — Anesthesiology
73BZC Computer, Pulmonary Function Data — Anesthesiology
73BZM Computer, Pulmonary Function Interpretator (Diagnostic) — Anesthesiology
73QMF Computer, Pulmonary Function Laboratory — Anesthesiology
73BTY Computer, Pulmonary Function, Predicted Values — Anesthesiology
90WKA Computer, Radiographic Data — Radiology
90UFD Computer, Radiographic Image Analysis — Radiology
74QMG Computer, Stress Exercise — Cardiovascular
90VHG Computer, Ultrasound — Radiology
74UER Electrocardiograph, Interpretive — Cardiovascular
80WQM Equipment/Service, Quality Control — General
84QUT Evoked Response Unit — Cns/Neurology
80VAW Form, Computer — General
73RLA Monitor, Physiological, Acute Care — Anesthesiology
74RLB Monitor, Physiological, Cardiac Catheterization — Cardiovascular
74RLC Monitor, Physiological, Stress Exercise — Cardiovascular
80WKM Mount, Equipment — General
80WUP Paper, Recording, Data — General
80WMT Printer, Bar Code — General
90UMF Radiographic Picture Archiving/Communication System (PACS) — Radiology
90TGL Radiographic Unit, Digital — Radiology
90VLE Radiographic Unit, Digital Subtraction Angiographic (DSA) — Radiology
90ROG Radiotherapy Treatment Planning Unit — Radiology
80WMS Reader, Bar Code — General
74DSH Recorder, Magnetic Tape/Disc — Cardiovascular
80TEF Recorder, Videotape/Videodisc — General
85MGK Scanner, Breast, Thermographic, Ultrasonic, Computer-Asstd. — Obstetrics/Gyn
90JAM Scanner, Magnetic Resonance (NMR/MRI) — Radiology
80VBS Service, Computer — General
84LEL Sleep Assessment Equipment — Cns/Neurology
81MMH Software, Blood Bank (Stand-Alone Products) — Hematology
81KSS Supplies, Blood Bank — Hematology
80SHI System, Drug Dispensing, Pharmacy, Automated — General
80WTV System, Robot — General
86MMQ Topographer, Corneal — Ophthalmology
90WOG Transmitter, Image & Data, Radiographic — Radiology

COMPUTER-ASSISTED

85MGK Scanner, Breast, Thermographic, Ultrasonic, Computer-Asstd. — Obstetrics/Gyn

CONCENTRATE

78KPO Concentrate, Dialysis, Hemodialysis (Liquid or Powder) — Gastro/Urology

CONCENTRATION

73VCC Analyzer, Blood Oxyhemoglobin Concentration — Anesthesiology
74JEE Analyzer, Concentration, Oxyhemoglobin, BP, Transcutaneous — Cardiovascular
91JFD Analyzer, Concentration, Oxyhemoglobin, Blood Phase — Toxicology

CONCENTRATION (cont'd)

73JED Analyzer, Oxyhemoglobin Concentration, Blood Phase, Indwell. — Anesthesiology
83LKS Analyzer, Parasite Concentration — Microbiology
73BXK Gas, Calibrated (Specified Concentration) — Anesthesiology
73BYF Mask, Oxygen, Low Concentration, Venturi — Anesthesiology
78LRI Meter, pH, Concentration, Ion, Hydrogen, Dialysis — Gastro/Urology
81MZJ System, Concentration, Hematopoietic Stem Cell — Hematology

CONCENTRATOR

75JJH Concentrator, Clinical Sample — Chemistry
73RJM Concentrator, Oxygen — Anesthesiology
75UHM Concentrator, Protein — Chemistry

CONDENSER

80WRU Capacitor, Defibrillator — General
76EKG Condenser, Amalgam And Foil, Operative — Dental And Oral
73BYD Condenser, Heat And Moisture (Artificial Nose) — Anesthesiology
88KEI Condenser, Microscope — Pathology
90IZR Generator, Radiographic, Capacitor Discharge — Radiology

CONDENSING

86HJL Lens, Condensing, Diagnostic — Ophthalmology

CONDITIONER

76DYH Adhesive, Bracket And Conditioner, Resin — Dental And Oral
74DRR Amplifier, Biopotential (W Signal Conditioner) — Cardiovascular
74DRQ Amplifier, Transducer Signal (W Signal Conditioner) — Cardiovascular
84GWK Conditioner, Signal, Physiological — Cns/Neurology
89RHJ Moist Therapy Pack Conditioner — Physical Med
76EBC Sealant, Pit And Fissure, And Conditioner, Resin — Dental And Oral

CONDITIONING

84HCB Device, Conditioning, Aversion — Cns/Neurology
84RWC Stimulator, Aversion Conditioning (Behavior Modification) — Cns/Neurology

CONDOM

78EXJ Appliance, Incontinence, Urosheath Type — Gastro/Urology
78QIS Catheter, Urinary, Condom — Gastro/Urology
85HIS Condom — Obstetrics/Gyn
85LTZ Condom With Nonoxynol-9 — Obstetrics/Gyn
85MOL Condom, Non-Latex — Obstetrics/Gyn
85LZL Micro-Condom — Obstetrics/Gyn
80FQT Prophylactic (Condom) — General

CONDUCTION

73BSO Catheter, Conduction, Anesthesia — Anesthesiology
84JXE Device, Measurement, Velocity, Conduction, Nerve — Cns/Neurology
74LPB Electrode, Ablation, Tissue, Conduction, Percutaneous — Cardiovascular
73BSN Filter, Conduction, Anesthesia — Anesthesiology
77LXB Hearing-Aid, Bone-Conduction — Ear/Nose/Throat
77MAH Hearing-Aid, Bone-Conduction, Implanted — Ear/Nose/Throat
77MKE Hearing-Aid, Bone-Conduction, Percutaneous — Ear/Nose/Throat
73CAZ Kit, Anesthesia, Conduction — Anesthesiology
73BSP Needle, Conduction, Anesthesia (W/Wo Introducer) — Anesthesiology

CONDUCTIVE

79QBK Apron, Conductive — Surgery
80QNA Cover, Mattress, Conductive — General
80QNE Cover, Shoe, Conductive — General
80QNF Cover, Shoe, Non-Conductive — General
80TCD Floor, Conductive — General
80QWU Footstool, Conductive — General
80QWV Footstool, Non-Conductive — General
73BRT Restraint, Patient, Conductive — Anesthesiology
73BWP Shoe And Shoe Cover, Conductive — Anesthesiology
79RSX Shoe, Conductive — Surgery
80SDL Tubing, Conductive — General
80SDO Tubing, Non-Conductive — General

CONDUCTIVITY

75LFP Conductivity Rate, Urea Nitrogen — Chemistry
75VCU Meter, Conductivity — Chemistry
78FLB Meter, Conductivity, Induction, Remote Type — Gastro/Urology
78FIZ Meter, Conductivity, Non-Remote — Gastro/Urology
78QPI Meter, Dialysate Conductivity — Gastro/Urology
78QZX Monitor, Hemodialysis Unit Conductivity — Gastro/Urology
78FKH Solution-Test, Standard-Conductivity, Dialysis — Gastro/Urology
80RZW Tester, Conductivity, Floor And Equipment — General
80RZX Tester, Conductivity, Shoe And Gown — General

CONDUCTORS

73BZT Stethoscope, Esophageal, With Electrical Conductors — Anesthesiology

CONDYLAR

87JDP Implant, Fixation Device, Condylar Plate — Orthopedics

CONDYLE

76MPL Prosthesis, Mandibular Condyle — Dental And Oral

CONE

90IZT Cone, Radiographic — Radiology

CONE *(cont'd)*

76EAH	Cone, Radiographic, Lead-Lined	Dental And Oral
85HDZ	Knife, Cervical Cone	Obstetrics/Gyn

CONFORMER

86HQN	Conformer, Ophthalmic	Ophthalmology

CONGENITAL

89IOZ	Splint, Abduction, Congenital Hip Dislocation	Physical Med

CONGO

88ICH	Stain, Congo Red	Pathology

CONJUGATED

83LIN	Antisera, Conjugated Fluorescent, Cytomegalovirus	Microbiology
75KWX	Radioimmunoassay, Conjugated Sulfalithocholic, Bile Acid	Chemistry

CONJUGATES

75JJB	Azo-Dyes, Colorimetric, Bilirubin And Conjugates	Chemistry

CONJUNCTIVAL

73LKE	Monitor, Oxygen, Conjunctival	Anesthesiology

CONNECTING

73BYY	Tube, Aspirating, Flexible, Connecting	Anesthesiology
80SCR	Tube, Connecting	General
80WSP	Tubing, Connecting	General
80VHQ	Tubing, Oxygen Connecting	General

CONNECTOR

79KGZ	Accessories, Catheter	Surgery
73CBJ	Airway, Bi-Nasopharyngeal (With Connector)	Anesthesiology
74WWW	Cable, Pacemaker	Cardiovascular
73CAI	Circuit, Breathing (W Connector, Adapter, Y Piece)	Anesthesiology
73BZA	Connector, Airway (Extension)	Anesthesiology
79GCD	Connector, Catheter	Surgery
84UAS	Connector, Hydrocephalic	Cns/Neurology
78FJQ	Connector, Shunt	Gastro/Urology
79SIP	Connector, Suction/Irrigation	Surgery
74WJY	Connector, Tubing, Blood	Cardiovascular
78FKB	Connector, Tubing, Blood, Infusion, T-Type	Gastro/Urology
78FKY	Connector, Tubing, Dialysate	Gastro/Urology
78EYK	Connector, Ureteral Catheter	Gastro/Urology
80SHM	Coupler, Optical, Laparoscopic	General
80QWK	Fitting, Luer	General
80QWL	Fitting, Quick Connect (Gas Connector)	General
79FSX	Light, Surgical, Connector	Surgery
73BTS	Tube, Bronchial (W/Wo Connector)	Anesthesiology
73BTO	Tube, Tracheostomy (W/Wo Connector)	Anesthesiology
78KQQ	Tubing, Dialysate (And Connector)	Gastro/Urology

CONSOLE

74DTQ	Console, Heart-Lung Machine, Cardiopulmonary Bypass	Cardiovascular
80RKA	Console, Patient Service	General

CONSTANT

75ULO	Bath, Dry (Constant Temperature)	Chemistry
75QCY	Bath, Water (Constant Temperature)	Chemistry
83UFT	Chamber, Constant Temperature (Environmental)	Microbiology

CONSTRAINED

87KXC	Prosthesis, Ankle, Non-Constrained	Orthopedics
87KMD	Prosthesis, Ankle, Semi-Constrained, Metal/Composite	Orthopedics
87HSN	Prosthesis, Ankle, Semi-Constrained, Metal/Polymer	Orthopedics
87JDC	Prosthesis, Elbow, Constrained	Orthopedics
87JDA	Prosthesis, Elbow, Non-Constrained, Unipolar	Orthopedics
87JDB	Prosthesis, Elbow, Semi-Constrained	Orthopedics
87LBC	Prosthesis, Finger, Constrained, Metal, Cemented	Orthopedics
87KWE	Prosthesis, Finger, Constrained, Metal, Uncemented	Orthopedics
87KWG	Prosthesis, Finger, Constrained, Metal/Polymer	Orthopedics
87KYJ	Prosthesis, Finger, Constrained, Polymer	Orthopedics
87KXD	Prosthesis, Hip, Constrained, Metal	Orthopedics
87KWZ	Prosthesis, Hip, Constrained, Metal/Polymer	Orthopedics
87MAZ	Prosthesis, Hip, Semi-Const., M/P, Por. Uncem., Calc./Phos.	Orthopedics
87LPH	Prosthesis, Hip, Semi-Const., Metal/Poly., Porous Uncemented	Orthopedics
87MIL	Prosthesis, Hip, Semi-Const., Uncem., M/P, Bone Morph. Prot.	Orthopedics
87MEH	Prosthesis, Hip, Semi-Const., Uncem., Non-P., M/P, Ca./Phos.	Orthopedics
87LZO	Prosthesis, Hip, Semi-Constr., Metal/Ceramic, Cemented/NC	Orthopedics
87JDL	Prosthesis, Hip, Semi-Constrained (Cemented Acetabular)	Orthopedics
87KWA	Prosthesis, Hip, Semi-Constrained Acetabular	Orthopedics
87JDI	Prosthesis, Hip, Semi-Constrained, Metal/Polymer	Orthopedics
87LWJ	Prosthesis, Hip, Semi-Constrained, Metal/Polymer, Uncemented	Orthopedics
87KMC	Prosthesis, Hip, Semi-constrained, Composite/metal	Orthopedics

CONSTRAINED *(cont'd)*

87MAY	Prosthesis, Hip, Semi-constrained, Metal/Ceramic/Polymer, Cemented or Non-porous Cemented, Osteophilic Finish	Orthopedics
87MBM	Prosthesis, Hip, Semi/Hemi-Const., M/PTFE Ctd./P, Cem./Unc.	Orthopedics
87KRN	Prosthesis, Knee, Femorotibial, Constrained, Metal	Orthopedics
87KRO	Prosthesis, Knee, Femorotibial, Constrained, Metal/Polymer	Orthopedics
87HSX	Prosthesis, Knee, Femorotibial, Non-Constrained	Orthopedics
87KTX	Prosthesis, Knee, Femorotibial, Non-Constrained, Metal	Orthopedics
87HRY	Prosthesis, Knee, Femorotibial, Semi-Constrained	Orthopedics
87KYK	Prosthesis, Knee, Femorotibial, Semi-Constrained, Metal	Orthopedics
87LGE	Prosthesis, Knee, Femorotibial, Semi-Constrained, Trunnion	Orthopedics
87KMB	Prosthesis, Knee, Non-Const. (M/C Reinf. Polyeth.) Cemented	Orthopedics
87KRR	Prosthesis, Knee, Patellofemoral, Semi-Constrained	Orthopedics
87KRP	Prosthesis, Knee, Patellofemorotibial, Constrained, Metal	Orthopedics
87KRQ	Prosthesis, Knee, Patellofemorotibial, Constrained, Polymer	Orthopedics
87JWH	Prosthesis, Knee, Patellofemorotibial, Semi-Constrained	Orthopedics
87MBV	Prosthesis, Knee, Patfem., S-C., UHMWPE, Pegged, Unc., P/M/P	Orthopedics
87MBH	Prosthesis, Knee, Patfem., S-C., Unc., Por., Ctd., P/M/P	Orthopedics
87MBA	Prosthesis, Knee, Patfem., Semi-Const., Unc., P/M/P, Osteo.	Orthopedics
87LXY	Prosthesis, Knee, Patfemotib., Semi-Const., P/M/P, Uncem.	Orthopedics
87KWR	Prosthesis, Shoulder, Constr., Metal/Metal or Polymer/Cem.	Orthopedics
87MJT	Prosthesis, Shoulder, Humeral, Bipol., Hemi-, Constr., M/P	Orthopedics
87KWT	Prosthesis, Shoulder, Non-Constrained, Metal/Polymer Cem.	Orthopedics
87KWS	Prosthesis, Shoulder, Semi-Constrained, Metal/Polymer Cem.	Orthopedics
87KYL	Prosthesis, Shoulder, Semi-Constrained, Uncemented	Orthopedics
87LZJ	Prosthesis, Toe (Metaphal.), Joint, Met./Poly., Semi-Const.	Orthopedics
87KWH	Prosthesis, Toe, Constrained, Polymer	Orthopedics
87KYN	Prosthesis, Wrist, Constrained, Metal	Orthopedics
87KIG	Prosthesis, Wrist, Constrained, Polymer	Orthopedics
87KWM	Prosthesis, Wrist, Semi-Constrained	Orthopedics

CONSTRICTOR

74WOZ	Occluder, Cardiovascular	Cardiovascular

CONSULTING

80VAS	Building Material	General
80WTQ	Service, Attorney, Patent	General
80VBN	Service, Consulting	General
80WIE	Service, Licensing, Device, Medical	General

CONSUMPTION

81GGQ	Test, Prothrombin Consumption	Hematology

CONTACT

80WQD	Accessories, Laser	General
86LYL	Accessories, Solution, Lens, Contact	Ophthalmology
86LRX	Case, Contact Lens	Ophthalmology
86LPN	Cleaner, Lens, Contact	Ophthalmology
85HGZ	Heater, Perineal, Direct Contact	Obstetrics/Gyn
85HHA	Heater, Perineal, Radiant, Non-Contact	Obstetrics/Gyn
86KYE	Inserter/Remover, Lens, Contact	Ophthalmology
78FHY	Jelly, Contact (For Transurethral Surgical Instrument)	Gastro/Urology
86HQD	Lens, Contact (Other Material)	Ophthalmology
86MWL	Lens, Contact(rigid Gas Permeable)-extended Wear	Ophthalmology
86ULH	Lens, Contact, Bifocal	Ophthalmology
86WIZ	Lens, Contact, Disposable	Ophthalmology
86ULD	Lens, Contact, Extended-Wear	Ophthalmology
86MRC	Lens, Contact, Gas-Permeable	Ophthalmology
86TGY	Lens, Contact, Hydrophilic	Ophthalmology
86HPX	Lens, Contact, Polymethylmethacrylate	Ophthalmology
86HJK	Lens, Contact, Polymethylmethacrylate, Diagnostic	Ophthalmology
86VJN	Lens, Contact, Tinted	Ophthalmology
86WZA	Lens, Contact, Trifocal	Ophthalmology
86LPL	Lenses, Soft Contact, Daily Wear	Ophthalmology
86LPM	Lenses, Soft Contact, Extended Wear	Ophthalmology
84HCS	Monitor, Temperature, Neurosurgery, Direct Contact, Powered	Cns/Neurology
88KIN	Stainer, Slide, Contact Type	Pathology
86LOH	System, Identification, Lens, Contact	Ophthalmology
86WNU	Unit, Examination, Lens, Contact	Ophthalmology

CONTAINED

80KLL	Monitor, Temperature (Self-Contained)	General

CONTAINER

81ULQ	Bag, Blood	Hematology
81KSR	Bag, Blood, Collection	Hematology
80WYL	Box, Transportation, Container, Specimen	General

CONTAINER *(cont'd)*
80WVU Cabinet, Storage, Catheter — General
80WUT Carrier, Container, Oxygen, Portable — General
86LRX Case, Contact Lens — Ophthalmology
83VFX Container, Cryobiological Storage — Microbiology
88KER Container, Embedding — Pathology
80TBL Container, Evacuated — General
80LPZ Container, Frozen Donor Tissue Storage — General
80KPE Container, IV — General
73VFY Container, Liquid Nitrogen — Anesthesiology
73VFZ Container, Liquid Oxygen — Anesthesiology
80KYW Container, Medication, Graduated Liquid — General
80WPQ Container, Medication, Home-Use — General
80MMK Container, Sharpes — General
83TDB Container, Slide Mailer — Microbiology
88KDT Container, Specimen Mailer And Storage — Pathology
88KDW Container, Specimen Mailer And Storage, Temperature Control — Pathology
80FMH Container, Specimen, All Types — General
79WYS Container, Specimen, Laparoscopic — Surgery
75MPQ Container, Specimen, Urine, Drugs Of Abuse, Over The Counter — Chemistry
80RVS Container, Sterilization (Tray) — General
90WJA Container, Substance, Radioactive — Radiology
79VEE Container, Surgical Instrument — Surgery
78KDK Container, Transport, Kidney — Gastro/Urology
80SEE Container, Urine Specimen — General
79QUA Cylinder, Carbon-Dioxide — Surgery
80RGZ Kit, Mid-Stream Collection — General
80WKH Monitor, Medication — General
80RVT Packaging, Sterilization — General
80KZD Pressure Infusor, IV Container — General
79SIO Rack, Instrument, Laparoscopy — Surgery
80LLC Supplementary Nitroglycerin Container — General
80WWJ Vial, Other — General
80FLH Washer, Receptacle, Waste, Body — General
80SFU Waste Receptacle, Contaminated — General

CONTAINING
88LDW Fixative, Acid Containing — Pathology
88LDZ Fixative, Alcohol Containing — Pathology
88LDY Fixative, Formalin Containing — Pathology
88LDX Fixative, Metallic Containing — Pathology
76MMT Resin, Filling, Root Canal (Containing Chloroform) — Dental And Oral
88KDX Solution, Pathology, Decalcifier, Acid Containing — Pathology

CONTAMINATED
80WVR Cart, Waste — General
80SFU Waste Receptacle, Contaminated — General

CONTAMINATION
80FRF Equipment, Cleaning, Air — General
80QDR Monitor, Biological (Contamination Testing) — General
80WIP Monitor, Contamination, Environmental, Personal — General

CONTENTS
78FJZ Tray, Declotting (Including Contents) — Gastro/Urology
78FKG Tray, Start/Stop (Including Contents), Dialysis — Gastro/Urology

CONTINENT
78KPH Catheter, Rectal, Ileostomy, Continent — Gastro/Urology
78KPG Continent Colostomy Magnet — Gastro/Urology

CONTINUOUS
75JJC Analyzer, Chemistry, Sequential Multiple, Continuous Flow — Chemistry
73RJI Analyzer, Gas, Oxygen, Continuous Controller — Anesthesiology
73RJJ Analyzer, Gas, Oxygen, Continuous Monitor — Anesthesiology
73CAT Cannula, Nasal, Oxygen — Anesthesiology
74KRA Catheter, Continuous Flush — Cardiovascular
79GBQ Catheter, Continuous Irrigation — Surgery
75UKI Centrifuge, Continuous Flow — Chemistry
73QMH Continuous Positive Airway Pressure Unit (CPAP, CPPB) — Anesthesiology
89IOO Exerciser, Passive, Non-Measuring (CPM Machine) — Physical Med
73RLV Monitor, Airway Pressure, Continuous — Anesthesiology
84GWM Monitor, Intracranial Pressure, Continuous — Cns/Neurology
79KFS Monitor, Po2, Continuous — Surgery
78RKL Peritoneal Dialysis Unit (CAPD) — Gastro/Urology
78FKX System, Peritoneal Dialysis, Automatic — Gastro/Urology
80FLL Thermometer, Electronic, Continuous — General
74QHI Valve, Catheter Flush, Continuous — Cardiovascular
73CBK Ventilator, Continuous (Respirator) — Anesthesiology
73MOD Ventilator, Continuous (Respirator), Accessory — Anesthesiology
73KLM Ventilator, Continuous, Hyperbaric — Anesthesiology
73MNT Ventilator, Continuous, Minimal Ventilatory Support, Facility Use — Anesthesiology
73MNS Ventilator, Continuous, Non-Life Supporting — Anesthesiology
73BZD Ventilator, Non-Continuous (Respirator) — Anesthesiology

CONTOUR
89LDK Sensor, Optical Contour, Physical Medicine — Physical Med

CONTOURING
76EKF Contouring, Instrument, Matrix, Operative — Dental And Oral
87HXP Instrument, Bending (Contouring) — Orthopedics

CONTRA-ANGLE
76EGS Handpiece, Contra- And Right-Angle Attachment, Dental — Dental And Oral

CONTRACEPTION
85MPT Calculator, Contraception — Obstetrics/Gyn

CONTRACEPTIVE
85HFY Band, Occlusion, Tubal — Obstetrics/Gyn
85HGB Clip, Tubal Occlusion — Obstetrics/Gyn
85HIS Condom — Obstetrics/Gyn
85LLQ Contraceptive Cervical Cap — Obstetrics/Gyn
85LLS Contraceptive Tubal Occlusion Device, Male — Obstetrics/Gyn
85MEE Device, Fertility, Contraceptive, Diagnostic — Obstetrics/Gyn
85HDW Diaphragm, Contraceptive — Obstetrics/Gyn
85RAL Hook, IUD Removal — Obstetrics/Gyn
85HHS Insert, Tubal Occlusion — Obstetrics/Gyn
85HDT Intrauterine Device, Contraceptive (IUD) And Introducer — Obstetrics/Gyn
85HDS Introducer, Contraceptive Diaphragm — Obstetrics/Gyn
85WSK Meter, Cavity, Intrauterine — Obstetrics/Gyn
85RKO Pessary, Diaphragm — Obstetrics/Gyn
85HHW Pessary, Vaginal — Obstetrics/Gyn
80FQT Prophylactic (Condom) — General
85HHF Remover, Intrauterine Device, Contraceptive (Hook Type) — Obstetrics/Gyn
85LLR Sponge, Contraceptive — Obstetrics/Gyn
85KNH Tubal Occlusive Device — Obstetrics/Gyn

CONTRACT
80VAS Building Material — General
80WUF Clamp, Tubing — General
80WKG Component, Electrical — General
80VAF Component, Electronic — General
80WOS Component, Metal, Other — General
80SHS Component, Optical — General
80WXA Component, Other — General
80VAE Component, Plastic — General
80VAL Component, Rubber — General
80VAM Component, Silicone — General
80WSN Computer Software, Industrial — General
80WVW Contract Assembly — General
80VAB Contract Laboratory — General
80VAC Contract Manufacturing — General
80WXH Contract Manufacturing, Pharmaceuticals/Chemicals — General
80WLY Contract Manufacturing, Product, Disposable — General
80WLX Contract Manufacturing, Product, Durable — General
80WLH Contract Manufacturing, Reagent — General
80VAO Contract Packaging — General
80VAN Contract R&D, Diagnostics — General
80WUH Contract R&D, Equipment — General
80VAD Contract Sterilization — General
80VAJ Equipment, Extruding/Molding — General
80WXE Equipment, Molding — General
80WJB Material, Raw, Production — General
80WYJ Molding, Injection — General
80VAP Production Equipment — General
80WVQ Service, Engraving — General
80WWR Service, Modification, Product — General
80WYM Service, Printing — General
80WYK Thermoforming, Extrusion, Custom — General

CONTRACTION
85HFM Monitor, Uterine Contraction, External — Obstetrics/Gyn

CONTRACTOR
79FZR Contractor, Surgical — Surgery

CONTRAST
85MGJ Contrast Echocardiograph — Obstetrics/Gyn
83RGS Contrast Enhancement Unit, Microscope — Microbiology
90IZQ Injector, Contrast Medium, Automatic — Radiology
84RCB Injector, Lymphangiographic — Cns/Neurology
90KTA Media, Contrast, Radiologic — Radiology
90MJS Media, Contrast, Ultrasound — Radiology
90UJW Media, Gastroenterographic Contrast (Barium Sulfate) — Radiology
90VGX Media, Radioactive Isotope Contrast — Radiology
90VGW Media, Radiographic Injectable Contrast — Radiology
88IBM Microscope, Phase Contrast — Pathology

CONTROL
79QTS Adapter, Unit, Electrosurgical, Hand-Controlled — Surgery
89LFF Aid, Control, Environmental, Controlled, Breath — Physical Med
82DBC Alpha 2, 2N-Glycoprotein, Antigen, Antiserum, Control — Immunology
82MGA Alpha-1 Microglobulin, Antigen, Antiserum, Control — Immunology
82LKL Alpha-1-Acid-Glycoprotein, Antigen, Antiserum, Control — Immunology
82DEX Alpha-1-B-Glycoprotein, Antigen, Antiserum, Control — Immunology
82DER Alpha-1-Lipoprotein, Antigen, Antiserum, Control — Immunology
82DEN Alpha-1-T-Glycoprotein, Antigen, Antiserum, Control — Immunology

CONTROL *(cont'd)*

82DAW	Alpha-2-AP-Glycoprotein, Antigen, Antiserum, Control	Immunology
82LRM	Anti-DNA Antibody (Enzyme-Labeled), Antigen, Control	Immunology
82LSW	Anti-DNA Antibody, Antigen and Control	Immunology
82LKO	Anti-RNP-Antibody, Antigen And Control	Immunology
82LKP	Anti-SM-Antibody, Antigen And Control	Immunology
82DCF	Antigen, Antiserum, Control, Albumin	Immunology
82DDZ	Antigen, Antiserum, Control, Albumin, FITC	Immunology
82DCM	Antigen, Antiserum, Control, Albumin, Fraction V	Immunology
82DFJ	Antigen, Antiserum, Control, Albumin, Rhodamine	Immunology
82DCO	Antigen, Antiserum, Control, Alpha Globulin	Immunology
82DFF	Antigen, Antiserum, Control, Alpha-1-Antichymotrypsin	Immunology
82DEM	Antigen, Antiserum, Control, Alpha-1-Antitrypsin	Immunology
82DEI	Antigen, Antiserum, Control, Alpha-1-Antitrypsin, FITC	Immunology
82DFB	Antigen, Antiserum, Control, Alpha-1-Antitrypsin, Rhodamine	Immunology
82DEJ	Antigen, Antiserum, Control, Alpha-2-Glycoproteins	Immunology
82DEF	Antigen, Antiserum, Control, Alpha-2-HS-Glycoprotein	Immunology
82DEB	Antigen, Antiserum, Control, Alpha-2-Macroglobulin	Immunology
82DDQ	Antigen, Antiserum, Control, Antithrombin III	Immunology
82CZQ	Antigen, Antiserum, Control, Bence-Jones Protein	Immunology
82DDN	Antigen, Antiserum, Control, Beta 2-Glycoprotein I	Immunology
82DCJ	Antigen, Antiserum, Control, Beta Globulin	Immunology
82DHX	Antigen, Antiserum, Control, Carcinoembryonic Antigen	Immunology
82DDB	Antigen, Antiserum, Control, Ceruloplasmin	Immunology
82DCY	Antigen, Antiserum, Control, Ceruloplasmin, FITC	Immunology
82DCT	Antigen, Antiserum, Control, Ceruloplasmin, Rhodamine	Immunology
82DAK	Antigen, Antiserum, Control, Complement C1q	Immunology
82DAI	Antigen, Antiserum, Control, Complement C1r	Immunology
82CZY	Antigen, Antiserum, Control, Complement C1s	Immunology
82CZW	Antigen, Antiserum, Control, Complement C3	Immunology
82DBI	Antigen, Antiserum, Control, Complement C4	Immunology
82DAY	Antigen, Antiserum, Control, Complement C5	Immunology
82DAG	Antigen, Antiserum, Control, Complement C8	Immunology
82DAE	Antigen, Antiserum, Control, Complement C9	Immunology
82DCE	Antigen, Antiserum, Control, FAB	Immunology
82DCB	Antigen, Antiserum, Control, FAB, FITC	Immunology
82DBY	Antigen, Antiserum, Control, FAB, Rhodamine	Immunology
82JZH	Antigen, Antiserum, Control, Factor B	Immunology
82DBT	Antigen, Antiserum, Control, Factor XIII A, S	Immunology
82DBF	Antigen, Antiserum, Control, Ferritin	Immunology
82DBD	Antigen, Antiserum, Control, Fibrin	Immunology
82DAZ	Antigen, Antiserum, Control, Fibrinogen And Split Products	Immunology
82DAJ	Antigen, Antiserum, Control, Free Secretory Component	Immunology
82DAH	Antigen, Antiserum, Control, Gamma Globulin	Immunology
82DAF	Antigen, Antiserum, Control, Gamma Globulin, FITC	Immunology
82DAD	Antigen, Antiserum, Control, Haptoglobin	Immunology
82DAB	Antigen, Antiserum, Control, Haptoglobin, FITC	Immunology
82CZZ	Antigen, Antiserum, Control, Haptoglobin, Rhodamine	Immunology
82CZX	Antigen, Antiserum, Control, Hemopexin	Immunology
82CZT	Antigen, Antiserum, Control, Hemopexin, FITC	Immunology
82CZR	Antigen, Antiserum, Control, Hemopexin, Rhodamine	Immunology
82CZP	Antigen, Antiserum, Control, IGA	Immunology
82CZN	Antigen, Antiserum, Control, IGA, FITC	Immunology
82CZL	Antigen, Antiserum, Control, IGA, Peroxidase	Immunology
82CZK	Antigen, Antiserum, Control, IGA, Rhodamine	Immunology
82CZJ	Antigen, Antiserum, Control, IGD	Immunology
82DGG	Antigen, Antiserum, Control, IGD, FITC	Immunology
82DGH	Antigen, Antiserum, Control, IGD, Peroxidase	Immunology
82DGE	Antigen, Antiserum, Control, IGD, Rhodamine	Immunology
82DGC	Antigen, Antiserum, Control, IGE	Immunology
82DGP	Antigen, Antiserum, Control, IGE, FITC	Immunology
82DGO	Antigen, Antiserum, Control, IGE, Peroxidase	Immunology
82DGL	Antigen, Antiserum, Control, IGE, Rhodamine	Immunology
82DEW	Antigen, Antiserum, Control, IGG	Immunology
82DFK	Antigen, Antiserum, Control, IGG (FAB Fragment Specific)	Immunology
82DAS	Antigen, Antiserum, Control, IGG (Fc Fragment Specific)	Immunology
82DFZ	Antigen, Antiserum, Control, IGG (Gamma Chain Specific)	Immunology
82DGK	Antigen, Antiserum, Control, IGG, FITC	Immunology
82DAA	Antigen, Antiserum, Control, IGG, Peroxidase	Immunology
82DFO	Antigen, Antiserum, Control, IGG, Rhodamine	Immunology
82DFT	Antigen, Antiserum, Control, IGM	Immunology
82DAO	Antigen, Antiserum, Control, IGM (Mu Chain Specific)	Immunology
82DFS	Antigen, Antiserum, Control, IGM, FITC	Immunology
82DEY	Antigen, Antiserum, Control, IGM, Peroxidase	Immunology
82DEZ	Antigen, Antiserum, Control, IGM, Rhodamine	Immunology
82CZO	Antigen, Antiserum, Control, Inter-Alpha Trypsin Inhibitor	Immunology
82DFH	Antigen, Antiserum, Control, Kappa	Immunology
82DEO	Antigen, Antiserum, Control, Kappa, FITC	Immunology
82DEK	Antigen, Antiserum, Control, Kappa, Rhodamine	Immunology
82DEG	Antigen, Antiserum, Control, Lactoferrin	Immunology
82DEH	Antigen, Antiserum, Control, Lambda	Immunology
82DES	Antigen, Antiserum, Control, Lambda, FITC	Immunology
82DFG	Antigen, Antiserum, Control, Lambda, Rhodamine	Immunology
82DFC	Antigen, Antiserum, Control, Lipoprotein, Low Density	Immunology
82DHP	Antigen, Antiserum, Control, Luteinizing Hormone	Immunology
82DGS	Antigen, Antiserum, Control, Lymphocyte Typing	Immunology

CONTROL *(cont'd)*

82DED	Antigen, Antiserum, Control, Lysozyme	Immunology
82DDR	Antigen, Antiserum, Control, Myoglobin	Immunology
82DGX	Antigen, Antiserum, Control, Ng1M(A)	Immunology
82WNJ	Antigen, Antiserum, Control, Other	Immunology
82DDX	Antigen, Antiserum, Control, Plasminogen	Immunology
82JZJ	Antigen, Antiserum, Control, Prealbumin	Immunology
82DDS	Antigen, Antiserum, Control, Prealbumin, FITC	Immunology
82DHL	Antigen, Antiserum, Control, Protein, Complement	Immunology
82DDF	Antigen, Antiserum, Control, Prothrombin	Immunology
81JZK	Antigen, Antiserum, Control, Red Cells	Hematology
82DFQ	Antigen, Antiserum, Control, Sperm	Immunology
82DFI	Antigen, Antiserum, Control, Spinal Fluid, Total	Immunology
82DDG	Antigen, Antiserum, Control, Transferrin	Immunology
82DDI	Antigen, Antiserum, Control, Transferrin, FITC	Immunology
82DDD	Antigen, Antiserum, Control, Transferrin, Rhodamine	Immunology
82DGR	Antigen, Antiserum, Control, Whole Human Serum	Immunology
83GOD	Antigen, CF (Including CF Control), Adenovirus 1-33	Microbiology
83GNG	Antigen, CF (Including CF Control), Coxsackievirus A 1-24	Microbiology
83GQH	Antigen, CF (Including CF Control), Cytomegalovirus	Microbiology
83GNL	Antigen, CF (Including CF Control), Echovirus 1-34	Microbiology
83GNQ	Antigen, CF (Including CF Control), Epstein-Barr Virus	Microbiology
83GQD	Antigen, CF (Including CF Control), Equine Encephalitis	Microbiology
83GNX	Antigen, CF (Including CF Control), Influenza Virus	Microbiology
83GRC	Antigen, CF (Including CF Control), Mumps Virus	Microbiology
83GQS	Antigen, CF (Including CF Control), Parainfluenza Virus	Microbiology
83GOH	Antigen, CF (Including CF Control), Poliovirus 1-3	Microbiology
83GQB	Antigen, CF (Including CF Control), Reovirus 1-3	Microbiology
83GON	Antigen, CF (Including CF Control), Rubella	Microbiology
83GRJ	Antigen, CF, (Including CF Control), Rubeola	Microbiology
83GQW	Antigen, CF, (Including CF Control), Varicella-Zoster	Microbiology
83GQN	Antigen, Cf (including Cf Control), Herpesvirus Hominis 1, 2	Microbiology
83GOB	Antigen, HA (Including HA Control), Adenovirus 1-33	Microbiology
83GNT	Antigen, HA (Including HA Control), Influenza Virus	Microbiology
83GQY	Antigen, HA (Including HA Control), Mumps Virus	Microbiology
83GQR	Antigen, HA (Including HA Control), Parainfluenza Virus	Microbiology
83GQA	Antigen, HA (Including HA Control), Reovirus 1-3	Microbiology
83GOL	Antigen, HA (Including HA Control), Rubella	Microbiology
83GRH	Antigen, HA (Including HA Control), Rubeola	Microbiology
83JWK	Antigen, Positive Control, Cryptococcus Neoformans	Microbiology
82LKJ	Antinuclear Antibody, Antigen, Control	Immunology
82DBJ	Antiparietal Antibody, Immunofluorescent, Antigen, Control	Immunology
83GPE	Antisera, Positive Control, Echinococcus SPP.	Microbiology
82DDY	Antiserum, Antigen, Control, FITC, Alpha-2-Macroglobulin	Immunology
83GMP	Antiserum, Control For Non-Treponemal Test	Microbiology
83GOK	Antiserum, HAI (Including HAI Control), Rubella	Microbiology
83GSN	Antiserum, Positive And Negative Febrile Antigen Control	Microbiology
83KFG	Antiserum, Positive Control, Aspergillus SPP.	Microbiology
83KFH	Antiserum, Positive Control, Blastomyces Dermatitidis	Microbiology
83GMH	Antiserum, Positive Control, Coccidioides Immitis	Microbiology
83GMK	Antiserum, Positive Control, Histoplasma Capsulatum	Microbiology
80TCV	Bag, Laundry, Infection Control	General
74DSP	Balloon, Intra-Aortic (With Control System)	Cardiovascular
90IWX	Barrier, Control Panel, X-Ray, Moveable	Radiology
82DDK	Beta-2-Glycoprotein III, Antigen, Antiserum, Control	Immunology
82DGM	Breast Milk, Antigen, Antiserum, Control	Immunology
82DGN	Breast Milk, FITC, Antigen, Antiserum, Control	Immunology
82DGI	Breast Milk, Rhodamine, Antigen, Antiserum, Control	Immunology
80QFG	Cabinet, Narcotic Control	General
82DDH	Carbonicanhydrase B, Antigen, Antiserum, Control	Immunology
82DDE	Carbonicanhydrase C, Antigen, Antiserum, Control	Immunology
91DCQ	Cholinesterase, Antigen, Antiserum, Control	Toxicology
82DGA	Cohn Fraction II, Antigen, Antiserum, Control	Immunology
82DGJ	Colostrum, Antigen, Antiserum, Control	Immunology
80VFR	Computer, Bar Code	General
88KDW	Container, Specimen Mailer And Storage, Temperature Control	Pathology
74DXX	Control System, Catheter, Steerable	Cardiovascular
80VBT	Control System, Energy	General
91DKC	Control, Alcohol	Toxicology
75JJX	Control, Analyte (Assayed And Unassayed)	Chemistry
82DAC	Control, Antiserum, Antigen, Activator, C3, Complement	Immunology
75JJS	Control, Blood Gas	Chemistry
81JCN	Control, Cell Counter, Normal And Abnormal	Hematology
81GGN	Control, Coagulation, Plasma	Hematology
81UJQ	Control, Coombs	Hematology
91DIF	Control, Drug Mixture	Toxicology
91LAS	Control, Drug Specific	Toxicology
75JJR	Control, Electrolyte (Assayed And Unassayed)	Chemistry
75JJT	Control, Enzyme (Assayed And Unassayed)	Chemistry
89KHZ	Control, Foot Driving, Automobile, Mechanical	Physical Med
89IPQ	Control, Hand Driving, Automobile, Mechanical	Physical Med
91DIE	Control, Heavy Metals	Toxicology
81GGM	Control, Hemoglobin	Hematology
81JCM	Control, Hemoglobin, Abnormal	Hematology
75JJY	Control, Multi Analyte, All Kinds (Assayed And Unassayed)	Chemistry

CONTROL (cont'd)

83LSC	Control, Neisseria	Microbiology
81GGC	Control, Plasma, Abnormal	Hematology
81GJP	Control, Platelet	Hematology
81GJR	Control, Red Cell	Hematology
75JJW	Control, Urinalysis (Assayed And Unassayed)	Chemistry
81GGL	Control, White Cell	Hematology
82DHF	D/KM-1, Antigen, Antiserum, Control	Immunology
89IQA	Environmental Control System, Powered	Physical Med
89ILR	Environmental Control System, Powered, Remote	Physical Med
82MLE	Enzyme, Immunoassay, Antipartietal, Antigen Control	Immunology
80WLA	Equipment, Control, Pollution	General
80WQM	Equipment/Service, Quality Control	General
82LLL	Extractable Antinuclear Antibody (Rnp/Sm), Antigen/Control	Immunology
82DBN	FC, Antigen, Antiserum, Control	Immunology
82DBK	FC, FITC, Antigen, Antiserum, Control	Immunology
82DBH	FC, Rhodamine, Antigen, Antiserum, Control	Immunology
82DBB	Fibrin, FITC, Antigen, Antiserum, Control	Immunology
81DAT	Fibrin. & Split Products, Peroxidase, Antigen, Antis., Cont.	Hematology
82DAN	Fibrinopeptide A, Antigen, Antiserum, Control	Immunology
82DAL	Fraction IV-5, Antigen, Antiserum, Control	Immunology
82KHT	Fraction V, Antigen, Antiserum, Control	Immunology
81GLK	Hematocrit Control	Hematology
81JPK	Hematology Quality Control Mixture	Hematology
82DAM	Hemoglobin, Chain Specific, Antigen, Antiserum, Control	Immunology
90LNE	Hyperthermia System, Automatic Control	Radiology
90LNF	Hyperthermia System, Manual Control	Radiology
82CZM	IGA, Ferritin, Antigen, Antiserum, Control	Immunology
82DFM	IGE, Ferritin, Antigen, Antiserum, Control	Immunology
82DAQ	IGG (FD Fragment Specific), Antigen, Antiserum, Control	Immunology
82DGD	IGG, Ferritin, Antigen, Antiserum, Control	Immunology
82DFL	IGM, Ferritin, Antigen, Antiserum, Control	Immunology
82DGT	INV-1, Antigen, Antiserum, Control	Immunology
82DEC	Inter-Alpha Trypsin, FITC, Antigen, Antiserum, Control	Immunology
82DFD	Kappa, Peroxidase, Antigen, Antiserum, Control	Immunology
83MKA	Kit, Direct Antigen, Negative Control	Microbiology
83MJZ	Kit, Direct Antigen, Positive Control	Microbiology
83JTR	Kit, Quality Control	Microbiology
81KSF	Kit, Quality Control, Blood Banking	Hematology
83MJY	Kit, Serological, Negative Control	Microbiology
83MJX	Kit, Serological, Positive Control	Microbiology
82DET	Lactic Dehydrogenase, Antigen, Antiserum, Control	Immunology
82DEP	Lambda, Peroxidase, Antigen, Antiserum, Control	Immunology
82DEL	Lipoprotein X, Antigen, Antiserum, Control	Immunology
80WKE	Mask, Face	General
91LAX	Material, Control, Lidocaine	Toxicology
91LAY	Methotrexate Control Materials	Toxicology
81GLQ	Mixture, Control, Indices, White and Red Cell	Hematology
79SIG	Module, Control, Electrosurgery	Surgery
90SGL	Monitor, X-Ray Film Processor Quality Control	Radiology
82DEA	Myoglobin, FITC, Antigen, Antiserum, Control	Immunology
82DDO	Myoglobin, Rhodamine, Antigen, Antiserum, Control	Immunology
91LAZ	N-Acetylprocainamide Control Materials	Toxicology
82DHI	NG3M(BO), Antigen, Antiserum, Control	Immunology
82DHQ	NG3M(G), Antigen, Antiserum, Control	Immunology
82DHY	NG4M(A), Antigen, Antiserum, Control	Immunology
81GIT	Partial Thromboplastin Time, Reagent, Control	Hematology
81GIL	Plasma, Control, Fibrinogen	Hematology
81GIZ	Plasma, Control, Normal	Hematology
82DFN	Platelets, Antigen, Antiserum, Control	Immunology
82JZI	Platelets, FITC, Antigen, Antiserum, Control	Immunology
82DFR	Platelets, Rhodamine, Antigen, Antiserum, Control	Immunology
80SHO	Polariscope	General
91LBA	Procainamide Control Materials	Toxicology
74DSO	Prosthesis, Heart, With Control System	Cardiovascular
80WRB	Reagent, Quality Control	General
81GGO	Reagent, Thromboplastin, With Control	Hematology
82DGF	Red Cells, FITC, Antigen, Antiserum, Control	Immunology
82DFW	Red Cells, Rhodamine, Antigen, Antiserum, Control	Immunology
82CZS	Retinol-Binding Protein, Antigen, Antiserum, Control	Immunology
82DGB	Seminal Fluid, Antigen, Antiserum, Control	Immunology
91DJK	Serum, Control, Digitoxin, RIA	Toxicology
91DMP	Serum, Control, Digoxin, RIA	Toxicology
83GMR	Serum, Reactive And Non-Specific Control, FTA-ABS Test	Microbiology
83LJG	Slide, Control, Quality	Microbiology
78VKQ	Solution, Ostomy, Odor Control	Gastro/Urology
82DFX	Sperm, FITC, Antigen, Antiserum, Control	Immunology
75UKC	Standard/Control, All Types	Chemistry
81GFK	Standard/Control, Fibrinogen Determination	Hematology
81GFS	Standard/Control, Hemoglobin, Normal/Abnormal	Hematology
78FLC	Station, Dialysis Control, Negative Pressure Type	Gastro/Urology
74MFZ	System, Pump & Control, Cardiac Assist, Axial Flow	Cardiovascular
91LAW	Theophylline Control Materials	Toxicology
82DEE	Thrombin, Antigen, Antiserum, Control	Immunology
82DDC	Thyroglobulin, Antigen, Antiserum, Control	Immunology
82DDJ	Thyroglobulin, FITC, Antigen, Antiserum, Control	Immunology
82DDL	Thyroglobulin, Rhodamine, Antigen, Antiserum, Control	Immunology

CONTROL (cont'd)

80WPL	Unit, Control, Bed, Patient, Powered	General
82DGQ	Whole Human Plasma, Antigen, Antiserum, Control	Immunology

CONTROLLED

79QTS	Adapter, Unit, Electrosurgical, Hand-Controlled	Surgery
89LFF	Aid, Control, Environmental, Controlled, Breath	Physical Med
90JAQ	Applicator, Radionuclide, Remote-Controlled	Radiology
79UEB	Electrode, Electrosurgical, Active, Foot Controlled	Surgery
80MEA	Pump, Infusion, Patient Controlled Analgesia (PCA)	General

CONTROLLER

73RJI	Analyzer, Gas, Oxygen, Continuous Controller	Anesthesiology
85HGG	Controller, Abortion Unit, Vacuum	Obstetrics/Gyn
76EBW	Controller, Foot, Handpiece And Cord	Dental And Oral
74DTX	Controller, Gas, Cardiopulmonary Bypass	Cardiovascular
80LHE	Controller, Glucose, Blood, Closed-Loop	General
78QZY	Controller, Hemodialysis Unit Single Needle	Gastro/Urology
74QMI	Controller, Infusion	Cardiovascular
80LDR	Controller, Infusion, Intravascular	General
74QMJ	Controller, Infusion, Intravenous	Cardiovascular
73BSC	Controller, Infusion, Manual	Anesthesiology
73CAJ	Controller, Infusion, Powered	Anesthesiology
74DQF	Controller, Injector, Angiographic	Cardiovascular
73QMK	Controller, Oxygen (Blender)	Anesthesiology
80LSX	Controller, Pressure, Blood, Closed-Loop	General
74DWA	Controller, Pump Speed, Cardiopulmonary Bypass	Cardiovascular
74DWD	Controller, Suction, Intracardiac, Cardiopulmonary Bypass	Cardiovascular
74DWC	Controller, Temperature, Cardiopulmonary Bypass	Cardiovascular
80QML	Controller, Temperature, Humidifier	General
80QMM	Controller, Temperature, Other	General
75VGA	Controller, Temperature, Programmable	Chemistry
90EGT	Controller, Temperature, Radiographic	Radiology
73SET	Controller, Ventilator IMV	Anesthesiology
75UHE	Controller, pH	Chemistry
74QMS	Counter, Intravenous Drop	Cardiovascular
73BZE	Heater, Breathing System W/Wo Controller	Anesthesiology
75JRR	Regulator, Temperature	Chemistry

CONTROLS

83GQG	Antigen, CF (Including CF Controls), Respiratory Syncytial	Microbiology
82LJM	Antinuclear Antibody (Enzyme-Labeled), Antigen, Controls	Immunology

CONVERSION

75JLG	Conversion Ferric Hydroxymates (Colorimetric), Fatty Acids	Chemistry
75JLA	Conversion To Creatinine, Creatine	Chemistry

CONVERTER

78QZZ	Converter, Unit, Hemodialysis, Single-Pass	Gastro/Urology

CONVERTING

75KQN	Radioassay, Angiotensin Converting Enzyme	Chemistry

CONVEYOR

80TGS	Conveyor, Guided Vehicle	General
80TFG	Conveyor, Tray	General
80TDT	Delivery System, Pneumatic Tube	General

CONVOLUTED

80RMC	Pad, Pressure, Foam Convoluted	General

COOLANT

89MLY	Refrigerant, Topical (Vapocoolant)	Physical Med

COOLER

78FBY	Cooler, Esophageal and Gastric	Gastro/Urology
78FBZ	Cooler, Prostatic	Gastro/Urology

COOLING

80TBU	Dispenser, Ice	General
75UFU	Plate, Cooling	Chemistry
79WOH	System, Cooling, Laser	Surgery
74WIU	Unit, Cooling, Cardiac	Cardiovascular

COOMBS

81KSM	Analyzer, Coombs, Automated	Hematology
83GMS	Anti-Human Globulin, FTA-ABS Test (Coombs)	Microbiology
81UJQ	Control, Coombs	Hematology

COPIER

90WUK	Copier, Image, Radiographic	Radiology

COPPER

75CFW	Copper Reduction, Glucose	Chemistry
75JKZ	Diethyldithiocarbamate (Colorimetric), Copper	Chemistry
82JFR	Indirect Copper Assay, Ceruloplasmin	Immunology
75JKY	Oxalydihydrazide (Spectroscopic), Copper	Chemistry
81KSL	Solution, Copper Sulfate, For Specific Gravity Test	Hematology

CORD

79WDY	Accessories, Electrical Power (Electrocautery)	Surgery
87HXF	Accessories, Traction (Cart, Frame, Cord, Weight)	Orthopedics

CORD *(cont'd)*
78FHC Adapter, Cord, Instrument, Surgical, Transurethral — Gastro/Urology
77MGF Collagen, Injectable (For Vocal Cord Augmentation) — Ear/Nose/Throat
80WKG Component, Electrical — General
76EBW Controller, Foot, Handpiece And Cord — Dental And Oral
78FFZ Cord, Electric, Endoscope — Gastro/Urology
78FBJ Cord, Electric, Instrument, Surgical, Transurethral — Gastro/Urology
76MVL Cord, Retraction — Dental And Oral
84LWC Device, Hypothermia, Injury, Cord, Spinal — Cns/Neurology
84LGW Stimulator, Cerebellar, Full Implant (Pain Relief) — Cns/Neurology
84LGT Stimulator, Cord, Spinal, Implantable (Motor Disorders) — Cns/Neurology
84LLE Stimulator, Cord, Spinal, Implantable (Periph. Vasc. Dis.) — Cns/Neurology
84GZB Stimulator, Spinal Cord, Implantable (Pain Relief) — Cns/Neurology
84GZD Stimulator, Spinal Cord, Implantable, Bladder Evacuator — Cns/Neurology
77MIX System, Vocal Cord Medialization — Ear/Nose/Throat
80SAD Tester, Resistance, Line Cord — General

CORDOTOMY
77RAJ Hook, Cordotomy — Ear/Nose/Throat

CORE
83LOM Hepatitis B Test (B Core, BE Antigen & Antibody, B Core IGM) — Microbiology

CORK
80WNN Stopper — General

CORKSCREW
87HWI Corkscrew — Orthopedics

CORNEA
86HRG Accessories, Engine, Trephine, AC-Powered — Ophthalmology
79HRF Accessories, Engine, Trephine, Battery-Powered — Surgery
79HLD Accessories, Engine, Trephine, Gas-Powered — Surgery
86WUA Implant, Scleral — Ophthalmology
86WQL Pachometer — Ophthalmology
86HNJ Punch, Corneo-Scleral — Ophthalmology

CORNEAL
86HQS Burr, Corneal, AC-Powered — Ophthalmology
86HOG Burr, Corneal, Battery-Powered — Ophthalmology
86HOF Burr, Corneal, Manual — Ophthalmology
86HLZ Electrode, Corneal — Ophthalmology
86VEX Elevator, Corneal — Ophthalmology
86LQE Implant, Corneal — Ophthalmology
86HJB Measurer, Corneal Radius — Ophthalmology
86LYX Media, Storage, Corneal — Ophthalmology
86RRD Scissors, Corneal — Ophthalmology
86WRV Shield, Corneal — Ophthalmology
86MOE Shield, Corneal, Collagen — Ophthalmology
86WXT System, Mapping, Corneal — Ophthalmology
86WQU Tissue, Corneal — Ophthalmology
86MMQ Topographer, Corneal — Ophthalmology
86HRH Trephine, Manual, Ophthalmic (Corneal) — Ophthalmology

CORNEO-SCLERAL
86HNJ Punch, Corneo-Scleral — Ophthalmology

CORNER
80TBM Bumper Guard, Corner — General

CORONARY
74MKG Balloon, Angioplasty, Coronary, Heated — Cardiovascular
74QFY Cannula, Coronary Artery — Cardiovascular
74LOX Catheter, Angioplasty, Coronary, Transluminal, Percut. Oper. — Cardiovascular
74MJR Catheter, Angioplasty, Coronary, Ultrasonic — Cardiovascular
74QHR Catheter, Coronary Perfusion — Cardiovascular
74MCX Catheter, Coronary, Atherectomy — Cardiovascular
74MGC Catheter, Myoplasty, Laser, Coronary — Cardiovascular
74DXS Gauge, Pressure, Coronary, Cardiopulmonary Bypass — Cardiovascular
74WTR Guide, Catheter — Cardiovascular
74LPC Laser, Angioplasty, Coronary — Cardiovascular
74WTT Legging, Compression, Inflatable, Sequential — Cardiovascular
74LPE System, Retroperfusion, Artery, Coronary — Cardiovascular

CORRECTIVE
89KNP Orthosis, Corrective Shoe — Physical Med

CORRIDOR
80TGZ Mirror, Corridor Safety — General

CORRUGATED
78EYT Sheath, Corrugated Rubber — Gastro/Urology
80SDM Tubing, Corrugated — General

CORSET
87QMN Corset — Orthopedics

CORTEX
84MFM Stimulator, Cortex, Visual, Implanted — Cns/Neurology

CORTICAL
84GYC Electrode, Cortical — Cns/Neurology
84MFO Electrode, Recording, Cortical, Implanted — Cns/Neurology
77MKP Hearing-Aid, Cortical, Shafer — Ear/Nose/Throat
84MHF Stimulator, Cortical, Implanted (Pain Relief) — Cns/Neurology

CORTICOIDS
75CHE Radioimmunoassay, Corticoids — Chemistry

CORTICOSTERONE
75CHA Radioimmunoassay, Corticosterone — Chemistry

CORTISOL
75JFT Fluorometric, Cortisol — Chemistry
75CGR Radioimmunoassay, Cortisol — Chemistry

CORYNEBACTERIUM
83KFI Corynebacterium Diphtheriae, Virulence Strip — Microbiology

COT
78EYX Drape, Pure Latex Sheet, With Self-Retaining Finger Cot — Gastro/Urology
80LZB Finger Cot — General
80WKO Stretcher, Collapsible — General
80FPP Stretcher, Hand-Carried — General
89INJ Stretcher, Wheeled, Mechanical — Physical Med

COTININE
91MRS Test System, Nicotine, Cotinine, Metabolites — Toxicology

COTTON
76DZQ Applicator, Cotton — Dental And Oral
80GDP Applicator, Cotton/Dye — General
80QMO Ball, Cotton — General
76EFN Cotton, Roll — Dental And Cral
80WVI Sock, Non-Compression — General
79RXW Suture, Cotton — Surgery
80RYH Swabs, Cotton — General
80RZH Tape, Cotton — General

COTTONOID
84HBA Paddie, Cottonoid — Cns/Neurology

COUCH
90JAI Couch, Radiation Therapy, Powered — Radiology

COUDE
78EZC Catheter, Coude — Gastro/Urology
78GBM Catheter, Urethral — Gastro/Urology

COULOMETRIC
78QJW Chloridimeter — Gastro/Urology
75CHS Coulometric Method, Carbon-Dioxide — Chemistry
75JFS Coulometric, Chloride — Chemistry
75JHB Uricase (Coulometric), Uric Acid — Chemistry

COUNT
81GJP Control, Platelet — Hematology
81JWD Count System — Hematology

COUNTER
81JCN Control, Cell Counter, Normal And Abnormal — Hematology
80VFK Counter, Air Ion — General
83QMP Counter, Bacteria — Microbiology
83QMQ Counter, Cell — Microbiology
81GKL Counter, Cell Or Particle, Automated — Hematology
81GKZ Counter, Cell, Differential Classifier, Automated — Hematology
81LKZ Counter, Cell, Photometric — Hematology
88IJY Counter, Chromosome — Pathology
83QMR Counter, Colony — Microbiology
83KZB Counter, Colony, Automated — Microbiology
83KZC Counter, Colony, Manual — Microbiology
81GKM Counter, Differential Hand Tally — Hematology
91DNR Counter, Gamma, General Use — Toxicology
91DNM Counter, Gamma, Radioimmunoassay (Manual) — Toxicology
74QMS Counter, Intravenous Drop — Cardiovascular
79QMT Counter, Needle — Surgery
80VDQ Counter, Pill — General
81GKX Counter, Platelet, Automated — Hematology
81GLG Counter, Platelet, Manual — Hematology
90RNU Counter, Radiation — Radiology
75QMU Counter, Scintillation — Chemistry
91DNY Counter, Scintillation, Liquid, Toxicology — Toxicology
79LWH Counter, Sponge, Surgical — Surgery
79VDL Counter, Surgical Instrument — Surgery
88LKM Counter, Urine Particle — Pathology
90JAN Counter, Whole Body, Nuclear — Radiology
75JJJ Detector, Beta/Gamma — Chemistry
86HPW Probe, Isotope, With Counter For Phosphorus 32 — Ophthalmology

COUNTERPRESSURE
74RLJ Suit, Pneumatic Counterpressure (Anti-Shock) — Cardiovascular

KEYWORD INDEX

CREATININE *(cont'd)*
75CGL Ion Electrode Based Enzymatic, Creatinine — Chemistry
75CGX Reagent, Creatinine (Test System) — Chemistry

CRESOL
75CIL Colorimetry, Cresol Red, Carbon-Dioxide — Chemistry

CRESOLPHTHALEIN
75CIC Complexone, Cresolphthalein, Calcium — Chemistry

CRESOLSULFONPHTHALEIN
75CJG Tetrabromo-M-Cresolsulfonphthalein, Albumin — Chemistry

CRESYL
81GHP Brilliant Cresyl Blue — Hematology
88KJN Stain, Brilliant Cresyl Blue — Pathology
88ICG Stain, Cresyl Violet Acetate — Pathology

CRIB
80FMS Bed, Pediatric (Crib) — General
80QNI Cover, Crib Top (Bubble) — General
80RPD Restraint, Crib — General

CRICOTHYROTOMY
73QNJ Kit, Cricothyrotomy — Anesthesiology

CRIMP
78FJY Pliers, Crimp — Gastro/Urology
78FJX Ring, Crimp — Gastro/Urology

CRIMPER
87HXQ Crimper, Pin — Orthopedics
77JXT Crimper, Wire, ENT — Ear/Nose/Throat

CRITICAL
73SEW Ventilator, Volume (Critical Care) — Anesthesiology

CROSSED
86HOR Simultan (Including Crossed Cylinder) — Ophthalmology

CROUPETTE
80RZS Tent, Mist — General

CROWN
76EBG Crown And Bridge, Temporary, Resin — Dental And Oral
76ELZ Crown, Preformed — Dental And Oral
76WKF Material, Acrylic, Dental — Dental And Oral
76EIS Remover, Crown — Dental And Oral
76EIR Scissors, Collar And Crown — Dental And Oral

CRUSHER
85HGA Cranioclast — Obstetrics/Gyn
80QNK Crusher, Pill — General
78FHH Crusher, Spur, Colostomy — Gastro/Urology
80QNL Crusher, Syringe — General
80WPN Crusher, Vial, Laboratory — General
80WTB Cutter, Pill — General
80QOG Cutter, Syringe And Needle — General

CRUSHING
78MET Lithotriptor, Mechanical, Non-Crushing — Gastro/Urology

CRUTCH
89UMM Attachment, Bag (Crutch, Walker, Wheelchair) — Physical Med
89IPR Crutch — Physical Med
86HJZ Crutch, Ptosis — Ophthalmology
89IMZ Holder, Crutch and Cane, Wheelchair — Physical Med
89INP Tips And Pads, Cane, Crutch And Walker — Physical Med

CRUZI
83GNF Antigen, CF, T. Cruzi — Microbiology
83GND Antigen, IHA, T. Cruzi — Microbiology
83GNE Antigen, Latex Agglutination, T. Cruzi — Microbiology
83MIU Enzyme Linked Immunoabsorbent Assay, T. Cruzi — Microbiology
83MIV Immunofluorescent Assay, T. Cruzi — Microbiology

CRYOBIOLOGICAL
83VFX Container, Cryobiological Storage — Microbiology

CRYOEXTRACTOR
86HPS Cryophthalmic Unit — Ophthalmology
86HRN Cryophthalmic Unit, AC-Powered — Ophthalmology
86QHF Extractor, Cataract — Ophthalmology

CRYOGENIC
80WRI Analgesia Unit, Cryogenic — General
81QNO Equipment, Bank, Blood, Cryogenic (Liquid Nitrogen) — Hematology
81KSE Freezer, Blood Storage — Hematology

CRYOMETER
79QNP Cryometer — Surgery

CRYOPHTHALMIC
86HPS Cryophthalmic Unit — Ophthalmology
86HRN Cryophthalmic Unit, AC-Powered — Ophthalmology

CRYOPHTHALMIC *(cont'd)*
86HQA Cryotherapy, Unit, Ophthalmic — Ophthalmology

CRYOSTAT
88IDP Microtome, Cryostat — Pathology

CRYOSURGICAL
80VLK Cartridge, Freon — General
79QNP Cryometer — Surgery
86HPS Cryophthalmic Unit — Ophthalmology
86HRN Cryophthalmic Unit, AC-Powered — Ophthalmology
79GEH Cryosurgical Unit — Surgery
85HGJ Cryosurgical Unit, Gynecologic — Obstetrics/Gyn
84GXH Cryosurgical Unit, Neurological — Cns/Neurology
79FAZ Cryosurgical, Unit, Urology — Surgery
86QHF Extractor, Cataract — Ophthalmology

CRYOTHERAPY
80WRI Analgesia Unit, Cryogenic — General
86HQA Cryotherapy, Unit, Ophthalmic — Ophthalmology
89WOK Equipment, Cryotherapy — Physical Med

CRYPTOCOCCAL
83MDE Reagent, DNA-Probe, Cryptococcal — Microbiology

CRYPTOCOCCUS
83MDU Antigen, Enzyme Linked Immunoabsorbent Assay, Cryptococcus — Microbiology
83JWK Antigen, Positive Control, Cryptococcus Neoformans — Microbiology
83GME Antiserum, Fluorescent, Cryptococcus Neoformans — Microbiology
83GMD Antiserum, Latex Agglutination, Cryptococcus Neoformans — Microbiology

CRYPTOSPORIDIUM
83MHJ Cryptosporidium Spp. — Microbiology

CRYSTAL
81GGD Crystal Violet — Hematology
88HYP Holzer Crystal Violet — Pathology
80KZA Locator, Vein, Liquid Crystal — General
88ICF Stain, Crystal Violet, Histology — Pathology
85LHM System, Thermographic, Liquid Crystal — Obstetrics/Gyn
80KPD Temperature Strip, Forehead, Liquid Crystal — General
90KXZ Thermographic Device, Liquid Crystal, Adjunctive — Radiology
90KYA Thermographic Device, Liquid Crystal, Non-Powered — Radiology
90LHR Thermographic Device, Liquid Crystal, Screen — Radiology

CRYSTALS
79FWR Thermometer, Liquid Crystals — Surgery

CSF
80CAQ Monitor, Cerebral Spinal Fluid Pressure (CSF) — General
80CAR Monitor, Cerebral Spinal Fluid Pressure, Electrical — General

CT
75JMY Citrulline, Arsenate, Nessler (Colorimetry), Ornithine CT — Chemistry
90VHB Phantom, Computed Axial Tomography (CAT, CT) — Radiology
90WMF Scanner, Computed Tomography, Cine — Radiology
84JXD Scanner, Computed Tomography, X-Ray (CAT, CT) — Cns/Neurology
90THS Scanner, Computed Tomography, X-Ray, Full Body — Radiology
90TEI Scanner, Computed Tomography, X-Ray, Head — Radiology
90JAK Scanner, Computed Tomography, X-Ray, Special Procedure — Radiology

CUBICLE
80QNY Curtain, Cubicle — General
80UEG Curtain, Cubicle, Disposable — General
80SBK Track And Carrier, Cubicle Curtain — General

CUFF
80WRS Bulb, Inflation — General
74DXQ Cuff, Blood Pressure — Cardiovascular
80FLZ Cuff, Inflation — General
84JXI Cuff, Nerve — Cns/Neurology
89INC Cuff, Pusher, Wheelchair — Physical Med
73BSK Cuff, Tracheal Tube, Inflatable — Anesthesiology
77JOH Cuff, Tracheostomy Tube — Ear/Nose/Throat
74MEY Cuff, Treatment, Varicose Vein, Implantable — Cardiovascular
80QNQ Inflator, Cuff — General
74WZC Monitor, Blood Pressure, Finger — Cardiovascular
74WOZ Occluder, Cardiovascular — Cardiovascular
74DYF Prosthesis, Vascular Graft, Less Than 6mm Diameter — Cardiovascular
74DSY Prosthesis, Vascular Graft, Of 6mm And Greater Diameter — Cardiovascular
80JOI Pump, Inflator — General
73CBG Spreader, Cuff — Anesthesiology
78FKF Tie Gun, Dialysis — Gastro/Urology
78FKE Tie, Dialysis — Gastro/Urology
80SBD Tourniquet — General
73BTR Tube, Tracheal (Endotracheal) — Anesthesiology

CUFFS
74WTT Legging, Compression, Inflatable, Sequential — Cardiovascular

KEYWORD INDEX

CUSTOM *(cont'd)*
80WNH Tray, Custom/Special Procedure — General

CUTANEOUS
80UDF Bilirubinometer, Cutaneous (Jaundice Meter) — General
84GXY Electrode, Cutaneous — Cns/Neurology
73TAJ Monitor, Blood Gas, Transcutaneous Carbon-Dioxide — Anesthesiology
73QEC Monitor, Blood Gas, Transcutaneous Oxygen — Anesthesiology
73LKD Monitor, Carbon-Dioxide, Cutaneous — Anesthesiology
73LPP Monitor, Oxygen, Cutan. (Not for Infant or Under Gas Anest.) — Anesthesiology
73KLK Monitor, Oxygen, Cutaneous — Anesthesiology
73ULU Monitor, Transcutaneous, Carbon-Dioxide — Anesthesiology
73ULV Monitor, Transcutaneous, Oxygen — Anesthesiology

CUTTER
86HRG Accessories, Engine, Trephine, AC-Powered — Ophthalmology
79HRF Accessories, Engine, Trephine, Battery-Powered — Surgery
79HLD Accessories, Engine, Trephine, Gas-Powered — Surgery
77KBH Adenotome — Ear/Nose/Throat
85HGE Amniotome — Obstetrics/Gyn
85HIN Coagulator/Cutter, Endoscopic, Bipolar — Obstetrics/Gyn
85KNF Coagulator/Cutter, Endoscopic, Unipolar — Obstetrics/Gyn
80QNL Crusher, Syringe — General
84JXJ Cutter, Bone, Ultrasonic — Cns/Neurology
87QGZ Cutter, Cast — Orthopedics
87LGH Cutter, Cast, AC-Powered — Orthopedics
84GZQ Cutter, Dowel — Cns/Neurology
79SIM Cutter, Linear, Laparoscopic — Surgery
76EKD Cutter, Operative — Dental And Oral
87HTZ Cutter, Orthopedic — Orthopedics
80WTB Cutter, Pill — General
80FNS Cutter, Ring — General
79RTO Cutter, Skin Graft — Surgery
79RTP Cutter, Skin Graft, Expanded Mesh — Surgery
79FZT Cutter, Surgical — Surgery
79UEN Cutter, Suture — Surgery
80QOG Cutter, Syringe And Needle — General
86HQE Cutter, Vitreous Aspiration, AC-Powered — Ophthalmology
86HKP Cutter, Vitreous Aspiration, Battery-Powered — Ophthalmology
86QOH Cutter, Vitreous Infusion Suction — Ophthalmology
87HXZ Cutter, Wire And Pin — Orthopedics
90TFP Cutter, X-Ray Film — Radiology
78TBS Cystotome — Gastro/Urology
86HNY Cystotome, Ophthalmic — Ophthalmology
79GFD Dermatome — Surgery
80TCA Extrication Equipment — General
77QZC Guillotine, Adenoid — Ear/Nose/Throat
87QZD Guillotine, Rib — Orthopedics
77KBO Guillotine, Tonsil — Ear/Nose/Throat
75RBN Immunodiffusion Equipment (Agar Cutter) — Chemistry
79SJR Irrigator/Coagulator/Cutter, Suction, Laparoscopic — Surgery
86HNO Keratome, AC-Powered — Ophthalmology
86HMY Keratome, Battery-Powered — Ophthalmology
86RCT Kit, Irrigation, Eye — Ophthalmology
79RDQ Knife, Skin Grafting — Surgery
84GXE Leukotome — Cns/Neurology
79HWM Osteotome (Orthopedic) — Surgery
79GFI Osteotome, Manual (Plastic Surgery) — Surgery
79RJX Papillotome — Surgery
80RRB Scissors, Bandage/Gauze/Plaster — General
86RRQ Sclerotome — Ophthalmology
87RZR Tenotome — Orthopedics
77KCA Tonsillectome — Ear/Nose/Throat
86HMZ Trabeculotome — Ophthalmology
78SEA Ureterotome — Gastro/Urology
78EZO Urethrotome — Gastro/Urology
87QGY Vacuum, Cast Cutter — Orthopedics
74MGZ Valvulotome — Cardiovascular

CUTTING
87QDU Blade, Bone Cutting — Orthopedics
87TAI Blade, Saw, Cast Cutting — Orthopedics
77JXS Block, Cutting, ENT — Ear/Nose/Throat
84HBS Clip, Instrument, Forming/Cutting — Cns/Neurology
79GEI Electrosurgical Unit, Cutting & Coagulation Device — Surgery
76KMW Handpiece, Rotary Bone Cutting — Dental And Oral
77JXY Jig, Piston Cutting, ENT — Ear/Nose/Throat
79SJW Needle, Cutting, Bipolar, Electrocauterization — Surgery
87HSO Saw, Bone Cutting — Orthopedics
87VHR Saw, Bone Cutting, Micro — Orthopedics
77JYA Scissors, Wire Cutting, ENT — Ear/Nose/Throat
87HWS Template, Femoral Angle Cutting — Orthopedics

CUVETTE
75TBQ Cuvette, Spectrophotometer — Chemistry
75JRI Cuvette, Thermostated — Chemistry

CYANOMETHEMOGLOBIN
81GKK Cyanomethemoglobin — Hematology
81GJZ Reagent, Cyanomethemoglobin, With Standard — Hematology

CYCLED
73SEU Ventilator, Pressure Cycled (IPPB Machine) — Anesthesiology
73SEV Ventilator, Time Cycled (Iron Lung) — Anesthesiology

CYCLIC
75CHO Radioimmunoassay, Cyclic AMP — Chemistry
75CGT Radioimmunoassay, Cyclic GMP — Chemistry

CYCLODESTRUCTIVE
86LZR Device, Cyclodestructive, Ultrasonic — Ophthalmology

CYCLODIALYSIS
86QGA Cannula, Cyclodialysis (Eye) — Ophthalmology

CYCLOSPORINE
91MAR Assay, Serum, Cyclosporine and Metabolites, TDX — Toxicology
91MKW Cyclosporine — Toxicology
75MGU Fluorescence Polarization, Immunoassay, Cyclosporine — Chemistry
75MGS High Performance Liquid Chromatography, Cyclosporine — Chemistry
75LTB Radioimmunoassay, Cyclosporine — Chemistry

CYCLOTRON
90IYG Betatron, Medical — Radiology
90IWK Cyclotron — Radiology
90JAE Microtron, Medical — Radiology
90IWM Synchrotron, Medical — Radiology

CYLINDER
80WUT Carrier, Container, Oxygen, Portable — General
73QXW Cart, Gas Cylinder (Carrier) — Anesthesiology
79QUA Cylinder, Carbon-Dioxide — Surgery
73ECX Cylinder, Compressed Gas, With Valve — Anesthesiology
73KGA Cylinder, Gas (Empty) — Anesthesiology
73VFF Cylinder, Oxygen — Anesthesiology
73BXH Gauge, Gas Pressure, Cylinder/Pipeline — Anesthesiology
73BSM Holder, Gas Cylinder — Anesthesiology
73CAN Regulator, Pressure, Gas Cylinder — Anesthesiology
86HOR Simultan (Including Crossed Cylinder) — Ophthalmology
73QXX Stand, Gas Cylinder — Anesthesiology

CYST
79RIJ Needle, Aspiration, Cyst, Laparoscopic — Surgery

CYSTIC
78QJW Chloridimeter — Gastro/Urology
78QOI Cystic Fibrosis System — Gastro/Urology
78RCP Iontophoresis Unit (Sweat Rate) — Gastro/Urology
89KTB Iontophoresis Unit, Physical Medicine — Physical Med
75VIP Test, Cystic Fibrosis — Chemistry

CYSTICERCOSIS
83MDJ Reagent, Cysticercosis — Microbiology

CYSTINE
75JLD Chromatographic, Cystine — Chemistry
75JLC Nitroprusside Reaction (Qualitative, Urine), Cystine — Chemistry

CYSTOLOGICAL
78RZA Table, Urological (Cystological) — Gastro/Urology
78EYH Table, Urological, Non-Electrical — Gastro/Urology
78UEE Table, Urological, Radiographic — Gastro/Urology

CYSTOMETER
78EXQ Cystometer, Electrical Recording — Gastro/Urology

CYSTOMETRIC
78FAO Cystometric Air Device — Gastro/Urology
78FAP Cystometric Gas (Carbon-Dioxide) Or Hydraulic Device — Gastro/Urology
78FEN Device, Cystometric, Hydraulic — Gastro/Urology
78MMZ Table, Cystometric, Electric — Gastro/Urology
78KQS Table, Cystometric, Non-Electrical — Gastro/Urology

CYSTOSCOPE
78FAJ Cystoscope — Gastro/Urology

CYSTOSCOPIC
78QSR Electrode, Cystoscopic — Gastro/Urology
78FBI Rongeur, Cystoscopic — Gastro/Urology
78KDO Rongeur, Cystoscopic, Hot — Gastro/Urology
78KGD Scissors, Cystoscopic — Gastro/Urology

CYSTOTOME
78TBS Cystotome — Gastro/Urology
86HNY Cystotome, Ophthalmic — Ophthalmology

CYSTOURETHROSCOPE
78FBO Cystourethroscope — Gastro/Urology

CYTOCENTRIFUGE
88IFB Cytocentrifuge — Pathology

CYTOKERATINS
82LYE Cytokeratins — Immunology

CYTOLOGICAL
85LTY Fluid, Collection, Cytological — Obstetrics/Gyn
88LEA Preservative, Cytological — Pathology

CYTOLOGY
80WKZ Brush, Cytology — General
78FDX Brush, Cytology, Endoscopic — Gastro/Urology
88MKQ Processor, Slide, Cytology, Automated — Pathology
88MNM Reader, Slide, Cytology, Cervical, Automated — Pathology
85RRS Scraper, Cytology (Cervical) — Obstetrics/Gyn
85HHT Spatula, Cervical, Cytology — Obstetrics/Gyn
83RTR Stainer, Slide, Cytology — Microbiology

CYTOMEGALOVIRUS
83LKQ Antibody Igm, If, Cytomegalovirus Virus — Microbiology
83GQH Antigen, CF (Including CF Control), Cytomegalovirus — Microbiology
83LJO Antigen, IHA, Cytomegalovirus — Microbiology
83LIN Antisera, Conjugated Fluorescent, Cytomegalovirus — Microbiology
83GQI Antiserum, CF, Cytomegalovirus — Microbiology
83LSO Cytomegalovirus, DNA Reagents — Microbiology
83LFZ Enzyme Linked Immunoabsorbent Assay, Cytomegalovirus — Microbiology

CYTOMETER
81JCN Control, Cell Counter, Normal And Abnormal — Hematology
83QMQ Counter, Cell — Microbiology
81GKL Counter, Cell Or Particle, Automated — Hematology
81GKZ Counter, Cell, Differential Classifier, Automated — Hematology
81ULS Hemacytometer — Hematology

CYTOPLASMIC
82MOB Test System, Antineutrophil Cytoplasmic Antibodies (ANCA) — Immunology

CYTOTOXIC
80SFU Waste Receptacle, Contaminated — General

DACRON
74DSX Pledget, Dacron, Teflon, Polypropylene — Cardiovascular
79GAS Suture, Non-Absorbable, Synthetic, Polyester — Surgery

DAILY
86LPL Lenses, Soft Contact, Daily Wear — Ophthalmology

DAM
76EEF Clamp, Rubber Dam — Dental And Oral
76QOK Dam, Dental — Dental And Oral
76EIE Dam, Rubber — Dental And Oral
76EJG Forceps, Rubber Dam Clamp — Dental And Oral
76EJE Frame, Rubber Dam — Dental And Oral
76RNK Punch, Dental, Rubber Dam — Dental And Oral
78EYS Ribdam — Gastro/Urology

DARKROOMS
90VGS Entrance, X-Ray Darkrooms — Radiology
90TGW Interlock System, X-Ray Darkrooms — Radiology

DARROW
88ICD Stain, Darrow Red — Pathology

DATA
85HEO Analyzer, Data, Obstetric — Obstetrics/Gyn
80WKP Camera, Other — General
80VBH Computer Software — General
80WLE Computer, Image, Endoscopic — General
90QMD Computer, Nuclear Medicine — Radiology
80VHN Computer, Patient Data Management — General
73BZC Computer, Pulmonary Function Data — Anesthesiology
90WKA Computer, Radiographic Data — Radiology
90UFD Computer, Radiographic Image Analysis — Radiology
90VHG Computer, Ultrasound — Radiology
80VAZ Microfilm/Microfiche Equipment — General
80QJP Paper, Chart, Record, Medical — General
80WUP Paper, Recording, Data — General
73WQI System, Recording, Data, Anesthesiology — Anesthesiology
90WOG Transmitter, Image & Data, Radiographic — Radiology

DAVIS
88IHD Irrigation, Davis Mailable Irrigation Kit — Pathology

DAYLIGHT
90UFC Handling Unit, Automatic Daylight X-Ray Film — Radiology

DC
74MPD Auxillary Power Supply, Low Energy Defibrillator (AC or DC) — Cardiovascular

DC-POWERED
79SJM Motor, Surgical Instrument, DC-Powered — Surgery
80FLW Stethoscope, DC-Powered — General

DEAF
77ESD Hearing-Aid — Ear/Nose/Throat
77LXB Hearing-Aid, Bone-Conduction — Ear/Nose/Throat
77MAH Hearing-Aid, Bone-Conduction, Implanted — Ear/Nose/Throat
77MKE Hearing-Aid, Bone-Conduction, Percutaneous — Ear/Nose/Throat
77KHL Hearing-Aid, Master — Ear/Nose/Throat
77LRB Hearing-Aid, Plate, Face — Ear/Nose/Throat
77EWE Protector, Hearing (Circumaural) — Ear/Nose/Throat
77EWD Protector, Hearing (Insert) — Ear/Nose/Throat
77LEZ Speech Training Aid, AC-Powered — Ear/Nose/Throat
77LFA Speech Training Aid, Battery-Powered — Ear/Nose/Throat

DEBRIDEMENT
74MEZ Device, Debridement, Ultrasonic, Heart Valve & HV Seat — Cardiovascular

DECALCIFICATION
88KDY Agent, Chelating, Decalcification — Pathology

DECALCIFIER
88KDZ Decalcifier Device, Electrolytic — Pathology
88IFF Decalcifier Solution, Electrolytic — Pathology
88KDX Solution, Pathology, Decalcifier, Acid Containing — Pathology

DECAPITATION
85HGA Cranioclast — Obstetrics/Gyn

DECLOTTING
78FJZ Tray, Declotting (Including Contents) — Gastro/Urology

DECOMPRESSION
78QIB Catheter, Jejunostomy — Gastro/Urology
85HEE Chamber, Decompression, Abdominal — Obstetrics/Gyn
84RPP Retractor, Brain Decompression — Cns/Neurology
80SCT Tube, Decompression — General
78FEG Tube, Double Lumen For Intestinal Decompression — Gastro/Urology
78VHP Tube, Gastrointestinal Decompression, Baker Jejunostomy — Gastro/Urology
78SDB Tube, Gastrointestinal Decompression, Cantor — Gastro/Urology
78SDC Tube, Gastrointestinal Decompression, Dennis — Gastro/Urology
78SDD Tube, Gastrointestinal Decompression, Miller-Abbott — Gastro/Urology

DECONGESTION
73BXQ Rhinoanemometer (Measurement Of Nasal Decongestion) — Anesthesiology

DECONTAMINATION
79MAC Decontamination Kit — Surgery
80WWK Washer/Disinfector — General

DECORATIVE
80VBQ Accessories, Decorative — General

DECUBITUS
89INX Bed, Air Fluidized — Physical Med
80UDH Bed, Flotation Therapy, Neonatal — General
89IOQ Bed, Flotation Therapy, Powered — Physical Med
89INY Bed, Patient Rotation, Manual — Physical Med
89IKZ Bed, Patient Rotation, Powered — Physical Med
89FNH Bed, Water Flotation, AC-Powered — Physical Med
80QJI Chair, Flotation Therapy — General
79KPJ Chamber, Oxygen, Topical, Extremity — Surgery
89IMP Cushion, Wheelchair (Pad) — Physical Med
80WKJ Dressing, Gel — General
80WSE Dressing, Layer, Charcoal — General
80WKL Dressing, Permeable, Moisture — General
80FNM Mattress, Air Flotation — General
89ILA Mattress, Alternating Pressure (Or Pads) — Physical Med
89IKY Mattress, Non-Powered Flotation Therapy — Physical Med
80WYO Mattress, Reduction, Pressure — General
80FNI Mattress, Silicone, And Chair Cushion — General
80RGI Mattress, Water — General
80FOH Mattress, Water, Temperature Regulated — General
80RLZ Pad, Pressure, Air — General
80RMA Pad, Pressure, Animal Skin — General
80RMB Pad, Pressure, Foam (Elbow, Heel) — General
80RMC Pad, Pressure, Foam Convoluted — General
80RMD Pad, Pressure, Gel — General
80WMD Pad, Pressure, Gel, Operating Table — General
80RME Pad, Pressure, Soft Rubber — General
80RMF Pad, Pressure, Water Cushion — General
80UCU Pressure Pad, Alternating, Disposable — General
80UCV Pressure Pad, Alternating, Reusable — General
80FMP Protector, Skin Pressure — General
80UBG Pump, Alternating Pressure Pad — General
79RTQ Sleeve, Topical Oxygen Therapy — Surgery
89WIN Stimulator, Wound Healing — Physical Med

DEDICATED
91DLK Chromatograph, HPL, Drugs of Abuse (Dedicated Instrument) — Toxicology
91DMM Flame Photometer, Pesticides (Dedicated Instruments) — Toxicology
91DOX Fluorometer, Lead (Dedicated Instruments) — Toxicology
91DLS Gas Chromatograph, Alcohol (Dedicated Instruments) — Toxicology

DEDICATED (cont'd)

91DMC Gas Chromatograph, Drugs of Abuse (Dedicated Instruments) — Toxicology
91DLM Photometer, Flame, Heavy Metals (Dedicated Instrument) — Toxicology
91JXP Thin Layer Chromatography, Drugs of Abuse (Dedicated Instr.) — Toxicology

DEEP

74QOM Detector, Deep Vein Thrombosis — Cardiovascular
90LNA Hyperthermia Applicator, Deep Heating, RF/Microwave — Radiology
90LNB Hyperthermia Applicator, Deep Heating, Ultrasound — Radiology
86MLZ Therapeutic Deep Heat Vitrectomy — Ophthalmology

DEFECT

82LOK Test, Neural Tube Defect, Alpha-Fetoprotein (AFP) — Immunology

DEFERANS

78EZZ Prosthesis, Vas Deferans — Gastro/Urology

DEFIBRILLATION

74MTE System, Pacing, Temporary, Acute, Internal Atrial Defibrillation — Cardiovascular

DEFIBRILLATOR

80WJN Analyzer, Battery — General
74MPD Auxillary Power Supply, Low Energy Defibrillator (AC or DC) — Cardiovascular
80WRU Capacitor, Defibrillator — General
80WSG Case, Protection, Equipment — General
80WJM Charger, Battery — General
74QOR Defibrillator, Battery-Powered — Cardiovascular
74DRK Defibrillator, Battery-Powered, High Energy — Cardiovascular
74LDD Defibrillator, Battery-Powered, Low Energy — Cardiovascular
74MKJ Defibrillator, External, Automatic — Cardiovascular
74LWS Defibrillator, Implantable, Automatic — Cardiovascular
74QOS Defibrillator, Line-Powered — Cardiovascular
74WJK Defibrillator, Transtelephonic — Cardiovascular
74QOO Defibrillator/Monitor, Battery-Powered — Cardiovascular
74QOP Defibrillator/Monitor, Line-Powered — Cardiovascular
74QSS Electrode, Defibrillator — Cardiovascular
74QOQ Pad, Defibrillator Paddle — Cardiovascular
74DRL Tester, Defibrillator — Cardiovascular

DEFICIENCY

81VJE Test, Antibody, Acquired Immune Deficiency Syndrome (AIDS) — Hematology
82MZF Test, Hiv Detection — Immunology
81GGP Test, Qualitative And Quantitative Factor Deficiency — Hematology

DEFICIENT

81GJT Plasma, Deficient, Factor, Coagulation — Hematology

DEFOAMER

74VCJ Bubble Defoamer, Cardiopulmonary Bypass — Cardiovascular
74DTP Defoamer, Cardiopulmonary Bypass — Cardiovascular

DEFORMITY

79MBR Silastic Elastomer (Angular Deformity Prevention) — Surgery

DEFROSTER

80SHJ Defroster, Drug, Frozen — General

DEGREASER

79KOY Degreaser, Skin, Surgical — Surgery
80TGV Solution, Skin Degreaser — General

DEHUMIDIFIER

80WUX Dehumidifier — General

DEHYDROEPIANDROSTERONE

75JKC Radioimmunoassay, Dehydroepiandrosterone (Free And Sulfate) — Chemistry

DEHYDROGENASE

75CER 2, 4-dinitrophenylhydrazine, Lactate Dehydrogenase — Chemistry
91DIC Alcohol Dehydrogenase, Spec. Reagent - Ethanol Enzyme — Toxicology
75CEX Chromatographic Separation, Lactate Dehydrogenase Isoenzyme — Chemistry
75JGF Differential Rate Method, Lactate Dehydrogenase Isoenzymes — Chemistry
81JLM Electrophoretic, Glucose-6-Phosphate Dehydrogenase — Hematology
75CFE Electrophoretic, Lactate Dehydrogenase Isoenzymes — Chemistry
91DMT Enzymatic Method, Alcohol Dehydrogenase, Ultraviolet — Toxicology
75LFR Glucose Dehydrogenase, Glucose — Chemistry
81JBJ Glucose-6-Phos. Dehydrogenase (Erythrocy.), Methemogl. Red. — Hematology
81JBH Glucose-6-Phos. Dehydrogenase (Erythrocytic), Micromethod — Hematology
81JBL Glucose-6-Phos. Dehydrogenase (Erythrocytic), Quantitative — Hematology
81JBK Glucose-6-Phos. Dehydrogenase (Erythrocytic), U.V. Kinetic — Hematology

DEHYDROGENASE (cont'd)

81JBI Glucose-6-Phosphate Dehydrogenase (Erythrocytic), Catalase — Hematology
81JBM Glucose-6-Phosphate Dehydrogenase (Erythrocytic), Electro — Hematology
81JBF Glucose-6-Phosphate Dehydrogenase (Erythrocytic), Screening — Hematology
81JBG Glucose-6-Phosphate Dehydrogenase (Erythrocytic), Spot — Hematology
75JKG L-Isocitrate And NADP (U.V.), Isocitric Dehydrogenase — Chemistry
82DET Lactic Dehydrogenase, Antigen, Antiserum, Control — Immunology
75CFJ NAD Reduction/NADH Oxidation, Lactate Dehydrogenase — Chemistry
81JMC NADP Reduction (U.V.), Glucose-6-Phosphate Dehydrogenase — Hematology
75JND NADP Reduction, 6-Phosphogluconate Dehydrogenase — Chemistry
81KQE Test, Erythrocytic Glucose-6-Phosphate Dehydrogenase — Hematology
75CFH Tetrazolium Int Dye-Diaphorase, Lactate Dehydrogenase — Chemistry
75CDQ Urease And Glutamic Dehydrogenase, Urea Nitrogen — Chemistry

DEIONIZATION

75QOU Demineralizer — Chemistry
75SFZ Purification System, Water, Deionization — Chemistry

DELAYED

91DIZ Delayed Analysis, Alcohol — Toxicology

DELIVERY

76EBX Bracket, Table Assembly, N2O Delivery System — Dental And Oral
80LDH Delivery System, Allergen And Vaccine — General
80TDT Delivery System, Pneumatic Tube — General
78FKQ Dialysate Delivery System, Central Multiple Patient — Gastro/Urology
78KPF Dialysate Delivery System, Peritoneal, Semi-Automatic — Gastro/Urology
78FIK Dialysate Delivery System, Recirculating — Gastro/Urology
78FIJ Dialysate Delivery System, Recirculating, Single Pass — Gastro/Urology
78FII Dialysate Delivery System, Sealed — Gastro/Urology
78FIL Dialysate Delivery System, Single Pass — Gastro/Urology
78FKP Dialysate Delivery System, Single Patient — Gastro/Urology
78FKT Dialysate Delivery System, Sorbent Regenerated — Gastro/Urology
74MOU Intravascular Radiation Delivery System — Cardiovascular
85MLS Kit, Labor and Delivery — Obstetrics/Gyn
85RGF Kit, Maternity — Obstetrics/Gyn
80WOL Patch, Transdermal — General
80WOI System, Delivery, Drug, Non-invasive — General
86WVM System, Delivery, Drug, Ocular — Ophthalmology
80SGR System, Delivery, Drug, Unit-Dose — General
80FPK Tubing, Fluid Delivery — General

DELTA

75JKK Acetylacetone (Colorimetric), Delta-Aminolevulinic Acid — Chemistry
91DIJ Acid, Levulinic, Amino, Delta, Lead — Toxicology
75JKL Column, Ion Exchange With Colorimetry, Delta-Aminolevulinic — Chemistry
83LQI Reagent, Serological, Delta, Hepatitis — Microbiology

DELTA-AMINOLEVULINIC

75JKK Acetylacetone (Colorimetric), Delta-Aminolevulinic Acid — Chemistry
75JKL Column, Ion Exchange With Colorimetry, Delta-Aminolevulinic — Chemistry

DEMAGNETIZER

80WIS Demagnetizer — General

DEMAND

73QWO Regulator, Intake, Oxygen — Anesthesiology
80FQB Resuscitator, Pulmonary, Manual (Demand Valve) — General
73WHT Valve, Breathing — Anesthesiology
73CBP Valve, Non-Rebreathing — Anesthesiology

DEMENTIA

83WSI Test, Dementia, Alzheimer's — Microbiology

DEMINERALIZER

75QOU Demineralizer — Chemistry
75SFZ Purification System, Water, Deionization — Chemistry

DENIS

89ITN Splint, Denis Brown — Physical Med

DENNIS

78SDC Tube, Gastrointestinal Decompression, Dennis — Gastro/Urology

DENSITOMETER

74DXM Densitometer — Cardiovascular
90WRK Densitometer, Bone, Dual Photon — Radiology
90KGI Densitometer, Bone, Single Photon — Radiology
75UKK Densitometer, Laboratory — Chemistry
90VGD Densitometer, Radiographic — Radiology
90WIR Densitometer, Radiography, Digital, Quantitative — Radiology
75JQT Densitometer/Scanner (Integrating, Reflectance, TLC, Radio) — Chemistry

DENSITOMETRIC

75JQJ Fractionation, Protein, Densitometric — Chemistry

KEYWORD INDEX

DEPRESSOR *(cont'd)*

80FMA	Depressor, Tongue	General
76EJC	Depressor, Tongue, Dental	Dental And Oral
77KBL	Depressor, Tongue, ENT, Metal	Ear/Nose/Throat
77EWF	Depressor, Tongue, ENT, Wood	Ear/Nose/Throat

DEPTH

84GZL	Electrode, Depth	Cns/Neurology
87HTJ	Gauge, Depth	Orthopedics
76EIL	Gauge, Depth, Instrument, Dental	Dental And Oral
86WQL	Pachometer	Ophthalmology

DERIVATIVE

75CFB	Chromatographic Derivative, Total Lipids	Chemistry
75JKH	Hydrazone Derivative Of Alpha-Ketogluterate (Colorimetry)	Chemistry
91DKW	Reagent, Test, Sulphanimide Derivative	Toxicology

DERMABRASION

79GFE	Brush, Dermabrasion	Surgery
79GED	Brush, Dermabrasion, Manual	Surgery
79QPC	Dermabrasion Unit	Surgery
79GFD	Dermatome	Surgery

DERMAL

79MDD	Device, Dermal Replacement	Surgery
79LMH	Implant, Collagen, Dermal (Aesthetic Use)	Surgery
79RNL	Punch, Dermal	Surgery

DERMATITIDIS

83LSH	Antigen, Blastomyces Dermatitidis, Other	Microbiology
83JWW	Antigen, CF, B. Dermatitidis	Microbiology
83LSI	Antiserum, Blastomyces Dermatitidis, Other	Microbiology
83KFH	Antiserum, Positive Control, Blastomyces Dermatitidis	Microbiology
83MDC	DNA-Probe, Blastomyces Dermatitidis	Microbiology
83MJL	EIA, Blastomyces Dermatitidis	Microbiology

DERMATOLOGIC

89LEJ	Booth, Sun Tan	Physical Med
80QQA	Disinfector, Pasteurization	General
79FTC	Light, Ultraviolet, Dermatologic	Surgery

DERMATOLOGICAL

90IYL	Collimator, Therapeutic X-Ray, Dermatological	Radiology
90IYH	Generator, Therapeutic X-Ray, Dermatological (Grenz Ray)	Radiology

DERMATOLOGY

90VHG	Computer, Ultrasound	Radiology

DERMATOME

79QPC	Dermabrasion Unit	Surgery
79GFD	Dermatome	Surgery
79RDI	Knife, Dermatome	Surgery

DERMATOPHYTE

83JSR	Kit, Identification, Dermatophyte	Microbiology

DESENSITIZER

73QPD	Desensitizer	Anesthesiology

DESICCATOR

75QPE	Desiccator	Chemistry
78FHZ	Desiccator, Transurethral	Gastro/Urology

DESIGN

80WXA	Component, Other	General
80WUH	Contract R&D, Equipment	General
87WIV	Service, Design, Implant, Custom	Orthopedics
80WND	Service, Engineering/Design	General
84LXL	Valve, Shunt, Fluid, CNS (Post-Amendment Design)	Cns/Neurology

DESK

75VIR	Analyzer, Chemistry, Desk-Top	Chemistry

DESK-TOP

75VIR	Analyzer, Chemistry, Desk-Top	Chemistry

DESOXYCORTICOSTERONE

75JLE	Radioimmunoassay, Desoxycorticosterone	Chemistry

DESTRUCTION

80MTV	Device, Needle Destruction	General

DESTRUCTIVE

85HGA	Cranioclast	Obstetrics/Gyn
85HDI	Hook, Destructive, Obstetrical	Obstetrics/Gyn
85KNB	Surgical Instrument, Obstetric, Destructive, Fetal	Obstetrics/Gyn

DETECTABLE

79GDY	Gauze, Non-Absorbable, X-Ray Detectable (Internal Sponge)	Surgery
79RVK	Sponge, X-Ray Detectable	Surgery

DETECTION

83LSG	Candida Species, Antibody Detection	Microbiology

DETECTION *(cont'd)*

83MKS	Device, Detection, Urinary Antibody	Microbiology
85TGQ	Kit, Breast Cancer Detection	Obstetrics/Gyn
83MAQ	Kit, DNA Detection, Human Papillomavirus	Microbiology
83TGR	Kit, Meningitis Detection	Microbiology
88KIW	Kit, Mycoplasma Detection	Pathology
85RJW	Kit, Pap Smear	Obstetrics/Gyn
88KIX	Media, Mycoplasma Detection	Pathology
74MWI	Monitor, Physiological, Patient(without Arrhythmia Detection Or Alarms)	Cardiovascular
88KPB	Mycoplasma Detection Media and Components	Pathology
76LXD	Optical Caries Detection Device	Dental And Oral
83UML	Reagent, Legionella Detection	Microbiology
88HZJ	Stain, Papanicolau	Pathology
83MYI	System, Test, Genotypic Detection, Resistant Markers, Staphylococcus Colonies	Microbiology
82NAH	System, Test, Tumor Marker, For Detection Of Bladder Cancer	Immunology
82VJL	Test, Cancer Detection, DNA-Probe	Immunology
82VJD	Test, Cancer Detection, Monoclonal Antibody	Immunology
81VIA	Test, Cancer Detection, Other	Hematology
82WUO	Test, Cancer Detection, QFI	Immunology
82MZF	Test, Hiv Detection	Immunology
82MTF	Total, Prostate Specific Antigen (noncomplexed & complexed) for Detection of Prostate Cancer	Immunology

DETECTOR

74DSM	Alarm, Leakage Current, Portable	Cardiovascular
74DRJ	Analyzer, Signal Isolation	Cardiovascular
90RNU	Counter, Radiation	Radiology
78FJF	Detector, Air Bubble	Gastro/Urology
78KQR	Detector, Air Or Foam	Gastro/Urology
74QZI	Detector, Air, Heart-Lung Bypass	Cardiovascular
74DSI	Detector, Arrhythmia Alarm	Cardiovascular
75JJJ	Detector, Beta/Gamma	Chemistry
74ULR	Detector, Blood Flow, Ultrasonic (Doppler)	Cardiovascular
78FJD	Detector, Blood Leakage	Gastro/Urology
78FJC	Detector, Blood Level	Gastro/Urology
74KRL	Detector, Bubble, Cardiopulmonary Bypass	Cardiovascular
76LFC	Detector, Caries	Dental And Oral
88IJW	Detector, Centromere	Pathology
74QOM	Detector, Deep Vein Thrombosis	Cardiovascular
78FJB	Detector, Dialysate Level	Gastro/Urology
91LEQ	Detector, Electrochemical, Chromatography, Liquid	Toxicology
80QTQ	Detector, Electrostatic Voltage	General
80UMV	Detector, Ethylene-Oxide Leakage	General
85QVO	Detector, Fetal Heart, Phono	Obstetrics/Gyn
78QZV	Detector, Hemodialysis Unit Air Bubble-Foam	Gastro/Urology
74RAD	Detector, His Bundle	Cardiovascular
80WPI	Detector, Leakage, Medical Gas	General
76VEL	Detector, Mercury	Dental And Oral
86RGN	Detector, Metal, Magnetic	Ophthalmology
90TDC	Detector, Metal, Ultrasonic	Radiology
80RGX	Detector, Microwave Leakage	General
84LEO	Detector, Radiation, Toftness	Cns/Neurology
90WQO	Detector, Radioisotope	Radiology
80RWM	Detector, Strain	General
76EAQ	Detector, Ultraviolet	Dental And Oral
80LJL	Detector/Remover, Lice	General
90QQI	Dosimeter, Radiation	Radiology
80REQ	Meter, Leakage Current (Ammeter)	General
80FLS	Monitor, Apnea	General
74DTW	Monitor, Cardiopulmonary Level Sensing	Cardiovascular
74QRX	Monitor, ECG, Arrhythmia	Cardiovascular
85MAA	Monitor, Fetal Doppler Ultrasound	Obstetrics/Gyn
74DRI	Monitor, Line Isolation	Cardiovascular
79RTA	Probe, Detector, Flow, Blood, Laparoscopy, Ultrasonic	Surgery

DETERGENT

81JCB	Detergent	Hematology

DETERMINATION

81GFK	Standard/Control, Fibrinogen Determination	Hematology
81KQJ	System, Determination, Fibrinogen	Hematology
81KHG	Whole Blood Hemoglobin Determination	Hematology

DEVELOPER

90VGU	Chemical, Film Processor	Radiology

DEVELOPING

91DKK	Tank, Developing, TLC	Toxicology

DEVELOPMENT

80VAN	Contract R&D, Diagnostics	General
80WUH	Contract R&D, Equipment	General

DEVICE

91DJZ	Alcohol Breath Trapping Device	Toxicology
77EWT	Anti-Choke Device, Suction	Ear/Nose/Throat
77EWW	Anti-Choke Device, Tongs	Ear/Nose/Throat

DEVICE *(cont'd)*

77KTH	Anti-Stammering Device	Ear/Nose/Throat
83LJF	Antimicrobial Drug Removal Device	Microbiology
74MOR	Battery, Rechargeable, Replacement for Class III Device	Cardiovascular
84HCC	Biofeedback Device	Cns/Neurology
74DWZ	Biopsy Device, Endomyocardial	Cardiovascular
81JCA	Bleeding Time Device	Hematology
80MDZ	Cleaner, Medical Device	General
85LLS	Contraceptive Tubal Occlusion Device, Male	Obstetrics/Gyn
78FAO	Cystometric Air Device	Gastro/Urology
78FAP	Cystometric Gas (Carbon-Dioxide) Or Hydraulic Device	Gastro/Urology
83MKT	DNA Device, Hepatitis B, Viral	Microbiology
88KDZ	Decalcifier Device, Electrolytic	Pathology
85MNB	Device, Ablation, Thermal, Endometrial	Obstetrics/Gyn
78MIK	Device, Ablation, Thermal, Ultrasonic	Gastro/Urology
74MNN	Device, Ablation, Varicose Vein	Cardiovascular
80LMQ	Device, Access, Peritoneal, Subcutaneous, Implantable	General
79SIW	Device, Anastomosis, Biofragmentable	Surgery
74MVR	Device, Anastomotic, Microvascular	Cardiovascular
77LRK	Device, Anti-Snoring	Ear/Nose/Throat
89IMR	Device, Anti-Tip, Wheelchair	Physical Med
74MUN	Device, Arterial, Temporary, For Embolization Prevention	Cardiovascular
73LYM	Device, Assist, CPR	Anesthesiology
77LZI	Device, Assistive Listening	Ear/Nose/Throat
79MJG	Device, Biopsy, Percutaneous	Surgery
74WYE	Device, Closure, Puncture, Hemostatic	Cardiovascular
84HCB	Device, Conditioning, Aversion	Cns/Neurology
86LZR	Device, Cyclodestructive, Ultrasonic	Ophthalmology
78FEN	Device, Cystometric, Hydraulic	Gastro/Urology
74MEZ	Device, Debridement, Ultrasonic, Heart Valve & HV Seat	Cardiovascular
79MDD	Device, Dermal Replacement	Surgery
83MKS	Device, Detection, Urinary Antibody	Microbiology
84MHM	Device, Diagnostic, Non-Physiological	Cns/Neurology
78LST	Device, Dysfunction, Erectile	Gastro/Urology
84HCG	Device, Embolization, Artificial	Cns/Neurology
84MFS	Device, Energy, Multiple Therapies, Non-Specific	Cns/Neurology
78LYW	Device, External, Management, Weight	Gastro/Urology
85MEE	Device, Fertility, Contraceptive, Diagnostic	Obstetrics/Gyn
84LBK	Device, Fragmentation and Aspiration, Neurosurgical	Cns/Neurology
78LNO	Device, Gastroplasty	Gastro/Urology
80MKB	Device, Germicidal, Ultraviolet	General
74MGB	Device, Hemostasis, Vascular	Cardiovascular
74BTE	Device, Hyperthermia (Blanket, Plumbing & Heat Exchanger)	Cardiovascular
84LWC	Device, Hypothermia, Injury, Cord, Spinal	Cns/Neurology
78LOA	Device, Hypothermia, Testicular	Gastro/Urology
78WLL	Device, Incontinence, Fecal	Gastro/Urology
78MIP	Device, Incontinence, Fecal, Implanted	Gastro/Urology
78EZY	Device, Incontinence, Mechanical/Hydraulic	Gastro/Urology
78MNG	Device, Incontinence, Occlusion, Urethral	Gastro/Urology
78EXI	Device, Incontinence, Paste-On	Gastro/Urology
77MJV	Device, Inflation, Middle Ear	Ear/Nose/Throat
90KPW	Device, Limiting, Beam, Diagnostic, X-Ray	Radiology
90KQA	Device, Limiting, Beam, Teletherapy	Radiology
90IWD	Device, Limiting, Beam, Teletherapy, Radionuclide	Radiology
78FFR	Device, Locking, Clamp, Instestinal	Gastro/Urology
84HCJ	Device, Measurement, Potential, Skin	Cns/Neurology
84JXE	Device, Measurement, Velocity, Conduction, Nerve	Cns/Neurology
78MKL	Device, Measuring, Blood Loss	Gastro/Urology
80MTV	Device, Needle Destruction	General
84MIT	Device, Nerve Repair, Resorbable	Cns/Neurology
74MLV	Device, Occlusion, Cardiac, Transcatheter	Cardiovascular
77MLJ	Device, Otoacoustic	Ear/Nose/Throat
79MBQ	Device, Peripheral Electromag. Field to Aid Wound Healing	Surgery
74MFA	Device, Removal, Pacemaker Electrode, Percutaneous	Cardiovascular
79MLB	Device, Repeat Access (Abdomen)	Surgery
76LQZ	Device, Repositioning, Jaw	Dental And Oral
74MMX	Device, Retrieval, Percutaneous	Cardiovascular
85MNA	Device, Semen Analysis	Obstetrics/Gyn
87MQP	Device, Spinal Vertebral Body Replacement	Orthopedics
74MWS	Device, Stabilizer, Heart	Cardiovascular
90LMB	Device, Storage, Image, Digital	Radiology
80KZG	Device, Suction, Enlargement, Breast	General
83MKR	Device, Susceptibility, Topical Antimicrobial	Microbiology
79MFJ	Device, Suturing, Endoscopic	Surgery
78LJR	Device, Thermal, Hemorrhoids	Gastro/Urology
78LKX	Device, Thermal, Hemorrhoids	Gastro/Urology
77LWI	Device, Ultrasound, Sinus	Ear/Nose/Throat
80MEC	Disinfector, Medical Device	General
79GEI	Electrosurgical Unit, Cutting & Coagulation Device	Surgery
74KRD	Embolization Device	Cardiovascular
80SHH	Equipment, Device Coating, Protective	General
80KZF	Examination Device, AC-Powered	General
85LHD	Fertility Diagnostic Device	Obstetrics/Gyn
76LQX	Finger-Sucking Device	Dental And Oral
86HPL	Fixation Device, AC-Powered, Ophthalmic	Ophthalmology
86HKJ	Fixation Device, Battery-Powered, Ophthalmic	Ophthalmology

DEVICE *(cont'd)*

87VKH	Fixation Device, Extra-Cranial (Head Frame)	Orthopedics
87TCT	Fixation Device, Jaw Fracture	Orthopedics
87UAP	Fixation Device, Spinal (External)	Orthopedics
73CBH	Fixation Device, Tracheal Tube	Anesthesiology
73KFY	Flushing Device, Automatic	Anesthesiology
80LDQ	General Medical Device	General
81LOQ	General Purpose Hematology Device	Hematology
83LIB	General Purpose Microbiology Diagnostic Device	Microbiology
80WXY	Guide, Device, Ultrasonic	General
81KSD	Heat-Sealing Device	Hematology
80LDS	Hot Water Pasteurization Device	General
87JDP	Implant, Fixation Device, Condylar Plate	Orthopedics
87JDO	Implant, Fixation Device, Proximal Femoral	Orthopedics
87JDN	Implant, Fixation Device, Spinal	Orthopedics
78FHW	Impotence Device, Mechanical/Hydraulic	Gastro/Urology
85HDT	Intrauterine Device, Contraceptive (IUD) And Introducer	Obstetrics/Gyn
76EGJ	Iontophoresis Device, Dental	Dental And Oral
80QPF	Label, Device	General
85HHJ	Locator, Intracorporeal Device, Ultrasonic	Obstetrics/Gyn
90LWN	Medical Radiographic Personal Monitoring Device	Radiology
83JTC	Microtiter Diluting/Dispensing Device	Microbiology
76LXD	Optical Caries Detection Device	Dental And Oral
83LGA	Oxidase Test Device for Gonorrhea	Microbiology
85HDM	Packer, Uterine	Obstetrics/Gyn
78FDY	Panendoscope Measuring Device	Gastro/Urology
89IQO	Prosthesis Alignment Device	Physical Med
85HHF	Remover, Intrauterine Device, Contraceptive (Hook Type)	Obstetrics/Gyn
79KGS	Retention Device, Suture	Surgery
80SHG	Service, Device Coating, Protective	General
80WIE	Service, Licensing, Device, Medical	General
79SIX	Sizer, Device, Anastomosis	Surgery
90IXL	Spot Film Device	Radiology
80MED	Sterilant, Medical Device	General
90VGY	Storage Device, Fluoroscopic Image	Radiology
74MFZ	System, Pump & Control, Cardiac Assist, Axial Flow	Cardiovascular
85LHM	System, Thermographic, Liquid Crystal	Obstetrics/Gyn
80QPG	Tag, Device Status	General
84MWT	Therapeutic Neurology Device, Magnet	Cns/Neurology
85SAG	Thermographic Device, Infrared	Obstetrics/Gyn
90KXZ	Thermographic Device, Liquid Crystal, Adjunctive	Radiology
90KYA	Thermographic Device, Liquid Crystal, Non-Powered	Radiology
90LHR	Thermographic Device, Liquid Crystal, Screen	Radiology
80FMR	Transfer Device, Patient, Manual	General
85KNH	Tubal Occlusive Device	Obstetrics/Gyn
84LLN	Vibration Threshold Measurement Device	Cns/Neurology

DEVICES

82MVJ	Devices, Measure, Antibodies to Glomerular Basement Membrane (gbm)	Immunology

DEWAR

75QPH	Flask, Dewar	Chemistry

DH

75JNK	Beta-D-Fructose & NADH Oxidation (U.V.), Sorbitol DH	Chemistry
75JMS	Oxalacetic Acid And NADH Oxidation (U.V.), Maleic DH	Chemistry

DHEA

75JKC	Radioimmunoassay, Dehydroepiandrosterone (Free And Sulfate)	Chemistry

DIABETES

78THN	Alarm, Hypoglycemia	Gastro/Urology
75CHZ	DI (O-Hydroxyphenylimine) Ethane, Calcium	Chemistry
80LZG	Infusion Pump, Insulin	General
78TCQ	Infusion System, Insulin, With Monitor	Gastro/Urology
78WRW	Injector, Insulin	Gastro/Urology
78TGM	Monitor, Blood Glucose (Test)	Gastro/Urology
75WXU	Monitor, Glucose, Blood, Non-Invasive	Chemistry
80WSZ	Sensor, Moisture	General
75WTX	Strip, Test	Chemistry
80RYR	Syringe, Insulin	General
75NBW	System, Test, Blood Glucose, Over-The-Counter	Chemistry

DIACETYL

75CDW	Diacetyl-Monoxime, Urea Nitrogen	Chemistry

DIACETYL-MONOXIME

75CDW	Diacetyl-Monoxime, Urea Nitrogen	Chemistry

DIAGNOSTIC

78MNZ	Analyzer, Diagnostic, Fiberoptic (Bladder)	Gastro/Urology
78MOA	Analyzer, Diagnostic, Fiberoptic (Colon)	Gastro/Urology
74DQO	Catheter, Intravascular, Diagnostic	Cardiovascular
78QIQ	Catheter, Urethral, Diagnostic	Gastro/Urology
81KSO	Centrifuge, Blood Bank, Diagnostic	Hematology
74DXG	Computer, Diagnostic, Pre-Programmed, Single-Function	Cardiovascular
74DQK	Computer, Diagnostic, Programmable	Cardiovascular
73BZM	Computer, Pulmonary Function Interpretator (Diagnostic)	Anesthesiology

DIAGNOSTIC *(cont'd)*

80WLH	Contract Manufacturing, Reagent	General
78FAJ	Cystoscope	Gastro/Urology
84MHM	Device, Diagnostic, Non-Physiological	Cns/Neurology
85MEE	Device, Fertility, Contraceptive, Diagnostic	Obstetrics/Gyn
90KPW	Device, Limiting, Beam, Diagnostic, X-Ray	Radiology
89IKT	Electrode, Needle, Diagnostic Electromyograph	Physical Med
89IKN	Electromyograph, Diagnostic	Physical Med
90UAD	Exerciser, Nuclear Diagnostic (Cardiac Stress Table)	Radiology
85LHD	Fertility Diagnostic Device	Obstetrics/Gyn
83LIB	General Purpose Microbiology Diagnostic Device	Microbiology
90VHL	Generator, Diagnostic X-Ray, High Voltage, 3-Phase	Radiology
90IZO	Generator, Diagnostic X-Ray, High Voltage, Single Phase	Radiology
90ITY	Housing, X-Ray Tube, Diagnostic	Radiology
86HJL	Lens, Condensing, Diagnostic	Ophthalmology
86HJK	Lens, Contact, Polymethylmethacrylate, Diagnostic	Ophthalmology
86HJJ	Lens, Fresnel, Flexible, Diagnostic	Ophthalmology
86HJI	Lens, Fundus, Hruby, Diagnostic	Ophthalmology
78FCQ	Light Source, Incandescent, Diagnostic	Gastro/Urology
79FSP	Loupe, Diagnostic/Surgical	Surgery
86HMC	Monitor, Eye Movement, Diagnostic	Ophthalmology
90IYB	Mount, X-Ray Tube, Diagnostic	Radiology
74WTO	Probe, Transesophageal	Cardiovascular
90KPR	Radiographic Unit, Diagnostic	Radiology
90QJT	Radiographic Unit, Diagnostic, Chest	Radiology
76RNY	Radiographic Unit, Diagnostic, Dental (X-Ray)	Dental And Oral
76EHD	Radiographic Unit, Diagnostic, Dental, Extraoral	Dental And Oral
90RNZ	Radiographic Unit, Diagnostic, Fixed (X-Ray)	Radiology
90TEA	Radiographic Unit, Diagnostic, Head	Radiology
76EAP	Radiographic Unit, Diagnostic, Intraoral	Dental And Oral
90IZH	Radiographic Unit, Diagnostic, Mammographic	Radiology
90IZK	Radiographic Unit, Diagnostic, Mobile, Explosion-Safe	Radiology
90IZG	Radiographic Unit, Diagnostic, Photofluorographic	Radiology
90VGJ	Radiographic Unit, Diagnostic, Pneumoencephalographic	Radiology
90VGK	Radiographic Unit, Diagnostic, Polytomographic	Radiology
90ROB	Radiographic Unit, Diagnostic, Portable (X-Ray)	Radiology
90VGL	Radiographic Unit, Diagnostic, Skeletal	Radiology
90IZF	Radiographic Unit, Diagnostic, Tomographic	Radiology
73BZG	Spirometer, Diagnostic (Respirometer)	Anesthesiology
89ISB	Stimulator, Muscle, Diagnostic	Physical Med
90IZL	System, X-Ray, Mobile	Radiology
90LHP	Telethermographic System (Sole Diagnostic Screen)	Radiology
83VLF	Test, Bacterial Diagnostic	Microbiology
75MGT	Test, Diagnostic, Bana Hydrolase, Dental Plaque	Chemistry
80LHA	Timer, Diagnostic Use	General
90ITX	Transducer, Ultrasonic, Diagnostic	Radiology
77ETK	Tube, Toynbee Diagnostic	Ear/Nose/Throat

DIAGNOSTICS

80VAN	Contract R&D, Diagnostics	General

DIALYSATE

78FKY	Connector, Tubing, Dialysate	Gastro/Urology
78FJB	Detector, Dialysate Level	Gastro/Urology
78FKQ	Dialysate Delivery System, Central Multiple Patient	Gastro/Urology
78KPF	Dialysate Delivery System, Peritoneal, Semi-Automatic	Gastro/Urology
78FIK	Dialysate Delivery System, Recirculating	Gastro/Urology
78FIJ	Dialysate Delivery System, Recirculating, Single Pass	Gastro/Urology
78FII	Dialysate Delivery System, Sealed	Gastro/Urology
78FIL	Dialysate Delivery System, Single Pass	Gastro/Urology
78FKP	Dialysate Delivery System, Single Patient	Gastro/Urology
78FKT	Dialysate Delivery System, Sorbent Regenerated	Gastro/Urology
78KPP	Filter, Peritoneal Dialysate	Gastro/Urology
78FIS	Flowmeter, Dialysate	Gastro/Urology
78QPI	Meter, Dialysate Conductivity	Gastro/Urology
78MNV	Strip, Indicator, pH, Dialysate	Gastro/Urology
78MSY	Strip, Test, Reagent, Residuals For Dialysate, Disinfectant	Gastro/Urology
78FID	Tube, Dialysate	Gastro/Urology
78KQQ	Tubing, Dialysate (And Connector)	Gastro/Urology
78MLW	Warmer, Dialysate, Peritoneal	Gastro/Urology

DIALYSIS

78KNZ	Accessories, AV Shunt	Gastro/Urology
78QGD	Cannula, Hemodialysis	Gastro/Urology
78LFK	Catheter, Femoral	Gastro/Urology
78MPB	Catheter, Hemodialysis	Gastro/Urology
78QIK	Catheter, Hemodialysis, Single-Needle	Gastro/Urology
78FKO	Catheter, Peritoneal Dialysis, Single-Use	Gastro/Urology
78WQV	Chair, Dialysis (With Scale)	Gastro/Urology
78FKS	Chair, Dialysis, Powered (Without Scale)	Gastro/Urology
78FIA	Chair, Dialysis, Unpowered (Without Scale)	Gastro/Urology
78UCO	Clamp, Hemodialysis Unit Blood Line	Gastro/Urology
78KPO	Concentrate, Dialysis, Hemodialysis (Liquid or Powder)	Gastro/Urology
78QZY	Controller, Hemodialysis Unit Single Needle	Gastro/Urology
78QZZ	Converter, Unit, Hemodialysis, Single-Pass	Gastro/Urology
78QZV	Detector, Hemodialysis Unit Air Bubble-Foam	Gastro/Urology
78FKP	Dialysate Delivery System, Single Patient	Gastro/Urology
78QPJ	Dialysis Unit Test Equipment	Gastro/Urology

DIALYSIS *(cont'd)*

78KDI	Dialyzer, High Permeability	Gastro/Urology
78FKJ	Filter, Blood, Dialysis	Gastro/Urology
78RAA	Hemodialysis Unit (Kidney Machine)	Gastro/Urology
78RAB	Hemofiltration Unit	Gastro/Urology
78FLD	Hemoperfusion System, Sorbent	Gastro/Urology
78FJT	Intracatheter, Dialysis	Gastro/Urology
78KDJ	Kit, Administration, Peritoneal Dialysis, Disposable	Gastro/Urology
78LBW	Kit, Dialysis, Single Needle (Co-Axial Flow)	Gastro/Urology
78FIF	Kit, Dialysis, Single Needle With Uni-Directional Pump	Gastro/Urology
78QZU	Kit, Hemodialysis Tubing	Gastro/Urology
78RKM	Kit, Tubing, Dialysis, Peritoneal	Gastro/Urology
78LRI	Meter, pH, Concentration, Ion, Hydrogen, Dialysis	Gastro/Urology
78QZX	Monitor, Hemodialysis Unit Conductivity	Gastro/Urology
78FLA	Monitor, Temperature, Dialysis	Gastro/Urology
78RIC	Needle, Dialysis	Gastro/Urology
78RKL	Peritoneal Dialysis Unit (CAPD)	Gastro/Urology
78FIB	Protector, Transducer, Dialysis	Gastro/Urology
78QZW	Pump, Blood, Hemodialysis Unit	Gastro/Urology
78FIP	Purification System, Water	Gastro/Urology
75SFZ	Purification System, Water, Deionization	Chemistry
75SGA	Purification System, Water, Reverse Osmosis	Chemistry
75SGB	Purification System, Water, Ultraviolet	Chemistry
80KOF	Scales, Dialysis	General
78RTB	Shunt, Arteriovenous	Gastro/Urology
78LLJ	Solution, Dialysis	Gastro/Urology
78FKH	Solution-Test, Standard-Conductivity, Dialysis	Gastro/Urology
78FLC	Station, Dialysis Control, Negative Pressure Type	Gastro/Urology
78FKX	System, Peritoneal Dialysis, Automatic	Gastro/Urology
78FIN	Tank, Holding, Dialysis	Gastro/Urology
78FKF	Tie Gun, Dialysis	Gastro/Urology
78FKE	Tie, Dialysis	Gastro/Urology
78FKG	Tray, Start/Stop (Including Contents), Dialysis	Gastro/Urology
80SDJ	Tube, Transfer	General

DIALYZER

75JQQ	Dialyzer	Chemistry
78LIF	Dialyzer Reprocessing System	Gastro/Urology
78FJI	Dialyzer, Capillary, Hollow Fiber (Hemodialysis)	Gastro/Urology
78FJH	Dialyzer, Disposable	Gastro/Urology
78KDI	Dialyzer, High Permeability	Gastro/Urology
75UFV	Dialyzer, Laboratory	Chemistry
78FJG	Dialyzer, Parallel Flow (Hemodialysis)	Gastro/Urology
75QPK	Dialyzer, Serum/Urine	Chemistry
78FHS	Dialyzer, Single Coil (Hemodialysis)	Gastro/Urology
78FJJ	Dialyzer, Twin Coil	Gastro/Urology
78VHO	Reprocessing Unit, Dialyzer	Gastro/Urology
78FKI	Set, Holder, Dialyzer	Gastro/Urology

DIAMETER

78WZV	Choledochoscope, Mini-Diameter (5mm or Less)	Gastro/Urology
74DYF	Prosthesis, Vascular Graft, Less Than 6mm Diameter	Cardiovascular
74DSY	Prosthesis, Vascular Graft, Of 6mm And Greater Diameter	Cardiovascular

DIAMOND

76DZP	Instrument, Diamond, Dental	Dental And Oral

DIAPER

80QPL	Diaper, Adult	General
80QPM	Diaper, Pediatric	General

DIAPHANOSCOPE

90LEK	Transilluminator (Diaphanoscope)	Radiology

DIAPHORASE

75CFH	Tetrazolium Int Dye-Diaphorase, Lactate Dehydrogenase	Chemistry

DIAPHRAGM

85HDW	Diaphragm, Contraceptive	Obstetrics/Gyn
85HDS	Introducer, Contraceptive Diaphragm	Obstetrics/Gyn
85RKO	Pessary, Diaphragm	Obstetrics/Gyn
84HTL	Stimulator, Diaphragm, Orthopedic	Cns/Neurology

DIAPHRAGMATIC

84GZE	Stimulator, Diaphragmatic/Phrenic Nerve, Implantable	Cns/Neurology

DIAPHYSIS

87HWG	Prosthesis, Diaphysis, Custom	Orthopedics

DIASTASE

88IBC	Diastase	Pathology

DIATHERMY

89VEM	Analyzer, Diathermy Unit, Shortwave	Physical Med
89IOA	Diathermy, Microwave	Physical Med
86HPH	Diathermy, Radiofrequency	Ophthalmology
89IMJ	Diathermy, Shortwave	Physical Med
90MWC	Diathermy, Shortwave (Non-heating)	Radiology
89ILX	Diathermy, Shortwave, Pulsed	Physical Med
89LXF	Diathermy, Ultrasonic (Non-Beep Heat)	Physical Med
89IMI	Diathermy, Ultrasonic (Physical Therapy)	Physical Med

DIATHERMY (cont'd)
89QST Electrode, Diathermy — Physical Med
79UCQ Electrosurgical Equipment, Special Purpose — Surgery
89IPF Stimulator, Muscle, Electrical-Powered (EMS) — Physical Med
89IMG Stimulator, Ultrasound, Muscle — Physical Med
86MLZ Therapeutic Deep Heat Vitrectomy — Ophthalmology

DIAZO
75JMT Diazo (Colorimetric), Nitrite (Urinary, Non-Quantitative) — Chemistry
75CJJ Diazo, ALT/SGPT — Chemistry
75CDF Diazo, P-Nitroaniline/Vanillin, Vanilmandelic Acid — Chemistry

DIAZONIUM
75CDM Diazonium Colorimetry, Urobilinogen (Urinary, Non-Quant.) — Chemistry

DICHROMATE
91DMI Potassium Dichromate Specific Reagent For Alcohol — Toxicology
91DOJ Potassium Dichromate, Alcohol — Toxicology

DIE
77JXW Die, Wire Bending, ENT — Ear/Nose/Throat

DIELECTRIC
80TDK Sealer, Packaging — General

DIETHYLDITHIOCARBAMATE
75JKZ Diethyldithiocarbamate (Colorimetric), Copper — Chemistry

DIFFERENTIAL
81GKZ Counter, Cell, Differential Classifier, Automated — Hematology
81GKM Counter, Differential Hand Tally — Hematology
83JSH Culture Media, Non-Selective And Differential — Microbiology
83JSG Culture Media, Non-Selective And Non-Differential — Microbiology
83JSI Culture Media, Selective And Differential — Microbiology
83JSJ Culture Media, Selective And Non-Differential — Microbiology
75JHS Differential Rate Kinetic Method, CPK Or Isoenzymes — Chemistry
75JGF Differential Rate Method, Lactate Dehydrogenase Isoenzymes — Chemistry
73BYR Transducer, Gas Pressure, Differential — Anesthesiology
73CBI Tube, Tracheal/Bronchial, Differential Ventilation — Anesthesiology

DIFFERENTIATION
83JTO Disc, Strip And Reagent, Microorganism Differentiation — Microbiology

DIFFICILE
83MCB Antigen, C. Difficile — Microbiology
83LLH Reagent, Clostridium Difficile Toxin — Microbiology

DIFFRACTOMETER
75QPO Diffractometer, X-Ray — Chemistry

DIFFUSION
91KZT Disc, Diffusion, Gel, Agar, Serum Level, Gentamicin — Toxicology
91KZW Disc, Diffusion, Gel, Agar, Serum Level, Kanamycin — Toxicology
91KZX Disc, Diffusion, Gel, Agar, Serum Level, Tobramycin — Toxicology
83JTP Kit, Disc Agar Gel Diffusion, Serum Level — Microbiology
84LME Monitor, Cerebral Blood Flow, Thermal Diffusion — Cns/Neurology
75CIK Radial Diffusion, Amylase — Chemistry

DIGITAL
90WIR Densitometer, Radiography, Digital, Quantitative — Radiology
90LMB Device, Storage, Image, Digital — Radiology
90VGB Kit, Angiographic, Digital — Radiology
90WNE Phantom, Digital Subtraction Angiography (DSA) — Radiology
90TGL Radiographic Unit, Digital — Radiology
90VLE Radiographic Unit, Digital Subtraction Angiographic (DSA) — Radiology
90VHC Radiographic/Fluoroscopic Unit, Angiographic, Digital — Radiology
86HMB Recorder, Analog/Digital, Ophthalmic — Ophthalmology
90LMD System, Communication, Image, Digital — Radiology
90MUH System, X-ray, Extraoral Source, Digital — Radiology
80SAK Thermometer, Electronic — General
90WOG Transmitter, Image & Data, Radiographic — Radiology

DIGITIZER
90LMA Image Digitizer — Radiology

DIGITOXIN
91DKQ Antiserum, Digitoxin — Toxicology
91LFM Enzyme Immunoassay, Digitoxin — Toxicology
91DND RIA, Digitoxin (125-I), Rabbit Antibody, Solid Phase Sep. — Toxicology
91DOW RIA, Digitoxin (3-H), Rabbit Antibody, Coated Tube — Toxicology
91LCW Radioimmunoassay, Digitoxin (125-I) — Toxicology
91DPL Radioimmunoassay, Digitoxin (125-I), Bovine, Charcoal — Toxicology
91DPG Radioimmunoassay, Digitoxin (125-I), Rabbit, Coated Tube — Toxicology
91DOB Radioimmunoassay, Digitoxin (3-H) — Toxicology
91DNW Radioimmunoassay, Digitoxin (3-H), Rabbit Antibody, Char. — Toxicology
91DJK Serum, Control, Digitoxin, RIA — Toxicology

DIGOXIN
91DKA Antiserum, Digoxin — Toxicology
91KXT Enzyme Immunoassay, Digoxin — Toxicology
91DNS RIA, Digoxin (125-I), Rabbit Antibody, Double Label Sep. — Toxicology

DIGOXIN (cont'd)
91DOY RIA, Digoxin (3-H), Goat Antibody, 2nd Antibody Sep. — Toxicology
91DNQ RIA, Digoxin (3-H), Rabbit Antibody, Coated Tube Sep. — Toxicology
91DPI Radioimmunoassay, Digoxin — Toxicology
91LCS Radioimmunoassay, Digoxin (125-I) — Toxicology
91DOA Radioimmunoassay, Digoxin (125-I), Goat Anion Exchange — Toxicology
91DNJ Radioimmunoassay, Digoxin (125-I), Goat, 2nd Antibody — Toxicology
91DNL Radioimmunoassay, Digoxin (125-I), Rabbit, 2nd Antibody — Toxicology
91DPB Radioimmunoassay, Digoxin (125-I), Rabbit, Charcoal — Toxicology
91DPO Radioimmunoassay, Digoxin (125-I), Rabbit, Coated Tube — Toxicology
91DOG Radioimmunoassay, Digoxin (125-I), Rabbit, Poly. Glycol — Toxicology
91DON Radioimmunoassay, Digoxin (125-I), Rabbit, Solid Phase — Toxicology
91LCT Radioimmunoassay, Digoxin (3-H) — Toxicology
91DOR Radioimmunoassay, Digoxin (3-H), Bovine, Charcoal — Toxicology
91DPD Radioimmunoassay, Digoxin (3-H), Rabbit, Charcoal — Toxicology
91DMP Serum, Control, Digoxin, RIA — Toxicology

DIHYDROTESTOSTERONE
75CDZ Radioimmunoassay, Testosterones And Dihydrotestosterone — Chemistry

DILATATION
78QIU Catheter, Balloon, Dilatation, Vessel — Gastro/Urology

DILATOMETER
78QPP Dilatometer — Gastro/Urology

DILATOR
77KCD Bougie, Esophageal, ENT — Ear/Nose/Throat
79WZY Dilator, Blunt — Surgery
79GCC Dilator, Catheter — Surgery
78EZN Dilator, Catheter, Ureteral — Gastro/Urology
85HDN Dilator, Cervical, Expandable — Obstetrics/Gyn
85HDQ Dilator, Cervical, Fixed Size — Obstetrics/Gyn
85MCR Dilator, Cervical, Hygroscopic, Synthetic — Obstetrics/Gyn
85HDY Dilator, Cervical, Hygroscopic-Laminaria — Obstetrics/Gyn
85HHG Dilator, Cervical, Vibratory — Obstetrics/Gyn
78QPR Dilator, Common Duct — Gastro/Urology
78KNQ Dilator, Esophageal — Gastro/Urology
78EZM Dilator, Esophageal (Metal Olive) Gastro-Urology — Gastro/Urology
77KCF Dilator, Esophageal, ENT — Ear/Nose/Throat
86MMC Dilator, Expansive Iris (Accessory) — Ophthalmology
79WZZ Dilator, Fascia, Umbilical — Surgery
86HNW Dilator, Lacrimal — Ophthalmology
77LWF Dilator, Nasal — Ear/Nose/Throat
79QPW Dilator, Other — Surgery
79SIN Dilator, Port, Laparoscopic — Surgery
73QPT Dilator, Pulmonary — Anesthesiology
78FFP Dilator, Rectal — Gastro/Urology
77VGE Dilator, Salivary Duct — Ear/Nose/Throat
77KCG Dilator, Tracheal — Ear/Nose/Throat
78QPU Dilator, Tubal — Gastro/Urology
78KOE Dilator, Urethral — Gastro/Urology
78FAH Dilator, Urethral, Mechanical — Gastro/Urology
85QPV Dilator, Uterine — Obstetrics/Gyn
85HDX Dilator, Vaginal — Obstetrics/Gyn
74QPQ Dilator, Vascular — Cardiovascular
78FKA Dilator, Vessel — Gastro/Urology
74DRE Dilator, Vessel, Percutaneous Catheterization — Cardiovascular
74DWP Dilator, Vessel, Surgical — Cardiovascular
85LOB Synthetic Osmotic Cervical Dilator — Obstetrics/Gyn

DILUENT
81GIF Diluent, Blood Cell — Hematology

DILUTER
75QPX Diluter — Chemistry
81GKH Diluter, Blood Cell, Automated — Hematology
81RLF Pipetter — Hematology

DILUTING
81JCG Fluid, Manual Cell Diluting — Hematology
81GJN Fluid, Red Cell Diluting — Hematology
81GGJ Fluid, White Cell Diluting — Hematology
83JTC Microtiter Diluting/Dispensing Device — Microbiology
81GGY Pipette, Diluting — Hematology
75JQW Pipetting And Diluting System, Automated — Chemistry

DILUTION
74UDP Cardiac Output Unit, Dye Dilution — Cardiovascular
74QGL Cardiac Output Unit, Indicator Dilution (Thermal) — Cardiovascular
74TBG Catheter, Dye Dilution (Cardiac Output Indicator) — Cardiovascular
74QIN Catheter, Thermal Dilution — Cardiovascular
74RCE Injector, Thermal Dilution — Cardiovascular
74RND Pump, Dye Dilution — Cardiovascular
75UIX Tray, Serial Dilution — Chemistry

DIMENSION
90UFD Computer, Radiographic Image Analysis — Radiology

DIMENSIONAL

74WYD	Equipment, Ultrasound, Intravascular, 3-Dimensional	Cardiovascular
79SGZ	System, Camera, 3-Dimensional	Surgery

DINITROFLUOROBENZENE

75JMW	2, 4-dinitrofluorobenzene (spectroscopic), Nitrogen (amino-nitrogen)	Chemistry

DINITROPHENYL

75JKF	Dinitrophenyl Hydrazone Measurement (Colorimetric), HBD	Chemistry

DIODE

79SJO	Laser, Diode, Laparoscopy	Surgery

DIOPTOMETER

86HKO	Refractometer, Ophthalmic	Ophthalmology

DIOXIDE

73CBL	Absorbent, Carbon-Dioxide	Anesthesiology
73BSF	Absorber, Carbon-Dioxide	Anesthesiology
73CCC	Analyzer, Gas, Carbon-Dioxide, Blood Phase, Indwelling	Anesthesiology
73CCK	Analyzer, Gas, Carbon-Dioxide, Gaseous Phase (Capnograph)	Anesthesiology
73BXZ	Analyzer, Gas, Carbon-Dioxide, Partial Pressure, Blood	Anesthesiology
75CIL	Colorimetry, Cresol Red, Carbon-Dioxide	Chemistry
75CHS	Coulometric Method, Carbon-Dioxide	Chemistry
79QUA	Cylinder, Carbon-Dioxide	Surgery
78FAP	Cystometric Gas (Carbon-Dioxide) Or Hydraulic Device	Gastro/Urology
73QSO	Electrode, Blood Gas, Carbon-Dioxide	Anesthesiology
73QTG	Electrode, Transcutaneous, Carbon-Dioxide	Anesthesiology
75KHS	Enzymatic, Carbon-Dioxide	Chemistry
78FCX	Insufflator, Carbon-Dioxide, Automatic (For Endoscope)	Gastro/Urology
85HES	Insufflator, Carbon-Dioxide, Uterotubal	Obstetrics/Gyn
77EWG	Laser, Carbon-Dioxide, Microsurgical, ENT	Ear/Nose/Throat
79UKZ	Laser, Carbon-Dioxide, Surgical	Surgery
73QEA	Monitor, Blood Gas, Carbon-Dioxide	Anesthesiology
73TAJ	Monitor, Blood Gas, Transcutaneous Carbon-Dioxide	Anesthesiology
73LKD	Monitor, Carbon-Dioxide, Cutaneous	Anesthesiology
80QUM	Monitor, Gas, Atmospheric, Environmental	General
73ULU	Monitor, Transcutaneous, Carbon-Dioxide	Anesthesiology
75KMS	Phenolphthalein Colorimetry, Carbon-Dioxide	Chemistry
75CHR	Titrimetric Phenol Red, Carbon-Dioxide	Chemistry
75CIE	Volumetric/Manometric, Carbon-Dioxide	Chemistry
75JFL	pH Rate Measurement, Carbon-Dioxide	Chemistry

DIPHENYL

75CHK	Mercuric Nitrate And Diphenyl Carbazone (Titrimetric)	Chemistry

DIPHENYLHYDANTOIN

91DIP	Enzyme Immunoassay, Diphenylhydantoin	Toxicology
91LGR	Fluorescence Polarization Immunoassay, Diphenylhydantoin	Toxicology
91LES	Fluorescent Immunoassay, Diphenylhydantoin	Toxicology
91DKH	Gas Chromatography, Diphenylhydantoin	Toxicology
91DOZ	Liquid Chromatography, Diphenylhydantoin	Toxicology
91LFO	Nephelometric Inhibition Immunoassay, Diphenylhydantoin	Toxicology
91DLP	Radioimmunoassay, Diphenylhydantoin	Toxicology
91DPE	Thin Layer Chromatography, Diphenylhydantoin	Toxicology
91LDC	U.V. Spectrometry, Diphenylhydantoin	Toxicology

DIPHOSPHATE

75CJC	Fructose-1, 6-Diphosphate And NADH (U.V.), Aldolase	Chemistry

DIPHTHERIAE

83GOS	Antiserum, Fluorescent, C. Diphtheriae	Microbiology
83KFI	Corynebacterium Diphtheriae, Virulence Strip	Microbiology

DIRECT

83LIC	Antiserum, Coagglutination (Direct) Neisseria Gonorrhoeae	Microbiology
83GTH	Antiserum, Fluorescent (Direct Test), N. Gonorrhoeae	Microbiology
83LRF	Candida SPP., Direct Antigen, ID	Microbiology
74QGK	Cardiac Output Unit, Direct Fick	Cardiovascular
79GCR	Endoscope, Direct Vision	Surgery
76EKX	Handpiece, Direct Drive, AC-Powered	Dental And Oral
85HGZ	Heater, Perineal, Direct Contact	Obstetrics/Gyn
73KFZ	Humidifier, Non-Direct Patient Interface (Home-Use)	Anesthesiology
73BTT	Humidifier, Respiratory Gas, (Direct Patient Interface)	Anesthesiology
83MKA	Kit, Direct Antigen, Negative Control	Microbiology
83MJZ	Kit, Direct Antigen, Positive Control	Microbiology
83LHL	Legionella Direct & Indirect Fluorescent Antibody Regents	Microbiology
74RLR	Monitor, Blood Pressure, Invasive (Arterial)	Cardiovascular
73CAA	Monitor, Blood Pressure, Invasive (Arterial), Anesthesia	Anesthesiology
84HCS	Monitor, Temperature, Neurosurgery, Direct Contact, Powered	Cns/Neurology
73CAF	Nebulizer, Direct Patient Interface	Anesthesiology
86RIV	Ophthalmoscope, Direct	Ophthalmology
75CIG	Reagent, Bilirubin (Total Or Direct Test System)	Chemistry
79FXD	Stethoscope, Direct (Acoustic), Ultrasonic	Surgery
83LLA	Test, Direct Agglutination, Toxoplasma Gondii	Microbiology

DIRECTED

74DYG	Catheter, Flow Directed	Cardiovascular

DIRECTIONAL

78FIF	Kit, Dialysis, Single Needle With Uni-Directional Pump	Gastro/Urology

DISABLED

89KNO	Accessories, Wheelchair	Physical Med
89IQG	Adapter, Holder, Syringe	Physical Med
89ILS	Adapter, Hygiene	Physical Med
89ILW	Adaptor, Grooming	Physical Med
89ILT	Adaptor, Recreational	Physical Med
77MCK	Amplifier, Voice	Ear/Nose/Throat
89IML	Armrest, Wheelchair	Physical Med
89UMM	Attachment, Bag (Crutch, Walker, Wheelchair)	Physical Med
89INB	Attachment, Commode, Wheelchair	Physical Med
89IMQ	Attachment, Narrowing, Wheelchair	Physical Med
80TDH	Attachment, Oxygen Canister/IV Pole, Wheelchair	General
89IQB	Belt, Wheelchair	Physical Med
89ILP	Communication System, Non-Powered	Physical Med
89ILQ	Communication System, Powered	Physical Med
89KHZ	Control, Foot Driving, Automobile, Mechanical	Physical Med
89IPQ	Control, Hand Driving, Automobile, Mechanical	Physical Med
89INC	Cuff, Pusher, Wheelchair	Physical Med
89IMP	Cushion, Wheelchair (Pad)	Physical Med
89ING	Elevator, Wheelchair	Physical Med
89IQA	Environmental Control System, Powered	Physical Med
89ILR	Environmental Control System, Powered, Remote	Physical Med
89WPB	Equipment, Therapy, Handicapped/Physical	Physical Med
89IMM	Footrest, Wheelchair	Physical Med
89IQZ	Hand, External Limb Component, Powered	Physical Med
77ESD	Hearing-Aid	Ear/Nose/Throat
89INA	Hill Holder, Wheelchair	Physical Med
89IQX	Hook, External Limb Component, Mechanical	Physical Med
89IQW	Hook, External Limb Component, Powered	Physical Med
80REY	Lift, Wheelchair	General
80TFY	Page Turner (Handicapped)	General
80UKQ	Ramp, Wheelchair	General
80TFZ	Reacher (Handicapped)	General
86HJY	Reader, Bar, Ophthalmic	Ophthalmology
86HJX	Reader, Prism, Ophthalmic	Ophthalmology
86HJG	Reading System, Closed-Circuit Television	Ophthalmology
80RPF	Restraint, Wheelchair	General
89INI	Scooter (Motorized 3-Wheeled Vehicle)	Physical Med
89INE	Sling, Overhead Suspension, Wheelchair	Physical Med
77LEZ	Speech Training Aid, AC-Powered	Ear/Nose/Throat
77LFA	Speech Training Aid, Battery-Powered	Ear/Nose/Throat
89IMS	Support, Head And Trunk, Wheelchair	Physical Med
89UME	Telephone, Handicapped Use	Physical Med
89IKX	Transfer Aid	Physical Med
89IMX	Tray, Wheelchair	Physical Med
89ILC	Utensil, Food	Physical Med
89IKW	Utensil, Handicapped Aid	Physical Med
80WMV	Vision Aid, Braille	General
86HPF	Vision Aid, Electronic, AC-Powered	Ophthalmology
86HPG	Vision Aid, Electronic, Battery-Powered	Ophthalmology
86HOT	Vision Aid, Image Intensification, Battery-Powered	Ophthalmology
86HPI	Vision Aid, Optical, AC-Powered	Ophthalmology
86HPE	Vision Aid, Optical, Battery-Powered	Ophthalmology
86WOM	Vision Aid, Ultrasonic	Ophthalmology
89IOR	Wheelchair, Manual	Physical Med
89ITI	Wheelchair, Powered	Physical Med
89IQC	Wheelchair, Special Grade	Physical Med
89IMK	Wheelchair, Stair Climbing	Physical Med
89IPL	Wheelchair, Standup	Physical Med
89KGH	Wrist, External Limb Component, Powered	Physical Med

DISC

91KZT	Disc, Diffusion, Gel, Agar, Serum Level, Gentamicin	Toxicology
91KZW	Disc, Diffusion, Gel, Agar, Serum Level, Kanamycin	Toxicology
91KZX	Disc, Diffusion, Gel, Agar, Serum Level, Tobramycin	Toxicology
83LTX	Disc, Elution	Microbiology
83JTO	Disc, Strip And Reagent, Microorganism Differentiation	Microbiology
83JTN	Disc, Susceptibility, Antimicrobial	Microbiology
83VCS	Dispenser, Disc, Sensitivity, Antibiotic	Microbiology
83JTP	Kit, Disc Agar Gel Diffusion, Serum Level	Microbiology
76MPJ	Prosthesis, Interarticular Disc (Interpositional Implant)	Dental And Oral
87MJO	Prosthesis, Spine, Intervertebral Disc	Orthopedics
87MQO	Prosthetic Disc Nucleus Device	Orthopedics
74DSH	Recorder, Magnetic Tape/Disc	Cardiovascular
75JQI	Rotating Disc, Plasma Viscometry	Chemistry

DISCECTOMY

87WYA	Equipment, Shaving, Disc, Spinal	Orthopedics

DISCHARGE

90IZR	Generator, Radiographic, Capacitor Discharge	Radiology

DISCLOSING
76EAW Kit, Plaque Disclosing — Dental And Oral

DISCONNECT
78FJR Forceps, Disconnect — Gastro/Urology

DISCRETE
75JJE Analyzer, Chemistry, Photometric, Discrete — Chemistry

DISCRIMINATION
84LQW Test, Discrimination, Temperature — Cns/Neurology

DISCRIMINATOR
84GWI Discriminator, Two-point — Cns/Neurology
84IKL Esthesiometer, Touch Discriminator — Cns/Neurology
84IKM Esthesiometer, Two Point Discriminator — Cns/Neurology

DISEASE
75LTC Assay, Disease, Membrane, Hyaline — Chemistry
90MOT Irradiator, Blood to Prevent Graft Vs Host Disease — Radiology
84LLE Stimulator, Cord, Spinal, Implantable (Periph. Vasc. Dis.) — Cns/Neurology
83WSI Test, Dementia, Alzheimer's — Microbiology
82WVP Test, Disease, Lyme — Immunology

DISH
83JTD Analyzer, Petri Dish — Microbiology
75QPY Dish, Petri — Chemistry
88KIZ Dish, Tissue Culture — Pathology

DISINFECTANT
78MSY Strip, Test, Reagent, Residuals For Dialysate, Disinfectant — Gastro/Urology

DISINFECTANTS
80LRJ Medical Disinfectants/Cleaners for Instruments — General

DISINFECTOR
80QKS Cleaner, Bedpan (Sterilizer) — General
80QPZ Disinfector, Liquid — General
80MEC Disinfector, Medical Device — General
80QQA Disinfector, Pasteurization — General
80RED Lamp, Ultraviolet, Germicidal — General
80LKB Pad, Alcohol — General
80RQL Sanitizer — General
76ECG Sterilizer, Boiling Water — Dental And Oral
80UDL Sterilizer, Bulk, Steam & Ethylene-Oxide — General
80KMH Sterilizer, Dry Heat — General
76ECF Sterilizer, Dry Heat, Dental — Dental And Oral
79WHQ Sterilizer, Electrolytic — Surgery
76KOK Sterilizer, Endodontic Dry Heat — Dental And Oral
80FLF Sterilizer, Ethylene-Oxide Gas — General
76ECE Sterilizer, Ethylene-Oxide Gas, Dental — Dental And Oral
79FSJ Sterilizer, Ethylene-Oxide Gas, Operating Room — Surgery
80UDJ Sterilizer, Ethylene-Oxide, Bulk — General
80UDK Sterilizer, Ethylene-Oxide, Table Top — General
85RVV Sterilizer, Formaldehyde — Obstetrics/Gyn
76ECC Sterilizer, Glass Bead — Dental And Oral
83UIM Sterilizer, Laboratory — Microbiology
80RVW Sterilizer, Liquid — General
80RVX Sterilizer, Radiation — General
86HRD Sterilizer, Soft Lens, Thermal, AC-Powered — Ophthalmology
80FLE Sterilizer, Steam (Autoclave) — General
76ECH Sterilizer, Steam (Autoclave), Dental — Dental And Oral
79FSI Sterilizer, Steam (Autoclave), Surgical — Surgery
80UCS Sterilizer, Steam, Bulk — General
80UCT Sterilizer, Steam, Table Top — General
86HKZ Sterilizer, Tonometer — Ophthalmology
80RVY Sterilizer, Ultraviolet — General
80RVZ Sterilizer, Vapor — General
80WWY Sterilizer/Compactor — General
80THI Sterilizer/Washer, Endoscope — General
80SFN Washer, Cart — General
80FLH Washer, Receptacle, Waste, Body — General
80SFR Washer, Utensil — General
80WWK Washer/Disinfector — General

DISINTEGRATOR
83UFW Disintegrator, Biological Cell — Microbiology

DISK
76EHJ Disk, Abrasive — Dental And Oral
86HKH Disk, Pinhole, Ophthalmic — Ophthalmology
76EEJ Guard, Disk — Dental And Oral
87RQD Rongeur, Intervertebral Disk — Orthopedics

DISLOCATION
89IOZ Splint, Abduction, Congenital Hip Dislocation — Physical Med

DISLODGER
78FFL Dislodger, Stone, Basket, Ureteral, Metal — Gastro/Urology
78FGO Dislodger, Stone, Flexible — Gastro/Urology
78LQR Dislodger, Store, Biliary — Gastro/Urology

DISODIUM
75CJX Disodium Phenyl Phosphate, Acid Phosphatase — Chemistry
75CJI Disodium Phenylphosphate, Alkaline Phosphatase Or Isoenzyme — Chemistry

DISORDER
80MIO Light, Therapy, Seasonal Affective Disorder (SAD) — General
84LEP Stimulator, Nerve, Transcutaneous Elec. (Speech Disorder) — Cns/Neurology

DISORDERS
84LGT Stimulator, Cord, Spinal, Implantable (Motor Disorders) — Cns/Neurology

DISPENSER
80WSA Accessories, Cart, Multipurpose — General
80WPQ Container, Medication, Home-Use — General
79QQB Dispenser, Brush — Surgery
87KIH Dispenser, Cement — Orthopedics
83VCS Dispenser, Disc, Sensitivity, Antibiotic — Microbiology
80TGU Dispenser, Fluid — General
80TBU Dispenser, Ice — General
79SJA Dispenser, Laparoscopic — Surgery
75VCT Dispenser, Liquid, Laboratory — Chemistry
80VDP Dispenser, Liquid, Unit-Dose — General
80KYX Dispenser, Medication, Liquid — General
76EHE Dispenser, Mercury And/Or Alloy — Dental And Oral
83JTB Dispenser, Microbiology Media — Microbiology
80QQC Dispenser, Narcotic — General
80WJO Dispenser, Other — General
88IDW Dispenser, Paraffin — Pathology
75WVX Dispenser, Pipette — Chemistry
90WJH Dispenser, Radiopharmaceuticals — Radiology
75QQD Dispenser, Slide — Chemistry
80TBV Dispenser, Soap — General
80WSB Dispenser, Syringe And Needle — General
74SIZ Dispenser, Thorascopic — Cardiovascular
80WIW Dispenser, Tissue, Toilet — General
80WIX Dispenser, Towel — General
76VLM Well, Amalgam — Dental And Oral

DISPENSING
83JTC Microtiter Diluting/Dispensing Device — Microbiology
80MWV Needles, Medicament Dispensing Tip & Irrigating — General
80SHI System, Drug Dispensing, Pharmacy, Automated — General

DISPERSIVE
79JOS Electrode, Electrosurgical, Return (Ground, Dispersive) — Surgery

DISPLAY
74DXJ Display, Cathode-Ray Tube — Cardiovascular

DISPOSABLE
78EXF Bag, Bile Collection — Gastro/Urology
80KYR Bag, Ice — General
78FGF Catheter, Ureteral Disposable (X-Ray) — Gastro/Urology
78FFH Collector, Urine, Disposable — Gastro/Urology
78EZS Colostomy Appliance, Disposable — Gastro/Urology
80WSM Component, Paper — General
80WLY Contract Manufacturing, Product, Disposable — General
80UEG Curtain, Cubicle, Disposable — General
80FMA Depressor, Tongue — General
78FJH Dialyzer, Disposable — Gastro/Urology
79FZJ Drape, Surgical, Disposable — Surgery
78EYY Drape, Urological, Disposable — Gastro/Urology
79RRV Dress, Scrub, Disposable — Surgery
78FFG Flowmeter, Urine, Disposable — Gastro/Urology
79FPH Gown, Operating Room, Disposable — Surgery
79FYB Gown, Patient — Surgery
80QYO Gown, Patient, Disposable — General
79FYA Gown, Surgical — Surgery
78KDJ Kit, Administration, Peritoneal Dialysis, Disposable — Gastro/Urology
78FCD Kit, Barium Enema, Disposable — Gastro/Urology
85QKG Kit, Circumcision, Disposable Tray — Obstetrics/Gyn
74SGT Kit, Disposable Procedure — Cardiovascular
78KDL Kit, Perfusion, Kidney, Disposable — Gastro/Urology
79KDD Kit, Surgical Instrument, Disposable — Surgery
75RDU Labware, Basic, Disposable — Chemistry
86WIZ Lens, Contact, Disposable — Ophthalmology
80RHF Mitt/Washcloth, Patient — General
79GAA Needle, Aspiration And Injection, Disposable — Surgery
79GAB Needle, Suture, Disposable — Surgery
89IMD Pack, Hot Or Cold, Disposable — Physical Med
80UCU Pressure Pad, Alternating, Disposable — General
80JOK Scissors, Disposable — General
79RSL Sheet, Drape, Disposable — Surgery
80RSM Sheet, Examination Table, Disposable — General
79RSO Sheet, Operating Room, Disposable — Surgery
80WKD Sheeting, Stretcher — General
73BWP Shoe And Shoe Cover, Conductive — Anesthesiology
79GAJ Stripper, Vein, Disposable — Surgery
79RRY Suit, Scrub, Disposable — Surgery

DISPOSABLE *(cont'd)*

79FXO	Suit, Surgical	Surgery
79KDC	Surgical Instrument, Disposable	Surgery
76KMT	Tray, Fluoride, Disposable	Dental And Oral

DISPOSAL

80WPN	Crusher, Vial, Laboratory	General
80WZH	Remover, Blade, Scalpel	General
80SFS	Waste Disposal Unit, Sharps	General
79KDB	Waste Disposal Unit, Surgical Instrument (Sharps)	Surgery
80SFT	Waste Disposal Unit, Syringe	General
90SFV	Waste Receptacle, Radioactive	Radiology

DISRUPTER

83VFS	Disrupter, Cell	Microbiology

DISSECTING

88WMB	Board, Dissecting	Pathology
79SIR	Forceps, Biopsy	Surgery
79QLE	Forceps, Grasping, Traumatic	Surgery
79WZD	Forceps, Laparoscopy, Electrosurgical	Surgery
79QQU	Instrument, Dissecting, Laparoscopic	Surgery
79QQY	Instrument, Dissecting, Myoma, Laparoscopic	Surgery
79SJB	Instrument, Separating, Nerve	Surgery
88QQE	Kit, Dissecting	Pathology
80RRI	Scissors, General Dissecting	General
79RRM	Scissors, Plastic Surgery (Dissecting)	Surgery
88RYV	Table, Autopsy	Pathology

DISSECTOR

79SJI	Balloon, Manipulation, Tissue	Surgery
79SJJ	Dissector, Balloon, Surgical	Surgery
79GDI	Dissector, Surgical, General & Plastic Surgery	Surgery
77KBM	Dissector, Tonsil	Ear/Nose/Throat
88RVD	Sponge, Dissector	Pathology

DISSOCIATION

86HJS	Test, Spectacle Dissociation, AC-Powered (Lancaster)	Ophthalmology
86HLO	Test, Spectacle Dissociation, Battery-Powered (Lancaster)	Ophthalmology

DISSOLUTION

78MEU	Agitator, Ultrasonic (Drug Dissolution)	Gastro/Urology
80MHD	Pump, Infusion, Gallstone Dissolution	General

DISSOLVING

76KZP	Solution, Cement Dissolving	Dental And Oral

DISTAL

79WZS	Cannula With Inflatable Balloon (Distal Tip)	Surgery
84UAQ	Catheter, Hydrocephalic, Distal	Cns/Neurology

DISTILLED

78TGB	Water, Distilled (Irrigation)	Gastro/Urology
83WKT	Water, Therapy, Respiratory	Microbiology

DISTILLING

75QQF	Distilling Unit	Chemistry
75UFX	Distilling Unit, Molecular	Chemistry
75UIA	Still, Solvent Recovery	Chemistry
75UIN	Still, Water	Chemistry

DISTOMETER

86HMM	Distometer	Ophthalmology

DISTRACTOR

76QQG	Distractor	Dental And Oral

DISTRIBUTION

87WQP	Analyzer, Distribution, Weight, Podiatric	Orthopedics

DITHIAZONE

91DJN	Mercury Dithiazone, Colorimetry, Barbiturate	Toxicology

DIVIDER

80WSA	Accessories, Cart, Multipurpose	General

DNA

88LNJ	Analyzer, Chromosome, Automated	Pathology
88JCZ	Analyzer, Karyotype	Pathology
82LRM	Anti-DNA Antibody (Enzyme-Labeled), Antigen, Control	Immunology
82LSW	Anti-DNA Antibody, Antigen and Control	Immunology
82KTL	Anti-DNA Indirect Immunofluorescent Solid Phase	Immunology
83LQO	Campylobacter SPP. DNA Reagents	Microbiology
83LSK	Chlamydia, DNA Reagents	Microbiology
83LSO	Cytomegalovirus, DNA Reagents	Microbiology
83MKT	DNA Device, Hepatitis B, Viral	Microbiology
83MCG	DNA-Probe, Agent, Listeria	Microbiology
83MDC	DNA-Probe, Blastomyces Dermatitidis	Microbiology
81MAO	DNA-Probe, Chromosome, Human	Hematology
83MJM	DNA-Probe, Gardnerella Vaginalis	Microbiology
82MMM	DNA-Probe, HER/NEU	Immunology
83MCC	DNA-Probe, Haemophilus SPP.	Microbiology
81MAM	DNA-Probe, Lymphocyte, B & T	Hematology

DNA *(cont'd)*

83MKZ	DNA-Probe, Nucleic Acid Amplification, Chlamydia	Microbiology
83MBT	DNA-Probe, Reagent	Microbiology
83MCS	DNA-Probe, Staphylococcus Aureus	Microbiology
83MCT	DNA-Probe, Strep Pneumoniae	Microbiology
83MJK	DNA-Probe, Trichomonas Vaginalis	Microbiology
83MLA	DNA-Probe, Yeast	Microbiology
83LSF	Epstein-Barr Virus, DNA Reagents	Microbiology
83UGH	Genetic Engineering	Microbiology
83MAQ	Kit, DNA Detection, Human Papillomavirus	Microbiology
83LQH	Legionella DNA Reagents	Microbiology
83WPR	Micro-Injector, Transplant, Gene	Microbiology
83LQF	Mycobacterium SPP. DNA Reagents	Microbiology
83LQG	Mycoplasma SPP. DNA Reagents	Microbiology
83LSL	Neisseria, DNA Reagents	Microbiology
83MDF	Reagent, DNA-Probe, Coccidioides Immitis	Microbiology
83MDE	Reagent, DNA-Probe, Cryptococcal	Microbiology
83MDK	Reagent, DNA-Probe, Streptococcal	Microbiology
83LSM	Salmonella SPP., DNA Reagents	Microbiology
83LSN	Shigella SPP., DNA Reagents	Microbiology
75WJI	Synthesizer, DNA	Chemistry
82VJL	Test, Cancer Detection, DNA-Probe	Immunology
83WNY	Test, DNA-Probe, Other	Microbiology

DNA-PROBE

83MCG	DNA-Probe, Agent, Listeria	Microbiology
83MDC	DNA-Probe, Blastomyces Dermatitidis	Microbiology
81MAO	DNA-Probe, Chromosome, Human	Hematology
83MJM	DNA-Probe, Gardnerella Vaginalis	Microbiology
82MMM	DNA-Probe, HER/NEU	Immunology
83MCC	DNA-Probe, Haemophilus SPP.	Microbiology
81MAM	DNA-Probe, Lymphocyte, B & T	Hematology
83MKZ	DNA-Probe, Nucleic Acid Amplification, Chlamydia	Microbiology
83MBT	DNA-Probe, Reagent	Microbiology
83MCS	DNA-Probe, Staphylococcus Aureus	Microbiology
83MCT	DNA-Probe, Strep Pneumoniae	Microbiology
83MJK	DNA-Probe, Trichomonas Vaginalis	Microbiology
83MLA	DNA-Probe, Yeast	Microbiology
83MDF	Reagent, DNA-Probe, Coccidioides Immitis	Microbiology
83MDE	Reagent, DNA-Probe, Cryptococcal	Microbiology
83MDK	Reagent, DNA-Probe, Streptococcal	Microbiology
82VJL	Test, Cancer Detection, DNA-Probe	Immunology
83WNY	Test, DNA-Probe, Other	Microbiology

DOCTOR'S

80RGJ	Bag, Medical, Physician	General

DOG

83UMA	Animal, Laboratory	Microbiology

DOME

80QQH	Dome, Pressure Transducer	General
80RLY	Kit, Pressure Monitoring (Air/Gas)	General

DONOR

80FML	Chair, Blood Donor	General
80LPZ	Container, Frozen Donor Tissue Storage	General
80QRA	Dressing, Skin Graft, Donor Site	General
81QDZ	Kit, Blood Donor	Hematology
81RHG	Mixer, Blood Bank, Donor Blood	Hematology
80WXG	Service, Tissue Bank	General
81RWS	Stripper, Donor Tube	Hematology
81RYW	Table, Blood Donor	Hematology
82MZE	Test, Donor, Cmv	Immunology

DOOR

90VGS	Entrance, X-Ray Darkrooms	Radiology
90TDY	Shield, X-Ray, Door	Radiology

DOPPLER

80TEU	Analyzer, Doppler Spectrum	General
74ULR	Detector, Blood Flow, Ultrasonic (Doppler)	Cardiovascular
74WSD	Doppler, Blood Flow, Transcranial	Cardiovascular
90VHA	Doppler, Flow Mapping	Radiology
85LQT	Equipment, Ultrasound, Doppler, Evaluation, Fetal	Obstetrics/Gyn
85LXE	Fetal Doppler Ultrasound	Obstetrics/Gyn
74WSR	Flowmeter, Blood, Other	Cardiovascular
78QWP	Flowmeter, Blood, Ultrasonic	Gastro/Urology
85HEP	Monitor, Blood Flow, Ultrasonic	Obstetrics/Gyn
85MAA	Monitor, Fetal Doppler Ultrasound	Obstetrics/Gyn
85KNG	Monitor, Fetal, Ultrasonic	Obstetrics/Gyn
80FLQ	Monitor, Neonatal, Blood Pressure, Ultrasonic/Doppler	General
79RTA	Probe, Detector, Flow, Blood, Laparoscopy, Ultrasonic	Surgery
90IYN	Scanner, Ultrasonic (Pulsed Doppler)	Radiology
90VCV	Scanner, Ultrasonic, Vascular	Radiology

DORSAL

84WHU	Electrode, TENS	Cns/Neurology
79ESS	Prosthesis, Nasal, Dorsal	Surgery
79ESR	Prosthesis, Rhinoplasty	Surgery

DRILL *(cont'd)*
84HBF *Drill, Powered Compound (With Burr, Trephine & Accessories)* Cns/Neurology
77ERL *Drill, Surgical, ENT (Electric Or Pneumatic)* *Ear/Nose/Throat*
76DZJ *Driver, Wire, And Bone Drill, Manual* *Dental And Oral*
87QZA *Guide, Drill* *Orthopedics*
87LXI *Guide, Drill, Ligament* *Orthopedics*
84HBD *Handpiece (Brace), Drill* *Cns/Neurology*
84HBC *Motor, Drill, Electric* *Cns/Neurology*
84HBB *Motor, Drill, Pneumatic* *Cns/Neurology*

DRINK
75MRV *Drink, Glucose Tolerance* *Chemistry*

DRIVE
76EKX *Handpiece, Direct Drive, AC-Powered* *Dental And Oral*

DRIVEN
76EFA *Handpiece, Belt and/or Gear Driven, Dental* *Dental And Oral*
74LWO *Single Chamber, Sensor Driven, Implantable Pulse Generator* Cardiovascular

DRIVER
76ECT *Driver, Band, Orthodontic* *Dental And Oral*
87QRO *Driver, Bone Staple* *Orthopedics*
87HXJ *Driver, Bone Staple, Powered* *Orthopedics*
87HWR *Driver, Prosthesis* *Orthopedics*
79GFC *Driver, Surgical, Pin* *Surgery*
87SGD *Driver, Wire* *Orthopedics*
76DZJ *Driver, Wire, And Bone Drill, Manual* *Dental And Oral*
87QRM *Driver/Extractor, Bone Nail/Pin* *Orthopedics*
87QRN *Driver/Extractor, Bone Plate* *Orthopedics*

DRIVING
89KHZ *Control, Foot Driving, Automobile, Mechanical* *Physical Med*
89IPQ *Control, Hand Driving, Automobile, Mechanical* *Physical Med*
89WHH *Vehicle, Handicapped* *Physical Med*

DROP
78TAQ *Calibrator, Drop-Rate, Infusion* *Gastro/Urology*
74QMS *Counter, Intravenous Drop* *Cardiovascular*

DROP-RATE
78TAQ *Calibrator, Drop-Rate, Infusion* *Gastro/Urology*

DROPPER
77KCM *Dropper, Ear* *Ear/Nose/Throat*
73BTP *Dropper, Ether* *Anesthesiology*
86QRP *Dropper, Eye* *Ophthalmology*
80QRQ *Dropper, Medicine* *General*
77QRR *Dropper, Nose* *Ear/Nose/Throat*

DRUG
78MEU *Agitator, Ultrasonic (Drug Dissolution)* *Gastro/Urology*
75ULK *Analyzer, Chemistry, Therapeutic Drug Monitor (TDM)* *Chemistry*
83LJF *Antimicrobial Drug Removal Device* *Microbiology*
91DKB *Calibrator, Drug Mixture* *Toxicology*
91DLJ *Calibrator, Drug Specific* *Toxicology*
91DLK *Chromatograph, HPL, Drugs of Abuse (Dedicated Instrument)* Toxicology
91MLK *Chromatography, Thin Layer, Tricyclic Antidepressant Drugs* Toxicology
80KYW *Container, Medication, Graduated Liquid* *General*
91DIF *Control, Drug Mixture* *Toxicology*
91LAS *Control, Drug Specific* *Toxicology*
80QNK *Crusher, Pill* *General*
80SHJ *Defroster, Drug, Frozen* *General*
90WJH *Dispenser, Radiopharmaceuticals* *Radiology*
79NAE *Dressing, Wound, Hydrogel W/out Drug And/or Biologic* *Surgery*
77LRD *ENT Drug Applicator* *Ear/Nose/Throat*
91DMC *Gas Chromatograph, Drugs of Abuse (Dedicated Instruments)* Toxicology
91LFI *High Pressure Liquid Chromatography, Tricyclic Drug* *Toxicology*
80QUB *Kit, Emergency Drug* *General*
80WKH *Monitor, Medication* *General*
91MHP *Monitor, Patch, Sudromed, Drug Abuse* *Toxicology*
80MXI *Nonabsorbable Gauze, Surgical Sponge, & Wound Dressing for External Use (with a Drug)* General
80WOL *Patch, Transdermal* *General*
80MQT *Pump, Drug Administration, Closed Loop* *General*
91LFG *Radioimmunoassay, Tricyclic Antidepressant Drugs* *Toxicology*
76DZF *Syringe, Drug, Luer-Lock* *Dental And Oral*
80WOI *System, Delivery, Drug, Non-invasive* *General*
86WVM *System, Delivery, Drug, Ocular* *Ophthalmology*
80SGR *System, Delivery, Drug, Unit-Dose* *General*
80SHI *System, Drug Dispensing, Pharmacy, Automated* *General*
80TGT *System, Infusion, Administration, Drug, Implantable* *General*
75MGX *System, Test, Drugs of Abuse* *Chemistry*
91LPX *Test, Radioreceptor, Neuroleptic Drugs* *Toxicology*
91DKE *Test, Tetrahydrocannabinol* *Toxicology*

DRUG *(cont'd)*
91JXP *Thin Layer Chromatography, Drugs of Abuse (Dedicated Instr.)* Toxicology
91LFH *U.V. Spectrometry, Tricyclic Antidepressant Drugs* *Toxicology*

DRUGS
75MPQ *Container, Specimen, Urine, Drugs Of Abuse, Over The Counter* Chemistry
91MVO *Kit, Test, Multiple, Drugs Of Abuse, Over The Counter* *Toxicology*

DRUM
86HMS *Drum, Eye Knife Test* *Ophthalmology*
86HOW *Drum, Opticokinetic* *Ophthalmology*
80RZU *Drum, Test* *General*

DRY
75ULO *Bath, Dry (Constant Temperature)* *Chemistry*
80VDK *Chest, Dry Ice* *General*
80TBU *Dispenser, Ice* *General*
75JIK *Dry Ash Method, Protein Bound Iodine* *Chemistry*
89LBG *Fluidized Therapy, Unit, Dry Heat* *Physical Med*
86THQ *Insert, Dry Eye* *Ophthalmology*
80KMH *Sterilizer, Dry Heat* *General*
76ECF *Sterilizer, Dry Heat, Dental* *Dental And Oral*
76KOK *Sterilizer, Endodontic Dry Heat* *Dental And Oral*
81SFH *Warmer, Blood, Dry Heat* *Hematology*

DRYER
76EGW *Dryer, Film, Radiographic* *Dental And Oral*
75TBY *Dryer, Labware* *Chemistry*
80WPV *Dryer, Respiratory/Anesthesia Equipment* *General*
80TCW *Laundry Equipment* *General*
80WPY *Washer, Respiratory/Anesthesia Equipment* *General*

DRYING
75JRJ *Drying Unit* *Chemistry*
75UGF *Freeze Drying Equipment* *Chemistry*
80QYG *Glove Processing Unit (Drying, Powdering)* *General*
75TDX *Rack, Drying* *Chemistry*

DSA
90WNE *Phantom, Digital Subtraction Angiography (DSA)* *Radiology*
90VLE *Radiographic Unit, Digital Subtraction Angiographic (DSA)* *Radiology*

DTNB
91JNI *Acetylcholine Iodine and DTNB, Pseudocholinesterase* *Toxicology*

DUAL
90WRK *Densitometer, Bone, Dual Photon* *Radiology*
74LWY *Dual Chamber, Anti-Tachycardia, Pulse Generator* *Cardiovascular*
74LWP *Dual Chamber, Implantable Pulse Generator* *Cardiovascular*
74ULJ *Pacemaker, Heart, Implantable, Dual Chamber* *Cardiovascular*

DUCT
78QPR *Dilator, Common Duct* *Gastro/Urology*
86HNW *Dilator, Lacrimal* *Ophthalmology*
77VGE *Dilator, Salivary Duct* *Ear/Nose/Throat*
78QXB *Forceps, Gallbladder (Biliary Duct)* *Gastro/Urology*
78QTO *Introducer, T-Tube* *Gastro/Urology*
78RMG *Probe, Common Duct* *Gastro/Urology*
86HNL *Probe, Lacrimal* *Ophthalmology*
86HNG *Rongeur, Lacrimal Sac* *Ophthalmology*
78RRR *Scoop, Common Duct* *Gastro/Urology*

DUCTOSCOPE
85MMN *Ductoscope, Breast* *Obstetrics/Gyn*

DUCTUS
79QKN *Clamp, Patent Ductus* *Surgery*
74MAE *Occluder, Patent Ductus, Arteriosus* *Cardiovascular*

DUODENOSCOPE
78FDT *Duodenoscope, Esophago/Gastro* *Gastro/Urology*

DUPLICATOR
90TFQ *Duplicator, X-Ray Film* *Radiology*
90RNW *Printer, Radiographic Duplicator* *Radiology*
90WTF *Unit, Imaging, Thermal* *Radiology*

DURA
84LEM *Dura Mater, Human, Lyophilized* *Cns/Neurology*
84GXQ *Dura-Substitute* *Cns/Neurology*
84RDJ *Knife, Dura Hook* *Cns/Neurology*
84UAV *Prosthesis, Nerve Sheath* *Cns/Neurology*
84RRK *Scissors, Neurosurgical (Dura)* *Cns/Neurology*
84RSB *Separator, Dural* *Cns/Neurology*

DURA-SUBSTITUTE
84GXQ *Dura-Substitute* *Cns/Neurology*
80RTE *Silicone Sheeting* *General*

DURABLE
80WLY *Contract Manufacturing, Product, Disposable* *General*

KEYWORD INDEX

ECHOCARDIOGRAPH
85MGJ Contrast Echocardiograph — Obstetrics/Gyn
74DXK Echocardiograph (Ultrasonic Scanner) — Cardiovascular
80WNI Table, Ultrasound — General

ECHOCARDIOGRAPHIC
74ROJ Recorder, Echocardiographic — Cardiovascular

ECHOENCEPHALOGRAPH
84GXW Echoencephalograph (Ultrasonic Scanner) — Cns/Neurology

ECHOOPHTHALMOGRAPH
90HPR Scanner, Ultrasonic, Ophthalmic — Radiology

ECHOVIRUS
83GNL Antigen, CF (Including CF Control), Echovirus 1-34 — Microbiology
83GNJ Antigen, HA, Echovirus 1-34 — Microbiology
83GRK Antisera, Fluorescent, Echovirus 1-34 — Microbiology
83GNK Antiserum, CF, Echovirus 1-34 — Microbiology
83GNI Antiserum, Neutralization, Echovirus 1-34 — Microbiology

ECT
84GXC Electroconvulsive Therapy Unit (Electroshock) — Cns/Neurology
84WJF Phantom, Therapy, Electroconvulsive — Cns/Neurology
90THG Scanner, Nuclear Emission Computed Tomography (ECT) — Radiology

EDEMA
80FQL Stocking, Elastic — General
89ILG Stocking, Elastic, Physical Medicine — Physical Med
80DWL Stocking, Support (Anti-Embolic) — General

EDTA
82JFQ P-Phenyl-Enediamine/EDTA (Spectrophotometric), Ceruloplasmi — Immunology
75CHW Titrimetric With EDTA And Indicator, Calcium — Chemistry

EEE
83GQC Antiserum, CF, Equine Encephalitis Virus, EEE, WEE — Microbiology

EEG
84GWS Analyzer, Spectrum, EEG Signal — Cns/Neurology
84VDF Cable/Lead, EEG — Cns/Neurology
80WTI Cart, Monitor — General
80QGT Cart, Multipurpose — General
84VKG Computer, Brain Mapping — Cns/Neurology
84QSU Electrode, Electroencephalographic — Cns/Neurology
84GWQ Electroencephalograph — Cns/Neurology
84BRR Monitor, EEG — Cns/Neurology
79FYX Monitor, EEG, Surgery — Surgery
85HGO Monitor, Electroencephalographic, Fetal — Obstetrics/Gyn
80VLR Paper, Recording, ECG/EEG — General
84RON Recorder, Long-Term, EEG — Cns/Neurology
84GZN Rheoencephalograph — Cns/Neurology
84VDD Scanner, Long-Term Recording, EEG — Cns/Neurology
84GWR Simulator, EEG Test Signal — Cns/Neurology
84RWF Stimulator, Visual — Cns/Neurology
84RZK Telemetry Unit, Physiological, EEG — Cns/Neurology
84GYA Tester, Electrode/Lead, Electroencephalograph — Cns/Neurology
84QSC Transmitter/Receiver, EEG, Telephone — Cns/Neurology

EFFORT
73MNR Recorder, Ventilatory Effort — Anesthesiology

EFFUSION
74SIZ Dispenser, Thorascopic — Cardiovascular

EGG
78MYE System, Electrogastrography(egg) — Gastro/Urology

EHRLICH'S
88KKT Hematoxylin, Ehrlich's — Pathology
75JNF Ion Exchange Resin, Ehrlich's Reagent, Porphobilinogen — Chemistry

EIA
83MJL EIA, Blastomyces Dermatitidis — Microbiology

EILEN
85MPS Eilen — Obstetrics/Gyn

EJECTOR
77QSD Ejector, Saliva — Ear/Nose/Throat
76DYN Mouthpiece, Saliva Ejector — Dental And Oral

EKC
74WWU Pad, Electrode — Cardiovascular

ELAPSED
80QLL Clock, Elapsed Time — General

ELASTIC
76ECI Band, Elastic, Orthodontic — Dental And Oral
80FQM Bandage, Elastic — General
80KMO Binder, Elastic — General

ELASTIC *(cont'd)*
80RPJ Retainer, Bandage (Elastic Net) — General
80FQL Stocking, Elastic — General
89ILG Stocking, Elastic, Physical Medicine — Physical Med
80DWL Stocking, Support (Anti-Embolic) — General

ELASTOMER
80WWD Elastomer, Other — General
79MDA Elastomer, Silicone (Scar Management) — Surgery
79MIB Elastomer, Silicone Block — Surgery
80QSE Elastomer, Silicone Rubber — General
77ESH Polymer, ENT Synthetic-PIFE, Silicon Elastomer — Ear/Nose/Throat
87MJU Prosthesis, Subtalar Plug, Polymer (Elastomer) — Orthopedics
79MBR Silastic Elastomer (Angular Deformity Prevention) — Surgery

ELASTOMERIC
80MEB Pump, Infusion, Elastomeric — General

ELBOW
89KFT Assembly, Shoulder/Elbow/Forearm/Wrist/Hand, Mechanical — Physical Med
89KFW Assembly, Shoulder/Elbow/Forearm/Wrist/Hand, Powered — Physical Med
87KRM Hemiprosthesis, Elbow (Humeral Resurfacing) — Orthopedics
87RBI Immobilizer, Elbow — Orthopedics
89IRD Joint, Elbow, External Limb Component, Mechanical — Physical Med
89IRE Joint, Elbow, External Limb Component, Powered — Physical Med
80RMB Pad, Pressure, Foam (Elbow, Heel) — General
87JDC Prosthesis, Elbow, Constrained — Orthopedics
87KWJ Prosthesis, Elbow, Hemi-, Humeral, Metal — Orthopedics
87KWI Prosthesis, Elbow, Hemi-, Radial, Polymer — Orthopedics
87UBN Prosthesis, Elbow, Humeral Component — Orthopedics
87JDA Prosthesis, Elbow, Non-Constrained, Unipolar — Orthopedics
87UBO Prosthesis, Elbow, Radial Component — Orthopedics
87JDB Prosthesis, Elbow, Semi-Constrained — Orthopedics
87UBM Prosthesis, Elbow, Total — Orthopedics
87UBP Prosthesis, Elbow, Ulna Component — Orthopedics
87RXF Support, Elbow — Orthopedics

ELECTRIC
80WJN Analyzer, Battery — General
80FNL Bed, Electric — General
80LLI Bed, Electric, Home-Use — General
80WJG Cable, Electric — General
89INO Chair, Position, Electric — Physical Med
80WJM Charger, Battery — General
78FFZ Cord, Electric, Endoscope — Gastro/Urology
78FBJ Cord, Electric, Instrument, Surgical, Transurethral — Gastro/Urology
77ERL Drill, Surgical, ENT (Electric Or Pneumatic) — Ear/Nose/Throat
78KGE Forceps, Biopsy, Electric — Gastro/Urology
78FCL Forceps, Biopsy, Non-Electric — Gastro/Urology
82MEM Generator, Electric Field (Aids Treatment) — Immunology
80KZE Injector, Fluid, Non-Electric — General
79FWA Locator, Electric — Surgery
86HRB Microscope, Operating, Non-Electric, Ophthalmic — Ophthalmology
84HBC Motor, Drill, Electric — Cns/Neurology
80MLX Pad, Medicated, Adhesive, Non-Electric — General
77KLY Photo-Electric Glottograph — Ear/Nose/Throat
74JOM Plethysmograph, Photo-Electric, Pneumatic Or Hydraulic — Cardiovascular
77JPW Pump, Nebulizer, Electric — Ear/Nose/Throat
87MCJ Pump, Vacuum, Electric, Suction-Type Electrode — Orthopedics
74DWI Saw, Electric — Cardiovascular
76DZH Saw, Electric Bone — Dental And Oral
77EWQ Saw, Surgical, ENT (Electric Or Pneumatic) — Ear/Nose/Throat
73MNC Stimulator, Abdominal, Electric — Anesthesiology
87HTM Stimulator, Osteogenesis, Electric, Invasive — Orthopedics
87WNT Stimulator, Osteogenesis, Electric, Non-Invasive — Orthopedics
78MMZ Table, Cystometric, Electric — Gastro/Urology
73BYK Tent, Oxygen, Electric — Anesthesiology
76LWM Unit, Anesthesia, Dental, Electric — Dental And Oral

ELECTRICAL
79WDY Accessories, Electrical Power (Electrocautery) — Surgery
74DSM Alarm, Leakage Current, Portable — Cardiovascular
80TAD Alarm, Voltage — General
80QSF Analyzer, Electrical Safety — General
78FFX Analyzer, Motility, Gastrointestinal, Electrical — Gastro/Urology
74DRJ Analyzer, Signal Isolation — Cardiovascular
79FZK Chair, Surgical, Non-Electrical — Surgery
78FGW Clamp, Electrical — Gastro/Urology
78FFN Clamp, Non-Electrical — Gastro/Urology
80UMS Column, Life Support (Electrical/Gas) — General
80WKG Component, Electrical — General
78EXQ Cystometer, Electrical Recording — Gastro/Urology
80QTQ Detector, Electrostatic Voltage — General
80SGQ Heater, Electrical Instrument — General
80REQ Meter, Leakage Current (Ammeter) — General
80CAR Monitor, Cerebral Spinal Fluid Pressure, Electrical — General
74DRI Monitor, Line Isolation — Cardiovascular
89FPG Pad, Heating, Electrical — Physical Med

KEYWORD INDEX

ELECTRICAL *(cont'd)*
80TDS Plug, Electrical — General
80TCS Power System, Isolated — General
80WMN Power Systems, Uninterruptible (UPS) — General
80TEE Receptacle, Electrical — General
80WMM Regulator, Line Voltage — General
78FAN Sigmoidoscope, Rigid, Electrical — Gastro/Urology
78KDM Sigmoidoscope, Rigid, Non-Electrical — Gastro/Urology
78FGX Snare, Non-Electrical — Gastro/Urology
86TEV Spud, Ophthalmic, Electrical — Ophthalmology
73BZT Stethoscope, Esophageal, With Electrical Conductors — Anesthesiology
78LNL Stimulator, Collection, Sperm, Electrical — Gastro/Urology
84LPY Stimulator, Electrical, Cranial, External — Cns/Neurology
84GWF Stimulator, Electrical, Evoked Response — Cns/Neurology
78EZW Stimulator, Electrical, For Incontinence — Gastro/Urology
84MEI Stimulator, Electrical, Implanted (Coma Arousal) — Cns/Neurology
84MHY Stimulator, Electrical, Implanted (Parkinsonian Tremor) — Cns/Neurology
89MPH Stimulator, Electrical, Muscle — Physical Med
78KPI Stimulator, Incontinence (Non-Implantable), Electrical — Gastro/Urology
89IPF Stimulator, Muscle, Electrical-Powered (EMS) — Physical Med
84LEP Stimulator, Nerve, Transcutaneous Elec. (Speech Disorder) — Cns/Neurology
84LEN Stimulator, Reduction, Anxiety, Electrical — Cns/Neurology
78KQS Table, Cystometric, Non-Electrical — Gastro/Urology
79GDC Table, Surgical, Electrical — Surgery
78EYH Table, Urological, Non-Electrical — Gastro/Urology
80RZW Tester, Conductivity, Floor And Equipment — General
80RZX Tester, Conductivity, Shoe And Gown — General
80QYV Tester, Ground Fault Circuit Interrupter — General
80QYX Tester, Ground Loop Impedance — General
80QYY Tester, Grounding System — General
80SAA Tester, Isolated Power System — General
80SAB Tester, Receptacle, Electrical — General
80SAD Tester, Resistance, Line Cord — General
84LSS Unit, Repair, Nerve, Implantable, Electric — Cns/Neurology
78EXS Urinometer, Electrical — Gastro/Urology
78EXT Urinometer, Non-Electrical — Gastro/Urology
80SGC Wattmeter — General

ELECTRICAL-POWERED
89IPF Stimulator, Muscle, Electrical-Powered (EMS) — Physical Med

ELECTRICITY
79SHL Generator, Power, Electrosurgical — Surgery

ELECTRO
81JBM Glucose-6-Phosphate Dehydrogenase (Erythrocytic), Electro — Hematology

ELECTRO-ANALGESIC
84UFF Stimulator, Electro-Analgesic — Cns/Neurology

ELECTRO-HYDRAULIC
78VKM Lithotriptor, Electro-Hydraulic, Extracorporeal — Gastro/Urology
78FFK Lithotriptor, Electro-Hydraulic, Percutaneous — Gastro/Urology

ELECTRO-OCULOGRAPH
86QTM Electro-Oculograph — Ophthalmology
86QSX Electrode, Electro-Oculograph — Ophthalmology
84RZM Telemetry Unit, Physiological, EOG — Cns/Neurology

ELECTROANALGESIC
84GYZ Stimulator, Intracerebral/Subcortical, Implantable — Cns/Neurology
84GZJ Stimulator, Nerve, Transcutaneous (Pain Relief, TENS) — Cns/Neurology
84GZF Stimulator, Peripheral Nerve, Implantable (Pain Relief) — Cns/Neurology
84GZB Stimulator, Spinal Cord, Implantable (Pain Relief) — Cns/Neurology

ELECTROANESTHESIA
73BWL Electroanesthesia Apparatus — Anesthesiology
73BSZ Gas-Machine, Anesthesia — Anesthesiology
73GZH Stimulator, Electroanesthesia — Anesthesiology

ELECTROCARDIOCONTOUROGRAPH
74QSG Electrocardiocontourograph — Cardiovascular

ELECTROCARDIOGRAM
74LOS Analyzer, ECG — Cardiovascular

ELECTROCARDIOGRAPH
74DRW Adapter, Lead Switching, Electrocardiograph — Cardiovascular
74LOS Analyzer, ECG — Cardiovascular
74DTC Analyzer, Pacemaker Generator Function — Cardiovascular
74REP Cable/Lead, ECG — Cardiovascular
74WLG Cable/Lead, ECG, Radiolucent — Cardiovascular
74DSA Cable/Lead, ECG, With Transducer And Electrode — Cardiovascular
74QMC Computer, ECG Interpretation (Arrhythmia) — Cardiovascular
74QMG Computer, Stress Exercise — Cardiovascular
74MLO Electrocardiograph, Ambulatory (With Analysis Algorithm) — Cardiovascular
74MWJ Electrocardiograph, Ambulatory(without Analysis) — Cardiovascular
74UER Electrocardiograph, Interpretive — Cardiovascular
74QSJ Electrocardiograph, Multi-Channel — Cardiovascular
74DPS Electrocardiograph, Single Channel — Cardiovascular

ELECTROCARDIOGRAPH *(cont'd)*
74WLP Electrode, ECG, Radiolucent — Cardiovascular
74DRX Electrode, Electrocardiograph — Cardiovascular
74WOW Electrode, Electrocardiograph, Long-Term — Cardiovascular
74MLN Electrode, Electrocardiograph, Multi-Function — Cardiovascular
74DYA Gel, Electrode, Electrocardiograph — Cardiovascular
74QRW Monitor, ECG — Cardiovascular
74TGX Monitor, ECG, Ambulatory, Real-Time — Cardiovascular
73BRS Monitor, ECG, Anesthesia — Anesthesiology
74QRX Monitor, ECG, Arrhythmia — Cardiovascular
79FYW Monitor, ECG, Surgery — Surgery
74QZN Monitor, Heart Rate, R-Wave (ECG) — Cardiovascular
80MLC Monitor, ST Segment — General
80MLD Monitor, ST Segment (With Alarm) — General
74ROL Recorder, Long-Term, ECG — Cardiovascular
74ROM Recorder, Long-Term, ECG, Portable (Holter Monitor) — Cardiovascular
74DSF Recorder, Paper Chart — Cardiovascular
74RQU Scanner, Long-Term, ECG, Recording — Cardiovascular
74RTH Simulator, ECG — Cardiovascular
90IXO Synchronizer, ECG/Respirator, Radiographic — Radiology
90IYY Synchronizer, Electrocardiograph, Nuclear — Radiology
74RZJ Telemetry Unit, Physiological, ECG — Cardiovascular
74QSI Tester, Electrocardiograph Cable — Cardiovascular
74KRC Tester, Electrode, Surface, Electrocardiograph — Cardiovascular
74QRY Transmitter/Receiver System, ECG, Telephone Multi-Channel — Cardiovascular
74QRZ Transmitter/Receiver System, ECG, Telephone Single-Channel — Cardiovascular

ELECTROCARDIOGRAPHIC
85HGQ Monitor, Electrocardiographic, Fetal — Obstetrics/Gyn

ELECTROCARDIOPHONE
74DQC Phonocardiograph — Cardiovascular

ELECTROCAUTERIZATION
79WWP Cover, Tip, Probe, Cauterization — Surgery
79SJK Equipment, Suction/Irrigation/Electrocautery, Laparoscopic — Surgery
79QLE Forceps, Grasping, Traumatic — Surgery
79QYU Laser, Nd:YAG, Laparoscopy — Surgery
79SJW Needle, Cutting, Bipolar, Electrocauterization — Surgery
79SJV Probe, Electrocauterization, Microlaparoscopy — Surgery
79QEZ Probe, Electrocauterization, Multi-Use — Surgery
79QHA Probe, Electrocauterization, Single-Use — Surgery
79QIJ Tip, Instrument, Electrocauterization, Monopolar — Surgery

ELECTROCAUTERY
79WDY Accessories, Electrical Power (Electrocautery) — Surgery
79SIH Blade, Electrosurgery, Laparoscopic — Surgery
86HQO Cautery, Thermal, AC-Powered — Ophthalmology
86HQP Cautery, Thermal, Battery-Powered — Ophthalmology
79QSK Electrocautery Unit, Battery-Powered — Surgery
85HIM Electrocautery Unit, Endoscopic — Obstetrics/Gyn
85HGI Electrocautery Unit, Gynecologic — Obstetrics/Gyn
79QSL Electrocautery Unit, Line-Powered — Surgery
79SII Electrode, Electrosurgery, Laparoscopic — Surgery
79SIF Handle, Instrument, Laparoscopic (Electrocautery) — Surgery
79SIJ Instrument, Electrosurgery, Laparoscopic — Surgery
79SIG Module, Control, Electrosurgery — Surgery
79SJC Probe, Electrosurgery, Endoscopy — Surgery
79SJE Scalpel, Ultrasonic — Surgery

ELECTROCHEMICAL
91LEQ Detector, Electrochemical, Chromatography, Liquid — Toxicology
80WXQ Equipment, Marking, Electrochemical — General

ELECTROCONVULSIVE
84GXC Electroconvulsive Therapy Unit (Electroshock) — Cns/Neurology
84WJF Phantom, Therapy, Electroconvulsive — Cns/Neurology

ELECTRODE
80RGO Amplifier, Microelectrode — General
85HGR Applicator, Electrode, Scalp, Fetal — Obstetrics/Gyn
74THD Belt, Electrode — Cardiovascular
89IKD Cable, Electrode — Physical Med
74DSA Cable/Lead, ECG, With Transducer And Electrode — Cardiovascular
74DRF Catheter, Electrode Recording, Or Probe — Cardiovascular
74MFA Device, Removal, Pacemaker Electrode, Percutaneous — Cardiovascular
74LPB Electrode, Ablation, Tissue, Conduction, Percutaneous — Cardiovascular
89IKA Electrode, Biopotential, Surface, Composite — Physical Med
89IKB Electrode, Biopotential, Surface, Metallic — Physical Med
73QSO Electrode, Blood Gas, Carbon-Dioxide — Anesthesiology
73QSP Electrode, Blood Gas, Oxygen — Anesthesiology
75CHL Electrode, Blood pH — Chemistry
74QSQ Electrode, Catheter Tip — Cardiovascular
85HGP Electrode, Circular (Spiral), Scalp And Applicator — Obstetrics/Gyn
85HIQ Electrode, Clip, Fetal Scalp (And Applicator) — Obstetrics/Gyn
86HLZ Electrode, Corneal — Ophthalmology
84GYC Electrode, Cortical — Cns/Neurology
84GXY Electrode, Cutaneous — Cns/Neurology

ELECTRODE *(cont'd)*

78QSR	Electrode, Cystoscopic	Gastro/Urology
74QSS	Electrode, Defibrillator	Cardiovascular
84GZL	Electrode, Depth	Cns/Neurology
89QST	Electrode, Diathermy	Physical Med
74WPX	Electrode, ECG, Hand-Held	Cardiovascular
74WLP	Electrode, ECG, Radiolucent	Cardiovascular
86QSX	Electrode, Electro-Oculograph	Ophthalmology
74DRX	Electrode, Electrocardiograph	Cardiovascular
74WOW	Electrode, Electrocardiograph, Long-Term	Cardiovascular
74MLN	Electrode, Electrocardiograph, Multi-Function	Cardiovascular
84QSU	Electrode, Electroencephalographic	Cns/Neurology
84QSV	Electrode, Electromyographic	Cns/Neurology
86QSW	Electrode, Electronystagmographic	Ophthalmology
79SII	Electrode, Electrosurgery, Laparoscopic	Surgery
79FAS	Electrode, Electrosurgical, Active (Blade)	Surgery
79UEB	Electrode, Electrosurgical, Active, Foot Controlled	Surgery
79JOS	Electrode, Electrosurgical, Return (Ground, Dispersive)	Surgery
84LHG	Electrode, Epidural, Spinal	Cns/Neurology
78QSY	Electrode, Esophageal	Gastro/Urology
85QSZ	Electrode, Fetal Scalp	Obstetrics/Gyn
78FEH	Electrode, Flexible Suction Coagulator	Gastro/Urology
74WOV	Electrode, Gel	Cardiovascular
74WOU	Electrode, Holter	Cardiovascular
80LJJ	Electrode, In Vivo Calcium Ion Selective	General
80LJI	Electrode, In Vivo Potassium Ion Selective	General
75JJP	Electrode, Ion Selective (Non-Specified)	Chemistry
75JIG	Electrode, Ion Specific, Ammonia	Chemistry
75JFP	Electrode, Ion Specific, Calcium	Chemistry
75CGZ	Electrode, Ion Specific, Chloride	Chemistry
75CFA	Electrode, Ion Specific, Magnesium	Chemistry
75CEM	Electrode, Ion Specific, Potassium	Chemistry
75JGS	Electrode, Ion Specific, Sodium	Chemistry
75CDS	Electrode, Ion Specific, Urea Nitrogen	Chemistry
75UHF	Electrode, Laboratory pH	Chemistry
89IKS	Electrode, Metallic With Soft Pad Covering	Physical Med
74QTA	Electrode, Myocardial	Cardiovascular
84GZK	Electrode, Nasopharyngeal	Cns/Neurology
84GXZ	Electrode, Needle	Cns/Neurology
84BWR	Electrode, Needle, Anesthesiology	Cns/Neurology
89IKT	Electrode, Needle, Diagnostic Electromyograph	Physical Med
84HMA	Electrode, Needle, Ophthalmic	Cns/Neurology
84QTB	Electrode, Neurological	Cns/Neurology
84QTC	Electrode, Neuromuscular Stimulator	Cns/Neurology
80QTI	Electrode, Other	General
74MIS	Electrode, Pacemaker, Esophageal	Cardiovascular
74QTD	Electrode, Pacemaker, External	Cardiovascular
74LDF	Electrode, Pacemaker, Temporary	Cardiovascular
74UCG	Electrode, Pacemaker, Transthoracic	Cardiovascular
84MFO	Electrode, Recording, Cortical, Implanted	Cns/Neurology
86QTE	Electrode, Retinographic	Ophthalmology
86HLY	Electrode, Skin Surface, Ophthalmic	Ophthalmology
75UFY	Electrode, Specific Ion	Chemistry
73BWY	Electrode, Surface	Anesthesiology
75QTF	Electrode, Sweat Test	Chemistry
84WHU	Electrode, TENS	Cns/Neurology
73QTG	Electrode, Transcutaneous, Carbon-Dioxide	Anesthesiology
73QTH	Electrode, Transcutaneous, Oxygen	Anesthesiology
78FFT	Electrode, pH	Gastro/Urology
80WKY	Garment, Electrode	General
74DYA	Gel, Electrode, Electrocardiograph	Cardiovascular
79JOT	Gel, Electrode, Electrosurgical	Surgery
76EAS	Gel, Electrode, Pulp Tester	Dental And Oral
84GYB	Gel, Electrode, Stimulator	Cns/Neurology
89IKC	Gel, Electrode, TENS	Physical Med
79QSM	Holder, Electrosurgical Electrode	Surgery
75CGL	Ion Electrode Based Enzymatic, Creatinine	Chemistry
74UCH	Lead, Pacemaker (Catheter)	Cardiovascular
74QIG	Lead, Pacemaker, Implantable Endocardial	Cardiovascular
74DTB	Lead, Pacemaker, Implantable Myocardial	Cardiovascular
80RGQ	Microelectrode	General
74WWU	Pad, Electrode	Cardiovascular
80RGP	Puller, Microelectrode	General
87MCJ	Pump, Vacuum, Electric, Suction-Type Electrode	Orthopedics
73RSA	Sensor, Oxygen	Anesthesiology
84LHY	Stabilized Epidural Spinal Electrode	Cns/Neurology
80QSN	Strap, Electrode	General
79SJQ	System, Monitoring, Electrode, Active, Electrosurgical	Surgery
80RZY	Tester, Electrode	General
74KRC	Tester, Electrode, Surface, Electrocardiograph	Cardiovascular
84GYA	Tester, Electrode/Lead, Electroencephalograph	Cns/Neurology
74DTA	Tester, Pacemaker Electrode Function	Cardiovascular

ELECTROENCEPHALOGRAPH

84GWS	Analyzer, Spectrum, EEG Signal	Cns/Neurology
84VDF	Cable/Lead, EEG	Cns/Neurology
84VKG	Computer, Brain Mapping	Cns/Neurology
84GWQ	Electroencephalograph	Cns/Neurology

ELECTROENCEPHALOGRAPH *(cont'd)*

84BRR	Monitor, EEG	Cns/Neurology
79FYX	Monitor, EEG, Surgery	Surgery
84GZN	Rheoencephalograph	Cns/Neurology
84VDD	Scanner, Long-Term Recording, EEG	Cns/Neurology
84GWR	Simulator, EEG Test Signal	Cns/Neurology
84GYA	Tester, Electrode/Lead, Electroencephalograph	Cns/Neurology

ELECTROENCEPHALOGRAPHIC

84QSU	Electrode, Electroencephalographic	Cns/Neurology
84BRR	Monitor, EEG	Cns/Neurology
85HGO	Monitor, Electroencephalographic, Fetal	Obstetrics/Gyn
84RON	Recorder, Long-Term, EEG	Cns/Neurology
84RZK	Telemetry Unit, Physiological, EEG	Cns/Neurology
84QSC	Transmitter/Receiver, EEG, Telephone	Cns/Neurology

ELECTROFOCUSING

75UFZ	Electrofocusing Equipment	Chemistry

ELECTROGASTROGRAPHY

78MYE	System, Electrogastrography(egg)	Gastro/Urology

ELECTROGLOTTOGRAPH

77KLX	Electroglottograph	Ear/Nose/Throat

ELECTROLYSIS

80WPK	Electrolysis Equipment, Other	General
86HPY	Electrolysis Unit, Battery-Powered, Ophthalmic	Ophthalmology
86HRO	Electrolysis Unit, Ophthalmic	Ophthalmology

ELECTROLYTE

75QTJ	Analyzer, Chemistry, Electrolyte	Chemistry
75VIN	Analyzer, Combination Chemistry/Hematology/Electrolyte	Chemistry
75JJR	Control, Electrolyte (Assayed And Unassayed)	Chemistry
75JJO	Photometer, Flame Emission	Chemistry
91DLM	Photometer, Flame, Heavy Metals (Dedicated Instrument)	Toxicology
75JIH	Photometer, Flame, Lithium	Chemistry
91DOQ	Photometer, Flame, Lithium, Toxicology	Toxicology
75JGM	Photometer, Flame, Potassium	Chemistry
75JGT	Photometer, Flame, Sodium	Chemistry

ELECTROLYTIC

88KDZ	Decalcifier Device, Electrolytic	Pathology
88IFF	Decalcifier Solution, Electrolytic	Pathology
79WHQ	Sterilizer, Electrolytic	Surgery

ELECTROMAGNETIC

79MBQ	Device, Peripheral Electromag. Field to Aid Wound Healing	Surgery
78FIT	Flowmeter, Blood, Non-Invasive Electromagnetic	Gastro/Urology
76LYD	Stimulator, Growth, Bone, Electromagnetic, Dental	Dental And Oral
81BSA	Warmer, Blood, Electromagnetic Radiation	Hematology
73BSB	Warmer, Blood, Non-Electromagnetic Radiation	Anesthesiology

ELECTROMANOMETER

80QTK	Electromanometer	General

ELECTROMETRY

91DOH	Electrometry, Cholinesterase	Toxicology

ELECTROMYOGRAPH

89IKT	Electrode, Needle, Diagnostic Electromyograph	Physical Med
89IKN	Electromyograph, Diagnostic	Physical Med
73CAB	Monitor, EMG	Anesthesiology
89GWP	Myograph	Physical Med

ELECTROMYOGRAPHIC

84QSV	Electrode, Electromyographic	Cns/Neurology
89RZL	Telemetry Unit, Physiological, EMG	Physical Med

ELECTRON-MICROSCOPY

88IFT	Glutaraldehyde (Fixative)	Pathology
83RGU	Microscope, Laboratory, Electron	Microbiology

ELECTRONIC

75QCF	Balance, Electronic	Chemistry
80VAF	Component, Electronic	General
89IKG	Dynamometer, Physical Medicine, Electronic	Physical Med
79VKP	Endoscope, Electronic (Videoendoscope)	Surgery
77ETS	Generator, Electronic Noise (For Audiometric Testing)	Ear/Nose/Throat
86HPM	Locator, Metal, Electronic	Ophthalmology
80THH	Sphygmomanometer, Electronic (Arterial Pressure)	General
80UDM	Sphygmomanometer, Electronic, Automatic	General
80UDN	Sphygmomanometer, Electronic, Manual	General
74DQD	Stethoscope, Electronic (Auscultoscope)	Cardiovascular
79FXC	Stethoscope, Electronic-Amplified	Surgery
80SAK	Thermometer, Electronic	General
80FLL	Thermometer, Electronic, Continuous	General
86HPF	Vision Aid, Electronic, AC-Powered	Ophthalmology
86HPG	Vision Aid, Electronic, Battery-Powered	Ophthalmology

ELECTRONIC-AMPLIFIED

79FXC	Stethoscope, Electronic-Amplified	Surgery

KEYWORD INDEX

EMBOLIC

79MFE	Agent, Injectable, Embolic	Surgery
74RWI	Stocking, Anti-Embolic, Pneumatic	Cardiovascular
80DWL	Stocking, Support (Anti-Embolic)	General

EMBOLISM

74QLZ	Compression Unit, Intermittent (Anti-Embolism Pump)	Cardiovascular
74QZI	Detector, Air, Heart-Lung Bypass	Cardiovascular
74ULR	Detector, Blood Flow, Ultrasonic (Doppler)	Cardiovascular
74KRL	Detector, Bubble, Cardiopulmonary Bypass	Cardiovascular
73CBA	Monitor, Air Embolism, Ultrasonic	Anesthesiology

EMBOLIZATION

79MAG	Agent, Embolization/Occlusion	Surgery
74MUN	Device, Arterial, Temporary, For Embolization Prevention	Cardiovascular
84HCG	Device, Embolization, Artificial	Cns/Neurology
74KRD	Embolization Device	Cardiovascular

EMBRYO

85VIK	Equipment, In Vitro Fertilization/Embryo Transfer	Obstetrics/Gyn

EMERGENCY

80QAO	Ambulance	General
80TFU	Ambulance, Air	General
80WNB	Amputation Protection Unit	General
77EWT	Anti-Choke Device, Suction	Ear/Nose/Throat
77EWW	Anti-Choke Device, Tongs	Ear/Nose/Throat
80QBQ	Aspirator, Emergency Suction	General
80LDI	Blanket, Fire	General
80QDV	Blanket, Rescue	General
73BZN	Cart, Emergency, Cardiopulmonary Resuscitation (Crash)	Anesthesiology
80WMY	Clothing, Protective	General
80WMR	Collar, Extrication	General
80VBO	Communication Equipment	General
80VFG	Communication System, Emergency Alert, Personal	General
77JOH	Cuff, Tracheostomy Tube	Ear/Nose/Throat
74QOR	Defibrillator, Battery-Powered	Cardiovascular
74QOS	Defibrillator, Line-Powered	Cardiovascular
74QOO	Defibrillator/Monitor, Battery-Powered	Cardiovascular
74QOP	Defibrillator/Monitor, Line-Powered	Cardiovascular
75TCG	Fountain, Eye Wash	Chemistry
73SBH	Holder, Tracheostomy Tube	Anesthesiology
86WKX	Irrigator, Ocular, Emergency	Ophthalmology
80QUB	Kit, Emergency Drug	General
80UDB	Kit, Emergency, Anaphylactic	General
80UDC	Kit, Emergency, Cardiopulmonary Resuscitation	General
80RCG	Kit, Emergency, Insect Sting	General
79LRR	Kit, First Aid	Surgery
88RSZ	Kit, Shroud	Pathology
73RGC	Mask, Tracheostomy, Aerosol Administration	Anesthesiology
80WLB	Mattress, Immobilization	General
73BWC	Needle, Emergency Airway	Anesthesiology
74QOQ	Pad, Defibrillator Paddle	Cardiovascular
80TCS	Power System, Isolated	General
80WMN	Power Systems, Uninterruptible (UPS)	General
80WMM	Regulator, Line Voltage	General
80WMZ	Rescue Equipment	General
73BTZ	Resuscitator, Cardiac, Mechanical, Compressor	Anesthesiology
76DZX	Resuscitator, Emergency Oxygen	Dental And Oral
73WJE	Resuscitator, Emergency, Protective, Infection	Anesthesiology
75TEP	Shower, Emergency	Chemistry
80VLO	Stretcher, Basket, Portable	General
80WKO	Stretcher, Collapsible	General
80WIG	Stretcher, Emergency, Other	General
80FPP	Stretcher, Hand-Carried	General
80VAT	Telephone Equipment	General
73BTO	Tube, Tracheostomy (W/Wo Connector)	Anesthesiology
73BTM	Ventilator, Emergency, Manual (Resuscitator)	Anesthesiology
73BTL	Ventilator, Emergency, Powered (Resuscitator)	Anesthesiology

EMESIS

80FNY	Basin, Emesis	General

EMG

84VDG	Cable/Lead, EMG	Cns/Neurology
84QSV	Electrode, Electromyographic	Cns/Neurology
89IKT	Electrode, Needle, Diagnostic Electromyograph	Physical Med
73CAB	Monitor, EMG	Anesthesiology
89GWP	Myograph	Physical Med
89RZL	Telemetry Unit, Physiological, EMG	Physical Med

EMISSION

80FRF	Equipment, Cleaning, Air	General
80WLA	Equipment, Control, Pollution	General
75JJO	Photometer, Flame Emission	Chemistry
90KPS	Scanner, Emission Computed Tomography	Radiology
90THG	Scanner, Nuclear Emission Computed Tomography (ECT)	Radiology
90ULI	Scanner, Positron Emission Tomography (PET)	Radiology

EMPHYSEMA

73RJM	Concentrator, Oxygen	Anesthesiology

EMPTY

73KGA	Cylinder, Gas (Empty)	Anesthesiology

EMS

89IPF	Stimulator, Muscle, Electrical-Powered (EMS)	Physical Med

EMULSIFIER

86HQC	Phacofragmentation Unit	Ophthalmology

EMULSION

75CFG	Emulsion, Oil, (Titrimetric), Lipase	Chemistry
75CET	Emulsion, Olive Oil (Turbidimetric), Lipase	Chemistry

ENCAPSULATOR

80WUM	Encapsulator, Fluid	General

ENCEPHALITIS

83GQD	Antigen, CF (Including CF Control), Equine Encephalitis	Microbiology
83GQC	Antiserum, CF, Equine Encephalitis Virus, EEE, WEE	Microbiology

ENCEPHALOGRAPH

84GXW	Echoencephalograph (Ultrasonic Scanner)	Cns/Neurology
84GWQ	Electroencephalograph	Cns/Neurology
84GZN	Rheoencephalograph	Cns/Neurology

ENCLOSURE

79FZI	Air Handling Apparatus, Enclosure	Surgery
75UHT	Enclosure, Bacteriological Safety	Chemistry

END

73BYE	Attachment, Breathing, Positive End Expiratory Pressure	Anesthesiology
73SEO	Valve, Positive End Expiratory Pressure (PEEP)	Anesthesiology

END-TIDAL

73CCK	Analyzer, Gas, Carbon-Dioxide, Gaseous Phase (Capnograph)	Anesthesiology

ENDARTERECTOMY

74RFH	Loop, Endarterectomy	Cardiovascular
74WWF	Shunt, Carotid	Cardiovascular

ENDOCAPSULAR

86MRJ	Ring, Endocapsular	Ophthalmology

ENDOCARDIAL

74QIG	Lead, Pacemaker, Implantable Endocardial	Cardiovascular
74UCI	Lead, Pacemaker, Temporary Endocardial	Cardiovascular

ENDOCERVICAL

85HFC	Aspirator, Endocervical	Obstetrics/Gyn

ENDODONTIC

76EKW	Broach, Endodontic	Dental And Oral
76EKT	Curette, Endodontic	Dental And Oral
76QUC	Endodontic Instrument	Dental And Oral
76EKS	File, Pulp Canal, Endodontic	Dental And Oral
76VEI	Kit, Endodontic	Dental And Oral
76EKR	Plugger, Root Canal, Endodontic	Dental And Oral
76EKN	Point, Paper, Endodontic	Dental And Oral
76EKL	Point, Silver, Endodontic	Dental And Oral
76EKQ	Preparer, Root Canal, Endodontic	Dental And Oral
76EKP	Reamer, Pulp Canal, Endodontic	Dental And Oral
76ELS	Splint, Endodontic Stabilizer	Dental And Oral
76EKK	Spreader, Pulp Canal Filling Material, Endodontic	Dental And Oral
76KOK	Sterilizer, Endodontic Dry Heat	Dental And Oral
76EIC	Syringe, Periodontic, Endodontic	Dental And Oral

ENDOILLUMINATOR

86MPA	Endoilluminator	Ophthalmology

ENDOLYMPHATIC

77UAG	Shunt, Endolymphatic	Ear/Nose/Throat
77ESZ	Tube, Shunt, Endolymphatic	Ear/Nose/Throat
77KLZ	Tube, Shunt, Endolymphatic, With Valve	Ear/Nose/Throat

ENDOMAGNETIC

78FCC	Retriever, Endomagnetic	Gastro/Urology

ENDOMETRIAL

85HFF	Aspirator, Endometrial	Obstetrics/Gyn
85HFE	Brush, Endometrial	Obstetrics/Gyn
85HHK	Curette, Suction, Endometrial	Obstetrics/Gyn
85MNB	Device, Ablation, Thermal, Endometrial	Obstetrics/Gyn
85RQI	Kit, Sampling, Endometrial	Obstetrics/Gyn
85HFD	Washer, Endometrial	Obstetrics/Gyn

ENDOMYOCARDIAL

74DWZ	Biopsy Device, Endomyocardial	Cardiovascular

ENDOMYSIAL

82MVM	Autoantibodies, Endomysial(tissue Transglutaminase)	Immunology

KEYWORD INDEX

ENDOPROSTHESIS

74MIR	Shunt, Portosystemic, Endoprosthesis	Cardiovascular

ENDORADIOSONDES

78EXW	Pill, Radio	Gastro/Urology

ENDOSCOPE

78MNK	Accessories, Bite Blocks (For Endoscope)	Gastro/Urology
78MNL	Accessories, Cleaning Brushes (For Endoscope)	Gastro/Urology
78FFY	Adapter, Bulb, Endoscope, Miscellaneous	Gastro/Urology
85HFA	Amnioscope, Transabdominal (Fetoscope)	Obstetrics/Gyn
74LYK	Angioscope	Cardiovascular
78FER	Anoscope, Non-Powered	Gastro/Urology
87HRX	Arthroscope	Orthopedics
77BTN	Bronchoscope, Non-Rigid	Ear/Nose/Throat
77EOQ	Bronchoscope, Rigid	Ear/Nose/Throat
73BTJ	Bronchoscope, Rigid, Non-Ventilating	Anesthesiology
73BTH	Bronchoscope, Rigid, Ventilating	Anesthesiology
78FCY	Bulb, Inflation (Endoscope)	Gastro/Urology
78WUJ	Cabinet, Storage, Endoscope	Gastro/Urology
78FBN	Choledochoscope, Flexible Or Rigid	Gastro/Urology
78FDF	Colonoscope, Gastro-Urology	Gastro/Urology
79FTJ	Colonoscope, General & Plastic Surgery	Surgery
85HEX	Colposcope	Obstetrics/Gyn
79SIP	Connector, Suction/Irrigation	Surgery
78FFZ	Cord, Electric, Endoscope	Gastro/Urology
85HEW	Culdoscope	Obstetrics/Gyn
78FAJ	Cystoscope	Gastro/Urology
78FBO	Cystourethroscope	Gastro/Urology
76WNX	Dentoscope	Dental And Oral
78FDT	Duodenoscope, Esophago/Gastro	Gastro/Urology
78KOG	Endoscope	Gastro/Urology
79GCP	Endoscope And Accessories, AC-Powered	Surgery
79GCS	Endoscope And Accessories, Battery-Powered	Surgery
79GCR	Endoscope, Direct Vision	Surgery
79VKP	Endoscope, Electronic (Videoendoscope)	Surgery
85HGK	Endoscope, Fetal Blood Sampling	Obstetrics/Gyn
79GDB	Endoscope, Fiberoptic	Surgery
78GCQ	Endoscope, Flexible	Gastro/Urology
84GWG	Endoscope, Neurological	Cns/Neurology
78KYH	Endoscope, Ophthalmic	Gastro/Urology
79GCM	Endoscope, Rigid	Surgery
85HEZ	Endoscope, Transcervical (Amnioscope)	Obstetrics/Gyn
78VJF	Endoscope, Ultrasonic Probe (Lithotriptor)	Gastro/Urology
78FDA	Enteroscope	Gastro/Urology
77EOX	Esophagoscope (Flexible Or Rigid)	Ear/Nose/Throat
78GCL	Esophagoscope, General & Plastic Surgery	Gastro/Urology
78FDW	Esophagoscope, Rigid, Gastro-Urology	Gastro/Urology
78QYC	Gastroscope, Flexible	Gastro/Urology
78FDS	Gastroscope, Gastro-Urology	Gastro/Urology
78GCK	Gastroscope, General & Plastic Surgery	Gastro/Urology
78QYD	Gastroscope, Rigid	Gastro/Urology
79QYN	Gown, Operating Room, Reusable	Surgery
85HIH	Hysteroscope	Obstetrics/Gyn
78FFS	Illuminator, Fiberoptic (For Endoscope)	Gastro/Urology
77WXV	Inflator, Sheet, Nasopharyngoscopic	Ear/Nose/Throat
78FCX	Insufflator, Carbon-Dioxide, Automatic (For Endoscope)	Gastro/Urology
79GCJ	Laparoscope, General & Plastic Surgery	Surgery
85HET	Laparoscope, Gynecologic	Obstetrics/Gyn
77EQN	Laryngoscope	Ear/Nose/Throat
73CAL	Laryngoscope, Flexible	Anesthesiology
73CCW	Laryngoscope, Rigid	Anesthesiology
79GCI	Laryngoscope, Surgical	Surgery
77EQL	Laryngostroboscope	Ear/Nose/Throat
79GCT	Light Source, Endoscope, Xenon Arc	Surgery
78TDA	Lumboscope	Gastro/Urology
77ESB	Magnifier, Aural (Pneumatic Otoscope)	Ear/Nose/Throat
79GCH	Mediastinoscope	Surgery
77EWY	Mediastinoscope, ENT	Ear/Nose/Throat
80TFB	Monitor, Video, Endoscope	General
84RHO	Myeloscope	Cns/Neurology
77EOB	Nasopharyngoscope (Flexible Or Rigid)	Ear/Nose/Throat
77RHS	Nasoscope	Ear/Nose/Throat
78RIM	Nephroscope, Flexible	Gastro/Urology
78RIN	Nephroscope, Rigid	Gastro/Urology
80RIP	Observerscope	General
77ERA	Otoscope	Ear/Nose/Throat
78FTK	Pancreatoscope, Biliary	Gastro/Urology
78FAK	Panendoscope (Gastroduodenoscope)	Gastro/Urology
78FAL	Panendoscope (Urethroscope)	Gastro/Urology
78GCG	Peritoneoscope	Gastro/Urology
77RKR	Pharyngoscope	Ear/Nose/Throat
79GCF	Proctoscope	Surgery
78RML	Proctosigmoidoscope	Gastro/Urology
90RNP	Pyeloscope	Radiology
78FJL	Resectoscope	Gastro/Urology
77RQB	Rhinoscope	Ear/Nose/Throat
73VDU	Scope, Fiberoptic Intubation	Anesthesiology

ENDOSCOPE *(cont'd)*

78FAM	Sigmoidoscope, Flexible	Gastro/Urology
78FAN	Sigmoidoscope, Rigid, Electrical	Gastro/Urology
78KDM	Sigmoidoscope, Rigid, Non-Electrical	Gastro/Urology
78FDR	Sphincteroscope	Gastro/Urology
80THI	Sterilizer/Washer, Endoscope	General
78FBP	Telescope, Rigid, Endoscopic	Gastro/Urology
74SAM	Thoracoscope	Cardiovascular
79GCW	Transformer, Endoscope	Surgery
78FGB	Ureteroscope	Gastro/Urology
78FGC	Urethroscope	Gastro/Urology
85SEL	Vaginoscope	Obstetrics/Gyn
79SHE	Warmer, Endoscope	Surgery

ENDOSCOPIC

78FEB	Accessories, Cleaning, Endoscopic	Gastro/Urology
79SJN	Accessories, Laser, Endoscopic	Surgery
78FEM	Accessories, Photographic, Endoscopic	Gastro/Urology
78FEJ	Attachment, Binocular, Endoscopic	Gastro/Urology
78QEE	Bottle, Endoscopic Wash	Gastro/Urology
78FCP	Box, Battery, Pocket (Endoscopic)	Gastro/Urology
78FCO	Box, Battery, Rechargeable (Endoscopic)	Gastro/Urology
78FDX	Brush, Cytology, Endoscopic	Gastro/Urology
79FTS	Camera, Cine, Endoscopic (With Audio)	Surgery
79FWL	Camera, Cine, Endoscopic (Without Audio)	Surgery
79FXM	Camera, Still, Endoscopic	Surgery
79FWG	Camera, Television, Endoscopic (With Audio)	Surgery
79FWF	Camera, Television, Endoscopic (Without Audio)	Surgery
80WQY	Camera, Video, Endoscopic	General
78FGS	Carrier, Sponge, Endoscopic	Gastro/Urology
85HIN	Coagulator/Cutter, Endoscopic, Bipolar	Obstetrics/Gyn
85KNF	Coagulator/Cutter, Endoscopic, Unipolar	Obstetrics/Gyn
80WLE	Computer, Image, Endoscopic	General
79MFJ	Device, Suturing, Endoscopic	Surgery
85HIM	Electrocautery Unit, Endoscopic	Obstetrics/Gyn
78FEI	Eyepiece, Lens, Non-Prescription, Endoscopic	Gastro/Urology
78FDZ	Eyepiece, Lens, Prescription, Endoscopic	Gastro/Urology
78QWY	Forceps, Endoscopic	Gastro/Urology
78QXC	Forceps, Grasping, Flexible Endoscopic	Gastro/Urology
78SJD	Kit, Gastrostomy, Endoscopic, Percutaneous	Gastro/Urology
79FTI	Lamp, Endoscopic, Incandescent	Surgery
85HIE	Light Source, Endoscopic	Obstetrics/Gyn
79FSW	Light, Surgical, Endoscopic	Surgery
79GCO	Mirror, Endoscopic	Surgery
78FBK	Needle, Endoscopic	Gastro/Urology
78FEC	Obturator, Endoscopic	Gastro/Urology
80QUD	Power Supply, Endoscopic, Battery-Operated	General
80QUE	Power Supply, Endoscopic, Line-Operated	General
79GCN	Prism, Endoscopic	Surgery
78FEQ	Pump, Air, Non-Manual, Endoscopic	Gastro/Urology
80QBN	Service, Repair, Endoscopic	General
78FED	Sheath, Endoscopic	Gastro/Urology
79ULT	Snare, Endoscopic	Surgery
78FET	Tape, Television & Video, Endoscopic	Gastro/Urology
78FEA	Teaching Attachment, Endoscopic	Gastro/Urology
78FBP	Telescope, Rigid, Endoscopic	Gastro/Urology
78FCZ	Tube, Smoke Removal, Endoscopic	Gastro/Urology

ENDOSCOPY

80WVY	Cart, Equipment, Video	General
79SHL	Generator, Power, Electrosurgical	Surgery
79SJC	Probe, Electrosurgery, Endoscopy	Surgery

ENDOSSEOUS

76DZE	Implant, Endosseous	Dental And Oral
76LYC	Implant, Endosseous (Bone Filling and/or Augmentation)	Dental And Oral

ENDOTHELIAL

74MFY	Kit, Cell Harvesting, Endothelial	Cardiovascular

ENDOTRACHEAL

73LNZ	Changer, Tube, Endotracheal	Anesthesiology
73BTR	Tube, Tracheal (Endotracheal)	Anesthesiology

ENDOVASCULAR

85UAN	Stent, Other	Obstetrics/Gyn
74MIH	System, Treatment, Aortic Aneurysm, Endovascular Graft	Cardiovascular

ENEDIAMINE

82JFQ	P-Phenyl-Enediamine/EDTA (Spectrophotometric), Ceruloplasmi	Immunology

ENEMA

80QUF	Bag, Enema	General
78FGD	Catheter, Retention, Barium Enema With Bag	Gastro/Urology
78FCD	Kit, Barium Enema, Disposable	Gastro/Urology
80QUG	Kit, Enema	General
78FCE	Kit, Enema (For Cleaning Purposes)	Gastro/Urology
80QUH	Tip, Enema	General
78SCU	Tube, Enema	Gastro/Urology

ENERGY

74MPD	Auxillary Power Supply, Low Energy Defibrillator (AC or DC)	Cardiovascular
74MPE	Auxillary Power Supply, Pacemaker, Cardiac, External Trans.	Cardiovascular
80WKG	Component, Electrical	General
80VBT	Control System, Energy	General
74DRK	Defibrillator, Battery-Powered, High Energy	Cardiovascular
74LDD	Defibrillator, Battery-Powered, Low Energy	Cardiovascular
84MFS	Device, Energy, Multiple Therapies, Non-Specific	Cns/Neurology
80TCS	Power System, Isolated	General
80WMN	Power Systems, Uninterruptible (UPS)	General

ENFLURANE

73QZE	Analyzer, Gas, Anesthetic	Anesthesiology
73CBQ	Analyzer, Gas, Enflurane, Gaseous Phase (Anesthetic Conc.)	Anesthesiology

ENG

86QTL	Electronystagmograph (ENG)	Ophthalmology

ENGINE

86HRG	Accessories, Engine, Trephine, AC-Powered	Ophthalmology
79HRF	Accessories, Engine, Trephine, Battery-Powered	Surgery
79HLD	Accessories, Engine, Trephine, Gas-Powered	Surgery
76QOV	Engine, Dental	Dental And Oral
76EIA	Operative Dental Treatment Unit	Dental And Oral

ENGINEERING

80WTN	Adapter, Cable, Equipment	General
74DSM	Alarm, Leakage Current, Portable	Cardiovascular
80TAD	Alarm, Voltage	General
89VEM	Analyzer, Diathermy Unit, Shortwave	Physical Med
80TEU	Analyzer, Doppler Spectrum	General
74LOS	Analyzer, ECG	Cardiovascular
80QSF	Analyzer, Electrical Safety	General
79QTT	Analyzer, Electrosurgical Unit	Surgery
80VLP	Analyzer, Infusion Pump	General
80REO	Analyzer, Lead	General
74DTC	Analyzer, Pacemaker Generator Function	Cardiovascular
74DRJ	Analyzer, Signal Isolation	Cardiovascular
84GWS	Analyzer, Spectrum, EEG Signal	Cns/Neurology
84RWA	Analyzer, Transcutaneous Nerve Stimulator	Cns/Neurology
80SDZ	Analyzer, Ultrasonic Unit	General
90IXD	Calibrator Source, Nuclear Sealed	Radiology
73QFN	Calibrator, Anesthesia Unit	Anesthesiology
77EWA	Calibrator, Audiometer	Ear/Nose/Throat
80WMK	Calibrator, Blood Gas	General
78TAQ	Calibrator, Drop-Rate, Infusion	Gastro/Urology
73BXX	Calibrator, Gas, Pressure	Anesthesiology
73BXW	Calibrator, Gas, Volume	Anesthesiology
80WML	Calibrator, Mass Spectrometer	General
73QFO	Calibrator, Pressure Transducer	Anesthesiology
90QFP	Calibrator, Radioisotope	Radiology
73QFQ	Calibrator, Respiratory Therapy Unit	Anesthesiology
86HLA	Calibrator, Tonometer	Ophthalmology
80UKP	Casters, Hospital Equipment	General
80WXA	Component, Other	General
80WUH	Contract R&D, Equipment	General
80QTQ	Detector, Electrostatic Voltage	General
78QPJ	Dialysis Unit Test Equipment	Gastro/Urology
73BXK	Gas, Calibrated (Specified Concentration)	Anesthesiology
83UGH	Genetic Engineering	Microbiology
74KFJ	Kit, Repair, Pacemaker	Cardiovascular
74DTG	Magnet, Test, Pacemaker	Cardiovascular
78QPI	Meter, Dialysate Conductivity	Gastro/Urology
80REQ	Meter, Leakage Current (Ammeter)	General
80SDX	Meter, Ultrasonic Power	General
74DRI	Monitor, Line Isolation	Cardiovascular
90IYP	Phantom, Anthropomorphic, Nuclear	Radiology
90IXG	Phantom, Anthropomorphic, Radiographic	Radiology
90VHB	Phantom, Computed Axial Tomography (CAT, CT)	Radiology
76VDR	Phantom, Dental, Radiographic	Dental And Oral
90IYQ	Phantom, Flood Source, Nuclear	Radiology
90VGI	Phantom, Mammographic	Radiology
90VKD	Phantom, NMR/MRI	Radiology
90VHI	Phantom, Radiotherapy	Radiology
84GXX	Phantom, Ultrasonic Scanner, Neurology	Cns/Neurology
90RKQ	Phantom, Ultrasound	Radiology
80TDS	Plug, Electrical	General
80TCS	Power System, Isolated	General
74KRG	Programmer, Pacemaker	Cardiovascular
80TEE	Receptacle, Electrical	General
80WND	Service, Engineering/Design	General
74RTF	Simulator, Arrhythmia	Cardiovascular
74RTG	Simulator, Blood Pressure	Cardiovascular
74RTH	Simulator, ECG	Cardiovascular
84GWR	Simulator, EEG Test Signal	Cns/Neurology
74RTI	Simulator, Heart Sound	Cardiovascular

ENGINEERING *(cont'd)*

73RTJ	Simulator, Lung	Anesthesiology
90RTL	Simulator, Radiotherapy	Radiology
90KPQ	Simulator, Radiotherapy, Special Purpose	Radiology
73RTK	Simulator, Respiration	Anesthesiology
80RTM	Simulator, Temperature	General
90IXF	Test Pattern, Radiographic	Radiology
90JAR	Test Pattern/Phantom, Radionuclide	Radiology
80QKC	Tester, Circuit Breaker	General
80RZW	Tester, Conductivity, Floor And Equipment	General
80RZX	Tester, Conductivity, Shoe And Gown	General
74DRL	Tester, Defibrillator	Cardiovascular
74QSI	Tester, Electrocardiograph Cable	Cardiovascular
80RZY	Tester, Electrode	General
84GYA	Tester, Electrode/Lead, Electroencephalograph	Cns/Neurology
80QYV	Tester, Ground Fault Circuit Interrupter	General
80QYX	Tester, Ground Loop Impedance	General
80QYY	Tester, Grounding System	General
80AZZ	Tester, Infusion Pump	General
80SAA	Tester, Isolated Power System	General
74DTA	Tester, Pacemaker Electrode Function	Cardiovascular
73RLK	Tester, Pneumatic	Anesthesiology
90LHO	Tester, Radiology	Radiology
90TDZ	Tester, Radiology Quality Assurance	Radiology
80SAB	Tester, Receptacle, Electrical	General
80SAC	Tester, Receptacle, Mechanical	General
80SAD	Tester, Resistance, Line Cord	General
80SAE	Tester, Surgical Glove	General
74DTF	Tools, Pacemaker Service	Cardiovascular
80SGC	Wattmeter	General

ENGRAVING

80WVQ	Service, Engraving	General

ENHANCEMENT

83RGS	Contrast Enhancement Unit, Microscope	Microbiology

ENLARGEMENT

80KZG	Device, Suction, Enlargement, Breast	General

ENOLASE

75MGW	Enzyme Immunoassay, Gamma Enolase	Chemistry

ENRICHED

83KZI	Culture Media, Enriched	Microbiology

ENT

77KCJ	Applicator, ENT	Ear/Nose/Throat
77KCK	Atomizer And Tip, ENT	Ear/Nose/Throat
77JPL	Block, Bite, ENT	Ear/Nose/Throat
77JXS	Block, Cutting, ENT	Ear/Nose/Throat
77KCL	Blower, Powder, ENT	Ear/Nose/Throat
77KCD	Bougie, Esophageal, ENT	Ear/Nose/Throat
77QFC	Cabinet, ENT Treatment	Ear/Nose/Throat
84WHW	Chair, Rotating	Cns/Neurology
77JXT	Crimper, Wire, ENT	Ear/Nose/Throat
77KBL	Depressor, Tongue, ENT, Metal	Ear/Nose/Throat
77EWF	Depressor, Tongue, ENT, Wood	Ear/Nose/Throat
77JXW	Die, Wire Bending, ENT	Ear/Nose/Throat
77KCF	Dilator, Esophageal, ENT	Ear/Nose/Throat
77ERY	Drape, Surgical, ENT	Ear/Nose/Throat
77ERL	Drill, Surgical, ENT (Electric Or Pneumatic)	Ear/Nose/Throat
77LRD	ENT Drug Applicator	Ear/Nose/Throat
77LRC	ENT Manual Surgical Instrument	Ear/Nose/Throat
77KAD	Elevator, ENT	Ear/Nose/Throat
77KAE	Forceps, ENT	Ear/Nose/Throat
77JXX	Forceps, Wire Closure, ENT	Ear/Nose/Throat
77ETQ	Fork, Tuning, ENT	Ear/Nose/Throat
77KAF	Headlight, ENT	Ear/Nose/Throat
77KAG	Holder, Speculum, ENT	Ear/Nose/Throat
77KCH	Hook, Tracheal, ENT	Ear/Nose/Throat
77JXY	Jig, Piston Cutting, ENT	Ear/Nose/Throat
77KTG	Knife, ENT	Ear/Nose/Throat
77EWG	Laser, Carbon-Dioxide, Microsurgical, ENT	Ear/Nose/Throat
77REM	Lavage Unit, ENT	Ear/Nose/Throat
77EWY	Mediastinoscope, ENT	Ear/Nose/Throat
77KAH	Microrule, ENT	Ear/Nose/Throat
77KAI	Mirror, ENT	Ear/Nose/Throat
77KAJ	Mobilizer, ENT	Ear/Nose/Throat
77ETO	Nystagmograph, ENT	Ear/Nose/Throat
77ESF	Polymer, ENT Composite Synthetic PTFE With Carbon-Fiber	Ear/Nose/Throat
77KHK	Polymer, ENT Natural Collagen Material	Ear/Nose/Throat
77KHJ	Polymer, ENT Synthetic Polyamide (Mesh Or Foil Material)	Ear/Nose/Throat
77JOF	Polymer, ENT Synthetic, Porous Polyethylene	Ear/Nose/Throat
77ESH	Polymer, ENT Synthetic-PIFE, Silicon Elastomer	Ear/Nose/Throat
77KTF	Punch, ENT	Ear/Nose/Throat
77KAL	Retractor, ENT (Thoracic)	Ear/Nose/Throat
77EWQ	Saw, Surgical, ENT (Electric Or Pneumatic)	Ear/Nose/Throat

ENZYME *(cont'd)*
74WYC System, Infusion, Enzyme, Thrombolytic — Cardiovascular

ENZYME-LABELED
82LRM Anti-DNA Antibody (Enzyme-Labeled), Antigen, Control — Immunology
82LJM Antinuclear Antibody (Enzyme-Labeled), Antigen, Controls — Immunology

EOA
73SBH Holder, Tracheostomy Tube — Anesthesiology

EOG
84RZM Telemetry Unit, Physiological, EOG — Cns/Neurology

EOSIN
88ICC Stain, Eosin B — Pathology
88HYB Stain, Eosin Y — Pathology
88KJS Stain, Ethyl Eosin — Pathology

EPI-BUTTON
86WQU Tissue, Corneal — Ophthalmology

EPIDURAL
85QFZ Cannula, Epidural — Obstetrics/Gyn
85QHT Catheter, Epidural — Obstetrics/Gyn
84LHG Electrode, Epidural, Spinal — Cns/Neurology
73QAW Kit, Anesthesia, Epidural — Anesthesiology
80MIA Needle, Spinal, Short-Term — General
84LHY Stabilized Epidural Spinal Electrode — Cns/Neurology

EPIKERATOPHAKIA
86WQT Phacoemulsification System — Ophthalmology
86WQU Tissue, Corneal — Ophthalmology

EPILATION
79QWZ Forceps, Epilation — Surgery

EPILATOR
79KCW Epilator, High-Frequency, Needle-Type — Surgery
79KCX Epilator, High-Frequency, Tweezer Type — Surgery

EPILEPSY
84LYJ Stimulator, Nerve, Autonomic, Implantable (Epilepsy) — Cns/Neurology
84LYI Stimulator, Subcortical, Implanted For Epilepsy — Cns/Neurology
84MBX Stimulator, Thalamic, Epilepsy, Implanted — Cns/Neurology
84MBY Stimulator, Vagus Nerve, Epilepsy, Implanted — Cns/Neurology

EPISIOTOMY
85HDK Scissors, Episiotomy — Obstetrics/Gyn

EPISTAXIS
77EMX Balloon, Epistaxis (Nasal) — Ear/Nose/Throat

EPITHELIAL
82LTK Test, Antigen (CA125), Tumor-Associated, Ovarian, Epithelial — Immunology

EPSTEIN-BARR
83LJN Antibody IGM, IF, Epstein-Barr Virus — Microbiology
83GNQ Antigen, CF (Including CF Control), Epstein-Barr Virus — Microbiology
83MCD Antigen, Epstein-Barr Virus, Capsid — Microbiology
83GNP Antiserum, CF, Epstein-Barr Virus — Microbiology
83JRY Antiserum, Fluorescent, Epstein-Barr Virus — Microbiology
83LSF Epstein-Barr Virus, DNA Reagents — Microbiology
83LSE Epstein-Barr Virus, Other — Microbiology
83LLM Test, Nuclear Antigen, Epstein-Barr Virus — Microbiology

EQUILIBRATION
75KMX Tonometer, Gas-Liquid Equilibration — Chemistry

EQUILIBRIUM
77LXV Analyzer, Apparatus, Vestibular — Ear/Nose/Throat

EQUINE
83GQD Antigen, CF (Including CF Control), Equine Encephalitis — Microbiology
83GQC Antiserum, CF, Equine Encephalitis Virus, EEE, WEE — Microbiology

EQUIPMENT
80WTN Adapter, Cable, Equipment — General
91KIE Apparatus, High Pressure Liquid Chromatography — Toxicology
89IQH Biofeedback Equipment, Myoelectric, Battery-Powered — Physical Med
89IRC Biofeedback Equipment, Myoelectric, Powered — Physical Med
80WVY Cart, Equipment, Video — General
79QZT Cart, Instrument/Equipment, Laparoscopy — Surgery
80WSG Case, Protection, Equipment — General
80UKP Casters, Hospital Equipment — General
75QJY Chromatography Equipment, Gas — Chemistry
91DJY Chromatography Equipment, Ion Exchange — Toxicology
75QJZ Chromatography Equipment, Liquid — Chemistry
75QKA Chromatography Equipment, Paper — Chemistry
91DPA Chromatography Equipment, Thin Layer — Toxicology
91MAS Chromatography, Liquid, Performance, High — Toxicology
80VAA Cleanroom Equipment — General
80VBO Communication Equipment — General
80VAX Computer Equipment — General

EQUIPMENT *(cont'd)*
80WLX Contract Manufacturing, Product, Durable — General
80WUH Contract R&D, Equipment — General
76WOJ Dental Laboratory Equipment — Dental And Oral
78QPJ Dialysis Unit Test Equipment — Gastro/Urology
80WPV Dryer, Respiratory/Anesthesia Equipment — General
75UFZ Electrofocusing Equipment — Chemistry
80WPK Electrolysis Equipment, Other — General
75UEO Electrophoresis Equipment, Cellulose Acetate Membrane — Chemistry
75UGG Electrophoresis Equipment, Gel — Chemistry
75JJN Electrophoresis Equipment, Liquid — Chemistry
75UHA Electrophoresis Equipment, Paper — Chemistry
75UIK Electrophoresis Equipment, Starch Block — Chemistry
75UIU Electrophoresis Equipment, Thin-Layer — Chemistry
82JZS Electrophoresis Instrumentation — Immunology
79UCP Electrosurgical Equipment, General Purpose — Surgery
79UCQ Electrosurgical Equipment, Special Purpose — Surgery
75UHG Equipment, Analysis, Photochemical — Chemistry
81VJC Equipment, Apheresis — Hematology
81QNO Equipment, Bank, Blood, Cryogenic (Liquid Nitrogen) — Hematology
80WRQ Equipment, Building Security — General
80FRF Equipment, Cleaning, Air — General
80WLA Equipment, Control, Pollution — General
89WOK Equipment, Cryotherapy — Physical Med
80SHH Equipment, Device Coating, Protective — General
80VAJ Equipment, Extruding/Molding — General
80WYN Equipment, Filtering, Air, ETO — General
82JZX Equipment, Immunoelectrophoresis, Rocket — Immunology
85VIK Equipment, In Vitro Fertilization/Embryo Transfer — Obstetrics/Gyn
75LXG Equipment, Laboratory, Gen. Purpose (Specific Medical Use) — Chemistry
80WYB Equipment, Management, Pain, Radiofrequency, Non-Invasive — General
80WXQ Equipment, Marking, Electrochemical — General
80WXE Equipment, Molding — General
87WRR Equipment, Screening, Scoliosis — Orthopedics
87WYA Equipment, Shaving, Disc, Spinal — Orthopedics
79WYP Equipment, Suction/Irrigation, Laparoscopic — Surgery
79SJK Equipment, Suction/Irrigation/Electrocautery, Laparoscopic — Surgery
83WKS Equipment, Test, Western Blot — Microbiology
73WLD Equipment, Therapy, Apnea — Anesthesiology
89WPB Equipment, Therapy, Handicapped/Physical — Physical Med
89ITH Equipment, Traction, Powered — Physical Med
85LQT Equipment, Ultrasound, Doppler, Evaluation, Fetal — Obstetrics/Gyn
74WYD Equipment, Ultrasound, Intravascular, 3-Dimensional — Cardiovascular
79SIV Equipment/Accessories, Laser, Laparoscopy — Surgery
80WQM Equipment/Service, Quality Control — General
80TCA Extrication Equipment — General
80WUC Facility, Equipment, Medical, Mobile — General
83UGA Fermentation Equipment — Microbiology
80VAV Foodservice Product/Equipment — General
75UGF Freeze Drying Equipment — Chemistry
80VBI Housekeeping Equipment — General
83UGN Hypothermic Equipment — Microbiology
75RBN Immunodiffusion Equipment (Agar Cutter) — Chemistry
82RBO Immunofluorescence Equipment — Immunology
91LDM Instrumentation, High Pressure Liquid Chromatography — Toxicology
75UGQ Iontophoresis Equipment — Chemistry
75UGR Isotachophoresis Equipment — Chemistry
80VAH Labeling Equipment — General
86WTY Laboratory Equipment, Ophthalmic — Ophthalmology
80TCW Laundry Equipment — General
80VAZ Microfilm/Microfiche Equipment — General
87JDZ Mixing Equipment, Cement — Orthopedics
75UGW Molecular Weight Equipment — Chemistry
80WTG Monitor, Utilization, Equipment — General
80WKM Mount, Equipment — General
75UGY Nuclear Magnetic Resonance Equipment, Laboratory — Chemistry
80VBG Office Equipment — General
80VAG Packaging Equipment — General
80VDO Packaging System, Unit-Dose — General
80VAP Production Equipment — General
75UHP Radioautographic Equipment — Chemistry
80WRN Rails, Equipment — General
83LHW Reag. & Equipment, Erythrocyte Suspension, Multi Species — Microbiology
80WWT Recovery Equipment, Gas — General
80VBL Recovery Equipment, Waste Heat — General
80VAQ Recovery Equipment, Water — General
80WMZ Rescue Equipment — General
75UHS Reverse Osmosis Membrane Equipment — Chemistry
75RDT Safety Equipment, Laboratory — Chemistry
80VAY Security Equipment/Supplies — General
80WMP Service, Equipment Leasing — General
80WMO Service, Used Equipment — General
90TER Silver Recovery Equipment — Radiology
84LEL Sleep Assessment Equipment — Cns/Neurology
75WKC Stand/Holder, Equipment, Laboratory — Chemistry

ETHOSUXIMIDE (cont'd)

91DNP	Thin Layer Chromatography, Ethosuximide	Toxicology

ETHYL

91DNN	Calibrator, Ethyl Alcohol	Toxicology
75JKW	N-Acetyl-L-Tyrosine Ethyl Ester (U.V.), Chymotrypsin	Chemistry
75JNO	N-Benzoyl-L-Arginine Ethyl Ester (U.V.), Trypsin	Chemistry
75JKX	N-Benzoyl-L-Tyrosine Ethyl Ester (U.V.), Chymotrypsin	Chemistry
88KJS	Stain, Ethyl Eosin	Pathology
91DMJ	Test, Ethyl Alcohol	Toxicology

ETHYLENE

80QUR	Analyzer, Ethylene-Oxide	General
80FLI	Cabinet, Aerator, Ethylene-Oxide Gas	General
76KOL	Carboxymethylcellulose Sodium/Ethylene-Oxide Homopolymer	Dental And Oral
80VLG	Cartridge, Ethylene-Oxide	General
80UMV	Detector, Ethylene-Oxide Leakage	General
80VDZ	Dosimeter, Ethylene-Oxide	General
76KXX	Homopolymer, Karaya and Ethylene-Oxide	Dental And Oral
80UDL	Sterilizer, Bulk, Steam & Ethylene-Oxide	General
80FLF	Sterilizer, Ethylene-Oxide Gas	General
76ECE	Sterilizer, Ethylene-Oxide Gas, Dental	Dental And Oral
79FSJ	Sterilizer, Ethylene-Oxide Gas, Operating Room	Surgery
80UDJ	Sterilizer, Ethylene-Oxide, Bulk	General
80UDK	Sterilizer, Ethylene-Oxide, Table Top	General
80WTH	Tubing, Polytetrafluoroethylene	General

ETHYLENE-OXIDE

80QUR	Analyzer, Ethylene-Oxide	General
80FLI	Cabinet, Aerator, Ethylene-Oxide Gas	General
76KOL	Carboxymethylcellulose Sodium/Ethylene-Oxide Homopolymer	Dental And Oral
80VLG	Cartridge, Ethylene-Oxide	General
80UMV	Detector, Ethylene-Oxide Leakage	General
80VDZ	Dosimeter, Ethylene-Oxide	General
80FRF	Equipment, Cleaning, Air	General
80WLA	Equipment, Control, Pollution	General
80WYN	Equipment, Filtering, Air, ETO	General
80WPE	Gas Mixtures, Sterilization	General
76KXX	Homopolymer, Karaya and Ethylene-Oxide	Dental And Oral
80QDR	Monitor, Biological (Contamination Testing)	General
80WIP	Monitor, Contamination, Environmental, Personal	General
80QUM	Monitor, Gas, Atmospheric, Environmental	General
80RVU	Sterilization Process Indicator, Chemical	General
80UDL	Sterilizer, Bulk, Steam & Ethylene-Oxide	General
80FLF	Sterilizer, Ethylene-Oxide Gas	General
76ECE	Sterilizer, Ethylene-Oxide Gas, Dental	Dental And Oral
79FSJ	Sterilizer, Ethylene-Oxide Gas, Operating Room	Surgery
80UDJ	Sterilizer, Ethylene-Oxide, Bulk	General
80UDK	Sterilizer, Ethylene-Oxide, Table Top	General

ETIOCHOLANOLONE

75JLF	Radioimmunoassay, Etiocholanolone	Chemistry

ETO

80WYN	Equipment, Filtering, Air, ETO	General
80WPE	Gas Mixtures, Sterilization	General
80WWT	Recovery Equipment, Gas	General
79FSJ	Sterilizer, Ethylene-Oxide Gas, Operating Room	Surgery

EUGENOL

76MZW	Dental Cement w/out Zinc-Oxide Eugenol as an Ulcer Covering for Pain Relief	Dental And Oral
76EMB	Zinc Oxide Eugenol	Dental And Oral

EUGLOBULIN

81JBO	Test, Euglobulin Lysis	Hematology

EUSTACHIAN

77KBI	Bougie, Eustachian (Ear)	Ear/Nose/Throat
79GBY	Catheter, Eustachian, General & Plastic Surgery	Surgery
77KBY	Filiform, Eustachian	Ear/Nose/Throat

EUTHYSCOPE

86HMK	Euthyscope, AC-Powered	Ophthalmology
86HML	Euthyscope, Battery-Powered	Ophthalmology

EVACUATED

80TAN	Bottle, Evacuated	General
80TBL	Container, Evacuated	General

EVACUATION

79VCN	System, Evacuation, Smoke, Laser	Surgery

EVACUATOR

80QBQ	Aspirator, Emergency Suction	General
85HFC	Aspirator, Endocervical	Obstetrics/Gyn
85HFF	Aspirator, Endometrial	Obstetrics/Gyn
78QBR	Aspirator, Low Volume (Gastric Suction)	Gastro/Urology
79QBU	Aspirator, Surgical	Surgery
74QBV	Aspirator, Thoracic (Suction Unit)	Cardiovascular

EVACUATOR (cont'd)

77QBW	Aspirator, Tracheal	Ear/Nose/Throat
80QBZ	Aspirator, Wound Suction Pump	General
74DWM	Canister, Suction	Cardiovascular
78FFD	Evacuator, Bladder, Manually Operated	Gastro/Urology
78FHF	Evacuator, Fluid	Gastro/Urology
75QXU	Evacuator, Fume	Chemistry
78KQT	Evacuator, Gastro-Urology	Gastro/Urology
76EHZ	Evacuator, Oral Cavity	Dental And Oral
87JDY	Evacuator, Vapor, Cement Monomer	Orthopedics
91RAG	Hood, Fume	Toxicology
85HHI	Pump, Abortion, Vacuum, Central System	Obstetrics/Gyn
76EBR	Pump, Suction Operatory	Dental And Oral
73QBA	Scavenger, Gas, Anesthesia Unit	Anesthesiology
84GZD	Stimulator, Spinal Cord, Implantable, Bladder Evacuator	Cns/Neurology
73BSS	Tube, Nasogastric	Anesthesiology
78SDI	Tube, Stomach Evacuator (Gastric Lavage)	Gastro/Urology

EVALUATION

82MLF	Computer Software, Prenatal Risk Evaluation	Immunology
85LQT	Equipment, Ultrasound, Doppler, Evaluation, Fetal	Obstetrics/Gyn
89IKK	Isokinetic Testing And Evaluation System	Physical Med
87REX	Unit, Evaluation, Height, Lift	Orthopedics

EVAPORATOR

75JRK	Evaporator	Chemistry

EVAPORIMETER

75JRK	Evaporator	Chemistry

EVERTING

84LJA	Catheter, Cerebrovascular, Everting	Cns/Neurology

EVIDENCE

88TCF	Kit, Forensic Evidence	Pathology
85QXO	Kit, Forensic Evidence, Sexual Assault	Obstetrics/Gyn

EVISCERATION

86UAZ	Prosthesis, Evisceration	Ophthalmology

EVOKED

84VKG	Computer, Brain Mapping	Cns/Neurology
84VDA	Evoked Potential Unit, Audiometric	Cns/Neurology
84QUT	Evoked Response Unit	Cns/Neurology
77ETZ	Evoked Response Unit, Auditory	Ear/Nose/Throat
84RWB	Stimulator, Audio	Cns/Neurology
84GWJ	Stimulator, Auditory, Evoked Response	Cns/Neurology
84GWF	Stimulator, Electrical, Evoked Response	Cns/Neurology
84GZP	Stimulator, Mechanical, Evoked Response	Cns/Neurology
79FXA	Stimulator, Neurological	Surgery
84GWE	Stimulator, Photic, Evoked Response	Cns/Neurology
84UFJ	Stimulator, Somatosensory	Cns/Neurology
84RWF	Stimulator, Visual	Cns/Neurology
77EWN	Unit, Measuring, Potential, Evoked, Auditory	Ear/Nose/Throat

EXAM

85MLT	Kit, Pelvic Exam	Obstetrics/Gyn

EXAMINATION

80FRK	Chair, Examination And Treatment	General
80KZF	Examination Device, AC-Powered	General
80WUC	Facility, Equipment, Medical, Mobile	General
88QYH	Glove, Autopsy	Pathology
80FMC	Glove, Patient Examination	General
80LYY	Glove, Patient Examination, Latex	General
80LZA	Glove, Patient Examination, Poly	General
80LZC	Glove, Patient Examination, Specialty	General
80LYZ	Glove, Patient Examination, Vinyl	General
80FME	Gown, Examination	General
79FYB	Gown, Patient	Surgery
80QYO	Gown, Patient, Disposable	General
80QYP	Gown, Patient, Reusable	General
80RDZ	Lamp, Examination (Light)	General
80TCY	Lamp, Examination, Ceiling Mounted (Light)	General
80KYT	Light, Examination, Battery-Powered	General
80LGX	Powered Medical Examination Table	General
80RSM	Sheet, Examination Table, Disposable	General
80RSJ	Sheeting, Examination Table	General
80RYX	Table, Examination/Treatment	General
86WNU	Unit, Examination, Lens, Contact	Ophthalmology
77ETF	Unit, Examining/Treatment, ENT	Ear/Nose/Throat

EXCAVATING

76QEW	Burr, Dental Excavating	Dental And Oral

EXCAVATOR

76EKC	Excavator, Dental, Operative	Dental And Oral
77JYH	Excavator, Ear	Ear/Nose/Throat

EXCHANGE

91DKO	Adsorbents, Ion Exchange	Toxicology
91DJY	Chromatography Equipment, Ion Exchange	Toxicology

EXTERNAL (cont'd)
74DTE Pacemaker, Heart, External — Cardiovascular
74JOQ Pacemaker, Heart, External, Programmable — Cardiovascular
85HER Pelvimeter, External — Obstetrics/Gyn
79KCZ Prosthesis, Breast, External — Surgery
78LKY Prosthesis, Penis, Rigid Rod, External — Gastro/Urology
79FYG Prosthesis, Splint, Nasal, External — Surgery
89ISS Prosthesis, Thigh Socket, External Component — Physical Med
74DRN Pump, Counterpulsating, External — Cardiovascular
78FES Recorder, External, Pressure, Amplifier & Transducer — Gastro/Urology
79FZF Splint, Extremity, Inflatable, External — Surgery
79FYH Splint, Extremity, Non-Inflatable, External — Surgery
79GER Sponge, External — Surgery
84HAY Sponge, External, Neurological — Cns/Neurology
79GEQ Sponge, External, Rubber — Surgery
79GEP Sponge, External, Synthetic — Surgery
84LPY Stimulator, Electrical, Cranial, External — Cns/Neurology
89IPP Stimulator, External, Neuromuscular, Functional — Physical Med
84GZI Stimulator, Neuromuscular, External Functional — Cns/Neurology
89ITC Stirrup, External Brace Component — Physical Med
74DWQ Stripper, Vein, External — Cardiovascular
73BYT Ventilator, External Body, Negative Pressure, (Cuirass) — Anesthesiology
86MML Weights, Eyelid, External — Ophthalmology
89KGH Wrist, External Limb Component, Powered — Physical Med

EXTRA-CRANIAL
87VKH Fixation Device, Extra-Cranial (Head Frame) — Orthopedics

EXTRA-LUMINAL
78FIR Pump, Blood, Extra-Luminal — Gastro/Urology
78FIH Pump, Infusion Or Syringe, Extra-Luminal — Gastro/Urology

EXTRA-OCULAR
86HQX Implant, Orbital, Extra-Ocular — Ophthalmology

EXTRACORPOREAL
78KXM Accessories, Extracorporeal System — Gastro/Urology
78LLB Blood System, Extracorporeal (With Accessories) — Gastro/Urology
78LQQ Column, Immunoadsorption, System, Extracorporeal — Gastro/Urology
78LNP Extracorporeal Hyperthermia System — Gastro/Urology
78LNR Extracorporeal Photopheresis System — Gastro/Urology
74QZM Heart-Lung Bypass Unit (Cardiopulmonary) — Cardiovascular
79QZP Heat Exchanger, Extracorporeal Perfusion — Surgery
78NAX Irradiator, Blood, Extracorporeal — Gastro/Urology
78VKM Lithotriptor, Electro-Hydraulic, Extracorporeal — Gastro/Urology
78LNS Lithotriptor, Extracorporeal Shock-wave, Urological — Gastro/Urology
78WUD Lithotriptor, Extracorporeal, Gallstone — Gastro/Urology
78WIL Lithotriptor, Multipurpose — Gastro/Urology
78RIZ Organ Preservation System — Gastro/Urology
73RJP Oxygenator, Extracorporeal Perfusion — Anesthesiology
74RNE Pump, Extracorporeal Perfusion — Cardiovascular

EXTRACTABLE
82LLL Extractable Antinuclear Antibody (Rnp/Sm), Antigen/Control — Immunology

EXTRACTION
79WZT Cannula, Extraction, Appendix — Surgery
75JMN Extraction/Chromatography, Ninhydrin, Hydroxyproline — Chemistry
75JOA Hexane Extraction And Trifluoroacetic Acid, Vitamin A — Chemistry
75JOB Hexane Extraction, Fluorescence, Vitamin E — Chemistry
87LZV System, Extraction, Cement Removal — Orthopedics

EXTRACTOR
87QRM Driver/Extractor, Bone Nail/Pin — Orthopedics
87QRN Driver/Extractor, Bone Plate — Orthopedics
86QHF Extractor, Cataract — Ophthalmology
78SIQ Extractor, Gall Bladder — Gastro/Urology
79QVF Extractor, Metal, Magnetic — Surgery
87HWB Extractor, Nail — Orthopedics
81QVG Extractor, Plasma — Hematology
85HDB Extractor, Vacuum, Fetal — Obstetrics/Gyn
78QXB Forceps, Gallbladder (Biliary Duct) — Gastro/Urology
85HDA Forceps, Obstetrical — Obstetrics/Gyn
76EMG Forceps, Tooth Extractor, Surgical — Dental And Oral
75UGE Fractionator, Polymer Extractor — Chemistry

EXTRAORAL
76EHC Film, X-Ray, Dental, Extraoral — Dental And Oral
76DZB Headgear, Extraoral, Orthodontic — Dental And Oral
76EHD Radiographic Unit, Diagnostic, Dental, Extraoral — Dental And Oral
90MUH System, X-ray, Extraoral Source, Digital — Radiology

EXTRAVASCULAR
74DPT Probe, Blood Flow, Extravascular — Cardiovascular
74DRS Transducer, Blood Pressure, Extravascular — Cardiovascular

EXTREMITY
79KPJ Chamber, Oxygen, Topical, Extremity — Surgery
74QLZ Compression Unit, Intermittent (Anti-Embolism Pump) — Cardiovascular
79FZF Splint, Extremity, Inflatable, External — Surgery
79FYH Splint, Extremity, Non-Inflatable, External — Surgery

EXTREMITY (cont'd)
84HTK Stimulator, Extremity, Internal, Peroneal — Cns/Neurology

EXTRICATION
80WMR Collar, Extrication — General
80TCA Extrication Equipment — General

EXTRUDING
80VAE Component, Plastic — General
80VAL Component, Rubber — General
80VAM Component, Silicone — General
80WSN Computer Software, Industrial — General
80VAJ Equipment, Extruding/Molding — General
80WNC Molding, Custom — General

EXTRUSION
80WYJ Molding, Injection — General
80WYK Thermoforming, Extrusion, Custom — General

EXUDATE
79KOZ Beads, Hydrophilic, Wound Exudate Absorption — Surgery

EYE
86QBG Applicator, Ophthalmic — Ophthalmology
86WKR Aspirator, Ophthalmic — Ophthalmology
86QEQ Brush, Ophthalmic — Ophthalmology
86NCK Button, Iris, Eye, Artificial — Ophthalmology
86QGA Cannula, Cyclodialysis (Eye) — Ophthalmology
86QGB Cannula, Lacrimal (Eye) — Ophthalmology
86HOX Chart, Visual Acuity — Ophthalmology
86HJZ Crutch, Ptosis — Ophthalmology
86LXQ Cup, Eye — Ophthalmology
86HNY Cystotome, Ophthalmic — Ophthalmology
86HNW Dilator, Lacrimal — Ophthalmology
86QRP Dropper, Eye — Ophthalmology
86HMS Drum, Eye Knife Test — Ophthalmology
86HQI Eye, Artificial, Custom — Ophthalmology
86HQH Eye, Artificial, Non-Custom — Ophthalmology
86QVI Eyeglasses — Ophthalmology
86QVJ Eyeglasses, Aphakic — Ophthalmology
86TCB Eyeglasses, Safety — Ophthalmology
75TCG Fountain, Eye Wash — Chemistry
86TCI Freezer, Eye Bank — Ophthalmology
86LPO Gas, Reattachment Procedure, Retinal — Ophthalmology
86WHZ Goggles, Protective, Eye — Ophthalmology
86KYF Implant, Eye Valve — Ophthalmology
86WJZ Implant, Retinal — Ophthalmology
86WUA Implant, Scleral — Ophthalmology
86THQ Insert, Dry Eye — Ophthalmology
86WKX Irrigator, Ocular, Emergency — Ophthalmology
86RCT Kit, Irrigation, Eye — Ophthalmology
86WTY Laboratory Equipment, Ophthalmic — Ophthalmology
86WMI Laser, Krypton, Ophthalmic — Ophthalmology
86WIZ Lens, Contact, Disposable — Ophthalmology
86RGA Mask, Eye, Phototherapy — Ophthalmology
80WKE Mask, Face — General
86HLL Monitor, Eye Movement — Ophthalmology
86HMC Monitor, Eye Movement, Diagnostic — Ophthalmology
86RID Needle, Ophthalmic — Ophthalmology
86WTA Ophthalmoscope, Laser — Ophthalmology
86WQL Pachometer — Ophthalmology
86HMP Pad, Eye — Ophthalmology
80FOK Pad, Neonatal Eye — General
86UET Patch, Eye — Ophthalmology
86HNL Probe, Lacrimal — Ophthalmology
86RMH Probe, Ophthalmic — Ophthalmology
79FWO Prosthesis, Eye, Internal (Sphere) — Surgery
86WNV Reducer, Pressure, Intraocular — Ophthalmology
86ULM Refrigerator, Eye Bank — Ophthalmology
86HNG Rongeur, Lacrimal Sac — Ophthalmology
86RRD Scissors, Corneal — Ophthalmology
86RRE Scissors, Enucleation — Ophthalmology
86RRF Scissors, Iris — Ophthalmology
86HNF Scissors, Ophthalmic — Ophthalmology
86RRH Scissors, Tenotomy — Ophthalmology
86WRV Shield, Corneal — Ophthalmology
86HOY Shield, Eye, Ophthalmic — Ophthalmology
90IWS Shield, Ophthalmic, Radiological — Radiology
86UBF Sleeve, Muscle, Ophthalmic — Ophthalmology
86HPZ Sphere, Ophthalmic (Implant) — Ophthalmology
86HOZ Sponge, Ophthalmic — Ophthalmology
86TEV Spud, Ophthalmic, Electrical — Ophthalmology
86WVM System, Delivery, Drug, Ocular — Ophthalmology
86WXT System, Mapping, Corneal — Ophthalmology
86HIT Tester, Color Vision — Ophthalmology
86SEN Valve, Ophthalmic — Ophthalmology

EYEBALL
76LZX Acid, Hyaluronic — Dental And Oral

KEYWORD INDEX

FEMORAL (cont'd)
87KWY	Prosthesis, Hip, Hemi-, Femoral, Metal/Polymer	Orthopedics
87JDH	Prosthesis, Hip, Hemi-, Trunnion-Bearing, Femoral	Orthopedics
87HSA	Prosthesis, Knee, Hemi-, Femoral	Orthopedics
87JDD	Prosthesis, Upper Femoral	Orthopedics
87HWP	Punch, Femoral Neck	Orthopedics
87HWS	Template, Femoral Angle Cutting	Orthopedics

FEMOROTIBIAL
87KRN	Prosthesis, Knee, Femorotibial, Constrained, Metal	Orthopedics
87KRO	Prosthesis, Knee, Femorotibial, Constrained, Metal/Polymer	Orthopedics
87HSX	Prosthesis, Knee, Femorotibial, Non-Constrained	Orthopedics
87KTX	Prosthesis, Knee, Femorotibial, Non-Constrained, Metal	Orthopedics
87HRY	Prosthesis, Knee, Femorotibial, Semi-Constrained	Orthopedics
87KYK	Prosthesis, Knee, Femorotibial, Semi-Constrained, Metal	Orthopedics
87LGE	Prosthesis, Knee, Femorotibial, Semi-Constrained, Trunnion	Orthopedics
87MBG	Prosthesis, Knee, Femotib., Unconst., Uncem., Unicond., M/P	Orthopedics
87MBD	Prosthesis, Knee, P/F, Unconst., Uncem., Por., Ctd., P/M/P	Orthopedics
87MBV	Prosthesis, Knee, Patfem., S-C., UHMWPE, Pegged, Unc., P/M/P	Orthopedics
87MBH	Prosthesis, Knee, Patfem., S-C., Unc., Por., Ctd., P/M/P	Orthopedics
87MBA	Prosthesis, Knee, Patfem., Semi-Const., Unc., P/M/P, Osteo.	Orthopedics

FERMENT
83JSW	Kit, Identification, Glucose (Non-Ferment)	Microbiology

FERMENTATION
83UGA	Fermentation Equipment	Microbiology
75UHW	Sampler, Fermentation	Chemistry

FERRIC
75LFQ	Acid Reduction Of Ferric Ion, Uric Acid	Chemistry
75JLG	Conversion Ferric Hydroxymates (Colorimetric), Fatty Acids	Chemistry
75JGK	Ferric Chloride, Phenylketones (Urinary, Non-Quantitative)	Chemistry
75CHD	Ferric Ion-Sulfuric Acid, Cholesterol	Chemistry

FERRICYANIDE
75CGD	Ferricyanide, Glucose	Chemistry

FERRITE
90MHG	Magnesium Ferrite	Radiology

FERRITIN
82DBF	Antigen, Antiserum, Control, Ferritin	Immunology
82CZM	IGA, Ferritin, Antigen, Antiserum, Control	Immunology
82DFM	IGE, Ferritin, Antigen, Antiserum, Control	Immunology
82DGD	IGG, Ferritin, Antigen, Antiserum, Control	Immunology
82DFL	IGM, Ferritin, Antigen, Antiserum, Control	Immunology
83JMG	Radioimmunoassay, Ferritin	Microbiology

FERROZINE
75JMO	Ferrozine (Colorimetric) Iron Binding Capacity	Chemistry

FERTILITY
82DFQ	Antigen, Antiserum, Control, Sperm	Immunology
85MEE	Device, Fertility, Contraceptive, Diagnostic	Obstetrics/Gyn
78LOA	Device, Hypothermia, Testicular	Gastro/Urology
85MNA	Device, Semen Analysis	Obstetrics/Gyn
85LHD	Fertility Diagnostic Device	Obstetrics/Gyn
78FHW	Impotence Device, Mechanical/Hydraulic	Gastro/Urology
85ULY	Kit, Sex Selection	Obstetrics/Gyn
85VDI	Monitor, Fertility	Obstetrics/Gyn
85HFJ	Prosthesis, Fallopian Tube	Obstetrics/Gyn
88LIY	Test, Cervical Mucous Penetration	Pathology
85VJM	Test, Fertility Monitoring	Obstetrics/Gyn
85LHZ	Viscometer, Mucus, Cervical	Obstetrics/Gyn

FERTILIZATION
85VIK	Equipment, In Vitro Fertilization/Embryo Transfer	Obstetrics/Gyn

FETAL
85HGR	Applicator, Electrode, Scalp, Fetal	Obstetrics/Gyn
74THD	Belt, Electrode	Cardiovascular
85HEN	Caliper, Fetal Head, Ultrasonic	Obstetrics/Gyn
85HGT	Cardiotachometer, Fetal, With Sensor	Obstetrics/Gyn
75JHG	Chromatographic Separation, Lecithin-Sphingomyelin Ratio	Chemistry
75JHF	Colorimetric Method, Lecithin-Sphingomyelin Ratio	Chemistry
85HGA	Cranioclast	Obstetrics/Gyn
85QVO	Detector, Fetal Heart, Phono	Obstetrics/Gyn
85HIQ	Electrode, Clip, Fetal Scalp (And Applicator)	Obstetrics/Gyn
85QSZ	Electrode, Fetal Scalp	Obstetrics/Gyn
75JHH	Electrophoretic Method, Lecithin-Sphingomyelin Ratio	Chemistry
85HGK	Endoscope, Fetal Blood Sampling	Obstetrics/Gyn
75MKV	Enzyme Immunoassay, Fetal Fibronectin	Chemistry
85LQT	Equipment, Ultrasound, Doppler, Evaluation, Fetal	Obstetrics/Gyn
85HDB	Extractor, Vacuum, Fetal	Obstetrics/Gyn

FETAL (cont'd)
85LXE	Fetal Doppler Ultrasound	Obstetrics/Gyn
85HDA	Forceps, Obstetrical	Obstetrics/Gyn
85HHX	Holograph, Fetal, Acoustical	Obstetrics/Gyn
85HGQ	Monitor, Electrocardiographic, Fetal	Obstetrics/Gyn
85HGO	Monitor, Electroencephalographic, Fetal	Obstetrics/Gyn
85QVQ	Monitor, Fetal	Obstetrics/Gyn
85MAA	Monitor, Fetal Doppler Ultrasound	Obstetrics/Gyn
85KXN	Monitor, Fetal, Cardiac	Obstetrics/Gyn
85KNG	Monitor, Fetal, Ultrasonic	Obstetrics/Gyn
85HEQ	Monitor, Fetal, Ultrasonic, Arterial Pressure	Obstetrics/Gyn
85HEL	Monitor, Fetal, Ultrasonic, Heart Rate	Obstetrics/Gyn
85HEK	Monitor, Fetal, Ultrasonic, Heart Sound	Obstetrics/Gyn
85HEI	Monitor, Heart Valve Movement, Fetal, Ultrasonic	Obstetrics/Gyn
85HFP	Monitor, Phonocardiographic, Fetal	Obstetrics/Gyn
90JAF	Monitor, Ultrasonic, Non-Fetal	Radiology
85LLT	Monitor, pH, Fetal	Obstetrics/Gyn
85MMA	Oximeter, Pulse, Fetal	Obstetrics/Gyn
85HGW	Sampler, Blood, Fetal	Obstetrics/Gyn
81GHQ	Stain, Fetal Hemoglobin	Hematology
85HGN	Stethoscope, Fetal	Obstetrics/Gyn
85MCP	Stimulator, Fetal, Acoustic	Obstetrics/Gyn
85KNB	Surgical Instrument, Obstetric, Destructive, Fetal	Obstetrics/Gyn
85VIL	Test, Chorionic Villi Sampling (Fetal Chromosome Analysis)	Obstetrics/Gyn
81LIM	Test, D Positive Fetal Rbc	Hematology
81KQI	Test, Fetal Hemoglobin	Hematology
75WHJ	Test, Maturity, Lung, Fetal	Chemistry
80VFH	Transmitter/Receiver System, Fetal Monitor, Telephone	General

FETOPROTEIN
82KTJ	Alpha-Fetoprotein RIA Test System	Immunology
82LOJ	Kit, Test, Alpha-fetoprotein For Testicular Cancer	Immunology
88UMR	Test, Alpha-Fetoprotein	Pathology
82LOK	Test, Neural Tube Defect, Alpha-Fetoprotein (AFP)	Immunology

FETOSCOPE
85HFA	Amnioscope, Transabdominal (Fetoscope)	Obstetrics/Gyn

FETUS
83GSP	Antiserum, Fluorescent, Campylobacter Fetus	Microbiology

FEVER
83GPS	Antigen, CF, Q Fever	Microbiology
83GPQ	Antigen, CF, Spotted Fever Group	Microbiology
83GPO	Antigen, CF, Typhus Fever Group	Microbiology
83GPR	Antiserum, CF, Q Fever	Microbiology
83GPJ	Antiserum, Fluorescent, Q Fever	Microbiology
83GPM	Antiserum, Murine Typhus Fever	Microbiology
83GPP	Antiserum, Rocky Mountain Spotted Fever	Microbiology
83GPN	Antiserum, Typhus Fever	Microbiology
80WXC	Band, Sweat	General

FIBER
78FJI	Dialyzer, Capillary, Hollow Fiber (Hemodialysis)	Gastro/Urology
80FRL	Fiber, Absorbent	General
77ESF	Polymer, ENT Composite Synthetic PTFE With Carbon-Fiber	Ear/Nose/Throat
79KDA	Prosthesis, PTFE/Carbon-Fiber	Surgery
77MQW	Transilluminator, Fiber Optic	Ear/Nose/Throat

FIBEROPTIC
78MNZ	Analyzer, Diagnostic, Fiberoptic (Bladder)	Gastro/Urology
78MOA	Analyzer, Diagnostic, Fiberoptic (Colon)	Gastro/Urology
80QFM	Cable, Fiberoptic	General
79ULX	Cable, Laser, Fiberoptic	Surgery
78FCS	Catheter, Light, Fiberoptic, Glass, Ureteral	Gastro/Urology
74DQE	Catheter, Oximeter, Fiberoptic	Cardiovascular
79GDB	Endoscope, Fiberoptic	Surgery
77EQH	Fiberoptic Light Source & Carrier	Ear/Nose/Throat
76THM	Handpiece, Fiberoptic	Dental And Oral
78FCT	Headlight, Fiberoptic Focusing	Gastro/Urology
78FFS	Illuminator, Fiberoptic (For Endoscope)	Gastro/Urology
84HBI	Illuminator, Fiberoptic, Surgical Field	Cns/Neurology
78FCW	Light Source, Fiberoptic, Routine	Gastro/Urology
78FCR	Light Source, Photographic, Fiberoptic	Gastro/Urology
76EAY	Light, Fiberoptic, Dental	Dental And Oral
79FST	Light, Surgical, Fiberoptic	Surgery
78FDG	Retractor, Fiberoptic	Gastro/Urology
73VDU	Scope, Fiberoptic Intubation	Anesthesiology
85HDG	Speculum, Vaginal, Metal, Fiberoptic	Obstetrics/Gyn
85HIC	Speculum, Vaginal, Non-Metal, Fiberoptic	Obstetrics/Gyn
80WTE	Thermometer, Fiberoptic	General
73RXA	Tip, Suction, Fiberoptic Illuminated	Anesthesiology

FIBRILLATOR
74QVT	Fibrillator	Cardiovascular
74LIW	Fibrillator, AC-Powered	Cardiovascular
74MDO	Fibrillator, AC-Powered, Internal	Cardiovascular

FIBRIN

82DBD	Antigen, Antiserum, Control, Fibrin	Immunology
81JBN	Fibrin Monomer Paracoagulation	Hematology
81GHH	Fibrin Split Products	Hematology
82DBB	Fibrin, FITC, Antigen, Antiserum, Control	Immunology

FIBRINOGEN

82DAZ	Antigen, Antiserum, Control, Fibrinogen And Split Products	Immunology
82DAP	Antigen, Antiserum, Fibrinogen And Fibrin Split Products	Immunology
82DAX	Antigen, Antiserum, Fibrinogen And Split Products, FITC	Immunology
82DAR	Antigen, Fibrinogen And Split Products, Rhodamine	Immunology
81DAT	Fibrin. & Split Products, Peroxidase, Antigen, Antis., Cont.	Hematology
81GIL	Plasma, Control, Fibrinogen	Hematology
81GFX	Standard, Fibrinogen	Hematology
81GFK	Standard/Control, Fibrinogen Determination	Hematology
81KQJ	System, Determination, Fibrinogen	Hematology
81GIS	Test, Fibrinogen	Hematology

FIBRINOPEPTIDE

82DAN	Fibrinopeptide A, Antigen, Antiserum, Control	Immunology

FIBROID

85HDE	Hook, Fibroid, Gynecological	Obstetrics/Gyn
85HHO	Screw, Fibroid, Gynecological	Obstetrics/Gyn

FIBROMETER

81GIE	Fibrometer	Hematology

FIBRONECTIN

75MKV	Enzyme Immunoassay, Fetal Fibronectin	Chemistry

FIBROSIS

78QJW	Chloridimeter	Gastro/Urology
78QOI	Cystic Fibrosis System	Gastro/Urology
89MLQ	Inhibitor, Peridural Fibrosis (Adhesion Barrier)	Physical Med
89MNY	Inhibitor, Post-Op Fibro., Carp. Tun. Syn.(Adhesion Barrier)	Physical Med
89MNX	Inhibitor, Post-Op Fibrosis, Tenolysis (Adhesion Barrier)	Physical Med
78RCP	Iontophoresis Unit (Sweat Rate)	Gastro/Urology
89KTB	Iontophoresis Unit, Physical Medicine	Physical Med
75VIP	Test, Cystic Fibrosis	Chemistry

FICK

74QGK	Cardiac Output Unit, Direct Fick	Cardiovascular

FIELD

79MBQ	Device, Peripheral Electromag. Field to Aid Wound Healing	Surgery
82MEM	Generator, Electric Field (Aids Treatment)	Immunology
84HBI	Illuminator, Fiberoptic, Surgical Field	Cns/Neurology
84MBZ	Instrument, Electrosurgical, Field Focused	Cns/Neurology
86HPJ	Laser, Field, Visual	Ophthalmology
86SFA	Plotter, Visual Field	Ophthalmology
90RSP	Shield, Magnetic Field	Radiology

FILE

87HTP	File	Orthopedics
76EMI	File, Bone, Surgical	Dental And Oral
79QVU	File, Callous	Surgery
76EKA	File, Margin Finishing, Operative	Dental And Oral
76EMR	File, Periodontic	Dental And Oral
76EKS	File, Pulp Canal, Endodontic	Dental And Oral
79GEO	File, Surgical, General & Plastic Surgery	Surgery
80QJP	Paper, Chart, Record, Medical	General

FILIFORM

77KBY	Filiform, Eustachian	Ear/Nose/Throat
78FBW	Filiform, With Filiform Follower	Gastro/Urology

FILLED

76KKO	Ring, Teething, Fluid-Filled	Dental And Oral
76MEF	Ring, Teething, Non-Fluid-Filled	Dental And Oral

FILLER

87MBE	Bone, Block, Filler, Metal, Porous, Uncemented	Orthopedics
89MBS	Filler, Bone Void, Non-Osteoinduction	Physical Med
89MBP	Filler, Bone Void, Osteoinduction	Physical Med
87MQV	Filler, Calcium Sulfate Preformed Pellets	Orthopedics

FILLING

76EBD	Coating, Filling Material, Resin	Dental And Oral
76EIY	Filling, Instrument Plastic, Dental	Dental And Oral
76LYC	Implant, Endosseous (Bone Filling and/or Augmentation)	Dental And Oral
76QOW	Material, Dental Filling	Dental And Oral
76MMT	Resin, Filling, Root Canal (Containing Chloroform)	Dental And Oral
76KIF	Resin, Root Canal Filling	Dental And Oral
76EKK	Spreader, Pulp Canal Filling Material, Endodontic	Dental And Oral

FILM

90IXA	Cassette, Radiographic Film	Radiology
90IZP	Changer Programmer, Radiographic Film/Cassette	Radiology
90IXS	Changer, Film, Radiographic	Radiology
90KPX	Changer, Radiographic Film/Cassette	Radiology
90VGU	Chemical, Film Processor	Radiology

FILM *(cont'd)*

90WZJ	Cover, Film, X-Ray	Radiology
90TFP	Cutter, X-Ray Film	Radiology
90QQI	Dosimeter, Radiation	Radiology
76EGW	Dryer, Film, Radiographic	Dental And Oral
90TFQ	Duplicator, X-Ray Film	Radiology
90WZI	Envelope, Film, X-Ray	Radiology
79FXT	Film, Camera	Surgery
90EAL	Film, X-Ray	Radiology
76EHC	Film, X-Ray, Dental, Extraoral	Dental And Oral
76EAO	Film, X-Ray, Dental, Intraoral	Dental And Oral
90VFL	Film, X-Ray, Instant	Radiology
90IWZ	Film, X-Ray, Special Purpose	Radiology
90UFC	Handling Unit, Automatic Daylight X-Ray Film	Radiology
76EGZ	Holder, X-Ray Film	Dental And Oral
90VGT	Holder, X-Ray Film Cassette, Vertical	Radiology
90IXC	Illuminator, Radiographic Film	Radiology
90JAG	Illuminator, Radiographic Film, Explosion-Proof	Radiology
90TGW	Interlock System, X-Ray Darkrooms	Radiology
90SGK	Labeler, X-Ray Film	Radiology
90TFR	Minifier, X-Ray Film (Reducer)	Radiology
90WHY	Mixer, Chemical, Film, X-Ray	Radiology
90SGL	Monitor, X-Ray Film Processor Quality Control	Radiology
90IXX	Processor, Cine Film	Radiology
90IXW	Processor, Radiographic Film, Automatic	Radiology
76EGY	Processor, Radiographic Film, Automatic, Dental	Dental And Oral
90JAH	Processor, Radiographic Film, Manual	Radiology
90VGV	Projector, X-Ray Film	Radiology
90TER	Silver Recovery Equipment	Radiology
90IXL	Spot Film Device	Radiology
90UAB	Storage Unit, X-Ray Film	Radiology
90JAC	System, Marking, Film, Radiographic	Radiology
90WTF	Unit, Imaging, Thermal	Radiology
90WUY	Viewer, Radiographic Film, Motorized	Radiology

FILMATED

80RVE	Sponge, Filmated	General

FILTER

75QVV	Filter Paper	Chemistry
80QVW	Filter, Air	General
79WIF	Filter, Aspirator	Surgery
80WOX	Filter, Bacteria, Pump, Breast	General
73CAH	Filter, Bacterial, Breathing Circuit	Anesthesiology
75UGC	Filter, Bacteriological, Laboratory	Chemistry
74DTM	Filter, Blood, Cardiopulmonary Bypass, Arterial Line	Cardiovascular
74JOD	Filter, Blood, Cardiotomy Suction Line, Cardiopulmonary	Cardiovascular
78FKJ	Filter, Blood, Dialysis	Gastro/Urology
88KET	Filter, Cell Collection, Tissue Processing	Pathology
73BSN	Filter, Conduction, Anesthesia	Anesthesiology
73QVX	Filter, Gas	Anesthesiology
80FPB	Filter, Infusion Line	General
74DTK	Filter, Intravascular, Cardiovascular	Cardiovascular
80QVY	Filter, Intravenous Tubing	General
78QVZ	Filter, Kidney Stone	Gastro/Urology
86WXB	Filter, Lens	Ophthalmology
75UGD	Filter, Membrane	Chemistry
78KPP	Filter, Peritoneal Dialysate	Gastro/Urology
74KRJ	Filter, Pre-Bypass, Cardiopulmonary Bypass	Cardiovascular
90QWA	Filter, Radiofrequency	Radiology
90VGF	Filter, Radiographic	Radiology
84QWB	Filter, Shunt, Hydrocephalic	Cns/Neurology
80QWC	Filter, Steam	General
80QWD	Filter, Syringe	General
73KHB	Filter, Tobacco Smoke (Attached)	Anesthesiology
73KHC	Filter, Tobacco Smoke (Unattached)	Anesthesiology
74QWE	Filter, Vena Cava	Cardiovascular
73QWF	Filter, Ventilator	Anesthesiology
75UGB	Gel, Filter	Chemistry
80WXR	Media, Filter	General
73CAK	Microfilter, Blood Transfusion	Anesthesiology
80VCQ	Needle, Filter	General
75SFX	Purification Filter, Water, Charcoal	Chemistry
75SFY	Purification Filter, Water, Particulate	Chemistry
75UIZ	Ultrafiltration Equipment	Chemistry
75JRL	Unit, Filter, Membrane	Chemistry

FILTERING

80WYN	Equipment, Filtering, Air, ETO	General

FINANCE

80WUE	Service, Finance	General

FINDER

80SER	Finder, Vein	General

FINGER

78EYX	Drape, Pure Latex Sheet, With Self-Retaining Finger Cot	Gastro/Urology
89JFA	Exerciser, Finger, Powered	Physical Med

FINGER *(cont'd)*

80LZB	Finger Cot	General
76LQX	Finger-Sucking Device	Dental And Oral
74WZC	Monitor, Blood Pressure, Finger	Cardiovascular
80VFN	Oximeter, Finger	General
87HSJ	Prosthesis, Finger	Orthopedics
87KQY	Prosthesis, Finger and Toe, Hemi-Arthroplasty	Orthopedics
87LBC	Prosthesis, Finger, Constrained, Metal, Cemented	Orthopedics
87KWE	Prosthesis, Finger, Constrained, Metal, Uncemented	Orthopedics
87KWG	Prosthesis, Finger, Constrained, Metal/Polymer	Orthopedics
87KYJ	Prosthesis, Finger, Constrained, Polymer	Orthopedics
87KWC	Prosthesis, Finger, Hemi	Orthopedics
87KWF	Prosthesis, Finger, Polymer	Orthopedics
87UBQ	Prosthesis, Finger, Total	Orthopedics
87QWH	Protector, Finger	Orthopedics
77JYB	Vise, Ossicular Finger	Ear/Nose/Throat

FINGER-SUCKING

76LQX	Finger-Sucking Device	Dental And Oral

FINGERNAIL

79QRH	Drill, Fingernail	Surgery

FINISH

87MBL	Prosthesis, Hip, Semi-, Uncemented, Osteophilic Finish	Orthopedics
87MAY	Prosthesis, Hip, Semi-constrained, Metal/Ceramic/Polymer, Cemented or Non-porous Cemented, Osteophilic Finish	Orthopedics

FINISHING

76EKA	File, Margin Finishing, Operative	Dental And Oral
76EJZ	Knife, Margin Finishing, Operative	Dental And Oral

FIRE

80LDI	Blanket, Fire	General
80WRQ	Equipment, Building Security	General

FIRST

79LRR	Kit, First Aid	Surgery
73WJE	Resuscitator, Emergency, Protective, Infection	Anesthesiology

FISSURE

76EBC	Sealant, Pit And Fissure, And Conditioner, Resin	Dental And Oral

FISTULA

78KNR	Adapter, AV Shunt Or Fistula	Gastro/Urology
78FKM	Adaptor, Fistula	Gastro/Urology
78FIE	Needle, Fistula	Gastro/Urology
78RMI	Probe, Fistula	Gastro/Urology

FITC

82DDZ	Antigen, Antiserum, Control, Albumin, FITC	Immunology
82DEI	Antigen, Antiserum, Control, Alpha-1-Antitrypsin, FITC	Immunology
82DCY	Antigen, Antiserum, Control, Ceruloplasmin, FITC	Immunology
82DCB	Antigen, Antiserum, Control, FAB, FITC	Immunology
82DAF	Antigen, Antiserum, Control, Gamma Globulin, FITC	Immunology
82DAB	Antigen, Antiserum, Control, Haptoglobin, FITC	Immunology
82CZT	Antigen, Antiserum, Control, Hemopexin, FITC	Immunology
82CZN	Antigen, Antiserum, Control, IGA, FITC	Immunology
82DGG	Antigen, Antiserum, Control, IGD, FITC	Immunology
82DGP	Antigen, Antiserum, Control, IGE, FITC	Immunology
82DGK	Antigen, Antiserum, Control, IGG, FITC	Immunology
82DFS	Antigen, Antiserum, Control, IGM, FITC	Immunology
82DEO	Antigen, Antiserum, Control, Kappa, FITC	Immunology
82DES	Antigen, Antiserum, Control, Lambda, FITC	Immunology
82DDS	Antigen, Antiserum, Control, Prealbumin, FITC	Immunology
82DDI	Antigen, Antiserum, Control, Transferrin, FITC	Immunology
82DAX	Antigen, Antiserum, Fibrinogen And Split Products, FITC	Immunology
82DDY	Antiserum, Antigen, Control, FITC, Alpha-2-Macroglobulin	Immunology
82DGN	Breast Milk, FITC, Antigen, Antiserum, Control	Immunology
82DBK	FC, FITC, Antigen, Antiserum, Control	Immunology
82DBB	Fibrin, FITC, Antigen, Antiserum, Control	Immunology
82DEC	Inter-Alpha Trypsin, FITC, Antigen, Antiserum, Control	Immunology
82DEA	Myoglobin, FITC, Antigen, Antiserum, Control	Immunology
82JZI	Platelets, FITC, Antigen, Antiserum, Control	Immunology
82DGF	Red Cells, FITC, Antigen, Antiserum, Control	Immunology
82DFX	Sperm, FITC, Antigen, Antiserum, Control	Immunology
82DCK	Test, C-Reactive Protein, FITC	Immunology
82DDJ	Thyroglobulin, FITC, Antigen, Antiserum, Control	Immunology

FITTING

75UIY	Fitting, Gas Chromatography Tube	Chemistry
80QWK	Fitting, Luer	General
80QWJ	Fitting, Other	General
80QWL	Fitting, Quick Connect (Gas Connector)	General
73ROW	Regulator, Anesthesia	Anesthesiology
80FQE	Regulator, Oxygen, Mechanical	General
73CAN	Regulator, Pressure, Gas Cylinder	Anesthesiology

FIXATION

87LYT	Accessories, Fixation, Orthopedic	Orthopedics

FIXATION *(cont'd)*

87LYP	Accessories, Fixation, Spinal Interlaminal	Orthopedics
87LYQ	Accessories, Fixation, Spinal Intervertebral Body	Orthopedics
83GNF	Antigen, CF, T. Cruzi	Microbiology
87LXT	Appliance, Fix., Nail/Blade/Plate Comb., Multiple Component	Orthopedics
87KWP	Appliance, Fixation, Spinal Interlaminal	Orthopedics
87KWQ	Appliance, Fixation, Spinal Intervertebral Body	Orthopedics
87HTN	Bolt, Nut, Washer	Orthopedics
87JDT	Cap, Bone	Orthopedics
77MLI	Cement, Bone, Ionomer	Ear/Nose/Throat
87JDQ	Cerclage, Fixation	Orthopedics
79WZW	Clamp, Fixation, Cholangiography	Surgery
79WZX	Clamp, Laparoscopy	Surgery
87MBJ	Fastener, Fixation, Biodegradable, Hard Tissue	Orthopedics
87MAI	Fastener, Fixation, Biodegradable, Soft Tissue	Orthopedics
87MBI	Fastener, Fixation, Non-Biodegradable, Soft Tissue	Orthopedics
87KTT	Fixation Appliance, Multiple Component	Orthopedics
87KTW	Fixation Appliance, Single Component	Orthopedics
86HPL	Fixation Device, AC-Powered, Ophthalmic	Ophthalmology
86HKJ	Fixation Device, Battery-Powered, Ophthalmic	Ophthalmology
87VKH	Fixation Device, Extra-Cranial (Head Frame)	Orthopedics
87TCT	Fixation Device, Jaw Fracture	Orthopedics
87UAP	Fixation Device, Spinal (External)	Orthopedics
73CBH	Fixation Device, Tracheal Tube	Anesthesiology
79QXA	Forceps, Fixation	Surgery
86RAO	Hook, Scleral Fixation	Ophthalmology
87JDP	Implant, Fixation Device, Condylar Plate	Orthopedics
87JDO	Implant, Fixation Device, Proximal Femoral	Orthopedics
87JDN	Implant, Fixation Device, Spinal	Orthopedics
86UBB	Lens, Intraocular, Iridocapsular Fixation	Ophthalmology
86UBC	Lens, Intraocular, Iris Fixation	Ophthalmology
87JDS	Nail, Fixation, Bone	Orthopedics
87MAT	Orthosis, Fixation, Cervical Intervertebral Body, Spinal	Orthopedics
87MNI	Orthosis, Fixation, Pedicle, Spinal	Orthopedics
87MNH	Orthosis, Fixation, Spinal, Spondylolisthesis	Orthopedics
87HTY	Pin, Fixation, Smooth	Orthopedics
87JDW	Pin, Fixation, Threaded	Orthopedics
80WMU	Pin, Safety	General
76JEY	Plate, Bone, Orthodontic	Dental And Oral
84RLI	Plate, Bone, Skull (Cranioplasty)	Cns/Neurology
84GWO	Plate, Bone, Skull, Preformed, Alterable	Cns/Neurology
84GXN	Plate, Bone, Skull, Preformed, Non-Alterable	Cns/Neurology
87HRS	Plate, Fixation, Bone	Orthopedics
87NDF	Plate, Fixation, Bone, Non-Spinal, Metallic	Orthopedics
87HSB	Rod, Fixation, Intramedullary	Orthopedics
84UAU	Screw, Cranioplasty Plate	Cns/Neurology
87HWC	Screw, Fixation, Bone	Orthopedics
87NDJ	Screw, Fixation, Bone, Non-Spinal, Metallic	Orthopedics
76DZL	Screw, Fixation, Intraosseous	Dental And Oral
87JDR	Staple, Fixation, Bone	Orthopedics
87MCV	System, Appliance, Fixation, Spinal Pedicle Screw	Orthopedics
76DZK	Wire, Fixation, Intraosseous	Dental And Oral

FIXATIVE

88LDW	Fixative, Acid Containing	Pathology
88LDZ	Fixative, Alcohol Containing	Pathology
88LDY	Fixative, Formalin Containing	Pathology
88LDX	Fixative, Metallic Containing	Pathology
88IFJ	Fixative, Richardson Glycol	Pathology
88IFT	Glutaraldehyde (Fixative)	Pathology

FIXED

75QKW	Analyzer, Chemistry, Multi-Channel, Fixed	Chemistry
80TBJ	Compactor, Fixed	General
85HDQ	Dilator, Cervical, Fixed Size	Obstetrics/Gyn
75RDW	Laminar Air Flow Unit, Fixed (Air Curtain)	Chemistry
90RNZ	Radiographic Unit, Diagnostic, Fixed (X-Ray)	Radiology
90QWR	Radiographic/Fluoroscopic Unit, Fixed	Radiology

FIXER

90VGU	Chemical, Film Processor	Radiology

FLAKE

80WPU	Soap	General

FLAKES

80TBU	Dispenser, Ice	General

FLAME

91DMM	Flame Photometer, Pesticides (Dedicated Instruments)	Toxicology
75JJO	Photometer, Flame Emission	Chemistry
91DMW	Photometer, Flame, General Use	Toxicology
91DLM	Photometer, Flame, Heavy Metals (Dedicated Instrument)	Toxicology
75JIH	Photometer, Flame, Lithium	Chemistry
91DOQ	Photometer, Flame, Lithium, Toxicology	Toxicology
75JGM	Photometer, Flame, Potassium	Chemistry
75JGT	Photometer, Flame, Sodium	Chemistry

KEYWORD INDEX

FLAMELESS
75JQS Atomizer, Flameless — Chemistry

FLASH
75RFC Light Source, Flash — Chemistry
80UCS Sterilizer, Steam, Bulk — General
80SFM Washer/Sterilizer — General

FLASHER
86HIZ Flasher, After-Image — Ophthalmology

FLASK
75QPH Flask, Dewar — Chemistry
88KJD Flask, Spinner — Pathology
88KJA Flask, Tissue Culture — Pathology
75WKC Stand/Holder, Equipment, Laboratory — Chemistry
80WNN Stopper — General

FLAT
90MQB Imager, X-Ray, Solid State (Flat Panel/Digital) — Radiology

FLAVOBACTERIUM
83GSW Antiserum, Flavobacterium Meningospeticum — Microbiology

FLEXIBLE
77BTN Bronchoscope, Non-Rigid — Ear/Nose/Throat
78WUJ Cabinet, Storage, Endoscope — Gastro/Urology
78FBN Choledochoscope, Flexible Or Rigid — Gastro/Urology
78FAJ Cystoscope — Gastro/Urology
78FGO Dislodger, Stone, Flexible — Gastro/Urology
78FEH Electrode, Flexible Suction Coagulator — Gastro/Urology
78GCQ Endoscope, Flexible — Gastro/Urology
77EOX Esophagoscope (Flexible Or Rigid) — Ear/Nose/Throat
78QXC Forceps, Grasping, Flexible Endoscopic — Gastro/Urology
78QYC Gastroscope, Flexible — Gastro/Urology
79QYN Gown, Operating Room, Reusable — Surgery
74QYZ Guidewire — Cardiovascular
74DQX Guidewire, Catheter — Cardiovascular
90JAJ Guidewire, Catheter, Radiological — Radiology
79WXI Laparoscope, Flexible — Surgery
73CAL Laryngoscope, Flexible — Anesthesiology
86HJJ Lens, Fresnel, Flexible, Diagnostic — Ophthalmology
77EOB Nasopharyngoscope (Flexible Or Rigid) — Ear/Nose/Throat
78RIM Nephroscope, Flexible — Gastro/Urology
79WRZ Retractor, Abdominal, Padded, Flexible — Surgery
78FAM Sigmoidoscope, Flexible — Gastro/Urology
78FDI Snare, Flexible — Gastro/Urology
80THI Sterilizer/Washer, Endoscope — General
73BYY Tube, Aspirating, Flexible, Connecting — Anesthesiology
73BYX Tubing, Flexible, Medical Gas, Low-Pressure — Anesthesiology

FLIERINGA
86HNH Ring, Ophthalmic (Flieringa) — Ophthalmology

FLOCCULATION
83GPI Antigen, Bentonite Flocculation, Trichinella Spiralis — Microbiology
83GPH Antiserum, Bentonite Flocculation, Trichinella Spiralis — Microbiology

FLOOD
90IYQ Phantom, Flood Source, Nuclear — Radiology

FLOOR
88QJA Centrifuge, Floor — Pathology
80TCC Floor Mat — General
80QWM Floor Mat, Antibacterial — General
80TCD Floor, Conductive — General
79FSS Light, Surgical, Floor Standing — Surgery
80WRN Rails, Equipment — General
80RZW Tester, Conductivity, Floor And Equipment — General

FLOORING
80VBC Flooring — General

FLOSS
76JES Floss, Dental — Dental And Oral

FLOTATION
83QCX Bath, Tissue Flotation — Microbiology
88IDY Bath, Tissue Flotation, Pathology — Pathology
80UDH Bed, Flotation Therapy, Neonatal — General
89IOQ Bed, Flotation Therapy, Powered — Physical Med
89FNH Bed, Water Flotation, AC-Powered — Physical Med
80QJI Chair, Flotation Therapy — General
89KIC Cushion, Flotation — Physical Med
89MOC Cushion, Flotation, Therapeutic — Physical Med
80FNM Mattress, Air Flotation — General
89IKY Mattress, Non-Powered Flotation Therapy — Physical Med

FLOW
75JJC Analyzer, Chemistry, Sequential Multiple, Continuous Flow — Chemistry
90WNR Angio-Dynograph — Radiology
84HBY Catheter, Angiographic — Cns/Neurology

FLOW *(cont'd)*
74DYG Catheter, Flow Directed — Cardiovascular
75UKI Centrifuge, Continuous Flow — Chemistry
80MJF Check Valve, Retrograde Flow (In-Line) — General
74ULR Detector, Blood Flow, Ultrasonic (Doppler) — Cardiovascular
78FJG Dialyzer, Parallel Flow (Hemodialysis) — Gastro/Urology
74WSD Doppler, Blood Flow, Transcranial — Cardiovascular
90VHA Doppler, Flow Mapping — Radiology
78QWP Flowmeter, Blood, Ultrasonic — Gastro/Urology
74JOR Generator, Pulsatile Flow, Cardiopulmonary Bypass — Cardiovascular
84HAP Guide, Wire, Angiographic (And Accessories) — Cns/Neurology
80RAH Hood, Isolation, Laminar Air Flow — General
74DXT Injector, Angiographic (Cardiac Catheterization) — Cardiovascular
90VGB Kit, Angiographic, Digital — Radiology
90VGC Kit, Angiographic, Special Procedure — Radiology
78LBW Kit, Dialysis, Single Needle (Co-Axial Flow) — Gastro/Urology
80FLJ Laminar Air Flow Unit — General
75RDW Laminar Air Flow Unit, Fixed (Air Curtain) — Chemistry
75RDX Laminar Air Flow Unit, Mobile — Chemistry
74WTT Legging, Compression, Inflatable, Sequential — Cardiovascular
80LLK Legging, Compression, Non-Inflatable — General
73BZH Meter, Peak Flow, Spirometry — Anesthesiology
85HEP Monitor, Blood Flow, Ultrasonic — Obstetrics/Gyn
84LME Monitor, Cerebral Blood Flow, Thermal Diffusion — Cns/Neurology
80FLN Monitor, Infusion, Gravity Flow — General
84HAQ Needle, Angiographic — Cns/Neurology
90RKT Phonoangiograph — Radiology
74DPT Probe, Blood Flow, Extravascular — Cardiovascular
79RTA Probe, Detector, Flow, Blood, Laparoscopy, Ultrasonic — Surgery
90VLE Radiographic Unit, Digital Subtraction Angiographic (DSA) — Radiology
90IZI Radiographic/Fluoroscopic Unit, Angiographic — Radiology
90VHC Radiographic/Fluoroscopic Unit, Angiographic, Digital — Radiology
90IYN Scanner, Ultrasonic (Pulsed Doppler) — Radiology
90IYO Scanner, Ultrasonic (Pulsed Echo) — Radiology
90VCV Scanner, Ultrasonic, Vascular — Radiology
74MFZ System, Pump & Control, Cardiac Assist, Axial Flow — Cardiovascular
75JNW Timed Flow in Capillary, Plasma Viscometry — Chemistry
73QWN Timer, Flow — Anesthesiology
73BXG Transducer, Blood Flow, Invasive — Anesthesiology
73BXF Transducer, Blood Flow, Non-Invasive — Anesthesiology
74WLT Transducer, Flow, Catheter Tip — Cardiovascular
73BXP Transducer, Gas Flow — Anesthesiology

FLOWMETER
76EFE Flowmeter, Anesthesia — Dental And Oral
73CAX Flowmeter, Back-Pressure Compensated, Thorpe Tube — Anesthesiology
74DPW Flowmeter, Blood, Intravenous — Cardiovascular
78FIT Flowmeter, Blood, Non-Invasive Electromagnetic — Gastro/Urology
74WSR Flowmeter, Blood, Other — Cardiovascular
78QWP Flowmeter, Blood, Ultrasonic — Gastro/Urology
74CAS Flowmeter, Blood, Ultrasonic, Transcutaneous (W/WO Calibr.) — Cardiovascular
78FIS Flowmeter, Dialysate — Gastro/Urology
73BXY Flowmeter, Gas (Oxygen), Calibrated — Anesthesiology
73CCN Flowmeter, Gas, Non-Back-Pressure Compensated, Bourdon Gauge — Anesthesiology
84UEW Flowmeter, Meter, Cerebral Blood, Xenon Clearance — Cns/Neurology
77ETL Flowmeter, Nasal — Ear/Nose/Throat
73VHT Flowmeter, Pulmonary Function — Anesthesiology
78FFG Flowmeter, Urine, Disposable — Gastro/Urology
74KFP Monitor, Cardiac Output, Flowmeter — Cardiovascular
73RLM Pneumotachograph — Anesthesiology
73ROW Regulator, Anesthesia — Anesthesiology
73QWO Regulator, Intake, Oxygen — Anesthesiology
80FQE Regulator, Oxygen, Mechanical — General
73CAN Regulator, Pressure, Gas Cylinder — Anesthesiology

FLUFF
80QWQ Fluff — General

FLUID
76LZX Acid, Hyaluronic — Dental And Oral
82DFI Antigen, Antiserum, Control, Spinal Fluid, Total — Immunology
91MAS Chromatography, Liquid, Performance, High — Toxicology
75WYT Chromatography, Supercritical Fluid (SFC) — Chemistry
80KPE Container, IV — General
80TGU Dispenser, Fluid — General
80WUM Encapsulator, Fluid — General
78FHF Evacuator, Fluid — Gastro/Urology
88IGN Fluid, Bouin's — Pathology
85LTY Fluid, Collection, Cytological — Obstetrics/Gyn
76MGG Fluid, Hylan (For TMJ Use) — Dental And Oral
86LWL Fluid, Intraocular — Ophthalmology
81JCG Fluid, Manual Cell Diluting — Hematology
81GJN Fluid, Red Cell Diluting — Hematology
81GGK Fluid, Red Cell Lysing — Hematology
81GGJ Fluid, White Cell Diluting — Hematology
85LTA Hysteroscopy Fluid — Obstetrics/Gyn

FLUID *(cont'd)*

80KZE	Injector, Fluid, Non-Electric	General
80FMJ	Manometer, Spinal Fluid	General
76JEO	Measurer, Gingival Fluid	Dental And Oral
80CAQ	Monitor, Cerebral Spinal Fluid Pressure (CSF)	General
80CAR	Monitor, Cerebral Spinal Fluid Pressure, Electrical	General
80QZS	Pad, Heating, Circulating Fluid	General
79QUQ	Probe, Suction, Irrigator/Aspirator, Laparoscopic	Surgery
84TEG	Reservoir, Spinal Fluid	Cns/Neurology
76KKO	Ring, Teething, Fluid-Filled	Dental And Oral
76MEF	Ring, Teething, Non-Fluid-Filled	Dental And Oral
85HIO	Sampler, Amniotic Fluid (Amniocentesis Tray)	Obstetrics/Gyn
82DGB	Seminal Fluid, Antigen, Antiserum, Control	Immunology
75WHJ	Test, Maturity, Lung, Fetal	Chemistry
79FWS	Thermometer, Fluid Column	Surgery
80LHI	Transfer Unit, IV Fluid	General
80FPK	Tubing, Fluid Delivery	General
84LXL	Valve, Shunt, Fluid, CNS (Post-Amendment Design)	Cns/Neurology
80LHF	Warmer, Infusion Fluid, Microwave	General
80LGZ	Warmer, Infusion Fluid, Thermal	General

FLUID-FILLED

76KKO	Ring, Teething, Fluid-Filled	Dental And Oral
76MEF	Ring, Teething, Non-Fluid-Filled	Dental And Oral

FLUIDIC

86MUS	Fluidic, Phacoemulsification/fragmentation	Ophthalmology

FLUIDIZED

89INX	Bed, Air Fluidized	Physical Med
89LBG	Fluidized Therapy, Unit, Dry Heat	Physical Med

FLUIDOTHERAPY

89LSB	Fluidotherapy Unit	Physical Med

FLUORESCEIN

79HJE	Lamp, Fluorescein, AC-Powered	Surgery
86KYC	Strip, Fluorescein	Ophthalmology

FLUORESCENCE

75UEI	Analyzer, Chemistry, Fluorescence Immunoassay	Chemistry
91LGJ	Fluorescence Polarization Immunoassay, Amibacin	Toxicology
91LGI	Fluorescence Polarization Immunoassay, Carbamazepine	Toxicology
91LGR	Fluorescence Polarization Immunoassay, Diphenylhydantoin	Toxicology
91LGQ	Fluorescence Polarization Immunoassay, Phenobarbital	Toxicology
91LGS	Fluorescence Polarization Immunoassay, Theophylline	Toxicology
91LFW	Fluorescence Polarization Immunoassay, Tobramycin	Toxicology
75MGU	Fluorescence Polarization, Immunoassay, Cyclosporine	Chemistry
75UIV	Fluorescence, Thin-Layer	Chemistry
81JMH	Fluorescence, Visual Observation (Qual., U.V.), Gsh	Hematology
75JOB	Hexane Extraction, Fluorescence, Vitamin E	Chemistry
83GMB	Light, Wood's, Fluorescence	Microbiology
88IBK	Microscope, Fluorescence/U.V.	Pathology
75RUL	Spectrophotometer, Fluorescence	Chemistry
82WUO	Test, Cancer Detection, QFI	Immunology

FLUORESCENT

91DKY	Alumina Fluorescent Indicator, TLC	Toxicology
87WQP	Analyzer, Distribution, Weight, Podiatric	Orthopedics
83GPD	Antigen, Fluorescent Antibody Test, Echinococcus Granulosus	Microbiology
83GNH	Antigen, Fluorescent Antibody Test, Schistosoma Mansoni	Microbiology
83LIN	Antisera, Conjugated Fluorescent, Cytomegalovirus	Microbiology
83GSY	Antisera, Fluorescent, All Globulins, Proteus SPP.	Microbiology
83GTN	Antisera, Fluorescent, All Types, Staphylococcus SPP.	Microbiology
83LKI	Antisera, Fluorescent, Chlamydia SPP.	Microbiology
83GNM	Antisera, Fluorescent, Coxsackievirus A 1-24, B 1-6	Microbiology
83GRK	Antisera, Fluorescent, Echovirus 1-34	Microbiology
83GQL	Antisera, Fluorescent, Herpesvirus Hominis 1, 2	Microbiology
83GOE	Antisera, Fluorescent, Poliovirus 1-3	Microbiology
83GSS	Antisera, Fluorescent, Pseudomonas Aeruginosa	Microbiology
83GTH	Antiserum, Fluorescent (Direct Test), N. Gonorrhoeae	Microbiology
83GMX	Antiserum, Fluorescent Antibody For FTA-ABS Test	Microbiology
83GNY	Antiserum, Fluorescent, Adenovirus 1-33	Microbiology
83GOO	Antiserum, Fluorescent, All Globulins, Salmonella SPP.	Microbiology
83JRW	Antiserum, Fluorescent, B. Parapertussis	Microbiology
83GOZ	Antiserum, Fluorescent, B. Pertussis	Microbiology
83GSM	Antiserum, Fluorescent, Brucella SPP.	Microbiology
83GOS	Antiserum, Fluorescent, C. Diphtheriae	Microbiology
83GSP	Antiserum, Fluorescent, Campylobacter Fetus	Microbiology
83LJP	Antiserum, Fluorescent, Chlamydia Trachomatis	Microbiology
83GME	Antiserum, Fluorescent, Cryptococcus Neoformans	Microbiology
83JRY	Antiserum, Fluorescent, Epstein-Barr Virus	Microbiology
83GSD	Antiserum, Fluorescent, Erysipelothrix Rhusiopathiae	Microbiology
83GMY	Antiserum, Fluorescent, Escherichia Coli	Microbiology
83GSJ	Antiserum, Fluorescent, Francisella Tularensis	Microbiology
83GTX	Antiserum, Fluorescent, Groups, Streptococcus SPP.	Microbiology
83GRO	Antiserum, Fluorescent, Hemophilus SPP.	Microbiology
83GML	Antiserum, Fluorescent, Histoplasma Capsulatum	Microbiology

FLUORESCENT *(cont'd)*

83GTB	Antiserum, Fluorescent, Klebsiella SPP.	Microbiology
83GRW	Antiserum, Fluorescent, Leptospira SPP.	Microbiology
83GSG	Antiserum, Fluorescent, Listeria Monocytogenes	Microbiology
83GRA	Antiserum, Fluorescent, Mumps Virus	Microbiology
83GRT	Antiserum, Fluorescent, Mycobacterium Tuberculosis	Microbiology
83GRZ	Antiserum, Fluorescent, Mycoplasma SPP.	Microbiology
83GTI	Antiserum, Fluorescent, N. Meningitidis	Microbiology
83GSR	Antiserum, Fluorescent, Pseudomonas Pseudomallei	Microbiology
83GPJ	Antiserum, Fluorescent, Q Fever	Microbiology
83GOI	Antiserum, Fluorescent, Rabies Virus	Microbiology
83GRE	Antiserum, Fluorescent, Rubeola	Microbiology
83GTD	Antiserum, Fluorescent, Shigella SPP., All Globulins	Microbiology
83GMA	Antiserum, Fluorescent, Sporothrix Schenekii	Microbiology
83GWB	Antiserum, Fluorescent, Streptococcus Pneumoniae	Microbiology
90WSH	Calculator, Technique, Radiographic	Radiology
91DJO	Cellulose Fluorescent Indicator, TLC	Toxicology
91LCQ	Fluorescent Immunoassay Gentamicin	Toxicology
91LES	Fluorescent Immunoassay, Diphenylhydantoin	Toxicology
91LET	Fluorescent Immunoassay, Phenobarbital	Toxicology
91LFT	Fluorescent Immunoassay, Primidone	Toxicology
91LER	Fluorescent Immunoassay, Theophylline	Toxicology
91LCR	Fluorescent Immunoassay, Tobramycin	Toxicology
75KQP	Fluorescent Proc. (Qual.), Galactose-1-Phosphate Uridyl	Chemistry
91WQE	Immunoassay, Other	Toxicology
83GWD	Indirect Fluorescent Antibody Test, Entamoeba Histolytica	Microbiology
83LHL	Legionella Direct & Indirect Fluorescent Antibody Regents	Microbiology
90JAO	Scanner, Fluorescent	Radiology
91DLO	Silica Gel Fluorescent Indicator, TLC	Toxicology

FLUORIDE

91DMA	Reagent, Test, Fluoride	Toxicology
76UDW	Tray, Fluoride	Dental And Oral
76KMT	Tray, Fluoride, Disposable	Dental And Oral

FLUORIMETRIC

75JNB	Ninhydrin And L-Leucyl-L-Alanine (Fluorimetric)	Chemistry

FLUORINATED

80WTH	Tubing, Polytetrafluoroethylene	General

FLUOROCARBON

80VLK	Cartridge, Freon	General

FLUOROGRAPHIC

90IZJ	Camera, X-Ray, Fluorographic, Cine Or Spot	Radiology

FLUOROIMMUNOASSAY

91LCB	Fluoroimmunoassay, Gentamicin	Toxicology

FLUOROMETER

82JZT	Fluorometer	Immunology
75KHO	Fluorometer, Chemistry	Chemistry
91DOX	Fluorometer, Lead (Dedicated Instruments)	Toxicology
91DPR	Fluorometer, Toxicology	Toxicology
90RKV	Photofluorometer	Radiology

FLUOROMETRIC

75CDR	1-Nitroso-2-Naphthol (Fluorometric), Free Tyrosine	Chemistry
75CHQ	Chromatographic/Fluorometric Method, Catecholamines	Chemistry
75JKJ	Fluorometric Measurement, Porphyrins	Chemistry
75JHD	Fluorometric Method, 17-Hydroxycorticosteroids	Chemistry
75JHX	Fluorometric Method, CPK Or Isoenzymes	Chemistry
75CGY	Fluorometric Method, Creatine Phosphokinase	Chemistry
75JGW	Fluorometric Method, Triglycerides	Chemistry
75JFT	Fluorometric, Cortisol	Chemistry
75JNZ	Fluorometric, Uroporphyrin	Chemistry
91DNX	Protoporphyrin Zinc Method, Fluorometric, Lead	Toxicology
91DMK	Protoporphyrin, Fluorometric, Lead	Toxicology

FLUOROMETRY

91DJJ	Fluorometry, Morphine	Toxicology

FLUOROPHOTOMETER

75VEC	Fluorophotometer	Chemistry

FLUOROSCOPE

90IZG	Radiographic Unit, Diagnostic, Photofluorographic	Radiology

FLUOROSCOPIC

90IYZ	Bed, Scanning, Nuclear/Fluoroscopic	Radiology
90WUK	Copier, Image, Radiographic	Radiology
90TCP	Image Intensification System	Radiology
90RKW	Photofluoroscope (Cardiac Catheterization)	Radiology
90IZI	Radiographic/Fluoroscopic Unit, Angiographic	Radiology
90VHC	Radiographic/Fluoroscopic Unit, Angiographic, Digital	Radiology
90QWR	Radiographic/Fluoroscopic Unit, Fixed	Radiology
90JAA	Radiographic/Fluoroscopic Unit, Image-Intensified	Radiology
90QWS	Radiographic/Fluoroscopic Unit, Mobile C-Arm	Radiology
90JAB	Radiographic/Fluoroscopic Unit, Non-Image-Intensified	Radiology
90THR	Radiographic/Fluoroscopic Unit, Special Procedure	Radiology
90VGY	Storage Device, Fluoroscopic Image	Radiology

KEYWORD INDEX

FORCEPS *(cont'd)*

87HYA	Forceps, Wire Holding	Orthopedics
87HRQ	Hemostat	Orthopedics
76EMD	Hemostat, Surgical	Dental And Oral
84GZX	Instrument, Microsurgical	Cns/Neurology
79RDB	Jar, Forceps	Surgery
80WXM	Pad, Forceps, Surgical	General
73JEI	Remover, Foreign Body, Bronchoscope (Non-Rigid)	Anesthesiology
86VKE	Surgical Instrument, Radial Keratotomy	Ophthalmology
79RZQ	Tenaculum, Other (Forceps)	Surgery

FOREARM

89KFT	Assembly, Shoulder/Elbow/Forearm/Wrist/Hand, Mechanical	Physical Med
89KFW	Assembly, Shoulder/Elbow/Forearm/Wrist/Hand, Powered	Physical Med

FOREHEAD

80KPD	Temperature Strip, Forehead, Liquid Crystal	General

FOREIGN

73JEI	Remover, Foreign Body, Bronchoscope (Non-Rigid)	Anesthesiology

FORENSIC

88TCF	Kit, Forensic Evidence	Pathology
85QXO	Kit, Forensic Evidence, Sexual Assault	Obstetrics/Gyn

FORK

87HXE	Fork	Orthopedics
84GWX	Fork, Tuning	Cns/Neurology
77ETQ	Fork, Tuning, ENT	Ear/Nose/Throat

FORM

80VAW	Form, Computer	General

FORMALDEHYDE

88IGG	Formaldehyde (Formalin, Formol)	Pathology
80QDR	Monitor, Biological (Contamination Testing)	General
80WIP	Monitor, Contamination, Environmental, Personal	General
88KEF	Paraformaldehyde	Pathology
85RVV	Sterilizer, Formaldehyde	Obstetrics/Gyn

FORMALIN

88LDY	Fixative, Formalin Containing	Pathology
88IGG	Formaldehyde (Formalin, Formol)	Pathology
88IFP	Formalin, Neutral Buffered	Pathology
88IGC	Formalin-Saline	Pathology
88IFY	Gelatin/Formalin	Pathology
88KEF	Paraformaldehyde	Pathology
88IGE	Solution, Formalin Ammonium Bromide	Pathology
88IGB	Solution, Formalin/Sodium Acetate	Pathology
88IGF	Solution, Pathology, Formalin-Alcohol-Acetic Acid	Pathology

FORMALIN-ALCOHOL-ACETIC

88IGF	Solution, Pathology, Formalin-Alcohol-Acetic Acid	Pathology

FORMALIN-SALINE

88IGC	Formalin-Saline	Pathology

FORMAT

90LMC	Camera, Multi Format	Radiology

FORMIMINOGLUTAMIC

75JLI	Tetrahydrofolate, Enzymatic (U.V.), Formiminoglutamic Acid	Chemistry

FORMING

84HBS	Clip, Instrument, Forming/Cutting	Cns/Neurology
84HBX	Instrument, Forming, Material, Cranioplasty	Cns/Neurology
91DMO	Reagent, Forming, Alkaloid, Microcrystalline	Toxicology
82VJK	Test, Chemotherapy Sensitivity (Tumor Colony Forming)	Immunology

FORMOL

88IGG	Formaldehyde (Formalin, Formol)	Pathology
88IGD	Solution, Pathology, Formol Calcium	Pathology

FORMS

80QXP	Forms, Medical And Patient	General

FORMULATIONS

88IFQ	Mercuric Chloride Formulations For Tissue	Pathology
88KEO	Paraffin, All Formulations	Pathology

FORNIXSCOPE

86HKG	Fornixscope	Ophthalmology

FOSSA

76MPI	Prosthesis, Glenoid Fossa	Dental And Oral

FOUNTAIN

75TCG	Fountain, Eye Wash	Chemistry

FPIA

91MHO	Teicoplanin, FPIA	Toxicology

FRACTION

82DCM	Antigen, Antiserum, Control, Albumin, Fraction V	Immunology
82DGA	Cohn Fraction II, Antigen, Antiserum, Control	Immunology
75QLS	Collector, Fraction	Chemistry
82DAL	Fraction IV-5, Antigen, Antiserum, Control	Immunology
82KHT	Fraction V, Antigen, Antiserum, Control	Immunology

FRACTIONATION

75CEF	Electrophoretic, Protein Fractionation	Chemistry
75JQJ	Fractionation, Protein, Densitometric	Chemistry
75JQK	Immunodiffusion, Protein Fractionation	Chemistry

FRACTIONATOR

83UFR	Fractionator, Cell	Microbiology
75UGE	Fractionator, Polymer Extractor	Chemistry

FRACTURE

80QDC	Bedpan, Fracture	General
79FYI	Facial Fracture Appliance, External	Surgery
87TCT	Fixation Device, Jaw Fracture	Orthopedics
89IPX	Orthosis, Rib Fracture, Soft	Physical Med
87RUB	Sock, Fracture	Orthopedics

FRAGILITY

81GKE	Test, Osmotic Fragility	Hematology

FRAGMENT

82DFK	Antigen, Antiserum, Control, IGG (FAB Fragment Specific)	Immunology
82DAS	Antigen, Antiserum, Control, IGG (Fc Fragment Specific)	Immunology
82DAQ	IGG (FD Fragment Specific), Antigen, Antiserum, Control	Immunology
81MIF	Prothrombin Fragment 1.2	Hematology

FRAGMENTATION

84LBK	Device, Fragmentation and Aspiration, Neurosurgical	Cns/Neurology

FRAME

87HXF	Accessories, Traction (Cart, Frame, Cord, Weight)	Orthopedics
89QVC	Exerciser, Trapeze	Physical Med
87VKH	Fixation Device, Extra-Cranial (Head Frame)	Orthopedics
79FXS	Frame, Camera, Surgical	Surgery
76EJE	Frame, Rubber Dam	Dental And Oral
86HQZ	Frame, Spectacle (Eyeglasses)	Ophthalmology
87QXQ	Frame, Traction	Orthopedics
86HPA	Frame, Trial, Ophthalmic	Ophthalmology
87QXR	Frame, Turning	Orthopedics
87WWB	Positioner, Spine, Surgical	Orthopedics

FRANCISELLA

83GSL	Antigen, Slide And Tube, Francisella Tularensis	Microbiology
83GSJ	Antiserum, Fluorescent, Francisella Tularensis	Microbiology
83GSK	Antiserum, Francisella Tularensis	Microbiology

FRAZIER

80WNO	Tube, Suction	General

FREE

75CDR	1-Nitroso-2-Naphthol (Fluorometric), Free Tyrosine	Chemistry
82DAJ	Antigen, Antiserum, Control, Free Secretory Component	Immunology
91DJL	Free Radical Assay, Amphetamine	Toxicology
91DIR	Free Radical Assay, Cocaine	Toxicology
91DPC	Free Radical Assay, Heavy Metals	Toxicology
91DOL	Free Radical Assay, LSD	Toxicology
91DPP	Free Radical Assay, Methadone	Toxicology
91DOK	Free Radical Assay, Morphine	Toxicology
91DKT	Free Radical Assay, Opiates	Toxicology
91DNG	Free Radical, Benzoylecgnonine	Toxicology
83UGI	Germ-Free Apparatus	Microbiology
79WWN	Glove, Surgical, Powder-Free	Surgery
75JKC	Radioimmunoassay, Dehydroepiandrosterone (Free And Sulfate)	Chemistry
75CEC	Radioimmunoassay, Free Thyroxine	Chemistry
80WZG	Set, Administration, Intravenous, Needle-Free	General
82MTG	Test, Prostate Specific Antigen, Free, (Noncomplexed) To Distinguish Prostate Cancer from Benign Conditions	Immunology

FREEZE

75UGF	Freeze Drying Equipment	Chemistry

FREEZER

81QNO	Equipment, Bank, Blood, Cryogenic (Liquid Nitrogen)	Hematology
81KSP	Freezer, Blood Cell	Hematology
81KSE	Freezer, Blood Storage	Hematology
87TCH	Freezer, Bone	Orthopedics
86TCI	Freezer, Eye Bank	Ophthalmology
75UKL	Freezer, Laboratory, Biological	Chemistry
75JRM	Freezer, Laboratory, General Purpose	Chemistry
75UKM	Freezer, Laboratory, Ultra-Low Temperature	Chemistry
75QXS	Monitor, Freezer	Chemistry

FREEZING

75ULP	Bath, Freezing	Chemistry

KEYWORD INDEX

FURNITURE *(cont'd)*

79FWW	Table, Operating Room, Pneumatic	Surgery
80RZB	Table, Other	General
80RYY	Table, Overbed	General
89JFB	Table, Physical Therapy	Physical Med
90IXQ	Table, Radiographic, Stationary Top	Radiology
90IXR	Table, Radiographic, Tilting	Radiology
88IEG	Table, Slide Warming	Pathology
79JEA	Table, Surgical With Orthopedic Accessories, AC-Powered	Surgery
79FWY	Table, Surgical, Hydraulic	Surgery
87RYZ	Table, Traction	Orthopedics
78RZA	Table, Urological (Cystological)	Gastro/Urology
78EYH	Table, Urological, Non-Electrical	Gastro/Urology
78UEE	Table, Urological, Radiographic	Gastro/Urology
77ETF	Unit, Examining/Treatment, ENT	Ear/Nose/Throat

FUSION

87MAX	Orthosis, Fusion, Intervertebral, Spinal	Orthopedics
86HLP	Target, Fusion/Stereoscopic	Ophthalmology

GAG

77KBN	Gag, Mouth	Ear/Nose/Throat

GAIT

87WQP	Analyzer, Distribution, Weight, Podiatric	Orthopedics
87VDV	Analyzer, Gait	Orthopedics
80WWG	Analyzer, Motion	General

GAL-I-P

75JLJ	UDP-Glucose, NAD (U.V.), Gal-I-P Uridyl Transperase	Chemistry

GALACTOSE

75JIC	Colorimetric Method, Galactose	Chemistry
75JIA	Enzymatic Method, Galactose	Chemistry
75KQP	Fluorescent Proc. (Qual.), Galactose-1-Phosphate Uridyl	Chemistry
75JIB	U.V. Method, Galactose	Chemistry

GALACTOSE-1-PHOSPHATE

75KQP	Fluorescent Proc. (Qual.), Galactose-1-Phosphate Uridyl	Chemistry

GALL

78SIQ	Extractor, Gall Bladder	Gastro/Urology

GALLBLADDER

78QXB	Forceps, Gallbladder (Biliary Duct)	Gastro/Urology
78MII	System, Gallbladder, Thermal Ablation	Gastro/Urology
78SCF	Trocar, Gallbladder	Gastro/Urology

GALLSTONE

78WUD	Lithotriptor, Extracorporeal, Gallstone	Gastro/Urology
78WSU	Lithotriptor, Laser	Gastro/Urology
78WIL	Lithotriptor, Multipurpose	Gastro/Urology
80MHD	Pump, Infusion, Gallstone Dissolution	General
78FHL	Scoop, Gallstone	Gastro/Urology

GALVANIC

84GZO	Monitor, Response, Skin, Galvanic	Cns/Neurology
89IPF	Stimulator, Muscle, Electrical-Powered (EMS)	Physical Med

GAMETE

85VIK	Equipment, In Vitro Fertilization/Embryo Transfer	Obstetrics/Gyn

GAMMA

82KTS	2nd Antibody (Species Specific Anti-Animal Gamma Globulin)	Immunology
82DAH	Antigen, Antiserum, Control, Gamma Globulin	Immunology
82DAF	Antigen, Antiserum, Control, Gamma Globulin, FITC	Immunology
82DFZ	Antigen, Antiserum, Control, IGG (Gamma Chain Specific)	Immunology
90IYX	Camera, Gamma (Nuclear/Scintillation)	Radiology
75JPZ	Colorimetric Method, Gamma-Glutamyl Transpeptidase	Chemistry
91DNR	Counter, Gamma, General Use	Toxicology
91DNM	Counter, Gamma, Radioimmunoassay (Manual)	Toxicology
75JJJ	Detector, Beta/Gamma	Chemistry
75JQA	Electrophoretic, Gamma-Glutamyl Transpeptidase Isoenzymes	Chemistry
75MGW	Enzyme Immunoassay, Gamma Enolase	Chemistry
75JQB	Kinetic Method, Gamma-Glutamyl Transpeptidase	Chemistry
90RYJ	Synchronizer, Nuclear Camera	Radiology
90RYK	Synchronizer, Radiographic Unit	Radiology
90JAD	Therapeutic X-Ray System	Radiology

GAMMA-GLUTAMYL

75JPZ	Colorimetric Method, Gamma-Glutamyl Transpeptidase	Chemistry
75JQA	Electrophoretic, Gamma-Glutamyl Transpeptidase Isoenzymes	Chemistry
75JQB	Kinetic Method, Gamma-Glutamyl Transpeptidase	Chemistry

GANTRY

90IYX	Camera, Gamma (Nuclear/Scintillation)	Radiology
90QMD	Computer, Nuclear Medicine	Radiology
90VCO	Gantry, Nuclear Imaging	Radiology
90THG	Scanner, Nuclear Emission Computed Tomography (ECT)	Radiology

GANTRY *(cont'd)*

90ULI	Scanner, Positron Emission Tomography (PET)	Radiology

GARBAGE

80VAU	Bag, Garbage	General

GARDNERELLA

83MJM	DNA-Probe, Gardnerella Vaginalis	Microbiology

GARMENT

80QDJ	Bib	General
80WKY	Garment, Electrode	General
78EYQ	Garment, Protective, For Incontinence	Gastro/Urology
80RTW	Slippers	General

GARREN-EDWARDS

78WNS	Balloon, Gastric	Gastro/Urology

GAS

75JQR	Accessories, Chromatography (Gas, Gel, Liquid, Thin Layer)	Chemistry
79HLD	Accessories, Engine, Trephine, Gas-Powered	Surgery
73TAC	Alarm, Central Gas System	Anesthesiology
73TAK	Analyzer, Blood Gas pH	Anesthesiology
73QZE	Analyzer, Gas, Anesthetic	Anesthesiology
73VCA	Analyzer, Gas, Argon	Anesthesiology
73JEG	Analyzer, Gas, Argon, Gaseous Phase	Anesthesiology
73CCC	Analyzer, Gas, Carbon-Dioxide, Blood Phase, Indwelling	Anesthesiology
73CCK	Analyzer, Gas, Carbon-Dioxide, Gaseous Phase (Capnograph)	Anesthesiology
73BXZ	Analyzer, Gas, Carbon-Dioxide, Partial Pressure, Blood	Anesthesiology
73CCJ	Analyzer, Gas, Carbon-Monoxide, Gaseous Phase	Anesthesiology
73VCB	Analyzer, Gas, Carbon-Monoxide, Non-Indwelling Blood Phase	Anesthesiology
91CCA	Analyzer, Gas, Carboxyhemoglobin, Blood Phase, Non-Indw.	Toxicology
73CBQ	Analyzer, Gas, Enflurane, Gaseous Phase (Anesthetic Conc.)	Anesthesiology
73CBS	Analyzer, Gas, Halothane, Gaseous Phase (Anesthetic Conc.)	Anesthesiology
73BSE	Analyzer, Gas, Helium, Gaseous Phase	Anesthesiology
73LXO	Analyzer, Gas, Hydrogen	Anesthesiology
73VCF	Analyzer, Gas, Neon	Anesthesiology
73JEF	Analyzer, Gas, Neon, Gaseous Phase	Anesthesiology
73CCI	Analyzer, Gas, Nitrogen, Gaseous Phase	Anesthesiology
73BSD	Analyzer, Gas, Nitrogen, Partial Pressure, Blood Phase (NI)	Anesthesiology
73CBR	Analyzer, Gas, Nitrous-Oxide, Gaseous Phase	Anesthesiology
73RJI	Analyzer, Gas, Oxygen, Continuous Controller	Anesthesiology
73RJJ	Analyzer, Gas, Oxygen, Continuous Monitor	Anesthesiology
73CCL	Analyzer, Gas, Oxygen, Gaseous Phase	Anesthesiology
73CCE	Analyzer, Gas, Oxygen, Partial Pr., Blood Phase, Indwelling	Anesthesiology
73CCD	Analyzer, Gas, Oxygen, Partial Pressure, Blood Phase	Anesthesiology
73RJK	Analyzer, Gas, Oxygen, Sampling	Anesthesiology
73BXA	Analyzer, Gas, Water Vapor, Gaseous Phase	Anesthesiology
79WTZ	Analyzer, Patient, Multiple Function (Surgery)	Surgery
73WSV	Analyzer, Trace Gas, Breath	Anesthesiology
80FLI	Cabinet, Aerator, Ethylene-Oxide Gas	General
80WMK	Calibrator, Blood Gas	General
73BXX	Calibrator, Gas, Pressure	Anesthesiology
73BXW	Calibrator, Gas, Volume	Anesthesiology
73QXW	Cart, Gas Cylinder (Carrier)	Anesthesiology
91KZQ	Chromatography (Gas), Clinical Use	Toxicology
75QJY	Chromatography Equipment, Gas	Chemistry
75JLR	Chromatography, Gas, Pregnanetriol	Chemistry
91DII	Column, GLC	Toxicology
80UMS	Column, Life Support (Electrical/Gas)	General
75JJS	Control, Blood Gas	Chemistry
74DTX	Controller, Gas, Cardiopulmonary Bypass	Cardiovascular
79QUA	Cylinder, Carbon-Dioxide	Surgery
73ECX	Cylinder, Compressed Gas, With Valve	Anesthesiology
73KGA	Cylinder, Gas (Empty)	Anesthesiology
73VFF	Cylinder, Oxygen	Anesthesiology
78FAP	Cystometric Gas (Carbon-Dioxide) Or Hydraulic Device	Gastro/Urology
80WPI	Detector, Leakage, Medical Gas	General
73QSO	Electrode, Blood Gas, Carbon-Dioxide	Anesthesiology
73QSP	Electrode, Blood Gas, Oxygen	Anesthesiology
80WRQ	Equipment, Building Security	General
80WLA	Equipment, Control, Pollution	General
80WYN	Equipment, Filtering, Air, ETO	General
73QVX	Filter, Gas	Anesthesiology
73QWF	Filter, Ventilator	Anesthesiology
75UIY	Fitting, Gas Chromatography Tube	Chemistry
80QWL	Fitting, Quick Connect (Gas Connector)	General
73BXY	Flowmeter, Gas (Oxygen), Calibrated	Anesthesiology
73CCN	Flowmeter, Gas, Non-Back-Pressure Compensated, Bourdon Gauge	Anesthesiology
91DLS	Gas Chromatograph, Alcohol (Dedicated Instruments)	Toxicology
91JKT	Gas Chromatograph, Carbon-Monoxide	Toxicology

GASTROENTEROLOGIC
78LNN Unit, Anastomosis, Gastroenterologic — Gastro/Urology

GASTROENTEROLOGY
78LNT Adhesive, Tissue, Gastroenterology/Urology — Gastro/Urology
78FAR Electrosurgical Unit, Gastroenterology — Gastro/Urology
78KNS Electrosurgical, Unit, Gastroenterology — Gastro/Urology
78LNK Laser, Gastroenterology/Urology — Gastro/Urology

GASTROESOPHAGEAL
78FDT Duodenoscope, Esophago/Gastro — Gastro/Urology
78LEI Implant, Anti-Gastroesophageal Reflux — Gastro/Urology
78UDE Prosthesis, Anti-Gastroesophageal Reflux — Gastro/Urology

GASTROINTESTINAL
78FFX Analyzer, Motility, Gastrointestinal, Electrical — Gastro/Urology
78FCF Biopsy Instrument, Mechanical, Gastrointestinal — Gastro/Urology
78FAT Bougie, Esophageal, And Gastrointestinal, Gastro-Urology — Gastro/Urology
78FFW Locator, Bleeding, Gastrointestinal, String And Tube — Gastro/Urology
78FGM Probe, Gastrointestinal — Gastro/Urology
78KNT Tube, Gastrointestinal — Gastro/Urology
78VHP Tube, Gastrointestinal Decompression, Baker Jejunostomy — Gastro/Urology
78SDB Tube, Gastrointestinal Decompression, Cantor — Gastro/Urology
78SDC Tube, Gastrointestinal Decompression, Dennis — Gastro/Urology
78SDD Tube, Gastrointestinal Decompression, Miller-Abbott — Gastro/Urology
78SCY Tube, Gastrointestinal, Kaslow — Gastro/Urology
78SCZ Tube, Gastrointestinal, Rehfuss — Gastro/Urology
78SDA Tube, Gastrointestinal, Wangensteen — Gastro/Urology

GASTROPLASTY
78LNO Device, Gastroplasty — Gastro/Urology

GASTROSCOPE
78QYC Gastroscope, Flexible — Gastro/Urology
78FDS Gastroscope, Gastro-Urology — Gastro/Urology
78GCK Gastroscope, General & Plastic Surgery — Gastro/Urology
78QYD Gastroscope, Rigid — Gastro/Urology

GASTROSTOMY
78FEW Catheter, Malecot (Gastrostomy Tube) — Gastro/Urology
78SJD Kit, Gastrostomy, Endoscopic, Percutaneous — Gastro/Urology

GAUGE
73CCN Flowmeter, Gas, Non-Back-Pressure Compensated, Bourdon Gauge — Anesthesiology
87HTJ Gauge, Depth — Orthopedics
76EIL Gauge, Depth, Instrument, Dental — Dental And Oral
73BXH Gauge, Gas Pressure, Cylinder/Pipeline — Anesthesiology
86HLN Gauge, Lens, Ophthalmic — Ophthalmology
77JYI Gauge, Mastoid — Ear/Nose/Throat
77JYJ Gauge, Measuring — Ear/Nose/Throat
80WVV Gauge, Pressure — General
74DXS Gauge, Pressure, Coronary, Cardiopulmonary Bypass — Cardiovascular
80RWN Gauge, Strain — General
79QQR Gauge, Thickness, Tissue — Surgery
86HJB Measurer, Corneal Radius — Ophthalmology
86HLF Measurer, Lens Radius, Ophthalmic — Ophthalmology
86HLM Measurer, Lens, AC-Powered — Ophthalmology
86HLC Measurer, Stereopsis — Ophthalmology
73CAP Monitor, Airway Pressure (Gauge/Alarm) — Anesthesiology
73RJV Pain Gauge, Transcutaneous — Anesthesiology
80CBB Regulator, Suction, Surgical — General

GAUSS
80WWL Gaussmeter — General
80RFP Magnetometer — General

GAUSSMETER
80WWL Gaussmeter — General

GAUZE
80QCI Bandage, Gauze — General
80QLX Compress, Gauze — General
80FRO Dressing, Other — General
80QQZ Dressing, Roller Gauze — General
79QYE Gauze Roll — Surgery
79GEM Gauze, Absorbable — Surgery
79GEL Gauze, Non-Absorbable, Medicated (Internal Sponge) — Surgery
79GEK Gauze, Non-Absorbable, Non-Medicated (Internal Sponge) — Surgery
79GDY Gauze, Non-Absorbable, X-Ray Detectable (Internal Sponge) — Surgery
79NAB Gauze/sponge, Nonresorbable For External Use — Surgery
79FTM Mesh, Surgical (Steel Gauze) — Surgery
80MXI Nonabsorbable Gauze, Surgical Sponge, & Wound Dressing for External Use (with a Drug) — General
80RJU Packer, Gauze — General
79RXO Packing, Surgical — Surgery
80RRB Scissors, Bandage/Gauze/Plaster — General
76EFQ Sponge, Gauze — Dental And Oral
80WMH Tape, Gauze, Adhesive — General

GAVAGE
78FHT Kit, Gavage, Infant, Sterile — Gastro/Urology

GEAR
76EFA Handpiece, Belt and/or Gear Driven, Dental — Dental And Oral

GEIGER
90RNU Counter, Radiation — Radiology

GEL
75JQR Accessories, Chromatography (Gas, Gel, Liquid, Thin Layer) — Chemistry
91KZR Chromatography (Liquid, Gel), Clinical Use — Toxicology
91KZT Disc, Diffusion, Gel, Agar, Serum Level, Gentamicin — Toxicology
91KZW Disc, Diffusion, Gel, Agar, Serum Level, Kanamycin — Toxicology
91KZX Disc, Diffusion, Gel, Agar, Serum Level, Tobramycin — Toxicology
80WKJ Dressing, Gel — General
80WKL Dressing, Permeable, Moisture — General
74WOV Electrode, Gel — Cardiovascular
75UGG Electrophoresis Equipment, Gel — Chemistry
74DYA Gel, Electrode, Electrocardiograph — Cardiovascular
79JOT Gel, Electrode, Electrosurgical — Surgery
76EAS Gel, Electrode, Pulp Tester — Dental And Oral
84GYB Gel, Electrode, Stimulator — Cns/Neurology
89IKC Gel, Electrode, TENS — Physical Med
75UGB Gel, Filter — Chemistry
82JZR Gel, Support — Immunology
89QYF Gel, Ultrasonic Coupling — Physical Med
80SDY Gel, Ultrasonic Transmission — General
78FHX Jelly, Lubricating, Transurethral Surgical Instrument — Gastro/Urology
83JTP Kit, Disc Agar Gel Diffusion, Serum Level — Microbiology
80WXR Media, Filter — General
80RMD Pad, Pressure, Gel — General
80WMD Pad, Pressure, Gel, Operating Table — General
80WKI Padding, Cast/Splint — General
91DKS Plate, Silica Gel, TLC — Toxicology
83TDG Separation Media — Microbiology
91DLO Silica Gel Fluorescent Indicator, TLC — Toxicology
80WLV Warmer, Gel — General

GELATIN
83JSK Culture Media, Supplements — Microbiology
88IEX Gelatin — Pathology
88IFZ Gelatin For Specimen Adhesion — Pathology
88IFY Gelatin/Formalin — Pathology
77ESI Polymer, Natural Absorbable Gelatin Material — Ear/Nose/Throat
77LBP Prosthesis, Ossicular (Stapes), Absorbable Gelatin Material — Ear/Nose/Throat
77LBO Prosthesis, Ossicular (Total), Absorbable Gelatin Material — Ear/Nose/Throat

GELFOAM
77JXZ Punch, Gelfoam — Ear/Nose/Throat

GENE
88LNJ Analyzer, Chromosome, Automated — Pathology
88JCZ Analyzer, Karyotype — Pathology
83UGH Genetic Engineering — Microbiology
83WPR Micro-Injector, Transplant, Gene — Microbiology
75WJI Synthesizer, DNA — Chemistry
85VIL Test, Chorionic Villi Sampling (Fetal Chromosome Analysis) — Obstetrics/Gyn
83WNY Test, DNA-Probe, Other — Microbiology

GENERAL
84KGG Adhesive, Tissue, General Neurosurgery — Cns/Neurology
75DOI Balance (General Use) — Chemistry
79GFA Blade, Surgical, Saw, General & Plastic Surgery — Surgery
79GEE Brush, Biopsy, General & Plastic Surgery — Surgery
79GFF Burr, Surgical, General & Plastic Surgery — Surgery
80TBA Cabinet Casework, General Purpose — General
79GEA Cannula, Surgical, General & Plastic Surgery — Surgery
79GCA Catheter, Biliary, General & Plastic Surgery — Surgery
79GBY Catheter, Eustachian, General & Plastic Surgery — Surgery
79GBO Catheter, Nephrostomy, General & Plastic Surgery — Surgery
79GBN Catheter, Pediatric, General & Plastic Surgery — Surgery
79GBL Catheter, Ureteral, General & Plastic Surgery — Surgery
79GBS Catheter, Ventricular, General & Plastic Surgery — Surgery
91DOT Centrifuge, General (Over 5,000 rpm) — Toxicology
88KDR Centrifuge, General (Up to 5,000 rpm) — Pathology
79GDJ Clamp, Surgical, General & Plastic Surgery — Surgery
79FTJ Colonoscope, General & Plastic Surgery — Surgery
75JJQ Colorimeter, General Use — Chemistry
91DNR Counter, Gamma, General Use — Toxicology
83JSC Culture Media, General Nutrient Broth — Microbiology
79GDI Dissector, Surgical, General & Plastic Surgery — Surgery
79UCP Electrosurgical Equipment, General Purpose — Surgery
79QTV Electrosurgical Unit, General Purpose (ESU) — Surgery
79GEG Elevator, Surgical, General & Plastic Surgery — Surgery
75LXG Equipment, Laboratory, Gen. Purpose (Specific Medical Use) — Chemistry
78GCL Esophagoscope, General & Plastic Surgery — Gastro/Urology
79GEO File, Surgical, General & Plastic Surgery — Surgery

GENERAL *(cont'd)*

79GEN	Forceps, General & Plastic Surgery	Surgery
75JRM	Freezer, Laboratory, General Purpose	Chemistry
80VBP	Furniture, General	General
78GCK	Gastroscope, General & Plastic Surgery	Gastro/Urology
88KQD	General Hematology Reagent	Pathology
80LDQ	General Medical Device	General
81LOQ	General Purpose Hematology Device	Hematology
83LIB	General Purpose Microbiology Diagnostic Device	Microbiology
79LRW	General Use Surgical Scissors	Surgery
79GDH	Gouge, Surgical, General & Plastic Surgery	Surgery
79GDG	Hook, Surgical, General & Plastic Surgery	Surgery
79MDM	Instrument, Manual, General Surgical	Surgery
79LRO	Kit, Surgical (General)	Surgery
79GCJ	Laparoscope, General & Plastic Surgery	Surgery
79GFJ	Mallet, Surgical, General & Plastic Surgery	Surgery
91DNB	Meter, pH, General Use	Toxicology
79FSO	Microscope, Surgical, General & Plastic Surgery	Surgery
79FTX	Mirror, General & Plastic Surgery	Surgery
91DMW	Photometer, Flame, General Use	Toxicology
80LKK	Pump, Infusion, Implantable, General	General
79GAC	Rasp, Surgical, General & Plastic Surgery	Surgery
88LDT	Reagent, General Purpose	Pathology
88UJH	Reagent, Virus, General	Pathology
90TEJ	Scanner, Ultrasonic, General Purpose	Radiology
80RRI	Scissors, General Dissecting	General
91UHZ	Serum, Biological, General	Toxicology
79GAF	Spatula, Surgical, General & Plastic Surgery	Surgery
91JXR	Spectrophotometer, Atomic Absorption, General Use	Toxicology
88UIG	Stain, Biological, General	Pathology
79FXB	Stimulator, Muscle, General & Plastic Surgery	Surgery
79MDW	Surgical Instrument, Manual (General Use)	Surgery
85KOH	Surgical Instrument, Obstetric/Gynecologic, General	Obstetrics/Gyn
81JBS	Timer, General Laboratory	Hematology
80UKO	Waste Receptacle, General Purpose	General

GENERATION

81GKQ	Test, Thromboplastin Generation	Hematology

GENERATOR

74DTC	Analyzer, Pacemaker Generator Function	Cardiovascular
74KRE	Analyzer, Pacemaker Generator Function, Indirect	Cardiovascular
74LWY	Dual Chamber, Anti-Tachycardia, Pulse Generator	Cardiovascular
74LWP	Dual Chamber, Implantable Pulse Generator	Cardiovascular
77QAH	Generator, Aerosol	Ear/Nose/Throat
90VHL	Generator, Diagnostic X-Ray, High Voltage, 3-Phase	Radiology
90IZO	Generator, Diagnostic X-Ray, High Voltage, Single Phase	Radiology
82MEM	Generator, Electric Field (Aids Treatment)	Immunology
77ETS	Generator, Electronic Noise (For Audiometric Testing)	Ear/Nose/Throat
83KZJ	Generator, Gas, Microbiology	Microbiology
90KPZ	Generator, High Voltage, X-Ray, Therapeutic	Radiology
73RCO	Generator, Ionized Air	Anesthesiology
90IWL	Generator, Neutron, Medical	Radiology
73RJN	Generator, Oxygen	Anesthesiology
73CAW	Generator, Oxygen, Portable	Anesthesiology
73RJR	Generator, Ozone	Anesthesiology
79SHL	Generator, Power, Electrosurgical	Surgery
74JOR	Generator, Pulsatile Flow, Cardiopulmonary Bypass	Cardiovascular
84GXD	Generator, Radiofrequency Lesion	Cns/Neurology
90IZR	Generator, Radiographic, Capacitor Discharge	Radiology
90IYR	Generator, Radionuclide	Radiology
90IYH	Generator, Therapeutic X-Ray, Dermatological (Grenz Ray)	Radiology
90IYF	Generator, Therapeutic X-Ray, High Voltage	Radiology
90IYD	Generator, Therapeutic X-Ray, Low Voltage	Radiology
90IYC	Generator, Therapeutic X-Ray, Orthovoltage	Radiology
74LOT	Module, Program, Generator, Pulse	Cardiovascular
74WST	Pacemaker, Heart, Implantable, Rate Responsive	Cardiovascular
80WMN	Power Systems, Uninterruptible (UPS)	General
74LWW	Single Chamber, Anti-Tachycardia, Pulse Generator	Cardiovascular
74LWO	Single Chamber, Sensor Driven, Implantable Pulse Generator	Cardiovascular
89IPF	Stimulator, Muscle, Electrical-Powered (EMS)	Physical Med

GENETIC

88LNJ	Analyzer, Chromosome, Automated	Pathology
88JCZ	Analyzer, Karyotype	Pathology
83UGH	Genetic Engineering	Microbiology
83WPR	Micro-Injector, Transplant, Gene	Microbiology
85VIL	Test, Chorionic Villi Sampling (Fetal Chromosome Analysis)	Obstetrics/Gyn
83WNY	Test, DNA-Probe, Other	Microbiology

GENITAL

85KXQ	Vibrator, Genital	Obstetrics/Gyn

GENOTYPIC

83MYI	System, Test, Genotypic Detection, Resistant Markers, Staphylococcus Colonies	Microbiology

GENTAMICIN

91DJI	Antiserum, Gentamicin	Toxicology
91DKD	Bacillus Subtilis, Microbiological Assay, Gentamicin	Toxicology
91KZT	Disc, Diffusion, Gel, Agar, Serum Level, Gentamicin	Toxicology
91KLO	Enzymatic Radiochemical Assay, Gentamicin	Toxicology
91LCD	Enzyme Immunoassay, Gentamicin	Toxicology
91LCQ	Fluorescent Immunoassay Gentamicin	Toxicology
91LCB	Fluoroimmunoassay, Gentamicin	Toxicology
91DNO	Hemagglutination Inhibition, Gentamicin	Toxicology
91DJB	Radioimmunoassay, Gentamicin (125-I), Second Antibody	Toxicology

GERIATRIC

80FRJ	Chair, Geriatric	General
80FRM	Chair, Geriatric, Wheeled	General
80QNV	Cup, Geriatric Feeding	General
89ILC	Utensil, Food	Physical Med

GERM

83UGI	Germ-Free Apparatus	Microbiology

GERM-FREE

83UGI	Germ-Free Apparatus	Microbiology

GERMAN-MEASLES

83GON	Antigen, CF (Including CF Control), Rubella	Microbiology
83GOL	Antigen, HA (Including HA Control), Rubella	Microbiology
83GOJ	Antisera, Neutralization, Rubella	Microbiology
83GOM	Antiserum, CF, Rubella	Microbiology
83GOK	Antiserum, HAI (Including HAI Control), Rubella	Microbiology
83LQN	Assay, Agglutination, Latex, Rubella	Microbiology
83LFX	Enzyme Linked Immunoabsorbent Assay, Rubella	Microbiology

GERMICIDAL

80MKB	Device, Germicidal, Ultraviolet	General
80QQW	Dressing, Germicidal	General
80RED	Lamp, Ultraviolet, Germicidal	General
80RVF	Sponge, Germicidal (Alcohol)	General

GGTP

75CGG	L-Glutamylnitroanilide/Glycylglycine, Ggtp	Chemistry

GIARDIA

83MHI	Giardia Spp.	Microbiology

GIEMSA

88HYF	Stain, Giemsa	Pathology
81GLP	Stain, Giemsa, Hematology	Hematology

GIGLI

87QZB	Guide, Gigli Saw	Orthopedics

GINGIVAL

76QER	Brush, Gum (Gingival)	Dental And Oral
76QLQ	Collar, Gingival	Dental And Oral
76VEG	Kit, Gingival Retraction	Dental And Oral
76JEO	Measurer, Gingival Fluid	Dental And Oral

GLAND

78QHO	Catheter, Bartholin Gland	Gastro/Urology
76LTF	Stimulator, Salivary System	Dental And Oral

GLARE

86WOO	Tester, Brightness Acuity	Ophthalmology

GLASS

80WOF	Breaker, Ampule	General
78FCS	Catheter, Light, Fiberoptic, Glass, Ureteral	Gastro/Urology
80VFE	Component, Ceramic	General
88KES	Coverslip, Microscope Slide	Pathology
76ECC	Sterilizer, Glass Bead	Dental And Oral

GLAUCOMA

86WVM	System, Delivery, Drug, Ocular	Ophthalmology
86WXL	System, Hyperthermia, Ultrasonic, Ophthalmic	Ophthalmology
86HPK	Tonograph	Ophthalmology
86HKX	Tonometer, AC-Powered	Ophthalmology
86HKY	Tonometer, Manual	Ophthalmology

GLC

91DII	Column, GLC	Toxicology
91DMS	Gas, GLC	Toxicology
91DLG	Liquid Coating, GLC	Toxicology
91JXQ	Monitor, U.V., GLC	Toxicology
91DJA	Support, Column, GLC	Toxicology

GLENNER'S

88HYG	Stain, Glenner's	Pathology

GLENOID

76MPI	Prosthesis, Glenoid Fossa	Dental And Oral
87KYM	Prosthesis, Shoulder, Hemi-, Glenoid, Metal	Orthopedics

GLIADIN

82MST	Antibodies, Gliadin	Immunology

GLOBE

86UAX	Cap, Ophthalmic, Quarter Globe	Ophthalmology

GLOBULIN

82KTS	2nd Antibody (Species Specific Anti-Animal Gamma Globulin)	Immunology
83GMS	Anti-Human Globulin, FTA-ABS Test (Coombs)	Microbiology
82DCO	Antigen, Antiserum, Control, Alpha Globulin	Immunology
82DCJ	Antigen, Antiserum, Control, Beta Globulin	Immunology
82DAH	Antigen, Antiserum, Control, Gamma Globulin	Immunology
82DAF	Antigen, Antiserum, Control, Gamma Globulin, FITC	Immunology
75CGH	Electrophoretic, Globulin	Chemistry
75JGD	Nephelometric Method, Globulin	Chemistry
75CEE	Radioimmunoassay, Thyroxine Binding Globulin	Chemistry
75JGE	Reagent, Globulin (Test System)	Chemistry
75JGC	Tryptophan Measurement (Colorimetric), Globulin	Chemistry

GLOBULINS

83GSY	Antisera, Fluorescent, All Globulins, Proteus SPP.	Microbiology
83GOO	Antiserum, Fluorescent, All Globulins, Salmonella SPP.	Microbiology
83GTD	Antiserum, Fluorescent, Shigella SPP., All Globulins	Microbiology

GLOMERULAR

82MVJ	Devices, Measure, Antibodies to Glomerular Basement Membrane (gbm)	Immunology

GLOSSOPHARYNGEAL

73QAX	Kit, Anesthesia, Glossopharyngeal	Anesthesiology

GLOTTOGRAPH

77KLY	Photo-Electric Glottograph	Ear/Nose/Throat

GLOVE

83JTM	Box, Glove	Microbiology
79KGQ	Cream, Surgical Gloving	Surgery
80WJO	Dispenser, Other	General
80QYG	Glove Processing Unit (Drying, Powdering)	General
88QYH	Glove, Autopsy	Pathology
80QYK	Glove, Other	General
80FMC	Glove, Patient Examination	General
80LYY	Glove, Patient Examination, Latex	General
80LZA	Glove, Patient Examination, Poly	General
80LZC	Glove, Patient Examination, Specialty	General
80LYZ	Glove, Patient Examination, Vinyl	General
90IWP	Glove, Protective, Radiographic	Radiology
80FPI	Glove, Surgical	General
80QYI	Glove, Surgical, Hypoallergenic	General
79KGO	Glove, Surgical, Plastic Surgery	Surgery
79WWN	Glove, Surgical, Powder-Free	Surgery
80QYJ	Glove, Utility	General
80WYZ	Liner, Glove	General
79FSN	Rack, Glove, Operating Room	Surgery
80SAE	Tester, Surgical Glove	General

GLOVING

79KGQ	Cream, Surgical Gloving	Surgery

GLUCAGON

75JME	Radioimmunoassay, Glucagon	Chemistry

GLUCOSE

75QYL	Analyzer, Glucose	Chemistry
80LHE	Controller, Glucose, Blood, Closed-Loop	General
75CFW	Copper Reduction, Glucose	Chemistry
75MRV	Drink, Glucose Tolerance	Chemistry
81JLM	Electrophoretic, Glucose-6-Phosphate Dehydrogenase	Hematology
75JIL	Enzymatic Method, Glucose (Urinary, Non-Quantitative)	Chemistry
75CGD	Ferricyanide, Glucose	Chemistry
75LFR	Glucose Dehydrogenase, Glucose	Chemistry
81JBJ	Glucose-6-Phos. Dehydrogenase (Erythrocy.), Methemogl. Red.	Hematology
81JBH	Glucose-6-Phos. Dehydrogenase (Erythrocytic), Micromethod	Hematology
81JBL	Glucose-6-Phos. Dehydrogenase (Erythrocytic), Quantitative	Hematology
81JBK	Glucose-6-Phos. Dehydrogenase (Erythrocytic), U.V. Kinetic	Hematology
75JNE	Glucose-6-Phosphate (Colorimetric), Phosphohexose Isomerase	Chemistry
81JBI	Glucose-6-Phosphate Dehydrogenase (Erythrocytic), Catalase	Hematology
81JBM	Glucose-6-Phosphate Dehydrogenase (Erythrocytic), Electro	Hematology
81JBF	Glucose-6-Phosphate Dehydrogenase (Erythrocytic), Screening	Hematology
81JBG	Glucose-6-Phosphate Dehydrogenase (Erythrocytic), Spot	Hematology
75CFR	Hexokinase, Glucose	Chemistry
83JSW	Kit, Identification, Glucose (Non-Ferment)	Microbiology
75JIM	Metallic Reduction Method, Glucose (Urinary, Non-Quant.)	Chemistry
78TGM	Monitor, Blood Glucose (Test)	Gastro/Urology

GLUCOSE (cont'd)

75WXU	Monitor, Glucose, Blood, Non-Invasive	Chemistry
81JMC	NADP Reduction (U.V.), Glucose-6-Phosphate Dehydrogenase	Hematology
75CGE	Orthotoluidine, Glucose	Chemistry
75CGA	Reagent, Glucose (Test System)	Chemistry
80MDS	Sensor, Glucose, Invasive	General
75WTX	Strip, Test	Chemistry
75NBW	System, Test, Blood Glucose, Over-The-Counter	Chemistry
81KQE	Test, Erythrocytic Glucose-6-Phosphate Dehydrogenase	Hematology
75JLJ	UDP-Glucose, NAD (U.V.), Gal-I-P Uridyl Transperase	Chemistry
81JMB	Visual, Semi-Quant. (Colorimetric), Glucose-6-Phosphate	Hematology

GLUCOSE-6-PHOSPHATE

81JLM	Electrophoretic, Glucose-6-Phosphate Dehydrogenase	Hematology
81JBJ	Glucose-6-Phos. Dehydrogenase (Erythrocy.), Methemogl. Red.	Hematology
81JBH	Glucose-6-Phos. Dehydrogenase (Erythrocytic), Micromethod	Hematology
81JBL	Glucose-6-Phos. Dehydrogenase (Erythrocytic), Quantitative	Hematology
81JBK	Glucose-6-Phos. Dehydrogenase (Erythrocytic), U.V. Kinetic	Hematology
75JNE	Glucose-6-Phosphate (Colorimetric), Phosphohexose Isomerase	Chemistry
81JBI	Glucose-6-Phosphate Dehydrogenase (Erythrocytic), Catalase	Hematology
81JBM	Glucose-6-Phosphate Dehydrogenase (Erythrocytic), Electro	Hematology
81JBF	Glucose-6-Phosphate Dehydrogenase (Erythrocytic), Screening	Hematology
81JBG	Glucose-6-Phosphate Dehydrogenase (Erythrocytic), Spot	Hematology
81JMC	NADP Reduction (U.V.), Glucose-6-Phosphate Dehydrogenase	Hematology
81KQE	Test, Erythrocytic Glucose-6-Phosphate Dehydrogenase	Hematology
81JMB	Visual, Semi-Quant. (Colorimetric), Glucose-6-Phosphate	Hematology

GLUE

80QAG	Adhesive, Liquid	General
87QIW	Cement, Orthopedic (Bone)	Orthopedics
79MFI	Glue, Surgical Tissue	Surgery

GLUTAMIC

75CDQ	Urease And Glutamic Dehydrogenase, Urea Nitrogen	Chemistry

GLUTAMYL

75JPZ	Colorimetric Method, Gamma-Glutamyl Transpeptidase	Chemistry
75JQA	Electrophoretic, Gamma-Glutamyl Transpeptidase Isoenzymes	Chemistry
75JQB	Kinetic Method, Gamma-Glutamyl Transpeptidase	Chemistry

GLUTAMYLNITROANILIDE

75CGG	L-Glutamylnitroanilide/Glycylglycine, Ggtp	Chemistry

GLUTARALDEHYDE

88IFT	Glutaraldehyde (Fixative)	Pathology
80QDR	Monitor, Biological (Contamination Testing)	General
80WIP	Monitor, Contamination, Environmental, Personal	General

GLUTATHIONE

75JLN	Chromatographic, Glutathione	Chemistry
75JLO	Enzymatic (Glutathione Reductase), Glutathione	Chemistry
81GII	Glutathione, Red Cell	Hematology
81KQF	Test, Glutathione Reductase	Hematology

GLYCERALDE

75JNY	Glyceralde-3-Phosphate, NADH (Enzymatic), Triose Phosphate	Chemistry

GLYCERALDE-3-PHOSPHATE

75JNY	Glyceralde-3-Phosphate, NADH (Enzymatic), Triose Phosphate	Chemistry

GLYCERINE

80VLI	Swabs, Oral Care	General

GLYCEROL

75CDT	Lipase Hydrolysis/Glycerol Kinase Enzyme, Triglycerides	Chemistry

GLYCEROPHOSPHATE

75CJL	Beta Glycerophosphate, Alkaline Phosphatase Or Isoenzymes	Chemistry
75CKH	Glycerophosphate, Beta, Phosphatase, Acid	Chemistry

GLYCOL

88IFJ	Fixative, Richardson Glycol	Pathology
88IER	Polyethylene Glycol (Carbowax)	Pathology
88IFL	Preservative, Polyethylene Glycol	Pathology
91DOG	Radioimmunoassay, Digoxin (125-I), Rabbit, Poly. Glycol	Toxicology

GLYCOPROTEIN

82DBC	Alpha 2, 2N-Glycoprotein, Antigen, Antiserum, Control	Immunology

KEYWORD INDEX

HANDLE (cont'd)

79RDE	Handle, Knife Blade	Surgery
79QWG	Handle, Knife, Laparoscopic	Surgery
79GDZ	Handle, Scalpel	Surgery
79QWI	Knife, Laparoscopic	Surgery

HANDLING

79FZI	Air Handling Apparatus, Enclosure	Surgery
79FZH	Air Handling Apparatus, Room	Surgery
79FZG	Air Handling, Apparatus, Bench	Surgery
90UFC	Handling Unit, Automatic Daylight X-Ray Film	Radiology

HANDPIECE

76EBW	Controller, Foot, Handpiece And Cord	Dental And Oral
84HBD	Handpiece (Brace), Drill	Cns/Neurology
76EFB	Handpiece, Air-Powered, Dental	Dental And Oral
76EFA	Handpiece, Belt and/or Gear Driven, Dental	Dental And Oral
76EGS	Handpiece, Contra- And Right-Angle Attachment, Dental	Dental And Oral
76EKX	Handpiece, Direct Drive, AC-Powered	Dental And Oral
76THM	Handpiece, Fiberoptic	Dental And Oral
76KMW	Handpiece, Rotary Bone Cutting	Dental And Oral
76EKY	Handpiece, Water-Powered	Dental And Oral

HANDRIM

89IMO	Handrim, Wheelchair	Physical Med

HANGER

80WVU	Cabinet, Storage, Catheter	General
80RCM	Hanger, Intravenous	General
78SEG	Hanger, Urologic	Gastro/Urology
90VHK	Hanger, X-Ray Tube	Radiology
80FOX	Infusion Stand	General

HAPLOSCOPE

86HJT	Haploscope	Ophthalmology

HAPTOGLOBIN

82DAD	Antigen, Antiserum, Control, Haptoglobin	Immunology
82DAB	Antigen, Antiserum, Control, Haptoglobin, FITC	Immunology
82CZZ	Antigen, Antiserum, Control, Haptoglobin, Rhodamine	Immunology

HARD

87MBJ	Fastener, Fixation, Biodegradable, Hard Tissue	Orthopedics

HARRIS'S

88HYK	Stain, Hematoxylin, Harris's	Pathology

HARVESTER

83UFS	Harvester, Cell	Microbiology

HARVESTING

74MFY	Kit, Cell Harvesting, Endothelial	Cardiovascular

HAZARD

80REQ	Meter, Leakage Current (Ammeter)	General
74DRI	Monitor, Line Isolation	Cardiovascular

HAZARDOUS

80WUN	Service, Waste Management	General

HBD

75JKF	Dinitrophenyl Hydrazone Measurement (Colorimetric), HBD	Chemistry

HCG

75JHJ	Agglutination Method, Human Chorionic Gonadotropin	Chemistry
75LCX	Kit, Pregnancy Test, Over The Counter, HCG	Chemistry
75JHI	Radioimmunoassay, Human Chorionic Gonadotropin	Chemistry
82JZN	Test, Human Chorionic Gonadotropin	Immunology
82DHA	Test, Human Chorionic Gonadotropin, Serum	Immunology

HDL

75LBT	Electrophoresis, Cholesterol Via Esterase-Oxidase, HDL	Chemistry
75KMZ	HDL Via LDL & VLDL Precipitation, Lipoproteins	Chemistry
75LBR	LDL & VLDL Precipitation, HDL	Chemistry
75NAQ	Lipoprotein, High Density, HDL, Over-The-Counter	Chemistry

HEAD

85HEN	Caliper, Fetal Head, Ultrasonic	Obstetrics/Gyn
79FYF	Cap, Surgical	Surgery
79RXN	Cover, Head, Surgical	Surgery
85HGA	Cranioclast	Obstetrics/Gyn
87VKH	Fixation Device, Extra-Cranial (Head Frame)	Orthopedics
89IRS	Halter, Head, Traction	Physical Med
87HSS	Halter, Head, Traction, Orthopedic	Orthopedics
79GFB	Hammer, Head, Surgical	Surgery
84HBM	Head Rest, Neurosurgical	Cns/Neurology
84HBL	Holder, Head, Neurosurgical (Skull Clamp)	Cns/Neurology
90IWY	Holder, Head, Radiographic	Radiology
79FXY	Hood, Surgical	Surgery
79MEP	Prosthesis, Craniofacial, Bone-Anchored	Surgery
87UCE	Prosthesis, Femoral Head	Orthopedics
87VCP	Prosthesis, Radial/Ulnar Head	Orthopedics
90TEA	Radiographic Unit, Diagnostic, Head	Radiology

HEAD (cont'd)

84JXD	Scanner, Computed Tomography, X-Ray (CAT, CT)	Cns/Neurology
90TEI	Scanner, Computed Tomography, X-Ray, Head	Radiology
73BTK	Strap, Head, Gas Mask	Anesthesiology
89IMS	Support, Head And Trunk, Wheelchair	Physical Med
77EPW	Support, Head, Surgical, ENT	Ear/Nose/Throat
73BZS	Transducer, Stethoscope	Anesthesiology

HEADBAND

77RHR	Headband, Nasogastric	Ear/Nose/Throat
79FSR	Light, Headband, Surgical	Surgery
86HKF	Mirror, Headband, Ophthalmic	Ophthalmology

HEADGEAR

76DZB	Headgear, Extraoral, Orthodontic	Dental And Oral

HEADLAMP

86HPQ	Headlamp, Operating, AC-Powered	Ophthalmology
86HPP	Headlamp, Operating, Battery-Operated	Ophthalmology

HEADLIGHT

79WRX	Camera, Video, Headlight, Surgical	Surgery
77KAF	Headlight, ENT	Ear/Nose/Throat
78FCT	Headlight, Fiberoptic Focusing	Gastro/Urology
86HBJ	Headlight, Neurosurgical	Ophthalmology
76EBA	Light, Surgical Headlight	Dental And Oral

HEADWALL

80RLO	Headwall System (Patient Room)	General

HEALING

79MBQ	Device, Peripheral Electromag. Field to Aid Wound Healing	Surgery
87VID	Indicator, Bone Healing	Orthopedics
79LXU	Laser, Healing, Wound	Surgery
90REI	Laser, Therapeutic	Radiology
89WIN	Stimulator, Wound Healing	Physical Med

HEALTH

75RGE	Mass Screening System	Chemistry

HEALTHCARE

80WVJ	Computer Software, Home Healthcare	General

HEARING

77LXV	Analyzer, Apparatus, Vestibular	Ear/Nose/Throat
77WOT	Battery, Hearing-Aid	Ear/Nose/Throat
77ETW	Calibrator, Hearing-Aid/Earphone And Analysis Systems	Ear/Nose/Throat
77WQJ	Computer, Audiometry	Ear/Nose/Throat
77ESD	Hearing-Aid	Ear/Nose/Throat
77LXB	Hearing-Aid, Bone-Conduction	Ear/Nose/Throat
77MAH	Hearing-Aid, Bone-Conduction, Implanted	Ear/Nose/Throat
77MKE	Hearing-Aid, Bone-Conduction, Percutaneous	Ear/Nose/Throat
77MKP	Hearing-Aid, Cortical, Shafer	Ear/Nose/Throat
77MMB	Hearing-Aid, External, Magnet, Membrane, Tympanic	Ear/Nose/Throat
77EPF	Hearing-Aid, Group, Or Auditory Trainer	Ear/Nose/Throat
77KHL	Hearing-Aid, Master	Ear/Nose/Throat
77LRB	Hearing-Aid, Plate, Face	Ear/Nose/Throat
77EWE	Protector, Hearing (Circumaural)	Ear/Nose/Throat
77EWD	Protector, Hearing (Insert)	Ear/Nose/Throat
77EWM	System, Analysis, Hearing-Aid	Ear/Nose/Throat
77LRA	Tactile Hearing-Aid	Ear/Nose/Throat
89UME	Telephone, Handicapped Use	Physical Med
77WXX	Unit, Testing, Hearing, Intraoperative	Ear/Nose/Throat

HEARING-AID

77EWO	Audiometer	Ear/Nose/Throat
77WOT	Battery, Hearing-Aid	Ear/Nose/Throat
77ETW	Calibrator, Hearing-Aid/Earphone And Analysis Systems	Ear/Nose/Throat
77EWC	Chamber, Acoustic, Testing	Ear/Nose/Throat
77ESD	Hearing-Aid	Ear/Nose/Throat
76MGE	Hearing-Aid, Audiodontic	Dental And Oral
77LXB	Hearing-Aid, Bone-Conduction	Ear/Nose/Throat
77MAH	Hearing-Aid, Bone-Conduction, Implanted	Ear/Nose/Throat
77MKE	Hearing-Aid, Bone-Conduction, Percutaneous	Ear/Nose/Throat
77MKP	Hearing-Aid, Cortical, Shafer	Ear/Nose/Throat
77MMB	Hearing-Aid, External, Magnet, Membrane, Tympanic	Ear/Nose/Throat
77EPF	Hearing-Aid, Group, Or Auditory Trainer	Ear/Nose/Throat
77KHL	Hearing-Aid, Master	Ear/Nose/Throat
77LRB	Hearing-Aid, Plate, Face	Ear/Nose/Throat
77EWM	System, Analysis, Hearing-Aid	Ear/Nose/Throat
77LRA	Tactile Hearing-Aid	Ear/Nose/Throat

HEART

74MIE	Allograft, Heart Valve	Cardiovascular
74QGJ	Board, Cardiac Compression	Cardiovascular
74DTQ	Console, Heart-Lung Machine, Cardiopulmonary Bypass	Cardiovascular
74QZI	Detector, Air, Heart-Lung Bypass	Cardiovascular
85QVO	Detector, Fetal Heart, Phono	Obstetrics/Gyn
74MEZ	Device, Debridement, Ultrasonic, Heart Valve & HV Seat	Cardiovascular
74MWS	Device, Stabilizer, Heart	Cardiovascular
74JOR	Generator, Pulsatile Flow, Cardiopulmonary Bypass	Cardiovascular

KEYWORD INDEX

HELLY
88IFS Solution, Pathology, Helly — Pathology

HELMET
79FXZ Helmet, Surgical — Surgery

HEMACYTOMETER
81ULS Hemacytometer — Hematology

HEMAGGLUTINATION
83LKC Antigen, Indirect Hemagglutination, Herpes Simplex Virus — Microbiology
91DLX Hemagglutination Inhibition, Barbiturate — Toxicology
91DNO Hemagglutination Inhibition, Gentamicin — Toxicology
91DIW Hemagglutination Inhibition, Methadone — Toxicology
91DLR Hemagglutination Inhibition, Morphine — Toxicology
91DKL Hemagglutination, Cocaine — Toxicology
91DLN Hemagglutination, Cocaine Metabolites (Benzoylecgnonine) — Toxicology
91DLT Hemagglutination, Opiates — Toxicology

HEMATEIN
88IDE Acid, Hematein — Pathology

HEMATIN
81GGF Acid Hematin — Hematology
81JCK Alkaline Hematin — Hematology

HEMATOCRIT
81WIT Brush, Centrifuge — Hematology
81KRZ Calibrator, Hemoglobin And Hematocrit Measurement — Hematology
81GKG Centrifuge, Hematocrit — Hematology
81GLK Hematocrit Control — Hematology
81GHY Hematocrit Tube, Rack, Sealer, Holder — Hematology
81GKF Hematocrit, Automated — Hematology
81JPI Hematocrit, Manual — Hematology

HEMATOFLUORIMETER
75VEO Hematofluorimeter (Bilirubinometer) — Chemistry

HEMATOLOGY
75VIN Analyzer, Combination Chemistry/Hematology/Electrolyte — Chemistry
81KSN Centrifuge, Cell Washing, Automated, Immuno-Hematology — Hematology
81JWS Computer, Hematology Analyzer — Hematology
88KQD General Hematology Reagent — Pathology
81LOQ General Purpose Hematology Device — Hematology
81JPK Hematology Quality Control Mixture — Hematology
81GJG Pipette, Quantitative, Hematology — Hematology
80WRA Reagent, Calibration — General
81VCW Sieve, Hematology — Hematology
81GLP Stain, Giemsa, Hematology — Hematology
88KQC Stain, Hematology — Pathology
81GFL Stain, Ponceau, Hematology — Hematology
81GIX Stain, Toluidine Blue, Hematology — Hematology
81GJK Stain, Wright's, Hematology — Hematology
81RTS Stainer, Slide, Hematology — Hematology
81GKD Stainer, Slide, Hematology, Automated — Hematology
80WPJ Vial, Hematology — General

HEMATOPOIETIC
81MZJ System, Concentration, Hematopoietic Stem Cell — Hematology

HEMATOXYLIN
88ICI Chrome Alum Hematoxylin — Pathology
88HYO Hematoxylin Weigert's — Pathology
88KKT Hematoxylin, Ehrlich's — Pathology
88HYJ Stain, Hematoxylin — Pathology
88HYK Stain, Hematoxylin, Harris's — Pathology
88HYL Stain, Hematoxylin, Mayer's — Pathology
88HZM Stain, Phosphotungstic Acid Hematoxylin — Pathology
88IAE Stain, Weigert's Iron Hematoxylin — Pathology

HEME
75JIZ Absorption, Atomic, Iron (Non-Heme) — Chemistry
75JIY Photometric Method, Iron (Non-Heme) — Chemistry
75JJA Radio-Labeled Iron Method, Iron (Non-Heme) — Chemistry

HEMI
87KWC Prosthesis, Finger, Hemi — Orthopedics

HEMI-
87LZY Hip, Hemi-, Femoral, Metal Ball — Orthopedics
87KWJ Prosthesis, Elbow, Hemi-, Humeral, Metal — Orthopedics
87KWI Prosthesis, Elbow, Hemi-, Radial, Polymer — Orthopedics
87KWB Prosthesis, Hip, Hemi-, Acetabular, Metal — Orthopedics
87KWL Prosthesis, Hip, Hemi-, Femoral, Metal — Orthopedics
87KWY Prosthesis, Hip, Hemi-, Femoral, Metal/Polymer — Orthopedics
87JDH Prosthesis, Hip, Hemi-, Trunnion-Bearing, Femoral — Orthopedics
87HSA Prosthesis, Knee, Hemi-, Femoral — Orthopedics
87HTG Prosthesis, Knee, Hemi-, Patellar Resurfacing, Uncemented — Orthopedics
87KRS Prosthesis, Knee, Hemi-, Tibial Resurfacing — Orthopedics
87HSH Prosthesis, Knee, Hemi-, Tibial Resurfacing, Uncemented — Orthopedics

HEMI- *(cont'd)*
87KYM Prosthesis, Shoulder, Hemi-, Glenoid, Metal — Orthopedics
87HSD Prosthesis, Shoulder, Hemi-, Humeral — Orthopedics
87MJT Prosthesis, Shoulder, Humeral, Bipol., Hemi-, Constr., M/P — Orthopedics
87KWD Prosthesis, Toe, Hemi-, Phalangeal — Orthopedics
87KXE Prosthesis, Wrist, Hemi-, Ulnar — Orthopedics

HEMI-ARTHROPLASTY
87KQY Prosthesis, Finger and Toe, Hemi-Arthroplasty — Orthopedics

HEMI-CONSTRAINED
87MBM Prosthesis, Hip, Semi/Hemi-Const., M/PTFE Ctd./P, Cem./Unc. — Orthopedics

HEMIC
85HEJ Monitor, Hemic Sound, Ultrasonic — Obstetrics/Gyn

HEMIPROSTHESIS
87KRM Hemiprosthesis, Elbow (Humeral Resurfacing) — Orthopedics

HEMOCONCENTRATOR
73CAC Autotransfusion Unit (Blood) — Anesthesiology
74UMG Hemoconcentrator — Cardiovascular
78RAB Hemofiltration Unit — Gastro/Urology

HEMOCYTOMETER
81GHO Hemocytometer — Hematology

HEMODETOXIFIER
81RAC Hemoperfusion System (Hemodetoxifier) — Hematology

HEMODIALYSIS
78KOC Accessories, Blood Circuit, Hemodialysis — Gastro/Urology
78QGD Cannula, Hemodialysis — Gastro/Urology
78LFK Catheter, Femoral — Gastro/Urology
78MPB Catheter, Hemodialysis — Gastro/Urology
78MSD Catheter, Hemodialysis, Implanted — Gastro/Urology
78QIK Catheter, Hemodialysis, Single-Needle — Gastro/Urology
78UCO Clamp, Hemodialysis Unit Blood Line — Gastro/Urology
78KPO Concentrate, Dialysis, Hemodialysis (Liquid or Powder) — Gastro/Urology
78QZY Controller, Hemodialysis Unit Single Needle — Gastro/Urology
78QZZ Converter, Unit, Hemodialysis, Single-Pass — Gastro/Urology
78QZV Detector, Hemodialysis Unit Air Bubble-Foam — Gastro/Urology
78FKQ Dialysate Delivery System, Central Multiple Patient — Gastro/Urology
78FKP Dialysate Delivery System, Single Patient — Gastro/Urology
78FJI Dialyzer, Capillary, Hollow Fiber (Hemodialysis) — Gastro/Urology
78FJG Dialyzer, Parallel Flow (Hemodialysis) — Gastro/Urology
78FHS Dialyzer, Single Coil (Hemodialysis) — Gastro/Urology
78MDQ Graft, Vascular, Biological, Hemodialysis Access — Gastro/Urology
78MCI Graft, Vascular, Synth./Bio. Composite, Hemodialysis Access — Gastro/Urology
78RAA Hemodialysis Unit (Kidney Machine) — Gastro/Urology
78RAB Hemofiltration Unit — Gastro/Urology
78QZU Kit, Hemodialysis Tubing — Gastro/Urology
78QZX Monitor, Hemodialysis Unit Conductivity — Gastro/Urology
78QZW Pump, Blood, Hemodialysis Unit — Gastro/Urology
78MQS System, Hemodialysis, Access Recirculation Monitoring — Gastro/Urology
78MON System, Hemodialysis, Remote Accessories — Gastro/Urology

HEMODYNAMIC
73VJA Monitor, Hemodynamic — Anesthesiology

HEMOFILTRATION
78RAB Hemofiltration Unit — Gastro/Urology
78MKM Monitor, Hemofiltration — Gastro/Urology

HEMOGLOBIN
75JKP 51 Chromium, Blood Volume — Chemistry
81KRZ Calibrator, Hemoglobin And Hematocrit Measurement — Hematology
81GGM Control, Hemoglobin — Hematology
81JCM Control, Hemoglobin, Abnormal — Hematology
74WWI Hemoglobin — Cardiovascular
81JPD Hemoglobin A2 Quantitation — Hematology
81MLL Hemoglobin C (Abnormal Hemoglobin Variant) — Hematology
81JPC Hemoglobin F Quantitation — Hematology
81JPB Hemoglobin M — Hematology
81GIQ Hemoglobin S — Hematology
82DAM Hemoglobin, Chain Specific, Antigen, Antiserum, Control — Immunology
81GHA Hemoglobin, Resistant, Alkali — Hematology
81GKA Quantitation, Hemoglobin, Abnormal — Hematology
81JBB Solubility, Hemoglobin, Abnormal — Hematology
81GHQ Stain, Fetal Hemoglobin — Hematology
81GFS Standard/Control, Hemoglobin, Normal/Abnormal — Hematology
81KQI Test, Fetal Hemoglobin — Hematology
81LCP Test, Glycosylated Hemoglobin Assay — Hematology
81LGL Test, Hemoglobin Bart's — Hematology
81KHG Whole Blood Hemoglobin Determination — Hematology

HEMOGLOBINOMETER
81GIG Hemoglobinometer — Hematology
81GKR Hemoglobinometer, Automated — Hematology
81JBD Hemoglobinometer, Electrophoretic Analysis System — Hematology

KEYWORD INDEX

HIP (cont'd)

87MEH	Prosthesis, Hip, Semi-Const., Uncem., Non-P., M/P, Ca./Phos.	Orthopedics
87LZO	Prosthesis, Hip, Semi-Constr., Metal/Ceramic, Cemented/NC	Orthopedics
87JDL	Prosthesis, Hip, Semi-Constrained (Cemented Acetabular)	Orthopedics
87KWA	Prosthesis, Hip, Semi-Constrained Acetabular	Orthopedics
87JDI	Prosthesis, Hip, Semi-Constrained, Metal/Polymer	Orthopedics
87LWJ	Prosthesis, Hip, Semi-Constrained, Metal/Polymer, Uncemented	Orthopedics
87KMC	Prosthesis, Hip, Semi-constrained, Composite/metal	Orthopedics
87MRA	Prosthesis, Hip, Semi-constrained, Metal/ Ceramic/ Ceramic/ Metal, Cemented or Uncemented	Orthopedics
87MAY	Prosthesis, Hip, Semi-constrained, Metal/Ceramic/Polymer, Cemented or Non-porous Cemented, Osteophilic Finish	Orthopedics
87MBM	Prosthesis, Hip, Semi/Hemi-Const., M/PTFE Ctd./P, Cem./Unc.	Orthopedics
89IOZ	Splint, Abduction, Congenital Hip Dislocation	Physical Med
87HSR	Traction Unit, Hip, Non-Powered, Non-Penetrating	Orthopedics

HIS

74RAD	Detector, His Bundle	Cardiovascular

HISTIDINE

75JMI	Chromatographic, Histidine	Chemistry
75JMJ	Microbiological, Histidine	Chemistry

HISTOLOGICAL

88LSP	Keratins, Histological	Pathology

HISTOLOGY

88ICF	Stain, Crystal Violet, Histology	Pathology
83RTT	Stainer, Slide, Histology	Microbiology
88KEY	Stainer, Tissue, Automated	Pathology
88SAV	Tissue Embedding Equipment/Reagent	Pathology

HISTOLYTICA

83KHW	Antigen, ID, HA, CEP, Entamoeba Histolytica	Microbiology
83GMO	Antigen, Latex Agglutination, Entamoeba Histolytica & Rel.	Microbiology
83GWD	Indirect Fluorescent Antibody Test, Entamoeba Histolytica	Microbiology

HISTOPLASMA

83GMJ	Antigen, Histoplasma Capsulatum, All	Microbiology
83GML	Antiserum, Fluorescent, Histoplasma Capsulatum	Microbiology
83GMK	Antiserum, Positive Control, Histoplasma Capsulatum	Microbiology
83MIZ	Enzyme Linked Immunoabsorbent Assay, Histoplasma Capsulatum	Microbiology

HIV

81MTL	Monitor, Test, Hiv-1	Hematology
81VJE	Test, Antibody, Acquired Immune Deficiency Syndrome (AIDS)	Hematology
82MZF	Test, Hiv Detection	Immunology

HIV-1

81MVX	Antibody, Monoclonal Blocking, Hiv-1	Hematology
81MWB	Kit, Test, Saliva, Hiv-1&2	Hematology
81MVW	Kit, Western Blot, Hiv-1	Hematology
81MVY	Monoclonal, Hiv-1	Hematology
81MVZ	System, Test, Home, Hiv-1	Hematology

HIV-2

81MWB	Kit, Test, Saliva, Hiv-1&2	Hematology

HLA

81MZH	Test, Quantitative, For Hla, Non-diagnostic	Hematology

HLA-DQB

81MVS	Kit, Typing, Hla-dqb	Hematology

HOE

76EMQ	Hoe, Periodontic	Dental And Oral

HOIST

80FSA	Lift, Bath, Non-AC-Powered	General
80FNG	Lift, Patient	General
90VET	Lift, Patient, Radiologic	Radiology
80REY	Lift, Wheelchair	General

HOLDER

89IQG	Adapter, Holder, Syringe	Physical Med
81GHY	Hematocrit Tube, Rack, Sealer, Holder	Hematology
89INA	Hill Holder, Wheelchair	Physical Med
79FXR	Holder, Camera, Surgical	Surgery
74WVD	Holder, Cardiac	Cardiovascular
78EYJ	Holder, Catheter	Gastro/Urology
89IMZ	Holder, Crutch and Cane, Wheelchair	Physical Med
77JYK	Holder, Ear Speculum	Ear/Nose/Throat
79QSM	Holder, Electrosurgical Electrode	Surgery
73BSM	Holder, Gas Cylinder	Anesthesiology
74DQW	Holder, Guide, Catheter	Cardiovascular

HOLDER (cont'd)

84HBL	Holder, Head, Neurosurgical (Skull Clamp)	Cns/Neurology
90IWY	Holder, Head, Radiographic	Radiology
74DTJ	Holder, Heart Valve Prosthesis	Cardiovascular
80FRP	Holder, Infant Position	General
79QNR	Holder, Instrument, Laparoscopic	Surgery
80KMK	Holder, Intravascular Catheter	General
79RDF	Holder, Knife	Surgery
85UEZ	Holder, Laparoscope	Obstetrics/Gyn
79UFB	Holder, Leg	Surgery
87THC	Holder, Leg, Arthroscopy	Orthopedics
80RGK	Holder, Medical Chart	General
78FHQ	Holder, Needle	Gastro/Urology
79QOJ	Holder, Needle, Curved, Laparoscopic	Surgery
79QNU	Holder, Needle, Laparoscopic	Surgery
87HXK	Holder, Needle, Orthopedic	Orthopedics
79RHW	Holder, Needle, Other	Surgery
90IXY	Holder, Radiographic Cassette, Wall-Mounted	Radiology
79WRE	Holder, Retractor	Surgery
79SIY	Holder, Ring, Anastomosis	Surgery
79WRY	Holder, Shoulder, Arthroscopy	Surgery
77KAG	Holder, Speculum, ENT	Ear/Nose/Throat
90IWR	Holder, Syringe, Leaded	Radiology
80SAI	Holder, Thermometer	General
73SBH	Holder, Tracheostomy Tube	Anesthesiology
73SBU	Holder, Transducer	Anesthesiology
76EGZ	Holder, X-Ray Film	Dental And Oral
90VGT	Holder, X-Ray Film Cassette, Vertical	Radiology
79QPN	Holder/Scissors, Needle, Laparoscopic	Surgery
79QRS	Instrument, Knot Tying, Suture, Laparoscopic	Surgery
79QPS	Instrument, Needle Holder/Knot Tying	Surgery
79QSH	Instrument, Passing, Suture, Laparoscopic	Surgery
87WWB	Positioner, Spine, Surgical	Orthopedics
80WME	Pouch, Telemetry	General
79RXS	Retractor, Fan-Type, Laparoscopy	Surgery
79RZZ	Retractor, Laparoscopy, Other	Surgery
78FKI	Set, Holder, Dialyzer	Gastro/Urology
75WKC	Stand/Holder, Equipment, Laboratory	Chemistry
73VDM	Strap, Tracheostomy Tube	Anesthesiology
90RNX	Support, Patient Position, Radiographic	Radiology

HOLDING

77JYF	Clamp, Ossicle Holding	Ear/Nose/Throat
87HYA	Forceps, Wire Holding	Orthopedics
78FIN	Tank, Holding, Dialysis	Gastro/Urology

HOLE

84GXR	Cover, Burr Hole (Cranial)	Cns/Neurology

HOLLOW

78FJI	Dialyzer, Capillary, Hollow Fiber (Hemodialysis)	Gastro/Urology
87HWL	Hollow Mill Set	Orthopedics

HOLMIUM

79WXW	Laser, Surgical, Holmium	Surgery

HOLOGRAPH

85HHX	Holograph, Fetal, Acoustical	Obstetrics/Gyn

HOLTER

74MLO	Electrocardiograph, Ambulatory (With Analysis Algorithm)	Cardiovascular
74WOU	Electrode, Holter	Cardiovascular
80WKY	Garment, Electrode	General
74TGX	Monitor, ECG, Ambulatory, Real-Time	Cardiovascular
84RMU	Prosthesis, Hydrocephalic (Holter Valve)	Cns/Neurology
74ROM	Recorder, Long-Term, ECG, Portable (Holter Monitor)	Cardiovascular
80ROP	Recorder, Long-Term, Trend	General
80WMC	Recorder, Long-Term, pH	General
74RQU	Scanner, Long-Term, ECG, Recording	Cardiovascular
84RTC	Shunt, Hydrocephalic	Cns/Neurology

HOLZER

88HYP	Holzer Crystal Violet	Pathology

HOME

81MVZ	System, Test, Home, Hiv-1	Hematology

HOME-USE

80VBQ	Accessories, Decorative	General
86LYL	Accessories, Solution, Lens, Contact	Ophthalmology
89ILZ	Accessories, Traction	Physical Med
87HXF	Accessories, Traction (Cart, Frame, Cord, Weight)	Orthopedics
89KNO	Accessories, Wheelchair	Physical Med
89IQG	Adapter, Holder, Syringe	Physical Med
89ILS	Adapter, Hygiene	Physical Med
89ILW	Adaptor, Grooming	Physical Med
89ILT	Adaptor, Recreational	Physical Med
89LFF	Aid, Control, Environmental, Controlled, Breath	Physical Med
74LIX	Aid, Resuscitation, Cardiopulmonary	Cardiovascular
73CBJ	Airway, Bi-Nasopharyngeal (With Connector)	Anesthesiology

HOME-USE *(cont'd)*

73BTQ	Airway, Nasopharyngeal (Breathing Tube)	Anesthesiology
74DSJ	Alarm, Blood Pressure	Cardiovascular
78THN	Alarm, Hypoglycemia	Gastro/Urology
89IRN	Alarm, Overload, External Limb, Powered	Physical Med
78FIW	Alarm, Pillow Pressure	Gastro/Urology
73RJJ	Analyzer, Gas, Oxygen, Continuous Monitor	Anesthesiology
89ISH	Ankle/Foot, External Limb Component	Physical Med
89QBC	Anklet	Physical Med
78EXJ	Appliance, Incontinence, Urosheath Type	Gastro/Urology
76DZQ	Applicator, Cotton	Dental And Oral
80FOR	Applicator, Tipped, Absorbent	General
89KNM	Applier, Pressure, Physical Medicine	Physical Med
89QBL	Arm Rest	Physical Med
89IML	Armrest, Wheelchair	Physical Med
89ISW	Assembly, Knee/Shank/Ankle/Foot, External	Physical Med
89KFT	Assembly, Shoulder/Elbow/Forearm/Wrist/Hand, Mechanical	Physical Med
89KFX	Assembly, Thigh/Knee/Shank/Ankle/Foot, External	Physical Med
77KCK	Atomizer And Tip, ENT	Ear/Nose/Throat
89UMM	Attachment, Bag (Crutch, Walker, Wheelchair)	Physical Med
89INB	Attachment, Commode, Wheelchair	Physical Med
89IMQ	Attachment, Narrowing, Wheelchair	Physical Med
80TDH	Attachment, Oxygen Canister/IV Pole, Wheelchair	General
78QQK	Bag, Drainage (Incontinence)	Gastro/Urology
80FON	Bag, Drainage, Ostomy (With Adhesive)	General
80QUF	Bag, Enema	General
80QVL	Bag, Enteral Feeding	General
80KYR	Bag, Ice	General
78FAQ	Bag, Leg	Gastro/Urology
80WNK	Bag, Plastic	General
80SEB	Bag, Urinary Collection	General
78EXG	Bag, Urinary Collection, Ureterostomy	Gastro/Urology
78EXH	Bag, Urinary, Ileostomy	Gastro/Urology
75QCG	Balance, Mechanical	Chemistry
80QMO	Ball, Cotton	General
89ISR	Band, Support, Pelvic	Physical Med
80WXC	Band, Sweat	General
79KGX	Bandage, Adhesive	Surgery
80QCH	Bandage, Butterfly	General
80MHW	Bandage, Compression	General
80FQM	Bandage, Elastic	General
80QCI	Bandage, Gauze	General
80QCO	Bandage, Other	General
80QCK	Bandage, Scultetus	General
80QCM	Bandage, Traction	General
80QCN	Bandage, Tubular	General
89IOE	Bars, Parallel, Exercise	Physical Med
89IRR	Bars, Parallel, Powered	Physical Med
89RJY	Bars, Parallel, Walking	Physical Med
87RVM	Bars, Spreader	Orthopedics
80WVN	Base, Roller, Tank, Oxygen	General
80FNY	Basin, Emesis	General
80QCS	Bassinet (Infant Bed)	General
89ILJ	Bath, Hydro-Massage (Whirlpool)	Physical Med
80TAG	Bath, Leg	General
89IMC	Bath, Paraffin	Physical Med
80QCU	Bath, Portable	General
89KTC	Bath, Sitz, Non-Powered	Physical Med
89ILM	Bath, Sitz, Physical Medicine	Physical Med
80QCW	Bath, Steam	General
80VKA	Bathtub	General
80QCZ	Bathtub, Portable	General
80VDY	Battery	General
77WOT	Battery, Hearing-Aid	Ear/Nose/Throat
74DSZ	Battery, Pacemaker	Cardiovascular
80QDA	Bed Cradle	General
89INX	Bed, Air Fluidized	Physical Med
80FNL	Bed, Electric	General
80LLI	Bed, Electric, Home-Use	General
80UDH	Bed, Flotation Therapy, Neonatal	General
89IOQ	Bed, Flotation Therapy, Powered	Physical Med
80FNJ	Bed, Manual	General
89INY	Bed, Patient Rotation, Manual	Physical Med
80FMS	Bed, Pediatric (Crib)	General
89FNH	Bed, Water Flotation, AC-Powered	Physical Med
80FOB	Bedpan	General
80QDC	Bedpan, Fracture	General
80QDD	Bedrail	General
78EXP	Belt, Abdominal	Gastro/Urology
87QDH	Belt, Lumbosacral	Orthopedics
87QDI	Belt, Rib (Support)	Orthopedics
85RQK	Belt, Sanitary	Obstetrics/Gyn
89ISQ	Belt, Support, Pelvic	Physical Med
89IRZ	Belt, Traction, Pelvic	Physical Med
87HSQ	Belt, Traction, Pelvic, Orthopedic	Orthopedics
89IQB	Belt, Wheelchair	Physical Med

HOME-USE *(cont'd)*

80QDJ	Bib	General
80FSD	Binder, Abdominal	General
85HFR	Binder, Abdominal, OB/GYN	Obstetrics/Gyn
87QDM	Binder, Ankle	Orthopedics
85HEF	Binder, Breast	Obstetrics/Gyn
80QDN	Binder, Chest	General
80KMO	Binder, Elastic	General
80FQK	Binder, Perineal	General
80QDO	Binder, Scultetus	General
87QDP	Binder, T	Orthopedics
87QDQ	Binder, Wrist	Orthopedics
84HCC	Biofeedback Device	Cns/Neurology
89IQH	Biofeedback Equipment, Myoelectric, Battery-Powered	Physical Med
89IRC	Biofeedback Equipment, Myoelectric, Powered	Physical Med
80QDW	Blanket, Infant	General
77JPL	Block, Bite, ENT	Ear/Nose/Throat
80FPS	Board, Bed	General
87QWT	Board, Foot	Orthopedics
89RNR	Board, Quadriceps (Exerciser)	Physical Med
89KNL	Board, Scooter, Prone	Physical Med
80QCT	Boot, Bath	General
73BYO	Bottle, Blow (Exerciser)	Anesthesiology
80FPF	Bottle, Hot/Cold Water	General
80VFT	Bottle, Medicine Spray	General
85TAO	Bottle, Nursing	Obstetrics/Gyn
89ITW	Brace, Joint, Ankle (External)	Physical Med
80RBE	Bracelet, Identification	General
85UKV	Brassiere, Maternity	Obstetrics/Gyn
76QEM	Bridges	Dental And Oral
80WVO	Brush, Other	General
80WRS	Bulb, Inflation	General
89ISN	Cable	Physical Med
84VDH	Cable/Lead, TENS	Cns/Neurology
89ITM	Cage, Knee	Physical Med
89IPS	Cane	Physical Med
89KHY	Cane, Safety Walk	Physical Med
73BYJ	Canister, Liquid Oxygen, Portable	Anesthesiology
73RJL	Canister, Oxygen	Anesthesiology
80FMM	Cannula, Nasal	General
73CAT	Cannula, Nasal, Oxygen	Anesthesiology
80WUT	Carrier, Container, Oxygen, Portable	General
73QXW	Cart, Gas Cylinder (Carrier)	Anesthesiology
73BZB	Catheter, Nasal, Oxygen (Tube)	Anesthesiology
78QIS	Catheter, Urinary, Condom	Gastro/Urology
89INN	Chair, Adjustable, Mechanical	Physical Med
80QJF	Chair, Bath	General
80FRJ	Chair, Geriatric	General
80FRM	Chair, Geriatric, Wheeled	General
80QJO	Chair, Other	General
80QJJ	Chair, Pediatric	General
80QJL	Chair, Rehabilitation	General
80UMP	Chair, Seat Lifting (Standing Aid)	General
80QJM	Chair, Shower	General
80QJN	Chair, Sitz Bath	General
76EFT	Cleaner, Denture	Dental And Oral
76JER	Cleaner, Denture, Mechanical	Dental And Oral
86LPN	Cleaner, Lens, Contact	Ophthalmology
73BXJ	Clip, Nose	Anesthesiology
80QLB	Clipper, Hair	General
80QLC	Clipper, Nail	General
80WMY	Clothing, Protective	General
87QLP	Collar, Cervical Neck	Orthopedics
80QLR	Collar, Ice	General
80QLV	Commode (Toilet)	General
80QLU	Commode Seat	General
80VBO	Communication Equipment	General
80VFG	Communication System, Emergency Alert, Personal	General
89ILP	Communication System, Non-Powered	Physical Med
89ILQ	Communication System, Powered	Physical Med
89IOD	Component, Exercise	Physical Med
87KQZ	Component, Traction, Non-Invasive	Orthopedics
89KNN	Component, Wheelchair	Physical Med
80QLW	Compress, Cold	General
80QLX	Compress, Gauze	General
89QLY	Compress, Moist Heat	Physical Med
80WVJ	Computer Software, Home Healthcare	General
73RJM	Concentrator, Oxygen	Anesthesiology
85HIS	Condom	Obstetrics/Gyn
73VFY	Container, Liquid Nitrogen	Anesthesiology
73VFZ	Container, Liquid Oxygen	Anesthesiology
80WPQ	Container, Medication, Home-Use	General
89KHZ	Control, Foot Driving, Automobile, Mechanical	Physical Med
89IPQ	Control, Hand Driving, Automobile, Mechanical	Physical Med
87QMN	Corset	Orthopedics
76EFN	Cotton, Roll	Dental And Oral
80VFA	Cover, Bedrail	General

HOME-USE *(cont'd)*

80KIA	Cover, Cast	General
89IPM	Cover, Limb	Physical Med
80FMW	Cover, Mattress	General
80QNB	Cover, Mattress, Waterproof	General
80WHO	Cover, Other	General
80WHM	Cover, Seat, Toilet, Sanitary	General
89IPR	Crutch	Physical Med
74DXQ	Cuff, Blood Pressure	Cardiovascular
89INC	Cuff, Pusher, Wheelchair	Physical Med
76QNT	Cup, Denture	Dental And Oral
86LXQ	Cup, Eye	Ophthalmology
80QNV	Cup, Geriatric Feeding	General
80QNW	Cup, Medicine	General
80TBP	Curtain, Shower	General
89KIC	Cushion, Flotation	Physical Med
87QNZ	Cushion, Foot	Orthopedics
80QOA	Cushion, Ring, Foam Rubber	General
80QOB	Cushion, Ring, Inflatable	General
89IMP	Cushion, Wheelchair (Pad)	Physical Med
80WTB	Cutter, Pill	General
73VFF	Cylinder, Oxygen	Anesthesiology
74WJK	Defibrillator, Transtelephonic	Cardiovascular
80WUX	Dehumidifier	General
76QPA	Dentifrice	Dental And Oral
76EKO	Denture, Preformed	Dental And Oral
80FMA	Depressor, Tongue	General
77EWF	Depressor, Tongue, ENT, Wood	Ear/Nose/Throat
84HCB	Device, Conditioning, Aversion	Cns/Neurology
78WLL	Device, Incontinence, Fecal	Gastro/Urology
80QPL	Diaper, Adult	General
80QPM	Diaper, Pediatric	General
85HDW	Diaphragm, Contraceptive	Obstetrics/Gyn
89IOA	Diathermy, Microwave	Physical Med
89IMJ	Diathermy, Shortwave	Physical Med
89ILX	Diathermy, Shortwave, Pulsed	Physical Med
89IMI	Diathermy, Ultrasonic (Physical Therapy)	Physical Med
80QPZ	Disinfector, Liquid	General
80WIW	Dispenser, Tissue, Toilet	General
85HED	Douche, Vaginal	Obstetrics/Gyn
80QQV	Dressing, Foam	General
80QQW	Dressing, Germicidal	General
80QQX	Dressing, Non-Adherent	General
80QQZ	Dressing, Roller Gauze	General
80QRC	Dressing, Universal	General
79MGP	Dressing, Wound and Burn, Occlusive	Surgery
77KCM	Dropper, Ear	Ear/Nose/Throat
86QRP	Dropper, Eye	Ophthalmology
80QRQ	Dropper, Medicine	General
77QRR	Dropper, Nose	Ear/Nose/Throat
89IKA	Electrode, Biopotential, Surface, Composite	Physical Med
89IKB	Electrode, Biopotential, Surface, Metallic	Physical Med
89IKS	Electrode, Metallic With Soft Pad Covering	Physical Med
84QTB	Electrode, Neurological	Cns/Neurology
84QTC	Electrode, Neuromuscular Stimulator	Cns/Neurology
84WHU	Electrode, TENS	Cns/Neurology
89ING	Elevator, Wheelchair	Physical Med
89ILR	Environmental Control System, Powered, Remote	Physical Med
80FRF	Equipment, Cleaning, Air	General
73WLD	Equipment, Therapy, Apnea	Anesthesiology
89WPB	Equipment, Therapy, Handicapped/Physical	Physical Med
89ITH	Equipment, Traction, Powered	Physical Med
74QUN	Ergometer, Bicycle	Cardiovascular
89QUU	Exercise Stair	Physical Med
89QUV	Exerciser, Arm	Physical Med
89QUW	Exerciser, Bicycle	Physical Med
89QUX	Exerciser, Chest	Physical Med
89JFA	Exerciser, Finger, Powered	Physical Med
89QUY	Exerciser, Hand	Physical Med
89SGS	Exerciser, Isorobic	Physical Med
89QUZ	Exerciser, Leg And Ankle	Physical Med
89ISD	Exerciser, Measuring	Physical Med
89ION	Exerciser, Non-Measuring	Physical Med
89QVE	Exerciser, Other	Physical Med
89ISC	Exerciser, Passive, Measuring	Physical Med
89IOO	Exerciser, Passive, Non-Measuring (CPM Machine)	Physical Med
73BXB	Exerciser, Powered	Anesthesiology
73QVA	Exerciser, Respiratory	Anesthesiology
89QVB	Exerciser, Shoulder	Physical Med
89QVC	Exerciser, Trapeze	Physical Med
89VLC	Exerciser, Wrist	Physical Med
86HQH	Eye, Artificial, Non-Custom	Ophthalmology
86QVI	Eyeglasses	Ophthalmology
86QVJ	Eyeglasses, Aphakic	Ophthalmology
86TCB	Eyeglasses, Safety	Ophthalmology
80QVK	Facial Tissue	General
80QVW	Filter, Air	General

HOME-USE *(cont'd)*

76JES	Floss, Dental	Dental And Oral
73CAX	Flowmeter, Back-Pressure Compensated, Thorpe Tube	Anesthesiology
89IMM	Footrest, Wheelchair	Physical Med
86HQZ	Frame, Spectacle (Eyeglasses)	Ophthalmology
87QXQ	Frame, Traction	Orthopedics
87QXR	Frame, Turning	Orthopedics
80TCJ	Furniture, Patient Room	General
78EYQ	Garment, Protective, For Incontinence	Gastro/Urology
79QYE	Gauze Roll	Surgery
89IKC	Gel, Electrode, TENS	Physical Med
89QYF	Gel, Ultrasonic Coupling	Physical Med
80SDY	Gel, Ultrasonic Transmission	General
77QAH	Generator, Aerosol	Ear/Nose/Throat
73RCO	Generator, Ionized Air	Anesthesiology
73CAW	Generator, Oxygen, Portable	Anesthesiology
73RJR	Generator, Ozone	Anesthesiology
80QYK	Glove, Other	General
80QYJ	Glove, Utility	General
80QYQ	Gown, Other	General
79FYB	Gown, Patient	Surgery
80QYO	Gown, Patient, Disposable	General
80QYP	Gown, Patient, Reusable	General
89IRS	Halter, Head, Traction	Physical Med
87HSS	Halter, Head, Traction, Orthopedic	Orthopedics
89IRA	Hand, External Limb Component, Mechanical	Physical Med
77ESD	Hearing-Aid	Ear/Nose/Throat
77LXB	Hearing-Aid, Bone-Conduction	Ear/Nose/Throat
77MAH	Hearing-Aid, Bone-Conduction, Implanted	Ear/Nose/Throat
77MKE	Hearing-Aid, Bone-Conduction, Percutaneous	Ear/Nose/Throat
89VFJ	Heater, Hot Pack	Physical Med
85HHA	Heater, Perineal, Radiant, Non-Contact	Obstetrics/Gyn
89IRQ	Heating Unit, Powered	Physical Med
89INA	Hill Holder, Wheelchair	Physical Med
80FOG	Hood, Oxygen, Infant	General
89IQX	Hook, External Limb Component, Mechanical	Physical Med
80VBI	Housekeeping Equipment	General
73RAU	Humidifier, Heat/Moisture Exchange	Anesthesiology
73RAV	Humidifier, Heated	Anesthesiology
73KFZ	Humidifier, Non-Direct Patient Interface (Home-Use)	Anesthesiology
73RAW	Humidifier, Non-Heated	Anesthesiology
73BTT	Humidifier, Respiratory Gas, (Direct Patient Interface)	Anesthesiology
73RAX	Hygrometer (Humidity Indicator)	Anesthesiology
80RAZ	Hypo/Hyperthermia Blanket	General
80RBC	Hypothermia Unit	General
80UEU	Identification, Alert, Medical	General
87RBF	Immobilizer, Ankle	Orthopedics
87RBG	Immobilizer, Arm	Orthopedics
87RBH	Immobilizer, Cervical	Orthopedics
87RBI	Immobilizer, Elbow	Orthopedics
87RBJ	Immobilizer, Infant (Circumcision Board)	Orthopedics
87RBK	Immobilizer, Knee	Orthopedics
87RBL	Immobilizer, Shoulder	Orthopedics
87RBM	Immobilizer, Wrist/Hand	Orthopedics
78FHW	Impotence Device, Mechanical/Hydraulic	Gastro/Urology
75CEN	Indicator, pH, Dye (Urinary, Non-Quantitative)	Chemistry
80LZG	Infusion Pump, Insulin	General
80FOX	Infusion Stand	General
78TCQ	Infusion System, Insulin, With Monitor	Gastro/Urology
77KCO	Inhaler, Nasal	Ear/Nose/Throat
78WRW	Injector, Insulin	Gastro/Urology
86KYE	Inserter/Remover, Lens, Contact	Ophthalmology
80KYS	Insoles, Medical	General
85HDS	Introducer, Contraceptive Diaphragm	Obstetrics/Gyn
87THB	Inversion Unit	Orthopedics
76EFS	Irrigator, Oral	Dental And Oral
80RFL	Jelly, Lubricating	General
89ITS	Joint, Hip, External Brace	Physical Med
89ITQ	Joint, Knee, External Brace	Physical Med
89ISY	Joint, Knee, External Limb Component	Physical Med
89ISZ	Joint, Wrist, External Limb Component, Mechanical	Physical Med
73RJH	Kit, Administration, Oxygen	Anesthesiology
78TGJ	Kit, Administration, Parenteral	Gastro/Urology
74QIX	Kit, Blood Pressure, Central Venous	Cardiovascular
76EBO	Kit, Denture Repair, OTC	Dental And Oral
80UDB	Kit, Emergency, Anaphylactic	General
80UDC	Kit, Emergency, Cardiopulmonary Resuscitation	General
80RCG	Kit, Emergency, Insect Sting	General
80QUG	Kit, Enema	General
80QVM	Kit, Feeding, Adult (Enteral)	General
80QVN	Kit, Feeding, Pediatric (Enteral)	General
79LRR	Kit, First Aid	Surgery
85TFV	Kit, Pregnancy Test	Obstetrics/Gyn
85ULY	Kit, Sex Selection	Obstetrics/Gyn
89HHC	Kit, Sitz Bath	Physical Med
80RTX	Kit, Snake Bite	General
80KYQ	Kit, Snake Bite, Chemical Cold Pack	General

HOME-USE *(cont'd)*

80KYP	Kit, Snake Bite, Suction	General
78RKM	Kit, Tubing, Dialysis, Peritoneal	Gastro/Urology
89RDN	Knife, Paraffin	Physical Med
80FOI	Lamp, Heat	General
89ILY	Lamp, Infrared	Physical Med
80REA	Lamp, Perineal Heat	General
80REB	Lamp, Sun, Incandescent	General
80REE	Lamp, Ultraviolet (Spectrum A)	General
89IOB	Lamp, Ultraviolet, Physical Medicine	Physical Med
77ESE	Larynx, Artificial Battery-Powered	Ear/Nose/Throat
80RER	Leg Rest	General
80LLK	Legging, Compression, Non-Inflatable	General
86HQD	Lens, Contact (Other Material)	Ophthalmology
86ULH	Lens, Contact, Bifocal	Ophthalmology
86ULD	Lens, Contact, Extended-Wear	Ophthalmology
86MRC	Lens, Contact, Gas-Permeable	Ophthalmology
86TGY	Lens, Contact, Hydrophilic	Ophthalmology
86HPX	Lens, Contact, Polymethylmethacrylate	Ophthalmology
86HRA	Lens, Spectacle/Eyeglasses, Custom (Prescription)	Ophthalmology
86HQG	Lens, Spectacle/Eyeglasses, Non-Custom	Ophthalmology
80FNG	Lift, Patient	General
80TFX	Lift, Stair Climbing	General
80REY	Lift, Wheelchair	General
80TCX	Light, Bilirubin (Phototherapy)	General
80RFF	Light, Overbed	General
80VLB	Lotion, Skin Care	General
80WVL	Manual, Policies	General
73BYG	Mask, Oxygen, Aerosol Administration	Anesthesiology
73KGB	Mask, Oxygen, Non-Rebreathing	Anesthesiology
80FQG	Mask, Oxygen, Other	General
80RFY	Mask, Oxygen, Partial Rebreathing	General
89IPD	Massager, Battery-Powered	Physical Med
89IRP	Massager, Powered Inflatable Tube	Physical Med
89ISA	Massager, Therapeutic	Physical Med
80FNM	Mattress, Air Flotation	General
89ILA	Mattress, Alternating Pressure (Or Pads)	Physical Med
80RGG	Mattress, Bed	General
89IKY	Mattress, Non-Powered Flotation Therapy	Physical Med
80WYO	Mattress, Reduction, Pressure	General
80FNI	Mattress, Silicone, And Chair Cushion	General
80RGI	Mattress, Water	General
80FOH	Mattress, Water, Temperature Regulated	General
73RJO	Meter, Oxygen	Anesthesiology
89RHD	Mirror, Posture	Physical Med
77RHE	Mirror, Speech	Ear/Nose/Throat
80RHF	Mitt/Washcloth, Patient	General
89RHK	Moist Therapy Pack	Physical Med
89RHJ	Moist Therapy Pack Conditioner	Physical Med
80RHL	Moleskin	General
80FLS	Monitor, Apnea	General
80QDB	Monitor, Bed Occupancy	General
78TGM	Monitor, Blood Glucose (Test)	Gastro/Urology
74JOE	Monitor, Blood Pressure, Indirect, Automatic	Cardiovascular
74DXN	Monitor, Blood Pressure, Indirect, Semi-Automatic	Cardiovascular
80QUM	Monitor, Gas, Atmospheric, Environmental	General
75WXU	Monitor, Glucose, Blood, Non-Invasive	Chemistry
80WKH	Monitor, Medication	General
73BWS	Monitor, Pulse Rate	Anesthesiology
73BWX	Monitor, Temperature (With Probe)	Anesthesiology
80WKM	Mount, Equipment	General
73BYP	Mouthpiece, Breathing	Anesthesiology
73CAF	Nebulizer, Direct Patient Interface	Anesthesiology
73RHT	Nebulizer, Heated	Anesthesiology
77EPN	Nebulizer, Medicinal	Ear/Nose/Throat
73CCQ	Nebulizer, Medicinal, Non-Ventilatory (Atomizer)	Anesthesiology
73RHU	Nebulizer, Non-Heated	Anesthesiology
73RHV	Nebulizer, Ultrasonic	Anesthesiology
80FNN	Nipple, Feeding	General
85QQJ	Nozzle, Douche	Obstetrics/Gyn
89KTD	Orthosis, Abdominal	Physical Med
89IQK	Orthosis, Cervical	Physical Med
89IQF	Orthosis, Cervical-Thoracic, Rigid	Physical Med
89KNP	Orthosis, Corrective Shoe	Physical Med
89IQI	Orthosis, Limb Brace	Physical Med
89IQE	Orthosis, Lumbar	Physical Med
89IPY	Orthosis, Lumbosacral	Physical Med
89RJB	Orthosis, Other	Physical Med
89IPX	Orthosis, Rib Fracture, Soft	Physical Med
89IPW	Orthosis, Sacroiliac, Soft	Physical Med
89IPT	Orthosis, Thoracic	Physical Med
78RJF	Ostomy Appliance (Ileostomy, Colostomy)	Gastro/Urology
80VFN	Oximeter, Finger	General
73WVK	Oxygen	Anesthesiology
80WRP	Pacifier	General
80QLO	Pack, Cold	General
80FRS	Pack, Cold, Chemical	General

HOME-USE *(cont'd)*

89IMD	Pack, Hot Or Cold, Disposable	Physical Med
89IME	Pack, Hot Or Cold, Reusable	Physical Med
89ILO	Pack, Hot Or Cold, Water Circulating	Physical Med
89IMA	Pack, Moist Heat	Physical Med
80LKB	Pad, Alcohol	General
85QEJ	Pad, Breast	Obstetrics/Gyn
80QQS	Pad, Dressing	General
74WWU	Pad, Electrode	Cardiovascular
86HMP	Pad, Eye	Ophthalmology
89UED	Pad, Heating, Chemical	Physical Med
80QZS	Pad, Heating, Circulating Fluid	General
89FPG	Pad, Heating, Electrical	Physical Med
89IRT	Pad, Heating, Powered	Physical Med
80RBU	Pad, Incontinence (Underpad)	General
80FNW	Pad, Kelly	General
80RGM	Pad, Medicated	General
85HHL	Pad, Menstrual, Scented	Obstetrics/Gyn
85HHD	Pad, Menstrual, Unscented	Obstetrics/Gyn
80RLZ	Pad, Pressure, Air	General
80RMA	Pad, Pressure, Animal Skin	General
80RMB	Pad, Pressure, Foam (Elbow, Heel)	General
80RMC	Pad, Pressure, Foam Convoluted	General
80RMD	Pad, Pressure, Gel	General
80RME	Pad, Pressure, Soft Rubber	General
80RMF	Pad, Pressure, Water Cushion	General
80TFY	Page Turner (Handicapped)	General
80RBV	Pant, Incontinence	General
86UET	Patch, Eye	Ophthalmology
80WOL	Patch, Transdermal	General
73BYI	Percussor, Powered	Anesthesiology
85RKO	Pessary, Diaphragm	Obstetrics/Gyn
80RKZ	Phototherapy Unit (Bilirubin Lamp)	General
80RLD	Pillow, Bath	General
87RLE	Pillow, Cervical	Orthopedics
77MYB	Pillow, Cervical(for Mild Sleep Apnea)	Ear/Nose/Throat
77QRU	Plug, Ear	Ear/Nose/Throat
80TDS	Plug, Electrical	General
78WHR	Plug, Ostomy	Gastro/Urology
89JFC	Pressure Measurement, System, Intermittent	Physical Med
80UCU	Pressure Pad, Alternating, Disposable	General
80UCV	Pressure Pad, Alternating, Reusable	General
80RMJ	Probe, Temperature	General
80FQT	Prophylactic (Condom)	General
78UDE	Prosthesis, Anti-Gastroesophageal Reflux	Gastro/Urology
87QWH	Protector, Finger	Orthopedics
76ELQ	Protector, Mouth Guard	Dental And Oral
80FMP	Protector, Skin Pressure	General
80UBG	Pump, Alternating Pressure Pad	General
85HGY	Pump, Breast, Non-Powered	Obstetrics/Gyn
85HGX	Pump, Breast, Powered	Obstetrics/Gyn
80RNF	Pump, Food (Enteral Feeding)	General
80JOI	Pump, Inflator	General
80VEZ	Pump, Infusion, Ambulatory	General
77JPT	Pump, Nebulizer, Manual	Ear/Nose/Throat
80FRA	Purifier, Air, Ultraviolet	General
80TEB	Rail, Bath	General
80TEC	Rail, Commode	General
80TED	Rail, Wall Side	General
80UKQ	Ramp, Wheelchair	General
80TFZ	Reacher (Handicapped)	General
86HJY	Reader, Bar, Ophthalmic	Ophthalmology
86HJX	Reader, Prism, Ophthalmic	Ophthalmology
86HJG	Reading System, Closed-Circuit Television	Ophthalmology
80TEE	Receptacle, Electrical	General
74ROK	Recorder, Long-Term, Blood Pressure, Portable	Cardiovascular
80ROP	Recorder, Long-Term, Trend	General
73QWO	Regulator, Intake, Oxygen	Anesthesiology
80FQE	Regulator, Oxygen, Mechanical	General
73CAN	Regulator, Pressure, Gas Cylinder	Anesthesiology
80RPD	Restraint, Crib	General
80FMQ	Restraint, Protective (Body)	General
80RPF	Restraint, Wheelchair	General
80RPG	Restraint, Wrist/Hand	General
73WJE	Resuscitator, Emergency, Protective, Infection	Anesthesiology
80RPJ	Retainer, Bandage (Elastic Net)	General
89RQF	Rowing Unit	Physical Med
80RQL	Sanitizer	General
80RQQ	Scale, Bed	General
80RQS	Scale, Chair	General
80FRW	Scale, Infant	General
89INF	Scale, Platform, Wheelchair	Physical Med
80FRI	Scale, Stand-On	General
80RRB	Scissors, Bandage/Gauze/Plaster	General
89INI	Scooter (Motorized 3-Wheeled Vehicle)	Physical Med
80VAY	Security Equipment/Supplies	General
80WSZ	Sensor, Moisture	General

HOME-USE *(cont'd)*

87RSE	Separator, Toe	Orthopedics
80VBS	Service, Computer	General
80VBN	Service, Consulting	General
85RSQ	Shield, Breast	Obstetrics/Gyn
87RSR	Shield, Bunion	Orthopedics
86HOY	Shield, Eye, Ophthalmic	Ophthalmology
85HFS	Shield, Nipple	Obstetrics/Gyn
89IPG	Shoe, Cast	Physical Med
87TEO	Shoe, Orthopedic	Orthopedics
89ILI	Sling, Arm	Physical Med
89ILE	Sling, Arm, Overhead Supported	Physical Med
87RTU	Sling, Knee	Orthopedics
87RTV	Sling, Leg	Orthopedics
89INE	Sling, Overhead Suspension, Wheelchair	Physical Med
80RTW	Slippers	General
80WPU	Soap	General
87RUA	Sock, Cast Toe	Orthopedics
87RUB	Sock, Fracture	Orthopedics
80WVI	Sock, Non-Compression	General
80WVH	Sock, Protective, Skin	General
80RUC	Sock, Stump Cover	General
78WWM	Solution, Nutrition, Enteral	Gastro/Urology
78TGK	Solution, Nutrition, Parenteral	Gastro/Urology
78VKQ	Solution, Ostomy, Odor Control	Gastro/Urology
77LEZ	Speech Training Aid, AC-Powered	Ear/Nose/Throat
77LFA	Speech Training Aid, Battery-Powered	Ear/Nose/Throat
80FLY	Sphygmomanometer, Aneroid (Arterial Pressure)	General
80THH	Sphygmomanometer, Electronic (Arterial Pressure)	General
80UDM	Sphygmomanometer, Electronic, Automatic	General
80UDN	Sphygmomanometer, Electronic, Manual	General
80FLX	Sphygmomanometer, Mercury (Arterial Pressure)	General
73BWF	Spirometer, Therapeutic (Incentive)	Anesthesiology
89IQJ	Splint, Clavicle	Physical Med
89ITN	Splint, Denis Brown	Physical Med
89ILH	Splint, Hand, And Component	Physical Med
87RUW	Splint, Molded, Aluminum	Orthopedics
87RUX	Splint, Molded, Plastic	Orthopedics
87RVC	Splint, Other	Orthopedics
87RUY	Splint, Padded Stays	Orthopedics
89IQM	Splint, Temporary Training	Physical Med
87HSP	Splint, Traction	Orthopedics
87RVB	Splint, Wire Board	Orthopedics
76EFQ	Sponge, Gauze	Dental And Oral
80RVF	Sponge, Germicidal (Alcohol)	General
73QXX	Stand, Gas Cylinder	Anesthesiology
86HRD	Sterilizer, Soft Lens, Thermal, AC-Powered	Ophthalmology
80FLT	Stethoscope, Mechanical	General
75UKD	Stick, Urinalysis Test	Chemistry
84UFF	Stimulator, Electro-Analgesic	Cns/Neurology
89IPP	Stimulator, External, Neuromuscular, Functional	Physical Med
89ISB	Stimulator, Muscle, Diagnostic	Physical Med
89IPF	Stimulator, Muscle, Electrical-Powered (EMS)	Physical Med
89LBF	Stimulator, Muscle, Low Intensity	Physical Med
84GZJ	Stimulator, Nerve, Transcutaneous (Pain Relief, TENS)	Cns/Neurology
84GZI	Stimulator, Neuromuscular, External Functional	Cns/Neurology
87WNT	Stimulator, Osteogenesis, Electric, Non-Invasive	Orthopedics
89IMG	Stimulator, Ultrasound, Muscle	Physical Med
84MBY	Stimulator, Vagus Nerve, Epilepsy, Implanted	Cns/Neurology
87RWH	Stockinette	Orthopedics
80FQL	Stocking, Elastic	General
89ILG	Stocking, Elastic, Physical Medicine	Physical Med
80DWL	Stocking, Support (Anti-Embolic)	General
89RWL	Stool, Exercise	Physical Med
79FPX	Strip, Adhesive	Surgery
75WTX	Strip, Test	Chemistry
89LBE	Stroller, Adaptive	Physical Med
86HQY	Sunglasses (Including Photosensitive)	Ophthalmology
89RXB	Support, Abdominal	Physical Med
87RXC	Support, Ankle	Orthopedics
89RXD	Support, Arch	Physical Med
89IOY	Support, Arm	Physical Med
87RXE	Support, Back	Orthopedics
87RXG	Support, Clavicle	Orthopedics
80WTK	Support, Cover, Bed	General
87RXF	Support, Elbow	Orthopedics
87RXH	Support, Foot	Orthopedics
87RXI	Support, Hand	Orthopedics
89IMS	Support, Head And Trunk, Wheelchair	Physical Med
78EXN	Support, Hernia	Gastro/Urology
89RXJ	Support, Knee	Physical Med
89RXK	Support, Leg	Physical Med
78EXO	Support, Scrotal	Gastro/Urology
80FQJ	Support, Scrotal, Therapeutic	General
89RXL	Support, Thigh	Physical Med
89RXM	Support, Wrist	Physical Med
80TGC	Swabs, Alcohol	General

HOME-USE *(cont'd)*

80RYG	Swabs, Antiseptic	General
80RYH	Swabs, Cotton	General
80VLI	Swabs, Oral Care	General
80RYI	Swabs, Specimen Collection	General
80RYR	Syringe, Insulin	General
78FKX	System, Peritoneal Dialysis, Automatic	Gastro/Urology
89INW	Table, Mechanical	Physical Med
80RYY	Table, Overbed	General
89JFB	Table, Physical Therapy	Physical Med
87RYZ	Table, Traction	Orthopedics
85HEB	Tampon, Menstrual, Unscented	Obstetrics/Gyn
80RZE	Tape, Adhesive	General
80RZF	Tape, Adhesive, Hypoallergenic	General
80RZG	Tape, Adhesive, Waterproof	General
80RZH	Tape, Cotton	General
80VAT	Telephone Equipment	General
89UME	Telephone, Handicapped Use	Physical Med
80KPD	Temperature Strip, Forehead, Liquid Crystal	General
80RZS	Tent, Mist	General
80RZT	Tent, Mist, Face	General
73BYL	Tent, Oxygen (Canopy)	Anesthesiology
80FNC	Tent, Pediatric Aerosol	General
90KYA	Thermographic Device, Liquid Crystal, Non-Powered	Radiology
80FQZ	Thermometer, Chemical Color Change	General
80SAK	Thermometer, Electronic	General
80FLL	Thermometer, Electronic, Continuous	General
79FWR	Thermometer, Liquid Crystals	Surgery
80FLK	Thermometer, Mercury	General
77WXS	Thermometer, Tympanic	Ear/Nose/Throat
80QUH	Tip, Enema	General
76JEW	Tip, Rubber, Oral-Hygiene	Dental And Oral
89INP	Tips And Pads, Cane, Crutch And Walker	Physical Med
80VBE	Tissue, Toilet	General
76EFW	Toothbrush, Manual	Dental And Oral
76JEQ	Toothbrush, Powered	Dental And Oral
80SBD	Tourniquet	General
80WNF	Towel/Towelette, Paper	General
87HSR	Traction Unit, Hip, Non-Powered, Non-Penetrating	Orthopedics
87HST	Traction Unit, Non-Powered	Orthopedics
87SBN	Traction Unit, Powered, Mobile	Orthopedics
87SBO	Traction Unit, Static, Bed	Orthopedics
87SBP	Traction Unit, Static, Chair	Orthopedics
87SBQ	Traction Unit, Static, Other	Orthopedics
89IKX	Transfer Aid	Physical Med
80FMR	Transfer Device, Patient, Manual	General
80UEL	Tray, Walker	General
89IMX	Tray, Wheelchair	Physical Med
89IOG	Treadmill, Mechanical	Physical Med
89IOL	Treadmill, Powered	Physical Med
78SCI	Truss, Hernia (Belt)	Gastro/Urology
85SCJ	Truss, Infant	Obstetrics/Gyn
80FPD	Tube, Feeding	General
73BTR	Tube, Tracheal (Endotracheal)	Anesthesiology
77EQK	Tube, Tracheostomy (Breathing Tube), ENT	Ear/Nose/Throat
80SDU	Tweezers	General
86WNU	Unit, Examination, Lens, Contact	Ophthalmology
89WWS	Unit, Pad, Heating, Portable	Physical Med
89QAP	Unit, Support, Ambulation	Physical Med
80FNP	Urinal	General
89ILC	Utensil, Food	Physical Med
89IKW	Utensil, Handicapped Aid	Physical Med
80SEQ	Vaporizer	General
73CAD	Vaporizer, Anesthesia, Non-Heated	Anesthesiology
89WHH	Vehicle, Handicapped	Physical Med
73SEU	Ventilator, Pressure Cycled (IPPB Machine)	Anesthesiology
73SEW	Ventilator, Volume (Critical Care)	Anesthesiology
89IRO	Vibrator, Therapeutic	Physical Med
80WMV	Vision Aid, Braille	General
86HPF	Vision Aid, Electronic, AC-Powered	Ophthalmology
86HPG	Vision Aid, Electronic, Battery-Powered	Ophthalmology
86HOT	Vision Aid, Image Intensification, Battery-Powered	Ophthalmology
86HPI	Vision Aid, Optical, AC-Powered	Ophthalmology
86HPE	Vision Aid, Optical, Battery-Powered	Ophthalmology
86WOM	Vision Aid, Ultrasonic	Ophthalmology
89ITJ	Walker, Mechanical	Physical Med
80SFF	Warmer, Blanket	General
80SFJ	Warmer, Radiant, Adult	General
89IOR	Wheelchair, Manual	Physical Med
89ITI	Wheelchair, Powered	Physical Med
89IQC	Wheelchair, Special Grade	Physical Med
89IMK	Wheelchair, Stair Climbing	Physical Med
89IPL	Wheelchair, Standup	Physical Med

HOMINIS

83WJS	Antibody, Herpes Virus	Microbiology
83GQN	Antigen, Cf (including Cf Control), Herpesvirus Hominis 1, 2	Microbiology

KEYWORD INDEX

HOMINIS (cont'd)

83GQO	Antisera, Cf, Herpesvirus Hominis 1, 2	Microbiology
83GQL	Antisera, Fluorescent, Herpesvirus Hominis 1, 2	Microbiology
83GQM	Antiserum, Neutralization, Herpes Virus Hominis	Microbiology

HOMOCYSTINE

75LPS	Urinary Homocystine (Non-Quantitative) Test System	Chemistry

HOMOGENIZER

83RAE	Homogenizer, Tissue	Microbiology

HOMOPOLYMER

76KOL	Carboxymethylcellulose Sodium/Ethylene-Oxide Homopolymer	Dental And Oral
76KXX	Homopolymer, Karaya and Ethylene-Oxide	Dental And Oral

HOOD

75QXU	Evacuator, Fume	Chemistry
90IXE	Hood and Exhaust, Nuclear	Radiology
75RAF	Hood, Chemical	Chemistry
91RAG	Hood, Fume	Toxicology
75JRN	Hood, Fume, Chemical	Chemistry
80RAH	Hood, Isolation, Laminar Air Flow	General
83RAI	Hood, Microbiological	Microbiology
80FOG	Hood, Oxygen, Infant	General
79FXY	Hood, Surgical	Surgery

HOOK

80RCM	Hanger, Intravenous	General
79KIK	Hook, Bone	Surgery
77RAJ	Hook, Cordotomy	Ear/Nose/Throat
85HDI	Hook, Destructive, Obstetrical	Obstetrics/Gyn
73BTB	Hook, Ether	Anesthesiology
89IQX	Hook, External Limb Component, Mechanical	Physical Med
89IQW	Hook, External Limb Component, Powered	Physical Med
85HDE	Hook, Fibroid, Gynecological	Obstetrics/Gyn
78FHB	Hook, Gastro-Urology	Gastro/Urology
85RAL	Hook, IUD Removal	Obstetrics/Gyn
77RAK	Hook, Incus	Ear/Nose/Throat
77JYL	Hook, Microsurgical Ear	Ear/Nose/Throat
86HNQ	Hook, Ophthalmic	Ophthalmology
79RAT	Hook, Other	Surgery
78RAM	Hook, Rectal	Gastro/Urology
79RAN	Hook, Rhinoplastic	Surgery
86RAO	Hook, Scleral Fixation	Ophthalmology
79RAP	Hook, Skin	Surgery
86RAQ	Hook, Strabismus	Ophthalmology
79GDG	Hook, Surgical, General & Plastic Surgery	Surgery
84RAR	Hook, Sympathectomy	Cns/Neurology
77KBP	Hook, Tonsil Suturing	Ear/Nose/Throat
77RAS	Hook, Tracheal	Ear/Nose/Throat
77KCH	Hook, Tracheal, ENT	Ear/Nose/Throat
84GZX	Instrument, Microsurgical	Cns/Neurology
84RDJ	Knife, Dura Hook	Cns/Neurology
85HHF	Remover, Intrauterine Device, Contraceptive (Hook Type)	Obstetrics/Gyn

HORMONE

82DHP	Antigen, Antiserum, Control, Luteinizing Hormone	Immunology
75CKG	Radioimmunoassay, ACTH	Chemistry
75CGJ	Radioimmunoassay, Follicle Stimulating Hormone	Chemistry
75CFL	Radioimmunoassay, Human Growth Hormone	Chemistry
75CEP	Radioimmunoassay, Luteinizing Hormone	Chemistry
75CEW	Radioimmunoassay, Parathyroid Hormone	Chemistry
75JLW	Radioimmunoassay, Thyroid Stimulating Hormone	Chemistry

HORSE

83JTL	Plasma, Coagulase, Human/Horse/Rabbit	Microbiology

HOSE

80FQL	Stocking, Elastic	General
89ILG	Stocking, Elastic, Physical Medicine	Physical Med
80DWL	Stocking, Support (Anti-Embolic)	General

HOSPITAL

80KMM	Bed, Adjustable Hospital	General
80UKP	Casters, Hospital Equipment	General
80VBH	Computer Software	General
80WSJ	Computer Software, Hospital/Nursing Management	General
80WOB	Meter, Patient Height	General
80TEQ	Sign, Hospital	General
80TES	Sink, Hospital	General
80WOE	System, Pipeline, Gas	General

HOST

90MOT	Irradiator, Blood to Prevent Graft Vs Host Disease	Radiology

HOT

80FPF	Bottle, Hot/Cold Water	General
89VFJ	Heater, Hot Pack	Physical Med
80LDS	Hot Water Pasteurization Device	General
89IMD	Pack, Hot Or Cold, Disposable	Physical Med

HOT (cont'd)

89IME	Pack, Hot Or Cold, Reusable	Physical Med
89ILO	Pack, Hot Or Cold, Water Circulating	Physical Med
80FRY	Pack, Hot, Chemical	General
75UGM	Plate, Hot	Chemistry
78KDO	Rongeur, Cystoscopic, Hot	Gastro/Urology
89UEC	Support, Hot/Cold Pack	Physical Med

HOUSE

80WIH	System, Transport, In-House	General

HOUSEKEEPING

80TAY	Cart, Housekeeping	General
80VBI	Housekeeping Equipment	General
80WNF	Towel/Towelette, Paper	General

HOUSING

90ITY	Housing, X-Ray Tube, Diagnostic	Radiology
90ITZ	Housing, X-Ray Tube, Therapeutic	Radiology

HPL

91DLK	Chromatograph, HPL, Drugs of Abuse (Dedicated Instrument)	Toxicology
75JMF	Radioimmunoassay, Human Placental Lactogen	Chemistry

HPLC

91MAS	Chromatography, Liquid, Performance, High	Toxicology
91LFI	High Pressure Liquid Chromatography, Tricyclic Drug	Toxicology

HRUBY

86HJI	Lens, Fundus, Hruby, Diagnostic	Ophthalmology

HS

82DEF	Antigen, Antiserum, Control, Alpha-2-HS-Glycoprotein	Immunology

HSV

83GQN	Antigen, Cf (including Cf Control), Herpesvirus Hominis 1, 2	Microbiology
83LKC	Antigen, Indirect Hemagglutination, Herpes Simplex Virus	Microbiology
83GQO	Antisera, Cf, Herpesvirus Hominis 1, 2	Microbiology
83GQL	Antisera, Fluorescent, Herpesvirus Hominis 1, 2	Microbiology
83GQM	Antiserum, Neutralization, Herpes Virus Hominis	Microbiology
83LGC	Enzyme Linked Immunoabsorbent Assay, Herpes Simplex Virus	Microbiology

HSV-1

83MXJ	Enzyme-Linked Immunosorbent Assay, Herpes Simplex Virus, HSV-1	Microbiology

HSV-2

83MYF	Enzyme-Linked Immunosorbent Assay, Herpes Simplex Virus, HSV-2	Microbiology

HTLV-1

81MTP	Antibody To HTLV-1, Elisa	Hematology

HTLV-III

81VJE	Test, Antibody, Acquired Immune Deficiency Syndrome (AIDS)	Hematology

HUB

74WTU	Adapter, Needle	Cardiovascular
80WSP	Tubing, Connecting	General

HUMAN

75JHJ	Agglutination Method, Human Chorionic Gonadotropin	Chemistry
83GMS	Anti-Human Globulin, FTA-ABS Test (Coombs)	Microbiology
81UJS	Anti-Human Serum, Manual	Hematology
82DGR	Antigen, Antiserum, Control, Whole Human Serum	Immunology
88KIR	Cultured Animal And Human Cells	Pathology
81MAO	DNA-Probe, Chromosome, Human	Hematology
84LEM	Dura Mater, Human, Lyophilized	Cns/Neurology
83MAQ	Kit, DNA Detection, Human Papillomavirus	Microbiology
83JTL	Plasma, Coagulase, Human/Horse/Rabbit	Microbiology
75JHI	Radioimmunoassay, Human Chorionic Gonadotropin	Chemistry
75CFL	Radioimmunoassay, Human Growth Hormone	Chemistry
75JMF	Radioimmunoassay, Human Placental Lactogen	Chemistry
88KPC	Serum, Human	Pathology
81KSX	Substance, Grouping, Blood (Non-Human Origin)	Hematology
75JZM	System, Gonadotropin, Chorionic, Human (Non-RIA)	Chemistry
81VJE	Test, Antibody, Acquired Immune Deficiency Syndrome (AIDS)	Hematology
82MZF	Test, Hiv Detection	Immunology
82JZN	Test, Human Chorionic Gonadotropin	Immunology
82DHA	Test, Human Chorionic Gonadotropin, Serum	Immunology
82DHT	Test, Human Placental Lactogen	Immunology
75LFS	Test, Radioreceptor, Human Chorionic Gonadotropin	Chemistry
75JHK	Titrimetric Method, Human Chorionic Gonadotropin	Chemistry
82DGQ	Whole Human Plasma, Antigen, Antiserum, Control	Immunology

HUMERAL

87KRM	Hemiprosthesis, Elbow (Humeral Resurfacing)	Orthopedics
87KWJ	Prosthesis, Elbow, Hemi-, Humeral, Metal	Orthopedics

HUMERAL (cont'd)
87UBN	Prosthesis, Elbow, Humeral Component	Orthopedics
87HSD	Prosthesis, Shoulder, Hemi-, Humeral	Orthopedics
87MJT	Prosthesis, Shoulder, Humeral, Bipol., Hemi-, Constr., M/P	Orthopedics

HUMIDIFIER
80QML	Controller, Temperature, Humidifier	General
80WUX	Dehumidifier	General
73RAU	Humidifier, Heat/Moisture Exchange	Anesthesiology
73RAV	Humidifier, Heated	Anesthesiology
73KFZ	Humidifier, Non-Direct Patient Interface (Home-Use)	Anesthesiology
73RAW	Humidifier, Non-Heated	Anesthesiology
73BTT	Humidifier, Respiratory Gas, (Direct Patient Interface)	Anesthesiology
73CAF	Nebulizer, Direct Patient Interface	Anesthesiology
73RHT	Nebulizer, Heated	Anesthesiology
77EPN	Nebulizer, Medicinal	Ear/Nose/Throat
73CCQ	Nebulizer, Medicinal, Non-Ventilatory (Atomizer)	Anesthesiology
73RHU	Nebulizer, Non-Heated	Anesthesiology
73RHV	Nebulizer, Ultrasonic	Anesthesiology
80SEQ	Vaporizer	General
73CAD	Vaporizer, Anesthesia, Non-Heated	Anesthesiology

HUMIDITY
73RAX	Hygrometer (Humidity Indicator)	Anesthesiology
80WSZ	Sensor, Moisture	General

HUMOR
76LZX	Acid, Hyaluoronic	Dental And Oral

HV
74MEZ	Device, Debridement, Ultrasonic, Heart Valve & HV Seat	Cardiovascular

HYALINE
75LTC	Assay, Disease, Membrane, Hyaline	Chemistry

HYALUORONIC
76LZX	Acid, Hyaluoronic	Dental And Oral

HYALURONIC
89MOZ	Acid, Hyaluronic, Intraarticular	Physical Med

HYALURONIDASE
88IBD	Hyaluronidase	Pathology

HYDRATE
91DJW	Reagent, Test, Chloral Hydrate	Toxicology

HYDRAULIC
80FNK	Bed, Hydraulic	General
90IYZ	Bed, Scanning, Nuclear/Fluoroscopic	Radiology
78FAP	Cystometric Gas (Carbon-Dioxide) Or Hydraulic Device	Gastro/Urology
78FEN	Device, Cystometric, Hydraulic	Gastro/Urology
78EZY	Device, Incontinence, Mechanical/Hydraulic	Gastro/Urology
80TCA	Extrication Equipment	General
78FHW	Impotence Device, Mechanical/Hydraulic	Gastro/Urology
78VKM	Lithotriptor, Electro-Hydraulic, Extracorporeal	Gastro/Urology
78FFK	Lithotriptor, Electro-Hydraulic, Percutaneous	Gastro/Urology
74JOM	Plethysmograph, Photo-Electric, Pneumatic Or Hydraulic	Cardiovascular
80TEW	Stretcher, Hydraulic	General
79FWY	Table, Surgical, Hydraulic	Surgery

HYDRAZINE
75JNS	Stannous Chloride - Hydrazine, Phospholipids	Chemistry

HYDRAZONE
75JKF	Dinitrophenyl Hydrazone Measurement (Colorimetric), HBD	Chemistry
75CJT	Hydrazone Colorimetry, Aldolase	Chemistry
75JKH	Hydrazone Derivative Of Alpha-Ketogluterate (Colorimetry)	Chemistry
75CDB	Porter Silber Hydrazone, 17-Hydroxycorticosteroids	Chemistry

HYDRO-MASSAGE
89ILJ	Bath, Hydro-Massage (Whirlpool)	Physical Med

HYDROCEPHALIC
84UCL	Catheter, Hydrocephalic	Cns/Neurology
84UBJ	Catheter, Hydrocephalic, Atrial	Cns/Neurology
84UAQ	Catheter, Hydrocephalic, Distal	Cns/Neurology
84UAR	Catheter, Hydrocephalic, Peritoneal	Cns/Neurology
84UCX	Catheter, Hydrocephalic, Ventricular	Cns/Neurology
84UAS	Connector, Hydrocephalic	Cns/Neurology
84QWB	Filter, Shunt, Hydrocephalic	Cns/Neurology
84RMU	Prosthesis, Hydrocephalic (Holter Valve)	Cns/Neurology
84UAT	Pump, Hydrocephalic	Cns/Neurology
84UCC	Reservoir, Hydrocephalic Catheter	Cns/Neurology
84RTC	Shunt, Hydrocephalic	Cns/Neurology

HYDROCEPHALUS
84LID	Ventriculo-Amniotic Shunt for Hydrocephalus	Cns/Neurology

HYDROCOLLATOR
89RHJ	Moist Therapy Pack Conditioner	Physical Med

HYDROGEL
80WKJ	Dressing, Gel	General
79MGQ	Dressing, Wound and Burn, Hydrogel	Surgery
79NAE	Dressing, Wound, Hydrogel W/out Drug And/or Biologic	Surgery

HYDROGEN
75UFP	Analyzer, Carbon Hydrogen	Chemistry
75UFQ	Analyzer, Carbon Hydrogen Nitrogen	Chemistry
73LXO	Analyzer, Gas, Hydrogen	Anesthesiology
73CBZ	Analyzer, Ion, Hydrogen-Ion (pH), Blood Phase, Indwelling	Anesthesiology
73CBY	Analyzer, Ion, Hydrogen-Ion pH, Blood Phase, Non-Indwelling	Anesthesiology
73WSV	Analyzer, Trace Gas, Breath	Anesthesiology
78LRI	Meter, pH, Concentration, Ion, Hydrogen, Dialysis	Gastro/Urology

HYDROGEN PEROXIDE
80RVZ	Sterilizer, Vapor	General

HYDROGEN-ION
73CBZ	Analyzer, Ion, Hydrogen-Ion (pH), Blood Phase, Indwelling	Anesthesiology
73CBY	Analyzer, Ion, Hydrogen-Ion pH, Blood Phase, Non-Indwelling	Anesthesiology

HYDROLASE
75MGT	Test, Diagnostic, Bana Hydrolase, Dental Plaque	Chemistry

HYDROLYSIS
75CDT	Lipase Hydrolysis/Glycerol Kinase Enzyme, Triglycerides	Chemistry

HYDROPHILIC
79KOZ	Beads, Hydrophilic, Wound Exudate Absorption	Surgery
76EBE	Coating, Denture Hydrophilic, Resin	Dental And Oral
79NAC	Dressing, Wound, Hydrophilic	Surgery
75UGD	Filter, Membrane	Chemistry
86WIZ	Lens, Contact, Disposable	Ophthalmology
86TGY	Lens, Contact, Hydrophilic	Ophthalmology

HYDROPHOBIC
75UGD	Filter, Membrane	Chemistry

HYDROTHERAPY
89ILJ	Bath, Hydro-Massage (Whirlpool)	Physical Med
80RZD	Tank, Full Body (Bath)	General

HYDROXIDE
76EJK	Liner, Cavity, Calcium Hydroxide	Dental And Oral
75JLK	Sodium Hydroxide/Phenol Red (Titrimetric), Gastric Acidity	Chemistry
88ICZ	Stain, Ammoniacal Silver Hydroxide Silver Nitrate	Pathology

HYDROXYAPATITE
79MGN	Cement, Hydroxyapatite	Surgery
87LMM	Ceramics, Triphos./Hydroxyapatite, Ca. (Load Bearing)	Orthopedics
87LMN	Ceramics, Triphos./Hydroxyapatite, Ca. (Non-Load Bearing)	Orthopedics
87QYR	Graft, Bone	Orthopedics
87WII	Hydroxyapatite	Orthopedics
84MHB	Hydroxyapatite (Cranioplasty)	Cns/Neurology

HYDROXYBUTYRIC
75JMK	Alpha-Ketobutyric Acid And NADH (U.V.), Hydroxybutyric	Chemistry

HYDROXYCORTICOSTEROIDS
75JHD	Fluorometric Method, 17-Hydroxycorticosteroids	Chemistry
75CDB	Porter Silber Hydrazone, 17-Hydroxycorticosteroids	Chemistry
75JHE	Radioassay, 17-Hydroxycorticosteroids	Chemistry

HYDROXYINDOLE
75CDA	Nitrous Acid & Nitrosonaphthol, 5-Hydroxyindole Acetic Acid	Chemistry

HYDROXYMATES
75JLG	Conversion Ferric Hydroxymates (Colorimetric), Fatty Acids	Chemistry

HYDROXYPHENYLIMINE
75CHZ	DI (O-Hydroxyphenylimine) Ethane, Calcium	Chemistry

HYDROXYPROGESTERONE
75JLX	Radioimmunoassay, 17-Hydroxyprogesterone	Chemistry

HYDROXYPROLINE
75JMM	Column, Chromatography, Hydroxyproline	Chemistry
75JMN	Extraction/Chromatography, Ninhydrin, Hydroxyproline	Chemistry

HYGIENE
89ILS	Adapter, Hygiene	Physical Med
80WHM	Cover, Seat, Toilet, Sanitary	General
76QOE	Cuspidor	Dental And Oral
80WIW	Dispenser, Tissue, Toilet	General
80WIX	Dispenser, Towel	General
80FQG	Mask, Oxygen, Other	General
80RHF	Mitt/Washcloth, Patient	General
78WHR	Plug, Ostomy	Gastro/Urology
76LCN	Scraper, Tongue	Dental And Oral

KEYWORD INDEX

IGD

82CZJ	Antigen, Antiserum, Control, IGD	Immunology
82DGG	Antigen, Antiserum, Control, IGD, FITC	Immunology
82DGH	Antigen, Antiserum, Control, IGD, Peroxidase	Immunology
82DGE	Antigen, Antiserum, Control, IGD, Rhodamine	Immunology

IGE

82DGC	Antigen, Antiserum, Control, IGE	Immunology
82DGP	Antigen, Antiserum, Control, IGE, FITC	Immunology
82DGO	Antigen, Antiserum, Control, IGE, Peroxidase	Immunology
82DGL	Antigen, Antiserum, Control, IGE, Rhodamine	Immunology
82DFM	IGE, Ferritin, Antigen, Antiserum, Control	Immunology

IGG

82DEW	Antigen, Antiserum, Control, IGG	Immunology
82DFK	Antigen, Antiserum, Control, IGG (FAB Fragment Specific)	Immunology
82DAS	Antigen, Antiserum, Control, IGG (Fc Fragment Specific)	Immunology
82DFZ	Antigen, Antiserum, Control, IGG (Gamma Chain Specific)	Immunology
82DGK	Antigen, Antiserum, Control, IGG, FITC	Immunology
82DAA	Antigen, Antiserum, Control, IGG, Peroxidase	Immunology
82DFO	Antigen, Antiserum, Control, IGG, Rhodamine	Immunology
83MYL	Assay, Enzyme Linked Immunosorbent, Parvovirus B19 Igg	Microbiology
82DAQ	IGG (FD Fragment Specific), Antigen, Antiserum, Control	Immunology
82KTO	IGG Immunoassay Reagents	Immunology
82DGD	IGG, Ferritin, Antigen, Antiserum, Control	Immunology
81LLG	Kit, Platelet Associated IGG	Hematology
82MLH	Strip, HAMA IGG, ELISA, In Vitro Test System	Immunology

IGM

83LJN	Antibody IGM, IF, Epstein-Barr Virus	Microbiology
83LKQ	Antibody Igm, If, Cytomegalovirus Virus	Microbiology
82DFT	Antigen, Antiserum, Control, IGM	Immunology
82DAO	Antigen, Antiserum, Control, IGM (Mu Chain Specific)	Immunology
82DFS	Antigen, Antiserum, Control, IGM, FITC	Immunology
82DEY	Antigen, Antiserum, Control, IGM, Peroxidase	Immunology
82DEZ	Antigen, Antiserum, Control, IGM, Rhodamine	Immunology
83MYM	Assay, Enzyme Linked Immunosorbent, Parvovirus B19 Igm	Microbiology
83LOM	Hepatitis B Test (B Core, BE Antigen & Antibody, B Core IGM)	Microbiology
82DFL	IGM, Ferritin, Antigen, Antiserum, Control	Immunology
83LOL	Test, Hepatitis A (Antibody and IGM Antibody)	Microbiology

IHA

83LJO	Antigen, IHA, Cytomegalovirus	Microbiology
83GND	Antigen, IHA, T. Cruzi	Microbiology
83GMM	Antigen, IHA, Toxoplasma Gondii	Microbiology
83LKC	Antigen, Indirect Hemagglutination, Herpes Simplex Virus	Microbiology

ILEOSTOMY

78EXH	Bag, Urinary, Ileostomy	Gastro/Urology
78KPH	Catheter, Rectal, Ileostomy, Continent	Gastro/Urology
78RJF	Ostomy Appliance (Ileostomy, Colostomy)	Gastro/Urology

ILLUMINATED

78FDG	Retractor, Fiberoptic	Gastro/Urology
79FXF	Speculum, Illuminated	Surgery
79FXE	Speculum, Non-Illuminated	Surgery
73RXA	Tip, Suction, Fiberoptic Illuminated	Anesthesiology

ILLUMINATOR

86HJD	Illuminator, Color Vision Plate	Ophthalmology
78FFS	Illuminator, Fiberoptic (For Endoscope)	Gastro/Urology
84HBI	Illuminator, Fiberoptic, Surgical Field	Cns/Neurology
79FTF	Illuminator, Non-Remote	Surgery
90IXC	Illuminator, Radiographic Film	Radiology
90JAG	Illuminator, Radiographic Film, Explosion-Proof	Radiology
79FTG	Illuminator, Remote	Surgery
76EAR	Illuminator, Ultraviolet	Dental And Oral
77SHF	Lamp, Laryngoscope	Ear/Nose/Throat
90WUY	Viewer, Radiographic Film, Motorized	Radiology

IMAGE

90TAS	Camera, Multi-Image	Radiology
80WKP	Camera, Other	General
80WZQ	Camera, Video, Multi-Image	General
90VGU	Chemical, Film Processor	Radiology
80WLE	Computer, Image, Endoscopic	General
90UFD	Computer, Radiographic Image Analysis	Radiology
90WUK	Copier, Image, Radiographic	Radiology
90LMB	Device, Storage, Image, Digital	Radiology
90TFQ	Duplicator, X-Ray Film	Radiology
86HIZ	Flasher, After-Image	Ophthalmology
90LMA	Image Digitizer	Radiology
90TCP	Image Intensification System	Radiology
90LLZ	Image Processing System	Radiology
80VAZ	Microfilm/Microfiche Equipment	General
80WLN	Printer, Image, Video	General
90RNW	Printer, Radiographic Duplicator	Radiology

IMAGE *(cont'd)*

74WTO	Probe, Transesophageal	Cardiovascular
90JAA	Radiographic/Fluoroscopic Unit, Image-Intensified	Radiology
90JAB	Radiographic/Fluoroscopic Unit, Non-Image-Intensified	Radiology
90ROQ	Recorder, Radiographic Video Tape	Radiology
90VFM	Recorder, X-Ray Image	Radiology
90LQA	Reusable Image Media	Radiology
90VGY	Storage Device, Fluoroscopic Image	Radiology
90LMD	System, Communication, Image, Digital	Radiology
82WUO	Test, Cancer Detection, QFI	Immunology
90WOG	Transmitter, Image & Data, Radiographic	Radiology
90IZE	Tube, Image Amplifier, X-Ray	Radiology
86HOT	Vision Aid, Image Intensification, Battery-Powered	Ophthalmology

IMAGE-INTENSIFIED

90JAA	Radiographic/Fluoroscopic Unit, Image-Intensified	Radiology
90JAB	Radiographic/Fluoroscopic Unit, Non-Image-Intensified	Radiology

IMAGER

90IXK	Imager, X-Ray, Electrostatic	Radiology
90MQB	Imager, X-Ray, Solid State (Flat Panel/Digital)	Radiology
90IYN	Scanner, Ultrasonic (Pulsed Doppler)	Radiology
90IYO	Scanner, Ultrasonic (Pulsed Echo)	Radiology
85RQW	Scanner, Ultrasonic, Breast (Mammographic)	Obstetrics/Gyn
85HEM	Scanner, Ultrasonic, Obstetrical/Gynecological	Obstetrics/Gyn
85RQX	Scanner, Ultrasonic, Obstetrical/Gynecological, Mobile	Obstetrics/Gyn
90HPR	Scanner, Ultrasonic, Ophthalmic	Radiology

IMAGING

90WNR	Angio-Dynograph	Radiology
84HBY	Catheter, Angiographic	Cns/Neurology
90WIO	Catheter, Imaging, Ultrasonic	Radiology
79WIY	Computer, Imaging, Presurgery	Surgery
90QMD	Computer, Nuclear Medicine	Radiology
90WKA	Computer, Radiographic Data	Radiology
90VCO	Gantry, Nuclear Imaging	Radiology
90WPG	Gas Mixtures, Magnetic Resonance Imaging	Radiology
84HAP	Guide, Wire, Angiographic (And Accessories)	Cns/Neurology
74DXT	Injector, Angiographic (Cardiac Catheterization)	Cardiovascular
90VGB	Kit, Angiographic, Digital	Radiology
90VGC	Kit, Angiographic, Special Procedure	Radiology
90WRT	Magnet, Permanent, MRI (Magnetic Resonance Imaging)	Radiology
90VIM	Magnet, Superconducting, MRI (Magnetic Resonance Imaging)	Radiology
84HAQ	Needle, Angiographic	Cns/Neurology
90LNH	Nuclear Magnetic Resonance Imaging System	Radiology
90VLE	Radiographic Unit, Digital Subtraction Angiographic (DSA)	Radiology
90IZI	Radiographic/Fluoroscopic Unit, Angiographic	Radiology
90VHC	Radiographic/Fluoroscopic Unit, Angiographic, Digital	Radiology
90WJP	Stand, Cardiovascular	Radiology
90WLW	Stand, Vascular	Radiology
90RYK	Synchronizer, Radiographic Unit	Radiology
90SIK	System, Imaging, Laparoscopy, Ultrasonic	Radiology
86WXT	System, Mapping, Corneal	Ophthalmology
90WTF	Unit, Imaging, Thermal	Radiology
90WJC	Videofluoroscopic Unit	Radiology

IMMERSION

83UGJ	Heater, Immersion	Microbiology
81GLF	Oil, Immersion	Hematology
88KIO	Stainer, Slide, Immersion Type	Pathology

IMMITIS

83GMI	Antigen, CF And/Or ID, Coccidioides Immitis	Microbiology
83GMG	Antigen, Latex Agglutination, Coccidioides Immitis	Microbiology
83GMH	Antiserum, Positive Control, Coccidioides Immitis	Microbiology
83MIY	Enzyme Linked Immunoabsorbent Assay, Coccidioides Immitis	Microbiology
83MDF	Reagent, DNA-Probe, Coccidioides Immitis	Microbiology

IMMOBILIZATION

80WLB	Mattress, Immobilization	General

IMMOBILIZER

90WJW	Accessories, Radiotherapy	Radiology
87QHE	Cast	Orthopedics
80WMR	Collar, Extrication	General
87RBF	Immobilizer, Ankle	Orthopedics
87RBG	Immobilizer, Arm	Orthopedics
87RBH	Immobilizer, Cervical	Orthopedics
87RBI	Immobilizer, Elbow	Orthopedics
87RBJ	Immobilizer, Infant (Circumcision Board)	Orthopedics
80RCJ	Immobilizer, Intravenous Catheter-Needle	General
87RBK	Immobilizer, Knee	Orthopedics
87RBL	Immobilizer, Shoulder	Orthopedics
90WUB	Immobilizer, Therapy, Radiation	Radiology
87WUW	Immobilizer, Upper Body	Orthopedics
87RBM	Immobilizer, Wrist/Hand	Orthopedics
80WLB	Mattress, Immobilization	General
80FMQ	Restraint, Protective (Body)	General

KEYWORD INDEX

IMMOBILIZER *(cont'd)*

89IPG	Shoe, Cast	Physical Med
87RUA	Sock, Cast Toe	Orthopedics
87WUU	Splint, Abduction, Shoulder	Orthopedics
79FZF	Splint, Extremity, Inflatable, External	Surgery
79FYH	Splint, Extremity, Non-Inflatable, External	Surgery
87RUW	Splint, Molded, Aluminum	Orthopedics
87RUX	Splint, Molded, Plastic	Orthopedics
73CCX	Support, Patient Position	Anesthesiology
90RNX	Support, Patient Position, Radiographic	Radiology

IMMUNE

81VJE	Test, Antibody, Acquired Immune Deficiency Syndrome (AIDS)	Hematology
82MZF	Test, Hiv Detection	Immunology

IMMUNITY

83NCD	Test, Immunity, Cell-Mediated, Mycobacterium Tuberculosis	Microbiology

IMMUNO-HEMATOLOGY

81KSN	Centrifuge, Cell Washing, Automated, Immuno-Hematology	Hematology

IMMUNOABSORBENT

83MDU	Antigen, Enzyme Linked Immunoabsorbent Assay, Cryptococcus	Microbiology
83LJC	Enzyme Linked Immunoabsorbent Assay, Chlamydia Group	Microbiology
83MIY	Enzyme Linked Immunoabsorbent Assay, Coccidioides Immitis	Microbiology
83LFZ	Enzyme Linked Immunoabsorbent Assay, Cytomegalovirus	Microbiology
83LGC	Enzyme Linked Immunoabsorbent Assay, Herpes Simplex Virus	Microbiology
83MIZ	Enzyme Linked Immunoabsorbent Assay, Histoplasma Capsulatum	Microbiology
83LJY	Enzyme Linked Immunoabsorbent Assay, Mumps Virus	Microbiology
83LJZ	Enzyme Linked Immunoabsorbent Assay, Mycoplasma SPP.	Microbiology
83LIR	Enzyme Linked Immunoabsorbent Assay, Neisseria Gonorrhoeae	Microbiology
83MCE	Enzyme Linked Immunoabsorbent Assay, Resp. Syncytial Virus	Microbiology
83LIQ	Enzyme Linked Immunoabsorbent Assay, Rotavirus	Microbiology
83LFX	Enzyme Linked Immunoabsorbent Assay, Rubella	Microbiology
83LJB	Enzyme Linked Immunoabsorbent Assay, Rubeola	Microbiology
83MIU	Enzyme Linked Immunoabsorbent Assay, T. Cruzi	Microbiology
83LGD	Enzyme Linked Immunoabsorbent Assay, Toxoplasma Gondii	Microbiology
83LIP	Enzyme Linked Immunoabsorbent Assay, Treponema Pallidum	Microbiology
83MDT	Enzyme Linked Immunoabsorbent Assay, Trichinella Spiralis	Microbiology
83LFY	Enzyme Linked Immunoabsorbent Assay, Varicella-Zoster	Microbiology

IMMUNOADSORPTION

80WON	Column, Immunoadsorption	General
78LQQ	Column, Immunoadsorption, System, Extracorporeal	Gastro/Urology

IMMUNOASSAY

75UJM	Analyzer, Chemistry, ELISA	Chemistry
75UEH	Analyzer, Chemistry, Enzyme Immunoassay	Chemistry
75UEI	Analyzer, Chemistry, Fluorescence Immunoassay	Chemistry
75WMG	Analyzer, Chemistry, Nephelometric Immunoassay	Chemistry
82KTK	Carbonic Anhydrase B And C Immunoassay Reagents	Immunology
91DKZ	Enzyme Immunoassay, Amphetamine	Toxicology
91DIS	Enzyme Immunoassay, Barbiturate	Toxicology
91JXM	Enzyme Immunoassay, Benzodiazepine	Toxicology
91LDJ	Enzyme Immunoassay, Cannabinoids	Toxicology
91KLT	Enzyme Immunoassay, Carbamazepine	Toxicology
91JXO	Enzyme Immunoassay, Cocaine	Toxicology
91DIO	Enzyme Immunoassay, Cocaine And Cocaine Metabolites	Toxicology
91LFM	Enzyme Immunoassay, Digitoxin	Toxicology
91KXT	Enzyme Immunoassay, Digoxin	Toxicology
91DIP	Enzyme Immunoassay, Diphenylhydantoin	Toxicology
91DLF	Enzyme Immunoassay, Ethosuximide	Toxicology
75MKV	Enzyme Immunoassay, Fetal Fibronectin	Chemistry
75MGW	Enzyme Immunoassay, Gamma Enolase	Chemistry
91LCD	Enzyme Immunoassay, Gentamicin	Toxicology
91KLR	Enzyme Immunoassay, Lidocaine	Toxicology
91DJR	Enzyme Immunoassay, Methadone	Toxicology
91LAO	Enzyme Immunoassay, Methotrexate	Toxicology
91LAN	Enzyme Immunoassay, N-Acetylprocainamide	Toxicology
91MKU	Enzyme Immunoassay, Nicotine and Nicotine Metabolites	Toxicology
75KLI	Enzyme Immunoassay, Non-Radiolabeled, Total Thyroxine	Chemistry
91DJG	Enzyme Immunoassay, Opiates	Toxicology
75VKK	Enzyme Immunoassay, Other	Chemistry
91LCM	Enzyme Immunoassay, Phencyclidine	Toxicology

IMMUNOASSAY *(cont'd)*

91DLZ	Enzyme Immunoassay, Phenobarbital	Toxicology
91DJD	Enzyme Immunoassay, Primidone	Toxicology
91LAR	Enzyme Immunoassay, Procainamide	Toxicology
91JXN	Enzyme Immunoassay, Propoxyphene	Toxicology
91LBZ	Enzyme Immunoassay, Quinidine	Toxicology
91MLM	Enzyme Immunoassay, Tacrolimus	Toxicology
91KLS	Enzyme Immunoassay, Theophylline	Toxicology
91LEG	Enzyme Immunoassay, Valproic Acid	Toxicology
82MLE	Enzyme, Immunoassay, Antipartietal, Antigen Control	Immunology
91LGJ	Fluorescence Polarization Immunoassay, Amibacin	Toxicology
91LGI	Fluorescence Polarization Immunoassay, Carbamazepine	Toxicology
91LGR	Fluorescence Polarization Immunoassay, Diphenylhydantoin	Toxicology
91LGQ	Fluorescence Polarization Immunoassay, Phenobarbital	Toxicology
91LGS	Fluorescence Polarization Immunoassay, Theophylline	Toxicology
91LFW	Fluorescence Polarization Immunoassay, Tobramycin	Toxicology
75MGU	Fluorescence Polarization, Immunoassay, Cyclosporine	Chemistry
91LCQ	Fluorescent Immunoassay Gentamicin	Toxicology
91LES	Fluorescent Immunoassay, Diphenylhydantoin	Toxicology
91LET	Fluorescent Immunoassay, Phenobarbital	Toxicology
91LFT	Fluorescent Immunoassay, Primidone	Toxicology
91LER	Fluorescent Immunoassay, Theophylline	Toxicology
91LCR	Fluorescent Immunoassay, Tobramycin	Toxicology
82KTO	IGG Immunoassay Reagents	Immunology
91WQE	Immunoassay, Other	Toxicology
91LFO	Nephelometric Inhibition Immunoassay, Diphenylhydantoin	Toxicology
91LFN	Nephelometric Inhibition Immunoassay, Phenobarbital	Toxicology
82KTP	Reagent, Immunoassay, Activator, C3, Complement	Immunology

IMMUNOCHEMICAL

82JKM	Immunochemical, Bence-Jones Protein	Immunology
82CHN	Immunochemical, Ceruloplasmin	Immunology
75JMR	Immunochemical, Lysozyme (Muramidase)	Chemistry
82JNL	Immunochemical, Thyroglobulin Autoantibody	Immunology
82JNM	Immunochemical, Transferrin	Immunology

IMMUNODEFICIENCY

82MZF	Test, Hiv Detection	Immunology

IMMUNODIFFUSION

75RBN	Immunodiffusion Equipment (Agar Cutter)	Chemistry
75CGM	Immunodiffusion Method, Immunoglobulins (G, A, M)	Chemistry
75JQK	Immunodiffusion, Protein Fractionation	Chemistry
82JZQ	Plate, Radial Immunodiffusion	Immunology
75CJQ	Radial Immunodiffusion, Albumin	Chemistry
75JHP	Radial Immunodiffusion, Lipoproteins	Chemistry
83WJV	Reader, Radial Immunodiffusion	Microbiology

IMMUNOELECTROPHORESIS

82JZX	Equipment, Immunoelectrophoresis, Rocket	Immunology

IMMUNOELECTROPHORETIC

75CFF	Immunoelectrophoretic, Immunoglobulins, (G, A, M)	Chemistry

IMMUNOFLUORESCENCE

82RBO	Immunofluorescence Equipment	Immunology

IMMUNOFLUORESCENT

82KTL	Anti-DNA Indirect Immunofluorescent Solid Phase	Immunology
82DBE	Antibody, Anti-Smooth Muscle, Indirect Immunofluorescent	Immunology
82WQF	Antibody, Anti-Thyroid, Indirect Immunofluorescent	Immunology
82DBM	Antibody, Antimitochondrial, Indirect Immunofluorescent	Immunology
82DHN	Antibody, Antinuclear, Indirect Immunofluorescent, Antigen	Immunology
82DBL	Antibody, Multiple Auto, Indirect Immunofluorescent	Immunology
83WJQ	Antibody, Treponema Pallidum	Microbiology
82DBJ	Antiparietal Antibody, Immunofluorescent, Antigen, Control	Immunology
82KTM	C3-Indirect Immunofluorescent Solid Phase	Immunology
83MIV	Immunofluorescent Assay, T. Cruzi	Microbiology

IMMUNOGLOBULINS

75CGM	Immunodiffusion Method, Immunoglobulins (G, A, M)	Chemistry
75CFF	Immunoelectrophoretic, Immunoglobulins, (G, A, M)	Chemistry
75CFN	Nephelometric Method, Immunoglobulins (G, A, M)	Chemistry
82JHR	Radioimmunoassay, Immunoglobulins (D, E)	Immunology
75CFQ	Radioimmunoassay, Immunoglobulins (G, A, M)	Chemistry

IMMUNOHISTOCHEMICAL

88LIJ	Stain, Peroxidase Anti-Peroxidase Immunohistochemical	Pathology

IMMUNOHISTOCHEMISTRY

88MYA	Immunohistochemistry Assay, Antibody, Estrogen Receptor	Pathology
88MXZ	Immunohistochemistry Assay, Antibody, Progesterone Receptor	Pathology

IMMUNOLOGICAL

82MID	System, Test, Anticardiolipin, Immunological	Immunology
82MOI	System, Test, Immunological, Antigen, Tumor	Immunology

IMMUNOLOGY

82JZS	Electrophoresis Instrumentation	Immunology

IMMUNOLOGY *(cont'd)*

82JZW	Nephelometer, Immunology	Immunology

IMMUNOPEROXIDASE

83LKH	Antisera, Immunoperoxidase, Chlamydia SPP.	Microbiology

IMMUNOREACTIVE

75CFP	Radioimmunoassay, Immunoreactive Insulin	Chemistry

IMMUNOSORBENT

83MZO	Assay, Enzyme Linked Immunosorbent, Hepatitis C Virus	Microbiology
83MYL	Assay, Enzyme Linked Immunosorbent, Parvovirus B19 Igg	Microbiology
83MYM	Assay, Enzyme Linked Immunosorbent, Parvovirus B19 Igm	Microbiology
75MMI	Enzymatic Method, Troponin Subunit	Chemistry
83MXJ	Enzyme-Linked Immunosorbent Assay, Herpes Simplex Virus, HSV-1	Microbiology
83MYF	Enzyme-Linked Immunosorbent Assay, Herpes Simplex Virus, HSV-2	Microbiology

IMPACTOR

87HWA	Impactor	Orthopedics

IMPEDANCE

80VDN	Analyzer, Composition, Weight, Patient	General
74RBP	Cardiograph, Impedance	Cardiovascular
79KFR	Monitor, Cardiac Output, Impedance Plethysmography	Surgery
73RBQ	Monitor, Impedance Pneumograph	Anesthesiology
74DQB	Phlebograph, Impedance	Cardiovascular
74DSB	Plethysmograph, Impedance	Cardiovascular
77ETY	Tester, Auditory Impedance	Ear/Nose/Throat
80QYX	Tester, Ground Loop Impedance	General

IMPLANT

78KNZ	Accessories, AV Shunt	Gastro/Urology
74MIE	Allograft, Heart Valve	Cardiovascular
87SHK	Assistant, Surgical, Orthopedic, Automated	Orthopedics
74DSW	Bag, Polymeric Mesh, Pacemaker	Cardiovascular
74DSZ	Battery, Pacemaker	Cardiovascular
87HTN	Bolt, Nut, Washer	Orthopedics
87MBB	Bone Cement, Antibiotic	Orthopedics
87JDT	Cap, Bone	Orthopedics
84UBI	Cap, Nerve	Cns/Neurology
86UAX	Cap, Ophthalmic, Quarter Globe	Ophthalmology
84UCL	Catheter, Hydrocephalic	Cns/Neurology
84UBJ	Catheter, Hydrocephalic, Atrial	Cns/Neurology
84UAQ	Catheter, Hydrocephalic, Distal	Cns/Neurology
84UAR	Catheter, Hydrocephalic, Peritoneal	Cns/Neurology
84UCX	Catheter, Hydrocephalic, Ventricular	Cns/Neurology
74MFC	Catheter, Occluding, Cardiovascular, Implantable	Cardiovascular
74DYD	Catheter, Vascular, Long-Term	Cardiovascular
77MLI	Cement, Bone, Ionomer	Ear/Nose/Throat
87JDQ	Cerclage, Fixation	Orthopedics
79MCH	Clip, Hemostatic	Surgery
79FZP	Clip, Implantable	Surgery
87JEC	Component, Traction, Invasive	Orthopedics
84UAS	Connector, Hydrocephalic	Cns/Neurology
80LPZ	Container, Frozen Donor Tissue Storage	General
78KDK	Container, Transport, Kidney	Gastro/Urology
84GXR	Cover, Burr Hole (Cranial)	Cns/Neurology
79RTO	Cutter, Skin Graft	Surgery
79RTP	Cutter, Skin Graft, Expanded Mesh	Surgery
74LWS	Defibrillator, Implantable, Automatic	Cardiovascular
78MIP	Device, Incontinence, Fecal, Implanted	Gastro/Urology
84MIT	Device, Nerve Repair, Resorbable	Cns/Neurology
79MLB	Device, Repeat Access (Abdomen)	Surgery
80QRA	Dressing, Skin Graft, Donor Site	General
84GXQ	Dura-Substitute	Cns/Neurology
74UCG	Electrode, Pacemaker, Transthoracic	Cardiovascular
79LCJ	Expander, Skin, Inflatable	Surgery
79FZW	Expander, Surgical, Skin Graft	Surgery
86HQI	Eye, Artificial, Custom	Ophthalmology
86HQH	Eye, Artificial, Non-Custom	Ophthalmology
87MBI	Fastener, Fixation, Non-Biodegradable, Soft Tissue	Orthopedics
79UKN	Felt	Surgery
74UAF	Felt, Cardiovascular	Cardiovascular
87TCT	Fixation Device, Jaw Fracture	Orthopedics
87UAP	Fixation Device, Spinal (External)	Orthopedics
86TCI	Freezer, Eye Bank	Ophthalmology
74WNZ	Graft, Bifurcation	Cardiovascular
87QYR	Graft, Bone	Orthopedics
79QYS	Graft, Bovine	Surgery
79QYT	Graft, Skin	Surgery
77MKE	Hearing-Aid, Bone-Conduction, Percutaneous	Ear/Nose/Throat
77MMB	Hearing-Aid, External, Magnet, Membrane, Tympanic	Ear/Nose/Throat
77LRB	Hearing-Aid, Plate, Face	Ear/Nose/Throat
86HQJ	Implant, Absorbable (Scleral Buckling Method)	Ophthalmology
78LEI	Implant, Anti-Gastroesophageal Reflux	Gastro/Urology

IMPLANT *(cont'd)*

77MHE	Implant, Auditory Brainstem	Ear/Nose/Throat
77MCM	Implant, Cochlear	Ear/Nose/Throat
79LMI	Implant, Collagen (Non-Aesthetic Use)	Surgery
79LMH	Implant, Collagen, Dermal (Aesthetic Use)	Surgery
86LQE	Implant, Corneal	Ophthalmology
76DZE	Implant, Endosseous	Dental And Oral
76LYC	Implant, Endosseous (Bone Filling and/or Augmentation)	Dental And Oral
86KYF	Implant, Eye Valve	Ophthalmology
85MCQ	Implant, Female Incontinence	Obstetrics/Gyn
87JDP	Implant, Fixation Device, Condylar Plate	Orthopedics
87JDO	Implant, Fixation Device, Proximal Femoral	Orthopedics
87JDN	Implant, Fixation Device, Spinal	Orthopedics
79MFH	Implant, Integrated Tissue	Surgery
86LZT	Implant, Intracorneal	Ophthalmology
78LTI	Implant, Intragastric, Obesity, Morbid	Gastro/Urology
76LZD	Implant, Joint, Temporomandibular	Dental And Oral
79MIC	Implant, Muscle, Pectoralis	Surgery
86HQX	Implant, Orbital, Extra-Ocular	Ophthalmology
77MKK	Implant, Phonosurgery	Ear/Nose/Throat
86WJZ	Implant, Retinal	Ophthalmology
86WUA	Implant, Scleral	Ophthalmology
76ELE	Implant, Subperiosteal	Dental And Oral
79MNF	Implant, Temporal	Surgery
76MDL	Implant, Transmandibular	Dental And Oral
86THQ	Insert, Dry Eye	Ophthalmology
84MBZ	Instrument, Electrosurgical, Field Focused	Cns/Neurology
85HDT	Intrauterine Device, Contraceptive (IUD) And Introducer	Obstetrics/Gyn
86HQK	Keratoprosthesis, Custom	Ophthalmology
86HQM	Keratoprosthesis, Non-Custom	Ophthalmology
86MLP	Keratoprosthesis, Temporary Implant, Surgical	Ophthalmology
79RDQ	Knife, Skin Grafting	Surgery
77ESE	Larynx, Artificial Battery-Powered	Ear/Nose/Throat
74UCH	Lead, Pacemaker (Catheter)	Cardiovascular
74QIG	Lead, Pacemaker, Implantable Endocardial	Cardiovascular
74UCI	Lead, Pacemaker, Temporary Endocardial	Cardiovascular
86HQL	Lens, Intraocular	Ophthalmology
86UBA	Lens, Intraocular, Anterior Chamber	Ophthalmology
86UBB	Lens, Intraocular, Iridocapsular Fixation	Ophthalmology
86UBC	Lens, Intraocular, Iris Fixation	Ophthalmology
86UBD	Lens, Intraocular, Posterior Chamber	Ophthalmology
79LZK	Malar Implant	Surgery
77ESG	Material, Metallic-Stainless Steel, Tantalum, Platinum	Ear/Nose/Throat
79KKY	Material, PTFE/Carbon, Maxillofacial	Surgery
80WUG	Material, Polymethylmethacrylate	General
74UAK	Mesh, Cardiovascular (Polymeric)	Cardiovascular
87UBH	Mesh, Orthopedic (Metallic)	Orthopedics
79FTM	Mesh, Surgical (Steel Gauze)	Surgery
79FTL	Mesh, Surgical, Polymeric	Surgery
87JDS	Nail, Fixation, Bone	Orthopedics
78RIZ	Organ Preservation System	Gastro/Urology
87MOO	Orthopedic Implant Material	Orthopedics
78EZT	Pacemaker, Bladder	Gastro/Urology
74UMI	Pacemaker, Heart, Implantable, Anti-Tachycardia	Cardiovascular
74ULJ	Pacemaker, Heart, Implantable, Dual Chamber	Cardiovascular
74DXY	Pacemaker, Heart, Implantable, Programmable	Cardiovascular
74WST	Pacemaker, Heart, Implantable, Rate Responsive	Cardiovascular
74UJO	Patch, Myocardial	Cardiovascular
87HTY	Pin, Fixation, Smooth	Orthopedics
87JDW	Pin, Fixation, Threaded	Orthopedics
84RLI	Plate, Bone, Skull (Cranioplasty)	Cns/Neurology
84GWO	Plate, Bone, Skull, Preformed, Alterable	Cns/Neurology
84GXN	Plate, Bone, Skull, Preformed, Non-Alterable	Cns/Neurology
87HRS	Plate, Fixation, Bone	Orthopedics
74DXZ	Pledget And Intracardiac Patch, PETP, PTFE, Polypropylene	Cardiovascular
74DSX	Pledget, Dacron, Teflon, Polypropylene	Cardiovascular
77ESF	Polymer, ENT Composite Synthetic PTFE With Carbon-Fiber	Ear/Nose/Throat
77JOF	Polymer, ENT Synthetic, Porous Polyethylene	Ear/Nose/Throat
77ESH	Polymer, ENT Synthetic-PIFE, Silicon Elastomer	Ear/Nose/Throat
77ESI	Polymer, Natural Absorbable Gelatin Material	Ear/Nose/Throat
80MHC	Port, Intraosseous, Implantable	General
74THP	Port, Vascular Access	Cardiovascular
87KXC	Prosthesis, Ankle, Non-Constrained	Orthopedics
87MBK	Prosthesis, Ankle, Semi-, Uncemented, Porous, Metal/Polymer	Orthopedics
87KMD	Prosthesis, Ankle, Semi-Constrained, Metal/Composite	Orthopedics
87HSN	Prosthesis, Ankle, Semi-Constrained, Metal/Polymer	Orthopedics
87UBK	Prosthesis, Ankle, Talar Component	Orthopedics
87UBL	Prosthesis, Ankle, Tibial Component	Orthopedics
78UDE	Prosthesis, Anti-Gastroesophageal Reflux	Gastro/Urology
87RMN	Prosthesis, Arm	Orthopedics
79FZC	Prosthesis, Arterial Graft, Bovine Carotid Artery	Surgery
79FZB	Prosthesis, Arterial Graft, Synthetic, Greater Than 6mm	Surgery
79JCP	Prosthesis, Arterial Graft, Synthetic, Less Than 6mm	Surgery
87UCR	Prosthesis, Bone Cerclage	Orthopedics

IMPLANT *(cont'd)*

76LTE	System, Implant, Tooth	Dental And Oral
80TGT	System, Infusion, Administration, Drug, Implantable	General
86WQU	Tissue, Corneal	Ophthalmology
77LBL	Tube, Tympanostomy, Porous Polyethylene	Ear/Nose/Throat
80WTH	Tubing, Polytetrafluoroethylene	General
87UBT	Wire, Bone	Orthopedics

IMPLANTABLE

74LOY	Cardioconverter, Implantable	Cardiovascular
80LMP	Catheter, Intraspinal, Subcutaneous, Implantable	General
74MFC	Catheter, Occluding, Cardiovascular, Implantable	Cardiovascular
79FZP	Clip, Implantable	Surgery
84HBP	Clip, Implantable, Malleable	Cns/Neurology
74MEY	Cuff, Treatment, Varicose Vein, Implantable	Cardiovascular
74LWS	Defibrillator, Implantable, Automatic	Cardiovascular
80LMQ	Device, Access, Peritoneal, Subcutaneous, Implantable	General
74LWP	Dual Chamber, Implantable Pulse Generator	Cardiovascular
74QIG	Lead, Pacemaker, Implantable Endocardial	Cardiovascular
74DTB	Lead, Pacemaker, Implantable Myocardial	Cardiovascular
84LII	Monitor, Pressure, Intracranial, Implantable	Cns/Neurology
74UMI	Pacemaker, Heart, Implantable, Anti-Tachycardia	Cardiovascular
74ULJ	Pacemaker, Heart, Implantable, Dual Chamber	Cardiovascular
74VHM	Pacemaker, Heart, Implantable, Non-Programmable	Cardiovascular
74DXY	Pacemaker, Heart, Implantable, Programmable	Cardiovascular
74WST	Pacemaker, Heart, Implantable, Rate Responsive	Cardiovascular
80MHC	Port, Intraosseous, Implantable	General
78THF	Pump, Infusion, Implantable	Gastro/Urology
80LKK	Pump, Infusion, Implantable, General	General
80MDY	Pump, Infusion, Implantable, Non-Programmable	General
74LWO	Single Chamber, Sensor Driven, Implantable Pulse Generator	Cardiovascular
79GDW	Staple, Implantable	Surgery
84GZA	Stimulator, Cerebral, Implantable	Cns/Neurology
84LGT	Stimulator, Cord, Spinal, Implantable (Motor Disorders)	Cns/Neurology
84LLE	Stimulator, Cord, Spinal, Implantable (Periph. Vasc. Dis.)	Cns/Neurology
84GZE	Stimulator, Diaphragmatic/Phrenic Nerve, Implantable	Cns/Neurology
78KPI	Stimulator, Incontinence (Non-Implantable), Electrical	Gastro/Urology
84GYZ	Stimulator, Intracerebral/Subcortical, Implantable	Cns/Neurology
84LYJ	Stimulator, Nerve, Autonomic, Implantable (Epilepsy)	Cns/Neurology
84GZF	Stimulator, Peripheral Nerve, Implantable (Pain Relief)	Cns/Neurology
84GZB	Stimulator, Spinal Cord, Implantable (Pain Relief)	Cns/Neurology
84GZD	Stimulator, Spinal Cord, Implantable, Bladder Evacuator	Cns/Neurology
84LYI	Stimulator, Subcortical, Implanted For Epilepsy	Cns/Neurology
80TGT	System, Infusion, Administration, Drug, Implantable	General
84LSS	Unit, Repair, Nerve, Implantable, Electric	Cns/Neurology

IMPLANTATION

86VEU	Clip, Lens Implantation	Ophthalmology
84GYK	Instrument, Implantation, Shunt	Cns/Neurology
87RNB	Prosthesis Implantation Instrument, Orthopedic	Orthopedics

IMPLANTED

78MSD	Catheter, Hemodialysis, Implanted	Gastro/Urology
80LJT	Catheter, Subcutaneous Intravascular, Implanted	General
80LKG	Catheter, Subcutaneous Intraventricular, Implanted	General
80LLD	Catheter, Subcutaneous Peritoneal, Implanted	General
78MIP	Device, Incontinence, Fecal, Implanted	Gastro/Urology
84MFO	Electrode, Recording, Cortical, Implanted	Cns/Neurology
77MAH	Hearing-Aid, Bone-Conduction, Implanted	Ear/Nose/Throat
80MDX	Port & Catheter, Infusion, Implanted, Subcut., Intraperit.	General
80MDV	Port & Catheter, Infusion, Implanted, Subcutaneous, Intraspinal	General
84MFR	Stimulator, Brain, Implanted (Behavior Modification)	Cns/Neurology
84MFM	Stimulator, Cortex, Visual, Implanted	Cns/Neurology
84MHF	Stimulator, Cortical, Implanted (Pain Relief)	Cns/Neurology
84MEI	Stimulator, Electrical, Implanted (Coma Arousal)	Cns/Neurology
84MHY	Stimulator, Electrical, Implanted (Parkinsonian Tremor)	Cns/Neurology
84MNQ	Stimulator, Hypoglossal Nerve, Implanted, Apnea	Cns/Neurology
84MFP	Stimulator, Nerve, Cranial, Implanted (Pain Relief)	Cns/Neurology
84GZC	Stimulator, Neuromuscular, Implanted	Cns/Neurology
84MQQ	Stimulator, Sacral Nerve, Implanted	Cns/Neurology
84MBX	Stimulator, Thalamic, Epilepsy, Implanted	Cns/Neurology
84MBY	Stimulator, Vagus Nerve, Epilepsy, Implanted	Cns/Neurology
84MUY	Stimulator, Vagus Nerve, Implanted (Coma And Vegetative State)	Cns/Neurology

IMPORT

80WMQ	Service, Import/Export	General
80WIE	Service, Licensing, Device, Medical	General

IMPOTENCE

78FHW	Impotence Device, Mechanical/Hydraulic	Gastro/Urology
78LIL	Monitor, Penile Tumescence	Gastro/Urology
78LKY	Prosthesis, Penis, Rigid Rod, External	Gastro/Urology

IMPRESSION

76VLL	Adhesive, Dental Impression	Dental And Oral
77LDG	Kit, Earmold Impression	Ear/Nose/Throat

IMPRESSION *(cont'd)*

76ELW	Material, Impression	Dental And Oral
76EBH	Material, Impression Tray, Resin	Dental And Oral
76KCQ	Matrix, Tube Impression	Dental And Oral
76EID	Syringe, Restorative And Impression Material	Dental And Oral
76EHY	Tray, Impression	Dental And Oral
87WPM	Tray, Impression, Foot	Orthopedics

IMV

73CBO	Attachment, Intermittent Mandatory Ventilation (IMV)	Anesthesiology
73SET	Controller, Ventilator IMV	Anesthesiology

IN-HOUSE

80WIH	System, Transport, In-House	General

IN-LINE

80MJF	Check Valve, Retrograde Flow (In-Line)	General
74DTY	Sensor, Blood Gas, In-Line, Cardiopulmonary Bypass	Cardiovascular
73MJJ	Valve, CPB Check, Retrograde, In-Line	Anesthesiology

INACTIVATOR

82DBA	Antigen, Antiserum, Complement C1 Inhibitor (Inactivator)	Immunology

INCANDESCENT

79FTI	Lamp, Endoscopic, Incandescent	Surgery
80REB	Lamp, Sun, Incandescent	General
79GBC	Lamp, Surgical, Incandescent	Surgery
78FCQ	Light Source, Incandescent, Diagnostic	Gastro/Urology

INCENTIVE

73BWF	Spirometer, Therapeutic (Incentive)	Anesthesiology

INCINERATOR

80TBJ	Compactor, Fixed	General
80TBK	Compactor, Portable	General
80VBK	Incinerator	General
80WUN	Service, Waste Management	General

INCISION

79WVZ	Drape, Incision, Surgical	Surgery
79RBS	Kit, Incision And Drainage	Surgery

INCLINOMETER

89LZW	Monitor, Spine Curvature	Physical Med

INCONTINENCE

78EXJ	Appliance, Incontinence, Urosheath Type	Gastro/Urology
78QQK	Bag, Drainage (Incontinence)	Gastro/Urology
78FAQ	Bag, Leg	Gastro/Urology
80SEB	Bag, Urinary Collection	General
78WSS	Balloon, Rectal	Gastro/Urology
78RBT	Clamp, Incontinence	Gastro/Urology
78WLL	Device, Incontinence, Fecal	Gastro/Urology
78MIP	Device, Incontinence, Fecal, Implanted	Gastro/Urology
78EZY	Device, Incontinence, Mechanical/Hydraulic	Gastro/Urology
78MNG	Device, Incontinence, Occlusion, Urethral	Gastro/Urology
78EXI	Device, Incontinence, Paste-On	Gastro/Urology
80QPL	Diaper, Adult	General
78EYQ	Garment, Protective, For Incontinence	Gastro/Urology
85MCQ	Implant, Female Incontinence	Obstetrics/Gyn
80RBU	Pad, Incontinence (Underpad)	General
80RBV	Pant, Incontinence	General
78WHR	Plug, Ostomy	Gastro/Urology
80VLU	Pump, Urinary Collection Bag	General
78EZW	Stimulator, Electrical, For Incontinence	Gastro/Urology
78KPI	Stimulator, Incontinence (Non-Implantable), Electrical	Gastro/Urology

INCREMENT

77ETR	Adapter, Index, Sensitivity, Increment, Short	Ear/Nose/Throat

INCUBATOR

83RBW	Incubator, Aerobic	Microbiology
83RBX	Incubator, Anaerobic	Microbiology
80FMZ	Incubator, Neonatal	General
80FPL	Incubator, Neonatal Transport	General
83RBY	Incubator, Test Tube, Portable	Microbiology
83RBZ	Incubator, Test Tube, Stationary	Microbiology
75JRH	Incubator/Water Bath	Chemistry
83JTQ	Incubator/Water Bath, Microbiology	Microbiology

INCUS

77RAK	Hook, Incus	Ear/Nose/Throat
77UBU	Prosthesis, Ossicular, Incus And Stapes	Ear/Nose/Throat

INDEX

77ETR	Adapter, Index, Sensitivity, Increment, Short	Ear/Nose/Throat
80QJP	Paper, Chart, Record, Medical	General

INDICATOR

91DKY	Alumina Fluorescent Indicator, TLC	Toxicology
74QGL	Cardiac Output Unit, Indicator Dilution (Thermal)	Cardiovascular
74TBG	Catheter, Dye Dilution (Cardiac Output Indicator)	Cardiovascular
91DJO	Cellulose Fluorescent Indicator, TLC	Toxicology

KEYWORD INDEX

INFORMATION *(cont'd)*

80VBH	Computer Software	General
80WSJ	Computer Software, Hospital/Nursing Management	General
75QMB	Computer, Clinical Laboratory	Chemistry
80VHN	Computer, Patient Data Management	General
90WKA	Computer, Radiographic Data	Radiology
80VAZ	Microfilm/Microfiche Equipment	General

INFRARED

75UGP	Analyzer, Chromatography Infrared	Chemistry
74WSR	Flowmeter, Blood, Other	Cardiovascular
75JNP	Infrared Spectroscopy Measurement, Urinary Calculi (Stone)	Chemistry
89ILY	Lamp, Infrared	Physical Med
75WHI	Spectrometer, Infrared	Chemistry
75RUM	Spectrophotometer, Infrared	Chemistry
85WSC	Spectroscope, Tumor Analysis, Mammary	Obstetrics/Gyn
85SAG	Thermographic Device, Infrared	Obstetrics/Gyn
80SAL	Thermometer, Infrared	General
77WXS	Thermometer, Tympanic	Ear/Nose/Throat
74MFL	Transmitter/Receiver, Physiological Signal, Infrared	Cardiovascular

INFUSER

80RLQ	Infuser, Pressure (Blood Pump)	General

INFUSION

80MRZ	Accessories, Pump, Infusion	General
74WTU	Adapter, Needle	Cardiovascular
80VLP	Analyzer, Infusion Pump	General
78TAQ	Calibrator, Drop-Rate, Infusion	Gastro/Urology
80QGT	Cart, Multipurpose	General
79JCY	Catheter, Infusion	Surgery
74WJY	Connector, Tubing, Blood	Cardiovascular
78FKB	Connector, Tubing, Blood, Infusion, T-Type	Gastro/Urology
74QMI	Controller, Infusion	Cardiovascular
80LDR	Controller, Infusion, Intravascular	General
74QMJ	Controller, Infusion, Intravenous	Cardiovascular
73BSC	Controller, Infusion, Manual	Anesthesiology
73CAJ	Controller, Infusion, Powered	Anesthesiology
74QMS	Counter, Intravenous Drop	Cardiovascular
86QOH	Cutter, Vitreous Infusion Suction	Ophthalmology
80WSB	Dispenser, Syringe And Needle	General
80FPB	Filter, Infusion Line	General
80RCM	Hanger, Intravenous	General
80LZF	Infusion Pump, Analytical Sampling	General
80LZH	Infusion Pump, Enteral	General
80LZG	Infusion Pump, Insulin	General
80FOX	Infusion Stand	General
78TCQ	Infusion System, Insulin, With Monitor	Gastro/Urology
90LLY	Infusion System, Radionuclide	Radiology
80RCD	Injector, Syringe	General
80WVF	Kit, Administration, Intra-Arterial	General
80FPA	Kit, Administration, Intravenous	General
78TGJ	Kit, Administration, Parenteral	Gastro/Urology
74QHL	Kit, Catheterization, Intravenous, Winged	Cardiovascular
80WLM	Lock, Catheter	General
80BYC	Monitor, Infusion Rate	General
80FLN	Monitor, Infusion, Gravity Flow	General
80RIL	Needle, Other	General
80MDX	Port & Catheter, Infusion, Implanted, Subcut., Intraperit.	General
80MDV	Port & Catheter, Infusion, Implanted, Subcutaneous, Intraspinal	General
74THP	Port, Vascular Access	Cardiovascular
80FRN	Pump, Infusion	General
78FIH	Pump, Infusion Or Syringe, Extra-Luminal	Gastro/Urology
80VEZ	Pump, Infusion, Ambulatory	General
80DWK	Pump, Infusion, Cardiovascular	General
80MEB	Pump, Infusion, Elastomeric	General
80MHD	Pump, Infusion, Gallstone Dissolution	General
78THF	Pump, Infusion, Implantable	Gastro/Urology
80LKK	Pump, Infusion, Implantable, General	General
80MDY	Pump, Infusion, Implantable, Non-Programmable	General
75UHO	Pump, Infusion, Laboratory	Chemistry
80MEA	Pump, Infusion, Patient Controlled Analgesia (PCA)	General
80RNG	Pump, Infusion, Syringe	General
74DQI	Pump, Withdrawal/Infusion	Cardiovascular
86WVM	System, Delivery, Drug, Ocular	Ophthalmology
80TGT	System, Infusion, Administration, Drug, Implantable	General
74WYC	System, Infusion, Enzyme, Thrombolytic	Cardiovascular
80AZZ	Tester, Infusion Pump	General
80LHF	Warmer, Infusion Fluid, Microwave	General
80LGZ	Warmer, Infusion Fluid, Thermal	General

INFUSOR

80KZD	Pressure Infusor, IV Container	General

INHALATION

73BZR	Mixer, Breathing Gases, Anesthesia Inhalation	Anesthesiology
83WKT	Water, Therapy, Respiratory	Microbiology

INHALATOR

73BYG	Mask, Oxygen, Aerosol Administration	Anesthesiology
80RPI	Resuscitator, Pulmonary, Gas	General

INHALER

77KCO	Inhaler, Nasal	Ear/Nose/Throat

INHIBITED

75JFH	Tartrate Inhibited, Acid Phosphatase (Prostatic)	Chemistry

INHIBITION

91DLX	Hemagglutination Inhibition, Barbiturate	Toxicology
91DNO	Hemagglutination Inhibition, Gentamicin	Toxicology
91DIW	Hemagglutination Inhibition, Methadone	Toxicology
91DLR	Hemagglutination Inhibition, Morphine	Toxicology
91LFO	Nephelometric Inhibition Immunoassay, Diphenylhydantoin	Toxicology
91LFN	Nephelometric Inhibition Immunoassay, Phenobarbital	Toxicology

INHIBITOR

82DBA	Antigen, Antiserum, Complement C1 Inhibitor (Inactivator)	Immunology
82CZO	Antigen, Antiserum, Control, Inter-Alpha Trypsin Inhibitor	Immunology
89MLQ	Inhibitor, Peridural Fibrosis (Adhesion Barrier)	Physical Med
89MNY	Inhibitor, Post-Op Fibro., Carp. Tun. Syn.(Adhesion Barrier)	Physical Med
89MNX	Inhibitor, Post-Op Fibrosis, Tenolysis (Adhesion Barrier)	Physical Med

INJECTABLE

78LNM	Agent, Bulking, Injectable (Gastro-Urology)	Gastro/Urology
79MFE	Agent, Injectable, Embolic	Surgery
77MGF	Collagen, Injectable (For Vocal Cord Augmentation)	Ear/Nose/Throat
79LWD	Irrigating Solution, Non-Injectable	Surgery
90VGW	Media, Radiographic Injectable Contrast	Radiology
76LTG	Paste, Injectable, Augmentation, Chord, Vocal	Dental And Oral
79KGM	Silicone, Liquid, Injectable	Surgery

INJECTION

78FGY	Cannula, Injection	Gastro/Urology
80QGT	Cart, Multipurpose	General
80WSB	Dispenser, Syringe And Needle	General
77KAA	Kit, Laryngeal Injection	Ear/Nose/Throat
80WYJ	Molding, Injection	General
79GAA	Needle, Aspiration And Injection, Disposable	Surgery
79GDM	Needle, Aspiration And Injection, Reusable	Surgery
80RIL	Needle, Other	General
80RSU	Shield, Wound, Injection Site	General
80WYK	Thermoforming, Extrusion, Custom	General

INJECTOR

85LKF	Cannula, Manipulator/Injector, Uterine	Obstetrics/Gyn
74DQF	Controller, Injector, Angiographic	Cardiovascular
80LDH	Delivery System, Allergen And Vaccine	General
85RCF	Injector & Accessories, Manipulator, Uterine	Obstetrics/Gyn
74DXT	Injector, Angiographic (Cardiac Catheterization)	Cardiovascular
90IZQ	Injector, Contrast Medium, Automatic	Radiology
80KZE	Injector, Fluid, Non-Electric	General
90VGZ	Injector, Hand-Held	Radiology
74DXL	Injector, Indicator	Cardiovascular
78WRW	Injector, Insulin	Gastro/Urology
76EGQ	Injector, Jet, Gas-Powered	Dental And Oral
76EGM	Injector, Jet, Mechanical-Powered	Dental And Oral
84RCB	Injector, Lymphangiographic	Cns/Neurology
80RCC	Injector, Medication (Inoculator)	General
75UHV	Injector, Sample	Chemistry
80RCD	Injector, Syringe	General
74RCE	Injector, Thermal Dilution	Cardiovascular
90VGB	Kit, Angiographic, Digital	Radiology
90VGC	Kit, Angiographic, Special Procedure	Radiology
83WPR	Micro-Injector, Transplant, Gene	Microbiology
84HAQ	Needle, Angiographic	Cns/Neurology
80RNG	Pump, Infusion, Syringe	General
83LIE	Reagent, Inoculator Calibration (Laboratory)	Microbiology

INJECTORS

86MSS	Folders and Injectors, Intraocular Lens (IOL)	Ophthalmology

INJURY

84LWC	Device, Hypothermia, Injury, Cord, Spinal	Cns/Neurology

INK

76KZO	Ink, Arch Tracing	Dental And Oral

INLAY

76EIS	Remover, Crown	Dental And Oral

INOCULATING

83RFI	Loop, Inoculating	Microbiology
83VLZ	Sterilizer, Loop, Inoculating	Microbiology

INOCULATOR

80LDH	Delivery System, Allergen And Vaccine	General
80RCC	Injector, Medication (Inoculator)	General
75WHL	Inoculator, Laboratory	Chemistry
80WOC	Microplate	General

INSUFFLATOR *(cont'd)*
85HIF Insufflator, Laparoscopic — Obstetrics/Gyn
79RCH Insufflator, Other — Surgery
85HEC Insufflator, Vaginal — Obstetrics/Gyn

INSULATION
80WRF Pad, Insulation, Cardiac — General

INSULIN
80LZG Infusion Pump, Insulin — General
78TCQ Infusion System, Insulin, With Monitor — Gastro/Urology
78WRW Injector, Insulin — Gastro/Urology
75WXU Monitor, Glucose, Blood, Non-Invasive — Chemistry
80LMY Monitor, Skin Resistance/skin Temperature, For Insulin Reactions — General
75CFP Radioimmunoassay, Immunoreactive Insulin — Chemistry
75WTX Strip, Test — Chemistry
80RYR Syringe, Insulin — General
80TGT System, Infusion, Administration, Drug, Implantable — General

INSURANCE
80VHN Computer, Patient Data Management — General
80VBR Service, Insurance — General

INTAKE
73QWO Regulator, Intake, Oxygen — Anesthesiology

INTEGRATED
79MFH Implant, Integrated Tissue — Surgery

INTEGRATING
75JQT Densitometer/Scanner (Integrating, Reflectance, TLC, Radio) — Chemistry

INTEGRITY
86HIY Brush, Haidinger, With Macular Integrity — Ophthalmology

INTELLIGENT
81WXZ Microscope, Intelligent, Automated — Hematology

INTENSIFICATION
90TCP Image Intensification System — Radiology
86HOT Vision Aid, Image Intensification, Battery-Powered — Ophthalmology

INTENSIFIED
90JAA Radiographic/Fluoroscopic Unit, Image-Intensified — Radiology
90JAB Radiographic/Fluoroscopic Unit, Non-Image-Intensified — Radiology

INTENSIFYING
90IXM Screen, Intensifying, Radiographic — Radiology
76EAM Screen, Intensifying, Radiographic, Dental — Dental And Oral

INTENSITY
90VHH Light, High Intensity — Radiology
89LBF Stimulator, Muscle, Low Intensity — Physical Med

INTER-ALPHA
82CZO Antigen, Antiserum, Control, Inter-Alpha Trypsin Inhibitor — Immunology
82DEC Inter-Alpha Trypsin, FITC, Antigen, Antiserum, Control — Immunology

INTERACTIVE
79MGR Dressing, Wound and Burn, Interactive — Surgery

INTERARTICULAR
76MPJ Prosthesis, Interarticular Disc (Interpositional Implant) — Dental And Oral

INTERCONNECTED
78FBS Sound, Metal, Interconnected — Gastro/Urology

INTERFACE
73KFZ Humidifier, Non-Direct Patient Interface (Home-Use) — Anesthesiology
73BTT Humidifier, Respiratory Gas, (Direct Patient Interface) — Anesthesiology
73CAF Nebulizer, Direct Patient Interface — Anesthesiology

INTERFERENTIAL
84LIH Unit, Therapy, Current, Interferential — Cns/Neurology

INTERFEROMETER
86WOO Tester, Brightness Acuity — Ophthalmology

INTERLAMINAL
87LYP Accessories, Fixation, Spinal Interlaminal — Orthopedics
87KWP Appliance, Fixation, Spinal Interlaminal — Orthopedics

INTERLEUKIN
81MAN Interleukin - 2 Assays — Hematology
82WPH Test, Receptor, Interleukin, Serum — Immunology

INTERLOCK
90TGW Interlock System, X-Ray Darkrooms — Radiology

INTERMITTENT
78QBR Aspirator, Low Volume (Gastric Suction) — Gastro/Urology
73CBO Attachment, Intermittent Mandatory Ventilation (IMV) — Anesthesiology
74QLZ Compression Unit, Intermittent (Anti-Embolism Pump) — Cardiovascular

INTERMITTENT *(cont'd)*
73SET Controller, Ventilator IMV — Anesthesiology
89JFC Pressure Measurement, System, Intermittent — Physical Med
78FKX System, Peritoneal Dialysis, Automatic — Gastro/Urology
73SEU Ventilator, Pressure Cycled (IPPB Machine) — Anesthesiology

INTERNAL
74MDO Fibrillator, AC-Powered, Internal — Cardiovascular
79GEL Gauze, Non-Absorbable, Medicated (Internal Sponge) — Surgery
79GEK Gauze, Non-Absorbable, Non-Medicated (Internal Sponge) — Surgery
79GDY Gauze, Non-Absorbable, X-Ray Detectable (Internal Sponge) — Surgery
74FYK Monitor, Pressure, Arterial, Internal — Cardiovascular
85LBX Pelvimeter, Internal — Obstetrics/Gyn
79FWM Prosthesis, Breast, Inflatable, Internal — Surgery
79FTR Prosthesis, Breast, Non-Inflatable, Internal — Surgery
79FWP Prosthesis, Chin, Internal — Surgery
79FZD Prosthesis, Ear, Internal — Surgery
79FWO Prosthesis, Eye, Internal (Sphere) — Surgery
79FZE Prosthesis, Nose, Internal — Surgery
79KGW Ring Drape Retention, Internal (Wound Protector) — Surgery
84HAZ Sponge, Internal — Cns/Neurology
84HTK Stimulator, Extremity, Internal, Peroneal — Cns/Neurology
74MTE System, Pacing, Temporary, Acute, Internal Atrial Defibrillation — Cardiovascular
79MCA Tape, Surgical, Internal — Surgery

INTERPOSITIONAL
76MPJ Prosthesis, Interarticular Disc (Interpositional Implant) — Dental And Oral

INTERPRETATION
74QMC Computer, ECG Interpretation (Arrhythmia) — Cardiovascular

INTERPRETATOR
73BZM Computer, Pulmonary Function Interpretator (Diagnostic) — Anesthesiology

INTERPRETIVE
74UER Electrocardiograph, Interpretive — Cardiovascular

INTERRUPTER
80QYW Interrupter, Ground Fault Circuit — General
80QYV Tester, Ground Fault Circuit Interrupter — General

INTERSTITIAL
90LMZ Hyperthermia Applicator, Interstitial — Radiology

INTERVERTEBRAL
87LYQ Accessories, Fixation, Spinal Intervertebral Body — Orthopedics
87KWQ Appliance, Fixation, Spinal Intervertebral Body — Orthopedics
87MAT Orthosis, Fixation, Cervical Intervertebral Body, Spinal — Orthopedics
87MAX Orthosis, Fusion, Intervertebral, Spinal — Orthopedics
87MJO Prosthesis, Spine, Intervertebral Disc — Orthopedics
87RQD Rongeur, Intervertebral Disk — Orthopedics

INTESTINAL
78QKM Clamp, Intestinal — Gastro/Urology
78FBF Clip, Suture, Stomach And Intestinal — Gastro/Urology
78FFR Device, Locking, Clamp, Instestinal — Gastro/Urology
78QXE Forceps, Intestinal (Clamps) — Gastro/Urology
78LNQ Stimulator, Intestinal — Gastro/Urology
78FHM Suture Apparatus, Stomach And Intestinal — Gastro/Urology
80RZN Telemetry Unit, Physiological, Pressure — General
78FEG Tube, Double Lumen For Intestinal Decompression — Gastro/Urology
78LCG Tube, Intestinal Splinting — Gastro/Urology

INTESTINE
79KGY Bag, Intestine — Surgery

INTRA-AORTIC
74DSP Balloon, Intra-Aortic (With Control System) — Cardiovascular
74QHY Catheter, Intra-Aortic Balloon — Cardiovascular
74QKE Circulatory Assist Unit, Intra-Aortic Balloon — Cardiovascular

INTRA-ARTERIAL
80WVF Kit, Administration, Intra-Arterial — General
74RIF Needle, Intra-Arterial — Cardiovascular

INTRAARTICULAR
89MOZ Acid, Hyaluronic, Intraarticular — Physical Med

INTRACARDIAC
74DWD Controller, Suction, Intracardiac, Cardiopulmonary Bypass — Cardiovascular
74QTA Electrode, Myocardial — Cardiovascular
74DQA Oximeter, Intracardiac — Cardiovascular
74DXZ Pledget And Intracardiac Patch, PETP, PTFE, Polypropylene — Cardiovascular
74DSX Pledget, Dacron, Teflon, Polypropylene — Cardiovascular

INTRACATHETER
78FJT Intracatheter, Dialysis — Gastro/Urology

INTRACAVITARY
74DXW Phonocatheter System, Intracavitary — Cardiovascular

KEYWORD INDEX

INVASIVE *(cont'd)*

73CCC	Analyzer, Gas, Carbon-Dioxide, Blood Phase, Indwelling	Anesthesiology
73FLM	Analyzer, Oxygen, Neonatal, Invasive	Anesthesiology
73JED	Analyzer, Oxyhemoglobin Concentration, Blood Phase, Indwell.	Anesthesiology
87JEC	Component, Traction, Invasive	Orthopedics
87KQZ	Component, Traction, Non-Invasive	Orthopedics
80WYB	Equipment, Management, Pain, Radiofrequency, Non-Invasive	General
78FIT	Flowmeter, Blood, Non-Invasive Electromagnetic	Gastro/Urology
74RLR	Monitor, Blood Pressure, Invasive (Arterial)	Cardiovascular
73CAA	Monitor, Blood Pressure, Invasive (Arterial), Anesthesia	Anesthesiology
74RLX	Monitor, Blood Pressure, Venous	Cardiovascular
79FYO	Monitor, Blood Pressure, Venous, Central	Surgery
79FYP	Monitor, Blood Pressure, Venous, Peripheral	Surgery
75WXU	Monitor, Glucose, Blood, Non-Invasive	Chemistry
80FLP	Monitor, Neonatal, Blood Pressure, Invasive	General
74DRO	Pacemaker, Cardiac, External Transcutaneous (Non-Invasive)	Cardiovascular
80MDS	Sensor, Glucose, Invasive	General
89MKC	Stimulator, Arthritis, Non-Invasive	Physical Med
87LOE	Stimulator, Growth, Bone, Invasive	Orthopedics
87LOF	Stimulator, Growth, Bone, Non-Invasive	Orthopedics
89MBN	Stimulator, Muscle, Powered, Invasive	Physical Med
89MKD	Stimulator, Neuromuscular, Functional Walking, Non-Invasive	Physical Med
87HTM	Stimulator, Osteogenesis, Electric, Invasive	Orthopedics
87WNT	Stimulator, Osteogenesis, Electric, Non-Invasive	Orthopedics
80WOI	System, Delivery, Drug, Non-invasive	General
73BXG	Transducer, Blood Flow, Invasive	Anesthesiology
73BXF	Transducer, Blood Flow, Non-Invasive	Anesthesiology
79GAZ	Tubing, Non-Invasive	Surgery

INVENTION

80WTQ	Service, Attorney, Patent	General

INVENTORY

80VAX	Computer Equipment	General
80VFR	Computer, Bar Code	General
80WNL	Label, Bar Code	General
80QPF	Label, Device	General
80WTG	Monitor, Utilization, Equipment	General
80WVQ	Service, Engraving	General
80QPG	Tag, Device Status	General

INVENTORY-CONTROL

80WMT	Printer, Bar Code	General
80WMS	Reader, Bar Code	General

INVERSION

87THB	Inversion Unit	Orthopedics

INVERTED

88IBL	Microscope, Inverted Stage, Tissue Culture	Pathology

INVESTMENT

76EGC	Material, Investment	Dental And Oral

IOAT

73CAC	Autotransfusion Unit (Blood)	Anesthesiology

IODINE

91JNI	Acetylcholine Iodine and DTNB, Pseudocholinesterase	Toxicology
75JIK	Dry Ash Method, Protein Bound Iodine	Chemistry
88IAL	Iodine (Tincture)	Pathology
88HYI	Stain, Grams Iodine	Pathology
75JIJ	Wet Ash Method, Protein Bound Iodine	Chemistry

ION

75LFQ	Acid Reduction Of Ferric Ion, Uric Acid	Chemistry
91DKO	Adsorbents, Ion Exchange	Toxicology
75QTJ	Analyzer, Chemistry, Electrolyte	Chemistry
73CBZ	Analyzer, Ion, Hydrogen-Ion (pH), Blood Phase, Indwelling	Anesthesiology
73CBY	Analyzer, Ion, Hydrogen-Ion pH, Blood Phase, Non-Indwelling	Anesthesiology
91DJY	Chromatography Equipment, Ion Exchange	Toxicology
75JKL	Column, Ion Exchange With Colorimetry, Delta-Aminolevulinic	Chemistry
80VFK	Counter, Air Ion	General
80LJJ	Electrode, In Vivo Calcium Ion Selective	General
80LJI	Electrode, In Vivo Potassium Ion Selective	General
75JJP	Electrode, Ion Selective (Non-Specified)	Chemistry
75JIG	Electrode, Ion Specific, Ammonia	Chemistry
75JFP	Electrode, Ion Specific, Calcium	Chemistry
75CGZ	Electrode, Ion Specific, Chloride	Chemistry
75CFA	Electrode, Ion Specific, Magnesium	Chemistry
75CEM	Electrode, Ion Specific, Potassium	Chemistry
75JGS	Electrode, Ion Specific, Sodium	Chemistry
75CDS	Electrode, Ion Specific, Urea Nitrogen	Chemistry
75UFY	Electrode, Specific Ion	Chemistry

ION *(cont'd)*

75CHD	Ferric Ion-Sulfuric Acid, Cholesterol	Chemistry
75CGL	Ion Electrode Based Enzymatic, Creatinine	Chemistry
75JIE	Ion Exchange Method, Ammonia	Chemistry
75JQE	Ion Exchange Resin, Ascorbic Acid, Colorimetry, Iron Bind	Chemistry
75JNF	Ion Exchange Resin, Ehrlich's Reagent, Porphobilinogen	Chemistry
75JQD	Ion Exchange Resin, Thioglycolic Acid, Colorimetry, Iron	Chemistry
78LRI	Meter, pH, Concentration, Ion, Hydrogen, Dialysis	Gastro/Urology
91DMG	Paper, Ion	Toxicology
88KEA	Resin, Ion-Exchange	Pathology
91DNH	Resins, Ion Exchange, Liquid Chromatography	Toxicology

ION-EXCHANGE

88KEA	Resin, Ion-Exchange	Pathology

ION-SULFURIC

75CHD	Ferric Ion-Sulfuric Acid, Cholesterol	Chemistry

IONIC

76MMD	Toothbrush, Ionic, Battery-Powered	Dental And Oral

IONIZATION

90RNU	Counter, Radiation	Radiology

IONIZED

73RCO	Generator, Ionized Air	Anesthesiology

IONOMER

77MLI	Cement, Bone, Ionomer	Ear/Nose/Throat

IONTOPHORESIS

75QTF	Electrode, Sweat Test	Chemistry
76EGJ	Iontophoresis Device, Dental	Dental And Oral
75UGQ	Iontophoresis Equipment	Chemistry
78RCP	Iontophoresis Unit (Sweat Rate)	Gastro/Urology
89KTB	Iontophoresis Unit, Physical Medicine	Physical Med
80WOI	System, Delivery, Drug, Non-invasive	General

IPPB

73SEU	Ventilator, Pressure Cycled (IPPB Machine)	Anesthesiology

IRIDIUM

90IWA	Source, Wire, Radioactive Iridium	Radiology

IRIDOCAPSULAR

86UBB	Lens, Intraocular, Iridocapsular Fixation	Ophthalmology

IRIS

86NCK	Button, Iris, Eye, Artificial	Ophthalmology
86HOC	Clip, Iris Retractor	Ophthalmology
86MMC	Dilator, Expansive Iris (Accessory)	Ophthalmology
86UBC	Lens, Intraocular, Iris Fixation	Ophthalmology
86RRF	Scissors, Iris	Ophthalmology

IRON

75JIZ	Absorption, Atomic, Iron (Non-Heme)	Chemistry
75RCQ	Analyzer, Iron	Chemistry
75JQF	Bathophenanthroline, Iron Binding Capacity	Chemistry
75JMO	Ferrozine (Colorimetric) Iron Binding Capacity	Chemistry
75JQE	Ion Exchange Resin, Ascorbic Acid, Colorimetry, Iron Bind	Chemistry
75JQD	Ion Exchange Resin, Thioglycolic Acid, Colorimetry, Iron	Chemistry
88HYQ	Iron Chloride-Weigert	Pathology
81JWQ	Iron Kinetics	Hematology
88HZD	Muller's Colloidal Iron	Pathology
75JIY	Photometric Method, Iron (Non-Heme)	Chemistry
75JJA	Radio-Labeled Iron Method, Iron (Non-Heme)	Chemistry
75JQG	Radiometric, Fe59, Iron Binding Capacity	Chemistry
75CFM	Reagent, Iron (Test System)	Chemistry
88GGH	Stain, Iron	Pathology
88IAE	Stain, Weigert's Iron Hematoxylin	Pathology
73SEV	Ventilator, Time Cycled (Iron Lung)	Anesthesiology

IRRADIATOR

90WIB	Irradiator	Radiology
90MOT	Irradiator, Blood to Prevent Graft Vs Host Disease	Radiology
78NAX	Irradiator, Blood, Extracorporeal	Gastro/Urology
80RVX	Sterilizer, Radiation	General

IRRIGATING

79LWD	Irrigating Solution, Non-Injectable	Surgery
80MWV	Needles, Medicament Dispensing Tip & Irrigating	General
80RYU	Syringe, Bulb	General
76DYY	Syringe, Bulb, Air Or Water	Dental And Oral
80KYZ	Syringe, Irrigating	General
76EIB	Syringe, Irrigating, Dental	Dental And Oral
80KYY	Syringe, Irrigating, Sterile	General

IRRIGATION

87WHX	Aspirator, Arthroscopy	Orthopedics
80WVO	Brush, Other	General
86HMX	Cannula, Ophthalmic	Ophthalmology
79WYX	Cannula, Suction/Irrigation, Laparoscopic	Surgery

KEYWORD INDEX

IV (cont'd)
80FMG Stopcock — General
80RWW Stylet, Intravenous — General
80LHI Transfer Unit, IV Fluid — General
80WTM Weight, IV Pole — General

IV-5
82DAL Fraction IV-5, Antigen, Antiserum, Control — Immunology

IVOX
73MEV Oxygenator, Intravascular — Anesthesiology

IVT
74MKH System, Renal Atherectomy, Ivt — Cardiovascular

JACKET
91DMA Reagent, Test, Fluoride — Toxicology
80RPE Restraint, Vest — General

JANUS
88KJW Stain, Janus Green B — Pathology

JAR
79RCY Jar, Applicator — Surgery
79RCZ Jar, Blade — Surgery
79RDA Jar, Dressing — Surgery
79RDB Jar, Forceps — Surgery
79FTE Jar, Operating Room — Surgery

JAUNDICE
80UDF Bilirubinometer, Cutaneous (Jaundice Meter) — General
80TCX Light, Bilirubin (Phototherapy) — General
80LMX Meter, Jaundice — General
80RKZ Phototherapy Unit (Bilirubin Lamp) — General

JAW
76LQZ Device, Repositioning, Jaw — Dental And Oral
87TCT Fixation Device, Jaw Fracture — Orthopedics
76LZD Implant, Joint, Temporomandibular — Dental And Oral
77JAZ Prosthesis, Facial, Mandibular Implant — Ear/Nose/Throat

JEJUNOSTOMY
78QIB Catheter, Jejunostomy — Gastro/Urology
78VHP Tube, Gastrointestinal Decompression, Baker Jejunostomy — Gastro/Urology

JELLY
78FHY Jelly, Contact (For Transurethral Surgical Instrument) — Gastro/Urology
80RFL Jelly, Lubricating — General
78FHX Jelly, Lubricating, Transurethral Surgical Instrument — Gastro/Urology
80TCZ Lubricant, Instrument — General

JENNER
88KJX Stain, Jenner Stain — Pathology

JET
78FFE Catheter, Water Jet, Renal — Gastro/Urology
76EGQ Injector, Jet, Gas-Powered — Dental And Oral
76EGM Injector, Jet, Mechanical-Powered — Dental And Oral
80RCC Injector, Medication (Inoculator) — General
80FQH Lavage Unit, Water Jet — General

JIG
77JXY Jig, Piston Cutting, ENT — Ear/Nose/Throat

JOBBS
80WMR Collar, Extrication — General

JOINT
89ITW Brace, Joint, Ankle (External) — Physical Med
76MGG Fluid, Hylan (For TMJ Use) — Dental And Oral
76LZD Implant, Joint, Temporomandibular — Dental And Oral
89IRD Joint, Elbow, External Limb Component, Mechanical — Physical Med
89IRE Joint, Elbow, External Limb Component, Powered — Physical Med
89ITS Joint, Hip, External Brace — Physical Med
89ISL Joint, Hip, External Limb Component — Physical Med
89ITQ Joint, Knee, External Brace — Physical Med
89ISY Joint, Knee, External Limb Component — Physical Med
89IQQ Joint, Shoulder, External Limb Component — Physical Med
89ISZ Joint, Wrist, External Limb Component, Mechanical — Physical Med
89LXM Plunger-Like Joint Manipulator — Physical Med
87HSN Prosthesis, Ankle, Semi-Constrained, Metal/Polymer — Orthopedics
87UBK Prosthesis, Ankle, Talar Component — Orthopedics
87UBL Prosthesis, Ankle, Tibial Component — Orthopedics
87JDC Prosthesis, Elbow, Constrained — Orthopedics
87UBN Prosthesis, Elbow, Humeral Component — Orthopedics
87JDA Prosthesis, Elbow, Non-Constrained, Unipolar — Orthopedics
87UBO Prosthesis, Elbow, Radial Component — Orthopedics
87JDB Prosthesis, Elbow, Semi-Constrained — Orthopedics
87UBM Prosthesis, Elbow, Total — Orthopedics
87UBP Prosthesis, Elbow, Ulna Component — Orthopedics
87HSJ Prosthesis, Finger — Orthopedics
87UBQ Prosthesis, Finger, Total — Orthopedics
87JDF Prosthesis, Hip (Metal Stem/Ceramic Self-Locking Ball) — Orthopedics

JOINT (cont'd)
87JDM Prosthesis, Hip, Acetabular Component, Metal, Non-Cemented — Orthopedics
87JDJ Prosthesis, Hip, Acetabular Mesh — Orthopedics
87JDK Prosthesis, Hip, Cement Restrictor — Orthopedics
87JDG Prosthesis, Hip, Femoral Component, Cemented, Metal — Orthopedics
87JDH Prosthesis, Hip, Hemi-, Trunnion-Bearing, Femoral — Orthopedics
87JDL Prosthesis, Hip, Semi-Constrained (Cemented Acetabular) — Orthopedics
87JDI Prosthesis, Hip, Semi-Constrained, Metal/Polymer — Orthopedics
87RMV Prosthesis, Joint, Other — Orthopedics
87HSX Prosthesis, Knee, Femorotibial, Non-Constrained — Orthopedics
87HRY Prosthesis, Knee, Femorotibial, Semi-Constrained — Orthopedics
87HSA Prosthesis, Knee, Hemi-, Femoral — Orthopedics
87HTG Prosthesis, Knee, Hemi-, Patellar Resurfacing, Uncemented — Orthopedics
87HSH Prosthesis, Knee, Hemi-, Tibial Resurfacing, Uncemented — Orthopedics
87HRZ Prosthesis, Knee, Hinged (Metal-Metal) — Orthopedics
87UCD Prosthesis, Knee, Patellar — Orthopedics
87JWH Prosthesis, Knee, Patellofemorotibial, Semi-Constrained — Orthopedics
87UBR Prosthesis, Knee, Total — Orthopedics
79JCR Prosthesis, Mandible — Surgery
87HSF Prosthesis, Shoulder — Orthopedics
87HSD Prosthesis, Shoulder, Hemi-, Humeral — Orthopedics
87UCM Prosthesis, Toe — Orthopedics
87LZJ Prosthesis, Toe (Metaphal.), Joint, Met./Poly., Semi-Const. — Orthopedics
87JWI Prosthesis, Wrist, 2 Part Metal-Plastic Articulation — Orthopedics
87JWJ Prosthesis, Wrist, 3 Part Metal-Plastic-Metal Articulation — Orthopedics
87KWO Prosthesis, Wrist, Carpal Scaphoid — Orthopedics
78FJW Ring, Joint — Gastro/Urology
76WLF Stethoscope, Dental — Dental And Oral

KANAMYCIN
91KZW Disc, Diffusion, Gel, Agar, Serum Level, Kanamycin — Toxicology
91KJI Radioimmunoassay, Kanamycin — Toxicology

KAPPA
82DFH Antigen, Antiserum, Control, Kappa — Immunology
82DEO Antigen, Antiserum, Control, Kappa, FITC — Immunology
82DEK Antigen, Antiserum, Control, Kappa, Rhodamine — Immunology
82DFD Kappa, Peroxidase, Antigen, Antiserum, Control — Immunology

KARAYA
76KOM Acacia And Karaya With Sodium Borate — Dental And Oral
76MMU Adhesive, Denture, Acacia & Karaya with Sodium Borate — Dental And Oral
76KOP Adhesive, Denture, Karaya — Dental And Oral
76KOR Adhesive, Denture, Karaya With Sodium Borate — Dental And Oral
76KXX Homopolymer, Karaya and Ethylene-Oxide — Dental And Oral

KARYOTYPE
88JCZ Analyzer, Karyotype — Pathology

KARYOTYPING
88LNJ Analyzer, Chromosome, Automated — Pathology

KASLOW
78SCY Tube, Gastrointestinal, Kaslow — Gastro/Urology

KEEL
77FWN Prosthesis, Larynx — Ear/Nose/Throat

KELLY
80FNW Pad, Kelly — General

KENDRIC
80TCA Extrication Equipment — General

KERATINS
88LSP Keratins, Histological — Pathology

KERATOME
86HNO Keratome, AC-Powered — Ophthalmology
86HMY Keratome, Battery-Powered — Ophthalmology
86RDK Knife, Keratome — Ophthalmology

KERATOMETER
86UEK Keratometer — Ophthalmology

KERATOMILEUSIS
86WQT Phacoemulsification System — Ophthalmology
86WQU Tissue, Corneal — Ophthalmology

KERATOPHAKIA
86WQT Phacoemulsification System — Ophthalmology
86WQU Tissue, Corneal — Ophthalmology

KERATOPROSTHESIS
86HQK Keratoprosthesis, Custom — Ophthalmology
86HQM Keratoprosthesis, Non-Custom — Ophthalmology
86MLP Keratoprosthesis, Temporary Implant, Surgical — Ophthalmology

KERATOSCOPE
86VED Keratoscope — Ophthalmology
86HLQ Keratoscope, AC-Powered — Ophthalmology

KERATOSCOPE *(cont'd)*
86HLR Keratoscope, Battery-Powered — Ophthalmology

KERATOTOMY
86VKE Surgical Instrument, Radial Keratotomy — Ophthalmology

KETOBUTYRIC
75JMK Alpha-Ketobutyric Acid And NADH (U.V.), Hydroxybutyric — Chemistry

KETOGENIC
75CDG Chromatographic Separation/Zimmerman 17-Ketogenic Steroids — Chemistry
75CCZ Zimmerman/Norymberski, 17-Ketogenic Steroids — Chemistry

KETOGLUTERATE
75JKH Hydrazone Derivative Of Alpha-Ketogluterate (Colorimetry) — Chemistry

KETONES
75JIN Nitroprusside, Ketones (Urinary, Non-Quantitative) — Chemistry

KETOSTEROIDS
75CDE Chromatographic Separation/Zimmerman, 17-Ketosteroids — Chemistry
75CCY Zimmerman (Spectrophotometric), 17-Ketosteroids — Chemistry

KICK
80RDC Liner, Kick Bucket — General
80RDD Waste Receptacle, Kick Bucket — General

KIDNEY
78MPB Catheter, Hemodialysis — Gastro/Urology
78KDK Container, Transport, Kidney — Gastro/Urology
78QPJ Dialysis Unit Test Equipment — Gastro/Urology
78FJI Dialyzer, Capillary, Hollow Fiber (Hemodialysis) — Gastro/Urology
78KDI Dialyzer, High Permeability — Gastro/Urology
78FJG Dialyzer, Parallel Flow (Hemodialysis) — Gastro/Urology
78FHS Dialyzer, Single Coil (Hemodialysis) — Gastro/Urology
78QVZ Filter, Kidney Stone — Gastro/Urology
78RAA Hemodialysis Unit (Kidney Machine) — Gastro/Urology
78KDL Kit, Perfusion, Kidney, Disposable — Gastro/Urology
78RKM Kit, Tubing, Dialysis, Peritoneal — Gastro/Urology
78UEP Lithotriptor — Gastro/Urology
78VKM Lithotriptor, Electro-Hydraulic, Extracorporeal — Gastro/Urology
78FFK Lithotriptor, Electro-Hydraulic, Percutaneous — Gastro/Urology
78LNS Lithotriptor, Extracorporeal Shock-wave, Urological — Gastro/Urology
78WSU Lithotriptor, Laser — Gastro/Urology
78WIL Lithotriptor, Multipurpose — Gastro/Urology
78QPI Meter, Dialysate Conductivity — Gastro/Urology
78RIM Nephroscope, Flexible — Gastro/Urology
78RIN Nephroscope, Rigid — Gastro/Urology
78RIZ Organ Preservation System — Gastro/Urology
78KDN Perfusion System, Kidney — Gastro/Urology
80FSB Perfusion Unit — General
78RKL Peritoneal Dialysis Unit (CAPD) — Gastro/Urology
78FKX System, Peritoneal Dialysis, Automatic — Gastro/Urology

KINASE
75JLB ATP and CK (Enzymatic), Creatine — Chemistry
75CDT Lipase Hydrolysis/Glycerol Kinase Enzyme, Triglycerides — Chemistry
75JNJ Phosphoenol Pyruvate, ADP, NADH, Pyruvate Kinase — Chemistry
75JFX Reagent, Kinase, Phosphate, Creatine — Chemistry

KINDS
75JJY Control, Multi Analyte, All Kinds (Assayed And Unassayed) — Chemistry

KINEMATIC
75UGS Bath, Kinematic Viscosity — Chemistry

KINESTHESIOMETER
87TCU Kinesthesiometer — Orthopedics

KINETIC
75JHS Differential Rate Kinetic Method, CPK Or Isoenzymes — Chemistry
81JBK Glucose-6-Phos. Dehydrogenase (Erythrocytic), U.V. Kinetic — Hematology
75JQB Kinetic Method, Gamma-Glutamyl Transpeptidase — Chemistry

KINETICS
81JWQ Iron Kinetics — Hematology

KIT
87QBO Arthrogram Kit — Orthopedics
80QCD Care Kit, Baby — General
80WLH Contract Manufacturing, Reagent — General
79MAC Decontamination Kit — Surgery
75LPJ Estrogen Receptor Assay Kit — Chemistry
79LRS IV Start Kit — Surgery
88IHD Irrigation, Davis Mailable Irrigation Kit — Pathology
73QAA Kit, Acupuncture — Anesthesiology
80QDX Kit, Administration, Blood — General
74UDD Kit, Administration, Cardioplegia Solution — Cardiovascular
78QUJ Kit, Administration, Enteral — Gastro/Urology
80WVF Kit, Administration, Intra-Arterial — General
80FPA Kit, Administration, Intravenous — General

KIT *(cont'd)*
73RJH Kit, Administration, Oxygen — Anesthesiology
78TGJ Kit, Administration, Parenteral — Gastro/Urology
78KDJ Kit, Administration, Peritoneal Dialysis, Disposable — Gastro/Urology
80RKC Kit, Admission (Patient Utensil) — General
73QAU Kit, Anesthesia, Brachial Plexus — Anesthesiology
73QAV Kit, Anesthesia, Caudal — Anesthesiology
73CAZ Kit, Anesthesia, Conduction — Anesthesiology
73QAW Kit, Anesthesia, Epidural — Anesthesiology
73QAX Kit, Anesthesia, Glossopharyngeal — Anesthesiology
85KNE Kit, Anesthesia, Obstetrical — Obstetrics/Gyn
73QAZ Kit, Anesthesia, Other — Anesthesiology
85HEH Kit, Anesthesia, Paracervical — Obstetrics/Gyn
85HEG Kit, Anesthesia, Pudendal — Obstetrics/Gyn
73QAY Kit, Anesthesia, Spinal — Anesthesiology
90VGB Kit, Angiographic, Digital — Radiology
90VGC Kit, Angiographic, Special Procedure — Radiology
82MEO Kit, Antigen, RIA, Prostatic Acid Phosphatase — Immunology
75LPI Kit, Assay, Receptor, Progesterone — Chemistry
74DQP Kit, Balloon Repair, Catheter — Cardiovascular
78FCD Kit, Barium Enema, Disposable — Gastro/Urology
80QDS Kit, Biopsy — General
78FCG Kit, Biopsy Needle — Gastro/Urology
78FCH Kit, Biopsy, Gastro-Urology — Gastro/Urology
80QDT Kit, Biopsy, Ultrasonic Aspiration — General
74RKS Kit, Blood Collection, Phlebotomy — Cardiovascular
81QDZ Kit, Blood Donor — Hematology
74QIX Kit, Blood Pressure, Central Venous — Cardiovascular
80BRZ Kit, Blood, Transfusion — General
78SIB Kit, Bowel — Gastro/Urology
85TGQ Kit, Breast Cancer Detection — Obstetrics/Gyn
80QEU Kit, Burn — General
80QHG Kit, Catheter Care — General
74QHK Kit, Catheterization, Cardiac — Cardiovascular
74QHL Kit, Catheterization, Intravenous, Winged — Cardiovascular
78FCM Kit, Catheterization, Sterile Urethral — Gastro/Urology
78QHM Kit, Catheterization, Urinary — Gastro/Urology
74MFY Kit, Cell Harvesting, Endothelial — Cardiovascular
80QJS Kit, Chest Drainage (Thoracentesis Tray) — General
78SHX Kit, Cholecystectomy — Gastro/Urology
88KIQ Kit, Chromosome Culture — Pathology
85QKG Kit, Circumcision, Disposable Tray — Obstetrics/Gyn
80LWE Kit, Collection/Transfusion, Marrow, Bone — General
73QNJ Kit, Cricothyrotomy — Anesthesiology
85QNS Kit, Culdocentesis — Obstetrics/Gyn
83MAQ Kit, DNA Detection, Human Papillomavirus — Microbiology
76RMM Kit, Dental Prophylaxis — Dental And Oral
76EBO Kit, Denture Repair, OTC — Dental And Oral
78LBW Kit, Dialysis, Single Needle (Co-Axial Flow) — Gastro/Urology
78FIF Kit, Dialysis, Single Needle With Uni-Directional Pump — Gastro/Urology
83MKA Kit, Direct Antigen, Negative Control — Microbiology
83MJZ Kit, Direct Antigen, Positive Control — Microbiology
83JTP Kit, Disc Agar Gel Diffusion, Serum Level — Microbiology
74SGT Kit, Disposable Procedure — Cardiovascular
88QQE Kit, Dissecting — Pathology
77LDG Kit, Earmold Impression — Ear/Nose/Throat
80QUB Kit, Emergency Drug — General
80UDB Kit, Emergency, Anaphylactic — General
80UDC Kit, Emergency, Cardiopulmonary Resuscitation — General
80RCG Kit, Emergency, Insect Sting — General
76VEI Kit, Endodontic — Dental And Oral
80QUG Kit, Enema — General
78FCE Kit, Enema (For Cleaning Purposes) — Gastro/Urology
83JST Kit, Fastidious Organism — Microbiology
80QVM Kit, Feeding, Adult (Enteral) — General
80QVN Kit, Feeding, Pediatric (Enteral) — General
79LRR Kit, First Aid — Surgery
88TCF Kit, Forensic Evidence — Pathology
85QXO Kit, Forensic Evidence, Sexual Assault — Obstetrics/Gyn
78SJD Kit, Gastrostomy, Endoscopic, Percutaneous — Gastro/Urology
78FHT Kit, Gavage, Infant, Sterile — Gastro/Urology
76VEG Kit, Gingival Retraction — Dental And Oral
83SGO Kit, Gonorrhoeae Test (Male Use) — Microbiology
78QZU Kit, Hemodialysis Tubing — Gastro/Urology
78SHY Kit, Herniorrhaphy — Gastro/Urology
85SHZ Kit, Hysterectomy — Obstetrics/Gyn
83JSP Kit, Identification, Anaerobic — Microbiology
83JSR Kit, Identification, Dermatophyte — Microbiology
83JSS Kit, Identification, Enterobacteriaceae — Microbiology
83JSW Kit, Identification, Glucose (Non-Ferment) — Microbiology
83JSX Kit, Identification, Neisseria Gonorrhoeae — Microbiology
83JSZ Kit, Identification, Pseudomonas — Microbiology
83JXB Kit, Identification, Yeast — Microbiology
79RBS Kit, Incision And Drainage — Surgery
79FTN Kit, Instruments and Accessories, Surgical — Surgery
80RCK Kit, Intravenous Extension Tubing — General
80RCI Kit, Intravenous, Administration, Buret — General

KIT *(cont'd)*

78RCR	Kit, Irrigation, Bladder	Gastro/Urology
77RCS	Kit, Irrigation, Ear	Ear/Nose/Throat
86RCT	Kit, Irrigation, Eye	Ophthalmology
77TCR	Kit, Irrigation, Oral	Ear/Nose/Throat
78RCU	Kit, Irrigation, Perineal	Gastro/Urology
78EYN	Kit, Irrigation, Sterile	Gastro/Urology
80RCW	Kit, Irrigation, Wound	General
85MLS	Kit, Labor and Delivery	Obstetrics/Gyn
78FDE	Kit, Laparoscopy	Gastro/Urology
77KAA	Kit, Laryngeal Injection	Ear/Nose/Throat
84RFM	Kit, Lumbar Puncture	Cns/Neurology
84RFN	Kit, Lymphangiographic	Cns/Neurology
85RGF	Kit, Maternity	Obstetrics/Gyn
83TGR	Kit, Meningitis Detection	Microbiology
80RGZ	Kit, Mid-Stream Collection	General
83JSY	Kit, Mycobacteria Identification	Microbiology
88KIW	Kit, Mycoplasma Detection	Pathology
84RHN	Kit, Myelogram	Cns/Neurology
85RJW	Kit, Pap Smear	Obstetrics/Gyn
85MLT	Kit, Pelvic Exam	Obstetrics/Gyn
79SIE	Kit, Pelviscopy	Surgery
78KDL	Kit, Perfusion, Kidney, Disposable	Gastro/Urology
76EAW	Kit, Plaque Disclosing	Dental And Oral
81LLG	Kit, Platelet Associated IGG	Hematology
85TFV	Kit, Pregnancy Test	Obstetrics/Gyn
75LCX	Kit, Pregnancy Test, Over The Counter, HCG	Chemistry
80RLP	Kit, Prep	General
80RLY	Kit, Pressure Monitoring (Air/Gas)	General
83JTR	Kit, Quality Control	Microbiology
81KSF	Kit, Quality Control, Blood Banking	Hematology
82MEL	Kit, RIA, Basic Protein, Myelin	Immunology
74KFJ	Kit, Repair, Pacemaker	Cardiovascular
73CBT	Kit, Sampling, Arterial Blood	Anesthesiology
80RQG	Kit, Sampling, Blood	General
80RQH	Kit, Sampling, Blood Gas	General
85RQI	Kit, Sampling, Endometrial	Obstetrics/Gyn
83JWX	Kit, Screening, Staphylococcus Aureus	Microbiology
83JXA	Kit, Screening, Urine	Microbiology
83MJY	Kit, Serological, Negative Control	Microbiology
83MJX	Kit, Serological, Positive Control	Microbiology
85ULY	Kit, Sex Selection	Obstetrics/Gyn
88RSZ	Kit, Shroud	Pathology
89HHC	Kit, Sitz Bath	Physical Med
80TFI	Kit, Skin Scrub	General
85MCO	Kit, Smear, Cervical	Obstetrics/Gyn
80RTX	Kit, Snake Bite	General
80KYQ	Kit, Snake Bite, Chemical Cold Pack	General
80KYP	Kit, Snake Bite, Suction	General
73CBE	Kit, Suction, Airway (Tracheal)	Anesthesiology
79LRQ	Kit, Suctioning, Tracheostomy and Nasal	Surgery
79LRO	Kit, Surgical (General)	Surgery
79KDD	Kit, Surgical Instrument, Disposable	Surgery
79RXR	Kit, Suture	Surgery
79MCZ	Kit, Suture Removal	Surgery
81MHS	Kit, Test, Coagglutinin	Hematology
91MVO	Kit, Test, Multiple, Drugs Of Abuse, Over The Counter	Toxicology
76MCL	Kit, Test, Periodontal, In Vitro	Dental And Oral
81MWB	Kit, Test, Saliva, Hiv-1&2	Hematology
73SBG	Kit, Tracheostomy Care	Anesthesiology
73SBJ	Kit, Tracheotomy	Anesthesiology
83JWZ	Kit, Trichomonas Screening	Microbiology
79SIA	Kit, Trocar	Surgery
78FJK	Kit, Tubing, Blood, Anti-Regurgitation	Gastro/Urology
78RKM	Kit, Tubing, Dialysis, Peritoneal	Gastro/Urology
81MVS	Kit, Typing, Hla-dqb	Hematology
75MPG	Kit, Urinary Carbohydrate Analysis	Chemistry
78FCN	Kit, Urinary Drainage Collection	Gastro/Urology
81MVW	Kit, Western Blot, Hiv-1	Hematology
80VFP	Kit, Wound Drainage	General
84SGF	Kit, Wound Drainage, Closed	Cns/Neurology
79MCY	Kit, Wound Dressing	Surgery
83JXC	Kit, Yeast Screening	Microbiology
80WNC	Molding, Custom	General
80WXF	Pack, Custom/Special Procedure	General
76LXX	Periodontal Test Kit	Dental And Oral
85HIO	Sampler, Amniotic Fluid (Amniocentesis Tray)	Obstetrics/Gyn
83MDB	System, Blood Culturing	Microbiology
80FLL	Thermometer, Electronic, Continuous	General
80WNH	Tray, Custom/Special Procedure	General
78LJH	Urological Irrigation System	Gastro/Urology

KITCHEN

80VAV	Foodservice Product/Equipment	General

KLEBSIELLA

83GTB	Antiserum, Fluorescent, Klebsiella SPP.	Microbiology
83GTC	Antiserum, Klebsiella SPP.	Microbiology

KNEE

89ISW	Assembly, Knee/Shank/Ankle/Foot, External	Physical Med
89KFX	Assembly, Thigh/Knee/Shank/Ankle/Foot, External	Physical Med
89ITM	Cage, Knee	Physical Med
87RBK	Immobilizer, Knee	Orthopedics
89ITQ	Joint, Knee, External Brace	Physical Med
89ISY	Joint, Knee, External Limb Component	Physical Med
87KRN	Prosthesis, Knee, Femorotibial, Constrained, Metal	Orthopedics
87KRO	Prosthesis, Knee, Femorotibial, Constrained, Metal/Polymer	Orthopedics
87HSX	Prosthesis, Knee, Femorotibial, Non-Constrained	Orthopedics
87KTX	Prosthesis, Knee, Femorotibial, Non-Constrained, Metal	Orthopedics
87HRY	Prosthesis, Knee, Femorotibial, Semi-Constrained	Orthopedics
87KYK	Prosthesis, Knee, Femorotibial, Semi-Constrained, Metal	Orthopedics
87LGE	Prosthesis, Knee, Femorotibial, Semi-Constrained, Trunnion	Orthopedics
87MBG	Prosthesis, Knee, Femotib., Unconst., Uncem., Unicond., M/P	Orthopedics
87HSA	Prosthesis, Knee, Hemi-, Femoral	Orthopedics
87HTG	Prosthesis, Knee, Hemi-, Patellar Resurfacing, Uncemented	Orthopedics
87KRS	Prosthesis, Knee, Hemi-, Tibial Resurfacing	Orthopedics
87HSH	Prosthesis, Knee, Hemi-, Tibial Resurfacing, Uncemented	Orthopedics
87HRZ	Prosthesis, Knee, Hinged (Metal-Metal)	Orthopedics
87KMB	Prosthesis, Knee, Non-Const. (M/C Reinf. Polyeth.) Cemented	Orthopedics
87MBD	Prosthesis, Knee, P/F, Unconst., Uncem., Por., Ctd., P/M/P	Orthopedics
87UCD	Prosthesis, Knee, Patellar	Orthopedics
87KRR	Prosthesis, Knee, Patellofemoral, Semi-Constrained	Orthopedics
87KRP	Prosthesis, Knee, Patellofemorotibial, Constrained, Metal	Orthopedics
87KRQ	Prosthesis, Knee, Patellofemorotibial, Constrained, Polymer	Orthopedics
87JWH	Prosthesis, Knee, Patellofemorotibial, Semi-Constrained	Orthopedics
87MBV	Prosthesis, Knee, Patfem., S-C., UHMWPE, Pegged, Unc., P/M/P	Orthopedics
87MBH	Prosthesis, Knee, Patfem., S-C., Unc., Por., Ctd., P/M/P	Orthopedics
87MBA	Prosthesis, Knee, Patfem., Semi-Const., Unc., P/M/P, Osteo.	Orthopedics
87LXY	Prosthesis, Knee, Patfemotib., Semi-Const., P/M/P, Uncem.	Orthopedics
87UBR	Prosthesis, Knee, Total	Orthopedics
87RTU	Sling, Knee	Orthopedics
89RXJ	Support, Knee	Physical Med
90RNX	Support, Patient Position, Radiographic	Radiology

KNIFE

79SIH	Blade, Electrosurgery, Laparoscopic	Surgery
79QVD	Blade, Knife, Laparoscopic	Surgery
79GES	Blade, Scalpel	Surgery
79SIM	Cutter, Linear, Laparoscopic	Surgery
79RTO	Cutter, Skin Graft	Surgery
86HMS	Drum, Eye Knife Test	Ophthalmology
79FAS	Electrode, Electrosurgical, Active (Blade)	Surgery
79GEI	Electrosurgical Unit, Cutting & Coagulation Device	Surgery
79RDE	Handle, Knife Blade	Surgery
79QWG	Handle, Knife, Laparoscopic	Surgery
79GDZ	Handle, Scalpel	Surgery
79RDF	Holder, Knife	Surgery
79QQU	Instrument, Dissecting, Laparoscopic	Surgery
79QQY	Instrument, Dissecting, Myoma, Laparoscopic	Surgery
79GDN	Knife, Amputation	Surgery
86RDH	Knife, Cataract	Ophthalmology
85HDZ	Knife, Cervical Cone	Obstetrics/Gyn
79RDI	Knife, Dermatome	Surgery
84RDJ	Knife, Dura Hook	Cns/Neurology
77KTG	Knife, ENT	Ear/Nose/Throat
77JYO	Knife, Ear	Ear/Nose/Throat
86RDK	Knife, Keratome	Ophthalmology
79QWI	Knife, Laparoscopic	Surgery
77JZY	Knife, Laryngeal	Ear/Nose/Throat
76EJZ	Knife, Margin Finishing, Operative	Dental And Oral
79RDL	Knife, Meniscus	Surgery
88RDM	Knife, Microtome	Pathology
77JYP	Knife, Myringotomy	Ear/Nose/Throat
77KAS	Knife, Nasal	Ear/Nose/Throat
86HNN	Knife, Ophthalmic	Ophthalmology
87HTS	Knife, Orthopedic	Orthopedics
79RDS	Knife, Other	Surgery
89RDN	Knife, Paraffin	Physical Med
76EMO	Knife, Periodontic	Dental And Oral
87RDO	Knife, Plaster	Orthopedics
79RDP	Knife, Scalpel	Surgery
79RDQ	Knife, Skin Grafting	Surgery
79RDR	Knife, Sternum	Surgery
76EMF	Knife, Surgical	Dental And Oral
77KBQ	Knife, Tonsil	Ear/Nose/Throat
79RDG	Needle, Knife	Surgery
79GDX	Scalpel, One-Piece (Knife)	Surgery

KEYWORD INDEX

LABWARE (cont'd)

81GIO	Tube, Capillary Blood Collection	Hematology
75SCP	Tube, Centrifuge	Chemistry
83SCS	Tube, Culture	Microbiology
81GHC	Tube, Sedimentation Rate	Hematology
75RZV	Tube, Test	Chemistry
88KJG	Tube, Tissue Culture	Pathology
81GIM	Tube, Vacuum Sample, With Anticoagulant	Hematology
75SFP	Washer, Labware	Chemistry

LACRIMAL

86QGB	Cannula, Lacrimal (Eye)	Ophthalmology
86HMX	Cannula, Ophthalmic	Ophthalmology
86HNW	Dilator, Lacrimal	Ophthalmology
86RCT	Kit, Irrigation, Eye	Ophthalmology
86HNL	Probe, Lacrimal	Ophthalmology
86HNG	Rongeur, Lacrimal Sac	Ophthalmology

LACTATE

75CER	2, 4-dinitrophenylhydrazine, Lactate Dehydrogenase	Chemistry
75CEX	Chromatographic Separation, Lactate Dehydrogenase Isoenzyme	Chemistry
75JGF	Differential Rate Method, Lactate Dehydrogenase Isoenzymes	Chemistry
75CFE	Electrophoretic, Lactate Dehydrogenase Isoenzymes	Chemistry
75CFJ	NAD Reduction/NADH Oxidation, Lactate Dehydrogenase	Chemistry
75CFH	Tetrazolium Int Dye-Diaphorase, Lactate Dehydrogenase	Chemistry

LACTIC

75KHP	Enzymatic Method, Lactic Acid	Chemistry
75JKI	L-Leucyl B-Naphthylamide, Lactic Acid	Chemistry
82DET	Lactic Dehydrogenase, Antigen, Antiserum, Control	Immunology

LACTOFERRIN

82DEG	Antigen, Antiserum, Control, Lactoferrin	Immunology

LACTOGEN

75JMF	Radioimmunoassay, Human Placental Lactogen	Chemistry
75CFT	Radioimmunoassay, Prolactin (Lactogen)	Chemistry
82DHT	Test, Human Placental Lactogen	Immunology

LACTOSE

73WSV	Analyzer, Trace Gas, Breath	Anesthesiology

LADDER

89QVB	Exerciser, Shoulder	Physical Med

LAL

83VJH	Test, Limulus Amebocyte Lysate (LAL)	Microbiology

LAMBDA

82DEH	Antigen, Antiserum, Control, Lambda	Immunology
82DES	Antigen, Antiserum, Control, Lambda, FITC	Immunology
82DFG	Antigen, Antiserum, Control, Lambda, Rhodamine	Immunology
82DEP	Lambda, Peroxidase, Antigen, Antiserum, Control	Immunology

LAMBS-WOOL

80RMA	Pad, Pressure, Animal Skin	General

LAMINAGRAPH

90IZF	Radiographic Unit, Diagnostic, Tomographic	Radiology
90TEJ	Scanner, Ultrasonic, General Purpose	Radiology

LAMINAR

80RAH	Hood, Isolation, Laminar Air Flow	General
80FLJ	Laminar Air Flow Unit	General
75RDW	Laminar Air Flow Unit, Fixed (Air Curtain)	Chemistry
75RDX	Laminar Air Flow Unit, Mobile	Chemistry

LAMINARIA

85HDY	Dilator, Cervical, Hygroscopic-Laminaria	Obstetrics/Gyn
80RDY	Tent, Laminaria	General

LAMINECTOMY

79RPS	Retractor, Laminectomy	Surgery

LAMP

86HPQ	Headlamp, Operating, AC-Powered	Ophthalmology
86HPP	Headlamp, Operating, Battery-Operated	Ophthalmology
77KAF	Headlight, ENT	Ear/Nose/Throat
78FCT	Headlight, Fiberoptic Focusing	Gastro/Urology
79FTI	Lamp, Endoscopic, Incandescent	Surgery
80RDZ	Lamp, Examination (Light)	General
80TCY	Lamp, Examination, Ceiling Mounted (Light)	General
79HJE	Lamp, Fluorescein, AC-Powered	Surgery
80FOI	Lamp, Heat	General
89ILY	Lamp, Infrared	Physical Med
77SHF	Lamp, Laryngoscope	Ear/Nose/Throat
88KEG	Lamp, Microscope	Pathology
80FQP	Lamp, Operating Room	General
80REF	Lamp, Other	General
80REA	Lamp, Perineal Heat	General
88IEH	Lamp, Slide Warming	Pathology

LAMP (cont'd)

86REC	Lamp, Slit	Ophthalmology
86HJO	Lamp, Slit, Biomicroscope, AC-Powered	Ophthalmology
80REB	Lamp, Sun, Incandescent	General
79FTD	Lamp, Surgical	Surgery
79GBC	Lamp, Surgical, Incandescent	Surgery
79FTB	Lamp, Surgical, Xenon	Surgery
80REE	Lamp, Ultraviolet (Spectrum A)	General
80RED	Lamp, Ultraviolet, Germicidal	General
89IOB	Lamp, Ultraviolet, Physical Medicine	Physical Med
80TCX	Light, Bilirubin (Phototherapy)	General
76RFD	Light, Dental	Dental And Oral
90VHH	Light, High Intensity	Radiology
80RFF	Light, Overbed	General
86HJP	Penlight, Battery-Powered	Ophthalmology
80RKZ	Phototherapy Unit (Bilirubin Lamp)	General
90VGO	Safelight, X-Ray	Radiology

LANCASTER

86HJS	Test, Spectacle Dissociation, AC-Powered (Lancaster)	Ophthalmology
86HLO	Test, Spectacle Dissociation, Battery-Powered (Lancaster)	Ophthalmology

LANCET

81JCA	Bleeding Time Device	Hematology
80FMK	Lancet, Blood	General

LAP

89IMX	Tray, Wheelchair	Physical Med

LAPAROSCOPE

79SIP	Connector, Suction/Irrigation	Surgery
79WZL	Cover, Laparoscope	Surgery
79QYN	Gown, Operating Room, Reusable	Surgery
85UEZ	Holder, Laparoscope	Obstetrics/Gyn
79WXI	Laparoscope, Flexible	Surgery
79GCJ	Laparoscope, General & Plastic Surgery	Surgery
85HET	Laparoscope, Gynecologic	Obstetrics/Gyn
79SJT	Laparoscope, Microlaparoscopy	Surgery

LAPAROSCOPIC

78WZN	Applier, Clip, Repair, Hernia, Laparoscopic	Gastro/Urology
79WZP	Bag, Specimen, Laparoscopic	Surgery
79SIH	Blade, Electrosurgery, Laparoscopic	Surgery
79QVD	Blade, Knife, Laparoscopic	Surgery
79WYX	Cannula, Suction/Irrigation, Laparoscopic	Surgery
85HFG	Coagulator, Laparoscopic, Unipolar	Obstetrics/Gyn
79WYS	Container, Specimen, Laparoscopic	Surgery
80SHM	Coupler, Optical, Laparoscopic	General
79SIM	Cutter, Linear, Laparoscopic	Surgery
79SIN	Dilator, Port, Laparoscopic	Surgery
79SJA	Dispenser, Laparoscopic	Surgery
79SII	Electrode, Electrosurgery, Laparoscopic	Surgery
79WYP	Equipment, Suction/Irrigation, Laparoscopic	Surgery
79SJK	Equipment, Suction/Irrigation/Electrocautery, Laparoscopic	Surgery
79SIF	Handle, Instrument, Laparoscopic (Electrocautery)	Surgery
79SJH	Handle, Instrument, Laparoscopic (Irrigation)	Surgery
79QWG	Handle, Knife, Laparoscopic	Surgery
79QNR	Holder, Instrument, Laparoscopic	Surgery
79QOJ	Holder, Needle, Curved, Laparoscopic	Surgery
79QNU	Holder, Needle, Laparoscopic	Surgery
79QPN	Holder/Scissors, Needle, Laparoscopic	Surgery
79QQU	Instrument, Dissecting, Laparoscopic	Surgery
79QQY	Instrument, Dissecting, Myoma, Laparoscopic	Surgery
79SIJ	Instrument, Electrosurgery, Laparoscopic	Surgery
79QRS	Instrument, Knot Tying, Suture, Laparoscopic	Surgery
79QSH	Instrument, Passing, Suture, Laparoscopic	Surgery
79SJP	Instrument, Removal, Myoma, Laparoscopic	Surgery
85HIF	Insufflator, Laparoscopic	Obstetrics/Gyn
79SJR	Irrigator/Coagulator/Cutter, Suction, Laparoscopic	Surgery
79QWI	Knife, Laparoscopic	Surgery
79SIL	Ligature, Laparoscopic	Surgery
78RCA	Lithotriptor, Laparoscopic	Gastro/Urology
79RIJ	Needle, Aspiration, Cyst, Laparoscopic	Surgery
79RKN	Needle, Insufflation, Laparoscopic	Surgery
79QUQ	Probe, Suction, Irrigator/Aspirator, Laparoscopic	Surgery
80WYR	Solution, Instrument, Laparoscopic, Anti-Fog	General
79WZO	Stapler, Laparoscopic	Surgery
79WYQ	Trocar, Laparoscopic	Surgery
79SHC	Videointerface, Laparoscopic, Non-Removable Rod	Surgery
79SHD	Videointerface, Laparoscopic, Removable Rod	Surgery

LAPAROSCOPY

79SJI	Balloon, Manipulation, Tissue	Surgery
79QZT	Cart, Instrument/Equipment, Laparoscopy	Surgery
79WZX	Clamp, Laparoscopy	Surgery
79SJJ	Dissector, Balloon, Surgical	Surgery
79SIV	Equipment/Accessories, Laser, Laparoscopy	Surgery
79SJX	Forceps, Laparoscopy, Bipolar, Electrosurgical	Surgery
79WZD	Forceps, Laparoscopy, Electrosurgical	Surgery

KEYWORD INDEX

LB

88HZQ	Stain, Red-Violet LB	Pathology

LDH

75CER	2, 4-dinitrophenylhydrazine, Lactate Dehydrogenase	Chemistry
75CEX	Chromatographic Separation, Lactate Dehydrogenase Isoenzyme	Chemistry
75JGF	Differential Rate Method, Lactate Dehydrogenase Isoenzymes	Chemistry
75CFE	Electrophoretic, Lactate Dehydrogenase Isoenzymes	Chemistry
75CFJ	NAD Reduction/NADH Oxidation, Lactate Dehydrogenase	Chemistry
75CFH	Tetrazolium Int Dye-Diaphorase, Lactate Dehydrogenase	Chemistry

LDL

74WTP	Column, Adsorption, Lipid	Cardiovascular
75KMZ	HDL Via LDL & VLDL Precipitation, Lipoproteins	Chemistry
75LBS	LDL & VLDL Precipitation, Cholesterol Via Esterase-Oxidase	Chemistry
75LBR	LDL & VLDL Precipitation, HDL	Chemistry

LEAD

91DOF	Absorption, Atomic, Lead	Toxicology
91DIJ	Acid, Levulinic, Amino, Delta, Lead	Toxicology
74DRW	Adapter, Lead Switching, Electrocardiograph	Cardiovascular
74DTD	Adapter, Lead, Pacemaker	Cardiovascular
80REO	Analyzer, Lead	General
76EAJ	Apron, Lead, Dental	Dental And Oral
90IWO	Apron, Lead, Radiographic	Radiology
74WWW	Cable, Pacemaker	Cardiovascular
74REP	Cable/Lead, ECG	Cardiovascular
74WLG	Cable/Lead, ECG, Radiolucent	Cardiovascular
74DSA	Cable/Lead, ECG, With Transducer And Electrode	Cardiovascular
84VDF	Cable/Lead, EEG	Cns/Neurology
84VDG	Cable/Lead, EMG	Cns/Neurology
84VDH	Cable/Lead, TENS	Cns/Neurology
76EAH	Cone, Radiographic, Lead-Lined	Dental And Oral
84WHU	Electrode, TENS	Cns/Neurology
91DOX	Fluorometer, Lead (Dedicated Instruments)	Toxicology
74UCH	Lead, Pacemaker (Catheter)	Cardiovascular
74QIG	Lead, Pacemaker, Implantable Endocardial	Cardiovascular
74DTB	Lead, Pacemaker, Implantable Myocardial	Cardiovascular
74UCI	Lead, Pacemaker, Temporary Endocardial	Cardiovascular
74WQA	Lead, Pacemaker, Temporary Myocardial	Cardiovascular
74WWX	Pacemaker, Temporary	Cardiovascular
91DNX	Protoporphyrin Zinc Method, Fluorometric, Lead	Toxicology
91DMK	Protoporphyrin, Fluorometric, Lead	Toxicology
90WPD	Shield, X-Ray, Lead-Plastic	Radiology
90VLA	Shield, X-Ray, Transparent	Radiology
84GYA	Tester, Electrode/Lead, Electroencephalograph	Cns/Neurology

LEAD-LINED

76EAH	Cone, Radiographic, Lead-Lined	Dental And Oral

LEAD-PLASTIC

90WPD	Shield, X-Ray, Lead-Plastic	Radiology

LEADED

90IWO	Apron, Lead, Radiographic	Radiology
90IWQ	Curtain, Protective, Radiographic	Radiology
90IWP	Glove, Protective, Radiographic	Radiology
90IWR	Holder, Syringe, Leaded	Radiology
90IWT	Shield, Gonadal	Radiology
90IWW	Shield, Vial	Radiology
90RSW	Shield, X-Ray	Radiology
90TDY	Shield, X-Ray, Door	Radiology
76EAK	Shield, X-Ray, Leaded	Dental And Oral
90TEN	Shield, X-Ray, Portable	Radiology

LEADS

74QNX	Current Limiter, Patient Leads	Cardiovascular

LEAKAGE

74DSM	Alarm, Leakage Current, Portable	Cardiovascular
80QSF	Analyzer, Electrical Safety	General
78FJD	Detector, Blood Leakage	Gastro/Urology
80UMV	Detector, Ethylene-Oxide Leakage	General
80WPI	Detector, Leakage, Medical Gas	General
80RGX	Detector, Microwave Leakage	General
80REQ	Meter, Leakage Current (Ammeter)	General

LEAN

80VDN	Analyzer, Composition, Weight, Patient	General

LEASING

80WMP	Service, Equipment Leasing	General
80WUE	Service, Finance	General

LECITHIN

75JHG	Chromatographic Separation, Lecithin-Sphingomyelin Ratio	Chemistry
75JHF	Colorimetric Method, Lecithin-Sphingomyelin Ratio	Chemistry
75JHH	Electrophoretic Method, Lecithin-Sphingomyelin Ratio	Chemistry

LECITHIN *(cont'd)*

75WHJ	Test, Maturity, Lung, Fetal	Chemistry

LECITHIN-SPHINGOMYELIN

75JHG	Chromatographic Separation, Lecithin-Sphingomyelin Ratio	Chemistry
75JHF	Colorimetric Method, Lecithin-Sphingomyelin Ratio	Chemistry
75JHH	Electrophoretic Method, Lecithin-Sphingomyelin Ratio	Chemistry
75WHJ	Test, Maturity, Lung, Fetal	Chemistry

LECTINS

81KSI	Lectins/Protectins	Hematology

LEFT

74DSQ	Circulatory Assist Unit, Left Ventricular	Cardiovascular

LEG

78FAQ	Bag, Leg	Gastro/Urology
80TAG	Bath, Leg	General
87WLZ	Custom Prosthesis	Orthopedics
89QUZ	Exerciser, Leg And Ankle	Physical Med
79UFB	Holder, Leg	Surgery
87THC	Holder, Leg, Arthroscopy	Orthopedics
80RER	Leg Rest	General
89LBD	Prosthesis, Inflatable Leg, And Pump	Physical Med
87RMX	Prosthesis, Leg	Orthopedics
87RTV	Sling, Leg	Orthopedics
89RXK	Support, Leg	Physical Med

LEGGING

74WTT	Legging, Compression, Inflatable, Sequential	Cardiovascular
80LLK	Legging, Compression, Non-Inflatable	General

LEGIONELLA

83LQH	Legionella DNA Reagents	Microbiology
83LHL	Legionella Direct & Indirect Fluorescent Antibody Regents	Microbiology
83MJH	Legionella, Spp., ELISA	Microbiology
83UML	Reagent, Legionella Detection	Microbiology

LEISHMANII

83LOO	Reagent, Leishmanii Serological	Microbiology

LENGTH

80WOB	Meter, Patient Height	General
80FRW	Scale, Infant	General

LENS

86LYL	Accessories, Solution, Lens, Contact	Ophthalmology
86LRX	Case, Contact Lens	Ophthalmology
86LPN	Cleaner, Lens, Contact	Ophthalmology
86VEU	Clip, Lens Implantation	Ophthalmology
86HPB	Clip, Lens, Trial, Ophthalmic	Ophthalmology
86RES	Expressor, Lens Loop	Ophthalmology
78FEI	Eyepiece, Lens, Non-Prescription, Endoscopic	Gastro/Urology
78FDZ	Eyepiece, Lens, Prescription, Endoscopic	Gastro/Urology
86WXB	Filter, Lens	Ophthalmology
86MSS	Folders and Injectors, Intraocular Lens (IOL)	Ophthalmology
86HLN	Gauge, Lens, Ophthalmic	Ophthalmology
86KYB	Guide, Intraocular Lens	Ophthalmology
86WJZ	Implant, Retinal	Ophthalmology
86WUA	Implant, Scleral	Ophthalmology
86KYE	Inserter/Remover, Lens, Contact	Ophthalmology
86WTY	Laboratory Equipment, Ophthalmic	Ophthalmology
86HPD	Lens, Bagolini	Ophthalmology
79FXQ	Lens, Camera, Surgical	Surgery
86HJL	Lens, Condensing, Diagnostic	Ophthalmology
86HQD	Lens, Contact (Other Material)	Ophthalmology
86MWL	Lens, Contact(rigid Gas Permeable)-extended Wear	Ophthalmology
86ULH	Lens, Contact, Bifocal	Ophthalmology
86WIZ	Lens, Contact, Disposable	Ophthalmology
86ULD	Lens, Contact, Extended-Wear	Ophthalmology
86MRC	Lens, Contact, Gas-Permeable	Ophthalmology
86TGY	Lens, Contact, Hydrophilic	Ophthalmology
86HPX	Lens, Contact, Polymethylmethacrylate	Ophthalmology
86HJK	Lens, Contact, Polymethylmethacrylate, Diagnostic	Ophthalmology
86VJN	Lens, Contact, Tinted	Ophthalmology
86WZA	Lens, Contact, Trifocal	Ophthalmology
86HJJ	Lens, Fresnel, Flexible, Diagnostic	Ophthalmology
86HJI	Lens, Fundus, Hruby, Diagnostic	Ophthalmology
86HQL	Lens, Intraocular	Ophthalmology
86UBA	Lens, Intraocular, Anterior Chamber	Ophthalmology
86UBB	Lens, Intraocular, Iridocapsular Fixation	Ophthalmology
86UBC	Lens, Intraocular, Iris Fixation	Ophthalmology
86MFK	Lens, Intraocular, Multifocal	Ophthalmology
86UBD	Lens, Intraocular, Posterior Chamber	Ophthalmology
86MJP	Lens, Intraocular, Toric	Ophthalmology
86HKR	Lens, Maddox	Ophthalmology
86REV	Lens, Other	Ophthalmology
86HPC	Lens, Set, Trial, Ophthalmic	Ophthalmology
86HRA	Lens, Spectacle/Eyeglasses, Custom (Prescription)	Ophthalmology
86HQG	Lens, Spectacle/Eyeglasses, Non-Custom	Ophthalmology

KEYWORD INDEX

LIGHT *(cont'd)*

76RFE	Light, Dental, Intraoral	Dental And Oral
80KYT	Light, Examination, Battery-Powered	General
76EAY	Light, Fiberoptic, Dental	Dental And Oral
79FSR	Light, Headband, Surgical	Surgery
90VHH	Light, High Intensity	Radiology
86HIX	Light, Maxwell Spot, AC-Powered	Ophthalmology
80RFG	Light, Other	General
80RFF	Light, Overbed	General
76EBA	Light, Surgical Headlight	Dental And Oral
76EAZ	Light, Surgical Operating, Dental	Dental And Oral
79FSZ	Light, Surgical, Carrier	Surgery
79FSY	Light, Surgical, Ceiling Mounted	Surgery
79FSX	Light, Surgical, Connector	Surgery
79FSW	Light, Surgical, Endoscopic	Surgery
79FST	Light, Surgical, Fiberoptic	Surgery
79FSS	Light, Surgical, Floor Standing	Surgery
79FSQ	Light, Surgical, Instrument	Surgery
80MIO	Light, Therapy, Seasonal Affective Disorder (SAD)	General
91DJS	Light, U.V., TLC	Toxicology
79FTC	Light, Ultraviolet, Dermatologic	Surgery
83GMB	Light, Wood's, Fluorescence	Microbiology
83RFB	Meter, Light, Photomicrographic	Microbiology
88IBJ	Microscope, Light	Pathology
90IWE	Monitor, Patient Position, Light Beam	Radiology
86HJP	Penlight, Battery-Powered	Ophthalmology
80RKZ	Phototherapy Unit (Bilirubin Lamp)	General
90VGO	Safelight, X-Ray	Radiology
85MPU	Source, Chemiluminescent Light	Obstetrics/Gyn
88HYS	Stain, Light Green	Pathology
84RWF	Stimulator, Visual	Cns/Neurology
79MYH	System, Non-coherent Light, Photodynamic Therapy	Surgery
86HJM	Transilluminator, AC-Powered, Ophthalmic	Ophthalmology
86ETJ	Transilluminator, AC-Powered, Other	Ophthalmology
86HJN	Transilluminator, Battery-Powered	Ophthalmology
75UIW	Transilluminator, Laboratory	Chemistry

LIGHT-MICROSCOPY

88LDW	Fixative, Acid Containing	Pathology
88LDZ	Fixative, Alcohol Containing	Pathology
88LDY	Fixative, Formalin Containing	Pathology
88LDX	Fixative, Metallic Containing	Pathology
88IFJ	Fixative, Richardson Glycol	Pathology

LIMB

89IRN	Alarm, Overload, External Limb, Powered	Physical Med
89ISH	Ankle/Foot, External Limb Component	Physical Med
89IPM	Cover, Limb	Physical Med
89IRA	Hand, External Limb Component, Mechanical	Physical Med
89IQZ	Hand, External Limb Component, Powered	Physical Med
89IQX	Hook, External Limb Component, Mechanical	Physical Med
89IQW	Hook, External Limb Component, Powered	Physical Med
89IRD	Joint, Elbow, External Limb Component, Mechanical	Physical Med
89IRE	Joint, Elbow, External Limb Component, Powered	Physical Med
89ISL	Joint, Hip, External Limb Component	Physical Med
89ISY	Joint, Knee, External Limb Component	Physical Med
89IQQ	Joint, Shoulder, External Limb Component	Physical Med
89ISZ	Joint, Wrist, External Limb Component, Mechanical	Physical Med
89IQI	Orthosis, Limb Brace	Physical Med
89MRI	Orthosis, Truncal/Limb	Physical Med
74JOW	Sleeve, Compressible Limb	Cardiovascular
89KGH	Wrist, External Limb Component, Powered	Physical Med

LIMITER

74QNX	Current Limiter, Patient Leads	Cardiovascular

LIMITING

90KPW	Device, Limiting, Beam, Diagnostic, X-Ray	Radiology
90KQA	Device, Limiting, Beam, Teletherapy	Radiology
90IWD	Device, Limiting, Beam, Teletherapy, Radionuclide	Radiology

LIMULUS

83VJH	Test, Limulus Amebocyte Lysate (LAL)	Microbiology

LINE

80MJF	Check Valve, Retrograde Flow (In-Line)	General
78UCO	Clamp, Hemodialysis Unit Blood Line	Gastro/Urology
78FKK	Clamp, Line	Gastro/Urology
74QOS	Defibrillator, Line-Powered	Cardiovascular
74QOP	Defibrillator/Monitor, Line-Powered	Cardiovascular
79QSL	Electrocautery Unit, Line-Powered	Surgery
74DTM	Filter, Blood, Cardiopulmonary Bypass, Arterial Line	Cardiovascular
74JOD	Filter, Blood, Cardiotomy Suction Line, Cardiopulmonary	Cardiovascular
80FPB	Filter, Infusion Line	General
74DRY	Monitor, Blood Gas, On-Line, Cardiopulmonary Bypass	Cardiovascular
74DRI	Monitor, Line Isolation	Cardiovascular
80QUE	Power Supply, Endoscopic, Line-Operated	General
80WMM	Regulator, Line Voltage	General
74DTY	Sensor, Blood Gas, In-Line, Cardiopulmonary Bypass	Cardiovascular

LINE *(cont'd)*

80SAD	Tester, Resistance, Line Cord	General
73MJJ	Valve, CPB Check, Retrograde, In-Line	Anesthesiology

LINE-OPERATED

80QUE	Power Supply, Endoscopic, Line-Operated	General

LINE-POWERED

74QOS	Defibrillator, Line-Powered	Cardiovascular
74QOP	Defibrillator/Monitor, Line-Powered	Cardiovascular
79QSL	Electrocautery Unit, Line-Powered	Surgery

LINEAR

90IYE	Accelerator, Linear, Medical	Radiology
90WIA	Afterloader, Radiotherapy	Radiology
79SIM	Cutter, Linear, Laparoscopic	Surgery
79WZO	Stapler, Laparoscopic	Surgery

LINED

76EAH	Cone, Radiographic, Lead-Lined	Dental And Oral

LINEN

80TCV	Bag, Laundry, Infection Control	General
80REJ	Bag, Laundry, Operating Room	General
80QDJ	Bib	General
80FMW	Cover, Mattress	General
86HMT	Drape, Patient, Ophthalmic	Ophthalmology
77ERY	Drape, Surgical, ENT	Ear/Nose/Throat
79QQQ	Drape, Surgical, Reusable	Surgery
80VBF	Linen	General
80KME	Linen, Bed	General
79RXP	Pack, Surgical (Drape)	Surgery
80WLC	Pillow	General
79RSK	Sheet, Drape	Surgery
79RSN	Sheet, Operating Room	Surgery
80RSJ	Sheeting, Examination Table	General
80WKD	Sheeting, Stretcher	General
79RXX	Suture, Linen	Surgery
80WIH	System, Transport, In-House	General
79SBE	Towel, Surgical	Surgery
80FRG	Wrap, Sterilization	General
80SGG	Wrapper, Surgical Instrument (Sterile)	General

LINER

76EJK	Liner, Cavity, Calcium Hydroxide	Dental And Oral
80WYZ	Liner, Glove	General
80RDC	Liner, Kick Bucket	General
80TCL	Liner, Laundry Hamper	General

LINGUAL

76KKN	Test, Acid, Ascorbic, Lingual	Dental And Oral

LINKED

83MDU	Antigen, Enzyme Linked Immunoabsorbent Assay, Cryptococcus	Microbiology
83MZO	Assay, Enzyme Linked Immunosorbent, Hepatitis C Virus	Microbiology
83MYL	Assay, Enzyme Linked Immunosorbent, Parvovirus B19 Igg	Microbiology
83MYM	Assay, Enzyme Linked Immunosorbent, Parvovirus B19 Igm	Microbiology
83LJC	Enzyme Linked Immunoabsorbent Assay, Chlamydia Group	Microbiology
83MIY	Enzyme Linked Immunoabsorbent Assay, Coccidioides Immitis	Microbiology
83LFZ	Enzyme Linked Immunoabsorbent Assay, Cytomegalovirus	Microbiology
83LGC	Enzyme Linked Immunoabsorbent Assay, Herpes Simplex Virus	Microbiology
83MIZ	Enzyme Linked Immunoabsorbent Assay, Histoplasma Capsulatum	Microbiology
83LJY	Enzyme Linked Immunoabsorbent Assay, Mumps Virus	Microbiology
83LJZ	Enzyme Linked Immunoabsorbent Assay, Mycoplasma SPP.	Microbiology
83LIR	Enzyme Linked Immunoabsorbent Assay, Neisseria Gonorrhoeae	Microbiology
83MCE	Enzyme Linked Immunoabsorbent Assay, Resp. Syncytial Virus	Microbiology
83LIQ	Enzyme Linked Immunoabsorbent Assay, Rotavirus	Microbiology
83LFX	Enzyme Linked Immunoabsorbent Assay, Rubella	Microbiology
83LJB	Enzyme Linked Immunoabsorbent Assay, Rubeola	Microbiology
83MIU	Enzyme Linked Immunoabsorbent Assay, T. Cruzi	Microbiology
83LGD	Enzyme Linked Immunoabsorbent Assay, Toxoplasma Gondii	Microbiology
83LIP	Enzyme Linked Immunoabsorbent Assay, Treponema Pallidum	Microbiology
83MDT	Enzyme Linked Immunoabsorbent Assay, Trichinella Spiralis	Microbiology
83LFY	Enzyme Linked Immunoabsorbent Assay, Varicella-Zoster	Microbiology
83MXJ	Enzyme-Linked Immunosorbent Assay, Herpes Simplex Virus, HSV-1	Microbiology

LOCATING

84UFH	Stimulator, Nerve Locating	Cns/Neurology
84UFI	Stimulator, Nerve Locating, Facial	Cns/Neurology

LOCATOR

73BWJ	Locator, Acupuncture Point	Anesthesiology
76LQY	Locator, Apex, Root	Dental And Oral
78FFW	Locator, Bleeding, Gastrointestinal, String And Tube	Gastro/Urology
81JOY	Locator, Cell, Automated	Hematology
79FWA	Locator, Electric	Surgery
85HHJ	Locator, Intracorporeal Device, Ultrasonic	Obstetrics/Gyn
79FTZ	Locator, Magnetic	Surgery
86HPM	Locator, Metal, Electronic	Ophthalmology
80KZA	Locator, Vein, Liquid Crystal	General

LOCATORS

88IJS	Locators, Metaphase Cell	Pathology

LOCK

80WLM	Lock, Catheter	General
76DYX	Lock, Wire, And Ligature, Intraoral	Dental And Oral
76DZF	Syringe, Drug, Luer-Lock	Dental And Oral

LOCKING

78FFR	Device, Locking, Clamp, Instestinal	Gastro/Urology
87JDF	Prosthesis, Hip (Metal Stem/Ceramic Self-Locking Ball)	Orthopedics

LONG

80LNY	Catheter, Intraspinal, Percutaneous, Long-Term	General
80LJS	Catheter, Intravascular, Therapeutic, Long-term Greater Than 30 Days	General
78FJS	Catheter, Peritoneal, Indwelling, Long-Term	Gastro/Urology
74DYD	Catheter, Vascular, Long-Term	Cardiovascular
74WOW	Electrode, Electrocardiograph, Long-Term	Cardiovascular
80WKY	Garment, Electrode	General
73BYS	Lung, Membrane (For Long-Term Respiratory Support)	Anesthesiology
75JMP	Radioimmunoassay, Long-Acting Thyroid Stimulator	Chemistry
74ROK	Recorder, Long-Term, Blood Pressure, Portable	Cardiovascular
74ROL	Recorder, Long-Term, ECG	Cardiovascular
74ROM	Recorder, Long-Term, ECG, Portable (Holter Monitor)	Cardiovascular
84RON	Recorder, Long-Term, EEG	Cns/Neurology
73ROO	Recorder, Long-Term, Oxygen	Anesthesiology
73VDC	Recorder, Long-Term, Respiration	Anesthesiology
80ROP	Recorder, Long-Term, Trend	General
80WMC	Recorder, Long-Term, pH	General
84VDD	Scanner, Long-Term Recording, EEG	Cns/Neurology
73VDB	Scanner, Long-Term Recording, Respiration	Anesthesiology
74RQU	Scanner, Long-Term, ECG, Recording	Cardiovascular

LONG-ACTING

75JMP	Radioimmunoassay, Long-Acting Thyroid Stimulator	Chemistry

LONG-TERM

80LNY	Catheter, Intraspinal, Percutaneous, Long-Term	General
80LJS	Catheter, Intravascular, Therapeutic, Long-term Greater Than 30 Days	General
78FJS	Catheter, Peritoneal, Indwelling, Long-Term	Gastro/Urology
74DYD	Catheter, Vascular, Long-Term	Cardiovascular
74WOW	Electrode, Electrocardiograph, Long-Term	Cardiovascular
73BYS	Lung, Membrane (For Long-Term Respiratory Support)	Anesthesiology
74ROK	Recorder, Long-Term, Blood Pressure, Portable	Cardiovascular
74ROL	Recorder, Long-Term, ECG	Cardiovascular
74ROM	Recorder, Long-Term, ECG, Portable (Holter Monitor)	Cardiovascular
84RON	Recorder, Long-Term, EEG	Cns/Neurology
73ROO	Recorder, Long-Term, Oxygen	Anesthesiology
73VDC	Recorder, Long-Term, Respiration	Anesthesiology
80ROP	Recorder, Long-Term, Trend	General
80WMC	Recorder, Long-Term, pH	General
84VDD	Scanner, Long-Term Recording, EEG	Cns/Neurology
73VDB	Scanner, Long-Term Recording, Respiration	Anesthesiology
74RQU	Scanner, Long-Term, ECG, Recording	Cardiovascular

LOOP

80LHE	Controller, Glucose, Blood, Closed-Loop	General
80LSX	Controller, Pressure, Blood, Closed-Loop	General
86RES	Expressor, Lens Loop	Ophthalmology
74RFH	Loop, Endarterectomy	Cardiovascular
83RFI	Loop, Inoculating	Microbiology
86RET	Loop, Lens	Ophthalmology
77RFJ	Loop, Tracheal	Ear/Nose/Throat
74RFK	Loop, Vascular	Cardiovascular
77JYQ	Loop, Wire	Ear/Nose/Throat
80MQT	Pump, Drug Administration, Closed Loop	General
83LIE	Reagent, Inoculator Calibration (Laboratory)	Microbiology
83VLZ	Sterilizer, Loop, Inoculating	Microbiology
80QYX	Tester, Ground Loop Impedance	General

LOOSE

79SGW	Suture, Laparoscopy, Loose	Surgery
79SGY	Suture, Laparoscopy, Pre-Tied	Surgery

LOSS

78MKL	Device, Measuring, Blood Loss	Gastro/Urology

LOTION

80VLB	Lotion, Skin Care	General
80WPU	Soap	General

LOUPE

86HJH	Loupe, Binocular, Low Power	Ophthalmology
79FSP	Loupe, Diagnostic/Surgical	Surgery
86HOH	Spectacle, Operating (Loupe), Ophthalmic	Ophthalmology

LOW

82DFC	Antigen, Antiserum, Control, Lipoprotein, Low Density	Immunology
78QBR	Aspirator, Low Volume (Gastric Suction)	Gastro/Urology
74MPD	Auxillary Power Supply, Low Energy Defibrillator (AC or DC)	Cardiovascular
90IYJ	Collimator, Therapeutic X-Ray, Low Voltage	Radiology
80LXW	Column, Adsorption, Lipoprotein, Low Density	General
74LDD	Defibrillator, Battery-Powered, Low Energy	Cardiovascular
75UKM	Freezer, Laboratory, Ultra-Low Temperature	Chemistry
90IYD	Generator, Therapeutic X-Ray, Low Voltage	Radiology
78MMY	Lipoprotein, Low Density, Removal	Gastro/Urology
86HJH	Loupe, Binocular, Low Power	Ophthalmology
86HJF	Magnifier, Hand-Held, Low-Vision	Ophthalmology
73BYF	Mask, Oxygen, Low Concentration, Venturi	Anesthesiology
78ROX	Regulator, Suction, Low Volume (Gastric)	Gastro/Urology
89LBF	Stimulator, Muscle, Low Intensity	Physical Med
86HKB	Telescope, Hand-Held, Low-Vision	Ophthalmology
86HKK	Telescope, Spectacle, Low-Vision	Ophthalmology
73BYX	Tubing, Flexible, Medical Gas, Low-Pressure	Anesthesiology

LOW-DENSITY

75MRR	System, Test, Low-Density, Lipoprotein	Chemistry

LOW-PRESSURE

73BYX	Tubing, Flexible, Medical Gas, Low-Pressure	Anesthesiology

LOW-VISION

86HJF	Magnifier, Hand-Held, Low-Vision	Ophthalmology
86HKC	Spectacle Microscope, Low-Vision	Ophthalmology
86HKB	Telescope, Hand-Held, Low-Vision	Ophthalmology
86HKK	Telescope, Spectacle, Low-Vision	Ophthalmology

LOWRY

75JGP	Lowry (Colorimetric), Total Protein	Chemistry

LSD

91DOL	Free Radical Assay, LSD	Toxicology
91DLB	Radioimmunoassay, LSD (125-I)	Toxicology

LUBRICANT

78FHY	Jelly, Contact (For Transurethral Surgical Instrument)	Gastro/Urology
80TCZ	Lubricant, Instrument	General
80KMJ	Lubricant, Patient	General
80MMS	Lubricant, Vaginal, Patient	General

LUBRICATING

80RFL	Jelly, Lubricating	General
78FHX	Jelly, Lubricating, Transurethral Surgical Instrument	Gastro/Urology

LUER

74WJY	Connector, Tubing, Blood	Cardiovascular
78FKB	Connector, Tubing, Blood, Infusion, T-Type	Gastro/Urology
80QWK	Fitting, Luer	General
80WLM	Lock, Catheter	General
76DZF	Syringe, Drug, Luer-Lock	Dental And Oral
80WSP	Tubing, Connecting	General

LUER-LOCK

80QWK	Fitting, Luer	General
76DZF	Syringe, Drug, Luer-Lock	Dental And Oral

LUGOL'S

88IAM	Solution, Pathology, Lugol's	Pathology

LUMBAR

84RFM	Kit, Lumbar Puncture	Cns/Neurology
80CAQ	Monitor, Cerebral Spinal Fluid Pressure (CSF)	General
89IQE	Orthosis, Lumbar	Physical Med

LUMBOSACRAL

87QDH	Belt, Lumbosacral	Orthopedics
89IPY	Orthosis, Lumbosacral	Physical Med
87RXE	Support, Back	Orthopedics

LUMBOSCOPE

78TDA	Lumboscope	Gastro/Urology

LUMEN

78FGH	Catheter, Double Lumen Female Urethrographic	Gastro/Urology
79GBP	Catheter, Multiple Lumen	Surgery
80FMI	Needle, Hypodermic, Single Lumen With Syringe	General

KEYWORD INDEX

MAINTENANCE (cont'd)
80WSO Pump, Industrial — General
80VBJ Service, Maintenance/Repair — General

MALACHITE
88KJY Stain, Malachite Green — Pathology

MALAR
79LZK Malar Implant — Surgery

MALE
78FGI Catheter, Urethrographic, Male — Gastro/Urology
85LLS Contraceptive Tubal Occlusion Device, Male — Obstetrics/Gyn
83SGO Kit, Gonorrhoeae Test (Male Use) — Microbiology

MALECOT
78FEW Catheter, Malecot (Gastrostomy Tube) — Gastro/Urology

MALEIC
75JMS Oxalacetic Acid And NADH Oxidation (U.V.), Maleic DH — Chemistry
76KQB PV Methylether Maleic Anhydride Copol./Carboxymethylcellul. — Dental And Oral
76KOO Polyvinyl Methylether Maleic Acid-Calcium-Sodium Dbl. Salt — Dental And Oral
76KOT Polyvinyl Methylether Maleic Acid/Carboxymethylcellulose — Dental And Oral
76KXY Polyvinyl Methylether Maleic Anhydride/Carboxymethylcellul. — Dental And Oral

MALLEABLE
84HBP Clip, Implantable, Malleable — Cns/Neurology

MALLET
79GFB Hammer, Head, Surgical — Surgery
84QZF Hammer, Neurological — Cns/Neurology
84QZG Hammer, Percussion — Cns/Neurology
79FZY Hammer, Surgical — Surgery
87HXL Mallet, Bone — Orthopedics
76RFR Mallet, Dental — Dental And Oral
79RFS Mallet, Other — Surgery
79GFJ Mallet, Surgical, General & Plastic Surgery — Surgery

MALLEUS
77JYR Nipper, Malleus — Ear/Nose/Throat

MALLORY'S
88HYW Stain, Mallory's Trichrome — Pathology

MAMMARY
85WJD Needle, Biopsy, Mammary — Obstetrics/Gyn
79KCZ Prosthesis, Breast, External — Surgery
79FWM Prosthesis, Breast, Inflatable, Internal — Surgery
79FTR Prosthesis, Breast, Non-Inflatable, Internal — Surgery
85WWA Retractor, Mammary — Obstetrics/Gyn
79MRD Sizer, Mammary, Breast Implant Volume — Surgery
85WSC Spectroscope, Tumor Analysis, Mammary — Obstetrics/Gyn

MAMMOGRAPHIC
90VGI Phantom, Mammographic — Radiology
90IZH Radiographic Unit, Diagnostic, Mammographic — Radiology
85RQW Scanner, Ultrasonic, Breast (Mammographic) — Obstetrics/Gyn
85WSC Spectroscope, Tumor Analysis, Mammary — Obstetrics/Gyn
85LHM System, Thermographic, Liquid Crystal — Obstetrics/Gyn
85SAG Thermographic Device, Infrared — Obstetrics/Gyn
90KXZ Thermographic Device, Liquid Crystal, Adjunctive — Radiology
90LHR Thermographic Device, Liquid Crystal, Screen — Radiology

MAMMOGRAPHY
85WJD Needle, Biopsy, Mammary — Obstetrics/Gyn

MANAGEMENT
82LTJ Antigen, Prostate-Specific (PSA), Management, Cancer — Immunology
80VAX Computer Equipment — General
80WSJ Computer Software, Hospital/Nursing Management — General
80VHN Computer, Patient Data Management — General
78LYW Device, External, Management, Weight — Gastro/Urology
79MDA Elastomer, Silicone (Scar Management) — Surgery
80WYB Equipment, Management, Pain, Radiofrequency, Non-Invasive — General
80WUN Service, Waste Management — General

MANDATORY
73CBO Attachment, Intermittent Mandatory Ventilation (IMV) — Anesthesiology
73SET Controller, Ventilator IMV — Anesthesiology

MANDIBLE
76LZD Implant, Joint, Temporomandibular — Dental And Oral
79JCR Prosthesis, Mandible — Surgery
76WLF Stethoscope, Dental — Dental And Oral

MANDIBULAR
77JAZ Prosthesis, Facial, Mandibular Implant — Ear/Nose/Throat
76MPL Prosthesis, Mandibular Condyle — Dental And Oral
76UEA Staple, Mandibular — Dental And Oral

MANDREL
76RFU Mandrel — Dental And Oral

MANIFOLD
74DTL Adapter, Stopcock, Manifold, Cardiopulmonary Bypass — Cardiovascular
75RFV Manifold, Gas — Chemistry
75RFW Manifold, Liquid — Chemistry
80FMG Stopcock — General
80WSP Tubing, Connecting — General

MANIKIN
80SBS Training Manikin, CPR (Resuscitation) — General
80TFF Training Manikin, Intravenous Arm — General
80SBT Training Manikin, Other — General
80TFO Training Manikin, Wound Moulage — General

MANIPULATION
79SJI Balloon, Manipulation, Tissue — Surgery
78QXJ Forceps, Stone Manipulation — Gastro/Urology

MANIPULATOR
85LKF Cannula, Manipulator/Injector, Uterine — Obstetrics/Gyn
85RCF Injector & Accessories, Manipulator, Uterine — Obstetrics/Gyn
80RGR Micromanipulator — General
89LXM Plunger-Like Joint Manipulator — Physical Med

MANOMETER
80QTK Electromanometer — General
74QIX Kit, Blood Pressure, Central Venous — Cardiovascular
75UGT Manometer, Laboratory — Chemistry
80FMJ Manometer, Spinal Fluid — General
78FJA Manometer, Water — Gastro/Urology
73BXR Monitor, Airway Pressure (Inspiratory Force) — Anesthesiology
73RLV Monitor, Airway Pressure, Continuous — Anesthesiology
74RLS Monitor, Blood Pressure, Indirect (Arterial) — Cardiovascular
73BXD Monitor, Blood Pressure, Indirect, Anesthesiology — Anesthesiology
74JOE Monitor, Blood Pressure, Indirect, Automatic — Cardiovascular
74DXN Monitor, Blood Pressure, Indirect, Semi-Automatic — Cardiovascular
79FYM Monitor, Blood Pressure, Indirect, Surgery — Surgery
79FYL Monitor, Blood Pressure, Indirect, Surgery, Powered — Surgery
73BZZ Monitor, Blood Pressure, Indirect, Transducer — Anesthesiology
74RLR Monitor, Blood Pressure, Invasive (Arterial) — Cardiovascular
73CAA Monitor, Blood Pressure, Invasive (Arterial), Anesthesia — Anesthesiology
74RLX Monitor, Blood Pressure, Venous — Cardiovascular
74KRK Monitor, Blood Pressure, Venous, Cardiopulmonary Bypass — Cardiovascular
79FYO Monitor, Blood Pressure, Venous, Central — Surgery
79FYP Monitor, Blood Pressure, Venous, Peripheral — Surgery
80CAQ Monitor, Cerebral Spinal Fluid Pressure (CSF) — General
78RLU Monitor, Esophageal Pressure — Gastro/Urology
84RLW Monitor, Intracranial Pressure — Cns/Neurology
84GWM Monitor, Intracranial Pressure, Continuous — Cns/Neurology
80FLY Sphygmomanometer, Aneroid (Arterial Pressure) — General
80THH Sphygmomanometer, Electronic (Arterial Pressure) — General
80UDM Sphygmomanometer, Electronic, Automatic — General
80UDN Sphygmomanometer, Electronic, Manual — General
80FLX Sphygmomanometer, Mercury (Arterial Pressure) — General

MANOMETRIC
75CIE Volumetric/Manometric, Carbon-Dioxide — Chemistry

MANSONI
83GNH Antigen, Fluorescent Antibody Test, Schistosoma Mansoni — Microbiology

MANTLE
83UGK Heating Mantle — Microbiology

MANUAL
73BXL Algesimeter, Manual — Anesthesiology
81QLN Analyzer, Coagulation, Manual — Hematology
81UJS Anti-Human Serum, Manual — Hematology
90IWJ Applicator, Radionuclide, Manual — Radiology
80FNJ Bed, Manual — General
89INY Bed, Patient Rotation, Manual — Physical Med
79GED Brush, Dermabrasion, Manual — Surgery
86HOF Burr, Corneal, Manual — Ophthalmology
86HMD Chair, Ophthalmic, Manual — Ophthalmology
79FZO Chisel, Surgical, Manual — Surgery
90IZX Collimator, Radiographic, Manual — Radiology
80FQD Compressor, External, Cardiac, Manual — General
73BSC Controller, Infusion, Manual — Anesthesiology
83KZC Counter, Colony, Manual — Microbiology
91DNM Counter, Gamma, Radioimmunoassay (Manual) — Toxicology
81GLG Counter, Platelet, Manual — Hematology
84HBG Drill, Manual (With Burr, Trephine & Accessories) — Cns/Neurology
76DZJ Driver, Wire, And Bone Drill, Manual — Dental And Oral
77LRC ENT Manual Surgical Instrument — Ear/Nose/Throat
81JCG Fluid, Manual Cell Diluting — Hematology
81JPI Hematocrit, Manual — Hematology
90LNF Hyperthermia System, Manual Control — Radiology
76QOY Instrument, Dental, Manual — Dental And Oral

MANUAL *(cont'd)*

79MDM	Instrument, Manual, General Surgical	Surgery
89HHC	Kit, Sitz Bath	Physical Med
80WVL	Manual, Policies	General
89LYG	Massager, Therapeutic, Manual	Physical Med
87LXH	Orthopedic Manual Surgical Instrument	Orthopedics
79GFI	Osteotome, Manual (Plastic Surgery)	Surgery
86HON	Perimeter, Manual	Ophthalmology
90JAH	Processor, Radiographic Film, Manual	Radiology
78FEQ	Pump, Air, Non-Manual, Endoscopic	Gastro/Urology
77JPT	Pump, Nebulizer, Manual	Ear/Nose/Throat
86HLH	Pupillometer, Manual	Ophthalmology
73WJE	Resuscitator, Emergency, Protective, Infection	Anesthesiology
80FQB	Resuscitator, Pulmonary, Manual (Demand Valve)	General
84GZW	Retractor, Manual	Cns/Neurology
84HAE	Rongeur, Manual, Neurosurgical	Cns/Neurology
79GDR	Saw, Manual, And Accessories	Surgery
84HAC	Saw, Manual, Neurological (With Accessories)	Cns/Neurology
80UDN	Sphygmomanometer, Electronic, Manual	General
74LDE	Stethoscope, Manual	Cardiovascular
78KOA	Surgical Instrument, G-U, Manual	Gastro/Urology
79MDW	Surgical Instrument, Manual (General Use)	Surgery
85HHP	Table, Obstetrical, Manual	Obstetrics/Gyn
86HRK	Table, Ophthalmic, Instrument, Manual	Ophthalmology
80FSE	Table, Surgical, Manual	General
86HKY	Tonometer, Manual	Ophthalmology
76EFW	Toothbrush, Manual	Dental And Oral
80FMR	Transfer Device, Patient, Manual	General
86HRH	Trephine, Manual, Ophthalmic (Corneal)	Ophthalmology
73BTM	Ventilator, Emergency, Manual (Resuscitator)	Anesthesiology
89IOR	Wheelchair, Manual	Physical Med

MANUALLY

78FFD	Evacuator, Bladder, Manually Operated	Gastro/Urology

MANUFACTURING

80VFE	Component, Ceramic	General
80WKG	Component, Electrical	General
80VAF	Component, Electronic	General
80WOS	Component, Metal, Other	General
80WSM	Component, Paper	General
80VAE	Component, Plastic	General
80VAL	Component, Rubber	General
80VAM	Component, Silicone	General
80WSN	Computer Software, Industrial	General
80WVW	Contract Assembly	General
80VAC	Contract Manufacturing	General
80WXH	Contract Manufacturing, Pharmaceuticals/Chemicals	General
80WLY	Contract Manufacturing, Product, Disposable	General
80WLX	Contract Manufacturing, Product, Durable	General
80WLH	Contract Manufacturing, Reagent	General
87WLZ	Custom Prosthesis	Orthopedics
80VAJ	Equipment, Extruding/Molding	General
80WQM	Equipment/Service, Quality Control	General
80WJB	Material, Raw, Production	General
80WYJ	Molding, Injection	General
80SHO	Polariscope	General
80VAP	Production Equipment	General
80WSO	Pump, Industrial	General
80WVQ	Service, Engraving	General
80WTV	System, Robot	General
80WYK	Thermoforming, Extrusion, Custom	General
80WWE	Tubing, Other	General

MAPPING

84VKG	Computer, Brain Mapping	Cns/Neurology
90VHA	Doppler, Flow Mapping	Radiology
86WXT	System, Mapping, Corneal	Ophthalmology

MARCESANS

83GTA	Antiserum, Serratia Marcesans	Microbiology

MARGIN

76EKA	File, Margin Finishing, Operative	Dental And Oral
76EJZ	Knife, Margin Finishing, Operative	Dental And Oral

MARKER

90WJW	Accessories, Radiotherapy	Radiology
90KXI	Anatomical Marker, Radionuclide	Radiology
82MMW	Antigen, Tumor Marker, Bladder (Basement Membrane Complexes)	Immunology
90SGK	Labeler, X-Ray Film	Radiology
74MAB	Marker, Cardiopulmonary Bypass (Vein Marker)	Cardiovascular
79MAW	Marker, Identification, Suture	Surgery
86HMR	Marker, Ocular	Ophthalmology
79KPK	Marker, Ostia, Aorto-Saphenous Vein	Surgery
76EMP	Marker, Periodontic	Dental And Oral
86HMQ	Marker, Sclera (Ocular)	Ophthalmology
79FZZ	Marker, Skin	Surgery

MARKER *(cont'd)*

90RFX	Marker, X-Ray	Radiology
86HRP	Pen, Marking, Surgical	Ophthalmology
86VKE	Surgical Instrument, Radial Keratotomy	Ophthalmology
82NAH	System, Test, Tumor Marker, For Detection Of Bladder Cancer	Immunology
81LJD	Test, B Lymphocyte Marker	Hematology
81LIZ	Test, T Lymphocyte Surface Marker	Hematology

MARKERS

83MYI	System, Test, Genotypic Detection, Resistant Markers, Staphylococcus Colonies	Microbiology

MARKING

80WXQ	Equipment, Marking, Electrochemical	General
86HRP	Pen, Marking, Surgical	Ophthalmology
80WVQ	Service, Engraving	General
90JAC	System, Marking, Film, Radiographic	Radiology
80WXP	System, Marking, Laser	General

MARROW

80LWE	Kit, Collection/Transfusion, Marrow, Bone	General
79SGU	Needle, Bone Marrow	Surgery

MARTIUS

88KJZ	Stain, Martius Yellow	Pathology

MASK

80WJO	Dispenser, Other	General
76UDX	Mask, Analgesia	Dental And Oral
86RGA	Mask, Eye, Phototherapy	Ophthalmology
80WKE	Mask, Face	General
73BSJ	Mask, Gas, Anesthesia	Anesthesiology
80RGD	Mask, Other	General
73BYG	Mask, Oxygen, Aerosol Administration	Anesthesiology
73BYF	Mask, Oxygen, Low Concentration, Venturi	Anesthesiology
73KGB	Mask, Oxygen, Non-Rebreathing	Anesthesiology
80FQG	Mask, Oxygen, Other	General
80RFY	Mask, Oxygen, Partial Rebreathing	General
73FSC	Mask, Oxygen, Venturi	Anesthesiology
73KHA	Mask, Scavenging	Anesthesiology
79FXX	Mask, Surgical	Surgery
77RGB	Mask, Tracheostomy	Ear/Nose/Throat
73RGC	Mask, Tracheostomy, Aerosol Administration	Anesthesiology
90VFC	Mask, X-Ray Shield	Radiology
86HOY	Shield, Eye, Ophthalmic	Ophthalmology
73BTK	Strap, Head, Gas Mask	Anesthesiology

MASKER

77KLW	Masker, Tinnitus	Ear/Nose/Throat

MASS

80WML	Calibrator, Mass Spectrometer	General
75RGE	Mass Screening System	Chemistry
91DOP	Mass Spectrometer, Clinical Use	Toxicology
75UGU	Spectrograph, Mass	Chemistry

MASSAGE

89ILJ	Bath, Hydro-Massage (Whirlpool)	Physical Med
89INW	Table, Mechanical	Physical Med

MASSAGER

89IPD	Massager, Battery-Powered	Physical Med
89IRP	Massager, Powered Inflatable Tube	Physical Med
89ISA	Massager, Therapeutic	Physical Med
89LYG	Massager, Therapeutic, Manual	Physical Med
86WNV	Reducer, Pressure, Intraocular	Ophthalmology

MASSAGING

76JET	Pick, Massaging	Dental And Oral

MAST

74RLJ	Suit, Pneumatic Counterpressure (Anti-Shock)	Cardiovascular

MASTECTOMY

79KCZ	Prosthesis, Breast, External	Surgery
79FWM	Prosthesis, Breast, Inflatable, Internal	Surgery
79FTR	Prosthesis, Breast, Non-Inflatable, Internal	Surgery
85VLD	Prosthesis, Nipple	Obstetrics/Gyn

MASTER

77KHL	Hearing-Aid, Master	Ear/Nose/Throat

MASTOID

77JYD	Chisel, Mastoid	Ear/Nose/Throat
77JYI	Gauge, Mastoid	Ear/Nose/Throat
77RPT	Retractor, Mastoid	Ear/Nose/Throat
77JZA	Rongeur, Mastoid	Ear/Nose/Throat
77JZC	Searcher, Mastoid	Ear/Nose/Throat

MAT

80TCC	Floor Mat	General
80QWM	Floor Mat, Antibacterial	General

MATER

84LEM	Dura Mater, Human, Lyophilized	Cns/Neurology
84UAV	Prosthesis, Nerve Sheath	Cns/Neurology

MATERIAL

76DYO	Band, Material, Orthodontic	Dental And Oral
80VAS	Building Material	General
76EBD	Coating, Filling Material, Resin	Dental And Oral
84HBX	Instrument, Forming, Material, Cranioplasty	Cns/Neurology
86HQD	Lens, Contact (Other Material)	Ophthalmology
76WKF	Material, Acrylic, Dental	Dental And Oral
76UDT	Material, Casting	Dental And Oral
91LAX	Material, Control, Lidocaine	Toxicology
76QOW	Material, Dental Filling	Dental And Oral
76LPG	Material, Dressing, Surgical, Acid, Polylactic	Dental And Oral
76ELW	Material, Impression	Dental And Oral
76EBH	Material, Impression Tray, Resin	Dental And Oral
76EGC	Material, Investment	Dental And Oral
77ESG	Material, Metallic-Stainless Steel, Tantalum, Platinum	Ear/Nose/Throat
79KKY	Material, PTFE/Carbon, Maxillofacial	Surgery
80WUG	Material, Polymethylmethacrylate	General
81KSC	Material, Preparation, Skin	Hematology
80WJB	Material, Raw, Production	General
79GBI	Material, Restoration, Aesthetic, External	Surgery
76EBF	Material, Tooth Shade, Resin	Dental And Oral
80VBD	Material, Training, Audiovisual	General
87MOO	Orthopedic Implant Material	Orthopedics
80VAI	Packaging Material	General
77KHK	Polymer, ENT Natural Collagen Material	Ear/Nose/Throat
77KHJ	Polymer, ENT Synthetic Polyamide (Mesh Or Foil Material)	Ear/Nose/Throat
77ESI	Polymer, Natural Absorbable Gelatin Material	Ear/Nose/Throat
80WTJ	Polymer, Synthetic, Other	General
77LBP	Prosthesis, Ossicular (Stapes), Absorbable Gelatin Material	Ear/Nose/Throat
77LBO	Prosthesis, Ossicular (Total), Absorbable Gelatin Material	Ear/Nose/Throat
80WWC	Resin, Other	General
76EKK	Spreader, Pulp Canal Filling Material, Endodontic	Dental And Oral
76EID	Syringe, Restorative And Impression Material	Dental And Oral

MATERIALS

91LAY	Methotrexate Control Materials	Toxicology
91LAZ	N-Acetylprocainamide Control Materials	Toxicology
91LBA	Procainamide Control Materials	Toxicology
91LAW	Theophylline Control Materials	Toxicology

MATERNAL

82LTQ	Calibrator, AFP, Serum, Maternal, Mid-Pregnancy	Immunology

MATERNITY

85UKV	Brassiere, Maternity	Obstetrics/Gyn
85RGF	Kit, Maternity	Obstetrics/Gyn

MATRIX

76UDY	Band, Matrix	Dental And Oral
76EKF	Contouring, Instrument, Matrix, Operative	Dental And Oral
76DZN	Matrix, Dental	Dental And Oral
76KCQ	Matrix, Tube Impression	Dental And Oral
76JEP	Retainer, Matrix	Dental And Oral

MATTRESS

89FNH	Bed, Water Flotation, AC-Powered	Physical Med
80FMW	Cover, Mattress	General
80QNA	Cover, Mattress, Conductive	General
80QNB	Cover, Mattress, Waterproof	General
80FNM	Mattress, Air Flotation	General
89ILA	Mattress, Alternating Pressure (Or Pads)	Physical Med
80RGG	Mattress, Bed	General
80WLB	Mattress, Immobilization	General
89IKY	Mattress, Non-Powered Flotation Therapy	Physical Med
80RGH	Mattress, Operating Table	General
80WYO	Mattress, Reduction, Pressure	General
80FNI	Mattress, Silicone, And Chair Cushion	General
80RGI	Mattress, Water	General
80FOH	Mattress, Water, Temperature Regulated	General
80RBU	Pad, Incontinence (Underpad)	General
80RMC	Pad, Pressure, Foam Convoluted	General
80RMD	Pad, Pressure, Gel	General
80RMF	Pad, Pressure, Water Cushion	General
80WLC	Pillow	General
80WKD	Sheeting, Stretcher	General

MATURITY

75JHG	Chromatographic Separation, Lecithin-Sphingomyelin Ratio	Chemistry
75JHF	Colorimetric Method, Lecithin-Sphingomyelin Ratio	Chemistry
75JHH	Electrophoretic Method, Lecithin-Sphingomyelin Ratio	Chemistry
75WHJ	Test, Maturity, Lung, Fetal	Chemistry

MAXILLA

79JCS	Prosthesis, Maxilla	Surgery

MAXILLOFACIAL

79KKY	Material, PTFE/Carbon, Maxillofacial	Surgery
79JCS	Prosthesis, Maxilla	Surgery
77LGK	Prosthesis, Maxillofacial	Ear/Nose/Throat

MAXWELL

86HIX	Light, Maxwell Spot, AC-Powered	Ophthalmology

MAYER'S

88HYL	Stain, Hematoxylin, Mayer's	Pathology

MAYO

79FSH	Stand, Operating Room Instrument (Mayo)	Surgery
79FZN	Table, Instrument, Surgical	Surgery

MEASLES

83GRJ	Antigen, CF, (Including CF Control), Rubeola	Microbiology
83GRH	Antigen, HA (Including HA Control), Rubeola	Microbiology
83GRF	Antiserum, CF, Rubeola	Microbiology
83GRE	Antiserum, Fluorescent, Rubeola	Microbiology
83GRG	Antiserum, HAI, Rubeola	Microbiology
83GRI	Antiserum, Neutralization, Rubeola	Microbiology
83LJB	Enzyme Linked Immunoabsorbent Assay, Rubeola	Microbiology

MEASURE

80SEC	Bag, Urinary Collection, Precision Measure (Urine Meter)	General
82MVJ	Devices, Measure, Antibodies to Glomerular Basement Membrane (gbm)	Immunology

MEASURED

81JBW	Red Cell Indices, Measured	Hematology

MEASUREMENT

81KRZ	Calibrator, Hemoglobin And Hematocrit Measurement	Hematology
90IWN	Cassette, Measurement, Ardran-Crooks	Radiology
84HCJ	Device, Measurement, Potential, Skin	Cns/Neurology
84JXE	Device, Measurement, Velocity, Conduction, Nerve	Cns/Neurology
75JKF	Dinitrophenyl Hydrazone Measurement (Colorimetric), HBD	Chemistry
75JKJ	Fluorometric Measurement, Porphyrins	Chemistry
75JNP	Infrared Spectroscopy Measurement, Urinary Calculi (Stone)	Chemistry
73JEZ	Monitor, Lung Water Measurement	Anesthesiology
89LZW	Monitor, Spine Curvature	Physical Med
89JFC	Pressure Measurement, System, Intermittent	Physical Med
73BXQ	Rhinoanemometer (Measurement Of Nasal Decongestion)	Anesthesiology
75JGC	Tryptophan Measurement (Colorimetric), Globulin	Chemistry
78SEF	Urodynamic Measurement System	Gastro/Urology
84LLN	Vibration Threshold Measurement Device	Cns/Neurology
75JFL	pH Rate Measurement, Carbon-Dioxide	Chemistry

MEASURER

86HLN	Gauge, Lens, Ophthalmic	Ophthalmology
86HJB	Measurer, Corneal Radius	Ophthalmology
76JEO	Measurer, Gingival Fluid	Dental And Oral
86HLF	Measurer, Lens Radius, Ophthalmic	Ophthalmology
86HLM	Measurer, Lens, AC-Powered	Ophthalmology
86HLC	Measurer, Stereopsis	Ophthalmology

MEASURING

90WSH	Calculator, Technique, Radiographic	Radiology
80KYW	Container, Medication, Graduated Liquid	General
78MKL	Device, Measuring, Blood Loss	Gastro/Urology
89ISD	Exerciser, Measuring	Physical Med
89ION	Exerciser, Non-Measuring	Physical Med
89ISC	Exerciser, Passive, Measuring	Physical Med
89IOO	Exerciser, Passive, Non-Measuring (CPM Machine)	Physical Med
77JYJ	Gauge, Measuring	Ear/Nose/Throat
81JWO	Meter, Volume, Blood	Hematology
78FDY	Panendoscope Measuring Device	Gastro/Urology
89KHX	Platform, Force-Measuring	Physical Med
77JYZ	Rod, Measuring Ear	Ear/Nose/Throat
79FTY	Tape, Measuring, Ruler And Caliper	Surgery
77EWN	Unit, Measuring, Potential, Evoked, Auditory	Ear/Nose/Throat

MECHANICAL

89KFT	Assembly, Shoulder/Elbow/Forearm/Wrist/Hand, Mechanical	Physical Med
75QCG	Balance, Mechanical	Chemistry
78FCF	Biopsy Instrument, Mechanical, Gastrointestinal	Gastro/Urology
89INN	Chair, Adjustable, Mechanical	Physical Med
76JER	Cleaner, Denture, Mechanical	Dental And Oral
89KHZ	Control, Foot Driving, Automobile, Mechanical	Physical Med
89IPQ	Control, Hand Driving, Automobile, Mechanical	Physical Med
90IZY	Cradle, Radiographic, Mechanical	Radiology
78EZY	Device, Incontinence, Mechanical/Hydraulic	Gastro/Urology
78FAH	Dilator, Urethral, Mechanical	Gastro/Urology
89IKQ	Goniometer, Mechanical	Physical Med
89IRA	Hand, External Limb Component, Mechanical	Physical Med
89IQX	Hook, External Limb Component, Mechanical	Physical Med
78FHW	Impotence Device, Mechanical/Hydraulic	Gastro/Urology
76EGM	Injector, Jet, Mechanical-Powered	Dental And Oral

MECHANICAL (cont'd)

89IRD	Joint, Elbow, External Limb Component, Mechanical	Physical Med
89ISZ	Joint, Wrist, External Limb Component, Mechanical	Physical Med
78LQC	Lithotriptor, Mechanical, Biliary	Gastro/Urology
78MET	Lithotriptor, Mechanical, Non-Crushing	Gastro/Urology
80FQE	Regulator, Oxygen, Mechanical	General
73BTZ	Resuscitator, Cardiac, Mechanical, Compressor	Anesthesiology
80FLT	Stethoscope, Mechanical	General
84GZP	Stimulator, Mechanical, Evoked Response	Cns/Neurology
89INJ	Stretcher, Wheeled, Mechanical	Physical Med
89INW	Table, Mechanical	Physical Med
79FWX	Table, Operating Room, Mechanical	Surgery
80SAC	Tester, Receptacle, Mechanical	General
89IOG	Treadmill, Mechanical	Physical Med
78EXR	Urinometer, Mechanical	Gastro/Urology
74LWQ	Valve, Heart, Mechanical	Cardiovascular
89ITJ	Walker, Mechanical	Physical Med

MECHANICAL-POWERED

76EGM	Injector, Jet, Mechanical-Powered	Dental And Oral

MEDIA

83JRZ	Culture Media, Amino Acid Assay	Microbiology
83JSL	Culture Media, Anaerobic Transport	Microbiology
83JSA	Culture Media, Antibiotic Assay	Microbiology
83MJE	Culture Media, Antifungal, Susceptibility Test	Microbiology
83JSO	Culture Media, Antimicrobial Susceptibility Test	Microbiology
83LKA	Culture Media, Antimicrobial Susceptibility Test	Microbiology
83MJD	Culture Media, Antimycobacteria, Susceptibility Test	Microbiology
83KZI	Culture Media, Enriched	Microbiology
83JTY	Culture Media, For Isolation Of Pathogenic Neisseria	Microbiology
83JSC	Culture Media, General Nutrient Broth	Microbiology
83JTZ	Culture Media, Mueller Hinton Agar Broth	Microbiology
83JSE	Culture Media, Multiple Biochemical Test	Microbiology
83JSM	Culture Media, Non-Propagating Transport	Microbiology
83JSH	Culture Media, Non-Selective And Differential	Microbiology
83JSG	Culture Media, Non-Selective And Non-Differential	Microbiology
83JSN	Culture Media, Propagating Transport	Microbiology
83JSI	Culture Media, Selective And Differential	Microbiology
83JSJ	Culture Media, Selective And Non-Differential	Microbiology
83JSD	Culture Media, Selective Broth	Microbiology
83JSF	Culture Media, Single Biochemical Test	Microbiology
83JSK	Culture Media, Supplements	Microbiology
88KIT	Culture Media, Synthetic Cell And Tissue	Pathology
83JSB	Culture Media, Vitamin Assay	Microbiology
83JTB	Dispenser, Microbiology Media	Microbiology
74DYA	Gel, Electrode, Electrocardiograph	Cardiovascular
79JOT	Gel, Electrode, Electrosurgical	Surgery
76EAS	Gel, Electrode, Pulp Tester	Dental And Oral
84GYB	Gel, Electrode, Stimulator	Cns/Neurology
89IKC	Gel, Electrode, TENS	Physical Med
89QYF	Gel, Ultrasonic Coupling	Physical Med
80SDY	Gel, Ultrasonic Transmission	General
90KTA	Media, Contrast, Radiologic	Radiology
90MJS	Media, Contrast, Ultrasound	Radiology
80WXR	Media, Filter	General
90UJW	Media, Gastroenterographic Contrast (Barium Sulfate)	Radiology
88LEB	Media, Mounting	Pathology
88KEQ	Media, Mounting, Water Soluble	Pathology
88KIX	Media, Mycoplasma Detection	Pathology
81KSG	Media, Potentiating	Hematology
90VGX	Media, Radioactive Isotope Contrast	Radiology
90VGW	Media, Radiographic Injectable Contrast	Radiology
85MQL	Media, Reproductive	Obstetrics/Gyn
86LYX	Media, Storage, Corneal	Ophthalmology
75UIO	Media, Supporting	Chemistry
74MFU	Media, Transport/Storage, Organ/Tissue	Cardiovascular
88KEP	Mounting Media, Oil Soluble	Pathology
88KPB	Mycoplasma Detection Media and Components	Pathology
83WNW	Plate, Culture	Microbiology
90LQA	Reusable Image Media	Radiology
83TDG	Separation Media	Microbiology

MEDIALIZATION

77MIX	System, Vocal Cord Medialization	Ear/Nose/Throat

MEDIASTINOSCOPE

79GCH	Mediastinoscope	Surgery
77EWY	Mediastinoscope, ENT	Ear/Nose/Throat

MEDICAL

90IYE	Accelerator, Linear, Medical	Radiology
80RGJ	Bag, Medical, Physician	General
90IYG	Betatron, Medical	Radiology
80MDR	Binder, Medical, Therapeutic	General
80KMN	Chair/Table, Medical	General
80MDZ	Cleaner, Medical Device	General
80FLG	Cleaner, Ultrasonic, Medical Instrument	General
80LNX	Computer and Software, Medical	General

MEDICAL (cont'd)

86LQB	Computer and Software, Medical, Ophthalmic Use	Ophthalmology
80WPI	Detector, Leakage, Medical Gas	General
80MEC	Disinfector, Medical Device	General
75LXG	Equipment, Laboratory, Gen. Purpose (Specific Medical Use)	Chemistry
80WUC	Facility, Equipment, Medical, Mobile	General
80QXP	Forms, Medical And Patient	General
80THJ	Gas Mixtures, Medical	General
80LDQ	General Medical Device	General
90IWL	Generator, Neutron, Medical	Radiology
80RGK	Holder, Medical Chart	General
80UEU	Identification, Alert, Medical	General
80KYS	Insoles, Medical	General
80LRJ	Medical Disinfectants/Cleaners for Instruments	General
90LWN	Medical Radiographic Personal Monitoring Device	Radiology
80WUL	Metal, Medical	General
90JAE	Microtron, Medical	Radiology
80QJP	Paper, Chart, Record, Medical	General
80LGX	Powered Medical Examination Table	General
80RGL	Rack, Medical Chart	General
80WIE	Service, Licensing, Device, Medical	General
80MED	Sterilant, Medical Device	General
90IWM	Synchrotron, Medical	Radiology
73BYX	Tubing, Flexible, Medical Gas, Low-Pressure	Anesthesiology
73CAM	Yoke, Medical Gas	Anesthesiology

MEDICAMENT

80MWV	Needles, Medicament Dispensing Tip & Irrigating	General

MEDICATED

79GEL	Gauze, Non-Absorbable, Medicated (Internal Sponge)	Surgery
79GEK	Gauze, Non-Absorbable, Non-Medicated (Internal Sponge)	Surgery
80RGM	Pad, Medicated	General
80MLX	Pad, Medicated, Adhesive, Non-Electric	General

MEDICATION

80KYW	Container, Medication, Graduated Liquid	General
80WPQ	Container, Medication, Home-Use	General
80QNK	Crusher, Pill	General
80WTB	Cutter, Pill	General
79SJA	Dispenser, Laparoscopic	Surgery
80KYX	Dispenser, Medication, Liquid	General
80WJO	Dispenser, Other	General
80RCC	Injector, Medication (Inoculator)	General
80WKH	Monitor, Medication	General
80WOL	Patch, Transdermal	General
80TFK	Vial, Medication	General

MEDICINAL

77EPN	Nebulizer, Medicinal	Ear/Nose/Throat
73CCQ	Nebulizer, Medicinal, Non-Ventilatory (Atomizer)	Anesthesiology

MEDICINE

89KNM	Applier, Pressure, Physical Medicine	Physical Med
89ILM	Bath, Sitz, Physical Medicine	Physical Med
80VFT	Bottle, Medicine Spray	General
80QFE	Cabinet, Medicine	General
80QGS	Cart, Medicine	General
89IKP	Chronaximeter, Physical Medicine	Physical Med
90QMD	Computer, Nuclear Medicine	Radiology
80QNW	Cup, Medicine	General
80LDH	Delivery System, Allergen And Vaccine	General
80QRQ	Dropper, Medicine	General
89IKG	Dynamometer, Physical Medicine, Electronic	Physical Med
89ITH	Equipment, Traction, Powered	Physical Med
89KTB	Iontophoresis Unit, Physical Medicine	Physical Med
89IOB	Lamp, Ultraviolet, Physical Medicine	Physical Med
89LDK	Sensor, Optical Contour, Physical Medicine	Physical Med
80VLJ	Spoon, Medicine	General
89ILG	Stocking, Elastic, Physical Medicine	Physical Med
90VHE	Table, Nuclear Medicine	Radiology
89INQ	Table, Physical Medicine, Powered	Physical Med
80SCA	Tray, Medicine	General

MEDIUM

90IZQ	Injector, Contrast Medium, Automatic	Radiology
81JCF	Medium, Lymphocyte Separation	Hematology
88KEO	Paraffin, All Formulations	Pathology
88IER	Polyethylene Glycol (Carbowax)	Pathology

MELTING

88IDT	Melting Point Apparatus, Paraffin	Pathology
88IDS	Melting Pot, Paraffin	Pathology

MEMBRANE

85MDH	Abruptio Placentae Catheter	Obstetrics/Gyn
82MMW	Antigen, Tumor Marker, Bladder (Basement Membrane Complexes)	Immunology
75LTC	Assay, Disease, Membrane, Hyaline	Chemistry

MEMBRANE *(cont'd)*

82MVJ	Devices, Measure, Antibodies to Glomerular Basement Membrane (gbm)	Immunology
75UEO	Electrophoresis Equipment, Cellulose Acetate Membrane	Chemistry
75UGD	Filter, Membrane	Chemistry
77MMB	Hearing-Aid, External, Magnet, Membrane, Tympanic	Ear/Nose/Throat
73BYS	Lung, Membrane (For Long-Term Respiratory Support)	Anesthesiology
75JNX	Oncometer, Plasma (Membrane Osmometry)	Chemistry
85RKH	Perforator, Amniotic Membrane	Obstetrics/Gyn
79TDU	Prosthesis, Membrane	Surgery
75UHS	Reverse Osmosis Membrane Equipment	Chemistry
78MDP	Separator, Blood Cell/Plasma, Therapeutic, Membrane, Auto.	Gastro/Urology
77KQL	Tube, Tympanostomy, With Semi-Permeable Membrane	Ear/Nose/Throat
75JRL	Unit, Filter, Membrane	Chemistry

MEMORY

83WSI	Test, Dementia, Alzheimer's	Microbiology

MENINGITIDIS

83GTI	Antiserum, Fluorescent, N. Meningitidis	Microbiology
83GTJ	Antiserum, N. Meningitidis	Microbiology

MENINGITIS

83TGR	Kit, Meningitis Detection	Microbiology

MENINGOSPETICUM

83GSW	Antiserum, Flavobacterium Meningospeticum	Microbiology

MENISCUS

79RDL	Knife, Meniscus	Surgery

MENSTRUAL

85HHE	Cup, Menstrual	Obstetrics/Gyn
85HHL	Pad, Menstrual, Scented	Obstetrics/Gyn
85HHD	Pad, Menstrual, Unscented	Obstetrics/Gyn
85HIL	Tampon, Menstrual, Scented	Obstetrics/Gyn
85HEB	Tampon, Menstrual, Unscented	Obstetrics/Gyn

MERCURIC

88IFQ	Mercuric Chloride Formulations For Tissue	Pathology
75CHK	Mercuric Nitrate And Diphenyl Carbazone (Titrimetric)	Chemistry

MERCURY

91DPH	Absorption, Atomic, Mercury	Toxicology
75WMX	Analyzer, Mercury	Chemistry
76VEL	Detector, Mercury	Dental And Oral
76EHE	Dispenser, Mercury And/Or Alloy	Dental And Oral
76ELY	Mercury	Dental And Oral
91DJN	Mercury Dithiazone, Colorimetry, Barbiturate	Toxicology
80FLX	Sphygmomanometer, Mercury (Arterial Pressure)	General
80FLK	Thermometer, Mercury	General
78FEF	Tube, Single Lumen, W Mercury Wt Balloon	Gastro/Urology

MERSILENE

79GAS	Suture, Non-Absorbable, Synthetic, Polyester	Surgery

MESH

74DSW	Bag, Polymeric Mesh, Pacemaker	Cardiovascular
79RTP	Cutter, Skin Graft, Expanded Mesh	Surgery
74UAK	Mesh, Cardiovascular (Polymeric)	Cardiovascular
78EZX	Mesh, Metal	Gastro/Urology
87UBH	Mesh, Orthopedic (Metallic)	Orthopedics
79FTM	Mesh, Surgical (Steel Gauze)	Surgery
79FTL	Mesh, Surgical, Polymeric	Surgery
77KHJ	Polymer, ENT Synthetic Polyamide (Mesh Or Foil Material)	Ear/Nose/Throat
87JDJ	Prosthesis, Hip, Acetabular Mesh	Orthopedics

METABOLISM

73QCP	Analyzer, Metabolism	Anesthesiology

METABOLITE

91KLN	Radioimmunoassay, Cocaine Metabolite	Toxicology

METABOLITES

91MAR	Assay, Serum, Cyclosporine and Metabolites, TDX	Toxicology
91DIO	Enzyme Immunoassay, Cocaine And Cocaine Metabolites	Toxicology
91MKU	Enzyme Immunoassay, Nicotine and Nicotine Metabolites	Toxicology
91DLN	Hemagglutination, Cocaine Metabolites (Benzoylecgnonine)	Toxicology
91LAC	High Pressure Liquid Chromatography, Cocaine & Metabolites	Toxicology
91MRS	Test System, Nicotine, Cotinine, Metabolites	Toxicology

METACRYLATE

84GXP	Metacrylate, Methyl, Cranioplasty	Cns/Neurology
84JXH	Methyl Metacrylate	Cns/Neurology

METAL

76EJS	Alloy, Precious Metal, For Clinical Use	Dental And Oral
87MBE	Bone, Block, Filler, Metal, Porous, Uncemented	Orthopedics
76EJF	Bracket, Metal, Orthodontic	Dental And Oral
80WOS	Component, Metal, Other	General
80WXA	Component, Other	General

METAL *(cont'd)*

80WLX	Contract Manufacturing, Product, Durable	General
77KBL	Depressor, Tongue, ENT, Metal	Ear/Nose/Throat
86RGN	Detector, Metal, Magnetic	Ophthalmology
90TDC	Detector, Metal, Ultrasonic	Radiology
78EZM	Dilator, Esophageal (Metal Olive) Gastro-Urology	Gastro/Urology
78FFL	Dislodger, Stone, Basket, Ureteral, Metal	Gastro/Urology
79QVF	Extractor, Metal, Magnetic	Surgery
87LZY	Hip, Hemi-, Femoral, Metal Ball	Orthopedics
86HPM	Locator, Metal, Electronic	Ophthalmology
78EZX	Mesh, Metal	Gastro/Urology
76EJH	Metal, Base	Dental And Oral
80WUL	Metal, Medical	General
87MBK	Prosthesis, Ankle, Semi-, Uncemented, Porous, Metal/Polymer	Orthopedics
87KMD	Prosthesis, Ankle, Semi-Constrained, Metal/Composite	Orthopedics
87HSN	Prosthesis, Ankle, Semi-Constrained, Metal/Polymer	Orthopedics
87KWJ	Prosthesis, Elbow, Hemi-, Humeral, Metal	Orthopedics
87LBC	Prosthesis, Finger, Constrained, Metal, Cemented	Orthopedics
87KWE	Prosthesis, Finger, Constrained, Metal, Uncemented	Orthopedics
87KWG	Prosthesis, Finger, Constrained, Metal/Polymer	Orthopedics
87JDF	Prosthesis, Hip (Metal Stem/Ceramic Self-Locking Ball)	Orthopedics
87JDM	Prosthesis, Hip, Acetabular Component, Metal, Non-Cemented	Orthopedics
87KXD	Prosthesis, Hip, Constrained, Metal	Orthopedics
87KWZ	Prosthesis, Hip, Constrained, Metal/Polymer	Orthopedics
87JDG	Prosthesis, Hip, Femoral Component, Cemented, Metal	Orthopedics
87KWB	Prosthesis, Hip, Hemi-, Acetabular, Metal	Orthopedics
87KWL	Prosthesis, Hip, Hemi-, Femoral, Metal	Orthopedics
87KWY	Prosthesis, Hip, Hemi-, Femoral, Metal/Polymer	Orthopedics
87KXB	Prosthesis, Hip, Pelvifemoral Resurfacing, Metal/polymer	Orthopedics
87MAZ	Prosthesis, Hip, Semi-Const., M/P, Por. Uncem., Calc./Phos.	Orthopedics
87LPF	Prosthesis, Hip, Semi-Const., Metal/Ceramic/Ceramic, Cem.	Orthopedics
87LPH	Prosthesis, Hip, Semi-Const., Metal/Poly., Porous Uncemented	Orthopedics
87MIL	Prosthesis, Hip, Semi-Const., Uncem., M/P, Bone Morph. Prot.	Orthopedics
87MEH	Prosthesis, Hip, Semi-Const., Uncem., Non-P., M/P, Ca./Phos.	Orthopedics
87LZO	Prosthesis, Hip, Semi-Constr., Metal/Ceramic, Cemented/NC	Orthopedics
87JDI	Prosthesis, Hip, Semi-Constrained, Metal/Polymer	Orthopedics
87LWJ	Prosthesis, Hip, Semi-Constrained, Metal/Polymer, Uncemented	Orthopedics
87KMC	Prosthesis, Hip, Semi-constrained, Composite/metal	Orthopedics
87MRA	Prosthesis, Hip, Semi-constrained, Metal/ Ceramic/ Ceramic/ Metal, Cemented or Uncemented	Orthopedics
87MAY	Prosthesis, Hip, Semi-constrained, Metal/Ceramic/Polymer, Cemented or Non-porous Cemented, Osteophilic Finish	Orthopedics
87MBM	Prosthesis, Hip, Semi/Hemi-Const., M/PTFE Ctd./P, Cem./Unc.	Orthopedics
87KRN	Prosthesis, Knee, Femorotibial, Constrained, Metal	Orthopedics
87KRO	Prosthesis, Knee, Femorotibial, Constrained, Metal/Polymer	Orthopedics
87KTX	Prosthesis, Knee, Femorotibial, Non-Constrained, Metal	Orthopedics
87KYK	Prosthesis, Knee, Femorotibial, Semi-Constrained, Metal	Orthopedics
87MBG	Prosthesis, Knee, Femotib., Unconst., Uncem., Unicond., M/P	Orthopedics
87HRZ	Prosthesis, Knee, Hinged (Metal-Metal)	Orthopedics
87KMB	Prosthesis, Knee, Non-Const. (M/C Reinf. Polyeth.) Cemented	Orthopedics
87MBD	Prosthesis, Knee, P/F, Unconst., Uncem., Por., Ctd., P/M/P	Orthopedics
87KRP	Prosthesis, Knee, Patellofemorotibial, Constrained, Metal	Orthopedics
87MBV	Prosthesis, Knee, Patfem., S-C., UHMWPE, Pegged, Unc., P/M/P	Orthopedics
87MBH	Prosthesis, Knee, Patfem., S-C., Unc., Por., Ctd., P/M/P	Orthopedics
87MBA	Prosthesis, Knee, Patfem., Semi-Const., Unc., P/M/P, Osteo.	Orthopedics
87LXY	Prosthesis, Knee, Patfemotib., Semi-Const., P/M/P, Uncem.	Orthopedics
87KWR	Prosthesis, Shoulder, Constr., Metal/Metal or Polymer/Cem.	Orthopedics
87KYM	Prosthesis, Shoulder, Hemi-, Glenoid, Metal	Orthopedics
87MJT	Prosthesis, Shoulder, Humeral, Bipol., Hemi-, Constr., M/P	Orthopedics
87MBF	Prosthesis, Shoulder, Metal/Polymer, Uncemented	Orthopedics
87KWT	Prosthesis, Shoulder, Non-Constrained, Metal/Polymer Cem.	Orthopedics
87KWS	Prosthesis, Shoulder, Semi-Constrained, Metal/Polymer Cem.	Orthopedics
87LZJ	Prosthesis, Toe (Metaphal.), Joint, Met./Poly., Semi-Const.	Orthopedics
87JWI	Prosthesis, Wrist, 2 Part Metal-Plastic Articulation	Orthopedics
87JWJ	Prosthesis, Wrist, 3 Part Metal-Plastic-Metal Articulation	Orthopedics
87KYN	Prosthesis, Wrist, Constrained, Metal	Orthopedics

KEYWORD INDEX

METHOD *(cont'd)*

75JPZ	Colorimetric Method, Gamma-Glutamyl Transpeptidase	Chemistry
75JHF	Colorimetric Method, Lecithin-Sphingomyelin Ratio	Chemistry
75JHM	Colorimetric Method, Lipoproteins	Chemistry
75JGY	Colorimetric Method, Triglycerides	Chemistry
75CHS	Coulometric Method, Carbon-Dioxide	Chemistry
75JHS	Differential Rate Kinetic Method, CPK Or Isoenzymes	Chemistry
75JGF	Differential Rate Method, Lactate Dehydrogenase Isoenzymes	Chemistry
75JIK	Dry Ash Method, Protein Bound Iodine	Chemistry
75CHT	Electrophoretic Method, Catecholamines	Chemistry
75JHH	Electrophoretic Method, Lecithin-Sphingomyelin Ratio	Chemistry
91DMT	Enzymatic Method, Alcohol Dehydrogenase, Ultraviolet	Toxicology
75JIF	Enzymatic Method, Ammonia	Chemistry
75JFM	Enzymatic Method, Bilirubin	Chemistry
75TGO	Enzymatic Method, Blood, Occcult, Fecal	Chemistry
75JIP	Enzymatic Method, Blood, Occult, Urinary	Chemistry
75JFY	Enzymatic Method, Creatinine	Chemistry
75JIA	Enzymatic Method, Galactose	Chemistry
75JIL	Enzymatic Method, Glucose (Urinary, Non-Quantitative)	Chemistry
75KHP	Enzymatic Method, Lactic Acid	Chemistry
75MMI	Enzymatic Method, Troponin Subunit	Chemistry
75JHD	Fluorometric Method, 17-Hydroxycorticosteroids	Chemistry
75JHX	Fluorometric Method, CPK Or Isoenzymes	Chemistry
75CGY	Fluorometric Method, Creatine Phosphokinase	Chemistry
75JGW	Fluorometric Method, Triglycerides	Chemistry
75CGM	Immunodiffusion Method, Immunoglobulins (G, A, M)	Chemistry
86HQJ	Implant, Absorbable (Scleral Buckling Method)	Ophthalmology
75JIR	Indicator Method, Protein Or Albumin (Urinary, Non-Quant.)	Chemistry
75JIE	Ion Exchange Method, Ammonia	Chemistry
75JFI	Isoenzyme, Phosphatase, Alkaline (Catalytic Method)	Chemistry
75JQB	Kinetic Method, Gamma-Glutamyl Transpeptidase	Chemistry
75JIM	Metallic Reduction Method, Glucose (Urinary, Non-Quant.)	Chemistry
75JHL	Microdensitometry Method, Lipoproteins	Chemistry
75CEQ	Molybdenum Blue Method, Phospholipids	Chemistry
75JGD	Nephelometric Method, Globulin	Chemistry
75CFN	Nephelometric Method, Immunoglobulins (G, A, M)	Chemistry
75JHQ	Nephelometric Method, Lipoproteins	Chemistry
75SHQ	Nephelometric Method, Myoglobin	Chemistry
75JFG	Phosphatase, Alkaline (Catalytic Method)	Chemistry
75JID	Photometric Method, Ammonia	Chemistry
75JIY	Photometric Method, Iron (Non-Heme)	Chemistry
75JGJ	Photometric Method, Magnesium	Chemistry
91DNX	Protoporphyrin Zinc Method, Fluorometric, Lead	Toxicology
75JJA	Radio-Labeled Iron Method, Iron (Non-Heme)	Chemistry
91DML	Reagent, NAD-NADH, Alcohol Enzyme Method	Toxicology
75JLP	Spectrophotometric Method, Pregnanediol	Chemistry
75JLQ	Spectrophotometric Method, Pregnanetriol	Chemistry
75JHK	Titrimetric Method, Human Chorionic Gonadotropin	Chemistry
75JHN	Turbidimetric Method, Lipoproteins	Chemistry
75SHR	Turbidimetric Method, Myoglobin	Chemistry
75JIQ	Turbidimetric Method, Protein Or Albumin (Urinary)	Chemistry
75JGX	Turbidimetric Method, Triglycerides	Chemistry
75JHW	U.V. Method, CPK Isoenzymes	Chemistry
75JIB	U.V. Method, Galactose	Chemistry
75JIJ	Wet Ash Method, Protein Bound Iodine	Chemistry

METHODS

75JGH	Catalytic Methods, Lipase	Chemistry

METHOTREXATE

91LAO	Enzyme Immunoassay, Methotrexate	Toxicology
91LAP	Enzyme Radioassay, Methotrexate	Toxicology
91LAY	Methotrexate Control Materials	Toxicology
91LAQ	Radioimmunoassay, Methotrexate	Toxicology

METHYL

84MYU	Accessory, Barium Sulfate, Methyl Methacrylate For Cranioplasty	Cns/Neurology
84GXP	Metacrylate, Methyl, Cranioplasty	Cns/Neurology
84JXH	Methyl Metacrylate	Cns/Neurology
75JNN	P-Toluenesulphonyl-L-Arginine Methyl Ester (U.V.), Trypsin	Chemistry
80WTJ	Polymer, Synthetic, Other	General
91DLA	Reagent, Test, Methyl Alcohol	Toxicology
88HZA	Stain, Methyl Green	Pathology
88KKA	Stain, Methyl Orange	Pathology
88KKB	Stain, Methyl Violet 2b	Pathology
88HZN	Stain, Picro Methyl Blue	Pathology

METHYLENE

88KFC	Stain, Methylene Blue	Pathology
88KKM	Stain, Methylene Blue Thiocyanate	Pathology
81GFR	Stain, Methylene Blue, New	Hematology
88KKC	Stain, Methylene Violet	Pathology

METHYLETHER

76KQB	PV Methylether Maleic Anhydride Copol./Carboxymethylcellul.	Dental And Oral

METHYLETHER *(cont'd)*

76KOO	Polyvinyl Methylether Maleic Acid-Calcium-Sodium Dbl. Salt	Dental And Oral
76KOT	Polyvinyl Methylether Maleic Acid/Carboxymethylcellulose	Dental And Oral
76KXY	Polyvinyl Methylether Maleic Anhydride/Carboxymethylcellul.	Dental And Oral

METHYLMALONIC

75LPT	System, Test, Acid, Methylmalonic, Urinary	Chemistry

METHYLTHYMOL

75CIA	Methylthymol Blue, Calcium	Chemistry

METREURYNTER

85HDN	Dilator, Cervical, Expandable	Obstetrics/Gyn
85HHQ	System, Abortion, Metreurynter-Balloon	Obstetrics/Gyn

METREURYNTER-BALLOON

85HHQ	System, Abortion, Metreurynter-Balloon	Obstetrics/Gyn

MICRO

75JJF	Analyzer, Chemistry, Micro	Chemistry
75UKF	Balance, Micro (0.001 mg Accuracy)	Chemistry
85LZL	Micro-Condom	Obstetrics/Gyn
83WPR	Micro-Injector, Transplant, Gene	Microbiology
80WOC	Microplate	General
75JRB	Mixer, Micro	Chemistry
75JRC	Pipette, Micro	Chemistry
80WOD	Reader, Microplate	General
87VHR	Saw, Bone Cutting, Micro	Orthopedics
83ULL	Tray, Micro (Mic Plate)	Microbiology

MICRO-CONDOM

85LZL	Micro-Condom	Obstetrics/Gyn

MICRO-INJECTOR

83WPR	Micro-Injector, Transplant, Gene	Microbiology

MICROBIAL

83JTA	Monitor, Microbial Growth	Microbiology

MICROBIOLOGICAL

91DKD	Bacillus Subtilis, Microbiological Assay, Gentamicin	Toxicology
83QFF	Cabinet, Microbiological	Microbiology
83KZI	Culture Media, Enriched	Microbiology
83RAI	Hood, Microbiological	Microbiology
75JMJ	Microbiological, Histidine	Chemistry
83JTS	Stain, Microbiological	Microbiology
83QCC	System, Automated, Microbiological	Microbiology

MICROBIOLOGY

83JTB	Dispenser, Microbiology Media	Microbiology
83LIB	General Purpose Microbiology Diagnostic Device	Microbiology
83KZJ	Generator, Gas, Microbiology	Microbiology
83JTQ	Incubator/Water Bath, Microbiology	Microbiology
80WRA	Reagent, Calibration	General
91DID	Test, Bacillus Subtilis Microbiology, Tobramycin	Toxicology

MICROCOLLECTION

75SCM	Tube, Blood Microcollection	Chemistry

MICROCRYSTALLINE

91DMO	Reagent, Forming, Alkaloid, Microcrystalline	Toxicology

MICRODENSITOMETRY

75JHL	Microdensitometry Method, Lipoproteins	Chemistry

MICROELECTRODE

80RGO	Amplifier, Microelectrode	General
80RGQ	Microelectrode	General
80RGP	Puller, Microelectrode	General

MICROFICHE

80VAZ	Microfilm/Microfiche Equipment	General

MICROFILM

80VAZ	Microfilm/Microfiche Equipment	General

MICROFILTER

73CAK	Microfilter, Blood Transfusion	Anesthesiology

MICROGLOBULIN

82MGA	Alpha-1 Microglobulin, Antigen, Antiserum, Control	Immunology
82JZG	Test, Beta 2 - Microglobulin	Immunology

MICROHEMATOCRIT

81QJB	Centrifuge, Microhematocrit	Hematology

MICROINJECTORS

85MQJ	Micromanipulators and Microinjectors, Assisted Reproduction	Obstetrics/Gyn

MICROLAPAROSCOPY

79SJS	Forceps, Microlaparoscopy	Surgery
79SJT	Laparoscope, Microlaparoscopy	Surgery

KEYWORD INDEX

MINIATURE
89IKE Transducer, Miniature Pressure — Physical Med

MINIFIER
90TFR Minifier, X-Ray Film (Reducer) — Radiology

MINIMAL
73MNT Ventilator, Continuous, Minimal Ventilatory Support, Facility Use — Anesthesiology

MIRROR
80SHS Component, Optical — General
80TGZ Mirror, Corridor Safety — General
77KAI Mirror, ENT — Ear/Nose/Throat
79GCO Mirror, Endoscopic — Surgery
79FTX Mirror, General & Plastic Surgery — Surgery
86HKF Mirror, Headband, Ophthalmic — Ophthalmology
77RHA Mirror, Laryngeal — Ear/Nose/Throat
77RHB Mirror, Middle Ear — Ear/Nose/Throat
76EAX Mirror, Mouth — Dental And Oral
85RHC Mirror, Obstetrical — Obstetrics/Gyn
89RHD Mirror, Posture — Physical Med
80VFD Mirror, Reversing — General
77RHE Mirror, Speech — Ear/Nose/Throat

MISCELLANEOUS
78FFY Adapter, Bulb, Endoscope, Miscellaneous — Gastro/Urology

MIST
80RZS Tent, Mist — General
80RZT Tent, Mist, Face — General

MITRAL
74RMO Prosthesis, Cardiac Valve — Cardiovascular

MITT
80RHF Mitt/Washcloth, Patient — General

MIXER
75JRO Blender/Mixer — Chemistry
73QMK Controller, Oxygen (Blender) — Anesthesiology
76VEF Mixer, Alginate — Dental And Oral
81RHG Mixer, Blood Bank, Donor Blood — Hematology
81GLE Mixer, Blood Tube — Hematology
73BZR Mixer, Breathing Gases, Anesthesia Inhalation — Anesthesiology
90WHY Mixer, Chemical, Film, X-Ray — Radiology
75RHH Mixer, Clinical Laboratory — Chemistry
75JRB Mixer, Micro — Chemistry
76VEN Mixer, Vacuum — Dental And Oral
81KSQ Mixer/Scale, Blood — Hematology
87JDZ Mixing Equipment, Cement — Orthopedics

MIXING
87JDZ Mixing Equipment, Cement — Orthopedics
76RHI Mixing Slab — Dental And Oral

MIXTURE
91DKB Calibrator, Drug Mixture — Toxicology
91DIF Control, Drug Mixture — Toxicology
81JPK Hematology Quality Control Mixture — Hematology
81GLQ Mixture, Control, Indices, White and Red Cell — Hematology
75JIX Multi Analyte Mixture, Calibrator — Chemistry

MIXTURES
80WPF Gas Mixtures, Laboratory — General
90WPG Gas Mixtures, Magnetic Resonance Imaging — Radiology
80THJ Gas Mixtures, Medical — General
80WPE Gas Mixtures, Sterilization — General

MMA
84MYU Accessory, Barium Sulfate, Methyl Methacrylate For Cranioplasty — Cns/Neurology

MOBILE
90VGM Battery, Mobile Radiographic Unit — Radiology
80WYG Courier, Supplies, Mobile, Automated — General
80WUC Facility, Equipment, Medical, Mobile — General
80RBB Hypo/Hyperthermia Unit, Mobile — General
75RDX Laminar Air Flow Unit, Mobile — Chemistry
90VGG Phototimer, Radiographic Mobile — Radiology
90IZK Radiographic Unit, Diagnostic, Mobile, Explosion-Safe — Radiology
90QWS Radiographic/Fluoroscopic Unit, Mobile C-Arm — Radiology
85RQX Scanner, Ultrasonic, Obstetrical/Gynecological, Mobile — Obstetrics/Gyn
80FPO Stretcher, Wheeled (Mobile) — General
90IZL System, X-Ray, Mobile — Radiology
87SBN Traction Unit, Powered, Mobile — Orthopedics

MOBILITY
89WHH Vehicle, Handicapped — Physical Med

MOBILIZER
77KAJ Mobilizer, ENT — Ear/Nose/Throat

MODEL
80TAE Anatomical Training Model — General
80WND Service, Engineering/Design — General

MODIFICATION
77LRE Instrument, Modification, Prosthesis, Ossicular Repl., Surg. — Ear/Nose/Throat
80WWR Service, Modification, Product — General
84RWC Stimulator, Aversion Conditioning (Behavior Modification) — Cns/Neurology
84MFR Stimulator, Brain, Implanted (Behavior Modification) — Cns/Neurology

MODIFIED
85MHT Tampon, Chemically Modified — Obstetrics/Gyn

MODULAR
80TBC Cabinet Casework, Modular — General

MODULE
79SIG Module, Control, Electrosurgery — Surgery
74LOT Module, Program, Generator, Pulse — Cardiovascular

MOIST
89IMB Cabinet, Moist Steam — Physical Med
89QLY Compress, Moist Heat — Physical Med
89RHK Moist Therapy Pack — Physical Med
89RHJ Moist Therapy Pack Conditioner — Physical Med
89IMA Pack, Moist Heat — Physical Med

MOISTURE
73BYD Condenser, Heat And Moisture (Artificial Nose) — Anesthesiology
80WKL Dressing, Permeable, Moisture — General
73RAU Humidifier, Heat/Moisture Exchange — Anesthesiology
80WSZ Sensor, Moisture — General

MOLD
77ETC Mold, Middle Ear — Ear/Nose/Throat
85HFK Mold, Vaginal — Obstetrics/Gyn

MOLDABLE
89MNE Orthosis, Moldable, Supportive, Skin Protective — Physical Med

MOLDED
87RUW Splint, Molded, Aluminum — Orthopedics
87RUX Splint, Molded, Plastic — Orthopedics

MOLDING
80VAJ Equipment, Extruding/Molding — General
80WXE Equipment, Molding — General
80WVT Foam, Plastic — General
80WNC Molding, Custom — General
80WYJ Molding, Injection — General
80WYK Thermoforming, Extrusion, Custom — General

MOLECULAR
75UFX Distilling Unit, Molecular — Chemistry
75UGW Molecular Weight Equipment — Chemistry

MOLESKIN
80RHL Moleskin — General

MOLYBDATE
75CEL Ammonium Molybdate And Ammonium Vanadate, Phospholipids — Chemistry

MOLYBDENUM
75CEQ Molybdenum Blue Method, Phospholipids — Chemistry

MONITOR
80WTN Adapter, Cable, Equipment — General
73TAK Analyzer, Blood Gas pH — Anesthesiology
75ULK Analyzer, Chemistry, Therapeutic Drug Monitor (TDM) — Chemistry
74LOS Analyzer, ECG — Cardiovascular
80QUR Analyzer, Ethylene-Oxide — General
73CCK Analyzer, Gas, Carbon-Dioxide, Gaseous Phase (Capnograph) — Anesthesiology
73BXZ Analyzer, Gas, Carbon-Dioxide, Partial Pressure, Blood — Anesthesiology
73CCJ Analyzer, Gas, Carbon-Monoxide, Gaseous Phase — Anesthesiology
73BSE Analyzer, Gas, Helium, Gaseous Phase — Anesthesiology
73CCI Analyzer, Gas, Nitrogen, Gaseous Phase — Anesthesiology
73CBR Analyzer, Gas, Nitrous-Oxide, Gaseous Phase — Anesthesiology
73RJI Analyzer, Gas, Oxygen, Continuous Controller — Anesthesiology
73RJJ Analyzer, Gas, Oxygen, Continuous Monitor — Anesthesiology
73CCL Analyzer, Gas, Oxygen, Gaseous Phase — Anesthesiology
73CCE Analyzer, Gas, Oxygen, Partial Pr., Blood Phase, Indwelling — Anesthesiology
73CCD Analyzer, Gas, Oxygen, Partial Pressure, Blood Phase — Anesthesiology
73RJK Analyzer, Gas, Oxygen, Sampling — Anesthesiology
75QYL Analyzer, Glucose — Chemistry
73CBZ Analyzer, Ion, Hydrogen-Ion (pH), Blood Phase, Indwelling — Anesthesiology
73CBY Analyzer, Ion, Hydrogen-Ion pH, Blood Phase, Non-Indwelling — Anesthesiology
73QCP Analyzer, Metabolism — Anesthesiology
78FFX Analyzer, Motility, Gastrointestinal, Electrical — Gastro/Urology
79WTZ Analyzer, Patient, Multiple Function (Surgery) — Surgery
73RNC Analyzer, Pulmonary Function — Anesthesiology

MONITOR *(cont'd)*

84HCC	Biofeedback Device	Cns/Neurology
89IQH	Biofeedback Equipment, Myoelectric, Battery-Powered	Physical Med
89IRC	Biofeedback Equipment, Myoelectric, Powered	Physical Med
78EXZ	Camera, Physiological, Function Monitor	Gastro/Urology
74RBP	Cardiograph, Impedance	Cardiovascular
80WVY	Cart, Equipment, Video	General
80WTI	Cart, Monitor	General
80WSG	Case, Protection, Equipment	General
73QME	Computer, Patient Monitor	Anesthesiology
74QOO	Defibrillator/Monitor, Battery-Powered	Cardiovascular
74QOP	Defibrillator/Monitor, Line-Powered	Cardiovascular
78FJF	Detector, Air Bubble	Gastro/Urology
74DSI	Detector, Arrhythmia Alarm	Cardiovascular
74ULR	Detector, Blood Flow, Ultrasonic (Doppler)	Cardiovascular
78FJD	Detector, Blood Leakage	Gastro/Urology
78FJC	Detector, Blood Level	Gastro/Urology
74QOM	Detector, Deep Vein Thrombosis	Cardiovascular
80QTQ	Detector, Electrostatic Voltage	General
80UMV	Detector, Ethylene-Oxide Leakage	General
78QZV	Detector, Hemodialysis Unit Air Bubble-Foam	Gastro/Urology
74RAD	Detector, His Bundle	Cardiovascular
80RGX	Detector, Microwave Leakage	General
74DXJ	Display, Cathode-Ray Tube	Cardiovascular
90QQI	Dosimeter, Radiation	Radiology
74BYQ	Ergometer, Treadmill	Cardiovascular
84QUT	Evoked Response Unit	Cns/Neurology
74WSR	Flowmeter, Blood, Other	Cardiovascular
84UEW	Flowmeter, Meter, Cerebral Blood, Xenon Clearance	Cns/Neurology
78TCQ	Infusion System, Insulin, With Monitor	Gastro/Urology
83UFL	Meter, Bacterial Culture Growth	Microbiology
73CBA	Monitor, Air Embolism, Ultrasonic	Anesthesiology
73CAP	Monitor, Airway Pressure (Gauge/Alarm)	Anesthesiology
73BXR	Monitor, Airway Pressure (Inspiratory Force)	Anesthesiology
73RLV	Monitor, Airway Pressure, Continuous	Anesthesiology
84GXS	Monitor, Alpha	Cns/Neurology
80FLS	Monitor, Apnea	General
80QDB	Monitor, Bed Occupancy	General
80KMI	Monitor, Bed Patient	General
80QDR	Monitor, Biological (Contamination Testing)	General
85HEP	Monitor, Blood Flow, Ultrasonic	Obstetrics/Gyn
73QEA	Monitor, Blood Gas, Carbon-Dioxide	Anesthesiology
74DRY	Monitor, Blood Gas, On-Line, Cardiopulmonary Bypass	Cardiovascular
73QEB	Monitor, Blood Gas, Oxygen	Anesthesiology
74UMH	Monitor, Blood Gas, Real-Time	Cardiovascular
73TAJ	Monitor, Blood Gas, Transcutaneous Carbon-Dioxide	Anesthesiology
73QEC	Monitor, Blood Gas, Transcutaneous Oxygen	Anesthesiology
78TGM	Monitor, Blood Glucose (Test)	Gastro/Urology
73TAM	Monitor, Blood Potassium	Anesthesiology
74KGJ	Monitor, Blood Pressure, Amplifier & Associated Electronics	Cardiovascular
74WZC	Monitor, Blood Pressure, Finger	Cardiovascular
74RLS	Monitor, Blood Pressure, Indirect (Arterial)	Cardiovascular
73BXD	Monitor, Blood Pressure, Indirect, Anesthesiology	Anesthesiology
74JOE	Monitor, Blood Pressure, Indirect, Automatic	Cardiovascular
74DXN	Monitor, Blood Pressure, Indirect, Semi-Automatic	Cardiovascular
79FYM	Monitor, Blood Pressure, Indirect, Surgery	Surgery
79FYL	Monitor, Blood Pressure, Indirect, Surgery, Powered	Surgery
73BZZ	Monitor, Blood Pressure, Indirect, Transducer	Anesthesiology
74RLR	Monitor, Blood Pressure, Invasive (Arterial)	Cardiovascular
73CAA	Monitor, Blood Pressure, Invasive (Arterial), Anesthesia	Anesthesiology
74BXE	Monitor, Blood Pressure, Transducer, Indwelling	Cardiovascular
74RLX	Monitor, Blood Pressure, Venous	Cardiovascular
74KRK	Monitor, Blood Pressure, Venous, Cardiopulmonary Bypass	Cardiovascular
79FYO	Monitor, Blood Pressure, Venous, Central	Surgery
79FYP	Monitor, Blood Pressure, Venous, Peripheral	Surgery
73LKD	Monitor, Carbon-Dioxide, Cutaneous	Anesthesiology
74DRT	Monitor, Cardiac (Cardiotachometer & Rate Alarm)	Cardiovascular
79KFO	Monitor, Cardiac Output, Dye (Central Venous & Arterial)	Surgery
74KFP	Monitor, Cardiac Output, Flowmeter	Cardiovascular
79KFR	Monitor, Cardiac Output, Impedance Plethysmography	Surgery
79KFN	Monitor, Cardiac Output, Thermal (Balloon Type Catheter)	Surgery
79KFQ	Monitor, Cardiac Output, Trend (Arterial Pressure Pulse)	Surgery
74DTW	Monitor, Cardiopulmonary Level Sensing	Cardiovascular
84LME	Monitor, Cerebral Blood Flow, Thermal Diffusion	Cns/Neurology
84QJE	Monitor, Cerebral Function	Cns/Neurology
80CAQ	Monitor, Cerebral Spinal Fluid Pressure (CSF)	General
80CAR	Monitor, Cerebral Spinal Fluid Pressure, Electrical	General
80WIP	Monitor, Contamination, Environmental, Personal	General
74QRW	Monitor, ECG	Cardiovascular
74TGX	Monitor, ECG, Ambulatory, Real-Time	Cardiovascular
73BRS	Monitor, ECG, Anesthesia	Anesthesiology
74QRX	Monitor, ECG, Arrhythmia	Cardiovascular
79FYW	Monitor, ECG, Surgery	Surgery
84BRR	Monitor, EEG	Cns/Neurology
79FYX	Monitor, EEG, Surgery	Surgery
73CAB	Monitor, EMG	Anesthesiology
85HGQ	Monitor, Electrocardiographic, Fetal	Obstetrics/Gyn

MONITOR *(cont'd)*

85HGO	Monitor, Electroencephalographic, Fetal	Obstetrics/Gyn
78KLA	Monitor, Esophageal Motility, And Tube	Gastro/Urology
78RLU	Monitor, Esophageal Pressure	Gastro/Urology
86HLL	Monitor, Eye Movement	Ophthalmology
86HMC	Monitor, Eye Movement, Diagnostic	Ophthalmology
85VDI	Monitor, Fertility	Obstetrics/Gyn
85QVQ	Monitor, Fetal	Obstetrics/Gyn
85MAA	Monitor, Fetal Doppler Ultrasound	Obstetrics/Gyn
85KXN	Monitor, Fetal, Cardiac	Obstetrics/Gyn
85KNG	Monitor, Fetal, Ultrasonic	Obstetrics/Gyn
85HEQ	Monitor, Fetal, Ultrasonic, Arterial Pressure	Obstetrics/Gyn
85HEL	Monitor, Fetal, Ultrasonic, Heart Rate	Obstetrics/Gyn
85HEK	Monitor, Fetal, Ultrasonic, Heart Sound	Obstetrics/Gyn
75QXS	Monitor, Freezer	Chemistry
80QUM	Monitor, Gas, Atmospheric, Environmental	General
75WXU	Monitor, Glucose, Blood, Non-Invasive	Chemistry
74QZO	Monitor, Heart Rate, Other	Cardiovascular
74QZN	Monitor, Heart Rate, R-Wave (ECG)	Cardiovascular
85HEI	Monitor, Heart Valve Movement, Fetal, Ultrasonic	Obstetrics/Gyn
85HEJ	Monitor, Hemic Sound, Ultrasonic	Obstetrics/Gyn
78QZX	Monitor, Hemodialysis Unit Conductivity	Gastro/Urology
73VJA	Monitor, Hemodynamic	Anesthesiology
78MKM	Monitor, Hemofiltration	Gastro/Urology
73RBQ	Monitor, Impedance Pneumograph	Anesthesiology
80BYC	Monitor, Infusion Rate	General
80FLN	Monitor, Infusion, Gravity Flow	General
84RLW	Monitor, Intracranial Pressure	Cns/Neurology
84GWM	Monitor, Intracranial Pressure, Continuous	Cns/Neurology
84GXT	Monitor, Lesion Temperature	Cns/Neurology
74DRI	Monitor, Line Isolation	Cardiovascular
73JEZ	Monitor, Lung Water Measurement	Anesthesiology
80WKH	Monitor, Medication	General
83JTA	Monitor, Microbial Growth	Microbiology
76KZM	Monitor, Muscle, Dental	Dental And Oral
85TDE	Monitor, Neonatal	Obstetrics/Gyn
80FLP	Monitor, Neonatal, Blood Pressure, Invasive	General
80FLQ	Monitor, Neonatal, Blood Pressure, Ultrasonic/Doppler	General
80FLO	Monitor, Neonatal, Heart Rate	General
85TDR	Monitor, Neonatal, Physiological	Obstetrics/Gyn
80SHT	Monitor, Oxygen	General
73BXC	Monitor, Oxygen (Ventilatory) W/Wo Alarm	Anesthesiology
84WYU	Monitor, Oxygen, Brain	Cns/Neurology
73LKE	Monitor, Oxygen, Conjunctival	Anesthesiology
73LPP	Monitor, Oxygen, Cutan. (Not for Infant or Under Gas Anest.)	Anesthesiology
73KLK	Monitor, Oxygen, Cutaneous	Anesthesiology
91MHP	Monitor, Patch, Sudromed, Drug Abuse	Toxicology
90IWE	Monitor, Patient Position, Light Beam	Radiology
78LIL	Monitor, Penile Tumescence	Gastro/Urology
85HGM	Monitor, Perinatal	Obstetrics/Gyn
85HFP	Monitor, Phonocardiographic, Fetal	Obstetrics/Gyn
73RLA	Monitor, Physiological, Acute Care	Anesthesiology
74RLB	Monitor, Physiological, Cardiac Catheterization	Cardiovascular
74MHX	Monitor, Physiological, Patient	Cardiovascular
74MWI	Monitor, Physiological, Patient(without Arrhythmia Detection Or Alarms)	Cardiovascular
74RLC	Monitor, Physiological, Stress Exercise	Cardiovascular
79KFS	Monitor, Po2, Continuous	Surgery
74FYK	Monitor, Pressure, Arterial, Internal	Cardiovascular
74FYQ	Monitor, Pressure, Cardiac, Atrial	Cardiovascular
74FYR	Monitor, Pressure, Cardiac, Ventricular	Cardiovascular
87LXC	Monitor, Pressure, Intracompartmental	Orthopedics
84LII	Monitor, Pressure, Intracranial, Implantable	Cns/Neurology
85KXO	Monitor, Pressure, Intrauterine	Obstetrics/Gyn
74FYS	Monitor, Pressure, Pulmonary Artery, Powered	Cardiovascular
74FYN	Monitor, Pressure, Venous, Central, Powered	Cardiovascular
73BWS	Monitor, Pulse Rate	Anesthesiology
90RNV	Monitor, Radiation	Radiology
79FYZ	Monitor, Respiratory	Surgery
84GZO	Monitor, Response, Skin, Galvanic	Cns/Neurology
80MLC	Monitor, ST Segment	General
80MLD	Monitor, ST Segment (With Alarm)	General
89LZW	Monitor, Spine Curvature	Physical Med
80KLL	Monitor, Temperature (Self-Contained)	General
73BWX	Monitor, Temperature (With Probe)	Anesthesiology
78FLA	Monitor, Temperature, Dialysis	Gastro/Urology
84HCS	Monitor, Temperature, Neurosurgery, Direct Contact, Powered	Cns/Neurology
79FZA	Monitor, Temperature, Surgery	Surgery
81MTL	Monitor, Test, Hiv-1	Hematology
73ULU	Monitor, Transcutaneous, Carbon-Dioxide	Anesthesiology
73ULV	Monitor, Transcutaneous, Oxygen	Anesthesiology
91JXQ	Monitor, U.V., GLC	Toxicology
90JAF	Monitor, Ultrasonic, Non-Fetal	Radiology
85HFM	Monitor, Uterine Contraction, External	Obstetrics/Gyn
80WTG	Monitor, Utilization, Equipment	General

MONITOR *(cont'd)*

73SES	Monitor, Ventilation	Anesthesiology
73BZQ	Monitor, Ventilatory Frequency	Anesthesiology
80TFB	Monitor, Video, Endoscope	General
90SGL	Monitor, X-Ray Film Processor Quality Control	Radiology
90VGH	Monitor, X-Ray Tube	Radiology
73RKP	Monitor, pH	Anesthesiology
85LLT	Monitor, pH, Fetal	Obstetrics/Gyn
80WKM	Mount, Equipment	General
80RHM	Mount, Monitor (Support)	General
84GWN	Nystagmograph	Cns/Neurology
80RJC	Oscilloscope	General
74DSB	Plethysmograph, Impedance	Cardiovascular
84JXF	Plethysmograph, Ocular	Cns/Neurology
74JOM	Plethysmograph, Photo-Electric, Pneumatic Or Hydraulic	Cardiovascular
73CCM	Plethysmograph, Pressure (Body)	Anesthesiology
73JEH	Plethysmograph, Volume	Anesthesiology
74ROJ	Recorder, Echocardiographic	Cardiovascular
74ROK	Recorder, Long-Term, Blood Pressure, Portable	Cardiovascular
74ROL	Recorder, Long-Term, ECG	Cardiovascular
74ROM	Recorder, Long-Term, ECG, Portable (Holter Monitor)	Cardiovascular
84RON	Recorder, Long-Term, EEG	Cns/Neurology
73ROO	Recorder, Long-Term, Oxygen	Anesthesiology
80ROP	Recorder, Long-Term, Trend	General
85HFO	Recorder, Pressure, Intrauterine	Obstetrics/Gyn
80RQQ	Scale, Bed	General
80RQS	Scale, Chair	General
80FRW	Scale, Infant	General
89INF	Scale, Platform, Wheelchair	Physical Med
74RQU	Scanner, Long-Term, ECG, Recording	Cardiovascular
80VAY	Security Equipment/Supplies	General
84LEL	Sleep Assessment Equipment	Cns/Neurology
80THH	Sphygmomanometer, Electronic (Arterial Pressure)	General
80UDM	Sphygmomanometer, Electronic, Automatic	General
80UDN	Sphygmomanometer, Electronic, Manual	General
73BZG	Spirometer, Diagnostic (Respirometer)	Anesthesiology
73BZK	Spirometer, Monitoring (Volumeter)	Anesthesiology
80FRC	Sterilization Process Indicator, Biological	General
80RVU	Sterilization Process Indicator, Chemical	General
80JOJ	Sterilization Process Indicator, Physical/Chemical	General
73UFG	Stimulator, Peripheral Nerve, Blockade Monitor	Anesthesiology
74RZJ	Telemetry Unit, Physiological, ECG	Cardiovascular
84RZK	Telemetry Unit, Physiological, EEG	Cns/Neurology
89RZL	Telemetry Unit, Physiological, EMG	Physical Med
84RZM	Telemetry Unit, Physiological, EOG	Cns/Neurology
80TEZ	Telemetry Unit, Physiological, Multiple Channel	General
84GYE	Telemetry Unit, Physiological, Neurological	Cns/Neurology
80RZN	Telemetry Unit, Physiological, Pressure	General
80RZO	Telemetry Unit, Physiological, Temperature	General
80TFC	Television Monitor, Microscope	General
80TFD	Television Monitor, Operating Room	General
80FLL	Thermometer, Electronic, Continuous	General
80WTE	Thermometer, Fiberoptic	General
79FWR	Thermometer, Liquid Crystals	Surgery
80VFH	Transmitter/Receiver System, Fetal Monitor, Telephone	General
80VFI	Transmitter/Receiver System, Pulmonary Monitor, Telephone	General
85LHZ	Viscometer, Mucus, Cervical	Obstetrics/Gyn

MONITORING

80WKY	Garment, Electrode	General
80RLY	Kit, Pressure Monitoring (Air/Gas)	General
90LWN	Medical Radiographic Personal Monitoring Device	Radiology
73BZK	Spirometer, Monitoring (Volumeter)	Anesthesiology
75WTX	Strip, Test	Chemistry
78MQS	System, Hemodialysis, Access Recirculation Monitoring	Gastro/Urology
79SJQ	System, Monitoring, Electrode, Active, Electrosurgical	Surgery
82NCW	System, Test, HER-2/NEU, Monitoring	Immunology
85VJM	Test, Fertility Monitoring	Obstetrics/Gyn

MONITORS

74MSX	System, Network And Communication, Physiological Monitors	Cardiovascular

MONOCHROMATOR

75JRP	Monochromator, for Clinical Use	Chemistry

MONOCLONAL

83TFW	Antibody, Monoclonal	Microbiology
81MVX	Antibody, Monoclonal Blocking, Hiv-1	Hematology
80WQZ	Antibody, Other	General
81MVY	Monoclonal, Hiv-1	Hematology
82VJD	Test, Cancer Detection, Monoclonal Antibody	Immunology

MONOCYTOGENES

83GSI	Antigen, Slide And Tube, Listeria Monocytogenes	Microbiology
83GSG	Antiserum, Fluorescent, Listeria Monocytogenes	Microbiology
83GSH	Antiserum, Listeria Monocytogenes	Microbiology

MONOFILAMENT

80WXR	Media, Filter	General
80WTJ	Polymer, Synthetic, Other	General
79GAQ	Suture, Non-Absorbable, Steel, Monofilament & Multifilament	Surgery
79RYC	Suture, Polypropylene Monofilament	Surgery

MONOMER

87JDY	Evacuator, Vapor, Cement Monomer	Orthopedics
81JBN	Fibrin Monomer Paracoagulation	Hematology

MONONUCLEOSIS

83LJN	Antibody IGM, IF, Epstein-Barr Virus	Microbiology
83GNQ	Antigen, CF (Including CF Control), Epstein-Barr Virus	Microbiology
83GNP	Antiserum, CF, Epstein-Barr Virus	Microbiology
83JRY	Antiserum, Fluorescent, Epstein-Barr Virus	Microbiology
83THL	Radioimmunoassay, Infectious Mononucleosis	Microbiology
82KTN	Test, Infectious Mononucleosis	Immunology

MONOPHOSPHATE

75CHO	Radioimmunoassay, Cyclic AMP	Chemistry
75CGT	Radioimmunoassay, Cyclic GMP	Chemistry
75CJR	Thymol Blue Monophosphate, Acid Phosphatase	Chemistry
75CJH	Thymol Blue Monophosphate, Alkaline Phosphatase/Isoenzymes	Chemistry
75CKE	Thymolphthalein Monophosphate, Acid Phosphatase	Chemistry
75CIO	Thymolphthalein Monophosphate, Alkaline Phosphatase	Chemistry

MONOPOLAR

79QIJ	Tip, Instrument, Electrocauterization, Monopolar	Surgery

MONOXIDE

73CCJ	Analyzer, Gas, Carbon-Monoxide, Gaseous Phase	Anesthesiology
73VCB	Analyzer, Gas, Carbon-Monoxide, Non-Indwelling Blood Phase	Anesthesiology
91JKT	Gas Chromatograph, Carbon-Monoxide	Toxicology
91JKS	Oxyhemoglobin/Carboxyhemoglobin Curve, Carbon-Monoxide	Toxicology
91DKM	Reagent, Test, Carbon Monoxide	Toxicology

MONOXIME

75CDW	Diacetyl-Monoxime, Urea Nitrogen	Chemistry

MORBID

78LTI	Implant, Intragastric, Obesity, Morbid	Gastro/Urology

MORCELLATION

79SJP	Instrument, Removal, Myoma, Laparoscopic	Surgery

MORGUE

88ROV	Refrigerator, Morgue, Walk-In	Pathology
88RYV	Table, Autopsy	Pathology

MORPHINE

91DJJ	Fluorometry, Morphine	Toxicology
91DOK	Free Radical Assay, Morphine	Toxicology
91DMY	Gas Chromatography, Morphine	Toxicology
91DLR	Hemagglutination Inhibition, Morphine	Toxicology
91DPK	Liquid Chromatography, Morphine	Toxicology
91DNA	RIA, Morphine-Barbiturate (125-I), Goat Antibody	Toxicology
91DOE	Radioimmunoassay, Morphine (125-I), Goat Antibody	Toxicology
91DIQ	Radioimmunoassay, Morphine (3-H), Ammonium Sulfate	Toxicology
91DNK	Thin Layer Chromatography, Morphine	Toxicology

MORPHINE-BARBITURATE

91DNA	RIA, Morphine-Barbiturate (125-I), Goat Antibody	Toxicology

MORPHOGENETIC

87MIL	Prosthesis, Hip, Semi-Const., Uncem., M/P, Bone Morph. Prot.	Orthopedics

MORTUARY

88RSZ	Kit, Shroud	Pathology
88RYV	Table, Autopsy	Pathology

MOSQUITO

79QXD	Forceps, Hemostatic	Surgery

MOTILITY

78FFX	Analyzer, Motility, Gastrointestinal, Electrical	Gastro/Urology
78KLA	Monitor, Esophageal Motility, And Tube	Gastro/Urology
78FGM	Probe, Gastrointestinal	Gastro/Urology

MOTION

80WWG	Analyzer, Motion	General
89IOO	Exerciser, Passive, Non-Measuring (CPM Machine)	Physical Med
74RLJ	Suit, Pneumatic Counterpressure (Anti-Shock)	Cardiovascular

MOTOR

84HBC	Motor, Drill, Electric	Cns/Neurology
84HBB	Motor, Drill, Pneumatic	Cns/Neurology
79GEY	Motor, Surgical Instrument, AC-Powered	Surgery
79SJM	Motor, Surgical Instrument, DC-Powered	Surgery

MOTOR *(cont'd)*

79GET	Motor, Surgical Instrument, Pneumatic-Powered	Surgery
84LGT	Stimulator, Cord, Spinal, Implantable (Motor Disorders)	Cns/Neurology
87HWE	Surgical Instrument, Orthopedic, AC-Powered Motor	Orthopedics

MOTORIZED

89INI	Scooter (Motorized 3-Wheeled Vehicle)	Physical Med
90WUY	Viewer, Radiographic Film, Motorized	Radiology

MOULAGE

80TFO	Training Manikin, Wound Moulage	General

MOUNT

80WKM	Mount, Equipment	General
80RHM	Mount, Monitor (Support)	General
79UMJ	Mount, Surgical Microscope	Surgery
80UMW	Mount, Television Set	General
90IYB	Mount, X-Ray Tube, Diagnostic	Radiology

MOUNTAIN

83GPP	Antiserum, Rocky Mountain Spotted Fever	Microbiology

MOUNTED

90IXY	Holder, Radiographic Cassette, Wall-Mounted	Radiology
80TCY	Lamp, Examination, Ceiling Mounted (Light)	General
79FSY	Light, Surgical, Ceiling Mounted	Surgery

MOUNTING

88LEB	Media, Mounting	Pathology
88KEQ	Media, Mounting, Water Soluble	Pathology
88KEP	Mounting Media, Oil Soluble	Pathology

MOUSE

83UMA	Animal, Laboratory	Microbiology

MOUTH

77KBN	Gag, Mouth	Ear/Nose/Throat
77KAI	Mirror, ENT	Ear/Nose/Throat
76EAX	Mirror, Mouth	Dental And Oral
76UDZ	Mouth Prop	Dental And Oral
76ELQ	Protector, Mouth Guard	Dental And Oral

MOUTHGUARD

76MQC	Mouthguard	Dental And Oral

MOUTHPIECE

73BYP	Mouthpiece, Breathing	Anesthesiology
76DYN	Mouthpiece, Saliva Ejector	Dental And Oral

MOVEABLE

90IWX	Barrier, Control Panel, X-Ray, Moveable	Radiology

MOVEMENT

86HLL	Monitor, Eye Movement	Ophthalmology
86HMC	Monitor, Eye Movement, Diagnostic	Ophthalmology
85HEI	Monitor, Heart Valve Movement, Fetal, Ultrasonic	Obstetrics/Gyn
89LXJ	Optical Position/Movement Recording System	Physical Med

MRI

90QMD	Computer, Nuclear Medicine	Radiology
90WPG	Gas Mixtures, Magnetic Resonance Imaging	Radiology
90WRT	Magnet, Permanent, MRI (Magnetic Resonance Imaging)	Radiology
90VIM	Magnet, Superconducting, MRI (Magnetic Resonance Imaging)	Radiology
90VKD	Phantom, NMR/MRI	Radiology
90JAM	Scanner, Magnetic Resonance (NMR/MRI)	Radiology
90WJP	Stand, Cardiovascular	Radiology
90WLW	Stand, Vascular	Radiology

MU

82DAO	Antigen, Antiserum, Control, IGM (Mu Chain Specific)	Immunology

MUCICARMINE

88HZC	Stain, Mucicarmine	Pathology

MUCOPOLYSACCHARIDES

75JQN	Colorimetric, Mucopolysaccharides	Chemistry

MUCOUS

88LIY	Test, Cervical Mucous Penetration	Pathology
73SBZ	Trap, Mucus	Anesthesiology
85LHZ	Viscometer, Mucus, Cervical	Obstetrics/Gyn

MUCUS

88LIY	Test, Cervical Mucous Penetration	Pathology
73SBZ	Trap, Mucus	Anesthesiology
85LHZ	Viscometer, Mucus, Cervical	Obstetrics/Gyn

MUELLER

83JTZ	Culture Media, Mueller Hinton Agar Broth	Microbiology

MULLER'S

88HZD	Muller's Colloidal Iron	Pathology

MULTI

90LMC	Camera, Multi Format	Radiology
75JJY	Control, Multi Analyte, All Kinds (Assayed And Unassayed)	Chemistry
75JIX	Multi Analyte Mixture, Calibrator	Chemistry
83LHW	Reag. & Equipment, Erythrocyte Suspension, Multi Species	Microbiology

MULTI-CHANNEL

75QKW	Analyzer, Chemistry, Multi-Channel, Fixed	Chemistry
75QKX	Analyzer, Chemistry, Multi-Channel, Programmable	Chemistry
74QSJ	Electrocardiograph, Multi-Channel	Cardiovascular
74QRY	Transmitter/Receiver System, ECG, Telephone Multi-Channel	Cardiovascular

MULTI-FUNCTION

74MLN	Electrode, Electrocardiograph, Multi-Function	Cardiovascular

MULTI-IMAGE

90TAS	Camera, Multi-Image	Radiology
80WZQ	Camera, Video, Multi-Image	General

MULTI-LUMEN

80WPT	Tubing, Multi-Lumen	General

MULTI-USE

79QEZ	Probe, Electrocauterization, Multi-Use	Surgery

MULTIFILAMENT

79RXY	Suture, Multifilament Steel	Surgery
79GAQ	Suture, Non-Absorbable, Steel, Monofilament & Multifilament	Surgery

MULTIFOCAL

86MFK	Lens, Intraocular, Multifocal	Ophthalmology

MULTIPHASIC

75RGE	Mass Screening System	Chemistry

MULTIPLE

75JJC	Analyzer, Chemistry, Sequential Multiple, Continuous Flow	Chemistry
79WTZ	Analyzer, Patient, Multiple Function (Surgery)	Surgery
82DBL	Antibody, Multiple Auto, Indirect Immunofluorescent	Immunology
87LXT	Appliance, Fix., Nail/Blade/Plate Comb., Multiple Component	Orthopedics
79GBP	Catheter, Multiple Lumen	Surgery
83JSE	Culture Media, Multiple Biochemical Test	Microbiology
84MFS	Device, Energy, Multiple Therapies, Non-Specific	Cns/Neurology
78FKQ	Dialysate Delivery System, Central Multiple Patient	Gastro/Urology
83GTP	Exoenzyme, Multiple, Streptococcal	Microbiology
87KTT	Fixation Appliance, Multiple Component	Orthopedics
91MVO	Kit, Test, Multiple, Drugs Of Abuse, Over The Counter	Toxicology
75UHK	Precipitator, Radioimmunoassay Multiple Sampling	Chemistry
80TEZ	Telemetry Unit, Physiological, Multiple Channel	General

MULTIPURPOSE

80WSA	Accessories, Cart, Multipurpose	General
81JPA	Analyzer, Coagulation, Multipurpose	Hematology
80QGT	Cart, Multipurpose	General
78WIL	Lithotriptor, Multipurpose	Gastro/Urology

MUMPS

83GRC	Antigen, CF (Including CF Control), Mumps Virus	Microbiology
83GQY	Antigen, HA (Including HA Control), Mumps Virus	Microbiology
83GRB	Antiserum, CF, Mumps Virus	Microbiology
83GRA	Antiserum, Fluorescent, Mumps Virus	Microbiology
83GRD	Antiserum, HAI, Mumps Virus	Microbiology
83GQZ	Antiserum, Neutralization, Mumps Virus	Microbiology
83LJY	Enzyme Linked Immunoabsorbent Assay, Mumps Virus	Microbiology

MURAMIDASE

75JMR	Immunochemical, Lysozyme (Muramidase)	Chemistry

MURINE

83GPM	Antiserum, Murine Typhus Fever	Microbiology

MUSCLE

82DBE	Antibody, Anti-Smooth Muscle, Indirect Immunofluorescent	Immunology
86HOB	Clamp, Muscle, Ophthalmic	Ophthalmology
84QTC	Electrode, Neuromuscular Stimulator	Cns/Neurology
79MIC	Implant, Muscle, Pectoralis	Surgery
76KZM	Monitor, Muscle, Dental	Dental And Oral
87RMY	Prosthesis, Muscle	Orthopedics
86UBF	Sleeve, Muscle, Ophthalmic	Ophthalmology
89MPH	Stimulator, Electrical, Muscle	Physical Med
89IPP	Stimulator, External, Neuromuscular, Functional	Physical Med
89ISB	Stimulator, Muscle, Diagnostic	Physical Med
89IPF	Stimulator, Muscle, Electrical-Powered (EMS)	Physical Med
79FXB	Stimulator, Muscle, General & Plastic Surgery	Surgery
89LBF	Stimulator, Muscle, Low Intensity	Physical Med
89MBN	Stimulator, Muscle, Powered, Invasive	Physical Med
89LPQ	Stimulator, Muscle, Ultrasonic (Non-Beep Heat)	Physical Med
85HII	Stimulator, Muscle, Vaginal	Obstetrics/Gyn
84GZI	Stimulator, Neuromuscular, External Functional	Cns/Neurology

MUSCLE (cont'd)
84GZC Stimulator, Neuromuscular, Implanted — Cns/Neurology
89IMG Stimulator, Ultrasound, Muscle — Physical Med
89WWS Unit, Pad, Heating, Portable — Physical Med

MUSHROOM
78QIC Catheter, Mushroom — Gastro/Urology

MUTASE
75JLZ Nadh, Phosphoglycerate Mutase, Atp (u.v.) 2, 3-diphosphoglyceric Acid — Chemistry
75JLY Phosphoglycerate Mutase (colorimetric), 2, 3-diphosphoglyceric Acid — Chemistry

MYCOBACTERIA
83JSY Kit, Mycobacteria Identification — Microbiology

MYCOBACTERIUM
83GRT Antiserum, Fluorescent, Mycobacterium Tuberculosis — Microbiology
83LQF Mycobacterium SPP. DNA Reagents — Microbiology
83NCD Test, Immunity, Cell-Mediated, Mycobacterium Tuberculosis — Microbiology

MYCOPLASMA
83WJT Antibody, Mycoplasma SPP. — Microbiology
83GSB Antigen, CF, Mycoplasma SPP. — Microbiology
83GRZ Antiserum, Fluorescent, Mycoplasma SPP. — Microbiology
83GSA Antiserum, Mycoplasma SPP. — Microbiology
83LJZ Enzyme Linked Immunoabsorbent Assay, Mycoplasma SPP. — Microbiology
88KIW Kit, Mycoplasma Detection — Pathology
88KIX Media, Mycoplasma Detection — Pathology
88KPB Mycoplasma Detection Media and Components — Pathology
83LQG Mycoplasma SPP. DNA Reagents — Microbiology

MYELIN
82MEL Kit, RIA, Basic Protein, Myelin — Immunology
82LTN Test, Myelin, Basic Protein — Immunology

MYELOGRAM
84RHN Kit, Myelogram — Cns/Neurology

MYELOSCOPE
84RHO Myeloscope — Cns/Neurology

MYOCARDIAL
74WTL Cleaner, Forceps, Biopsy — Cardiovascular
74QTA Electrode, Myocardial — Cardiovascular
74DTB Lead, Pacemaker, Implantable Myocardial — Cardiovascular
74WQA Lead, Pacemaker, Temporary Myocardial — Cardiovascular
74UJO Patch, Myocardial — Cardiovascular
75VIQ Test, Myocardial Infarction (Heart Attack) — Chemistry

MYOELECTRIC
89IQH Biofeedback Equipment, Myoelectric, Battery-Powered — Physical Med
89IRC Biofeedback Equipment, Myoelectric, Powered — Physical Med

MYOGLOBIN
82DDR Antigen, Antiserum, Control, Myoglobin — Immunology
82DEA Myoglobin, FITC, Antigen, Antiserum, Control — Immunology
82DDO Myoglobin, Rhodamine, Antigen, Antiserum, Control — Immunology
75SHQ Nephelometric Method, Myoglobin — Chemistry
75SHR Turbidimetric Method, Myoglobin — Chemistry

MYOGRAPH
89GWP Myograph — Physical Med

MYOMA
79QQY Instrument, Dissecting, Myoma, Laparoscopic — Surgery
79SJP Instrument, Removal, Myoma, Laparoscopic — Surgery

MYOPLASTY
74MGC Catheter, Myoplasty, Laser, Coronary — Cardiovascular

MYRINGOTOMY
77JYM Inserter, Myringotomy Tube — Ear/Nose/Throat
77JYP Knife, Myringotomy — Ear/Nose/Throat
77SDE Tube, Myringotomy — Ear/Nose/Throat

N-ACETYL-L-TYROSINE
75JKW N-Acetyl-L-Tyrosine Ethyl Ester (U.V.), Chymotrypsin — Chemistry

N-ACETYLPROCAINAMIDE
91LAN Enzyme Immunoassay, N-Acetylprocainamide — Toxicology
91LAZ N-Acetylprocainamide Control Materials — Toxicology

N-BENZOYL-L-ARGININE
75JNO N-Benzoyl-L-Arginine Ethyl Ester (U.V.), Trypsin — Chemistry

N-BENZOYL-L-TYROSINE
75JKX N-Benzoyl-L-Tyrosine Ethyl Ester (U.V.), Chymotrypsin — Chemistry

N. MENINGITIDIS
83GTI Antiserum, Fluorescent, N. Meningitidis — Microbiology

N. MENINGITIDIS (cont'd)
83GTJ Antiserum, N. Meningitidis — Microbiology

N2O
73CBR Analyzer, Gas, Nitrous-Oxide, Gaseous Phase — Anesthesiology
76EBX Bracket, Table Assembly, N2O Delivery System — Dental And Oral
73VEA Dosimeter, Nitrous-Oxide — Anesthesiology

NAD
75KLJ NAD Reduction (U.V.), Phosphohexose Isomerase — Chemistry
75CGS NAD Reduction/NADH Oxidation, CPK Or Isoenzymes — Chemistry
75CFJ NAD Reduction/NADH Oxidation, Lactate Dehydrogenase — Chemistry
75CIT NADH Oxidation/NAD Reduction, AST/SGOT — Chemistry
91DML Reagent, NAD-NADH, Alcohol Enzyme Method — Toxicology
75JLJ UDP-Glucose, NAD (U.V.), Gal-I-P Uridyl Transperase — Chemistry

NAD-NADH
91DML Reagent, NAD-NADH, Alcohol Enzyme Method — Toxicology

NADH
75JMK Alpha-Ketobutyric Acid And NADH (U.V.), Hydroxybutyric — Chemistry
75JNK Beta-D-Fructose & NADH Oxidation (U.V.), Sorbitol DH — Chemistry
75CJC Fructose-1, 6-Diphosphate And NADH (U.V.), Aldolase — Chemistry
75JNY Glyceralde-3-Phosphate, NADH (Enzymatic), Triose Phosphate — Chemistry
75CGS NAD Reduction/NADH Oxidation, CPK Or Isoenzymes — Chemistry
75CFJ NAD Reduction/NADH Oxidation, Lactate Dehydrogenase — Chemistry
75CIT NADH Oxidation/NAD Reduction, AST/SGOT — Chemistry
75JLZ Nadh, Phosphoglycerate Mutase, Atp (u.v.) 2, 3-diphosphoglyceric Acid — Chemistry
75JMS Oxalacetic Acid And NADH Oxidation (U.V.), Maleic DH — Chemistry
75JNJ Phosphoenol Pyruvate, ADP, NADH, Pyruvate Kinase — Chemistry
91DML Reagent, NAD-NADH, Alcohol Enzyme Method — Toxicology

NADP
75JKG L-Isocitrate And NADP (U.V.), Isocitric Dehydrogenase — Chemistry
81JMC NADP Reduction (U.V.), Glucose-6-Phosphate Dehydrogenase — Hematology
75JND NADP Reduction, 6-Phosphogluconate Dehydrogenase — Chemistry

NAIL
87LXT Appliance, Fix., Nail/Blade/Plate Comb., Multiple Component — Orthopedics
80QLC Clipper, Nail — General
87QRM Driver/Extractor, Bone Nail/Pin — Orthopedics
87HWB Extractor, Nail — Orthopedics
87JDS Nail, Fixation, Bone — Orthopedics
87KWK Nail/Blade/Plate Appliance — Orthopedics
79MQZ Prosthesis, Nail — Surgery

NAPHTHOL
75CDR 1-Nitroso-2-Naphthol (Fluorometric), Free Tyrosine — Chemistry

NAPHTHYL
75CJO Alpha-Naphthyl Phosphate, Alkaline Phosphatase Or Isoenzyme — Chemistry
75CKB Naphthyl Phosphate, Acid Phosphatase — Chemistry

NAPHTHYLAMIDE
75JKI L-Leucyl B-Naphthylamide, Lactic Acid — Chemistry
75CDC L-Leucyl B-Naphthylamide, Leucine Aminopeptidase — Chemistry

NARCOLEPTIC
73BSZ Gas-Machine, Anesthesia — Anesthesiology

NARCOTIC
80QFG Cabinet, Narcotic Control — General
80QQC Dispenser, Narcotic — General

NARROWING
89IMQ Attachment, Narrowing, Wheelchair — Physical Med

NASAL
77QBT Aspirator, Nasal — Ear/Nose/Throat
77EMX Balloon, Epistaxis (Nasal) — Ear/Nose/Throat
77LFB Button, Nasal Septal — Ear/Nose/Throat
80FMM Cannula, Nasal — General
73CAT Cannula, Nasal, Oxygen — Anesthesiology
73BZB Catheter, Nasal, Oxygen (Tube) — Anesthesiology
73WLJ Catheter, Oxygen, Tracheal — Anesthesiology
77KAN Chisel, Nasal — Ear/Nose/Throat
77KAP Curette, Nasal — Ear/Nose/Throat
77LWF Dilator, Nasal — Ear/Nose/Throat
77ETL Flowmeter, Nasal — Ear/Nose/Throat
77KAQ Gouge, Nasal — Ear/Nose/Throat
77KCO Inhaler, Nasal — Ear/Nose/Throat
77KMA Irrigator, Powered Nasal — Ear/Nose/Throat
79LRQ Kit, Suctioning, Tracheostomy and Nasal — Surgery
77KAS Knife, Nasal — Ear/Nose/Throat
79RXO Packing, Surgical — Surgery
79ESS Prosthesis, Nasal, Dorsal — Surgery
79ESR Prosthesis, Rhinoplasty — Surgery

NASAL *(cont'd)*
79FYG Prosthesis, Splint, Nasal, External — Surgery
77KAY Punch, Nasal — Ear/Nose/Throat
77KBA Rasp, Nasal — Ear/Nose/Throat
77RPA Regulator, Suction, Tracheal (Nasal, Oral) — Ear/Nose/Throat
73BXQ Rhinoanemometer (Measurement Of Nasal Decongestion) — Anesthesiology
77KBB Rongeur, Nasal — Ear/Nose/Throat
77KBC Saw, Nasal — Ear/Nose/Throat
77KBD Scissors, Nasal — Ear/Nose/Throat
77KBE Snare, Nasal — Ear/Nose/Throat
77RUR Speculum, Nasal — Ear/Nose/Throat
77EPP Splint, Nasal — Ear/Nose/Throat
77SCK Truss, Nasal — Ear/Nose/Throat

NASOBILIARY
78QAN Drain, Nasobiliary — Gastro/Urology

NASOGASTRIC
80WOQ Bag, Drainage, Nasogastric — General
77RHR Headband, Nasogastric — Ear/Nose/Throat
78SCV Tube, Esophageal, Blakemore — Gastro/Urology
73BSS Tube, Nasogastric — Anesthesiology

NASOGRAPH
77ENL Nasograph — Ear/Nose/Throat

NASOJEJUNAL
78QUJ Kit, Administration, Enteral — Gastro/Urology
80FPD Tube, Feeding — General

NASOPHARYNGEAL
73CBJ Airway, Bi-Nasopharyngeal (With Connector) — Anesthesiology
73BTQ Airway, Nasopharyngeal (Breathing Tube) — Anesthesiology
77ENW Catheter, Nasopharyngeal — Ear/Nose/Throat
84GZK Electrode, Nasopharyngeal — Cns/Neurology

NASOPHARYNGOSCOPE
77EOB Nasopharyngoscope (Flexible Or Rigid) — Ear/Nose/Throat

NASOPHARYNGOSCOPIC
77WXV Inflator, Sheet, Nasopharyngoscopic — Ear/Nose/Throat

NASOSCOPE
77RHS Nasoscope — Ear/Nose/Throat

NATRIUM
75QTJ Analyzer, Chemistry, Electrolyte — Chemistry

NATURAL
77KHK Polymer, ENT Natural Collagen Material — Ear/Nose/Throat
77ESI Polymer, Natural Absorbable Gelatin Material — Ear/Nose/Throat
79GAL Suture, Absorbable, Natural — Surgery

ND:YAG
79SIV Equipment/Accessories, Laser, Laparoscopy — Surgery
80WQS Laser, Combination — General
79QYU Laser, Nd:YAG, Laparoscopy — Surgery
79ULA Laser, Nd:YAG, Surgical — Surgery

NEARPOINT
86HLE Ruler, Nearpoint (Punctometer) — Ophthalmology

NEBULIZER
77KCK Atomizer And Tip, ENT — Ear/Nose/Throat
73RAU Humidifier, Heat/Moisture Exchange — Anesthesiology
73RAV Humidifier, Heated — Anesthesiology
73KFZ Humidifier, Non-Direct Patient Interface (Home-Use) — Anesthesiology
73RAW Humidifier, Non-Heated — Anesthesiology
73BTT Humidifier, Respiratory Gas, (Direct Patient Interface) — Anesthesiology
77KCO Inhaler, Nasal — Ear/Nose/Throat
73CAF Nebulizer, Direct Patient Interface — Anesthesiology
73RHT Nebulizer, Heated — Anesthesiology
77EPN Nebulizer, Medicinal — Ear/Nose/Throat
73CCQ Nebulizer, Medicinal, Non-Ventilatory (Atomizer) — Anesthesiology
73RHU Nebulizer, Non-Heated — Anesthesiology
73RHV Nebulizer, Ultrasonic — Anesthesiology
77JPW Pump, Nebulizer, Electric — Ear/Nose/Throat
77JPT Pump, Nebulizer, Manual — Ear/Nose/Throat
80SEQ Vaporizer — General
73CAD Vaporizer, Anesthesia, Non-Heated — Anesthesiology
83WKT Water, Therapy, Respiratory — Microbiology

NECK
87QLP Collar, Cervical Neck — Orthopedics
80WMR Collar, Extrication — General
87HWP Punch, Femoral Neck — Orthopedics
78FHK Spreader, Bladder Neck — Gastro/Urology

NEEDLE
74WTU Adapter, Needle — Cardiovascular
78QIK Catheter, Hemodialysis, Single-Needle — Gastro/Urology
80QKU Cleaner, Needle — General
78QZY Controller, Hemodialysis Unit Single Needle — Gastro/Urology

NEEDLE *(cont'd)*
79QMT Counter, Needle — Surgery
80QOG Cutter, Syringe And Needle — General
80MTV Device, Needle Destruction — General
80WSB Dispenser, Syringe And Needle — General
84QSU Electrode, Electroencephalographic — Cns/Neurology
84GXZ Electrode, Needle — Cns/Neurology
84BWR Electrode, Needle, Anesthesiology — Cns/Neurology
89IKT Electrode, Needle, Diagnostic Electromyograph — Physical Med
84HMA Electrode, Needle, Ophthalmic — Cns/Neurology
79KCW Epilator, High-Frequency, Needle-Type — Surgery
79QQR Gauge, Thickness, Tissue — Surgery
80WXY Guide, Device, Ultrasonic — General
79TDD Guide, Needle — Surgery
79GDF Guide, Surgical, Needle — Surgery
78FHQ Holder, Needle — Gastro/Urology
79QOJ Holder, Needle, Curved, Laparoscopic — Surgery
79QNU Holder, Needle, Laparoscopic — Surgery
87HXK Holder, Needle, Orthopedic — Orthopedics
79RHW Holder, Needle, Other — Surgery
79QPN Holder/Scissors, Needle, Laparoscopic — Surgery
80RCJ Immobilizer, Intravenous Catheter-Needle — General
79QRS Instrument, Knot Tying, Suture, Laparoscopic — Surgery
79QPS Instrument, Needle Holder/Knot Tying — Surgery
79QSH Instrument, Passing, Suture, Laparoscopic — Surgery
73BWD Introducer, Spinal Needle — Anesthesiology
80KZH Introducer, Syringe Needle — General
78FCG Kit, Biopsy Needle — Gastro/Urology
74QHK Kit, Catheterization, Cardiac — Cardiovascular
74QHL Kit, Catheterization, Intravenous, Winged — Cardiovascular
78LBW Kit, Dialysis, Single Needle (Co-Axial Flow) — Gastro/Urology
78FIF Kit, Dialysis, Single Needle With Uni-Directional Pump — Gastro/Urology
73BWI Needle, Acupuncture — Anesthesiology
80MQX Needle, Acupuncture, Single Use — General
84HAQ Needle, Angiographic — Cns/Neurology
79GAA Needle, Aspiration And Injection, Disposable — Surgery
79GDM Needle, Aspiration And Injection, Reusable — Surgery
79RIJ Needle, Aspiration, Cyst, Laparoscopic — Surgery
85MQE Needle, Assisted Reproduction — Obstetrics/Gyn
74DWO Needle, Biopsy, Cardiovascular — Cardiovascular
85WJD Needle, Biopsy, Mammary — Obstetrics/Gyn
80RHY Needle, Blood Collection — General
80RHZ Needle, Blunt — General
79SGU Needle, Bone Marrow — Surgery
74RIA Needle, Cardiac — Cardiovascular
79GCB Needle, Catheter — Surgery
85HDH Needle, Cerclage, Gynecological — Obstetrics/Gyn
74RIB Needle, Cholangiography — Cardiovascular
73BSP Needle, Conduction, Anesthesia (W/Wo Introducer) — Anesthesiology
79SJW Needle, Cutting, Bipolar, Electrocauterization — Surgery
76DZM Needle, Dental — Dental And Oral
78RIC Needle, Dialysis — Gastro/Urology
73BWC Needle, Emergency Airway — Anesthesiology
78FBK Needle, Endoscopic — Gastro/Urology
80VCQ Needle, Filter — General
78FIE Needle, Fistula — Gastro/Urology
78FHR Needle, Gastro-Urology — Gastro/Urology
80RIE Needle, Hypodermic — General
80FMI Needle, Hypodermic, Single Lumen With Syringe — General
79RKN Needle, Insufflation, Laparoscopic — Surgery
74RIF Needle, Intra-Arterial — Cardiovascular
80RIG Needle, Intravenous — General
90IWF Needle, Isotope, Gold, Titanium, Platinum — Radiology
79RDG Needle, Knife — Surgery
85MHK Needle, Oocyte Aspiration — Obstetrics/Gyn
86RID Needle, Ophthalmic — Ophthalmology
80RIL Needle, Other — General
78FHP Needle, Pneumoperitoneum, Simple — Gastro/Urology
78FHO Needle, Pneumoperitoneum, Spring Loaded — Gastro/Urology
79SIS Needle, Puncture — Surgery
90RIH Needle, Radiographic — Radiology
84RII Needle, Scalp — Cns/Neurology
80MIA Needle, Spinal, Short-Term — General
87WUR Needle, Suture, Arthroscopy — Orthopedics
79GAB Needle, Suture, Disposable — Surgery
84HAS Needle, Suture, Neurosurgical — Cns/Neurology
86HNM Needle, Suture, Ophthalmic — Ophthalmology
79GDL Needle, Suture, Reusable — Surgery
80RIK Needle, Tine Test — General
77KBR Needle, Tonsil Suture — Ear/Nose/Throat
79MIJ Needle, Tumor Localization — Surgery
80WUI Protector, Puncture, Needle — General
80WZG Set, Administration, Intravenous, Needle-Free — General
80RSI Sharpener, Needle — General
80RWX Stylet, Needle — General
86VKE Surgical Instrument, Radial Keratotomy — Ophthalmology
80MEG Syringe, Antistick — General

NEEDLE (cont'd)

80RYQ	Syringe, Hypodermic	General
85SCD	Trocar, Amniotic	Obstetrics/Gyn
74DRC	Trocar, Cardiovascular	Cardiovascular
80SCH	Trocar, Other	General
80WHK	Tubing, Hypodermic	General
80SFT	Waste Disposal Unit, Syringe	General

NEEDLE-FREE

80WZG	Set, Administration, Intravenous, Needle-Free	General

NEEDLE-TYPE

79KCW	Epilator, High-Frequency, Needle-Type	Surgery

NEEDLES

80MWV	Needles, Medicament Dispensing Tip & Irrigating	General

NEGATIVE

83GSN	Antiserum, Positive And Negative Febrile Antigen Control	Microbiology
83MKA	Kit, Direct Antigen, Negative Control	Microbiology
83MJY	Kit, Serological, Negative Control	Microbiology
83LQM	Panel, Identification, Gram Negative	Microbiology
78FLC	Station, Dialysis Control, Negative Pressure Type	Gastro/Urology
73BYT	Ventilator, External Body, Negative Pressure, (Cuirass)	Anesthesiology

NEISSERIA

83LIC	Antiserum, Coagglutination (Direct) Neisseria Gonorrhoeae	Microbiology
83LSC	Control, Neisseria	Microbiology
83JTY	Culture Media, For Isolation Of Pathogenic Neisseria	Microbiology
83LIR	Enzyme Linked Immunoabsorbent Assay, Neisseria Gonorrhoeae	Microbiology
83JSX	Kit, Identification, Neisseria Gonorrhoeae	Microbiology
83LSL	Neisseria, DNA Reagents	Microbiology
83LTS	Test, Reagent, Biochemical, Neisseria Gonorrhoeae	Microbiology

NELATON

78QID	Catheter, Nelaton	Gastro/Urology
78GBM	Catheter, Urethral	Gastro/Urology

NEODYMIUM

79SIV	Equipment/Accessories, Laser, Laparoscopy	Surgery
80WQS	Laser, Combination	General
79QYU	Laser, Nd:YAG, Laparoscopy	Surgery
79ULA	Laser, Nd:YAG, Surgical	Surgery
86LOI	Laser, Neodymium:YAG (Excl. Post. Capstmy./Pupilloplasty)	Ophthalmology
86LXS	Laser, Neodymium:YAG, Ophthalmic (Post. Capsulotomy)	Ophthalmology
85LLW	Laser, Neodymium:YAG, Surgical, Gynecologic	Obstetrics/Gyn
73LLO	Laser, Neodymium:YAG, Surgical, Pulmonary	Anesthesiology
79WOH	System, Cooling, Laser	Surgery

NEODYMIUM:YAG

86LOI	Laser, Neodymium:YAG (Excl. Post. Capstmy./Pupilloplasty)	Ophthalmology
86LXS	Laser, Neodymium:YAG, Ophthalmic (Post. Capsulotomy)	Ophthalmology
85LLW	Laser, Neodymium:YAG, Surgical, Gynecologic	Obstetrics/Gyn
73LLO	Laser, Neodymium:YAG, Surgical, Pulmonary	Anesthesiology

NEOFORMANS

83JWK	Antigen, Positive Control, Cryptococcus Neoformans	Microbiology
83GME	Antiserum, Fluorescent, Cryptococcus Neoformans	Microbiology
83GMD	Antiserum, Latex Agglutination, Cryptococcus Neoformans	Microbiology

NEON

73VCF	Analyzer, Gas, Neon	Anesthesiology
73JEF	Analyzer, Gas, Neon, Gaseous Phase	Anesthesiology

NEONATAL

73FLM	Analyzer, Oxygen, Neonatal, Invasive	Anesthesiology
80UDH	Bed, Flotation Therapy, Neonatal	General
74WPX	Electrode, ECG, Hand-Held	Cardiovascular
80FMZ	Incubator, Neonatal	General
80FPL	Incubator, Neonatal Transport	General
80FLS	Monitor, Apnea	General
85TDE	Monitor, Neonatal	Obstetrics/Gyn
80FLP	Monitor, Neonatal, Blood Pressure, Invasive	General
80FLQ	Monitor, Neonatal, Blood Pressure, Ultrasonic/Doppler	General
80FLO	Monitor, Neonatal, Heart Rate	General
85TDR	Monitor, Neonatal, Physiological	Obstetrics/Gyn
80FOK	Pad, Neonatal Eye	General
80LBI	Phototherapy Unit, Neonatal	General
80FQC	Ventilator, Neonatal Respirator	General

NEONATE

75MQM	Bilirubin (Total and Unbound) Neonate Test System	Chemistry

NEPHELOMETER

75JQX	Nephelometer	Chemistry
82JZW	Nephelometer, Immunology	Immunology

NEPHELOMETRIC

75WMG	Analyzer, Chemistry, Nephelometric Immunoassay	Chemistry

NEPHELOMETRIC (cont'd)

91LFO	Nephelometric Inhibition Immunoassay, Diphenylhydantoin	Toxicology
91LFN	Nephelometric Inhibition Immunoassay, Phenobarbital	Toxicology
75JGD	Nephelometric Method, Globulin	Chemistry
75CFN	Nephelometric Method, Immunoglobulins (G, A, M)	Chemistry
75JHQ	Nephelometric Method, Lipoproteins	Chemistry
75SHQ	Nephelometric Method, Myoglobin	Chemistry
75KHM	Nephelometric, Amylase	Chemistry

NEPHROSCOPE

78FAJ	Cystoscope	Gastro/Urology
78FFK	Lithotriptor, Electro-Hydraulic, Percutaneous	Gastro/Urology
78FGA	Nephroscope Set	Gastro/Urology
78RIM	Nephroscope, Flexible	Gastro/Urology
78RIN	Nephroscope, Rigid	Gastro/Urology
90RNP	Pyeloscope	Radiology

NEPHROSTOMY

78LJE	Catheter, Nephrostomy	Gastro/Urology
79GBO	Catheter, Nephrostomy, General & Plastic Surgery	Surgery
78FFK	Lithotriptor, Electro-Hydraulic, Percutaneous	Gastro/Urology
78SDF	Tube, Nephrostomy	Gastro/Urology

NERVE

84RWA	Analyzer, Transcutaneous Nerve Stimulator	Cns/Neurology
84UBI	Cap, Nerve	Cns/Neurology
84JXI	Cuff, Nerve	Cns/Neurology
84JXE	Device, Measurement, Velocity, Conduction, Nerve	Cns/Neurology
84MIT	Device, Nerve Repair, Resorbable	Cns/Neurology
79SJB	Instrument, Separating, Nerve	Surgery
84UAV	Prosthesis, Nerve Sheath	Cns/Neurology
84JXG	Shunt, Central Nerve, With Component	Cns/Neurology
74DSR	Stimulator, Carotid Sinus Nerve	Cardiovascular
84GZE	Stimulator, Diaphragmatic/Phrenic Nerve, Implantable	Cns/Neurology
84MNQ	Stimulator, Hypoglossal Nerve, Implanted, Apnea	Cns/Neurology
84UFH	Stimulator, Nerve Locating	Cns/Neurology
84UFI	Stimulator, Nerve Locating, Facial	Cns/Neurology
73BXM	Stimulator, Nerve, AC-Powered	Anesthesiology
73KOI	Stimulator, Nerve, Anesthesia	Anesthesiology
84LYJ	Stimulator, Nerve, Autonomic, Implantable (Epilepsy)	Cns/Neurology
73BXN	Stimulator, Nerve, Battery-Powered	Anesthesiology
84MFP	Stimulator, Nerve, Cranial, Implanted (Pain Relief)	Cns/Neurology
77ETN	Stimulator, Nerve, ENT	Ear/Nose/Throat
84GZJ	Stimulator, Nerve, Transcutaneous (Pain Relief, TENS)	Cns/Neurology
84LEP	Stimulator, Nerve, Transcutaneous Elec. (Speech Disorder)	Cns/Neurology
79FXA	Stimulator, Neurological	Surgery
73UFG	Stimulator, Peripheral Nerve, Blockade Monitor	Anesthesiology
84GZF	Stimulator, Peripheral Nerve, Implantable (Pain Relief)	Cns/Neurology
84MQQ	Stimulator, Sacral Nerve, Implanted	Cns/Neurology
84MBY	Stimulator, Vagus Nerve, Epilepsy, Implanted	Cns/Neurology
84MUY	Stimulator, Vagus Nerve, Implanted (Coma And Vegetative State)	Cns/Neurology
84LSS	Unit, Repair, Nerve, Implantable, Electric	Cns/Neurology

NESSLER

75JMY	Citrulline, Arsenate, Nessler (Colorimetry), Ornithine CT	Chemistry

NET

74WVD	Holder, Cardiac	Cardiovascular
80RPJ	Retainer, Bandage (Elastic Net)	General

NETILMICIN

91LCE	Radioimmunoassay, Netilmicin (125-I)	Toxicology

NETWORK

74MSX	System, Network And Communication, Physiological Monitors	Cardiovascular

NEURAL

82LOK	Test, Neural Tube Defect, Alpha-Fetoprotein (AFP)	Immunology

NEURAMININASE

88IBE	Neuraminidase (Sialidase)	Pathology

NEUROLEPTIC

91LPX	Test, Radioreceptor, Neuroleptic Drugs	Toxicology

NEUROLOGICAL

84GXH	Cryosurgical Unit, Neurological	Cns/Neurology
84QTB	Electrode, Neurological	Cns/Neurology
84HAM	Electrosurgical Unit, Neurological	Cns/Neurology
84GWG	Endoscope, Neurological	Cns/Neurology
84QZF	Hammer, Neurological	Cns/Neurology
84HAC	Saw, Manual, Neurological (With Accessories)	Cns/Neurology
84HAY	Sponge, External, Neurological	Cns/Neurology
79FXA	Stimulator, Neurological	Surgery
84GYE	Telemetry Unit, Physiological, Neurological	Cns/Neurology

NEUROLOGY

84HBK	Chair, Pneumoencephalographic, Neurology	Cns/Neurology
84WHW	Chair, Rotating	Cns/Neurology
84GXX	Phantom, Ultrasonic Scanner, Neurology	Cns/Neurology

NOISE
77ETS Generator, Electronic Noise (For Audiometric Testing) — Ear/Nose/Throat

NON-ABSORBABLE
79LMG Agent, Hemostatic, Non-Absorbable, Collagen-Based — Surgery
79GEL Gauze, Non-Absorbable, Medicated (Internal Sponge) — Surgery
79GEK Gauze, Non-Absorbable, Non-Medicated (Internal Sponge) — Surgery
79GDY Gauze, Non-Absorbable, X-Ray Detectable (Internal Sponge) — Surgery
79SGX Suture, Laparoscopy — Surgery
79SGW Suture, Laparoscopy, Loose — Surgery
79SGY Suture, Laparoscopy, Pre-Tied — Surgery
79GAO Suture, Non-Absorbable — Surgery
86HMN Suture, Non-Absorbable, Ophthalmic — Ophthalmology
79GAP Suture, Non-Absorbable, Silk — Surgery
79GAQ Suture, Non-Absorbable, Steel, Monofilament & Multifilament — Surgery
79GAR Suture, Non-Absorbable, Synthetic, Polyamide — Surgery
79GAS Suture, Non-Absorbable, Synthetic, Polyester — Surgery
79GAT Suture, Non-Absorbable, Synthetic, Polyethylene — Surgery
79GAW Suture, Non-Absorbable, Synthetic, Polypropylene — Surgery

NON-AC-POWERED
80FSA Lift, Bath, Non-AC-Powered — General

NON-ADHERENT
80QQX Dressing, Non-Adherent — General

NON-AESTHETIC
79LMI Implant, Collagen (Non-Aesthetic Use) — Surgery

NON-ALTERABLE
84GXN Plate, Bone, Skull, Preformed, Non-Alterable — Cns/Neurology

NON-BACK-PRESSURE
73CCN Flowmeter, Gas, Non-Back-Pressure Compensated, Bourdon Gauge — Anesthesiology

NON-BEEP
89LXF Diathermy, Ultrasonic (Non-Beep Heat) — Physical Med
89LPQ Stimulator, Muscle, Ultrasonic (Non-Beep Heat) — Physical Med

NON-BIODEGRADABLE
87MBI Fastener, Fixation, Non-Biodegradable, Soft Tissue — Orthopedics

NON-CEMENTED
87JDM Prosthesis, Hip, Acetabular Component, Metal, Non-Cemented — Orthopedics
87LZO Prosthesis, Hip, Semi-Constr., Metal/Ceramic, Cemented/NC — Orthopedics

NON-COHERENT
79MYH System, Non-coherent Light, Photodynamic Therapy — Surgery

NON-COMPRESSION
80WVI Sock, Non-Compression — General

NON-CONDUCTIVE
80QNF Cover, Shoe, Non-Conductive — General
80QWV Footstool, Non-Conductive — General
80SDO Tubing, Non-Conductive — General

NON-CONSTRAINED
87KXC Prosthesis, Ankle, Non-Constrained — Orthopedics
87JDA Prosthesis, Elbow, Non-Constrained, Unipolar — Orthopedics
87HSX Prosthesis, Knee, Femorotibial, Non-Constrained — Orthopedics
87KTX Prosthesis, Knee, Femorotibial, Non-Constrained, Metal — Orthopedics
87KMB Prosthesis, Knee, Non-Const. (M/C Reinf. Polyeth.) Cemented — Orthopedics
87KWT Prosthesis, Shoulder, Non-Constrained, Metal/Polymer Cem. — Orthopedics

NON-CONTACT
85HHA Heater, Perineal, Radiant, Non-Contact — Obstetrics/Gyn

NON-CONTINUOUS
73BZD Ventilator, Non-Continuous (Respirator) — Anesthesiology

NON-CRUSHING
78MET Lithotriptor, Mechanical, Non-Crushing — Gastro/Urology

NON-CUSTOM
86HQH Eye, Artificial, Non-Custom — Ophthalmology
86HQM Keratoprosthesis, Non-Custom — Ophthalmology
86HQG Lens, Spectacle/Eyeglasses, Non-Custom — Ophthalmology

NON-DIAGNOSTIC
81MZH Test, Quantitative, For Hla, Non-diagnostic — Hematology

NON-DIFFERENTIAL
83JSG Culture Media, Non-Selective And Non-Differential — Microbiology
83JSJ Culture Media, Selective And Non-Differential — Microbiology

NON-DIRECT
73KFZ Humidifier, Non-Direct Patient Interface (Home-Use) — Anesthesiology

NON-ELECTRIC
78FCL Forceps, Biopsy, Non-Electric — Gastro/Urology
80KZE Injector, Fluid, Non-Electric — General
86HRB Microscope, Operating, Non-Electric, Ophthalmic — Ophthalmology
80MLX Pad, Medicated, Adhesive, Non-Electric — General

NON-ELECTRICAL
79FZK Chair, Surgical, Non-Electrical — Surgery
78FFN Clamp, Non-Electrical — Gastro/Urology
78KDM Sigmoidoscope, Rigid, Non-Electrical — Gastro/Urology
78FGX Snare, Non-Electrical — Gastro/Urology
78KQS Table, Cystometric, Non-Electrical — Gastro/Urology
78EYH Table, Urological, Non-Electrical — Gastro/Urology
78EXT Urinometer, Non-Electrical — Gastro/Urology

NON-ELECTROMAGNETIC
73BSB Warmer, Blood, Non-Electromagnetic Radiation — Anesthesiology

NON-FERMENT
83JSW Kit, Identification, Glucose (Non-Ferment) — Microbiology

NON-FETAL
90JAF Monitor, Ultrasonic, Non-Fetal — Radiology

NON-FLUID-FILLED
76MEF Ring, Teething, Non-Fluid-Filled — Dental And Oral

NON-HEATED
73RAW Humidifier, Non-Heated — Anesthesiology
73RHU Nebulizer, Non-Heated — Anesthesiology
73CAD Vaporizer, Anesthesia, Non-Heated — Anesthesiology

NON-HEATING
90MWC Diathermy, Shortwave (Non-heating) — Radiology

NON-HEME
75JIZ Absorption, Atomic, Iron (Non-Heme) — Chemistry
75JIY Photometric Method, Iron (Non-Heme) — Chemistry
75JJA Radio-Labeled Iron Method, Iron (Non-Heme) — Chemistry

NON-HUMAN
81KSX Substance, Grouping, Blood (Non-Human Origin) — Hematology

NON-ILLUMINATED
79FXE Speculum, Non-Illuminated — Surgery

NON-IMAGE-INTENSIFIED
90JAB Radiographic/Fluoroscopic Unit, Non-Image-Intensified — Radiology

NON-IMPLANTABLE
78KPI Stimulator, Incontinence (Non-Implantable), Electrical — Gastro/Urology

NON-INDWELLING
91JFD Analyzer, Concentration, Oxyhemoglobin, Blood Phase — Toxicology
73VCB Analyzer, Gas, Carbon-Monoxide, Non-Indwelling Blood Phase — Anesthesiology
91CCA Analyzer, Gas, Carboxyhemoglobin, Blood Phase, Non-Indw. — Toxicology
73BSD Analyzer, Gas, Nitrogen, Partial Pressure, Blood Phase (NI) — Anesthesiology
73CBY Analyzer, Ion, Hydrogen-Ion pH, Blood Phase, Non-Indwelling — Anesthesiology
73BXF Transducer, Blood Flow, Non-Invasive — Anesthesiology

NON-INFLATABLE
80LLK Legging, Compression, Non-Inflatable — General
79FTR Prosthesis, Breast, Non-Inflatable, Internal — Surgery
79FYH Splint, Extremity, Non-Inflatable, External — Surgery

NON-INJECTABLE
79LWD Irrigating Solution, Non-Injectable — Surgery

NON-INVASIVE
87MHH Analyzer, Bone, Sonic, Non-Invasive — Orthopedics
87KQZ Component, Traction, Non-Invasive — Orthopedics
74QTD Electrode, Pacemaker, External — Cardiovascular
80WYB Equipment, Management, Pain, Radiofrequency, Non-Invasive — General
78FIT Flowmeter, Blood, Non-Invasive Electromagnetic — Gastro/Urology
74WSR Flowmeter, Blood, Other — Cardiovascular
75WXU Monitor, Glucose, Blood, Non-Invasive — Chemistry
74DRO Pacemaker, Cardiac, External Transcutaneous (Non-Invasive) — Cardiovascular
89MKC Stimulator, Arthritis, Non-Invasive — Physical Med
87LOF Stimulator, Growth, Bone, Non-Invasive — Orthopedics
89MKD Stimulator, Neuromuscular, Functional Walking, Non-Invasive — Physical Med
87WNT Stimulator, Osteogenesis, Electric, Non-Invasive — Orthopedics
80WOI System, Delivery, Drug, Non-invasive — General
73BXF Transducer, Blood Flow, Non-Invasive — Anesthesiology
79GAZ Tubing, Non-Invasive — Surgery

NOURISHMENT

80UMU	Station, Nourishment	General

NOZZLE

85QQJ	Nozzle, Douche	Obstetrics/Gyn

NUCLEAR

90WIA	Afterloader, Radiotherapy	Radiology
90IYZ	Bed, Scanning, Nuclear/Fluoroscopic	Radiology
90IXD	Calibrator Source, Nuclear Sealed	Radiology
90IYX	Camera, Gamma (Nuclear/Scintillation)	Radiology
90QMD	Computer, Nuclear Medicine	Radiology
90WJA	Container, Substance, Radioactive	Radiology
90JAN	Counter, Whole Body, Nuclear	Radiology
90WJH	Dispenser, Radiopharmaceuticals	Radiology
90UAD	Exerciser, Nuclear Diagnostic (Cardiac Stress Table)	Radiology
90VCO	Gantry, Nuclear Imaging	Radiology
90WPG	Gas Mixtures, Magnetic Resonance Imaging	Radiology
90IXE	Hood and Exhaust, Nuclear	Radiology
75UGY	Nuclear Magnetic Resonance Equipment, Laboratory	Chemistry
90LNH	Nuclear Magnetic Resonance Imaging System	Radiology
90LNI	Nuclear Magnetic Resonance Spectroscopic System	Radiology
90IYP	Phantom, Anthropomorphic, Nuclear	Radiology
90IYQ	Phantom, Flood Source, Nuclear	Radiology
90IZD	Probe, Uptake, Nuclear	Radiology
90JAM	Scanner, Magnetic Resonance (NMR/MRI)	Radiology
90THG	Scanner, Nuclear Emission Computed Tomography (ECT)	Radiology
90IYW	Scanner, Nuclear, Rectilinear	Radiology
90JWM	Scanner, Nuclear, Tomographic	Radiology
90ULI	Scanner, Positron Emission Tomography (PET)	Radiology
75RUJ	Spectrometer, Nuclear	Chemistry
88HZF	Stain, Nuclear Fast Red	Pathology
90WJP	Stand, Cardiovascular	Radiology
90WLW	Stand, Vascular	Radiology
90IYY	Synchronizer, Electrocardiograph, Nuclear	Radiology
90RYJ	Synchronizer, Nuclear Camera	Radiology
90RYK	Synchronizer, Radiographic Unit	Radiology
90VHE	Table, Nuclear Medicine	Radiology
83LLM	Test, Nuclear Antigen, Epstein-Barr Virus	Microbiology
90SFV	Waste Receptacle, Radioactive	Radiology

NUCLEIC

83MKZ	DNA-Probe, Nucleic Acid Amplification, Chlamydia	Microbiology
82MVD	System, Test, Her-2/Neu, Nucleic Acid Or Serum	Immunology

NUCLEOTIDASE

75CED	5-AMP-Phosphate Release (Colorimetric), 5'-Nucleotidase	Chemistry

NUCLEOTIDE

81KHF	Adenine Nucleotide Quantitation	Hematology

NUCLEUS

87MQO	Prosthetic Disc Nucleus Device	Orthopedics

NURSE

80QYQ	Gown, Other	General
80RIO	Nurse Call System	General

NURSING

85TAO	Bottle, Nursing	Obstetrics/Gyn
80VBH	Computer Software	General
80WSJ	Computer Software, Hospital/Nursing Management	General
80FNN	Nipple, Feeding	General
80TBD	Station, Nursing	General

NUT

87HTN	Bolt, Nut, Washer	Orthopedics

NUTRIENT

83JSC	Culture Media, General Nutrient Broth	Microbiology

NUTRITION

80QVM	Kit, Feeding, Adult (Enteral)	General
80QVN	Kit, Feeding, Pediatric (Enteral)	General
78WWM	Solution, Nutrition, Enteral	Gastro/Urology
78TGK	Solution, Nutrition, Parenteral	Gastro/Urology
80UMU	Station, Nourishment	General
80FPD	Tube, Feeding	General

NUTRITIONAL

80RNF	Pump, Food (Enteral Feeding)	General

NYLON

80WXR	Media, Filter	General
80WTJ	Polymer, Synthetic, Other	General
79GAR	Suture, Non-Absorbable, Synthetic, Polyamide	Surgery
80SDP	Tubing, Nylon	General

NYSTAGMOGRAPH

86QTL	Electronystagmograph (ENG)	Ophthalmology
84GWN	Nystagmograph	Cns/Neurology

NYSTAGMOGRAPH *(cont'd)*

77ETO	Nystagmograph, ENT	Ear/Nose/Throat

NYSTAGMUS

86HKD	Tape, Nystagmus	Ophthalmology

O-HYDROXYPHENYLIMINE

75CHZ	DI (O-Hydroxyphenylimine) Ethane, Calcium	Chemistry

O-PHTHALALDEHYDE

75JGZ	O-Phthalaldehyde, Urea Nitrogen	Chemistry

OBESE

80VDN	Analyzer, Composition, Weight, Patient	General
78WNS	Balloon, Gastric	Gastro/Urology
80TAH	Bed, Obese	General

OBESITY

78SAP	Elevator, Wall, Abdominal	Gastro/Urology
78LTI	Implant, Intragastric, Obesity, Morbid	Gastro/Urology

OBSERVATION

81JMH	Fluorescence, Visual Observation (Qual., U.V.), Gsh	Hematology

OBSERVERSCOPE

80RIP	Observerscope	General

OBSTETRIC

85HEO	Analyzer, Data, Obstetric	Obstetrics/Gyn
85KNB	Surgical Instrument, Obstetric, Destructive, Fetal	Obstetrics/Gyn
85KNA	Surgical Instrument, Obstetric/Gynecologic	Obstetrics/Gyn
85KOH	Surgical Instrument, Obstetric/Gynecologic, General	Obstetrics/Gyn
85LNW	pH Paper, Obstetric	Obstetrics/Gyn

OBSTETRICAL

85HFR	Binder, Abdominal, OB/GYN	Obstetrics/Gyn
85HDA	Forceps, Obstetrical	Obstetrics/Gyn
85HDI	Hook, Destructive, Obstetrical	Obstetrics/Gyn
85KNE	Kit, Anesthesia, Obstetrical	Obstetrics/Gyn
85MLS	Kit, Labor and Delivery	Obstetrics/Gyn
85RHC	Mirror, Obstetrical	Obstetrics/Gyn
85HEM	Scanner, Ultrasonic, Obstetrical/Gynecological	Obstetrics/Gyn
85RQX	Scanner, Ultrasonic, Obstetrical/Gynecological, Mobile	Obstetrics/Gyn
85KNC	Table, Obstetrical	Obstetrics/Gyn
85HDD	Table, Obstetrical, AC-Powered	Obstetrics/Gyn
85HHP	Table, Obstetrical, Manual	Obstetrics/Gyn
80WNI	Table, Ultrasound	General
85HGL	Transducer, Ultrasonic, Obstetrical	Obstetrics/Gyn

OBSTRUCTION

80QAJ	Airway, Obstruction Removal (Choke Saver)	General

OBTURATOR

73CAO	Airway, Esophageal (Obturator)	Anesthesiology
77LFB	Button, Nasal Septal	Ear/Nose/Throat
87LZN	Obturator, Cement	Orthopedics
77UCZ	Obturator, Cleft Palate	Ear/Nose/Throat
78FEC	Obturator, Endoscopic	Gastro/Urology
74DTI	Sizer, Heart Valve Prosthesis	Cardiovascular

OCCLUDER

76TDF	Occluder	Dental And Oral
74WOZ	Occluder, Cardiovascular	Cardiovascular
74DQT	Occluder, Catheter Tip	Cardiovascular
86HKE	Occluder, Ophthalmic	Ophthalmology
74MAE	Occluder, Patent Ductus, Arteriosus	Cardiovascular
80FOD	Occluder, Umbilical	General
74LWT	Vena Cava Balloon Occluder	Cardiovascular

OCCLUDING

84HBZ	Catheter, Intravascular Occluding	Cns/Neurology
74MJN	Catheter, Intravascular Occluding, Temporary	Cardiovascular
74MFC	Catheter, Occluding, Cardiovascular, Implantable	Cardiovascular

OCCLUSION

79MAG	Agent, Embolization/Occlusion	Surgery
84LHH	Balloon, Occlusion, Cerebrovascular	Cns/Neurology
85HFY	Band, Occlusion, Tubal	Obstetrics/Gyn
74QIE	Catheter, Occlusion	Cardiovascular
85HGB	Clip, Tubal Occlusion	Obstetrics/Gyn
85LLS	Contraceptive Tubal Occlusion Device, Male	Obstetrics/Gyn
78MNG	Device, Incontinence, Occlusion, Urethral	Gastro/Urology
74MLV	Device, Occlusion, Cardiac, Transcatheter	Cardiovascular
85HHS	Insert, Tubal Occlusion	Obstetrics/Gyn
74DXP	Transducer, Vessel Occlusion	Cardiovascular
85HDO	Valve, Tubal Occlusion	Obstetrics/Gyn

OCCLUSIVE

79MSA	Dressing, Wound And Burn, Occlusive, Heated	Surgery
79MGP	Dressing, Wound and Burn, Occlusive	Surgery
79NAD	Dressing, Wound, Occlusive	Surgery
85KNH	Tubal Occlusive Device	Obstetrics/Gyn

OCCULT
81JIO Colorimetric, Occult Blood in Urine — Hematology
75TGO Enzymatic Method, Blood, Occcult, Fecal — Chemistry
75JIP Enzymatic Method, Blood, Occult, Urinary — Chemistry
81GGG Reagent, Guaiac — Hematology
81KHE Reagent, Occult Blood — Hematology

OCCUPANCY
80QDB Monitor, Bed Occupancy — General

OCULAR
86LCC Applicator, Ocular Pressure — Ophthalmology
86HQX Implant, Orbital, Extra-Ocular — Ophthalmology
86KYG Irrigator, Ocular Surgery — Ophthalmology
86WKX Irrigator, Ocular, Emergency — Ophthalmology
86HMR Marker, Ocular — Ophthalmology
86HMQ Marker, Sclera (Ocular) — Ophthalmology
86MQU Ocular Peg — Ophthalmology
86HLB Ophthalmodynamometer — Ophthalmology
84JXF Plethysmograph, Ocular — Cns/Neurology
86WVM System, Delivery, Drug, Ocular — Ophthalmology

OCULOGRAPH
86QTM Electro-Oculograph — Ophthalmology
86QSX Electrode, Electro-Oculograph — Ophthalmology
84RZM Telemetry Unit, Physiological, EOG — Cns/Neurology

OCULOPLETHYSMOGRAPH
84JXF Plethysmograph, Ocular — Cns/Neurology

ODOR
78VKQ Solution, Ostomy, Odor Control — Gastro/Urology

ODYNOMETER
73RJV Pain Gauge, Transcutaneous — Anesthesiology

OFFICE
80VBG Office Equipment — General
80VBM Office Product — General

OIL
88IJZ Clearing Oil — Pathology
75CFG Emulsion, Oil, (Titrimetric), Lipase — Chemistry
75CET Emulsion, Olive Oil (Turbidimetric), Lipase — Chemistry
88KEP Mounting Media, Oil Soluble — Pathology
81GLF Oil, Immersion — Hematology
88HZG Stain, Oil Red O — Pathology

OLEOPHOBIC
75UGD Filter, Membrane — Chemistry

OLFACTOMETER
80RIR Olfactometer — General

OLIVE
78QIF Catheter, Olive Tip — Gastro/Urology
78EZM Dilator, Esophageal (Metal Olive) Gastro-Urology — Gastro/Urology
75CET Emulsion, Olive Oil (Turbidimetric), Lipase — Chemistry

OMNICARDIOGRAPH
74RIS Omnicardiograph (Cardiointegraph) — Cardiovascular

ON-LINE
74DRY Monitor, Blood Gas, On-Line, Cardiopulmonary Bypass — Cardiovascular

ONCOMETER
83RIT Oncometer — Microbiology
75UGZ Oncometer, Laboratory — Chemistry
75JJK Oncometer, Plasma — Chemistry
75JNX Oncometer, Plasma (Membrane Osmometry) — Chemistry

ONE
79GDX Scalpel, One-Piece (Knife) — Surgery

ONE-PIECE
79GDX Scalpel, One-Piece (Knife) — Surgery

OOCYTE
85MHK Needle, Oocyte Aspiration — Obstetrics/Gyn

OPAQUE
74JAP Catheter, Vascular, Opaque — Cardiovascular

OPENER
78QAR Opener, Ampule — Gastro/Urology

OPENING
78FDJ Snare, Rigid Self-Opening — Gastro/Urology

OPERATED
78FFD Evacuator, Bladder, Manually Operated — Gastro/Urology
86HPP Headlamp, Operating, Battery-Operated — Ophthalmology
80QUD Power Supply, Endoscopic, Battery-Operated — General
80QUE Power Supply, Endoscopic, Line-Operated — General

OPERATING
79FWZ Accessories, Operating Room, Table — Surgery
80REJ Bag, Laundry, Operating Room — General
79GEC Brush, Scrub, Operating Room — Surgery
79FSK Cart, Supply, Operating Room — Surgery
79FXP Cover, Shoe, Operating Room — Surgery
79FZL Footstool, Operating Room — Surgery
79FPH Gown, Operating Room, Disposable — Surgery
79QYN Gown, Operating Room, Reusable — Surgery
86HPQ Headlamp, Operating, AC-Powered — Ophthalmology
86HPP Headlamp, Operating, Battery-Operated — Ophthalmology
79FTE Jar, Operating Room — Surgery
80FQP Lamp, Operating Room — General
76EAZ Light, Surgical Operating, Dental — Dental And Oral
79RFQ Magnifier, Operating — Surgery
80RGH Mattress, Operating Table — General
86HRM Microscope, Operating, AC-Powered, Ophthalmic — Ophthalmology
86HRB Microscope, Operating, Non-Electric, Ophthalmic — Ophthalmology
80WMD Pad, Pressure, Gel, Operating Table — General
79FSN Rack, Glove, Operating Room — Surgery
79FSF Rack, Sponge, Operating Room — Surgery
80WRN Rails, Equipment — General
79RSN Sheet, Operating Room — Surgery
79RSO Sheet, Operating Room, Disposable — Surgery
79FXW Shoe, Operating Room — Surgery
86HOH Spectacle, Operating (Loupe), Ophthalmic — Ophthalmology
79FSH Stand, Operating Room Instrument (Mayo) — Surgery
79FSJ Sterilizer, Ethylene-Oxide Gas, Operating Room — Surgery
79FZM Stool, Operating Room, Adjustable — Surgery
79GCX Suction Apparatus, Operating Room, Wall Vacuum-Powered — Surgery
79FQO Table, Operating Room, AC-Powered — Surgery
79FWX Table, Operating Room, Mechanical — Surgery
79FWW Table, Operating Room, Pneumatic — Surgery
80TFD Television Monitor, Operating Room — General
80WTM Weight, IV Pole — General

OPERATIVE
76EKJ Burnisher, Operative, Dental — Dental And Oral
76EKI Carrier, Amalgam, Operative — Dental And Oral
76EKH Carver, Dental Amalgam, Operative — Dental And Oral
74LOX Catheter, Angioplasty, Coronary, Transluminal, Percut. Oper. — Cardiovascular
76EFG Chair, Operative — Dental And Oral
76EKG Condenser, Amalgam And Foil, Operative — Dental And Oral
76EKF Contouring, Instrument, Matrix, Operative — Dental And Oral
76EKE Curette, Operative — Dental And Oral
76EKD Cutter, Operative — Dental And Oral
76QOV Engine, Dental — Dental And Oral
76EKC Excavator, Dental, Operative — Dental And Oral
76EKB Explorer, Operative — Dental And Oral
76EKA File, Margin Finishing, Operative — Dental And Oral
76EJZ Knife, Margin Finishing, Operative — Dental And Oral
76EIA Operative Dental Treatment Unit — Dental And Oral
76EJY Pliers, Operative — Dental And Oral

OPERATORY
76EBR Pump, Suction Operatory — Dental And Oral

OPHTHALMIC
86LZQ Adhesive, Tissue, Ophthalmology — Ophthalmology
86QBG Applicator, Ophthalmic — Ophthalmology
86WKR Aspirator, Ophthalmic — Ophthalmology
86WQG Astigmometer — Ophthalmology
86HKW Bar, Prism, Ophthalmic — Ophthalmology
86QEQ Brush, Ophthalmic — Ophthalmology
86HRE Cabinet, Instrument, AC-Powered, Ophthalmic — Ophthalmology
86HOE Caliper, Ophthalmic — Ophthalmology
86HKI Camera, Ophthalmic, AC-Powered (Fundus) — Ophthalmology
86QGA Cannula, Cyclodialysis (Eye) — Ophthalmology
86QGB Cannula, Lacrimal (Eye) — Ophthalmology
86HMX Cannula, Ophthalmic — Ophthalmology
86MXY Cannula, Ophthalmic, Posterior Capsular Polishing, Polyvinyl Acetal — Ophthalmology
86UAX Cap, Ophthalmic, Quarter Globe — Ophthalmology
86HME Chair, Ophthalmic, AC-Powered — Ophthalmology
86HMD Chair, Ophthalmic, Manual — Ophthalmology
86HOX Chart, Visual Acuity — Ophthalmology
86HOD Clamp, Eyelid, Ophthalmic — Ophthalmology
86HOB Clamp, Muscle, Ophthalmic — Ophthalmology
86HPB Clip, Lens, Trial, Ophthalmic — Ophthalmology
86HQW Clip, Tantalum, Ophthalmic — Ophthalmology
86LQB Computer and Software, Medical, Ophthalmic Use — Ophthalmology
86HQN Conformer, Ophthalmic — Ophthalmology
86HQA Cryotherapy, Unit, Ophthalmic — Ophthalmology
86HNZ Curette, Ophthalmic — Ophthalmology
86HNY Cystotome, Ophthalmic — Ophthalmology
86HKH Disk, Pinhole, Ophthalmic — Ophthalmology
86HMW Drape, Microscope, Ophthalmic — Ophthalmology

OPHTHALMIC *(cont'd)*

86HMT	Drape, Patient, Ophthalmic	Ophthalmology
84HMA	Electrode, Needle, Ophthalmic	Cns/Neurology
86HLY	Electrode, Skin Surface, Ophthalmic	Ophthalmology
86HPY	Electrolysis Unit, Battery-Powered, Ophthalmic	Ophthalmology
86HRO	Electrolysis Unit, Ophthalmic	Ophthalmology
78KYH	Endoscope, Ophthalmic	Gastro/Urology
78FDZ	Eyepiece, Lens, Prescription, Endoscopic	Gastro/Urology
86HPL	Fixation Device, AC-Powered, Ophthalmic	Ophthalmology
86HKJ	Fixation Device, Battery-Powered, Ophthalmic	Ophthalmology
86UAY	Foil, Ophthalmic	Ophthalmology
86HNR	Forceps, Ophthalmic	Ophthalmology
86HPA	Frame, Trial, Ophthalmic	Ophthalmology
86TCI	Freezer, Eye Bank	Ophthalmology
86HLN	Gauge, Lens, Ophthalmic	Ophthalmology
86HNQ	Hook, Ophthalmic	Ophthalmology
86KYF	Implant, Eye Valve	Ophthalmology
86WUA	Implant, Scleral	Ophthalmology
86THQ	Insert, Dry Eye	Ophthalmology
86WKX	Irrigator, Ocular, Emergency	Ophthalmology
86RCT	Kit, Irrigation, Eye	Ophthalmology
86HNN	Knife, Ophthalmic	Ophthalmology
86WTY	Laboratory Equipment, Ophthalmic	Ophthalmology
79ULC	Laser, Dye, Surgical	Surgery
86WMI	Laser, Krypton, Ophthalmic	Ophthalmology
86LXS	Laser, Neodymium:YAG, Ophthalmic (Post. Capsulotomy)	Ophthalmology
86HQF	Laser, Ophthalmic	Ophthalmology
86HPC	Lens, Set, Trial, Ophthalmic	Ophthalmology
86HLF	Measurer, Lens Radius, Ophthalmic	Ophthalmology
86HRM	Microscope, Operating, AC-Powered, Ophthalmic	Ophthalmology
86HRB	Microscope, Operating, Non-Electric, Ophthalmic	Ophthalmology
86HKF	Mirror, Headband, Ophthalmic	Ophthalmology
86HLL	Monitor, Eye Movement	Ophthalmology
86RID	Needle, Ophthalmic	Ophthalmology
86HNM	Needle, Suture, Ophthalmic	Ophthalmology
86HKE	Occluder, Ophthalmic	Ophthalmology
86WQL	Pachometer	Ophthalmology
86HMP	Pad, Eye	Ophthalmology
80FOK	Pad, Neonatal Eye	General
86HLT	Preamplifier, AC-Powered, Ophthalmic	Ophthalmology
86HLW	Preamplifier, Battery-Powered, Ophthalmic	Ophthalmology
86HKT	Prism, Fresnel, Ophthalmic	Ophthalmology
86HKQ	Prism, Rotary, Ophthalmic	Ophthalmology
86RMH	Probe, Ophthalmic	Ophthalmology
86HOS	Projector, Ophthalmic	Ophthalmology
86RMQ	Prosthesis, Eyelid	Ophthalmology
86HJY	Reader, Bar, Ophthalmic	Ophthalmology
86HJX	Reader, Prism, Ophthalmic	Ophthalmology
86HMB	Recorder, Analog/Digital, Ophthalmic	Ophthalmology
86HKO	Refractometer, Ophthalmic	Ophthalmology
86HKN	Refractor, Ophthalmic	Ophthalmology
86HNI	Retractor, Ophthalmic	Ophthalmology
86HNH	Ring, Ophthalmic (Flieringa)	Ophthalmology
90HPR	Scanner, Ultrasonic, Ophthalmic	Radiology
86RRD	Scissors, Corneal	Ophthalmology
86RRE	Scissors, Enucleation	Ophthalmology
86RRF	Scissors, Iris	Ophthalmology
86HNF	Scissors, Ophthalmic	Ophthalmology
86RRH	Scissors, Tenotomy	Ophthalmology
86WRV	Shield, Corneal	Ophthalmology
86HOY	Shield, Eye, Ophthalmic	Ophthalmology
90IWS	Shield, Ophthalmic, Radiological	Radiology
86UBF	Sleeve, Muscle, Ophthalmic	Ophthalmology
86HND	Spatula, Ophthalmic	Ophthalmology
86HOH	Spectacle, Operating (Loupe), Ophthalmic	Ophthalmology
86HNC	Speculum, Ophthalmic	Ophthalmology
86HPZ	Sphere, Ophthalmic (Implant)	Ophthalmology
86HOZ	Sponge, Ophthalmic	Ophthalmology
86HNB	Spoon, Ophthalmic	Ophthalmology
86HNA	Spud, Ophthalmic	Ophthalmology
86TEV	Spud, Ophthalmic, Electrical	Ophthalmology
86HMF	Stand, Instrument, AC-Powered, Ophthalmic	Ophthalmology
86HMG	Stand, Instrument, Ophthalmic	Ophthalmology
86HMO	Suture, Absorbable, Ophthalmic	Ophthalmology
86HMN	Suture, Non-Absorbable, Ophthalmic	Ophthalmology
86HKA	Syringe, Ophthalmic	Ophthalmology
86WXL	System, Hyperthermia, Ultrasonic, Ophthalmic	Ophthalmology
86LZS	System, Laser, Excimer, Ophthalmic	Ophthalmology
86WXT	System, Mapping, Corneal	Ophthalmology
86HRK	Table, Ophthalmic, Instrument, Manual	Ophthalmology
86HRJ	Table, Ophthalmic, Instrument, Powered	Ophthalmology
86HIT	Tester, Color Vision	Ophthalmology
86MMQ	Topographer, Corneal	Ophthalmology
86HJM	Transilluminator, AC-Powered, Ophthalmic	Ophthalmology
86HRH	Trephine, Manual, Ophthalmic (Corneal)	Ophthalmology
86HRL	Unit, Radiation, Beta, Ophthalmic	Ophthalmology
86SEN	Valve, Ophthalmic	Ophthalmology

OPHTHALMODYNAMOGRAPH

84HMI	Ophthalmodynamograph	Cns/Neurology

OPHTHALMODYNAMOMETER

86HLB	Ophthalmodynamometer	Ophthalmology

OPHTHALMOLOGY

86LZQ	Adhesive, Tissue, Ophthalmology	Ophthalmology
86WQK	Computer, Ophthalmology	Ophthalmology

OPHTHALMOMETER

86HLS	Exophthalmometer	Ophthalmology
86UEK	Keratometer	Ophthalmology

OPHTHALMOSCOPE

86QXV	Funduscope	Ophthalmology
86HLI	Ophthalmoscope, AC-Powered	Ophthalmology
86HLJ	Ophthalmoscope, Battery-Powered	Ophthalmology
86RIV	Ophthalmoscope, Direct	Ophthalmology
86RIW	Ophthalmoscope, Indirect	Ophthalmology
86WTA	Ophthalmoscope, Laser	Ophthalmology
86HKL	Retinoscope, AC-Powered	Ophthalmology
86HKM	Retinoscope, Battery-Powered	Ophthalmology

OPHTHALMOTONOMETER

86HKX	Tonometer, AC-Powered	Ophthalmology
86HKY	Tonometer, Manual	Ophthalmology

OPHTHALMOTROPOMETER

86RIX	Ophthalmotropometer	Ophthalmology

OPIATES

91DJG	Enzyme Immunoassay, Opiates	Toxicology
91DKT	Free Radical Assay, Opiates	Toxicology
91DJF	Gas Chromatography, Opiates	Toxicology
91DLT	Hemagglutination, Opiates	Toxicology
91LAH	High Pressure Liquid Chromatography, Opiates	Toxicology
91LAI	Thin Layer Chromatography, Opiates	Toxicology

OPTIC

77MQW	Transilluminator, Fiber Optic	Ear/Nose/Throat

OPTICAL

81JBY	Aggregometer, Platelet, Photo-Optical Scanning	Hematology
80SHS	Component, Optical	General
80SHM	Coupler, Optical, Laparoscopic	General
86WXB	Filter, Lens	Ophthalmology
83RGV	Microscope, Laboratory, Optical	Microbiology
76LXD	Optical Caries Detection Device	Dental And Oral
89LXJ	Optical Position/Movement Recording System	Physical Med
86HQB	Photocoagulator	Ophthalmology
89LDK	Sensor, Optical Contour, Physical Medicine	Physical Med
86HPI	Vision Aid, Optical, AC-Powered	Ophthalmology
86HPE	Vision Aid, Optical, Battery-Powered	Ophthalmology

OPTICOKINETIC

86HOW	Drum, Opticokinetic	Ophthalmology

OPTOKINETIC

84RWE	Stimulator, Optokinetic	Cns/Neurology

ORAL

76EJR	Agent, Polishing, Abrasive, Oral Cavity	Dental And Oral
77MSC	Barrier, Std, Oral Sex	Ear/Nose/Throat
80KYX	Dispenser, Medication, Liquid	General
76QRK	Drill, Oral Surgery	Dental And Oral
76EHZ	Evacuator, Oral Cavity	Dental And Oral
76EFS	Irrigator, Oral	Dental And Oral
80QVN	Kit, Feeding, Pediatric (Enteral)	General
77TCR	Kit, Irrigation, Oral	Ear/Nose/Throat
77REL	Lavage Unit, Oral	Ear/Nose/Throat
73MEX	Meter, Oxygen, Oral	Anesthesiology
80LEY	Oral Administration Set	General
77RPA	Regulator, Suction, Tracheal (Nasal, Oral)	Ear/Nose/Throat
76EGN	Scissors, Surgical Tissue, Dental (Oral)	Dental And Oral
77KBW	Screw, Oral	Ear/Nose/Throat
80VLI	Swabs, Oral Care	General

ORAL-HYGIENE

76QEP	Brush, Dental Plate (Denture)	Dental And Oral
76JER	Cleaner, Denture, Mechanical	Dental And Oral
76QPA	Dentifrice	Dental And Oral
76JES	Floss, Dental	Dental And Oral
76JEW	Tip, Rubber, Oral-Hygiene	Dental And Oral
76EFW	Toothbrush, Manual	Dental And Oral
76JEQ	Toothbrush, Powered	Dental And Oral

ORANGE

80RIY	Orange Stick	General
88IDC	Stain, Acridine Orange	Pathology
88KKA	Stain, Methyl Orange	Pathology
88HZH	Stain, Orange G	Pathology

KEYWORD INDEX

OSSICULAR

77LRE	Instrument, Modification, Prosthesis, Ossicular Repl., Surg.	Ear/Nose/Throat
79FZD	Prosthesis, Ear, Internal	Surgery
77ETB	Prosthesis, Ossicular	Ear/Nose/Throat
77LBP	Prosthesis, Ossicular (Stapes), Absorbable Gelatin Material	Ear/Nose/Throat
77LBO	Prosthesis, Ossicular (Total), Absorbable Gelatin Material	Ear/Nose/Throat
77UBU	Prosthesis, Ossicular, Incus And Stapes	Ear/Nose/Throat
77LBM	Prosthesis, Ossicular, Porous Polyethylene	Ear/Nose/Throat
77ETA	Prosthesis, Ossicular, Total	Ear/Nose/Throat
77LBN	Prosthesis, Ossicular, Total, Porous Polyethylene	Ear/Nose/Throat
77UBV	Prosthesis, Ossicular, Total, Silicone	Ear/Nose/Throat
77JYB	Vise, Ossicular Finger	Ear/Nose/Throat

OSTEOARTHRITIS

80WYB	Equipment, Management, Pain, Radiofrequency, Non-Invasive	General

OSTEOGENESIS

87HTM	Stimulator, Osteogenesis, Electric, Invasive	Orthopedics
87WNT	Stimulator, Osteogenesis, Electric, Non-Invasive	Orthopedics

OSTEOINDUCTION

89MBS	Filler, Bone Void, Non-Osteoinduction	Physical Med
89MBP	Filler, Bone Void, Osteoinduction	Physical Med

OSTEOPHILIC

87MBL	Prosthesis, Hip, Semi-, Uncemented, Osteophilic Finish	Orthopedics
87MAY	Prosthesis, Hip, Semi-constrained, Metal/Ceramic/Polymer, Cemented or Non-porous Cemented, Osteophilic Finish	Orthopedics
87MBA	Prosthesis, Knee, Patfem., Semi-Const., Unc., P/M/P, Osteo.	Orthopedics

OSTEOPOROSIS

90WRK	Densitometer, Bone, Dual Photon	Radiology
90KGI	Densitometer, Bone, Single Photon	Radiology
90WIR	Densitometer, Radiography, Digital, Quantitative	Radiology

OSTEOTOME

79KDG	Chisel (Osteotome)	Surgery
76EMM	Chisel, Osteotome, Surgical	Dental And Oral
79HWM	Osteotome (Orthopedic)	Surgery
79GFI	Osteotome, Manual (Plastic Surgery)	Surgery
79RJE	Osteotome, Other	Surgery
76EGR	Osteotome, Roto With Blade	Dental And Oral

OSTIA

79KPK	Marker, Ostia, Aorto-Saphenous Vein	Surgery

OSTOMY

80FON	Bag, Drainage, Ostomy (With Adhesive)	General
78EZR	Cement, Stomal Appliance, Ostomy	Gastro/Urology
78EXB	Collector, Ostomy	Gastro/Urology
78EZS	Colostomy Appliance, Disposable	Gastro/Urology
78EXD	Irrigator, Ostomy	Gastro/Urology
78RJF	Ostomy Appliance (Ileostomy, Colostomy)	Gastro/Urology
78WHR	Plug, Ostomy	Gastro/Urology
78EZQ	Pouch, Colostomy	Gastro/Urology
78EXE	Protector, Ostomy	Gastro/Urology
78EZP	Rod, Colostomy	Gastro/Urology
78EXA	Selector, Size, Ostomy	Gastro/Urology
78VKQ	Solution, Ostomy, Odor Control	Gastro/Urology

OTC

76EBM	Adhesive, Denture, OTC	Dental And Oral
75MPQ	Container, Specimen, Urine, Drugs Of Abuse, Over The Counter	Chemistry
76EHS	Cushion, Denture, OTC	Dental And Oral
76EBO	Kit, Denture Repair, OTC	Dental And Oral
91MVO	Kit, Test, Multiple, Drugs Of Abuse, Over The Counter	Toxicology
75NAQ	Lipoprotein, High Density, HDL, Over-The-Counter	Chemistry
76EHR	Pad, Denture, OTC	Dental And Oral
76EBP	Reliner, Denture, OTC	Dental And Oral
75NBW	System, Test, Blood Glucose, Over-The-Counter	Chemistry

OTHER

80WQZ	Antibody, Other	General
82WNJ	Antigen, Antiserum, Control, Other	Immunology
83LSH	Antigen, Blastomyces Dermatitidis, Other	Microbiology
83LSJ	Antigen, Rubella, Other	Microbiology
83LSI	Antiserum, Blastomyces Dermatitidis, Other	Microbiology
80QBI	Applicator, Other	General
80QCO	Bandage, Other	General
80WVO	Brush, Other	General
79QEY	Burr, Other	Surgery
80QFL	Cabinet, Other	General
80WKP	Camera, Other	General
80QGI	Cannula, Other	General
74QGM	Cardiac Output Unit, Other	Cardiovascular
80QGW	Cart, Other	General
78QIV	Catheter, Other	Gastro/Urology

OTHER (cont'd)

80QJO	Chair, Other	General
79QJV	Chisel, Other	Surgery
79QKR	Clamp, Other	Surgery
79QLK	Clip, Other	Surgery
80WSY	Closure, Other	General
80WOS	Component, Metal, Other	General
80WXA	Component, Other	General
80QMM	Controller, Temperature, Other	General
80WHO	Cover, Other	General
80QOD	Cushion, Other	General
79QPW	Dilator, Other	Surgery
80WJO	Dispenser, Other	General
80FRO	Dressing, Other	General
84GWH	Dynamometer, Other	Cns/Neurology
80WWD	Elastomer, Other	General
80QTI	Electrode, Other	General
80WPK	Electrolysis Equipment, Other	General
80QTZ	Elevator, Other	General
75VKK	Enzyme Immunoassay, Other	Chemistry
83LSE	Epstein-Barr Virus, Other	Microbiology
73QUO	Ergometer, Other	Anesthesiology
89QVE	Exerciser, Other	Physical Med
80QWJ	Fitting, Other	General
74WSR	Flowmeter, Blood, Other	Cardiovascular
80QYK	Glove, Other	General
80QYQ	Gown, Other	General
79RHW	Holder, Needle, Other	Surgery
79RAT	Hook, Other	Surgery
91WQE	Immunoassay, Other	Toxicology
79RCH	Insufflator, Other	Surgery
73QAZ	Kit, Anesthesia, Other	Anesthesiology
79RDS	Knife, Other	Surgery
80REF	Lamp, Other	General
86HQD	Lens, Contact (Other Material)	Ophthalmology
86REV	Lens, Other	Ophthalmology
80RFG	Light, Other	General
79RFS	Mallet, Other	Surgery
80RGD	Mask, Other	General
80FQG	Mask, Oxygen, Other	General
74QZO	Monitor, Heart Rate, Other	Cardiovascular
80RIL	Needle, Other	General
89RJB	Orthosis, Other	Physical Med
79RJE	Osteotome, Other	Surgery
79RKI	Perforator, Other	Surgery
80WTJ	Polymer, Synthetic, Other	General
80RMK	Probe, Other	General
87RMV	Prosthesis, Joint, Other	Orthopedics
79RNO	Punch, Other	Surgery
75VKJ	Radioimmunoassay, Other	Chemistry
75JMD	Radioimmunoassay, Total Estrogen, Other	Chemistry
79ROI	Rasp, Other	Surgery
80WPW	Reagent, Other	General
88UJH	Reagent, Virus, General	Pathology
80WWC	Resin, Other	General
79RZZ	Retractor, Laparoscopy, Other	Surgery
79RPY	Retractor, Other	Surgery
83LSQ	Rickettsia Serological Reagents, Other	Microbiology
79RQE	Rongeur, Other	Surgery
83LSD	Rubella, Other Assays	Microbiology
79RQO	Saw, Other	Surgery
90RQZ	Scanner, Ultrasonic, Other	Radiology
79RTZ	Snare, Other	Surgery
79RUH	Spatula, Other	Surgery
80RUS	Speculum, Other	General
87RVC	Splint, Other	Orthopedics
80RVL	Sponge, Other	General
79RVQ	Spreader, Other	Surgery
88WRC	Stain, Other	Pathology
85UAN	Stent, Other	Obstetrics/Gyn
80WIG	Stretcher, Emergency, Other	General
79RWU	Stripper, Other	Surgery
79RYF	Suture, Other	Surgery
80WVE	Syringe, Other	General
80RZB	Table, Other	General
79RZQ	Tenaculum, Other (Forceps)	Surgery
81VIA	Test, Cancer Detection, Other	Hematology
83WNY	Test, DNA-Probe, Other	Microbiology
87SBQ	Traction Unit, Static, Other	Orthopedics
80SBT	Training Manikin, Other	General
86ETJ	Transilluminator, AC-Powered, Other	Ophthalmology
80WNH	Tray, Custom/Special Procedure	General
80SCH	Trocar, Other	General
80WWE	Tubing, Other	General
75UJD	Valve, Other	Chemistry
73SEX	Ventilator, Other	Anesthesiology
80WWJ	Vial, Other	General

OXYGEN (cont'd)

73LKE	Monitor, Oxygen, Conjunctival	Anesthesiology
73LPP	Monitor, Oxygen, Cutan. (Not for Infant or Under Gas Anest.)	Anesthesiology
73KLK	Monitor, Oxygen, Cutaneous	Anesthesiology
73ULV	Monitor, Transcutaneous, Oxygen	Anesthesiology
74DPZ	Oximeter, Ear	Cardiovascular
74DQA	Oximeter, Intracardiac	Cardiovascular
80WOR	Oximeter, Pulse	General
73WVK	Oxygen	Anesthesiology
73ROO	Recorder, Long-Term, Oxygen	Anesthesiology
73QWO	Regulator, Intake, Oxygen	Anesthesiology
80FQE	Regulator, Oxygen, Mechanical	General
76DZX	Resuscitator, Emergency Oxygen	Dental And Oral
73RSA	Sensor, Oxygen	Anesthesiology
79RTQ	Sleeve, Topical Oxygen Therapy	Surgery
80RZS	Tent, Mist	General
73BYL	Tent, Oxygen (Canopy)	Anesthesiology
73BYK	Tent, Oxygen, Electric	Anesthesiology
80VHQ	Tubing, Oxygen Connecting	General
75JHC	Uricase (Oxygen Rate), Uric Acid	Chemistry

OXYGEN-UPTAKE

73BZL	Computer, Oxygen-Uptake	Anesthesiology

OXYGENATOR

74DTZ	Oxygenator, Cardiopulmonary Bypass	Cardiovascular
73RJP	Oxygenator, Extracorporeal Perfusion	Anesthesiology
73MEV	Oxygenator, Intravascular	Anesthesiology
79UAA	Oxygenator, Organ Preservation	Surgery
73RJQ	Oxygenator, Regional Perfusion	Anesthesiology

OXYHEMOGLOBIN

73VCC	Analyzer, Blood Oxyhemoglobin Concentration	Anesthesiology
74JEE	Analyzer, Concentration, Oxyhemoglobin, BP, Transcutaneous	Cardiovascular
91JFD	Analyzer, Concentration, Oxyhemoglobin, Blood Phase	Toxicology
73JED	Analyzer, Oxyhemoglobin Concentration, Blood Phase, Indwell.	Anesthesiology
81GGZ	Oxyhemoglobin	Hematology
91JKS	Oxyhemoglobin/Carboxyhemoglobin Curve, Carbon-Monoxide	Toxicology

OXYTOCIN

85UDG	Pump, Syringe, Oxytocin	Obstetrics/Gyn

OZONE

73RJR	Generator, Ozone	Anesthesiology

P-BROMOANILINE

75JQM	P-Bromoaniline, Xylose	Chemistry

P-NITROANILINE

75CDF	Diazo, P-Nitroaniline/Vanillin, Vanilmandelic Acid	Chemistry

P-PHENYL-ENEDIAMINE

82JFQ	P-Phenyl-Enediamine/EDTA (Spectrophotometric), Ceruloplasmi	Immunology

P-TOLUENESULPHONYL-L-ARGININE

75JNN	P-Toluenesulphonyl-L-Arginine Methyl Ester (U.V.), Trypsin	Chemistry

PACEMAKER

74DTD	Adapter, Lead, Pacemaker	Cardiovascular
74DTC	Analyzer, Pacemaker Generator Function	Cardiovascular
74KRE	Analyzer, Pacemaker Generator Function, Indirect	Cardiovascular
74MPE	Auxillary Power Supply, Pacemaker, Cardiac, External Trans.	Cardiovascular
74DSW	Bag, Polymeric Mesh, Pacemaker	Cardiovascular
74DSZ	Battery, Pacemaker	Cardiovascular
74WWW	Cable, Pacemaker	Cardiovascular
74KRF	Charger, Pacemaker	Cardiovascular
74MFA	Device, Removal, Pacemaker Electrode, Percutaneous	Cardiovascular
74MIS	Electrode, Pacemaker, Esophageal	Cardiovascular
74QTD	Electrode, Pacemaker, External	Cardiovascular
74LDF	Electrode, Pacemaker, Temporary	Cardiovascular
74UCG	Electrode, Pacemaker, Transthoracic	Cardiovascular
74KFJ	Kit, Repair, Pacemaker	Cardiovascular
74UCH	Lead, Pacemaker (Catheter)	Cardiovascular
74QIG	Lead, Pacemaker, Implantable Endocardial	Cardiovascular
74DTB	Lead, Pacemaker, Implantable Myocardial	Cardiovascular
74UCI	Lead, Pacemaker, Temporary Endocardial	Cardiovascular
74WQA	Lead, Pacemaker, Temporary Myocardial	Cardiovascular
74DTG	Magnet, Test, Pacemaker	Cardiovascular
78EZT	Pacemaker, Bladder	Gastro/Urology
74DRO	Pacemaker, Cardiac, External Transcutaneous (Non-Invasive)	Cardiovascular
74DTE	Pacemaker, Heart, External	Cardiovascular
74JOQ	Pacemaker, Heart, External, Programmable	Cardiovascular
74UMI	Pacemaker, Heart, Implantable, Anti-Tachycardia	Cardiovascular
74ULJ	Pacemaker, Heart, Implantable, Dual Chamber	Cardiovascular

PACEMAKER (cont'd)

74VHM	Pacemaker, Heart, Implantable, Non-Programmable	Cardiovascular
74DXY	Pacemaker, Heart, Implantable, Programmable	Cardiovascular
74WST	Pacemaker, Heart, Implantable, Rate Responsive	Cardiovascular
79RJT	Pacemaker, Respiratory	Surgery
74WWX	Pacemaker, Temporary	Cardiovascular
74KRG	Programmer, Pacemaker	Cardiovascular
84GZE	Stimulator, Diaphragmatic/Phrenic Nerve, Implantable	Cns/Neurology
78EZW	Stimulator, Electrical, For Incontinence	Gastro/Urology
78UAE	Stimulator, Urinary	Gastro/Urology
74DTA	Tester, Pacemaker Electrode Function	Cardiovascular
74DTF	Tools, Pacemaker Service	Cardiovascular
74QRZ	Transmitter/Receiver System, ECG, Telephone Single-Channel	Cardiovascular

PACER

84CCP	Pacer, Electrophrenic	Cns/Neurology

PACHOMETER

79VDT	Pachometer	Surgery
86WQL	Pachometer	Ophthalmology

PACIFIER

80WRP	Pacifier	General

PACING

74MGD	Catheter, Pacing, Esophageal	Cardiovascular
74LPD	System, Pacing, Anti-Tachycardia	Cardiovascular
74LPA	System, Pacing, Esophageal	Cardiovascular
74MTE	System, Pacing, Temporary, Acute, Internal Atrial Defibrillation	Cardiovascular

PACK

89VFJ	Heater, Hot Pack	Physical Med
88RSZ	Kit, Shroud	Pathology
80KYQ	Kit, Snake Bite, Chemical Cold Pack	General
89RHK	Moist Therapy Pack	Physical Med
89RHJ	Moist Therapy Pack Conditioner	Physical Med
80QLO	Pack, Cold	General
80FRS	Pack, Cold, Chemical	General
80WXF	Pack, Custom/Special Procedure	General
89IMD	Pack, Hot Or Cold, Disposable	Physical Med
89IME	Pack, Hot Or Cold, Reusable	Physical Med
89ILO	Pack, Hot Or Cold, Water Circulating	Physical Med
80FRY	Pack, Hot, Chemical	General
89IMA	Pack, Moist Heat	Physical Med
79KCT	Pack, Sterilization Wrapper (Bag And Accessories)	Surgery
79RXP	Pack, Surgical (Drape)	Surgery
85HDM	Packer, Uterine	Obstetrics/Gyn
79RXO	Packing, Surgical	Surgery
89UEC	Support, Hot/Cold Pack	Physical Med
80WNH	Tray, Custom/Special Procedure	General
89MPO	Warmer, Heel, Infant	Physical Med

PACKAGE

88KDT	Container, Specimen Mailer And Storage	Pathology
88KDW	Container, Specimen Mailer And Storage, Temperature Control	Pathology

PACKAGING

80WNK	Bag, Plastic	General
80WVW	Contract Assembly	General
80VAO	Contract Packaging	General
80WYN	Equipment, Filtering, Air, ETO	General
80WVT	Foam, Plastic	General
81KSD	Heat-Sealing Device	Hematology
79KCT	Pack, Sterilization Wrapper (Bag And Accessories)	Surgery
80VAG	Packaging Equipment	General
80VAI	Packaging Material	General
80VDO	Packaging System, Unit-Dose	General
80RVT	Packaging, Sterilization	General
80TDK	Sealer, Packaging	General

PACKER

80RJU	Packer, Gauze	General
85HDM	Packer, Uterine	Obstetrics/Gyn

PACKING

85HDM	Packer, Uterine	Obstetrics/Gyn
79RXO	Packing, Surgical	Surgery

PACS

90UMF	Radiographic Picture Archiving/Communication System (PACS)	Radiology

PAD

80VFA	Cover, Bedrail	General
80QOD	Cushion, Other	General
80QOC	Cushion, Stool	General
89IMP	Cushion, Wheelchair (Pad)	Physical Med
78WLL	Device, Incontinence, Fecal	Gastro/Urology

PAD *(cont'd)*

80WKJ	Dressing, Gel	General
80WKL	Dressing, Permeable, Moisture	General
79JOS	Electrode, Electrosurgical, Return (Ground, Dispersive)	Surgery
89IKS	Electrode, Metallic With Soft Pad Covering	Physical Med
80LKB	Pad, Alcohol	General
85QEJ	Pad, Breast	Obstetrics/Gyn
79WUZ	Pad, Clamp	Surgery
74QOQ	Pad, Defibrillator Paddle	Cardiovascular
76EHR	Pad, Denture, OTC	Dental And Oral
80QQS	Pad, Dressing	General
74WWU	Pad, Electrode	Cardiovascular
86HMP	Pad, Eye	Ophthalmology
80WXM	Pad, Forceps, Surgical	General
89UED	Pad, Heating, Chemical	Physical Med
80QZS	Pad, Heating, Circulating Fluid	General
89FPG	Pad, Heating, Electrical	Physical Med
89IRT	Pad, Heating, Powered	Physical Med
80RBU	Pad, Incontinence (Underpad)	General
80WRF	Pad, Insulation, Cardiac	General
80FNW	Pad, Kelly	General
80RGM	Pad, Medicated	General
80MLX	Pad, Medicated, Adhesive, Non-Electric	General
85HHL	Pad, Menstrual, Scented	Obstetrics/Gyn
85HHD	Pad, Menstrual, Unscented	Obstetrics/Gyn
80FOK	Pad, Neonatal Eye	General
84RKG	Pad, Percussion	Cns/Neurology
80RLZ	Pad, Pressure, Air	General
80RMA	Pad, Pressure, Animal Skin	General
80RMB	Pad, Pressure, Foam (Elbow, Heel)	General
80RMC	Pad, Pressure, Foam Convoluted	General
80RMD	Pad, Pressure, Gel	General
80WMD	Pad, Pressure, Gel, Operating Table	General
80RME	Pad, Pressure, Soft Rubber	General
80RMF	Pad, Pressure, Water Cushion	General
80SEJ	Pad, Vacuum Stabilized	General
80WKI	Padding, Cast/Splint	General
80UCU	Pressure Pad, Alternating, Disposable	General
80UCV	Pressure Pad, Alternating, Reusable	General
80FMP	Protector, Skin Pressure	General
80UBG	Pump, Alternating Pressure Pad	General
86HOY	Shield, Eye, Ophthalmic	Ophthalmology
87RVA	Splint, Vacuum	Orthopedics
89INP	Tips And Pads, Cane, Crutch And Walker	Physical Med
89WWS	Unit, Pad, Heating, Portable	Physical Med

PADDED

79WRZ	Retractor, Abdominal, Padded, Flexible	Surgery
87RUY	Splint, Padded Stays	Orthopedics

PADDIE

84HBA	Paddie, Cottonoid	Cns/Neurology

PADDING

80WKI	Padding, Cast/Splint	General

PADDLE

74QOQ	Pad, Defibrillator Paddle	Cardiovascular

PADS

89ILA	Mattress, Alternating Pressure (Or Pads)	Physical Med

PAGE

80TFY	Page Turner (Handicapped)	General

PAGER

80TDN	Pager, Non-Radio	General
80TDM	Pager, Radio	General
80VDJ	Pager, Visual	General

PAIN

73BXL	Algesimeter, Manual	Anesthesiology
73BSI	Algesimeter, Powered	Anesthesiology
84GWT	Chronaximeter	Cns/Neurology
76MZW	Dental Cement w/out Zinc-Oxide Eugenol as an Ulcer Covering for Pain Relief	Dental And Oral
84WHU	Electrode, TENS	Cns/Neurology
80WYB	Equipment, Management, Pain, Radiofrequency, Non-Invasive	General
84LLP	Laser, Therapy, Pain	Cns/Neurology
73RJV	Pain Gauge, Transcutaneous	Anesthesiology
84LGW	Stimulator, Cerebellar, Full Implant (Pain Relief)	Cns/Neurology
84MHF	Stimulator, Cortical, Implanted (Pain Relief)	Cns/Neurology
84UFF	Stimulator, Electro-Analgesic	Cns/Neurology
84MFP	Stimulator, Nerve, Cranial, Implanted (Pain Relief)	Cns/Neurology
84GZJ	Stimulator, Nerve, Transcutaneous (Pain Relief, TENS)	Cns/Neurology
84GZF	Stimulator, Peripheral Nerve, Implantable (Pain Relief)	Cns/Neurology
84GZB	Stimulator, Spinal Cord, Implantable (Pain Relief)	Cns/Neurology

PALATE

77UCZ	Obturator, Cleft Palate	Ear/Nose/Throat

PALLIDUM

83WJQ	Antibody, Treponema Pallidum	Microbiology
83GMT	Antigen, HA, Treponema Pallidum	Microbiology
83JWL	Antigen, Treponema Pallidum For FTA-ABS Test	Microbiology
83LIP	Enzyme Linked Immunoabsorbent Assay, Treponema Pallidum	Microbiology

PAN

80FOB	Bedpan	General
80QDC	Bedpan, Fracture	General

PANCREAS

88ICI	Chrome Alum Hematoxylin	Pathology

PANCREATIC

75VIJ	Test, Pancreatic Insufficiency	Chemistry

PANCREATOSCOPE

78FTK	Pancreatoscope, Biliary	Gastro/Urology

PANEL

90IWX	Barrier, Control Panel, X-Ray, Moveable	Radiology
81UJR	Identification Panel, Blood Cell	Hematology
83LQM	Panel, Identification, Gram Negative	Microbiology
83LQL	Panel, Identification, Gram Positive	Microbiology
88MHQ	Panel, Tumor, Undifferentiated	Pathology

PANEL/DIGITAL

90MQB	Imager, X-Ray, Solid State (Flat Panel/Digital)	Radiology

PANELS

83LTT	Susceptibility Test Panels, Antimicrobial	Microbiology

PANENDOSCOPE

78FAK	Panendoscope (Gastroduodenoscope)	Gastro/Urology
78FAL	Panendoscope (Urethroscope)	Gastro/Urology
78FDY	Panendoscope Measuring Device	Gastro/Urology

PANORAMIC

76RNY	Radiographic Unit, Diagnostic, Dental (X-Ray)	Dental And Oral

PANT

78WLL	Device, Incontinence, Fecal	Gastro/Urology
80RBV	Pant, Incontinence	General

PANTOGRAPH

76KCS	Pantograph	Dental And Oral

PANTS

74RLJ	Suit, Pneumatic Counterpressure (Anti-Shock)	Cardiovascular

PAP

85RJW	Kit, Pap Smear	Obstetrics/Gyn
88HZJ	Stain, Papanicolau	Pathology
88LIJ	Stain, Peroxidase Anti-Peroxidase Immunohistochemical	Pathology

PAPAIN

88IBF	Papain	Pathology

PAPANICOLAU

85RJW	Kit, Pap Smear	Obstetrics/Gyn
88HZJ	Stain, Papanicolau	Pathology

PAPER

76KHR	Absorber, Saliva, Paper	Dental And Oral
75QKA	Chromatography Equipment, Paper	Chemistry
75JNC	Column Or Paper Chromatography Plus Ninhydrin, Phenylalanin	Chemistry
80WSM	Component, Paper	General
80QPL	Diaper, Adult	General
80WIW	Dispenser, Tissue, Toilet	General
80WIX	Dispenser, Towel	General
75UHA	Electrophoresis Equipment, Paper	Chemistry
75QVV	Filter Paper	Chemistry
76EFK	Forceps, Articulation Paper	Dental And Oral
91DNC	Paper Strip, Salicylate	Toxicology
76EFH	Paper, Articulation	Dental And Oral
80QJP	Paper, Chart, Record, Medical	General
91DMG	Paper, Ion	Toxicology
80WMJ	Paper, Photographic	General
80WUP	Paper, Recording, Data	General
80VLR	Paper, Recording, ECG/EEG	General
76EKN	Point, Paper, Endodontic	Dental And Oral
74DSF	Recorder, Paper Chart	Cardiovascular
80RSJ	Sheeting, Examination Table	General
91DIG	Test Paper, Cholinesterase	Toxicology
80VBE	Tissue, Toilet	General
80WNF	Towel/Towelette, Paper	General
80TFM	Wallpaper, Antibacterial	General
85LNW	pH Paper, Obstetric	Obstetrics/Gyn

PAPILLOMAVIRUS
83MAQ Kit, DNA Detection, Human Papillomavirus — Microbiology

PAPILLOTOME
79RJX Papillotome — Surgery

PARACERVICAL
85HEH Kit, Anesthesia, Paracervical — Obstetrics/Gyn

PARACOAGULATION
81JBN Fibrin Monomer Paracoagulation — Hematology

PARAFFIN
89IMC Bath, Paraffin — Physical Med
88IDW Dispenser, Paraffin — Pathology
89RDN Knife, Paraffin — Physical Med
88IDT Melting Point Apparatus, Paraffin — Pathology
88IDS Melting Pot, Paraffin — Pathology
88IDR Oven, Paraffin — Pathology
88KEO Paraffin, All Formulations — Pathology

PARAFORMALDEHYDE
88KEF Paraformaldehyde — Pathology

PARAINFLUENZA
83GQS Antigen, CF (Including CF Control), Parainfluenza Virus — Microbiology
83GQR Antigen, HA (Including HA Control), Parainfluenza Virus — Microbiology
83GQT Antiserum, CF, Parainfluenza Virus 1-4 — Microbiology
83GQQ Antiserum, HAI, Parainfluenza Virus 1-4 — Microbiology
83GQP Antiserum, Neutralization, Parainfluenza Virus 1-4 — Microbiology

PARALLEL
89IOE Bars, Parallel, Exercise — Physical Med
89IRR Bars, Parallel, Powered — Physical Med
89RJY Bars, Parallel, Walking — Physical Med
78FJG Dialyzer, Parallel Flow (Hemodialysis) — Gastro/Urology

PARALLELOMETER
76EGI Parallelometer — Dental And Oral

PARAMETER
73RLA Monitor, Physiological, Acute Care — Anesthesiology

PARANASAL
77UBY Prosthesis, Paranasal — Ear/Nose/Throat

PARAPERTUSSIS
83GOT Antigen, B. Parapertussis — Microbiology
83GOW Antiserum, Agglutinating, B. Parapertussis — Microbiology
83JRW Antiserum, Fluorescent, B. Parapertussis — Microbiology

PARAPLEGIC
89LFF Aid, Control, Environmental, Controlled, Breath — Physical Med

PARAQUAT
75LTD Paraquat Assay — Chemistry

PARASITE
83LKS Analyzer, Parasite Concentration — Microbiology
83GNF Antigen, CF, T. Cruzi — Microbiology
83GND Antigen, IHA, T. Cruzi — Microbiology
83GNE Antigen, Latex Agglutination, T. Cruzi — Microbiology

PARATHYROID
75CEW Radioimmunoassay, Parathyroid Hormone — Chemistry

PARENTERAL
78TGJ Kit, Administration, Parenteral — Gastro/Urology
78TGK Solution, Nutrition, Parenteral — Gastro/Urology
80FPD Tube, Feeding — General

PARIS
87LGF Component, Cast — Orthopedics

PARKINSONIAN
84MHY Stimulator, Electrical, Implanted (Parkinsonian Tremor) — Cns/Neurology

PAROVIRUS
83MYL Assay, Enzyme Linked Immunosorbent, Parvovirus B19 Igg — Microbiology
83MYM Assay, Enzyme Linked Immunosorbent, Parvovirus B19 Igm — Microbiology

PART
87JWI Prosthesis, Wrist, 2 Part Metal-Plastic Articulation — Orthopedics
87JWJ Prosthesis, Wrist, 3 Part Metal-Plastic-Metal Articulation — Orthopedics
80WSO Pump, Industrial — General

PARTIAL
73BXZ Analyzer, Gas, Carbon-Dioxide, Partial Pressure, Blood — Anesthesiology
73BSD Analyzer, Gas, Nitrogen, Partial Pressure, Blood Phase (NI) — Anesthesiology
73CCE Analyzer, Gas, Oxygen, Partial Pr., Blood Phase, Indwelling — Anesthesiology
73CCD Analyzer, Gas, Oxygen, Partial Pressure, Blood Phase — Anesthesiology
80RFY Mask, Oxygen, Partial Rebreathing — General
79KFS Monitor, Po2, Continuous — Surgery

PARTIAL *(cont'd)*
81GGW Partial Thromboplastin Time — Hematology
81GIT Partial Thromboplastin Time, Reagent, Control — Hematology
81GFO Thromboplastin, Activated Partial — Hematology

PARTICLE
75UHB Analyzer, Particle — Chemistry
81GKL Counter, Cell Or Particle, Automated — Hematology
88LKM Counter, Urine Particle — Pathology
90LHN Radiotherapy Unit, Charged-Particle — Radiology

PARTICULATE
75UGD Filter, Membrane — Chemistry
75SFY Purification Filter, Water, Particulate — Chemistry
79UMK Remover, Particulate — Surgery
80WWH Sampler, Particulate — General

PARTITION
80RRU Screen, Bedside — General

PARTS
90TEK Scanner, Ultrasonic, Small Parts — Radiology
80WTD Service, Parts, Repair — General

PAS
88HZK Stain, Periodic Acid Schiff (PAS) — Pathology

PASS
80QFH Cabinet, Pass Through — General
78QZZ Converter, Unit, Hemodialysis, Single-Pass — Gastro/Urology
78FIJ Dialysate Delivery System, Recirculating, Single Pass — Gastro/Urology
78FIL Dialysate Delivery System, Single Pass — Gastro/Urology

PASSER
87HWQ Passer — Orthopedics
87HXI Passer, Wire, Orthopedic — Orthopedics

PASSING
84HCF Instrument, Passing, Ligature, Knot Tying — Cns/Neurology
79QSH Instrument, Passing, Suture, Laparoscopic — Surgery

PASSIVE
89ISC Exerciser, Passive, Measuring — Physical Med
89IOO Exerciser, Passive, Non-Measuring (CPM Machine) — Physical Med
87HXA Prosthesis, Tendon, Passive — Orthopedics

PASTE
76LTG Paste, Injectable, Augmentation, Chord, Vocal — Dental And Oral

PASTE-ON
78EXI Device, Incontinence, Paste-On — Gastro/Urology

PASTEUR
81GJW Pipette, Pasteur — Hematology

PASTEURIZATION
80QQA Disinfector, Pasteurization — General
80LDS Hot Water Pasteurization Device — General

PATCH
91MHP Monitor, Patch, Sudromed, Drug Abuse — Toxicology
86UET Patch, Eye — Ophthalmology
74UJO Patch, Myocardial — Cardiovascular
74MFX Patch, Pericardial — Cardiovascular
80WOL Patch, Transdermal — General
74DXZ Pledget And Intracardiac Patch, PETP, PTFE, Polypropylene — Cardiovascular
74DSX Pledget, Dacron, Teflon, Polypropylene — Cardiovascular
86HOY Shield, Eye, Ophthalmic — Ophthalmology
80SGR System, Delivery, Drug, Unit-Dose — General

PATELLAR
87HTG Prosthesis, Knee, Hemi-, Patellar Resurfacing, Uncemented — Orthopedics
87UCD Prosthesis, Knee, Patellar — Orthopedics

PATELLOFEMORAL
87KRR Prosthesis, Knee, Patellofemoral, Semi-Constrained — Orthopedics

PATELLOFEMOROTIBIAL
87MBD Prosthesis, Knee, P/F, Unconst., Uncem., Por., Ctd., P/M/P — Orthopedics
87KRP Prosthesis, Knee, Patellofemorotibial, Constrained, Metal — Orthopedics
87KRQ Prosthesis, Knee, Patellofemorotibial, Constrained, Polymer — Orthopedics
87JWH Prosthesis, Knee, Patellofemorotibial, Semi-Constrained — Orthopedics
87MBV Prosthesis, Knee, Patfem., S-C., UHMWPE, Pegged, Unc., P/M/P — Orthopedics
87MBH Prosthesis, Knee, Patfem., S-C., Unc., Por., Ctd., P/M/P — Orthopedics
87MBA Prosthesis, Knee, Patfem., Semi-Const., Unc., P/M/P, Osteo. — Orthopedics
87LXY Prosthesis, Knee, Patfemotib., Semi-Const., P/M/P, Uncem. — Orthopedics

KEYWORD INDEX

PENILE
78FHA Clamp, Penile — Gastro/Urology
78LIL Monitor, Penile Tumescence — Gastro/Urology
78FAE Prosthesis, Penile — Gastro/Urology

PENIS
78QLG Clip, Penis — Gastro/Urology
79JCW Prosthesis, Penis, Inflatable — Surgery
79FTQ Prosthesis, Penis, Rigid Rod — Surgery
78LKY Prosthesis, Penis, Rigid Rod, External — Gastro/Urology

PENLIGHT
80KYT Light, Examination, Battery-Powered — General
86HJP Penlight, Battery-Powered — Ophthalmology

PENROSE
78QQL Drain, Penrose — Gastro/Urology

PEPTIDE
75UHY Analyzer, Peptide & Protein Sequence — Chemistry
75WJI Synthesizer, DNA — Chemistry
75UIP Synthesizer, Peptide & Protein — Chemistry

PEPTIDES
75UHC Peptides — Chemistry
75JKD Radioimmunoassay, C Peptides Of Proinsulin — Chemistry

PERCHA
76EKM Gutta Percha — Dental And Oral

PERCUSSION
84QZG Hammer, Percussion — Cns/Neurology
84RKG Pad, Percussion — Cns/Neurology

PERCUSSOR
84GWZ Percussor — Cns/Neurology
73BYI Percussor, Powered — Anesthesiology
89IRO Vibrator, Therapeutic — Physical Med

PERCUTANEOUS
74LOX Catheter, Angioplasty, Coronary, Transluminal, Percut. Oper. — Cardiovascular
80LNY Catheter, Intraspinal, Percutaneous, Long-Term — General
80MAJ Catheter, Intraspinal, Percutaneous, Short-Term — General
80LJS Catheter, Intravascular, Therapeutic, Long-term Greater Than 30 Days — General
74DQY Catheter, Percutaneous — Cardiovascular
74MAD Catheter, Percutaneous (Valvuloplasty) — Cardiovascular
79MJG Device, Biopsy, Percutaneous — Surgery
74MFA Device, Removal, Pacemaker Electrode, Percutaneous — Cardiovascular
74MMX Device, Retrieval, Percutaneous — Cardiovascular
74DRE Dilator, Vessel, Percutaneous Catheterization — Cardiovascular
74LPB Electrode, Ablation, Tissue, Conduction, Percutaneous — Cardiovascular
77MKE Hearing-Aid, Bone-Conduction, Percutaneous — Ear/Nose/Throat
78SJD Kit, Gastrostomy, Endoscopic, Percutaneous — Gastro/Urology
78FFK Lithotriptor, Electro-Hydraulic, Percutaneous — Gastro/Urology
74WTW Syringe, Angioplasty — Cardiovascular

PERFORATOR
85HGE Amniotome — Obstetrics/Gyn
84QRL Drill, Perforator — Cns/Neurology
85RKH Perforator, Amniotic Membrane — Obstetrics/Gyn
77KAT Perforator, Antrum — Ear/Nose/Throat
77QRT Perforator, Ear — Ear/Nose/Throat
77JYS Perforator, Ear-Lobe — Ear/Nose/Throat
79RKI Perforator, Other — Surgery

PERFORMANCE
91MAS Chromatography, Liquid, Performance, High — Toxicology
75MGS High Performance Liquid Chromatography, Cyclosporine — Chemistry
84LQD Recorder, Attention Task Performance — Cns/Neurology

PERFUSION
74QHR Catheter, Coronary Perfusion — Cardiovascular
74QIH Catheter, Perfusion — Cardiovascular
74QZM Heart-Lung Bypass Unit (Cardiopulmonary) — Cardiovascular
79QZP Heat Exchanger, Extracorporeal Perfusion — Surgery
79QZR Heat Exchanger, Regional Perfusion — Surgery
81RAC Hemoperfusion System (Hemodetoxifier) — Hematology
78KDL Kit, Perfusion, Kidney, Disposable — Gastro/Urology
78RIZ Organ Preservation System — Gastro/Urology
73RJP Oxygenator, Extracorporeal Perfusion — Anesthesiology
73RJQ Oxygenator, Regional Perfusion — Anesthesiology
88KJH Perfusion Apparatus — Pathology
78KDN Perfusion System, Kidney — Gastro/Urology
80FSB Perfusion Unit — General
74RNE Pump, Extracorporeal Perfusion — Cardiovascular

PERICARDIAL
74MFX Patch, Pericardial — Cardiovascular

PERICARDIUM
74QII Catheter, Pericardium Drainage — Cardiovascular

PERIDURAL
89MLQ Inhibitor, Peridural Fibrosis (Adhesion Barrier) — Physical Med

PERIMETER
86HOO Perimeter, AC-Powered — Ophthalmology
86HPT Perimeter, Automatic, AC-Powered — Ophthalmology
86HON Perimeter, Manual — Ophthalmology

PERINATAL
85HGM Monitor, Perinatal — Obstetrics/Gyn

PERINEAL
80FQK Binder, Perineal — General
85KND Heater, Perineal — Obstetrics/Gyn
85HGZ Heater, Perineal, Direct Contact — Obstetrics/Gyn
85HHA Heater, Perineal, Radiant, Non-Contact — Obstetrics/Gyn
78RCX Irrigator, Perineal — Gastro/Urology
78RCU Kit, Irrigation, Perineal — Gastro/Urology
80REA Lamp, Perineal Heat — General

PERINEOMETER
85HIR Perineometer — Obstetrics/Gyn

PERIODATE
88KKR Potassium Periodate — Pathology
88KKQ Sodium Periodate — Pathology

PERIODIC
88KKS Periodic Acid — Pathology
88HZK Stain, Periodic Acid Schiff (PAS) — Pathology
88GGI Stain, Schiff, Periodic Acid — Pathology

PERIODONTAL
76TBW Dressing, Periodontal — Dental And Oral
76MCL Kit, Test, Periodontal, In Vitro — Dental And Oral
76RKJ Periodontal Instrument — Dental And Oral
76LXX Periodontal Test Kit — Dental And Oral

PERIODONTIC
76EMS Curette, Periodontic — Dental And Oral
76WNX Dentoscope — Dental And Oral
76EMR File, Periodontic — Dental And Oral
76ELA Hand Instrument, Calculus Removal — Dental And Oral
76EMQ Hoe, Periodontic — Dental And Oral
76EMO Knife, Periodontic — Dental And Oral
76EMP Marker, Periodontic — Dental And Oral
76EIX Probe, Periodontic — Dental And Oral
76EMN Scaler, Periodontic — Dental And Oral
76EIC Syringe, Periodontic, Endodontic — Dental And Oral

PERIPHERAL
86RKK Analyzer, Peripheral Vision — Ophthalmology
86SFB Analyzer, Visual Function — Ophthalmology
74MKF Balloon, Angioplasty, Peripheral, Heated — Cardiovascular
74MJQ Catheter, Angioplasty, Peripheral, Ultrasonic — Cardiovascular
74LIT Catheter, Angioplasty, Transluminal, Peripheral — Cardiovascular
74MCW Catheter, Peripheral, Atherectomy — Cardiovascular
74QKO Clamp, Peripheral Vascular — Cardiovascular
79MBQ Device, Peripheral Electromag. Field to Aid Wound Healing — Surgery
74MKI Guidewire, Peripheral, Ablative — Cardiovascular
74LWX Laser, Angioplasty, Peripheral — Cardiovascular
79FYP Monitor, Blood Pressure, Venous, Peripheral — Surgery
84LLE Stimulator, Cord, Spinal, Implantable (Periph. Vasc. Dis.) — Cns/Neurology
73UFG Stimulator, Peripheral Nerve, Blockade Monitor — Anesthesiology
84GZF Stimulator, Peripheral Nerve, Implantable (Pain Relief) — Cns/Neurology
74WTW Syringe, Angioplasty — Cardiovascular

PERISTALTIC
80FRN Pump, Infusion — General

PERITONEAL
84UAR Catheter, Hydrocephalic, Peritoneal — Cns/Neurology
79GBW Catheter, Peritoneal — Surgery
78FKO Catheter, Peritoneal Dialysis, Single-Use — Gastro/Urology
78FJS Catheter, Peritoneal, Indwelling, Long-Term — Gastro/Urology
80LLD Catheter, Subcutaneous Peritoneal, Implanted — General
80LMQ Device, Access, Peritoneal, Subcutaneous, Implantable — General
78KPF Dialysate Delivery System, Peritoneal, Semi-Automatic — Gastro/Urology
78FKP Dialysate Delivery System, Single Patient — Gastro/Urology
78KPP Filter, Peritoneal Dialysate — Gastro/Urology
78KDJ Kit, Administration, Peritoneal Dialysis, Disposable — Gastro/Urology
78RKM Kit, Tubing, Dialysis, Peritoneal — Gastro/Urology
78RKL Peritoneal Dialysis Unit (CAPD) — Gastro/Urology
78KPM Shunt, Peritoneal — Gastro/Urology
78FKX System, Peritoneal Dialysis, Automatic — Gastro/Urology
80SDJ Tube, Transfer — General
78MLW Warmer, Dialysate, Peritoneal — Gastro/Urology

PHASE *(cont'd)*

73CBS	Analyzer, Gas, Halothane, Gaseous Phase (Anesthetic Conc.)	Anesthesiology
73BSE	Analyzer, Gas, Helium, Gaseous Phase	Anesthesiology
73JEF	Analyzer, Gas, Neon, Gaseous Phase	Anesthesiology
73CCI	Analyzer, Gas, Nitrogen, Gaseous Phase	Anesthesiology
73BSD	Analyzer, Gas, Nitrogen, Partial Pressure, Blood Phase (NI)	Anesthesiology
73CBR	Analyzer, Gas, Nitrous-Oxide, Gaseous Phase	Anesthesiology
73CCL	Analyzer, Gas, Oxygen, Gaseous Phase	Anesthesiology
73CCE	Analyzer, Gas, Oxygen, Partial Pr., Blood Phase, Indwelling	Anesthesiology
73CCD	Analyzer, Gas, Oxygen, Partial Pressure, Blood Phase	Anesthesiology
73BXA	Analyzer, Gas, Water Vapor, Gaseous Phase	Anesthesiology
73CBZ	Analyzer, Ion, Hydrogen-Ion (pH), Blood Phase, Indwelling	Anesthesiology
73CBY	Analyzer, Ion, Hydrogen-Ion pH, Blood Phase, Non-Indwelling	Anesthesiology
73JED	Analyzer, Oxyhemoglobin Concentration, Blood Phase, Indwell.	Anesthesiology
82KTL	Anti-DNA Indirect Immunofluorescent Solid Phase	Immunology
82KTM	C3-Indirect Immunofluorescent Solid Phase	Immunology
90VHL	Generator, Diagnostic X-Ray, High Voltage, 3-Phase	Radiology
90IZO	Generator, Diagnostic X-Ray, High Voltage, Single Phase	Radiology
88IBM	Microscope, Phase Contrast	Pathology
91DND	RIA, Digitoxin (125-I), Rabbit Antibody, Solid Phase Sep.	Toxicology
91DON	Radioimmunoassay, Digoxin (125-I), Rabbit, Solid Phase	Toxicology
75UIL	Stationary Liquid Phase	Chemistry

PHENCYCLIDINE

91LCM	Enzyme Immunoassay, Phencyclidine	Toxicology
91LCL	Radioimmunoassay, Phencyclidine	Toxicology
91LCK	Thin Layer Chromatography, Phencyclidine	Toxicology

PHENOBARBITAL

91DLZ	Enzyme Immunoassay, Phenobarbital	Toxicology
91LGQ	Fluorescence Polarization Immunoassay, Phenobarbital	Toxicology
91LET	Fluorescent Immunoassay, Phenobarbital	Toxicology
91DJH	Gas Chromatography, Phenobarbital	Toxicology
91DOO	Liquid Chromatography, Phenobarbital	Toxicology
91LFN	Nephelometric Inhibition Immunoassay, Phenobarbital	Toxicology
91DKP	Radioimmunoassay, Phenobarbital	Toxicology
91DIX	Thin Layer Chromatography, Phenobarbital	Toxicology
91LDA	U.V. Spectrometry, Phenobarbital	Toxicology

PHENOL

75JLK	Sodium Hydroxide/Phenol Red (Titrimetric), Gastric Acidity	Chemistry
75CHR	Titrimetric Phenol Red, Carbon-Dioxide	Chemistry

PHENOLPHTHALEIN

75KMS	Phenolphthalein Colorimetry, Carbon-Dioxide	Chemistry
75CJK	Phenolphthalein Phosphate, Alkaline Phosphatase	Chemistry

PHENOTHIAZINE

91DJQ	Reagent, Test, Phenothiazine	Toxicology

PHENYL

75CJX	Disodium Phenyl Phosphate, Acid Phosphatase	Chemistry
82JFQ	P-Phenyl-Enediamine/EDTA (Spectrophotometric), Ceruloplasmi	Immunology

PHENYLALANIN

75JNC	Column Or Paper Chromatography Plus Ninhydrin, Phenylalanin	Chemistry

PHENYLKETONES

75CES	Chromogenesis, Phenylketones (Urinary, Non-Quantitative)	Chemistry
75JGK	Ferric Chloride, Phenylketones (Urinary, Non-Quantitative)	Chemistry

PHENYLPHOSPHATE

75CJI	Disodium Phenylphosphate, Alkaline Phosphatase Or Isoenzyme	Chemistry
75CKF	Phenylphosphate, Alkaline Phosphatase Or Isoenzymes	Chemistry

PHLEBOGRAPH

74DQB	Phlebograph, Impedance	Cardiovascular

PHLEBOGRAPHY

80RIE	Needle, Hypodermic	General

PHLEBOTOMY

80WZB	Chair, Blood Drawing	General
74RKS	Kit, Blood Collection, Phlebotomy	Cardiovascular

PHLOXINE

88HZL	Stain, Phloxine B	Pathology

PHONO

85QVO	Detector, Fetal Heart, Phono	Obstetrics/Gyn

PHONOANGIOGRAPH

90RKT	Phonoangiograph	Radiology

PHONOCARDIOGRAPH

74DQC	Phonocardiograph	Cardiovascular

PHONOCARDIOGRAPHIC

85HFP	Monitor, Phonocardiographic, Fetal	Obstetrics/Gyn

PHONOCATHETER

74DXW	Phonocatheter System, Intracavitary	Cardiovascular
73BZW	Stethoscope, Esophageal	Anesthesiology

PHONOSTETHOGRAPH

74RKU	Phonostethograph	Cardiovascular

PHONOSURGERY

77MKK	Implant, Phonosurgery	Ear/Nose/Throat

PHOROPTER

75RKX	Photometer	Chemistry

PHOSPHATASE

75CJO	Alpha-Naphthyl Phosphate, Alkaline Phosphatase Or Isoenzyme	Chemistry
75CJL	Beta Glycerophosphate, Alkaline Phosphatase Or Isoenzymes	Chemistry
75CJX	Disodium Phenyl Phosphate, Acid Phosphatase	Chemistry
75CJI	Disodium Phenylphosphate, Alkaline Phosphatase Or Isoenzyme	Chemistry
75CIN	Electrophoretic Separation, Alkaline Phosphatase Isoenzymes	Chemistry
75CKH	Glycerophosphate, Beta, Phosphatase, Acid	Chemistry
75JFI	Isoenzyme, Phosphatase, Alkaline (Catalytic Method)	Chemistry
82MEO	Kit, Antigen, RIA, Prostatic Acid Phosphatase	Immunology
81GHD	Leukocyte Alkaline Phosphatase	Hematology
75CKB	Naphthyl Phosphate, Acid Phosphatase	Chemistry
75CJN	Nitrophenylphosphate, Acid Phosphatase	Chemistry
75CJE	Nitrophenylphosphate, Alkaline Phosphatase Or Isoenzymes	Chemistry
75CJK	Phenolphthalein Phosphate, Alkaline Phosphatase	Chemistry
75CKF	Phenylphosphate, Alkaline Phosphatase Or Isoenzymes	Chemistry
81JCI	Phosphatase, Acid	Hematology
81JCJ	Phosphatase, Alkaline	Hematology
75JFG	Phosphatase, Alkaline (Catalytic Method)	Chemistry
75JFH	Tartrate Inhibited, Acid Phosphatase (Prostatic)	Chemistry
75CJR	Thymol Blue Monophosphate, Acid Phosphatase	Chemistry
75CJH	Thymol Blue Monophosphate, Alkaline Phosphatase/Isoenzymes	Chemistry
75CKE	Thymolphthalein Monophosphate, Acid Phosphatase	Chemistry
75CIO	Thymolphthalein Monophosphate, Alkaline Phosphatase	Chemistry

PHOSPHATE

75CED	5-AMP-Phosphate Release (Colorimetric), 5'-Nucleotidase	Chemistry
75CJO	Alpha-Naphthyl Phosphate, Alkaline Phosphatase Or Isoenzyme	Chemistry
75CJX	Disodium Phenyl Phosphate, Acid Phosphatase	Chemistry
81JLM	Electrophoretic, Glucose-6-Phosphate Dehydrogenase	Hematology
75KQP	Fluorescent Proc. (Qual.), Galactose-1-Phosphate Uridyl	Chemistry
81JBJ	Glucose-6-Phos. Dehydrogenase (Erythrocy.), Methemogl. Red.	Hematology
81JBH	Glucose-6-Phos. Dehydrogenase (Erythrocytic), Micromethod	Hematology
81JBL	Glucose-6-Phos. Dehydrogenase (Erythrocytic), Quantitative	Hematology
81JBK	Glucose-6-Phos. Dehydrogenase (Erythrocytic), U.V. Kinetic	Hematology
75JNE	Glucose-6-Phosphate (Colorimetric), Phosphohexose Isomerase	Chemistry
81JBI	Glucose-6-Phosphate Dehydrogenase (Erythrocytic), Catalase	Hematology
81JBM	Glucose-6-Phosphate Dehydrogenase (Erythrocytic), Electro	Hematology
81JBF	Glucose-6-Phosphate Dehydrogenase (Erythrocytic), Screening	Hematology
81JBG	Glucose-6-Phosphate Dehydrogenase (Erythrocytic), Spot	Hematology
75JNY	Glyceralde-3-Phosphate, NADH (Enzymatic), Triose Phosphate	Chemistry
81JMC	NADP Reduction (U.V.), Glucose-6-Phosphate Dehydrogenase	Hematology
75CKB	Naphthyl Phosphate, Acid Phosphatase	Chemistry
75CJK	Phenolphthalein Phosphate, Alkaline Phosphatase	Chemistry
87MAZ	Prosthesis, Hip, Semi-Const., M/P, Por. Uncem., Calc./Phos.	Orthopedics
87MEH	Prosthesis, Hip, Semi-Const., Uncem., Non-P., M/P, Ca./Phos.	Orthopedics
75JFX	Reagent, Kinase, Phosphate, Creatine	Chemistry
81KQE	Test, Erythrocytic Glucose-6-Phosphate Dehydrogenase	Hematology
76LPK	Tricalcium Phosphate Granules for Dental Bone Repair	Dental And Oral
81JMB	Visual, Semi-Quant. (Colorimetric), Glucose-6-Phosphate	Hematology

PHOSPHATIDYLGLYCEROL

75WHJ	Test, Maturity, Lung, Fetal	Chemistry

PHRENIC

84GZE	Stimulator, Diaphragmatic/Phrenic Nerve, Implantable	Cns/Neurology

PHTHALALDEHYDE

75JGZ	O-Phthalaldehyde, Urea Nitrogen	Chemistry

PHYSICAL

89KNM	Applier, Pressure, Physical Medicine	Physical Med
89ILM	Bath, Sitz, Physical Medicine	Physical Med
89IKP	Chronaximeter, Physical Medicine	Physical Med
89IMI	Diathermy, Ultrasonic (Physical Therapy)	Physical Med
89IKG	Dynamometer, Physical Medicine, Electronic	Physical Med
89WPB	Equipment, Therapy, Handicapped/Physical	Physical Med
89ITH	Equipment, Traction, Powered	Physical Med
89KTB	Iontophoresis Unit, Physical Medicine	Physical Med
89IOB	Lamp, Ultraviolet, Physical Medicine	Physical Med
89LDK	Sensor, Optical Contour, Physical Medicine	Physical Med
80JOJ	Sterilization Process Indicator, Physical/Chemical	General
89ILG	Stocking, Elastic, Physical Medicine	Physical Med
89INQ	Table, Physical Medicine, Powered	Physical Med
89JFB	Table, Physical Therapy	Physical Med

PHYSICIAN

80RGJ	Bag, Medical, Physician	General
80TDQ	Physician Registry	General

PHYSIOLOGICAL

84GWL	Amplifier, Physiological Signal	Cns/Neurology
84HCC	Biofeedback Device	Cns/Neurology
89IQH	Biofeedback Equipment, Myoelectric, Battery-Powered	Physical Med
89IRC	Biofeedback Equipment, Myoelectric, Powered	Physical Med
78EXZ	Camera, Physiological, Function Monitor	Gastro/Urology
74QMG	Computer, Stress Exercise	Cardiovascular
84GWK	Conditioner, Signal, Physiological	Cns/Neurology
84MHM	Device, Diagnostic, Non-Physiological	Cns/Neurology
74BYQ	Ergometer, Treadmill	Cardiovascular
85TDR	Monitor, Neonatal, Physiological	Obstetrics/Gyn
73RLA	Monitor, Physiological, Acute Care	Anesthesiology
74RLB	Monitor, Physiological, Cardiac Catheterization	Cardiovascular
74MHX	Monitor, Physiological, Patient	Cardiovascular
74MWI	Monitor, Physiological, Patient(without Arrhythmia Detection Or Alarms)	Cardiovascular
74RLC	Monitor, Physiological, Stress Exercise	Cardiovascular
80ROP	Recorder, Long-Term, Trend	General
74MSX	System, Network And Communication, Physiological Monitors	Cardiovascular
74RZJ	Telemetry Unit, Physiological, ECG	Cardiovascular
84RZK	Telemetry Unit, Physiological, EEG	Cns/Neurology
89RZL	Telemetry Unit, Physiological, EMG	Physical Med
84RZM	Telemetry Unit, Physiological, EOG	Cns/Neurology
80TEZ	Telemetry Unit, Physiological, Multiple Channel	General
84GYE	Telemetry Unit, Physiological, Neurological	Cns/Neurology
80RZN	Telemetry Unit, Physiological, Pressure	General
80RZO	Telemetry Unit, Physiological, Temperature	General
74DRG	Transmitter/Receiver System, Physiological, Radiofrequency	Cardiovascular
74DXH	Transmitter/Receiver System, Physiological, Telephone	Cardiovascular
74MFL	Transmitter/Receiver, Physiological Signal, Infrared	Cardiovascular

PHYTOHEMAGLUTININ

88IBB	Phytohemaglutinin M	Pathology

PICK

76JET	Pick, Massaging	Dental And Oral
77JYT	Pick, Microsurgical Ear	Ear/Nose/Throat

PICRO

88HZN	Stain, Picro Methyl Blue	Pathology

PICRO-FUCHSIN

88IAD	Van Gieson's Picro-Fuchsin	Pathology

PICTURE

90UMF	Radiographic Picture Archiving/Communication System (PACS)	Radiology

PIECE

73CAI	Circuit, Breathing (W Connector, Adapter, Y Piece)	Anesthesiology
79GDX	Scalpel, One-Piece (Knife)	Surgery

PIERCER

84GXB	Esthesiometer	Cns/Neurology

PIERCING

77QRT	Perforator, Ear	Ear/Nose/Throat
77JYS	Perforator, Ear-Lobe	Ear/Nose/Throat

PIFE

77ESH	Polymer, ENT Synthetic-PIFE, Silicon Elastomer	Ear/Nose/Throat

PIG

83UMA	Animal, Laboratory	Microbiology

PILL

80WPQ	Container, Medication, Home-Use	General
80VDQ	Counter, Pill	General
80QNK	Crusher, Pill	General
80WTB	Cutter, Pill	General
90WJH	Dispenser, Radiopharmaceuticals	Radiology
80WKH	Monitor, Medication	General
80VDO	Packaging System, Unit-Dose	General
78EXW	Pill, Radio	Gastro/Urology

PILLOW

78FIW	Alarm, Pillow Pressure	Gastro/Urology
80VBF	Linen	General
80WLC	Pillow	General
80RLD	Pillow, Bath	General
87RLE	Pillow, Cervical	Orthopedics
77MYB	Pillow, Cervical(for Mild Sleep Apnea)	Ear/Nose/Throat

PIN

87HXQ	Crimper, Pin	Orthopedics
87HXZ	Cutter, Wire And Pin	Orthopedics
79GFC	Driver, Surgical, Pin	Surgery
87QRM	Driver/Extractor, Bone Nail/Pin	Orthopedics
87HTY	Pin, Fixation, Smooth	Orthopedics
87JDW	Pin, Fixation, Threaded	Orthopedics
76EBL	Pin, Retentive And Splinting	Dental And Oral
80WMU	Pin, Safety	General
80WYV	Pin, Transfer, Solution	General

PINHOLE

86HKH	Disk, Pinhole, Ophthalmic	Ophthalmology

PINWHEEL

84GWY	Pinwheel	Cns/Neurology

PIPELINE

73BXH	Gauge, Gas Pressure, Cylinder/Pipeline	Anesthesiology
80WOE	System, Pipeline, Gas	General

PIPETTE

75WVX	Dispenser, Pipette	Chemistry
75WKU	Pipette	Chemistry
75TGI	Pipette Tip	Chemistry
81GGY	Pipette, Diluting	Hematology
75JRC	Pipette, Micro	Chemistry
81GJW	Pipette, Pasteur	Hematology
81GJG	Pipette, Quantitative, Hematology	Hematology
81GGX	Pipette, Sahli	Hematology
88IHB	Pipette, Vaginal Pool Smear	Pathology
81RLF	Pipetter	Hematology
83LIE	Reagent, Inoculator Calibration (Laboratory)	Microbiology
75WKC	Stand/Holder, Equipment, Laboratory	Chemistry
75SFQ	Washer, Pipette	Chemistry
75UJA	Washer, Pipette, Ultrasonic	Chemistry

PIPETTER

81RLF	Pipetter	Hematology

PIPETTING

75JQW	Pipetting And Diluting System, Automated	Chemistry
75JRD	Station Pipetting	Chemistry

PISTON

77JXY	Jig, Piston Cutting, ENT	Ear/Nose/Throat
80FMF	Syringe, Piston	General

PIT

76EBC	Sealant, Pit And Fissure, And Conditioner, Resin	Dental And Oral

PLACENTAE

85MDH	Abruptio Placentae Catheter	Obstetrics/Gyn

PLACENTAL

85HDA	Forceps, Obstetrical	Obstetrics/Gyn
75JMF	Radioimmunoassay, Human Placental Lactogen	Chemistry
82DHT	Test, Human Placental Lactogen	Immunology

PLANCHET

75UHH	Planchet	Chemistry

PLANE

80TFU	Ambulance, Air	General

PLANNING

90ROG	Radiotherapy Treatment Planning Unit	Radiology
90MUJ	System, Planning, Radiation Therapy Treatment	Radiology

PLANOGRAPH

90IZF	Radiographic Unit, Diagnostic, Tomographic	Radiology

PLAQUE

76ELA	Hand Instrument, Calculus Removal	Dental And Oral
76EAW	Kit, Plaque Disclosing	Dental And Oral

KEYWORD INDEX

PLETHYSMOGRAPH *(cont'd)*
84JXF Plethysmograph, Ocular — Cns/Neurology
74JOM Plethysmograph, Photo-Electric, Pneumatic Or Hydraulic — Cardiovascular
73CCM Plethysmograph, Pressure (Body) — Anesthesiology
73JEH Plethysmograph, Volume — Anesthesiology

PLETHYSMOGRAPHY
79KFR Monitor, Cardiac Output, Impedance Plethysmography — Surgery

PLEURAL
74QBV Aspirator, Thoracic (Suction Unit) — Cardiovascular
74SIZ Dispenser, Thorascopic — Cardiovascular

PLEXUS
73QAU Kit, Anesthesia, Brachial Plexus — Anesthesiology

PLIERS
78FJY Pliers, Crimp — Gastro/Urology
76EJY Pliers, Operative — Dental And Oral
76JEX Pliers, Orthodontic — Dental And Oral
87HTC Pliers, Surgical — Orthopedics
78FJO Pliers, Tube — Gastro/Urology

PLINTH
89INT Plinth — Physical Med

PLOSS
73JFE Valve, Switching (Ploss) — Anesthesiology

PLOTTER
86SFA Plotter, Visual Field — Ophthalmology

PLUG
73SBI Button, Tracheostomy Tube — Anesthesiology
80WSY Closure, Other — General
80WKG Component, Electrical — General
78QHJ Plug, Catheter — Gastro/Urology
77QRU Plug, Ear — Ear/Nose/Throat
80TDS Plug, Electrical — General
78WHR Plug, Ostomy — Gastro/Urology
86LZU Plug, Punctum — Ophthalmology
87MJW Prosthesis, Subtalar Plug, Polymer — Orthopedics
87MJU Prosthesis, Subtalar Plug, Polymer (Elastomer) — Orthopedics
86LXP Scleral Plug — Ophthalmology

PLUGGER
76EKR Plugger, Root Canal, Endodontic — Dental And Oral

PLUMBING
74BTE Device, Hyperthermia (Blanket, Plumbing & Heat Exchanger) — Cardiovascular
73BTF Hypothermia Unit (Blanket, Plumbing & Heat Exchanger) — Anesthesiology

PLUNGER
89LXM Plunger-Like Joint Manipulator — Physical Med

PLUNGER-LIKE
89LXM Plunger-Like Joint Manipulator — Physical Med

PMMA
80WUG Material, Polymethylmethacrylate — General
80WTJ Polymer, Synthetic, Other — General

PNEUMATACHOGRAPH
73RLL Pneumograph — Anesthesiology

PNEUMATIC
74QLZ Compression Unit, Intermittent (Anti-Embolism Pump) — Cardiovascular
80TDT Delivery System, Pneumatic Tube — General
77ERL Drill, Surgical, ENT (Electric Or Pneumatic) — Ear/Nose/Throat
80QWJ Fitting, Other — General
87HSZ Instrument, Surgical, Powered, Pneumatic — Orthopedics
77ESB Magnifier, Aural (Pneumatic Otoscope) — Ear/Nose/Throat
84HBB Motor, Drill, Pneumatic — Cns/Neurology
79GET Motor, Surgical Instrument, Pneumatic-Powered — Surgery
89IPO Orthosis, Pneumatic Structure, Rigid — Physical Med
74JOM Plethysmograph, Photo-Electric, Pneumatic Or Hydraulic — Cardiovascular
87RQN Saw, Bone, Pneumatic — Orthopedics
77EWQ Saw, Surgical, ENT (Electric Or Pneumatic) — Ear/Nose/Throat
87RUZ Splint, Pneumatic — Orthopedics
74RWI Stocking, Anti-Embolic, Pneumatic — Cardiovascular
74RLJ Suit, Pneumatic Counterpressure (Anti-Shock) — Cardiovascular
79FWW Table, Operating Room, Pneumatic — Surgery
73RLK Tester, Pneumatic — Anesthesiology
79GAX Tourniquet, Non-Pneumatic, Surgical — Surgery
79KCY Tourniquet, Pneumatic — Surgery

PNEUMATIC-POWERED
79GET Motor, Surgical Instrument, Pneumatic-Powered — Surgery

PNEUMATICALLY
79KFK Saw, Pneumatically Powered — Surgery

PNEUMOCYSTIS
83LYF Pneumocystis Carinii — Microbiology

PNEUMOENCEPHALOGRAPHIC
90IZN Chair, Pneumoencephalographic — Radiology
84HBK Chair, Pneumoencephalographic, Neurology — Cns/Neurology
90VGJ Radiographic Unit, Diagnostic, Pneumoencephalographic — Radiology

PNEUMOGRAPH
73RBQ Monitor, Impedance Pneumograph — Anesthesiology
73RLL Pneumograph — Anesthesiology
73BZG Spirometer, Diagnostic (Respirometer) — Anesthesiology
73BZK Spirometer, Monitoring (Volumeter) — Anesthesiology

PNEUMONIAE
83GWB Antiserum, Fluorescent, Streptococcus Pneumoniae — Microbiology
83GWC Antiserum, Streptococcus Pneumoniae — Microbiology
83MCT DNA-Probe, Strep Pneumoniae — Microbiology

PNEUMONITIS
82DGW Test, Hypersensitivity Pneumonitis — Immunology

PNEUMOPERITONEUM
79QUA Cylinder, Carbon-Dioxide — Surgery
79RKN Needle, Insufflation, Laparoscopic — Surgery
78FHP Needle, Pneumoperitoneum, Simple — Gastro/Urology
78FHO Needle, Pneumoperitoneum, Spring Loaded — Gastro/Urology
78FDP Pneumoperitoneum Apparatus, Automatic — Gastro/Urology

PNEUMOPHILIA
83UML Reagent, Legionella Detection — Microbiology

PNEUMOTACHOGRAPH
73RNC Analyzer, Pulmonary Function — Anesthesiology
73RLM Pneumotachograph — Anesthesiology

PNEUMOTACHOMETER
73QFQ Calibrator, Respiratory Therapy Unit — Anesthesiology
73JAX Pneumotachometer — Anesthesiology

PO2
79KFS Monitor, Po2, Continuous — Surgery

POCKET
78FCP Box, Battery, Pocket (Endoscopic) — Gastro/Urology

PODIATRIC
87WQP Analyzer, Distribution, Weight, Podiatric — Orthopedics
87VDV Analyzer, Gait — Orthopedics
87QEX Burr, Podiatric — Orthopedics
87QJK Chair, Podiatric — Orthopedics

PODOSCOPE
87WQP Analyzer, Distribution, Weight, Podiatric — Orthopedics

POINT
84GWI Discriminator, Two-point — Cns/Neurology
84IKM Esthesiometer, Two Point Discriminator — Cns/Neurology
75JMZ Freezing Point, Osmolality — Chemistry
73BWJ Locator, Acupuncture Point — Anesthesiology
88IDT Melting Point Apparatus, Paraffin — Pathology
76EHL Point, Abrasive — Dental And Oral
76EKN Point, Paper, Endodontic — Dental And Oral
76EKL Point, Silver, Endodontic — Dental And Oral

POLARIMETER
75JQZ Polarimeter — Chemistry

POLARISCOPE
80SHO Polariscope — General

POLARIZATION
91LGJ Fluorescence Polarization Immunoassay, Amibacin — Toxicology
91LGI Fluorescence Polarization Immunoassay, Carbamazepine — Toxicology
91LGR Fluorescence Polarization Immunoassay, Diphenylhydantoin — Toxicology
91LGQ Fluorescence Polarization Immunoassay, Phenobarbital — Toxicology
91LGS Fluorescence Polarization Immunoassay, Theophylline — Toxicology
91LFW Fluorescence Polarization Immunoassay, Tobramycin — Toxicology
75MGU Fluorescence Polarization, Immunoassay, Cyclosporine — Chemistry

POLE
80TDH Attachment, Oxygen Canister/IV Pole, Wheelchair — General
80RCM Hanger, Intravenous — General
80FOX Infusion Stand — General
80WTM Weight, IV Pole — General

POLICIES
80WVL Manual, Policies — General

POLIOVIRUS
83GOH Antigen, CF (Including CF Control), Poliovirus 1-3 — Microbiology
83GOE Antisera, Fluorescent, Poliovirus 1-3 — Microbiology
83GOG Antiserum, CF, Poliovirus 1-3 — Microbiology

POLYTETRAFLUOROETHYLENE *(cont'd)*

77ESF	Polymer, ENT Composite Synthetic PTFE With Carbon-Fiber	Ear/Nose/Throat
87MBM	Prosthesis, Hip, Semi/Hemi-Const., M/PTFE Ctd./P, Cem./Unc.	Orthopedics
79KDA	Prosthesis, PTFE/Carbon-Fiber	Surgery
79WLR	Suture, Polytetrafluoroethylene	Surgery
80WTH	Tubing, Polytetrafluoroethylene	General

POLYTOMOGRAPHIC

90VGK	Radiographic Unit, Diagnostic, Polytomographic	Radiology

POLYURETHANE

80WWD	Elastomer, Other	General
80WWC	Resin, Other	General
80WWE	Tubing, Other	General
80VKF	Tubing, Urethane	General

POLYVALENT

83GTF	Antiserum, Bethesda-Ballerup Polyvalent, Citrobacter SPP.	Microbiology

POLYVINYL

86MXY	Cannula, Ophthalmic, Posterior Capsular Polishing, Polyvinyl Acetal	Ophthalmology
76KOO	Polyvinyl Methylether Maleic Acid-Calcium-Sodium Dbl. Salt	Dental And Oral
76KOT	Polyvinyl Methylether Maleic Acid/Carboxymethylcellulose	Dental And Oral
76KXY	Polyvinyl Methylether Maleic Anhydride/Carboxymethylcellul.	Dental And Oral
80SDR	Tubing, Polyvinyl Chloride	General

PONCEAU

88HZO	Stain, Ponceau	Pathology
81GFL	Stain, Ponceau, Hematology	Hematology

POOL

79WZU	Cannula, Suction, Pool-Tip	Surgery
88IHB	Pipette, Vaginal Pool Smear	Pathology

POOL-TIP

79WZU	Cannula, Suction, Pool-Tip	Surgery

POOLE

79ULE	Tip, Suction Tube (Yankauer, Poole, Etc.)	Surgery
80WNO	Tube, Suction	General

PORCELAIN

76VEJ	Furnace, Porcelain	Dental And Oral
76EIH	Powder, Porcelain	Dental And Oral
76ELL	Teeth, Porcelain	Dental And Oral

PORCINE

79KGN	Dressing, Burn, Porcine	Surgery

POROUS

87MBE	Bone, Block, Filler, Metal, Porous, Uncemented	Orthopedics
77JOF	Polymer, ENT Synthetic, Porous Polyethylene	Ear/Nose/Throat
87MBK	Prosthesis, Ankle, Semi-, Uncemented, Porous, Metal/Polymer	Orthopedics
87MAZ	Prosthesis, Hip, Semi-Const., M/P, Por. Uncem., Calc./Phos.	Orthopedics
87LPH	Prosthesis, Hip, Semi-Const., Metal/Poly., Porous Uncemented	Orthopedics
87MEH	Prosthesis, Hip, Semi-Const., Uncem., Non-P., M/P, Ca./Phos.	Orthopedics
87MAY	Prosthesis, Hip, Semi-constrained, Metal/Ceramic/Polymer, Cemented or Non-porous Cemented, Osteophilic Finish	Orthopedics
87MBD	Prosthesis, Knee, P/F, Unconst., Uncem., Por., Ctd., P/M/P	Orthopedics
87MBH	Prosthesis, Knee, Patfem., S-C., Unc., Por., Ctd., P/M/P	Orthopedics
77LBM	Prosthesis, Ossicular, Porous Polyethylene	Ear/Nose/Throat
77LBN	Prosthesis, Ossicular, Total, Porous Polyethylene	Ear/Nose/Throat
77LBL	Tube, Tympanostomy, Porous Polyethylene	Ear/Nose/Throat

PORPHOBILINOGEN

75JNF	Ion Exchange Resin, Ehrlich's Reagent, Porphobilinogen	Chemistry

PORPHYRINS

75JKJ	Fluorometric Measurement, Porphyrins	Chemistry

PORT

79SIN	Dilator, Port, Laparoscopic	Surgery
79SIA	Kit, Trocar	Surgery
80MDX	Port & Catheter, Infusion, Implanted, Subcut., Intraperit.	General
80MDV	Port & Catheter, Infusion, Implanted, Subcutaneous, Intraspinal	General
80MHC	Port, Intraosseous, Implantable	General
74THP	Port, Vascular Access	Cardiovascular
79SHV	Sleeve, Trocar	Surgery
79SID	Thread, Stability, Trocar	Surgery

PORT *(cont'd)*

78SCC	Trocar, Abdominal	Gastro/Urology
79WYQ	Trocar, Laparoscopic	Surgery
80SCH	Trocar, Other	General
79SHB	Trocar, Short	Surgery
74SCG	Trocar, Thoracic	Cardiovascular

PORTABLE

74DSM	Alarm, Leakage Current, Portable	Cardiovascular
80WVN	Base, Roller, Tank, Oxygen	General
80QCU	Bath, Portable	General
80QCZ	Bathtub, Portable	General
73BYJ	Canister, Liquid Oxygen, Portable	Anesthesiology
80WUT	Carrier, Container, Oxygen, Portable	General
80WSG	Case, Protection, Equipment	General
80TBK	Compactor, Portable	General
73BTI	Compressor, Air, Portable	Anesthesiology
73CAW	Generator, Oxygen, Portable	Anesthesiology
83RBY	Incubator, Test Tube, Portable	Microbiology
78WRW	Injector, Insulin	Gastro/Urology
75JQY	Meter, pH, Portable	Chemistry
73BTA	Pump, Aspiration, Portable	Anesthesiology
90ROB	Radiographic Unit, Diagnostic, Portable (X-Ray)	Radiology
74ROK	Recorder, Long-Term, Blood Pressure, Portable	Cardiovascular
74ROM	Recorder, Long-Term, ECG, Portable (Holter Monitor)	Cardiovascular
90TEN	Shield, X-Ray, Portable	Radiology
80UAC	Sink, Portable	General
80VLO	Stretcher, Basket, Portable	General
79GCY	Suction Apparatus, Single Patient, Portable, Non-Powered	Surgery
79JCX	Suction Apparatus, Ward Use, Portable, AC-Powered	Surgery
90IZL	System, X-Ray, Mobile	Radiology
89WWS	Unit, Pad, Heating, Portable	Physical Med
73SEX	Ventilator, Other	Anesthesiology

PORTER

75CDB	Porter Silber Hydrazone, 17-Hydroxycorticosteroids	Chemistry

PORTION

80WTB	Cutter, Pill	General

PORTOSYSTEMIC

74MIR	Shunt, Portosystemic, Endoprosthesis	Cardiovascular

POSITION

89INO	Chair, Position, Electric	Physical Med
90IWY	Holder, Head, Radiographic	Radiology
80FRP	Holder, Infant Position	General
90IWE	Monitor, Patient Position, Light Beam	Radiology
89LXJ	Optical Position/Movement Recording System	Physical Med
90SGN	Sand Bag, X-Ray	Radiology
73CCX	Support, Patient Position	Anesthesiology
90RNX	Support, Patient Position, Radiographic	Radiology

POSITIONER

87KIL	Positioner, Socket	Orthopedics
87WWB	Positioner, Spine, Surgical	Orthopedics
76KMY	Positioner, Tooth, Preformed	Dental And Oral

POSITIVE

83JWK	Antigen, Positive Control, Cryptococcus Neoformans	Microbiology
83GPE	Antisera, Positive Control, Echinococcus SPP.	Microbiology
83GSN	Antiserum, Positive And Negative Febrile Antigen Control	Microbiology
83KFG	Antiserum, Positive Control, Aspergillus SPP.	Microbiology
83KFH	Antiserum, Positive Control, Blastomyces Dermatitidis	Microbiology
83GMH	Antiserum, Positive Control, Coccidioides Immitis	Microbiology
83GMK	Antiserum, Positive Control, Histoplasma Capsulatum	Microbiology
73BYE	Attachment, Breathing, Positive End Expiratory Pressure	Anesthesiology
73CAT	Cannula, Nasal, Oxygen	Anesthesiology
73QMH	Continuous Positive Airway Pressure Unit (CPAP, CPPB)	Anesthesiology
83MJZ	Kit, Direct Antigen, Positive Control	Microbiology
83MJX	Kit, Serological, Positive Control	Microbiology
83LQL	Panel, Identification, Gram Positive	Microbiology
81LIM	Test, D Positive Fetal Rbc	Hematology
73SEO	Valve, Positive End Expiratory Pressure (PEEP)	Anesthesiology
73SEU	Ventilator, Pressure Cycled (IPPB Machine)	Anesthesiology

POSITRON

90IZC	Camera, Positron	Radiology
90ULI	Scanner, Positron Emission Tomography (PET)	Radiology

POST

76ELR	Post, Root Canal	Dental And Oral
89ISM	Pylon, Post Surgical	Physical Med
84LXL	Valve, Shunt, Fluid, CNS (Post-Amendment Design)	Cns/Neurology

POST-AMENDMENT

84LXL	Valve, Shunt, Fluid, CNS (Post-Amendment Design)	Cns/Neurology

POSTERIOR

86MXY	Cannula, Ophthalmic, Posterior Capsular Polishing, Polyvinyl Acetal	Ophthalmology

POSTERIOR *(cont'd)*
86LOI Laser, Neodymium:YAG (Excl. Post. Capstmy./Pupilloplasty) Ophthalmology
86LXS Laser, Neodymium:YAG, Ophthalmic (Post. Capsulotomy) Ophthalmology
86UBD Lens, Intraocular, Posterior Chamber Ophthalmology
76ELJ Teeth, Artificial, Posterior With Metal Insert Dental And Oral

POSTOPERATIVE
89MNY Inhibitor, Post-Op Fibro., Carp. Tun. Syn.(Adhesion Barrier) Physical Med
89MNX Inhibitor, Post-Op Fibrosis, Tenolysis (Adhesion Barrier) Physical Med

POSTURE
80WWG Analyzer, Motion General
78EXP Belt, Abdominal Gastro/Urology
73BYN Chair, Posture, For Cardiac And Pulmonary Treatment Anesthesiology
87QJR Chart, Posture Orthopedics
87WRR Equipment, Screening, Scoliosis Orthopedics
89RHD Mirror, Posture Physical Med

POT
88IDS Melting Pot, Paraffin Pathology

POTASSIUM
75QTJ Analyzer, Chemistry, Electrolyte Chemistry
80LJI Electrode, In Vivo Potassium Ion Selective General
75CEM Electrode, Ion Specific, Potassium Chemistry
73TAM Monitor, Blood Potassium Anesthesiology
75JGM Photometer, Flame, Potassium Chemistry
91DMI Potassium Dichromate Specific Reagent For Alcohol Toxicology
91DOJ Potassium Dichromate, Alcohol Toxicology
88KKR Potassium Periodate Pathology
75CEJ Tetraphenyl Borate, Colorimetry, Potassium Chemistry

POTENTIAL
84VKG Computer, Brain Mapping Cns/Neurology
84HCJ Device, Measurement, Potential, Skin Cns/Neurology
84VDA Evoked Potential Unit, Audiometric Cns/Neurology
77ETZ Evoked Response Unit, Auditory Ear/Nose/Throat
84RWB Stimulator, Audio Cns/Neurology
84UFJ Stimulator, Somatosensory Cns/Neurology
84RWF Stimulator, Visual Cns/Neurology
77EWN Unit, Measuring, Potential, Evoked, Auditory Ear/Nose/Throat

POTENTIATING
81KSG Media, Potentiating Hematology

POTENTIATOR
81UJP Potentiator, Blood Antibody Hematology

POTENTIOMETER
75UHJ Potentiometer Chemistry

POUCH
80WNK Bag, Plastic General
80SEB Bag, Urinary Collection General
80SEC Bag, Urinary Collection, Precision Measure (Urine Meter) General
79KCT Pack, Sterilization Wrapper (Bag And Accessories) Surgery
80RVT Packaging, Sterilization General
78EZQ Pouch, Colostomy Gastro/Urology
85MBU Pouch, Intravaginal Obstetrics/Gyn
80WME Pouch, Telemetry General

POWDER
76VLN Amalgam, Dental, Powder Dental And Oral
77KCL Blower, Powder, ENT Ear/Nose/Throat
78KPO Concentrate, Dialysis, Hemodialysis (Liquid or Powder) Gastro/Urology
79KGP Dusting Powder, Surgical Surgery
79WWN Glove, Surgical, Powder-Free Surgery
76EIH Powder, Porcelain Dental And Oral
83JTT Sensitivity Test Powder, Antimicrobial Microbiology
88LEF Stain, Dye Powder Pathology

POWDER-FREE
79WWN Glove, Surgical, Powder-Free Surgery

POWDERING
80QYG Glove Processing Unit (Drying, Powdering) General

POWDERS
83MJA Powders, Antimycobacterial Susceptibility Test Microbiology

POWER
79WDY Accessories, Electrical Power (Electrocautery) Surgery
80WTN Adapter, Cable, Equipment General
80WJN Analyzer, Battery General
74MPD Auxillary Power Supply, Low Energy Defibrillator (AC or DC) Cardiovascular
74MPE Auxillary Power Supply, Pacemaker, Cardiac, External Trans. Cardiovascular
80VDY Battery General
80WJG Cable, Electric General
80WJM Charger, Battery General

POWER *(cont'd)*
80WKG Component, Electrical General
79SHL Generator, Power, Electrosurgical Surgery
86HJH Loupe, Binocular, Low Power Ophthalmology
80SDX Meter, Ultrasonic Power General
80TDS Plug, Electrical General
80QUD Power Supply, Endoscopic, Battery-Operated General
80QUE Power Supply, Endoscopic, Line-Operated General
80TCS Power System, Isolated General
80WMN Power Systems, Uninterruptible (UPS) General
80TEE Receptacle, Electrical General
80WMM Regulator, Line Voltage General
80SAA Tester, Isolated Power System General

POWERED
86HRG Accessories, Engine, Trephine, AC-Powered Ophthalmology
79HRF Accessories, Engine, Trephine, Battery-Powered Surgery
79HLD Accessories, Engine, Trephine, Gas-Powered Surgery
84HBE Accessories, Powered Drill Cns/Neurology
89IRN Alarm, Overload, External Limb, Powered Physical Med
73BSI Algesimeter, Powered Anesthesiology
76EFD Amalgamator, Dental, AC-Powered Dental And Oral
78FER Anoscope, Non-Powered Gastro/Urology
89KFW Assembly, Shoulder/Elbow/Forearm/Wrist/Hand, Powered Physical Med
89IRR Bars, Parallel, Powered Physical Med
89KTC Bath, Sitz, Non-Powered Physical Med
89IOQ Bed, Flotation Therapy, Powered Physical Med
89IKZ Bed, Patient Rotation, Powered Physical Med
89FNH Bed, Water Flotation, AC-Powered Physical Med
89IQH Biofeedback Equipment, Myoelectric, Battery-Powered Physical Med
89IRC Biofeedback Equipment, Myoelectric, Powered Physical Med
86HQS Burr, Corneal, AC-Powered Ophthalmology
86HOG Burr, Corneal, Battery-Powered Ophthalmology
86HRE Cabinet, Instrument, AC-Powered, Ophthalmic Ophthalmology
86HKI Camera, Ophthalmic, AC-Powered (Fundus) Ophthalmology
86HOP Campimeter, Stereo, Battery-Powered Ophthalmology
86HQR Cautery, Radiofrequency, AC-Powered Ophthalmology
86HQQ Cautery, Radiofrequency, Battery-Powered Ophthalmology
86HQO Cautery, Thermal, AC-Powered Ophthalmology
86HQP Cautery, Thermal, Battery-Powered Ophthalmology
78FKS Chair, Dialysis, Powered (Without Scale) Gastro/Urology
86HME Chair, Ophthalmic, AC-Powered Ophthalmology
79GBB Chair, Surgical, AC-Powered Surgery
89ILP Communication System, Non-Powered Physical Med
89ILQ Communication System, Powered Physical Med
80FQI Compressor, External, Cardiac, Powered General
73CAJ Controller, Infusion, Powered Anesthesiology
90JAI Couch, Radiation Therapy, Powered Radiology
90IZM Cradle, Radiographic, Powered Radiology
86HRN Cryophthalmic Unit, AC-Powered Ophthalmology
87LGH Cutter, Cast, AC-Powered Orthopedics
86HQE Cutter, Vitreous Aspiration, AC-Powered Ophthalmology
86HKP Cutter, Vitreous Aspiration, Battery-Powered Ophthalmology
74QOR Defibrillator, Battery-Powered Cardiovascular
74DRK Defibrillator, Battery-Powered, High Energy Cardiovascular
74LDD Defibrillator, Battery-Powered, Low Energy Cardiovascular
74QOS Defibrillator, Line-Powered Cardiovascular
74QOO Defibrillator/Monitor, Battery-Powered Cardiovascular
74QOP Defibrillator/Monitor, Line-Powered Cardiovascular
76DZI Drill, Bone, Powered Dental And Oral
84HBF Drill, Powered Compound (With Burr, Trephine & Accessories) Cns/Neurology
87HXJ Driver, Bone Staple, Powered Orthopedics
87LBB Dynamometer, AC-Powered Orthopedics
87HRW Dynamometer, Non-Powered Orthopedics
79QSK Electrocautery Unit, Battery-Powered Surgery
79QSL Electrocautery Unit, Line-Powered Surgery
86HPY Electrolysis Unit, Battery-Powered, Ophthalmic Ophthalmology
79GCP Endoscope And Accessories, AC-Powered Surgery
79GCS Endoscope And Accessories, Battery-Powered Surgery
89IQA Environmental Control System, Powered Physical Med
89ILR Environmental Control System, Powered, Remote Physical Med
89ITH Equipment, Traction, Powered Physical Med
86HMK Euthyscope, AC-Powered Ophthalmology
86HML Euthyscope, Battery-Powered Ophthalmology
80KZF Examination Device, AC-Powered General
89JFA Exerciser, Finger, Powered Physical Med
73BXB Exerciser, Powered Anesthesiology
74LIW Fibrillator, AC-Powered Cardiovascular
74MDO Fibrillator, AC-Powered, Internal Cardiovascular
86HPL Fixation Device, AC-Powered, Ophthalmic Ophthalmology
86HKJ Fixation Device, Battery-Powered, Ophthalmic Ophthalmology
87KQW Goniometer, Non-Powered Orthopedics
89IKO Hammer, Reflex, Powered Physical Med
89IQZ Hand, External Limb Component, Powered Physical Med
76EFB Handpiece, Air-Powered, Dental Dental And Oral
76EKX Handpiece, Direct Drive, AC-Powered Dental And Oral
76EKY Handpiece, Water-Powered Dental And Oral

POWERED *(cont'd)*

86HPQ	Headlamp, Operating, AC-Powered	Ophthalmology
74QZQ	Heat Exchanger, Heart-Lung Bypass, AC-Powered	Cardiovascular
89IRQ	Heating Unit, Powered	Physical Med
89IQW	Hook, External Limb Component, Powered	Physical Med
76EGQ	Injector, Jet, Gas-Powered	Dental And Oral
76EGM	Injector, Jet, Mechanical-Powered	Dental And Oral
87HSZ	Instrument, Surgical, Powered, Pneumatic	Orthopedics
77KMA	Irrigator, Powered Nasal	Ear/Nose/Throat
89IRE	Joint, Elbow, External Limb Component, Powered	Physical Med
86HNO	Keratome, AC-Powered	Ophthalmology
86HMY	Keratome, Battery-Powered	Ophthalmology
86HLQ	Keratoscope, AC-Powered	Ophthalmology
86HLR	Keratoscope, Battery-Powered	Ophthalmology
79HJE	Lamp, Fluorescein, AC-Powered	Surgery
86HJO	Lamp, Slit, Biomicroscope, AC-Powered	Ophthalmology
77ESE	Larynx, Artificial Battery-Powered	Ear/Nose/Throat
80FSA	Lift, Bath, Non-AC-Powered	General
80KYT	Light, Examination, Battery-Powered	General
86HIX	Light, Maxwell Spot, AC-Powered	Ophthalmology
86HPO	Magnet, AC-Powered	Ophthalmology
89IPD	Massager, Battery-Powered	Physical Med
89IRP	Massager, Powered Inflatable Tube	Physical Med
89IKY	Mattress, Non-Powered Flotation Therapy	Physical Med
86HLM	Measurer, Lens, AC-Powered	Ophthalmology
89IKI	Meter, Skin Resistance, AC-Powered	Physical Med
89IKJ	Meter, Skin Resistance, Battery-Powered	Physical Med
86HRM	Microscope, Operating, AC-Powered, Ophthalmic	Ophthalmology
79FYL	Monitor, Blood Pressure, Indirect, Surgery, Powered	Surgery
74FYS	Monitor, Pressure, Pulmonary Artery, Powered	Cardiovascular
74FYN	Monitor, Pressure, Venous, Central, Powered	Cardiovascular
84HCS	Monitor, Temperature, Neurosurgery, Direct Contact, Powered	Cns/Neurology
79GEY	Motor, Surgical Instrument, AC-Powered	Surgery
79GET	Motor, Surgical Instrument, Pneumatic-Powered	Surgery
86HLI	Ophthalmoscope, AC-Powered	Ophthalmology
86HLJ	Ophthalmoscope, Battery-Powered	Ophthalmology
89IRT	Pad, Heating, Powered	Physical Med
80FRZ	Patient Transfer Unit, Powered	General
86HJP	Penlight, Battery-Powered	Ophthalmology
73BYI	Percussor, Powered	Anesthesiology
86HOO	Perimeter, AC-Powered	Ophthalmology
86HPT	Perimeter, Automatic, AC-Powered	Ophthalmology
86HLX	Photostimulator, AC-Powered	Ophthalmology
80LGX	Powered Medical Examination Table	General
86HLT	Preamplifier, AC-Powered, Ophthalmic	Ophthalmology
86HLW	Preamplifier, Battery-Powered, Ophthalmic	Ophthalmology
78EXX	Probe, Rectal, Non-Powered	Gastro/Urology
85HGY	Pump, Breast, Non-Powered	Obstetrics/Gyn
85HGX	Pump, Breast, Powered	Obstetrics/Gyn
86HLG	Pupillometer, AC-Powered	Ophthalmology
86HKL	Retinoscope, AC-Powered	Ophthalmology
86HKM	Retinoscope, Battery-Powered	Ophthalmology
84HAD	Rongeur, Powered	Cns/Neurology
79KFK	Saw, Pneumatically Powered	Surgery
84HAB	Saw, Powered, And Accessories	Cns/Neurology
86HOM	Screen, Tangent, AC-Powered (Campimeter)	Ophthalmology
86HOK	Screen, Tangent, Projection, AC-Powered	Ophthalmology
86HMJ	Screen, Tangent, Projection, Battery-Powered	Ophthalmology
86HLK	Screen, Tangent, Target, Battery-Powered	Ophthalmology
77LEZ	Speech Training Aid, AC-Powered	Ear/Nose/Throat
77LFA	Speech Training Aid, Battery-Powered	Ear/Nose/Throat
86HMF	Stand, Instrument, AC-Powered, Ophthalmic	Ophthalmology
86HJQ	Stereoscope, AC-Powered	Ophthalmology
86HJR	Stereoscope, Battery-Powered	Ophthalmology
86HRD	Sterilizer, Soft Lens, Thermal, AC-Powered	Ophthalmology
86HRC	Sterilizer, Soft Lens, Thermal, Battery-Powered	Ophthalmology
80FLW	Stethoscope, DC-Powered	General
89IPF	Stimulator, Muscle, Electrical-Powered (EMS)	Physical Med
89MBN	Stimulator, Muscle, Powered, Invasive	Physical Med
73BXM	Stimulator, Nerve, AC-Powered	Anesthesiology
73BXN	Stimulator, Nerve, Battery-Powered	Anesthesiology
89INK	Stretcher, Wheeled, Powered	Physical Med
79GCX	Suction Apparatus, Operating Room, Wall Vacuum-Powered	Surgery
79GCY	Suction Apparatus, Single Patient, Portable, Non-Powered	Surgery
79JCX	Suction Apparatus, Ward Use, Portable, AC-Powered	Surgery
84HAO	Surgical Instrument, Non-Powered, Neurosurgical	Cns/Neurology
87HWE	Surgical Instrument, Orthopedic, AC-Powered Motor	Orthopedics
79KIJ	Surgical Instrument, Orthopedic, Battery-Powered	Surgery
85HDD	Table, Obstetrical, AC-Powered	Obstetrics/Gyn
79FQO	Table, Operating Room, AC-Powered	Surgery
86HRJ	Table, Ophthalmic, Instrument, Powered	Ophthalmology
89INQ	Table, Physical Medicine, Powered	Physical Med
90IZZ	Table, Radiographic, Non-Tilting, Powered	Radiology
79JEA	Table, Surgical With Orthopedic Accessories, AC-Powered	Surgery
86HJS	Test, Spectacle Dissociation, AC-Powered (Lancaster)	Ophthalmology
86HLO	Test, Spectacle Dissociation, Battery-Powered (Lancaster)	Ophthalmology

POWERED *(cont'd)*

90KYA	Thermographic Device, Liquid Crystal, Non-Powered	Radiology
86HKX	Tonometer, AC-Powered	Ophthalmology
76MMD	Toothbrush, Ionic, Battery-Powered	Dental And Oral
76JEQ	Toothbrush, Powered	Dental And Oral
87HSR	Traction Unit, Hip, Non-Powered, Non-Penetrating	Orthopedics
87HST	Traction Unit, Non-Powered	Orthopedics
87SBN	Traction Unit, Powered, Mobile	Orthopedics
86HJM	Transilluminator, AC-Powered, Ophthalmic	Ophthalmology
86ETJ	Transilluminator, AC-Powered, Other	Ophthalmology
86HJN	Transilluminator, Battery-Powered	Ophthalmology
89ILK	Transport, Patient, Powered	Physical Med
89IOL	Treadmill, Powered	Physical Med
80WPL	Unit, Control, Bed, Patient, Powered	General
84LIH	Unit, Therapy, Current, Interferential	Cns/Neurology
73BTL	Ventilator, Emergency, Powered (Resuscitator)	Anesthesiology
89IPE	Vibrator, Battery-Powered	Physical Med
85HIJ	Vibrator, Vaginal, AC-Powered	Obstetrics/Gyn
85HIK	Vibrator, Vaginal, Battery-Powered	Obstetrics/Gyn
86HPF	Vision Aid, Electronic, AC-Powered	Ophthalmology
86HPG	Vision Aid, Electronic, Battery-Powered	Ophthalmology
86HOT	Vision Aid, Image Intensification, Battery-Powered	Ophthalmology
86HPI	Vision Aid, Optical, AC-Powered	Ophthalmology
86HPE	Vision Aid, Optical, Battery-Powered	Ophthalmology
89ITI	Wheelchair, Powered	Physical Med
89KGH	Wrist, External Limb Component, Powered	Physical Med

PRADER

80WXO	Orchidometer	General

PRE-BYPASS

74KRJ	Filter, Pre-Bypass, Cardiopulmonary Bypass	Cardiovascular

PRE-PROGRAMMED

74DXG	Computer, Diagnostic, Pre-Programmed, Single-Function	Cardiovascular

PRE-TIED

79SGX	Suture, Laparoscopy	Surgery
79SGW	Suture, Laparoscopy, Loose	Surgery
79SGY	Suture, Laparoscopy, Pre-Tied	Surgery

PREALBUMIN

82JZJ	Antigen, Antiserum, Control, Prealbumin	Immunology
82DDS	Antigen, Antiserum, Control, Prealbumin, FITC	Immunology

PREAMPLIFIER

86HLT	Preamplifier, AC-Powered, Ophthalmic	Ophthalmology
86HLW	Preamplifier, Battery-Powered, Ophthalmic	Ophthalmology

PRECIOUS

76EJS	Alloy, Precious Metal, For Clinical Use	Dental And Oral
80WUL	Metal, Medical	General

PRECIPITATION

75KMZ	HDL Via LDL & VLDL Precipitation, Lipoproteins	Chemistry
75JKN	Heat-Precipitation, Bence-Jones Protein	Chemistry
75LBS	LDL & VLDL Precipitation, Cholesterol Via Esterase-Oxidase	Chemistry
75LBR	LDL & VLDL Precipitation, HDL	Chemistry

PRECIPITATOR

75UHK	Precipitator, Radioimmunoassay Multiple Sampling	Chemistry

PRECISION

76EGG	Attachment, Precision	Dental And Oral
80SEC	Bag, Urinary Collection, Precision Measure (Urine Meter)	General

PRECURSOR

82MME	Proteins, Amyloid And Precursor	Immunology

PREDICTED

73BTY	Computer, Pulmonary Function, Predicted Values	Anesthesiology

PREFORMED

76EJX	Anchor, Preformed	Dental And Oral
76ECM	Band, Preformed, Orthodontic	Dental And Oral
76EHO	Bar, Preformed	Dental And Oral
76EHP	Clasp, Preformed	Dental And Oral
76ELZ	Crown, Preformed	Dental And Oral
76EHQ	Cusp, Preformed	Dental And Oral
76EKO	Denture, Preformed	Dental And Oral
87MQV	Filler, Calcium Sulfate Preformed Pellets	Orthopedics
76DYT	Maintainer, Space Preformed, Orthodontic	Dental And Oral
84GWO	Plate, Bone, Skull, Preformed, Alterable	Cns/Neurology
84GXN	Plate, Bone, Skull, Preformed, Non-Alterable	Cns/Neurology
76KMY	Positioner, Tooth, Preformed	Dental And Oral
84GXO	Strip, Craniosynostosis, Preformed	Cns/Neurology

PREGNANCY

85MDH	Abruptio Placentae Catheter	Obstetrics/Gyn
75JHJ	Agglutination Method, Human Chorionic Gonadotropin	Chemistry
82LTQ	Calibrator, AFP, Serum, Maternal, Mid-Pregnancy	Immunology

PREGNANCY *(cont'd)*
85VIK Equipment, In Vitro Fertilization/Embryo Transfer Obstetrics/Gyn
85TFV Kit, Pregnancy Test Obstetrics/Gyn
75LCX Kit, Pregnancy Test, Over The Counter, HCG Chemistry
75JHI Radioimmunoassay, Human Chorionic Gonadotropin Chemistry
75CHM Radioimmunoassay, Total Estrogens In Pregnancy Chemistry
82JZN Test, Human Chorionic Gonadotropin Immunology
82DHA Test, Human Chorionic Gonadotropin, Serum Immunology
85HFN Transducer, Pressure, Intrauterine Obstetrics/Gyn

PREGNANEDIOL
75JLP Spectrophotometric Method, Pregnanediol Chemistry

PREGNANETRIOL
75JLR Chromatography, Gas, Pregnanetriol Chemistry
75JLQ Spectrophotometric Method, Pregnanetriol Chemistry

PREGNENOLONE
75JNG Radioimmunoassay, Pregnenolone Chemistry

PRENATAL
82MLF Computer Software, Prenatal Risk Evaluation Immunology

PREP
80WPK Electrolysis Equipment, Other General
80RLP Kit, Prep General
80TGG Solution, Patient Preparation General

PREPARATION
79WVZ Drape, Incision, Surgical Surgery
81KSC Material, Preparation, Skin Hematology
80TGG Solution, Patient Preparation General

PREPARER
76EKQ Preparer, Root Canal, Endodontic Dental And Oral

PRESCRIPTION
78FEI Eyepiece, Lens, Non-Prescription, Endoscopic Gastro/Urology
78FDZ Eyepiece, Lens, Prescription, Endoscopic Gastro/Urology
86WTY Laboratory Equipment, Ophthalmic Ophthalmology
86HRA Lens, Spectacle/Eyeglasses, Custom (Prescription) Ophthalmology

PRESERVATION
78RIZ Organ Preservation System Gastro/Urology
79UAA Oxygenator, Organ Preservation Surgery

PRESERVATIVE
88LEA Preservative, Cytological Pathology
88IFL Preservative, Polyethylene Glycol Pathology

PRESS
77JYW Press, Vein Ear/Nose/Throat

PRESSURE
74DSJ Alarm, Blood Pressure Cardiovascular
78FIW Alarm, Pillow Pressure Gastro/Urology
73BXZ Analyzer, Gas, Carbon-Dioxide, Partial Pressure, Blood Anesthesiology
73BSD Analyzer, Gas, Nitrogen, Partial Pressure, Blood Phase (NI) Anesthesiology
73CCD Analyzer, Gas, Oxygen, Partial Pressure, Blood Phase Anesthesiology
79WTZ Analyzer, Patient, Multiple Function (Surgery) Surgery
91KIE Apparatus, High Pressure Liquid Chromatography Toxicology
86LCC Applicator, Ocular Pressure Ophthalmology
89KNM Applier, Pressure, Physical Medicine Physical Med
73BYE Attachment, Breathing, Positive End Expiratory Pressure Anesthesiology
80MHW Bandage, Compression General
80WRS Bulb, Inflation General
73BXX Calibrator, Gas, Pressure Anesthesiology
73QFO Calibrator, Pressure Transducer Anesthesiology
73CAT Cannula, Nasal, Oxygen Anesthesiology
74DSK Computer, Blood Pressure Cardiovascular
73QMH Continuous Positive Airway Pressure Unit (CPAP, CPPB) Anesthesiology
80LSX Controller, Pressure, Blood, Closed-Loop General
74DXQ Cuff, Blood Pressure Cardiovascular
80QQH Dome, Pressure Transducer General
73CAX Flowmeter, Back-Pressure Compensated, Thorpe Tube Anesthesiology
73CCN Flowmeter, Gas, Non-Back-Pressure Compensated, Bourdon Gauge Anesthesiology
86LPO Gas, Reattachment Procedure, Retinal Ophthalmology
73BXH Gauge, Gas Pressure, Cylinder/Pipeline Anesthesiology
80WVV Gauge, Pressure General
74DXS Gauge, Pressure, Coronary, Cardiopulmonary Bypass Cardiovascular
74JOR Generator, Pulsatile Flow, Cardiopulmonary Bypass Cardiovascular
91KZY High Pressure Liquid Chromatography, Barbiturate Toxicology
91LAA High Pressure Liquid Chromatography, Benzodiazepine Toxicology
91LAC High Pressure Liquid Chromatography, Cocaine & Metabolites Toxicology
91LAE High Pressure Liquid Chromatography, Codeine Toxicology
91LAG High Pressure Liquid Chromatography, Methamphetamine Toxicology
91LAH High Pressure Liquid Chromatography, Opiates Toxicology
91LAK High Pressure Liquid Chromatography, Propoxyphene Toxicology
91LAM High Pressure Liquid Chromatography, Quinine Toxicology
91LFI High Pressure Liquid Chromatography, Tricyclic Drug Toxicology

PRESSURE *(cont'd)*
80RLQ Infuser, Pressure (Blood Pump) General
91LDM Instrumentation, High Pressure Liquid Chromatography Toxicology
74QIX Kit, Blood Pressure, Central Venous Cardiovascular
84RFM Kit, Lumbar Puncture Cns/Neurology
80RLY Kit, Pressure Monitoring (Air/Gas) General
89ILA Mattress, Alternating Pressure (Or Pads) Physical Med
80WYO Mattress, Reduction, Pressure General
73CAP Monitor, Airway Pressure (Gauge/Alarm) Anesthesiology
73BXR Monitor, Airway Pressure (Inspiratory Force) Anesthesiology
73RLV Monitor, Airway Pressure, Continuous Anesthesiology
74KGJ Monitor, Blood Pressure, Amplifier & Associated Electronics Cardiovascular
74WZC Monitor, Blood Pressure, Finger Cardiovascular
74RLS Monitor, Blood Pressure, Indirect (Arterial) Cardiovascular
73BXD Monitor, Blood Pressure, Indirect, Anesthesiology Anesthesiology
74JOE Monitor, Blood Pressure, Indirect, Automatic Cardiovascular
74DXN Monitor, Blood Pressure, Indirect, Semi-Automatic Cardiovascular
79FYM Monitor, Blood Pressure, Indirect, Surgery Surgery
79FYL Monitor, Blood Pressure, Indirect, Surgery, Powered Surgery
73BZZ Monitor, Blood Pressure, Indirect, Transducer Anesthesiology
74RLR Monitor, Blood Pressure, Invasive (Arterial) Cardiovascular
73CAA Monitor, Blood Pressure, Invasive (Arterial), Anesthesia Anesthesiology
74BXE Monitor, Blood Pressure, Transducer, Indwelling Cardiovascular
74RLX Monitor, Blood Pressure, Venous Cardiovascular
74KRK Monitor, Blood Pressure, Venous, Cardiopulmonary Bypass Cardiovascular
79FYO Monitor, Blood Pressure, Venous, Central Surgery
79FYP Monitor, Blood Pressure, Venous, Peripheral Surgery
79KFQ Monitor, Cardiac Output, Trend (Arterial Pressure Pulse) Surgery
80CAQ Monitor, Cerebral Spinal Fluid Pressure (CSF) General
80CAR Monitor, Cerebral Spinal Fluid Pressure, Electrical General
78RLU Monitor, Esophageal Pressure Gastro/Urology
85HEQ Monitor, Fetal, Ultrasonic, Arterial Pressure Obstetrics/Gyn
84RLW Monitor, Intracranial Pressure Cns/Neurology
84GWM Monitor, Intracranial Pressure, Continuous Cns/Neurology
80FLP Monitor, Neonatal, Blood Pressure, Invasive General
80FLQ Monitor, Neonatal, Blood Pressure, Ultrasonic/Doppler General
79KFS Monitor, Po2, Continuous Surgery
74FYK Monitor, Pressure, Arterial, Internal Cardiovascular
74FYQ Monitor, Pressure, Cardiac, Atrial Cardiovascular
74FYR Monitor, Pressure, Cardiac, Ventricular Cardiovascular
87LXC Monitor, Pressure, Intracompartmental Orthopedics
84LII Monitor, Pressure, Intracranial, Implantable Cns/Neurology
85KXO Monitor, Pressure, Intrauterine Obstetrics/Gyn
74FYS Monitor, Pressure, Pulmonary Artery, Powered Cardiovascular
74FYN Monitor, Pressure, Venous, Central, Powered Cardiovascular
80RLZ Pad, Pressure, Air General
80RMA Pad, Pressure, Animal Skin General
80RMB Pad, Pressure, Foam (Elbow, Heel) General
80RMC Pad, Pressure, Foam Convoluted General
80RMD Pad, Pressure, Gel General
80WMD Pad, Pressure, Gel, Operating Table General
80RME Pad, Pressure, Soft Rubber General
80RMF Pad, Pressure, Water Cushion General
73CCM Plethysmograph, Pressure (Body) Anesthesiology
80KZD Pressure Infusor, IV Container General
89JFC Pressure Measurement, System, Intermittent Physical Med
80UCU Pressure Pad, Alternating, Disposable General
80UCV Pressure Pad, Alternating, Reusable General
80FMP Protector, Skin Pressure General
80UBG Pump, Alternating Pressure Pad General
80JOI Pump, Inflator General
78FES Recorder, External, Pressure, Amplifier & Transducer Gastro/Urology
74ROK Recorder, Long-Term, Blood Pressure, Portable Cardiovascular
85HFO Recorder, Pressure, Intrauterine Obstetrics/Gyn
86WNV Reducer, Pressure, Intraocular Ophthalmology
73CAN Regulator, Pressure, Gas Cylinder Anesthesiology
74RTG Simulator, Blood Pressure Cardiovascular
80FLY Sphygmomanometer, Aneroid (Arterial Pressure) General
80THH Sphygmomanometer, Electronic (Arterial Pressure) General
80UDM Sphygmomanometer, Electronic, Automatic General
80UDN Sphygmomanometer, Electronic, Manual General
80FLX Sphygmomanometer, Mercury (Arterial Pressure) General
78FLC Station, Dialysis Control, Negative Pressure Type Gastro/Urology
80RZN Telemetry Unit, Physiological, Pressure General
86HPK Tonograph Ophthalmology
86HKX Tonometer, AC-Powered Ophthalmology
86HKY Tonometer, Manual Ophthalmology
80SBD Tourniquet General
87HTA Tourniquet, Air Pressure Orthopedics
80SBW Transducer, Blood Pressure General
74DXO Transducer, Blood Pressure, Catheter Tip Cardiovascular
74DRS Transducer, Blood Pressure, Extravascular Cardiovascular
73BXO Transducer, Gas Pressure Anesthesiology
73BYR Transducer, Gas Pressure, Differential Anesthesiology
89IKE Transducer, Miniature Pressure Physical Med
85HFN Transducer, Pressure, Intrauterine Obstetrics/Gyn
73BYX Tubing, Flexible, Medical Gas, Low-Pressure Anesthesiology

PRESSURE *(cont'd)*

73SEO	Valve, Positive End Expiratory Pressure (PEEP)	Anesthesiology
74MNJ	Valve, Pressure Relief, Cardiopulmonary Bypass	Cardiovascular
75JNA	Vapor Pressure, Osmolality Of Serum & Urine	Chemistry
73BYT	Ventilator, External Body, Negative Pressure, (Cuirass)	Anesthesiology
73SEU	Ventilator, Pressure Cycled (IPPB Machine)	Anesthesiology

PRESSURE-SENSITIVE

80RZE	Tape, Adhesive	General

PRESURGERY

79WIY	Computer, Imaging, Presurgery	Surgery

PREVENT

90MOT	Irradiator, Blood to Prevent Graft Vs Host Disease	Radiology

PREVENTION

74MUN	Device, Arterial, Temporary, For Embolization Prevention	Cardiovascular
79MBR	Silastic Elastomer (Angular Deformity Prevention)	Surgery

PRIMARY

75JIS	Calibrator, Primary, Clinical Chemistry	Chemistry

PRIMER

76EBJ	Primer, Cavity, Resin	Dental And Oral

PRIMIDONE

91DJD	Enzyme Immunoassay, Primidone	Toxicology
91LFT	Fluorescent Immunoassay, Primidone	Toxicology
91DMQ	Gas Chromatography, Primidone	Toxicology
91DPQ	Liquid Chromatography, Primidone	Toxicology
91DIL	Radioimmunoassay, Primidone	Toxicology
91DOS	Thin Layer Chromatography, Primidone	Toxicology
91LCZ	U.V. Spectrometry, Primidone	Toxicology

PRINTER

80VFR	Computer, Bar Code	General
90TFQ	Duplicator, X-Ray Film	Radiology
80WNL	Label, Bar Code	General
80WMT	Printer, Bar Code	General
80WLN	Printer, Image, Video	General
90RNW	Printer, Radiographic Duplicator	Radiology

PRINTING

80WYM	Service, Printing	General

PRISM

86HKW	Bar, Prism, Ophthalmic	Ophthalmology
86HKS	Gonioscope (Prism)	Ophthalmology
79GCN	Prism, Endoscopic	Surgery
86HKT	Prism, Fresnel, Ophthalmic	Ophthalmology
86HKQ	Prism, Rotary, Ophthalmic	Ophthalmology
86HJX	Reader, Prism, Ophthalmic	Ophthalmology

PROBE

74TAV	Cardiac Output Unit, Radioisotope Probe	Cardiovascular
74DRF	Catheter, Electrode Recording, Or Probe	Cardiovascular
79WHN	Cover, Probe, Transducer	Surgery
80QND	Cover, Thermometer	General
79WWP	Cover, Tip, Probe, Cauterization	Surgery
83MCG	DNA-Probe, Agent, Listeria	Microbiology
83MDC	DNA-Probe, Blastomyces Dermatitidis	Microbiology
81MAO	DNA-Probe, Chromosome, Human	Hematology
83MJM	DNA-Probe, Gardnerella Vaginalis	Microbiology
82MMM	DNA-Probe, HER/NEU	Immunology
83MCC	DNA-Probe, Haemophilus SPP.	Microbiology
81MAM	DNA-Probe, Lymphocyte, B & T	Hematology
83MKZ	DNA-Probe, Nucleic Acid Amplification, Chlamydia	Microbiology
83MBT	DNA-Probe, Reagent	Microbiology
83MCS	DNA-Probe, Staphylococcus Aureus	Microbiology
83MCT	DNA-Probe, Strep Pneumoniae	Microbiology
83MJK	DNA-Probe, Trichomonas Vaginalis	Microbiology
83MLA	DNA-Probe, Yeast	Microbiology
78VJF	Endoscope, Ultrasonic Probe (Lithotriptor)	Gastro/Urology
78QXB	Forceps, Gallbladder (Biliary Duct)	Gastro/Urology
89IRQ	Heating Unit, Powered	Physical Med
84GZX	Instrument, Microsurgical	Cns/Neurology
73BWX	Monitor, Temperature (With Probe)	Anesthesiology
87HXB	Probe	Orthopedics
74DPT	Probe, Blood Flow, Extravascular	Cardiovascular
78RMG	Probe, Common Duct	Gastro/Urology
79RTA	Probe, Detector, Flow, Blood, Laparoscopy, Ultrasonic	Surgery
79SJV	Probe, Electrocauterization, Microlaparoscopy	Surgery
79QEZ	Probe, Electrocauterization, Multi-Use	Surgery
79QHA	Probe, Electrocauterization, Single-Use	Surgery
79SJC	Probe, Electrosurgery, Endoscopy	Surgery
78RMI	Probe, Fistula	Gastro/Urology
78FGM	Probe, Gastrointestinal	Gastro/Urology
86HPW	Probe, Isotope, With Counter For Phosphorus 32	Ophthalmology
86HNL	Probe, Lacrimal	Ophthalmology
86RMH	Probe, Ophthalmic	Ophthalmology

PROBE *(cont'd)*

80RMK	Probe, Other	General
76EIX	Probe, Periodontic	Dental And Oral
84GXI	Probe, Radiofrequency Lesion	Cns/Neurology
78EXX	Probe, Rectal, Non-Powered	Gastro/Urology
77KAK	Probe, Sinus	Ear/Nose/Throat
79QUQ	Probe, Suction, Irrigator/Aspirator, Laparoscopic	Surgery
80RMJ	Probe, Temperature	General
74LXN	Probe, Test, Valve, Heart	Cardiovascular
74KRB	Probe, Thermodilution	Cardiovascular
86HNK	Probe, Trabeculotomy	Ophthalmology
74WTO	Probe, Transesophageal	Cardiovascular
90VCR	Probe, Ultrasonic	Radiology
90IZD	Probe, Uptake, Nuclear	Radiology
73DQZ	Probe, pH Catheter	Anesthesiology
83MDF	Reagent, DNA-Probe, Coccidioides Immitis	Microbiology
83MDE	Reagent, DNA-Probe, Cryptococcal	Microbiology
83MDK	Reagent, DNA-Probe, Streptococcal	Microbiology
73RSA	Sensor, Oxygen	Anesthesiology
90SIK	System, Imaging, Laparoscopy, Ultrasonic	Radiology
82VJL	Test, Cancer Detection, DNA-Probe	Immunology
83WNY	Test, DNA-Probe, Other	Microbiology
79QIJ	Tip, Instrument, Electrocauterization, Monopolar	Surgery
73BXG	Transducer, Blood Flow, Invasive	Anesthesiology
73BXF	Transducer, Blood Flow, Non-Invasive	Anesthesiology
73BXP	Transducer, Gas Flow	Anesthesiology
73BXO	Transducer, Gas Pressure	Anesthesiology
74JOP	Transducer, Ultrasonic	Cardiovascular
90ITX	Transducer, Ultrasonic, Diagnostic	Radiology
85HGL	Transducer, Ultrasonic, Obstetrical	Obstetrics/Gyn

PROCAINAMIDE

91LAR	Enzyme Immunoassay, Procainamide	Toxicology
91LBA	Procainamide Control Materials	Toxicology

PROCEDURE

75JPY	Catalytic Procedure, CPK Isoenzymes	Chemistry
86LPO	Gas, Reattachment Procedure, Retinal	Ophthalmology
90VGC	Kit, Angiographic, Special Procedure	Radiology
74SGT	Kit, Disposable Procedure	Cardiovascular
80WXF	Pack, Custom/Special Procedure	General
90THR	Radiographic/Fluoroscopic Unit, Special Procedure	Radiology
90JAK	Scanner, Computed Tomography, X-Ray, Special Procedure	Radiology
80WNH	Tray, Custom/Special Procedure	General

PROCESS

80MRB	Indicator, Biological, Liquid Chemical Steril. Process	General
80FRC	Sterilization Process Indicator, Biological	General
80RVU	Sterilization Process Indicator, Chemical	General
80JOJ	Sterilization Process Indicator, Physical/Chemical	General
80WLS	Test, Equipment, Sterilization	General

PROCESSED

79LMO	Allograft, Processed	Surgery

PROCESSING

88KET	Filter, Cell Collection, Tissue Processing	Pathology
80QYG	Glove Processing Unit (Drying, Powdering)	General
90LLZ	Image Processing System	Radiology
90WHY	Mixer, Chemical, Film, X-Ray	Radiology

PROCESSOR

90VGU	Chemical, Film Processor	Radiology
90TGW	Interlock System, X-Ray Darkrooms	Radiology
90SGL	Monitor, X-Ray Film Processor Quality Control	Radiology
90IXX	Processor, Cine Film	Radiology
81KSW	Processor, Frozen Blood	Hematology
90IXW	Processor, Radiographic Film, Automatic	Radiology
76EGY	Processor, Radiographic Film, Automatic, Dental	Dental And Oral
90JAH	Processor, Radiographic Film, Manual	Radiology
88MKQ	Processor, Slide, Cytology, Automated	Pathology
80THI	Sterilizer/Washer, Endoscope	General
88SAW	Tissue Processor (Infiltrator)	Pathology
88IEO	Tissue Processor, Automated	Pathology
90WTF	Unit, Imaging, Thermal	Radiology
81SFO	Washer, Cell (Frozen Blood Processor)	Hematology

PROCONVERTIN

81JPF	Prothrombin-Proconvertin And Thrombotest	Hematology

PROCTOSCOPE

79GCF	Proctoscope	Surgery

PROCTOSCOPIC

78QBH	Applicator, Proctoscopic	Gastro/Urology

PROCTOSIGMOIDOSCOPE

78RML	Proctosigmoidoscope	Gastro/Urology

KEYWORD INDEX

PROSTHESIS *(cont'd)*

87MBK	Prosthesis, Ankle, Semi-, Uncemented, Porous, Metal/Polymer	Orthopedics
87KMD	Prosthesis, Ankle, Semi-Constrained, Metal/Composite	Orthopedics
87HSN	Prosthesis, Ankle, Semi-Constrained, Metal/Polymer	Orthopedics
87UBK	Prosthesis, Ankle, Talar Component	Orthopedics
87UBL	Prosthesis, Ankle, Tibial Component	Orthopedics
78UDE	Prosthesis, Anti-Gastroesophageal Reflux	Gastro/Urology
87RMN	Prosthesis, Arm	Orthopedics
79FZC	Prosthesis, Arterial Graft, Bovine Carotid Artery	Surgery
79FZB	Prosthesis, Arterial Graft, Synthetic, Greater Than 6mm	Surgery
79JCP	Prosthesis, Arterial Graft, Synthetic, Less Than 6mm	Surgery
84LIK	Prosthesis, Baroreflex	Cns/Neurology
87UCR	Prosthesis, Bone Cerclage	Orthopedics
79KCZ	Prosthesis, Breast, External	Surgery
79FWM	Prosthesis, Breast, Inflatable, Internal	Surgery
79FTR	Prosthesis, Breast, Non-Inflatable, Internal	Surgery
74RMO	Prosthesis, Cardiac Valve	Cardiovascular
74DYE	Prosthesis, Cardiac Valve, Biological	Cardiovascular
87HSM	Prosthesis, Carpal	Orthopedics
79FWP	Prosthesis, Chin, Internal	Surgery
77UAI	Prosthesis, Cochlear	Ear/Nose/Throat
77JBA	Prosthesis, Craniofacial	Ear/Nose/Throat
79MEP	Prosthesis, Craniofacial, Bone-Anchored	Surgery
76RMP	Prosthesis, Dental	Dental And Oral
87HWG	Prosthesis, Diaphysis, Custom	Orthopedics
79FZD	Prosthesis, Ear, Internal	Surgery
87JDC	Prosthesis, Elbow, Constrained	Orthopedics
87KWJ	Prosthesis, Elbow, Hemi-, Humeral, Metal	Orthopedics
87KWI	Prosthesis, Elbow, Hemi-, Radial, Polymer	Orthopedics
87UBN	Prosthesis, Elbow, Humeral Component	Orthopedics
87JDA	Prosthesis, Elbow, Non-Constrained, Unipolar	Orthopedics
87UBO	Prosthesis, Elbow, Radial Component	Orthopedics
87JDB	Prosthesis, Elbow, Semi-Constrained	Orthopedics
87UBM	Prosthesis, Elbow, Total	Orthopedics
87UBP	Prosthesis, Elbow, Ulna Component	Orthopedics
77ESW	Prosthesis, Esophageal	Ear/Nose/Throat
79JCQ	Prosthesis, Esophagus	Surgery
86UAZ	Prosthesis, Evisceration	Ophthalmology
79FWO	Prosthesis, Eye, Internal (Sphere)	Surgery
86RMQ	Prosthesis, Eyelid	Ophthalmology
77JAZ	Prosthesis, Facial, Mandibular Implant	Ear/Nose/Throat
85HFJ	Prosthesis, Fallopian Tube	Obstetrics/Gyn
87HSW	Prosthesis, Femoral	Orthopedics
87UCE	Prosthesis, Femoral Head	Orthopedics
87HSJ	Prosthesis, Finger	Orthopedics
87KQY	Prosthesis, Finger and Toe, Hemi-Arthroplasty	Orthopedics
87LBC	Prosthesis, Finger, Constrained, Metal, Cemented	Orthopedics
87KWE	Prosthesis, Finger, Constrained, Metal, Uncemented	Orthopedics
87KWG	Prosthesis, Finger, Constrained, Metal/Polymer	Orthopedics
87KYJ	Prosthesis, Finger, Constrained, Polymer	Orthopedics
87KWC	Prosthesis, Finger, Hemi	Orthopedics
87KWF	Prosthesis, Finger, Polymer	Orthopedics
87UBQ	Prosthesis, Finger, Total	Orthopedics
87RMR	Prosthesis, Foot	Orthopedics
87UCN	Prosthesis, Foot Arch	Orthopedics
76MPI	Prosthesis, Glenoid Fossa	Dental And Oral
87RMS	Prosthesis, Hand	Orthopedics
74RMT	Prosthesis, Heart	Cardiovascular
74DSO	Prosthesis, Heart, With Control System	Cardiovascular
87JDF	Prosthesis, Hip (Metal Stem/Ceramic Self-Locking Ball)	Orthopedics
87JDM	Prosthesis, Hip, Acetabular Component, Metal, Non-Cemented	Orthopedics
87JDJ	Prosthesis, Hip, Acetabular Mesh	Orthopedics
87JDK	Prosthesis, Hip, Cement Restrictor	Orthopedics
87KXD	Prosthesis, Hip, Constrained, Metal	Orthopedics
87KWZ	Prosthesis, Hip, Constrained, Metal/Polymer	Orthopedics
87JDG	Prosthesis, Hip, Femoral Component, Cemented, Metal	Orthopedics
87KXA	Prosthesis, Hip, Femoral, Resurfacing	Orthopedics
87KWB	Prosthesis, Hip, Hemi-, Acetabular, Metal	Orthopedics
87KWL	Prosthesis, Hip, Hemi-, Femoral, Metal	Orthopedics
87KWY	Prosthesis, Hip, Hemi-, Femoral, Metal/Polymer	Orthopedics
87JDH	Prosthesis, Hip, Hemi-, Trunnion-Bearing, Femoral	Orthopedics
87KXB	Prosthesis, Hip, Pelvifemoral Resurfacing, Metal/polymer	Orthopedics
87MBL	Prosthesis, Hip, Semi-, Uncemented, Osteophilic Finish	Orthopedics
87MEJ	Prosthesis, Hip, Semi-Const., Composite/Polymer	Orthopedics
87MAZ	Prosthesis, Hip, Semi-Const., M/P, Por. Uncem., Calc./Phos.	Orthopedics
87LPF	Prosthesis, Hip, Semi-Const., Metal/Ceramic/Ceramic, Cem.	Orthopedics
87LPH	Prosthesis, Hip, Semi-Const., Metal/Poly., Porous Uncemented	Orthopedics
87MIL	Prosthesis, Hip, Semi-Const., Uncem., M/P, Bone Morph. Prot.	Orthopedics
87MEH	Prosthesis, Hip, Semi-Const., Uncem., Non-P., M/P, Ca./Phos.	Orthopedics
87LZO	Prosthesis, Hip, Semi-Constr., Metal/Ceramic, Cemented/NC	Orthopedics
87JDL	Prosthesis, Hip, Semi-Constrained (Cemented Acetabular)	Orthopedics
87KWA	Prosthesis, Hip, Semi-Constrained Acetabular	Orthopedics
87JDI	Prosthesis, Hip, Semi-Constrained, Metal/Polymer	Orthopedics
87LWJ	Prosthesis, Hip, Semi-Constrained, Metal/Polymer, Uncemented	Orthopedics
87KMC	Prosthesis, Hip, Semi-constrained, Composite/metal	Orthopedics
87MRA	Prosthesis, Hip, Semi-constrained, Metal/ Ceramic/ Ceramic/ Metal, Cemented or Uncemented	Orthopedics
87MAY	Prosthesis, Hip, Semi-constrained, Metal/Ceramic/Polymer, Cemented or Non-porous Cemented, Osteophilic Finish	Orthopedics
87MBM	Prosthesis, Hip, Semi/Hemi-Const., M/PTFE Ctd./P, Cem./Unc.	Orthopedics
84RMU	Prosthesis, Hydrocephalic (Holter Valve)	Cns/Neurology
89LBD	Prosthesis, Inflatable Leg, And Pump	Physical Med
76MPJ	Prosthesis, Interarticular Disc (Interpositional Implant)	Dental And Oral
87RMV	Prosthesis, Joint, Other	Orthopedics
87KRN	Prosthesis, Knee, Femorotibial, Constrained, Metal	Orthopedics
87KRO	Prosthesis, Knee, Femorotibial, Constrained, Metal/Polymer	Orthopedics
87HSX	Prosthesis, Knee, Femorotibial, Non-Constrained	Orthopedics
87KTX	Prosthesis, Knee, Femorotibial, Non-Constrained, Metal	Orthopedics
87HRY	Prosthesis, Knee, Femorotibial, Semi-Constrained	Orthopedics
87KYK	Prosthesis, Knee, Femorotibial, Semi-Constrained, Metal	Orthopedics
87LGE	Prosthesis, Knee, Femorotibial, Semi-Constrained, Trunnion	Orthopedics
87MBG	Prosthesis, Knee, Femotib., Unconst., Uncem., Unicond., M/P	Orthopedics
87HSA	Prosthesis, Knee, Hemi-, Femoral	Orthopedics
87HTG	Prosthesis, Knee, Hemi-, Patellar Resurfacing, Uncemented	Orthopedics
87KRS	Prosthesis, Knee, Hemi-, Tibial Resurfacing	Orthopedics
87HSH	Prosthesis, Knee, Hemi-, Tibial Resurfacing, Uncemented	Orthopedics
87HRZ	Prosthesis, Knee, Hinged (Metal-Metal)	Orthopedics
87KMB	Prosthesis, Knee, Non-Const. (M/C Reinf. Polyeth.) Cemented	Orthopedics
87MBD	Prosthesis, Knee, P/F, Unconst., Uncem., Por., Ctd., P/M/P	Orthopedics
87UCD	Prosthesis, Knee, Patellar	Orthopedics
87KRR	Prosthesis, Knee, Patellofemoral, Semi-Constrained	Orthopedics
87KRP	Prosthesis, Knee, Patellofemorotibial, Constrained, Metal	Orthopedics
87KRQ	Prosthesis, Knee, Patellofemorotibial, Constrained, Polymer	Orthopedics
87JWH	Prosthesis, Knee, Patellofemorotibial, Semi-Constrained	Orthopedics
87MBV	Prosthesis, Knee, Patfem., S-C., UHMWPE, Pegged, Unc., P/M/P	Orthopedics
87MBH	Prosthesis, Knee, Patfem., S-C., Unc., Por., Ctd., P/M/P	Orthopedics
87MBA	Prosthesis, Knee, Patfem., Semi-Const., Unc., P/M/P, Osteo.	Orthopedics
87LXY	Prosthesis, Knee, Patfemotib., Semi-Const., P/M/P, Uncem.	Orthopedics
87UBR	Prosthesis, Knee, Total	Orthopedics
77EWL	Prosthesis, Laryngeal (Taub)	Ear/Nose/Throat
77FWN	Prosthesis, Larynx	Ear/Nose/Throat
87RMX	Prosthesis, Leg	Orthopedics
87HWF	Prosthesis, Ligament	Orthopedics
87LWA	Prosthesis, Ligament (PTFE)	Orthopedics
79JCR	Prosthesis, Mandible	Surgery
76MPL	Prosthesis, Mandibular Condyle	Dental And Oral
79JCS	Prosthesis, Maxilla	Surgery
77LGK	Prosthesis, Maxillofacial	Ear/Nose/Throat
79TDU	Prosthesis, Membrane	Surgery
87RMY	Prosthesis, Muscle	Orthopedics
79MQZ	Prosthesis, Nail	Surgery
79ESS	Prosthesis, Nasal, Dorsal	Surgery
84UAV	Prosthesis, Nerve Sheath	Cns/Neurology
85VLD	Prosthesis, Nipple	Obstetrics/Gyn
79FZE	Prosthesis, Nose, Internal	Surgery
86UBX	Prosthesis, Orbital Rim	Ophthalmology
77ETB	Prosthesis, Ossicular	Ear/Nose/Throat
77LBP	Prosthesis, Ossicular (Stapes), Absorbable Gelatin Material	Ear/Nose/Throat
77LBO	Prosthesis, Ossicular (Total), Absorbable Gelatin Material	Ear/Nose/Throat
77UBU	Prosthesis, Ossicular, Incus And Stapes	Ear/Nose/Throat
77LBM	Prosthesis, Ossicular, Porous Polyethylene	Ear/Nose/Throat
77ETA	Prosthesis, Ossicular, Total	Ear/Nose/Throat
77LBN	Prosthesis, Ossicular, Total, Porous Polyethylene	Ear/Nose/Throat
77UBV	Prosthesis, Ossicular, Total, Silicone	Ear/Nose/Throat
77ESY	Prosthesis, Otoplasty	Ear/Nose/Throat
79KDA	Prosthesis, PTFE/Carbon-Fiber	Surgery
77UBY	Prosthesis, Paranasal	Ear/Nose/Throat
78FAE	Prosthesis, Penile	Gastro/Urology
79JCW	Prosthesis, Penis, Inflatable	Surgery
79FTQ	Prosthesis, Penis, Rigid Rod	Surgery
78LKY	Prosthesis, Penis, Rigid Rod, External	Gastro/Urology
87VCP	Prosthesis, Radial/Ulnar Head	Orthopedics

PROSTHESIS (cont'd)

79ESR	Prosthesis, Rhinoplasty	Surgery
87MDI	Prosthesis, Rib Replacement	Orthopedics
84MHN	Prosthesis, Sensory	Cns/Neurology
87HSF	Prosthesis, Shoulder	Orthopedics
87KWR	Prosthesis, Shoulder, Constr., Metal/Metal or Polymer/Cem.	Orthopedics
87KYM	Prosthesis, Shoulder, Hemi-, Glenoid, Metal	Orthopedics
87HSD	Prosthesis, Shoulder, Hemi-, Humeral	Orthopedics
87MJT	Prosthesis, Shoulder, Humeral, Bipol., Hemi-, Constr., M/P	Orthopedics
87MBF	Prosthesis, Shoulder, Metal/Polymer, Uncemented	Orthopedics
87KWT	Prosthesis, Shoulder, Non-Constrained, Metal/Polymer Cem.	Orthopedics
87KWS	Prosthesis, Shoulder, Semi-Constrained, Metal/Polymer Cem.	Orthopedics
87KYL	Prosthesis, Shoulder, Semi-Constrained, Uncemented	Orthopedics
79UCY	Prosthesis, Soft Tissue	Surgery
87MJO	Prosthesis, Spine, Intervertebral Disc	Orthopedics
79FYG	Prosthesis, Splint, Nasal, External	Surgery
87MJW	Prosthesis, Subtalar Plug, Polymer	Orthopedics
87MJU	Prosthesis, Subtalar Plug, Polymer (Elastomer)	Orthopedics
85HHY	Prosthesis, Suture, Cerclage	Obstetrics/Gyn
79FTP	Prosthesis, Tendon	Surgery
87HXA	Prosthesis, Tendon, Passive	Orthopedics
78FAF	Prosthesis, Testicle	Gastro/Urology
79FTO	Prosthesis, Testicle, Surgical	Surgery
89ISS	Prosthesis, Thigh Socket, External Component	Physical Med
87RNA	Prosthesis, Tibial	Orthopedics
87UCM	Prosthesis, Toe	Orthopedics
87LZJ	Prosthesis, Toe (Metaphal.), Joint, Met./Poly., Semi-Const.	Orthopedics
87KWH	Prosthesis, Toe, Constrained, Polymer	Orthopedics
87KWD	Prosthesis, Toe, Hemi-, Phalangeal	Orthopedics
79JCT	Prosthesis, Trachea	Surgery
87JDD	Prosthesis, Upper Femoral	Orthopedics
78FAG	Prosthesis, Urethral Sphincter	Gastro/Urology
78EZZ	Prosthesis, Vas Deferans	Gastro/Urology
74MUX	Prosthesis, Vascular	Cardiovascular
74DYF	Prosthesis, Vascular Graft, Less Than 6mm Diameter	Cardiovascular
74DSY	Prosthesis, Vascular Graft, Of 6mm And Greater Diameter	Cardiovascular
74MIM	Prosthesis, Venous Valve	Cardiovascular
87JWI	Prosthesis, Wrist, 2 Part Metal-Plastic Articulation	Orthopedics
87JWJ	Prosthesis, Wrist, 3 Part Metal-Plastic-Metal Articulation	Orthopedics
87KWN	Prosthesis, Wrist, Carpal Lunate	Orthopedics
87KWO	Prosthesis, Wrist, Carpal Scaphoid	Orthopedics
87KYI	Prosthesis, Wrist, Carpal Trapezium	Orthopedics
87KYN	Prosthesis, Wrist, Constrained, Metal	Orthopedics
87KIG	Prosthesis, Wrist, Constrained, Polymer	Orthopedics
87KXE	Prosthesis, Wrist, Hemi-, Ulnar	Orthopedics
87KWM	Prosthesis, Wrist, Semi-Constrained	Orthopedics
77UCA	Prosthesis, Zygomatic	Ear/Nose/Throat
80WXG	Service, Tissue Bank	General
87TEO	Shoe, Orthopedic	Orthopedics
84RTC	Shunt, Hydrocephalic	Cns/Neurology
74DTI	Sizer, Heart Valve Prosthesis	Cardiovascular
86HPZ	Sphere, Ophthalmic (Implant)	Ophthalmology
73WLI	Stent, Tracheal	Anesthesiology
74WLQ	Stent, Vascular	Cardiovascular
84MBY	Stimulator, Vagus Nerve, Epilepsy, Implanted	Cns/Neurology
89ISP	Valve, Prosthesis	Physical Med
80WMV	Vision Aid, Braille	General
86HPF	Vision Aid, Electronic, AC-Powered	Ophthalmology
86HPG	Vision Aid, Electronic, Battery-Powered	Ophthalmology
86HOT	Vision Aid, Image Intensification, Battery-Powered	Ophthalmology
86HPI	Vision Aid, Optical, AC-Powered	Ophthalmology
86HPE	Vision Aid, Optical, Battery-Powered	Ophthalmology

PROSTHETIC

87MQO	Prosthetic Disc Nucleus Device	Orthopedics
74MOP	Rotator, Prosthetic Heart Valve	Cardiovascular

PROTAMINE

81GFT	Protamine Sulphate	Hematology

PROTARGOL

88KKG	Protargol S	Pathology

PROTECTINS

81KSI	Lectins/Protectins	Hematology

PROTECTION

80WNB	Amputation Protection Unit	General
80WSG	Case, Protection, Equipment	General
80WRQ	Equipment, Building Security	General
86WHZ	Goggles, Protective, Eye	Ophthalmology
90RSW	Shield, X-Ray	Radiology
90RSV	Shield, X-Ray, Brick	Radiology
90TDY	Shield, X-Ray, Door	Radiology
90WPD	Shield, X-Ray, Lead-Plastic	Radiology
76EAK	Shield, X-Ray, Leaded	Dental And Oral

PROTECTION (cont'd)

90TEN	Shield, X-Ray, Portable	Radiology
90VGQ	Shield, X-Ray, Throat	Radiology
90VLA	Shield, X-Ray, Transparent	Radiology

PROTECTIVE

90IWO	Apron, Lead, Radiographic	Radiology
80QDJ	Bib	General
80WMY	Clothing, Protective	General
79MIW	Clothing, Protective, Sun	Surgery
80MMP	Cover, Barrier, Protective	General
80VFA	Cover, Bedrail	General
80WHM	Cover, Seat, Toilet, Sanitary	General
90IWQ	Curtain, Protective, Radiographic	Radiology
80SHH	Equipment, Device Coating, Protective	General
86TCB	Eyeglasses, Safety	Ophthalmology
78EYQ	Garment, Protective, For Incontinence	Gastro/Urology
80QYK	Glove, Other	General
90IWP	Glove, Protective, Radiographic	Radiology
86WHZ	Goggles, Protective, Eye	Ophthalmology
80WYZ	Liner, Glove	General
80WKE	Mask, Face	General
80FQG	Mask, Oxygen, Other	General
89MNE	Orthosis, Moldable, Supportive, Skin Protective	Physical Med
80WUI	Protector, Puncture, Needle	General
80FMQ	Restraint, Protective (Body)	General
73WJE	Resuscitator, Emergency, Protective, Infection	Anesthesiology
80SHG	Service, Device Coating, Protective	General
90KPY	Shield, Protective, Personnel	Radiology
80WVH	Sock, Protective, Skin	General
80WTK	Support, Cover, Bed	General
80MEG	Syringe, Antistick	General

PROTECTOR

80VLY	Cap, Tip, Syringe	General
80TDS	Plug, Electrical	General
73BRW	Protector, Dental	Anesthesiology
87QWH	Protector, Finger	Orthopedics
77EWE	Protector, Hearing (Circumaural)	Ear/Nose/Throat
77EWD	Protector, Hearing (Insert)	Ear/Nose/Throat
80KIB	Protector, Heel	General
76ELQ	Protector, Mouth Guard	Dental And Oral
78EXE	Protector, Ostomy	Gastro/Urology
80WUI	Protector, Puncture, Needle	General
76EFX	Protector, Silicate	Dental And Oral
80FMP	Protector, Skin Pressure	General
79UEM	Protector, Surgical Instrument	Surgery
78FIB	Protector, Transducer, Dialysis	Gastro/Urology
78EYF	Protector, Wound, Plastic	Gastro/Urology
79KGW	Ring Drape Retention, Internal (Wound Protector)	Surgery

PROTEIN

75UHY	Analyzer, Peptide & Protein Sequence	Chemistry
75UHL	Analyzer, Protein	Chemistry
82CZQ	Antigen, Antiserum, Control, Bence-Jones Protein	Immunology
82DHL	Antigen, Antiserum, Control, Protein, Complement	Immunology
75UHM	Concentrator, Protein	Chemistry
75JIK	Dry Ash Method, Protein Bound Iodine	Chemistry
75CEF	Electrophoretic, Protein Fractionation	Chemistry
75JQJ	Fractionation, Protein, Densitometric	Chemistry
75JKN	Heat-Precipitation, Bence-Jones Protein	Chemistry
82JKM	Immunochemical, Bence-Jones Protein	Immunology
75JQK	Immunodiffusion, Protein Fractionation	Chemistry
75JIR	Indicator Method, Protein Or Albumin (Urinary, Non-Quant.)	Chemistry
82MEL	Kit, RIA, Basic Protein, Myelin	Immunology
75JGP	Lowry (Colorimetric), Total Protein	Chemistry
87MIL	Prosthesis, Hip, Semi-Const., Uncem., M/P, Bone Morph. Prot.	Orthopedics
82MME	Proteins, Amyloid And Precursor	Immunology
75CEK	Reagent, Protein, Total	Chemistry
75JRE	Refractometer	Chemistry
75JGR	Refractometric, Total Protein	Chemistry
82CZS	Retinol-Binding Protein, Antigen, Antiserum, Control	Immunology
75UHN	Separator, Protein	Chemistry
83LHJ	Staphylococcus Aureus Protein A Insoluble	Microbiology
75UIP	Synthesizer, Peptide & Protein	Chemistry
82DCN	Test, C-Reactive Protein	Immunology
82DCK	Test, C-Reactive Protein, FITC	Immunology
82DCH	Test, C-Reactive Protein, Rhodamine	Immunology
82LTN	Test, Myelin, Basic Protein	Immunology
75JIQ	Turbidimetric Method, Protein Or Albumin (Urinary)	Chemistry
75JGQ	Turbidimetric, Total Protein	Chemistry
75JIJ	Wet Ash Method, Protein Bound Iodine	Chemistry

PROTEUS

83GSY	Antisera, Fluorescent, All Globulins, Proteus SPP.	Microbiology

PROTHROMBIN

82DDF	Antigen, Antiserum, Control, Prothrombin	Immunology

PROTHROMBIN (cont'd)

81MIF	Prothrombin Fragment 1.2	Hematology
81GJS	Prothrombin Time	Hematology
81JPF	Prothrombin-Proconvertin And Thrombotest	Hematology
81GGQ	Test, Prothrombin Consumption	Hematology

PROTHROMBIN-PROCONVERTIN

81JPF	Prothrombin-Proconvertin And Thrombotest	Hematology

PROTHROMETER

81GLR	Prothrometer	Hematology

PROTOPORPHYRIN

91DNX	Protoporphyrin Zinc Method, Fluorometric, Lead	Toxicology
91DMK	Protoporphyrin, Fluorometric, Lead	Toxicology

PROTOTYPE

80WTQ	Service, Attorney, Patent	General
80WND	Service, Engineering/Design	General

PROTRACTOR

87HTH	Protractor	Orthopedics

PROXIMAL

87JDO	Implant, Fixation Device, Proximal Femoral	Orthopedics

PSA

82LTJ	Antigen, Prostate-Specific (PSA), Management, Cancer	Immunology
82MGY	Radioimmunoassay, Prostate-Specific Antigen (PSA)	Immunology
82MTG	Test, Prostate Specific Antigen, Free, (Noncomplexed) To Distinguish Prostate Cancer from Benign Conditions	Immunology
82MTF	Total, Prostate Specific Antigen (noncomplexed & complexed) for Detection of Prostate Cancer	Immunology

PSEUDOCHOLINESTERASE

91JNI	Acetylcholine Iodine and DTNB, Pseudocholinesterase	Toxicology
91DLI	Reagent, Acetylcholine Chloride	Toxicology

PSEUDOMALLEI

83GSR	Antiserum, Fluorescent, Pseudomonas Pseudomallei	Microbiology
83GST	Antiserum, Pseudomonas Pseudomallei	Microbiology

PSEUDOMONAS

83GSS	Antisera, Fluorescent, Pseudomonas Aeruginosa	Microbiology
83GSR	Antiserum, Fluorescent, Pseudomonas Pseudomallei	Microbiology
83GST	Antiserum, Pseudomonas Pseudomallei	Microbiology
83JSZ	Kit, Identification, Pseudomonas	Microbiology

PSITTACOSIS

83GPW	Antigen, CF, Psittacosis (Chlamydia Group)	Microbiology
83GPT	Antiserum, CF, Psittacosis (Chlamydia Group)	Microbiology

PTCA

78QIU	Catheter, Balloon, Dilatation, Vessel	Gastro/Urology

PTFE

79KKY	Material, PTFE/Carbon, Maxillofacial	Surgery
74DXZ	Pledget And Intracardiac Patch, PETP, PTFE, Polypropylene	Cardiovascular
77ESF	Polymer, ENT Composite Synthetic PTFE With Carbon-Fiber	Ear/Nose/Throat
87MBM	Prosthesis, Hip, Semi/Hemi-Const., M/PTFE Ctd./P, Cem./Unc.	Orthopedics
87LWA	Prosthesis, Ligament (PTFE)	Orthopedics
79KDA	Prosthesis, PTFE/Carbon-Fiber	Surgery
79WLR	Suture, Polytetrafluoroethylene	Surgery
80WTH	Tubing, Polytetrafluoroethylene	General

PTOSIS

86HJZ	Crutch, Ptosis	Ophthalmology

PUBLIC

80TDL	Public Address System	General

PUBLICATION

80WNM	Service, Publication Acquisition	General

PUDENDAL

85HEG	Kit, Anesthesia, Pudendal	Obstetrics/Gyn

PULLER

80RGP	Puller, Microelectrode	General

PULMONARY

73RNC	Analyzer, Pulmonary Function	Anesthesiology
74MFT	Band, Pulmonary Artery	Cardiovascular
73WVG	Catheter, Culture, Pulmonary	Anesthesiology
73BYN	Chair, Posture, For Cardiac And Pulmonary Treatment	Anesthesiology
73BZC	Computer, Pulmonary Function Data	Anesthesiology
73BZM	Computer, Pulmonary Function Interpretator (Diagnostic)	Anesthesiology
73QMF	Computer, Pulmonary Function Laboratory	Anesthesiology
73BTY	Computer, Pulmonary Function, Predicted Values	Anesthesiology
73QPT	Dilator, Pulmonary	Anesthesiology

PULMONARY (cont'd)

73WLD	Equipment, Therapy, Apnea	Anesthesiology
73VHT	Flowmeter, Pulmonary Function	Anesthesiology
73LLO	Laser, Neodymium:YAG, Surgical, Pulmonary	Anesthesiology
80FQG	Mask, Oxygen, Other	General
80FLS	Monitor, Apnea	General
74FYS	Monitor, Pressure, Pulmonary Artery, Powered	Cardiovascular
79FYZ	Monitor, Respiratory	Surgery
73SES	Monitor, Ventilation	Anesthesiology
73RLM	Pneumotachograph	Anesthesiology
73JAX	Pneumotachometer	Anesthesiology
80RPI	Resuscitator, Pulmonary, Gas	General
80FQB	Resuscitator, Pulmonary, Manual (Demand Valve)	General
73BWF	Spirometer, Therapeutic (Incentive)	Anesthesiology
73WWO	Surfactometer	Anesthesiology
80VFI	Transmitter/Receiver System, Pulmonary Monitor, Telephone	General
73WHT	Valve, Breathing	Anesthesiology
73CBP	Valve, Non-Rebreathing	Anesthesiology

PULP

76EKS	File, Pulp Canal, Endodontic	Dental And Oral
76EAS	Gel, Electrode, Pulp Tester	Dental And Oral
76EKP	Reamer, Pulp Canal, Endodontic	Dental And Oral
76EKK	Spreader, Pulp Canal Filling Material, Endodontic	Dental And Oral
76EAT	Tester, Pulp	Dental And Oral

PULSATILE

74JOR	Generator, Pulsatile Flow, Cardiopulmonary Bypass	Cardiovascular

PULSE

74LWY	Dual Chamber, Anti-Tachycardia, Pulse Generator	Cardiovascular
74LWP	Dual Chamber, Implantable Pulse Generator	Cardiovascular
74LOT	Module, Program, Generator, Pulse	Cardiovascular
79KFQ	Monitor, Cardiac Output, Trend (Arterial Pressure Pulse)	Surgery
73BWS	Monitor, Pulse Rate	Anesthesiology
80WOR	Oximeter, Pulse	General
85MMA	Oximeter, Pulse, Fetal	Obstetrics/Gyn
74WST	Pacemaker, Heart, Implantable, Rate Responsive	Cardiovascular
84JXF	Plethysmograph, Ocular	Cns/Neurology
74LWW	Single Chamber, Anti-Tachycardia, Pulse Generator	Cardiovascular
74LWO	Single Chamber, Sensor Driven, Implantable Pulse Generator	Cardiovascular

PULSED

89ILX	Diathermy, Shortwave, Pulsed	Physical Med
90IYN	Scanner, Ultrasonic (Pulsed Doppler)	Radiology
90IYO	Scanner, Ultrasonic (Pulsed Echo)	Radiology
90VCV	Scanner, Ultrasonic, Vascular	Radiology

PULSEMETER

73BWS	Monitor, Pulse Rate	Anesthesiology

PUMP

80MRZ	Accessories, Pump, Infusion	General
80VLP	Analyzer, Infusion Pump	General
87WHX	Aspirator, Arthroscopy	Orthopedics
80QBQ	Aspirator, Emergency Suction	General
85HFC	Aspirator, Endocervical	Obstetrics/Gyn
85HFF	Aspirator, Endometrial	Obstetrics/Gyn
78QBR	Aspirator, Low Volume (Gastric Suction)	Gastro/Urology
79QBU	Aspirator, Surgical	Surgery
74QBV	Aspirator, Thoracic (Suction Unit)	Cardiovascular
80QBZ	Aspirator, Wound Suction Pump	General
73CAC	Autotransfusion Unit (Blood)	Anesthesiology
74DWM	Canister, Suction	Cardiovascular
74QKE	Circulatory Assist Unit, Intra-Aortic Balloon	Cardiovascular
74QLZ	Compression Unit, Intermittent (Anti-Embolism Pump)	Cardiovascular
85HGG	Controller, Abortion Unit, Vacuum	Obstetrics/Gyn
74DWA	Controller, Pump Speed, Cardiopulmonary Bypass	Cardiovascular
78FHF	Evacuator, Fluid	Gastro/Urology
76EHZ	Evacuator, Oral Cavity	Dental And Oral
85HDB	Extractor, Vacuum, Fetal	Obstetrics/Gyn
79WIF	Filter, Aspirator	Surgery
80WOX	Filter, Bacteria, Pump, Breast	General
74JOR	Generator, Pulsatile Flow, Cardiopulmonary Bypass	Cardiovascular
74QZM	Heart-Lung Bypass Unit (Cardiopulmonary)	Cardiovascular
80RLQ	Infuser, Pressure (Blood Pump)	General
80LZF	Infusion Pump, Analytical Sampling	General
80LZH	Infusion Pump, Enteral	General
80LZG	Infusion Pump, Insulin	General
78TCQ	Infusion System, Insulin, With Monitor	Gastro/Urology
74DXT	Injector, Angiographic (Cardiac Catheterization)	Cardiovascular
80RCD	Injector, Syringe	General
78FKL	Insert, Blood Pump	Gastro/Urology
78FIF	Kit, Dialysis, Single Needle With Uni-Directional Pump	Gastro/Urology
89LBD	Prosthesis, Inflatable Leg, And Pump	Physical Med
85HGF	Pump, Abortion Unit, Vacuum	Obstetrics/Gyn
85HHI	Pump, Abortion, Vacuum, Central System	Obstetrics/Gyn

KEYWORD INDEX

PYRUVATE (cont'd)
75CIF Vanillin Pyruvate, AST/SGOT — Chemistry

PYRUVIC
75JLT Enzymatic (U.V.), Pyruvic Acid — Chemistry

Q-TIP
80FOR Applicator, Tipped, Absorbent — General

QDR
90WIR Densitometer, Radiography, Digital, Quantitative — Radiology

QFI
82WUO Test, Cancer Detection, QFI — Immunology

QUADRICEPS
89RNR Board, Quadriceps (Exerciser) — Physical Med

QUADRIPLEGIC
89LFF Aid, Control, Environmental, Controlled, Breath — Physical Med

QUALITATIVE
81JMH Fluorescence, Visual Observation (Qual., U.V.), Gsh — Hematology
75KQP Fluorescent Proc. (Qual.), Galactose-1-Phosphate Uridyl — Chemistry
75JLC Nitroprusside Reaction (Qualitative, Urine), Cystine — Chemistry
75JNQ Qualitative Chemical Reactions, Urinary Calculi (Stone) — Chemistry
81GGP Test, Qualitative And Quantitative Factor Deficiency — Hematology

QUALITY
80WUH Contract R&D, Equipment — General
80WQM Equipment/Service, Quality Control — General
81JPK Hematology Quality Control Mixture — Hematology
83JTR Kit, Quality Control — Microbiology
81KSF Kit, Quality Control, Blood Banking — Hematology
90SGL Monitor, X-Ray Film Processor Quality Control — Radiology
80SHO Polariscope — General
80WRB Reagent, Quality Control — General
83LJG Slide, Control, Quality — Microbiology
80WZF Tester, Alignment, Laser Beam — General
90TDZ Tester, Radiology Quality Assurance — Radiology

QUANTIFIED
84GWQ Electroencephalograph — Cns/Neurology

QUANTITATION
81KHF Adenine Nucleotide Quantitation — Hematology
81JPD Hemoglobin A2 Quantitation — Hematology
81JPC Hemoglobin F Quantitation — Hematology
81JBQ Quantitation, Antithrombin III — Hematology
81GKA Quantitation, Hemoglobin, Abnormal — Hematology

QUANTITATIVE
75CES Chromogenesis, Phenylketones (Urinary, Non-Quantitative) — Chemistry
90WIR Densitometer, Radiography, Digital, Quantitative — Radiology
75JMT Diazo (Colorimetric), Nitrite (Urinary, Non-Quantitative) — Chemistry
75CDM Diazonium Colorimetry, Urobilinogen (Urinary, Non-Quant.) — Chemistry
75JIL Enzymatic Method, Glucose (Urinary, Non-Quantitative) — Chemistry
75JGK Ferric Chloride, Phenylketones (Urinary, Non-Quantitative) — Chemistry
81JBL Glucose-6-Phos. Dehydrogenase (Erythrocytic), Quantitative — Hematology
75JIR Indicator Method, Protein Or Albumin (Urinary, Non-Quant.) — Chemistry
75CEN Indicator, pH, Dye (Urinary, Non-Quantitative) — Chemistry
75JIM Metallic Reduction Method, Glucose (Urinary, Non-Quant.) — Chemistry
75JIN Nitroprusside, Ketones (Urinary, Non-Quantitative) — Chemistry
81GJG Pipette, Quantitative, Hematology — Hematology
82WUO Test, Cancer Detection, QFI — Immunology
81GGP Test, Qualitative And Quantitative Factor Deficiency — Hematology
81MZH Test, Quantitative, For Hla, Non-diagnostic — Hematology
75LPS Urinary Homocystine (Non-Quantitative) Test System — Chemistry

QUARTER
86UAX Cap, Ophthalmic, Quarter Globe — Ophthalmology

QUICK
80QWL Fitting, Quick Connect (Gas Connector) — General

QUINIDINE
91LBZ Enzyme Immunoassay, Quinidine — Toxicology

QUININE
91LAL Gas Chromatography, Quinine — Toxicology
91LAM High Pressure Liquid Chromatography, Quinine — Toxicology
91DIK Thin Layer Chromatography, Quinine — Toxicology

R&D
80VAN Contract R&D, Diagnostics — General
80WUH Contract R&D, Equipment — General
83UGH Genetic Engineering — Microbiology

R-WAVE
74QZN Monitor, Heart Rate, R-Wave (ECG) — Cardiovascular

RABBIT
83UMA Animal, Laboratory — Microbiology
83JTL Plasma, Coagulase, Human/Horse/Rabbit — Microbiology
91DND RIA, Digitoxin (125-I), Rabbit Antibody, Solid Phase Sep. — Toxicology
91DOW RIA, Digitoxin (3-H), Rabbit Antibody, Coated Tube — Toxicology
91DNS RIA, Digoxin (125-I), Rabbit Antibody, Double Label Sep. — Toxicology
91DNQ RIA, Digoxin (3-H), Rabbit Antibody, Coated Tube Sep. — Toxicology
91DPG Radioimmunoassay, Digitoxin (125-I), Rabbit, Coated Tube — Toxicology
91DNW Radioimmunoassay, Digitoxin (3-H), Rabbit Antibody, Char. — Toxicology
91DNL Radioimmunoassay, Digoxin (125-I), Rabbit, 2nd Antibody — Toxicology
91DPB Radioimmunoassay, Digoxin (125-I), Rabbit, Charcoal — Toxicology
91DPO Radioimmunoassay, Digoxin (125-I), Rabbit, Coated Tube — Toxicology
91DOG Radioimmunoassay, Digoxin (125-I), Rabbit, Poly. Glycol — Toxicology
91DON Radioimmunoassay, Digoxin (125-I), Rabbit, Solid Phase — Toxicology
91DPD Radioimmunoassay, Digoxin (3-H), Rabbit, Charcoal — Toxicology

RABIES
83GOI Antiserum, Fluorescent, Rabies Virus — Microbiology

RACK
80WVU Cabinet, Storage, Catheter — General
81GHY Hematocrit Tube, Rack, Sealer, Holder — Hematology
80RNS Rack, Bedpan — General
84HBR Rack, Clip — Cns/Neurology
75TDX Rack, Drying — Chemistry
79FSN Rack, Glove, Operating Room — Surgery
79SIO Rack, Instrument, Laparoscopy — Surgery
80RGL Rack, Medical Chart — General
86HMH Rack, Skiascopic — Ophthalmology
79FSF Rack, Sponge, Operating Room — Surgery
79FSG Rack, Surgical Instrument — Surgery
75RNT Rack, Test Tube — Chemistry

RADIAL
82JZQ Plate, Radial Immunodiffusion — Immunology
87KWI Prosthesis, Elbow, Hemi-, Radial, Polymer — Orthopedics
87UBO Prosthesis, Elbow, Radial Component — Orthopedics
87VCP Prosthesis, Radial/Ulnar Head — Orthopedics
75CIK Radial Diffusion, Amylase — Chemistry
75CJQ Radial Immunodiffusion, Albumin — Chemistry
75JHP Radial Immunodiffusion, Lipoproteins — Chemistry
83WJV Reader, Radial Immunodiffusion — Microbiology
86VKE Surgical Instrument, Radial Keratotomy — Ophthalmology

RADIANT
85HHA Heater, Perineal, Radiant, Non-Contact — Obstetrics/Gyn
80SFJ Warmer, Radiant, Adult — General
80FMT Warmer, Radiant, Infant — General
80SFK Warmer, Radiant, Infant, Transport — General

RADIATION
90WJW Accessories, Radiotherapy — Radiology
90WIA Afterloader, Radiotherapy — Radiology
90THK Alarm, Radiation — Radiology
90WKV Block, Therapy, Radiation — Radiology
90JAI Couch, Radiation Therapy, Powered — Radiology
90RNU Counter, Radiation — Radiology
75QMU Counter, Scintillation — Chemistry
84LEO Detector, Radiation, Toftness — Cns/Neurology
90QQI Dosimeter, Radiation — Radiology
80WLA Equipment, Control, Pollution — General
80WUC Facility, Equipment, Medical, Mobile — General
90WUB Immobilizer, Therapy, Radiation — Radiology
74MOU Intravascular Radiation Delivery System — Cardiovascular
90WIB Irradiator — Radiology
80WIP Monitor, Contamination, Environmental, Personal — General
90RNV Monitor, Radiation — Radiology
90RSW Shield, X-Ray — Radiology
90RSV Shield, X-Ray, Brick — Radiology
90TDY Shield, X-Ray, Door — Radiology
90WPD Shield, X-Ray, Lead-Plastic — Radiology
76EAK Shield, X-Ray, Leaded — Dental And Oral
90TEN Shield, X-Ray, Portable — Radiology
90VGQ Shield, X-Ray, Throat — Radiology
90VLA Shield, X-Ray, Transparent — Radiology
80RVX Sterilizer, Radiation — General
90MUJ System, Planning, Radiation Therapy Treatment — Radiology
86HRL Unit, Radiation, Beta, Ophthalmic — Ophthalmology
81BSA Warmer, Blood, Electromagnetic Radiation — Hematology
73BSB Warmer, Blood, Non-Electromagnetic Radiation — Anesthesiology

RADICAL
91DJL Free Radical Assay, Amphetamine — Toxicology
91DIR Free Radical Assay, Cocaine — Toxicology
91DPC Free Radical Assay, Heavy Metals — Toxicology
91DOL Free Radical Assay, LSD — Toxicology
91DPP Free Radical Assay, Methadone — Toxicology
91DOK Free Radical Assay, Morphine — Toxicology

RADIOGRAPHIC *(cont'd)*

90LHN	Radiotherapy Unit, Charged-Particle	Radiology
90ROQ	Recorder, Radiographic Video Tape	Radiology
90VFM	Recorder, X-Ray Image	Radiology
90SGN	Sand Bag, X-Ray	Radiology
90WMF	Scanner, Computed Tomography, Cine	Radiology
84JXD	Scanner, Computed Tomography, X-Ray (CAT, CT)	Cns/Neurology
90THS	Scanner, Computed Tomography, X-Ray, Full Body	Radiology
90TEI	Scanner, Computed Tomography, X-Ray, Head	Radiology
90JAK	Scanner, Computed Tomography, X-Ray, Special Procedure	Radiology
90IXM	Screen, Intensifying, Radiographic	Radiology
76EAM	Screen, Intensifying, Radiographic, Dental	Dental And Oral
90VGP	Sensitometer, Radiographic	Radiology
76EAK	Shield, X-Ray, Leaded	Dental And Oral
90VLA	Shield, X-Ray, Transparent	Radiology
90TER	Silver Recovery Equipment	Radiology
90IXL	Spot Film Device	Radiology
90WJP	Stand, Cardiovascular	Radiology
90WLW	Stand, Vascular	Radiology
90TEY	Stretcher, Radiographic	Radiology
90RNX	Support, Patient Position, Radiographic	Radiology
90IXO	Synchronizer, ECG/Respirator, Radiographic	Radiology
90RYJ	Synchronizer, Nuclear Camera	Radiology
90RYK	Synchronizer, Radiographic Unit	Radiology
90JAC	System, Marking, Film, Radiographic	Radiology
85LHM	System, Thermographic, Liquid Crystal	Obstetrics/Gyn
90IZL	System, X-Ray, Mobile	Radiology
90KXJ	Table, Radiographic	Radiology
90IZZ	Table, Radiographic, Non-Tilting, Powered	Radiology
90IXQ	Table, Radiographic, Stationary Top	Radiology
90IXR	Table, Radiographic, Tilting	Radiology
78UEE	Table, Urological, Radiographic	Gastro/Urology
90IWB	Teletherapy System, Radionuclide	Radiology
90IXF	Test Pattern, Radiographic	Radiology
90JAD	Therapeutic X-Ray System	Radiology
85SAG	Thermographic Device, Infrared	Obstetrics/Gyn
90SAS	Timer, Radiographic	Radiology
90WOG	Transmitter, Image & Data, Radiographic	Radiology
90VHF	Tube, X-Ray	Radiology
80WNG	Tubing, Radiopaque	General
90WTF	Unit, Imaging, Thermal	Radiology
90WJC	Videofluoroscopic Unit	Radiology
90WUY	Viewer, Radiographic Film, Motorized	Radiology

RADIOGRAPHY

74QMA	Computer, Cardiac Catheterization Laboratory	Cardiovascular
90WIR	Densitometer, Radiography, Digital, Quantitative	Radiology
80TCS	Power System, Isolated	General
80WMN	Power Systems, Uninterruptible (UPS)	General

RADIOIMMUNOASSAY

82KTJ	Alpha-Fetoprotein RIA Test System	Immunology
75LCI	Analyzer, Chemistry, Radioimmunoassay	Chemistry
75ROC	Analyzer, Chemistry, Radioimmunoassay, Automated	Chemistry
75CJB	Chromatographic Separation/Radioimmunoassay, Aldosterone	Chemistry
91DNM	Counter, Gamma, Radioimmunoassay (Manual)	Toxicology
75UHK	Precipitator, Radioimmunoassay Multiple Sampling	Chemistry
91DNA	RIA, Morphine-Barbiturate (125-I), Goat Antibody	Toxicology
75JLX	Radioimmunoassay, 17-Hydroxyprogesterone	Chemistry
75CKG	Radioimmunoassay, ACTH	Chemistry
75CJM	Radioimmunoassay, Aldosterone	Chemistry
91KLQ	Radioimmunoassay, Amikacin	Toxicology
91DJP	Radioimmunoassay, Amphetamine	Toxicology
75CIZ	Radioimmunoassay, Androstenedione	Chemistry
75CIY	Radioimmunoassay, Androsterone	Chemistry
75CIB	Radioimmunoassay, Angiotensin I And Renin	Chemistry
75KHN	Radioimmunoassay, Angiotensin II	Chemistry
91DKN	Radioimmunoassay, Barbiturate	Toxicology
75JKD	Radioimmunoassay, C Peptides Of Proinsulin	Chemistry
75JKR	Radioimmunoassay, Calcitonin	Chemistry
91LAT	Radioimmunoassay, Cannabinoid (S)	Toxicology
75KWW	Radioimmunoassay, Cholyglycine, Bile Acids	Chemistry
91KLN	Radioimmunoassay, Cocaine Metabolite	Toxicology
75JKB	Radioimmunoassay, Compound S (11-Deoxycortisol)	Chemistry
75KWX	Radioimmunoassay, Conjugated Sulfalithocholic, Bile Acid	Chemistry
75CHE	Radioimmunoassay, Corticoids	Chemistry
75CHA	Radioimmunoassay, Corticosterone	Chemistry
75CGR	Radioimmunoassay, Cortisol	Chemistry
75CHO	Radioimmunoassay, Cyclic AMP	Chemistry
75CGT	Radioimmunoassay, Cyclic GMP	Chemistry
75LTB	Radioimmunoassay, Cyclosporine	Chemistry
75JKC	Radioimmunoassay, Dehydroepiandrosterone (Free And Sulfate)	Chemistry
75JLE	Radioimmunoassay, Desoxycorticosterone	Chemistry
91LCW	Radioimmunoassay, Digitoxin (125-I)	Toxicology
91DPL	Radioimmunoassay, Digitoxin (125-I), Bovine, Charcoal	Toxicology

RADIOIMMUNOASSAY *(cont'd)*

91DPG	Radioimmunoassay, Digitoxin (125-I), Rabbit, Coated Tube	Toxicology
91DOB	Radioimmunoassay, Digitoxin (3-H)	Toxicology
91DNW	Radioimmunoassay, Digitoxin (3-H), Rabbit Antibody, Char.	Toxicology
91DPI	Radioimmunoassay, Digoxin	Toxicology
91LCS	Radioimmunoassay, Digoxin (125-I)	Toxicology
91DOA	Radioimmunoassay, Digoxin (125-I), Goat Anion Exchange	Toxicology
91DNJ	Radioimmunoassay, Digoxin (125-I), Goat, 2nd Antibody	Toxicology
91DNL	Radioimmunoassay, Digoxin (125-I), Rabbit, 2nd Antibody	Toxicology
91DPB	Radioimmunoassay, Digoxin (125-I), Rabbit, Charcoal	Toxicology
91DPO	Radioimmunoassay, Digoxin (125-I), Rabbit, Coated Tube	Toxicology
91DOG	Radioimmunoassay, Digoxin (125-I), Rabbit, Poly. Glycol	Toxicology
91DON	Radioimmunoassay, Digoxin (125-I), Rabbit, Solid Phase	Toxicology
91LCT	Radioimmunoassay, Digoxin (3-H)	Toxicology
91DOR	Radioimmunoassay, Digoxin (3-H), Bovine, Charcoal	Toxicology
91DPD	Radioimmunoassay, Digoxin (3-H), Rabbit, Charcoal	Toxicology
91DLP	Radioimmunoassay, Diphenylhydantoin	Toxicology
75CHP	Radioimmunoassay, Estradiol	Chemistry
75CGI	Radioimmunoassay, Estriol	Chemistry
75CGF	Radioimmunoassay, Estrone	Chemistry
91DJX	Radioimmunoassay, Ethosuximide	Toxicology
75JLF	Radioimmunoassay, Etiocholanolone	Chemistry
83JMG	Radioimmunoassay, Ferritin	Microbiology
75CGN	Radioimmunoassay, Folic Acid	Chemistry
75CGJ	Radioimmunoassay, Follicle Stimulating Hormone	Chemistry
75CEC	Radioimmunoassay, Free Thyroxine	Chemistry
75CGC	Radioimmunoassay, Gastrin	Chemistry
91DJB	Radioimmunoassay, Gentamicin (125-I), Second Antibody	Toxicology
75JME	Radioimmunoassay, Glucagon	Chemistry
75JHI	Radioimmunoassay, Human Chorionic Gonadotropin	Chemistry
75CFL	Radioimmunoassay, Human Growth Hormone	Chemistry
75JMF	Radioimmunoassay, Human Placental Lactogen	Chemistry
82JHR	Radioimmunoassay, Immunoglobulins (D, E)	Immunology
75CFQ	Radioimmunoassay, Immunoglobulins (G, A, M)	Chemistry
75CFP	Radioimmunoassay, Immunoreactive Insulin	Chemistry
83THL	Radioimmunoassay, Infectious Mononucleosis	Microbiology
91KJI	Radioimmunoassay, Kanamycin	Toxicology
91DLB	Radioimmunoassay, LSD (125-I)	Toxicology
75JMP	Radioimmunoassay, Long-Acting Thyroid Stimulator	Chemistry
75CEP	Radioimmunoassay, Luteinizing Hormone	Chemistry
91KXS	Radioimmunoassay, Methaqualone	Toxicology
91LAQ	Radioimmunoassay, Methotrexate	Toxicology
91DOE	Radioimmunoassay, Morphine (125-I), Goat Antibody	Toxicology
91DIQ	Radioimmunoassay, Morphine (3-H), Ammonium Sulfate	Toxicology
91LCE	Radioimmunoassay, Netilmicin (125-I)	Toxicology
75VKJ	Radioimmunoassay, Other	Chemistry
75CEW	Radioimmunoassay, Parathyroid Hormone	Chemistry
91LCL	Radioimmunoassay, Phencyclidine	Toxicology
91DKP	Radioimmunoassay, Phenobarbital	Toxicology
81LCO	Radioimmunoassay, Platelet Factor 4	Hematology
75JNG	Radioimmunoassay, Pregnenolone	Chemistry
91DIL	Radioimmunoassay, Primidone	Toxicology
75JLS	Radioimmunoassay, Progesterone	Chemistry
75CFT	Radioimmunoassay, Prolactin (Lactogen)	Chemistry
82MGY	Radioimmunoassay, Prostate-Specific Antigen (PSA)	Immunology
91LBY	Radioimmunoassay, Sisomicin	Toxicology
75CDY	Radioimmunoassay, T3 Uptake	Chemistry
75UKB	Radioimmunoassay, T4	Chemistry
75CDZ	Radioimmunoassay, Testosterones And Dihydrotestosterone	Chemistry
91LCA	Radioimmunoassay, Theophylline	Toxicology
75JLW	Radioimmunoassay, Thyroid Stimulating Hormone	Chemistry
75CEE	Radioimmunoassay, Thyroxine Binding Globulin	Chemistry
91KLB	Radioimmunoassay, Tobramycin	Toxicology
75JMD	Radioimmunoassay, Total Estrogen, Other	Chemistry
75CHM	Radioimmunoassay, Total Estrogens In Pregnancy	Chemistry
75CDX	Radioimmunoassay, Total Thyroxine	Chemistry
75CDP	Radioimmunoassay, Total Triiodothyronine	Chemistry
91LFG	Radioimmunoassay, Tricyclic Antidepressant Drugs	Toxicology
91LEH	Radioimmunoassay, Vancomycin	Toxicology
75CDD	Radioimmunoassay, Vitamin B12	Chemistry
91DJK	Serum, Control, Digitoxin, RIA	Toxicology
91DMP	Serum, Control, Digoxin, RIA	Toxicology
75VKI	Test, Radioreceptor	Chemistry

RADIOISOTOPE

90QFP	Calibrator, Radioisotope	Radiology
74TAV	Cardiac Output Unit, Radioisotope Probe	Cardiovascular
90WQO	Detector, Radioisotope	Radiology
75UIC	Source, Radioisotope Reference	Chemistry
90ROD	Transfer Unit, Radioisotope	Radiology

RADIOLABELED

75KLI	Enzyme Immunoassay, Non-Radiolabeled, Total Thyroxine	Chemistry

RADIOLOGIC

90VET	Lift, Patient, Radiologic	Radiology

RAY (cont'd)

90IYC	Generator, Therapeutic X-Ray, Orthovoltage	Radiology
90UFC	Handling Unit, Automatic Daylight X-Ray Film	Radiology
90VHK	Hanger, X-Ray Tube	Radiology
76EGZ	Holder, X-Ray Film	Dental And Oral
90VGT	Holder, X-Ray Film Cassette, Vertical	Radiology
90ITY	Housing, X-Ray Tube, Diagnostic	Radiology
90ITZ	Housing, X-Ray Tube, Therapeutic	Radiology
90IXC	Illuminator, Radiographic Film	Radiology
90IXK	Imager, X-Ray, Electrostatic	Radiology
90TGW	Interlock System, X-Ray Darkrooms	Radiology
90SGK	Labeler, X-Ray Film	Radiology
90RFX	Marker, X-Ray	Radiology
90VFC	Mask, X-Ray Shield	Radiology
90TFR	Minifier, X-Ray Film (Reducer)	Radiology
90WHY	Mixer, Chemical, Film, X-Ray	Radiology
90SGL	Monitor, X-Ray Film Processor Quality Control	Radiology
90VGH	Monitor, X-Ray Tube	Radiology
90IYB	Mount, X-Ray Tube, Diagnostic	Radiology
90VGV	Projector, X-Ray Film	Radiology
76RNY	Radiographic Unit, Diagnostic, Dental (X-Ray)	Dental And Oral
90RNZ	Radiographic Unit, Diagnostic, Fixed (X-Ray)	Radiology
90ROB	Radiographic Unit, Diagnostic, Portable (X-Ray)	Radiology
90VFM	Recorder, X-Ray Image	Radiology
90VGO	Safelight, X-Ray	Radiology
90SGN	Sand Bag, X-Ray	Radiology
84JXD	Scanner, Computed Tomography, X-Ray (CAT, CT)	Cns/Neurology
90THS	Scanner, Computed Tomography, X-Ray, Full Body	Radiology
90TEI	Scanner, Computed Tomography, X-Ray, Head	Radiology
90JAK	Scanner, Computed Tomography, X-Ray, Special Procedure	Radiology
90RSW	Shield, X-Ray	Radiology
90RSV	Shield, X-Ray, Brick	Radiology
90TDY	Shield, X-Ray, Door	Radiology
90WPD	Shield, X-Ray, Lead-Plastic	Radiology
76EAK	Shield, X-Ray, Leaded	Dental And Oral
90TEN	Shield, X-Ray, Portable	Radiology
90VGQ	Shield, X-Ray, Throat	Radiology
90VLA	Shield, X-Ray, Transparent	Radiology
79RVK	Sponge, X-Ray Detectable	Surgery
90UAB	Storage Unit, X-Ray Film	Radiology
90IZL	System, X-Ray, Mobile	Radiology
90JAD	Therapeutic X-Ray System	Radiology
90IZE	Tube, Image Amplifier, X-Ray	Radiology
90VHF	Tube, X-Ray	Radiology

RAYON

80RVI	Sponge, Rayon Cellulose	General

RAZOR

80QLB	Clipper, Hair	General
80RLP	Kit, Prep	General
79LWK	Surgical, Razor	Surgery

RBC

81JPH	Analyzer, Sedimentation Rate, Erythrocyte	Hematology
81JZK	Antigen, Antiserum, Control, Red Cells	Hematology
81KSA	Calibrator, Red Cell And White Cell Counting	Hematology
81GJR	Control, Red Cell	Hematology
81JBE	Enzyme, Cell (Erythrocytic And Leukocytic)	Hematology
81GJN	Fluid, Red Cell Diluting	Hematology
81GGK	Fluid, Red Cell Lysing	Hematology
81JBM	Glucose-6-Phosphate Dehydrogenase (Erythrocytic), Electro	Hematology
81JBF	Glucose-6-Phosphate Dehydrogenase (Erythrocytic), Screening	Hematology
81JBG	Glucose-6-Phosphate Dehydrogenase (Erythrocytic), Spot	Hematology
81KQH	Red Cell Indices	Hematology
81JPJ	Red Cell Indices, Calculated	Hematology
81LIM	Test, D Positive Fetal Rbc	Hematology
81KQE	Test, Erythrocytic Glucose-6-Phosphate Dehydrogenase	Hematology

REACHER

80TFZ	Reacher (Handicapped)	General

REACTION

75JLC	Nitroprusside Reaction (Qualitative, Urine), Cystine	Chemistry
83UHQ	Reaction Apparatus	Microbiology

REACTIONS

80LMY	Monitor, Skin Resistance/skin Temperature, For Insulin Reactions	General
75JNQ	Qualitative Chemical Reactions, Urinary Calculi (Stone)	Chemistry

REACTIVE

83GMR	Serum, Reactive And Non-Specific Control, FTA-ABS Test	Microbiology
82DCN	Test, C-Reactive Protein	Immunology
82DCK	Test, C-Reactive Protein, FITC	Immunology
82DCH	Test, C-Reactive Protein, Rhodamine	Immunology

READER

80VFR	Computer, Bar Code	General
80WMS	Reader, Bar Code	General
86HJY	Reader, Bar, Ophthalmic	Ophthalmology
80WOD	Reader, Microplate	General
86HJX	Reader, Prism, Ophthalmic	Ophthalmology
83WJV	Reader, Radial Immunodiffusion	Microbiology
88MNM	Reader, Slide, Cytology, Cervical, Automated	Pathology
83KZK	Reader, Zone, Automated	Microbiology
80WLU	Washer, Microplate	General

READING

86HJG	Reading System, Closed-Circuit Television	Ophthalmology

REAGENT

75CER	2, 4-dinitrophenylhydrazine, Lactate Dehydrogenase	Chemistry
91DIC	Alcohol Dehydrogenase, Spec. Reagent - Ethanol Enzyme	Toxicology
80WLH	Contract Manufacturing, Reagent	General
80VAN	Contract R&D, Diagnostics	General
83MBT	DNA-Probe, Reagent	Microbiology
83JTO	Disc, Strip And Reagent, Microorganism Differentiation	Microbiology
88KQD	General Hematology Reagent	Pathology
75JNF	Ion Exchange Resin, Ehrlich's Reagent, Porphobilinogen	Chemistry
91DMR	M-Nitrophenol Solution, Specific Reagent For Cholinesterase	Toxicology
81GIT	Partial Thromboplastin Time, Reagent, Control	Hematology
75CEO	Phosphorus Reagent (Test System)	Chemistry
91DMI	Potassium Dichromate Specific Reagent For Alcohol	Toxicology
75JRT	Purification System, Water, Reverse Osmosis, Reagent Grade	Chemistry
83LHW	Reag. & Equipment, Erythrocyte Suspension, Multi Species	Microbiology
91DLI	Reagent, Acetylcholine Chloride	Toxicology
75CJZ	Reagent, Albumin, Colorimetric	Chemistry
75CJA	Reagent, Amylase, Colorimetric	Chemistry
83UFK	Reagent, Analyzer, Amino Acid	Microbiology
83GTQ	Reagent, Antistreptolysin-Titer/Streptolysin O	Microbiology
75CIG	Reagent, Bilirubin (Total Or Direct Test System)	Chemistry
80WRG	Reagent, Blood Gas/pH	General
75UMB	Reagent, Blood Urea Nitrogen (BUN)	Chemistry
81JCO	Reagent, Bothrops Atrox	Hematology
75JFO	Reagent, Calcium (Test System)	Chemistry
80WRA	Reagent, Calibration	General
75CHJ	Reagent, Chloride (Test System)	Chemistry
75CGO	Reagent, Cholesterol (Total Test System)	Chemistry
83LLH	Reagent, Clostridium Difficile Toxin	Microbiology
75CGX	Reagent, Creatinine (Test System)	Chemistry
81GJZ	Reagent, Cyanomethemoglobin, With Standard	Hematology
83MDJ	Reagent, Cysticercosis	Microbiology
83MDF	Reagent, DNA-Probe, Coccidioides Immitis	Microbiology
83MDE	Reagent, DNA-Probe, Cryptococcal	Microbiology
83MDK	Reagent, DNA-Probe, Streptococcal	Microbiology
91DMO	Reagent, Forming, Alkaloid, Microcrystalline	Toxicology
88LDT	Reagent, General Purpose	Pathology
75JGE	Reagent, Globulin (Test System)	Chemistry
75CGA	Reagent, Glucose (Test System)	Chemistry
81GGG	Reagent, Guaiac	Hematology
83LIE	Reagent, Inoculator Calibration (Laboratory)	Microbiology
75CFM	Reagent, Iron (Test System)	Chemistry
75JFX	Reagent, Kinase, Phosphate, Creatine	Chemistry
83UML	Reagent, Legionella Detection	Microbiology
83LOO	Reagent, Leishmanii Serological	Microbiology
91DML	Reagent, NAD-NADH, Alcohol Enzyme Method	Toxicology
81KHE	Reagent, Occult Blood	Hematology
80WPW	Reagent, Other	General
81GHR	Reagent, Platelet Aggregation	Hematology
75CEK	Reagent, Protein, Total	Chemistry
80WRB	Reagent, Quality Control	General
81GIR	Reagent, Russel Viper Venom	Hematology
83LQI	Reagent, Serological, Delta, Hepatitis	Microbiology
83GTS	Reagent, Streptolysin O/Antistreptolysin-Titer	Microbiology
91DKM	Reagent, Test, Carbon Monoxide	Toxicology
91DJW	Reagent, Test, Chloral Hydrate	Toxicology
91DMA	Reagent, Test, Fluoride	Toxicology
91DLA	Reagent, Test, Methyl Alcohol	Toxicology
91DKI	Reagent, Test, Ouabain	Toxicology
91DJQ	Reagent, Test, Phenothiazine	Toxicology
91DKW	Reagent, Test, Sulphanimide Derivative	Toxicology
81GGO	Reagent, Thromboplastin, With Control	Hematology
88UJH	Reagent, Virus, General	Pathology
91DLE	Reagents, Test, Bromides	Toxicology
88HZT	Stain, Reagent, Schiff	Pathology
75WTX	Strip, Test	Chemistry
78MSY	Strip, Test, Reagent, Residuals For Dialysate, Disinfectant	Gastro/Urology
83LTS	Test, Reagent, Biochemical, Neisseria Gonorrhoeae	Microbiology
88SAV	Tissue Embedding Equipment/Reagent	Pathology

KEYWORD INDEX

RECTAL *(cont'd)*

78KPH	Catheter, Rectal, Ileostomy, Continent	Gastro/Urology
78QKP	Clamp, Rectal	Gastro/Urology
78FFP	Dilator, Rectal	Gastro/Urology
78RAM	Hook, Rectal	Gastro/Urology
78EXX	Probe, Rectal, Non-Powered	Gastro/Urology
78RPV	Retractor, Rectal	Gastro/Urology
78RRN	Scissors, Rectal	Gastro/Urology
78FFQ	Speculum, Rectal	Gastro/Urology
78SDH	Tube, Rectal	Gastro/Urology

RECTILINEAR

90IYW	Scanner, Nuclear, Rectilinear	Radiology

RECYCLING

80VBL	Recovery Equipment, Waste Heat	General
80VAQ	Recovery Equipment, Water	General
90TER	Silver Recovery Equipment	Radiology
75UIA	Still, Solvent Recovery	Chemistry

RED

81JPH	Analyzer, Sedimentation Rate, Erythrocyte	Hematology
81JZK	Antigen, Antiserum, Control, Red Cells	Hematology
81KSA	Calibrator, Red Cell And White Cell Counting	Hematology
75CIL	Colorimetry, Cresol Red, Carbon-Dioxide	Chemistry
81GJP	Control, Platelet	Hematology
81GJR	Control, Red Cell	Hematology
81JBE	Enzyme, Cell (Erythrocytic And Leukocytic)	Hematology
81GJN	Fluid, Red Cell Diluting	Hematology
81GGK	Fluid, Red Cell Lysing	Hematology
81JBM	Glucose-6-Phosphate Dehydrogenase (Erythrocytic), Electro	Hematology
81JBF	Glucose-6-Phosphate Dehydrogenase (Erythrocytic), Screening	Hematology
81JBG	Glucose-6-Phosphate Dehydrogenase (Erythrocytic), Spot	Hematology
81GII	Glutathione, Red Cell	Hematology
81GLQ	Mixture, Control, Indices, White and Red Cell	Hematology
81KQH	Red Cell Indices	Hematology
81JPJ	Red Cell Indices, Calculated	Hematology
81JBW	Red Cell Indices, Measured	Hematology
81JWP	Red Cell Survival Test	Hematology
82DGF	Red Cells, FITC, Antigen, Antiserum, Control	Immunology
82DFW	Red Cells, Rhodamine, Antigen, Antiserum, Control	Immunology
88HZY	Sirius Red	Pathology
75JLK	Sodium Hydroxide/Phenol Red (Titrimetric), Gastric Acidity	Chemistry
88IDD	Stain, Alizarin Red	Pathology
88ICH	Stain, Congo Red	Pathology
88ICD	Stain, Darrow Red	Pathology
88HYD	Stain, Fast Red Salt B	Pathology
88KFE	Stain, Neutral Red	Pathology
88HZF	Stain, Nuclear Fast Red	Pathology
88HZG	Stain, Oil Red O	Pathology
88HZQ	Stain, Red-Violet LB	Pathology
81LIM	Test, D Positive Fetal Rbc	Hematology
81KQE	Test, Erythrocytic Glucose-6-Phosphate Dehydrogenase	Hematology
75CHR	Titrimetric Phenol Red, Carbon-Dioxide	Chemistry

RED-VIOLET

88HZQ	Stain, Red-Violet LB	Pathology

REDUCER

90TFR	Minifier, X-Ray Film (Reducer)	Radiology
86WNV	Reducer, Pressure, Intraocular	Ophthalmology

REDUCTASE

75JLO	Enzymatic (Glutathione Reductase), Glutathione	Chemistry
81KQF	Test, Glutathione Reductase	Hematology

REDUCTION

75LFQ	Acid Reduction Of Ferric Ion, Uric Acid	Chemistry
78WNS	Balloon, Gastric	Gastro/Urology
75CFW	Copper Reduction, Glucose	Chemistry
81JBJ	Glucose-6-Phos. Dehydrogenase (Erythrocy.), Methemogl. Red.	Hematology
80WYO	Mattress, Reduction, Pressure	General
75JIM	Metallic Reduction Method, Glucose (Urinary, Non-Quant.)	Chemistry
75KLJ	NAD Reduction (U.V.), Phosphohexose Isomerase	Chemistry
75CGS	NAD Reduction/NADH Oxidation, CPK Or Isoenzymes	Chemistry
75CFJ	NAD Reduction/NADH Oxidation, Lactate Dehydrogenase	Chemistry
75CIT	NADH Oxidation/NAD Reduction, AST/SGOT	Chemistry
81JMC	NADP Reduction (U.V.), Glucose-6-Phosphate Dehydrogenase	Hematology
75JND	NADP Reduction, 6-Phosphogluconate Dehydrogenase	Chemistry
75CJD	Nitrosalicylate Reduction, Amylase	Chemistry
75CDH	Phosphotungstate Reduction, Uric Acid	Chemistry
84LEN	Stimulator, Reduction, Anxiety, Electrical	Cns/Neurology

REFERENCE

80WRA	Reagent, Calibration	General
80WRB	Reagent, Quality Control	General

REFERENCE *(cont'd)*

75UIC	Source, Radioisotope Reference	Chemistry
75UJC	Standard, Ultraviolet Reference	Chemistry

REFLECTANCE

75QYL	Analyzer, Glucose	Chemistry
75JQT	Densitometer/Scanner (Integrating, Reflectance, TLC, Radio)	Chemistry
78TGM	Monitor, Blood Glucose (Test)	Gastro/Urology
75VFU	Photometer, Reflectance	Chemistry

REFLEX

89IKO	Hammer, Reflex, Powered	Physical Med

REFLUX

78LEI	Implant, Anti-Gastroesophageal Reflux	Gastro/Urology
78UDE	Prosthesis, Anti-Gastroesophageal Reflux	Gastro/Urology

REFRACTIVE

86HLB	Ophthalmodynamometer	Ophthalmology

REFRACTOMETER

75JRE	Refractometer	Chemistry
86HKO	Refractometer, Ophthalmic	Ophthalmology

REFRACTOMETRIC

75JGR	Refractometric, Total Protein	Chemistry

REFRACTOR

86HKN	Refractor, Ophthalmic	Ophthalmology

REFRIGERANT

89MLY	Refrigerant, Topical (Vapocoolant)	Physical Med

REFRIGERATED

88QJC	Centrifuge, Refrigerated	Pathology

REFRIGERATOR

81QAM	Alarm, Refrigerator	Hematology
83ROS	Refrigerator, Biological	Microbiology
81ROT	Refrigerator, Blood Bank	Hematology
87ULN	Refrigerator, Bone	Orthopedics
75ROU	Refrigerator, Explosion-Proof	Chemistry
86ULM	Refrigerator, Eye Bank	Ophthalmology
80UKW	Refrigerator, Foodservice	General
80WRM	Refrigerator, Laboratory	General
88ROV	Refrigerator, Morgue, Walk-In	Pathology
80WRL	Refrigerator, Pharmacy	General

REFURBISH

80WMO	Service, Used Equipment	General

REGENERATED

78FKT	Dialysate Delivery System, Sorbent Regenerated	Gastro/Urology

REGENTS

83LHL	Legionella Direct & Indirect Fluorescent Antibody Regents	Microbiology

REGIONAL

79QZR	Heat Exchanger, Regional Perfusion	Surgery
73RJQ	Oxygenator, Regional Perfusion	Anesthesiology

REGISTRATION

80WVL	Manual, Policies	General
80WTQ	Service, Attorney, Patent	General
80WIE	Service, Licensing, Device, Medical	General

REGISTRY

80TDQ	Physician Registry	General

REGULATED

80FOH	Mattress, Water, Temperature Regulated	General

REGULATOR

80WMK	Calibrator, Blood Gas	General
80WML	Calibrator, Mass Spectrometer	General
80QWL	Fitting, Quick Connect (Gas Connector)	General
76EFE	Flowmeter, Anesthesia	Dental And Oral
73CAX	Flowmeter, Back-Pressure Compensated, Thorpe Tube	Anesthesiology
73BXY	Flowmeter, Gas (Oxygen), Calibrated	Anesthesiology
73CCN	Flowmeter, Gas, Non-Back-Pressure Compensated, Bourdon Gauge	Anesthesiology
73ROW	Regulator, Anesthesia	Anesthesiology
73QWO	Regulator, Intake, Oxygen	Anesthesiology
80WMM	Regulator, Line Voltage	General
80FQE	Regulator, Oxygen, Mechanical	General
73CAN	Regulator, Pressure, Gas Cylinder	Anesthesiology
78ROX	Regulator, Suction, Low Volume (Gastric)	Gastro/Urology
80CBB	Regulator, Suction, Surgical	General
73ROZ	Regulator, Suction, Thoracic	Anesthesiology
77RPA	Regulator, Suction, Tracheal (Nasal, Oral)	Ear/Nose/Throat
75JRR	Regulator, Temperature	Chemistry
74DWJ	Regulator, Thermal, Cardiopulmonary Bypass	Cardiovascular
80KDP	Regulator, Vacuum	General

RESECTOSCOPE

78FJL	Resectoscope	Gastro/Urology
78FDC	Resectoscope Working Element	Gastro/Urology

RESERVOIR

73BTC	Bag, Reservoir (Blood)	Anesthesiology
74DTN	Reservoir, Blood, Cardiopulmonary Bypass	Cardiovascular
84UCC	Reservoir, Hydrocephalic Catheter	Cns/Neurology
84TEG	Reservoir, Spinal Fluid	Cns/Neurology

RESIDUALS

78MSY	Strip, Test, Reagent, Residuals For Dialysate, Disinfectant	Gastro/Urology

RESIN

76DYH	Adhesive, Bracket And Conditioner, Resin	Dental And Oral
76KXR	Applicator, Resin	Dental And Oral
76EBI	Base, Denture, Relining, Repairing, Rebasing, Resin	Dental And Oral
76EBE	Coating, Denture Hydrophilic, Resin	Dental And Oral
76EBD	Coating, Filling Material, Resin	Dental And Oral
76EBG	Crown And Bridge, Temporary, Resin	Dental And Oral
80WWD	Elastomer, Other	General
75JQE	Ion Exchange Resin, Ascorbic Acid, Colorimetry, Iron Bind	Chemistry
75JNF	Ion Exchange Resin, Ehrlich's Reagent, Porphobilinogen	Chemistry
75JQD	Ion Exchange Resin, Thioglycolic Acid, Colorimetry, Iron	Chemistry
76EBH	Material, Impression Tray, Resin	Dental And Oral
76EBF	Material, Tooth Shade, Resin	Dental And Oral
76EBJ	Primer, Cavity, Resin	Dental And Oral
76MMT	Resin, Filling, Root Canal (Containing Chloroform)	Dental And Oral
88KEA	Resin, Ion-Exchange	Pathology
80WWC	Resin, Other	General
80VAK	Resin, Plastic	General
76KIF	Resin, Root Canal Filling	Dental And Oral
76EBC	Sealant, Pit And Fissure, And Conditioner, Resin	Dental And Oral
76KLE	Tooth Bonding Agent, Resin Restoration	Dental And Oral
80WTH	Tubing, Polytetrafluoroethylene	General

RESINOUS

76VLQ	Compound, Resinous, Composite	Dental And Oral
76UDV	Resinous Compound	Dental And Oral
84UCK	Resinous Compound, Cranial	Cns/Neurology

RESINS

91DNH	Resins, Ion Exchange, Liquid Chromatography	Toxicology

RESISTANCE

89IQH	Biofeedback Equipment, Myoelectric, Battery-Powered	Physical Med
89IRC	Biofeedback Equipment, Myoelectric, Powered	Physical Med
89IKI	Meter, Skin Resistance, AC-Powered	Physical Med
89IKJ	Meter, Skin Resistance, Battery-Powered	Physical Med
80LMY	Monitor, Skin Resistance/skin Temperature, For Insulin Reactions	General
80RZW	Tester, Conductivity, Floor And Equipment	General
80RZX	Tester, Conductivity, Shoe And Gown	General
80SAD	Tester, Resistance, Line Cord	General

RESISTANT

81GHA	Hemoglobin, Resistant, Alkali	Hematology
83MYI	System, Test, Genotypic Detection, Resistant Markers, Staphylococcus Colonies	Microbiology

RESISTIVITY

75VCY	Meter, Resistivity	Chemistry

RESONANCE

90MOS	Coil, Magnetic Resonance, Specialty	Radiology
90QMD	Computer, Nuclear Medicine	Radiology
90WPG	Gas Mixtures, Magnetic Resonance Imaging	Radiology
90WRT	Magnet, Permanent, MRI (Magnetic Resonance Imaging)	Radiology
90VIM	Magnet, Superconducting, MRI (Magnetic Resonance Imaging)	Radiology
75UGY	Nuclear Magnetic Resonance Equipment, Laboratory	Chemistry
90LNH	Nuclear Magnetic Resonance Imaging System	Radiology
90LNI	Nuclear Magnetic Resonance Spectroscopic System	Radiology
90VKD	Phantom, NMR/MRI	Radiology
90JAM	Scanner, Magnetic Resonance (NMR/MRI)	Radiology
90RYK	Synchronizer, Radiographic Unit	Radiology

RESORBABLE

84MIT	Device, Nerve Repair, Resorbable	Cns/Neurology

RESORCIN

88HZR	Resorcin Fuchsin	Pathology

RESPIRATION

73VDC	Recorder, Long-Term, Respiration	Anesthesiology
73VDB	Scanner, Long-Term Recording, Respiration	Anesthesiology
73RTK	Simulator, Respiration	Anesthesiology

RESPIRATOR

90IXO	Synchronizer, ECG/Respirator, Radiographic	Radiology
73CBK	Ventilator, Continuous (Respirator)	Anesthesiology

RESPIRATOR *(cont'd)*

73LSZ	Ventilator, High-Frequency	Anesthesiology
80FQC	Ventilator, Neonatal Respirator	General
73BZD	Ventilator, Non-Continuous (Respirator)	Anesthesiology
73SEX	Ventilator, Other	Anesthesiology
73SEU	Ventilator, Pressure Cycled (IPPB Machine)	Anesthesiology
73SEV	Ventilator, Time Cycled (Iron Lung)	Anesthesiology
73SEW	Ventilator, Volume (Critical Care)	Anesthesiology

RESPIRATOR)

73MOD	Ventilator, Continuous (Respirator), Accessory	Anesthesiology

RESPIRATORY

73RNC	Analyzer, Pulmonary Function	Anesthesiology
83GQG	Antigen, CF (Including CF Controls), Respiratory Syncytial	Microbiology
83GQF	Antiserum, Neutralization, Respiratory Syncytial Virus	Microbiology
73QFQ	Calibrator, Respiratory Therapy Unit	Anesthesiology
75QMB	Computer, Clinical Laboratory	Chemistry
80WPV	Dryer, Respiratory/Anesthesia Equipment	General
83MCE	Enzyme Linked Immunoabsorbent Assay, Resp. Syncytial Virus	Microbiology
73WLD	Equipment, Therapy, Apnea	Anesthesiology
73QVA	Exerciser, Respiratory	Anesthesiology
73BTT	Humidifier, Respiratory Gas, (Direct Patient Interface)	Anesthesiology
73BYS	Lung, Membrane (For Long-Term Respiratory Support)	Anesthesiology
80FLS	Monitor, Apnea	General
73RBQ	Monitor, Impedance Pneumograph	Anesthesiology
79FYZ	Monitor, Respiratory	Surgery
73WVK	Oxygen	Anesthesiology
79RJT	Pacemaker, Respiratory	Surgery
83LKT	Respiratory Syncytial Virus, Antigen, Antibody, IFA	Microbiology
80QAI	Sampler, Air	General
84GZE	Stimulator, Diaphragmatic/Phrenic Nerve, Implantable	Cns/Neurology
80WPY	Washer, Respiratory/Anesthesia Equipment	General
83WKT	Water, Therapy, Respiratory	Microbiology

RESPIROMETER

73BZG	Spirometer, Diagnostic (Respirometer)	Anesthesiology

RESPONSE

80VFG	Communication System, Emergency Alert, Personal	General
84VKG	Computer, Brain Mapping	Cns/Neurology
84QUT	Evoked Response Unit	Cns/Neurology
77ETZ	Evoked Response Unit, Auditory	Ear/Nose/Throat
84GZO	Monitor, Response, Skin, Galvanic	Cns/Neurology
81MMG	Response Test, Antithrombin III (ATIII)	Hematology
84GWJ	Stimulator, Auditory, Evoked Response	Cns/Neurology
84GWF	Stimulator, Electrical, Evoked Response	Cns/Neurology
84GZP	Stimulator, Mechanical, Evoked Response	Cns/Neurology
84GWE	Stimulator, Photic, Evoked Response	Cns/Neurology

RESPONSIVE

74WST	Pacemaker, Heart, Implantable, Rate Responsive	Cardiovascular

REST

89QBL	Arm Rest	Physical Med
80QCE	Back Rest	General
84HBM	Head Rest, Neurosurgical	Cns/Neurology
87THC	Holder, Leg, Arthroscopy	Orthopedics
79WRY	Holder, Shoulder, Arthroscopy	Surgery
80RER	Leg Rest	General

RESTORATION

79GBI	Material, Restoration, Aesthetic, External	Surgery
76KLE	Tooth Bonding Agent, Resin Restoration	Dental And Oral

RESTORATIVE

76EID	Syringe, Restorative And Impression Material	Dental And Oral

RESTRAINING

80RWQ	Strap, Restraining	General

RESTRAINT

87RBF	Immobilizer, Ankle	Orthopedics
87RBG	Immobilizer, Arm	Orthopedics
87RBH	Immobilizer, Cervical	Orthopedics
87RBI	Immobilizer, Elbow	Orthopedics
87RBJ	Immobilizer, Infant (Circumcision Board)	Orthopedics
87RBK	Immobilizer, Knee	Orthopedics
87RBL	Immobilizer, Shoulder	Orthopedics
90WUB	Immobilizer, Therapy, Radiation	Radiology
87WUW	Immobilizer, Upper Body	Orthopedics
87RBM	Immobilizer, Wrist/Hand	Orthopedics
89KID	Restraint	Physical Med
80RPB	Restraint, Ankle/Foot	General
80RPC	Restraint, Arm	General
80RPD	Restraint, Crib	General
73BRT	Restraint, Patient, Conductive	Anesthesiology
80FMQ	Restraint, Protective (Body)	General
80RPE	Restraint, Vest	General
80RPF	Restraint, Wheelchair	General

RESTRAINT *(cont'd)*
80RPG Restraint, Wrist/Hand General

RESTRICTOR
87JDK Prosthesis, Hip, Cement Restrictor Orthopedics
87UCF Restrictor, Orthopedic Cement Orthopedics

RESURFACING
87KRM Hemiprosthesis, Elbow (Humeral Resurfacing) Orthopedics
87KXA Prosthesis, Hip, Femoral, Resurfacing Orthopedics
87KXB Prosthesis, Hip, Pelvifemoral Resurfacing, Metal/polymer Orthopedics
87HTG Prosthesis, Knee, Hemi-, Patellar Resurfacing, Uncemented Orthopedics
87KRS Prosthesis, Knee, Hemi-, Tibial Resurfacing Orthopedics
87HSH Prosthesis, Knee, Hemi-, Tibial Resurfacing, Uncemented Orthopedics

RESUSCITATION
74LIX Aid, Resuscitation, Cardiopulmonary Cardiovascular
80KMP Board (Bed and Cardiopulmonary Resuscitation) General
80FOA Board, Cardiopulmonary Resuscitation General
73BZN Cart, Emergency, Cardiopulmonary Resuscitation (Crash) Anesthesiology
73LYM Device, Assist, CPR Anesthesiology
80UDC Kit, Emergency, Cardiopulmonary Resuscitation General
80SBS Training Manikin, CPR (Resuscitation) General

RESUSCITATOR
80FQG Mask, Oxygen, Other General
73BTZ Resuscitator, Cardiac, Mechanical, Compressor Anesthesiology
74RPH Resuscitator, Cardiopulmonary Cardiovascular
76DZX Resuscitator, Emergency Oxygen Dental And Oral
73WJE Resuscitator, Emergency, Protective, Infection Anesthesiology
80RPI Resuscitator, Pulmonary, Gas General
80FQB Resuscitator, Pulmonary, Manual (Demand Valve) General
74LOR Resuscitator, Trans-Telephone Cardiovascular
73WHT Valve, Breathing Anesthesiology
73CBP Valve, Non-Rebreathing Anesthesiology
73BTM Ventilator, Emergency, Manual (Resuscitator) Anesthesiology
73BTL Ventilator, Emergency, Powered (Resuscitator) Anesthesiology

RETAINER
79QNR Holder, Instrument, Laparoscopic Surgery
80RPJ Retainer, Bandage (Elastic Net) General
76RPK Retainer, Dental Dental And Oral
76JEP Retainer, Matrix Dental And Oral
76DYJ Retainer, Screw Expansion, Orthodontic Dental And Oral
79GCZ Retainer, Surgical Surgery
79RPL Retainer, Visceral Surgery
79WRZ Retractor, Abdominal, Padded, Flexible Surgery

RETAINING
78EYX Drape, Pure Latex Sheet, With Self-Retaining Finger Cot Gastro/Urology
78FGN Retractor, Non-Self-Retaining Gastro/Urology
78FFO Retractor, Self-Retaining Gastro/Urology
84GZT Retractor, Self-Retaining, Neurology Cns/Neurology

RETENTION
78EZK Catheter, Retention Type Gastro/Urology
78EZL Catheter, Retention Type, Balloon Gastro/Urology
78FGD Catheter, Retention, Barium Enema With Bag Gastro/Urology
79KGS Retention Device, Suture Surgery
79KGW Ring Drape Retention, Internal (Wound Protector) Surgery

RETENTIVE
76EBL Pin, Retentive And Splinting Dental And Oral

RETICULOCYTE
81GJH Stain, Reticulocyte Hematology

RETINAL
86LOG Catheter, Balloon, Reattachment, Retinal Ophthalmology
86LPO Gas, Reattachment Procedure, Retinal Ophthalmology
86WJZ Implant, Retinal Ophthalmology

RETINOGRAPHIC
86QTE Electrode, Retinographic Ophthalmology

RETINOL
82CZS Retinol-Binding Protein, Antigen, Antiserum, Control Immunology

RETINOL-BINDING
82CZS Retinol-Binding Protein, Antigen, Antiserum, Control Immunology

RETINOSCOPE
86HKL Retinoscope, AC-Powered Ophthalmology
86HKM Retinoscope, Battery-Powered Ophthalmology

RETRACTION
76MVL Cord, Retraction Dental And Oral
76VEG Kit, Gingival Retraction Dental And Oral

RETRACTOR
76EIF Accessories, Retractor, Dental Dental And Oral
79SJI Balloon, Manipulation, Tissue Surgery

RETRACTOR *(cont'd)*
86HOC Clip, Iris Retractor Ophthalmology
79WRE Holder, Retractor Surgery
87HXM Retractor Orthopedics
79RPM Retractor, Abdominal Surgery
79WRZ Retractor, Abdominal, Padded, Flexible Surgery
76EIG Retractor, All Types Dental And Oral
78RPN Retractor, Bladder Gastro/Urology
84RPO Retractor, Brain Cns/Neurology
84RPP Retractor, Brain Decompression Cns/Neurology
74RPQ Retractor, Cardiac Cardiovascular
77KAL Retractor, ENT (Thoracic) Ear/Nose/Throat
79RXS Retractor, Fan-Type, Laparoscopy Surgery
78FDG Retractor, Fiberoptic Gastro/Urology
79RPS Retractor, Laminectomy Surgery
79RZZ Retractor, Laparoscopy, Other Surgery
85WWA Retractor, Mammary Obstetrics/Gyn
84GZW Retractor, Manual Cns/Neurology
77RPT Retractor, Mastoid Ear/Nose/Throat
78FGN Retractor, Non-Self-Retaining Gastro/Urology
86HNI Retractor, Ophthalmic Ophthalmology
79RPU Retractor, Orbital Surgery
79RPY Retractor, Other Surgery
78RPV Retractor, Rectal Gastro/Urology
87RPW Retractor, Rib Orthopedics
78FFO Retractor, Self-Retaining Gastro/Urology
84GZT Retractor, Self-Retaining, Neurology Cns/Neurology
79GAD Retractor, Surgical Surgery
85HDL Retractor, Vaginal Obstetrics/Gyn
74RPX Retractor, Vessel Cardiovascular
84RSB Separator, Dural Cns/Neurology
78RSC Separator, Pylorus Gastro/Urology
77RSD Separator, Stapes Ear/Nose/Throat

RETRIEVAL
78TEH Basket, Biliary Stone Retrieval Gastro/Urology
74MMX Device, Retrieval, Percutaneous Cardiovascular

RETRIEVER
78FCC Retriever, Endomagnetic Gastro/Urology

RETROGRADE
80MJF Check Valve, Retrograde Flow (In-Line) General
73MJJ Valve, CPB Check, Retrograde, In-Line Anesthesiology

RETROPERFUSION
84MBW Cranial Retroperfusion (Stroke Treatment) Cns/Neurology
74LPE System, Retroperfusion, Artery, Coronary Cardiovascular

RETURN
74QKF Circulatory Assist Unit, Venous Return Cardiovascular
79JOS Electrode, Electrosurgical, Return (Ground, Dispersive) Surgery
74DTS Sucker, Cardiotomy Return, Cardiopulmonary Bypass Cardiovascular
78FDL Wristlet, Patient Return Gastro/Urology

REUSABLE
79QQQ Drape, Surgical, Reusable Surgery
79RRW Dress, Scrub, Reusable Surgery
79QYN Gown, Operating Room, Reusable Surgery
79FYB Gown, Patient Surgery
80QYP Gown, Patient, Reusable General
79FYA Gown, Surgical Surgery
75RDV Labware, Basic, Reusable Chemistry
80RHF Mitt/Washcloth, Patient General
79GDM Needle, Aspiration And Injection, Reusable Surgery
79GDL Needle, Suture, Reusable Surgery
89IME Pack, Hot Or Cold, Reusable Physical Med
80UCV Pressure Pad, Alternating, Reusable General
90LQA Reusable Image Media Radiology
73BWP Shoe And Shoe Cover, Conductive Anesthesiology
79RSX Shoe, Conductive Surgery
79FXW Shoe, Operating Room Surgery
79GAI Stripper, Vein, Reusable Surgery
79RRZ Suit, Scrub, Reusable Surgery
79FXO Suit, Surgical Surgery
85QKH Tray, Circumcision, Reusable Obstetrics/Gyn

REVASCULARIZATION
74MNO System, Laser, Transmyocardial Revascularization Cardiovascular

REVERSE
75SGA Purification System, Water, Reverse Osmosis Chemistry
75JRT Purification System, Water, Reverse Osmosis, Reagent Grade Chemistry
81UJT Reverse Grouping Cells Hematology
75UHS Reverse Osmosis Membrane Equipment Chemistry

REVERSING
80VFD Mirror, Reversing General

RF

90LNA	*Hyperthermia Applicator, Deep Heating, RF/Microwave*	*Radiology*
90LNC	*Hyperthermia Applicator, Superficial, RF/Microwave*	*Radiology*
90LOC	*System, Cancer Treatment, Hyperthermia, RF/Microwave*	*Radiology*
78MEQ	*System, Hyperthermia, Rf/microwave (benign* Prostatic Hyperplasia), Thermotherapy	Gastro/Urology

RH

81SEY	*View Box, Rh Typing*	*Hematology*

RHEOENCEPHALOGRAPH

84GZN	*Rheoencephalograph*	*Cns/Neurology*

RHEUMATISM

89WOK	*Equipment, Cryotherapy*	*Physical Med*

RHEUMATOID

82WVP	*Test, Disease, Lyme*	*Immunology*
82DHR	*Test, Rheumatoid Factor*	*Immunology*

RHINOANEMOMETER

73BXQ	*Rhinoanemometer (Measurement Of Nasal Decongestion)*	*Anesthesiology*

RHINOMANOMETER

73RQA	*Rhinomanometer*	*Anesthesiology*

RHINOPLASTIC

79RAN	*Hook, Rhinoplastic*	*Surgery*

RHINOPLASTY

79ESR	*Prosthesis, Rhinoplasty*	*Surgery*

RHINOSCOPE

77RQB	*Rhinoscope*	*Ear/Nose/Throat*

RHINOVIRUS

83GQE	*Antisera, Neutralization, All Types, Rhinovirus*	*Microbiology*

RHODAMINE

82DDT	*Antigen, Antiserum, Alpha-2-Macroglobulin, Rhodamine*	*Immunology*
82DFJ	*Antigen, Antiserum, Control, Albumin, Rhodamine*	*Immunology*
82DFB	*Antigen, Antiserum, Control, Alpha-1-Antitrypsin,* Rhodamine	Immunology
82DCT	*Antigen, Antiserum, Control, Ceruloplasmin, Rhodamine*	*Immunology*
82DBY	*Antigen, Antiserum, Control, FAB, Rhodamine*	*Immunology*
82CZZ	*Antigen, Antiserum, Control, Haptoglobin, Rhodamine*	*Immunology*
82CZR	*Antigen, Antiserum, Control, Hemopexin, Rhodamine*	*Immunology*
82CZK	*Antigen, Antiserum, Control, IGA, Rhodamine*	*Immunology*
82DGE	*Antigen, Antiserum, Control, IGD, Rhodamine*	*Immunology*
82DGL	*Antigen, Antiserum, Control, IGE, Rhodamine*	*Immunology*
82DFO	*Antigen, Antiserum, Control, IGG, Rhodamine*	*Immunology*
82DEZ	*Antigen, Antiserum, Control, IGM, Rhodamine*	*Immunology*
82DEK	*Antigen, Antiserum, Control, Kappa, Rhodamine*	*Immunology*
82DFG	*Antigen, Antiserum, Control, Lambda, Rhodamine*	*Immunology*
82DDD	*Antigen, Antiserum, Control, Transferrin, Rhodamine*	*Immunology*
82DAR	*Antigen, Fibrinogen And Split Products, Rhodamine*	*Immunology*
82DGI	*Breast Milk, Rhodamine, Antigen, Antiserum, Control*	*Immunology*
82DBH	*FC, Rhodamine, Antigen, Antiserum, Control*	*Immunology*
82DDO	*Myoglobin, Rhodamine, Antigen, Antiserum, Control*	*Immunology*
82DFR	*Platelets, Rhodamine, Antigen, Antiserum, Control*	*Immunology*
82DFW	*Red Cells, Rhodamine, Antigen, Antiserum, Control*	*Immunology*
82DCH	*Test, C-Reactive Protein, Rhodamine*	*Immunology*
82DDL	*Thyroglobulin, Rhodamine, Antigen, Antiserum, Control*	*Immunology*

RHUSIOPATHIAE

83GSF	*Antigen, Erysipelothrix Rhusiopathiae*	*Microbiology*
83GSE	*Antiserum, Erysipelothrix Rhusiopathiae*	*Microbiology*
83GSD	*Antiserum, Fluorescent, Erysipelothrix Rhusiopathiae*	*Microbiology*

RIA

82KTJ	*Alpha-Fetoprotein RIA Test System*	*Immunology*
75ROC	*Analyzer, Chemistry, Radioimmunoassay, Automated*	*Chemistry*
91DNM	*Counter, Gamma, Radioimmunoassay (Manual)*	*Toxicology*
82MEO	*Kit, Antigen, RIA, Prostatic Acid Phosphatase*	*Immunology*
82MEL	*Kit, RIA, Basic Protein, Myelin*	*Immunology*
91DPJ	*RIA, Amphetamine (125-I), Goat Antibody, Ammonia*	*Toxicology*
91DND	*RIA, Digitoxin (125-I), Rabbit Antibody, Solid Phase Sep.*	*Toxicology*
91DOW	*RIA, Digitoxin (3-H), Rabbit Antibody, Coated Tube*	*Toxicology*
91DNS	*RIA, Digoxin (125-I), Rabbit Antibody, Double Label Sep.*	*Toxicology*
91DOY	*RIA, Digoxin (3-H), Goat Antibody, 2nd Antibody Sep.*	*Toxicology*
91DNQ	*RIA, Digoxin (3-H), Rabbit Antibody, Coated Tube Sep.*	*Toxicology*
91DNA	*RIA, Morphine-Barbiturate (125-I), Goat Antibody*	*Toxicology*
91DJK	*Serum, Control, Digitoxin, RIA*	*Toxicology*
91DMP	*Serum, Control, Digoxin, RIA*	*Toxicology*
75JZM	*System, Gonadotropin, Chorionic, Human (Non-RIA)*	*Chemistry*

RIB

87QDI	*Belt, Rib (Support)*	*Orthopedics*
87QZD	*Guillotine, Rib*	*Orthopedics*
89IPX	*Orthosis, Rib Fracture, Soft*	*Physical Med*
87MDI	*Prosthesis, Rib Replacement*	*Orthopedics*
87RPW	*Retractor, Rib*	*Orthopedics*

RIB *(cont'd)*

78EYS	*Ribdam*	*Gastro/Urology*
87HTX	*Rongeur, Rib*	*Orthopedics*
87RVO	*Spreader, Rib*	*Orthopedics*

RIBDAM

78EYS	*Ribdam*	*Gastro/Urology*

RICHARDSON

88IFJ	*Fixative, Richardson Glycol*	*Pathology*

RICKETTSIA

83LSQ	*Rickettsia Serological Reagents, Other*	*Microbiology*

RICKETTSIALPOX

83GPK	*Antiserum, Rickettsialpox*	*Microbiology*

RID

83WJV	*Reader, Radial Immunodiffusion*	*Microbiology*

RIGHT

76EGS	*Handpiece, Contra- And Right-Angle Attachment, Dental*	*Dental And Oral*

RIGHT-ANGLE

76EGS	*Handpiece, Contra- And Right-Angle Attachment, Dental*	*Dental And Oral*

RIGID

77BTN	*Bronchoscope, Non-Rigid*	*Ear/Nose/Throat*
77EOQ	*Bronchoscope, Rigid*	*Ear/Nose/Throat*
73BTJ	*Bronchoscope, Rigid, Non-Ventilating*	*Anesthesiology*
73BTH	*Bronchoscope, Rigid, Ventilating*	*Anesthesiology*
73BTG	*Brush, Biopsy, Bronchoscope (Non-Rigid)*	*Anesthesiology*
78FBN	*Choledochoscope, Flexible Or Rigid*	*Gastro/Urology*
73BST	*Curette, Biopsy, Bronchoscope (Non-Rigid)*	*Anesthesiology*
73JEL	*Curette, Biopsy, Bronchoscope (Rigid)*	*Anesthesiology*
78FAJ	*Cystoscope*	*Gastro/Urology*
79GCM	*Endoscope, Rigid*	*Surgery*
77EOX	*Esophagoscope (Flexible Or Rigid)*	*Ear/Nose/Throat*
78FDW	*Esophagoscope, Rigid, Gastro-Urology*	*Gastro/Urology*
73BWH	*Forceps, Biopsy, Bronchoscope (Non-Rigid)*	*Anesthesiology*
73JEK	*Forceps, Biopsy, Bronchoscope (Rigid)*	*Anesthesiology*
78QYD	*Gastroscope, Rigid*	*Gastro/Urology*
73CAL	*Laryngoscope, Flexible*	*Anesthesiology*
73CCW	*Laryngoscope, Rigid*	*Anesthesiology*
86MWL	*Lens, Contact(rigid Gas Permeable)-extended Wear*	*Ophthalmology*
77EOB	*Nasopharyngoscope (Flexible Or Rigid)*	*Ear/Nose/Throat*
78RIN	*Nephroscope, Rigid*	*Gastro/Urology*
89IQF	*Orthosis, Cervical-Thoracic, Rigid*	*Physical Med*
89IPO	*Orthosis, Pneumatic Structure, Rigid*	*Physical Med*
79FTQ	*Prosthesis, Penis, Rigid Rod*	*Surgery*
78LKY	*Prosthesis, Penis, Rigid Rod, External*	*Gastro/Urology*
73JEI	*Remover, Foreign Body, Bronchoscope (Non-Rigid)*	*Anesthesiology*
78FAN	*Sigmoidoscope, Rigid, Electrical*	*Gastro/Urology*
78KDM	*Sigmoidoscope, Rigid, Non-Electrical*	*Gastro/Urology*
78FDJ	*Snare, Rigid Self-Opening*	*Gastro/Urology*
80THI	*Sterilizer/Washer, Endoscope*	*General*
78FBP	*Telescope, Rigid, Endoscopic*	*Gastro/Urology*
77KTR	*Tube, Aspirating, Rigid Bronchoscope Aspirating*	*Ear/Nose/Throat*

RIGIDITY

84GZM	*Analyzer, Rigidity*	*Cns/Neurology*

RIM

86UBX	*Prosthesis, Orbital Rim*	*Ophthalmology*

RING

85HFX	*Clamp, Circumcision*	*Obstetrics/Gyn*
80QOA	*Cushion, Ring, Foam Rubber*	*General*
80QOB	*Cushion, Ring, Inflatable*	*General*
80FNS	*Cutter, Ring*	*General*
79SIY	*Holder, Ring, Anastomosis*	*Surgery*
80WRP	*Pacifier*	*General*
79KGW	*Ring Drape Retention, Internal (Wound Protector)*	*Surgery*
74KRH	*Ring, Annuloplasty*	*Cardiovascular*
78FJX	*Ring, Crimp*	*Gastro/Urology*
76QOZ	*Ring, Dental (Casting)*	*Dental And Oral*
86MRJ	*Ring, Endocapsular*	*Ophthalmology*
78FJW	*Ring, Joint*	*Gastro/Urology*
78FHI	*Ring, Laparotomy*	*Gastro/Urology*
86HNH	*Ring, Ophthalmic (Flieringa)*	*Ophthalmology*
79RXT	*Ring, Suture*	*Surgery*
86UBE	*Ring, Symblepharon*	*Ophthalmology*
76KKO	*Ring, Teething, Fluid-Filled*	*Dental And Oral*
76MEF	*Ring, Teething, Non-Fluid-Filled*	*Dental And Oral*

RISK

82MLF	*Computer Software, Prenatal Risk Evaluation*	*Immunology*

RNA

88LNJ	*Analyzer, Chromosome, Automated*	*Pathology*
88JCZ	*Analyzer, Karyotype*	*Pathology*
83UGH	*Genetic Engineering*	*Microbiology*

RUBEOLA *(cont'd)*

83GRG	Antiserum, HAI, Rubeola	Microbiology
83GRI	Antiserum, Neutralization, Rubeola	Microbiology
83LJB	Enzyme Linked Immunoabsorbent Assay, Rubeola	Microbiology

RULER

86HLE	Ruler, Nearpoint (Punctometer)	Ophthalmology
79FTY	Tape, Measuring, Ruler And Caliper	Surgery

RUPTURE

85MDH	Abruptio Placentae Catheter	Obstetrics/Gyn

RUSSEL

81GIR	Reagent, Russel Viper Venom	Hematology

SAC

86HNG	Rongeur, Lacrimal Sac	Ophthalmology

SACCHAROGENIC

75CIJ	Saccharogenic, Amylase	Chemistry

SACCULOTOMY

77JYN	Inserter, Sacculotomy Tack	Ear/Nose/Throat
77ESX	Tack, Sacculotomy (Cody)	Ear/Nose/Throat

SACRAL

84MQQ	Stimulator, Sacral Nerve, Implanted	Cns/Neurology

SACROILIAC

89IPW	Orthosis, Sacroiliac, Soft	Physical Med

SAD

80MIO	Light, Therapy, Seasonal Affective Disorder (SAD)	General

SAFE

90IZK	Radiographic Unit, Diagnostic, Mobile, Explosion-Safe	Radiology
90JAS	Safe, Radionuclide	Radiology

SAFELIGHT

90VGO	Safelight, X-Ray	Radiology

SAFETY

74DSM	Alarm, Leakage Current, Portable	Cardiovascular
90THK	Alarm, Radiation	Radiology
80QSF	Analyzer, Electrical Safety	General
80QUR	Analyzer, Ethylene-Oxide	General
80RBE	Bracelet, Identification	General
80WOF	Breaker, Ampule	General
89KHY	Cane, Safety Walk	Physical Med
78FJD	Detector, Blood Leakage	Gastro/Urology
80QTQ	Detector, Electrostatic Voltage	General
80UMV	Detector, Ethylene-Oxide Leakage	General
80RGX	Detector, Microwave Leakage	General
75UHT	Enclosure, Bacteriological Safety	Chemistry
86TCB	Eyeglasses, Safety	Ophthalmology
75TCG	Fountain, Eye Wash	Chemistry
80UEU	Identification, Alert, Medical	General
80REQ	Meter, Leakage Current (Ammeter)	General
80TGZ	Mirror, Corridor Safety	General
80WMU	Pin, Safety	General
80TDS	Plug, Electrical	General
80TCS	Power System, Isolated	General
80WMN	Power Systems, Uninterruptible (UPS)	General
80WSO	Pump, Industrial	General
80TEE	Receptacle, Electrical	General
75RDT	Safety Equipment, Laboratory	Chemistry
80VAY	Security Equipment/Supplies	General
75TEP	Shower, Emergency	Chemistry
79SJQ	System, Monitoring, Electrode, Active, Electrosurgical	Surgery
80QYV	Tester, Ground Fault Circuit Interrupter	General
80QYY	Tester, Grounding System	General
80WTM	Weight, IV Pole	General

SAFRANIN

88HZS	Stain, Safranin	Pathology

SAHLI

81GGX	Pipette, Sahli	Hematology

SALICYLATE

91DKJ	Colorimetry, Salicylate	Toxicology
91DIM	Gas Chromatography, Salicylate	Toxicology
91DMX	Liquid Chromatography, Salicylate	Toxicology
91DNC	Paper Strip, Salicylate	Toxicology
91DJE	Thin Layer Chromatography, Salicylate	Toxicology

SALINE

88IGC	Formalin-Saline	Pathology
79MUG	Solution, Saline(wound Dressing)	Surgery

SALIVA

76KHR	Absorber, Saliva, Paper	Dental And Oral
76QOE	Cuspidor	Dental And Oral

SALIVA *(cont'd)*

77QSD	Ejector, Saliva	Ear/Nose/Throat
81MWB	Kit, Test, Saliva, Hiv-1&2	Hematology
76DYN	Mouthpiece, Saliva Ejector	Dental And Oral
76LFD	Saliva, Artificial	Dental And Oral

SALIVARY

77VGE	Dilator, Salivary Duct	Ear/Nose/Throat
76LTF	Stimulator, Salivary System	Dental And Oral

SALMONELLA

83GNC	Antigen, Febrile, Slide And Tube, Salmonella	Microbiology
83GRL	Antigen, Salmonella SPP.	Microbiology
83GOO	Antiserum, Fluorescent, All Globulins, Salmonella SPP.	Microbiology
83GRM	Antiserum, Salmonella SPP.	Microbiology
83LSM	Salmonella SPP., DNA Reagents	Microbiology

SALPINGEAL

77KBK	Curette, Salpingeal	Ear/Nose/Throat

SALPINGOGRAPHY

85MOV	Catheter, Salpingography	Obstetrics/Gyn

SALT

76KOO	Polyvinyl Methylether Maleic Acid-Calcium-Sodium Dbl. Salt	Dental And Oral
88KIP	Solution, Balanced Salt	Pathology
88HYD	Stain, Fast Red Salt B	Pathology

SAMPLE

75UHU	Applicator, Sample	Chemistry
79WZP	Bag, Specimen, Laparoscopic	Surgery
80WKZ	Brush, Cytology	General
73WVG	Catheter, Culture, Pulmonary	Anesthesiology
75JJH	Concentrator, Clinical Sample	Chemistry
75UHV	Injector, Sample	Chemistry
79QQU	Instrument, Dissecting, Laparoscopic	Surgery
79QQY	Instrument, Dissecting, Myoma, Laparoscopic	Surgery
81GIM	Tube, Vacuum Sample, With Anticoagulant	Hematology

SAMPLER

78FDX	Brush, Cytology, Endoscopic	Gastro/Urology
80QAI	Sampler, Air	General
85HIO	Sampler, Amniotic Fluid (Amniocentesis Tray)	Obstetrics/Gyn
85HGW	Sampler, Blood, Fetal	Obstetrics/Gyn
75UHW	Sampler, Fermentation	Chemistry
75QXY	Sampler, Gas	Chemistry
80WWH	Sampler, Particulate	General

SAMPLING

73RJK	Analyzer, Gas, Oxygen, Sampling	Anesthesiology
85LLX	Catheter, Sampling, Chorionic Villus	Obstetrics/Gyn
83QMQ	Counter, Cell	Microbiology
85HGK	Endoscope, Fetal Blood Sampling	Obstetrics/Gyn
80LZF	Infusion Pump, Analytical Sampling	General
74RKS	Kit, Blood Collection, Phlebotomy	Cardiovascular
73CBT	Kit, Sampling, Arterial Blood	Anesthesiology
80RQG	Kit, Sampling, Blood	General
80RQH	Kit, Sampling, Blood Gas	General
85RQI	Kit, Sampling, Endometrial	Obstetrics/Gyn
75UHK	Precipitator, Radioimmunoassay Multiple Sampling	Chemistry
80WUI	Protector, Puncture, Needle	General
80FRC	Sterilization Process Indicator, Biological	General
80RVU	Sterilization Process Indicator, Chemical	General
80JOJ	Sterilization Process Indicator, Physical/Chemical	General
85VIL	Test, Chorionic Villi Sampling (Fetal Chromosome Analysis)	Obstetrics/Gyn

SAND

90RQJ	Sand Bag	Radiology
90SGN	Sand Bag, X-Ray	Radiology

SANITARY

85RQK	Belt, Sanitary	Obstetrics/Gyn
80WHM	Cover, Seat, Toilet, Sanitary	General
80WIW	Dispenser, Tissue, Toilet	General
80WIX	Dispenser, Towel	General
80VBI	Housekeeping Equipment	General
80VBE	Tissue, Toilet	General

SANITATION

76MCF	Unit, Sanitation/Sterilization, Toothbrush, Ultraviolet	Dental And Oral

SANITIZER

80QKS	Cleaner, Bedpan (Sterilizer)	General
80RQL	Sanitizer	General
80THI	Sterilizer/Washer, Endoscope	General
80SFN	Washer, Cart	General
80SFR	Washer, Utensil	General
80SFM	Washer/Sterilizer	General

SAPHENOUS

79KPK	Marker, Ostia, Aorto-Saphenous Vein	Surgery

KEYWORD INDEX

SATURATION

74MUD	Oximeter, Tissue Saturation	Cardiovascular

SAVER

80QAJ	Airway, Obstruction Removal (Choke Saver)	General

SAW

87TAI	Blade, Saw, Cast Cutting	Orthopedics
74DWH	Blade, Saw, Surgical, Cardiovascular	Cardiovascular
79GFA	Blade, Surgical, Saw, General & Plastic Surgery	Surgery
87QZB	Guide, Gigli Saw	Orthopedics
88RQM	Saw, Autopsy	Pathology
87HSO	Saw, Bone Cutting	Orthopedics
87VHR	Saw, Bone Cutting, Micro	Orthopedics
87RQN	Saw, Bone, Pneumatic	Orthopedics
74DWI	Saw, Electric	Cardiovascular
76DZH	Saw, Electric Bone	Dental And Oral
77JZZ	Saw, Laryngeal	Ear/Nose/Throat
79GDR	Saw, Manual, And Accessories	Surgery
84HAC	Saw, Manual, Neurological (With Accessories)	Cns/Neurology
77KBC	Saw, Nasal	Ear/Nose/Throat
79RQO	Saw, Other	Surgery
79KFK	Saw, Pneumatically Powered	Surgery
84HAB	Saw, Powered, And Accessories	Cns/Neurology
77EWQ	Saw, Surgical, ENT (Electric Or Pneumatic)	Ear/Nose/Throat

SCALE

80VDN	Analyzer, Composition, Weight, Patient	General
75QCF	Balance, Electronic	Chemistry
75UKH	Balance, Macro (0.1 mg Accuracy)	Chemistry
75QCG	Balance, Mechanical	Chemistry
75UKF	Balance, Micro (0.001 mg Accuracy)	Chemistry
75UKG	Balance, Semimicro (0.01 mg Accuracy)	Chemistry
75UKE	Balance, Ultramicro (0.0001 mg Accuracy)	Chemistry
78WQV	Chair, Dialysis (With Scale)	Gastro/Urology
78FKS	Chair, Dialysis, Powered (Without Scale)	Gastro/Urology
78FIA	Chair, Dialysis, Unpowered (Without Scale)	Gastro/Urology
80WOB	Meter, Patient Height	General
81KSQ	Mixer/Scale, Blood	Hematology
88RQP	Scale, Autopsy	Pathology
80RQQ	Scale, Bed	General
81RQR	Scale, Blood	Hematology
80RQS	Scale, Chair	General
80WXD	Scale, Chair, Transfer	General
80FRW	Scale, Infant	General
75RQT	Scale, Laboratory	Chemistry
89INF	Scale, Platform, Wheelchair	Physical Med
80FRI	Scale, Stand-On	General
80FQA	Scale, Surgical Sponge	General

SCALER

76EMN	Scaler, Periodontic	Dental And Oral
76ELB	Scaler, Rotary	Dental And Oral
76ELC	Scaler, Ultrasonic	Dental And Oral

SCALES

80KOF	Scales, Dialysis	General

SCALP

85HGR	Applicator, Electrode, Scalp, Fetal	Obstetrics/Gyn
84UCL	Catheter, Hydrocephalic	Cns/Neurology
84HBO	Clip, Scalp	Cns/Neurology
85HGP	Electrode, Circular (Spiral), Scalp And Applicator	Obstetrics/Gyn
85HIQ	Electrode, Clip, Fetal Scalp (And Applicator)	Obstetrics/Gyn
85QSZ	Electrode, Fetal Scalp	Obstetrics/Gyn
84RII	Needle, Scalp	Cns/Neurology
84GZT	Retractor, Self-Retaining, Neurology	Cns/Neurology

SCALPEL

79QVD	Blade, Knife, Laparoscopic	Surgery
79GES	Blade, Scalpel	Surgery
79FAS	Electrode, Electrosurgical, Active (Blade)	Surgery
79RDE	Handle, Knife Blade	Surgery
79QWG	Handle, Knife, Laparoscopic	Surgery
79GDZ	Handle, Scalpel	Surgery
79RDF	Holder, Knife	Surgery
86RDH	Knife, Cataract	Ophthalmology
85HDZ	Knife, Cervical Cone	Obstetrics/Gyn
79RDI	Knife, Dermatome	Surgery
84RDJ	Knife, Dura Hook	Cns/Neurology
86RDK	Knife, Keratome	Ophthalmology
79QWI	Knife, Laparoscopic	Surgery
79RDL	Knife, Meniscus	Surgery
77KAS	Knife, Nasal	Ear/Nose/Throat
86HNN	Knife, Ophthalmic	Ophthalmology
79RDS	Knife, Other	Surgery
79RDP	Knife, Scalpel	Surgery
77KBQ	Knife, Tonsil	Ear/Nose/Throat
79RDG	Needle, Knife	Surgery
80WZH	Remover, Blade, Scalpel	General

SCALPEL *(cont'd)*

79GDX	Scalpel, One-Piece (Knife)	Surgery
79SJE	Scalpel, Ultrasonic	Surgery
79SEP	Scissors with Removable Tips, Laparoscopy	Surgery
79SAZ	Scissors, Laparoscopy	Surgery
79SJL	Scissors, Laparoscopy, Bipolar, Electrosurgical	Surgery
79SGV	Scissors, Laparoscopy, Unipolar, Electrosurgical	Surgery

SCAN

90UEY	Television System, Slow Scan	Radiology

SCANNER

74QBM	Arteriographic Unit, Ultrasonic	Cardiovascular
90IYX	Camera, Gamma (Nuclear/Scintillation)	Radiology
90QMD	Computer, Nuclear Medicine	Radiology
75JQT	Densitometer/Scanner (Integrating, Reflectance, TLC, Radio)	Chemistry
74WSD	Doppler, Blood Flow, Transcranial	Cardiovascular
74DXK	Echocardiograph (Ultrasonic Scanner)	Cardiovascular
84GXW	Echoencephalograph (Ultrasonic Scanner)	Cns/Neurology
80WNL	Label, Bar Code	General
86WTA	Ophthalmoscope, Laser	Ophthalmology
84GXX	Phantom, Ultrasonic Scanner, Neurology	Cns/Neurology
85MGK	Scanner, Breast, Thermographic, Ultrasonic, Computer-Asstd.	Obstetrics/Gyn
76KZN	Scanner, Color	Dental And Oral
90WMF	Scanner, Computed Tomography, Cine	Radiology
84JXD	Scanner, Computed Tomography, X-Ray (CAT, CT)	Cns/Neurology
90THS	Scanner, Computed Tomography, X-Ray, Full Body	Radiology
90TEI	Scanner, Computed Tomography, X-Ray, Head	Radiology
90JAK	Scanner, Computed Tomography, X-Ray, Special Procedure	Radiology
90KPS	Scanner, Emission Computed Tomography	Radiology
90JAO	Scanner, Fluorescent	Radiology
84VDD	Scanner, Long-Term Recording, EEG	Cns/Neurology
73VDB	Scanner, Long-Term Recording, Respiration	Anesthesiology
74RQU	Scanner, Long-Term, ECG, Recording	Cardiovascular
90JAM	Scanner, Magnetic Resonance (NMR/MRI)	Radiology
90THG	Scanner, Nuclear Emission Computed Tomography (ECT)	Radiology
90IYW	Scanner, Nuclear, Rectilinear	Radiology
90JWM	Scanner, Nuclear, Tomographic	Radiology
90ULI	Scanner, Positron Emission Tomography (PET)	Radiology
75JRF	Scanner, Radiochromatogram	Chemistry
90IYN	Scanner, Ultrasonic (Pulsed Doppler)	Radiology
90IYO	Scanner, Ultrasonic (Pulsed Echo)	Radiology
90RQV	Scanner, Ultrasonic, Abdominal	Radiology
85RQW	Scanner, Ultrasonic, Breast (Mammographic)	Obstetrics/Gyn
90VHD	Scanner, Ultrasonic, Compound B	Radiology
90TEJ	Scanner, Ultrasonic, General Purpose	Radiology
85HEM	Scanner, Ultrasonic, Obstetrical/Gynecological	Obstetrics/Gyn
85RQX	Scanner, Ultrasonic, Obstetrical/Gynecological, Mobile	Obstetrics/Gyn
90HPR	Scanner, Ultrasonic, Ophthalmic	Radiology
90RQZ	Scanner, Ultrasonic, Other	Radiology
90RQY	Scanner, Ultrasonic, Pediatric	Radiology
90TEK	Scanner, Ultrasonic, Small Parts	Radiology
79UMD	Scanner, Ultrasonic, Surgical	Surgery
90VCV	Scanner, Ultrasonic, Vascular	Radiology
75UHX	Scanner, Ultraviolet	Chemistry
85WSC	Spectroscope, Tumor Analysis, Mammary	Obstetrics/Gyn
90WJP	Stand, Cardiovascular	Radiology
90WLW	Stand, Vascular	Radiology

SCANNING

81JBY	Aggregometer, Platelet, Photo-Optical Scanning	Hematology
90IYZ	Bed, Scanning, Nuclear/Fluoroscopic	Radiology
83UEV	Microscope, Laser, Scanning, Acoustic	Microbiology

SCAPHOID

87KWO	Prosthesis, Wrist, Carpal Scaphoid	Orthopedics

SCAR

79MDA	Elastomer, Silicone (Scar Management)	Surgery

SCARIFIER

80RRA	Scarifier	General

SCARLET

88ICN	Stain, Biebrich Scarlet	Pathology

SCAVENGER

73CBN	Scavenger, Gas	Anesthesiology
73QBA	Scavenger, Gas, Anesthesia Unit	Anesthesiology

SCAVENGING

73KHA	Mask, Scavenging	Anesthesiology

SCENTED

85HHL	Pad, Menstrual, Scented	Obstetrics/Gyn
85HIL	Tampon, Menstrual, Scented	Obstetrics/Gyn

SCHEDULING

80WSJ	Computer Software, Hospital/Nursing Management	General
80VHN	Computer, Patient Data Management	General

SCHENEKII

83GMA	Antiserum, Fluorescent, Sporothrix Schenekii	Microbiology

SCHIFF

88HZK	Stain, Periodic Acid Schiff (PAS)	Pathology
88HZT	Stain, Reagent, Schiff	Pathology
88GGI	Stain, Schiff, Periodic Acid	Pathology

SCHILLING'S

81JWN	Schilling's Test	Hematology

SCHIRMER

86KYD	Strip, Schirmer	Ophthalmology

SCHISTOSOMA

83GNH	Antigen, Fluorescent Antibody Test, Schistosoma Mansoni	Microbiology

SCINTILLATION

90IYX	Camera, Gamma (Nuclear/Scintillation)	Radiology
75QMU	Counter, Scintillation	Chemistry
91DNY	Counter, Scintillation, Liquid, Toxicology	Toxicology
80WPN	Crusher, Vial, Laboratory	General
75UJF	Vial, Liquid Scintillation Counting	Chemistry

SCISSORS

79QVD	Blade, Knife, Laparoscopic	Surgery
77KBM	Dissector, Tonsil	Ear/Nose/Throat
79LRW	General Use Surgical Scissors	Surgery
79QWG	Handle, Knife, Laparoscopic	Surgery
79QPN	Holder/Scissors, Needle, Laparoscopic	Surgery
79QQU	Instrument, Dissecting, Laparoscopic	Surgery
79QQY	Instrument, Dissecting, Myoma, Laparoscopic	Surgery
84GZX	Instrument, Microsurgical	Cns/Neurology
79QWI	Knife, Laparoscopic	Surgery
79SEP	Scissors with Removable Tips, Laparoscopy	Surgery
80RRB	Scissors, Bandage/Gauze/Plaster	General
74RRC	Scissors, Cardiovascular	Cardiovascular
76EIR	Scissors, Collar And Crown	Dental And Oral
86RRD	Scissors, Corneal	Ophthalmology
78KGD	Scissors, Cystoscopic	Gastro/Urology
80JOK	Scissors, Disposable	General
77JZB	Scissors, Ear	Ear/Nose/Throat
86RRE	Scissors, Enucleation	Ophthalmology
85HDK	Scissors, Episiotomy	Obstetrics/Gyn
80RRI	Scissors, General Dissecting	General
85RRJ	Scissors, Gynecological	Obstetrics/Gyn
86RRF	Scissors, Iris	Ophthalmology
79SAZ	Scissors, Laparoscopy	Surgery
79SJL	Scissors, Laparoscopy, Bipolar, Electrosurgical	Surgery
79WZE	Scissors, Laparoscopy, Electrosurgical	Surgery
79SGV	Scissors, Laparoscopy, Unipolar, Electrosurgical	Surgery
79SJU	Scissors, Microlaparoscopy	Surgery
77KBD	Scissors, Nasal	Ear/Nose/Throat
84RRK	Scissors, Neurosurgical (Dura)	Cns/Neurology
86HNF	Scissors, Ophthalmic	Ophthalmology
87HRR	Scissors, Orthopedic	Orthopedics
80RRL	Scissors, Pediatric	General
79RRM	Scissors, Plastic Surgery (Dissecting)	Surgery
78RRN	Scissors, Rectal	Gastro/Urology
76EGN	Scissors, Surgical Tissue, Dental (Oral)	Dental And Oral
79RRO	Scissors, Suture	Surgery
86RRH	Scissors, Tenotomy	Ophthalmology
74RRP	Scissors, Thoracic	Cardiovascular
85HDJ	Scissors, Umbilical	Obstetrics/Gyn
77JYA	Scissors, Wire Cutting, ENT	Ear/Nose/Throat
79WVB	Sharpener, Instrument, Surgical	Surgery

SCLERA

86HMQ	Marker, Sclera (Ocular)	Ophthalmology

SCLERAL

86RAO	Hook, Scleral Fixation	Ophthalmology
86HQJ	Implant, Absorbable (Scleral Buckling Method)	Ophthalmology
86WUA	Implant, Scleral	Ophthalmology
86HNJ	Punch, Corneo-Scleral	Ophthalmology
86TEL	Scleral Buckling Instrument	Ophthalmology
86LXP	Scleral Plug	Ophthalmology
86HQT	Shell, Scleral	Ophthalmology
86HOZ	Sponge, Ophthalmic	Ophthalmology

SCLEROTOME

86RRQ	Sclerotome	Ophthalmology

SCOLIOSIS

80WWG	Analyzer, Motion	General
87WRR	Equipment, Screening, Scoliosis	Orthopedics
89VIH	Stimulator, Scoliosis (Orthosis)	Physical Med

SCOLIOSIS *(cont'd)*

87LWB	Stimulator, Scoliosis, Neuromuscular, Functional	Orthopedics

SCOOP

78RRR	Scoop, Common Duct	Gastro/Urology
78FHL	Scoop, Gallstone	Gastro/Urology

SCOOTER

89KNL	Board, Scooter, Prone	Physical Med
89INI	Scooter (Motorized 3-Wheeled Vehicle)	Physical Med

SCOPE

74LYK	Angioscope	Cardiovascular
86HIW	Anomaloscope	Ophthalmology
78FER	Anoscope, Non-Powered	Gastro/Urology
87HRX	Arthroscope	Orthopedics
77BTN	Bronchoscope, Non-Rigid	Ear/Nose/Throat
77EOQ	Bronchoscope, Rigid	Ear/Nose/Throat
73BTJ	Bronchoscope, Rigid, Non-Ventilating	Anesthesiology
73BTH	Bronchoscope, Rigid, Ventilating	Anesthesiology
78FBN	Choledochoscope, Flexible Or Rigid	Gastro/Urology
78WZV	Choledochoscope, Mini-Diameter (5mm or Less)	Gastro/Urology
78FDF	Colonoscope, Gastro-Urology	Gastro/Urology
79FTJ	Colonoscope, General & Plastic Surgery	Surgery
85HEY	Colpomicroscope	Obstetrics/Gyn
85HEX	Colposcope	Obstetrics/Gyn
85HEW	Culdoscope	Obstetrics/Gyn
78FAJ	Cystoscope	Gastro/Urology
78FBO	Cystourethroscope	Gastro/Urology
76WNX	Dentoscope	Dental And Oral
85MMN	Ductoscope, Breast	Obstetrics/Gyn
78FDT	Duodenoscope, Esophago/Gastro	Gastro/Urology
78KOG	Endoscope	Gastro/Urology
79GCP	Endoscope And Accessories, AC-Powered	Surgery
79GCS	Endoscope And Accessories, Battery-Powered	Surgery
79GCR	Endoscope, Direct Vision	Surgery
79VKP	Endoscope, Electronic (Videoendoscope)	Surgery
85HGK	Endoscope, Fetal Blood Sampling	Obstetrics/Gyn
79GDB	Endoscope, Fiberoptic	Surgery
78GCQ	Endoscope, Flexible	Gastro/Urology
84GWG	Endoscope, Neurological	Cns/Neurology
78KYH	Endoscope, Ophthalmic	Gastro/Urology
79GCM	Endoscope, Rigid	Surgery
85HEZ	Endoscope, Transcervical (Amnioscope)	Obstetrics/Gyn
78VJF	Endoscope, Ultrasonic Probe (Lithotriptor)	Gastro/Urology
78FDA	Enteroscope	Gastro/Urology
86QUK	Entoptoscope	Ophthalmology
77EOX	Esophagoscope (Flexible Or Rigid)	Ear/Nose/Throat
78GCL	Esophagoscope, General & Plastic Surgery	Gastro/Urology
78FDW	Esophagoscope, Rigid, Gastro-Urology	Gastro/Urology
86HMK	Euthyscope, AC-Powered	Ophthalmology
86HML	Euthyscope, Battery-Powered	Ophthalmology
86HKG	Fornixscope	Ophthalmology
86QXV	Funduscope	Ophthalmology
78QYC	Gastroscope, Flexible	Gastro/Urology
78FDS	Gastroscope, Gastro-Urology	Gastro/Urology
79WXI	Laparoscope, Flexible	Surgery
79GCJ	Laparoscope, General & Plastic Surgery	Surgery
85HET	Laparoscope, Gynecologic	Obstetrics/Gyn
79SJT	Laparoscope, Microlaparoscopy	Surgery
88IBL	Microscope, Inverted Stage, Tissue Culture	Pathology
86HLI	Ophthalmoscope, AC-Powered	Ophthalmology
86HLJ	Ophthalmoscope, Battery-Powered	Ophthalmology
86RIV	Ophthalmoscope, Direct	Ophthalmology
86RIW	Ophthalmoscope, Indirect	Ophthalmology
86WTA	Ophthalmoscope, Laser	Ophthalmology
78FTK	Pancreatoscope, Biliary	Gastro/Urology
78FAK	Panendoscope (Gastroduodenoscope)	Gastro/Urology
78FAL	Panendoscope (Urethroscope)	Gastro/Urology
78GCG	Peritoneoscope	Gastro/Urology
80TDP	Phaneroscope	General
77RKR	Pharyngoscope	Ear/Nose/Throat
90RKW	Photofluoroscope (Cardiac Catheterization)	Radiology
86HJA	Photokeratoscope	Ophthalmology
80SHO	Polariscope	General
79GCF	Proctoscope	Surgery
78RML	Proctosigmoidoscope	Gastro/Urology
90RNP	Pyeloscope	Radiology
78FJL	Resectoscope	Gastro/Urology
86HKL	Retinoscope, AC-Powered	Ophthalmology
86HKM	Retinoscope, Battery-Powered	Ophthalmology
77RQB	Rhinoscope	Ear/Nose/Throat
73VDU	Scope, Fiberoptic Intubation	Anesthesiology
78FAM	Sigmoidoscope, Flexible	Gastro/Urology
78FAN	Sigmoidoscope, Rigid, Electrical	Gastro/Urology
78KDM	Sigmoidoscope, Rigid, Non-Electrical	Gastro/Urology
86HKC	Spectacle Microscope, Low-Vision	Ophthalmology
85WSC	Spectroscope, Tumor Analysis, Mammary	Obstetrics/Gyn

SCOPE *(cont'd)*
78FDR Sphincteroscope — Gastro/Urology
86HJQ Stereoscope, AC-Powered — Ophthalmology
86HJR Stereoscope, Battery-Powered — Ophthalmology
80VKO Stethoscope, Amplified — General
80FLW Stethoscope, DC-Powered — General
76WLF Stethoscope, Dental — Dental And Oral
79FXD Stethoscope, Direct (Acoustic), Ultrasonic — Surgery
74DQD Stethoscope, Electronic (Auscultoscope) — Cardiovascular
79FXC Stethoscope, Electronic-Amplified — Surgery
73BZW Stethoscope, Esophageal — Anesthesiology
73BZT Stethoscope, Esophageal, With Electrical Conductors — Anesthesiology
85HGN Stethoscope, Fetal — Obstetrics/Gyn
74LDE Stethoscope, Manual — Cardiovascular
80FLT Stethoscope, Mechanical — General
83RZC Tachistoscope — Microbiology
86HKB Telescope, Hand-Held, Low-Vision — Ophthalmology
77ENZ Telescope, Laryngeal-Bronchial — Ear/Nose/Throat
78FBP Telescope, Rigid, Endoscopic — Gastro/Urology
86HKK Telescope, Spectacle, Low-Vision — Ophthalmology
74SAM Thoracoscope — Cardiovascular
77JOG Tympanoscope — Ear/Nose/Throat
78QIL Ureteroendoscope — Gastro/Urology
78FGB Ureteroscope — Gastro/Urology
78FGC Urethroscope — Gastro/Urology
85SEL Vaginoscope — Obstetrics/Gyn
85MOK Vaginoscope and Accessories — Obstetrics/Gyn

SCRAPER
80WKZ Brush, Cytology — General
85RRS Scraper, Cytology (Cervical) — Obstetrics/Gyn
79LXK Scraper, Specimen, Skin — Surgery
76LCN Scraper, Tongue — Dental And Oral

SCREEN
80WKP Camera, Other — General
73RRT Screen, Anesthesia — Anesthesiology
80RRU Screen, Bedside — General
90IXM Screen, Intensifying, Radiographic — Radiology
76EAM Screen, Intensifying, Radiographic, Dental — Dental And Oral
86HOM Screen, Tangent, AC-Powered (Campimeter) — Ophthalmology
86HOL Screen, Tangent, Felt (Campimeter) — Ophthalmology
86HOK Screen, Tangent, Projection, AC-Powered — Ophthalmology
86HMJ Screen, Tangent, Projection, Battery-Powered — Ophthalmology
86HOJ Screen, Tangent, Target — Ophthalmology
86HLK Screen, Tangent, Target, Battery-Powered — Ophthalmology
90LHP Telethermographic System (Sole Diagnostic Screen) — Radiology
90LHR Thermographic Device, Liquid Crystal, Screen — Radiology

SCREENER
77ETY Tester, Auditory Impedance — Ear/Nose/Throat

SCREENING
87WRR Equipment, Screening, Scoliosis — Orthopedics
81JBF Glucose-6-Phosphate Dehydrogenase (Erythrocytic), Screening — Hematology
83JWX Kit, Screening, Staphylococcus Aureus — Microbiology
83JXA Kit, Screening, Urine — Microbiology
83JWZ Kit, Trichomonas Screening — Microbiology
83JXC Kit, Yeast Screening — Microbiology
75RGE Mass Screening System — Chemistry
81UJU Serum, Screening, Blood — Hematology
77ETY Tester, Auditory Impedance — Ear/Nose/Throat

SCREW
84HBW Fastener, Cranioplasty Plate — Cns/Neurology
76DYJ Retainer, Screw Expansion, Orthodontic — Dental And Oral
84UAU Screw, Cranioplasty Plate — Cns/Neurology
85HHO Screw, Fibroid, Gynecological — Obstetrics/Gyn
87HWC Screw, Fixation, Bone — Orthopedics
87NDJ Screw, Fixation, Bone, Non-Spinal, Metallic — Orthopedics
76DZL Screw, Fixation, Intraosseous — Dental And Oral
77KBW Screw, Oral — Ear/Nose/Throat
77KBX Screw, Tonsil — Ear/Nose/Throat
87HWD Starter, Bone Screw — Orthopedics
87MCV System, Appliance, Fixation, Spinal Pedicle Screw — Orthopedics
87MRW System, Facet Screw Spinal Device — Orthopedics

SCREWDRIVER
87HXX Screwdriver — Orthopedics
84GXL Screwdriver, Skullplate — Cns/Neurology
79LRZ Screwdriver, Surgical — Surgery

SCROTAL
78EXO Support, Scrotal — Gastro/Urology
80FQJ Support, Scrotal, Therapeutic — General

SCRUB
79LYU Accessories, Apparel, Surgical — Surgery
79GEC Brush, Scrub, Operating Room — Surgery

SCRUB *(cont'd)*
79RRV Dress, Scrub, Disposable — Surgery
79RRW Dress, Scrub, Reusable — Surgery
79FPH Gown, Operating Room, Disposable — Surgery
79QYN Gown, Operating Room, Reusable — Surgery
80TFI Kit, Skin Scrub — General
79RRX Scrub Machine, Surgical — Surgery
80TGD Solution, Surgical Scrub — General
79RVJ Sponge, Scrub — Surgery
79RRY Suit, Scrub, Disposable — Surgery
79RRZ Suit, Scrub, Reusable — Surgery
79VLW Timer, Scrub Station — Surgery

SCULTETUS
80QCK Bandage, Scultetus — General
80QDO Binder, Scultetus — General

SEAL
73CCS Drain, Thoracic, Water Seal — Anesthesiology

SEALANT
76EBC Sealant, Pit And Fissure, And Conditioner, Resin — Dental And Oral

SEALED
90IXD Calibrator Source, Nuclear Sealed — Radiology
78FII Dialysate Delivery System, Sealed — Gastro/Urology
90IWI Source, Isotope, Sealed, Gold, Titanium, Platinum — Radiology

SEALER
81KSD Heat-Sealing Device — Hematology
81GHY Hematocrit Tube, Rack, Sealer, Holder — Hematology
88KIM Sealer, Microsection — Pathology
80TDK Sealer, Packaging — General

SEALING
81KSD Heat-Sealing Device — Hematology

SEARCHER
77JZC Searcher, Mastoid — Ear/Nose/Throat

SEASONAL
80MIO Light, Therapy, Seasonal Affective Disorder (SAD) — General

SEAT
80UMP Chair, Seat Lifting (Standing Aid) — General
80QLU Commode Seat — General
80WHM Cover, Seat, Toilet, Sanitary — General
74MEZ Device, Debridement, Ultrasonic, Heart Valve & HV Seat — Cardiovascular

SECOND
82KTS 2nd Antibody (Species Specific Anti-Animal Gamma Globulin) — Immunology
91DJB Radioimmunoassay, Gentamicin (125-I), Second Antibody — Toxicology

SECONDARY
75JIT Calibrator, Secondary, Clinical Chemistry — Chemistry

SECRETORY
82DAJ Antigen, Antiserum, Control, Free Secretory Component — Immunology

SECURITY
80RBE Bracelet, Identification — General
80WRQ Equipment, Building Security — General
80UEU Identification, Alert, Medical — General
80VAY Security Equipment/Supplies — General

SEDIMENTATION
81GKB Analyzer, Sedimentation Rate, Automated — Hematology
81JPH Analyzer, Sedimentation Rate, Erythrocyte — Hematology
81GHC Tube, Sedimentation Rate — Hematology

SEDIMENTOMETER
81GKB Analyzer, Sedimentation Rate, Automated — Hematology
81JPH Analyzer, Sedimentation Rate, Erythrocyte — Hematology

SEED
90IWG Seed, Isotope, Gold, Titanium, Platinum — Radiology

SEGMENT
80MLC Monitor, ST Segment — General
80MLD Monitor, ST Segment (With Alarm) — General

SELECTION
85ULY Kit, Sex Selection — Obstetrics/Gyn

SELECTIVE
75QTJ Analyzer, Chemistry, Electrolyte — Chemistry
83JSH Culture Media, Non-Selective And Differential — Microbiology
83JSG Culture Media, Non-Selective And Non-Differential — Microbiology
83JSI Culture Media, Selective And Differential — Microbiology
83JSJ Culture Media, Selective And Non-Differential — Microbiology
83JSD Culture Media, Selective Broth — Microbiology
80LJJ Electrode, In Vivo Calcium Ion Selective — General
80LJI Electrode, In Vivo Potassium Ion Selective — General

SELECTIVE *(cont'd)*
75JJP Electrode, Ion Selective (Non-Specified) — Chemistry

SELECTOR
78EXA Selector, Size, Ostomy — Gastro/Urology

SELF
78EYX Drape, Pure Latex Sheet, With Self-Retaining Finger Cot — Gastro/Urology
80KLL Monitor, Temperature (Self-Contained) — General
87JDF Prosthesis, Hip (Metal Stem/Ceramic Self-Locking Ball) — Orthopedics
78FGN Retractor, Non-Self-Retaining — Gastro/Urology
78FFO Retractor, Self-Retaining — Gastro/Urology
84GZT Retractor, Self-Retaining, Neurology — Cns/Neurology
78FDJ Snare, Rigid Self-Opening — Gastro/Urology

SELF-CONTAINED
80KLL Monitor, Temperature (Self-Contained) — General

SELF-LOCKING
87JDF Prosthesis, Hip (Metal Stem/Ceramic Self-Locking Ball) — Orthopedics

SELF-OPENING
78FDJ Snare, Rigid Self-Opening — Gastro/Urology

SELF-RETAINING
78EYX Drape, Pure Latex Sheet, With Self-Retaining Finger Cot — Gastro/Urology
79WRE Holder, Retractor — Surgery
78FGN Retractor, Non-Self-Retaining — Gastro/Urology
78FFO Retractor, Self-Retaining — Gastro/Urology
84GZT Retractor, Self-Retaining, Neurology — Cns/Neurology

SEMEN
82DFQ Antigen, Antiserum, Control, Sperm — Immunology
85MNA Device, Semen Analysis — Obstetrics/Gyn

SEMI-
87MBK Prosthesis, Ankle, Semi-, Uncemented, Porous, Metal/Polymer — Orthopedics
87MBL Prosthesis, Hip, Semi-, Uncemented, Osteophilic Finish — Orthopedics

SEMI-AUTOMATED
81KQG Analyzer, Coagulation, Semi-Automated — Hematology

SEMI-AUTOMATIC
78KPF Dialysate Delivery System, Peritoneal, Semi-Automatic — Gastro/Urology
74DXN Monitor, Blood Pressure, Indirect, Semi-Automatic — Cardiovascular

SEMI-CONSTRAINED
87KMD Prosthesis, Ankle, Semi-Constrained, Metal/Composite — Orthopedics
87HSN Prosthesis, Ankle, Semi-Constrained, Metal/Polymer — Orthopedics
87JDB Prosthesis, Elbow, Semi-Constrained — Orthopedics
87MEJ Prosthesis, Hip, Semi-Const., Composite/Polymer — Orthopedics
87MAZ Prosthesis, Hip, Semi-Const., M/P, Por. Uncem., Calc./Phos. — Orthopedics
87LPF Prosthesis, Hip, Semi-Const., Metal/Ceramic/Ceramic, Cem. — Orthopedics
87LPH Prosthesis, Hip, Semi-Const., Metal/Poly., Porous Uncemented — Orthopedics
87MIL Prosthesis, Hip, Semi-Const., Uncem., M/P, Bone Morph. Prot. — Orthopedics
87MEH Prosthesis, Hip, Semi-Const., Uncem., Non-P., M/P, Ca./Phos. — Orthopedics
87LZO Prosthesis, Hip, Semi-Constr., Metal/Ceramic, Cemented/NC — Orthopedics
87JDL Prosthesis, Hip, Semi-Constrained (Cemented Acetabular) — Orthopedics
87KWA Prosthesis, Hip, Semi-Constrained Acetabular — Orthopedics
87JDI Prosthesis, Hip, Semi-Constrained, Metal/Polymer — Orthopedics
87LWJ Prosthesis, Hip, Semi-Constrained, Metal/Polymer, Uncemented — Orthopedics
87KMC Prosthesis, Hip, Semi-constrained, Composite/metal — Orthopedics
87MRA Prosthesis, Hip, Semi-constrained, Metal/ Ceramic/ Ceramic/ Metal, Cemented or Uncemented — Orthopedics
87MAY Prosthesis, Hip, Semi-constrained, Metal/Ceramic/Polymer, Cemented or Non-porous Cemented, Osteophilic Finish — Orthopedics
87MBM Prosthesis, Hip, Semi/Hemi-Const., M/PTFE Ctd./P, Cem./Unc. — Orthopedics
87HRY Prosthesis, Knee, Femorotibial, Semi-Constrained — Orthopedics
87KYK Prosthesis, Knee, Femorotibial, Semi-Constrained, Metal — Orthopedics
87LGE Prosthesis, Knee, Femorotibial, Semi-Constrained, Trunnion — Orthopedics
87KRR Prosthesis, Knee, Patellofemoral, Semi-Constrained — Orthopedics
87JWH Prosthesis, Knee, Patellofemorotibial, Semi-Constrained — Orthopedics
87MBV Prosthesis, Knee, Patfem., S-C., UHMWPE, Pegged, Unc., P/M/P — Orthopedics
87MBH Prosthesis, Knee, Patfem., S-C., Unc., Por., Ctd., P/M/P — Orthopedics
87MBA Prosthesis, Knee, Patfem., Semi-Const., Unc., P/M/P, Osteo. — Orthopedics
87LXY Prosthesis, Knee, Patfemotib., Semi-Const., P/M/P, Uncem. — Orthopedics
87KWS Prosthesis, Shoulder, Semi-Constrained, Metal/Polymer Cem. — Orthopedics

SEMI-CONSTRAINED *(cont'd)*
87KYL Prosthesis, Shoulder, Semi-Constrained, Uncemented — Orthopedics
87LZJ Prosthesis, Toe (Metaphal.), Joint, Met./Poly., Semi-Const. — Orthopedics
87KWM Prosthesis, Wrist, Semi-Constrained — Orthopedics

SEMI-FLEXIBLE
79QYN Gown, Operating Room, Reusable — Surgery

SEMI-PERMANENT
78MES Stent, Urethral, Bulbous, Permanent/Semi-Permanent — Gastro/Urology
78MER Stent, Urethral, Prostatic, Permanent/Semi-Permanent — Gastro/Urology

SEMI-PERMEABLE
77KQL Tube, Tympanostomy, With Semi-Permeable Membrane — Ear/Nose/Throat

SEMIMICRO
75UKG Balance, Semimicro (0.01 mg Accuracy) — Chemistry

SEMINAL
82DGB Seminal Fluid, Antigen, Antiserum, Control — Immunology

SENGSTAKEN
78SCX Tube, Esophageal, Sengstaken — Gastro/Urology

SENSING
74DTW Monitor, Cardiopulmonary Level Sensing — Cardiovascular

SENSITIVITY
77ETR Adapter, Index, Sensitivity, Increment, Short — Ear/Nose/Throat
83VCS Dispenser, Disc, Sensitivity, Antibiotic — Microbiology
83JTT Sensitivity Test Powder, Antimicrobial — Microbiology
82VJK Test, Chemotherapy Sensitivity (Tumor Colony Forming) — Immunology

SENSITOMETER
90VGP Sensitometer, Radiographic — Radiology

SENSOR
85HGT Cardiotachometer, Fetal, With Sensor — Obstetrics/Gyn
74DTY Sensor, Blood Gas, In-Line, Cardiopulmonary Bypass — Cardiovascular
80MDS Sensor, Glucose, Invasive — General
80WSZ Sensor, Moisture — General
89LDK Sensor, Optical Contour, Physical Medicine — Physical Med
73RSA Sensor, Oxygen — Anesthesiology
74LWO Single Chamber, Sensor Driven, Implantable Pulse Generator — Cardiovascular
73BXG Transducer, Blood Flow, Invasive — Anesthesiology
73BXF Transducer, Blood Flow, Non-Invasive — Anesthesiology
80SBW Transducer, Blood Pressure — General
74WLT Transducer, Flow, Catheter Tip — Cardiovascular
73BXP Transducer, Gas Flow — Anesthesiology
73BXO Transducer, Gas Pressure — Anesthesiology

SENSORY
84MHN Prosthesis, Sensory — Cns/Neurology

SEPARATING
79SJB Instrument, Separating, Nerve — Surgery

SEPARATION
75JHT Chromatographic Separation, CPK Isoenzymes — Chemistry
75CEX Chromatographic Separation, Lactate Dehydrogenase Isoenzyme — Chemistry
75JHG Chromatographic Separation, Lecithin-Sphingomyelin Ratio — Chemistry
75CJB Chromatographic Separation/Radioimmunoassay, Aldosterone — Chemistry
75CDG Chromatographic Separation/Zimmerman 17-Ketogenic Steroids — Chemistry
75CDE Chromatographic Separation/Zimmerman, 17-Ketosteroids — Chemistry
75CIN Electrophoretic Separation, Alkaline Phosphatase Isoenzymes — Chemistry
75JHO Electrophoretic Separation, Lipoproteins — Chemistry
75CDK Electrophoretic Separation, Vanilmandelic Acid — Chemistry
81JCF Medium, Lymphocyte Separation — Hematology
83TDG Separation Media — Microbiology
81UJN Serum Separation System — Hematology
75CEA Triglyceride, Separation, Chromatographic, TLC — Chemistry

SEPARATOR
80WON Column, Immunoadsorption — General
79GAD Retractor, Surgical — Surgery
81GKT Separator, Blood Cell, Automated — Hematology
78LKN Separator, Blood Cell/Plasma, Therapeutic — Gastro/Urology
78MDP Separator, Blood Cell/Plasma, Therapeutic, Membrane, Auto. — Gastro/Urology
84RSB Separator, Dural — Cns/Neurology
75UHN Separator, Protein — Chemistry
78RSC Separator, Pylorus — Gastro/Urology
77RSD Separator, Stapes — Ear/Nose/Throat
87RSE Separator, Toe — Orthopedics
88KEX Sorter, Cell (Separator) — Pathology

SEPTAL
77LFB Button, Nasal Septal — Ear/Nose/Throat

KEYWORD INDEX

SHAFER
77MKP Hearing-Aid, Cortical, Shafer — Ear/Nose/Throat

SHAKER
75VLS Shaker, Waterbath — Chemistry
75JRQ Shaker/Stirrer — Chemistry

SHANK
89ISW Assembly, Knee/Shank/Ankle/Foot, External — Physical Med
89KFX Assembly, Thigh/Knee/Shank/Ankle/Foot, External — Physical Med

SHAPE
90WKV Block, Therapy, Radiation — Radiology

SHAPING
90IXI Block, Beam Shaping, Radionuclide — Radiology

SHARPENER
76RSF Sharpener, Dental — Dental And Oral
79WVB Sharpener, Instrument, Surgical — Surgery
79RSG Sharpener, Knife — Surgery
88RSH Sharpener, Microtome Blade — Pathology
80RSI Sharpener, Needle — General

SHARPES
80MMK Container, Sharpes — General

SHARPS
80TBJ Compactor, Fixed — General
80TBK Compactor, Portable — General
80WZH Remover, Blade, Scalpel — General
80WWY Sterilizer/Compactor — General
80SFS Waste Disposal Unit, Sharps — General
79KDB Waste Disposal Unit, Surgical Instrument (Sharps) — Surgery

SHAVE
80RLP Kit, Prep — General

SHAVING
87WYA Equipment, Shaving, Disc, Spinal — Orthopedics

SHEARLING
80RMA Pad, Pressure, Animal Skin — General

SHEARS
80RRB Scissors, Bandage/Gauze/Plaster — General

SHEATH
78EXJ Appliance, Incontinence, Urosheath Type — Gastro/Urology
78QIS Catheter, Urinary, Condom — Gastro/Urology
80QND Cover, Thermometer — General
84UAV Prosthesis, Nerve Sheath — Cns/Neurology
78EYT Sheath, Corrugated Rubber — Gastro/Urology
78FED Sheath, Endoscopic — Gastro/Urology

SHEEP
80RMA Pad, Pressure, Animal Skin — General

SHEET
90WZJ Cover, Film, X-Ray — Radiology
78EYX Drape, Pure Latex Sheet, With Self-Retaining Finger Cot — Gastro/Urology
79MGP Dressing, Wound and Burn, Occlusive — Surgery
77WXV Inflator, Sheet, Nasopharyngoscopic — Ear/Nose/Throat
80VBF Linen — General
80KME Linen, Bed — General
90IXW Processor, Radiographic Film, Automatic — Radiology
80FPY Sheet, Burn — General
84UAW Sheet, Cranioplasty — Cns/Neurology
79RSK Sheet, Drape — Surgery
79RSL Sheet, Drape, Disposable — Surgery
80RSM Sheet, Examination Table, Disposable — General
79RSN Sheet, Operating Room — Surgery
79RSO Sheet, Operating Room, Disposable — Surgery
80RSJ Sheeting, Examination Table — General
80WKD Sheeting, Stretcher — General

SHEETING
76EIE Dam, Rubber — Dental And Oral
79UCB Reconstructive Sheeting, Plastic Surgery — Surgery
80RSJ Sheeting, Examination Table — General
80WKD Sheeting, Stretcher — General
80RTE Silicone Sheeting — General

SHELF
80WSA Accessories, Cart, Multipurpose — General
80VKB Bin, Storage — General

SHELL
86HQT Shell, Scleral — Ophthalmology

SHELLAC
76EEA Plate, Base, Shellac — Dental And Oral

SHELVING
80TBA Cabinet Casework, General Purpose — General

SHIELD
76EAJ Apron, Lead, Dental — Dental And Oral
90IWO Apron, Lead, Radiographic — Radiology
90IWQ Curtain, Protective, Radiographic — Radiology
90IWP Glove, Protective, Radiographic — Radiology
90IWR Holder, Syringe, Leaded — Radiology
80WKE Mask, Face — General
90VFC Mask, X-Ray Shield — Radiology
90TEM Shield Radio Frequency — Radiology
85RSQ Shield, Breast — Obstetrics/Gyn
87RSR Shield, Bunion — Orthopedics
78FHJ Shield, Circumcision — Gastro/Urology
86WRV Shield, Corneal — Ophthalmology
86MOE Shield, Corneal, Collagen — Ophthalmology
86HOY Shield, Eye, Ophthalmic — Ophthalmology
90IWT Shield, Gonadal — Radiology
80RSS Shield, Heat, Infant — General
90RSP Shield, Magnetic Field — Radiology
85HFS Shield, Nipple — Obstetrics/Gyn
90IWS Shield, Ophthalmic, Radiological — Radiology
90KPY Shield, Protective, Personnel — Radiology
80RST Shield, Syringe — General
90IWW Shield, Vial — Radiology
80RSU Shield, Wound, Injection Site — General
90RSW Shield, X-Ray — Radiology
90RSV Shield, X-Ray, Brick — Radiology
90TDY Shield, X-Ray, Door — Radiology
90WPD Shield, X-Ray, Lead-Plastic — Radiology
76EAK Shield, X-Ray, Leaded — Dental And Oral
90TEN Shield, X-Ray, Portable — Radiology
90VGQ Shield, X-Ray, Throat — Radiology
90VLA Shield, X-Ray, Transparent — Radiology

SHIGELLA
83LIA Antigen, All Groups, Shigella SPP. — Microbiology
83GTD Antiserum, Fluorescent, Shigella SPP., All Globulins — Microbiology
83GNB Antiserum, Shigella SPP. — Microbiology
83LSN Shigella SPP., DNA Reagents — Microbiology

SHOCK
78LNS Lithotriptor, Extracorporeal Shock-wave, Urological — Gastro/Urology
78WUD Lithotriptor, Extracorporeal, Gallstone — Gastro/Urology
80REQ Meter, Leakage Current (Ammeter) — General
74RLJ Suit, Pneumatic Counterpressure (Anti-Shock) — Cardiovascular
73LHX Trousers, Anti-Shock — Anesthesiology

SHOCK-WAVE
78VKM Lithotriptor, Electro-Hydraulic, Extracorporeal — Gastro/Urology
78LNS Lithotriptor, Extracorporeal Shock-wave, Urological — Gastro/Urology

SHOE
80QNE Cover, Shoe, Conductive — General
80QNF Cover, Shoe, Non-Conductive — General
79FXP Cover, Shoe, Operating Room — Surgery
80KYS Insoles, Medical — General
89KNP Orthosis, Corrective Shoe — Physical Med
73BWP Shoe And Shoe Cover, Conductive — Anesthesiology
89IPG Shoe, Cast — Physical Med
79RSX Shoe, Conductive — Surgery
79FXW Shoe, Operating Room — Surgery
87TEO Shoe, Orthopedic — Orthopedics
80RTW Slippers — General
80RZX Tester, Conductivity, Shoe And Gown — General
87WPM Tray, Impression, Foot — Orthopedics

SHORT
77ETR Adapter, Index, Sensitivity, Increment, Short — Ear/Nose/Throat
80MAJ Catheter, Intraspinal, Percutaneous, Short-Term — General
80MIA Needle, Spinal, Short-Term — General
79SHB Trocar, Short — Surgery

SHORT-TERM
80MAJ Catheter, Intraspinal, Percutaneous, Short-Term — General
80MIA Needle, Spinal, Short-Term — General

SHORTWAVE
89VEM Analyzer, Diathermy Unit, Shortwave — Physical Med
89IMJ Diathermy, Shortwave — Physical Med
90MWC Diathermy, Shortwave (Non-heating) — Radiology
89ILX Diathermy, Shortwave, Pulsed — Physical Med

SHOULDER
89KFT Assembly, Shoulder/Elbow/Forearm/Wrist/Hand, Mechanical — Physical Med
89KFW Assembly, Shoulder/Elbow/Forearm/Wrist/Hand, Powered — Physical Med
87WRR Equipment, Screening, Scoliosis — Orthopedics
89QVB Exerciser, Shoulder — Physical Med

SHOULDER *(cont'd)*
79WRY Holder, Shoulder, Arthroscopy — Surgery
87RBL Immobilizer, Shoulder — Orthopedics
89IQQ Joint, Shoulder, External Limb Component — Physical Med
87HSF Prosthesis, Shoulder — Orthopedics
87KWR Prosthesis, Shoulder, Constr., Metal/Metal or Polymer/Cem. — Orthopedics
87KYM Prosthesis, Shoulder, Hemi-, Glenoid, Metal — Orthopedics
87HSD Prosthesis, Shoulder, Hemi-, Humeral — Orthopedics
87MJT Prosthesis, Shoulder, Humeral, Bipol., Hemi-, Constr., M/P — Orthopedics
87MBF Prosthesis, Shoulder, Metal/Polymer, Uncemented — Orthopedics
87KWT Prosthesis, Shoulder, Non-Constrained, Metal/Polymer Cem. — Orthopedics
87KWS Prosthesis, Shoulder, Semi-Constrained, Metal/Polymer Cem. — Orthopedics
87KYL Prosthesis, Shoulder, Semi-Constrained, Uncemented — Orthopedics
87WUU Splint, Abduction, Shoulder — Orthopedics
87WUS System, Traction, Arthroscopy — Orthopedics

SHOWER
80QJM Chair, Shower — General
80TBP Curtain, Shower — General
75TEP Shower, Emergency — Chemistry

SHREDDER
80QNL Crusher, Syringe — General
80SFS Waste Disposal Unit, Sharps — General
79KDB Waste Disposal Unit, Surgical Instrument (Sharps) — Surgery
80SFT Waste Disposal Unit, Syringe — General

SHROUD
88RSZ Kit, Shroud — Pathology

SHUNT
78KNZ Accessories, AV Shunt — Gastro/Urology
78KNR Adapter, AV Shunt Or Fistula — Gastro/Urology
78FKN Adapter, Shunt — Gastro/Urology
78FIQ Cannula, AV Shunt — Gastro/Urology
84UCL Catheter, Hydrocephalic — Cns/Neurology
84UBJ Catheter, Hydrocephalic, Atrial — Cns/Neurology
84UAQ Catheter, Hydrocephalic, Distal — Cns/Neurology
84UAR Catheter, Hydrocephalic, Peritoneal — Cns/Neurology
84UCX Catheter, Hydrocephalic, Ventricular — Cns/Neurology
78FJQ Connector, Shunt — Gastro/Urology
84QWB Filter, Shunt, Hydrocephalic — Cns/Neurology
78FJM Guard, Shunt — Gastro/Urology
84GYK Instrument, Implantation, Shunt — Cns/Neurology
78RTB Shunt, Arteriovenous — Gastro/Urology
74WWF Shunt, Carotid — Cardiovascular
84JXG Shunt, Central Nerve, With Component — Cns/Neurology
77UAG Shunt, Endolymphatic — Ear/Nose/Throat
84RTC Shunt, Hydrocephalic — Cns/Neurology
86WQB Shunt, Intraocular — Ophthalmology
78KPM Shunt, Peritoneal — Gastro/Urology
74RTD Shunt, Peritoneo-Venous — Cardiovascular
74MIR Shunt, Portosystemic, Endoprosthesis — Cardiovascular
78FJN Stabilizer, Shunt — Gastro/Urology
77ESZ Tube, Shunt, Endolymphatic — Ear/Nose/Throat
77KLZ Tube, Shunt, Endolymphatic, With Valve — Ear/Nose/Throat
84LXL Valve, Shunt, Fluid, CNS (Post-Amendment Design) — Cns/Neurology
84LID Ventriculo-Amniotic Shunt for Hydrocephalus — Cns/Neurology

SIALIC
82MEN Assay, Serum, Sialic Acid — Immunology

SIALIDASE
88IBE Neuramininase (Sialidase) — Pathology

SIALOGLYCOPROTEIN
78WXJ Catheter, Sialoglycoprotein — Gastro/Urology

SICKLE
81GHM Test, Sickle Cell — Hematology

SIDE
80TED Rail, Wall Side — General

SIDERAIL
80QDD Bedrail — General

SIEVE
81VCW Sieve, Hematology — Hematology
88IDX Sieve, Tissue — Pathology

SIGHT
86WIZ Lens, Contact, Disposable — Ophthalmology

SIGMOIDOSCOPE
78FAM Sigmoidoscope, Flexible — Gastro/Urology
78FAN Sigmoidoscope, Rigid, Electrical — Gastro/Urology
78KDM Sigmoidoscope, Rigid, Non-Electrical — Gastro/Urology

SIGN
80TEQ Sign, Hospital — General

SIGNAL
74DRR Amplifier, Biopotential (W Signal Conditioner) — Cardiovascular
84GWL Amplifier, Physiological Signal — Cns/Neurology
74DRQ Amplifier, Transducer Signal (W Signal Conditioner) — Cardiovascular
74DRJ Analyzer, Signal Isolation — Cardiovascular
84GWS Analyzer, Spectrum, EEG Signal — Cns/Neurology
84GWK Conditioner, Signal, Physiological — Cns/Neurology
84GWR Simulator, EEG Test Signal — Cns/Neurology
74MFL Transmitter/Receiver, Physiological Signal, Infrared — Cardiovascular

SILASTIC
79MBR Silastic Elastomer (Angular Deformity Prevention) — Surgery

SILBER
75CDB Porter Silber Hydrazone, 17-Hydroxycorticosteroids — Chemistry

SILICA
91DKS Plate, Silica Gel, TLC — Toxicology
91DLO Silica Gel Fluorescent Indicator, TLC — Toxicology

SILICATE
84MLG Cement, Silicate (Cranioplasty) — Cns/Neurology
76EFX Protector, Silicate — Dental And Oral

SILICON
77ESH Polymer, ENT Synthetic-PIFE, Silicon Elastomer — Ear/Nose/Throat

SILICONE
80VAM Component, Silicone — General
79MDA Elastomer, Silicone (Scar Management) — Surgery
79MIB Elastomer, Silicone Block — Surgery
80QSE Elastomer, Silicone Rubber — General
80FNI Mattress, Silicone, And Chair Cushion — General
77UBV Prosthesis, Ossicular, Total, Silicone — Ear/Nose/Throat
80RTE Silicone Sheeting — General
79KGM Silicone, Liquid, Injectable — Surgery
80SDS Tubing, Silicone — General

SILK
79GAP Suture, Non-Absorbable, Silk — Surgery
79RYD Suture, Silk — Surgery

SILVER
80WUL Metal, Medical — General
76EKL Point, Silver, Endodontic — Dental And Oral
88HZX Silver Nitrate — Pathology
90TER Silver Recovery Equipment — Radiology
88HYE Solution, Pathology, Fontanna Silver — Pathology
88KKP Solution, Silver Carbonate — Pathology
88ICZ Stain, Ammoniacal Silver Hydroxide Silver Nitrate — Pathology
88HYZ Stain, Methenamine Silver — Pathology

SIMPLE
78FHP Needle, Pneumoperitoneum, Simple — Gastro/Urology

SIMPLEX
83WJS Antibody, Herpes Virus — Microbiology
83LKC Antigen, Indirect Hemagglutination, Herpes Simplex Virus — Microbiology
83LGC Enzyme Linked Immunoabsorbent Assay, Herpes Simplex Virus — Microbiology
83MXJ Enzyme-Linked Immunosorbent Assay, Herpes Simplex Virus, HSV-1 — Microbiology
83MYF Enzyme-Linked Immunosorbent Assay, Herpes Simplex Virus, HSV-2 — Microbiology

SIMULATION
79SHA Trainer, Laparoscopy — Surgery

SIMULATOR
74LOS Analyzer, ECG — Cardiovascular
73QFN Calibrator, Anesthesia Unit — Anesthesiology
73QFO Calibrator, Pressure Transducer — Anesthesiology
73QFQ Calibrator, Respiratory Therapy Unit — Anesthesiology
74RTF Simulator, Arrhythmia — Cardiovascular
74RTG Simulator, Blood Pressure — Cardiovascular
74RTH Simulator, ECG — Cardiovascular
84GWR Simulator, EEG Test Signal — Cns/Neurology
74RTI Simulator, Heart Sound — Cardiovascular
73RTJ Simulator, Lung — Anesthesiology
90RTL Simulator, Radiotherapy — Radiology
90KPQ Simulator, Radiotherapy, Special Purpose — Radiology
73RTK Simulator, Respiration — Anesthesiology
80RTM Simulator, Temperature — General

SIMULTAN
86HOR Simultan (Including Crossed Cylinder) — Ophthalmology

SINGLE
75QKY Analyzer, Chemistry, Single Channel, Programmable — Chemistry
78QIK Catheter, Hemodialysis, Single-Needle — Gastro/Urology

SINGLE *(cont'd)*
78FKO	Catheter, Peritoneal Dialysis, Single-Use	Gastro/Urology
74DXG	Computer, Diagnostic, Pre-Programmed, Single-Function	Cardiovascular
78QZY	Controller, Hemodialysis Unit Single Needle	Gastro/Urology
78QZZ	Converter, Unit, Hemodialysis, Single-Pass	Gastro/Urology
83JSF	Culture Media, Single Biochemical Test	Microbiology
90KGI	Densitometer, Bone, Single Photon	Radiology
78FIJ	Dialysate Delivery System, Recirculating, Single Pass	Gastro/Urology
78FIL	Dialysate Delivery System, Single Pass	Gastro/Urology
78FKP	Dialysate Delivery System, Single Patient	Gastro/Urology
78FHS	Dialyzer, Single Coil (Hemodialysis)	Gastro/Urology
74DPS	Electrocardiograph, Single Channel	Cardiovascular
87KTW	Fixation Appliance, Single Component	Orthopedics
90IZO	Generator, Diagnostic X-Ray, High Voltage, Single Phase	Radiology
78LBW	Kit, Dialysis, Single Needle (Co-Axial Flow)	Gastro/Urology
78FIF	Kit, Dialysis, Single Needle With Uni-Directional Pump	Gastro/Urology
80MQX	Needle, Acupuncture, Single Use	General
80FMI	Needle, Hypodermic, Single Lumen With Syringe	General
74WST	Pacemaker, Heart, Implantable, Rate Responsive	Cardiovascular
79QHA	Probe, Electrocauterization, Single-Use	Surgery
74LWW	Single Chamber, Anti-Tachycardia, Pulse Generator	Cardiovascular
74LWO	Single Chamber, Sensor Driven, Implantable Pulse Generator	Cardiovascular
79GCY	Suction Apparatus, Single Patient, Portable, Non-Powered	Surgery
74QRZ	Transmitter/Receiver System, ECG, Telephone Single-Channel	Cardiovascular
78FEF	Tube, Single Lumen, W Mercury Wt Balloon	Gastro/Urology

SINGLE-CHANNEL
74QRZ	Transmitter/Receiver System, ECG, Telephone Single-Channel	Cardiovascular

SINGLE-FUNCTION
74DXG	Computer, Diagnostic, Pre-Programmed, Single-Function	Cardiovascular

SINGLE-NEEDLE
78QIK	Catheter, Hemodialysis, Single-Needle	Gastro/Urology

SINGLE-PASS
78QZZ	Converter, Unit, Hemodialysis, Single-Pass	Gastro/Urology

SINGLE-USE
78FKO	Catheter, Peritoneal Dialysis, Single-Use	Gastro/Urology
79QHA	Probe, Electrocauterization, Single-Use	Surgery

SINK
79RRX	Scrub Machine, Surgical	Surgery
80TES	Sink, Hospital	General
75TET	Sink, Laboratory	Chemistry
80UAC	Sink, Portable	General
80WHP	Sink, Sonic	General

SINUS
77KAM	Cannula, Sinus	Ear/Nose/Throat
77LWI	Device, Ultrasound, Sinus	Ear/Nose/Throat
77KAR	Irrigator, Sinus	Ear/Nose/Throat
77KAK	Probe, Sinus	Ear/Nose/Throat
77KAZ	Rasp, Frontal-Sinus	Ear/Nose/Throat
74DSR	Stimulator, Carotid Sinus Nerve	Cardiovascular
77KBF	Trephine, Sinus	Ear/Nose/Throat
77KBG	Trocar, Sinus	Ear/Nose/Throat

SIREN
80WRQ	Equipment, Building Security	General

SIRIUS
88HZY	Sirius Red	Pathology

SISOMICIN
91LBY	Radioimmunoassay, Sisomicin	Toxicology

SITE
80QRA	Dressing, Skin Graft, Donor Site	General
80RSU	Shield, Wound, Injection Site	General

SITUATIONAL
84GZG	Stimulator, Cranial Electrotherapy (Situational Anxiety)	Cns/Neurology

SITZ
89KTC	Bath, Sitz, Non-Powered	Physical Med
89ILM	Bath, Sitz, Physical Medicine	Physical Med
80QJN	Chair, Sitz Bath	General
89HHC	Kit, Sitz Bath	Physical Med

SIZE
83TBH	Analyzer, Cell Size	Microbiology
85HDQ	Dilator, Cervical, Fixed Size	Obstetrics/Gyn
78EXA	Selector, Size, Ostomy	Gastro/Urology

SIZER
79SIX	Sizer, Device, Anastomosis	Surgery
74DTI	Sizer, Heart Valve Prosthesis	Cardiovascular
79MRD	Sizer, Mammary, Breast Implant Volume	Surgery

SKELETAL
90VGL	Radiographic Unit, Diagnostic, Skeletal	Radiology

SKELETON
87UFE	Training Aid	Orthopedics

SKIASCOPE
86HKL	Retinoscope, AC-Powered	Ophthalmology
86HKM	Retinoscope, Battery-Powered	Ophthalmology
90IZL	System, X-Ray, Mobile	Radiology

SKIASCOPIC
86HMH	Rack, Skiascopic	Ophthalmology

SKID
87HWO	Skid, Bone	Orthopedics

SKIN
89IQH	Biofeedback Equipment, Myoelectric, Battery-Powered	Physical Med
89IRC	Biofeedback Equipment, Myoelectric, Powered	Physical Med
79GFE	Brush, Dermabrasion	Surgery
79GED	Brush, Dermabrasion, Manual	Surgery
79FZQ	Clip, Removable (Skin)	Surgery
79RTO	Cutter, Skin Graft	Surgery
79RTP	Cutter, Skin Graft, Expanded Mesh	Surgery
78QOI	Cystic Fibrosis System	Gastro/Urology
79KOY	Degreaser, Skin, Surgical	Surgery
79QPC	Dermabrasion Unit	Surgery
79GFD	Dermatome	Surgery
84HCJ	Device, Measurement, Potential, Skin	Cns/Neurology
80QRA	Dressing, Skin Graft, Donor Site	General
86HLY	Electrode, Skin Surface, Ophthalmic	Ophthalmology
79LCJ	Expander, Skin, Inflatable	Surgery
79FZW	Expander, Surgical, Skin Graft	Surgery
79QYT	Graft, Skin	Surgery
79LZM	Guard, Graft, Skin	Surgery
79RAP	Hook, Skin	Surgery
80TFI	Kit, Skin Scrub	General
79RDI	Knife, Dermatome	Surgery
79RDQ	Knife, Skin Grafting	Surgery
79FTC	Light, Ultraviolet, Dermatologic	Surgery
80VLB	Lotion, Skin Care	General
79FZZ	Marker, Skin	Surgery
81KSC	Material, Preparation, Skin	Hematology
89IKI	Meter, Skin Resistance, AC-Powered	Physical Med
89IKJ	Meter, Skin Resistance, Battery-Powered	Physical Med
84GZO	Monitor, Response, Skin, Galvanic	Cns/Neurology
80LMY	Monitor, Skin Resistance/skin Temperature, For Insulin Reactions	General
89MNE	Orthosis, Moldable, Supportive, Skin Protective	Physical Med
80RMA	Pad, Pressure, Animal Skin	General
80FMP	Protector, Skin Pressure	General
79RNL	Punch, Dermal	Surgery
79LXK	Scraper, Specimen, Skin	Surgery
80WVH	Sock, Protective, Skin	General
80TGV	Solution, Skin Degreaser	General
79GDT	Staple, Removable (Skin)	Surgery
89WIN	Stimulator, Wound Healing	Physical Med
79FPX	Strip, Adhesive	Surgery
79MKY	System, Skin Closure	Surgery

SKINFOLD
80QFR	Caliper, Skinfold	General

SKULL
84GXM	Anvil, Skull Plate	Cns/Neurology
84QKQ	Clamp, Skull	Cns/Neurology
84WVA	Craniotome	Cns/Neurology
84HBL	Holder, Head, Neurosurgical (Skull Clamp)	Cns/Neurology
84RLI	Plate, Bone, Skull (Cranioplasty)	Cns/Neurology
84GWO	Plate, Bone, Skull, Preformed, Alterable	Cns/Neurology
84GXN	Plate, Bone, Skull, Preformed, Non-Alterable	Cns/Neurology
84GXJ	Punch, Skull	Cns/Neurology
84SBB	Tongs, Skull	Cns/Neurology
84HAX	Tongs, Skull, Traction	Cns/Neurology
84SCB	Trephine, Skull	Cns/Neurology

SKULLPLATE
84GXL	Screwdriver, Skullplate	Cns/Neurology

SLAB
76RHI	Mixing Slab	Dental And Oral

SLEEP
73WLD	Equipment, Therapy, Apnea	Anesthesiology
77MYB	Pillow, Cervical(for Mild Sleep Apnea)	Ear/Nose/Throat
84LEL	Sleep Assessment Equipment	Cns/Neurology

SLEEVE
79SIN	Dilator, Port, Laparoscopic	Surgery
74JOW	Sleeve, Compressible Limb	Cardiovascular

KEYWORD INDEX

SLEEVE *(cont'd)*
86UBF Sleeve, Muscle, Ophthalmic — Ophthalmology
79RTQ Sleeve, Topical Oxygen Therapy — Surgery
79SHV Sleeve, Trocar — Surgery

SLIDE
83GNC Antigen, Febrile, Slide And Tube, Salmonella — Microbiology
83GSL Antigen, Slide And Tube, Francisella Tularensis — Microbiology
83GSI Antigen, Slide And Tube, Listeria Monocytogenes — Microbiology
80WRH Cabinet, Storage, Slide — General
88KIY Chamber, Slide Culture — Pathology
83TDB Container, Slide Mailer — Microbiology
88KES Coverslip, Microscope Slide — Pathology
75QQD Dispenser, Slide — Chemistry
75TBY Dryer, Labware — Chemistry
88WSW Guard, Stain (Slide) — Pathology
88IEH Lamp, Slide Warming — Pathology
88MKQ Processor, Slide, Cytology, Automated — Pathology
88MNM Reader, Slide, Cytology, Cervical, Automated — Pathology
81GJO Slide And Coverslip — Hematology
88WSX Slide, Cell Adhesive — Pathology
83LJG Slide, Control, Quality — Microbiology
88KEW Slide, Microscope — Pathology
81GKJ Spinner, Slide, Automated — Hematology
88KPA Stainer, Slide, Automated — Pathology
88KIN Stainer, Slide, Contact Type — Pathology
83RTR Stainer, Slide, Cytology — Microbiology
81RTS Stainer, Slide, Hematology — Hematology
81GKD Stainer, Slide, Hematology, Automated — Hematology
83RTT Stainer, Slide, Histology — Microbiology
88KIO Stainer, Slide, Immersion Type — Pathology
88IEG Table, Slide Warming — Pathology

SLIDING
88KFL Microtome, Sliding — Pathology

SLING
74WVD Holder, Cardiac — Cardiovascular
89ILI Sling, Arm — Physical Med
89ILE Sling, Arm, Overhead Supported — Physical Med
87RTU Sling, Knee — Orthopedics
87RTV Sling, Leg — Orthopedics
89INE Sling, Overhead Suspension, Wheelchair — Physical Med

SLIPPERS
80RTW Slippers — General

SLIT
86REC Lamp, Slit — Ophthalmology
86HJO Lamp, Slit, Biomicroscope, AC-Powered — Ophthalmology

SLOW
90UEY Television System, Slow Scan — Radiology

SLUSH
80TBU Dispenser, Ice — General

SM
82LKP Anti-SM-Antibody, Antigen And Control — Immunology
82LLL Extractable Antinuclear Antibody (Rnp/Sm), Antigen/Control — Immunology

SMALL
90TEK Scanner, Ultrasonic, Small Parts — Radiology

SMEAR
85RJW Kit, Pap Smear — Obstetrics/Gyn
85MCO Kit, Smear, Cervical — Obstetrics/Gyn
88IHB Pipette, Vaginal Pool Smear — Pathology
88IFI Sprays, Synthetic, Smear — Pathology

SMOKE
73KHB Filter, Tobacco Smoke (Attached) — Anesthesiology
73KHC Filter, Tobacco Smoke (Unattached) — Anesthesiology
79VCN System, Evacuation, Smoke, Laser — Surgery
78FCZ Tube, Smoke Removal, Endoscopic — Gastro/Urology

SMOOTH
82DBE Antibody, Anti-Smooth Muscle, Indirect Immunofluorescent — Immunology
87HTY Pin, Fixation, Smooth — Orthopedics

SNAKE
80RTX Kit, Snake Bite — General
80KYQ Kit, Snake Bite, Chemical Cold Pack — General
80KYP Kit, Snake Bite, Suction — General

SNARE
73JEI Remover, Foreign Body, Bronchoscope (Non-Rigid) — Anesthesiology
77JZD Snare, Ear — Ear/Nose/Throat
79ULT Snare, Endoscopic — Surgery
86HNE Snare, Enucleating — Ophthalmology
78FDI Snare, Flexible — Gastro/Urology
77KBE Snare, Nasal — Ear/Nose/Throat

SNARE *(cont'd)*
78FGX Snare, Non-Electrical — Gastro/Urology
79RTZ Snare, Other — Surgery
79RTY Snare, Polyp — Surgery
78FDJ Snare, Rigid Self-Opening — Gastro/Urology
79GAE Snare, Surgical — Surgery
77KBZ Snare, Tonsil — Ear/Nose/Throat

SNELLEN
86HOX Chart, Visual Acuity — Ophthalmology

SNORING
77LRK Device, Anti-Snoring — Ear/Nose/Throat

SOAP
80TBV Dispenser, Soap — General
80WPU Soap — General

SOCK
87RUA Sock, Cast Toe — Orthopedics
87RUB Sock, Fracture — Orthopedics
80WVI Sock, Non-Compression — General
80WVH Sock, Protective, Skin — General
80RUC Sock, Stump Cover — General

SOCKET
87KIL Positioner, Socket — Orthopedics
89ISS Prosthesis, Thigh Socket, External Component — Physical Med
87HXO Pusher, Socket — Orthopedics

SODIUM
76KOM Acacia And Karaya With Sodium Borate — Dental And Oral
76MMU Adhesive, Denture, Acacia & Karaya with Sodium Borate — Dental And Oral
76KOR Adhesive, Denture, Karaya With Sodium Borate — Dental And Oral
75QTJ Analyzer, Chemistry, Electrolyte — Chemistry
76KXW Carboxymethylcellulose Sodium — Dental And Oral
76KOS Carboxymethylcellulose Sodium & Cationic Polyacrylamide — Dental And Oral
76KOQ Carboxymethylcellulose Sodium (40-100%) — Dental And Oral
76KOL Carboxymethylcellulose Sodium/Ethylene-Oxide Homopolymer — Dental And Oral
75JGS Electrode, Ion Specific, Sodium — Chemistry
75JGT Photometer, Flame, Sodium — Chemistry
76KOO Polyvinyl Methylether Maleic Acid-Calcium-Sodium Dbl. Salt — Dental And Oral
75JLK Sodium Hydroxide/Phenol Red (Titrimetric), Gastric Acidity — Chemistry
88KKQ Sodium Periodate — Pathology
88IGB Solution, Formalin/Sodium Acetate — Pathology
75CEI Uranyl Acetate/Zinc Acetate, Sodium — Chemistry

SOFT
79MPN Adhesive, Soft Tissue Approximation — Surgery
89IKS Electrode, Metallic With Soft Pad Covering — Physical Med
87MAI Fastener, Fixation, Biodegradable, Soft Tissue — Orthopedics
87MBI Fastener, Fixation, Non-Biodegradable, Soft Tissue — Orthopedics
86LPL Lenses, Soft Contact, Daily Wear — Ophthalmology
86LPM Lenses, Soft Contact, Extended Wear — Ophthalmology
89IPX Orthosis, Rib Fracture, Soft — Physical Med
89IPW Orthosis, Sacroiliac, Soft — Physical Med
80RME Pad, Pressure, Soft Rubber — General
77LBP Prosthesis, Ossicular (Stapes), Absorbable Gelatin Material — Ear/Nose/Throat
79UCY Prosthesis, Soft Tissue — Surgery
86HRD Sterilizer, Soft Lens, Thermal, AC-Powered — Ophthalmology
86HRC Sterilizer, Soft Lens, Thermal, Battery-Powered — Ophthalmology

SOFTWARE
80VAX Computer Equipment — General
80VBH Computer Software — General
80WVJ Computer Software, Home Healthcare — General
80WSJ Computer Software, Hospital/Nursing Management — General
80WSN Computer Software, Industrial — General
82MLF Computer Software, Prenatal Risk Evaluation — Immunology
80LNX Computer and Software, Medical — General
86LQB Computer and Software, Medical, Ophthalmic Use — Ophthalmology
75QMB Computer, Clinical Laboratory — Chemistry
87WIV Service, Design, Implant, Custom — Orthopedics
81MMH Software, Blood Bank (Stand-Alone Products) — Hematology
81MTQ Software, Blood Virus Applications — Hematology

SOLE
90LHP Telethermographic System (Sole Diagnostic Screen) — Radiology

SOLID
82KTL Anti-DNA Indirect Immunofluorescent Solid Phase — Immunology
82KTM C3-Indirect Immunofluorescent Solid Phase — Immunology
90MQB Imager, X-Ray, Solid State (Flat Panel/Digital) — Radiology
91DND RIA, Digitoxin (125-I), Rabbit Antibody, Solid Phase Sep. — Toxicology
91DON Radioimmunoassay, Digoxin (125-I), Rabbit, Solid Phase — Toxicology

SOLIDIFYING
83JSK Culture Media, Supplements — Microbiology

SOLUBILITY
81JBB	Solubility, Hemoglobin, Abnormal	Hematology

SOLUBLE
88KEQ	Media, Mounting, Water Soluble	Pathology
88KEP	Mounting Media, Oil Soluble	Pathology

SOLUTION
86LYL	Accessories, Solution, Lens, Contact	Ophthalmology
80QAF	Adhesive, Aerosol	General
80QAG	Adhesive, Liquid	General
80QEF	Bottle, Sterile Solution	General
80QEG	Bowl, Solution	General
88IFF	Decalcifier Solution, Electrolytic	Pathology
79LWD	Irrigating Solution, Non-Injectable	Surgery
74UDD	Kit, Administration, Cardioplegia Solution	Cardiovascular
91DMR	M-Nitrophenol Solution, Specific Reagent For Cholinesterase	Toxicology
80WYV	Pin, Transfer, Solution	General
83LIE	Reagent, Inoculator Calibration (Laboratory)	Microbiology
80TGE	Solution, Antibacterial Cleaner	General
83LOP	Solution, Antimicrobial	Microbiology
88KIP	Solution, Balanced Salt	Pathology
76KZP	Solution, Cement Dissolving	Dental And Oral
88IGK	Solution, Clarke's	Pathology
81KSL	Solution, Copper Sulfate, For Specific Gravity Test	Hematology
78LLJ	Solution, Dialysis	Gastro/Urology
88IGE	Solution, Formalin Ammonium Bromide	Pathology
88IGB	Solution, Formalin/Sodium Acetate	Pathology
80TGF	Solution, Instrument Cleaner	General
80WYR	Solution, Instrument, Laparoscopic, Anti-Fog	General
80TGA	Solution, Intravenous	General
81JCE	Solution, Isotonic	Hematology
78WWM	Solution, Nutrition, Enteral	Gastro/Urology
78TGK	Solution, Nutrition, Parenteral	Gastro/Urology
78VKQ	Solution, Ostomy, Odor Control	Gastro/Urology
88IGM	Solution, Pathology, Carnoy's	Pathology
88KDX	Solution, Pathology, Decalcifier, Acid Containing	Pathology
88HYE	Solution, Pathology, Fontanna Silver	Pathology
88IGF	Solution, Pathology, Formalin-Alcohol-Acetic Acid	Pathology
88IGD	Solution, Pathology, Formol Calcium	Pathology
88IFS	Solution, Pathology, Helly	Pathology
88IAM	Solution, Pathology, Lugol's	Pathology
88IFO	Solution, Pathology, Newcomer's	Pathology
88IFN	Solution, Pathology, Orth's	Pathology
88IFH	Solution, Pathology, Zenker's	Pathology
80TGG	Solution, Patient Preparation	General
76LMW	Solution, Removal, Caries	Dental And Oral
79MUG	Solution, Saline(wound Dressing)	Surgery
88KKP	Solution, Silver Carbonate	Pathology
80TGV	Solution, Skin Degreaser	General
81KSK	Solution, Stabilized Enzyme	Hematology
76LFE	Solution, Sterilizing, Cold	Dental And Oral
80TGD	Solution, Surgical Scrub	General
75UHD	Solution, pH Buffer	Chemistry
78FKH	Solution-Test, Standard-Conductivity, Dialysis	Gastro/Urology
79KOX	Solvent, Adhesive Tape	Surgery
88LED	Stain, Chemical Solution	Pathology
88LEE	Stain, Dye Solution	Pathology
88GHZ	Stain, Gugol Blue Solution	Pathology
80LHC	Warmer, Irrigation Solution	General
75SFL	Warmer, Solution	Chemistry

SOLUTION-TEST
78FKH	Solution-Test, Standard-Conductivity, Dialysis	Gastro/Urology

SOLVENT
75UIB	Solvent	Chemistry
79KOX	Solvent, Adhesive Tape	Surgery
75UIE	Solvent, Spectrophotometer	Chemistry
75UIA	Still, Solvent Recovery	Chemistry

SOMATIC
83LHT	Antigen, Somatic, Staphylococcus Aureus	Microbiology

SOMATOSENSORY
84UFJ	Stimulator, Somatosensory	Cns/Neurology

SOMNOGRAPH
84LEL	Sleep Assessment Equipment	Cns/Neurology

SONIC
87MHH	Analyzer, Bone, Sonic, Non-Invasive	Orthopedics
80WHP	Sink, Sonic	General
87JDX	Surgical Instrument, Sonic	Orthopedics

SONOMETER
90MUA	Sonometer, Bone	Radiology

SORBENT
78FKT	Dialysate Delivery System, Sorbent Regenerated	Gastro/Urology

SORBENT *(cont'd)*
78FLD	Hemoperfusion System, Sorbent	Gastro/Urology
83GMW	Sorbent, FTA-ABS Test	Microbiology

SORBITOL
75JNK	Beta-D-Fructose & NADH Oxidation (U.V.), Sorbitol DH	Chemistry

SORE
80WYO	Mattress, Reduction, Pressure	General

SORTER
88KEX	Sorter, Cell (Separator)	Pathology

SOUND
85HEK	Monitor, Fetal, Ultrasonic, Heart Sound	Obstetrics/Gyn
85HEJ	Monitor, Hemic Sound, Ultrasonic	Obstetrics/Gyn
74RTI	Simulator, Heart Sound	Cardiovascular
78FBS	Sound, Metal, Interconnected	Gastro/Urology
78FBX	Sound, Urethral, Metal Or Plastic	Gastro/Urology
85HHM	Sound, Uterine	Obstetrics/Gyn
74JOO	Transducer, Heart Sound	Cardiovascular
86WOM	Vision Aid, Ultrasonic	Ophthalmology

SOURCE
90IXD	Calibrator Source, Nuclear Sealed	Radiology
77EQH	Fiberoptic Light Source & Carrier	Ear/Nose/Throat
79GCT	Light Source, Endoscope, Xenon Arc	Surgery
85HIE	Light Source, Endoscopic	Obstetrics/Gyn
78FCW	Light Source, Fiberoptic, Routine	Gastro/Urology
75RFC	Light Source, Flash	Chemistry
78FCQ	Light Source, Incandescent, Diagnostic	Gastro/Urology
78FCR	Light Source, Photographic, Fiberoptic	Gastro/Urology
90IYQ	Phantom, Flood Source, Nuclear	Radiology
90KXK	Source, Brachytherapy, Radionuclide	Radiology
85MPU	Source, Chemiluminescent Light	Obstetrics/Gyn
76EEG	Source, Heat, Bleaching, Teeth, Dental	Dental And Oral
90IWI	Source, Isotope, Sealed, Gold, Titanium, Platinum	Radiology
75UIC	Source, Radioisotope Reference	Chemistry
90IWH	Source, Teletherapy, Radionuclide	Radiology
90IWA	Source, Wire, Radioactive Iridium	Radiology

SPA
90WRK	Densitometer, Bone, Dual Photon	Radiology
90KGI	Densitometer, Bone, Single Photon	Radiology

SPACE
76DYT	Maintainer, Space Preformed, Orthodontic	Dental And Oral

SPACER
87LTO	Spacer, Cement	Orthopedics
87UBS	Spacer, Tendon	Orthopedics

SPATULA
84RUD	Spatula, Brain	Cns/Neurology
76RUE	Spatula, Cement	Dental And Oral
85HHT	Spatula, Cervical, Cytology	Obstetrics/Gyn
79RUF	Spatula, Lung	Surgery
77RUG	Spatula, Middle Ear	Ear/Nose/Throat
86HND	Spatula, Ophthalmic	Ophthalmology
87HXR	Spatula, Orthopedic	Orthopedics
79RUH	Spatula, Other	Surgery
79GAF	Spatula, Surgical, General & Plastic Surgery	Surgery

SPEAKING
77WRO	Valve, Speaking, Tracheal	Ear/Nose/Throat

SPEAR
86HOZ	Sponge, Ophthalmic	Ophthalmology

SPECIAL
79UCQ	Electrosurgical Equipment, Special Purpose	Surgery
90IWZ	Film, X-Ray, Special Purpose	Radiology
90VGC	Kit, Angiographic, Special Procedure	Radiology
80WXF	Pack, Custom/Special Procedure	General
90THR	Radiographic/Fluoroscopic Unit, Special Procedure	Radiology
90JAK	Scanner, Computed Tomography, X-Ray, Special Procedure	Radiology
90KPQ	Simulator, Radiotherapy, Special Purpose	Radiology
85KXP	Stent, Vaginal, Special Purpose	Obstetrics/Gyn
80WNH	Tray, Custom/Special Procedure	General
89IQC	Wheelchair, Special Grade	Physical Med

SPECIALTY
90MOS	Coil, Magnetic Resonance, Specialty	Radiology
80LZC	Glove, Patient Examination, Specialty	General

SPECIES
82KTS	2nd Antibody (Species Specific Anti-Animal Gamma Globulin)	Immunology
83LSG	Candida Species, Antibody Detection	Microbiology
83LHW	Reag. & Equipment, Erythrocyte Suspension, Multi Species	Microbiology

KEYWORD INDEX

SPHERE
86HNP *Introducer, Sphere* — *Ophthalmology*
79FWO *Prosthesis, Eye, Internal (Sphere)* — *Surgery*
86HPZ *Sphere, Ophthalmic (Implant)* — *Ophthalmology*

SPHINCTER
78FAG *Prosthesis, Urethral Sphincter* — *Gastro/Urology*

SPHINCTEROSCOPE
78FDR *Sphincteroscope* — *Gastro/Urology*

SPHINGOMYELIN
75JHG *Chromatographic Separation, Lecithin-Sphingomyelin Ratio* — *Chemistry*
75JHF *Colorimetric Method, Lecithin-Sphingomyelin Ratio* — *Chemistry*
75JHH *Electrophoretic Method, Lecithin-Sphingomyelin Ratio* — *Chemistry*
75WHJ *Test, Maturity, Lung, Fetal* — *Chemistry*

SPHYGMOGRAPH
74RUU *Sphygmograph (Recorder)* — *Cardiovascular*

SPHYGMOMANOMETER
80WRS *Bulb, Inflation* — *General*
74WZC *Monitor, Blood Pressure, Finger* — *Cardiovascular*
74RLS *Monitor, Blood Pressure, Indirect (Arterial)* — *Cardiovascular*
73BXD *Monitor, Blood Pressure, Indirect, Anesthesiology* — *Anesthesiology*
74JOE *Monitor, Blood Pressure, Indirect, Automatic* — *Cardiovascular*
74DXN *Monitor, Blood Pressure, Indirect, Semi-Automatic* — *Cardiovascular*
79FYM *Monitor, Blood Pressure, Indirect, Surgery* — *Surgery*
79FYL *Monitor, Blood Pressure, Indirect, Surgery, Powered* — *Surgery*
73BZZ *Monitor, Blood Pressure, Indirect, Transducer* — *Anesthesiology*
80JOI *Pump, Inflator* — *General*
80FLY *Sphygmomanometer, Aneroid (Arterial Pressure)* — *General*
80THH *Sphygmomanometer, Electronic (Arterial Pressure)* — *General*
80UDM *Sphygmomanometer, Electronic, Automatic* — *General*
80UDN *Sphygmomanometer, Electronic, Manual* — *General*
80FLX *Sphygmomanometer, Mercury (Arterial Pressure)* — *General*
80SBD *Tourniquet* — *General*

SPILL
80WUM *Encapsulator, Fluid* — *General*

SPINAL
87LYP *Accessories, Fixation, Spinal Interlaminal* — *Orthopedics*
87LYQ *Accessories, Fixation, Spinal Intervertebral Body* — *Orthopedics*
82DFI *Antigen, Antiserum, Control, Spinal Fluid, Total* — *Immunology*
87KWP *Appliance, Fixation, Spinal Interlaminal* — *Orthopedics*
87KWQ *Appliance, Fixation, Spinal Intervertebral Body* — *Orthopedics*
84LWC *Device, Hypothermia, Injury, Cord, Spinal* — *Cns/Neurology*
87MQP *Device, Spinal Vertebral Body Replacement* — *Orthopedics*
84LHG *Electrode, Epidural, Spinal* — *Cns/Neurology*
87WYA *Equipment, Shaving, Disc, Spinal* — *Orthopedics*
87UAP *Fixation Device, Spinal (External)* — *Orthopedics*
87JDN *Implant, Fixation Device, Spinal* — *Orthopedics*
73BWD *Introducer, Spinal Needle* — *Anesthesiology*
73QAY *Kit, Anesthesia, Spinal* — *Anesthesiology*
84RFM *Kit, Lumbar Puncture* — *Cns/Neurology*
80FMJ *Manometer, Spinal Fluid* — *General*
80CAQ *Monitor, Cerebral Spinal Fluid Pressure (CSF)* — *General*
80CAR *Monitor, Cerebral Spinal Fluid Pressure, Electrical* — *General*
80MIA *Needle, Spinal, Short-Term* — *General*
87MAT *Orthosis, Fixation, Cervical Intervertebral Body, Spinal* — *Orthopedics*
87MNI *Orthosis, Fixation, Pedicle, Spinal* — *Orthopedics*
87MNH *Orthosis, Fixation, Spinal, Spondylolisthesis* — *Orthopedics*
87MAX *Orthosis, Fusion, Intervertebral, Spinal* — *Orthopedics*
84TEG *Reservoir, Spinal Fluid* — *Cns/Neurology*
84LHY *Stabilized Epidural Spinal Electrode* — *Cns/Neurology*
84LGW *Stimulator, Cerebellar, Full Implant (Pain Relief)* — *Cns/Neurology*
84LGT *Stimulator, Cord, Spinal, Implantable (Motor Disorders)* — *Cns/Neurology*
84LLE *Stimulator, Cord, Spinal, Implantable (Periph. Vasc. Dis.)* — *Cns/Neurology*
84RWD *Stimulator, Dorsal Column* — *Cns/Neurology*
84UFF *Stimulator, Electro-Analgesic* — *Cns/Neurology*
84GZB *Stimulator, Spinal Cord, Implantable (Pain Relief)* — *Cns/Neurology*
84GZD *Stimulator, Spinal Cord, Implantable, Bladder Evacuator* — *Cns/Neurology*
87MCV *System, Appliance, Fixation, Spinal Pedicle Screw* — *Orthopedics*
87MRW *System, Facet Screw Spinal Device* — *Orthopedics*

SPINE
87RUV *Board, Spine* — *Orthopedics*
80WMR *Collar, Extrication* — *General*
89LZW *Monitor, Spine Curvature* — *Physical Med*
87WWB *Positioner, Spine, Surgical* — *Orthopedics*
87MJO *Prosthesis, Spine, Intervertebral Disc* — *Orthopedics*
84RWD *Stimulator, Dorsal Column* — *Cns/Neurology*
84UFF *Stimulator, Electro-Analgesic* — *Cns/Neurology*

SPINNER
88KJD *Flask, Spinner* — *Pathology*
88KJE *Spinner System, Cell Culture* — *Pathology*
81GKJ *Spinner, Slide, Automated* — *Hematology*

SPIRAL
85HGP *Electrode, Circular (Spiral), Scalp And Applicator* — *Obstetrics/Gyn*

SPIRALIS
83GPI *Antigen, Bentonite Flocculation, Trichinella Spiralis* — *Microbiology*
83GPG *Antigen, Latex Agglutination, Trichinella Spiralis* — *Microbiology*
83GPH *Antiserum, Bentonite Flocculation, Trichinella Spiralis* — *Microbiology*
83MDT *Enzyme Linked Immunoabsorbent Assay, Trichinella Spiralis* — Microbiology

SPIROMETER
73QFQ *Calibrator, Respiratory Therapy Unit* — *Anesthesiology*
73QXZ *Gasometer* — *Anesthesiology*
73SES *Monitor, Ventilation* — *Anesthesiology*
80WUP *Paper, Recording, Data* — *General*
73RLL *Pneumograph* — *Anesthesiology*
73BZG *Spirometer, Diagnostic (Respirometer)* — *Anesthesiology*
73BZK *Spirometer, Monitoring (Volumeter)* — *Anesthesiology*
73BWF *Spirometer, Therapeutic (Incentive)* — *Anesthesiology*
73WTC *Syringe, Calibration Testing, Spirometer* — *Anesthesiology*

SPIROMETRY
73BZH *Meter, Peak Flow, Spirometry* — *Anesthesiology*

SPITTOON
76QOE *Cuspidor* — *Dental And Oral*

SPLINT
87RBF *Immobilizer, Ankle* — *Orthopedics*
87RBG *Immobilizer, Arm* — *Orthopedics*
87RBH *Immobilizer, Cervical* — *Orthopedics*
87RBI *Immobilizer, Elbow* — *Orthopedics*
87RBJ *Immobilizer, Infant (Circumcision Board)* — *Orthopedics*
87RBK *Immobilizer, Knee* — *Orthopedics*
87RBL *Immobilizer, Shoulder* — *Orthopedics*
87RBM *Immobilizer, Wrist/Hand* — *Orthopedics*
80SEJ *Pad, Vacuum Stabilized* — *General*
80WKI *Padding, Cast/Splint* — *General*
79FYG *Prosthesis, Splint, Nasal, External* — *Surgery*
89IOZ *Splint, Abduction, Congenital Hip Dislocation* — *Physical Med*
87WUU *Splint, Abduction, Shoulder* — *Orthopedics*
89IQJ *Splint, Clavicle* — *Physical Med*
89ITN *Splint, Denis Brown* — *Physical Med*
76ELS *Splint, Endodontic Stabilizer* — *Dental And Oral*
79FZF *Splint, Extremity, Inflatable, External* — *Surgery*
79FYH *Splint, Extremity, Non-Inflatable, External* — *Surgery*
89ILH *Splint, Hand, And Component* — *Physical Med*
87RUW *Splint, Molded, Aluminum* — *Orthopedics*
87RUX *Splint, Molded, Plastic* — *Orthopedics*
77EPP *Splint, Nasal* — *Ear/Nose/Throat*
87RVC *Splint, Other* — *Orthopedics*
87RUY *Splint, Padded Stays* — *Orthopedics*
87RUZ *Splint, Pneumatic* — *Orthopedics*
77LYA *Splint, Septal, Intranasal* — *Ear/Nose/Throat*
89IQM *Splint, Temporary Training* — *Physical Med*
87HSP *Splint, Traction* — *Orthopedics*
78FAD *Splint, Ureteral* — *Gastro/Urology*
87RVA *Splint, Vacuum* — *Orthopedics*
87RVB *Splint, Wire Board* — *Orthopedics*

SPLINTING
76EBL *Pin, Retentive And Splinting* — *Dental And Oral*
78LCG *Tube, Intestinal Splinting* — *Gastro/Urology*

SPLIT
82DAZ *Antigen, Antiserum, Control, Fibrinogen And Split Products* — *Immunology*
82DAP *Antigen, Antiserum, Fibrinogen And Fibrin Split Products* — *Immunology*
82DAX *Antigen, Antiserum, Fibrinogen And Split Products, FITC* — *Immunology*
82DAR *Antigen, Fibrinogen And Split Products, Rhodamine* — *Immunology*
81GHH *Fibrin Split Products* — *Hematology*
81DAT *Fibrin. & Split Products, Peroxidase, Antigen, Antis., Cont.* — *Hematology*

SPLITTER
80WTB *Cutter, Pill* — *General*

SPONDYLOLISTHESIS
87MNH *Orthosis, Fixation, Spinal, Spondylolisthesis* — *Orthopedics*

SPONGE
80QCR *Basin, Sponge* — *General*
80QEH *Bowl, Sponge* — *General*
78FGS *Carrier, Sponge, Endoscopic* — *Gastro/Urology*
79LWH *Counter, Sponge, Surgical* — *Surgery*
80FRO *Dressing, Other* — *General*
79QXH *Forceps, Sponge* — *Surgery*
79GEL *Gauze, Non-Absorbable, Medicated (Internal Sponge)* — *Surgery*
79GEK *Gauze, Non-Absorbable, Non-Medicated (Internal Sponge)* — *Surgery*
79GDY *Gauze, Non-Absorbable, X-Ray Detectable (Internal Sponge)* — Surgery
79NAB *Gauze/sponge, Nonresorbable For External Use* — *Surgery*

SPONGE *(cont'd)*
80MXI Nonabsorbable Gauze, Surgical Sponge, & Wound Dressing for External Use (with a Drug) General
79RXO Packing, Surgical Surgery
79FSF Rack, Sponge, Operating Room Surgery
80FQA Scale, Surgical Sponge General
85LLR Sponge, Contraceptive Obstetrics/Gyn
88RVD Sponge, Dissector Pathology
79GER Sponge, External Surgery
84HAY Sponge, External, Neurological Cns/Neurology
79GEQ Sponge, External, Rubber Surgery
79GEP Sponge, External, Synthetic Surgery
80RVE Sponge, Filmated General
76EFQ Sponge, Gauze Dental And Oral
80RVF Sponge, Germicidal (Alcohol) General
79THO Sponge, Hemostatic, Absorbable Collagen Surgery
84HAZ Sponge, Internal Cns/Neurology
79RVG Sponge, Laparotomy Surgery
84RVH Sponge, Neuro Cns/Neurology
86HOZ Sponge, Ophthalmic Ophthalmology
80RVL Sponge, Other General
80RVI Sponge, Rayon Cellulose General
79RVJ Sponge, Scrub Surgery
79RVK Sponge, X-Ray Detectable Surgery
80SFU Waste Receptacle, Contaminated General
80RDD Waste Receptacle, Kick Bucket General

SPOON
77JZE Spoon, Ear Ear/Nose/Throat
86REU Spoon, Lens Ophthalmology
80VLJ Spoon, Medicine General
86HNB Spoon, Ophthalmic Ophthalmology
89ILC Utensil, Food Physical Med

SPOROTHRIX
83GMA Antiserum, Fluorescent, Sporothrix Schenekii Microbiology

SPOT
90IXH Camera, Focal Spot, Radiographic Radiology
90IZJ Camera, X-Ray, Fluorographic, Cine Or Spot Radiology
81JBG Glucose-6-Phosphate Dehydrogenase (Erythrocytic), Spot Hematology
86HIX Light, Maxwell Spot, AC-Powered Ophthalmology
90IXL Spot Film Device Radiology

SPOTTED
83GPQ Antigen, CF, Spotted Fever Group Microbiology
83GPP Antiserum, Rocky Mountain Spotted Fever Microbiology

SPP.
83WJT Antibody, Mycoplasma SPP. Microbiology
83GTR Antideoxyribonuclease, Streptococcus SPP. Microbiology
83GSO Antigen, (Febrile), Agglutination, Brucella SPP. Microbiology
83GPF Antigen, Agglutinating, Echinococcus SPP. Microbiology
83LIA Antigen, All Groups, Shigella SPP. Microbiology
83JWT Antigen, CF, Aspergillus SPP. Microbiology
83GSB Antigen, CF, Mycoplasma SPP. Microbiology
83GMO Antigen, Latex Agglutination, Entamoeba Histolytica & Rel. Microbiology
83GRY Antigen, Leptospira SPP. Microbiology
83GRL Antigen, Salmonella SPP. Microbiology
83GTY Antigen, Streptococcus SPP. Microbiology
83GSY Antisera, Fluorescent, All Globulins, Proteus SPP. Microbiology
83GTN Antisera, Fluorescent, All Types, Staphylococcus SPP. Microbiology
83LKI Antisera, Fluorescent, Chlamydia SPP. Microbiology
83LKH Antisera, Immunoperoxidase, Chlamydia SPP. Microbiology
83GPE Antisera, Positive Control, Echinococcus SPP. Microbiology
83GTE Antiserum, Arizona SPP. Microbiology
83GTF Antiserum, Bethesda-Ballerup Polyvalent, Citrobacter SPP. Microbiology
83GOO Antiserum, Fluorescent, All Globulins, Salmonella SPP. Microbiology
83GSM Antiserum, Fluorescent, Brucella SPP. Microbiology
83GTX Antiserum, Fluorescent, Groups, Streptococcus SPP. Microbiology
83GRO Antiserum, Fluorescent, Hemophilus SPP. Microbiology
83GTB Antiserum, Fluorescent, Klebsiella SPP. Microbiology
83GRW Antiserum, Fluorescent, Leptospira SPP. Microbiology
83GRZ Antiserum, Fluorescent, Mycoplasma SPP. Microbiology
83GTD Antiserum, Fluorescent, Shigella SPP., All Globulins Microbiology
83GTC Antiserum, Klebsiella SPP. Microbiology
83GRX Antiserum, Leptospira SPP. Microbiology
83GSA Antiserum, Mycoplasma SPP. Microbiology
83KFG Antiserum, Positive Control, Aspergillus SPP. Microbiology
83GRM Antiserum, Salmonella SPP. Microbiology
83GNB Antiserum, Shigella SPP. Microbiology
83GTZ Antiserum, Streptococcus SPP. Microbiology
83LQP Campylobacter SPP. Microbiology
83LQO Campylobacter SPP. DNA Reagents Microbiology
83LRF Candida SPP., Direct Antigen, ID Microbiology
83MHJ Cryptosporidium Spp. Microbiology
83MCC DNA-Probe, Haemophilus SPP. Microbiology
83LJZ Enzyme Linked Immunoabsorbent Assay, Mycoplasma SPP. Microbiology

SPP. *(cont'd)*
83MHI Giardia Spp. Microbiology
83MJH Legionella, Spp., ELISA Microbiology
83LQF Mycobacterium SPP. DNA Reagents Microbiology
83LQG Mycoplasma SPP. DNA Reagents Microbiology
83LSM Salmonella SPP., DNA Reagents Microbiology
83LSN Shigella SPP., DNA Reagents Microbiology

SPRAY
80VFT Bottle, Medicine Spray General

SPRAYER
75UIF Sprayer, Thin Layer Chromatography Chemistry

SPRAYS
88IFI Sprays, Synthetic, Smear Pathology

SPREADER
87RVM Bars, Spreader Orthopedics
80TCA Extrication Equipment General
78FHK Spreader, Bladder Neck Gastro/Urology
73CBG Spreader, Cuff Anesthesiology
79RVQ Spreader, Other Surgery
87RVN Spreader, Plaster (Cast) Orthopedics
76EKK Spreader, Pulp Canal Filling Material, Endodontic Dental And Oral
87RVO Spreader, Rib Orthopedics
74RVP Spreader, Vein Cardiovascular
86VKE Surgical Instrument, Radial Keratotomy Ophthalmology

SPRING
78FHO Needle, Pneumoperitoneum, Spring Loaded Gastro/Urology
76ECO Spring, Orthodontic Dental And Oral

SPRINKLER
80WRQ Equipment, Building Security General

SPUD
86HNA Spud, Ophthalmic Ophthalmology
86TEV Spud, Ophthalmic, Electrical Ophthalmology

SPUR
78FHH Crusher, Spur, Colostomy Gastro/Urology

SPUTUM
88IHJ Blender, Sputum Pathology
73WVG Catheter, Culture, Pulmonary Anesthesiology
73QLT Collector, Sputum Anesthesiology

SQUAMOUS
81MAP Test, Squamous Cell Carcinoma Hematology

SQUEEZE
73BSH Dynamometer, Grip-Strength (Squeeze) Anesthesiology

ST
80MLC Monitor, ST Segment General
80MLD Monitor, ST Segment (With Alarm) General

STABILITY
79SID Thread, Stability, Trocar Surgery

STABILIZED
80SEJ Pad, Vacuum Stabilized General
81KSK Solution, Stabilized Enzyme Hematology
84LHY Stabilized Epidural Spinal Electrode Cns/Neurology

STABILIZER
74MWS Device, Stabilizer, Heart Cardiovascular
80WMM Regulator, Line Voltage General
76ELS Splint, Endodontic Stabilizer Dental And Oral
78FJN Stabilizer, Shunt Gastro/Urology
80LBJ Stabilizer, Vein General

STAFF
80WSJ Computer Software, Hospital/Nursing Management General

STAGE
88IBL Microscope, Inverted Stage, Tissue Culture Pathology
88KEJ Stage, Microscope Pathology
81JPE Test, Antithrombin III, Two Stage Clotting Time Hematology

STAIN
76MAU Eraser, Dental Stain Dental And Oral
88WSW Guard, Stain (Slide) Pathology
88IDF Stain, Acid Fuchsin Pathology
88IDC Stain, Acridine Orange Pathology
88IDA Stain, Alcian Blue Pathology
88IDB Stain, Aldehyde Fuchsin Pathology
88IDD Stain, Alizarin Red Pathology
88ICZ Stain, Ammoniacal Silver Hydroxide Silver Nitrate Pathology
88KFD Stain, Aniline Blue Pathology
88KJK Stain, Auramine O Pathology
88ICT Stain, Azan Counterstain Pathology
88ICR Stain, Azocarmine B Pathology

STAIN *(cont'd)*

88ICS	Stain, Azocarmine G	Pathology
88ICQ	Stain, Azure A	Pathology
88KJL	Stain, Azure C	Pathology
88ICO	Stain, Best's Carmine	Pathology
88ICN	Stain, Biebrich Scarlet	Pathology
88UIG	Stain, Biological, General	Pathology
88KJM	Stain, Bismarck Brown Y	Pathology
88KJN	Stain, Brilliant Cresyl Blue	Pathology
88KJO	Stain, Brilliant Green	Pathology
88ICM	Stain, Brilliant Yellow	Pathology
88ICL	Stain, Carbol Fuchsin	Pathology
88ICJ	Stain, Carbol Night Blue	Pathology
88KJP	Stain, Carmine	Pathology
88LED	Stain, Chemical Solution	Pathology
88KJQ	Stain, Chlorazol Black E	Pathology
88ICH	Stain, Congo Red	Pathology
88ICG	Stain, Cresyl Violet Acetate	Pathology
88ICF	Stain, Crystal Violet, Histology	Pathology
88ICD	Stain, Darrow Red	Pathology
88LEF	Stain, Dye Powder	Pathology
88LEE	Stain, Dye Solution	Pathology
88ICC	Stain, Eosin B	Pathology
88HYB	Stain, Eosin Y	Pathology
88KJR	Stain, Erythrosin B	Pathology
88KJS	Stain, Ethyl Eosin	Pathology
88HYC	Stain, Fast Green	Pathology
88HYD	Stain, Fast Red Salt B	Pathology
81GHQ	Stain, Fetal Hemoglobin	Hematology
88HYF	Stain, Giemsa	Pathology
81GLP	Stain, Giemsa, Hematology	Hematology
88HYG	Stain, Glenner's	Pathology
88HYH	Stain, Gold Chloride	Pathology
88HYI	Stain, Grams Iodine	Pathology
88GHZ	Stain, Gugol Blue Solution	Pathology
81GJJ	Stain, Heinz Body	Hematology
88KQC	Stain, Hematology	Pathology
88HYJ	Stain, Hematoxylin	Pathology
88HYK	Stain, Hematoxylin, Harris's	Pathology
88HYL	Stain, Hematoxylin, Mayer's	Pathology
88KJT	Stain, Indigocarmine	Pathology
88GGH	Stain, Iron	Pathology
88KJW	Stain, Janus Green B	Pathology
88KJX	Stain, Jenner Stain	Pathology
88HYR	Stain, Leuco-Patent Blue	Pathology
88HYS	Stain, Light Green	Pathology
88HYT	Stain, Luxol Fast Blue	Pathology
88KJY	Stain, Malachite Green	Pathology
88HYW	Stain, Mallory's Trichrome	Pathology
88KJZ	Stain, Martius Yellow	Pathology
88HYY	Stain, Metanil Yellow	Pathology
88HYZ	Stain, Methenamine Silver	Pathology
88HZA	Stain, Methyl Green	Pathology
88KKA	Stain, Methyl Orange	Pathology
88KKB	Stain, Methyl Violet 2b	Pathology
88KFC	Stain, Methylene Blue	Pathology
88KKM	Stain, Methylene Blue Thiocyanate	Pathology
81GFR	Stain, Methylene Blue, New	Hematology
88KKC	Stain, Methylene Violet	Pathology
83JTS	Stain, Microbiological	Microbiology
88HZC	Stain, Mucicarmine	Pathology
88KFE	Stain, Neutral Red	Pathology
88KKD	Stain, Nigrosin	Pathology
88HZE	Stain, Nile Blue	Pathology
88HZF	Stain, Nuclear Fast Red	Pathology
88HZG	Stain, Oil Red O	Pathology
88HZH	Stain, Orange G	Pathology
88KKE	Stain, Orange II	Pathology
88WRC	Stain, Other	Pathology
88HZJ	Stain, Papanicolau	Pathology
88HZK	Stain, Periodic Acid Schiff (PAS)	Pathology
88LIJ	Stain, Peroxidase Anti-Peroxidase Immunohistochemical	Pathology
88HZL	Stain, Phloxine B	Pathology
88HZM	Stain, Phosphotungstic Acid Hematoxylin	Pathology
88HZN	Stain, Picro Methyl Blue	Pathology
88HZO	Stain, Ponceau	Pathology
81GFL	Stain, Ponceau, Hematology	Hematology
88HZP	Stain, Pyronin	Pathology
88HZT	Stain, Reagent, Schiff	Pathology
88HZQ	Stain, Red-Violet LB	Pathology
81GJH	Stain, Reticulocyte	Hematology
81GJL	Stain, Romanowsky	Hematology
88KKI	Stain, Rose Bengal	Pathology
88HZS	Stain, Safranin	Pathology
88GGI	Stain, Schiff, Periodic Acid	Pathology
88HZZ	Stain, Sudan Black B	Pathology
88IAA	Stain, Titan Yellow	Pathology

STAIN *(cont'd)*

88IAB	Stain, Toluidine Blue	Pathology
81GIX	Stain, Toluidine Blue, Hematology	Hematology
88LGY	Stain, Trypan Blue	Pathology
88IAC	Stain, Van Gieson's	Pathology
88IAE	Stain, Weigert's Iron Hematoxylin	Pathology
88IAF	Stain, Wright's	Pathology
81GJK	Stain, Wright's, Hematology	Hematology

STAINER

88KPA	Stainer, Slide, Automated	Pathology
88KIN	Stainer, Slide, Contact Type	Pathology
83RTR	Stainer, Slide, Cytology	Microbiology
81RTS	Stainer, Slide, Hematology	Hematology
81GKD	Stainer, Slide, Hematology, Automated	Hematology
83RTT	Stainer, Slide, Histology	Microbiology
88KIO	Stainer, Slide, Immersion Type	Pathology
88KEY	Stainer, Tissue, Automated	Pathology

STAINLESS

76ELO	Cusp, Gold And Stainless Steel	Dental And Oral
77ESG	Material, Metallic-Stainless Steel, Tantalum, Platinum	Ear/Nose/Throat
79RYE	Suture, Stainless Steel	Surgery
80WHK	Tubing, Hypodermic	General

STAIR

89QUU	Exercise Stair	Physical Med
80TFX	Lift, Stair Climbing	General
89IMK	Wheelchair, Stair Climbing	Physical Med

STAMMERING

77KTH	Anti-Stammering Device	Ear/Nose/Throat

STAND

73QXW	Cart, Gas Cylinder (Carrier)	Anesthesiology
80FOX	Infusion Stand	General
80FRI	Scale, Stand-On	General
80QCQ	Stand, Basin	General
90WJP	Stand, Cardiovascular	Radiology
87UES	Stand, Casting	Orthopedics
73QXX	Stand, Gas Cylinder	Anesthesiology
86HMF	Stand, Instrument, AC-Powered, Ophthalmic	Ophthalmology
86HMG	Stand, Instrument, Ophthalmic	Ophthalmology
80TCM	Stand, Laundry Hamper	General
79FSH	Stand, Operating Room Instrument (Mayo)	Surgery
90WLW	Stand, Vascular	Radiology
75WKC	Stand/Holder, Equipment, Laboratory	Chemistry
79FZN	Table, Instrument, Surgical	Surgery

STAND-ON

80FRI	Scale, Stand-On	General

STANDARD

81GJZ	Reagent, Cyanomethemoglobin, With Standard	Hematology
78FKH	Solution-Test, Standard-Conductivity, Dialysis	Gastro/Urology
75UIH	Standard, Amino Acid	Chemistry
75UII	Standard, Carbohydrate	Chemistry
81GFX	Standard, Fibrinogen	Hematology
75UIJ	Standard, Lipid	Chemistry
75UJC	Standard, Ultraviolet Reference	Chemistry
75UKC	Standard/Control, All Types	Chemistry
81GFK	Standard/Control, Fibrinogen Determination	Hematology
81GFS	Standard/Control, Hemoglobin, Normal/Abnormal	Hematology

STANDARD-CONDUCTIVITY

78FKH	Solution-Test, Standard-Conductivity, Dialysis	Gastro/Urology

STANDBY

80TCS	Power System, Isolated	General
80WMN	Power Systems, Uninterruptible (UPS)	General

STANDING

80UMP	Chair, Seat Lifting (Standing Aid)	General
79FSS	Light, Surgical, Floor Standing	Surgery

STANDUP

89IPL	Wheelchair, Standup	Physical Med

STANNOUS

75JNS	Stannous Chloride - Hydrazine, Phospholipids	Chemistry

STAPES

77LBP	Prosthesis, Ossicular (Stapes), Absorbable Gelatin Material	Ear/Nose/Throat
77LBO	Prosthesis, Ossicular (Total), Absorbable Gelatin Material	Ear/Nose/Throat
77UBU	Prosthesis, Ossicular, Incus And Stapes	Ear/Nose/Throat
77RSD	Separator, Stapes	Ear/Nose/Throat

STAPHYLOCOCCAL

83GTK	Enterotoxins, All Types, Staphylococcal	Microbiology
83GTL	Phages, Staphylococcal Typing, All Types	Microbiology

STAPHYLOCOCCUS

83LHT	Antigen, Somatic, Staphylococcus Aureus	Microbiology

KEYWORD INDEX

STERILE *(cont'd)*

78EYN	Kit, Irrigation, Sterile	Gastro/Urology
79LYV	Label/Tag, Sterile	Surgery
80LKB	Pad, Alcohol	General
80KYY	Syringe, Irrigating, Sterile	General
73BYZ	Trap, Sterile Specimen	Anesthesiology
80SGG	Wrapper, Surgical Instrument (Sterile)	General

STERILIZATION

80RVS	Container, Sterilization (Tray)	General
79VEE	Container, Surgical Instrument	Surgery
80VAD	Contract Sterilization	General
79WZL	Cover, Laparoscope	Surgery
80WPV	Dryer, Respiratory/Anesthesia Equipment	General
80WYN	Equipment, Filtering, Air, ETO	General
80WPE	Gas Mixtures, Sterilization	General
90WIB	Irradiator	Radiology
79KCT	Pack, Sterilization Wrapper (Bag And Accessories)	Surgery
80RVT	Packaging, Sterilization	General
79SIO	Rack, Instrument, Laparoscopy	Surgery
80WWT	Recovery Equipment, Gas	General
79LRT	Sterilization Indicator	Surgery
80FRC	Sterilization Process Indicator, Biological	General
80RVU	Sterilization Process Indicator, Chemical	General
80JOJ	Sterilization Process Indicator, Physical/Chemical	General
80WLS	Test, Equipment, Sterilization	General
79SIC	Tray, Sterilization, Instrument	Surgery
76MCF	Unit, Sanitation/Sterilization, Toothbrush, Ultraviolet	Dental And Oral
80WPY	Washer, Respiratory/Anesthesia Equipment	General
80WWK	Washer/Disinfector	General
80FRG	Wrap, Sterilization	General

STERILIZER

79LZZ	Bath, Sterilizer	Surgery
80VLG	Cartridge, Ethylene-Oxide	General
80QKS	Cleaner, Bedpan (Sterilizer)	General
80QPZ	Disinfector, Liquid	General
80QXI	Forceps, Sterilizer Transfer	General
83UGI	Germ-Free Apparatus	Microbiology
80RED	Lamp, Ultraviolet, Germicidal	General
80QDR	Monitor, Biological (Contamination Testing)	General
80WIP	Monitor, Contamination, Environmental, Personal	General
80RQL	Sanitizer	General
76ECG	Sterilizer, Boiling Water	Dental And Oral
80UDL	Sterilizer, Bulk, Steam & Ethylene-Oxide	General
80MLR	Sterilizer, Chemical	General
80KMH	Sterilizer, Dry Heat	General
76ECF	Sterilizer, Dry Heat, Dental	Dental And Oral
79WHQ	Sterilizer, Electrolytic	Surgery
76KOK	Sterilizer, Endodontic Dry Heat	Dental And Oral
80FLF	Sterilizer, Ethylene-Oxide Gas	General
76ECE	Sterilizer, Ethylene-Oxide Gas, Dental	Dental And Oral
79FSJ	Sterilizer, Ethylene-Oxide Gas, Operating Room	Surgery
80UDJ	Sterilizer, Ethylene-Oxide, Bulk	General
80UDK	Sterilizer, Ethylene-Oxide, Table Top	General
85RVV	Sterilizer, Formaldehyde	Obstetrics/Gyn
76ECC	Sterilizer, Glass Bead	Dental And Oral
83UIM	Sterilizer, Laboratory	Microbiology
80RVW	Sterilizer, Liquid	General
83VLZ	Sterilizer, Loop, Inoculating	Microbiology
80RVX	Sterilizer, Radiation	General
86HRD	Sterilizer, Soft Lens, Thermal, AC-Powered	Ophthalmology
86HRC	Sterilizer, Soft Lens, Thermal, Battery-Powered	Ophthalmology
80FLE	Sterilizer, Steam (Autoclave)	General
76ECH	Sterilizer, Steam (Autoclave), Dental	Dental And Oral
79FSI	Sterilizer, Steam (Autoclave), Surgical	Surgery
80UCS	Sterilizer, Steam, Bulk	General
80UCT	Sterilizer, Steam, Table Top	General
86HKZ	Sterilizer, Tonometer	Ophthalmology
80RVY	Sterilizer, Ultraviolet	General
80RVZ	Sterilizer, Vapor	General
80WWY	Sterilizer/Compactor	General
80THI	Sterilizer/Washer, Endoscope	General
80SFN	Washer, Cart	General
80SFR	Washer, Utensil	General
80SFM	Washer/Sterilizer	General

STERILIZING

76LFE	Solution, Sterilizing, Cold	Dental And Oral

STERNUM

79RDR	Knife, Sternum	Surgery

STEROIDS

75CDG	Chromatographic Separation/Zimmerman 17-Ketogenic Steroids	Chemistry
75CCZ	Zimmerman/Norymberski, 17-Ketogenic Steroids	Chemistry

STEROTAXIC

84RVR	Sterotaxic Unit	Cns/Neurology

STETHOGRAPH

74DQC	Phonocardiograph	Cardiovascular
74RKU	Phonostethograph	Cardiovascular

STETHOSCOPE

85QVO	Detector, Fetal Heart, Phono	Obstetrics/Gyn
74RKU	Phonostethograph	Cardiovascular
80VKO	Stethoscope, Amplified	General
80FLW	Stethoscope, DC-Powered	General
76WLF	Stethoscope, Dental	Dental And Oral
79FXD	Stethoscope, Direct (Acoustic), Ultrasonic	Surgery
74DQD	Stethoscope, Electronic (Auscultoscope)	Cardiovascular
79FXC	Stethoscope, Electronic-Amplified	Surgery
73BZW	Stethoscope, Esophageal	Anesthesiology
73BZT	Stethoscope, Esophageal, With Electrical Conductors	Anesthesiology
85HGN	Stethoscope, Fetal	Obstetrics/Gyn
74LDE	Stethoscope, Manual	Cardiovascular
80FLT	Stethoscope, Mechanical	General
73BZS	Transducer, Stethoscope	Anesthesiology

STICK

80RIY	Orange Stick	General
80WZG	Set, Administration, Intravenous, Needle-Free	General
75UKD	Stick, Urinalysis Test	Chemistry

STIFF-NECK

80WMR	Collar, Extrication	General

STILL

79FXM	Camera, Still, Endoscopic	Surgery
79FTH	Camera, Still, Microsurgical	Surgery
79FTT	Camera, Still, Surgical	Surgery
75QQF	Distilling Unit	Chemistry
75UIA	Still, Solvent Recovery	Chemistry
75UIN	Still, Water	Chemistry

STIMULATING

75CGJ	Radioimmunoassay, Follicle Stimulating Hormone	Chemistry
75JLW	Radioimmunoassay, Thyroid Stimulating Hormone	Chemistry

STIMULATION

87LMJ	Xenograft for Bone Growth/Stimulation	Orthopedics

STIMULATOR

84RWA	Analyzer, Transcutaneous Nerve Stimulator	Cns/Neurology
84HCB	Device, Conditioning, Aversion	Cns/Neurology
89IOA	Diathermy, Microwave	Physical Med
89IMJ	Diathermy, Shortwave	Physical Med
89ILX	Diathermy, Shortwave, Pulsed	Physical Med
89IMI	Diathermy, Ultrasonic (Physical Therapy)	Physical Med
84QTC	Electrode, Neuromuscular Stimulator	Cns/Neurology
84WHU	Electrode, TENS	Cns/Neurology
84QUT	Evoked Response Unit	Cns/Neurology
84GYB	Gel, Electrode, Stimulator	Cns/Neurology
78FHW	Impotence Device, Mechanical/Hydraulic	Gastro/Urology
78RCP	Iontophoresis Unit (Sweat Rate)	Gastro/Urology
78EZT	Pacemaker, Bladder	Gastro/Urology
74DTE	Pacemaker, Heart, External	Cardiovascular
74JOQ	Pacemaker, Heart, External, Programmable	Cardiovascular
74UMI	Pacemaker, Heart, Implantable, Anti-Tachycardia	Cardiovascular
74ULJ	Pacemaker, Heart, Implantable, Dual Chamber	Cardiovascular
74DXY	Pacemaker, Heart, Implantable, Programmable	Cardiovascular
74WST	Pacemaker, Heart, Implantable, Rate Responsive	Cardiovascular
79RJT	Pacemaker, Respiratory	Surgery
74WWX	Pacemaker, Temporary	Cardiovascular
74WWU	Pad, Electrode	Cardiovascular
80RKY	Photostimulator	General
86HLX	Photostimulator, AC-Powered	Ophthalmology
75JMP	Radioimmunoassay, Long-Acting Thyroid Stimulator	Chemistry
73MNC	Stimulator, Abdominal, Electric	Anesthesiology
73UKR	Stimulator, Acupuncture	Anesthesiology
89MKC	Stimulator, Arthritis, Non-Invasive	Physical Med
84RWB	Stimulator, Audio	Cns/Neurology
84GWJ	Stimulator, Auditory, Evoked Response	Cns/Neurology
84RWC	Stimulator, Aversion Conditioning (Behavior Modification)	Cns/Neurology
84MFR	Stimulator, Brain, Implanted (Behavior Modification)	Cns/Neurology
77KHH	Stimulator, Caloric Air	Ear/Nose/Throat
77ETP	Stimulator, Caloric Water	Ear/Nose/Throat
74DSR	Stimulator, Carotid Sinus Nerve	Cardiovascular
84LKR	Stimulator, Cerebellar, Full Implant	Cns/Neurology
84LGW	Stimulator, Cerebellar, Full Implant (Pain Relief)	Cns/Neurology
84GZA	Stimulator, Cerebral, Implantable	Cns/Neurology
78LNL	Stimulator, Collection, Sperm, Electrical	Gastro/Urology
84LGT	Stimulator, Cord, Spinal, Implantable (Motor Disorders)	Cns/Neurology
84LLE	Stimulator, Cord, Spinal, Implantable (Periph. Vasc. Dis.)	Cns/Neurology
84MFM	Stimulator, Cortex, Visual, Implanted	Cns/Neurology
84MHF	Stimulator, Cortical, Implanted (Pain Relief)	Cns/Neurology

KEYWORD INDEX

STIMULATOR *(cont'd)*

84JXK	Stimulator, Cranial Electrotherapy	Cns/Neurology
84GZG	Stimulator, Cranial Electrotherapy (Situational Anxiety)	Cns/Neurology
84HTL	Stimulator, Diaphragm, Orthopedic	Cns/Neurology
84GZE	Stimulator, Diaphragmatic/Phrenic Nerve, Implantable	Cns/Neurology
84RWD	Stimulator, Dorsal Column	Cns/Neurology
84LPY	Stimulator, Electrical, Cranial, External	Cns/Neurology
84GWF	Stimulator, Electrical, Evoked Response	Cns/Neurology
78EZW	Stimulator, Electrical, For Incontinence	Gastro/Urology
84MEI	Stimulator, Electrical, Implanted (Coma Arousal)	Cns/Neurology
84MHY	Stimulator, Electrical, Implanted (Parkinsonian Tremor)	Cns/Neurology
89MPH	Stimulator, Electrical, Muscle	Physical Med
84UFF	Stimulator, Electro-Analgesic	Cns/Neurology
73BWK	Stimulator, Electro/Acupuncture	Anesthesiology
73GZH	Stimulator, Electroanesthesia	Anesthesiology
89IPP	Stimulator, External, Neuromuscular, Functional	Physical Med
84HTK	Stimulator, Extremity, Internal, Peroneal	Cns/Neurology
85MCP	Stimulator, Fetal, Acoustic	Obstetrics/Gyn
76LYD	Stimulator, Growth, Bone, Electromagnetic, Dental	Dental And Oral
87LOE	Stimulator, Growth, Bone, Invasive	Orthopedics
87LOF	Stimulator, Growth, Bone, Non-Invasive	Orthopedics
84MNQ	Stimulator, Hypoglossal Nerve, Implanted, Apnea	Cns/Neurology
78KPI	Stimulator, Incontinence (Non-Implantable), Electrical	Gastro/Urology
78LNQ	Stimulator, Intestinal	Gastro/Urology
84GYZ	Stimulator, Intracerebral/Subcortical, Implantable	Cns/Neurology
84GZP	Stimulator, Mechanical, Evoked Response	Cns/Neurology
89ISB	Stimulator, Muscle, Diagnostic	Physical Med
89IPF	Stimulator, Muscle, Electrical-Powered (EMS)	Physical Med
79FXB	Stimulator, Muscle, General & Plastic Surgery	Surgery
89LBF	Stimulator, Muscle, Low Intensity	Physical Med
89MBN	Stimulator, Muscle, Powered, Invasive	Physical Med
89LPQ	Stimulator, Muscle, Ultrasonic (Non-Beep Heat)	Physical Med
85HII	Stimulator, Muscle, Vaginal	Obstetrics/Gyn
84UFH	Stimulator, Nerve Locating	Cns/Neurology
84UFI	Stimulator, Nerve Locating, Facial	Cns/Neurology
73BXM	Stimulator, Nerve, AC-Powered	Anesthesiology
73KOI	Stimulator, Nerve, Anesthesia	Anesthesiology
84LYJ	Stimulator, Nerve, Autonomic, Implantable (Epilepsy)	Cns/Neurology
73BXN	Stimulator, Nerve, Battery-Powered	Anesthesiology
84MFP	Stimulator, Nerve, Cranial, Implanted (Pain Relief)	Cns/Neurology
77ETN	Stimulator, Nerve, ENT	Ear/Nose/Throat
84GZJ	Stimulator, Nerve, Transcutaneous (Pain Relief, TENS)	Cns/Neurology
84LEP	Stimulator, Nerve, Transcutaneous Elec. (Speech Disorder)	Cns/Neurology
79FXA	Stimulator, Neurological	Surgery
84GZI	Stimulator, Neuromuscular, External Functional	Cns/Neurology
89MKD	Stimulator, Neuromuscular, Functional Walking, Non-Invasive	Physical Med
84GZC	Stimulator, Neuromuscular, Implanted	Cns/Neurology
84RWE	Stimulator, Optokinetic	Cns/Neurology
87HTM	Stimulator, Osteogenesis, Electric, Invasive	Orthopedics
87WNT	Stimulator, Osteogenesis, Electric, Non-Invasive	Orthopedics
73UFG	Stimulator, Peripheral Nerve, Blockade Monitor	Anesthesiology
84GZF	Stimulator, Peripheral Nerve, Implantable (Pain Relief)	Cns/Neurology
84GWE	Stimulator, Photic, Evoked Response	Cns/Neurology
84LEN	Stimulator, Reduction, Anxiety, Electrical	Cns/Neurology
84MQQ	Stimulator, Sacral Nerve, Implanted	Cns/Neurology
76LTF	Stimulator, Salivary System	Dental And Oral
89VIH	Stimulator, Scoliosis (Orthosis)	Physical Med
87LWB	Stimulator, Scoliosis, Neuromuscular, Functional	Orthopedics
84UFJ	Stimulator, Somatosensory	Cns/Neurology
84GZB	Stimulator, Spinal Cord, Implantable (Pain Relief)	Cns/Neurology
84GZD	Stimulator, Spinal Cord, Implantable, Bladder Evacuator	Cns/Neurology
84LYI	Stimulator, Subcortical, Implanted For Epilepsy	Cns/Neurology
84MBX	Stimulator, Thalamic, Epilepsy, Implanted	Cns/Neurology
77EPG	Stimulator, Transdermal	Ear/Nose/Throat
89IMG	Stimulator, Ultrasound, Muscle	Physical Med
78UAE	Stimulator, Urinary	Gastro/Urology
84MBY	Stimulator, Vagus Nerve, Epilepsy, Implanted	Cns/Neurology
84MUY	Stimulator, Vagus Nerve, Implanted (Coma And Vegetative State)	Cns/Neurology
84MHZ	Stimulator, Vestibular Acceleration, Therapeutic	Cns/Neurology
84RWF	Stimulator, Visual	Cns/Neurology
89WIN	Stimulator, Wound Healing	Physical Med
89WWS	Unit, Pad, Heating, Portable	Physical Med

STING

80RCG	Kit, Emergency, Insect Sting	General

STIRRER

75JRQ	Shaker/Stirrer	Chemistry
75RWG	Stirrer	Chemistry

STIRRUP

87QMZ	Cover, Heel Stirrup	Orthopedics
78EYD	Stirrup	Gastro/Urology
89ITC	Stirrup, External Brace Component	Physical Med

STOCKINETTE

87RWH	Stockinette	Orthopedics

STOCKINETTE *(cont'd)*

87QHB	Stockinette, Cast	Orthopedics

STOCKING

80LLK	Legging, Compression, Non-Inflatable	General
74RWI	Stocking, Anti-Embolic, Pneumatic	Cardiovascular
80FQL	Stocking, Elastic	General
89ILG	Stocking, Elastic, Physical Medicine	Physical Med
80DWL	Stocking, Support (Anti-Embolic)	General
89RXK	Support, Leg	Physical Med

STOMA

73SBI	Button, Tracheostomy Tube	Anesthesiology

STOMACH

78FBF	Clip, Suture, Stomach And Intestinal	Gastro/Urology
78FHM	Suture Apparatus, Stomach And Intestinal	Gastro/Urology
73BSS	Tube, Nasogastric	Anesthesiology
78SDI	Tube, Stomach Evacuator (Gastric Lavage)	Gastro/Urology

STOMAL

79GDS	Bag, Stomal	Surgery
78EZR	Cement, Stomal Appliance, Ostomy	Gastro/Urology

STONE

78TEH	Basket, Biliary Stone Retrieval	Gastro/Urology
78FFL	Dislodger, Stone, Basket, Ureteral, Metal	Gastro/Urology
78FGO	Dislodger, Stone, Flexible	Gastro/Urology
78QVZ	Filter, Kidney Stone	Gastro/Urology
78QXJ	Forceps, Stone Manipulation	Gastro/Urology
75JNP	Infrared Spectroscopy Measurement, Urinary Calculi (Stone)	Chemistry
78LNS	Lithotriptor, Extracorporeal Shock-wave, Urological	Gastro/Urology
78WSU	Lithotriptor, Laser	Gastro/Urology
75JNQ	Qualitative Chemical Reactions, Urinary Calculi (Stone)	Chemistry
78FGK	Tripsor, Stone, Bladder	Gastro/Urology

STOOL

80QNG	Cover, Stool	General
80QOC	Cushion, Stool	General
75TGO	Enzymatic Method, Blood, Occcult, Fecal	Chemistry
80QWU	Footstool, Conductive	General
80QWV	Footstool, Non-Conductive	General
79FZL	Footstool, Operating Room	Surgery
81KHE	Reagent, Occult Blood	Hematology
73BRX	Stool, Anesthetist's	Anesthesiology
80RWJ	Stool, Bedside	General
76RWK	Stool, Dental	Dental And Oral
89RWL	Stool, Exercise	Physical Med
79FZM	Stool, Operating Room, Adjustable	Surgery

STOP

78FKG	Tray, Start/Stop (Including Contents), Dialysis	Gastro/Urology

STOPCOCK

74DTL	Adapter, Stopcock, Manifold, Cardiopulmonary Bypass	Cardiovascular
75RFW	Manifold, Liquid	Chemistry
80FMG	Stopcock	General
80WSP	Tubing, Connecting	General
73WHT	Valve, Breathing	Anesthesiology
73CBP	Valve, Non-Rebreathing	Anesthesiology
73SEO	Valve, Positive End Expiratory Pressure (PEEP)	Anesthesiology

STOPPER

80WSY	Closure, Other	General
80WNN	Stopper	General

STORAGE

80WNK	Bag, Plastic	General
80VKB	Bin, Storage	General
80WYL	Box, Transportation, Container, Specimen	General
80TBA	Cabinet Casework, General Purpose	General
80WVU	Cabinet, Storage, Catheter	General
78WUJ	Cabinet, Storage, Endoscope	Gastro/Urology
80WRH	Cabinet, Storage, Slide	General
81KSH	Chamber, Environmental, Platelet Storage	Hematology
80WLE	Computer, Image, Endoscopic	General
83VFX	Container, Cryobiological Storage	Microbiology
80LPZ	Container, Frozen Donor Tissue Storage	General
88KDT	Container, Specimen Mailer And Storage	Pathology
88KDW	Container, Specimen Mailer And Storage, Temperature Control	Pathology
90WJA	Container, Substance, Radioactive	Radiology
90LMB	Device, Storage, Image, Digital	Radiology
80WJO	Dispenser, Other	General
80WSB	Dispenser, Syringe And Needle	General
90WZI	Envelope, Film, X-Ray	Radiology
81KSE	Freezer, Blood Storage	Hematology
86LYX	Media, Storage, Corneal	Ophthalmology
74MFU	Media, Transport/Storage, Organ/Tissue	Cardiovascular
80VAZ	Microfilm/Microfiche Equipment	General

STORAGE (cont'd)
80WKM Mount, Equipment — General
79SIO Rack, Instrument, Laparoscopy — Surgery
90VGY Storage Device, Fluoroscopic Image — Radiology
90UAB Storage Unit, X-Ray Film — Radiology

STORE
78LQR Dislodger, Store, Biliary — Gastro/Urology

STRABISMUS
86RAQ Hook, Strabismus — Ophthalmology
86WNQ Synoptophore — Ophthalmology

STRAIGHT
78EZD Catheter, Straight — Gastro/Urology

STRAIN
80RWM Detector, Strain — General
80WVV Gauge, Pressure — General
80RWN Gauge, Strain — General

STRAIT
80RPE Restraint, Vest — General

STRAP
79UFB Holder, Leg — Surgery
80RWO Strap, Cable — General
87RWP Strap, Clavicle — Orthopedics
80QSN Strap, Electrode — General
73BTK Strap, Head, Gas Mask — Anesthesiology
80RWQ Strap, Restraining — General
73VDM Strap, Tracheostomy Tube — Anesthesiology

STREAM
80RGZ Kit, Mid-Stream Collection — General

STRENGTH
87LBB Dynamometer, AC-Powered — Orthopedics
73BSH Dynamometer, Grip-Strength (Squeeze) — Anesthesiology
87HRW Dynamometer, Non-Powered — Orthopedics
84GWH Dynamometer, Other — Cns/Neurology
89IKG Dynamometer, Physical Medicine, Electronic — Physical Med
86HLB Ophthalmodynamometer — Ophthalmology

STREP
83MCT DNA-Probe, Strep Pneumoniae — Microbiology

STREPTOCOCCAL
83GTP Exoenzyme, Multiple, Streptococcal — Microbiology
83MDK Reagent, DNA-Probe, Streptococcal — Microbiology

STREPTOCOCCUS
83GTR Antideoxyribonuclease, Streptococcus SPP. — Microbiology
83GTY Antigen, Streptococcus SPP. — Microbiology
83GTX Antiserum, Fluorescent, Groups, Streptococcus SPP. — Microbiology
83GWB Antiserum, Fluorescent, Streptococcus Pneumoniae — Microbiology
83GWC Antiserum, Streptococcus Pneumoniae — Microbiology
83GTZ Antiserum, Streptococcus SPP. — Microbiology

STREPTOKINASE
83GTO Anti-Streptokinase — Microbiology

STREPTOLYSIN
83GTQ Reagent, Antistreptolysin-Titer/Streptolysin O — Microbiology
83GTS Reagent, Streptolysin O/Antistreptolysin-Titer — Microbiology
88IBA Streptolysin O — Pathology

STRESS
74LOS Analyzer, ECG — Cardiovascular
74QMC Computer, ECG Interpretation (Arrhythmia) — Cardiovascular
74QMG Computer, Stress Exercise — Cardiovascular
74QUN Ergometer, Bicycle — Cardiovascular
74BYQ Ergometer, Treadmill — Cardiovascular
90UAD Exerciser, Nuclear Diagnostic (Cardiac Stress Table) — Radiology
74RLC Monitor, Physiological, Stress Exercise — Cardiovascular
89IOG Treadmill, Mechanical — Physical Med
89IOL Treadmill, Powered — Physical Med

STRETCHER
73BWM Cart, Patient (Stretcher) — Anesthesiology
80RKB Patient Transfer Unit — General
80WKD Sheeting, Stretcher — General
80VLO Stretcher, Basket, Portable — General
80WKO Stretcher, Collapsible — General
80WIG Stretcher, Emergency, Other — General
80FPP Stretcher, Hand-Carried — General
80TEW Stretcher, Hydraulic — General
87TEX Stretcher, Orthopedic — Orthopedics
90TEY Stretcher, Radiographic — Radiology
79FSL Stretcher, Transfer — Surgery
80FPO Stretcher, Wheeled (Mobile) — General
89INJ Stretcher, Wheeled, Mechanical — Physical Med
89INK Stretcher, Wheeled, Powered — Physical Med

STRETCHER (cont'd)
88RYV Table, Autopsy — Pathology
89IKX Transfer Aid — Physical Med
80FMR Transfer Device, Patient, Manual — General
89ILK Transport, Patient, Powered — Physical Med

STRING
78FFW Locator, Bleeding, Gastrointestinal, String And Tube — Gastro/Urology

STRIP
80QAC Adhesive Strip, Hypoallergenic — General
80QAD Adhesive Strip, Waterproof — General
83KFI Corynebacterium Diphtheriae, Virulence Strip — Microbiology
83JTO Disc, Strip And Reagent, Microorganism Differentiation — Microbiology
91DNC Paper Strip, Salicylate — Toxicology
79FPX Strip, Adhesive — Surgery
84GXO Strip, Craniosynostosis, Preformed — Cns/Neurology
86KYC Strip, Fluorescein — Ophthalmology
82MLH Strip, HAMA IGG, ELISA, In Vitro Test System — Immunology
78MNV Strip, Indicator, pH, Dialysate — Gastro/Urology
76EHM Strip, Polishing Agent — Dental And Oral
86KYD Strip, Schirmer — Ophthalmology
75WTX Strip, Test — Chemistry
78MSY Strip, Test, Reagent, Residuals For Dialysate, Disinfectant — Gastro/Urology
80KPD Temperature Strip, Forehead, Liquid Crystal — General
91MIG Test Strip, Isoniazid — Toxicology

STRIPPER
74DWX Stripper, Artery, Intraluminal — Cardiovascular
81RWS Stripper, Donor Tube — Hematology
79RWU Stripper, Other — Surgery
87HRT Stripper, Surgical — Orthopedics
79RWT Stripper, Tendon — Surgery
79GAJ Stripper, Vein, Disposable — Surgery
74DWQ Stripper, Vein, External — Cardiovascular
79GAI Stripper, Vein, Reusable — Surgery

STROKE
84MBW Cranial Retroperfusion (Stroke Treatment) — Cns/Neurology
84QTB Electrode, Neurological — Cns/Neurology

STROLLER
89LBE Stroller, Adaptive — Physical Med

STRUCTURE
79SJB Instrument, Separating, Nerve — Surgery
89IPO Orthosis, Pneumatic Structure, Rigid — Physical Med

STUDY
81JBZ Adhesive Study, Platelet — Hematology

STUMP
80WNB Amputation Protection Unit — General
80RUC Sock, Stump Cover — General

STYLET
77RWV Stylet, Bronchial — Ear/Nose/Throat
74DRB Stylet, Catheter — Cardiovascular
78EZB Stylet, Catheter, Gastro-Urology — Gastro/Urology
80RWW Stylet, Intravenous — General
80RWX Stylet, Needle — General
79GAH Stylet, Surgical — Surgery
73BSR Stylet, Tracheal Tube — Anesthesiology
78EYA Stylet, Ureteral — Gastro/Urology

SUBCLAVIAN
74LFJ Catheter, Subclavian — Cardiovascular

SUBCORTICAL
84GYZ Stimulator, Intracerebral/Subcortical, Implantable — Cns/Neurology
84LYI Stimulator, Subcortical, Implanted For Epilepsy — Cns/Neurology

SUBCUT.
80MDX Port & Catheter, Infusion, Implanted, Subcut., Intraperit. — General

SUBCUTANEOUS
80LMP Catheter, Intraspinal, Subcutaneous, Implantable — General
80LJT Catheter, Subcutaneous Intravascular, Implanted — General
80LKG Catheter, Subcutaneous Intraventricular, Implanted — General
80LLD Catheter, Subcutaneous Peritoneal, Implanted — General
80LMQ Device, Access, Peritoneal, Subcutaneous, Implantable — General
80MDV Port & Catheter, Infusion, Implanted, Subcutaneous, Intraspinal — General
79WVC Tunneler, Surgical — Surgery

SUBPERIOSTEAL
76ELE Implant, Subperiosteal — Dental And Oral

SUBSTANCE
90WJA Container, Substance, Radioactive — Radiology
81KSX Substance, Grouping, Blood (Non-Human Origin) — Hematology

SUBSTITUTE
84GXQ Dura-Substitute — Cns/Neurology
89MBO Substitute, Graft, Bone — Physical Med

SUBTALAR
87MJW Prosthesis, Subtalar Plug, Polymer — Orthopedics
87MJU Prosthesis, Subtalar Plug, Polymer (Elastomer) — Orthopedics

SUBTILIS
91DKD Bacillus Subtilis, Microbiological Assay, Gentamicin — Toxicology
91DID Test, Bacillus Subtilis Microbiology, Tobramycin — Toxicology

SUBTRACTION
90WNE Phantom, Digital Subtraction Angiography (DSA) — Radiology
90VLE Radiographic Unit, Digital Subtraction Angiographic (DSA) — Radiology

SUBUNIT
75MMI Enzymatic Method, Troponin Subunit — Chemistry

SUCKER
74DTS Sucker, Cardiotomy Return, Cardiopulmonary Bypass — Cardiovascular
79ULE Tip, Suction Tube (Yankauer, Poole, Etc.) — Surgery

SUCKING
76LQX Finger-Sucking Device — Dental And Oral

SUCTION
77EWT Anti-Choke Device, Suction — Ear/Nose/Throat
87WHX Aspirator, Arthroscopy — Orthopedics
80QBQ Aspirator, Emergency Suction — General
85HFC Aspirator, Endocervical — Obstetrics/Gyn
85HFF Aspirator, Endometrial — Obstetrics/Gyn
78QBR Aspirator, Low Volume (Gastric Suction) — Gastro/Urology
77QBT Aspirator, Nasal — Ear/Nose/Throat
86WKR Aspirator, Ophthalmic — Ophthalmology
79QBU Aspirator, Surgical — Surgery
74QBV Aspirator, Thoracic (Suction Unit) — Cardiovascular
77QBW Aspirator, Tracheal — Ear/Nose/Throat
80QBZ Aspirator, Wound Suction Pump — General
78FCK Biopsy Instrument, Suction — Gastro/Urology
80KDQ Bottle, Collection, Vacuum (Aspirator) — General
74DWM Canister, Suction — Cardiovascular
79WZU Cannula, Suction, Pool-Tip — Surgery
85HGH Cannula, Suction, Uterine — Obstetrics/Gyn
79WYX Cannula, Suction/Irrigation, Laparoscopic — Surgery
73BSY Catheter, Suction (Tracheal Aspirating Tube) — Anesthesiology
80JOL Catheter, Suction, With Tip — General
79SIP Connector, Suction/Irrigation — Surgery
74DWD Controller, Suction, Intracardiac, Cardiopulmonary Bypass — Cardiovascular
85HHK Curette, Suction, Endometrial — Obstetrics/Gyn
86QOH Cutter, Vitreous Infusion Suction — Ophthalmology
80KZG Device, Suction, Enlargement, Breast — General
79QCL Drain, Suction, Closed — Surgery
78FEH Electrode, Flexible Suction Coagulator — Gastro/Urology
79WYP Equipment, Suction/Irrigation, Laparoscopic — Surgery
79SJK Equipment, Suction/Irrigation/Electrocautery, Laparoscopic — Surgery
78FHF Evacuator, Fluid — Gastro/Urology
76EHZ Evacuator, Oral Cavity — Dental And Oral
74JOD Filter, Blood, Cardiotomy Suction Line, Cardiopulmonary — Cardiovascular
79QXK Forceps, Suction — Surgery
79SJH Handle, Instrument, Laparoscopic (Irrigation) — Surgery
80RWY Irrigator, Suction — General
79SJR Irrigator/Coagulator/Cutter, Suction, Laparoscopic — Surgery
80KYP Kit, Snake Bite, Suction — General
73CBE Kit, Suction, Airway (Tracheal) — Anesthesiology
79SIS Needle, Puncture — Surgery
79SJC Probe, Electrosurgery, Endoscopy — Surgery
79QUQ Probe, Suction, Irrigator/Aspirator, Laparoscopic — Surgery
85HHI Pump, Abortion, Vacuum, Central System — Obstetrics/Gyn
76EBR Pump, Suction Operatory — Dental And Oral
78ROX Regulator, Suction, Low Volume (Gastric) — Gastro/Urology
80CBB Regulator, Suction, Surgical — General
73ROZ Regulator, Suction, Thoracic — Anesthesiology
77RPA Regulator, Suction, Tracheal (Nasal, Oral) — Ear/Nose/Throat
79GCX Suction Apparatus, Operating Room, Wall Vacuum-Powered — Surgery
79GCY Suction Apparatus, Single Patient, Portable, Non-Powered — Surgery
79JCX Suction Apparatus, Ward Use, Portable, AC-Powered — Surgery
73BSQ Tip, Suction — Anesthesiology
79ULE Tip, Suction Tube (Yankauer, Poole, Etc.) — Surgery
79RWZ Tip, Suction, Electrosurgical — Surgery
73RXA Tip, Suction, Fiberoptic Illuminated — Anesthesiology
77JZF Tube, Ear Suction — Ear/Nose/Throat
80WNO Tube, Suction — General
77KCB Tube, Tonsil Suction — Ear/Nose/Throat
79SIT Tubing, Irrigation — Surgery

SUCTION-TYPE
87MCJ Pump, Vacuum, Electric, Suction-Type Electrode — Orthopedics

SUCTIONING
79LRQ Kit, Suctioning, Tracheostomy and Nasal — Surgery

SUDAN
88HZZ Stain, Sudan Black B — Pathology
88KKJ Sudan III — Pathology
88KKK Sudan IV — Pathology

SUDROMED
91MHP Monitor, Patch, Sudromed, Drug Abuse — Toxicology

SUGAR
78TGM Monitor, Blood Glucose (Test) — Gastro/Urology
75WTX Strip, Test — Chemistry

SUIT
79RRV Dress, Scrub, Disposable — Surgery
79RRW Dress, Scrub, Reusable — Surgery
79FYE Dress, Surgical — Surgery
79FPH Gown, Operating Room, Disposable — Surgery
79QYN Gown, Operating Room, Reusable — Surgery
74RLJ Suit, Pneumatic Counterpressure (Anti-Shock) — Cardiovascular
79RRY Suit, Scrub, Disposable — Surgery
79RRZ Suit, Scrub, Reusable — Surgery
79FXO Suit, Surgical — Surgery

SULFALITHOCHOLIC
75KWX Radioimmunoassay, Conjugated Sulfalithocholic, Bile Acid — Chemistry

SULFATE
84MYU Accessory, Barium Sulfate, Methyl Methacrylate For Cranioplasty — Cns/Neurology
87MQV Filler, Calcium Sulfate Preformed Pellets — Orthopedics
90UJW Media, Gastroenterographic Contrast (Barium Sulfate) — Radiology
75JKC Radioimmunoassay, Dehydroepiandrosterone (Free And Sulfate) — Chemistry
91DIQ Radioimmunoassay, Morphine (3-H), Ammonium Sulfate — Toxicology
81KSL Solution, Copper Sulfate, For Specific Gravity Test — Hematology

SULFHEMOGLOBIN
81GJC Test, Sulfhemoglobin — Hematology

SULFONATE
75CID Alizarin Sulfonate, Calcium — Chemistry
75JQH Trinitrobenzene Sulfonate (Spectroscopic), Nitrogen — Chemistry

SULFOPHOSPHOVANILLIN
75CFD Sulfophosphovanillin, Colorimetry, Total Lipids — Chemistry

SULFURIC
75CHD Ferric Ion-Sulfuric Acid, Cholesterol — Chemistry

SULPHANIMIDE
91DKW Reagent, Test, Sulphanimide Derivative — Toxicology

SULPHATE
81GFT Protamine Sulphate — Hematology

SUMP
78QQM Drain, Sump — Gastro/Urology

SUN
89LEJ Booth, Sun Tan — Physical Med
79MIW Clothing, Protective, Sun — Surgery
80REB Lamp, Sun, Incandescent — General

SUNGLASSES
86HQY Sunglasses (Including Photosensitive) — Ophthalmology

SUPERCONDUCTING
90VIM Magnet, Superconducting, MRI (Magnetic Resonance Imaging) — Radiology

SUPERCRITICAL
91MAS Chromatography, Liquid, Performance, High — Toxicology
75WYT Chromatography, Supercritical Fluid (SFC) — Chemistry

SUPERFICIAL
90LNC Hyperthermia Applicator, Superficial, RF/Microwave — Radiology
90LND Hyperthermia Applicator, Superficial, Ultrasound — Radiology

SUPPLEMENTARY
80LLC Supplementary Nitroglycerin Container — General

SUPPLEMENTS
83JSK Culture Media, Supplements — Microbiology

SUPPLIES
80WYG Courier, Supplies, Mobile, Automated — General
80VAY Security Equipment/Supplies — General
81KSS Supplies, Blood Bank — Hematology

SUPPLY
74MPD Auxillary Power Supply, Low Energy Defibrillator (AC or DC) — Cardiovascular

SUPPLY *(cont'd)*

74MPE	Auxillary Power Supply, Pacemaker, Cardiac, External Trans.	Cardiovascular
87QGU	Cart, Orthopedic Supply (Cast)	Orthopedics
80TAW	Cart, Supply	General
79FSK	Cart, Supply, Operating Room	Surgery
80QUD	Power Supply, Endoscopic, Battery-Operated	General
80QUE	Power Supply, Endoscopic, Line-Operated	General

SUPPORT

89ISR	Band, Support, Pelvic	Physical Med
80QDA	Bed Cradle	General
89INX	Bed, Air Fluidized	Physical Med
87QDI	Belt, Rib (Support)	Orthopedics
89ISQ	Belt, Support, Pelvic	Physical Med
89ITW	Brace, Joint, Ankle (External)	Physical Med
80UMS	Column, Life Support (Electrical/Gas)	General
82JZR	Gel, Support	Immunology
84HBM	Head Rest, Neurosurgical	Cns/Neurology
90IWY	Holder, Head, Radiographic	Radiology
87THC	Holder, Leg, Arthroscopy	Orthopedics
79WRY	Holder, Shoulder, Arthroscopy	Surgery
90WUB	Immobilizer, Therapy, Radiation	Radiology
73BYS	Lung, Membrane (For Long-Term Respiratory Support)	Anesthesiology
80RHM	Mount, Monitor (Support)	General
79UMJ	Mount, Surgical Microscope	Surgery
80UMW	Mount, Television Set	General
90SGN	Sand Bag, X-Ray	Radiology
74RWI	Stocking, Anti-Embolic, Pneumatic	Cardiovascular
80FQL	Stocking, Elastic	General
89ILG	Stocking, Elastic, Physical Medicine	Physical Med
80DWL	Stocking, Support (Anti-Embolic)	General
89RXB	Support, Abdominal	Physical Med
87RXC	Support, Ankle	Orthopedics
89RXD	Support, Arch	Physical Med
89IOY	Support, Arm	Physical Med
87RXE	Support, Back	Orthopedics
73JAY	Support, Breathing Tube	Anesthesiology
87RXG	Support, Clavicle	Orthopedics
91DJA	Support, Column, GLC	Toxicology
80WTK	Support, Cover, Bed	General
87RXF	Support, Elbow	Orthopedics
87RXH	Support, Foot	Orthopedics
87RXI	Support, Hand	Orthopedics
89IMS	Support, Head And Trunk, Wheelchair	Physical Med
77EPW	Support, Head, Surgical, ENT	Ear/Nose/Throat
78EXN	Support, Hernia	Gastro/Urology
89UEC	Support, Hot/Cold Pack	Physical Med
89RXJ	Support, Knee	Physical Med
89RXK	Support, Leg	Physical Med
73CCX	Support, Patient Position	Anesthesiology
90RNX	Support, Patient Position, Radiographic	Radiology
78EXO	Support, Scrotal	Gastro/Urology
80FQJ	Support, Scrotal, Therapeutic	General
89RXL	Support, Thigh	Physical Med
75WID	Support, Tube, Test	Chemistry
89RXM	Support, Wrist	Physical Med
89QAP	Unit, Support, Ambulation	Physical Med
73MNT	Ventilator, Continuous, Minimal Ventilatory Support, Facility Use	Anesthesiology

SUPPORTED

89ILE	Sling, Arm, Overhead Supported	Physical Med

SUPPORTING

75UIO	Media, Supporting	Chemistry
73MNS	Ventilator, Continuous, Non-Life Supporting	Anesthesiology

SUPPORTIVE

89MNE	Orthosis, Moldable, Supportive, Skin Protective	Physical Med

SUPPRESSION

74RLJ	Suit, Pneumatic Counterpressure (Anti-Shock)	Cardiovascular

SUPRAPUBIC

78FBM	Cannula, Suprapubic, With Trocar	Gastro/Urology
78KOB	Catheter, Suprapubic	Gastro/Urology
78FEZ	Catheter, Suprapubic, With Tube	Gastro/Urology
78FFA	Tube, Drainage	Gastro/Urology

SURFACE

89IKA	Electrode, Biopotential, Surface, Composite	Physical Med
89IKB	Electrode, Biopotential, Surface, Metallic	Physical Med
86HLY	Electrode, Skin Surface, Ophthalmic	Ophthalmology
73BWY	Electrode, Surface	Anesthesiology
81LIZ	Test, T Lymphocyte Surface Marker	Hematology
74KRC	Tester, Electrode, Surface, Electrocardiograph	Cardiovascular

SURFACTOMETER

73WWO	Surfactometer	Anesthesiology

SURGERY

79WTZ	Analyzer, Patient, Multiple Function (Surgery)	Surgery
86WKR	Aspirator, Ophthalmic	Ophthalmology
79GFA	Blade, Surgical, Saw, General & Plastic Surgery	Surgery
79GEE	Brush, Biopsy, General & Plastic Surgery	Surgery
79GFF	Burr, Surgical, General & Plastic Surgery	Surgery
79GEA	Cannula, Surgical, General & Plastic Surgery	Surgery
80WVY	Cart, Equipment, Video	General
79GCA	Catheter, Biliary, General & Plastic Surgery	Surgery
79GBY	Catheter, Eustachian, General & Plastic Surgery	Surgery
79GBO	Catheter, Nephrostomy, General & Plastic Surgery	Surgery
79GBN	Catheter, Pediatric, General & Plastic Surgery	Surgery
79GBL	Catheter, Ureteral, General & Plastic Surgery	Surgery
79GBS	Catheter, Ventricular, General & Plastic Surgery	Surgery
79GDJ	Clamp, Surgical, General & Plastic Surgery	Surgery
79FTJ	Colonoscope, General & Plastic Surgery	Surgery
75QMB	Computer, Clinical Laboratory	Chemistry
80WLE	Computer, Image, Endoscopic	General
79WIY	Computer, Imaging, Presurgery	Surgery
90UFD	Computer, Radiographic Image Analysis	Radiology
90WQO	Detector, Radioisotope	Radiology
80TBU	Dispenser, Ice	General
79GDI	Dissector, Surgical, General & Plastic Surgery	Surgery
80WKJ	Dressing, Gel	General
80WKL	Dressing, Permeable, Moisture	General
77QRJ	Drill, Middle Ear Surgery	Ear/Nose/Throat
76QRK	Drill, Oral Surgery	Dental And Oral
79GEG	Elevator, Surgical, General & Plastic Surgery	Surgery
78GCL	Esophagoscope, General & Plastic Surgery	Gastro/Urology
79GEO	File, Surgical, General & Plastic Surgery	Surgery
79GEN	Forceps, General & Plastic Surgery	Surgery
78GCK	Gastroscope, General & Plastic Surgery	Gastro/Urology
79KGO	Glove, Surgical, Plastic Surgery	Surgery
79GDH	Gouge, Surgical, General & Plastic Surgery	Surgery
87THC	Holder, Leg, Arthroscopy	Orthopedics
79WRY	Holder, Shoulder, Arthroscopy	Surgery
79GDG	Hook, Surgical, General & Plastic Surgery	Surgery
86KYG	Irrigator, Ocular Surgery	Ophthalmology
80RLP	Kit, Prep	General
79GCJ	Laparoscope, General & Plastic Surgery	Surgery
73LLO	Laser, Neodymium:YAG, Surgical, Pulmonary	Anesthesiology
79GFJ	Mallet, Surgical, General & Plastic Surgery	Surgery
79FSO	Microscope, Surgical, General & Plastic Surgery	Surgery
79FTX	Mirror, General & Plastic Surgery	Surgery
79FYM	Monitor, Blood Pressure, Indirect, Surgery	Surgery
79FYL	Monitor, Blood Pressure, Indirect, Surgery, Powered	Surgery
79FYW	Monitor, ECG, Surgery	Surgery
79FYX	Monitor, EEG, Surgery	Surgery
79FZA	Monitor, Temperature, Surgery	Surgery
79GFI	Osteotome, Manual (Plastic Surgery)	Surgery
79GAC	Rasp, Surgical, General & Plastic Surgery	Surgery
79UAO	Reconstruction Block, Plastic Surgery	Surgery
79UCB	Reconstructive Sheeting, Plastic Surgery	Surgery
79RRM	Scissors, Plastic Surgery (Dissecting)	Surgery
87WIV	Service, Design, Implant, Custom	Orthopedics
79GAF	Spatula, Surgical, General & Plastic Surgery	Surgery
79FXB	Stimulator, Muscle, General & Plastic Surgery	Surgery
74WIU	Unit, Cooling, Cardiac	Cardiovascular

SURGICAL

79LYU	Accessories, Apparel, Surgical	Surgery
80WQD	Accessories, Laser	General
79FTA	Accessories, Light, Surgical	Surgery
79FWZ	Accessories, Operating Room, Table	Surgery
79KQM	Accessories, Surgical Camera	Surgery
78FHC	Adapter, Cord, Instrument, Surgical, Transurethral	Gastro/Urology
79GEF	Applier, Surgical Staple	Surgery
79GDO	Applier, Surgical, Clip	Surgery
79GDA	Apron, Surgical	Surgery
87WHX	Aspirator, Arthroscopy	Orthopedics
79QBU	Aspirator, Surgical	Surgery
87SHK	Assistant, Surgical, Orthopedic, Automated	Orthopedics
79GFG	Bit, Surgical	Surgery
74DWH	Blade, Saw, Surgical, Cardiovascular	Cardiovascular
79GFA	Blade, Surgical, Saw, General & Plastic Surgery	Surgery
79QEI	Brassiere, Surgical	Surgery
79GFF	Burr, Surgical, General & Plastic Surgery	Surgery
79GEB	Button, Surgical	Surgery
79FWI	Camera, Cine, Surgical (With Audio)	Surgery
79FWH	Camera, Cine, Surgical (Without Audio)	Surgery
79FTT	Camera, Still, Surgical	Surgery
79FWC	Camera, Television, Surgical (With Audio)	Surgery
79FWB	Camera, Television, Surgical (Without Audio)	Surgery
79WRX	Camera, Video, Headlight, Surgical	Surgery
79FXN	Camera, Videotape, Surgical	Surgery
86HMX	Cannula, Ophthalmic	Ophthalmology
79GEA	Cannula, Surgical, General & Plastic Surgery	Surgery
79FYF	Cap, Surgical	Surgery

KEYWORD INDEX

SURGICAL (cont'd)

Code	Description	Category
79GEJ	Carrier, Ligature	Surgery
78GBM	Catheter, Urethral	Gastro/Urology
86HQR	Cautery, Radiofrequency, AC-Powered	Ophthalmology
86HQQ	Cautery, Radiofrequency, Battery-Powered	Ophthalmology
86HQO	Cautery, Thermal, AC-Powered	Ophthalmology
86HQP	Cautery, Thermal, Battery-Powered	Ophthalmology
79GBB	Chair, Surgical, AC-Powered	Surgery
79FZK	Chair, Surgical, Non-Electrical	Surgery
76EML	Chisel, Bone, Surgical	Dental And Oral
79LWH	Counter, Sponge, Surgical	Surgery
79VDL	Counter, Surgical Instrument	Surgery
79RXN	Cover, Head, Surgical	Surgery
79KGQ	Cream, Surgical Gloving	Surgery
86HRN	Cryophthalmic Unit, AC-Powered	Ophthalmology
79FZS	Curette, Surgical	Surgery
76EMK	Curette, Surgical, Dental	Dental And Oral
79LWG	Cushion, Table, Surgical	Surgery
79FZT	Cutter, Surgical	Surgery
86HQE	Cutter, Vitreous Aspiration, AC-Powered	Ophthalmology
86HKP	Cutter, Vitreous Aspiration, Battery-Powered	Ophthalmology
86QOH	Cutter, Vitreous Infusion Suction	Ophthalmology
79KOY	Degreaser, Skin, Surgical	Surgery
74DWP	Dilator, Vessel, Surgical	Cardiovascular
79WVZ	Drape, Incision, Surgical	Surgery
79KKX	Drape, Surgical	Surgery
79WQC	Drape, Surgical Instrument, Magnetic	Surgery
79FZJ	Drape, Surgical, Disposable	Surgery
77ERY	Drape, Surgical, ENT	Ear/Nose/Throat
79QQQ	Drape, Surgical, Reusable	Surgery
79FYE	Dress, Surgical	Surgery
77ERL	Drill, Surgical, ENT (Electric Or Pneumatic)	Ear/Nose/Throat
79GFC	Driver, Surgical, Pin	Surgery
79KGP	Dusting Powder, Surgical	Surgery
77LRC	ENT Manual Surgical Instrument	Ear/Nose/Throat
79QSK	Electrocautery Unit, Battery-Powered	Surgery
85HIM	Electrocautery Unit, Endoscopic	Obstetrics/Gyn
85HGI	Electrocautery Unit, Gynecologic	Obstetrics/Gyn
79QSL	Electrocautery Unit, Line-Powered	Surgery
76EMJ	Elevator, Surgical, Dental	Dental And Oral
79FXT	Film, Camera	Surgery
76EMH	Forceps, Rongeur, Surgical	Dental And Oral
85HCZ	Forceps, Surgical, Gynecological	Obstetrics/Gyn
76EMG	Forceps, Tooth Extractor, Surgical	Dental And Oral
79FXS	Frame, Camera, Surgical	Surgery
79LRW	General Use Surgical Scissors	Surgery
80FPI	Glove, Surgical	General
80QYI	Glove, Surgical, Hypoallergenic	General
79KGO	Glove, Surgical, Plastic Surgery	Surgery
79WWN	Glove, Surgical, Powder-Free	Surgery
79MFI	Glue, Surgical Tissue	Surgery
79GDH	Gouge, Surgical, General & Plastic Surgery	Surgery
79FYC	Gown, Isolation, Surgical	Surgery
80QYQ	Gown, Other	General
79FYA	Gown, Surgical	Surgery
79FZY	Hammer, Surgical	Surgery
79FXZ	Helmet, Surgical	Surgery
76EMD	Hemostat, Surgical	Dental And Oral
79FXR	Holder, Camera, Surgical	Surgery
79RHW	Holder, Needle, Other	Surgery
79WRE	Holder, Retractor	Surgery
79FXY	Hood, Surgical	Surgery
79GDG	Hook, Surgical, General & Plastic Surgery	Surgery
84HBI	Illuminator, Fiberoptic, Surgical Field	Cns/Neurology
79MDM	Instrument, Manual, General Surgical	Surgery
77LRE	Instrument, Modification, Prosthesis, Ossicular Repl., Surg.	Ear/Nose/Throat
87HSZ	Instrument, Surgical, Powered, Pneumatic	Orthopedics
80FRT	Isolation Unit, Surgical	General
78FHY	Jelly, Contact (For Transurethral Surgical Instrument)	Gastro/Urology

SURGICAL (cont'd)

Code	Description	Category
78FHX	Jelly, Lubricating, Transurethral Surgical Instrument	Gastro/Urology
86MLP	Keratoprosthesis, Temporary Implant, Surgical	Ophthalmology
79FTN	Kit, Instruments and Accessories, Surgical	Surgery
86RCT	Kit, Irrigation, Eye	Ophthalmology
79LRO	Kit, Surgical (General)	Surgery
79KDD	Kit, Surgical Instrument, Disposable	Surgery
79RDQ	Knife, Skin Grafting	Surgery
76EMF	Knife, Surgical	Dental And Oral
79FTD	Lamp, Surgical	Surgery
79GBC	Lamp, Surgical, Incandescent	Surgery
79FTB	Lamp, Surgical, Xenon	Surgery
79GCI	Laryngoscope, Surgical	Surgery
79ULB	Laser, Argon, Surgical	Surgery
79UKZ	Laser, Carbon-Dioxide, Surgical	Surgery
79ULC	Laser, Dye, Surgical	Surgery
79VIC	Laser, Excimer, Surgical	Surgery
79ULA	Laser, Nd:YAG, Surgical	Surgery
79GEX	Laser, Surgical	Surgery
79WXW	Laser, Surgical, Holmium	Surgery
79REN	Lavage Unit, Surgical	Surgery
79FXQ	Lens, Camera, Surgical	Surgery
86LQJ	Lens, Surgical, Laser	Ophthalmology
79FSR	Light, Headband, Surgical	Surgery
76EBA	Light, Surgical Headlight	Dental And Oral
76EAZ	Light, Surgical Operating, Dental	Dental And Oral
79FSZ	Light, Surgical, Carrier	Surgery
79FSY	Light, Surgical, Ceiling Mounted	Surgery
79FSX	Light, Surgical, Connector	Surgery
79FSW	Light, Surgical, Endoscopic	Surgery
79FST	Light, Surgical, Fiberoptic	Surgery
79FSS	Light, Surgical, Floor Standing	Surgery
79FSQ	Light, Surgical, Instrument	Surgery
79FSP	Loupe, Diagnostic/Surgical	Surgery
79GFJ	Mallet, Surgical, General & Plastic Surgery	Surgery
79FXX	Mask, Surgical	Surgery
76LPG	Material, Dressing, Surgical, Acid, Polylactic	Dental And Oral
79FTM	Mesh, Surgical (Steel Gauze)	Surgery
79FTL	Mesh, Surgical, Polymeric	Surgery
79UMJ	Mount, Surgical Microscope	Surgery
80MXI	Nonabsorbable Gauze, Surgical Sponge, & Wound Dressing for External Use (with a Drug)	General
87LXH	Orthopedic Manual Surgical Instrument	Orthopedics
80WXF	Pack, Custom/Special Procedure	General
79RXP	Pack, Surgical (Drape)	Surgery
79RXO	Packing, Surgical	Surgery
80WXM	Pad, Forceps, Surgical	General
86HRP	Pen, Marking, Surgical	Ophthalmology
87HTC	Pliers, Surgical	Orthopedics
87WWB	Positioner, Spine, Surgical	Orthopedics
74WTO	Probe, Transesophageal	Cardiovascular
79FTO	Prosthesis, Testicle, Surgical	Surgery
79UEM	Protector, Surgical Instrument	Surgery
76EME	Punch, Biopsy, Surgical	Dental And Oral
79LRY	Punch, Surgical	Surgery
89ISM	Pylon, Post Surgical	Physical Med
79FSG	Rack, Surgical Instrument	Surgery
79GAC	Rasp, Surgical, General & Plastic Surgery	Surgery
80CBB	Regulator, Suction, Surgical	General
79VLT	Remover, Staple, Surgical	Surgery
79GCZ	Retainer, Surgical	Surgery
79WRZ	Retractor, Abdominal, Padded, Flexible	Surgery
79GAD	Retractor, Surgical	Surgery
77EWQ	Saw, Surgical, ENT (Electric Or Pneumatic)	Ear/Nose/Throat
80FQA	Scale, Surgical Sponge	General
79UMD	Scanner, Ultrasonic, Surgical	Surgery
76EGN	Scissors, Surgical Tissue, Dental (Oral)	Dental And Oral
79LRZ	Screwdriver, Surgical	Surgery
79RRX	Scrub Machine, Surgical	Surgery
79WVB	Sharpener, Instrument, Surgical	Surgery
73BWP	Shoe And Shoe Cover, Conductive	Anesthesiology
79RSX	Shoe, Conductive	Surgery
79FXW	Shoe, Operating Room	Surgery
79GAE	Snare, Surgical	Surgery
80TGD	Solution, Surgical Scrub	General
79GAF	Spatula, Surgical, General & Plastic Surgery	Surgery
79GAG	Stapler, Surgical	Surgery
79FSI	Sterilizer, Steam (Autoclave), Surgical	Surgery
87HRT	Stripper, Surgical	Orthopedics

www.mdrweb.com

I-219

SURGICAL (cont'd)

79GAH	Stylet, Surgical	Surgery
79RRY	Suit, Scrub, Disposable	Surgery
79RRZ	Suit, Scrub, Reusable	Surgery
79FXO	Suit, Surgical	Surgery
77EPW	Support, Head, Surgical, ENT	Ear/Nose/Throat
79LSA	Surgical Bench Vise	Surgery
74DWS	Surgical Instrument, Cardiovascular	Cardiovascular
79KDC	Surgical Instrument, Disposable	Surgery
78KOA	Surgical Instrument, G-U, Manual	Gastro/Urology
79MDW	Surgical Instrument, Manual (General Use)	Surgery
84HAO	Surgical Instrument, Non-Powered, Neurosurgical	Cns/Neurology
85KNB	Surgical Instrument, Obstetric, Destructive, Fetal	Obstetrics/Gyn
85KNA	Surgical Instrument, Obstetric/Gynecologic	Obstetrics/Gyn
85KOH	Surgical Instrument, Obstetric/Gynecologic, General	Obstetrics/Gyn
87HWE	Surgical Instrument, Orthopedic, AC-Powered Motor	Orthopedics
79KIJ	Surgical Instrument, Orthopedic, Battery-Powered	Surgery
86VKE	Surgical Instrument, Radial Keratotomy	Ophthalmology
87JDX	Surgical Instrument, Sonic	Orthopedics
79LFL	Surgical Instrument, Ultrasonic	Surgery
79LWK	Surgical, Razor	Surgery
76UDU	System, Coding, Color, Instrument	Dental And Oral
79FZN	Table, Instrument, Surgical	Surgery
79JEA	Table, Surgical With Orthopedic Accessories, AC-Powered	Surgery
79GDC	Table, Surgical, Electrical	Surgery
79FWY	Table, Surgical, Hydraulic	Surgery
80FSE	Table, Surgical, Manual	General
87JEB	Table, Surgical, Orthopedic	Orthopedics
79MCA	Tape, Surgical, Internal	Surgery
80SAE	Tester, Surgical Glove	General
79GAX	Tourniquet, Non-Pneumatic, Surgical	Surgery
79SBE	Towel, Surgical	Surgery
80WNH	Tray, Custom/Special Procedure	General
79LRP	Tray, Surgical	Surgery
79FSM	Tray, Surgical Instrument	Surgery
77MMO	Tray, Surgical, ENT	Ear/Nose/Throat
79WVC	Tunneler, Surgical	Surgery
86LZP	Viscoelastic Surgical Aid	Ophthalmology
79KDB	Waste Disposal Unit, Surgical Instrument (Sharps)	Surgery
87LRN	Wire, Surgical	Orthopedics
80SGG	Wrapper, Surgical Instrument (Sterile)	General

SURROGATE

75JIW	Calibrator, Surrogate, Clinical Chemistry	Chemistry

SURVIVAL

81JWP	Red Cell Survival Test	Hematology

SUSCEPTIBILITY

83QBD	Analyzer, Antibiotic Susceptibility	Microbiology
83LRG	Analyzer, Overnight Suscept. System, Automated	Microbiology
83MJE	Culture Media, Antifungal, Susceptibility Test	Microbiology
83JSO	Culture Media, Antimicrobial Susceptibility Test	Microbiology
83LKA	Culture Media, Antimicrobial Susceptibility Test	Microbiology
83MJD	Culture Media, Antimycobacteria, Susceptibility Test	Microbiology
83MKR	Device, Susceptibility, Topical Antimicrobial	Microbiology
83JTN	Disc, Susceptibility, Antimicrobial	Microbiology
83MJA	Powders, Antimycobacterial Susceptibility Test	Microbiology
83LTW	Susceptibility Test Cards, Antimicrobial	Microbiology
83LTT	Susceptibility Test Panels, Antimicrobial	Microbiology
83LON	Test System, Antimicrobial Susceptibility, Automated	Microbiology
83UJX	Test, Antibiotic Susceptibility	Microbiology
83JWY	Test, Antimicrobial Susceptibility	Microbiology

SUSPENSION

83LHW	Reag. & Equipment, Erythrocyte Suspension, Multi Species	Microbiology
89INE	Sling, Overhead Suspension, Wheelchair	Physical Med
88KJF	Suspension System, Cell Culture	Pathology

SUTURE

78WZN	Applier, Clip, Repair, Hernia, Laparoscopic	Gastro/Urology
79SJF	Applier, Ligature Clip	Surgery
79RXQ	Bolster, Suture (Bumper)	Surgery
79SJG	Clip, Ligature	Surgery
79QLH	Clip, Suture	Surgery
78FBF	Clip, Suture, Stomach And Intestinal	Gastro/Urology
79UEN	Cutter, Suture	Surgery
79QQR	Gauge, Thickness, Tissue	Surgery
79QOJ	Holder, Needle, Curved, Laparoscopic	Surgery
79QNU	Holder, Needle, Laparoscopic	Surgery
79QPN	Holder/Scissors, Needle, Laparoscopic	Surgery
79QRS	Instrument, Knot Tying, Suture, Laparoscopic	Surgery
79QPS	Instrument, Needle Holder/Knot Tying	Surgery
79QSH	Instrument, Passing, Suture, Laparoscopic	Surgery
79RXR	Kit, Suture	Surgery
79MCZ	Kit, Suture Removal	Surgery
79MAW	Marker, Identification, Suture	Surgery
87WUR	Needle, Suture, Arthroscopy	Orthopedics
79GAB	Needle, Suture, Disposable	Surgery

SUTURE (cont'd)

84HAS	Needle, Suture, Neurosurgical	Cns/Neurology
86HNM	Needle, Suture, Ophthalmic	Ophthalmology
79GDL	Needle, Suture, Reusable	Surgery
77KBR	Needle, Tonsil Suture	Ear/Nose/Throat
85HHY	Prosthesis, Suture, Cerclage	Obstetrics/Gyn
79VLT	Remover, Staple, Surgical	Surgery
79KGS	Retention Device, Suture	Surgery
79RXT	Ring, Suture	Surgery
86HNF	Scissors, Ophthalmic	Ophthalmology
79RRO	Scissors, Suture	Surgery
79WZO	Stapler, Laparoscopic	Surgery
79GAG	Stapler, Surgical	Surgery
78FHM	Suture Apparatus, Stomach And Intestinal	Gastro/Urology
79GAK	Suture, Absorbable	Surgery
79GAL	Suture, Absorbable, Natural	Surgery
86HMO	Suture, Absorbable, Ophthalmic	Ophthalmology
79GAN	Suture, Absorbable, Synthetic	Surgery
79GAM	Suture, Absorbable, Synthetic, Polyglycolic Acid	Surgery
74DTH	Suture, Cardiovascular	Cardiovascular
79RXV	Suture, Catgut	Surgery
79RXW	Suture, Cotton	Surgery
76DZG	Suture, Dental	Dental And Oral
79SGX	Suture, Laparoscopy	Surgery
79SGW	Suture, Laparoscopy, Loose	Surgery
79SGY	Suture, Laparoscopy, Pre-Tied	Surgery
79RXX	Suture, Linen	Surgery
79RXY	Suture, Multifilament Steel	Surgery
79GAO	Suture, Non-Absorbable	Surgery
86HMN	Suture, Non-Absorbable, Ophthalmic	Ophthalmology
79GAP	Suture, Non-Absorbable, Silk	Surgery
79GAQ	Suture, Non-Absorbable, Steel, Monofilament & Multifilament	Surgery
79GAR	Suture, Non-Absorbable, Synthetic, Polyamide	Surgery
79GAS	Suture, Non-Absorbable, Synthetic, Polyester	Surgery
79GAT	Suture, Non-Absorbable, Synthetic, Polyethylene	Surgery
79GAW	Suture, Non-Absorbable, Synthetic, Polypropylene	Surgery
79RYF	Suture, Other	Surgery
79RYC	Suture, Polypropylene Monofilament	Surgery
79WLR	Suture, Polytetrafluoroethylene	Surgery
79RYD	Suture, Silk	Surgery
79RYE	Suture, Stainless Steel	Surgery
78LNN	Unit, Anastomosis, Gastroenterologic	Gastro/Urology
79SGE	Wire, Ligature	Surgery
79UKY	Zipper, Wound Closure	Surgery

SUTURING

79MFJ	Device, Suturing, Endoscopic	Surgery
77KBP	Hook, Tonsil Suturing	Ear/Nose/Throat

SWABS

80TGC	Swabs, Alcohol	General
80RYG	Swabs, Antiseptic	General
80RYH	Swabs, Cotton	General
80VLI	Swabs, Oral Care	General
80RYI	Swabs, Specimen Collection	General

SWAN-GANZ

74GBR	Catheter, Cardiovascular, Balloon Type	Cardiovascular
74QIN	Catheter, Thermal Dilution	Cardiovascular

SWEAT

80WXC	Band, Sweat	General
75VCX	Collector, Sweat	Chemistry
75QTF	Electrode, Sweat Test	Chemistry
78RCP	Iontophoresis Unit (Sweat Rate)	Gastro/Urology
89KTB	Iontophoresis Unit, Physical Medicine	Physical Med
80WSZ	Sensor, Moisture	General

SWITCHING

74DRW	Adapter, Lead Switching, Electrocardiograph	Cardiovascular
73JFE	Valve, Switching (Ploss)	Anesthesiology

SYMBLEPHARON

86UBE	Ring, Symblepharon	Ophthalmology

SYMPATHECTOMY

84RAR	Hook, Sympathectomy	Cns/Neurology

SYNCHRONIZER

90IXO	Synchronizer, ECG/Respirator, Radiographic	Radiology
90IYY	Synchronizer, Electrocardiograph, Nuclear	Radiology
90RYJ	Synchronizer, Nuclear Camera	Radiology
90RYK	Synchronizer, Radiographic Unit	Radiology

SYNCHROTRON

90IWM	Synchrotron, Medical	Radiology

SYNCYTIAL

83GQG	Antigen, CF (Including CF Controls), Respiratory Syncytial	Microbiology
83GQF	Antiserum, Neutralization, Respiratory Syncytial Virus	Microbiology

SYNCYTIAL *(cont'd)*
83MCE Enzyme Linked Immunoabsorbent Assay, Resp. Syncytial Virus — Microbiology
83LKT Respiratory Syncytial Virus, Antigen, Antibody, IFA — Microbiology

SYNDROME
89MNY Inhibitor, Post-Op Fibro., Carp. Tun. Syn.(Adhesion Barrier) — Physical Med
81VJE Test, Antibody, Acquired Immune Deficiency Syndrome (AIDS) — Hematology
82MZF Test, Hiv Detection — Immunology

SYNOPTOPHORE
86WNQ Synoptophore — Ophthalmology

SYNTHESIZER
88LNJ Analyzer, Chromosome, Automated — Pathology
80VBO Communication Equipment — General
75WJI Synthesizer, DNA — Chemistry
75UIP Synthesizer, Peptide & Protein — Chemistry
75UIQ Synthesizer, Polynucleotide — Chemistry

SYNTHETIC
88KIT Culture Media, Synthetic Cell And Tissue — Pathology
85MCR Dilator, Cervical, Hygroscopic, Synthetic — Obstetrics/Gyn
78MCI Graft, Vascular, Synth./Bio. Composite, Hemodialysis Access — Gastro/Urology
74MAL Graft, Vascular, Synthetic/Biological Composite — Cardiovascular
77ESF Polymer, ENT Composite Synthetic PTFE With Carbon-Fiber — Ear/Nose/Throat
77KHJ Polymer, ENT Synthetic Polyamide (Mesh Or Foil Material) — Ear/Nose/Throat
77JOF Polymer, ENT Synthetic, Porous Polyethylene — Ear/Nose/Throat
77ESH Polymer, ENT Synthetic-PIFE, Silicon Elastomer — Ear/Nose/Throat
80WTJ Polymer, Synthetic, Other — General
79FZB Prosthesis, Arterial Graft, Synthetic, Greater Than 6mm — Surgery
79JCP Prosthesis, Arterial Graft, Synthetic, Less Than 6mm — Surgery
79GEP Sponge, External, Synthetic — Surgery
88IFI Sprays, Synthetic, Smear — Pathology
79GAN Suture, Absorbable, Synthetic — Surgery
79GAM Suture, Absorbable, Synthetic, Polyglycolic Acid — Surgery
79GAR Suture, Non-Absorbable, Synthetic, Polyamide — Surgery
79GAS Suture, Non-Absorbable, Synthetic, Polyester — Surgery
79GAT Suture, Non-Absorbable, Synthetic, Polyethylene — Surgery
79GAW Suture, Non-Absorbable, Synthetic, Polypropylene — Surgery
87MBC Synthetic Ligaments & Tendons, Absorbable — Orthopedics
87LML Synthetic Ligaments and Tendons — Orthopedics
85LOB Synthetic Osmotic Cervical Dilator — Obstetrics/Gyn

SYNTHETIC-PIFE
77ESH Polymer, ENT Synthetic-PIFE, Silicon Elastomer — Ear/Nose/Throat

SYPHILIS
83WJQ Antibody, Treponema Pallidum — Microbiology
83GMT Antigen, HA, Treponema Pallidum — Microbiology
83JWL Antigen, Treponema Pallidum For FTA-ABS Test — Microbiology
83LIP Enzyme Linked Immunoabsorbent Assay, Treponema Pallidum — Microbiology
83UMO Test, Syphilis (RPR or VDRL) — Microbiology

SYRINGE
89IQG Adapter, Holder, Syringe — Physical Med
74WTU Adapter, Needle — Cardiovascular
80RYL Adapter, Syringe — General
80VLY Cap, Tip, Syringe — General
80QKV Cleaner, Syringe — General
80QNL Crusher, Syringe — General
80QOG Cutter, Syringe And Needle — General
80KYX Dispenser, Medication, Liquid — General
80WSB Dispenser, Syringe And Needle — General
80QWD Filter, Syringe — General
90IWR Holder, Syringe, Leaded — Radiology
74DXT Injector, Angiographic (Cardiac Catheterization) — Cardiovascular
80RCC Injector, Medication (Inoculator) — General
80RCD Injector, Syringe — General
74RCE Injector, Thermal Dilution — Cardiovascular
80KZH Introducer, Syringe Needle — General
77KAR Irrigator, Sinus — Ear/Nose/Throat
77RCS Kit, Irrigation, Ear — Ear/Nose/Throat
80RCW Kit, Irrigation, Wound — General
80RIE Needle, Hypodermic — General
80FMI Needle, Hypodermic, Single Lumen With Syringe — General
80WUI Protector, Puncture, Needle — General
78FIH Pump, Infusion Or Syringe, Extra-Luminal — Gastro/Urology
80RNG Pump, Infusion, Syringe — General
85UDG Pump, Syringe, Oxytocin — Obstetrics/Gyn
80RST Shield, Syringe — General
76ECB Syringe Unit, Air And/Or Water — Dental And Oral
82WKW Syringe, Allergy — Immunology
73RYM Syringe, Anesthesia — Anesthesiology
84RYN Syringe, Angiographic — Cns/Neurology
74WTW Syringe, Angioplasty — Cardiovascular

SYRINGE *(cont'd)*
80MEG Syringe, Antistick — General
87VIF Syringe, Arterial Blood Gas — Orthopedics
74MAV Syringe, Balloon Inflation — Cardiovascular
80RYU Syringe, Bulb — General
76DYY Syringe, Bulb, Air Or Water — Dental And Oral
73WTC Syringe, Calibration Testing, Spirometer — Anesthesiology
76EJI Syringe, Cartridge — Dental And Oral
80RYO Syringe, Catheter — General
76RYP Syringe, Dental — Dental And Oral
76DZF Syringe, Drug, Luer-Lock — Dental And Oral
77KCP Syringe, Ear — Ear/Nose/Throat
80RYQ Syringe, Hypodermic — General
80RYR Syringe, Insulin — General
80KYZ Syringe, Irrigating — General
76EIB Syringe, Irrigating, Dental — Dental And Oral
80KYY Syringe, Irrigating, Sterile — General
75UIR Syringe, Laboratory — Chemistry
86HKA Syringe, Ophthalmic — Ophthalmology
80WVE Syringe, Other — General
76EIC Syringe, Periodontic, Endodontic — Dental And Oral
80FMF Syringe, Piston — General
76EID Syringe, Restorative And Impression Material — Dental And Oral
80RYT Syringe, Tuberculin — General
80SFT Waste Disposal Unit, Syringe — General

SYRUP
88IAT Apathy's Gum Syrup — Pathology

SYSTEM
75CER 2, 4-dinitrophenylhydrazine, Lactate Dehydrogenase — Chemistry
78KXM Accessories, Extracorporeal System — Gastro/Urology
73TAC Alarm, Central Gas System — Anesthesiology
82KTJ Alpha-Fetoprotein RIA Test System — Immunology
83LRH Analyzer, Overnight Microorganism I.D. System, Automated — Microbiology
83LRG Analyzer, Overnight Suscept. System, Automated — Microbiology
74DSP Balloon, Intra-Aortic (With Control System) — Cardiovascular
75MQM Bilirubin (Total and Unbound) Neonate Test System — Chemistry
78LLB Blood System, Extracorporeal (With Accessories) — Gastro/Urology
73CBD Bottle, Collection, Breathing System (Calibrated) — Anesthesiology
73CBC Bottle, Collection, Breathing System (Uncalibrated) — Anesthesiology
76EBX Bracket, Table Assembly, N2O Delivery System — Dental And Oral
78LQQ Column, Immunoadsorption, System, Extracorporeal — Gastro/Urology
80VFG Communication System, Emergency Alert, Personal — General
89ILP Communication System, Non-Powered — Physical Med
89ILQ Communication System, Powered — Physical Med
80THE Communication System, Room Status — General
74DXX Control System, Catheter, Steerable — Cardiovascular
80VBT Control System, Energy — General
81JWD Count System — Hematology
78QOI Cystic Fibrosis System — Gastro/Urology
80LDH Delivery System, Allergen And Vaccine — General
80TDT Delivery System, Pneumatic Tube — General
78FKQ Dialysate Delivery System, Central Multiple Patient — Gastro/Urology
78KPF Dialysate Delivery System, Peritoneal, Semi-Automatic — Gastro/Urology
78FIK Dialysate Delivery System, Recirculating — Gastro/Urology
78FIJ Dialysate Delivery System, Recirculating, Single Pass — Gastro/Urology
78FII Dialysate Delivery System, Sealed — Gastro/Urology
78FIL Dialysate Delivery System, Single Pass — Gastro/Urology
78FKP Dialysate Delivery System, Single Patient — Gastro/Urology
78FKT Dialysate Delivery System, Sorbent Regenerated — Gastro/Urology
78LIF Dialyzer Reprocessing System — Gastro/Urology
78EYZ Drainage System, Urine, Closed — Gastro/Urology
89IQA Environmental Control System, Powered — Physical Med
89ILR Environmental Control System, Powered, Remote — Physical Med
80UDO Exhaust System, Body — General
79FYD Exhaust System, Surgical — Surgery
78LNP Extracorporeal Hyperthermia System — Gastro/Urology
78LNR Extracorporeal Photopheresis System — Gastro/Urology
80RLO Headwall System (Patient Room) — General
73BZE Heater, Breathing System W/Wo Controller — Anesthesiology
81JBD Hemoglobinometer, Electrophoretic Analysis System — Hematology
81RAC Hemoperfusion System (Hemodetoxifier) — Hematology
78FLD Hemoperfusion System, Sorbent — Gastro/Urology
90LNE Hyperthermia System, Automatic Control — Radiology
90LNF Hyperthermia System, Manual Control — Radiology
90LNG Hyperthermia System, Whole-Body — Radiology
90TCP Image Intensification System — Radiology
90LLZ Image Processing System — Radiology
78TCQ Infusion System, Insulin, With Monitor — Gastro/Urology
90LLY Infusion System, Radionuclide — Radiology
90TGW Interlock System, X-Ray Darkrooms — Radiology
74MOU Intravascular Radiation Delivery System — Cardiovascular
89IKK Isokinetic Testing And Evaluation System — Physical Med
75RGE Mass Screening System — Chemistry
90LNH Nuclear Magnetic Resonance Imaging System — Radiology
90LNI Nuclear Magnetic Resonance Spectroscopic System — Radiology

SYSTEM *(cont'd)*

80RIO	Nurse Call System	General
89LXJ	Optical Position/Movement Recording System	Physical Med
78RIZ	Organ Preservation System	Gastro/Urology
75LPW	Oxalate Test System	Chemistry
80VDO	Packaging System, Unit-Dose	General
78KDN	Perfusion System, Kidney	Gastro/Urology
86WQT	Phacoemulsification System	Ophthalmology
74DXW	Phonocatheter System, Intracavitary	Cardiovascular
75CEO	Phosphorus Reagent (Test System)	Chemistry
75JQW	Pipetting And Diluting System, Automated	Chemistry
80TCS	Power System, Isolated	General
89JFC	Pressure Measurement, System, Intermittent	Physical Med
74DSO	Prosthesis, Heart, With Control System	Cardiovascular
80TDL	Public Address System	General
85HHI	Pump, Abortion, Vacuum, Central System	Obstetrics/Gyn
78FIP	Purification System, Water	Gastro/Urology
75SFZ	Purification System, Water, Deionization	Chemistry
75SGA	Purification System, Water, Reverse Osmosis	Chemistry
75JRT	Purification System, Water, Reverse Osmosis, Reagent Grade	Chemistry
75SGB	Purification System, Water, Ultraviolet	Chemistry
90UMF	Radiographic Picture Archiving/Communication System (PACS)	Radiology
86HJG	Reading System, Closed-Circuit Television	Ophthalmology
75CIG	Reagent, Bilirubin (Total Or Direct Test System)	Chemistry
75JFO	Reagent, Calcium (Test System)	Chemistry
75CHJ	Reagent, Chloride (Test System)	Chemistry
75CGO	Reagent, Cholesterol (Total Test System)	Chemistry
75CGX	Reagent, Creatinine (Test System)	Chemistry
75JGE	Reagent, Globulin (Test System)	Chemistry
75CGA	Reagent, Glucose (Test System)	Chemistry
75CFM	Reagent, Iron (Test System)	Chemistry
90IYT	Rebreathing System, Radionuclide	Radiology
81UJN	Serum Separation System	Hematology
88KJE	Spinner System, Cell Culture	Pathology
76LTF	Stimulator, Salivary System	Dental And Oral
82MLH	Strip, HAMA IGG, ELISA, In Vitro Test System	Immunology
88KJF	Suspension System, Cell Culture	Pathology
85HHQ	System, Abortion, Metreurynter-Balloon	Obstetrics/Gyn
77EWM	System, Analysis, Hearing-Aid	Ear/Nose/Throat
87MCV	System, Appliance, Fixation, Spinal Pedicle Screw	Orthopedics
88MHR	System, Assay, Chemoresponse	Pathology
83QCC	System, Automated, Microbiological	Microbiology
83MDB	System, Blood Culturing	Microbiology
79SGZ	System, Camera, 3-Dimensional	Surgery
90LOC	System, Cancer Treatment, Hyperthermia, RF/Microwave	Radiology
85MDG	System, Cannula, Intrafallopian	Obstetrics/Gyn
74MFW	System, Cardiomyoplasty	Cardiovascular
74MKX	System, Carotid Atherectomy	Cardiovascular
76UDU	System, Coding, Color, Instrument	Dental And Oral
73BXT	System, Collection, Gas	Anesthesiology
90LMD	System, Communication, Image, Digital	Radiology
81MZJ	System, Concentration, Hematopoietic Stem Cell	Hematology
79WOH	System, Cooling, Laser	Surgery
80WOI	System, Delivery, Drug, Non-invasive	General
86WVM	System, Delivery, Drug, Ocular	Ophthalmology
80SGR	System, Delivery, Drug, Unit-Dose	General
81KQJ	System, Determination, Fibrinogen	Hematology
80SHI	System, Drug Dispensing, Pharmacy, Automated	General
78MYE	System, Electrogastrography(egg)	Gastro/Urology
79VCN	System, Evacuation, Smoke, Laser	Surgery
87LZV	System, Extraction, Cement Removal	Orthopedics
87MRW	System, Facet Screw Spinal Device	Orthopedics
78MII	System, Gallbladder, Thermal Ablation	Gastro/Urology
78MQS	System, Hemodialysis, Access Recirculation Monitoring	Gastro/Urology
78MON	System, Hemodialysis, Remote Accessories	Gastro/Urology
78MEQ	System, Hyperthermia, Rf/microwave (benign Prostatic Hyperplasia), Thermotherapy	Gastro/Urology
86WXL	System, Hyperthermia, Ultrasonic, Ophthalmic	Ophthalmology
86LOH	System, Identification, Lens, Contact	Ophthalmology
90SIK	System, Imaging, Laparoscopy, Ultrasonic	Radiology
76LTE	System, Implant, Tooth	Dental And Oral
80TGT	System, Infusion, Administration, Drug, Implantable	General
74WYC	System, Infusion, Enzyme, Thrombolytic	Cardiovascular
86LZS	System, Laser, Excimer, Ophthalmic	Ophthalmology
79MVF	System, Laser, Photodynamic Therapy	Surgery
74MNO	System, Laser, Transmyocardial Revascularization	Cardiovascular
86WXT	System, Mapping, Corneal	Ophthalmology
90JAC	System, Marking, Film, Radiographic	Radiology
80WXP	System, Marking, Laser	General
79MWY	System, Microwave, Hair Removal	Surgery
79SJQ	System, Monitoring, Electrode, Active, Electrosurgical	Surgery
74MSX	System, Network And Communication, Physiological Monitors	Cardiovascular
79MYH	System, Non-coherent Light, Photodynamic Therapy	Surgery
88MJI	System, Orientation, Identification, Specimen/Tissue	Pathology
74LPD	System, Pacing, Anti-Tachycardia	Cardiovascular
74LPA	System, Pacing, Esophageal	Cardiovascular
74MTE	System, Pacing, Temporary, Acute, Internal Atrial Defibrillation	Cardiovascular
78FKX	System, Peritoneal Dialysis, Automatic	Gastro/Urology
80WOE	System, Pipeline, Gas	General
90MUJ	System, Planning, Radiation Therapy Treatment	Radiology
74MFZ	System, Pump & Control, Cardiac Assist, Axial Flow	Cardiovascular
73WQI	System, Recording, Data, Anesthesiology	Anesthesiology
74MKH	System, Renal Atherectomy, Ivt	Cardiovascular
74MFB	System, Reprocessing, Catheter, Balloon Angioplasty	Cardiovascular
74LPE	System, Retroperfusion, Artery, Coronary	Cardiovascular
80WTV	System, Robot	General
79MKY	System, Skin Closure	Surgery
75LPT	System, Test, Acid, Methylmalonic, Urinary	Chemistry
82MSV	System, Test, Antibodies, B2 - Glycoprotein I (b2 - Gpi)	Immunology
82MID	System, Test, Anticardiolipin, Immunological	Immunology
75NBW	System, Test, Blood Glucose, Over-The-Counter	Chemistry
75MGX	System, Test, Drugs of Abuse	Chemistry
83MYI	System, Test, Genotypic Detection, Resistant Markers, Staphylococcus Colonies	Microbiology
82NCW	System, Test, HER-2/NEU, Monitoring	Immunology
82MVD	System, Test, Her-2/Neu, Nucleic Acid Or Serum	Immunology
81MVZ	System, Test, Home, Hiv-1	Hematology
82MOI	System, Test, Immunological, Antigen, Tumor	Immunology
75MRR	System, Test, Low-Density, Lipoprotein	Chemistry
82MSW	System, Test, Thyroglobulin	Immunology
91MSL	System, Test, Topiramatee	Toxicology
82NAH	System, Test, Tumor Marker, For Detection Of Bladder Cancer	Immunology
85LHM	System, Thermographic, Liquid Crystal	Obstetrics/Gyn
87WUS	System, Traction, Arthroscopy	Orthopedics
80WIH	System, Transport, In-House	General
74MIH	System, Treatment, Aortic Aneurysm, Endovascular Graft	Cardiovascular
84MHA	System, Treatment, Brain Tumor, Hyperthermia, Ultrasonic	Cns/Neurology
77MIX	System, Vocal Cord Medialization	Ear/Nose/Throat
85MTW	System, Water, Reproduction, Assisted, And Purification	Obstetrics/Gyn
90IZL	System, X-Ray, Mobile	Radiology
90MUH	System, X-ray, Extraoral Source, Digital	Radiology
90IWB	Teletherapy System, Radionuclide	Radiology
90IYM	Telethermographic System	Radiology
90LHQ	Telethermographic System (Adjunctive Use)	Radiology
90LHP	Telethermographic System (Sole Diagnostic Screen)	Radiology
90UEY	Television System, Slow Scan	Radiology
83LON	Test System, Antimicrobial Susceptibility, Automated	Microbiology
82MOB	Test System, Antineutrophil Cytoplasmic Antibodies (ANCA)	Immunology
91MRS	Test System, Nicotine, Cotinine, Metabolites	Toxicology
80QYY	Tester, Grounding System	General
80SAA	Tester, Isolated Power System	General
90JAD	Therapeutic X-Ray System	Radiology
90VGR	Thyroid Uptake System	Radiology
74QRY	Transmitter/Receiver System, ECG, Telephone Multi-Channel	Cardiovascular
74QRZ	Transmitter/Receiver System, ECG, Telephone Single-Channel	Cardiovascular
80VFH	Transmitter/Receiver System, Fetal Monitor, Telephone	General
74DRG	Transmitter/Receiver System, Physiological, Radiofrequency	Cardiovascular
74DXH	Transmitter/Receiver System, Physiological, Telephone	Cardiovascular
80VFI	Transmitter/Receiver System, Pulmonary Monitor, Telephone	General
83JTW	Transport System, Aerobic	Microbiology
83JTX	Transport System, Anaerobic	Microbiology
90LSY	Ultrasound, Hyperthermia, Cancer Treatment	Radiology
75LPS	Urinary Homocystine (Non-Quantitative) Test System	Chemistry
78SEF	Urodynamic Measurement System	Gastro/Urology
78LJH	Urological Irrigation System	Gastro/Urology
75UJE	Venting System, Gas Chromatography	Chemistry
73SGH	Xenon System	Anesthesiology

SYSTEMIC

82DHC	Test, Systemic Lupus Erythematosus	Immunology

SYSTEMS

77ETW	Calibrator, Hearing-Aid/Earphone And Analysis Systems	Ear/Nose/Throat
80WMN	Power Systems, Uninterruptible (UPS)	General
80WMM	Regulator, Line Voltage	General
75JZM	System, Gonadotropin, Chorionic, Human (Non-RIA)	Chemistry
82DCL	Test, Hemolytic Systems	Immunology

T-TUBE

78QTO	Introducer, T-Tube	Gastro/Urology

T-TYPE

74WJY	Connector, Tubing, Blood	Cardiovascular
78FKB	Connector, Tubing, Blood, Infusion, T-Type	Gastro/Urology

T. CRUZI
83GNF Antigen, CF, T. Cruzi — Microbiology
83GND Antigen, IHA, T. Cruzi — Microbiology
83GNE Antigen, Latex Agglutination, T. Cruzi — Microbiology
83MIU Enzyme Linked Immunoabsorbent Assay, T. Cruzi — Microbiology
83MIV Immunofluorescent Assay, T. Cruzi — Microbiology

T3
75KHQ Radioassay, Triiodothyronine Uptake — Chemistry
75CDY Radioimmunoassay, T3 Uptake — Chemistry
75CDP Radioimmunoassay, Total Triiodothyronine — Chemistry

T4
75KLI Enzyme Immunoassay, Non-Radiolabeled, Total Thyroxine — Chemistry
75CEC Radioimmunoassay, Free Thyroxine — Chemistry
75UKB Radioimmunoassay, T4 — Chemistry
75CEE Radioimmunoassay, Thyroxine Binding Globulin — Chemistry
75CDX Radioimmunoassay, Total Thyroxine — Chemistry

TABLE
79FWZ Accessories, Operating Room, Table — Surgery
76EBX Bracket, Table Assembly, N2O Delivery System — Dental And Oral
80QFA Cabinet, Bedside — General
73BRY Cabinet, Table And Tray, Anesthesia — Anesthesiology
85QJG Chair, Birthing — Obstetrics/Gyn
80KMN Chair/Table, Medical — General
79LWG Cushion, Table, Surgical — Surgery
90UAD Exerciser, Nuclear Diagnostic (Cardiac Stress Table) — Radiology
80RGH Mattress, Operating Table — General
80WMD Pad, Pressure, Gel, Operating Table — General
80LGX Powered Medical Examination Table — General
80RSM Sheet, Examination Table, Disposable — General
80RSJ Sheeting, Examination Table — General
86HMF Stand, Instrument, AC-Powered, Ophthalmic — Ophthalmology
86HMG Stand, Instrument, Ophthalmic — Ophthalmology
80UDK Sterilizer, Ethylene-Oxide, Table Top — General
80UCT Sterilizer, Steam, Table Top — General
73BWN Table, Anesthetist's — Anesthesiology
88RYV Table, Autopsy — Pathology
81RYW Table, Blood Donor — Hematology
78MMZ Table, Cystometric, Electric — Gastro/Urology
78KQS Table, Cystometric, Non-Electrical — Gastro/Urology
80RYX Table, Examination/Treatment — General
79FZN Table, Instrument, Surgical — Surgery
89INW Table, Mechanical — Physical Med
90VHE Table, Nuclear Medicine — Radiology
85KNC Table, Obstetrical — Obstetrics/Gyn
85HDD Table, Obstetrical, AC-Powered — Obstetrics/Gyn
85HHP Table, Obstetrical, Manual — Obstetrics/Gyn
79FQO Table, Operating Room, AC-Powered — Surgery
79FWX Table, Operating Room, Mechanical — Surgery
79FWW Table, Operating Room, Pneumatic — Surgery
86HRK Table, Ophthalmic, Instrument, Manual — Ophthalmology
86HRJ Table, Ophthalmic, Instrument, Powered — Ophthalmology
80RZB Table, Other — General
80RYY Table, Overbed — General
89INQ Table, Physical Medicine, Powered — Physical Med
89JFB Table, Physical Therapy — Physical Med
90KXJ Table, Radiographic — Radiology
90IZZ Table, Radiographic, Non-Tilting, Powered — Radiology
90IXQ Table, Radiographic, Stationary Top — Radiology
90IXR Table, Radiographic, Tilting — Radiology
88IEG Table, Slide Warming — Pathology
79JEA Table, Surgical With Orthopedic Accessories, AC-Powered — Surgery
79GDC Table, Surgical, Electrical — Surgery
79FWY Table, Surgical, Hydraulic — Surgery
80FSE Table, Surgical, Manual — General
87JEB Table, Surgical, Orthopedic — Orthopedics
87RYZ Table, Traction — Orthopedics
80WNI Table, Ultrasound — General
78RZA Table, Urological (Cystological) — Gastro/Urology
78EYH Table, Urological, Non-Electrical — Gastro/Urology
78UEE Table, Urological, Radiographic — Gastro/Urology
77ETF Unit, Examining/Treatment, ENT — Ear/Nose/Throat

TABLET
80QNK Crusher, Pill — General
80WTB Cutter, Pill — General
88KKH Resazurin Tablet — Pathology

TABLETOP
88QJD Centrifuge, Tabletop — Pathology

TACHISTOSCOPE
83RZC Tachistoscope — Microbiology

TACHOMETER
74DPW Flowmeter, Blood, Intravenous — Cardiovascular
78FIT Flowmeter, Blood, Non-Invasive Electromagnetic — Gastro/Urology
74QZN Monitor, Heart Rate, R-Wave (ECG) — Cardiovascular

TACHOMETER *(cont'd)*
73JAX Pneumotachometer — Anesthesiology
80UKT Tachometer — General

TACHYCARDIA
74LWY Dual Chamber, Anti-Tachycardia, Pulse Generator — Cardiovascular
74UMI Pacemaker, Heart, Implantable, Anti-Tachycardia — Cardiovascular
74LWW Single Chamber, Anti-Tachycardia, Pulse Generator — Cardiovascular
74LPD System, Pacing, Anti-Tachycardia — Cardiovascular

TACK
77JYN Inserter, Sacculotomy Tack — Ear/Nose/Throat
77ESX Tack, Sacculotomy (Cody) — Ear/Nose/Throat

TACROLIMUS
91MLM Enzyme Immunoassay, Tacrolimus — Toxicology

TACTILE
77LRA Tactile Hearing-Aid — Ear/Nose/Throat

TAG
80QPF Label, Device — General
79LYV Label/Tag, Sterile — Surgery
80QPG Tag, Device Status — General

TALAR
87UBK Prosthesis, Ankle, Talar Component — Orthopedics

TALLY
81GKM Counter, Differential Hand Tally — Hematology

TAMP
87HXG Tamp — Orthopedics

TAMPON
79RXO Packing, Surgical — Surgery
85MHT Tampon, Chemically Modified — Obstetrics/Gyn
85HIL Tampon, Menstrual, Scented — Obstetrics/Gyn
85HEB Tampon, Menstrual, Unscented — Obstetrics/Gyn

TAN
89LEJ Booth, Sun Tan — Physical Med

TANGENT
86HOM Screen, Tangent, AC-Powered (Campimeter) — Ophthalmology
86HOL Screen, Tangent, Felt (Campimeter) — Ophthalmology
86HOK Screen, Tangent, Projection, AC-Powered — Ophthalmology
86HMJ Screen, Tangent, Projection, Battery-Powered — Ophthalmology
86HOJ Screen, Tangent, Target — Ophthalmology
86HLK Screen, Tangent, Target, Battery-Powered — Ophthalmology

TANGENTIAL
87WQP Analyzer, Distribution, Weight, Podiatric — Orthopedics

TANK
80WVN Base, Roller, Tank, Oxygen — General
73BYJ Canister, Liquid Oxygen, Portable — Anesthesiology
73RJL Canister, Oxygen — Anesthesiology
73VFY Container, Liquid Nitrogen — Anesthesiology
73VFZ Container, Liquid Oxygen — Anesthesiology
73ECX Cylinder, Compressed Gas, With Valve — Anesthesiology
73VFF Cylinder, Oxygen — Anesthesiology
73RJH Kit, Administration, Oxygen — Anesthesiology
91DKK Tank, Developing, TLC — Toxicology
80RZD Tank, Full Body (Bath) — General
78FIN Tank, Holding, Dialysis — Gastro/Urology

TANTALUM
86HQW Clip, Tantalum, Ophthalmic — Ophthalmology
77ESG Material, Metallic-Stainless Steel, Tantalum, Platinum — Ear/Nose/Throat

TAP
87HWX Tap, Bone — Orthopedics

TAPE
79KGX Bandage, Adhesive — Surgery
90WSH Calculator, Technique, Radiographic — Radiology
74MCU Cassette, Audio Tape — Cardiovascular
80WXA Component, Other — General
74DSH Recorder, Magnetic Tape/Disc — Cardiovascular
90ROQ Recorder, Radiographic Video Tape — Radiology
79KOX Solvent, Adhesive Tape — Surgery
80RVU Sterilization Process Indicator, Chemical — General
80RZE Tape, Adhesive — General
80RZF Tape, Adhesive, Hypoallergenic — General
80RZG Tape, Adhesive, Waterproof — General
80RZH Tape, Cotton — General
80WMH Tape, Gauze, Adhesive — General
79FTY Tape, Measuring, Ruler And Caliper — Surgery
86HKD Tape, Nystagmus — Ophthalmology
87HXT Tape, Orthopedic — Orthopedics
79MCA Tape, Surgical, Internal — Surgery
78FET Tape, Television & Video, Endoscopic — Gastro/Urology

TAPE (cont'd)
80RZI Tape, Umbilical — General

TARGET
86HOJ Screen, Tangent, Target — Ophthalmology
86HLK Screen, Tangent, Target, Battery-Powered — Ophthalmology
86HLP Target, Fusion/Stereoscopic — Ophthalmology

TARTAR
76ELA Hand Instrument, Calculus Removal — Dental And Oral

TARTRATE
75JFH Tartrate Inhibited, Acid Phosphatase (Prostatic) — Chemistry

TASK
84LQD Recorder, Attention Task Performance — Cns/Neurology

TASTE
75VII Test, Taste Acuity — Chemistry

TAUB
77EWL Prosthesis, Laryngeal (Taub) — Ear/Nose/Throat

TDD
89UME Telephone, Handicapped Use — Physical Med

TDM
75ULK Analyzer, Chemistry, Therapeutic Drug Monitor (TDM) — Chemistry

TDX
91MAR Assay, Serum, Cyclosporine and Metabolites, TDX — Toxicology

TEACHING
80RIP Observerscope — General
78FEA Teaching Attachment, Endoscopic — Gastro/Urology
79SHA Trainer, Laparoscopy — Surgery
87UFE Training Aid — Orthopedics
74VCZ Training Aid, Arrhythmia Recognition — Cardiovascular

TEAR
86HNW Dilator, Lacrimal — Ophthalmology
86HNL Probe, Lacrimal — Ophthalmology
86HNG Rongeur, Lacrimal Sac — Ophthalmology

TECHNIQUE
90WSH Calculator, Technique, Radiographic — Radiology

TEE
73BYH Drain, Tee (Water Trap) — Anesthesiology

TEETH
76ELN Denture, Gold — Dental And Oral
76ELM Denture, Plastic, Teeth — Dental And Oral
76EKO Denture, Preformed — Dental And Oral
76EEG Source, Heat, Bleaching, Teeth, Dental — Dental And Oral
76ELK Teeth, Artificial, Backing And Facing — Dental And Oral
76ELJ Teeth, Artificial, Posterior With Metal Insert — Dental And Oral
76ELL Teeth, Porcelain — Dental And Oral

TEETHING
80WRP Pacifier — General
76KKO Ring, Teething, Fluid-Filled — Dental And Oral
76MEF Ring, Teething, Non-Fluid-Filled — Dental And Oral

TEFLON
79KKY Material, PTFE/Carbon, Maxillofacial — Surgery
74DXZ Pledget And Intracardiac Patch, PETP, PTFE, Polypropylene — Cardiovascular
74DSX Pledget, Dacron, Teflon, Polypropylene — Cardiovascular
77ESF Polymer, ENT Composite Synthetic PTFE With Carbon-Fiber — Ear/Nose/Throat
79KDA Prosthesis, PTFE/Carbon-Fiber — Surgery
79WLR Suture, Polytetrafluoroethylene — Surgery
80WTH Tubing, Polytetrafluoroethylene — General

TEICOPLANIN
91MHO Teicoplanin, FPIA — Toxicology

TELECONFERENCE
90UEY Television System, Slow Scan — Radiology

TELEMETRY
74DTC Analyzer, Pacemaker Generator Function — Cardiovascular
80WME Pouch, Telemetry — General
74RZJ Telemetry Unit, Physiological, ECG — Cardiovascular
84RZK Telemetry Unit, Physiological, EEG — Cns/Neurology
89RZL Telemetry Unit, Physiological, EMG — Physical Med
84RZM Telemetry Unit, Physiological, EOG — Cns/Neurology
80TEZ Telemetry Unit, Physiological, Multiple Channel — General
84GYE Telemetry Unit, Physiological, Neurological — Cns/Neurology
80RZN Telemetry Unit, Physiological, Pressure — General
80RZO Telemetry Unit, Physiological, Temperature — General
74DRG Transmitter/Receiver System, Physiological, Radiofrequency — Cardiovascular

TELEPHONE
80VBO Communication Equipment — General
74LOR Resuscitator, Trans-Telephone — Cardiovascular
80VAT Telephone Equipment — General
89UME Telephone, Handicapped Use — Physical Med
90WOG Transmitter, Image & Data, Radiographic — Radiology
74QRY Transmitter/Receiver System, ECG, Telephone Multi-Channel — Cardiovascular
74QRZ Transmitter/Receiver System, ECG, Telephone Single-Channel — Cardiovascular
80VFH Transmitter/Receiver System, Fetal Monitor, Telephone — General
74DXH Transmitter/Receiver System, Physiological, Telephone — Cardiovascular
80VFI Transmitter/Receiver System, Pulmonary Monitor, Telephone — General
84QSC Transmitter/Receiver, EEG, Telephone — Cns/Neurology

TELERADIOLOGY
90UEY Television System, Slow Scan — Radiology
90WOG Transmitter, Image & Data, Radiographic — Radiology

TELESCOPE
86HKB Telescope, Hand-Held, Low-Vision — Ophthalmology
77ENZ Telescope, Laryngeal-Bronchial — Ear/Nose/Throat
78FBP Telescope, Rigid, Endoscopic — Gastro/Urology
86HKK Telescope, Spectacle, Low-Vision — Ophthalmology

TELETHERAPY
90KQA Device, Limiting, Beam, Teletherapy — Radiology
90IWD Device, Limiting, Beam, Teletherapy, Radionuclide — Radiology
90ROG Radiotherapy Treatment Planning Unit — Radiology
90LHN Radiotherapy Unit, Charged-Particle — Radiology
90RTL Simulator, Radiotherapy — Radiology
90KPQ Simulator, Radiotherapy, Special Purpose — Radiology
90IWH Source, Teletherapy, Radionuclide — Radiology
90IWB Teletherapy System, Radionuclide — Radiology
90JAD Therapeutic X-Ray System — Radiology

TELETHERMOGRAPHIC
90IYM Telethermographic System — Radiology
90LHQ Telethermographic System (Adjunctive Use) — Radiology
90LHP Telethermographic System (Sole Diagnostic Screen) — Radiology

TELETYPEWRITER
89UME Telephone, Handicapped Use — Physical Med

TELEVISION
79FWG Camera, Television, Endoscopic (With Audio) — Surgery
79FWF Camera, Television, Endoscopic (Without Audio) — Surgery
79FWE Camera, Television, Microsurgical (With Audio) — Surgery
79FWD Camera, Television, Microsurgical (Without Audio) — Surgery
79FWC Camera, Television, Surgical (With Audio) — Surgery
79FWB Camera, Television, Surgical (Without Audio) — Surgery
74DXJ Display, Cathode-Ray Tube — Cardiovascular
80KMI Monitor, Bed Patient — General
80UMW Mount, Television Set — General
86HJG Reading System, Closed-Circuit Television — Ophthalmology
78FET Tape, Television & Video, Endoscopic — Gastro/Urology
80TFC Television Monitor, Microscope — General
80TFD Television Monitor, Operating Room — General
90UEY Television System, Slow Scan — Radiology
80TFA Television, Patient Room — General

TEMPERATURE
79WTZ Analyzer, Patient, Multiple Function (Surgery) — Surgery
75ULO Bath, Dry (Constant Temperature) — Chemistry
75QCY Bath, Water (Constant Temperature) — Chemistry
83UFT Chamber, Constant Temperature (Environmental) — Microbiology
88KDW Container, Specimen Mailer And Storage, Temperature Control — Pathology
74DWC Controller, Temperature, Cardiopulmonary Bypass — Cardiovascular
80QML Controller, Temperature, Humidifier — General
80QMM Controller, Temperature, Other — General
75VGA Controller, Temperature, Programmable — Chemistry
90EGT Controller, Temperature, Radiographic — Radiology
80QND Cover, Thermometer — General
80TBU Dispenser, Ice — General
75UKM Freezer, Laboratory, Ultra-Low Temperature — Chemistry
80FOH Mattress, Water, Temperature Regulated — General
84GXT Monitor, Lesion Temperature — Cns/Neurology
80LMY Monitor, Skin Resistance/skin Temperature, For Insulin Reactions — General
80KLL Monitor, Temperature (Self-Contained) — General
73BWX Monitor, Temperature (With Probe) — Anesthesiology
78FLA Monitor, Temperature, Dialysis — Gastro/Urology
84HCS Monitor, Temperature, Neurosurgery, Direct Contact, Powered — Cns/Neurology
79FZA Monitor, Temperature, Surgery — Surgery
80RMJ Probe, Temperature — General
75JRR Regulator, Temperature — Chemistry
80RTM Simulator, Temperature — General

KEYWORD INDEX

TEST *(cont'd)*

82DDZ	Antigen, Antiserum, Control, Albumin, FITC	Immunology
82DCM	Antigen, Antiserum, Control, Albumin, Fraction V	Immunology
82DFJ	Antigen, Antiserum, Control, Albumin, Rhodamine	Immunology
82DCO	Antigen, Antiserum, Control, Alpha Globulin	Immunology
82DFF	Antigen, Antiserum, Control, Alpha-1-Antichymotrypsin	Immunology
82DEM	Antigen, Antiserum, Control, Alpha-1-Antitrypsin	Immunology
82DEI	Antigen, Antiserum, Control, Alpha-1-Antitrypsin, FITC	Immunology
82DFB	Antigen, Antiserum, Control, Alpha-1-Antitrypsin, Rhodamine	Immunology
82DEJ	Antigen, Antiserum, Control, Alpha-2-Glycoproteins	Immunology
82DEF	Antigen, Antiserum, Control, Alpha-2-HS-Glycoprotein	Immunology
82DEB	Antigen, Antiserum, Control, Alpha-2-Macroglobulin	Immunology
82DDQ	Antigen, Antiserum, Control, Antithrombin III	Immunology
82CZQ	Antigen, Antiserum, Control, Bence-Jones Protein	Immunology
82DDN	Antigen, Antiserum, Control, Beta 2-Glycoprotein I	Immunology
82DCJ	Antigen, Antiserum, Control, Beta Globulin	Immunology
82DHX	Antigen, Antiserum, Control, Carcinoembryonic Antigen	Immunology
82DDB	Antigen, Antiserum, Control, Ceruloplasmin	Immunology
82DCY	Antigen, Antiserum, Control, Ceruloplasmin, FITC	Immunology
82DCT	Antigen, Antiserum, Control, Ceruloplasmin, Rhodamine	Immunology
82DAK	Antigen, Antiserum, Control, Complement C1q	Immunology
82DAI	Antigen, Antiserum, Control, Complement C1r	Immunology
82CZY	Antigen, Antiserum, Control, Complement C1s	Immunology
82CZW	Antigen, Antiserum, Control, Complement C3	Immunology
82DBI	Antigen, Antiserum, Control, Complement C4	Immunology
82DAY	Antigen, Antiserum, Control, Complement C5	Immunology
82DAG	Antigen, Antiserum, Control, Complement C8	Immunology
82DAE	Antigen, Antiserum, Control, Complement C9	Immunology
82DCE	Antigen, Antiserum, Control, FAB	Immunology
82DCB	Antigen, Antiserum, Control, FAB, FITC	Immunology
82DBY	Antigen, Antiserum, Control, FAB, Rhodamine	Immunology
82JZH	Antigen, Antiserum, Control, Factor B	Immunology
82DBT	Antigen, Antiserum, Control, Factor XIII A, S	Immunology
82DBF	Antigen, Antiserum, Control, Ferritin	Immunology
82DBD	Antigen, Antiserum, Control, Fibrin	Immunology
82DAZ	Antigen, Antiserum, Control, Fibrinogen And Split Products	Immunology
82DAJ	Antigen, Antiserum, Control, Free Secretory Component	Immunology
82DAH	Antigen, Antiserum, Control, Gamma Globulin	Immunology
82DAF	Antigen, Antiserum, Control, Gamma Globulin, FITC	Immunology
82DAD	Antigen, Antiserum, Control, Haptoglobin	Immunology
82DAB	Antigen, Antiserum, Control, Haptoglobin, FITC	Immunology
82CZZ	Antigen, Antiserum, Control, Haptoglobin, Rhodamine	Immunology
82CZX	Antigen, Antiserum, Control, Hemopexin	Immunology
82CZT	Antigen, Antiserum, Control, Hemopexin, FITC	Immunology
82CZR	Antigen, Antiserum, Control, Hemopexin, Rhodamine	Immunology
82CZP	Antigen, Antiserum, Control, IGA	Immunology
82CZN	Antigen, Antiserum, Control, IGA, FITC	Immunology
82CZL	Antigen, Antiserum, Control, IGA, Peroxidase	Immunology
82CZK	Antigen, Antiserum, Control, IGA, Rhodamine	Immunology
82CZJ	Antigen, Antiserum, Control, IGD	Immunology
82DGG	Antigen, Antiserum, Control, IGD, FITC	Immunology
82DGH	Antigen, Antiserum, Control, IGD, Peroxidase	Immunology
82DGE	Antigen, Antiserum, Control, IGD, Rhodamine	Immunology
82DGC	Antigen, Antiserum, Control, IGE	Immunology
82DGP	Antigen, Antiserum, Control, IGE, FITC	Immunology
82DGO	Antigen, Antiserum, Control, IGE, Peroxidase	Immunology
82DGL	Antigen, Antiserum, Control, IGE, Rhodamine	Immunology
82DEW	Antigen, Antiserum, Control, IGG	Immunology
82DFK	Antigen, Antiserum, Control, IGG (FAB Fragment Specific)	Immunology
82DAS	Antigen, Antiserum, Control, IGG (Fc Fragment Specific)	Immunology
82DFZ	Antigen, Antiserum, Control, IGG (Gamma Chain Specific)	Immunology
82DGK	Antigen, Antiserum, Control, IGG, FITC	Immunology
82DAA	Antigen, Antiserum, Control, IGG, Peroxidase	Immunology
82DFO	Antigen, Antiserum, Control, IGG, Rhodamine	Immunology
82DFT	Antigen, Antiserum, Control, IGM	Immunology
82DAO	Antigen, Antiserum, Control, IGM (Mu Chain Specific)	Immunology
82DFS	Antigen, Antiserum, Control, IGM, FITC	Immunology
82DEY	Antigen, Antiserum, Control, IGM, Peroxidase	Immunology
82DEZ	Antigen, Antiserum, Control, IGM, Rhodamine	Immunology
82CZO	Antigen, Antiserum, Control, Inter-Alpha Trypsin Inhibitor	Immunology
82DFH	Antigen, Antiserum, Control, Kappa	Immunology
82DEO	Antigen, Antiserum, Control, Kappa, FITC	Immunology
82DEK	Antigen, Antiserum, Control, Kappa, Rhodamine	Immunology
82DEG	Antigen, Antiserum, Control, Lactoferrin	Immunology
82DEH	Antigen, Antiserum, Control, Lambda	Immunology
82DES	Antigen, Antiserum, Control, Lambda, FITC	Immunology
82DFG	Antigen, Antiserum, Control, Lambda, Rhodamine	Immunology
82DFC	Antigen, Antiserum, Control, Lipoprotein, Low Density	Immunology
82DHP	Antigen, Antiserum, Control, Luteinizing Hormone	Immunology
82DGS	Antigen, Antiserum, Control, Lymphocyte Typing	Immunology
82DED	Antigen, Antiserum, Control, Lysozyme	Immunology
82DDR	Antigen, Antiserum, Control, Myoglobin	Immunology
82DGX	Antigen, Antiserum, Control, Ng1M(A)	Immunology
82DDX	Antigen, Antiserum, Control, Plasminogen	Immunology
82JZJ	Antigen, Antiserum, Control, Prealbumin	Immunology
82DDS	Antigen, Antiserum, Control, Prealbumin, FITC	Immunology

TEST *(cont'd)*

82DHL	Antigen, Antiserum, Control, Protein, Complement	Immunology
82DDF	Antigen, Antiserum, Control, Prothrombin	Immunology
81JZK	Antigen, Antiserum, Control, Red Cells	Hematology
82DFQ	Antigen, Antiserum, Control, Sperm	Immunology
82DFI	Antigen, Antiserum, Control, Spinal Fluid, Total	Immunology
82DDG	Antigen, Antiserum, Control, Transferrin	Immunology
82DDI	Antigen, Antiserum, Control, Transferrin, FITC	Immunology
82DDD	Antigen, Antiserum, Control, Transferrin, Rhodamine	Immunology
82DGR	Antigen, Antiserum, Control, Whole Human Serum	Immunology
82DAP	Antigen, Antiserum, Fibrinogen And Fibrin Split Products	Immunology
82DAX	Antigen, Antiserum, Fibrinogen And Split Products, FITC	Immunology
83GOT	Antigen, B. Parapertussis	Microbiology
83GOX	Antigen, B. Pertussis	Microbiology
83GPI	Antigen, Bentonite Flocculation, Trichinella Spiralis	Microbiology
83GOD	Antigen, CF (Including CF Control), Adenovirus 1-33	Microbiology
83GNG	Antigen, CF (Including CF Control), Coxsackievirus A 1-24	Microbiology
83GQH	Antigen, CF (Including CF Control), Cytomegalovirus	Microbiology
83GNL	Antigen, CF (Including CF Control), Echovirus 1-34	Microbiology
83GNQ	Antigen, CF (Including CF Control), Epstein-Barr Virus	Microbiology
83GQD	Antigen, CF (Including CF Control), Equine Encephalitis	Microbiology
83GNX	Antigen, CF (Including CF Control), Influenza Virus	Microbiology
83GRC	Antigen, CF (Including CF Control), Mumps Virus	Microbiology
83GQS	Antigen, CF (Including CF Control), Parainfluenza Virus	Microbiology
83GOH	Antigen, CF (Including CF Control), Poliovirus 1-3	Microbiology
83GQB	Antigen, CF (Including CF Control), Reovirus 1-3	Microbiology
83GON	Antigen, CF (Including CF Control), Rubella	Microbiology
83GQG	Antigen, CF (Including CF Controls), Respiratory Syncytial	Microbiology
83GMI	Antigen, CF And/Or ID, Coccidioides Immitis	Microbiology
83GRJ	Antigen, CF, (Including CF Control), Rubeola	Microbiology
83GQW	Antigen, CF, (Including CF Control), Varicella-Zoster	Microbiology
83JWT	Antigen, CF, Aspergillus SPP.	Microbiology
83JWW	Antigen, CF, B. Dermatitidis	Microbiology
83GQK	Antigen, CF, Lymphocytic Choriomeningitis Virus	Microbiology
83GSB	Antigen, CF, Mycoplasma SPP.	Microbiology
83GPW	Antigen, CF, Psittacosis (Chlamydia Group)	Microbiology
83GPS	Antigen, CF, Q Fever	Microbiology
83GPQ	Antigen, CF, Spotted Fever Group	Microbiology
83GNF	Antigen, CF, T. Cruzi	Microbiology
83GMN	Antigen, CF, Toxoplasma Gondii	Microbiology
83GPO	Antigen, CF, Typhus Fever Group	Microbiology
82LTL	Antigen, Carbohydrate (CA19-9)	Immunology
83GQN	Antigen, Cf (including Cf Control), Herpesvirus Hominis 1, 2	Microbiology
83GSF	Antigen, Erysipelothrix Rhusiopathiae	Microbiology
83GSZ	Antigen, Febrile	Microbiology
83GNC	Antigen, Febrile, Slide And Tube, Salmonella	Microbiology
82DAR	Antigen, Fibrinogen And Split Products, Rhodamine	Immunology
83GPD	Antigen, Fluorescent Antibody Test, Echinococcus Granulosus	Microbiology
83GNH	Antigen, Fluorescent Antibody Test, Schistosoma Mansoni	Microbiology
83GOB	Antigen, HA (Including HA Control), Adenovirus 1-33	Microbiology
83GNT	Antigen, HA (Including HA Control), Influenza Virus	Microbiology
83GQY	Antigen, HA (Including HA Control), Mumps Virus	Microbiology
83GQR	Antigen, HA (Including HA Control), Parainfluenza Virus	Microbiology
83GQA	Antigen, HA (Including HA Control), Reovirus 1-3	Microbiology
83GOL	Antigen, HA (Including HA Control), Rubella	Microbiology
83GRH	Antigen, HA (Including HA Control), Rubeola	Microbiology
83GNJ	Antigen, HA, Echovirus 1-34	Microbiology
83GMT	Antigen, HA, Treponema Pallidum	Microbiology
83GMJ	Antigen, Histoplasma Capsulatum, All	Microbiology
83KHW	Antigen, ID, HA, CEP, Entamoeba Histolytica	Microbiology
83GLZ	Antigen, IF, Toxoplasma Gondii	Microbiology
83LJO	Antigen, IHA, Cytomegalovirus	Microbiology
83GND	Antigen, IHA, T. Cruzi	Microbiology
83GMM	Antigen, IHA, Toxoplasma Gondii	Microbiology
83LKC	Antigen, Indirect Hemagglutination, Herpes Simplex Virus	Microbiology
83GMG	Antigen, Latex Agglutination, Coccidioides Immitis	Microbiology
83GMO	Antigen, Latex Agglutination, Entamoeba Histolytica & Rel.	Microbiology
83GNE	Antigen, Latex Agglutination, T. Cruzi	Microbiology
83GPG	Antigen, Latex Agglutination, Trichinella Spiralis	Microbiology
83GRY	Antigen, Leptospira SPP.	Microbiology
83GMQ	Antigen, Non-Treponemal, All	Microbiology
83JWK	Antigen, Positive Control, Cryptococcus Neoformans	Microbiology
83GRL	Antigen, Salmonella SPP.	Microbiology
83GSL	Antigen, Slide And Tube, Francisella Tularensis	Microbiology
83GSI	Antigen, Slide And Tube, Listeria Monocytogenes	Microbiology
83LHT	Antigen, Somatic, Staphylococcus Aureus	Microbiology
83GTY	Antigen, Streptococcus SPP.	Microbiology
83JWL	Antigen, Treponema Pallidum For FTA-ABS Test	Microbiology
82LJM	Antinuclear Antibody (Enzyme-Labeled), Antigen, Controls	Immunology
82LKJ	Antinuclear Antibody, Antigen, Control	Immunology
82DBJ	Antiparietal Antibody, Immunofluorescent, Antigen, Control	Immunology
83GSX	Antisera, Acinetobacter Calcoaceticus, All Varieties	Microbiology
83KLH	Antisera, C. Acnes	Microbiology
83GQO	Antisera, Cf, Herpesvirus Hominis 1, 2	Microbiology
83LIN	Antisera, Conjugated Fluorescent, Cytomegalovirus	Microbiology

KEYWORD INDEX

TEST *(cont'd)*

Code	Description	Category
83GSY	Antisera, Fluorescent, All Globulins, Proteus SPP.	Microbiology
82KTM	C3-Indirect Immunofluorescent Solid Phase	Immunology
91DNN	Calibrator, Ethyl Alcohol	Toxicology
82KTK	Carbonic Anhydrase B And C Immunoassay Reagents	Immunology
82DDH	Carbonicanhydrase B, Antigen, Antiserum, Control	Immunology
82DDE	Carbonicanhydrase C, Antigen, Antiserum, Control	Immunology
75JFK	Catalytic Method, AST/SGOT	Chemistry
75JFJ	Catalytic Method, Amylase	Chemistry
75JFW	Catalytic Method, Creatine Phosphokinase	Chemistry
75JPY	Catalytic Procedure, CPK Isoenzymes	Chemistry
91DJO	Cellulose Fluorescent Indicator, TLC	Toxicology
83JSQ	Chromatographic Bacterial Identification	Microbiology
91DKX	Chromatographic Barbiturate Identification (Thin Layer)	Toxicology
75CFB	Chromatographic Derivative, Total Lipids	Chemistry
75JHT	Chromatographic Separation, CPK Isoenzymes	Chemistry
75JOC	Colorimetric, Xylose	Chemistry
91LDP	Colorimetry, Acetaminophen	Toxicology
91DIH	Colorimetry, Cholinesterase	Toxicology
75CIL	Colorimetry, Cresol Red, Carbon-Dioxide	Chemistry
91DKJ	Colorimetry, Salicylate	Toxicology

TEST *(cont'd)*

82DGJ	Colostrum, Antigen, Antiserum, Control	Immunology
75JNC	Column Or Paper Chromatography Plus Ninhydrin, Phenylalanin	Chemistry
75JMM	Column, Chromatography, Hydroxyproline	Chemistry
82KTQ	Complement	Immunology
75CIC	Complexone, Cresolphthalein, Calcium	Chemistry
80WLH	Contract Manufacturing, Reagent	General
80VAN	Contract R&D, Diagnostics	General
80WUH	Contract R&D, Equipment	General
82DAC	Control, Antiserum, Antigen, Activator, C3, Complement	Immunology
91LAS	Control, Drug Specific	Toxicology
81GJP	Control, Platelet	Hematology
81GJR	Control, Red Cell	Hematology
75JLG	Conversion Ferric Hydroxymates (Colorimetric), Fatty Acids	Chemistry
75JLA	Conversion To Creatinine, Creatine	Chemistry
75CFW	Copper Reduction, Glucose	Chemistry
83KFI	Corynebacterium Diphtheriae, Virulence Strip	Microbiology
75CHS	Coulometric Method, Carbon-Dioxide	Chemistry
75JFS	Coulometric, Chloride	Chemistry
83MJE	Culture Media, Antifungal, Susceptibility Test	Microbiology
83JSO	Culture Media, Antimicrobial Susceptibility Test	Microbiology
83LKA	Culture Media, Antimicrobial Susceptibility Test	Microbiology
83MJD	Culture Media, Antimycobacteria, Susceptibility Test	Microbiology
83JSE	Culture Media, Multiple Biochemical Test	Microbiology
83JSF	Culture Media, Single Biochemical Test	Microbiology
75CHZ	DI (O-Hydroxyphenylimine) Ethane, Calcium	Chemistry
91DIZ	Delayed Analysis, Alcohol	Toxicology
91LEQ	Detector, Electrochemical, Chromatography, Liquid	Toxicology
75CDW	Diacetyl-Monoxime, Urea Nitrogen	Chemistry
78QPJ	Dialysis Unit Test Equipment	Gastro/Urology
75JMT	Diazo (Colorimetric), Nitrite (Urinary, Non-Quantitative)	Chemistry
75CJJ	Diazo, ALT/SGPT	Chemistry
75CDF	Diazo, P-Nitroaniline/Vanillin, Vanilmandelic Acid	Chemistry
75CDM	Diazonium Colorimetry, Urobilinogen (Urinary, Non-Quant.)	Chemistry
75JKZ	Diethyldithiocarbamate (Colorimetric), Copper	Chemistry
75JHS	Differential Rate Kinetic Method, CPK Or Isoenzymes	Chemistry
75JGF	Differential Rate Method, Lactate Dehydrogenase Isoenzymes	Chemistry
75JKF	Dinitrophenyl Hydrazone Measurement (Colorimetric), HBD	Chemistry
75CJX	Disodium Phenyl Phosphate, Acid Phosphatase	Chemistry
75CJI	Disodium Phenylphosphate, Alkaline Phosphatase Or Isoenzyme	Chemistry
86HMS	Drum, Eye Knife Test	Ophthalmology
80RZU	Drum, Test	General
75JIK	Dry Ash Method, Protein Bound Iodine	Chemistry
75CIX	Dye-Binding, Albumin, Bromcresol, Green	Chemistry
75CJW	Dye-Binding, Albumin, Bromcresol, Purple	Chemistry
75QTF	Electrode, Sweat Test	Chemistry
91DOH	Electrometry, Cholinesterase	Toxicology
75CHT	Electrophoretic Method, Catecholamines	Chemistry
75JHH	Electrophoretic Method, Lecithin-Sphingomyelin Ratio	Chemistry
75CIN	Electrophoretic Separation, Alkaline Phosphatase Isoenzymes	Chemistry
75JHO	Electrophoretic Separation, Lipoproteins	Chemistry
75CDK	Electrophoretic Separation, Vanilmandelic Acid	Chemistry
75JQA	Electrophoretic, Gamma-Glutamyl Transpeptidase Isoenzymes	Chemistry
75CGH	Electrophoretic, Globulin	Chemistry
81JLM	Electrophoretic, Glucose-6-Phosphate Dehydrogenase	Hematology
75CFE	Electrophoretic, Lactate Dehydrogenase Isoenzymes	Chemistry
75CEF	Electrophoretic, Protein Fractionation	Chemistry
75CFG	Emulsion, Oil, (Titrimetric), Lipase	Chemistry
75CET	Emulsion, Olive Oil (Turbidimetric), Lipase	Chemistry
75JLO	Enzymatic (Glutathione Reductase), Glutathione	Chemistry
75JLT	Enzymatic (U.V.), Pyruvic Acid	Chemistry
75CHH	Enzymatic Esterase-Oxidase, Cholesterol	Chemistry
91DMT	Enzymatic Method, Alcohol Dehydrogenase, Ultraviolet	Toxicology
75JIF	Enzymatic Method, Ammonia	Chemistry
75JFM	Enzymatic Method, Bilirubin	Chemistry
75TGO	Enzymatic Method, Blood, Occcult, Fecal	Chemistry
75JIP	Enzymatic Method, Blood, Occult, Urinary	Chemistry
75JFY	Enzymatic Method, Creatinine	Chemistry
75JIA	Enzymatic Method, Galactose	Chemistry
75JIL	Enzymatic Method, Glucose (Urinary, Non-Quantitative)	Chemistry
91LDN	Enzymatic Radiochemical Assay, Amikacin	Toxicology
91KLO	Enzymatic Radiochemical Assay, Gentamicin	Toxicology
91LDO	Enzymatic Radiochemical Assay, Tobramycin	Toxicology
91DKZ	Enzyme Immunoassay, Amphetamine	Toxicology
91DIS	Enzyme Immunoassay, Barbiturate	Toxicology
91JXM	Enzyme Immunoassay, Benzodiazepine	Toxicology
91LDJ	Enzyme Immunoassay, Cannabinoids	Toxicology
91KLT	Enzyme Immunoassay, Carbamazepine	Toxicology
91JXO	Enzyme Immunoassay, Cocaine	Toxicology
91DIO	Enzyme Immunoassay, Cocaine And Cocaine Metabolites	Toxicology
91LFM	Enzyme Immunoassay, Digitoxin	Toxicology

TEST *(cont'd)*

91KXT	Enzyme Immunoassay, Digoxin	Toxicology
91DIP	Enzyme Immunoassay, Diphenylhydantoin	Toxicology
91DLF	Enzyme Immunoassay, Ethosuximide	Toxicology
91LCD	Enzyme Immunoassay, Gentamicin	Toxicology
91KLR	Enzyme Immunoassay, Lidocaine	Toxicology
91DJR	Enzyme Immunoassay, Methadone	Toxicology
91LAO	Enzyme Immunoassay, Methotrexate	Toxicology
91LAN	Enzyme Immunoassay, N-Acetylprocainamide	Toxicology
75KLI	Enzyme Immunoassay, Non-Radiolabeled, Total Thyroxine	Chemistry
91DJG	Enzyme Immunoassay, Opiates	Toxicology
75VKK	Enzyme Immunoassay, Other	Chemistry
91DLZ	Enzyme Immunoassay, Phenobarbital	Toxicology
91DJD	Enzyme Immunoassay, Primidone	Toxicology
91LAR	Enzyme Immunoassay, Procainamide	Toxicology
91JXN	Enzyme Immunoassay, Propoxyphene	Toxicology
91LBZ	Enzyme Immunoassay, Quinidine	Toxicology
91KLS	Enzyme Immunoassay, Theophylline	Toxicology
91LEG	Enzyme Immunoassay, Valproic Acid	Toxicology
83LJC	Enzyme Linked Immunoabsorbent Assay, Chlamydia Group	Microbiology
83LFZ	Enzyme Linked Immunoabsorbent Assay, Cytomegalovirus	Microbiology
83LGC	Enzyme Linked Immunoabsorbent Assay, Herpes Simplex Virus	Microbiology
83LJY	Enzyme Linked Immunoabsorbent Assay, Mumps Virus	Microbiology
83LJZ	Enzyme Linked Immunoabsorbent Assay, Mycoplasma SPP.	Microbiology
83LIR	Enzyme Linked Immunoabsorbent Assay, Neisseria Gonorrhoeae	Microbiology
83LIQ	Enzyme Linked Immunoabsorbent Assay, Rotavirus	Microbiology
83LFX	Enzyme Linked Immunoabsorbent Assay, Rubella	Microbiology
83LJB	Enzyme Linked Immunoabsorbent Assay, Rubeola	Microbiology
83LGD	Enzyme Linked Immunoabsorbent Assay, Toxoplasma Gondii	Microbiology
83LIP	Enzyme Linked Immunoabsorbent Assay, Treponema Pallidum	Microbiology
83LFY	Enzyme Linked Immunoabsorbent Assay, Varicella-Zoster	Microbiology
91LAP	Enzyme Radioassay, Methotrexate	Toxicology
83WKS	Equipment, Test, Western Blot	Microbiology
83GTP	Exoenzyme, Multiple, Streptococcal	Microbiology
82LLL	Extractable Antinuclear Antibody (Rnp/Sm), Antigen/Control	Immunology
75JMN	Extraction/Chromatography, Ninhydrin, Hydroxyproline	Chemistry
82DBN	FC, Antigen, Antiserum, Control	Immunology
82DBK	FC, FITC, Antigen, Antiserum, Control	Immunology
82DBH	FC, Rhodamine, Antigen, Antiserum, Control	Immunology
75JGK	Ferric Chloride, Phenylketones (Urinary, Non-Quantitative)	Chemistry
75CHD	Ferric Ion-Sulfuric Acid, Cholesterol	Chemistry
75CGD	Ferricyanide, Glucose	Chemistry
75JMO	Ferrozine (Colorimetric) Iron Binding Capacity	Chemistry
81JBN	Fibrin Monomer Paracoagulation	Hematology
82DAN	Fibrinopeptide A, Antigen, Antiserum, Control	Immunology
91LGJ	Fluorescence Polarization Immunoassay, Amibacin	Toxicology
91LGI	Fluorescence Polarization Immunoassay, Carbamazepine	Toxicology
91LGR	Fluorescence Polarization Immunoassay, Diphenylhydantoin	Toxicology
91LGQ	Fluorescence Polarization Immunoassay, Phenobarbital	Toxicology
91LGS	Fluorescence Polarization Immunoassay, Theophylline	Toxicology
91LFW	Fluorescence Polarization Immunoassay, Tobramycin	Toxicology
81JMH	Fluorescence, Visual Observation (Qual., U.V.), Gsh	Hematology
91LCQ	Fluorescent Immunoassay Gentamicin	Toxicology
91LES	Fluorescent Immunoassay, Diphenylhydantoin	Toxicology
91LET	Fluorescent Immunoassay, Phenobarbital	Toxicology
91LFT	Fluorescent Immunoassay, Primidone	Toxicology
91LER	Fluorescent Immunoassay, Theophylline	Toxicology
91LCR	Fluorescent Immunoassay, Tobramycin	Toxicology
91DOX	Fluorometer, Lead (Dedicated Instruments)	Toxicology
75JHD	Fluorometric Method, 17-Hydroxycorticosteroids	Chemistry
75JHX	Fluorometric Method, CPK Or Isoenzymes	Chemistry
75CGY	Fluorometric Method, Creatine Phosphokinase	Chemistry
75JGW	Fluorometric Method, Triglycerides	Chemistry
75JFT	Fluorometric, Cortisol	Chemistry
75JNZ	Fluorometric, Uroporphyrin	Chemistry
91DJJ	Fluorometry, Morphine	Toxicology
82DAL	Fraction IV-5, Antigen, Antiserum, Control	Immunology
75JQJ	Fractionation, Protein, Densitometric	Chemistry
91DJL	Free Radical Assay, Amphetamine	Toxicology
91DIR	Free Radical Assay, Cocaine	Toxicology
91DOL	Free Radical Assay, LSD	Toxicology
91DPP	Free Radical Assay, Methadone	Toxicology
91DOK	Free Radical Assay, Morphine	Toxicology
91DKT	Free Radical Assay, Opiates	Toxicology
91DNG	Free Radical, Benzoylecgnonine	Toxicology
75JMZ	Freezing Point, Osmolality	Chemistry
75CJC	Fructose-1, 6-Diphosphate And NADH (U.V.), Aldolase	Chemistry
91DLH	Gas Chromatography, Alcohol	Toxicology
91DOD	Gas Chromatography, Amphetamine	Toxicology

TEST *(cont'd)*

91KZZ Gas Chromatography, Benzodiazepine — Toxicology
91DIN Gas Chromatography, Cocaine — Toxicology
91LAD Gas Chromatography, Codeine — Toxicology
91DKH Gas Chromatography, Diphenylhydantoin — Toxicology
91DIY Gas Chromatography, Ethosuximide — Toxicology
91DMB Gas Chromatography, Methadone — Toxicology
91LAF Gas Chromatography, Methamphetamine — Toxicology
91DMY Gas Chromatography, Morphine — Toxicology
91DJF Gas Chromatography, Opiates — Toxicology
91DJH Gas Chromatography, Phenobarbital — Toxicology
91DMQ Gas Chromatography, Primidone — Toxicology
91LAJ Gas Chromatography, Propoxyphene — Toxicology
91LAL Gas Chromatography, Quinine — Toxicology
91DIM Gas Chromatography, Salicylate — Toxicology
91DMF Gas Liquid Chromatography, Barbiturate — Toxicology
82JZR Gel, Support — Immunology
75JNE Glucose-6-Phosphate (Colorimetric), Phosphohexose Isomerase — Chemistry
75JNY Glyceralde-3-Phosphate, NADH (Enzymatic), Triose Phosphate — Chemistry
75CKH Glycerophosphate, Beta, Phosphatase, Acid — Chemistry
91JKQ Gold Chloride (Colorimetric), Bromide — Toxicology
91DLX Hemagglutination Inhibition, Barbiturate — Toxicology
91DNO Hemagglutination Inhibition, Gentamicin — Toxicology
91DIW Hemagglutination Inhibition, Methadone — Toxicology
91DLR Hemagglutination Inhibition, Morphine — Toxicology
91DKL Hemagglutination, Cocaine — Toxicology
91DLN Hemagglutination, Cocaine Metabolites (Benzoylecgnonine) — Toxicology
91DLT Hemagglutination, Opiates — Toxicology
81JPD Hemoglobin A2 Quantitation — Hematology
82DAM Hemoglobin, Chain Specific, Antigen, Antiserum, Control — Immunology
81JBR Heparin Neutralization Test — Hematology
83LOM Hepatitis B Test (B Core, BE Antigen & Antibody, B Core IGM) — Microbiology
75JOA Hexane Extraction And Trifluoroacetic Acid, Vitamin A — Chemistry
75JOB Hexane Extraction, Fluorescence, Vitamin E — Chemistry
75CFR Hexokinase, Glucose — Chemistry
91KZY High Pressure Liquid Chromatography, Barbiturate — Toxicology
91LAA High Pressure Liquid Chromatography, Benzodiazepine — Toxicology
91LAC High Pressure Liquid Chromatography, Cocaine & Metabolites — Toxicology
91LAE High Pressure Liquid Chromatography, Codeine — Toxicology
91LAG High Pressure Liquid Chromatography, Methamphetamine — Toxicology
91LAH High Pressure Liquid Chromatography, Opiates — Toxicology
91LAK High Pressure Liquid Chromatography, Propoxyphene — Toxicology
91LAM High Pressure Liquid Chromatography, Quinine — Toxicology
91LFI High Pressure Liquid Chromatography, Tricyclic Drug — Toxicology
75CJT Hydrazone Colorimetry, Aldolase — Chemistry
75JKH Hydrazone Derivative Of Alpha-Ketogluterate (Colorimetry) — Chemistry
82DAQ IGG (FD Fragment Specific), Antigen, Antiserum, Control — Immunology
75JMR Immunochemical, Lysozyme (Muramidase) — Chemistry
75CGM Immunodiffusion Method, Immunoglobulins (G, A, M) — Chemistry
75JQK Immunodiffusion, Protein Fractionation — Chemistry
75CFF Immunoelectrophoretic, Immunoglobulins, (G, A, M) — Chemistry
83RBY Incubator, Test Tube, Portable — Microbiology
83RBZ Incubator, Test Tube, Stationary — Microbiology
75JIR Indicator Method, Protein Or Albumin (Urinary, Non-Quant.) — Chemistry
75CEN Indicator, pH, Dye (Urinary, Non-Quantitative) — Chemistry
83GWD Indirect Fluorescent Antibody Test, Entamoeba Histolytica — Microbiology
75CDL Indophenol, Berthelot, Urea Nitrogen — Chemistry
75JNP Infrared Spectroscopy Measurement, Urinary Calculi (Stone) — Chemistry
75CGL Ion Electrode Based Enzymatic, Creatinine — Chemistry
75JIE Ion Exchange Method, Ammonia — Chemistry
75JQE Ion Exchange Resin, Ascorbic Acid, Colorimetry, Iron Bind — Chemistry
75JNF Ion Exchange Resin, Ehrlich's Reagent, Porphobilinogen — Chemistry
75JQD Ion Exchange Resin, Thioglycolic Acid, Colorimetry, Iron — Chemistry
82LTM Islet Cell Antibody (ICA) Test — Immunology
75JQB Kinetic Method, Gamma-Glutamyl Transpeptidase — Chemistry
85TGQ Kit, Breast Cancer Detection — Obstetrics/Gyn
83JST Kit, Fastidious Organism — Microbiology
83SGO Kit, Gonorrhoeae Test (Male Use) — Microbiology
83JSP Kit, Identification, Anaerobic — Microbiology
83JSR Kit, Identification, Dermatophyte — Microbiology
83JSS Kit, Identification, Enterobacteriaceae — Microbiology
83JSW Kit, Identification, Glucose (Non-Ferment) — Microbiology
83JSX Kit, Identification, Neisseria Gonorrhoeae — Microbiology
83JSZ Kit, Identification, Pseudomonas — Microbiology
83JXB Kit, Identification, Yeast — Microbiology
85RJW Kit, Pap Smear — Obstetrics/Gyn
85TFV Kit, Pregnancy Test — Obstetrics/Gyn
75LCX Kit, Pregnancy Test, Over The Counter, HCG — Chemistry
83JWX Kit, Screening, Staphylococcus Aureus — Microbiology
83JXA Kit, Screening, Urine — Microbiology
82LOJ Kit, Test, Alpha-fetoprotein For Testicular Cancer — Immunology

TEST *(cont'd)*

81MHS Kit, Test, Coagglutinin — Hematology
91MVO Kit, Test, Multiple, Drugs Of Abuse, Over The Counter — Toxicology
76MCL Kit, Test, Periodontal, In Vitro — Dental And Oral
81MWB Kit, Test, Saliva, Hiv-1&2 — Hematology
75CGG L-Glutamylnitroanilide/Glycylglycine, Ggtp — Chemistry
75JKG L-Isocitrate And NADP (U.V.), Isocitric Dehydrogenase — Chemistry
75JGG L-Leucine-4-Nitroanilide (Colorimetric), Leucine — Chemistry
75JKI L-Leucyl B-Naphthylamide, Lactic Acid — Chemistry
75CDC L-Leucyl B-Naphthylamide, Leucine Aminopeptidase — Chemistry
82DET Lactic Dehydrogenase, Antigen, Antiserum, Control — Immunology
83GMB Light, Wood's, Fluorescence — Microbiology
75CDT Lipase Hydrolysis/Glycerol Kinase Enzyme, Triglycerides — Chemistry
75CHI Lipase-Esterase, Enzymatic, Photometric, Lipase — Chemistry
82DEL Lipoprotein X, Antigen, Antiserum, Control — Immunology
91DNI Liquid Chromatography, Amphetamine — Toxicology
91DOZ Liquid Chromatography, Diphenylhydantoin — Toxicology
91DNF Liquid Chromatography, Ethosuximide — Toxicology
91DNT Liquid Chromatography, Methadone — Toxicology
91DPK Liquid Chromatography, Morphine — Toxicology
91DOO Liquid Chromatography, Phenobarbital — Toxicology
91DPQ Liquid Chromatography, Primidone — Toxicology
91DMX Liquid Chromatography, Salicylate — Toxicology
75JGP Lowry (Colorimetric), Total Protein — Chemistry
91DMR M-Nitrophenol Solution, Specific Reagent For Cholinesterase — Toxicology
75JMQ M. Lysodeikticus Cells (Spectrophotometric), Lysozyme — Chemistry
74DTG Magnet, Test, Pacemaker — Cardiovascular
75CHK Mercuric Nitrate And Diphenyl Carbazone (Titrimetric) — Chemistry
91DJN Mercury Dithiazone, Colorimetry, Barbiturate — Toxicology
75JIM Metallic Reduction Method, Glucose (Urinary, Non-Quant.) — Chemistry
75CIA Methylthymol Blue, Calcium — Chemistry
75JMJ Microbiological, Histidine — Chemistry
75JHL Microdensitometry Method, Lipoproteins — Chemistry
75CEQ Molybdenum Blue Method, Phospholipids — Chemistry
78TGM Monitor, Blood Glucose (Test) — Gastro/Urology
81MTL Monitor, Test, Hiv-1 — Hematology
75JKW N-Acetyl-L-Tyrosine Ethyl Ester (U.V.), Chymotrypsin — Chemistry
75JNO N-Benzoyl-L-Arginine Ethyl Ester (U.V.), Trypsin — Chemistry
75JKX N-Benzoyl-L-Tyrosine Ethyl Ester (U.V.), Chymotrypsin — Chemistry
75CGS NAD Reduction/NADH Oxidation, CPK Or Isoenzymes — Chemistry
75CFJ NAD Reduction/NADH Oxidation, Lactate Dehydrogenase — Chemistry
75CIT NADH Oxidation/NAD Reduction, AST/SGOT — Chemistry
81JMC NADP Reduction (U.V.), Glucose-6-Phosphate Dehydrogenase — Hematology
75JND NADP Reduction, 6-Phosphogluconate Dehydrogenase — Chemistry
75JLZ Nadh, Phosphoglycerate Mutase, Atp (u.v.) 2, 3-diphosphoglyceric Acid — Chemistry
75CKB Naphthyl Phosphate, Acid Phosphatase — Chemistry
80RIK Needle, Tine Test — General
91LFO Nephelometric Inhibition Immunoassay, Diphenylhydantoin — Toxicology
91LFN Nephelometric Inhibition Immunoassay, Phenobarbital — Toxicology
75JGD Nephelometric Method, Globulin — Chemistry
75CFN Nephelometric Method, Immunoglobulins (G, A, M) — Chemistry
75JHQ Nephelometric Method, Lipoproteins — Chemistry
75JNB Ninhydrin And L-Leucyl-L-Alanine (Fluorimetric) — Chemistry
75JMX Ninhydrin, Nitrogen (Amino-Nitrogen) — Chemistry
75CJN Nitrophenylphosphate, Acid Phosphatase — Chemistry
75CJE Nitrophenylphosphate, Alkaline Phosphatase Or Isoenzymes — Chemistry
75JLC Nitroprusside Reaction (Qualitative, Urine), Cystine — Chemistry
75JIN Nitroprusside, Ketones (Urinary, Non-Quantitative) — Chemistry
75CJD Nitrosalicylate Reduction, Amylase — Chemistry
75CDA Nitrous Acid & Nitrosonaphthol, 5-Hydroxyindole Acetic Acid — Chemistry
75JGZ O-Phthalaldehyde, Urea Nitrogen — Chemistry
75CGE Orthotoluidine, Glucose — Chemistry
75JMS Oxalacetic Acid And NADH Oxidation (U.V.), Maleic DH — Chemistry
75LPW Oxalate Test System — Chemistry
75JKY Oxalydihydrazide (Spectroscopic), Copper — Chemistry
83LGA Oxidase Test Device for Gonorrhea — Micrcbiology
91JKS Oxyhemoglobin/Carboxyhemoglobin Curve, Carbon-Monoxide — Toxicology
75JQM P-Bromoaniline, Xylose — Chemistry
82JFQ P-Phenyl-Enediamine/EDTA (Spectrophotometric), Ceruloplasmi — Immunology
75JNN P-Toluenesulphonyl-L-Arginine Methyl Ester (U.V.), Trypsin — Chemistry
91DNC Paper Strip, Salicylate — Toxicology
76LXX Periodontal Test Kit — Dental And Oral
83GTL Phages, Staphylococcal Typing, All Types — Microbiology
75CJK Phenolphthalein Phosphate, Alkaline Phosphatase — Chemistry
75CKF Phenylphosphate, Alkaline Phosphatase Or Isoenzymes — Chemistry
75JNJ Phosphoenol Pyruvate, ADP, NADH, Pyruvate Kinase — Chemistry
75JLY Phosphoglycerate Mutase (colorimetric), 2, 3-diphosphoglyceric Acid — Chemistry
75CHG Phosphoric-Tungstic Acid (Spectrophotometric), Chloride — Chemistry
75CEO Phosphorus Reagent (Test System) — Chemistry

TEST *(cont'd)*

75CDH	Phosphotungstate Reduction, Uric Acid	Chemistry
75JID	Photometric Method, Ammonia	Chemistry
75JIY	Photometric Method, Iron (Non-Heme)	Chemistry
75JGJ	Photometric Method, Magnesium	Chemistry
82JZP	Plate, Agar, Ouchterlony	Immunology
91DLY	Plate, Alumina, TLC	Toxicology
83WNW	Plate, Culture	Microbiology
91DKS	Plate, Silica Gel, TLC	Toxicology
75CDB	Porter Silber Hydrazone, 17-Hydroxycorticosteroids	Chemistry
91DMI	Potassium Dichromate Specific Reagent For Alcohol	Toxicology
91DOJ	Potassium Dichromate, Alcohol	Toxicology
83MJA	Powders, Antimycobacterial Susceptibility Test	Microbiology
74LXN	Probe, Test, Valve, Heart	Cardiovascular
81JPF	Prothrombin-Proconvertin And Thrombotest	Hematology
91DNX	Protoporphyrin Zinc Method, Fluorometric, Lead	Toxicology
91DMK	Protoporphyrin, Fluorometric, Lead	Toxicology
75JNQ	Qualitative Chemical Reactions, Urinary Calculi (Stone)	Chemistry
81JBQ	Quantitation, Antithrombin III	Hematology
81GKA	Quantitation, Hemoglobin, Abnormal	Hematology
91DPJ	RIA, Amphetamine (125-I), Goat Antibody, Ammonia	Toxicology
91DNA	RIA, Morphine-Barbiturate (125-I), Goat Antibody	Toxicology
75RNT	Rack, Test Tube	Chemistry
75CIK	Radial Diffusion, Amylase	Chemistry
75CJQ	Radial Immunodiffusion, Albumin	Chemistry
75JHP	Radial Immunodiffusion, Lipoproteins	Chemistry
75JJA	Radio-Labeled Iron Method, Iron (Non-Heme)	Chemistry
75JHE	Radioassay, 17-Hydroxycorticosteroids	Chemistry
75KHQ	Radioassay, Triiodothyronine Uptake	Chemistry
75JLX	Radioimmunoassay, 17-Hydroxyprogesterone	Chemistry
75CKG	Radioimmunoassay, ACTH	Chemistry
75CJM	Radioimmunoassay, Aldosterone	Chemistry
91KLQ	Radioimmunoassay, Amikacin	Toxicology
91DJP	Radioimmunoassay, Amphetamine	Toxicology
75CIZ	Radioimmunoassay, Androstenedione	Chemistry
75CIY	Radioimmunoassay, Androsterone	Chemistry
75CIB	Radioimmunoassay, Angiotensin I And Renin	Chemistry
91DKN	Radioimmunoassay, Barbiturate	Toxicology
75JKD	Radioimmunoassay, C Peptides Of Proinsulin	Chemistry
75JKR	Radioimmunoassay, Calcitonin	Chemistry
91LAT	Radioimmunoassay, Cannabinoid (S)	Toxicology
91KLN	Radioimmunoassay, Cocaine Metabolite	Toxicology
75JKB	Radioimmunoassay, Compound S (11-Deoxycortisol)	Chemistry
75CHE	Radioimmunoassay, Corticoids	Chemistry
75CHA	Radioimmunoassay, Corticosterone	Chemistry
75CGR	Radioimmunoassay, Cortisol	Chemistry
75CHO	Radioimmunoassay, Cyclic AMP	Chemistry
75CGT	Radioimmunoassay, Cyclic GMP	Chemistry
75JKC	Radioimmunoassay, Dehydroepiandrosterone (Free And Sulfate)	Chemistry
75JLE	Radioimmunoassay, Desoxycorticosterone	Chemistry
91LCW	Radioimmunoassay, Digitoxin (125-I)	Toxicology
91DPL	Radioimmunoassay, Digitoxin (125-I), Bovine, Charcoal	Toxicology
91DPG	Radioimmunoassay, Digitoxin (125-I), Rabbit, Coated Tube	Toxicology
91DOB	Radioimmunoassay, Digitoxin (3-H)	Toxicology
91DNW	Radioimmunoassay, Digitoxin (3-H), Rabbit Antibody, Char.	Toxicology
91DPI	Radioimmunoassay, Digoxin	Toxicology
91LCS	Radioimmunoassay, Digoxin (125-I)	Toxicology
91DOA	Radioimmunoassay, Digoxin (125-I), Goat Anion Exchange	Toxicology
91DNJ	Radioimmunoassay, Digoxin (125-I), Goat, 2nd Antibody	Toxicology
91DNL	Radioimmunoassay, Digoxin (125-I), Rabbit, 2nd Antibody	Toxicology
91DPB	Radioimmunoassay, Digoxin (125-I), Rabbit, Charcoal	Toxicology
91DPO	Radioimmunoassay, Digoxin (125-I), Rabbit, Coated Tube	Toxicology
91DOG	Radioimmunoassay, Digoxin (125-I), Rabbit, Poly. Glycol	Toxicology
91DON	Radioimmunoassay, Digoxin (125-I), Rabbit, Solid Phase	Toxicology
91LCT	Radioimmunoassay, Digoxin (3-H)	Toxicology
91DOR	Radioimmunoassay, Digoxin (3-H), Bovine, Charcoal	Toxicology
91DPD	Radioimmunoassay, Digoxin (3-H), Rabbit, Charcoal	Toxicology
91DLP	Radioimmunoassay, Diphenylhydantoin	Toxicology
75CHP	Radioimmunoassay, Estradiol	Chemistry
75CGI	Radioimmunoassay, Estriol	Chemistry
75CGF	Radioimmunoassay, Estrone	Chemistry
91DJX	Radioimmunoassay, Ethosuximide	Toxicology
75JLF	Radioimmunoassay, Etiocholanolone	Chemistry
83JMG	Radioimmunoassay, Ferritin	Microbiology
75CGN	Radioimmunoassay, Folic Acid	Chemistry
75CGJ	Radioimmunoassay, Follicle Stimulating Hormone	Chemistry
75CEC	Radioimmunoassay, Free Thyroxine	Chemistry
75CGC	Radioimmunoassay, Gastrin	Chemistry
91DJB	Radioimmunoassay, Gentamicin (125-I), Second Antibody	Toxicology
75JME	Radioimmunoassay, Glucagon	Chemistry
75JHI	Radioimmunoassay, Human Chorionic Gonadotropin	Chemistry
75CFL	Radioimmunoassay, Human Growth Hormone	Chemistry
75JMF	Radioimmunoassay, Human Placental Lactogen	Chemistry
82JHR	Radioimmunoassay, Immunoglobulins (D, E)	Immunology
75CFQ	Radioimmunoassay, Immunoglobulins (G, A, M)	Chemistry

TEST *(cont'd)*

75CFP	Radioimmunoassay, Immunoreactive Insulin	Chemistry
83THL	Radioimmunoassay, Infectious Mononucleosis	Microbiology
91KJI	Radioimmunoassay, Kanamycin	Toxicology
91DLB	Radioimmunoassay, LSD (125-I)	Toxicology
75CEP	Radioimmunoassay, Luteinizing Hormone	Chemistry
91KXS	Radioimmunoassay, Methaqualone	Toxicology
91LAQ	Radioimmunoassay, Methotrexate	Toxicology
91DOE	Radioimmunoassay, Morphine (125-I), Goat Antibody	Toxicology
91DIQ	Radioimmunoassay, Morphine (3-H), Ammonium Sulfate	Toxicology
91LCE	Radioimmunoassay, Netilmicin (125-I)	Toxicology
75VKJ	Radioimmunoassay, Other	Chemistry
75CEW	Radioimmunoassay, Parathyroid Hormone	Chemistry
91LCL	Radioimmunoassay, Phencyclidine	Toxicology
91DKP	Radioimmunoassay, Phenobarbital	Toxicology
75JNG	Radioimmunoassay, Pregnenolone	Chemistry
91DIL	Radioimmunoassay, Primidone	Toxicology
75JLS	Radioimmunoassay, Progesterone	Chemistry
75CFT	Radioimmunoassay, Prolactin (Lactogen)	Chemistry
91LBY	Radioimmunoassay, Sisomicin	Toxicology
75CDY	Radioimmunoassay, T3 Uptake	Chemistry
75UKB	Radioimmunoassay, T4	Chemistry
75CDZ	Radioimmunoassay, Testosterones And Dihydrotestosterone	Chemistry
91LCA	Radioimmunoassay, Theophylline	Toxicology
75JLW	Radioimmunoassay, Thyroid Stimulating Hormone	Chemistry
75CEE	Radioimmunoassay, Thyroxine Binding Globulin	Chemistry
75JMD	Radioimmunoassay, Total Estrogen, Other	Chemistry
75CHM	Radioimmunoassay, Total Estrogens In Pregnancy	Chemistry
75CDX	Radioimmunoassay, Total Thyroxine	Chemistry
75CDP	Radioimmunoassay, Total Triiodothyronine	Chemistry
91LFG	Radioimmunoassay, Tricyclic Antidepressant Drugs	Toxicology
91LEH	Radioimmunoassay, Vancomycin	Toxicology
75CDD	Radioimmunoassay, Vitamin B12	Chemistry
75JQG	Radiometric, Fe59, Iron Binding Capacity	Chemistry
91DLI	Reagent, Acetylcholine Chloride	Toxicology
75CJZ	Reagent, Albumin, Colorimetric	Chemistry
75CJA	Reagent, Amylase, Colorimetric	Chemistry
75CIG	Reagent, Bilirubin (Total Or Direct Test System)	Chemistry
75JFO	Reagent, Calcium (Test System)	Chemistry
75CHJ	Reagent, Chloride (Test System)	Chemistry
75CGO	Reagent, Cholesterol (Total Test System)	Chemistry
75CGX	Reagent, Creatinine (Test System)	Chemistry
75JGE	Reagent, Globulin (Test System)	Chemistry
75CGA	Reagent, Glucose (Test System)	Chemistry
81GGG	Reagent, Guaiac	Hematology
82KTP	Reagent, Immunoassay, Activator, C3, Complement	Immunology
75CFM	Reagent, Iron (Test System)	Chemistry
75JFX	Reagent, Kinase, Phosphate, Creatine	Chemistry
83UML	Reagent, Legionella Detection	Microbiology
91DML	Reagent, NAD-NADH, Alcohol Enzyme Method	Toxicology
81KHE	Reagent, Occult Blood	Hematology
75CEK	Reagent, Protein, Total	Chemistry
91DKM	Reagent, Test, Carbon Monoxide	Toxicology
91DJW	Reagent, Test, Chloral Hydrate	Toxicology
91DMA	Reagent, Test, Fluoride	Toxicology
91DLA	Reagent, Test, Methyl Alcohol	Toxicology
91DKI	Reagent, Test, Ouabain	Toxicology
91DJQ	Reagent, Test, Phenothiazine	Toxicology
91DKW	Reagent, Test, Sulphanimide Derivative	Toxicology
91DLE	Reagents, Test, Bromides	Toxicology
81JWP	Red Cell Survival Test	Hematology
75JGR	Refractometric, Total Protein	Chemistry
83LKT	Respiratory Syncytial Virus, Antigen, Antibody, IFA	Microbiology
81MMG	Response Test, Antithrombin III (ATIII)	Hematology
82CZS	Retinol-Binding Protein, Antigen, Antiserum, Control	Immunology
75CIS	SGOT, Colorimetric	Chemistry
75CIQ	SGOT, Ultraviolet	Chemistry
75CKD	SGPT, Colorimetric	Chemistry
75CKA	SGPT, Ultraviolet	Chemistry
75CIJ	Saccharogenic, Amylase	Chemistry
81JWN	Schilling's Test	Hematology
82DGB	Seminal Fluid, Antigen, Antiserum, Control	Immunology
83JTT	Sensitivity Test Powder, Antimicrobial	Microbiology
83TDG	Separation Media	Microbiology
91DJK	Serum, Control, Digitoxin, RIA	Toxicology
91DMP	Serum, Control, Digoxin, RIA	Toxicology
83GMR	Serum, Reactive And Non-Specific Control, FTA-ABS Test	Microbiology
91DLO	Silica Gel Fluorescent Indicator, TLC	Toxicology
84GWR	Simulator, EEG Test Signal	Cns/Neurology
75JLK	Sodium Hydroxide/Phenol Red (Titrimetric), Gastric Acidity	Chemistry
81KSL	Solution, Copper Sulfate, For Specific Gravity Test	Hematology
78FKH	Solution-Test, Standard-Conductivity, Dialysis	Gastro/Urology
83GMW	Sorbent, FTA-ABS Test	Microbiology
75JLP	Spectrophotometric Method, Pregnanediol	Chemistry
75JLQ	Spectrophotometric Method, Pregnanetriol	Chemistry
75JQL	Spectrophotometric, Uroporphyrin	Chemistry

KEYWORD INDEX

TEST (cont'd)

75CFO	Titrimetric, Magnesium	Chemistry
75CEA	Triglyceride, Separation, Chromatographic, TLC	Chemistry
75JQH	Trinitrobenzene Sulfonate (Spectroscopic), Nitrogen	Chemistry
75JGC	Tryptophan Measurement (Colorimetric), Globulin	Chemistry
75RZV	Tube, Test	Chemistry
75JLL	Tubeless Analysis, Gastric Acidity	Chemistry
82LTR	Tumor-Associated Antigen, Tennagen Test	Immunology
75JHN	Turbidimetric Method, Lipoproteins	Chemistry
75JIQ	Turbidimetric Method, Protein Or Albumin (Urinary)	Chemistry
75JGX	Turbidimetric Method, Triglycerides	Chemistry
75JGQ	Turbidimetric, Total Protein	Chemistry
75JHW	U.V. Method, CPK Isoenzymes	Chemistry
75JIB	U.V. Method, Galactose	Chemistry
91LDB	U.V. Spectrometry, Carbamazepine	Toxicology
91LDC	U.V. Spectrometry, Diphenylhydantoin	Toxicology
91LDA	U.V. Spectrometry, Phenobarbital	Toxicology
91LCZ	U.V. Spectrometry, Primidone	Toxicology
91LCY	U.V. Spectrometry, Theophylline	Toxicology
91LFH	U.V. Spectrometry, Tricyclic Antidepressant Drugs	Toxicology
75JLJ	UDP-Glucose, NAD (U.V.), Gal-I-P Uridyl Transperase	Chemistry
75CEI	Uranyl Acetate/Zinc Acetate, Sodium	Chemistry
75CDQ	Urease And Glutamic Dehydrogenase, Urea Nitrogen	Chemistry
75CDN	Urease, Photometric, Urea Nitrogen	Chemistry
75JHB	Uricase (Coulometric), Uric Acid	Chemistry
75JHA	Uricase (Gasometric), Uric Acid	Chemistry
75JHC	Uricase (Oxygen Rate), Uric Acid	Chemistry
75CDO	Uricase (U.V.), Uric Acid	Chemistry
75LPS	Urinary Homocystine (Non-Quantitative) Test System	Chemistry
75CKC	Vanillin Pyruvate, ALT/SGPT	Chemistry
75CIF	Vanillin Pyruvate, AST/SGOT	Chemistry
75JNA	Vapor Pressure, Osmolality Of Serum & Urine	Chemistry
81JMB	Visual, Semi-Quant. (Colorimetric), Glucose-6-Phosphate	Hematology
75CIE	Volumetric/Manometric, Carbon-Dioxide	Chemistry
75JIJ	Wet Ash Method, Protein Bound Iodine	Chemistry
81KHG	Whole Blood Hemoglobin Determination	Hematology
82DGQ	Whole Human Plasma, Antigen, Antiserum, Control	Immunology
75CCY	Zimmerman (Spectrophotometric), 17-Ketosteroids	Chemistry
75CCZ	Zimmerman/Norymberski, 17-Ketogenic Steroids	Chemistry
91DJM	Zinc, Test Reagents	Toxicology
75JFL	pH Rate Measurement, Carbon-Dioxide	Chemistry

TESTER

80TEU	Analyzer, Doppler Spectrum	General
74LOS	Analyzer, ECG	Cardiovascular
79QTT	Analyzer, Electrosurgical Unit	Surgery
80QUR	Analyzer, Ethylene-Oxide	General
80VLP	Analyzer, Infusion Pump	General
80REO	Analyzer, Lead	General
84GWS	Analyzer, Spectrum, EEG Signal	Cns/Neurology
84RWA	Analyzer, Transcutaneous Nerve Stimulator	Cns/Neurology
80SDZ	Analyzer, Ultrasonic Unit	General
86HLA	Calibrator, Tonometer	Ophthalmology
76EAS	Gel, Electrode, Pulp Tester	Dental And Oral
78QPI	Meter, Dialysate Conductivity	Gastro/Urology
80SDX	Meter, Ultrasonic Power	General
90IYP	Phantom, Anthropomorphic, Nuclear	Radiology
90IXG	Phantom, Anthropomorphic, Radiographic	Radiology
90IYQ	Phantom, Flood Source, Nuclear	Radiology
84GXX	Phantom, Ultrasonic Scanner, Neurology	Cns/Neurology
90RKQ	Phantom, Ultrasound	Radiology
74RTF	Simulator, Arrhythmia	Cardiovascular
74RTG	Simulator, Blood Pressure	Cardiovascular
74RTH	Simulator, ECG	Cardiovascular
84GWR	Simulator, EEG Test Signal	Cns/Neurology
74RTI	Simulator, Heart Sound	Cardiovascular
90RTL	Simulator, Radiotherapy	Radiology
73RTK	Simulator, Respiration	Anesthesiology
77EWM	System, Analysis, Hearing-Aid	Ear/Nose/Throat
90IXF	Test Pattern, Radiographic	Radiology
90JAR	Test Pattern/Phantom, Radionuclide	Radiology
80WZF	Tester, Alignment, Laser Beam	General
77ETY	Tester, Auditory Impedance	Ear/Nose/Throat
86WOO	Tester, Brightness Acuity	Ophthalmology
80QKC	Tester, Circuit Breaker	General
86HIT	Tester, Color Vision	Ophthalmology
80RZW	Tester, Conductivity, Floor And Equipment	General
80RZX	Tester, Conductivity, Shoe And Gown	General
74DRL	Tester, Defibrillator	Cardiovascular
74QSI	Tester, Electrocardiograph Cable	Cardiovascular
80RZY	Tester, Electrode	General
74KRC	Tester, Electrode, Surface, Electrocardiograph	Cardiovascular
84GYA	Tester, Electrode/Lead, Electroencephalograph	Cns/Neurology
80QYV	Tester, Ground Fault Circuit Interrupter	General
80QYX	Tester, Ground Loop Impedance	General
80QYY	Tester, Grounding System	General
80AZZ	Tester, Infusion Pump	General
80SAA	Tester, Isolated Power System	General

TESTER (cont'd)

74DTA	Tester, Pacemaker Electrode Function	Cardiovascular
73RLK	Tester, Pneumatic	Anesthesiology
76EAT	Tester, Pulp	Dental And Oral
90LHO	Tester, Radiology	Radiology
90TDZ	Tester, Radiology Quality Assurance	Radiology
80SAB	Tester, Receptacle, Electrical	General
80SAC	Tester, Receptacle, Mechanical	General
80SAD	Tester, Resistance, Line Cord	General
80SAE	Tester, Surgical Glove	General

TESTICLE

80WXO	Orchidometer	General
78FAF	Prosthesis, Testicle	Gastro/Urology
79FTO	Prosthesis, Testicle, Surgical	Surgery

TESTICULAR

78LOA	Device, Hypothermia, Testicular	Gastro/Urology
82LOJ	Kit, Test, Alpha-fetoprotein For Testicular Cancer	Immunology

TESTING

77EWC	Chamber, Acoustic, Testing	Ear/Nose/Throat
77ETT	Cushion, Earphone (For Audiometric Testing)	Ear/Nose/Throat
77ETS	Generator, Electronic Noise (For Audiometric Testing)	Ear/Nose/Throat
89IKK	Isokinetic Testing And Evaluation System	Physical Med
80QDR	Monitor, Biological (Contamination Testing)	General
90VHB	Phantom, Computed Axial Tomography (CAT, CT)	Radiology
73WTC	Syringe, Calibration Testing, Spirometer	Anesthesiology
77WXX	Unit, Testing, Hearing, Intraoperative	Ear/Nose/Throat

TESTOSTERONES

75CDZ	Radioimmunoassay, Testosterones And Dihydrotestosterone	Chemistry

TETRABROMO

75CJG	Tetrabromo-M-Cresolsulfonphthalein, Albumin	Chemistry

TETRABROMO-M-CRESOLSULFONPHTHALEIN

75CJG	Tetrabromo-M-Cresolsulfonphthalein, Albumin	Chemistry

TETRABROMOPHENOLPHTHALEIN

75CJF	Tetrabromophenolphthalein, Albumin	Chemistry

TETRAHYDROCANNABINOL

91DKE	Test, Tetrahydrocannabinol	Toxicology

TETRAHYDROFOLATE

75JLI	Tetrahydrofolate, Enzymatic (U.V.), Formiminoglutamic Acid	Chemistry

TETRAPHENYL

75CEJ	Tetraphenyl Borate, Colorimetry, Potassium	Chemistry

TETRAZOLIUM

75CFH	Tetrazolium Int Dye-Diaphorase, Lactate Dehydrogenase	Chemistry

TETROXIDE

88KEE	Osmium Tetroxide	Pathology

THALAMIC

84MBX	Stimulator, Thalamic, Epilepsy, Implanted	Cns/Neurology

THEOPHYLLINE

91KLS	Enzyme Immunoassay, Theophylline	Toxicology
91LGS	Fluorescence Polarization Immunoassay, Theophylline	Toxicology
91LER	Fluorescent Immunoassay, Theophylline	Toxicology
91LCA	Radioimmunoassay, Theophylline	Toxicology
91LAW	Theophylline Control Materials	Toxicology
91LEW	Thin Layer Chromatography, Theophylline	Toxicology
91LCY	U.V. Spectrometry, Theophylline	Toxicology

THERAPEUTIC

90IYE	Accelerator, Linear, Medical	Radiology
90WIA	Afterloader, Radiotherapy	Radiology
75ULK	Analyzer, Chemistry, Therapeutic Drug Monitor (TDM)	Chemistry
80MDR	Binder, Medical, Therapeutic	General
90IYL	Collimator, Therapeutic X-Ray, Dermatological	Radiology
90IYK	Collimator, Therapeutic X-Ray, High Voltage	Radiology
90IYJ	Collimator, Therapeutic X-Ray, Low Voltage	Radiology
90IYI	Collimator, Therapeutic X-Ray, Orthovoltage	Radiology
89MOC	Cushion, Flotation, Therapeutic	Physical Med
80QTW	Electrotherapeutic Unit	General
90KPZ	Generator, High Voltage, X-Ray, Therapeutic	Radiology
90IYH	Generator, Therapeutic X-Ray, Dermatological (Grenz Ray)	Radiology
90IYF	Generator, Therapeutic X-Ray, High Voltage	Radiology
90IYD	Generator, Therapeutic X-Ray, Low Voltage	Radiology
90IYC	Generator, Therapeutic X-Ray, Orthovoltage	Radiology
90ITZ	Housing, X-Ray Tube, Therapeutic	Radiology
90REI	Laser, Therapeutic	Radiology
89RFO	Magnetic Unit, Therapeutic	Physical Med
89ISA	Massager, Therapeutic	Physical Med
89LYG	Massager, Therapeutic, Manual	Physical Med
78LKN	Separator, Blood Cell/Plasma, Therapeutic	Gastro/Urology

THERAPEUTIC *(cont'd)*
78MDP Separator, Blood Cell/Plasma, Therapeutic, Membrane, Auto. — Gastro/Urology
73BWF Spirometer, Therapeutic (Incentive) — Anesthesiology
84MHZ Stimulator, Vestibular Acceleration, Therapeutic — Cns/Neurology
80FQJ Support, Scrotal, Therapeutic — General
86MLZ Therapeutic Deep Heat Vitrectomy — Ophthalmology
84MWT Therapeutic Neurology Device, Magnet — Cns/Neurology
90JAD Therapeutic X-Ray System — Radiology
84LIH Unit, Therapy, Current, Interferential — Cns/Neurology
89IRO Vibrator, Therapeutic — Physical Med

THERAPIES
84MFS Device, Energy, Multiple Therapies, Non-Specific — Cns/Neurology

THERAPY
90WJW Accessories, Radiotherapy — Radiology
80TDH Attachment, Oxygen Canister/IV Pole, Wheelchair — General
89RJY Bars, Parallel, Walking — Physical Med
80UDH Bed, Flotation Therapy, Neonatal — General
89IOQ Bed, Flotation Therapy, Powered — Physical Med
90WKV Block, Therapy, Radiation — Radiology
73QFQ Calibrator, Respiratory Therapy Unit — Anesthesiology
80QJI Chair, Flotation Therapy — General
75QMB Computer, Clinical Laboratory — Chemistry
90JAI Couch, Radiation Therapy, Powered — Radiology
89IMI Diathermy, Ultrasonic (Physical Therapy) — Physical Med
84GXC Electroconvulsive Therapy Unit (Electroshock) — Cns/Neurology
80QTW Electrotherapeutic Unit — General
89WOK Equipment, Cryotherapy — Physical Med
73WLD Equipment, Therapy, Apnea — Anesthesiology
89WPB Equipment, Therapy, Handicapped/Physical — Physical Med
89LBG Fluidized Therapy, Unit, Dry Heat — Physical Med
90RAY Hyperthermia Unit, Microwave — Radiology
90WUB Immobilizer, Therapy, Radiation — Radiology
84LLP Laser, Therapy, Pain — Cns/Neurology
80MIO Light, Therapy, Seasonal Affective Disorder (SAD) — General
89RFO Magnetic Unit, Therapeutic — Physical Med
89IKY Mattress, Non-Powered Flotation Therapy — Physical Med
89RHK Moist Therapy Pack — Physical Med
89RHJ Moist Therapy Pack Conditioner — Physical Med
80WKH Monitor, Medication — General
73WVK Oxygen — Anesthesiology
80WOL Patch, Transdermal — General
84WJF Phantom, Therapy, Electroconvulsive — Cns/Neurology
90ROG Radiotherapy Treatment Planning Unit — Radiology
79RTQ Sleeve, Topical Oxygen Therapy — Surgery
77RUT Speech Therapy Unit (Trainer) — Ear/Nose/Throat
77LEZ Speech Training Aid, AC-Powered — Ear/Nose/Throat
77LFA Speech Training Aid, Battery-Powered — Ear/Nose/Throat
79MVF System, Laser, Photodynamic Therapy — Surgery
79MYH System, Non-coherent Light, Photodynamic Therapy — Surgery
90MUJ System, Planning, Radiation Therapy Treatment — Radiology
89JFB Table, Physical Therapy — Physical Med
90JAD Therapeutic X-Ray System — Radiology
80QDG Unit, Therapy, Behavior — General
84LIH Unit, Therapy, Current, Interferential — Cns/Neurology
77SAT Unit, Therapy, Tinnitus — Ear/Nose/Throat
83WKT Water, Therapy, Respiratory — Microbiology

THERMAL
74QGL Cardiac Output Unit, Indicator Dilution (Thermal) — Cardiovascular
74QIN Catheter, Thermal Dilution — Cardiovascular
86HQO Cautery, Thermal, AC-Powered — Ophthalmology
86HQP Cautery, Thermal, Battery-Powered — Ophthalmology
85MNB Device, Ablation, Thermal, Endometrial — Obstetrics/Gyn
78MIK Device, Ablation, Thermal, Ultrasonic — Gastro/Urology
78LJR Device, Thermal, Hemorrhoids — Gastro/Urology
78LKX Device, Thermal, Hemorrhoids — Gastro/Urology
79QSK Electrocautery Unit, Battery-Powered — Surgery
85HIM Electrocautery Unit, Endoscopic — Obstetrics/Gyn
85HGI Electrocautery Unit, Gynecologic — Obstetrics/Gyn
79QSL Electrocautery Unit, Line-Powered — Surgery
74RCE Injector, Thermal Dilution — Cardiovascular
79KFN Monitor, Cardiac Output, Thermal (Balloon Type Catheter) — Surgery
84LME Monitor, Cerebral Blood Flow, Thermal Diffusion — Cns/Neurology
74DWJ Regulator, Thermal, Cardiopulmonary Bypass — Cardiovascular
86HRD Sterilizer, Soft Lens, Thermal, AC-Powered — Ophthalmology
86HRC Sterilizer, Soft Lens, Thermal, Battery-Powered — Ophthalmology
78MII System, Gallbladder, Thermal Ablation — Gastro/Urology
90WTF Unit, Imaging, Thermal — Radiology
80LGZ Warmer, Infusion Fluid, Thermal — General

THERMISTOR
80SAF Thermistor — General
80SAK Thermometer, Electronic — General
80FLL Thermometer, Electronic, Continuous — General

THERMODILUTION
74QHP Catheter, Cardiac Thermodilution — Cardiovascular
74KRB Probe, Thermodilution — Cardiovascular

THERMOFORMING
80VAO Contract Packaging — General
80WNC Molding, Custom — General
80WYJ Molding, Injection — General
80WYK Thermoforming, Extrusion, Custom — General

THERMOGRAPHIC
90IZH Radiographic Unit, Diagnostic, Mammographic — Radiology
85MGK Scanner, Breast, Thermographic, Ultrasonic, Computer-Asstd. — Obstetrics/Gyn
85WSC Spectroscope, Tumor Analysis, Mammary — Obstetrics/Gyn
85LHM System, Thermographic, Liquid Crystal — Obstetrics/Gyn
85SAG Thermographic Device, Infrared — Obstetrics/Gyn
90KXZ Thermographic Device, Liquid Crystal, Adjunctive — Radiology
90KYA Thermographic Device, Liquid Crystal, Non-Powered — Radiology
90LHR Thermographic Device, Liquid Crystal, Screen — Radiology

THERMOGRAVIMETRIC
75UIS Thermogravimetric Analysis Equipment — Chemistry

THERMOMETER
80QND Cover, Thermometer — General
80SAI Holder, Thermometer — General
73BWX Monitor, Temperature (With Probe) — Anesthesiology
79FZA Monitor, Temperature, Surgery — Surgery
80RNQ Pyrometer — General
80KPD Temperature Strip, Forehead, Liquid Crystal — General
80SAF Thermistor — General
80FQZ Thermometer, Chemical Color Change — General
80SAK Thermometer, Electronic — General
80FLL Thermometer, Electronic, Continuous — General
80WTE Thermometer, Fiberoptic — General
79FWS Thermometer, Fluid Column — Surgery
80SAL Thermometer, Infrared — General
75UIT Thermometer, Laboratory — Chemistry
80VLX Thermometer, Laboratory, Recording — General
79FWR Thermometer, Liquid Crystals — Surgery
80FLK Thermometer, Mercury — General
77WXS Thermometer, Tympanic — Ear/Nose/Throat

THERMOPLASTIC
80WTJ Polymer, Synthetic, Other — General

THERMOPLASTIC ELASTOMER
80WWD Elastomer, Other — General

THERMOPLASTIC VULCANIZATE
80WWD Elastomer, Other — General

THERMOREGULATOR
80RBA Hypo/Hyperthermia Unit, Central — General
80RBB Hypo/Hyperthermia Unit, Mobile — General

THERMOSTATED
75JRI Cuvette, Thermostated — Chemistry

THICKNESS
79QQR Gauge, Thickness, Tissue — Surgery
86WQL Pachometer — Ophthalmology

THIGH
89KFX Assembly, Thigh/Knee/Shank/Ankle/Foot, External — Physical Med
89ISS Prosthesis, Thigh Socket, External Component — Physical Med
89RXL Support, Thigh — Physical Med

THIN
75JQR Accessories, Chromatography (Gas, Gel, Liquid, Thin Layer) — Chemistry
91DKX Chromatographic Barbiturate Identification (Thin Layer) — Toxicology
91KZS Chromatography (Thin Layer), Clinical Use — Toxicology
91DPA Chromatography Equipment, Thin Layer — Toxicology
91MLK Chromatography, Thin Layer, Tricyclic Antidepressant Drugs — Toxicology
75UIU Electrophoresis Equipment, Thin-Layer — Chemistry
75UIV Fluorescence, Thin-Layer — Chemistry
75UIF Sprayer, Thin Layer Chromatography — Chemistry
91DIT Thin Layer Chromatography, Amphetamine — Toxicology
91LAB Thin Layer Chromatography, Benzodiazepine — Toxicology
91DOM Thin Layer Chromatography, Benzoylecgnonine — Toxicology
91DMN Thin Layer Chromatography, Cocaine — Toxicology
91DLD Thin Layer Chromatography, Codeine — Toxicology
91DPE Thin Layer Chromatography, Diphenylhydantoin — Toxicology
91JXP Thin Layer Chromatography, Drugs of Abuse (Dedicated Instr.) — Toxicology
91DNP Thin Layer Chromatography, Ethosuximide — Toxicology
91DJC Thin Layer Chromatography, Metamphetamine — Toxicology
91DKR Thin Layer Chromatography, Methadone — Toxicology
91DNK Thin Layer Chromatography, Morphine — Toxicology

THIN *(cont'd)*

91LAI	Thin Layer Chromatography, Opiates	Toxicology
91LCK	Thin Layer Chromatography, Phencyclidine	Toxicology
91DIX	Thin Layer Chromatography, Phenobarbital	Toxicology
91DOS	Thin Layer Chromatography, Primidone	Toxicology
91DPN	Thin Layer Chromatography, Propoxyphene	Toxicology
91DIK	Thin Layer Chromatography, Quinine	Toxicology
91DJE	Thin Layer Chromatography, Salicylate	Toxicology
91LEW	Thin Layer Chromatography, Theophylline	Toxicology

THIN-LAYER

75UIU	Electrophoresis Equipment, Thin-Layer	Chemistry
75UIV	Fluorescence, Thin-Layer	Chemistry

THIOCYANATE

88KKM	Stain, Methylene Blue Thiocyanate	Pathology

THIOGLYCOLIC

75JQD	Ion Exchange Resin, Thioglycolic Acid, Colorimetry, Iron	Chemistry

THIONIN

88KKL	Thionin	Pathology

THORACENTESIS

80QJS	Kit, Chest Drainage (Thoracentesis Tray)	General

THORACIC

74QBV	Aspirator, Thoracic (Suction Unit)	Cardiovascular
73QQO	Drain, Thoracic (Chest)	Anesthesiology
73CCS	Drain, Thoracic, Water Seal	Anesthesiology
89IQF	Orthosis, Cervical-Thoracic, Rigid	Physical Med
89IPT	Orthosis, Thoracic	Physical Med
73ROZ	Regulator, Suction, Thoracic	Anesthesiology
77KAL	Retractor, ENT (Thoracic)	Ear/Nose/Throat
74RQU	Scanner, Long-Term, ECG, Recording	Cardiovascular
74RRP	Scissors, Thoracic	Cardiovascular
74SCG	Trocar, Thoracic	Cardiovascular
78FFA	Tube, Drainage	Gastro/Urology

THORACOSCOPE

74SAM	Thoracoscope	Cardiovascular

THORASCOPIC

74SIZ	Dispenser, Thorascopic	Cardiovascular

THORPE

73CAX	Flowmeter, Back-Pressure Compensated, Thorpe Tube	Anesthesiology
73BYM	Tube, Thorpe, Uncompensated	Anesthesiology

THREAD

79SID	Thread, Stability, Trocar	Surgery

THREADED

87JDW	Pin, Fixation, Threaded	Orthopedics

THRESHOLD

84LLN	Vibration Threshold Measurement Device	Cns/Neurology

THROAT

90VGQ	Shield, X-Ray, Throat	Radiology

THROMBECTOMY

74QIO	Catheter, Thrombectomy	Cardiovascular

THROMBIN

81GJA	Test, Thrombin Time	Hematology
81GJB	Thrombin	Hematology
82DEE	Thrombin, Antigen, Antiserum, Control	Immunology

THROMBOKINETOGRAM

81GKW	Aggregometer, Platelet, Thrombokinetogram	Hematology

THROMBOLYTIC

74WYC	System, Infusion, Enzyme, Thrombolytic	Cardiovascular

THROMBOMETER

81TFE	Thrombometer	Hematology

THROMBOPLASTIN

81GGW	Partial Thromboplastin Time	Hematology
81GIT	Partial Thromboplastin Time, Reagent, Control	Hematology
81GGO	Reagent, Thromboplastin, With Control	Hematology
81GKQ	Test, Thromboplastin Generation	Hematology
81GFO	Thromboplastin, Activated Partial	Hematology

THROMBOSIS

74QOM	Detector, Deep Vein Thrombosis	Cardiovascular
80FQL	Stocking, Elastic	General
89ILG	Stocking, Elastic, Physical Medicine	Physical Med
80DWL	Stocking, Support (Anti-Embolic)	General
74WYC	System, Infusion, Enzyme, Thrombolytic	Cardiovascular

THROMBOTEST

81JPF	Prothrombin-Proconvertin And Thrombotest	Hematology

THYMOL

75CJR	Thymol Blue Monophosphate, Acid Phosphatase	Chemistry
75CJH	Thymol Blue Monophosphate, Alkaline Phosphatase/Isoenzymes	Chemistry

THYMOLPHTHALEIN

75CKE	Thymolphthalein Monophosphate, Acid Phosphatase	Chemistry
75CIO	Thymolphthalein Monophosphate, Alkaline Phosphatase	Chemistry

THYROGLOBULIN

82JNL	Immunochemical, Thyroglobulin Autoantibody	Immunology
82MSW	System, Test, Thyroglobulin	Immunology
82DDC	Thyroglobulin, Antigen, Antiserum, Control	Immunology
82DDJ	Thyroglobulin, FITC, Antigen, Antiserum, Control	Immunology
82DDL	Thyroglobulin, Rhodamine, Antigen, Antiserum, Control	Immunology

THYROID

82WQF	Antibody, Anti-Thyroid, Indirect Immunofluorescent	Immunology
75JMP	Radioimmunoassay, Long-Acting Thyroid Stimulator	Chemistry
75JLW	Radioimmunoassay, Thyroid Stimulating Hormone	Chemistry
78RZP	Tenaculum, Thyroid	Gastro/Urology
82JZO	Test, Thyroid Autoantibody	Immunology
75SAO	Thyroid Function Unit	Chemistry
90VGR	Thyroid Uptake System	Radiology

THYROTROPIN

75JLW	Radioimmunoassay, Thyroid Stimulating Hormone	Chemistry

THYROXINE

75KLI	Enzyme Immunoassay, Non-Radiolabeled, Total Thyroxine	Chemistry
75CEC	Radioimmunoassay, Free Thyroxine	Chemistry
75UKB	Radioimmunoassay, T4	Chemistry
75CEE	Radioimmunoassay, Thyroxine Binding Globulin	Chemistry
75CDX	Radioimmunoassay, Total Thyroxine	Chemistry

TIBIAL

87UBL	Prosthesis, Ankle, Tibial Component	Orthopedics
87KRS	Prosthesis, Knee, Hemi-, Tibial Resurfacing	Orthopedics
87HSH	Prosthesis, Knee, Hemi-, Tibial Resurfacing, Uncemented	Orthopedics
87RNA	Prosthesis, Tibial	Orthopedics

TICK

82WVP	Test, Disease, Lyme	Immunology

TIE

78FKF	Tie Gun, Dialysis	Gastro/Urology
78FKE	Tie, Dialysis	Gastro/Urology

TIED

79SGX	Suture, Laparoscopy	Surgery
79SGW	Suture, Laparoscopy, Loose	Surgery
79SGY	Suture, Laparoscopy, Pre-Tied	Surgery

TIEMAN

78GBM	Catheter, Urethral	Gastro/Urology

TILT

89JFB	Table, Physical Therapy	Physical Med

TILTING

90IZZ	Table, Radiographic, Non-Tilting, Powered	Radiology
90IXR	Table, Radiographic, Tilting	Radiology

TIME

81JBP	Activated Whole Blood Clotting Time	Hematology
81JCA	Bleeding Time Device	Hematology
80QLL	Clock, Elapsed Time	General
74UMH	Monitor, Blood Gas, Real-Time	Cardiovascular
74TGX	Monitor, ECG, Ambulatory, Real-Time	Cardiovascular
80WTG	Monitor, Utilization, Equipment	General
81GGW	Partial Thromboplastin Time	Hematology
81GIT	Partial Thromboplastin Time, Reagent, Control	Hematology
81GJS	Prothrombin Time	Hematology
81JPE	Test, Antithrombin III, Two Stage Clotting Time	Hematology
81KFF	Test, Heparin (Clotting Time)	Hematology
81GJA	Test, Thrombin Time	Hematology
73SEV	Ventilator, Time Cycled (Iron Lung)	Anesthesiology

TIMECLOCK

80VBA	Timeclock	General

TIMED

75JNW	Timed Flow in Capillary, Plasma Viscometry	Chemistry

TIMER

81GKP	Analyzer, Coagulation	Hematology
81QLM	Analyzer, Coagulation, Automated	Hematology
81QLN	Analyzer, Coagulation, Manual	Hematology
81JPA	Analyzer, Coagulation, Multipurpose	Hematology
81KQG	Analyzer, Coagulation, Semi-Automated	Hematology
74DQF	Controller, Injector, Angiographic	Cardiovascular
80LHB	Timer, Apgar	General
81GKN	Timer, Clot, Automated	Hematology

KEYWORD INDEX

TOBACCO *(cont'd)*

73KHC	Filter, Tobacco Smoke (Unattached)	Anesthesiology

TOBRAMYCIN

91KZX	Disc, Diffusion, Gel, Agar, Serum Level, Tobramycin	Toxicology
91LDO	Enzymatic Radiochemical Assay, Tobramycin	Toxicology
91LFW	Fluorescence Polarization Immunoassay, Tobramycin	Toxicology
91LCR	Fluorescent Immunoassay, Tobramycin	Toxicology
91KLB	Radioimmunoassay, Tobramycin	Toxicology
91DID	Test, Bacillus Subtilis Microbiology, Tobramycin	Toxicology

TOE

87KQY	Prosthesis, Finger and Toe, Hemi-Arthroplasty	Orthopedics
87UCM	Prosthesis, Toe	Orthopedics
87LZJ	Prosthesis, Toe (Metaphal.), Joint, Met./Poly., Semi-Const.	Orthopedics
87KWH	Prosthesis, Toe, Constrained, Polymer	Orthopedics
87KWD	Prosthesis, Toe, Hemi-, Phalangeal	Orthopedics
87RSE	Separator, Toe	Orthopedics
87RUA	Sock, Cast Toe	Orthopedics

TOFTNESS

84LEO	Detector, Radiation, Toftness	Cns/Neurology

TOILET

80QLV	Commode (Toilet)	General
80WHM	Cover, Seat, Toilet, Sanitary	General
80WIW	Dispenser, Tissue, Toilet	General
80WIX	Dispenser, Towel	General
80VBE	Tissue, Toilet	General

TOKODYNAMOMETER

85LQK	Tokodynamometer	Obstetrics/Gyn

TOLERANCE

75MRV	Drink, Glucose Tolerance	Chemistry

TOLUENESULPHONYL

75JNN	P-Toluenesulphonyl-L-Arginine Methyl Ester (U.V.), Trypsin	Chemistry

TOLUIDINE

88IAB	Stain, Toluidine Blue	Pathology
81GIX	Stain, Toluidine Blue, Hematology	Hematology

TOMOGRAPHIC

90IZF	Radiographic Unit, Diagnostic, Tomographic	Radiology
90JAM	Scanner, Magnetic Resonance (NMR/MRI)	Radiology
90JWM	Scanner, Nuclear, Tomographic	Radiology

TOMOGRAPHY

90QMD	Computer, Nuclear Medicine	Radiology
90VHB	Phantom, Computed Axial Tomography (CAT, CT)	Radiology
90WMF	Scanner, Computed Tomography, Cine	Radiology
84JXD	Scanner, Computed Tomography, X-Ray (CAT, CT)	Cns/Neurology
90THS	Scanner, Computed Tomography, X-Ray, Full Body	Radiology
90TEI	Scanner, Computed Tomography, X-Ray, Head	Radiology
90JAK	Scanner, Computed Tomography, X-Ray, Special Procedure	Radiology
90KPS	Scanner, Emission Computed Tomography	Radiology
90THG	Scanner, Nuclear Emission Computed Tomography (ECT)	Radiology
90ULI	Scanner, Positron Emission Tomography (PET)	Radiology
90RYK	Synchronizer, Radiographic Unit	Radiology

TONGS

77EWW	Anti-Choke Device, Tongs	Ear/Nose/Throat
87SBA	Tongs, Bone	Orthopedics
84SBB	Tongs, Skull	Cns/Neurology
84HAX	Tongs, Skull, Traction	Cns/Neurology

TONGUE

79FWQ	Blade, Tongue	Surgery
80FMA	Depressor, Tongue	General
76EJC	Depressor, Tongue, Dental	Dental And Oral
77KBL	Depressor, Tongue, ENT, Metal	Ear/Nose/Throat
77EWF	Depressor, Tongue, ENT, Wood	Ear/Nose/Throat
76LCN	Scraper, Tongue	Dental And Oral

TONOGRAPH

86HPK	Tonograph	Ophthalmology

TONOMETER

86HLA	Calibrator, Tonometer	Ophthalmology
86HKZ	Sterilizer, Tonometer	Ophthalmology
86HPK	Tonograph	Ophthalmology
75LCH	Tonometer (Calibration And Q.C. Of Blood Gas Instruments)	Chemistry
86HKX	Tonometer, AC-Powered	Ophthalmology
75KMX	Tonometer, Gas-Liquid Equilibration	Chemistry
86HKY	Tonometer, Manual	Ophthalmology

TONSIL

77KBM	Dissector, Tonsil	Ear/Nose/Throat
77QXM	Forceps, Tonsil	Ear/Nose/Throat
77KBO	Guillotine, Tonsil	Ear/Nose/Throat

TONSIL *(cont'd)*

77KBP	Hook, Tonsil Suturing	Ear/Nose/Throat
77KBQ	Knife, Tonsil	Ear/Nose/Throat
77KBR	Needle, Tonsil Suture	Ear/Nose/Throat
77KBT	Punch, Tonsil	Ear/Nose/Throat
80RRI	Scissors, General Dissecting	General
77KBX	Screw, Tonsil	Ear/Nose/Throat
77KBZ	Snare, Tonsil	Ear/Nose/Throat
77KCB	Tube, Tonsil Suction	Ear/Nose/Throat

TONSILLECTOME

77KCA	Tonsillectome	Ear/Nose/Throat

TOOLS

74DTF	Tools, Pacemaker Service	Cardiovascular

TOOTH

76DYH	Adhesive, Bracket And Conditioner, Resin	Dental And Oral
76EMG	Forceps, Tooth Extractor, Surgical	Dental And Oral
76EBF	Material, Tooth Shade, Resin	Dental And Oral
76KMY	Positioner, Tooth, Preformed	Dental And Oral
76LTE	System, Implant, Tooth	Dental And Oral
76KLE	Tooth Bonding Agent, Resin Restoration	Dental And Oral

TOOTHBRUSH

76MMD	Toothbrush, Ionic, Battery-Powered	Dental And Oral
76EFW	Toothbrush, Manual	Dental And Oral
76JEQ	Toothbrush, Powered	Dental And Oral
76MCF	Unit, Sanitation/Sterilization, Toothbrush, Ultraviolet	Dental And Oral

TOOTHPASTE

76QPA	Dentifrice	Dental And Oral

TOP

75VIR	Analyzer, Chemistry, Desk-Top	Chemistry
80QNI	Cover, Crib Top (Bubble)	General
80UDK	Sterilizer, Ethylene-Oxide, Table Top	General
80UCT	Sterilizer, Steam, Table Top	General
90IXQ	Table, Radiographic, Stationary Top	Radiology

TOPICAL

73CCT	Applicator (Laryngo-Tracheal), Topical Anesthesia	Anesthesiology
79KPJ	Chamber, Oxygen, Topical, Extremity	Surgery
83MKR	Device, Susceptibility, Topical Antimicrobial	Microbiology
89MLY	Refrigerant, Topical (Vapocoolant)	Physical Med
79RTQ	Sleeve, Topical Oxygen Therapy	Surgery

TOPIRAMATEE

91MSL	System, Test, Topiramatee	Toxicology

TOPOGRAPHER

86MMQ	Topographer, Corneal	Ophthalmology

TORIC

86MJP	Lens, Intraocular, Toric	Ophthalmology

TOTAL

82DFI	Antigen, Antiserum, Control, Spinal Fluid, Total	Immunology
75MQM	Bilirubin (Total and Unbound) Neonate Test System	Chemistry
75CFB	Chromatographic Derivative, Total Lipids	Chemistry
75KLI	Enzyme Immunoassay, Non-Radiolabeled, Total Thyroxine	Chemistry
75JGP	Lowry (Colorimetric), Total Protein	Chemistry
87UBM	Prosthesis, Elbow, Total	Orthopedics
87UBQ	Prosthesis, Finger, Total	Orthopedics
87UBR	Prosthesis, Knee, Total	Orthopedics
77LBO	Prosthesis, Ossicular (Total), Absorbable Gelatin Material	Ear/Nose/Throat
77ETA	Prosthesis, Ossicular, Total	Ear/Nose/Throat
77LBN	Prosthesis, Ossicular, Total, Porous Polyethylene	Ear/Nose/Throat
77UBV	Prosthesis, Ossicular, Total, Silicone	Ear/Nose/Throat
75JMD	Radioimmunoassay, Total Estrogen, Other	Chemistry
75CHM	Radioimmunoassay, Total Estrogens In Pregnancy	Chemistry
75CDX	Radioimmunoassay, Total Thyroxine	Chemistry
75CDP	Radioimmunoassay, Total Triiodothyronine	Chemistry
75CIG	Reagent, Bilirubin (Total Or Direct Test System)	Chemistry
75CGO	Reagent, Cholesterol (Total Test System)	Chemistry
75CEK	Reagent, Protein, Total	Chemistry
75JRE	Refractometer	Chemistry
75JGR	Refractometric, Total Protein	Chemistry
75CFD	Sulfophosphovanillin, Colorimetry, Total Lipids	Chemistry
75JGQ	Turbidimetric, Total Protein	Chemistry

TOUCH

84IKL	Esthesiometer, Touch Discriminator	Cns/Neurology
80WTK	Support, Cover, Bed	General

TOURNIQUET

74JOW	Sleeve, Compressible Limb	Cardiovascular
80SBD	Tourniquet	General
87HTA	Tourniquet, Air Pressure	Orthopedics
74DRP	Tourniquet, Automatic Rotating	Cardiovascular
79EYR	Tourniquet, Gastro-Urology	Surgery
79GAX	Tourniquet, Non-Pneumatic, Surgical	Surgery

TOURNIQUET *(cont'd)*

79KCY Tourniquet, Pneumatic — Surgery

TOWEL

79QLI Clip, Towel — Surgery
80WIX Dispenser, Towel — General
80VBF Linen — General
79SBE Towel, Surgical — Surgery
80WNF Towel/Towelette, Paper — General

TOWELETTE

80WNF Towel/Towelette, Paper — General

TOXIC

80FRF Equipment, Cleaning, Air — General

TOXICOLOGY

91DNY Counter, Scintillation, Liquid, Toxicology — Toxicology
91DPR Fluorometer, Toxicology — Toxicology
91DOQ Photometer, Flame, Lithium, Toxicology — Toxicology

TOXIN

83LLH Reagent, Clostridium Difficile Toxin — Microbiology

TOXOPLASMA

83WJR Antibody, Toxoplasma Gondii — Microbiology
83GMN Antigen, CF, Toxoplasma Gondii — Microbiology
83GLZ Antigen, IF, Toxoplasma Gondii — Microbiology
83GMM Antigen, IHA, Toxoplasma Gondii — Microbiology
83LJK Antisera, IF, Toxoplasma Gondii — Microbiology
83LGD Enzyme Linked Immunoabsorbent Assay, Toxoplasma Gondii — Microbiology
83LLA Test, Direct Agglutination, Toxoplasma Gondii — Microbiology

TOYNBEE

77ETK Tube, Toynbee Diagnostic — Ear/Nose/Throat

TPA

82LTP Test, Tissue Polypeptide Antigen (TPA) — Immunology

TPE

80WWD Elastomer, Other — General

TPV

80WWD Elastomer, Other — General

TRABECULOTOME

86HMZ Trabeculotome — Ophthalmology

TRABECULOTOMY

86HNK Probe, Trabeculotomy — Ophthalmology

TRACE

73WSV Analyzer, Trace Gas, Breath — Anesthesiology
74DQG Microsphere, Trace — Cardiovascular

TRACHEA

79JCT Prosthesis, Trachea — Surgery

TRACHEAL

73SBF Adapter, Tube, Tracheal — Anesthesiology
73CCT Applicator (Laryngo-Tracheal), Topical Anesthesia — Anesthesiology
77QBW Aspirator, Tracheal — Ear/Nose/Throat
77KCC Bistoury, Tracheal — Ear/Nose/Throat
77EPE Brush, Cleaning, Tracheal Tube — Ear/Nose/Throat
73SBI Button, Tracheostomy Tube — Anesthesiology
73WLJ Catheter, Oxygen, Tracheal — Anesthesiology
73BSY Catheter, Suction (Tracheal Aspirating Tube) — Anesthesiology
73BSK Cuff, Tracheal Tube, Inflatable — Anesthesiology
77KCG Dilator, Tracheal — Ear/Nose/Throat
73CBH Fixation Device, Tracheal Tube — Anesthesiology
77RAS Hook, Tracheal — Ear/Nose/Throat
77KCH Hook, Tracheal, ENT — Ear/Nose/Throat
73CBE Kit, Suction, Airway (Tracheal) — Anesthesiology
77RFJ Loop, Tracheal — Ear/Nose/Throat
77RPA Regulator, Suction, Tracheal (Nasal, Oral) — Ear/Nose/Throat
73WLI Stent, Tracheal — Anesthesiology
73BSR Stylet, Tracheal Tube — Anesthesiology
77KCI Trocar, Tracheal — Ear/Nose/Throat
73BTR Tube, Tracheal (Endotracheal) — Anesthesiology
73CBI Tube, Tracheal/Bronchial, Differential Ventilation — Anesthesiology
77WRO Valve, Speaking, Tracheal — Ear/Nose/Throat

TRACHEOSTOMY

73SBI Button, Tracheostomy Tube — Anesthesiology
77QGF Cannula, Tracheostomy — Ear/Nose/Throat
77JOH Cuff, Tracheostomy Tube — Ear/Nose/Throat
77QRB Dressing, Tracheostomy Tube — Ear/Nose/Throat
73SBH Holder, Tracheostomy Tube — Anesthesiology
79LRQ Kit, Suctioning, Tracheostomy and Nasal — Surgery
73SBG Kit, Tracheostomy Care — Anesthesiology
73SBJ Kit, Tracheotomy — Anesthesiology
77RGB Mask, Tracheostomy — Ear/Nose/Throat

TRACHEOSTOMY *(cont'd)*

73RGC Mask, Tracheostomy, Aerosol Administration — Anesthesiology
73VDM Strap, Tracheostomy Tube — Anesthesiology
77EQK Tube, Tracheostomy (Breathing Tube), ENT — Ear/Nose/Throat
73BTO Tube, Tracheostomy (W/Wo Connector) — Anesthesiology
77WRO Valve, Speaking, Tracheal — Ear/Nose/Throat

TRACHEOTOME

73LJW Tracheotome — Anesthesiology

TRACHEOTOMY

73SBJ Kit, Tracheotomy — Anesthesiology

TRACHOMATIS

83LJP Antiserum, Fluorescent, Chlamydia Trachomatis — Microbiology
83MGM Chlamydia Trachomatis — Microbiology

TRACING

76KZO Ink, Arch Tracing — Dental And Oral
87VDE Tracing Unit, Arch — Orthopedics

TRACK

80SBK Track And Carrier, Cubicle Curtain — General
80SBL Track And Carrier, Intravenous — General

TRACT

78EYC Catheter, Upper Urinary Tract — Gastro/Urology

TRACTION

89ILZ Accessories, Traction — Physical Med
87HXF Accessories, Traction (Cart, Frame, Cord, Weight) — Orthopedics
87KRT Accessories, Traction, Invasive — Orthopedics
80QCM Bandage, Traction — General
89IRZ Belt, Traction, Pelvic — Physical Med
87HSQ Belt, Traction, Pelvic, Orthopedic — Orthopedics
87QGV Cart, Traction — Orthopedics
87JEC Component, Traction, Invasive — Orthopedics
87KQZ Component, Traction, Non-Invasive — Orthopedics
89ITH Equipment, Traction, Powered — Physical Med
89QVC Exerciser, Trapeze — Physical Med
87QXQ Frame, Traction — Orthopedics
89IRS Halter, Head, Traction — Physical Med
87HSS Halter, Head, Traction, Orthopedic — Orthopedics
87HSP Splint, Traction — Orthopedics
87WUS System, Traction, Arthroscopy — Orthopedics
87RYZ Table, Traction — Orthopedics
84HAX Tongs, Skull, Traction — Cns/Neurology
87HSR Traction Unit, Hip, Non-Powered, Non-Penetrating — Orthopedics
87HST Traction Unit, Non-Powered — Orthopedics
87SBN Traction Unit, Powered, Mobile — Orthopedics
87SBO Traction Unit, Static, Bed — Orthopedics
87SBP Traction Unit, Static, Chair — Orthopedics
87SBQ Traction Unit, Static, Other — Orthopedics

TRAINER

77EPF Hearing-Aid, Group, Or Auditory Trainer — Ear/Nose/Throat
77RUT Speech Therapy Unit (Trainer) — Ear/Nose/Throat
78FEA Teaching Attachment, Endoscopic — Gastro/Urology
77SBR Trainer, Auditory — Ear/Nose/Throat
79SHA Trainer, Laparoscopy — Surgery

TRAINING

80TAE Anatomical Training Model — General
80UKS Chart, Anatomical Training — General
80VBD Material, Training, Audiovisual — General
80RIP Observerscope — General
77LEZ Speech Training Aid, AC-Powered — Ear/Nose/Throat
77LFA Speech Training Aid, Battery-Powered — Ear/Nose/Throat
89IQM Splint, Temporary Training — Physical Med
78FEA Teaching Attachment, Endoscopic — Gastro/Urology
87UFE Training Aid — Orthopedics
74VCZ Training Aid, Arrhythmia Recognition — Cardiovascular
80SBS Training Manikin, CPR (Resuscitation) — General
80TFF Training Manikin, Intravenous Arm — General
80SBT Training Manikin, Other — General
80TFO Training Manikin, Wound Moulage — General

TRANS-TELEPHONE

74LOR Resuscitator, Trans-Telephone — Cardiovascular

TRANSABDOMINAL

85HFA Amnioscope, Transabdominal (Fetoscope) — Obstetrics/Gyn

TRANSCATHETER

74MLV Device, Occlusion, Cardiac, Transcatheter — Cardiovascular

TRANSCERVICAL

85MKN Catheter, Transcervical, Balloon Tuboplasty — Obstetrics/Gyn
85HEZ Endoscope, Transcervical (Amnioscope) — Obstetrics/Gyn

TRANSCRANIAL

74ULR Detector, Blood Flow, Ultrasonic (Doppler) — Cardiovascular

TRANSCRANIAL *(cont'd)*

74WSD	Doppler, Blood Flow, Transcranial	Cardiovascular

TRANSCUTANEOUS

74JEE	Analyzer, Concentration, Oxyhemoglobin, BP, Transcutaneous	Cardiovascular
84RWA	Analyzer, Transcutaneous Nerve Stimulator	Cns/Neurology
74MPE	Auxillary Power Supply, Pacemaker, Cardiac, External Trans.	Cardiovascular
74QTD	Electrode, Pacemaker, External	Cardiovascular
73QTG	Electrode, Transcutaneous, Carbon-Dioxide	Anesthesiology
73QTH	Electrode, Transcutaneous, Oxygen	Anesthesiology
74CAS	Flowmeter, Blood, Ultrasonic, Transcutaneous (W/WO Calibr.)	Cardiovascular
80WKY	Garment, Electrode	General
73TAJ	Monitor, Blood Gas, Transcutaneous Carbon-Dioxide	Anesthesiology
73QEC	Monitor, Blood Gas, Transcutaneous Oxygen	Anesthesiology
73LKD	Monitor, Carbon-Dioxide, Cutaneous	Anesthesiology
73KLK	Monitor, Oxygen, Cutaneous	Anesthesiology
73ULU	Monitor, Transcutaneous, Carbon-Dioxide	Anesthesiology
73ULV	Monitor, Transcutaneous, Oxygen	Anesthesiology
74DRO	Pacemaker, Cardiac, External Transcutaneous (Non-Invasive)	Cardiovascular
73RJV	Pain Gauge, Transcutaneous	Anesthesiology
84GZJ	Stimulator, Nerve, Transcutaneous (Pain Relief, TENS)	Cns/Neurology
84LEP	Stimulator, Nerve, Transcutaneous Elec. (Speech Disorder)	Cns/Neurology

TRANSDERMAL

80WOL	Patch, Transdermal	General
77EPG	Stimulator, Transdermal	Ear/Nose/Throat
80WOI	System, Delivery, Drug, Non-invasive	General
80RZE	Tape, Adhesive	General

TRANSDUCER

80WTN	Adapter, Cable, Equipment	General
74DRQ	Amplifier, Transducer Signal (W Signal Conditioner)	Cardiovascular
74DSA	Cable/Lead, ECG, With Transducer And Electrode	Cardiovascular
73QFO	Calibrator, Pressure Transducer	Anesthesiology
79WHN	Cover, Probe, Transducer	Surgery
80QQH	Dome, Pressure Transducer	General
80WKY	Garment, Electrode	General
73SBU	Holder, Transducer	Anesthesiology
80RLY	Kit, Pressure Monitoring (Air/Gas)	General
73BZZ	Monitor, Blood Pressure, Indirect, Transducer	Anesthesiology
74BXE	Monitor, Blood Pressure, Transducer, Indwelling	Cardiovascular
78FGM	Probe, Gastrointestinal	Gastro/Urology
80RMK	Probe, Other	General
78FIB	Protector, Transducer, Dialysis	Gastro/Urology
78FES	Recorder, External, Pressure, Amplifier & Transducer	Gastro/Urology
73RSA	Sensor, Oxygen	Anesthesiology
74JON	Transducer, Apex Cardiographic	Cardiovascular
73BXG	Transducer, Blood Flow, Invasive	Anesthesiology
73BXF	Transducer, Blood Flow, Non-Invasive	Anesthesiology
80SBW	Transducer, Blood Pressure	General
74DXO	Transducer, Blood Pressure, Catheter Tip	Cardiovascular
74DRS	Transducer, Blood Pressure, Extravascular	Cardiovascular
74WLT	Transducer, Flow, Catheter Tip	Cardiovascular
80SBV	Transducer, Force	General
73BXP	Transducer, Gas Flow	Anesthesiology
73BXO	Transducer, Gas Pressure	Anesthesiology
73BYR	Transducer, Gas Pressure, Differential	Anesthesiology
74JOO	Transducer, Heart Sound	Cardiovascular
89IKE	Transducer, Miniature Pressure	Physical Med
85HFN	Transducer, Pressure, Intrauterine	Obstetrics/Gyn
73BZS	Transducer, Stethoscope	Anesthesiology
84GYD	Transducer, Tremor	Cns/Neurology
74JOP	Transducer, Ultrasonic	Cardiovascular
90ITX	Transducer, Ultrasonic, Diagnostic	Radiology
85WOP	Transducer, Ultrasonic, Intravaginal	Obstetrics/Gyn
85HGL	Transducer, Ultrasonic, Obstetrical	Obstetrics/Gyn
74DXP	Transducer, Vessel Occlusion	Cardiovascular

TRANSESOPHAGEAL

74WTO	Probe, Transesophageal	Cardiovascular

TRANSFER

90QFK	Cabinet, X-Ray Transfer	Radiology
85MHL	Catheter, Transfer, Intrafallopian	Obstetrics/Gyn
80QTZ	Elevator, Other	General
85VIK	Equipment, In Vitro Fertilization/Embryo Transfer	Obstetrics/Gyn
80QXI	Forceps, Sterilizer Transfer	General
80RKB	Patient Transfer Unit	General
80FRZ	Patient Transfer Unit, Powered	General
80WYV	Pin, Transfer, Solution	General
80WXD	Scale, Chair, Transfer	General
80VLO	Stretcher, Basket, Portable	General
80WIG	Stretcher, Emergency, Other	General
79FSL	Stretcher, Transfer	Surgery
89IKX	Transfer Aid	Physical Med

TRANSFER *(cont'd)*

80FMR	Transfer Device, Patient, Manual	General
81KSB	Transfer Unit, Blood	Hematology
80LHI	Transfer Unit, IV Fluid	General
90ROD	Transfer Unit, Radioisotope	Radiology
80SDJ	Tube, Transfer	General

TRANSFERRIN

82DDG	Antigen, Antiserum, Control, Transferrin	Immunology
82DDI	Antigen, Antiserum, Control, Transferrin, FITC	Immunology
82DDD	Antigen, Antiserum, Control, Transferrin, Rhodamine	Immunology
82JNM	Immunochemical, Transferrin	Immunology

TRANSFORMER

79GCW	Transformer, Endoscope	Surgery

TRANSFUSION

80BRZ	Kit, Blood, Transfusion	General
80LWE	Kit, Collection/Transfusion, Marrow, Bone	General
73CAK	Microfilter, Blood Transfusion	Anesthesiology
81KSS	Supplies, Blood Bank	Hematology

TRANSGLUTAMINASE

82MVM	Autoantibodies, Endomysial(tissue Transglutaminase)	Immunology

TRANSIENT

80ROR	Recorder, Transient	General

TRANSILLUMINATOR

80TDP	Phaneroscope	General
90LEK	Transilluminator (Diaphanoscope)	Radiology
86HJM	Transilluminator, AC-Powered, Ophthalmic	Ophthalmology
86ETJ	Transilluminator, AC-Powered, Other	Ophthalmology
86HJN	Transilluminator, Battery-Powered	Ophthalmology
77MQW	Transilluminator, Fiber Optic	Ear/Nose/Throat
75UIW	Transilluminator, Laboratory	Chemistry

TRANSLUCENT

74WLG	Cable/Lead, ECG, Radiolucent	Cardiovascular
74WLP	Electrode, ECG, Radiolucent	Cardiovascular

TRANSLUMINAL

74LOX	Catheter, Angioplasty, Coronary, Transluminal, Percut. Oper.	Cardiovascular
74LIT	Catheter, Angioplasty, Transluminal, Peripheral	Cardiovascular

TRANSMANDIBULAR

76MDL	Implant, Transmandibular	Dental And Oral

TRANSMISSION

80SDY	Gel, Ultrasonic Transmission	General

TRANSMITTER

74DTC	Analyzer, Pacemaker Generator Function	Cardiovascular
90WOG	Transmitter, Image & Data, Radiographic	Radiology
74QRY	Transmitter/Receiver System, ECG, Telephone Multi-Channel	Cardiovascular
74QRZ	Transmitter/Receiver System, ECG, Telephone Single-Channel	Cardiovascular
80VFH	Transmitter/Receiver System, Fetal Monitor, Telephone	General
74DRG	Transmitter/Receiver System, Physiological, Radiofrequency	Cardiovascular
74DXH	Transmitter/Receiver System, Physiological, Telephone	Cardiovascular
80VFI	Transmitter/Receiver System, Pulmonary Monitor, Telephone	General
84QSC	Transmitter/Receiver, EEG, Telephone	Cns/Neurology
74MFL	Transmitter/Receiver, Physiological Signal, Infrared	Cardiovascular

TRANSMYOCARDIAL

74MNO	System, Laser, Transmyocardial Revascularization	Cardiovascular

TRANSPARENT

90VLA	Shield, X-Ray, Transparent	Radiology

TRANSPEPTIDASE

75JPZ	Colorimetric Method, Gamma-Glutamyl Transpeptidase	Chemistry
75JQA	Electrophoretic, Gamma-Glutamyl Transpeptidase Isoenzymes	Chemistry
75JQB	Kinetic Method, Gamma-Glutamyl Transpeptidase	Chemistry

TRANSPERASE

75JLJ	UDP-Glucose, NAD (U.V.), Gal-I-P Uridyl Transperase	Chemistry

TRANSPLANT

80LPZ	Container, Frozen Donor Tissue Storage	General
78KDK	Container, Transport, Kidney	Gastro/Urology
86TCI	Freezer, Eye Bank	Ophthalmology
83WPR	Micro-Injector, Transplant, Gene	Microbiology
78RIZ	Organ Preservation System	Gastro/Urology
79RNN	Punch, Hair Transplant	Surgery

TRANSPORT

80LGN	Chamber, Isolation, Patient Transport	General

KEYWORD INDEX

TRANSPORT *(cont'd)*

90WJA	Container, Substance, Radioactive	Radiology
78KDK	Container, Transport, Kidney	Gastro/Urology
80WYG	Courier, Supplies, Mobile, Automated	General
83JSL	Culture Media, Anaerobic Transport	Microbiology
83JSM	Culture Media, Non-Propagating Transport	Microbiology
83JSN	Culture Media, Propagating Transport	Microbiology
80FPL	Incubator, Neonatal Transport	General
74MFU	Media, Transport/Storage, Organ/Tissue	Cardiovascular
80WKO	Stretcher, Collapsible	General
80FPP	Stretcher, Hand-Carried	General
89INJ	Stretcher, Wheeled, Mechanical	Physical Med
80WIH	System, Transport, In-House	General
83JTW	Transport System, Aerobic	Microbiology
83JTX	Transport System, Anaerobic	Microbiology
89ILK	Transport, Patient, Powered	Physical Med
74MFV	Unit, Transport, Organ	Cardiovascular
80SFK	Warmer, Radiant, Infant, Transport	General

TRANSPORTATION

80QAO	Ambulance	General
80TFU	Ambulance, Air	General
80WYL	Box, Transportation, Container, Specimen	General
80QTZ	Elevator, Other	General

TRANSTELEPHONIC

74WJK	Defibrillator, Transtelephonic	Cardiovascular

TRANSTHORACIC

74UCG	Electrode, Pacemaker, Transthoracic	Cardiovascular

TRANSURETHRAL

78FHC	Adapter, Cord, Instrument, Surgical, Transurethral	Gastro/Urology
78FBJ	Cord, Electric, Instrument, Surgical, Transurethral	Gastro/Urology
78FHZ	Desiccator, Transurethral	Gastro/Urology
78FHY	Jelly, Contact (For Transurethral Surgical Instrument)	Gastro/Urology
78FHX	Jelly, Lubricating, Transurethral Surgical Instrument	Gastro/Urology
78WYF	Unit, Microwave, Transurethral	Gastro/Urology

TRANSVENOUS

74QIG	Lead, Pacemaker, Implantable Endocardial	Cardiovascular

TRANSVERSE

89IQP	Rotator, Transverse	Physical Med

TRAP

73CBD	Bottle, Collection, Breathing System (Calibrated)	Anesthesiology
73CBC	Bottle, Collection, Breathing System (Uncalibrated)	Anesthesiology
80KDQ	Bottle, Collection, Vacuum (Aspirator)	General
73QLT	Collector, Sputum	Anesthesiology
73BYH	Drain, Tee (Water Trap)	Anesthesiology
74SBY	Trap, Bubble	Cardiovascular
73SBZ	Trap, Mucus	Anesthesiology
73BYZ	Trap, Sterile Specimen	Anesthesiology

TRAPEZE

89QVC	Exerciser, Trapeze	Physical Med

TRAPEZIUM

87KYI	Prosthesis, Wrist, Carpal Trapezium	Orthopedics

TRAPPING

91DJZ	Alcohol Breath Trapping Device	Toxicology

TRAUMATIC

79QKT	Forceps, Grasping, Atraumatic	Surgery
79QLE	Forceps, Grasping, Traumatic	Surgery
79QQR	Gauge, Thickness, Tissue	Surgery

TRAY

79FWZ	Accessories, Operating Room, Table	Surgery
73BRY	Cabinet, Table And Tray, Anesthesia	Anesthesiology
80RVS	Container, Sterilization (Tray)	General
79VEE	Container, Surgical Instrument	Surgery
80TFG	Conveyor, Tray	General
78FCH	Kit, Biopsy, Gastro-Urology	Gastro/Urology
78FCM	Kit, Catheterization, Sterile Urethral	Gastro/Urology
80QJS	Kit, Chest Drainage (Thoracentesis Tray)	General
85QKG	Kit, Circumcision, Disposable Tray	Obstetrics/Gyn
78EYN	Kit, Irrigation, Sterile	Gastro/Urology
80TFI	Kit, Skin Scrub	General
76EBH	Material, Impression Tray, Resin	Dental And Oral
80WNC	Molding, Custom	General
80WXF	Pack, Custom/Special Procedure	General
79SIO	Rack, Instrument, Laparoscopy	Surgery
85HIO	Sampler, Amniotic Fluid (Amniocentesis Tray)	Obstetrics/Gyn
81GJE	Tray, Blood Collection	Hematology
85QKH	Tray, Circumcision, Reusable	Obstetrics/Gyn
80WNH	Tray, Custom/Special Procedure	General
78FJZ	Tray, Declotting (Including Contents)	Gastro/Urology
76UDW	Tray, Fluoride	Dental And Oral
76KMT	Tray, Fluoride, Disposable	Dental And Oral

TRAY *(cont'd)*

80TFH	Tray, Foodservice	General
76EHY	Tray, Impression	Dental And Oral
87WPM	Tray, Impression, Foot	Orthopedics
80SCA	Tray, Medicine	General
83ULL	Tray, Micro (Mic Plate)	Microbiology
75UIX	Tray, Serial Dilution	Chemistry
78FKG	Tray, Start/Stop (Including Contents), Dialysis	Gastro/Urology
79SIC	Tray, Sterilization, Instrument	Surgery
79LRP	Tray, Surgical	Surgery
79FSM	Tray, Surgical Instrument	Surgery
77MMO	Tray, Surgical, ENT	Ear/Nose/Throat
80UEL	Tray, Walker	General
89IMX	Tray, Wheelchair	Physical Med

TREADMILL

74BYQ	Ergometer, Treadmill	Cardiovascular
89IOG	Treadmill, Mechanical	Physical Med
89IOL	Treadmill, Powered	Physical Med

TREATMENT

77QFC	Cabinet, ENT Treatment	Ear/Nose/Throat
80QFI	Cabinet, Treatment, Ultraviolet	General
80FRK	Chair, Examination And Treatment	General
80UDI	Chair, Infant Treatment	General
73BYN	Chair, Posture, For Cardiac And Pulmonary Treatment	Anesthesiology
84MBW	Cranial Retroperfusion (Stroke Treatment)	Cns/Neurology
74MEY	Cuff, Treatment, Varicose Vein, Implantable	Cardiovascular
89WOK	Equipment, Cryotherapy	Physical Med
80WUC	Facility, Equipment, Medical, Mobile	General
82MEM	Generator, Electric Field (Aids Treatment)	Immunology
76EIA	Operative Dental Treatment Unit	Dental And Oral
90ROG	Radiotherapy Treatment Planning Unit	Radiology
90LOC	System, Cancer Treatment, Hyperthermia, RF/Microwave	Radiology
74MIH	System, Treatment, Aortic Aneurysm, Endovascular Graft	Cardiovascular
84MHA	System, Treatment, Brain Tumor, Hyperthermia, Ultrasonic	Cns/Neurology
80RYX	Table, Examination/Treatment	General
90LSY	Ultrasound, Hyperthermia, Cancer Treatment	Radiology
77ETF	Unit, Examining/Treatment, ENT	Ear/Nose/Throat

TREMOR

84MHY	Stimulator, Electrical, Implanted (Parkinsonian Tremor)	Cns/Neurology
84GYD	Transducer, Tremor	Cns/Neurology

TREND

79KFQ	Monitor, Cardiac Output, Trend (Arterial Pressure Pulse)	Surgery
80ROP	Recorder, Long-Term, Trend	General

TREPHINE

86HRG	Accessories, Engine, Trephine, AC-Powered	Ophthalmology
79HRF	Accessories, Engine, Trephine, Battery-Powered	Surgery
79HLD	Accessories, Engine, Trephine, Gas-Powered	Surgery
84HBG	Drill, Manual (With Burr, Trephine & Accessories)	Cns/Neurology
84HBF	Drill, Powered Compound (With Burr, Trephine & Accessories)	Cns/Neurology
87HWK	Trephine, Bone	Orthopedics
86HRH	Trephine, Manual, Ophthalmic (Corneal)	Ophthalmology
77KBF	Trephine, Sinus	Ear/Nose/Throat
84SCB	Trephine, Skull	Cns/Neurology

TREPONEMA

83WJQ	Antibody, Treponema Pallidum	Microbiology
83GMT	Antigen, HA, Treponema Pallidum	Microbiology
83JWL	Antigen, Treponema Pallidum For FTA-ABS Test	Microbiology
83LIP	Enzyme Linked Immunoabsorbent Assay, Treponema Pallidum	Microbiology
83UMO	Test, Syphilis (RPR or VDRL)	Microbiology

TREPONEMAL

83GMQ	Antigen, Non-Treponemal, All	Microbiology
83GMP	Antiserum, Control For Non-Treponemal Test	Microbiology

TRIAL

86HPB	Clip, Lens, Trial, Ophthalmic	Ophthalmology
86HPA	Frame, Trial, Ophthalmic	Ophthalmology
86HPC	Lens, Set, Trial, Ophthalmic	Ophthalmology

TRICALCIUM

76LPK	Tricalcium Phosphate Granules for Dental Bone Repair	Dental And Oral

TRICHINELLA

83GPI	Antigen, Bentonite Flocculation, Trichinella Spiralis	Microbiology
83GPG	Antigen, Latex Agglutination, Trichinella Spiralis	Microbiology
83GPH	Antiserum, Bentonite Flocculation, Trichinella Spiralis	Microbiology
83MDT	Enzyme Linked Immunoabsorbent Assay, Trichinella Spiralis	Microbiology

TRICHOLABION

79QWZ	Forceps, Epilation	Surgery

TRICHOMONAS

83MJK	DNA-Probe, Trichomonas Vaginalis	Microbiology

TRICHOMONAS *(cont'd)*
83JWZ Kit, Trichomonas Screening — Microbiology

TRICHROME
88HYW Stain, Mallory's Trichrome — Pathology

TRICYCLIC
91MLK Chromatography, Thin Layer, Tricyclic Antidepressant Drugs — Toxicology
91LFI High Pressure Liquid Chromatography, Tricyclic Drug — Toxicology
91LFG Radioimmunoassay, Tricyclic Antidepressant Drugs — Toxicology
91LFH U.V. Spectrometry, Tricyclic Antidepressant Drugs — Toxicology

TRIFLUOROACETIC
75JOA Hexane Extraction And Trifluoroacetic Acid, Vitamin A — Chemistry

TRIFOCAL
86WZA Lens, Contact, Trifocal — Ophthalmology

TRIGLYCERIDE
75CEA Triglyceride, Separation, Chromatographic, TLC — Chemistry

TRIGLYCERIDES
75JGY Colorimetric Method, Triglycerides — Chemistry
75JGW Fluorometric Method, Triglycerides — Chemistry
75CDT Lipase Hydrolysis/Glycerol Kinase Enzyme, Triglycerides — Chemistry
75JGX Turbidimetric Method, Triglycerides — Chemistry

TRIIODOTHYRONINE
75KHQ Radioassay, Triiodothyronine Uptake — Chemistry
75CDY Radioimmunoassay, T3 Uptake — Chemistry
75CDP Radioimmunoassay, Total Triiodothyronine — Chemistry

TRINITROBENZENE
75JQH Trinitrobenzene Sulfonate (Spectroscopic), Nitrogen — Chemistry

TRIOSE
75JNY Glyceralde-3-Phosphate, NADH (Enzymatic), Triose Phosphate — Chemistry

TRIPHOSPHATE
81JWR ATP Release (Luminescence) — Hematology
75JLB ATP and CK (Enzymatic), Creatine — Chemistry
87LMM Ceramics, Triphos./Hydroxyapatite, Ca. (Load Bearing) — Orthopedics
87LMN Ceramics, Triphos./Hydroxyapatite, Ca. (Non-Load Bearing) — Orthopedics

TRIPSOR
78FGK Tripsor, Stone, Bladder — Gastro/Urology

TROCAR
79SJI Balloon, Manipulation, Tissue — Surgery
78FBM Cannula, Suprapubic, With Trocar — Gastro/Urology
79SIN Dilator, Port, Laparoscopic — Surgery
79SJJ Dissector, Balloon, Surgical — Surgery
79SIA Kit, Trocar — Surgery
79SHV Sleeve, Trocar — Surgery
79SID Thread, Stability, Trocar — Surgery
78SCC Trocar, Abdominal — Gastro/Urology
85SCD Trocar, Amniotic — Obstetrics/Gyn
77SCE Trocar, Antrum — Ear/Nose/Throat
74DRC Trocar, Cardiovascular — Cardiovascular
77KTE Trocar, ENT — Ear/Nose/Throat
78SCF Trocar, Gallbladder — Gastro/Urology
78FBQ Trocar, Gastro-Urology — Gastro/Urology
79WYQ Trocar, Laparoscopic — Surgery
77KAB Trocar, Laryngeal — Ear/Nose/Throat
80SCH Trocar, Other — General
79SHB Trocar, Short — Surgery
77KBG Trocar, Sinus — Ear/Nose/Throat
74SCG Trocar, Thoracic — Cardiovascular
77KCI Trocar, Tracheal — Ear/Nose/Throat
80WHK Tubing, Hypodermic — General

TROLLEY
80TGS Conveyor, Guided Vehicle — General

TROPONIN
75MMI Enzymatic Method, Troponin Subunit — Chemistry

TROUSERS
74RLJ Suit, Pneumatic Counterpressure (Anti-Shock) — Cardiovascular
73LHX Trousers, Anti-Shock — Anesthesiology

TRUNCAL
89MRI Orthosis, Truncal/Limb — Physical Med

TRUNK
89IMS Support, Head And Trunk, Wheelchair — Physical Med

TRUNNION
87JDH Prosthesis, Hip, Hemi-, Trunnion-Bearing, Femoral — Orthopedics
87LGE Prosthesis, Knee, Femorotibial, Semi-Constrained, Trunnion — Orthopedics

TRUNNION-BEARING
87JDH Prosthesis, Hip, Hemi-, Trunnion-Bearing, Femoral — Orthopedics

TRUSS
78SCI Truss, Hernia (Belt) — Gastro/Urology
85SCJ Truss, Infant — Obstetrics/Gyn
77SCK Truss, Nasal — Ear/Nose/Throat
78EXM Truss, Umbilical — Gastro/Urology

TRYPAN
88LGY Stain, Trypan Blue — Pathology

TRYPANOSOMA
83GNF Antigen, CF, T. Cruzi — Microbiology
83GND Antigen, IHA, T. Cruzi — Microbiology
83GNE Antigen, Latex Agglutination, T. Cruzi — Microbiology

TRYPSIN
82CZO Antigen, Antiserum, Control, Inter-Alpha Trypsin Inhibitor — Immunology
82DEC Inter-Alpha Trypsin, FITC, Antigen, Antiserum, Control — Immunology
75JNO N-Benzoyl-L-Arginine Ethyl Ester (U.V.), Trypsin — Chemistry
75JNN P-Toluenesulphonyl-L-Arginine Methyl Ester (U.V.), Trypsin — Chemistry
88IBG Trypsin — Pathology

TRYPTOPHAN
75JGC Tryptophan Measurement (Colorimetric), Globulin — Chemistry

TSH
75JLW Radioimmunoassay, Thyroid Stimulating Hormone — Chemistry

TUBAL
85HFY Band, Occlusion, Tubal — Obstetrics/Gyn
85HGB Clip, Tubal Occlusion — Obstetrics/Gyn
85LLS Contraceptive Tubal Occlusion Device, Male — Obstetrics/Gyn
78QPU Dilator, Tubal — Gastro/Urology
85HHS Insert, Tubal Occlusion — Obstetrics/Gyn
85KNH Tubal Occlusive Device — Obstetrics/Gyn
85HDO Valve, Tubal Occlusion — Obstetrics/Gyn

TUBE
75QIY Adapter, Centrifuge Tube — Chemistry
73SBF Adapter, Tube, Tracheal — Anesthesiology
73CAO Airway, Esophageal (Obturator) — Anesthesiology
73BTQ Airway, Nasopharyngeal (Breathing Tube) — Anesthesiology
80QAJ Airway, Obstruction Removal (Choke Saver) — General
73CAE Airway, Oropharyngeal, Anesthesia — Anesthesiology
83GNC Antigen, Febrile, Slide And Tube, Salmonella — Microbiology
83GSL Antigen, Slide And Tube, Francisella Tularensis — Microbiology
83GSI Antigen, Slide And Tube, Listeria Monocytogenes — Microbiology
77EPE Brush, Cleaning, Tracheal Tube — Ear/Nose/Throat
73SBI Button, Tracheostomy Tube — Anesthesiology
86QGB Cannula, Lacrimal (Eye) — Ophthalmology
80FMM Cannula, Nasal — General
78FEW Catheter, Malecot (Gastrostomy Tube) — Gastro/Urology
78QIC Catheter, Mushroom — Gastro/Urology
73BZB Catheter, Nasal, Oxygen (Tube) — Anesthesiology
73BSY Catheter, Suction (Tracheal Aspirating Tube) — Anesthesiology
78FEZ Catheter, Suprapubic, With Tube — Gastro/Urology
73LNZ Changer, Tube, Endotracheal — Anesthesiology
73CAI Circuit, Breathing (W Connector, Adapter, Y Piece) — Anesthesiology
73QEL Circuit, Breathing, Ventilator — Anesthesiology
73BSK Cuff, Tracheal Tube, Inflatable — Anesthesiology
77JOH Cuff, Tracheostomy Tube — Ear/Nose/Throat
80TDT Delivery System, Pneumatic Tube — General
74DXJ Display, Cathode-Ray Tube — Cardiovascular
73QQO Drain, Thoracic (Chest) — Anesthesiology
77QRB Dressing, Tracheostomy Tube — Ear/Nose/Throat
75UIY Fitting, Gas Chromatography Tube — Chemistry
73CBH Fixation Device, Tracheal Tube — Anesthesiology
73CAX Flowmeter, Back-Pressure Compensated, Thorpe Tube — Anesthesiology
73BWB Forceps, Tube Introduction — Anesthesiology
90VHK Hanger, X-Ray Tube — Radiology
81GHY Hematocrit Tube, Rack, Sealer, Holder — Hematology
73SBH Holder, Tracheostomy Tube — Anesthesiology
90ITY Housing, X-Ray Tube, Diagnostic — Radiology
90ITZ Housing, X-Ray Tube, Therapeutic — Radiology
83RBY Incubator, Test Tube, Portable — Microbiology
83RBZ Incubator, Test Tube, Stationary — Microbiology
77JYM Inserter, Myringotomy Tube — Ear/Nose/Throat
78QTO Introducer, T-Tube — Gastro/Urology
78QUJ Kit, Administration, Enteral — Gastro/Urology
80FPA Kit, Administration, Intravenous — General
74QHL Kit, Catheterization, Intravenous, Winged — Cardiovascular
80QVM Kit, Feeding, Adult (Enteral) — General
80QVN Kit, Feeding, Pediatric (Enteral) — General
78QZU Kit, Hemodialysis Tubing — Gastro/Urology
80RCK Kit, Intravenous Extension Tubing — General
78RKM Kit, Tubing, Dialysis, Peritoneal — Gastro/Urology
78FFW Locator, Bleeding, Gastrointestinal, String And Tube — Gastro/Urology
73RGC Mask, Tracheostomy, Aerosol Administration — Anesthesiology

TUBE *(cont'd)*
89IRP *Massager, Powered Inflatable Tube* Physical Med
76KCQ *Matrix, Tube Impression* Dental And Oral
81GLE *Mixer, Blood Tube* Hematology
78KLA *Monitor, Esophageal Motility, And Tube* Gastro/Urology
90VGH *Monitor, X-Ray Tube* Radiology
90IYB *Mount, X-Ray Tube, Diagnostic* Radiology
78FJO *Pliers, Tube* Gastro/Urology
85HFJ *Prosthesis, Fallopian Tube* Obstetrics/Gyn
91DOW *RIA, Digitoxin (3-H), Rabbit Antibody, Coated Tube* Toxicology
91DNQ *RIA, Digoxin (3-H), Rabbit Antibody, Coated Tube Sep.* Toxicology
75RNT *Rack, Test Tube* Chemistry
91DPG *Radioimmunoassay, Digitoxin (125-I), Rabbit, Coated Tube* Toxicology
91DPO *Radioimmunoassay, Digoxin (125-I), Rabbit, Coated Tube* Toxicology
75WKC *Stand/Holder, Equipment, Laboratory* Chemistry
80WNN *Stopper* General
73VDM *Strap, Tracheostomy Tube* Anesthesiology
81RWS *Stripper, Donor Tube* Hematology
73BSR *Stylet, Tracheal Tube* Anesthesiology
73JAY *Support, Breathing Tube* Anesthesiology
75WID *Support, Tube, Test* Chemistry
83UKA *Test, Agar Tube* Microbiology
82LOK *Test, Neural Tube Defect, Alpha-Fetoprotein (AFP)* Immunology
73BSQ *Tip, Suction* Anesthesiology
79ULE *Tip, Suction Tube (Yankauer, Poole, Etc.)* Surgery
80SCH *Trocar, Other* General
73BYY *Tube, Aspirating, Flexible, Connecting* Anesthesiology
77KTR *Tube, Aspirating, Rigid Bronchoscope Aspirating* Ear/Nose/Throat
80SCL *Tube, Autoclaving* General
75SCN *Tube, Blood Collection* Chemistry
75SCM *Tube, Blood Microcollection* Chemistry
73BTS *Tube, Bronchial (W/Wo Connector)* Anesthesiology
73JEJ *Tube, Bronchoscope* Anesthesiology
73JEM *Tube, Bronchoscope, Aspirating* Anesthesiology
75SCO *Tube, Capillary* Chemistry
81GIO *Tube, Capillary Blood Collection* Hematology
87KII *Tube, Cement Ventilation* Orthopedics
75SCP *Tube, Centrifuge* Chemistry
78SCQ *Tube, Colon* Gastro/Urology
78MIQ *Tube, Colostomy* Gastro/Urology
80SCR *Tube, Connecting* General
83SCS *Tube, Culture* Microbiology
80SCT *Tube, Decompression* General
78FID *Tube, Dialysate* Gastro/Urology
78FEG *Tube, Double Lumen For Intestinal Decompression* Gastro/Urology
78FFA *Tube, Drainage* Gastro/Urology
77JZF *Tube, Ear Suction* Ear/Nose/Throat
78SCU *Tube, Enema* Gastro/Urology
78SCV *Tube, Esophageal, Blakemore* Gastro/Urology
78SCW *Tube, Esophageal, Replogle* Gastro/Urology
78SCX *Tube, Esophageal, Sengstaken* Gastro/Urology
80FPD *Tube, Feeding* General
78KGC *Tube, Gastro-Enterostomy* Gastro/Urology
78KNT *Tube, Gastrointestinal* Gastro/Urology
78VHP *Tube, Gastrointestinal Decompression, Baker Jejunostomy* Gastro/Urology
78SDB *Tube, Gastrointestinal Decompression, Cantor* Gastro/Urology
78SDC *Tube, Gastrointestinal Decompression, Dennis* Gastro/Urology
78SDD *Tube, Gastrointestinal Decompression, Miller-Abbott* Gastro/Urology
78SCY *Tube, Gastrointestinal, Kaslow* Gastro/Urology
78SCZ *Tube, Gastrointestinal, Rehfuss* Gastro/Urology
78SDA *Tube, Gastrointestinal, Wangensteen* Gastro/Urology
90IZE *Tube, Image Amplifier, X-Ray* Radiology
78LCG *Tube, Intestinal Splinting* Gastro/Urology
77KAC *Tube, Laryngectomy* Ear/Nose/Throat
80FRQ *Tube, Levine* General
77SDE *Tube, Myringotomy* Ear/Nose/Throat
73BSS *Tube, Nasogastric* Anesthesiology
78SDF *Tube, Nephrostomy* Gastro/Urology
76DZD *Tube, Orthodontic* Dental And Oral
74DWE *Tube, Pump, Cardiopulmonary Bypass* Cardiovascular
73SDG *Tube, Rebreathing* Anesthesiology
78SDH *Tube, Rectal* Gastro/Urology
81GHC *Tube, Sedimentation Rate* Hematology
77ESZ *Tube, Shunt, Endolymphatic* Ear/Nose/Throat
77KLZ *Tube, Shunt, Endolymphatic, With Valve* Ear/Nose/Throat
78FEF *Tube, Single Lumen, W Mercury Wt Balloon* Gastro/Urology
78FCZ *Tube, Smoke Removal, Endoscopic* Gastro/Urology
78SDI *Tube, Stomach Evacuator (Gastric Lavage)* Gastro/Urology
80WNO *Tube, Suction* General
75RZV *Tube, Test* Chemistry
73BYM *Tube, Thorpe, Uncompensated* Anesthesiology
88KJG *Tube, Tissue Culture* Pathology
77KCB *Tube, Tonsil Suction* Ear/Nose/Throat
77ETK *Tube, Toynbee Diagnostic* Ear/Nose/Throat
73BTR *Tube, Tracheal (Endotracheal)* Anesthesiology
73CBI *Tube, Tracheal/Bronchial, Differential Ventilation* Anesthesiology
77EQK *Tube, Tracheostomy (Breathing Tube), ENT* Ear/Nose/Throat

TUBE *(cont'd)*
73BTO *Tube, Tracheostomy (W/Wo Connector)* Anesthesiology
80SDJ *Tube, Transfer* General
77ETD *Tube, Tympanostomy* Ear/Nose/Throat
77LBL *Tube, Tympanostomy, Porous Polyethylene* Ear/Nose/Throat
77KQL *Tube, Tympanostomy, With Semi-Permeable Membrane* Ear/Nose/Throat
81GIM *Tube, Vacuum Sample, With Anticoagulant* Hematology
90VHF *Tube, X-Ray* Radiology
79WVC *Tunneler, Surgical* Surgery
89ILC *Utensil, Food* Physical Med
77WRO *Valve, Speaking, Tracheal* Ear/Nose/Throat
76EFC *Warmer, Anesthesia Tube* Dental And Oral
73CAM *Yoke, Medical Gas* Anesthesiology

TUBELESS
75JLL *Tubeless Analysis, Gastric Acidity* Chemistry

TUBERCULIN
80RYT *Syringe, Tuberculin* General

TUBERCULOSIS
83GRT *Antiserum, Fluorescent, Mycobacterium Tuberculosis* Microbiology
83JSY *Kit, Mycobacteria Identification* Microbiology
83NCD *Test, Immunity, Cell-Mediated, Mycobacterium Tuberculosis* Microbiology

TUBING
79KGZ *Accessories, Catheter* Surgery
73WLJ *Catheter, Oxygen, Tracheal* Anesthesiology
73QEL *Circuit, Breathing, Ventilator* Anesthesiology
80WUF *Clamp, Tubing* General
78FIG *Clamp, Tubing, Blood, Automatic* Gastro/Urology
74WJY *Connector, Tubing, Blood* Cardiovascular
78FKB *Connector, Tubing, Blood, Infusion, T-Type* Gastro/Urology
78FKY *Connector, Tubing, Dialysate* Gastro/Urology
80VAC *Contract Manufacturing* General
80WLX *Contract Manufacturing, Product, Durable* General
80VAJ *Equipment, Extruding/Molding* General
80QVY *Filter, Intravenous Tubing* General
78QZU *Kit, Hemodialysis Tubing* Gastro/Urology
80RCK *Kit, Intravenous Extension Tubing* General
78FJK *Kit, Tubing, Blood, Anti-Regurgitation* Gastro/Urology
78RKM *Kit, Tubing, Dialysis, Peritoneal* Gastro/Urology
80WLM *Lock, Catheter* General
80WNC *Molding, Custom* General
78FID *Tube, Dialysate* Gastro/Urology
74DWE *Tube, Pump, Cardiopulmonary Bypass* Cardiovascular
80SDK *Tubing, Braided* General
80SDL *Tubing, Conductive* General
80WSP *Tubing, Connecting* General
80SDM *Tubing, Corrugated* General
78KQQ *Tubing, Dialysate (And Connector)* Gastro/Urology
73BYX *Tubing, Flexible, Medical Gas, Low-Pressure* Anesthesiology
80FPK *Tubing, Fluid Delivery* General
80WHK *Tubing, Hypodermic* General
79SIT *Tubing, Irrigation* Surgery
80SDN *Tubing, Latex* General
80WPT *Tubing, Multi-Lumen* General
80SDO *Tubing, Non-Conductive* General
79GAZ *Tubing, Non-Invasive* Surgery
80SDP *Tubing, Nylon* General
80WWE *Tubing, Other* General
80VHQ *Tubing, Oxygen Connecting* General
80VKN *Tubing, Plastic* General
80SDQ *Tubing, Polyethylene* General
80WPS *Tubing, Polypropylene* General
80WTH *Tubing, Polytetrafluoroethylene* General
80SDR *Tubing, Polyvinyl Chloride* General
80WNG *Tubing, Radiopaque* General
80SDS *Tubing, Silicone* General
80VKF *Tubing, Urethane* General
73BZO *Tubing, Ventilator* Anesthesiology
80SDT *Tubing, Vinyl* General

TUBOPLASTY
85MKN *Catheter, Transcervical, Balloon Tuboplasty* Obstetrics/Gyn

TUBULAR
80QCN *Bandage, Tubular* General

TUCKER
76ECP *Tucker, Ligature, Orthodontic* Dental And Oral

TULARENSIS
83GSL *Antigen, Slide And Tube, Francisella Tularensis* Microbiology
83GSJ *Antiserum, Fluorescent, Francisella Tularensis* Microbiology
83GSK *Antiserum, Francisella Tularensis* Microbiology

TUMESCENCE
78LIL *Monitor, Penile Tumescence* Gastro/Urology

TUMOR

82MMW	Antigen, Tumor Marker, Bladder (Basement Membrane Complexes)	Immunology
85WJD	Needle, Biopsy, Mammary	Obstetrics/Gyn
79MIJ	Needle, Tumor Localization	Surgery
88MHQ	Panel, Tumor, Undifferentiated	Pathology
85WSC	Spectroscope, Tumor Analysis, Mammary	Obstetrics/Gyn
82MOI	System, Test, Immunological, Antigen, Tumor	Immunology
82NAH	System, Test, Tumor Marker, For Detection Of Bladder Cancer	Immunology
84MHA	System, Treatment, Brain Tumor, Hyperthermia, Ultrasonic	Cns/Neurology
82LTK	Test, Antigen (CA125), Tumor-Associated, Ovarian, Epithelial	Immunology
82VJK	Test, Chemotherapy Sensitivity (Tumor Colony Forming)	Immunology
82LTR	Tumor-Associated Antigen, Tennagen Test	Immunology

TUMOR-ASSOCIATED

82LTK	Test, Antigen (CA125), Tumor-Associated, Ovarian, Epithelial	Immunology
82LTR	Tumor-Associated Antigen, Tennagen Test	Immunology

TUNGSTIC

75CHG	Phosphoric-Tungstic Acid (Spectrophotometric), Chloride	Chemistry

TUNING

84GWX	Fork, Tuning	Cns/Neurology
77ETQ	Fork, Tuning, ENT	Ear/Nose/Throat

TUNNEL

89MNY	Inhibitor, Post-Op Fibro., Carp. Tun. Syn.(Adhesion Barrier)	Physical Med

TUNNELER

74QPQ	Dilator, Vascular	Cardiovascular
74DWP	Dilator, Vessel, Surgical	Cardiovascular
79WVC	Tunneler, Surgical	Surgery

TURBIDIMETER

75JJQ	Colorimeter, General Use	Chemistry

TURBIDIMETRIC

75CET	Emulsion, Olive Oil (Turbidimetric), Lipase	Chemistry
75JHN	Turbidimetric Method, Lipoproteins	Chemistry
75SHR	Turbidimetric Method, Myoglobin	Chemistry
75JIQ	Turbidimetric Method, Protein Or Albumin (Urinary)	Chemistry
75JGX	Turbidimetric Method, Triglycerides	Chemistry
75JGQ	Turbidimetric, Total Protein	Chemistry

TURNER

80TFY	Page Turner (Handicapped)	General

TURNING

87QXR	Frame, Turning	Orthopedics

TUSSILATOR

88IGT	Tussilator	Pathology

TV

80KMI	Monitor, Bed Patient	General

TWEEZER

79KCX	Epilator, High-Frequency, Tweezer Type	Surgery

TWEEZERS

80SDU	Tweezers	General

TWIN

78FJJ	Dialyzer, Twin Coil	Gastro/Urology

TWISTER

89ITO	Twister, Brace Setting	Physical Med
87HXS	Twister, Wire	Orthopedics

TWO

84GWI	Discriminator, Two-point	Cns/Neurology
84IKM	Esthesiometer, Two Point Discriminator	Cns/Neurology
81JPE	Test, Antithrombin III, Two Stage Clotting Time	Hematology

TWO-POINT

84GWI	Discriminator, Two-point	Cns/Neurology

TYING

79QOJ	Holder, Needle, Curved, Laparoscopic	Surgery
79QNU	Holder, Needle, Laparoscopic	Surgery
79QPN	Holder/Scissors, Needle, Laparoscopic	Surgery
79QRS	Instrument, Knot Tying, Suture, Laparoscopic	Surgery
79QPS	Instrument, Needle Holder/Knot Tying	Surgery
84HCF	Instrument, Passing, Ligature, Knot Tying	Cns/Neurology

TYMPANIC

77MMB	Hearing-Aid, External, Magnet, Membrane, Tympanic	Ear/Nose/Throat
77WXS	Thermometer, Tympanic	Ear/Nose/Throat

TYMPANOMETER

77RGY	Analyzer, Middle Ear	Ear/Nose/Throat

TYMPANOMETER *(cont'd)*

80WUP	Paper, Recording, Data	General

TYMPANOSCOPE

77JOG	Tympanoscope	Ear/Nose/Throat

TYMPANOSTOMY

77ETD	Tube, Tympanostomy	Ear/Nose/Throat
77LBL	Tube, Tympanostomy, Porous Polyethylene	Ear/Nose/Throat
77KQL	Tube, Tympanostomy, With Semi-Permeable Membrane	Ear/Nose/Throat

TYPE

78EXJ	Appliance, Incontinence, Urosheath Type	Gastro/Urology
79GBA	Catheter, Balloon (Foley Type)	Surgery
74GBR	Catheter, Cardiovascular, Balloon Type	Cardiovascular
74DXE	Catheter, Embolectomy (Fogarty Type)	Cardiovascular
78EZK	Catheter, Retention Type	Gastro/Urology
78EZL	Catheter, Retention Type, Balloon	Gastro/Urology
78FKB	Connector, Tubing, Blood, Infusion, T-Type	Gastro/Urology
79KCW	Epilator, High-Frequency, Needle-Type	Surgery
79KCX	Epilator, High-Frequency, Tweezer Type	Surgery
78FLB	Meter, Conductivity, Induction, Remote Type	Gastro/Urology
79KFN	Monitor, Cardiac Output, Thermal (Balloon Type Catheter)	Surgery
74KFM	Pump, Blood, Cardiopulmonary Bypass, Non-Roller Type	Cardiovascular
74DWB	Pump, Blood, Cardiopulmonary Bypass, Roller Type	Cardiovascular
85HHF	Remover, Intrauterine Device, Contraceptive (Hook Type)	Obstetrics/Gyn
79RXS	Retractor, Fan-Type, Laparoscopy	Surgery
88KIN	Stainer, Slide, Contact Type	Pathology
88KIO	Stainer, Slide, Immersion Type	Pathology
78FLC	Station, Dialysis Control, Negative Pressure Type	Gastro/Urology

TYPES

83GMZ	Antigen, All Types, Escherichia Coli	Microbiology
83GTN	Antisera, Fluorescent, All Types, Staphylococcus SPP.	Microbiology
83GQE	Antisera, Neutralization, All Types, Rhinovirus	Microbiology
80FMH	Container, Specimen, All Types	General
83GTK	Enterotoxins, All Types, Staphylococcal	Microbiology
83GTL	Phages, Staphylococcal Typing, All Types	Microbiology
76EIG	Retractor, All Types	Dental And Oral
75UKC	Standard/Control, All Types	Chemistry

TYPHUS

83GPO	Antigen, CF, Typhus Fever Group	Microbiology
83GPM	Antiserum, Murine Typhus Fever	Microbiology
83GPN	Antiserum, Typhus Fever	Microbiology

TYPING

82DGS	Antigen, Antiserum, Control, Lymphocyte Typing	Immunology
81UJY	Antiserum, ABO Blood Grouping	Hematology
81MVS	Kit, Typing, Hla-dqb	Hematology
83GTL	Phages, Staphylococcal Typing, All Types	Microbiology
88HYJ	Stain, Hematoxylin	Pathology
88HYK	Stain, Hematoxylin, Harris's	Pathology
88HYL	Stain, Hematoxylin, Mayer's	Pathology
81LGO	Test, Leukocyte Typing	Hematology
81SEY	View Box, Rh Typing	Hematology

TYROSINE

75CDR	1-Nitroso-2-Naphthol (Fluorometric), Free Tyrosine	Chemistry
75JKW	N-Acetyl-L-Tyrosine Ethyl Ester (U.V.), Chymotrypsin	Chemistry
75JKX	N-Benzoyl-L-Tyrosine Ethyl Ester (U.V.), Chymotrypsin	Chemistry

TYVEK

80WMY	Clothing, Protective	General

U.V.

76EBZ	Activator, Ultraviolet, Polymerization	Dental And Oral
75JMK	Alpha-Ketobutyric Acid And NADH (U.V.), Hydroxybutyric	Chemistry
75UJB	Analyzer, Ultraviolet	Chemistry
75JNK	Beta-D-Fructose & NADH Oxidation (U.V.), Sorbitol DH	Chemistry
89LEJ	Booth, Sun Tan	Physical Med
75UJG	Cabinet, Chromatography (U.V.) Viewing	Chemistry
80QFI	Cabinet, Treatment, Ultraviolet	General
75UHI	Chamber, Ultraviolet Polymerization	Chemistry
76EAQ	Detector, Ultraviolet	Dental And Oral
80QQA	Disinfector, Pasteurization	General
75JLT	Enzymatic (U.V.), Pyruvic Acid	Chemistry
91DMT	Enzymatic Method, Alcohol Dehydrogenase, Ultraviolet	Toxicology
81JMH	Fluorescence, Visual Observation (Qual., U.V.), Gsh	Hematology
75CJC	Fructose-1, 6-Diphosphate And NADH (U.V.), Aldolase	Chemistry
81JBK	Glucose-6-Phos. Dehydrogenase (Erythrocytic), U.V. Kinetic	Hematology
76EAR	Illuminator, Ultraviolet	Dental And Oral
75JKG	L-Isocitrate And NADP (U.V.), Isocitric Dehydrogenase	Chemistry
80REE	Lamp, Ultraviolet (Spectrum A)	General
80RED	Lamp, Ultraviolet, Germicidal	General
89IOB	Lamp, Ultraviolet, Physical Medicine	Physical Med
91DJS	Light, U.V., TLC	Toxicology
79FTC	Light, Ultraviolet, Dermatologic	Surgery
88IBK	Microscope, Fluorescence/U.V.	Pathology

KEYWORD INDEX
80FLG	Cleaner, Ultrasonic, Medical Instrument	General
90VHG	Computer, Ultrasound	Radiology
90WUK	Copier, Image, Radiographic	Radiology
84JXJ	Cutter, Bone, Ultrasonic	Cns/Neurology

ULTRASONIC *(cont'd)*

74ULR	Detector, Blood Flow, Ultrasonic (Doppler)	Cardiovascular
90TDC	Detector, Metal, Ultrasonic	Radiology
78MIK	Device, Ablation, Thermal, Ultrasonic	Gastro/Urology
86LZR	Device, Cyclodestructive, Ultrasonic	Ophthalmology
74MEZ	Device, Debridement, Ultrasonic, Heart Valve & HV Seat	Cardiovascular
89LXF	Diathermy, Ultrasonic (Non-Beep Heat)	Physical Med
89IMI	Diathermy, Ultrasonic (Physical Therapy)	Physical Med
83VFS	Disrupter, Cell	Microbiology
74WSD	Doppler, Blood Flow, Transcranial	Cardiovascular
74DXK	Echocardiograph (Ultrasonic Scanner)	Cardiovascular
84GXW	Echoencephalograph (Ultrasonic Scanner)	Cns/Neurology
78VJF	Endoscope, Ultrasonic Probe (Lithotriptor)	Gastro/Urology
78QWP	Flowmeter, Blood, Ultrasonic	Gastro/Urology
74CAS	Flowmeter, Blood, Ultrasonic, Transcutaneous (W/WO Calibr.)	Cardiovascular
89QYF	Gel, Ultrasonic Coupling	Physical Med
80SDY	Gel, Ultrasonic Transmission	General
80WXY	Guide, Device, Ultrasonic	General
83RAE	Homogenizer, Tissue	Microbiology
80QDT	Kit, Biopsy, Ultrasonic Aspiration	General
78WIL	Lithotriptor, Multipurpose	Gastro/Urology
78FEO	Lithotriptor, Ultrasonic	Gastro/Urology
85HHJ	Locator, Intracorporeal Device, Ultrasonic	Obstetrics/Gyn
80SDX	Meter, Ultrasonic Power	General
73CBA	Monitor, Air Embolism, Ultrasonic	Anesthesiology
80WHP	Sink, Sonic	General
79FXD	Stethoscope, Direct (Acoustic), Ultrasonic	Surgery
89LPQ	Stimulator, Muscle, Ultrasonic (Non-Beep Heat)	Physical Med
87JDX	Surgical Instrument, Sonic	Orthopedics
85WOP	Transducer, Ultrasonic, Intravaginal	Obstetrics/Gyn
85HGL	Transducer, Ultrasonic, Obstetrical	Obstetrics/Gyn
90WTF	Unit, Imaging, Thermal	Radiology
86WOM	Vision Aid, Ultrasonic	Ophthalmology
80WLV	Warmer, Gel	General
75UJA	Washer, Pipette, Ultrasonic	Chemistry

ULTRASOUND

90WPC	Calibrator, Beam	Radiology
74QMA	Computer, Cardiac Catheterization Laboratory	Cardiovascular
90WKA	Computer, Radiographic Data	Radiology
90VHG	Computer, Ultrasound	Radiology
79WHN	Cover, Probe, Transducer	Surgery
86LZR	Device, Cyclodestructive, Ultrasonic	Ophthalmology
77LWI	Device, Ultrasound, Sinus	Ear/Nose/Throat
85LQT	Equipment, Ultrasound, Doppler, Evaluation, Fetal	Obstetrics/Gyn
74WYD	Equipment, Ultrasound, Intravascular, 3-Dimensional	Cardiovascular
85LXE	Fetal Doppler Ultrasound	Obstetrics/Gyn

ULTRASOUND *(cont'd)*

90LNB	Hyperthermia Applicator, Deep Heating, Ultrasound	Radiology
90LND	Hyperthermia Applicator, Superficial, Ultrasound	Radiology
90MJS	Media, Contrast, Ultrasound	Radiology
85MAA	Monitor, Fetal Doppler Ultrasound	Obstetrics/Gyn
90RKQ	Phantom, Ultrasound	Radiology
89IMG	Stimulator, Ultrasound, Muscle	Physical Med
80WNI	Table, Ultrasound	General
90LSY	Ultrasound, Hyperthermia, Cancer Treatment	Radiology

ULTRAVIOLET

76EBZ	Activator, Ultraviolet, Polymerization	Dental And Oral
75JMK	Alpha-Ketobutyric Acid And NADH (U.V.), Hydroxybutyric	Chemistry
75UJB	Analyzer, Ultraviolet	Chemistry
75JNK	Beta-D-Fructose & NADH Oxidation (U.V.), Sorbitol DH	Chemistry
89LEJ	Booth, Sun Tan	Physical Med
75UJG	Cabinet, Chromatography (U.V.) Viewing	Chemistry
80QFI	Cabinet, Treatment, Ultraviolet	General
75UHI	Chamber, Ultraviolet Polymerization	Chemistry
76EAQ	Detector, Ultraviolet	Dental And Oral
80MKB	Device, Germicidal, Ultraviolet	General
80QQA	Disinfector, Pasteurization	General
75JLT	Enzymatic (U.V.), Pyruvic Acid	Chemistry
91DMT	Enzymatic Method, Alcohol Dehydrogenase, Ultraviolet	Toxicology
81JMH	Fluorescence, Visual Observation (Qual., U.V.), Gsh	Hematology
75CJC	Fructose-1, 6-Diphosphate And NADH (U.V.), Aldolase	Chemistry
86WHZ	Goggles, Protective, Eye	Ophthalmology
76EAR	Illuminator, Ultraviolet	Dental And Oral
75JKG	L-Isocitrate And NADP (U.V.), Isocitric Dehydrogenase	Chemistry
80REE	Lamp, Ultraviolet (Spectrum A)	General
80RED	Lamp, Ultraviolet, Germicidal	General
89IOB	Lamp, Ultraviolet, Physical Medicine	Physical Med
91DJS	Light, U.V., TLC	Toxicology
79FTC	Light, Ultraviolet, Dermatologic	Surgery
88IBK	Microscope, Fluorescence/U.V.	Pathology
91JXQ	Monitor, U.V., GLC	Toxicology
75JKW	N-Acetyl-L-Tyrosine Ethyl Ester (U.V.), Chymotrypsin	Chemistry
75JNO	N-Benzoyl-L-Arginine Ethyl Ester (U.V.), Trypsin	Chemistry
75JKX	N-Benzoyl-L-Tyrosine Ethyl Ester (U.V.), Chymotrypsin	Chemistry
75KLJ	NAD Reduction (U.V.), Phosphohexose Isomerase	Chemistry
81JMC	NADP Reduction (U.V.), Glucose-6-Phosphate Dehydrogenase	Hematology
75JLZ	Nadh, Phosphoglycerate Mutase, Atp (u.v.) 2, 3-diphosphoglyceric Acid	Chemistry
75JMS	Oxalacetic Acid And NADH Oxidation (U.V.), Maleic DH	Chemistry
75JNN	P-Toluenesulphonyl-L-Arginine Methyl Ester (U.V.), Trypsin	Chemistry
75SGB	Purification System, Water, Ultraviolet	Chemistry
80FRA	Purifier, Air, Ultraviolet	General
80VDS	Radiometer, Ultraviolet	General
75CIQ	SGOT, Ultraviolet	Chemistry
75CKA	SGPT, Ultraviolet	Chemistry
75UHX	Scanner, Ultraviolet	Chemistry
75RUO	Spectrophotometer, U.V./Visible	Chemistry
75RUN	Spectrophotometer, Ultraviolet	Chemistry
75UJC	Standard, Ultraviolet Reference	Chemistry
80RVY	Sterilizer, Ultraviolet	General
75JLI	Tetrahydrofolate, Enzymatic (U.V.), Formiminoglutamic Acid	Chemistry
75JHW	U.V. Method, CPK Isoenzymes	Chemistry
91LDB	U.V. Spectrometry, Carbamazepine	Toxicology
91LDC	U.V. Spectrometry, Diphenylhydantoin	Toxicology
91LDA	U.V. Spectrometry, Phenobarbital	Toxicology
91LCZ	U.V. Spectrometry, Primidone	Toxicology
91LCY	U.V. Spectrometry, Theophylline	Toxicology
91LFH	U.V. Spectrometry, Tricyclic Antidepressant Drugs	Toxicology
75JLJ	UDP-Glucose, NAD (U.V.), Gal-I-P Uridyl Transperase	Chemistry
76MCF	Unit, Sanitation/Sterilization, Toothbrush, Ultraviolet	Dental And Oral
75CDO	Uricase (U.V.), Uric Acid	Chemistry
80KMG	Water Purifier, Ultraviolet	General

UMBILICAL

80FOS	Catheter, Umbilical Artery	General
85HFW	Clamp, Umbilical	Obstetrics/Gyn
79WZZ	Dilator, Fascia, Umbilical	Surgery
85REZ	Ligator, Umbilical	Obstetrics/Gyn
80FOD	Occluder, Umbilical	General
85HDJ	Scissors, Umbilical	Obstetrics/Gyn
80RZI	Tape, Umbilical	General
78EXM	Truss, Umbilical	Gastro/Urology

UNASSAYED

75JJX	Control, Analyte (Assayed And Unassayed)	Chemistry
75JJR	Control, Electrolyte (Assayed And Unassayed)	Chemistry
75JJT	Control, Enzyme (Assayed And Unassayed)	Chemistry
75JJY	Control, Multi Analyte, All Kinds (Assayed And Unassayed)	Chemistry
75JJW	Control, Urinalysis (Assayed And Unassayed)	Chemistry

UNATTACHED

73KHC	Filter, Tobacco Smoke (Unattached)	Anesthesiology

UNBOUND

75MQM	Bilirubin (Total and Unbound) Neonate Test System	Chemistry

UNCALIBRATED

73CBC	Bottle, Collection, Breathing System (Uncalibrated)	Anesthesiology

UNCEMENTED

87MBE	Bone, Block, Filler, Metal, Porous, Uncemented	Orthopedics
87MBK	Prosthesis, Ankle, Semi-, Uncemented, Porous, Metal/Polymer	Orthopedics
87KWE	Prosthesis, Finger, Constrained, Metal, Uncemented	Orthopedics
87MBL	Prosthesis, Hip, Semi-, Uncemented, Osteophilic Finish	Orthopedics
87MAZ	Prosthesis, Hip, Semi-Const., M/P, Por. Uncem., Calc./Phos.	Orthopedics
87LPH	Prosthesis, Hip, Semi-Const., Metal/Poly., Porous Uncemented	Orthopedics
87MIL	Prosthesis, Hip, Semi-Const., Uncem., M/P, Bone Morph. Prot.	Orthopedics
87MEH	Prosthesis, Hip, Semi-Const., Uncem., Non-P., M/P, Ca./Phos.	Orthopedics
87LWJ	Prosthesis, Hip, Semi-Constrained, Metal/Polymer, Uncemented	Orthopedics
87MRA	Prosthesis, Hip, Semi-constrained, Metal/ Ceramic/ Ceramic/ Metal, Cemented or Uncemented	Orthopedics
87MBM	Prosthesis, Hip, Semi/Hemi-Const., M/PTFE Ctd./P, Cem./Unc.	Orthopedics
87MBG	Prosthesis, Knee, Femotib., Unconst., Uncem., Unicond., M/P	Orthopedics
87HTG	Prosthesis, Knee, Hemi-, Patellar Resurfacing, Uncemented	Orthopedics
87KRS	Prosthesis, Knee, Hemi-, Tibial Resurfacing	Orthopedics
87HSH	Prosthesis, Knee, Hemi-, Tibial Resurfacing, Uncemented	Orthopedics
87MBD	Prosthesis, Knee, P/F, Unconst., Uncem., Por., Ctd., P/M/P	Orthopedics
87MBV	Prosthesis, Knee, Patfem., S-C., UHMWPE, Pegged, Unc., P/M/P	Orthopedics
87MBH	Prosthesis, Knee, Patfem., S-C., Unc., Por., Ctd., P/M/P	Orthopedics
87MBA	Prosthesis, Knee, Patfem., Semi-Const., Unc., P/M/P, Osteo.	Orthopedics
87LXY	Prosthesis, Knee, Patfemotib., Semi-Const., P/M/P, Uncem.	Orthopedics
87MBF	Prosthesis, Shoulder, Metal/Polymer, Uncemented	Orthopedics
87KYL	Prosthesis, Shoulder, Semi-Constrained, Uncemented	Orthopedics

UNCOMPENSATED

73BYM	Tube, Thorpe, Uncompensated	Anesthesiology

UNCONSTRAINED

87MBG	Prosthesis, Knee, Femotib., Unconst., Uncem., Unicond., M/P	Orthopedics
87MBD	Prosthesis, Knee, P/F, Unconst., Uncem., Por., Ctd., P/M/P	Orthopedics

UNDERPAD

80RBU	Pad, Incontinence (Underpad)	General

UNDIFFERENTIATED

88MHQ	Panel, Tumor, Undifferentiated	Pathology

UNI-DIRECTIONAL

78FIF	Kit, Dialysis, Single Needle With Uni-Directional Pump	Gastro/Urology

UNICONDYLER

87MBG	Prosthesis, Knee, Femotib., Unconst., Uncem., Unicond., M/P	Orthopedics

UNIFORM

79FYF	Cap, Surgical	Surgery
80WMY	Clothing, Protective	General
80VKC	Coat, Laboratory	General
79RXN	Cover, Head, Surgical	Surgery
79FXP	Cover, Shoe, Operating Room	Surgery
79RRV	Dress, Scrub, Disposable	Surgery
79RRW	Dress, Scrub, Reusable	Surgery
79FYE	Dress, Surgical	Surgery
88QYH	Glove, Autopsy	Pathology
80FPI	Glove, Surgical	General
80QYI	Glove, Surgical, Hypoallergenic	General
79KGO	Glove, Surgical, Plastic Surgery	Surgery
80QYJ	Glove, Utility	General
80FME	Gown, Examination	General
79FYC	Gown, Isolation, Surgical	Surgery
79FPH	Gown, Operating Room, Disposable	Surgery
79QYN	Gown, Operating Room, Reusable	Surgery
80QYQ	Gown, Other	General
79FYA	Gown, Surgical	Surgery
79FXY	Hood, Surgical	Surgery
73BWP	Shoe And Shoe Cover, Conductive	Anesthesiology
79RSX	Shoe, Conductive	Surgery
79FXW	Shoe, Operating Room	Surgery

UNIFORM *(cont'd)*
79RRY Suit, Scrub, Disposable — Surgery
79RRZ Suit, Scrub, Reusable — Surgery
79FXO Suit, Surgical — Surgery

UNINTERRUPTIBLE
80WMN Power Systems, Uninterruptible (UPS) — General
80WMM Regulator, Line Voltage — General

UNIPOLAR
85HFG Coagulator, Laparoscopic, Unipolar — Obstetrics/Gyn
85KNF Coagulator/Cutter, Endoscopic, Unipolar — Obstetrics/Gyn
87JDA Prosthesis, Elbow, Non-Constrained, Unipolar — Orthopedics
79SGV Scissors, Laparoscopy, Unipolar, Electrosurgical — Surgery

UNIT
79QTR Adapter, Electrosurgical Unit, Cable — Surgery
79QTS Adapter, Unit, Electrosurgical, Hand-Controlled — Surgery
80WNB Amputation Protection Unit — General
80WRI Analgesia Unit, Cryogenic — General
89VEM Analyzer, Diathermy Unit, Shortwave — Physical Med
79QTT Analyzer, Electrosurgical Unit — Surgery
80SDZ Analyzer, Ultrasonic Unit — General
74QBM Arteriographic Unit, Ultrasonic — Cardiovascular
74QBV Aspirator, Thoracic (Suction Unit) — Cardiovascular
73CAC Autotransfusion Unit (Blood) — Anesthesiology
90VGM Battery, Mobile Radiographic Unit — Radiology
79QTU Cable, Electrosurgical Unit — Surgery
73QFN Calibrator, Anesthesia Unit — Anesthesiology
73QFQ Calibrator, Respiratory Therapy Unit — Anesthesiology
74QGK Cardiac Output Unit, Direct Fick — Cardiovascular
74UDP Cardiac Output Unit, Dye Dilution — Cardiovascular
74QGL Cardiac Output Unit, Indicator Dilution (Thermal) — Cardiovascular
74QGM Cardiac Output Unit, Other — Cardiovascular
74TAV Cardiac Output Unit, Radioisotope Probe — Cardiovascular
76QHD Casting Unit, Dental — Dental And Oral
76KLC Chair, Dental (With Unit) — Dental And Oral
89IMF Chilling Unit — Physical Med
74QKD Circulatory Assist Unit, Cardiac — Cardiovascular
74QKE Circulatory Assist Unit, Intra-Aortic Balloon — Cardiovascular
74DSQ Circulatory Assist Unit, Left Ventricular — Cardiovascular
74QKF Circulatory Assist Unit, Venous Return — Cardiovascular
78UCO Clamp, Hemodialysis Unit Blood Line — Gastro/Urology
74QLZ Compression Unit, Intermittent (Anti-Embolism Pump) — Cardiovascular
73QMH Continuous Positive Airway Pressure Unit (CPAP, CPPB) — Anesthesiology
83RGS Contrast Enhancement Unit, Microscope — Microbiology
85HGG Controller, Abortion Unit, Vacuum — Obstetrics/Gyn
78QZY Controller, Hemodialysis Unit Single Needle — Gastro/Urology
78QZZ Converter, Unit, Hemodialysis, Single-Pass — Gastro/Urology
86HPS Cryophthalmic Unit — Ophthalmology
86HRN Cryophthalmic Unit, AC-Powered — Ophthalmology
79GEH Cryosurgical Unit — Surgery
85HGJ Cryosurgical Unit, Gynecologic — Obstetrics/Gyn
84GXH Cryosurgical Unit, Neurological — Cns/Neurology
79FAZ Cryosurgical, Unit, Urology — Surgery
86HQA Cryotherapy, Unit, Ophthalmic — Ophthalmology
76VEH Curing Unit, Acrylic — Dental And Oral
79QPC Dermabrasion Unit — Surgery
78QZV Detector, Hemodialysis Unit Air Bubble-Foam — Gastro/Urology
78LOA Device, Hypothermia, Testicular — Gastro/Urology
78QPJ Dialysis Unit Test Equipment — Gastro/Urology
80VDP Dispenser, Liquid, Unit-Dose — General
75QQF Distilling Unit — Chemistry
75UFX Distilling Unit, Molecular — Chemistry
80SED Drainage Unit, Urinary — General
75JRJ Drying Unit — Chemistry
79QSK Electrocautery Unit, Battery-Powered — Surgery
85HIM Electrocautery Unit, Endoscopic — Obstetrics/Gyn
85HGI Electrocautery Unit, Gynecologic — Obstetrics/Gyn
79QSL Electrocautery Unit, Line-Powered — Surgery
84GXC Electroconvulsive Therapy Unit (Electroshock) — Cns/Neurology
86HPY Electrolysis Unit, Battery-Powered, Ophthalmic — Ophthalmology
86HRO Electrolysis Unit, Ophthalmic — Ophthalmology
79BWA Electrosurgical Unit, Anesthesiology Accessories — Surgery
74DWG Electrosurgical Unit, Cardiovascular — Cardiovascular
79GEI Electrosurgical Unit, Cutting & Coagulation Device — Surgery
76EKZ Electrosurgical Unit, Dental — Dental And Oral
78FAR Electrosurgical Unit, Gastroenterology — Gastro/Urology
79QTV Electrosurgical Unit, General Purpose (ESU) — Surgery
84HAM Electrosurgical Unit, Neurological — Cns/Neurology
78KNS Electrosurgical, Unit, Gastroenterology — Gastro/Urology
80QTW Electrotherapeutic Unit — General
89ITH Equipment, Traction, Powered — Physical Med
84VDA Evoked Potential Unit, Audiometric — Cns/Neurology
84QUT Evoked Response Unit — Cns/Neurology
77ETZ Evoked Response Unit, Auditory — Ear/Nose/Throat
89LBG Fluidized Therapy, Unit, Dry Heat — Physical Med
89LSB Fluidotherapy Unit — Physical Med

UNIT *(cont'd)*
73ELI Gas-Machine, Analgesia — Anesthesiology
73BSZ Gas-Machine, Anesthesia — Anesthesiology
74JOR Generator, Pulsatile Flow, Cardiopulmonary Bypass — Cardiovascular
80QYG Glove Processing Unit (Drying, Powdering) — General
90UFC Handling Unit, Automatic Daylight X-Ray Film — Radiology
74QZM Heart-Lung Bypass Unit (Cardiopulmonary) — Cardiovascular
89IRQ Heating Unit, Powered — Physical Med
78RAA Hemodialysis Unit (Kidney Machine) — Gastro/Urology
78RAB Hemofiltration Unit — Gastro/Urology
90RAY Hyperthermia Unit, Microwave — Radiology
80RBA Hypo/Hyperthermia Unit, Central — General
80RBB Hypo/Hyperthermia Unit, Mobile — General
80RBC Hypothermia Unit — General
73BTF Hypothermia Unit (Blanket, Plumbing & Heat Exchanger) — Anesthesiology
87THB Inversion Unit — Orthopedics
78RCP Iontophoresis Unit (Sweat Rate) — Gastro/Urology
89KTB Iontophoresis Unit, Physical Medicine — Physical Med
80FRT Isolation Unit, Surgical — General
80FLJ Laminar Air Flow Unit — General
75RDW Laminar Air Flow Unit, Fixed (Air Curtain) — Chemistry
75RDX Laminar Air Flow Unit, Mobile — Chemistry
78REK Lavage Unit — Gastro/Urology
77REM Lavage Unit, ENT — Ear/Nose/Throat
77REL Lavage Unit, Oral — Ear/Nose/Throat
79REN Lavage Unit, Surgical — Surgery
80FQH Lavage Unit, Water Jet — General
89RFO Magnetic Unit, Therapeutic — Physical Med
74DTW Monitor, Cardiopulmonary Level Sensing — Cardiovascular
78QZX Monitor, Hemodialysis Unit Conductivity — Gastro/Urology
80WKH Monitor, Medication — General
76EIA Operative Dental Treatment Unit — Dental And Oral
80VDO Packaging System, Unit-Dose — General
80RKB Patient Transfer Unit — General
80FRZ Patient Transfer Unit, Powered — General
80FSB Perfusion Unit — General
78RKL Peritoneal Dialysis Unit (CAPD) — Gastro/Urology
86HQC Phacofragmentation Unit — Ophthalmology
80RKZ Phototherapy Unit (Bilirubin Lamp) — General
80LBI Phototherapy Unit, Neonatal — General
76DZY Prophylaxis Unit, Ultrasonic, Dental — Dental And Oral
85HGF Pump, Abortion Unit, Vacuum — Obstetrics/Gyn
78QZW Pump, Blood, Hemodialysis Unit — Gastro/Urology
90KPR Radiographic Unit, Diagnostic — Radiology
90QJT Radiographic Unit, Diagnostic, Chest — Radiology
76RNY Radiographic Unit, Diagnostic, Dental (X-Ray) — Dental And Oral
76EHD Radiographic Unit, Diagnostic, Dental, Extraoral — Dental And Oral
90RNZ Radiographic Unit, Diagnostic, Fixed (X-Ray) — Radiology
90TEA Radiographic Unit, Diagnostic, Head — Radiology
76EAP Radiographic Unit, Diagnostic, Intraoral — Dental And Oral
90IZH Radiographic Unit, Diagnostic, Mammographic — Radiology
90IZK Radiographic Unit, Diagnostic, Mobile, Explosion-Safe — Radiology
90IZG Radiographic Unit, Diagnostic, Photofluorographic — Radiology
90VGJ Radiographic Unit, Diagnostic, Pneumoencephalographic — Radiology
90VGK Radiographic Unit, Diagnostic, Polytomographic — Radiology
90ROB Radiographic Unit, Diagnostic, Portable (X-Ray) — Radiology
90VGL Radiographic Unit, Diagnostic, Skeletal — Radiology
90IZF Radiographic Unit, Diagnostic, Tomographic — Radiology
90TGL Radiographic Unit, Digital — Radiology
90VLE Radiographic Unit, Digital Subtraction Angiographic (DSA) — Radiology
90IZI Radiographic/Fluoroscopic Unit, Angiographic — Radiology
90VHC Radiographic/Fluoroscopic Unit, Angiographic, Digital — Radiology
90QWR Radiographic/Fluoroscopic Unit, Fixed — Radiology
90JAA Radiographic/Fluoroscopic Unit, Image-Intensified — Radiology
90QWS Radiographic/Fluoroscopic Unit, Mobile C-Arm — Radiology
90JAB Radiographic/Fluoroscopic Unit, Non-Image-Intensified — Radiology
90THR Radiographic/Fluoroscopic Unit, Special Procedure — Radiology
90ROG Radiotherapy Treatment Planning Unit — Radiology
90LHN Radiotherapy Unit, Charged-Particle — Radiology
73BYW Rebreathing Unit — Anesthesiology
78VHO Reprocessing Unit, Dialyzer — Gastro/Urology
89RQF Rowing Unit — Physical Med
73QBA Scavenger, Gas, Anesthesia Unit — Anesthesiology
77RUT Speech Therapy Unit (Trainer) — Ear/Nose/Throat
79GAG Stapler, Surgical — Surgery
84RVR Sterotaxic Unit — Cns/Neurology
90UAB Storage Unit, X-Ray Film — Radiology
90RYK Synchronizer, Radiographic Unit — Radiology
76ECB Syringe Unit, Air And/Or Water — Dental And Oral
90LOC System, Cancer Treatment, Hyperthermia, RF/Microwave — Radiology
80SGR System, Delivery, Drug, Unit-Dose — General
90IZL System, X-Ray, Mobile — Radiology
74RZJ Telemetry Unit, Physiological, ECG — Cardiovascular
84RZK Telemetry Unit, Physiological, EEG — Cns/Neurology
89RZL Telemetry Unit, Physiological, EMG — Physical Med
84RZM Telemetry Unit, Physiological, EOG — Cns/Neurology
80TEZ Telemetry Unit, Physiological, Multiple Channel — General

UNIT *(cont'd)*

84GYE	Telemetry Unit, Physiological, Neurological	Cns/Neurology
80RZN	Telemetry Unit, Physiological, Pressure	General
80RZO	Telemetry Unit, Physiological, Temperature	General
77ETY	Tester, Auditory Impedance	Ear/Nose/Throat
90JAD	Therapeutic X-Ray System	Radiology
75SAO	Thyroid Function Unit	Chemistry
87VDE	Tracing Unit, Arch	Orthopedics
87HSR	Traction Unit, Hip, Non-Powered, Non-Penetrating	Orthopedics
87HST	Traction Unit, Non-Powered	Orthopedics
87SBN	Traction Unit, Powered, Mobile	Orthopedics
87SBO	Traction Unit, Static, Bed	Orthopedics
87SBP	Traction Unit, Static, Chair	Orthopedics
87SBQ	Traction Unit, Static, Other	Orthopedics
81KSB	Transfer Unit, Blood	Hematology
80LHI	Transfer Unit, IV Fluid	General
90ROD	Transfer Unit, Radioisotope	Radiology
74DWE	Tube, Pump, Cardiopulmonary Bypass	Cardiovascular
78LNN	Unit, Anastomosis, Gastroenterologic	Gastro/Urology
76LWM	Unit, Anesthesia, Dental, Electric	Dental And Oral
80WPL	Unit, Control, Bed, Patient, Powered	General
74WIU	Unit, Cooling, Cardiac	Cardiovascular
87REX	Unit, Evaluation, Height, Lift	Orthopedics
86WNU	Unit, Examination, Lens, Contact	Ophthalmology
77ETF	Unit, Examining/Treatment, ENT	Ear/Nose/Throat
75JRL	Unit, Filter, Membrane	Chemistry
90WTF	Unit, Imaging, Thermal	Radiology
77EWN	Unit, Measuring, Potential, Evoked, Auditory	Ear/Nose/Throat
78WYF	Unit, Microwave, Transurethral	Gastro/Urology
89WWS	Unit, Pad, Heating, Portable	Physical Med
86HRL	Unit, Radiation, Beta, Ophthalmic	Ophthalmology
84LSS	Unit, Repair, Nerve, Implantable, Electric	Cns/Neurology
76MCF	Unit, Sanitation/Sterilization, Toothbrush, Ultraviolet	Dental And Oral
89QAP	Unit, Support, Ambulation	Physical Med
77WXX	Unit, Testing, Hearing, Intraoperative	Ear/Nose/Throat
80QDG	Unit, Therapy, Behavior	General
84LIH	Unit, Therapy, Current, Interferential	Cns/Neurology
77SAT	Unit, Therapy, Tinnitus	Ear/Nose/Throat
74MFV	Unit, Transport, Organ	Cardiovascular
73QBB	Ventilator, Anesthesia Unit	Anesthesiology
90WJC	Videofluoroscopic Unit	Radiology
80SFS	Waste Disposal Unit, Sharps	General
79KDB	Waste Disposal Unit, Surgical Instrument (Sharps)	Surgery
80SFT	Waste Disposal Unit, Syringe	General

UNIT-DOSE

80VDP	Dispenser, Liquid, Unit-Dose	General
80VDO	Packaging System, Unit-Dose	General
80SGR	System, Delivery, Drug, Unit-Dose	General

UNIVERSAL

80QRC	Dressing, Universal	General

UNLOADER

80WVS	Unloader, Cart	General

UNPOWERED

78FIA	Chair, Dialysis, Unpowered (Without Scale)	Gastro/Urology

UNSCENTED

85HHD	Pad, Menstrual, Unscented	Obstetrics/Gyn
85HEB	Tampon, Menstrual, Unscented	Obstetrics/Gyn

UPPER

78EYC	Catheter, Upper Urinary Tract	Gastro/Urology
87WUW	Immobilizer, Upper Body	Orthopedics
87JDD	Prosthesis, Upper Femoral	Orthopedics

UPS

80WMN	Power Systems, Uninterruptible (UPS)	General
80WMM	Regulator, Line Voltage	General

UPTAKE

73BZL	Computer, Oxygen-Uptake	Anesthesiology
90IZD	Probe, Uptake, Nuclear	Radiology
75KHQ	Radioassay, Triiodothyronine Uptake	Chemistry
75CDY	Radioimmunoassay, T3 Uptake	Chemistry
90VGR	Thyroid Uptake System	Radiology

URANYL

75CEI	Uranyl Acetate/Zinc Acetate, Sodium	Chemistry

UREA

75QES	Analyzer, BUN (Blood Urea Nitrogen)	Chemistry
75LFP	Conductivity Rate, Urea Nitrogen	Chemistry
75CDW	Diacetyl-Monoxime, Urea Nitrogen	Chemistry
75CDS	Electrode, Ion Specific, Urea Nitrogen	Chemistry
75CDL	Indophenol, Berthelot, Urea Nitrogen	Chemistry
75JGZ	O-Phthalaldehyde, Urea Nitrogen	Chemistry
75UMB	Reagent, Blood Urea Nitrogen (BUN)	Chemistry
83MSQ	Test, Urea (Breath or Blood)	Microbiology

UREASE

75CDQ	Urease And Glutamic Dehydrogenase, Urea Nitrogen	Chemistry
75CDN	Urease, Photometric, Urea Nitrogen	Chemistry

URETERAL

78EYI	Adapter, Catheter, Ureteral	Gastro/Urology
78FCS	Catheter, Light, Fiberoptic, Glass, Ureteral	Gastro/Urology
78FGF	Catheter, Ureteral Disposable (X-Ray)	Gastro/Urology
78EYB	Catheter, Ureteral, Gastro-Urology	Gastro/Urology
79GBL	Catheter, Ureteral, General & Plastic Surgery	Surgery
78EYK	Connector, Ureteral Catheter	Gastro/Urology
78EZN	Dilator, Catheter, Ureteral	Gastro/Urology
78FFL	Dislodger, Stone, Basket, Ureteral, Metal	Gastro/Urology
78WSU	Lithotriptor, Laser	Gastro/Urology
78FAB	Replacer, Ureteral	Gastro/Urology
78FAD	Splint, Ureteral	Gastro/Urology
85UAN	Stent, Other	Obstetrics/Gyn
78UAM	Stent, Ureteral	Gastro/Urology
78EYA	Stylet, Ureteral	Gastro/Urology

URETEROENDOSCOPE

78QIL	Ureteroendoscope	Gastro/Urology

URETEROSCOPE

78QIL	Ureteroendoscope	Gastro/Urology
78FGB	Ureteroscope	Gastro/Urology

URETEROSTOMY

78EXG	Bag, Urinary Collection, Ureterostomy	Gastro/Urology

URETEROTOME

78SEA	Ureterotome	Gastro/Urology

URETEROVESICLE

78FAC	Valve, Ureterovesicle	Gastro/Urology

URETHANE

80VKF	Tubing, Urethane	General

URETHRAL

78GBM	Catheter, Urethral	Gastro/Urology
78QIQ	Catheter, Urethral, Diagnostic	Gastro/Urology
78MNG	Device, Incontinence, Occlusion, Urethral	Gastro/Urology
78KOE	Dilator, Urethral	Gastro/Urology
78FAH	Dilator, Urethral, Mechanical	Gastro/Urology
78FCM	Kit, Catheterization, Sterile Urethral	Gastro/Urology
78FAG	Prosthesis, Urethral Sphincter	Gastro/Urology
78FAA	Replacer, Urethral	Gastro/Urology
78FBX	Sound, Urethral, Metal Or Plastic	Gastro/Urology
85UAN	Stent, Other	Obstetrics/Gyn
78MES	Stent, Urethral, Bulbous, Permanent/Semi-Permanent	Gastro/Urology
78MER	Stent, Urethral, Prostatic, Permanent/Semi-Permanent	Gastro/Urology

URETHROGRAPHIC

78FGH	Catheter, Double Lumen Female Urethrographic	Gastro/Urology
78FGI	Catheter, Urethrographic, Male	Gastro/Urology

URETHROMETER

78FBR	Urethrometer	Gastro/Urology

URETHROSCOPE

78FAL	Panendoscope (Urethroscope)	Gastro/Urology
78QIL	Ureteroendoscope	Gastro/Urology
78FGC	Urethroscope	Gastro/Urology

URETHROTOME

78EZO	Urethrotome	Gastro/Urology

URIC

75LFQ	Acid Reduction Of Ferric Ion, Uric Acid	Chemistry
75CDH	Phosphotungstate Reduction, Uric Acid	Chemistry

URICASE

75KNK	Uricase (Colorimetric), Uric Acid	Chemistry
75JHB	Uricase (Coulometric), Uric Acid	Chemistry
75JHA	Uricase (Gasometric), Uric Acid	Chemistry
75JHC	Uricase (Oxygen Rate), Uric Acid	Chemistry
75CDO	Uricase (U.V.), Uric Acid	Chemistry

URIDYL

75KQP	Fluorescent Proc. (Qual.), Galactose-1-Phosphate Uridyl	Chemistry
75JLJ	UDP-Glucose, NAD (U.V.), Gal-I-P Uridyl Transperase	Chemistry

URINAL

80QNH	Cover, Urinal	General
80FNP	Urinal	General

URINALYSIS

75KQO	Analyzer, Chemistry, Urinalysis	Chemistry
75JJZ	Analyzer, Chemistry, Urinalysis, Automated	Chemistry
75JJW	Control, Urinalysis (Assayed And Unassayed)	Chemistry
75UKD	Stick, Urinalysis Test	Chemistry

KEYWORD INDEX

URINARY
80FON	Bag, Drainage, Ostomy (With Adhesive)	General
78FAQ	Bag, Leg	Gastro/Urology
78QIT	Catheter, Urinary, Irrigation	Gastro/Urology
75CES	Chromogenesis, Phenylketones (Urinary, Non-Quantitative)	Chemistry
83MKS	Device, Detection, Urinary Antibody	Microbiology
75JMT	Diazo (Colorimetric), Nitrite (Urinary, Non-Quantitative)	Chemistry
75CDM	Diazonium Colorimetry, Urobilinogen (Urinary, Non-Quant.)	Chemistry
80SED	Drainage Unit, Urinary	General
75JIP	Enzymatic Method, Blood, Occult, Urinary	Chemistry
75JIL	Enzymatic Method, Glucose (Urinary, Non-Quantitative)	Chemistry
75JGK	Ferric Chloride, Phenylketones (Urinary, Non-Quantitative)	Chemistry
75JIR	Indicator Method, Protein Or Albumin (Urinary, Non-Quant.)	Chemistry
75CEN	Indicator, pH, Dye (Urinary, Non-Quantitative)	Chemistry
75JNP	Infrared Spectroscopy Measurement, Urinary Calculi (Stone)	Chemistry
78QHM	Kit, Catheterization, Urinary	Gastro/Urology
75MPG	Kit, Urinary Carbohydrate Analysis	Chemistry
78FCN	Kit, Urinary Drainage Collection	Gastro/Urology
75JIM	Metallic Reduction Method, Glucose (Urinary, Non-Quant.)	Chemistry
75JIN	Nitroprusside, Ketones (Urinary, Non-Quantitative)	Chemistry
80VLU	Pump, Urinary Collection Bag	General
75JNQ	Qualitative Chemical Reactions, Urinary Calculi (Stone)	Chemistry
84GZD	Stimulator, Spinal Cord, Implantable, Bladder Evacuator	Cns/Neurology
78UAE	Stimulator, Urinary	Gastro/Urology
75LPT	System, Test, Acid, Methylmalonic, Urinary	Chemistry
75JIQ	Turbidimetric Method, Protein Or Albumin (Urinary)	Chemistry
75LPS	Urinary Homocystine (Non-Quantitative) Test System	Chemistry
78SEF	Urodynamic Measurement System	Gastro/Urology
78LJH	Urological Irrigation System	Gastro/Urology

URINE
75VEP	Analyzer, Chemistry, Urine	Chemistry
80FOC	Bag, Collection, Urine, Newborn	General
80SEC	Bag, Urinary Collection, Precision Measure (Urine Meter)	General
78KNX	Collector, Urine	Gastro/Urology
78FFH	Collector, Urine, Disposable	Gastro/Urology
81JIO	Colorimetric, Occult Blood in Urine	Hematology
75MPQ	Container, Specimen, Urine, Drugs Of Abuse, Over The Counter	Chemistry
80SEE	Container, Urine Specimen	General
88LKM	Counter, Urine Particle	Pathology
75QPK	Dialyzer, Serum/Urine	Chemistry
78EYZ	Drainage System, Urine, Closed	Gastro/Urology
80WUM	Encapsulator, Fluid	General
75JIP	Enzymatic Method, Blood, Occult, Urinary	Chemistry
78FFG	Flowmeter, Urine, Disposable	Gastro/Urology
80RGZ	Kit, Mid-Stream Collection	General
83JXA	Kit, Screening, Urine	Microbiology
75JLC	Nitroprusside Reaction (Qualitative, Urine), Cystine	Chemistry
81KHE	Reagent, Occult Blood	Hematology
75JRE	Refractometer	Chemistry
75WTX	Strip, Test	Chemistry
78EXY	Uroflowmeter	Gastro/Urology

UROBILINOGEN
75CDM	Diazonium Colorimetry, Urobilinogen (Urinary, Non-Quant.)	Chemistry

URODYNAMIC
78SEF	Urodynamic Measurement System	Gastro/Urology

UROFLOWMETER
78EXY	Uroflowmeter	Gastro/Urology

UROGRAPHY
90RNP	Pyeloscope	Radiology

UROLOGIC
78SEG	Hanger, Urologic	Gastro/Urology

UROLOGICAL
78KNY	Accessories, Catheter, G-U	Gastro/Urology
78UEE	Table, Urological, Radiographic	Gastro/Urology
78LJH	Urological Irrigation System	Gastro/Urology

UROLOGY
78LNT	Adhesive, Tissue, Gastroenterology/Urology	Gastro/Urology
78LNM	Agent, Bulking, Injectable (Gastro-Urology)	Gastro/Urology
78FGZ	Applicator, Gastro-Urology	Gastro/Urology
78FAT	Bougie, Esophageal, And Gastrointestinal, Gastro-Urology	Gastro/Urology
79FAZ	Cryosurgical, Unit, Urology	Surgery
78EZM	Dilator, Esophageal (Metal Olive) Gastro-Urology	Gastro/Urology
78FHR	Needle, Gastro-Urology	Gastro/Urology
78FGM	Probe, Gastrointestinal	Gastro/Urology
78EZB	Stylet, Catheter, Gastro-Urology	Gastro/Urology
78KOA	Surgical Instrument, G-U, Manual	Gastro/Urology
79EYR	Tourniquet, Gastro-Urology	Surgery
78FBQ	Trocar, Gastro-Urology	Gastro/Urology

UROPORPHYRIN
75JNZ	Fluorometric, Uroporphyrin	Chemistry
75JQL	Spectrophotometric, Uroporphyrin	Chemistry

UROSHEATH
78EXJ	Appliance, Incontinence, Urosheath Type	Gastro/Urology

USE
76EJT	Alloy, Gold Based, For Clinical Use	Dental And Oral
76EJS	Alloy, Precious Metal, For Clinical Use	Dental And Oral
75DOI	Balance (General Use)	Chemistry
91KZQ	Chromatography (Gas), Clinical Use	Toxicology
91KZR	Chromatography (Liquid, Gel), Clinical Use	Toxicology
91KZS	Chromatography (Thin Layer), Clinical Use	Toxicology
75JJQ	Colorimeter, General Use	Chemistry
86LQB	Computer and Software, Medical, Ophthalmic Use	Ophthalmology
91DNR	Counter, Gamma, General Use	Toxicology
75LXG	Equipment, Laboratory, Gen. Purpose (Specific Medical Use)	Chemistry
76MGG	Fluid, Hylan (For TMJ Use)	Dental And Oral
79LRW	General Use Surgical Scissors	Surgery
79LMI	Implant, Collagen (Non-Aesthetic Use)	Surgery
79LMH	Implant, Collagen, Dermal (Aesthetic Use)	Surgery
83SGO	Kit, Gonorrhoeae Test (Male Use)	Microbiology
91DOP	Mass Spectrometer, Clinical Use	Toxicology
91DNB	Meter, pH, General Use	Toxicology
75JRP	Monochromator, for Clinical Use	Chemistry
80MQX	Needle, Acupuncture, Single Use	General
91DMW	Photometer, Flame, General Use	Toxicology
91JXR	Spectrophotometer, Atomic Absorption, General Use	Toxicology
79JCX	Suction Apparatus, Ward Use, Portable, AC-Powered	Surgery
79MDW	Surgical Instrument, Manual (General Use)	Surgery
89UME	Telephone, Handicapped Use	Physical Med
90LHQ	Telethermographic System (Adjunctive Use)	Radiology
80LHA	Timer, Diagnostic Use	General

USED
80WMO	Service, Used Equipment	General

UTENSIL
80RKC	Kit, Admission (Patient Utensil)	General
89ILC	Utensil, Food	Physical Med
89IKW	Utensil, Handicapped Aid	Physical Med
80SFR	Washer, Utensil	General

UTERINE
85HHH	Cannula, Insufflation, Uterine	Obstetrics/Gyn
85LKF	Cannula, Manipulator/Injector, Uterine	Obstetrics/Gyn
85HGH	Cannula, Suction, Uterine	Obstetrics/Gyn
85HGC	Clamp, Uterine	Obstetrics/Gyn
85HCY	Curette, Uterine	Obstetrics/Gyn
85QPV	Dilator, Uterine	Obstetrics/Gyn
85HDP	Elevator, Uterine	Obstetrics/Gyn
85RCF	Injector & Accessories, Manipulator, Uterine	Obstetrics/Gyn
85WSK	Meter, Cavity, Intrauterine	Obstetrics/Gyn
85HFM	Monitor, Uterine Contraction, External	Obstetrics/Gyn
85HDM	Packer, Uterine	Obstetrics/Gyn
85HHI	Pump, Abortion, Vacuum, Central System	Obstetrics/Gyn
85HHM	Sound, Uterine	Obstetrics/Gyn

UTERINE *(cont'd)*

85HDC	Tenaculum, Uterine	Obstetrics/Gyn

UTEROTUBAL

85HES	Insufflator, Carbon-Dioxide, Uterotubal	Obstetrics/Gyn

UTILITY

79QXN	Forceps, Utility	Surgery
80QYJ	Glove, Utility	General

UTILIZATION

80WTG	Monitor, Utilization, Equipment	General

UVA

80REE	Lamp, Ultraviolet (Spectrum A)	General

VACCINE

80LDH	Delivery System, Allergen And Vaccine	General

VACUUM

80KDQ	Bottle, Collection, Vacuum (Aspirator)	General
74WTL	Cleaner, Forceps, Biopsy	Cardiovascular
81KST	Collector, Blood, Vacuum-Assisted	Hematology
85HGG	Controller, Abortion Unit, Vacuum	Obstetrics/Gyn
76EHZ	Evacuator, Oral Cavity	Dental And Oral
85HDB	Extractor, Vacuum, Fetal	Obstetrics/Gyn
76VEN	Mixer, Vacuum	Dental And Oral
80SEJ	Pad, Vacuum Stabilized	General
85HGF	Pump, Abortion Unit, Vacuum	Obstetrics/Gyn
85HHI	Pump, Abortion, Vacuum, Central System	Obstetrics/Gyn
73SEI	Pump, Vacuum, Central	Anesthesiology
87MCJ	Pump, Vacuum, Electric, Suction-Type Electrode	Orthopedics
80KDP	Regulator, Vacuum	General
87RVA	Splint, Vacuum	Orthopedics
79GCX	Suction Apparatus, Operating Room, Wall Vacuum-Powered	Surgery
80WVE	Syringe, Other	General
81GIM	Tube, Vacuum Sample, With Anticoagulant	Hematology
87QGY	Vacuum, Cast Cutter	Orthopedics

VACUUM-ASSISTED

81KST	Collector, Blood, Vacuum-Assisted	Hematology

VACUUM-POWERED

79GCX	Suction Apparatus, Operating Room, Wall Vacuum-Powered	Surgery

VAGINAL

85HGD	Applicator, Vaginal	Obstetrics/Gyn
85HDX	Dilator, Vaginal	Obstetrics/Gyn
85HED	Douche, Vaginal	Obstetrics/Gyn
85HEC	Insufflator, Vaginal	Obstetrics/Gyn
80MMS	Lubricant, Vaginal, Patient	General
85HFK	Mold, Vaginal	Obstetrics/Gyn
79RXO	Packing, Surgical	Surgery
85HHW	Pessary, Vaginal	Obstetrics/Gyn
88IHB	Pipette, Vaginal Pool Smear	Pathology
85HDL	Retractor, Vaginal	Obstetrics/Gyn
85HDF	Speculum, Vaginal, Metal	Obstetrics/Gyn
85HDG	Speculum, Vaginal, Metal, Fiberoptic	Obstetrics/Gyn
85HIB	Speculum, Vaginal, Non-Metal	Obstetrics/Gyn
85HIC	Speculum, Vaginal, Non-Metal, Fiberoptic	Obstetrics/Gyn
85KXP	Stent, Vaginal, Special Purpose	Obstetrics/Gyn
85HII	Stimulator, Muscle, Vaginal	Obstetrics/Gyn
85WOP	Transducer, Ultrasonic, Intravaginal	Obstetrics/Gyn
85HIJ	Vibrator, Vaginal, AC-Powered	Obstetrics/Gyn
85HIK	Vibrator, Vaginal, Battery-Powered	Obstetrics/Gyn

VAGINALIS

83MJM	DNA-Probe, Gardnerella Vaginalis	Microbiology
83MJK	DNA-Probe, Trichomonas Vaginalis	Microbiology

VAGINOMETER

85SEK	Vaginometer	Obstetrics/Gyn

VAGINOSCOPE

85SEL	Vaginoscope	Obstetrics/Gyn
85MOK	Vaginoscope and Accessories	Obstetrics/Gyn

VAGUS

84MBY	Stimulator, Vagus Nerve, Epilepsy, Implanted	Cns/Neurology
84MUY	Stimulator, Vagus Nerve, Implanted (Coma And Vegetative State)	Cns/Neurology

VALPROIC

91LEG	Enzyme Immunoassay, Valproic Acid	Toxicology

VALUES

73BTY	Computer, Pulmonary Function, Predicted Values	Anesthesiology

VALVE

74KRI	Accessories, Cardiopulmonary Bypass	Cardiovascular
79KGZ	Accessories, Catheter	Surgery
74MIE	Allograft, Heart Valve	Cardiovascular
80MJF	Check Valve, Retrograde Flow (In-Line)	General

VALVE *(cont'd)*

73ECX	Cylinder, Compressed Gas, With Valve	Anesthesiology
74MEZ	Device, Debridement, Ultrasonic, Heart Valve & HV Seat	Cardiovascular
74DTJ	Holder, Heart Valve Prosthesis	Cardiovascular
86KYF	Implant, Eye Valve	Ophthalmology
85HEI	Monitor, Heart Valve Movement, Fetal, Ultrasonic	Obstetrics/Gyn
74LXN	Probe, Test, Valve, Heart	Cardiovascular
74RMO	Prosthesis, Cardiac Valve	Cardiovascular
74DYE	Prosthesis, Cardiac Valve, Biological	Cardiovascular
84RMU	Prosthesis, Hydrocephalic (Holter Valve)	Cns/Neurology
74MIM	Prosthesis, Venous Valve	Cardiovascular
80RPI	Resuscitator, Pulmonary, Gas	General
80FQB	Resuscitator, Pulmonary, Manual (Demand Valve)	General
74MOP	Rotator, Prosthetic Heart Valve	Cardiovascular
80WZG	Set, Administration, Intravenous, Needle-Free	General
84RTC	Shunt, Hydrocephalic	Cns/Neurology
74DTI	Sizer, Heart Valve Prosthesis	Cardiovascular
80FMG	Stopcock	General
77KLZ	Tube, Shunt, Endolymphatic, With Valve	Ear/Nose/Throat
73WHT	Valve, Breathing	Anesthesiology
73MJJ	Valve, CPB Check, Retrograde, In-Line	Anesthesiology
74QHH	Valve, Catheter Flush	Cardiovascular
74QHI	Valve, Catheter Flush, Continuous	Cardiovascular
77SEM	Valve, Ear	Ear/Nose/Throat
74LWQ	Valve, Heart, Mechanical	Cardiovascular
74LWR	Valve, Heart, Tissue	Cardiovascular
75WYH	Valve, Laboratory	Chemistry
73CBP	Valve, Non-Rebreathing	Anesthesiology
86SEN	Valve, Ophthalmic	Ophthalmology
75UJD	Valve, Other	Chemistry
73SEO	Valve, Positive End Expiratory Pressure (PEEP)	Anesthesiology
74MNJ	Valve, Pressure Relief, Cardiopulmonary Bypass	Cardiovascular
89ISP	Valve, Prosthesis	Physical Med
84LXL	Valve, Shunt, Fluid, CNS (Post-Amendment Design)	Cns/Neurology
77WRO	Valve, Speaking, Tracheal	Ear/Nose/Throat
73JFE	Valve, Switching (Ploss)	Anesthesiology
85HDO	Valve, Tubal Occlusion	Obstetrics/Gyn
78FAC	Valve, Ureterovesicle	Gastro/Urology

VALVULOPLASTY

74LIT	Catheter, Angioplasty, Transluminal, Peripheral	Cardiovascular
78QIU	Catheter, Balloon, Dilatation, Vessel	Gastro/Urology
74MAD	Catheter, Percutaneous (Valvuloplasty)	Cardiovascular

VALVULOTOME

74MGZ	Valvulotome	Cardiovascular

VAN

80QAO	Ambulance	General
89WHH	Vehicle, Handicapped	Physical Med

VAN GIESON'S

88IAC	Stain, Van Gieson's	Pathology
88IAD	Van Gieson's Picro-Fuchsin	Pathology

VANADATE

75CEL	Ammonium Molybdate And Ammonium Vanadate, Phospholipids	Chemistry

VANCOMYCIN

91LEH	Radioimmunoassay, Vancomycin	Toxicology

VANILLIN

75CDF	Diazo, P-Nitroaniline/Vanillin, Vanilmandelic Acid	Chemistry
75CKC	Vanillin Pyruvate, ALT/SGPT	Chemistry
75CIF	Vanillin Pyruvate, AST/SGOT	Chemistry

VANILMANDELIC

75CDF	Diazo, P-Nitroaniline/Vanillin, Vanilmandelic Acid	Chemistry
75CDK	Electrophoretic Separation, Vanilmandelic Acid	Chemistry

VAPOCOOLANT

89MLY	Refrigerant, Topical (Vapocoolant)	Physical Med

VAPOR

73BXA	Analyzer, Gas, Water Vapor, Gaseous Phase	Anesthesiology
73VCH	Analyzer, Water Vapor	Anesthesiology
87JDY	Evacuator, Vapor, Cement Monomer	Orthopedics
80RVZ	Sterilizer, Vapor	General
75JNA	Vapor Pressure, Osmolality Of Serum & Urine	Chemistry

VAPORIZER

73RAU	Humidifier, Heat/Moisture Exchange	Anesthesiology
73RAV	Humidifier, Heated	Anesthesiology
73KFZ	Humidifier, Non-Direct Patient Interface (Home-Use)	Anesthesiology
73RAW	Humidifier, Non-Heated	Anesthesiology
73BTT	Humidifier, Respiratory Gas, (Direct Patient Interface)	Anesthesiology
80SEQ	Vaporizer	General
73CAD	Vaporizer, Anesthesia, Non-Heated	Anesthesiology

VARIANT

81MLL	Hemoglobin C (Abnormal Hemoglobin Variant)	Hematology

VARICELLA-ZOSTER
83WJU Antibody, Varicella-Zoster Microbiology
83GQW Antigen, CF, (Including CF Control), Varicella-Zoster Microbiology
83GQX Antiserum, CF, Varicella-Zoster Microbiology
83LFY Enzyme Linked Immunoabsorbent Assay, Varicella-Zoster Microbiology

VARICOSE
74MEY Cuff, Treatment, Varicose Vein, Implantable Cardiovascular
74MNN Device, Ablation, Varicose Vein Cardiovascular

VARICOSIS
80LLK Legging, Compression, Non-Inflatable General
80FQL Stocking, Elastic General
89ILG Stocking, Elastic, Physical Medicine Physical Med
80DWL Stocking, Support (Anti-Embolic) General

VARIETIES
83GSX Antisera, Acinetobacter Calcoaceticus, All Varieties Microbiology

VARNISH
76EMC Varnish Dental And Oral
76LBH Varnish, Cavity Dental And Oral
76KLF Varnish, With Additive Dental And Oral
76KLG Varnish, Without Additive Dental And Oral

VAS
78EZZ Prosthesis, Vas Deferans Gastro/Urology

VASCULAR
90WNR Angio-Dynograph Radiology
84HBY Catheter, Angiographic Cns/Neurology
74DWF Catheter, Vascular, Cardiopulmonary Bypass Cardiovascular
74DYD Catheter, Vascular, Long-Term Cardiovascular
74JAP Catheter, Vascular, Opaque Cardiovascular
74QKO Clamp, Peripheral Vascular Cardiovascular
74DXC Clamp, Vascular Cardiovascular
74DSS Clip, Vascular Cardiovascular
74ULR Detector, Blood Flow, Ultrasonic (Doppler) Cardiovascular
74MGB Device, Hemostasis, Vascular Cardiovascular
74QPQ Dilator, Vascular Cardiovascular
74DXK Echocardiograph (Ultrasonic Scanner) Cardiovascular
78QWP Flowmeter, Blood, Ultrasonic Gastro/Urology
74MAK Graft, Vascular, Biological Cardiovascular
78MDQ Graft, Vascular, Biological, Hemodialysis Access Gastro/Urology
78MCI Graft, Vascular, Synth./Bio. Composite, Hemodialysis Access Gastro/Urology
74MAL Graft, Vascular, Synthetic/Biological Composite Cardiovascular
84HAP Guide, Wire, Angiographic (And Accessories) Cns/Neurology
74QYZ Guidewire Cardiovascular
74DQX Guidewire, Catheter Cardiovascular
90JAJ Guidewire, Catheter, Radiological Radiology
74DXT Injector, Angiographic (Cardiac Catheterization) Cardiovascular
90VGB Kit, Angiographic, Digital Radiology
90VGC Kit, Angiographic, Special Procedure Radiology
74WTT Legging, Compression, Inflatable, Sequential Cardiovascular
80LLK Legging, Compression, Non-Inflatable General
74RFK Loop, Vascular Cardiovascular
85HEP Monitor, Blood Flow, Ultrasonic Obstetrics/Gyn
90RKT Phonoangiograph Radiology
74THP Port, Vascular Access Cardiovascular
74WTO Probe, Transesophageal Cardiovascular
79FZC Prosthesis, Arterial Graft, Bovine Carotid Artery Surgery
79FZB Prosthesis, Arterial Graft, Synthetic, Greater Than 6mm Surgery
79JCP Prosthesis, Arterial Graft, Synthetic, Less Than 6mm Surgery
74MUX Prosthesis, Vascular Cardiovascular
74DYF Prosthesis, Vascular Graft, Less Than 6mm Diameter Cardiovascular
74DSY Prosthesis, Vascular Graft, Of 6mm And Greater Diameter Cardiovascular
90VLE Radiographic Unit, Digital Subtraction Angiographic (DSA) Radiology
90IZI Radiographic/Fluoroscopic Unit, Angiographic Radiology
90VHC Radiographic/Fluoroscopic Unit, Angiographic, Digital Radiology
90IYN Scanner, Ultrasonic (Pulsed Doppler) Radiology
90IYO Scanner, Ultrasonic (Pulsed Echo) Radiology
90VCV Scanner, Ultrasonic, Vascular Radiology
90WJP Stand, Cardiovascular Radiology
90WLW Stand, Vascular Radiology
85UAN Stent, Other Obstetrics/Gyn
74WLQ Stent, Vascular Cardiovascular
84LLE Stimulator, Cord, Spinal, Implantable (Periph. Vasc. Dis.) Cns/Neurology
74WTW Syringe, Angioplasty Cardiovascular
78LTH Vascular Access Graft Gastro/Urology

VASODILATOR
80WXN Vasodilator General

VDRL
83UMO Test, Syphilis (RPR or VDRL) Microbiology

VECTORCARDIOGRAPH
74DYC Vectorcardiograph Cardiovascular

VEGETATIVE
84MUY Stimulator, Vagus Nerve, Implanted (Coma And Vegetative State) Cns/Neurology

VEHICLE
80QAO Ambulance General
80TGS Conveyor, Guided Vehicle General
89INI Scooter (Motorized 3-Wheeled Vehicle) Physical Med
89WHH Vehicle, Handicapped Physical Med
80SHN Vehicle/Equipment, Recreational (Handicapped) General

VEIN
84UCL Catheter, Hydrocephalic Cns/Neurology
74MEY Cuff, Treatment, Varicose Vein, Implantable Cardiovascular
74QOM Detector, Deep Vein Thrombosis Cardiovascular
74MNN Device, Ablation, Varicose Vein Cardiovascular
80SER Finder, Vein General
80KZA Locator, Vein, Liquid Crystal General
74MAB Marker, Cardiopulmonary Bypass (Vein Marker) Cardiovascular
79KPK Marker, Ostia, Aorto-Saphenous Vein Surgery
77JYW Press, Vein Ear/Nose/Throat
74RVP Spreader, Vein Cardiovascular
80LBJ Stabilizer, Vein General
79GAJ Stripper, Vein, Disposable Surgery
74DWQ Stripper, Vein, External Cardiovascular
79GAI Stripper, Vein, Reusable Surgery
74WTW Syringe, Angioplasty Cardiovascular

VELCRO
79MDN Burr, Artificial (Velcro Fastener - Temp. Abdominal Closure) Surgery

VELOCITY
84JXE Device, Measurement, Velocity, Conduction, Nerve Cns/Neurology

VENA
74QGG Cannula, Vena Cava Cardiovascular
74DST Clip, Vena Cava Cardiovascular
74QWE Filter, Vena Cava Cardiovascular
74LWT Vena Cava Balloon Occluder Cardiovascular

VENEER
76VDX Veneer, Dental Dental And Oral

VENOM
81GIR Reagent, Russel Viper Venom Hematology

VENOUS
74QGH Cannula, Venous Cardiovascular
80WQH Catheter, Central Venous General
78UBW Catheter, Peritoneo-Venous Gastro/Urology
74QKF Circulatory Assist Unit, Venous Return Cardiovascular
74QIX Kit, Blood Pressure, Central Venous Cardiovascular
74RLX Monitor, Blood Pressure, Venous Cardiovascular
74KRK Monitor, Blood Pressure, Venous, Cardiopulmonary Bypass Cardiovascular
79FYO Monitor, Blood Pressure, Venous, Central Surgery
79FYP Monitor, Blood Pressure, Venous, Peripheral Surgery
79KFO Monitor, Cardiac Output, Dye (Central Venous & Arterial) Surgery
74FYN Monitor, Pressure, Venous, Central, Powered Cardiovascular
74MIM Prosthesis, Venous Valve Cardiovascular
74RTD Shunt, Peritoneo-Venous Cardiovascular

VENT
78QQP Drain, Vent Gastro/Urology
75UGD Filter, Membrane Chemistry

VENTILATING
73BTJ Bronchoscope, Rigid, Non-Ventilating Anesthesiology
73BTH Bronchoscope, Rigid, Ventilating Anesthesiology

VENTILATION
73CBO Attachment, Intermittent Mandatory Ventilation (IMV) Anesthesiology
73SES Monitor, Ventilation Anesthesiology
87KII Tube, Cement Ventilation Orthopedics
73CBI Tube, Tracheal/Bronchial, Differential Ventilation Anesthesiology

VENTILATOR
73QAK Alarm, Breathing Circuit Anesthesiology
73QEL Circuit, Breathing, Ventilator Anesthesiology
73QMK Controller, Oxygen (Blender) Anesthesiology
73SET Controller, Ventilator IMV Anesthesiology
80WPV Dryer, Respiratory/Anesthesia Equipment General
73QWF Filter, Ventilator Anesthesiology
73BZO Tubing, Ventilator Anesthesiology
73WHT Valve, Breathing Anesthesiology
73CBP Valve, Non-Rebreathing Anesthesiology
73QBB Ventilator, Anesthesia Unit Anesthesiology
73CBK Ventilator, Continuous (Respirator) Anesthesiology
73MOD Ventilator, Continuous (Respirator), Accessory Anesthesiology
73KLM Ventilator, Continuous, Hyperbaric Anesthesiology
73MNT Ventilator, Continuous, Minimal Ventilatory Support, Facility Use Anesthesiology
73MNS Ventilator, Continuous, Non-Life Supporting Anesthesiology

VENTILATOR *(cont'd)*

73BTM	Ventilator, Emergency, Manual (Resuscitator)	Anesthesiology
73BTL	Ventilator, Emergency, Powered (Resuscitator)	Anesthesiology
73BYT	Ventilator, External Body, Negative Pressure, (Cuirass)	Anesthesiology
73LSZ	Ventilator, High-Frequency	Anesthesiology
80FQC	Ventilator, Neonatal Respirator	General
73BZD	Ventilator, Non-Continuous (Respirator)	Anesthesiology
73SEX	Ventilator, Other	Anesthesiology
73SEU	Ventilator, Pressure Cycled (IPPB Machine)	Anesthesiology
73SEV	Ventilator, Time Cycled (Iron Lung)	Anesthesiology
73SEW	Ventilator, Volume (Critical Care)	Anesthesiology
80WPY	Washer, Respiratory/Anesthesia Equipment	General

VENTILATORY

73BXC	Monitor, Oxygen (Ventilatory) W/Wo Alarm	Anesthesiology
73BZQ	Monitor, Ventilatory Frequency	Anesthesiology
73CCQ	Nebulizer, Medicinal, Non-Ventilatory (Atomizer)	Anesthesiology
73MNR	Recorder, Ventilatory Effort	Anesthesiology
73BZG	Spirometer, Diagnostic (Respirometer)	Anesthesiology
73BZK	Spirometer, Monitoring (Volumeter)	Anesthesiology
73MNT	Ventilator, Continuous, Minimal Ventilatory Support, Facility Use	Anesthesiology

VENTING

75UJE	Venting System, Gas Chromatography	Chemistry

VENTRICULAR

84HCD	Cannula, Ventricular	Cns/Neurology
84UCX	Catheter, Hydrocephalic, Ventricular	Cns/Neurology
84HCA	Catheter, Ventricular	Cns/Neurology
79GBS	Catheter, Ventricular, General & Plastic Surgery	Surgery
74DSQ	Circulatory Assist Unit, Left Ventricular	Cardiovascular
74FYR	Monitor, Pressure, Cardiac, Ventricular	Cardiovascular
74RMT	Prosthesis, Heart	Cardiovascular
84RTC	Shunt, Hydrocephalic	Cns/Neurology

VENTRICULO-AMNIOTIC

84LID	Ventriculo-Amniotic Shunt for Hydrocephalus	Cns/Neurology

VENTURI

73BYF	Mask, Oxygen, Low Concentration, Venturi	Anesthesiology
73FSC	Mask, Oxygen, Venturi	Anesthesiology

VERRES

78FHP	Needle, Pneumoperitoneum, Simple	Gastro/Urology
78FHO	Needle, Pneumoperitoneum, Spring Loaded	Gastro/Urology

VERTEBRAL

87MQP	Device, Spinal Vertebral Body Replacement	Orthopedics

VERTICAL

90VGT	Holder, X-Ray Film Cassette, Vertical	Radiology

VESSEL

78QIU	Catheter, Balloon, Dilatation, Vessel	Gastro/Urology
90WIO	Catheter, Imaging, Ultrasonic	Radiology
78FKA	Dilator, Vessel	Gastro/Urology
74DRE	Dilator, Vessel, Percutaneous Catheterization	Cardiovascular
74DWP	Dilator, Vessel, Surgical	Cardiovascular
73KGK	Gas, Collecting Vessel	Anesthesiology
79SJB	Instrument, Separating, Nerve	Surgery
74WOZ	Occluder, Cardiovascular	Cardiovascular
79FZC	Prosthesis, Arterial Graft, Bovine Carotid Artery	Surgery
79FZB	Prosthesis, Arterial Graft, Synthetic, Greater Than 6mm	Surgery
79JCP	Prosthesis, Arterial Graft, Synthetic, Less Than 6mm	Surgery
74DYF	Prosthesis, Vascular Graft, Less Than 6mm Diameter	Cardiovascular
74DSY	Prosthesis, Vascular Graft, Of 6mm And Greater Diameter	Cardiovascular
74RPX	Retractor, Vessel	Cardiovascular
78FKW	Tip, Vessel	Gastro/Urology
74DXP	Transducer, Vessel Occlusion	Cardiovascular

VEST

87WUW	Immobilizer, Upper Body	Orthopedics
80RPE	Restraint, Vest	General

VESTIBULAR

77LXV	Analyzer, Apparatus, Vestibular	Ear/Nose/Throat
84WHW	Chair, Rotating	Cns/Neurology
84MHZ	Stimulator, Vestibular Acceleration, Therapeutic	Cns/Neurology

VHP

80RVZ	Sterilizer, Vapor	General

VIAL

80WPN	Crusher, Vial, Laboratory	General
80SHJ	Defroster, Drug, Frozen	General
90IWW	Shield, Vial	Radiology
80WPJ	Vial, Hematology	General
75UJF	Vial, Liquid Scintillation Counting	Chemistry
80TFK	Vial, Medication	General
80WWJ	Vial, Other	General

VIBRATION

84LLN	Vibration Threshold Measurement Device	Cns/Neurology

VIBRATOR

84GWZ	Percussor	Cns/Neurology
73BYI	Percussor, Powered	Anesthesiology
77TFL	Vibrator, Audiometric Bone	Ear/Nose/Throat
89IPE	Vibrator, Battery-Powered	Physical Med
85KXQ	Vibrator, Genital	Obstetrics/Gyn
89IRO	Vibrator, Therapeutic	Physical Med
85HIJ	Vibrator, Vaginal, AC-Powered	Obstetrics/Gyn
85HIK	Vibrator, Vaginal, Battery-Powered	Obstetrics/Gyn

VIBRATORY

85HHG	Dilator, Cervical, Vibratory	Obstetrics/Gyn

VIBRIO

83GSQ	Antiserum, Vibrio Cholerae	Microbiology

VIBROCARDIOGRAPH

74DQH	Cardiograph, Apex (Vibrocardiograph)	Cardiovascular

VIBROPHONOCARDIOGRAPH

74DXR	Ballistocardiograph	Cardiovascular

VICOSIMETER

75UJI	Viscometer	Chemistry

VIDEO

80WKP	Camera, Other	General
80WQX	Camera, Video	General
80WQY	Camera, Video, Endoscopic	General
79WRX	Camera, Video, Headlight, Surgical	Surgery
80WZQ	Camera, Video, Multi-Image	General
80WVY	Cart, Equipment, Video	General
79WIY	Computer, Imaging, Presurgery	Surgery
80SHM	Coupler, Optical, Laparoscopic	General
80TFB	Monitor, Video, Endoscope	General
80WLN	Printer, Image, Video	General
90ROQ	Recorder, Radiographic Video Tape	Radiology
79SGZ	System, Camera, 3-Dimensional	Surgery
86WXT	System, Mapping, Corneal	Ophthalmology
78FET	Tape, Television & Video, Endoscopic	Gastro/Urology
90WTF	Unit, Imaging, Thermal	Radiology
90WJC	Videofluoroscopic Unit	Radiology

VIDEOCAMERA

80WWG	Analyzer, Motion	General

VIDEODISC

80TEF	Recorder, Videotape/Videodisc	General

VIDEOENDOSCOPE

79VKP	Endoscope, Electronic (Videoendoscope)	Surgery
80WLN	Printer, Image, Video	General

VIDEOFLUOROSCOPIC

90WJC	Videofluoroscopic Unit	Radiology

VIDEOINTERFACE

79SHC	Videointerface, Laparoscopic, Non-Removable Rod	Surgery
79SHD	Videointerface, Laparoscopic, Removable Rod	Surgery

VIDEOTAPE

79FXN	Camera, Videotape, Surgical	Surgery
80TEF	Recorder, Videotape/Videodisc	General

VIEW

90IXC	Illuminator, Radiographic Film	Radiology
90JAG	Illuminator, Radiographic Film, Explosion-Proof	Radiology
81KSY	View Box, Blood Grouping	Hematology
83WHV	View Box, Microtiter	Microbiology
81SEY	View Box, Rh Typing	Hematology
90WUY	Viewer, Radiographic Film, Motorized	Radiology

VIEWER

90WUY	Viewer, Radiographic Film, Motorized	Radiology
90SGP	Viewer/Analyzer, 35mm Angio	Radiology
81GLO	Viewer/Magnifier	Hematology

VIEWING

75UJG	Cabinet, Chromatography (U.V.) Viewing	Chemistry

VILLI

85VIL	Test, Chorionic Villi Sampling (Fetal Chromosome Analysis)	Obstetrics/Gyn

VILLUS

85LLX	Catheter, Sampling, Chorionic Villus	Obstetrics/Gyn

VINYL

80VAE	Component, Plastic	General
80LYZ	Glove, Patient Examination, Vinyl	General
80SDT	Tubing, Vinyl	General

KEYWORD INDEX

VITRECTOMY
86HQE Cutter, Vitreous Aspiration, AC-Powered — Ophthalmology
86HKP Cutter, Vitreous Aspiration, Battery-Powered — Ophthalmology
86QOH Cutter, Vitreous Infusion Suction — Ophthalmology
86MLZ Therapeutic Deep Heat Vitrectomy — Ophthalmology

VITRECTOR
86HQE Cutter, Vitreous Aspiration, AC-Powered — Ophthalmology
86HKP Cutter, Vitreous Aspiration, Battery-Powered — Ophthalmology

VITREOUS
76LZX Acid, Hyaluronic — Dental And Oral
86HMX Cannula, Ophthalmic — Ophthalmology
86HQE Cutter, Vitreous Aspiration, AC-Powered — Ophthalmology
86HKP Cutter, Vitreous Aspiration, Battery-Powered — Ophthalmology
86QOH Cutter, Vitreous Infusion Suction — Ophthalmology
86RCT Kit, Irrigation, Eye — Ophthalmology

VITRO
85VIK Equipment, In Vitro Fertilization/Embryo Transfer — Obstetrics/Gyn
76MCL Kit, Test, Periodontal, In Vitro — Dental And Oral
82MLH Strip, HAMA IGG, ELISA, In Vitro Test System — Immunology

VIVO
80LJJ Electrode, In Vivo Calcium Ion Selective — General
80LJI Electrode, In Vivo Potassium Ion Selective — General

VLDL
74WTP Column, Adsorption, Lipid — Cardiovascular
75KMZ HDL Via LDL & VLDL Precipitation, Lipoproteins — Chemistry
75LBS LDL & VLDL Precipitation, Cholesterol Via Esterase-Oxidase — Chemistry
75LBR LDL & VLDL Precipitation, HDL — Chemistry

VOCAL
77MGF Collagen, Injectable (For Vocal Cord Augmentation) — Ear/Nose/Throat
76LTG Paste, Injectable, Augmentation, Chord, Vocal — Dental And Oral
77MIX System, Vocal Cord Medialization — Ear/Nose/Throat

VOICE
89LFF Aid, Control, Environmental, Controlled, Breath — Physical Med
77MCK Amplifier, Voice — Ear/Nose/Throat
80VBO Communication Equipment — General

VOID
89MBS Filler, Bone Void, Non-Osteoinduction — Physical Med
89MBP Filler, Bone Void, Osteoinduction — Physical Med

VOLTAGE
80TAD Alarm, Voltage — General
90IYK Collimator, Therapeutic X-Ray, High Voltage — Radiology
90IYJ Collimator, Therapeutic X-Ray, Low Voltage — Radiology
80QTQ Detector, Electrostatic Voltage — General
90VHL Generator, Diagnostic X-Ray, High Voltage, 3-Phase — Radiology
90IZO Generator, Diagnostic X-Ray, High Voltage, Single Phase — Radiology
90KPZ Generator, High Voltage, X-Ray, Therapeutic — Radiology
90IYF Generator, Therapeutic X-Ray, High Voltage — Radiology
90IYD Generator, Therapeutic X-Ray, Low Voltage — Radiology
80WMM Regulator, Line Voltage — General

VOLTMETER
75SFD Voltmeter — Chemistry

VOLUME
75JKP 51 Chromium, Blood Volume — Chemistry
78QBR Aspirator, Low Volume (Gastric Suction) — Gastro/Urology
73BXW Calibrator, Gas, Volume — Anesthesiology
78WYI Instrument, Volume, Bladder — Gastro/Urology
81JWO Meter, Volume, Blood — Hematology
73JEH Plethysmograph, Volume — Anesthesiology
78ROX Regulator, Suction, Low Volume (Gastric) — Gastro/Urology
79MRD Sizer, Mammary, Breast Implant Volume — Surgery
73SEW Ventilator, Volume (Critical Care) — Anesthesiology

VOLUMETER
73BZK Spirometer, Monitoring (Volumeter) — Anesthesiology
75UJK Volumeter — Chemistry

VOLUMETRIC
80FRN Pump, Infusion — General
75CIE Volumetric/Manometric, Carbon-Dioxide — Chemistry

WALK
89KHY Cane, Safety Walk — Physical Med
89KNP Orthosis, Corrective Shoe — Physical Med
88ROV Refrigerator, Morgue, Walk-In — Pathology
87TEO Shoe, Orthopedic — Orthopedics
86WOM Vision Aid, Ultrasonic — Ophthalmology

WALK-IN
88ROV Refrigerator, Morgue, Walk-In — Pathology

WALKER
80WYY Accessories, Walker — General
89UMM Attachment, Bag (Crutch, Walker, Wheelchair) — Physical Med
89INP Tips And Pads, Cane, Crutch And Walker — Physical Med
80UEL Tray, Walker — General
89ITJ Walker, Mechanical — Physical Med

WALKING
89RJY Bars, Parallel, Walking — Physical Med
87QHC Cast Walking Heel — Orthopedics
89MKD Stimulator, Neuromuscular, Functional Walking, Non-Invasive — Physical Med

WALL
78SAP Elevator, Wall, Abdominal — Gastro/Urology
80RCM Hanger, Intravenous — General
90IXY Holder, Radiographic Cassette, Wall-Mounted — Radiology
80TED Rail, Wall Side — General
80WRN Rails, Equipment — General
79GCX Suction Apparatus, Operating Room, Wall Vacuum-Powered — Surgery
80TFM Wallpaper, Antibacterial — General

WALL-MOUNTED
90IXY Holder, Radiographic Cassette, Wall-Mounted — Radiology

WALLPAPER
80TFM Wallpaper, Antibacterial — General

WANGENSTEEN
78SDA Tube, Gastrointestinal, Wangensteen — Gastro/Urology

WARBURG
75UJL Warburg Apparatus — Chemistry

WARD
79JCX Suction Apparatus, Ward Use, Portable, AC-Powered — Surgery

WARMER
76EFC Warmer, Anesthesia Tube — Dental And Oral
80SFE Warmer, Bedpan — General
80SFF Warmer, Blanket — General
81KZL Warmer, Blood and Plasma — Hematology
81SFG Warmer, Blood, Coil — Hematology
81SFH Warmer, Blood, Dry Heat — Hematology
81BSA Warmer, Blood, Electromagnetic Radiation — Hematology
81SFI Warmer, Blood, Microwave — Hematology
73BSB Warmer, Blood, Non-Electromagnetic Radiation — Anesthesiology
81VLV Warmer, Blood, Water Bath — Hematology
78MLW Warmer, Dialysate, Peritoneal — Gastro/Urology
79SHE Warmer, Endoscope — Surgery
80WLV Warmer, Gel — General
89MPO Warmer, Heel, Infant — Physical Med
80LHF Warmer, Infusion Fluid, Microwave — General
80LGZ Warmer, Infusion Fluid, Thermal — General
80LHC Warmer, Irrigation Solution — General
80SFJ Warmer, Radiant, Adult — General
80FMT Warmer, Radiant, Infant — General
80SFK Warmer, Radiant, Infant, Transport — General
75SFL Warmer, Solution — Chemistry

WARMING
80QFJ Cabinet, Warming — General
88IEH Lamp, Slide Warming — Pathology
88IEG Table, Slide Warming — Pathology

WASH
80TAF Basin, Wash — General
78QEE Bottle, Endoscopic Wash — Gastro/Urology
86LXQ Cup, Eye — Ophthalmology
75TCG Fountain, Eye Wash — Chemistry

WASHCLOTH
80VBF Linen — General
80RHF Mitt/Washcloth, Patient — General

WASHER
87HTN Bolt, Nut, Washer — Orthopedics
80QKS Cleaner, Bedpan (Sterilizer) — General
80FLG Cleaner, Ultrasonic, Medical Instrument — General
80WPV Dryer, Respiratory/Anesthesia Equipment — General
80QYG Glove Processing Unit (Drying, Powdering) — General
80TCW Laundry Equipment — General
76ECG Sterilizer, Boiling Water — Dental And Oral
80UDL Sterilizer, Bulk, Steam & Ethylene-Oxide — General
79FSJ Sterilizer, Ethylene-Oxide Gas, Operating Room — Surgery
76ECH Sterilizer, Steam (Autoclave), Dental — Dental And Oral
79FSI Sterilizer, Steam (Autoclave), Surgical — Surgery
80UCS Sterilizer, Steam, Bulk — General
80UCT Sterilizer, Steam, Table Top — General
80THI Sterilizer/Washer, Endoscope — General
80SFN Washer, Cart — General
81SFO Washer, Cell (Frozen Blood Processor) — Hematology

WASHER *(cont'd)*

85HFD	Washer, Endometrial	Obstetrics/Gyn
75SFP	Washer, Labware	Chemistry
80TFN	Washer, Laundry	General
80WLU	Washer, Microplate	General
75SFQ	Washer, Pipette	Chemistry
75UJA	Washer, Pipette, Ultrasonic	Chemistry
80FLH	Washer, Receptacle, Waste, Body	General
80WPY	Washer, Respiratory/Anesthesia Equipment	General
80SFR	Washer, Utensil	General
80WWK	Washer/Disinfector	General
80SFM	Washer/Sterilizer	General

WASHING

81JQC	Centrifuge, Cell Washing	Hematology
81KSN	Centrifuge, Cell Washing, Automated, Immuno-Hematology	Hematology

WASTE

80WVR	Cart, Waste	General
80TBJ	Compactor, Fixed	General
80TBK	Compactor, Portable	General
79LWH	Counter, Sponge, Surgical	Surgery
80WPN	Crusher, Vial, Laboratory	General
80WLA	Equipment, Control, Pollution	General
80VBK	Incinerator	General
80VBL	Recovery Equipment, Waste Heat	General
80WUN	Service, Waste Management	General
80WWY	Sterilizer/Compactor	General
80WIH	System, Transport, In-House	General
80FLH	Washer, Receptacle, Waste, Body	General
80SFS	Waste Disposal Unit, Sharps	General
79KDB	Waste Disposal Unit, Surgical Instrument (Sharps)	Surgery
80SFT	Waste Disposal Unit, Syringe	General
80SFU	Waste Receptacle, Contaminated	General
80UKO	Waste Receptacle, General Purpose	General
80RDD	Waste Receptacle, Kick Bucket	General
90SFV	Waste Receptacle, Radioactive	Radiology

WATCH

80SHP	Aid, Living, Handicapped	General

WATER

73BXA	Analyzer, Gas, Water Vapor, Gaseous Phase	Anesthesiology
73VCH	Analyzer, Water Vapor	Anesthesiology
75QCY	Bath, Water (Constant Temperature)	Chemistry
89FNH	Bed, Water Flotation, AC-Powered	Physical Med
80FPF	Bottle, Hot/Cold Water	General
78FFE	Catheter, Water Jet, Renal	Gastro/Urology
75SFW	Circulator, Water Bath	Chemistry
75QOU	Demineralizer	Chemistry
75QQF	Distilling Unit	Chemistry
73BYH	Drain, Tee (Water Trap)	Anesthesiology
73CCS	Drain, Thoracic, Water Seal	Anesthesiology
76EKY	Handpiece, Water-Powered	Dental And Oral
80LDS	Hot Water Pasteurization Device	General
75JRH	Incubator/Water Bath	Chemistry
83JTQ	Incubator/Water Bath, Microbiology	Microbiology
80FQH	Lavage Unit, Water Jet	General
78VKM	Lithotriptor, Electro-Hydraulic, Extracorporeal	Gastro/Urology
78FJA	Manometer, Water	Gastro/Urology
80RGI	Mattress, Water	General
80FOH	Mattress, Water, Temperature Regulated	General
88KEQ	Media, Mounting, Water Soluble	Pathology
73JEZ	Monitor, Lung Water Measurement	Anesthesiology
89ILO	Pack, Hot Or Cold, Water Circulating	Physical Med
80RMF	Pad, Pressure, Water Cushion	General
75SFX	Purification Filter, Water, Charcoal	Chemistry
75SFY	Purification Filter, Water, Particulate	Chemistry
78FIP	Purification System, Water	Gastro/Urology
75SFZ	Purification System, Water, Deionization	Chemistry
75SGA	Purification System, Water, Reverse Osmosis	Chemistry
75JRT	Purification System, Water, Reverse Osmosis, Reagent Grade	Chemistry
75SGB	Purification System, Water, Ultraviolet	Chemistry
75JRS	Purifier, Water	Chemistry
80VAQ	Recovery Equipment, Water	General
80WWH	Sampler, Particulate	General
76ECG	Sterilizer, Boiling Water	Dental And Oral
75UIN	Still, Water	Chemistry
77ETP	Stimulator, Caloric Water	Ear/Nose/Throat
75WID	Support, Tube, Test	Chemistry
76ECB	Syringe Unit, Air And/Or Water	Dental And Oral
76DYY	Syringe, Bulb, Air Or Water	Dental And Oral
79WOH	System, Cooling, Laser	Surgery
85MTW	System, Water, Reproduction, Assisted, And Purification	Obstetrics/Gyn
81VLV	Warmer, Blood, Water Bath	Hematology
80KMG	Water Purifier, Ultraviolet	General
78TGB	Water, Distilled (Irrigation)	Gastro/Urology

WATER *(cont'd)*

83WKT	Water, Therapy, Respiratory	Microbiology

WATER-POWERED

76EKY	Handpiece, Water-Powered	Dental And Oral

WATERBATH

75VLS	Shaker, Waterbath	Chemistry

WATERPROOF

80QAD	Adhesive Strip, Waterproof	General
80QNB	Cover, Mattress, Waterproof	General
80RZG	Tape, Adhesive, Waterproof	General

WATTMETER

80SGC	Wattmeter	General

WAVE

78LNS	Lithotriptor, Extracorporeal Shock-wave, Urological	Gastro/Urology
78WUD	Lithotriptor, Extracorporeal, Gallstone	Gastro/Urology
74QZN	Monitor, Heart Rate, R-Wave (ECG)	Cardiovascular

WAX

76EIT	Applicator, Rapid Wax, Dental	Dental And Oral
76EIK	Carver, Wax, Dental	Dental And Oral
79MTJ	Wax, Bone	Surgery
76EGD	Wax, Dental	Dental And Oral

WEAR

86MWL	Lens, Contact(rigid Gas Permeable)-extended Wear	Ophthalmology
86ULD	Lens, Contact, Extended-Wear	Ophthalmology
86LPL	Lenses, Soft Contact, Daily Wear	Ophthalmology
86LPM	Lenses, Soft Contact, Extended Wear	Ophthalmology

WEDGES

76UMQ	Wedges	Dental And Oral

WEE

83GQC	Antiserum, CF, Equine Encephalitis Virus, EEE, WEE	Microbiology

WEIGERT

88HYQ	Iron Chloride-Weigert	Pathology

WEIGERT'S

88HYO	Hematoxylin Weigert's	Pathology
88IAE	Stain, Weigert's Iron Hematoxylin	Pathology

WEIGHT

87HXF	Accessories, Traction (Cart, Frame, Cord, Weight)	Orthopedics
80VDN	Analyzer, Composition, Weight, Patient	General
87WQP	Analyzer, Distribution, Weight, Podiatric	Orthopedics
75QCF	Balance, Electronic	Chemistry
75UKH	Balance, Macro (0.1 mg Accuracy)	Chemistry
75QCG	Balance, Mechanical	Chemistry
75UKF	Balance, Micro (0.001 mg Accuracy)	Chemistry
75UKG	Balance, Semimicro (0.01 mg Accuracy)	Chemistry
75UKE	Balance, Ultramicro (0.0001 mg Accuracy)	Chemistry
78WNS	Balloon, Gastric	Gastro/Urology
78LYW	Device, External, Management, Weight	Gastro/Urology
89QUV	Exerciser, Arm	Physical Med
89QUX	Exerciser, Chest	Physical Med
89QUY	Exerciser, Hand	Physical Med
89QUZ	Exerciser, Leg And Ankle	Physical Med
89QVB	Exerciser, Shoulder	Physical Med
89VLC	Exerciser, Wrist	Physical Med
75UGW	Molecular Weight Equipment	Chemistry
88RQP	Scale, Autopsy	Pathology
80RQQ	Scale, Bed	General
81RQR	Scale, Blood	Hematology
80RQS	Scale, Chair	General
80WXD	Scale, Chair, Transfer	General
80FRW	Scale, Infant	General
75RQT	Scale, Laboratory	Chemistry
89INF	Scale, Platform, Wheelchair	Physical Med
80FRI	Scale, Stand-On	General
80FQA	Scale, Surgical Sponge	General
80WTM	Weight, IV Pole	General
86MML	Weights, Eyelid, External	Ophthalmology

WELDING

76WOJ	Dental Laboratory Equipment	Dental And Oral

WELL

80WOC	Microplate	General
80WOD	Reader, Microplate	General
76VLM	Well, Amalgam	Dental And Oral

WESTERN

83WKS	Equipment, Test, Western Blot	Microbiology
81MVW	Kit, Western Blot, Hiv-1	Hematology

WET

75JIJ	Wet Ash Method, Protein Bound Iodine	Chemistry

WHEEL
89QVB Exerciser, Shoulder — Physical Med
76EJQ Wheel, Polishing Agent — Dental And Oral

WHEELCHAIR
89KNO Accessories, Wheelchair — Physical Med
89IMY Armboard, Wheelchair — Physical Med
89IML Armrest, Wheelchair — Physical Med
89UMM Attachment, Bag (Crutch, Walker, Wheelchair) — Physical Med
89INB Attachment, Commode, Wheelchair — Physical Med
89IMQ Attachment, Narrowing, Wheelchair — Physical Med
80TDH Attachment, Oxygen Canister/IV Pole, Wheelchair — General
89IQB Belt, Wheelchair — Physical Med
89IMW Brake, Extension, Wheelchair — Physical Med
80WJM Charger, Battery — General
89IMN Climber, Curb, Wheelchair — Physical Med
89KNN Component, Wheelchair — Physical Med
89INC Cuff, Pusher, Wheelchair — Physical Med
89IMP Cushion, Wheelchair (Pad) — Physical Med
89IMR Device, Anti-Tip, Wheelchair — Physical Med
89ING Elevator, Wheelchair — Physical Med
89IMM Footrest, Wheelchair — Physical Med
89IMO Handrim, Wheelchair — Physical Med
89INA Hill Holder, Wheelchair — Physical Med
89IMZ Holder, Crutch and Cane, Wheelchair — Physical Med
80REY Lift, Wheelchair — General
80UKQ Ramp, Wheelchair — General
80RPF Restraint, Wheelchair — General
89INF Scale, Platform, Wheelchair — Physical Med
89INI Scooter (Motorized 3-Wheeled Vehicle) — Physical Med
89INE Sling, Overhead Suspension, Wheelchair — Physical Med
89IMS Support, Head And Trunk, Wheelchair — Physical Med
89IMX Tray, Wheelchair — Physical Med
89IOR Wheelchair, Manual — Physical Med
89ITI Wheelchair, Powered — Physical Med
89IQC Wheelchair, Special Grade — Physical Med
89IMK Wheelchair, Stair Climbing — Physical Med
89IPL Wheelchair, Standup — Physical Med

WHEELED
80FRM Chair, Geriatric, Wheeled — General
89INI Scooter (Motorized 3-Wheeled Vehicle) — Physical Med
80FPO Stretcher, Wheeled (Mobile) — General
89INJ Stretcher, Wheeled, Mechanical — Physical Med
89INK Stretcher, Wheeled, Powered — Physical Med

WHIRLPOOL
89ILJ Bath, Hydro-Massage (Whirlpool) — Physical Med

WHITE
81KSA Calibrator, Red Cell And White Cell Counting — Hematology
81GJP Control, Platelet — Hematology
81GGL Control, White Cell — Hematology
81JBE Enzyme, Cell (Erythrocytic And Leukocytic) — Hematology
81GGJ Fluid, White Cell Diluting — Hematology
81GHD Leukocyte Alkaline Phosphatase — Hematology
81GIA Leukocyte Peroxidase — Hematology
81GLQ Mixture, Control, Indices, White and Red Cell — Hematology
81LJX Test, Urine Leukocyte — Hematology

WHOLE
81JBP Activated Whole Blood Clotting Time — Hematology
81SAN Analyzer, Coagulation, Whole Blood — Hematology
82DGR Antigen, Antiserum, Control, Whole Human Serum — Immunology
90JAN Counter, Whole Body, Nuclear — Radiology
90LNG Hyperthermia System, Whole-Body — Radiology
81GLY Oximeter, Whole Blood — Hematology
81KHG Whole Blood Hemoglobin Determination — Hematology
82DGQ Whole Human Plasma, Antigen, Antiserum, Control — Immunology

WHOLE-BODY
90LNG Hyperthermia System, Whole-Body — Radiology

WICK
86HOZ Sponge, Ophthalmic — Ophthalmology
77KCN Wick, Ear — Ear/Nose/Throat

WINGED
74QHL Kit, Catheterization, Intravenous, Winged — Cardiovascular

WIPE
80LKB Pad, Alcohol — General
80TGC Swabs, Alcohol — General
80RYG Swabs, Antiseptic — General
80WPO Wipe, Instrument — General

WIRE
76ECN Clamp, Wire, Orthodontic — Dental And Oral
76EJW Clasp, Wire — Dental And Oral
77JXT Crimper, Wire, ENT — Ear/Nose/Throat
87HXZ Cutter, Wire And Pin — Orthopedics

WIRE *(cont'd)*
77JXW Die, Wire Bending, ENT — Ear/Nose/Throat
87SGD Driver, Wire — Orthopedics
76DZJ Driver, Wire, And Bone Drill, Manual — Dental And Oral
77JXX Forceps, Wire Closure, ENT — Ear/Nose/Throat
87HYA Forceps, Wire Holding — Orthopedics
74WTR Guide, Catheter — Cardiovascular
84HAP Guide, Wire, Angiographic (And Accessories) — Cns/Neurology
74QYZ Guidewire — Cardiovascular
74DQX Guidewire, Catheter — Cardiovascular
90JAJ Guidewire, Catheter, Radiological — Radiology
76DYX Lock, Wire, And Ligature, Intraoral — Dental And Oral
77JYQ Loop, Wire — Ear/Nose/Throat
87HXI Passer, Wire, Orthopedic — Orthopedics
77JYA Scissors, Wire Cutting, ENT — Ear/Nose/Throat
90IWA Source, Wire, Radioactive Iridium — Radiology
87RVB Splint, Wire Board — Orthopedics
74DRB Stylet, Catheter — Cardiovascular
78EZB Stylet, Catheter, Gastro-Urology — Gastro/Urology
80RWW Stylet, Intravenous — General
80RWX Stylet, Needle — General
79GAH Stylet, Surgical — Surgery
73BSR Stylet, Tracheal Tube — Anesthesiology
78EYA Stylet, Ureteral — Gastro/Urology
79GAQ Suture, Non-Absorbable, Steel, Monofilament & Multifilament — Surgery
79RYE Suture, Stainless Steel — Surgery
87HXS Twister, Wire — Orthopedics
87UBT Wire, Bone — Orthopedics
76DZK Wire, Fixation, Intraosseous — Dental And Oral
79SGE Wire, Ligature — Surgery
76DZC Wire, Orthodontic — Dental And Oral
87LRN Wire, Surgical — Orthopedics

WIRING
80WJG Cable, Electric — General

WITHDRAWAL
74DQI Pump, Withdrawal/Infusion — Cardiovascular

WOOD
77EWF Depressor, Tongue, ENT, Wood — Ear/Nose/Throat

WOOD'S
83GMB Light, Wood's, Fluorescence — Microbiology

WORKING
78FDC Resectoscope Working Element — Gastro/Urology

WOUND
79MGO Adhesive, Wound Closure — Surgery
80QBZ Aspirator, Wound Suction Pump — General
79KOZ Beads, Hydrophilic, Wound Exudate Absorption — Surgery
79QLJ Clip, Wound — Surgery
79MBQ Device, Peripheral Electromag. Field to Aid Wound Healing — Surgery
80WKJ Dressing, Gel — General
80WKL Dressing, Permeable, Moisture — General
80QRA Dressing, Skin Graft, Donor Site — General
79MSA Dressing, Wound And Burn, Occlusive, Heated — Surgery
79MGQ Dressing, Wound and Burn, Hydrogel — Surgery
79MGR Dressing, Wound and Burn, Interactive — Surgery
79MGP Dressing, Wound and Burn, Occlusive — Surgery
79NAE Dressing, Wound, Hydrogel W/out Drug And/or Biologic — Surgery
79NAC Dressing, Wound, Hydrophilic — Surgery
79NAD Dressing, Wound, Occlusive — Surgery
80RCW Kit, Irrigation, Wound — General
80VFP Kit, Wound Drainage — General
84SGF Kit, Wound Drainage, Closed — Cns/Neurology
79MCY Kit, Wound Dressing — Surgery
79LXU Laser, Healing, Wound — Surgery
90REI Laser, Therapeutic — Radiology
80MXI Nonabsorbable Gauze, Surgical Sponge, & Wound Dressing for External Use (with a Drug) — General
78EYF Protector, Wound, Plastic — Gastro/Urology
79KGW Ring Drape Retention, Internal (Wound Protector) — Surgery
80RSU Shield, Wound, Injection Site — General
79MUG Solution, Saline(wound Dressing) — Surgery
89WIN Stimulator, Wound Healing — Physical Med
80RZE Tape, Adhesive — General
80TFO Training Manikin, Wound Moulage — General
79UKY Zipper, Wound Closure — Surgery

WOVEN
80WXA Component, Other — General

WRAP
88RSZ Kit, Shroud — Pathology
79KCT Pack, Sterilization Wrapper (Bag And Accessories) — Surgery
80FRG Wrap, Sterilization — General

KEYWORD INDEX

Y-TYPE
74WJY Connector, Tubing, Blood — Cardiovascular

YAG
79SIV Equipment/Accessories, Laser, Laparoscopy — Surgery
80WQS Laser, Combination — General
79QYU Laser, Nd:YAG, Laparoscopy — Surgery
79ULA Laser, Nd:YAG, Surgical — Surgery
86LOI Laser, Neodymium:YAG (Excl. Post. Capstmy./Pupilloplasty) — Ophthalmology
86LXS Laser, Neodymium:YAG, Ophthalmic (Post. Capsulotomy) — Ophthalmology
85LLW Laser, Neodymium:YAG, Surgical, Gynecologic — Obstetrics/Gyn
73LLO Laser, Neodymium:YAG, Surgical, Pulmonary — Anesthesiology
79WOH System, Cooling, Laser — Surgery

YANKAUER
79ULE Tip, Suction Tube (Yankauer, Poole, Etc.) — Surgery
80WNO Tube, Suction — General

YEAST
83LHK Antigen, ID, Candida Albicans — Microbiology
83MLA DNA-Probe, Yeast — Microbiology
83JXB Kit, Identification, Yeast — Microbiology
83JXC Kit, Yeast Screening — Microbiology

YELLOW
88ICM Stain, Brilliant Yellow — Pathology
88KJZ Stain, Martius Yellow — Pathology
88HYY Stain, Metanil Yellow — Pathology
88IAA Stain, Titan Yellow — Pathology

YOKE
73CAM Yoke, Medical Gas — Anesthesiology

ZENKER'S
88IFH Solution, Pathology, Zenker's — Pathology

ZIMMERMAN
75CDG Chromatographic Separation/Zimmerman 17-Ketogenic Steroids — Chemistry
75CDE Chromatographic Separation/Zimmerman, 17-Ketosteroids — Chemistry
75CCY Zimmerman (Spectrophotometric), 17-Ketosteroids — Chemistry
75CCZ Zimmerman/Norymberski, 17-Ketogenic Steroids — Chemistry

ZINC
76MZW Dental Cement w/out Zinc-Oxide Eugenol as an Ulcer Covering for Pain Relief — Dental And Oral
91DNX Protoporphyrin Zinc Method, Fluorometric, Lead — Toxicology
75CEI Uranyl Acetate/Zinc Acetate, Sodium — Chemistry
76EMB Zinc Oxide Eugenol — Dental And Oral
91DJM Zinc, Test Reagents — Toxicology

ZIPPER
80WSY Closure, Other — General
79UKY Zipper, Wound Closure — Surgery

ZONE
83KZK Reader, Zone, Automated — Microbiology

ZYGOMATIC
77UCA Prosthesis, Zygomatic — Ear/Nose/Throat

11-DEOXYCORTISOL
75JKB Radioimmunoassay, Compound S (11-Deoxycortisol) — Chemistry

125-I
91DPJ RIA, Amphetamine (125-I), Goat Antibody, Ammonia — Toxicology
91DND RIA, Digitoxin (125-I), Rabbit Antibody, Solid Phase Sep. — Toxicology
91DNS RIA, Digoxin (125-I), Rabbit Antibody, Double Label Sep. — Toxicology
91DNA RIA, Morphine-Barbiturate (125-I), Goat Antibody — Toxicology
91LCW Radioimmunoassay, Digitoxin (125-I) — Toxicology
91DPL Radioimmunoassay, Digitoxin (125-I), Bovine, Charcoal — Toxicology
91DPG Radioimmunoassay, Digitoxin (125-I), Rabbit, Coated Tube — Toxicology
91LCS Radioimmunoassay, Digoxin (125-I) — Toxicology
91DOA Radioimmunoassay, Digoxin (125-I), Goat Anion Exchange — Toxicology
91DNJ Radioimmunoassay, Digoxin (125-I), Goat, 2nd Antibody — Toxicology
91DNL Radioimmunoassay, Digoxin (125-I), Rabbit, 2nd Antibody — Toxicology
91DPB Radioimmunoassay, Digoxin (125-I), Rabbit, Charcoal — Toxicology
91DPO Radioimmunoassay, Digoxin (125-I), Rabbit, Coated Tube — Toxicology
91DOG Radioimmunoassay, Digoxin (125-I), Rabbit, Poly. Glycol — Toxicology
91DON Radioimmunoassay, Digoxin (125-I), Rabbit, Solid Phase — Toxicology
91DJB Radioimmunoassay, Gentamicin (125-I), Second Antibody — Toxicology
91DLB Radioimmunoassay, LSD (125-I) — Toxicology
91DOE Radioimmunoassay, Morphine (125-I), Goat Antibody — Toxicology
91LCE Radioimmunoassay, Netilmicin (125-I) — Toxicology

17-HYDROXYCORTICOSTEROIDS
75JHD Fluorometric Method, 17-Hydroxycorticosteroids — Chemistry
75CDB Porter Silber Hydrazone, 17-Hydroxycorticosteroids — Chemistry
75JHE Radioassay, 17-Hydroxycorticosteroids — Chemistry

17-HYDROXYPROGESTERONE
75JLX Radioimmunoassay, 17-Hydroxyprogesterone — Chemistry

17-KETOGENIC
75CDG Chromatographic Separation/Zimmerman 17-Ketogenic Steroids — Chemistry
75CCZ Zimmerman/Norymberski, 17-Ketogenic Steroids — Chemistry

17-KETOSTEROIDS
75CDE Chromatographic Separation/Zimmerman, 17-Ketosteroids — Chemistry
75CCY Zimmerman (Spectrophotometric), 17-Ketosteroids — Chemistry

2-GLYCOPROTEIN
82DDN Antigen, Antiserum, Control, Beta 2-Glycoprotein I — Immunology

2B
88KKB Stain, Methyl Violet 2b — Pathology

2N-GLYCOPROTEIN
82DBC Alpha 2, 2N-Glycoprotein, Antigen, Antiserum, Control — Immunology

3-DIMENSIONAL
90UFD Computer, Radiographic Image Analysis — Radiology
74WYD Equipment, Ultrasound, Intravascular, 3-Dimensional — Cardiovascular
79SGZ System, Camera, 3-Dimensional — Surgery

3-DPG
75JLY Phosphoglycerate Mutase (colorimetric), 2, 3-diphosphoglyceric Acid — Chemistry

3-H
91DOW RIA, Digitoxin (3-H), Rabbit Antibody, Coated Tube — Toxicology
91DOY RIA, Digoxin (3-H), Goat Antibody, 2nd Antibody Sep. — Toxicology
91DNQ RIA, Digoxin (3-H), Rabbit Antibody, Coated Tube Sep. — Toxicology
91DOB Radioimmunoassay, Digitoxin (3-H) — Toxicology
91DNW Radioimmunoassay, Digitoxin (3-H), Rabbit Antibody, Char. — Toxicology
91LCT Radioimmunoassay, Digoxin (3-H) — Toxicology
91DOR Radioimmunoassay, Digoxin (3-H), Bovine, Charcoal — Toxicology
91DPD Radioimmunoassay, Digoxin (3-H), Rabbit, Charcoal — Toxicology
91DIQ Radioimmunoassay, Morphine (3-H), Ammonium Sulfate — Toxicology

3-PHASE
90VHL Generator, Diagnostic X-Ray, High Voltage, 3-Phase — Radiology

3-WHEELED
89INI Scooter (Motorized 3-Wheeled Vehicle) — Physical Med

35MM
90SGP Viewer/Analyzer, 35mm Angio — Radiology

4-DINITROFLUOROBENZENE
75JMW 2, 4-dinitrofluorobenzene (spectroscopic), Nitrogen (amino-nitrogen) — Chemistry

5'-NUCLEOTIDASE
75CED 5-AMP-Phosphate Release (Colorimetric), 5'-Nucleotidase — Chemistry

5-AMP-PHOSPHATE
75CED 5-AMP-Phosphate Release (Colorimetric), 5'-Nucleotidase — Chemistry

5-HYDROXYINDOLE
75CDA Nitrous Acid & Nitrosonaphthol, 5-Hydroxyindole Acetic Acid — Chemistry

5MM
78WZV Choledochoscope, Mini-Diameter (5mm or Less) — Gastro/Urology

6-DIPHOSPHATE
75CJC Fructose-1, 6-Diphosphate And NADH (U.V.), Aldolase — Chemistry

6-PHOSPHOGLUCONATE
75JND NADP Reduction, 6-Phosphogluconate Dehydrogenase — Chemistry

6MM
79FZB Prosthesis, Arterial Graft, Synthetic, Greater Than 6mm — Surgery
79JCP Prosthesis, Arterial Graft, Synthetic, Less Than 6mm — Surgery
74DYF Prosthesis, Vascular Graft, Less Than 6mm Diameter — Cardiovascular
74DSY Prosthesis, Vascular Graft, Of 6mm And Greater Diameter — Cardiovascular
74LXA Tissue Graft of 6mm and Greater — Cardiovascular
74LWZ Tissue Graft of Less than 6mm — Cardiovascular

Section II

Product Directory

Purpose of this Section

Allows you to identify all manufacturers of a particular product, and to compare products among the different manufacturers.

Features

- Each FDA/*MDR* standard medical product category is listed in alphabetical order, followed by the medical specialty area and the specific five-character product code. Before using this section, consult the Keyword Index to be sure you have the correct FDA/*MDR* standard product category name.

- Under each product category, each manufacturer of that product is listed, with the manufacturer's address, phone number, and any more-detailed product information or descriptions the company has submitted. For many products, specifications and prices can be compared among manufacturers, on a summary basis.

- Additional product information is available in advertisements within the section, including display ads and enhanced listings.

- Users who cannot locate a particular product or manufacturer can obtain assistance from the *MDR* staff, who will search for the latest information. Please call 215-944-9836.

Health Resources from Grey House Publishing

The HMO/PPO Directory

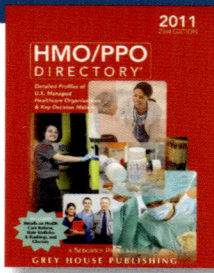

This comprehensive directory details more information about more managed health care organizations than ever before. Over 1,100 HMOs, PPOs and affiliated companies are listed, arranged alphabetically by state. Detailed listings include Key Contact Information, Drug Benefits, Enrollment, Geographical Areas served, Affiliated Physicians & Hospitals, Federal Qualifications, Status, Year Founded, Managed Care Partners, Employer References, Fees & Payment Information and more. *The HMO/PPO Directory* provides the most comprehensive information on the most companies available on the market place today.

600 pages; Softcover ISBN 978-1-59237-587-5, $325.00
Online & Directory Combo: $800.00
Online Database (Single User): $650.00

Medical Device Register

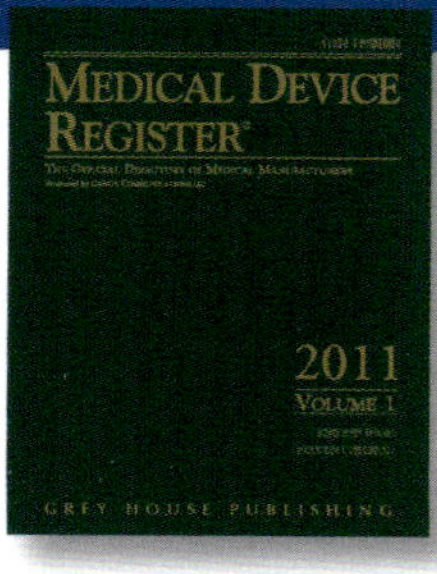

Offers fast access to over 13,000 companies - and more than 65,000 products. Volume I: Products, provides the essential information you need when purchasing or specifying medical supplies on every medical device, supply, and diagnostic available in the US. Listings provide FDA codes, Federal Procurement Eligibility, Contact information, Prices and Product Specifications. Volume 2: Suppliers, details the most complete and important data about Suppliers, Manufacturers and Distributors, with Key Executives, Contact Information along with their medical products and specialties. *Medical Device Register* is your only one-stop source for locating suppliers and products; looking for new manufacturers or hard-to-find medical devices; comparing products; know who's selling what and who to buy from cost effectively.

3,000 pages; Two Volumes; Hardcover ISBN 978-1-59237-588-2, $350.00
Online Database & Print Combo, $1,295.00

The Directory of Hospital Personnel

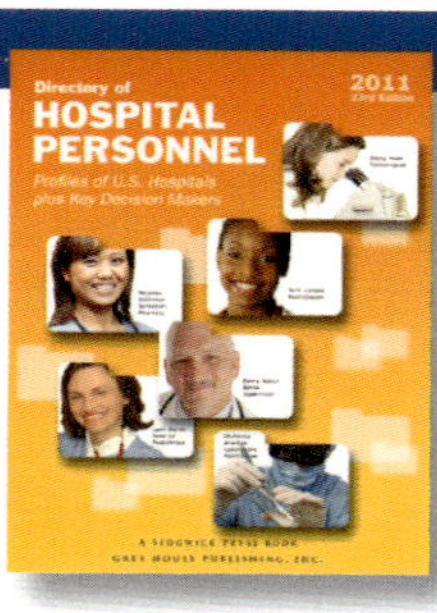

The Directory of Hospital Personnel is the best resource you can have at your fingertips when researching or marketing a product or service to the hospital market. A "Who's Who" of the hospital universe, this directory puts you in touch with over 150,000 key decision-makers. Every hospital in the U.S. is profiled, listed alphabetically by city within state. *The Directory of Hospital Personnel* is the only complete source for key hospital decision-makers by name. Whether you want to define or restructure sales territories... locate hospitals with the purchasing power to accept your proposals... or find information on which insurance plans are accepted, *The Directory of Hospital Personnel* gives you the information you need – easily, efficiently, effectively and accurately.

2,500 pages; Softcover ISBN 978-1-59237-738-1, $325.00
Online & Directory Combo: $800.00 | Online Database (Single User): $650.00

The Directory of Health Care Group Purchasing Organizations

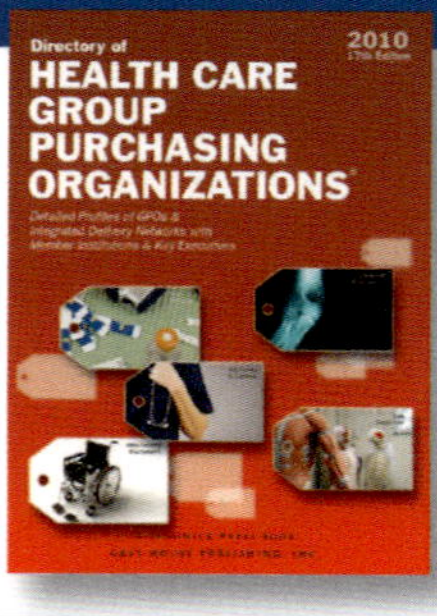

By providing in-depth information on this growing market and its members, *The Directory of Health Care Group Purchasing Organizations* fills a major need for the most accurate and comprehensive information on over 800 GPOs – Mailing Address, Phone & Fax Numbers, E-mail Addresses, Key Contacts, Purchasing Agents, Group Descriptions, Membership Categorization, Standard Vendor Proposal Requirements, Membership Fees & Terms, Expanded Services, Total Member Beds & Outpatient Visits represented and more. With its comprehensive and detailed information on each purchasing organization, *The Directory of Health Care Group Purchasing Organizations* is the go-to source for anyone looking to target this market.

1,000 pages; Softcover ISBN 978-1-59237-541-7, $325.00
Online & Directory Combo: $800.00 | Online Database (Single User): $650.00

The Comparative Guide to American Hospitals

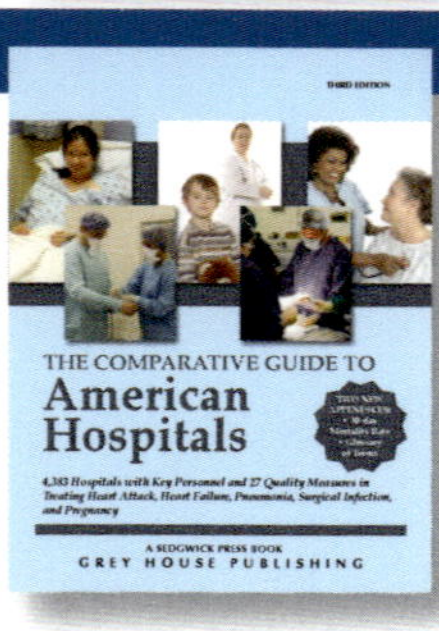

This important resource illustrates how the nation's hospitals rate when providing 24 different treatments within four broad categories: Heart Attack Care, Heart Failure Care, Surgical Infection Prevention, and Pregnancy Care. Each profile includes the raw percentage for that hospital, the state and US averages and data on the top hospital. Most importantly, *The Comparative Guide to American Hospitals* provides easy-to-use Regional State by State Statistical Summary Tables for each of the data elements to allow the user to quickly locate hospitals with the best level of service. Plus, a new 30-Day Mortality Chart, Glossary of Terms and Regional Hospital Profile Index make this a must-have source. This new, expanded edition will be a must for the reference collection at all public, medical and academic libraries.

2,000 pages; Four Volume Set; Softcover ISBN 978-1-59237-838-8, $350.00

(800) 562-2139 • www.greyhouse.com

PRODUCT DIRECTORY

ABERROMETER, OPHTHALMIC *(Ophthalmology) 86NCF*

Amo Wavefront Sciences Llc 714-247-8656
14820 Central Ave SE, Albuquerque, NM 87123
Ophthalmic refractometer.

Digital Vision, Inc 678-222-5200
301 Perimeter Ctr N Ste 600, Atlanta, GA 30346
Aberrometer, ophthalmic.

Ophthonix Inc. 760-842-5772
1491 Poinsettia Ave, Vista, CA 92081
Aberrometer.

Tracey Technologies Corp. 281-445-1666
16720 Hedgecroft Dr Ste 208, Houston, TX 77060
Wave front aberrometer.

Wavetec Vision 949-273-5970
6 Cromwell Ste 102, Irvine, CA 92618

Wavetec Vision Systems, Inc. 949-273-5970
66 Argonaut Ste 170, Aliso Viejo, CA 92656

ABSORBENT, CARBON-DIOXIDE *(Anesthesiology) 73CBL*

A-M Systems, Inc. 800-426-1306
131 Business Park Loop, Sequim, WA 98382
4 types-from $11.13/3lb Sodalime to $175.48/500 gr Ascarite; $7.54 ea. to $16.00 ea. for prefilled, disposable drying columns (4 types).

Allied Healthcare Products, Inc. 314-268-1683
46 New St., Stuyvesant Falls, NY 12174
Absorbent carbon dioxide.

Allied Healthcare Products, Inc. 800-444-3954
1720 Sublette Ave, Saint Louis, MO 63110

Darex Container Products 617-498-4357
6050 W 51st St, Chicago, IL 60638
Sodasorb.

Intersurgical Inc. 315-451-2900
417 Electronics Pkwy, Liverpool, NY 13088
SPHERASORB Soda Lime, carbon dioxide absorbent.

Optimize Mfg. Co. 520-287-4605
Apdo Postal 205-A,, Parque Industrial San Ramon
Nogales, Sonora Mexico
An-trol ii co2 absorber

UBM Canon 800-442-4200
11444 W Olympic Blvd Ste 900, Los Angeles, CA 90064

ABSORBER, CARBON-DIOXIDE *(Anesthesiology) 73BSF*

Anesthesia Associates, Inc. 760-744-6561
460 Enterprise St, San Marcos, CA 92078
Adult and Pediatric sizes. Complete with scavenger valve, inspiratory/expiratory valves, bag mount, fresh gas inlet, and pressure gauge. Constructed of Chrome Plated Brass. PN 00-720A and 00-720

Datex-Ohmeda Inc. 608-221-1551
3030 Ohmeda Dr, Madison, WI 53718
Various.

Hacker Industries, Inc. 803-712-6100
1132 Kincaid Bridge Rd, Winnsboro, SC 29180
Downdraft fume extractor.

ABSORBER, CARBON-DIOXIDE *(cont'd)*

Optimize Mfg. Co. 520-287-4605
Apdo Postal 205-A,, Parque Industrial San Ramon
Nogales, Sonora Mexico
An-trol ii co2 absorber

ABSORBER, SALIVA, PAPER *(Dental And Oral) 76KHR*

Coltene/Whaledent Inc. 330-916-8858
235 Ascot Pkwy, Cuyahoga Falls, OH 44223
Dam napkins.

Crosstex International, Inc. 516-482-9001
621 Hurricane Shoals Rd NW Ste G, Lawrenceville, GA 30046

Dental Health Products, Inc. 716-754-2696
4011 Creek Rd, Youngstown, NY 14174
Various types of thin absorbant cellulose triangles.

Garrison Dental Solutions 616-842-2244
110 Dewitt Ln, Spring Lake, MI 49456
Paper rolls, cotton rolls, dry angles.

George Taub Products & Fusion Co., Inc. 800-828-2634
277 New York Ave, Jersey City, NJ 07307
Sal-Dri, is absorbent paper dry angles used to maintain a dry field during sealing procedures and protect the cheek from being scratched by dental instruments. One size. Rounded edges. Absorbent on both sides.

Lorvic Corp. 800-325-1881
13705 Shoreline Ct E, Earth City, MO 63045
Dri Aid Absorbent protective wafer.

Statsure Diagnostic Systems, Inc. 508-872-2625
1881 Worcester Rd, Framingham, MA 01701

Tidi Products, Llc 920-751-4380
570 Enterprise Dr, Neenah, WI 54956
Dental towel (bib).

United Medical Enterprises 757-224-0177
4049 Allen Station Rd, Augusta, GA 30906
Cotton dental rolls.

ABSORPTION, ATOMIC, ANTIMONY *(Toxicology) 91DNE*

Celsis Laboratory Group 800-523-5227
165 Fieldcrest Ave, Edison, NJ 08837

ABSORPTION, ATOMIC, ARSENIC *(Toxicology) 91DNZ*

Celsis Laboratory Group 800-523-5227
165 Fieldcrest Ave, Edison, NJ 08837

ABSORPTION, ATOMIC, CALCIUM *(Chemistry) 75JFN*

Celsis Laboratory Group 800-523-5227
165 Fieldcrest Ave, Edison, NJ 08837

ABSORPTION, ATOMIC, IRON (NON-HEME) *(Chemistry) 75JIZ*

Celsis Laboratory Group 800-523-5227
165 Fieldcrest Ave, Edison, NJ 08837

ABSORPTION, ATOMIC, LEAD *(Toxicology) 91DOF*

Celsis Laboratory Group 800-523-5227
165 Fieldcrest Ave, Edison, NJ 08837

ABSORPTION, ATOMIC, LITHIUM *(Toxicology) 91JII*

Carolina Liquid Chemistries Corp. 800-471-7272
510 W Central Ave Ste C, Brea, CA 92821
Lithium reagent.

Celsis Laboratory Group 800-523-5227
165 Fieldcrest Ave, Edison, NJ 08837

Diazyme Laboratories 858-455-4761
12889 Gregg Ct, Poway, CA 92064
Lithium enzymatic assay.

ABSORPTION, ATOMIC, MAGNESIUM *(Chemistry) 75JGI*

Celsis Laboratory Group 800-523-5227
165 Fieldcrest Ave, Edison, NJ 08837

ABSORPTION, ATOMIC, MERCURY *(Toxicology) 91DPH*

Celsis Laboratory Group 800-523-5227
165 Fieldcrest Ave, Edison, NJ 08837

ABUTMENT, IMPLANT, DENTAL, ENDOSSEOUS
(Dental And Oral) 76NHA

Implant Direct Llc 818-444-3300
27030 Malibu Hills Rd, Calabasas Hills, CA 91301
Various types of sterile and non sterile dental implants, abutments, and accesso.

Nobel Biocare Usa, Llc 800-579-6515
22715/22725 Savi Ranch Parkway, Yorba Linda, CA 92887
Abutment, implant, dental, endosseous.

Straumann Manufacturing, Inc. 978-747-2575
60 Minuteman Rd, Andover, MA 01810
Coping, occlusal & closure screws, healing caps.

Swiss Implants, Inc. 805-781-8700
567 Marsh St, San Luis Obispo, CA 93401
Dental implants in flat top or hex top with abutments.

ACACIA AND KARAYA WITH SODIUM BORATE
(Dental And Oral) 76KOM

Chewrite Co., A Subsidiary Of Magnesia Products, I 513-746-5509
265 Pioneer Blvd., Springboro, OH 45066
Denture adhesive.

ACCELERATOR, LINEAR, MEDICAL *(Radiology) 90IYE*

.Decimal, Inc. 407-330-3300
121 Central Park Pl, Sanford, FL 32771
Blocking tray.

Accuray, Inc. 888-522-3740
1310 Chesapeake Ter, Sunnyvale, CA 94089
Medical linear accelerator.

Calypso Medical Technologies Inc 206-254-0600
2101 4th Ave Ste 500, Seattle, WA 98121
Patient localization system.

Capintec, Inc. 800-631-3826
6 Arrow Rd, Ramsey, NJ 07446
292 THERARAD Measurements can be performed in total mode and rate mode. Display of exposure/exposure rate, dose/dose rate available, up to 100 measured results can be stored.

Computerized Medical Systems, Inc. 468-587-2550
1145 Corporate Lake Dr, Olivette, MO 63132
Patient positioning system.

Direx Systems Corp. 339-502-6013
437 Turnpike St, Canton, MA 02021
Acculeaf.

Elekta Inc. 800-535-7355
4775 Peachtree Industrial Blvd, Bldg. 300, Suite 300
Norcross, GA 30092

Elekta, Inc. 800-535-7355
4775 Peachtree Industrial Blvd, Building 300, Suite 300
Norcross, GA 30092
Radiation therapy devices. Radiotherapy networking system.

Impac Medical Systems, Inc. 888-464-6722
100 W Evelyn Ave, Mountain View, CA 94041
Oncology Management Software.

International Radiographic, Inc. 404-405-7909
395 Grand Teton Cir, Fayetteville, GA 30215
Reconditioned linear accelerators for radiation oncology.

K&S Assoc., Inc. 615-883-9760
1926 Elm Tree Dr, Nashville, TN 37210
K & s setup program for dos and windows.

ACCELERATOR, LINEAR, MEDICAL *(cont'd)*

L-3 Communications Electron Devices 650-591-8411
960 Industrial Rd, San Carlos, CA 94070
Klystrons (component of accelerator, linear, medical).

Larson Medical Products, Inc. 614-235-9100
2844 Banwick Rd, Columbus, OH 43232
Klarity thermoplastic.

Medical Devices International 504-455-8311
3724 Severn Ave, Metairie, LA 70002
pre owned Varian , Elekta

Medical Dosimetry Services, Inc. 405-680-5222
1601 SW 89th St Ste E100, Oklahoma City, OK 73159
Monitor unit calculation program.

Medicalibration Physics Consultant Services, Inc. 209-524-6789
558 Van Dyken Way, Ripon, CA 95366
3d treatment planning system.

Medtec 800-842-8688
1401 8th St SE, PO Box 320, Orange City, IA 51041
Testicle separator.

Melton And Associates 800-831-8221
PO Box 947, Manassas, VA 20113
Various patient immobilization devices for breast, head, neck treatment.

Mpi Medical Products, Inc. 321-676-1299
1631 Elmhurst Cir SE, Palm Bay, FL 32909
Breast board.

Multidata Systems International Corp. 314-968-6880
9801 Manchester Rd, Saint Louis, MO 63119
Dosimetry system.

Northwest Medical Physics Equipment, Inc. 319-656-4447
21031 67th Ave W, Lynnwood, WA 98036
Hardware for stereotactic radiotherapy;software for stereotactic radiotherapy.

Oncology Services International 800-445-4516
500 N Franklin Tpke, Ramsey, NJ 07446
Linear accelerator.

Pro-Comm, Inc. 800-920-1476
1105 Industrial Pkwy, Brick, NJ 08724
2856 MHz, 2999 MHz, 3000 MHz RF Driver portion of Klystron linear accelerators (including high energy type) from $20,000 new. Also rebuild @ $5K to $8K.

Radiological Imaging Technology, Inc. 719-590-1077
5065 List Dr, Colorado Springs, CO 80919
Rit 113 film dosimetry system; rit 113 film analysis system.

S & S X-Ray Products, Inc. 800-231-1747
10625 Telge Rd, Houston, TX 77095
Medical linear accelerator (vacuum fixation device).

Sicel Technologies, Inc. 919-465-2236
3800 Gateway Centre Blvd Ste 308, Morrisville, NC 27560
Radiation dosimeter.

Standard Imaging, Inc. 608-831-0025
3120 Deming Way, Middleton, WI 53562
Various types of qa software.

Sun Nuclear Corp. 321-259-6862
425 Pineda Ct Ste A, Melbourne, FL 32940
Dosimetry electrometer and monitors: model 1010,1131,1133,& 1135.

The Phantom Laboratory, Inc. 800-525-1190
PO Box 511, Salem, NY 12865

The Soule Co., Inc. 813-907-6000
4322 Pet Ln, Lutz, FL 33559
Patient positioning system.

Tomotherapy Incorporated 608-824-2800
1209 Deming Way, Madison, WI 53717
Radiation therapy device.

Varian Medical Systems 800-544-4636
3100 Hansen Way, Palo Alto, CA 94304
Trilogy(tm) and Clinac(R) medical linear accelerators. Models with 4 to 22 MV x-ray energy; 200-500 rad/min max x-ray output and 500 rad/min max electron output at S.A.D. Trilogy medical linear accelerator is optimized for conventional, conformal, IMRT, and stereotactic radiotherapies.

Varian Medical Systems, Oncology Systems 800 278-2747
911 Hansen Way, Bldg.3 M/S C-165, Palo Alto, CA 94304
Medical linear accelerator, accessories.

ACCELEROMETER *(Chemistry) 75TAA*

Analog Devices, Inc. 800-262-5643
1 Technology Way, P. O. Box 9106, Norwood, MA 02062
ADXL345 ultra-low-power digital accelerometer measures tilt, shock and acceleration. The device operates at a primary supply voltage down to 1.8 V and uses less than 25 uA of power, yet has a resolution high enough to detect inclination changes as small as 0.25 degrees. The ADXL345 has an output data range that scales from 0.1 Hz to 3.2 kHz, unlike competing devices, which have fixed 100-Hz, 400-Hz, or 1-kHz data rates.

Apollo Research Corporation 800-418-1718
2300 Walden Ave Ste 200, Buffalo, NY 14225
Small, lightweight piezoelectric motion sensors. Available in single and multi versions.

Kistler Instrument Corp. 716-691-5100
75 John Glenn Dr, Amherst, NY 14228

U.F.I. 805-772-1203
545 Main St Ste C2, Morro Bay, CA 93442
$170.00 for Model 1110.

ACCESSORIES, APPAREL, SURGICAL *(Surgery) 79LYU*

A Plus International, Inc 909-591-5168
5138 Eucalyptus Ave, Chino, CA 91710
Non woven apparel.

Ahlstrom Windsor Locks Llc 860-654-8300
2 Elm St, Windsor Locks, CT 06096

Alphaprotech, Inc. 229-242-1931
1287 W Fairway Dr, Nogales, AZ 85621

Amd-Ritmed, Inc. 800-445-0340
295 Firetower Road, Tonawanda, NY 14150

American Health Care Apparel Ltd. 800-252-0584
302 Town Center Blvd, Easton, PA 18040
Assistive dressing apparel.

Angelica Image Apparel 800-222-3112
700 Rosedale Ave, Saint Louis, MO 63112

Biomed Resource, Inc. 310-323-3888
3388 Rosewood Ave, Los Angeles, CA 90066
Face mask, lab coat, coverall.

Brennen Medical, Llc 651-429-7413
1290 Hammond Rd, Saint Paul, MN 55110
Water repellent apron.

Busse Hospital Disposables, Inc. 631-435-4711
75 Arkay Dr, Hauppauge, NY 11788
Lab coats and coveralls.

Clinetics 518-477-6886
25 Hy Dr, East Schodack, NY 12063
Dispoaable, splash, face shield.

Coast Scientific 800-445-1544
1445 Engineer St, Vista, CA 92081
Polypropylene apparel, ear-loop/tie-on mask, cone mask, ear-loop/tie-on mask with protective shield, polypropylene bouffant caps. Surgical caps, polypropylene beard covers, polypropylene shoe covers, polylatex shoe covers.

Customed, Inc. 787-801-0101
Calle Igualdad #7, Fajardo, PR 00738
Male ambulatory kit.

Dale Medical Products, Inc. 800-343-3980
7 Cross St, Plainville, MA 02762
Post Surgical Bra: 701 small 32-34 in. A,B.; 702 Med 34-36 in. B,C.; 703 Large 36-38 in. C,D; 704 X-Large 38-44 in. C,D; 705 XX-Large 40-44 in. DD

Dental/Medical Optics Mfg., Inc. 516-889-5857
4217 Austin Blvd, Island Park, NY 11558
Full face protective shield.

Depuy Orthopaedics, Inc. 800-473-3789
700 Orthopaedic Dr, P.O. Box 988, Warsaw, IN 46582
Various types of surgical apparel accessories.

Innovamed, Inc. 801-885-9085
13524 Oakridge Dr, Alpine, UT 84004
External fixator protective cover.

Kentron Health Care, Inc. 615-384-0573
3604 Kelton Jackson Rd, P.o. Box 120, Springfield, TN 37172
Face shield.

Kerma Medical Products, Inc. 757-398-8400
400 Port Centre Pkwy, Portsmouth, VA 23704
Face shield, sweatbands.

ACCESSORIES, APPAREL, SURGICAL *(cont'd)*

Lakeland De Mexico S.A. De C.V. 516-981-9700
Rancho La Soledad Lote No. 2, Fracc. Poniente C.p. Celaya, Guajuato Mexico
Surgical apparel accessory items

Lexamed 419-693-5307
705 Front St, Northwood, OH 43605
Sterile towels.

Microtek Medical, Inc 800-936-9248
512 N Lehmberg Rd, Columbus, MS 39702
CleanOp system consists of an entire line of products and supplies designed to efficiently and effectively clean a procedural room and prepare it for subsequent use.

Oto-Med, Inc. 800-433-7703
1090 Empire Dr, Lake Havasu City, AZ 86404
Sheehy Bone Dust Pate collector: Easy-to-use bone-collecting device used in the suction line.

Polyconversions, Inc. 888-893-3330
505 E Condit Dr, Rantoul, IL 61866
Thumbloop, open-back, polyethylene infection control gowns.

Pro-Tex International, Inc. 209-545-1691
5038 Salida Blvd, Salida, CA 95368
Face shield, face protector, plastic & designer support frames.

Products For Medicine 800-333-3087
1201 E Ball Rd Ste H, Anaheim, CA 92805
Face shield.

Sloan Corp. 402-597-5700
13316 A St, Omaha, NE 68144
Bootleg legging,pant protector.

Standard Textile 800-999-0400
1 Knollcrest Dr, Cincinnati, OH 45237

Surgical Tools, Inc. 800-774-2040
1106 Monroe St, Bedford, VA 24523

Tapeless Wound Care Products, Llc. 866-714-9199
PO Box 4515, Englewood, CO 80155
G- tube holder with variably located pocket

Techstyles Manufacturing Division 800-826-4490
16415 Addison Rd Ste 660, Addison, TX 75001
Non-sterile disposable protective apparel.

Tradewinds Rehabilitation Center, Inc. 219-949-4000
5901 W 7th Ave, Gary, IN 46406
Coat, laboratory.

Watkins-Witt Group, Llc 714-368-0790
15731 Pasadena Ave Apt 10, Tustin, CA 92780
Patient bed socks,accessory,surgical.

White Knight Engineered Products 888-743-4700
7422 Carmel Executive Park, Suite 310, Charlotte, NC 28226
Polar Pack personal cooling vests.

White Knight Healthcare 800-851-4431
Calle 16, Number 780, Agua Prieta, Sonora Mexico
Surgeons vest

ACCESSORIES, ARTHROSCOPE *(Orthopedics) 87VIE*

Future Medical Systems, Inc. 800-367-6021
504 McCormick Dr Ste T, Glen Burnie, MD 21061
FMS-DUO, FMS-SOLO pumps, shavers, cannulas

Integral Design Inc. 781-740-2036
52 Burr Rd, Hingham, MA 02043

Karl Storz Endoscopy-America Inc. 800-421-0837
600 Corporate Pointe, Culver City, CA 90230
Full line of both diagnostic and operative models in various sizes.

Microtek Medical, Inc 800-936-9248
512 N Lehmberg Rd, Columbus, MS 39702
Camera drapes, specialty arthroscopy patient drapes.

Mizuho Osi 800-777-4674
30031 Ahern Ave, Union City, CA 94587
Arthroscopic positioning devices.

Plastic And Metal Center, Inc. 949-770-8230
23162 La Cadena Dr, Laguna Hills, CA 92653

Richard Wolf Medical Instruments Corp. 800-323-9653
353 Corporate Woods Pkwy, Vernon Hills, IL 60061

Smith & Nephew, Inc., Endoscopy Division 800-343-8386
150 Minuteman Rd, Andover, MA 01810
Cannulae, trocars, obturators, couplers and beamsplitters.

Smith & Nephew, Inc., Endoscopy Division 800-343-8386
130 Forbes Blvd, Mansfield, MA 02048

ACCESSORIES, ARTHROSCOPE *(cont'd)*

Symmetry Tnco 888-447-6661
15 Colebrook Blvd, Whitman, MA 02382
Punches, graspers and scissors.

ACCESSORIES, ARTHROSCOPIC *(Orthopedics) 87NBH*

Arthrex Manufacturing 239-643-5553
1958 Trade Center Way, Naples, FL 34109
Scope,dilator,c-mount adaptor,arthroscopy sheath.

Arthrex, Inc. 239-643-5553
1370 Creekside Blvd, Naples, FL 34108
Obturators, sheaths.

Ascent Healthcare Solutions 480-763-5300
10232 S 51st St, Phoenix, AZ 85044
Orthopedic cannulas and trocars.

Medisiss 866-866-7477
2747 SW 6th St, Redmond, OR 97756
Orthopedic arthroscopic accessories, sterile.

Medtronic Sofamor Danek Instrument Manufacturing 901-396-3133
7375 Adrianne Pl, Bartlett, TN 38133
Arthroscope.

Medtronic Sofamor Danek Usa, Inc. 901-396-3133
4340 Swinnea Rd, Memphis, TN 38118
Arthroscope.

Nuvasive, Inc. 800-475-9131
7475 Lusk Blvd, San Diego, CA 92121
Surgical instruments.

Osseon Therapeutics, Inc. 877-567-7366
2330 Circadian Way, Santa Rosa, CA 95407
OsseoFlex 1.0 Steerable Needle

Sohniks Endoscopy, Inc. 651-452-4059
930 Blue Gentian Rd Ste 1400, Eagan, MN 55121
Rigid telescope.

Spine Wave, Inc. 203-944-9494
2 Enterprise Dr Ste 302, Shelton, CT 06484
Various types of cannulas.

Sterilmed, Inc. 763-488-3400
11400 73rd Ave N Ste 100, Maple Grove, MN 55369
Obturators, sheaths.

Synthes San Diego 858-452-1266
6244 Ferris Sq Ste B, San Diego, CA 92121
Various arthroscopic accessories.

Warsaw Orthopedic, Inc. 901-396-3133
2500 Silveus Xing, Warsaw, IN 46582
Arthroscope.

ACCESSORIES, AV SHUNT *(Gastro/Urology) 78KNZ*

Angiodynamics, Inc. 800-472-5221
1 Horizon Way, Manchester, GA 31816
Connectors, adapters, and other accessories from the A-V shunt products line.

Lifemed Of California 800-543-3633
1216 S Allec St, Anaheim, CA 92805

ACCESSORIES, BITE BLOCKS (FOR ENDOSCOPE)

(Gastro/Urology) 78MNK

Encompas Unlimited, Inc. 800-825-7701
PO Box 516, Tallevast, FL 34270
$2.20 for disposable bite block used during endoscopy. BB-30, KB-40. Latex-free versions of all Endo Bit Blocks are now available.

Endo-Therapeutics, Inc. 888-294-2377
15251 Roosevelt Blvd Ste 204, Clearwater, FL 33760

Schueler & Company, Inc. 516-487-1500
PO Box 528, Stratford, CT 06615

ACCESSORIES, BLOOD CIRCUIT, HEMODIALYSIS

(Gastro/Urology) 78KOC

Apheresis Technologies, Inc. 800-749-9284
PO Box 2081, Palm Harbor, FL 34682
Plasma discard bag.

Erika De Reynosa, S.A. De C.V. 781-402-9068
Brecha E99 Sur; Parque, Industrial Reynos, Bldg. Ii Cd, Reynosa, Tamps Mexico
Various types of blood tubing sets (sterile fluid path)

Hema Metrics Inc. 800-546-5463
695 N Kays Dr, Kaysville, UT 84037

ACCESSORIES, BLOOD CIRCUIT, HEMODIALYSIS *(cont'd)*

Innovations For Access, Inc. 800-297-8485
1815 NW 169th Pl Ste 6030, Beaverton, OR 97006
Hemoban.

Interventional Hemostasis Products, Inc. 503-638-9743
1815 NW 169th Pl Ste 6030, Beaverton, OR 97006
Pressure band,dialysis pressure band.

Lee Medical International, Inc. 800-433-8950
612 Distributors Row, Harahan, LA 70123
Bloodlines.

Medisystems Corporation 800-369-6334
439 S Union St Fl 5, Lawrence, MA 01843
Blood tubing sets for all machines.

Molded Products Inc. 800-435-8957
1112 Chatburn Ave, Harlan, IA 51537
Luer to Luer Adapter Lines

Nxstage Medical, Inc. 866-697-8243
439 S Union St Fl 5, Lawrence, MA 01843
Multiple

Rismed Oncology Systems 256-534-6993
2494 Washington St NW, Huntsville, AL 35811
Blood Line Tubing (BLT), pre and post pump, 6mm & 8mm.

Sorb Technology, Inc. 405-682-1993
3631 SW 54th St, Oklahoma City, OK 73119
Hemodialysis accessories.

Terumo Cardiovascular Systems (Tcvs) 800-283-7866
28 Howe St, Ashland, MA 01721
Transducer protector.

ACCESSORIES, CARDIOPULMONARY BYPASS

(Cardiovascular) 74KRI

Allen Medical Systems, Inc. 800-433-5774
1 Post Office Sq, Acton, MA 01720
Frogger pad naturally flexes legs and offers a stable platform on which to perform saphenous vein removal.

Atek Medical 800-253-1540
620 Watson St SW, Grand Rapids, MI 49504
Tourniquet set, coronary artery probes, coronary artery occluders.

Chase Medical, Lp 972-783-0644
1876 Firman Dr, Richardson, TX 75081
Temperature monitoring probe.

Cp Medical Corporation 800-950-2763
803 NE 25th Ave, Portland, OR 97232
Bone Wax and Cotton Umbilical Tape

International Biophysics Corp. 512-326-3244
2101 E Saint Elmo Rd Ste 275, Austin, TX 78744
Tubing organizer.

Jostra Bentley, Inc. 302-454-9959
Rd. 402 N. Km 1.4, Industrial Park, Anasco, PR 00610-1577
Various types of cardiopulmonary bypass device holder.

Medtronic Perfusion Systems 800-854-3570
7611 Northland Dr N, Brooklyn Park, MN 55428

Mmj S.A. De C.V. 314-654-2000
716 Ponciano Arriaga, Cd. Juarez, Chih. Mexico
Myocardial temperature sensor

Plastic And Metal Center, Inc. 949-770-8230
23162 La Cadena Dr, Laguna Hills, CA 92653

Terumo Cardiovascular Systems (Tcvs) 800-283-7866
28 Howe St, Ashland, MA 01721
Pressure relief valve.

Terumo Cardiovascular Systems, Corp 800-521-2818
6200 Jackson Rd, Ann Arbor, MI 48103

ACCESSORIES, CART, MULTIPURPOSE *(General) 80WSA*

Alimed, Inc. 800-225-2610
297 High St, Dedham, MA 02026

Allen Medical Systems, Inc. 800-433-5774
1 Post Office Sq, Acton, MA 01720
Storage cart for accessories

American Innovations, Inc. 800-223-3913
123 N Main St, Dublin, PA 18917
Dishwasher-safe rigid caddy captures food/beverage containers, preventing spills to the floor, and organizes daily needed items. Attaches to virtually all mobility devices.

PRODUCT DIRECTORY

ACCESSORIES, CART, MULTIPURPOSE *(cont'd)*

Armstrong Medical Industries, Inc. 800-323-4220
575 Knightsbridge Pkwy, Lincolnshire, IL 60069
Drawer trays, movable dividers and shelving units; SCOPESAFE locking fiber optic scope storage cabinet.

Blue Bell Bio-Medical 800-258-3235
1260 Industrial Dr, Van Wert, OH 45891
Combination push-button lock eliminates the need for keys.

Custom Comfort Medtek 800-749-0933
3939 Forsyth Rd Ste A, Winter Park, FL 32792
A wide range of carts, including polymer carts offering light weight and ease of use for those on a tight budget as well as tough, versatile, custom-built aluminum mobile supply carts. Adjustable-height mobile workstations come with trays, drawers, and laptop-computer space. Classic cabinets are offered with a choice of eighteen Formica colors to match any decor.

Eagle Mhc 800-637-5100
100 Industrial Blvd, Clayton, DE 19938
Exchange Carts- With various shelving configurations, caster styles, accessory packages, and various sizes, Eagle exchange carts are the ultimate in versatility.

Exchange Cart Accessories 800-823-1490
1 Commerce Dr, Freeburg, IL 62243

Gi Supply 800-451-5797
200 Grandview Ave, Camp Hill, PA 17011
UNITY, procedure cart with multiple optional attachments.

Homak Manufacturing Company Inc. 800-874-6625
1605 Old Route 18 Ste 4-36, Wampum, PA 16157
Drawer trays with dividers, coat racks (mounted to back of medical carts) for gowns or coats, and breakaway aluminum seals (used instead of padlock and key).

Home Aid Products 888-823-7605
111 Esna Park Dr., Unit 9, Markham, ONT L3R-1H2 Canada
A strong, all-purpose utility cart designed for people who are unsteady on their feet. Strong and stable enough for users to lean on and aid their balance.

Livingston Products, Inc. 800-822-2156
260 Holbrook Dr Unit A, Wheeling, IL 60090
GlideBoard is a patient transfer assistance board to bridge gaps between patinet bed and gurney to make transfer much less stressful on EMT and hospital personnel. It is also a great help in transfer of heavy patients because two boards can be combined to transfer a heavier load with safety. The board provides safety traction on the two adjoing surfaces to keep patients from falling thru the gap when transfering from one surface to another by sliding the patient easily accross the slick surface.

Mcclure Industries, Inc. 800-752-2821
9051 SE 55th Ave, Portland, OR 97206
Casters, conveyors, covers, tow systems, unloaders, washers.

Mel R. Manufacturas 956-655-1380
417 E Coma Ave Ste 534, Hidalgo, TX 78557
general subcontractor assembly services

National Systems Co. 877-672-4278
31B Durward Pl., Waterloo N2J 3Z9 Canada
A-Z index dividers (poly), alphabetic plastic dividers, plastic dietary and medication bin cards.

Stackbin Corporation 800-333-1603
29 Powder Hill Rd, Lincoln, RI 02865
Stackfiles for storage of medical records or x-rays; combination units also available.

Steelcraft, Inc. 800-225-7710
115 W Main St, Millbury, MA 01527

Valley Craft 800-328-1480
2001 S Highway 61, Lake City, MN 55041

Waterloo Healthcare, Llc 800-833-4419
3730 E Southern Ave, Phoenix, AZ 85040
Priced from $10 - $800. Packages Available. Please visit waterloohaethcare.com for a list of accessories and pictures.

Youngs, Inc. 800-523-5454
55 E Cherry Ln, Souderton, PA 18964

ACCESSORIES, CATHETER *(Surgery) 79KGZ*

Angiodynamics, Inc. 800-472-5221
1 Horizon Way, Manchester, GA 31816
Wide array of accessories including guidewires, introducer needles, dilators, caps, clips, ties/tie guns, fluid barriers, and forceps.

Bacterin International Inc. 406-388-0480
664 Cruiser Ln, Belgrade, MT 59714
Sterile closed surgical wound drains.

ACCESSORIES, CATHETER *(cont'd)*

Baxter Healthcare Corporation, Renal 888-229-0001
1620 S Waukegan Rd, Waukegan, IL 60085
Dialysis catheter accessories: IMMOBILIZER catheter stabilizing device, locking titanium adapter. BETA-CAP adapter, locking cap for Baxter peritoneal dialysis catheter adapter.

Becton Dickinson Infusion Therapy Systems, Inc. 888-237-2762
9450 S State St, Sandy, UT 84070
Continuous flush and other catheter accessories.

Better Parts Co.
219 W 90th St, Minneapolis, MN 55420
#444 catheter clamp.

Bioderm, Inc. 800-373-7006
12320 73rd Ct, Largo, FL 33773
Tube holder.

Blue Sky Medical Group Incorporated 727-392-1261
5924 Balfour Ct Ste 102, Carlsbad, CA 92008
Drainage catheter.

Boston Scientific - Maple Grove 800-553-5878
1 Scimed Pl, Maple Grove, MN 55311

Boston Scientific Corporation 508-652-5578
780 Brookside Dr, Spencer, IN 47460

Brentwood Industries, Inc. 610-374-5109
610 Morgantown Rd, Reading, PA 19611
Catheter trays up to 66in. long.

C. R. Bard, Inc., Bard Medical Div. 800-526-4455
8195 Industrial Blvd NE, Covington, GA 30014

C. R. Bard, Inc., Bard Urological Div. 888-367-2273
13183 Harland Dr NE, Covington, GA 30014

Catheter Connections Inc. 1-888-706-8883
615 Arapeen Dr Ste 302A, Salt Lake City, UT 84108
DualCap

Centurion Medical Products Corp. 517-545-1135
3310 S Main St, Salisbury, NC 28147

Dj Orthopedics De Mexico, S.A. De C.V. 690-727-1280
Blvd., Delagacion La Presa, Tijuana 22397 Mexico
Catheter straps

Dj Orthopedics De Mexico, S.A. De C.V. 690-727-1280
Ave. Venustiano Carranza 6802, Castillo, Tijuana 22100 Mexico
Catheter straps

Dma Med-Chem Corporation 800-362-1833
49 Watermill Ln, Great Neck, NY 11021
Cholangiogram Catheters

Excel Medical Products, Llc 810-714-4775
3145 Copper Ave, Fenton, MI 48430
PTCA accessory kit includes Excel-9 large bore hemostatic y-connector, guidewire insertion tool and torque device.

Exelint International Co. 800-940-3935
5840 W Centinela Ave, Los Angeles, CA 90045

Filtrona Extrusion, Inc./Pexcor Medical Products Div. 800-755-7528
764 S Athol Rd, P.O. Box 659, Athol, MA 01331

Genpore, A Division Of General Polymeric Corp. 800-654-4391
1136 Morgantown Rd, Reading, PA 19607
IV catheter vent.

Gish Biomedical, Inc. 800-938-0531
22942 Arroyo Vis, Rancho Santa Margarita, CA 92688

Haemonetics Corp. 800-225-5242
400 Wood Rd, P.O. Box 9114, Braintree, MA 02184

Halkey-Roberts Corp. 800-303-4384
2700 Halkey Roberts Pl N, Saint Petersburg, FL 33716
Valves for Foley catheters, endotracheal tubes, and I.V. applications.

Intersurgical Inc. 315-451-2900
417 Electronics Pkwy, Liverpool, NY 13088
Catheter mounts and patient elbow connections.

Intravascular Incorporated 800-917-3234
3600 Burwood Dr, Waukegan, IL 60085
FloStar Needleless Connector - patented 'dual-valve' needle free connector for use on venous or arterial lines with luer lock or luer slip in intravenous therapy. Available stand alone or on extension sets.

Johnson & Johnson De Monterrey, Sa De Cv 817-262-5211
Carretera Miguel Aleman,km21.7, Apodaca, Monterrey Mexico
Jelco intermittent injection cap*

ACCESSORIES, CATHETER *(cont'd)*

Kentron Health Care, Inc. 615-384-0573
3604 Kelton Jackson Rd, P.o. Box 120, Springfield, TN 37172
Catheter insertion trays.

Kmi Kolster Methods, Inc. 909-737-5476
3185 Palisades Dr, Corona, CA 92880
Aspiration/infiltration tubing.

Lifemed Of California 800-543-3633
1216 S Allec St, Anaheim, CA 92805

M & I Medical Sales, Inc. 305-663-6444
4711 SW 72nd Ave, Miami, FL 33155

Medicus Technologies 800-762-1574
105 Morgan Ln, Plainsboro, NJ 08536

Medovations, Inc. 800-558-6408
102 E Keefe Ave, Milwaukee, WI 53212

Merlin's Medical Supply 800-639-9322
699 Mobil Ave, Camarillo, CA 93010
Quick Snap(tm) Connector Set; Alows for a quick connect/disconnect of the GeeWhiz Condom Catheter, as well as a tubing connector for other medical and consumer product uses.

Micor, Inc. 412-487-1113
2855 Oxford Blvd, Allison Park, PA 15101
Touhy burst adapters, and catheter and needle guards (LDPE, HDPE, PVC).

Navilyst Medical 800-833-9973
100 Boston Scientific Way, Marlborough, MA 01752
Various sterile catheter accessories.

Navion Biomedical Corp. 781-341-8058
312 Tosca Dr, Stoughton, MA 02072
NAVIGATOR hand-held battery-operated catheter locating instrument displays position and direction of Navion sensor stylets and sensor guidewires.

Neo Medical Inc. 888-450-3334
42514 Albrae St, Fremont, CA 94538
Accessories, catheter.

Novosci Corp. 281-363-4949
2828 N Crescentridge Dr, The Woodlands, TX 77381
Connectors - KWIK-OFF, parallel Ys, Ys, straight and reducers.

Rose Technologies Company 616-233-3000
1440 Front Ave NW, Grand Rapids, MI 49504

Smith & Nephew, Inc. 800-876-1261
970 Lake Carillon Dr Ste 110, Saint Petersburg, FL 33716
DERMIVEX

St. Jude Medical, Inc. 800-328-9634
1 Saint Jude Medical Dr, Saint Paul, MN 55117
Connectors; ICDs.

Telios Pharmaceuticals 800-762-1574
105 Morgan Ln, Plainsboro, NJ 08536

Thomas Medical Products, Inc. 866-446-3003
65 Great Valley Pkwy, Malvern, PA 19355
Contamination / repositioning sleeve.

Tri-State Hospital Supply Corp. 517-545-1135
3173 E 43rd St, Yuma, AZ 85365

Tua Systems, Inc. 321-453-3200
3645 N Courtenay Pkwy, Merritt Island, FL 32953
HYDRO-SLIK, a hydrophobical hydrophylic coating for catheter guidewires and any device where invasive lubricity is required. All natural ionic hydrophilic, of fatty acids and amino acids especially effective on silicones, latex, natural rubber guidewires, catheters and other devices. IONIC-PTFE is a surface treatment which provides the ultimate in release and lubricity qualities to the surface to which it has been applied. The treatment may be sterilized by steam, gamma, E-beam or EtO. HYDRO-SILK, all natural hydrophillic compound formulated form fatty acids and amino acids. One-step process, material thickness of 0.0001. Used on catheters, guidewires, stylets, balloons.

Vernay Laboratories, Inc. 800-666-5227
120 E South College St, Yellow Springs, OH 45387

Vygon Corp. 800-544-4907
2495 General Armistead Ave, Norristown, PA 19403
Catheter removal kits.

ACCESSORIES, CATHETER, G-U *(Gastro/Urology) 78KNY*

Angiodynamics, Inc. 800-472-5221
1 Horizon Way, Manchester, GA 31816
Wide array of accessories including guidewires, introducer needles, dilators, caps, clips, ties/tie guns, fluid barriers, and forceps.

ACCESSORIES, CATHETER, G-U *(cont'd)*

B. Braun Of Puerto Rico, Inc. 610-691-5400
215.7 Insular Rd., Sabana Grande, PR 00637
Sterile catheter adapter and accessories.

Boston Scientific Corporation 800-225-2732
1 Boston Scientific Pl, Natick, MA 01760

Health Care Logistics, Inc. 800-848-1633
450 Town St, PO Box 25, Circleville, OH 43113
Various.

Medovations, Inc. 800-558-6408
102 E Keefe Ave, Milwaukee, WI 53212

Microcision Llc 800-264-3811
5805 Keystone St, Philadelphia, PA 19135
Stainless-steel catheter connectors.

Nbs Medical Products Inc. 888-800-8192
257 Livingston Ave, New Brunswick, NJ 08901
General urologic accessories.

Percutaneous Systems, Incorporated 650-493-4200
3260 Hillview Ave Ste 100, Palo Alto, CA 94304
Introducer sheath.

Rtc Inc.-Memcath Technologies Llc
1777 Oakdale Ave, West St Paul, MN 55118
Introducer.

Southside Biotechnology 440-974-4074
8780 Tyler Blvd, Mentor, OH 44060
Silicone Rubber Bolsters, Silicone Rubber Spacers, Silicone Rubber YPort Adaptors

ACCESSORIES, CHROMATOGRAPHY (GAS, GEL, LIQUID, THIN LAYER) *(Chemistry) 75JQR*

Aura Industries, Inc. 800-551-2872
545 8th Ave Rm 5W, New York, NY 10018

Beckman Coulter, Inc. 800-742-2345
250 S Kraemer Blvd, PO Box 8000, Brea, CA 92821

Bio-Rad Laboratories, Life Science Group 800-424-6723
2000 Alfred Nobel Dr, Hercules, CA 94547
Monoclonal antibody purification systems Byhplc and column chromatography - liquid and thin layer only.

Cadence Science Inc. 888-717-7677
1979 Marcus Ave Ste 215, New Hyde Park, NY 11042

Camag Scientific, Inc. 800-334-3909
515 Cornelius Harnett Dr, Wilmington, NC 28401

Cobert Associates, Inc. 800-972-4766
2302 Weldon Pkwy, Saint Louis, MO 63146

Frontier Scientific, Inc., 453-753-1901
PO Box 31, Logan, UT 84323
$62.68 per kit (12 vials) of CMK-IA porphyrin acids - chromatographic markers; $54.50 per kit (12 vials) of CMK-IE porphyrin esters - $57.39 for chromatographic markers.

Kontes Glass Co. 888-546-2531
1022 Spruce St, Vineland, NJ 08360

Polymer Laboratories, Now A Part Of Varian, Inc. 800-767-3963
160 Old Farm Rd, Amherst Fields Research Park, Amherst, MA 01002

Scientific Instrument Services, Inc. 908-788-5550
1027 Old York Rd, Ringoes, NJ 08551
Short path thermal desorption unit for the analysis of volatile and semi-volatile organics by GC, GC/MS and GC/FTIR.

Spectrum Laboratories, Inc. 800-634-3300
18617 S Broadwick St, Rancho Dominguez, CA 90220

Waters Corp. 800-252-4752
34 Maple St, Milford, MA 01757
Gel and liquid chromatography columns and supplies.

ACCESSORIES, CLEANING BRUSHES (FOR ENDOSCOPE) *(Gastro/Urology) 78MNL*

Cook Endoscopy 336-744-0157
4900 Bethania Station Rd # &, 5951 Grassy Creek Blvd.
Winston Salem, NC 27105
Endoscope cleaning brush.

Encision Inc. 303-444-2600
6797 Winchester Cir, Boulder, CO 80301
AEM Cleaning Brush

Endo-Therapeutics, Inc. 888-294-2377
15251 Roosevelt Blvd Ste 204, Clearwater, FL 33760

ACCESSORIES, CLEANING BRUSHES (FOR ENDOSCOPE)

(cont'd)

Endochoice Inc. 888-682-3636
11810 Wills Rd Ste 100, Alpharetta, GA 30009
Hedgehog

Gyrus Acmi, Inc. 508-804-2739
93 N Pleasant St, Norwalk, OH 44857
Accessories, cleaning brushes, for endoscope.

Hmb Endoscopy Products 800-659-5743
3746 SW 30th Ave, Fort Lauderdale, FL 33312
all accessories including biopsy, foreign body removal tools, snares, injector needles, etc.

Max Endoscopy Inc. 330-425-7041
1410 Highland Rd E Ste 6, Macedonia, OH 44056

Omnitech Systems, Inc. 866-266-9490
450 Campbell St Ste 2, Valparaiso, IN 46385
Cleaning Brushes for endoscopes

Primed Instruments, Inc. 877-565-0565
1080 Tristar Dr., Unit 14, Mississauga, ONTAR L5T 1P1 Canada
Reusable cleaning brush.Disposable Endoscope Cleaning Brushes

ACCESSORIES, CLEANING, ENDOSCOPIC

(Gastro/Urology) 78FEB

Aesculap Implant Systems Inc. 1-800-234-9179
3773 Corporate Pkwy, Center Valley, PA 18034

Ballard Medical Products 770-587-7835
12050 Lone Peak Pkwy, Draper, UT 84020
Baskets, forceps, snares.

Coopersurgical, Inc. 800-243-2974
95 Corporate Dr, Trumbull, CT 06611
$25.00-$995.00.

Electro Surgical Instrument Co., Inc. 888-464-2784
37 Centennial St, Rochester, NY 14611
Various cleaning tools and brushes for endoscope cleaning.

Encompas Unlimited, Inc. 800-825-7701
PO Box 516, Tallevast, FL 34270
$350/endoscope gas autoclaving trays; $99.00-$138.50/soaking trays; ultrasonic cleaners; Disposable endoscopic scrubs/50 for $55.00

Hmb Endoscopy Products 800-659-5743
3746 SW 30th Ave, Fort Lauderdale, FL 33312
Scope Reprocessors and Disinfectors

Justman Brush Co. • 800-800-6940
828 Crown Point Ave, Omaha, NE 68110
Endoscopic cleaning brush.

Karl Storz Endoscopy-America Inc. 800-421-0837
600 Corporate Pointe, Culver City, CA 90230

Mahe International Inc. 800-294-7946
468 Craighead St, Nashville, TN 37204

Medical Engineering Laboratory, Inc. 704-487-0166
108 W Warren St Ste 207, Shelby, NC 28150
Channel cleaning brushes/ non disposable/ peg brushes-disposable.

Miele Professional Products Group 800-843-7231
9 Independence Way, Princeton, NJ 08540
Endoscopic washer.

N.M. Beale Co. Inc. 978-456-6990
89 Old Shirley Rd, PO Box 494, Harvard, MA 01451
Endoscopic water bottle.

North American Marketing, Inc. 208-524-4949
3005 N 4th E, Idaho Falls, ID 83401
KLEER VU - external lens anti-fog solution. Anti-Fog Cleaner for all lenses, eyeglasses scopes, dental mirrors etc..'NEW' Non-smearing cleaner for anti-reflective(Teflon UV, Transition etc.) eyeglass lenses.

Pentax Medical Company 800-431-5880
102 Chestnut Ridge Rd, Montvale, NJ 07645
Cleaning brush, suction cylinder cleaning brush and curette.

Preservation Solutions, Inc. 262-723-6715
980 Proctor Dr, Elkhorn, WI 53121
ClearIt TM - Anti-Fog Solution

Richard Wolf Medical Instruments Corp. 800-323-9653
353 Corporate Woods Pkwy, Vernon Hills, IL 60061

Ultracell Medical Technologies, Inc. 877-SPO-NGE1
183 Providence New London Tpke, North Stonington, CT 06359
ULTRACELL VENUS Cleaning kits

Welch Allyn, Inc. 800-535-6663
4341 State Street Rd, Skaneateles Falls, NY 13153

ACCESSORIES, DECORATIVE *(General) 80VBQ*

Covoc Corp. 800-725-3266
1194 E Valencia Dr, Fullerton, CA 92831
Cubicle curtains, cubicle track, I.V. ceiling track & I.V. trees; venetian and vertical blinds, window draperies, window shades

Extra Packaging, Corp. 800-872-7548
631 Golden Harbour Dr, Boca Raton, FL 33432
We offer a large selection of solid brass cremation urns for adults, children and even pets.

Rockaway Chairs 800-256-6601
111 Alexander Rd Apt 11, West Monroe, LA 71291
Fabrics; All window treatments, drapery and upholstery. 100% cotton and poly-cotton flame retardant or laminated at roll pricing of $17.00 per yard, fabric ring available, all vinyls also available.

Vergason Technology, Inc. 607-589-4429
166 State Route 224, Van Etten, NY 14889
VTI's coating services group has provided hard coatings and metalizing coatings since 1987. We utilize our patented Cat Arc® optimum temperature PVD methods and sputtering processes to supply a wide variety of quality coating solutions. VTI supplies strippable CrN coatings for plastic injection molds, as well as TiN, TiAlN/AlTiN, TiB2, ZrN and TiCN for aerospace, electronic, machine tools, components and other applications.

ACCESSORIES, ELECTRICAL POWER (ELECTROCAUTERY)

(Surgery) 79WDY

Aesculap Implant Systems Inc. 1-800-234-9179
3773 Corporate Pkwy, Center Valley, PA 18034

Aubrey Group 949-581-0188
6 Cromwell Ste 100, Irvine, CA 92618

ACCESSORIES, EXTRACORPOREAL SYSTEM

(Gastro/Urology) 78KXM

Organogenesis Inc. 888-432-5232
150 Dan Rd, Canton, MA 02021
Liver Assist Device, extracorporeal device using living liver cells to provide liver function until or instead of transplantation; currently in animal studies.

ACCESSORIES, FIXATION, ORTHOPEDIC *(Orthopedics) 87LYT*

Allen Medical Systems, Inc. 800-433-5774
1 Post Office Sq, Acton, MA 01720

Back Support Systems 800-669-2225
67684 San Andreas St, Desert Hot Springs, CA 92240
POSTURITE orthopedic seating device made from medical quality, high density foam that allows correct posture while seated in any chair. Comes with oil and water resistant cover.

Bolt Bethel, Llc 763-434-5900
23530 University Avenue Ext NW, PO Box 135, Bethel, MN 55005

Cmo, Inc. 800-344-0011
PO Box 147, Barberton, OH 44203
CMORTHO Derma Dry orthopedic soft goods contain no adhesives, and the 90%-chemical-free, non-neoprene, open- cell material lets perspiration evaporate.

Crystal Medical Technology 205-733-0901
153 Cahaba Valley Pkwy, Pelham, AL 35124
Various screws and instruments

Depuy Ace, A Johnson & Johnson Company 800-473-3789
700 Orthopaedic Dr, Warsaw, IN 46582

Depuy Orthopaedics, Inc. 800-473-3789
700 Orthopaedic Dr, P.O. Box 988, Warsaw, IN 46582
Various types of fixation accessories.

DJO Inc. 800-336-6569
1430 Decision St, Vista, CA 92081
Softgoods and Neoprene, general accommodative orthopedic bracing.

Holmed Corporation 508-238-3351
40 Norfolk Ave, South Easton, MA 02375

Kerr Group 800-524-3577
1400 Holcomb Bridge Rd, Roswell, GA 30076

Quatro Composites 858-513-4300
13250 Gregg St Ste A1, Poway, CA 92064

Rogers Foam Corp. 714-538-3033
808 W Nicolas Ave, Orange, CA 92868
Manufacturer of orthopedic devices.

Synthes (Usa) 610-719-5000
35 Airport Rd, Horseheads, NY 14845
Various types and sizes of fixation accessories.

ACCESSORIES, FIXATION, ORTHOPEDIC *(cont'd)*

Telos Medical Equipment (Austin & Assoc., Inc.) 800-934-3029
1109 Sturbridge Rd, Fallston, MD 21047
TELOS O.R. table accessories, standard and custom made.

Truform Orthotics & Prosthetics 800-888-0458
3960 Rosslyn Dr, Cincinnati, OH 45209
Lower-extremity prosthetic accessories.

ACCESSORIES, FIXATION, SPINAL INTERLAMINAL
(Orthopedics) 87LYP

Holmed Corporation 508-238-3351
40 Norfolk Ave, South Easton, MA 02375

Warsaw Orthopedic, Inc. 901-396-3133
2500 Silveus Xing, Warsaw, IN 46582
Spinal implant fixation device.

ACCESSORIES, FIXATION, SPINAL INTERVERTEBRAL BODY
(Orthopedics) 87LYQ

Holmed Corporation 508-238-3351
40 Norfolk Ave, South Easton, MA 02375

Implex Corp. 800-613-6131
1800 W Center St, Warsaw, IN 46580

Warsaw Orthopedic, Inc. 901-396-3133
2500 Silveus Xing, Warsaw, IN 46582
Spinal implant fixation devices.

ACCESSORIES, GERMICIDE, CLEANING, FOR ENDOSCOPES
(Gastro/Urology) 78NZA

Steris Corporation 440-354-2600
6515 Hopkins Rd, Mentor, OH 44060
Endoscope and accessories, disinfector.

ACCESSORIES, IMPLANT, DENTAL, ENDOSSEOUS
(Dental And Oral) 76NDP

Altiva Corp. 866-425-8482
9800 Southern Pine Blvd Ste I, Charlotte, NC 28273
Various endosseous dental implant accessories and kits.

Etkon Usa, Inc. 978-747-2575
916 113th St Ste A, Arlington, TX 76011

H & H Co. 909-390-0373
4435 E Airport Dr Ste 108, Ontario, CA 91761
Accessories, implant, dental all types.

Nobel Biocare Usa, Llc 800-579-6515
22715/22725 Savi Ranch Parkway, Yorba Linda, CA 92887
Endosseous dental implant accessories and laboratory accessories.

Quantum Bioengineering, Ltd. 954-474-4707
7951 SW 6th St, Plantation, FL 33324
Dental implant accessories & instrumentation.

Steiner Laboratories 808-371-2700
590 Farrington Hwy, #1010 Suite 7, Kapolei, HI 96707
Stainless steel rods.

Straumann Manufacturing, Inc. 978-747-2575
60 Minuteman Rd, Andover, MA 01810
Implant analog.

ACCESSORIES, LASER *(General) 80WQD*

Aura Lens Products, Inc. 800-281-2872
51 8th St N, PO Box 763, St. Cloud,, Sauk Rapids, MN 56379
Laser protective eyeglasses, prescription and non-prescription type.

Awi Industries (Usa), Inc. 909-597-0808
14502 Central Ave, Chino, CA 91710
A.W.I. laser pointers and laser modules.

Biolitec, Inc. 800-934-2377
515 Shaker Rd, East Longmeadow, MA 01028
Optical fibers for use with excimer, argon, KTP, HeNe, YAG, Holmium and CO2 lasers.

Buffalo Filter, A Division Of Medtek Devices Inc. 800-343-2324
595 Commerce Dr, Amherst, NY 14228
VIROSAFE Filters, PLUMESAFE Smoke Evacuation Systems, laser & electrsurgical accessories for smoke evacuation.

Burkhart Roentgen Intl. Inc. 800-USA-XRAY
5201 8th Ave S, Gulfport, FL 33707
Extremity rulers.

Cardiofocus, Inc. 508-658-7200
500 Nickerson Rd Ste 500-200, Marlborough, MA 01752
Fiber-optic laser diffusors. Cylindrical, hemicylindrical, spherical, and micro lens.

ACCESSORIES, LASER *(cont'd)*

Coherent, Inc. 800-527-3786
5100 Patrick Henry Dr, Santa Clara, CA 95054

Conoptics, Inc. 800-748-3349
19 Eagle Rd, Danbury, CT 06810

Convergent Laser Technologies 800-848-8200
1660 S Loop Rd, Alameda, CA 94502
ROTALASE XT angle delivery fibers for surgical YAG laser for urology and other applications. OPTILITE fiberoptic delivery systems, probes, handpieces, sheaths, scopes, etc. ROTALASE SPECTRA Quartz cap delivery fibers for surgical YAG laser for urology and other applications. OPTICON II Adapters for SLT and Laserscope surgical lasers. Model number AR3000 and AR3030.

Coopersurgical, Inc. 800-243-2974
95 Corporate Dr, Trumbull, CT 06611
90 items, including smoke filters, tubing, steel instruments.

Cynosure, Inc. 800-886-2966
5 Carlisle Rd, Westford, MA 01886
(Used in treating vascular lesions) Alexandrite, pulsed-dye, solid-state diode-pumped.

Gam Laser Inc 407-851-8999
6901 Tpc Dr Ste 300, Orlando, FL 32822
Excimer lasers, UV lasers

Infrared Fiber Systems, Inc. 301-622-7131
2301 Broadbirch Dr Ste A, Silver Spring, MD 20904
Infrared transmitting optical fibers for remote sensing and medical laser surgery.

Iridex Corporation 800-388-4747
1212 Terra Bella Ave, Mountain View, CA 94043
Aesthetic lasers, Apex 800 for hair removal, DioLite 532 for vascular and pigmented skin lesions.

Labsphere, Inc. 603-927-4266
231 Shaker St., North Sutton, NH 03260-9986
Laser power meters for lasers, laser diodes, and laser-driven fiber optics.

Lase-R Shield, A Bacou-Dalloz Company 800-288-1164
7011 Prospect Pl NE, Albuquerque, NM 87110
Priced from $28.00; Eye protection, prescription and non-prescription all wavelengths. Visitor, professional, staff members. Protection film; price depends on size and application.

Laser, Inc. 800-367-5694
27831 Commercial Park Ln, Tomball, TX 77375

Linos Photonics, Inc 800-334-5678
459 Fortune Blvd, Milford, MA 01757
Lens tubes.

Medical Energy, Inc. 850-469-1727
225 E Zaragoza St, Pensacola, FL 32502
LASER 'American' Irrigator System. Dual trumpet suction/irrigation instrument with large 10mm chamber and 5mm cannula with laser fiber working port.

Microtek Medical, Inc 800-936-9248
512 N Lehmberg Rd, Columbus, MS 39702
Laser and microscope drapes.

Novosci Corp. 281-363-4949
2828 N Crescentridge Dr, The Woodlands, TX 77381
Laser fibers; smoke evacuator (tubing and filters); in-line filters; safety eyewear.

Ocular Instruments, Inc. 800-888-6616
2255 116th Ave NE, Bellevue, WA 98004
Hand-held contact lenses for laser therapy.

Ophir Optronics, Inc. 800-820-0814
260A Fordham Rd, Wilmington, MA 01887
Laser power/energy meters.

Pharmaceutical Innovations, Inc. 973-242-2900
897 Frelinghuysen Ave, Newark, NJ 07114
Photon Transmitting Gel is specifically designed, tested and approved for Laser and Pulsed Light procedures. Ultra clear, Photon Transmitting Gel effeciently transmits light energy while absorbing thermal energy from the skin's surface. It protects the patient's skin form heat and burns and does not liquify form the salts in perspiration. One application remains thick, lubricating and heat absorbent. It stays in place and is non-staining and hypoallergenic.

Quatronix 800-289-7707
41 Research Way, East Setauket, NY 11733

Reliant Technologies, Inc. 650-473-0200
260 Sheridan Ave Ste 300, Palo Alto, CA 94306
Laser handpiece.

ACCESSORIES, LASER *(cont'd)*

Scientech, Inc. 303-444-1361
5649 Arapahoe Ave, Boulder, CO 80303
Laser power and energy meters.

Surgical Laser Technologies, Inc. 800-366-4758
147 Keystone Dr, Montgomeryville, PA 18936
Contact fiber delivery systems for laders producing 532 nm to 1064 nm wavelengths. This includes KTP, 810 diode, 980 diode, and Nd:YAG lasers.

Telsar Laboratories Inc 800-255-9938
1 Enviro Way Ste 100, Wood River, IL 62095
Physician's arm rest for ophthalmic laser surgery & auxiliary safety equipment.

Transamerican Technologies International 800-322-7373
2246 Camino Ramon, San Ramon, CA 94583
ACCU-BEAM, CO2 laser laparoscopy kits, CO2 universal laser micromanipulators, and CO2 laser focusing handpiece. Fiber optic handpieces, and suction/irrigation cannulas for laser fiber delivery.

Trimedyne, Inc. 800-733-5273
15091 Bake Pkwy, Irvine, CA 92618
Arthroscopic laser handpieces. The Omni switchtip system with multi-use handpiece and interchangeable tips, and the Tapertip reusable holmium arthroscopic handpieces for use with the Omnipulse holmium laser. Complete line of FlexMAX optical fibers for use in lithotripsy.

Vorum Research Corporation 800-461-4353
8765 Ash St., Ste. 6, Vancouver, BC V6P-6T3 Canada
Portable Hand held scanner

ACCESSORIES, LASER, ENDOSCOPIC *(Surgery) 79SJN*

Novosci Corp. 281-363-4949
2828 N Crescentridge Dr, The Woodlands, TX 77381

Oto-Med, Inc. 800-433-7703
1090 Empire Dr, Lake Havasu City, AZ 86404
SafeTrap, Sterile in-line specimen collection device used in any surgery with powered instruments.

Schueler & Company, Inc. 516-487-1500
PO Box 528, Stratford, CT 06615

Surgical Laser Technologies, Inc. 800-366-4758
147 Keystone Dr, Montgomeryville, PA 18936

Thomas Medical Inc. 800-556-0349
5610 West 82 2nd Street, Indianpolis, IN 46278
Re-usable instruments for endoscopic procedures. Scissors, graspers, clamps, suction irrigation canals, T20 cars with safety shield, dissectors, retractors, needle holders, biopsy forceps, suction coagulators.

World Of Medicine Usa, Inc. 407-438-8810
4531 36th St, Orlando, FL 32811
W.O.M. Products Minimally Invasive Surgery and Urology: Laser 'Freddy' Lithotripsy laser/Uropower uroflow device (urodynamics), cameras, light sources, monitors, pumps (orthopedic and hysteroscopy), insufflators. Gamma Finder: defeats markers for locating lymph nodes, cordless.

Xodus Medical, Inc. 800-963-8776
702 Prominence Dr, Westmoreland Business & Research Park
New Kensington, PA 15068
Anti-Fog Solution

ACCESSORIES, LIGHT, SURGICAL *(Surgery) 79FTA*

Advanced Medical Innovations, Inc. 888-367-2641
9410 De Soto Ave Ste J, Chatsworth, CA 91311
Light Handle Cover (Surgery) - Disposable Light Handle Cover for all Surgical Lights including free Universal handles.

Bulbworks, Inc. 800-334-2852
80 N Dell Ave Unit 5, Kenvil, NJ 07847
Replacement Lamps For All Types Of Surgical Equipment

Burton Medical Products, Inc. 800-444-9909
21100 Lassen St, Chatsworth, CA 91311

Embo-Optics, Llc. 887-885-6400
100 Cummings Ctr # 326B, Beverly, MA 01915
IV illuminator with lighted monitoring feature aids medical personnel in assuring that all IV solutions and medications are infusing properly and at the correct infusion rate. Greatly enhance patient safety in aiding to prevent any adverse events during infusion.

General Scientific Corp. 800-959-0153
77 Enterprise Dr, Ann Arbor, MI 48103

ACCESSORIES, LIGHT, SURGICAL *(cont'd)*

Getinge Usa, Inc. 800-475-9040
1777 E Henrietta Rd, Rochester, NY 14623
MAQUET surgical lighting systems deliver precisely focused, evenly distributed illumination onto the surgical site.

John Cudia And Associates, Inc. 408-782-2628
18440 Technology Dr Ste 110, Morgan Hill, CA 95037

Mahe International Inc. 800-294-7946
468 Craighead St, Nashville, TN 37204

Maquet, Inc. 843-552-8652
7371 Spartan Blvd E, N Charleston, SC 29418
Sterile light handles.

Medical Action Industries, Inc. 800-645-7042
25 Heywood Rd, Arden, NC 28704
Light shields.

Medical Illumination International 800-831-1222
547 Library St, San Fernando, CA 91340
Sterilizable handles.

Solos Endoscopy 800-388-6445
65 Sprague St # B, Boston/dedham Commerce Park, Boston, MA 02136
Various light source accessories.

Sterion, Incorporated 800-328-7958
13828 Lincoln St NE, Ham Lake, MN 55304
Cautery Tip Cleaner, abrasive foam pad used to clean cautery probes.

Syris Scientific 800-714-1374
22 Shaker Rd, Gray, ME 04039
Syris v600

Transamerican Technologies International 800-322-7373
2246 Camino Ramon, San Ramon, CA 94583
ACCU-BEAM, high energy flashtubes for use with Zeiss fundus cameras and slit lamps. Filled with xenon gas and set in non-conductive ceramic base.

Welch Allyn, Inc. 800-535-6663
4341 State Street Rd, Skaneateles Falls, NY 13153
MICRO ILLIMINATION single-fiber technology to replace bulky fiber bundles.

Whittemore Enterprises, Inc. 800-999-2452
11149 Arrow Rte, Rancho Cucamonga, CA 91730

Wisap America 800-233-8448
8231 Melrose Dr, Lenexa, KS 66214
Laparoscopic Xenon Light Source: 100W, 180W and 300W

ACCESSORIES, MICROTOME *(Pathology) 88IDL*

Boeckeler Instruments, Inc. 800-552-2262
4650 S Butterfield Dr, Tucson, AZ 85714
a full range of microtome and EM Sample Prep accessories

C. L. Sturkey, Inc. 717-274-9441
824 Cumberland St, Lebanon, PA 17042
Accessory to microtome.

Crescent Manufacturing Company 419-332-6484
4615 Progress Dr, Columbus, IN 47201
Microtome blade.

Crescent Mfg. Co. 800-537-1330
1310 Majestic Dr, Fremont, OH 43420
DURAEDGE Microtome Blades.

Richard-Allan Scientific 269-544-5628
4481 Campus Dr, Kalamazoo, MI 49008
Microtome accessories.

ACCESSORIES, OPERATING ROOM, TABLE *(Surgery) 79FWZ*

Advanced Medical Innovations, Inc. 888-367-2641
9410 De Soto Ave Ste J, Chatsworth, CA 91311
MAGNI-GUARD, splash prevention products. Surgical splash prevention handle/guard with a clear lense for ultimate protection from blood borne pathogens during surgery. Different sizes for cardiovascular, orthopedic and general surgery. Available sterile or through the kit and tray assemblers.

Aegis Medical 203-838-9081
10 Wall St, Norwalk, CT 06850
Disposable, custom procedure trays.

Alimed, Inc. 800-225-2610
297 High St, Dedham, MA 02026
Clark and side-rail sockets fit all American-made tables with side rails. Combo-Clamp attaches anywhere to an operating-room table side rail and does not have to slide to the end to be removed.

ACCESSORIES, OPERATING ROOM, TABLE *(cont'd)*

Allen Medical Systems, Inc. 800-433-5774
1 Post Office Sq, Acton, MA 01720
Allen Medical focuses on improving patient outcomes and caregiver safety, while enhancing customers' efficiency through the development of technologically advanced surgical positioning accessories. Allen offers a range of spine, GYN, orthopedic, and pressure management OR accessories.

American Pacific Plastic Fabricators, Inc. 714-891-3191
7274 Lampson Ave, Garden Grove, CA 92841
Surgical patient positioner.

Arthrex Manufacturing 239-643-5553
1958 Trade Center Way, Naples, FL 34109
Leg holder, strap.

Arthrex, Inc. 239-643-5553
1370 Creekside Blvd, Naples, FL 34108
Arthroscopy leg holder.

Bemis Mfg. Co. 920-467-5206
Hwy. Pp West, Sheboygan Falls, WI 53085
Reuseable positioning system.

Birkova Products 888-567-4502
809 4th St, Gothenburg, NE 69138
Surgical table accessories, leg holders, stirrups, replacement cushions, pads, Clark sockets, and more.

Bryton Corp. 800-567-9500
4310 Guion Rd, Indianapolis, IN 46254
Accessories for all types of surgical procedures, including all types of arm supports, head rests, restraint straps, leg holders, stirrups, kidney horn, x-ray panels and imaging attachments.

Camtec 410-228-1156
1959 Church Creek Rd, Cambridge, MD 21613
Table accessories operating room.

Composiflex, Inc. 800-673-2544
8100 Hawthorne Dr, Erie, PA 16509
Accesories for surgical procedures. Armboards, arm/hand tables, headholders, leg extensions and imaging attachments

Depuy Spine, Inc. 800-227-6633
325 Paramount Dr, Raynham, MA 02767
Surgical positioning board.

Elite Medical Equipment 719-659-7926
5470 Kates Dr, Colorado Springs, CO 80919
Hand table.

General Hospital Supply Corp. 704-225-9500
2844 Gray Fox Rd, Monroe, NC 28110
Instrument organizer with stabilizer post.

Griff Industries, Inc. 800-709-4743
19761 Bahama St, Northridge, CA 91324
Essentials positioning foam--reusable foam positioners. Instrument Organizers

Health Supply Company Inc., The 770-452-0090
2902 Marlin Cir, Atlanta, GA 30341
Midkiff GEOSTATIC Clamp. Each clamping function independent and silent, helpful in lithotomy positioning. Clamp may remain on OR table while transferring patient. 'LIL MAC Accessory Clamp, Midkiff GEOSTATIC Clamp, TKO Multi-Position Armboard, TKO Telescoping Stirrups.

Integra Lifesciences Of Ohio 800-654-2873
4900 Charlemar Dr Bldg A, Cincinnati, OH 45227
Various table accessories.

Invuity, Inc. 760-744-4447
334 Via Vera Cruz Ste 255, San Marcos, CA 92078
Surgical or diagnostic instrument holder.

Invuity, Inc. 415-655-2100
39 Stillman St, San Francisco, CA 94107

Kinetic Concepts, Inc. 800-275-4524
8023 Vantage Dr, San Antonio, TX 78230
Operating table pad.

Lex-Ton Orthopedics 615-890-6969
1133 White Cliff Rd, Lawrenceburg, TN 38464
Spinal surgery frame.

Maquet, Inc. 843-552-8652
7371 Spartan Blvd E, N Charleston, SC 29418
Shampaine orthopedic attachment.

Mcconnell Orthopedic Mfg. Co. 513-573-0085
1324 East Interstate 30 Bldg. B, Floyd, TX 75401
No common name listed.

ACCESSORIES, OPERATING ROOM, TABLE *(cont'd)*

Medi-Tech International, Inc. 305-593-9373
2924 NW 109th Ave, Doral, FL 33172
Operating lamps and tables by SKYTRON

Medrecon, Inc. 877-526-4323
257 South Ave, Garwood, NJ 07027
New, remanufactured and custom applications.

Modular Cutting Systems, Inc. 203-336-3526
650 Clinton Ave, Bridgeport, CT 06605
Accessories,operating room table.

Nds Surgical Imaging, Inc. 866-637-5237
5750 Hellyer Ave, San Jose, CA 95138
Hard, non-porous Surface disinfection products

Nimbic Systems, Llc 281-565-5700
4910 Wright Rd Ste 170, Stafford, TX 77477
Patient positioning device.

North American Scientific, Inc. 818-734-8600
8300 Aurora Ave N, Seattle, WA 98103
Various accessories, operating room table.

Olympic Medical Corp. 206-767-3500
5900 1st Ave S, Seattle, WA 98108
$1739.50 for extremities operating-room table.

P And G Engineering, Incorporated 978-263-6254
20 Main St Ste E, Acton, MA 01720
Various types of operating-room, table accessories.

Phelan Manufacturing Corp. 800-328-2358
2523 Minnehaha Ave, Minneapolis, MN 55404

Quatro Composites 858-513-4300
13250 Gregg St Ste A1, Poway, CA 92064

Schuerch Corp. 617-773-0927
48 Oval Rd, Quincy, MA 02170
Various.

Scientek Medical Equipment 604-273-9094
11151 Bridgeport Rd., Richmond, BC V6X 1T3 Canada

Simple Orthopaedic Solutions, Llc 317-414-1558
9337 N 700 E, Darlington, IN 47940
Hand table, armboard, short board.

Tekquest Industries 800-327-7175
4200 Saint Johns Pkwy, Sanford, FL 32771
No common name listed.

Tempur-Medical, Inc. 888-255-3302
1713 Jaggie Fox Way, Lexington, KY 40511
Tempur-Med OR table pad.

Tenet Medical Engineering, Inc. 888-836-3863
5540 1A St. SW, Calgary, ALB T2H 0E7 Canada
Shoulder surgery positioner

ACCESSORIES, PHOTOGRAPHIC, ENDOSCOPIC
(Gastro/Urology) 78FEM

Ams Innovative Center-San Jose 800-356-7600
3070 Orchard Dr, San Jose, CA 95134

Clarus Medical, Llc. 763-525-8400
1000 Boone Ave N Ste 300, Minneapolis, MN 55427
Endoscope console.

Coopersurgical, Inc. 800-243-2974
95 Corporate Dr, Trumbull, CT 06611

Hmb Endoscopy Products 800-659-5743
3746 SW 30th Ave, Fort Lauderdale, FL 33312
Video Cameras and Image Capture Devices

Karl Storz Endoscopy-America Inc. 800-421-0837
600 Corporate Pointe, Culver City, CA 90230

Mahe International Inc. 800-294-7946
468 Craighead St, Nashville, TN 37204

Microtek Medical, Inc 800-936-9248
512 N Lehmberg Rd, Columbus, MS 39702
Camera drapes.

Omex Technologies, Inc. 847-564-0206
3665 Woodhead Dr, Northbrook, IL 60062
Accessory to an endoscope, video coupler lens for relaying endoscope image to camera

Reznik Instrument, Inc. 847-673-3444
7337 Lawndale Ave, Skokie, IL 60076
Photographic equipment (camera, lenses, flash unit).

Richard Wolf Medical Instruments Corp. 800-323-9653
353 Corporate Woods Pkwy, Vernon Hills, IL 60061

ACCESSORIES, PHOTOGRAPHIC, ENDOSCOPIC *(cont'd)*

Transamerican Technologies International 800-322-7373
2246 Camino Ramon, San Ramon, CA 94583
ACCU-BEAM, microsurgical video adapters for surgical microscopes. Endoscopic video adaptors.

Vision Systems Group, A Division Of Viking Systems 508-366-3668
134 Flanders Rd, Westborough, MA 01581
Endoscopy video camera; stereo viewing system.

Volpi Manufacturing Usa Co., Inc. 315-255-1737
5 Commerce Way, Auburn, NY 13021
Accessory to an endoscope fiberoptic light source.

ACCESSORIES, POWERED DRILL *(Cns/Neurology) 84HBE*

Acra Cut, Inc. 978-263-0250
989 Main St, Acton, MA 01720
Cranio blade.

Biomet Microfixation Inc. 800-874-7711
1520 Tradeport Dr, Jacksonville, FL 32218
Twist drill.

Brasseler Usa - Komet Medical 800-535-6638
1 Brasseler Blvd, Savannah, GA 31419
XK-95 high-speed motor drill system, high-speed drill and components, high-speed drill system.

Brasseler Usa - Medical 805-650-5209
4837 McGrath St Ste J, Ventura, CA 93003
Surgical Instrument System

Medtronic Powered Surgical Solutions 800-643-2773
4620 N Beach St, Haltom City, TX 76137
Various models of (ah) sterile/non-sterile burrs/acces.

Strenumed, Inc. 805-477-1000
1833 Portola Rd Unit K, Ventura, CA 93003
Development

Tava Surgical Instruments 805-650-5209
4837 McGrath St Ste J, Ventura, CA 93003
Surgical Instrument System.

ACCESSORIES, PUMP, INFUSION *(General) 80MRZ*

Aiv, Inc. (Formerly American Iv) 800-990-2911
7485 Shipley Ave, Harmans, MD 21077
AC Adapters for leading syringe and ambulatory pumps.

Cardinal Health 303,Inc. 858-458-7830
1515 Ivac Way, Creedmoor, NC 27522
Infusion pump accessories.

Clarus Medical, Llc. 763-525-8400
1000 Boone Ave N Ste 300, Minneapolis, MN 55427
Endoscopy pump.

Curlin Medical, Inc. 714-893-2200
15751 Graham St, Huntington Beach, CA 92649
Various infusion pump accessories.

Glucotec, Inc. 864-370-3297
14 Pelham Ridge Dr # D, Greenville, SC 29615
Dosing calcutor, for glucose, insulin, and saline.

Integra Lifesciences Corp. 609-275-0500
311 Enterprise Dr, Plainsboro, NJ 08536
Accessories.

Zoll Medical Corp. 800-348-9011
269 Mill Rd, Chelmsford, MA 01824
Power Infuser

ACCESSORIES, RADIOTHERAPY *(Radiology) 90WJW*

Burkhart Roentgen Intl. Inc. 800-USA-XRAY
5201 8th Ave S, Gulfport, FL 33707

Capintec, Inc. 800-631-3826
6 Arrow Rd, Ramsey, NJ 07446

Composiflex, Inc. 800-673-2544
8100 Hawthorne Dr, Erie, PA 16509
Carbon fiber couch tops, carbon fiber head holders, carbon fiber patient support systems.

Frank Barker Assoc, Inc. 800-222-7537
33 Jacksonville Rd Ste 1, Towaco, NJ 07082
Finesse Patient Positioning Frames; BEBIG Block Cutter System

Impac Medical Systems, Inc. 888-464-6722
100 W Evelyn Ave, Mountain View, CA 94041
Practice management for oncology electronic medical records for radiation oncology.

ACCESSORIES, RADIOTHERAPY *(cont'd)*

Owens Scientific Inc. 281-394-2311
23230 Sandsage Ln, Katy, TX 77494
Radiation therapy equipment and accessories.

Pro-Comm, Inc. 800-920-1476
1105 Industrial Pkwy, Brick, NJ 08724
2856 MHz, 2999 MHz, 3000 MHz RF Driver portion of Klystron linear accelerators (including high energy type) from $20,000 new. Also rebuild @ $5K to $8K.

Varian Medical Systems 800-544-4636
3100 Hansen Way, Palo Alto, CA 94304
The On-Board Imager(tm) device for image-guided radiotherapy; multileaf collimators; electronic portal imaging devices, Exact treatment couch, RPM respiratory gating.

Waldmann Lighting 800-634-0007
9 Century Dr, Wheeling, IL 60090

Whiting & Davis Company, Inc. 800-876-6374
200 John L Dietsch Blvd, Attleboro Falls, MA 02763
Bolus flexible brass metal fabric for use in Tangential Chest Wall Irradiation. This bolus conveniently conforms to the body contours, eliminating air spaces between the bolus and skin surface.

ACCESSORIES, RETRACTOR, DENTAL *(Dental And Oral) 76EIF*

Alltec Integrated Manufacturing,Inc. 805-595-3500
4330 Old Santa Fe Rd, San Luis Obispo, CA 93401
Dental ruler.

Biomet Microfixation Inc. 800-874-7711
1520 Tradeport Dr, Jacksonville, FL 32218
Various types of retractors.

Glenroe Technologies 800-237-4060
1912 44th Ave E, Bradenton, FL 34203
Cheek expander.

H & H Co. 909-390-0373
4435 E Airport Dr Ste 108, Ontario, CA 91761
Accessories, retractor, dental.

Hager Worldwide, Inc. 800-328-2335
13322 Byrd Dr, Odessa, FL 33556
SPANDEX/MIRAHOLD (autoclavable) and LIP-EX(cold sterilizable).

Lmi 714-349-5386
2324 Raintree Dr, Brea, CA 92821
Mini-prop dental hand instrument.

Miltex Dental Technologies, Inc. 516-576-6022
589 Davies Dr, York, PA 17402
Various lip and cheek retractors,mouth props,and tongue guards.

Oraceutical Llc 413-528-5070
815 Pleasant St, Lee, MA 01238
Cheek retractor-accessory to photographic procedure.

Oscar, Inc. 317-849-2618
11793 Technology Ln, Fishers, IN 46038
Cheek retractor.

Pac-Dent Intl., Inc. 909-839-0888
21078 Commerce Point Dr, Walnut, CA 91789
Bur block.

Pascal Co., Inc. 425-602-3633
2929 Northup Way, Bellevue, WA 98004
Gingival retraction cord.

Prosurge Instruments, Inc. 866-832-7874
199 Laidlaw Ave, Jersey City, NJ 07306

Pulpdent Corp. 800-343-4342
80 Oakland St, Watertown, MA 02472
No common name listed.

Ultradent Products, Inc. 801-553-4586
505 W 10200 S, South Jordan, UT 84095
Retraction cord.

Westside Packaging, Llc. 909-570-3508
1700 S Baker Ave Ste A, Ontario, CA 91761
Dental retractors

ACCESSORIES, SOLUTION, LENS, CONTACT
(Ophthalmology) 86LYL

Altaire Pharmaceuticals, Inc. 631-722-5988
311 West Ln., Aquebogue, NY 11931
Cleaning, disinfecting & storage solution by altaire.

Bausch & Lomb 585-338-6000
1 Bausch and Lomb Pl, Rochester, NY 14604

ACCESSORIES, SOLUTION, LENS, CONTACT *(cont'd)*

Bausch & Lomb, Vision Care 800-553-5340
1400 Goodman St N, Rochester, NY 14609
RENU rewetting drops, sensitive eye drops and sterile lens lubricating drops.

Ciba Vision Corporation 800-875-3001
11460 Johns Creek Pkwy, Duluth, GA 30097

Mectra Labs, Inc. 800-323-3968
PO Box 350, Two Quality Way, Bloomfield, IN 47424
MISTER CLEAR, reduces fogging of endoscopes.

Niagara Pharmaceuticals Div. 905-690-6277
60 Innovation Dr., Flamborough, ONT L9H-7P3 Canada
HEALTHSAVER contact lens disinfecttion solutions.

Oms, 177108 Canada Inc. 800-461-6637
97 Columbus, Pointe Claire, QUE H9R-4K3 Canada
OMS coating materials for ophthalmic lenses. MICRO-TINTS ophthalmic lens tinting in microwave oven. Clean in office process up to 100X faster than the conventional method.

Onyx Medical Inc./Face-It 800-333-5773
445 Coloma St, Sausalito, CA 94965
FOG anti-fog solution is an optically clear spray that dries within minutes. FOG is for use on lenses, loupes, mirrors, goggles, glasses and visors. No cross contamination. Will not wash off under air or water spray. Available sterile.

Optikem International, Inc. 800-525-1752
2172 S Jason St, Denver, CO 80223
SEREINE Contact lens care solutions.

The Lifestyle Co. Inc. 800-622-0777
1800 State Route 34 Ste 401, Wall Township, NJ 07719
PuriLens Plus-- contact lens cleaning and disinfection device

Tua Systems, Inc. 321-453-3200
3645 N Courtenay Pkwy, Merritt Island, FL 32953
HYDRO-SILK IPT, hydrophillic treatment specifically formulated for use on RGP, soft contact lenses, and IOLs. Treated contact lenses exhibit enhanced comfort and visual acuity.

ACCESSORIES, SPECULUM *(Surgery) 79FXG*

Electro Surgical Instrument Co., Inc. 888-464-2784
37 Centennial St, Rochester, NY 14611
Various types styles and sizes of nasal and vaginal specula with fiberoptic light.

Olsen Medical 800-297-6344
3001 W Kentucky St, Louisville, KY 40211
Graves speculum, with and without smoke tubes. Open-sided speculum.

Pedia Pals, Llc 888-733-4272
965 Highway 169 N, Plymouth, MN 55441
Tip dispenser & otoscope specula.

ACCESSORIES, SURGICAL CAMERA *(Surgery) 79KQM*

Airway Cam Technologies, Inc. 610-341-9560
205 Spruce Tree Rd, Radnor, PA 19087
Airway cam.

Dma Med-Chem Corporation 800-362-1833
49 Watermill Ln, Great Neck, NY 11021

Emr Tools, Llc 602-579-2694
4814 W Laurel Ln, Glendale, AZ 85304
Imageacquire.

Femsuite, Llc 415-561-2565
220 Halleck St Ste 120B, San Francisco, CA 94129
Video camera.

Genicon 800-936-1020
6869 Stapoint Ct Ste 114, Winter Park, FL 32792
Single and Three Chip Camera Systems

Gyrus Acmi, Inc. 508-804-2739
93 N Pleasant St, Norwalk, OH 44857
Camera,surgical and accessories.

Gyrus Acmi, Inc. 508-804-2739
300 Stillwater P.o.box 1971, Stamford, CT 06902
Camera,surgical and accessories.

Gyrus Ent L.L.C., Sub. Of Gyrus Acmi, Inc. 508-804-2739
2925 Appling Rd, Bartlett, TN 38133
Multiple.

Jedmed Instruments Co. 314-845-3770
5416 Jedmed Ct, Saint Louis, MO 63129

Kelleher Medical, Inc. 804-378-9956
3049 St Marys Way, Powhatan, VA 23139

ACCESSORIES, SURGICAL CAMERA *(cont'd)*

Lighthouse Imaging Corp. 207-253-5350
477 Congress St, Portland, ME 04101

Med X Change, Inc. 941-794-9977
525 8th St W, Bradenton, FL 34205
Accessories to surgical camera.

Nds Surgical Imaging, Inc. 866-637-5237
5750 Hellyer Ave, San Jose, CA 95138
Surgical Flat Panels designed for Minimally Invasive Surgery, Cardiology, Radiology and bedside monitoring applications

Olympus America, Inc. 800-645-8160
3500 Corporate Pkwy, PO Box 610, Center Valley, PA 18034

Provation Medical, Inc. 612-313-1564
800 Washington Ave N Ste 400, Minneapolis, MN 55401
Medical procedure documentation and coding compliance sofware.

Smith & Nephew Inc., Endoscopy Div. 978-749-1000
76 S Meridian Ave, Oklahoma City, OK 73107
Various.

Solos Endoscopy 800-388-6445
65 Sprague St # B, Boston/dedham Commerce Park, Boston, MA 02136
Various surgical camera accessories.

Sony Electronics, Inc., Medical Systems Div. 800-686-7669
1 Sony Dr, Park Ridge, NJ 07656

Sunoptic Technologies 877-677-2832
6018 Bowdendale Ave, Jacksonville, FL 32216
CD documentation system with up to 80 minutes digital video recording on CD-ROM. VCD, DVD and PC compatibility. Easy operation including remote conrol. Free software package including video editing and still image extraction.

Tidi Products, Llc 920-751-4380
570 Enterprise Dr, Neenah, WI 54956
Drape for arthroscopic camera.

Transamerican Technologies International 800-322-7373
2246 Camino Ramon, San Ramon, CA 94583
ACCU-Beam microscope and endoscope adaptors for digital still image capture cameras.Image Capture System - 8MP camera, microscope adaptor,image capture software with secure patent filing.

Vts Medical Systems, Inc. 516-249-1703
40 Melville Park Rd, Melville, NY 11747
Display, lcd monitor.

Wisap America 800-233-8448
8231 Melrose Dr, Lenexa, KS 66214
Digital Video System: 1 CCD, 3 CCD, digital enhancement, digital zoom, auto white balance.

ACCESSORIES, TRACTION *(Physical Med) 89ILZ*

Biomet, Inc. 574-267-6639
56 E Bell Dr, PO Box 587, Warsaw, IN 46582
Various types of traction accessories.

Bird & Cronin, Inc. 651-683-1111
1200 Trapp Rd, Saint Paul, MN 55121
Spreader bar; knee sling for traction.

Chattanooga Group 800-592-7329
4717 Adams Rd, Hixson, TN 37343
TX cervical halters and lumbar belts.

Chi'Am International 727-647-3940
4155 Grandchamp Cir, Palm Harbor, FL 34685
Export management company for products manufactured by Pneumex, Inc. which includes unweighting, traction, scoliosis treament, vibration.

Circular Traction Supply, Inc. 800-247-6535
7602 Talbert Ave Ste 9, Huntington Beach, CA 92648
Non-powered spinal traction device.

Core Products International, Inc. 800-365-3047
808 Prospect Ave, Osceola, WI 54020

Depuy Mitek, Inc. 800-451-2006
325 Paramount Dr, Raynham, MA 02767
Traction pins.

Dj Orthopedics De Mexico, S.A. De C.V. 690-727-1280
Blvd., Delagacion La Presa, Tijuana 22397 Mexico
Knee and other stings

Dj Orthopedics De Mexico, S.A. De C.V. 690-727-1280
Ave. Venustiano Carranza 6802, Castillo, Tijuana 22100 Mexico
Knee and other stings

DJO Inc. 800-336-6569
1430 Decision St, Vista, CA 92081

ACCESSORIES, TRACTION *(cont'd)*

Dynatronics Corp. Chattanooga Operations 801-568-7000
6607 Mountain View Rd, Ooltewah, TN 37363
Traction accessories.

Erp Group Professional Products Ltd. 800-361-3537
3232 Autoroute Laval W., Laval, QC H7T 2H6 Canada

Florida Manufacturing Corp. 800-447-2372
501 Beville Rd, South Daytona, FL 32119

Inland Specialties, Inc. 800-741-0022
7655 Matoaka Rd, Sarasota, FL 34243
Traction spreader plates for buck's style traction.

John Evans Sons, Inc. 215-368-7700
1 Spring Ave, Lansdale, PA 19446
Medical reel.

Larkotex Company 800-972-3037
1002 Olive St, Texarkana, TX 75501

Medical Depot 516-998-4600
99 Seaview Blvd, Port Washington, NY 11050
Accessories, traction.

Mizuho Osi 800-777-4674
30031 Ahern Ave, Union City, CA 94587
Full line of frames, halters, weights, belts, etc.

Primo, Inc. 770-486-7394
417 Dividend Dr Ste B, Peachtree City, GA 30269
Buck's traction boot.

The Saunders Group 800-445-9836
4250 Norex Dr, Chaska, MN 55318
Traction belt, harness.

Truform Orthotics & Prosthetics 800-888-0458
3960 Rosslyn Dr, Cincinnati, OH 45209

Tuff Orthopedic Products 925-595-7053
776 W Lumsden Rd Ste 104, Brandon, FL 33511
Traction boot.

Warsaw Orthopedic, Inc. 901-396-3133
2500 Silveus Xing, Warsaw, IN 46582
Various types of traction bars, wire tighteners.

Zimmer Holdings, Inc. 800-613-6131
1800 W Center St, PO Box 708, Warsaw, IN 46580

ACCESSORIES, TRACTION (CART, FRAME, CORD, WEIGHT)
(Orthopedics) 87HXF

Florida Manufacturing Corp. 800-447-2372
501 Beville Rd, South Daytona, FL 32119

Freeman Manufacturing Company 800-253-2091
900 W Chicago Rd, PO Box J, Sturgis, MI 49091
Head halters, spreader bars, weight bags, traction stands.

Kronner Medical 800-706-3533
1443 Upper Cleveland Rapids Rd, Roseburg, OR 97471
Kronner Colles-Forearm Frame - external fixator for the colles or forearm fractures.

Larkotex Company 800-972-3037
1002 Olive St, Texarkana, TX 75501

Mizuho Osi 800-777-4674
30031 Ahern Ave, Union City, CA 94587
Full line of frames, halters, weights, belts, etc.

Morrison Medical 800-438-6677
3735 Paragon Dr, Columbus, OH 43228
Ankle hitch traction accessory.

Stryker Medical 800-869-0770
3800 E Centre Ave, Portage, MI 49002

Val Med 800-242-5355
3700 Desire Pkwy, Ace Bayou Group, New Orleans, LA 70126
Knee pillow.

Zimmer Holdings, Inc. 800-613-6131
1800 W Center St, PO Box 708, Warsaw, IN 46580

ACCESSORIES, TRACTION, INVASIVE *(Orthopedics) 87KRT*

Frantz Medical Development Ltd. 440-255-1155
7740 Metric Dr, Mentor, OH 44060
Invasive disposable surgical devices used for MIS procedures.

ACCESSORIES, WALKER *(General) 80WYY*

Alimed, Inc. 800-225-2610
297 High St, Dedham, MA 02026

ACCESSORIES, WALKER *(cont'd)*

American Innovations, Inc. 800-223-3913
123 N Main St, Dublin, PA 18917
Dishwasher-safe rigid caddy captures food/beverage containers, preventing spills to the floor, and organizes daily needed items. Attaches to walker interior or exterior. Also, available for crutches, wheelchairs, canes, and bed rails.

C.J.T. Enterprises, Inc. 714-751-6295
PO Box 10028, Costa Mesa, CA 92627
Similiar to a mobile cain the New AT Flash has been enhaced with larger front wheels, an optional breaking system and a easy to use quick release system. Perferect for carrying AAC devices, notebook computers and much more.

Can-Dan Rehatec Ltd. 9056487522
3-1378 Sandhill Dr., Ancaster, ONT L9G-4V5 Canada
MEYWALK Gait Trainer. (spring assist system) Miniwalk Gait Trainer. (spring assist system) KM-SP Ring Walkers. Camilla Multi-Rollator (push and reverse walker)

Colonial Scientific Ltd. 902-468-1811
201 Brownlow Ave., Unit 52, Dartmouth, NS B3B-1W2 Canada

Crestline Products Inc. 407-859-6428
PO Box 2108, Orlando, FL 32802
EASY-UP Handle - assists in rising from sitting position to standing position from chairs, beds, sofas, and autos when using walkers.

Invacare Corporation 800-333-6900
1 Invacare Way, Elyria, OH 44035
INVACARE.

Kaye Products, Inc. 919-732-6444
535 Dimmocks Mill Rd, Hillsborough, NC 27278
Walker, pelvic stabilizer, add to Kaye posture walkers; walker supports for forearms and hands, add to all Kaye posture control walkers.

Mobility Transfer Systems 800-854-4687
PO Box 253, Medford, MA 02155
HandyBar personal support handle to get in and out of your car safely and comfortably.

O&M Enterprise 847-258-4515
641 Chelmsford Ln, Elk Grove Village, IL 60007
Walkers

Optimal Healthcare Products 800-364-8574
11444 W Olympic Blvd Ste 900, Los Angeles, CA 90064

Parsons A.D.L. Inc. 800-263-1281
R.R. #2, 1986 Sideroad 15, Tottenham, ONT L0G 1W0 Canada
Walker Bags and baskets, trays, cane / crutch holders, padded grips

Sunrise Medical 800-333-4000
7477 Dry Creek Pkwy, Longmont, CO 80503

Tuffcare 800-367-6160
3999 E La Palma Ave, Anaheim, CA 92807

Wenzelite Rehab Supplies, Llc 800-706-9255
220 36th St, 99 Seaview Blvd, Brooklyn, NY 11232
SAFETY ROLLER, is a four-wheeled walker with natural action braking system and variable resistance. Adult, pediatric, bariatric anterior and posterior models are available in a choice of colors. Forearm Platform, Walker Accessory is an adjustable forearm platform that rotates 360 degrees and tilts forward and back. It can be custom fit to patients' needs. Posterior Pediatric Walker is a posterior walker that supoorts a child from behind and requires child to adjust to a more upright position; constructed of heavy duty steel.

ACCESSORIES, WHEELCHAIR *(Physical Med) 89KNO*

A.R.C. Distributors 800-296-8724
PO Box 599, Centreville, MD 21617
CLEAR-VIEW POUCH = clear vinyl pouch for back of wheelchair; NO MORE LOST CHARTS! COLORED POUCH = match your wheelchair upolstery. CADDY = wheeled wheelchair accessory with dual baskets (upper and lower) to store and transfer patient's belongings, attaches to back of most wheelchairs simply and securely, non-folding so it reduces theft. INVACARE IV POLES = portable, permanent & removable. 02 HOLDERS = permanent, removable, wheeled, stand alone; single & multi. ANTI-FOLD BARS = reduces wheelchair theft. Anti-Theft Hoops = over-head hoops discourges wheelchair theft. SEAT BELTS = increased patient safety, WHEELCHAIR RAMPS = to help ease wheelchair transports. HANDLEBAR EXTENSIONS = for wheelchair handles. POLECATS = POLECAT I.V. transport system for wheelchair and stretcher patients. POLECAT facilitates moving patients using infusion pumps mounted on portable (wheeled) IV poles. Forms a single unit for improved safety and productivity. FAST, SAFE AND EASY! PREVENTS INJURIES TO PATIENT & TRANSPORTERS TOO!

ACCESSORIES, WHEELCHAIR *(cont'd)*

Accessible Designs, Inc. 210-341-0008
401 Isom Rd Ste 520, San Antonio, TX 78216
Carbon-fiber wheelchair back replacement system.

Action Bag Co. 800-490-8830
1001 Entry Dr, Bensenville, IL 60106
Tinted Equipment Covers

Adlib, Inc. 714-895-9529
5142 Bolsa Ave Ste 106, Huntington Beach, CA 92649
Wheelchair beverage holder.

Advantage Bag Co. 800-556-6307
22633 Ellinwood Dr, Torrance, CA 90505
Backpacks, Totes, Pouches and Cargo nets(Catch-alls) for your clients carrying solutions.

Air Movement Technologies, Inc. 800-317-9582
320 Gateway Park Dr, Syracuse, NY 13212
Wheelchair brake.

Alimed, Inc. 800-225-2610
297 High St, Dedham, MA 02026

Alternative Products 904-378-9081
5351 Ramona Blvd Ste 7, Jacksonville, FL 32205
Arm rest.

American Innovations, Inc. 800-223-3913
123 N Main St, Dublin, PA 18917
Dishwasher-safe rigid caddy captures food/beverage containers, preventing spills to the floor, and organizes daily needed items. Easily transfers to crutch, cane, scooter, walker, or bed rail.

Arcmate Mfg. Corp. 888-637-1926
637 S Vinewood St, Escondido, CA 92029

Assistance Products Lp 972-240-4279
3710 S Country Club Rd, Garland, TX 75043
Wheelchair accessory.

Blue Chip Medical Products, Inc. 800-795-6115
7-11 Suffern Pl Ste 2, Suffern, NY 10901

Blue Earth, Inc. 518-237-5585
31 Ontario St, 2nd Floor - Front, Cohoes, NY 12047
Various wheelchair accessories.

Body Tech 1 Nw 866-315-0640
10727 47th Pl W, Mukilteo, WA 98275
Accessories, wheelchair.

Bodypoint, Inc. 800-547-5716
558 1st Ave S Ste 300, Seattle, WA 98104
Wheelchair seating accessories.

Borel Enterprises Llc 337-583-3448
3664 A Miller Rd, Lake Charles, LA 70605
Wheelchair seat lift.

Bower, Inc. 205-884-7918
830 Pine Harbor Rd, Pell City, AL 35128
Wheelchair leg sling.

C.J.T. Enterprises, Inc. 714-751-6295
PO Box 10028, Costa Mesa, CA 92627
The Profiler mounting system's streamline body and unique design enabling the mount to be attached to round and non-round tubing. Easy to install, light weight and durable the Profiler mount goes beyond traditional expectations. The Profiler supports all AAC devices, notebook computers, tablets and LCD screens.

Care Electronics, Inc. 303-444-2273
4700 Sterling Dr Ste D, Boulder, CO 80301
Care Mobility Monitor portable wheelchair alarm that notifies staff if a client attempts to get up from the chair.

Convaquip Industries, Inc. 800-637-8436
4834 Derrick Dr, PO Box 3417, Abilene, TX 79601
CONVAQUIP IND., INC. 926 XL, 928 XL, 930 XL. Bariatric folding wheelchairs, available in 26-, 28-, or 30-in.-wide seat with 700 lb. capacity.

Crosley Medical Products, Inc. 631-595-2547
60 S 2nd St Ste E, Deer Park, NY 11729

Dallas Trim Industries Corp. 972-278-3598
2511 National Dr, Garland, TX 75041
No-sorz.

David Zeller's Wheelchair Brake & Attachment Brkt. 610-759-5134
182 Bath Pike, Nazareth, PA 18064
Wheelchair brake & attachment bracket.

ACCESSORIES, WHEELCHAIR *(cont'd)*

Diestco Manufacturing Corp. 800-795-2392
PO Box 6504, Chico, CA 95927
WEATHERBREAKER, canopy attaches to any wheelchair or scooter to provide protection from heat/rain/sun. WEATHERBEE, scooter/wheelchair cover protects your vehicle when being stored or transported. WEATHERMUFF, hand and controls' shield protects your scooter, tiller or power chair joystick. WEATHERCHAPS, lap, leg and feet covers provide waterproof protection for lower body. MEGATRAY, polycarbonate wheelchair tray. MINITRAY, flip up tray for scooters. BUDDY SYSTEM, 3-in-1 utility kit. Includes cupholder, tray/clipboard, and utility pouch. Also includes mounting receptor for wheelchair and storage bag. Assortment of wheelchair bags. EZRAMP, rubber threshold ramps. Wheelchair cupholders, armrests and armrest pads and wheelchair cushions also available.

Dj Orthopedics De Mexico, S.A. De C.V. 690-727-1280
Blvd., Delagacion La Presa, Tijuana 22397 Mexico
Wheelchair accessories

Dj Orthopedics De Mexico, S.A. De C.V. 690-727-1280
Ave. Venustiano Carranza 6802, Castillo, Tijuana 22100 Mexico
Wheelchair accessories

Dynatronics Corp. Chattanooga Operations 801-568-7000
6607 Mountain View Rd, Ooltewah, TN 37363
Aluminum reachers.

Ease Of Life Products, Llc 914-834-3480
515 Larchmont Acres Apt D, Larchmont, NY 10538
Assistive devices, wheelchair accessories.

Electric Mobility Corporation 800-718-2082
591 Mantua Blvd, PO Box 450, Sewell, NJ 08080

Feiter's Inc 414-355-7575
8700 W Port Ave, Milwaukee, WI 53224
Accessories, wheelchair.

Fortress Scientifique Du Quebec Ltee. 418-847-5225
2160 Rue De Celles, Quebec G2C 1X8 Canada
Various accessories for a wheelchair

Freedom Designs, Inc. 800-331-8551
2241 N Madera Rd, Simi Valley, CA 93065
Positing systems for wheelchair.

Frog Legs, Inc. 319-472-4972
500 E 6th St, Vinton, IA 52349
Shock absorbing, suspension caster forks.

Genadyne Biotechnologies, Inc. 516-487-8787
65 Watermill Ln, Great Neck, NY 11021
Wheel chair accessory.

Gendron, Inc. 800-537-2521
400 E Lugbill Rd, Archbold, OH 43502
Priced at $3500. add on power pack to motorize a manual wheelchair.

Gerber Chair Mates, Inc. 814-269-9531
1171 Ringling Ave, Johnstown, PA 15902
$310.00 - $345.00 SWING-AWAY amputee stump support attaches to front rigging of the wheelchair, has horizontal adjustment for varied stump length, vertical adjustment for cushion thickness and swing-away action for ease in transfer.

Greenco Industries, Inc. 608-328-8311
1601 4th Ave W, Monroe, WI 53566
Wheelchair pads.

Gunnell, Inc. 800-551-0055
8440 State Rd, Millington, MI 48746
Seating, footrest pad, hip belt.

Hatch Corporation 800-347-1200
42374 Avenida Alvarado Ste A, Temecula, CA 92590
Full line of wheelchair gloves for specific levels of disability as well as wheelchair seat pads. Gloves for rehab, work hardening, and edema control. (See Glove, other.)

Helping Hand Trays 303-781-4019
4351 S Galapago St, Englewood, CO 80110
Adapter for the Helping Hands Tray, allowing it to fit on wheelchairs and open arm chairs.

Helvetia Development Co. Llc. 269-345-1620
225 Parcom St, Kalamazoo, MI 49048
Wheel chair cushions, back cushions.

ACCESSORIES, WHEELCHAIR *(cont'd)*

Homecare Products, Inc. 800-451-1903
1704 B St NW Ste 110, Auburn, WA 98001
EZ-ACCESSORIES features a line of packs and pouches designed primarily for use with walkers, wheelchairs, and bathing related products. Designed for simple attachment and are intended to carry everything from oxygen tanks, portable phones, keys, and even shampoo to the shower!

Inglis Foundation 215-581-0725
2600 Belmont Ave, Phila, PA 19131
Water bottle.

Intarsia Ltd. 203-355-1357
14 Martha Ln, Gaylordsville, CT 06755
Medial & lateral thigh supports, lateral pelvic support, armrest.

Invacare Corporation 800-333-6900
1 Invacare Way, Elyria, OH 44035
INVACARE.

Invaquest 406-543-4228
3116 Old Pond Rd, Missoula, MT 59802
Accessory leverage device for wheelchair assistance.

Kareco International, Inc. 800-8KA-RECO
299 Rte. 22 E., Green Brook, NJ 08812-1714
Anti-tipping attachments and air pumps.

Kayjae Mfg. Co. Inc. 888-452-9523
PO Box 95, Rte. 198 at Chapel Creek Road, Cobbs Creek, VA 23035
This product is a portable table that can be used both under the legs of a wheelchair user, or on top of a wheelchair tray. The easy to use knobs allows the table top to be adjusted for level or slanted use. This versa-table is the most comfortable to use since it is also ergonomically designed.

Kenda American Airless 800-248-4737
7120 Americana Pkwy, Reynoldsburg, OH 43068
Airless inner tubes for wheelchair tires, airless tires for wheelchairs, SUPERLITE combination caster wheel tire & bearing, standard pneumatic wheelchair tires (all sizes), INNTERTHANES for 3 & 4 wheel carts.

Kristi-Care, Inc. 207-637-2672
110 Millturn Rd, Limington, ME 04049
Anterior trunk support.

L.P.A. Medical, Inc. 888-845-6447
460 Desrochers, Ste. 150D, Vanier, QUEBE G1M 1C2 Canada

Lester Electrical Of Nebraska, Inc. 402-477-8988
625 W A St, Lincoln, NE 68522
LESTRONIC II fully automatic wheelchair battery charger, 24 volt, 8 amp with fully automated shut-off.

Maddak Inc. 800-443-4926
661 State Route 23, Wayne, NJ 07470

Marken International, Inc. 800-564-9248
W231N2811 Roundy Cir E Ste 100, Pewaukee, WI 53072
Various.

Matamatic Inc. 800-603-4050
230 Westec Dr, Mount Pleasant, PA 15666
Seat sensor.

Medical Depot 516-998-4600
99 Seaview Blvd, Port Washington, NY 11050
Wheelchairs, accessories.

Metalcraft Industries, Inc. 608-835-3232
399 N Burr Oak Ave, Fitchburg, WI 53575
Wheelchair seating accessories.

Metro Medical Equipment, Inc. 734-522-8400
12985 Wayne Rd, Livonia, MI 48150
Stump Support System for amputees, 'Sit-Rite' Seating and Positioning for wheelchairs

Miller's Adaptive Technologies 800-837-4544
2023 Romig Rd, Akron, OH 44320
Many specialized hardware components for use on a wheelchair. Footrest devices and foot cradles to arm supports. Including Dynamic Hardware.

Nurse Assist ,Inc. 800-649-6800
3400 Northern Cross Blvd, Fort Worth, TX 76137
Wheelchair alarm. Fall prevention monitor with disposable sensor pad. 9 volt battery powered. Monitor $120.00, Package of 10 disposable pads $180.00.

ACCESSORIES, WHEELCHAIR *(cont'd)*

Obus Forme Ltd. 888-225-7378
550 Hopewell Ave., Toronto, ON M6E 2S6 Canada
Flexible seat has been engineered to distribute body weight more evenly and eliminiate pressure points for longer sitting comfort. It is ideal for wheelchairs and comes in nine colors.

Ocelco, Inc. 800-328-5343
1111 Industrial Park Rd SW, Brainerd, MN 56401

Parsons A.D.L. Inc. 800-263-1281
R.R. #2, 1986 Sideroad 15, Tottenham, ONT L0G 1W0 Canada
Molded transparent or solid beige tray, padded positioning belts, bags, pouches, cup holders, ashtrays, ponchos, cane/crutch holders, transfer accessories, cushions

Patterson Medical Supply, Inc. 262-387-8720
W68N158 Evergreen Blvd, Cedarburg, WI 53012
Wheelchair accessories.

Pediatric Seating Dist., Inc. 416-604-9219
2833 Dundas St W, Toronto M6P 1Y6 Canada
Pediatric seating system

Ramsey Machine 724-787-3059
1392 Darlington Rd, Ligonier, PA 15658
Exercise equipment.

Rhamdec Inc. 800-4-MYDESC
PO Box 4296, Santa Clara, CA 95056
MYDESC Portable, ergonomic desktop with infinite positions, built-in height adjustment swings down to the side for transfer, mounts to vertical or horizontal frame of wheelchair. Adapts to beds, sofas, and scooters.

Richardson Products, Inc. 888-928-7297
9408 Gulfstream Rd, Frankfort, IL 60423
Wheelchair accessories.

Safeslideboard.Com 770-675-2978
56 Strickland Dr SW, Mableton, GA 30126
Safeslide board.

Skil-Care Corp. 800-431-2972
29 Wells Ave, Yonkers, NY 10701
Reclining wheelchair backrest converts standard wheelchair to reclining back wheelchair.

Skyway Machine, Inc 530-243-5151
4451 Caterpillar Rd, Redding, CA 96003
Wheels.

Slawner Ltd., J. 514-731-3378
5713 Cote Des Neiges Rd., Montreal, QUE H3S 1Y7 Canada

Stealth Products 800-965-9229
103 John Kelly St, Burnet, TX 78611
Headrest.

Sunrise Medical 800-333-4000
7477 Dry Creek Pkwy, Longmont, CO 80503
Positioning accessories for wheelchairs; wheelchair back; wheelchair-adjustable solid seat.

Sunrise Medical Hhg Inc 303-218-4505
7128 Ambassador Rd, Baltimore, MD 21244
Mounting hardware,various types and sizes for seats & pads.

Sunrise Medical Hhg Inc 303-218-4505
2010 E Spruce Cir, Olathe, KS 66062
Custom wheelchair seats.

Sunrise Medical Hhg Inc 303-218-4505
6724 Preston Ave # 1, Livermore, CA 94551

Sunrise Medical Hhg Inc 303-218-4505
2615 W Casino Rd # 2B, Everett, WA 98204

Sunrise Medical Hhg Inc 303-218-4505
2842 N Business Park Ave, Fresno, CA 93727

Superquad, Llc 800-659-4548
8265 Sierra College Blvd Ste 316, Roseville, CA 95661
Manual wheelchair driver & braking system.

Tamarack Habilitation Technologies, Inc. 763-795-0057
1670 94th Ln NE, Blaine, MN 55449
Micro shell.

Tempur Production Usa, Inc. 276-431-7174
203 Tempur Pedic Dr Ste 102, Duffield, VA 24244
Wheelchair cushion.

The Aftermarket Group 888-TAG-8200
10173 Croydon Way, Sacramento, CA 95827
Accessories, wheelchair.

Theradyne Products Division 800-328-4014
395 Ervin Industrial Dr, Jordan, MN 55352

ACCESSORIES, WHEELCHAIR *(cont'd)*

Therafin Corporation 800-843-7234
19747 Wolf Rd, Mokena, IL 60448
Various wheelchair accessories.

Thompson Medical Specialties 800-777-4949
3404 Library Ln, Saint Louis Park, MN 55426
Support vests for children and adults. Transfer belts, solid insert seats and backs, padded calf panels.

Three Rivers Holdings, Llc 480-833-1829
1826 W Broadway Rd Ste 43, Mesa, AZ 85202
Wheelchair handrim.

Transilwrap Co., Inc. 847-678-1800
9201 Belmont Ave, Franklin Park, IL 60131
Wheelchair patient monitoring alarm.

Trayco 512-341-3709
1101 Pecan St W, Pflugerville, TX 78660
Wheelchair, accessories.

Tub Master Lc 800-833-0260
413 Virginia Dr, Orlando, FL 32803
Barrier-free, adaptable, folding shower doors for wheelchair entry.

Tuffcare 800-367-6160
3999 E La Palma Ave, Anaheim, CA 92807

Tumble Forms, Inc. 262-387-8720
1013 Barker Rd, Dolgeville, NY 13329
Seat cover.

United Plastic Molders, Inc. 601-353-3193
105 E Rankin St, Jackson, MS 39201
Accessories, wheelchair.

ACCESSORY - FILM DOSIMETRY SYSTEM *(Radiology) 90MWW*

Agile Radiological Technologies 513-985-9877
11180 Reed Hartman Hwy, Cincinnati, OH 45242
Radiation analyzer (ray).

3cognition Llc 516-458-2905
1 Portico Ct Apt 302, Great Neck, NY 11021
Radiotherapy film dosimetry system.

ACCESSORY, ASSISTED REPRODUCTION *(Obstetrics/Gyn) 85MQG*

Cook Ob/Gyn 800-541-5591
1100 W Morgan St, Spencer, IN 47460

Genx International 888-GEN-XNOW
393 Soundview Rd, Guilford, CT 06437

Mid-Atlantic Diagnostics Inc., Custom Products Div 856-762-2000
77 Elbo Ln, Mount Laurel, NJ 08054
Ivf-1.

Penetrating Innovations, Inc. 608-845-3270
415 Venture Ct, Verona, WI 53593
Temperature control unit for a heated microscope stage.

Thermo Fisher Scientific (Asheville) Llc 740-373-4763
Millcreek Rd., Marietta, OH 45750
Various models of ivf incubators and controlled rate freezers.

Zander Medical Supplies, Inc. / Zander Ivf, Inc. 800-820-3029
755 8th Ct Ste 4, Vero Beach, FL 32962
Cryopreservation instrumentation - Rectangular or triangular plastic cassettes used for holding cryo-straws during cryopreservation. Stage Warmer - MTG and Tokai Hit - Heated stages and inserts for inverted, upright and stereo

ACCESSORY, BARIUM SULFATE, METHYL METHACRYLATE FOR CRANIOPLASTY *(Cns/Neurology) 84MYU*

Sciarra Laboratories, Inc 516-933-7853
485 S Broadway Ste 09, Hicksville, NY 11801
Barium sulfate.

ACETONE *(Chemistry) 75UJV*

Biomerieux Inc. 800-682-2666
100 Rodolphe St, Durham, NC 27712

Honeywell Burdick & Jackson 800-368-0050
1953 Harvey St, Muskegon, MI 49442

Poly Scientific R&D Corp. 800-645-5825
70 Cleveland Ave, Bay Shore, NY 11706

Polysciences, Inc. 800-523-2575
400 Valley Rd, Warrington, PA 18976

ACID, HEMATEIN *(Pathology) 88IDE*

Sci Gen, Inc. 310-324-6576
333 E Gardena Blvd, Gardena, CA 90248
FDA: Medical Device Manufacturing and packaging. Focus on Histology, Cytology, Analytical and General purpose Reagents, Chemistry, and Sterling and Disinfecting agents.

ACID, HYALUORONIC *(Dental And Oral) 76LZX*

Allergan 800-366-6554
2525 Dupont Dr, Irvine, CA 92612
Balanced salt solution in 500cc and 30cc bottles.

Anika Therapeutics 781-457-9000
32 Wiggins Ave, Bedford, MA 01730
Orthovisc injection for treatment of osteoarthritis of the knee.

Biomet, Inc. 574-267-6639
56 E Bell Dr, PO Box 587, Warsaw, IN 46582
Hyaluronic acid.

Genzyme 800-332-1042
500 Kendall St, Cambridge, MA 02142
Medical grade hyaluronic acid.

Lifecore Biomedical, Inc. 952-368-4300
3515 Lyman Blvd, Chaska, MN 55318
Sodium hyaluronate pharmaceutical-grade viscoelastic biomaterial and cosmetic-grade sodium hyaluronate.

Seikagaku America, Inc. 800-848-3248
124 Bernard St. Jean Dr., East Falmouth, MA 02536-4445
Hyaluronic Acid Binding Protein. Binds specifically and strongly to hyaluronic acid, similar to an antibody. Can be used to stain tissue sections or measure H acid concentration in fluid by ELISA.

Staar Surgical Co. 626-3037-902
27121 Aliso Creek Rd, Suite #100,105, 110 & 115
Aliso Viejo, CA 92656
Viscoelastic.

ACID, HYALURONIC, INTRAARTICULAR *(Physical Med) 89MOZ*

Genzyme Corporation 617-252-7500
1125 Pleasantview Ter, Ridgefield, NJ 07657
Hylan g-f 20.

Lifecore Biomedical, Inc. 952-368-4300
3515 Lyman Blvd, Chaska, MN 55318
Sodium hyaluronate pharmaceutical-grade viscoelastic biomaterial and cosmetic-grade sodium hyaluronate.

ACTIVATED WHOLE BLOOD CLOTTING TIME *(Hematology) 81JBP*

Abbott Point Of Care Inc. 609-443-9300
104 Windsor Center Dr, East Windsor, NJ 08520
I-stat system (various panels of tests).

Analytical Control Systems, Inc. 317-841-0458
9058 Technology Dr, Fishers, IN 46038
ACT-TROL Simulated Whole Blood Coagulation Controls, Levels I, II, AND III. A quality control procedure for activated clotting time instruments. Simple and consistent instructions. 8 hour reconstituted, unrefrigerated stability. No incubation period. Same lot available for up to 2 years.

International Technidyne Corp. 800-631-5945
23 Nevsky St, Edison, NJ 08820

International Technidyne Corporation 732-548-5700
8 Olsen Ave, Edison, NJ 08820
Microcoagulation activated clotting time plus test cuvette.

Medtronic Blood Management 612-514-4000
18501 E Plaza Dr, Parker, CO 80134
Invitro diagnostic cartridge & controls.

ACTIVATOR, ULTRAVIOLET, POLYMERIZATION *(Dental And Oral) 76EBZ*

Bisco, Inc. 847-534-6000
1100 W Irving Park Rd, Schaumburg, IL 60193
Dental curing light.

Cao Group, Inc. 801-256-9282
4628 Skyhawk Dr, West Jordan, UT 84084
Led dental curing light.

Coltene/Whaledent Inc. 330-916-8858
235 Ascot Pkwy, Cuyahoga Falls, OH 44223
Curing light.

Dentlight Inc. 972-889-8857
1411 E Campbell Rd Ste 500, Richardson, TX 75081
Dental curing light.

ACTIVATOR, ULTRAVIOLET, POLYMERIZATION *(cont'd)*

Dentsply Canada, Ltd. 800-263-1437
161 Vinyl Ct., Woodbridge, ONT L4L 4A3 Canada

Dp Manufacture Corp. 305-640-9894
1460 NW 107th Ave Ste H, Doral, FL 33172
Various models of curing lights.

Eele Laboratories, Llc 631-244-0051
50 Orville Dr, Bohemia, NY 11716
Dental curing light.

Forestadent Usa 314-878-5985
2315 Weldon Pkwy, Saint Louis, MO 63146
Ultraviolet activator for polymerization.

Ivoclar Vivadent, Inc. 800-533-6825
175 Pineview Dr, Amherst, NY 14228
ASTRALIS.

Kerr Corp. 949-255-8766
3225 Deming Way Ste 190, Middleton, WI 53562
Dental curing light.

Milestone Scientific Inc. 800-862-1125
45 Knightsbridge Rd, Piscataway, NJ 08854
cool blue cordless curing light

Milestone Scientific Inc. 800-862-1125
220 S Orange Ave, Livingston, NJ 07039
cool blue cordless curing light

Nova Ranger, Inc. 858-452-7300
9885 Mesa Rim Rd Ste 127, San Diego, CA 92121
Cordless curing light.

Pac-Dent Intl., Inc. 909-839-0888
21078 Commerce Point Dr, Walnut, CA 91789
Curing light.

Pentron Clinical Technologies 203-265-7397
68-70 North Plains Industrial, Road, Wallingford, CT 06492
Activator,ultraviolet,for polymerization.

Tpc Advanced Technology, Inc. 626-810-4337
18525 Gale Ave, City Of Industry, CA 91748
Advance 320 and Advance 500 Curing Lights--dental UV curing lights.

Ultradent Products, Inc. 801-553-4586
505 W 10200 S, South Jordan, UT 84095
Intraoral light cure unit.

Usa Think, Inc. 605-787-7717
13030 Homer Smith Rd, Piedmont, SD 57769
Dental curing light.

Westside Packaging, Llc. 909-570-3508
1700 S Baker Ave Ste A, Ontario, CA 91761
Dental curing light.

ADAPTER, ANESTHESIA *(Anesthesiology) 73QAT*

Cadence Science Inc. 888-717-7677
1979 Marcus Ave Ste 215, New Hyde Park, NY 11042

Globalmed Inc. 613-394-9844
155 N. Murray St., Trenton, ONT K8V-5R5 Canada
Various-diameter anesthesia circuit adaptors.

Instrumentation Industries, Inc. 800-633-8577
2990 Industrial Blvd, Bethel Park, PA 15102

Intersurgical Inc. 315-451-2900
417 Electronics Pkwy, Liverpool, NY 13088

Mercury Medical 800-237-6418
11300 49th St N, Clearwater, FL 33762

Southmedic Inc. 800-463-7146
50 Alliance Blvd., Barrie, ONT L4M-5K3 Canada
Aluminum and injection molded nylon VAPOFIL vaporizer filling device; also nylon VAPOFIL HOLDER, mountable storage device for VAPOFIL.

Sunmed Healthcare 727-531-7266
12393 Belcher Rd S Ste 460, Largo, FL 33773

Trudell Medical Marketing Ltd. 800-265-5494
926 Leathorne St., London, ON N5Z-3M5 Canada

Vascular Technology Incorporated 800-550-0856
12 Murphy Dr, Nashua, NH 03062
VTI-976. T-adaptor (1/4 in. OD x 1/4 in. OD x 15 mm ID).

ADAPTER, AV SHUNT OR FISTULA *(Gastro/Urology) 78KNR*

Angiodynamics, Inc. 800-472-5221
1 Horizon Way, Manchester, GA 31816
Shunt adapter set (12/package) from the broadest line of A-V shunt products available.

ADAPTER, BULB, ENDOSCOPE, MISCELLANEOUS
(Gastro/Urology) 78FFY

Boston Scientific Corporation 508-652-5578
780 Brookside Dr, Spencer, IN 47460

Cook Endoscopy 336-744-0157
4900 Bethania Station Rd # &, 5951 Grassy Creek Blvd. Winston Salem, NC 27105
Endoscope holder.

Gyrus Acmi, Inc. 508-804-2739
93 N Pleasant St, Norwalk, OH 44857
Adaptor, bulbs, miscellaneous, for endoscope.

Medical Innovations International Inc. 507-289-0761
6256 34th Ave NW, Rochester, MN 55901
Endo X Trainer™ trays with ex-vivo animal tissue service for endoscopic training.

Pentax Medical Company 800-431-5880
102 Chestnut Ridge Rd, Montvale, NJ 07645
A full line of light source adaptors for other manufacturers' scopes to PENTAX lightsources or PENTAX scopes to other manufacturers' lightsources. Also a full line of scope eyepiece direct couplers or beamsplitters for other manufacturers' scopes to PENTAX eyepiece mount or PENTAX scopes to other manufacturers' eyepiece mount.

ADAPTER, CABLE, EQUIPMENT *(General) 80WTN*

Aiv, Inc. (Formerly American Iv) 800-990-2911
7485 Shipley Ave, Harmans, MD 21077
Pulse oximeter adapter cables connecting sensors to leading patient monitors.

Bicron Electronics 800-624-2766
50 Barlow St, Canaan, CT 06018
Toroidal transformers. Specially, magnetics, current sensors, solenoids (open frame), tubular, rotary, Mag-Latch.

Btx Tech 800-666-0996
5 Skyline Dr, Hawthorne, NY 10532
Connectors, cable assemblies, power supplies and tools.

Dwfritz Automation, Inc. 503-598-9393
17750 SW Upper Boones Ferry Rd, Portland, OR 97224

O&M Enterprise 847-258-4515
641 Chelmsford Ln, Elk Grove Village, IL 60007
ECG MACHINE ADAPTER,CABLE, EQUIPMENT

ADAPTER, CATHETER *(Surgery) 79GCE*

Addto, Inc. 773-278-0294
816 N Kostner Ave, Chicago, IL 60651

Baxter Healthcare Corporation, Renal 888-229-0001
1620 S Waukegan Rd, Waukegan, IL 60085
Locking cap for Baxter peritoneal dialysis catheter adapter.

Cadence Science Inc. 888-717-7677
1979 Marcus Ave Ste 215, New Hyde Park, NY 11042

Hospira, Inc. 877-946-7747
Hwy. 301 North, Rocky Mount, NC 27801
Various.

Medical Action Industries, Inc. 800-645-7042
25 Heywood Rd, Arden, NC 28704
Tubing connectors.

Mercury Medical 800-237-6418
11300 49th St N, Clearwater, FL 33762

Vygon Corp. 800-544-4907
2495 General Armistead Ave, Norristown, PA 19403

ADAPTER, CATHETER, URETERAL *(Gastro/Urology) 78EYI*

Boston Scientific Corporation 508-652-5578
780 Brookside Dr, Spencer, IN 47460

Cook Urological, Inc. 800-457-4500
1100 W Morgan St, P.O. Box 227, Spencer, IN 47460

ADAPTER, CENTRIFUGE TUBE *(Chemistry) 75QIY*

Nalge Nunc International 800-625-4327
75 Panorama Creek Dr, Rochester, NY 14625
NALGENE centrifuge accessories.

ADAPTER, ELECTROSURGICAL UNIT, CABLE *(Surgery) 79QTR*

Cameron-Miller, Inc. 800-621-0142
5410 W Roosevelt Rd, Road #241, Chicago, IL 60644

Elmed, Inc. 630-543-2792
60 W Fay Ave, Addison, IL 60101

ADAPTER, ELECTROSURGICAL UNIT, CABLE *(cont'd)*

Gyrus Medical, Inc. 800-852-9361
6655 Wedgwood Rd N Ste 105, Maple Grove, MN 55311
Connects Everest medical instruments to most common electrosurgical generators.

Kirwan Surgical Products, Inc. 888-547-9267
180 Enterprise Dr, PO Box 427, Marshfield, MA 02050
Electrosurgical tips.

Olsen Medical 800-297-6344
3001 W Kentucky St, Louisville, KY 40211
Bipolar and Monopolar Cables, Including Stortz Style and Kleppinger Instruments

ADAPTER, HOLDER, SYRINGE *(Physical Med) 89IQG*

Biomet Microfixation Inc. 800-874-7711
1520 Tradeport Dr, Jacksonville, FL 32218
Various types of syringes.

Cook Endoscopy 336-744-0157
4900 Bethania Station Rd # &, 5951 Grassy Creek Blvd. Winston Salem, NC 27105
Various types of syringe holders.

Engineers Express, Inc. 800-255-8823
7 Industrial Park Rd, Medway, MA 02053

Hospira, Inc. 877-946-7747
1776 Centennial Dr, McPherson, KS 67460
Various types.

Precision Sclero 727-517-0729
12408 Chickasaw Trl, Largo, FL 33774
Syringe holder.

ADAPTER, HYGIENE *(Physical Med) 89ILS*

Dynatronics Corp. Chattanooga Operations 801-568-7000
6607 Mountain View Rd, Ooltewah, TN 37363
Shower benches and transfer benches.

Ergounlimited, Inc. 205-591-9977
5401 9th Ave S, Birmingham, AL 35212
Enema board.

Ginacor, Inc. 206-860-1595
513 31st Ave, Seattle, WA 98122
SQUATTING DEVICE, DAILY ACTIVITY ASSIST DEVICE. FDA 510K exempt. approved as an aid to proper elimination

Great Lakes Innovation Inc 248-680-8671
1103 Winthrop Dr, Troy, MI 48083
Innolife portable commode.

Health Care Logistics, Inc. 800-848-1633
450 Town St, PO Box 25, Circleville, OH 43113
Daily activity assist devices.

Higgs Medical Products, Llc 973-625-4424
21 Pine St Ste 109, Rockaway, NJ 07866
Bath bench.

Hospital Therapy Products, Inc. 630-766-7101
757 N Central Ave, Wood Dale, IL 60191
Spray bathing.

Liftseat Corporation 630-424-2840
158 Eisenhower Ln S, Lombard, IL 60148
Daily activity assist device.

Lotus Hygiene Systems Inc. 714-259-8805
15042 Parkway Loop Ste B, Tustin, CA 92780
Toilet seat,bidet.

Maddak Inc. 800-443-4926
661 State Route 23, Wayne, NJ 07470

Medical Depot 516-998-4600
99 Seaview Blvd, Port Washington, NY 11050
Hygiene and personal assist adaptors.

Medical Products Of Milwaukee, Llc. 414-281-8713
2500 W Layton Ave Ste 250, Milwaukee, WI 53221
Hair washing apparatus.

Mobility Inc. 858-456-8121
5726 La Jolla Blvd Ste 104, La Jolla, CA 92037
Hydraulic toilet seat.

Parsons A.D.L. Inc. 800-263-1281
R.R. #2, 1986 Sideroad 15, Tottenham, ONT L0G 1W0 Canada

Patterson Medical Supply, Inc. 262-387-8720
W68N158 Evergreen Blvd, Cedarburg, WI 53012
Hygiene aid, daily activity assist device.

ADAPTER, HYGIENE *(cont'd)*

Richardson Products, Inc. 888-928-7297
9408 Gulfstream Rd, Frankfort, IL 60423
Hygiene aids.

Therafin Corporation 800-843-7234
19747 Wolf Rd, Mokena, IL 60448
Various types of hygiene aids.

Tumble Forms, Inc. 262-387-8720
1013 Barker Rd, Dolgeville, NY 13329
Toileting system.

ADAPTER, LEAD SWITCHING, ELECTROCARDIOGRAPH *(Cardiovascular) 74DRW*

Vital Connections, Inc. 937-667-3880
955 N 3rd St, Phoneton, OH 45371
Ecg cable/ lead wires.

ADAPTER, LEAD, PACEMAKER *(Cardiovascular) 74DTD*

Alto Development Corp. 732-938-2266
5206 Asbury Rd, Wall Township, NJ 07727

Ela Medical, Inc. 800-352-6466
2950 Xenium Ln N, Plymouth, MN 55441

Enpath Medical, Inc. 800-559-2613
2300 Berkshire Ln N, Minneapolis, MN 55441

Maquet Puerto Rico Inc. 408-635-3900
No. 12, Rd. #698, Dorado, PR 00646
Various models of lead adapters.

Oscor, Inc. 800-726-7267
3816 Desoto Blvd, Palm Harbor, FL 34683
Lead adaptors. Permanent pacing leads.

St. Jude Medical Cardiac Rhythm Management Div. 800-777-2237
15900 Valley View Ct, Sylmar, CA 91342
Subclavian cardiac pacing lead introducer sets available in single pack, single sheath/dilator 8-13Fr; single pack, dual sheath/dilator 8-10Fr. and 10 pack dispenser box 8-13Fr.

ADAPTER, NEEDLE *(Cardiovascular) 74WTU*

Engineers Express, Inc. 800-255-8823
7 Industrial Park Rd, Medway, MA 02053

Premier Medical Products 888-PREMUSA
1710 Romano Dr, Plymouth Meeting, PA 19462

ADAPTER, SHUNT *(Gastro/Urology) 78FKN*

Codman & Shurtleff, Inc 800-225-0460
325 Paramount Dr, Raynham, MA 02767

Lifemed Of California 800-543-3633
1216 S Allec St, Anaheim, CA 92805

ADAPTER, STOPCOCK, MANIFOLD, CARDIOPULMONARY BYPASS *(Cardiovascular) 74DTL*

Abbott Vascular, Cardiac Therapies 800-227-9902
26531 Ynez Rd, Mailing P.O. Box 9018, Temecula, CA 92591
Hemostatic valve.

Angiodynamics, Inc. 518-795-1400
14 Plaza Drive, Latham, NY 12110
High Pressure Connecting Lines

Argon Medical Devices Inc. 903-675-9321
1445 Flat Creek Rd, Athens, TX 75751
Various.

Atek Medical 800-253-1540
620 Watson St SW, Grand Rapids, MI 49504
Various types of rapid prime set, multiple perfusion set, decanting set, pressure.

Bard Electro Physiology 800-824-8724
55 Technology Dr, Lowell, MA 01851

Boston Scientific - Maple Grove 800-553-5878
1 Scimed Pl, Maple Grove, MN 55311

C. R. Bard, Inc., Bard Urological Div. 888-367-2273
13183 Harland Dr NE, Covington, GA 30014

Cadence Science Inc. 888-717-7677
1979 Marcus Ave Ste 215, New Hyde Park, NY 11042

Edwards Lifesciences Research Medical 949-250-2500
6864 Cottonwood St, Midvale, UT 84047
Various types of monitoring, infusion & delivery set.

Elcam Medical, Inc. 800-530-2441
2 University Plz Ste 620, Hackensack, NJ 07601

ADAPTER, STOPCOCK, MANIFOLD, CARDIOPULMONARY BYPASS *(cont'd)*

Engineers Express, Inc. 800-255-8823
7 Industrial Park Rd, Medway, MA 02053
Cardiopulmonary bypass, 316L stainles steel, luer fittings to the new ANSI standards.

Icu Medical (Ut), Inc 949-366-2183
4455 Atherton Dr, Salt Lake City, UT 84123
Three-way stopcock with male locking luer ada.

Medtronic Dlp 616-643-5200
620 Watson St SW, Grand Rapids, MI 49504

Medtronic Perfusion Systems 800-854-3570
7611 Northland Dr N, Brooklyn Park, MN 55428

Medtronic Vascular 707-525-0111
3576 Unocal Pl, Santa Rosa, CA 95403
Adapter, stopcock, fitting

Merit Medical Systems, Inc. 800-356-3748
1600 Merit Pkwy, South Jordan, UT 84095
MARQUIS SERIES stopcocks and manifolds.

Navilyst Medical 800-833-9973
100 Boston Scientific Way, Marlborough, MA 01752
Various types of check valves, stopcocks, manifolds, y-adaptors, kits.

Smiths Medical Asd, Inc. 800-848-1757
6250 Shier Rings Rd, Dublin, OH 43016

Sorin Group Usa 800-289-5759
14401 W 65th Way, Arvada, CO 80004

Terumo Cardiovascular Systems (Tcvs) 800-283-7866
28 Howe St, Ashland, MA 01721
Adaptor, stopcock, manifold, & fitting.

Terumo Cardiovascular Systems, Corp 800-521-2818
6200 Jackson Rd, Ann Arbor, MI 48103

Total Molding Services, Inc. 215-538-9613
354 East Broad St., Trumbauersville, PA 18970
Male luer adaptor.

Vygon Corp. 800-544-4907
2495 General Armistead Ave, Norristown, PA 19403

ADAPTER, SYRINGE *(General) 80RYL*

Cadence Science Inc. 888-717-7677
1979 Marcus Ave Ste 215, New Hyde Park, NY 11042

Engineers Express, Inc. 800-255-8823
7 Industrial Park Rd, Medway, MA 02053

Hospira Inc. 877-946-7747
275 N Field Dr, Lake Forest, IL 60045
HOSPIRA CARPUJECT HOLDER

RamÇ-Hart, Inc. 973-448-0305
95 Allen St, PO Box 400, Netcong, NJ 07857
Semi-auto device to install stoppers in syringes.

Vygon Corp. 800-544-4907
2495 General Armistead Ave, Norristown, PA 19403

ADAPTER, TUBE, TRACHEAL *(Anesthesiology) 73SBF*

A-M Systems, Inc. 800-426-1306
131 Business Park Loop, Sequim, WA 98382
19 types, autoclavable, plastic, or plexiglas.

Bausch & Lomb Surgical 636-255-5051
3365 Tree Court Ind Blvd, Saint Louis, MO 63122

Bunnell Incorporated 800-800-4358
436 Lawndale Dr, Salt Lake City, UT 84115
Endotracheal tube, 15mm jet ventilator E.T. tube adapter. 2.5mm - 5.5 mm.

Globalmed Inc. 613-394-9844
155 N. Murray St., Trenton, ONT K8V-5R5 Canada
Catheter mounts and patient connections.

Instrumentation Industries, Inc. 800-633-8577
2990 Industrial Blvd, Bethel Park, PA 15102
Swivel adapters for endotube/trach tube.

Mercury Medical 800-237-6418
11300 49th St N, Clearwater, FL 33762

ADAPTER, TUBE, TRACHEAL *(cont'd)*

Passy-Muir Inc. 800-634-5397
4521 Campus Dr, Irvine, CA 92612
Passy-Muir™ closed-position 'no leak' Tracheostomy & Ventilator Swallowing and Speaking valves (PMVs.) The only swallowing & speaking valves that are interchangeable for use on or off the ventilator (with the exception of the PMV™ 2020 for metal trach tubes.) Independent research has shown that the closed position PMV improves swallowing, reduces aspiration, facilitates secretion management, and reduces weaning and decannulation time. Reimbursable by Medicare, Medicaid, MediCal, and CCS.

Southmedic Inc. 800-463-7146
50 Alliance Blvd., Barrie, ONT L4M-5K3 Canada
AEROSOL-T respiratory care connector allowing administration of cannister agents directly into the endotracheal tube.

ADAPTER, UNIT, ELECTROSURGICAL, HAND-CONTROLLED
(Surgery) 79QTS

Buffalo Filter, A Division Of Medtek Devices Inc. 800-343-2324
595 Commerce Dr, Amherst, NY 14228
PenAdapt Electrosurgical Pencil Adapter for capture of smoke plume generated from ESU procedures; fits all ESU pencils.

Cameron-Miller, Inc. 800-621-0142
5410 W Roosevelt Rd, Road #241, Chicago, IL 60644

Elmed, Inc. 630-543-2792
60 W Fay Ave, Addison, IL 60101

ADAPTER, Y *(Gastro/Urology) 78FJP*

Boston Scientific - Maple Grove 800-553-5878
1 Scimed Pl, Maple Grove, MN 55311

Directmed, Inc. 516-656-3377
150 Pratt Oval, Glen Cove, NY 11542

Respironics California, Inc. 724-387-4559
2271 Cosmos Ct, Carlsbad, CA 92011
Various sizes of adapters.

Respironics Novametrix, Llc. 724-387-4559
5 Technology Dr, Wallingford, CT 06492
Various sizes of adapters.

Total Molding Services, Inc. 215-538-9613
354 East Broad St., Trumbauersville, PA 18970
Large Y Bore Connector.

Vygon Corp. 800-544-4907
2495 General Armistead Ave, Norristown, PA 19403

ADAPTOMETER (BIOPHOTOMETER) *(Ophthalmology) 86HJW*

Lkc Technologies, Inc. 800-638-7055
2 Professional Dr Ste 222, Gaithersburg, MD 20879
Dark adaptometer. Scotopic sensitivity tester SST-1.

ADAPTOR, DRESSING *(Physical Med) 89ILD*

Assisted Access-Nfss, Inc. 800-950-9655
822 Preston Ct, Lake Villa, IL 60046

Bsn-Jobst 704-554-9933
5825 Carnegie Blvd, Charlotte, NC 28209
Cotton lined PVC gloves.

Dynatronics Corp. Chattanooga Operations 801-568-7000
6607 Mountain View Rd, Ooltewah, TN 37363
Dressing adaptor.

Mecanaids Co., Inc. 800-227-0877
21 Hampden Dr, South Easton, MA 02375
Handicapped dressing and reaching aids. Variety of daily living aids.

Patterson Medical Supply, Inc. 262-387-8720
W68N158 Evergreen Blvd, Cedarburg, WI 53012
Dressing aid, daily activity assist device.

Preferred Solutions Llc 757-224-0177
467 Swan Ave, Hohenwald, TN 38462
Daily activity assist device.

Richardson Products, Inc. 888-928-7297
9408 Gulfstream Rd, Frankfort, IL 60423
Dressing aids.

Therafin Corporation 800-843-7234
19747 Wolf Rd, Mokena, IL 60448
Various types of dressing aids.

ADAPTOR, GROOMING *(Physical Med) 89ILW*

Designs For Comfort, Inc. 800-443-9226
PO Box 671044, Marietta, GA 30066
$15/25 HEADLINER soft fabric cap with separate hair piece, both in various colors (washable) to resemble original hair. $25/25 HEADLINER PLUS-2 soft fabric cap with tails to wrap or tie in bow, separate hair, etc. $15/25 HEADLINER TURBAN classic turban with separate hair, etc. Sleep cap, swim cap, baseball cap, scrunch hat. HEADLINER Hoop of Hair is a circle of hair that leaves sensitive scalp untouched. For women bald from chemotherapy.

Dynatronics Corp. Chattanooga Operations 801-568-7000
6607 Mountain View Rd, Ooltewah, TN 37363
Grooming adaptor.

Maddak Inc. 800-443-4926
661 State Route 23, Wayne, NJ 07470

Mecanaids Co., Inc. 800-227-0877
21 Hampden Dr, South Easton, MA 02375
Handicapped dressing and reaching aids. Variety of daily living aids.

P.R.I.D.E. Foundation 800-332-9122
391 Long Hill Rd, Groton, CT 06340
Clothing instructions and patterns to sew, modify or adapt garments for the blind, arthritic, physically impaired children and handicapped adults. Educational literature about the above is available. Sample fashions, sample devices to aid in bathing, dressing, grooming. Books and literature.

Parsons A.D.L. Inc. 800-263-1281
R.R. #2, 1986 Sideroad 15, Tottenham, ONT L0G 1W0 Canada
Grooming Aids for the physically challenged

Patterson Medical Supply, Inc. 262-387-8720
W68N158 Evergreen Blvd, Cedarburg, WI 53012
Grooming aid, daily activity assist device.

Richardson Products, Inc. 888-928-7297
9408 Gulfstream Rd, Frankfort, IL 60423
Grooming aids.

Therafin Corporation 800-843-7234
19747 Wolf Rd, Mokena, IL 60448
Fingernail clippers.

ADAPTOR, RECREATIONAL *(Physical Med) 89ILT*

Adlib, Inc. 714-895-9529
5142 Bolsa Ave Ste 106, Huntington Beach, CA 92649
Various types of mouthsticks.

Generations, Inc. 360-840-6550
22895 E Apple Ln, Sedro Woolley, WA 98284
Tension release book holder.

Maddak Inc. 800-443-4926
661 State Route 23, Wayne, NJ 07470

Patterson Medical Supply, Inc. 262-387-8720
W68N158 Evergreen Blvd, Cedarburg, WI 53012
Recreational aid, a daily activity assist device.

Reha Partner Inc. 866-282-4558
530 Means St NW Ste 120, Atlanta, GA 30318
PEPPINO, the 3 in 1 talent. The PEPPINO system features a light weight seating shell, designed for use as a car seat, in a stroller and with an high-low indoor base.

Richardson Products, Inc. 888-928-7297
9408 Gulfstream Rd, Frankfort, IL 60423
Recreational rehab devices.

Tetra Computer Systems, Llc 856-728-6835
328 Bryn Mawr Dr, Williamstown, NJ 08094
Computer system.

The Steady-Arm Company, Inc. 570-358-3632
RR 1 Box 353, Ulster, PA 18850
Easy glide kit.

Therafin Corporation 800-843-7234
19747 Wolf Rd, Mokena, IL 60448
Bowling ball pusher.

ADENOTOME *(Ear/Nose/Throat) 77KBH*

Aesculap Implant Systems Inc. 1-800-234-9179
3773 Corporate Pkwy, Center Valley, PA 18034

Bausch & Lomb Surgical 636-255-5051
3365 Tree Court Ind Blvd, Saint Louis, MO 63122

Biomet Microfixation Inc. 800-874-7711
1520 Tradeport Dr, Jacksonville, FL 32218
Adenotome.

Clinimed, Incorporated 877-CLINIMED
303 Markus Ct, Sandy Brae Industrial Park, Newark, DE 19713

ADENOTOME *(cont'd)*

Precision Medical Manufacturing Corporation 866-633-4626
852 Seton Ct, Wheeling, IL 60090
Different types of adenotome blades specificaly made in sizes:infant,small,medium and large.Positive cutting blades will not buckle or bend.

ADHESIVE STRIP, HYPOALLERGENIC *(General) 80QAC*

Brady Corporation 800-541-1686
6555 W Good Hope Rd, PO Box 571, Milwaukee, WI 53223
Wound-closure devices, manufactured to customer specifications. TruMed specializes in multi-layer laminating, incorporating hydrogels, tapes, and liners. Skin-testing strips, occlusive and semi-occlusive, are available as single-site and five-site designs.

E-Med Corp. 800-974-3633
8307 Marigold Ln, Maineville, OH 45039
I. V. STRIP 2 x 6 in., non-occlusive with non-stick gauze pad, moisture resistant, resealable for IV securement and hypoallergenic. TUBE STRIP, 1 x 6 in. resealable, hypoallergenic, moisture resistant for securing Foley catheters, miscellaneous tubing, etc. P.D. STRIP, non-occlusive resealable dressing and immobilizer for peritoneal dialysis and hemodialysis catheters.

Johnson & Johnson Medical Division Of Ethicon, Inc. 800-423-4018
2500 E Arbrook Blvd, Arlington, TX 76014

Meddev Corporation 800-543-2789
730 N Pastoria Ave, Sunnyvale, CA 94085
EYECLOSE adhesive strips for use with EYECLOSE external eyelid weights.

Tailored Label Products, Inc. 800-727-1344
W165N5731 Ridgewood Dr, Menomonee Falls, WI 53051

ADHESIVE STRIP, WATERPROOF *(General) 80QAD*

Border Opportunity Saver Systems, Inc. 830-775-0992
10 Finegan Rd, Del Rio, TX 78840

Brady Corporation 800-541-1686
6555 W Good Hope Rd, PO Box 571, Milwaukee, WI 53223
Custom manufactured adhesive devices, manufactured to customer specifications.

Closure Medical 888-257-7633
5250 Greens Dairy Rd, Raleigh, NC 27616
LIQUIDERM

Johnson & Johnson Medical Division Of Ethicon, Inc. 800-423-4018
2500 E Arbrook Blvd, Arlington, TX 76014

Smith & Nephew, Inc. 800-876-1261
11775 Starkey Rd, Largo, FL 33773
UNIFLEX adhesive dressing.

Tailored Label Products, Inc. 800-727-1344
W165N5731 Ridgewood Dr, Menomonee Falls, WI 53051

Urocare Products, Inc. 800-423-4441
2735 Melbourne Ave, Pomona, CA 91767
Single sided UROFOAM 1 adhesive strip (50/box), double sided UROFOAM 2 adhesive strip (50/box).

ADHESIVE, AEROSOL *(General) 80QAF*

Kik Custom Products 574-295-0000
1919 Superior St, PO Box 2988, Elkhart, IN 46516
For prosthetiic devices, surgical dressings and pads.

ADHESIVE, ALBUMIN BASED *(Pathology) 88KEL*

Alpha-Tec Systems, Inc. 800-221-6058
12019 NE 99th St Ste 1780, Vancouver, WA 98682
Mayer's albumin fixative.

American Mastertech Scientific, Inc. 209-368-4031
1330 Thurman St, Lodi, CA 95240
Multiple.

E K Industries, Inc. 877-EKI-CHEM
1403 Herkimer St, Joliet, IL 60432

Poly Scientific R&D Corp. 800-645-5825
70 Cleveland Ave, Bay Shore, NY 11706

ADHESIVE, BRACKET AND CONDITIONER, RESIN *(Dental And Oral) 76DYH*

Align Technology, Inc. 408-470-1000
881 Martin Ave, Santa Clara, CA 95050
Adhesive,bracket and tooth conditioner,resin.

ADHESIVE, BRACKET AND CONDITIONER, RESIN *(cont'd)*

American Dental Products, Inc. 800-846-7120
603 Country Club Dr Ste B, Bensenville, IL 60106
American dental products,fluoride releasing glass ionomer band cement.

Bisco, Inc. 847-534-6000
1100 W Irving Park Rd, Schaumburg, IL 60193
Orthodontic direct bonding adhesive.

Classone Orthodontics, Inc. 806-799-0608
5064 50th St, Lubbock, TX 79414
Various types of adhesives and conditioners.

Den-Mat Holdings, Llc 805-922-8491
2727 Skyway Dr, Santa Maria, CA 93455
No common name listed.

Dent Zar, Inc. 800-444-1241
6362 Hollywood Blvd Ste 214, Los Angeles, CA 90028
Bracket adhesive.

Dental Technologies, Inc. 847-677-5500
6901 N Hamlin Ave, Lincolnwood, IL 60712
Adhesive, bracket & conditioner resin.

Forestadent Usa 314-878-5985
2315 Weldon Pkwy, Saint Louis, MO 63146
Bracket adhesive resin and tooth conditioner.

G & H Wire Co. 800-526-1026
2165 Earlywood Dr, Franklin, IN 46131

Glenroe Technologies 800-237-4060
1912 44th Ave E, Bradenton, FL 34203
Gel etch.

Gresco Products, Inc. 800-527-3250
13391 Murphy Rd, P.o. Box 865, Stafford, TX 77477
Phosphoric acid etching gel for enamel.

Ivoclar Vivadent, Inc. 800-533-6825
175 Pineview Dr, Amherst, NY 14228
Heliosit Orthodontic

Kerr Corp. 949-255-8766
1717 W Collins Ave, Orange, CA 92867
Dental adhesive.

Lancer Orthodontics, Inc. 760-304-2705
253 Pawnee St, San Marcos, CA 92078
Orthodontic bonding adhesive.

Medental Intl. 760-727-5889
3008 Palm Hill Dr, Vista, CA 92084
Various.

Novocol, Inc. 303-665-7535
416 S Taylor Ave, Louisville, CO 80027
Orthodontic bracket adhesive, tooth conditioner, porcelain primer.

Ortho Organizers, Inc. 760-448-8730
1822 Aston Ave, Carlsbad, CA 92008
Orthodontic bonding adhesive and cement.

Orthodontic Design And Production, Inc. 760-734-3995
1370 Decision St Ste D, Vista, CA 92081
Orhtodontic bracket adhesive and tooth conditioner.

Pentron Laboratory Technologies 203-265-7397
53 N Plains Industrial Rd, Wallingford, CT 06492
Visible light curing polymer resin.

Pulpdent Corp. 800-343-4342
80 Oakland St, Watertown, MA 02472
Various.

Scientific Pharmaceuticals, Inc. 800-634-3047
3221 Producer Way, Pomona, CA 91768
$85.00 for 20-g kit with accessories.

Ultradent Products, Inc. 801-553-4586
505 W 10200 S, South Jordan, UT 84095
Ortho bracket bonding agent.

Water Pik, Inc. 970-221-6129
1730 E Prospect Rd, Fort Collins, CO 80525
Gel etchant, enamel conditioner.

3m Espe Dental Products 949-863-1360
2111 McGaw Ave, Irvine, CA 92614
$223.35 per unit.

3m Unitek 800-634-5300
2724 Peck Rd, Monrovia, CA 91016

ADHESIVE, DENTAL *(Dental And Oral) 76UDQ*

American Diversified Dental Systems 800-637-2330
22991 La Cadena Dr, Laguna Hills, CA 92653
QX-4 Premium Quality Cyanoacrylate Adhesive. ADDS-IT Base, 1/2 & 1 oz E-Z squeeze Bottle. ADDS-Hesive 1 & 2 Fast & Regular set Adhesive. ADDS-Tex Articulator Adhesive.

Cooley & Cooley, Ltd. 800-215-4487
8550 Westland West Blvd, Houston, TX 77041
SNAPBOND is one step Dentin bonding adhesive systems. It bonds, desensitizes and adheres. Ideal for composites and veneers, light cure for hard to reach areas. Doc's Red Copper Cement: A dental cement that is reported to prevent decay from around composite, gold, and ceramic restorations. It can be used as a cement for orthodontic bands.

Danville Materials 800-827-7940
3420 Fostoria Way Ste A200, San Ramon, CA 94583
Prelude self-etch adhesive. Full strength to uncut enamel. Bond to self/dual cure composits. Fast to use high bond strengths.

Harry J. Bosworth Company 800-323-4352
7227 Hamlin Ave, Skokie, IL 60076

J. Morita Usa, Inc. 888-566-7482
9 Mason, Irvine, CA 92618
M-BOND Adhesive Resin Cement's newly developed technology combines superior bond strength with the convenience and proven results of iself-etchingî primers. This revolutionary new product offers clinicians exceptional bond strengths, reduced steps, extended working time, and decreased setting time. The excellent physical and handling properties are unmatched by any 4-META systems.

Mds Products, Inc. 800-637-2330
22991 La Cadena Dr, Laguna Hills, CA 92653
QX-4 Cyanoacrylate Adhesive, 1 oz.

Parkell, Inc. 800-243-7446
300 Executive Dr, Edgewood, NY 11717
Brush&Bond

Tp Orthodontics, Inc. 800-348-8856
100 Center Plz, La Porte, IN 46350
Right-On, 1-To-1, Python, CrossLink, Turbo Bond.

3m Espe Dental Products 949-863-1360
2111 McGaw Ave, Irvine, CA 92614
$168.20 per unit

3m Unitek 800-634-5300
2724 Peck Rd, Monrovia, CA 91016
Orthodontic adhesives; light cured bracket adhesive and light cured lingual retail adhesive.

ADHESIVE, DENTAL IMPRESSION *(Dental And Oral) 76VLL*

Denplus Inc. 800-344-4424
205 - 1221 Labadie, Longueuil, QUE J4N 1E2 Canada

Sterngold 800-243-9942
23 Frank Mossberg Dr, PO Box 2967, Attleboro, MA 02703
Stern Vantage Monophase - Medium to heavy viscosity, polyvinyl siloxane precision impression material in automixing cartridges.

ADHESIVE, DENTURE, KARAYA *(Dental And Oral) 76KOP*

Ameripac, Inc. 972-660-6633
904 Fountain Pkwy, Grand Prairie, TX 75050
Denture adhesive, over the counter.

Regent Labs, Inc. 954-426-4403
700 W Hillsboro Blvd Ste 2-206, Deerfield Bch, FL 33441
Types of denture adhesives.

ADHESIVE, DENTURE, OTC *(Dental And Oral) 76EBM*

Harry J. Bosworth Company 800-323-4352
7227 Hamlin Ave, Skokie, IL 60076
Cora-Caine denture adhesive and analgesic.

Moyco Technologies, Inc. 800-331-8837
200 Commerce Dr, Montgomeryville, PA 18936
$3.00 per 3oz.

ADHESIVE, LIQUID *(General) 80QAG*

Ca Plus Adhesives, Inc. 803-772-4138
701 Kingsbridge Rd, Columbia, SC 29210
Medical-grade adhesives with USP Class VI certification.

Ldb Medical, Inc. 800-243-2554
2909 Langford Rd Ste B500, Norcross, GA 30071
LAPIDES.

ADHESIVE, LIQUID *(cont'd)*

Master Bond, Inc. 201-343-8983
154 Hobart St, Hackensack, NJ 07601
EP30R adhesive for high performance structural bonding, comprised of an aramid fiber reinforced epoxy.

Smith & Nephew, Inc. 800-876-1261
11775 Starkey Rd, Largo, FL 33773
SKIN BOND cement.

Smiths Medical Asd 800-424-8662
5700 W 23rd Ave, Gary, IN 46406
Liquid silicone adhesive(pressure sensitive adhesive) for tracheostome valves.

Titertek Instruments, Inc. 256-859-8600
330 Wynn Dr NW, Huntsville, AL 35805

Torbot Group, Inc. 800-545-4254
1367 Elmwood Ave, Cranston, RI 02910

ADHESIVE, PROSTHESIS, EXTERNAL *(Surgery) 79GBJ*

Avery Dennison Corporation 626-304-2000
150 N Orange Grove Blvd, Pasadena, CA 91103
PSA-based adhesive materials for wound care, electrodes, surgical drapes, diagnostics, and drug delivery systems.

DAW Industries 800-252-2828
5737 Pacific Center Blvd, San Diego, CA 92121
External Components prosthesis and orthodics.

Harry J. Bosworth Company 800-323-4352
7227 Hamlin Ave, Skokie, IL 60076

Ldb Medical, Inc. 800-243-2554
2909 Langford Rd Ste B500, Norcross, GA 30071
LAPIDES.

Nearly Me Technologies, Inc. 800-887-3370
3630 South I 35, Suite A, Waco, TX 76702-1475
Silicone adhesive.

ADHESIVE, SOFT TISSUE APPROXIMATION *(Surgery) 79MPN*

Medisav Services, Inc. 905-201-1313
B-56 Elson St, Markham L3S 1Y7 Canada
Tissue adhesive for repair of minor cuts & lacerations

Praxis, Llc. 508-400-3969
1110 Washington St, Holliston, MA 01746
Tissue adhesive.

ADHESIVE, TISSUE, OPHTHALMOLOGY *(Ophthalmology) 86LZQ*

Closure Medical 888-257-7633
5250 Greens Dairy Rd, Raleigh, NC 27616
NEXACRYL; n-Butyl cyanoacrylate for treatment of corneal ulcerations.

ADHESIVE, WOUND CLOSURE *(Surgery) 79MGO*

Brady Precision Converting, Llc 214-275-9595
1801 Big Town Blvd Ste 100, Mesquite, TX 75149
Reinforced wound closure strips made to customer specifications.

Classone Orthodontics, Inc. 806-799-0608
5064 50th St, Lubbock, TX 79414
Various types of adhesive wound closures.

Closure Medical 888-257-7633
5250 Greens Dairy Rd, Raleigh, NC 27616
DERMABOND topical skin adhesive. NEXABAND FAMILY n-Butyl Cyanacrylate and 2-Octyl Cyanoacrylate for closure of nicks, cuts, abrasions and incisions.

K. W. Griffen Co. 203-846-1923
100 Pearl St, Norwalk, CT 06850
Wound closure strips.

Kerr Group 800-524-3577
1400 Holcomb Bridge Rd, Roswell, GA 30076

Starsurgical, Inc. 888-609-2470
7781 Lakeview Dr, Burlington, WI 53105
Wittmann Patch for temporary bridging of abdominal wall openings where primary closure is not possible and or repeat abdominal entries are necessary.

Tailored Label Products, Inc. 800-727-1344
W165N5731 Ridgewood Dr, Menomonee Falls, WI 53051

ADSORBENTS, ION EXCHANGE *(Toxicology) 91DKO*

Alltech Associates, Inc. 847-282-2090
17434 Mojave St, Hesperia, CA 92345

Reflex Industries, Inc. 619-562-1821
9530 Pathway St Ste 105, Santee, CA 92071
A separation agent for radioassay.

ADSORBENTS, LIQUID CHROMATOGRAPHY
(Toxicology) 91DMZ

Alltech Associates, Inc. 847-282-2090
17434 Mojave St, Hesperia, CA 92345

Buck Scientific, Inc. 800-562-5566
58 Fort Point St, Norwalk, CT 06855
HPLC Isocratic Liquid Chromatographs. BLC-10 Fixed Wavelength Isocratic HPLC System; BLC-20 Variable Wavelength Isocratic HPLC System; BLC-20G Binary Gradient Variable Wavelength HPLC.

AESTHESIOMETER *(Ophthalmology) 86HJC*

Western Ophthalmics Corporation 800-426-9938
19019 36th Ave W Ste G, Lynnwood, WA 98036

AFTERLOADER, RADIOTHERAPY *(Radiology) 90WIA*

Varian Medical Systems 800-544-4636
3100 Hansen Way, Palo Alto, CA 94304
GammaMed and VariSource HDR afterloaders.

AGENT, BULKING, INJECTABLE (GASTRO-UROLOGY)
(Gastro/Urology) 78LNM

Bioform Medical, Inc. 262-835-3323
4133 Courtney Rd Ste 10, Franksville, WI 53126
Uretheral bulking agent.

AGENT, CHELATING, DECALCIFICATION *(Pathology) 88KDY*

American Mastertech Scientific, Inc. 209-368-4031
1330 Thurman St, Lodi, CA 95240
Multiple.

Sci Gen, Inc. 310-324-6576
333 E Gardena Blvd, Gardena, CA 90248
FDA: Medical Device Manufacturing and packaging. Focus on Histology, Cytology, Analytical and General purpose Reagents, Chemistry, and Sterling and Disinfecting agents.

AGENT, EMBOLIZATION/OCCLUSION *(Surgery) 79MAG*

Ivalon, Inc. 800-948-2566
1015 Cordova St, San Diego, CA 92107

AGENT, HEMOSTATIC, ABSORBABLE, COLLAGEN-BASED
(Surgery) 79LMF

Baxter Healthcare Corporation, Medication Delivery 949-851-9066
17511 Armstrong Ave, Irvine, CA 92614
Sterile hemostatic sealant kit.

Cryolife, Inc. 800-438-8285
1655 Roberts Blvd NW, Kennesaw, GA 30144
BioFoam Surgical Matrix

Datascope Interventional Products Division 800-225-5827
1300 MacArthur Blvd, Mahwah, NJ 07430
First stop.

Davol Inc., Sub. C.R. Bard, Inc. 800-556-6275
100 Crossings Blvd, Warwick, RI 02886
Microfibriller collagen hemostat(mch) flour microfibrillar non-woven.

Dma Med-Chem Corporation 800-362-1833
49 Watermill Ln, Great Neck, NY 11021
Hemostasis Devices

Ethicon, Llc. 908-218-2887
Rd. 183, Km. 8.3,, Industrial Area Hato, San Lorenzo, PR 00754
Sterile absorbable hemostatic, collagen based.

Johnson & Johnson Medical Division Of Ethicon, Inc. 800-423-4018
2500 E Arbrook Blvd, Arlington, TX 76014

Medchem Products, Inc. 908-277-8000
160 New Boston St, Woburn, MA 01801
Microfibriller collagen hemostat(mch) flour microfibrillar non-woven.

Medchem Products, Inc. 800-451-4716
160 New Boston St, Woburn, MA 01801
AVITENE Microfibrillar Collagen Hemostat available now in pre-loaded syringe applicators: 1 gm syringe AVITENE, 5mm Neuro AVITENE and 5mm ENT AVITENE. ENDO-AVITENE and 10mm Endo-Avitine. ACTIFOAM Collagen Hemostatic Sponge.

Medicus Technologies 800-762-1574
105 Morgan Ln, Plainsboro, NJ 08536

Medtronic Sofamor Danek Usa, Inc. 901-396-3133
4340 Swinnea Rd, Memphis, TN 38118
Collagen sponge.

AGENT, HEMOSTATIC, ABSORBABLE, COLLAGEN-BASED *(cont'd)*

Orthovita, Inc. 610-640-1775
77 Great Valley Pkwy, Malvern, PA 19355
Sterile surgical hemostat.

Telios Pharmaceuticals 800-762-1574
105 Morgan Ln, Plainsboro, NJ 08536

Zimmer Dental, Inc. 800-854-7019
1900 Aston Ave, Carlsbad, CA 92008
BioMend® absorbable collagen membrane is a compressed, non-friable Type I collagen matrix derived from bovine Achilles tendon. The BioMend membrane becomes translucent when hydrated but remains non-slippery and adaptable to the tooth root facilitating easy placement. During manufacture, potentially antigenic portions of the collagen molecule are removed, resulting in a product that is highly biocompatible and well-tolerated by the tissue. Lack of immune response was verified during clinical investigation through over 350 dermal patch tests and blood serum analysis1. Each manufacturing lot of BioMend is certified nonpyrogenic. By creating an environment where the wound can heal, the BioMend membrane helps stabilize and maintain the blood clot in the defect site. BioMend absorbs completely into surrounding gingival connective tissue through enzyme (collagenase) degradation. BioMend's three-dimensional matrix allows for the integration of connective tissue flaps as well as passage of essential nutrients, reducing the likelihood of membrane exposure and gingival recession. BioMend eliminates the need for a second surgical procedure for membrane removal. Because the absorption rate is controlled by the degree of cross-linking, BioMend is designed to remain intact for at least four weeks, functioning as a barrier during the critical period of wound healing. The membrane has an average retention of six to seven weeks. It is then fully absorbed by host enzymes into the surrounding tissue within eight weeks. BioMend Extend™, a longer-lasting membrane, has the same benefits as BioMend, with the additional advantages of greater thickness and it maintains an effective barrier longer for greater regenerative results - it is fully absorbed within 18 weeks. BioMend is supplied in sheet form in three different sizes: 15mm x 20mm, 20mm x 30mm, and 30mm x 40mm, packaged as a single unit within a sterile template envelope. CollaCote(R), CollaTape(R) and CollaPlug(R) wound dressings for dental surgery outperformed traditional periodontal wound packing in clinical tests by a wide margin. These products control bleeding and stabilize blood clots as well as protect the wound bed while accelerating the healing process. All Colla products are fully absorbed in 10 to 14 days. CollaCote: Palatal donor sites; Mucosal flaps. CollaTape: Minor oral wounds; Closure of grafted sites; Repair of Schneiderian Membranes. Each Colla product is sold in boxes of 10 dressings.

AGENT, HEMOSTATIC, NON-ABSORBABLE, COLLAGEN-BASED *(Surgery) 79LMG*

Ethicon, Llc. 908-218-2887
Rd. 183, Km. 8.3,, Industrial Area Hato, San Lorenzo, PR 00754
Oxidized regenerated cellulose-absorbable hemostat.

Gramsmed, Llc 800-366-1976
2225 Dakota Dr, Grafton, WI 53024
Suture.

Johnson & Johnson Medical Division Of Ethicon, Inc. 800-423-4018
2500 E Arbrook Blvd, Arlington, TX 76014

Noramco, Inc. 706-353-4400
1440 Olympic Dr, Athens, GA 30601
Oxidized regenerated cellulose, usp.

Pharmacia & Upjohn Co. 212-573-1000
7000 Portage Rd, Kalamazoo, MI 49001
Absorbable gelatin sponge, usp and powder.

Superstat Corp. 800-487-3786
2001 E University Dr, Rancho Dominguez, CA 90220
Agent, absorbable hemostatic, non-collagen based.

Wortham Laboratories Inc 423-296-0090
6340 Bonny Oaks Dr, Chattanooga, TN 37416
Hemostatic agent.

AGENT, INJECTABLE, EMBOLIC *(Surgery) 79MFE*

Carbon Medical Technologies, Inc. 877-277-1788
1290 Hammond Rd, Saint Paul, MN 55110
Injectable bulking agent.

Cordis Neurovascular, Inc. 800-327-7714
14201 NW 60th Ave, Miami Lakes, FL 33014
Liquid embolic agent.

AGENT, INJECTABLE, EMBOLIC *(cont'd)*

Ev3 Neurovascular 800-716-6700
9775 Toledo Way, Irvine, CA 92618
Injectable embolic agent.

AGENT, POLISHING, ABRASIVE, ORAL CAVITY *(Dental And Oral) 76EJR*

Abrasive Technology, Inc. 740-548-4100
8400 Green Meadows Dr N, Lewis Center, OH 43035
Oral cavity abrasive polishing agent.

Cadco Dental Products 800-833-8267
600 E Hueneme Rd, Oxnard, CA 93033
$4.00 for 380g jar Prophy Paste.

Dedeco International, Inc. 888-433-3326
Route 97, Long Eddy, NY 12760

Dedeco Intl., Inc. 845-887-4840
11617 Route 97, Long Eddy, NY 12760
Various types of polishing agents.

Deepak Products, Inc. 305-482-9669
5220 NW 72nd Ave Ste 15, Miami, FL 33166
Prophylaxis paste.

Den-Mat Holdings, Llc 805-922-8491
2727 Skyway Dr, Santa Maria, CA 93455
No common name listed.

Dent Zar, Inc. 800-444-1241
6362 Hollywood Blvd Ste 214, Los Angeles, CA 90028
Omega dental polishing paste.

Dental Resources 717-866-7571
52 King St, Myerstown, PA 17067
Prophy paste.

Dental Technologies, Inc. 847-677-5500
6901 N Hamlin Ave, Lincolnwood, IL 60712
Abrasive polishing paste, prophylaxis paste.

Denticator International, Inc. 800-325-1881
13705 Shoreline Ct E, Earth City, MO 63045
$19.95 per box of 200 (2 gram) doses.

Dshealthcare Inc. 201-871-1232
85 W Forest Ave, Englewood, NJ 07631
Various prophylaxis powder & paste.

Dux Dental 800-833-8267
600 E Hueneme Rd, Oxnard, CA 93033
$4.00 for 380g jar Prophy Paste.

Foremost Dental Llc. 201-894-5500
242 S Dean St, Englewood, NJ 07631
Oral polishing abrasives with-without naf (prophy paste).

G & H Wire Co. 800-526-1026
2165 Earlywood Dr, Franklin, IN 46131

George Taub Products & Fusion Co., Inc. 800-828-2634
277 New York Ave, Jersey City, NJ 07307
Insta-Glaze and Insta-Glaze HYB are diamond filled polishing pastes for chairside polishing of composite and porcelain surfaces, as well as lab side. Makes the porcelain look as polished as if it were fired.

Gresco Products, Inc. 800-527-3250
13391 Murphy Rd, P.o. Box 865, Stafford, TX 77477
Composite polishing paste.

Harry J. Bosworth Company 800-323-4352
7227 Hamlin Ave, Skokie, IL 60076

Ivoclar Vivadent, Inc. 800-533-6825
175 Pineview Dr, Amherst, NY 14228
Proxyt

Kerr Corp. 714-516-7400
28200 Wick Rd, Romulus, MI 48174
Primer.

Kerr Corp. 949-255-8766
1717 W Collins Ave, Orange, CA 92867
Abrasive polishing agents-prpphy paste.

Medical Products Laboratories, Inc. 215-677-2700
9990 Global Rd, Philadelphia, PA 19115
Oral polishing abrasives with and without naf (prophy paste).

Micro-Vac, Inc. 800-729-1020
5905 E 5th St, Tucson, AZ 85711
PROPHY-EZ AIR POLISHING SPEARMENT FLAVORED POWDER for prophy jet cleaning machines.

Miltex Dental Technologies, Inc. 516-576-6022
589 Davies Dr, York, PA 17402
Various intra-oral abrasive pastes and powders.

AGENT, POLISHING, ABRASIVE, ORAL CAVITY *(cont'd)*

Motloid Company 800-662-5021
300 N Elizabeth St, Chicago, IL 60607
Polishing compounds. RAPID GLAZE diamond porcelain polishinig paste.

Moyco Technologies, Inc. 800-331-8837
200 Commerce Dr, Montgomeryville, PA 18936
$9.95 per 100g.

Nomax, Inc. 314-961-2500
40 N Rock Hill Rd, Saint Louis, MO 63119
Prophylaxis paste mix.

Pac-Dent Intl., Inc. 909-839-0888
21078 Commerce Point Dr, Walnut, CA 91789
Prophy paste, prophy powder.

Pascal Co., Inc. 425-602-3633
2929 Northup Way, Bellevue, WA 98004
Abrasive polishing paste containing sodium fluoride.

Preventive Technologies, Inc. 704-849-2416
1150 Crews Rd Ste H, Matthews, NC 28105
Disposable prophy angle.

Pulpdent Corp. 800-343-4342
80 Oakland St, Watertown, MA 02472
No common name listed.

Scientific Pharmaceuticals, Inc. 800-634-3047
3221 Producer Way, Pomona, CA 91768
$20.00 for 25 g.

Shofu Dental Corporation 800-827-4638
1225 Stone Dr, San Marcos, CA 92078
DURA-WHITE, DURA-GREEN, LAB SERIES STONES, CERAMISTE, CERAMISTE SOFT, CERAMASTER, COREMASTER, ULTRA II POLISHING PASTE, BROWNIE, GREENIE, SUPER GREENIE, ONEGLOSS, SUPERBUFF, SUPERSNAP, ACRYPOINT, HARDIE, COMPOSITE, COMPOSITE FINE, COMPOMASTER, ONEGLOSS, ONEGLOSS PS, COMPOSITE POLISHING PASTE

Span Packaging Services Llc. 864-627-4155
4611A Dairy Dr, Greenville, SC 29607
Dentrifice, toothpaste.

Ultradent Products, Inc. 801-553-4586
505 W 10200 S, South Jordan, UT 84095
Microabrasion paste.

Water Pik, Inc. 970-221-6129
1730 E Prospect Rd, Fort Collins, CO 80525
Various grits and flavors prophy paste.

Westside Packaging, Llc. 909-570-3508
1700 S Baker Ave Ste A, Ontario, CA 91761
Oral cavity abrasive polishing agent.

Young Colorado, Llc. 800-325-1881
13705 Shoreline Ct E, Earth City, MO 63045
Oral cavity abrasive polishing agent.

Young Dental Manufacturing Co 1, Llc 800-325-1881
4401 Paredes Line Rd, Brownsville, TX 78526
Prophylaxis paste.

Young Innovations, Inc. 800-325-1881
13705 Shoreline Ct E, Earth City, MO 63045
Prophy paste.

Zila, Inc. 800-228-5595
701 Centre Ave, Fort Collins, CO 80526
MULTIPLE; PRO-FLEX PROPHY PASTE

AGGLUTINATION METHOD, HUMAN CHORIONIC GONADOTROPIN *(Chemistry) 75JHJ*

Biomerieux Inc. 800-682-2666
100 Rodolphe St, Durham, NC 27712

Carter-Horner, Inc. 800-387-2130
6600 Kitimat Rd., Mississauga L5N-1L9 Canada
At-home pregnancy test kit

Immunostics, Inc. 800-722-7505
3505 Sunset Ave, Ocean, NJ 07712

Teco Diagnostics 714-693-7788
1268 N Lakeview Ave, Anaheim, CA 92807
Monoclonal b-hcg pregnancy test (indirect).

Wampole Laboratories 800-257-9525
2 Research Way, Princeton, NJ 08540
Broad line, urine/serum, 0.2-2.0 IuhCG/ml.

AGGREGOMETER, PLATELET *(Hematology) 81JBX*

Chrono-Log Corp. 800-247-6665
2 W Park Rd, Havertown, PA 19083
Impedance for Whole Blood, Optical for PRP and Luminescence for ATP Secretion, Calcium and Superoxides.

Payton Scientific Inc. 716-876-1813
964 Kenmore Ave, Buffalo, NY 14216

AGGREGOMETER, PLATELET, PHOTO-OPTICAL SCANNING *(Hematology) 81JBY*

Chrono-Log Corp. 800-247-6665
2 W Park Rd, Havertown, PA 19083

AGGREGOMETER, PLATELET, THROMBOKINETOGRAM *(Hematology) 81GKW*

American Labor 800-424-0443
3329 Durham Chapel Hill Blvd Ste 200, Durham, NC 27707
Manual & automated.

Bio/Data Corp. 215-441-4000
155 Gibraltar Rd, Horsham, PA 19044
Platelet aggregometer.

AID, CONTROL, ENVIRONMENTAL, CONTROLLED, BREATH *(Physical Med) 89LFF*

Action Bag Co. 800-490-8830
1001 Entry Dr, Bensenville, IL 60106
Foil Liner and Foil Foam Liner Pouches

Airex, Inc. 425-222-3665
13704 SE 17th St, Bellevue, WA 98005
M100 mobile ultra-clean air delivery system with attachable enclosures providing both positive and negative controlled pressurized patient environments

Assistive Technology, Inc. 800-793-9227
333 Elm St Ste 115, Dedham, MA 02026

Prentke Romich Company 800-262-1984
1022 Heyl Rd, Wooster, OH 44691
HeadMaster computer access device for use by handicapped who cannot use their hands.

AID, LIVING, HANDICAPPED *(General) 80SHP*

Alumiramp, Inc. 800-800-3864
855 E Chicago Rd, Quincy, MI 49082
Prefabricated, aluminum modular commercial ramping for institutional, commercial, and educational use; complies with all codes, including BOCA & CABO. Specifications and drawings provided at no charge.

Colonial Scientific Ltd. 902-468-1811
201 Brownlow Ave., Unit 52, Dartmouth, NS B3B-1W2 Canada
Aids for the handicapped.

Complete Medical Supplies, Inc. 800-242-2674
10 Ford Products Rd, Valley Cottage, NY 10989
Aid to daily living, blood pressure, cast products, diabetic, diagnostic, doctor's supplies, electrotherapy, emergency, exercise, foot care, health care, home care, orthopedic, ostomy, physical therapy, physician's supplies, respiratory, skin care, stocking, traction, urologicals, wheelchairs, wound care.

Eastman Medical Products Inc. 800-373-4410
2000 Powell St Ste 1540, Emeryville, CA 94608
ILE-SORB--polymer that solidifies body fluids. For use by ileostomates.

Home Aid Products 888-823-7605
111 Esna Park Dr., Unit 9, Markham, ONT L3R-1H2 Canada
Transfer poles. Full line of grab bars and bath safety rails. Perching stool. Three-wheeled mobile stool. Over-bed tables. Toilet safety frames. Raised toilet seats.

Laszlo Corp. 314-830-3222
2573 Millvalley Dr, Florissant, MO 63031
Swing Tray can be placed on any standard wheel chair arm and will swing in front of patient for eating purposes and then swings out to the side of the wheel chair and acts as an end table for medicine, water, snacks etc.

O&M Enterprise 847-258-4515
641 Chelmsford Ln, Elk Grove Village, IL 60007
HANDICAPPED AIDS

Rifton Equipment 800-571-8198
PO Box 260, Rifton, NY 12471
The Rifton Anchors offer comfortable stabilization to an upper extremity with a secure suction cup. Increases functional use of the hand and arm that is free.

AID, LIVING, HANDICAPPED *(cont'd)*

Sunrise Medical 800-333-4000
7477 Dry Creek Pkwy, Longmont, CO 80503

Tub Master Lc 800-833-0260
413 Virginia Dr, Orlando, FL 32803
Safety Grab Bars - Available in Different Textures, Colors, and Sizes. (ADA-compliant)

AID, RESUSCITATION, CARDIOPULMONARY
(Cardiovascular) 74LIX

Cft, Inc./Life Mask 800-331-8844
14602 N Cave Creek Rd Ste B, Phoenix, AZ 85022
Safety device for giving CPR without direct mouth-to-mouth contact. LIFE MASK face shield is a CPR Life Mask Face Shield with 3M Filtrete filter.

Great Plains Ballistics Inc. 888-265-2226
PO Box 16385, Lubbock, TX 79490
BECK Tracheal Whistle; Endotracheal intubation assist/aid device that converts airflow to sound. Greatly facilitates blind nasal or oral tracheal intubation.

Marco Products Company 800-572-USA1
12860 San Fernando Rd, Sylmar, CA 91342
Portable CPR device.

Medical Devices International, Div. Of Plasco, Inc. 800-438-7634
512 N Lehmberg Rd, Columbus, MS 39702
CPR MICROSHIELD first response physical barrier with anti-reflux valve, for single person CPR or mouth-to-mouth resuscitation.

AIR HANDLING APPARATUS, ENCLOSURE *(Surgery) 79FZI*

Airex, Inc. 425-222-3665
13704 SE 17th St, Bellevue, WA 98005
M100 mobile self-contained HEPA air contamination/infection control system. Attachable EIU portable neg/pos pressure patient isolation chamber. Positive pressure patient enclosure.

Aqua Products Company, Inc. 800-849-4264
14301 C R Koon Hwy, Newberry, SC 29108
AQUA CHILLER air-cool package chiller modules, 2 to 20 tons.

AIR HANDLING, APPARATUS, BENCH *(Surgery) 79FZG*

Airex, Inc. 425-222-3665
13704 SE 17th St, Bellevue, WA 98005
M100 mobile self-contained certifiable clean bench alternative with attachable portable exclosures

AIRBRUSH *(Dental And Oral) 76KOJ*

Air Techniques, Inc. 800-247-8324
1295 Walt Whitman Rd, Melville, NY 11747
Airdent II

American Diversified Dental Systems 800-637-2330
22991 La Cadena Dr, Laguna Hills, CA 92653
5100-2000 Spray Gun 2000 (Badger)

American Medical Technologies, Inc. 361-289-1145
5655 Bear Ln, Corpus Christi, TX 78405
KCP Brand Air Abrasive Instrument. KCP (Kinetic Cavity Preparation) 1000 air abrasive instrument used for hard tissue procedures, primarily for cavity preparations.

Asi Medical, Inc. 303-766-3646
14550 E Easter Ave Ste 700, Centennial, CO 80112
Air abrasion.

Bisco, Inc. 847-534-6000
1100 W Irving Park Rd, Schaumburg, IL 60193
Oral sandblaster-various types.

Buffalo Dental Mfg. Co., Inc. 516-496-7200
159 Lafayette Dr, Syosset, NY 11791
Intraoral sandblaster.

Crystalmark Dental Systems, Inc. 818-240-7596
621 Ruberta Ave, Glendale, CA 91201
Micro abrasive sandblaster.

Danville Materials 800-827-7940
3420 Fostoria Way Ste A200, San Ramon, CA 94583
Microetcher intra oral sandblaster is ideal for etching to increase bond u to 400%

Groman Inc. 954-649-8008
4900 NW 15th St Unit 4494, Margate, FL 33063
Disposable dental air abrasion handpiece.

Kavo Dental Corp. 800-323-8029
340 East Route 22, Lake Zurich, IL 60047
KAVO RONDOflex Handpiece 2013: air abrasion or air brush using aluminum oxide as an abrasive material.

AIRBRUSH *(cont'd)*

Lares Research 800-347-3289
295 Lockheed Ave, Chico, CA 95973
Air abrasion cavity preparation systems

Mds Products, Inc. 800-637-2330
22991 La Cadena Dr, Laguna Hills, CA 92653
Spray Gun 2000.

Ultradent Products, Inc. 801-553-4586
505 W 10200 S, South Jordan, UT 84095
Intra oral sandblaster.

AIRWAY, BI-NASOPHARYNGEAL (WITH CONNECTOR)
(Anesthesiology) 73CBJ

Covidien Lp 508-261-8000
15 Hampshire St, Mansfield, MA 02048

Neotech Products, Inc. 800-966-0500
27822 Fremont Ct, Valencia, CA 91355
BINASAL AIRWAY: NCPAP prongs made of soft silicone. Ideal for neonatal patients. Held gently in place with the NeoBar.

Smiths Medical Asd 800-424-8662
5700 W 23rd Ave, Gary, IN 46406
Connectors, Airway management. 15mm 150 connectors, disconnect wedges, side-port connector, SAF-T-FLO connector; swivel connector.

AIRWAY, ESOPHAGEAL (OBTURATOR) *(Anesthesiology) 73CAO*

Armstrong Medical Industries, Inc. 800-323-4220
575 Knightsbridge Pkwy, Lincolnshire, IL 60069

Brunswick Laboratories 800-362-3482
50 Commerce Way, Norton, MA 02766
Used in the first responder environment. Requires little training.

Covidien Lp 508-261-8000
15 Hampshire St, Mansfield, MA 02048

Dixie Ems Supply 800-347-3494
385 Union Ave, Brooklyn, NY 11211
$320.00 per 10 (90mm).

K. W. Griffen Co. 203-846-1923
100 Pearl St, Norwalk, CT 06850
Airway.

Rockford Medical & Safety Co. 800-435-9451
2420 Harrison Ave, PO Box 5646, Rockford, IL 61108

AIRWAY, NASOPHARYNGEAL (BREATHING TUBE)
(Anesthesiology) 73BTQ

Aesculap Implant Systems Inc. 1-800-234-9179
3773 Corporate Pkwy, Center Valley, PA 18034

Alliant Healthcare Products 269-629-0300
8850 M89, Richland, MI 49083
Nasopharyngeal airway.

Anesthesia Associates, Inc. 760-744-6561
460 Enterprise St, San Marcos, CA 92078
Available in a variety of sizes and styles.

Armstrong Medical Industries, Inc. 800-323-4220
575 Knightsbridge Pkwy, Lincolnshire, IL 60069

Covidien Lp 508-261-8000
15 Hampshire St, Mansfield, MA 02048

Dale Medical Products, Inc. 800-343-3980
7 Cross St, Plainville, MA 02762
Naso-Gastric Tube Holder #160.

Eastmed Enterprises, Inc. 856-797-0131
11 Brandywine Dr, Marlton, NJ 08053
Robertazzi nasopharyngeal airway.

Kentron Health Care, Inc. 615-384-0573
3604 Kelton Jackson Rd, P.o. Box 120, Springfield, TN 37172
Nasopharyngeal airways.

Rtech, Inc. 877-783-2446
739 Brandywine Dr, Moorestown, NJ 08057
Various types and sizes of nasopharyngeal airways.

Sharn, Inc. 800-325-3671
4517 George Rd Ste 200, Tampa, FL 33634
Adjustable latex-free airway.

Smiths Medical Asd 800-424-8662
5700 W 23rd Ave, Gary, IN 46406
AIRE-CUF, FOME-CUF & TTS Epistaxis catheters and endotracheal tubes; Silicone; adult/pediatric.

AIRWAY, NASOPHARYNGEAL (BREATHING TUBE) *(cont'd)*

Sun-Med 800-433-2797
12393 Belcher Rd S Ste 450, Largo, FL 33773
sterile package of 10 units; Oral=Guedel, Berman. Nasal=Blue latex, Green latex-free and Latex-free adjustable flange.

Sunmed Healthcare 727-531-7266
12393 Belcher Rd S Ste 460, Largo, FL 33773

AIRWAY, OBSTRUCTION REMOVAL (CHOKE SAVER)
(General) 80QAJ

Cook Inc. 800-457-4500
PO Box 489, Bloomington, IN 47402

O&M Enterprise 847-258-4515
641 Chelmsford Ln, Elk Grove Village, IL 60007
AIRWAY

Unisplint Corp. 770-271-0646
4485 Commerce Dr Ste 106, Buford, GA 30518
Wall suction airway.

AIRWAY, OROPHARYNGEAL, ANESTHESIA
(Anesthesiology) 73CAE

Ac Healthcare Supply, Inc. 905-448-4706
11651 230th St, Cambria Heights, NY 11411
Oropharyngeal airway.

Achi Corp. 408-321-9581
2168 Ringwood Ave, San Jose, CA 95131
The ChouAirway is an adjustable oropharyngeal airway for routine and difficult airway management.

Ambu A/S 457-225-2210
6740 Baymeadow Dr, Glen Burnie, MD 21060
Laryngeal mask.

Ambu, Inc. 800-262-8462
6740 Baymeadow Dr, Glen Burnie, MD 21060
AuraOnce and Aura40 Laryngeal Mask

Anesthesia Associates, Inc. 760-744-6561
460 Enterprise St, San Marcos, CA 92078
Available in a variety of sizes and styles.

Anesthesia Equipment Supply, Inc. 253-631-8008
24301 Roberts Dr, Black Diamond, WA 98010
Various.

Arc Medical, Inc. 800-950-ARC1
4296 Cowan Rd, Tucker, GA 30084
SLIPA, Cuffless supralaryngeal airway for routine instrumentation of the airway during anesthesia.

Cookgas Llc 314-781-5700
1167 Hillside Dr, Saint Louis, MO 63117
Laryngeal mask airway (lma).

E-Global Medical Equipment, L.L.C. 866-422-1845
2f 500 Lincoln St., Allston, MA 02134
Laryngeal airway, la & laryngeal airway shield, las.

Eastmed Enterprises, Inc. 856-797-0131
11 Brandywine Dr, Marlton, NJ 08053
Guedel and Berman airways.

Green Field Medical Sourcing, Inc. 512-894-3002
14141 W Highway 290 Ste 410, Austin, TX 78737
Cpr barrier mask.

Health Care Logistics, Inc. 800-848-1633
450 Town St, PO Box 25, Circleville, OH 43113
Various sizes.

Idm Plastics 904-734-4740
1813 Patterson Ave, Deland, FL 32724
Airway, oropharyngeal, anesthesiology.

Intersurgical Inc. 315-451-2900
417 Electronics Pkwy, Liverpool, NY 13088
Guedel oral airways.

Kentron Health Care, Inc. 615-384-0573
3604 Kelton Jackson Rd, P.o. Box 120, Springfield, TN 37172
Airway.

Mainline Medical, Inc. 800-366-2084
3250 Peachtree Corners Cir Ste J, Norcross, GA 30092
Color coded individually wrapped Guedel and Berman oral Airways,along with the Williams pink Intubating Airway. Latex-free.

Medical Action Industries, Inc. 800-645-7042
25 Heywood Rd, Arden, NC 28704
Airways.

Medline Industries, Inc. 800-633-5886
1 Medline Pl, Mundelein, IL 60060

AIRWAY, OROPHARYNGEAL, ANESTHESIA *(cont'd)*

Medline Manufacturing And Services Llc 847-837-2759
1 Medline Pl, Mundelein, IL 60060
Oropharyngeal airway.

Mercury Medical 800-237-6418
11300 49th St N, Clearwater, FL 33762

Numask, Inc. 818-596-2100
6320 Canoga Ave Ste 1502, Woodland Hills, CA 91367
Oropharyngeal airway.

Primary Medical Co., Inc. 727-520-1920
6541 44th St N Ste 6003, Pinellas Park, FL 33781
Berman, Guedel, various sizes, non-sterile.

Quadromed Inc. 800-363-0192
5776 Thimens Ave., St-Laurent, QUE H4R 2K9 Canada

Seven Harvest Intl. Import & Export 765-456-3584
108 N Dixon Rd, Kokomo, IN 46901
Airways '6'.

Sharn, Inc. 800-325-3671
4517 George Rd Ste 200, Tampa, FL 33634
Berman, Guedel and Williams disposable airways.

Smiths Medical Asd Inc. 800-258-5361
10 Bowman Dr, Keene, NH 03431
Oropheryngeal airway.

Sterilmed, Inc. 763-488-3400
11400 73rd Ave N Ste 100, Maple Grove, MN 55369
Laryngeal airway.

Surgical Technology Laboratories Inc. 803-462-1714
610 Clemson Rd, Columbia, SC 29229
Straith tongue retracting airway.

ALARM, BREATHING CIRCUIT *(Anesthesiology) 73QAK*

Precision Medical, Inc. 800-272-7285
300 Held Dr, Northampton, PA 18067

ALARM, CENTRAL GAS SYSTEM *(Anesthesiology) 73TAC*

Aga Linde Healthcare P.R. Inc. 787-622-7900
PO Box 363868, GPO Box 364727, San Juan, PR 00936
Anesth/Pul Med.

Allied Healthcare Products, Inc. 800-444-3954
1720 Sublette Ave, Saint Louis, MO 63110

Enmet Corp. 734-761-1270
PO Box 979, Ann Arbor, MI 48106
Gas detectors for toxic gas, combustible gas, oxygen deficiency.

Enviro Guard, Inc. 800-438-1152
201 Shannon Oaks Cir Ste 115, Cary, NC 27511

ALARM, ENURESIS *(Gastro/Urology) 78KPN*

Enuresis Solutions, Llc 912-353-7675
51 W Fairmont Ave Ste 2, Savannah, GA 31406
Various types of enuresis solution.

Ideas For Living 303-440-8517
1285 N Cedar Brook Rd, Boulder, CO 80304
Bedwetting alarm.

Jonas, Inc. 302-478-1375
1113 Faun Rd, Wilmington, DE 19803
HEALTHSHIELD, automatic incontinence detector/alarm, miniature reusable detector and alarm for monitoring urinary incontinence (UI).

Nytone Medical Products 801-973-4090
2424 S 900 W, Salt Lake City, UT 84119

Pacific Intl. Co. 715-886-4550
555 Birch St, Nekoosa, WI 54457
No common name listed.

Palco Labs, Inc. 800-346-4488
8030 Soquel Ave Ste 104, Santa Cruz, CA 95062
WET-STOP small, wearable enuresis alarm.

Potty Md, Llc 865-584-6700
6512 Baum Dr Ste 14, Knoxville, TN 37919
Enuresis alarm.

Starchild Labs 805-564-7194
57 Tierra Cielo Ln, Santa Barbara, CA 93105
Enuresis alarm.

Z-Pack, Inc. 818-887-4924
6215 Oakdale Ave, Woodland Hills, CA 91367
Bedwetting alarm.

ALARM, HYPOGLYCEMIA *(Gastro/Urology) 78THN*

Diabetes Sentry Products 360-738-1200
1200 Dupont St Ste 1D, Bellingham, WA 98225
SLEEP SENTRY: Wrist alarm for nighttime use for people with insulin dependent diabetes; detects presence of moisture or decrease of skin temperature.

ALARM, LEAKAGE CURRENT, PORTABLE *(Cardiovascular) 74DSM*

Biotek Instruments, Inc. 802-655-4040
100 Tigan St, Highland Park, Winooski, VT 05404
Iso-tester (model 12).

ALARM, OVERLOAD, EXTERNAL LIMB, POWERED *(Physical Med) 89IRN*

E. Q., Inc. 215-997-1765
3469 Limekiln Pike, Chalfont, PA 18914
Limb load monitor.

Patterson Medical Supply, Inc. 262-387-8720
W68N158 Evergreen Blvd, Cedarburg, WI 53012
Device, warning, overload, external limb, powered.

Planet Llc 800-338-2010
1212 Fourier Dr, Madison, WI 53717
PedAlert Monitor - for patients with lower limb weight-bearing limitations. Sensor constantly monitors weight and sounds a warning tone and light when the weight threshold is met or exceeded.

ALARM, OXYGEN DEPLETION *(Anesthesiology) 73QAL*

Vascular Technology Incorporated 800-550-0856
12 Murphy Dr, Nashua, NH 03062
VTI-102, oxygen monitor.

ALARM, RADIATION *(Radiology) 90THK*

Ludlum Measurements, Inc. 800-622-0828
501 Oak St, Sweetwater, TX 79556

ALARM, REFRIGERATOR *(Hematology) 81QAM*

Cmt, Inc. 800-659-9140
PO Box 297, Hamilton, MA 01936

Kendro Laboratory Products 800-252-7100
308 Ridgefield Ct, Asheville, NC 28806

ALCOHOL BREATH TRAPPING DEVICE *(Toxicology) 91DJZ*

Alcohol Countermeasure Systems Corp. 905-670-2288
14-975 Midway Blvd., Mississauga, ONT L5T-2C6 Canada

Cmi, Inc. 270-685-6200
316 E 9th St, Owensboro, KY 42303
Various models of breath-alcohol test systems.

Intoximeters, Inc. 800-451-8639
8110 Lackland Rd, Saint Louis, MO 63114
Breath Alcohol testing equipment.

Omegapoint Systems, Llc 513-241-7540
1077 Celestial St Ste 400, Cincinnati, OH 45202
Breath alcohol tester,breathalyzer.

Sirchie Finger Print Laboratories 800-356-7311
100 Hunter Pl, Youngsville, NC 27596

ALCOHOL DEHYDROGENASE, SPEC. REAGENT - ETHANOL ENZYME *(Toxicology) 91DIC*

Carolina Liquid Chemistries Corp. 800-471-7272
510 W Central Ave Ste C, Brea, CA 92821
Ethanol reagent.

Warner Graham Co., The 800-872-2300
160 Church Ln, Cockeysville, MD 21030

ALIGNER, BEAM, X-RAY (COLLIMATOR) *(Dental And Oral) 76EHA*

Americomp, Inc. 800-458-1782
2901 W Lawrence Ave, Chicago, IL 60625

Margraf Dental Manufacturing, Inc. 800-762-2641
611 Harper Ave, Jenkintown, PA 19046
Cephalometric.

Water Pik, Inc. 970-221-6129
1730 E Prospect Rd, Fort Collins, CO 80525
Dental transcranial headholder.

Wehmer Corporation 800-323-0229
1151 N Main St, Lombard, IL 60148
$295.00

Whip Mix Corp. 502-637-1451
1730 E Prospect Rd Ste 101, Fort Collins, CO 80525

ALIGNER, BRACKET, ORTHODONTIC *(Dental And Oral) 76ECQ*

Coltene/Whaledent Inc. 330-916-8858
235 Ascot Pkwy, Cuyahoga Falls, OH 44223
Tweezers.

G & H Wire Co. 800-526-1026
2165 Earlywood Dr, Franklin, IN 46131
Zand Gauges and Bracket Positioners.

Glenroe Technologies 800-237-4060
1912 44th Ave E, Bradenton, FL 34203
Dental hand instrument, bracket aligner.

Masel Co., Inc. 800-423-8227
2701 Bartram Rd, Bristol, PA 19007

Orthodontic Design And Production, Inc. 760-734-3995
1370 Decision St Ste D, Vista, CA 92081
Type of orthodontic hand instrument.

Oscar, Inc. 317-849-2618
11793 Technology Ln, Fishers, IN 46038
Bracket height gauge.

Progressive Dental Supply/Progressive Orthodontics Seminars 800-443-3106
1701 E Edinger Ave Ste C1, Santa Ana, CA 92705

Progressive Technology, Inc. 916-632-6715
4130 Citrus Ave Ste 17, Rocklin, CA 95677
Ceramic dental bracket.

3m Unitek 800-634-5300
2724 Peck Rd, Monrovia, CA 91016

ALIGNER, SEQUENTIAL *(Dental And Oral) 76NXC*

Align Technology, Inc. 408-470-1000
881 Martin Ave, Santa Clara, CA 95050
Plastic aligners.

Allesee Orthodontic Appliances 714-516-7484
13931 Spring St, Sturtevant, WI 53177
Plastic retainers.

Allesee Orthodontic Appliances (Calexico) 714-516-7400
341 E 1st St, Calexico, CA 92231
Plastic retainers.

Allesee Orthodontic Appliances, Inc. - Connecticut 949-255-8766
6 Niblick Rd, Enfield, CT 06082
Plastic retainers.

ALLOGRAFT, HEART VALVE *(Cardiovascular) 74MIE*

Alabama Tissue Center, Inc. 205-934-4314
1900 University Blvd, 855 Tinsley Harrison Tower
Birmingham, AL 35233
Aortic human allograft heart valve/pulmonary human allograft heart valve.

American Red Cross National Tissue Services 202-303-4280
3535 Hyland Ave, Costa Mesa, CA 92626
Heart valve.

Cryolife, Inc. 800-438-8285
1655 Roberts Blvd NW, Kennesaw, GA 30144
CRYOVALVE cryopreserved allograft human heart valve.

ALLOGRAFT, PROCESSED *(Surgery) 79LMO*

Lifecell Corp. 800-367-5737
1 Millennium Way, Branchburg, NJ 08876
ALLODERM Dermal Transplant/Implant. Repliform and Cymetra.

Zimmer Dental, Inc. 800-854-7019
1900 Aston Ave, Carlsbad, CA 92008
Puros is an allograft bone grafting material. Puros is manufactured by Tutogen Medical, Inc., which utilizes its patented Tutoplast® process for tissue preservation and viral inactivation to ensure that the product is safe and effective. This same process has been used for years to preserve tissue and manufacture bioimplants for neurological, orthopedic, reconstructive and general surgical indications. Unlike other grafting materials, Puros retains the mineralized content as well as the native collagen, which facilitates strong, natural bone growth and results in excellent handling characteristics.

ALLOY, AMALGAM *(Dental And Oral) 76EJJ*

Den-Mat Holdings, Llc 805-922-8491
2727 Skyway Dr, Santa Maria, CA 93455
No common name listed.

Foremost Dental Llc. 201-894-5500
242 S Dean St, Englewood, NJ 07631
Amalgam alloy.

ALLOY, AMALGAM *(cont'd)*

Kerr Corp. 714-516-7400
28200 Wick Rd, Romulus, MI 48174
Silver alloy.

Pulpdent Corp. 800-343-4342
80 Oakland St, Watertown, MA 02472
Amalgam well.

Wilkinson Company, Inc. 208-777-8332
590 S Clearwater Loop Ste C, Post Falls, ID 83854
Non-amalgam. For use in manufacturing dental implant parts.

Wykle Research, Inc. 775-887-7500
2222 College Pkwy, Carson City, NV 89706
Alloy for dental amalgam.

Zenith/Dmg Brand 800-662-6383
242 S Dean St, Division of Foremost Dental LLC, Englewood, NJ 07631

ALLOY, GOLD BASED, FOR CLINICAL USE
(Dental And Oral) 76EJT

Argen Corp. 800-375-9077
5855 Oberlin Dr, San Diego, CA 92121

Aurident, Inc. 714-523-5544
610 S State College Blvd, Fullerton, CA 92831
Various gold based alloys for clinical use.

D. Sign Dental Lab, Inc. 757-224-0177
690 W Fremont Ave Ste 9C, Sunnyvale, CA 94087
Gold metal alloy.

Golden Triangle Dental Laboratory Inc. 972-910-9912
7475 Las Colinas Blvd Ste A, Irving, TX 75063
Crown/bridges, inlay/onlay.

Heraeus Kulzer, Inc. 800-431-1785
99 Business Park Dr, Armonk, NY 10504
Gold based porcelain to metal, crown and bridge dental alloys.

Hong Kong Dental Lab 415-330-9099
9 Silliman St Ste C, San Francisco, CA 94134
Alloy, gold based noble metal.

Imagen (An Ex One Company) 724-863-9663
8075 Pennsylvania Ave, Irwin, PA 15642
Porcelain fused metal.

Ivoclar Vivadent, Inc. 800-533-6825
175 Pineview Dr, Amherst, NY 14228
Large array of ceramic and C&B alloys

Jensen Industries, Inc. 203-239-2090
50 Stillman Rd, North Haven, CT 06473
Dental alloys.

Kodent Inc. 562-404-8466
13340 Firestone Blvd Ste J, Santa Fe Springs, CA 90670
Implant alloy using ucla abutment.

Lloyd Baum Dental Center 909-796-2152
25742 Hinckley St, Loma Linda, CA 92354
E-Z GOLD direct filling gold. E-Z GOLD is powdered gold wrapped inside a thin gold leaf. This is heated in an alcohol flame, carried to the cavity of the tooth, and condensed. In this manner, several pellets are packed together to form a solid-gold filling. E-Z GOLD is available in 1/10- and 1/20-oz bottles.

Metalor Technologies Usa 800-554-5504
255 John L Dietsch Blvd, PO Box 255, North Attleboro, MA 02763
Casting gold.

Motloid Company 800-662-5021
300 N Elizabeth St, Chicago, IL 60607
Gold plating equipment and supplies.

Mountain Medico, Inc. 909-931-0688
600 N Mountain Ave Ste D204, Upland, CA 91786

Pentron Laboratory Technologies 203-265-7397
53 N Plains Industrial Rd, Wallingford, CT 06492
Gold base, yellow ceramic alloy.

Prince & Izant Nutec Metal Joining 216-362-7000
12999 Plaza Dr, Cleveland, OH 44130
Noble metal alloy.

Product Development Industries, Inc. 520-881-2556
4500 E Speedway Blvd Ste 50, Tucson, AZ 85712
Alloy, gold based, for clinical use.

Recigno Laboratories Inc. 215-659-7755
509 Davisville Rd, Willow Grove, PA 19090
High noble metal crown/bridge with porcelain.

ALLOY, GOLD BASED, FOR CLINICAL USE *(cont'd)*

Sterngold 800-243-9942
23 Frank Mossberg Dr, PO Box 2967, Attleboro, MA 02703
ADA certified and complete line available.

W.E. Mowrey Co. 651-646-1895
1435 University Ave W, Saint Paul, MN 55104
Mowrey dental alloys.

Wilkinson Company, Inc. 208-777-8332
590 S Clearwater Loop Ste C, Post Falls, ID 83854

ALLOY, PRECIOUS METAL, FOR CLINICAL USE
(Dental And Oral) 76EJS

A Plus Dental Lab 215-996-4177
1700 Horizon Dr, --suite 104, Chalfont, PA 18914
Crowns, bridges, dentures.

Aalba Dent, Inc. 707-864-3334
400 Watt Dr, Fairfield, CA 94534
Alloy, non-precious, dental, for crowns and bridges.

American Dental Designs Inc. 215-643-3232
1116 Horsham Rd, North Wales, PA 19454
Crown & bridge.

American Micro Products, Inc. 800-479-2193
4288 Armstrong Blvd, Batavia, OH 45103
Manufacture and assembly of precision engineered medical devices as a contract manufacturer. Full prototyping and process development available. Materials include all types of titanium, stainless steel, aluminum, precious metals and super alloys.

Argen Corp. 800-375-9077
5855 Oberlin Dr, San Diego, CA 92121
Full range of precious, semiprecious and non-precious dental alloys. Dental alloys for fabrication of porcelain-to-metal and full-cast crowns.

Aurident, Inc. 714-523-5544
610 S State College Blvd, Fullerton, CA 92831
Various precious metal alloys for clinical use.

Den-Mat Holdings, Llc 805-922-8491
2727 Skyway Dr, Santa Maria, CA 93455
No common name listed.

Dentalium Dental Ceramics, Inc. 949-440-2600
4141 MacArthur Blvd, Newport Beach, CA 92660

Dentsply Canada, Ltd. 800-263-1437
161 Vinyl Ct., Woodbridge, ONT L4L 4A3 Canada

Etkon Usa, Inc. 978-747-2575
916 113th St Ste A, Arlington, TX 76011

Eurotech Dental Laboratory, Inc. 307-234-6808
301 N McKinley St, Casper, WY 82601
Porcelain crowns, bridges, gold crowns.

Global Dentech Inc. 215-654-1237
1116 Horsham Rd, North Wales, PA 19454
Crown, pfm, bridges.

Golden Triangle Dental Laboratory Inc. 972-910-9912
7475 Las Colinas Blvd Ste A, Irving, TX 75063
Crown/bridges, inlay/onlay.

Heraeus Kulzer, Inc. 800-431-1785
99 Business Park Dr, Armonk, NY 10504
Palladium based alloys for porcelain to metal, crown and bridge dental alloys.

Ivoclar Vivadent, Inc. 800-533-6825
175 Pineview Dr, Amherst, NY 14228
Large array of ceramic and C&B alloys

Jensen Industries, Inc. 203-239-2090
50 Stillman Rd, North Haven, CT 06473
Dental gasting alloy.

Matech, Inc. 818-367-2472
13000 San Fernando Rd, Sylmar, CA 91342
Hi bond non-precious alloy.

Metalor Technologies Usa 800-554-5504
255 John L Dietsch Blvd, PO Box 255, North Attleboro, MA 02763
Casting alloy, semiprecious.

Mountain Medico, Inc. 909-931-0688
600 N Mountain Ave Ste D204, Upland, CA 91786

Moyco Technologies, Inc. 800-331-8837
200 Commerce Dr, Montgomeryville, PA 18936

Pentron Laboratory Technologies 203-265-7397
53 N Plains Industrial Rd, Wallingford, CT 06492
Precious metal ceramic alloy.

ALLOY, PRECIOUS METAL, FOR CLINICAL USE *(cont'd)*

Prince & Izant Nutec Metal Joining 216-362-7000
12999 Plaza Dr, Cleveland, OH 44130
Noble metal alloy.

Read Dental Lab 337-496-3706
1508 Ford St, Lake Charles, LA 70601
Gold based alloy for clinical use.

Recigno Laboratories Inc. 215-659-7755
509 Davisville Rd, Willow Grove, PA 19090
Noble metal crown/bridge.

Somerset Dental Products (Pentron Ceramics, Inc.) 800-496-9600
500 Memorial Dr, Somerset, NJ 08873
Types of dental casting metals.

Sterngold 800-243-9942
23 Frank Mossberg Dr, PO Box 2967, Attleboro, MA 02703
Full line of various compositions.

Stevens Metallurgical Corp. 800-794-7887
239 E 79th St, New York, NY 10075
Compounds, crystals, powders and solutions. Gold, iridium, osmium, palladium, platinum, phodium, ruthenium, and silver.

Talladium, Inc. 661-295-0900
27360 Muirfield Ln, Valencia, CA 91355
Precious metal alloy (talladium).

Temrex Corp. 516-868-6221
112 Albany Ave, P.o. Box 182, Freeport, NY 11520
Silver alloy for repairing of partial dentures.

Vident 800-828-3839
3150 E Birch St, Brea, CA 92821
Palladius V+.

Wilkinson Company, Inc. 208-777-8332
590 S Clearwater Loop Ste C, Post Falls, ID 83854
Gold, platimun, silver, palladium; wire & foil.

ALPHA-1 MICROGLOBULIN, ANTIGEN, ANTISERUM, CONTROL
(Immunology) 82MGA

Binding Site, Inc., The 800-633-4484
5889 Oberlin Dr Ste 101, San Diego, CA 92121

United Biotech, Inc. 650-961-2910
211 S Whisman Rd Ste E, Mountain View, CA 94041
ELISA quantitative for Beta-2-Microglobulin.

ALPHA-1-ACID-GLYCOPROTEIN, ANTIGEN, ANTISERUM, CONTROL *(Immunology) 82LKL*

Beckman Coulter, Inc. 800-742-2345
250 S Kraemer Blvd, PO Box 8000, Brea, CA 92821

Binding Site, Inc., The 800-633-4484
5889 Oberlin Dr Ste 101, San Diego, CA 92121

Biocell Laboratories, Inc. 800-222-8382
2001 E University Dr, Rancho Dominguez, CA 90220

Dako North America, Inc 805-566-6655
6392 Via Real, Carpinteria, CA 93013

International Immunology Corp. 800-843-2853
PO Box 972, Murrieta, CA 92564
Goat antiserum to Human Alpha-1-Acid Glycoprotein and General Immunology Human Calibrator/Control Serum.

ALPHA-1-LIPOPROTEIN, ANTIGEN, ANTISERUM, CONTROL
(Immunology) 82DER

Carolina Liquid Chemistries Corp. 800-471-7272
510 W Central Ave Ste C, Brea, CA 92821
Lipoprotein.

Raichem, Division Of Hemagen Diagnostics, Inc. 800-438-6100
8225 Mercury Ct, San Diego, CA 92111
Apolipoprotein A-1 determination, liquid ready-to-use immunological reagent, turbidimetric.

ALPHA-1-T-GLYCOPROTEIN, ANTIGEN, ANTISERUM, CONTROL *(Immunology) 82DEN*

Binding Site, Inc., The 800-633-4484
5889 Oberlin Dr Ste 101, San Diego, CA 92121

ALPHA-2-AP-GLYCOPROTEIN, ANTIGEN, ANTISERUM, CONTROL *(Immunology) 82DAW*

Binding Site, Inc., The 800-633-4484
5889 Oberlin Dr Ste 101, San Diego, CA 92121

ALPHA-FETOPROTEIN RIA TEST SYSTEM *(Immunology) 82KTJ*

Ameritek Usa, Inc. 425-379-2580
125 130th St SE Ste 200, Everett, WA 98208
Afp test kit.

Princeton Biomeditech Corp. 732-274-1000
4242 US Highway 1, Monmouth Junction, NJ 08852
Rapid one-step AFP test.

ALPHA-KETOBUTYRIC ACID AND NADH (U.V.), HYDROXYBUTYRIC *(Chemistry) 75JMK*

Biomerieux Inc. 800-682-2666
100 Rodolphe St, Durham, NC 27712

Dade Behring, Inc. 800-948-3233
1717 Deerfield Rd, Deerfield, IL 60015

Health Chem Diagnostics Llc 954-979-3845
3341 W McNab Rd, Pompano Beach, FL 33069
Acid, alpha-ketobutyric and nadh (u.v.), hydroxybutyric dehydrogenase.

Polymer Technology Systems, Inc. 317-870-5610
7736 Zionsville Rd, Indianapolis, IN 46268
Ketone test.

ALPHA-NAPHTHYL PHOSPHATE, ALKALINE PHOSPHATASE OR ISOENZYME *(Chemistry) 75CJO*

Health Chem Diagnostics Llc 954-979-3845
3341 W McNab Rd, Pompano Beach, FL 33069
Alpha-naphthyl phosphate, alkaline phosphatase or isoenzymes.

AMALGAM, DENTAL, POWDER *(Dental And Oral) 76VLN*

Ivoclar Vivadent, Inc. 800-533-6825
175 Pineview Dr, Amherst, NY 14228
Valiant

Starmet Corporation 978-369-5410
2229 Main St, Concord, MA 01742
Titanium Cobalt Alloy Powders, spherical metal powders used as coating on dental and orthopedic implants.

AMALGAMATOR, DENTAL, AC-POWERED
(Dental And Oral) 76EFD

A-Dec, Inc. 800-547-1883
2601 Crestview Dr, Newberg, OR 97132
Amalgamator.

Bristol-Myers Squibb Medical Imaging 978-671-8350
331 Treble Cove Rd, North Billerica, MA 01862
Vialmix.

Dentsply Canada, Ltd. 800-263-1437
161 Vinyl Ct., Woodbridge, ONT L4L 4A3 Canada

Dp Manufacture Corp. 305-640-9894
1460 NW 107th Ave Ste H, Doral, FL 33172
Dental amalgamator.

Ivoclar Vivadent, Inc. 800-533-6825
175 Pineview Dr, Amherst, NY 14228
SILIMAT PLUS.

Kerr Corp. 949-255-8766
3225 Deming Way Ste 190, Middleton, WI 53562
Dental amalgamator.

Kerr Corp. 714-516-7400
28200 Wick Rd, Romulus, MI 48174
Dental amalgamator.

Lantheus Medical Imaging, Inc. 1-800-362-2668
331 Treble Cove Rd Bldg 200-2, North Billerica, MA 01862
VIALMIX

Pelton & Crane 704-588-2126
11727 Fruehauf Dr, Charlotte, NC 28273
Amalgamator.

Rite-Dent Manufacturing Corp. 305-693-8626
3750 E 10th Ct, Hialeah, FL 33013
Various types of dental amalgamator.

Tpc Advanced Technology, Inc. 626-810-4337
18525 Gale Ave, City Of Industry, CA 91748
Amalgamator M-250 and M-500 dental amalgamator.

Wykle Research, Inc. 775-887-7500
2222 College Pkwy, Carson City, NV 89706
Dental amalgamator.

Zenith/Dmg Brand 800-662-6383
242 S Dean St, Division of Foremost Dental LLC, Englewood, NJ 07631

AMBULANCE *(General) 80QAO*

American Emergency Vehicles 800-374-9749
165 American Way, Jefferson, NC 28640
Ambulances: type I, II, and III.

Braun Industries, Inc. 800-222-7286
1170 Production Dr, Van Wert, OH 45891

Braun Northwest, Inc. 800-245-6303
PO Box 1204, Chehalis, WA 98532
Custom manufactured ambulance or specialty vehicle designed and built to meet customer requirements.

Business Aviation Services 800-888-1646
3501 N Aviation Ave, Sioux Falls, SD 57104
Manufacturing and retrofitting of dedicated air ambulance aeromedical interiors. Meets all F.A.A standards. STC'd for dedicated; PMA-authorized for interior components.

Calmaquip Engineering Corp. 305-592-4510
7240 NW 12th St, Miami, FL 33126

Dynacon, Inc. 573-594-3813
4924 Pike 451, Curryville, MO 63339
Ambulances

Embo-Optics, Llc. 887-885-6400
100 Cummings Ctr # 326B, Beverly, MA 01915
Portable IV illuminator with lighted monitoring feature aids medical personnel in assuring that all IV solutions and medications are infusing properly and at the correct infusion rate. Greatly enhance patient safety in aiding to prevent any adverse events during infusion.

Emergency Medical International 305-362-6050
6065 NW 167th St Ste B18, Hialeah, FL 33015
Type I, II, and III rescue vehicles & equipment.

Excellance, Inc. 800-882-9799
453 Lanier Rd, Madison, AL 35758
Modular ambulances, mobile ICU/neonatal units, rescue trucks, mobile clinics.

Horton Emergency Vehicles 614-539-8181
3800 McDowell Rd, Grove City, OH 43123

Medical Coaches, Inc. 607-432-1333
399 County Highway 58, P.O. Box 129, Oneonta, NY 13820
$100,000 & up, including mobile medical clinics, dental clinics, X-ray clinics, audiometric clinics, magnetic resonance imaging (MRI) trailers, positron emission tomography (PET), positron emission tomography/computed tomography (PET/CT) trailers, and lithotripsy units.

Medtec Ambulance Corp. 866-263-3832
2429 Lincolnway E, Goshen, IN 46526
3 types of EMS van/modulars, paramedic vehicles, neonatal, critical care and rescue vehicles.

Metronix 813-972-1212
12421 N Florida Ave Ste D201, Tampa, FL 33612
Ambulances Type I, II, and III. Also, fire trucks, mobile clinics, and mobile kitchens.

Microtek Medical, Inc 800-936-9248
512 N Lehmberg Rd, Columbus, MS 39702
EMT/EMS products such as masks, splints, & Microshield®.

Miller Coach Co., Inc. 800-824-9643
1744 W College St, Springfield, MO 65806

National Ambulance Builders, Inc. 800-747-0064
230 N Ortman Dr, Orlando, FL 32805
Adult, pediatric & neo-natal transport.

Plano Molding Co. 800-451-2122
431 E South St, Plano, IL 60545
6133 M Plano Medical Box: This 3 tray medical box features 29-39 adjustable compartments and bottom storage area. Dimensions: 19.25 'L x 10 'W x 9.75 'H

Tri-Star Industries Ltd. 902-742-9254
P.O. Box 486, Yarmouth, NS B5A 4B4 Canada

Wheeled Coach Industries, Inc. 800-422-8206
2737 Forsyth Rd, Winter Park, FL 32792

AMBULANCE, AIR *(General) 80TFU*

Agusta Aerospace Corporation 888-AGUSTA-2
3050 Red Lion Rd, Philadelphia, PA 19114
Sales and support of the A109 series EMS helicopters including the latest models - A109 power with superior speed and cat. 'A' performance, A109K2 has excellent hot and high capabilities and new in 1999 the A119 single engine Koala (8 place, 1000+SHP).

Business Aviation Services 800-888-1646
3501 N Aviation Ave, Sioux Falls, SD 57104

AMBULANCE, AIR *(cont'd)*

Embo-Optics, Llc. 887-885-6400
100 Cummings Ctr # 326B, Beverly, MA 01915
Portable IV illuminator with lighted monitoring feature aids medical personnel in assuring that all IV solutions and medications are infusing properly and at the correct infusion rate. Greatly enhance patient safety in aiding to prevent any adverse events during infusion.

National Air Ambulance 800-327-3710
3495 SW 9th Ave, Fort Lauderdale, FL 33315

Rocky Mountain Helicopters 801-375-1124
800 S 3110 W, Provo, UT 84601
Aircraft accessories and ground support equipment.

AMNIOSCOPE, TRANSABDOMINAL (FETOSCOPE)
(Obstetrics/Gyn) 85HFA

Allen Medical Instruments Corp. 949-646-3215
177 Riverside Ave Ste F602, Newport Beach, CA 92663

Mahe International Inc. 800-294-7946
468 Craighead St, Nashville, TN 37204

AMNIOTOME *(Obstetrics/Gyn) 85HGE*

Busse Hospital Disposables, Inc. 631-435-4711
75 Arkay Dr, Hauppauge, NY 11788
Amniontic hook.

Rocket Medical Plc. 800-707-7625
150 Recreation Park Dr Ste 3, Hingham, MA 02043

Utah Medical Products, Inc. 800-533-4984
7043 Cottonwood St, Midvale, UT 84047
AROM-COT, non-latex instrument for amniotomy with a finger cot hook on the end.

AMPLIFIER, BIOPOTENTIAL (W SIGNAL CONDITIONER)
(Cardiovascular) 74DRR

Grass Technologies, An Astro-Med, Inc. Product Gro 401-828-4002
53 Airport Park Drive, Rockland, MA 02370
Eeg average reference.

Lds Life Science (Formerly Gould Instrument Systems Inc.) 216-328-7000
5525 Cloverleaf Pkwy, Valley View, OH 44125

Lechnologies Research, Inc.. 866-321-2342
N64W24801 Main St Ste 107, Sussex, WI 53089
Cardiac event recorder.

U.F.I. 805-772-1203
545 Main St Ste C2, Morro Bay, CA 93442
$655.00 for Model 2122.

AMPLIFIER, MICROELECTRODE *(General) 80RGO*

Bak Electronics, Inc. 800-894-6000
PO Box 623, Mount Airy, MD 21771
Micro iontophoresis equipment.

Bio-Feedback Systems, Inc. 303-444-1411
2736 47th St, Boulder, CO 80301
$545.00 per unit (standard).

AMPLIFIER, PHYSIOLOGICAL SIGNAL *(Cns/Neurology) 84GWL*

Barrett Engineering 714-246-4388
606 L St, Fortuna, CA 95540
Signal amplifier for botox.

Bio-Feedback Systems, Inc. 303-444-1411
2736 47th St, Boulder, CO 80301
Multi-channel, isolated AC amplifier.

Cardinal Healthcare 209, Inc. 610-862-0800
5225 Verona Rd, Fitchburg, WI 53711
Amplifier system.

Cyberkinetics Neurotechnology Systems, Inc. 508-549-9981
100 Foxboro Blvd Ste 240, Foxborough, MA 02035
Physiological signal amplifier.

Grass Technologies, An Astro-Med, Inc. Product Gro 401-828-4002
53 Airport Park Drive, Rockland, MA 02370
Dc physiological amplifier.

Hospira Sedation, Inc. 877-946-7747
5 Billerica Ave, 101 Billerica Avenue, North Billerica, MA 01862
Eeg amplifier.

Nellcor Puritan Bennett (Melville) Ltd. 613-238-1840
700-141 Laurier Ave W, Ottawa K1P 5J3 Canada
Physiologic signal amplifier

AMPLIFIER, PHYSIOLOGICAL SIGNAL *(cont'd)*

U.F.I. 805-772-1203
545 Main St Ste C2, Morro Bay, CA 93442
$655.00 for Model 2122.

AMPLIFIER, TRANSDUCER SIGNAL (W SIGNAL CONDITIONER)
(Cardiovascular) 74DRQ

C. R. Bard, Inc., Bard Urological Div. 888-367-2273
13183 Harland Dr NE, Covington, GA 30014

Draeger Medical Systems, Inc. 215-660-2626
16 Electronics Ave, Danvers, MA 01923
Amplifier and signal conditioner, transducer signal.

Grass Technologies, An Astro-Med, Inc. Product Gro 401-828-4002
53 Airport Park Drive, Rockland, MA 02370
Oximeter coupler.

Lds Life Science (Formerly Gould Instrument Systems Inc.) 216-328-7000
5525 Cloverleaf Pkwy, Valley View, OH 44125
Plug-in, universal and carrier amplifiers.

Soltec Corp. 800-423-2344
12977 Arroyo St, San Fernando, CA 91340

U.F.I. 805-772-1203
545 Main St Ste C2, Morro Bay, CA 93442
$655.00 for Model 2122.

AMPLIFIER, VOICE *(Ear/Nose/Throat) 77MCK*

Doc's Proplugs, Inc. 800-521-2982
719 Swift St Ste 100, Santa Cruz, CA 95060
Doc's Promold used for music monitors and cell phones to block ambient noise and to hold the ear bud securely in the auricle.

Hitec Group Intl. 800-288-8303
8160 S Madison St, Burr Ridge, IL 60527

Luminaud, Inc. 800-255-3408
8688 Tyler Blvd, Mentor, OH 44060
4 models of voice amplifiers - price ranging from $160.00 to $500.00.

Park Surgical Co., Inc. 800-633-7878
5001 New Utrecht Ave, Brooklyn, NY 11219

Prentke Romich Company 800-262-1984
1022 Heyl Rd, Wooster, OH 44691
Speech-output communication device.

Sennheiser Electronic Corp. 877-736-6434
1 Enterprise Dr, Old Lyme, CT 06371
AUDIOPORT A 200 personal amplifier for one-on-one communications with hearing impaired clients.

AMPULE *(Gastro/Urology) 78QAS*

Aidlab, Inc. 416-410-5377
60 5th Street., Toronto, ONT M2N-6N1 Canada
AIDPAK Type I Borosilicate amber and clear ampules. Funnel top, long or short stem, scorebreak.

J. G. Finneran Associates, Inc. 800-552-3696
3600 Reilly Ct, Vineland, NJ 08360

ANALGESIA UNIT, CRYOGENIC *(General) 80WRI*

Zimmer Medizinsystems 800-327-3576
25 Mauchly Ste 300, Irvine, CA 92618
CRYO 5 ice wind cryotherapy unit. Ice wind therapy is the latest innovation in cryotherapy. For pain relief and inflammation reduction for 1-3 hours following a 30 sec. to 3 min. treatment.

ANALYZER, ALCOHOL *(Toxicology) 91DMH*

Akers Biosciences, Inc. 800-451-8378
201 Grove Rd, West Deptford, NJ 08086
Alcohol (check): Disposable breath alcohol test. Approved to test at .02 level by U.S. Department of Transportation. Breath Alcohol (check): Disposable version that tests for .02 & .08 on the same test (called the Graded Scale Breath Alcohol (check) Test); also have tests for .03, .04, .05, .06, .07, .08, .09 & .10, but these are not standard.

Alcohol Countermeasure Systems Corp. 905-670-2288
14-975 Midway Blvd., Mississauga, ONT L5T-2C6 Canada

Alcohol Countermeasure Systems, Inc. 303-366-5699
1670 Jasper St Unit G, Aurora, CO 80011

Alcopro 800-227-9890
2547 Sutherland Ave, Knoxville, TN 37919

ANALYZER, AMINO ACID *(Microbiology) 83QAQ*

Applied Biosystems 800-345-5724
850 Lincoln Centre Dr, Foster City, CA 94404
$36,000 for model 130A PTH amino acid analyzer; $85,000 for model 420A.

Basi (Bioanalytical Systems, Inc.) 800-845-4246
2701 Kent Ave, West Lafayette, IN 47906

Beckman Coulter, Inc. 800-742-2345
250 S Kraemer Blvd, PO Box 8000, Brea, CA 92821

Bio-Rad Laboratories, Life Science Group 800-424-6723
2000 Alfred Nobel Dr, Hercules, CA 94547

Bomem Inc. 800-858-FTIR
585 Charest Blvd. East, Suite 300, Quebec City, QUE G1K-9H4 Canada

Hitachi High Technologies America, Inc. 800-548-9001
3100 N 1st St, San Jose, CA 95134
For extensive use in the fields of biochemistry, food, medical, and pharmaceutical research and analysis, Hitachi's Amino Acid Analyzers offer outstanding performance as well as high-speed throughput.

Waters Corp. 800-252-4752
34 Maple St, Milford, MA 01757

ANALYZER, APPARATUS, VESTIBULAR *(Ear/Nose/Throat) 77LXV*

Gn Otometrics North America 800-289-2150
125 Commerce Dr, Schaumburg, IL 60173
Rotary vestibular test system.

Micromedical Technologies, Inc. 800-334-4154
10 Kemp Dr, Chatham, IL 62629
Meta-4 computerized ENG system with 4-channel programmable EOG amplifier for recording both horizontal and vertical eye movement; quadlight calibration bar, PC compatible computer with two disk drives, monitor and laserjet printer. Also, auto-rotational test hard- and software plus VORTEQ tuning fork transducer, Rotational Vestibular Chair.

Neuro Kinetics 412-963-6649
128 Gamma Dr, Pittsburgh, PA 15238
Rotary chair system.

Neurocom International, Inc. 503-653-2144
9570 SE Lawnfield Rd, Clackamas, OR 97015
Various models of posturography apparatus.

ANALYZER, AUDIO SPECTRUM *(Ear/Nose/Throat) 77RUQ*

Kaypentax 800-289-5297
2 Bridgewater Ln, Lincoln Park, NJ 07035
COMPUTERIZED SPEECH LAB (CSL) and MULTI-SPEECH, computerized systems for analyzing acoustic signals.

ANALYZER, BATTERY *(General) 80WJN*

Access Battery Inc. 800-654-9845
12104 W Carmen Ave, Division of Alpha Source, Inc. Milwaukee, WI 53225
Nickel-cadmium and sealed lead-acid battery analyzers.

Fecom Corporation 800-292-3362
12 Stults Rd Ste 103, Dayton, NJ 08810
Digital Key-chain battery tester with LCD indicator for hearing aid batteries and household battery tester that tester sizes D, C, AA, AAA, 9 volt, and Lithium all in one unit

Jbm Service Limited 800-663-2280
1405 Menu Road, Westbank, BC V4T-2R9 Canada
CADEX analyzer addresses the special needs of rechargeable batteries. Weak batteries are identified and automatically reconditioned. Good batteries are exercised to maintain peak performance. Comes in 2 and 4 channel versions.

W&W Manufacturing Co. 800-221-0732
800 S Broadway, Hicksville, NY 11801
ANALYZER I, III, & VI, single 3 station & 6 station analyzer/conditioner that analyzes N.cd & N.mtt batteries. Easy to use. Over 200 adapter cups available.

ANALYZER, BLOOD GAS PH *(Anesthesiology) 73TAK*

Allegro Biodiesel Corporation 800-949-4762
6245 Bristol Pkwy Ste 263, Culver City, CA 90230
IRMA, IRMA SL measures pC02, p02, Na+, k+, iCa, Hct, Cl-, BUN, Glucose. Portable, handheld.

Fisher Healthcare 800-766-7000
9999 Veterans Memorial Dr, Houston, TX 77038

ANALYZER, BLOOD GAS PH *(cont'd)*

Medica Corp. 800-777-5983
5 Oak Park Dr, Bedford, MA 01730
EASY BLOOD Gas Analyzer measures pH, PCO2 and PO2 on 100 microliter whole blood (syringe), 75 microliter whole blood capillaries.

Medical Sales & Service Group 888-357-6520
10 Woodchester Dr, Acton, MA 01720

Myco Instrumentation Source, Inc. 425-228-4239
PO Box 354, Renton, WA 98057

Nova Biomedical 800-458-5813
200 Prospect St, Waltham, MA 02453
Analyzers, Blood Gas/Critical Care. STAT PROFILE pHOx SERIES models from $12,000 to $32,000 per unit. Three test pHOx Basic offers pH, pO2 and PO2. Six test pHOx adds Hct, Hb and measured SO2%. Ten test pHOx Plus adds glucose, Na, K and a choice of Cl or ionized Ca. Eleven test pHOx Plus C offers both Cl and ionized Ca. Eleven test pHOx Plus L adds lactate to pHOx Plus menu. Companion co-oximeter provides a more comprehensive hemoglobin profile. STAT PROFILE Critical Care Xpress from $25,000 to $59,000. Provides a comprehensive test menu consisting of 19 measured and 29 calculated tests. Measures blood gases, electrolytes, chemistry, hemotology, and co-oximetry with on-board data management 'all in one' single, compact instrument. Measured tests include pH, PCO2, PO2, SO2%, hematocrit and hemoglobin, sodium, potassium, chloride, ionized calcium, ionized magnesium, glucose, BUN, creatinine, lactate, deoxyhemoglobin, oxyhemoglobin, methemoglobin, and carboxyhemoglobin. Thirteen standard models provide a choice of popular critical care assays.

Radiometer America, Inc. 800-736-0600
810 Sharon Dr, Westlake, OH 44145
ABL automated measurement of pH, pO2, and pCO2; some models also measure blood oximetry (co-ox) parameters, electrolytes, glucose, and lactate. NPT7 efficient, easy-to-use, point-of-care analyzer.

Spectron Corp. 425-827-9317
934 S Burlington Blvd # 603, Burlington, WA 98233
Reconditioned equipment.

Tecnomed International S.A. De C.V. 52-55-5519-7234
Andalucia 25, Alamos, Ciudad De Mexico, DF 03400 Mexico
OSMETECH OPTI CCA, ROCHE/AVL, AVL blood-gas analyzer.

ANALYZER, BLOOD GROUPING *(Hematology) 81TAL*

Daxor Corporation 212-244-0805
350 5th Ave Ste 7120, New York, NY 10118
DAXOR MAX 100 - 'BVA-100', blood volume analyzer. The BVA-100 is the first semi-automated instrument patented for direct measurement of blood volume, red cell volume and plasma volume. The system includes an injection-collection kit for a multi-sample blood volume. The system permits easy, rapid (within 18-36 minutes) precise total blood volume measurement with accuracy of 98%. Preliminary results are available in less than 20 minutes for use in acute blood loss situations. The instrument, also, calculates the normal blood volume for a specific individual. Measurement of blood volume can be used in medical and surgical conditions including hypertension, congestive heart failure, blood transfusion therapy, anemia, orthostatic hypertension and syncope.

Dms Laboratories, Inc. 800-567-4367
2 Darts Mill Rd, Flemington, NJ 08822
RAPIDVET-H Canine 1.1 blood group determination system (agglutination cards, diluent and controls) for identifying DEA 1.1 positive and DEA 1.1 negative dogs. 2, 5, or 20 tests per kit. RAPIDVET-H Feline blood group determination system (agglutination cards, diluent and optional controls)for identifying types A, B and AB cats. 2, 5, or 15 tests per kit.

ANALYZER, BLOOD GROUPING/ANTIBODY, AUTOMATED *(Hematology) 81KSZ*

Biomerieux Inc. 800-682-2666
100 Rodolphe St, Durham, NC 27712

Immucor, Inc. 800-829-2553
3130 Gateway Dr, PO Box 5625, Norcross, GA 30071
ABS2000 fully automated to perform the routine blood transfusion compatibility tests currently done manually by blood bank technologists.

Micro Typing Systems, Inc. 908-218-8177
1295 SW 29th Ave, Pompano Beach, FL 33069
Analyzer.

ANALYZER, BODY COMPOSITION *(Cardiovascular) 74MNW*

Life Measurement, Inc. 925-676-6002
1850 Bates Ave, Concord, CA 94520
Bod pod.

Promed Technologies Inc. 877-977-6633
P.O. Box 2070, Richmond Hill, ONT L4E-1A3 Canada

Sunbeam Products, Inc. 561-912-4100
2381 NW Executive Center Dr, Boca Raton, FL 33431
Body fat scale.

Tanita Corporation Of America, Inc. 877-682-6482
2625 S Clearbrook Dr, Arlington Heights, IL 60005
Body composition analyzer / Body fat monitor

ANALYZER, BONE, SONIC, NON-INVASIVE *(Orthopedics) 87MHH*

Imsi, Integrated Modular Systems Inc. 800-220-9729
2500 W Township Line Rd, PO Box 616, Havertown, PA 19083
Ortho Image Viewing Sytem. Full Functionality. Standard Software (MS) and Hardware Components. Cost Effective Licensing.

ANALYZER, BUN (BLOOD UREA NITROGEN) *(Chemistry) 75QES*

Beckman Coulter, Inc. 800-742-2345
250 S Kraemer Blvd, PO Box 8000, Brea, CA 92821

ANALYZER, CARBON HYDROGEN NITROGEN *(Chemistry) 75UFQ*

Spectro Analytical Instruments Inc. 800-548-5809
160 Authority Dr, Fitchburg, MA 01420

ANALYZER, CELL SIZE *(Microbiology) 83TBH*

Immunicon Corporation 215-830-0777
3401 Masons Mill Rd Ste 100, Huntingdon Valley, PA 19006
The EasyCount System is a simple cell counter that is designed to replace manual hemocytometers.

Koaman International 909-983-4888
656 E D St, Ontario, CA 91764

Moll Industries, Inc. 972-663-6900
13455 Noel Rd Ste 1310, Dallas, TX 75240
Cell replication unit

ANALYZER, CHEMISTRY, CENTRIFUGE *(Chemistry) 75JJG*

Beckman Coulter, Inc. 800-635-3497
740 W 83rd St, Hialeah, FL 33014

Beckman Coulter, Inc. 800-742-2345
250 S Kraemer Blvd, PO Box 8000, Brea, CA 92821

Fiberlite Centrifuge Inc. 408-988-1103
422 Aldo Ave, Santa Clara, CA 95054
Carbon composite science rotor.

Sarstedt, Inc. 800-257-5101
PO Box 468, 1025, St. James Church Road, Newton, NC 28658

ANALYZER, CHEMISTRY, DESK-TOP *(Chemistry) 75VIR*

Abaxis, Inc. 800-822-2947
3240 Whipple Rd, Union City, CA 94587

Analytical Spectral Devices, Inc. 303-444-6522
2555 55th St Ste A, Boulder, CO 80301

Antek Instruments, Inc. 281-580-0339
300 Bammel Westfield Rd, Houston, TX 77090
Total nitrogen analyzer. Also, nitric oxide, (nitrite/nitrate) fluoride, total sulfur and total nitrogen, and sulfur analyzers. Puro-chemiluminescent.

Beckman Coulter, Inc. 800-742-2345
250 S Kraemer Blvd, PO Box 8000, Brea, CA 92821

ANALYZER, CHEMISTRY, ELECTROLYTE *(Chemistry) 75QTJ*

Abaxis, Inc. 800-822-2947
3240 Whipple Rd, Union City, CA 94587

Alfa Wassermann, Inc. 800-220-4488
4 Henderson Dr, West Caldwell, NJ 07006
STARLYTE III; Sodium/Potassium/Chloride.

Basi (Bioanalytical Systems, Inc.) 800-845-4246
2701 Kent Ave, West Lafayette, IN 47906
Voltammographs and Polarographs, $1000 to $25,000.

Beckman Coulter, Inc. 800-635-3497
740 W 83rd St, Hialeah, FL 33014
$16,000 for FLEXLYTE 6; $9,000 for FLEXLYTE 3.

Beckman Coulter, Inc. 800-742-2345
250 S Kraemer Blvd, PO Box 8000, Brea, CA 92821

Biomerieux Inc. 800-682-2666
100 Rodolphe St, Durham, NC 27712

ANALYZER, CHEMISTRY, ELECTROLYTE *(cont'd)*

Buck Scientific, Inc. 800-562-5566
58 Fort Point St, Norwalk, CT 06855
Lithium 10 ppt BUCK 300 0.1 PPB sodium analyzer, 7-second reading time - also, model 404 oil in water analyzers.

Medica Corp. 800-777-5983
5 Oak Park Dr, Bedford, MA 01730
Na & K analysis in whole blood, serum, plasma, urine; $3,625.00 Na K & Cl analysis in whole blood, serum, plasma, urine; sodium/potassium/lithium analysis in whole blood, serum or plasma; Na K Ca pH analysis in whole blood, serum or plasma.

Medical Sales & Service Group 888-357-6520
10 Woodchester Dr, Acton, MA 01720

Nova Biomedical 800-458-5813
200 Prospect St, Waltham, MA 02453
16 models - from $10,192 to $25,500 for NOVA 1 through 16 line. Parameters: Na, K, Cl, TCO2, Li, ionized Mg, ionized Ca, total Ca, glucose, creatinine, BUN, Hct, and pH.

Radiometer America, Inc. 800-736-0600
810 Sharon Dr, Westlake, OH 44145
EML ion-specific electrodes unit, providing 60-sec STAT response.

ANALYZER, CHEMISTRY, ELISA *(Chemistry) 75UJM*

Accurate Chemical & Scientific Corp. 800-645-6264
300 Shames Dr, Westbury, NY 11590
Tests for diagnosis and management of patients with antineutrophil cytoplasmic autoantibody-associated diseases, particularly pulmonary-renal syndromes and rapidly progressive glomerulonephritis.

American Laboratory Products Co. 800-592-5726
26 Keewaydin Dr Ste G, Salem, NH 03079
Adrenocorticotropic hormone. Quantitative ELISA to determine ACTH in plasma.

Beckman Coulter, Inc. 800-742-2345
250 S Kraemer Blvd, PO Box 8000, Brea, CA 92821

Dade Behring, Inc. 800-948-3233
1717 Deerfield Rd, Deerfield, IL 60015
STRATUS immunoassay system (fluorometric).

Diagnostic Specialties 732-549-4011
4 Leonard St, Metuchen, NJ 08840
ENZIP Urinary Microalbumin Kit. ELISA (96 wELL) for albumin in urine

Drg International, Inc. 800-321-1167
1167 US Highway 22, Mountainside, NJ 07092
MTPL ELISA readers: E-LizaMat 3000, E-LizaMat 3200; fully automated ELIZAMAT 8882 (2-plate) and ELIZAMAT 8884 (4-plate)

Elabsupply 714-446-8740
1001 Starbuck St Apt C306, Fullerton, CA 92833
Extensive line of Microtiter ELISA tests for Thyroid Gland Function, Steroids, Fertility, Hormones, and Tumor Markers.

Meridian Bioscience, Inc. 800-696-0739
3471 River Hills Dr, Cincinnati, OH 45244
HPSA, Premier type-specific HSV-11gG ELISA test. EHEC Premier Type-Specific HSV-21gG ELISA Test.

Oncogene Research Products 800-854-3417
10394 Pacific Center Ct, San Diego, CA 92121
ELISA kit

Zymark Corporation 508-435-9500
68 Elm St, Hopkinton, MA 01748

ANALYZER, CHEMISTRY, ENZYME *(Chemistry) 75JJI*

Abaxis, Inc. 800-822-2947
3240 Whipple Rd, Union City, CA 94587

Beckman Coulter, Inc. 800-635-3497
740 W 83rd St, Hialeah, FL 33014
DACOS system.

Beckman Coulter, Inc. 800-742-2345
250 S Kraemer Blvd, PO Box 8000, Brea, CA 92821

Bio-Rad Laboratories Inc., Clinical Systems Div. 800-224-6723
4000 Alfred Nobel Dr, Hercules, CA 94547
Automated eia analyzer.

Biomerieux Inc. 800-682-2666
100 Rodolphe St, Durham, NC 27712

Biozyme Laboratories International Ltd. 800-423-8199
9939 Hibert St Ste 101, San Diego, CA 92131
Clinical & diagnostic enzymes.

ANALYZER, CHEMISTRY, ENZYME *(cont'd)*

Clinical Data Inc 800-937-5449
1 Gateway Ctr Ste 702, Newton, MA 02458
Clinical chemistry analyzer; immunochemistry analyzer.

Dade Behring, Inc. 800-948-3233
1717 Deerfield Rd, Deerfield, IL 60015

Helena Laboratories 409-842-3714
PO Box 752, Beaumont, TX 77704

Olympus America, Inc. 800-645-8160
3500 Corporate Pkwy, PO Box 610, Center Valley, PA 18034

ANALYZER, CHEMISTRY, ENZYME IMMUNOASSAY
(Chemistry) 75UEH

Beckman Coulter Inc. 800-231-7970
445 Medical Center Blvd, Webster, TX 77598
Inhibin-A ELISA

Beckman Coulter, Inc. 800-742-2345
250 S Kraemer Blvd, PO Box 8000, Brea, CA 92821

Dade Behring, Inc. 800-948-3233
1717 Deerfield Rd, Deerfield, IL 60015
STRATUS immunoassay system (fluorometric).

Global Focus (G.F.M.D. Ltd.) 800-527-2320
2280 Springlake Rd Ste 106, Dallas, TX 75234
Automated slide and ELISA processor.

Meridian Bioscience, Inc. 800-696-0739
3471 River Hills Dr, Cincinnati, OH 45244
IMMUNOCARD: Rapid membrane enzyme immunosorbent assay products. IMMUNOCARD STAT, E.coli 0157:H7.

Nuclin Diagnostics, Inc. 847-498-5210
3322 Commercial Ave, Northbrook, IL 60062

ANALYZER, CHEMISTRY, FLUORESCENCE IMMUNOASSAY
(Chemistry) 75UEI

Astoria-Pacific,Inc. 800-536-3111
PO Box 830, Clackamas, OR 97015

Bio-Medical Products Corp. 800-543-7427
10 Halstead Rd, Mendham, NJ 07945
i-chroma fluorometer for rapid quantative test result in 5 minutes.

Sea Horse Bio Science 800-671-0633
16 Esquire Rd, North Billerica, MA 01862
Thermogenic Imaging, the company that îmeasures the heat of life,î manufactures ultra-sensitive infrared imaging systems to measure unique thermal signatures in cells and animals that are indicative of disease, genetic variations or drug function. Thermal Signature Analysis (TSA) is a real-time measurement of metabolic activity, toxic reactions and other biological processes that produce or consume minute changes in heat.

ANALYZER, CHEMISTRY, MICRO *(Chemistry) 75JJF*

Beckman Coulter, Inc. 800-635-3497
740 W 83rd St, Hialeah, FL 33014
DACOS system.

Beckman Coulter, Inc. 800-742-2345
250 S Kraemer Blvd, PO Box 8000, Brea, CA 92821

Biokinetix Corp. 203-327-7893
33 Parker Ave, Stamford, CT 06906
Ministat-s chemistry analyzer.

Cst Technologies, Inc. 800-448-4407
55 Northern Blvd Ste 200, Great Neck, NY 11021
ENZDIL, $195.00 per liter, enzyme diluent for enzyme controls.

Idaho Technology, Inc. 1-800-735-6544
390 Wakara Way, Salt Lake City, UT 84108
Real-time polymerase chain reaction (pcr) amplification and detection system.

Labworld, Inc. 800-447-2428
471 Page St Ste 4, Stoughton, MA 02072
We sell chemistry and hematology analyzers. Roche, Bayer, Beckman Coulter are a few of the manufacturers' instruments we sell.

Roche Molecular Systems, Inc. 925-730-8110
4300 Hacienda Dr, Pleasanton, CA 94588
Nucleic acid chemistry analyzer.

Synermed Intl., Inc. 317-896-1565
17408 Tiller Ct Ste 1900, Westfield, IN 46074
Various models chemistry analyzers.

ANALYZER, CHEMISTRY, MULTI-CHANNEL, FIXED
(Chemistry) 75QKW

Beckman Coulter, Inc. 800-742-2345
250 S Kraemer Blvd, PO Box 8000, Brea, CA 92821

Berkeley Nucleonics Corp. 800-234-7858
2955 Kerner Blvd, San Rafael, CA 94901
Berkeley Nucleonics Model 565 Digital Delay Pulse Generator and 505 Pulse Generator expand the boundaries of pulse generator and digital delay capabilities. They provide up to eight independent pulse generator outputs or up to 16 digital delay generator edges in one instrument. As a pulse generator they provide rate, delay, width, and output adjustability with each of the channels. As a digital delay generator with fine resolution timing they provide multiple pulses from an external, internal, or software trigger.

Cds Analytical, Inc. 800-541-6593
465 Limestone Rd, Oxford, PA 19363

Dade Behring, Inc. 800-948-3233
1717 Deerfield Rd, Deerfield, IL 60015

Medical Sales & Service Group 888-357-6520
10 Woodchester Dr, Acton, MA 01720

Myco Instrumentation Source, Inc. 425-228-4239
PO Box 354, Renton, WA 98057

Olympus America, Inc. 800-645-8160
3500 Corporate Pkwy, PO Box 610, Center Valley, PA 18034

Spectron Corp. 425-827-9317
934 S Burlington Blvd # 603, Burlington, WA 98233
Reconditioned equipment.

ANALYZER, CHEMISTRY, MULTI-CHANNEL, PROGRAMMABLE
(Chemistry) 75QKX

Alfa Wassermann, Inc. 800-220-4488
4 Henderson Dr, West Caldwell, NJ 07006
ACE, clinical chemistry system. NEXCT, clinical chemisty system, is an automated, random access, discrete centrifugal benchtop analyzer designed for lower volume & specialty testing.

Beckman Coulter, Inc. 800-635-3497
740 W 83rd St, Hialeah, FL 33014
$155,000 for DACOS XL.

Beckman Coulter, Inc. 800-742-2345
250 S Kraemer Blvd, PO Box 8000, Brea, CA 92821

Cds Analytical, Inc. 800-541-6593
465 Limestone Rd, Oxford, PA 19363

Esa, Inc. 800-959-5095
22 Alpha Rd, Chelmsford, MA 01824
Eight-channel array analyzer.

Helena Laboratories 409-842-3714
PO Box 752, Beaumont, TX 77704
Four channel, programmable chemical analzyer. Performs platelet aggregation, ristocetin co-factor and chromogenic testing.

ANALYZER, CHEMISTRY, NEPHELOMETRIC IMMUNOASSAY
(Chemistry) 75WMG

Beckman Coulter, Inc. 800-742-2345
250 S Kraemer Blvd, PO Box 8000, Brea, CA 92821

ANALYZER, CHEMISTRY, PHOTOMETRIC, BICHROMATIC
(Chemistry) 75JJD

Abaxis, Inc. 800-822-2947
3240 Whipple Rd, Union City, CA 94587

ANALYZER, CHEMISTRY, PHOTOMETRIC, DISCRETE
(Chemistry) 75JJE

Abbott Diagnostics Div. 847-937-7988
1921 Hurd Dr, Irving, TX 75038
Various.

Abbott Diagnostics Div. 626-440-0700
820 Mission St, South Pasadena, CA 91030
Various models of bichromatic photometric analyzers.

Alfa Wassermann, Inc. 800-220-4488
4 Henderson Dr, West Caldwell, NJ 07006
ACE, NEXCT, clinical chemistry systems.

Beckman Coulter, Inc. 800-635-3497
740 W 83rd St, Hialeah, FL 33014
DACOS XL, $69,500 for OPTICHEM 120; $89,500 for OPTICHEM 180.

Chemdev Instruments, Inc. 408-541-8535
1289 Reamwood Ave Ste B, Sunnyvale, CA 94089
Eco chem 300 chemistry system.

ANALYZER, CHEMISTRY, PHOTOMETRIC, DISCRETE *(cont'd)*

Diamond Diagnostics, Inc. 508-429-0450
333 Fiske St, Holliston, MA 01746

Kodak Canada Inc., Health Imaging Division 800-295-5526
3500 Eglinton Ave. W., Toronto, ONT M6M 1V3 Canada

Lab-Interlink, Inc. 705-860-1220
8950 J St, Omaha, NE 68127
Awcc-automated workcell control system.

Mgm Instruments 800-551-1415
925 Sherman Ave, Hamden, CT 06514
Luminometer with Injector Systems; $6,240 to $7,600 for OPTOCOMP I semiautomatic; $14,160 to $15,520 for OPTOCOMP II 250-sample. All luminometers include built-in printer and data reduction software.

Ortho-Clinical Diagnostics, Inc. 908-218-8177
Route 202, Raritan, NJ 08869
Discrete photometric chemistry analyzer for clinical use.

Ortho-Clinical Diagnostics, Inc. 585-453-3768
1000 Lee Rd, Rochester, NY 14606
Discrete photometric chemistry analyzer for clinical use.

Ortho-Clinical Diagnostics, Inc. 800-828-6316
513 Technology Blvd, Rochester, NY 14626
Microplate assay test procedure processing system.

Ortho-Clinical Diagnostics, Inc. 585-453-3768
100 Indigo Creek Dr, Rochester, NY 14626
VITROS 350 Chemistry System; VITROS 5,1 FS Chemistry System; VITROS DT60II Chemistry System

Sparton Medical Systems 440-878-4630
22740 Lunn Rd, Strongsville, OH 44149
Discrete photometric chem. analyzer for clin. use.

Teco Diagnostics 714-693-7788
1268 N Lakeview Ave, Anaheim, CA 92807
Chemistry analyzer.

ANALYZER, CHEMISTRY, RADIOIMMUNOASSAY
(Chemistry) 75LCI

Diasorin Inc 800-328-1482
1951 Northwestern Ave S, PO Box 285, Stillwater, MN 55082
ETI MAX 4 plate Elisa Microplate Analyzer for Hepatitis, Infectious Disease and Autoimmune testing. Liaison automated chemiluminescence analyzer for Hepatitis, Infectious Disease, Autoimmune, Steroid, Bone and Mineral Metabolism and Transplant Monitoring testing.

Medical Sales & Service Group 888-357-6520
10 Woodchester Dr, Acton, MA 01720

Stryker Puerto Rico, Ltd. 939-307-2500
Hwy. 3, Km. 131.2, Las Guasimas Ind. Park, Arroyo, PR 00714
Insufflator tubing w/ filter.

ANALYZER, CHEMISTRY, RADIOIMMUNOASSAY, AUTOMATED
(Chemistry) 75ROC

Beckman Coulter, Inc. 800-742-2345
250 S Kraemer Blvd, PO Box 8000, Brea, CA 92821

Capintec, Inc. 800-631-3826
6 Arrow Rd, Ramsey, NJ 07446

ANALYZER, CHEMISTRY, SEQUENTIAL MULTIPLE, CONTINUOUS FLOW *(Chemistry) 75JJC*

Amresco Inc. 800-366-1313
30175 Solon Industrial Pkwy, Solon, OH 44139
Random Access Liquid

Astoria-Pacific,Inc. 800-536-3111
PO Box 830, Clackamas, OR 97015
Various models of chemistry analyzers for clinical use.

Diamond Diagnostics, Inc. 508-429-0450
333 Fiske St, Holliston, MA 01746

ANALYZER, CHEMISTRY, SINGLE CHANNEL, PROGRAMMABLE
(Chemistry) 75QKY

Beckman Coulter, Inc. 800-742-2345
250 S Kraemer Blvd, PO Box 8000, Brea, CA 92821

Cds Analytical, Inc. 800-541-6593
465 Limestone Rd, Oxford, PA 19363

Esa, Inc. 800-959-5095
22 Alpha Rd, Chelmsford, MA 01824
Single-channel chemistry analyzer.

Helena Laboratories 409-842-3714
PO Box 752, Beaumont, TX 77704

ANALYZER, CHEMISTRY, SINGLE CHANNEL, PROGRAMMABLE *(cont'd)*

Medical Sales & Service Group 888-357-6520
10 Woodchester Dr, Acton, MA 01720

Myco Instrumentation Source, Inc. 425-228-4239
PO Box 354, Renton, WA 98057

Olympus America, Inc. 800-645-8160
3500 Corporate Pkwy, PO Box 610, Center Valley, PA 18034

Spectron Corp. 425-827-9317
934 S Burlington Blvd # 603, Burlington, WA 98233
Reconditioned equipment.

Zymark Corporation 508-435-9500
68 Elm St, Hopkinton, MA 01748
Robotic arm can be programmed to prepare & process samples for analysis by any analyzer - $26,000.00.

ANALYZER, CHEMISTRY, THERAPEUTIC DRUG MONITOR (TDM) *(Chemistry) 75ULK*

Beckman Coulter, Inc. 800-635-3497
740 W 83rd St, Hialeah, FL 33014
DACOS XL.

Dade Behring, Inc. 800-948-3233
1717 Deerfield Rd, Deerfield, IL 60015
STRATUS TDM system.

ANALYZER, CHEMISTRY, URINALYSIS *(Chemistry) 75KQO*

Arkray Factory Usa, Inc. 952-646-3168
5182 W 76th St, Minneapolis, MN 55439
Urine chemistry analyzer.

Arkray Usa 800-818-8877
5198 W 76th St, Edina, MN 55439
DIASCREEN 50 URINE CHEMISTRY ANALYZER-Virtually eliminates transcription errors with an easy-to-read printout. Minimizes variability between operators. Throughput of up to 50 samples per hour.

Bayer Healthcare Llc 914-524-2955
555 White Plains Rd Fl 5, Tarrytown, NY 10591
Automated urinalysis system.

Bayer Healthcare, Llc 574-256-3430
430 S Beiger St, Mishawaka, IN 46544
Automated urinalysis system.

Clin-Chem Mfg. Llc. 800-359-9691
2560 Business Pkwy Ste C, Minden, NV 89423
For control of urine assays.

Elabsupply 714-446-8740
1001 Starbuck St Apt C306, Fullerton, CA 92833
Uritek 720+ Urine Strip Reader to run 720 tests per hour, 2,000 test memory capacity, PC and barcode interface, and compatible with 110/220 voltage sources.

Garren Scientific, Inc. 800-342-3725
15916 Blythe St Unit A, Van Nuys, CA 91406
Urinalysis system.

Iris Diagnostics 800-776-4747
9172 Eton Ave, Chatsworth, CA 91311
Automated urinalysis workstation.

Sparton Medical Systems 440-878-4630
22740 Lunn Rd, Strongsville, OH 44149
Automated urinalysis system.

Teco Diagnostics 714-693-7788
1268 N Lakeview Ave, Anaheim, CA 92807
Urine strip reader.

ANALYZER, CHEMISTRY, URINALYSIS, AUTOMATED *(Chemistry) 75JJZ*

Iris International, Inc. 800-776-4747
9162 Eton Ave, Chatsworth, CA 91311
IRIS MODEL 500 URINE/FLUIDS WORKSTATION and IRIS MODEL 300 URINALYSIS WORKSTATION for complete laboratory urinalysis profile including microscopic examination, chemistry and specific gravity. IRIS 900UDX URINE PATHOLOGY SYSTEM is a walkaway, fully automated system for complete routine urinalysis including chemistry, sediment microscopy, specific gravity, color, and clarity.

ANALYZER, CHEMISTRY, URINE *(Chemistry) 75VEP*

Elabsupply 714-446-8740
1001 Starbuck St Apt C306, Fullerton, CA 92833
Urine Reagent Strips for testing Blood, Glucose, Proten, Ketone, pH, Specific Gravity, Bilirubin, Urobilinogen, Leukocyte, Nitrite and Asorbic Acid.

ANALYZER, CHEMISTRY, URINE *(cont'd)*

Globe Scientific, Inc. 800-394-4562
610 Winters Ave, Paramus, NJ 07652
URI-PAK urine collection system: 12mL urine tubes, caps, collection cups and patient-ID labels. Optional rack.

Medical Sales & Service Group 888-357-6520
10 Woodchester Dr, Acton, MA 01720

ANALYZER, CHROMATOGRAPHY INFRARED *(Chemistry) 75UGP*

Jasco, Inc. 800-333-5272
8649 Commerce Dr, Easton, MD 21601

ANALYZER, CHROMOSOME, AUTOMATED *(Pathology) 88LNJ*

Invitrogen Corporation 800-955-6288
101 Lincoln Centre Dr, Foster City, CA 94404

Koaman International 909-983-4888
656 E D St, Ontario, CA 91764

ANALYZER, COAGULATION *(Hematology) 81GKP*

American Labor 800-424-0443
3329 Durham Chapel Hill Blvd Ste 200, Durham, NC 27707
Manual & automated.

Bio/Data Corp. 215-441-4000
155 Gibraltar Rd, Horsham, PA 19044
Coagulation instrument.

Biomerieux Inc. 800-682-2666
100 Rodolphe St, Durham, NC 27712
COAG-A-MATE: Coagulation instrumentation. COAG-A-MATE MTX II is a fully automated bench top random access analyzer for the performance of clotting and chromogenic assays.

Dade Behring, Inc. 800-948-3233
1717 Deerfield Rd, Deerfield, IL 60015

Diagnostica Stago, Inc. 800-222-COAG
5 Century Dr, Parsippany, NJ 07054
STA-C and STA-R hemostasis systems.

Haemoscope Corp. 800-438-2834
6231 W Howard St, Niles, IL 60714
Thrombelastograph (TEG) Hemostasis Analyzer performs a global evaluation of coagulation kinetics, clot formation, strength, stability and lysis using whole blood. It is used world-wide to monitor hemorrhagic and thrombotic risks and to evaluate the efficacy of blood product replacement, anticoagulant therapy and antifibrinolytic and fibrinolytic agents, pre-, peri- and post-operatively. The data is transferred to the PC which instantaneously measures the patient's coagulation parameters and computes coagulation and fibrinolytic indices; displays the patient data, and normal ranges; and stores and retrieves all information.

Helena Laboratories 409-842-3714
PO Box 752, Beaumont, TX 77704

Medicos Laboratories, Inc. (Mdt) 800-724-4003
801 Montrose Ave, South Plainfield, NJ 07080

Mettler Toledo Lasentec Products (Lasentec) 425-881-7117
14833 NE 87th St, Redmond, WA 98052

ANALYZER, COAGULATION, AUTOMATED *(Hematology) 81QLM*

American Labor 800-424-0443
3329 Durham Chapel Hill Blvd Ste 200, Durham, NC 27707

Biomerieux Inc. 800-682-2666
100 Rodolphe St, Durham, NC 27712
2 models: COAG-A-MATE RA4 performs PT, APTT, TT, fibrinogen, and factor assays on plasma samples. In random access, 12 sample maximum load.

Dade Behring, Inc. 800-948-3233
1717 Deerfield Rd, Deerfield, IL 60015

International Technidyne Corp. 800-631-5945
23 Nevsky St, Edison, NJ 08820
Whole blood coagulation timer, dual-well version (test tube). Microsample whole blood congulation time (cartridge). Anticoagulation monitor for home use. HEMOCHRON RESPONSE, whole blood coagulation timer with integrated data management. PROTIME 3, Anticoagulation monitor for professional and home use.

Medtronic Perfusion Systems 800-328-3320
7611 Northland Dr N, Brooklyn Park, MN 55428
4 models - from $3,400.00 to $11,500.00; up to 4 channels, Heparin & ACT measurement.

ANALYZER, COAGULATION, AUTOMATED *(cont'd)*

Sienco, Inc. 800-432-1624
7985 Vance Dr Ste 104, Arvada, CO 80003
SONOCLOT Coagulation & Platelet Function Analyzer: Ultrasensitve detection system measures hemostatic changes in whole blood. Automated graphical results characterize blood viscosity, initial clot formation time, rate of fibrin formation and clot retraction (platelet function) $9,358.00 for continuously recording system using 0.4ml sample size and time stirring, includes thermal graphics printer.

ANALYZER, COAGULATION, MANUAL *(Hematology) 81QLN*

American Labor 800-424-0443
3329 Durham Chapel Hill Blvd Ste 200, Durham, NC 27707

Biomerieux Inc. 800-682-2666
100 Rodolphe St, Durham, NC 27712
COAG-A-MATE XM performs PT, APTT, TT, fibrinogen, factor assays and semi-quantitative (SQF) fibrinogen on plasma samples.

Medical Innovations International Inc. 507-289-0761
6256 34th Ave NW, Rochester, MN 55901
Rochester Fistula Training Arm™ with artificial blood, veins and arm.

ANALYZER, COAGULATION, MULTIPURPOSE
(Hematology) 81JPA

Bio/Data Corp. 215-441-4000
155 Gibraltar Rd, Horsham, PA 19044
Calcium chloride; imidazole buffer; tris buffered saline.

Farallon Medical, Inc. 510-785-0800
3521 Investment Blvd Ste 1, Hayward, CA 94545
Immedia.

International Technidyne Corp. 800-631-5945
23 Nevsky St, Edison, NJ 08820

International Technidyne Corporation 732-548-5700
8 Olsen Ave, Edison, NJ 08820
Blood coagulation analyzer and electronic quality control.

ANALYZER, COAGULATION, SEMI-AUTOMATED
(Hematology) 81KQG

Biosearch Medical Products, Inc. 908-722-5000
35 Industrial Pkwy, Branchburg, NJ 08876
Bipolar coagulation probe.

Clinical Diagnostic Solutions, Inc. 954-791-1773
1800 NW 65th Ave, Plantation, FL 33313
Instrument, coagulation.

International Technidyne Corporation 732-548-5700
8 Olsen Ave, Edison, NJ 08820
Hemochron jr. analyzer.

ANALYZER, COAGULATION, WHOLE BLOOD
(Hematology) 81SAN

Biomerieux Inc. 800-682-2666
100 Rodolphe St, Durham, NC 27712
MDA analyzer, coagulation automated. MDA 180 is a fully automated, random access analyzer for clotting, chronogenic, and immunoassay procedures. Key features include cap piercing, bar code ID, and LIS interface capabilities. Other options include 180 tests per hour, touch screen, bidirectional ITS interface, automated bar-code scanning.

Haemoscope Corp. 800-438-2834
6231 W Howard St, Niles, IL 60714
Thrombelastograph (TEG) Hemostasis Analyzer performs a global evaluation of coagulation kinetics, clot formation, strength, stability and lysis using whole blood. It is used world-wide to monitor hemorrhagic and thrombotic risks and to evaluate the efficacy of blood product replacement, anticoagulant therapy and antifibrinolytic and fibrinolytic agents, pre-, peri- and post-operatively. The data is transferred to the PC which instantaneously measures the patient's coagulation parameters and computes coagulation and fibrinolytic indices; displays the patient data, and normal ranges; and stores and retrieves all information.

Omni Medical Supply Inc. 800-860-6664
4153 Pioneer Dr, Commerce Township, MI 48390

Roche Diagnostics 800-361-2070
201 Armand-Frappier Blvd., Laval, QUE H7V 4A2 Canada
Retail Price of monitors range from $2,800 (plus) to $1,300 CDN. Retail price of cartridge is $150 CDN.

ANALYZER, COMBINATION CHEMISTRY/HEMATOLOGY/ELECTROLYTE *(Chemistry) 75VIN*

Beckman Coulter, Inc. 800-742-2345
250 S Kraemer Blvd, PO Box 8000, Brea, CA 92821

ANALYZER, COMBINATION CHEMISTRY/HEMATOLOGY/ELECTROLYTE *(cont'd)*

Elabsupply 714-446-8740
1001 Starbuck St Apt C306, Fullerton, CA 92833
Complete line of Hematology blood analysis solutions in powder and liquid format for Beckman Coulter, Coulter/Stks and Sysmex analyzers.

Harvey, R.J. Instrument Corp. 201-664-1380
123 Patterson St, Hillsdale, NJ 07642
DISCOVERY f2 chemistry, coagulation, electrolyte & hematology analyzer.

ANALYZER, COMPOSITION, WEIGHT, PATIENT
(General) 80VDN

Bioanalogics 503-626-8000
7909 SW Cirrus Dr # 27, Beaverton, OR 97008
Body composition analyzer.

Creative Health Products, Inc. 800-742-4478
5148 Saddle Ridge Rd, Plymouth, MI 48170
Bodyfat Analyzer/Scale, Bio Impedance; TANITA from basic model $128.00 to $1516.00 professional model with printer output for % bodyfat, fat mass, total body water, BMR. Can interface with computer. From CHP.

Detecto Scale Co. 800-641-2008
203 E Daugherty St, PO Box 151, Webb City, MO 64870

Monarch Art Plastics, Llc. 856-235-5151
3838 Church Rd, Mount Laurel, NJ 08054
Body Mass Index (BMI)Calculator

Novel Products, Inc. 800-323-5143
PO Box 408, Rockton, IL 61072
Hydrostatic weight system.

Trademark Medical Llc 800-325-9044
449 Soverign Ct, St. Louis, MO 63011
TANITA scales, complete line of wieght scales and body composition analyzers.

ANALYZER, CONCENTRATION, OXYHEMOGLOBIN, BLOOD PHASE *(Toxicology) 91JFD*

Radiometer America, Inc. 800-736-0600
810 Sharon Dr, Westlake, OH 44145
OSM3.

ANALYZER, CONCENTRATION, OXYHEMOGLOBIN, BP, TRANSCUTANEOUS *(Cardiovascular) 74JEE*

Mcdalt Medical Corp. 800-841-5774
2225 Prestonwood Dr Ste 100-A, Arlington, TX 76012
AVOXimeter 1000-E for O2 Sats, Concentration, Total Hemoglobin. Results in less than 10 Seconds.

ANALYZER, DIAGNOSTIC, FIBEROPTIC (COLON)
(Gastro/Urology) 78MOA

Spectrascience, Inc. 858-847-0200
11568 Sorrento Valley Rd Ste 11, San Diego, CA 92121
Laser induced fluoroscopy.

ANALYZER, DISTRIBUTION, WEIGHT, PODIATRIC
(Orthopedics) 87WQP

Advanced Mechanical Technology, Inc. (Amti) 800-422-AMTI
176 Waltham St, Watertown, MA 02472
6-component force/torque platform for gait, balance and sports analysis

ANALYZER, DOPPLER SPECTRUM *(General) 80TEU*

Md International, Inc. 305-669-9003
11300 NW 41st St, Doral, FL 33178

New Life Systems, Inc. 954-972-4600
PO Box 8767, Coral Springs, FL 33075

Perimed, Inc. 877-374-3589
6785 Wallings Rd Ste 2C-2D, North Royalton, OH 44133
Laser Doppler Blood Perfusion Imager

ANALYZER, ECG *(Cardiovascular) 74LOS*

Agfa Healthcare Corp. 864-421-1815
1 Crosswind Dr, Westerly, RI 02891
Ecg management system.

Capintec, Inc. 800-631-3826
6 Arrow Rd, Ramsey, NJ 07446
Cardiac function evaluation system detects, records, and analyzes left ventricular function.

ANALYZER, ECG *(cont'd)*

Cardiac Science Corp. 800-777-1777
500 Burdick Pkwy, Deerfield, WI 53531
Vision and Vision Premier

Compumed, Inc. 800-421-3395
5777 W Century Blvd Ste 360, Los Angeles, CA 90045
Electrocardiograph.

Drg International, Inc. 800-321-1167
1167 US Highway 22, Mountainside, NJ 07092

Fukuda Denshi Usa, Inc. 800-365-6668
17725 NE 65th St Ste C, Redmond, WA 98052
System, ecg analysis.

Futuremed America, Inc. 800-222-6780
15700 Devonshire St, Granada Hills, CA 91344
FUTUREMED ECG resting and stress from $1,300 to $15,000.

Galix Biomedical Instrumentation, Inc. 305-534-5905
2555 Collins Ave Ste C-5, Miami Beach, FL 33140
New, fast, and accurate Windows-based ECG Holter analyzer, model WinTer, with automatic diagnostics report and printing. All patient information can now be stored on a memory card to ensure patient data and study identification, while patient diary is automatically printed. Real-time ECG waveform from the recorder can now be monitored at the computer's display. Proprietary noise-analysis algorithm software, dramatically improves arrhythmia-detection accuracy. Short- and long-term heart-rate-variability analysis with time and frequency domain standards. Unlimited patient database report storing, with the possibility to export and import complete studies via Internet, satellite, CD, etc.

Ge Medical Systems Information Technologies 800-643-6439
8200 W Tower Ave, Milwaukee, WI 53223
MUSE System for cardiology management; capable of on-line ECG interpretations, serial comparisons, editing, retrieval, management reports, interface to hospital information systems and database search. Provides storage for most cardiology data including: resting ECGs, pacemaker ECG data, Holter final reports, stress final reports, vector cardiography and signal averaging, and late potential reports. System storage can be configured to provide online data storage of one million resting ECGs.

J.M. Baragano Biomedical P.M. And Consulting, Inc. 787-722-4007
808 Ave Fernandez Juncos, San Juan, PR 00907
Metron Biomedical Test Equipment, Dale Biomedical and Electrical test equipment. EKG simulation equipment and electrical safety analyzers.

Lds Life Science (Formerly Gould Instrument Systems Inc.) 216-328-7000
5525 Cloverleaf Pkwy, Valley View, OH 44125

Midmark Diagnostics Group 800-624-8950
3300 Fujita St, Torrance, CA 90505
IQmark Digital ECG--The IQmark Digital ECG is a compact, portable device that easily connects to a Windows computer. It features full interpretations, pediatrics to adults, using the Telemed® Analysis algorithm; 12-channel monitoring, storage, review and serial comparison of ECG waveforms and measurements; lead-off detection; local or network database, archive and email capabilities; printed reports on plain paper; and a weight of 11 oz., with no moving parts.

Nasiff Assoc., Inc. 315-676-2346
841 County Route 37 # 1, Central Square, NY 13036
Cardio-card.

Omni Medical Supply Inc. 800-860-6664
4153 Pioneer Dr, Commerce Township, MI 48390

Pace Tech, Inc. 800-722-3024
510 N Garden Ave, Clearwater, FL 33755

ANALYZER, ELECTRICAL SAFETY *(General) 80QSF*

Bender, Inc. 800-356-4266
700 Fox Chase, Highlands Corp. Center, Coatesville, PA 19320
UNIMET 1100 tests according to IEC 607.7 (European Standards), microprocessor based with PCMCIA card to upload the lastest standards.

Fluke Biomedical 800-648-7952
6920 Seaway Blvd, Everett, WA 98203
5 models-from $895 to $5,500.00. Models vary with (&) calibration feature, external voltmeter, automatic patient lead sequencing.

ANALYZER, ELECTRICAL SAFETY *(cont'd)*

Krohn-Hite Corporation 877-549-7781
15 Jonathan Dr Ste 4, Brockton, MA 02301
Measures/records watts, volts, amps, cos angle, K Var, K Varh. Resistance calibrators. Also, standards for true passive resistance and electricity, AC/DC/voltage/current.

Netech, Corp. 800-547-6557
110 Toledo St, Farmingdale, NY 11735
A series of electrical safety analyzers is available with different features for various medical requirements. The LKG 601 is a basic analyzer designed for non-ECG medical equipment. The LKG 2000 has 5 patient leads and the new LKG 610 is a full function analyzer with 10 patient leads. The MULTIPRO 2000 is a comprehensive tester with some automatic functions and a built- in 12 lead ECG/arrhythmia/performance waveform simulator. Each model is complete with a carrying case, manual, test cable, and NIST Certificate of Calibration.

ANALYZER, ELECTROSURGICAL UNIT *(Surgery) 79QTT*

Fluke Biomedical 800-648-7952
6920 Seaway Blvd, Everett, WA 98203
2 models - output tester & RF measurement analyzer incl. digital display, watts, RF current.

ANALYZER, ETHYLENE-OXIDE *(General) 80QUR*

Advanced Chemical Sensors Inc. 561-338-3116
3201 N Dixie Hwy Ste 3, Boca Raton, FL 33431
Electronic instruments and monitoring badges. Electronic instruments provide real time measurement and alarm with data logging capability. Monitoring badges provide a written record from an independent laboratory.

Cea Instruments, Inc. 888-893-9640
16 Chestnut St, Emerson, NJ 07630

Enmet Corp. 734-761-1270
PO Box 979, Ann Arbor, MI 48106
Solid state, semiconductor.

Guided Wave Inc. 916-939-4300
5190 Golden Foothill Pkwy, El Dorado Hills, CA 95762
NIR Analyzer for Ethylene Oxide. 412 L model.

Interscan Corp. 800-458-6153
21700 Nordhoff St, P.O. Box 2496, Chatsworth, CA 91311
$1,990.00 ea. for portable survey units, and $2750.00 and up for fixed systems. Full data acquisition/archiving/reporting system available.

Kem Medical Products Corp. 800-553-0330
75 Price Pkwy, Farmingdale, NY 11735
EO-TRAK Passive diffusion monitoring badges for ethylene oxide gas, and VAPOR-TRAL toxic gas monitors for formaldehyde, xylene, and nitrous oxide.

ANALYZER, GAIT *(Orthopedics) 87VDV*

Advanced Mechanical Technology, Inc. (Amti) 800-422-AMTI
176 Waltham St, Watertown, MA 02472
Gait and Balance analysis software, bio electronics data acquisition software.

Minisun, Llc 559-439-4600
935 E Mill Creek Dr, Fresno, CA 93720
Portable Gait Analyzer, size of a pager, low cost. Measures all major gait parameters automatically, anywhere, anytime (from a few steps to multiple days).

Pedifix, Inc. 800-424-5561
310 Guinea Rd, Brewster, NY 10509
ORTHOPRINT.

Tekscan, Inc. 800-248-3669
307 W 1st St, South Boston, MA 02127
F-SCAN or F-SCAN Mobile, computerized gait analysis system, insole system. MATSCAN or HR (High-Resolution) MAT, computerized gait analysis system, pressure mapping floor mat.

ANALYZER, GAS, ANESTHETIC *(Anesthesiology) 73QZE*

Andros, Inc. 510-837-3500
870 Harbour Way S, Richmond, CA 94804
Unit measures level of halogenated anesthetic gases (used in surgery) as well as CO2 and N2O. The Model 4800 will, in addition, identify and measure ethanol and identify acetone.

Aspect Medical Systems, Inc. 617-559-7000
141 Needham St, Newton, MA 02464
BIS Bispectral Index directly measures effects of anesthesia on the conscious state of patients.

ANALYZER, GAS, ARGON, GASEOUS PHASE
(Anesthesiology) 73JEG

Ge Medical Systems Information Technologies 800-643-6439
8200 W Tower Ave, Milwaukee, WI 53223
MGA-1100 Mass Spectrometer. Capable of simultaneously measuring up to 8 gas channels within a dynamic range of 2 to 120 atomic mass units (AMU). Configurability of the MGA-1000 allows for use in many applications such as pulmonary functions, stress testing, anesthesia, ICU, CCU, hyperbaric studies, and veterinarian clinics. Complete self-contained, cost depending upon options selected. The MGA-1100 utilizes a fixed magnetic sector analyzer. RAMS Quadrupole Mass Spectrometer. Capable of simultaneous measuring of up to 10 gas channels within a dynamic range of 1-250 AMU. This unit is configurable and allows for use in many applications such as anesthesia, stress testing, pulmonary function, hyperbaric studies and research applications. The unit is software controlled and can be reprogrammed to measure new gases for different applications.

Industrial Welding Supplies Of Hattiesburg, Inc. 601-545-1800
1924 Byron St, Hattiesburg, MS 39402
Clinical blood gas mixtures.

ANALYZER, GAS, CARBON-DIOXIDE, BLOOD PHASE, INDWELLING *(Anesthesiology) 73CCC*

Ge Medical Systems Information Technologies 800-643-6439
8200 W Tower Ave, Milwaukee, WI 53223

Maine Oxy-Acetylene Supply Co. 207-784-5788
22 Albiston Way, Auburn, ME 04210
Various mixtures.

Spec Connection Intl Inc. 813-618-0400
34310 State Road 54, Zephyrhills, FL 33543
Lung diffusion.

ANALYZER, GAS, CARBON-DIOXIDE, GASEOUS PHASE (CAPNOGRAPH) *(Anesthesiology) 73CCK*

Advanced Chemical Sensors Inc. 561-338-3116
3201 N Dixie Hwy Ste 3, Boca Raton, FL 33431
Electronic instruments that provide real time measurement and alarm with data logging capability.

Aei Technologies Inc. 630-548-3545
300 William Pitt Way, Pittsburgh, PA 15238
Carbon dioxide analyzer.

Andros, Inc. 510-837-3500
870 Harbour Way S, Richmond, CA 94804
Continuous monitor of CO2, N2O and O2 levels (used in surgery). On-airway CO2 analyzer.

Draeger Medical Systems, Inc. 215-660-2626
16 Electronics Ave, Danvers, MA 01923
Et c02 module.

Fukuda Denshi Usa, Inc. 800-365-6668
17725 NE 65th St Ste C, Redmond, WA 98052
Analyzer, gas, carbon-dioxide, gaseous-phase.

Ge Medical Systems Information Technologies 800-643-6439
8200 W Tower Ave, Milwaukee, WI 53223
SAM Module (multigas) infrared monitor which utilizes the near- and mid-band infrared analysis of anesthetic agents. Carbon dioxide, nitrous oxide, and oxygen paramagnetic. This module is an accessory for the Tramscope and Solar vital-signs-monitoring products.

Invivo Corporation 425-487-7000
12601 Research Pkwy, Orlando, FL 32826
Side-stream end-tidal co2 monitor.

Lifegas Llc 866-543-3427
1500 Indian Trail Lilburn Rd, Norcross, GA 30093

LumaSense Technologies Inc. 408-727-1600
3301 Leonard Ct, Santa Clara, CA 95054
Andros Analyzers Airway Adapter

Oridion Medical Inc. 888-674-3466
140 Towne& Country Drive, SuiteB, Danville, CA 94526
MEDICO2 OEM capnography module measures inspired/expired carbon dioxide and respiratory rate via serial/digital interface. MICROCAP portable capnograph continuously measures end tidal carbon dioxide and respiratory rate. MICROSTREAM CO2 Circuits separate liquids and vapor from the breath sample maintaining accurate real time readings and waveforms. VitalCap capnograph interfaces with HP central monitoring systems.

ANALYZER, GAS, CARBON-DIOXIDE, GASEOUS PHASE (CAPNOGRAPH) *(cont'd)*

Pace Tech, Inc. 800-722-3024
510 N Garden Ave, Clearwater, FL 33755
VITALMAX 4000-C. $8995 to $10,495. ECG/capnometer w/NIBP, temp., resp. and pulse oximeter - EL display - optional strip chart recorder.

Promedic, Inc. 239-498-2155
3460 Pointe Creek Ct Apt 102, Bonita Springs, FL 34134
Gas-sampling catheter for obtaining a high-quality end-tidal sample for pediatric anesthesia.

Respironics California, Inc. 724-387-4559
2271 Cosmos Ct, Carlsbad, CA 92011
Tidalwave monitor.

Respironics Novametrix, Llc. 724-387-4559
5 Technology Dr, Wallingford, CT 06492
Tidalwave monitor.

Smiths Medical Asd, Inc. 610-578-9600
9255 Customhouse Plz Ste N, San Diego, CA 92154
Gas sampling lines,connectors and gas sampling filters.(accessories for gas anal.

Smiths Medical Pm, Inc. 800-558-2345
N7W22025 Johnson Dr, Waukesha, WI 53186
Capnocheck Plus, stand-alone, bedside or transportable capnograph with optional pulse oximetry and FiO2. The Capnocheck Sleep Capnograph/Oximeter, designed specifically for sleep screening and lab-based sleep studies, provides reliable measurements of CO2 and SpO2 in one unit.

Spacelabs Healthcare 800-522-7025
5150 220th Ave SE, Issaquah, WA 98029
Ultraview SL Capnograph Module

Spacelabs Medical Inc. 800-522-7212
5150 220th Ave SE, Issaquah, WA 98029
Multigas analyzers and accessories.

Treymed, Inc. 262-820-1294
N56W24790 N Corporate Cir Ste C, Sussex, WI 53089
Capnograph.

Vacumed 800-235-3333
4538 Westinghouse St, Ventura, CA 93003
Oxygen Analyzer, 'Gold Edition', precision side-stream, paramagnetic, with pump and nafion gas dryer. Has digital display and analog output.

Welch Allyn Protocol Inc. 800-289-2500
8500 SW Creekside Pl, Beaverton, OR 97008
CO2 monitor.

ANALYZER, GAS, CARBON-DIOXIDE, PARTIAL PRESSURE, BLOOD *(Anesthesiology) 73BXZ*

Ge Medical Systems Information Technologies 800-643-6439
8200 W Tower Ave, Milwaukee, WI 53223

Radiometer America, Inc. 800-736-0600
810 Sharon Dr, Westlake, OH 44145
ABL pH, pCO2, pO2 on micro or macro samples.

Respironics, Inc 800-345-6443
1010 Murry Ridge Ln, Murrysville, PA 15668
CO2SMO is a combined mainstream capnograph/pulse oximeter. CAPNOGARD is mainstream capnograph. Both monitors utilize the capnostat III solid state, mainstream CO2 sensor.

ANALYZER, GAS, CARBON-MONOXIDE, GASEOUS PHASE
(Anesthesiology) 73CCJ

Advanced Chemical Sensors Inc. 561-338-3116
3201 N Dixie Hwy Ste 3, Boca Raton, FL 33431
Electronic instruments that provide real time measurement and alarm with data logging capability.

Aim Safe Air Products Ltd. 604-244-7272
170-13151 Vanier Pl, Richmond V6V 2J1 Canada
Carbon monoxide monitor

Breathe E-Z Systems, Inc. 800-490-5061
12702 Cherokee Ln, Leawood, KS 66209
Carbon monoxide moniter.

Draeger Safety, Inc. 800-922-5518
101 Technology Dr, Pittsburgh, PA 15275

ANALYZER, GAS, CARBON-MONOXIDE, GASEOUS PHASE
(cont'd)

Ge Medical Systems Information Technologies 800-643-6439
8200 W Tower Ave, Milwaukee, WI 53223
MGA-1100 medical mass spectrometer, capable of simultaneous measurement of 8 gas channels within a dynamic range of 2-135 atomic mass units (AMU). Configurability of the MGA-1100 allows for use in many applications such as pulmonary function, stress testing, anesthesia, ICU/CCU, hyperbaric studies and veterinary clinics. Completely self-contained and portable. Cost per unit depends on options selected.

Industrial Welding Supplies Of Hattiesburg, Inc. 601-545-1800
1924 Byron St, Hattiesburg, MS 39402
Lung diffusion gas mixtures.

Natus Medical Inc. 800-255-3901
1501 Industrial Rd, San Carlos, CA 94070
CO-STAT End Tidal Breath Analyzer passively and non-invasively measures end tidal carbon-monoxide concentration corrected for background carbon monoxide (ETCOc) as an indicator of bilirubin production and hemolysis. It also provides end tidal carbon-dioxide concentration and respiratory rate.

Vitalograph, Inc. 800-255-6626
13310 W 99th St, Lenexa, KS 66215
$1,050.00 for BREATHCO, expired CO for smoking cessation and fire victims.

ANALYZER, GAS, CARBOXYHEMOGLOBIN, BLOOD PHASE, NON-INDW. *(Toxicology) 91CCA*

Radiometer America, Inc. 800-736-0600
810 Sharon Dr, Westlake, OH 44145
OSM3.

ANALYZER, GAS, ENFLURANE, GASEOUS PHASE (ANESTHETIC CONC.) *(Anesthesiology) 73CBQ*

Baxter Healthcare Corporation, Baxter Pharmaceuticals And Technologies 800-667-0959
95 Spring St, New Providence, NJ 07974

Pace Tech, Inc. 800-722-3024
510 N Garden Ave, Clearwater, FL 33755
$12,495-13.995 for Vitalmax 4100-G. Anesthetic agent monitor.

ANALYZER, GAS, HALOTHANE, GASEOUS PHASE (ANESTHETIC CONC.) *(Anesthesiology) 73CBS*

Criticare Systems, Inc. 262-798-5361
20925 Crossroads Cir, Waukesha, WI 53186
Various models.

Ge Medical Systems Information Technologies 800-643-6439
8200 W Tower Ave, Milwaukee, WI 53223
SAM Module, (multigas), infrared monitor which utilizes the near- and mid-band infrared analysis of anesthetic agents. Carbon dioxide, nitrous oxide, and oxygen paramagnetic. This module is an accessory for the Tramscope and Solar vital signs monitoring products. MGA-1100 Mass Spectrometer is cable of simultaneously measuring up to 8 gas channels within a dynamic range of 2 to 120 atomic mass units (AMU). Configurability of the MGA-1100 allows for use in many applications such as pulmonary functions, stress testing, anesthesia, ICU, CCU, hyperbaric studies, and veterinarian clinics. Complete self-contained, cost depending upon options selected. The MGA-1100 uses a fixed magnetic-sector analyzer. RAMS Quadrupole Mass Spectrometer is capable of simultaneous measuring of up to 10 gas channels within a dynamic range of 1-250 AMU. This unit is configurable and allows for use in many applications such as anesthesia, stress testing, pulmonary function, hyperbaric studies, and research applications. The unit is software controlled and can be reprogrammed to measure new gases for different applications.

Pace Tech, Inc. 800-722-3024
510 N Garden Ave, Clearwater, FL 33755
VITALMAX 4100-G. $12,495-13,995. ECG/anesthetic agent monitor/capnometer w/NIBP, temp., resp., and pulse oximeter.

ANALYZER, GAS, HELIUM, GASEOUS PHASE
(Anesthesiology) 73BSE

Ge Medical Systems Information Technologies 800-643-6439
8200 W Tower Ave, Milwaukee, WI 53223
MGA-1100 Mass Spectrometer, capable of simultaneous measuring up to 8 gas channels within a dynamic range of 2-120 atomic mass units (AMU). Configurability of the MGA-1100 allows for use in many applications such as pulmonary function, stress testing, anesthesia, ICU/CCU, hyperbaric studies and veterinary clinics. Complete self-contained, cost depending upon options selected. A fixed magnetic-sector analyzer. RAMS Quadrupole Mass Spectrometer, capable of simultaneous measuring of up to 10 gas channels within a dynamic range of 1-250 AMU. This unit is configurable and allows for use in many applications such as anesthesia, stress testing, pulmonary function, hyperbaric studies, and research applications. The unit is software controlled and can be reprogrammed to measure new gases for different applications.

Lifegas Llc 866-543-3427
1500 Indian Trail Lilburn Rd, Norcross, GA 30093

Ulvac Technologies, Inc. 800-998-5822
401 Griffin Brook Dr, Methuen, MA 01844
Portable helium leak detectors.

ANALYZER, GAS, HYDROGEN *(Anesthesiology) 73LXO*

Breathe E-Z Systems, Inc. 800-490-5061
12702 Cherokee Ln, Leawood, KS 66209
Hydrogen breath moniter.

ANALYZER, GAS, NEON, GASEOUS PHASE
(Anesthesiology) 73JEF

Ge Medical Systems Information Technologies 800-643-6439
8200 W Tower Ave, Milwaukee, WI 53223

ANALYZER, GAS, NITROGEN, GASEOUS PHASE
(Anesthesiology) 73CCI

Ge Medical Systems Information Technologies 800-643-6439
8200 W Tower Ave, Milwaukee, WI 53223
MGA-1100 Mass Spectrometer, capable of simultaneous measurement of 8 gas channels within a dynamic range of 2-120 atomic mass units (AMU). Configurability of the MGA-1100 allows for use in many applications such as pulmonary function, stress testing, anesthesia, ICU/CCU, hyperbaric studies and veterinary clinics. Complete self-contained, cost depending upon options selected. A fixed magnetic sector analyzer. RAMS Quadrupole Mass Spectrometer, capable of simultaneous measuring of up to 10 gas channels within a dynamic range of 1-250 AMU. This unit is configurable and allows for use in many applications such as anesthesia, stress testing, pulmonary function, hyperbaric studies, and research applications. The unit is software controlled and can be reprogrammed to measure new gases for different applications.

ANALYZER, GAS, NITROUS-OXIDE, GASEOUS PHASE
(Anesthesiology) 73CBR

Advanced Chemical Sensors Inc. 561-338-3116
3201 N Dixie Hwy Ste 3, Boca Raton, FL 33431
Electronic instruments and monitoring badges. Electronic instruments provide real time measurement and alarm with data logging capability. Monitoring badges provide a written record from an independent laboratory.

Andros, Inc. 510-837-3500
870 Harbour Way S, Richmond, CA 94804
Continuous monitor of N2, CO2, and O2 levels (used in surgery).

Cea Instruments, Inc. 888-893-9640
16 Chestnut St, Emerson, NJ 07630
TG-KA Series, portable and AC powered gas monitors available for formaldehyde or glutaraldehyde. CEA 266, Nitrous Oxide Infrared Monitor, available for 0-5% up to 0-100% monitoring of nitrous oxide.

Invivo Corporation 425-487-7000
12601 Research Pkwy, Orlando, FL 32826
Side-stream mean n20 monitor.

Pace Tech, Inc. 800-722-3024
510 N Garden Ave, Clearwater, FL 33755
VITALMAX 4100-CN. $9,495-10,995. ECG/capnometer w/NIBP, temp, resp and pulse oximeter - EL display.

Spacelabs Healthcare 800-522-7025
5150 220th Ave SE, Issaquah, WA 98029
Ultraview SL Multigas Analyzer

Spacelabs Medical Inc. 800-522-7212
5150 220th Ave SE, Issaquah, WA 98029
Multigas analyzers and accessories.

ANALYZER, GAS, OXYGEN, CONTINUOUS CONTROLLER
(Anesthesiology) 73RJI

Maxtec, Inc. 800-748-5355
6526 Cottonwood St, Salt Lake City, UT 84107
OXY threshold monitor to protect against failure of oxygen concentrators.

ANALYZER, GAS, OXYGEN, CONTINUOUS MONITOR
(Anesthesiology) 73RJJ

Datascope Corp. 800-288-2121
14 Philips Pkwy, Montvale, NJ 07645
Gas Module II gas analysis monitor featuring CO2, N2O, fst O2 and 5 agent analysis.

Datex-Ohmeda (Canada) 800-268-1472
1093 Meyerside Dr., Unit 2, Mississauga, ONT L5T-1J6 Canada

Maxtec, Inc. 800-748-5355
6526 Cottonwood St, Salt Lake City, UT 84107
MAXO2(OM-25 Series) Oxygen analyzers and monitor for homecare and hospital use. Also available is the HANDI ultra-lightweight compact oxygen analyzer.

Respironics Georgia, Inc. 724-387-4559
175 Chastain Meadows Ct NW, Kennesaw, GA 30144
Oximeters.

Vascular Technology Incorporated 800-550-0856
12 Murphy Dr, Nashua, NH 03062
VTI oxygen analyzer/monitor.

ANALYZER, GAS, OXYGEN, GASEOUS PHASE
(Anesthesiology) 73CCL

Advanced Chemical Sensors Inc. 561-338-3116
3201 N Dixie Hwy Ste 3, Boca Raton, FL 33431
Electronic instruments that provide real time measurement and alarm with data logging capability.

Aei Technologies Inc. 630-548-3545
300 William Pitt Way, Pittsburgh, PA 15238
Oxygen analyzer.

Analytical Industries, Inc. 909-392-6900
2855 Metropolitan Pl, Pomona, CA 91767
Electrochemical oxygen gas sensor--percent oxygen analyzer. An electrochemical transducer specific to oxygen that generates current output proportional to the oxygen concentration present in the gas stream sampled.

Draeger Medical Systems, Inc. 215-660-2626
16 Electronics Ave, Danvers, MA 01923
Monitor.

Keene Medical Products, Inc. 603-448-5290
240 Meriden Rd, Lebanon, NH 03766
Oxygen medical gas.

Mercury Medical 800-237-6418
11300 49th St N, Clearwater, FL 33762
Replacement oxygen sensors.

O2 Technologies, Inc. 804-897-8555
11341 Business Center Dr Ste C, Richmond, VA 23236
Oxygen indicator.

Oxigraf, Inc. 650-237-0155
1170 Terra Bella Ave, Mountain View, CA 94043
Oxygen gas analyzer.

Pace Tech, Inc. 800-722-3024
510 N Garden Ave, Clearwater, FL 33755
$12,495-13,995 for Vitalmax 4100G. Non-invasive, oxygen.

Respironics Novametrix, Llc. 724-387-4559
5 Technology Dr, Wallingford, CT 06492
Oxicheck.

Salter Labs 805-854-3166
220 W C St, Tehachapi, CA 93561
Oxygen gas analyzer.

Spacelabs Healthcare 800-522-7025
5150 220th Ave SE, Issaquah, WA 98029
Ultraview SL Capnograph Module

Spacelabs Medical Inc. 800-522-7212
5150 220th Ave SE, Issaquah, WA 98029
Multigas analyzers and accessories.

Teledyne Analytical Instruments 888-789-8168
16830 Chestnut St, City Of Industry, CA 91748
MDL AX 300, MX 300

ANALYZER, GAS, OXYGEN, GASEOUS PHASE *(cont'd)*

Vacumed 800-235-3333
4538 Westinghouse St, Ventura, CA 93003
CO2 Analyzer, 'Gold Edition' carbon dioxide analyzer, precision side-stream, infrared type, with pump and nafion dryer. Has digital display and analog output of both normal and end-tidal CO2.

Vascular Technology Incorporated 800-550-0856
12 Murphy Dr, Nashua, NH 03062
VTI-200, oxygen analyzer.

ANALYZER, GAS, OXYGEN, PARTIAL PR., BLOOD PHASE, INDWELLING *(Anesthesiology) 73CCE*

Respironics California, Inc. 724-387-4559
2271 Cosmos Ct, Carlsbad, CA 92011
Transcutaneous monitor.

Respironics Novametrix, Llc. 724-387-4559
5 Technology Dr, Wallingford, CT 06492
Transcutaneous monitor.

Terumo Cardiovascular Systems (Tcvs) 714-258-8001
1311 Valencia Ave, Tustin, CA 92780
Intravascular blood gas monitoring system.

ANALYZER, GAS, OXYGEN, PARTIAL PRESSURE, BLOOD PHASE *(Anesthesiology) 73CCD*

Ge Medical Systems Information Technologies 800-643-6439
8200 W Tower Ave, Milwaukee, WI 53223

Radiometer America, Inc. 800-736-0600
810 Sharon Dr, Westlake, OH 44145
ABL pH, pCO2, pO2 on micro samples.

Respironics, Inc 800-345-6443
1010 Murry Ridge Ln, Murrysville, PA 15668
The model 840 provides continuous display of O2 and CO2. The 840 can utilize a dual O2/CO2 or single O0 or CO2 sensor.

Tcs Scientific Corp. 215-862-3910
6467 Stoney Hill Rd, New Hope, PA 18938
HEMOX-ANALYZER, model B from $20,300.00. Blood Oxygen Equilibrium analyzer for plotting the physiological important assocation curve and the p50 value.

ANALYZER, GAS, OXYGEN, SAMPLING *(Anesthesiology) 73RJK*

Airsep Corp. 800-874-0202
401 Creekside Dr, Amherst, NY 14228

Myco Instrumentation Source, Inc. 425-228-4239
PO Box 354, Renton, WA 98057

Spectron Corp. 425-827-9317
934 S Burlington Blvd # 603, Burlington, WA 98233
Reconditioned equipment.

ANALYZER, GAS, SEVOFLURANE, GASEOUS-PHASE (ANESTHETIC CONCENTRATION) *(Anesthesiology) 73NHP*

Draeger Medical Systems, Inc. 215-660-2626
16 Electronics Ave, Danvers, MA 01923
Gas monitor.

ANALYZER, GAS, WATER VAPOR, GASEOUS PHASE
(Anesthesiology) 73BXA

Ge Medical Systems Information Technologies 800-643-6439
8200 W Tower Ave, Milwaukee, WI 53223
MGA-1100 Mass Spectrometer, capable of simultaneously measuring up to 8 gas channels within a dynamic range of 2 to 120 atomic mass units (AMU). Configurability of the MGA-1100 allows for use in many applications such as pulmonary functions, stress testing, anesthesia, ICU/CCU, hyperbaric studies, and veterinarian clinics. Complete self-contained, cost depending upon options selected. The MGA-1100 utilizes a fixed magnetic sector analyzer. RAMS Quadrupole Mass Spectrometer, capable of simultaneous measuring of up to 10 gas channels within a dynamic range of 1-250 AMU. This unit is configurable and allows for use in many applications such as anesthesia, stress testing, pulmonary function, hyperbaric studies, and research applications. The unit is software controlled and can be reprogrammed to measure new gases for different applications.

ANALYZER, GLUCOSE *(Chemistry) 75QYL*

Beckman Coulter, Inc. 800-742-2345
250 S Kraemer Blvd, PO Box 8000, Brea, CA 92821

ANALYZER, GLUCOSE *(cont'd)*
Nova Biomedical 800-458-5813
200 Prospect St, Waltham, MA 02453
Analyzers, Glucose. STATSTRIP Point-of-Care Glucose Monitoring System. Patented Multi-Well measuring technology eliminates interferences from hematocrit, maltose, oxygen, acetominophen, ascorbic acid, uric acid. Eliminates calibration codes. Results in 6 seconds. Uses only 1.2 microliters of sample. Accepts capillary, venous, arterial samples. Advanced meter has color touch screen, provides flexible POC control, facilitates hospital-wide connectivity.

ANALYZER, HEPARIN, AUTOMATED *(Hematology) 81JOX*
Medtronic Blood Management 612-514-4000
18501 E Plaza Dr, Parker, CO 80134
Invitro diagnostic heparin analyzer & controls.

Medtronic Perfusion Systems 800-328-3320
7611 Northland Dr N, Brooklyn Park, MN 55428
3 models - $3,400.00 to $11,500.00; for use in operating room, recovery room, or clinical lab. $7,500.00 for unit reading circulating heparin level optically.

ANALYZER, INFUSION PUMP *(General) 80VLP*
Fluke Biomedical 800-648-7952
6920 Seaway Blvd, Everett, WA 98203
Battery powered, digital display, multi-range pressure analyzer. 1 to 4 simultaneous channels.

Medved Products, Inc. 651-482-8413
PO Box 120883, Saint Paul, MN 55112
Infusion Pump Cage Mount, pump hanger for use with veterinary animal cages.

ANALYZER, ION, HYDROGEN-ION (PH), BLOOD PHASE, INDWELLING *(Anesthesiology) 73CBZ*
Terumo Cardiovascular Systems (Tcvs) 714-258-8001
1311 Valencia Ave, Tustin, CA 92780
Indwelling ph monitor.

ANALYZER, ION, HYDROGEN-ION PH, BLOOD PHASE, NON-INDWELLING *(Anesthesiology) 73CBY*
Radiometer America, Inc. 800-736-0600
810 Sharon Dr, Westlake, OH 44145
ABL pH, pCO2, pO2 on micro samples; some models also measure blood oximetry (co-ox) parameters.

Waters Corp. 800-252-4752
34 Maple St, Milford, MA 01757

ANALYZER, KARYOTYPE *(Pathology) 88JCZ*
Illumina, Inc. 1.800.809.4566
9885 Towne Centre Dr, San Diego, CA 92121
HiScanSQ

Koaman International 909-983-4888
656 E D St, Ontario, CA 91764

Vysis 800-553-7042
3100 Woodcreek Dr, Downers Grove, IL 60515
QUIPS KARYOTYPE.

ANALYZER, LEAD *(General) 80REO*
Esa, Inc. 800-959-5095
22 Alpha Rd, Chelmsford, MA 01824

ANALYZER, MEDICAL IMAGE *(Radiology) 90MYN*
Hologic|r2, Inc 866-243-2533
2585 Augustine Dr, Santa Clara, CA 95054
Imagechecker.

Icad Inc. 866-280-2239
98 Spit Brook Rd Ste 100, Nashua, NH 03062
Computer-aided detection system.

Proven Process Medical Devices, Inc. 508-261-0806
110 Forbes Blvd, Mansfield, MA 02048
Computer-aided detection system.

Riverain Medical Group 800-990-3387
3020 S Tech Blvd, Miamisburg, OH 45342
Computer aided detection systems (cad).

ANALYZER, MERCURY *(Chemistry) 75WMX*
Advanced Chemical Sensors Inc. 561-338-3116
3201 N Dixie Hwy Ste 3, Boca Raton, FL 33431
Monitoring badges for a written record from an independent laboratory.

Buck Scientific, Inc. 800-562-5566
58 Fort Point St, Norwalk, CT 06855
Buck 400. Complete system; manual operation.

ANALYZER, MERCURY *(cont'd)*
Thermo - Industrial Hygiene Division 508-520-0430
27 Forge Pkwy, Franklin, MA 02038

ANALYZER, METABOLISM *(Anesthesiology) 73QCP*
Cardinal Health 207, Inc. 800-231-2466
22745 Savi Ranch Pkwy, Yorba Linda, CA 92887
$20,000-$60,000 for metabolic measurement system incl. mixing chamber & BXB analysis. $30,000-$60,000 for metabolic stress testing analyzer and measures expired gas during exercise.

Equilibrated Bio Systems, Inc. 800-327-9490
22 Lawrence Ave Ste LL2, Smithtown, NY 11787

Phipps & Bird, Inc. 800-955-7621
1519 Summit Ave, Richmond, VA 23230
Small animal metabolism apparatus for student education.

Vacumed 800-235-3333
4538 Westinghouse St, Ventura, CA 93003
O2 consumption, etc.

ANALYZER, MIDDLE EAR *(Ear/Nose/Throat) 77RGY*
Md International, Inc. 305-669-9003
11300 NW 41st St, Doral, FL 33178

Micro Audiometrics Corp. 800-729-9509
655 Keller Rd, Murphy, NC 28906
$1,695.00-$2,395.00 for EARSCAN impedance microprocessor audiometer.

Tsi Medical Ltd. 800-661-7263
47 Athabascan Ave., Unit 105, Sherwood Park, AB T8A-4H3 Canada

Welch Allyn, Inc. 800-535-6663
4341 State Street Rd, Skaneateles Falls, NY 13153

ANALYZER, MOTILITY, GASTROINTESTINAL, ELECTRICAL *(Gastro/Urology) 78FFX*
Cook Endoscopy 336-744-0157
4900 Bethania Station Rd # &, 5951 Grassy Creek Blvd. Winston Salem, NC 27105
Various gastrointestinal motility catheters.

Imsi, Integrated Modular Systems Inc. 800-220-9729
2500 W Township Line Rd, PO Box 616, Havertown, PA 19083
RADIN GI Image Viewing. Full Functionality. Very Cost Effective Licensing.

Konsyl Pharmaceuticals, Inc. 800-356-6795
8050 Industrial Park Rd, Easton, MD 21601
Radiopaque markers.

Medtronic Neuromodulation 763-514-4000
710 Medtronic Pkwy, Minneapolis, MN 55432
Various types of gastrointestinal motility systems (electrical).

Sandhill Scientific, Inc. 800-468-4556
9150 Commerce Center Cir Ste 500, Highlands Ranch, CO 80129
Small bowel, biliary and anal-rectal motility analyzers.

Sierra Scientific Instruments, Inc. 310-641-8492
5757 W Century Blvd Ste 660, Los Angeles, CA 90045
Gastrointestional manometry system.

Unisensor Usa, Inc. 603-926-5200
1 Park Ave Ste 6, Hampton, NH 03842
Catheter pressure transducer.

ANALYZER, MOTION *(General) 80WWG*
Advanced Mechanical Technology, Inc. (Amti) 800-422-AMTI
176 Waltham St, Watertown, MA 02472
Hip/Knee Simulator Wear Tester - Simulate loading/motion of hip and knee joints - osteolysis studies.

Biodex Medical Systems, Inc. 800-224-6339
20 Ramsey Rd, Shirley, NY 11967
BIODEX Balance System SD, assesses dynamic postural stability on an unstable surface by measuring degree of angle from 0 degrees center. $9,995.

Brytech Inc. 613-731-5800
600 Peter Morand Crescent, Suite 240, Ottawa, ONT K1G-5Z3 Canada
Personal alarm transmitter: detects motion and movement using optical based sensors; home health care.

Dynatronics Corp. 800-874-6251
7030 Park Centre Dr, Salt Lake City, UT 84121
DYNATRON EQUALIZER Posture analyzer.

Myotronics-Noromed, Inc. 206-243-4214
5870 S 194th St, Kent, WA 98032
NOROTRACK 360 Range of Motion System. Records real time motion of spine and extremities rapidly and accurately.

ANALYZER, OVERNIGHT MICROORGANISM I.D. SYSTEM, AUTOMATED *(Microbiology) 83LRH*

Dade Behring, Inc. 800-948-3233
1717 Deerfield Rd, Deerfield, IL 60015
WalkAway system; AutoSCAN-4 system.

ANALYZER, OVERNIGHT SUSCEPT. SYSTEM, AUTOMATED *(Microbiology) 83LRG*

Trek Diagnostic Systems 800-871-8909
982 Keynote Cir Ste 6, Cleveland, OH 44131

ANALYZER, OXYHEMOGLOBIN CONCENTRATION, BLOOD PHASE, INDWELL. *(Anesthesiology) 73JED*

Maine Oxy-Acetylene Supply Co. 207-784-5788
22 Albiston Way, Auburn, ME 04210
Various mixtures.

ANALYZER, PACEMAKER GENERATOR FUNCTION *(Cardiovascular) 74DTC*

Biotek Instruments, Inc. 802-655-4040
100 Tigan St, Highland Park, Winooski, VT 05404
Same.

Cardiac Pacemakers, Inc. 800-227-3422
4100 Hamline Ave N, P.O. Box 64079, Saint Paul, MN 55112

Ela Medical, Inc. 800-352-6466
2950 Xenium Ln N, Plymouth, MN 55441
SCE 22.

Meridian Medical Technologies 800-638-8093
10240 Old Columbia Rd, Columbia, MD 21046
CARDIOBEEPER ECG transmitter.

Oscor, Inc. 800-726-7267
3816 Desoto Blvd, Palm Harbor, FL 34683
Pacemaker system analyzer.

Pace Medical, Inc. 781-890-5656
391 Totten Pond Rd, Waltham, MA 02451
Pacing system analyzer, dual chamber modes AOO, AAI, VOO, VVI, DOO, DVI, DDD.

ANALYZER, PACEMAKER GENERATOR FUNCTION, INDIRECT *(Cardiovascular) 74KRE*

Instromedix, A Card Guard Co. 800-633-3361
10255 W Higgins Rd Ste 100, Rosemont, IL 60018

Medtronic Inc, Paceart 763-514-4000
4265 Lexington Ave N, Arden Hills, MN 55126
Pacemaker analyzer and 12 lead electrode.

Omni Medical Supply Inc. 800-860-6664
4153 Pioneer Dr, Commerce Township, MI 48390

ANALYZER, PARASITE CONCENTRATION *(Microbiology) 83LKS*

Hardy Diagnostics 800-226-2222
1430 W McCoy Ln, Santa Maria, CA 93455
ParaKit Fecal Concentration Kit.

Meridian Bioscience, Inc. 800-696-0739
3471 River Hills Dr, Cincinnati, OH 45244
MACRO CON and CON-TRATE For the concentration of eggs, larvae and protozoa from preserved fecal specimens.

Para Scientific, Inc. 503-636-4121
17170 Wall St, Lake Oswego, OR 97034
Parasite concentration kit.

United Biotech, Inc. 650-961-2910
211 S Whisman Rd Ste E, Mountain View, CA 94041
ELISAs detecting: Chagas, Cysticercosis, Leishmania

ANALYZER, PARTICLE *(Chemistry) 75UHB*

Beckman Coulter, Inc. 800-635-3497
740 W 83rd St, Hialeah, FL 33014
Particle size analyzers and counters available.

Matec Instrument Companies, Inc. 508-393-0155
56 Hudson St, Northborough, MA 01532
Zeta Potential analyzers. Ultrasonic Test Equipment.

Quantachrome 800-989-2476
1900 Corporate Dr, Boynton Beach, FL 33426
Laser diffraction analyzer that measures particles from 500 micrometers down to 0.1 micrometers. Also available particle characterization instruments.

ANALYZER, PARTICLE *(cont'd)*

Tsi Incorporated 800-874-2811
500 Cardigan Rd, Shoreview, MN 55126
The PSD 3603 Particle Size Distribution Analyzer is a high-speed, easy-to-use instrument that gives you high-resolution aerodynamic size measurments of dry powders in the range from 0.3 to 500 micrometers, and medical aerosols from 0.3 to 700 micrometers. Ultraviolet Aerodynamic Particle Sizer spectrometer provides three measurements: aerodynamic size and scattered-light intensity in the range from 0.5 to 15 micrometers, as well as particle fluorescence. The instrument distinguishes biological aerosol particles from inanimate materials in real time. The Aerosol Time-of-Flight Mass Spectrometer determines size and chemical composition of individual aerosol particles in the range from 0.3 to 3 micrometers in near real time. The Aero-Flow Powder Flowability Analyzer provides an objective, quantitative measurement of powder cohesivity.

ANALYZER, PATIENT, MULTIPLE FUNCTION (SURGERY) *(Surgery) 79WTZ*

American Bio-Medical Service Corporation (Abmsc) 800-755-9055
631 W Covina Blvd, Sales,Service and Refurbishing Center
San Dimas, CA 91773

ANALYZER, PEPTIDE & PROTEIN SEQUENCE *(Chemistry) 75UHY*

Applied Biosystems 800-345-5724
850 Lincoln Centre Dr, Foster City, CA 94404
$175,000 for model 477A protein/peptide sequencing system. $92,500 for model 370A DNA sequencing system. $98,500 for model 471A protein/peptide sequencing system.

ANALYZER, PERIPHERAL VISION *(Ophthalmology) 86RKK*

Stereo Optical Co., Inc. 800-344-9500
3539 N Kenton Ave, Chicago, IL 60641

ANALYZER, PLATELET AGGREGATION *(Hematology) 81RLG*

Chrono-Log Corp. 800-247-6665
2 W Park Rd, Havertown, PA 19083
Variety of models for whole blood or PRP testing and luminescence for measuring ATP secretion, calcium and superoxides.

Payton Scientific Inc. 716-876-1813
964 Kenmore Ave, Buffalo, NY 14216
$4,500.00 for manual system single sample unit $6,000.00 for manual system dual sample unit. $7,500.00 for the dual automatic and $3,500.00 for the single automatic.

ANALYZER, PLATELET AGGREGATION, AUTOMATED *(Hematology) 81JOZ*

Accumetrics, Inc. 858-404-8247
3985 Sorrento Valley Blvd, San Diego, CA 92121
Ultegra rpfa-asa kit.

Chrono-Log Corp. 800-247-6665
2 W Park Rd, Havertown, PA 19083
Chrono-log Whole Blood Aggregometer (WBA) small low cost platelet aggregometer, with automatic zero and gain setting, for fast and accurate testing of platelet aggregation in whole blood. Available in one or two channels. Now available with disposable electrodes.

Payton Scientific Inc. 716-876-1813
964 Kenmore Ave, Buffalo, NY 14216
$10,400.00 for system with internal 10 in. recorder - 4 other models available, $10,350.00 to $14,900.00 (Lumiaggregation).

ANALYZER, PROTEIN *(Chemistry) 75UHL*

Antek Instruments, Inc. 281-580-0339
300 Bammel Westfield Rd, Houston, TX 77090
Total nitrogen and total sulfur analyzers.

Beckman Coulter, Inc. 800-742-2345
250 S Kraemer Blvd, PO Box 8000, Brea, CA 92821

Bio-Rad Laboratories, Life Science Group 800-424-6723
2000 Alfred Nobel Dr, Hercules, CA 94547

Tsi Incorporated 800-874-2811
500 Cardigan Rd, Shoreview, MN 55126
GEMMA Macromolecule Analyzer offers a new method for the analysis of large molecules. Offers a wide molecular weight range, high sensitivity, fast results, and long-term stability.

ANALYZER, PULMONARY FUNCTION *(Anesthesiology) 73RNC*

Cardiac Science Corp. 800-777-1777
500 Burdick Pkwy, Deerfield, WI 53531
Sensaire.

ANALYZER, PULMONARY FUNCTION *(cont'd)*

Cardinal Health 207, Inc. 800-231-2466
22745 Savi Ranch Pkwy, Yorba Linda, CA 92887
$4,000-$43,000 for screening system & full PFT lab.

Circadian Systems 800-669-7001
8099 Savage Way, Valley Springs, CA 95252
Circadian pulmonary function module is fully computerized, automatically provides all calculations; parameters include FVC, FEV1, FEVc, FMEF25.75, MVV as applied to three predicted values: Knudson, Morris, Pulgar. This model exceeds most Social Security and other regulatory requirements. Equipment designed for office physician and for use by nontechnical staff.

Covidien Lp 508-261-8000
15 Hampshire St, Mansfield, MA 02048
Battery-powered pulmonary function monitor, measures simultaneously FUC, FEV, FEF and PF.

Midmark Diagnostics Group 800-624-8950
3300 Fujita St, Torrance, CA 90505
The IQmark Digital Spirometer has met or exceeded the requirements of the ATS. All standard spirometry measurements are available including FEV6, as recommended by the NLHEP. Full-loop, FVC, SVC, MVV, and pre/post BD tests are easily performed on this computer-based spirometer. It is lightweight, weighing only 10 oz., and has no moving parts.

Morgan Scientific Inc. 800-525-5002
151 Essex St, Haverhill, MA 01832
We have two models of PFT system: (1) Trans'Air (pneumotach-based) PFT System. Instrument for the measurement of Spirometry (Dynamic and Static), Lung Volumes (nitrogen dilution), DLCO, Membrane Diffusion and Capillary Blood Volume, Bronchial Challenge and Respiratory Pressures. Interfaced to PC running ComPAS SQL Software (full network or stand-alone).(2) Spiro'Air spirometer (rolling seal) PFT system. Instrument for the measurement of Spirometry (Dynamic and Static), Lung Volumes (by helium dilution and/or nitrogen dilution), DLCO, Membrane Diffusion and Capillary Blood Volume, Bronchial Challenge and Respiratory Pressures. Interfaced to PC running ComPAS SQL Software (full network or stand-alone).

New Life Systems, Inc. 954-972-4600
PO Box 8767, Coral Springs, FL 33075

Nspire Health, Inc 800-574-7374
1830 Lefthand Cir, Longmont, CO 80501
KEYSTONE III, uses a direct displacement spirometer which determines lung volume measurements by helium dilution and diffusion analysis by the single breath method. Also measures spirometry, methacholine challenge and maximum respiratory pressures.

Omni Medical Supply Inc. 800-860-6664
4153 Pioneer Dr, Commerce Township, MI 48390

Promed Technologies Inc. 877-977-6633
P.O. Box 2070, Richmond Hill, ONT L4E-1A3 Canada

Vacumed 800-235-3333
4538 Westinghouse St, Ventura, CA 93003
FRC & DLCO.

ANALYZER, SEDIMENTATION RATE, AUTOMATED
(Hematology) 81GKB

Beckman Coulter, Inc. 800-526-3821
11800 SW 147th Ave, Miami, FL 33196
Automated sedimentation rate device.

Sarstedt, Inc. 800-257-5101
PO Box 468, 1025, St. James Church Road, Newton, NC 28658

Streck Laboratories, Inc. 800-843-0912
7002 S 109th St, Ralston, NE 68128
ESR-Auto Plus, a 10 position ESR analyzer designed to accurately and precisely measure the sedimentation rate of erythrocytes in a 1.2ml vacuum tube. Results available in 30 minutes.

Vital Diagnostics Inc. 714-672-3553
27 Wellington Rd, Lincoln, RI 02865

ANALYZER, SEDIMENTATION RATE, ERYTHROCYTE
(Hematology) 81JPH

Arkray Usa 800-818-8877
5198 W 76th St, Edina, MN 55439
DISPETTE, DISPETTE 2-Westergren standard pipette offers a triple plugged pipette tube and transparent reservoir. Conforms with NCCLS guidelines for ESR testing. WINPETTE-designed for the Wintrobe ESR system. Only 0.6 ml of blood is required.

ANALYZER, SEDIMENTATION RATE, ERYTHROCYTE *(cont'd)*

Bio-Rad Laboratories, Diagnostic Group 800-224-6723
524 Stone Rd Ste A, Benicia, CA 94510
Esr control.

Globe Scientific, Inc. 800-394-4562
610 Winters Ave, Paramus, NJ 07652
SEDI-RATE and SEDIGREN erythrocyte-sedimentation-rate systems for Westergren sedimentation-rate determination.

Hematechnologies, Inc. 877-436-2835
291 Rte. 22, Suite 12, Lebanon, NJ 08833
Automated, direct read. 25-microliter sample volume. Results in 4 minutes. Additional feature includes a direct read hematocrit

Life Science Technologies, Ltd. 888-511-0600
898 W King St, Boone, NC 28607
Various.

Sarstedt, Inc. 800-257-5101
PO Box 468, 1025, St. James Church Road, Newton, NC 28658

Statspin, Inc. 800-782-8774
60 Glacier Dr, Westwood, MA 02090
The ESRA-10 provides results in 30 minutes. Analyzes up to 20 amples an hour, and offers random access to any of 10 measuring channels - no waiting for prior analyses to complete and no need to batch tubes. Samples are collected in 1.6-ml primary vacuum collection tubes. Speed, accuracy and automation in a compact, economical package.

ANALYZER, SIGNAL ISOLATION *(Cardiovascular) 74DRJ*

Bio-Feedback Systems, Inc. 303-444-1411
2736 47th St, Boulder, CO 80301
Multi-channel, isolated AC amplifier.

Grass Technologies, An Astro-Med, Inc. Product Gro 401-828-4002
53 Airport Park Drive, Rockland, MA 02370
Patient isolator.

Soltec Corp. 800-423-2344
12977 Arroyo St, San Fernando, CA 91340

ANALYZER, SPECTRUM, EEG SIGNAL *(Cns/Neurology) 84GWS*

Bio-Logic Systems Corp. 800-323-8326
1 Bio Logic Plz, Mundelein, IL 60060
CEEGRAPH, models provides up to 32 channels; color, high resolution display, on-line data compression, remote monitoring, long-term video, real-time networking and more.

Cardinal Healthcare 209, Inc. 610-862-0800
5225 Verona Rd, Fitchburg, WI 53711
Eeg topographycial mapping system.

Draeger Medical Systems, Inc. 215-660-2626
16 Electronics Ave, Danvers, MA 01923
Monitor.

Lexicor Medical Technology, Inc. 706-447-1074
2840 Wilderness Pl Ste E, Boulder, CO 80301
Electroencephalogram signal spectrum analyzer.

Persyst Development Corp. 928-708-0705
1060 Sandretto Dr Ste E2, Prescott, AZ 86305
EEG review & analysis software.

Soltec Corp. 800-423-2344
12977 Arroyo St, San Fernando, CA 91340

Stellate Systems 514-486-1306
300-345 Av Victoria, Westmount H3Z 2N2 Canada
Digital eeg recording & analysis software

ANALYZER, TRACE GAS, BREATH *(Anesthesiology) 73WSV*

Quintron Instrument Company 800-542-4448
3712 W Pierce St, Milwaukee, WI 53215
BreathTracker Model SC MicroLyzer measures H2, CH4, and CO2, self-correcting for sample contamination. BreathTracker MicroLyzer DP, analyzes breath H2 and CH4. BreathTracker Model 12i PLUS measures H2 and CO2, self correcting for sample comtamination. BreathTracker 12i MicroLyzer, analyzes breath H2 only. Used primarily in gastroenterology as a diagnostic aid to determine, carbohydrate malabsorption, SIBO (snamll bowel bacterial overgrowth) and IBS (irritable bowel syndrome).

ANALYZER, TRANSCUTANEOUS NERVE STIMULATOR
(Cns/Neurology) 84RWA

Whalen Biomedical Incorporated 617-868-4433
11 Miller St, Somerville, MA 02143
TRANS POWER - This device transfers electrical power to implanted devices through intact skin.

ANALYZER, ULTRASONIC UNIT *(General) 80SDZ*

Dedicated Distribution 800-325-8367
640 Miami Ave, Kansas City, KS 66105

ANALYZER, ULTRAVIOLET *(Chemistry) 75UJB*

Advanced American Biotechnology (Aab) 714-870-0290
1166 E Valencia Dr Unit 6C, Fullerton, CA 92831
UV Imager.

ANALYZER, VISUAL FUNCTION *(Ophthalmology) 86SFB*

Good-Lite Co. 800-362-3860
865 Muirfield Dr, Bartlett, IL 60133
INSTRA-LINE - precise vision screening instrument for testing visual activity, muscle imbalance.

Mast/Keystone View 800-806-6569
2200 Dickerson Rd, Reno, NV 89503
VS II; Automated vision screener use 8 drum mounted stereo test targets illuminated by reflected light to test acuity, phoria, fusion and color/depth perception, $1450.00.

Schumann Inc., A. 978-369-6782
167 Hayward Mill Rd, Concord, MA 01742
$1200.00 for Prontograph screen for exact diagnosis of central field of vision.

Stereo Optical Co., Inc. 800-344-9500
3539 N Kenton Ave, Chicago, IL 60641
Vision screeners.

Titmus Optical Inc. 800-446-1802
690 Hp Way, 3811 CorPOrate Drive, Chester, VA 23836
3 base models for general use. $1,600.00-$2,100.00 for vision screening instrument (children or adults).

ANALYZER, WATER VAPOR *(Anesthesiology) 73VCH*

Quantachrome 800-989-2476
1900 Corporate Dr, Boynton Beach, FL 33426
HYDROSORB - water vapor sorption analyzer.

ANATOMICAL TRAINING MODEL *(General) 80TAE*

Alimed, Inc. 800-225-2610
297 High St, Dedham, MA 02026

Armstrong Medical Industries, Inc. 800-323-4220
575 Knightsbridge Pkwy, Lincolnshire, IL 60069

Biomedical Models Llc 800-635-4801
327 7th St S, Hudson, WI 54016
300+ different models of the human body including skeletons.

Dixie Ems Supply 800-347-3494
385 Union Ave, Brooklyn, NY 11211
$1,100.00 per unit (standard).

Galloway Plastics, Inc. 847-615-8900
940 W North Shore Dr, Lake Bluff, IL 60044

Gwb International, Ltd. 888-436-4826
PO Box 370, 76 Prospect Street, Marshfield Hills, MA 02051
Model practice eye for ophthalmology.

Hager Worldwide, Inc. 800-328-2335
13322 Byrd Dr, Odessa, FL 33556
BRUSH-N-FLOSS (study model).

Health Edco 800-299-3366
PO Box 21207, Waco, TX 76702

Kilgore International, Inc. 800-892-9999
36 W Pearl St, Coldwater, MI 49036

Mammatech Corp. 800-626-2273
930 NW 8th Ave, Gainesville, FL 32601

Medcom, Inc. 800-877-1443
6060 Phyllis Dr, Cypress, CA 90630
T-3 training, testing, and tracking system with over 500 online courses.

Medi-Tech International, Inc. 305-593-9373
2924 NW 109th Ave, Doral, FL 33172
NASCO

ANATOMICAL TRAINING MODEL *(cont'd)*

Medical Plastics Laboratory, Inc. 800-433-5539
226 FM 116, Industrial Air Park, PO Box 38, Gatesville, TX 76528
Detailed anatomical reproductions including skeletons (radio-opaque) and models of the heart, arterial system, viscera and joints. Life-size, 2x life-size and 3x life-size heart models are available to depict electrophysiology, bypass, coronary occlusions, cardiovascular catheters and stents. Pacemaker Heart features patent SVC to allow passage of pacer lead into right ventricle and window in right ventricle allows placement of pacer lead. ECG Heart features plexiglas overlay of electrocardiographic surface referencing ECG leads around axis of heart. Angiogram Sam, a life-size reproduction of the upper arterial system made of clear plastic with hollow passageways to allow the tracking and deployment of transluminal cardiovascular catheters, stents and guidewires, is x-ray imagable. Venous Sam and Pacemaker Pete models also available. Full-spine models are available, as well as various models showing cervical, thoracic or lumbar vertebrae. Models featuring abnormalities such as spondylolysis, spondylolisthesis, pseudoarthrosis, scoliosis and a herniated disc are also available.

Medsim-Eagle Simulation Inc. 607-779-6000
151 Court St, Binghamton, NY 13901
Medical Training Simulator, a full-body, computer controlled patient mannequin with lifelike qualities. The simulation software models cardiovascular and pulmonary functions, metabolic effects and drug reactions-simulating the mannequin, anesthesia machine and monitors to provide information. The simulator realistically simulates the look, feel, symptoms and responses of a human patient in an O.R./E.R./C.C. or I.C.U. environment.

O&M Enterprise 847-258-4515
641 Chelmsford Ln, Elk Grove Village, IL 60007
ANATOMICAL MODELS

Pacific Research Laboratories, Inc. 206-463-5551
10221 SW 188th St, PO Box 409, Vashon, WA 98070
Cortical bone models: $24.00 to $30.00 for upper extremity, lower extremity, long bones; knee models-$27.00 to $45.00; pelvis-$40.00 to $75.00. Sawbones are designed with a hard cortical shell & cancellous material in the core to replicate real bone. Composite bone models available that have the same physical strength as real bone for use in biomechanical testing.

Passy-Muir Inc. 800-634-5397
4521 Campus Dr, Irvine, CA 92612
Tracheostomy T. O. M.™ (Tracheostomy Tube Observation Model) is a portable, durable polyurethane model designed for instructors and clinicians for hands-on demonstration of tracheostomy care and discussion of tracheostomy and nasogastric tube-placement issues.

Pinnacle Technology Group, Inc. 800-345-5123
7076 Schnipke Dr, Ottawa Lake, MI 49267
$430 for Model AT-35 Arrhythmia TUTOR provides a quick and effective way to teach arrhythmia recognition and has built-in menus; $415 for Model TUTOR I - data selector presents recordings from hospital patients and digitalizes actual patient ECGs into plug-in modules; $935 for TUTOR IV - data selector includes 3 three channel hemodynamic & ECG modules with display of hemodynamics through cables at transducer receptable; $1035 for ST2 Sounds TUTOR includes 2 built-in Sounders; $1300 HS-2 Heart Sounds TUTOR includes 2 built-in and 2 extra Sounders and carrying case; also, accessory items and plug-in modules are available to be ordered separately.

Pocket Nurse Enterprises, Inc. 800-225-1600
200 1st St, Ambridge, PA 15003
Variety of training aids for colleges and universities

Radiology Support Devices 800-221-0527
1904 E Dominguez St, Long Beach, CA 90810

Wrs Group, Ltd. 800-299-3366
5045 Franklin Ave, Waco, TX 76710
Anatomical and patient care models.

ANCHOR, PREFORMED *(Dental And Oral) 76EJX*

Dentsply Canada, Ltd. 800-263-1437
161 Vinyl Ct., Woodbridge, ONT L4L 4A3 Canada

Moss Tubes, Inc. 800-827-0470
749 Columbia Tpke, East Greenbush, NY 12061
Anchor guns.

ANCHOR, SUTURE, BONE FIXATION, METALLIC *(Orthopedics) 87NOV*

C-Axis P.R., Inc.
Parque Industrial Valle Polima, Edif Multifabril 14-a-2, Caguas, PR 00727
Various types of bone anchors, various types of bone fixation.

ANGIOSCOPE *(Cardiovascular) 74LYK*
Edwards Lifesciences, Llc. 800-424-3278
1 Edwards Way, Irvine, CA 92614
Mahe International Inc. 800-294-7946
468 Craighead St, Nashville, TN 37204
Olympus America, Inc. 800-645-8160
3500 Corporate Pkwy, PO Box 610, Center Valley, PA 18034

ANILINE ACID FUCHSIN *(Pathology) 88ICY*
American Mastertech Scientific, Inc. 209-368-4031
1330 Thurman St, Lodi, CA 95240
Multiple types of fuchsin aniline acid.

ANIMAL, LABORATORY *(Microbiology) 83UMA*
Bd Diagnostic Systems 800-675-0908
7 Loveton Cir, Sparks, MD 21152
Bio Breeders, Inc. 617-926-5278
116 Temperton Parkway, Watertown, MA 02472
Produces and sells genetic-defined inbred, hybrid and mutant Syrian hamsters for research in cardiomyopathy, carcinogenesis, aging and athereosclerosis. These are animal models for human diseases.
Zivic Laboratories 800-422-5227
178 Toll Gate School Road, Zelienople, PA 16063
SD/maximum barrier maintained SD rodents.

ANKLE/FOOT, EXTERNAL LIMB COMPONENT
(Physical Med) 89ISH
Bioquest Prosthetics 661-325-3338
4615 Shepard St, Bakersfield, CA 93313
Various types of external limb prosthetic components.
Brown Medical Industries 800-843-4395
1300 Lundberg Dr W, Spirit Lake, IA 51360
STEADY STEP TOE HOLD foot splint, prevents lateral drift of hallux and stabilizes hallux valgus after surgery.
Endolite North America, Ltd. 937-291-3636
105 Westpark Rd, Centerville, OH 45459
Prosthetic foot.
Energy Prosthetics 818-675-5083
20438 Acre St, Winnetka, CA 91306
Push,magnetic valve.
Freedom Innovations, Inc. 888-818-6777
30 Fairbanks Ste 114, Irvine, CA 92618
Various types of external limb prosthetic components.
Freedom Innovations, Llc 435-528-7199
425 East 400 North, Gunnison, UT 84634
Various external limb prosthetic devices & components.
Hartford Walking Systems Inc. 315-735-1659
22 Pearl St, New Hartford, NY 13413
External limb prosthetic component.
Hosmer Dorrance Corp. 408-379-5151
561 Division St, Campbell, CA 95008
Cone shaped comesis.
Lifeline Usa 800-553-6633
3201 Syene Rd, Madison, WI 53713
Foot attachment.
Ohio Willow Wood Company 800-848-4930
15441 Scioto Darby Rd, Mount Sterling, OH 43143
Structural components for ankle, foot, knee and thigh prostheses.
Ossur Americas 517-629-8890
910 Burstein Dr, Albion, MI 49224
Otto Bock Healthcare 763-489-5106
3820 Great Lakes Dr, Salt Lake City, UT 84120
Various artificial foot kits.
Otto Bock Healthcare, Lp 763-489-5106
9420 Delegates Dr Ste 100, Orlando, FL 32837
Various types of ankle/foot components/accessories.
Otto Bock Technical Center 763-489-5106
14800 28th Ave N Ste 110, Minneapolis, MN 55447
Scott Specialties, Inc. 785-527-5627
1827 Meadowlark Rd, Clay Center, KS 67432
Various types of limb, ankle, foot orthosis.
Scott Specialties, Inc. 785-527-5627
1820 E 7th St, Concordia, KS 66901
Trulife, Inc. 360-697-5656
26296 12 Trees Ln NW, Poulsbo, WA 98370
Prosthetic foot & attachment components (assorted).

ANKLET *(Physical Med) 89QBC*
Paramedical Distributors 800-245-3278
2020 Grand Blvd, Kansas City, MO 64108

ANOMALOSCOPE *(Ophthalmology) 86HIW*
Multi-Tronics Corp. 817-246-5821
8400 White Settlement Rd, Fort Worth, TX 76108
Anomaloscope.

ANOSCOPE, NON-POWERED *(Gastro/Urology) 78FER*
Cameron-Miller, Inc. 800-621-0142
5410 W Roosevelt Rd, Road #241, Chicago, IL 60644
Codman & Shurtleff, Inc 800-225-0460
325 Paramount Dr, Raynham, MA 02767
Electro Surgical Instrument Co., Inc. 888-464-2784
37 Centennial St, Rochester, NY 14611
Various types, styles and sizes of lighted and not lighted anoscopes.
Mahe International Inc. 800-294-7946
468 Craighead St, Nashville, TN 37204
Miltex Inc. 800-645-8000
589 Davies Dr, York, PA 17402
Precision Medical Manufacturing Corporation 866-633-4626
852 Seton Ct, Wheeling, IL 60090
Princeton Medical Group, Inc. 800-875-0869
1189 Royal Links Dr, Mt Pleasant, SC 29466
Welch Allyn, Inc. 800-535-6663
4341 State Street Rd, Skaneateles Falls, NY 13153

ANTI-CHOKE DEVICE, SUCTION *(Ear/Nose/Throat) 77EWT*
Mada, Inc. 800-526-6370
625 Washington Ave, Carlstadt, NJ 07072
Precious Life Saving Products, Inc. 416-644-0011
101-200 Ronson Dr, Toronto M9W 5Z9 Canada
Choke reliever

ANTI-DNA ANTIBODY (ENZYME-LABELED), ANTIGEN, CONTROL *(Immunology) 82LRM*
American Laboratory Products Co. 800-592-5726
26 Keewaydin Dr Ste G, Salem, NH 03079
Utilizes recombinant human antigen to semi-quantitate anti-dsDNA in plasma and serum with high level of diagnostic efficiency.
Binding Site, Inc., The 800-633-4484
5889 Oberlin Dr Ste 101, San Diego, CA 92121
Bio-Rad Laboratories Inc., Clinical Systems Div. 800-224-6723
4000 Alfred Nobel Dr, Hercules, CA 94547
Enzyme immunoassay anti-dna antibody test.
Corgenix, Inc. 800-729-5661
12061 Tejon St, Westminster, CO 80234
Anti-ds DNA semi-quantitative test kit.
Global Focus (G.F.M.D. Ltd.) 800-527-2320
2280 Springlake Rd Ste 106, Dallas, TX 75234
Immuno Concepts Colorzyme assay.
Hycor Biomedical, Inc. 800-382-2527
7272 Chapman Ave, Garden Grove, CA 92841
Anti-ds-dna autoimmune kit.
Innominata dba GENBIO 800-288-4368
15222 Avenue of Science Ste A, San Diego, CA 92128
Enzyme - linked immunoassay - for dsdna antibodies.
Micro Detect, Inc. 714-832-8234
2852 Walnut Ave Ste H1, Tustin, CA 92780
Mdi ds-dna test.
Theratest Laboratories, Inc. 800-441-0771
1111 N Main St, Lombard, IL 60148
High sensitivity/specificity phage DNA based, 96 wells ELISA kits
United Biotech, Inc. 650-961-2910
211 S Whisman Rd Ste E, Mountain View, CA 94041
ELISA for detecting Anti ds-DNA.

ANTI-DNA ANTIBODY, ANTIGEN AND CONTROL
(Immunology) 82LSW
Antibodies, Inc. 800-824-8540
PO Box 1560, Davis, CA 95617
DNA diagnostic test kit for autoimmune diseases.
Binding Site, Inc., The 800-633-4484
5889 Oberlin Dr Ste 101, San Diego, CA 92121
Diamedix Corp. 800-327-4565
2140 N Miami Ave, Miami, FL 33127
Is-anti-ds-DNA catalog #720-700.

ANTI-DNA ANTIBODY, ANTIGEN AND CONTROL *(cont'd)*

Medica, Inc. 800-845-6496
336 Encinitas Blvd Ste 200, Encinitas, CA 92024
48 & 96-test kits, Crithidia luciliae, A-nDNA.48&96 test kits, monkey esophagus sections,ASA.

Quest Intl., Inc. 305-592-6991
8127 NW 29th St, Doral, FL 33122
Anti-dsdna serological reagents, elisa.

ANTI-DNA INDIRECT IMMUNOFLUORESCENT SOLID PHASE
(Immunology) 82KTL

Binding Site, Inc., The 800-633-4484
5889 Oberlin Dr Ste 101, San Diego, CA 92121

Global Focus (G.F.M.D. Ltd.) 800-527-2320
2280 Springlake Rd Ste 106, Dallas, TX 75234
Immuno Concepts.

Hemagen Diagnostics, Inc. 800-436-2436
9033 Red Branch Rd, Columbia, MD 21045
Anti-ndna.

Immuno Concepts N.A. Ltd. 800-251-5115
9779 Business Park Dr, Sacramento, CA 95827

ANTI-HUMAN GLOBULIN, FTA-ABS TEST (COOMBS)
(Microbiology) 83GMS

Wampole Laboratories 800-257-9525
2 Research Way, Princeton, NJ 08540
Zeus Scientific Double stain test also available. Not Coombs.

ANTI-HUMAN SERUM, MANUAL *(Hematology) 81UJS*

Antibodies, Inc. 800-824-8540
PO Box 1560, Davis, CA 95617
Various anti-human antisera and labeled conjugates. Various purifications available.

Dade Behring, Inc. 800-948-3233
1717 Deerfield Rd, Deerfield, IL 60015

Rockland Immunochemicals, Inc. 800-656-ROCK
PO Box 326, Gilbertsville, PA 19525
Customized antisera.

ANTI-RNP-ANTIBODY, ANTIGEN AND CONTROL
(Immunology) 82LKO

Binding Site, Inc., The 800-633-4484
5889 Oberlin Dr Ste 101, San Diego, CA 92121

Bio-Rad Laboratories Inc., Clinical Systems Div. 800-224-6723
4000 Alfred Nobel Dr, Hercules, CA 94547
Enzyme immunoassay anti-smrnp antibody test kit.

Corgenix Medical Corporation 800-729-5661
11575 Main St, Broomfield, CO 80020
Multiple

Diamedix Corp. 800-327-4565
2140 N Miami Ave, Miami, FL 33127
Is-Sm/RNP catalog #720-270.

Global Focus (G.F.M.D. Ltd.) 800-527-2320
2280 Springlake Rd Ste 106, Dallas, TX 75234
Immuno Concepts Auto I.D. immunodiffusion and RELISA assays.

Hycor Biomedical, Inc. 800-382-2527
7272 Chapman Ave, Garden Grove, CA 92841
Rnp/sm autoimmune kit.

Innominata dba GENBIO 800-288-4368
15222 Avenue of Science Ste A, San Diego, CA 92128
Enzyme - linked immunoassay - for rnp/sm antibodies.

Quest Intl., Inc. 305-592-6991
8127 NW 29th St, Doral, FL 33122
Anti-sm/rnp serological reagents, elisa.

ANTI-SM-ANTIBODY, ANTIGEN AND CONTROL
(Immunology) 82LKP

Binding Site, Inc., The 800-633-4484
5889 Oberlin Dr Ste 101, San Diego, CA 92121

Bio-Rad Laboratories Inc., Clinical Systems Div. 800-224-6723
4000 Alfred Nobel Dr, Hercules, CA 94547
Enzyme immunoassay anti-sm antibody test kit.

Corgenix Medical Corporation 800-729-5661
11575 Main St, Broomfield, CO 80020
Multiple

Diamedix Corp. 800-327-4565
2140 N Miami Ave, Miami, FL 33127
Is-Sm catalog #720-240.

ANTI-SM-ANTIBODY, ANTIGEN AND CONTROL *(cont'd)*

Global Focus (G.F.M.D. Ltd.) 800-527-2320
2280 Springlake Rd Ste 106, Dallas, TX 75234
Immuno Concepts Auto I.D. immunodiffusion and RELISA assays.

Hycor Biomedical, Inc. 800-382-2527
7272 Chapman Ave, Garden Grove, CA 92841
Anti sm autoimmune kit.

Innominata dba GENBIO 800-288-4368
15222 Avenue of Science Ste A, San Diego, CA 92128
Enzyme - linked immunoassay - for sm antibodies.

Quest Intl., Inc. 305-592-6991
8127 NW 29th St, Doral, FL 33122
Anti-sm, serological reagents, elisa.

Wampole Laboratories 800-257-9525
2 Research Way, Princeton, NJ 08540
Autoimmune disease ELISA kits.

ANTI-STAMMERING DEVICE *(Ear/Nose/Throat) 77KTH*

Griffin Laboratories 800-330-5969
43391 Business Park Dr Ste C5, Temecula, CA 92590
Speech fluency system.

Janus Development Group, Inc. 866-551-9042
112 Staton Rd, Greenville, NC 27834
Anti-stuttering device.

Speecheasy International, Llc 252-551-9042
112 Staton Rd, Greenville, NC 27834

ANTI-STREPTOKINASE *(Microbiology) 83GTO*

Immunostics, Inc. 800-722-7505
3505 Sunset Ave, Ocean, NJ 07712

Pulse Scientific, Inc. 800-363-7907
5100 S. Service Rd., Unit 18, Burlington, ONT L7L-6A5 Canada
ASO Latex Test, Latex Agglutination Test to detect the presence of ASO as an aid to diagnosis of Streptococci infection.

ANTIBODIES, ANTI-RIBOSOMAL P *(Immunology) 82MQA*

Binding Site, Inc., The 800-633-4484
5889 Oberlin Dr Ste 101, San Diego, CA 92121

Bio-Rad Laboratories Inc., Clinical Systems Div. 800-224-6723
4000 Alfred Nobel Dr, Hercules, CA 94547
Ana screening test.

ANTIBODIES, GLIADIN *(Immunology) 82MST*

Binding Site, Inc., The 800-633-4484
5889 Oberlin Dr Ste 101, San Diego, CA 92121

Epitope Diagnostics, Inc. 858-693-7877
8940 Activity Rd Ste G, San Diego, CA 92126
Gliadin immunolgical test system.

Micro Detect, Inc. 714-832-8234
2852 Walnut Ave Ste H1, Tustin, CA 92780
Mdi gliadin igg test kit.

Seracare Life Sciences 800-676-1881
37 Birch St, Milford, MA 01757

ANTIBODY IGM, IF, CYTOMEGALOVIRUS VIRUS
(Microbiology) 83LKQ

Bbi Diagnostics, A Division Of Seracare Life Scien 508-244-6428
375 West St, West Bridgewater, MA 02379
Accurun 146 cmv igm positive control.

Hemagen Diagnostics, Inc. 800-436-2436
9033 Red Branch Rd, Columbia, MD 21045
Cmv ifa.

Wampole Laboratories 800-257-9525
2 Research Way, Princeton, NJ 08540
Zeus Scientific IgG and IgM. Cytomegalovirus IgG and Cytomegalovirus IgM.

Zeus Scientific, Inc. 800-286-2111
PO Box 38, Raritan, NJ 08869
100-test kit, indirect IgM immunofluorescent cytomegalovirus antibody.

ANTIBODY IGM, IF, EPSTEIN-BARR VIRUS *(Microbiology) 83LJN*

Immuno Concepts N.A. Ltd. 800-251-5115
9779 Business Park Dr, Sacramento, CA 95827
EBV antibody test systems or antigen controls.

Innominata dba GENBIO 800-288-4368
15222 Avenue of Science Ste A, San Diego, CA 92128
Immunowell ebv vca igm test.

ANTIBODY IGM, IF, EPSTEIN-BARR VIRUS *(cont'd)*

Meridian Bioscience, Inc. 800-696-0739
3471 River Hills Dr, Cincinnati, OH 45244
Enzyme immunoassay for the detection of IgM and IsG antibodies to the EBNA antigens of EBV.

Quest Intl., Inc. 305-592-6991
8127 NW 29th St, Doral, FL 33122
Anti-eb vca igm serological reagents, elisa.

Wampole Laboratories 800-257-9525
2 Research Way, Princeton, NJ 08540
Zeus Scientific VCA IgG and Igm, nuclear antigen, early antigen.

Zeus Scientific, Inc. 800-286-2111
PO Box 38, Raritan, NJ 08869
50-test IFA kit, Indirect Immunofluorescent Antibody-IgM, EBV-VCA.

ANTIBODY, ANTI-SMOOTH MUSCLE, INDIRECT IMMUNOFLUORESCENT *(Immunology) 82DBE*

Binding Site, Inc., The 800-633-4484
5889 Oberlin Dr Ste 101, San Diego, CA 92121

Biomedical Technologies, Inc. 781-344-9942
378 Page St, Stoughton, MA 02072

Hemagen Diagnostics, Inc. 800-436-2436
9033 Red Branch Rd, Columbia, MD 21045
Ifa.

Medica, Inc. 800-845-6496
336 Encinitas Blvd Ste 200, Encinitas, CA 92024
48 & 96-test kits, rat or mouse stomach sections, ASMA.

Scimedx Corporation 800-221-5598
100 Ford Rd Ste 100-08, Denville, NJ 07834

Wampole Laboratories 800-257-9525
2 Research Way, Princeton, NJ 08540
Zeus Scientific.

Zeus Scientific, Inc. 800-286-2111
PO Box 38, Raritan, NJ 08869
48-test IFA kit.

ANTIBODY, ANTI-THYROID, INDIRECT IMMUNOFLUORESCENT *(Immunology) 82WQF*

Binding Site, Inc., The 800-633-4484
5889 Oberlin Dr Ste 101, San Diego, CA 92121

Biomerica, Inc. 800-854-3002
17571 Von Karman Ave, Irvine, CA 92614
Anti-thyroid peroxidase, anti-TPO ELISA test, cat #7016. Also, anti-thyroid quality control (liquid) for anti-Tg and anti-TPO, 2 levels.

Medica, Inc. 800-845-6496
336 Encinitas Blvd Ste 200, Encinitas, CA 92024
48 & 96-test kits, monkey thyroid sections, ATA., MI (Microsomal). 48 & 96-test kits, monkey thyroid sections, ATA, TA (Thyroglobulin).

Wampole Laboratories 800-257-9525
2 Research Way, Princeton, NJ 08540
Autoimmune disease ELISA kits.

ANTIBODY, ANTIMITOCHONDRIAL, INDIRECT IMMUNOFLUORESCENT *(Immunology) 82DBM*

Binding Site, Inc., The 800-633-4484
5889 Oberlin Dr Ste 101, San Diego, CA 92121

Bio-Rad Laboratories, Inc. 425-881-8300
14620 NE North Woodinville Way, Way, Suite 200
Woodinville, WA 98072
Various hep-2 autoimmune ifa kits, components, and controls.

Global Focus (G.F.M.D. Ltd.) 800-527-2320
2280 Springlake Rd Ste 106, Dallas, TX 75234
Medica tissue slides.

Hemagen Diagnostics, Inc. 800-436-2436
9033 Red Branch Rd, Columbia, MD 21045
Ama ifa.

Hycor Biomedical, Inc. 800-382-2527
7272 Chapman Ave, Garden Grove, CA 92841
Mitochondria autoimmune kit.

Medica, Inc. 800-845-6496
336 Encinitas Blvd Ste 200, Encinitas, CA 92024
48 & 96-test kits, rat or mouse kidney sections, AMA.

Scimedx Corporation 800-221-5598
100 Ford Rd Ste 100-08, Denville, NJ 07834

Zeus Scientific, Inc. 800-286-2111
PO Box 38, Raritan, NJ 08869
48-test IFA kit.

ANTIBODY, ANTINUCLEAR, INDIRECT IMMUNOFLUORESCENT, ANTIGEN *(Immunology) 82DHN*

Antibodies, Inc. 800-824-8540
PO Box 1560, Davis, CA 95617
ANA/DNA diagnostics for autoimmune diseases.

Binding Site, Inc., The 800-633-4484
5889 Oberlin Dr Ste 101, San Diego, CA 92121

Bio-Rad Laboratories, Inc. 425-881-8300
14620 NE North Woodinville Way, Way, Suite 200
Woodinville, WA 98072
Various mouse stomach kidney and crithidia autoimmune ifa kits, components, and.

Dako North America, Inc 805-566-6655
6392 Via Real, Carpinteria, CA 93013

Diagnostic Technology, Inc. 631-582-4949
175 Commerce Dr Ste L, Hauppauge, NY 11788
Rapid latex slide test for detection of antinuclear antibodies.

Global Focus (G.F.M.D. Ltd.) 800-527-2320
2280 Springlake Rd Ste 106, Dallas, TX 75234
Immuno Concepts HEp-2 and HEp-2000 assays.

Hemagen Diagnostics, Inc. 800-436-2436
9033 Red Branch Rd, Columbia, MD 21045
Various.

Immco Diagnostics, Inc. 800-537-8378
60 Pineview Dr, Buffalo, NY 14228
IMMUGLO 48 and 96 determination kits.

Immuno Concepts N.A. Ltd. 800-251-5115
9779 Business Park Dr, Sacramento, CA 95827

Medica, Inc. 800-845-6496
336 Encinitas Blvd Ste 200, Encinitas, CA 92024
48 & 96-test kits, rat liver, mouse kidney or HEp-2 cells, ANA. Indirect Immunofluorescence Anti-Endomysial Anti-body Test Kit, 48 & 96 test kits, monkey esophagus (distal) sections AEMA.

Scimedx Corporation 800-221-5598
100 Ford Rd Ste 100-08, Denville, NJ 07834

Wampole Laboratories 800-257-9525
2 Research Way, Princeton, NJ 08540
Zeus Scientific Mouse kidney, rat liver or human epithelial (HEp-2) substrate.

Zeus Scientific, Inc. 800-286-2111
PO Box 38, Raritan, NJ 08869
Antinuclear Antibody, IFA (Hep-2 Substrate), and IFA rat liver test system (9 x 6 well)

ANTIBODY, HERPES VIRUS *(Microbiology) 83WJS*

Wampole Laboratories 800-257-9525
2 Research Way, Princeton, NJ 08540
Zeus Scientific Herpes simplex fluorescent antibody, IgG and IgM.

Zeus Scientific, Inc. 800-286-2111
PO Box 38, Raritan, NJ 08869
100-test HSV-1 kit or HSV 2 100-test IF-Antibody kit.

ANTIBODY, MONOCLONAL *(Microbiology) 83TFW*

Accurate Chemical & Scientific Corp. 800-645-6264
300 Shames Dr, Westbury, NY 11590
Le-a-01, Le-b-01, P-k-002, RAMOL (unlabelled or biotinylated).

American Diagnostica, Inc. 888-234-4435
500 West Ave, Stamford, CT 06902
Monoclonal antibody to hemostasis antigens; ACTICHROME chromogenic substrate kits for AT-III, plsg, fxa and heparin; SPECTORZYME chromogenic substrates. Imubind ELISA kits for cancer prognosis.

American Qualex, Inc. 800-772-1776
920 Calle Negocio Ste A, San Clemente, CA 92673

Amgen Inc. 206-265-7000
1201 Amgen Ct W, Seattle, WA 98119

Antibodies, Inc. 800-824-8540
PO Box 1560, Davis, CA 95617
Monoclonal antibodies from your hybridoma line, by in-vivo ascites, or in-vitro tissue culture.

Bachem Bioscience, Inc. 800-634-3183
3700 Horizon Dr, King Of Prussia, PA 19406

Beckman Coulter, Inc. 800-635-3497
740 W 83rd St, Hialeah, FL 33014
Available in 25, 50 & 100 test sizes as COULTER CLONES.

Beckman Coulter, Inc. 800-742-2345
250 S Kraemer Blvd, PO Box 8000, Brea, CA 92821

ANTIBODY, MONOCLONAL *(cont'd)*

Biogenex Laboratories 800-421-4149
4600 Norris Canyon Rd, San Ramon, CA 94583
Murine monoclonal antibodies and kits for tumor-associated cell surface antigens, cancer-associated antigens and cellular antigens, hormones and immunoglobulins.

Biotest Diagnostic Corp. 800-522-0090
400 Commons Way, Rockaway, NJ 07866
Monoclonal blood-typing sera; monoclonal antibodies for cancer research.

Braton Biotech, Inc. 301-762-5301
1 Taft Ct Ste 101, Rockville, MD 20850

Cedarlane Laboratories Ltd. 800-268-5058
5516 8th Line R.R. 2, Hornby, ONT L0P 1E0 Canada
ANTI-SERA for medical research.

Cliniqa Corporation 800-728-9558
774 N Twin Oaks Valley Rd Ste C, San Marcos, CA 92069
For drugs of abuse, hormones, HIV, hepatitis, cardiac enzymes.

Covance Research Products Inc. 800-223-0796
180 Rustcraft Rd Ste 140, Dedham, MA 02026
Monoclonal antibodies to tumor antigens and immunopathology reagents (mono abs.)Neuroscience, Alzheimers, Prion Disease antibodies and assay kits. Multidrug resistance markers. ABP26 assay for Sepsis and related diseases.

Cytogen Corp. 800-833-3533
600 College Rd E Ste 3100, Princeton, NJ 08540
ONCOSCINT for colorectal and ovarian cancer imaging and tumor-targeted radioimmunoscintigraphy.

Dade Behring, Inc. 800-948-3233
1717 Deerfield Rd, Deerfield, IL 60015

Dako North America, Inc 805-566-6655
6392 Via Real, Carpinteria, CA 93013

Dominion Biologicals Ltd. 800-565-0653
5 Isnor Dr., Dartmouth, NS B3B 1M1 Canada

Drg International, Inc. 800-321-1167
1167 US Highway 22, Mountainside, NJ 07092

Enzo Biochem, Inc. 212-583-0100
527 Madison Ave, New York, NY 10022
Monoclonal antibodies for immunopathology, intermediate filaments, anti muscle, anti melanoma, anti neuroendocrine, anti macrophage, anti-smooth muscle.

Genzyme 800-332-1042
500 Kendall St, Cambridge, MA 02142
Laboratory reagent formulations of cytokines for research use (mono and polyclonal).

Intracel Corporation 301-668-8400
93 Monocacy Blvd Ste A8, Frederick, MD 21701

Kamiya Biomedical Company 206-575-8068
12779 Gateway Dr S, Tukwila, WA 98168

Meridian Bioscience, Inc. 800-696-0739
3471 River Hills Dr, Cincinnati, OH 45244
$100.00 for 25 Giardia lamblia/Cryptosporidium DFA test detection kits.

Nanoprobes, Inc. 877-447-6266
95 Horseblock Rd, Yaphank, NY 11980

One Lambda, Inc. 800-822-8824
21001 Kittridge St, Canoga Park, CA 91303
HLA monoclonal antibodies; FITC conjugated; dual tag, lyophilized.

Peregrine Pharmaceuticals, Inc. 714-508-6000
14282 Franklin Ave, Tustin, CA 92780
Defined serum free media-in vitro diagnostic test kits.

Pierce Biotechnology 800-487-4885
30 Commerce Way, Woburn, MA 01801
Monoclanal antibodies to human, mouse, rat, pig and rabbit cytokines.

Promega Corp. 800-356-9526
2800 Woods Hollow Rd, Fitchburg, WI 53711

Qed Bioscience, Inc. 800-929-2114
10919 Technology Pl Ste C, San Diego, CA 92127
Therapeutic drugs, infectious disease agents, enzymes and inhibitors, hormones and serum proteins, coagulation factors, immunoglobulins, DNA, retinoblastoma protein, cancer research, neuroscience, signal transduction, protein transcription, apoptosis, adhesion molecules, cell matrix proteins, and biowarfare agents.

Seikagaku America, Inc. 800-848-3248
124 Bernard St. Jean Dr., East Falmouth, MA 02536-4445

ANTIBODY, MONOCLONAL *(cont'd)*

Seradyn, Inc. 800-428-4072
7998 Georgetown Rd Ste 1000, Indianapolis, IN 46268

Tanox Biosystems, Inc. 713-664-2288
10301 Stella Link Rd Ste 110, Houston, TX 77025
Development of monoclonal antibodies for research uses.

Zeptometrix Corporation 800-274-5487
872 Main St, Buffalo, NY 14202
Monoclonal antibodies for HIV-1 and HTLV-1 proteins.

ANTIBODY, MULTIPLE AUTO, INDIRECT IMMUNOFLUORESCENT *(Immunology) 82DBL*

Bio-Rad Laboratories, Inc. 425-881-8300
14620 NE North Woodinville Way, Way, Suite 200
Woodinville, WA 98072
Kallestad mouse kidney kits and components.

Drg International, Inc. 800-321-1167
1167 US Highway 22, Mountainside, NJ 07092

Global Focus (G.F.M.D. Ltd.) 800-527-2320
2280 Springlake Rd Ste 106, Dallas, TX 75234
Immuno Concepts HEp-2, HEp-2000, Auto I.D. immunodiffusion and RELISA assays

Medica, Inc. 800-845-6496
336 Encinitas Blvd Ste 200, Encinitas, CA 92024
48- and 96-test kits, rat or mouse (liver, kidney, stomach), rat or mouse (kidney, stomach) sections, ANA, AMA, ASMA, APCA. 48- and 96-test kits with monkey esophagus substrate (section) with controls, conjugate, PBS, and mounting medium.

Meridian Bioscience, Inc. 800-696-0739
3471 River Hills Dr, Cincinnati, OH 45244
MERIFLUOR: Immunofluorescent products.

Scimedx Corporation 800-221-5598
100 Ford Rd Ste 100-08, Denville, NJ 07834

Wampole Laboratories 800-257-9525
2 Research Way, Princeton, NJ 08540
Zeus Scientific Autoantibody screen by IFA (ANA, AMA, ASMA, & PCA).

ANTIBODY, MYCOPLASMA SPP. *(Microbiology) 83WJT*

Zeus Scientific, Inc. 800-286-2111
PO Box 38, Raritan, NJ 08869
100 IgG test kit or IgM mycoplasma pneumonia by IFA.

ANTIBODY, OTHER *(General) 80WQZ*

American Qualex, Inc. 800-772-1776
920 Calle Negocio Ste A, San Clemente, CA 92673
Antibodies to drugs and infectious diseases.

Antibodies, Inc. 800-824-8540
PO Box 1560, Davis, CA 95617
Polyclonal and monoclonal antibodies from genes, proteins, other antigens. Contract and catalog antisera production, purification, labeling, and packaging.

Beckman Coulter, Inc. 800-742-2345
250 S Kraemer Blvd, PO Box 8000, Brea, CA 92821

Binding Site, Inc., The 800-633-4484
5889 Oberlin Dr Ste 101, San Diego, CA 92121
Antigen specific IgG and subclass EIA kits for C. Tetani, S. Pneumonia, Hemophilus Influenza.

Covance Research Products Inc. 800-223-0796
180 Rustcraft Rd Ste 140, Dedham, MA 02026
Multi-drug resistance markers--p-glycoprotein and non-p-glycoprotein monoclonal antibodies for tissue, flow cytometry, Western blot, others. Monoclonal antibodies for neuroscience--4G8, 6E10, Alzheimer's disease, prion disease markers.

Cst Technologies, Inc. 800-448-4407
55 Northern Blvd Ste 200, Great Neck, NY 11021
ABCOAT, $195 per liter for antibody and enzyme coating.

Home Access Health Corp. 800-HIV-TEST
2401 Hassell Rd Ste 1510, Hoffman Estates, IL 60169
Home Access Hepatitis C Check. A blood specimen collection and transportation device intended for home use to obtain a dried blood spot (DES) to be tested for antibodies to hepatitis C virus at a laboratory site.

Invitrogen Corporation 800-955-6288
101 Lincoln Centre Dr, Foster City, CA 94404

Kent Laboratories, Inc. 360-398-8641
777 Jorgensen Pl, Bellingham, WA 98226
Full line of fluorescein and peroxidase conjugated antibodies.

ANTIBODY, OTHER *(cont'd)*

Kronus, Inc. 800-822-6999
12554 W Bridger St Ste 108, Boise, ID 83713
Acetylcholine Receptor Ab (AChRAb) test kits for myasthenia gravis diagnosis. Voltage-Gated Calcium Channel (VGCC) Ab test kits for Lambert-Eaton Myasthenic Syndrome (LEMS). TSH Receptor Ab test kit for Graves' disease. Thyroglobulin (Tg) Ab and Thyroid Peroxidase (TPO) Ab direct RIA and ELISA test kits for various autoimmune thyroid diseases (AID), including Hashimoto's disease. Serum Thyroglobulin (Tg) test kits. Glumatic Acid Decarboxylase (GAD65) Ab, IA-2 Ab, and Insulin Ab test kits - useful in the diagnosis and management of Type I diabetes. 21-Hydroxylase (21-OH) Ab test kits - useful in the prediction and diagnosis of autoimmune Addison's disease.

Medica, Inc. 800-845-6496
336 Encinitas Blvd Ste 200, Encinitas, CA 92024
Custom made slides for research with up to 4 sections per well using rat, mouse, monkey, crithidia luciliae or HEp-2, all slides of 4,6, or 8 wells.

Meridian Life Science, Inc. 888-530-0140
60 Industrial Park Rd, Saco, ME 04072
Assay development reagents, animal sera, apolipoproteins, autoimmune, cancer related reagents, cardiac markers, cd markers, collagens, hormone and steroids, immunoglobulins, human proteins, infectious disease reagents, cancer markers, turbidimetric/neph reagents.

PerkinElmer 800-762-4000
940 Winter St, Waltham, MA 02451
Monocloral antibody; detects presence of hemoglobin.

Pierce Biotechnology 800-487-4885
30 Commerce Way, Woburn, MA 01801
Antibodies to human T Cell receptors; human, rat and mouse cell adhesion molecules; human apoptosis markers; and human, mouse and rat chemokines.

Promega Corp. 800-356-9526
2800 Woods Hollow Rd, Fitchburg, WI 53711

Scimedx Corporation 800-221-5598
100 Ford Rd Ste 100-08, Denville, NJ 07834
ANCA (anti-neutrophil cytoplasm antibody) indirect immunofluorescent test system. AUTOPOINT ENA screen - antibody detection. AUTOPOINT - vascular disease panel detection for antibodies to ANCA, MPO, GMB.

Vector Laboratories, Inc. 800-227-6666
30 Ingold Rd, Burlingame, CA 94010
$85.00 for 1mg Phycoerythrin Anti-Mouse IgG (H+L), made in horse. $70.00 for 1.5mg Texas Red Anti-Rabbit IgG (H+L), made in goat.

Zeus Scientific, Inc. 800-286-2111
PO Box 38, Raritan, NJ 08869
48 test IFA kit (monkey esophagus substrate) anti-skin antibody (pemphigus and bullous pemphigoid).

ANTIBODY, POLYCLONAL *(Microbiology) 83WJL*

American Qualex, Inc. 800-772-1776
920 Calle Negocio Ste A, San Clemente, CA 92673

Amresco Inc. 800-366-1313
30175 Solon Industrial Pkwy, Solon, OH 44139
Enzyme-conjugated antibodies provide ultrahigh-specificity detection in immunohistochemistry, ELISA and Western blotting applications.

Bachem Bioscience, Inc. 800-634-3183
3700 Horizon Dr, King Of Prussia, PA 19406

Bd Lee Laboratories 800-732-9150
1475 Athens Hwy, Grayson, GA 30017

Beckman Coulter, Inc. 800-742-2345
250 S Kraemer Blvd, PO Box 8000, Brea, CA 92821

Biogenex Laboratories 800-421-4149
4600 Norris Canyon Rd, San Ramon, CA 94583
Polyclonal antibodies and kits for tumor-associated cell surface antigens, cancer-associated antigens and cellular antigens, hormones and immunoglobulins.

Braton Biotech, Inc. 301-762-5301
1 Taft Ct Ste 101, Rockville, MD 20850

Cedarlane Laboratories Ltd. 800-268-5058
5516 8th Line R.R. 2, Hornby, ONT L0P 1E0 Canada
Custom antibody production service - custom polyclonal antibody production in rabbits, goats, and sheep.

Cliniqa Corporation 800-728-9558
774 N Twin Oaks Valley Rd Ste C, San Marcos, CA 92069
Serum proteins and immunoglobulins, lipoproteins and HIV/SIV antibodies.

ANTIBODY, POLYCLONAL *(cont'd)*

Diamed, Inc. 207-892-7521
2 Inland Farm Rd, Windham, ME 04062

Genzyme 800-332-1042
500 Kendall St, Cambridge, MA 02142
Laboratory reagent formulations of cytokines for research use (mono and polyclonal).

Nanoprobes, Inc. 877-447-6266
95 Horseblock Rd, Yaphank, NY 11980

Pierce Biotechnology 800-487-4885
30 Commerce Way, Woburn, MA 01801
Polyclonal antibodies to human, mouse, rat, pig and rabbit cytokines.

Quality Bioresources, Inc. 888-674-7224
1015 N Austin St, Seguin, TX 78155
OEM, Liquid or Lyophilized

Rockland Immunochemicals, Inc. 800-656-ROCK
PO Box 326, Gilbertsville, PA 19525

ANTIBODY, TOXOPLASMA GONDII *(Microbiology) 83WJR*

United Biotech, Inc. 650-961-2910
211 S Whisman Rd Ste E, Mountain View, CA 94041
Antibody, Toxoplasma Gondii

Wampole Laboratories 800-257-9525
2 Research Way, Princeton, NJ 08540
Zeus Scientific IgG and IgM.

Zeus Scientific, Inc. 800-286-2111
PO Box 38, Raritan, NJ 08869
120-test IFA kit, indirect Toxoplasma gondii immunofluorescent antibody for IgG or IgM.

ANTIBODY, TREPONEMA PALLIDUM *(Microbiology) 83WJQ*

Bd Diagnostic Systems 800-675-0908
7 Loveton Cir, Sparks, MD 21152

United Biotech, Inc. 650-961-2910
211 S Whisman Rd Ste E, Mountain View, CA 94041
Antibody, Treponema Pallidum

Zeus Scientific, Inc. 800-286-2111
PO Box 38, Raritan, NJ 08869
100-test kit, Indirect Treponema pallidum immunofluorescent antibody for FTA-ABS test.

ANTIBODY, VARICELLA-ZOSTER *(Microbiology) 83WJU*

Zeus Scientific, Inc. 800-286-2111
PO Box 38, Raritan, NJ 08869
100-test system Varicella-zoster IgG IFA.

ANTIDEOXYRIBONUCLEASE, STREPTOCOCCUS SPP. *(Microbiology) 83GTR*

Wampole Laboratories 800-257-9525
2 Research Way, Princeton, NJ 08540
Zeus Scientific.

ANTIGEN, (FEBRILE), AGGLUTINATION, BRUCELLA SPP. *(Microbiology) 83GSO*

Bd Diagnostic Systems 800-675-0908
7 Loveton Cir, Sparks, MD 21152

Bd Lee Laboratories 800-732-9150
1475 Athens Hwy, Grayson, GA 30017

Germaine Laboratories, Inc. 210-692-4192
4139 Gardendale St Ste 101, San Antonio, TX 78229
Various types.

Immuno Resources, Inc. 830-537-6199
415 Sisterdale Rd, Boerne, TX 78006
Various.

Immunostics, Inc. 800-722-7505
3505 Sunset Ave, Ocean, NJ 07712

Sa Scientific, Inc. 800-272-2710
4919 Golden Quail, San Antonio, TX 78240
Brucella SPP (slide and tube agglutination test).

ANTIGEN, ALL GROUPS, SHIGELLA SPP. *(Microbiology) 83LIA*

Immunostics, Inc. 800-722-7505
3505 Sunset Ave, Ocean, NJ 07712

ANTIGEN, ALL TYPES, ESCHERICHIA COLI *(Microbiology) 83GMZ*

Ivd Research, Inc. 760-929-7744
5909 Sea Lion Pl Ste D, Carlsbad, CA 92010
E. coli 0157 stool antigen elisa.

ANTIGEN, ALL TYPES, ESCHERICHIA COLI *(cont'd)*

Oxoid, Inc. 800-567-8378
800 Proctor Ave, Ogdensburg, NY 13669
Latex test kit, Staph.

Sa Scientific, Inc. 800-272-2710
4919 Golden Quail, San Antonio, TX 78240

ANTIGEN, ANTISERUM, ALPHA-2-MACROGLOBULIN, RHODAMINE *(Immunology) 82DDT*

Binding Site, Inc., The 800-633-4484
5889 Oberlin Dr Ste 101, San Diego, CA 92121

ANTIGEN, ANTISERUM, COMPLEMENT C1 INHIBITOR (INACTIVATOR) *(Immunology) 82DBA*

Binding Site, Inc., The 800-633-4484
5889 Oberlin Dr Ste 101, San Diego, CA 92121

Kent Laboratories, Inc. 360-398-8641
777 Jorgensen Pl, Bellingham, WA 98226
2 ml antiserum (antigen, antiserum, complement C1 esterase inhibitor) R.I.D. kit.

Quidel Corp. 858-552-1100
2981 Copper Rd, Santa Clara, CA 95051
Complement c1 inhibitor (inactivator), antigen, antiserum, control.

ANTIGEN, ANTISERUM, CONTROL, ALBUMIN *(Immunology) 82DCF*

Access Bio Incorporate 732-297-2222
2033 Rt. 130 Unit H, Monmouth Junction, NJ 08852
Urinary albumin test.

American International Chemical 800-238-0001
135 Newbury St, Framingham, MA 01701

Antibodies, Inc. 800-824-8540
PO Box 1560, Davis, CA 95617

Binding Site, Inc., The 800-633-4484
5889 Oberlin Dr Ste 101, San Diego, CA 92121

Biocell Laboratories, Inc. 800-222-8382
2001 E University Dr, Rancho Dominguez, CA 90220

Dade Behring, Inc. 800-948-3233
1717 Deerfield Rd, Deerfield, IL 60015

Dako North America, Inc 805-566-6655
6392 Via Real, Carpinteria, CA 93013

Exocell, Inc. 800-234-3962
1880 John F Kennedy Blvd Ste 200, Philadelphia, PA 19103
Enzyme linked immunosorbent assay (elisa).

Health Chem Diagnostics Llc 954-979-3845
3341 W McNab Rd, Pompano Beach, FL 33069
Albumin, antigen, antiserum, control.

Immucor, Inc. 800-829-2553
3130 Gateway Dr, PO Box 5625, Norcross, GA 30071
CAPTURE-R solid phase for detection of donor antibodies. REACT micro-bead assay for antibody detection, identification and crossmatch.

Immuno Diagnostic Center, Inc. 214-351-1231
9978 Monroe Dr Ste 303, Dallas, TX 75220
Microalbumin kit.

International Immunology Corp. 800-843-2853
PO Box 972, Murrieta, CA 92564
Goat antiserum to Human Albumin and General Immunology Human Calibrator/Control Serum.

United Biotech, Inc. 650-961-2910
211 S Whisman Rd Ste E, Mountain View, CA 94041
ELISA quantitative for detecting Micro Albumin in human urine.

ANTIGEN, ANTISERUM, CONTROL, ALBUMIN, FITC *(Immunology) 82DDZ*

Antibodies, Inc. 800-824-8540
PO Box 1560, Davis, CA 95617

Binding Site, Inc., The 800-633-4484
5889 Oberlin Dr Ste 101, San Diego, CA 92121

Dako North America, Inc 805-566-6655
6392 Via Real, Carpinteria, CA 93013

ANTIGEN, ANTISERUM, CONTROL, ALBUMIN, FRACTION V *(Immunology) 82DCM*

Biocell Laboratories, Inc. 800-222-8382
2001 E University Dr, Rancho Dominguez, CA 90220

ANTIGEN, ANTISERUM, CONTROL, ALPHA-1-ANTICHYMOTRYPSIN *(Immunology) 82DFF*

Binding Site, Inc., The 800-633-4484
5889 Oberlin Dr Ste 101, San Diego, CA 92121

Dako North America, Inc 805-566-6655
6392 Via Real, Carpinteria, CA 93013

ANTIGEN, ANTISERUM, CONTROL, ALPHA-1-ANTITRYPSIN *(Immunology) 82DEM*

Dako North America, Inc 805-566-6655
6392 Via Real, Carpinteria, CA 93013

Health Chem Diagnostics Llc 954-979-3845
3341 W McNab Rd, Pompano Beach, FL 33069
Alpha-1-antitrypsin, antigen, antiserum, control.

International Immunology Corp. 800-843-2853
PO Box 972, Murrieta, CA 92564
Goat antiserum to Human Alpha-1-Antitrypsin and General Immunology Human Calibrator/Control Serum.

Kent Laboratories, Inc. 360-398-8641
777 Jorgensen Pl, Bellingham, WA 98226
Radial immunodiffusion kit.

Ventana Medical Systems, Inc. 800-227-2155
1910 E Innovation Park Dr, Oro Valley, AZ 85755
Various alpha-1-antitrypsin immunological test systems.

ANTIGEN, ANTISERUM, CONTROL, ALPHA-2-GLYCOPROTEINS *(Immunology) 82DEJ*

Binding Site, Inc., The 800-633-4484
5889 Oberlin Dr Ste 101, San Diego, CA 92121

ANTIGEN, ANTISERUM, CONTROL, ALPHA-2-HS-GLYCOPROTEIN *(Immunology) 82DEF*

Binding Site, Inc., The 800-633-4484
5889 Oberlin Dr Ste 101, San Diego, CA 92121

ANTIGEN, ANTISERUM, CONTROL, ALPHA-2-MACROGLOBULIN *(Immunology) 82DEB*

Binding Site, Inc., The 800-633-4484
5889 Oberlin Dr Ste 101, San Diego, CA 92121

Biocell Laboratories, Inc. 800-222-8382
2001 E University Dr, Rancho Dominguez, CA 90220

International Immunology Corp. 800-843-2853
PO Box 972, Murrieta, CA 92564
Goat antiserum to Human Alpha-2-Macroglobulin and General Immunology Human Calibrator/Control Serum.

ANTIGEN, ANTISERUM, CONTROL, ANTITHROMBIN III *(Immunology) 82DDQ*

Binding Site, Inc., The 800-633-4484
5889 Oberlin Dr Ste 101, San Diego, CA 92121

Dako North America, Inc 805-566-6655
6392 Via Real, Carpinteria, CA 93013

International Immunology Corp. 800-843-2853
PO Box 972, Murrieta, CA 92564
Goat antiserum to Human Antithrombin III

Kent Laboratories, Inc. 360-398-8641
777 Jorgensen Pl, Bellingham, WA 98226
2ml antiserum; radial immunodiffusion kit.

ANTIGEN, ANTISERUM, CONTROL, BENCE-JONES PROTEIN *(Immunology) 82CZQ*

Binding Site, Inc., The 800-633-4484
5889 Oberlin Dr Ste 101, San Diego, CA 92121

Invitrogen Corporation 800-955-6288
101 Lincoln Centre Dr, Foster City, CA 94404

Kent Laboratories, Inc. 360-398-8641
777 Jorgensen Pl, Bellingham, WA 98226
2 ml antiserum.

ANTIGEN, ANTISERUM, CONTROL, BETA GLOBULIN *(Immunology) 82DCJ*

United Biotech, Inc. 650-961-2910
211 S Whisman Rd Ste E, Mountain View, CA 94041
ELISA quantitative for Beta-2-Microglobulin.

ANTIGEN, ANTISERUM, CONTROL, CARCINOEMBRYONIC ANTIGEN *(Immunology) 82DHX*

Ameritek Usa, Inc. 425-379-2580
125 130th St SE Ste 200, Everett, WA 98208
Cea test kit.

ANTIGEN, ANTISERUM, CONTROL, CARCINOEMBRYONIC ANTIGEN *(cont'd)*

Biocheck, Inc. 650-573-1968
323 Vintage Park Dr, Foster City, CA 94404
Carcinoembryonic antigen eia test kit.

Dako North America, Inc 805-566-6655
6392 Via Real, Carpinteria, CA 93013

ANTIGEN, ANTISERUM, CONTROL, CERULOPLASMIN
(Immunology) 82DDB

Binding Site, Inc., The 800-633-4484
5889 Oberlin Dr Ste 101, San Diego, CA 92121

Dako North America, Inc 805-566-6655
6392 Via Real, Carpinteria, CA 93013

ANTIGEN, ANTISERUM, CONTROL, COMPLEMENT C1Q
(Immunology) 82DAK

Binding Site, Inc., The 800-633-4484
5889 Oberlin Dr Ste 101, San Diego, CA 92121

Dako North America, Inc 805-566-6655
6392 Via Real, Carpinteria, CA 93013

Kent Laboratories, Inc. 360-398-8641
777 Jorgensen Pl, Bellingham, WA 98226
2 ml antiserum, R.I.D. kit.

Quidel Corp. 858-552-1100
2981 Copper Rd, Santa Clara, CA 95051
Igg enzyme immunoassay.

ANTIGEN, ANTISERUM, CONTROL, COMPLEMENT C1R
(Immunology) 82DAI

Binding Site, Inc., The 800-633-4484
5889 Oberlin Dr Ste 101, San Diego, CA 92121

ANTIGEN, ANTISERUM, CONTROL, COMPLEMENT C1S
(Immunology) 82CZY

Binding Site, Inc., The 800-633-4484
5889 Oberlin Dr Ste 101, San Diego, CA 92121

ANTIGEN, ANTISERUM, CONTROL, COMPLEMENT C3
(Immunology) 82CZW

Abbott Diagnostics Div. 626-440-0700
820 Mission St, South Pasadena, CA 91030
Complement 3.

Binding Site, Inc., The 800-633-4484
5889 Oberlin Dr Ste 101, San Diego, CA 92121

Biocell Laboratories, Inc. 800-222-8382
2001 E University Dr, Rancho Dominguez, CA 90220

Carolina Liquid Chemistries Corp. 800-471-7272
510 W Central Ave Ste C, Brea, CA 92821
Complement c3 reagent.

Dako North America, Inc 805-566-6655
6392 Via Real, Carpinteria, CA 93013

Diasorin Inc 800-328-1482
1951 Northwestern Ave S, PO Box 285, Stillwater, MN 55082

International Immunology Corp. 800-843-2853
PO Box 972, Murrieta, CA 92564
Goat antiserum to Human Complement C3 and Goat antiserum to Human Complement C3 gamma fractionated and General Immunology Human Calibrator/Control Serum.

Kent Laboratories, Inc. 360-398-8641
777 Jorgensen Pl, Bellingham, WA 98226
2 ml C3b inactivator antiserum.

ANTIGEN, ANTISERUM, CONTROL, COMPLEMENT C4
(Immunology) 82DBI

Abbott Diagnostics Div. 626-440-0700
820 Mission St, South Pasadena, CA 91030
Complement 4.

Binding Site, Inc., The 800-633-4484
5889 Oberlin Dr Ste 101, San Diego, CA 92121

Biocell Laboratories, Inc. 800-222-8382
2001 E University Dr, Rancho Dominguez, CA 90220

Carolina Liquid Chemistries Corp. 800-471-7272
510 W Central Ave Ste C, Brea, CA 92821
Complement c4 reagent.

Dako North America, Inc 805-566-6655
6392 Via Real, Carpinteria, CA 93013

Diasorin Inc 800-328-1482
1951 Northwestern Ave S, PO Box 285, Stillwater, MN 55082

ANTIGEN, ANTISERUM, CONTROL, COMPLEMENT C4 *(cont'd)*

International Immunology Corp. 800-843-2853
PO Box 972, Murrieta, CA 92564
Goat antiserum to Human Complement C4 and Goat antiserum to Human Complement C4 gamma fractionated and General Immunology Human Calibrator/Control Serum.

Kent Laboratories, Inc. 360-398-8641
777 Jorgensen Pl, Bellingham, WA 98226
2ml antiserum; $79.88 for C-4 (BIE) radial immunodiffusion kit.

ANTIGEN, ANTISERUM, CONTROL, COMPLEMENT C5
(Immunology) 82DAY

Binding Site, Inc., The 800-633-4484
5889 Oberlin Dr Ste 101, San Diego, CA 92121

Dako North America, Inc 805-566-6655
6392 Via Real, Carpinteria, CA 93013

Kent Laboratories, Inc. 360-398-8641
777 Jorgensen Pl, Bellingham, WA 98226
2 ml antiserum, R.I.D. kit.

ANTIGEN, ANTISERUM, CONTROL, COMPLEMENT C8
(Immunology) 82DAG

Binding Site, Inc., The 800-633-4484
5889 Oberlin Dr Ste 101, San Diego, CA 92121

ANTIGEN, ANTISERUM, CONTROL, COMPLEMENT C9
(Immunology) 82DAE

Binding Site, Inc., The 800-633-4484
5889 Oberlin Dr Ste 101, San Diego, CA 92121

ANTIGEN, ANTISERUM, CONTROL, FAB *(Immunology) 82DCE*

Invitrogen Corporation 800-955-6288
101 Lincoln Centre Dr, Foster City, CA 94404

ANTIGEN, ANTISERUM, CONTROL, FAB, FITC
(Immunology) 82DCB

Invitrogen Corporation 800-955-6288
101 Lincoln Centre Dr, Foster City, CA 94404

ANTIGEN, ANTISERUM, CONTROL, FAB, RHODAMINE
(Immunology) 82DBY

Invitrogen Corporation 800-955-6288
101 Lincoln Centre Dr, Foster City, CA 94404

Kent Laboratories, Inc. 360-398-8641
777 Jorgensen Pl, Bellingham, WA 98226

ANTIGEN, ANTISERUM, CONTROL, FACTOR B
(Immunology) 82JZH

Binding Site, Inc., The 800-633-4484
5889 Oberlin Dr Ste 101, San Diego, CA 92121

Dako North America, Inc 805-566-6655
6392 Via Real, Carpinteria, CA 93013

Kent Laboratories, Inc. 360-398-8641
777 Jorgensen Pl, Bellingham, WA 98226
2 ml antiserum, R.I.D. kit.

ANTIGEN, ANTISERUM, CONTROL, FERRITIN
(Immunology) 82DBF

Ameritek Usa, Inc. 425-379-2580
125 130th St SE Ste 200, Everett, WA 98208
Ferritin test kit.

Dako North America, Inc 805-566-6655
6392 Via Real, Carpinteria, CA 93013

Kent Laboratories, Inc. 360-398-8641
777 Jorgensen Pl, Bellingham, WA 98226
2 ml antiserum.

Rockland Immunochemicals, Inc. 800-656-ROCK
PO Box 326, Gilbertsville, PA 19525

United Biotech, Inc. 650-961-2910
211 S Whisman Rd Ste E, Mountain View, CA 94041
ELISA quantitative for Ferritin.

ANTIGEN, ANTISERUM, CONTROL, FIBRINOGEN AND SPLIT PRODUCTS *(Immunology) 82DAZ*

Dako North America, Inc 805-566-6655
6392 Via Real, Carpinteria, CA 93013

ANTIGEN, ANTISERUM, CONTROL, FREE SECRETORY COMPONENT *(Immunology) 82DAJ*

Binding Site, Inc., The 800-633-4484
5889 Oberlin Dr Ste 101, San Diego, CA 92121

ANTIGEN, ANTISERUM, CONTROL, FREE SECRETORY COMPONENT *(cont'd)*

Dako North America, Inc 805-566-6655
6392 Via Real, Carpinteria, CA 93013

ANTIGEN, ANTISERUM, CONTROL, GAMMA GLOBULIN
(Immunology) 82DAH

Antibodies, Inc. 800-824-8540
PO Box 1560, Davis, CA 95617

Binding Site, Inc., The 800-633-4484
5889 Oberlin Dr Ste 101, San Diego, CA 92121

Dako North America, Inc 805-566-6655
6392 Via Real, Carpinteria, CA 93013

ANTIGEN, ANTISERUM, CONTROL, GAMMA GLOBULIN, FITC
(Immunology) 82DAF

Antibodies, Inc. 800-824-8540
PO Box 1560, Davis, CA 95617

Binding Site, Inc., The 800-633-4484
5889 Oberlin Dr Ste 101, San Diego, CA 92121

Dako North America, Inc 805-566-6655
6392 Via Real, Carpinteria, CA 93013

ANTIGEN, ANTISERUM, CONTROL, HAPTOGLOBIN
(Immunology) 82DAD

Abbott Diagnostics Div. 626-440-0700
820 Mission St, South Pasadena, CA 91030
Haptoglobin.

Binding Site, Inc., The 800-633-4484
5889 Oberlin Dr Ste 101, San Diego, CA 92121

Biocell Laboratories, Inc. 800-222-8382
2001 E University Dr, Rancho Dominguez, CA 90220

Biomerieux Inc. 800-682-2666
100 Rodolphe St, Durham, NC 27712

Carolina Liquid Chemistries Corp. 800-471-7272
510 W Central Ave Ste C, Brea, CA 92821
Haptoglobin reagent.

Dako North America, Inc 805-566-6655
6392 Via Real, Carpinteria, CA 93013

Helena Laboratories 409-842-3714
PO Box 752, Beaumont, TX 77704

International Immunology Corp. 800-843-2853
PO Box 972, Murrieta, CA 92564
Goat antiserum to Human Haptoglobin and General Immunology Human Calibrator/Control Serum.

Kent Laboratories, Inc. 360-398-8641
777 Jorgensen Pl, Bellingham, WA 98226
Radial immunodiffusion kit.

ANTIGEN, ANTISERUM, CONTROL, HEMOPEXIN
(Immunology) 82CZX

Dako North America, Inc 805-566-6655
6392 Via Real, Carpinteria, CA 93013

ANTIGEN, ANTISERUM, CONTROL, IGA *(Immunology) 82CZP*

Abbott Diagnostics Div. 626-440-0700
820 Mission St, South Pasadena, CA 91030
Immunoglobulin a.

Accurate Chemical & Scientific Corp. 800-645-6264
300 Shames Dr, Westbury, NY 11590

Antibodies, Inc. 800-824-8540
PO Box 1560, Davis, CA 95617

Binding Site, Inc., The 800-633-4484
5889 Oberlin Dr Ste 101, San Diego, CA 92121

Biocell Laboratories, Inc. 800-222-8382
2001 E University Dr, Rancho Dominguez, CA 90220

Dako North America, Inc 805-566-6655
6392 Via Real, Carpinteria, CA 93013

Diasorin Inc 800-328-1482
1951 Northwestern Ave S, PO Box 285, Stillwater, MN 55082

Health Chem Diagnostics Llc 954-979-3845
3341 W McNab Rd, Pompano Beach, FL 33069
Iga, antigen, antiserum, control.

Helena Laboratories 409-842-3714
PO Box 752, Beaumont, TX 77704

ANTIGEN, ANTISERUM, CONTROL, IGA *(cont'd)*

International Immunology Corp. 800-843-2853
PO Box 972, Murrieta, CA 92564
Goat antiserum to Human IgA and Goat antiserum to Human IgA gamma fractionated and Goat antibodies to Human IgA affinity-purified and General Immunology Human Calibrator/Control Sera.

Invitrogen Corporation 800-955-6288
101 Lincoln Centre Dr, Foster City, CA 94404

Kent Laboratories, Inc. 360-398-8641
777 Jorgensen Pl, Bellingham, WA 98226
2 ml antiserum.

ANTIGEN, ANTISERUM, CONTROL, IGA, FITC
(Immunology) 82CZN

Antibodies, Inc. 800-824-8540
PO Box 1560, Davis, CA 95617

Binding Site, Inc., The 800-633-4484
5889 Oberlin Dr Ste 101, San Diego, CA 92121

Dako North America, Inc 805-566-6655
6392 Via Real, Carpinteria, CA 93013

Diasorin Inc 800-328-1482
1951 Northwestern Ave S, PO Box 285, Stillwater, MN 55082

Invitrogen Corporation 800-955-6288
101 Lincoln Centre Dr, Foster City, CA 94404

ANTIGEN, ANTISERUM, CONTROL, IGA, PEROXIDASE
(Immunology) 82CZL

Binding Site, Inc., The 800-633-4484
5889 Oberlin Dr Ste 101, San Diego, CA 92121

Dako North America, Inc 805-566-6655
6392 Via Real, Carpinteria, CA 93013

Diasorin Inc 800-328-1482
1951 Northwestern Ave S, PO Box 285, Stillwater, MN 55082

Invitrogen Corporation 800-955-6288
101 Lincoln Centre Dr, Foster City, CA 94404

ANTIGEN, ANTISERUM, CONTROL, IGA, RHODAMINE
(Immunology) 82CZK

Dako North America, Inc 805-566-6655
6392 Via Real, Carpinteria, CA 93013

ANTIGEN, ANTISERUM, CONTROL, IGD *(Immunology) 82CZJ*

Binding Site, Inc., The 800-633-4484
5889 Oberlin Dr Ste 101, San Diego, CA 92121

Dako North America, Inc 805-566-6655
6392 Via Real, Carpinteria, CA 93013

Health Chem Diagnostics Llc 954-979-3845
3341 W McNab Rd, Pompano Beach, FL 33069
Igd, antigen, antiserum, control.

Helena Laboratories 409-842-3714
PO Box 752, Beaumont, TX 77704

International Immunology Corp. 800-843-2853
PO Box 972, Murrieta, CA 92564
Goat antiserum to Human IgD, gamma fractionated

Invitrogen Corporation 800-955-6288
101 Lincoln Centre Dr, Foster City, CA 94404

Kent Laboratories, Inc. 360-398-8641
777 Jorgensen Pl, Bellingham, WA 98226
Radial immunodiffusion kit.

ANTIGEN, ANTISERUM, CONTROL, IGD, FITC
(Immunology) 82DGG

Dako North America, Inc 805-566-6655
6392 Via Real, Carpinteria, CA 93013

Invitrogen Corporation 800-955-6288
101 Lincoln Centre Dr, Foster City, CA 94404

ANTIGEN, ANTISERUM, CONTROL, IGD, PEROXIDASE
(Immunology) 82DGH

Dako North America, Inc 805-566-6655
6392 Via Real, Carpinteria, CA 93013

Invitrogen Corporation 800-955-6288
101 Lincoln Centre Dr, Foster City, CA 94404

ANTIGEN, ANTISERUM, CONTROL, IGD, RHODAMINE
(Immunology) 82DGE

Dako North America, Inc 805-566-6655
6392 Via Real, Carpinteria, CA 93013

ANTIGEN, ANTISERUM, CONTROL, IGE *(Immunology) 82DGC*

Alerchek, Inc. 877-282-9542
203 Anderson St, Portland, ME 04101
Elisa based microwell assays for total IgE, IgG, IgM, IgA, Apo AI, Apo B, Lp(a), C-Reactive Protein, Allergen-specific IgE (400 allergens).

Ameritek Usa, Inc. 425-379-2580
125 130th St SE Ste 200, Everett, WA 98208
Ige test kit.

Antibodies, Inc. 800-824-8540
PO Box 1560, Davis, CA 95617

Binding Site, Inc., The 800-633-4484
5889 Oberlin Dr Ste 101, San Diego, CA 92121

Dako North America, Inc 805-566-6655
6392 Via Real, Carpinteria, CA 93013

Health Chem Diagnostics Llc 954-979-3845
3341 W McNab Rd, Pompano Beach, FL 33069
Ige, antigen, antiserum, control.

Helena Laboratories 409-842-3714
PO Box 752, Beaumont, TX 77704

International Immunology Corp. 800-843-2853
PO Box 972, Murrieta, CA 92564
Goat antiserum to Human IgE and Goat antiserum to Human IgE, gamma fractionated and Goat antibodies to Human IgE, affinity purified

Invitrogen Corporation 800-955-6288
101 Lincoln Centre Dr, Foster City, CA 94404

Kent Laboratories, Inc. 360-398-8641
777 Jorgensen Pl, Bellingham, WA 98226
2 ml antiserum.

United Biotech, Inc. 650-961-2910
211 S Whisman Rd Ste E, Mountain View, CA 94041
ELISA for detecting IgE

ANTIGEN, ANTISERUM, CONTROL, IGE, FITC *(Immunology) 82DGP*

Antibodies, Inc. 800-824-8540
PO Box 1560, Davis, CA 95617

Dako North America, Inc 805-566-6655
6392 Via Real, Carpinteria, CA 93013

Invitrogen Corporation 800-955-6288
101 Lincoln Centre Dr, Foster City, CA 94404

ANTIGEN, ANTISERUM, CONTROL, IGE, PEROXIDASE *(Immunology) 82DGO*

Binding Site, Inc., The 800-633-4484
5889 Oberlin Dr Ste 101, San Diego, CA 92121

Dako North America, Inc 805-566-6655
6392 Via Real, Carpinteria, CA 93013

Health Chem Diagnostics Llc 954-979-3845
3341 W McNab Rd, Pompano Beach, FL 33069
Ige, peroxidase, antigen, antiserum, control.

Invitrogen Corporation 800-955-6288
101 Lincoln Centre Dr, Foster City, CA 94404

ANTIGEN, ANTISERUM, CONTROL, IGG *(Immunology) 82DEW*

Abbott Diagnostics Div. 626-440-0700
820 Mission St, South Pasadena, CA 91030
Immunoglobulin g.

Beckman Coulter, Inc. 800-635-3497
740 W 83rd St, Hialeah, FL 33014

Binding Site, Inc., The 800-633-4484
5889 Oberlin Dr Ste 101, San Diego, CA 92121
Human IgG subclass quantitation kits, IgG, A, M; poly-/monoclonal RID and EIA kits and nephelometric/turbidimetric kits.

Biocell Laboratories, Inc. 800-222-8382
2001 E University Dr, Rancho Dominguez, CA 90220

Biogenex Laboratories 800-421-4149
4600 Norris Canyon Rd, San Ramon, CA 94583

Dako North America, Inc 805-566-6655
6392 Via Real, Carpinteria, CA 93013

Diasorin Inc 800-328-1482
1951 Northwestern Ave S, PO Box 285, Stillwater, MN 55082

Health Chem Diagnostics Llc 954-979-3845
3341 W McNab Rd, Pompano Beach, FL 33069
Igg, antigen, antiserum, control.

ANTIGEN, ANTISERUM, CONTROL, IGG *(cont'd)*

Kent Laboratories, Inc. 360-398-8641
777 Jorgensen Pl, Bellingham, WA 98226
Radial immunodiffusion kit.

Rockland Immunochemicals, Inc. 800-656-ROCK
PO Box 326, Gilbertsville, PA 19525

Vector Laboratories, Inc. 800-227-6666
30 Ingold Rd, Burlingame, CA 94010
$215.00 for VECTASTAIN ABC horseradish peroxidase, alkaline phosphatase or glucose oxidase (with biotinylated anti-immunoglobulin). $75.00 for 0.5-1.5mg unconjugated anti-immunoglobulins.

ANTIGEN, ANTISERUM, CONTROL, IGG (FAB FRAGMENT SPECIFIC) *(Immunology) 82DFK*

Antibodies, Inc. 800-824-8540
PO Box 1560, Davis, CA 95617

Diasorin Inc 800-328-1482
1951 Northwestern Ave S, PO Box 285, Stillwater, MN 55082

Invitrogen Corporation 800-955-6288
101 Lincoln Centre Dr, Foster City, CA 94404

ANTIGEN, ANTISERUM, CONTROL, IGG (FC FRAGMENT SPECIFIC) *(Immunology) 82DAS*

Antibodies, Inc. 800-824-8540
PO Box 1560, Davis, CA 95617

Dako North America, Inc 805-566-6655
6392 Via Real, Carpinteria, CA 93013

International Immunology Corp. 800-843-2853
PO Box 972, Murrieta, CA 92564
Goat antiserum to Human IgG, Fc and Goat antiserum to Human IgG, Fc - gamma fractionated and Goat antibodies to Human IgG, Fc - affinity purified and General Immunology Human Calibrator/Control Serum

ANTIGEN, ANTISERUM, CONTROL, IGG (GAMMA CHAIN SPECIFIC) *(Immunology) 82DFZ*

Antibodies, Inc. 800-824-8540
PO Box 1560, Davis, CA 95617

Binding Site, Inc., The 800-633-4484
5889 Oberlin Dr Ste 101, San Diego, CA 92121

Dako North America, Inc 805-566-6655
6392 Via Real, Carpinteria, CA 93013

Helena Laboratories 409-842-3714
PO Box 752, Beaumont, TX 77704

Invitrogen Corporation 800-955-6288
101 Lincoln Centre Dr, Foster City, CA 94404

ANTIGEN, ANTISERUM, CONTROL, IGG, FITC *(Immunology) 82DGK*

Antibodies, Inc. 800-824-8540
PO Box 1560, Davis, CA 95617

Beckman Coulter, Inc. 800-635-3497
740 W 83rd St, Hialeah, FL 33014

Dako North America, Inc 805-566-6655
6392 Via Real, Carpinteria, CA 93013

Hemagen Diagnostics, Inc. 800-436-2436
9033 Red Branch Rd, Columbia, MD 21045
Conjugates, ifa.

Immco Diagnostics, Inc. 800-537-8378
60 Pineview Dr, Buffalo, NY 14228

Invitrogen Corporation 800-955-6288
101 Lincoln Centre Dr, Foster City, CA 94404

Rockland Immunochemicals, Inc. 800-656-ROCK
PO Box 326, Gilbertsville, PA 19525

Vector Laboratories, Inc. 800-227-6666
30 Ingold Rd, Burlingame, CA 94010
$80.00 for fluorescent Avidin sample kit (0.5mg ea. of fluorescein, AMCA, and Texas Red conjugated to Avidin D). $65.00 to $75.00 for 1-5mg flurochrome avidins (AMCA, fluorescein, rhodamine, Texas Red, phycoerythrin). $70.00 for either 1.5mg fluorescein anti-goat IgG (H+L), made in rabbit; 1.5mg fluorescein anti-human IgG (H+L), made in goat; $70.00, 0.5mg fluorescein anti-mouse IgM (mu chain specific), made in goat; 1.5mg fluorescein anti-rat IgG (H+L), made in rabbit; 1.5mg fluorescein anti-guinea pig IgG (H+L), made in goat; or 1.5mg fluorescein anti-sheep IgG (H+L), made in rabbit.

ANTIGEN, ANTISERUM, CONTROL, IGG, PEROXIDASE
(Immunology) 82DAA

Antibodies, Inc. 800-824-8540
PO Box 1560, Davis, CA 95617

Dako North America, Inc 805-566-6655
6392 Via Real, Carpinteria, CA 93013

Invitrogen Corporation 800-955-6288
101 Lincoln Centre Dr, Foster City, CA 94404

Rockland Immunochemicals, Inc. 800-656-ROCK
PO Box 326, Gilbertsville, PA 19525
Peroxidase, anti-peroxidase soluble complexes.

Vector Laboratories, Inc. 800-227-6666
30 Ingold Rd, Burlingame, CA 94010
$65.00 for 1mg horseradish peroxidase anti-human IgG (H+L), made in goat; or for 1mg horseradish peroxidase anti-rabbit IgG (H+L), made in goat; or for 1mg horseradish peroxidase anti-mouse IgG (H+L), made in horse. $215.00 for VECTASTAIN ABC horseradish peroxidase kit, - $235.00 for the elite version.

ANTIGEN, ANTISERUM, CONTROL, IGG, RHODAMINE
(Immunology) 82DFO

Dako North America, Inc 805-566-6655
6392 Via Real, Carpinteria, CA 93013

Invitrogen Corporation 800-955-6288
101 Lincoln Centre Dr, Foster City, CA 94404

Rockland Immunochemicals, Inc. 800-656-ROCK
PO Box 326, Gilbertsville, PA 19525

ANTIGEN, ANTISERUM, CONTROL, IGM *(Immunology) 82DFT*

Abbott Diagnostics Div. 626-440-0700
820 Mission St, South Pasadena, CA 91030
Immunoglobulin m.

Antibodies, Inc. 800-824-8540
PO Box 1560, Davis, CA 95617

Beckman Coulter, Inc. 800-635-3497
740 W 83rd St, Hialeah, FL 33014

Biocell Laboratories, Inc. 800-222-8382
2001 E University Dr, Rancho Dominguez, CA 90220

Dako North America, Inc 805-566-6655
6392 Via Real, Carpinteria, CA 93013

Diasorin Inc 800-328-1482
1951 Northwestern Ave S, PO Box 285, Stillwater, MN 55082

Health Chem Diagnostics Llc 954-979-3845
3341 W McNab Rd, Pompano Beach, FL 33069
Igm, antigen, antiserum, control.

Kent Laboratories, Inc. 360-398-8641
777 Jorgensen Pl, Bellingham, WA 98226
Radial immunodiffusion kit.

Vector Laboratories, Inc. 800-227-6666
30 Ingold Rd, Burlingame, CA 94010
$215.00 for Vectastain ABC-Horseradish Peroxidase, ABC-Glucose Oxidase and ABC-Alkaline Phosphatase kit (human IgM).

ANTIGEN, ANTISERUM, CONTROL, IGM (MU CHAIN SPECIFIC)
(Immunology) 82DAO

Antibodies, Inc. 800-824-8540
PO Box 1560, Davis, CA 95617

Beckman Coulter, Inc. 800-635-3497
740 W 83rd St, Hialeah, FL 33014

Dako North America, Inc 805-566-6655
6392 Via Real, Carpinteria, CA 93013

Helena Laboratories 409-842-3714
PO Box 752, Beaumont, TX 77704

International Immunology Corp. 800-843-2853
PO Box 972, Murrieta, CA 92564
Goat antiserum to Human IgM and Goat antiserum to Human IgM, gamma fractionated and Goat antibodies to Human IgM, affinity purified and General Immunology Human Calibrator/Control Serum

Invitrogen Corporation 800-955-6288
101 Lincoln Centre Dr, Foster City, CA 94404

Vector Laboratories, Inc. 800-227-6666
30 Ingold Rd, Burlingame, CA 94010
$60.00 for 0.5mg anti-human and anti-mouse IgM, mu chain specific, made in goat.

ANTIGEN, ANTISERUM, CONTROL, IGM, FITC
(Immunology) 82DFS

Antibodies, Inc. 800-824-8540
PO Box 1560, Davis, CA 95617

Beckman Coulter, Inc. 800-635-3497
740 W 83rd St, Hialeah, FL 33014

Dako North America, Inc 805-566-6655
6392 Via Real, Carpinteria, CA 93013

Invitrogen Corporation 800-955-6288
101 Lincoln Centre Dr, Foster City, CA 94404

ANTIGEN, ANTISERUM, CONTROL, IGM, PEROXIDASE
(Immunology) 82DEY

Dako North America, Inc 805-566-6655
6392 Via Real, Carpinteria, CA 93013

Invitrogen Corporation 800-955-6288
101 Lincoln Centre Dr, Foster City, CA 94404

Ventana Medical Systems, Inc. 800-227-2155
1910 E Innovation Park Dr, Oro Valley, AZ 85755
Various igm peroxidase antigen antiserum controls.

ANTIGEN, ANTISERUM, CONTROL, IGM, RHODAMINE
(Immunology) 82DEZ

Dako North America, Inc 805-566-6655
6392 Via Real, Carpinteria, CA 93013

Invitrogen Corporation 800-955-6288
101 Lincoln Centre Dr, Foster City, CA 94404

ANTIGEN, ANTISERUM, CONTROL, INTER-ALPHA TRYPSIN INHIBITOR *(Immunology) 82CZO*

Dako North America, Inc 805-566-6655
6392 Via Real, Carpinteria, CA 93013

ANTIGEN, ANTISERUM, CONTROL, KAPPA *(Immunology) 82DFH*

Dako North America, Inc 805-566-6655
6392 Via Real, Carpinteria, CA 93013

Health Chem Diagnostics Llc 954-979-3845
3341 W McNab Rd, Pompano Beach, FL 33069
Kappa, antigen, antiserum, control.

Helena Laboratories 409-842-3714
PO Box 752, Beaumont, TX 77704

International Immunology Corp. 800-843-2853
PO Box 972, Murrieta, CA 92564
Goat antiserum to Human Kappa (Free & Bound), gamma fractionated

Invitrogen Corporation 800-955-6288
101 Lincoln Centre Dr, Foster City, CA 94404

Kent Laboratories, Inc. 360-398-8641
777 Jorgensen Pl, Bellingham, WA 98226
2 ml antiserum.

ANTIGEN, ANTISERUM, CONTROL, KAPPA, FITC
(Immunology) 82DEO

Dako North America, Inc 805-566-6655
6392 Via Real, Carpinteria, CA 93013

Invitrogen Corporation 800-955-6288
101 Lincoln Centre Dr, Foster City, CA 94404

ANTIGEN, ANTISERUM, CONTROL, KAPPA, RHODAMINE
(Immunology) 82DEK

Dako North America, Inc 805-566-6655
6392 Via Real, Carpinteria, CA 93013

ANTIGEN, ANTISERUM, CONTROL, LACTOFERRIN
(Immunology) 82DEG

Dako North America, Inc 805-566-6655
6392 Via Real, Carpinteria, CA 93013

Techlab, Inc. 800-832-4522
2001 Kraft Dr, Blacksburg, VA 24060
IBD-CHEK is an enzyme immunoassay for the detection of elevated levels of lactoferrin, a stable marker of intestinal inflammation. The test can distinguish between Inflammatory Bowel Disease and Irritable Bowel Syndrome after other causes of inflammation have been ruled out.

ANTIGEN, ANTISERUM, CONTROL, LAMBDA
(Immunology) 82DEH

Dako North America, Inc 805-566-6655
6392 Via Real, Carpinteria, CA 93013

ANTIGEN, ANTISERUM, CONTROL, LAMBDA *(cont'd)*

Health Chem Diagnostics Llc 954-979-3845
3341 W McNab Rd, Pompano Beach, FL 33069
Lambda, antigen, antiserum, control.

Helena Laboratories 409-842-3714
PO Box 752, Beaumont, TX 77704

International Immunology Corp. 800-843-2853
PO Box 972, Murrieta, CA 92564
Goat antiserum to Human Lambda (Free & Bound), gamma fractionated

Invitrogen Corporation 800-955-6288
101 Lincoln Centre Dr, Foster City, CA 94404

Kent Laboratories, Inc. 360-398-8641
777 Jorgensen Pl, Bellingham, WA 98226
2 ml antiserum.

Ventana Medical Systems, Inc. 800-227-2155
1910 E Innovation Park Dr, Oro Valley, AZ 85755
Keratin antibody.

ANTIGEN, ANTISERUM, CONTROL, LAMBDA, FITC
(Immunology) 82DES

Dako North America, Inc 805-566-6655
6392 Via Real, Carpinteria, CA 93013

Invitrogen Corporation 800-955-6288
101 Lincoln Centre Dr, Foster City, CA 94404

ANTIGEN, ANTISERUM, CONTROL, LAMBDA, RHODAMINE
(Immunology) 82DFG

Dako North America, Inc 805-566-6655
6392 Via Real, Carpinteria, CA 93013

ANTIGEN, ANTISERUM, CONTROL, LIPOPROTEIN, LOW DENSITY *(Immunology) 82DFC*

Biomedical Technologies, Inc. 781-344-9942
378 Page St, Stoughton, MA 02072

Carolina Liquid Chemistries Corp. 800-471-7272
510 W Central Ave Ste C, Brea, CA 92821
Lp(a) calibrator and control.

Creative Laboratory Products, Inc. 317-293-2991
6420 Guion Rd, Indianapolis, IN 46268
Lipoproteins - human low density and human high density, cholesterol lipoproteins and lipid controls.

Diadexus, Inc. 650-246-6400
343 Oyster Point Blvd, South San Francisco, CA 94080
Lp-pla2 test.

Raichem, Division Of Hemagen Diagnostics, Inc. 800-438-6100
8225 Mercury Ct, San Diego, CA 92111
SPIA Apolipoprotein B determination, liquid ready-to-use immunological reagent, Immunoturbidimetric.

Strategic Diagnostics, Inc. 302-456-6785
111 Pencader Dr, Newark, DE 19702
Lp(a) test kit; lipoprotein (a) test kit.

ANTIGEN, ANTISERUM, CONTROL, LUTEINIZING HORMONE
(Immunology) 82DHP

Biomerica, Inc. 800-854-3002
17571 Von Karman Ave, Irvine, CA 92614
#1050 One step 5 min. test for determination of LH surge (EZ-LH). #50001 One step home test for determination of LH surge (Fortel).

Dako North America, Inc 805-566-6655
6392 Via Real, Carpinteria, CA 93013

ANTIGEN, ANTISERUM, CONTROL, LYMPHOCYTE TYPING
(Immunology) 82DGS

Advanced Biotechnologies, Inc. 800-426-0764
9108 Guilford Rd, Rivers Park II, Columbia, MD 21046
Viral antigens, viral antibodies, proteins and DNA/RNA controls.

Amgen Inc. 206-265-7000
1201 Amgen Ct W, Seattle, WA 98119

Dako North America, Inc 805-566-6655
6392 Via Real, Carpinteria, CA 93013

Genzyme 800-332-1042
500 Kendall St, Cambridge, MA 02142
Laboratory reagent formulations of lymphokines to cytokines.

Invitrogen Corporation 800-955-6288
101 Lincoln Centre Dr, Foster City, CA 94404

ANTIGEN, ANTISERUM, CONTROL, LYSOZYME
(Immunology) 82DED

Biomedical Technologies, Inc. 781-344-9942
378 Page St, Stoughton, MA 02072

Dako North America, Inc 805-566-6655
6392 Via Real, Carpinteria, CA 93013

ANTIGEN, ANTISERUM, CONTROL, MYOGLOBIN
(Immunology) 82DDR

Ameritek Usa, Inc. 425-379-2580
125 130th St SE Ste 200, Everett, WA 98208
Myoglobin test kit.

Biosite Incorporated 888-246-7483
9975 Summers Ridge Rd, San Diego, CA 92121
Fluorescence immunoassay for ckmb, troponini and myoglobin.

Dako North America, Inc 805-566-6655
6392 Via Real, Carpinteria, CA 93013

International Immunology Corp. 800-843-2853
PO Box 972, Murrieta, CA 92564
Goat antibodies to Human Myoglobin, IgG fractionated and Goat antibodies to Human Myoglobin, affinity purified

Nano-Ditech Corporation 609-409-0700
7 Clarke Dr, Cranbury, NJ 08512
Myoglobin, antigen, antiserum control.

ANTIGEN, ANTISERUM, CONTROL, OTHER *(Immunology) 82WNJ*

American Diagnostica, Inc. 888-234-4435
500 West Ave, Stamford, CT 06902

Antibodies, Inc. 800-824-8540
PO Box 1560, Davis, CA 95617
Contract and catalog antisera production, purification, labeling and packaging.

Cedarlane Laboratories Ltd. 800-268-5058
5516 8th Line R.R. 2, Hornby, ONT L0P 1E0 Canada
Anti-HLA antiserum.

Immucor, Inc. 800-829-2553
3130 Gateway Dr, PO Box 5625, Norcross, GA 30071
CAPTURE-P solid phase IA for detection of antibodies to platelets. CAPTURE-S solid phase for detection of syphilis in donors.

International Immunology Corp. 800-843-2853
PO Box 972, Murrieta, CA 92564
Goat antiserum/antibodies to Human apolipoproteins A1, B, A2, C2, C3, Apo(a). Goat antiserum/antibodies to Human Troponin I and CKMM and Dual Apolipoprotein (AI+B)Human Calibrator and Goat antiserum to Human CRP and Goat antiserum to Human CRP, gamma fractionated and Goat antiserum to Human CRP, affinity purified and CRP Human Calibrator/Control Serum.

Kent Laboratories, Inc. 360-398-8641
777 Jorgensen Pl, Bellingham, WA 98226
2ml C-1 Esterase Inhibitor antiserum.

Kronus, Inc. 800-822-6999
12554 W Bridger St Ste 108, Boise, ID 83713
Calibrators and control sera for use in autoimmune disease diagnostic kits.

United Biotech, Inc. 650-961-2910
211 S Whisman Rd Ste E, Mountain View, CA 94041
ELISA detecting Protein C.

Vector Laboratories, Inc. 800-227-6666
30 Ingold Rd, Burlingame, CA 94010
$60.00 for either 0.5mg anti-human IgA, alpha chain specific, made in goat; 0.5mg anti-human kappa chain, made in goat; or for 0.5mg anti-human lambda chain, made in goat. $75.00 for either 0.5mg anti-mouse IgG, gamma chain specific, made in horse; or for 0.5mg biotinylated anti-sheep IgG, gamma chain specific, made in rabbit.

ANTIGEN, ANTISERUM, CONTROL, PLASMINOGEN
(Immunology) 82DDX

Dako North America, Inc 805-566-6655
6392 Via Real, Carpinteria, CA 93013

ANTIGEN, ANTISERUM, CONTROL, PREALBUMIN
(Immunology) 82JZJ

Abbott Diagnostics Div. 626-440-0700
820 Mission St, South Pasadena, CA 91030
Prealbumin.

Dako North America, Inc 805-566-6655
6392 Via Real, Carpinteria, CA 93013

Diasorin Inc 800-328-1482
1951 Northwestern Ave S, PO Box 285, Stillwater, MN 55082

ANTIGEN, ANTISERUM, CONTROL, PREALBUMIN *(cont'd)*

Helena Laboratories 409-842-3714
PO Box 752, Beaumont, TX 77704

Immucor, Inc. 800-829-2553
3130 Gateway Dr, PO Box 5625, Norcross, GA 30071
CAPTURE-CMV solid phase for detection of CMV.

Jas Diagnostics, Inc. 305-418-2320
7220 NW 58th St, Miami, FL 33166
Prealbumin.

ANTIGEN, ANTISERUM, CONTROL, PREALBUMIN, FITC
(Immunology) 82DDS

Carolina Liquid Chemistries Corp. 800-471-7272
510 W Central Ave Ste C, Brea, CA 92821
Prealbumin reagent.

ANTIGEN, ANTISERUM, CONTROL, PROTEIN, COMPLEMENT
(Immunology) 82DHL

Aalto Scientific Ltd. 760-431-7922
1959 Kellogg Ave, Carlsbad, CA 92008
Multiple

Dako North America, Inc 805-566-6655
6392 Via Real, Carpinteria, CA 93013

ANTIGEN, ANTISERUM, CONTROL, PROTHROMBIN
(Immunology) 82DDF

Biomerieux Inc. 800-682-2666
100 Rodolphe St, Durham, NC 27712
Prothrombin time test reagent, simplastin products are thromboplastin reagent for PT determinations; used to monitor oral anticoagulant therapy and detect factor deficiencies.

Dako North America, Inc 805-566-6655
6392 Via Real, Carpinteria, CA 93013

Immucor, Inc. 800-829-2553
3130 Gateway Dr, PO Box 5625, Norcross, GA 30071

ANTIGEN, ANTISERUM, CONTROL, RED CELLS
(Hematology) 81JZK

Immucor, Inc. 800-829-2553
3130 Gateway Dr, PO Box 5625, Norcross, GA 30071

ANTIGEN, ANTISERUM, CONTROL, SPINAL FLUID, TOTAL
(Immunology) 82DFI

Clin-Chem Mfg. Llc. 800-359-9691
2560 Business Pkwy Ste C, Minden, NV 89423
For control of spinal fluid assays.

Health Chem Diagnostics Llc 954-979-3845
3341 W McNab Rd, Pompano Beach, FL 33069
Total spinal-fluid, antigen, antiserum, control.

Hycor Biomedical, Inc. 800-382-2527
7272 Chapman Ave, Garden Grove, CA 92841
Spinal fluid (microscopic) control.

Kenlor Industries, Inc. 714-647-0770
1560 E Edinger Ave Ste A1, Santa Ana, CA 92705
Kenlor human spinal fluid control liquid.

ANTIGEN, ANTISERUM, CONTROL, TRANSFERRIN
(Immunology) 82DDG

Abbott Diagnostics Div. 626-440-0700
820 Mission St, South Pasadena, CA 91030
Transferrin.

Accurate Chemical & Scientific Corp. 800-645-6264
300 Shames Dr, Westbury, NY 11590

Biocell Laboratories, Inc. 800-222-8382
2001 E University Dr, Rancho Dominguez, CA 90220

Carolina Liquid Chemistries Corp. 800-471-7272
510 W Central Ave Ste C, Brea, CA 92821
Transferrin reagent.

Dako North America, Inc 805-566-6655
6392 Via Real, Carpinteria, CA 93013

International Immunology Corp. 800-843-2853
PO Box 972, Murrieta, CA 92564
Goat antiserum to Human Transferrin and General Immunology Human Calibrator/Control Serum.

Kent Laboratories, Inc. 360-398-8641
777 Jorgensen Pl, Bellingham, WA 98226
Radial immunodiffusion kit.

ANTIGEN, ANTISERUM, CONTROL, WHOLE HUMAN SERUM
(Immunology) 82DGR

Advanced Biotechnologies, Inc. 800-426-0764
9108 Guilford Rd, Rivers Park II, Columbia, MD 21046

Biocell Laboratories, Inc. 800-222-8382
2001 E University Dr, Rancho Dominguez, CA 90220

Cst Technologies, Inc. 800-448-4407
55 Northern Blvd Ste 200, Great Neck, NY 11021
$145 per liter of SERASUB HSA, BSA, outdated plasma substitute.

Dako North America, Inc 805-566-6655
6392 Via Real, Carpinteria, CA 93013

Health Chem Diagnostics Llc 954-979-3845
3341 W McNab Rd, Pompano Beach, FL 33069
Whole human serum, antigen, antiserum, control.

Helena Laboratories 409-842-3714
PO Box 752, Beaumont, TX 77704

International Immunology Corp. 800-843-2853
PO Box 972, Murrieta, CA 92564
Goat antiserum to Whole Human Serum

Kent Laboratories, Inc. 360-398-8641
777 Jorgensen Pl, Bellingham, WA 98226
2 ml antiserum.

Ortho-Clinical Diagnostics, Inc. 800-828-6316
513 Technology Blvd, Rochester, NY 14626
Control reagent for all blood grouping reagent for rh slide test.

Theratest Laboratories, Inc. 800-441-0771
1111 N Main St, Lombard, IL 60148
Normal human serum controls, 100 donor set with demographics.

Valley Biomedical Products/Ser., Inc. 540-868-0800
121 Industrial Dr, Winchester, VA 22602
Dental curing light.

ANTIGEN, ANTISERUM, FIBRINOGEN AND FIBRIN SPLIT PRODUCTS *(Immunology) 82DAP*

Biomerieux Inc. 800-682-2666
100 Rodolphe St, Durham, NC 27712

Biosite Incorporated 888-246-7483
9975 Summers Ridge Rd, San Diego, CA 92121
Fluorescence immunoassay for ckmb,tnl,myoglobin,onp & d-dimer.

Clinical Controls International 805-528-4039
1236 Los Osos Valley Rd Ste T, Los Osos, CA 93402
Fibrinogen fdp control.

Dako North America, Inc 805-566-6655
6392 Via Real, Carpinteria, CA 93013

More Diagnostics, Inc. 800-758-0978
PO Box 6714, Los Osos, CA 93412
D-dimer/FDP Control, 2 levels, assayed values for Dade Behring Stratus CS.

ANTIGEN, ANTISERUM, FIBRINOGEN AND SPLIT PRODUCTS, FITC *(Immunology) 82DAX*

Dako North America, Inc 805-566-6655
6392 Via Real, Carpinteria, CA 93013

ANTIGEN, B. PARAPERTUSSIS *(Microbiology) 83GOT*

Bd Diagnostic Systems 800-675-0908
7 Loveton Cir, Sparks, MD 21152

ANTIGEN, B. PERTUSSIS *(Microbiology) 83GOX*

Bd Diagnostic Systems 800-675-0908
7 Loveton Cir, Sparks, MD 21152

ANTIGEN, C. DIFFICILE *(Microbiology) 83MCB*

Ivd Research, Inc. 760-929-7744
5909 Sea Lion Pl Ste D, Carlsbad, CA 92010
Clostridium difficile a & b stool antigen elisa.

Wampole Laboratories 800-257-9525
2 Research Way, Princeton, NJ 08540
C. difficile Toxin A and C. difficile Toxin B.

ANTIGEN, CANCER 549 *(Immunology) 82MJB*

Biocheck, Inc. 650-573-1968
323 Vintage Park Dr, Foster City, CA 94404
Myoglobin eia test kit.

ANTIGEN, CARBOHYDRATE (CA19-9) *(Immunology) 82LTL*

Fujirebio Diagnostics, Inc. (Fdi) 877-861-7246
201 Great Valley Pkwy, Malvern, PA 19355
In vitro diagnostic test for the quantitative measurement of CA 19-9 tumor-associated antigen in human serum or plasma. This test is indicated for the serial measurement of CA 19-9 to aid in the management of patients diagnosed with cancers of the exocrine pancreas. The test is useful as an aid in monitoring of disease status in those patients having confirmed pancreatic cancer who have levels of serum and plasma Ca 19-9 above the cutoff at the time of diagnosis.

United Biotech, Inc. 650-961-2910
211 S Whisman Rd Ste E, Mountain View, CA 94041
ELISA Cancer Marker for CA-199 Pancreatic & Gastro-Intestinal Cancer (P&GC)Quantitative test.

ANTIGEN, CF (INCLUDING CF CONTROL), ADENOVIRUS 1-33 *(Microbiology) 83GOD*

Rapid Pathogen Screening, Inc. 941-556-1850
101 Phillips Park Dr, S Williamsport, PA 17702
Adeno detector.

ANTIGEN, CF (INCLUDING CF CONTROL), COXSACKIEVIRUS A 1-24 *(Microbiology) 83GNG*

Lonza Walkersville, Inc. 201-316-9200
8830 Biggs Ford Rd, Walkersville, MD 21793
Coxsackievirus cf antigen, b 1-6.

ANTIGEN, CF (INCLUDING CF CONTROL), CYTOMEGALOVIRUS *(Microbiology) 83GQH*

Innominata dba GENBIO 800-288-4368
15222 Avenue of Science Ste A, San Diego, CA 92128
Enzyme-linked dot-blot immunoassay-cmv.

ANTIGEN, CF (INCLUDING CF CONTROL), EPSTEIN-BARR VIRUS *(Microbiology) 83GNQ*

Innominata dba GENBIO 800-288-4368
15222 Avenue of Science Ste A, San Diego, CA 92128
Enzyme-linked dot-blot immunoassay-im.

ANTIGEN, CF (INCLUDING CF CONTROL), HERPESVIRUS HOMINIS 1, 2 *(Microbiology) 83GQN*

Diagnostic Hybrids, Inc. 740-589-3300
1055 E State St Ste 100, Athens, OH 45701
Various herpes culture/identification test.

Innominata dba GENBIO 800-288-4368
15222 Avenue of Science Ste A, San Diego, CA 92128
Enzyme-linked dot-blot immunoassay-hsv.

ANTIGEN, CF (INCLUDING CF CONTROL), INFLUENZA VIRUS *(Microbiology) 83GNX*

Genzyme Diagnostics 617-252-7500
6659 Top Gun St, San Diego, CA 92121
Osom flu test.

Lonza Walkersville, Inc. 201-316-9200
8830 Biggs Ford Rd, Walkersville, MD 21793
Influenza cf antigen, a -b.

ANTIGEN, CF (INCLUDING CF CONTROL), PARAINFLUENZA VIRUS *(Microbiology) 83GQS*

Lonza Walkersville, Inc. 201-316-9200
8830 Biggs Ford Rd, Walkersville, MD 21793
Parainfluenza 3 cf antigen.

ANTIGEN, CF AND/OR ID, COCCIDIOIDES IMMITIS *(Microbiology) 83GMI*

Immuno-Mycologics, Inc. 800-654-3639
PO Box 1151, Norman, OK 73070

Meridian Bioscience, Inc. 800-696-0739
3471 River Hills Dr, Cincinnati, OH 45244
$140.00 for 50-test latex agglutination system; $130.00 for 48-test immunodiffusion system.

ANTIGEN, CF, (INCLUDING CF CONTROL), VARICELLA-ZOSTER *(Microbiology) 83GQW*

Hemagen Diagnostics, Inc. 800-436-2436
9033 Red Branch Rd, Columbia, MD 21045
Vzv ifa.

ANTIGEN, CF, ASPERGILLUS SPP. *(Microbiology) 83JWT*

Immuno-Mycologics, Inc. 800-654-3639
PO Box 1151, Norman, OK 73070

ANTIGEN, CF, B. DERMATITIDIS *(Microbiology) 83JWW*

Immuno-Mycologics, Inc. 800-654-3639
PO Box 1151, Norman, OK 73070

ANTIGEN, CF, MYCOPLASMA SPP. *(Microbiology) 83GSB*

Lonza Walkersville, Inc. 201-316-9200
8830 Biggs Ford Rd, Walkersville, MD 21793
Mycoplasma pneumoniae serological reagents.

Meridian Bioscience, Inc. 800-696-0739
3471 River Hills Dr, Cincinnati, OH 45244
Latex agglutination assay for the detection of IgM and IgG to Mycoplasma pneumoniae in serum.

ANTIGEN, CF, T. CRUZI *(Microbiology) 83GNF*

United Biotech, Inc. 650-961-2910
211 S Whisman Rd Ste E, Mountain View, CA 94041
Antigen for T. Cruzi

ANTIGEN, CF, TOXOPLASMA GONDII *(Microbiology) 83GMN*

Ameritek Usa, Inc. 425-379-2580
125 130th St SE Ste 200, Everett, WA 98208
Toxo test kit.

ANTIGEN, CF, TYPHUS FEVER GROUP *(Microbiology) 83GPO*

Protatek Reference Laboratory 602-545-8499
574 E Alamo Dr Ste 90, Chandler, AZ 85225
Rickettsia spotted fever-typhus group antigen slides.

ANTIGEN, ENZYME LINKED IMMUNOABSORBENT ASSAY, CRYPTOCOCCUS *(Microbiology) 83MDU*

Calbiotech, Inc. 619-660-6162
10461 Austin Dr Ste G, Spring Valley, CA 91978
Invitro diagnostic kits.

Meridian Bioscience, Inc. 800-696-0739
3471 River Hills Dr, Cincinnati, OH 45244
Enzyme immunoassay for detection of Cryptococcal antigen in serum and CSF.

Qed Bioscience, Inc. 800-929-2114
10919 Technology Pl Ste C, San Diego, CA 92127
Extensive panel of infectious disease antigens suitable for ELISA.

ANTIGEN, EPSTEIN-BARR VIRUS, CAPSID *(Microbiology) 83MCD*

Meridian Life Science, Inc. 800-327-6299
5171 Wilfong Rd, Memphis, TN 38134
Affinity-purified gp125.

Virotech International, Inc. 301-924-3000
12 Meem Ave Ste C, Gaithersburg, MD 20877
Ebv.

ANTIGEN, FEBRILE *(Microbiology) 83GSZ*

Bd Diagnostic Systems 800-675-0908
7 Loveton Cir, Sparks, MD 21152

Bd Lee Laboratories 800-732-9150
1475 Athens Hwy, Grayson, GA 30017

Immuno Resources, Inc. 830-537-6199
415 Sisterdale Rd, Boerne, TX 78006
Proteus agglutinating antigens.

Immunostics, Inc. 800-722-7505
3505 Sunset Ave, Ocean, NJ 07712

Sa Scientific, Inc. 800-272-2710
4919 Golden Quail, San Antonio, TX 78240
Febrile (slide and tube agglutination test).

ANTIGEN, FEBRILE, SLIDE AND TUBE, SALMONELLA *(Microbiology) 83GNC*

Bd Diagnostic Systems 800-675-0908
7 Loveton Cir, Sparks, MD 21152

Bd Lee Laboratories 800-732-9150
1475 Athens Hwy, Grayson, GA 30017

Germaine Laboratories, Inc. 210-692-4192
4139 Gardendale St Ste 101, San Antonio, TX 78229
Various types.

Immuno Resources, Inc. 830-537-6199
415 Sisterdale Rd, Boerne, TX 78006
Various.

Immunostics, Inc. 800-722-7505
3505 Sunset Ave, Ocean, NJ 07712

ANTIGEN, FLUORESCENT ANTIBODY TEST, ECHINOCOCCUS GRANULOSUS *(Microbiology) 83GPD*

Ivd Research, Inc. 760-929-7744
5909 Sea Lion Pl Ste D, Carlsbad, CA 92010
Echinococcus serum elisa.

ANTIGEN, HA (INCLUDING HA CONTROL), RUBELLA *(Microbiology) 83GOL*

Innominata dba GENBIO 800-288-4368
15222 Avenue of Science Ste A, San Diego, CA 92128
Enzyme-linked dot-blot immunoassay, torch.

Wampole Laboratories 800-257-9525
2 Research Way, Princeton, NJ 08540
WAMPOLE Rubella virus antibody latex agglutination test.

ANTIGEN, HISTOPLASMA CAPSULATUM, ALL *(Microbiology) 83GMJ*

Immuno-Mycologics, Inc. 800-654-3639
PO Box 1151, Norman, OK 73070

ANTIGEN, ID, CANDIDA ALBICANS *(Microbiology) 83LHK*

Biomerica, Inc. 800-854-3002
17571 Von Karman Ave, Irvine, CA 92614
#7003 Candiquant (candida albican antibody test).

Immuno-Mycologics, Inc. 800-654-3639
PO Box 1151, Norman, OK 73070

Ramco Laboratories, Inc. 281-313-1200
4100 Greenbriar Dr Ste 200, Stafford, TX 77477
Detection of antigen associated with systemic candidiasis using latex agglutination technology.

ANTIGEN, ID, HA, CEP, ENTAMOEBA HISTOLYTICA *(Microbiology) 83KHW*

Biovir Laboratories, Inc. 707-747-5906
685 Stone Rd Ste 6, Benicia, CA 94510
Direct fluorescent antibody reagent kit for giardia lamlia.

Wampole Laboratories 800-257-9525
2 Research Way, Princeton, NJ 08540
Enteric disease diagnostic assays.

ANTIGEN, IF, TOXOPLASMA GONDII *(Microbiology) 83GLZ*

Hemagen Diagnostics, Inc. 800-436-2436
9033 Red Branch Rd, Columbia, MD 21045
Toxo ifa.

Innominata dba GENBIO 800-288-4368
15222 Avenue of Science Ste A, San Diego, CA 92128
Enzyme-linked dot-blot immunoassay-toxoplasma.

ANTIGEN, IHA, TOXOPLASMA GONDII *(Microbiology) 83GMM*

Sa Scientific, Inc. 800-272-2710
4919 Golden Quail, San Antonio, TX 78240

ANTIGEN, INDIRECT HEMAGGLUTINATION, HERPES SIMPLEX VIRUS *(Microbiology) 83LKC*

Hemagen Diagnostics, Inc. 800-436-2436
9033 Red Branch Rd, Columbia, MD 21045
Hsv Ag.

ANTIGEN, LATEX AGGLUTINATION, COCCIDIOIDES IMMITIS *(Microbiology) 83GMG*

Immuno-Mycologics, Inc. 800-654-3639
PO Box 1151, Norman, OK 73070

J&S Medical Associates 800-229-6000
35 Tripp St Ste 1, Framingham, MA 01702
ACCUTEX, full line of latex agglutination tests for ASO, SLE, RF, CRP and Mono.

Meridian Bioscience, Inc. 800-696-0739
3471 River Hills Dr, Cincinnati, OH 45244
Coccidioides Latex Agglutination System for the detection of antibodies to Coccidioides immitis in serum.

ANTIGEN, LATEX AGGLUTINATION, ENTAMOEBA HISTOLYTICA & REL. *(Microbiology) 83GMO*

Biosite Incorporated 888-246-7483
9975 Summers Ridge Rd, San Diego, CA 92121
Visual immunoassay system for detection of entabmoeba histolytica,giardia,crypto.

Ivd Research, Inc. 760-929-7744
5909 Sea Lion Pl Ste D, Carlsbad, CA 92010
Toxocara serum elisa.

ANTIGEN, NON-TREPONEMAL, ALL *(Microbiology) 83GMQ*

Bd Diagnostic Systems 800-675-0908
7 Loveton Cir, Sparks, MD 21152

Bd Lee Laboratories 800-732-9150
1475 Athens Hwy, Grayson, GA 30017

Beacon Biologicals, Inc. 561-395-1862
5139 Point Alexis, Boca Raton, FL 33486
The toluidine red unheated serum test.

Immunostics, Inc. 800-722-7505
3505 Sunset Ave, Ocean, NJ 07712

Pulse Scientific, Inc. 800-363-7907
5100 S. Service Rd., Unit 18, Burlington, ONT L7L-6A5 Canada
RPR Antigen Test as a screening test for Syphilis.

ANTIGEN, POSITIVE CONTROL, CRYPTOCOCCUS NEOFORMANS *(Microbiology) 83JWK*

Wampole Laboratories 800-257-9525
2 Research Way, Princeton, NJ 08540
CRYPTO-LA Serum/CSF cryptococcus latex agglutination antigen.

ANTIGEN, PROSTATE-SPECIFIC (PSA), MANAGEMENT, CANCER *(Immunology) 82LTJ*

Akers Biosciences, Inc. 800-451-8378
201 Grove Rd, West Deptford, NJ 08086
HEALTHTEST, prostate specific antigen.

Alfa Scientific Designs, Inc. 877-204-5071
13200 Gregg St, Poway, CA 92064
Psa serum cassette test.

Bio-Medical Products Corp. 800-543-7427
10 Halstead Rd, Mendham, NJ 07945
Prostate specific antigen PSA screening strip. 5 minute test. Blood serum immunochromatographic test.

Biocheck, Inc. 650-573-1968
323 Vintage Park Dr, Foster City, CA 94404
Free prostate specific antigen (psa) eia test kit.

Biomerica, Inc. 800-854-3002
17571 Von Karman Ave, Irvine, CA 92614
EZ-PSA, one-step 10 minute test for detection of prostate specific cancer.

Chembio Diagnostic Systems, Inc. 631-924-1135
3661 Horseblock Rd, Medford, NY 11763
Immunochromatographic assay for the visual detection of prostate specific antige.

Qualigen, Inc. 760-918-9165
2042 Corte Del Nogal, Carlsbad, CA 92011
Various.

St. Paul Biotech 714-903-1000
11555 Monarch St, Garden Grove, CA 92841
Psa test.

ANTIGEN, RUBELLA, OTHER *(Microbiology) 83LSJ*

Bio-Med U.S.A. Inc. 973-278-5222
111 Ellison St, Paterson, NJ 07505
BIO-ACCU RUBELLA Rapid Rubella Antigent test kit, $1.80-$2.40 per kit included accessaries.

Meridian Life Science, Inc. 800-327-6299
5171 Wilfong Rd, Memphis, TN 38134
Rubella Grades I-IV, Chagas, CMV, HAV, HSV-1&2, Rubeola, Mumps, TOXO, VZV

ANTIGEN, SALMONELLA SPP. *(Microbiology) 83GRL*

Bd Diagnostic Systems 800-675-0908
7 Loveton Cir, Sparks, MD 21152

Biomerieux Inc. 800-682-2666
100 Rodolphe St, Durham, NC 27712
Salmonella-Tek ELISA to screen foods and feeds for the presence of Salmonella species.

Calbiotech, Inc. 619-660-6162
10461 Austin Dr Ste G, Spring Valley, CA 91978
Salmonella igg elisa.

Germaine Laboratories, Inc. 210-692-4192
4139 Gardendale St Ste 101, San Antonio, TX 78229
Various types.

Immuno Resources, Inc. 830-537-6199
415 Sisterdale Rd, Boerne, TX 78006
Various.

Immunostics, Inc. 800-722-7505
3505 Sunset Ave, Ocean, NJ 07712

ANTIGEN, SALMONELLA SPP. *(cont'd)*

Medical & Clinical Consortium (Mcc) 877-622-8378
13740 Nelson Ave, City Of Industry, CA 91746
Instant Test Kits for E-Coli & Salmonella, in just minutes.

Sa Scientific, Inc. 800-272-2710
4919 Golden Quail, San Antonio, TX 78240
Salmonella (slide and tube agglutination test).

ANTIGEN, SLIDE AND TUBE, FRANCISELLA TULARENSIS
(Microbiology) 83GSL

Bd Diagnostic Systems 800-675-0908
7 Loveton Cir, Sparks, MD 21152

Bd Lee Laboratories 800-732-9150
1475 Athens Hwy, Grayson, GA 30017

Germaine Laboratories, Inc. 210-692-4192
4139 Gardendale St Ste 101, San Antonio, TX 78229
Francisella tularensis antigen.

Immuno Resources, Inc. 830-537-6199
415 Sisterdale Rd, Boerne, TX 78006
Francisella tularensis antigen.

Sa Scientific, Inc. 800-272-2710
4919 Golden Quail, San Antonio, TX 78240

ANTIGEN, SLIDE AND TUBE, LISTERIA MONOCYTOGENES
(Microbiology) 83GSI

Bd Diagnostic Systems 800-675-0908
7 Loveton Cir, Sparks, MD 21152

ANTIGEN, SOMATIC, STAPHYLOCOCCUS AUREUS
(Microbiology) 83LHT

Oxoid, Inc. 800-567-8378
800 Proctor Ave, Ogdensburg, NY 13669

ANTIGEN, STREPTOCOCCUS SPP. *(Microbiology) 83GTY*

Access Bio Incorporate 732-297-2222
2033 Rt. 130 Unit H, Monmouth Junction, NJ 08852
Strep a test.

Ameritek Usa, Inc. 425-379-2580
125 130th St SE Ste 200, Everett, WA 98208
Strep a test kit.

Antibodies, Inc. 800-824-8540
PO Box 1560, Davis, CA 95617

Bd Diagnostic Systems 800-675-0908
7 Loveton Cir, Sparks, MD 21152

Bd Lee Laboratories 800-732-9150
1475 Athens Hwy, Grayson, GA 30017

Chembio Diagnostic Systems, Inc. 631-924-1135
3661 Horseblock Rd, Medford, NY 11763
Immunochromatographic assay for the visual detection of step b antigen.

Culture Kits, Inc. 888-680-6853
14 Prentice St, PO Box 748, Norwich, NY 13815
Streptococcus screening kit.

Genzyme Diagnostics 617-252-7500
6659 Top Gun St, San Diego, CA 92121
Group a streptococcus antigen test.

Germaine Laboratories, Inc. 210-692-4192
4139 Gardendale St Ste 101, San Antonio, TX 78229
Various types, streptococcus test kit.

Immuno Resources, Inc. 830-537-6199
415 Sisterdale Rd, Boerne, TX 78006
Various types of streptococcus antigens.

Innovacon, Inc. 858-535-2030
4106 Sorrento Valley Blvd, San Diego, CA 92121
Strep a test.

Inverness Medical Professional Diagnostics-San Die 858-535-2030
4106 Sorrento Valley Blvd, San Diego, CA 92121
Strep a test.

J&S Medical Associates 800-229-6000
35 Tripp St Ste 1, Framingham, MA 01702
Presumptive ID for Enterococcus and group A Streptococcus.

Lifesign 800-526-2125
71 Veronica Ave, Somerset, NJ 08873
STATUS STREPA - EIA Test for Strep A Antigen.

ANTIGEN, STREPTOCOCCUS SPP. *(cont'd)*

Meridian Bioscience, Inc. 800-696-0739
3471 River Hills Dr, Cincinnati, OH 45244
Coagglutination procedure for the identification of beta-hemolytic streptococci based on serogroups described by Lancefield.

Oxoid, Inc. 800-567-8378
800 Proctor Ave, Ogdensburg, NY 13669
Streptococcal grouping kit A,B,C,D,F,G.

Princeton Biomeditech Corp. 732-274-1000
4242 US Highway 1, Monmouth Junction, NJ 08852
BioSign Strep A and BioStrep A, direct antigen detection from throat swab in 7 min. Simplified 2-step procedure.

Sa Scientific, Inc. 800-272-2710
4919 Golden Quail, San Antonio, TX 78240
SAS; A rapid test for the detection of Group A strep antigen from throat swabs.

Thermo Biostar, Inc. 800-637-3717
331 S 104th St, Louisville, CO 80027
Strep A OIA rapid test (less than 10 minutes) for the identification of Group A Strep antigen. The sensitivity and specificity has proven to be superior to routine agarculture and equivalent to broth enhanced culture. Strep B OIA rapid test (less than 30 minutes) for the identification of Group B Strep antigen which has a sensitivity equivalent to routine culture.

ANTIGEN, TREPONEMA PALLIDUM FOR FTA-ABS TEST
(Microbiology) 83JWL

Bd Diagnostic Systems 800-675-0908
7 Loveton Cir, Sparks, MD 21152

Bd Lee Laboratories 800-732-9150
1475 Athens Hwy, Grayson, GA 30017
SYPHILIGEN r15, & r17 and r47, recombinant antigens for syphilis. Three recombinant antigens for detection of syphilis.

ANTIGEN, TUMOR MARKER, BLADDER (BASEMENT MEMBRANE COMPLEXES) *(Immunology) 82MMW*

Abbott Molecular, Inc. 847-937-6100
1300 E Touhy Ave, Des Plaines, IL 60018
Fluorescence in situ hybridization (fish) reagents.

C. R. Bard, Inc., Bard Urological Div. 888-367-2273
13183 Harland Dr NE, Covington, GA 30014

United Biotech, Inc. 650-961-2910
211 S Whisman Rd Ste E, Mountain View, CA 94041
ELISA quantitative detecting PAP Prostatic Acid Phophatase (PAP)

ANTINUCLEAR ANTIBODY (ENZYME-LABELED), ANTIGEN, CONTROLS *(Immunology) 82LJM*

Bio-Rad Laboratories Inc., Clinical Systems Div. 800-224-6723
4000 Alfred Nobel Dr, Hercules, CA 94547
Various.

Corgenix Medical Corporation 800-729-5661
11575 Main St, Broomfield, CO 80020
Multiple

Corgenix, Inc. 800-729-5661
12061 Tejon St, Westminster, CO 80234
Anti-nuclear antibody (ANA) semi-quantitative test kit.

Dako North America, Inc 805-566-6655
6392 Via Real, Carpinteria, CA 93013

Hycor Biomedical, Inc. 800-382-2527
7272 Chapman Ave, Garden Grove, CA 92841
Histone autoimmune kit.

Innominata dba GENBIO 800-288-4368
15222 Avenue of Science Ste A, San Diego, CA 92128
Immunodot autoimmunity screening panel 1.

Micro Detect, Inc. 714-832-8234
2852 Walnut Ave Ste H1, Tustin, CA 92780
Mdi ss-a test.

Quest Intl., Inc. 305-592-6991
8127 NW 29th St, Doral, FL 33122
Anti-ssa serological reagents, elisa.

Quidel Corp. 858-552-1100
2981 Copper Rd, Santa Clara, CA 95051
Antinuclear antibody, indirect immunofluorescent, antigen, control.

Theratest Laboratories, Inc. 800-441-0771
1111 N Main St, Lombard, IL 60148
Specific,multiple autoantibodies, panels and screening, ELISA kits

ANTINUCLEAR ANTIBODY (ENZYME-LABELED), ANTIGEN, CONTROLS *(cont'd)*

Tripath Imaging, Inc. 919-206-7140
780 Plantation Dr, Burlington, NC 27215
Antinuclear antibody immunological test system.

United Biotech, Inc. 650-961-2910
211 S Whisman Rd Ste E, Mountain View, CA 94041
ELISA for detecting ANA

Zeus Scientific, Inc. 800-286-2111
PO Box 38, Raritan, NJ 08869
ANA Screen; ENA Screen; SSA (Ro); SSA (La); Sm; Sm/RNP; Scl-70; Jo-1; Cardiolipin IgG; Microsomal (TPO); Thyroglobulin 96 tests ELISA IgG only. ds DNA 96 tests ELISA. Cardiolipin IgM 96 tests ELISA IgM only. Cardiolipin IgA 96 tests ELISA IgA only. ENA Profile-4 192 tests ELISA.

ANTINUCLEAR ANTIBODY, ANTIGEN, CONTROL
(Immunology) 82LKJ

Antibodies, Inc. 800-824-8540
PO Box 1560, Davis, CA 95617
ANA diagnostic test kits for autoimmune diseases.

Bio-Rad Laboratories Inc., Clinical Systems Div. 800-224-6723
4000 Alfred Nobel Dr, Hercules, CA 94547
Enzyme immunoassay antinuclear antibody screening test kit.

Bio-Rad Laboratories, Inc. 425-881-8300
14620 NE North Woodinville Way, Way, Suite 200
Woodinville, WA 98072
Multi-analyte detection system-ana screen.

Hycor Biomedical, Inc. 800-382-2527
7272 Chapman Ave, Garden Grove, CA 92841
Autoimmune ss-a & ss-b kits.

Immuno Concepts N.A. Ltd. 800-251-5115
9779 Business Park Dr, Sacramento, CA 95827
Extractable nuclear antigen test systems or controls.

Innominata dba GENBIO 800-288-4368
15222 Avenue of Science Ste A, San Diego, CA 92128
Enzyme-linked dot-blot immunoassay antinuclear antibodies.

ANTIPARIETAL ANTIBODY, IMMUNOFLUORESCENT, ANTIGEN, CONTROL *(Immunology) 82DBJ*

Hemagen Diagnostics, Inc. 800-436-2436
9033 Red Branch Rd, Columbia, MD 21045
Ifa.

Immco Diagnostics, Inc. 800-537-8378
60 Pineview Dr, Buffalo, NY 14228
IMMUGLO.

Medica, Inc. 800-845-6496
336 Encinitas Blvd Ste 200, Encinitas, CA 92024
48 & 96-test kits, rat or mouse stomach sections, APCA.

ANTISERA, CONJUGATED FLUORESCENT, CYTOMEGALOVIRUS *(Microbiology) 83LIN*

Diasorin Inc 800-328-1482
1951 Northwestern Ave S, PO Box 285, Stillwater, MN 55082

Meridian Bioscience, Inc. 800-696-0739
3471 River Hills Dr, Cincinnati, OH 45244
Direct immunofluorescent procedure for the detection of Cytomegalovirus in cell culture.

ANTISERA, FLUORESCENT, ALL GLOBULINS, PROTEUS SPP.
(Microbiology) 83GSY

Germaine Laboratories, Inc. 210-692-4192
4139 Gardendale St Ste 101, San Antonio, TX 78229
Various types of proteus antisera.

Immuno Resources, Inc. 830-537-6199
415 Sisterdale Rd, Boerne, TX 78006
Various.

Sa Scientific, Inc. 800-272-2710
4919 Golden Quail, San Antonio, TX 78240

ANTISERA, FLUORESCENT, CHLAMYDIA SPP.
(Microbiology) 83LKI

Focus Diagnostics, Inc. 714-220-1900
10703 Progress Way, Cypress, CA 90630
Various.

Meridian Bioscience, Inc. 800-696-0739
3471 River Hills Dr, Cincinnati, OH 45244
Direct immunofluorescent procedure for the detection of Chlamydia in McCoy cells.

ANTISERA, FLUORESCENT, COXSACKIEVIRUS A 1-24, B 1-6
(Microbiology) 83GNM

Cepheid 408-400-8460
904 E Caribbean Dr, Sunnyvale, CA 94089
Nucleic acid amplification test.

Diagnostic Hybrids, Inc. 740-589-3300
1055 E State St Ste 100, Athens, OH 45701
Various enteroviruses culture-id tests.

ANTISERA, FLUORESCENT, ECHOVIRUS 1-34
(Microbiology) 83GRK

Diagnostic Hybrids, Inc. 740-589-3300
1055 E State St Ste 100, Athens, OH 45701
Various enteroviruses culture-id tests.

ANTISERA, FLUORESCENT, HERPESVIRUS HOMINIS 1, 2
(Microbiology) 83GQL

Bio-Rad Laboratories, Inc. 425-881-8300
14620 NE North Woodinville Way, Way, Suite 200
Woodinville, WA 98072
Kallestad hsv 1&2 direct antigen detection kits and components.

Dako North America, Inc 805-566-6655
6392 Via Real, Carpinteria, CA 93013

Hemagen Diagnostics, Inc. 800-436-2436
9033 Red Branch Rd, Columbia, MD 21045
Hsv-1/hsv-2.

ANTISERA, FLUORESCENT, POLIOVIRUS 1-3
(Microbiology) 83GOE

Diagnostic Hybrids, Inc. 740-589-3300
1055 E State St Ste 100, Athens, OH 45701
Various enteroviruses culture-id tests.

ANTISERA, IF, TOXOPLASMA GONDII *(Microbiology) 83LJK*

Bbi Diagnostics, A Division Of Seracare Life Scien 508-244-6428
375 West St, West Bridgewater, MA 02379
Accurun 135 toxoplasma igg positive control.

ANTISERUM, ABO BLOOD GROUPING *(Hematology) 81UJY*

Dade Behring, Inc. 800-948-3233
1717 Deerfield Rd, Deerfield, IL 60015

ANTISERUM, AGGLUTINATING, B. PARAPERTUSSIS
(Microbiology) 83GOW

Bd Diagnostic Systems 800-675-0908
7 Loveton Cir, Sparks, MD 21152

ANTISERUM, AGGLUTINATING, B. PERTUSSIS, ALL
(Microbiology) 83GOY

Bd Diagnostic Systems 800-675-0908
7 Loveton Cir, Sparks, MD 21152

ANTISERUM, CF, COXSACKIEVIRUS A 1-24, B 1-6
(Microbiology) 83GNO

Lonza Walkersville, Inc. 201-316-9200
8830 Biggs Ford Rd, Walkersville, MD 21793
Coxsackievirus cf antisera, b 1-6.

ANTISERUM, CF, EQUINE ENCEPHALITIS VIRUS, EEE, WEE
(Microbiology) 83GQC

Chembio Diagnostic Systems, Inc. 631-924-1135
3661 Horseblock Rd, Medford, NY 11763
Immunochromatogrphic assay for visual detection of antibodies to dengue virus.

Focus Diagnostics, Inc. 714-220-1900
10703 Progress Way, Cypress, CA 90630
Flavivirus or west nile virus serological reagents.

ANTISERUM, CF, INFLUENZA VIRUS A, B, C
(Microbiology) 83GNW

Diagnostic Hybrids, Inc. 740-589-3300
1055 E State St Ste 100, Athens, OH 45701
Respiratory virus direct fluroescent monoclonal antibodies kit.

Lonza Walkersville, Inc. 201-316-9200
8830 Biggs Ford Rd, Walkersville, MD 21793
Influenza cf antisera, a-b.

ANTISERUM, CF, PARAINFLUENZA VIRUS 1-4
(Microbiology) 83GQT

Lonza Walkersville, Inc. 201-316-9200
8830 Biggs Ford Rd, Walkersville, MD 21793
Parainfluenza 3 cf antisera.

ANTISERUM, CF, RUBELLA *(Microbiology) 83GOM*

Princeton Biomeditech Corp. 732-274-1000
4242 US Highway 1, Monmouth Junction, NJ 08852
BioSign Rubella IgG antibody test, one step, 5 minutes, results from whole blood, serum, or plasma.

ANTISERUM, CONTROL FOR NON-TREPONEMAL TEST
(Microbiology) 83GMP

Bd Diagnostic Systems 800-675-0908
7 Loveton Cir, Sparks, MD 21152

Bd Lee Laboratories 800-732-9150
1475 Athens Hwy, Grayson, GA 30017

Immunostics, Inc. 800-722-7505
3505 Sunset Ave, Ocean, NJ 07712

ANTISERUM, DIGITOXIN *(Toxicology) 91DKQ*

Health Chem Diagnostics Llc 954-979-3845
3341 W McNab Rd, Pompano Beach, FL 33069
Antiserum, digitoxin.

ANTISERUM, ESCHERICHIA COLI *(Microbiology) 83GNA*

Bd Diagnostic Systems 800-675-0908
7 Loveton Cir, Sparks, MD 21152

Bd Lee Laboratories 800-732-9150
1475 Athens Hwy, Grayson, GA 30017

Dako North America, Inc 805-566-6655
6392 Via Real, Carpinteria, CA 93013

Immuno Resources, Inc. 830-537-6199
415 Sisterdale Rd, Boerne, TX 78006
Various types of escherichia coli antisera.

Ivd Research, Inc. 760-929-7744
5909 Sea Lion Pl Ste D, Carlsbad, CA 92010
Verotoxin stool antigen elisa.

Meridian Bioscience, Inc. 800-696-0739
3471 River Hills Dr, Cincinnati, OH 45244
PREMIER H. pylori, enzyme immunoasary for Enterohemorrhagic E. coli Toxin.

Sa Scientific, Inc. 800-272-2710
4919 Golden Quail, San Antonio, TX 78240

ANTISERUM, FLUORESCENT ANTIBODY FOR FTA-ABS TEST
(Microbiology) 83GMX

Bd Diagnostic Systems 800-675-0908
7 Loveton Cir, Sparks, MD 21152

Hemagen Diagnostics, Inc. 800-436-2436
9033 Red Branch Rd, Columbia, MD 21045
Fta-abs ifa.

Wampole Laboratories 800-257-9525
2 Research Way, Princeton, NJ 08540
Zeus Scientific.

ANTISERUM, FLUORESCENT, ADENOVIRUS 1-33
(Microbiology) 83GNY

Ivd Research, Inc. 760-929-7744
5909 Sea Lion Pl Ste D, Carlsbad, CA 92010
Adenovirus stool antigen elisa.

Prodesse, Inc. 888-589-6974
W229N1870 Westwood Dr, Waukesha, WI 53186
Adenoplex® - Multiplex PCR Reagents for simultaneous detection and subtyping of adenovirus subtypes A, B, C D, E, F. - Research Use Only

ANTISERUM, FLUORESCENT, B. PARAPERTUSSIS
(Microbiology) 83JRW

Bd Diagnostic Systems 800-675-0908
7 Loveton Cir, Sparks, MD 21152

ANTISERUM, FLUORESCENT, B. PERTUSSIS
(Microbiology) 83GOZ

Bd Diagnostic Systems 800-675-0908
7 Loveton Cir, Sparks, MD 21152

Cytovax Biotechnologies, Inc. 800-661-1426
8925 51 Ave NW, Ste. 308, Edmonton, AB T6E 5J3 Canada
ACCU-MAB.

ANTISERUM, FLUORESCENT, BRUCELLA SPP.
(Microbiology) 83GSM

Germaine Laboratories, Inc. 210-692-4192
4139 Gardendale St Ste 101, San Antonio, TX 78229
Various types of brucella antisera.

Immuno Resources, Inc. 830-537-6199
415 Sisterdale Rd, Boerne, TX 78006
Various.

ANTISERUM, FLUORESCENT, CHLAMYDIA TRACHOMATIS
(Microbiology) 83LJP

Bio-Rad Laboratories, Inc. 425-881-8300
14620 NE North Woodinville Way, Way, Suite 200
Woodinville, WA 98072
Various chlamydia fa kits.

Hemagen Diagnostics, Inc. 800-436-2436
9033 Red Branch Rd, Columbia, MD 21045
C.trach ifa.

Meridian Bioscience, Inc. 800-696-0739
3471 River Hills Dr, Cincinnati, OH 45244

ANTISERUM, FLUORESCENT, CRYPTOCOCCUS NEOFORMANS *(Microbiology) 83GME*

Meridian Bioscience, Inc. 800-696-0739
3471 River Hills Dr, Cincinnati, OH 45244
Cryptococcus neoformans EIA test.

ANTISERUM, FLUORESCENT, EPSTEIN-BARR VIRUS
(Microbiology) 83JRY

Diagnostic Technology, Inc. 631-582-4949
175 Commerce Dr Ste L, Hauppauge, NY 11788
Epstein-barr viral capsid antigen slide.

ANTISERUM, FLUORESCENT, GROUPS, STREPTOCOCCUS SPP. *(Microbiology) 83GTX*

Antibodies, Inc. 800-824-8540
PO Box 1560, Davis, CA 95617

Bd Diagnostic Systems 800-675-0908
7 Loveton Cir, Sparks, MD 21152

Biomerieux Inc. 800-682-2666
100 Rodolphe St, Durham, NC 27712

ANTISERUM, FLUORESCENT, HEMOPHILUS SPP.
(Microbiology) 83GRO

Biomerieux Inc. 800-682-2666
100 Rodolphe St, Durham, NC 27712

ANTISERUM, FLUORESCENT, MUMPS VIRUS
(Microbiology) 83GRA

Hemagen Diagnostics, Inc. 800-436-2436
9033 Red Branch Rd, Columbia, MD 21045
Mumps virus.

ANTISERUM, FLUORESCENT, MYCOBACTERIUM TUBERCULOSIS *(Microbiology) 83GRT*

Ameritek Usa, Inc. 425-379-2580
125 130th St SE Ste 200, Everett, WA 98208
M.tuberculosis test kit.

Bio-Medical Products Corp. 800-543-7427
10 Halstead Rd, Mendham, NJ 07945
Rapid serum TB test, 10 minutes. $8.00 per test.

Chembio Diagnostic Systems, Inc. 631-924-1135
3661 Horseblock Rd, Medford, NY 11763
Immunochromatographic assay for the visual detection of tb antibodies.

St. Paul Biotech 714-903-1000
11555 Monarch St, Garden Grove, CA 92841
Tuberculosis test.

ANTISERUM, FLUORESCENT, RUBEOLA *(Microbiology) 83GRE*

Hemagen Diagnostics, Inc. 800-436-2436
9033 Red Branch Rd, Columbia, MD 21045
Measles ifa.

Zeus Scientific, Inc. 800-286-2111
PO Box 38, Raritan, NJ 08869
100 test IFA kit for IgG.

ANTISERUM, FLUORESCENT, STREPTOCOCCUS PNEUMONIAE *(Microbiology) 83GWB*

Antibodies, Inc. 800-824-8540
PO Box 1560, Davis, CA 95617
Detect-A-Strep diagnostic test kit for direct detection from throat swabs.

ANTISERUM, FRANCISELLA TULARENSIS *(Microbiology) 83GSK*

Bd Diagnostic Systems 800-675-0908
7 Loveton Cir, Sparks, MD 21152

Germaine Laboratories, Inc. 210-692-4192
4139 Gardendale St Ste 101, San Antonio, TX 78229
Francisella tularensis.

Immuno Resources, Inc. 830-537-6199
415 Sisterdale Rd, Boerne, TX 78006
Francisella tularensis antiserum.

ANTISERUM, H. INFLUENZAE *(Microbiology) 83GRP*

Bd Diagnostic Systems 800-675-0908
7 Loveton Cir, Sparks, MD 21152

Sa Scientific, Inc. 800-272-2710
4919 Golden Quail, San Antonio, TX 78240

ANTISERUM, LATEX AGGLUTINATION, CRYPTOCOCCUS NEOFORMANS *(Microbiology) 83GMD*

Immuno-Mycologics, Inc. 800-654-3639
PO Box 1151, Norman, OK 73070
Latex cryptococcal Antigen Detection System.

Meridian Bioscience, Inc. 800-696-0739
3471 River Hills Dr, Cincinnati, OH 45244
CALAS Latex agglutination assay for the detection of Cryptococcus neoformans antigens in serum and CSF.

Ramco Laboratories, Inc. 281-313-1200
4100 Greenbriar Dr Ste 200, Stafford, TX 77477
Detection of Candida antigen using a latex agglutination system.

ANTISERUM, LEPTOSPIRA SPP. *(Microbiology) 83GRX*

Access Bio Incorporate 732-297-2222
2033 Rt. 130 Unit H, Monmouth Junction, NJ 08852
Leptospira test.

ANTISERUM, LISTERIA MONOCYTOGENES *(Microbiology) 83GSH*

Bd Diagnostic Systems 800-675-0908
7 Loveton Cir, Sparks, MD 21152

Immuno Resources, Inc. 830-537-6199
415 Sisterdale Rd, Boerne, TX 78006
Listeria monocytogenes antiseria.

Sa Scientific, Inc. 800-272-2710
4919 Golden Quail, San Antonio, TX 78240

ANTISERUM, MYCOPLASMA SPP. *(Microbiology) 83GSA*

Lonza Walkersville, Inc. 201-316-9200
8830 Biggs Ford Rd, Walkersville, MD 21793
Mycoplasma pneumoniae serological reagents.

ANTISERUM, N. MENINGITIDIS *(Microbiology) 83GTJ*

Bd Diagnostic Systems 800-675-0908
7 Loveton Cir, Sparks, MD 21152

Sa Scientific, Inc. 800-272-2710
4919 Golden Quail, San Antonio, TX 78240

ANTISERUM, NEUTRALIZATION, HERPES VIRUS HOMINIS *(Microbiology) 83GQM*

Zeus Scientific, Inc. 800-286-2111
PO Box 38, Raritan, NJ 08869

ANTISERUM, NEUTRALIZATION, RESPIRATORY SYNCYTIAL VIRUS *(Microbiology) 83GQF*

Bio-Rad Laboratories, Inc. 425-881-8300
6565 185th Ave NE, Redmond, WA 98052
No common name listed.

ANTISERUM, POSITIVE AND NEGATIVE FEBRILE ANTIGEN CONTROL *(Microbiology) 83GSN*

Bd Diagnostic Systems 800-675-0908
7 Loveton Cir, Sparks, MD 21152

Germaine Laboratories, Inc. 210-692-4192
4139 Gardendale St Ste 101, San Antonio, TX 78229
Various.

ANTISERUM, POSITIVE AND NEGATIVE FEBRILE ANTIGEN CONTROL *(cont'd)*

Health Chem Diagnostics Llc 954-979-3845
3341 W McNab Rd, Pompano Beach, FL 33069
Antiserum, positive and negative febrile antigen control serum.

Immuno Resources, Inc. 830-537-6199
415 Sisterdale Rd, Boerne, TX 78006
Various.

Immunostics, Inc. 800-722-7505
3505 Sunset Ave, Ocean, NJ 07712

Sa Scientific, Inc. 800-272-2710
4919 Golden Quail, San Antonio, TX 78240

ANTISERUM, POSITIVE CONTROL, BLASTOMYCES DERMATITIDIS *(Microbiology) 83KFH*

Immuno-Mycologics, Inc. 800-654-3639
PO Box 1151, Norman, OK 73070

ANTISERUM, POSITIVE CONTROL, COCCIDIOIDES IMMITIS *(Microbiology) 83GMH*

Immuno-Mycologics, Inc. 800-654-3639
PO Box 1151, Norman, OK 73070

ANTISERUM, POSITIVE CONTROL, HISTOPLASMA CAPSULATUM *(Microbiology) 83GMK*

Immuno-Mycologics, Inc. 800-654-3639
PO Box 1151, Norman, OK 73070

ANTISERUM, SALMONELLA SPP. *(Microbiology) 83GRM*

Bd Diagnostic Systems 800-675-0908
7 Loveton Cir, Sparks, MD 21152

Bd Lee Laboratories 800-732-9150
1475 Athens Hwy, Grayson, GA 30017

Germaine Laboratories, Inc. 210-692-4192
4139 Gardendale St Ste 101, San Antonio, TX 78229
Various types of salmonella antisera.

Immuno Resources, Inc. 830-537-6199
415 Sisterdale Rd, Boerne, TX 78006
Various.

Sa Scientific, Inc. 800-272-2710
4919 Golden Quail, San Antonio, TX 78240

ANTISERUM, SERRATIA MARCESANS *(Microbiology) 83GTA*

Advanced Biotechnologies, Inc. 800-426-0764
9108 Guilford Rd, Rivers Park II, Columbia, MD 21046

ANTISERUM, SHIGELLA SPP. *(Microbiology) 83GNB*

Bd Diagnostic Systems 800-675-0908
7 Loveton Cir, Sparks, MD 21152

Bd Lee Laboratories 800-732-9150
1475 Athens Hwy, Grayson, GA 30017

Immuno Resources, Inc. 830-537-6199
415 Sisterdale Rd, Boerne, TX 78006
Various types of shigella antisera.

Sa Scientific, Inc. 800-272-2710
4919 Golden Quail, San Antonio, TX 78240

ANTISERUM, STREPTOCOCCUS PNEUMONIAE *(Microbiology) 83GWC*

Antibodies, Inc. 800-824-8540
PO Box 1560, Davis, CA 95617
Detect-A-Strep diagnostic test kit for direct detection from throat swabs.

Bd Diagnostic Systems 800-675-0908
7 Loveton Cir, Sparks, MD 21152

ANTISERUM, STREPTOCOCCUS SPP. *(Microbiology) 83GTZ*

Ameritek Usa, Inc. 425-379-2580
125 130th St SE Ste 200, Everett, WA 98208
Strep b test kit.

Antibodies, Inc. 800-824-8540
PO Box 1560, Davis, CA 95617
Detect-A-Strep diagnostic test kit for direct detection from throat swabs.

Bd Diagnostic Systems 800-675-0908
7 Loveton Cir, Sparks, MD 21152

Bd Lee Laboratories 800-732-9150
1475 Athens Hwy, Grayson, GA 30017

Genzyme Diagnostics 617-252-7500
6659 Top Gun St, San Diego, CA 92121
Group a streptococcal antigen test.

ANTISERUM, STREPTOCOCCUS SPP. *(cont'd)*

Immuno Resources, Inc. 830-537-6199
415 Sisterdale Rd, Boerne, TX 78006
Streptococcus grouping antisera.

Jant Pharmacal Corp. 800-676-5565
16255 Ventura Blvd Ste 505, Encino, CA 91436
Rapid diagnostic immunoassay for the qualitative detection of group A streptoccu.

Lifesign 800-526-2125
71 Veronica Ave, Somerset, NJ 08873

Meridian Bioscience, Inc. 800-696-0739
3471 River Hills Dr, Cincinnati, OH 45244
Enzyme immunoassay for the detection of Group A streptococcal antigen form throat swabs.

Myers-Stevens Group, Inc. 903-566-6696
2931 Vail Ave, Commerce, CA 90040
Eia test for the detection of strep-a.

Sa Scientific, Inc. 800-272-2710
4919 Golden Quail, San Antonio, TX 78240

ANTISERUM, VIBRIO CHOLERAE *(Microbiology) 83GSQ*

Bd Diagnostic Systems 800-675-0908
7 Loveton Cir, Sparks, MD 21152

Immuno Resources, Inc. 830-537-6199
415 Sisterdale Rd, Boerne, TX 78006
Vibrio cholerae antisera.

Sa Scientific, Inc. 800-272-2710
4919 Golden Quail, San Antonio, TX 78240

APPARATUS, AUDIOMETRIC, REINFORCEMENT, VISUAL *(Ear/Nose/Throat) 77LYN*

Monitor Instruments Inc. 800-853-6785
437 Dimmocks Mill Rd, Hillsborough, NC 27278

APPARATUS, NITRIC OXIDE DELIVERY *(Anesthesiology) 73MRN*

Datex-Ohmeda Inc. 608-221-1551
3030 Ohmeda Dr, Madison, WI 53718
Nitric oxide delivery system.

Pulmonox Medical Corporation 888-464-8742
5243-53 Ave, Tofield, ALB T0B 4J0 Canada
Nitric oxide delivery and analysis system

APPLIANCE, FIX., NAIL/BLADE/PLATE COMB., MULTIPLE COMPONENT *(Orthopedics) 87LXT*

Amedica Corporation 801-839-3500
1885 W 2100 S, Salt Lake City, UT 84119
Valeo CP

Biomet, Inc. 574-267-6639
56 E Bell Dr, PO Box 587, Warsaw, IN 46582
Various types of fixation appliances.

Biopro, Inc. 800-252-7707
2929 Lapeer Rd, Port Huron, MI 48060
Wujin #3 Plating System

Depuy Orthopaedics, Inc. 800-473-3789
700 Orthopaedic Dr, P.O. Box 988, Warsaw, IN 46582
Various types of fixation appliances, nail/blade/plate combination,multicomponet.

Nutek Orthopaedics, Llc 954-779-1400
301 S.w. 7th St., Ft. Lauderdale, FL 33301
Nbx non-bridging external fixator.

Synthes (Usa) 610-719-5000
35 Airport Rd, Horseheads, NY 14845
Various types and sizes of multiple component, metal composite, fixation devices.

APPLIANCE, FIXATION, SPINAL INTERLAMINAL *(Orthopedics) 87KWP*

Abbott Spine, Inc. 847-937-6100
12708 Riata Vista Cir Ste B-100, Austin, TX 78727
Bacfix system.

Aesculap Implant Systems, Inc. 610-984-9074
9999 Hamilton Blvd Bldg 8, Breinigsville, PA 18031
Spinal interlaminal orthosis.

Allez Spine, Llc 949-752-7885
2301 Dupont Dr Ste 510, Irvine, CA 92612
Spinal fixation system.

Alphatec Spine, Inc. 760-494-6769
5818 El Camino Real, Carlsbad, CA 92008
Pedicle screw system.

APPLIANCE, FIXATION, SPINAL INTERLAMINAL *(cont'd)*

Centinel Spine Inc. 952-885-0500
505 Park Ave Fl 14, New York, NY 10022
Titanium Hartshill System

Depuy Spine, Inc. 800-227-6633
325 Paramount Dr, Raynham, MA 02767
Pedicle screw.

Integra Lifesciences Of Ohio 800-654-2873
4900 Charlemar Dr Bldg A, Cincinnati, OH 45227
Cervical spinal implant.

K2m, Inc. 866-526-4171
751 Miller Dr SE Ste F1, Leesburg, VA 20175
Spinal fixator.

Lanx Inc. 303-443-7500
390 Interlocken Cres, Broomfield, CO 80021
Aspen; Lanx Spinal Fixation System

Medtronic Sofamor Danek Usa, Inc. 901-396-3133
4340 Swinnea Rd, Memphis, TN 38118
Interlaminal clamp.

Nuvasive, Inc. 800-475-9131
7475 Lusk Blvd, San Diego, CA 92121
Spinal implants.

Orthotec, Llc 800-557-2988
9595 Wilshire Blvd Ste 502, Beverly Hills, CA 90212
Various.

Scient'X Usa, Inc. 407-571-2550
1015 Maitland Center Commons Blvd Ste 10, Maitland, FL 32751
Anterior cervical plate.

Spinecraft Llc 708-531-9700
2215 Enterprise Dr, Westchester, IL 60154
Spinal fixation system.

Synthes (Usa) 610-719-5000
35 Airport Rd, Horseheads, NY 14845
Various types and sizes of spinal interlaminal fixation devices.

Us Spine Inc. 561-367-7463
3600 Fau Blvd Ste 101, Boca Raton, FL 33431
Pedicle screw system.

Warsaw Orthopedic, Inc. 901-396-3133
2500 Silveus Xing, Warsaw, IN 46582
Spinal implant fixation devices.

Zimmer Spine, Inc. 800-655-2614
7375 Bush Lake Rd, Minneapolis, MN 55439
Rod, hook, and screw spinal devices.

APPLIANCE, FIXATION, SPINAL INTERVERTEBRAL BODY *(Orthopedics) 87KWQ*

Abbott Spine, Inc. 847-937-6100
12708 Riata Vista Cir Ste B-100, Austin, TX 78727
Bone fixation plate.

Advanced Spine Technology, Inc. 415-241-2400
457 Mariposa St, San Francisco, CA 94107
Anterior locking plate.

Allez Spine, Llc 949-752-7885
2301 Dupont Dr Ste 510, Irvine, CA 92612
Spinal fixation system.

Alphatec Spine, Inc. 760-494-6769
5818 El Camino Real, Carlsbad, CA 92008
Deltaloc anterior cervical plate system.

Atlas Spine Inc. 561-741-1108
1555 Jupiter Park Dr Ste 4, Jupiter, FL 33458
Anterior cervical plate.

Centinel Spine Inc. 952-885-0500
505 Park Ave Fl 14, New York, NY 10022
Hartshill Rect & Wires, Spinal Fixa

Depuy Spine, Inc. 800-227-6633
325 Paramount Dr, Raynham, MA 02767
Anterior spine bone plate.

Depuy-Raynham, A Div. Of Depuy Orthopaedics 800-451-2006
325 Paramount Dr, Raynham, MA 02767
Anterior cervical spine plate.

Innovasis, Inc. 801-261-2236
614 E 3900 S, Salt Lake City, UT 84107
Cervical plate.

K2m, Inc. 866-526-4171
751 Miller Dr SE Ste F1, Leesburg, VA 20175
Anterior cervical plate.

APPLIANCE, FIXATION, SPINAL INTERVERTEBRAL BODY (cont'd)

Lanx Inc. 303-443-7500
390 Interlocken Cres, Broomfield, CO 80021
Anterior cervical spine (acp) system.

Macropore Biosurgery, Inc. 858-458-0900
6740 Top Gun St, San Diego, CA 92121
Spinal intervertebral body fixation orthosis.

Medtronic Puerto Rico Operations Co.,Med Rel 763-514-4000
Road 909, Km. 0.4., Barrio Mariana, Humacao, PR 00792
Anterior fixation devices.

Medtronic Sofamor Danek Usa, Inc. 901-396-3133
4340 Swinnea Rd, Memphis, TN 38118
Anterior fixation devices.

Nuvasive, Inc. 800-475-9131
7475 Lusk Blvd, San Diego, CA 92121
Spinal implants.

Orthotec, Llc 800-557-2988
9595 Wilshire Blvd Ste 502, Beverly Hills, CA 90212
Anterior spine plates, cervical spine plates.

Paramount Surgicals, Inc. 956-541-1220
942 Wildrose Ln Ste B, Brownsville, TX 78520
Cervical plate.

Pisharodi Surgicals, Inc. 956-541-6725
3475 W Alton Gloor Blvd, Brownsville, TX 78520
Cervical plate.

Rsb Spine Llc. 866-241-2104
2530 Superior Ave E Ste 703, Cleveland, OH 44114
Cervical plate.

Scient'X Usa, Inc. 407-571-2550
1015 Maitland Center Commons Blvd Ste 10, Maitland, FL 32751
Anterior plate.

Spinal Elements, Inc. 760-607-0121
2744 Loker Ave W Ste 100, Carlsbad, CA 92010
Anterior cervical plate system.

Trans1 Incorporated 910-332-1700
411 Landmark Dr, Wilmington, NC 28412
Anterior spinal fixation device.

Us Spine Inc. 561-367-7463
3600 Fau Blvd Ste 101, Boca Raton, FL 33431
Pedicle screw system.

Ussc Puerto Rico, Inc. 203-845-1000
Building 911-67, Sabanetas Industrial Park, Ponce, PR 00731
Spinal fusion system.

Vertebron, Inc. 203-380-9340
400 Long Beach Blvd, Stratford, CT 06615
Cervical plate.

Warsaw Orthopedic, Inc. 901-396-3133
2500 Silveus Xing, Warsaw, IN 46582
Anterior implant fixation devices.

Zimmer Spine, Inc. 800-655-2614
7375 Bush Lake Rd, Minneapolis, MN 55439
Spinal intervertebral body fixation orthosis.

APPLIANCE, INCONTINENCE, UROSHEATH TYPE

(Gastro/Urology) 78EXJ

Bioderm, Inc. 800-373-7006
12320 73rd Ct, Largo, FL 33773
External male continence device.

Coloplast Manufacturing Us, Llc 612-302-4992
1185 Willow Lake Blvd, Vadnais Heights, MN 55110
Various types of sterile male external catheters.

Kelsar, S.A. 508-261-8000
Blvd. Insurgentes, Libriamento a La, Tijuana 22450 Mexico
Texas catheter, external catheter, and accessories

Ldb Medical, Inc. 800-243-2554
2909 Langford Rd Ste B500, Norcross, GA 30071
WEIMER.

Leading Edge Innovations 805-388-7669
699 Mobil Ave, Camarillo, CA 93010
Offerings include a range of devices and accessories for male urinary incontinence.

Medline Industries, Inc. 800-633-5886
1 Medline Pl, Mundelein, IL 60060

APPLIANCE, INCONTINENCE, UROSHEATH TYPE (cont'd)

Mentor Corp. 800-525-0245
201 Mentor Dr, Santa Barbara, CA 93111
Self-adhesive, male, external catheters, leg bags, catheter straps. Female catheters, connecting tubing.

Perma Type Company, Inc. 860-747-9999
83 Northwest Dr, Plainville, CT 06062
Male incontinent device.

Reach Global Industries, Inc. (Reachgood) 888-518-8389
8 Corporate Park Ste 300, Irvine, CA 92606
Male external catheter.

Rochester Medical Corp. 800-615-2364
1 Rochester Medical Dr NW, Stewartville, MN 55976
External catheter.

APPLICATOR (LARYNGO-TRACHEAL), TOPICAL ANESTHESIA

(Anesthesiology) 73CCT

Allergan 800-366-6554
2525 Dupont Dr, Irvine, CA 92612

Hemaedics, Inc. 310-471-2719
3411 Mandeville Canyon Rd, Los Angeles, CA 90049
yopical applicator device

Wolfe Tory Medical, Inc. 801-281-3000
79 W 4500 S Ste 18, Salt Lake City, UT 84107
Applicator (caryngo-tracheal), topical anesthesia.

APPLICATOR, ANTISEPTIC *(General) 80QBE*

Enturia, Inc. (Formerly Medi-Flex) 800-523-0502
11400 Tomahawk Creek Pkwy Ste 310, Leawood, KS 66211
Medi-Flex, Inc. designs, develops and manufactures clinically superior aseptic skin preparation products. Our unique applicators; Sepp, Frepp and ChloraPrep applicators provide a hands free delivery system with no mess to the patient. Our applicators are available in several antiseptic solutions to include 2% Chlorhexidine Gluconate in 70% Isopropyl Alcohol (which has been recognized by the Center for Disease Control and Prevention as being more effective at reducing bacteria than other antiseptics) 2% Tincture of Iodine, 10% Povidone Iodine and 70% Isopropyl Alcohol. We also offer Compound Tincture of Benzoin as an adhesive adjunct.

Medco Supply Company 800-556-3326
500 Fillmore Ave, Tonawanda, NY 14150
Cotton tipped & cotton mini-tipped.

Niagara Pharmaceuticals Div. 905-690-6277
60 Innovation Dr., Flamborough, ONT L9H-7P3 Canada
HEALTH SAVER antiseptic skin cleanser for killing harmful bacteria and germs.

Norpak Manufacturing Inc. 905-427-0960
85 Chambers Dr., Unit 4, Ajax, ONT L1Z-1E2 Canada
Pad Plus povidone-iodine No-Touch infection control applicator for replacement of prep pads and swab sticks. Alcohol preps are available in medium and large sizes, both non-sterile and sterile. Institutional boxes of 200 and retail boxes of 100.

APPLICATOR, CLIP (FORCEPS) *(General) 80QBF*

Codman & Shurtleff, Inc 800-225-0460
325 Paramount Dr, Raynham, MA 02767

O&M Enterprise 847-258-4515
641 Chelmsford Ln, Elk Grove Village, IL 60007
FORCEPS

Prosurge Instruments, Inc. 866-832-7874
199 Laidlaw Ave, Jersey City, NJ 07306

Richard Wolf Medical Instruments Corp. 800-323-9653
353 Corporate Woods Pkwy, Vernon Hills, IL 60061
HULKA forceps.

Wisap America 800-233-8448
8231 Melrose Dr, Lenexa, KS 66214

Zimmer Holdings, Inc. 800-613-6131
1800 W Center St, PO Box 708, Warsaw, IN 46580

APPLICATOR, COTTON *(Dental And Oral) 76DZQ*

Puritan Medical Products Company Llc 800-321-2313
31 School St., Guilford, ME 04443-0149
Plastic or wood shaft.

Ross Disposable Products 800-649-6526
401 Traders Blvd E, Unit 10, Mississauga, ON L4Z 2H8 Canada

Solon Manufacturing Co. 800-341-6640
338 Madison Ave Ste 7, Skowhegan, ME 04976
3- and 6-in. sterile and non-sterile. Available in assorted packs with wood or plastic shafts.

APPLICATOR, ELECTRODE, SCALP, FETAL
(Obstetrics/Gyn) 85HGR

Rocket Medical Plc. 800-707-7625
150 Recreation Park Dr Ste 3, Hingham, MA 02043

APPLICATOR, ENT *(Ear/Nose/Throat) 77KCJ*

Aesculap Implant Systems Inc. 1-800-234-9179
3773 Corporate Pkwy, Center Valley, PA 18034

Amsino International, Inc. 800-MD-AMSINO
855 Towne Center Dr, Pomona, CA 91767
Non-sterile 3- or 6-in. applicators. Item #AS026.

Apdyne Medical Company 800-457-6853
1049 S Vine St, Denver, CO 80209
Disposable phenol applicator kit used by ENT physicians for in-office myringotomies.

Bausch & Lomb Surgical 636-255-5051
3365 Tree Court Ind Blvd, Saint Louis, MO 63122

Biomet Microfixation Inc. 800-874-7711
1520 Tradeport Dr, Jacksonville, FL 32218
Various types of tubes, tonsil suction.

Clinimed, Incorporated 877-CLINIMED
303 Markus Ct, Sandy Brae Industrial Park, Newark, DE 19713

Gyrus Ent L.L.C., Sub. Of Gyrus Acmi, Inc. 508-804-2739
2925 Appling Rd, Bartlett, TN 38133
Various types and sizes of ent applicator.

Micromedics 800-624-5662
1270 Eagan Industrial Rd, Saint Paul, MN 55121
Biomaterials applicators and delivery systems

Puritan Medical Products Company Llc 800-321-2313
31 School St., Guilford, ME 04443-0149

Solon Manufacturing Co. 800-341-6640
338 Madison Ave Ste 7, Skowhegan, ME 04976
3- and 6-in. cotton, rayon, polyester and calcium alginate; sterile and non-sterile with plastic, wood or wire shafts.

APPLICATOR, OCULAR PRESSURE *(Ophthalmology) 86LCC*

Eyetech Ltd. 847-470-1777
9408 Normandy Ave, Morton Grove, IL 60053
Tonometry eye model for ocular pressure simulation/teaching and demonstration device for applanation tonometers like: Goldman Tonometer, Tonopen

Jedmed Instruments Co. 314-845-3770
5416 Jedmed Ct, Saint Louis, MO 63129

Microsurgical Technology, Inc. 425-556-0544
PO Box 2679, Redmond, WA 98073
MCINTYRE OCULO-PRESSOR oculopression device.

APPLICATOR, OTHER *(General) 80QBI*

Arzol Chemical Co. 603-352-5242
12 Norway Ave Ste 2, Keene, NH 03431
Silver nitrate applicators.

Best Medical International, Inc. 800-336-4970
7643 Fullerton Rd, Springfield, VA 22153
Isotope-Manual; various types; Flexi-Needles, Template Needles, Implant Needles, Afterloading Tubes, Bronchial Tubes, Esophageal Applicator and Brain Implant Kit.

C.B. Fleet Company Inc. 804-528-4000
PO Box 11349, 4615 Murray Place, Lynchburg, VA 24506
Liquid Glycerin Suppositories. Liquid glycerin suppositories; disposable, pre-filled dispensers; 4/carton, 12/case. Child size, 6/carton, 12/case.

Coopersurgical, Inc. 800-243-2974
95 Corporate Dr, Trumbull, CT 06611
Applicator for endo-ligature of bleeding vessels and 3-mm needle holder.

Micromedics 800-624-5662
1270 Eagan Industrial Rd, Saint Paul, MN 55121
FibriJet Delivery Systems offers a controlled delivery of biologic components through dual and single lumen applicator tips. Six syringe sizes and a variety of specialized tips, including micro, endoscopic, flexible catheter, blending and both manual and air assisted spray, you may conveniently apply the appropriate amount of material to a specified site with simple one-handed operation.

Mml Diagnostics Packaging, Inc. 800-826-7186
1625 NW Sundial Rd, P.O. Box 458, Troutdale, OR 97060
Collection swab, stainless steel/plastic shaft; Collection swab, plastic shaft.

APPLICATOR, OTHER *(cont'd)*

Puritan Medical Products Company Llc 800-321-2313
31 School St., Guilford, ME 04443-0149
Calcium alginate, rayon, polyester and plain wood applicator.

Spectra Medical Devices, Inc. 978-657-0889
260H Fordham Rd, Wilmington, MA 01887
sponge applicators

Spectra Medical Devices, Inc. 866-938-8649
4C Henshaw St, Woburn, MA 01801
Sponge.

Surgipath Medical Industries, Inc. 800-225-3035
PO Box 528, 5205 Route 12, Richmond, IL 60071

Tmp Technologies, Inc. 716-895-6100
1200 Northland Ave, Buffalo, NY 14215
Foam-tipped applicators.

APPLICATOR, PROCTOSCOPIC *(Gastro/Urology) 78QBH*

Puritan Medical Products Company Llc 800-321-2313
31 School St., Guilford, ME 04443-0149

Solon Manufacturing Co. 800-341-6640
338 Madison Ave Ste 7, Skowhegan, ME 04976
16-in. rayon-tipped applicator with polypropylene shaft, non-sterile with assorted packs.

APPLICATOR, RADIONUCLIDE, MANUAL *(Radiology) 90IWJ*

Alpha-Omega Services, Inc. 800-346-7894
9156 Rose St, Bellflower, CA 90706
Manual radionuclide applicator system.

Bard Reynosa S.A. De C.V. 908-277-8000
Blvd. Montebello #1, Parque Industrial Colonial
Reynosa, Tamaulipas Mexico
System, applicator, radionuclide, manual

Best Medical International, Inc. 800-336-4970
7643 Fullerton Rd, Springfield, VA 22153

Computerized Medical Systems, Inc. 468-587-2550
1145 Corporate Lake Dr, Olivette, MO 63132
Stepping and stabilizing system.

Cytyc Surgical Products 800-442-9892
250 Campus Dr, Marlborough, MA 01752
System, applicator, radionuclide, manual.

Envisioneering Medical Technologies 314-429-7367
1982 Innerbelt Business Center Dr, Drive, Overland, MO 63114
Stabilizer.

International Brachytherapy, Inc. 770-582-0662
6000 Live Oak Pkwy Ste 107, Norcross, GA 30093
Brachytherapy needle.

Liberty Medical Llc 888-257-2408
10 Acacia Ln, Sterling, VA 20166
Various sterile and non-sterile manual radionuclide applicators.

Mcdalt Medical Corp. 800-841-5774
2225 Prestonwood Dr Ste 100-A, Arlington, TX 76012
Brachytherapy prostate seeding needles.

Micro Tool Engineering, Inc. 561-842-7381
7575 Central Industrial Dr, West Palm Beach, FL 33404

Mills Biopharmaceuticals, Llc 405-523-1868
120 NE 26th St, Oklahoma City, OK 73105
Seedvue.

Mpi Medical Products, Inc. 321-676-1299
1631 Elmhurst Cir SE, Palm Bay, FL 32909
Seeding needle.

North American Scientific, Inc. 818-734-8600
8300 Aurora Ave N, Seattle, WA 98103
Various system applicator radionuclide, manual.

Promex Technologies, Llc 317-736-0128
3049 Hudson St, Franklin, IN 46131
Prostate seeding needle.

APPLICATOR, RADIONUCLIDE, REMOTE-CONTROLLED
(Radiology) 90JAQ

Cianna Medical, Inc. 866-920-9444
6 Journey Ste 125, Aliso Viejo, CA 92656
BIOLUCENT APPLICATOR KIT

Cytyc Surgical Products 800-442-9892
250 Campus Dr, Marlborough, MA 01752
Radiation therapy system.

APPLICATOR, RADIONUCLIDE, REMOTE-CONTROLLED *(cont'd)*

Mills Biopharmaceuticals, Llc 405-523-1868
120 NE 26th St, Oklahoma City, OK 73105
Isocartridge.

Mpi Medical Products, Inc. 321-676-1299
1631 Elmhurst Cir SE, Palm Bay, FL 32909
6 french catheter.

APPLICATOR, RAPID WAX, DENTAL *(Dental And Oral) 76EIT*

Almore International, Inc. 503-643-6633
PO Box 25214, Portland, OR 97298
$185.00 to $355.00 for electric waxing unit.

APPLICATOR, RESIN *(Dental And Oral) 76KXR*

Denbur, Inc. 630-969-6865
433 Plaza Dr Ste 4, Westmont, IL 60559
Applicator, dental.

Foremost Dental Llc. 201-894-5500
242 S Dean St, Englewood, NJ 07631
Resin applicator brush.

Nagl Manufacturing Co. 423-587-2199
3626 Martha St, Omaha, NE 68105
Applicator brushes, handles, and brush tips.

Pentron Clinical Technologies 203-265-7397
68-70 North Plains Industrial, Road, Wallingford, CT 06492
Resin applicator.

Ultradent Products, Inc. 801-553-4586
505 W 10200 S, South Jordan, UT 84095
Brush tip.

Wykle Research, Inc. 775-887-7500
2222 College Pkwy, Carson City, NV 89706
Applicator brush.

APPLICATOR, SAMPLE *(Chemistry) 75UHU*

Cetac Technologies, Inc. 800-369-2822
14306 Industrial Rd, Omaha, NE 68144

Leap Technologies 800-229-8814
PO Box 969, Carrboro, NC 27510

Porex Corporation 800-241-0195
500 Bohannon Rd, Fairburn, GA 30213
Custom manufactured.

APPLICATOR, TIPPED, ABSORBENT *(General) 80FOR*

Bioseal 800-441-7325
167 W Orangethorpe Ave, Placentia, CA 92870
Sterile, various, precounted quantities.

Birchwood Laboratories, Inc. 800-328-6156
7900 Fuller Rd, Eden Prairie, MN 55344
SCOPETTES, sized and non-sized 8 in. x 12 box (100), 8 in. x 500, 16 in. x 12 box (100),16 in. x 500, 8 in. OB/GYN swab, 16 in. procto swab, 12 in. x 12 box (100)

Covidien Lp 508-261-8000
15 Hampshire St, Mansfield, MA 02048
Single tipped applicators with soft, absorbent tips.

Hospira 800-441-4100
268 E 4th St, Ashland, OH 44805
Sponge applicator.

Puritan Medical Products Company Llc 800-321-2313
31 School St., Guilford, ME 04443-0149

Solon Manufacturing Co. 800-341-6640
338 Madison Ave Ste 7, Skowhegan, ME 04976
3- and 6-in. cotton, rayon, polyester and calcium alginate tips in assorted packs with wood, plastic or wire shafts. Available in sterile or non-sterile.

Ultracell Medical Technologies, Inc. 877-SPO-NGE1
183 Providence New London Tpke, North Stonington, CT 06359
ULTRACELL P.V.A. and cellulose surgical spears and points and LASIK spears.

APPLICATOR, TIPPED, ABSORBENT, NON-STERILE *(General) 80KXF*

American Fiber & Finishing, Inc. 800-522-2438
PO Box 2488, Albemarle, NC 28002
Cotton balls.

Citmed 251-866-5519
18601 S Main St, Citronelle, AL 36522
Absorbent tipped applicator.

APPLICATOR, TIPPED, ABSORBENT, NON-STERILE *(cont'd)*

Customs Hospital Products, Inc 800-426-2780
6336 SE 107th Ave, Portland, OR 97266
Cotton tipped applicators-non sterile.

Dukal Corporation 800-243-0741
5 Plant Ave, Hauppauge, NY 11788
Single cotton-tipped applicators, wooden shaft only, various sizes.

Healer Products, Llc 914-663-6300
427 Commerce Ln Ste 1, West Berlin, NJ 08091
Cotton tipped applicators.

Icp Medical 314-429-1000
10486 Baur Blvd, Saint Louis, MO 63132
Oral swan.

Inter-Med, Inc. 877-418-4782
2200 Northwestern Ave, Racine, WI 53404
Cotton tipped applicator.

Kentron Health Care, Inc. 615-384-0573
3604 Kelton Jackson Rd, P.o. Box 120, Springfield, TN 37172
Cotton tipped applicators.

Medical Action Industries, Inc. 800-645-7042
25 Heywood Rd, Arden, NC 28704
Applicators.

Nagl Manufacturing Co. 423-587-2199
3626 Martha St, Omaha, NE 68105
Oral swab.

Purfybr, Inc. 800-947-9227
9384 Calumet Ave, Munster, IN 46321
Specimen collection swab.

Puritan Medical Products Company Llc 800-321-2313
31 School St., Guilford, ME 04443-0149

Qfc Plastics, Inc. 817-649-7400
728 111th St, Arlington, TX 76011
Applicator.

Solstice Corp. 207-874-7922
68 Marginal Way Fl 4, Portland, ME 04101
Various size non-sterile absorbent tipped applicators.

Statsure Diagnostic Systems, Inc. 508-872-2625
1881 Worcester Rd, Framingham, MA 01701

Teartec 816-518-8626
7400 NW Whipple Ln, Kansas City, MO 64152
Applicator strips.

APPLICATOR, TIPPED, ABSORBENT, STERILE *(General) 80KXG*

Celera Corporation 510-749-4219
1401 Harbor Bay Pkwy, Alameda, CA 94502

Centurion Medical Products Corp. 517-545-1135
3310 S Main St, Salisbury, NC 28147

Citmed 251-866-5519
18601 S Main St, Citronelle, AL 36522
Cotton tipped or absorbent tipped applicator sterile.

Covidien Lp 508-261-8000
15 Hampshire St, Mansfield, MA 02048

Demetech Corp. 888-324-2447
3530 NW 115th Ave, Doral, FL 33178
Cotton applicator.

Diagnostic Hybrids, Inc. 740-589-3300
1055 E State St Ste 100, Athens, OH 45701
Specimen collection device.

Dukal Corporation 800-243-0741
5 Plant Ave, Hauppauge, NY 11788
Single cotton-tipped applicator, wooden and plastic shaft, various sizes available.

First Aid Bandage Co., Inc. 888-813-8214
3 State Pier Rd, New London, CT 06320

Kentron Health Care, Inc. 615-384-0573
3604 Kelton Jackson Rd, P.o. Box 120, Springfield, TN 37172
Cotton tipped applicators.

Norwood Promotional Products, Inc. 651-388-1298
5151 Moundview Dr, Red Wing, MN 55066
Providone-iodine swabstick.

Purfybr, Inc. 800-947-9227
9384 Calumet Ave, Munster, IN 46321
Specimen collection swab.

Puritan Medical Products Company Llc 800-321-2313
31 School St., Guilford, ME 04443-0149

APPLICATOR, TIPPED, ABSORBENT, STERILE *(cont'd)*

Qiagen Gaithersburg, Inc. 800-344-3631
1201 Clopper Rd, Gaithersburg, MD 20878
Swab collection kit.

Tri-State Hospital Supply Corp. 517-545-1135
3173 E 43rd St, Yuma, AZ 85365

Ultracell Medical Technologies, Inc. 877-SPO-NGE1
183 Providence New London Tpke, North Stonington, CT 06359
ULTRACELL, P.V.A. cellulose surgical spears and points, LASIK spears.

APPLICATOR, VAGINAL *(Obstetrics/Gyn) 85HGD*

Birchwood Laboratories, Inc. 800-328-6156
7900 Fuller Rd, Eden Prairie, MN 55344
PREP AID; SCOPETTES (R); SCOPETTES JR (R)

Centurion Medical Products Corp. 517-545-1135
3310 S Main St, Salisbury, NC 28147

Confluent Surgical,Inc 888-734-2583
101A 1st Ave, Waltham, MA 02451
Applicator.

Genesis Instruments, Inc. 715-639-9209
200 Main St., Elmwood, WI 54740
Vaginal applicator.

Health Care Logistics, Inc. 800-848-1633
450 Town St, PO Box 25, Circleville, OH 43113
Vaginal applicator.

Heinke Technoogy, Inc. (Hti Plastics) 800-824-0607
5120 NW 38th St, Lincoln, NE 68524
Vaginal cream, tablet, suppository, gel, or foam applicators. Cream available in 3.0-, 4.0-, 5.5-, 6.0-, or 7.0-ml applicators. Tablet applicators available in two sizes. Suppository applicators available in three sizes. New products include prefilled applicators also available in various dose sizes.

Janler Corporation 773-774-0166
6545 N Avondale Ave, Chicago, IL 60631
Applicator, vaginal.

Ortho-Mcneil-Janssen Pharmaceuticals, Inc. 800-526-7736
1000 US Highway 202, Raritan, NJ 08869

Puritan Medical Products Company Llc 800-321-2313
31 School St., Guilford, ME 04443-0149
Non-sterile and sterile.

Radium Accessories Service, Inc. 305-289-1361
34 Coco Plum Dr, Marathon, FL 33050
Various types and models of vaginal applicators.

Solon Manufacturing Co. 800-341-6640
338 Madison Ave Ste 7, Skowhegan, ME 04976
8-in. rayon-tipped OB-GYN applicator with paper shaft in non-sterile. Sterile available with a polystyrene shaft. Assorted packs.

Src Medical, Inc. 781-826-9100
263 Winter St, Hanover, MA 02339
Various vaginal applicators.

Tri-State Hospital Supply Corp. 517-545-1135
3173 E 43rd St, Yuma, AZ 85365

Wisap America 800-233-8448
8231 Melrose Dr, Lenexa, KS 66214

APPLIER, ANEURYSM CLIP *(Cns/Neurology) 84HCI*

Aesculap Implant Systems Inc. 1-800-234-9179
3773 Corporate Pkwy, Center Valley, PA 18034
Various aneurysm clip appliers: Caspar, Yasargil, Vario.

Mizuho America Inc. 800-699-2547
133 Brimbal Ave, Beverly, MA 01915

APPLIER, CAST *(Orthopedics) 87LGG*

Biomet, Inc. 574-267-6639
56 E Bell Dr, PO Box 587, Warsaw, IN 46582
Various types of manual cast removel instruments.

Cmt Inc. 910-497-3172
26 Mockingbird Ln, Spring Lake, NC 28390
Universal casting stand.

Ortho-Med, Inc. 800-547-5571
3208 SE 13th Ave, Portland, OR 97202

W.L. Gore & Associates,Inc 928-526-3030
1505 North Fourth St., Flagstaff, AZ 86004
Cast removal aid.

APPLIER, CERCLAGE *(Orthopedics) 87HXN*

Arthrex, Inc. 239-643-5553
1370 Creekside Blvd, Naples, FL 34108
Applier, cerclage.

Biomet, Inc. 574-267-6639
56 E Bell Dr, PO Box 587, Warsaw, IN 46582
Parham band clamp.

Zimmer Holdings, Inc. 800-613-6131
1800 W Center St, PO Box 708, Warsaw, IN 46580

APPLIER, CLIP, LAPAROSCOPIC *(Surgery) 79WZM*

Aesculap Implant Systems Inc. 1-800-234-9179
3773 Corporate Pkwy, Center Valley, PA 18034

Coopersurgical, Inc. 800-243-2974
95 Corporate Dr, Trumbull, CT 06611

Ethicon Endo-Surgery, Inc. 800-USE-ENDO
4545 Creek Rd, Cincinnati, OH 45242
LIGACLIP multiple clip applier, with rotating shaft and rotating 10mm shaft, 20 titanium (med) and (lg), 20/20; reload multiple clip applier, 20 titanium (med), 20/20.

APPLIER, CLIP, REPAIR, HERNIA, LAPAROSCOPIC *(Gastro/Urology) 78WZN*

Coopersurgical, Inc. 800-243-2974
95 Corporate Dr, Trumbull, CT 06611

Covidien Lp 508-261-8000
15 Hampshire St, Mansfield, MA 02048
Absorbable ligating clip.

APPLIER, HEMOSTATIC CLIP *(Cns/Neurology) 84HBT*

Biomet Microfixation Inc. 800-874-7711
1520 Tradeport Dr, Jacksonville, FL 32218
Various types of clips.

Ethicon Endo-Surgery, Inc. 877-384-4266
3801 University Blvd SE, Albuquerque, NM 87106
Various types of clip appliers.

Kmedic 800-955-0559
190 Veterans Dr, Northvale, NJ 07647

Medisiss 866-866-7477
2747 SW 6th St, Redmond, OR 97756
Various hemostatic clip appliers,sterile.

Sterilmed, Inc. 763-488-3400
11400 73rd Ave N Ste 100, Maple Grove, MN 55369
Hemostatic clip applier.

APPLIER, LIGATURE CLIP *(Surgery) 79SJF*

Okay Industries, Inc. 860-225-8707
200 Ellis St, P.O. Box 2470, New Britain, CT 06051

APPLIER, PRESSURE, PHYSICAL MEDICINE *(Physical Med) 89KNM*

Bionix Development Corp. 800-551-7096
5154 Enterprise Blvd, Toledo, OH 43612
Shotblocker.

Helio Medical Supplies, Inc. 408-433-3355
606 Charcot Ave, San Jose, CA 95131
Cupping jar, cupping cup set.

Plexus Biomedical Inc. 901-763-2900
7495 Highway 64, Oakland, TN 38060
Pressure-applying device.

Therafin Corporation 800-843-7234
19747 Wolf Rd, Mokena, IL 60448
Squeeze machine.

APPLIER, SURGICAL STAPLE *(Surgery) 79GEF*

Depuy Mitek, A Johnson & Johnson Company 800-451-2006
50 Scotland Blvd, Bridgewater, MA 02324
Inserter.

Medisiss 866-866-7477
2747 SW 6th St, Redmond, OR 97756
Various surgical staple appliers,sterile.

Putnam Precision Products 845-278-2141
3859 Danbury Rd, Brewster, NY 10509

Roboz Surgical Instrument Co., Inc. 800-424-2984
PO Box 10710, Gaithersburg, MD 20898

Temedco, Ltd. 210-798-0978
1141 N Loop 1604 E Ste 105, Box 418, San Antonio, TX 78232
Stapler.

APPLIER, SURGICAL STAPLE *(cont'd)*

Total Molding Services, Inc. 215-538-9613
354 East Broad St., Trumbauersville, PA 18970
Anvil parts & staple retainers for intraluminal staplers.

Zimmer Holdings, Inc. 800-613-6131
1800 W Center St, PO Box 708, Warsaw, IN 46580

APPLIER, SURGICAL, CLIP *(Surgery) 79GDO*

Acra Cut, Inc. 978-263-0250
989 Main St, Acton, MA 01720
Scalp clip gun.

Aesculap Implant Systems Inc. 1-800-234-9179
3773 Corporate Pkwy, Center Valley, PA 18034

Biomet Microfixation Inc. 800-874-7711
1520 Tradeport Dr, Jacksonville, FL 32218
Various types of clamps.

Biomet, Inc. 574-267-6639
56 E Bell Dr, PO Box 587, Warsaw, IN 46582
Stichs wound clip.

Ethicon Endo-Surgery, Inc. 800-USE-ENDO
4545 Creek Rd, Cincinnati, OH 45242
LIGACLIP single clip applier, 5.75in. and 7.5in. for (sm); 3.5 alligator for (sm); 5.75in., 7.5in and 10.5in. for (med); 10.5in. r-angle for (med); 5in. and 7in. alligator for (med); 7.5in. and 10in. for (med/lg); 14in. alligator for (med/lg); 10.5in. r-angle for (med.Lg); 7.5in and 10.5in. for (lg); 10.5in. r-angle for (lg), all reuseable. ABSOLOCK single clip applier, 5.5in. and 7.5 for (sm); 7.5in. and 10.5in. for (med); 7.5in. and 10.5 for (med/lg); 7.5in. and 10.5in. for (lg); all reuseable. 10mm shaft (med/lg) reuseable.

Genicon 800-936-1020
6869 Stapoint Ct Ste 114, Winter Park, FL 32792
Disposable 10mm Clip Applier

International Plastics, Llc 262-781-2270
4965 N. Campbell Dr., Menomonee Falls, WI 53051
Sterile specimen marker for radiology analysis.

Karl Storz Endoscopy-America Inc. 800-421-0837
600 Corporate Pointe, Culver City, CA 90230
For thorascopic procedures.

Kelsar, S.A. 508-261-8000
Blvd. Insurgentes, Libriamento a La, Tijuana 22450 Mexico
Ligating clip, applier

Mikron Precision, Inc. 310-515-6221
1558 W 139th St Ste C, Gardena, CA 90249
Wound clip applier.

Okay Industries, Inc. 860-225-8707
200 Ellis St, P.O. Box 2470, New Britain, CT 06051

Putnam Precision Products 845-278-2141
3859 Danbury Rd, Brewster, NY 10509

Roboz Surgical Instrument Co., Inc. 800-424-2984
PO Box 10710, Gaithersburg, MD 20898

Teleflex Medical 800-334-9751
2917 Weck Drive, Research Triangle Park, NC 27709
Horizon, Hemoclip Traditional, Hemoclip Plus, ATRAUCLIP.

Tuzik Boston 800-886-6363
104 Longwater Dr, Assinippi Park, Norwell, MA 02061

Ussc Puerto Rico, Inc. 203-845-1000
Building 911-67, Sabanetas Industrial Park, Ponce, PR 00731
Various sizes and types of surgical clipping instruments.

Zimmer Holdings, Inc. 800-613-6131
1800 W Center St, PO Box 708, Warsaw, IN 46580

APRON, CONDUCTIVE *(Surgery) 79QBK*

General Scientific Safety Equipment Co. 800-523-0166
2553 E Somerset St Fl 1, Philadelphia, PA 19134

APRON, LABORATORY *(Chemistry) 75QBJ*

Adi Medical Division Of Asia Dynamics (Group) Inc. 877-647-7699
1565 S Shields Dr, Waukegan, IL 60085

Alimed, Inc. 800-225-2610
297 High St, Dedham, MA 02026

Brain Power, Inc. 800-327-2250
4470 SW 74th Ave, Miami, FL 33155
$54.00 per box of 100 and $247.50 per case of 6 boxes of Kimwear Aprons. 3-gauge embossed plastic, tough and liquid-resistant.

Cole-Parmer Instrument Inc. 800-323-4340
625 E Bunker Ct, Vernon Hills, IL 60061

APRON, LABORATORY *(cont'd)*

General Scientific Safety Equipment Co. 800-523-0166
2553 E Somerset St Fl 1, Philadelphia, PA 19134

Kerr Group 800-524-3577
1400 Holcomb Bridge Rd, Roswell, GA 30076
Nonwoven disposable.

Maddak Inc. 800-443-4926
661 State Route 23, Wayne, NJ 07470
ABLEWARE 36in x 27in size apron.

Pharaoh Trading Company 866-929-4913
9701 Brookpark Rd, Knollwood Plaza, Suite 241, Cleveland, OH 44129
Polyethylene apron.

Postcraft Co. 800-528-4844
625 W Rillito St, Tucson, AZ 85705
Synthetic aprons.

Quincy Specialties Co. 217-222-4057
631 Vermont St, Quincy, IL 62301
Laboratory coats.

Rockford Medical & Safety Co. 800-435-9451
2420 Harrison Ave, PO Box 5646, Rockford, IL 61108

Ross Disposable Products 800-649-6526
401 Traders Blvd E, Unit 10, Mississauga, ON L4Z 2H8 Canada

APRON, LEAD, DENTAL *(Dental And Oral) 76EAJ*

Aadco Medical, Inc. 800-225-9014
2279 VT Route 66, Randolph, VT 05060
X-ray protective aprons & accessories.

Burlington Medical Supplies, Inc. 800-221-3466
3 Elmhurst St, PO Box 3194, Newport News, VA 23603

Cadco Dental Products 800-833-8267
600 E Hueneme Rd, Oxnard, CA 93033
35 types - from $17.50 to $60.00 each.

Clive Craig Co. 805-488-1122
600 E Hueneme Rd, Oxnard, CA 93033
Apron, leaded, various.

Davis Lead Apron, Inc. 800-483-3979
4560 W 34th St, PO Box 924585, Houston, TX 77092
Aprons, apron racks.

Dux Dental 800-833-8267
600 E Hueneme Rd, Oxnard, CA 93033
35 types - from $17.50 to $60.00 each.

Fabrite Laminating Corp. 973-777-1406
70 Passaic St, Wood Ridge, NJ 07075

Gammadirect Medical Division 847-267-5929
PO Box 383, Lake Forest, IL 60045
Aukulyte radiation protective aprons.

Lite Tech, Inc. 610-650-8690
975 Madison Ave, Norristown, PA 19403
Lead & lead-free x-ray aprons, dental x-ray aprons.

Rf Design, Inc. 810-632-6000
10143 Bergin Rd, Howell, MI 48843
Lead protection aprons.

Shielding Intl., Inc. 541-475-7211
2150 N.w. Andrews Dr., Madras, OR 97741
X-ray protective garment.

Star X-Ray Co., Inc. 800-374-2163
63 Ranick Dr S, Amityville, NY 11701
$59.40 per unit (standard).

APRON, LEAD, RADIOGRAPHIC *(Radiology) 90IWO*

Alimed, Inc. 800-225-2610
297 High St, Dedham, MA 02026

Americomp, Inc. 800-458-1782
2901 W Lawrence Ave, Chicago, IL 60625

Bar-Ray Products, Inc. 800-359-6115
95 Monarch St, Littlestown, PA 17340

Brennen Medical, Llc 651-429-7413
1290 Hammond Rd, Saint Paul, MN 55110
Water repellent apron.

Burkhart Roentgen Intl. Inc. 800-USA-XRAY
5201 8th Ave S, Gulfport, FL 33707
Complete line of x-ray protective leaded clothing for doctors, technicians and patients.

Burlington Medical Supplies, Inc. 800-221-3466
3 Elmhurst St, PO Box 3194, Newport News, VA 23603
Custom x-ray aprons.

APRON, LEAD, RADIOGRAPHIC *(cont'd)*

Busse Hospital Disposables, Inc. 631-435-4711
75 Arkay Dr, Hauppauge, NY 11788
Plastic apron.

Carr Corporation 800-952-2398
1547 11th St, Santa Monica, CA 90401

Cone Instruments, Inc. 800-321-6964
5201 Naiman Pkwy, Solon, OH 44139

Davis Lead Apron, Inc. 800-483-3979
4560 W 34th St, PO Box 924585, Houston, TX 77092
Aprons, apron racks.

Frank Scholz X-Ray Corp. 508-586-8308
244 Liberty St, Brockton, MA 02301
$285.00 per unit (standard).

Gammadirect Medical Division 847-267-5929
PO Box 383, Lake Forest, IL 60045
Aukulyte is the world's first non-Lead apron. Safe for the environment. Available in standard or custom sizes.

Infab Corp. 805-987-5255
3651 Via Pescador, Camarillo, CA 93012
Large selection of models, colors, and custom designs.

Lite Tech, Inc. 610-650-8690
975 Madison Ave, Norristown, PA 19403
Lead & lead-free x-ray aprons.

Marconi Medical Systems. 800-323-0550
595 Miner Rd, Cleveland, OH 44143

Mcdalt Medical Corp. 800-841-5774
2225 Prestonwood Dr Ste 100-A, Arlington, TX 76012
A complete line of quality lead protective aprons and protective lead shielded glasses.

Medlink Imaging, Inc. 800-456-7800
200 Clearbrook Rd, Elmsford, NY 10523

Occk, Inc. 800-526-9731
1710 W Schilling Rd, Salina, KS 67401
Disposable apron.

Owens Scientific Inc. 281-394-2311
23230 Sandsage Ln, Katy, TX 77494

Palmero Health Care 800-344-6424
120 Goodwin Pl, Stratford, CT 06615
CLING SHIELD X-ray protective aprons for radiology, .3mm and .5mm.

Protech Leaded Eyewear 561-627-9769
4087 Burns Rd, Palm Beach Gardens, FL 33410
Radiation protective lead and non-lead aprons and apparel.

Pulse Medical Inc. 800-342-5973
4131 SW 47th Ave Ste 1404, Davie, FL 33314
Custom made with a large selection of color, design and comfort. Available in lightweight lead as well. Also, unique, portable, lead apron racks which will not tip over with excess weight.

S&S Technology 281-815-1300
10625 Telge Rd, Houston, TX 77095
Many sizes , tie-wrap or Velcro closure, special procedure and apron and glove rack.

Schueler & Company, Inc. 516-487-1500
PO Box 528, Stratford, CT 06615

Shielding International, Inc. 800-292-2247
PO Box Z, 2150 NW Andrews Drive, Madras, OR 97741
Full and fontal protection, medical, dental and veterinarian, 0.5-mm Pb equiv. protection. Many options to choose from.

Shielding Intl., Inc. 541-475-7211
2150 N.w. Andrews Dr., Madras, OR 97741
X-ray protective garment.

Star X-Ray Co., Inc. 800-374-2163
63 Ranick Dr S, Amityville, NY 11701
$108.00 per unit (standard).

Techno-Aide, Inc. 800-251-2629
7117 Centennial Blvd, Nashville, TN 37209
Full-line protective apparel.

Wolf X-Ray Corporation 800-356-9729
100 W Industry Ct, Deer Park, NY 11729
Easy wrap, front closing, or bib style.

Xma (X-Ray Marketing Associates, Inc.) 800-325-8880
1205 W Lakeview Ct, Windham Lakes Business Park
Romeoville, IL 60446

APRON, SURGICAL *(Surgery) 79GDA*

Alimed, Inc. 800-225-2610
297 High St, Dedham, MA 02026

Brant-Wald Surgicals, Inc. 865-483-5230
368 E Tennessee Ave, Oak Ridge, TN 37830
TUR APRON SYSTEM: Sterile Disposable trans-urethral resection apron with and reusable receptor kit. Quickly and easily installed and dismantled on any type table. Very time and cost effective. Can also be used for ablation procedure.

General Econopak, Inc. 888-871-8568
1725 N 6th St, Philadelphia, PA 19122
Surgeon's aprons and sleeves, sterile and non-sterile.

Global Concepts, Ltd. 818-363-7195
19464 Eagle Ridge Ln, Northridge, CA 91326

Kerr Group 800-524-3577
1400 Holcomb Bridge Rd, Roswell, GA 30076
Nonwoven disposable.

Mi-Co Company 516-481-7775
564 Warren Blvd, Garden City, NY 11530

Tartan Orthopedics, Ltd. 888-287-1456
10651 Irma Dr Unit C, Northglenn, CO 80233
$140.00 per 10 units.

ARM REST *(Physical Med) 89QBL*

Alimed, Inc. 800-225-2610
297 High St, Dedham, MA 02026

Bryton Corp. 800-567-9500
4310 Guion Rd, Indianapolis, IN 46254
Arm support and positioning devices for all surgical tables and surgical procedures. Arm and hand surgery tables.

Cloward Instrument Corporation 808-734-3511
3787 Diamond Head Rd, Honolulu, HI 96816
CLOWARD Disposable arm rests and face rests.

Gunnell, Inc. 800-551-0055
8440 State Rd, Millington, MI 48746
#735 Heavy Duty Swing Up Armrest assists in patient transfers. The armrests can be placed on any 7/8-inch uprights and they adjust along any point on the uprights.

Invacare Corporation 800-333-6900
1 Invacare Way, Elyria, OH 44035
Standard wheelchairs.

Telsar Laboratories Inc 800-255-9938
1 Enviro Way Ste 100, Wood River, IL 62095
Physician's arm rest for ophthalmic laser surgery.

ARMBOARD, WHEELCHAIR *(Physical Med) 89IMY*

Daher Mfg., Inc. 204-663-3299
Mazenod Rd, Winnipeg R2J 4H2 Canada
Various

Rk Froom & Co., Inc. 310-327-5125
903 Cunningham Ln S, Salem, OR 97302
Arm rest.

Tarry Manufacturing 800-688-2779
22 Shelter Rock Ln, Danbury, CT 06810
IV Armboard.

Therafin Corporation 800-843-7234
19747 Wolf Rd, Mokena, IL 60448
Various armrest trays.

ARMREST, WHEELCHAIR *(Physical Med) 89IML*

Alimed, Inc. 800-225-2610
297 High St, Dedham, MA 02026

Emergencia 2000, Inc. 757-224-0177
8160 NW 66th St, Miami, FL 33166
Medical devices: wheelchair.

Feiter's Inc 414-355-7575
8700 W Port Ave, Milwaukee, WI 53224
Armrest, wheelchair.

Genadyne Biotechnologies, Inc. 516-487-8787
65 Watermill Ln, Great Neck, NY 11021
Gentrack std/lx/dx.

Leeder Group, Inc. 305-436-5030
8508 NW 66th St, Miami, FL 33166
Wheelchair arm rest.

Patterson Medical Supply, Inc. 262-387-8720
W68N158 Evergreen Blvd, Cedarburg, WI 53012
Various types of wheelchair armrests.

ARMREST, WHEELCHAIR *(cont'd)*

Richardson Products, Inc. 888-928-7297
9408 Gulfstream Rd, Frankfort, IL 60423
Wheelchair armrest.

Sheepskin Ranch, Inc. 800-366-9950
3408 Indale Rd, Fort Worth, TX 76116
$32.00 for one pair of SOFSHEEP lamb or sheep armrest covers.

Sunrise Medical Hhg Inc 303-218-4505
2842 N Business Park Ave, Fresno, CA 93727

Tuffcare 800-367-6160
3999 E La Palma Ave, Anaheim, CA 92807

ARTHROGRAM KIT *(Orthopedics) 87QBO*

Marconi Medical Systems 800-323-0550
595 Miner Rd, Cleveland, OH 44143

ARTHROMETER *(Orthopedics) 87LYH*

Medmetric Corp. 800-995-6066
7542 Trade St, San Diego, CA 92121
Knee Ligament ARTHROMETER System-KT2000 with X-Y Plotter, $7,700.00; Knee Ligament ARTHROMETER-KT2000 CompuKT, $7,700.00; Knee Ligament ARTHROMETER-KT1000, $3,900.00; Intraoperative ARTHROMETER-KT1000/S $4,200.00.

ARTHROSCOPE *(Orthopedics) 87HRX*

Accellent El Paso 915-771-9112
31 Butterfield Trail Blvd Ste C, El Paso, TX 79906
Arthroscopic irrigation sets

Advanced Endoscopy Devices, Inc. 818-227-2720
22134 Sherman Way, Canoga Park, CA 91303
1.9mm-5mm sizes available. Compatible to any manufacturer's sheaths.

Arthrex, Inc. 239-643-5553
1370 Creekside Blvd, Naples, FL 34108
Various.

Arthro Kinetics Inc. 49-711-30511070
8 Faneuil Hall Sq Fl 3, Boston, MA 02109
Endoscopic spine system.

Arthronet Medical, Inc. 949-254-3343
520 Broadway Ste 350, Santa Monica, CA 90401
Various.

Arthroplastics, Inc. 440-247-5131
34 W Washington St, P.o. Box 332, Chagrin Falls, OH 44022
Distractor.

Ascent Healthcare Solutions 480-763-5300
10232 S 51st St, Phoenix, AZ 85044
Arthroscopic shavers and burs.

Biomet Sports Medicine 530-226-5800
6704 Lockheed Dr, Redding, CA 96002
Powertek ii with various accessories.

Biomet, Inc. 574-267-6639
56 E Bell Dr, PO Box 587, Warsaw, IN 46582
Arthroscope.

Clarus Medical, Llc. 763-525-8400
1000 Boone Ave N Ste 300, Minneapolis, MN 55427
2600 series, working channel endoscope.

Cortek Endoscopy, Inc. 847-526-2266
260 Jamie Ln Ste D, Wauconda, IL 60084
Orthopedics.

Davol Inc., Sub. C.R. Bard, Inc. 800-556-6275
100 Crossings Blvd, Warwick, RI 02886
Arthroscope and accessories.

Depuy Mitek, A Johnson & Johnson Company 800-451-2006
50 Scotland Blvd, Bridgewater, MA 02324
Suture bone fastener instrument set.

Depuy Spine, Inc. 800-227-6633
325 Paramount Dr, Raynham, MA 02767
Manual endoscopic instruments.

Dixon Medical Inc 770-457-0602
3710 Longview Dr, Atlanta, GA 30341

Ebi Patient Care, Inc. 973-299-9300
1 Electro-biology Blvd., Guaynabo, PR 00657
Spinal endoscopic system.

Global Endoscopy, Inc. 888-434-3398
914 Estes Ct, Schaumburg, IL 60193
Arthroscope.

Henke Sass Wolf Of America, Inc. 508-671-9300
135 Schofield Ave, Dudley, MA 01571

ARTHROSCOPE *(cont'd)*

Instratek, Inc. 281-890-8020
210 Spring Hill Dr Ste 130, Spring, TX 77386

Karl Storz Endoscopy-America Inc. 800-421-0837
600 Corporate Pointe, Culver City, CA 90230
Full line of both diagnostic and operative models in various sizes.

Medifix, Inc 847-965-1898
8727 Narragansett Ave, Morton Grove, IL 60053
Arthroscope.

Medisiss 866-866-7477
2747 SW 6th St, Redmond, OR 97756
Various arthroscopic & accessories, sterile.

Medivision Endoscopy 800-349-5367
1210 N Jefferson St, Anaheim, CA 92807
Independent service center specializing in rigid endoscope repairs and sales. Quality Control Department on premises. Provide customized maintenance reports to customers and distributors. Conduct technical training seminars and in-service programs. Manufacturer of new endoscopes. An endoscope that can be attached directly to a video camera. This product is available.

Medtec Applications, Inc. 630-628-0444
50 W Fay Ave, Addison, IL 60101
Arthroscope and accessories.

Minrad, Inc. 716-855-1068
50 Cobham Dr, Orchard Park, NY 14127
Arthroscope.

Myelotec, Inc. 770-664-4656
4000 Northfield Way Ste 900, Roswell, GA 30076
Flexible arthroscope and accessories.

Nuvasive, Inc. 800-475-9131
7475 Lusk Blvd, San Diego, CA 92121
Various.

Olympus America, Inc. 800-645-8160
3500 Corporate Pkwy, PO Box 610, Center Valley, PA 18034

Precision Optics Corp. 800-447-2812
22 E Broadway, Gardner, MA 01440

Regen Biologics, Inc. 415-562-0800
411 Hackensack Ave, Hackensack, NJ 07601
Suture passer and cannulas.

Rei Rotolux Enterprises, Inc. 888-773-7611
4145 North Service Rd, Ste. 200, Burlington, ON L7L 6A3 Canada
From 2.7mm to 4mm in diameter, autoclavable. Custom configurations are available.

Richard Wolf Medical Instruments Corp. 800-323-9653
353 Corporate Woods Pkwy, Vernon Hills, IL 60061

Romc, Inc. 508-829-4602
37 Kris Alan Dr, Holden, MA 01520

Rx Honing Machine Corporation 800-346-6464
1301 E 5th St, Mishawaka, IN 46544
RX Honing Machines: System II sharpening machine with surgical set #92701/11 easily maintains and restores arthroscopic instruments. Video and detailed manual included.

Smith & Nephew Inc., Endoscopy Div. 978-749-1000
76 S Meridian Ave, Oklahoma City, OK 73107
Dyonics ep-1 shaver system.

Smith & Nephew, Inc., Endoscopy Division 800-343-8386
150 Minuteman Rd, Andover, MA 01810
2 diagnostic models, 4.0mm diameter, 76mm insertion length, rod-lens optics with 30deg. and 70deg. view or as 1.7mm diam., 55mm length, 15deg. model. Also available: arthroscopy accessories/powered surgical instruments.

Smith & Nephew, Inc., Endoscopy Division 800-343-8386
130 Forbes Blvd, Mansfield, MA 02048

Solos Endoscopy 800-388-6445
65 Sprague St # B, Boston/dedham Commerce Park, Boston, MA 02136
Arthroscope and accessories.

Sterilmed, Inc. 763-488-3400
11400 73rd Ave N Ste 100, Maple Grove, MN 55369
Arthroscopy instruments.

Stryker Corp. 800-726-2725
2825 Airview Blvd, Portage, MI 49002

Stryker Endoscopy 800-435-0220
5900 Optical Ct, San Jose, CA 95138

Stryker Puerto Rico, Ltd. 939-307-2500
Hwy. 3, Km. 131.2, Las Guasimas Ind. Park, Arroyo, PR 00714
Various arthroscopic instruments.

ARTHROSCOPE *(cont'd)*

Symmetry Tnco 888-447-6661
15 Colebrook Blvd, Whitman, MA 02382
Orthopedic manual surgical instruments: rasp, drills, graspers, scissors, punches.

Trans1 Incorporated 910-332-1700
411 Landmark Dr, Wilmington, NC 28412
Arthroscope/orthopedic.

Ussc Puerto Rico, Inc. 203-845-1000
Building 911-67, Sabanetas Industrial Park, Ponce, PR 00731
Arthroscopic instruments.

Warsaw Orthopedic, Inc. 901-396-3133
2500 Silveus Xing, Warsaw, IN 46582
Arthroscopic system.

Wisap America 800-233-8448
8231 Melrose Dr, Lenexa, KS 66214

Zimmer Spine 508-643-0983
23 W Bacon St, Plainville, MA 02762
FLEXPOSURE Endo-Retractor for increased visualization and access to the disc in endoscopic posterior spine procedures.

Zimmer Spine, Inc. 800-655-2614
7375 Bush Lake Rd, Minneapolis, MN 55439
Laparoscopic spinal fusion instrumentation.

ARTICULATORS *(Dental And Oral) 76EJP*

Almore International, Inc. 503-643-6633
PO Box 25214, Portland, OR 97298
$250.00 per unit (standard).

Alrand, Inc./Boca Dental Supply, Inc. 800-5004908
3401 N Federal Hwy Ste 203, Boca Raton, FL 33431
Various types.

American Dental Designs Inc. 215-643-3232
1116 Horsham Rd, North Wales, PA 19454
Disposible - articulator.

American Diversified Dental Systems 800-637-2330
22991 La Cadena Dr, Laguna Hills, CA 92653
Artex Articulators

Biomet Microfixation Inc. 800-874-7711
1520 Tradeport Dr, Jacksonville, FL 32218
Types of articulators.

Buffalo Dental Mfg. Co., Inc. 516-496-7200
159 Lafayette Dr, Syosset, NY 11791
Articulator.

Dental Resources 717-866-7571
52 King St, Myerstown, PA 17067
Plasterless articulator.

Dentsply Canada, Ltd. 800-263-1437
161 Vinyl Ct., Woodbridge, ONT L4L 4A3 Canada

Hager Worldwide, Inc. 800-328-2335
13322 Byrd Dr, Odessa, FL 33556
ATOMIC, BALANCE & COMBITEC.

Ivoclar Vivadent, Inc. 800-533-6825
175 Pineview Dr, Amherst, NY 14228
STRATOS 200 A semi-adjustible, state of the art articulator.

L.A.K. Enterprises, Inc. 800-824-3112
423 Broadway Ste 501, Millbrae, CA 94030
Articular, anterior and posterior.

Mds Products, Inc. 800-637-2330
22991 La Cadena Dr, Laguna Hills, CA 92653
Artex, Plastic Articulators, Bag of 100.

Mycone Dental Supply Co. Inc. T/A Keystone Ind-Myerstown 717-866-7571
52 King St, Myerstown, PA 17067
Plasterless articulator, model holder.

Myotronics-Noromed, Inc. 206-243-4214
5870 S 194th St, Kent, WA 98032
$495.00 for standard unit.

ARTICULATORS *(cont'd)*

Panadent Corp. 800-368-9777
22573 Barton Rd, Grand Terrace, CA 92313
The PCH articulator is a precision articulator which allows the transfer of dental casts from one PCH or PSH articulator to another. The model PCH has a curced incisal pin calibrated in degrees. The curved pin holder allows the tip of the pin to stay in the same location on the incisal table when the vertical dimension is changed on the articulator. The positive centic latch depressed the centric pin to keep the articulator in perfect centric relation for mounting procedures or the pin can be depressed by hand to verify the centric position. The unique Dyna-Links keep the upper and lower frames joined together during excursive movements.

Perfect Fit, L.P. 972-955-6836
6315 Riverview Ln, Dallas, TX 75248
Articulator.

Shofu Dental Corporation 800-827-4638
1225 Stone Dr, San Marcos, CA 92078
HANDY-SERIES, PROARCH

Water Pik, Inc. 970-221-6129
1730 E Prospect Rd, Fort Collins, CO 80525
Various models of dental articulators, kits.

Whip Mix Corp. 502-637-1451
1730 E Prospect Rd Ste 101, Fort Collins, CO 80525

Whip-Mix Corporation 800-626-5651
361 Farmington Ave, PO Box 17183, Louisville, KY 40209

ASPIRATOR, EMERGENCY SUCTION *(General) 80QBQ*

Allied Healthcare Products, Inc. 800-444-3954
1720 Sublette Ave, Saint Louis, MO 63110

Ambu, Inc. 800-262-8462
6740 Baymeadow Dr, Glen Burnie, MD 21060
UNI-SUCTION pump.

Dixie Ems Supply 800-347-3494
385 Union Ave, Brooklyn, NY 11211
$60.70 per unit (standard).

Farley Inc., W.T. 800-327-5397
931 Via Alondra, Camarillo, CA 93012
$399.00 for oxygen powered Model 5-100 DU-O-VAC suction for crash carts and transport.

Mada, Inc. 800-526-6370
625 Washington Ave, Carlstadt, NJ 07072
Aspirator - oxygen powered.

Mckesson General Medical 800-446-3008
8741 Landmark Rd, Richmond, VA 23228

Medi-Tech International, Inc. 305-593-9373
2924 NW 109th Ave, Doral, FL 33172
SORENSEN

O&M Enterprise 847-258-4515
641 Chelmsford Ln, Elk Grove Village, IL 60007
ASPIRATOR

Ohio Medical Corp. 800-662-5822
1111 Lakeside Dr, Gurnee, IL 60031
TOTE-L-VAC battery powered emergency aspirator for transport use; CARE-E-VAC AC/DC aspirator for crash carts, E.R., E.M.S., or ward use.

Phipps & Bird, Inc. 800-955-7621
1519 Summit Ave, Richmond, VA 23230
0-22 in. Hg 1000cc collection bottle; overflow protected, U.L. listed. Weighs 16 lbs.

Rockford Medical & Safety Co. 800-435-9451
2420 Harrison Ave, PO Box 5646, Rockford, IL 61108

Sscor 800-434-5211
11064 Randall St, Sun Valley, CA 91352

Trademark Medical Llc 800-325-9044
449 Soverign Ct, St. Louis, MO 63011
RES-Q-VAC portable hand-powered emergency suction unit.

Trudell Medical Marketing Ltd. 800-265-5494
926 Leathorne St., London, ON N5Z-3M5 Canada
Tester for ambulance emergency suction aspirator.

U O Equipment Co. 800-231-6372
5863 W 34th St, Houston, TX 77092

Vitalograph, Inc. 800-255-6626
13310 W 99th St, Lenexa, KS 66215
$205.00 per unit, manual powered, 450mmHg.

ASPIRATOR, ENDOCERVICAL *(Obstetrics/Gyn) 85HFC*

Genx International 888-GEN-XNOW
393 Soundview Rd, Guilford, CT 06437

Ipas 919-967-7052
PO Box 5027, Chapel Hill, NC 27514

Medical Systems, Inc. 800-441-1973
30 Winter Sport Ln, PO Box 966, Williston, VT 05495
Cervical mucus sampling device.

Milex Products, Inc. 800-621-1278
4311 N Normandy Ave, Chicago, IL 60634
$7.50 (less than 25) per unit (standard) in boxes of 25 units; $156.20/box.

Rocket Medical Plc. 800-707-7625
150 Recreation Park Dr Ste 3, Hingham, MA 02043

Select Medical Systems 800-441-1973
30 Winter Sport Ln, PO Box 966, Williston, VT 05495
SELECTMUCUS.

Thomas Medical Inc. 800-556-0349
5610 West 82 2nd Street, Indianpolis, IN 46278

ASPIRATOR, ENDOMETRIAL *(Obstetrics/Gyn) 85HFF*

Ipas 919-967-7052
PO Box 5027, Chapel Hill, NC 27514

Milex Products, Inc. 800-621-1278
4311 N Normandy Ave, Chicago, IL 60634
Various devices ranging in price from $3 to $15 each.

Rocket Medical Plc. 800-707-7625
150 Recreation Park Dr Ste 3, Hingham, MA 02043

Thomas Medical Inc. 800-556-0349
5610 West 82 2nd Street, Indianpolis, IN 46278
Endometrial aspirator: Zinnanti Endometrial Curette, disposable endometrial suction curette.

ASPIRATOR, INFANT *(General) 80QBS*

Hospira 800-441-4100
268 E 4th St, Ashland, OH 44805
1-oz. volume, vinyl.

Medi-Tech International, Inc. 305-593-9373
2924 NW 109th Ave, Doral, FL 33172
SORENSEN

Utah Medical Products, Inc. 800-533-4984
7043 Cottonwood St, Midvale, UT 84047
MUC-X mucus trap, available in two sizes, 8FR and 10FR.

ASPIRATOR, LIPOSUCTION *(Surgery) 79MFF*

Adivamed 703-729-8836
44141 Bristow Cir, Ashburn, VA 20147
Apiration Tubing

Byron Medical 800-777-3434
602 W Rillito St, Tucson, AZ 85705
PSI-TEC Liposuction aspirator and aspiration pump.

Reliance Medical Corp. 800-633-8423
23392 Connecticut St, Hayward, CA 94545
RM2000-TITAN: The quiestest in the industry!

Sound Surgical Technologies Llc 888-471-4777
357 McCaslin Blvd Ste 100, Louisville, CO 80027
VentX™ suction and infusion system for accurate, variable speed/volume infusion and aspiration of fluids in surgical sites. Precision Fluid Managment System allows rapid, accurate filling of breast implants and sizers. Accurate +/- 1cc any volume.

Wells Johnson Co. 800-528-1597
8000 S Kolb Rd, Tucson, AZ 85756
Hercules or Whisperator

ASPIRATOR, LOW VOLUME (GASTRIC SUCTION) *(Gastro/Urology) 78QBR*

Allied Healthcare Products, Inc. 800-444-3954
1720 Sublette Ave, Saint Louis, MO 63110

Andersen Products, Inc., 800-523-1276
3202 Caroline Dr, Health Science Park, Haw River, NC 27258
SUMP PUMP electric motor with glass or plastic collection container; disposable and reuseable models available.

Medela, Inc. 800-435-8316
1101 Corporate Dr, McHenry, IL 60050
BASIC 30 - high vacuum high flow suction pump for endoscopy, operating room, physician practice -638mmHg, 30 l/min.

Medovations, Inc. 800-558-6408
102 E Keefe Ave, Milwaukee, WI 53212

ASPIRATOR, LOW VOLUME (GASTRIC SUCTION) *(cont'd)*

Ohio Medical Corp. 800-662-5822
1111 Lakeside Dr, Gurnee, IL 60031
Moblvac III multi purpose suction system, constant or intermittent procedures: Intermittent Gastrointestinal decompression. Instavac II ideal for gastroenterology.

ASPIRATOR, NASAL *(Ear/Nose/Throat) 77QBT*

Invacare Corporation 800-333-6900
1 Invacare Way, Elyria, OH 44035

Ohio Medical Corp. 800-662-5822
1111 Lakeside Dr, Gurnee, IL 60031

Vetter Pharma-Turm, Inc. 215-321-6930
1790 Yardley Langhorne Rd, Heston Hall/Carriage House, Suite 203 Yardley, PA 19067

ASPIRATOR, OPHTHALMIC *(Ophthalmology) 86WKR*

Bausch & Lomb Surgical 636-255-5051
3365 Tree Court Ind Blvd, Saint Louis, MO 63122

Oasis Medical, Inc. 800-528-9786
514 S Vermont Ave, Glendora, CA 91741
Manual irrigating/aspirating system.

Rhein Medical, Inc. 800-637-4346
5460 Beaumont Center Blvd Ste 500, Suite 500, Tampa, FL 33634
Irrigation/aspiration handpieces.

ASPIRATOR, SURGICAL *(Surgery) 79QBU*

Allied Healthcare Products, Inc. 800-444-3954
1720 Sublette Ave, Saint Louis, MO 63110

Biomedics, Inc. 949-458-1998
23322 Peralta Dr Ste 11, Laguna Hills, CA 92653

Dean Medical Instruments, Inc. 714-893-2772
15502 Commerce Ln, Huntington Beach, CA 92649
Multi-purpose aspirators.

Grams Medical Inc 949-548-7337
2443 Norse Ave, Costa Mesa, CA 92627

Jedmed Instruments Co. 314-845-3770
5416 Jedmed Ct, Saint Louis, MO 63129

Medela, Inc. 800-435-8316
1101 Corporate Dr, McHenry, IL 60050
VARIO 18 - high vacuum low flow portable suction pump for patient transfer, crash cart, gastric suction, ENT, endoscopy for hospital, nursing home, home use -563mmHg, 18 l/min. DOMINANT 35/ci - high vacuum medium flow intermittent suction pump for wound drainage, gastric suction, operating room, ENT -380mmHg 35 l/min. DOMINANT 50 - high vacuum high flow suction pump for plastic surgery, emergency, operating room, general surgery -675mmHg, 50 l/min.

Medical Device Resource Corporation 800-633-8423
23392 Connecticut St, Hayward, CA 94545
LS1000 surgical aspirator

Ohio Medical Corp. 800-662-5822
1111 Lakeside Dr, Gurnee, IL 60031
MOBLVAC III CS; quiet, high vacuum and flow for sugical backup or primary suction source.

Quality Aspirators 800-858-2121
1419 Godwin Ln, Duncanville, TX 75116
Aspirators for oral surgery, implantalogy, periodontics, endodontics and general dentistry. Soft tip screen fits over standard HUE tips and prevents grabbing of the tounge, cheek and soft tissue.

Richard Wolf Medical Instruments Corp. 800-323-9653
353 Corporate Woods Pkwy, Vernon Hills, IL 60061

Surgimark, Inc. 800-228-1186
2516 W Washington Ave, Yakima, WA 98903

Tulip Medical Products 800-325-6526
PO Box 7368, San Diego, CA 92167
High powered, deep vacuum aspirators for all soft tissue surgery. Silent & powerful. The most technically advanced surgical suction aspirators available today. Featuring state of the art pneumatic footswitch.

Valleylab 800-255-8522
5920 Longbow Dr, Boulder, CO 80301
Handswitching and footswitching monopolar suction coagulators.

Wisap America 800-233-8448
8231 Melrose Dr, Lenexa, KS 66214
Aspiration Cannula

ASPIRATOR, THORACIC (SUCTION UNIT)
(Cardiovascular) 74QBV

Allied Healthcare Products, Inc. 800-444-3954
1720 Sublette Ave, Saint Louis, MO 63110

Andersen Products, Inc., 800-523-1276
3202 Caroline Dr, Health Science Park, Haw River, NC 27258
THOROVAC electric thoracic aspirator, sterile, for water-seal drainage of chest cavity, disposable and reuseable models available.

Medela, Inc. 800-435-8316
1101 Corporate Dr, McHenry, IL 60050
VARIO 8 - low vacuum low flow portable thoracic drainage pump for hospital, nursing home, home use -68mmHg, 8 l/min

Ohio Medical Corp. 800-662-5822
1111 Lakeside Dr, Gurnee, IL 60031
Moblvac III multi-purpose suction system, constant or intermittent procedures, wall vacuum performance, thoracic drainage.

Richard Wolf Medical Instruments Corp. 800-323-9653
353 Corporate Woods Pkwy, Vernon Hills, IL 60061

Smiths Medical Asd 800-424-8662
5700 W 23rd Ave, Gary, IN 46406
NU-THOR emergency thoracostomy device. PEDIA-THOR emergency thoracostomy device for children.

ASPIRATOR, TRACHEAL *(Ear/Nose/Throat) 77QBW*

Allied Healthcare Products, Inc. 800-444-3954
1720 Sublette Ave, Saint Louis, MO 63110

Invacare Corporation 800-333-6900
1 Invacare Way, Elyria, OH 44035

Medela, Inc. 800-435-8316
1101 Corporate Dr, McHenry, IL 60050
CLARIO Portable - maintenance-free airway suctioning up to -550mmHg, 15 l/min.

O-Two Systems International Inc. 800-387-3405
7575 Kimbel St., Mississauga, ONT L5S 1C8 Canada
STATVAC II - 01AS9500 oxygen-powered aspirator for emergency use.

Ohio Medical Corp. 800-662-5822
1111 Lakeside Dr, Gurnee, IL 60031
MOBLVAC III CS; for O.R. or E.R. use, wall vacuum backup or as primary suction source; high vacuum and flow.

Rico Suction Labs, Inc. 800-845-8490
326 MacArthur Ln, Burlington, NC 27217

Schueler & Company, Inc. 516-487-1500
PO Box 528, Stratford, CT 06615
Schueler Model 2200 Aspirator. Compact budget-priced suction pump for use in the hospital, nursing home, doctors' clinic or home-use environment. Vacuum can be regulated for tracheal suction or E.N.T. drainage.

ASPIRATOR, ULTRASONIC *(Obstetrics/Gyn) 85MGI*

Misonix, Inc. 800-694-9612
1938 New Hwy, Farmingdale, NY 11735
FS1000RF Ultrasonic Surgical Aspirator for neurosurgery, spinal surgery, thoracic surgery, general surgery.

Mydent International 800-275-0020
80 Suffolk Ct, Hauppauge, NY 11788
DEFEND Ultrasonic/Enzymatic Cleaning Tablet effervescent tablet with water makes ultrasonic cleaning solution for ultrasonic cleaners.

ASPIRATOR, WOUND SUCTION PUMP *(General) 80QBZ*

Andersen Products, Inc., 800-523-1276
3202 Caroline Dr, Health Science Park, Haw River, NC 27258
SUMP PUMP electric surgical aspirator with glass or plastic collection container; disposable or reusable models available.

Covidien Lp 508-261-8000
15 Hampshire St, Mansfield, MA 02048

Hospira 800-441-4100
268 E 4th St, Ashland, OH 44805
1-, 2-, 3-oz vinyl bulb.

Medela, Inc. 800-435-8316
1101 Corporate Dr, McHenry, IL 60050
VARIO 18 c/i - high vacuum low flow portable suction pump for use in the operating room or at the patient's bedside for hospital, nursing home, home use -380mmHg, 18 l/min.

Medi-Tech International, Inc. 305-593-9373
2924 NW 109th Ave, Doral, FL 33172
SORENSEN

ASPIRATOR, WOUND SUCTION PUMP *(cont'd)*

Zimmer Holdings, Inc. 800-613-6131
1800 W Center St, PO Box 708, Warsaw, IN 46580

Zimmer Orthopaedic Surgical Products 800-321-5533
PO Box 10, 200 West Ohio Ave., Dover, OH 44622
HEMOVAC.

ASSAY, AGGLUTINATION, LATEX, RUBELLA
(Microbiology) 83LQN

Biokit Usa, Inc. 800-926-3353
101 Hartwell Ave, Lexington, MA 02421
MONOGEN Mononucleosis, RHEUMAJET RF Rheumatoid Factor, RHEUMAJET ASO, RHEUMAJET CRP, RUBAGEN Rubella, SURE-VUE Serology Kits.

Lifesign 800-526-2125
71 Veronica Ave, Somerset, NJ 08873
RUBALEX. Latex agglutination for rubella antibodies. 10 IU sensitivity. 245/500 Test. 1100/500 Test.

ASSAY, ENTEROVIRUS NUCLEIC ACID *(Microbiology) 83OAI*

Cepheid 408-541-4191
904 E Caribbean Dr, Sunnyvale, CA 94089

ASSAY, ENZYME LINKED IMMUNOSORBENT, HEPATITIS C VIRUS *(Microbiology) 83MZO*

St. Paul Biotech 714-903-1000
11555 Monarch St, Garden Grove, CA 92841
Hepatitis c virus test.

Virotech International, Inc. 301-924-8000
12 Meem Ave Ste C, Gaithersburg, MD 20877
Hcv.

ASSAY, ENZYME LINKED IMMUNOSORBENT, PARVOVIRUS B19 IGG *(Microbiology) 83MYL*

Cameron-Miller, Inc. 800-621-0142
5410 W Roosevelt Rd, Road #241, Chicago, IL 60644

ASSAY, HYBRIDIZATION AND/OR NUCLEIC ACID AMPLIFICATION FOR DETECTION OF HEPATITIS C RNA, HEPATITIS C VIRUS *(Microbiology) 83MZP*

Abbott Molecular, Inc. 847-937-6100
1300 E Touhy Ave, Des Plaines, IL 60018
Pcr hcv assay.

Roche Molecular Systems, Inc. 925-730-8110
4300 Hacienda Dr, Pleasanton, CA 94588
Various hepatitis c virus tests.

ASSAY, PORPHYRIN, SPECTROPHOTOMETRY, LITHIUM
(Toxicology) 91NDW

Absorption Systems 610-280-7300
436 Creamery Way, Exton, PA 19341

ASSAY, PROLIFERATION, IN VITRO, T LYMPHOCYTE
(Hematology) 81NID

Cylex, Inc. 410-964-0236
8980 State Route 108, Columbia, MD 21045
Cd4 cell stimulation assay.

ASSAY, SERUM, CYCLOSPORINE AND METABOLITES, TDX
(Toxicology) 91MAR

Abbott Diagnostics Intl, Biotechnology Ltd 787-846-3500
Road #2 KM. 58.0 , PO Box 278, Cruce Davila, Barceloneta, PR 00617
Fluorescence polarization immunoassay to quantitative cyclosporine in human seru.

ASSEMBLY, KNEE/SHANK/ANKLE/FOOT, EXTERNAL
(Physical Med) 89ISW

Exactech, Inc. 800-392-2832
2320 NW 66th Ct, Gainesville, FL 32653
OPTETRAK Comprehensive Total Knee System.

Lifeline Usa 800-553-6633
3201 Syene Rd, Madison, WI 53713
Foot attachment.

Valley Institute Of Prosthetics And Orthotics, Inc 661-322-1005
1524 21st St Ste B, Bakersfield, CA 93301
External assembled lower limb prosthesis.

ASSEMBLY, SHOULDER/ELBOW/FOREARM/WRIST/HAND, MECHANICAL *(Physical Med) 89KFT*

Biomet, Inc. 574-267-6639
56 E Bell Dr, PO Box 587, Warsaw, IN 46582
Miracle mechanical arms and hands.

ASSEMBLY, SHOULDER/ELBOW/FOREARM/WRIST/HAND, MECHANICAL *(cont'd)*

Caguas Orthopedic Center, Inc. 787-744-2325
FF4 Calle 11, Villa Del Rey, Caguas, PR 00727
Upper extremity prosthesis.

Hosmer Dorrance Corp. 408-379-5151
561 Division St, Campbell, CA 95008
Various.

ASSEMBLY, SHOULDER/ELBOW/FOREARM/WRIST/HAND, POWERED *(Physical Med) 89KFW*

Hosmer Dorrance Corp. 408-379-5151
561 Division St, Campbell, CA 95008
Various.

ASSEMBLY, THIGH/KNEE/SHANK/ANKLE/FOOT, EXTERNAL *(Physical Med) 89KFX*

Care Apparel Industries 800-326-6262
12709 91st Ave, Richmond Hill, NY 11418
For edema and diabetic foot conditions. Slippers for those with edema or diabetic condition.

ASSISTANT, SURGICAL, ORTHOPEDIC, AUTOMATED *(Orthopedics) 87SHK*

Integrated Surgical Systems 530-792-2600
1850 Research Park Dr, Davis, CA 95618
The ROBODOC System assists orthopedic surgeons perform major joint replacements (Hip and Knee joints) surgeries.

ASTIGMOMETER *(Ophthalmology) 86WQG*

Oasis Medical, Inc. 800-528-9786
514 S Vermont Ave, Glendora, CA 91741
Terry-Schanzlin Vacuum Speculum Astigmatome to make arcuate incisions of a controlled length and depth to correct astigmatism.

ATOMIZER AND TIP, ENT *(Ear/Nose/Throat) 77KCK*

Aesculap Implant Systems Inc. 1-800-234-9179
3773 Corporate Pkwy, Center Valley, PA 18034

Micromedics 800-624-5662
1270 Eagan Industrial Rd, Saint Paul, MN 55121
Rhino-Guard, a single-use tip, designed to prevent cross contamination. Fits most commonly used atomziers. Helps keep tip in nasal passage. Reduces trauma and splash back.

Richard Wolf Medical Instruments Corp. 800-323-9653
353 Corporate Woods Pkwy, Vernon Hills, IL 60061

ATP AND CK (ENZYMATIC), CREATINE *(Chemistry) 75JLB*

Raichem, Division Of Hemagen Diagnostics, Inc. 800-438-6100
8225 Mercury Ct, San Diego, CA 92111

ATP RELEASE (LUMINESCENCE) *(Hematology) 81JWR*

Laboratory Technologies, Inc. 800-542-1123
43 W 900 Rte. 64, Maple Park, IL 60151

Quality Bioresources, Inc. 888-674-7224
1015 N Austin St, Seguin, TX 78155
Luciferin/luciferase reagents, lyophilized ATP controls, lyophilized.

ATTACHMENT, BAG (CRUTCH, WALKER, WHEELCHAIR) *(Physical Med) 89UMM*

A.R.C. Distributors 800-296-8724
PO Box 599, Centreville, MD 21617
CLEAR-VIEW WHEELCHAIR POUCH = Clear vinyl pouch to fit all size wheelchairs or stretchers for patient information storage. Eliminates time wasted searching for lost patient charts. COLORED WHEELCHAIR POUCH = match your wheelchairs upolstery, assures patient records confidentiality!

Advantage Bag Co. 800-556-6307
22633 Ellinwood Dr, Torrance, CA 90505
Bags and straps. Millenium Pac Bac Pac optional strap system.

Diestco Manufacturing Corp. 800-795-2392
PO Box 6504, Chico, CA 95927
Monster Bag is an extra-large seatback bag. Front Bag extends from the armrest. Saddle Bag hangs from the side of the armrest. 25 different types of bags available for wheelchairs, scooters and walkers.

Kareco International, Inc. 800-8KA-RECO
299 Rte. 22 E., Green Brook, NJ 08812-1714

Medcovers, Inc 800-948-8917
500 W Goldsboro St, Kenly, NC 27542
Lined beverage bag.

Profex Medical Products 800-325-0196
2224 E Person Ave, Memphis, TN 38114

ATTACHMENT, BAG (CRUTCH, WALKER, WHEELCHAIR) *(cont'd)*

Thompson Medical Specialties 800-777-4949
3404 Library Ln, Saint Louis Park, MN 55426
For walkers and wheelchairs only.

Tuffcare 800-367-6160
3999 E La Palma Ave, Anaheim, CA 92807

Ventura Enterprises 317-745-2989
35 Lawton Ave, Danville, IN 46122
Vinyl bags for attachment to handicapped mobility devices.

ATTACHMENT, BINOCULAR, ENDOSCOPIC *(Gastro/Urology) 78FEJ*

Manico Bloomington 812-336-2567
PO Box 5504, Bloomington, IN 47407
Translid binocular interactor (tbi).

ATTACHMENT, BREATHING, POSITIVE END EXPIRATORY PRESSURE *(Anesthesiology) 73BYE*

Airon Corporation 888-448-1238
751 North Dr Ste 6, Melbourne, FL 32934
MACS CPAP System

Ambu A/S 457-225-2210
6740 Baymeadow Dr, Glen Burnie, MD 21060
Single patient use peep value,various models.

Ambu, Inc. 800-262-8462
6740 Baymeadow Dr, Glen Burnie, MD 21060
RMT-PEP valves.

Armstrong Medical Industries, Inc. 800-323-4220
575 Knightsbridge Pkwy, Lincolnshire, IL 60069

Corpak Medsystems, Inc. 800-323-6305
100 Chaddick Dr, Wheeling, IL 60090
Peep valve.

Dhd Healthcare Corporation 800-847-8000
PO Box 6, One Madison Street, Wampsville, NY 13163
Oxy-PEEP High Flow O2 with PEEP

Instrumentation Industries, Inc. 800-633-8577
2990 Industrial Blvd, Bethel Park, PA 15102
PEEP, Adjustable and pre-set (magnetic) PEEP valves. Non-rebreathing T with speaking attachment.

Matrx 716-662-6650
145 Mid County Dr, Orchard Park, NY 14127
Peep valve.

Mercury Medical 800-237-6418
11300 49th St N, Clearwater, FL 33762
RESISTEX Respiratory PEP Therapy Device with monometer port.

Respironics Colorado 800-345-6443
12301 Grant St Unit 190, Thornton, CO 80241
$767.00 for custom nasal mask kit for CPAP.

Respironics Novametrix, Llc. 724-387-4559
5 Technology Dr, Wallingford, CT 06492
Whisperflow,system 22 peep valve.

Smiths Medical Asd Inc. 800-258-5361
10 Bowman Dr, Keene, NH 03431
Peep value.

Ventlab Corp. 336-753-5000
155 Boyce Dr, Mocksville, NC 27028
Peep valve.

ATTACHMENT, COMMODE, WHEELCHAIR *(Physical Med) 89INB*

Activeaid, Inc. 800-533-5330
101 Activeaid Rd, Redwood Falls, MN 56283

Alex Orthopedic, Inc. 800-544-2539
PO Box 201442, Arlington, TX 76006
Three-in-one commode.

Creative Foam Medical Systems 800-446-4644
405 Industrial Dr, Bremen, IN 46506
Various coated foam commode attachments for wheelchair.

Essential Medical Supply, Inc. 800-826-8423
6420 Hazeltine National Dr, Orlando, FL 32822

Laszlo Corp. 314-830-3222
2573 Millvalley Dr, Florissant, MO 63031
Attachment for wheeled chair.

Nuprodx, Inc. 888-288-5653
4 Malone Ln, San Rafael, CA 94903
Tub/Slider System

ATTACHMENT, COMMODE, WHEELCHAIR *(cont'd)*

Perfect Care 718-805-7800
8927 126th St, Richmond Hill, NY 11418
Commode.

Triaid, Inc. 301-759-3525
637 N Centre St, Cumberland, MD 21502
Hygea chair.

Tubular Fabricators Industry, Inc. 804-733-4000
600 W Wythe St, Petersburg, VA 23803
Various models of commodes.

Tuffcare 800-367-6160
3999 E La Palma Ave, Anaheim, CA 92807

Uplift Technologies, Inc. 800-387-0896
125-11 Morris Dr., Dartmouth, NS B3B 1M2 Canada
Commode accessory

ATTACHMENT, INTERMITTENT MANDATORY VENTILATION (IMV) *(Anesthesiology) 73CBO*

Instrumentation Industries, Inc. 800-633-8577
2990 Industrial Blvd, Bethel Park, PA 15102
IMV/CPAP assembly (reusable).

Smiths Medical Asd Inc. 800-258-5361
10 Bowman Dr, Keene, NH 03431
Imv set-up.

ATTACHMENT, NARROWING, WHEELCHAIR
(Physical Med) 89IMQ

Alimed, Inc. 800-225-2610
297 High St, Dedham, MA 02026

Jaeco Orthopedic Specialties, Inc. 501-623-5944
214 Drexel St, Hot Springs, AR 71901

Patterson Medical Supply, Inc. 262-387-8720
W68N158 Evergreen Blvd, Cedarburg, WI 53012
Wheelchair narrows bolster.

Primo, Inc. 770-486-7394
417 Dividend Dr Ste B, Peachtree City, GA 30269
Wrist support, wrist immobilizer, wrist restraint.

ATTACHMENT, OXYGEN CANISTER/IV POLE, WHEELCHAIR
(General) 80TDH

A.R.C. Distributors 800-296-8724
PO Box 599, Centreville, MD 21617
POLECATS = POLECAT I.V. transport system for wheelchair and stretcher patients. POLECAT facilitates moving patients using infusion pumps mounted on portable (wheeled) IV poles. Forms a single unit for improved safety and productivity. FAST, SAFE AND EASY!! PREVENTS INJURIES TO PATIENT & TRANSPORTERS TOO!!!!!!

Farley Inc., W.T. 800-327-5397
931 Via Alondra, Camarillo, CA 93012
$90.00 for oxygen holder/IV pole (Model IV02); $95.00 for OXY-IV-TOTER to simplify moving wheelchair patient and oxygen cylinder cart and IV pole together. Model HW200.

Kareco International, Inc. 800-8KA-RECO
299 Rte. 22 E., Green Brook, NJ 08812-1714

Pryor Products 800-854-2280
1819 Peacock Blvd, Oceanside, CA 92056
Accessories are available such as oxygen tank holders, power strips, baskets, special IV top poles and hook tops, IV bag hangers, and support wheels.

Sunrise Medical 800-333-4000
7477 Dry Creek Pkwy, Longmont, CO 80503

Tagg Industries L.L.C. 800-548-3514
23210 Del Lago Dr, Laguna Hills, CA 92653
Cylinder with adjustable clamp can be attached to the side, back, or hand grip of a wheelchair, bedrail, cot or stretcher.

Wenzelite Rehab Supplies, Llc 800-706-9255
220 36th St, 99 Seaview Blvd, Brooklyn, NY 11232
Oxygen Tank holder and IV Pole are available accessories that will mount on all Wenzelite adult, bariatric and pediatric anterior and posterior Safety Rollers.

ATTACHMENT, PRECISION *(Dental And Oral) 76EGG*

Argen Corp. 800-375-9077
5855 Oberlin Dr, San Diego, CA 92121
ARGEN ATTACHMENTS

ATTACHMENT, PRECISION *(cont'd)*

Biomet 3i 800-342-5454
4555 Riverside Dr, Palm Beach Gardens, FL 33410
LOCATOR® OverdentSURE Abutment - The LOCATOR Abutment is ideal for overdenture restorations.

Coltene/Whaledent Inc. 330-916-8858
235 Ascot Pkwy, Cuyahoga Falls, OH 44223
Attachment.

Heraeus Kulzer, Inc. 800-431-1785
99 Business Park Dr, Armonk, NY 10504
Dental attachments.

Metalor Technologies Usa 800-554-5504
255 John L Dietsch Blvd, PO Box 255, North Attleboro, MA 02763
Dental connector, precision attachment.

Oco Inc. 800-228-0477
600 Paisano St NE Ste A, Albuquerque, NM 87123
Attachment.

Preat Corp. 800-232-7732
2976 Long Valley Rd, P.O. Box 1030, Santa Ynez, CA 93460

Sterngold 800-243-9942
23 Frank Mossberg Dr, PO Box 2967, Attleboro, MA 02703
ERA, STERN, C&M, HADER and others available.

AUDIOMETER *(Ear/Nose/Throat) 77EWO*

Allen Medical Technologies Llc 520-232-4221
15088 S Camino Rio Puerco, Sahuarita, AZ 85629

Ambco Electronics 800-345-1079
15052 Red Hill Ave Ste D, Tustin, CA 92780
MODEL 650A $735.00 for portable threshold audiometer with 5 yr. warranty, 6 lbs. MODEL 1000+ $795.00, digital LED displays with 5 yr. warranty, membrane switches. MODEL 2500 $2300.00 automatic audiometer, storage, with printer and 5 yr. warranty.

Audiphone Hearing Instruments 800-721-9611
3333 Kingman St Ste 205, Metairie, LA 70006

Benson Medical Instruments Co. 612-827-2222
310 4th Ave S Ste 5000, Minneapolis, MN 55415
Automatic audiometer and software for occupational hearing conservation.

Cardinal Healthcare 209, Inc. 610-862-0800
5225 Verona Rd, Fitchburg, WI 53711
Audiometer.

Dac Inc./Diagnostic Audiology Corp. 800-551-3277
351 Bank St Ste 105, Southlake, TX 76092
Ilo.

Diagnostic Group Llc 952-278-4457
7625 Golden Triangle Dr Ste F, Eden Prairie, MN 55344
Various.

Digital Hearing Systems Corp. 479-925-7700
9679 E High Meadows Dr, Rogers, AR 72756
Audiometer, ENT.

Eckstein Brothers, Inc. 800-432-4913
2807 Oregon Ct Ste D5, Torrance, CA 90503
3 portable models - $1,085.00 for 350-1, wght. 9lbs. $1,170.00 for 390, 10lbs. $1,495.00 for 390 MB with bone vibrator; 10lbs. Infant screening; Model EB23 microprocessor hearing screening, TETRATONE II, $625.00. TETRATONE II model EB47 is a 4 frequency rapid screening audiometer 5 levels of intensity-microprocessor.

Everest Biomedical Instruments Co. 636-305-9900
1732 Gilsinn Ln, Fenton, MO 63026
Otoacoustic emissions test instrument.

Frye Electronics, Inc. 800-547-8209
9826 SW Tigard St, Tigard, OR 97223
FONIX FA-10 Hearing Evaluator audiometer with master hearing aid air/bone/speech. $3295 standard pricing. FONIX FA-12 Hearing Evaluator audiometer with master hearing and air/bone/speech. $3295 standard pricing.

Hti, Inc. 800-685-2997
500 W Wilson Bridge Rd Ste 105, Worthington, OH 43085
Audiometer.

Intelligent Hearing Systems, Corp. 800-447-9783
6860 SW 81st St, Miami, FL 33143
SMARTDPOAE and SMARTTrOAE, otoacoustic emissions (OAE) testing and screening system. SmartAudiometer, screening audiometer testing system.

Maico Diagnostics 888-941-4201
7625 Golden Triangle Dr, Eden Prairie, MN 55344
THE DIGITAL PILOT TEST child hearing screening audiometer.

AUDIOMETER *(cont'd)*

Md International, Inc. 305-669-9003
11300 NW 41st St, Doral, FL 33178

Medrx, Inc. 727-584-9600
1200 Starkey Rd Ste 105, Largo, FL 33771
Audiometer and real ear analyzer.

Micro Audiometrics Corp. 800-729-9509
655 Keller Rd, Murphy, NC 28906
$695.00 for DSP Pure Tone audiometer with battery operation, $1,095.00 EARSCAN Microprocessor Pure Tone Audiometer. $1,495 for EARSCAN with data output. $1,695.00-$2,395.00 for EARSCAN Impedance Microprocessor Pure Tone Audiometer. $1995.00 for MicroLab industrial audiometer.

Mimosa Acoustics, Inc. 217-367-9740
60 Hazelwood Dr Ste 209, Champaign, IL 61820
Distortion product otoacoustic emission (dpoae) measurement system.

Monitor Instruments Inc. 800-853-6785
437 Dimmocks Mill Rd, Hillsborough, NC 27278
MODEL MI-5000, microprocessor audiometer. Microprocessor audiometer testing at 500-8000 Hz, HTL range 0-90 dB with Hugheson Westlake test paradigm manual overide, RS-232 port, attached case portable. Model MI-7000 has a printer, storage capacity of 200+ tests, RS-232 port, keypad & real-time clock with battery.

Occupational Hearing Services 800-622-3277
300 S Chester Rd Ste 301, Swarthmore, PA 19081
Telephone hearing screening test system.

Otovation, Llc 866-OTOVATION
1001 W 9th Ave Ste A, King Of Prussia, PA 19406
Pocket Hearo is an ANSI-compliant screening and threshold audiometer that runs on a handheld PC. It provides quick and efficient screening and full reimbursable testing for physicians, audiologists and other speech and hearing professionals, hearing aid dispensers, schools, and occupational health testing markets. The Pocket Hearo is affordably priced and offers portability and features found in no other audiometer.

Precision Cast Plastic Parts, Llc. 530-241-5189
2278 Crescent Moon Dr, Redding, CA 96001
Precision probe tubes.

Singer Medical Products Inc., Md Systems Div. 630-860-6500
3800 Buckner St, El Paso, TX 79925
Screening audiometer & impedance analyzer.

Singer Medical Products, Inc. 800-222-2572
790 Maple Ln, Bensenville, IL 60106
$2,495 for portable impedance tester & audiometer MD-1, $1,995 for portable impedance tester MD-2, $3,195 for desk-top impedance tester & audiometer with printer model MD-3, $395 for MD-P printer for MD-1 or MD-2, $725 for portable audiometer MD-4, $1,095 for portable audiometer with printer, $3,700 for automatic screening audiometer MD-5 with built-in printer.

Starkey Florida 800-327-7939
2200 N Commerce Pkwy, Weston, FL 33326

Starkey Laboratories, Inc. 800-328-8602
6700 Washington Ave S, Eden Prairie, MN 55344
$2,950 for Tinnitus Research Audiometer with master & subject consoles.

Tremetrics 800-825-0121
7625 Golden Triangle Dr, Eden Prairie, MN 55344
$2,295 for RA 300 6lbs; 2 tabletop models, $4,295.00 for RA 500, 9.5 lbs; Hearing conservation software for data management system for employee testing. HT-WIZARD Audiometer, touch-screen hearing testing system conducts automated tests in seven languages, portable with 2000 audiogram storage and interfaces to safety & health software; $5,250.00.

Tsi Medical Ltd. 800-661-7263
47 Athabascan Ave., Unit 105, Sherwood Park, AB T8A-4H3 Canada

Vestibular Technologies, Llc 307-637-5711
205 County Road 128a, Suite 200, Cheyenne, WY 82007-1831
Various models of audiometers.

Welch Allyn, Inc. 800-535-6663
4341 State Street Rd, Skaneateles Falls, NY 13153

AUTOANTIBODIES, ENDOMYSIAL(TISSUE TRANSGLUTAMINASE) *(Immunology) 82MVM*

Medica, Inc. 800-845-6496
336 Encinitas Blvd Ste 200, Encinitas, CA 92024
Anti-endomysial antibody test kit, ESD test kit. 48- and 96-test kit of monkey endomysial distal substrate (sections) with controls, conjugate, PBS, mounting medium.

AUTOMATED DIGITAL IMAGE MANUAL INTERPRETATION MICROSCOPE *(Hematology) 81OEO*

Aperio Technologies Inc. 866-478-4111
1360 Park Center Dr, Vista, CA 92081
ScanScope XT System

AUTOTRANSFUSION UNIT (BLOOD) *(Anesthesiology) 73CAC*

Atrium Medical Corp. 800-528-7486
5 Wentworth Dr, Hudson, NH 03051
ATRIUM 2050 and 3650 blood-recovery systems. Disposable autotransfusion systems also available.

Boehringer Laboratories, Inc. 800-642-4945
500 E Washington St, Norristown, PA 19401
Postoperative and intraoperative autotransfusion systems.

Covidien Lp 508-261-8000
15 Hampshire St, Mansfield, MA 02048
Disposable autotransfusion systems.

Cytori Therapeutics, Inc. 877-470-8000
3020 Callan Rd, San Diego, CA 92121
Transfusion apparatus.

Davol Inc., Sub. C.R. Bard, Inc. 800-556-6275
100 Crossings Blvd, Warwick, RI 02886
Post-operative autotransfusion system.

Gish Biomedical, Inc. 800-938-0531
22942 Arroyo Vis, Rancho Santa Margarita, CA 92688
Blood reinfusion/autotransfusion reservoir; orthopedic autotransfusion reservoir.

Haemonetics Corp. 800-225-5242
400 Wood Rd, P.O. Box 9114, Braintree, MA 02184
ORTHOPAT Autotransfusion System Autotransfusion Apparatus salvages blood during and after orthopedic surgery.

Harvest Technologies, Corp. 508-732-7500
40 Grissom Rd Ste 100, Plymouth, MA 02360
Autotransfusion system.

Icu Medical (Ut), Inc 949-366-2183
4455 Atherton Dr, Salt Lake City, UT 84123
Receptal a.t.s. mediastinal liner.

Jostra Bentley, Inc. 302-454-9959
Rd. 402 N. Km 1.4, Industrial Park, Anasco, PR 00610-1577
Pleural drainage/autotransfusion system.

Medtronic Blood Management 612-514-4000
18501 E Plaza Dr, Parker, CO 80134
Autotransfusion.

Medtronic Perfusion Systems 800-328-3320
7611 Northland Dr N, Brooklyn Park, MN 55428
AT1000/AT750EF for high volume blood processing and AT500P/ELMD-500 for transportable applications. All systems are capable of performing red cell processing and platelet-rich plasma sequestration for total autologous blood conservation. AUTOLOG autotransfusion system.

Sorin Group Usa 800-289-5759
14401 W 65th Way, Arvada, CO 80004
BRAT autologous blood transfusion unit.

Stryker Puerto Rico, Ltd. 939-307-2500
Hwy. 3, Km. 131.2, Las Guasimas Ind. Park, Arroyo, PR 00714
Various.

Terumo Cardiovascular Systems (Tcvs) 800-283-7866
28 Howe St, Ashland, MA 01721
Blood recovery device.

The Tech Group Tempe 480-281-4400
640 S Rockford Dr, Tempe, AZ 85281
Blood cell separator disposable bowl.

Zimmer Holdings, Inc. 800-613-6131
1800 W Center St, PO Box 708, Warsaw, IN 46580
Disposable autotransfusion systems.

Zimmer Orthopaedic Surgical Products 800-321-5533
PO Box 10, 200 West Ohio Ave., Dover, OH 44622
HEMOVAC; Autotransfusion system.

AWL *(Orthopedics) 87HWJ*

Abbott Spine, Inc. 847-937-6100
12708 Riata Vista Cir Ste B-100, Austin, TX 78727
Awl.

Biomet Microfixation Inc. 800-874-7711
1520 Tradeport Dr, Jacksonville, FL 32218
Various types of screws.

Biomet, Inc. 574-267-6639
56 E Bell Dr, PO Box 587, Warsaw, IN 46582
Various types of awl.

Centinel Spine Inc. 952-885-0500
505 Park Ave Fl 14, New York, NY 10022
STALIF C 4.5 Flexible Awl Guide

Depuy Mitek, A Johnson & Johnson Company 800-451-2006
50 Scotland Blvd, Bridgewater, MA 02324
Various awls, non-sterile.

Depuy Spine, Inc. 800-227-6633
325 Paramount Dr, Raynham, MA 02767
Orthopaedic awl.

DJO Inc. 800-336-6569
1430 Decision St, Vista, CA 92081

George Tiemann & Co. 800-843-6266
25 Plant Ave, Hauppauge, NY 11788

Hu-Friedy Manufacturing Co., Inc. 800-483-7433
3232 N Rockwell St, Chicago, IL 60618
$50.00 to $51.00 for orthognathic surgery.

Integral Design Inc. 781-740-2036
52 Burr Rd, Hingham, MA 02043

K2m, Inc. 866-526-4171
751 Miller Dr SE Ste F1, Leesburg, VA 20175
Awl.

Kirwan Surgical Products, Inc. 888-547-9267
180 Enterprise Dr, PO Box 427, Marshfield, MA 02050
Bankart shoulder repair instruments.

Kls-Martin L.P. 800-625-1557
11239-1 St. John`s Industrial, Parkway South
Jacksonville, FL 32250
Mandibular awl, maxillary awl, zygomatic arch awl.

Kmedic 800-955-0559
190 Veterans Dr, Northvale, NJ 07647

Lenox-Maclaren Surgical Corp. 720-890-9660
657 S Taylor Ave Ste A, Colorado Technology Center
Louisville, CO 80027
Awl / all different.

Medtronic Sofamor Danek Usa, Inc. 901-396-3133
4340 Swinnea Rd, Memphis, TN 38118
Awl.

Spine Wave, Inc. 203-944-9494
2 Enterprise Dr Ste 302, Shelton, CT 06484
Awl.

Surgical Implant Generation Network (Sign) 509-371-1107
451 Hills St, Richland, WA 99354
Awl.

Symmetry Medical Usa, Inc. 574-267-8700
486 W 350 N, Warsaw, IN 46582
Rc awl.

Synthes San Diego 858-452-1266
6244 Ferris Sq Ste B, San Diego, CA 92121
Various awls.

Warsaw Orthopedic, Inc. 901-396-3133
2500 Silveus Xing, Warsaw, IN 46582
Awl.

Zimmer Holdings, Inc. 800-613-6131
1800 W Center St, PO Box 708, Warsaw, IN 46580

Zimmer Spine, Inc. 800-655-2614
7375 Bush Lake Rd, Minneapolis, MN 55439
Awl.

Zimmer Trabecular Metal Technology 800-613-6131
10 Pomeroy Rd, Parsippany, NJ 07054
Starter awl.

AZO-DYE, CALCIUM *(Chemistry) 75CJY*

Abbott Diagnostics Div. 626-440-0700
820 Mission St, South Pasadena, CA 91030
Calcium.

AZO-DYE, CALCIUM *(cont'd)*

Jas Diagnostics, Inc. 305-418-2320
7220 NW 58th St, Miami, FL 33166
Calcium-arsenazo iii.

Synermed Intl., Inc. 317-896-1565
17408 Tiller Ct Ste 1900, Westfield, IN 46074
Calcium reagent kit.

Vital Diagnostics Inc. 714-672-3553
1075 W Lambert Rd Ste D, Brea, CA 92821
Various total calcium reagents.

AZO-DYES, COLORIMETRIC, BILIRUBIN AND CONJUGATES *(Chemistry) 75JJB*

American Qualex, Inc. 800-772-1776
920 Calle Negocio Ste A, San Clemente, CA 92673
Antibody conjugates.

Arkray Factory Usa, Inc. 952-646-3168
5182 W 76th St, Minneapolis, MN 55439
Urine test strips.

Arkray Usa 800-818-8877
5198 W 76th St, Edina, MN 55439
DIASCREEN REAGENT STRIPS FOR URINALYSIS- high quality strips available in 15 different configurations. reagens include glucose, protein, ketone, pH, blood, bilirubin, urobilinogen, nitrite, specific gravity, and leukocytes.

Bayer Healthcare Llc 914-524-2955
555 White Plains Rd Fl 5, Tarrytown, NY 10591
Test for bilirubin in urine.

Raichem, Division Of Hemagen Diagnostics, Inc. 800-438-6100
8225 Mercury Ct, San Diego, CA 92111

BACK REST *(General) 80QCE*

Freeman Manufacturing Company 800-253-2091
900 W Chicago Rd, PO Box J, Sturgis, MI 49091
Sacro-ease.

Mccarty's Sacro-Ease Llc 800-635-3557
3329 Industrial Ave S, Coeur D Alene, ID 83815
SACRO-EASE support.

Obus Forme Ltd. 888-225-7378
550 Hopewell Ave., Toronto, ON M6E 2S6 Canada
$79 and $101 for low back, wide back, and highback backrest support. CUSTOM AIR

Pyramid Industries, Llc 888-343-3352
3911 Schaad Rd Unit 102, Knoxville, TN 37921
BACK CUSHION, FOAM,for general use with wheelchair for back support and positioning. Available in three sizes with or w/o stabilization board.

BAG, BILE COLLECTION *(Gastro/Urology) 78EXF*

Cook Inc. 800-457-4500
PO Box 489, Bloomington, IN 47402

Cook Urological, Inc. 800-457-4500
1100 W Morgan St, P.O. Box 227, Spencer, IN 47460

Marlen Manufacturing & Development Co. 216-292-7060
5150 Richmond Rd, Bedford, OH 44146

Redi-Tech Medical Products,Llc 800-824-1793
529 Front St Ste 125, Berea, OH 44017

BAG, BLOOD *(Hematology) 81ULQ*

Atrium Medical Corp. 800-528-7486
5 Wentworth Dr, Hudson, NH 03051
ATRIUM #2450 self-filling and #2550 in-line ATS blood bags to be used with ATRIUM autotransfusion chest-drainage systems.

Charter Medical Ltd. 866-458-3116
3948 Westpoint Blvd Ste A, Winston Salem, NC 27103

Command Medical Products, Inc. 386-672-8116
15 Signal Ave, Ormond Beach, FL 32174
Contract assembly.

Fenwal Inc. 800-766-1077
3 Corporate Dr, Lake Zurich, IL 60047
Pooling bag.

Harmac Medical Products, Inc. 716-897-4500
2201 Bailey Ave, Buffalo, NY 14211
OEM and private-labeled products. RF heat-sealed bags and sets. Contract manufacturer. Class 100,000 cleanrooms.

Millipore Corporation 877-246-2247
290 Concord Rd, Billerica, MA 01821
For animal blood only.

BAG, BLOOD *(cont'd)*

Stericon, Inc. 708-865-8790
2315 Gardner Rd, Broadview, IL 60155
Blood and blood component freezing bags and accessories.

The Metrix Co. 800-752-3148
4400 Chavenelle Rd, Dubuque, IA 52002
Custom contract manufacturer.

BAG, BLOOD, COLLECTION *(Hematology) 81KSR*

Achilles Usa, Inc. 425-353-7000
1407 80th St SW, Everett, WA 98203
Development of vinyls and plastics for the medical industry.

Baxter Healthcare Corp., Renal Division 847-948-2000
7511 114th Ave, Largo, FL 33773
Various sterile & non-sterile empty containers & accessories.

Caridianbct Inc. 800-525-2623
10810 W Collins Ave, Lakewood, CO 80215
TRIMA - Automated blood collection system for red blood cells, plasma, or platelets.

Charter Medical, Ltd. 336-768-6447
3948 Westpoint Blvd Ste A, Winston Salem, NC 27103
Transfer packs, empty.

Citizens Development Center 214-637-2911
8800 Ambassador Row, Dallas, TX 75247
Dental mask; gauze, disposable.

Diasol, Inc. 800-366-0546
13212 Raymer St, North Hollywood, CA 91605
Safesting--Blood Collection Device: Protected blood collection device that allows full control over the rate of blood flow, though avoiding hemolysis, foaming. Comes in 19-256A or needleless access.

Ethox International 800-521-1022
251 Seneca St, Buffalo, NY 14204
Empty container,blood processing.

Fenwal Inc. 800-766-1077
3 Corporate Dr, Lake Zurich, IL 60047
Automated BLOOD PACK System. BLOOD PACK Units. CPDA-1 blood pack unit.

Fenwal International, Inc. 847-550-7908
Road 357, Km. 0.8, Maricao, PR 00606
Various sterile & non-sterile empty containers & accessories used in collect.

Haemonetics Corp. 781-848-7100
400 Wood Rd, P.O.Box 9114, Braintree, MA 02184
Plastic plasma bottle.

Medsep Corp., A Subsidiary Of Pall Corp. 516-484-5400
1630 W Industrial Park St, Covina, CA 91722
Various.

Medtronic Blood Management 612-514-4000
18501 E Plaza Dr, Parker, CO 80134
Blood transfer bar.

Micro Typing Systems, Inc. 908-218-8177
1295 SW 29th Ave, Pompano Beach, FL 33069
Container, empty, for collection & processing of blood & blood components.

Terumo Cardiovascular Systems (Tcvs) 800-283-7866
28 Howe St, Ashland, MA 01721
Collection or transfer bag.

The Metrix Co. 800-752-3148
4400 Chavenelle Rd, Dubuque, IA 52002
Custom contract manufacturer.

Total Molding Services, Inc. 215-538-9613
354 East Broad St., Trumbauersville, PA 18970
Cuvette for blood collection.

BAG, BODY *(General) 80WNA*

Adi Medical Division Of Asia Dynamics (Group) Inc. 877-647-7699
1565 S Shields Dr, Waukegan, IL 60085

Centennial Products Inc. 888-604-1004
6900 Philips Hwy Ste 45, Jacksonville, FL 32216
Hospital, medical examiner, coroner body bags. Complete line of pouches from light hospital to heavy duty transport bags with handles. Also, complete line of infection control products for medical examiners coroners, etc.

BAG, BODY *(cont'd)*

Extra Packaging, Corp. 800-872-7548
631 Golden Harbour Dr, Boca Raton, FL 33432
We provide body bags. Custom sizes and applications available. We have a chlorine free line for safe cremation and a transport line for helicopter transport and water recovery.

General Econopak, Inc. 888-871-8568
1725 N 6th St, Philadelphia, PA 19122
Zippered, standard color: white, isolation: safety yellow.

Global Healthcare 800-601-3880
1495 Hembree Rd Ste 700, Roswell, GA 30076
Curved and straight styles.

Jero Medical Equipment & Supplies, Inc. 800-457-0644
1701 W 13th St, Chicago, IL 60608
Biohazardous Body Bag.

Medi-Tech International, Inc. 305-593-9373
2924 NW 109th Ave, Doral, FL 33172
FERNO

O&M Enterprise 847-258-4515
641 Chelmsford Ln, Elk Grove Village, IL 60007
BODY BAG

Precision Dynamics Corp. 800-772-1122
13880 Del Sur St, San Fernando, CA 91340

Total Care 800-334-3802
PO Box 1661, Rockville, MD 20849
sales 'only' to hospitals,nursing homes, state,municipal and federal govt.facilities /purchase authorization required/

Tri-State Hospital Supply Corp. 800-248-4058
301 Catrell Dr, PO Box 170, Howell, MI 48843
Extra large.

Walkers, Inc., E. C. 800-494-8589
#1 515 Milner Ave., Toronto, ONT M1B-2K4 Canada

BAG, BREATHING *(Anesthesiology) 73QEK*

A-M Systems, Inc. 800-426-1306
131 Business Park Loop, Sequim, WA 98382
$25.68 for case of 10 3-liter conductive bags.

Alimed, Inc. 800-225-2610
297 High St, Dedham, MA 02026
Disposable resuscitator bag.

Csi International, Inc. 303-795-8273
4301 S Federal Blvd Ste 116, Englewood, CO 80110

Directmed, Inc. 516-656-3377
150 Pratt Oval, Glen Cove, NY 11542

Dixie Ems Supply 800-347-3494
385 Union Ave, Brooklyn, NY 11211
$98.00 per unit (2000ml).

Hi-Tech Rubber, Inc. 800-924-4832
3191 E La Palma Ave, Anaheim, CA 92806

Hospira 800-441-4100
268 E 4th St, Ashland, OH 44805
Latex-dipped, natural, and synthetic rubber.

Instrumentation Industries, Inc. 800-633-8577
2990 Industrial Blvd, Bethel Park, PA 15102

Intersurgical Inc. 315-451-2900
417 Electronics Pkwy, Liverpool, NY 13088

Kent Elastomer Products, Inc. 800-331-4762
1500 Saint Clair Ave, PO Box 668, Kent, OH 44240
Non-Latex

Matrx By Midmark 800-847-1000
145 Mid County Dr, Orchard Park, NY 14127

Medcovers, Inc 800-948-8917
500 W Goldsboro St, Kenly, NC 27542
Universal Oxygen Bag; Fits all types of conservers, available with M-6, D, C, E cylinders and CR-50, EX 2005, and other new ones.

Mercury Medical 800-237-6418
11300 49th St N, Clearwater, FL 33762
Hyperinflation Bag - family of gas (oxygen) powered resuscitation system featuring patented pressure manometer. CCK, CAP carbon dioxide gas analyzer

Morris Latex Products, Inc. 405-872-3486
1101 E Maguire Rd, Noble, OK 73068

Nano Mask Inc. 888-656-3697
175 Cassia Way Ste A115, Henderson, NV 89014
E.L.V.I.S. - BVM Bag with nebulizer port

BAG, BREATHING *(cont'd)*

Sun-Med 800-433-2797
12393 Belcher Rd S Ste 450, Largo, FL 33773

Sunmed Healthcare 727-531-7266
12393 Belcher Rd S Ste 460, Largo, FL 33773

Vacumed 800-235-3333
4538 Westinghouse St, Ventura, CA 93003
20 models.

BAG, COLLECTION, URINE, NEWBORN *(General) 80FOC*

Avail Medical Products, Inc. 858-635-2206
1225 N. 28th Avenue, Suite 500, Dallas, TX 75261
Various types of fluid collection pouches.

Enova Medical Technologies 866-773-0539
1839 Buerkle Rd, Saint Paul, MN 55110
P.V.C. Bags, R.F. bag manufacturing for collection bags in custom sizes.

Microtek Medical, Inc 800-936-9248
512 N Lehmberg Rd, Columbus, MS 39702
Various fluid containment bags.

O&M Enterprise 847-258-4515
641 Chelmsford Ln, Elk Grove Village, IL 60007
URINE COLLECTION BAG

Precision Dynamics Corp. 800-772-1122
13880 Del Sur St, San Fernando, CA 91340

Ross Disposable Products 800-649-6526
401 Traders Blvd E, Unit 10, Mississauga, ON L4Z 2H8 Canada

Vygon Corp. 800-544-4907
2495 General Armistead Ave, Norristown, PA 19403

BAG, DRAINAGE (INCONTINENCE) *(Gastro/Urology) 78QQK*

Achilles Usa, Inc. 425-353-7000
1407 80th St SW, Everett, WA 98203

Coloplast Manufacturing Us, Llc 800-533-0464
1840 W Oak Pkwy, Marietta, GA 30062
CONVEEN 1500 ml drainage bag with pre-attached adjustable, anti-kink tubing; soft cloth backing; anti-reflux valve.

Command Medical Products, Inc. 386-672-8116
15 Signal Ave, Ormond Beach, FL 32174
Contract assembly.

Covidien Lp 508-261-8000
15 Hampshire St, Mansfield, MA 02048
Dover urological products.

Ldb Medical, Inc. 800-243-2554
2909 Langford Rd Ste B500, Norcross, GA 30071

Medi Inc 800-225-8634
75 York Ave, P.O. Box 302, Randolph, MA 02368

Precision Dynamics Corp. 800-772-1122
13880 Del Sur St, San Fernando, CA 91340
UR-ASSURE Urinary Drainage Bag; 2000ml drainage bag with graduations and drain port.

Skil-Care Corp. 800-431-2972
29 Wells Ave, Yonkers, NY 10701

Smith & Nephew, Inc. 800-876-1261
11775 Starkey Rd, Largo, FL 33773

Smith & Nephew, Inc. 800-876-1261
970 Lake Carillon Dr Ste 110, Saint Petersburg, FL 33716
WITH ADHESIVE, OSTOMY - BANISH II LIQUID DEODORANT; Tincture Benzoin; URI-KLEEN DETERGENT

Torbot Group, Inc. 800-545-4254
1367 Elmwood Ave, Cranston, RI 02910

Uresil, Llc 800-538-7374
5418 Touhy Ave, Skokie, IL 60077
TRU-CLOSE gravity drainage reservoirs.

BAG, DRAINAGE, NASOGASTRIC *(General) 80WOQ*

Command Medical Products, Inc. 386-672-8116
15 Signal Ave, Ormond Beach, FL 32174
Contract assembly.

Harmac Medical Products, Inc. 716-897-4500
2201 Bailey Ave, Buffalo, NY 14211
Contract manufacturer of custom RF-welded bags and sets. OEM and private-labeled products.

Towic Medical, Inc. 847-823-2215
303 S Clifton Ave, PO Box 883, Park Ridge, IL 60068
Disposable, see-through bag for collection of fluids from a nasogastric tube draining by gravity.

BAG, DRAINAGE, OSTOMY (WITH ADHESIVE) *(General) 80FON*

Amd-Ritmed, Inc. 800-445-0340
295 Firetower Road, Tonawanda, NY 14150

Blanchard Ostomy Products 818-242-6789
1510 Raymond Ave, Glendale, CA 91201
Karaya seals, ostomy appliances and pouches

Command Medical Products, Inc. 386-672-8116
15 Signal Ave, Ormond Beach, FL 32174
Contract assembly.

Marlen Manufacturing & Development Co. 216-292-7060
5150 Richmond Rd, Bedford, OH 44146

Mentor Corp. 800-525-0245
201 Mentor Dr, Santa Barbara, CA 93111

Organics Corporation Of America 973-890-9002
55 W End Rd, Paterson, NJ 07512
Perry drug denture adhesive.

Perma Type Company, Inc. 860-747-9999
83 Northwest Dr, Plainville, CT 06062
Ostomy appliance.

Smith & Nephew, Inc. 800-876-1261
11775 Starkey Rd, Largo, FL 33773
BONGORT odor barrier drain.

Urocare Products, Inc. 800-423-4441
2735 Melbourne Ave, Pomona, CA 91767

BAG, ENEMA *(General) 80QUF*

C.B. Fleet Company Inc. 804-528-4000
PO Box 11349, 4615 Murray Place, Lynchburg, VA 24506
Bagenema. 1500 cc enema.

BAG, ENTERAL FEEDING *(General) 80QVL*

Abbott Laboratories 800-624-7677
1033 Kingsmill Pkwy, Columbus, OH 43229
Case of 24 pcs. FLEXITAINER 1L with 40mm screw-on top feeding bags; case of 24 pcs. of FLEXITAINER 500 bags (500ml with 40mm screw-on top); case of 24 pcs. FLEXIFLO bags (top-fill, 1000ml with spike port on bottom of bag, rigid neck); and TOPTAINER, 1000ml with spike port on bottom of bag.

Harmac Medical Products, Inc. 716-897-4500
2201 Bailey Ave, Buffalo, NY 14211
Contract manufacturer of custom RF-welded bags and sets.

Omni Medical Supply Inc. 800-860-6664
4153 Pioneer Dr, Commerce Township, MI 48390

Zinetics Medical, Inc. 800-648-4070
1050 E South Temple, Salt Lake City, UT 84102
Enteral feeding system.

BAG, GARBAGE *(General) 80VAU*

Medical Safety Systems Inc. 888-803-9303
230 White Pond Dr, Akron, OH 44313
Infectious waste.

Mi-Co Company 516-481-7775
564 Warren Blvd, Garden City, NY 11530

Silverstone Packaging, Inc.-Your One Stop Supplier 800-413-1108
1401 Lakeland Ave, Bohemia, NY 11716

Spectra Medical Devices, Inc. 866-938-8649
4C Henshaw St, Woburn, MA 01801
Bag-biohazard.

BAG, ICE *(General) 80KYR*

Advanced Materials, Inc. 310-537-5444
20211 S Susana Rd, East Rancho Dominguez, CA 90221
Ice pack.

Afassco, Inc. 800-441-6774
2244 Park Pl Ste C, Minden, NV 89423
Large and small cold packs.

Bagco 800-533-1931
1650 Airport Rd NW Ste 104, Kennesaw, GA 30144
ICE BAGS 67, biohazard ice bags for hospitals and clinics. A bottom gusset ziplock bag printed w/biohazard logo on front.

Breg, Inc., An Orthofix Company 800-897-BREG
2611 Commerce Way, Vista, CA 92081
Ice bag.

Bruder Healthcare Company 888-827-8337
3150 Engineering Pkwy, Alpharetta, GA 30004
Latex Free Ice Bags

BAG, ICE *(cont'd)*

Busse Hospital Disposables, Inc. 631-435-4711
75 Arkay Dr, Hauppauge, NY 11788
Ice bag.

Certified Safety Manufacturing 800-854-7474
1400 Chestnut Ave, Kansas City, MO 64127
CERTI-COOL INSTANT.

Electro Medical Equipment Co., Inc. 800-423-2926
12015 Industriplex Blvd, Baton Rouge, LA 70809

Frontier Medical Products, Inc. 800-367-6828
140 S Park St, Port Washington, WI 53074

Global Healthcare 800-601-3880
1495 Hembree Rd Ste 700, Roswell, GA 30076
Large and Small size, disposable

Hospira 800-441-4100
268 E 4th St, Ashland, OH 44805
6-, 9-, 11-in. ice bag.

Hospital Marketing Svcs. Company, Inc. 800-786-5094
162 Great Hill Rd./ Ind. Park, Naugatuck, CT 06770
HMS COL-PRESS instant cold compress - large (6in. x 10in.), cat. no. 6627, 24/case, Col-Press JR. Cat. No 6527 24/case (4in. x 7in.). 6000-080 - 7in. x 8in. soft and dry zip lock, ice bag with ties and large mouth. 6000-110 - 7in. x 11in. soft and dry zip lock ice bag with 4 ties, large EZ fill mouth.

Kentron Health Care, Inc. 615-384-0573
3604 Kelton Jackson Rd, P.o. Box 120, Springfield, TN 37172
Ice bag.

Kerma Medical Products, Inc. 757-398-8400
400 Port Centre Pkwy, Portsmouth, VA 23704
Ice bag.

Kerr Group 800-524-3577
1400 Holcomb Bridge Rd, Roswell, GA 30076

Medi Inc 800-225-8634
75 York Ave, P.O. Box 302, Randolph, MA 02368
Instant ice bag.

O&M Enterprise 847-258-4515
641 Chelmsford Ln, Elk Grove Village, IL 60007
BAG ICE

Occk, Inc. 800-526-9731
1710 W Schilling Rd, Salina, KS 67401
Ice bag.

Sunbeam Products, Inc. 561-912-4100
2381 NW Executive Center Dr, Boca Raton, FL 33431
Ice bag.

Tapeless Wound Care Products, Llc. 866-714-9199
PO Box 4515, Englewood, CO 80155
Ice bag and holder.

Tetra Medical Supply Corp. 800-621-4041
6364 W Gross Point Rd, Niles, IL 60714

Velcro Usa, Inc. 603-669-4880
406 Brown Ave, Manchester, NH 03103
Ice bag.

Vonco Products, Inc. 800-323-9077
201 Park Ave, Lake Villa, IL 60046

BAG, INTESTINE *(Surgery) 79KGY*

Firehouse Medical, Inc. 714-688-1575
1045 N Armando St Ste D, Anaheim, CA 92806
Sterile amputation kit.

BAG, LAUNDRY, INFECTION CONTROL *(General) 80TCV*

Approved Medical Systems 951-353-2453
7101 Jurupa Ave Ste 4, Riverside, CA 92504
Sterilization, decontamination and water soluble, meets OSHA regulations & CDC guidelines.

Atd-American Co. 800-523-2300
135 Greenwood Ave, Wyncote, PA 19095

Bussard & Son Inc., R.D. 800-252-2692
415 25th Ave SW, Albany, OR 97322
Leakproof hamper bags available in different sizes and styles.

Iron Duck, A Div. Of Fleming Industries, Inc. 800-669-6900
20 Veterans Dr, Chicopee, MA 01022
Fluidproof hamper bag, meets OSHA guidelines. Available in 6 sizes.

Medical Safety Systems Inc. 888-803-9303
230 White Pond Dr, Akron, OH 44313

Medline Industries, Inc. 800-633-5886
1 Medline Pl, Mundelein, IL 60060

BAG, LAUNDRY, INFECTION CONTROL *(cont'd)*

Mip Inc. 800-361-4964
9100 Ray Lawson Blvd., Montreal, QC H1J-1K8 Canada
Leakproof soiled laundry bag.

Spectra Medical Devices, Inc. 978-657-0889
260H Fordham Rd, Wilmington, MA 01887
biohazard bags, disposable

Uniflex Inc., Medical Packaging Division 800-223-0564
383 W John St, Hicksville, NY 11801

Webb Manufacturing Co. 800-932-2634
1241 Carpenter St, Philadelphia, PA 19147

BAG, LAUNDRY, OPERATING ROOM *(General) 80REJ*

Angelica Image Apparel 800-222-3112
700 Rosedale Ave, Saint Louis, MO 63112

Atd-American Co. 800-523-2300
135 Greenwood Ave, Wyncote, PA 19095

Best Manufacturing Group Llc 800-843-3233
1633 Broadway Fl 18, New York, NY 10019
Impervious, color coded.

Standard Textile Co., Inc. 888-999-0400
PO Box 371805, Cincinnati, OH 45222

BAG, LEG *(Gastro/Urology) 78FAQ*

American Innotek, Inc. 760-741-6600
501 S Andreasen Dr, Escondido, CA 92029
Various.

Browning Enterprises, Inc. 616-849-2420
1234 Zoschke Rd, Benton Harbor, MI 49022
The male bag.

California Medical Innovations 800-229-5871
873 E Arrow Hwy, Pomona, CA 91767
Latex leg bags.

Centurion Medical Products Corp. 517-545-1135
3310 S Main St, Salisbury, NC 28147

Coloplast Manufacturing Us, Llc 800-533-0464
1840 W Oak Pkwy, Marietta, GA 30062

Cook Endoscopy 336-744-0157
4900 Bethania Station Rd # &, 5951 Grassy Creek Blvd.
Winston Salem, NC 27105
Irrigation/drainage system.

Cypress Medical Products 800-334-3646
1202 S. Rte. 31, McHenry, IL 60050
Available in medium (600 cc) or large (800 cc), both with twist valve.

Farmatap S.A. De C.V.
117 Alfonso Esparza Oteo, Mexico Df 01020 Mexico
No common name listed

Hollister, Inc. 847-680-2849
366 Draft Ave, Stuarts Draft, VA 24477

Kelsar, S.A. 508-261-8000
Blvd. Insurgentes, Libriamento a La, Tijuana 22450 Mexico
Various

Kentron Health Care, Inc. 615-384-0573
3604 Kelton Jackson Rd, P.o. Box 120, Springfield, TN 37172
Urine collection leg bag.

Ldb Medical, Inc. 800-243-2554
2909 Langford Rd Ste B500, Norcross, GA 30071

Marlen Manufacturing & Development Co. 216-292-7060
5150 Richmond Rd, Bedford, OH 44146

Medi Inc 800-225-8634
75 York Ave, P.O. Box 302, Randolph, MA 02368

Medical Devices International, Div. Of Plasco, Inc. 800-438-7634
512 N Lehmberg Rd, Columbus, MS 39702
Leg bags (3 styles) with integral button attach, twist drain valve; available in deluxe, medium and large.

Medical Plastic Devices (Mpd), Inc. 866-633-9835
161 Oneida Dr., Pointe Claire, QUE H9R 1A9 Canada

Medline Industries, Inc. 800-633-5886
1 Medline Pl, Mundelein, IL 60060

Medline Manufacturing And Services Llc 847-837-2759
1 Medline Pl, Mundelein, IL 60060
Drainbag.

Precision Dynamics Corp. 800-772-1122
13880 Del Sur St, San Fernando, CA 91340
UR-Assure connector tubing set.

BAG, LEG *(cont'd)*

R. D. Equipment, Inc. 508-362-7498
230 Percival Dr, West Barnstable, MA 02668
Electric leg bag emptier.

The Hygenic Corp. 800-321-2135
1245 Home Ave, Akron, OH 44310
Leg strap for holding urinary bag to leg.

Tri-State Hospital Supply Corp. 517-545-1135
3173 E 43rd St, Yuma, AZ 85365

Unomedical, Inc. 800-634-6003
5701 S Ware Rd Ste 1, McAllen, TX 78503

Urocare Products, Inc. 800-423-4441
2735 Melbourne Ave, Pomona, CA 91767
Reusable latex leg bag, disposable leg bag and adjustable Velcro leg strap.

Vygon Corp. 800-544-4907
2495 General Armistead Ave, Norristown, PA 19403

Welcon, Inc. 800-877-0923
7409 Pebble Dr, Fort Worth, TX 76118

Work, Inc. 800-898-0301
3 Arlington St, Quincy, MA 02171
MEDIUM & LARGE SIZE URINARY COLLECTION BAGS

BAG, MEDICAL, PHYSICIAN *(General) 80RGJ*

Air Lift Unlimited Inc. 800-776-6771
1212 Kerr Gulch Rd, Evergreen, CO 80439
AIR LIFT nursing bags feature functional design and superior quality to ensure compliance with certification protocols & HIPAA requirements. Multiple pockets allow easy organization of contents and segregation of sterile supplies. Silk screening & embroidery available on all bags.Three styles and two colors.

Biotek, Inc. 800-269-2918
PO Box 2216, West Lafayette, IN 47996
Carrying cases for paramedics and EMS personnel.

Ch Ellis Company Inc. 800-466-3351
2432 Southeastern Ave, Indianapolis, IN 46201
Nurse's Aide Bag.

Hartwell Medical Corp. 800-633-5900
6352 Corte Del Abeto Ste J, Carlsbad, CA 92011
BIO-HOOP Collection bag. Bio-Hoop waste and emesis bag (disposable); leak-proof for blood and urine samples, waste, and trash.

Iron Duck, A Div. Of Fleming Industries, Inc. 800-669-6900
20 Veterans Dr, Chicopee, MA 01022
Emergency medical bags and equipment. Precaution bags made of autoclavable, wipe-clean material.

Uniflex Inc., Medical Packaging Division 800-223-0564
383 W John St, Hicksville, NY 11801
Complete line of personal belongings and patient courtesy bags.

Western Case, Inc. 877-593-2182
14351 Chambers Rd, Tustin, CA 92780
Plastic carrying cases.

Whitney Products, Inc. 800-338-4237
6153 W Mulford St Ste C, Niles, IL 60714
TERMINAL Biohazard bags & containers available in printed red or plain blue, autoclavable, 4 different sizes.

BAG, PLASTIC *(General) 80WNK*

A.R.C. Distributors 800-296-8724
PO Box 599, Centreville, MD 21617
CLEAR-VIEW WHEELCHAIR POUCH - Clear vinyl pouch to fit all size wheelchairs or stretchers for patient information storage. Eliminates time wasted searching for lost patient charts. Assures patient records confidentiality!

Action Bag Co. 800-490-8830
1001 Entry Dr, Bensenville, IL 60106
Reclosable, lab transport bag.

Adi Medical Division Of Asia Dynamics (Group) Inc. 877-647-7699
1565 S Shields Dr, Waukegan, IL 60085

American Fluoroseal Corp. 800-360-1050
431 E Diamond Ave Ste A, Gaithersburg, MD 20877
VueLife FEP (Teflon) tissue culture bags for cryogenics, cell culture and reagent storage. From 2 ml to 3, 500 ml; priced from $12 to $98.

BAG, PLASTIC *(cont'd)*

Bagco 800-533-1931
1650 Airport Rd NW Ste 104, Kennesaw, GA 30144
Zip-locking bags with wide, white zipper and double teeth closure tracks; open-ended full gauged bottom sealed bags; PRN medication bags for medication on demand; zip-locking white block write-on bags; chemotherapy bags for disposal of contaminated clothing. Polyethylene (LDPE) & polypropylene. TEARZONE, Safeguard specimen handling bags. Tamper evident specimen bags, ice bags. Free samples are available. All packed in convenient soft-packed dispenser bags. Biohazard Trash Bags, custom order or stock in red w/ black print. Patient Belonging Bags, with draw string, drawer tape and die cut handles.

Berghof/America 800-544-5004
3773 NW 126th Ave Bldg 1, Coral Springs, FL 33065
Various fluoropolymer and telar gas and liquid sampling bags and liners.

Donovan Industries 800-334-4404
13401 McCormick Dr, Tampa, FL 33626
Zip-lock bag (reclosable bags) and bags for patient belongings with drawstring.

Dravon Medical, Inc. 503-656-6600
11465 SE Highway 212, PO Box 69, Clackamas, OR 97015
Custom medical grade bags; uses range from blood handling to drainage to fluid adminstration.

Extra Packaging, Corp. 800-872-7548
631 Golden Harbour Dr, Boca Raton, FL 33432
AQUATANK, Emergency water storage bags for emergencies and preparedness.

Gi Supply 800-451-5797
200 Grandview Ave, Camp Hill, PA 17011
SCOPETOTE, for transport of clean or soiled scopes. CLEAN-UP, bags to contain soiled accessories.

Harmac Medical Products, Inc. 716-897-4500
2201 Bailey Ave, Buffalo, NY 14211
Contract manufacturer of all types of RF-welded and heat-sealed medical device bags and sets, including blood bags, enteral bags, medication bags, drainage bags, irrigation bags, and sets. OEM and private-labeled products. Class 100,000 cleanrooms.

Medela, Inc. 800-435-8316
1101 Corporate Dr, McHenry, IL 60050
CSF Breastmilk Collection Bag - individually sterile disposable bags for collecting, storing and freezing breastmilk. PUMP & SAVE Breastmilk Collection Bag - individually sterile disposable bags for collecting, storing, and freezing breastmilk.

Medi-Dose, Inc. 800-523-8966
70 Industrial Dr, Ivyland, PA 18974
Resealable bags; ultraviolet inhibitant bags for protection of medication.

Medical Plastic Devices (Mpd), Inc. 866-633-9835
161 Oneida Dr., Pointe Claire, QUE H9R 1A9 Canada

Mes, Inc. 800-423-2215
1968 E US Highway 90, Seguin, TX 78155
Drawstring bags for respiratory set-up, flat poly bags and dust covers, can liners, recloseable bags, etc

New World Imports 800-329-1903
160 Athens Way, Nashville, TN 37228
Personal belongings bags, rigid handle and drawstring; diaper bags of PVC or cloth and rayon canvas bags; sewing kits.

Origen Biomedical, Inc. 512-474-7278
4020 S Industrial Dr Ste 160, Austin, TX 78744
Cell-culture and freezing bags.

Polyzen, Inc. 919-319-9599
1041 Classic Rd, Apex, NC 27539
Custom Bags: Polyurethane organ bags, endoscopic bags, tissue bags. Laparoscopic specimen bag, semen collection, etc.

Stericon, Inc. 708-865-8790
2315 Gardner Rd, Broadview, IL 60155
Blood and blood component freezing bags and accessories; volume bags for culture media storage.

Swisslog Translogic Corporation 800-525-1841
10825 E 47th Ave, Denver, CO 80239
ZIP N FOLD Secondary containment transport pouches.

Uniflex Inc., Medical Packaging Division 800-223-0564
383 W John St, Hicksville, NY 11801
Personal belongins, pharmaceutical transport, specimen transport, respiratory therapy, kit packaging, custom imprinting, dressing disposed.

BAG, PLASTIC *(cont'd)*

Veriad 800-423-4643
650 Columbia St, Brea, CA 92821
Liquid tight specimen transport bags.

BAG, POLYMERIC MESH, PACEMAKER *(Cardiovascular) 74DSW*

Bard Shannon Limited 908-277-8000
San Geronimo Industrial Park, Lot # 1, Road # 3, Km 79.7
Humacao, PR 00791
Mesh bags.

Plastic And Metal Center, Inc. 949-770-8230
23162 La Cadena Dr, Laguna Hills, CA 92653

BAG, RESERVOIR (BLOOD) *(Anesthesiology) 73BTC*

Hans Rudolph, Inc. 816-363-5522
7200 Wyandotte St, Kansas City, MO 64114
Reservoir bag.

Integra Neurosciences 800-762-1574
5955 Pacific Center Blvd, San Diego, CA 92121
Ventricular drainage bag.

Johnson & Johnson Medical Division Of Ethicon, Inc. 800-423-4018
2500 E Arbrook Blvd, Arlington, TX 76014

Matrx 716-662-6650
145 Mid County Dr, Orchard Park, NY 14127
Oxygen reservoir.

Medi Inc 800-225-8634
75 York Ave, P.O. Box 302, Randolph, MA 02368
Blood and bone marrow freezing bags.

Medtronic Perfusion Systems 800-328-3320
7611 Northland Dr N, Brooklyn Park, MN 55428
Blood collection/cardiovascular reservoirs.

Mount Olive Manufacturing, Inc. 317-279-2152
923 Whitaker Rd Ste E, Plainfield, IN 46168
Oxygen reservoir bag.

Smiths Medical Asd Inc. 800-258-5361
10 Bowman Dr, Keene, NH 03431
Various types and sizes of anesthesia bags.

Stericon, Inc. 708-865-8790
2315 Gardner Rd, Broadview, IL 60155
Blood and blood component freezing bags and accessories.

BAG, SPECIMEN, LAPAROSCOPIC *(Surgery) 79WZP*

Approved Medical Systems 951-353-2453
7101 Jurupa Ave Ste 4, Riverside, CA 92504

Ethicon Endo-Surgery, Inc. 800-USE-ENDO
4545 Creek Rd, Cincinnati, OH 45242
ENDOPOUCH specimen retrieval bag, 5in. x 7in with introducer.

Pare Surgical, Inc. 303-689-0187
7332 S Alton Way Ste H, Centennial, CO 80112
BERT Laparoscopic Retrieval Bag offered in three sizes, Nubert 120nl, Albert 900ml and Hubert 3,000ml.

Uniflex Inc., Medical Packaging Division 800-223-0564
383 W John St, Hicksville, NY 11801
SPECI-GARD specimen transport bags.

United States Endoscopy Group 800-769-8226
5976 Heisley Rd, Mentor, OH 44060
Ponsky ENDO-SOCK disposable specimen retrieval pouch, 10mm.

Zenith Medical Inc. 800-747-0216
10064 Mesa Ridge Ct Ste 218, San Diego, CA 92121
ENDOSAC Seamless Specimen Collection Pouch used in laparoscopic surgeries to remove tissues from the body.

BAG, STOMAL *(Surgery) 79GDS*

Coloplast Manufacturing Us, Llc 800-533-0464
1840 W Oak Pkwy, Marietta, GA 30062
Open and closed end ostomy pouches with attached skin barrier.

Hollister, Inc. 847-680-2849
366 Draft Ave, Stuarts Draft, VA 24477

Marlen Manufacturing & Development Co. 216-292-7060
5150 Richmond Rd, Bedford, OH 44146

BAG, URINARY COLLECTION *(General) 80SEB*

Briggs Corporation 800-247-2343
PO Box 1698, 7300 Westown Pkwy., Des Moines, IA 50306

BAG, URINARY COLLECTION *(cont'd)*

Clarke Health Care Products, Inc. 888-347-4537
1003 International Dr, Oakdale, PA 15071
Cleanis Care Bag, contains GelMax super absorbent pad, converts liquid to solid gel and eliminates odors. Polyethylene bags in sizes to line collection pails, bedpans or for personal use. Simply use attached ties to secure bag and dispose in trash.

Coloplast Manufacturing Us, Llc 800-533-0464
1840 W Oak Pkwy, Marietta, GA 30062
CONVEEN urine bags include pre-attached, adjustable, anti-kink tubing; cloth backing, anti-reflux valve.

Covidien Lp 508-261-8000
15 Hampshire St, Mansfield, MA 02048

Csi International, Inc. 303-795-8273
4301 S Federal Blvd Ste 116, Englewood, CO 80110

Cypress Medical Products 800-334-3646
1202 S. Rte. 31, McHenry, IL 60050
2000CC., Velcro hanger, anti-reflux and sampling port.

Dma Med-Chem Corporation 800-362-1833
49 Watermill Ln, Great Neck, NY 11021

Gkr Industries, Inc. 800-526-7879
13653 Kenton Ave, Crestwood, IL 60445
Midstream Urine Collection Kit, U.T. Bag System, unique bag for urine collection and strip testing. Patented inner valve seals urine in, extra-wide 6' rigid funnel opening is three times wider than the typical collection jar, only one hand required for use and patented outer sleeve gives added protection from infectious fluids.
VOID-EASE, collection bag with easy transfer to a test tube which is attached right to the bag.

Ldb Medical, Inc. 800-243-2554
2909 Langford Rd Ste B500, Norcross, GA 30071

Medi Inc 800-225-8634
75 York Ave, P.O. Box 302, Randolph, MA 02368

Medical Devices International, Div. Of Plasco, Inc. 800-438-7634
512 N Lehmberg Rd, Columbus, MS 39702
6 models of urinary collection bags, available with and without reflux, with and without sample port.

Mediseal Products Ltd. 416-744-2011
375 Rexdale Blvd., Etobicoke, ONT M9W 1S1 Canada
Urinary leg bag.

Mentor Corp. 800-525-0245
201 Mentor Dr, Santa Barbara, CA 93111

Ross Disposable Products 800-649-6526
401 Traders Blvd E, Unit 10, Mississauga, ON L4Z 2H8 Canada

Smith & Nephew, Inc. 800-876-1261
11775 Starkey Rd, Largo, FL 33773
FEATHER-LITE urinary collection bag.

Torbot Group, Inc. 800-545-4254
1367 Elmwood Ave, Cranston, RI 02910

Unomedical, Inc. 800-634-6003
5701 S Ware Rd Ste 1, McAllen, TX 78503
Drainage.

Urocare Products, Inc. 800-423-4441
2735 Melbourne Ave, Pomona, CA 91767
Male urinal kit. Three sizes available: large, standard and small.

Vygon Corp. 800-544-4907
2495 General Armistead Ave, Norristown, PA 19403

BAG, URINARY COLLECTION, URETEROSTOMY
(Gastro/Urology) 78EXG

Ac Healthcare Supply, Inc. 905-448-4706
11651 230th St, Cambria Heights, NY 11411
Ostomy pouch and accessories.

Cook Urological, Inc. 800-457-4500
1100 W Morgan St, P.O. Box 227, Spencer, IN 47460

Hollister, Inc. 847-680-2849
366 Draft Ave, Stuarts Draft, VA 24477

Imed Technology, Inc. 972-732-7333
17408 Tamaron Dr, Dallas, TX 75287
Uring leg bags - sterile.

Marlen Manufacturing & Development Co. 216-292-7060
5150 Richmond Rd, Bedford, OH 44146
Ileostomy, urostomy and colostomy appliances.

Urocare Products, Inc. 800-423-4441
2735 Melbourne Ave, Pomona, CA 91767
Sterile, 2000cc drainage bag.

BAG, URINARY, ILEOSTOMY *(Gastro/Urology) 78EXH*

Coloplast Manufacturing Us, Llc 800-533-0464
1840 W Oak Pkwy, Marietta, GA 30062
COLOPLAST, ASSURA one or two piece drainable pouches include soft backing, anti-reflux valve, secure closure. Available in transparent or opaque.

Cook Urological, Inc. 800-457-4500
1100 W Morgan St, P.O. Box 227, Spencer, IN 47460

Ldb Medical, Inc. 800-243-2554
2909 Langford Rd Ste B500, Norcross, GA 30071

Marlen Manufacturing & Development Co. 216-292-7060
5150 Richmond Rd, Bedford, OH 44146
Ileostomy, urostomy and colostomy appliances.

North American Latex Corp. 812-268-6608
49 Industrial Park Dr, Sullivan, IN 47882
Urinal leg bag, latex.

Smith & Nephew, Inc. 800-876-1261
11775 Starkey Rd, Largo, FL 33773

Torbot Group, Inc. 800-545-4254
1367 Elmwood Ave, Cranston, RI 02910

Urocare Products, Inc. 800-423-4441
2735 Melbourne Ave, Pomona, CA 91767

BAG, URINE COLLECTION, LEG, FOR EXTERNAL USE, NON-STERILE *(Gastro/Urology) 78NNW*

Ac Healthcare Supply, Inc. 905-448-4706
11651 230th St, Cambria Heights, NY 11411
Urine collector and accessories.

Arcus Medical Llc 704-332-3424
2327 Distribution St, Charlotte, NC 28203
Leg bag.

Hollister, Inc. 847-680-2849
366 Draft Ave, Stuarts Draft, VA 24477

BALANCE (GENERAL USE) *(Chemistry) 75DOI*

Precisa Balances Usa Inc. 877-PRE-CISA
540 Powder Springs St Ste 8, Marietta, GA 30064
Top loading and precision industrial; statistics, check-weighing, and animal-weighing programs standard.

BALANCE, ANALYTICAL *(Chemistry) 75JQO*

A&D Medical 800-726-7099
1756 Automation Pkwy, San Jose, CA 95131

Advanced Mechanical Technology, Inc. (Amti) 800-422-AMTI
176 Waltham St, Watertown, MA 02472
Accusway - Balance/Postural Sway analysis.

Clean Air Engineering 800-627-0033
500 W Wood St, Palatine, IL 60067

Gilson Company, Inc. 800-444-1508
PO Box 200, Lewis Center, OH 43035

Intersciences Inc. 800-661-6431
169 Idema Rd., Markham, ONT L3R 1A9 Canada

Koehler Instrument Co., Inc. 800-878-9070
1595 Sycamore Ave, Bohemia, NY 11716
CE Mark. 30 Models available with maximum capacities from 80 g to 12,000 g and readabilities from 0.1 mg to 0.1 g. Auto calibration.

Mehlrose Associates 410-730-0263
11660 Little Patuxent Pkwy Apt 304, Columbia, MD 21044
Analytical balance.

Mg Scientific, Inc. 800-343-8338
8500 107th St, Pleasant Prairie, WI 53158

Precisa Balances Usa Inc. 877-PRE-CISA
540 Powder Springs St Ste 8, Marietta, GA 30064
Analytical up to 404 g; semi-micro to 92 g. Check-weighing program standard, options include Smartbox with program for 200+ product check-weigh and piece count.

Preiser Scientific, Inc. 800-624-8285
94 Oliver St, P.O. Box 1330, Saint Albans, WV 25177

Rice Lake Weighing Systems 800-472-6703
230 W Coleman St, Rice Lake, WI 54868
High precision analytical and top loading balances available in a variety of weighing ranges and readabilities, prices from $2,800.

Sepor, Inc. 800-753-6463
718 N Fries Ave, P.O. Box 578, Wilmington, CA 90744

Utech Products, Inc. 800-828-8324
135 Broadway, Schenectady, NY 12305
SARTORIUS, OHAUS, DENVER, SCALTEC, & ACCULAB Scales.

BALANCE, ELECTRONIC *(Chemistry) 75QCF*

Algen Scale Corp. 800-836-8445
68 Enter Ln, Islandia, NY 11749
Battery operated or plug-in electric. All capacities and resolutions.

Csc Scientific Co. 800-621-4778
2810 Old Lee Hwy, Fairfax, VA 22031
Top loading & analytical, RS-232 interface, multiple weighing modes, automatic calibration, full range taring.

Edmund Industrial Optics 800-363-1992
101 E Gloucester Pike, Barrington, NJ 08007

Mettler-Toledo, Inc. 800-METTLER
1900 Polaris Pkwy, Columbus, OH 43240

Precisa Balances Usa Inc. 877-PRE-CISA
540 Powder Springs St Ste 8, Marietta, GA 30064
Product line ranges from 62.00001 g to 60000 g. All balances have Precisa's exclusive anti-theft-code protection preventing unautorized use and most have password protection preventing unauthorized reprogramming. Education and government discounts available.

Rice Lake Weighing Systems 800-472-6703
230 W Coleman St, Rice Lake, WI 54868
Electronic precision balances.

Schueler & Company, Inc. 516-487-1500
PO Box 528, Stratford, CT 06615

Scientech, Inc. 303-444-1361
5649 Arapahoe Ave, Boulder, CO 80303
17 models priced from $995 to $3,495 with capacities from 150 to 12000 g.

BALANCE, MACRO (0.1 MG ACCURACY) *(Chemistry) 75UKH*

A&D Medical 800-726-7099
1756 Automation Pkwy, San Jose, CA 95131

Cole-Parmer Instrument Inc. 800-323-4340
625 E Bunker Ct, Vernon Hills, IL 60061

Mettler-Toledo, Inc. 800-METTLER
1900 Polaris Pkwy, Columbus, OH 43240
Electronic unit with capacity up to 504g.

Scientech, Inc. 303-444-1361
5649 Arapahoe Ave, Boulder, CO 80303
8 electronic models priced from $1395 to $3995, with capacities from 80 to 500 g.

BALANCE, MECHANICAL *(Chemistry) 75QCG*

Algen Scale Corp. 800-836-8445
68 Enter Ln, Islandia, NY 11749

Edmund Industrial Optics 800-363-1992
101 E Gloucester Pike, Barrington, NJ 08007
Digital.

Jayza Corp. 305-477-1136
7215 NW 41st St Ste A, Miami, FL 33166

Rice Lake Weighing Systems 800-472-6703
230 W Coleman St, Rice Lake, WI 54868
The manufacturing process MASSTAR weights undergo is specifically designed to reduce the magnetic field strength and magnetic susceptibility of the weights in order to gain more accurate weighments. In addition, when a set of weights for callibration is received, they are tested for magnetic field strength before the calibration process and the owner is notified if the magnetic properties are too high to gain consistent measurements.

Schueler & Company, Inc. 516-487-1500
PO Box 528, Stratford, CT 06615

Troemner Llc 800-352-7705
201 Wolf Dr, PO Box 87, West Deptford, NJ 08086
Precision calibration weights.

BALANCE, MICRO (0.001 MG ACCURACY) *(Chemistry) 75UKF*

Intersciences Inc. 800-661-6431
169 Idema Rd., Markham, ONT L3R 1A9 Canada

Mettler-Toledo, Inc. 800-METTLER
1900 Polaris Pkwy, Columbus, OH 43240
Electronic unit with capacity up to 5.1g.

Orion Research, Inc. 800-225-1480
166 Cummings Ctr, Beverly, MA 01915

U.V. Process Supply, Inc. 800-621-1296
1229 W Cortland St, Chicago, IL 60614

BALANCE, SEMIMICRO (0.01 MG ACCURACY)
(Chemistry) 75UKG

A&D Medical 800-726-7099
1756 Automation Pkwy, San Jose, CA 95131

Cole-Parmer Instrument Inc. 800-323-4340
625 E Bunker Ct, Vernon Hills, IL 60061

Mettler-Toledo, Inc. 800-METTLER
1900 Polaris Pkwy, Columbus, OH 43240
Electronic unit with capacity up to 220g.

Precisa Balances Usa Inc. 877-PRE-CISA
540 Powder Springs St Ste 8, Marietta, GA 30064
Two models available: 262SMA-FR (202 g/0.1mg with a 62/0.01mg range that repeats with each tare); 92SM-202A dualrange (92 g/0.01 mg; 202 g/0.1mg). For a limited time, both models include a free pH900 meter.

Scientech, Inc. 303-444-1361
5649 Arapahoe Ave, Boulder, CO 80303
Four models with capacities from 50g to 120g and pricing from $2,995.00

BALANCE, ULTRAMICRO (0.0001 MG ACCURACY)
(Chemistry) 75UKE

Mettler-Toledo, Inc. 800-METTLER
1900 Polaris Pkwy, Columbus, OH 43240
Electronic unit with capacity up to 2.1g.

BALL, COTTON *(General) 80QMO*

Amd-Ritmed, Inc. 800-445-0340
295 Firetower Road, Tonawanda, NY 14150
Strung or unstrung, x-ray or non-x-ray detectable.

Bioseal 800-441-7325
167 W Orangethorpe Ave, Placentia, CA 92870
Sterile and precounted.

Border Opportunity Saver Systems, Inc. 830-775-0992
10 Finegan Rd, Del Rio, TX 78840
Sterilized cotton balls.

Carolina Absorbent Cotton Co. 800-277-0377
1100 Hawthorne Ln, Charlotte, NC 28205
Cotton, Rayon and Polyester Pharmaceutical Coil (pharmaceutical).

Custom Healthcare Systems, Inc. 804-421-5959
4205 Eubank Rd, Richmond, VA 23231

Ross Disposable Products 800-649-6526
401 Traders Blvd E, Unit 10, Mississauga, ON L4Z 2H8 Canada

Silverstone Packaging, Inc.-Your One Stop Supplier 800-413-1108
1401 Lakeland Ave, Bohemia, NY 11716

BALLOON, ANGIOPLASTY, CORONARY, HEATED
(Cardiovascular) 74MKG

Advanced Polymers, Inc. 603-327-0600
29 Northwestern Dr, Salem, NH 03079
Custom angioplasty, high pressure non-compliant PET balloons available in any length. Optically clear with diameters as small as 0.5mm and wall thickness down to 0.00025 in. Burst pressures up to 30 atm.

Biosensors International - Usa 949-553-8300
20280 SW Acacia St Ste 300, Newport Beach, CA 92660
Powerline PTCA Balloon featuring Slip-X Hydrophilic Coating; swaged marker bands; silk-50 balloon, and EztTrek Tip for optimal tracking (not available for sale in US).

Cardio-Nef, S.A. De C.V. 01-800-024-0240
Rio Grijalva 186, Col. Mitras Norte, Monterrey, N.L. 64320 Mexico

Cardiovascular Research, Inc. 813-832-6222
4810 W Gandy Blvd, Tampa, FL 33611
Sheath for balloon pump (under development), Ballon pumping can be hazardous in women with small arteries or older people with arteriosclerosis of femoral vessels. The danger of amputation is significant in this group of people. This device directs oxygenated blood to lower leg, preventing amputations.

Embo-Optics, Llc. 887-885-6400
100 Cummings Ctr # 326B, Beverly, MA 01915
IV illuminator with lighted monitoring feature aids medical personnel in assuring that all IV solutions and medications are infusing properly and at the correct infusion rate. Greatly enhance patient safety in aiding to prevent any adverse events during infusion.

BALLOON, ANGIOPLASTY, PERIPHERAL, HEATED
(Cardiovascular) 74MKF

Cardio-Nef, S.A. De C.V. 01-800-024-0240
Rio Grijalva 186, Col. Mitras Norte, Monterrey, N.L. 64320 Mexico

Consumaquip Corporation 305-592-4510
7240 NW 12th St, Miami, FL 33126

M & I Medical Sales, Inc. 305-663-6444
4711 SW 72nd Ave, Miami, FL 33155

BALLOON, EPISTAXIS (NASAL) *(Ear/Nose/Throat) 77EMX*

Applied Therapeutics, Inc. 877-682-2777
3104 Cherry Palm Dr Ste 220, Tampa, FL 33619
Hemostatic hydrocolloid gel and gentle tamponade, available in multiple sizes.

Armstrong Medical Industries, Inc. 800-323-4220
575 Knightsbridge Pkwy, Lincolnshire, IL 60069

Arthrocare Corp. 800-797-6520
680 Vaqueros Ave, Sunnyvale, CA 94085
Balloon epistaxis.

Bausch & Lomb Surgical 636-255-5051
3365 Tree Court Ind Blvd, Saint Louis, MO 63122

Bridger Biomed, Inc. 908-277-8000
2430 N 7th Ave, Bozeman, MT 59715
Medical packing-film, sterile, post operative.

Gyrus Ent L.L.C., Sub. Of Gyrus Acmi, Inc. 508-804-2739
2925 Appling Rd, Bartlett, TN 38133
Various.

Invotec Intl. 800-998-8580
6833 Phillips Industrial Blvd, Jacksonville, FL 32256
Epistatis balloon.

Ultracell Medical Technologies, Inc. 877-SPO-NGE1
183 Providence New London Tpke, North Stonington, CT 06359
ULTRACELL Anterior/posterior or epistaxis catheter.

BALLOON, INTRA-AORTIC (WITH CONTROL SYSTEM)
(Cardiovascular) 74DSP

Abiomed, Inc. 800-422-8666
22 Cherry Hill Dr, Danvers, MA 01923

Arrow International, Inc. 800-523-8446
9 Plymouth St, Everett, MA 02149
Various sterile intra-aortic balloon catheters and pumps.

Arrow International, Inc. 800-523-8446
2400 Bernville Rd, Reading, PA 19605

Arrow Medical Products, Ltd. 800-387-7819
2300 Bristol Circle Unit 1, Oakville, ONT L6H-5S3 Canada
ARROW Intra-Aortic Balloons

Boston Scientific Corporation 800-225-2732
1 Boston Scientific Pl, Natick, MA 01760

Datascope Cardiac Assist Div. 800-777-4222
15 Law Dr, Fairfield, NJ 07004
INTROSTAT-DL.

Datascope Corp., Cardiac Assist Division 201-307-5400
1300 MacArthur Blvd, Mahwah, NJ 07430
Intra-aortic balloon catheter.

Drg International, Inc. 800-321-1167
1167 US Highway 22, Mountainside, NJ 07092

Orqis (Tm) Medical 888-723-7277
14 Orchard Ste 100, Lake Forest, CA 92630
Various.

Peter Schiff Enterprise 931-537-6505
4900 Forrest Hill Rd, Cookeville, TN 38506
Various sizes of intra-aortic balloons, with acessories.

BALLOON, MIDDLE EAR *(Ear/Nose/Throat) 77MGL*

Almat, Inc. 423-928-6861
215 E Watauga Ave, Johnson City, TN 37601
Device for Inflating the Middle Ear Space

BALLOON, OCCLUSION, CEREBROVASCULAR
(Cns/Neurology) 84LHH

Telemed Systems Inc. 800-481-6718
8 Kane Industrial Dr, Hudson, MA 01749
DURALON, occlusion balloons.

BAND, ELASTIC, ORTHODONTIC *(Dental And Oral) 76ECI*

Align Technology, Inc. 408-470-1000
881 Martin Ave, Santa Clara, CA 95050
Band,elastic,orthodontic.

BAND, ELASTIC, ORTHODONTIC *(cont'd)*

American Eagle Instruments, Inc. 406-549-7451
6575 Butler Creek Rd, Missoula, MT 59808
Band, elastic, orthodontic.

American Orthodontics Corp. 800-558-7687
1714 Cambridge Ave, Sheboygan, WI 53081

Auradonics Incorporated 856-764-8866
439 Saint Mihiel Dr, Delran, NJ 08075
Elastics.

Barnhart Industries, Inc. 800-325-9973
3690 Highway M, Imperial, MO 63052
Traction band.

Bioseal 800-441-7325
167 W Orangethorpe Ave, Placentia, CA 92870
Sterile rubber bands.

Classone Orthodontics, Inc. 806-799-0608
5064 50th St, Lubbock, TX 79414
Elastomeric ligature tie.

D.C.A. (Dental Corporation Of America) 800-638-6684
889 S Matlack St, West Chester, PA 19382
$29.65 per box of 10,000, discounts available for quantity purchases.

Dexta Corporation 800-733-3982
962 Kaiser Rd, Napa, CA 94558

Fairdale Orthodontic Co., Inc. 513-421-2620
312 W 4th St, Cincinnati, OH 45202
Orthodontic xtra oral appliances.

Forestadent Usa 314-878-5985
2315 Weldon Pkwy, Saint Louis, MO 63146
Orthodontic elastic band.

G & H Wire Co. 800-526-1026
2165 Earlywood Dr, Franklin, IN 46131
Intraoral elastics.

Glenroe Technologies 800-237-4060
1912 44th Ave E, Bradenton, FL 34203
Orthodontic impression protector.

Highland Metals, Inc. 800-368-6484
419 Perrymont Ave, San Jose, CA 95125
Various.

Lancer Orthodontics, Inc. 760-304-2705
253 Pawnee St, San Marcos, CA 92078
Various sizes of orthodontic elastic bands.

Lee Pharmaceuticals 626-442-3141
1434 Santa Anita Ave, El Monte, CA 91733
Elastic ligature thread.

Masel Co., Inc. 800-423-8227
2701 Bartram Rd, Bristol, PA 19007

Mathison Industries, Inc. 775-284-1020
220 Coney Island Dr, Sparks, NV 89431
Orthodontic elastics.

Ortho Organizers, Inc. 760-448-8730
1822 Aston Ave, Carlsbad, CA 92008
Various orthodontic elastic tubing, thread, tissue guard and lip protectors.

Orthoband Company, Inc. 800-325-9973
3690 Highway M, Imperial, MO 63052

Orthodontic Design And Production, Inc. 760-734-3995
1370 Decision St Ste D, Vista, CA 92081
Orthodontic elastic bands.

Oscar, Inc. 317-849-2618
11793 Technology Ln, Fishers, IN 46038
Orthodontic elastic bands.

Pyramid Orthodontics 800-752-8884
4328 Redwood Hwy Ste 100, San Rafael, CA 94903
Rebound - polyurethane ligature ties.

Tap Express, Inc. 305-468-0038
8424 NW 61st St, Miami, FL 33166
Orthodontic chains.

The Hygenic Corp. 800-321-2135
1245 Home Ave, Akron, OH 44310
Orthodontic Elastics - Various Sizes

3m Unitek 800-634-5300
2724 Peck Rd, Monrovia, CA 91016

BAND, MATERIAL, ORTHODONTIC *(Dental And Oral) 76DYO*

American Orthodontics Corp. 800-558-7687
1714 Cambridge Ave, Sheboygan, WI 53081

BAND, MATERIAL, ORTHODONTIC *(cont'd)*

Biomet Microfixation Inc. 800-874-7711
1520 Tradeport Dr, Jacksonville, FL 32218
Various types of ortho band material.

Cdb Corporation 910-383-6464
9201 Industrial Blvd NE, Leland, NC 28451

Classone Orthodontics, Inc. 806-799-0608
5064 50th St, Lubbock, TX 79414
Various types of bands.

Ortho-Tain, Inc.
Carr 861 # KM5.0, Pinas, Toa Alta, PR 00953
Orthodontic appliance.

Oscar, Inc. 317-849-2618
11793 Technology Ln, Fishers, IN 46038
Orthodontic band material.

Pulpdent Corp. 800-343-4342
80 Oakland St, Watertown, MA 02472
No common name listed.

Tp Orthodontics, Inc. 800-348-8856
100 Center Plz, La Porte, IN 46350
Pre-Fit, GripTite.

Unisplint Corp. 770-271-0646
4485 Commerce Dr Ste 106, Buford, GA 30518
Latex bands 3/32 inch, 12 Pks. per pkg., $15.00/pkg.

3m Unitek 800-634-5300
2724 Peck Rd, Monrovia, CA 91016

BAND, MATRIX *(Dental And Oral) 76UDY*

Denovo Dental, Inc. 800-854-7949
5130 Commerce Dr, Baldwin Park, CA 91706

Hager Worldwide, Inc. 800-328-2335
13322 Byrd Dr, Odessa, FL 33556

Hu-Friedy Manufacturing Co., Inc. 800-483-7433
3232 N Rockwell St, Chicago, IL 60618
5 types.

J.R. Rand Corp. 800-526-7111
100 S. Jeffryn Blvd. E., Deer Park, NY 11729

Miltex Inc. 800-645-8000
589 Davies Dr, York, PA 17402

Moyco Technologies, Inc. 800-331-8837
200 Commerce Dr, Montgomeryville, PA 18936

BAND, PREFORMED, ORTHODONTIC *(Dental And Oral) 76ECM*

American Orthodontics Corp. 800-558-7687
1714 Cambridge Ave, Sheboygan, WI 53081

Classone Orthodontics, Inc. 806-799-0608
5064 50th St, Lubbock, TX 79414
Molar bands.

Forestadent Usa 314-878-5985
2315 Weldon Pkwy, Saint Louis, MO 63146
Preformed orthodontic band.

G & H Wire Co. 800-526-1026
2165 Earlywood Dr, Franklin, IN 46131

Lancer Orthodontics, Inc. 760-304-2705
253 Pawnee St, San Marcos, CA 92078
Various sizes and types of orthodontic preformed bands.

Ortho Organizers, Inc. 760-448-8730
1822 Aston Ave, Carlsbad, CA 92008
Preformed orthodontic metal bands.

Ortho-Tain, Inc.
Carr 861 # KM5.0, Pinas, Toa Alta, PR 00953
Various sizes of preformed activator positioners orthodontic.

Orthodontic Design And Production, Inc. 760-734-3995
1370 Decision St Ste D, Vista, CA 92081
Various types of band, preformed orthodontic.

3m Unitek 800-634-5300
2724 Peck Rd, Monrovia, CA 91016

BAND, SUPPORT, PELVIC *(Physical Med) 89ISR*

A&A Orthopedics, Incorporated 757-224-0177
12250 SW 129th Ct Bldg 1, Miami, FL 33186
Pelvic traction support.

Aztec Heart, Inc. 530-533-7069
2445 Oro Dam Blvd E Ste 7, Oroville, CA 95966
Chest and rib support.

BAND, SUPPORT, PELVIC *(cont'd)*

Barjan Mfg., Ltd. 631-420-5588
28 Baiting Place Rd, Farmingdale, NY 11735
No common name listed.

Biomet, Inc. 574-267-6639
56 E Bell Dr, PO Box 587, Warsaw, IN 46582
Various types of pelvic support belts.

Coopercare Lastrap Inc 416-741-9675
Highway H, Koopman Ln., Elkhorn, WI 53121
Lastrap braces for repetitive strain/soft tissue injuries.

Hipsavers, Inc. 800-358-4477
7 Hubbard St, Canton, MA 02021

Ita-Med Co. 888-9IT-AMED
310 Littlefield Ave, South San Francisco, CA 94080
Complete range.

Patterson Medical Supply, Inc. 262-387-8720
W68N158 Evergreen Blvd, Cedarburg, WI 53012
Altus support belt.

Serola Biomechanics, Inc. 815-636-2780
5281 Zenith Pkwy, Loves Park, IL 61111

The Saunders Group 800-445-9836
4250 Norex Dr, Chaska, MN 55318
Back support.

Therafin Corporation 800-843-7234
19747 Wolf Rd, Mokena, IL 60448
Various pelvic positioning products.

BAND, SWEAT *(General) 80WXC*

General Econopak, Inc. 888-871-8568
1725 N 6th St, Philadelphia, PA 19122
Highly absorbent, non-allergenic, universal size.

Ultracell Medical Technologies, Inc. 877-SPO-NGE1
183 Providence New London Tpke, North Stonington, CT 06359
ULTRACELL, P.V.A. headband.

BANDAGE, ADHESIVE *(Surgery) 79KGX*

Access Business Group Llc 616-787-4964
7575 E Fulton St, Ada, MI 49355
Magnet adhesive.

Advanced Wound Systems, Llc. 541-867-4726
4909 S. Coast Hwy. Suite 245, Newport, OR 97365
Transparent adhesive bandage, semi-transparent adhesive bandage.

Afassco, Inc. 800-441-6774
2244 Park Pl Ste C, Minden, NV 89423
All sizes plastic and elastic adhesive bandages, including Hydrocolloids.

Ambu A/S 457-225-2210
6740 Baymeadow Dr, Glen Burnie, MD 21060
Adhesive tape and bandage.

American White Cross - Houston 609-514-4744
15200 North Fwy, Houston, TX 77090
Various types of adhesive bandages and tapes.

Argentum Medical Llc 708-927-9398
424 Stamp Creek Rd Ste F, Salem, SC 29676
Medical adhesive tape and adhesive bandage.

Arthrex, Inc. 239-643-5553
1370 Creekside Blvd, Naples, FL 34108
Bandage.

Aso Corporation 941-379-0300
300 Sarasota Center Blvd, Sarasota, FL 34240
Various shapes and sizes of Plastic, Sheer, Clear, Fabric, Foam and Decorated adhesive bandages.

Aso Llc 941-379-0300
12120 Esther Lama Dr Ste 112, El Paso, TX 79936
Adhesive bandages.

Avent S.A. De C.V. 602-748-6900
Camino De Libramiento, Km. 1.5, Nogales, Sonora Mexico
Vaious sizes and colors of elastic bandages of medical uses

Beacon Promotions, Inc. 507-354-3900
2121 S Bridge St, New Ulm, MN 56073
Various types of medical adhesive tape and bandage.

Beekley Corp. 860-583-4700
150 Dolphin Rd, Bristol, CT 06010
Adhesive cover, various sizes.

Brady Precision Converting, Llc 214-275-9595
1801 Big Town Blvd Ste 100, Mesquite, TX 75149
Custom manufactured bandages with a variety of sizes and shapes.

BANDAGE, ADHESIVE *(cont'd)*

Brennen Medical, Llc 651-429-7413
1290 Hammond Rd, Saint Paul, MN 55110
Wound closure tape.

Briggs Corporation 800-247-2343
PO Box 1698, 7300 Westown Pkwy., Des Moines, IA 50306

Bsn-Jobst 704-554-9933
5825 Carnegie Blvd, Charlotte, NC 28209
Island dressing.

C.B. Medical L.L.C. 860-693-2103
26 Center St, Collinsville, CT 06019
Various types & styles of sterile adhesive tape and bandages.

Certified Safety Manufacturing 800-854-7474
1400 Chestnut Ave, Kansas City, MO 64127
CERTI-STRIPS, all sizes.

Concept Health, Llc 215-364-3600
3600 Boundbrook Ave, Trevose, PA 19053
Wound dressing.

Cytyc Surgical Products 800-442-9892
250 Campus Dr, Marlborough, MA 01752
Medical adhesive tape and adhesive bandage.

Dexcom, Inc. 858-200-0200
6340 Sequence Dr, San Diego, CA 92121
Medical adhesive.

Dixie Ems Supply 800-347-3494
385 Union Ave, Brooklyn, NY 11211
$38.60 per 1000 (1in x 3in).

Dumex Medical Surgical Products Ltd. 800-463-9613
104 Shorting Rd., Scarborough, ONT M1S 3S4 Canada
DuBoot 2 layer system: medical adhesive tape and bandages.

Etchells Technology Corp. 413-587-3922
82 Industrial Dr, Northampton, MA 01060
Various.

Eye Care And Cure 800-486-6169
4646 S Overland Dr, Tucson, AZ 85714
Adhesive tape.

Facet Technologies, Llc 800-526-2387
112 Townpark Dr NW Ste 300, Kennesaw, GA 30144

Ferndale Laboratories, Inc. 248-548-0900
780 W 8 Mile Rd, Detroit, MI 48220
Adhesive liquid-glue gauze to skin.

First Response Solutions 310-537-3300
2015 E University Dr, Rancho Dominguez, CA 90220
Bandaid.

Global Medicaid Products Inc. 905-339-0666
3-1100 Invicta Dr, Oakville L6H 2K9 Canada
'bandaid'

Hartmann-Conco Inc. 800-243-2294
481 Lakeshore Pkwy, Rock Hill, SC 29730
Non-adhesive. Cohesive Medirip co-wrap. Econo-Paste conforming paste bandage. AC Tape-Plus elastic adhesive bandage. Omnifix non-woven dressing retention tape. Econo-Paste conforming paste bandage - provides moderate compression and soothing comfort for edema, lymphatic edema, dermal, vascular, and diabetic vecus, dermatitis and lower-leg trauma. Omnifix non-woven dressing retention tape - quick and secure. Complete-cover non-woven wound retention dressing that is permeable to air and water vapor. AC-Tape Plus elastic adhesive tape for maximum compression support and fixation.

Hawaii Medical, Llc 781-826-5565
750 Corporate Park Dr, Pembroke, MA 02359

Healer Products, Llc 914-663-6300
427 Commerce Ln Ste 1, West Berlin, NJ 08091
Adhesive tape.

Homecare Clinical Emergencies, Inc. 416-665-7373
21-1111 Flint Rd, North York M3J 3C7 Canada
Adhesives for application to the skin

I.Z.I. Medical Products, Inc. 800-231-1499
7020 Tudsbury Rd, Baltimore, MD 21244
Non-invasive radiographic skin markers, non-sterile.

Innova Corp. 860-242-3210
68 E Dudley Town Rd, Bloomfield, CT 06002

Johnson & Johnson Consumer Products, Inc. 800-526-3967
199 Grandview Rd, Skillman, NJ 08558
BAND-AID brand sheer, extra large, brand children's, brand plastic, brand flexible and brand medicated.

BANDAGE, ADHESIVE *(cont'd)*

Johnson & Johnson Medical Division Of Ethicon, Inc. 800-423-4018
2500 E Arbrook Blvd, Arlington, TX 76014

Jones Speciality Products 314-845-6850
4010 Nottingham Estates Dr, Saint Louis, MO 63129
Moisture barrier, aqua ban-self adhesive polyethylene.

K. W. Griffen Co. 203-846-1923
100 Pearl St, Norwalk, CT 06850
Adhesive tape.

Kentron Health Care, Inc. 615-384-0573
3604 Kelton Jackson Rd, P.o. Box 120, Springfield, TN 37172
Adhesive bandages and surgical tapes.

Kern Surgical Supply, Inc. 800-582-3939
2823 Gibson St, Bakersfield, CA 93308

Kerr Corp. 949-255-8766
1717 W Collins Ave, Orange, CA 92867
Oral bandage.

Kree Technologies Usa, Inc. 450-676-9444
11429 53rd St N, Clearwater, FL 33760
Pink tape.

Legend Aerospace, Inc. 305-883-8804
8300 NW South River Dr, Medley, FL 33166

Lemaitre Vascular, Inc. 781-221-2266
63 2nd Ave, Burlington, MA 01803
GLOW 'N TELL TAPE radiopaque, adhesive, tape ruler in 30cm length. LEMAITRE STENT GUIDE, radiopaque adhesive tape for stent implantations. 270 millimeter length. GLOW'N TELL TAPE FOR DORSAL PLACEMENT, radiopaque, flexible, adhesive tape with centimeter marking for easy reading and precise location. Stent graft guide, radiopaque, flexible, adhesive tape with unique bifurcated design for angioplasty, stent and stent graft procedures. Easy to measure vessel sizes, place stents and insert balloons.

Lifescience Plus, Inc. 650-565-8172
473 Sapena Ct Ste 7, Santa Clara, CA 95054
Bandage.

Lohmann & Rauscher, Inc. 800-279-3863
6001 SW 6th Ave Ste 101, Topeka, KS 66615

Marine Polymer Technologies, Inc. 888-666-2560
461 Boston St Unit B5, Topsfield, MA 01983
Adhesive bandage.

Marlen Manufacturing & Development Co. 216-292-7060
5150 Richmond Rd, Bedford, OH 44146
SKIN-TITE adhesive skin barrier.

Maxpak, Llc 863-682-0123
2808 New Tampa Hwy, Lakeland, FL 33815
Waterproof tape, adhesive bandages.

Medi Inc 800-225-8634
75 York Ave, P.O. Box 302, Randolph, MA 02368
Flexible bandages & underwrap.

Medical Action Industries, Inc. 800-645-7042
25 Heywood Rd, Arden, NC 28704
Tape.

Medspring Group, Inc. 801-295-9750
533 W 2600 S Ste 105, Bountiful, UT 84010
Bandage.

Medtronic Ep Systems 763-514-4000
8299 Central Ave NE, Spring Lake Park, Minneapolis, MN 55432
Medical adhesive tape and adhesive bandage.

Medtronic Vascular 707-525-0111
3576 Unocal Pl, Santa Rosa, CA 95403
Wound dressing

Miami Medical Equipment & Supply Corp. 305-592-0111
2150 NW 93rd Ave, Doral, FL 33172

Microstim Technology, Inc. 772-283-0408
1849 SW Crane Creek Ave, Palm City, FL 34990
Injection site dressing.

Mine Safety Appliances Company 866-MSA-1001
121 Gamma Dr, Pittsburgh, PA 15238

Mowbray Co., Inc. 800-325-5787
706 Sheridan Rd, Waterloo, IA 50701
Pre-tape or dressing adhesive.

Nearly Me Technologies, Inc. 800-887-3370
3630 South I 35, Suite A, Waco, TX 76702-1475
Adhesive tape.

BANDAGE, ADHESIVE *(cont'd)*

Normed 800-288-8200
PO Box 3644, Seattle, WA 98124
Various adhesive/non-adhesive, sterile/non-sterile bandages.

North Safety Products 401-943-4400
1101 B Calle Neutron, Parque Industrial Maran, Mexicali, B.c. Mexico
Adhesive tape

Norwood Promotional Products, Inc. 651-388-1298
5151 Moundview Dr, Red Wing, MN 55066
Finger bandage.

Omega Medical Products Corp. 888-837-TAPE
494 Saw Mill River Rd, Yonkers, NY 10701
Medical Adhesive Tape

Orange-Sol Medical Products, Inc. 800-877-7771
1400 N Fiesta Blvd Ste 100, Gilbert, AZ 85233

Ossur Americas 949-268-3155
742 Pancho Rd, Camarillo, CA 93012

P M Assoc. 828-324-5739
826 Airport Road, Hickory, NC 28601
Leukotape combo kit-item 76103001. Packaging and labeling only.

Parker Anderson Llc 888-799-4289
5030 Paradise Rd Ste A214, Las Vegas, NV 89119
Medical adhesive tape and adhesive bandage.

Premier Brands Of America, Inc. 914-667-6200
120 Pearl St, Mount Vernon, NY 10550
Various wart, callus, and corn removers.

Quadris Medical 507-389-4319
2030 Lookout Dr, North Mankato, MN 56003
Various styles and types of adhesive tapes,adhesive skin closures,surgical tapes.

Raleigh Lions Clinic For The Blind, Inc. 919-256-4220
3200 Bush St, Raleigh, NC 27609
Adhesive tape, surgical.

Respond Industries, Inc. 1-800-523-8999
9500 Woodend Rd, Edwardsville, KS 66111
Various sizes & styles of adhesive bandages & tape.

Schering-Plough Healthcare Products, Inc. 862-245-5115
4207 Michigan Avenue Rd NE, Cleveland, TN 37323
Blister cushions.

Scivolutions, Inc. 704-853-0100
2260 Raeford Ct, Gastonia, NC 28052
Adhesive bandages.

Smi 920-876-3361
Industrial Park, 544 Sohn Drive, Elkhart Lake, WI 53020

Smith & Nephew, Inc. 800-876-1261
11775 Starkey Rd, Largo, FL 33773
UNIFLEX transparent dressing.

Span Packaging Services Llc. 864-627-4155
4611A Dairy Dr, Greenville, SC 29607
Gelocast unna's boot bandage.

Sun Glitz Corp. 800-287-0911
111 S McVicker Dr, Energy, IL 62933
Polyvinyl foam self-sticking non adhesive, latex free bandage.

Sunmed Usa Llc. 310-531-8222
841 Apollo St Ste 334, El Segundo, CA 90245

Tailored Label Products, Inc. 800-727-1344
W165N5731 Ridgewood Dr, Menomonee Falls, WI 53051

Tampa Work Services 813-663-9555
5602 E Columbus Dr, Tampa, FL 33619
Waterproof tape; adhesive bandages.

Tellus Medical Products, Inc. 760-200-9772
77971 Wildcat Dr Ste C, Palm Desert, CA 92211
Fabric adhesive bandage.

Uresil, Llc 800-538-7374
5418 Touhy Ave, Skokie, IL 60077
TRU-FIX external catheter fixation systems.

Vector Firstaid, Inc. 800-999-4423
316 N Corona Ave, Ontario, CA 91764

Vonex Medical Supplies Inc. 888-866-3920
29-601 Magnetic Dr., Toronto M3J 3J2 Canada
Various types of sterile band-aids

Webtec Converting, Llc. 865-246-4342
5900 Middleview Way, Knoxville, TN 37909
Finger bandage.

BANDAGE, ADHESIVE *(cont'd)*

Western Medical, Ltd. 800-628-8276
214 Carnegie Ctr Ste 100, Princeton, NJ 08540
FLEXOPLAST elastic adhesive bandage.

3m Company 651-733-4365
601 22nd Ave S, Brookings, SD 57006

3m Hutchinson 320-234-2000
905 Adams St SE, Hutchinson, MN 55350
Various types & styles of adhesive tape,surgical tape,bandages & dispenser tapes.

BANDAGE, BUTTERFLY *(General) 80QCH*

Brady Corporation 800-541-1686
6555 W Good Hope Rd, PO Box 571, Milwaukee, WI 53223
Custom butterfly bandages manufactured to customer specifications.

Durden Enterprises 800-554-5673
1317 4th Ave, P.O. Box 909, Auburn, GA 30011
7007B Butterfly Dressing - butterfly shape pressure dressing for use on femoral puncture site after angioplasty or any other biopsy puncture site.

Smi 920-876-3361
Industrial Park, 544 Sohn Drive, Elkhart Lake, WI 53020

Tailored Label Products, Inc. 800-727-1344
W165N5731 Ridgewood Dr, Menomonee Falls, WI 53051

BANDAGE, CAST *(Physical Med) 89ITG*

Bct Midwest, Inc. 785-856-1414
1220 Wagon Wheel Rd, Lawrence, KS 66049
Cast tape,synthetic.

Bsn Medical, Inc 800-552-1157
5825 Carnegie Blvd, Charlotte, NC 28209
M-PACT® PLASTER is designed for rapid wetting and excellent lamination. The bright, white plaster has a creamy texture for a smooth finish.

Carolina Narrow Fabric Co. 336-631-3000
1100 Patterson Ave, Winston Salem, NC 27101
Various.

Centurion Medical Products Corp. 517-545-1135
3310 S Main St, Salisbury, NC 28147

Custom Healthcare Systems, Inc. 804-421-5959
4205 Eubank Rd, Richmond, VA 23231

Customs Hospital Products, Inc 800-426-2780
6336 SE 107th Ave, Portland, OR 97266
Multiple-non-sterile.

Debusk Orthopedic Casting (Doc) 865-362-2334
420 Straight Creek Rd Ste 1, New Tazewell, TN 37825
Various types of cast bandages.

Degasa, S.A. De C.V. 525-5-483 31
Prolongacion Canal De, Miramontes #3775 Col. Ex-Hacienda San Juan Del. Tlalpan Mexico
(multiple 3) protec sponge gauze, protec gauze bandage & protec gauze roll

Depuy Orthopaedics, Inc. 800-473-3789
700 Orthopaedic Dr, P.O. Box 988, Warsaw, IN 46582
Various types of cast bandages.

Depuy-Raynham, A Div. Of Depuy Orthopaedics 800-451-2006
325 Paramount Dr, Raynham, MA 02767
Various types of cast bandages.

DJO Inc. 800-336-6569
1430 Decision St, Vista, CA 92081
Stockinette in various sizes.

Ebi Patient Care, Inc. 973-299-9300
1 Electro-biology Blvd., Guaynabo, PR 00657
Cast, bandage.

Elwyn Industries Products. 610-364-3551
2047 Bridgewater Rd, Aston, PA 19014

Great Lakes Innovation Inc 248-680-8671
1103 Winthrop Dr, Troy, MI 48083
Innolife stair climbing walker.

Hartmann-Conco Inc. 800-243-2294
481 Lakeshore Pkwy, Rock Hill, SC 29730
Dema-Pad--non-woven padding bandage used for extra protection to delicate and traumatized skin.

Just Packaging Inc. 908-753-6700
450 Oak Tree Ave, South Plainfield, NJ 07080
Various types of casting material.

BANDAGE, CAST *(cont'd)*

Kendall De Mexico, S.A. De C.V. 508-261-8000
Piniente 44, No. 3401, 16 D.f, Co. San Salvador Xochimanca Mexico City Mexico
Cast bandage

Lohmann & Rauscher, Inc. 800-279-3863
6001 SW 6th Ave Ste 101, Topeka, KS 66615

Mizuho Osi 800-777-4674
30031 Ahern Ave, Union City, CA 94587

Ossur Americas 949-268-3155
742 Pancho Rd, Camarillo, CA 93012

Paramedical Distributors 800-245-3278
2020 Grand Blvd, Kansas City, MO 64108

Polygell Llc. 973-884-8995
30 Leslie Ct, Whippany, NJ 07981
Various type of non-medicated toe, callace, bunion pad.

Rx Textiles, Inc. 704-283-9787
3107 Chamber Dr, Monroe, NC 28110
Prosthetic and orthotic accessories.

Smith & Nephew Casting & Bandaging Sa. De Cv 012-82-61774
Ave.de Los Encinos S/n Esq.ave, Del Parque,parque Ind. Villa Florida, Reynosa Tamaulipas Mexico
Various

Smith & Nephew Inc. 800-463-7439
2100 52nd Ave., Lachine, QUE H8T 2Y5 Canada
GYPSONA plaster of paris and DYNACAST XR fibreglass cast bandages.

Sturges Manufacturing Company, Inc. 315-732-6159
2030 Sunset Ave, Utica, NY 13502
Leg sling.

Tri-State Hospital Supply Corp. 517-545-1135
3173 E 43rd St, Yuma, AZ 85365

BANDAGE, COMPRESSION *(General) 80MHW*

Afassco, Inc. 800-441-6774
2244 Park Pl Ste C, Minden, NV 89423

Anodyne Therapy, Llc 813-645-2855
13570 Wright Cir, Tampa, FL 33626
Compression dressing.

Biacare Corporation 616-931-1267
140 W Washington Ave Ste 100, Zeeland, MI 49464
Foam rubber bandage and sheets.

Coloplast Manufacturing Us, Llc 800-533-0464
1840 W Oak Pkwy, Marietta, GA 30062
CIRCAID, CIRCPLUS and THERA-BOOT non-elastic, adjustable, reusable leggings for lower leg venous disorders.

Datascope Interventional Products Division 800-225-5827
1300 MacArthur Blvd, Mahwah, NJ 07430
Safeguard pressure-assisted dressing is used to maintain hemostasis once it's been achieved. A clear window allows for visualization of puncture site. .

Dr. Len's Medical Products Llc 678-908-8180
412 Atwood Rd, Erdenheim, PA 19038
Abrams therapeutic foam sleeve.

Facet Technologies, Llc 800-526-2387
112 Townpark Dr NW Ste 300, Kennesaw, GA 30144

Gomez Packaging Corp. 973-569-9500
75 Wood St, Paterson, NJ 07524
Elastic bandage.

Hartmann-Conco Inc. 800-243-2294
481 Lakeshore Pkwy, Rock Hill, SC 29730
Shur-Band latex-free high quality reinforced elastic support and compression bandage with a self-closure flap. Lopress high-quality cotton bandage that delivers maximum compression. Conco Fourpress four-layer bandage, system containing one padding layer, one crepe bandage, one compression bandage, and one cohesive bandage. Ideal for venous siasis ulcers and related conditions.

Healer Products, Llc 914-663-6300
427 Commerce Ln Ste 1, West Berlin, NJ 08091
Bandage compress.

Hospital Marketing Svcs. Company, Inc. 800-786-5094
162 Great Hill Rd./ Ind. Park, Naugatuck, CT 06770
HMS TEMP-WRAP - large (6' wide x 30'long) cat. no. 7636, 12/case; small (4' wide x 30' long) cat. no. 7634, 12/case.

BANDAGE, COMPRESSION *(cont'd)*

Kmi Kolster Methods, Inc. 909-737-5476
3185 Palisades Dr, Corona, CA 92880
Compression dressing.

Lohmann & Rauscher, Inc. 800-279-3863
6001 SW 6th Ave Ste 101, Topeka, KS 66615

Telesto Medtech Llc 831-621-8011
635 E Rockwell St, Arlington Heights, IL 60005
Compression garment.

Tz Medical Inc. 800-944-0187
7272 SW Durham Rd Ste 800, Portland, OR 97224
Pressure pad band.

Vascular Solutions, Inc. 888-240-6001
6464 Sycamore Ct N, Maple Grove, MN 55369
Topical hemostat.

Vascular Solutions, Inc. 763-656-4300
5025 Cheshire Ln N, Plymouth, MN 55446
Topical hemostat.

BANDAGE, ELASTIC *(General) 80FQM*

A&A Orthopedics, Incorporated 757-224-0177
12250 SW 129th Ct Bldg 1, Miami, FL 33186
Elastic bandage.

Alex Orthopedic, Inc. 800-544-2539
PO Box 201442, Arlington, TX 76006

Alimed, Inc. 800-225-2610
297 High St, Dedham, MA 02026

Asheboro Elastics Corp. 336-629-2626
150 N Park St, PO Box 1143, Asheboro, NC 27203

Aso Llc 941-379-0300
12120 Esther Lama Dr Ste 112, El Paso, TX 79936
Stretch gauze.

Biacare Corporation 616-931-1267
140 W Washington Ave Ste 100, Zeeland, MI 49464
Short stretch bandage.

Biomet, Inc. 574-267-6639
56 E Bell Dr, PO Box 587, Warsaw, IN 46582
Various types of elastic bandage.

Bioseal 800-441-7325
167 W Orangethorpe Ave, Placentia, CA 92870
Sterile various styles.

Bird & Cronin, Inc. 651-683-1111
1200 Trapp Rd, Saint Paul, MN 55121
Elastic bandage.

Brennen Medical, Llc 651-429-7413
1290 Hammond Rd, Saint Paul, MN 55110
Tubular elastic bandage.

Briggs Corporation 800-247-2343
PO Box 1698, 7300 Westown Pkwy., Des Moines, IA 50306

Bsn Medical, Inc 800-552-1157
5825 Carnegie Blvd, Charlotte, NC 28209
M-PACT Elastic Bandage gives exceptional conformability for those complex anatomies or difficult casting procedures.

Bsn-Jobst 704-554-9933
5825 Carnegie Blvd, Charlotte, NC 28209
Elastic tube bandage.

Carrington Laboratories, Inc. 800-527-5216
2001 W Walnut Hill Ln, Irving, TX 75038

Centurion Medical Products Corp. 517-545-1135
3310 S Main St, Salisbury, NC 28147

Core Products International, Inc. 800-365-3047
808 Prospect Ave, Osceola, WI 54020

Covidien Lp 508-261-8000
15 Hampshire St, Mansfield, MA 02048

Cropper Medical, Inc./Bio Skin 800-541-2455
240 E Hersey St Ste 2, Ashland, OR 97520
Orthopedic compression support.

Custom Healthcare Systems, Inc. 804-421-5959
4205 Eubank Rd, Richmond, VA 23231

Cypress Medical Products 800-334-3646
1202 S. Rte. 31, McHenry, IL 60050
Rubber elastic bandages, 2in., 3in., 4in., or 6in. Five boxes per case.

Debusk Orthopedic Casting (Doc) 865-362-2334
420 Straight Creek Rd Ste 1, New Tazewell, TN 37825
Elastic bandage.

BANDAGE, ELASTIC *(cont'd)*

Degasa, S.A. De C.V. 525-5-483 31
Prolongacion Canal De, Miramontes #3775 Col. Ex-Hacienda San Juan Del. Tlalpan Mexico
Bandage, elastic

Demetech Corp. 888-324-2447
3530 NW 115th Ave, Doral, FL 33178
Elastic cohesive bandage.

Depuy Orthopaedics, Inc. 800-473-3789
700 Orthopaedic Dr, P.O. Box 988, Warsaw, IN 46582
Various types of elastic bandages.

DJO Inc. 800-336-6569
1430 Decision St, Vista, CA 92081
Various types and sizes of bandages.

Dome Publishing Company, Inc. 401-738-7900
10 New England Way, Warwick, RI 02886
Athletic tape/bandage.

Dukal Corporation 800-243-0741
5 Plant Ave, Hauppauge, NY 11788

Dumex Medical Surgical Products Ltd. 800-463-9613
104 Shorting Rd., Scarborough, ONT M1S 3S4 Canada
DUFLEX Conforming bandage - gentle elasticity provides secure fir, minimizes bunching. Dufore 4 Layer System: four layer compression system. Tresflex 3 Layer System: three layer compresion system

Dynarex Corp. 888-356-2739
10 Glenshaw St, Orangeburg, NY 10962
Poly-wrapped, available in four sizes.

Elastic Corporation Of America 704-328-5381
455 Highway 70, Columbiana, AL 35051
Various sizes of elastic bandages.

First Aid Bandage Co., Inc. 888-813-8214
3 State Pier Rd, New London, CT 06320
Ortho-Flex latex-free elastic bandage.

Fulflex Of Vermont, Inc. 802-257-5256
32 Justin Holden Dr, Brattleboro, VT 05301
Esmark medical bandage-sterile and non-sterile.

Gelsmart Llc 973-884-8995
30 Leslie Ct Ste B-202, Whippany, NJ 07981
Various types of elastic braces for arch and ankle.

Gf Health Products, Inc. 678-291-3288
131 Clay St, Central Falls, RI 02863

Global Healthcare 800-601-3880
1495 Hembree Rd Ste 700, Roswell, GA 30076
Various sizes.

H & H Associates, Inc. 757-224-0177
4173 G.w. Memorial Highway, Ordinary, VA 23131
Elastic bandage.

Hartmann-Conco Inc. 800-243-2294
481 Lakeshore Pkwy, Rock Hill, SC 29730
Contex LF, Deluxe, REB elastic bandages. Eze-Band latex-free double-Velcro rubber elastic bandage. Co-Lastic high-quality cohesive elastic wrap, versatile enough to use as a securing protective compression and support bandage. Flexitube tubular gauze bandage--holds dressings securely in place.

Healer Products, Llc 914-663-6300
427 Commerce Ln Ste 1, West Berlin, NJ 08091
Elastic bandage.

Health Care Logistics, Inc. 800-848-1633
450 Town St, PO Box 25, Circleville, OH 43113
Sterile elastic bandage.

Home-Aid-Healthcare, Inc. 888-297-9109
PO Box 801764, Santa Clarita, CA 91380
WRAP-AID, non-sterile elastic bandages in 2', 3', 4' and 6' width by 4.5 yrds stretched. Available with clips or Velcro closures (similar to Ace brand elastic bandage).

Hospital Marketing Svcs. Company, Inc. 800-786-5094
162 Great Hill Rd./ Ind. Park, Naugatuck, CT 06770
HMS TEMP-WRAP 30in. long bandage with pocket for cold packs - large (6in. wide), cat. no. 7666, 12/case; small (4in. wide), cat. no. 7665, 12/case.

Hydro-Med Products, Inc. 214-350-5100
3400 Royalty Row, Irving, TX 75062
Bandage, elastic.

Innova Corp. 860-242-3210
68 E Dudley Town Rd, Bloomfield, CT 06002

BANDAGE, ELASTIC *(cont'd)*

Innovate Medical, L.L.C. 423-854-9694
225 White Top Rd. Ext., Bluff City, TN 37618
Various types of latex and latex free elastic bandages.elastic bandages or esma.

Ita-Med Co. 888-9IT-AMED
310 Littlefield Ave, South San Francisco, CA 94080

Johnson & Johnson Medical Division Of Ethicon, Inc. 800-423-4018
2500 E Arbrook Blvd, Arlington, TX 76014

Judah Mfg. Corp. 800-618-9792
13657 Jupiter Rd Ste 100, Dallas, TX 75238
Compression orthoisis (back brace).

K. W. Griffen Co. 203-846-1923
100 Pearl St, Norwalk, CT 06850
Elastic bandage.

Kennedy Center, Inc. 203-365-8522
2440 Reservoir Ave, Trumbull, CT 06611
Elastic bandage.

Kentron Health Care, Inc. 615-384-0573
3604 Kelton Jackson Rd, P.o. Box 120, Springfield, TN 37172
Elastic bandage.

Kerma Medical Products, Inc. 757-398-8400
400 Port Centre Pkwy, Portsmouth, VA 23704
Bandage, various sizes.

Laboratorios Jaloma, S.A. De C.V. 3-617-5010
Aquiles Serdan No. 438, Guadalajara, Jalisco Mexico
Bandage, elastic

Legend Aerospace, Inc. 305-883-8804
8300 NW South River Dr, Medley, FL 33166

Levine Health Products 800-426-6763
21101 NE 108th St, Redmond, WA 98053
Elastic bandages with clips and elastic bandages with velcro.

Lohmann & Rauscher, Inc. 800-279-3863
6001 SW 6th Ave Ste 101, Topeka, KS 66615

Maxpak, Llc 863-682-0123
2808 New Tampa Hwy, Lakeland, FL 33815
Stretch gauze.

Medi-Tech International Corp. 800-333-0109
26 Court St, Brooklyn, NY 11242
Open netted tubular elastic dressing retainer.

Medicom 800-361-2862
9404 Cote de Liesse, Lachine, QUE H8T 1A1 Canada

Medikmark Inc. 800-424-8520
3600 Burwood Dr, Waukegan, IL 60085

Medline Manufacturing And Services Llc 847-837-2759
1 Medline Pl, Mundelein, IL 60060
Bandages,various sizes.

Normed 800-288-8200
PO Box 3644, Seattle, WA 98124
Various types & sizes of elastic bandges.

Omni Medical Supply Inc. 800-860-6664
4153 Pioneer Dr, Commerce Township, MI 48390

Orange-Sol Medical Products, Inc. 800-877-7771
1400 N Fiesta Blvd Ste 100, Gilbert, AZ 85233

Ortho-Med, Inc. 800-547-5571
3208 SE 13th Ave, Portland, OR 97202
Elastic soft goods.

Ossur Americas 949-268-3155
742 Pancho Rd, Camarillo, CA 93012

Paramedical Distributors 800-245-3278
2020 Grand Blvd, Kansas City, MO 64108
COMPRESSOPAW tubular elastic bandage for post-declaw surgery in pets.

Patterson Medical Supply, Inc. 262-387-8720
W68N158 Evergreen Blvd, Cedarburg, WI 53012
Hapla stockinette; foam padding; countor foam polycushion.

Pedifix, Inc. 800-424-5561
310 Guinea Rd, Brewster, NY 10509

Pedinol Pharmacal, Inc. 800-733-4665
30 Banfi Plz N, Farmingdale, NY 11735

Polygell Llc. 973-884-8995
30 Leslie Ct, Whippany, NJ 07981
Various type of elastic braces for arch and ankle.

BANDAGE, ELASTIC *(cont'd)*

Qmd Medical 800-665-9950
9800 Clark St., Montreal, QUE H3L 2R3 Canada
Rubber elastic bandages.

Respond Industries, Inc. 1-800-523-8999
9500 Woodend Rd, Edwardsville, KS 66111
Various sizes & styles of elastic bandages & bandage compresses.

Richardson Products, Inc. 888-928-7297
9408 Gulfstream Rd, Frankfort, IL 60423
Bandage.

Rush Medical 401-461-9132
18 Gallup Ave, Cranston, RI 02910
Wrist strap.

Rx Textiles, Inc. 704-283-9787
3107 Chamber Dr, Monroe, NC 28110
Elastic bandage.

Sanax Protective Products, Inc. 800-379-9929
236 Upland Ave, Newton Highlands, MA 02461

Shelby Elastics, Llc Of North Carolina 800-562-4507
639 N Post Rd, Shelby, NC 28150
Elastic bandage-various types.

Sportsbands, Inc. 302-322-1148
181 S Dupont Hwy, New Castle, DE 19720
Various elastic patches,pads, bandages, wraps, muscle wraps & bands.

Tape-O-Corporation 800-752-4944
35 Crosby Rd, Dover, NH 03820
COHERE, all nylon, cohesive elastic bandage wrap, latex and latex-free. Comprable to Coban and Coflex. COTEAR, all cotton, cohesive elastic bandage wrap, latex and latex-free. Comparable to Medi-rip and Powerflex.

Tapeless Wound Care Products, Llc. 866-714-9199
PO Box 4515, Englewood, CO 80155
Tapeless wound dressing holder.

Tellus Medical Products, Inc. 760-200-9772
77971 Wildcat Dr Ste C, Palm Desert, CA 92211
Elastic bandage.

Tetra Medical Supply Corp. 800-621-4041
6364 W Gross Point Rd, Niles, IL 60714

Tillotson Healthcare Corp. 888-335-7500
10 Glenshaw St, Orangeburg, NY 10962
POLY STRETCH, sterile and non-sterile, rayon/poly blend stretch conforming bandage. Features a comfortable stretch to conform to body contours with moderate compression allowing ease of movement.

Tri-Fi Knitting, Llc 423-855-0501
4641 Shallowford Rd, Chattanooga, TN 37411
Elastic bandage.

Tri-State Hospital Supply Corp. 517-545-1135
3173 E 43rd St, Yuma, AZ 85365

Web-Tex, Inc. 888-633-2723
5445 De Gaspe Ave., Ste. 702, Montreal, QC H2T 3B2 Canada

Western Medical, Ltd. 800-628-8276
214 Carnegie Ctr Ste 100, Princeton, NJ 08540

Zimmer Holdings, Inc. 800-613-6131
1800 W Center St, PO Box 708, Warsaw, IN 46580

Zimmer Orthopaedic Surgical Products 800-321-5533
PO Box 10, 200 West Ohio Ave., Dover, OH 44622
ZIM-FLEX.

3m Company 651-733-4365
601 22nd Ave S, Brookings, SD 57006

BANDAGE, GAUZE *(General) 80QCI*

Afassco, Inc. 800-441-6774
2244 Park Pl Ste C, Minden, NV 89423

Amd-Ritmed, Inc. 800-445-0340
295 Firetower Road, Tonawanda, NY 14150

Brasel Products, Inc. 630-879-3759
715 Hunter Dr, Batavia, IL 60510
BANTEX cohesive bandages & tapes.

Briggs Corporation 800-247-2343
PO Box 1698, 7300 Westown Pkwy., Des Moines, IA 50306

Crosstex International 800-223-2497
10 Ranick Rd, Hauppauge, NY 11788
Nonwoven Gauze,All Gauze, & Cotton Filled

BANDAGE, GAUZE *(cont'd)*

Crosstex International Ltd., W. Region 800-707-2737
14059 Stage Rd, Santa Fe Springs, CA 90670

Crosstex International,Inc. 888-276-7783
10 Ranick Rd, Hauppauge, NY 11788
CROSSTEX.

Csi Holdings 615-452-9633
170 Commerce Way, Gallatin, TN 37066

Dermapac, Inc. 203-924-7148
PO Box 852, Shelton, CT 06484

Dixie Ems Supply 800-347-3494
385 Union Ave, Brooklyn, NY 11211
$15.23 per 10 (3in x 10yds).

Dukal Corporation 800-243-0741
5 Plant Ave, Hauppauge, NY 11788
Stringed-indexed gauze, various sizes and plys available.

Dumex Medical Surgical Products Ltd. 800-463-9613
104 Shorting Rd., Scarborough, ONT M1S 3S4 Canada
THALAFIX, sea salt guaze dressing. Natural sea salt impregnated guaze dressing.

Dynarex Corp. 888-356-2739
10 Glenshaw St, Orangeburg, NY 10962
Two ply construction, available in four sizes.

Gentell 800-840-9041
3600 Boundbrook Ave, Trevose, PA 19053
GENTELL Hydrogel Impregnated Gauze dressings are pre-cut, pre-saturated, 12 ply gauze pads ready for use. Using the same aloe-barbadenisis, aloe-vera based hydrating gel, these dressings provide the and maintain the moist environment necessary to enhance the wound healing process. Available in 2' x 2' and 4' x 4' sizes.

Hartmann-Conco Inc. 800-243-2294
481 Lakeshore Pkwy, Rock Hill, SC 29730
Flexicon elastic gauze bandage. Also available, Flexi-Paste, a quality stretch-gauze bandage designed to provide moderate compression and soothing comfort when used for edema, lymphatic edema, dermal, vascular and diabetic ulcers, dermatitis and lower-leg trauma. Conco Medical Bulky Gauze, used to pad and protect wounds, very absorbent.

Home-Aid-Healthcare, Inc. 888-297-9109
PO Box 801764, Santa Clarita, CA 91380
CONFORM-A-GAUZE, non-sterile conforming stretch gauze bandage in 2', 3', 4' and 6' width by 4.1 yrds stretched.

Innova Corp. 860-242-3210
68 E Dudley Town Rd, Bloomfield, CT 06002

Johnson & Johnson Medical Division Of Ethicon, Inc. 800-423-4018
2500 E Arbrook Blvd, Arlington, TX 76014

Lohmann & Rauscher, Inc. 800-279-3863
6001 SW 6th Ave Ste 101, Topeka, KS 66615

Mine Safety Appliances Company 866-MSA-1001
121 Gamma Dr, Pittsburgh, PA 15238

Omni Medical Supply Inc. 800-860-6664
4153 Pioneer Dr, Commerce Township, MI 48390

Qmd Medical 800-665-9950
9800 Clark St., Montreal, QUE H3L 2R3 Canada
Conforming gauze bandages, sterile and non-sterile

Schueler & Company, Inc. 516-487-1500
PO Box 528, Stratford, CT 06615

Web-Tex, Inc. 888-633-2723
5445 De Gaspe Ave., Ste. 702, Montreal, QC H2T 3B2 Canada

Western Medical, Ltd. 800-628-8276
214 Carnegie Ctr Ste 100, Princeton, NJ 08540
PRIMER 3in. and 4in. UNNA boot. PRIMER UNNA-PAK bandage with Co-Press self-adherent bandages. 3in. and 4in. available.

BANDAGE, LIQUID *(Surgery) 79KMF*

Ac Healthcare Supply, Inc. 905-448-4706
11651 230th St, Cambria Heights, NY 11411
Liquid bandage.

Adhezion Biomedical, Llc 610-431-2398
506 Pine Mountain Rd, Hudson, NC 28638
Liquid bandage.

American Spraytech, L.L.C. 908-725-6060
205 Meister Ave, Branchburg, NJ 08876
Adhesive aid, tincture benzoin compound aerosol.

BANDAGE, LIQUID *(cont'd)*

Argentum Medical Llc 708-927-9398
424 Stamp Creek Rd Ste F, Salem, SC 29676
Sterile wound dressing.

Aso Corporation 941-379-0300
300 Sarasota Center Blvd, Sarasota, FL 34240

Biocore Medical Technologies, Inc. 301-740-1893
13851 90th St, Oskaloosa, KS 66066
Sterile wound care dressings.

Cardinal Health 200, Inc. 913-451-0880
1550 Northwestern Dr, El Paso, TX 79912
Compound benzoin tincture usp sepp.

Chemence Medical Products Inc. 770-664-6624
185 Bluegrass Valley Pkwy Ste 100, Alpharetta, GA 30005
Sterile liquid occlusive wound bandage.

Del Pharmaceuticals, Inc. 516-844-2020
1830 Carver Dr, Rocky Point, NC 28457
Liquid bandage.

Derma Sciences 609-514-4744
214 Carnegie Ctr Ste 300, Princeton, NJ 08540
DERMAGRAN wound cleanser with zinc.

Dumex Medical Surgical Products Ltd. 800-463-9613
104 Shorting Rd., Scarborough, ONT M1S 3S4 Canada
Thalafix Natural Seasalt Dressing: dry dressing impregnated with crystalline sea water. Dumex Pak-Its non-woven dressing impregnated with sodium chloride, for paking wounds.

Epikeia, Inc. 210-313-4600
500 Sandau Rd Ste 200, San Antonio, TX 78216
Liquid skin protectant.

Hanson Medical, Inc. 800-771-2215
825 Riverside Ave Ste 2, Paso Robles, CA 93446
Scarfade, scar gel;

Hemcon Medical Technologies, Inc. 877-247-0196
10575 SW Cascade Ave Ste 130, Portland, OR 97223
Hemostatic wound dressing for control of moderate and severe external hemorrhage.

Johnson & Johnson Medical Division Of Ethicon, Inc. 800-423-4018
2500 E Arbrook Blvd, Arlington, TX 76014

Kentron Health Care, Inc. 615-384-0573
3604 Kelton Jackson Rd, P.o. Box 120, Springfield, TN 37172
Adhesive aid, tincture benzoin compound aerosol.

Marine Polymer Technologies, Inc. 888-666-2560
461 Boston St Unit B5, Topsfield, MA 01983
Liquide bandage.

Medchem Products, Inc. 908-277-8000
160 New Boston St, Woburn, MA 01801
Primary wound dressing, sterile.

Medtronic Ep Systems 763-514-4000
8299 Central Ave NE, Spring Lake Park, Minneapolis, MN 55432
Liquid bandge.

Revalesio Corporation 253-922-2600
5102 20th St E Ste 100, Fife, WA 98424
Sterile saline solution.

Rynel, Inc. 207-882-0200
11 Twin Rivers Dr, Wiscasset, ME 04578
Hydrophilic polyurethane dressing.

Xennovate Medical Llc 765-939-2037
1080 University Blvd, Richmond, IN 47374
Hydrocolloid wound dressing.

BANDAGE, OTHER *(General) 80QCO*

Amd-Ritmed, Inc. 800-445-0340
295 Firetower Road, Tonawanda, NY 14150

Bovie Medical Corp. 800-537-2790
5115 Ulmerton Rd, Clearwater, FL 33760
Eye bubble.

Brasel Products, Inc. 630-879-3759
715 Hunter Dr, Batavia, IL 60510
PROTECTAPE; Cohesive bandages and tapes.

Crosswell International Corporation 305-648-0777
101 Madeira Ave, Coral Gables, FL 33134

Cypress Medical Products 800-334-3646
1202 S. Rte. 31, McHenry, IL 60050
Esmark bandages, sterile and individually wrapped.

BANDAGE, OTHER *(cont'd)*

Dumex Medical Surgical Products Ltd. 800-463-9613
104 Shorting Rd., Scarborough, ONT M1S 3S4 Canada
GAZETEX Washed cotton bandage - 100% cotton, Rymple weave, low lint for superior performance. Bandage rolls, 100% cotton, low lint, high absorbancy. Also available, DUFORM conforming bandage is a rayon/nylon blend that provides elasticity, maximizes absorbency ans ensures a virtually lint free bandage.

Exelint International Co. 800-940-3935
5840 W Centinela Ave, Los Angeles, CA 90045
EXEL Zorband pressure bandage.

Ferris Mfg Corp. 800-765-9636
16 W300 83rd St., Burr Ridge, IL 60527-5848
PolyMem Wound Care Dressings, The Pink Dressing. A unique patented formula in 28 sizes and configurations include, non-adhesives, Island Dressings, Strips, Cavity Fillers, Calcium Alginates, Super Thick and Silver dressings

Gentell 800-840-9041
3600 Boundbrook Ave, Trevose, PA 19053
GENTELL BORDERED GAUZE is a multi-purpose, all inclusive wound dressing that saves nursing time and is gentle to delicate skin. A non-adherent pad is paired with a conforming beveled spun lace tape to create a secure, comfortable dressing that stays in place. GENTELL BORDERED GAUZE can be used as a primar or secondary dressing. GENTELL BORDERED GAUZE is available in 4'x4' and 6'x6' size.

Hartmann-Conco Inc. 800-243-2294
481 Lakeshore Pkwy, Rock Hill, SC 29730
CEB all cotton bandage.

Hermell Products, Inc. 800-233-2342
9 Britton Dr, PO Box 7345, Bloomfield, CT 06002
Self-adhering pressure pads, finger and toe protective bandages.

Hospital Marketing Svcs. Company, Inc. 800-786-5094
162 Great Hill Rd./ Ind. Park, Naugatuck, CT 06770
HMS TEMP-WRAP 30in. long bandage with COL-PRESS instant cold pack - large (6in. wide), cat. no. 7626, 12/case; small (4in. wide), cat. no. 7624, 12/case.

Innova Corp. 860-242-3210
68 E Dudley Town Rd, Bloomfield, CT 06002
Hydrogel.

Lohmann & Rauscher, Inc. 800-279-3863
6001 SW 6th Ave Ste 101, Topeka, KS 66615

Medi-Tech International Corp. 800-333-0109
26 Court St, Brooklyn, NY 11242
Open netted tubular elastic dressing retainer.

Medicom 800-361-2862
9404 Cote de Liesse, Lachine, QUE H8T 1A1 Canada
Conforming, non-sterile bandages.

Morrison Medical 800-438-6677
3735 Paragon Dr, Columbus, OH 43228
Triangular bandages (large cloth, or Tyvek by DuPont).

Park Surgical Co., Inc. 800-633-7878
5001 New Utrecht Ave, Brooklyn, NY 11219

Pedifix, Inc. 800-424-5561
310 Guinea Rd, Brewster, NY 10509

Pepin Manufacturing, Inc. 800-291-6505
1875 S Highway 61, Lake City, MN 55041
Specialty die-cut adhesive bandages for medical field. Also, wound dressings, hydrocolloids.

Romaine, Inc. D.B.A. Koldcare 800-294-7101
2026 Sterling Ave, Elkhart, IN 46516
KOLDWRAP Gelled water bandages for sprains, swelling, insect bites, headaches. Cools by evaporation like cold pack. 3 in. x 72 in., 2 in. x 48 in., 1 in. x 24 in., and 4 in. x 4 in. In wraps or pads.

Smith & Nephew, Inc. 800-876-1261
970 Lake Carillon Dr Ste 110, Saint Petersburg, FL 33716
LIQUID - IODOFLEX PADS, SKIN PREP, No-Sting Skin Prep, Flexigel, Replicare Ultra

Tapeless Wound Care Products, Llc. 866-714-9199
PO Box 4515, Englewood, CO 80155
Anatomically designed wound dressing holders for commonly located radiation wound problems.

BANDAGE, TUBULAR *(General) 80QCN*

Brecon Knitting Mills, Inc. 800-841-2821
PO Box 478, Talladega, AL 35161
Tubular compression bandage.

BANDAGE, TUBULAR *(cont'd)*

Hartmann-Conco Inc. 800-243-2294
481 Lakeshore Pkwy, Rock Hill, SC 29730
Comperm tubular elastic bandage. Eze-Net tubular netting for retention of wound dressings.

Knit-Rite, Inc. 800-821-3094
120 Osage Ave, Kansas City, KS 66105
COMPRESSOGRIP.

Lohmann & Rauscher, Inc. 800-279-3863
6001 SW 6th Ave Ste 101, Topeka, KS 66615

Medi-Tech International Corp. 800-333-0109
26 Court St, Brooklyn, NY 11242
Open netted tubular elastic dressing retainer.

Medical Equipment Specialists, Inc. 800-795-6641
107 Otis St, Northborough, MA 01532
NEWBAND, tubular elastic material; dimensions 9 in., 33 ft long, and 11 in., 33 ft long, designed to hold steady fetal monitor transducers and probes.

O&M Enterprise 847-258-4515
641 Chelmsford Ln, Elk Grove Village, IL 60007
BANDAGE TUBULAR

Paramedical Distributors 800-245-3278
2020 Grand Blvd, Kansas City, MO 64108
COMPRESSOGRIP knit tubular elastic bandage.

Tetra Medical Supply Corp. 800-621-4041
6364 W Gross Point Rd, Niles, IL 60714

Western Medical, Ltd. 800-628-8276
214 Carnegie Ctr Ste 100, Princeton, NJ 08540
SURGITUBE tubular gauze bandages, SURGILAST tubular elastic net, SURGILAST Latex-Free tubular elastic net, BANDNET tubular elastic net.

BAR, PREFORMED *(Dental And Oral) 76EHO*

Biomet 3i 800-342-5454
4555 Riverside Dr, Palm Beach Gardens, FL 33410
CAM StructSURE® Precision Milled Bars -The Foundations For Great Restorations.

BAR, PRISM, OPHTHALMIC *(Ophthalmology) 86HKW*

Astron International Inc. 239-435-0136
3410 Westview Dr, Naples, FL 34104
Prism, bar, ophthalmic.

Gulden Ophthalmics 800-659-2250
225 Cadwalader Ave, Elkins Park, PA 19027

Newport Optical Laboratories, Inc. 714-484-3200
10564C Fern Ave, Stanton, CA 90680

Western Ophthalmics Corporation 800-426-9938
19019 36th Ave W Ste G, Lynnwood, WA 98036

BARRIER, ADHESION, ABSORBABLE *(Obstetrics/Gyn) 85MCN*

Dma Med-Chem Corporation 800-362-1833
49 Watermill Ln, Great Neck, NY 11021
Sepra Film

Ethicon, Inc. 800-4-ETHICON
Route 22 West, Somerville, NJ 08876

Ethicon, Llc. 908-218-2887
Rd. 183, Km. 8.3,, Industrial Area Hato, San Lorenzo, PR 00754
Oxidized regenerated cellulose.

Genzyme Corp. 617-252-7500
51 New York Ave. 1 Mountain Rd, 76-80 New York Avenue Framingham, MA 01701
Adhesion barrier.

Johnson & Johnson Medical Division Of Ethicon, Inc. 800-423-4018
2500 E Arbrook Blvd, Arlington, TX 76014

Noramco, Inc. 706-353-4400
1440 Olympic Dr, Athens, GA 30601
Oxidized regenerated cellulose, usp.

BARRIER, CONTROL PANEL, X-RAY, MOVEABLE *(Radiology) 90IWX*

Aadco Medical, Inc. 800-225-9014
2279 VT Route 66, Randolph, VT 05060
X-ray protective barriers, movable.

Alimed, Inc. 800-225-2610
297 High St, Dedham, MA 02026

BARRIER, CONTROL PANEL, X-RAY, MOVEABLE *(cont'd)*

Fziomed, Inc. 805-546-0610
231 Bonetti Dr, San Luis Obispo, CA 93401
Adhesion barrier film.

Phillips Safety Products 516-482-9001
123 Lincoln Blvd, Middlesex, NJ 08846

Protech Leaded Eyewear 561-627-9769
4087 Burns Rd, Palm Beach Gardens, FL 33410
Radiation filtering barriers.

Renick Ent., Inc. 561-863-4183
1211 W 13th St, Riviera Beach, FL 33404
Moveable clear barriers: see-through barriers, lead-filled acrylics.

Supertech, Inc. 800-654-1054
PO Box 186, Elkhart, IN 46515
CLEAR-PB leaded plastic modular and mobile for shielding of medical personnel from scattered radiation.

Xma (X-Ray Marketing Associates, Inc.) 800-325-8880
1205 W Lakeview Ct, Windham Lakes Business Park
Romeoville, IL 60446

BARS, PARALLEL, EXERCISE *(Physical Med) 89IOE*

Alimed, Inc. 800-225-2610
297 High St, Dedham, MA 02026

Biomet, Inc. 574-267-6639
56 E Bell Dr, PO Box 587, Warsaw, IN 46582
Adjustable folding parallel bars.

Erp Group Professional Products Ltd. 800-361-3537
3232 Autoroute Laval W., Laval, QC H7T 2H6 Canada

Hausmann Industries, Inc. 888-428-7626
130 Union St, Northvale, NJ 07647
$1,186.00 per unit (10ft).

S&W By Hausmann 888-428-7626
130 Union St, Northvale, NJ 07647

Tri W-G Group 800-437-8011
215 12th Ave NE, PO Box 905, Valley City, ND 58072
Floor and platform mounted manual adjustment.

BARS, PARALLEL, POWERED *(Physical Med) 89IRR*

Activeaid, Inc. 800-533-5330
101 Activeaid Rd, Redwood Falls, MN 56283

Alimed, Inc. 800-225-2610
297 High St, Dedham, MA 02026

Tri W-G Group 800-437-8011
215 12th Ave NE, PO Box 905, Valley City, ND 58072
Motorized height and motorized height and width.

BARS, PARALLEL, WALKING *(Physical Med) 89RJY*

Alimed, Inc. 800-225-2610
297 High St, Dedham, MA 02026

Hausmann Industries, Inc. 888-428-7626
130 Union St, Northvale, NJ 07647
$1,658.00 per unit (10ft).

N-K Products Company, Div. Of I-Rep,Inc. 800-462-6509
508 Chaney St Ste B, Lake Elsinore, CA 92530
Economy (height adjust) and Deluxe (height and width adjust)parallel bars. Both are available in folding or floor mount designs.

Prime Engineering 800-827-8263
4202 W Sierra Madre Ave, Fresno, CA 93722
Original Lift Walker: Lifts the client to their feet and allows the client to gait as they would in fixed parallel bars while holding client upright

BARS, SPREADER *(Orthopedics) 87RVM*

Freeman Manufacturing Company 800-253-2091
900 W Chicago Rd, PO Box J, Sturgis, MI 49091

Inland Specialties, Inc. 800-741-0022
7655 Matoaka Rd, Sarasota, FL 34243
Available in 8in., 12in., and 22in. sizes.

Paramedical Distributors 800-245-3278
2020 Grand Blvd, Kansas City, MO 64108

Surgical Appliance Industries 800-888-0458
3960 Rosslyn Dr, Cincinnati, OH 45209

Truform Orthotics & Prosthetics 800-888-0458
3960 Rosslyn Dr, Cincinnati, OH 45209

Zimmer Holdings, Inc. 800-613-6131
1800 W Center St, PO Box 708, Warsaw, IN 46580

Zimmer Orthopaedic Surgical Products 800-321-5533
PO Box 10, 200 West Ohio Ave., Dover, OH 44622
ZIMCODE.

BASE, DENTURE, RELINING, REPAIRING, REBASING, RESIN

(Dental And Oral) 76EBI

Aci 913-384-7390
5830 Woodson Rd Ste 3, Mission, KS 66202
Denture.

Almore International, Inc. 503-643-6633
PO Box 25214, Portland, OR 97298
$9.00 to $15.00/box.

American Dental Products, Inc. 800-846-7120
603 Country Club Dr Ste B, Bensenville, IL 60106
Tissue conditioner & temporary reliner.

American Tooth Industries 800-235-4639
1200 Stellar Dr, Oxnard, CA 93033
JUSTI.

Astron Dental Corporation 847-726-8787
815 Oakwood Rd Ste G, Lake Zurich, IL 60047
Acrylic denture material.

Biomedical Composites, Ltd. 805-644-4892
4526 Telephone Rd Ste 204, Ventura, CA 93003
Reinforcing fiber.

Biosoft International Corp. 215-295-0088
102 W Bridge St # 4, Morrisville, PA 19067
Biosoft denture base resin.

Bisco, Inc. 847-534-6000
1100 W Irving Park Rd, Schaumburg, IL 60193
Fiber reinforcement material.

Buffalo Dental Mfg. Co., Inc. 516-496-7200
159 Lafayette Dr, Syosset, NY 11791
Base plate material.

Cmp Industries Llc 800-888-5868
413 N Pearl St, Albany, NY 12207
$13.60 per 10 units.

Co-Oral-Ite Dental Mfg. Co. 530-621-4913
6635 Merchandise Way, Diamond Springs, CA 95619
Dental resin.

Coltene/Whaledent Inc. 330-916-8858
235 Ascot Pkwy, Cuyahoga Falls, OH 44223
Denture base resin.

Comfort Acrylics, Inc. 360-834-9218
2103 NE 272nd Ave, Camas, WA 98607
Talon.

Denplus Inc. 800-344-4424
205 - 1221 Labadie, Longueuil, QUE J4N 1E2 Canada

Dental Resources 717-866-7571
52 King St, Myerstown, PA 17067
Denture material.

Dentalez Group 866-DTE-INFO
101 Lindenwood Dr Ste 225, Valleybrooke Corporate Center
Malvern, PA 19355

Dentsply Canada, Ltd. 800-263-1437
161 Vinyl Ct., Woodbridge, ONT L4L 4A3 Canada

Fricke Dental Manufacturing Co. 800-537-4253
208 W Ridge Rd, Villa Park, IL 60181

General Dental Products, Inc. 888-367-6212
201 Ogden Ave, Ely, NV 89301
POLY-TONE (R) & Tru-Pak (TM)

Harry J. Bosworth Company 800-323-4352
7227 Hamlin Ave, Skokie, IL 60076
IMPACT 2000, IMPACT 750, SOFTONE, TRUSOFT, New TRULINER, Original TRULINER, LIGHTLINER (hard and soft), IMPACT 1500, DENTUSIL, TruRepair, Duz-All.

Ivoclar Vivadent, Inc. 800-533-6825
175 Pineview Dr, Amherst, NY 14228
IVOCAP Denture Base. An encapaulated denture base material with a methylmethacrylate base. Indicated for full and partial dentures, occlusal splints. PROBASE. Denture-repair materials.

BASE, DENTURE, RELINING, REPAIRING, REBASING, RESIN
(cont'd)

J. Morita Usa, Inc. 888-566-7482
9 Mason, Irvine, CA 92618
SOFRELINER TOUGH is an addition-cured silicone chairside soft lining material for dentures. This new resilient denture liner is manufactured by Tokuyama Dental and distributed by J. Morita USA. Sofreliner Tough has no odor or taste and offers strong adhesion, exceptional durability, and high resistance to tear, abrasion and discoloration. Capable of withstanding wear up to 3 years, Sofreliner Tough is preferred especially when the primary concern is durability. The material cures in 5 minutes intraorally or 20 minutes at room temperature. Sofreliner Tough comes in both kit and refill forms. Separately-sold Silicone Remover helps to easily remove silicone denture liner from the acrylic denture.

J.B.C And Co. 702-914-8842
7980 W Torino Ave, Las Vegas, NV 89113
Orthodontic acrylic resin powders- colored tints.

Kay See Dental Mfg. Co. 816-842-2817
124 Missouri Ave, Kansas City, MO 64106
Hydro-cast or kayon or kay see (various).

Lang Dental Manufacturing Co., Inc. 800-222-5264
175 Messner Dr, Wheeling, IL 60090
Premium heat cure denture resins in a variety of sizes and colors available.

Mds Products, Inc. 800-637-2330
22991 La Cadena Dr, Laguna Hills, CA 92653
ADDS-IT Base, Block-out & Splinting Material, 1/2 & 1 oz.

Nobel Biocare Usa, Llc 800-579-6515
22715/22725 Savi Ranch Parkway, Yorba Linda, CA 92887
Carbon fiber bridge.

Pentron Clinical Technologies 203-265-7397
68-70 North Plains Industrial, Road, Wallingford, CT 06492
Resin,denture,relining,repairing,rebasing.

Pentron Laboratory Technologies 203-265-7397
53 N Plains Industrial Rd, Wallingford, CT 06492
Visible light cure glaze/sealant.

Plastodent 718-792-3554
2881 Middletown Rd, Bronx, NY 10461

Preat Corp. 800-232-7732
2976 Long Valley Rd, P.O. Box 1030, Santa Ynez, CA 93460

Protech Professional Products, Inc. 561-493-9818
2900 Commerce Park Dr Ste 10, Boynton Beach, FL 33426
Denture acrylic, repair acrylic, soft reline acrylic.

Reliance Dental Mfg., Co. 708-597-6694
5805 W 117th Pl, Alsip, IL 60803
Various types of base and rebase acrylics.

Rite-Dent Manufacturing Corp. 305-693-8626
3750 E 10th Ct, Hialeah, FL 33013
Various types of reline system.

Sterngold 800-243-9942
23 Frank Mossberg Dr, PO Box 2967, Attleboro, MA 02703
QuickLine-Permanent soft reline material for complete and partial denture.

Talon Acrylics, Inc. 888-433-2551
850 NE 102nd Ave, Portland, OR 97220
REVERE ®. Used in fabrication of Liners/Relines for Complete and Partial Dentures, Overdentures / Gaskets, and other appliances as prescribed.

Thermoplastic Comfort Systems, Inc. 562-426-2970
2619 Lime Ave, Signal Hill, CA 90755
Dental,base polymer,relining material.

Trans-Atlantic Dental 609-695-0168
46 Arctic Pkwy, Ewing, NJ 08638
Flexible nylon denture base material.

Valplast Intl. Corp. 718-361-7440
3430 31st St, Long Island City, NY 11106
Flexible denture base material.

Vident 800-828-3839
3150 E Birch St, Brea, CA 92821
V.R.S. Denture Resin System (Dentimex). Fabrication of denture bases.

Vynacron Dental Resins, Inc. 732-780-6728
1751 US Highway 9, Howell, NJ 07731
Acrylic and vinyl acrylic dental resins.

BASE, ROLLER, TANK, OXYGEN *(General) 80WVN*

Clinimed, Incorporated 877-CLINIMED
303 Markus Ct, Sandy Brae Industrial Park, Newark, DE 19713

BASIN, EMESIS *(General) 80FNY*

Alimed, Inc. 800-225-2610
297 High St, Dedham, MA 02026

Alpha Scientific Corp. 800-242-5989
287 Great Valley Pkwy, Malvern, PA 19355
Irrigation basin for containing effluent.

Argon Medical Devices Inc. 903-675-9321
1445 Flat Creek Rd, Athens, TX 75751
Guidewire bowl.

Biomet Microfixation Inc. 800-874-7711
1520 Tradeport Dr, Jacksonville, FL 32218
Restraint, protective.

Care Products Inc. 757-224-0177
10701 N Ware Rd, McAllen, TX 78504
Various models of emesis basins.

Centurion Medical Products Corp. 517-545-1135
3310 S Main St, Salisbury, NC 28147

Dornoch Medical Systems, Inc. 816-505-2226
4032 NW Riverside Dr, Riverside, MO 64150
Suction canister.

Gkr Industries, Inc. 800-526-7879
13653 Kenton Ave, Crestwood, IL 60445
Convenience Bag, has many unique features; a large rigid funnel to direct flow of vomitus, a one way valve to prevent fluid from spilling and hand protection features in white opaque and clear graduated models.

Health Care Logistics, Inc. 800-848-1633
450 Town St, PO Box 25, Circleville, OH 43113
Emesis bag / convenience bag.

Jones-Zylon Company 800-848-8160
305 N Center St, West Lafayette, OH 43845
8- and 10-in. sizes, autoclavable and disposable.

Kentron Health Care, Inc. 615-384-0573
3604 Kelton Jackson Rd, P.o. Box 120, Springfield, TN 37172
Emesis basin.

Lsl Industries, Inc. 888-225-5575
5535 N Wolcott Ave, Chicago, IL 60640
$20.00 for 250 units.

Medegen Medical Products, Llc 800-233-1987
209 Medegen Drive, Gallaway, TN 38036-0228
MED-ASSIST Disp. 10in. graduated 700cc basins.

O&M Enterprise 847-258-4515
641 Chelmsford Ln, Elk Grove Village, IL 60007
BASIN EMESIS

Polar Plastic Ltd. 514-331-0207
4210 Thimens Blvd., St. Laurent, QUE H4R 2B9 Canada
POLAR RX. 500cc, 700cc various colors.

Polar Ware Co. 800-237-3655
2806 N 15th St, Sheboygan, WI 53083
Stainless steel, reusable plastic.

Ross Disposable Products 800-649-6526
401 Traders Blvd E, Unit 10, Mississauga, ON L4Z 2H8 Canada

Stryker Puerto Rico, Ltd. 939-307-2500
Hwy. 3, Km. 131.2, Las Guasimas Ind. Park, Arroyo, PR 00714
Irrigation tray.

Synergy Technologies, Inc. 218-879-4610
240 Erkkila Rd, Esko, MN 55733
Emesis containment bottle with handle and attached lid. Multi-use body fluid containment: extra wide opening can be urinal or emesis container. Ideal for ambulances, emergency rooms, recovery rooms, drug and alcohol treatment centers, home health care.

Tri-State Hospital Supply Corp. 517-545-1135
3173 E 43rd St, Yuma, AZ 85365

BASIN, SPONGE *(General) 80QCR*

Clinimed, Incorporated 877-CLINIMED
303 Markus Ct, Sandy Brae Industrial Park, Newark, DE 19713

Medegen Medical Products, Llc 800-233-1987
209 Medegen Drive, Gallaway, TN 38036-0228
MED-ASSIST.

Polar Ware Co. 800-237-3655
2806 N 15th St, Sheboygan, WI 53083
Stainless steel, reusable plastic.

BASIN, WASH *(General) 80TAF*

Alimed, Inc. 800-225-2610
297 High St, Dedham, MA 02026

American Specialties, Inc. 914-476-9000
441 Saw Mill River Rd, Yonkers, NY 10701
Washroom accessories.

Homecare Products, Inc. 800-451-1903
1704 B St NW Ste 110, Auburn, WA 98001
EZ-SHAMPOO, the original inflatable shampoo basin. Made of heavy-duty vinyl. Inflates to 24î wide x 20î long x 8î deep. Features inflatable headrest for added comfort and includes drain hose and stopper.

Jones-Zylon Company 800-848-8160
305 N Center St, West Lafayette, OH 43845
3 1/2- and 4 1/2-quart sizes; autoclavable.

Lsl Industries, Inc. 888-225-5575
5535 N Wolcott Ave, Chicago, IL 60640
$24.00 for 50 rectangular wash basins, $24.00 for 50 round units.

Medegen Medical Products, Llc 800-233-1987
209 Medegen Drive, Gallaway, TN 38036-0228
ROOM-MATES Disposable and reusable.

O&M Enterprise 847-258-4515
641 Chelmsford Ln, Elk Grove Village, IL 60007
BASIN WASH, SPONGES

Polar Ware Co. 800-237-3655
2806 N 15th St, Sheboygan, WI 53083
Stainless steel, resuable plastic.

World Dryer Corp. 800-323-0701
5700 McDermott Dr, Berkeley, IL 60163
Employee wash stations and automatic faucets.

BASKET, BILIARY STONE RETRIEVAL *(Gastro/Urology) 78TEH*

Boston Scientific Corporation 800-225-2732
1 Boston Scientific Pl, Natick, MA 01760
Segura baskets

C. R. Bard, Inc., Bard Urological Div. 888-367-2273
13183 Harland Dr NE, Covington, GA 30014

Cathguide, Division Of Scilogy Corp. 305-269-0500
9135 Fontainebleau Blvd Apt 5, Miami, FL 33172

Cook Inc. 800-457-4500
PO Box 489, Bloomington, IN 47402

Medi-Globe Corporation 800-966-1431
110 W Orion St Ste 136, Tempe, AZ 85283
Baskets to catch and retrieve gallstones.

Telemed Systems Inc. 800-481-6718
8 Kane Industrial Dr, Hudson, MA 01749

BASSINET (INFANT BED) *(General) 80QCS*

Alimed, Inc. 800-225-2610
297 High St, Dedham, MA 02026

Atlantic Medco, Inc. 800-203-8444
166 Bloomfield Ave, Verona, NJ 07044
$300 to $1,000.

Blickman 800-247-5070
39 Robinson Rd, Lodi, NJ 07644
4 models, all stainless steel.Model 8044SS has two shelves, 8047SS has a shelf and drawer, 8048SS has a two-door cabinet, 8049SS has an open cabinet. Infant basket and mattress pad sold separately. Optional pullout shelf available on all models except 8044SS.

Hill-Rom Holdings, Inc. 800-445-3730
1069 State Road 46 E, Batesville, IN 47006

Lic Care 800-323-5232
2935A Northeast Pkwy, Atlanta, GA 30360

Mastercraft Products Corporation 800-874-6094
PO Box 117, De Leon Springs, FL 32130

Medi-Tech International, Inc. 305-593-9373
2924 NW 109th Ave, Doral, FL 33172
BLICKMAN, NK

Nk Medical Products Inc. 800-274-2742
10123 Main St, PO Box 627, Clarence, NY 14031
Stainless Steel and Woodtone Versions

O&M Enterprise 847-258-4515
641 Chelmsford Ln, Elk Grove Village, IL 60007
BASSINET INFANT BED

BASSINET (INFANT BED) *(cont'd)*

Pedicraft, Inc. 800-223-7649
4134 Saint Augustine Rd, Jacksonville, FL 32207
$785.00 complete with mattress and acrylic basket.

Pedigo Products 360-695-3500
4000 SE Columbia Way, Vancouver, WA 98661
Stainless steel or chrome style with options.

Stryker Medical 800-869-0770
3800 E Centre Ave, Portage, MI 49002

United Metal Fabricators, Inc. 800-638-5322
1316 Eisenhower Blvd, Johnstown, PA 15904
All stainless steel or enamel with optional retractable work surface. Optional bassinet basket and pad.

BATH, DRY (CONSTANT TEMPERATURE) *(Chemistry) 75ULO*

Omega Engineering, Inc. 800-848-4286
1 Omega Dr, Stamford, CT 06907
The design, thermistor temperature sensor, and solid-state circuitry of the Series HDB dry-heat baths provide constant temperature uniformity.

Thermo Fisher Scientific Inc. 563-556-2241
2555 Kerper Blvd, Dubuque, IA 52001

BATH, HYDRO-MASSAGE (WHIRLPOOL) *(Physical Med) 89ILJ*

Alimed, Inc. 800-225-2610
297 High St, Dedham, MA 02026

Apollo Corporation 800-247-5490
PO Box 219, Somerset, WI 54025
APOLLO BATH, Space Performer II, whirlpool bathing system with reservoir prefill, level glide transfer/carrier device, and dispensing system. Also, Serenity assisted-living bathing system.

Arjo Canada, Inc. 800-665-4831
1575 South Gateway Rd., Unit C, Mississauga, ONT L4W-5J1 Canada

Arjo, Inc. 800-323-1245
50 Gary Ave Ste A, Roselle, IL 60172
Bathtubs with stretcher lift/transfer unit featuring computer controlled water temperature, shampoo dispensing system (optional), hot water alarm and shut-off, plus multiple whirlpool outlets for thorough cleaning of the perineal and other less accessible body areas. Can be retrofitted with electronic, digital readout patient scale.

Bath-Tec Whirlpool Bath 800-526-3301
5142 W Highway 34, Ennis, TX 75119

Bathease Inc. 888-747-7845
3815 Darston St, Palm Harbor, FL 34685

Colonial Scientific Ltd. 902-468-1811
201 Brownlow Ave., Unit 52, Dartmouth, NS B3B-1W2 Canada

Enneking Medical Inc. 816-300-4279
1801 Guinotte Ave, Kansas City, MO 64120
Various models of whirlpool bathing systems.

Ferno-Washington, Inc. 800-733-3766
70 Weil Way, Wilmington, OH 45177

Grimm Scientific Ind., Inc. 800-223-5395
1403 Pike St, PO Box 2143, Marietta, OH 45750
CRYOTherm $13,900-$43,500 for refrigerated single- and dual-tank hyrdotherapy consoles. In-ground systems priced per specific installation.

Homedics Inc. 800-333-8282
3000 N Pontiac Trl, Commerce Township, MI 48390
Jet spas, aqua skates and fountains.

Hospital Therapy Products, Inc. 630-766-7101
757 N Central Ave, Wood Dale, IL 60191
Various types of liners.

Hygiene Specialties, Inc./Andermac, Inc. 800-824-0214
2626 Live Oak Blvd, Yuba City, CA 95991
Hygenique-the standard of care whirlpool, hydrotherapy, and heat therapy bidet and sitz bath system for post partum care, episiotomy care, UTI, prevention, stimulation of voiding, perineal care and general personal hygiene.

Jacuzzi, Bath Division 800-288-4002
14880 Monte Vista Ave Ste 550, Chino, CA 91710
J-SHA II - ancient, innovative therapy of Shiatsu massage is at the core of this state-of-the-art whirlpool bath. It has two recessed channels in the backrest which feature 32 hydrotherapeutic Shiatsu micro jets.

Kohler Co. 800-456-4537
444 Highland Dr, Kohler, WI 53044

BATH, HYDRO-MASSAGE (WHIRLPOOL) *(cont'd)*

Medi-Man Rehabilitation Products, Inc. 800-268-4256
6200A Tomken Rd., Mississauga, ONT L5T-1X7 Canada
MEDI-BATHER, MALIBU, GENESIS, VENTURA, RIVIERA, MONTEGO, BELAIR, SIERRA, DAYTONA, MADEIRA, MONTEREY, DELRAY, CATALINA. Supine, stationary, hi-low and sit-in type whirlpool bathing systems.

Medi-Tech International, Inc. 305-593-9373
2924 NW 109th Ave, Doral, FL 33172
FERNO.

Medical Depot 516-998-4600
99 Seaview Blvd, Port Washington, NY 11050
Tub water jet.

Nor-Am Patient Care Products, Inc. 800-387-7103
2388 Speers Rd., Oakville, ONT L6L 5M2 Canada
Porpoise bath

Noram Solutions 800-387-7103
PO Box 543, Lewiston, NY 14092
Dolphin Hi-lo recumbent and fixed height sit tub available. Also available, Millenium 200 bath with built in sliding seat. Little Milli side entry assisted living sit tub with built-in seat.

Penner Manufacturing Inc 800-732-0717
102 Grant St, PO Box 523, Aurora, NE 68818
Theraputic bathing system (therapy tub with lift and chair).

Portacare Llc 509-928-0650
13023 E Tall Tree Rd, Spokane Valley, WA 99216
Bathing or shower enclosure.

Sanijet Corp. 972-745-2283
1461 S Belt Line Rd Ste 100, Coppell, TX 75019
Various models of hydro-massage systems.

Spectrum Aquatics 406-542-9781
7100 Spectrum Ln, Missoula, MT 59808
Therapy pool.

Thera-Tronics, Inc. 800-267-6211
623 Mamaroneck Ave, Mamaroneck, NY 10543
And pools. Hot/cold fluid therapy.

Tr Group, Inc. 800-752-6900
903 Wedel Ln, Glenview, IL 60025
Various.

Whitehall Manufacturing 800-782-7706
15125 Proctor Ave, City Of Industry, CA 91746
43 stationary/mobile/stationary with legs/stationary with a pedestal/mobile with undercarriage models divided up into Podiatry/Extremity/Hi-Boy/Lo-Boy/Sports Series, ranging in model numbers form P-10-M (Podiatry-10gal-Mobile) to S-110-S (Sports-110gal-Stationary) to full body immersion 'burn' tanks.

Whitehall/A Division Of Acorn Engineering Co. 626-336-4561
15125 Proctor Ave, City Of Industry, CA 91746
Hydor-massage bath.

BATH, ICE *(Microbiology) 83UGO*

Streck Laboratories, Inc. 800-843-0912
7002 S 109th St, Ralston, NE 68128
The Kryorack is a sealed unit containing an aqueous solution which, when frozen provides ice-bath temperatures for up to eight hours at room temperature. Four sizes are available.

BATH, KINEMATIC VISCOSITY *(Chemistry) 75UGS*

Cannon Instrument Co. 800-676-6232
PO Box 16, State College, PA 16804
CT-500, priced at $3,360.00 per unit.

Koehler Instrument Co., Inc. 800-878-9070
1595 Sycamore Ave, Bohemia, NY 11716
New constant-temperature-bath series with advanced temperature-control circuitry and integrated timing features for convenient, accurate glass capillary viscometry determinations. Microprocessor PID circuitry assures precise, reliable temperature control within ASTM-specified tolerances throughout the operating range of the bath.

Petrolab Company 518-783-5133
874 Albany Shaker Rd, Latham, NY 12110
TV 4000 visibility baths.

Thermo Fisher Scientific 877-843-7668
81 Wyman St, Waltham, MA 02451

BATH, PARAFFIN *(Physical Med) 89IMC*

Alimed, Inc. 800-225-2610
297 High St, Dedham, MA 02026

BATH, PARAFFIN *(cont'd)*

Grimm Scientific Ind., Inc. 800-223-5395
1403 Pike St, PO Box 2143, Marietta, OH 45750
PARATherm $199.00 for Deluxe paraffin bath and $139.00 for Personal paraffin bath.

Plomeria Especializada De Baja California, S.A. De 626-336-4561
Calle Maquiladoras No. 322, Seccion Dorada
Nueva Tijuana, Baja California Mexico
Various

The Hygenic Corp. 800-321-2135
1245 Home Ave, Akron, OH 44310
Thera-band paraffin bath.

Thermo Electric Company 800-523-2002
1193 McDermott Dr, West Chester, PA 19380
Paraffin baths.

Whitehall Manufacturing 800-782-7706
15125 Proctor Ave, City Of Industry, CA 91746
50 lb. cap. 'New' 6 lb. capacity and 18 lb. capacity.

Whitehall/A Division Of Acorn Engineering Co. 626-336-4561
15125 Proctor Ave, City Of Industry, CA 91746
Various.

Wr Medical Electronics Co. 800-321-6387
123 2nd St N, Stillwater, MN 55082
$175 for basic THERABATH model.

BATH, PORTABLE *(General) 80QCU*

Blevins Medical Inc 866-783-3056
207 Broad St, Marion, VA 24354

Galaxy Aquatics, Inc. 713-464-0303
1075 W Sam Houston Pkwy N Ste 210, Houston, TX 77043
All tile, fiberglass pools & spas. Custom designed to fit client requirements. Special equipment packages available through distributor or subsidiary.

Innovative Health Care Products, Inc. 678-320-0009
6850 Peachtree Dunwoody Rd NE Apt 402, Atlanta, GA 30328
NoRinse shampoo and body bath

Noram Solutions 800-387-7103
PO Box 543, Lewiston, NY 14092
Dolphin Shower Trolley, a highly mobile and versatile shower trolley. Designed with a rugged X-frame for maximum stability during recumbent showering the Dolphin Shower Trolley has a unique & luxurious closed-cell foam mattress that offers ultimate safety in a hygienic bathing environment.

Organomation Associates, Inc. 978-838-7300
266 River Rd W, Berlin, MA 01503
OA-SYS industrial-duty, thermostatically controlled stainless steel baths designed for handling water, oil-based liquids and dry media. Available with volumes ranging from two quarts to five gallons. Can be constructed in standard sizes ranging from 8.5 in. to 18 in. with depths from 4.5 in. to 12 in. and custom sizes.

P-Ryton Corp. 800-221-9840
504 50th Ave, Long Island City, NY 11101
SETMA Spa equipment. Hydro therapy tub(U.L. approved), (5 head)Vichy shower, swiss shower, spa tables(wet tables) available.

Sundance Spas, Inc. 800-883-7727
14525 Monte Vista Ave, Chino, CA 91710
Portable spas.

Wheelchair Sales And Service Co., Inc. 877-736-0376
315 Main St, West Springfield, MA 01089
Lumex; T.F.I.; Invacare; API.

BATH, SITZ, NON-POWERED *(Physical Med) 89KTC*

Centurion Medical Products Corp. 517-545-1135
3310 S Main St, Salisbury, NC 28147

Drummond Industries, Inc. 260-356-6837
254 W McCrum St, Huntington, IN 46750
Sit-n-bathe.

Medical Depot 516-998-4600
99 Seaview Blvd, Port Washington, NY 11050
Commodes and accessories.

Tri-State Hospital Supply Corp. 517-545-1135
3173 E 43rd St, Yuma, AZ 85365

West Coast Surgical Llc. 650-728-8095
141 California Ave Ste 101, Half Moon Bay, CA 94019
Calipers for measuring bone grafts and implant size.

BATH, SITZ, PHYSICAL MEDICINE *(Physical Med) 89ILM*

Arjo, Inc. 800-323-1245
50 Gary Ave Ste A, Roselle, IL 60172

BATH, SITZ, PHYSICAL MEDICINE *(cont'd)*

Hospital Therapy Products, Inc. 630-766-7101
757 N Central Ave, Wood Dale, IL 60191
Barrier gowns.

Kohler Co. 800-456-4537
444 Highland Dr, Kohler, WI 53044

Medegen Medical Products, Llc 800-233-1987
209 Medegen Drive, Gallaway, TN 38036-0228
ROOM-MATES Disposable baths.

Medi Inc 800-225-8634
75 York Ave, P.O. Box 302, Randolph, MA 02368

North Coast Medical, Inc. 800-821-9319
18305 Sutter Blvd, Morgan Hill, CA 95037
Hygenique Plus is a bidet/sitz bath system intended for persons having trouble with personal hygiene or needing heat therapy to promote healing.

Penner Manufacturing Inc 800-732-0717
102 Grant St, PO Box 523, Aurora, NE 68818
Various models of hydrobaths.

Polar Ware Co. 800-237-3655
2806 N 15th St, Sheboygan, WI 53083
Single-patient plastic.

BATH, STEAM *(General) 80QCW*

Electro-Steam Generator Corp. 888-783-2624
1000 Bernard St, Alexandria, VA 22314
Steam generator.

BATH, TISSUE FLOTATION *(Microbiology) 83QCX*

Boekel Scientific 800-336-6929
855 Pennsylvania Blvd, Feasterville Trevose, PA 19053
product specialty is for Hematology and histology for slide preparation

Fts Systems 800-824-0400
PO Box 158, 3538 Main Street,, Stone Ridge, NY 12484

Phipps & Bird, Inc. 800-955-7621
1519 Summit Ave, Richmond, VA 23230
Isolated organ & tissue bath for student education.

Thermo Fisher Scientific 877-843-7668
81 Wyman St, Waltham, MA 02451

BATH, TISSUE FLOTATION, PATHOLOGY *(Pathology) 88IDY*

Bayer Healthcare Llc 914-524-2955
555 White Plains Rd Fl 5, Tarrytown, NY 10591
Water bath.

Surgipath Medical Industries, Inc. 800-225-3035
PO Box 528, 5205 Route 12, Richmond, IL 60071

BATH, VISCOSITY *(Chemistry) 75UJJ*

Thermal Product Solutions 800-216-7725
2121 Reach Rd, Williamsport, PA 17701

Thermo Fisher Scientific 877-843-7668
81 Wyman St, Waltham, MA 02451

BATH, WATER (CONSTANT TEMPERATURE)
(Chemistry) 75QCY

Almore International, Inc. 503-643-6633
PO Box 25214, Portland, OR 97298
$355.00 per set.

Brinkmann Instruments, Inc. 800-645-3050
PO Box 1019, Westbury, NY 11590

Cole-Parmer Instrument Inc. 800-323-4340
625 E Bunker Ct, Vernon Hills, IL 60061

Fisher Healthcare 800-766-7000
9999 Veterans Memorial Dr, Houston, TX 77038

Pro Scientific Inc. 800-584-3776
99 Willenbrock Rd, Oxford, CT 06478
Memmert water baths, from 10-100 degrees Celsius are available in 6 sizes from 7-45l. Standard features; high grade stainless steel, microprocessor PID control, integral self-diagnostics, digital timer, digital temperature display, overtemperature protection and corrosion proof large-area heating system on three sides of the working space ensuring optimum temperature uniformity.

Science-Electronics, Inc. 937-224-4444
521 Kiser St, Dayton, OH 45404

Thermal Product Solutions 800-216-7725
2121 Reach Rd, Williamsport, PA 17701

BATHTUB *(General) 80VKA*

Aqua Bath Co., Inc. 800-232-2284
921 Cherokee Ave, Nashville, TN 37207
Acrylic tub/shower ID 60x32x84, acrylic showers ID 36x36x84, ID 60x36x84 and 60x30x84-all ADA compliant.

Aqua Glass Corporation 800-632-0911
320 Industrial Park Rd, Adamsville, TN 38310
Two models tub/shower: $1,950 for 60 acrylic; $1,224 for 60 gelcoat tub/shower. $2,000 for 48-inch acrylic shower (low threshold); $1,170 for 48 gelcoat shower; $1,172 for gelcoat shower; $1,380 for acrylic corner shower number SC 4584. Also available, SPECIAL CARE 60 in. by 32 in. special-care shower. Ideal for remodeling projects. Comes complete with wraparound bar and transfer seat.

Arjo, Inc. 800-323-1245
50 Gary Ave Ste A, Roselle, IL 60172

Bathease Inc. 888-747-7845
3815 Darston St, Palm Harbor, FL 34685
Acrylic bathtub/shower with door of standard size, residential-style, and universal design. Options include walls, dome, whirlpool, and colors. BATHEASE Convertible Shower Model #6034TS, full-size acrylic shower measuring 60 x 34 x 84 in. that may be converted to an accessible bathtub with the addition of a front wall with door.

Colonial Scientific Ltd. 902-468-1811
201 Brownlow Ave., Unit 52, Dartmouth, NS B3B-1W2 Canada
bathing systems

Jetta Corporation 800-288-7771
425 Centennial Blvd, Edmond, OK 73013
Hydrotherapy Bath Systems

North Coast Medical, Inc. 800-821-9319
18305 Sutter Blvd, Morgan Hill, CA 95037

BATHTUB, PORTABLE *(General) 80QCZ*

Activeaid, Inc. 800-533-5330
101 Activeaid Rd, Redwood Falls, MN 56283
Folding tub transfer bench.

Arjo, Inc. 800-323-1245
50 Gary Ave Ste A, Roselle, IL 60172

Homecare Products, Inc. 800-451-1903
1704 B St NW Ste 110, Auburn, WA 98001
EZ-BATHE™ Inflatable tub with accessories. Enjoy bathing the way it's meant to be - soaking wet! The EZ-BATHE allows clients to enjoy a bath or shower without leaving their bed. The reinforced tub with its new streamlined design is longer & deeper with a new double tube design to prevent splashes and spills. Inside dimensions of inflated tub are 71î long x 31î wide x 13¾î deep (accommodates individuals up to 6' 2î). Fits all beds. Complete with the following: Inflatable pillow, 25' reinforced drain hose with on/off valve, 25' hose with shower head, shower accessories, wet & dry vacuum, and one (1) year limited warranty.

BATTERIES, RECHARGEABLE, CLASS II DEVICES
(Cardiovascular) 74MOX

Amco International Manufacturing & Design, Inc. 303-646-3583
10 Conselyea St, Brooklyn, NY 11211
Battery, box, rechargeable.

BATTERY *(General) 80VDY*

Access Battery Inc. 800-654-9845
12104 W Carmen Ave, Division of Alpha Source, Inc.
Milwaukee, WI 53225
Life, King, Gold Premium, Lite full line of nickel-cadmium, nickel-metal hydride, sealed lead-acid and lithium batteries for monitors, defibrillators, infusion pumps, thermometers, holter recorders, ECG, TENS, radiology, ventilators, etc., with 18-month warranty on Gold Premium nickel-cadmium packs, and 1 year or 2 year warranty options on radiology batteries, not pro-rated. Master distributor for original Motorola brand batteries and accessories for Motorola radios, pagers and cellular products.

Anton/Bauer - Custom Power Systems 800-422-3473
14 Progress Dr, Shelton, CT 06484

Astralite Corporation 800-345-7703
PO Box 689, Somerset, CA 95684
Rechargeable; for OTO/OPH power handles, replacements for Statham, Burton, Astralite. C & AA batteries available.

Battery Specialties 800-854-5759
3530 Cadillac Ave, Costa Mesa, CA 92626
Ni-Cad, NiMH, Lion, Sealed Lead Acid, Alkaline, Mercury, Lithium, Carbon Zinc, Zinc-Air.

Brasseler Usa - Komet Medical 800-535-6638
1 Brasseler Blvd, Savannah, GA 31419
Replacement batteries, rechargers and testers.

BATTERY *(cont'd)*

Concorde Battery 626-813-1234
2009 W San Bernardino Rd, West Covina, CA 91790
Wheelchair batteries (valve regulated sealed lead acid) built maintenance free and long lasting for deep cycle requirements.

Enersys 610-208-1991
2366 Bernville Rd, Reading, PA 19605
Genesis Pure Lead, Genesis NP and CYCLON sealed rechargeable lead-acid batteries for reliable back-up power for critical applications

Engineered Assemblies Corporation 201-288-4477
380 North St, Teterboro, NJ 07608
Battery design, manufacturing and distribution service and charging systems for rechargeable batteries.

Eveready Battery Co. 314-985-1569
Checkerboard Sq, Saint Louis, MO 63164
EVEREADY Full line supplier of batteries, including AA and 9V lithium and flashlights to the medical industry.

Greatbatch Inc 716-759-5600
10000 Wehrle Dr, Clarence, NY 14031

Hal-Hen Company, Inc. 800-242-5436
180 Atlantic Ave, Garden City Park, NY 11040
Complete line of batteries for hearing aids.

Maxwell Technologies Power Systems 877-511-4324
9244 Balboa Ave, San Diego, CA 92123
Ultracapacitor, high power density, long 10 year life for short term energy storage seconds to minutes or burst power requirements. 5 fared to 2700 fared capacitors.

Micro Power Electronics, Inc. 800-576-6177
13955 SW Millikan Way, Beaverton, OR 97005
Smart battery pack for portable equipment

Mk Battery 800-372-9253
1645 S Sinclair St, Anaheim, CA 92806
Sealed lead acid batteries, GEL and AGM, for the HME market for wheelchairs, scooters and respiratory equipment.

Moltech Power Systems Inc 800-677-6937
1908 NW 67th Pl, Gainesville, FL 32653
Rechargeable cells and battery packs for medical applications. 1.2 V, capacities from 180 mA to 5700 mAh.

Nica-Power Battery Corp. 800-565-6422
5155 Spectrum Way, Mississauga, ON L4W 5A1 Canada
Complete line of batteries for replacement to biomedical instruments.

Ovonic Battery Company 248-293-0440
2968 Waterview Dr, Rochester Hills, MI 48309
Rechargeable batteries.

Physio-Control, Inc. 800-442-1142
11811 Willows Rd NE, Redmond, WA 98052
Replacement battery packs.

Plainview Batteries, Inc. 800-642-2354
23 Newtown Rd, Plainview, NY 11803
Electrolaryn, custom prosthesis, and wheelchair batteries, custom battery packs, computer memory back-up batteries, and TENS Unit 9 V. Also all alkaline and lithium batteries. ENERGEX BATTERIES for professional video cameras and recorders.

Rayovac 800-331-4522
601 Rayovac Drive, Madison, WI 53744-4960
Lithium coin cells, lithium batteries and battery holder, RAYOVAC Maximum Plus Alkaline, heavy-duty zinc carbon batteries, zinc air-button cells, and I-C3 15-minute-rechargeable NiMH cells, Varta Lithium Batteries

Rozinn By Scottcare Corporation 800-243-9412
4791 W 150th St, Cleveland, OH 44135
Batteries for Holter monitors, refurbishment of battery packs, new and reconditioned battery packs and chargers, and new battery pack adaptors. Rechargeable Battery is good for 1000 Holter studies when used with the RR151 Holter Recorder.

Sentry Battery Corp. 800-747-0199
62 Colin Dr, Manchester, NH 03103
PM BATTERY. Complete line of sealed-lead rechargeable batteries for back-up power and medical applications.

Standard Supply Co. 800-453-7036
3424 S Main St, Salt Lake City, UT 84115
Custom and standard nickel cadmium, lead acid and lithium battery packs; also nickel metal hydride battery packs.

BATTERY *(cont'd)*

Storage Battery Systems, Inc. 800-554-2243
N56W16665 Ridgewood Dr, Menomonee Falls, WI 53051
SBS DEEP CYCLE wheelchair and gel CELL batteries, SBS and Interacter chargers, battery fuel gauges and battery water level indicators.

Tungstone Power Inc 800-232-3557
623 Main St, Woburn, MA 01801
Customized battery packs.

Ultralife Batteries, Inc. 800-332-5000
2000 Technology Pkwy, Newark, NY 14513
ULTRALIFE, ULTRALIFE THIN CELL, ULTRALIFE POLYMER batteries. ULTRALIFE 9-volt lithium battery is ideal for use in telemetry systems, ambulatory infusion pumps, and any device requiring long, reliable battery life. ULTRALIFE THIN CELL batteries are flat-profile primary batteries as thin as 2 mm. ULTRALIFE POLYMER BATTERIES are thin li-ion rechargeable batteries with high-energy density; flat-profile, prismatic construction for outstanding design flexibility; solid electrolyte for safety.

VARTA Microbattery Inc. 800-468-2782
1311 Mamaroneck Ave Ste 120, White Plains, NY 10605
Lithium, Polymer, lithium ion, nickel metal hydride, zinc air, silver oxide, etc. Customized battery packs. Nickel metal Hydride 9V battery, V7/8H, 180mAh.

W&W Manufacturing Co. 800-221-0732
800 S Broadway, Hicksville, NY 11801
Replacement battery packs for communication equipment and bar code scanners.

BATTERY, HEARING-AID *(Ear/Nose/Throat) 77WOT*

Fecom Corporation 800-292-3362
12 Stults Rd Ste 103, Dayton, NJ 08810
Digital Key-chain battery tester with LCD indicator for hearing aid batteries and household battery tester that tester sizes D, C, AA, AAA, 9 volt, and Lithium all in one unit

Harc Mercantile Ltd. 800-445-9968
1111 W Centre Ave, Portage, MI 49024

Hitec Group Intl. 800-288-8303
8160 S Madison St, Burr Ridge, IL 60527

Nica-Power Battery Corp. 800-565-6422
5155 Spectrum Way, Mississauga, ON L4W 5A1 Canada

Nu-Ear Electronics 800-626-8327
6769 Mesa Ridge Rd Ste 100, San Diego, CA 92121

Plainview Batteries, Inc. 800-642-2354
23 Newtown Rd, Plainview, NY 11803
Rechargeable hearing aid batteries with companion charger. (One for size 13 battery, one for size 675 battery.)

Rayovac 800-331-4522
601 Rayovac Drive, Madison, WI 53744-4960
Rayovac Zinc-Air Hearing Aid Batteries, Varta Lithium Batteries, Medical batteries.

Rayovac Canada, Inc. 800-268-0425
5448 Timberlea Blvd., Mississauga, ONT L4W-2T7 Canada

Spectrum-Brands 800-237-6541
601 Rayovac Drive, Madison, WI 53711-2497
Zinc air hearing-aid batteries in private-label packaging.

Starkey Laboratories, Inc. 800-328-8602
6700 Washington Ave S, Eden Prairie, MN 55344

VARTA Microbattery Inc. 800-468-2782
1311 Mamaroneck Ave Ste 120, White Plains, NY 10605
Rechargeable.

BATTERY, MOBILE RADIOGRAPHIC UNIT *(Radiology) 90VGM*

Access Battery Inc. 800-654-9845
12104 W Carmen Ave, Division of Alpha Source, Inc.
Milwaukee, WI 53225
Full line of King and Life lead-acid Retrokit batteries for all portable x-ray units; includes 1 year and 2 year warranty options. One-hour installation, no electronic module required, no space taken from cassette drawer.

Advanced Battery Systems, Inc. 800-227-7090
1300 19th St Ste 170, East Moline, IL 61244

Burkhart Roentgen Intl. Inc. 800-USA-XRAY
5201 8th Ave S, Gulfport, FL 33707
Field service on radiographic units. C.T. systems and processors.

Xma (X-Ray Marketing Associates, Inc.) 800-325-8880
1205 W Lakeview Ct, Windham Lakes Business Park
Romeoville, IL 60446

BATTERY, RECHARGEABLE, REPLACEMENT FOR CLASS III DEVICE *(Cardiovascular) 74MOR*

Anton/Bauer - Custom Power Systems 800-422-3473
14 Progress Dr, Shelton, CT 06484

BATTERY, REPLACEMENT, RECHARGEABLE *(Surgery) 79MOQ*

Bioplate, Inc. 310-815-2100
3643 Lenawee Ave, Los Angeles, CA 90016
Battery powered screwdriver-replacement battery.

BEADS, HYDROPHILIC, WOUND EXUDATE ABSORPTION *(Surgery) 79KOZ*

Gentell 800-840-9041
3600 Boundbrook Ave, Trevose, PA 19053
DERMATELL HYDROCOLLOID DRESSING; consists of a hydrocolloid wafer paired with a polyurethane foam. This combination enhances patient comfort and protection while promoting moist wound healing by absorbing exudate and allowing natural debridemnt. Dermatell will not break down into the wound upon saturation and will resist contamination. Dressing may remain on the patient for 3 to 7 days. DERMATELL is available in 4.5'x4.5' size.

Johnson & Johnson Medical Division Of Ethicon, Inc. 800-423-4018
2500 E Arbrook Blvd, Arlington, TX 76014

Lendell Mfg., Inc. 800-566-8569
5301 S Graham Rd, Saint Charles, MI 48655
Hydrophilic foam.

Medicus Technologies 800-762-1574
105 Morgan Ln, Plainsboro, NJ 08536

Telios Pharmaceuticals 800-762-1574
105 Morgan Ln, Plainsboro, NJ 08536

BEAKER (LABORATORY) *(Chemistry) 75TGH*

Berghof/America 800-544-5004
3773 NW 126th Ave Bldg 1, Coral Springs, FL 33065
Teflon beakers with broad spouts, pouring spouts, thin wall or thick wall. Lids also available.

Cargille Laboratories 973-239-6633
55 Commerce Rd, Cedar Grove, NJ 07009
Graduated beakers in polypropylene, 4oz. $28.00 per 1000, 17oz $43.50 per 1000, 4oz.; in paper, $17.50 per 1000, 4oz.

Kimble Glass, Inc. 888-546-2531
537 Crystal Ave, Vineland, NJ 08360
KIMAX.

Medegen Medical Products, Llc 800-233-1987
209 Medegen Drive, Gallaway, TN 38036-0228
LAB-CHOICE Reusable 1qt. translucent, sterilizable and translucent graduated measure/beakers. 1qt. sterile, disposable, graduated measure/beakers.

Nalge Nunc International 800-625-4327
75 Panorama Creek Dr, Rochester, NY 14625
NALGENE available in transparent polymethylpentene, translucent polypropylene and chemical resistant, high purity Teflon FEP. Sizes from 30ml to 4L.

Quartz Scientific, Inc. 800-229-2186
819 East St, Fairport Harbor, OH 44077

Simport Plastics Ltd. 450-464-1723
2588 Bernard-Pilon, Beloeil, QUE J3G 4S5 Canada
TRICORN polypropylene, unbreakable and suitable for use with commonly used acids, alkalies and solvents.

BED CRADLE *(General) 80QDA*

Clinimed, Incorporated 877-CLINIMED
303 Markus Ct, Sandy Brae Industrial Park, Newark, DE 19713

Home Aid Products 888-823-7605
111 Esna Park Dr., Unit 9, Markham, ONT L3R-1H2 Canada
Blanket supports.

J. T. Posey Co. 800-447-6739
5635 Peck Rd, Arcadia, CA 91006

Mayo Medical, S.A. De C.V. 800-715-3872
Edison 1141 Nte., Col. Talleres, Monterrey N.L. 64480 Mexico

Zimmer Holdings, Inc. 800-613-6131
1800 W Center St, PO Box 708, Warsaw, IN 46580

BED, ADJUSTABLE HOSPITAL *(General) 80KMM*

Alex Orthopedic, Inc. 800-544-2539
PO Box 201442, Arlington, TX 76006

BED, ADJUSTABLE HOSPITAL *(cont'd)*

Carroll Healthcare Inc. 800-668-2337
994 Hargrieve Rd., London, ONT N6E-1P5 Canada
The world's first and only hospital low bed with a travel range from 8 1/2' to 34'.

Colonial Scientific Ltd. 902-468-1811
201 Brownlow Ave., Unit 52, Dartmouth, NS B3B-1W2 Canada

Gaymar Industries, Inc. 800-828-7341
10 Centre Dr, Orchard Park, NY 14127
Specialty beds.

Mayo Medical, S.A. De C.V. 800-715-3872
Edison 1141 Nte., Col. Talleres, Monterrey N.L. 64480 Mexico

Med-Rent, Inc. 800-233-7345
435 Bethany Rd, Burbank, CA 91504

Sunrise Medical 800-333-4000
7477 Dry Creek Pkwy, Longmont, CO 80503

Tuffcare 800-367-6160
3999 E La Palma Ave, Anaheim, CA 92807

BED, AIR FLUIDIZED *(Physical Med) 89INX*

Asi Medical Equipment, Ltd. 800-527-0443
1735 N Interstate 35E, Carrollton, TX 75006
Air support therapy bed with sixteen zones of pressure relief with the MAPP pressure profiling system. The support surface can be customized according to patient's needs.

Dynamedics Corp. 519-433-7474
30 Adelaide St N, Ste. 205, London, ONT N6B 3N5 Canada
Low air loss mattress system

Hill-Rom Manufacturing, Inc. 800-638-2546
4349 Corporate Rd, Charleston, SC 29405
Microsphere air fluidized beds. CLINITRON RITE-HITE air fluidized therapy.

Kinetic Concepts, Inc. 800-275-4524
8023 Vantage Dr, San Antonio, TX 78230
Air fluidized bead bed.

Reditac Medical Usa, Llc
1555 Cottondale Dr Ste 4, Baton Rouge, LA 70815
Air fluidized bed.

Thermo Electric Company 800-523-2002
1193 McDermott Dr, West Chester, PA 19380
Fluido-therapy.

BED, BIRTHING *(General) 80QDE*

Bryton Corp. 800-567-9500
4310 Guion Rd, Indianapolis, IN 46254
Birthing Beds, replacement matresses, mattress Comfi-Toppers, etc

Calmaquip Engineering Corp. 305-592-4510
7240 NW 12th St, Miami, FL 33126

Hill-Rom Holdings, Inc. 800-445-3730
1069 State Road 46 E, Batesville, IN 47006

Lic Care 800-323-5232
2935A Northeast Pkwy, Atlanta, GA 30360

Smith & Nephew Inc. 800-463-7439
2100 52nd Ave., Lachine, QUE H8T 2Y5 Canada

Stryker Medical 800-869-0770
3800 E Centre Ave, Portage, MI 49002

BED, ELECTRIC *(General) 80FNL*

Adden Furniture, Inc. 800-625-3876
26 Jackson St, Lowell, MA 01852

Aggressive Solutions, Inc. 972-242-2164
1735 N Interstate 35E, Carrollton, TX 75006
Hospital bed, tilting table.

Allied Medco, Inc. 631-447-0093
25 Corporate Dr, Holtsville, NY 11742
Electric hospital bed.

American Biomed Instruments, Inc. 718-235-8900
11 Wyona St, Brooklyn, NY 11207

American Of Martinsville 276-632-2061
128 E Church St, Martinsville, VA 24112

Asi Medical Equipment, Ltd. 800-527-0443
1735 N Interstate 35E, Carrollton, TX 75006
ICU and air support therapy.

Basic American Medical Products 800-849-6664
2935A Northeast Pkwy, Atlanta, GA 30360
Medical equipment. Furniture for nursing homes.

BED, ELECTRIC *(cont'd)*

Blevins Medical Inc 866-783-3056
207 Broad St, Marion, VA 24354

Calmaquip Engineering Corp. 305-592-4510
7240 NW 12th St, Miami, FL 33126

Camtec 410-228-1156
1959 Church Creek Rd, Cambridge, MD 21613
Bariatric bed.

Colonial Scientific Ltd. 902-468-1811
201 Brownlow Ave., Unit 52, Dartmouth, NS B3B-1W2 Canada
Electric hospital beds

Curbell Electronics Inc. 716-667-3377
20 Centre Dr, Orchard Park, NY 14127
Headboards, footboards, bed control pendants, bed cables.

Elite Mattress Manufacturing 800-332-5878
4999 Rear Fyler Avenue, St. Louis, MO 63139

Evermed Corp. 714-777-9997
4999 E La Palma Ave, Anaheim, CA 92807
Home care bed.

Extended Care Air Therapy Systems, Inc. 740-697-0845
7165 Payne Rd, Roseville, OH 43777
Bed enclosure.

Flex-A-Bed, Inc. 800-421-2277
1825 Hillsdale Rd, La Fayette, GA 30728
Two models of Semi-electric beds, as well as one model of fully-electric bed with Hi-Low function in twin, full, and queen size. Optional safety side rails mount on all FLEX-A-BEDS & most other adjustable beds.

Golden Technologies, Inc. 800-624-6374
401 Bridge St, Old Forge, PA 18518
Luxury electric adjustable beds, feating heat and massage options.

Hard Manufacturing Co. 800-873-4273
230 Grider St, Buffalo, NY 14215
$2,575 for Model 2000 w/ solid pan; bed height 19-28in.; weight 355 lbs. Pendant-type patient controls with 6 functions.

Hbr Healthcare Company, Inc. 765-966-1400
2211 Williamsburg Pike, Richmond, IN 47374
Hospital beds.

Heritage Medical Products, Inc 417-256-3628
10380 County Road 6310, West Plains, MO 65775
Various types of ultrasound beds.

Hill-Rom Holdings, Inc. 800-445-3730
1069 State Road 46 E, Batesville, IN 47006

Hill-Rom, Inc. 812-934-7777
4115 Dorchester Rd Unit 600, North Charleston, SC 29405
Various models of electric hospital beds.

International Hospital Supply Co. 800-398-9450
6914 Canby Ave Ste 105, Reseda, CA 91335

Invacare Corporation 800-333-6900
1 Invacare Way, Elyria, OH 44035
INVACARE.

Kinetic Concepts, Inc. 800-275-4524
8023 Vantage Dr, San Antonio, TX 78230
Bariatric bed.

Kma Remarketing Corp. 814-371-5242
302 Aspen Way, Dubois, PA 15801
Electric hospital bed.

Lic Care 800-323-5232
2935A Northeast Pkwy, Atlanta, GA 30360
ICU, CCU, recovery, labor, or transport models, electric and non-electric.

M.C. Healthcare Products, Inc. 800-268-8671
4658 Ontario St., Beamsville, ONT L0R 1B4 Canada
Full-function, three-motor subacute-hospital and long-term care beds or semielectric. Low-height adjustable electric beds. 7 7/8 to 25 in.

Mat Automotive 847-821-9630
355 W Crossroads Pkwy Ste A, Bolingbrook, IL 60440
Hospital bed.

Md International, Inc. 305-669-9003
11300 NW 41st St, Doral, FL 33178

Med-Mizer, Inc 812-932-2345
80 Commerce Dr, Batesville, IN 47006
Electric bed.

Medical Depot 516-998-4600
99 Seaview Blvd, Port Washington, NY 11050
Electrical bed.

BED, ELECTRIC *(cont'd)*

Nk Medical Products Inc. 800-274-2742
10123 Main St, PO Box 627, Clarence, NY 14031
Adult and Youth Size Beds

Noa Medical Industries 800-633-6068
801 Terry Ln, Washington, MO 63090
A. P. RISER, a three-function electric low bed that raises from 7 to 26 in. with optional Trendelenburg, Reverse Trendelenburg, and Cardio Chair.

Schueler & Company, Inc. 516-487-1500
PO Box 528, Stratford, CT 06615

Scott Technology Llc 203-888-2783
1 Jacks Hill Rd, Oxford, CT 06478
Powered hospital bed,bariatric bed.

Stryker Medical 800-869-0770
3800 E Centre Ave, Portage, MI 49002

Symphony Medical Products 877-470-9995
6320 NW 84th Ave, Miami, FL 33166
Hospital bed.

Tele-Made Disposables, Inc. 888-822-4299
3215 Huffman Eastgate Rd, Huffman, TX 77336
Electric hospital bed.

The Neurological Research And Development Group 800-327-6759
115 Rotary Dr, West Hazleton, PA 18202
Double & queen size hospital bed.Can accommodate up to 1000 lbs. Excellent for Sleep Disorder Labs and Clinics.

BED, ELECTRIC, HOME-USE *(General) 80LLI*

Basic American Medical Products 800-849-6664
2935A Northeast Pkwy, Atlanta, GA 30360

Convaquip Industries, Inc. 800-637-8436
4834 Derrick Dr, PO Box 3417, Abilene, TX 79601
ConvaQuip offers both semi-electric and fully Bariatric electric beds with capacities of 750 lbs. to 1000 lbs.

Invacare Corporation 800-333-6900
1 Invacare Way, Elyria, OH 44035
INVACARE - Comfort Solutions homecare beds.

Sunrise Medical 800-333-4000
7477 Dry Creek Pkwy, Longmont, CO 80503

Tuffcare 800-367-6160
3999 E La Palma Ave, Anaheim, CA 92807

Ultrassage, Inc. 514-344-1083
5680 Rue Pare, Mont-Royal, QUEBE H4P 2M2 Canada
Electrical adustable bed, massage furniture.

BED, FLOTATION THERAPY, NEONATAL *(General) 80UDH*

Howard Medical Company 800-443-1444
1690 N Elston Ave, Chicago, IL 60642
Waffle neonate water/air mattress for premature infant flotation therapy. $59.00 for two compartment set (12 x 24).

BED, FLOTATION THERAPY, POWERED *(Physical Med) 89IOQ*

Electronic Mfg. Co. 813-855-4068
13440 Wright Cir, Tampa, FL 33626
Air sac bed.

Gaymar Industries, Inc. 800-828-7341
10 Centre Dr, Orchard Park, NY 14127
CLINI.FLOAT allows patient to be semi-immersed in a temperature-controlled fluid-like environment for pressure management needs.

Healing Solutions, Llc. 636-376-8100
2112 Penta Dr, High Ridge, MO 63049
Low air loss bed.

Hill-Rom Holdings, Inc. 800-445-3730
1069 State Road 46 E, Batesville, IN 47006
Therapy bed, nonflotation, nonpowered.

Hill-Rom Manufacturing, Inc. 800-638-2546
4349 Corporate Rd, Charleston, SC 29405
PRIME-AIRE therapy surface, FLEXICAIR Low Airloss Therapy.

Hill-Rom, Inc. 812-934-7777
4115 Dorchester Rd Unit 600, North Charleston, SC 29405
Air floatation mattress.

Huntleigh Healthcare Llc. 800-223-1218
40 Christopher Way, Eatontown, NJ 07724

Invacare Corporation 800-333-6900
1 Invacare Way, Elyria, OH 44035
INVACARE microAIR, Turn-Q, Turn-Q Plus, LTM, APM low air loss.

BED, FLOTATION THERAPY, POWERED *(cont'd)*

Kap Medical 951-340-4360
1395 Pico St, Corona, CA 92881
Low air loss mattress system.

Kinetic Concepts, Inc. 800-275-4524
8023 Vantage Dr, San Antonio, TX 78230
Low air loss bed.

Numotech, Inc. 818-772-1579
9420 Reseda Blvd Ste 504, Northridge, CA 91324
Generic total contact seat.

Scott Technology Llc 203-888-2783
1 Jacks Hill Rd, Oxford, CT 06478
Low air loss mattress.

Sentech Medical Systems, Inc. 954-340-0500
4200 NW 120th Ave, Coral Springs, FL 33065
Floatation low air loss mattress.

BED, HYDRAULIC *(General) 80FNK*

Amelife Llc 302-476-2631
702 N West St Ste 101, Wilmington, DE 19801

Asi Medical Equipment, Ltd. 800-527-0443
1735 N Interstate 35E, Carrollton, TX 75006
Intensive care beds.

Griffin Medical Products, Inc. 800-366-6870
80 Manheim Ave, PO Box 457, Bridgeton, NJ 08302
Underpad adult briefs, washcloths, adult liners.

Kma Remarketing Corp. 814-371-5242
302 Aspen Way, Dubois, PA 15801
Hydraulic hospital bed.

Lic Care 800-323-5232
2935A Northeast Pkwy, Atlanta, GA 30360

Medical Depot 516-998-4600
99 Seaview Blvd, Port Washington, NY 11050
Beds and acc.

Stryker Medical 800-869-0770
3800 E Centre Ave, Portage, MI 49002

Symphony Medical Products 877-470-9995
6320 NW 84th Ave, Miami, FL 33166
Hydraulic hospital bed.

Wheelchair Sales And Service Co., Inc. 877-736-0376
315 Main St, West Springfield, MA 01089
Mobilite (Invacare); Sunrise Medical.

BED, MANUAL *(General) 80FNJ*

American Biomed Instruments, Inc. 718-235-8900
11 Wyona St, Brooklyn, NY 11207

Asi Medical Equipment, Ltd. 800-527-0443
1735 N Interstate 35E, Carrollton, TX 75006
Critical care beds.

Atd-American Co. 800-523-2300
135 Greenwood Ave, Wyncote, PA 19095

B & T Davis Electric Inc. 812-644-7615
Rr4 Box 150a, Washington, IN 47501
Dignity bed.

Basic American Metal Products 800-365-2338
336 Trowbridge Dr, PO Box 907, Fond Du Lac, WI 54937

Better Health, Inc. 866-BED-BLOX
4117 E Emory Rd Ste 601, Knoxville, TN 37938
Head-of-bed elevators (risers).

Calmaquip Engineering Corp. 305-592-4510
7240 NW 12th St, Miami, FL 33126

Clinimed, Incorporated 877-CLINIMED
303 Markus Ct, Sandy Brae Industrial Park, Newark, DE 19713

Concept Plastics, Inc. 336-889-2001
1210 Hickory Chapel Rd, High Point, NC 27260
Bed elevaton blocks.

Cw Medical, Inc. 909-591-5220
5595 Daniels St Ste E, Chino, CA 91710
Easy Transboard is a waterproof, antistatic, antiseptic, and mold-resistant product for transfering up to 550-lb patients from one bed to another. Easy Transboard can help prevent secondary injuries due to handling of patients, and can even be operated by one person alone.

Cyr Designs, Llc 207-723-6766
112 New York St, Millinocket, ME 04462
Manual bed.

BED, MANUAL *(cont'd)*

Footent, Llc 757-224-0177
3392 W 8600 S, West Jordan, UT 84088
Bed clothes elevator.

Hard Manufacturing Co. 800-873-4273
230 Grider St, Buffalo, NY 14215
$1,750 for Model S2030 Trendelenburg 3 crank bed; $373 for Model 4189 3-crank nursing home bed; $267 for COMFORTCARE fixed-height bed; and $549 for SECURECARE 3-crank Model S3089 multi-height bed.

Hill-Rom Holdings, Inc. 800-445-3730
1069 State Road 46 E, Batesville, IN 47006

Hill-Rom, Inc. 812-934-7777
4115 Dorchester Rd Unit 600, North Charleston, SC 29405
Various models of manual hilow beds.

Invacare Corporation 800-333-6900
1 Invacare Way, Elyria, OH 44035
INVACARE.

Kma Remarketing Corp. 814-371-5242
302 Aspen Way, Dubois, PA 15801
Manual hospital bed.

M.C. Healthcare Products, Inc. 800-268-8671
4658 Ontario St., Beamsville, ONT L0R 1B4 Canada
Full-function subacute-hospital and long-term care beds for adults and youths; dormitory beds, fixed height, steel construction flat, head gatch, and head and foot gatch.

Marken International, Inc. 800-564-9248
W231N2811 Roundy Cir E Ste 100, Pewaukee, WI 53072
Various.

Mat Automotive 847-821-9630
355 W Crossroads Pkwy Ste A, Bolingbrook, IL 60440
Manual hospital bed.

Md International, Inc. 305-669-9003
11300 NW 41st St, Doral, FL 33178

Medical Depot 516-998-4600
99 Seaview Blvd, Port Washington, NY 11050
Bed.

Mjm International Corporation 956-781-5000
2003 N Veterans Blvd Ste 10, San Juan, TX 78589
Various models of low beds.

Nk Medical Products Inc. 800-274-2742
10123 Main St, PO Box 627, Clarence, NY 14031
Adult and Youth Size Beds

Noa Medical Industries 800-633-6068
801 Terry Ln, Washington, MO 63090
$320.00 to $360.00 for rib-deck resident bed.

Rite Time Corporation 800-266-2924
2950 E Dover St, Mesa, AZ 85213
Face-prone bed-extension system.

Schueler & Company, Inc. 516-487-1500
PO Box 528, Stratford, CT 06615

Sunrise Medical 800-333-4000
7477 Dry Creek Pkwy, Longmont, CO 80503

Symphony Medical Products 877-470-9995
6320 NW 84th Ave, Miami, FL 33166
Manual hospital bed.

Taylor's Mfg. 336-886-4192
524 Barker Ave, High Point, NC 27262
Pillow-hold.

The Anthros Medical Group 785-544-6592
807 E Spring St, Highland, KS 66035
Low bed.

Tuffcare 800-367-6160
3999 E La Palma Ave, Anaheim, CA 92807

Unilab, Inc. 9058559093
2355 Royal Windsor Dr., Unit 3, Mississauga, ON L5M-5R5 Canada
E.C.G. beds and E.C.G. stands.

Wheelchair Sales And Service Co., Inc. 877-736-0376
315 Main St, West Springfield, MA 01089
Mobilite (Invacare); Sunrise Medical.

BED, OBESE *(General) 80TAH*

Alimed, Inc. 800-225-2610
297 High St, Dedham, MA 02026

BED, OBESE *(cont'd)*

Gendron, Inc. 800-537-2521
400 E Lugbill Rd, Archbold, OH 43502
MAXI-REST Bariatric Beds.

Medi-Tech International, Inc. 305-593-9373
2924 NW 109th Ave, Doral, FL 33172
GENDRON

Tuffcare 800-367-6160
3999 E La Palma Ave, Anaheim, CA 92807

Wheelchairs Of Kansas 800-537-6454
204 W 2nd St, Ellis, KS 67637
DIAMOND HOMECARE BED, HOMECARE ADVANTAGE BED & MIGHTY REST REHAB BED: Diamond Homecare Bed is available in semi-electric or 8-function, full electric with Trendelenburg and Reverse Trendelenburg; Frame splits easily for transport; 600 lb. weight capacity; The frame is constructed of durable, heavy-duty steel with the deck made up of a thermoformed (fire retardant) plastic; This bed is offered in two widths - 39' & 48'. The HOMECARE ADVANTAGE BED is designed specifically for the bariatric individual; Constructed with durable, heavby-duty steel, this bed will hold up to 850 lbs. This full electric bed will operate the head section, foot section, a variety of height positions and a Comfort Chair position; 39' frame with optional 48' deck-wing kit to expand existing frame. The MIGHTY REST REHAB BED offers superior performance for bariatric individuals weighing up to 1,000 lbs.; This bed is offered in semi and full electric models with multiple functions for the head and foot sections as well as bed height adjustability; It comes in four width sizes and an extra-tall length; Frame splits easily for transportation.

BED, ORTHOPEDIC *(Orthopedics) 87QDF*

Jobri Llc 800-432-2225
520 N Division St, Konawa, OK 74849
Memory foam mattress and toppers

BED, PATIENT ROTATION, MANUAL *(Physical Med) 89INY*

Biomet, Inc. 574-267-6639
56 E Bell Dr, PO Box 587, Warsaw, IN 46582
Orthopedic turning frame.

Stryker Medical 800-869-0770
3800 E Centre Ave, Portage, MI 49002

BED, PATIENT ROTATION, POWERED *(Physical Med) 89IKZ*

Aggressive Solutions, Inc. 972-242-2164
1735 N Interstate 35E, Carrollton, TX 75006
Patient rotation mattress system.

Amf Support Surfaces, Inc. 951-549-6800
1691 N Delilah St, Corona, CA 92879
Continuous lateral rotation & alternating pressure mattress.

Gaymar Industries, Inc. 800-828-7341
10 Centre Dr, Orchard Park, NY 14127
The Clini-Dyne and O2 Zoned lateral turning mattresses additionally provide low air loss therapy. Small, quiet and portable control units.

Hill-Rom Holdings, Inc. 800-445-3730
1069 State Road 46 E, Batesville, IN 47006

Hill-Rom Manufacturing, Inc. 800-638-2546
4349 Corporate Rd, Charleston, SC 29405
EFICA CC Dynamic Air Therapy unit. V-CUE Dynamic Air Therapy Unit. PULMON EX Dynamic Air Therapy Unit.

Kap Medical 951-340-4360
1395 Pico St, Corona, CA 92881
Rotating low air loss mattress system.

Kinetic Concepts, Inc. 800-275-4524
8023 Vantage Dr, San Antonio, TX 78230
Various.

Lba Technology, Inc. 252-757-0279
3400 Tupper Dr, Greenville, NC 27834
Patient rotation.

Pro Bed Medical Techonogies, Inc. 800-816-8243
602-30930 Wheel Ave., Abbotsford, BC V2T 6G7 Canada
The Freedom Bed--lateral-rotation therapy system.

Sentech Medical Systems, Inc. 954-340-0500
4200 NW 120th Ave, Coral Springs, FL 33065
Rotating low air loss mattress overlay.

Stryker Medical 800-869-0770
3800 E Centre Ave, Portage, MI 49002

Tempur Production Usa, Inc. 276-431-7174
203 Tempur Pedic Dr Ste 102, Duffield, VA 24244
Continuous lateral rotation and alterating pressure mattress.

BED, PATIENT ROTATION, POWERED *(cont'd)*

Tempur-Medical, Inc. 888-255-3302
1713 Jaggie Fox Way, Lexington, KY 40511
Tempur-Plus3

BED, PEDIATRIC (CRIB) *(General) 80FMS*

Atlantic Medco, Inc. 800-203-8444
166 Bloomfield Ave, Verona, NJ 07044
$500 to $2000.

Basic American Medical Products 800-849-6664
2935A Northeast Pkwy, Atlanta, GA 30360

Bennett Industries, Inc. 931-432-4011
1805 Burgess Falls Rd, Cookeville, TN 38506
Pediatrics crib.

Hard Manufacturing Co. 800-873-4273
230 Grider St, Buffalo, NY 14215
$1,265 for crib Model C1913IL infant crib; $1,790 for Model 1073MG youth bed; $2,055 to $5,090 for Springfield Crib (135 models); $595 for D1230E crib Plexiglas end panels.

Hill-Rom, Inc. 812-934-7777
4115 Dorchester Rd Unit 600, North Charleston, SC 29405
Various models of bassinets.

Imperial Surgical Ltd. 800-661-5432
581 Orly Ave., Dorval, ONT H9P-1G1 Canada
$2,175 per unit.

Kinetic Concepts, Inc. 800-275-4524
8023 Vantage Dr, San Antonio, TX 78230
Pediatric low air loss bed.

Lic Care 800-323-5232
2935A Northeast Pkwy, Atlanta, GA 30360
Mobile unit.

M.C. Healthcare Products, Inc. 800-268-8671
4658 Ontario St., Beamsville, ONT L0R 1B4 Canada
Chrome, epoxy, sizes child, youth and adult.

Major Lab. Manufacturing 800-598-2621
4408 N Sewell Ave, Oklahoma City, OK 73118
Several models - $402.00 to $1,502.00 each.

Mayo Medical, S.A. De C.V. 800-715-3872
Edison 1141 Nte., Col. Talleres, Monterrey N.L. 64480 Mexico

Md International, Inc. 305-669-9003
11300 NW 41st St, Doral, FL 33178

Nk Medical Products Inc. 800-274-2742
10123 Main St, PO Box 627, Clarence, NY 14031
Over 30 sizes and styles.

O&M Enterprise 847-258-4515
641 Chelmsford Ln, Elk Grove Village, IL 60007
BED CRIBS-PEDIATRIC

Pedicraft, Inc. 800-223-7649
4134 Saint Augustine Rd, Jacksonville, FL 32207
PEDI-CRIB BED; $2,380 per unit (standard 60in.). ROVER Pediatric Stretcher Crib, $5,125 full crib height side rails on hydraulic stretcher base; $3,800 for fixed height. All four sides drop below mattress level for 100% patient access.

Schaerer Mayfield Usa 800-755-6381
4900 Charlemar Dr, Cincinnati, OH 45227
500 Pediatric Stretcher.

Symphony Medical Products 877-470-9995
6320 NW 84th Ave, Miami, FL 33166
Pediatric open hospital bed.

Trace Medical Equipment, Inc. 800-323-3786
5000 Varsity Dr, Lisle, IL 60532
Newborn Beds and Bassinets, wooden

BED, SCANNING, NUCLEAR/FLUOROSCOPIC *(Radiology) 90IYZ*

Asi Medical Equipment, Ltd. 800-527-0443
1735 N Interstate 35E, Carrollton, TX 75006
Intensive care beds.

Composiflex, Inc. 800-673-2544
8100 Hawthorne Dr, Erie, PA 16509
low absorption, high strength carbon fiber table tops

Jpl Electronics Corp. 631-345-9700
27 Scouting Blvd, Medford, NY 11763
Various models and types of scanning and imaging tables.

Marconi Medical Systems 800-323-0550
595 Miner Rd, Cleveland, OH 44143

BED, SCANNING, NUCLEAR/FLUOROSCOPIC *(cont'd)*

Mie America, Inc. 847-981-6100
420 Bennett Rd, Elk Grove Village, IL 60007
Nuclear scanning bed, gamma camera.

BEDPAN *(General) 80FOB*

American Bantex Corp. 800-633-4839
1815 Rollins Rd, Burlingame, CA 94010

Arcus Medical Llc 704-332-3424
2327 Distribution St, Charlotte, NC 28203
Male incontinence management system.

Centurion Medical Products Corp. 517-545-1135
3310 S Main St, Salisbury, NC 28147

Church Products Co. 800-317-8161
12 Briarglenn, Aliso Viejo, CA 92656
The Comfortpan is an improved, patented, adult bedpan, that is also ideal for bariatric patients.

Feiter's Inc 414-355-7575
8700 W Port Ave, Milwaukee, WI 53224
Bedpan.

Jones-Zylon Company 800-848-8160
305 N Center St, West Lafayette, OH 43845
Adult and pediatric sizes; autoclavable and disposable.

Kentron Health Care, Inc. 615-384-0573
3604 Kelton Jackson Rd, P.o. Box 120, Springfield, TN 37172
Bed pan.

Lsl Industries, Inc. 888-225-5575
5535 N Wolcott Ave, Chicago, IL 60640
$18.00 for 20 single use bed pans, $45.00 for 50 single use bed pans, all stackable. $20.00 for pontoon bedpan.

Medegen Medical Products, Llc 800-233-1987
209 Medegen Drive, Gallaway, TN 38036-0228
ROOM-MATES Disposable, sterilizable plastic & stainless steel.

Parsons A.D.L. Inc. 800-263-1281
R.R. #2, 1986 Sideroad 15, Tottenham, ONT L0G 1W0 Canada
A variety of male and female bedpans

Phillips Environmental Products, Inc. 406-388-5999
290 Arden Dr, Belgrade, MT 59714
Wag bags,waste kits, human waste bag kits.

Polar Ware Co. 800-237-3655
2806 N 15th St, Sheboygan, WI 53083
Stainless steel, reusable plastic.

Sunrise Medical 800-333-4000
7477 Dry Creek Pkwy, Longmont, CO 80503

Tidi Products, Llc 920-751-4380
570 Enterprise Dr, Neenah, WI 54956
Bedside bag.

Tri-State Hospital Supply Corp. 517-545-1135
3173 E 43rd St, Yuma, AZ 85365

BEDPAN, FRACTURE *(General) 80QDC*

Lsl Industries, Inc. 888-225-5575
5535 N Wolcott Ave, Chicago, IL 60640
$12.00 for 12 single use bed pans.

Medegen Medical Products, Llc 800-233-1987
209 Medegen Drive, Gallaway, TN 38036-0228
ROOM-MATES Disposable, sterilizable plastic & stainless steel.

O&M Enterprise 847-258-4515
641 Chelmsford Ln, Elk Grove Village, IL 60007
BEDPAN FRACTURE

Polar Ware Co. 800-237-3655
2806 N 15th St, Sheboygan, WI 53083
Stainless steel, resuable plastic.

BEDRAIL *(General) 80QDD*

Adden Furniture, Inc. 800-625-3876
26 Jackson St, Lowell, MA 01852

Alimed, Inc. 800-225-2610
297 High St, Dedham, MA 02026

American Innovations, Inc. 800-223-3913
123 N Main St, Dublin, PA 18917
Dishwasher-safe rigid caddy captures food/beverage containers, preventing spills to the floor, and organizes daily necessities. Transfers easily to wheelchair, walker, scooter, or crutch/cane.

Basic American Medical Products 800-849-6664
2935A Northeast Pkwy, Atlanta, GA 30360
Safety bed rails, telescoping and swing down models.

BEDRAIL *(cont'd)*

Basic American Metal Products 800-365-2338
336 Trowbridge Dr, PO Box 907, Fond Du Lac, WI 54937

Brown Engineering Corp. 800-726-4233
289 Chesterfield Rd, Westhampton, MA 01027
BED-BAR is an enabling device that promotes restraint-free mobility. The sturdiest and most cost-effective product available to assist with bed mobility. Used in rehabilitation centers and in clients' homes throughout North America.

Country Craft Furniture, Inc. 800-569-1968
5318 Railroad Ave, Flowery Branch, GA 30542

Crest Healthcare Supply 800-328-8908
195 3rd St, Dassel, MN 55325
Grab bars and security rails.

Formedica Ltd. 800-361-9671
1481 Rue Begin, St Laurent, QUE H4R 1V8 Canada
Bedrail padding only.

Hard Manufacturing Co. 800-873-4273
230 Grider St, Buffalo, NY 14215
$119 to $270 for 1/2, 3/4 or full length bedrails.

Home Aid Products 888-823-7605
111 Esna Park Dr., Unit 9, Markham, ONT L3R-1H2 Canada
Adjustable bed rails for beds with box spring and mattress. Bed assist rails.

Invacare Corporation 800-333-6900
1 Invacare Way, Elyria, OH 44035
INVACARE.

Larkotex Company 800-972-3037
1002 Olive St, Texarkana, TX 75501

Maddak Inc. 800-443-4926
661 State Route 23, Wayne, NJ 07470
ABLEWARE Able Rise Bed Rails with roomy storage areas. Single, double, fit twin, full & queen.

Mobility Transfer Systems 800-854-4687
PO Box 253, Medford, MA 02155
The Helping Hand Bedrail. Fits any style or size home bed. Installs easily between mattress & box springs. Strong and Stable; no tools required. Also available for hospital beds. Freedom Grip helps when getting out of bed.

Noa Medical Industries 800-633-6068
801 Terry Ln, Washington, MO 63090
Multiple bedrail options.

Sunrise Medical 800-333-4000
7477 Dry Creek Pkwy, Longmont, CO 80503

Tuffcare 800-367-6160
3999 E La Palma Ave, Anaheim, CA 92807

BELT, ABDOMINAL *(Gastro/Urology) 78EXP*

Alimed, Inc. 800-225-2610
297 High St, Dedham, MA 02026

Dale Medical Products, Inc. 800-343-3980
7 Cross St, Plainville, MA 02762
2 panel 6' wide: 28-50'; 3 panel 9' wide: #410 30-45', #411 46-62', #418 60-75' 4 panel 12' wide: #810 30-45', #811 46-62', #818 60-75', #819 72-84', #820 82-94' 5 panel 15 in. wide: #920 82-94 in.

Freeman Manufacturing Company 800-253-2091
900 W Chicago Rd, PO Box J, Sturgis, MI 49091

Hospital Marketing Svcs. Company, Inc. 800-786-5094
162 Great Hill Rd./ Ind. Park, Naugatuck, CT 06770
HMS FLEXITONE DUO Velcro closure post-operative abdominal belt - 9in. (three panels) wide, cat. no. 7350 (size 26in. to 49in.), and cat. no. 7364 (size 48in. to 64in.;)12in. (four panels) wide, cat. no. 7450 (size 26in. to 49in; and cat. no. 7464 (size 48in. to 64in.)

Ita-Med Co. 888-9IT-AMED
310 Littlefield Ave, South San Francisco, CA 94080
Support girdles, warming support girdles, and abdominal binders; 12-in. wide/4 panels, and 9-in. wide/3 panels.

Larkotex Company 800-972-3037
1002 Olive St, Texarkana, TX 75501

Ldb Medical, Inc. 800-243-2554
2909 Langford Rd Ste B500, Norcross, GA 30071
LAPIDES.

Lohmann & Rauscher, Inc. 800-279-3863
6001 SW 6th Ave Ste 101, Topeka, KS 66615

Tartan Orthopedics, Ltd. 888-287-1456
10651 Irma Dr Unit C, Northglenn, CO 80233
$132.50 per 10 (med).

BELT, ABDOMINAL *(cont'd)*

Zimmer Holdings, Inc. 800-613-6131
1800 W Center St, PO Box 708, Warsaw, IN 46580

BELT, ELECTRODE *(Cardiovascular) 74THD*

Electro Therapeutic Devices Inc. 800-268-3834
570 Hood Rd., Ste. 14, Markham, ONT L3R 4G7 Canada

BELT, LUMBOSACRAL *(Orthopedics) 87QDH*

Formedica Ltd. 800-361-9671
1481 Rue Begin, St Laurent, QUE H4R 1V8 Canada
$300.00 per 10 (med).

Freeman Manufacturing Company 800-253-2091
900 W Chicago Rd, PO Box J, Sturgis, MI 49091

Hospital Marketing Svcs. Company, Inc. 800-786-5094
162 Great Hill Rd./ Ind. Park, Naugatuck, CT 06770
HMS FLEXITONE UNIVERSAL sized for 24-62in. waist, one size fits all - 9in. (three panels) wide, cat. no. 7333 12in. (four panels) wide, cat. no. 7444; 15in. (five panels) wide, cat. no. 7555.

Larkotex Company 800-972-3037
1002 Olive St, Texarkana, TX 75501

Lohmann & Rauscher, Inc. 800-279-3863
6001 SW 6th Ave Ste 101, Topeka, KS 66615

Orthosource, Inc. 800-649-5525
17374 W Sunset Blvd, Pacific Palisades, CA 90272
Textile and Neoprene support belts; Industrial Safety Back Support belt with or without suspenders

Paramedical Distributors 800-245-3278
2020 Grand Blvd, Kansas City, MO 64108
Back support. Assorted styles and sizes available.

Scott Specialties, Inc./Cmo Inc./Ginny Inc. 800-255-7136
512 M St, Belleville, KS 66935
DURAFOAM.

Slawner Ltd., J. 514-731-3378
5713 Cote Des Neiges Rd., Montreal, QUE H3S 1Y7 Canada

Tetra Medical Supply Corp. 800-621-4041
6364 W Gross Point Rd, Niles, IL 60714

Truform Orthotics & Prosthetics 800-888-0458
3960 Rosslyn Dr, Cincinnati, OH 45209

Zimmer Holdings, Inc. 800-613-6131
1800 W Center St, PO Box 708, Warsaw, IN 46580

Zimmer Orthopaedic Surgical Products 800-321-5533
PO Box 10, 200 West Ohio Ave., Dover, OH 44622

BELT, RIB (SUPPORT) *(Orthopedics) 87QDI*

Alex Orthopedic, Inc. 800-544-2539
PO Box 201442, Arlington, TX 76006

Corflex, Inc. 800-426-7353
669 E Industrial Park Dr, Manchester, NH 03109

Dale Medical Products, Inc. 800-343-3980
7 Cross St, Plainville, MA 02762
2 panel 6 in. Female #425 28-50', #427 46-60'; 2 panel 6' Male #525 28-50' #527 46-60'

Fla Orthopedics, Inc. 800-327-4110
2881 Corporate Way, Miramar, FL 33025

Formedica Ltd. 800-361-9671
1481 Rue Begin, St Laurent, QUE H4R 1V8 Canada
$70.00 per 10 (med).

Frank Stubbs Co., Inc 800-223-1713
2100 Eastman Ave Ste B, Oxnard, CA 93030

Freeman Manufacturing Company 800-253-2091
900 W Chicago Rd, PO Box J, Sturgis, MI 49091

Hermell Products, Inc. 800-233-2342
9 Britton Dr, PO Box 7345, Bloomfield, CT 06002
Male (straight) or female.

Hospital Marketing Svcs. Company, Inc. 800-786-5094
162 Great Hill Rd./ Ind. Park, Naugatuck, CT 06770
HMS UNIVERSAL - 6in. (two panels) wide, one size fits 28-60in. waist - male (cat. no. 0909) and female (cat. no. 0908.)

Jobri Llc 800-432-2225
520 N Division St, Konawa, OK 74849
MOR-LOC, EZ-FIT.

Larkotex Company 800-972-3037
1002 Olive St, Texarkana, TX 75501

Lohmann & Rauscher, Inc. 800-279-3863
6001 SW 6th Ave Ste 101, Topeka, KS 66615

BELT, RIB (SUPPORT) *(cont'd)*

Orthosource, Inc. 800-649-5525
17374 W Sunset Blvd, Pacific Palisades, CA 90272
Universal or sized. Many belts are specific for either men or women, while some can fit either gender.

Paramedical Distributors 800-245-3278
2020 Grand Blvd, Kansas City, MO 64108

Scott Specialties, Inc./Cmo Inc./Ginny Inc. 800-255-7136
512 M St, Belleville, KS 66935
ADAM AND EVE.

Sroufe Healthcare Products Llc 888-894-4171
PO Box 347, 601 Sroufe St., Ligonier, IN 46767

Surgical Appliance Industries 800-888-0458
3960 Rosslyn Dr, Cincinnati, OH 45209

Tetra Medical Supply Corp. 800-621-4041
6364 W Gross Point Rd, Niles, IL 60714

Truform Orthotics & Prosthetics 800-888-0458
3960 Rosslyn Dr, Cincinnati, OH 45209

Zimmer Holdings, Inc. 800-613-6131
1800 W Center St, PO Box 708, Warsaw, IN 46580

Zimmer Orthopaedic Surgical Products 800-321-5533
PO Box 10, 200 West Ohio Ave., Dover, OH 44622

BELT, SANITARY *(Obstetrics/Gyn) 85RQK*

Atd-American Co. 800-523-2300
135 Greenwood Ave, Wyncote, PA 19095

R Medical Supply 800-882-7578
620 Valley Forge Rd Ste F, Hillsborough, NC 27278

BELT, SUPPORT, PELVIC *(Physical Med) 89ISQ*

Activeaid, Inc. 800-533-5330
101 Activeaid Rd, Redwood Falls, MN 56283

Alimed, Inc. 800-225-2610
297 High St, Dedham, MA 02026

Hospital Marketing Svcs. Company, Inc. 800-786-5094
162 Great Hill Rd./ Ind. Park, Naugatuck, CT 06770
HMS FLEXITONE pelvic traction belt, single or double pull - waist size 26-48in., cat. no. 7340; waist size 48-64in., cat. no. 7345.

Ita-Med Co. 888-9IT-AMED
310 Littlefield Ave, South San Francisco, CA 94080
GABRIALLA maternity collection support products for women during and after pregnancy. Products include elastic support belt, graduated compression maternity pantyhose, support girdles, and replenishing body cream.

Pro Orthopedic Devices, Inc. 800-523-5611
2884 E Ganley Rd, Tucson, AZ 85706
PRO Neoprene rubber joint sleeves and supports.

Tartan Orthopedics, Ltd. 888-287-1456
10651 Irma Dr Unit C, Northglenn, CO 80233
$145.00 per 10 (med); industrial support belt, $15.90/unit.

Zimmer Orthopaedic Surgical Products 800-321-5533
PO Box 10, 200 West Ohio Ave., Dover, OH 44622

BELT, TRACTION, PELVIC *(Physical Med) 89IRZ*

DJO Inc. 800-336-6569
1430 Decision St, Vista, CA 92081

Hospital Marketing Svcs. Company, Inc. 800-786-5094
162 Great Hill Rd./ Ind. Park, Naugatuck, CT 06770
Single or double pull, 26-48in. long pelvic traction belt, cat. no. 7340.

Lohmann & Rauscher, Inc. 800-279-3863
6001 SW 6th Ave Ste 101, Topeka, KS 66615

Lossing Orthopedic 800-328-5216
PO Box 6224, Minneapolis, MN 55406
LOSSING pelvic tilt belt constructed of non-slip fabric for customized fit; available in four different sizes: small, medium, large, extra-large.

Mizuho Osi 800-777-4674
30031 Ahern Ave, Union City, CA 94587

Rehabilitation Technical Components, Corp. 919-732-1705
3913 Devonwood Rd, Hillsborough, NC 27278
Eleva streckbandage.

Scott Specialties, Inc./Cmo Inc./Ginny Inc. 800-255-7136
512 M St, Belleville, KS 66935
DURAFOAM.

Surgical Appliance Industries 800-888-0458
3960 Rosslyn Dr, Cincinnati, OH 45209

BELT, TRACTION, PELVIC, ORTHOPEDIC *(Orthopedics) 87HSQ*

A&A Orthopedics, Incorporated 757-224-0177
12250 SW 129th Ct Bldg 1, Miami, FL 33186
Pelvic traction set?.

American Orthopedic Supply Co., Inc.
37017 State Highway 79, Cleveland, AL 35049
Pelvic belt.

Biomet, Inc. 574-267-6639
56 E Bell Dr, PO Box 587, Warsaw, IN 46582
Various types of pelvic traction belt.

Bird & Cronin, Inc. 651-683-1111
1200 Trapp Rd, Saint Paul, MN 55121
Pelvic traction belt.

Chattanooga Group 800-592-7329
4717 Adams Rd, Hixson, TN 37343
Universal size.

Core Products International, Inc. 800-365-3047
808 Prospect Ave, Osceola, WI 54020
Orthopedic belt available.

Dj Orthopedics De Mexico, S.A. De C.V. 690-727-1280
Blvd., Delagacion La Presa, Tijuana 22397 Mexico
Pelvic traction belts

Dj Orthopedics De Mexico, S.A. De C.V. 690-727-1280
Ave. Venustiano Carranza 6802, Castillo, Tijuana 22100 Mexico
Pelvic traction belts

DJO Inc. 800-336-6569
1430 Decision St, Vista, CA 92081

Elastic Corporation Of America 704-328-5381
455 Highway 70, Columbiana, AL 35051
Transducer/fetal monitor belt.

Freeman Manufacturing Company 800-253-2091
900 W Chicago Rd, PO Box J, Sturgis, MI 49091

Hospital Marketing Svcs. Company, Inc. 800-786-5094
162 Great Hill Rd./ Ind. Park, Naugatuck, CT 06770
Single or double pull, size 48-64in., cat. no. 7345.

Jobri Llc 800-432-2225
520 N Division St, Konawa, OK 74849
MOR-LOC.

Kenad Sg Medical, Inc. 800-825-0606
2692 Huntley Dr, Memphis, TN 38132
Pelvic traction belt.

Larkotex Company 800-972-3037
1002 Olive St, Texarkana, TX 75501

Lohmann & Rauscher, Inc. 800-279-3863
6001 SW 6th Ave Ste 101, Topeka, KS 66615

Lossing Orthopedic 800-328-5216
PO Box 6224, Minneapolis, MN 55406
LOSSING maternity pelvic tilt belt is custom designed with a separate, removable panel to accommodate growth. This belt will gently reverse the heavy curve in the lower back and help neutralize lordosis caused by pregnancy.

Mizuho Osi 800-777-4674
30031 Ahern Ave, Union City, CA 94587

Orthofix Inc. 800-535-4492
1720 Bray Central Dr, McKinney, TX 75069
Pneumatic Bracing

Paramedical Distributors 800-245-3278
2020 Grand Blvd, Kansas City, MO 64108

Scott Specialties, Inc. 785-527-5627
1827 Meadowlark Rd, Clay Center, KS 67432
Various types of pelvic traction belts.

Scott Specialties, Inc. 785-527-5627
1820 E 7th St, Concordia, KS 66901

Scott Specialties, Inc./Cmo Inc./Ginny Inc. 800-255-7136
512 M St, Belleville, KS 66935
DURAFOAM.

Shamrock Medical, Inc. 503-233-5055
3620 SE Powell Blvd, Portland, OR 97202
Single pull traction belts.

Slawner Ltd., J. 514-731-3378
5713 Cote Des Neiges Rd., Montreal, QUE H3S 1Y7 Canada

Tartan Orthopedics, Ltd. 888-287-1456
10651 Irma Dr Unit C, Northglenn, CO 80233
$145.00 per 10 (med).

BELT, TRACTION, PELVIC, ORTHOPEDIC *(cont'd)*

Tetra Medical Supply Corp. 800-621-4041
6364 W Gross Point Rd, Niles, IL 60714

Truform Orthotics & Prosthetics 800-888-0458
3960 Rosslyn Dr, Cincinnati, OH 45209

Val Med 800-242-5355
3700 Desire Pkwy, Ace Bayou Group, New Orleans, LA 70126
Universal pelvic belt.

Warsaw Orthopedic, Inc. 901-396-3133
2500 Silveus Xing, Warsaw, IN 46582
Various types of pelvic traction belts.

Zimmer Holdings, Inc. 800-613-6131
1800 W Center St, PO Box 708, Warsaw, IN 46580

Zimmer Orthopaedic Surgical Products 800-321-5533
PO Box 10, 200 West Ohio Ave., Dover, OH 44622

BELT, WHEELCHAIR *(Physical Med) 89IQB*

Alimed, Inc. 800-225-2610
297 High St, Dedham, MA 02026

Bird & Cronin, Inc. 651-683-1111
1200 Trapp Rd, Saint Paul, MN 55121
Wheel chair belt.

Blue Earth, Inc. 518-237-5585
31 Ontario St, 2nd Floor - Front, Cohoes, NY 12047
Heel/toe loops, lap belt.

Bodypoint, Inc. 800-547-5716
558 1st Ave S Ste 300, Seattle, WA 98104

Daher Mfg., Inc. 204-663-3299
Mazenod Rd, Winnipeg R2J 4H2 Canada
Various

E.J. Wagner & Associates, Inc. 814-849-9983
716 N. 67nd St., Mesa, AZ 85205
Wheelchair torso support.

Humane Restraint Co Inc 800-356-7472
912 Bethel Cir, Waunakee, WI 53597

Innovative Concepts 800-676-5030
300 N State St, Girard, OH 44420
Seat belts, ankle straps for wheelchairs.

Intarsia Ltd. 203-355-1357
14 Martha Ln, Gaylordsville, CT 06755
Lapbelt, pelvic belt, pelvic stabilizer, ankle straps, toe straps, chestp.

Kareco International, Inc. 800-8KA-RECO
299 Rte. 22 E., Green Brook, NJ 08812-1714

Ocelco, Inc. 800-328-5343
1111 Industrial Park Rd SW, Brainerd, MN 56401

Sunrise Medical Hhg Inc 303-218-4505
7128 Ambassador Rd, Baltimore, MD 21244
Pelvic positioning belts,various sizes.

Sunrise Medical Hhg Inc 303-218-4505
2010 E Spruce Cir, Olathe, KS 66062
Wheelchair belt.

Sunrise Medical Hhg Inc 303-218-4505
6724 Preston Ave # 1, Livermore, CA 94551

Sunrise Medical Hhg Inc 303-218-4505
2615 W Casino Rd # 2B, Everett, WA 98204

Sunrise Medical Hhg Inc 303-218-4505
2842 N Business Park Ave, Fresno, CA 93727

Thompson Medical Specialties 800-777-4949
3404 Library Ln, Saint Louis Park, MN 55426

Tuffcare 800-367-6160
3999 E La Palma Ave, Anaheim, CA 92807

BENDER *(Orthopedics) 87HXW*

Biomet, Inc. 574-267-6639
56 E Bell Dr, PO Box 587, Warsaw, IN 46582
Brace bending iron.

Bioquest 480-350-9944
2211 W 1st St Ste 106, Tempe, AZ 85281
Rod bender.

Holmed Corporation 508-238-3351
40 Norfolk Ave, South Easton, MA 02375

K2m, Inc. 866-526-4171
751 Miller Dr SE Ste F1, Leesburg, VA 20175
Bender.

BENDER *(cont'd)*

Kmedic 800-955-0559
190 Veterans Dr, Northvale, NJ 07647
GRATLOCH wire bender for stabilizing and bending a Kirschner wire simultaneously.

Medtronic Sofamor Danek Usa, Inc. 901-396-3133
4340 Swinnea Rd, Memphis, TN 38118
Various benders.

Rush-Berivon, Inc. 800-251-7874
1010 19th St, P.O. Box 1851, Meridian, MS 39301
$127.00 for 2mm thru 6mm pin usage.

Spine Wave, Inc. 203-944-9494
2 Enterprise Dr Ste 302, Shelton, CT 06484
Various types of rod benders.

Symmetry Medical Usa, Inc. 574-267-8700
486 W 350 N, Warsaw, IN 46582
Orthopedic manual surgical instrument.

Warsaw Orthopedic, Inc. 901-396-3133
2500 Silveus Xing, Warsaw, IN 46582
Various benders.

Zimmer Holdings, Inc. 800-613-6131
1800 W Center St, PO Box 708, Warsaw, IN 46580

BIB *(General) 80QDJ*

Atd-American Co. 800-523-2300
135 Greenwood Ave, Wyncote, PA 19095

Best Manufacturing Group Llc 800-843-3233
1633 Broadway Fl 18, New York, NY 10019
Adult and childrens' bibs, 100% cotton, ties, colors.

Chagrin Safety Supply, Inc. 800-227-0468
8227 Washington St # 1, Chagrin Falls, OH 44023

Crosstex International 800-223-2497
10 Ranick Rd, Hauppauge, NY 11788
Dental bibs,professional towels,10 colors

Crosstex International Ltd., W. Region 800-707-2737
14059 Stage Rd, Santa Fe Springs, CA 90670
Dental bibs.

Crosstex International,Inc. 888-276-7783
10 Ranick Rd, Hauppauge, NY 11788
CROSSTEX Dental bibs. POLYBACK, ECONOBACK, POLYGARD, PROBACK, PROFESSIONAL ULTRAGARD.

Fabrite Laminating Corp. 973-777-1406
70 Passaic St, Wood Ridge, NJ 07075

Freestyle Medical Supplies, Inc. 800-841-5330
336 Green Rd, Stoney Creek, ON L8E 2B2 Canada
FREESTYLE bibs. Protect outer clothing from moisture and staining. Two sizes, frontal coverage bib with foot catch-all, and extra long bib for frontal and lap coverage.

Geri-Care Products 201-440-0409
250 Moonachie Ave, Moonachie, NJ 07074
Terry & Designer pattern bibs

Gi Supply 800-451-5797
200 Grandview Ave, Camp Hill, PA 17011
ENDOBIB, disposable absorbant patient bib with catch pocket.

Graham Medical Products/Div. Of Little Rapids Corp 866-429-1408
2273 Larsen Rd, Green Bay, WI 54303

Hager Worldwide, Inc. 800-328-2335
13322 Byrd Dr, Odessa, FL 33556
'SUPER' BIB CLIP (patient bib holder) autoclavable.

Health-Pak, Inc. 315-724-8370
2005 Beechgrove Pl, Utica, NY 13501

Hos-Pillow Corp. 800-468-7874
1011 Campus Dr, Mundelein, IL 60060
Cotton and disposable.

Jms Converters Inc Dba Sabee Products & Stanford Prof Prod 215-396-3302
67 Buck Rd Ste B7, Huntingdon Valley, PA 19006
Disposable bibs.

Lew Jan Textile 800-899-0531
366 Veterans Memorial Hwy Ste 4, Commack, NY 11725
Adult bibs in terry solids, terry stripes, plaid flannel with various closure systems.

Maddak Inc. 800-443-4926
661 State Route 23, Wayne, NJ 07470
ABLEWARE (med) vinyl.

BIB *(cont'd)*

Mip Inc. 800-361-4964
9100 Ray Lawson Blvd., Montreal, QC H1J-1K8 Canada
Adult bibs.

Pharaoh Trading Company 866-929-4913
9701 Brookpark Rd, Knollwood Plaza, Suite 241, Cleveland, OH 44129

Postcraft Co. 800-528-4844
625 W Rillito St, Tucson, AZ 85705
Synthetic bibs.

Ross Disposable Products 800-649-6526
401 Traders Blvd E, Unit 10, Mississauga, ON L4Z 2H8 Canada

Salk Inc. 800-343-4497
119 Braintree St Ste 701, 4th Floor, Boston, MA 02134
Adult Bib, Terry cloth & Flannel bibs.

Viscot Medical, Llc 800-221-0658
32 West St, PO Box 351, East Hanover, NJ 07936
Tissue or tissue/poly dental bibs.

BILIRUBIN (TOTAL AND UNBOUND) NEONATE TEST SYSTEM
(Chemistry) 75MQM

Abbott Diagnostics Div. 626-440-0700
820 Mission St, South Pasadena, CA 91030
Neonatal bilirubin.

BILIRUBINOMETER *(Chemistry) 75QDL*

Advanced Instruments Inc. 800-225-4034
2 Technology Way, Norwood, MA 02062
$3969.00 for tabletop model. BR 2 measures infant total and direct bilirubin by direct spectrophotometry and Malloy-Evelyn methods.

Hematechnologies, Inc. 877-436-2835
291 Rte. 22, Suite 12, Lebanon, NJ 08833
One-step direct read. 25-microliter heel stick. Bilirubin+hematocrit in 5 minutes.

International Light Technologies, Inc. 978-818-6180
10 Technology Dr, Peabody, MA 01960
IL has just released the new low cost specialist series radiometer, IL74, for a low cost alternative for bilirubin testing. IL has a broad range of radiometers which can be used for phototherapy. By selecting either the IL1400 or IL1700 series radiometer and either/all of the UVA, UVB or Hyperbilirubinemia sensors, you can use one meter to make all of your phototherapy measurement.

Spectronics Corporation 800-274-8888
956 Brush Hollow Rd, Westbury, NY 11590
Hyperbilirubinemia radiometer.

Wako Chemicals Usa, Inc. 877-714-1924
1600 Bellwood Rd, Richmond, VA 23237
Instrument used to measure neonatal bilirubin levels in capillary tube.

BILIRUBINOMETER, CUTANEOUS (JAUNDICE METER)
(General) 80UDF

Medi-Tech International, Inc. 305-593-9373
2924 NW 109th Ave, Doral, FL 33172
OLYMPIC

BIN, STORAGE *(General) 80VKB*

Akro-Mils, Inc. 800-253-2467
1293 S Main St, Akron, OH 44301
Storage bins and accessories.

Armstrong Medical Industries, Inc. 800-323-4220
575 Knightsbridge Pkwy, Lincolnshire, IL 60069
Tilt bin organizers available in four sizes, from three to six bins across.

Cargille Laboratories 973-239-6633
55 Commerce Rd, Cedar Grove, NJ 07009
Tissue files, storage for 100 histopathology tissue blocks, $29.00 each; microslide files storage for 48 3- x 1-in. slides, $28.50 each.

Cryo-Cell International, Inc. 800-786-7235
700 Brooker Creek Blvd Ste 1800, Oldsmar, FL 34677
Cryogenic cellular storage unit capable of storing 35,000 5cc vials under optimal conditions, robotic insertion and retrieval process.

Frank Scholz X-Ray Corp. 508-586-8308
244 Liberty St, Brockton, MA 02301
$400.00 for radiation protection storage units, X-ray room accessories for apron wall mount brackets for apron storage.

Freund Container 800-363-9822
4200 Commerce Ct Ste 206, Corporate Center II, Lisle, IL 60532

Healthmark Industries 800-521-6224
22522 E 9 Mile Rd, Saint Clair Shores, MI 48080
Over 100 sizes of general storage containers.

BIN, STORAGE *(cont'd)*

Ideal Products 800-321-5490
1287 County Road 623, Broseley, MO 63932
Storage racks for therapeutic and rehabilitation cuff weights, dumbells and therapy balls.

Intermetro Industries Corp. 800-441-2714
651 N Washington St, Wilkes Barre, PA 18705
METROTOTES, bins and tote box storage.

Kardex Systems, Inc. 800-234-3654
114 Westview Ave, Marietta, OH 45750
Movable shelving.

Lewis Bins+ 877-97L-EWIS
PO Box 389, Oconomowoc, WI 53066
High-performance storage containers/bins and metal systems for improved inventory control and space optimization. Hopper-front bins are also available to facilitate easy visual and physical access to parts. Available in ESD-safe materials to protect sensitive medical devices during storage and transport.

Medical Packaging Corporation 800-792-0600
941 Avenida Acaso, Camarillo, CA 93012
Storage filing system for slides or tissue blocks.

Orbis Corporation 800-890-7292
1055 Corporate Center Dr, PO Box 389, Oconomowoc, WI 53066
Handheld containers which stack; nest and collapse when not in use. Products are available with custom dunnage and interiors in a wide variety of colors.

Rycor Medical, Inc. 800-227-9267
2053 Atwater Dr, North Port, FL 34288
RYCOR U.S. 300, storage device capable of holding one set of stirrurps, two armboards, and various O.R. table clamps.

Spacesaver Corporation 800-492-3434
1450 Janesville Ave, Fort Atkinson, WI 53538
PHARMASTOR, STOREFRONT and QUICKSPACE, high-density mobile storage systems.

Stackbin Corporation 800-333-1603
29 Powder Hill Rd, Lincoln, RI 02865
Stackbins/plastic bins for storage of medical components and products.

White Systems, Inc. 800-275-1442
30 Boright Ave, Kenilworth, NJ 07033
Stockroom carousel systems.

Wire Crafters L.L.C. 800-924-9473
6208 Strawberry Ln, Louisville, KY 40214
STYLE 840 WOVENWIRE PARTITION. Can be used to make cages to store class III, IV, and V controlled substances, or anything that needs to be stored (ie. equipment, maintenance supplies, etc.).

BINDER, ABDOMINAL *(General) 80FSD*

A&A Orthopedics, Incorporated 757-224-0177
12250 SW 129th Ct Bldg 1, Miami, FL 33186
Abdominal binder.

Azmec, Inc. 877-862-9632
519 N Smith Ave Ste 110, Corona, CA 92880
Abdominal binders.

Baron Medical Supply 888-702-2766
709 Grand St, Brooklyn, NY 11211

Best Orthopedic And Medical Services, Inc. 800-344-5279
2356B Springs Rd NE, Hickory, NC 28601

Biomet, Inc. 574-267-6639
56 E Bell Dr, PO Box 587, Warsaw, IN 46582
Various types of abdominal binder.

Bird & Cronin, Inc. 651-683-1111
1200 Trapp Rd, Saint Paul, MN 55121
Abdominal binder.

Centurion Medical Products Corp. 517-545-1135
3310 S Main St, Salisbury, NC 28147

Corflex, Inc. 800-426-7353
669 E Industrial Park Dr, Manchester, NH 03109

Dale Medical Products, Inc. 800-343-3980
7 Cross St, Plainville, MA 02762
2 panel 6' wide: 28-50'; 3 panel 9' wide: #410 30-45', #411 46-62', #418 60-75' 4 panel 12' wide: #810 30-45', #811 46-62', #818 60-75', #819 72-84', #820 82-94' 5 panel 15 in. wide: #920 82-94 in.

Dj Orthopedics De Mexico, S.A. De C.V. 690-727-1280
Blvd., Delagacion La Presa, Tijuana 22397 Mexico
Binder, abdominal

BINDER, ABDOMINAL *(cont'd)*

Dj Orthopedics De Mexico, S.A. De C.V. 690-727-1280
Ave. Venustiano Carranza 6802, Castillo, Tijuana 22100 Mexico
Binder, abdominal

DJO Inc. 800-336-6569
1430 Decision St, Vista, CA 92081
Various abdominal binders and supports.

Dowling Textiles 770-957-3981
615 Macon Rd, McDonough, GA 30253
Various types of abdominal binders.

Fla Orthopedics, Inc. 800-327-4110
2881 Corporate Way, Miramar, FL 33025

Formedica Ltd. 800-361-9671
1481 Rue Begin, St Laurent, QUE H4R 1V8 Canada
$120.00 per 10 (10in, med).

Frank Stubbs Co., Inc 800-223-1713
2100 Eastman Ave Ste B, Oxnard, CA 93030

Frederick Lee Inc 787-834-4880
191 Calle Balboa, PO Box 3287, Mayaguez, PR 00680

Freeman Manufacturing Company 800-253-2091
900 W Chicago Rd, PO Box J, Sturgis, MI 49091

Geen Healthcare Inc. 800-565-4336
931 Progress Ave. Ste.13, Scarborough, ONT M1G 3V5 Canada

Hanson Medical, Inc. 800-771-2215
825 Riverside Ave Ste 2, Paso Robles, CA 93446
Various.

Hospital Marketing Svcs. Company, Inc. 800-786-5094
162 Great Hill Rd./ Ind. Park, Naugatuck, CT 06770
No. 7350 DUO FLEXITONE universal binder, cat. no. 7333, size 24-62in., 9in. wide rib belt, cat. nos. 0908 and 0909. Assorted sizes of binders. Single pelvic traction belt, cat. no. 7340. Double unit, cat. no. 7345.

Jeunique International, Inc. 800-628-7747
19501 E Walnut Dr S, City Of Industry, CA 91748
Jeunique back-to-normal.

Kenad Sg Medical, Inc. 800-825-0606
2692 Huntley Dr, Memphis, TN 38132
Adominal binder.

Kentron Health Care, Inc. 615-384-0573
3604 Kelton Jackson Rd, P.o. Box 120, Springfield, TN 37172
Abdominal binder.

Kmi Kolster Methods, Inc. 909-737-5476
3185 Palisades Dr, Corona, CA 92880
Abdominal binders.

Lac-Mac Ltd. 800-461-0001
425 Rectory St., London, ONT N5W 3W5 Canada

Larkotex Company 800-972-3037
1002 Olive St, Texarkana, TX 75501

Leading Lady, Inc. 216-464-5490
24050 Commerce Park Dr., Beachwood, OH 44122
Abdominal binder.

Lohmann & Rauscher, Inc. 800-279-3863
6001 SW 6th Ave Ste 101, Topeka, KS 66615

Medline Industries, Inc. 800-633-5886
1 Medline Pl, Mundelein, IL 60060

Moore Products, A Sale Proprietorship 650-592-1822
596 Teredo Dr, Redwood City, CA 94065
Maternity supporter.

Morris Designs, Inc. 757-463-9400
2212 Commerce Pkwy, Virginia Beach, VA 23454
Various girdle circumpress.

My True Image Mfg. 510-231-5253
999 Marina Way S, Richmond, CA 94804
Abdominal binder.

Ny Orthopedic Usa, Inc. 718-852-5330
63 Flushing Ave Unit 333, Brooklyn, NY 11205
Abdominal binder.

O&M Enterprise 847-258-4515
641 Chelmsford Ln, Elk Grove Village, IL 60007
BINDER - ABDOMINAL/CHEST/ELASTIC

Ossur Americas 949-268-3155
742 Pancho Rd, Camarillo, CA 93012

Scott Specialties, Inc. 785-527-5627
1827 Meadowlark Rd, Clay Center, KS 67432
Binder, abdominal.

BINDER, ABDOMINAL *(cont'd)*

Scott Specialties, Inc. 785-527-5627
1820 E 7th St, Concordia, KS 66901

Scott Specialties, Inc./Cmo Inc./Ginny Inc. 800-255-7136
512 M St, Belleville, KS 66935

Tartan Orthopedics, Ltd. 888-287-1456
10651 Irma Dr Unit C, Northglenn, CO 80233
$132.50 per 10 (10in, med).

Tetra Medical Supply Corp. 800-621-4041
6364 W Gross Point Rd, Niles, IL 60714

Tri-State Hospital Supply Corp. 517-545-1135
3173 E 43rd St, Yuma, AZ 85365

Truform Orthotics & Prosthetics 800-888-0458
3960 Rosslyn Dr, Cincinnati, OH 45209

Warsaw Orthopedic, Inc. 901-396-3133
2500 Silveus Xing, Warsaw, IN 46582
Various abdominal binders.

Zimmer Holdings, Inc. 800-613-6131
1800 W Center St, PO Box 708, Warsaw, IN 46580

BINDER, ABDOMINAL, OB/GYN *(Obstetrics/Gyn) 85HFR*

Body Therapeutics, Div. Of I-Rep, Inc. 800-530-3722
508 Chaney St Ste 13, Lake Elsinore, CA 92530

Dale Medical Products, Inc. 800-343-3980
7 Cross St, Plainville, MA 02762
2 panel 6' wide: 28-50'; 3 panel 9' wide: #410 30-45', #411 46-62', #418 60-75' 4 panel 12' wide: #810 30-45', #811 46-62', #818 60-75', #819 72-84', #820 82-94' 5 panel 15 in. wide: #920 82-94 in.

Hospital Marketing Svcs. Company, Inc. 800-786-5094
162 Great Hill Rd./ Ind. Park, Naugatuck, CT 06770
9in. wide, 24-62in. long, cat. nos. 7333, 7444 or 7555.

Lohmann & Rauscher, Inc. 800-279-3863
6001 SW 6th Ave Ste 101, Topeka, KS 66615
Mom-EZ Maternity Support

BINDER, ANKLE *(Orthopedics) 87QDM*

Formedica Ltd. 800-361-9671
1481 Rue Begin, St Laurent, QUE H4R 1V8 Canada
$40.00 per 10 (med).

Hospital Marketing Svcs. Company, Inc. 800-786-5094
162 Great Hill Rd./ Ind. Park, Naugatuck, CT 06770
FLEXITONE trauma wrap - cat. no. 7614.

Larkotex Company 800-972-3037
1002 Olive St, Texarkana, TX 75501

Paramedical Distributors 800-245-3278
2020 Grand Blvd, Kansas City, MO 64108

Tetra Medical Supply Corp. 800-621-4041
6364 W Gross Point Rd, Niles, IL 60714

Zimmer Orthopaedic Surgical Products 800-321-5533
PO Box 10, 200 West Ohio Ave., Dover, OH 44622

BINDER, BREAST *(Obstetrics/Gyn) 85HEF*

Aztec Heart, Inc. 530-533-7069
2445 Oro Dam Blvd E Ste 7, Oroville, CA 95966
Support bra.

Bsn-Jobst 704-554-9933
5825 Carnegie Blvd, Charlotte, NC 28209
Mammarry support bra.

Centurion Medical Products Corp. 517-545-1135
3310 S Main St, Salisbury, NC 28147

General Cardiac Technology, Inc. 831-471-2940
15814 Winchester Blvd Ste 105, Los Gatos, CA 95030
Heart hugger sternum support harness.

Golda, Inc. 800-321-4804
24050 Commerce Park, Cleveland, OH 44122
SURGI-BRA Bra/binders used for compression and support for post-mastectomy, thoracic and chest surgeries. New products include the SURGI-VEST, which provides substantial post-surgical support to immobilize ribs, sternum, and breast tissue after heart/chest surgeries, especially those complicated by obesity, large breasts, and/or excess fatty tissue.

Hospital Marketing Svcs. Company, Inc. 800-786-5094
162 Great Hill Rd./ Ind. Park, Naugatuck, CT 06770
Cat no. 7350.

Lac-Mac Ltd. 800-461-0001
425 Rectory St., London, ONT N5W 3W5 Canada

BINDER, BREAST *(cont'd)*

Leading Lady, Inc. 216-464-5490
24050 Commerce Park Dr., Beachwood, OH 44122
Breast wrap, augmentation band.

Medi-Garb Co., Inc. 800-233-2463
216 W Broad St, Statesville, NC 28677
Breast Binder for lactation suppression for mothers who will not be nursing their infants. Also used as compression bandage for chest edema, cardiac, and breast surgery post op.

Morris Designs, Inc. 757-463-9400
2212 Commerce Pkwy, Virginia Beach, VA 23454
Bra.

My True Image Mfg. 510-231-5253
999 Marina Way S, Richmond, CA 94804
Support bra.

Scott Specialties, Inc. 785-527-5627
1827 Meadowlark Rd, Clay Center, KS 67432
Various types of breast binders.

Scott Specialties, Inc. 785-527-5627
1820 E 7th St, Concordia, KS 66901

Tartan Orthopedics, Ltd. 888-287-1456
10651 Irma Dr Unit C, Northglenn, CO 80233
$132.50 per 10 (med).

Tri-State Hospital Supply Corp. 517-545-1135
3173 E 43rd St, Yuma, AZ 85365

BINDER, CHEST *(General) 80QDN*

Alimed, Inc. 800-225-2610
297 High St, Dedham, MA 02026

Dale Medical Products, Inc. 800-343-3980
7 Cross St, Plainville, MA 02762
2 panel 6' wide: 28-50'; 3 panel 9' wide: #410 30-45', #411 46-62', #418 60-75' 4 panel 12' wide: #810 30-45', #811 46-62', #818 60-75', #819 72-84', #820 82-94' 5 panel 15 in. wide: #920 82-94 in.

Hospital Marketing Svcs. Company, Inc. 800-786-5094
162 Great Hill Rd./ Ind. Park, Naugatuck, CT 06770
9in. wide, 20-62in. long, cat. no. 0320-0458.

Medical Specialties, Inc. 800-582-4040
4600 Lebanon Rd, Mint Hill, NC 28227

BINDER, ELASTIC *(General) 80KMO*

Biacare Corporation 616-931-1267
140 W Washington Ave Ste 100, Zeeland, MI 49464
Binder, elastic.

Byron Medical 800-777-3434
602 W Rillito St, Tucson, AZ 85705
Post-Surgical compression garment.

Centurion Medical Products Corp. 517-545-1135
3310 S Main St, Salisbury, NC 28147

Compression Design 616-931-1267
140 W Washington Ave Ste 200, Zeeland, MI 49464
Compression sleeve.

Dj Orthopedics De Mexico, S.A. De C.V. 690-727-1280
Blvd., Delagacion La Presa, Tijuana 22397 Mexico
Binder

Dj Orthopedics De Mexico, S.A. De C.V. 690-727-1280
Ave. Venustiano Carranza 6802, Castillo, Tijuana 22100 Mexico
Binder

Freeman Manufacturing Company 800-253-2091
900 W Chicago Rd, PO Box J, Sturgis, MI 49091

Hospital Marketing Svcs. Company, Inc. 800-786-5094
162 Great Hill Rd./ Ind. Park, Naugatuck, CT 06770
SURGIMED Velcro and hook & eye elastic binders, fits male or female, 9in. and 12in. widths, waist/hip sizes 20-64in.

Ita-Med Co. 888-9IT-AMED
310 Littlefield Ave, South San Francisco, CA 94080

Lohmann & Rauscher, Inc. 800-279-3863
6001 SW 6th Ave Ste 101, Topeka, KS 66615

My True Image Mfg. 510-231-5253
999 Marina Way S, Richmond, CA 94804
Universal band.

Rubicor Medical, Inc. 650-587-3446
600 Chesapeake Dr, Redwood City, CA 94063
Binder, elastic.

Scott Specialties, Inc. 785-527-5627
1827 Meadowlark Rd, Clay Center, KS 67432
Various types of abdominal binders.

BINDER, ELASTIC *(cont'd)*

Scott Specialties, Inc. 785-527-5627
1820 E 7th St, Concordia, KS 66901

Tri-State Hospital Supply Corp. 517-545-1135
3173 E 43rd St, Yuma, AZ 85365

Vascular Solutions, Inc. 763-656-4300
5025 Cheshire Ln N, Plymouth, MN 55446
Belly support system.

BINDER, MEDICAL, THERAPEUTIC *(General) 80MDR*

Anodyne Therapy, Llc 813-645-2855
13570 Wright Cir, Tampa, FL 33626
Compression sleeve.

Avazzia, Inc. 214-575-2820
13154 Coit Rd Ste 200, Dallas, TX 75240
Gloves, sleeves, socks, leg sleeves, wraps, finger electrode.

Biacare Corporation 616-931-1267
140 W Washington Ave Ste 100, Zeeland, MI 49464
Binder, medical, therapeutic.

Dr. Len's Medical Products Llc 678-908-8180
412 Atwood Rd, Erdenheim, PA 19038
Back or abdominal brace.

Farrow Medical Innovations, Inc. 877-417-5187
801 N Bryan Ave, Bryan, TX 77803
Various types of therapeutic binders for the body.

Gemtech Products, Inc. 281-469-4042
10623 Tower Oaks Blvd, Houston, TX 77070
Mott binder.

Judah Mfg. Corp. 800-618-9792
13657 Jupiter Rd Ste 100, Dallas, TX 75238
Form fit conductive garments. over 20 styles of one size fits all electrotherapy garments.

My True Image Mfg. 510-231-5253
999 Marina Way S, Richmond, CA 94804
Plastic surgery girdle.

North Safety Products 401-943-4400
1101 B Calle Neutron, Parque Industrial Maran, Mexicali, B.c. Mexico
Self adherent gauze

Peninsula Medical, Inc. 831-430-9066
108 Whispering Pines Dr Ste 115, Santa Cruz, CA 95066
Reidsleeve.

Solaris, Inc. 414-918-9180
6737 W Washington St Ste 3260, West Allis, WI 53214
Binder, medical, therapeutic.

Thermotek Inc. 877-242-3232
1454 Halsey Way, Carrollton, TX 75007
Various.

Torbot Group Inc., Jobskin Division 800-207-1074
653 Miami St, Toledo, OH 43605
Plastic Surgery Girdle/Bra

Tri-D Corp.
19625 62nd Ave S Ste B101, Kent, WA 98032
Bandage liner.

BINDER, PERINEAL *(General) 80FQK*

Amd-Ritmed, Inc. 800-445-0340
295 Firetower Road, Tonawanda, NY 14150

Birchwood Laboratories, Inc. 800-328-6156
7900 Fuller Rd, Eden Prairie, MN 55344
FULLER SHIELD, anorectal protective garment, case of 12 boxes.

Hospital Marketing Svcs. Company, Inc. 800-786-5094
162 Great Hill Rd./ Ind. Park, Naugatuck, CT 06770
Cat no. 6300, 6300-S4, 6300-S6, HMS Peri-Plus Extra Absorbent Perineal Cold-Post-Partum Therapy with self-adhesive strip; Kits with disposable mesh pants to hold product in place.

Patient's Pride, Inc. 209-839-2255
28421 S Chrisman Rd Ste 3, Tracy, CA 95304
Peritoneal dialysis security band, pd security band.

BINDER, SCULTETUS *(General) 80QDO*

Geen Healthcare Inc. 800-565-4336
931 Progress Ave. Ste.13, Scarborough, ONT M1G 3V5 Canada

Lac-Mac Ltd. 800-461-0001
425 Rectory St., London, ONT N5W 3W5 Canada

BINDER, WRIST *(Orthopedics) 87QDQ*

Hermell Products, Inc. 800-233-2342
9 Britton Dr, PO Box 7345, Bloomfield, CT 06002
Also wrist binder with thumb lock.

Hospital Marketing Svcs. Company, Inc. 800-786-5094
162 Great Hill Rd./ Ind. Park, Naugatuck, CT 06770

Larkotex Company 800-972-3037
1002 Olive St, Texarkana, TX 75501

Tartan Orthopedics, Ltd. 888-287-1456
10651 Irma Dr Unit C, Northglenn, CO 80233
$115.00 per 10 (med).

Tetra Medical Supply Corp. 800-621-4041
6364 W Gross Point Rd, Niles, IL 60714

Zimmer Orthopaedic Surgical Products 800-321-5533
PO Box 10, 200 West Ohio Ave., Dover, OH 44622

BIOFEEDBACK DEVICE *(Cns/Neurology) 84HCC*

American Imex 800-521-8286
16520 Aston, Irvine, CA 92606
EMG Biofeedback (electromyographic feedback) Myoexorciser II/Myoexorciser II Dual biofeedback - single & dual channels. Provides visual and audio feedback. Also provides documentation for reimbursement by downloading to P.C. or directly to a printer. The Educator: Visual biofeedback device that teaches correct pelvic floor contraction.

Avazzia, Inc. 214-575-2820
13154 Coit Rd Ste 200, Dallas, TX 75240
Biofeedback device.

Bio-Feedback Systems, Inc. 303-444-1411
2736 47th St, Boulder, CO 80301
18 models - from $175 to $3,500 each.

Bio-Medical Instruments, Inc. 800-521-4640
2387 E 8 Mile Rd, Warren, MI 48091
Biofeedback-disposable supplies and accessories and replacement parts.

Bio. Works Corp. 208-772-5509
12611 N Chicken Point Rd, Hayden, ID 83835
Gsr biofeed back to pc device.

Biocomp Research Institute 800-246-3526
6542 Hayes Dr, Los Angeles, CA 90048
$8,999 for BIOCOMP 2001 microprocessor-based system. BIOCOMP 2010-4 reduced price unit 4995 4 channel. BIOCOMP 2010-2 2 channel.

Biofeedback Instrument Corp. 212-222-5665
255 W 98th St Apt 3D, New York, NY 10025
Five models - $850 for galvanic skin unit, single channel EMG, temperature unit, $1550 for stand-alone EEG, $795 for dual channel EMG, $3,000 for computerized biofeedback system, $4,000 for computerized muscle scanner EMG, Resp, Temp, SCL, HR. Also, Procomp Infiniti 8 channel computerized biofeedback system, $5700, Heart Tracker - $395.00, HeartScanner - $1495; U-control for incontinence $350.

Biomation 888-667-2324
335 Perth St., P.O. Box 156, Almonte, ON K0A 1A0 Canada
EMG Trainer. Biofeedback equipment. Distribute physical therapy and psychotherapy equipment including biofeedback, muscle testing, electrical stimulation and psychotherapy.

Biosearch Medical Products, Inc. 908-722-5000
35 Industrial Pkwy, Branchburg, NJ 08876
Biofeedback.

Biosentient Corporation
700 Gemini St Ste 210, Houston, TX 77058
Multi-parameter ambulatory physiologial monitor.

Biosig Instruments, Inc. 800-463-5470
PO Box 860, Champlain, NY 12919
ANTENSE Fitness Device teaches the user how to relax face/neck/scalp/shoulder muscles.

Cardinal Healthcare 209, Inc. 610-862-0800
5225 Verona Rd, Fitchburg, WI 53711
Biofeedback device.

Care Rehab And Orthopaedic Products, Inc. 703-448-9644
3930 Horseshoe Bend Rd, Keysville, VA 23947
Biofeedback device.

Casa Futura Technologies 303-417-9752
720 31st St, Boulder, CO 80303
Speech aids, speech training for the speech impaired, (ac-powered and patient-co.

BIOFEEDBACK DEVICE *(cont'd)*

Delsys, Inc. 617-236-0599
650 Beacon St Fl 6, Boston, MA 02215
Myomonitor emg system.

Discovery Engineering Intl., Inc. 785-272-3781
3115 SW Westwood Dr, Topeka, KS 66614
Eeg biofeedback.

Empi 651-415-9000
Clear Lake Industrial Park, Clear Lake, SD 57226
Semg biofeedback device.

Enhanced Mobility Technologies 612-310-4408
1615 Aquila Ave N, Golden Valley, MN 55427
Biorehab system.

Eumedic Incorporated
1369 Forest Park Cir Ste 100, Lafayette, CO 80026
Biofeedback.

Fasstech 978-663-2800
76 Treble Cove Rd Ste 3, North Billerica, MA 01862
PSI 220 dual EMG Hand-held surface EMG with SMART SENSORS. FOCUS EMG Computerized multi-channel surface EMG.

Human Measurement Systems 626-201-2437
1159 N Conwell Ave Apt 311, P.o. Box 2442, Covina, CA 91722
Lifestress temperature trainer, stress control.

Ibm Integrated Tool Technology Center 507-253-5215
3605 Highway 52 N, Rochester, MN 55901

Industrial & Biomedical Sensors Corp. 781-891-4201
1377 Main St, Waltham, MA 02451
$799 and up for biofeedback monitor that measures pulse rate, blood flow, ECG and EMG.

J&J Engineering Inc. 888-550-8300
22797 Holgar Ct NE, Poulsbo, WA 98370

L.D. Technology, Llc 305-777-0336
100 Biscayne Blvd, Miami, FL 33132
Biofeedback device.

Lafayette Instrument Company 800-428-7545
PO Box 5729, 3700 Sagamore Pkwy,, Lafayette, IN 47903
Computer based ambulaory and standalone biofeedback systems.

Lexicor Medical Technology, Inc. 706-447-1074
2840 Wilderness Pl Ste E, Boulder, CO 80301
Biofeedback device.

Life-Tech, Inc. 281-491-6600
4235 Greenbriar Dr, Stafford, TX 77477
Consys II surface EMG/Biofeedback system for pelvic floor retraining.

Living Information Systems Llc 315-469-7399
886 E Brighton Ave, Syracuse, NY 13205
Biofeedback system.

Made On Earth 831-475-7352
5044B Wilder Dr, Soquel, CA 95073
Various types and models of eeg biofeedback devices.

Manufacturing Technology, Inc. 850-664-6070
70 Ready Ave NW, Fort Walton Beach, FL 32548
Biofeedback device.

Myotronics-Noromed, Inc. 206-243-4214
5870 S 194th St, Kent, WA 98032
NORODYN 2000 & 8000 Surface EMG. Static and dynamic EMG evaluation of soft tissue and muscles.

Neuro Resource Group, Inc. 972-665-1810
1100 Jupiter Rd Ste 190, Plano, TX 75074
Biofeedback device.

Neurocybernetics, Inc. 516-482-9001
21601 Vanowen St Ste 100, Canoga Park, CA 91303
Biofeedback devic.

Neurodyne Medical Corp. 800-963-8633
186 Alewife Brook Pkwy, Cambridge, MA 02138
MEDAC System/3 for relaxation and muscle reeducation; provides surface EMG, skin conductance level and response, temperature, respiration, heart rate, and peripheral blood flow. New EKG option available. Biofeedback System/3 for relaxation and muscle reeducation; provides surface EMG, skin conductance level and response, skin temperature, and respiration. M44 Clinical Series dual-channel desk-top surface EMG device with light bar and meter displays as well as multiple audio-feedback modes. M4 Monitor Series single-channel surface EMG biofeedback device suitable for clinical and patient home use.

BIOFEEDBACK DEVICE *(cont'd)*

Neurosync Llc 425-605-8694
12215 NE 39th St, Bellevue, WA 98005
Prescription battery powered device indicated for relaxation training and muscle.

Neurotone Systems, Inc. 972-271-1978
510 Nesbit Dr, Garland, TX 75041
Biofeedback.

Noraxon Usa, Inc. 800-364-8985
13430 N Scottsdale Rd Ste 104, Scottsdale, AZ 85254
The MyoTrace™ Plus is a 2-in-1 handheld system for biofeedback training or data collection and analysis. It allows clinicians or researchers to collect and store two channels of SEMG and up to four channels of analog data to create reports and use for biofeedback.

Precision Biometrics, Inc. 650-508-2600
981 Industrial Rd Ste A, San Carlos, CA 94070
Myovision 8000.

Restorative Therapies Inc. 800-609-9166
907 S Lakewood Ave, Baltimore, MD 21224

Scenar Training Center 248-318-2001
12222 Merit Dr Ste 955, Dallas, TX 75251
Biofeedback devices.

Self Regulation Systems, Inc. 800-345-5642
8672 154th Ave NE Bldg F, Redmond, WA 98052
ORION Platinum/PC & REGAIN DESKTOP/2020; state-of-the-art and standard clinical biofeedback instrument systems for muscle reeducation, including pelvic floor rehabilitation related to incontinence.

Self-Programmed Control Center 800-782-2256
11949 Jefferson Blvd Ste 104, Culver City, CA 90230
Stress biofeedback card.

Sharn, Inc. 800-325-3671
4517 George Rd Ste 200, Tampa, FL 33634
DERMATHERM flexible band or strip indicates skin temperature for biofeedback thermographic mapping, vascular assessment, diagnosis of chronic pain syndromes and more.

Star Tech Health Services, Llc. 801-229-1114
1219 S 1840 W, Orem, UT 84058
Eq4 dcm.

Stoelting Co. 630-860-9700
620 Wheat Ln, Wood Dale, IL 60191
Eeg monitor.

The Prometheus Group 603-749-0733
1 Washington St Ste 303, Dover, NH 03820
Various models of surface electromyographs.

Therapeutic Alliances, Inc. 937-879-0734
333 N Broad St, Fairborn, OH 45324
Powered myoelectric biofeedback equipment.

Thought Technology Ltd. 800-361-3651
2180 Belgrave Ave., Montreal, QUE H4A 2L8 Canada
ProComp Infiniti™ with BioGraph®Infiniti Software is a powerful clinical tool, designed in conjunction with some of the leading clinicians in the field. The system comes packaged with the Legacy and Multimodality Suites providing you with a variety of options for your client, with just one database. With this 8-channel system you can record EEG, EKG, EMG, Temperature, Skin Conductance, Heart Rate/Blood Volume Pulse, Respiration and Voltage, providing you with the most complete view of your client’s physiology. The system offers a variety of screens with an array of animations and audio feedbacks that you can change on the fly. The highly integrated system’s new features are high-speed channels, automatic sensor recognition, impedance checking and compact flash memory. The ability to switch between five screens during a session provides your client with the ultimate training experience. Powerful new audio features include split midi tracks, which allow your client’s brain to control a virtual orchestra instrument by instrument. EEG Coherence, video, event counters, discrete feedback and reward animations, and powerful trend reports are all part of the infinite ways you can evaluate and train your patients.*

Zynex Inc. 800-495-6670
9990 Park Meadows Dr, Lone Tree, CO 80124
NeuroMove NM900

BIOFEEDBACK EQUIPMENT, MYOELECTRIC, BATTERY-POWERED *(Physical Med) 89IQH*

Bio-Feedback Systems, Inc. 303-444-1411
2736 47th St, Boulder, CO 80301
4 models - $425, $495, $945, or $1,095.

BIOFEEDBACK EQUIPMENT, MYOELECTRIC, BATTERY-POWERED *(cont'd)*

Bio-Medical Instruments, Inc. 800-521-4640
2387 E 8 Mile Rd, Warren, MI 48091

Biofeedback Instrument Corp. 212-222-5665
255 W 98th St Apt 3D, New York, NY 10025
Models - $850 for galvanic skin unit, single channel EMG, temperature unit, $1550 for stand-alone EEG, $795 for dual channel EMG, $3,000 for computerized biofeedback system, $4,000 for computerized muscle scanner EMG, Resp, Temp, SCL, HR. Also, Procomp Infiniti 8 channel computerized biofeedback system, $5700, Heart Tracker - $395.00, HeartScanner - $1495; U-control for incontinence $350. Mindset QEEG - $2195. U-control EMG for incontinence-$350.

Biomation 888-667-2324
335 Perth St., P.O. Box 156, Almonte, ON K0A 1A0 Canada
NeuroMove NM 900 EMG-Controlled Stimulator for stroke and spinal chord rehab. NeuroGym trainer for muscle rehab and balance training.

Thought Technology Ltd. 800-361-3651
2180 Belgrave Ave., Montreal, QUE H4A 2L8 Canada
MYOTRAC $499.00 for hand-held unit measuring 0.08-2,000uV with bargraph, tone feedback and active sensor with 1,000,000 meg ohms input impedance.

BIOFEEDBACK EQUIPMENT, MYOELECTRIC, POWERED
(Physical Med) 89IRC

Bio-Feedback Systems, Inc. 303-444-1411
2736 47th St, Boulder, CO 80301
$3500 for research model.

Bio-Medical Instruments, Inc. 800-521-4640
2387 E 8 Mile Rd, Warren, MI 48091

Biocomp Research Institute 800-246-3526
6542 Hayes Dr, Los Angeles, CA 90048
$8,999 for BIOCOMP 2002 microprocessor-based system.

Myotronics-Noromed, Inc. 206-243-4214
5870 S 194th St, Kent, WA 98032
MES-9000/SEMG and MES-9000/NT360 Musculoskeletal evaluation system

Noraxon Usa, Inc. 800-364-8985
13430 N Scottsdale Rd Ste 104, Scottsdale, AZ 85254
The Multi-Mode FootSwitch system provides real time foot-strike data via four contact sensors per foot included in the system. It easily connects to all of Noraxon's artifact-free EMG systems and is comprised of a belt-worn amplifier and cables with pluggable sensors for eight locations (4 per foot).

BIOPSY DEVICE, ENDOMYOCARDIAL *(Cardiovascular) 74DWZ*

Aesculap Implant Systems Inc. 1-800-234-9179
3773 Corporate Pkwy, Center Valley, PA 18034

Argon Medical Devices Inc. 903-675-9321
1445 Flat Creek Rd, Athens, TX 75751
Jawz.

Atc Technologies, Inc. 781-939-0725
30B Upton Dr, Wilmington, MA 01887
SPARROWHAWK 1.5mm, 1.8mm + 2.2mm OD biopsy forceps with fenestrated or non-fenestrated jaws, coated or uncoated, straight or pre-curved, disposable or reusable devices.

Fehling Surgical Instruments 800-FEHLING
509 Broadstone Ln NW, Acworth, GA 30101
Reusable and disposable.

Scholten Surgical Instruments, Inc. 209-365-1393
170 Commerce St Ste 101, Lodi, CA 95240
BIOPTOME, Reusable Endomyocardial Biopsy Forceps: Right Ventricular: 9 Fr, 2.8mm head diam.x 50cm long; 8 Fr, 2.5mm head diam.x 50cm long; 6.5 Fr, 2.1mm head diam.x 50cm long; 5 Fr, 1.6mm head diam.x 40cm long), Left Ventricular: 6.5 Fr, 2.1mm head diam.x 100cm long), pediatric (#6.5 french, 2.1mm head diam.x 50cm long - Most Bioptomes $825.00 - Custom catheter length avail. at no extra cost. Service:$150.00 per reconditioning. Accessories:Storage Plate: $30.00 for RV and $50.00 for LV storage plate.

Vlv Associates, Inc. 973-428-2884
30C Ridgedale Ave, East Hanover, NJ 07936
Super core biopsy needle.

BIOPSY INSTRUMENT *(Gastro/Urology) 78KNW*

Abbott Spine, Inc. 847-937-6100
12708 Riata Vista Cir Ste B-100, Austin, TX 78727
Vertebral body biopsy needle.

BIOPSY INSTRUMENT *(cont'd)*

Aesculap Implant Systems Inc. 1-800-234-9179
3773 Corporate Pkwy, Center Valley, PA 18034

Anchor Products Company 800-323-5134
52 W Official Rd, Addison, IL 60101
$542.00 for case of 20/soft tissue biopsy device.

Atrion Medical Products, Inc. 800-343-9334
1426 Curt Francis Rd NW, Arab, AL 35016
Biopsy device.

Avantis Medical Systems, Inc. 408-733-1901
263 Santa Ana Ct, Sunnyvale, CA 94085
Endoscope.

Bard Access Systems, Inc. 800-545-0890
605 N 5600 W, Salt Lake City, UT 84116
Portable, battery powered ultrasound scanners.

Bard Shannon Limited 908-277-8000
San Geronimo Industrial Park, Lot # 1, Road # 3, Km 79.7
Humacao, PR 00791
Biopsy systems.

Biomet Microfixation Inc. 800-874-7711
1520 Tradeport Dr, Jacksonville, FL 32218
Biopsy instruments.

Busse Hospital Disposables, Inc. 631-435-4711
75 Arkay Dr, Hauppauge, NY 11788
Bone marrow biopsy tray and j-style needles.

C. R. Bard, Inc., Bard Urological Div. 888-367-2273
13183 Harland Dr NE, Covington, GA 30014

Cook Urological, Inc. 800-457-4500
1100 W Morgan St, P.O. Box 227, Spencer, IN 47460

Cytyc Surgical Products 800-442-9892
250 Campus Dr, Marlborough, MA 01752
Gastroenterology-urology biopsy instrument.

Devicor Medical Products Inc. 262-857-9300
10505 Corporate Dr Ste 207, Pleasant Prairie, WI 53158
Mammotome Biopsy System; Mammotome EX Hand Held System; Mammotome EX Hand Held System;Biopsy Needle

Ethicon Endo-Surgery, Inc. 877-384-4266
3801 University Blvd SE, Albuquerque, NM 87106
Various types of sterile and non sterile biopsy instrument.

Gi Supply 800-451-5797
200 Grandview Ave, Camp Hill, PA 17011
HpOne: One-hour rapid urease test for presumptive identification of h. pylori via gastric biopsy.

Havel's Inc. 800-638-4770
3726 Lonsdale St, Cincinnati, OH 45227

Inrad 800-558-4647
4375 Donkers Ct SE, Kentwood, MI 49512
Automated core biopsy device, sterile.

Mcdalt Medical Corp. 800-841-5774
2225 Prestonwood Dr Ste 100-A, Arlington, TX 76012
Disposable and reusable devices.'HS Medical'Inc.

Mcpherson Enterprises, Inc. 813-931-4201
3851 62nd Ave N Ste A, Pinellas Park, FL 33781
Soft tissue biopsy.

Medical Device Technologies, Inc. (Md Tech) 800-338-0440
3600 SW 47th Ave, Gainesville, FL 32608
TRU-CORE, PRO-MAG, SUPER-CORE, MANAN. MD TECH.

Medtronic, Inc. 800-633-8766
710 Medtronic Pkwy, Minneapolis, MN 55432
ACCUCORE, ACCUMARK, ACCUPLACE.

Minnetronix Inc. 888-301-1025
1635 Energy Park Dr, Saint Paul, MN 55108
EN BLOC BIOPSY SYSTEM, Intact Breast Lesion Excision System

Minrad, Inc. 716-855-1068
50 Cobham Dr, Orchard Park, NY 14127
Core tissue biopsy needle.

Neomatrix, Llc 949-753-7844
16 Technology Dr Ste 118, Irvine, CA 92618
Breast aspirator.

Orthovita, Inc. 610-640-1775
77 Great Valley Pkwy, Malvern, PA 19355
Bone marrow aspiration needle.

BIOPSY INSTRUMENT *(cont'd)*

Personna Medical/Div. Of American Safety Razor Co. 800-457-2222
1 Razor Blade Ln, Verona, VA 24482
DERMABLADE is a one piece shave biopsy instrument. DERMABLADE's flexible design can be used to remove surface protuberances, as well as deep lesions, while reducing ragged skin edges. Sterile, single use.

Pneumrx Inc 650-625-8910
530 Logue Ave, Mountain View, CA 94043
Sterile and non-sterile instrument, biopsy.

Promex Technologies, Llc 317-736-0128
3049 Hudson St, Franklin, IN 46131
Manual bone marrow biopsy device, bone biopsy needle, trocar, introducer needle,.

Rubicor Medical, Inc. 650-587-3446
600 Chesapeake Dr, Redwood City, CA 94063
Biopsy instrument.

Sanarus Medical, Inc. 925-460-5730
4696 Willow Rd, Pleasanton, CA 94588
Core tissue biopsy system.

Senorx, Inc. 949-362-4800
11 Columbia, Aliso Viejo, CA 92656
Lesion localiztion device-sterile.

Sterylab Usa, Llc 390-293-5084
2916 N Graham Rd Ste C, Franklin, IN 46131
Biopsy instrument.

Stryker Puerto Rico, Ltd. 939-307-2500
Hwy. 3, Km. 131.2, Las Guasimas Ind. Park, Arroyo, PR 00714
Biopsy needles.

Suros Surgical Systems, Inc 877-887-8767
6100 Technology Center Dr, Indianapolis, IN 46278
Vacuum assisted core biopsy device.

Ussc Puerto Rico, Inc. 203-845-1000
Building 911-67, Sabanetas Industrial Park, Ponce, PR 00731
Biopsy instrument.

Webb Manufacturing Co. 800-932-2634
1241 Carpenter St, Philadelphia, PA 19147
E-Z GRID (FAST FIND) is a CT grid for needle biopsy.

BIOPSY INSTRUMENT, MECHANICAL, GASTROINTESTINAL
(Gastro/Urology) 78FCF

Aesculap Implant Systems Inc. 1-800-234-9179
3773 Corporate Pkwy, Center Valley, PA 18034

Ballard Medical Products 770-587-7835
12050 Lone Peak Pkwy, Draper, UT 84020
Instrument, biopsy, mechanical, gastrointestinal.

Cathguide, Division Of Scilogy Corp. 305-269-0500
9135 Fontainebleau Blvd Apt 5, Miami, FL 33172

Inrad 800-558-4647
4375 Donkers Ct SE, Kentwood, MI 49512
Instrument, biopsy, mechanical, gastrointestinal.

International Hospital Supply Co. 800-398-9450
6914 Canby Ave Ste 105, Reseda, CA 91335

Mahe International Inc. 800-294-7946
468 Craighead St, Nashville, TN 37204

Richard Wolf Medical Instruments Corp. 800-323-9653
353 Corporate Woods Pkwy, Vernon Hills, IL 60061

Surgi-Aid Endoscopics, Inc. 480-988-0916
3553 E Wildhorse Dr, Gilbert, AZ 85297
Gastrointestinal biopsy instrument.

Vidacare Corp. 800-680-4911
4350 Lockhill Selma Rd Ste 150, Shavano Park, TX 78249
OnControl

BIOPSY INSTRUMENT, SUCTION *(Gastro/Urology) 78FCK*

Aesculap Implant Systems Inc. 1-800-234-9179
3773 Corporate Pkwy, Center Valley, PA 18034

Mahe International Inc. 800-294-7946
468 Craighead St, Nashville, TN 37204

Pmt Corp. 800-626-5463
1500 Park Rd, Chanhassen, MN 55317

Richard Wolf Medical Instruments Corp. 800-323-9653
353 Corporate Woods Pkwy, Vernon Hills, IL 60061

BIOSENSOR, IMMUNOASSAY, CPK OR ISOENZYMES
(Chemistry) 75MYT

Abbott Point Of Care Inc. 609-443-9300
104 Windsor Center Dr, East Windsor, NJ 08520
Creatine kinase mb.

BIOSENSOR, IMMUNOASSAY, MYOGLOBIN
(Immunology) 82MVE

Immuno Diagnostic Center, Inc. 214-351-1231
9978 Monroe Dr Ste 303, Dallas, TX 75220
Myoglobin kit.

BISTOURY, TRACHEAL *(Ear/Nose/Throat) 77KCC*

Aesculap Implant Systems Inc. 1-800-234-9179
3773 Corporate Pkwy, Center Valley, PA 18034

BIT, DRILL *(Orthopedics) 87HTW*

Abbott Spine, Inc. 847-937-6100
12708 Riata Vista Cir Ste B-100, Austin, TX 78727
Drill.

American Medical Specialties, Inc. 800-808-2877
10650 77th St., Suite 405, Largo, FL 33777
drills to fit synthes and other power equipment.

Arthrex Manufacturing 239-643-5553
1958 Trade Center Way, Naples, FL 34109
Drill, drill bit.

Arthrex, Inc. 239-643-5553
1370 Creekside Blvd, Naples, FL 34108
Drill (various size drill bits).

Ascent Healthcare Solutions 480-763-5300
10232 S 51st St, Phoenix, AZ 85044
Drill bit.

Biomedical Enterprises, Inc. 800-880-6528
14785 Omicron Dr Ste 205, San Antonio, TX 78245
Unique drill bit engineered for use in applications where removing drill cuttings from the drill hole is critical.

Biomet Microfixation Inc. 800-874-7711
1520 Tradeport Dr, Jacksonville, FL 32218
Various types of drills.

Biomet, Inc. 574-267-6639
56 E Bell Dr, PO Box 587, Warsaw, IN 46582
Various types of drill bits.

Bonutti Research, Inc. 217-342-3412
2600 S Raney St, Effingham, IL 62401
Various.

Depuy Mitek, A Johnson & Johnson Company 800-451-2006
50 Scotland Blvd, Bridgewater, MA 02324
Drill.

Depuy Spine, Inc. 800-227-6633
325 Paramount Dr, Raynham, MA 02767
Various sizes of surgical drill bits.

DJO Inc. 800-336-6569
1430 Decision St, Vista, CA 92081
Various orthopedic surgical hand drills and bits.

Greystone Of Lincoln, Inc. 401-333-0444
7 Wellington Rd, Lincoln, RI 02865
Cranial drill bit.

Hand Biomechanics Lab, Inc. 800-522-5778
77 Scripps Dr Ste 104, Sacramento, CA 95825

Integra Lifesciences Of Ohio 800-654-2873
4900 Charlemar Dr Bldg A, Cincinnati, OH 45227
Various sizes and styles for drill bits.

Integral Design Inc. 781-740-2036
52 Burr Rd, Hingham, MA 02043

Internal Fixation Systems, Inc. 305-491-9133
10100 NW 116th Way Ste 18, Medley, FL 33178
Drill bit.

Interphase Implants, Inc. 248-442-1460
19928 Farmington Rd, Livonia, MI 48152
Various types of drill bits.

Interventional Spine, Inc. 800-497-0484
13700 Alton Pkwy Ste 160, Irvine, CA 92618
Various types of drill bits.

K2m, Inc. 866-526-4171
751 Miller Dr SE Ste F1, Leesburg, VA 20175
Drill bit.

BIT, DRILL *(cont'd)*

Kls-Martin L.P. 800-625-1557
11239-1 St. John`s Industrial, Parkway South
Jacksonville, FL 32250

Kmedic 800-955-0559
190 Veterans Dr, Northvale, NJ 07647

Medcon Llc 410-744-8367
1002 Frederick Rd, Catonsville, MD 21228
Drill bit.

Medisiss 866-866-7477
2747 SW 6th St, Redmond, OR 97756
Various drill bits,sterile.

Medtronic Puerto Rico Operations Co.,Med Rel 763-514-4000
Road 909, Km. 0.4., Barrio Mariana, Humacao, PR 00792
Various drill bits.

Medtronic Sofamor Danek Instrument Manufacturing 901-396-3133
7375 Adrianne Pl, Bartlett, TN 38133
Various twist, bit drills.

Medtronic Sofamor Danek Usa, Inc. 901-396-3133
4340 Swinnea Rd, Memphis, TN 38118
Various twist, bit drills.

Medtronic Spine Llc 877-690-5353
1221 Crossman Ave, Sunnyvale, CA 94089
Various.

Mekanika, Inc. 561-417-7244
3998 Fau Blvd Ste 210, Boca Raton, FL 33431
Bone drill bit.

Onyx Medical Corp. 901-323-6699
152 Collins St, Memphis, TN 38112

Richard Wolf Medical Instruments Corp. 800-323-9653
353 Corporate Woods Pkwy, Vernon Hills, IL 60061
Pneumatic drill for ACL reconstruction.

Salumedica, L.L.C. 404-589-1727
4451 Atlanta Rd SE Ste 138, Smyrna, GA 30080
Bit, drill.

Sim Medical Sales 574-268-0341
PO Box 895, Warsaw, IN 46581

Simpex Medical, Inc. 800-851-9753
401 E Prospect Ave, Mount Prospect, IL 60056

Small Bone Innovations, Inc. 215-428-1791
1380 S Pennsylvania Ave, Morrisville, PA 19067
Bit, drill.

Spineworks Medical Inc. 408-986-8950
1735 N 1st St Ste 245, San Jose, CA 95112

Sterilmed, Inc. 763-488-3400
11400 73rd Ave N Ste 100, Maple Grove, MN 55369
Drill bit.

Stryker Spine 866-457-7463
2 Pearl Ct, Allendale, NJ 07401

Surgical Implant Generation Network (Sign) 509-371-1107
451 Hills St, Richland, WA 99354
Various sizes of drill bits.

Warsaw Orthopedic, Inc. 901-396-3133
2500 Silveus Xing, Warsaw, IN 46582
Various twist, bit drills.

Zimmer Holdings, Inc. 800-613-6131
1800 W Center St, PO Box 708, Warsaw, IN 46580

Zimmer Trabecular Metal Technology 800-613-6131
10 Pomeroy Rd, Parsippany, NJ 07054
Drill bit.

BIT, SURGICAL *(Surgery) 79GFG*

American Medical Specialties, Inc. 800-808-2877
10650 77th St., Suite 405, Largo, FL 33777
Disposable wire pass drills and cranio blades for powered equipment of major manufacturers.

Biomet, Inc. 574-267-6639
56 E Bell Dr, PO Box 587, Warsaw, IN 46582
Various types of surgical bits.

Depuy Mitek, A Johnson & Johnson Company 800-451-2006
50 Scotland Blvd, Bridgewater, MA 02324
Drill bits.

Depuy Orthopaedics, Inc. 800-473-3789
700 Orthopaedic Dr, P.O. Box 988, Warsaw, IN 46582
Various types of surgical drill bits.

BIT, SURGICAL *(cont'd)*

Depuy-Raynham, A Div. Of Depuy Orthopaedics 800-451-2006
325 Paramount Dr, Raynham, MA 02767
Various types of surgical drill bits.

Kirwan Surgical Products, Inc. 888-547-9267
180 Enterprise Dr, PO Box 427, Marshfield, MA 02050
Disposable cranio blades and wire pass drills.

minSURG International, Inc. 727-466-4550
611 Druid Rd E, Suite 200, Clearwater, FL 33756

Musculoskeletal Transplant Foundation 732-661-0202
1232 Mid Valley Dr, Jessup, PA 18434

Symmetry Medical Usa, Inc. 574-267-8700
486 W 350 N, Warsaw, IN 46582
Bit drill.

BLADE, BONE CUTTING *(Orthopedics) 87QDU*

American Medical Specialties, Inc. 800-808-2877
10650 77th St., Suite 405, Largo, FL 33777
Quality and value in replacement cutting tools for powered surgical equipment of all major instrument manufacturers.

Becton Dickinson And Co. 866-906-8080
411 Waverley Oaks Rd, Waltham, MA 02452

Brasseler Usa - Komet Medical 800-535-6638
1 Brasseler Blvd, Savannah, GA 31419
MicroLine Small Bone High Speed Power System

Incisiontech 800-213-7809
9 Technology Dr, Staunton, VA 24401

Micro-Aire Surgical Instruments, Inc. 800-722-0822
1641 Edlich Dr, Charlottesville, VA 22911

Sim Medical Sales 574-268-0341
PO Box 895, Warsaw, IN 46581

Smith & Nephew, Inc., Endoscopy Division 800-343-8386
130 Forbes Blvd, Mansfield, MA 02048
Bone Cutter, the high performance blade that replaces a blade and burr combination. Resects both soft tissue and bone with one blade. Ideal for notchplasty and acromioplasty procedures.

Vilex, Inc. 800-872-4911
345 Old Curry Hollow Rd, Pittsburgh, PA 15236
$7.95 through $14.75 each. Small bone oscillating, sagittal, and reciprocating.

BLADE, ELECTROSURGERY, LAPAROSCOPIC *(Surgery) 79SIH*

Okay Industries, Inc. 860-225-8707
200 Ellis St, P.O. Box 2470, New Britain, CT 06051

Olsen Medical 800-297-6344
3001 W Kentucky St, Louisville, KY 40211
Laparoscopic Electrodes available with Standard Hook, J Hook, L Hook, Hockey Stick and Spatula Tip. All styles available with Pen, Cable and Hex connectors.

Wisap America 800-233-8448
8231 Melrose Dr, Lenexa, KS 66214

BLADE, KNIFE, LAPAROSCOPIC *(Surgery) 79QVD*

Crescent Mfg. Co. 800-537-1330
1310 Majestic Dr, Fremont, OH 43420
Duraedge. Laparoscopic Surgical Blades.

Elmed, Inc. 630-543-2792
60 W Fay Ave, Addison, IL 60101

Incisiontech 800-213-7809
9 Technology Dr, Staunton, VA 24401

Lyons Tool And Die Company 800-422-9363
185 Research Pkwy, Meriden, CT 06450
Rapid prototyping. Production of medical devices in class 10,000 clean rooms. Medical knives and scissors. Precision metal stamping. Engineering services.

Okay Industries, Inc. 860-225-8707
200 Ellis St, P.O. Box 2470, New Britain, CT 06051

Sable Industries 800-890-0251
4751 Oceanside Blvd Ste G, Oceanside, CA 92056

Wisap America 800-233-8448
8231 Melrose Dr, Lenexa, KS 66214

BLADE, SAW, CAST CUTTING *(Orthopedics) 87TAI*

American Medical Specialties, Inc. 800-808-2877
10650 77th St., Suite 405, Largo, FL 33777
Quality and value in replacement blades for all major cast cutting saws.

Brasseler Usa - Komet Medical 800-535-6638
1 Brasseler Blvd, Savannah, GA 31419

BLADE, SAW, CAST CUTTING *(cont'd)*

Bsn Medical, Inc 800-552-1157
5825 Carnegie Blvd, Charlotte, NC 28209
M-PACT blades for cutting plaster or synthetic materials. Hexagonal drive provides 6 blades rotations . Pin drive provides 4 blades rotations. 'Universal Hub' fits most popular brands of cast cutters. Five types of blades available.

Micro-Aire Surgical Instruments, Inc. 800-722-0822
1641 Edlich Dr, Charlottesville, VA 22911

Omni Medical Supply Inc. 800-860-6664
4153 Pioneer Dr, Commerce Township, MI 48390

Protectair Inc. 800-235-7932
59 Eisenhower Ln S, Lombard, IL 60148

BLADE, SAW, SURGICAL, CARDIOVASCULAR
(Cardiovascular) 74DWH

Aesculap Implant Systems Inc. 1-800-234-9179
3773 Corporate Pkwy, Center Valley, PA 18034

American Medical Specialties, Inc. 800-808-2877
10650 77th St., Suite 405, Largo, FL 33777
Quality and value in blades for all powered equipment.

Ascent Healthcare Solutions 480-763-5300
10232 S 51st St, Phoenix, AZ 85044
Cardiovascular surgical saw blade.

Clinimed, Incorporated 877-CLINIMED
303 Markus Ct, Sandy Brae Industrial Park, Newark, DE 19713

Medisiss 866-866-7477
2747 SW 6th St, Redmond, OR 97756
Various types of cardiovascular saw blades.

Medtronic Powered Surgical Solutions 800-643-2773
4620 N Beach St, Haltom City, TX 76137
Various models motors & various models of sterile & non sterile accessories.

Terumo Cardiovascular Systems (Tcvs) 800-283-7866
28 Howe St, Ashland, MA 01721
Sternal saw.

Terumo Cardiovascular Systems, Corp 800-521-2818
6200 Jackson Rd, Ann Arbor, MI 48103

BLADE, SCALPEL *(Surgery) 79GES*

Advanced Medical Innovations, Inc. 888-367-2641
9410 De Soto Ave Ste J, Chatsworth, CA 91311
Retractable SAF-T-Scalpel™ Pat. Pending: Retractable Safety Scalpel is a safe replacement for standard scalpels used during surgery. This innovative product has been specifically designed to protect the practitioner's hands during surgery. It is the ultimate in safety since it is a fool-proof design using a spring to retract the blade fully during passing. There is no partially exposed blade when the Practitioner's guard is off. Activation is a simple push by the finger and retraction requires pushing two buttons simultaneously, therefore there are no accidental retractions. The blade is very stable and the scalpel comes in a weighted version too. It has a unique and permanent locking mechanism for final disposal; the ultimate in safety and effectiveness. It is the only full proof product on the market today.

American Safety Razor Co. 540-248-8000
1 Razor Blade Ln, Verona, VA 24482
Sterile stainless or carbon steel surgical blades.

Argon Medical Devices Inc. 903-675-9321
1445 Flat Creek Rd, Athens, TX 75751
Scalpel.

Arista Surgical Supply Co. Inc. 800-223-1984
297 High St, Dedham, MA 02026

Bd Caribe, Ltd. 201-847-4298
Rd. 183, Km. 20.3, Las Piedras, PR 00771
Scalpel blade.

Becton Dickinson And Co. 866-906-8080
411 Waverley Oaks Rd, Waltham, MA 02452

Becton Dickinson And Company 800-284-6845
1 Becton Dr, Franklin Lakes, NJ 07417
BD Beaver; MULTIPLE; MULTIPLE - BLADE SCALPEL; NONE

Biomet Microfixation Inc. 800-874-7711
1520 Tradeport Dr, Jacksonville, FL 32218
Various types of blades.

C & A Scientific Co. Inc. 703-330-1413
7241 Gabe Ct, Manassas, VA 20109
PREMIERE Sterile, high carbon, & stainless steel.

BLADE, SCALPEL *(cont'd)*

Carl Heyer, Inc. 800-284-5550
1872 Bellmore Ave, North Bellmore, NY 11710

Chagrin Safety Supply, Inc. 800-227-0468
8227 Washington St # 1, Chagrin Falls, OH 44023

Cincinnati Surgical Company 800-544-3100
11256 Cornell Park Dr, Cincinnati, OH 45242
Cincinnati Surgical & Lance brand, & Swann-Morton; also miniature, myringotomy, special orthopedic and post mortem, miniature edgeblades.

Curetteblade, Inc. 866-287-3883
20 Cedar Blvd Ste 410, Pittsburgh, PA 15228
Single use, stainless steel surgical curette blade.

Demetech Corp. 888-324-2447
3530 NW 115th Ave, Doral, FL 33178
Dental blade.

Dgh Technology, Inc. 800-722-3883
110 Summit Dr Ste B, Exton, PA 19341
Surgical diamond blades.

E.A. Beck & Co. 949-645-4072
657 W 19th St Ste E, P O Box 10857, Costa Mesa, CA 92627
Blade.

Eagle Laboratories 800-782-6534
10201 Trademark St Ste A, Rancho Cucamonga, CA 91730

Exelint International Co. 800-940-3935
5840 W Centinela Ave, Los Angeles, CA 90045
Exel surgical blades and scalpels.

Fortrad Eye Instruments Corp. 973-543-2371
8 Franklin Rd, Mendham, NJ 07945
Blade breaker blades, double edged, stainless steel.

George Tiemann & Co. 800-843-6266
25 Plant Ave, Hauppauge, NY 11788

Global Healthcare 800-601-3880
1495 Hembree Rd Ste 700, Roswell, GA 30076
Carbon and stainless steel.

Havel's Inc. 800-638-4770
3726 Lonsdale St, Cincinnati, OH 45227

Health Care Logistics, Inc. 800-848-1633
450 Town St, PO Box 25, Circleville, OH 43113
Sterile and non-sterile accessory to scalpel blade.

Her-Mar, Inc. 800-327-8209
8550 NW 30th Ter, Doral, FL 33122
$30.00/box of 100 sterile and stainless surgical blades.

Hospital Marketing Svcs. Company, Inc. 800-786-5094
162 Great Hill Rd./ Ind. Park, Naugatuck, CT 06770
HMS SURGIBLADE disposable - box of 50 (#10, 11, 20, 21, 15); box of 50 (#12, 22, 23).

Hu-Friedy Manufacturing Co., Inc. 800-483-7433
3232 N Rockwell St, Chicago, IL 60618
$68.25 to $111.50 per box of 100, 12 sizes.

Incisiontech 800-213-7809
9 Technology Dr, Staunton, VA 24401
Special purpose and custom-made surgical blades.

Jaisons International, Inc. 203-261-1653
22 Bittersweet Ln, Trumbull, CT 06611

Katena Products, Inc. 800-225-1195
4 Stewart Ct, Denville, NJ 07834
Assorted disposable blades with and without handles.

Km Instruments, Llc 520-529-8455
5941 E Fort Crittendon Trl, Tucson, AZ 85750
Multi-bladed scalpel.

Lampac International Ltd. 636-797-3659
230 N Lake Dr, Hillsboro, MO 63050
Stainless and carbon steel.

Magnaplan Corp. 800-361-1192
1320 Rte. 9, Champlain, NY 12919-5007
Handles made of nickel-silver alloy. Blades are easily attached with a simple sliding motion. Push-button type handles make blade changing even simpler and faster. Contour blades made of .005 inches stainless steel.

Medical Sterile Products, Inc. 800-292-2887
Road 413 Km. 0.2 BO. Ensenada, Rincon, PR 00743
Miniature edged blade, oral-perio blade, arthro blade, podiatry blade, ENT-micro blade, ophthalmology blade.

PRODUCT DIRECTORY

BLADE, SCALPEL *(cont'd)*

Medisiss 866-866-7477
2747 SW 6th St, Redmond, OR 97756
Various scalpel blades,sterile.

Miltex Inc. 800-645-8000
589 Davies Dr, York, PA 17402

Molecular Metallurgy, Inc. 619-596-7444
11649 Riverside Dr Ste 139, Lakeside, CA 92040
Various types of sterile scalpel blades.

Myco Medical 800-454-6926
158 Towerview Ct, Cary, NC 27513
General surgery and specialty blades, disposable safety scalpels, handles and prep razors.

Personna Medical/Div. Of American Safety Razor Co. 800-457-2222
1 Razor Blade Ln, Verona, VA 24482
PERSONNA PLUS Safety Scalpel System an innovative plastic sheath, coupled a dedicated PERSONNA PLUS Safety Metal Handle, you never have to touch the blade whether you are loading or unloading. Cartridges are available in 5 sizes and feature the PERSONNA PLUS surgical blades. PERSONNA PLUS Safety Metal Handle is available in 5 sizes, with the same weight as most traditional scalpels. PERSONNA PLUS scalpel blades with MicroCoat: 10 sizes available. PERSONNA stainless blades come in 4 sizes and Single and double edge prep blades, scalpel handles, disposable scalpels and mini-scalpels are also available.

PI Medical Co., Llc. 800-874-0120
321 Ellis St, New Britain, CT 06051
Surgical blades/disposable safety scalpels, stainless steel and high carbon steel - all regular sizes; Sterling.

Propper Manufacturing Co., Inc. 800-832-4300
3604 Skillman Ave, Long Island City, NY 11101

Rhein Mfg., Inc. 314-997-1775
2269 Grissom Dr, Saint Louis, MO 63146
General surgical instrument.

Roboz Surgical Instrument Co., Inc. 800-424-2984
PO Box 10710, Gaithersburg, MD 20898

Sable Industries 800-890-0251
4751 Oceanside Blvd Ste G, Oceanside, CA 92056

Salvin Dental Specialties, Inc. 800-535-6566
3450 Latrobe Dr, Charlotte, NC 28211
Various types of surgical scalpel blades.

Schueler & Company, Inc. 516-487-1500
PO Box 528, Stratford, CT 06615

Spectra Medical Devices, Inc. 978-657-0889
260H Fordham Rd, Wilmington, MA 01887
disposable scalpels

Spectra Medical Devices, Inc. 866-938-8649
4C Henshaw St, Woburn, MA 01801
Disposable.

Statlab Medical Products, Inc. 800-442-3573
106 Hillside Dr, Lewisville, TX 75057
Various sizes, especially for grassing and autopsy.

Stephens Instruments, Inc. 800-354-7848
2500 Sandersville Rd, Lexington, KY 40511

Surgical Tools, Inc. 800-774-2040
1106 Monroe St, Bedford, VA 24523

Surgipath Medical Industries, Inc. 800-225-3035
PO Box 528, 5205 Route 12, Richmond, IL 60071

Symmetry Medical Usa, Inc. 574-267-8700
486 W 350 N, Warsaw, IN 46582
Manual surgical instrument for general use.

Tuzik Boston 800-886-6363
104 Longwater Dr, Assinippi Park, Norwell, MA 02061

Unique Technologies, Inc. 610-775-9191
111 Chestnut St, Mohnton, PA 19540
Microsurgical knife.

V.I.R. Engineering, Inc. 805-964-0553
5951 Encina Rd Ste 209, Goleta, CA 93117
Scapel blade remover.

Zimcor Corporation 616-813-2699
6414 Skyridge Dr NE, Belmont, MI 49306
Laparoscopic scalpel.

BLADE, SURGICAL, SAW, GENERAL & PLASTIC SURGERY

(Surgery) 79GFA

American Medical Specialties, Inc. 800-808-2877
10650 77th St., Suite 405, Largo, FL 33777
Qualtiy and value in replacement blades for Zimmer, Stryker, 3M, and others.

Arthrex Manufacturing 239-643-5553
1958 Trade Center Way, Naples, FL 34109
Blade, saw.

Arthrex, Inc. 239-643-5553
1370 Creekside Blvd, Naples, FL 34108
Various.

Ascent Healthcare Solutions 480-763-5300
10232 S 51st St, Phoenix, AZ 85044
Saw blade.

Bausch & Lomb Surgical 636-255-5051
3365 Tree Court Ind Blvd, Saint Louis, MO 63122

Becton Dickinson And Co. 866-906-8080
411 Waverley Oaks Rd, Waltham, MA 02452

Biomet Microfixation Inc. 800-874-7711
1520 Tradeport Dr, Jacksonville, FL 32218
Various types of blades.

Brasseler Usa - Komet Medical 800-535-6638
1 Brasseler Blvd, Savannah, GA 31419
Sagittal, reciprocating and oscillating sawblades.

Brasseler Usa - Medical 805-650-5209
4837 McGrath St Ste J, Ventura, CA 93003
Sawblade.

Cincinnati Surgical Company 800-544-3100
11256 Cornell Park Dr, Cincinnati, OH 45242
Cincinnati Surgical & Lance brand, & Swann-Morton.

Crescent Mfg. Co. 800-537-1330
1310 Majestic Dr, Fremont, OH 43420

E-Global Medical Equipment, L.L.C. 866-422-1845
2f 500 Lincoln St., Allston, MA 02134
Morcellator.

Eagle Laboratories 800-782-6534
10201 Trademark St Ste A, Rancho Cucamonga, CA 91730
EAGLE TALON scleral, spoon, ear, and slit (phaco) blades.

Grace Manufacturing, Inc. 479-968-5455
614 Sr 247, Russellville, AR 72802

Havel's Inc. 800-638-4770
3726 Lonsdale St, Cincinnati, OH 45227

Lasersight Technologies, Inc. 630-530-9700
6848 Stapoint Ct, Winter Park, FL 32792
Keratome blade.

Medisiss 866-866-7477
2747 SW 6th St, Redmond, OR 97756
Various saw blades,sterile.

Micro-Aire Surgical Instruments, Inc. 800-722-0822
1641 Edlich Dr, Charlottesville, VA 22911
Neuro blades also available.

Microaire Surgical Instruments, Llc 434-975-8000
1641 Edlich Dr, Charlottesville, VA 22911

Microspecialties, Inc. 877-874-1933
264 Quarry Rd, PO Box 3030, Milford, CT 06460
Keratome blade with holder.

Miltex Inc. 800-645-8000
589 Davies Dr, York, PA 17402

Minnesota Bramstedt Surgical, Inc. 800-456-5052
1835 Energy Park Dr, Saint Paul, MN 55108

Molecular Metallurgy, Inc. 619-596-7444
11649 Riverside Dr Ste 139, Lakeside, CA 92040
Various types of sterile bone saw blades.

Nuell, Inc. 800-829-7694
PO Box 55, 312 East Van Buren St., Leesburg, IN 46538
Dermatome blade.

Omega Surgical Instruments 800-656-6342
G-8305 Saginaw St., Suite 6, Grand Blanc, MI 48439

Pharaoh Trading Company 866-929-4913
9701 Brookpark Rd, Knollwood Plaza, Suite 241, Cleveland, OH 44129

Ross Disposable Products 800-649-6526
401 Traders Blvd E, Unit 10, Mississauga, ON L4Z 2H8 Canada

BLADE, SURGICAL, SAW, GENERAL & PLASTIC SURGERY *(cont'd)*

Signal Medical Corporation 800-246-6324
1000 Des Peres Rd Ste 140, Saint Louis, MO 63131
Stryker standard, 2000, and zimmer.

Sim Medical Sales 574-268-0341
PO Box 895, Warsaw, IN 46581

Smith & Nephew, Inc., Endoscopy Division 800-343-8386
150 Minuteman Rd, Andover, MA 01810
38 styles; disposable.

Sterilmed, Inc. 763-488-3400
11400 73rd Ave N Ste 100, Maple Grove, MN 55369
Saw blade.

Symmetry Medical Usa, Inc. 574-267-8700
486 W 350 N, Warsaw, IN 46582
Saw blade.

Tava Surgical Instruments 805-650-5209
4837 McGrath St Ste J, Ventura, CA 93003
Sawblade.

Tuzik Boston 800-886-6363
104 Longwater Dr, Assinippi Park, Norwell, MA 02061

Vilex, Inc. 931-474-7550
111 Moffitt St, McMinnville, TN 37110

Zimmer Spine, Inc. 800-655-2614
7375 Bush Lake Rd, Minneapolis, MN 55439
Saw blade, general and plastic surgery.

BLADE, TONGUE *(Surgery) 79FWQ*

Puritan Medical Products Company Llc 800-321-2313
31 School St., Guilford, ME 04443-0149

BLANKET, FIRE *(General) 80LDI*

Burnfree Products Division 888-909-2876
9382 S 670 W, Sandy, UT 84070
A gel coated fire blanket for rescue, escape, and transport of burn victims.

Carolina Biological Supply Co. 800-334-5551
2700 York Rd, Burlington, NC 27215

Medi-Tech International, Inc. 305-593-9373
2924 NW 109th Ave, Doral, FL 33172
FERNO

Newtex Industries, Inc. 585-924-9135
8050 Victor Mendon Rd, Victor, NY 14564

Romaine, Inc. D.B.A. Koldcare 800-294-7101
2026 Sterling Ave, Elkhart, IN 46516
BURN BLANKET. Made from 100% polyester and a water based gel. Product is not wet or messy. Sterile, non-toxic, non-adhering and non-irritating. Available in three sizes: 24' x 36', 50' x 72' and 68' x 72'. Blankets are fire resistant and can be used to estinguish flames or escape from a fire, as well as treat burns.

Water-Jel Technologies 800-275-3433
50 Broad St, Carlstadt, NJ 07072
Blankets & Dressings soaked in a water-based gel. Stops the burn progression, cools the burn - not the patient, relieves pain and prevents contamination. Ideal pre-hospital preparation for all types of burns.

BLANKET, INFANT *(General) 80QDW*

Best Manufacturing Group Llc 800-843-3233
1633 Broadway Fl 18, New York, NY 10019
30 x 40, 100% cotton: solid prints, pink and blue, BDR stripe colors.

General Econopak, Inc. 888-871-8568
1725 N 6th St, Philadelphia, PA 19122

Global Healthcare 800-601-3880
1495 Hembree Rd Ste 700, Roswell, GA 30076
Disposable Baby Blankets and Baby Shirts

Riegel Consumer Products Div. 800-845-2232
PO Box E, 51 Riegel Road, Johnston, SC 29832

Standard Textile Co., Inc. 888-999-0400
PO Box 371805, Cincinnati, OH 45222

BLANKET, RESCUE *(General) 80QDV*

American Woolen Company 305-635-4000
4000 NW 30th Ave, Miami, FL 33142

Armstrong Medical Industries, Inc. 800-323-4220
575 Knightsbridge Pkwy, Lincolnshire, IL 60069

General Econopak, Inc. 888-871-8568
1725 N 6th St, Philadelphia, PA 19122

BLANKET, RESCUE *(cont'd)*

General Scientific Safety Equipment Co. 800-523-0166
2553 E Somerset St Fl 1, Philadelphia, PA 19134

Protector Canada Inc. 800-268-6594
1111 Flint Rd., Unit 23, Toronto, ON M3J 3C7 Canada

Rockford Medical & Safety Co. 800-435-9451
2420 Harrison Ave, PO Box 5646, Rockford, IL 61108

BLEEDING TIME DEVICE *(Hematology) 81JCA*

Biomerieux Inc. 800-682-2666
100 Rodolphe St, Durham, NC 27712
SIMPLATE bleeding time device.

International Technidyne Corp. 800-631-5945
23 Nevsky St, Edison, NJ 08820
Disposable incision maker incl. stainless steel blade #11 making a 5x1mm deep horizontal incision; retracts blade automatically after incision.

International Technidyne Corporation 732-548-5700
8 Olsen Ave, Edison, NJ 08820
Incision device.

Medtronic Perfusion Systems 800-328-3320
7611 Northland Dr N, Brooklyn Park, MN 55428

BLENDER/MIXER *(Chemistry) 75JRO*

Alfa Laval Inc. 866-253-2528
5400 International Trade Dr, Richmond, VA 23231

Brinkmann Instruments, Inc. 800-645-3050
PO Box 1019, Westbury, NY 11590

Carolina Biological Supply Co. 800-334-5551
2700 York Rd, Burlington, NC 27215

Eberbach Corp. 800-422-2558
505 S Maple Rd, Ann Arbor, MI 48103

Fisher Healthcare 800-766-7000
9999 Veterans Memorial Dr, Houston, TX 77038

Pro Scientific Inc. 800-584-3776
99 Willenbrock Rd, Oxford, CT 06478
The VSN-5 Nutating Mixer can be used for a variety of applications including mixing or resuspenision of specimens, tissue culture, immunoblots, etc. Variable speed at 5-40 rpm and operates at a 20 degree tilt angle and fits either a 5' x 9' or 8' x 8' table. The VSM-3 Vortex Mixer features continuous operation or touch start/stop and provides vortexing action for variable speeds up to 3000 rpm or in a continuous mixing mode. The VSM-3 mixer has a variety of adaptors available and includes a cap for single test tubes and 3' platform head.

Sarstedt, Inc. 800-257-5101
PO Box 468, 1025, St. James Church Road, Newton, NC 28658

Scientific Industries, Inc. 888-850-6208
70 Orville Dr, Bohemia, NY 11716

Solutek Corp. 800-403-0770
94 Shirley St, Roxbury, MA 02119
Chemical mixing & replenishment system.

Vulcon Technologies 816-966-1212
718 Main St, Grandview, MO 64030
Rotator/mixer.

Waring Products, Div. Conair Corp. 203-351-9000
1 Crystal Dr, Mc Connellsburg, PA 17233
Blender.

Whip-Mix Corporation 800-626-5651
361 Farmington Ave, PO Box 17183, Louisville, KY 40209

BLOCK, BEAM SHAPING, RADIONUCLIDE *(Radiology) 90IXI*

.Decimal, Inc. 407-330-3300
121 Central Park Pl, Sanford, FL 32771
Radiation therapy beam shaping block, range compensator.

Akribeia, Inc. 256-564-7450
1251 Washington St NW, Huntsville, AL 35801
Various types of radiotherapy accessories.

Best Nomos Corp. 800-70-NOMOS
1 Best Dr, Pittsburgh, PA 15202
Radiation therapy beam shaping block. Multileaf intensity modulating collimator (MIMiC).

Computerized Medical Systems, Inc. 468-587-2550
1145 Corporate Lake Dr, Olivette, MO 63132
Compensating filter.

Huestis Medical 800-972-9222
68 Buttonwood St, Bristol, RI 02809
SELECTABLE, x-ray collimator.

BLOCK, BEAM SHAPING, RADIONUCLIDE *(cont'd)*

Innocure, Llc 480-966-0980
1045 E Sandpiper Dr, Tempe, AZ 85283
Compensator.

Oncology Tech, Llc 210-497-2100
5608 Business Park, San Antonio, TX 78218
Compensators.

BLOCK, BITE *(Cns/Neurology) 84JXL*

Biomet Microfixation Inc. 800-874-7711
1520 Tradeport Dr, Jacksonville, FL 32218
Block, bite.

Common Sense Dental Inc. 616-837-1231
12261 Cleveland St Ste D, Nunica, MI 49448
Bite block.

Electro Surgical Instrument Co., Inc. 888-464-2784
37 Centennial St, Rochester, NY 14611
Bite block.

Ethox International 800-521-1022
251 Seneca St, Buffalo, NY 14204
Block,bite intubation.

Gi Supply 800-451-5797
200 Grandview Ave, Camp Hill, PA 17011
Six different disposable bite blocks: GENERA BLOC, OMNI BLOC, ULTIMA BLOC, PEDIA BLOC, MAX BLOC, OXYBLOC, MAX BLOC for endoscopic procedures.

Omni Medical Supply Inc. 800-860-6664
4153 Pioneer Dr, Commerce Township, MI 48390
Disposable bite block.

Somatics, Llc 847-234-6761
910 Sherwood Dr Ste 23, Lake Bluff, IL 60044
Bite block; mouth prop.

Temrex Corp. 516-868-6221
112 Albany Ave, P.o. Box 182, Freeport, NY 11520
Bite sticks.

BLOCK, BITE, ENT *(Ear/Nose/Throat) 77JPL*

Aesculap Implant Systems Inc. 1-800-234-9179
3773 Corporate Pkwy, Center Valley, PA 18034

BLOCK, BITE, INTUBATION *(Anesthesiology) 73BTW*

Aesculap Implant Systems Inc. 1-800-234-9179
3773 Corporate Pkwy, Center Valley, PA 18034

Armstrong Medical Industries, Inc. 800-323-4220
575 Knightsbridge Pkwy, Lincolnshire, IL 60069

Sunmed Healthcare 727-531-7266
12393 Belcher Rd S Ste 460, Largo, FL 33773

BLOCK, CUTTING, ENT *(Ear/Nose/Throat) 77JXS*

Bausch & Lomb Surgical 636-255-5051
3365 Tree Court Ind Blvd, Saint Louis, MO 63122

Gyrus Ent L.L.C., Sub. Of Gyrus Acmi, Inc. 508-804-2739
2925 Appling Rd, Bartlett, TN 38133
Various types and sizes of ent cutting blocks.

Oto-Med, Inc. 800-433-7703
1090 Empire Dr, Lake Havasu City, AZ 86404
Teflon cutting blocks. Standard sise: 2 7/8' x 2 1/2' x 3/8'. Custom sizes by request.

BLOCK, HEATING *(Chemistry) 75JRG*

Barnstead International 412-490-8425
2555 Kerper Blvd, Dubuque, IA 52001
Various.

Certol International, Llc 303-799-9401
6120 E 58th Ave, Commerce City, CO 80022
Dry block incubator.

Diagnostic Hybrids, Inc. 740-589-3300
1055 E State St Ste 100, Athens, OH 45701
Heat block.

Iris Sample Processing 800-782-8774
60 Glacier Dr, Westwood, MA 02090
Denaturation and hybridization system.

Matrix Technologies Corporation 800-345-0206
12 Executive Dr, Hudson, NH 03051

Statspin, Inc. 800-782-8774
60 Glacier Dr, Westwood, MA 02090
The THERMOBRITE is a slide Denaturation/Hybridization processing system used for (F)ISH assays, used in research or genetics laboratories.

BLOCK, HEATING *(cont'd)*

Thermo Fisher Scientific Inc. 563-556-2241
2555 Kerper Blvd, Dubuque, IA 52001
$436.00 per unit (standard).

Troemner Llc 800-352-7705
201 Wolf Dr, PO Box 87, West Deptford, NJ 08086

BLOCK, THERAPY, RADIATION *(Radiology) 90WKV*

Diacor, Inc. 800-342-2679
3191 Valley St Ste 100A, Salt Lake City, UT 84109
$35,850.00 for PORTALCAST radiotherapy block cutting & casting system for customized blocks.

S&S Technology 281-815-1300
10625 Telge Rd, Houston, TX 77095

Samco Scientific Corporation 800-522-3359
1050 Arroyo St, San Fernando, CA 91340
Disposable pipette and polyethylene pipette.

BLOOD AND URINE COLLECTION KIT (EXCLUDES HIV TESTING) *(Chemistry) 75OIB*

Endochoice Inc. 888-682-3636
11810 Wills Rd Ste 100, Alpharetta, GA 30009

BLOOD SYSTEM, EXTRACORPOREAL (WITH ACCESSORIES) *(Gastro/Urology) 78LLB*

Castle Pines Medical, Inc. 303-442-4514
14883 E Hinsdale Ave Ste 2, Centennial, CO 80112
Vented dialysate port cap.

Hema Metrics Inc. 800-546-5463
695 N Kays Dr, Kaysville, UT 84037
CRITLINE disposable extracorporeal conduit for blood constituent monitoring.

BLOWER, POWDER, ENT *(Ear/Nose/Throat) 77KCL*

Brailsford & Co., Inc. 603-588-2880
15 Elm Ave, Antrim, NH 03440
Brushless D.C. fans and blowers.

Oto-Med, Inc. 800-433-7703
1090 Empire Dr, Lake Havasu City, AZ 86404
Powder Insufflator: simple method for dry powder treatment.

BOARD, ARM *(Anesthesiology) 73BTX*

Alimed, Inc. 800-225-2610
297 High St, Dedham, MA 02026
Pivoting, lateral, and surgical. Pivoting used for general and specific surgical procedures for the patient in the supine position. Lateral set allows variations in adjustments to be made easily. Surgical model may be inclined from below horizontal to a completely vertical position.

Bryton Corp. 800-567-9500
4310 Guion Rd, Indianapolis, IN 46254
Arm boards for a variety of surgical procedures.

Cas Medical Systems, Inc. 800-227-4414
44 E Industrial Rd, Branford, CT 06405
Neonatal limb board immobilizes I.V. site.

Dale Medical Products, Inc. 800-343-3980
7 Cross St, Plainville, MA 02762
DALE Bendable Armboard. Large #650 fits most adults. Medium #651 fits pediatrics. Small # 652 fits infant.

Fpp, Inc. 352-622-4595
6800 SW 66th St, Ocala, FL 34476
Reusable armboard strap.

Hausmann Industries, Inc. 888-428-7626
130 Union St, Northvale, NJ 07647

Health Supply Company Inc., The 770-452-0090
2902 Marlin Cir, Atlanta, GA 30341
TKO Multi-Position Armboard, used with virtually any rail clamp; when used with the Midkiff GEOSTATIC Clamp, greater positioning flexibility and allocation is achieved.

J. T. Posey Co. 800-447-6739
5635 Peck Rd, Arcadia, CA 91006

Kentec Medical Inc. 800-825-5996
17871 Fitch, Irvine, CA 92614
Ameritus Neonatal and Pediatric limb boards designed to stabilize the hand and foot for IV securement and other applications.

Kentron Health Care, Inc. 615-384-0573
3604 Kelton Jackson Rd, P.o. Box 120, Springfield, TN 37172
Arm board.

Lac-Mac Ltd. 800-461-0001
425 Rectory St., London, ONT N5W 3W5 Canada

BOARD, ARM *(cont'd)*

Lundy Medical Product, Llc 480-473-7330
9376 E Bahia Dr Ste D101, Scottsdale, AZ 85260
Vinyl covered foam. Disposable/reusable. Item no. 1012.

Medrecon, Inc. 877-526-4323
257 South Ave, Garwood, NJ 07027

Mizuho Osi 800-777-4674
30031 Ahern Ave, Union City, CA 94587
Lateral, pivoting & surgical (radiolucent).

Morrison Medical 800-438-6677
3735 Paragon Dr, Columbus, OH 43228
Premie, newborn, neonatal to adult models, disposable or reusable: 1x4, 1.5x3, 2x4, 2x6, 2x9, 3x6, 3x9, 3x12, 3x18, 4x9, & 4x18in.

Pedicraft, Inc. 800-223-7649
4134 Saint Augustine Rd, Jacksonville, FL 32207
PEDI-BOARD $2.52 to $6.90 for 3, 4, 6, 8, and 15 in. sizes.

Ross Disposable Products 800-649-6526
401 Traders Blvd E, Unit 10, Mississauga, ON L4Z 2H8 Canada
Intravenous arm board.

Telos Medical Equipment (Austin & Assoc., Inc.) 800-934-3029
1109 Sturbridge Rd, Fallston, MD 21047
TELOS anesthesia/general purpose radiolucent arm board. Fits any Clark Socket and may be used for hand and shoulder surgery.

BOARD, BED *(General) 80FPS*

Biomet, Inc. 574-267-6639
56 E Bell Dr, PO Box 587, Warsaw, IN 46582
Slated bed board.

Bird & Cronin, Inc. 651-683-1111
1200 Trapp Rd, Saint Paul, MN 55121
Bed board.

Dixie Ems Supply 800-347-3494
385 Union Ave, Brooklyn, NY 11211
$119.00 per unit (standard).

Medical Depot 516-998-4600
99 Seaview Blvd, Port Washington, NY 11050
Board, bed.

Mrc Industries Inc. 516-328-6900
85 Denton Ave, New Hyde Park, NY 11040
Bed, bed board.

Ortho Development Corp. 800-429-8339
12187 Business Park Dr, Draper, UT 84020
Patil Stereotactic System II. Center of the arc stereotactic head frame, both CT & MRI compatible.

Warsaw Orthopedic, Inc. 901-396-3133
2500 Silveus Xing, Warsaw, IN 46582
Bed board.

BOARD, CARDIAC COMPRESSION *(Cardiovascular) 74QGJ*

Armstrong Medical Industries, Inc. 800-323-4220
575 Knightsbridge Pkwy, Lincolnshire, IL 60069

Rockford Medical & Safety Co. 800-435-9451
2420 Harrison Ave, PO Box 5646, Rockford, IL 61108

BOARD, CARDIOPULMONARY RESUSCITATION *(General) 80FOA*

Dixie Ems Supply 800-347-3494
385 Union Ave, Brooklyn, NY 11211
$49.75 per unit (standard).

Health Care Logistics, Inc. 800-848-1633
450 Town St, PO Box 25, Circleville, OH 43113
Cardiac compression board.

Homak Manufacturing Company Inc. 800-874-6625
1605 Old Route 18 Ste 4-36, Wampum, PA 16157

Protector Canada Inc. 800-268-6594
1111 Flint Rd., Unit 23, Toronto, ON M3J 3C7 Canada

BOARD, DISSECTING *(Pathology) 88WMB*

Carolina Biological Supply Co. 800-334-5551
2700 York Rd, Burlington, NC 27215

Marketing International, Inc. 800-447-0173
PO Box 4835, Topeka, KS 66604
Disposable and reusable cutting boards.

Scientek Medical Equipment 604-273-9094
11151 Bridgeport Rd., Richmond, BC V6X 1T3 Canada
Dissecting Table.

BOARD, FOOT *(Orthopedics) 87QWT*

Ergodyne 800-225-8238
1021 Bandana Blvd E Ste 220, Saint Paul, MN 55108
Adjustable foot rest.

J. T. Posey Co. 800-447-6739
5635 Peck Rd, Arcadia, CA 91006

Remington Products Company Llc 800-491-1571
961 Seville Rd, Wadsworth, OH 44281
Diabetic insole that will mold to foot. Tri-laminate packages. Fabricated from the company's ProCell, a closed-cell, specially formulated, nonabrasive EVA blend.

Zimmer Holdings, Inc. 800-613-6131
1800 W Center St, PO Box 708, Warsaw, IN 46580

BOARD, QUADRICEPS (EXERCISER) *(Physical Med) 89RNR*

Hausmann Industries, Inc. 888-428-7626
130 Union St, Northvale, NJ 07647
$82.90 per unit (standard).

BOARD, SCOOTER, PRONE *(Physical Med) 89KNL*

Community Products, Llc 845-658-7723
2032 Route 213, Rifton, NY 12471
Stander with wheels.

Therafin Corporation 800-843-7234
19747 Wolf Rd, Mokena, IL 60448
Various types of standers.

Tumble Forms, Inc. 262-387-8720
1013 Barker Rd, Dolgeville, NY 13329
Multiple.

BOARD, SPINE *(Orthopedics) 87RUV*

Allied Healthcare Products, Inc. 800-444-3954
1720 Sublette Ave, Saint Louis, MO 63110

Armstrong Medical Industries, Inc. 800-323-4220
575 Knightsbridge Pkwy, Lincolnshire, IL 60069

Bound Tree Medical 800-533-0523
PO Box 8023, Dublin, OH 43016

Bound Tree Medical, Llc 800-533-0523
5200 Rings Rd Ste A, Dublin, OH 43017
Baltic Birch wood backboards are available with or without runners and pins. Also available are short extrication boards and pediatric backboards.

Composiflex, Inc. 800-673-2544
8100 Hawthorne Dr, Erie, PA 16509
Low x-ray absorption, high strength carbon fiber cervical/spinal boards.

Composites Horizons, Inc. 626-331-0861
1471 W Industrial Park St, Covina, CA 91722
JELSMA radiolucent spinal fracture/multiple injuries board to eliminate need for multiple transfers of patient for radiographic evaluation, using CT, MRI, myelographic, fluoroscopic & other radiographic equipment ($2,350 for JELSMA 1 board with attachment for cervical traction, $1,450 for JELSMA 2 board w/o attachment).

Dixie Ems Supply 800-347-3494
385 Union Ave, Brooklyn, NY 11211
$94.50 per unit (standard).

Ferno-Washington, Inc. 800-733-3766
70 Weil Way, Wilmington, OH 45177

Iron Duck, A Div. Of Fleming Industries, Inc. 800-669-6900
20 Veterans Dr, Chicopee, MA 01022
Plastic backboard, measuring 72x16x1.75 in; also available, 14-ply wood backboard.

Profex Medical Products 800-325-0196
2224 E Person Ave, Memphis, TN 38114

Rockford Medical & Safety Co. 800-435-9451
2420 Harrison Ave, PO Box 5646, Rockford, IL 61108

Schueler & Company, Inc. 516-487-1500
PO Box 528, Stratford, CT 06615

Skedco, Inc. 503-639-2119
16420 SW 72nd Ave, PO Box 230487, Portland, OR 97224
OREGON SPINE SPLINT II vest-type short back board for immobilization and extrication.

BOLSTER, SUTURE (BUMPER) *(Surgery) 79RXQ*

Covidien Lp 508-261-8000
15 Hampshire St, Mansfield, MA 02048
Retention suture bolsters.

BOLT, NUT, WASHER *(Orthopedics) 87HTN*

Arthrex Manufacturing 239-643-5553
1958 Trade Center Way, Naples, FL 34109
Washer.

Arthrex, Inc. 239-643-5553
1370 Creekside Blvd, Naples, FL 34108
Various types of washers.

Biomet, Inc. 574-267-6639
56 E Bell Dr, PO Box 587, Warsaw, IN 46582
Various types of bolts, nuts, and washers.

Depuy Mitek, A Johnson & Johnson Company 800-451-2006
50 Scotland Blvd, Bridgewater, MA 02324
Various sizes of spiked washers.

Depuy Orthopaedics, Inc. 800-473-3789
700 Orthopaedic Dr, P.O. Box 988, Warsaw, IN 46582
Various types of washers, bolts, nuts.

Depuy Spine, Inc. 800-227-6633
325 Paramount Dr, Raynham, MA 02767
Washer, nut, bolt.

Depuy-Raynham, A Div. Of Depuy Orthopaedics 800-451-2006
325 Paramount Dr, Raynham, MA 02767
Various types of washers, bolts, nuts.

DJO Inc. 800-336-6569
1430 Decision St, Vista, CA 92081

Interventional Spine, Inc. 800-497-0484
13700 Alton Pkwy Ste 160, Irvine, CA 92618
Washer.

Koros Usa, Inc. 805-529-0825
610 Flinn Ave, Moorpark, CA 93021
316l washer.

Warsaw Orthopedic, Inc. 901-396-3133
2500 Silveus Xing, Warsaw, IN 46582
Various bolts and nuts.

Zimmer Holdings, Inc. 800-613-6131
1800 W Center St, PO Box 708, Warsaw, IN 46580

BONE CEMENT *(Orthopedics) 87LOD*

Advanced Biomaterial Systems, Inc. 973-635-9040
100 Passaic Ave, Chatham, NJ 07928
Polymethylmethacrylate (pmma) bone cement.

Biomet, Inc. 574-267-6639
56 E Bell Dr, PO Box 587, Warsaw, IN 46582
Pmma bone cement.

Dentsply Canada, Ltd. 800-263-1437
161 Vinyl Ct., Woodbridge, ONT L4L 4A3 Canada

Depuy Orthopaedics, Inc. 800-473-3789
700 Orthopaedic Dr, P.O. Box 988, Warsaw, IN 46582
Various.

Osteotech, Inc. 800-537-9842
51 James Way, Eatontown, NJ 07724
GRAFTON matrix putty for packing and filling voids. Grafton DBM putty, DBM flex, DBM gel and DBM crunch.

BONE CEMENT, ANTIBIOTIC *(Orthopedics) 87MBB*

Biomet, Inc. 574-267-6639
56 E Bell Dr, PO Box 587, Warsaw, IN 46582
Various types of bone cement.

Depuy Orthopaedics, Inc. 800-473-3789
700 Orthopaedic Dr, P.O. Box 988, Warsaw, IN 46582
Various types of antibiotic bone cement.

BONE GRAFTING MATERIAL, ANIMAL SOURCE *(Dental And Oral) 76NPM*

Collagen Matrix, Inc. 201-405-1477
509 Commerce St, Franklin Lakes, NJ 07417
Tricalcium phosphate granules for dental bone repair.

BONE GRAFTING MATERIAL, DENTAL, WITH BIOLOGIC COMPONENT *(Dental And Oral) 76NPZ*

Dentsply Friadent Ceramed 717-849-4229
12860 W Cedar Dr Ste 110, Lakewood, CO 80228
Dental bone grafting material.

BONE GRAFTING MATERIAL, HUMAN SOURCE *(Dental And Oral) 76NUN*

Musculoskeletal Transplant Foundation 800-433-6576
125 May St Ste 300, Edison Corp Ctr, Edison, NJ 08837
Bone void filler containing human demineralized bone matrix (dbm).

BONE MILL *(Orthopedics) 87LYS*

Biomedical Composites, Ltd. 805-644-4892
4526 Telephone Rd Ste 204, Ventura, CA 93003
Manual bone mill.

Biomet Microfixation Inc. 800-874-7711
1520 Tradeport Dr, Jacksonville, FL 32218
Bio comp mini mill.

Depuy Orthopaedics, Inc. 800-473-3789
700 Orthopaedic Dr, P.O. Box 988, Warsaw, IN 46582
Various types of bone mills.

H & H Co. 909-390-0373
4435 E Airport Dr Ste 108, Ontario, CA 91761
Bone crusher, all types.

Ika-Works, Inc. 800-733-3037
2635 Northchase Pkwy SE, Wilmington, NC 28405
Analytical mills designed to reduce dry, hard and brittle materials including bone and teeth for analytical evaluation.

Lenox-Maclaren Surgical Corp. 720-890-9660
657 S Taylor Ave Ste A, Colorado Technology Center
Louisville, CO 80027
Bone mill.

Lighthouse Industries 219-879-1550
107 Eastwood Rd, Po Box 8905, Michigan City, IN 46360

Symmetry Medical Usa, Inc. 574-267-8700
486 W 350 N, Warsaw, IN 46582
Orthopedic manual surgical instrument.

Tracer Designs, Inc. 805-933-2616
333 S 11th St, Santa Paula, CA 93060
Bone mill.

BONE PARTICLE COLLECTOR *(Ear/Nose/Throat) 77MXP*

H & H Co. 909-390-0373
4435 E Airport Dr Ste 108, Ontario, CA 91761
Bone carrier.

BOOTH, SUN TAN *(Physical Med) 89LEJ*

Avex Industries, Ltd.
27 Allen St, Hudson Falls, NY 12839
Peacock.

Creative Marketing Concepts, Inc. 978-532-7517
96 Audubon Rd, Wakefield, MA 01880
The sun capsule.

Esb Enterprises, Llc 847-429-9990
1490 Crispin Dr, Elgin, IL 60123
Tanning beds.

Ets, Inc. 317-554-3500
7445 Company Dr, Indianapolis, IN 46237
Tanning beds, tanning booths, portable sunlamp products.

Heartland Tanning, Inc. 816-795-1414
4251 NE Port Dr, Lees Summit, MO 64064
Tanning bed.

Helio Balance 425-453-9849
13000 Bel Red Rd Ste 207, Bellevue, WA 98005
Various.

Hollywood Tanning Systems, Inc. 856-914-9090
11 Enterprise Ct, Sewell, NJ 08080
Suntanning booth.

International Design & Marketing Incorporated 978-921-0638
140 Elliott St, Rt. 62 Business Center, Bldg E, Beverly, MA 01915
Indoor suntanning booth.

J&B Products, Ltd. 800-556-3201
2201 S Michigan Ave, Saginaw, MI 48602

Jk Products & Services, Inc. 870-268-2852
1 Walter Kratz Dr, Jonesboro, AR 72401
Tanning bed.

Light Sources, Inc. 203-234-7338
37 Robinson Blvd, Orange, CT 06477
Uva tanning lamps.

M&R Printing Equipment, Inc. 630-858-6101
1 N 372 Main Street, Glen Ellyn, IL 60137
Tanning booth.

Nova Companies 217-763-9016
209 E South St, Po Box 139, Cerro Gordo, IL 61818
Sun lamp.

Photoclear, Inc. 888-789-3784
8819 Hoskins Rd, Freeport, TX 77541

BOOTH, SUN TAN *(cont'd)*

Precision Plastic Molding, Inc. 865-982-5552
28035 US Highway 31, Jemison, AL 35085
Sun tan booth.

Prosun Tanning International, Llc. 800-874-2776
2442 23rd St N, Saint Petersburg, FL 33713
Tanning beds, Tanning booth, SunShower.

Sol Enterprises, Inc. 800-510-8267
3101 Northside Ave, Richmond, VA 23228
Tanning bed.

Sun Technologies, Inc. 865-982-5552
154 Frog Level Rd Ste 2, Gray, TN 37615

Tan Source Supply, Inc. 913-451-7000
12142A State Line Rd, Leawood, KS 66209
Sun tan booth.

Ultra-Derm Systems 989-792-6110
2201 S Michigan Ave, Saginaw, MI 48602
Uvb booth.

BOTTLE, BLOW (EXERCISER) *(Anesthesiology) 73BYO*

Ac Healthcare Supply, Inc. 905-448-4706
11651 230th St, Cambria Heights, NY 11411
Blow bottle.

Covidien Lp 508-261-8000
15 Hampshire St, Mansfield, MA 02048

Instrumentation Industries, Inc. 800-633-8577
2990 Industrial Blvd, Bethel Park, PA 15102
Component, exercise, inspiratory, variable-resistance.

Medi Inc 800-225-8634
75 York Ave, P.O. Box 302, Randolph, MA 02368

BOTTLE, COLLECTION, BREATHING SYSTEM (UNCALIBRATED) *(Anesthesiology) 73CBC*

Datex-Ohmeda Inc. 608-221-1551
3030 Ohmeda Dr, Madison, WI 53718
Overflow safety trap bottle.

Ventlab Corp. 336-753-5000
155 Boyce Dr, Mocksville, NC 27028
Bottle, collection, drain & trap tee.

BOTTLE, COLLECTION, VACUUM (ASPIRATOR) *(General) 80KDQ*

Allied Healthcare Products, Inc. 800-444-3954
1720 Sublette Ave, Saint Louis, MO 63110

Ambu A/S 457-225-2210
6740 Baymeadow Dr, Glen Burnie, MD 21060
Collection bottle.

Amerivac Usa Inc. 908-486-5200
1207 Pennsylvania Ave, Linden, NJ 07036
Suction canister.

Axiom Medical, Inc. 800-221-8569
19320 Van Ness Ave, Torrance, CA 90501
Multiple

Bemis Mfg. Co. 920-467-5206
Hwy. Pp West, Sheboygan Falls, WI 53085
Suction catheter.

Buffalo Filter, A Division Of Medtek Devices Inc. 800-343-2324
595 Commerce Dr, Amherst, NY 14228
REPLACEMENT FILTERS; VIROSAFE FILTER

Dhd Healthcare Corporation 800-847-8000
PO Box 6, One Madison Street, Wampsville, NY 13163
VACON.

H2or, Inc. 918-744-4267
1638 S Main St, Tulsa, OK 74119
Suction canister.

Huntington Mechanical Laboratories, Inc. 800-227-8059
1040 La Avenida St, Mountain View, CA 94043
Ultra high vaccum components.

J. H. Emerson Co. 800-252-1414
22 Cottage Park Ave, Cambridge, MA 02140
System, drainage, thoracic, waterseal.

Jedmed Instruments Co. 314-845-3770
5416 Jedmed Ct, Saint Louis, MO 63129

Kelsar, S.A. 508-261-8000
Blvd. Insurgentes, Libriamento a La, Tijuana 22450 Mexico
Thoracic catheter - straight/angled, mediastinal

BOTTLE, COLLECTION, VACUUM (ASPIRATOR) *(cont'd)*

M D Technologies, Inc. 800-201-3060
PO Box 60, Galena, IL 61036
Environ-Mate DM6000 Series Suction-Drain Systems. Three versions: DM6000 (SPD/general), DM6000-2 (Endoscopy) and DM6000-2A (Surgery/Urology).

Maquet, Inc. 843-552-8652
7371 Spartan Blvd E, N Charleston, SC 29418
Various types of vacuum collection apparatus.

Matrx 716-662-6650
145 Mid County Dr, Orchard Park, NY 14127
Vacuum bottle.

Medtek Devices, Inc. 716-835-7000
595 Commerce Dr, 155 Pineview Dr., Amherst, NY 14228
Smoke filters.

Ohio Medical Corp. 800-662-5822
1111 Lakeside Dr, Gurnee, IL 60031
1/2 gallon glass reusable collection bottle with associated mounting brackets, disposable cap and float assemblies.

Ohmeda Medical 800-345-2700
8880 Gorman Rd, Laurel, MD 20723

Rico Suction Labs, Inc. 800-845-8490
326 MacArthur Ln, Burlington, NC 27217

Scanlan International, Inc. 800-328-9458
1 Scanlan Plz, Saint Paul, MN 55107
Suction instruments.

Stryker Puerto Rico, Ltd. 939-307-2500
Hwy. 3, Km. 131.2, Las Guasimas Ind. Park, Arroyo, PR 00714
Various vacuum collection bottles,sterile.

Terumo Cardiovascular Systems (Tcvs) 800-283-7866
28 Howe St, Ashland, MA 01721
Thoracic drain device.

The Metrix Co. 800-752-3148
4400 Chavenelle Rd, Dubuque, IA 52002
250ml, 500ml, 1000ml and 2000ml sterile evacuated bottles.

Ubimed 310-556-0624
1180 S Beverly Dr Ste 400, Los Angeles, CA 90035
Vacuum-powered bodyfluid suction asparatus.

BOTTLE, EVACUATED *(General) 80TAN*

Baxter Healthcare Corporation, Global Drug Delivery 888-229-0001
25212 W Il Route 120, Round Lake, IL 60073
Evacuated glass containers.

The Metrix Co. 800-752-3148
4400 Chavenelle Rd, Dubuque, IA 52002
250ml, 500ml and 1000ml sterile evacuated glass containers with 43mm necks; 500ml and 2000ml with 28mm necks also.

BOTTLE, HOT/COLD WATER *(General) 80FPF*

Aqua-Cel Corp. 888-254-HEAT
17137 Sparkleberry St, Fountain Valley, CA 92708
$15 for back and cervical size, microwavable hot & cold water pad.

Bruder Healthcare Company 888-827-8337
3150 Engineering Pkwy, Alpharetta, GA 30004
Latex Free Hot/Cold Water Bottle

Hospira 800-441-4100
268 E 4th St, Ashland, OH 44805

Northern Falls, Llc 616-975-0733
4460 44th St SE Ste A, Kentwood, MI 49512
Bottle water.

Sunbeam Products, Inc. 561-912-4100
2381 NW Executive Center Dr, Boca Raton, FL 33431
Hot/cold water bottle.

Telemed Systems Inc. 800-481-6718
8 Kane Industrial Dr, Hudson, MA 01749
View-thru water bottle available.

BOTTLE, MEDICINE SPRAY *(General) 80VFT*

Medi-Dose, Inc. 800-523-8966
70 Industrial Dr, Ivyland, PA 18974
Bottle, sterile, dropping - 3,7,15 ml sizes. Also, bottle, sterile, spraying, 30 ml.

BOTTLE, MEDICINE SPRAY *(cont'd)*

Safetec Of America, Inc. 800-456-7077
887 Kensington Ave, Buffalo, NY 14215
Safetec CUT & SCRAPE CLEANER provides temporary pain relief and aids in preventing infection in minor cuts, scrapes and abrasions. Contains Benzocaine. Packaging: individually wrapped, pre-moistened 1 x 5-in wipe or 2-oz spray bottle. Hydrogen PEROXIDE SPRAY provides painless, antiseptic treatment to cuts, scrapes, and abrasions. 2-oz 'no touch' spray. Isopropyl ALCOHOL SPRAY provides a convenient method for cleaning and sanitizing. 2-oz 'no touch' spray.

The Hymed Group Corp. 610-865-9876
1890 Bucknell Dr, Bethlehem, PA 18015
Collasate spray with bitrex to deter licking and biting of wounds in the veterinary market.

BOTTLE, NURSING *(Obstetrics/Gyn) 85TAO*

Gerber Products Co. 800-430-0150
120 N Commercial St Fl 4, Neenah, WI 54956

Medi-Dose, Inc. 800-523-8966
70 Industrial Dr, Ivyland, PA 18974

BOTTLE, STERILE SOLUTION *(General) 80QEF*

Baxter Healthcare Corporation, Global Drug Delivery 888-229-0001
25212 W Il Route 120, Round Lake, IL 60073
Irrigating solutions in plastic pour bottles.

Blairex Laboratories, Inc. 800-252-4739
PO Box 2127, 1600 Brian Drive, Columbus, IN 47202
WOUND WASH SALINE, sterile saline solution 0.9%, unique 360 degree dispensing allows any position during dispensing and eliminates waste by using only what is needed for each individual patient. BRONCHO SALINE, metered dispensing, 1cc at a time, is push-button easy. No measuring mistakes and no possibility of bulk saline contamination. Sealed, pressurized container protects product sterility up to two years.

Meditron Inc D.B.A. Medcare Usa 800-243-2442
3435 Montee Gagnon, Terrebonne, QUEBE J6Y-1J4 Canada
Sterile water/saline.

Nalge Nunc International 800-625-4327
75 Panorama Creek Dr, Rochester, NY 14625
NALGENE sterile square PETG bottles. Non-pyrogenic. Sizes from 30ml to 2L.

Pennsylvania Glass Products Co. 412-621-2853
430 N Craig St, Pittsburgh, PA 15213
Perfection.

Therakos, Inc., A Johnson & Johnson Company 877-865-6850
437 Creamery Way, Exton, PA 19341
UVADEX is liquid methoxsalen (sterile solution).

BOTTLE, TISSUE CULTURE, ROLLER *(Pathology) 88KJC*

Bd Biosciences Discovery Labware 978-901-7431
1 Becton Cir, Durham, NC 27712
Various styles of sterile and non-sterile disposable tissue culture roller bottl.

Sarstedt, Inc. 800-257-5101
PO Box 468, 1025, St. James Church Road, Newton, NC 28658

Thermo Fisher Scientific (Rochester) 585-899-7600
75 Panorama Creek Dr, Panorama, NY 14625
Various tc roller bottles.

BOUGIE, ESOPHAGEAL, AND GASTROINTESTINAL, GASTRO-UROLOGY *(Gastro/Urology) 78FAT*

Medovations, Inc. 800-558-6408
102 E Keefe Ave, Milwaukee, WI 53212
INNERVISION-Lighted Bougie (Fiberoptic cable with detachable, disposable tip)

BOUGIE, ESOPHAGEAL, ENT *(Ear/Nose/Throat) 77KCD*

Karl Storz Endoscopy-America Inc. 800-421-0837
600 Corporate Pointe, Culver City, CA 90230

Medovations, Inc. 800-558-6408
102 E Keefe Ave, Milwaukee, WI 53212
Maloney and Hurst styles. Mercury filled and mercury free.

Sunmed Healthcare 727-531-7266
12393 Belcher Rd S Ste 460, Largo, FL 33773

BOUGIE, UROLOGICAL *(Gastro/Urology) 78FAX*

Codman & Shurtleff, Inc 800-225-0460
325 Paramount Dr, Raynham, MA 02767

BOUGIE, UROLOGICAL *(cont'd)*

Greenwald Surgical Co., Inc. 219-962-1604
2688 Dekalb St, Gary, IN 46405
Various types of urethral bougies a boule.

Karl Storz Endoscopy-America Inc. 800-421-0837
600 Corporate Pointe, Culver City, CA 90230
Range of styles and sizes available.

BOWL, SOLUTION *(General) 80QEG*

Clinimed, Incorporated 877-CLINIMED
303 Markus Ct, Sandy Brae Industrial Park, Newark, DE 19713

Lsl Industries, Inc. 888-225-5575
5535 N Wolcott Ave, Chicago, IL 60640
$30.25 per 75 16oz. bowls, $30.00 per 50 32oz. bowls; all sterile and individually packed.

Medegen Medical Products, Llc 800-233-1987
209 Medegen Drive, Gallaway, TN 38036-0228
MED-ASSIST Disposable 6qt. units.

Polar Ware Co. 800-237-3655
2806 N 15th St, Sheboygan, WI 53083
Stainless steel, resuable plastic.

Primesource Healthcare, Inc. 888-842-6999
3708 E Columbia St Ste 100, Tucson, AZ 85714
Anti-Fog Solution.

Terriss-Consolidated Industries 800-342-1611
807 Summerfield Ave, Asbury Park, NJ 07712
Stainless steel.

BOWL, SPONGE *(General) 80QEH*

Medegen Medical Products, Llc 800-233-1987
209 Medegen Drive, Gallaway, TN 38036-0228
MED-ASSIST Sterilizable 1.3/8qt. units.

Polar Ware Co. 800-237-3655
2806 N 15th St, Sheboygan, WI 53083
Stainless steel, reusable plastic.

BOX, BATTERY, POCKET (ENDOSCOPIC) *(Gastro/Urology) 78FCP*

Electro Surgical Instrument Co., Inc. 888-464-2784
37 Centennial St, Rochester, NY 14611
Battery case, portable in various types, styles and sizes.

BOX, BATTERY, RECHARGEABLE (ENDOSCOPIC) *(Gastro/Urology) 78FCO*

Access Battery Inc. 800-654-9845
12104 W Carmen Ave, Division of Alpha Source, Inc. Milwaukee, WI 53225
Full line of nickel-cadmium, nickel-metal hydride, sealed lead-acid and lithium batteries for monitors, defibrillators, infusion pumps, thermometers, Holter recorders, ECG, TENS, radiology, ventilators, etc., with 18-month warranty on premium nickel-cadmium packs, and 1 year, no, 2 year warranty options on radiology batteries, not pro-rated.

Qed, Inc. 859-231-0338
750 Enterprise Dr, Lexington, KY 40510
Rechargeable battery pack.

R & D Batteries, Inc. 800-950-1945
3300 Corporate Center Dr, Burnsville, MN 55306
Rechargeable batteries.

BOX, GLOVE *(Microbiology) 83JTM*

Air Control, Inc. 252-492-2300
237 Raleigh Rd, Henderson, NC 27536
HYDROVOID.

Coy Laboratory Products, Inc. 734-475-2200
14500 Coy Dr, Grass Lake, MI 49240

Encompass Medical 800-826-4490
16415 Addison Rd Ste 660, Addison, TX 75001
Disposable.

Labconco Corp. 800-821-5525
8811 Prospect Ave, Kansas City, MO 64132
PROTECTOR Controlled Atmosphere and Multi-Hazard Glove Boxes. Stainless Steel or Fiberglass lined.

Matheson Tri-Gas, Inc. 972-893-5600
8200 Washington St NE, Albuquerque, NM 87113
Anaerobic gas mixture.

Nuaire, Inc. 800-328-3352
2100 Fernbrook Ln N, Plymouth, MN 55447

BOX, GLOVE *(cont'd)*

Omnimed, Inc. (Beam Products) 800-257-2326
800 Glen Ave, Moorestown, NJ 08057

Pm Gloves, Inc. 800-788-9486
13808 Magnolia Ave, Chino, CA 91710
Vinyl and latex, powdered and powder free.

Polar Cryogenics, Inc. 503-239-5252
2734 SE Raymond St, Portland, OR 97202
Anaerobic gas mixture.

Purified Micro Environments, Div. Of Germfree Laboratories 800-888-5357
11 Aviator Way, Ormond Beach, FL 32174
Glovebox Class III.

Thermo Fisher Scientific (Asheville) Llc 740-373-4763
Millcreek Rd., Marietta, OH 45750
Anaerobic glove box.

Trademark Medical Llc 800-325-9044
449 Soverign Ct, St. Louis, MO 63011
Glove box holder.

Vacuum Atmospheres Co. 310-644-0255
4652 W Rosecrans Ave, Hawthorne, CA 90250

BOX, TRANSPORTATION, CONTAINER, SPECIMEN
(General) 80WYL

Medical Action Industries, Inc 800-645-7042
500 Express Dr S, Brentwood, NY 11717
Laboratory specimen transport bags. Separate pocket for paper work, resealable adhesive for specimen pocket.

Packaging Products Corp. 800-225-0484
198 Herman Melville Blvd, New Bedford, MA 02740
STANDALONE ARCTIC BOX molded foam insulated shippers.

Phoenix Metal Products, Inc. 516-546-4200
35 Hanse Ave, Freeport, NY 11520
Courier pick-up; non-transportation, container. Metal route collection box, available in floor or hanging models, are insulated, lockable, constructed of galvanized steel.

Sonoco 513-874-7655
4633 Dues Dr, Cincinnati, OH 45246
DRY ICE SHIPPER Affordable united nations class 9 certified dry ice containers for transport and mail of temprature sensitive class6.2 certified container for transport and mail of infectious substances and diagnostic specimens.

Tagg Industries L.L.C. 800-548-3514
23210 Del Lago Dr, Laguna Hills, CA 92653
Dual door lockboxes designed for 24-hour pick-up and delivery.

The Mason Box Company 800-225-2708
521 Mount Hope St, PO Box 129, North Attleboro, MA 02760
Reusable alleregy vial transport packaging. Soft foam cavities securely hold and protect glass vials during transit. Sturdy outer cardboard ensures against breakage.

BRACE, DRILL *(Orthopedics) 87HXY*

Biomet, Inc. 574-267-6639
56 E Bell Dr, PO Box 587, Warsaw, IN 46582
Various types of brace.

K2m, Inc. 866-526-4171
751 Miller Dr SE Ste F1, Leesburg, VA 20175
Drill guide.

Princeton Medical Group, Inc. 800-875-0869
1189 Royal Links Dr, Mt Pleasant, SC 29466

Small Bone Innovations, Inc. 215-428-1791
1380 S Pennsylvania Ave, Morrisville, PA 19067
Brace, drill.

Spine Smith Partners L.P. 512-206-0770
8140 N MO Pac Expy Bldg 120, Austin, TX 78759
Drill guide.

Warsaw Orthopedic, Inc. 901-396-3133
2500 Silveus Xing, Warsaw, IN 46582
Drill brace.

Zimmer Holdings, Inc. 800-613-6131
1800 W Center St, PO Box 708, Warsaw, IN 46580

Zimmer Trabecular Metal Technology 800-613-6131
10 Pomeroy Rd, Parsippany, NJ 07054
Drill guide.

BRACE, JOINT, ANKLE (EXTERNAL) *(Physical Med) 89ITW*

Active Ankle Systems, Inc. 812-258-0663
233 Quartermaster Ct, Jeffersonville, IN 47130
Active ankle brace.

Air A Med, Inc. 239-936-5590
2049 Beacon Manor Dr, Fort Myers, FL 33907
Joint, ankle, external brace.

Alimed, Inc. 800-225-2610
297 High St, Dedham, MA 02026

Allsport Dynamics, Inc. 800-594-5350
2724 SE Stallings Dr, Nacogdoches, TX 75961
Allsport ankle.

American Orthopedic Supply Co., Inc.
37017 State Highway 79, Cleveland, AL 35049
Ankle brace.

Anatomical Concepts, Inc. 800-837-3888
1399 E Western Reserve Rd, Poland, OH 44514
Pressure-relief ankle/foot orthosis.

Anodyne Therapy, Llc 813-645-2855
13570 Wright Cir, Tampa, FL 33626
External brace.

Bauerfeind Usa, Inc. 800-423-3405
55 Chastain Rd NW Ste 112, Kennesaw, GA 30144
MALLEOLOC ankle-joint stabilizer.

Becker Orthopedic Appliance Co. 248-588-7480
635 Executive Dr, Troy, MI 48083
Various ankle orthoses and orthosis components.

Benik Corp. 360-692-5601
11871 Silverdale Way NW Ste 107, Silverdale, WA 98383
Ankle support.

Biomet, Inc. 574-267-6639
56 E Bell Dr, PO Box 587, Warsaw, IN 46582
Various types of ankle braces.

Bird & Cronin, Inc. 651-683-1111
1200 Trapp Rd, Saint Paul, MN 55121
Ankle splint.

Breg, Inc., An Orthofix Company 800-897-BREG
2611 Commerce Way, Vista, CA 92081
Limb orthosis.

Brown Medical Industries 800-843-4395
1300 Lundberg Dr W, Spirit Lake, IA 51360
STEADY STEP PERFORM 8 lateral ankle stabilizer, available in four sizes.

Capstone Therapeutics 800-937-5520
1275 W Washington St, Tempe, AZ 85281
TALON ACL brace and SPORTLITE 2 step.

Cramer Products, Inc. 800-255-6621
153 W Warren St, Gardner, KS 66030
$15.20 per #75 padded ankle stabilizer.

Dalco International, Inc. 888-354-5515
8433 Glazebrook Ave, Richmond, VA 23228

Darco International, Inc. 800-999-8866
810 Memorial Blvd, Huntington, WV 25701
DARCOGEL.

Dj Orthopedics De Mexico, S.A. De C.V. 690-727-1280
Blvd., Delagacion La Presa, Tijuana 22397 Mexico
Ankle braces

Dj Orthopedics De Mexico, S.A. De C.V. 690-727-1280
Ave. Venustiano Carranza 6802, Castillo, Tijuana 22100 Mexico
Ankle braces

DJO Inc. 800-336-6569
1430 Decision St, Vista, CA 92081
Functional custom and off-the-shelf ankle braces. Post surgical/rehabilitation ankle brace.

Dynatronics Corp. Chattanooga Operations 801-568-7000
6607 Mountain View Rd, Ooltewah, TN 37363
Joint, ankle, external brace.

Elite Orthopaedics, Inc. 800-284-1688
1535 Santa Anita Ave, South El Monte, CA 91733

Evs Sports Protection 800-229-4EVS
2146 E Gladwick St, Rancho Dominguez, CA 90220

Frank Stubbs Co., Inc 800-223-1713
2100 Eastman Ave Ste B, Oxnard, CA 93030

BRACE, JOINT, ANKLE (EXTERNAL) *(cont'd)*

Freeman Manufacturing Company 800-253-2091
900 W Chicago Rd, PO Box J, Sturgis, MI 49091
Elastic, leather and neoprene braces.

Gillette Children's Specialty Healthcare 612-229-3805
200 University Ave E, Saint Paul, MN 55101
Multiple.

Health Ent., Inc. 508-695-0727
90 George Leven Dr, North Attleboro, MA 02760
Ankle brace.

Hosmer Dorrance Corp. 408-379-5151
561 Division St, Campbell, CA 95008
Various.

I.M.K. Distributors, Inc. 800-878-5552
19 W 34th St Rm 915, New York, NY 10001
Stabilcast patented ankle brace. A fully immobilizing and supporting ankle-sprain brace system with dual air patented chambers, bladders.

Ita-Med Co. 888-9IT-AMED
310 Littlefield Ave, South San Francisco, CA 94080
Designed to prevent and treat common ankle injuries.

J.T. Enterprises, Llc 800-452-0631
5729 Bowmiller Rd, Lockport, NY 14094
The strassburg sock.

Just Packaging Inc. 908-753-6700
450 Oak Tree Ave, South Plainfield, NJ 07080
Various types of ankle joint kits.

K-Fit Orthotics Llc 516-293-6400
1464 Old Country Rd, Plainview, NY 11803
Custom ankle brace.

Kenad Sg Medical, Inc. 800-825-0606
2692 Huntley Dr, Memphis, TN 38132
Ankle brace.

Kern Surgical Supply, Inc. 800-582-3939
2823 Gibson St, Bakersfield, CA 93308

Leeder Group, Inc. 305-436-5030
8508 NW 66th St, Miami, FL 33166
Foot splint.

Lohmann & Rauscher, Inc. 800-279-3863
6001 SW 6th Ave Ste 101, Topeka, KS 66615
Various types of ankle braces.

Maramed Orthopedic Systems 800-327-5830
2480 W 82nd St, No. 8, Hialeah, FL 33016

Medi Usa 800-633-6334
6481 Franz Warner Pkwy, Whitsett, NC 27377
Anatomically knitted supports with silicone inserts for treatment of ankle and Achilles tendon injuries.

Medical Industries Of America Llc. 203-254-8080
1735 Post Rd Ste 6, Fairfield, CT 06824
External fixation of a limb to support,prevent deformities (more).

Mizuho Osi 800-777-4674
30031 Ahern Ave, Union City, CA 94587

Neumed Inc. 800-367-1238
800 Silvia St, Ewing, NJ 08628
STIMPRENE Electrotherapy Braces support the back, knee, ankle, wrist, elbow and thigh which supply electrotherapy treatment from stimulation modalities such as TENS, NMES, and HVPC.

Orthotic & Prosthetic Lab, Inc. 314-968-8555
748 Marshall Ave, Webster Groves, MO 63119
O&p ankle foot orthosis.

Orthotics Choice Llc. 407-321-0454
451 E Airport Blvd, Sanford, FL 32773
Various types of ankle joint external braces/accessories.

Ossur Americas 949-268-3155
742 Pancho Rd, Camarillo, CA 93012

Otto Bock Healthcare, Lp 763-489-5106
9420 Delegates Dr Ste 100, Orlando, FL 32837
Various types of ankle joints/accessories.

Patterson Medical Supply, Inc. 262-387-8720
W68N158 Evergreen Blvd, Cedarburg, WI 53012
Sta-bil angle brace.

Pfs Med, Inc. 541-349-9646
3295 Cross St, Eugene, OR 97402
Pfs.

BRACE, JOINT, ANKLE (EXTERNAL) *(cont'd)*

Pine Tree Orthopedic Lab L.L.C. 207-524-2079
2120 Route 106, Leeds, ME 04263
Limb orthosis.

Primo, Inc. 770-486-7394
417 Dividend Dr Ste B, Peachtree City, GA 30269
Ankle brace or ankle support.

Pro Custom Labs 866-776-5227
190 Resolute Ln, Port Ludlow, WA 98365
Various types of below knee orthosis.

Pro Orthopedic Devices, Inc. 800-523-5611
2884 E Ganley Rd, Tucson, AZ 85706
PRO Neoprene rubber joint sleeves and supports.

Scott Orthotic Labs, Inc. 800-821-5795
1831 E Mulberry St, Fort Collins, CO 80524
Ankle foot orthotic.

Spinal Solutions, Inc. 770-922-2434
1971 Old Covington Rd NE Ste 103, Conyers, GA 30013
Carbon fiber ankle foot orthosis.

Star Medical Systems 800-626-3006
8301 Torresdale Ave Ste 13, Philadelphia, PA 19136

Surgical Appliance Industries 800-888-0458
3960 Rosslyn Dr, Cincinnati, OH 45209

Swede-O, Inc. 651-674-8301
6459 Ash St, North Branch, MN 55056
Various types of ankle braces.

Tamarack Habilitation Technologies, Inc. 763-795-0057
1670 94th Ln NE, Blaine, MN 55449
Flexure joint for ankle-foot-orthosis.

Tartan Orthopedics, Ltd. 888-287-1456
10651 Irma Dr Unit C, Northglenn, CO 80233
$20.00 per unit (med).

Therafirm, A Knit Rite Company 800-562-2701
120 Osage Ave, Kansas City, KS 66105
THERAFIRM Tubular knit, one piece, two-way stretch.

Tiburon Medical Enterprises 909-654-2333
915 Industrial Way, San Jacinto, CA 92582
Various.

Top Shelf Manufacturing, Llc 209-834-8185
1851 Paradise Rd Ste B, Tracy, CA 95304
Various types of ankle supports.

Unique Sports Products, Inc. 800-554-3707
840 McFarland Pkwy, Alpharetta, GA 30004
Ankle support.

Vq Orthocare
1390 Decision St Ste A, Vista, CA 92081
Limb orthosis.

Warsaw Orthopedic, Inc. 901-396-3133
2500 Silveus Xing, Warsaw, IN 46582
Various types of ankle splints and braces.

Zimmer Holdings, Inc. 800-613-6131
1800 W Center St, PO Box 708, Warsaw, IN 46580

BRACELET, IDENTIFICATION *(General) 80RBE*

Achilles Usa, Inc. 425-353-7000
1407 80th St SW, Everett, WA 98203
Development of vinyls and plastics for the medical industry.

Avondale Badge Co 800-874-2551
4114 Herschel St Ste 101, Jacksonville, FL 32210
Clincher armbands, temp cards, ID cards, equipment and supplies.

Bio-Logics Products, Inc. 800-426-7577
PO Box 505, West Jordan, UT 84084
Complete patient ID and specimen labeling systems ranging from blood bank to hospital-wide bar code systems.

Care Electronics, Inc. 303-444-2273
4700 Sterling Dr Ste D, Boulder, CO 80301
WANDERCARE electronic supervision system that alerts institutional staff of patients tending to wander off the premises or grounds. Long distance tracking is included. Home Care System notifies at-home care-giver and central monitoring facility of patients tending to wander from home. Long distance tracking is included.

Fenwal Inc. 800-766-1077
3 Corporate Dr, Lake Zurich, IL 60047
Blood. TYPENEX Blood-recipient.

BRACELET, IDENTIFICATION *(cont'd)*

Global Healthcare 800-601-3880
1495 Hembree Rd Ste 700, Roswell, GA 30076
Write-on and card insert types.

Health Enterprises 800-633-4243
90 George Leven Dr, North Attleboro, MA 02760
Necklaces, bracelets and wallet cards.

Instantel Inc. 800-267-9111
309 Legget Dr., Kanata, ON K2K 3A3 Canada
Wandering patient tracking device and monitoring equipment for healthcare facilities and home use, the latter includes a medical alert system. WATCHMATE is designed to protect residents long term care facilities who have a tendency to wander.

Levine Health Products 800-426-6763
21101 NE 108th St, Redmond, WA 98053
Medical Id Jewelry bracelets and necklaces stainless steel with raised symbols.

Medic Id's International 800-926-3342
PO Box 571687, Tarzana, CA 91357
Luxurious Medical Identification Bracelets and Pendants, in Goldtone $12.00 and up, Sterling Silver $25.00 - $300.00, Goldfilled $38.00 - $200.00 , 14k,18kt Soild Gold - $59.00 - $2000.00,

Nbs Technologies Inc. 800-524-0419
70 Eisenhower Dr, Paramus, NJ 07652
Embossing equipment, portable imprinter & non-impact printer (computer controlled). Also, patient card issuance systems.

O&M Enterprise 847-258-4515
641 Chelmsford Ln, Elk Grove Village, IL 60007
I.D. BAND PED/ADULT

Omnimed, Inc. (Beam Products) 800-257-2326
800 Glen Ave, Moorestown, NJ 08057

Precision Dynamics Corp. 800-772-1122
13880 Del Sur St, San Fernando, CA 91340
SECURLINE, SENTRY, SUPERBAND 43 styles, 16 colors, custom prints available, imprinter, insert and write on versions, plastic snap or adhesive closure.

Products International Co. 800-521-5123
2320 W Holly St, Phoenix, AZ 85009
TABBAND SHIELD, patient identification that accepts a pre-printed label, covers the label with a plastic shield, protecting label. TABBAND IMPRINT, patient identification for card imprinters or direct write-on. Available in colors. TABBAND STAT, patient identification bracelet for color coding and rapid identification in emergency rooms.

Secure Care Products, Inc. 800-451-7917
39 Chenell Dr, Concord, NH 03301
Waterproof ankle bracelet for disoriented patients alerting staff when patient passes through monitored exits.

BRACKET, CERAMIC, ORTHODONTIC *(Dental And Oral) 76NJM*

Classone Orthodontics, Inc. 806-799-0608
5064 50th St, Lubbock, TX 79414
Various types of ceramic brackets.

Ortho Organizers, Inc. 760-448-8730
1822 Aston Ave, Carlsbad, CA 92008
Various types of ceramic orthodontic brackets.

Orthodontic Design And Production, Inc. 760-734-3995
1370 Decision St Ste D, Vista, CA 92081
Orthodontic ceramic bracket.

BRACKET, METAL, ORTHODONTIC *(Dental And Oral) 76EJF*

Allodex Systems 561-477-3154
19940 Dinner Key Dr, Boca Raton, FL 33498
Pre-emergent tooth correction system.

American Orthodontics Corp. 800-558-7687
1714 Cambridge Ave, Sheboygan, WI 53081

Auradonics Incorporated 856-764-8866
439 Saint Mihiel Dr, Delran, NJ 08075
Brackets.

Cdb Corp. 910-383-6464
9201 Industrial Blvd NE, Leland, NC 28451
Ceramic dental brackets, stainless steel dental brackets.

Classone Orthodontics, Inc. 806-799-0608
5064 50th St, Lubbock, TX 79414
Metal bracket.

Dentlight Inc. 972-889-8857
1411 E Campbell Rd Ste 500, Richardson, TX 75081
Dental brackets.

BRACKET, METAL, ORTHODONTIC *(cont'd)*

Forestadent Usa 314-878-5985
2315 Weldon Pkwy, Saint Louis, MO 63146
Orthodontic metal bracket.

G & H Wire Co. 800-526-1026
2165 Earlywood Dr, Franklin, IN 46131

Glenroe Technologies 800-237-4060
1912 44th Ave E, Bradenton, FL 34203
Metal orthodontic braclet.

Gold'N Braces, Inc. 800-785-1970
2595 Tampa Rd Ste 1, Palm Harbor, FL 34684
Gold-plated orthodontic bracket.

Herbsthelp, Corp. 702-245-6958
2917 Linkview Dr, Las Vegas, NV 89134
Herbst appliance accessory, telescoping rod/tube actuating assembly.

Lancer Orthodontics, Inc. 760-304-2705
253 Pawnee St, San Marcos, CA 92078
Metal orthodontic bracket.

Lee Pharmaceuticals 626-442-3141
1434 Santa Anita Ave, El Monte, CA 91733
Orthodontic metal brackets and lingual buttons.

Ormco Corp. 800-672-5068
1332 S Lone Hill Ave, Glendora, CA 91740

Ortho Organizers, Inc. 760-448-8730
1822 Aston Ave, Carlsbad, CA 92008
Various.

Orthodontic Design And Production, Inc. 760-734-3995
1370 Decision St Ste D, Vista, CA 92081
Various types of metal orthodontic brackets.

Orthodontic Supply & Equipment Co., Inc. 800-638-4003
7851 Airpark Rd Ste 202, Gaithersburg, MD 20879

Oscar, Inc. 317-849-2618
11793 Technology Ln, Fishers, IN 46038
Orthodontic brackets.

Pyramid Orthodontics 800-752-8884
4328 Redwood Hwy Ste 100, San Rafael, CA 94903
PRESTIGE nickel free appliance. PRESTIGE nickel free dual-purpose for banding or bonding of molar teeth.

Strite Industries Ltd. 800-267-7333
298 Shepherd Ave., Cambridge, ON N3C 1V1 Canada
$4.55 per bracket.

Tp Orthodontics, Inc. 800-348-8856
100 Center Plz, La Porte, IN 46350
Advant-Edge, Straight-Edge, Tip-Edge PLUS, Twin-Edge, Nu-Edge.

Ultradent Products, Inc. 801-553-4586
505 W 10200 S, South Jordan, UT 84095
Orthodontic metal bracket.

World Class Technology Corporation 503-472-8320
1300 NE Alpha Dr, McMinnville, OR 97128
Bracket, metal, orthodontic.

3m Unitek 800-634-5300
2724 Peck Rd, Monrovia, CA 91016

BRACKET, PLASTIC, ORTHODONTIC *(Dental And Oral) 76DYW*

Align Technology, Inc. 408-470-1000
881 Martin Ave, Santa Clara, CA 95050
Bracket,plastic,orthodontic.

American Orthodontics Corp. 800-558-7687
1714 Cambridge Ave, Sheboygan, WI 53081

Cdb Corp. 910-383-6464
9201 Industrial Blvd NE, Leland, NC 28451
Polyure thane dental brackets.

G & H Wire Co. 800-526-1026
2165 Earlywood Dr, Franklin, IN 46131

Glenroe Technologies 800-237-4060
1912 44th Ave E, Bradenton, FL 34203
Orthodontic ceramic bracket.

Lar Mfg., Llc. 727-846-7860
6828 Commerce Ave, Port Richey, FL 34668
Various.

Lee Pharmaceuticals 626-442-3141
1434 Santa Anita Ave, El Monte, CA 91733
Plastic orthodontic brackets.

BRACKET, PLASTIC, ORTHODONTIC *(cont'd)*

Ortho Organizers, Inc. 760-448-8730
1822 Aston Ave, Carlsbad, CA 92008
Various types of plastic and composite brackets.

Pyramid Orthodontics 800-752-8884
4328 Redwood Hwy Ste 100, San Rafael, CA 94903
ICE and ICECUBE.

Stelrema Corp. 814-422-8892
4055 E 250 N, Knox, IN 46534
Orthodontic brackets.

Ultradent Products, Inc. 801-553-4586
505 W 10200 S, South Jordan, UT 84095
Plastic orthodontic bracket.

BRACKET, TABLE ASSEMBLY, N2O DELIVERY SYSTEM
(Dental And Oral) 76EBX

Midmark Corporation 800-643-6275
60 Vista Dr, P.O. Box 286, Versailles, OH 45380

BRAKE, EXTENSION, WHEELCHAIR *(Physical Med) 89IMW*

Alimed, Inc. 800-225-2610
297 High St, Dedham, MA 02026

Sunrise Medical Hhg Inc 303-218-4505
2842 N Business Park Ave, Fresno, CA 93727

Tuffcare 800-367-6160
3999 E La Palma Ave, Anaheim, CA 92807

BRASSIERE, MATERNITY *(Obstetrics/Gyn) 85UKV*

Airway Division Of Surgical Appliance Industries, Inc. 800-888-0458
3960 Rosslyn Dr, Cincinnati, OH 45209
MY TIME Maternity girdle.

Atd-American Co. 800-523-2300
135 Greenwood Ave, Wyncote, PA 19095

BRASSIERE, SURGICAL *(Surgery) 79QEI*

Allergan 800-624-4261
71 S Los Carneros Rd, Goleta, CA 93117
Post-operative brassiere.

Freeman Manufacturing Company 800-253-2091
900 W Chicago Rd, PO Box J, Sturgis, MI 49091
Mastectomy bras.

Ladies First, Inc. 800-497-8285
PO Box 4400, Salem, OR 97302
Post-mastectomy bras and garments

Truform Orthotics & Prosthetics 800-888-0458
3960 Rosslyn Dr, Cincinnati, OH 45209

BRILLIANT CRESYL BLUE *(Hematology) 81GHP*

Medical Chemical Corp. 800-424-9394
19430 Van Ness Ave, Torrance, CA 90501
$12.00 per 100mL.

Rocky Mountain Reagents,Inc. 303-762-0800
3207 W Hampden Ave, Englewood, CO 80110

BROACH *(Orthopedics) 87HTQ*

Biomet, Inc. 574-267-6639
56 E Bell Dr, PO Box 587, Warsaw, IN 46582
Various types of broachs.

Depuy Spine, Inc. 800-227-6633
325 Paramount Dr, Raynham, MA 02767
Various sizes of broaches.

Small Bone Innovations, Inc. 215-428-1791
1380 S Pennsylvania Ave, Morrisville, PA 19067
Broach.

Zimmer Holdings, Inc. 800-613-6131
1800 W Center St, PO Box 708, Warsaw, IN 46580

Zimmer Trabecular Metal Technology 800-613-6131
10 Pomeroy Rd, Parsippany, NJ 07054
Femoral stem broach.

BROACH, ENDODONTIC *(Dental And Oral) 76EKW*

Biolase Technology, Inc. 888-424-6527
4 Cromwell, Irvine, CA 92618

Biomet Microfixation Inc. 800-874-7711
1520 Tradeport Dr, Jacksonville, FL 32218
Curette, endodontic.

D&S Dental, Llc 423-928-1299
3111 Hanover Rd, Johnson City, TN 37604
Endodontic broach.

BROACH, ENDODONTIC *(cont'd)*

Js Dental Mfg., Inc. 800-284-3368
196 N Salem Rd, Ridgefield, CT 06877
Broach, barbed broach, nerve broach, rat-tail file.

Medidenta International, Inc. 800-221-0750
3923 62nd St, PO Box 409, Woodside, NY 11377

Miltex Dental Technologies, Inc. 516-576-6022
589 Davies Dr, York, PA 17402
Barbed broach.

Moyco Technologies, Inc. 800-331-8837
200 Commerce Dr, Montgomeryville, PA 18936
Endo files and broaches.

Pulpdent Corp. 800-343-4342
80 Oakland St, Watertown, MA 02472
No common name listed.

BRONCHOSCOPE, NON-RIGID *(Ear/Nose/Throat) 77BTN*

Asthmatx, Inc. 1-877-810-6060
888 Ross Dr Ste 100, Sunnyvale, CA 94089
Alair Bronchial Thermoplasty System

Karl Storz Endoscopy-America Inc. 800-421-0837
600 Corporate Pointe, Culver City, CA 90230
Fiberoptic bronchoscopes for white-light and autofluorescence (AF) bronchoscopy procedures; 2-way tip deflection.

Mahe International Inc. 800-294-7946
468 Craighead St, Nashville, TN 37204

Olympus America, Inc. 800-645-8160
3500 Corporate Pkwy, PO Box 610, Center Valley, PA 18034

Pentax Medical Company 800-431-5880
102 Chestnut Ridge Rd, Montvale, NJ 07645
$12,495.00 to $13,020.00 per unit for several fiberoptic models with various distal tip diameters (2.7 to 6.2mm) and channel sizes (1.2 to 3.2mm). $9,450.00 for several fiberoptic bronchoscopes with a portable battery powered light source with various distal tip diameters (4.8 to 5.9mm) and channel sizes (2.0 to 2.6mm). $22,470.00 to $22,575.00 per unit for video bronchoscopes with built-in CCD chip at distal tip. Four models available, with various distal tip diameters (5.3 to 6.3mm) and channel sizes (2.0 to 2.8mm). All models are fully immersible.

Richard Wolf Medical Instruments Corp. 800-323-9653
353 Corporate Woods Pkwy, Vernon Hills, IL 60061

Vision-Sciences, Inc. 800-874-9975
40 Ramland Rd S Ste 1, Orangeburg, NY 10962
Disposable protective cover for proprietary bronchoscopic system.

BRONCHOSCOPE, RIGID *(Ear/Nose/Throat) 77EOQ*

Asthmatx, Inc. 1-877-810-6060
888 Ross Dr Ste 100, Sunnyvale, CA 94089
Catheter.

Boehm Surgical Instrument Corp. 716-436-6584
966 Chili Ave, Rochester, NY 14611
Bronchoscope.

Bryan Corp. 800-343-7711
4 Plympton St, Woburn, MA 01801
Universal Rigid Bronchoscope System, available for adult and pediatric.

Electro Surgical Instrument Co., Inc. 888-464-2784
37 Centennial St, Rochester, NY 14611
Various types, styles and sizes of fiberoptic bronchoscopes.

Gyrus Ent L.L.C., Sub. Of Gyrus Acmi, Inc. 508-804-2739
2925 Appling Rd, Bartlett, TN 38133
Laryngoscopes.

Karl Storz Endoscopy-America Inc. 800-421-0837
600 Corporate Pointe, Culver City, CA 90230

Mahe International Inc. 800-294-7946
468 Craighead St, Nashville, TN 37204

Pentax Southern Region Service Center 201-571-2300
8934 Kirby Dr, Houston, TX 77054
Bronchoscope.

Pentax West Coast Service Center 800-431-5880
10410 Pioneer Blvd Ste 2, Santa Fe Springs, CA 90670
Pentax bronchoscope.

Richard Wolf Medical Instruments Corp. 800-323-9653
353 Corporate Woods Pkwy, Vernon Hills, IL 60061
Bronchoscopy CO2 laser system.

BRONCHOSCOPE, RIGID, NON-VENTILATING
(Anesthesiology) 73BTJ

Bryan Corp. 800-343-7711
4 Plympton St, Woburn, MA 01801
5 sizes available for use with basic Bryan-Dumon Bronchoscope system.

Karl Storz Endoscopy-America Inc. 800-421-0837
600 Corporate Pointe, Culver City, CA 90230

Richard Wolf Medical Instruments Corp. 800-323-9653
353 Corporate Woods Pkwy, Vernon Hills, IL 60061

BRONCHOSCOPE, RIGID, VENTILATING *(Anesthesiology) 73BTH*

Bryan Corp. 800-343-7711
4 Plympton St, Woburn, MA 01801
8 sizes available (including 3 pediatric) for use with basic Bryan-Dumon Bronchoscope system.

Karl Storz Endoscopy-America Inc. 800-421-0837
600 Corporate Pointe, Culver City, CA 90230
Rigid bronchoscope and laser bronchoscope with extra catheter channels, suction catheter, anesthesia connector etc.; also video bronchoscopes.

Mahe International Inc. 800-294-7946
468 Craighead St, Nashville, TN 37204

Richard Wolf Medical Instruments Corp. 800-323-9653
353 Corporate Woods Pkwy, Vernon Hills, IL 60061

BRUSH, BIOPSY, BRONCHOSCOPE (NON-RIGID)
(Anesthesiology) 73BTG

Cook Endoscopy 336-744-0157
4900 Bethania Station Rd # &, 5951 Grassy Creek Blvd. Winston Salem, NC 27105
Brush, biopsy, bronchoscope.

Olympus America, Inc. 800-645-8160
3500 Corporate Pkwy, PO Box 610, Center Valley, PA 18034

Sanderson-Macleod, Inc. 866-522-3481
1199 S Main St, P.O. Box 50, Palmer, MA 01069

BRUSH, BIOPSY, GENERAL & PLASTIC SURGERY
(Surgery) 79GEE

Medchannel Llc 617-314-9861
1241 Adams St Apt 110, Dorchester Center, MA 02124
Brush.

Medisiss 866-866-7477
2747 SW 6th St, Redmond, OR 97756
Various biopsy brushes,sterile.

Vilex, Inc. 931-474-7550
111 Moffitt St, McMinnville, TN 37110

BRUSH, BURR CLEANING *(Dental And Oral) 76QEO*

Comco, Inc. 800-796-6626
2151 N Lincoln St, Burbank, CA 91504
Micro-abrasive blasting equipment for dental lab applications including devesting, surface preparation, removal of oxides, selective texturing, and shaping tooth anatomy.

Key Surgical, Inc. 800-541-7995
8101 Wallace Rd Ste 100, Eden Prairie, MN 55344

Sanderson-Macleod, Inc. 866-522-3481
1199 S Main St, P.O. Box 50, Palmer, MA 01069

BRUSH, CENTRIFUGE *(Hematology) 81WIT*

Justman Brush Co. 800-800-6940
828 Crown Point Ave, Omaha, NE 68110

BRUSH, CLEANING, TRACHEAL TUBE *(Ear/Nose/Throat) 77EPE*

Centurion Medical Products Corp. 517-545-1135
3310 S Main St, Salisbury, NC 28147

Datex-Ohmeda (Canada) 800-268-1472
1093 Meyerside Dr., Unit 2, Mississauga, ONT L5T-1J6 Canada

Gyrus Acmi, Inc. 508-804-2739
93 N Pleasant St, Norwalk, OH 44857
Various types of cleaning brushes.

Justman Brush Co. 800-800-6940
828 Crown Point Ave, Omaha, NE 68110
Test tube cleaning brush.

Kelsar, S.A. 508-261-8000
Blvd. Insurgentes, Libriamento a La, Tijuana 22450 Mexico
Tracheostomy care set

Medical Action Industries, Inc. 800-645-7042
25 Heywood Rd, Arden, NC 28704
Brush.

BRUSH, CLEANING, TRACHEAL TUBE *(cont'd)*

Sanderson-Macleod, Inc. 866-522-3481
1199 S Main St, P.O. Box 50, Palmer, MA 01069

Tri-State Hospital Supply Corp. 517-545-1135
3173 E 43rd St, Yuma, AZ 85365

BRUSH, CYTOLOGY *(General) 80WKZ*

American Catheter Corp. 800-345-6714
13047 S Highway 475, Ocala, FL 34480

Birchwood Laboratories, Inc. 800-328-6156
7900 Fuller Rd, Eden Prairie, MN 55344
CYTETTE, Endocervical cytology brush.

Directmed, Inc. 516-656-3377
150 Pratt Oval, Glen Cove, NY 11542

Globe Scientific, Inc. 800-394-4562
610 Winters Ave, Paramus, NJ 07652
ENDO-BRUSH for collecting endocervical cells from the endocervical canal.

Medical Packaging Corporation 800-792-0600
941 Avenida Acaso, Camarillo, CA 93012
Cytology brush for cellular collection, sterile or non-sterile.

Puritan Medical Products Company Llc 800-321-2313
31 School St., Guilford, ME 04443-0149
CERVISOFT alternative cytology brush is made of non-abrasive foam securely bonded to a 7-inch long plastic shaft. Foam construction makes it gentler than the traditional cytology brush.

Rocket Medical Plc. 800-707-7625
150 Recreation Park Dr Ste 3, Hingham, MA 02043

Solon Manufacturing Co. 800-341-6640
338 Madison Ave Ste 7, Skowhegan, ME 04976
8-in. non-sterile or sterile brush with soft nylon bristles secured by surgical stainless steel. Made in the USA.

Statlab Medical Products, Inc. 800-442-3573
106 Hillside Dr, Lewisville, TX 75057
ANAPATH for endocervical cell collection, hex handle, U.S. made.

Telemed Systems Inc. 800-481-6718
8 Kane Industrial Dr, Hudson, MA 01749
Bronchial.

BRUSH, CYTOLOGY, ENDOSCOPIC *(Gastro/Urology) 78FDX*

Annex Medical, Inc. 952-942-7576
6018 Blue Circle Dr, Minnetonka, MN 55343
3.0 Fr. or smaller biopsy brush with metal bristles.

Cook Endoscopy 336-744-0157
4900 Bethania Station Rd # &, 5951 Grassy Creek Blvd. Winston Salem, NC 27105
Brush, cytology, endoscopic.

Cook Urological, Inc. 800-457-4500
1100 W Morgan St, P.O. Box 227, Spencer, IN 47460

Gyrus Acmi, Inc. 508-804-2739
93 N Pleasant St, Norwalk, OH 44857
Various sizes and kinds of endoscope cytology brushes.

Gyrus Acmi, Inc. 508-804-2739
300 Stillwater P.o.box 1971, Stamford, CT 06902
Various sizes and kinds of endoscope cytology brushes.

Hobbs Medical, Inc. 860-684-5875
8 Spring St, Stafford Springs, CT 06076
Sheath brush.

Karl Storz Endoscopy-America Inc. 800-421-0837
600 Corporate Pointe, Culver City, CA 90230

Olympus America, Inc. 800-645-8160
3500 Corporate Pkwy, PO Box 610, Center Valley, PA 18034

Omni Medical Supply Inc. 800-860-6664
4153 Pioneer Dr, Commerce Township, MI 48390
Disposable endoscope cleaning brush 1.7 mm diameter with 230 cm length.

Richard Wolf Medical Instruments Corp. 800-323-9653
353 Corporate Woods Pkwy, Vernon Hills, IL 60061

Sanderson-Macleod, Inc. 866-522-3481
1199 S Main St, P.O. Box 50, Palmer, MA 01069

United States Endoscopy Group 800-769-8226
5976 Heisley Rd, Mentor, OH 44060
HARVEST BRUSH, Disposable cytology brushes for flexible endoscopes.

BRUSH, DENTAL PLATE (DENTURE) *(Dental And Oral) 76QEP*

Almore International, Inc. 503-643-6633
PO Box 25214, Portland, OR 97298
Washout brush and cleaning pic. $4.95/each.

BRUSH, DERMABRASION *(Surgery) 79GFE*

Advanced Dermal Systems Llc 847-451-0145
9109 Medill Ave, Franklin Park, IL 60131
Microdermabrasion machine.

Advanced Microderm, Inc. 630-980-3300
904 S Roselle Rd # 302, Schaumburg, IL 60193
Micro dermabrasion machine.

Apex Medical Corp. 903-314-1217
6406 Prestige Ln, Texarkana, TX 75503
Microdermabrasion machine.

Bella Products, Inc. 877-550-5655
27136 Burbank, Foothill Ranch, CA 92610
Various.

Dermasweep, Inc. 916-772-9134
7251 Galilee Rd Ste 160, Roseville, CA 95678

Dermatec Industries, Llc 765-427-0092
970 Cape Marco Dr Apt 405, Marco Island, FL 34145
Various types of dermabrasion systems.

Dms 410-757-8400
530 College Pkwy Ste D, Annapolis, MD 21409
Dermoabrader. Also available is the Dermocell skin-toner device. New products include the Dermocell body toner, a skin toner device.

Dusouth Industries 707-745-5117
651 Stone Rd, Benicia, CA 94510
Microdermabrasion.

Edge Systems Corporation 800-603-4996
2277 Redondo Ave, Signal Hill, CA 90755
Microdermabrasion systems & HydraFacial skin resurfacing system.

Imagederm, Inc. 818-500-9034
3032 Dolores St, Los Angeles, CA 90065
Micro-derma brasion machine.

International Business Solutions, Inc. 901-861-7144
350 Poplar View Pkwy, Collierville, TN 38017
International business solutions, inc.

Lifeline Medical, Inc. 800-452-4566
22 Shelter Rock Ln, Danbury, CT 06810
Microdermabrasion.

Mednet Locator, Inc. 800-754-5070
7000 Shadow Oaks Dr, Memphis, TN 38125
Hydroxylapetite (ha) trimmer.

Mei Beauty Products, Inc. 909-861-7575
1971 W Holt Ave, Pomona, CA 91768
Microdermabrasion machine.

P-Ryton Corp. 800-221-9840
504 50th Ave, Long Island City, NY 11101

Pretika Corporation, North America Market Headquarters 949-481-8818
16 Salermo, Laguna Niguel, CA 92677
Dermabrasion device.

Skinscience Labs, Inc. 212-265-4600
330 W 58th St Ste 211, New York, NY 10019
Microdermabrader.

Vibraderm, Inc. 301-279-2899
2100 N Highway 360 Ste 1502, Grand Prairie, TX 75050
Dermabrasion device.

BRUSH, DERMABRASION, MANUAL *(Surgery) 79GED*

Cardinal Health, Snowden Pencer Products 847-689-8410
5175 S Royal Atlanta Dr, Tucker, GA 30084
Manual surgical instrument for general use.

United States Pumice Co. 818-882-0300
20219 Bahama St, Chatsworth, CA 91311
Footstone.

BRUSH, ENDOMETRIAL *(Obstetrics/Gyn) 85HFE*

Berkeley Medevices, Inc. 800-227-2388
1330 S 51st St, Richmond, CA 94804
Cytosmear cytology brush.

Rms Medical Products 800-624-9600
24 Carpenter Rd, Chester, NY 10918

BRUSH, OPHTHALMIC *(Ophthalmology) 86QEQ*

Alger Equipment Company, Inc. 800-320-1043
320 Flightline Rd, Lago Vista, TX 78645
Algerbrush II, for Corneal Rust Ring Removal and assistance on Pterygiectomies

BRUSH, OTHER *(General) 80WVO*

Adi Medical Division Of Asia Dynamics (Group) Inc. 877-647-7699
1565 S Shields Dr, Waukegan, IL 60085

Amson Products 718-435-3728
1401 42nd St, Brooklyn, NY 11219
Hairbrushes and combs.

Case Medical, Inc. 888-227-2273
65 Railroad Ave, Ridgefield, NJ 07657
for cleaning micro, general, and endoscopic instruments

Centrix, Inc. 800-235-5862
770 River Rd, Shelton, CT 06484
Disposable brushes.

Cytogen Corp. 800-833-3533
600 College Rd E Ste 3100, Princeton, NJ 08540
QUADRAMET is a radio pharmaceutral preparation to treat bone pain associated with cancers thta have spreed to the bone. Relief of pain in patients with confirmed osteoblastic metastatic bone lesions tht enhance on radionuclide bone scan.

Damas Corp. 609-695-9121
1977 N Olden Avenue Ext Ste 289, Ewing, NJ 08618
Ethylene oxide gas scrubbers.

Healthmark Industries 800-521-6224
22522 E 9 Mile Rd, Saint Clair Shores, MI 48080
FLEXISTEM Instrument Cleaners, brush-like cleaners for cleaning surgical instruments.

Hygolet Usa 800-494-6538
349 SE 2nd Ave, Deerfield Beach, FL 33441
ASTRO BRUSH Toilet brush set mounts to the wall for easy cleaning of restroom floors. Brush has a refillable head.

Justman Brush Co. 800-800-6940
828 Crown Point Ave, Omaha, NE 68110
Various cleaning brushes for surgical instruments.

K W Griffen Company 800-424-5556
100 Pearl St, Norwalk, CT 06850
Disposable scrub.

Key Surgical, Inc. 800-541-7995
8101 Wallace Rd Ste 100, Eden Prairie, MN 55344
Assorted brushes for cleaning instruments and sterilizers.

Milex Products, Inc. 800-621-1278
4311 N Normandy Ave, Chicago, IL 60634
Endocervical brushes. Sterile. (50/bag), $0.30 to $0.44 each. Nonsterile $0.15 to $0.35

Miltex Inc. 800-645-8000
589 Davies Dr, York, PA 17402
Surgical instrument cleaning brushes.

Moyco Technologies, Inc. 800-331-8837
200 Commerce Dr, Montgomeryville, PA 18936
Steel wire scratch brushes bound in plastic handle for cleaning endodontic instruments and burs.

New World Imports 800-329-1903
160 Athens Way, Nashville, TN 37228
Hairbrushes for adults and children, 7 and 5 in. combs, Mini Pik handle combs and dresser combs.

O&M Enterprise 847-258-4515
641 Chelmsford Ln, Elk Grove Village, IL 60007
BRUSH - CYTOLOGY/HAIR/NAIL/TOOTH

Omni Medical Supply Inc. 800-860-6664
4153 Pioneer Dr, Commerce Township, MI 48390

Puritan Medical Products Company Llc 800-321-2313
31 School St., Guilford, ME 04443-0149
HISTOBRUSH for the collection of specimens from the endocervical region of the body.

Sanderson-Macleod, Inc. 866-522-3481
1199 S Main St, P.O. Box 50, Palmer, MA 01069
Pap smear and instrument cleaning brushes.

Sharn, Inc. 800-325-3671
4517 George Rd Ste 200, Tampa, FL 33634
SHARN, full line of brushes for cleaning virtually all devices from scopes to instruments to sterilizers. Featuring brushes for cleaning LMA(s).

BRUSH, OTHER *(cont'd)*

Wisap America 800-233-8448
8231 Melrose Dr, Lenexa, KS 66214
Brushes and Laparoscopic Brushes.

Young Innovations, Inc. 800-325-1881
13705 Shoreline Ct E, Earth City, MO 63045
Prophy brush.

BRUSH, SCRUB, OPERATING ROOM *(Surgery) 79GEC*

Ac Healthcare Supply, Inc. 905-448-4706
11651 230th St, Cambria Heights, NY 11411
Scrub brush.

Alimed, Inc. 800-225-2610
297 High St, Dedham, MA 02026

Ballard Medical Products 770-587-7835
12050 Lone Peak Pkwy, Draper, UT 84020
Scrub brush.

Covidien Lp 508-261-8000
15 Hampshire St, Mansfield, MA 02048

Gift Sales Co. 316-267-0671
517 S Saint Francis St, Wichita, KS 67202
Gsc soft scrub brush.

Ivry 305-448-9858
216 Catalonia Ave Ste 106, Coral Gables, FL 33134
Sponge and bristle (sterile).

K. W. Griffen Co. 203-846-1923
100 Pearl St, Norwalk, CT 06850
Dry sterile scrub brush.

Lampac International Ltd. 636-797-3659
230 N Lake Dr, Hillsboro, MO 63050
Brush, scrub, operating room. Scrub brush-sponge with nail pick, either dry sterile or impregnated with PVI, PCMX or CHG wet packs.

Lsl Industries, Inc. 888-225-5575
5535 N Wolcott Ave, Chicago, IL 60640
Various configurations - Mostly Price ranging from $50 to $75 for 20 scrub trays

Nbm Llc 502-895-7503
2604 River Green Cir, Louisville, KY 40206
Scrub brush-sponge, dry or chg or pcmx or pvp.

Purdue Frederick Company 800-877-5666
1 Stamford Forum, Stamford, CT 06901
Betadine Surgical Scrub.

Small Bone Innovations, Inc. 215-428-1791
1380 S Pennsylvania Ave, Morrisville, PA 19067
Brush.

Sunstar Butler 800-J BUTLER
4635 W Foster Ave, Chicago, IL 60630

Team Technologies, Inc. 423-587-2199
5949 Commerce Blvd, Morristown, TN 37814
Surgical scrub brush.

Vygon Corp. 800-544-4907
2495 General Armistead Ave, Norristown, PA 19403

BUFFER, PH *(Hematology) 81JCC*

Beckman Coulter, Inc. 800-742-2345
250 S Kraemer Blvd, PO Box 8000, Brea, CA 92821

Bio-Scientific Specialty Products, Inc. 516-868-2553
197 N Main St # 99, P.o. Box 521, Freeport, NY 11520
Giordano buffer ph 6.4.

Bionostics, Inc. 978-772-7070
7 Jackson Rd, Devens, MA 01434
Precisions buffers for blood gas analyzers.

Biotecx Laboratories, Inc. 800-535-6286
15225 Gulf Hwy, #F106, Houston, TX 77034
Hybridization buffer.

Caledon Laboratories Ltd. 877-cal-edon
40 Armstrong Ave., Georgetown, ONT L7G 4R9 Canada

Diagnostic Biosystems 925-484-3350
1020 Serpentine Ln Ste 114, Pleasanton, CA 94566

Ease Labs, Inc. 650-872-7788
338 N Canal St Ste 9, South San Francisco, CA 94080
Blocking buffer.

Helena Laboratories 409-842-3714
PO Box 752, Beaumont, TX 77704
Citrate, Electa B1, Electra HR, Owen's Veronal, sodium acetate, SupreHeme, Tris-Triscine, Titan Gel High Res.

BUFFER, PH *(cont'd)*

Labchem, Inc. 412-826-5230
200 William Pitt Way, Pittsburgh, PA 15238
Buffer solution, giordano (lc12590).

Mg Scientific, Inc. 800-343-8338
8500 107th St, Pleasant Prairie, WI 53158

Motloid Company 800-662-5021
300 N Elizabeth St, Chicago, IL 60607
DUAL LUSTRE & MOLDENT Buffing compounds.

Nerl Diagnostics Llc. 401-824-2046
14 Almeida Ave, East Providence, RI 02914
Ph buffer.

Orion Research, Inc. 800-225-1480
166 Cummings Ctr, Beverly, MA 01915
ORION $9.50 per 475ml bottle.

Pochemco, Inc. 413-536-2900
724 Main St, Holyoke, MA 01040
Ph buffer.

Richard-Allan Scientific 269-544-5628
4481 Campus Dr, Kalamazoo, MI 49008
Ph buffer.

Scytek Laboratories, Inc. 435-755-9848
205 S 600 W, Logan, UT 84321
Ph buffer.

Tripath Imaging, Inc. 919-206-7140
780 Plantation Dr, Burlington, NC 27215
Buffer solution.

Ventana Medical Systems, Inc. 800-227-2155
1910 E Innovation Park Dr, Oro Valley, AZ 85755
Various ph buffers.

Volu-Sol, Inc. 801-974-9474
2100 South 5095 West, Salt Lake City, UT 84121

BUILDING MATERIAL *(General) 80VAS*

Clean Air Technology, Inc. 800 459 6320
41105 Capital Dr, Canton, MI 48187
Cleanroom Modular wall panels and load bearing air return wall and srtructural top teck systems and cleanroom ceilings, sealed cleanroon lights and HEPA filters.

Sloan Valve Co. 800-9VA-LVE9
10500 Seymour Ave, Franklin Park, IL 60131
Flush valves, shower heads, electronic faucets, hand dryers.

BULB, INFLATION *(General) 80WRS*

American Diagnostic Corporation (Adc) 800-232-2670
55 Commerce Dr, Hauppauge, NY 11788

Carolina Biological Supply Co. 800-334-5551
2700 York Rd, Burlington, NC 27215

Schueler & Company, Inc. 516-487-1500
PO Box 528, Stratford, CT 06615

Trimline Medical Products Corp. 800-526-3538
34 Columbia Rd, Branchburg, NJ 08876
Available in regular and extra large sizes, all latex-free.

BULB, INFLATION (ENDOSCOPE) *(Gastro/Urology) 78FCY*

Richard Wolf Medical Instruments Corp. 800-323-9653
353 Corporate Woods Pkwy, Vernon Hills, IL 60061

Tools For Surgery, Llc 631-444-4448
1339 Stony Brook Rd, Stony Brook, NY 11790
Anastomotic leak tester.

BUMPER GUARD, CORNER *(General) 80TBM*

Children's Medical Ventures, Inc. 800-345-6443
191 Wyngate Dr, Monroeville, PA 15146

Construction Specialties Inc. 800-233-8493
6696 Route. 405, Muncy, PA 17756
Wall guards for corners and bumper.

Hamilton Caster & Mfg. Co. 888-699-7164
1637 Dixie Hwy, Hamilton, OH 45011
Protective bumpers for hand carts, etc.

Independent Solutions, Inc. 847-498-0500
900 Skokie Blvd Ste 118, Northbrook, IL 60062
Aluminum, vinyl or stainless steel. Surface or flush wall mounted. Boston Bumper and Sani Rail.

Iron Duck, A Div. Of Fleming Industries, Inc. 800-669-6900
20 Veterans Dr, Chicopee, MA 01022

BUMPER GUARD, CORNER *(cont'd)*

Pawling Corp., Architectural Prod. Div. 800-431-3456
32 Nelson Hill Rd, PO Box 200, Wassaic, NY 12592
Complete line of impact protection for walls, corners and doors. Handrails that meet ADA requirements. Sixty standard colors, plus custom colors and wood finishes. Thousands of combinations available to protect all areas, from the basement to the lobby to the parking garage.

R.C.A. Rubber Company, The 800-321-2340
1833 E Market St, P.O. Box 9240, Akron, OH 44305

BUR, DIAMOND COATED, REPROCESSED
(Dental And Oral) 76NME

Ascent Healthcare Solutions 480-763-5300
10232 S 51st St, Phoenix, AZ 85044
Dental burs and blades, reprocessed.

BUR, ENT, DIAMOND COATED, SINGLE USE, REPROCESSED
(Ear/Nose/Throat) 77NLZ

Ascent Healthcare Solutions 480-763-5300
10232 S 51st St, Phoenix, AZ 85044
Ent bur, reprocessed.

BURET *(Chemistry) 75QET*

Analyticon Instruments Corp. 973-379-6771
99 Morris Ave, P.O. Box 92, Springfield, NJ 07081

Brinkmann Instruments (Canada) Ltd. 800-263-8715
6670 Campobello Rd., Mississauga, ONT L5N 2L8 Canada
Automatic burets with digital readout and microprocessor control of the motor-driven piston.

Brinkmann Instruments, Inc. 800-645-3050
PO Box 1019, Westbury, NY 11590

Carolina Biological Supply Co. 800-334-5551
2700 York Rd, Burlington, NC 27215

Corning Inc., Science Products Division 800-492-1110
45 Nagog Park, Acton, MA 01720

Kimble Glass, Inc. 888-546-2531
537 Crystal Ave, Vineland, NJ 08360
KIMAX.

Kontes Glass Co. 888-546-2531
1022 Spruce St, Vineland, NJ 08360

Lamotte Co. 800-344-3100
802 Washington Ave, PO Box 329, Chestertown, MD 21620

Mg Scientific, Inc. 800-343-8338
8500 107th St, Pleasant Prairie, WI 53158

Nalge Nunc International 800-625-4327
75 Panorama Creek Dr, Rochester, NY 14625
NALGENE transparent, break-resistant acrylic burets. Self-zeroing burets available. Sizes from 10 to 10ml.

Tudor Scientific Glass Co., Inc. 800-336-4666
555 Edgefield Rd, Belvedere, SC 29841

BURNER *(Chemistry) 75UFM*

Bethlehem Apparatus Co., Inc. 610-838-7034
890 Front St, Hellertown, PA 18055

Gilson Company, Inc. 800-444-1508
PO Box 200, Lewis Center, OH 43035

Mg Scientific, Inc. 800-343-8338
8500 107th St, Pleasant Prairie, WI 53158

Wall Lenk Corp. 252-527-4186
PO Box 3349, Kinston, NC 28502
Portable lab burner with replaceable butane fuel container.

BURNISHER, OPERATIVE, DENTAL *(Dental And Oral) 76EKJ*

Dental Usa, Inc. 815-363-8003
5005 McCullom Lake Rd, McHenry, IL 60050
Various types of burnishers.

Hu-Friedy Manufacturing Co., Inc. 800-483-7433
3232 N Rockwell St, Chicago, IL 60618
$21.00 to $26.45 each, 11 types.

Micro-Dent Inc. 866-526-1166
379 Hollow Hill Rd, Wauconda, IL 60084
Burnisher.

Motloid Company 800-662-5021
300 N Elizabeth St, Chicago, IL 60607
CHROMETAL #2 & CHROMETAL #1 Burnishing agents.

Nordent Manufacturing, Inc. 800-966-7336
610 Bonnie Ln, Elk Grove Village, IL 60007
$15.75 per unit (standard).

BURNISHER, OPERATIVE, DENTAL *(cont'd)*

Pac-Dent Intl., Inc. 909-839-0888
21078 Commerce Point Dr, Walnut, CA 91789
Various types of burnisher.

Premier Dental Products Co. 888-670-6100
1710 Romano Dr, PO Box 4500, Plymouth Meeting, PA 19462

Sci-Dent, Inc. 800-323-4145
210 Dowdle St Ste 2, Algonquin, IL 60102

Suter Dental Manufacturing Company, Inc. 800-368-8376
632 Cedar St, Chico, CA 95928

Ultradent Products, Inc. 801-553-4586
505 W 10200 S, South Jordan, UT 84095
Syringe covers.

Wykle Research, Inc. 775-887-7500
2222 College Pkwy, Carson City, NV 89706
Operative burnisher.

BURR *(Ear/Nose/Throat) 77EQJ*

Acumed Instruments Corp. 800-234-5045
5286 Evanwood Ave, Oak Park, CA 91377

American Medical Specialties, Inc. 800-808-2877
10650 77th St., Suite 405, Largo, FL 33777
Quality and value in cutting tools for powered surgical equipment of Zimmer, Stryker, 3M, Midas Rex and others.

Biomet Microfixation Inc. 800-874-7711
1520 Tradeport Dr, Jacksonville, FL 32218
Various types of burrs.

Brasseler Usa - Medical 805-650-5209
4837 McGrath St Ste J, Ventura, CA 93003
Sterile bur.

Gyrus Ent L.L.C., Sub. Of Gyrus Acmi, Inc. 508-804-2739
2925 Appling Rd, Bartlett, TN 38133
Various.

Lasco Diamond Products 800-621-4726
PO Box 4657, 9950 Canoga Avenue, Unit A-8, Chatsworth, CA 91313
Diamond Coated Burrs

Medtronic Powered Surgical Solutions 800-643-2773
4620 N Beach St, Haltom City, TX 76137
Various models of sterile & non sterile burs.

Micromedics 800-624-5662
1270 Eagan Industrial Rd, Saint Paul, MN 55121
Amorphous diamond coated burs

Motloid Company 800-662-5021
300 N Elizabeth St, Chicago, IL 60607
Carbide lab and fissure burs; also tungsten steel.

Sim Medical Sales 574-268-0341
PO Box 895, Warsaw, IN 46581
Sterile packed burrs.

Tava Surgical Instruments 805-650-5209
4837 McGrath St Ste J, Ventura, CA 93003
Sterile bur.

Warsaw Orthopedic, Inc. 901-396-3133
2500 Silveus Xing, Warsaw, IN 46582
Bur.

Wecom, Inc. 800-628-4115
20 Warrick Ave, Glassboro, NJ 08028
Holder, dental bur, aluminum.

BURR, CORNEAL, AC-POWERED *(Ophthalmology) 86HQS*

Optimal Healthcare Products 800-364-8574
11444 W Olympic Blvd Ste 900, Los Angeles, CA 90064
For the eyes.

BURR, CORNEAL, BATTERY-POWERED *(Ophthalmology) 86HOG*

Bovie Medical Corp. 800-537-2790
5115 Ulmerton Rd, Clearwater, FL 33760
Replacement burr, ten per box.

Eagle Vision, Inc. 800-222-7584
8500 Wolf Lake Dr Ste 110, Memphis, TN 38133
Corneal rust ring remover.

Fortrad Eye Instruments Corp. 973-543-2371
8 Franklin Rd, Mendham, NJ 07945

Innovative Excimer Solutions, Inc. 416-410-1868
3340a Yonge St, Toronto M4N 2M4 Canada
Epithelial scrubber

BURR, CORNEAL, BATTERY-POWERED *(cont'd)*

Western Ophthalmics Corporation 800-426-9938
19019 36th Ave W Ste G, Lynnwood, WA 98036
Alger Brush, OrthoBurr, and Aaron Burr

BURR, CORNEAL, MANUAL *(Ophthalmology) 86HOF*

Bausch & Lomb Surgical 636-255-5051
3365 Tree Court Ind Blvd, Saint Louis, MO 63122

Bovie Medical Corp. 800-537-2790
5115 Ulmerton Rd, Clearwater, FL 33760

Fortrad Eye Instruments Corp. 973-543-2371
8 Franklin Rd, Mendham, NJ 07945

Katena Products, Inc. 800-225-1195
4 Stewart Ct, Denville, NJ 07834

BURR, CRANIAL *(Cns/Neurology) 84QEV*

American Medical Specialties, Inc. 800-808-2877
10650 77th St., Suite 405, Largo, FL 33777
Quality value in replacement cutting tools for powered surgical equipment of Aesculap, Codman, Zimmer, Stryker and others.

Brasseler Usa - Komet Medical 800-535-6638
1 Brasseler Blvd, Savannah, GA 31419
Tapered and wire pass drills.

Codman & Shurtleff, Inc 800-225-0460
325 Paramount Dr, Raynham, MA 02767

Sim Medical Sales 574-268-0341
PO Box 895, Warsaw, IN 46581

BURR, DENTAL *(Dental And Oral) 76EJL*

Aesculap Implant Systems Inc. 1-800-234-9179
3773 Corporate Pkwy, Center Valley, PA 18034

Align Technology, Inc. 408-470-1000
881 Martin Ave, Santa Clara, CA 95050
Bur,dental.

Arnel Healthcare, Inc. 516-783-1939
1523 Dewey Ave, North Bellmore, NY 11710
Diamond burs.

Arnold Tuber Industries 716-648-3363
97 Main St, Hamburg, NY 14075
Dental burs.

Blue Sky Bio, Llc 847-548-8499
888 E Belvidere Rd Ste 212, Grayslake, IL 60030
Bur, dental.

Brasseler Usa - Komet Medical 800-535-6638
1 Brasseler Blvd, Savannah, GA 31419

Brasseler Usa - Medical 805-650-5209
4837 McGrath St Ste J, Ventura, CA 93003
Dental bur.

Buffalo Dental Mfg. Co., Inc. 516-496-7200
159 Lafayette Dr, Syosset, NY 11791
Dental bur.

Calibur Dental Technologies, Inc. 905-833-5122
2189 King Rd, Po Box 520, King City L7B 1A7 Canada
Calibur

Coltene/Whaledent Inc. 330-916-8858
235 Ascot Pkwy, Cuyahoga Falls, OH 44223
Dental bur.

Cutting Edge Instruments Inc. 330-916-8858
312 River Rd., Bridgewater Corners, VT 05035
Dental bur.

Dedeco Intl., Inc. 845-887-4840
11617 Route 97, Long Eddy, NY 12760
Various types of burs.

Dentalez Group 866-DTE-INFO
101 Lindenwood Dr Ste 225, Valleybrooke Corporate Center
Malvern, PA 19355

Dentalez Group, Stardental Division 717-291-1161
1816 Colonial Village Ln, Lancaster, PA 17601
Carbide bur.

Ditec Mfg. 800-332-7083
1019 Mark Ave, Carpinteria, CA 93013
Diamond-plated.

G & H Wire Co. 800-526-1026
2165 Earlywood Dr, Franklin, IN 46131

Grobet File Co. 800-847-4188
1912 Whitney Rd, Cheyenne, WY 82007
Dental burr.

BURR, DENTAL *(cont'd)*

H & H Co. 909-390-0373
4435 E Airport Dr Ste 108, Ontario, CA 91761
Dental bur, all types.

Hager Worldwide, Inc. 800-328-2335
13322 Byrd Dr, Odessa, FL 33556
INTER COOL (implantology).

Havel's Inc. 800-638-4770
3726 Lonsdale St, Cincinnati, OH 45227

Hu-Friedy Manufacturing Co., Inc. 800-483-7433
3232 N Rockwell St, Chicago, IL 60618
$18.50 to $66.60, 16 types.

Impladent Ltd. 800-526-9343
19845 Foothill Ave, Hollis, NY 11423
76EJC Profiler Class I. The Profiler is a universal, time saving, rotary instrument which can be used with many implant systems in your contra-angle, designed to accomplish 6 functions. It serves as a Crestal Reduction Rotary Instrument, Osteotomy Locator, Osteotomy Lateral Redirector, Osteotomy Drill, Countersink, and an Osteocompressive Rotary Osteotome.

Lasco Diamond Products 800-621-4726
PO Box 4657, 9950 Canoga Avenue, Unit A-8, Chatsworth, CA 91313
Diamond FG, Surgical, and Laboratory Burrs; Specialty burrs for Porcelain Veneers, Rotary Gingival Curettage, Micron Finishing Diamonds, Depth Cutters, and more.

Menlo Tool Co., Inc. 810-756-6010
22760 Dequindre Rd, Warren, MI 48091

Miltex Dental Technologies, Inc. 516-576-6022
589 Davies Dr, York, PA 17402
Various dental burs.

Miltex Inc. 800-645-8000
589 Davies Dr, York, PA 17402

Nobel Biocare Usa, Llc 800-579-6515
22715/22725 Savi Ranch Parkway, Yorba Linda, CA 92887
Bur, dental.

Oco Inc. 800-228-0477
600 Paisano St NE Ste A, Albuquerque, NM 87123
Dental, bur.

Oratronics, Inc. 212-986-0050
405 Lexington Ave, New York, NY 10174
Implant channeling burr.

Pac-Dent Intl., Inc. 909-839-0888
21078 Commerce Point Dr, Walnut, CA 91789
Carbide bur, diamond bur.

Pentron Clinical Technologies 203-265-7397
68-70 North Plains Industrial, Road, Wallingford, CT 06492
Dental bur.

Prodrive Systems, Inc. 866-937-8882
812 Commerce Dr., Ogdensburg, NY 13669
Bur for dental handpiece.

Promident Llc 845-634-3997
242 N Main St, New City, NY 10956

Rite-Dent Manufacturing Corp. 305-693-8626
3750 E 10th Ct, Hialeah, FL 33013
Various types of dental bur.

S.S. White Burs Inc. 800-535-2877
1145 Towbin Ave, Lakewood, NJ 08701
Cone flat or round end, pointed end, cylinder round end, flame, round, inlay, straight fissure, finishing, taper fissure, curretage, TDA diamonds and tungsten carbide burrs. Burr blocks with 36 holes for holding and storing dental rotary cutting instruments (sterilizable).

Salvin Dental Specialties, Inc. 800-535-6566
3450 Latrobe Dr, Charlotte, NC 28211
Various types of dental burs.

Spring Health Products, Inc. 800-800-1680
705 General Washington Ave Ste 701, Norristown, PA 19403

Sterngold 800-243-9942
23 Frank Mossberg Dr, PO Box 2967, Attleboro, MA 02703
Laboratory diamonds and carbides.

Tava Surgical Instruments 805-650-5209
4837 McGrath St Ste J, Ventura, CA 93003
Dental burr.

BURR, DENTAL *(cont'd)*

Tri Hawk Corporation 866-874-4295
150 Highland Rd, Massena, NY 13662
$79.00 per roll of 100, disposable, Dental carbide burs and dental diamond burs. Also available TRI HAWK and KRONOS dental rotary instruments.

Ultradent Products, Inc. 801-553-4586
505 W 10200 S, South Jordan, UT 84095
Diamond/carbide bur.

BURR, DENTAL EXCAVATING *(Dental And Oral) 76QEW*

Brasseler Usa - Komet Medical 800-535-6638
1 Brasseler Blvd, Savannah, GA 31419

Dentalez Group 866-DTE-INFO
101 Lindenwood Dr Ste 225, Valleybrooke Corporate Center
Malvern, PA 19355

Miltex Inc. 800-645-8000
589 Davies Dr, York, PA 17402

Pfingst & Company, Inc. 908-561-6400
105 Snyder Rd, South Plainfield, NJ 07080

S.S. White Burs Inc. 800-535-2877
1145 Towbin Ave, Lakewood, NJ 08701
Cone flat or round end, pointed end, cylinder round end, flame, round, inlay, straight fissure, finishing, taper fissure, curretage, TDA diamonds and tungsten carbide burrs. Burr blocks with 36 holes for holding and storing dental rotary cutting instruments (sterilizable).

BURR, ORTHOPEDIC *(Orthopedics) 87HTT*

American Medical Specialties, Inc. 800-808-2877
10650 77th St., Suite 405, Largo, FL 33777
Qualtiy value in replacement cutting tools for powered surgical equipment of Zimmer, Stryker, 3M and others.

Ascent Healthcare Solutions 480-763-5300
10232 S 51st St, Phoenix, AZ 85044
Burr.

Biomet Microfixation Inc. 800-874-7711
1520 Tradeport Dr, Jacksonville, FL 32218
Various types of burrs.

Biomet, Inc. 574-267-6639
56 E Bell Dr, PO Box 587, Warsaw, IN 46582
Various types of burr.

Brasseler Usa - Komet Medical 800-535-6638
1 Brasseler Blvd, Savannah, GA 31419
Full range of shapes, sizes and lengths.

DJO Inc. 800-336-6569
1430 Decision St, Vista, CA 92081

Grace Engineering Corp. 810-392-2181
34775 Potter St, Memphis, MI 48041
Surgical burr.

Hydrocision, Inc. 888-747-7470
22 Linnell Cir Ste 102, Billerica, MA 01821
Arthroscopic hydrosurgery system for bone burring and soft-tissue management.

Medisiss 866-866-7477
2747 SW 6th St, Redmond, OR 97756
Various orthopedic burrs,sterile.

Micro-Aire Surgical Instruments, Inc. 800-722-0822
1641 Edlich Dr, Charlottesville, VA 22911

Sim Medical Sales 574-268-0341
PO Box 895, Warsaw, IN 46581

Small Bone Innovations, Inc. 215-428-1791
1380 S Pennsylvania Ave, Morrisville, PA 19067
Orthopedic burr.

BURR, OTHER *(Surgery) 79QEY*

American Medical Specialties, Inc. 800-808-2877
10650 77th St., Suite 405, Largo, FL 33777
Neuro blades, wire pass drills, revision tools.

Brasseler Usa - Komet Medical 800-535-6638
1 Brasseler Blvd, Savannah, GA 31419
ENT, neuro and oral burrs.

Comco, Inc. 800-796-6626
2151 N Lincoln St, Burbank, CA 91504
MICROBLASTER, is a micro-abrasive precision blaster for medical applications such as deburring, deflashing, beveling, coating removal, and surface prep/cleaning.

BURR, OTHER *(cont'd)*

Micro-Aire Surgical Instruments, Inc. 800-722-0822
1641 Edlich Dr, Charlottesville, VA 22911
Neuro burrs.

Sim Medical Sales 574-268-0341
PO Box 895, Warsaw, IN 46581

BURR, PODIATRIC *(Orthopedics) 87QEX*

American Medical Specialties, Inc. 800-808-2877
10650 77th St., Suite 405, Largo, FL 33777
Quality and value in cutting tools for powered surgical equipment.

Brasseler Usa - Komet Medical 800-535-6638
1 Brasseler Blvd, Savannah, GA 31419

Menlo Tool Co., Inc. 810-756-6010
22760 Dequindre Rd, Warren, MI 48091

Micro-Aire Surgical Instruments, Inc. 800-722-0822
1641 Edlich Dr, Charlottesville, VA 22911

Sim Medical Sales 574-268-0341
PO Box 895, Warsaw, IN 46581

Vilex, Inc. 800-872-4911
345 Old Curry Hollow Rd, Pittsburgh, PA 15236

BURR, SURGICAL, GENERAL & PLASTIC SURGERY *(Surgery) 79GFF*

Abrasive Technology, Inc. 740-548-4100
8400 Green Meadows Dr N, Lewis Center, OH 43035
Various instruments for podiatry or dermatolgy.

American Medical Specialties, Inc. 800-808-2877
10650 77th St., Suite 405, Largo, FL 33777
Quality and value in cutting tools for powered surgical equipment.

Arthrex Manufacturing 239-643-5553
1958 Trade Center Way, Naples, FL 34109
Bur.

Arthrex, Inc. 239-643-5553
1370 Creekside Blvd, Naples, FL 34108
Bur.

Ascent Healthcare Solutions 480-763-5300
10232 S 51st St, Phoenix, AZ 85044
Bur.

Bausch & Lomb Surgical 636-255-5051
3365 Tree Court Ind Blvd, Saint Louis, MO 63122

Biomet, Inc. 574-267-6639
56 E Bell Dr, PO Box 587, Warsaw, IN 46582
Various types of general and plastic surgical burs.

Brasseler Usa - Komet Medical 800-535-6638
1 Brasseler Blvd, Savannah, GA 31419

Brasseler Usa - Medical 805-650-5209
4837 McGrath St Ste J, Ventura, CA 93003
Surgical bur.

Ditec Mfg. 800-332-7083
1019 Mark Ave, Carpinteria, CA 93013
Diamond-plated.

Grace Engineering Corp. 810-392-2181
34775 Potter St, Memphis, MI 48041
Surgical bur.

Lasco Diamond Products 800-621-4726
PO Box 4657, 9950 Canoga Avenue, Unit A-8, Chatsworth, CA 91313
Diamond Coated Burrs

Medisiss 866-866-7477
2747 SW 6th St, Redmond, OR 97756
Various surgical burs,sterile.

Medtronic Powered Surgical Solutions 800-643-2773
4620 N Beach St, Haltom City, TX 76137
Electric high speed motor & various sterile & non sterile accessories.

Mekanika, Inc. 561-417-7244
3998 Fau Blvd Ste 210, Boca Raton, FL 33431
Bone drill bit.

Musculoskeletal Transplant Foundation 732-661-0202
1232 Mid Valley Dr, Jessup, PA 18434

Nuell, Inc. 800-829-7694
PO Box 55, 312 East Van Buren St., Leesburg, IN 46538
Surgical burs.

Omega Surgical Instruments 800-656-6342
G-8305 Saginaw St., Suite 6, Grand Blanc, MI 48439

BURR, SURGICAL, GENERAL & PLASTIC SURGERY *(cont'd)*

Sterilmed, Inc. 763-488-3400
11400 73rd Ave N Ste 100, Maple Grove, MN 55369
Bur.

Stryker Puerto Rico, Ltd. 939-307-2500
Hwy. 3, Km. 131.2, Las Guasimas Ind. Park, Arroyo, PR 00714
Surgical shaver, bur, accessories.

Tava Surgical Instruments 805-650-5209
4837 McGrath St Ste J, Ventura, CA 93003
Surgical burr.

Tri Hawk Corporation 866-874-4295
150 Highland Rd, Massena, NY 13662

BUTTON, IRIS, EYE, ARTIFICIAL *(Ophthalmology) 86NCK*

Danz Inc. 973-783-2955
460 Bloomfield Ave Ste 302, Montclair, NJ 07042

Erickson Labs Northwest 425-823-1861
12911 120th Ave NE Ste C10, Kirkland, WA 98034
Artificial eye.

Eyetech Ltd. 847-470-1777
9408 Normandy Ave, Morton Grove, IL 60053
Practice eye for laser's (Argon, Yag) procedures demostration

Ocular Concepts Llc. 503-699-7700
4035 Mercantile Dr Ste 208, Lake Oswego, OR 97035
Corneal button or iris button.

Randal Minor Ocular Prosthetics Inc. 813-949-2500
1628 Dale Mabry Hwy Ste 110, Lutz, FL 33548
Eye, artificial, plastic, custom made.

BUTTON, NASAL SEPTAL *(Ear/Nose/Throat) 77LFB*

Boston Medical Products, Inc. 800-433-2674
117 Flanders Rd, Westborough, MA 01581
SALMAN stent designed to help prevent complications resulting from functional endoscopic sinus surgery.

E. Benson Hood Laboratories, Inc. 800-942-5227
575 Washington St, Pembroke, MA 02359
Three sizes 30mm, 40mm, and 50mm.

Invotec Intl. 800-998-8580
6833 Phillips Industrial Blvd, Jacksonville, FL 32256
Septal button.

Medical Innovations International Inc. 507-289-0761
6256 34th Ave NW, Rochester, MN 55901
Rochester Nasal Septal Button™.

Micromedics 800-624-5662
1270 Eagan Industrial Rd, Saint Paul, MN 55121
Two sizes available for nonsurgical closure of septal perforations.

Shippert Medical Technologies Corp. 800-888-8663
6248 S Troy Cir Ste A, Centennial, CO 80111
Full line of Internal Nasal Splinting Devices

Silmed, Inc. 435-753-7307
97 West 300 South, Millville, UT 84326-0438
Nasal septal button.

BUTTON, SURGICAL *(Surgery) 79GEB*

Codman & Shurtleff, Inc 800-225-0460
325 Paramount Dr, Raynham, MA 02767

Ethicon, Inc. 800-4-ETHICON
Route 22 West, Somerville, NJ 08876
Polypropylene buttons, 36 to a box.

BUTTON, TRACHEOSTOMY TUBE *(Anesthesiology) 73SBI*

E. Benson Hood Laboratories, Inc. 800-942-5227
575 Washington St, Pembroke, MA 02359
Stoma stent with accessories, including speaking valves.

Gulden Ophthalmics 800-659-2250
225 Cadwalader Ave, Elkins Park, PA 19027

Medical Innovations International Inc. 507-289-0761
6256 34th Ave NW, Rochester, MN 55901
Barton-Mayo Tracheostoma Button™.

Olympic Medical Corp. 206-767-3500
5900 1st Ave S, Seattle, WA 98108
$98.95 each.

Smiths Medical Asd 800-424-8662
5700 W 23rd Ave, Gary, IN 46406
Tracheostome Vent, silicone, 15mm, 17.5mm and 20 mm OD with and without voice prosthesis.

Unomedical, Inc. 800-634-6003
5701 S Ware Rd Ste 1, McAllen, TX 78503

CABINET CASEWORK, GENERAL PURPOSE *(General) 80TBA*

Cif Furniture Ltd. 905-738-5821
56 Edilcan Dr., Concord, ONT L4K-3S6 Canada
General purpose.

Colonial Scientific Ltd. 902-468-1811
201 Brownlow Ave., Unit 52, Dartmouth, NS B3B-1W2 Canada
Utility carts and shelving.

Continental Metal Products Co., Inc. 800-221-4439
35 Olympia Ave, Woburn, MA 01801
Stainless steel.

DURHAM MANUFACTURING COMPANY 800-243-3774
201 Main St, Durham, CT 06422
Wire shelving.

Ethicon, Inc. 800-4-ETHICON
Route 22 West, Somerville, NJ 08876

Fleetwood Group, Incorporated 800-257-6390
PO Box 1259, Holland, MI 49422
Storage cabinets, mobile or with base.

General Devices Co., Inc. 800-626-9484
1410 S Post Rd, PO Box 39100, Indianapolis, IN 46239
Accessories, cooling modules, sliding shelves, etc. for mounting in cabinetry.

Getinge Usa, Inc. 800-475-9040
1777 E Henrietta Rd, Rochester, NY 14623
GETINGE, operating room storage modules.

Gillis Associated Industries 800-397-1675
750 Pinecrest Dr, Prospect Heights, IL 60070
Rolling steel office and warehouse ladders, mail carts, wire shelving, rivet rack decking, pallet rack decking, security carts (both mobile and immobile), steel shelving, rivet rack and benches.

Homak Manufacturing Company Inc. 800-874-6625
1605 Old Route 18 Ste 4-36, Wampum, PA 16157
Medical storage cabinet may be wall mounted or set under workstation. Cylinder lock with two keys; spring clip door latch.

Independent Solutions, Inc. 847-498-0500
900 Skokie Blvd Ste 118, Northbrook, IL 60062
UNICELL molded plastic. IEI & Alir stainless steel. Alir & Mott painted steel. CIF plastic laminate & wood

Intermetro Industries Corp. 800-441-2714
651 N Washington St, Wilkes Barre, PA 18705
STARSYS, storage shelving. Modular mobile/stationary workstations.

Invincible Office Furniture Co. 800-558-4417
PO Box 1117, Manitowoc, WI 54221

Jaece Industries, Inc. 716-694-2811
908 Niagara Falls Blvd, North Tonawanda, NY 14120
Foam bench, drawer and shelf liners, general-purpose surface cushion; non-absorbent. Bench liners, general-purpose non-absorbent surface.

Lab Safety Supply, Inc. 800-356-0783
401 S Wright Rd, Janesville, WI 53546

Medical Design Systems, Inc. 800-593-1900
10035 Lakeview Ave, Lenexa, KS 66219
MASS cabinets come in 16 or 22 in. configuration. Modular items available include FIFOGLIDES, bins, SLOTSHELVES, baskets, LOKSHELVES, hanger bars, and more.

Mmi Of Mississippi, Inc. 800-448-5918
PO Box 488, Crystal Springs, MS 39059
Pharmaceutical; hospital

Omnimed, Inc. (Beam Products) 800-257-2326
800 Glen Ave, Moorestown, NJ 08057
Cabinets designed for personal protection equipment (PPE). Can accommodate most gowns, gloves, masks, etc.

Pedigo Products 360-695-3500
4000 SE Columbia Way, Vancouver, WA 98661
Operating Room storage cabinets, various sizes, available as free-standing, built-in or caster base models.

Penco Products Inc. 800-562-1000
PO Box 378, 99 Brower Ave., Oaks, PA 19456
CLIPPER steel shelving, clip type shelving; RIVETRITE rivet shelving, boltless shelving.

Rem Systems 305-499-4800
625 E 10th Ave, Hialeah, FL 33010
Storage shelving and boxes for archival storage systems; Quik-View cabinet with see-through doors; Stor-Mor mobile storage system.

CABINET CASEWORK, GENERAL PURPOSE *(cont'd)*

Richards-Wilcox, Inc. 800-253-5668
600 S Lake St, Aurora, IL 60506
The Times-2 Step Up Step Down is a unique bank of cabinets suitable for medical filing and storage. The four cabinets feature two taller units on the outside and two shorter cabinets in the center with a countertop task area. Store medical equipment, color coded files, personal items, and office supplies. Use the countertop area to hold printers, fax machines or postage meters. Available in an antimicrobial powder coat finish, the Times-2 Step Up Step Down is a perfect solution for the busy medical or dental office.

Spacesaver Corporation 800-492-3434
1450 Janesville Ave, Fort Atkinson, WI 53538
PHARMASTOR, high density mobile storage systems.

Stackbin Corporation 800-333-1603
29 Powder Hill Rd, Lincoln, RI 02865
Stacktracks - mobile storage systems for x-ray files and medical records.

Suburban Surgical Co., Inc. 800-323-7366
275 12th St, Wheeling, IL 60090

Tecni-Quip 800-826-1245
960 Crossroads Blvd, PO Box 2050, Seguin, TX 78155
TECNI-QUIP General purpose shelving. The Husky line of shelving available with wire or solid metal shelves. Mobile or stationary units. Variety of sizes.

Thermo Scientific Hamilton 920-794-6800
1316 18th St, Two Rivers, WI 54241

Valley Craft 800-328-1480
2001 S Highway 61, Lake City, MN 55041

Western Case, Inc. 877-593-2182
14351 Chambers Rd, Tustin, CA 92780

Wheelit, Inc. 800-523-7508
440 Arco Dr, Toledo, OH 43607
$127.00 to $335.00 for twelve models of computer cabinets.

Ziamatic Corp. 800-711-FIRE
10 W College Ave, Yardley, PA 19067
Wall-mounted storage cabinets for self contained breathing apparatus, respirators and fire extinguishers.

CABINET CASEWORK, LABORATORY *(Chemistry) 75TBB*

American Seating 616-732-6600
401 American Seating Ctr NW, Grand Rapids, MI 49504

Bedcolab Ltd. 800-461-6414
2305 Francis Hughes, Laval, QUE H7S 1N5 Canada
Complete installations.

Blickman 800-247-5070
39 Robinson Rd, Lodi, NJ 07644
All stainless steel cabinets include base, wall, and high cabinets. Recessed cabinets.

Carolina Biological Supply Co. 800-334-5551
2700 York Rd, Burlington, NC 27215

Carr Corporation 800-952-2398
1547 11th St, Santa Monica, CA 90401
CARR stainless steel surgical casework.

Cif Furniture Ltd. 905-738-5821
56 Edilcan Dr., Concord, ONT L4K-3S6 Canada
Laboratory furniture.

Colonial Scientific Ltd. 902-468-1811
201 Brownlow Ave., Unit 52, Dartmouth, NS B3B-1W2 Canada

Hemco Corp. 816-796-2900
111 S Powell Rd, Independence, MO 64056
Enameled steel modular base cabinets are offered in a wide selection of sizes and drawer/door combinations.

Independent Solutions, Inc. 847-498-0500
900 Skokie Blvd Ste 118, Northbrook, IL 60062
UNICELL molded plastic. Alir & IEI stainless steel. Alir painted steel. LABCONCO fiberglass. CIF wood.

Jamestown Metal Products 716-665-5313
178 Blackstone Ave, Jamestown, NY 14701
In painted or stainless steel.

Kewaunee Scientific Corp. 704-873-7202
2700 W Front St, PO Box 1842, Statesville, NC 28677
Signature (wood) and steel.

Lab Fabricators Company 888-431-5444
1802 E 47th St, Cleveland, OH 44103
A complete line of base, wall and tall storage cabinets are available in painted steel and stainless steel constructions.

CABINET CASEWORK, LABORATORY *(cont'd)*

Lab Safety Supply, Inc. 800-356-0783
401 S Wright Rd, Janesville, WI 53546

Lista International Corp. 800-722-3020
106 Lowland St, Holliston, MA 01746
Electric static dissipative (ESD) workbenches and technical workbenches.

Nuaire, Inc. 800-328-3352
2100 Fernbrook Ln N, Plymouth, MN 55447
Polypropylene.

R.C. Smith Company 800-747-7648
14200 Southcross Dr W, Burnsville, MN 55306
Modular laboratory casework. Laboratory design service is also available. Installation of casework.

Scientek Medical Equipment 604-273-9094
11151 Bridgeport Rd., Richmond, BC V6X 1T3 Canada

Suburban Surgical Co., Inc. 800-323-7366
275 12th St, Wheeling, IL 60090
Laminated modular units.

Thermo Scientific Hamilton 920-794-6800
1316 18th St, Two Rivers, WI 54241

CABINET CASEWORK, MODULAR *(General) 80TBC*

Akro-Mils, Inc. 800-253-2467
1293 S Main St, Akron, OH 44301

Armstrong Medical Industries, Inc. 800-323-4220
575 Knightsbridge Pkwy, Lincolnshire, IL 60069

Atlantic Medco, Inc. 800-203-8444
166 Bloomfield Ave, Verona, NJ 07044
$500.00 to $2,000.00.

Bio-Safe America Corp. 800-767-4284
3250 S Susan St Ste B, Sterilaire Medical Division
Santa Ana, CA 92704
Sterilaire Medical unit. Sterilaire Medical HEPA units.

Cif Furniture Ltd. 905-738-5821
56 Edilcan Dr., Concord, ONT L4K-3S6 Canada

Continental Metal Products Co., Inc. 800-221-4439
35 Olympia Ave, Woburn, MA 01801
Stainless steel.

Getinge Usa, Inc. 800-475-9040
1777 E Henrietta Rd, Rochester, NY 14623
GETINGE, operating room storage modules.

Hill-Rom Holdings, Inc. 800-445-3730
1069 State Road 46 E, Batesville, IN 47006
Modular wall systems.

Independent Solutions, Inc. 847-498-0500
900 Skokie Blvd Ste 118, Northbrook, IL 60062
UNICELL molded plastic. Alir, IEI & Mott stainless steel. Alir & Mott painted steel. Collegedale & CIF plastic laminate & wood. CSI ULTRAFLEX.

Intermetro Industries Corp. 800-441-2714
651 N Washington St, Wilkes Barre, PA 18705
STARSYS modular/moveable casework.

Invincible Office Furniture Co. 800-558-4417
PO Box 1117, Manitowoc, WI 54221

Jamestown Metal Products 716-665-5313
178 Blackstone Ave, Jamestown, NY 14701
In painted or stainless steel.

Lionville Systems, Inc. 800-523-7114
501 Gunnard Carlson Dr, Coatesville, PA 19320
Modular, free-standing cabinetry and shelving units exclusively designed for pharmacy applications, supported by free professional design with detailed drawings.

Lista International Corp. 800-722-3020
106 Lowland St, Holliston, MA 01746
Drawer storage cabinets suitable for labs, Central Supply, sterile instrument processing, ORs, maintenance dept.

Md International, Inc. 305-669-9003
11300 NW 41st St, Doral, FL 33178

Midmark Corporation 800-643-6275
60 Vista Dr, P.O. Box 286, Versailles, OH 45380

Nevin Laboratories, Inc 800-544-5337
5000 S Halsted St, Chicago, IL 60609
Modular steel cabinets.

R.C. Smith Company 800-747-7648
14200 Southcross Dr W, Burnsville, MN 55306

CABINET CASEWORK, MODULAR *(cont'd)*

Suburban Surgical Co., Inc. 800-323-7366
275 12th St, Wheeling, IL 60090
Laminated modular units.

Thermo Scientific Hamilton 920-794-6800
1316 18th St, Two Rivers, WI 54241

United Metal Fabricators, Inc. 800-638-5322
1316 Eisenhower Blvd, Johnstown, PA 15904
Modular cabinetry for examining room and clinics, all metal and color coordinated.

Valley Craft 800-328-1480
2001 S Highway 61, Lake City, MN 55041

CABINET CASEWORK, PATIENT ROOM *(General) 80TBE*

Independent Solutions, Inc. 847-498-0500
900 Skokie Blvd Ste 118, Northbrook, IL 60062
BWM wood or plastic laminate.

Jamestown Metal Products 716-665-5313
178 Blackstone Ave, Jamestown, NY 14701
In painted or stainless steel.

Kewaunee Scientific Corp. 704-873-7202
2700 W Front St, PO Box 1842, Statesville, NC 28677
Signature (wood) and steel.

Newschoff Chairs, Inc. 800-203-8916
909 N.E. St., Sheboygan, WI 53081

S&W By Hausmann 888-428-7626
130 Union St, Northvale, NJ 07647

CABINET CASEWORK, PHARMACY *(General) 80TBF*

Bio-Safe America Corp. 800-767-4284
3250 S Susan St Ste B, Sterilaire Medical Division
Santa Ana, CA 92704
Class 10 prefabricated pharmacy.

Independent Solutions, Inc. 847-498-0500
900 Skokie Blvd Ste 118, Northbrook, IL 60062
UNICELL molded plastic. CIF plastic laminate & wood.

Intermetro Industries Corp. 800-441-2714
651 N Washington St, Wilkes Barre, PA 18705
STARSYS pharmacy casework.

Jamestown Metal Products 716-665-5313
178 Blackstone Ave, Jamestown, NY 14701
In painted or stainless steel.

R.C. Smith Company 800-747-7648
14200 Southcross Dr W, Burnsville, MN 55306
Modular pharmacy casework system with over 3,000 installations worldwide. Pharmacy design service is also available along with installation of the casework product.

Valley Craft 800-328-1480
2001 S Highway 61, Lake City, MN 55041

CABINET, AERATOR, ETHYLENE-OXIDE GAS *(General) 80FLI*

Andersen Products, Inc., 800-523-1276
3202 Caroline Dr, Health Science Park, Haw River, NC 27258

Environmental Tectonics Corp. 215-355-9100
125 James Way, Southampton, PA 18966

CABINET, BEDSIDE *(General) 80QFA*

Adden Furniture, Inc. 800-625-3876
26 Jackson St, Lowell, MA 01852

Clinimed, Incorporated 877-CLINIMED
303 Markus Ct, Sandy Brae Industrial Park, Newark, DE 19713

Colonial Scientific Ltd. 902-468-1811
201 Brownlow Ave., Unit 52, Dartmouth, NS B3B-1W2 Canada

Hard Manufacturing Co. 800-873-4273
230 Grider St, Buffalo, NY 14215
$311.00 for model S92295 bedside cabinet with steel frame, wood grain; $330.00 for model 92245 three drawer chest; $458.00 for model 95255 four drawer chest; $555.00 for model 96145 desk chest combination; $122.50 for wood cabinet W92295.

Hausmann Industries, Inc. 888-428-7626
130 Union St, Northvale, NJ 07647
$216.00 per unit (standard).

Hill-Rom Holdings, Inc. 800-445-3730
1069 State Road 46 E, Batesville, IN 47006

Independent Solutions, Inc. 847-498-0500
900 Skokie Blvd Ste 118, Northbrook, IL 60062
BWM wood or plastic laminate.

CABINET, BEDSIDE *(cont'd)*

Intermetro Industries Corp. 800-441-2714
651 N Washington St, Wilkes Barre, PA 18705
STARSYS bedside cabinet or cart.

M.C. Healthcare Products, Inc. 800-268-8671
4658 Ontario St., Beamsville, ONT L0R 1B4 Canada
H.P.L. laminates and veneers, Prestige series, plastic removable drawers. 3 drawer & door & drawer - laminate top & drawer fronts.

Mayo Medical, S.A. De C.V. 800-715-3872
Edison 1141 Nte., Col. Talleres, Monterrey N.L. 64480 Mexico

Newschoff Chairs, Inc. 800-203-8916
909 N.E. St., Sheboygan, WI 53081

Radix Corp. 204-697-2349
#2-572 South Fifth St., Pembina, ND 58271
TEMPO, WOODLANDS, CAMBRIDGE series. Bedside cabinets, hutch, four-drawer chests, wardrobes, mirrors, armoires, head/footboard sets.

Rockaway Chairs 800-256-6601
111 Alexander Rd Apt 11, West Monroe, LA 71291

S&W By Hausmann 888-428-7626
130 Union St, Northvale, NJ 07647

Stryker Medical 800-869-0770
3800 E Centre Ave, Portage, MI 49002

Suburban Surgical Co., Inc. 800-323-7366
275 12th St, Wheeling, IL 60090

CABINET, CHROMATOGRAPHY (U.V.) VIEWING
(Chemistry) 75UJG

Camag Scientific, Inc. 800-334-3909
515 Cornelius Harnett Dr, Wilmington, NC 28401

Spectronics Corporation 800-274-8888
956 Brush Hollow Rd, Westbury, NY 11590
7 models: short, medium or long wave UV, and visible light combinations.

Uvp, Llc 800-452-6788
2066 W 11th St, Upland, CA 91786
CHROMATO-VUE UV Viewing Cabinets.

CABINET, DENTAL *(Dental And Oral) 76QFB*

Danville Materials 800-827-7940
3420 Fostoria Way Ste A200, San Ramon, CA 94583
Dental dust cabinet.

Dentalez Group 866-DTE-INFO
101 Lindenwood Dr Ste 225, Valleybrooke Corporate Center
Malvern, PA 19355

Dntlworks Equipment Corporation 800-847-0694
7300 S Tucson Way, Centennial, CO 80112
Many models. From sophisticated, self-contained dental delivery systems to basic delivery units.

Handler Manufacturing Co. 800-274-2635
612 North Ave E, Westfield, NJ 07090
Dental laboratory cabinetry.

Health Science Products, Inc. 800-237-5794
1489 Hueytown Rd, Hueytown, AL 35023
A complete line of operatory modular cabinets for closed or open bay operatories and a line of mobile cabinets. Custom cabinets are optional.

Independent Solutions, Inc. 847-498-0500
900 Skokie Blvd Ste 118, Northbrook, IL 60062

Mastercraft Dental Co. Of Texas 972-775-8757
880 Eastgate Rd, P.O. Box 882, Midlothian, TX 76065
Mobile orthodontic cabinets.

Moyco Technologies, Inc. 800-331-8837
200 Commerce Dr, Montgomeryville, PA 18936

CABINET, ENT TREATMENT *(Ear/Nose/Throat) 77QFC*

HAAG-STREIT USA, INC. 800-787-5426
3535 Kings Mills Rd, Mason, OH 45040
$2,495 for ENT treatment cabinet.

Jedmed Instruments Co. 314-845-3770
5416 Jedmed Ct, Saint Louis, MO 63129

Medical Technology Industries, Inc. 800-924-4655
3555 W 1500 S, Salt Lake City, UT 84104
Surgery/Examination Chairs and Tables and Treatment Cabinets

Tsi Medical Ltd. 800-661-7263
47 Athabascan Ave., Unit 105, Sherwood Park, AB T8A-4H3 Canada

CABINET, INSTRUMENT *(General) 80QFD*

Alimed, Inc. 800-225-2610
297 High St, Dedham, MA 02026

Altech Corporation 908-806-9400
35 Royal Rd, Flemington, NJ 08822

Atlantic Medco, Inc. 800-203-8444
166 Bloomfield Ave, Verona, NJ 07044
$1000 to $2000 Surgical instrument cabinets.

Blickman 800-247-5070
39 Robinson Rd, Lodi, NJ 07644
Freestanding stainless steel cabinets in four models with glass or stainless steel shelves. One available with stainless steel pegboard. Custom designs available.

Colonial Scientific Ltd. 902-468-1811
201 Brownlow Ave., Unit 52, Dartmouth, NS B3B-1W2 Canada
Stainless steel stands and tables.

Enochs Examining Room Furniture, Inc. 800-428-2305
PO Box 50559, Indianapolis, IN 46250
$822.00 per unit (standard).

Florida Life Systems 727-321-9554
3446 5th Ave N, Saint Petersburg, FL 33713
Stainless steel O.R. cabinetry.

General Devices Co., Inc. 800-626-9484
1410 S Post Rd, PO Box 39100, Indianapolis, IN 46239
Telescoping slides: solid-bearing, roller-bearing, and bottom-mount slides that are installed in cabinets or enclosures for mounting equipment.

Gerstner & Sons Inc. 937-228-1662
20 Gerstner Way, Dayton, OH 45402
$350 to $4000 for dental cabinets and portable instrument cases with drawers. $250.00 to $650.00 for dental hygiene cases. Also available are tool chests and wood chests/cases. Many standard sizes are offered, as are lockable models. Custom sizes are considered.

Hausmann Industries, Inc. 888-428-7626
130 Union St, Northvale, NJ 07647
$216.00 per unit (standard).

Imperial Surgical Ltd. 800-661-5432
581 Orly Ave., Dorval, ONT H9P-1G1 Canada
Various models available.

Independent Solutions, Inc. 847-498-0500
900 Skokie Blvd Ste 118, Northbrook, IL 60062
Alir & Blickman stainless steel. Alir painted steel. MASS plastic laminate.

Intermetro Industries Corp. 800-441-2714
651 N Washington St, Wilkes Barre, PA 18705
STARSYS sterile-instrument cabinet.

International Hospital Supply Co. 800-398-9450
6914 Canby Ave Ste 105, Reseda, CA 91335

Md International, Inc. 305-669-9003
11300 NW 41st St, Doral, FL 33178

Midmark Corporation 800-643-6275
60 Vista Dr, P.O. Box 286, Versailles, OH 45380

Penco Products Inc. 800-562-1000
PO Box 378, 99 Brower Ave., Oaks, PA 19456

Scientek Medical Equipment 604-273-9094
11151 Bridgeport Rd., Richmond, BC V6X 1T3 Canada

Stanley Vidmar 800-523-9462
11 Grammes Rd, Allentown, PA 18103

United Metal Fabricators, Inc. 800-638-5322
1316 Eisenhower Blvd, Johnstown, PA 15904
Enameled or stainless steel in 16in., 25in. and 32in. widths with glass door. Drawer and door arrangements variable.

Valley Craft 800-328-1480
2001 S Highway 61, Lake City, MN 55041

Vector Electronics & Technology, Inc. 800-423-5659
11115 Vanowen St, North Hollywood, CA 91605

CABINET, INSTRUMENT, AC-POWERED, OPHTHALMIC
(Ophthalmology) 86HRE

Medical Technology Industries, Inc. 800-924-4655
3555 W 1500 S, Salt Lake City, UT 84104
Treatment cabinet ENT and OPH.

Varitronics, Inc. 800-345-1244
620 Park Way, Broomall, PA 19008

CABINET, LABORATORY *(Chemistry) 75TAP*

Akro-Mils, Inc. 800-253-2467
1293 S Main St, Akron, OH 44301

Altech Corporation 908-806-9400
35 Royal Rd, Flemington, NJ 08822

American Seating 616-732-6600
401 American Seating Ctr NW, Grand Rapids, MI 49504

Carolina Biological Supply Co. 800-334-5551
2700 York Rd, Burlington, NC 27215

Electra-Tec Inc. 800-225-3532
PO Box 17, Otsego, MI 49078

Genie Scientific, Inc. 800-545-8816
17430 Mount Cliffwood Cir, Fountain Valley, CA 92708

Hemco Corp. 816-796-2900
111 S Powell Rd, Independence, MO 64056
Enameled steel modular base cabinets are offered in a wide selection of sizes and drawer/door combinations.

Independent Solutions, Inc. 847-498-0500
900 Skokie Blvd Ste 118, Northbrook, IL 60062
Vacuum bottle storage coves (recessed wall mounted or headwall mounted); molded plastic or stainless steel; loose or framed. Alir painted & IEI stainless steel. CIF wood & plam. Class 1 Kydex molded.

Kewaunee Scientific Corp. 704-873-7202
2700 W Front St, PO Box 1842, Statesville, NC 28677
Signature (wood) and steel.

Lab Fabricators Company 888-431-5444
1802 E 47th St, Cleveland, OH 44103
Base, wall and tall storage cabinets are available in painted steel and stainless steel constructions.

Lab Safety Supply, Inc. 800-356-0783
401 S Wright Rd, Janesville, WI 53546

Nuaire, Inc. 800-328-3352
2100 Fernbrook Ln N, Plymouth, MN 55447
Biological safety cabinets.

Scientek Medical Equipment 604-273-9094
11151 Bridgeport Rd., Richmond, BC V6X 1T3 Canada

Stanley Vidmar 800-523-9462
11 Grammes Rd, Allentown, PA 18103

Terriss-Consolidated Industries 800-342-1611
807 Summerfield Ave, Asbury Park, NJ 07712
Stainless steel.

Thermo Scientific Hamilton 920-794-6800
1316 18th St, Two Rivers, WI 54241

CABINET, MEDICINE *(General) 80QFE*

Akro-Mils, Inc. 800-253-2467
1293 S Main St, Akron, OH 44301

Atlantic Medco, Inc. 800-203-8444
166 Bloomfield Ave, Verona, NJ 07044
$200 to $1000.

Colonial Scientific Ltd. 902-468-1811
201 Brownlow Ave., Unit 52, Dartmouth, NS B3B-1W2 Canada
Drug storage cabinets.

Lionville Systems, Inc. 800-523-7114
501 Gunnard Carlson Dr, Coatesville, PA 19320
DOCUMED Pharmacy Cabinet, an economical, after-hours med cabinet for facilities without a 24-hour pharmacy including correctional healthcare facilities. This automated cabinet issues single-dose medication packs while recording who, what, and when the med was removed.

Mayo Medical, S.A. De C.V. 800-715-3872
Edison 1141 Nte., Col. Talleres, Monterrey N.L. 64480 Mexico
Showcase or single door cabinets with three glass shelves.

Protectoseal Co. 800-323-2268
225 Foster Ave, Bensenville, IL 60106

S&W By Hausmann 888-428-7626
130 Union St, Northvale, NJ 07647

Schueler & Company, Inc. 516-487-1500
PO Box 528, Stratford, CT 06615

Stanley Vidmar 800-523-9462
11 Grammes Rd, Allentown, PA 18103

Suburban Surgical Co., Inc. 800-323-7366
275 12th St, Wheeling, IL 60090

Valley Craft 800-328-1480
2001 S Highway 61, Lake City, MN 55041

CABINET, MICROBIOLOGICAL *(Microbiology) 83QFF*

Microzone Corporation 877-252-7746
86 Harry Douglas Drive, Ottawa, ONT K2S 2C7 Canada
Class II, Type A2 NSF49 certified

CABINET, MOIST STEAM *(Physical Med) 89IMB*

Vanny Corp. 310-556-1170
10390 Santa Monica Blvd Ste 270, Los Angeles, CA 90025
Pulsed-air heater.

CABINET, NARCOTIC CONTROL *(General) 80QFG*

Armstrong Medical Industries, Inc. 800-323-4220
575 Knightsbridge Pkwy, Lincolnshire, IL 60069

Atlantic Medco, Inc. 800-203-8444
166 Bloomfield Ave, Verona, NJ 07044
$400.00 to $2,000.00.

Blickman 800-247-5070
39 Robinson Rd, Lodi, NJ 07644
Stainless steel narcotic lockers are available with or without jeweled warning light. Individual keyed cylinder cam locks on both doors.

Homak Manufacturing Company Inc. 800-874-6625
1605 Old Route 18 Ste 4-36, Wampum, PA 16157
Narcotic cabinet features extra-heavy-duty 18 guage steel exterior and coded tubular cam lock with spring clip door catch for superior strength and security.

Imperial Surgical Ltd. 800-661-5432
581 Orly Ave., Dorval, ONT H9P-1G1 Canada
Various models available.

Independent Solutions, Inc. 847-498-0500
900 Skokie Blvd Ste 118, Northbrook, IL 60062
Blickman & UMF stainless steel or enamel steel, two-lock, with or without warning light, one or two door.

Medi-Dose, Inc. 800-523-8966
70 Industrial Dr, Ivyland, PA 18974

Omnimed, Inc. (Beam Products) 800-257-2326
800 Glen Ave, Moorestown, NJ 08057

Protectoseal Co. 800-323-2268
225 Foster Ave, Bensenville, IL 60106

Stanley Vidmar 800-523-9462
11 Grammes Rd, Allentown, PA 18103

Sunroc / Telkee, Inc. 800-478-6762
60 Starlifter Ave, Kent County Aero Park, Dover, DE 19901
$715.00 each (retail); Simplex lock model SMTC, 5 3/16 in. x 3/4 in.; dual-compartment system.

Valley Craft 800-328-1480
2001 S Highway 61, Lake City, MN 55041

CABINET, OTHER *(General) 80QFL*

Abbott Associates 203-878-2370
620 West Ave, Milford, CT 06461
Sterile Field Organizers; 6- and 3-compartment, PVC, multi pockets.

Altech Corporation 908-806-9400
35 Royal Rd, Flemington, NJ 08822

Atlantic Medco, Inc. 800-203-8444
166 Bloomfield Ave, Verona, NJ 07044
$500.00 to $2,000.00.

Capintec, Inc. 800-631-3826
6 Arrow Rd, Ramsey, NJ 07446

Clinimed, Incorporated 877-CLINIMED
303 Markus Ct, Sandy Brae Industrial Park, Newark, DE 19713

Custom Comfort 800-749-0933
PO Box 4779, Winter Park, FL 32793
Custom Comfort offers a wide selection of supply cabinets to meet both your facility and portable needs that are designed to be functional yet cost effective. Since all of the cabinets are equipped with casters, new room configurations are easily created. All 'SC' series cabinets are available with WilsonArt platinum gray top and sides. A secondary accent color for the drawer/door fronts may also be selected at no extra cost.

Custom Comfort Medtek 800-749-0933
3939 Forsyth Rd Ste A, Winter Park, FL 32792
Sturdy cabinets are designed so customers can mix and match from a wide assortment of drawer and door combinations. A folding table can be added to one or both sides for additional work space. All cabinets feature easy-roll casters. Eighteen Formica colors are available to match any decor.

CABINET, OTHER *(cont'd)*

Deflecto Corp. 800-428-4328
7035 E 86th St, Indianapolis, IN 46250
Interlocking Tilt Bin Storage System. Versatile units feature clear bins that tilt out for easy access. Interlocking capabilites allow you to connect different sizes creating a customized system. Stack on desktop or hang on wall with hardware included. Each bin comes with identification labels. Great for medical and dental settings for tongue depressors, cotton balls, gauze, dental floss, latex gloves and smaller first aid supplies. Tilt Bins can also be used in administrative areas for handy storage of office supplies.

Diacor, Inc. 800-342-2679
3191 Valley St Ste 100A, Salt Lake City, UT 84109
Cerrobend Blocking tray storage cabinet $695.00 to $4540.00. Provides storage spaces for blocking trays used in radiation therapy treatments.

Enochs Examining Room Furniture, Inc. 800-428-2305
PO Box 50559, Indianapolis, IN 46250
$716.00 per unit (standard), $403.00 for wall unit.

General Devices Co., Inc. 800-626-9484
1410 S Post Rd, PO Box 39100, Indianapolis, IN 46239
VENT RAK for electronics and telecommunications equipment. Standard and custom cabinetry and racks for housing or test equipment.

Independent Solutions, Inc. 847-498-0500
900 Skokie Blvd Ste 118, Northbrook, IL 60062
Stainless steel or enamel steel or wood or plastic laminate or plastic or phenolic resin.

Intermetro Industries Corp. 800-441-2714
651 N Washington St, Wilkes Barre, PA 18705
STARSYS suture, catheter, scope, or general supply cabinets.

Justrite Manufacturing Co., L.L.C. 800-798-9250
2454 E Dempster St, Des Plaines, IL 60016
Justrite cabinets are available in over 42 flammable models and over 11 acid models with the Sure Grip® handle or Lever handle. The cabinets are available in manual, self-closing or sliding doors. Our cabinets have FM approval, UL listing and conform with OSHA & NFPA regulations.

Kadan Co. Inc., D.A. 800-325-2326
1 Brigadoon Ln, Waxhaw, NC 28173

Knox Company 800-552-5669
1601 W Deer Valley Rd, Phoenix, AZ 85027
Armored cabinets used for storage of haz-mat data sheets; key control; storage of blue prints and evacuation plans.

Lionville Systems, Inc. 800-523-7114
501 Gunnard Carlson Dr, Coatesville, PA 19320
Wall-mounted cabinets for patient rooms to store meds, charts, supplies, etc. Narcotic cabinets for nursing units and pharmacies.

Medical Design Systems, Inc. 800-593-1900
10035 Lakeview Ave, Lenexa, KS 66219
Cabinets and endoscope storage. MASS scope storage system features customized nesting bracket to secure scope heads. Padded back wall prevents damage to distal tips. Four, nine and eighteen scope models with FLEXLOK Door for security. Pass-Through Scope Cabinet installed in wall holds eight scopes. MASS Modular cabinets come in 16 or 22 in. deep configuration. Modular items available include FIFOGLIDES, bins, SLOTSHELVES, baskets, LOKSHELVES, hanger bars and more. Cabinets can be secured with MASS FLEXLOK overhead door, solid hinged doors, or hinged doors with glass inserts. MASS countertop and above counter storage systems have unlimited applications. Maximize working surfaces and create additional secure storage space to blend with your decor.

Nevin Laboratories, Inc 800-544-5337
5000 S Halsted St, Chicago, IL 60609
Medical office cabinets.

Omnimed, Inc. (Beam Products) 800-257-2326
800 Glen Ave, Moorestown, NJ 08057

Pryor Products 800-854-2280
1819 Peacock Blvd, Oceanside, CA 92056
Storage cabinets; Specialty storage carts.

S&S Technology 281-815-1300
10625 Telge Rd, Houston, TX 77095
Darkroom cabinets.

Spacesaver Corporation 800-492-3434
1450 Janesville Ave, Fort Atkinson, WI 53538
PHARMASTOR, high density mobile storage systems.

CABINET, OTHER *(cont'd)*

Spectronics Corporation 800-274-8888
956 Brush Hollow Rd, Westbury, NY 11590
SPECTROLINE model CM-26 UV viewing cabinet provides both long-wave and short-wave UV irradiance.

Spin-Cast Plastics, Inc. 800-422-3625
3300 N Kenmore St, South Bend, IN 46628

Stanley Vidmar 800-523-9462
11 Grammes Rd, Allentown, PA 18103
Central supply, operating room, biomedical engineering.

Tower Medical System, Ltd. 631-699-3200
917 Lincoln Ave Ste 11, Holbrook, NY 11741
Lead-Lined Cabinets

Valley Craft 800-328-1480
2001 S Highway 61, Lake City, MN 55041

White Systems, Inc. 800-275-1442
30 Boright Ave, Kenilworth, NJ 07033
Medical records, pharmacy storage units.

Winsted Corp. 800-447-2257
10901 Hampshire Ave S, Minneapolis, MN 55438
Racks, cabinets, consoles.

Wire Crafters L.L.C. 800-924-9473
6208 Strawberry Ln, Louisville, KY 40214

CABINET, PASS THROUGH *(General) 80QFH*

Clean Air Technology, Inc. 800 459 6320
41105 Capital Dr, Canton, MI 48187
Cleanroom pass-through cabinets, custom sizes in laminate, aluminum and stainless steel finishes.

Independent Solutions, Inc. 847-498-0500
900 Skokie Blvd Ste 118, Northbrook, IL 60062
IEI & CMP stainless steel. Alir painted steel. ASI & Bobrick.

Justrite Manufacturing Co., L.L.C. 800-798-9250
2454 E Dempster St, Des Plaines, IL 60016
Safety cabinets with Pass-through systems are available from Justrite

Liberty Industries, Inc. 800-828-5656
133 Commerce St, East Berlin, CT 06023
Standard and custom sizes available.

Lm Air Technology, Inc. 866-381-8200
1467 Pinewood St, Cleanroom & Lab Equipment - Mfger
Rahway, NJ 07065
Stainless or painted steel, laminated, polypropylene construction. Also includes cart Pass-Thru's

Scientek Medical Equipment 604-273-9094
11151 Bridgeport Rd., Richmond, BC V6X 1T3 Canada

CABINET, PHOTOTHERAPY (PUVA) *(Surgery) 79KGL*

National Biological Corp. 800-338-5045
1532 Enterprise Pkwy, Twinsburg, OH 44087
Ultraviolet light phototherapy devices (UVA, UVB & UVBNB).

Ultralite Enterprises, Inc. 800-241-7506
390 Farmer Ct, Lawrenceville, GA 30046

CABINET, STORAGE, CATHETER *(General) 80WVU*

Intermetro Industries Corp. 800-441-2714
651 N Washington St, Wilkes Barre, PA 18705
STARSYS catheter storage cabinets or carts.

Medical Design Systems, Inc. 800-593-1900
10035 Lakeview Ave, Lenexa, KS 66219
Cabinet, catheters - Keep catheters, wires, balloons, stents and other supplies secure and handy. Create just the right cabinet for your specific procedures and protocols. Catheter, storage - MASS cabinets and carts will keep your catheters, wires, balloons, stents, and other supplies handy and secure. Create just the right storage for your specific procedures and protocols.

S&S Technology 281-815-1300
10625 Telge Rd, Houston, TX 77095
Mobile and Modular.

Stanley Vidmar 800-523-9462
11 Grammes Rd, Allentown, PA 18103
Modular storage cabinet for cardiac catheters up to 55 1/2in. in length.

Tulox Plastics Corp. 800-234-1118
PO Box 984, 401 S. Miller Ave., Marion, IN 46952
Clear containers for catheters.

Youngs, Inc. 800-523-5454
55 E Cherry Ln, Souderton, PA 18964

CABINET, STORAGE, ENDOSCOPE *(Gastro/Urology) 78WUJ*

Custom Ultrasonics, Inc. 215-364-1477
144 Railroad Dr, Hartsville, PA 18974
DRYLOCK uniquely designed forced air system for the drying and safe storage of endoscopic instruments and accessories.

Elmed, Inc. 630-543-2792
60 W Fay Ave, Addison, IL 60101

Encompas Unlimited, Inc. 800-825-7701
PO Box 516, Tallevast, FL 34270
BC-99, Endo Bottom Cover, protects fragile end of endoscopes during storage and transport. Also available is the MF-10 Endo Work Tray, with a design that fits snugly between mattress and gurney for even support and provides a hands-free shelf during procedures.

Intermetro Industries Corp. 800-441-2714
651 N Washington St, Wilkes Barre, PA 18705
STARSYS scope-storage cabinet.

CABINET, STORAGE, SLIDE *(General) 80WRH*

Boekel Scientific 800-336-6929
855 Pennsylvania Blvd, Feasterville Trevose, PA 19053

Carolina Biological Supply Co. 800-334-5551
2700 York Rd, Burlington, NC 27215

Jaece Industries, Inc. 716-694-2811
908 Niagara Falls Blvd, North Tonawanda, NY 14120
Slide holders, holds glass slides for drying or draining.

Mccrone Microscopes & Accessories 800-622-8122
850 Pasquinelli Dr, Westmont, IL 60559
Includes organizers, tool holders, and slide boxes.

Negafile Systems 800-523-5474
1560 Industry Rd, Hatfield, PA 19440
Photographic archival preserves for photo-microscopy.

Phoenix Metal Products, Inc. 516-546-4200
35 Hanse Ave, Freeport, NY 11520
Microscope slide storage cabinets, 6 drawers with card holder to facilitate easy retrieval of 1' x 3' glass slides. Each cabinet is painted with chip-resistant powder paint, has a capacity of 4,500+ glass slides and is stackable. Cabinet, Storage, 35mm slides. Steel storage cabinets; 3 drawers; holds approximately 2,250 standard 2' x 2' cardboard mounted 35mm slides. Each cabinet is painted with chip-resistant power paint and is stackable.

CABINET, TABLE AND TRAY, ANESTHESIA
(Anesthesiology) 73BRY

Abbott Laboratories 800-223-2064
100 Abbott Park Rd, Abbott Park, IL 60064

Alimed, Inc. 800-225-2610
297 High St, Dedham, MA 02026

Cameron-Miller, Inc. 800-621-0142
5410 W Roosevelt Rd, Road #241, Chicago, IL 60644

Dencraft 800-328-9729
PO Box 57, Moorestown, NJ 08057

Integra Lifesciences Corp. 609-275-0500
311 Enterprise Dr, Plainsboro, NJ 08536
Epidural tray.

Maquet, Inc. 843-552-8652
7371 Spartan Blvd E, N Charleston, SC 29418
Various models of ceiling mounted gas, vacuum,and power delivery systems.

Skytron 800-759-8766
5085 Corporate Exchange Blvd SE, Grand Rapids, MI 49512
POWER BOOM Sky Boom, ceiling-mounted providing medical gas, electric, and communications utilities and equipment storage for anesthesia, indoscopic, endoscopic, emergency, and ICU departments.

Stanley Vidmar 800-523-9462
11 Grammes Rd, Allentown, PA 18103

Suburban Surgical Co., Inc. 800-323-7366
275 12th St, Wheeling, IL 60090

United Metal Fabricators, Inc. 800-638-5322
1316 Eisenhower Blvd, Johnstown, PA 15904

CABINET, TREATMENT, ULTRAVIOLET *(General) 80QFI*

National Biological Corp. 800-338-5045
1532 Enterprise Pkwy, Twinsburg, OH 44087
UV home & office treatment panels & cabinets. (UVA, UVB & UVBNB phototherapy systems.)

CABINET, WARMING *(General) 80QFJ*

Atlantic Medco, Inc. 800-203-8444
166 Bloomfield Ave, Verona, NJ 07044
$1,900.00 to $2,175.00.

Blickman 800-247-5070
39 Robinson Rd, Lodi, NJ 07644
Twelve different models are offered, in dimensions measuring 24 or 30 in. wide; 18, 20, or 26 in. deep; and 24, 36, 60, or 74 in. high. Cabinets feature double-wall insulated construction of Type 304, nonmagnetic stainless steel; magnetic-closure gasket systems on all doors; and double-panel, tempered, insulated glass. Control panels feature a set temperature button, which the operator can set from 90 to 160 degrees Fahrenheit, in one-degree increments (Celsius setting and read-out optional). The units are furnished with tubular heating assemblies and a circulating fan for even distribution. All units have a visual and audible alarm, and an automatic safety switch. A 1/32 DIN electronic controller contains operating switches and a digital temperature display.

Continental Metal Products Co., Inc. 800-221-4439
35 Olympia Ave, Woburn, MA 01801
Solution-warming cabinet.

Enthermics Medical Systems, Inc. 800-862-9276
W164N9221 Water St, Menomonee Falls, WI 53051
EC2180, EC2060, EC1540, EC770, EC340, EC230 Upright warming cabinets to heat blankets used to relieve symptoms of hypothermia in patient recovering from surgery. Mobile, durable stainless steel construction, electronic control. EC770L, EC1730BL, EC1540BL, EC340L, EC230L warming cabinets to heat irrigation or injection fluids to recommended storage temperatures. Mobile, durable stainless steel construction, electronic control.

Getinge Usa, Inc. 800-475-9040
1777 E Henrietta Rd, Rochester, NY 14623
GETINGE.

Imperial Surgical Ltd. 800-661-5432
581 Orly Ave., Dorval, ONT H9P-1G1 Canada
Various models available.

Independent Solutions, Inc. 847-498-0500
900 Skokie Blvd Ste 118, Northbrook, IL 60062
Blickman electronic stainless steel, digital.

Medical Technologies Co. 800-280-3220
1728 W Park Center Dr Ste A, Fenton, MO 63026
Solution/blanket warmer.

Pedigo Products 360-695-3500
4000 SE Columbia Way, Vancouver, WA 98661
Warming cabinet, various sizes and models of blanket and fluid warming cabinets.

Scientek Medical Equipment 604-273-9094
11151 Bridgeport Rd., Richmond, BC V6X 1T3 Canada
Mechanically convected electric or steam heat, thermostatic temperature control, dial thermometer, stainless steel constr.

Skytron 800-759-8766
5085 Corporate Exchange Blvd SE, Grand Rapids, MI 49512
Blanket and solution warming cabinets provide evenly distributed consistent heat throughout the cabinet.

CABINET, X-RAY SYSTEM *(Radiology) 90MWP*

Bioptics, Inc. 520-514-2298
4605 S Palo Verde Rd Ste 605, Tucson, AZ 85714
Cabinet, x-ray system.

X-Ray Imaging Solutions Inc. 847-878-0867
641 Industrial Dr Ste D, Cary, IL 60013
Various types of x-ray systems.

CABINET, X-RAY TRANSFER *(Radiology) 90QFK*

Bar-Ray Products, Inc. 800-359-6115
95 Monarch St, Littlestown, PA 17340

Carr Corporation 800-952-2398
1547 11th St, Santa Monica, CA 90401

Colonial Scientific Ltd. 902-468-1811
201 Brownlow Ave., Unit 52, Dartmouth, NS B3B-1W2 Canada
x-ray shelving

Independent Solutions, Inc. 847-498-0500
900 Skokie Blvd Ste 118, Northbrook, IL 60062
S&S.

Marconi Medical Systems 800-323-0550
595 Miner Rd, Cleveland, OH 44143

Rem Systems 305-499-4800
625 E 10th Ave, Hialeah, FL 33010
X-ray transport cart.

CABINET, X-RAY TRANSFER *(cont'd)*

S&S Technology 281-815-1300
10625 Telge Rd, Houston, TX 77095
Full line of transfer cabinets, other darkroom cabinets, and x-ray filing systems.

Wolf X-Ray Corporation 800-356-9729
100 W Industry Ct, Deer Park, NY 11729
6 models of cassette transfer boxes.

Xma (X-Ray Marketing Associates, Inc.) 800-325-8880
1205 W Lakeview Ct, Windham Lakes Business Park
Romeoville, IL 60446

CABLE *(Physical Med) 89ISN*

Callcare 800-345-9414
1370 Arcadia Rd, Lancaster, PA 17601

Csi International, Inc. 303-795-8273
4301 S Federal Blvd Ste 116, Englewood, CO 80110

Ep Medsystems, Inc. 609-753-8533
575 N Route 73 Bldg D, West Berlin, NJ 08091
PROCATH disposable and reusable threshold cables.

Epic Medical Equipment Services, Inc. 800-327-3742
1800 10th St Ste 300, Plano, TX 75074
For pulse oximeters and fetal monitoring.

Lake Region Manufacturing, Inc. 952-448-5111
340 Lake Hazeltine Dr, Chaska, MN 55318
OEM Custom contract manufacturing.

Ludlow Technological Products 800-445-5025
2 Ludlow Park Dr, Chicopee, MA 01022
Lead wire and cable.

Ludlum Measurements, Inc. 800-622-0828
501 Oak St, Sweetwater, TX 79556

Medical Cables, Inc. 800-314-51111
1365 Logan Ave, Costa Mesa, CA 92626

Minnesota Wire & Cable Co. 800-258-6922
1835 Energy Park Dr, Saint Paul, MN 55108
Manufacturer of custom wire and cable assemblies for the medical device industry.

Nurse Assist ,Inc. 800-649-6800
3400 Northern Cross Blvd, Fort Worth, TX 76137
QUANTUM Electrosurgical Connecting Cables.

Progeny, Inc. 847-415-9800
675 Heathrow Dr, Lincolnshire, IL 60069
High voltage cables.

Signal Medical Corporation 800-246-6324
1000 Des Peres Rd Ste 140, Saint Louis, MO 63131
CoCR low profile cables. Also cable instruments set, cable passer, tensioner, crimper/cutter, twister/passer, and sterilization case.

Warsaw Orthopedic, Inc. 901-396-3133
2500 Silveus Xing, Warsaw, IN 46582
Cable.

CABLE, ELECTRIC *(General) 80WJG*

American Biosurgical 770-416-1992
1850 Beaver Ridge Cir Ste B, Norcross, GA 30071
Including electrosurgical bipolar cable, monopolar cables, patient plate cables and monopolar cable subassemblies.

Crest Healthcare Supply 800-328-8908
195 3rd St, Dassel, MN 55325
TV-antenna jumper cables. Electrical wiring components.

Minnesota Wire & Cable Co. 800-258-6922
1835 Energy Park Dr, Saint Paul, MN 55108
Custom or standard, all types, designed to customer specifications.

CABLE, ELECTRODE *(Physical Med) 89IKD*

Ballard Medical Products 770-587-7835
12050 Lone Peak Pkwy, Draper, UT 84020
Cable, electrode.

Bard Electro Physiology 800-824-8724
55 Technology Dr, Lowell, MA 01851

Cardima, Inc. 888-354-0300
47266 Benicia St, Fremont, CA 94538
Various.

Dynatronics Corp. Chattanooga Operations 801-568-7000
6607 Mountain View Rd, Ooltewah, TN 37363
Electrode cable.

Evergreen Sales & Marketing, Inc. 651-222-2885
1010 University Ave W Ste 211, Saint Paul, MN 55104
Molded Cable & Lead Wire Assemblies

CABLE, ELECTRODE *(cont'd)*

Invivo Corporation 425-487-7000
12601 Research Pkwy, Orlando, FL 32826
Ecg cable.

Medtronic Neuromodulation 763-514-4000
710 Medtronic Pkwy, Minneapolis, MN 55432
Cable, electrode.

Minnesota Wire & Cable Co. 800-258-6922
1835 Energy Park Dr, Saint Paul, MN 55108
Reusable or disposable.

Mmj S.A. De C.V. 314-654-2000
716 Ponciano Arriaga, Cd. Juarez, Chih. Mexico
Cables

National Cable Molding 323-225-5611
136 N San Fernando Rd, Los Angeles, CA 90031
Various types of patient electrode cables and other contract manufacturing.

Navilyst Medical 800-833-9973
100 Boston Scientific Way, Marlborough, MA 01752
Same.

Nuvasive, Inc. 800-475-9131
7475 Lusk Blvd, San Diego, CA 92121
Electrode cable.

Peter Schiff Enterprise 931-537-6505
4900 Forrest Hill Rd, Cookeville, TN 38506
Electrode cables/pads.

Plastics One, Inc. 540-772-7950
6591 Merriman Rd, Roanoke, VA 24018

Primary Care Physician Platform Llc Dba Qrs Diagnostic 763-559-8492
14755 27th Ave N, Minneapolis, MN 55447

Respiratory Diagnostics, Inc. 425-881-8300
47987 Fremont Blvd, Fremont, CA 94538
Electrode cable.

Rochester Electro Medical, Inc. 813-963-2933
4212 Cypress Gulch Dr, Lutz, FL 33559
Connection, adaptors, clip and snap electrodes (detachable lead wires).

Sterilmed, Inc. 763-488-3400
11400 73rd Ave N Ste 100, Maple Grove, MN 55369
Electrode cable.

Tyco Electronics/Precision Interconnect 503-673-5027
10025 SW Freeman Dr, Wilsonville, OR 97070
Cables & leadwires for electrodes.

CABLE, ELECTROSURGICAL UNIT *(Surgery) 79QTU*

Alto Development Corp. 732-938-2266
5206 Asbury Rd, Wall Township, NJ 07727

Cameron-Miller, Inc. 800-621-0142
5410 W Roosevelt Rd, Road #241, Chicago, IL 60644

Elmed, Inc. 630-543-2792
60 W Fay Ave, Addison, IL 60101

Evergreen Sales & Marketing, Inc. 651-222-2885
1010 University Ave W Ste 211, Saint Paul, MN 55104
Custom Molded Cable & Lead Wire Assemblies

Kirwan Surgical Products, Inc. 888-547-9267
180 Enterprise Dr, PO Box 427, Marshfield, MA 02050
Disposable electrosurgical bipolar cables.

Minnesota Wire & Cable Co. 800-258-6922
1835 Energy Park Dr, Saint Paul, MN 55108
For active and dispersive electrodes.

Richard Wolf Medical Instruments Corp. 800-323-9653
353 Corporate Woods Pkwy, Vernon Hills, IL 60061

CABLE, FIBEROPTIC *(General) 80QFM*

Advanced Endoscopy Devices, Inc. 818-227-2720
22134 Sherman Way, Canoga Park, CA 91303
Universal cable adapts to any manufacturer's scope lightsource.

Automated Medical Products Corp. 800-832-4567
PO Box 2508, Edison, NJ 08818

Biolitec, Inc. 800-934-2377
515 Shaker Rd, East Longmeadow, MA 01028
Manufacture PCS hard clad and all-silica optical fiber (248um to 2.1 micron) and medical fiber optic assemblies (25 to 100 watts).

Clinimed, Incorporated 877-CLINIMED
303 Markus Ct, Sandy Brae Industrial Park, Newark, DE 19713

CABLE, FIBEROPTIC *(cont'd)*

Codman & Shurtleff, Inc 800-225-0460
325 Paramount Dr, Raynham, MA 02767

Coopersurgical, Inc. 800-243-2974
95 Corporate Dr, Trumbull, CT 06611
Cables can be special ordered in any length.

Elmed, Inc. 630-543-2792
60 W Fay Ave, Addison, IL 60101

Integra Luxtec, Inc. 800-325-8966
99 Hartwell St, West Boylston, MA 01583

Karl Storz Endoscopy-America Inc. 800-421-0837
600 Corporate Pointe, Culver City, CA 90230

Keeler Instruments Inc. 800-523-5620
456 Park Way, Broomall, PA 19008

Rei Rotolux Enterprises, Inc. 888-773-7611
4145 North Service Rd, Ste. 200, Burlington, ON L7L 6A3 Canada
5mm in diameter, made of pure silica glass, autoclavable with universal adaptors. Custom lengths are available.

Smith & Nephew, Inc., Endoscopy Division 800-343-8386
150 Minuteman Rd, Andover, MA 01810

Sunoptic Technologies 877-677-2832
6018 Bowdendale Ave, Jacksonville, FL 32216
High performance fiberoptic cables and adaptors, all types, sizes and lengths, autoclavable.

CABLE, LASER, FIBEROPTIC *(Surgery) 79ULX*

Biolitec, Inc. 800-934-2377
515 Shaker Rd, East Longmeadow, MA 01028
Manufacture contact laser fibers to customer specifications. Shaped tips available with or without optional handpieces; diameters range from 200-1000 microns. Gas or liquid cooled delivery systems also available (1.8 or 2.2 mm). 248nm to 2.1 micron wavelength; 25 to 100 watts power.

Medical Energy, Inc. 850-469-1727
225 E Zaragoza St, Pensacola, FL 32502
LASER-POWER TOUCH: disposable contact/non-contact Nd:YAG delivery FIBER. UROLITE: Radial emission contact/non- contact. ND:YAG and 980nm delivery fiber.

Novosci Corp. 281-363-4949
2828 N Crescentridge Dr, The Woodlands, TX 77381
Quartz fibers for contact and non-contact light energy from 488nm to 1064nm and 2010nm for medical applications.

Photovac Laser Corp., Inc. 614-875-3300
3513 Farm Bank Way, Grove City, OH 43123

Schott Glass Technologies, Inc. 570-457-7485
400 York Ave, Duryea, PA 18642

Vitalcor, Inc. 800-874-8358
100 Chestnut Ave, Westmont, IL 60559
Applied Fiberoptics fiber-optic cables for surgical headlight systems.

CABLE, PACEMAKER *(Cardiovascular) 74WWW*

St. Jude Medical Atrial Fibrillation 800-328-3873
14901 Deveau Pl, Minnetonka, MN 55345
Disposable pacing/threshold cables for connecting temporary pacemakers and pacing analyzers to pacing leads.

CABLE/LEAD, ECG *(Cardiovascular) 74REP*

Cardiac Pacemakers, Inc. 800-227-3422
4100 Hamline Ave N, P.O. Box 64079, Saint Paul, MN 55112

Cone Instruments, Inc. 800-321-6964
5201 Naiman Pkwy, Solon, OH 44139

Cp Medical Corporation 800-950-2763
803 NE 25th Ave, Portland, OR 97232
ECG Cable/Lead

Crest Healthcare Supply 800-328-8908
195 3rd St, Dassel, MN 55325

Elmed, Inc. 630-543-2792
60 W Fay Ave, Addison, IL 60101

Evergreen Sales & Marketing, Inc. 651-222-2885
1010 University Ave W Ste 211, Saint Paul, MN 55104
Custom Molded Cable & Lead Wire Assemblies

Ge Medical Systems Information Technologies 800-643-6439
8200 W Tower Ave, Milwaukee, WI 53223
A unique patient cable and leadwire system. The leadwire sets are common to the patient cable for bedside monitoring and to the telemetry transmitter. The system cables and leadwires are electrically shielded to protect the integrity of the ECG signal, are resistant to a wide range of commonly used hospital cleaning agents, and yet remain highly flexible for patient comfort.

CABLE/LEAD, ECG *(cont'd)*

Maguire Enterprises, Inc. 800-548-9686
10289 NW 46th St, Sunrise, FL 33351
Sync/Slave cables (ECG/IBP) from bedside monitor to/from defibrillators, balloon pumps, and ultrasound units. Device Activated Nurse Call Alarm Cables.

Minnesota Wire & Cable Co. 800-258-6922
1835 Energy Park Dr, Saint Paul, MN 55108
ECG cable assemblies for all applications; custom or standard.

Plastics One, Inc. 540-772-7950
6591 Merriman Rd, Roanoke, VA 24018

Pulse Biomedical Inc. 610-666-5510
1305 Catfish Ln, Norristown, PA 19403
Lead Wire

Tsi Medical Ltd. 800-661-7263
47 Athabascan Ave., Unit 105, Sherwood Park, AB T8A-4H3 Canada

CABLE/LEAD, ECG, RADIOLUCENT *(Cardiovascular) 74WLG*

Minnesota Wire & Cable Co. 800-258-6922
1835 Energy Park Dr, Saint Paul, MN 55108
Specialized high-strength carbon fiber.

CABLE/LEAD, ECG, WITH TRANSDUCER AND ELECTRODE *(Cardiovascular) 74DSA*

Advantage Medical Electronics, Inc. 954-345-9800
10630 Wiles Rd, Coral Springs, FL 33076
Cable, transducer and electrode, patient, (including connector).

Affinity Medical Technologies Llc 949-477-9495
1732 Reynolds Ave, Irvine, CA 92614
ECG patient cables and leadwires.

Cardima, Inc. 888-354-0300
47266 Benicia St, Fremont, CA 94538
Various.

Curbell Electronics Inc. 716-667-3377
20 Centre Dr, Orchard Park, NY 14127
Electrode clip.

Docxs Biomedical Products And Accessories 707-462-2351
564 S Dora St Ste A-1, Ukiah, CA 95482
Patient cable, lead wires, custom lead wires.

Evergreen Sales & Marketing, Inc. 651-222-2885
1010 University Ave W Ste 211, Saint Paul, MN 55104
Custom Molded Cable & Lead Wire Assemblies

Grass Technologies, An Astro-Med, Inc. Product Gro 401-828-4002
53 Airport Park Drive, Rockland, MA 02370
Strain gage coupler.

Masimo Corp. 800-326-4890
40 Parker, Irvine, CA 92618
Senors (oximetry) and cables.

Medical Cables, Inc. 800-314-51111
1365 Logan Ave, Costa Mesa, CA 92626
ECG leads, ECG cable, transducer and electrode, patient connector.

Minnesota Wire & Cable Co. 800-258-6922
1835 Energy Park Dr, Saint Paul, MN 55108

Pace Medical, Inc. 781-890-5656
391 Totten Pond Rd, Waltham, MA 02451
8ft. sterile cable with alligator clips on one end.

Quality Cable Assembly, Llc 248-236-9915
3204 Adventure Ln, Oxford, MI 48371
Electrical connectors.

Respiratory Diagnostics, Inc. 425-881-8300
47987 Fremont Blvd, Fremont, CA 94538
Electrosurgical ground pad.

Tyco Electronics/Precision Interconnect 503-673-5027
10025 SW Freeman Dr, Wilsonville, OR 97070
Various types of cable & leadwire systems.

Vital Connections, Inc. 937-667-3880
955 N 3rd St, Phoneton, OH 45371
Egg cables, leadwires and accessories.

CABLE/LEAD, EEG *(Cns/Neurology) 84VDF*

Ad-Tech Medical Instrument Corp. 800-776-1555
1901 William St, Racine, WI 53404
TECH-ATTACH; CABRIO EEG connecting cables.

Evergreen Sales & Marketing, Inc. 651-222-2885
1010 University Ave W Ste 211, Saint Paul, MN 55104
Custom Molded Cable & Lead Wire Assemblies

CABLE/LEAD, EEG *(cont'd)*

Minnesota Wire & Cable Co. 800-258-6922
1835 Energy Park Dr, Saint Paul, MN 55108
Sized to smallest available; flexible high strength #36 AWG.

Plastics One, Inc. 540-772-7950
6591 Merriman Rd, Roanoke, VA 24018

Pmt Corp. 800-626-5463
1500 Park Rd, Chanhassen, MN 55317

Quadromed Inc. 800-363-0192
5776 Thimens Ave., St-Laurent, QUE H4R 2K9 Canada

CABLE/LEAD, EMG *(Cns/Neurology) 84VDG*

Evergreen Sales & Marketing, Inc. 651-222-2885
1010 University Ave W Ste 211, Saint Paul, MN 55104
Custom Molded Cable & Lead Wire Assemblies

Minnesota Wire & Cable Co. 800-258-6922
1835 Energy Park Dr, Saint Paul, MN 55108
Sized to smallest available; flexible high strength; #36 AWG.

Plastics One, Inc. 540-772-7950
6591 Merriman Rd, Roanoke, VA 24018

The Electrode Store 360-829-0400
PO Box 188, Enumclaw, WA 98022

CABLE/LEAD, TENS *(Cns/Neurology) 84VDH*

Electro Therapeutic Devices Inc. 800-268-3834
570 Hood Rd., Ste. 14, Markham, ONT L3R 4G7 Canada

Evergreen Sales & Marketing, Inc. 651-222-2885
1010 University Ave W Ste 211, Saint Paul, MN 55104
Custom Molded Cable & Lead Wire Assemblies

Medical Science Products, Inc. 800-456-1971
517 Elm Ridge Ave, P.O. Box 381, Canal Fulton, OH 44614
MSP TENS lead wires with flexible PVC wire and pin- or snap-type compatibility.

Minnesota Wire & Cable Co. 800-258-6922
1835 Energy Park Dr, Saint Paul, MN 55108
Large selection available of molded terminators.

Plastics One, Inc. 540-772-7950
6591 Merriman Rd, Roanoke, VA 24018

CAGE, ANIMAL *(Microbiology) 83THA*

Carolina Biological Supply Co. 800-334-5551
2700 York Rd, Burlington, NC 27215

Nalge Nunc International 800-625-4327
75 Panorama Creek Dr, Rochester, NY 14625
NALGENE plastic domicile and metabolic cages for rodents; activity wheels; racks and accessories.

Suburban Surgical Co., Inc. 800-323-7366
275 12th St, Wheeling, IL 60090
Stainless steel cages and runs to accommodate mice, rats, dogs, cats, rabbits, guinea pigs, primates.

CAGE, KNEE *(Physical Med) 89ITM*

Bird & Cronin, Inc. 651-683-1111
1200 Trapp Rd, Saint Paul, MN 55121
Knee splint, post-op.

Caguas Orthopedic Center, Inc. 787-744-2325
FF4 Calle 11, Villa Del Rey, Caguas, PR 00727
Cage, knee.

Dj Orthopedics De Mexico, S.A. De C.V. 690-727-1280
Blvd., Delagacion La Presa, Tijuana 22397 Mexico
Functional knee brace

Dj Orthopedics De Mexico, S.A. De C.V. 690-727-1280
Ave. Venustiano Carranza 6802, Castillo, Tijuana 22100 Mexico
Functional knee brace

Orthotic & Prosthetic Lab, Inc. 314-968-8555
748 Marshall Ave, Webster Groves, MO 63119
O&p knee cage.

Tartan Orthopedics, Ltd. 888-287-1456
10651 Irma Dr Unit C, Northglenn, CO 80233
$50.00 per unit (standard).

Truform Orthotics & Prosthetics 800-888-0458
3960 Rosslyn Dr, Cincinnati, OH 45209

CALCULATOR, DRUG DOSE *(Surgery) 79NDC*

Glucotec, Inc. 864-370-3297
14 Pelham Ridge Dr # D, Greenville, SC 29615
Glucommander.

CALCULATOR, DRUG DOSE *(cont'd)*

Lewis Pharmaceutical Information, Llc 423-942-9445
534 Spears Rd, Kimball, TN 37347
Dosebuster renal function dose calculator, lpi pharmacy advisor.

Md Scientific Llc 704-335-1300
2815 Coliseum Centre Dr, --suite 250, Charlotte, NC 28217
Drug dose calculator.

CALCULATOR, TECHNIQUE, RADIOGRAPHIC *(Radiology) 90WSH*

Supertech, Inc. 800-654-1054
PO Box 186, Elkhart, IN 46515
$150 for X-ray technique calculator kit which gives combinations of KV, time, screens, distance and filtrations. Corrects for all causes of light or dark film and can be used for all screens including rare earth. Also Software download to Palm.

CALIBRATOR SOURCE, NUCLEAR SEALED *(Radiology) 90IXD*

Ballard Medical Products 770-587-7835
12050 Lone Peak Pkwy, Draper, UT 84020
Pytest, standard test.

Biodex Medical Systems, Inc. 800-224-6339
20 Ramsey Rd, Shirley, NY 11967

Bristol-Myers Squibb Medical Imaging 978-671-8350
331 Treble Cove Rd, North Billerica, MA 01862
Samarium sm-153 calibration source, various sizes and configurations threrof.

Capintec, Inc. 800-631-3826
6 Arrow Rd, Ramsey, NJ 07446

Diagnostix Plus, Inc. 516-536-2670
100 N Village Ave Ste 33, Rockville Centre, NY 11570
Many new and used accessory items for setting up a nuclear hot lab.

Dome Imaging Systems, Inc. 866-752-6271
400 5th Ave, Waltham, MA 02451
Luminance calibration.

Eckert & Ziegler Isotope Products 661-309-1034
24937 Avenue Tibbitts, Valencia, CA 91355
Various types of calibration sources with multiple nuclides.

International Isotopes Inc. 800-699-3108
4137 Commerce Cir, Idaho Falls, ID 83401

Isotope Products Laboratories, Inc. 661-309-1010
24937 Avenue Tibbitts, Valencia, CA 91355

Lantheus Medical Imaging, Inc. 1-800-362-2668
331 Treble Cove Rd Bldg 200-2, North Billerica, MA 01862
SAMARIUM SM-153

Marconi Medical Systems 800-323-0550
595 Miner Rd, Cleveland, OH 44143

Qsa-Global Inc. 781-272-2000
40 North Ave, Burlington, MA 01803
Source, calibration, sealed, nuclear.

Sanders Medical Products, Inc. 865-588-8998
520 Bearden Park Cir, Knoxville, TN 37919
Calibration source.

CALIBRATOR, AUDIOMETER *(Ear/Nose/Throat) 77EWA*

Ambco Electronics 800-345-1079
15052 Red Hill Ave Ste D, Tustin, CA 92780

Monitor Instruments Inc. 800-853-6785
437 Dimmocks Mill Rd, Hillsborough, NC 27278
MI-300 Calibration Monitor performs a quick and efficient daily biological calibration check of your audiometer. Lightweight and durable construction ensures years of trouble-free operation. 3 LED indicators, left response, right response, power, automatic power off when not in use.

Tremetrics 800-825-0121
7625 Golden Triangle Dr, Eden Prairie, MN 55344
$545.00 for portable battery operated OSCAR 6 Electro-Acoustic Ear which tests frequencies of 250 HZ-8000 HZ.

CALIBRATOR, BEAM *(Radiology) 90WPC*

Capintec, Inc. 800-631-3826
6 Arrow Rd, Ramsey, NJ 07446

CALIBRATOR, BLOOD GAS *(General) 80WMK*

Aga Linde Healthcare P.R. Inc. 787-622-7900
PO Box 363868, GPO Box 364727, San Juan, PR 00936
General.

CALIBRATOR, BLOOD GAS *(cont'd)*

Rna Medical, A Division Of Bionostics, Inc. 800-533-6162
7 Jackson Rd, Devens, MA 01434
Calibration Verification Control/Linearity Material for Blood Gas Instruments and CO-Oximeters.

Thermo Fisher Scientific Inc. 781-622-1000
81 Wyman St, Waltham, MA 02451

CALIBRATOR, CELL INDICES *(Hematology) 81KRX*

Biosure, Inc. 800-345-2267
12301 Loma Rica Dr Unit G, Grass Valley, CA 95945
Flow cytometry contols for DNA and instrument calibration. Chicken, trout and calf thymocyte nuclei for checking instrument linearty, cell cycle analysis and as internal controls. Just add control to your stain and analyze.

Clinical Diagnostic Solutions, Inc. 954-791-1773
1800 NW 65th Ave, Plantation, FL 33313
Calibrator for use on automated hematology analyzers.

Horiba Abx 888-903-5001
34 Bunsen, Irvine, CA 92618
Calibrator for cell indices.

R & D Systems, Inc. 1-800-343-7475
614 McKinley Pl NE, Minneapolis, MN 55413
Impedance and laser calibrators.

CALIBRATOR, DOSE, RADIONUCLIDE *(Radiology) 90KPT*

Biodex Medical Systems, Inc. 800-224-6339
20 Ramsey Rd, Shirley, NY 11967
ATOMLAB 300 Simplifies compliance with built-in constancy reports, clock/calendar and generates peel-n-stick syringe labels. Price $6,600.

Capintec, Inc. 800-631-3826
6 Arrow Rd, Ramsey, NJ 07446

Diagnostix Plus, Inc. 516-536-2670
100 N Village Ave Ste 33, Rockville Centre, NY 11570
New and used dose calibrators.

Mills Biopharmaceuticals, Llc 405-523-1868
120 NE 26th St, Oklahoma City, OK 73105
Automatic needle loading system.

Qsa-Global Inc. 781-272-2000
40 North Ave, Burlington, MA 01803
Calibrator, dose, radionuclide.

Standard Imaging, Inc. 608-831-0025
3120 Deming Way, Middleton, WI 53562
Well chamber.

Sun Nuclear Corp. 321-259-6862
425 Pineda Ct Ste A, Melbourne, FL 32940
Various atomlab dose calibrators:models 1070,1071,1072 and 1076.

CALIBRATOR, DRUG MIXTURE *(Toxicology) 91DKB*

Mps Acacia 800-486-6677
785 Challenger St, Brea, CA 92821

Verichem Laboratories, Inc. 401-461-0180
90 Narragansett Ave, Providence, RI 02907
No common name listed.

CALIBRATOR, DRUG SPECIFIC *(Toxicology) 91DLJ*

Bayer Healthcare, Llc 574-256-3430
430 S Beiger St, Mishawaka, IN 46544
Calibrator.

Biochemical Diagnostics, Inc. 800-223-4835
180 Heartland Blvd, Edgewood, NY 11717
Urinary calibrators for toxicology proficiency.

Lin-Zhi International, Inc. 408-732-3856
687 N Pastoria Ave, Sunnyvale, CA 94085
Phencyclidine calibrators, opiate caibrators, cocaine calibrators & amphetamines.

Opus Diagnostics, Inc. 877-944-1777
1 Parker Plz, Fort Lee, NJ 07024
Innofluor Amikacin; Carbamazepine; Digitoxin; Digoxin; Gentamicin; Phenobarbital; Phenytoin; Quinidine; Theophylline; Tobramycin; Valproic Acid; Vancomycin; Topiramate; Teicoplanin calibrator sets.

Oxis International, Inc. 800-547-3686
468 N Camden Dr Fl 2, Beverly Hills, CA 90210
1-ml theophylline, phenytoin, phenobarbital, gentamicin, tobramycin, or vancomycin fluorescence polarization calibrator for immunoassay. Also, Amikacin, Carbamazepine, Digoxin, Quinidine, and Valproic Acid.

CALIBRATOR, ETHYL ALCOHOL *(Toxicology) 91DNN*

Jas Diagnostics, Inc. 305-418-2320
7220 NW 58th St, Miami, FL 33166
Ethanol calibrator/ controls.

Nerl Diagnostics Llc. 401-824-2046
14 Almeida Ave, East Providence, RI 02914
Ethyl alcohol calibrators.

Verichem Laboratories, Inc. 401-461-0180
90 Narragansett Ave, Providence, RI 02907
No common name listed.

CALIBRATOR, GAS, PRESSURE *(Anesthesiology) 73BXX*

Aga Linde Healthcare P.R. Inc. 787-622-7900
PO Box 363868, GPO Box 364727, San Juan, PR 00936
Anesth/ Pul Med.

Allied Healthcare Products, Inc. 800-444-3954
1720 Sublette Ave, Saint Louis, MO 63110

Netech, Corp. 800-547-6557
110 Toledo St, Farmingdale, NY 11735
Several Models of Pressure/Vacuum Meters are available with different accuracies, pressure ranges, and features to meet any medical requirement. All models are powered by one 9 Volt alkaline battery or an optional AC adapter. The small Digimano 1000 series have an accuracy of 0.25% full scale and display two ranges. A Luer lock connector and data output are standard. The Digimano 2000 series offers accuracies of 0.1% or 0.05% FS and display 5 engineering units, in several ranges. A UL version is available. The Unimano series is the most comprehensive model with the display of 8 engineering units, multiple ranges, and a temperature option.

Thermo Fisher Scientific Inc. 781-622-1000
81 Wyman St, Waltham, MA 02451
Calibrated gas, (specific concentration).

CALIBRATOR, GAS, VOLUME *(Anesthesiology) 73BXW*

Allied Healthcare Products, Inc. 800-444-3954
1720 Sublette Ave, Saint Louis, MO 63110

Caldyne, Inc. 215-830-3076
2425 Maryland Rd, Willow Grove, PA 19090

Hans Rudolph, Inc. 816-363-5522
7200 Wyandotte St, Kansas City, MO 64114
Dlco simulator.

CALIBRATOR, HEARING-AID/EARPHONE AND ANALYSIS SYSTEMS *(Ear/Nose/Throat) 77ETW*

Cardinal Healthcare 209, Inc. 610-862-0800
5225 Verona Rd, Fitchburg, WI 53711
Dpoae system.

Etymonic Design Inc. 800-265-2093
41 Byron Ave., Dorchester, ONT N0L 1G0 Canada
REAL EAR measurement system. VERIFIT Real-Ear Hearing-Aid Analyzer.

Starkey Laboratories, Inc. 800-328-8602
6700 Washington Ave S, Eden Prairie, MN 55344

CALIBRATOR, HEMOGLOBIN AND HEMATOCRIT MEASUREMENT *(Hematology) 81KRZ*

Bio-Rad Laboratories Inc., Clinical Systems Div. 800-224-6723
4000 Alfred Nobel Dr, Hercules, CA 94547
Hemoglobin a1c program.

Horiba Abx 888-903-5001
34 Bunsen, Irvine, CA 92618
Multi-parameter whole blood calibrator.

R & D Systems, Inc. 1-800-343-7475
614 McKinley Pl NE, Minneapolis, MN 55413
Impedance and laser calibrators.

Vegamed, Inc. 787-807-0392
39 Calle Las Flores, Edificio Multifabril #5, Vega Baja, PR 00693
Calibrator for hematocrit and hemoglobin.

Wampole Laboratories 800-257-9525
2 Research Way, Princeton, NJ 08540
Spuncrit Hematocrit/Hemoglobin Analyzer measures hematocrit and provides estimated hemoglobin from fingerstick blood.

CALIBRATOR, MASS SPECTROMETER *(General) 80WML*

Jeol Usa, Inc. 978-536-2270
11 Dearborn Rd, Peabody, MA 01960

Kratos Analytical Inc. 800-935-0213
100 Red Schoolhouse Rd Bldg A, Spring Valley, NY 10977
High performance GC-MS and LC-MS.

CALIBRATOR, PLATELET COUNTING *(Hematology) 81KRY*

Horiba Abx 888-903-5001
34 Bunsen, Irvine, CA 92618
Multi-parameter whole blood calibrator.

R & D Systems, Inc. 1-800-343-7475
614 McKinley Pl NE, Minneapolis, MN 55413

CALIBRATOR, PRESSURE TRANSDUCER *(Anesthesiology) 73QFO*

Dresser Inc., Dresser Measurement Division 203-426-3115
PO Box 5605, Newtown, CT 06470
HEISE Lightweight, pressure calibrator with interchangeable modules for measurement of pressure. Ideal for performing preventive maintenance on infusion pumps, anesthesia equipment, sterilizers, utility supplies.

Kistler Instrument Corp. 716-691-5100
75 John Glenn Dr, Amherst, NY 14228

CALIBRATOR, PRIMARY, CLINICAL CHEMISTRY *(Chemistry) 75JIS*

Beckman Coulter, Inc. 800-742-2345
250 S Kraemer Blvd, PO Box 8000, Brea, CA 92821

Carolina Liquid Chemistries Corp. 800-471-7272
510 W Central Ave Ste C, Brea, CA 92821
Lipid calibrator.

Dade Behring, Inc. 800-948-3233
1717 Deerfield Rd, Deerfield, IL 60015

Diazyme Laboratories 858-455-4761
12889 Gregg Ct, Poway, CA 92064
Hba1c enzymatic assay.

Health Chem Diagnostics Llc 954-979-3845
3341 W McNab Rd, Pompano Beach, FL 33069
Calibrator, primary.

Hemagen Diagnostics, Inc. 800-436-2436
9033 Red Branch Rd, Columbia, MD 21045
Various primary calibrators.

Jas Diagnostics, Inc. 305-418-2320
7220 NW 58th St, Miami, FL 33166
C-reactive protein calibrator set.

Maine Standards Company, Llc 800-377-9684
765 Roosevelt Trl Ste 9A, Windham, ME 04062
Various chemistry calibrator kits.

More Diagnostics, Inc. 800-758-0978
PO Box 6714, Los Osos, CA 93412
Cyclosporine C2 Calibrator, whole-blood, 6 levels

Nerl Diagnostics Llc. 401-824-2046
14 Almeida Ave, East Providence, RI 02914
Primary calibrator.

Scantibodies Laboratory, Inc. 619-258-9300
9336 Abraham Way, Santee, CA 92071
Serum calibrator.

Streck Laboratories, Inc. 800-843-0912
7002 S 109th St, Ralston, NE 68128
The VC-100 is a UL approved acid-based titration system for verifying the volume that a pipet of dilutor delivers (1µl to 5,000 µl). Economical and rapidly tests both accuracy and precision.

Teco Diagnostics 714-693-7788
1268 N Lakeview Ave, Anaheim, CA 92807
Direct hdl cholesterol reagent.

Verichem Laboratories, Inc. 401-461-0180
90 Narragansett Ave, Providence, RI 02907
No common name listed.

Vital Diagnostics Inc. 714-672-3553
1075 W Lambert Rd Ste D, Brea, CA 92821
Various calibration standards.

CALIBRATOR, RADIOISOTOPE *(Radiology) 90QFP*

Capintec, Inc. 800-631-3826
6 Arrow Rd, Ramsey, NJ 07446

Lnd, Inc. 516-678-6141
3230 Lawson Blvd, Oceanside, NY 11572

Marconi Medical Systems 800-323-0550
595 Miner Rd, Cleveland, OH 44143

Owens Scientific Inc. 281-394-2311
23230 Sandsage Ln, Katy, TX 77494

Radiology Support Devices 800-221-0527
1904 E Dominguez St, Long Beach, CA 90810

CALIBRATOR, RED CELL AND WHITE CELL COUNTING
(Hematology) 81KSA

Clinical Diagnostic Solutions, Inc. 954-791-1773
1800 NW 65th Ave, Plantation, FL 33313
Latron, latex calibrator.

Horiba Abx 888-903-5001
34 Bunsen, Irvine, CA 92618
Multi-parameter whole blood calibrator.

R & D Systems, Inc. 1-800-343-7475
614 McKinley Pl NE, Minneapolis, MN 55413
Impedance and laser calibrators.

CALIBRATOR, RESPIRATORY THERAPY UNIT
(Anesthesiology) 73QFQ

A-M Systems, Inc. 800-426-1306
131 Business Park Loop, Sequim, WA 98382
Volume calibration syringe Aluminum and Acrylic (Adjustable, 2, 3, or 4 L) - $240.75 to $347.75

Cis-Us, Inc. 800-221-7554
10 Deangelo Dr, Bedford, MA 01730
Aerotech delivery system: nebulizer, nuclear medicine and repiratory therapy.

Jones Medical Instrument Co. 800-323-7336
200 Windsor Dr, Oak Brook, IL 60523
Digitally displays both volume and flow data. $945.00.

Sensidyne, Inc. • 800-451-9444
16333 Bay Vista Dr, Clearwater, FL 33760
GILIBRATOR 2 piston cell calibration unit for air sampling pumps.

CALIBRATOR, SECONDARY, CLINICAL CHEMISTRY
(Chemistry) 75JIT

Alden Medical Llc 413-747-9717
360 Cold Spring Ave, West Springfield, MA 01089
Conductivity/ph.

Biosite Incorporated 888-246-7483
9975 Summers Ridge Rd, San Diego, CA 92121
Bnp calibrators.

Hemagen Diagnostics, Inc. 800-436-2436
9033 Red Branch Rd, Columbia, MD 21045
Various secondary calibrators.

Jas Diagnostics, Inc. 305-418-2320
7220 NW 58th St, Miami, FL 33166
Multi calibrator two levels.

Mission Diagnostics 508-429-0450
333 Fiske St, Holliston, MA 01746
Various types of calibrators for blood gas & electrolyte analyzers.

Nerl Diagnostics Llc. 401-824-2046
14 Almeida Ave, East Providence, RI 02914
Conductivity/ph.

Qualigen, Inc. 760-918-9165
2042 Corte Del Nogal, Carlsbad, CA 92011
Calibrators.

Thermo Fisher Scientific Inc. 781-622-1000
81 Wyman St, Waltham, MA 02451

Verichem Laboratories, Inc. 401-461-0180
90 Narragansett Ave, Providence, RI 02907
No common name listed.

Vital Diagnostics Inc. 714-672-3553
1075 W Lambert Rd Ste D, Brea, CA 92821
Various calibrators.

CALIBRATOR, SURROGATE, CLINICAL CHEMISTRY
(Chemistry) 75JIW

Bayer Healthcare, Llc 574-256-3430
430 S Beiger St, Mishawaka, IN 46544
Calibrator.

CALIBRATOR, TONOMETER *(Ophthalmology) 86HLA*

Gulden Ophthalmics 800-659-2250
225 Cadwalader Ave, Elkins Park, PA 19027

CALIPER *(Orthopedics) 87KTZ*

Abbott Spine, Inc. 847-937-6100
12708 Riata Vista Cir Ste B-100, Austin, TX 78727
Caliper.

Accu-Measure, Llc 303-799-4721
PO Box 4411, Englewood, CO 80155
'Accu-measure.'

CALIPER *(cont'd)*

Alimed, Inc. 800-225-2610
297 High St, Dedham, MA 02026

Arthrex, Inc. 239-643-5553
1370 Creekside Blvd, Naples, FL 34108
Sizing block.

Biomet, Inc. 574-267-6639
56 E Bell Dr, PO Box 587, Warsaw, IN 46582
Various types of caliper.

Dalzell Usa Medical Systems 540-253-7715
PO Box 162, Marshall, VA 20116
Caliper/orchometer.

Dental Usa, Inc. 815-363-8003
5005 McCullom Lake Rd, McHenry, IL 60050
Caliper.

Depuy Spine, Inc. 800-227-6633
325 Paramount Dr, Raynham, MA 02767
Caliper.

Healthtronics Service Center 800-464-3795
300 Townpark Dr NW Ste 260, Kennesaw, GA 30144
DIGITAL. Stores and totalise patient's individual measurements (up to 19 per patient) and store up to 255 patients.

In'Tech Medical, Incorporated 757-224-0177
2851 Lamb Pl Ste 15, Memphis, TN 38118
Caliper.

K2m, Inc. 866-526-4171
751 Miller Dr SE Ste F1, Leesburg, VA 20175
Caliper.

Motloid Company 800-662-5021
300 N Elizabeth St, Chicago, IL 60607
Calipers for metal or wax.

Mydent International 800-275-0020
80 Suffolk Ct, Hauppauge, NY 11788
DEFEND.

Nk Biotechnical Corp. 612-541-0411
701 Decatur Ave N Ste 111A, Golden Valley, MN 55427
Caliper for medical use.

Salvin Dental Specialties, Inc. 800-535-6566
3450 Latrobe Dr, Charlotte, NC 28211
Various types of calipers and measuring devices.

West Coast Surgical Llc. 650-728-8095
141 California Ave Ste 101, Half Moon Bay, CA 94019
Calipers for measuring bone grafts and implant size.

Zimmer Trabecular Metal Technology 800-613-6131
10 Pomeroy Rd, Parsippany, NJ 07054
Caliper.

CALIPER, OPHTHALMIC *(Ophthalmology) 86HOE*

Accutome, Inc. 610-889-0200
3222 Phoenixville Pike, Malvern, PA 19355
Marker.

B. Graczyk, Inc. 269-782-2100
27826 Burmax Park, Dowagiac, MI 49047
Various types of calipers.

Bausch & Lomb Surgical 636-255-5051
3365 Tree Court Ind Blvd, Saint Louis, MO 63122

Demetech Corp. 888-324-2447
3530 NW 115th Ave, Doral, FL 33178
Ophthalmic caliper, ruler, degree gauge.

Diamond Edge Co. 727-586-2927
928 W Bay Dr, Largo, FL 33770
Calipers.

Edmund Industrial Optics 800-363-1992
101 E Gloucester Pike, Barrington, NJ 08007

Elmed, Inc. 630-543-2792
60 W Fay Ave, Addison, IL 60101

Eye Care And Cure 800-486-6169
4646 S Overland Dr, Tucson, AZ 85714
Caliper.

Fibra-Sonics, A Division Of Misonix, Inc. 631-694-9555
1938 New Hwy, Farmingdale, NY 11735
Phacofragmentor and vacuum pump.

Fortrad Eye Instruments Corp. 973-543-2371
8 Franklin Rd, Mendham, NJ 07945

CALIPER, OPHTHALMIC *(cont'd)*

Gyrus Ent L.L.C., Sub. Of Gyrus Acmi, Inc. 508-804-2739
2925 Appling Rd, Bartlett, TN 38133
Various.

Hai Laboratories, Inc. 781-862-9884
320 Massachusetts Ave, Lexington, MA 02420
Ophthalmic caliper - various types.

Katena Products, Inc. 800-225-1195
4 Stewart Ct, Denville, NJ 07834

Stephens Instruments, Inc. 800-354-7848
2500 Sandersville Rd, Lexington, KY 40511
$95.00 per unit (standard).

Total Titanium, Inc. 618-473-2429
140 East Monroe St., Hecker, IL 62248
Various types of ophthalmic calipers.

CALIPER, ORTHOPEDIC *(Orthopedics) 87HSY*

Elmed, Inc. 630-543-2792
60 W Fay Ave, Addison, IL 60101

Kmedic 800-955-0559
190 Veterans Dr, Northvale, NJ 07647

Wolf X-Ray Corporation 800-356-9729
100 W Industry Ct, Deer Park, NY 11729

Zimmer Holdings, Inc. 800-613-6131
1800 W Center St, PO Box 708, Warsaw, IN 46580

CALIPER, SKINFOLD *(General) 80QFR*

Alimed, Inc. 800-225-2610
297 High St, Dedham, MA 02026

Creative Health Products, Inc. 800-742-4478
5148 Saddle Ridge Rd, Plymouth, MI 48170
SLIM GUIDE; $29.95 each for SLIM GUIDE skinfold body fat calipers with instruction book. HARPENDEN, $364.00 each for HARPENDEN skinfold body fat calipers with instruction book and hard cover case. LANGE skinfold caliper, $198.00 each with instruction book and hard cover case.

Fitness Motivation Institute Of America, Inc. 800-538-7790
26685 Sussex Hwy Ste A, Seaford, DE 19973
$59.95 per unit (60mm) & video.

Novel Products, Inc. 800-323-5143
PO Box 408, Rockton, IL 61072
Plastic and spring-loaded.

Seritex Inc. 973-472-4200
1 Madison St, East Rutherford, NJ 07073
Caliper for assessing body fat content.

CALORIMETER *(Chemistry) 75UFN*

Gilson Company, Inc. 800-444-1508
PO Box 200, Lewis Center, OH 43035

Harris Products Group 800-241-0804
2345 Murphy Blvd, Gainesville, GA 30504

Ika-Works, Inc. 800-733-3037
2635 Northchase Pkwy SE, Wilmington, NC 28405
IKA Calorimeter C5000 allows the user to select adiabatic, isoperibolic and time reduced isoperibolic from unit menu.

Linseis, Inc. 800-732-6733
PO Box 666, Princeton Junction, NJ 08550
Model L 63 DDK (DSC) differential micro calorimeter has high resolution, stable baseline and is easy to calibrate.

Medicos Laboratories, Inc. (Mdt) 800-724-4003
801 Montrose Ave, South Plainfield, NJ 07080

Mg Scientific, Inc. 800-343-8338
8500 107th St, Pleasant Prairie, WI 53158

Netzsch Instruments, Inc. 800-688-6738
37 North Ave, Burlington, MA 01803
Full line of advanced Differential Scanning Calorimeters and simultaneous DSC/TGA instruments

Parr Instrument Co. 800-872-7720
211 53rd St, Moline, IL 61265
Semi-automatic oxygen bomb calorimeter for measuring the heats of combustion of solid and liquid fuels, combustible wastes and foods rapidly and precisely.

Preiser Scientific, Inc. 800-624-8285
94 Oliver St, P.O. Box 1330, Saint Albans, WV 25177

Scientech, Inc. 303-444-1361
5649 Arapahoe Ave, Boulder, CO 80303

Standard Instrumentation, Div. Preiser Scientific 800-624-8285
94 Oliver St, Saint Albans, WV 25177

CALORIMETER *(cont'd)*

Ta Instruments 302-427-4000
109 Lukens Dr, New Castle, DE 19720

Ulvac Technologies, Inc. 800-998-5822
401 Griffin Brook Dr, Methuen, MA 01844

Utech Products, Inc. 800-828-8324
135 Broadway, Schenectady, NY 12305

CAMERA, CINE, ENDOSCOPIC (WITH AUDIO) *(Surgery) 79FTS*

Smith & Nephew, Inc., Endoscopy Division 800-343-8386
150 Minuteman Rd, Andover, MA 01810

CAMERA, CINE, ENDOSCOPIC (WITHOUT AUDIO)
(Surgery) 79FWL

Arthrex, Inc. 239-643-5553
1370 Creekside Blvd, Naples, FL 34108
S-vhs video camera-soakable.

JVC Americas Corp. 973-315-5000
1700 Valley Rd, Wayne, NJ 07470

Smith & Nephew, Inc., Endoscopy Division 800-343-8386
150 Minuteman Rd, Andover, MA 01810

CAMERA, CINE, MICROSURGICAL (WITH AUDIO)
(Surgery) 79FWK

Jedmed Instruments Co. 314-845-3770
5416 Jedmed Ct, Saint Louis, MO 63129

CAMERA, CINE, SURGICAL (WITHOUT AUDIO)
(Surgery) 79FWH

JVC Americas Corp. 973-315-5000
1700 Valley Rd, Wayne, NJ 07470
High definition television, standard.

CAMERA, FOCAL SPOT, RADIOGRAPHIC *(Radiology) 90IXH*

Rti Electronics, Inc. 800-222-7537
1275 Bloomfield Ave, Building 5, Unit 29A, Fairfield, NJ 07004
RFM

CAMERA, GAMMA (NUCLEAR/SCINTILLATION)
(Radiology) 90IYX

Diagnostix Plus, Inc. 516-536-2670
100 N Village Ave Ste 33, Rockville Centre, NY 11570
Remanufactured and used SPECT and planar radionuclide gamma cameras.

Digirad Corp. 800-947-6134
13950 Stowe Dr, Poway, CA 92064
Gamma camera.

Dilon Technologies Llc 877-GO-DILON
12050 Jefferson Ave, Newport News, VA 23606
The Dilon 6800, a small field-of-view, high resolution, portable gamma camera for anatomic-specific imaging such as for the breast.

Gamma Medica-Ideas, Inc 877-426-2633
19355 Business Center Dr Ste 8, Northridge, CA 91324
Designs, builds, and markets high-resolution, dedicated, small field-of-view gamma cameras. For breast imaging, LumaGEM 3200S/12K delivers high-resolution solid-state nuclear medicine technology to the breast clinic as an adjunct to traditional mammography. For preclinical imaging, the FLEX Pre-Clinical Platform speeds advances in drug discovery and cancer and genetics research.

Gvi Technology Partners 330-963-4083
1470 Enterprise Pkwy, Twinsburg, OH 44087
Cardiac first pass imaging system.

Health Care Exports, Inc. 800-847-0173
5701 NW 74th Ave, Miami, FL 33166
Refurbished and used spect and planar radionuclide gamma cameras.

Marconi Medical Systems 800-323-0550
595 Miner Rd, Cleveland, OH 44143
Digital Dynacamera with single, 16.25" diam. crystal, comp. with picker computer, weighs 1,800lbs.

CAMERA, GAMMA (NUCLEAR/SCINTILLATION) *(cont'd)*

Medx Incorporated 800-323-6339
3456 N Ridge Ave Ste 100, Arlington Heights, IL 60004
Our mission is to provide high quality Nuclear Medicine equipment, service, support and parts to the medical community. MEDX is the nation's leading remanufacturer of high quality GE, Siemens and Philips gamma cameras since 1973 and has delivered over 3,000 systems and computers worldwide. We offer complete nuclear medicine coverage including facility licensing, ICANL/ACR accreditation, radiation physics, hot lab equipment, cardiac SPECT cameras, new NuQuest computers, installation/relocation, training, upgrades and replacement.

Medx, Inc. 847-463-2020
3456 N Ridge Ave Ste 100, Arlington Heights, IL 60004
Gamma camera and accessories.

Mie America, Inc. 847-981-6100
420 Bennett Rd, Elk Grove Village, IL 60007
Gamma camera (various models).

Myco Instrumentation Source, Inc. 425-228-4239
PO Box 354, Renton, WA 98057

Proportional Technologies, Inc. 713-747-7324
8022 El Rio St, Houston, TX 77054
Multiwire gamma camera.

Spectron Corp. 425-827-9317
934 S Burlington Blvd # 603, Burlington, WA 98233
Reconditioned equipment.

Transphoton Corporation 305-234-0836
14350 SW 142nd Ave, Miami, FL 33186
Gamma camera.

Vanderbilt University 615-343-0068
2201 W End Ave, Nashville, TN 37235
Software for internal dose calculations.

CAMERA, IDENTIFICATION *(General) 80QFT*

Laminex, Inc. 800-438-8850
9900 Brookford St, Charlotte, NC 28273

Nikon Instruments Inc. 800-52-Nikon
1300 Walt Whitman Rd, Melville, NY 11747

CAMERA, MICROSCOPE *(Microbiology) 83TAR*

Carl Zeiss Surgical, Inc. 800-442-4020
1 Zeiss Dr, Thornwood, NY 10594

Carolina Biological Supply Co. 800-334-5551
2700 York Rd, Burlington, NC 27215

Dage-MTI, Inc. 219-872-5514
701 N Roeske Ave, Michigan City, IN 46360

Diagnostic Instruments Inc. 586-731-6000
6540 Burroughs Ave, Sterling Heights, MI 48314
SPOT Digital Cameras, designed specifically for microscope use.

Edmund Industrial Optics 800-363-1992
101 E Gloucester Pike, Barrington, NJ 08007
Video microscope (cameras and monitors).

Hitachi Kokusai Electric America, Ltd. 516-921-7200
150 Crossways Park Dr, Woodbury, NY 11797
VCC-151 - small color camera with Y/C output. KPD - 580 - cooled color camera with 8 second in integration.

JVC Americas Corp. 973-315-5000
1700 Valley Rd, Wayne, NJ 07470

Leica Microsystems (Canada) Inc. 800-205-3422
400 - 111 Granton Drive, Richmond Hill, ONT L4B 1L5 Canada
Analog & Digital Microsocpe Camera's

Micromanipulator Co., Inc., The 800-972-4032
1555 Forrest Way, Carson City, NV 89706
Products and accessories to aid in embryo recovery, grading, splitting, injection, micromanipulation and photomicrography.

Navitar, Inc. 800-828-6778
200 Commerce Dr, Rochester, NY 14623
Video microscope/inspection system.

Nikon Canada Inc., Instrument Div. 905-625-9910
1366 Aerowood Dr., Mississauga, ONT L4W-1C1 Canada

Nikon Instruments Inc. 800-52-Nikon
1300 Walt Whitman Rd, Melville, NY 11747

Sony Electronics, Inc., Medical Systems Div. 800-686-7669
1 Sony Dr, Park Ridge, NJ 07656
High resolution video cameras for surgical and compound microscopes.

Unitron Ltd 631-589-6666
120 Wilbur Pl Ste C, Bohemia, NY 11716

CAMERA, MICROSCOPE *(cont'd)*

Western Scientific Co., Inc. 877-489-3726
4104 24th St # 183, San Francisco, CA 94114
Complete line of video and digital imaging systems.

CAMERA, MULTI FORMAT *(Radiology) 90LMC*

Afp Imaging Corp. 800-592-6666
250 Clearbrook Rd, Elmsford, NY 10523

Agfa Corporation 877-777-2432
PO Box 19048, 10 South Academy Street, Greenville, SC 29602

Atlas Medical Technologies 909-923-7887
1137 E Philadelphia St, Ontario, CA 91761
Atlas sells multi-format cameras in conjuction with our equipment sale. Wet or dry units, new or used.

Carestream Health, Inc. 888-777-2072
150 Verona St, Rochester, NY 14608
Various types of laser printers and accessories.

Codonics 800-444-1198
17991 Englewood Dr, Middleburg Heights, OH 44130
Codonics EP-1000 Color Medical Imager is a desktop network printer, providing the highest image quality of any color medical class printer at a very economical price. It's dye-diffusion technology is the only output to truly rival conventional color photographic film.

Dejarnette Research Systems 410-583-0680
401 Washington Ave Ste 1010, Towson, MD 21204
Accessory to a medical image hard copy device.

Frantz Imaging, Inc. 440-255-1155
7740 Metric Dr, Mentor, OH 44060
Under $30,000.00 for LASERSTAR laser imager, 8x10 automatic film handling from 100 sheet bins; 2200x2750 pixels.

Fujifilm Medical Systems Usa, Inc. 800-431-1850
419 West Ave, Stamford, CT 06902

Multi Imager Service, Inc 800-400-4549
13865 Magnolia Ave Bldg C, Chino, CA 91710
Multiformat and compact video imaging camera. New, used and refurbished video imaging cameras, printers and supplies, and accessories. Buy, sell, trade, lease.

CAMERA, MULTI-IMAGE *(Radiology) 90TAS*

Afp Imaging Corp. 800-592-6666
250 Clearbrook Rd, Elmsford, NY 10523
Multi-format radiology camera.

American Diagnostic Medicine, Inc. 800-262-9645
960 N Industrial Dr Ste 7, Elmhurst, IL 60126
Turnkey Imaging programs specializing in MRI, Nuclear Medicine, PET, and CT. Alternative financing solutions and operating leases

Atlas Medical Technologies 909-923-7887
1137 E Philadelphia St, Ontario, CA 91761

Diagnostix Plus, Inc. 516-536-2670
100 N Village Ave Ste 33, Rockville Centre, NY 11570
Multi-imagers and multi-format cameras, new and used.

Frantz Imaging, Inc. 440-255-1155
7740 Metric Dr, Mentor, OH 44060
Three models - $8,950.00 for SPACEMISER 8-10; $35,500.00 for SPACEMISER 8-17 bulk load; $22,500.00 for SPACEMISER 8-17 cassette load.

Multi Imager Service, Inc 800-400-4549
13865 Magnolia Ave Bldg C, Chino, CA 91710
Multiformat and compact video imaging camera. New, used and refurbished video imaging cameras, printers and supplies, and accessories. Buy, sell, trade, lease.

CAMERA, OPHTHALMIC, AC-POWERED (FUNDUS) *(Ophthalmology) 86HKI*

Canon Development Americas, Inc 949-932-3100
15955 Alton Pkwy, Irvine, CA 92618
CF-60DSi mydriatic fundus camera, CR-DGi all digital non-mydriatic retinal camera (no pupil dilation needed). CF-60UD mydriatic fundus camera, two angles (60, 40), SP switch. Canon Eye Imaging System: Eye Q PRIME: Bundled with Canon's best-selling CR-DGi non-mydriatic retinal camera and the Canon digital EOS 20D, the true Digital Retinal Imaging system, Eye Q PRIME provides great image resolution--8.2 mega pixels--which is perfectly suitable for diabetic retinopathy screening to detect the subtle changes on retina.

Carl Zeiss Surgical, Inc. 800-442-4020
1 Zeiss Dr, Thornwood, NY 10594

CAMERA, OPHTHALMIC, AC-POWERED (FUNDUS) *(cont'd)*

Clarity Medical Systems 925-463-7984
5775 W Las Positas Blvd Ste 200, Pleasanton, CA 94588
Fundus camera.

Escalon Trek Medical 800-433-8197
2440 S 179th St, New Berlin, WI 53146
Camera opththalmic(ac-powered.

Eye Expert, Llc. 252-758-2402
2501 Stantonsburg Rd, Greenville, NC 27834
Digital angiography system for ophthalmic use.

Eyetel Imaging, Inc. 781-890-9989
9130 Guilford Rd, Columbia, MD 21046
Opthalmic camera.

Nidek Inc. 800-223-9044
47651 Westinghouse Dr, Fremont, CA 94539
NIDEK NM-200D digital non-mydriatic handheld portable fundus camera; Model NM-1000D digital non-mydriatic fundus camera.

Nidek, Inc. 510-226-5700
47651 Westinghouse Dr, Fremont, CA 94539
Ophthalmic camera.

Topcon Medical Systems, Inc. 800-223-1130
37 W Century Rd, Paramus, NJ 07652
Four models of retinal cameras: $21,490.00 and $25,990.00 for non-mydriatic cameras; $31,610.00 for mydriatic fluorescein camera; $38,600 for mydriatic fluorescein/ICG camera. Non-contact specular microscope. Also, a complete family of IMAGEnet digital imaging products (please call for current pricing).

CAMERA, OTHER *(General) 80WKP*

American Medical Technologies, Inc. 361-289-1145
5655 Bear Ln, Corpus Christi, TX 78405
UltraCam Intra-Oral Camera. Provides crystal clear, effortless images without the burden of another footcontrol.

Analogic Corporation 978-326-4000
8 Centennial Dr, Peabody, MA 01960
Ultrasound digital film camera.

Briggs Corporation 800-247-2343
PO Box 1698, 7300 Westown Pkwy., Des Moines, IA 50306
Polaroid & Macro V.

Codonics 800-444-1198
17991 Englewood Dr, Middleburg Heights, OH 44130
Horizon Multi-media Dry Medical Imagers print diagnostic film, color paper and grayscale paper at the same time, all automatically. Models available to suit every need and budget, the versatile imageris small enough to fit on a countertop and is the perfect solution in a PACS environment.

Frantz Imaging, Inc. 440-255-1155
7740 Metric Dr, Mentor, OH 44060
Laser cameras.

Isotope Products Laboratories, Inc. 661-309-1010
24937 Avenue Tibbitts, Valencia, CA 91355
Flood Source, Cobalt-57, sealed source for uniformity testing of gamma and spect nuclear cameras. Germanium-68 Phantoms, sealed source for uniformity testing of gamma and spect nuclear cameras.

Itm Partners, Ltd. 210-651-9066
5925 Corridor Pkwy, Schertz, TX 78154
X-ray moire cameras and x-ray imaging and contouring cameras.

Labsphere, Inc. 603-927-4266
231 Shaker St., North Sutton, NH 03260-9986
Integrating-sphere based uniform source systems for camera calibration and characterization.

Nidek Inc. 800-223-9044
47651 Westinghouse Dr, Fremont, CA 94539
3DX stereo disc fundus camera; Models 3DX, 3DXF, and 3DX digital.

CAMERA, OTHER *(cont'd)*

Ophthalmic Imaging Systems 800-338-8436
221 Lathrop Way Ste I, Sacramento, CA 95815
OIS capabilities have expanded significantly in the past few years, beyond traditional high-resolution digital FA and color fundus imaging. For example, OIS now has the ability to automatically import other clinical test and report data directly-tests like OCT, Humphrey visual fields, corneal topography, HRT, etc. These imports do not require the technicians to do anything different than current clinical protocols-OIS simply intercepts the data on its way to the printer and automatically creates an electronic version and adds to the patient database. The Ophthalmology Office™ solution is the integration of imaging, electronic medical records, and practice management. It has the ability to collect data from a variety of other ophthalmic diagnostic devices (like autorefractors, etc.), and also has extensive templates for tech exams and physician exams for the various specialties. The system is also very flexible to adapt to the specific needs of a given physician, while still maintaining a consistent standard database. The knowledgebase is very ophthalmic-specific and is rich in content to cover a variety of ophthalmic specialties.

Pulnix America Inc. 800-445-5444
1330 Orleans Dr, Sunnyvale, CA 94089
Pulnix America CCD cameras, high-resolution CCD cameras, CMOS cameras.

Smith & Nephew, Inc., Endoscopy Division 800-343-8386
130 Forbes Blvd, Mansfield, MA 02048
Dyonics Vision 325Z digital 3-chip camera. Exceptional resolution & color reproduction, 2.5x digital zoom, superior detail. Dyonics Vision 625 digital capture system. 250 MB Zip disk storage capacity, features automatic motion correction, reduces blurring and other image artifacts.

Spectral Instruments, Inc. 520-884-8821
420 N Bonita Ave, Tucson, AZ 85745
Low light level CCD cooled camera.

Surgical Tools, Inc. 800-774-2040
1106 Monroe St, Bedford, VA 24523

CAMERA, POSITRON *(Radiology) 90IZC*

Diagnostix Plus, Inc. 516-536-2670
100 N Village Ave Ste 33, Rockville Centre, NY 11570

Positron Corporation 800-766-2984
1304 Langham Creek Dr Ste 300, Houston, TX 77084
Posicam HZ/HZL and mPower whole body positron tomography system for oncology, neurology and cardiology applications. High sensitivity, dynamic capability, fast throughput.

CAMERA, RADIOGRAPHIC PHOTOSPOT *(Radiology) 90VER*

Ti-Ba Enterprises, Inc. 585-247-1212
25 Hytec Cir, Rochester, NY 14606
Ti-Ba sells FILMSTATION dry laser printer by SONY Medical.

CAMERA, STILL, ENDOSCOPIC *(Surgery) 79FXM*

Coopersurgical, Inc. 800-243-2974
95 Corporate Dr, Trumbull, CT 06611

Karl Storz Endoscopy-America Inc. 800-421-0837
600 Corporate Pointe, Culver City, CA 90230
Single-chip and three-chip models. Digital auto exposure, multi format outputs - optional title generation. Image processing module.

Mahe International Inc. 800-294-7946
468 Craighead St, Nashville, TN 37204

Richard Wolf Medical Instruments Corp. 800-323-9653
353 Corporate Woods Pkwy, Vernon Hills, IL 60061

Smith & Nephew, Inc., Endoscopy Division 800-343-8386
150 Minuteman Rd, Andover, MA 01810

CAMERA, STILL, SURGICAL *(Surgery) 79FTT*

Nikon Instruments Inc. 800-52-Nikon
1300 Walt Whitman Rd, Melville, NY 11747

Richard Wolf Medical Instruments Corp. 800-323-9653
353 Corporate Woods Pkwy, Vernon Hills, IL 60061

4d Medical Systems, Inc. / Ortiz 865-483-5145
1020 Commerce Park Dr Ste B, Oak Ridge, TN 37830

CAMERA, TELEVISION, ENDOSCOPIC (WITH AUDIO) *(Surgery) 79FWG*

Biomet Sports Medicine 530-226-5800
6704 Lockheed Dr, Redding, CA 96002
Camera, various sizes and types, endoscopic.

Mahe International Inc. 800-294-7946
468 Craighead St, Nashville, TN 37204

CAMERA, TELEVISION, ENDOSCOPIC (WITH AUDIO) *(cont'd)*

Medcam Technology, Inc. 888-829-2848
4586 N Hiatus Rd, Sunrise, FL 33351
The Medcam Pro Plus is a high resolution soakable CCD color video camera/light source comination product with UL 2601 classification & CE mark

Nds Surgical Imaging, Inc. 866-637-5237
5750 Hellyer Ave, San Jose, CA 95138

Smith & Nephew, Inc., Endoscopy Division 800-343-8386
150 Minuteman Rd, Andover, MA 01810

CAMERA, TELEVISION, ENDOSCOPIC (WITHOUT AUDIO)

(Surgery) 79FWF

Clarus Medical, Llc. 763-525-8400
1000 Boone Ave N Ste 300, Minneapolis, MN 55427
Camera/light source.

D & D Video Specialists, Llc 405-720-3180
6444 NW Expressway Ste 209, Oklahoma City, OK 73132

Karl Storz Endoscopy-America Inc. 800-421-0837
600 Corporate Pointe, Culver City, CA 90230

Pentax Southern Region Service Center 201-571-2300
8934 Kirby Dr, Houston, TX 77054
Add-on camera.

Pentax West Coast Service Center 800-431-5880
10410 Pioneer Blvd Ste 2, Santa Fe Springs, CA 90670
Pentax add-on camera.

Richard Wolf Medical Instruments Corp. 800-323-9653
353 Corporate Woods Pkwy, Vernon Hills, IL 60061

Seitz Technical Products, Inc. 610-268-2228
729 Newark Rd, Avondale, PA 19311

Smith & Nephew Inc., Endoscopy Div. 978-749-1000
76 S Meridian Ave, Oklahoma City, OK 73107
No common name listed.

Smith & Nephew, Inc., Endoscopy Division 800-343-8386
150 Minuteman Rd, Andover, MA 01810

Solos Endoscopy 800-388-6445
65 Sprague St # B, Boston/dedham Commerce Park, Boston, MA 02136
Various models of endoscopic cameras.

Thales Components Corporation 973-812-9000
40G Commerce Way, PO Box 540, Totowa, NJ 07512
ATC3000 3-chip CCD camera with various coupler configurations and video output formats.

Tulip Medical Products 800-325-6526
PO Box 7368, San Diego, CA 92167
The TULIP LCI 300 integrated endoscopic imaging system. This integrated and miniaturized video imager combines the patented HiLUX lamp developed by Welch Allyn with Sony's HyperHAD camera architecture in a superior performance endoscopic imaging system that weighs less than 5 lbs. and is easily affordable.

Vision Systems Group, A Division Of Viking Systems 508-366-3668
134 Flanders Rd, Westborough, MA 01581
Various monitors.

Welch Allyn, Inc. 800-535-6663
4341 State Street Rd, Skaneateles Falls, NY 13153

Wisap America 800-233-8448
8231 Melrose Dr, Lenexa, KS 66214

CAMERA, TELEVISION, MICROSURGICAL (WITH AUDIO)

(Surgery) 79FWE

Jedmed Instruments Co. 314-845-3770
5416 Jedmed Ct, Saint Louis, MO 63129

CAMERA, TELEVISION, MICROSURGICAL (WITHOUT AUDIO)

(Surgery) 79FWD

Coopersurgical, Inc. 800-243-2974
95 Corporate Dr, Trumbull, CT 06611

Jedmed Instruments Co. 314-845-3770
5416 Jedmed Ct, Saint Louis, MO 63129

Seitz Technical Products, Inc. 610-268-2228
729 Newark Rd, Avondale, PA 19311

CAMERA, TELEVISION, SURGICAL (WITH AUDIO)

(Surgery) 79FWC

Hitachi Kokusai Electric America, Ltd. 516-921-7200
150 Crossways Park Dr, Woodbury, NY 11797

Karl Storz Endoscopy-America Inc. 800-421-0837
600 Corporate Pointe, Culver City, CA 90230

CAMERA, TELEVISION, SURGICAL (WITH AUDIO) *(cont'd)*

Nds Surgical Imaging, Inc. 866-637-5237
5750 Hellyer Ave, San Jose, CA 95138
ZeroWire

Stryker Endoscopy 800-435-0220
5900 Optical Ct, San Jose, CA 95138

CAMERA, TELEVISION, SURGICAL (WITHOUT AUDIO)

(Surgery) 79FWB

Coopersurgical, Inc. 800-243-2974
95 Corporate Dr, Trumbull, CT 06611

Isolux Llc 239-514-7475
1045 Collier Center Way Ste 6, Naples, FL 34110
Camera headlight system.

Nds Surgical Imaging, Inc. 866-637-5237
5750 Hellyer Ave, San Jose, CA 95138
OR overhead camera, inline camera for Surgical Lights

Progeny, Inc. 847-415-9800
675 Heathrow Dr, Lincolnshire, IL 60069
Surgical camera.

Qed, Inc. 859-231-0338
750 Enterprise Dr, Lexington, KY 40510
Bfw headlight/video camera system.

Vts Medical Systems, Inc. 516-249-1703
40 Melville Park Rd, Melville, NY 11747
Camera.

Welch Allyn, Inc. 800-535-6663
4341 State Street Rd, Skaneateles Falls, NY 13153

CAMERA, VIDEO *(General) 80WQX*

Advanced American Biotechnology (Aab) 714-870-0290
1166 E Valencia Dr Unit 6C, Fullerton, CA 92831
$6,995 for video camera, IBM programs and simple microscope. $26,500 for color video camera, 80Mb disk 286 IBM. $4,995 for video camera, IBM program for colony counter or particle size analyzer; also, $5,995 for image analysis video camera, frame grabber and software. Video Densitometry Station: Video camera, stand, grabber & 1D software. Plus high tech scanner to read 35x45 X-ray film...$8,995. Frame Grabber, Video Capturing Card: color-monochrome, for PC 286 or better, Pentium Windows 3.1, 95, NT, Resolution 1,260x986. NTSC, PAL, RGB...$1,495. Colonyj Counting Sorting: Video camera, lens, stand, transilluminator and software with background correction, automatic or manual. User-defined sorting dark, faint or translucent, size, area, perimeter, circularity. For microbial and tissue culture, cell count, Ames test, microscope attachment...$7,995. Core Facility: Gel documentation, chemiluminescence & color microscopy, CF: Integrating CCD monochrome video camera, lens, frame grabber, dark room, transilluminator & color printer. Color video camera, microscope, c-adapter, big-sample scanner, two 18-sets of software. Available only from AAB...$16,950. Gel Documentation & Chemiluminescence: Chem-1; Integrating CCD video camera, (Sensitivity 1 Femtogram proteins, 1pg DNA), lens, frame grabber, dark room, transilluminator, color printer, ELISA & Universal 1D s...$12,995.

Cardiovascular Research, Inc. 813-832-6222
4810 W Gandy Blvd, Tampa, FL 33611
Videotape: technique of cannulation.

Carl Zeiss Meditec Inc. 877-486-7473
5160 Hacienda Dr, Dublin, CA 94568
ZEISS VIDEO DOCUMENTATION SYSTEM - The Zeiss Video Documentation System enables practitioners to explain more clearly to their patients the examination findings and treatment options. The combination of superior Zeiss optics with the miniature high resolution, low-light CCD Camera with integrated optical beam splitter creates a system with the shortest working distance between examiner and patient.

Carolina Biological Supply Co. 800-334-5551
2700 York Rd, Burlington, NC 27215

Deknatel Snowden-Pencer 800-367-7874
5175 S Royal Atlanta Dr, Tucker, GA 30084

Hitachi Kokusai Electric America, Ltd. 516-921-7200
150 Crossways Park Dr, Woodbury, NY 11797
HV-C20 color video camera designed for the industrial user is light weight, cost-effective and ideal for video conferencing, image processing, and microscope appications.

Integra Luxtec, Inc. 800-325-8966
99 Hartwell St, West Boylston, MA 01583

Jedmed Instruments Co. 314-845-3770
5416 Jedmed Ct, Saint Louis, MO 63129

CAMERA, VIDEO *(cont'd)*

Kelleher Medical, Inc. 804-378-9956
3049 St Marys Way, Powhatan, VA 23139

Ken-A-Vision Manufacturing Co., Inc. 800-627-1953
5615 Raytown Rd, Raytown, MO 64133
VIDEO FLEX Imaging device on full 25 inch flexible gooseneck. Focusing as close as 1/4' (6mm) to infinity. $595.00 to $1,495.00.

Lw Scientific 800-726-7345
865 Marathon Pkwy, Lawrenceville, GA 30046
MiniVID eyepiece camera works on any microscope. BioVID medical camera attaches to microscopes, endoscopes, odoscopes, colposcopes, and slit lamps.

Multi Imager Service, Inc 800-400-4549
13865 Magnolia Ave Bldg C, Chino, CA 91710
Multiformat and compact video imaging camera. New, used and refurbished video imaging cameras, printers and supplies, and accessories. Buy, sell, trade, lease.

Peripheral Dynamics Inc. 800-253-0253
5150 Campus Dr, Plymouth Meeting, PA 19462

Photon Technology International, Inc. 609-894-4420
300 Birmingham Road, Birmingham, NJ 08011-0272
IC-200 and IC 300 intensified CCD video camera for low light imaging applications.

Progeny Dental 888-924-3800
1407 Barclay Blvd, Buffalo Grove, IL 60089
Progeny Dental is a leading provider of dental imaging products. Products include: The JB-70 Intraoral X-ray System, Micro and MicroPlus Series Intraoral Cameras, and CygnusRay MPS Digital X-Ray System.

Seitz Technical Products, Inc. 610-268-2228
729 Newark Rd, Avondale, PA 19311

Sleepmed Incorporated 800-334-5085
200 Corporate Pl Ste 5-B, Peabody, MA 01960
DigiTrace Video System is a time synchronized self-contained color video system designed for in-home use.

Smith & Nephew, Inc., Endoscopy Division 800-343-8386
150 Minuteman Rd, Andover, MA 01810
For surgical use. Single chip and three chip technology.

Sony Electronics, Inc., Medical Systems Div. 800-686-7669
1 Sony Dr, Park Ridge, NJ 07656
Video cameras for wide-range of medical applications.

Starkey Florida 800-327-7939
2200 N Commerce Pkwy, Weston, FL 33326
Video autoscope

Vicon Industries Inc. 800-645-9116
89 Arkay Dr, Hauppauge, NY 11788
Video surveillance equipment incl. cameras, lenses, monitors, etc. Also Available, SURVEYOR 99 mini dome systems. A high-speed motorized domed camera/housing system.

Western Scientific Co., Inc. 877-489-3726
4104 24th St # 183, San Francisco, CA 94114
Complete line of video and digital imaging systems.

Wisap America 800-233-8448
8231 Melrose Dr, Lenexa, KS 66214
Single Chip, Three Chip and Eco-cam.

CAMERA, VIDEO, ENDOSCOPIC *(General) 80WQY*

Bryan Corp. 800-343-7711
4 Plympton St, Woburn, MA 01801
Panasonic CCd video camera has automatic white balance with 35mm 6ns endoscopic coupler.

Clinimed, Incorporated 877-CLINIMED
303 Markus Ct, Sandy Brae Industrial Park, Newark, DE 19713

Coopersurgical, Inc. 800-243-2974
95 Corporate Dr, Trumbull, CT 06611
$8,995 for soakable endoscopic video camera and $3,995 for non-soakable endoscopic video camera.

Elmed, Inc. 630-543-2792
60 W Fay Ave, Addison, IL 60101

Endoscopy Support Services, Inc. 800-349-3636
3 Fallsview Ln, Brewster, NY 10509

Innervision Inc. 901-682-0417
6258 E Shady Grove Rd, Memphis, TN 38120

Integra Luxtec, Inc. 800-325-8966
99 Hartwell St, West Boylston, MA 01583

Jedmed Instruments Co. 314-845-3770
5416 Jedmed Ct, Saint Louis, MO 63129

CAMERA, VIDEO, ENDOSCOPIC *(cont'd)*

Karl Storz Endoscopy-America Inc. 800-421-0837
600 Corporate Pointe, Culver City, CA 90230
Completely digital camera systems with large selection of camera heads, including autoclavable models.

Labsphere, Inc. 603-927-4266
231 Shaker St., North Sutton, NH 03260-9986
Uniform source systems for camera calibration and characterization. Luminometers/Radiometers for measuring flux output of endoscopic illuminators.

Mahe International Inc. 800-294-7946
468 Craighead St, Nashville, TN 37204

Md International, Inc. 305-669-9003
11300 NW 41st St, Doral, FL 33178

Olympus America, Inc. 800-645-8160
3500 Corporate Pkwy, PO Box 610, Center Valley, PA 18034

Pentax Medical Company 800-431-5880
102 Chestnut Ridge Rd, Montvale, NJ 07645
$7,135.00 for ultra-miniature solid state add-on color video camera for endoscopic applications. Immersible camera (with 1/3' CCD) weighs only 3 oz. (85g). Packages including color video monitors and direct couplers and/or beamsplitters for all type endoscopes as well as hard copy devices. Medical Grade & Broadcast grade color TV monitors and hard copy devices are also available separately.

Richard Wolf Medical Instruments Corp. 800-323-9653
353 Corporate Woods Pkwy, Vernon Hills, IL 60061

Smith & Nephew, Inc., Endoscopy Division 800-343-8386
150 Minuteman Rd, Andover, MA 01810

Sony Electronics, Inc., Medical Systems Div. 800-686-7669
1 Sony Dr, Park Ridge, NJ 07656

Surgicorp, Inc. 727-934-5000
40347 US Highway 19 N Ste 121, Tarpon Springs, FL 34689
Video cameras, monitors, printers and recorders.

Welch Allyn, Inc. 800-535-6663
4341 State Street Rd, Skaneateles Falls, NY 13153

Whittemore Enterprises, Inc. 800-999-2452
11149 Arrow Rte, Rancho Cucamonga, CA 91730

CAMERA, VIDEO, HEADLIGHT, SURGICAL *(Surgery) 79WRX*

Bulbworks, Inc. 800-334-2852
80 N Dell Ave Unit 5, Kenvil, NJ 07847
Replacement Lamps For All Types Of Cameras, Video, Headlight, And Surgical Equipment

CAMERA, VIDEO, MULTI-IMAGE *(General) 80WZQ*

Ams Innovative Center-San Jose 800-356-7600
3070 Orchard Dr, San Jose, CA 95134

Multi Imager Service, Inc 800-400-4549
13865 Magnolia Ave Bldg C, Chino, CA 91710
Multiformat and compact video imaging camera. New, used and refurbished video imaging cameras, printers and supplies, and accessories. Buy, sell, trade, lease.

Pentax Medical Company 800-431-5880
102 Chestnut Ridge Rd, Montvale, NJ 07645
Video endoscope system features advanced black and white chip technology, compact size and design, documentation ability, and split/live feature for continuous viewing. Color video endoscope system features advanced color chip technology, compact size and design, documentation ability, and split/live feature for continuous viewing.

Smith & Nephew, Inc., Endoscopy Division 800-343-8386
150 Minuteman Rd, Andover, MA 01810

Sony Electronics, Inc., Medical Systems Div. 800-686-7669
1 Sony Dr, Park Ridge, NJ 07656

Welch Allyn, Inc. 800-535-6663
4341 State Street Rd, Skaneateles Falls, NY 13153

CAMERA, VIDEOTAPE, SURGICAL *(Surgery) 79FXN*

Hitachi Kokusai Electric America, Ltd. 516-921-7200
150 Crossways Park Dr, Woodbury, NY 11797

JVC Americas Corp. 973-315-5000
1700 Valley Rd, Wayne, NJ 07470
Multipurpose 3-CCD color video camera.

Sony Electronics, Inc., Medical Systems Div. 800-686-7669
1 Sony Dr, Park Ridge, NJ 07656

Stryker Endoscopy 800-435-0220
5900 Optical Ct, San Jose, CA 95138

CAMERA, VIDEOTAPE, SURGICAL *(cont'd)*

Verg, Inc. 800-563-7676
55 Henlow Bay, #3, Winnipeg, MANIT R3G-1L1 Canada
VeV MD wound-measurement system (Verge Videometer).

CAMERA, X-RAY, FLUOROGRAPHIC, CINE OR SPOT
(Radiology) 90IZJ

Frantz Imaging, Inc. 440-255-1155
7740 Metric Dr, Mentor, OH 44060
2 models - $8,950.00 for SPACEMISER 8-10; $35,500.00 for SPACEMISER 8-17.

Marconi Medical Systems 800-323-0550
595 Miner Rd, Cleveland, OH 44143

Precise Optics/Pme, Inc. 800-242-6604
239 S Fehr Way, Bay Shore, NY 11706

Radiographic And Data Solutions, Inc. 612-379-7152
2101 Kennedy St NE Ste 190, Minneapolis, MN 55413
Fluoroscopic system.

Stallion Technologies, Inc. 315-476-4330
1201 E Fayette St, Syracuse, NY 13210

Thales Components Corporation 973-812-9000
40G Commerce Way, PO Box 540, Totowa, NJ 07512
TH8740 and TH8730 CCD Cameras and Video-kits (optics included) provide for the capture of fluorographic images in 1k x 1k format at up to 60fps.

CAMPYLOBACTER PYLORI *(Microbiology) 83LYR*

Accuech, Llc 760-599-6555
2641 La Mirada Dr, Vista, CA 92081
H. pylori test.

Alfa Scientific Designs, Inc. 877-204-5071
13200 Gregg St, Poway, CA 92064
H.pylori serum cassette.

Ameritek Usa, Inc. 425-379-2580
125 130th St SE Ste 200, Everett, WA 98208
H.pylori test kit.

Ballard Medical Products 770-587-7835
12050 Lone Peak Pkwy, Draper, UT 84020
Ph indicator agar.

Beckman Coulter, Inc. Primary Care Diagnostics 714-961-3712
606 Elmwood Ave, Elmwood Court Three, Sharon Hill, PA 19079
Serological test for helicobacter pylori.

Bio-Medical Products Corp. 800-543-7427
10 Halstead Rd, Mendham, NJ 07945
Helicobactor strip. H. pylori one-step antibody test strip (30 per package). Blood serum 10 minute test. Immunochromatographic test.

Biocheck, Inc. 650-573-1968
323 Vintage Park Dr, Foster City, CA 94404
H.pylori igg quantitative eia test kit.

Biomerica, Inc. 800-854-3002
17571 Von Karman Ave, Irvine, CA 92614
GAP-IGG, clinical lab test for detection of Helicobacter pylori. IgA and IgM test also available; non-campylobacter.

Chembio Diagnostic Systems, Inc. 631-924-1135
3661 Horseblock Rd, Medford, NY 11763
Immunochromatographic assay for visual detection of h. pylori antibodies.

Germaine Laboratories, Inc. 210-692-4192
4139 Gardendale St Ste 101, San Antonio, TX 78229
H. pylori test device, h. pylori dipstick test.

Gi Supply 800-451-5797
200 Grandview Ave, Camp Hill, PA 17011
HPFAST rapid urease test for the prescriptive identification of Helicobacter pylori via gastric biopsy.

Hycor Biomedical, Inc. 800-382-2527
7272 Chapman Ave, Garden Grove, CA 92841
H.pylori iga test.

Immunospec Corporation 818-717-1840
9428 Eton Ave Ste O, Chatsworth, CA 91311
H. pylori igg.

Innovacon, Inc. 858-535-2030
4106 Sorrento Valley Blvd, San Diego, CA 92121
H. pylori immunological test.

CAMPYLOBACTER PYLORI *(cont'd)*

Inverness Medical Professional Diagnostics-San Die 858-535-2030
4106 Sorrento Valley Blvd, San Diego, CA 92121
H. pylori immunological test.

Kenlor Industries, Inc. 714-647-0770
1560 E Edinger Ave Ste A1, Santa Ana, CA 92705
H. pylori serum control (positive & negative).

Meridian Bioscience, Inc. 800-696-0739
3471 River Hills Dr, Cincinnati, OH 45244
PREMIER H. pylori, enzyme immunoasary for H. pylori antibody. PREMIER PLATINUM HpSA, H. pylori specific antigen test detects the presence of H. pylori in system using a non-invasive method.

Micro Detect, Inc. 714-832-8234
2852 Walnut Ave Ste H1, Tustin, CA 92780
H.pylori iga elisa test kit.

Quest Intl., Inc. 305-592-6991
8127 NW 29th St, Doral, FL 33122
H. pylori antibody.

Radient Pharmaceuticals 714-505-4460
2492 Walnut Ave Ste 100, Tustin, CA 92780
Enzyme immunoassay for H. Pylori antibodies in serum.

Serim Research Corp. 574-264-3440
3506 Reedy Dr, Elkhart, IN 46514
Test for helicobacter pylori urease in gastric biopsy specimens.

St. Paul Biotech 714-903-1000
11555 Monarch St, Garden Grove, CA 92841
H. pylori test.

United Biotech, Inc. 650-961-2910
211 S Whisman Rd Ste E, Mountain View, CA 94041
ELISA for detecting Helicobactor pylori IgG.

Wampole Laboratories 800-257-9525
2 Research Way, Princeton, NJ 08540
H. pylori IgG.

Washington Biotechnology, Inc. 206-292-9734
562 1st Ave S Fl 7, Seattle, WA 98104
Helicobacter serology.

Zeus Scientific, Inc. 800-286-2111
PO Box 38, Raritan, NJ 08869

CAMPYLOBACTER SPP. *(Microbiology) 83LQP*

Gen-Probe, Inc. 800-523-5001
10210 Genetic Center Dr, San Diego, CA 92121
AccuProbe CAMPYLOBACTER Culture Identification Test - For the identification of Campylobacter jejuni, C.coli, and C. lari isolated from culture.

CANDIDA SPECIES, ANTIBODY DETECTION
(Microbiology) 83LSG

Sa Scientific, Inc. 800-272-2710
4919 Golden Quail, San Antonio, TX 78240

CANE *(Physical Med) 89IPS*

A&A Orthopedics, Incorporated 757-224-0177
12250 SW 129th Ct Bldg 1, Miami, FL 33186
Wood and aluminum cane.

A.M.G. Medical, Inc. 888-396-1213
8505 Dalton Rd., Montreal, QUE H4T-IV5 Canada

Access Mobility, Inc. 800-336-1147
5240 Elmwood Ave, Indianapolis, IN 46203

Alex Orthopedic, Inc. 800-544-2539
PO Box 201442, Arlington, TX 76006

Alimed, Inc. 800-225-2610
297 High St, Dedham, MA 02026

Ambutech Inc. 800-561-3340
34 DeBaets St., Winnipeg, MAN R2J-3S9 Canada
Adjustable canes (contoured handle, Helix adjustment system) and fixed length canes (contoured handle, wooden shaft), 6 pcs. per carton. Canes for the blind or vision impaired, folding and rigid mobility cane, and folding identification cane.

Assisted Access-Nfss, Inc. 800-950-9655
822 Preston Ct, Lake Villa, IL 60046

Biomet, Inc. 574-267-6639
56 E Bell Dr, PO Box 587, Warsaw, IN 46582
Various types of cane.

Bird & Cronin, Inc. 651-683-1111
1200 Trapp Rd, Saint Paul, MN 55121
Cane.

CANE *(cont'd)*

Colored Plastics, Llc 888-807-9554
6002 NE 72nd St, Bondurant, IA 50035
Colored plastic cane.

Convaquip Industries, Inc. 800-637-8436
4834 Derrick Dr, PO Box 3417, Abilene, TX 79601
Bariatric Quad or single points. Weight certified to 500 lbs.

Dynatronics Corp. Chattanooga Operations 801-568-7000
6607 Mountain View Rd, Ooltewah, TN 37363
Adjustable cane, quad cane, stand assist cane.

Essential Medical Supply, Inc. 800-826-8423
6420 Hazeltine National Dr, Orlando, FL 32822
SPRING GARDEN, STEPPIN' OUT, HIGH SOCIETY, SURE GRIP. DESIGNER OFFSET CANES, DELUXE QUAD CANES - CAT'S MEOW SPECIALTY CANES, WHITE GLOVE SERIES.

Flaghouse, Inc. 800-793-7900
601 US Highway 46 W, Hasbrouck Heights, NJ 07604

Freeman Manufacturing Company 800-253-2091
900 W Chicago Rd, PO Box J, Sturgis, MI 49091
Adjustable black aluminum.

G. Hirsch And Co., Inc. 650-692-8770
870 Mahler Rd, Burlingame, CA 94010
Various types of canes.

Kaye Products, Inc. 919-732-6444
535 Dimmocks Mill Rd, Hillsborough, NC 27278
Pediatric quad canes, handgrip rotates to accommodate developing forearm, two base sizes for small children, three sizes available.

Larkotex Company 800-972-3037
1002 Olive St, Texarkana, TX 75501

Lofstrand Co. 800-221-0142
3435 Collins Pl, Flushing, NY 11354
$7.00 TO $15.00 350 different styles.

Medical Depot 516-998-4600
99 Seaview Blvd, Port Washington, NY 11050
Canes.

Melet Plastics, Inc. 204-667-6635
34 De Baets St, Winnipeg R2J 3S9 Canada
Various models of adjustable, orthopedic canes

Momentum Medical 208-523-3600
1330 Enterprise St, Idaho Falls, ID 83402
Quad cane.

Ortho-Med, Inc. 800-547-5571
3208 SE 13th Ave, Portland, OR 97202
Wooden and aluminium canes.

Paramedical Distributors 800-245-3278
2020 Grand Blvd, Kansas City, MO 64108
Wood and/or aluminum canes, and tips.

Parsons A.D.L. Inc. 800-263-1281
R.R. #2, 1986 Sideroad 15, Tottenham, ONT L0G 1W0 Canada
Light weight walking canes with orthopaedic grips and slip resistant tips.

Pathlighter, Inc. 877-728-4544
105 Riverside Dr, Ormond Beach, FL 32176
Lighted safety cane.

Patterson Medical Supply, Inc. 262-387-8720
W68N158 Evergreen Blvd, Cedarburg, WI 53012
Cane.

Perfect Care 718-805-7800
8927 126th St, Richmond Hill, NY 11418
Cane.

Productos Rubbermaid, Sociedad Anonima De Capital 540-542-8363
Kmi-Ote, Carretera Cadereyta-Allende
Cadereyta Jimenez 67450 Mexico
Various

Secure Products 469-233-0385
914 Thistle Green Ln, Duncanville, TX 75137
Lapstand.

Truform Orthotics & Prosthetics 800-888-0458
3960 Rosslyn Dr, Cincinnati, OH 45209

Tubular Fabricators Industry, Inc. 804-733-4000
600 W Wythe St, Petersburg, VA 23803
Various models of canes.

Tuffcare 800-367-6160
3999 E La Palma Ave, Anaheim, CA 92807

CANE *(cont'd)*

Wheelchairs Of Kansas 800-537-6454
204 W 2nd St, Ellis, KS 67637
The variety of CANES offered for the bariatric individual consists of wood canes, offset canes and quad canes; The offset canes and quad cane are constructed out of heavy-duty steel; The wood canes have an elegant sleek appearance and are offered in a black or walnut finish; Soft, vinyl hand grips on the offset and quad; Customized height for the wood canes; Adjustable height offered on the offset and quad canes; 500 lb. weight capacity.

CANE, SAFETY WALK *(Physical Med) 89KHY*

Assisted Access-Nfss, Inc. 800-950-9655
822 Preston Ct, Lake Villa, IL 60046

Bio-Medic Health Services, Inc. 800-525-0072
5041B Benois Rd Bldg B, Roanoke, VA 24018

In Home Products, Inc. 800-810-8475
12015 Shiloh Rd Ste 158-B, Dallas, TX 75228
Foldable cane with new non-slip tip and CANEKEEPER, which keeps cane attached to body while it is being used.

Invacare Corporation 800-333-6900
1 Invacare Way, Elyria, OH 44035
INVACARE.

Keen Mobility Company 503-285-9090
6500 NE Halsey St Ste B, Portland, OR 97213

Merry Walker Corp. 847-837-9580
21350 Sylvan Dr S Unit 9, Mundelein, IL 60060
MERRY MOVER PD visual stimulation cane for Parkinson's disease patients. Standard cane with lever that lowers to the floor to engage patient in walking, helping eliminate 'freezing' syndrome.

Momentum Medical 208-523-3600
1330 Enterprise St, Idaho Falls, ID 83402
Cane.

Orthotic Mobility Systems, Inc. 301-949-2444
10421 Metropolitan Ave, Kensington, MD 20895
Cane.

Productos Rubbermaid, Sociedad Anonima De Capital 540-542-8363
Kmi-Ote, Carretera Cadereyta-Allende
Cadereyta Jimenez 67450 Mexico
Various

Tuffcare 800-367-6160
3999 E La Palma Ave, Anaheim, CA 92807

CANISTER, COIL *(Gastro/Urology) 78FKD*

Medrad, Inc. 800-633-7231
100 Global View Dr, Warrendale, PA 15086
MR Body surface coils for neurovascular, knee, multi-purpose, extremity and torso. Gore Cardiovascular Array: Cardiovascular Array, MR Body Surface Coil.

CANISTER, LIQUID OXYGEN, PORTABLE *(Anesthesiology) 73BYJ*

Allied Medco, Inc. 631-447-0093
25 Corporate Dr, Holtsville, NY 11742

Caire, Inc. 800-482-2473
1800 Sandy Plains Industrial Parkway, Suite 316, Marietta, GA 30066
STROLLER, STROLLER SPRINT, Spirit 300/600/1200, Portable liquid oxygen unit.

Essex Cryogenics Of Missouri, Inc. 314-832-8077
8007 Chivvis Dr, Saint Louis, MO 63123
Portable therapeutic liquid oxygen unit.

Home Care Express & Mass Bay Respiratory 781-740-9797
85 Research Rd, Hingham, MA 02043
Medical grade gases & other devices.

Inovo, Inc. 239-643-6577
2975 Horseshoe Dr S Ste 600, Naples, FL 34104
Portable & stationary liquid oxygen system.

Medcovers, Inc 800-948-8917
500 W Goldsboro St, Kenly, NC 27542

Puritan Bennett Corp. 925-463-4371
2800 Airwest Blvd, Plainfield, IN 46168
Lox units.

Respond Industries, Inc. 1-800-523-8999
9500 Woodend Rd, Edwardsville, KS 66111
Oxygen unit, portable.

CANISTER, OXYGEN *(Anesthesiology) 73RJL*

Allied Healthcare Products, Inc. 800-444-3954
1720 Sublette Ave, Saint Louis, MO 63110

CANISTER, OXYGEN *(cont'd)*

Erie Medical 800-932-2293
10225 82nd Ave, Lakeview Corporate Park, Pleasant Prairie, WI 53158
Aluminum medical oxygen cylinders supplied in 164-, 247-, 406-, 682-, 1750-, and 3500-liter sizes.

Farley Inc., W.T. 800-327-5397
931 Via Alondra, Camarillo, CA 93012
MRI non-magnetic oxygen regulator. 2-15 Liters/min. Model 3-300A $250.00 MR non-magnetic oxygen regulator 50 PSI Preset, Model 3-250A $250.00.

Life Corporation 800-700-0202
1776 N Water St, Milwaukee, WI 53202
LIFE, OxygenPac Portable emergency oxygen units, clear cover and wall-mounted, off/on lever control, resuscitation mask with one-way valve for hygiene, 6lpm 90min. supply, refillable. Also available 6 & 12 lpm NORM & HIGH, 0-25 lpm variable, and demand-valve for 100% oxygen resuscitation. GSA Federal Supply Schedule.

Mada, Inc. 800-526-6370
625 Washington Ave, Carlstadt, NJ 07072

U O Equipment Co. 800-231-6372
5863 W 34th St, Houston, TX 77092

CANISTER, SUCTION *(Cardiovascular) 74DWM*

Allied Healthcare Products, Inc. 800-444-3954
1720 Sublette Ave, Saint Louis, MO 63110

Bemis Mfg. Co. 800-558-7651
300 Mill St, Sheboygan Falls, WI 53085
Hi-Flow and Hydrophobic rigid plastic suction canisters: Quick-Fit Suction Liner System.

Medela, Inc. 800-435-8316
1101 Corporate Dr, McHenry, IL 60050
Collection canisters autoclavable and not-autoclavable from .25 to 5 liter sizes.

Ohio Medical Corp. 800-662-5822
1111 Lakeside Dr, Gurnee, IL 60031
Disposable canisters in 800 and 1200 cc sizes.

Ohmeda Medical 800-345-2700
8880 Gorman Rd, Laurel, MD 20723

Stryker Puerto Rico, Ltd. 939-307-2500
Hwy. 3, Km. 131.2, Las Guasimas Ind. Park, Arroyo, PR 00714
Blood conversation reservoir.

CANNULA WITH INFLATABLE BALLOON (DISTAL TIP) *(Surgery) 79WZS*

Rocket Medical Plc. 800-707-7625
150 Recreation Park Dr Ste 3, Hingham, MA 02043

CANNULA, AORTIC *(Cardiovascular) 74TAT*

Avalon Laboratories, Inc. 866-938-6613
2610 Homestead Pl, Rancho Dominguez, CA 90220
Pediatric/femoral.

Diablo Sales & Marketing, Inc. 925-648-1611
PO Box 3219, Danville, CA 94526
Custom design and manufacturing of catheters and specialty guidewires. Guiding catheters; stent delivery and drug delivery systems.

Rocket Medical Plc. 800-707-7625
150 Recreation Park Dr Ste 3, Hingham, MA 02043

CANNULA, ARTERIAL *(Cardiovascular) 74QFV*

Alimed, Inc. 800-225-2610
297 High St, Dedham, MA 02026

Cadence Science Inc. 888-717-7677
1979 Marcus Ave Ste 215, New Hyde Park, NY 11042

Ispg, Inc. 860-355-8511
517 Litchfield Rd, New Milford, CT 06776
Ground cannulae

CANNULA, ASPIRATING *(Cardiovascular) 74QFW*

Atc Technologies, Inc. 781-939-0725
30B Upton Dr, Wilmington, MA 01887

Cadence Science Inc. 888-717-7677
1979 Marcus Ave Ste 215, New Hyde Park, NY 11042

Ispg, Inc. 860-355-8511
517 Litchfield Rd, New Milford, CT 06776
Ground cannulae

Medovations, Inc. 800-558-6408
102 E Keefe Ave, Milwaukee, WI 53212

Novosci Corp. 281-363-4949
2828 N Crescentridge Dr, The Woodlands, TX 77381

CANNULA, AV SHUNT *(Gastro/Urology) 78FIQ*

Angiodynamics, Inc. 800-472-5221
1 Horizon Way, Manchester, GA 31816
Full range of shunts and vessel tips including S-300 Series, Allen-Brown, pediatric, and ST-Series with integral tips.

Icu Medical (Ut), Inc 949-366-2183
4455 Atherton Dr, Salt Lake City, UT 84123
Various.

CANNULA, BRAIN *(Cns/Neurology) 84QFX*

Cadence Science Inc. 888-717-7677
1979 Marcus Ave Ste 215, New Hyde Park, NY 11042

Codman & Shurtleff, Inc 800-225-0460
325 Paramount Dr, Raynham, MA 02767

Diablo Sales & Marketing, Inc. 925-648-1611
PO Box 3219, Danville, CA 94526
Custom design and manufacturing of catheters and specialty guidewires. Guiding catheters; stent delivery and drug delivery systems.

Miltex Inc. 800-645-8000
589 Davies Dr, York, PA 17402

CANNULA, BRONCHIAL *(Ear/Nose/Throat) 77KCE*

Bausch & Lomb Surgical 636-255-5051
3365 Tree Court Ind Blvd, Saint Louis, MO 63122

Electro Surgical Instrument Co., Inc. 888-464-2784
37 Centennial St, Rochester, NY 14611
Various types, styles and sizes of aspirating tubes.

Laprostop, Llc 858-705-3838
1845 Newport Avenue, San Diego, CA 92107
Trocar accessory.

CANNULA, CATHETER *(Cardiovascular) 74DQR*

Angiodynamics, Inc. 518-795-1400
14 Plaza Drive, Latham, NY 12110

Argon Medical Devices Inc. 903-675-9321
1445 Flat Creek Rd, Athens, TX 75751
Translumbar aortography needle catheter.

Cadence Science Inc. 888-717-7677
1979 Marcus Ave Ste 215, New Hyde Park, NY 11042

Cardiac Assist, Inc. 412-963-7770
240 Alpha Dr, Pittsburgh, PA 15238
Transseptal cannula.

Diablo Sales & Marketing, Inc. 925-648-1611
PO Box 3219, Danville, CA 94526
Custom design and manufacturing of catheters and specialty guidewires. Guiding catheters; stent delivery and drug delivery systems.

Edwards Lifesciences Research Medical 949-250-2500
6864 Cottonwood St, Midvale, UT 84047
Cannula.

Edwards Lifesciences, Llc. 800-424-3278
1 Edwards Way, Irvine, CA 92614

Insitu Technologies, Inc. 651-389-1017
5810 Blackshire Path, Inver Grove Heights, MN 55076
Guide and angiography catheters.

Ispg, Inc. 860-355-8511
517 Litchfield Rd, New Milford, CT 06776
Ground cannulae

Medovations, Inc. 800-558-6408
102 E Keefe Ave, Milwaukee, WI 53212

Medtronic, Inc. 800-633-8766
710 Medtronic Pkwy, Minneapolis, MN 55432
VC2.

Orqis (Tm) Medical 888-723-7277
14 Orchard Ste 100, Lake Forest, CA 92630
Cannula.

Rose Technologies Company 616-233-3000
1440 Front Ave NW, Grand Rapids, MI 49504

Sorin Group Usa 800-289-5759
14401 W 65th Way, Arvada, CO 80004

United States Endoscopy Group 800-769-8226
5976 Heisley Rd, Mentor, OH 44060
Disposable angulated guide sleeve. 2.5 mm cannula with angled tip; pass cholangiocatheter through the angulated guide sleeve and direct the flexible catheter into the cystic duct.

CANNULA, CATHETER *(cont'd)*

Vitalcor, Inc. 800-874-8358
100 Chestnut Ave, Westmont, IL 60559
Cardiovascular cannula.

CANNULA, CORONARY ARTERY *(Cardiovascular) 74QFY*

Avalon Laboratories, Inc. 866-938-6613
2610 Homestead Pl, Rancho Dominguez, CA 90220

CANNULA, CYCLODIALYSIS (EYE) *(Ophthalmology) 86QGA*

Bausch & Lomb Surgical 636-255-5051
3365 Tree Court Ind Blvd, Saint Louis, MO 63122

Kmi Surgical Ltd. 800-528-2900
110 Hopewell Rd, Laird Professional Building, Downingtown, PA 19335
Disposable cannula.

Stephens Instruments, Inc. 800-354-7848
2500 Sandersville Rd, Lexington, KY 40511
$10.00 each.

Western Ophthalmics Corporation 800-426-9938
19019 36th Ave W Ste G, Lynnwood, WA 98036

CANNULA, DRAINAGE, ARTHROSCOPY *(Orthopedics) 87TAU*

Integral Design Inc. 781-740-2036
52 Burr Rd, Hingham, MA 02043

Karl Storz Endoscopy-America Inc. 800-421-0837
600 Corporate Pointe, Culver City, CA 90230

Mahe International Inc. 800-294-7946
468 Craighead St, Nashville, TN 37204

Richard Wolf Medical Instruments Corp. 800-323-9653
353 Corporate Woods Pkwy, Vernon Hills, IL 60061

Smith & Nephew, Inc., Endoscopy Division 800-343-8386
150 Minuteman Rd, Andover, MA 01810

CANNULA, EAR *(Ear/Nose/Throat) 77JYC*

Aesculap Implant Systems Inc. 1-800-234-9179
3773 Corporate Pkwy, Center Valley, PA 18034

Bausch & Lomb Surgical 636-255-5051
3365 Tree Court Ind Blvd, Saint Louis, MO 63122

Clinimed, Incorporated 877-CLINIMED
303 Markus Ct, Sandy Brae Industrial Park, Newark, DE 19713

Jedmed Instruments Co. 314-845-3770
5416 Jedmed Ct, Saint Louis, MO 63129

Miltex Inc. 800-645-8000
589 Davies Dr, York, PA 17402

CANNULA, EPIDURAL *(Obstetrics/Gyn) 85QFZ*

B. Braun Oem Division, B. Braun Medical Inc. 866-8-BBRAUN
824 12th Ave, Bethlehem, PA 18018

Cadence Science Inc. 888-717-7677
1979 Marcus Ave Ste 215, New Hyde Park, NY 11042
11 types.

Gvs Filter Technology Inc. 317-471-3700
5353 W 79th St, Indianapolis, IN 46268
Epicare Adult is our 0.2µm filter for epidural anesthesia. Double luer lock fittings. Can be vented or non-vented. We also offer Epicare Baby. All Epicare filters have our new high pressure rating of 8.5 bar. Available only on an OEM basis.

Ispg, Inc. 860-355-8511
517 Litchfield Rd, New Milford, CT 06776

Ranfac Corp. 800-2RANFAC
30 Doherty Ave, Avon Industrial Park, Avon, MA 02322
$18.00 to $20.00 each.

Tegra Medical Inc. 508-541-4200
9 Forge Pkwy, Franklin, MA 02038

Vygon Corp. 800-544-4907
2495 General Armistead Ave, Norristown, PA 19403

CANNULA, EXTRACTION, APPENDIX *(Surgery) 79WZT*

Boss Instruments, Ltd. 800-210-2677
395 Reas Ford Rd Ste 120, Earlysville, VA 22936

Richard Wolf Medical Instruments Corp. 800-323-9653
353 Corporate Woods Pkwy, Vernon Hills, IL 60061

Wisap America 800-233-8448
8231 Melrose Dr, Lenexa, KS 66214

CANNULA, FEMORAL *(Gastro/Urology) 78QGC*

Novosci Corp. 281-363-4949
2828 N Crescentridge Dr, The Woodlands, TX 77381

CANNULA, HEMODIALYSIS *(Gastro/Urology) 78QGD*

Kawasumi Laboratories America, Inc. 800-529-2786
4723 Oak Fair Blvd, Tampa, FL 33610
AV Fistula needles and Blood Tubing Lines

Medisystems Corporation 800-369-6334
439 S Union St Fl 5, Lawrence, MA 01843
AV fistula needle.

Rismed Oncology Systems 256-534-6993
2494 Washington St NW, Huntsville, AL 35811
A. V. Fistula neddle set with fixed and rotating wing.

CANNULA, INJECTION *(Gastro/Urology) 78FGY*

Ac Healthcare Supply, Inc. 905-448-4706
11651 230th St, Cambria Heights, NY 11411
Introduction/drainage catheter and accessories.

Aesculap Implant Systems Inc. 1-800-234-9179
3773 Corporate Pkwy, Center Valley, PA 18034

Atek Medical 800-253-1540
620 Watson St SW, Grand Rapids, MI 49504
Cannula insertion kit.

Becton, Dickinson & Co. 308-872-6811
150 S 1st Ave, Broken Bow, NE 68822
Needleless cannula.

Cadence Science Inc. 888-717-7677
1979 Marcus Ave Ste 215, New Hyde Park, NY 11042

Connecticut Hypodermics, Inc. 203-265-4881
519 Main St, Yalesville, CT 06492
Custom made.

Cook Endoscopy 336-744-0157
4900 Bethania Station Rd # &, 5951 Grassy Creek Blvd. Winston Salem, NC 27105
Ercp cannula.

Hobbs Medical, Inc. 860-684-5875
8 Spring St, Stafford Springs, CT 06076
Ercp cannula.

Ispg, Inc. 860-355-8511
517 Litchfield Rd, New Milford, CT 06776
Ground cannulae

Molded Products Inc. 800-435-8957
1112 Chatburn Ave, Harlan, IA 51537
Latex-free injection sites.

Tegra Medical Inc. 508-541-4200
9 Forge Pkwy, Franklin, MA 02038

CANNULA, INSUFFLATION, UTERINE *(Obstetrics/Gyn) 85HHH*

Premier Medical Products 888-PREMUSA
1710 Romano Dr, Plymouth Meeting, PA 19462

Rocket Medical Plc. 800-707-7625
150 Recreation Park Dr Ste 3, Hingham, MA 02043

CANNULA, INTRAUTERINE INSEMINATION *(Obstetrics/Gyn) 85MFD*

Cook Ob/Gyn 800-541-5591
1100 W Morgan St, Spencer, IN 47460

Irvine Scientific 800-437-5706
2511 Daimler St, Santa Ana, CA 92705
Wallace IUI and embryo transfer Catheters.Sureview transfer catheters.

Medical Systems, Inc. 800-441-1973
30 Winter Sport Ln, PO Box 966, Williston, VT 05495
Intrauterine insemination catheter.

Redi-Tech Medical Products,Llc 800-824-1793
529 Front St Ste 125, Berea, OH 44017
Used for Intrauterine Insemination. 20/bx

Rocket Medical Plc. 800-707-7625
150 Recreation Park Dr Ste 3, Hingham, MA 02043

Select Medical Systems 800-441-1973
30 Winter Sport Ln, PO Box 966, Williston, VT 05495
SELECT1U1 dual-opening intrauterine insemination catheter. MINISPACE 1U1 ultra-low residual volume intrauterine insemination catheter.THECURVE small diameter with smooth end opening and pre curve to facilitates insertion.

CANNULA, LACRIMAL (EYE) *(Ophthalmology) 86QGB*

Bausch & Lomb Surgical 636-255-5051
3365 Tree Court Ind Blvd, Saint Louis, MO 63122

Becton Dickinson And Co. 866-906-8080
411 Waverley Oaks Rd, Waltham, MA 02452

CANNULA, LACRIMAL (EYE) *(cont'd)*

Cadence Science Inc. 888-717-7677
1979 Marcus Ave Ste 215, New Hyde Park, NY 11042
8 sizes.

Eagle Laboratories 800-782-6534
10201 Trademark St Ste A, Rancho Cucamonga, CA 91730

Elmed, Inc. 630-543-2792
60 W Fay Ave, Addison, IL 60101

Fortrad Eye Instruments Corp. 973-543-2371
8 Franklin Rd, Mendham, NJ 07945

Jedmed Instruments Co. 314-845-3770
5416 Jedmed Ct, Saint Louis, MO 63129

Kmi Surgical Ltd. 800-528-2900
110 Hopewell Rd, Laird Professional Building, Downingtown, PA 19335
Disposable unit.

Oasis Medical, Inc. 800-528-9786
514 S Vermont Ave, Glendora, CA 91741
Lacrimal intubation sets.

Stephens Instruments, Inc. 800-354-7848
2500 Sandersville Rd, Lexington, KY 40511
$10.00 each.

Western Ophthalmics Corporation 800-426-9938
19019 36th Ave W Ste G, Lynnwood, WA 98036

CANNULA, MANIPULATOR/INJECTOR, UTERINE
(Obstetrics/Gyn) 85LKF

Apple Medical Corp. 508-357-2700
28 Lord Rd Ste 135, Marlborough, MA 01752
Uterine manipulator and injector with accessory.

Ob Specialties, Inc. 800-325-6644
1799 Northwood Ct, Oakland, CA 94611

Rocket Medical Plc. 800-707-7625
150 Recreation Park Dr Ste 3, Hingham, MA 02043

CANNULA, NASAL *(General) 80FMM*

Bausch & Lomb Surgical 636-255-5051
3365 Tree Court Ind Blvd, Saint Louis, MO 63122

Dixie Ems Supply 800-347-3494
385 Union Ave, Brooklyn, NY 11211
$12.80 per 10 (7in).

Filtrona Extrusion, Inc./Pexcor Medical Products Div. 800-755-7528
764 S Athol Rd, P.O. Box 659, Athol, MA 01331

Invacare Corporation 800-333-6900
1 Invacare Way, Elyria, OH 44035
INVACARE.

Salter Labs 800-235-4203
100 Sycamore Rd, Arvin, CA 93203

Sunrise Medical 800-333-4000
7477 Dry Creek Pkwy, Longmont, CO 80503

CANNULA, NASAL, OXYGEN *(Anesthesiology) 73CAT*

A-M Systems, Inc. 800-426-1306
131 Business Park Loop, Sequim, WA 98382
$49.22 for case of 50.

Afton Medical Llc 707-577-0685
3137 Swetzer Rd Ste C, Loomis, CA 95650
Oxygen nasal cannula.

Allied Healthcare Products, Inc. 800-444-3954
1720 Sublette Ave, Saint Louis, MO 63110

American Medical Products, Inc. 800-279-1999
713 S Darrow Dr, Tempe, AZ 85281
Oxy-Ears Nasal Cannula, Oxy-ears, Oxy-Nose

Caplugs West 310-537-2300
18704 S Ferris Pl, Rancho Dominguez, CA 90220
Cannula.

Comfort Strap Co. 605-997-3810
212 E 2nd St, Egan, SD 57024
Strap accessory to cannula tubes.

Covidien Lp 508-261-8000
15 Hampshire St, Mansfield, MA 02048

Delta Systems De Mexico 702-331-1890
Prolongacion Las Lomas No. 16, Tijuana, B.c. Mexico
Oxygen cannula

Directmed, Inc. 516-656-3377
150 Pratt Oval, Glen Cove, NY 11542

CANNULA, NASAL, OXYGEN *(cont'd)*

Gi Supply 800-451-5797
200 Grandview Ave, Camp Hill, PA 17011
OXYBLOC disposable bite block with nasal cannula.

Kelsar, S.A. 508-261-8000
Blvd. Insurgentes, Libriamento a La, Tijuana 22450 Mexico
Cpap nasal cannula

Kentron Health Care, Inc. 615-384-0573
3604 Kelton Jackson Rd, P.o. Box 120, Springfield, TN 37172
Nasal cannula.

Lampac International Ltd. 636-797-3659
230 N Lake Dr, Hillsboro, MO 63050

Life Corporation 800-700-0202
1776 N Water St, Milwaukee, WI 53202
LIFE cannulas.

Mada, Inc. 800-526-6370
625 Washington Ave, Carlstadt, NJ 07072
Box of 25 in 7ft. or 25ft. length.

Medicomp 763-389-4473
12535 316th Ave, Princeton, MN 55371
No common name listed.

Medline Industries, Inc. 800-633-5886
1 Medline Pl, Mundelein, IL 60060

Omni Medical Supply Inc. 800-860-6664
4153 Pioneer Dr, Commerce Township, MI 48390

Oxy-View, Inc. 877-699-8439
109 Inverness Dr E Ste C, Englewood, CO 80112
Oxy-view nasal cannula.

Rockford Medical & Safety Co. 800-435-9451
2420 Harrison Ave, PO Box 5646, Rockford, IL 61108

Salter Labs 800-235-4203
100 Sycamore Rd, Arvin, CA 93203

Smiths Medical Asd Inc. 800-258-5361
10 Bowman Dr, Keene, NH 03431
Various types of oxygen cannulas.

Smiths Medical Asd, Inc. 847-793-0135
330 Corporate Woods Pkwy, Vernon Hills, IL 60061
Nasal cannula.

Superior Products, Inc. 216-651-9400
3786 Ridge Rd, Cleveland, OH 44144
Nasal cannula.

Vygon Corp. 800-544-4907
2495 General Armistead Ave, Norristown, PA 19403

CANNULA, OPHTHALMIC *(Ophthalmology) 86HMX*

Ac Healthcare Supply, Inc. 905-448-4706
11651 230th St, Cambria Heights, NY 11411
Nasal oxygen cannula.

Accutome, Inc. 610-889-0200
3222 Phoenixville Pike, Malvern, PA 19355
Cannulas.

Akorn, Inc. 800-535-7155
2500 Millbrook Dr, Buffalo Grove, IL 60089
Disposable and reusable cannula plus diamond knives and titanium instruments; also, disposable cannulas.

Alcon Manufacturing, Ltd. 817-551-6813
714 Columbia Ave, Sinking Spring, PA 19608
Various types of ophthalmic cannulas.

American Surgical Instrument Corp. 800-628-2879
26 Plaza Dr, Westmont, IL 60559
Pars plana cannula.

B. Graczyk, Inc. 269-782-2100
27826 Burmax Park, Dowagiac, MI 49047
Various sizes of sterile & non-sterile cannula.

Bausch & Lomb Surgical 636-255-5051
3365 Tree Court Ind Blvd, Saint Louis, MO 63122

Becton Dickinson And Co. 866-906-8080
411 Waverley Oaks Rd, Waltham, MA 02452

Demetech Corp. 888-324-2447
3530 NW 115th Ave, Doral, FL 33178
Ophthalmic cannulae.

Diamond Edge Co. 727-586-2927
928 W Bay Dr, Largo, FL 33770
Cannula.

CANNULA, OPHTHALMIC *(cont'd)*

Dutch Ophthalmic Usa, Inc. 800-753-8824
10 Continental Dr Bldg 1, Exeter, NH 03833
Various models of backflush needles, infusion cannulas, etc.

Eagle Laboratories 800-782-6534
10201 Trademark St Ste A, Rancho Cucamonga, CA 91730
Disposable instruments for ophthalmic microsurgery; Retrobulbars/peribulbars, Double I/A cannulas, retinal cannulas, and ECCE kits, ETC.

Elmed, Inc. 630-543-2792
60 W Fay Ave, Addison, IL 60101

Escalon Trek Medical 800-433-8197
2440 S 179th St, New Berlin, WI 53146
Syringe and cannula.

Fortrad Eye Instruments Corp. 973-543-2371
8 Franklin Rd, Mendham, NJ 07945

Hai Laboratories, Inc. 781-862-9884
320 Massachusetts Ave, Lexington, MA 02420
Ophthalmic cannula - various types.

Harvey Precision Instruments 707-793-2600
217 Fairway Rd, Cape Haze, FL 33947
Straight, curved, angled, air injection, aspiration, etc. cannula.

Hurricane Medical 941-751-0588
5315 Lena Rd, Bradenton, FL 34211
Ophthalmic cannula.

Jedmed Instruments Co. 314-845-3770
5416 Jedmed Ct, Saint Louis, MO 63129

Katena Products, Inc. 800-225-1195
4 Stewart Ct, Denville, NJ 07834

Kmi Surgical Ltd. 800-528-2900
110 Hopewell Rd, Laird Professional Building, Downingtown, PA 19335
Disposable cannula.

Mediflex Surgical Products 800-879-7575
250 Gibbs Rd, Islandia, NY 11749
Weiss Retinal Microcannula for the treatment of Central Retinal Vein and Artery Occlusion.

Medone Surgical, Inc. 941-359-3129
670 Tallevast Rd, Sarasota, FL 34243
Various.

Micro Medical Instruments 314-845-3663
123 Cliff Cave Rd, Saint Louis, MO 63129
Ophthalmic cannulas.

Microsurgical Technology, Inc. 425-556-0544
PO Box 2679, Redmond, WA 98073

Microvision, Inc. 603-474-5566
34 Folly Mill Rd, Seabrook, NH 03874
Disposable infusion cannula.

Mira, Inc. 508-278-7877
414 Quaker Hwy, Uxbridge, MA 01569
Manual surgical instrument.

Oasis Medical, Inc. 800-528-9786
514 S Vermont Ave, Glendora, CA 91741
Retrobulbar and peribulbar cannulas.

Ocusoft, Inc. 281-342-3350
PO Box 429, Richmond, TX 77406
Ophthalmic cannula.

Peregrine Surgical, Ltd. 215-348-0456
51 Britain Dr, Doylestown, PA 18901
Cannula.

Psi/Eye-Ko, Inc. 636-447-1010
804 Corporate Centre Dr, O Fallon, MO 63368
Disposable sterile surgical instruments for opthalmology.

Ranfac Corp. 800-2RANFAC
30 Doherty Ave, Avon Industrial Park, Avon, MA 02322
13 types - from $7.50 to $16.00 each.

Solos Endoscopy 800-388-6445
65 Sprague St # B, Boston/dedham Commerce Park, Boston, MA 02136
Manual opthalmic surgical instrument.

Stephens Instruments, Inc. 800-354-7848
2500 Sandersville Rd, Lexington, KY 40511
$12.00 each.

Surgical Instrument Manufacturers, Inc. 800-521-2985
1650 Headland Dr, Fenton, MO 63026

CANNULA, OPHTHALMIC *(cont'd)*

Synergetics Usa, Inc. 800-600-0565
3845 Corporate Centre Dr, O Fallon, MO 63368
Various.

Tegra Medical Inc. 508-541-4200
9 Forge Pkwy, Franklin, MA 02038

Total Titanium, Inc. 618-473-2429
140 East Monroe St., Hecker, IL 62248
Various types of ophthalmic cannulas.

CANNULA, OPHTHALMIC, POSTERIOR CAPSULAR POLISHING, POLYVINYL ACETAL *(Ophthalmology) 86MXY*

Alcon Manufacturing, Ltd. 817-551-6813
714 Columbia Ave, Sinking Spring, PA 19608
Various types of ophthalmic capsule polishers.

Hai Laboratories, Inc. 781-862-9884
320 Massachusetts Ave, Lexington, MA 02420
Various types.

John F. Steinman Ltd. 419-893-1740
2330 Detroit Ave, Maumee, OH 43537
Dental polisher.

CANNULA, OTHER *(General) 80QGI*

Applied Medical Technology, Inc. 800-869-7382
8000 Katherine Blvd, Brecksville, OH 44141
SURGICAL, GENERAL & PLASTIC SURGERY - SOFT SUCTION ADAPTER

Cadence Science Inc. 888-717-7677
1979 Marcus Ave Ste 215, New Hyde Park, NY 11042

Cardiovascular Research, Inc. 813-832-6222
4810 W Gandy Blvd, Tampa, FL 33611
Razi's Cannula Introducer.

Dedicated Distribution 800-325-8367
640 Miami Ave, Kansas City, KS 66105
Respiratory supplies.

Future Medical Systems, Inc. 800-367-6021
504 McCormick Dr Ste T, Glen Burnie, MD 21061
Arthroscopic.

Gyrus Medical, Inc. 800-852-9361
6655 Wedgwood Rd N Ste 105, Maple Grove, MN 55311
Model 5890 tapered-tip ERCP cannula; leakproof injection over .035 guidewire; 7F Teflon catheter.

Ispg, Inc. 860-355-8511
517 Litchfield Rd, New Milford, CT 06776
Stainless steel, custom geometrics, huber, low-coring bent tip, double point.

Plastics One, Inc. 540-772-7950
6591 Merriman Rd, Roanoke, VA 24018

Ranfac Corp. 800-2RANFAC
30 Doherty Ave, Avon Industrial Park, Avon, MA 02322
Galactography infusion unit, available with various needle sizes.

Roboz Surgical Instrument Co., Inc. 800-424-2984
PO Box 10710, Gaithersburg, MD 20898
Fastbreak cannula; cannula and cannula catheter set; catheter-introducer system.

Smith & Nephew, Inc., Endoscopy Division 800-343-8386
150 Minuteman Rd, Andover, MA 01810
Reusable and disposable.

Tegra Medical Inc. 508-541-4200
9 Forge Pkwy, Franklin, MA 02038

Telemed Systems Inc. 800-481-6718
8 Kane Industrial Dr, Hudson, MA 01749
ERCP Cannula available.

Tulip Medical Products 800-325-6526
PO Box 7368, San Diego, CA 92167
TULIP brand syringe instrumentation for soft tissue surgery.

Vita Needle Company 781-444-1780
919 Great Plain Ave, Needham, MA 02492
Stainless steel cannula. Moderate and long runs; short lead times; second operations; gauges 3-34, ss304/316 all stock; custom tubing sizes.

Y.I. Ventures, Llc 314-344-0010
2260 Wendt St, Algonquin, IL 60102
Endoscopy liposuction cannulae.

Zimmer Holdings, Inc. 800-613-6131
1800 W Center St, PO Box 708, Warsaw, IN 46580
Cannulated screws.

CANNULA, SINUS *(Ear/Nose/Throat) 77KAM*

Acclarent, Inc. 877-775-2789
1525B Obrien Dr, Menlo Park, CA 94025
Guide/lavage catheter; guidewire; adapter; sinus spacer.

Aesculap Implant Systems Inc. 1-800-234-9179
3773 Corporate Pkwy, Center Valley, PA 18034

Bausch & Lomb Surgical 636-255-5051
3365 Tree Court Ind Blvd, Saint Louis, MO 63122

E. Benson Hood Laboratories, Inc. 800-942-5227
575 Washington St, Pembroke, MA 02359
Maxillary Antrum Sinus Tube (M.A.S.T.): a flexible tube with an anchoring member at its distal end. It is used to provide access to the maxillary sinus cavity. Jacobs Frontal Sinus Cannula: developed to provide temporary postoperative stenting of the frontal sinus outflow tract.

Gyrus Ent L.L.C., Sub. Of Gyrus Acmi, Inc. 508-804-2739
2925 Appling Rd, Bartlett, TN 38133
Multiple.

Lfi, Inc-Laser Fare, Inc. 401-231-4400
1 Industrial Dr S, Lan-Rex Industrial Pk., Smithfield, RI 02917

Miltex Inc. 800-645-8000
589 Davies Dr, York, PA 17402

Stryker Puerto Rico, Ltd. 939-307-2500
Hwy. 3, Km. 131.2, Las Guasimas Ind. Park, Arroyo, PR 00714
Irrigation cannula.

CANNULA, SUCTION, POOL-TIP *(Surgery) 79WZU*

Elmed, Inc. 630-543-2792
60 W Fay Ave, Addison, IL 60101

Transamerican Technologies International 800-322-7373
2246 Camino Ramon, San Ramon, CA 94583
ACCU-SURG, suction/irrigation cannula for laparoscopic surgery.

Wells Johnson Co. 800-528-1597
8000 S Kolb Rd, Tucson, AZ 85756

CANNULA, SUCTION, UTERINE *(Obstetrics/Gyn) 85HGH*

Berkeley Medevices, Inc. 800-227-2388
1330 S 51st St, Richmond, CA 94804
Vacuum curettage equipment and supplies (curettes, tubing, etc.)

Biomet Microfixation Inc. 800-874-7711
1520 Tradeport Dr, Jacksonville, FL 32218
Various types of suction•cannula.

Busse Hospital Disposables, Inc. 631-435-4711
75 Arkay Dr, Hauppauge, NY 11788
Various sizes, sterile uterine cannula.

Cardinal Healthcare 209, Inc. 610-862-0800
5225 Verona Rd, Fitchburg, WI 53711
Test monitor.

Ipas 919-967-7052
PO Box 5027, Chapel Hill, NC 27514
Karman flexible cannulae, sizes 4-12mm.

Kmi Kolster Methods, Inc. 909-737-5476
3185 Palisades Dr, Corona, CA 92880
Cannula.

Premier Medical Products 888-PREMUSA
1710 Romano Dr, Plymouth Meeting, PA 19462

R Medical Supply 800-882-7578
620 Valley Forge Rd Ste F, Hillsborough, NC 27278
Sterile, disposable, sizes 5 through 14.

Richard Wolf Medical Instruments Corp. 800-323-9653
353 Corporate Woods Pkwy, Vernon Hills, IL 60061

Rocket Medical Plc. 800-707-7625
150 Recreation Park Dr Ste 3, Hingham, MA 02043

Sun Medical, Inc. 800-678-6633
2607 Aero Dr, Grand Prairie, TX 75052

CANNULA, SUCTION/IRRIGATION, LAPAROSCOPIC
(Surgery) 79WYX

Deknatel Snowden-Pencer 800-367-7874
5175 S Royal Atlanta Dr, Tucker, GA 30084
ENDO-VALUE reusable cannula available in 60mm and 10mm cannula lengths, and 5.5mm, 10/11mm and 12/13mm diameters.

Genicon 800-936-1020
6869 Stapoint Ct Ste 114, Winter Park, FL 32792
Disposable Laparoscopic Suction Irrigation products

Mediflex Surgical Products 800-879-7575
250 Gibbs Rd, Islandia, NY 11749

CANNULA, SUCTION/IRRIGATION, LAPAROSCOPIC *(cont'd)*

Transamerican Technologies International 800-322-7373
2246 Camino Ramon, San Ramon, CA 94583
ACCU-Surg suction / irrigation cannula for laparoscopic surgery.

Wells Johnson Co. 800-528-1597
8000 S Kolb Rd, Tucson, AZ 85756

Wisap America 800-233-8448
8231 Melrose Dr, Lenexa, KS 66214

CANNULA, SUPRAPUBIC, WITH TROCAR
(Gastro/Urology) 78FBM

Aesculap Implant Systems Inc. 1-800-234-9179
3773 Corporate Pkwy, Center Valley, PA 18034
Cannula and tracer, suprapubic, non-disposable.

Cardinal Health, Snowden Pencer Products 847-689-8410
5175 S Royal Atlanta Dr, Tucker, GA 30084
Various types of reusable cannulas and trocars.

E-Global Medical Equipment, L.L.C. 866-422-1845
2f 500 Lincoln St., Allston, MA 02134
Trocar.

Gibbons Surgical Corp. 800-959-1989
1112 Jensen Dr Ste 101, Virginia Beach, VA 23451

Greenwald Surgical Co., Inc. 219-962-1604
2688 Dekalb St, Gary, IN 46405
Various types of suprapubic trocars.

Karl Storz Endoscopy-America Inc. 800-421-0837
600 Corporate Pointe, Culver City, CA 90230
Reusable trocar/cannula kits.

Kmi Kolster Methods, Inc. 909-737-5476
3185 Palisades Dr, Corona, CA 92880
Cannulas and trocars.

Koros Usa, Inc. 805-529-0825
610 Flinn Ave, Moorpark, CA 93021
Discectomy cannula system.

Mahe International Inc. 800-294-7946
468 Craighead St, Nashville, TN 37204

New Innovations Inc. 765-668-7470
125 E Bradford St, Marion, IN 46952
Non disposable trocar needles.

Reznik Instrument, Inc. 847-673-3444
7337 Lawndale Ave, Skokie, IL 60076
Trocar and trocar sleeves.

Richard Wolf Medical Instruments Corp. 800-323-9653
353 Corporate Woods Pkwy, Vernon Hills, IL 60061

Solos Endoscopy 800-388-6445
65 Sprague St # B, Boston/dedham Commerce Park, Boston, MA 02136
Urologic catheter & accessories.

Surgistar Inc. 800-995-7086
2310 La Mirada Dr, Vista, CA 92081
Trocars.

Synectic Medical Product Development 203-877-8488
60 Commerce Park, Milford, CT 06460

Tegra Medical Inc. 508-541-4200
9 Forge Pkwy, Franklin, MA 02038

CANNULA, SURGICAL, GENERAL & PLASTIC SURGERY
(Surgery) 79GEA

Abbott Spine, Inc. 847-937-6100
12708 Riata Vista Cir Ste B-100, Austin, TX 78727
Cannula.

Bausch & Lomb Surgical 636-255-5051
3365 Tree Court Ind Blvd, Saint Louis, MO 63122

Biomet Microfixation Inc. 800-874-7711
1520 Tradeport Dr, Jacksonville, FL 32218
Cannula, surgical, general & plastic surgery.

Boston Scientific - Marina Bay Customer Fulfillment Center 617-689-6000
500 Commander Shea Blvd, Quincy, MA 02171
Various.

Byron Medical 800-777-3434
602 W Rillito St, Tucson, AZ 85705

Cadence Science Inc. 888-717-7677
1979 Marcus Ave Ste 215, New Hyde Park, NY 11042

Centurion Medical Products Corp. 517-545-1135
3310 S Main St, Salisbury, NC 28147

CANNULA, SURGICAL, GENERAL & PLASTIC SURGERY *(cont'd)*

Chase Medical, Lp 972-783-0644
1876 Firman Dr, Richardson, TX 75081
Disposable suction cannula.

Depuy Mitek, A Johnson & Johnson Company 800-451-2006
50 Scotland Blvd, Bridgewater, MA 02324
Various cannulas.

Depuy Spine, Inc. 800-227-6633
325 Paramount Dr, Raynham, MA 02767
Bone funnel.

Ethicon Endo-Surgery, Inc. 877-384-4266
3801 University Blvd SE, Albuquerque, NM 87106
Various types of sterile surgical trocars.

Evera Medical, Inc. 650-287-2884
353 Vintage Park Dr Ste F, Foster City, CA 94404
Trocar.

Invuity, Inc. 760-744-4447
334 Via Vera Cruz Ste 255, San Marcos, CA 92078
Cannula.

Invuity, Inc. 415-655-2100
39 Stillman St, San Francisco, CA 94107

Kmi Kolster Methods, Inc. 909-737-5476
3185 Palisades Dr, Corona, CA 92880
Suction cannula.

Laprostop, Llc 858-705-3838
1845 Newport Avenue, San Diego, CA 92107
Trocar accessory.

Medical Device Resource Corporation 800-633-8423
23392 Connecticut St, Hayward, CA 94545

Medovations, Inc. 800-558-6408
102 E Keefe Ave, Milwaukee, WI 53212

Medtronic Dlp 616-643-5200
620 Watson St SW, Grand Rapids, MI 49504

Medtronic Spine Llc 877-690-5353
1221 Crossman Ave, Sunnyvale, CA 94089
Various.

nContact Surgical, Inc. 919-466-9810
1001 Aviation Pkwy Ste 400, Morrisville, NC 27560
Cannula, surgical, general & plastic surgery.

Orthopaedic Development, Llc 561-827-8006
1300 Corporate Center Way, Wellington, FL 33414
Various cannulas or introducers.

Osseon Therapeutics, Inc. 877-567-7366
2330 Circadian Way, Santa Rosa, CA 95407
OsseoFlex 1.0 Steerable Needle

Pac-Dent Intl., Inc. 909-839-0888
21078 Commerce Point Dr, Walnut, CA 91789
Suction adapter.

Putnam Precision Products 845-278-2141
3859 Danbury Rd, Brewster, NY 10509

Renick Ent., Inc. 561-863-4183
1211 W 13th St, Riviera Beach, FL 33404
custom Cannula's

Sanarus Medical, Inc. 925-460-5730
4696 Willow Rd, Pleasanton, CA 94588
Sanarus biopsy cannula.

Shippert Medical Technologies Corp. 800-888-8663
6248 S Troy Cir Ste A, Centennial, CO 80111
New Biplane Ergonomic Liposuction Handle. Full line of handles and cannulas with 40 different hole patterns.

Shoney Scientific, Inc. 262-970-0170
West 223 North 720 Saratoga Drive,, Suite 120, Waukesha, WI 53186
Cannula, surgical, general & plastic surgery.

Sound Surgical Technologies Llc 888-471-4777
357 McCaslin Blvd Ste 100, Louisville, CO 80027
VentX™ aspiration cannulae for body sculpting. Various diameters, lengths and hole patterns.

Surgical Implant Generation Network (Sign) 509-371-1107
451 Hills St, Richland, WA 99354
Cannula.

Symmetry Medical Usa, Inc. 574-267-8700
486 W 350 N, Warsaw, IN 46582
Manual surgical instrument for general use.

CANNULA, SURGICAL, GENERAL & PLASTIC SURGERY *(cont'd)*

Tl Tate Mfg, Inc. 765-452-8283
1500 N Webster St, Kokomo, IN 46901
Operating-room tools.

Tri-State Hospital Supply Corp. 517-545-1135
3173 E 43rd St, Yuma, AZ 85365

Tulip Medical Products 800-325-6526
PO Box 7368, San Diego, CA 92167
TULIP brand syringe instrumentation for soft tissue surgery. Cell-Friendly, extraction and injection cannulas specifically treated to provide maximum cell viability for autotransportation.

Zimmer Spine, Inc. 800-655-2614
7375 Bush Lake Rd, Minneapolis, MN 55439
Surgical cannula.

CANNULA, TRACHEOSTOMY *(Ear/Nose/Throat) 77QGF*

Bausch & Lomb Surgical 636-255-5051
3365 Tree Court Ind Blvd, Saint Louis, MO 63122

Boston Medical Products, Inc. 800-433-2674
117 Flanders Rd, Westborough, MA 01581
Montgomery silicone tracheal cannulas, sizes 4, 6, 8 and 10, in 6 lengths.

E. Benson Hood Laboratories, Inc. 800-942-5227
575 Washington St, Pembroke, MA 02359
Stoma cannula system, T-tubes, stents and speaking valves.

Mahe International Inc. 800-294-7946
468 Craighead St, Nashville, TN 37204

Smiths Medical Asd 800-424-8662
5700 W 23rd Ave, Gary, IN 46406
AIRE-CUF, FOME-CUF & TTS Adult and Pediatric fixed and adjustable neck flange; silicone.

CANNULA, VENA CAVA *(Cardiovascular) 74QGG*

Novosci Corp. 281-363-4949
2828 N Crescentridge Dr, The Woodlands, TX 77381

CANNULA, VENOUS *(Cardiovascular) 74QGH*

Avalon Laboratories, Inc. 866-938-6613
2610 Homestead Pl, Rancho Dominguez, CA 90220

Connecticut Hypodermics, Inc. 203-265-4881
519 Main St, Yalesville, CT 06492
Custom made to your design.

Ispg, Inc. 860-355-8511
517 Litchfield Rd, New Milford, CT 06776
Ground cannulae

Novosci Corp. 281-363-4949
2828 N Crescentridge Dr, The Woodlands, TX 77381
Saphenous vein cannula.

Rocket Medical Plc. 800-707-7625
150 Recreation Park Dr Ste 3, Hingham, MA 02043

Rose Technologies Company 616-233-3000
1440 Front Ave NW, Grand Rapids, MI 49504

Tegra Medical Inc. 508-541-4200
9 Forge Pkwy, Franklin, MA 02038

CANNULA, VENTRICULAR *(Cns/Neurology) 84HCD*

Diablo Sales & Marketing, Inc. 925-648-1611
PO Box 3219, Danville, CA 94526
Custom design and manufacturing of catheters and specialty guidewires. Guiding catheters; stent delivery and drug delivery systems.

Innerspace, Inc. 877.HUM.BIRD
1622 Edinger Ave Ste C, Tustin, CA 92780
Hummingbird Ventricular - Integrated ICP with Ventricular Drainage

Integra Neurosciences Pr 800-654-2873
Road 402 North, Km 1.2, Anasco, PR 00610
Various.

Tegra Medical Inc. 508-541-4200
9 Forge Pkwy, Franklin, MA 02038

CAP, BONE *(Orthopedics) 87JDT*

Martin Technology, Llc 901-682-1006
1505 S Perkins Rd, Memphis, TN 38117
Bone cap.

CAP, CERVICAL *(Obstetrics/Gyn) 85HDR*

Cervical Barrier Advancement Society
P.O. Box 38203, Cambridge, MA 02238-2031

CAP, CERVICAL *(cont'd)*

Cook Ob/Gyn 800-541-5591
1100 W Morgan St, Spencer, IN 47460
Insemination catheters.

Milex Products, Inc. 800-621-1278
4311 N Normandy Ave, Chicago, IL 60634
OLIGOSPERMIA CUP at $17.00 per unit (standard) for insemination cervical cap.

CAP, NERVE *(Cns/Neurology) 84UBI*

Electro-Cap International, Inc. 800-527-2193
1011 W Lexington Rd, PO Box 87, Eaton, OH 45320
ELECTRO CAP, a cap containing EEG electrodes.

CAP, OPHTHALMIC, QUARTER GLOBE *(Ophthalmology) 86UAX*

Oculo Plastik Inc. 888-381-3292
200 Sauve West, Montreal, QUE H3L-1Y9 Canada
Surgical protective ocular shields in plastic or stainless steel. 2 autoclavable models in black or clear, or stainless steel. The stainless, non-glare is for use with the laser. Also patient external laser shields.

CAP, SURGICAL *(Surgery) 79FYF*

Alphaprotech, Inc. 229-242-1931
1287 W Fairway Dr, Nogales, AZ 85621

Angelica Image Apparel 800-222-3112
700 Rosedale Ave, Saint Louis, MO 63112

Atd-American Co. 800-523-2300
135 Greenwood Ave, Wyncote, PA 19095

Becton Dickinson Infusion Therapy Systems, Inc. 888-237-2762
9450 S State St, Sandy, UT 84070
Male Luer-Lok dead end cap.

Busse Hospital Disposables, Inc. 631-435-4711
75 Arkay Dr, Hauppauge, NY 11788
Variuos sizes & styles.

Cellucap Manufacturing Co. 800-523-3814
4626 N 15th St, Philadelphia, PA 19140
Disposable headwear products, hairnets and beard restraints for the O.R. and kitchen.

Chagrin Safety Supply, Inc. 800-227-0468
8227 Washington St # 1, Chagrin Falls, OH 44023

Clean Esd Products, Inc. 510-257-5080
48340 Milmont Dr, Fremont, CA 94538
Model number BC-201-24 x 24 in. Bouffant caps priced at $6.00/bag, 50pcs/bag.

Cleanwear Products Ltd. 416-438-4831
54 Crockford Rd., Toronto, ON M1R-3C3 Canada
Disposable surgeon caps and hoods plus bouffant caps.

Cms Worldwide, Inc. 800-426-4633
30011 Ivy Glenn Dr Ste 215, Laguna Niguel, CA 92677
Spun-bonded caps, blue or white. 500 per carton.

Cypress Medical Products 800-334-3646
1202 S. Rte. 31, McHenry, IL 60050
Nurse's caps, available in blue, white, or green, 21in. or 24in. 100 per box, 50 boxes per case.

Dowling Textiles 770-957-3981
615 Macon Rd, McDonough, GA 30253
Various types of surgeon and nurse caps.

Global Healthcare 800-601-3880
1495 Hembree Rd Ste 700, Roswell, GA 30076
Nurses' and surgeon's caps.

Grand Medical Products 800-521-2055
7222 Ertel Ln, Houston, TX 77040

Health-Pak, Inc. 315-724-8370
2005 Beechgrove Pl, Utica, NY 13501
Nonwoven poly spunbonded.

Jero Medical Equipment & Supplies, Inc. 800-457-0644
1701 W 13th St, Chicago, IL 60608
Various.

Johnson & Johnson Medical Division Of Ethicon, Inc. 800-423-4018
2500 E Arbrook Blvd, Arlington, TX 76014

Kentron Health Care, Inc. 615-384-0573
3604 Kelton Jackson Rd, P.o. Box 120, Springfield, TN 37172
Surgical cap.

Kerr Group 800-524-3577
1400 Holcomb Bridge Rd, Roswell, GA 30076

CAP, SURGICAL *(cont'd)*

Lakeland De Mexico S.A. De C.V. 516-981-9700
Rancho La Soledad Lote No. 2, Fracc. Poniente C.p. Celaya, Guajuato Mexico
Surgical cap

Maquilas Teta-Kawi, S.A. De C.V. 413-593-6400
Carretera Internacional, Km 1969, Enpalme, Sonora Mexico
Surgical cap

Maytex Corp. 800-462-9839
23521 Foley St, Hayward, CA 94545
Fluid-resistant, 21 or 24 in. available, latex free.

Medical Action Industries, Inc. 800-645-7042
25 Heywood Rd, Arden, NC 28704
Cap.

New York Hospital Disposables, Inc. 718-384-1620
101 Richardson St, Brooklyn, NY 11211

Pfb Inter-Apparel Corp. 800-828-7629
1930 Harrison St Ste 304, Hollywood, FL 33020

Precept Medical Products, Inc. 800-438-5827
PO Box 2400, 370 Airport Road/, Arden, NC 28704

R. Sabee Company 920-882-7350
1718 W 8th St, Appleton, WI 54914

Ross Disposable Products 800-649-6526
401 Traders Blvd E, Unit 10, Mississauga, ON L4Z 2H8 Canada

Sanax Protective Products, Inc. 800-379-9929
236 Upland Ave, Newton Highlands, MA 02461

Total Molding Services, Inc. 215-538-9613
354 East Broad St., Trumbauersville, PA 18970
Cap for end of pin in knee replacement.

U-Ten Corporation 630-289-8058
1286 Humbracht Cir, Bartlett, IL 60103
Bouffant caps and surgeon's caps.

White Knight Healthcare 800-851-4431
Calle 16, Number 780, Agua Prieta, Sonora Mexico
Various types of surgical caps

CAP, TIP, SYRINGE *(General) 80VLY*

Air-Tite Products Co., Inc. 800-231-7762
565 Central Dr Ste 101, Virginia Beach, VA 23454
PALMERO Palco syringe tip cover for use with air/water gun. Various sterile and unsterile syringe caps (luer).

Baxa Corporation 800-567-2292
9540 S Maroon Circle, Suite 400, Englewood, CO 80112
DISC PAC, sterile luer/injectable syringe tip caps.

Baxter Healthcare Corporation, Global Drug Delivery 888-229-0001
25212 W Il Route 120, Round Lake, IL 60073
SQUIRT CAP irrigation cap with syringe tip.

Cadence Science Inc. 888-717-7677
1979 Marcus Ave Ste 215, New Hyde Park, NY 11042

Covidien Lp 508-261-8000
15 Hampshire St, Mansfield, MA 02048

Csi International, Inc. 303-795-8273
4301 S Federal Blvd Ste 116, Englewood, CO 80110

Hoover Precision Products, Inc 906-632-7310
1390 Industrial Park Dr, Sault S Marie, MI 49783
MagCap Sample Protection System. Magnetic ball caps for archiving.

Medi-Dose, Inc. 800-523-8966
70 Industrial Dr, Ivyland, PA 18974

Molded Products Inc. 800-435-8957
1112 Chatburn Ave, Harlan, IA 51537
Luer-lock caps.

Sterion, Incorporated 800-328-7958
13828 Lincoln St NE, Ham Lake, MN 55304
One-handed syringe handling system to extract cap and to re-cap.

Total Molding Services, Inc. 215-538-9613
354 East Broad St., Trumbauersville, PA 18970
Oral Syringe Cap.

CAPACITOR, DEFIBRILLATOR *(General) 80WRU*

American Biomed Instruments, Inc. 718-235-8900
11 Wyona St, Brooklyn, NY 11207

CAPSULE, DENTAL, AMALGAM *(Dental And Oral) 76DZS*

Arnel, Inc. 516-486-7098
73 High St, Hempstead, NY 11550
Various.

CAPSULE, DENTAL, AMALGAM *(cont'd)*

Dentalez Group 866-DTE-INFO
101 Lindenwood Dr Ste 225, Valleybrooke Corporate Center Malvern, PA 19355

Dentsply Canada, Ltd. 800-263-1437
161 Vinyl Ct., Woodbridge, ONT L4L 4A3 Canada

Foremost Dental Llc. 201-894-5500
242 S Dean St, Englewood, NJ 07631
Dental amalgam capsule.

Ivoclar Vivadent, Inc. 800-533-6825
175 Pineview Dr, Amherst, NY 14228
Ultrasonically sealed with Valiant amalgam products

Kerr Corp. 714-516-7400
28200 Wick Rd, Romulus, MI 48174
Dental amalgam capsules.

Wykle Research, Inc. 775-887-7500
2222 College Pkwy, Carson City, NV 89706
Capsule.

Zenith/Dmg Brand 800-662-6383
242 S Dean St, Division of Foremost Dental LLC, Englewood, NJ 07631

CARBOXYMETHYLCELLULOSE SODIUM
(Dental And Oral) 76KXW

U.S. Medical Systems, Inc. 512-347-8800
3160 Bee Caves Rd Ste 300C, Austin, TX 78746
Denture adhesive.

CARBOXYMETHYLCELLULOSE SODIUM (40-100%)
(Dental And Oral) 76KOQ

Perfect Smile Corporation 800-520-1906
29313 Clemens Rd Ste 2E, Westlake, OH 44145
Oragrip denture adhesive.

CARBOXYMETHYLCELLULOSE SODIUM/ETHYLENE-OXIDE HOMOPOLYMER *(Dental And Oral) 76KOL*

Block Drug Co., Inc. 973-889-2578
2149 Harbor Ave., Memphis, TN 38113
Ethylene oxide homopolymer & cmc sodium denture adhesive.

CARD, IDENTIFICATION *(General) 80WZK*

Arthur Blank & Co., Inc. 800-776-7333
225 Rivermoor St, Boston, MA 02132
Printed hospital data cards, plastic patient ID cards and name badges, RFID cards.

Avondale Badge Co 800-874-2551
4114 Herschel St Ste 101, Jacksonville, FL 32210
Clincher armbands, temp. cards, ID cards, equipment and supplies.

Datacard Group 800-621-6972
11111 Bren Rd W, Minnetonka, MN 55343
Plastic patient ID cards that can be embossed, encoded, or bar coded.

Health Enterprises 800-633-4243
90 George Leven Dr, North Attleboro, MA 02760
Necklaces, bracelets and wallet cards.

Newbold Corporation 800-552-3282
450 Weaver St, Rocky Mount, VA 24151
ADDRESSOGRAPH MDL 610 Plastic card embosser, electronic card embosser for healthcare patient data system.

R&Da Co. 508-747-5803
37 Dwight Ave, Plymouth, MA 02360
MEDEK Medical Emergency Data Card - two-sided. The back contains 3,000 bytes (characters; =1 1/2 pages) in code, decodable by a flatbed scanner. Front is ID with picture and icons for quick appraisal of problem by EMT. By special order only.

Sound Feelings 818-757-0600
18375 Ventura Blvd # 8000, Tarzana, CA 91356
Emergency Contact Card, for listing of life-saving information and contacts.

Wolf X-Ray Corporation 800-356-9729
100 W Industry Ct, Deer Park, NY 11729
Cards and printers.

CARDIAC ALLOGRAFT GENE EXPRESSION PROFILING TEST SYSTEM *(Cardiovascular) 74OJQ*

XDx Expression Diagnostics 415-287-2300
3260 Bayshore Blvd, Brisbane, CA 94005
AlloMap Test

CARDIAC OUTPUT UNIT, INDICATOR DILUTION (THERMAL)
(Cardiovascular) 74QGL

Ge Medical Systems Information Technologies 800-643-6439
8200 W Tower Ave, Milwaukee, WI 53223
Measuring arterial, pulmonary artery, venous, left atrial, or intracranial pressure. Displays systolic, diastolic, and mean pressures with label. PAW measurement program calculates end-expiration wedge. Thermodilution cardiac output method displays and averages up to 5 washout curves. Stores 30 sets of cardiac calculations.

Hospira, Inc. 877-946-7747
755 Jarvis Dr, Morgan Hill, CA 95037
$3,950 for model 03950-00. Displays CO, PA, injection temps. Optional recorder. Operating instructions and table of compensation factors on top cover.

Mennen Medical Corp. 800-223-2201
2540 Metropolitan Dr, Trevose, PA 19053
HORIZON SE, HORIZON LITE, HORIZON COMPACT, cath-lab information systems; HORIZON ANGIO interventional peripheral vascular analysis system; ENVOY patient monitor.

CARDIAC OUTPUT UNIT, OTHER *(Cardiovascular) 74QGM*

Advanced Biomedical Devices, Inc. (Abd, Inc.) 978-470-1177
Dundee Park, Bldg. 17, Andover, MA 01810
OMP 210000 gas dsipenser for balloon inflation with CO2.

Capintec, Inc. 800-631-3826
6 Arrow Rd, Ramsey, NJ 07446

Intellectual Property, Llc 608-798-0904
8030 Stagecoach Rd, Cross Plains, WI 53528
Ambulatory long-term recording of Cardiac Output or bedside monitoring of Cardiac Output. Both methods require 5 spot electrodes. Patented method yields accurate determinations.

Md International, Inc. 305-669-9003
11300 NW 41st St, Doral, FL 33178
9600, 7600 Uroview, cardiac cath. lab, orthopedic, cardiac, neuro, urology, GYN imaging equipment for fluoroscopy.

Vasomedical Inc. 800-455-3327
180 Linden Ave, Westbury, NY 11590
Enhanced external counterpulsation device to treat patients suffering from angina.

CARDIAC OUTPUT UNIT, RADIOISOTOPE PROBE
(Cardiovascular) 74TAV

Capintec, Inc. 800-631-3826
6 Arrow Rd, Ramsey, NJ 07446

CARDIOGRAPH, APEX (VIBROCARDIOGRAPH)
(Cardiovascular) 74DQH

U.F.I. 805-772-1203
545 Main St Ste C2, Morro Bay, CA 93442
$105.00 for Model 1010.

CARDIOGRAPH, IMPEDANCE *(Cardiovascular) 74RBP*

Elmed, Inc. 630-543-2792
60 W Fay Ave, Addison, IL 60101

U.F.I. 805-772-1203
545 Main St Ste C2, Morro Bay, CA 93442
$6,250 for 1-channel unit, $10,250 for 4-channel unit.

CARE KIT, BABY *(General) 80QCD*

Apothecary Products, Inc. 800-328-2742
11750 12th Ave S, Burnsville, MN 55337
Baby Solutions brand.

Carex Health Brands 800-526-8051
921 E Amidon St, PO Box 2526, Sioux Falls, SD 57104
Pediatric Kit contains everything a customer needs to care for a new baby: 1 nasal aspirator, 1 medicine nurser, 1 super dropper, 1 digital thermometer, 5 probe covers and 1 oral syringe (small).

General Econopak, Inc. 888-871-8568
1725 N 6th St, Philadelphia, PA 19122
Baby hats and shirts, crib liners.

Johnson & Johnson Consumer Products, Inc. 800-526-3967
199 Grandview Rd, Skillman, NJ 08558

CARIES DETECTOR, LASER LIGHT, TRANSMISSION
(Dental And Oral) 76NTK

Electro-Optical Sciences, Inc. 800-729-8849
1 Bridge St Ste 15, Irvington, NY 10533
Dental examination system.

CARPETING *(General) 80VBB*

Sprayway, Inc. 800-332-9000
484 S Vista Ave, Addison, IL 60101
Cleaner. Chewing-gum remover, foaming cleaner sprays.

CARRIER, AMALGAM, OPERATIVE *(Dental And Oral) 76EKI*

Biomet Microfixation Inc. 800-874-7711
1520 Tradeport Dr, Jacksonville, FL 32218
Various types of carriers.

Buffalo Dental Mfg. Co., Inc. 516-496-7200
159 Lafayette Dr, Syosset, NY 11791
Amalgam carrier.

Dental Usa, Inc. 815-363-8003
5005 McCullom Lake Rd, McHenry, IL 60050
Amalgam carrier.

Hager Worldwide, Inc. 800-328-2335
13322 Byrd Dr, Odessa, FL 33556
DEL JECT (plastic, autoclavable).

Hu-Friedy Manufacturing Co., Inc. 800-483-7433
3232 N Rockwell St, Chicago, IL 60618
$56.85 to $59.90, 6 models.

Miltex Dental Technologies, Inc. 516-576-6022
589 Davies Dr, York, PA 17402
Various amalgam carriers.

Moyco Technologies, Inc. 800-331-8837
200 Commerce Dr, Montgomeryville, PA 18936

Nordent Manufacturing, Inc. 800-966-7336
610 Bonnie Ln, Elk Grove Village, IL 60007
$43.00 per unit (standard).

Premier Dental Products Co. 888-670-6100
1710 Romano Dr, PO Box 4500, Plymouth Meeting, PA 19462

Pulpdent Corp. 800-343-4342
80 Oakland St, Watertown, MA 02472
Amalgam carrier.

CARRIER, CONTAINER, OXYGEN, PORTABLE *(General) 80WUT*

Air Lift Unlimited Inc. 800-776-6771
1212 Kerr Gulch Rd, Evergreen, CO 80439
AIR LIFT oxygen carriers offer a full line of carriers for portable liquid and cylinder oxygen systems. These versatile carriers meet the needs of oxygen-dependent individuals and parents with oxygen-dependent children seeking more comfortable and convenient ways to transport oxygen. Carriers include fanny packs; backpacks; shoulder/hand carriers; carriers for wheelchairs, scooters and walkers; and a universal conserving device pouch. All carriers feature nonflammable, washable fabric and adjustable straps; liquid carriers feature breathable mesh pouches. Silk screening or embroidery available on all bags.

Armstrong Medical Industries, Inc. 800-323-4220
575 Knightsbridge Pkwy, Lincolnshire, IL 60069

Chad Therapeutics, Inc. 800-423-8870
21622 Plummer St, Chatsworth, CA 91311
Portable oxygen system.

Cryofab, Inc. 800-426-2186
540 N Michigan Ave, Kenilworth, NJ 07033
Van-mounted tanks for delivery of liquid oxygen to homes.

Farley Inc., W.T. 800-327-5397
931 Via Alondra, Camarillo, CA 93012
$225.00 for Model OS100A, MRI ventilator stand/oxygen cylinder holder, 5 legged aluminum ventilator stand holds two oxygen cylinders.

Lewis Bins+ 877-97L-EWIS
PO Box 389, Oconomowoc, WI 53066

Life Corporation 800-700-0202
1776 N Water St, Milwaukee, WI 53202
LIFE, OxygenPac Portable emergency oxygen units, clear cover and wall-mounted, off/on lever control, resuscitation mask with one-way valve for hygiene, 6lpm 90min. supply, refillable. Also available 6 & 12 lpm NORM & HIGH, 0-25 lpm variable, and demand-valve for 100% oxygen resuscitation. GSA Federal Supply Schedule.

Medcovers, Inc 800-948-8917
500 W Goldsboro St, Kenly, NC 27542

Michigan Instruments, Inc. 800-530-9939
4717 Talon Ct SE, Grand Rapids, MI 49512
MOC mobile oxygen carrier consists of a durable and lightweight canvas bag, high quality regulators with 70 psi outles, easy to read gauges, compact dual carrier for either 'D' or 'E' size cylinders, and quick connect ports.

CARRIER, CONTAINER, OXYGEN, PORTABLE *(cont'd)*

Orbis Corporation 800-890-7292
1055 Corporate Center Dr, PO Box 389, Oconomowoc, WI 53066

Sunrise Medical 800-333-4000
7477 Dry Creek Pkwy, Longmont, CO 80503

U O Equipment Co. 800-231-6372
5863 W 34th St, Houston, TX 77092

CARRIER, LIGATURE *(Surgery) 79GEJ*

Alliant Healthcare Products 269-629-0300
8850 M89, Richland, MI 49083
Tubing organizer-suture guide.

Biomet Microfixation Inc. 800-874-7711
1520 Tradeport Dr, Jacksonville, FL 32218
Various types of ligature.

Codman & Shurtleff, Inc 800-225-0460
325 Paramount Dr, Raynham, MA 02767

Integral Design Inc. 781-740-2036
52 Burr Rd, Hingham, MA 02043

Island Biosurgical, Llc 425-251-3455
18 Meadow Ln, Mercer Island, WA 98040
Suture carrier for accurate placement of endopelvic fascia bolster.

Kelsar, S.A. 508-261-8000
Blvd. Insurgentes, Libriamento a La, Tijuana 22450 Mexico
Ligature carrier

Kirwan Surgical Products, Inc. 888-547-9267
180 Enterprise Dr, PO Box 427, Marshfield, MA 02050
Bankart shoulder repair instruments.

Marina Medical Instruments, Inc. 800-697-1119
955 Shotgun Rd, Sunrise, FL 33326
Various.

Solos Endoscopy 800-388-6445
65 Sprague St # B, Boston/dedham Commerce Park, Boston, MA 02136
Manual surgical instruments for general use.

Tuzik Boston 800-886-6363
104 Longwater Dr, Assinippi Park, Norwell, MA 02061

Zimmer Holdings, Inc. 800-613-6131
1800 W Center St, PO Box 708, Warsaw, IN 46580

CARRIER, SPONGE, ENDOSCOPIC *(Gastro/Urology) 78FGS*

Aesculap Implant Systems Inc. 1-800-234-9179
3773 Corporate Pkwy, Center Valley, PA 18034

Electro Surgical Instrument Co., Inc. 888-464-2784
37 Centennial St, Rochester, NY 14611
Cotton carrier-various styles, type and sizes.

Richard Wolf Medical Instruments Corp. 800-323-9653
353 Corporate Woods Pkwy, Vernon Hills, IL 60061

CART, ANESTHETIST'S *(Anesthesiology) 73QGO*

ARMSTRONG MEDICAL INDUSTRIES, INC. 800-323-4220
575 Knightsbridge Pkwy, Lincolnshire, IL 60069
Five- and six-drawer (key-locking, auto-locking with optional proximity reader and push-button locking) lightweight, aluminum models with deep bottom drawer; ball-bearing drawer slides; interchangeable drawers; twin safety push handles; moveable drawer dividers and drug tray stock exchange system; available in 14 colors and more than 100 accessories; custom drawer arrangements available.

Atlantic Medco, Inc. 800-203-8444
166 Bloomfield Ave, Verona, NJ 07044
$500.00 to $1,000.00.

Blickman 800-247-5070
39 Robinson Rd, Lodi, NJ 07644
Stainless steel cart with your choice of 1- to 4-drawers, guard rails on three or four sides, travels on two-inch ballbearing swivel casters.

Blue Bell Bio-Medical 800-258-3235
1260 Industrial Dr, Van Wert, OH 45891
Four sizes, several styles, 75 different accessories, dividers & shelves for equipment. SURE CLAMP mounting system customizes each unit to meet specific needs plus transfer tray system allows total exchange of drawer contents. Difficult Airway Cart includes Fiberoptic Scope Cabinet (for one scope) and shelving system as well as multi-outlet strip and O2 brackets.

DURHAM MANUFACTURING COMPANY 800-243-3774
201 Main St, Durham, CT 06422

A-SMART®
AUTO-LOCKING CART
With Optional Proximity Reader

Simply wave the card in front of the reader to open. Lock the cart by pressing the lock button or set the Auto-Lock Timer for anywhere from 1 to 998 minutes. The Proximity Reader will read most low frequency HID™ Prox Cards (125 kHz).

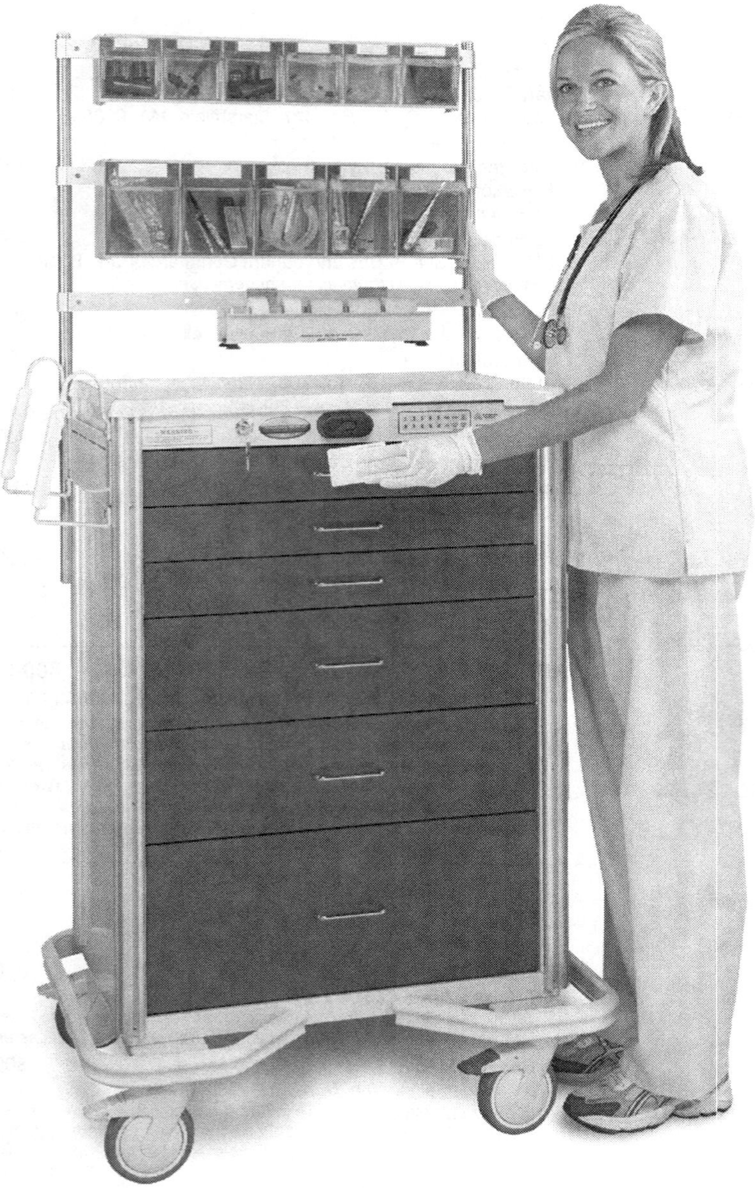

Also, our Auto-Locking Carts feature SureSeal™ Drawers. Once within approximately an inch of being shut, the SureSeal™ Drawers close automatically, so you don't need to worry if they are fully closed or if they will lock properly.

We offer several different sizes of Auto-Locking Carts. Choose from full-sized 24" or 30" Carts, Mini Cart, or Narrow Cart.

Other features include lightweight aluminum construction, many colors to choose from, master code for all programming, access code for daily use, up to 250 user codes possible,manual or automatic locking, an Auto-Lock Timer that can be set from 1 to 998 minutes or shut off so that the cart never auto-locks, and battery operation (never needs to be plugged into an outlet).Other features include lightweight aluminum construction, master code for all programming, access code for daily use, up to 250 user codes possible, manual or automatic locking, an Auto-Lock Timer that can be set from 1 to 998 minutes or shut off so that the cart never auto-locks, and battery operation (never needs to be plugged into an outlet)

Armstrong Medical
800/323-4220
FAX: 847/913-0138
www.armstrongmedical.com
csr@armstrongmedical.com

CART, ANESTHETIST'S *(cont'd)*

Harloff Company, Inc. 800-433-4064
650 Ford St, Colorado Springs, CO 80915
$1,000 to $2,000.00 list price for carts adapted to requirements of anesthesiology departments. Standard and custom drawer configurations, ball-bearing drawer slides, keylocking cabinets. Twelve cart colors, numerous storage rails and drawer divider accessories; five-year warranty.

Homak Manufacturing Company Inc. 800-874-6625
1605 Old Route 18 Ste 4-36, Wampum, PA 16157

Imperial Surgical Ltd. 800-661-5432
581 Orly Ave., Dorval, ONT H9P-1G1 Canada
Various models available.

Mayo Medical, S.A. De C.V. 800-715-3872
Edison 1141 Nte., Col. Talleres, Monterrey N.L. 64480 Mexico

Midwest Products & Engineering, Inc. 800-266-1687
10597 W Glenbrook Ct, Milwaukee, WI 53224
Carts custom designed and produced to unique OEM requirements; standard designs available from stock.

S&S Technology 281-815-1300
10625 Telge Rd, Houston, TX 77095

Waterloo Healthcare, Llc 800-833-4419
3730 E Southern Ave, Phoenix, AZ 85040
$580.00 to $2000.00 for Steel or Lightweight Aluminum crash construction. Available in three sizes with hundreds of drawer configurations to choose from. Three exterior color options; All Red, All Electric Blue, or All Gray and 18 drawer front colors to choose from. Four available locking options including our new fully-automated electronic locking system. Equipment shelves and various accessories are also available.

CART, DRESSING *(General) 80QGP*

Armstrong Medical Industries, Inc. 800-323-4220
575 Knightsbridge Pkwy, Lincolnshire, IL 60069
Five- and six-drawer (key-locking, auto-locking with optional proximity reader and push-button locking), lightweight, aluminum models with interchangeable drawers; ball bearing drawing slides, moveable drawer dividers; available in 14 colors with more than 100 accessories.

Blue Bell Bio-Medical 800-258-3235
1260 Industrial Dr, Van Wert, OH 45891
Four sizes available plus accessories.

Eagle Mhc 800-637-5100
100 Industrial Blvd, Clayton, DE 19938
Sterile wrap carts. Provide a safe and convenient place to hang, store or transport sterile wraps.

Intermetro Industries Corp. 800-441-2714
651 N Washington St, Wilkes Barre, PA 18705
STARSYS, METROFLEX or METROBASIX dressing cart.

Medikmark Inc. 800-424-8520
3600 Burwood Dr, Waukegan, IL 60085
CVC/dressing change tray. Central line dressing change tray and kits. Chloraprep.

S&S Technology 281-815-1300
10625 Telge Rd, Houston, TX 77095

Waterloo Healthcare, Llc 800-833-4419
3730 E Southern Ave, Phoenix, AZ 85040
$525.00 to $800.00 for 2 models: 3 deep drawers, 2 drawer adjustable shelf, lock/latch door.

CART, EMERGENCY, CARDIOPULMONARY RESUSCITATION (CRASH) *(Anesthesiology) 73BZN*

Ambu, Inc. 800-262-8462
6740 Baymeadow Dr, Glen Burnie, MD 21060

Armstrong Medical Industries, Inc. 800-323-4220
575 Knightsbridge Pkwy, Lincolnshire, IL 60069
Four- and six-drawer lightweight aluminum models with single seal breakaway lock, auto-locking with optional proximity reader and push-button locking,interchangeable drawers; available in 14 colors. Ball bearing drawer slides. Custom arrangements available.

Blue Bell Bio-Medical 800-258-3235
1260 Industrial Dr, Van Wert, OH 45891
Four sizes, several styles, 75 different accessories, dividers and shelves. Transfer tray system allows total exchange of drawer contents. Swing away defibrillator shelf clears top of cart for workspace.

Care Products Inc. 757-224-0177
10701 N Ware Rd, McAllen, TX 78504
Various models of cardiopulmonary emergency carts.

CART, EMERGENCY, CARDIOPULMONARY RESUSCITATION (CRASH) *(cont'd)*

Carlisle Street Llc 610-821-4222
321 S Carlisle St, Allentown, PA 18109
Carlisle systems.

Crest Healthcare Supply 800-328-8908
195 3rd St, Dassel, MN 55325

Dixie Ems Supply 800-347-3494
385 Union Ave, Brooklyn, NY 11211
$755.00 per unit (standard).

DURHAM MANUFACTURING COMPANY 800-243-3774
201 Main St, Durham, CT 06422

Harloff Company, Inc. 800-433-4064
650 Ford St, Colorado Springs, CO 80915
Full range of crash carts and accessory packages in industry-standard configurations. Carts featuring interchangeable drawers with ball-bearing drawer slides, standard and specialty packages, breakaway locking on all drawers, drawer divider options; five-year warranty. List prices range from $500 to $1500 depending on configuration, accessories, etc. Sold through Allegiance, GM, Owens and Minor, and other distributors.

Health Care Logistics, Inc. 800-848-1633
450 Town St, PO Box 25, Circleville, OH 43113
Emergency crash carts.

Healthfirst Corp. 425-771-5733
22316 70th Ave W Ste A, Mountlake Terrace, WA 98043
Cpr crash cart.

Homak Manufacturing Company Inc. 800-874-6625
1605 Old Route 18 Ste 4-36, Wampum, PA 16157

Intermetro Industries Corp. 800-441-2714
651 N Washington St, Wilkes Barre, PA 18705
LIFELINE, METROFLEX or METROBASIX emergency cart.

Life Corporation 800-700-0202
1776 N Water St, Milwaukee, WI 53202
LIFE, OxygenPac Portable emergency oxygen units, clear cover and wall-mounted, off/on lever control, resuscitation mask with one-way valve for hygiene, 6lpm 90min. supply, refillable. Also available 6 & 12 lpm NORM & HIGH, 0-25 lpm variable, and demand-valve for 100% oxygen resuscitation. GSA Federal Supply Schedule.

Mada, Inc. 800-526-6370
625 Washington Ave, Carlstadt, NJ 07072

Major Lab. Manufacturing 800-598-2621
4408 N Sewell Ave, Oklahoma City, OK 73118
3 models - from $422 to $627, with 35" or 39" working height. Optional Mayo tray, exam light, drop-leaf extension.

Midwest Products & Engineering, Inc. 800-266-1687
10597 W Glenbrook Ct, Milwaukee, WI 53224
Carts custom designed and produced to unique requirements; standard designs available from stock.

Mjm International Corporation 956-781-5000
2003 N Veterans Blvd Ste 10, San Juan, TX 78589
Various models of crash carts.

Promedica, Inc. 800-899-5278
114 Douglas Rd E, Oldsmar, FL 34677
Medical equipment carts.

S&S Technology 281-815-1300
10625 Telge Rd, Houston, TX 77095

Stanley Vidmar 800-523-9462
11 Grammes Rd, Allentown, PA 18103

Suburban Surgical Co., Inc. 800-323-7366
275 12th St, Wheeling, IL 60090

T+d Metal Products 757-224-0177
602 E Walnut St, Watseka, IL 60970
Emergency crash cart.

Tekna Solutions, Inc. 269-978-3500
3400 Tech Cir, Kalamazoo, MI 49008
Medical equipment carts.

The Anthros Medical Group 785-544-6592
807 E Spring St, Highland, KS 66035
Emergency cart.

CART, EMERGENCY, CARDIOPULMONARY RESUSCITATION (CRASH) *(cont'd)*

Waterloo Healthcare, Llc 800-833-4419
3730 E Southern Ave, Phoenix, AZ 85040
560.00 - $2,200.00 for Steel or Lightweight Aluminum crash construction. Available in three sizes with hundreds of drawer configurations to choose from. Three exterior color options; All Red, All Electric Blue, or All Gray and 18 drawer front colors to choose from. Supply/drug trays and various accessories available. Full access, emergency adult, pediatric and clinic models available. Ask about our new secure FAST PASS option available on any of our Light Weight Aluminum carts! www.waterloohealthcare.com

Youngs, Inc. 800-523-5454
55 E Cherry Ln, Souderton, PA 18964

CART, EQUIPMENT, VIDEO *(General) 80WVY*

Ams Innovative Center-San Jose 800-356-7600
3070 Orchard Dr, San Jose, CA 95134

Anthro Corporation 800-325-3841
10450 SW Manhasset Dr, Tualatin, OR 97062
Medical equipment rack.

Atd-American Co. 800-523-2300
135 Greenwood Ave, Wyncote, PA 19095

Blue Bell Bio-Medical 800-258-3235
1260 Industrial Dr, Van Wert, OH 45891

Carolina Biological Supply Co. 800-334-5551
2700 York Rd, Burlington, NC 27215

Clinimed, Incorporated 877-CLINIMED
303 Markus Ct, Sandy Brae Industrial Park, Newark, DE 19713

Custom Comfort Medtek 800-749-0933
3939 Forsyth Rd Ste A, Winter Park, FL 32792
Complete PC/entertainment center allows patients to work on MS Word documents or Excel spread sheets, send and receive e-mails, surf the Web, listen to music, and watch DVDs. The compact e-Chair self-contained unit will be available in the summer of 2003.

Deknatel Snowden-Pencer 800-367-7874
5175 S Royal Atlanta Dr, Tucker, GA 30084

Elmed, Inc. 630-543-2792
60 W Fay Ave, Addison, IL 60101

Encompas Unlimited, Inc. 800-825-7701
PO Box 516, Tallevast, FL 34270

Exchange Cart Accessories 800-823-1490
1 Commerce Dr, Freeburg, IL 62243

Intermetro Industries Corp. 800-441-2714
651 N Washington St, Wilkes Barre, PA 18705
STARSYS, SUPER ADJUSTABLE SUPER ERECTA or METROMAX video-equipment cart.

Karl Storz Endoscopy-America Inc. 800-421-0837
600 Corporate Pointe, Culver City, CA 90230
Laparoscopic video carts.

Northeast Medical Systems Corp. 856-910-8111
901 Beechwood Ave, Cherry Hill, NJ 08002
Mobile carts for cassettes or film files. Various sizes to accomodate customers' needs.

Pentax Medical Company 800-431-5880
102 Chestnut Ridge Rd, Montvale, NJ 07645
A complete line of carts for the endoscopy environment; available with optional scope holders, keyboard trays, shelves, drawers, power strips, etc.

Peter Pepper Products, Inc. 800-496-0204
17929 S Susana Rd, PO Box 5769, Compton, CA 90221

Richard Wolf Medical Instruments Corp. 800-323-9653
353 Corporate Woods Pkwy, Vernon Hills, IL 60061
Laparoscopic video carts.

S&S Technology 281-815-1300
10625 Telge Rd, Houston, TX 77095

Smith & Nephew, Inc., Endoscopy Division 800-343-8386
150 Minuteman Rd, Andover, MA 01810
Laparoscopic video carts.

Sony Electronics, Inc., Medical Systems Div. 800-686-7669
1 Sony Dr, Park Ridge, NJ 07656

Surgicorp, Inc. 727-934-5000
40347 US Highway 19 N Ste 121, Tarpon Springs, FL 34689
CARTSMART.

Valley Craft 800-328-1480
2001 S Highway 61, Lake City, MN 55041

CART, FOODSERVICE *(General) 80TAX*

Aladdin Synergetics, Inc. 800-888-8018
250 E Main St, Hendersonville, TN 37075
Various capabilities of pellet and insulated tray stainless steel delivery carts are available.

Carter-Hoffmann 800-323-9793
1551 McCormick Blvd, Mundelein, IL 60060
Tray delivery, heated banquet, mobile cafeteria and heated and refrigerated holding carts, self-leveling dispensers, slow cook and hold ovens.

DURHAM MANUFACTURING COMPANY 800-243-3774
201 Main St, Durham, CT 06422

Intermetro Industries Corp. 800-441-2714
651 N Washington St, Wilkes Barre, PA 18705
Super Erecta Super Adjustable, MetroMax, MetroMax Q, Polyerecta.

Piper Products, Inc. 800-492-3431
300 S 84th Ave, Wausau, WI 54401

Servolift/Eastern Corp. 800-727-3786
266 Hancock St, Dorchester, MA 02125
Tray delivery carts.

Suburban Surgical Co., Inc. 800-323-7366
275 12th St, Wheeling, IL 60090
Open or closed - either stainless steel or aluminum.

Tecni-Quip 800-826-1245
960 Crossroads Blvd, PO Box 2050, Seguin, TX 78155
TECNI-QUIP Many carts available, open and closed models, variety of sizes. Custom carts available to accommodate your requirements.

CART, GAS CYLINDER (CARRIER) *(Anesthesiology) 73QXW*

Air Products And Chemicals, Inc. 800-654-4567
7201 Hamilton Blvd, Allentown, PA 18195

Alimed, Inc. 800-225-2610
297 High St, Dedham, MA 02026

Contemporary Products, Inc. 800-424-2444
530 Riverside Industrial Pkwy, Portland, ME 04103

Dixie Ems Supply 800-347-3494
385 Union Ave, Brooklyn, NY 11211
$46.15 per unit (standard).

DURHAM MANUFACTURING COMPANY 800-243-3774
201 Main St, Durham, CT 06422

Eagle Mhc 800-637-5100
100 Industrial Blvd, Clayton, DE 19938
Inhalation therapy cart. Twelve 4 1/2 in. square compartments allow for any combination of D & E cylinder storage.

Farley Inc., W.T. 800-327-5397
931 Via Alondra, Camarillo, CA 93012
$67.00 Single/multiple carts; wheelchair oxygen transport, bed and gurney oxygen transport. $99.00 for double cart holding 2 cylinders plus mounting adapters for transport ventilator and blender. H tank cylinder cart, model HC400, $167.00

Intermetro Industries Corp. 800-441-2714
651 N Washington St, Wilkes Barre, PA 18705
SUPERERECTA.

Life Corporation 800-700-0202
1776 N Water St, Milwaukee, WI 53202
LIFE, OxygenPac Portable emergency oxygen units, clear cover and wall-mounted, off/on lever control, resuscitation mask with one-way valve for hygiene, 6lpm 90min. supply, refillable. Also available 6 & 12 lpm NORM & HIGH, 0-25 lpm variable, and demand-valve for 100% oxygen resuscitation. GSA Federal Supply Schedule.

Mada, Inc. 800-526-6370
625 Washington Ave, Carlstadt, NJ 07072

Mes, Inc. 800-423-2215
1968 E US Highway 90, Seguin, TX 78155
Carts for individual 'E' cylinders with gurney hook or tubing hook, dual 'E' cylinder carts, multiple (12 or 20) 'E' cylinder carts, 'H' cylinder carts, Wheelchair 'E' cylinder brackets

Troemner Llc 800-352-7705
201 Wolf Dr, PO Box 87, West Deptford, NJ 08086
Gas cylinder stands and holders.

U O Equipment Co. 800-231-6372
5863 W 34th St, Houston, TX 77092

Youngs, Inc. 800-523-5454
55 E Cherry Ln, Souderton, PA 18964

CART, HOUSEKEEPING *(General) 80TAY*

Approved Medical Systems 951-353-2453
7101 Jurupa Ave Ste 4, Riverside, CA 92504
Priced under $70 each, hampers for solid linen, trash are available with or without foot pedal.

Bennett Manufacturing Co., Inc. 800-345-2142
13315 Railroad St, Alden, NY 14004

Crest Healthcare Supply 800-328-8908
195 3rd St, Dassel, MN 55325

Geerpres 800-253-0373
1780 Harvey St, Muskegon, MI 49442
ESCORT, ESCORT RX, and WAGON MASTER housekeeping carts.

Ideal Products 800-321-5490
1287 County Road 623, Broseley, MO 63932

Intermetro Industries Corp. 800-441-2714
651 N Washington St, Wilkes Barre, PA 18705
SUPERERECTA, METROMAX, STARSYS, Metro Lodgix.

Lakeside Manufacturing Co., Inc. 800-558-8565
4900 W Electric Ave, West Milwaukee, WI 53219
Single and 2 bucket capacity in Stainless Steel and Epoxy Powder Coat. Fixed and fold up platforms.

Mcclure Industries, Inc. 800-752-2821
9051 SE 55th Ave, Portland, OR 97206
Fire-retardant Models TC35, L55, L55DL, SC700.

Medegen Medical Products, Llc 800-233-1987
209 Medegen Drive, Gallaway, TN 38036-0228
ROOM-MATES.

Meese Orbitron Dunne Co. 800-829-3230
535 N Midland Ave, Saddle Brook, NJ 07663

Mit Poly-Cart Corp. 800-234-7659
211 Central Park W, New York, NY 10024
Large capacity (60 cu ft.) waste handling cart suitable for separation and safe handling of medical home waste and regular trash.

Mobile-Tronics Co., Inc. 800-368-8181
28570 Marguerite Pkwy Ste 227, Mission Viejo, CA 92692

Omnimed, Inc. (Beam Products) 800-257-2326
800 Glen Ave, Moorestown, NJ 08057

Royce Rolls Ringer Co. 800-253-9638
PO Box 1831, 16 Riverview Terrace, Grand Rapids, MI 49501
Stainless steel seven models of wet-mopping carts ($300.00 to $900.00).

Tecni-Quip 800-826-1245
960 Crossroads Blvd, PO Box 2050, Seguin, TX 78155
TECNI-QUIP Many models for the collection or waste, biohazardous waste and recycling. Fiberglass and metal construction. Variety of sizes.

Youngs, Inc. 800-523-5454
55 E Cherry Ln, Souderton, PA 18964

CART, INSTRUMENT *(Surgery) 79QGQ*

Alimed, Inc. 800-225-2610
297 High St, Dedham, MA 02026

Armstrong Medical Industries, Inc. 800-323-4220
575 Knightsbridge Pkwy, Lincolnshire, IL 60069
Lightweight aluminum carts available with SCOPESAFE locking fiber optic scope storage cabinet attached.

Blickman 800-247-5070
39 Robinson Rd, Lodi, NJ 07644
Open and closed case carts in various sizes and configurations for transport of instruments and supplies used in surgery.

Blue Bell Bio-Medical 800-258-3235
1260 Industrial Dr, Van Wert, OH 45891
Four sizes, several styles, and various options available.

Bond Caster And Wheel Corporation 800-233-2663
230 S Penn St, PO Box 339, Manheim, PA 17545
Custom cart manufacturing in a variety of mateials.

Cameron-Miller, Inc. 800-621-0142
5410 W Roosevelt Rd, Road #241, Chicago, IL 60644

Dntlworks Equipment Corporation 800-847-0694
7300 S Tucson Way, Centennial, CO 80112
A variety of configurations includes doctor's delivery carts, assistant's carts, and complete, self-contained delivery units.

DURHAM MANUFACTURING COMPANY 800-243-3774
201 Main St, Durham, CT 06422

CART, INSTRUMENT *(cont'd)*

Eagle Mhc 800-637-5100
100 Industrial Blvd, Clayton, DE 19938
Suture cart. Open wire slanted shelves provide quick and easy access to sutures.

Harloff Company, Inc. 800-433-4064
650 Ford St, Colorado Springs, CO 80915
$300 to $600 for carts featuring interchangeable drawers with ball-bearing drawer slides, three cabinet models, standard and specialty packages, keylocking cabinets, eight cart colors, plastic tops; five-year warranty.

Healthmark Industries 800-521-6224
22522 E 9 Mile Rd, Saint Clair Shores, MI 48080
Hushkarts - decorative colors.

Homak Manufacturing Company Inc. 800-874-6625
1605 Old Route 18 Ste 4-36, Wampum, PA 16157

Ideal Products 800-321-5490
1287 County Road 623, Broseley, MO 63932
Specialty equipment carts designed to fit a variety of instruments and devices.

Intermetro Industries Corp. 800-441-2714
651 N Washington St, Wilkes Barre, PA 18705
SUPERERECTA, METROMAX, METROMAXQ, STARSYS Super Adjustable.

Kadan Co. Inc., D.A. 800-325-2326
1 Brigadoon Ln, Waxhaw, NC 28173
Mobile utility carts model #313, 314 and 315.

KnÅrr Usa Inc. 800-465-6877
1890 Voyager Ave, Simi Valley, CA 93063
DACOMOBILE modular mobile workstation. Heavy duty aesthetic design for uses in all aspects of the medical market. Flat Screen mounting, and a wide variety of accessories. Custom configurations & colors. Available with integrated 19' rack system. Metra Mobil economical modular mobile workstation with add-on options.

Labconco Corp. 800-821-5525
8811 Prospect Ave, Kansas City, MO 64132
16 Different Laboratory Carts and Mobile Benches

Md International, Inc. 305-669-9003
11300 NW 41st St, Doral, FL 33178

Midmark Corporation 800-643-6275
60 Vista Dr, P.O. Box 286, Versailles, OH 45380

Midwest Products & Engineering, Inc. 800-266-1687
10597 W Glenbrook Ct, Milwaukee, WI 53224
Carts designed and produced to unique OEM requirements; standard designs available from stock.

Mobile-Tronics Co., Inc. 800-368-8181
28570 Marguerite Pkwy Ste 227, Mission Viejo, CA 92692

Pedigo Products 360-695-3500
4000 SE Columbia Way, Vancouver, WA 98661
Instrument Container Wash Cart: Model CDS-160, an all stainless steel mobile cart designed specifically for washing instrument containers in an automatic cart washer. Holds up to 20 instrument containers.

Pentax Medical Company 800-431-5880
102 Chestnut Ridge Rd, Montvale, NJ 07645
Mobile cart for endoscopic procedures.

S&S Technology 281-815-1300
10625 Telge Rd, Houston, TX 77095

S&W By Hausmann 888-428-7626
130 Union St, Northvale, NJ 07647

Scientek Medical Equipment 604-273-9094
11151 Bridgeport Rd., Richmond, BC V6X 1T3 Canada

Stanley Vidmar 800-523-9462
11 Grammes Rd, Allentown, PA 18103
Surgical instruments.

Suburban Surgical Co., Inc. 800-323-7366
275 12th St, Wheeling, IL 60090

Waterloo Healthcare, Llc 800-833-4419
3730 E Southern Ave, Phoenix, AZ 85040
$525.00 to $800.00 for two models: 3, 4, 5, 6 drawers, drawer trays.

Wheelit, Inc. 800-523-7508
440 Arco Dr, Toledo, OH 43607
Instrumentation carts: $224.00 to $440.00 (folding); $209.00 to $379.00 (nonfolding).

CART, INSTRUMENT/EQUIPMENT, LAPAROSCOPY
(Surgery) 79QZT

Armstrong Medical Industries, Inc. 800-323-4220
575 Knightsbridge Pkwy, Lincolnshire, IL 60069
Carts available with SCOPESAFE locking fiber optic scope storage cabinet attached.

Dma Med-Chem Corporation 800-362-1833
49 Watermill Ln, Great Neck, NY 11021

Elmed, Inc. 630-543-2792
60 W Fay Ave, Addison, IL 60101

Exchange Cart Accessories 800-823-1490
1 Commerce Dr, Freeburg, IL 62243

Intermetro Industries Corp. 800-441-2714
651 N Washington St, Wilkes Barre, PA 18705
STARSY, METROFLEX, or METROBASIX laparoscopy cart.

Seitz Technical Products, Inc. 610-268-2228
729 Newark Rd, Avondale, PA 19311

Tapco Medical, Inc. 818-225-5376
23981 Craftsman Rd, Calabasas, CA 91302
Cool Cart

Taut, Inc. 800-231-8288
2571 Kaneville Ct, Geneva, IL 60134
Self adjustable check valve prevents loss of insufflation gas.

Wisap America 800-233-8448
8231 Melrose Dr, Lenexa, KS 66214

CART, ISOLATION *(General) 80QGR*

Approved Medical Systems 951-353-2453
7101 Jurupa Ave Ste 4, Riverside, CA 92504
Priced under $70 each, hampers for infectious, biohazard waste and linen, available with or without a foot pedal.

Armstrong Medical Industries, Inc. 800-323-4220
575 Knightsbridge Pkwy, Lincolnshire, IL 60069
Four different lightweight aluminum models available.

Exchange Cart Accessories 800-823-1490
1 Commerce Dr, Freeburg, IL 62243

Homak Manufacturing Company Inc. 800-874-6625
1605 Old Route 18 Ste 4-36, Wampum, PA 16157

Intermetro Industries Corp. 800-441-2714
651 N Washington St, Wilkes Barre, PA 18705
STARSYS, METROFLEX or METROBASIX isolation cart.

S&S Technology 281-815-1300
10625 Telge Rd, Houston, TX 77095

Waterloo Healthcare, Llc 800-833-4419
3730 E Southern Ave, Phoenix, AZ 85040
$560.00 to $800.00 Steel or Lightweight Aluminum crash construction. Available in three sizes with hundreds of drawer configurations to choose from. Drawers are available in 18 colors including 'Sunshine Yellow' the most popular for isolation departments.

CART, LAUNDRY *(General) 80TAZ*

Alimed, Inc. 800-225-2610
297 High St, Dedham, MA 02026

Approved Medical Systems 951-353-2453
7101 Jurupa Ave Ste 4, Riverside, CA 92504
For infectious and soiled linen; also usable with water soluble bags and liners.

Atd-American Co. 800-523-2300
135 Greenwood Ave, Wyncote, PA 19095

Atlantic Medco, Inc. 800-203-8444
166 Bloomfield Ave, Verona, NJ 07044
$1,000.00 to $1,500.00.

Duralife, Inc. 800-443-5433
195 Phillips Park Dr, Williamsport, PA 17702

Innovative Products Unlimited, Inc. 800-833-2826
2120 Industrial Dr, Niles, MI 49120
$570.00 for PVC 3 shelf w/cover linen cart.

Intermetro Industries Corp. 800-441-2714
651 N Washington St, Wilkes Barre, PA 18705
SUPERERECTA, METROTRUX.

Mayo Medical, S.A. De C.V. 800-715-3872
Edison 1141 Nte., Col. Talleres, Monterrey N.L. 64480 Mexico

Mcclure Industries, Inc. 800-752-2821
9051 SE 55th Ave, Portland, OR 97206
Fire-retardant Models L55, L55DL, 240, 400, 440, 600, 610, 630, 650, 2460.

CART, LAUNDRY *(cont'd)*

Meese Orbitron Dunne Co. 800-829-3230
535 N Midland Ave, Saddle Brook, NJ 07663

Mip Inc. 800-361-4964
9100 Ray Lawson Blvd., Montreal, QC H1J-1K8 Canada
MED-I-CART laundry cart.

Mit Poly-Cart Corp. 800-234-7659
211 Central Park W, New York, NY 10024
Pilfer-proof security provided by the patented Roll-Top door.

Pedigo Products 360-695-3500
4000 SE Columbia Way, Vancouver, WA 98661
Stainless steel, various styles and sizes.

R&B Wire Products, Inc. 800-634-0555
2902 W Garry Ave, Santa Ana, CA 92704
Heavy gauge wire basket; 2 1/2 and 4 bushel capacity.

Royce Rolls Ringer Co. 800-253-9638
PO Box 1831, 16 Riverview Terrace, Grand Rapids, MI 49501
Stainless steel two models of laundry-linen carts.

Secure Care Products, Inc. 800-451-7917
39 Chenell Dr, Concord, NH 03301
Mobile handwashing and laundry cart designed to prevent spread of infectants when changing linen and and handling high-risk patients.

Steele Canvas Basket Co., Inc. 800-541-8929
201 Williams St, Chelsea, MA 02150

Suburban Surgical Co., Inc. 800-323-7366
275 12th St, Wheeling, IL 60090
Open stainless steel.

Tecni-Quip 800-826-1245
960 Crossroads Blvd, PO Box 2050, Seguin, TX 78155
TECNI-QUIP Aluminum, fiberglass, poly and wire carts. Open or closed models available in a variety of sizes. Laundry processing and linen delivery custom manufacturing.

Youngs, Inc. 800-523-5454
55 E Cherry Ln, Souderton, PA 18964

CART, MEDICINE *(General) 80QGS*

Armstrong Medical Industries, Inc. 800-323-4220
575 Knightsbridge Pkwy, Lincolnshire, IL 60069

Artromick International, Inc. 800-848-6462
4800 Hilton Corporate Dr, Columbus, OH 43232
Medication carts with digital electronic locking option and alarm feature. Single-sided or dual-sided, with cable lock and color-code system. PC models exclusively for punch card drug applications. 9 cart models available.

Atlantic Medco, Inc. 800-203-8444
166 Bloomfield Ave, Verona, NJ 07044
Three models: $849.00 to $1,015.00 for FOREST 9200-6 oral/syringe model with 24 to 36 med cups; $1,217.00 to $1,234.00 for MEDI-SERV MS 18:30 unit dose model with 18:30 med drawers; $1,701.00 to $1,737.00 for MEDI-SERV MS-36:60 unit dose model with 36:60 drawers.

Colonial Scientific Ltd. 902-468-1811
201 Brownlow Ave., Unit 52, Dartmouth, NS B3B-1W2 Canada

Crest Healthcare Supply 800-328-8908
195 3rd St, Dassel, MN 55325

Flo Healthcare 877-356-4040
5801 Goshen Springs Rd Ste A, Norcross, GA 30071

Harloff Company, Inc. 800-433-4064
650 Ford St, Colorado Springs, CO 80915
Full line of medication delivery carts for unit-dose, cassette-exchange, or bingo-card pharmacy systems. List prices range from $ 1900 to $ 2800. Features include dual-locking narc drawer for compliance with JCAHO, high-capacity design, wrap-around bumper, ball-bearing drawer slides. Custom configurations to suit patient needs. Available in twelve cart colors with five-year warranty. New model features electronic lock with proximity sensor that can be used as a badge scanner.

Homak Manufacturing Company Inc. 800-874-6625
1605 Old Route 18 Ste 4-36, Wampum, PA 16157

Imperial Surgical Ltd. 800-661-5432
581 Orly Ave., Dorval, ONT H9P-1G1 Canada
$1,250 per unit.

Lionville Systems, Inc. 800-523-7114
501 Gunnard Carlson Dr, Coatesville, PA 19320
Several styles with a patented drawer grabber locking mechanism to ensure that drawers that look locked are locked. Cart options include automatic relocking, keyless entry, keyless 'narcotic' drawers, and a full array of computer-related accessories.

CART, MEDICINE *(cont'd)*

Metronix 813-972-1212
12421 N Florida Ave Ste D201, Tampa, FL 33612
Rehab equipment.

O&M Enterprise 847-258-4515
641 Chelmsford Ln, Elk Grove Village, IL 60007
CARTS MEDICINE/MULTIPURPOSE

S&S Medcart 800-231-1747
10625 Telge Rd, Houston, TX 77095
A highly adaptable medication storage to complement state-of-the-art mobile computer solutions. The Q-Pack Battery maintains power to computer and single monitor. 2000 user-ID access codes provide a silent partner audit trail.

S&S Technology 281-815-1300
10625 Telge Rd, Houston, TX 77095

Waterloo Healthcare, Llc 800-833-4419
3730 E Southern Ave, Phoenix, AZ 85040
$1,370.00 to $2,800.00 for Long Term or Acute Care medication carts. Available as a single sided or dual sided medical carts. Optional patient bins, exchange cassettes available in 3 sizes. Medication drawers, bin/tray systems and accessories.

CART, MONITOR *(General) 80WTI*

Armstrong Medical Industries, Inc. 800-323-4220
575 Knightsbridge Pkwy, Lincolnshire, IL 60069

Blue Bell Bio-Medical 800-258-3235
1260 Industrial Dr, Van Wert, OH 45891
Four sizes available with SURE CLAMP mounting system with large selection of accessories and various styles of shelving.

Flo Healthcare 877-356-4040
5801 Goshen Springs Rd Ste A, Norcross, GA 30071

Gcx Corp. 800-228-2555
3875 Cypress Dr, Petaluma, CA 94954
POLYMOUNT rollstands for patient monitor and other medical devices.

Harloff Company, Inc. 800-433-4064
650 Ford St, Colorado Springs, CO 80915
Carts have choice of overhead shelves, interchangeable drawers with ball-bearing drawer slides, key-locking cabinets, nine cart colors, hospital-grade electrical outlet, drawer divider accessories; five-year warranty. Custom configurations also available.

Intermetro Industries Corp. 800-441-2714
651 N Washington St, Wilkes Barre, PA 18705
STARSYS, METROFLEX or METROBASIX monitor cart.

Medical Design Systems, Inc. 800-593-1900
10035 Lakeview Ave, Lenexa, KS 66219
Cart, Monitoring - configure carts to suit your own specific requirements. Modular items available include FIFOGLIDES, SLOTSHELVES, baskets, bins, LOKSHELVES, hanger bars and more.

Medved Products, Inc. 651-482-8413
PO Box 120883, Saint Paul, MN 55112
Roll stands for monitors

Midwest Products & Engineering, Inc. 800-266-1687
10597 W Glenbrook Ct, Milwaukee, WI 53224
Carts custom designed and produced to unique OEM requirements; standard designs available from stock.

Pentax Medical Company 800-431-5880
102 Chestnut Ridge Rd, Montvale, NJ 07645
Various models available for monitors ranging in sizes.

Purdy Electronics Corp. 408-523-8201
720 Palomar Ave, Sunnyvale, CA 94085
AND Displays liquid crystal displays - high bright IFC color monitors and modules - 1,000 displays.

S&S Technology 281-815-1300
10625 Telge Rd, Houston, TX 77095

CART, MULTIPURPOSE *(General) 80QGT*

Anthro Corporation 800-325-3841
10450 SW Manhasset Dr, Tualatin, OR 97062
ANTHROCART, available in different widths, heights and depths. Over 75 accessories to add for all types of equipment.

CART, MULTIPURPOSE *(cont'd)*

Armstrong Medical Industries, Inc. 800-323-4220
575 Knightsbridge Pkwy, Lincolnshire, IL 60069
Key-locking, breakaway locking, auto-locking with optional proximity reader and push-button locking, lightweight aluminum customized workstations, interchangeable drawers, deep bottom drawer, twin push safety handles, shelving units and wide variety of accessories. Movable, adjustable drawer dividers, drawer trays, and organizers. Available in 14 colors and accessories.

Atlantic Medco, Inc. 800-203-8444
166 Bloomfield Ave, Verona, NJ 07044
$500.00 to 1,000.00.

Blickman 800-247-5070
39 Robinson Rd, Lodi, NJ 07644
Model 7534SS stainless steel general purpose utility cart 16'x24'. Larger carts such as par level, supply/exchange carts are available in three styles and six sizes and come with a wire mesh back screen, full length chrome wire shelves, totes.

Blue Bell Bio-Medical 800-258-3235
1260 Industrial Dr, Van Wert, OH 45891
Four sizes available with SURE CLAMP mounting system, and over 75 accessories, shelves and dividers. Complete system of adjustable dividers and organizers for crash carts, anesthesia carts and other mobile storage units. Trays hold dividers for quick exchange of drawer contents. (Also, transport covers and bags.)

Brandt Industries, Inc. 800-221-8031
4461 Bronx Blvd, Bronx, NY 10470
36410: for use with pumps, ECG, scalers, and other units. 36411: with roll. Variety with drawers, slanted tops, without drawers. 34241: stand with drawer, ECG.

Cole-Parmer Instrument Inc. 800-323-4340
625 E Bunker Ct, Vernon Hills, IL 60061

Contemporary Products, Inc. 800-424-2444
530 Riverside Industrial Pkwy, Portland, ME 04103

DURHAM MANUFACTURING COMPANY 800-243-3774
201 Main St, Durham, CT 06422
Stainless steel cart.

Ethicon, Inc. 800-4-ETHICON
Route 22 West, Somerville, NJ 08876

Gi Supply 800-451-5797
200 Grandview Ave, Camp Hill, PA 17011
UNITY procedure cart with multiple optional attachments. To aid in endoscopic procedure organization, processing biopsies, and cleanup.

Gillis Associated Industries 800-397-1675
750 Pinecrest Dr, Prospect Heights, IL 60070
Open wire all-purpose carts made of heavy-duty, self-cleaning wire mesh.

Hamilton Caster & Mfg. Co. 888-699-7164
1637 Dixie Hwy, Hamilton, OH 45011
Variety of non-powered carts and platform trucks.

Harloff Company, Inc. 800-433-4064
650 Ford St, Colorado Springs, CO 80915
$800.00 to $1000.00 list price for multi-treat carts featuring interchangeable drawers with ball-bearing drawer slides, choice of locking systems, twelve cart colors, numerous accessories, drawer-divider accessories; five-year warranty (customize to requirement). Storage space with 21-in. key-locking door.

Hausmann Industries, Inc. 888-428-7626
130 Union St, Northvale, NJ 07647
$268.00 per unit (standard).

Healthmark Industries 800-521-6224
22522 E 9 Mile Rd, Saint Clair Shores, MI 48080
$1,400.00 per unit (standard); custom designed carts and racks available.

Hill-Rom Holdings, Inc. 800-445-3730
1069 State Road 46 E, Batesville, IN 47006

Homak Manufacturing Company Inc. 800-874-6625
1605 Old Route 18 Ste 4-36, Wampum, PA 16157

Intermetro Industries Corp. 800-441-2714
651 N Washington St, Wilkes Barre, PA 18705
METROFLEX, STARSYS, METROMAX, SUPERERECTA, supply/procedure carts.

Labconco Corp. 800-821-5525
8811 Prospect Ave, Kansas City, MO 64132

CART, MULTIPURPOSE *(cont'd)*

Lakeside Manufacturing Co., Inc. 800-558-8565
4900 W Electric Ave, West Milwaukee, WI 53219
Welded stainless steel construction. Four shelf sizes, weight capacities of 300, 500, 700, & 1000#. Ergo and Traditional style.

Lionville Systems, Inc. 800-523-7114
501 Gunnard Carlson Dr, Coatesville, PA 19320
The Healthcare cart line is designed to support anesthesia, emergency, isolation, treatments, and a variety of other multipurpose applications. Available in two different heights, cart options include automatic re-locking, keyless entry, keyless 'narcotic' drawers, and an array of storage accessories.

Mayo Medical, S.A. De C.V. 800-715-3872
Edison 1141 Nte., Col. Talleres, Monterrey N.L. 64480 Mexico

Mcclure Industries, Inc. 800-752-2821
9051 SE 55th Ave, Portland, OR 97206
Fire-retardant Models L55, L55DL, 240, 400, 440, 600, 610, 630, 650.

Medical Safety Systems Inc. 888-803-9303
230 White Pond Dr, Akron, OH 44313
Bloodborne compliance guide wall chart.

Midwest Products & Engineering, Inc. 800-266-1687
10597 W Glenbrook Ct, Milwaukee, WI 53224
Carts designed and produced to unique OEM requirements; standard designs available from stock.

Penco Products Inc. 800-562-1000
PO Box 378, 99 Brower Ave., Oaks, PA 19456

Pentax Medical Company 800-431-5880
102 Chestnut Ridge Rd, Montvale, NJ 07645
A full line of procedure carts is available.

R&B Wire Products, Inc. 800-634-0555
2902 W Garry Ave, Santa Ana, CA 92704
Trucks and utility carts; 8 x 12 bushel trucks with vinyl/nylon laminate liner; can be shipped UPS; utility cart for supplies, mail, etc.

Rem Systems 305-499-4800
625 E 10th Ave, Hialeah, FL 33010
X-Ray carts - line of x-ray film and cassette transports.

S&S Technology 281-815-1300
10625 Telge Rd, Houston, TX 77095

Stackbin Corporation 800-333-1603
29 Powder Hill Rd, Lincoln, RI 02865
Stacktracks - mobile storage systems for x-ray files and medical records.

Suburban Surgical Co., Inc. 800-323-7366
275 12th St, Wheeling, IL 60090

Tecni-Quip 800-826-1245
960 Crossroads Blvd, PO Box 2050, Seguin, TX 78155
Various models: linen, laundry, waste, central supply and custom designed carts.

Valley Craft 800-328-1480
2001 S Highway 61, Lake City, MN 55041

Waterloo Healthcare, Llc 800-833-4419
3730 E Southern Ave, Phoenix, AZ 85040
$300.00 to $1200.00 for 3, 4, 5, or 6 drawer units.

Wheelit, Inc. 800-523-7508
440 Arco Dr, Toledo, OH 43607
$127.00 to $599.00 per unit; 28 models.

Windquest 800-562-4257
3311 Windquest Dr, Holland, MI 49424

Youngs, Inc. 800-523-5454
55 E Cherry Ln, Souderton, PA 18964

CART, ORTHOPEDIC SUPPLY (CAST) *(Orthopedics) 87QGU*

Bsn Medical, Inc 800-552-1157
5825 Carnegie Blvd, Charlotte, NC 28209
M-PACT® MOBILE PLASTER VENDOR has a stainless steel work surface that unfolds to a convenient height with a large enough area to prepare most casts and splints. Ample storage keeps instruments and supplies within easy reach.

Harloff Company, Inc. 800-433-4064
650 Ford St, Colorado Springs, CO 80915
Cast carts designed in conjunction with orthopedic technicians for effective storage of supplies. Stainless-steel construction, numerous options. List prices range from $1,800 to $2,600.

Imperial Surgical Ltd. 800-661-5432
581 Orly Ave., Dorval, ONT H9P-1G1 Canada
$3,000 each.

CART, ORTHOPEDIC SUPPLY (CAST) *(cont'd)*

Intermetro Industries Corp. 800-441-2714
651 N Washington St, Wilkes Barre, PA 18705
STARSYS, METROFLEX or METROBASIX cast cart.

Suburban Surgical Co., Inc. 800-323-7366
275 12th St, Wheeling, IL 60090

Zimmer Holdings, Inc. 800-613-6131
1800 W Center St, PO Box 708, Warsaw, IN 46580

CART, OTHER *(General) 80QGW*

A.R.C. Distributors 800-296-8724
PO Box 599, Centreville, MD 21617
TRANSCART wheelchair and cart. Because of its size, it discourages theft; anti-fold wheelchair cart, ultramodern design. Wheelchair for patient, cart for belongings. Weight limit 500 lbs. Caddy: a dual basket wheelchair accessory, reduces theft. Stretchair is a wheelchair that easily converts into a strecher. Weight capacity 250lb, 400lb, 600lb and 800lb. PhaseChair & CareChair is a wheelchair that converts into a stretcher. Weight Capacity 400lb 650lb & 850lb.

Akro-Mils, Inc. 800-253-2467
1293 S Main St, Akron, OH 44301

Appropriate Technical Resources, Inc. 800-827-5931
9157 Whiskey Bottom Rd, PO Box 460, Laurel, MD 20723
Custom Laboratory Cart.

Artromick International, Inc. 800-848-6462
4800 Hilton Corporate Dr, Columbus, OH 43232
Medication/Narcotics carts with digital electronic locking and alarm option. Single-sided or dual-sided, with cable lock and color-code system. PC models exclusively for punch card drug applications. Over 30 cart models available. New products include the AVALO medical/hospital cart series as well as a line of keyless, automatic-relocking hospital carts.

Atlantic Medco, Inc. 800-203-8444
166 Bloomfield Ave, Verona, NJ 07044
$950 to $1100 Case carts.

Best Manufacturing Group Llc 800-843-3233
1633 Broadway Fl 18, New York, NY 10019
Linen carts and covers.

Blue Bell Bio-Medical 800-258-3235
1260 Industrial Dr, Van Wert, OH 45891
Emergency malignant hyperthermia cart: including refrigerator and freezer, cold packs, drawers for supplies, and sealing system. Also divider and drug transfer systems; adjustable, flexible, customized, drawers and trays for emergency, anesthesia carts and others.

Bunnell Incorporated 800-800-4358
436 Lawndale Dr, Salt Lake City, UT 84115
Four shelf equipment cart.

C.J.T. Enterprises, Inc. 714-751-6295
PO Box 10028, Costa Mesa, CA 92627
Adjustable Floor Stand is perfect for achieving multiple positions in a single location. A simple design and extremely effective, the Floor Stand starts with a 5 legged base for stability and strength. Two telescoping tubes allow you to achieve the height you need. Easy to move around and adjust the Floor stand can hold notebook comuters, LCD screens and all AAC devices.

Case Medical, Inc. 888-227-2273
65 Railroad Ave, Ridgefield, NJ 07657
transport and store sterilization containers

Colonial Scientific Ltd. 902-468-1811
201 Brownlow Ave., Unit 52, Dartmouth, NS B3B-1W2 Canada
Crash carts.

Da-Lite Screen Co., Inc. 800-622-3737
3100 N Detroit St, PO Box 137, Warsaw, IN 46582
Computer carts, all metal, adjustable with monitor shelf, 25 x 36 in. work surface.

Diacor, Inc. 800-342-2679
3191 Valley St Ste 100A, Salt Lake City, UT 84109
$1,295.00 for blocking tray cart.

Duralife, Inc. 800-443-5433
195 Phillips Park Dr, Williamsport, PA 17702
Lightweight, durable ice cart features large worktop area skirt, storage shelf, 25qt. removable ice chest, scoop and scoop holder.

DURHAM MANUFACTURING COMPANY 800-243-3774
201 Main St, Durham, CT 06422

Eagle Mhc 800-637-5100
100 Industrial Blvd, Clayton, DE 19938
Catheter procedure carts hold all types of catheter packages. Also, a variety of cassette transport carts carry 8 cassettes.

CART, OTHER *(cont'd)*

Ergotron, Inc. 800-888-8458
1181 Trapp Rd, Saint Paul, MN 55121
The StyleView point-of-care computer cart offers 20î height adjustment, UL 60601 listed and open architecture. It offers easy to use straight up and down movement on a small stable base. Also included are an oversized work surface, internal cable management and equipment locks for increased hardware security.

Exchange Cart Accessories 800-823-1490
1 Commerce Dr, Freeburg, IL 62243
Catheter cart.

Farley Inc., W.T. 800-327-5397
931 Via Alondra, Camarillo, CA 93012
MRI Non-Aluminum magnetic oxygen cylinder carts. Model HC100A single cylinder cart $175.00. Model HC200A dual cylinder cart $225.00. MOBILOX 6 cylinder transport cart, ES106W $140.00, MOBILOX 20 cylinder, ES120W, $237.00.

Gcx Corp. 800-228-2555
3875 Cypress Dr, Petaluma, CA 94954
POLYMOUNT rollstands for mobile information technology (IT) hardware coponents including keyboard or other input devices, display, CPU, and UPS units.

Gillis Associated Industries 800-397-1675
750 Pinecrest Dr, Prospect Heights, IL 60070
Mail carts, security carts (both mobile and immobile), chart and record carts. Also sterile wrap cart, linen carts, Exchange carts and suture carts.

Homak Manufacturing Company Inc. 800-874-6625
1605 Old Route 18 Ste 4-36, Wampum, PA 16157

Hos-Pillow Corp. 800-468-7874
1011 Campus Dr, Mundelein, IL 60060
Stem caster wire and solid carts.

Ideal Products 800-321-5490
1287 County Road 623, Broseley, MO 63932
Unique carts designed to fit special equipment or needs.

Imperial Surgical Ltd. 800-661-5432
581 Orly Ave., Dorval, ONT H9P-1G1 Canada
Surgical case cart, various models.

Infab Corp. 805-987-5255
3651 Via Pescador, Camarillo, CA 93012
Lightweight, sturdy carts for cassette and film transport.

Innovative Products Unlimited, Inc. 800-833-2826
2120 Industrial Dr, Niles, MI 49120
Utility treatment, ice and emergency carts, $390 for insulated ice delivery cart.

Intermetro Industries Corp. 800-441-2714
651 N Washington St, Wilkes Barre, PA 18705
Linen, catheter, suture and surgical carts.

Leader Instruments Corp. 800-645-5104
6484 Commerce Dr, Cypress, CA 90630
Technical instrument carts.

Leeco Industries, Inc. 662-551-1025
540 S Industrial Park Rd, Holly Springs, MS 38635
Mobile filing carts.

Leisure-Lift, Inc. 800-255-0285
1800 Merriam Ln, Kansas City, KS 66106
$1,700 to $2,800 for 3- and 4-wheeled battery-powered mobility carts.

Lionville Systems, Inc. 800-523-7114
501 Gunnard Carlson Dr, Coatesville, PA 19320
Patient-care centers with built-in cart components; pharmacy master carts; restock carts for medication 'ATM's; and anesthesia carts that re-lock automatically.

Lista International Corp. 800-722-3020
106 Lowland St, Holliston, MA 01746
Mobile drawer and shelf carts.

Lm Air Technology, Inc. 866-381-8200
1467 Pinewood St, Cleanroom & Lab Equipment - Mfger Rahway, NJ 07065
Stainless steel or chrome plated.

Mcclure Industries, Inc. 800-752-2821
9051 SE 55th Ave, Portland, OR 97206
Fire-retardant standard and custom designed carts.

CART, OTHER *(cont'd)*

Medical Design Systems, Inc. 800-593-1900
10035 Lakeview Ave, Lenexa, KS 66219
Modular Supply Carts to create just the right cart for your specific procedures and protocols or an entire customized mobile storage system. Unique interior modules to precisely accommodate catheters, guidewires, balloons, stents and all types of supply packaging with no wasted space. Interior modules include FIFOGLIDES, SLOTSHELVES, baskets, bins, LOKSHELVES, hanger bars and numerous accessories. Unlimited design options for every department. Fifth wheel design for maximum maneuverability. Catheter carts, Angioplasty carts, Stent Carts, ERCP Carts, Monitor carts, Cysto carts, Vascular Surgery carts, Biopsy carts, Anesthesia Supply carts, Orthopedic Supply carts, General Surgery Supply carts, IV carts, Computer carts, and more.

Medin Corporation 800-922-0476
90 Dayton Ave, Bldg. 16 C, Passaic, NJ 07055
Sterilization carts and baskets.

Medirecord Systems 800-561-9791
P.O. Box 6201 Station A, Saint John, NB E2L 4R6 Canada
X-ray records, medical charts and records carts.

Midwest Products & Engineering, Inc. 800-266-1687
10597 W Glenbrook Ct, Milwaukee, WI 53224
Carts custom designed and produced to unique OEM requirements; standard designs available from stock.

Mit Poly-Cart Corp. 800-234-7659
211 Central Park W, New York, NY 10024
Recycling Cart

Mobile-Tronics Co., Inc. 800-368-8181
28570 Marguerite Pkwy Ste 227, Mission Viejo, CA 92692

Omnimed, Inc. (Beam Products) 800-257-2326
800 Glen Ave, Moorestown, NJ 08057

Peter Pepper Products, Inc. 800-496-0204
17929 S Susana Rd, PO Box 5769, Compton, CA 90221
Gift display. Audio Visual, Mobile Chart Cart.

Phelan Manufacturing Corp. 800-328-2358
2523 Minnehaha Ave, Minneapolis, MN 55404
$247.00 for step stand cart.

Physio-Control, Inc. 800-442-1142
11811 Willows Rd NE, Redmond, WA 98052
LIFECART and QUIK-CART emergency carts.

R&B Wire Products, Inc. 800-634-0555
2902 W Garry Ave, Santa Ana, CA 92704
Trucks and utility carts; 8 x 12 bushel trucks with vinyl/nylon laminate liner; can be shipped UPS; utility cart for supplies, mail, etc.

Rem Systems 305-499-4800
625 E 10th Ave, Hialeah, FL 33010
Film Transfer, Mobile Cassette & film & X-Ray Transport.

Ross Disposable Products 800-649-6526
401 Traders Blvd E, Unit 10, Mississauga, ON L4Z 2H8 Canada

Royce Rolls Ringer Co. 800-253-9638
PO Box 1831, 16 Riverview Terrace, Grand Rapids, MI 49501
Open shelf cart and stainless steel utility carry-all cart.

S&S Technology 281-815-1300
10625 Telge Rd, Houston, TX 77095
X-ray cassette and film carts with four models to choose from. Two- and three-shelf carts plus a full line of illuminations, motorized viewers, darkroom cabinets, and x-ray storage.

Servolift/Eastern Corp. 800-727-3786
266 Hancock St, Dorchester, MA 02125

Steelcraft, Inc. 800-225-7710
115 W Main St, Millbury, MA 01527

United Metal Fabricators, Inc. 800-638-5322
1316 Eisenhower Blvd, Johnstown, PA 15904

Valley Craft 800-328-1480
2001 S Highway 61, Lake City, MN 55041

Wes-Pak, Inc. 1-800-493-7725
11610 Vimy Ridge Rd, Alexander, AR 72002
Custom cart systems designed to meet the needs of clinical customers.

Wheelit, Inc. 800-523-7508
440 Arco Dr, Toledo, OH 43607
28 folding and rigid models.

Windquest 800-562-4257
3311 Windquest Dr, Holland, MI 49424
Portable modular storage carts for ICU, endoscopy, I.V. therapy, phlebotomy, dialysis, and fetal monitoring.

CART, OTHER *(cont'd)*

Youngs, Inc. 800-523-5454
55 E Cherry Ln, Souderton, PA 18964
Medical.

CART, PATIENT (STRETCHER) *(Anesthesiology) 73BWM*

A.R.C. Distributors 800-296-8724
PO Box 599, Centreville, MD 21617
GENDRON, Prone Stretcher Cart self propelled stretcher with pad. Series 1000 General Transfer and Transport; Series 600 Folding Transfer and Emergency. Stretchair: a wheelchair that easily converts into a stretcher; weight capacity 200lb, 400lb, 600lb, and 800lb. Phase Chair/Care Chair wheelchair and stretcher combination; weight capacity 400lb (manual), 600lb and 850lb (electric).

Colonial Scientific Ltd. 902-468-1811
201 Brownlow Ave., Unit 52, Dartmouth, NS B3B-1W2 Canada

Gendron, Inc. 800-537-2521
400 E Lugbill Rd, Archbold, OH 43502
Prone cart/self-propelled stretcher. $910.00. Patient can propel in prone position.

Mayo Medical, S.A. De C.V. 800-715-3872
Edison 1141 Nte., Col. Talleres, Monterrey N.L. 64480 Mexico

Morrison Medical 800-438-6677
3735 Paragon Dr, Columbus, OH 43228
SHAMU Soft Stretcher is extra large for carrying large people. It is 60 x 80' and will hold up to 1500 pounds. It has 8 handles. 2 smaller sizes available.

Scientek Medical Equipment 604-273-9094
11151 Bridgeport Rd., Richmond, BC V6X 1T3 Canada
Mobile dissection table and body tray, stainless steel, 800 pounds capacity/cart.

Stryker Medical 800-869-0770
3800 E Centre Ave, Portage, MI 49002

CART, SUPPLY *(General) 80TAW*

Alimed, Inc. 800-225-2610
297 High St, Dedham, MA 02026

Armstrong Medical Industries, Inc. 800-323-4220
575 Knightsbridge Pkwy, Lincolnshire, IL 60069

Atd-American Co. 800-523-2300
135 Greenwood Ave, Wyncote, PA 19095

Atlantic Medco, Inc. 800-203-8444
166 Bloomfield Ave, Verona, NJ 07044
$500.00 to $1,000.00.

Blue Bell Bio-Medical 800-258-3235
1260 Industrial Dr, Van Wert, OH 45891
Four sizes available with SURE CLAMP mounting system, and over 75 accessories, shelves and dividers. Complete system of adjustable dividers and organizers for crash carts, anesthesia carts and other mobile storage units. Trays hold dividers for quick exchange of drawer contents. (Also, transport covers and bags.)

Brewer Company, The 888-873-9371
N88W13901 Main St, Menomonee Falls, WI 53051
#63500: Stainless Steel Cart, #63400: Multi-Purpose Utility Cart, #63530: Plastic Utility Cart

Chem-Tainer Industries, Inc. 800-ASK-CHEM
361 Neptune Ave, West Babylon, NY 11704
Material handling.

Contemporary Products, Inc. 800-424-2444
530 Riverside Industrial Pkwy, Portland, ME 04103

Custom Comfort 800-749-0933
PO Box 4779, Winter Park, FL 32793
Custom Comfort's mobile supply cart series is perfect for any development where portable lockable storage is needed to conform to current and future regulations. The carts are fully customizable to meet your exact requirements.

Custom Comfort Medtek 800-749-0933
3939 Forsyth Rd Ste A, Winter Park, FL 32792
Custom-built supply carts with options that include glove-box holders, phlebotomy trays, folding trays or tables, sliding drawers, and lockable fixtures.

DURHAM MANUFACTURING COMPANY 800-243-3774
201 Main St, Durham, CT 06422

Eagle Mhc 800-637-5100
100 Industrial Blvd, Clayton, DE 19938
Clinic treatment cart holds supplies & instruments. Stainless steel construction w/pull out tray. Also, security carts. Provide secure storage for costly goods.

CART, SUPPLY *(cont'd)*

Ergotron, Inc. 800-888-8458
1181 Trapp Rd, Saint Paul, MN 55121
ERGOTRON Medical Carts organize computer equipment into self-contained WorkCenters on wheels that take computing to any room.

Exchange Cart Accessories 800-823-1490
1 Commerce Dr, Freeburg, IL 62243

Gillis Associated Industries 800-397-1675
750 Pinecrest Dr, Prospect Heights, IL 60070

Homak Manufacturing Company Inc. 800-874-6625
1605 Old Route 18 Ste 4-36, Wampum, PA 16157

Ideal Products 800-321-5490
1287 County Road 623, Broseley, MO 63932
Stainless steel or new lightweight poly-carts in 4 colors, 3 or 4 shelves, cabinets or drawers.

Intermetro Industries Corp. 800-441-2714
651 N Washington St, Wilkes Barre, PA 18705
SUPERERECTA, METROMAX, METROMAXQ, Super Adjustable, STARSYS, general storage supply.

Lakeside Manufacturing Co., Inc. 800-558-8565
4900 W Electric Ave, West Milwaukee, WI 53219
Flapped opening nylon cover included. Four shelves, three sizes. Welded stainless steel construction.

Mayo Medical, S.A. De C.V. 800-715-3872
Edison 1141 Nte., Col. Talleres, Monterrey N.L. 64480 Mexico

Meese Orbitron Dunne Co. 800-829-3230
535 N Midland Ave, Saddle Brook, NJ 07663

Mobile-Tronics Co., Inc. 800-368-8181
28570 Marguerite Pkwy Ste 227, Mission Viejo, CA 92692

Rem Systems 305-499-4800
625 E 10th Ave, Hialeah, FL 33010

Suburban Surgical Co., Inc. 800-323-7366
275 12th St, Wheeling, IL 60090
Tubular stainless steel exchange cart with solid, perforated, or wire shelf; includes drawer dividers, retaining rods, covers and all other accessories.

Tecni-Quip 800-826-1245
960 Crossroads Blvd, PO Box 2050, Seguin, TX 78155
TECNI-QUIP Carts for every delivery requirement. Open and closed models in a variety of sizes. Custom manufacturing available.

Total Care 800-334-3802
PO Box 1661, Rockville, MD 20849

Valley Craft 800-328-1480
2001 S Highway 61, Lake City, MN 55041

Windquest 800-562-4257
3311 Windquest Dr, Holland, MI 49424
Procedure and medication with customer specified interiors.

CART, SUPPLY, OPERATING ROOM *(Surgery) 79FSK*

Armstrong Medical Industries, Inc. 800-323-4220
575 Knightsbridge Pkwy, Lincolnshire, IL 60069
Lightweight aluminum carts available with optional SCOPESAFE fiber optic scope storage cabinet. Also, wide carts with spacious drawers for instruments, small scopes and surgical supplies.

Blue Bell Bio-Medical 800-258-3235
1260 Industrial Dr, Van Wert, OH 45891
Four sizes available with SURE CLAMP mounting system and over 75 accessories, shelves and dividers to create special procedure carts. Complete system of adjustable dividers and organizers. Trays hold dividers for quick exchange of drawer contents. (Also, transport covers and bags.)

Eagle Mhc 800-637-5100
100 Industrial Blvd, Clayton, DE 19938
Open and closed surgical case carts. Used to transport individual case equipment to O.R.

Exchange Cart Accessories 800-823-1490
1 Commerce Dr, Freeburg, IL 62243

Harloff Company, Inc. 800-433-4064
650 Ford St, Colorado Springs, CO 80915
$1,400 to $1,800 for surgical case carts constructed to facilitate cleaning and drainage. Stainless steel, extension shelves. Wrap-around bumper, tracking caster set, and adjustable-height shelf. Three sizes or custom-built.

Homak Manufacturing Company Inc. 800-874-6625
1605 Old Route 18 Ste 4-36, Wampum, PA 16157

CART, SUPPLY, OPERATING ROOM *(cont'd)*

Imperial Surgical Ltd. 800-661-5432
581 Orly Ave., Dorval, ONT H9P-1G1 Canada
Various models available.

Intermetro Industries Corp. 800-441-2714
651 N Washington St, Wilkes Barre, PA 18705
Open and closed Case Carts. STARSYS enclosed supply cart. SUPER ADJUSTABLE SUPER ERECTA open wire supply carts. METROMAX open polymer supply carts.

Meese Orbitron Dunne Co. 800-829-3230
535 N Midland Ave, Saddle Brook, NJ 07663

Mobility Matters Incorporated 812-459-4584
3588 Katalla Dr, Newburgh, IN 47630

Pedigo Products 360-695-3500
4000 SE Columbia Way, Vancouver, WA 98661
Stainless steel, enclosed or open styles, various sizes.

S&S Technology 281-815-1300
10625 Telge Rd, Houston, TX 77095

Scientek Medical Equipment 604-273-9094
11151 Bridgeport Rd., Richmond, BC V6X 1T3 Canada

Suburban Surgical Co., Inc. 800-323-7366
275 12th St, Wheeling, IL 60090
Open or closed stainless steel.

Waterloo Healthcare, Llc 800-833-4419
3730 E Southern Ave, Phoenix, AZ 85040
$560.00 to $1800.00 for Steel or Lightweight Aluminum crash construction. Available in three sizes with hundreds of drawer configurations to choose from. Drawers are available in 18 colors.

Windquest 800-562-4257
3311 Windquest Dr, Holland, MI 49424
General and specific supplies; several models available.

CART, TISSUE *(General) 80VFB*

Gi Supply 800-451-5797
200 Grandview Ave, Camp Hill, PA 17011
UNITY BX STATION Specially designed counter for processing biopsies.

Intermetro Industries Corp. 800-441-2714
651 N Washington St, Wilkes Barre, PA 18705
Sterile wrap rack cart.

CART, TRACTION *(Orthopedics) 87QGV*

Zimmer Holdings, Inc. 800-613-6131
1800 W Center St, PO Box 708, Warsaw, IN 46580

Zimmer Orthopaedic Surgical Products 800-321-5533
PO Box 10, 200 West Ohio Ave., Dover, OH 44622

CART, WASTE *(General) 80WVR*

Approved Medical Systems 951-353-2453
7101 Jurupa Ave Ste 4, Riverside, CA 92504
Priced under $70 each, KOMPACT KART infectious & biohazard waste carts, available with or without foot pedal.

Bio-Logics Products, Inc. 800-426-7577
PO Box 505, West Jordan, UT 84084
Bio Bag, used for water, laundry, or biochemical waste.

Gi Supply 800-451-5797
200 Grandview Ave, Camp Hill, PA 17011
UNITY CLEANUP portable waste recepticle.

Mcclure Industries, Inc. 800-752-2821
9051 SE 55th Ave, Portland, OR 97206
Fire-retardant fire-extinguishing Models TC-35FL, TC35FLX and TC-600FL. GS-96 Fire-retardant, fiberglass cart suitable for hippa regulation, regulated waste and general waste.

Tecni-Quip 800-826-1245
960 Crossroads Blvd, PO Box 2050, Seguin, TX 78155
TECNI-QUIP Carts for collection of waste, biohazardous, recycling, automatic dumping. Variety of models in fiberglass or metal. Custom manufacturing available. Fire-retardant.

Toter, Inc. 800-772-0071
841 Meacham Rd, PO Box 5338, Statesville, NC 28677
Provide carts for bio-hazardous waste and building maintenance/janitorial.

CARTRIDGE, ETHYLENE-OXIDE *(General) 80VLG*

Andersen Products, Inc., 800-523-1276
3202 Caroline Dr, Health Science Park, Haw River, NC 27258
EOGAS 100% EO unit-dose cartridge system employs gas-diffusion technology to reduce gas consumption; for use with the ANDERSEN EOGAS System.

CARVER, DENTAL AMALGAM, OPERATIVE
(Dental And Oral) 76EKH

Aesculap Implant Systems Inc. 1-800-234-9179
3773 Corporate Pkwy, Center Valley, PA 18034

American Eagle Instruments, Inc. 406-549-7451
6575 Butler Creek Rd, Missoula, MT 59808
Various sizes & styles of operative instruments.

Den-Mat Holdings, Llc 805-922-8491
2727 Skyway Dr, Santa Maria, CA 93455
No common name listed.

Dental Usa, Inc. 815-363-8003
5005 McCullom Lake Rd, McHenry, IL 60050
Carver.

Dentalez Group 866-DTE-INFO
101 Lindenwood Dr Ste 225, Valleybrooke Corporate Center
Malvern, PA 19355

Dentalez Group, Stardental Division 717-291-1161
1816 Colonial Village Ln, Lancaster, PA 17601
Explorer, operative.

E.A. Beck & Co. 949-645-4072
657 W 19th St Ste E, P O Box 10857, Costa Mesa, CA 92627
Carver.

Hu-Friedy Manufacturing Co., Inc. 800-483-7433
3232 N Rockwell St, Chicago, IL 60618
$22.00 to $23.60 each, 20 types.

Micro-Dent Inc. 866-526-1166
379 Hollow Hill Rd, Wauconda, IL 60084
Carver.

Nordent Manufacturing, Inc. 800-966-7336
610 Bonnie Ln, Elk Grove Village, IL 60007
$19.00 per unit (standard).

Premier Dental Products Co. 888-670-6100
1710 Romano Dr, PO Box 4500, Plymouth Meeting, PA 19462

Sci-Dent, Inc. 800-323-4145
210 Dowdle St Ste 2, Algonquin, IL 60102

Suter Dental Manufacturing Company, Inc. 800-368-8376
632 Cedar St, Chico, CA 95928

Ultradent Products, Inc. 801-553-4586
505 W 10200 S, South Jordan, UT 84095
Carver.

Wykle Research, Inc. 775-887-7500
2222 College Pkwy, Carson City, NV 89706
Dental amalgam carver.

CARVER, WAX, DENTAL *(Dental And Oral) 76EIK*

Almore International, Inc. 503-643-6633
PO Box 25214, Portland, OR 97298
$77.50 for set of 5.

American Eagle Instruments, Inc. 406-549-7451
6575 Butler Creek Rd, Missoula, MT 59808
Various types of wax carvers.

Arnold Tuber Industries 716-648-3363
97 Main St, Hamburg, NY 14075
Carver, wax, dental, dental hand instruments.

Buffalo Dental Mfg. Co., Inc. 516-496-7200
159 Lafayette Dr, Syosset, NY 11791
Dental wax carver.

Dental Usa, Inc. 815-363-8003
5005 McCullom Lake Rd, McHenry, IL 60050
Dental wax.

E.A. Beck & Co. 949-645-4072
657 W 19th St Ste E, P O Box 10857, Costa Mesa, CA 92627
Wax carver.

George Taub Products & Fusion Co., Inc. 800-828-2634
277 New York Ave, Jersey City, NJ 07307
George Taub Products offers sets of wax carvers for dental technician. Some are light weight, made with a plastic handle and will not tire out the wrist from constant use.

Hager Worldwide, Inc. 800-328-2335
13322 Byrd Dr, Odessa, FL 33556

Hu-Friedy Manufacturing Co., Inc. 800-483-7433
3232 N Rockwell St, Chicago, IL 60618
$20.00 to $35.50, 26 types.

Mds Products, Inc. 800-637-2330
22991 La Cadena Dr, Laguna Hills, CA 92653
Production Dipwax, Green & Red, 6 & 16 oz. 'James Pitre'

CARVER, WAX, DENTAL *(cont'd)*

Pac-Dent Intl., Inc. 909-839-0888
21078 Commerce Point Dr, Walnut, CA 91789
Various types of carver.

Premier Dental Products Co. 888-670-6100
1710 Romano Dr, PO Box 4500, Plymouth Meeting, PA 19462

Productivity Training Company 800-448-8855
360 Cochrane Cir # A, Morgan Hill, CA 95037

Pulpdent Corp. 800-343-4342
80 Oakland St, Watertown, MA 02472
Wax carver.

Suter Dental Manufacturing Company, Inc. 800-368-8376
632 Cedar St, Chico, CA 95928

CASE, CONTACT LENS *(Ophthalmology) 86LRX*

Atrion Medical Products, Inc. 800-343-9334
1426 Curt Francis Rd NW, Arab, AL 35016
Side by Side LGM Storage Cases. Cylindrical Cup Lens Disinfection Cases for chemical disinfection.

Bausch & Lomb 585-338-6000
1 Bausch and Lomb Pl, Rochester, NY 14604

Nomax, Inc. 314-961-2500
40 N Rock Hill Rd, Saint Louis, MO 63119
Amcon deepwell flat pack.

Pelican Products, Llc 864-699-4181
209 Jones Rd, Spartanburg, SC 29307
Various types of contact lens cases.

Shamir Insight, Inc. 877-514-833
9938 Via Pasar, San Diego, CA 92126
contact lenses

Western Ophthalmics Corporation 800-426-9938
19019 36th Ave W Ste G, Lynnwood, WA 98036
Cases available in single quantities, significant discounts for volume purchases

CASE, PROTECTION, EQUIPMENT *(General) 80WSG*

Air Lift Unlimited Inc. 800-776-6771
1212 Kerr Gulch Rd, Evergreen, CO 80439
AIR LIFT custom cases can be designed and manufactured to meet the any technology or medical device carrying and protective needs. With over 40 years experience in innovative design, AIR LIFT is well positioned to meet your custom case or carrier needs.

Case Design Corp. 800-847-4176
333 School Ln, Telford, PA 18969
Stock and custom-made carrying and shipping cases.

Case Medical, Inc. 888-227-2273
65 Railroad Ave, Ridgefield, NJ 07657
Custom engineered carrying cases and customized medical equipment, & cabinets.

Ch Ellis Company Inc. 800-466-3351
2432 Southeastern Ave, Indianapolis, IN 46201
Carrying cases for variety of medical equipment, such as dialysis

Fieldtex Products, Inc. 800-772-4816
3055 Brighton-Henrietta Tl Rd, Rochester, NY 14623
Custom manufacturer of soft-sided carrying cases for portable instruments, offering a wide range of fabrics and foams.

Gemini, Inc. 800-533-3631
103 Mensing Way, Cannon Falls, MN 55009
Customized and standard cases for electronics and instrumentation: transit, sample/demo, rotationally molded, or shock and rack-mount cases. Also, reusable shipping containers.

Mobile Dental Equipment Corp.(M-Dec) 425-747-5424
13300 SE 30th St Ste 101, Bellevue, WA 98005
Portable dental instrument case. $625.00.

Mushield Company, Inc., The 888-669-3539
9 Ricker Ave, Londonderry, NH 03053
GB ENCLOSURE MRI monitor enclosure. Eliminates EMI interference up to 30 gauss. Custom and off-the-shelf designs.

Platt Luggage, Inc. 800-222-1555
4051 W 51st St, Chicago, IL 60632
Cases for demo, display, carrying, and shipping applications. Molded plastic, ATA, watertight, and sewn fabric cases. Complete in-house design, water-jet cut custom foam inserts, and logos available.

CASE, PROTECTION, EQUIPMENT *(cont'd)*

Princeton Case Co., Inc. 908-687-1750
667 Lehigh Ave, Union, NJ 07083
Carrying cases in standard sizes and custom manufactured. Line includes vacuum-formed, blow-molded, injection-molded and soft-sided cases. Interiors finished with fabricated foam inserts. Medical instrumentation cases available.

Stanley Supply & Services, Inc 800-225-5370
335 Willow St, North Andover, MA 01845
Shipping and storage, high density polyethylene cases.

Star Case Manufacturing Co., Inc. 800-822-7827
648 Superior Ave, Munster, IN 46321
Heavy-duty carrying and shipping cases and containers custom and standard designs for all medical, computer, and diagnostic devices.

Tcp Reliable, Inc. 888-TCP-3393
551 Raritan Center Pkwy, Edison, NJ 08837
TEM-PAK insulated containers.

Tegrant Corporation, Protexic Brands 800-289-9966
800 5th Ave, P.O. Box 448, New Brighton, PA 15066
Protective packaging for medical devices

Tegrant Corporation, Thermosafe Brands 847-398-0110
3930 N Ventura Dr Ste 450, Arlington Heights, IL 60004
Protective packaging fo medical devices

Zero Manufacturing, Inc. 800-500-9376
500 W 200 N, North Salt Lake, UT 84054
Tempered-aluminum-alloy, high-density-polyethylene, and ABS-plastic carrying and shipping cases and enclosures.

CASSETTE, AUDIO TAPE *(Cardiovascular) 74MCU*

Print Media, Inc. 800-994-3318
9002 NW 105th Way, Medley, FL 33178
Full Line of brand name audio, video and digital recording media available.

CASSETTE, RADIOGRAPHIC FILM *(Radiology) 90IXA*

Agfa Corp. 800-581-2432
100 Challenger Rd, Ridgefield Park, NJ 07660

Agfa Corporation 877-777-2432
PO Box 19048, 10 South Academy Street, Greenville, SC 29602

Americomp, Inc. 800-458-1782
2901 W Lawrence Ave, Chicago, IL 60625

Burkhart Roentgen Intl. Inc. 800-USA-XRAY
5201 8th Ave S, Gulfport, FL 33707

Composiflex, Inc. 800-673-2544
8100 Hawthorne Dr, Erie, PA 16509
Carbon fiber film cassettes.

Fujifilm Medical Systems Usa, Inc. 800-431-1850
419 West Ave, Stamford, CT 06902

Marconi Medical Systems 800-323-0550
595 Miner Rd, Cleveland, OH 44143

Mci Optonix, Div. Of Usr Optonix Inc. 800-678-6649
253 E Washington Ave, Washington, NJ 07882

Medlink Imaging, Inc. 800-456-7800
200 Clearbrook Rd, Elmsford, NY 10523

Pl Medical Co., Llc. 800-874-0120
321 Ellis St, New Britain, CT 06051

Schueler & Company, Inc. 516-487-1500
PO Box 528, Stratford, CT 06615

Soyee Products, Inc. 800-574-4743
459 Thompson Rd, Thompson, CT 06277

Spectronics Corporation 800-274-8888
956 Brush Hollow Rd, Westbury, NY 11590
FOUR SQUARE , MONOTEC, and VALUE radiographic film, grids cassette.

Umi Intl. 888-511-8655
2 E Union Ave, PO Box 170, East Rutherford, NJ 07073
Various.

Wolf X-Ray Corporation 800-356-9729
100 W Industry Ct, Deer Park, NY 11729
Over 100 different types.

Xma (X-Ray Marketing Associates, Inc.) 800-325-8880
1205 W Lakeview Ct, Windham Lakes Business Park
Romeoville, IL 60446

CASSETTE, TISSUE *(Pathology) 88IDZ*

Leica Biosystems - St. Louis, Llc 847-317-7209
12100A Prichard Farm Rd, Maryland Heights, MO 63043
Tissue processing equipment.

CASSETTE, TISSUE *(cont'd)*

Polysciences, Inc. 800-523-2575
400 Valley Rd, Warrington, PA 18976

Richard-Allan Scientific 269-544-5628
4481 Campus Dr, Kalamazoo, MI 49008
Various.

Sakura Finetek U.S.A., Inc. 800-725-8723
1750 W 214th St, Torrance, CA 90501
TISSUE-TEK, UNI-CASSETTE tissue cassette for surgical specimens. BIOPSY CASSETTE tissue cassette for biopsies.

Simport Plastics Ltd. 450-464-1723
2588 Bernard-Pilon, Beloeil, QUE J3G 4S5 Canada

Statlab Medical Products, Inc. 800-442-3573
106 Hillside Dr, Lewisville, TX 75057
ANAPATH histological cassettes with or w/o lids in various colors, also biopsy cassettes.

Surgipath Medical Industries, Inc. 800-225-3035
PO Box 528, 5205 Route 12, Richmond, IL 60071

CAST *(Orthopedics) 87QHE*

Aegis Medical 203-838-9081
10 Wall St, Norwalk, CT 06850

Bsn Medical, Inc 800-552-1157
5825 Carnegie Blvd, Charlotte, NC 28209
OCL® FIBERGLASS CASTING TAPE provides effortless application due to easy unrolling saves you time and prevents tight molds and casts. The easy to open package eliminates frustration while enabling the user to turn out cast after cast when time is critical. OCL® FLEXIBLE CASTING TAPE remains semi-rigid and resilient, even in its cured state. Provides semi-rigid support of the limb, while allowing some degree of joint movement.

Mueller Sports Medicine 800-356-9522
1 Quench Dr, P.O. Box 99, Prairie Du Sac, WI 53578
Limb support.

Omni Medical Supply Inc. 800-860-6664
4153 Pioneer Dr, Commerce Township, MI 48390

Ortho-Med, Inc. 800-547-5571
3208 SE 13th Ave, Portland, OR 97202
Post-op braces.

Paramedical Distributors 800-245-3278
2020 Grand Blvd, Kansas City, MO 64108
Casting supplies.

Xero Products 888-937-6769
6702 Netherlands Dr, Wilmington, NC 28405
XEROSOX Cast, bandage protector. The XEROSOX is the only truly waterproof protector in the world with the patented vacuum seal. Just a few pumps of the attached bulb creates the perfect watertight seal.

Zimmer Orthopaedic Surgical Products 800-321-5533
PO Box 10, 200 West Ohio Ave., Dover, OH 44622

CAST WALKING HEEL *(Orthopedics) 87QHC*

Bsn Medical, Inc 800-552-1157
5825 Carnegie Blvd, Charlotte, NC 28209
M-PACT® WALKING HEELS are available in 4 styles. Resiliency and long wear from a specialized synthetic rubber. Deep tread provides good patient comfort and stability by allowing regular heel-toe walking.

Darco International, Inc. 800-999-8866
810 Memorial Blvd, Huntington, WV 25701
BODY ARMOR short leg walker.

Dm Systems, Inc. 800-254-5438
1316 Sherman Ave, Evanston, IL 60201
CASTWALKER® CAST SOLE is a new and innovative way to prepare a cast for ambulation. The Walker was designed to perform two important functions: to improve the gait of the patient wearing the cast and reduce the time and cost of its application.

Mizuho Osi 800-777-4674
30031 Ahern Ave, Union City, CA 94587

Zimmer Holdings, Inc. 800-613-6131
1800 W Center St, PO Box 708, Warsaw, IN 46580

CASTERS, HOSPITAL EQUIPMENT *(General) 80UKP*

Bond Caster And Wheel Corporation 800-233-2663
230 S Penn St, PO Box 339, Manheim, PA 17545
Casters and wheels to suit any OEM application and service center need.

CASTERS, HOSPITAL EQUIPMENT *(cont'd)*

Colson Caster Corporation 800-643-5515
3700 Airport Rd, Jonesboro, AR 72401
Complete line of casters, bumpers and wheels designed for hospitals and institutions.

Crest Healthcare Supply 800-328-8908
195 3rd St, Dassel, MN 55325

Curbell, Inc. Electronics 800-235-7500
7 Cobham Dr, Orchard Park, NY 14127
Hospital-grade casters and wheels for beds and medical equipment.

Darnell-Rose Casters 800-327-6355
17915 Railroad St, City Of Industry, CA 91748
Carpetmaster 2: Swivel caster for medical equipment, IV stands. Caster has 2-inch neoprene rubber wheel, chrome-plated fender and a 110-lb load capacity. Three-year factory warranty applies.

Hamilton Caster & Mfg. Co. 888-699-7164
1637 Dixie Hwy, Hamilton, OH 45011
Light- and medium-duty casters and stainless-steel casters.

Healthmark Industries 800-521-6224
22522 E 9 Mile Rd, Saint Clair Shores, MI 48080
High quality German bearing casters.

Jero Medical Equipment & Supplies, Inc. 800-457-0644
1701 W 13th St, Chicago, IL 60608
Various sizes.

Jilson Group, Inc. 800-969-5400
20 Industrial Rd, Lodi, NJ 07644
Casters specifically designed for medical applications include; stainless steel, total locking, steering lock and central locking types. New Series 550 / 551 twin-wheel casters offer designer appearance with increased mobility.

Magnus Mobility Systems 800-858-7801
1912 W Business Center Dr, Orange, CA 92867
CASTER-PRO casters and wheels available in all sizes and attachments. Conductive and antistatic, all options and wheel materials and in-stock program for immediate shipment. Also available are STABILUS gas springs for positioning, dampening or controlling motion. All sizes, forces and attachments. In-stock program for immediate shipment. Levelers (glides) from 100 to 43,000 lbs. capacity are also available. Made of stainless or carbon steel; imperial or metric; non-skid, nylon or steel bases. In stock program for immediate shipment.

Shepherd Caster Corporation 800-253-0868
203 Kerth St, Saint Joseph, MI 49085
Casters, IV poles and chair bases.

Steelcraft, Inc. 800-225-7710
115 W Main St, Millbury, MA 01527

Tente Casters, Inc. 800-783-2470
2266 S Park Dr, Hebron, KY 41048

Youngs, Inc. 800-523-5454
55 E Cherry Ln, Souderton, PA 18964

CASTING UNIT, DENTAL *(Dental And Oral) 76QHD*

Dencraft 800-328-9729
PO Box 57, Moorestown, NJ 08057
USDI

Mds Products, Inc. 800-637-2330
22991 La Cadena Dr, Laguna Hills, CA 92653
Spiracast Ringless Casting System

CATALYTIC METHOD, AMYLASE *(Chemistry) 75JFJ*

Abbott Diagnostics Div. 626-440-0700
820 Mission St, South Pasadena, CA 91030
Amylase.

Carolina Liquid Chemistries Corp. 800-471-7272
510 W Central Ave Ste C, Brea, CA 92821
Amylase reagent.

Genzyme Corp. 800-325-2436
160 Christian St, Oxford, CT 06478
Amylase, CNPG3.

Hemagen Diagnostics, Inc. 800-436-2436
9033 Red Branch Rd, Columbia, MD 21045
Various amylase methods.

Intersect Systems, Inc. 360-577-1062
1152 3rd Avenue, Suite D & E, Longview, WA 98632
Catalytic methods, amylase, Liquid Direct Amylase.

Jas Diagnostics, Inc. 305-418-2320
7220 NW 58th St, Miami, FL 33166
Amylase.

CATALYTIC METHOD, AMYLASE *(cont'd)*

Synermed Intl., Inc. 317-896-1565
17408 Tiller Ct Ste 1900, Westfield, IN 46074
Amylase analysis system.

Teco Diagnostics 714-693-7788
1268 N Lakeview Ave, Anaheim, CA 92807
Amylase liquid reagent, amylase, kinetic.

Vital Diagnostics Inc. 714-672-3553
1075 W Lambert Rd Ste D, Brea, CA 92821
Alpha-amylase reagent.

CATALYTIC METHOD, CREATINE PHOSPHOKINASE
(Chemistry) 75JFW

Dade Behring, Inc. 800-948-3233
1717 Deerfield Rd, Deerfield, IL 60015

CATALYTIC PROCEDURE, CPK ISOENZYMES
(Chemistry) 75JPY

Dade Behring, Inc. 800-948-3233
1717 Deerfield Rd, Deerfield, IL 60015

CATHETER AND ACCESSORIES, UROLOGICAL
(Gastro/Urology) 78MJC

C. R. Bard, Inc., Bard Urological Div. 888-367-2273
13183 Harland Dr NE, Covington, GA 30014

Datascope Corp. 800-288-2121
14 Philips Pkwy, Montvale, NJ 07645
Staged Guidewire extra stiff guidewire designed to facilitate sheathless IAB insertion. Sold with True Sheatless insertion kit or separately in boxes of 10 ea.

Memcath Technologies Llc 651-450-7400
1777 Oakdale Ave, Saint Paul, MN 55118

Rochester Medical Corp. 800-615-2364
1 Rochester Medical Dr NW, Stewartville, MN 55976
Antibacterial foley catheter.

CATHETER, ANGIOGRAPHIC *(Cns/Neurology) 84HBY*

Angiodynamics, Inc. 518-795-1400
14 Plaza Drive, Latham, NY 12110
AngioDynamics' product listings go far beyond the Angiographic Catheter. Following are AngioDynamics' products (along with FDA codes), designed for interventionalists treating PVD, currently listed on the company web site (www.angiodynamics.com) as of August 2004: Angiographic Catheters (DQO); Angiographic Accessories - Guidewires (DQX); Angiographic Accessories - Needles (DYB); Hemodialysis Catheters & Accessories (MSD); PTA Products (DQY); Embolization Products (HCG); Thrombolytic Products (KRA); Vein Laser (GEX); Drainage Products - Biliary (FGE); Drainage Products - General (GBX); Biliary Stents (FGE); Transjugular Access Products (DYB); Flow Measurement System (DPW).

Boston Scientific - Maple Grove 800-553-5878
1 Scimed Pl, Maple Grove, MN 55311

Boston Scientific Corp. 800-323-6472
5905 Nathan Ln N, Minneapolis, MN 55442
SOFTIP angiographic catheters.

Boston Scientific Corporation 800-225-2732
1 Boston Scientific Pl, Natick, MA 01760
IMAGER catheters and accessories for angiography.

Cook Inc. 800-457-4500
PO Box 489, Bloomington, IN 47402

Marconi Medical Systems 800-323-0550
595 Miner Rd, Cleveland, OH 44143

Mmi 800-999-4664
PO Box 5396, Vernon Hills, IL 60061
Mobile/modular cardiac cath/angio; short and long term rental of mobile/modular angiography and/or cardiac cath labs.

Tfx Medical Oem 800-548-6600
50 Plantation Dr, Jaffrey, NH 03452

CATHETER, ANGIOGRAPHY, REPROCESSED
(Cardiovascular) 74NLI

Sterilmed, Inc. 763-488-3400
11400 73rd Ave N Ste 100, Maple Grove, MN 55369
Imaging catheter.

CATHETER, ANGIOPLASTY, CORONARY, TRANSLUMINAL, PERCUT. OPER. *(Cardiovascular) 74LOX*

Abbott Vascular, Cardiac Therapies 800-227-9902
3200 Lakeside Dr, Santa Clara, CA 95054
Ptca catheters.

CATHETER, ANGIOPLASTY, CORONARY, TRANSLUMINAL, PERCUT. OPER. *(cont'd)*

Abbott Vascular, Cardiac Therapies 800-227-9902
26531 Ynez Rd, Mailing P.O. Box 9018, Temecula, CA 92591
Ptca catheters.

Atrium Medical Corp. 800-528-7486
5 Wentworth Dr, Hudson, NH 03051
ATRIUM HYPERLITE coronary angioplasty balloon catheters, and FLYER balloon-expandable coronary stents and Advanta V-12 peripheral PTFE-covered stent graft systems.

Avantec Vascular Corp. 408-329-5425
605 W California Ave, Sunnyvale, CA 94086
Percutaneous transluminal coronary angioplasty catheter.

Bolton Medical, Inc. 954-838-9699
799 International Pkwy, Sunrise, FL 33325
Ptca catheters - various types.

Boston Scientific - Maple Grove 800-553-5878
1 Scimed Pl, Maple Grove, MN 55311
Disposable medical devices, principally coronary and peripheral angioplasty catheters, for non-surgical treatment of cardiovascular disease.

Boston Scientific - Marina Bay Customer Fulfillment Center 617-689-6000
500 Commander Shea Blvd, Quincy, MA 02171
Percutaneous, transluminal coronary angioplasty catheters.

Boston Scientific Corp. 800-323-6472
5905 Nathan Ln N, Minneapolis, MN 55442
SOFTRAC-PTA peripheral dilatation catheter; MONORAIL PICOLINO coronary dilatation catheter.

Boston Scientific Corporation 800-225-2732
1 Boston Scientific Pl, Natick, MA 01760

Cardiac Pacemakers, Inc. 800-227-3422
4100 Hamline Ave N, P.O. Box 64079, Saint Paul, MN 55112
Coronary dilatation catheter offers extended pressure balloon material.

Cardio-Nef, S.A. De C.V. 01-800-024-0240
Rio Grijalva 186, Col. Mitras Norte, Monterrey, N.L. 64320 Mexico

Cook Inc. 800-457-4500
PO Box 489, Bloomington, IN 47402

Drg International, Inc. 800-321-1167
1167 US Highway 22, Mountainside, NJ 07092

Insitu Technologies, Inc. 651-389-1017
5810 Blackshire Path, Inver Grove Heights, MN 55076
Ptca catheter.

Intella Interventional Systems, Inc. 408-737-7121
870 Hermosa Ave, Sunnyvale, CA 94085
Various.

Medtronic, Inc. 800-633-8766
710 Medtronic Pkwy, Minneapolis, MN 55432
14K, 18K, OMNIFLEX, THRUFLEX, THRUFLEX II, MAINE GUIDE, SPIRIT, SAFETIP, SHERPA.

Numed Canada, Inc. 613-936-2592
45, Second Street West, Cornwall, ONT K6J 1G3 Canada

Volcano Corporation 800-228-4728
3661 Valley Centre Dr Ste 200, San Diego, CA 92130
Ptca catheter.

CATHETER, ANGIOPLASTY, CORONARY, ULTRASONIC
(Cardiovascular) 74MJR

Embo-Optics, Llc. 887-885-6400
100 Cummings Ctr # 326B, Beverly, MA 01915
IV illuminator with lighted monitoring feature aids medical personnel in assuring that all IV solutions and medications are infusing properly and at the correct infusion rate. Greatly enhance patient safety in aiding to prevent any adverse events during infusion.

Mmsi 503-538-3270
PO Box 3005, Newberg, OR 97132
Wire and Cable Machinery, Extrusion Ancillary Machinery,

CATHETER, ANGIOPLASTY, PERIPHERAL, TRANSLUMINAL, DUAL-BALLOON *(Cardiovascular) 74NVM*

Hotspur Technologies Inc. 650-969-3150
880 Maude Ave Ste A, Mountain View, CA 94043
GPS Cath PTA Balloon Catheter

CATHETER, ANGIOPLASTY, TRANSLUMINAL, PERIPHERAL
(Cardiovascular) 74LIT

Abbott Vascular, Cardiac Therapies 800-227-9902
3200 Lakeside Dr, Santa Clara, CA 95054
Peripheral catheter.

Abbott Vascular, Cardiac Therapies 800-227-9902
26531 Ynez Rd, Mailing P.O. Box 9018, Temecula, CA 92591
Peripheral catheter.

Abbott Vascular, Vascular Solutions 800-227-9902
26531 Ynez Rd, Temecula, CA 92591
Peripheral catheter.

Angioscore, Inc. 877-264-4692
5055 Brandin Ct, Fremont, CA 94538
Catheter.

Atrium Medical Corp. 800-528-7486
5 Wentworth Dr, Hudson, NH 03051
Atrium Hyperlite Angioplasty Balloon.

Bipore, Inc. 201-767-1993
31 Industrial Pkwy, Northvale, NJ 07647
BIPORE, PTA Balloons.

Bolton Medical, Inc. 954-838-9699
799 International Pkwy, Sunrise, FL 33325
Pta catheter.

Cardio-Nef, S.A. De C.V. 01-800-024-0240
Rio Grijalva 186, Col. Mitras Norte, Monterrey, N.L. 64320 Mexico

Cook Inc. 800-457-4500
PO Box 489, Bloomington, IN 47402

Insitu Technologies, Inc. 651-389-1017
5810 Blackshire Path, Inver Grove Heights, MN 55076
Pta balloon catheter.

Kensey Nash Corporation 484-713-2100
735 Pennsylvania Dr, Exton, PA 19341
TriActiv Embolic Protection System combines balloon protection, active flush and automated extraction to treat occluded saphenous vein grafts.

Navilyst Medical 800-833-9973
100 Boston Scientific Way, Marlborough, MA 01752
Various types of angioplasty accessories.

Norfolk Medical Products, Inc. 847-674-7075
7350 Ridgeway Ave, Skokie, IL 60076
Catheters.

Numed, Inc. 315-328-4491
2880 Main St., Hopkinton, NY 12965
Pediatric PTV catheter.

Radius Medical Technologies, Inc. 978-263-4466
15 Craig Rd, Acton, MA 01720
Guidewire.

Thomas Medical Products, Inc. 866-446-3003
65 Great Valley Pkwy, Malvern, PA 19355
Hemostatic wye connector.

CATHETER, ARTERIAL *(Cardiovascular) 74QHN*

Angiodynamics, Inc. 800-472-5221
1 Horizon Way, Manchester, GA 31816
Central venous silicone in single, double, and triple lumen configurations, with or without placement kits.

Arrow International, Inc. 800-523-8446
2400 Bernville Rd, Reading, PA 19605
Adult and pediatric sizes.

Becton Dickinson Infusion Therapy Systems, Inc. 888-237-2762
9450 S State St, Sandy, UT 84070

Diablo Sales & Marketing, Inc. 925-648-1611
PO Box 3219, Danville, CA 94526
Custom design and manufacturing of catheters and specialty guidewires. Guiding catheters; stent delivery and drug delivery systems.

Hospira, Inc. 877-946-7747
755 Jarvis Dr, Morgan Hill, CA 95037

Lemaitre Vascular, Inc. 781-221-2266
63 2nd Ave, Burlington, MA 01803
LeMaitre Catheter, high performance latex catheters for arterial emborectomy, venous mombectomy, gallstone extrication and irrigation.

Marconi Medical Systems 800-323-0550
595 Miner Rd, Cleveland, OH 44143

CATHETER, ARTERIAL *(cont'd)*

Rose Technologies Company 616-233-3000
1440 Front Ave NW, Grand Rapids, MI 49504

Smiths Medical Asd, Inc. 800-433-5832
1265 Grey Fox Rd, Saint Paul, MN 55112

CATHETER, ASPIRATION *(Surgery) 79KDH*

Ballard Medical Products 770-587-7835
12050 Lone Peak Pkwy, Draper, UT 84020
Pediatric/adult lavage kit.

Covidien Lp 508-261-8000
15 Hampshire St, Mansfield, MA 02048

Ethox International 800-521-1022
251 Seneca St, Buffalo, NY 14204
Irrigation/aspiration catheter.

Kelsar, S.A. 508-261-8000
Blvd. Insurgentes, Libriamento a La, Tijuana 22450 Mexico
Gastrointestinal tubes and accessories and kits

Medtec Applications, Inc. 630-628-0444
50 W Fay Ave, Addison, IL 60101
Irrigator.

CATHETER, ASSISTED REPRODUCTION *(Obstetrics/Gyn) 85MQF*

Conceptus, Inc. 650-962-4000
331 E Evelyn Ave, Mountain View, CA 94041

Cook Ob/Gyn 800-541-5591
1100 W Morgan St, Spencer, IN 47460

Genx International 888-GEN-XNOW
393 Soundview Rd, Guilford, CT 06437

Inntec, Inc. 608-444-4544
401 E Edgewater St, Portage, WI 53901
Embryo transfer catheter.

Rocket Medical Plc. 800-707-7625
150 Recreation Park Dr Ste 3, Hingham, MA 02043

CATHETER, BALLOON (FOLEY TYPE) *(Surgery) 79GBA*

Arrow International, Inc. 800-523-8446
2400 Bernville Rd, Reading, PA 19605

Axiom Medical, Inc. 800-221-8569
19320 Van Ness Ave, Torrance, CA 90501

Boston Scientific-Neurovascular 510-440-7700
47900 Bayside Pkwy, Fremont, CA 94538
Balloon catheter.

California Medical Innovations 800-229-5871
873 E Arrow Hwy, Pomona, CA 91767
Custom balloon catheters.

Cianna Medical, Inc. 866-920-9444
6 Journey Ste 125, Aliso Viejo, CA 92656
SAVI Preparation Device

Clinical Instruments Intl., Inc. 508-764-2200
278 Worcester St, Southbridge, MA 01550
Introducers.

Cook Endoscopy 336-744-0157
4900 Bethania Station Rd # &, 5951 Grassy Creek Blvd. Winston Salem, NC 27105
Various balloon extraction and dilation catheters.

Covidien Lp 508-261-8000
15 Hampshire St, Mansfield, MA 02048

Datascope Cardiac Assist Div. 800-777-4222
15 Law Dr, Fairfield, NJ 07004
Intra-aortic balloon catheter.

Degania Silicone, Inc. 401-333-8199
1226 Mendon Rd, Cumberland, RI 02864
Foley catheters and Foley temperature sensor catheters sterile packaged under customer's private label.

Ethicon Endo-Surgery, Inc. 800-USE-ENDO
4545 Creek Rd, Cincinnati, OH 45242
ENDOPATH cholangiogram with balloon, 50cm with 14g, 2.25in. with introducer; cholangiogram, 50cm with 14g, 2.25in. with introducer.

Global Healthcare 800-601-3880
1495 Hembree Rd Ste 700, Roswell, GA 30076
Disposable, 2-way, 3-way, various French and balloon volume.

Gynecare 888-GYN-ECAR
235 Constitution Dr, Menlo Park, CA 94025
Balloon catheter, endometrial ablation system which is an office-based procedure for the treatment of menorrhagia (dysfunctional uterine bleeding in women).

CATHETER, BALLOON (FOLEY TYPE) *(cont'd)*

Hobbs Medical, Inc. 860-684-5875
8 Spring St, Stafford Springs, CT 06076
Endoscopic dilation balloon.

Lampac International Ltd. 636-797-3659
230 N Lake Dr, Hillsboro, MO 63050
Available in latex, silicone. Elastomer coated latex and 100% silicone.

Manufacturing & Research, Inc.(Dba Mri Medical) 520-882-7794
4700 S Overland Dr, Tucson, AZ 85714
Including tri-lumen and temperature monitoring, 6-30Fr., silicone.

Medi Inc 800-225-8634
75 York Ave, P.O. Box 302, Randolph, MA 02368

Mentor Corp. 800-525-0245
201 Mentor Dr, Santa Barbara, CA 93111

Merit Medical Systems, Inc. 801-253-1600
1111 S Velasco St, Angleton, TX 77515
Percutataneous transluminal angioplasty catheter.

Navilyst Medical 800-833-9973
100 Boston Scientific Way, Marlborough, MA 01752
Pneumatic hand pump.

Novamed, Llc 800-425-3535
4 Westchester Plz, Elmsford, NY 10523
NovaTemp Foley Catheters with Temperature 100% Silicone -- Available in Sterile Packaging -- Sizes 8FR, 10FR, 12FR, 14FR, 16FR, 18FR. Packaged 10/ Box; 40/ case.

Optimal Healthcare Products 800-364-8574
11444 W Olympic Blvd Ste 900, Los Angeles, CA 90064
Nice balloon

Tacpro, Inc. 408-364-7100
13845 Industrial Park Blvd, Plymouth, MN 55441

Tactx Medical/Produxx, Inc. 408-364-7100
1353 Dell Ave, Campbell, CA 95008

Unomedical, Inc. 800-634-6003
5701 S Ware Rd Ste 1, McAllen, TX 78503

CATHETER, BALLOON, DILATATION, VESSEL
(Gastro/Urology) 78QIU

Advanced Polymers, Inc. 603-327-0600
29 Northwestern Dr, Salem, NH 03079
Heat transfer, custom design and fabrication of unique catheters for both heating and cooling therapies including cryosurgery.

Atrion Medical Products, Inc. 800-343-9334
1426 Curt Francis Rd NW, Arab, AL 35016
Inflation Device Angio Plasty & PTCA. QL1030, QL1455, QL2030, QL2540, QL4015, QL6015, inflation devices.

Boston Scientific Interventional Technologies 858-268-4488
3574 Ruffin Rd, San Diego, CA 92123
Cutting balloon, infiltrator drug delivery

Cook Inc. 800-457-4500
PO Box 489, Bloomington, IN 47402

Cook Urological, Inc. 800-457-4500
1100 W Morgan St, P.O. Box 227, Spencer, IN 47460

Diseno Y Desarrollo Medico S.A. De C.V. 5-584-1483
San Luis Potosi 96, Roma, Ciudad De Mexico, DF 06700 Mexico
PTCA Range of Products.

M & I Medical Sales, Inc. 305-663-6444
4711 SW 72nd Ave, Miami, FL 33155

Telemed Systems Inc. 800-481-6718
8 Kane Industrial Dr, Hudson, MA 01749
SURE-FLEX, dilatation balloon catheters, esophageal and biliary, GI tract.

CATHETER, BALLOON, REATTACHMENT, RETINAL
(Ophthalmology) 86LOG

Howard Instruments, Inc. 205-553-4453
4749 Appletree Ln, Tuscaloosa, AL 35405

CATHETER, BARTHOLIN GLAND *(Gastro/Urology) 78QHO*

Berkeley Medevices, Inc. 800-227-2388
1330 S 51st St, Richmond, CA 94804
Word Bartholin-gland catheter.

R Medical Supply 800-882-7578
620 Valley Forge Rd Ste F, Hillsborough, NC 27278

CATHETER, BILIARY *(Gastro/Urology) 78FGE*

Abbott Vascular Inc. 800-227-9902
400 Saginaw Dr, Redwood City, CA 94063
Biliary catheter and accessories.

CATHETER, BILIARY *(cont'd)*

Abbott Vascular, Cardiac Therapies 800-227-9902
3200 Lakeside Dr, Santa Clara, CA 95054
Biliary stent.

Abbott Vascular, Cardiac Therapies 800-227-9902
26531 Ynez Rd, Mailing P.O. Box 9018, Temecula, CA 92591
Biliary stent.

Abbott Vascular, Vascular Solutions 800-227-9902
26531 Ynez Rd, Temecula, CA 92591
Biliary stent.

Ballard Medical Products 770-587-7835
12050 Lone Peak Pkwy, Draper, UT 84020
Various ercp catheters.

Bentec Medical, Inc. 757-224-0177
1380 E Beamer St, Woodland, CA 95776
Biliary catheter.

Biosearch Medical Products, Inc. 908-722-5000
35 Industrial Pkwy, Branchburg, NJ 08876
Biliary stent.

Boston Scientific - Marina Bay Customer Fulfillment Center 617-689-6000
500 Commander Shea Blvd, Quincy, MA 02171
Biliary stent.

Boston Scientific Corporation 800-225-2732
1 Boston Scientific Pl, Natick, MA 01760
Biliary drainage catheters for use in radiology.

C. R. Bard, Inc., Bard Urological Div. 888-367-2273
13183 Harland Dr NE, Covington, GA 30014

Cook Endoscopy 336-744-0157
4900 Bethania Station Rd # &, 5951 Grassy Creek Blvd. Winston Salem, NC 27105
Various types of sterile biliary catheters including biliary and.

Cook Inc. 800-457-4500
PO Box 489, Bloomington, IN 47402

Covidien Lp 508-261-8000
15 Hampshire St, Mansfield, MA 02048
CHOLE-CATH biliary catheter.

Edwards Lifesciences, Llc. 800-424-3278
1 Edwards Way, Irvine, CA 92614

Endochoice Inc. 888-682-3636
11810 Wills Rd Ste 100, Alpharetta, GA 30009
Bonastent Biliary by Sewoon Medical; Bonastent Biliary designed by SST; Bonastent manufactured by Sewoon; EndoChoice Bonastent Biliary stent

Ev3 Inc. 800-716-6700
4600 Nathan Ln N, Plymouth, MN 55442
Biliary stent.

Hobbs Medical, Inc. 860-684-5875
8 Spring St, Stafford Springs, CT 06076
Biliary stent set.

Lucas Medical, Inc. 714-938-0233
1751 S Douglass Rd, Anaheim, CA 92806
Biliary catheter.

Orbusneich Medical, Inc. 852-280-2228
5363 NW 35th Ave, Ft Lauderdale, FL 33309
Biliary stent system.

Specialty Surgical Products, Inc. 406-961-0102
1131 US Highway 93 N, Victor, MT 59875
Biliary stent.

Uresil, Llc 800-538-7374
5418 Touhy Ave, Skokie, IL 60077
CHOLE-CATH percutaneous.

W.L. Gore & Associates,Inc 928-526-3030
1505 North Fourth St., Flagstaff, AZ 86004
Biliary stent.

CATHETER, BILIARY, GENERAL & PLASTIC SURGERY
(Surgery) 79GCA

Ballard Medical Products 770-587-7835
12050 Lone Peak Pkwy, Draper, UT 84020
Wilteck biliary stent set, wiltek pancreatic stent set.

Consumaquip Corporation 305-592-4510
7240 NW 12th St, Miami, FL 33126

CATHETER, BILIARY, GENERAL & PLASTIC SURGERY *(cont'd)*

Cook Endoscopy 336-744-0157
4900 Bethania Station Rd # &, 5951 Grassy Creek Blvd.
Winston Salem, NC 27105
Balloon stone extractor.

Geneva Medical Inc. 630-232-2507
2571 Kaneville Ct, Geneva, IL 60134
Balloon dilation catheter.

Gml, Inc. 651-486-3691
500 Oak Grove Pkwy, Saint Paul, MN 55127
Blood glucose test strips.

Rocket Medical Plc. 800-707-7625
150 Recreation Park Dr Ste 3, Hingham, MA 02043

CATHETER, BILIARY, REPROCESSED *(Gastro/Urology) 78NML*

Sterilmed, Inc. 763-488-3400
11400 73rd Ave N Ste 100, Maple Grove, MN 55369
Ercp cannula.

CATHETER, CARDIAC THERMODILUTION
(Cardiovascular) 74QHP

Biosensors International - Usa 949-553-8300
20280 SW Acacia St Ste 300, Newport Beach, CA 92660
Thermodilution catheters featuring Safetywedge. Device to virtually eliminate the risk of PA rupture.

Ge Industrial, Sensing 800-833-9438
1100 Technology Park Dr, Billerica, MA 01821

M & I Medical Sales, Inc. 305-663-6444
4711 SW 72nd Ave, Miami, FL 33155

CATHETER, CARDIOVASCULAR *(Surgery) 79GBK*

Boston Scientific Corp. 800-323-6472
5905 Nathan Ln N, Minneapolis, MN 55442
SOFTIP cardiovascular catheter for angiographic and angioplasty procedures.

Catheter Research, Inc. (Cri) 317-872-0074
5610 W 82nd St, Indianapolis, IN 46278

Ep Medsystems, Inc. 609-753-8533
575 N Route 73 Bldg D, West Berlin, NJ 08091
PROCATH temporary pacing catheter.

Heartport 888-478-7678
700 Bay Rd, Redwood City, CA 94063
EndoCPB catheter system to perform Port-Access minimally invasive cardiac surgery, coronary artery bypass grafting and other cardiac surgeries.

Hospira, Inc. 877-946-7747
755 Jarvis Dr, Morgan Hill, CA 95037

M & I Medical Sales, Inc. 305-663-6444
4711 SW 72nd Ave, Miami, FL 33155

Medovations, Inc. 800-558-6408
102 E Keefe Ave, Milwaukee, WI 53212

Millar Instruments, Inc. 800.669.2343
6001 Gulf Fwy Ste A, Houston, TX 77023

CATHETER, CARDIOVASCULAR, BALLOON TYPE
(Cardiovascular) 74GBR

Arrow International, Inc. 800-523-8446
2400 Bernville Rd, Reading, PA 19605
Wedge pressure catheter, bipolar balloon pacing catheter, balloon thermodilution catheter, and Berman angiographic catheters. Balloon occlusion femoral angiography.

Boston Scientific - Maple Grove 800-553-5878
1 Scimed Pl, Maple Grove, MN 55311

C. R. Bard, Inc., Bard Urological Div. 888-367-2273
13183 Harland Dr NE, Covington, GA 30014

Cook Inc. 800-457-4500
PO Box 489, Bloomington, IN 47402

Manufacturing & Research, Inc.(Dba Mri Medical) 520-882-7794
4700 S Overland Dr, Tucson, AZ 85714
Custom silicone catheters.

Millar Instruments, Inc. 800.669.2343
6001 Gulf Fwy Ste A, Houston, TX 77023

Oscor, Inc. 800-726-7267
3816 Desoto Blvd, Palm Harbor, FL 34683
Balloon catheter.

CATHETER, CARDIOVASCULAR, BALLOON TYPE *(cont'd)*

Polyzen, Inc. 919-319-9599
1041 Classic Rd, Apex, NC 27539
BALLOONS , Low pressure and specialty balloons non-latex balloons. Polyurethane, silicone, cardiac, trachea, spinal, epistaxis, gastric, GI, gynecology and sleeve balloons. Compliant & Non-compliant. Sleeves and pre-shaped.

CATHETER, CAROTID, TEMPORARY, FOR EMBOLIZATION CAPTURE *(Cardiovascular) 74NTE*

Abbott Vascular, Vascular Solutions 800-227-9902
26531 Ynez Rd, Temecula, CA 92591
Embolic protection device.

Embrella Cardiovascular, Inc. 610-783-1100
880 E Swedesford Rd Ste 220, Wayne, PA 19087
Embrella Embolic Deflector

Ev3 Inc. 800-716-6700
4600 Nathan Ln N, Plymouth, MN 55442
Embolic protection device.

Lumen Biomedical, Inc. 763-577-9600
14505 21st Ave N Ste 212, Plymouth, MN 55447
Percutaneous catheter.

CATHETER, CENTRAL VENOUS *(General) 80WQH*

Angiodynamics, Inc. 800-472-5221
1 Horizon Way, Manchester, GA 31816
Central venous silicone in single, double and triple lumen configurations, with or without placement kits.

Arrow International, Inc. 800-523-8446
2400 Bernville Rd, Reading, PA 19605
Single-lumen central venous catheter.

B. Braun Oem Division, B. Braun Medical Inc. 866-8-BBRAUN
824 12th Ave, Bethlehem, PA 18018
The Introcan Safety IV Catheter incorporates a passive design to minimize needlestick injuries without requiring user activation. The safety clip is pre-assembled in the catheter hub, and is automatically engaged when the needle bevel exits the catheter hub.

Becton Dickinson Infusion Therapy Systems, Inc. 888-237-2762
9450 S State St, Sandy, UT 84070

Diablo Sales & Marketing, Inc. 925-648-1611
PO Box 3219, Danville, CA 94526
Custom design and manufacturing of catheters and specialty guidewires. Guiding catheters; stent delivery and drug delivery systems.

Lsl Industries, Inc. 888-225-5575
5535 N Wolcott Ave, Chicago, IL 60640
Dressing kits

Medi Inc 800-225-8634
75 York Ave, P.O. Box 302, Randolph, MA 02368

CATHETER, CHOLANGIOGRAPHY *(Surgery) 79GBZ*

American Catheter Corp. 800-345-6714
13047 S Highway 475, Ocala, FL 34480

Arrow International, Inc. 800-523-8446
2400 Bernville Rd, Reading, PA 19605
Laparoscopic cholangiography catheters.

Cook Endoscopy 336-744-0157
4900 Bethania Station Rd # &, 5951 Grassy Creek Blvd.
Winston Salem, NC 27105
Ercp catheters.

Cook Inc. 800-457-4500
PO Box 489, Bloomington, IN 47402

Dma Med-Chem Corporation 800-362-1833
49 Watermill Ln, Great Neck, NY 11021

Edwards Lifesciences Technology Sarl 949-250-2500
State Rd. 402 N.km 1.4, Anasco, PR 00610-1577
Cholangiography catheter.

Edwards Lifesciences, Llc. 800-424-3278
1 Edwards Way, Irvine, CA 92614

Geneva Medical Inc. 630-232-2507
2571 Kaneville Ct, Geneva, IL 60134
Sterile cholangiogram catheter.

Lemaitre Vascular, Inc. 781-221-2266
63 2nd Ave, Burlington, MA 01803
Features a ribbed balloon design for stable catheter baloon design for stable catheter placement without clamping.

CATHETER, CHOLANGIOGRAPHY *(cont'd)*

Medchannel Llc 617-314-9861
1241 Adams St Apt 110, Dorchester Center, MA 02124
Irrigation catheter.

Navilyst Medical 800-833-9973
100 Boston Scientific Way, Marlborough, MA 01752
Tuohy-borst adaptor.

Novosci Corp. 281-363-4949
2828 N Crescentridge Dr, The Woodlands, TX 77381
Rigid needle stock with oval injection port angled to enter cystic duct and clipped for no leakage.

Ranfac Corp. 800-2RANFAC
30 Doherty Ave, Avon Industrial Park, Avon, MA 02322
Catheter set with cannula, tubing, and stopcock; also, disposable laporoscopic cholangiography catheter.

Taut, Inc. 800-231-8288
2571 Kaneville Ct, Geneva, IL 60134
Smooth polished tip, rear shoulder, and support tube require minimal intubation for successful cholangiography; models M55, M56 and M57 available.

United States Endoscopy Group 800-769-8226
5976 Heisley Rd, Mentor, OH 44060
Ponsky disposable cholangiography catheter with guidewire, standard catheters without guidewires.

Utah Pioneer Medical, Inc. 801-280-1053
8173 Summit Valley Dr, West Jordan, UT 84088
Cholangiography catheter 4.5 French with introducer and two labeled syringes. Patented valve system (automatic stopcocks) facilitates fluoroscopy.

CATHETER, CONDUCTION, ANESTHESIA *(Anesthesiology) 73BSO*

Arrow International, Inc. 800-523-8446
2400 Bernville Rd, Reading, PA 19605

Axiom Medical, Inc. 800-221-8569
19320 Van Ness Ave, Torrance, CA 90501
Pleural Anaesthesia Catheter, chest tube to allow administration of anaesthetic for pain management while draining. Various sizes, multipostion entry port.

Cardiomed Supplies Inc. 800-387-9757
5 Gormley Industrial Ave., P.O. Box 575
Gormley, ONT L0H 1 Canada
$60.00 for anesthesia catheter.

Embo-Optics, Llc. 887-885-6400
100 Cummings Ctr # 326B, Beverly, MA 01915
IV Illuminator with lighted monitoring feature aids medical personnel in assuring that all IV solutions and medications are infusing properly and at the correct infusion rate. Greatly enhance patient safety in aiding to prevent any adverse events during infusion.

I-Flow Corporation 800-448-3569
20202 Windrow Dr, Lake Forest, CA 92630
SOAKER CATHETER, designed to infuse drugs into large incisions to relieve postoperative pain; catheter length FDA approved up to 12.5 cm.

Micor, Inc. 412-487-1113
2855 Oxford Blvd, Allison Park, PA 15101
19- to 28-ga epidural with or without radiopaque stripe. Also, spinal catheters.

Smiths Medical Asd, Inc. 610-578-9600
9255 Customhouse Plz Ste N, San Diego, CA 92154
Various.

Stryker Puerto Rico, Ltd. 939-307-2500
Hwy. 3, Km. 131.2, Las Guasimas Ind. Park, Arroyo, PR 00714
Various anesthesia conduction catheters.

CATHETER, CONTINUOUS FLUSH *(Cardiovascular) 74KRA*

Argon Medical Devices Inc. 903-675-9321
1445 Flat Creek Rd, Athens, TX 75751
Steriflo.

Bacchus Vascular, Inc. 408-980-8300
3110 Coronado Dr, Santa Clara, CA 95054
Continious flush catheter.

Boston Scientific - Maple Grove 800-553-5878
1 Scimed Pl, Maple Grove, MN 55311

Boston Scientific-Neurovascular 510-440-7700
47900 Bayside Pkwy, Fremont, CA 94538
Catheter.

CATHETER, CONTINUOUS FLUSH *(cont'd)*

Clinical Instruments Intl., Inc. 508-764-2200
278 Worcester St, Southbridge, MA 01550
Introducers.

Cordis Neurovascular, Inc. 800-327-7714
14201 NW 60th Ave, Miami Lakes, FL 33014
Infusion catheters.

Edwards Lifesciences Technology Sarl 949-250-2500
State Rd. 402 N.km 1.4, Anasco, PR 00610-1577
Catheter, continuous flush.

Edwards Lifesciences, Llc. 800-424-3278
1 Edwards Way, Irvine, CA 92614

Ekos Corp. 888-400-3567
11911 N Creek Pkwy S, Bothell, WA 98011
Various types of ultrasound infusion catheter systems.

Ev3 Neurovascular 800-716-6700
9775 Toledo Way, Irvine, CA 92618
Continuous flush catheter.

Flowmedica, Inc. 866-671-9500
46563 Fremont Blvd, Fremont, CA 94538
Continuous flush catheter.

Hospira, Inc. 877-946-7747
755 Jarvis Dr, Morgan Hill, CA 95037

Icu Medical (Ut), Inc 949-366-2183
4455 Atherton Dr, Salt Lake City, UT 84123
Various continuous flush devices.

Impact Medical Technologies, Llc 770-817-3300
311 Curie Dr, Alpharetta, GA 30005
Various types of microcatheters.

Medical Murray Inc. 847-620-7990
400 N Rand Rd, North Barrington, IL 60010

Mercator Medsystems, Inc. 510-614-4550
3077 Teagarden St, San Leandro, CA 94577
Microsyringe.

Merit Medical Systems, Inc. 800-356-3748
1600 Merit Pkwy, South Jordan, UT 84095
Thrombolytic catheters. Fountain Series Catheters.

Smiths Medical Asd, Inc. 800-848-1757
6250 Shier Rings Rd, Dublin, OH 43016

Vascular Insights LLC 203-376-3775
395 Boston Post Rd, Madison, CT 06443

CATHETER, CONTINUOUS IRRIGATION *(Surgery) 79GBQ*

Armm, Inc. 714-848-8190
17744 Sampson Ln, Huntington Beach, CA 92647

Clinical Instruments Intl., Inc. 508-764-2200
278 Worcester St, Southbridge, MA 01550
Introducers.

Cook Endoscopy 336-744-0157
4900 Bethania Station Rd # &, 5951 Grassy Creek Blvd.
Winston Salem, NC 27105
Oral gastric tube.

Medline Industries, Inc. 800-633-5886
1 Medline Pl, Mundelein, IL 60060

Utah Medical Products, Inc. 800-533-4984
7043 Cottonwood St, Midvale, UT 84047
General procedure catheterization tray, specialized tray for minor surgical procedures: umbilical catheter placements, cut downs, circumcisions, etc.

CATHETER, CORONARY, ATHERECTOMY
(Cardiovascular) 74MCX

Abbott Vascular, Cardiac Therapies 800-227-9902
26531 Ynez Rd, Mailing P.O. Box 9018, Temecula, CA 92591
Coronary atherectomy catheter.

Boston Scientific - Marina Bay Customer Fulfillment Center 617-689-6000
500 Commander Shea Blvd, Quincy, MA 02171
Rotational angioplasty system guide wires.

Boston Scientific-Neurovascular 510-440-7700
47900 Bayside Pkwy, Fremont, CA 94538
Rotablator console.

Minnetronix Inc. 888-301-1025
1635 Energy Park Dr, Saint Paul, MN 55108
Angiojet Ultra Thrombectomy Console

CATHETER, COUDE *(Gastro/Urology) 78EZC*

Benlan Inc. 905-829-5004
2760 Brighton Rd., Oakville, ONT L6H 5T4 Canada

Coloplast Manufacturing Us, Llc 612-302-4992
1185 Willow Lake Blvd, Vadnais Heights, MN 55110
Coude catheter sterile.

Coloplast Manufacturing Us, Llc 800-533-0464
1840 W Oak Pkwy, Marietta, GA 30062
CONVEEN sterile with frosted surface and smooth tip for ease of use, lateral eyelets for maximum drainage.

CATHETER, ELECTRODE RECORDING, OR PROBE *(Cardiovascular) 74DRF*

Arrow International, Inc. 800-523-8446
2 Berry Dr, Mount Holly, NJ 08060
Various types of sterile electrophysiology catheters & accessories.

Biosense Webster, Inc 800-729-9010
3333 S Diamond Canyon Rd, Diamond Bar, CA 91765
Diagnostic electrophysiology catheters.

Boston Scientific Corporation 800-225-2732
1 Boston Scientific Pl, Natick, MA 01760

Cardima, Inc. 888-354-0300
47266 Benicia St, Fremont, CA 94538
Various.

Catheffects, Llc. 916-677-1790
1100 Melody Ln, Roseville, CA 95678
Electrophysiology mapping catheter & cable.

Ep Medsystems, Inc. 609-753-8533
575 N Route 73 Bldg D, West Berlin, NJ 08091
PROCATH electrode/electrophysiology catheter.

Ep Technologies, Inc. 888-272-1001
2710 Orchard Pkwy, San Jose, CA 95134
Various.

Medtronic Ep Systems 763-514-4000
8299 Central Ave NE, Spring Lake Park, Minneapolis, MN 55432
Cardiac electrophysiology catheters.

Medtronic Puerto Rico Operations Co., Villalba 763-514-4000
PO Box 6001, Rd. 149, Km. 56.3, Villalba, PR 00766
Cardiac electrophysiology catheters.

Millar Instruments, Inc. 800.669.2343
6001 Gulf Fwy Ste A, Houston, TX 77023
EPR-800 Ultra-Miniature Catheter for Electrophysiology Research -- Animal Use Only

Numed, Inc. 315-328-4491
2880 Main St., Hopkinton, NY 12965
Temporary ballon pacing probe.

Prorhythm, Inc. 631-981-3907
105 Comac St, Ronkonkoma, NY 11779
Sterile electrophysiology catheter and connection cable.

St. Jude Medical Atrial Fibrillation 800-328-3873
14901 Deveau Pl, Minnetonka, MN 55345

CATHETER, EMBOLECTOMY (FOGARTY TYPE) *(Cardiovascular) 74DXE*

Arrow Internacional De Mexico, S.A. De C.V. 610-378-0131
Modulo 1, Circuito 5, Parque Industrias De America
Col. Panamericana, Chihuahua Mexico
Multiple

Biosensors International - Usa 949-553-8300
20280 SW Acacia St Ste 300, Newport Beach, CA 92660
Embolectomy catheters featuring a complete line of springed tipped and standard latex balloon catheters (2F-7F) in convenient tube packs.

Clinical Instruments Intl., Inc. 508-764-2200
278 Worcester St, Southbridge, MA 01550
Carotid bypass shunt.

Covidien Lp 508-261-8000
15 Hampshire St, Mansfield, MA 02048
VASCU-FLO silicone embolectomy balloon catheter.

Edwards Lifesciences Technology Sarl 949-250-2500
State Rd. 402 N.km 1.4, Anasco, PR 00610-1577
Embolectomy catheter.

Genesis Medical Interventional, Inc. 650-367-7667
652 Bair Island Rd Ste 103, Redwood City, CA 94063
Embolectomy catheter.

CATHETER, EMBOLECTOMY (FOGARTY TYPE) *(cont'd)*

Hotspur Technologies Inc. 650-969-3150
880 Maude Ave Ste A, Mountain View, CA 94043
Keeper Embolectomy Catheter; IQ Cath PTA Balloon Catheter

Lucas Medical, Inc. 714-938-0233
1751 S Douglass Rd, Anaheim, CA 92806
Various.

Lumen Biomedical, Inc. 763-577-9600
14505 21st Ave N Ste 212, Plymouth, MN 55447
Catheter, embolectomy.

Manufacturing & Research, Inc.(Dba Mri Medical) 520-882-7794
4700 S Overland Dr, Tucson, AZ 85714
Custom silicone balloon catheters.

Medtronic Vascular 707-525-0111
3576 Unocal Pl, Santa Rosa, CA 95403
Aspiration catheter.

Omnisonics Medical Technologies 978-657-9980
66 Concord St Ste A, Wilmington, MA 01887
Same.

Radius Medical Technologies, Inc. 978-263-4466
15 Craig Rd, Acton, MA 01720
Embolectomy catheter.

Vascular Solutions, Inc. 888-240-6001
6464 Sycamore Ct N, Maple Grove, MN 55369
Pronto LP Extraction Catheter

Vascular Solutions, Inc. 763-656-4300
5025 Cheshire Ln N, Plymouth, MN 55446
Thrombus removal catheter, embolectomy catheter.

CATHETER, EPIDURAL *(Obstetrics/Gyn) 85QHT*

Arrow International, Inc. 800-523-8446
2400 Bernville Rd, Reading, PA 19605
Single-shot or continuous (intermittent) anesthesia kits.

B. Braun Oem Division, B. Braun Medical Inc. 866-8-BBRAUN
824 12th Ave, Bethlehem, PA 18018

Cardiomed Supplies Inc. 800-387-9757
5 Gormley Industrial Ave., P.O. Box 575
Gormley, ONT L0H 1 Canada
BODYSOFT Tray assembly

Covidien Lp 508-261-8000
15 Hampshire St, Mansfield, MA 02048

Dma Med-Chem Corporation 800-362-1833
49 Watermill Ln, Great Neck, NY 11021

Epimed International, Inc. 800-866-3342
141 Sal Landrio Dr, Crossroads Business Park, Johnstown, NY 12095

Micor, Inc. 412-487-1113
2855 Oxford Blvd, Allison Park, PA 15101
18-, 19-, 20-ga, pediatric 24-ga with dispenser.

Pain Products International 800-359-5756
4763 Hamilton Wolfe Rd # 210, San Antonio, TX 78229

Pmt Corp. 800-626-5463
1500 Park Rd, Chanhassen, MN 55317
Epidural infusion catheter.

Spectra Medical Devices, Inc. 866-938-8649
4C Henshaw St, Woburn, MA 01801

Tfx Medical Oem 800-548-6600
50 Plantation Dr, Jaffrey, NH 03452

Vygon Corp. 800-544-4907
2495 General Armistead Ave, Norristown, PA 19403

CATHETER, EUSTACHIAN, GENERAL & PLASTIC SURGERY *(Surgery) 79GBY*

Mcpherson Enterprises, Inc. 813-931-4201
3851 62nd Ave N Ste A, Pinellas Park, FL 33781
Thoracentesis tray.

CATHETER, FEMORAL *(Gastro/Urology) 78LFK*

Angiodynamics, Inc. 800-472-5221
1 Horizon Way, Manchester, GA 31816
Dual and single lumen for hemodialysis, and CAVH catheters for continuous hemofiltration.

Clinical Instruments Intl., Inc. 508-764-2200
278 Worcester St, Southbridge, MA 01550
Introducers.

Medron, Inc. 801-974-3010
1518 Gladiola St, Salt Lake City, UT 84104
Cavh catheter.

CATHETER, FLOW DIRECTED *(Cardiovascular) 74DYG*

Argon Medical Devices Inc. 903-675-9321
1445 Flat Creek Rd, Athens, TX 75751
Various catheter kits including protective sleeves.

Arrow International, Inc. 800-523-8446
2 Berry Dr, Mount Holly, NJ 08060
Various.

Biosensors International - Usa 949-553-8300
20280 SW Acacia St Ste 300, Newport Beach, CA 92660
Thermodilution catheters, PA monitoring catheters, and Paceport catheters with patented SafetyWedge.

Clinical Instruments Intl., Inc. 508-764-2200
278 Worcester St, Southbridge, MA 01550
Introducers.

Edwards Lifesciences Technology Sarl 949-250-2500
State Rd. 402 N.km 1.4, Anasco, PR 00610-1577
Various.

Edwards Lifesciences, Llc. 800-424-3278
1 Edwards Way, Irvine, CA 92614

Hantel Technologies 510-487-1561
721 Sandoval Way, Hayward, CA 94544
Flow-directed catheter.

Hospira, Inc. 877-946-7747
755 Jarvis Dr, Morgan Hill, CA 95037

Icu Medical (Ut), Inc 949-366-2183
4455 Atherton Dr, Salt Lake City, UT 84123
Various types of flow directed catheter.

Vitalcor, Inc. 800-874-8358
100 Chestnut Ave, Westmont, IL 60559
Balloon-type cardiovascular catheter.

CATHETER, HEMODIALYSIS *(Gastro/Urology) 78MPB*

Angiodynamics, Inc. 800-472-5221
1 Horizon Way, Manchester, GA 31816
Single and double lumen catheters for acute and chronic use.

Excelsior Medical Corp. 732-776-7525
1933 Heck Ave, Neptune, NJ 07753
Heparin lock syringe.

Lee Medical International, Inc. 800-433-8950
612 Distributors Row, Harahan, LA 70123
Fistula needles.

Medcomp (Medical Components, Inc.) 800-220-3791
1499 Delp Dr, Harleysville, PA 19438
Dialysis, infusion, and specialty CVC catheters.

Smiths Medical Asd, Inc. 800-433-5832
1265 Grey Fox Rd, Saint Paul, MN 55112
TruFlow short- and long-term hemodialysis catheters.

CATHETER, HEMODIALYSIS, IMPLANTED *(Gastro/Urology) 78MSD*

Navilyst Medical 800-833-9973
100 Boston Scientific Way, Marlborough, MA 01752
Dialysis catheters and dialysis catheter kits.

CATHETER, HEMODIALYSIS, SINGLE-NEEDLE *(Gastro/Urology) 78QIK*

Angiodynamics, Inc. 800-472-5221
1 Horizon Way, Manchester, GA 31816
Dual lumen fistula needle provides single puncture access for continuous flow hemodialysis, CVVH, plasmapheresis, and apheresis, plus acute care catheters.

Medisystems Corporation 800-369-6334
439 S Union St Fl 5, Lawrence, MA 01843

CATHETER, HYDROCEPHALIC, ATRIAL *(Cns/Neurology) 84UBJ*

Novosci Corp. 281-363-4949
2828 N Crescentridge Dr, The Woodlands, TX 77381

CATHETER, IMAGING, ULTRASONIC *(Radiology) 90WIO*

Boston Scientific - Maple Grove 800-553-5878
1 Scimed Pl, Maple Grove, MN 55311
SONICATH.

Boston Scientific Corporation 800-225-2732
1 Boston Scientific Pl, Natick, MA 01760
SONICATH.

CATHETER, IMAGING, ULTRASONIC *(cont'd)*

Diablo Sales & Marketing, Inc. 925-648-1611
PO Box 3219, Danville, CA 94526
Custom design and manufacturing of catheters and specialty guidewires. Guiding catheters; stent delivery and drug delivery systems.

Embo-Optics, Llc. 887-885-6400
100 Cummings Ctr # 326B, Beverly, MA 01915
IV illuminator with lighted monitoring feature aids medical personnel in assuring that all IV solutions and medications are infusing properly and at the correct infusion rate. Greatly enhance patient safety in aiding to prevent any adverse events during infusion.

Redi-Tech Medical Products,Llc 800-824-1793
529 Front St Ste 125, Berea, OH 44017

Rocket Medical Plc. 800-707-7625
150 Recreation Park Dr Ste 3, Hingham, MA 02043

CATHETER, INFUSION *(Surgery) 79JCY*

Ac Healthcare Supply, Inc. 905-448-4706
11651 230th St, Cambria Heights, NY 11411
Various types of sizes of catheters.

Arrow International, Inc. 800-523-8446
2400 Bernville Rd, Reading, PA 19605
Emergency infusion device, peripheral emergency infusion device, rapid infusion catheter exchange set, high-flow fluid administration set, emergency/trauma catheter and peritoneal lavage kit.

Boston Scientific-Neurovascular 510-440-7700
47900 Bayside Pkwy, Fremont, CA 94538
Infusion catheter.

Cardiomed Supplies Inc. 800-387-9757
5 Gormley Industrial Ave., P.O. Box 575
Gormley, ONT L0H 1 Canada
$18.00 Nova catheter 1 and 2.

Clinical Instruments Intl., Inc. 508-764-2200
278 Worcester St, Southbridge, MA 01550
Introducers.

Cook Inc. 800-457-4500
PO Box 489, Bloomington, IN 47402

Covidien Lp 508-261-8000
15 Hampshire St, Mansfield, MA 02048

E-Z-Em, Inc. 516-333-8230
750 Summa Ave, Westbury, NY 11590
Infusion catheter.

Edwards Lifesciences, Llc. 800-424-3278
1 Edwards Way, Irvine, CA 92614

Hospira, Inc. 877-946-7747
755 Jarvis Dr, Morgan Hill, CA 95037

Intravascular Incorporated 800-917-3234
3600 Burwood Dr, Waukegan, IL 60085
FloStar Needleless Connector - patented 'dual-valve' needle free connector for use on venous or arterial lines with luer lock or luer slip in intravenous therapy. Available stand alone or on extension sets.

Medi Inc 800-225-8634
75 York Ave, P.O. Box 302, Randolph, MA 02368

Medtronic Minimed 800-933-3322
18000 Devonshire St, Northridge, CA 91325
SOF-SET subcutaneous non-needle infusion set.

Ranfac Corp. 800-2RANFAC
30 Doherty Ave, Avon Industrial Park, Avon, MA 02322

CATHETER, INTRA-AORTIC BALLOON *(Cardiovascular) 74QHY*

Arrow International, Inc. 800-523-8446
2400 Bernville Rd, Reading, PA 19605

Datascope Cardiac Assist Div. 800-777-4222
15 Law Dr, Fairfield, NJ 07004
PERCOR STAT-DL.

Datascope Corp. 800-288-2121
14 Philips Pkwy, Montvale, NJ 07645
Intra-aortic Balloon Catheter. Percor-Stat DL. Dual Lumen IAB Catheter available in 34, 40, 50cc (9.5 & 10.5 Fr). Also available is True Sheathless, an intra-aortic catheter (9.5 Fr.) volume 25, 34, 40cc. IAB catheter designed especially to facilitate sheathless IAB catheter insertion. Also available Profile 8 Fr first fully functional co-lumen IAB catheter small enough to be inserted through an 8 Fr sheath, 34, 40cc (8 Fr).

CATHETER, INTRACARDIAC MAPPING, HIGH-DENSITY ARRAY
(Cardiovascular) 74MTD

Ep Technologies, Inc. 888-272-1001
2710 Orchard Pkwy, San Jose, CA 95134
Various.

St. Jude Medical Atrial Fibrillation (Endocardial Solutions) 800-374-8038
1350 Energy Ln Ste 110, Saint Paul, MN 55108
Ensite multi-electrode diagnostic catheter.

CATHETER, INTRASPINAL, PERCUTANEOUS, SHORT-TERM
(General) 80MAJ

Diablo Sales & Marketing, Inc. 925-648-1611
PO Box 3219, Danville, CA 94526
Custom design and manufacturing of catheters and specialty guidewires. Guiding catheters; stent delivery and drug delivery systems.

Medtronic Neurosurgery 800-468-9710
125 Cremona Dr, Goleta, CA 93117
Analgesia delivery catheter, externalized.

Neo Medical Inc. 888-450-3334
42514 Albrae St, Fremont, CA 94538
Percutaneous intraspinal short term catheter.

CATHETER, INTRASPINAL, SUBCUTANEOUS, IMPLANTABLE
(General) 80LMP

Smiths Medical Asd, Inc. 800-433-5832
1265 Grey Fox Rd, Saint Paul, MN 55112

Vygon Corp. 800-544-4907
2495 General Armistead Ave, Norristown, PA 19403

CATHETER, INTRAUTERINE, WITH INTRODUCER
(Obstetrics/Gyn) 85HGS

Clinical Innovations, Inc. 888-268-6222
747 W 4170 S, Murray, UT 84123
KOALA Intrauterine pressure system is a sensor-tip catheter designed with a small, soft tip for safe and easy insertion. Cables and telemetry system available.

Conceptus, Inc. 650-962-4000
331 E Evelyn Ave, Mountain View, CA 94041

Gish Biomedical, Inc. 800-938-0531
22942 Arroyo Vis, Rancho Santa Margarita, CA 92688
Amnio infusion and uterine pressure-monitoring catheter.

Memcath Technologies Llc 651-450-7400
1777 Oakdale Ave, Saint Paul, MN 55118
Sizes 8-22 FR, each available in 5,7,9,11,and 13 cm sheath lengths.

Rocket Medical Plc. 800-707-7625
150 Recreation Park Dr Ste 3, Hingham, MA 02043

Utah Medical Products, Inc. 800-533-4984
7043 Cottonwood St, Midvale, UT 84047
INTRAN trasducer-tipped intra-uterine pressure catheter for uterine monitoring during labor; also, a complete line of transducer-tipped and fluid-filled catheters.

CATHETER, INTRAVASCULAR OCCLUDING
(Cns/Neurology) 84HBZ

Clinical Instruments Intl., Inc. 508-764-2200
278 Worcester St, Southbridge, MA 01550
Introducers.

Diablo Sales & Marketing, Inc. 925-648-1611
PO Box 3219, Danville, CA 94526
Custom micro-catheter design and manufacturing. Platinum coils or machined components and drug delivery systems.

Edwards Lifesciences Technology Sarl 949-250-2500
State Rd. 402 N.km 1.4, Anasco, PR 00610-1577
Occlusion catheter.

Edwards Lifesciences, Llc. 800-424-3278
1 Edwards Way, Irvine, CA 92614

Uresil, Llc 800-538-7374
5418 Touhy Ave, Skokie, IL 60077
VASCU-FLO silicone balloon carotid shunt.

CATHETER, INTRAVASCULAR OCCLUDING, TEMPORARY
(Cardiovascular) 74MJN

Aga Medical Corporation. 888-546-4407
5050 Nathan Ln N, Plymouth, MN 55442
Sterile sizing balloon.

CATHETER, INTRAVASCULAR OCCLUDING, TEMPORARY
(cont'd)

Boston Scientific Corp. 408-935-3400
150 Baytech Dr, San Jose, CA 95134
Occluding shunt.

Chase Medical, Lp 972-783-0644
1876 Firman Dr, Richardson, TX 75081
Vessel occluder.

Coaxia, Inc. 763-315-8395
10900 73rd Ave N, Maple Grove, MN 55369
Peripheral occlusion catheter.

Edwards Lifesciences Technology Sarl 949-250-2500
State Rd. 402 N.km 1.4, Anasco, PR 00610-1577
Occlusion catheter.

Ev3 Neurovascular 800-716-6700
9775 Toledo Way, Irvine, CA 92618
Occlusion balloon catheter.

Numed, Inc. 315-328-4491
2880 Main St., Hopkinton, NY 12965
Sizing catheter.

CATHETER, INTRAVASCULAR, DIAGNOSTIC
(Cardiovascular) 74DQO

Abbott Vascular, Cardiac Therapies 800-227-9902
3200 Lakeside Dr, Santa Clara, CA 95054
Various types of catheters.

Abbott Vascular, Cardiac Therapies 800-227-9902
26531 Ynez Rd, Mailing P.O. Box 9018, Temecula, CA 92591
Various types of catheters.

Abiomed, Inc. 800-422-8666
22 Cherry Hill Dr, Danvers, MA 01923
Impella 2.5; MPC and Power Supply; Quick Set-up Kit

Argon Medical Devices Inc. 903-675-9321
1445 Flat Creek Rd, Athens, TX 75751
Digital subtraction procedure trays.

Biocardia, Inc. 650-624-0900
384 Oyster Point Blvd, S San Fran, CA 94080
Guide catheter.

Biosphere Medical, Inc. 781-681-7900
1050 Hingham St, Rockland, MA 02370
Infusion catheter.

Boston Scientific - Maple Grove 800-553-5878
1 Scimed Pl, Maple Grove, MN 55311

Boston Scientific-Neurovascular 510-440-7700
47900 Bayside Pkwy, Fremont, CA 94538
Endovascular snare catheter.

Cardio-Nef, S.A. De C.V. 01-800-024-0240
Rio Grijalva 186, Col. Mitras Norte, Monterrey, N.L. 64320 Mexico

Clinical Instruments Intl., Inc. 508-764-2200
278 Worcester St, Southbridge, MA 01550
Detergent reagent.

Concentric Medical, Inc. 650-938-2100
301 E Evelyn Ave, Mountain View, CA 94041
Diagnostic intravascular catheter.

E-Z-Em, Inc. 516-333-8230
750 Summa Ave, Westbury, NY 11590
Angiographic catheters.

Edwards Lifesciences Research Medical 949-250-2500
6864 Cottonwood St, Midvale, UT 84047
Atrial pressure monitoring catheter.

Edwards Lifesciences Technology Sarl 949-250-2500
State Rd. 402 N.km 1.4, Anasco, PR 00610-1577
Angiography catheters, various.

Edwards Lifesciences, Llc. 800-424-3278
1 Edwards Way, Irvine, CA 92614

Eyesupply Usa, Inc. 800-521-5257
10770 N 46th St Ste C700, Tampa, FL 33617
AngioPAK: Fluorescein angiography kit for Ophthalmology

Hospira, Inc. 877-946-7747
755 Jarvis Dr, Morgan Hill, CA 95037

Irvine Biomedical, Inc. 888-IBI-9876
2375 Morse Ave, Irvine, CA 92614
Electrophysiology (diagnostic/mapping) catheter.

Kelsar, S.A. 508-261-8000
Blvd. Insurgentes, Libriamento a La, Tijuana 22450 Mexico
Silicone left ventricular catheter

CATHETER, INTRAVASCULAR, DIAGNOSTIC *(cont'd)*

LightLab Imaging Inc. 978-399-1000
1 Technology Park Dr, Westford, MA 01886
C7 Dragonfly; ImageWire 1.5, 1.8

Lucas Medical, Inc. 714-938-0233
1751 S Douglass Rd, Anaheim, CA 92806
Silicone carotid shunt catheter, carotid catheter, carotid shunt.

Medtronic Vascular 707-525-0111
3576 Unocal Pl, Santa Rosa, CA 95403
Angiographic diagnostic catheter

Merit Medical Systems, Inc. 801-253-1600
1111 S Velasco St, Angleton, TX 77515
Various catheters.

Merit Medical Systems, Inc. 800-356-3748
1600 Merit Pkwy, South Jordan, UT 84095
Performa, Softouch, Impress

Micrus Endovascular Corporation 888-550-4120
821 Fox Ln, San Jose, CA 95131
Catheter.

Millar Instruments, Inc. 800.669.2343
6001 Gulf Fwy Ste A, Houston, TX 77023

Navilyst Medical 800-833-9973
100 Boston Scientific Way, Marlborough, MA 01752
Various types of angiographic accessories, closed systems/kits.

Neuro Vasx, Inc. 763-315-0013
7351 Kirkwood Ln N Ste 112, Maple Grove, MN 55369
Sterile, infusion catheter.

Numed, Inc. 315-328-4491
2880 Main St., Hopkinton, NY 12965
Septostomy catheter and angiographic catheter.

Therox, Inc. 949-757-1999
17500 Cartwright Rd Ste 100, Irvine, CA 92614
Infusion catheter, sterile.

Transoma Medical 651-481-7429
4211 Lexington Ave N Ste 2244, Saint Paul, MN 55126
Sterile blood pressure measurement catheter and system.

Vascular Solutions, Inc. 763-656-4300
5025 Cheshire Ln N, Plymouth, MN 55446
Pigtail catheter, dual lumen catheter, diagnostic catheter.

Vitalcor, Inc. 800-874-8358
100 Chestnut Ave, Westmont, IL 60559
Cardiovascular catheter.

Volcano Corporation 800-228-4728
3661 Valley Centre Dr Ste 200, San Diego, CA 92130
Ultrasound imaging catheter.

CATHETER, INTRAVASCULAR, PLAQUE MORPHOLOGY EVALUATION *(Cardiovascular) 74OGZ*

InfraRedRx 888-680-7339
34 3rd Ave, Burlington, MA 01803
LipiScan Coronary Imaging System

CATHETER, INTRAVASCULAR, THERAPEUTIC, LONG-TERM GREATER THAN 30 DAYS *(General) 80LJS*

Angiodynamics, Inc. 800-472-5221
1 Horizon Way, Manchester, GA 31816
Long-term silicone dialysis and critical care catheters in varying lumen configurations, lengths, and french sizes.

Arrow Internacional De Mexico, S.A. De C.V. 610-378-0131
Modulo 1, Circuito 5, Parque Industrias De America
Col. Panamericana, Chihuahua Mexico
Sterile needleless injection hub

Bard Reynosa S.A. De C.V. 908-277-8000
Blvd. Montebello #1, Parque Industrial Colonial
Reynosa, Tamaulipas Mexico
Various styles & sizes of long term catheters

Bard Shannon Limited 908-277-8000
San Geronimo Industrial Park, Lot # 1, Road # 3, Km 79.7
Humacao, PR 00791
Catheters.

Becton Dickinson And Company 800-284-6845
1 Becton Dr, Franklin Lakes, NJ 07417

Catheter Innovations, Inc. 800-418-2828
3598 W 1820 S, Salt Lake City, UT 84104
Various.

CATHETER, INTRAVASCULAR, THERAPEUTIC, LONG-TERM GREATER THAN 30 DAYS *(cont'd)*

Corpak Medsystems, Inc. 800-323-6305
100 Chaddick Dr, Wheeling, IL 60090
Catheter positioning locating instrument and accesories.

Crs Medical Diagnostics Inc. 262-264-0047
662 Capitol Dr, Pewaukee, WI 53072
Endoluminal brush.

Embo-Optics, Llc. 887-885-6400
100 Cummings Ctr # 326B, Beverly, MA 01915
IV illuminator with lighted monitoring feature aids medical personnel in assuring that all IV solutions and medications are infusing properly and at the correct infusion rate. Greatly enhance patient safety in aiding to prevent any adverse events during infusion.

Johnson & Johnson De Monterrey, Sa De Cv 817-262-5211
Carretera Miguel Aleman,km21.7, Apodaca, Monterrey Mexico
Peripherally inserted central catheter

Medtronic Neurosurgery 800-468-9710
125 Cremona Dr, Goleta, CA 93117
Vascular catheter.

Navilyst Medical 800-833-9973
100 Boston Scientific Way, Marlborough, MA 01752
Central venous catheters and catheter accessories.

Neo Medical Inc. 888-450-3334
42514 Albrae St, Fremont, CA 94538
Chemo-cath subclavian.

Neo-Care Arrow International 800-640-6428
5714 Epsilon, San Antonio, TX 78249
NEO PICC (Peripherally Inserted Central Catheter).

Qualitel Corporation 425-423-8388
4608 150th Ave NE, Redmond, WA 98052
Catheter.

Utah Medical Products, Inc. 800-533-4984
7043 Cottonwood St, Midvale, UT 84047
PICC-NATE®, a PICC used specifically in neonatal patients for administration of medications for a long duration of time.

CATHETER, INTRAVASCULAR, THERAPEUTIC, SHORT-TERM LESS THAN 30 DAYS *(General) 80FOZ*

All Star Orthodontics, Llc 812-314-0804
4570 Progress Dr, Columbus, IN 47201
Various models of orthodontic products.

Alsius Corp. 949-453-0150
15770 Laguna Canyon Rd Ste 150, Irvine, CA 92618
Various central lines sterile.

Amsino Medical Usa 615-332-9959
5209 Linbar Dr Ste 640, Nashville, TN 37211
Flush syringes.

Argon Medical Devices Inc. 903-675-9321
1445 Flat Creek Rd, Athens, TX 75751
Central catheter, central venous catheter, kit & tray.

Arkray Factory Usa, Inc. 952-646-3168
5182 W 76th St, Minneapolis, MN 55439
Intravascular catheter.

Arrow Internacional De Mexico, S.A. De C.V. 610-378-0131
Modulo 1, Circuito 5, Parque Industrias De America
Col. Panamericana, Chihuahua Mexico
Various intravascular catheters

B. Braun Medical Inc., Renal Therapies Div. 800-854-6851
824 12th Ave, Bethlehem, PA 18018

Bard Reynosa S.A. De C.V. 908-277-8000
Blvd. Montebello #1, Parque Industrial Colonial
Reynosa, Tamaulipas Mexico
Various

Becton Dickinson And Company 800-284-6845
1 Becton Dr, Franklin Lakes, NJ 07417
0.9% SODIUM CHLORIDE INJECTION ; BD Posiflush Saline

Becton Dickinson Medical Systems 201-847-6800
9630 S 54th St, Franklin, WI 53132
Catheter, intravascular, short term.

Bentec Medical, Inc. 757-224-0177
1380 E Beamer St, Woodland, CA 95776
Infusion catheter.

Catalent Pharma Solutions 866-720-3148
2200 Lake Shore Dr, Woodstock, IL 60098
Multiple

CATHETER, INTRAVASCULAR, THERAPEUTIC, SHORT-TERM LESS THAN 30 DAYS *(cont'd)*

Catheter Research, Inc. (Cri) 317-872-0074
5610 W 82nd St, Indianapolis, IN 46278

Centurion Medical Products Corp. 517-545-1135
3310 S Main St, Salisbury, NC 28147

Cook Inc. 800-457-4500
PO Box 489, Bloomington, IN 47402

Covidien Lp 508-261-8000
15 Hampshire St, Mansfield, MA 02048

Diablo Sales & Marketing, Inc. 925-648-1611
PO Box 3219, Danville, CA 94526
Custom design and manufacturing of catheters and specialty guidewires. Guiding catheters; stent delivery and drug delivery systems.

Edwards Lifesciences Technology Sarl 949-250-2500
State Rd. 402 N.km 1.4, Anasco, PR 00610-1577
Central venous catheter kit.

Edwards Lifesciences, Llc. 800-424-3278
1 Edwards Way, Irvine, CA 92614
Therapeutic, short-term (less than 30 days).

Ev3 Neurovascular 800-716-6700
9775 Toledo Way, Irvine, CA 92618
Various types of sterile infusion catheter & accessories.

Excelsior Medical Corp. 732-776-7525
1933 Heck Ave, Neptune, NJ 07753
Pre-filled saline flush syringe.

Haemonetics Corp. 800-225-5242
400 Wood Rd, P.O. Box 9114, Braintree, MA 02184
Needle

Hospira Inc. 877-946-7747
275 N Field Dr, Lake Forest, IL 60045
Multiple

Hospira, Inc. 877-946-7747
755 Jarvis Dr, Morgan Hill, CA 95037

Johnson & Johnson De Monterrey, Sa De Cv 817-262-5211
Carretera Miguel Aleman,km21.7, Apodaca, Monterrey Mexico
Various

Kollsut Scientific Corporation 630-290-5746
3286 N 29th Ct, Hollywood, FL 33020
Catheter, iv, therapeutic, short-term less than 30 days.

Medefil, Inc. 630-682-4600
250 Windy Point Dr, Glendale Heights, IL 60139
Normal Saline & Heparin I. V. Flush Syringe (in diff. volumes) - prefilled syringe for single use

Millar Instruments, Inc. 800.669.2343
6001 Gulf Fwy Ste A, Houston, TX 77023

Navilyst Medical 800-833-9973
100 Boston Scientific Way, Marlborough, MA 01752
Peripherally inserted central catheters and placement kits.

Neo Medical Inc. 888-450-3334
42514 Albrae St, Fremont, CA 94538
Intravenous silicone catheter.

Neo-Care Arrow International 800-640-6428
5714 Epsilon, San Antonio, TX 78249
Neonatal, dual lumen umbilical catheter; pediatric PICC and umbilical catheterization kit.

Terumo Medical Corporation 800-283-7866
950 Elkton Blvd, P.O.Box 605, Elkton, MD 21921
Intravascular catheter.

Thomas Medical Products, Inc. 866-446-3003
65 Great Valley Pkwy, Malvern, PA 19355
Over-the-needle catheter.

Tri-State Hospital Supply Corp. 517-545-1135
3173 E 43rd St, Yuma, AZ 85365

CATHETER, INTRAVENOUS *(Cardiovascular) 74QHZ*

Air-Tite Products Co., Inc. 800-231-7762
565 Central Dr Ste 101, Virginia Beach, VA 23454
Terumo Medical Corp. 14G to 24G I.V. catheters. Thin wall needles, color coded, double bevel with flashback chamber.

Becton Dickinson Infusion Therapy Systems, Inc. 888-237-2762
9450 S State St, Sandy, UT 84070
INSYTE AUTOGUARD shielded catheter with wings.

Bipore, Inc. 201-767-1993
31 Industrial Pkwy, Northvale, NJ 07647

CATHETER, INTRAVENOUS *(cont'd)*

Charter Medical Ltd. 866-458-3116
3948 Westpoint Blvd Ste A, Winston Salem, NC 27103

Covidien Lp 508-261-8000
15 Hampshire St, Mansfield, MA 02048

Diablo Sales & Marketing, Inc. 925-648-1611
PO Box 3219, Danville, CA 94526
Custom design and manufacturing of catheters and specialty guidewires. Guiding catheters; stent delivery and drug delivery systems.

Exelint International Co. 800-940-3935
5840 W Centinela Ave, Los Angeles, CA 90045
Safelet IV catheter.

Globe Medical Tech, Inc. 713-365-9595
1766 W Sam Houston Pkwy N, Houston, TX 77043
IV sets; burettes, blood sets also available.

Medi Inc 800-225-8634
75 York Ave, P.O. Box 302, Randolph, MA 02368

Myco Medical 800-454-6926
158 Towerview Ct, Cary, NC 27513
Radiopaque IV cannula with catheter.

Taut, Inc. 800-231-8288
2571 Kaneville Ct, Geneva, IL 60134

Vygon Corp. 800-544-4907
2495 General Armistead Ave, Norristown, PA 19403
Central venous and intravenous.

CATHETER, INTRAVENOUS, CENTRAL *(Cardiovascular) 74QIA*

Covidien Lp 508-261-8000
15 Hampshire St, Mansfield, MA 02048

Gish Biomedical, Inc. 800-938-0531
22942 Arroyo Vis, Rancho Santa Margarita, CA 92688
Subclavian and jugular central-venous catheters for pressure monitoring and anesthesia.

Vygon Corp. 800-544-4907
2495 General Armistead Ave, Norristown, PA 19403
Percutaneous intravenous central catheters.

CATHETER, IRRIGATION *(Surgery) 79GBX*

Ac Healthcare Supply, Inc. 905-448-4706
11651 230th St, Cambria Heights, NY 11411
Introduction/drainage catheter & accessories.

Angiodynamics, Inc. 518-795-1400
14 Plaza Drive, Latham, NY 12110

Armm, Inc. 714-848-8190
17744 Sampson Ln, Huntington Beach, CA 92647

Autovage 412-653-5888
1631 Citation Dr, South Park, PA 15129
Endotracheal medication catheter.

Axiom Medical, Inc. 800-221-8569
19320 Van Ness Ave, Torrance, CA 90501
Drain system with detachable trocar and various collection devices for draining cysts, hematomata through single site. Multiple sizes single & multiple lumen blunt & sharp trocars.

Ballard Medical Products 770-587-7835
12050 Lone Peak Pkwy, Draper, UT 84020
Irrigation catheter.

Bentec Medical, Inc. 757-224-0177
1380 E Beamer St, Woodland, CA 95776
Irrigation/infusion catheter.

Biomet, Inc. 574-267-6639
56 E Bell Dr, PO Box 587, Warsaw, IN 46582
Irrigation catheter.

Clinical Instruments Intl., Inc. 508-764-2200
278 Worcester St, Southbridge, MA 01550
Introducers.

Edwards Lifesciences Technology Sarl 949-250-2500
State Rd. 402 N.km 1.4, Anasco, PR 00610-1577
Irrigation catheter.

Edwards Lifesciences, Llc. 800-424-3278
1 Edwards Way, Irvine, CA 92614

Hollister, Inc. 847-680-2849
366 Draft Ave, Stuarts Draft, VA 24477

Kentron Health Care, Inc. 615-384-0573
3604 Kelton Jackson Rd, P.o. Box 120, Springfield, TN 37172
Irrigation tray.

CATHETER, IRRIGATION *(cont'd)*

Lucas Medical, Inc. 714-938-0233
1751 S Douglass Rd, Anaheim, CA 92806
Bi-lumen irrigation catheter.

Smith & Nephew, Inc. 800-876-1261
11775 Starkey Rd, Largo, FL 33773

Stryker Puerto Rico, Ltd. 939-307-2500
Hwy. 3, Km. 131.2, Las Guasimas Ind. Park, Arroyo, PR 00714
Handpiece and tubing set.

CATHETER, JEJUNOSTOMY *(Gastro/Urology) 78QIB*

Abbott Laboratories 800-624-7677
1033 Kingsmill Pkwy, Columbus, OH 43229
Jejunostomy tubes in various sizes (8Fr, 10Fr). Also, over-the-guidewire J-tubes (8Fr, 10Fr).

Cook Inc. 800-457-4500
PO Box 489, Bloomington, IN 47402

CATHETER, LIGHT, FIBEROPTIC, GLASS, URETERAL
(Gastro/Urology) 78FCS

Apple Medical Corp. 508-357-2700
28 Lord Rd Ste 135, Marlborough, MA 01752
Ureteral illuminator.

Hospira, Inc. 877-946-7747
755 Jarvis Dr, Morgan Hill, CA 95037
$95 for arterial fiberoptic catheter.

CATHETER, MALECOT (GASTROSTOMY TUBE)
(Gastro/Urology) 78FEW

Abbott Laboratories 800-624-7677
1033 Kingsmill Pkwy, Columbus, OH 43229

Cook Inc. 800-457-4500
PO Box 489, Bloomington, IN 47402

Cook Urological, Inc. 800-457-4500
1100 W Morgan St, P.O. Box 227, Spencer, IN 47460

Dumex Medical Surgical Products Ltd. 800-463-9613
104 Shorting Rd., Scarborough, ONT M1S 3S4 Canada

Novartis Nutrition 800-333-3785
1600 Utica Ave S Ste 600, PO Box 370, Minneapolis, MN 55416
Surgical; balloon gastrostomy.

Omni Medical Supply Inc. 800-860-6664
4153 Pioneer Dr, Commerce Township, MI 48390

Technical Products, Inc. 800-226-8434
805 Marathon Pkwy Ste 150, Lawrenceville, GA 30046
Silicone malecot catheter available in 20,24 and 32 fr sizes. Latex free; not normally used as a gastroscopy tube.

CATHETER, MAPPING, INTRACARDIAC, REPROCESSED
(Cardiovascular) 74NLG

Ascent Healthcare Solutions 480-763-5300
10232 S 51st St, Phoenix, AZ 85044
Electrophysiology catheters, reprocessed.

CATHETER, MULTIPLE LUMEN *(Surgery) 79GBP*

Angiodynamics, Inc. 800-472-5221
1 Horizon Way, Manchester, GA 31816
Double and triple lumen acute care and chronic dialysis catheters, and multiple lumen critical care central venous catheters. PHERES-FLOW Apheresis/BMT Catheter has triple-lumen, high flow catheter specfically designed for the apheresis/BMT procedure.

Argon Medical Devices Inc. 903-675-9321
1445 Flat Creek Rd, Athens, TX 75751
Multiple lumen catheter.

Armm, Inc. 714-848-8190
17744 Sampson Ln, Huntington Beach, CA 92647

Arndorfer Medical Specialties 414-425-1661
5656 Grove Ter, Greendale, WI 53129
The ams esophageal manometry catheters.

Arrow International, Inc. 800-523-8446
2400 Bernville Rd, Reading, PA 19605
Adult and pediatric sizes, 2- and 3-lumen tubing.

Arrow Medical Products, Ltd. 800-387-7819
2300 Bristol Circle Unit 1, Oakville, ONT L6H-5S3 Canada
Kits and sets available. Priced from $50.00 up.

Atek Medical 800-253-1540
620 Watson St SW, Grand Rapids, MI 49504
Multi lumen catheter.

CATHETER, MULTIPLE LUMEN *(cont'd)*

B. Braun Oem Division, B. Braun Medical Inc. 866-8-BBRAUN
824 12th Ave, Bethlehem, PA 18018

Becton Dickinson Infusion Therapy Systems, Inc. 888-237-2762
9450 S State St, Sandy, UT 84070

Cardiomed Supplies Inc. 800-387-9757
5 Gormley Industrial Ave., P.O. Box 575
Gormley, ONT L0H 1 Canada
$22.00 double and single trays only.

Clinical Instruments Intl., Inc. 508-764-2200
278 Worcester St, Southbridge, MA 01550
Introducers.

Coloplast Manufacturing Us, Llc 612-302-4992
1185 Willow Lake Blvd, Vadnais Heights, MN 55110
Ileal conduit sampling catheter (sterile).

Gish Biomedical, Inc. 800-938-0531
22942 Arroyo Vis, Rancho Santa Margarita, CA 92688

Hospira, Inc. 877-946-7747
755 Jarvis Dr, Morgan Hill, CA 95037

Icu Medical (Ut), Inc 949-366-2183
4455 Atherton Dr, Salt Lake City, UT 84123
Various types.

Manufacturing & Research, Inc.(Dba Mri Medical) 520-882-7794
4700 S Overland Dr, Tucson, AZ 85714
6-30 Fr., silicone.

Smiths Medical Asd, Inc. 800-433-5832
1265 Grey Fox Rd, Saint Paul, MN 55112

Sunlite Plastics, Inc. 262-253-0600
W194N11340 McCormick Dr, Germantown, WI 53022

Tools For Surgery, Llc 631-444-4448
1339 Stony Brook Rd, Stony Brook, NY 11790
Rectal/colon irrigator.

Vygon Corp. 800-544-4907
2495 General Armistead Ave, Norristown, PA 19403

CATHETER, NASAL, OXYGEN (TUBE) *(Anesthesiology) 73BZB*

Allied Healthcare Products, Inc. 800-444-3954
1720 Sublette Ave, Saint Louis, MO 63110

Applied Medical Technology, Inc. 800-869-7382
8000 Katherine Blvd, Brecksville, OH 44141

Covidien Lp 508-261-8000
15 Hampshire St, Mansfield, MA 02048

Mada, Inc. 800-526-6370
625 Washington Ave, Carlstadt, NJ 07072
For use with #1543 Aspirator.

Medline Industries, Inc. 800-633-5886
1 Medline Pl, Mundelein, IL 60060

Vygon Corp. 800-544-4907
2495 General Armistead Ave, Norristown, PA 19403

CATHETER, NASOPHARYNGEAL *(Ear/Nose/Throat) 77ENW*

Anesthesia Associates, Inc. 760-744-6561
460 Enterprise St, San Marcos, CA 92078
Available in a variety of sizes and styles.

Medline Industries, Inc. 800-633-5886
1 Medline Pl, Mundelein, IL 60060

Micromedics 800-624-5662
1270 Eagan Industrial Rd, Saint Paul, MN 55121
RhinoCath a nasal catheter and tampon for intra- and post-operative nasal bleeding.

CATHETER, NEPHROSTOMY *(Gastro/Urology) 78LJE*

Bentec Medical, Inc. 757-224-0177
1380 E Beamer St, Woodland, CA 95776
Nephrostomy catheter.

C. R. Bard, Inc., Bard Urological Div. 888-367-2273
13183 Harland Dr NE, Covington, GA 30014

Cook Inc. 800-457-4500
PO Box 489, Bloomington, IN 47402

Cook Urological, Inc. 800-457-4500
1100 W Morgan St, P.O. Box 227, Spencer, IN 47460

Manufacturing & Research, Inc.(Dba Mri Medical) 520-882-7794
4700 S Overland Dr, Tucson, AZ 85714
Silicone catheters.

CATHETER, NEPHROSTOMY *(cont'd)*

Uresil, Llc 800-538-7374
5418 Touhy Ave, Skokie, IL 60077
NEPHRO-CATH percutaneous. Nephro-Ureteral Stent system for percutaneous internal/external nephroureteral drainage.

CATHETER, NEPHROSTOMY, GENERAL & PLASTIC SURGERY
(Surgery) 79GBO

Boston Scientific Corporation 508-652-5578
780 Brookside Dr, Spencer, IN 47460

Rocket Medical Plc. 800-707-7625
150 Recreation Park Dr Ste 3, Hingham, MA 02043

CATHETER, NEURO-VASCULATURE, OCCLUDING BALLON
(Cns/Neurology) 84NUF

Coaxia, Inc. 763-315-8395
10900 73rd Ave N, Maple Grove, MN 55369
Intravascular occluding catheter.

CATHETER, OCCLUDING, CARDIOVASCULAR, IMPLANTABLE
(Cardiovascular) 74MFC

Cath-Labs Corp. 201-883-0008
282 Hudson St, Hackensack, NJ 07601
Catheters, cardiovascular.

CATHETER, OCCLUSION *(Cardiovascular) 74QIE*

Boston Scientific Corporation 800-225-2732
1 Boston Scientific Pl, Natick, MA 01760
Occlusion balloon catheter.

Catheter Research, Inc. (Cri) 317-872-0074
5610 W 82nd St, Indianapolis, IN 46278

Covidien Lp 508-261-8000
15 Hampshire St, Mansfield, MA 02048
VASCU-FLO silicone occlusion balloon catheter.

Lemaitre Vascular, Inc. 781-221-2266
63 2nd Ave, Burlington, MA 01803
For safe, rapid control of bleeding without clamping.

Telemed Systems Inc. 800-481-6718
8 Kane Industrial Dr, Hudson, MA 01749

CATHETER, OLIVE TIP *(Gastro/Urology) 78QIF*

Coloplast Manufacturing Us, Llc 800-533-0464
1840 W Oak Pkwy, Marietta, GA 30062
CONVEEN sterile with frosted surface and smooth tip for ease of use, lateral eyelets for maximum drainage.

Compex Technologies, Inc. 866-676-6489
1811 Old Highway 8 NW, New Brighton, MN 55112

CATHETER, OTHER *(Gastro/Urology) 78QIV*

Angiodynamics, Inc. 800-472-5221
1 Horizon Way, Manchester, GA 31816
Custom dialysis and critical care catheters including acute care, silicone, peritoneal, and central venous.

Arlon Engineered Coated Products 800-232-7181
6110 Rittiman Rd, San Antonio, TX 78218
Catheter Strips, catheter tape for attachment.

Arrow International, Inc. 800-523-8446
2400 Bernville Rd, Reading, PA 19605
Two-lumen peripheral catheterization set; thoracentesis, pneumothorax, cavity drainage and peripheral multiple-lumen catheters. Also, H.I.S. bundle mapping catheters.

Atrium Medical Corp. 800-528-7486
5 Wentworth Dr, Hudson, NH 03051
Thoracic catheters: straight, right-angle, trocar configurations. ATRIUM heparine-coated thoracic catheters. Hydra-Glide technology to improve catheter performance. Also available, PVC and silicone thoracic catheters.

Axiom Medical, Inc. 800-221-8569
19320 Van Ness Ave, Torrance, CA 90501
Adult & pediatric catheters, cannulae, chest tubes, sumps & multilumen tubing, drainage collection devices, closed wound units, seroma & epyema catheters, penrose, continuous tubing, coatings, sheeting.

Bard Electro Physiology 800-824-8724
55 Technology Dr, Lowell, MA 01851

Biosense Webster, Inc 800-729-9010
3333 S Diamond Canyon Rd, Diamond Bar, CA 91765
The NAVI-STAR, a 4mm large-dome defectable catheter, is used to indicate various mapping points from within the heart and send them back to the EP Navigation system.

CATHETER, OTHER *(cont'd)*

Boston Scientific Corporation 800-225-2732
1 Boston Scientific Pl, Natick, MA 01760
Valvuloplasty and electronpnysiology catheters.

Cardiomed Supplies Inc. 800-387-9757
5 Gormley Industrial Ave., P.O. Box 575
Gormley, ONT L0H 1 Canada
Catheters for cath lab.

Catheter Research, Inc. (Cri) 317-872-0074
5610 W 82nd St, Indianapolis, IN 46278
Steerable vessel occlusion catheter system for peripheral in-situ bypass.

Cook Ob/Gyn 800-541-5591
1100 W Morgan St, Spencer, IN 47460
CVS catheter.

Covidien Lp 508-261-8000
15 Hampshire St, Mansfield, MA 02048

David Scott Company 800-804-0333
59 Fountain St, Framingham, MA 01702
Thoracic catheters and drains.

Janin Group, Inc. 800-323-5389
14A Stonehill Rd, Oswego, IL 60543
FLEX-NECK, peritoneal dialysis catheters. Also, ASH ADVANTAGE peritoneal dialysis catheter.

Manufacturing & Research, Inc.(Dba Mri Medical) 520-882-7794
4700 S Overland Dr, Tucson, AZ 85714
6-18 Fr. silicone balloon catheters.

Medi-Globe Corporation 800-966-1431
110 W Orion St Ste 136, Tempe, AZ 85283
E.R.C.P. catheters.

Medovations, Inc. 800-558-6408
102 E Keefe Ave, Milwaukee, WI 53212
Thoracic catheter.

Memcath Technologies Llc 651-450-7400
1777 Oakdale Ave, Saint Paul, MN 55118

Milex Products, Inc. 800-621-1278
4311 N Normandy Ave, Chicago, IL 60634
WORD catheter at $95.00 per 6 Word catheters.

Mui Scientific 800-303-6611
145 Traders Blvd. E., Unit 34, Mississauga, ONT L4Z 3L3 Canada
$84.00 to $300.00 for Manometric Catheters; accessory for above device.

Ranfac Corp. 800-2RANFAC
30 Doherty Ave, Avon Industrial Park, Avon, MA 02322
Disposable galactography infusion unit.

Seecor, Inc. 972-288-3278
844 Dalworth Dr Ste 6, Mesquite, TX 75149
STAT-CATH: Bipolar pacing catheter; adult or pedi.

Smiths Medical Asd, Inc. 800-848-1757
6250 Shier Rings Rd, Dublin, OH 43016
Including catheters and introducers.

Specialty Manufacturing, Inc. 800-269-6204
2210 Midland Rd, Saginaw, MI 48603

St. Jude Medical Atrial Fibrillation 800-328-3873
14901 Deveau Pl, Minnetonka, MN 55345
Multi-electrode electrophysiology catheters available in 5 & 6 sizes.

St. Jude Medical, Inc. 800-328-9634
1 Saint Jude Medical Dr, Saint Paul, MN 55117
EP catheters.

Tfx Medical Oem 800-548-6600
50 Plantation Dr, Jaffrey, NH 03452

Unomedical, Inc. 800-634-6003
5701 S Ware Rd Ste 1, McAllen, TX 78503
UNO-PLAST PHARMA-PLAST PVC catheters for urology, gastro-enterology, pediatrics, anaesthetics, and surgery.

Zinetics Medical, Inc. 800-648-4070
1050 E South Temple, Salt Lake City, UT 84102
Esophageal manometric catheter.

CATHETER, OXIMETER, FIBEROPTIC *(Cardiovascular) 74DQE*

Edwards Lifesciences Technology Sarl 949-250-2500
State Rd. 402 N.km 1.4, Anasco, PR 00610-1577
Catheter, oximeter, fiberoptic.

Edwards Lifesciences, Llc. 800-424-3278
1 Edwards Way, Irvine, CA 92614

CATHETER, OXIMETER, FIBEROPTIC *(cont'd)*

Hospira, Inc. 877-946-7747
755 Jarvis Dr, Morgan Hill, CA 95037
$1,050 for fiberoptic catheter oximeter system.

Icu Medical (Ut), Inc 949-366-2183
4455 Atherton Dr, Salt Lake City, UT 84123
Various fiberoptic oximeter catheters.

CATHETER, OXYGEN, TRACHEAL *(Anesthesiology) 73WLJ*

Covidien Lp 508-261-8000
15 Hampshire St, Mansfield, MA 02048

Filtrona Extrusion, Inc./Pexcor Medical Products Div. 800-755-7528
764 S Athol Rd, P.O. Box 659, Athol, MA 01331

Passy-Muir Inc. 800-634-5397
4521 Campus Dr, Irvine, CA 92612
Passy-Muir™ PMA™ 2000 O2 adapter allows for easy inhalation of supplemental low-flow oxygen and humidity through the Low Profile PMV™ 2000 Series Speaking Valves. The Passy-Muir PMA 2000 O2 Adapter is small, lightweight, clear in color, and clips onto both the PMV 2000 (Clear) and PMV 2001 (Purple™) Swallowing & Speaking Valves. It is easily removed when not in use. Oxygen is delivered in front of the diaphragm of the PMV to avoid complications associated with devices that provide continuous flow behind the diaphragm of a speaking valve such as air trapping, drying of secretions, and possible cilia damage.

Transtracheal Systems, Inc. 800-527-2667
109 Inverness Dr E Ste C, Englewood, CO 80112
SCOOP transtracheal systems oxygen catheter has a proven clinical record of successfully treating chronic hypoxemia through the application of 24 hour oxygen therapy. Over 120 professional publications have documented the clinical benefits of SCOOP. These benefits include: reduction in the work of breathing, greater exercise capacity, reduced hospitalizations, shorter lengths of stay and significantly lower average cost per discharge than similar nasal cannula patients. FAST TRACK Procedure Kit. The Fast Track Kit is designed to support fast tract, a surgical procedure for the placement of a scoop oxygen catheter into the trachea of an oxygen dependent patient. It offers several clinical/patient benefits not available with the Modified Seldinger Technique currently used for catheter placement. These include: SCOOP oxygen delivery within 24 hours of the procedure and a reduction in tract maturation from 6-8 weeks to about 2 weeks. The kit features a special tracheal punch and stent. It also contains several additional devices and items required for post surgical patient care and the stent to SCOOP conversion the next day. The objective is to assist the otolaryngologist in providing consistent, high quality patient outcomes.

Vitaid Ltd. 800-267-9301
300 International Dr, Williamsville, NY 14221
Boussignac Oxygen Bougie

CATHETER, PEDIATRIC, GENERAL & PLASTIC SURGERY
(Surgery) 79GBN

Axiom Medical, Inc. 800-221-8569
19320 Van Ness Ave, Torrance, CA 90501

Memcath Technologies Llc 651-450-7400
1777 Oakdale Ave, Saint Paul, MN 55118

Smiths Medical Asd, Inc. 800-433-5832
1265 Grey Fox Rd, Saint Paul, MN 55112
CliniCath peripherally inserted catheters with a full line of catheter sizes and lengths, including adult central and midline placement.

Vygon Corp. 800-544-4907
2495 General Armistead Ave, Norristown, PA 19403

CATHETER, PERCUTANEOUS *(Cardiovascular) 74DQY*

Abbott Vascular, Cardiac Therapies 800-227-9902
3200 Lakeside Dr, Santa Clara, CA 95054
Percutaneous catheter.

Abbott Vascular, Cardiac Therapies 800-227-9902
26531 Ynez Rd, Mailing P.O. Box 9018, Temecula, CA 92591
Percutaneous catheter.

Abbott Vascular, Vascular Solutions 800-227-9902
26531 Ynez Rd, Temecula, CA 92591
Retriever device, catheter.

Acumen Medical, Inc. 408-530-1810
275 Santa Ana Ct, Sunnyvale, CA 94085
Percutaneous catheter.

Aga Medical Corporation. 888-546-4407
5050 Nathan Ln N, Plymouth, MN 55442
Amplatzer delivery system.

CATHETER, PERCUTANEOUS *(cont'd)*

Argon Medical Devices Inc. 903-675-9321
1445 Flat Creek Rd, Athens, TX 75751
Sniper guide wire.

Ascent Healthcare Solutions 480-763-5300
10232 S 51st St, Phoenix, AZ 85044
Pericardiocentesis tray.

Avinger Inc. 650-363-2400
400 Chesapeake Dr, Redwood City, CA 94063
Wildcat

Boston Scientific - Maple Grove 800-553-5878
1 Scimed Pl, Maple Grove, MN 55311

Boston Scientific - Marina Bay Customer Fulfillment Center 617-689-6000
500 Commander Shea Blvd, Quincy, MA 02171
Sterling.

Boston Scientific Corp. 800-323-6472
5905 Nathan Ln N, Minneapolis, MN 55442

Brevet, Inc. 949-474-7000
16661 Jamboree Rd, Irvine, CA 92606

BridgePoint Medical 763-225-8500
2800 Campus Dr Ste 50, Plymouth, MN 55441
Stingray Catheter; CrossBoss

Candela Corp. 800-733-8550
530 Boston Post Rd, Wayland, MA 01778

Cardima, Inc. 888-354-0300
47266 Benicia St, Fremont, CA 94538
Various.

Concentric Medical, Inc. 650-938-2100
301 E Evelyn Ave, Mountain View, CA 94041
Percutaneous catheter.

Cordis Neurovascular, Inc. 800-327-7714
14201 NW 60th Ave, Miami Lakes, FL 33014
Various types of sterile percutaneous catheter.

Edwards Lifesciences Technology Sarl 949-250-2500
State Rd. 402 N.km 1.4, Anasco, PR 00610-1577
Introducer kit.

Edwards Lifesciences, Llc. 800-424-3278
1 Edwards Way, Irvine, CA 92614

Endologix, Inc. 800-983-2284
11 Studebaker, Irvine, CA 92618
Dual Lumen Catheter

Ev3 Inc. 800-716-6700
9600 54th Ave N, Plymouth, MN 55442
Catheter, percutaneous.

Ev3 Inc. 800-716-6700
4600 Nathan Ln N, Plymouth, MN 55442
Catheter,percutaneous.

Flowcardia, Inc. 408-617-0352
745 N Pastoria Ave, Sunnyvale, CA 94085
High frequency mechanical chronic total occlusion recanalization system.

Invatec +1 877 446 8283
3101 Emrick Blvd Ste 113, Bethlehem, PA 18020

Lumend, Inc. 650-364-1400
400 Chesapeake Dr, Redwood City, CA 94063
Various types of sterile percutaneous catheters.

Medical Murray Inc. 847-620-7990
400 N Rand Rd, North Barrington, IL 60010

Medtronic Ep Systems 763-514-4000
8299 Central Ave NE, Spring Lake Park, Minneapolis, MN 55432
Percutaneous catheter.

Medtronic Vascular 707-525-0111
3576 Unocal Pl, Santa Rosa, CA 95403
Pioneer.

Micrus Design Technology, Inc. 408-433-1460
9344 NW 13th St, Doral, FL 33172
Guiding catheters.

Millar Instruments, Inc. 800.669.2343
6001 Gulf Fwy Ste A, Houston, TX 77023

Neo Medical Inc. 888-450-3334
42514 Albrae St, Fremont, CA 94538
Sterile peripherally inserted central catheter (picc) tray and accessories.

CATHETER, PERCUTANEOUS *(cont'd)*

Numed Canada, Inc. 613-936-2592
45, Second Street West, Cornwall, ONT K6J 1G3 Canada

Numed, Inc. 315-328-4491
2880 Main St., Hopkinton, NY 12965
Percutaneous transluminal angioplasty catheter.

Orqis (Tm) Medical 888-723-7277
14 Orchard Ste 100, Lake Forest, CA 92630
Catheter.

Penumbra, Inc. 510-618-3223
1351 Harbor Bay Pkwy, Alameda, CA 94502
Balloon guide catheter.

Smiths Medical Asd, Inc. 800-433-5832
1265 Grey Fox Rd, Saint Paul, MN 55112
VENTRA percutaneous intravenous catheters. The one-piece radiopaque silicone catheters are available in single, dual and triple lumen configurations.

Spectrascience, Inc. 858-847-0200
11568 Sorrento Valley Rd Ste 11, San Diego, CA 92121
Pta balloon catheter.

Thomas Medical Products, Inc. 866-446-3003
65 Great Valley Pkwy, Malvern, PA 19355
Percutaneous introducer kit.

TriReme Medical Inc. 925-931-1300
7060 Koll Center Pkwy Ste 300, Pleasanton, CA 94566
Glider

Uresil, Llc 800-538-7374
5418 Touhy Ave, Skokie, IL 60077
GP, TRU-FLO drainage catheters.

Ussc Puerto Rico, Inc. 203-845-1000
Building 911-67, Sabanetas Industrial Park, Ponce, PR 00731
Tunneler.

Vascular Solutions, Inc. 763-656-4300
5025 Cheshire Ln N, Plymouth, MN 55446
Intravascular catheter.

W.L. Gore & Associates,Inc 928-526-3030
1505 North Fourth St., Flagstaff, AZ 86004
Balloon catheter.

CATHETER, PERCUTANEOUS (VALVULOPLASTY)
(Cardiovascular) 74MAD

Boston Scientific - Maple Grove 800-553-5878
1 Scimed Pl, Maple Grove, MN 55311

Cardio-Nef, S.A. De C.V. 01-800-024-0240
Rio Grijalva 186, Col. Mitras Norte, Monterrey, N.L. 64320 Mexico

Numed, Inc. 315-328-4491
2880 Main St., Hopkinton, NY 12965

Toray International America Inc. 800-662-1777
140 Cypress Station Dr Ste 210, Houston, TX 77090
INOUE-BALLOON percutaneous mitral valvuloplasty catheter (PTMC).

CATHETER, PERFUSION *(Cardiovascular) 74QIH*

Covidien Lp 508-261-8000
15 Hampshire St, Mansfield, MA 02048

Diablo Sales & Marketing, Inc. 925-648-1611
PO Box 3219, Danville, CA 94526
Custom design and manufacturing of catheters and specialty guidewires. Guiding catheters; stent delivery and drug delivery systems.

Quest Medical, Inc. 800-627-0226
1 Allentown Pkwy, Allen, TX 75002

Rocket Medical Plc. 800-707-7625
150 Recreation Park Dr Ste 3, Hingham, MA 02043

Vygon Corp. 800-544-4907
2495 General Armistead Ave, Norristown, PA 19403

CATHETER, PERICARDIUM DRAINAGE *(Cardiovascular) 74QII*

Armm, Inc. 714-848-8190
17744 Sampson Ln, Huntington Beach, CA 92647
MedDrain Mediastinal Drain. Silicone.

Axiom Medical, Inc. 800-221-8569
19320 Van Ness Ave, Torrance, CA 90501
Mediastinal, non-pericardium, pericardial, closed sump, round sumps.

Boston Scientific Corporation 800-225-2732
1 Boston Scientific Pl, Natick, MA 01760

CATHETER, PERICARDIUM DRAINAGE *(cont'd)*

Cook Inc. 800-457-4500
PO Box 489, Bloomington, IN 47402

CATHETER, PERIPHERAL, ATHERECTOMY
(Cardiovascular) 74MCW

Abbott Vascular, Cardiac Therapies 800-227-9902
26531 Ynez Rd, Mailing P.O. Box 9018, Temecula, CA 92591
Peripheral atherectomy catheter.

Bacchus Vascular, Inc. 408-980-8300
3110 Coronado Dr, Santa Clara, CA 95054
Peripheral atherectomy catheter.

Cardiovascular Systems, Inc. 877-CSI-0360
651 Campus Dr, Saint Paul, MN 55112
Diamondback 360; Orbital atherectomy controller,sterile orbital atherectomy device.

Edwards Lifesciences Technology Sarl 949-250-2500
State Rd. 402 N.km 1.4, Anasco, PR 00610-1577
Percutaneous mechanical thrombectomy (pmt).

Edwards Lifesciences, Llc. 800-424-3278
1 Edwards Way, Irvine, CA 92614

Ev3 Inc. 800-716-6700
9600 54th Ave N, Plymouth, MN 55442
Thrombectomy catheter.

Ev3 Inc. 800-716-6700
4600 Nathan Ln N, Plymouth, MN 55442
Thrombectomy catheter.

Ev3 Neurovascular 800-716-6700
9775 Toledo Way, Irvine, CA 92618
Thrombolytic brush catheter.

Idev Technologies, Inc. 866-806-4338
253 Medical Center Blvd, Webster, TX 77598
Eliminator.

Minnetronix Inc. 888-301-1025
1635 Energy Park Dr, Saint Paul, MN 55108
Diamondback 360 Orbital Atherectomy

Smiths Medical Asd, Inc. 800-433-5832
1265 Grey Fox Rd, Saint Paul, MN 55112

CATHETER, PERITONEAL *(Surgery) 79GBW*

Access Llc 800-973-0355
11 W End Rd, Totowa, NJ 07512
Capd cather support undergarment.

Angiodynamics, Inc. 800-472-5221
1 Horizon Way, Manchester, GA 31816
Neonatal, pediatric, adult, and custom configurations in 16 silicone models including coiled, straight, and variable, with one universal placement kit.

Geneva Medical Inc. 630-232-2507
2571 Kaneville Ct, Geneva, IL 60134
Intraducer.

Integra Neurosciences Pr 800-654-2873
Road 402 North, Km 1.2, Anasco, PR 00610
Various sites and configurations.

Kent Elastomer Products, Inc 330-628-1802
3890 Mogadore Industrial Pkwy, Mogadore, OH 44260
Penrose drain, non-latex.

Smiths Medical Asd, Inc. 800-433-5832
1265 Grey Fox Rd, Saint Paul, MN 55112

Taut, Inc. 800-231-8288
2571 Kaneville Ct, Geneva, IL 60134
P.I.-104 New rigid design provides easy extracorporeal maneuverability of catheters. The 8.9 cm. length and 2.7 mm I.D. will accommodate all Taut catheters and a wide variety of instrumentation. P.I.-128 The PI-128's 3.3 internal diameter and 20.3 cm length will guide Taut cholangiogram catheters and other instrumentation directly to the cystic duct. The new rigid design provides easy extracorporal maneuverability of catheters, and is an excellent access site for Lap CBDE equipment including 2mm and 3mm instruments and choledochoscopes.

W.L. Gore & Associates,Inc 928-526-3030
1505 North Fourth St., Flagstaff, AZ 86004
Gore-tex peritoneal catheter.

CATHETER, PERITONEAL DIALYSIS, SINGLE-USE
(Gastro/Urology) 78FKO

Argon Medical Devices Inc. 903-675-9321
1445 Flat Creek Rd, Athens, TX 75751
Acute hemodialysis kit.

B. Braun Of Puerto Rico, Inc. 610-691-5400
215.7 Insular Rd., Sabana Grande, PR 00637
Sterile peritoneal dialysis catheter.

Corpak Medsystems, Inc. 800-323-6305
100 Chaddick Dr, Wheeling, IL 60090
Peritoneal dialysis catheter.

Lifemed Of California 800-543-3633
1216 S Allec St, Anaheim, CA 92805

Vygon Corp. 800-544-4907
2495 General Armistead Ave, Norristown, PA 19403

CATHETER, PERITONEAL, INDWELLING, LONG-TERM
(Gastro/Urology) 78FJS

Angiodynamics, Inc. 800-472-5221
1 Horizon Way, Manchester, GA 31816
Neonatal, pediatric, adult, and custom configurations in 16 silicone models including coiled, straight, and variable, with one universal placement kit.

Bard Reynosa S.A. De C.V. 908-277-8000
Blvd. Montebello #1, Parque Industrial Colonial
Reynosa, Tamaulipas Mexico
Various

Lifemed Of California 800-543-3633
1216 S Allec St, Anaheim, CA 92805

CATHETER, RECORDING, ELECTRODE, REPROCESSED
(Cardiovascular) 74NLH

Ascent Healthcare Solutions 480-763-5300
10232 S 51st St, Phoenix, AZ 85044
Electrophysiology catheter.

Sterilmed, Inc. 763-488-3400
11400 73rd Ave N Ste 100, Maple Grove, MN 55369
Electrophysiology catheters.

CATHETER, RECTAL *(Surgery) 79GBT*

Benlan Inc. 905-829-5004
2760 Brighton Rd., Oakville, ONT L6H 5T4 Canada

Kelsar, S.A. 508-261-8000
Blvd. Insurgentes, Libriamento a La, Tijuana 22450 Mexico
Rectal tube

Neo Medical Inc. 888-450-3334
42514 Albrae St, Fremont, CA 94538
Rectal irrigation tube-sterile.

Vygon Corp. 800-544-4907
2495 General Armistead Ave, Norristown, PA 19403

CATHETER, RECTAL, ILEOSTOMY, CONTINENT
(Gastro/Urology) 78KPH

Ac Healthcare Supply, Inc. 905-448-4706
11651 230th St, Cambria Heights, NY 11411
Continent iliostomy catheter.

Coloplast Manufacturing Us, Llc 612-302-4992
1185 Willow Lake Blvd, Vadnais Heights, MN 55110
Sterile rectal catheter for continent ileostomy.

Zassi Medical Evolutions, Inc. 904-261-2169
1886 S 14th St Ste 6, Fernandina Beach, FL 32034
A catheter system designed to safely and reliably divert, collect, and contain potentially harmful and contaminated gastrointestinal waste from bedridden and immobilized patients in hospitals, rehabilitation centers, nursing homes, and home-care settings.

CATHETER, RETENTION TYPE *(Gastro/Urology) 78EZK*

Cook Urological, Inc. 800-457-4500
1100 W Morgan St, P.O. Box 227, Spencer, IN 47460

Tmp Technologies, Inc. 716-895-6100
1200 Northland Ave, Buffalo, NY 14215
Catheter pads

CATHETER, RETENTION TYPE, BALLOON
(Gastro/Urology) 78EZL

Coloplast Manufacturing Us, Llc 612-302-4992
1185 Willow Lake Blvd, Vadnais Heights, MN 55110
Urinary catheter.

CATHETER, RETENTION TYPE, BALLOON *(cont'd)*

Cook Urological, Inc. 800-457-4500
1100 W Morgan St, P.O. Box 227, Spencer, IN 47460

Covidien Lp 508-261-8000
15 Hampshire St, Mansfield, MA 02048

Degania Silicone, Inc. 401-333-8199
1226 Mendon Rd, Cumberland, RI 02864
Gastrostomy tubes under private label.

Kelsar, S.A. 508-261-8000
Blvd. Insurgentes, Libriamento a La, Tijuana 22450 Mexico
Foley catheters-silicone, teflon coatef, latex, silicone elastomer coated

Kentron Health Care, Inc. 615-384-0573
3604 Kelton Jackson Rd, P.o. Box 120, Springfield, TN 37172
Foley catheters.

Manufacturing & Research, Inc.(Dba Mri Medical) 520-882-7794
4700 S Overland Dr, Tucson, AZ 85714
Silicone balloon.

Medline Industries, Inc. 800-633-5886
1 Medline Pl, Mundelein, IL 60060

Medline Manufacturing And Services Llc 847-837-2759
1 Medline Pl, Mundelein, IL 60060
Foley catheters.

Mmj S.A. De C.V. 314-654-2000
716 Ponciano Arriaga, Cd. Juarez, Chih. Mexico
Foley catheters

Opticon Medical 614-336-2000
7001 Post Rd Ste 100, Dublin, OH 43016
Urinary catheter and accessories.

Rochester Medical Corp. 800-615-2364
1 Rochester Medical Dr NW, Stewartville, MN 55976
Various.

CATHETER, RETENTION, BARIUM ENEMA WITH BAG
(Gastro/Urology) 78FGD

Manufacturing & Research, Inc.(Dba Mri Medical) 520-882-7794
4700 S Overland Dr, Tucson, AZ 85714
Custom silicone balloon catheters.

CATHETER, SALPINGOGRAPHY *(Obstetrics/Gyn) 85MOV*

Redi-Tech Medical Products,Llc 800-824-1793
529 Front St Ste 125, Berea, OH 44017
These catheters are used for Hystersalpongography,ans Salpingography.

Rocket Medical Plc. 800-707-7625
150 Recreation Park Dr Ste 3, Hingham, MA 02043

CATHETER, SAMPLING, CHORIONIC VILLUS
(Obstetrics/Gyn) 85LLX

Rocket Medical Plc. 800-707-7625
150 Recreation Park Dr Ste 3, Hingham, MA 02043

CATHETER, SEPTOSTOMY *(Cardiovascular) 74DXF*

Cook Inc. 800-457-4500
PO Box 489, Bloomington, IN 47402

Edwards Lifesciences Technology Sarl 949-250-2500
State Rd. 402 N.km 1.4, Anasco, PR 00610-1577
Atrioseptostomy catheter.

Edwards Lifesciences, Llc. 800-424-3278
1 Edwards Way, Irvine, CA 92614

Medtronic Vascular 707-525-0111
3576 Unocal Pl, Santa Rosa, CA 95403

Numed, Inc. 315-328-4491
2880 Main St., Hopkinton, NY 12965

CATHETER, SIALOGLYCOPROTEIN *(Gastro/Urology) 78WXJ*

Ranfac Corp. 800-2RANFAC
30 Doherty Ave, Avon Industrial Park, Avon, MA 02322
Disposable sialography catheters.

CATHETER, STEERABLE *(Cardiovascular) 74DRA*

Boston Scientific Corporation 800-225-2732
1 Boston Scientific Pl, Natick, MA 01760
Steerable catheter systems.

Catheter Research, Inc. (Cri) 317-872-0074
5610 W 82nd St, Indianapolis, IN 46278

CATHETER, STEERABLE *(cont'd)*

Diablo Sales & Marketing, Inc. 925-648-1611
PO Box 3219, Danville, CA 94526
Custom design and manufacturing of catheters and specialty guidewires. Guiding catheters; stent delivery and drug delivery systems.

Enpath Medical, Inc. 800-559-2613
2300 Berkshire Ln N, Minneapolis, MN 55441

Intraluminal Therapeutics, Inc. 800-513-4458
6354 Corte Del Abeto Ste A, Carlsbad, CA 92011
Straight and angled support catheters for a variety of clinical applications.

Maquet Puerto Rico Inc. 408-635-3900
No. 12, Rd. #698, Dorado, PR 00646
Various models of steerable catheters.

Oscor, Inc. 800-726-7267
3816 Desoto Blvd, Palm Harbor, FL 34683
RF Ablation Catheter

CATHETER, STEERABLE, REPROCESSED
(Cardiovascular) 74NKS

Ascent Healthcare Solutions 480-763-5300
10232 S 51st St, Phoenix, AZ 85044
Steerable electrophysiology catheter.

CATHETER, STRAIGHT *(Gastro/Urology) 78EZD*

Busse Hospital Disposables, Inc. 631-435-4711
75 Arkay Dr, Hauppauge, NY 11788
Urine catheter kit.

Clinical Instruments Intl., Inc. 508-764-2200
278 Worcester St, Southbridge, MA 01550
Introducers.

Cook Urological, Inc. 800-457-4500
1100 W Morgan St, P.O. Box 227, Spencer, IN 47460

Covidien Lp 508-261-8000
15 Hampshire St, Mansfield, MA 02048

Neo-Care Arrow International 800-640-6428
5714 Epsilon, San Antonio, TX 78249
Urological neonatal catheter and urological drainage kit.

Percutaneous Systems, Incorporated 650-493-4200
3260 Hillview Ave Ste 100, Palo Alto, CA 94304
Urology catheter.

CATHETER, SUBCLAVIAN *(Cardiovascular) 74LFJ*

Angiodynamics, Inc. 800-472-5221
1 Horizon Way, Manchester, GA 31816
Dual and single lumen acute care, and dual lumen chronic silicone catheters in varying styles and lengths.

Arrow International, Inc. 800-523-8446
2400 Bernville Rd, Reading, PA 19605

Cardiomed Supplies Inc. 800-387-9757
5 Gormley Industrial Ave., P.O. Box 575
Gormley, ONT L0H 1 Canada
Dual lumen dialysis/homofiltration catheter.

Hospira, Inc. 877-946-7747
755 Jarvis Dr, Morgan Hill, CA 95037

CATHETER, SUBCUTANEOUS INTRAVASCULAR, IMPLANTED
(General) 80LJT

B. Braun Oem Division, B. Braun Medical Inc. 866-8-BBRAUN
824 12th Ave, Bethlehem, PA 18018
New Introcan Safety IV Catheter with a passive design to minimize needlestick injuries without requiring change in technique.

Bard Reynosa S.A. De C.V. 908-277-8000
Blvd. Montebello #1, Parque Industrial Colonial
Reynosa, Tamaulipas Mexico
Implanted ports

Catheter Innovations, Inc. 800-418-2828
3598 W 1820 S, Salt Lake City, UT 84104
Intravasular implanted port.

Cook Vascular, Incorporated 800-457-4500
1186 Montgomery Ln, Vandergrift, PA 15690
VITAL-PORT Vascular Access System - Complete infusion port product line including: silicone or polyurethane catheters, titanium or MRI (polymer based) housing, sized from mini peripheral port through dual-chamber models. Winged infusion sets included.

Medtronic Neurosurgery 800-468-9710
125 Cremona Dr, Goleta, CA 93117
Vascular access port and catheter.

CATHETER, SUBCUTANEOUS INTRAVASCULAR, IMPLANTED *(cont'd)*

Navilyst Medical 800-833-9973
100 Boston Scientific Way, Marlborough, MA 01752
Various types of implanted vascular access ports and vascular access port kits.

Neo Medical Inc. 888-450-3334
42514 Albrae St, Fremont, CA 94538
Subcutaneous intravascular access device.

Norfolk Medical Products, Inc. 847-674-7075
7350 Ridgeway Ave, Skokie, IL 60076
Catheters.

Ussc Puerto Rico, Inc. 203-845-1000
Building 911-67, Sabanetas Industrial Park, Ponce, PR 00731
Infusion port and catheter.

CATHETER, SUBCUTANEOUS PERITONEAL, IMPLANTED
(General) 80LLD

B. Braun Oem Division, B. Braun Medical Inc. 866-8-BBRAUN
824 12th Ave, Bethlehem, PA 18018

CATHETER, SUCTION (TRACHEAL ASPIRATING TUBE)
(Anesthesiology) 73BSY

Ac Healthcare Supply, Inc. 905-448-4706
11651 230th St, Cambria Heights, NY 11411
Tracheobronchial suction catheter.

Amsino International, Inc. 800-MD-AMSINO
855 Towne Center Dr, Pomona, CA 91767
AMSINO catheters and kits are available with control ports in a full range of French sizes.

Ballard Medical Products 770-587-7835
12050 Lone Peak Pkwy, Draper, UT 84020
Suction catheter.

Benlan Inc. 905-829-5004
2760 Brighton Rd., Oakville, ONT L6H 5T4 Canada

Centurion Medical Products Corp. 517-545-1135
3310 S Main St, Salisbury, NC 28147

Corpak Medsystems, Inc. 800-323-6305
100 Chaddick Dr, Wheeling, IL 60090
Various types of sterile suction catheters and accessories.

Filtrona Extrusion, Inc./Pexcor Medical Products Div. 800-755-7528
764 S Athol Rd, P.O. Box 659, Athol, MA 01331

Global Healthcare 800-601-3880
1495 Hembree Rd Ste 700, Roswell, GA 30076
Suction catheters, thumb and vacuum control connectors.

Kelsar, S.A. 508-261-8000
Blvd. Insurgentes, Libriamento a La, Tijuana 22450 Mexico
Suction catheters and suction catheter kits (various)

Kentron Health Care, Inc. 615-384-0573
3604 Kelton Jackson Rd, P.o. Box 120, Springfield, TN 37172
Catheters, suction tracheobronchial.

Medi Inc 800-225-8634
75 York Ave, P.O. Box 302, Randolph, MA 02368

Meditron Inc D.B.A. Medcare Usa 800-243-2442
3435 Montee Gagnon, Terrebonne, QUEBE J6Y-1J4 Canada
ACCS Airway Catheter Cartridge System. Modular closed suction system that reduces dissaturation. Prevents pressure spires and addresses infection control by maintaining a closed system for up to one week. AEROCARE Specialty Suction Catheter. Automatic specialty suction catheter designed to address patients who can not tolerate. Delete and whistle tip catheters.

Medline Industries, Inc. 800-633-5886
1 Medline Pl, Mundelein, IL 60060

Medline Manufacturing And Services Llc 847-837-2759
1 Medline Pl, Mundelein, IL 60060
Suction catheters.

Repro-Med Systems, Inc. 845-469-2042
24 Carpenter Rd, Chester, NY 10918

Richard Wolf Medical Instruments Corp. 800-323-9653
353 Corporate Woods Pkwy, Vernon Hills, IL 60061

Rico Suction Labs, Inc. 800-845-8490
326 MacArthur Ln, Burlington, NC 27217

Rockford Medical & Safety Co. 800-435-9451
2420 Harrison Ave, PO Box 5646, Rockford, IL 61108

CATHETER, SUCTION (TRACHEAL ASPIRATING TUBE) *(cont'd)*

Shoney Scientific, Inc. 262-970-0170
West 223 North 720 Saratoga Drive,, Suite 120, Waukesha, WI 53186
Suction catheter.

Smiths Medical Asd Inc. 800-258-5361
10 Bowman Dr, Keene, NH 03431
Meconium aspirator.

Stryker Puerto Rico, Ltd. 939-307-2500
Hwy. 3, Km. 131.2, Las Guasimas Ind. Park, Arroyo, PR 00714
Pmma bone cement.

Team Technologies, Inc. 423-587-2199
5949 Commerce Blvd, Morristown, TN 37814
Suction catheter.

Terumo Cardiovascular Systems (Tcvs) 800-283-7866
28 Howe St, Ashland, MA 01721
Specimen trap.

Tnc Devices, Inc. 504-286-7794
50 McDonald Blvd, Aston, PA 19014
Tnc suction holder.

Tri-State Hospital Supply Corp. 517-545-1135
3173 E 43rd St, Yuma, AZ 85365

Trinity Sterile, Inc. 410-860-5123
201 Kiley Dr, Salisbury, MD 21801

Unomedical, Inc. 800-634-6003
5701 S Ware Rd Ste 1, McAllen, TX 78503

Virtec Enterprises, Llc 440-352-8970
11351 Prouty Rd, Painesville, OH 44077
Hand-operated emergency suction device, 'Suction Easy.'

Vygon Corp. 800-544-4907
2495 General Armistead Ave, Norristown, PA 19403

CATHETER, SUCTION, WITH TIP *(General) 80JOL*

American Catheter Corp. 800-345-6714
13047 S Highway 475, Ocala, FL 34480

Ballard Medical Products 770-587-7835
12050 Lone Peak Pkwy, Draper, UT 84020
Oral suction catheter.

Bausch & Lomb Surgical 636-255-5051
3365 Tree Court Ind Blvd, Saint Louis, MO 63122

Benlan Inc. 905-829-5004
2760 Brighton Rd., Oakville, ONT L6H 5T4 Canada
Bulk assembled.

Biomet Microfixation Inc. 800-874-7711
1520 Tradeport Dr, Jacksonville, FL 32218
Catheter and tip, suction (rigid).

Catalent Pharma Solutions 866-720-3148
2200 Lake Shore Dr, Woodstock, IL 60098
Multiple

Dma Med-Chem Corporation 800-362-1833
49 Watermill Ln, Great Neck, NY 11021

E.A. Beck & Co. 949-645-4072
657 W 19th St Ste E, P O Box 10857, Costa Mesa, CA 92627
Suction tip.

Engineered Medical Solutions Co. Llc. 908-213-9001
85 Industrial Rd Bldg B, Phillipsburg, NJ 08865
Suction.

Hygo Plastic, Inc. 414-375-4011
1376 Cheyenne Ave, Grafton, WI 53024
Hve tips.

Implantech Associates, Inc. 800-733-0833
6025 Nicolle St Ste B, Ventura, CA 93003
Attachment to electrocautery pencil to evaluate smake and aspirate fluids.

Kelsar, S.A. 508-261-8000
Blvd. Insurgentes, Libriamento a La, Tijuana 22450 Mexico
Various types

Kentron Health Care, Inc. 615-384-0573
3604 Kelton Jackson Rd, P.o. Box 120, Springfield, TN 37172
Yankaur suction handle.

Medical Depot 516-998-4600
99 Seaview Blvd, Port Washington, NY 11050
Suction device.

Medline Manufacturing And Services Llc 847-837-2759
1 Medline Pl, Mundelein, IL 60060
Suction catheters.

CATHETER, SUCTION, WITH TIP *(cont'd)*

O&M Enterprise 847-258-4515
641 Chelmsford Ln, Elk Grove Village, IL 60007
CATHETER SUCTION TIP

Pmt Corp. 800-626-5463
1500 Park Rd, Chanhassen, MN 55317

Primary Care Solutions, Inc. 888-212-5336
40420 Free Fall Ave, Zephyrhills, FL 33542
Sterile water, sterile saline.

Stryker Puerto Rico, Ltd. 939-307-2500
Hwy. 3, Km. 131.2, Las Guasimas Ind. Park, Arroyo, PR 00714
Irrigation tips.

Terumo Cardiovascular Systems (Tcvs) 800-283-7866
28 Howe St, Ashland, MA 01721
Suction assembly.

Trinity Sterile, Inc. 410-860-5123
201 Kiley Dr, Salisbury, MD 21801

Tuzik Boston 800-886-6363
104 Longwater Dr, Assinippi Park, Norwell, MA 02061

Vygon Corp. 800-544-4907
2495 General Armistead Ave, Norristown, PA 19403

Wel Industries, Inc. 805-985-2462
5114 Terramar Way, Oxnard, CA 93035
Various.

Wells Johnson Co. 800-528-1597
8000 S Kolb Rd, Tucson, AZ 85756

CATHETER, SUPRAPUBIC *(Gastro/Urology) 78KOB*

C. R. Bard, Inc., Bard Urological Div. 888-367-2273
13183 Harland Dr NE, Covington, GA 30014

Cook Urological, Inc. 800-457-4500
1100 W Morgan St, P.O. Box 227, Spencer, IN 47460

Covidien Lp 508-261-8000
15 Hampshire St, Mansfield, MA 02048

Gyrus Acmi, Inc. 508-804-2739
93 N Pleasant St, Norwalk, OH 44857
Catheter, suprapubic (and accessories).

Laborie Medical Technologies Inc. 888-522-6743
6415 Northwest Dr., Units 7-14, Mississauga, ONT L4V-1X1 Canada
Priced $178.00 for a box of ten; available in sizes 16, 12 FR. Trocar and cannula only. Packaged sterile.

Manufacturing & Research, Inc.(Dba Mri Medical) 520-882-7794
4700 S Overland Dr, Tucson, AZ 85714
10-14 Fr., silicone.

CATHETER, SUPRAPUBIC, WITH TUBE *(Gastro/Urology) 78FEZ*

Cook Urological, Inc. 800-457-4500
1100 W Morgan St, P.O. Box 227, Spencer, IN 47460

Covidien Lp 508-261-8000
15 Hampshire St, Mansfield, MA 02048

CATHETER, TENCKHOFF *(Gastro/Urology) 78QIM*

Angiodynamics, Inc. 800-472-5221
1 Horizon Way, Manchester, GA 31816
Neonatal, pediatric, adult, and custom configurations with one or two Dacron cuffs and one universal placement kit.

Lifemed Of California 800-543-3633
1216 S Allec St, Anaheim, CA 92805

Redi-Tech Medical Products,Llc 800-824-1793
529 Front St Ste 125, Berea, OH 44017

CATHETER, THERMAL DILUTION *(Cardiovascular) 74QIN*

Biosensors International - Usa 949-553-8300
20280 SW Acacia St Ste 300, Newport Beach, CA 92660
Safetywedge. Device to virtually eliminate the risk of PA rupture.

Cardiomed Supplies Inc. 800-387-9757
5 Gormley Industrial Ave., P.O. Box 575
Gormley, ONT L0H 1 Canada
4 & 5 Lumens thermodilution catheter

Dma Med-Chem Corporation 800-362-1833
49 Watermill Ln, Great Neck, NY 11021

Manufacturing & Research, Inc.(Dba Mri Medical) 520-882-7794
4700 S Overland Dr, Tucson, AZ 85714
Thermodilution Catheter, all silicone, available in 7Fr, 110 cm height with 1.5 cc balloon.

CATHETER, THROMBECTOMY *(Cardiovascular) 74QIO*

Possis Medical, Inc. 888-848-7677
9055 Evergreen Blvd NW, Minneapolis, MN 55433
AngioJet Rheolytic Thrombectomy System approved for native coronary arteries, saphenous vein coronary bypass grafts, av access grafts and fistulas.

CATHETER, THROMBUS RETRIEVER *(Cardiovascular) 74NRY*

Concentric Medical, Inc. 650-938-2100
301 E Evelyn Ave, Mountain View, CA 94041
Thrombus retriever.

CATHETER, TRANSCERVICAL, BALLOON TUBOPLASTY *(Obstetrics/Gyn) 85MKN*

Conceptus, Inc. 650-962-4000
331 E Evelyn Ave, Mountain View, CA 94041

CATHETER, TRANSFER, INTRAFALLOPIAN *(Obstetrics/Gyn) 85MHL*

Rocket Medical Plc. 800-707-7625
150 Recreation Park Dr Ste 3, Hingham, MA 02043

CATHETER, UMBILICAL ARTERY *(General) 80FOS*

Health Care Logistics, Inc. 800-848-1633
450 Town St, PO Box 25, Circleville, OH 43113
Accessory to intravascular catheter.

Utah Medical Products, Inc. 800-533-4984
7043 Cottonwood St, Midvale, UT 84047
UMBILI-CATH, umbilical vessel & umbilical artery catheters used for administration of meds & monitoring blood pressure invasively. Many sizes, both silicone & polyurethane.

Vygon Corp. 800-544-4907
2495 General Armistead Ave, Norristown, PA 19403

CATHETER, UPPER URINARY TRACT *(Gastro/Urology) 78EYC*

Biosearch Medical Products, Inc. 908-722-5000
35 Industrial Pkwy, Branchburg, NJ 08876
Intermittent urinary catheter.

Cook Urological, Inc. 800-457-4500
1100 W Morgan St, P.O. Box 227, Spencer, IN 47460

CATHETER, URETERAL DISPOSABLE (X-RAY) *(Gastro/Urology) 78FGF*

Cook Urological, Inc. 800-457-4500
1100 W Morgan St, P.O. Box 227, Spencer, IN 47460

Covidien Lp 508-261-8000
15 Hampshire St, Mansfield, MA 02048

CATHETER, URETERAL, GASTRO-UROLOGY *(Gastro/Urology) 78EYB*

Axiom Medical, Inc. 800-221-8569
19320 Van Ness Ave, Torrance, CA 90501
Available with exclusive ATRAUM Coating

Bard Canada, Inc. 800-268-2862
2345 Stanfield Rd, Mississauga, ONT L4Y 3Y3 Canada

Cook Urological, Inc. 800-457-4500
1100 W Morgan St, P.O. Box 227, Spencer, IN 47460

Medikmark Inc. 800-424-8520
3600 Burwood Dr, Waukegan, IL 60085
Foley, Uretheral, & Irrigation Kits & Tray

Medline Manufacturing And Services Llc 847-837-2759
1 Medline Pl, Mundelein, IL 60060
Catheters.

Millar Instruments, Inc. 800.669.2343
6001 Gulf Fwy Ste A, Houston, TX 77023

Mmj S.A. De C.V. 314-654-2000
716 Ponciano Arriaga, Cd. Juarez, Chih. Mexico
Foley-temp ureteral catheter

Reach Global Industries, Inc. (Reachgood) 888-518-8389
8 Corporate Park Ste 300, Irvine, CA 92606
Ureteral catheter.

CATHETER, URETERAL, GENERAL & PLASTIC SURGERY *(Surgery) 79GBL*

Degania Silicone, Inc. 401-333-8199
1226 Mendon Rd, Cumberland, RI 02864
Standard and custom designed silicone catheters. Capabilities include silicone extrusion, liquid injection molding, balloon manufacturing, catheter printing, perforations, tipping and packaging,

CATHETER, URETERAL, GENERAL & PLASTIC SURGERY *(cont'd)*

Memcath Technologies Llc 651-450-7400
1777 Oakdale Ave, Saint Paul, MN 55118

CATHETER, URETHRAL *(Gastro/Urology) 78GBM*

Apogee Medical, Llc 919-570-9605
90 Weathers Ct, Youngsville, NC 27596
Urological catheter.

Benlan Inc. 905-829-5004
2760 Brighton Rd., Oakville, ONT L6H 5T4 Canada
Bulk assembled.

Busse Hospital Disposables, Inc. 631-435-4711
75 Arkay Dr, Hauppauge, NY 11788
Urine catheter kit.

Covidien Lp 508-261-8000
15 Hampshire St, Mansfield, MA 02048

Kelsar, S.A. 508-261-8000
Blvd. Insurgentes, Libriamento a La, Tijuana 22450 Mexico
Urethral catherter and kits

Life-Tech, Inc. 281-491-6600
4235 Greenbriar Dr, Stafford, TX 77477

Medi Inc 800-225-8634
75 York Ave, P.O. Box 302, Randolph, MA 02368

Medline Manufacturing And Services Llc 847-837-2759
1 Medline Pl, Mundelein, IL 60060
Catheter,urethral,sterile.

Medtronic Blood Management 612-514-4000
18501 E Plaza Dr, Parker, CO 80134
Urethral catheter.

Memcath Technologies Llc 651-450-7400
1777 Oakdale Ave, Saint Paul, MN 55118

Miltex Inc. 800-645-8000
589 Davies Dr, York, PA 17402

Momentum Medical 208-523-3600
1330 Enterprise St, Idaho Falls, ID 83402
Male external catheter system.

Reach Global Industries, Inc. (Reachgood) 888-518-8389
8 Corporate Park Ste 300, Irvine, CA 92606
Foley catheter.

Rochester Medical Corp. 800-615-2364
1 Rochester Medical Dr NW, Stewartville, MN 55976
Various sizes of nelaton-type urethral catheters.

CATHETER, URETHRAL, DIAGNOSTIC *(Gastro/Urology) 78QIQ*

Memcath Technologies Llc 651-450-7400
1777 Oakdale Ave, Saint Paul, MN 55118

Mentor Corp. 800-525-0245
201 Mentor Dr, Santa Barbara, CA 93111
Urethral red-rubber catheters.

Timm Medical Technologies, Inc. 800-966-2796
6585 City West Pkwy, Eden Prairie, MN 55344
Also available, C3 Male Continence Device, an external occlusive disposable device.

CATHETER, URINARY *(Gastro/Urology) 78QIR*

Axiom Medical, Inc. 800-221-8569
19320 Van Ness Ave, Torrance, CA 90501

Benlan Inc. 905-829-5004
2760 Brighton Rd., Oakville, ONT L6H 5T4 Canada

Coloplast Manufacturing Us, Llc 800-533-0464
1840 W Oak Pkwy, Marietta, GA 30062
CONVEEN sterile, non-latex, Intermittent catheters, in female, long, coude and olive tip coude styles, include frosted surface and smooth tip, lateral eyelits for maximum drainage. Male external catheters, one-or two-piece styles include adhesive and easy application.

Covidien Lp 508-261-8000
15 Hampshire St, Mansfield, MA 02048

Invacare Supply Group, An Invacare Co. 800-225-4792
75 October Hill Rd, Holliston, MA 01746
Carry full lines of urologicals from: Bard, Convatec, Kendall, Mentor, Hollister, Rochester, Rusch.

Life-Tech, Inc. 281-491-6600
4235 Greenbriar Dr, Stafford, TX 77477

Lsl Industries, Inc. 888-225-5575
5535 N Wolcott Ave, Chicago, IL 60640
$20.00 for 50 individually packed male external catheters.

CATHETER, URINARY *(cont'd)*

Manufacturing & Research, Inc.(Dba Mri Medical) 520-882-7794
4700 S Overland Dr, Tucson, AZ 85714
6-30 Fr., silicone.

Medi Inc 800-225-8634
75 York Ave, P.O. Box 302, Randolph, MA 02368

Memcath Technologies Llc 651-450-7400
1777 Oakdale Ave, Saint Paul, MN 55118

Mentor Corp. 800-525-0245
201 Mentor Dr, Santa Barbara, CA 93111
100% silicone; Foley catheters.

CATHETER, URINARY, CONDOM *(Gastro/Urology) 78QIS*

Coloplast Manufacturing Us, Llc 800-533-0464
1840 W Oak Pkwy, Marietta, GA 30062
Male external catheters with skin protective adhesive strip.

Leading Edge Innovations 805-388-7669
699 Mobil Ave, Camarillo, CA 93010
External Male Condom Catheter with new patented technology for creating a water tight seal. Also a uniques connector with a quick connect/disconnect feature.

Medi Inc 800-225-8634
75 York Ave, P.O. Box 302, Randolph, MA 02368

Merlin's Medical Supply 800-639-9322
699 Mobil Ave, Camarillo, CA 93010
GEE WHIZ(R) male urinary incontinent device. A male urinary collection system for males who have urinary incontinent problems. Designed for minor leakage to total loss of urine control. Ideal for Incontinent people, urgency needs, pilots, hunters, etc.

Smith & Nephew, Inc. 800-876-1261
11775 Starkey Rd, Largo, FL 33773

Urocare Products, Inc. 800-423-4441
2735 Melbourne Ave, Pomona, CA 91767
URO-CON, external catheter, Texas style 50pcs/box.

CATHETER, URINARY, IRRIGATION *(Gastro/Urology) 78QIT*

Axiom Medical, Inc. 800-221-8569
19320 Van Ness Ave, Torrance, CA 90501

Cook Urological, Inc. 800-457-4500
1100 W Morgan St, P.O. Box 227, Spencer, IN 47460

Covidien Lp 508-261-8000
15 Hampshire St, Mansfield, MA 02048

Manufacturing & Research, Inc.(Dba Mri Medical) 520-882-7794
4700 S Overland Dr, Tucson, AZ 85714
16-30 Fr., silicone.

Memcath Technologies Llc 651-450-7400
1777 Oakdale Ave, Saint Paul, MN 55118

CATHETER, UROLOGICAL *(Gastro/Urology) 78KOD*

Apogee Medical, Llc 919-570-9605
90 Weathers Ct, Youngsville, NC 27596
Closed system intermittent catheterization kit.

Apple Medical Corp. 508-357-2700
28 Lord Rd Ste 135, Marlborough, MA 01752
Infusion/aspiration device.

Argon Medical Devices Inc. 903-675-9321
1445 Flat Creek Rd, Athens, TX 75751
Gastroenterology catheter.

Biosearch Medical Products, Inc. 908-722-5000
35 Industrial Pkwy, Branchburg, NJ 08876
Intermittent urinary catheter.

C. R. Bard, Inc., Bard Urological Div. 888-367-2273
13183 Harland Dr NE, Covington, GA 30014

Coloplast Manufacturing Us, Llc 612-302-4992
1185 Willow Lake Blvd, Vadnais Heights, MN 55110
Urethral catheterization system.

Coloplast Manufacturing Us, Llc 800-533-0464
1840 W Oak Pkwy, Marietta, GA 30062
CONVEEN sterile, non-latex. Intermittent catheters, in female, long, coude and olive tip coude styles, include frosted surface and smooth tip, lateral eyelets for maximum drainage. Male external catheters, one- or two-piece styles include adhesive and easy application.

Cook Urological, Inc. 800-457-4500
1100 W Morgan St, P.O. Box 227, Spencer, IN 47460

Health Care Logistics, Inc. 800-848-1633
450 Town St, PO Box 25, Circleville, OH 43113
Securement accessories for catheter holder.

CATHETER, UROLOGICAL *(cont'd)*

Healthtronics Inc. 888-252-6575
9825 Spectrum Dr Bldg B, Austin, TX 78717

Kelsar, S.A. 508-261-8000
Blvd. Insurgentes, Libriamento a La, Tijuana 22450 Mexico
Foley catheters, and kits (all types)

Life-Tech, Inc. 281-491-6600
4235 Greenbriar Dr, Stafford, TX 77477

Manufacturing & Research, Inc.(Dba Mri Medical) 520-882-7794
4700 S Overland Dr, Tucson, AZ 85714
6-30 Fr., silicone.

Memcath Technologies Llc 651-450-7400
1777 Oakdale Ave, Saint Paul, MN 55118
Sizes 8-18 FR.

Mentor Corp. 800-525-0245
201 Mentor Dr, Santa Barbara, CA 93111
Urethral, 2-way, 3-way and pediatric.

Mmj S.A. De C.V. 314-654-2000
716 Ponciano Arriaga, Cd. Juarez, Chih. Mexico
Drainage catheter, urological catheter

Navilyst Medical 800-833-9973
100 Boston Scientific Way, Marlborough, MA 01752
Fluid administration accessory.

Utah Medical Products, Inc. 800-533-4984
7043 Cottonwood St, Midvale, UT 84047
URI-CATH silicone urinary drainage catheter for collection of urine & accurate output measurement, available as part of a set or separately.

CATHETER, VASCULAR, CARDIOPULMONARY BYPASS
(Cardiovascular) 74DWF

Alliant Healthcare Products 269-629-0300
8850 M89, Richland, MI 49083
Vein graft vessel cannula.

Atek Medical 800-253-1540
620 Watson St SW, Grand Rapids, MI 49504
Various types of shunts, nerve pads, cardioplegia, and aspirating needles.

Bard Shannon Limited 908-277-8000
San Geronimo Industrial Park, Lot # 1, Road # 3, Km 79.7
Humacao, PR 00791
Carotid bypass shunt,shunts.

California Medical Laboratories, Inc. 714-556-7365
1570 Sunland Ln, Costa Mesa, CA 92626
Cardiovascular catheter, cannula and tubing; vascular cardiopulmonary bypass.

Cardeon Corp. 408-253-3319
10600 N Tantau Ave, Cupertino, CA 95014
Various.

Cascade Life Solutions, Llc 616-977-2505
3710 Sysco Ct SE, Grand Rapids, MI 49512
Cardioplegia cannula.

Chase Medical, Lp 972-783-0644
1876 Firman Dr, Richardson, TX 75081
Various models of perfusion cannula, vessel shunt, vent valve, vessel cannula.

Circulatory Technology, Inc. 516-624-2424
21 Singworth St, Oyster Bay, NY 11771
The 'better-venter'.

Clinical Instruments Intl., Inc. 508-764-2200
278 Worcester St, Southbridge, MA 01550
Carotid bypass shunt.

Cook Inc. 800-457-4500
PO Box 489, Bloomington, IN 47402

Covidien Lp 508-261-8000
15 Hampshire St, Mansfield, MA 02048

Edwards Lifesciences Research Medical 949-250-2500
6864 Cottonwood St, Midvale, UT 84047
Various sizes & types of sterile catheters & cannulae.

Edwards Lifesciences, Llc. 800-424-3278
1 Edwards Way, Irvine, CA 92614

Integra Neurosciences Pr 800-654-2873
Road 402 North, Km 1.2, Anasco, PR 00610
Various cardiopulmonary bypass vascular catheter.

CATHETER, VASCULAR, CARDIOPULMONARY BYPASS *(cont'd)*

Jostra Bentley, Inc. 302-454-9959
Rd. 402 N. Km 1.4, Industrial Park, Anasco, PR 00610-1577
Cardiopulmonary bypass catheters, cannula and tubing.

Kelsar, S.A. 508-261-8000
Blvd. Insurgentes, Libriamento a La, Tijuana 22450 Mexico
Parallel 'y' connector, perfusion adaptor, vena caval catheter artey shunts, per

Medtronic Blood Management 612-514-4000
18501 E Plaza Dr, Parker, CO 80134
Catheter, cannula and tubing.

Medtronic Dlp 616-643-5200
620 Watson St SW, Grand Rapids, MI 49504

Origen Biomedical, Inc. 512-474-7278
4020 S Industrial Dr Ste 160, Austin, TX 78744
ORIGEN perfusion catheters.

Pemco, Inc. - Medical Div. 216-524-2990
5663 Brecksville Rd, Cleveland, OH 44131

Shelhigh, Inc. 908-206-8706
650 Liberty Ave, Union, NJ 07083
Aortic perfusion cannula and tubing.

Smiths Medical Asd, Inc. 800-433-5832
1265 Grey Fox Rd, Saint Paul, MN 55112

Surge Medical Solutions, Llc. 616-977-2516
3710 Sysco Ct SE, Grand Rapids, MI 49512
Left vent safety valve.

Terumo Cardiovascular Systems (Tcvs) 800-283-7866
125 Blue Ball Rd, Elkton, MD 21921
Circuit tubing.

Terumo Cardiovascular Systems (Tcvs) 800-283-7866
28 Howe St, Ashland, MA 01721
Catheters, cannulas, tubing, and accessories.

Terumo Cardiovascular Systems, Corp 800-521-2818
6200 Jackson Rd, Ann Arbor, MI 48103

Vitalcor, Inc. 800-874-8358
100 Chestnut Ave, Westmont, IL 60559
Various types of thoracic, venous, and vena cava catheters.

Voss Medical Products 210-650-3124
4235 Centergate St, San Antonio, TX 78217
Coronary cannula.

CATHETER, VASCULAR, LONG-TERM *(Cardiovascular) 74DYD*

Angiodynamics, Inc. 800-472-5221
1 Horizon Way, Manchester, GA 31816
Long-term silicone dialysis and critical care catheters in varying lumen configurations, lengths, and french sizes.

Gish Biomedical, Inc. 800-938-0531
22942 Arroyo Vis, Rancho Santa Margarita, CA 92688
Single- and double-lumen, silicone, tunneled. Single-lumen non-adhesive, double-lumen adhesive repair kit.

Millar Instruments, Inc. 800.669.2343
6001 Gulf Fwy Ste A, Houston, TX 77023

St. Jude Medical, Inc. 800-328-9634
1 Saint Jude Medical Dr, Saint Paul, MN 55117
Cardiology/vascular access products; vascular closure devices.

CATHETER, VENTRICULAR *(Cns/Neurology) 84HCA*

Codman & Shurtleff, Inc 800-225-0460
325 Paramount Dr, Raynham, MA 02767

Innerspace, Inc. 877.HUM.BIRD
1622 Edinger Ave Ste C, Tustin, CA 92780
Hummingbird Multi-Parameter with OxiPort. Provides concurrent monitoring of ICP, Oxygen, Temperature while providing ventricular drainage through a single burr-hole.

Integra Neurosciences Pr 800-654-2873
Road 402 North, Km 1.2, Anasco, PR 00610
Various sites and configurations.

Medtronic Image-Guided Neurologics, Inc. 800-707-0933
2290 W Eau Gallie Blvd, Melbourne, FL 32935
Aspiration/irrigation catheter.

Medtronic Neurosurgery 800-468-9710
125 Cremona Dr, Goleta, CA 93117
Ventricular catheter, flanged.

Millar Instruments, Inc. 800.669.2343
6001 Gulf Fwy Ste A, Houston, TX 77023

CATHETER, VENTRICULAR, GENERAL & PLASTIC SURGERY
(Surgery) 79GBS

Medtronic, Inc. 800-633-8766
710 Medtronic Pkwy, Minneapolis, MN 55432
ATAKR.

CAUTERY, RADIOFREQUENCY, AC-POWERED
(Ophthalmology) 86HQR

Acuderm Inc. 800-327-0015
5370 NW 35th Ter Ste 106, Fort Lauderdale, FL 33309
Acu-E-Surg. Full-featured ESU with up to 120 W of power for cutting, blending, desiccation, fulguration, and coagulation. Autoclavable and cold-sterilizable handpieces.

Bausch & Lomb Surgical 636-255-5051
3365 Tree Court Ind Blvd, Saint Louis, MO 63122

Hospira, Inc. 877-946-7747
755 Jarvis Dr, Morgan Hill, CA 95037
$3,600.00 for heated-blade electronic surgical system.

Mira, Inc. 508-278-7877
414 Quaker Hwy, Uxbridge, MA 01569
Accessory handle and cable for diathermy console.

Neomedix Corp. 949-258-8355
15042 Parkway Loop Ste A, Tustin, CA 92780
Electrosurgical bipolar handpiece.

Ophthalmic Technologies, Inc. 416-631-9123
12-37 Kodiak Cres, Downsview M3J 3E5 Canada
Ophthalmic diathermy system.

Refractec, Inc. 949-784-2600
5 Jenner Ste 150, Irvine, CA 92618
Electrosurgical device.

Synergetics Usa, Inc. 800-600-0565
3845 Corporate Centre Dr, O Fallon, MO 63368
Three function manipulator.

CAUTERY, RADIOFREQUENCY, BATTERY-POWERED
(Ophthalmology) 86HQQ

Mira, Inc. 508-278-7877
414 Quaker Hwy, Uxbridge, MA 01569
Accessory handle and cable for diathermy console.

CAUTERY, THERMAL, AC-POWERED *(Ophthalmology) 86HQO*

Dermatologic Lab & Supply, Inc. 800-831-6273
608 13th Ave, Council Bluffs, IA 51501
Thermal Cautery Unit

Geiger Medical Technologies 800-320-9612
608 13th Ave, Council Bluffs, IA 51501
GEIGER line-powered thermal cautery unit utilizes reusable handpiece and electrodes.

Hospira, Inc. 877-946-7747
755 Jarvis Dr, Morgan Hill, CA 95037
$3,600.00 for heated-blade electronic surgical system.

Starion Instruments 800-782-7466
775 Palomar Ave, Sunnyvale, CA 94085
Various models of ac powered thermal cautery units.

Western Ophthalmics Corporation 800-426-9938
19019 36th Ave W Ste G, Lynnwood, WA 98036

CAUTERY, THERMAL, BATTERY-POWERED
(Ophthalmology) 86HQP

Acuderm Inc. 800-327-0015
5370 NW 35th Ter Ste 106, Fort Lauderdale, FL 33309
Acu-Dispo-Cautery. High-temperature ((2200 degrees F) disposable cautery with fine or loop tip. Fingertip control, safety cap, sterile. Also available in 1300- and 650-deg F models and a high-temp (2200-deg F) model.

Bausch & Lomb Surgical 636-255-5051
3365 Tree Court Ind Blvd, Saint Louis, MO 63122

Bovie Medical Corp. 800-537-2790
5115 Ulmerton Rd, Clearwater, FL 33760
Micro-variable temperature.

Hospira, Inc. 877-946-7747
755 Jarvis Dr, Morgan Hill, CA 95037
$350.00 for heated-blade unit.

Kirwan Surgical Products, Inc. 888-547-9267
180 Enterprise Dr, PO Box 427, Marshfield, MA 02050
Non-stick ophthalmic bipolar cautery pencils.

CAUTERY, THERMAL, BATTERY-POWERED *(cont'd)*

Medtronic Heart Valves 800-227-3191
8299 Central Ave NE, Spring Lake Park, MN 55432
Disposable cautery.

Oasis Medical, Inc. 800-528-9786
514 S Vermont Ave, Glendora, CA 91741

Starion Instruments 800-782-7466
775 Palomar Ave, Sunnyvale, CA 94085
Various.

Western Ophthalmics Corporation 800-426-9938
19019 36th Ave W Ste G, Lynnwood, WA 98036

CELL, SPECTROPHOTOMETER *(Chemistry) 75UID*

Beckman Coulter, Inc. 800-742-2345
250 S Kraemer Blvd, PO Box 8000, Brea, CA 92821

Harrick Scientific Products, Inc. 800-248-3847
141 Tomkins Avenue, Pleasantville, N 10570 United

International Crystal Laboratories 973-478-8944
11 Erie St, Garfield, NJ 07026

Jasco, Inc. 800-333-5272
8649 Commerce Dr, Easton, MD 21601

Nsg Precision Cells, Inc. 631-249-7474
195 Central Ave Ste G, Farmingdale, NY 11735

Thermo Spectronic 800-654-9955
820 Linden Ave, Rochester, NY 14625
BioMATE UV-visible spectrometers. AquaMATE UV-visible spectrophotometers. UV Senes UV-visible spectrophotometers.

CELLOIDIN *(Pathology) 88IEZ*

Polysciences, Inc. 800-523-2575
400 Valley Rd, Warrington, PA 18976
23% solids solution in ethyl acetate

CEMENT, BONE, PRE-FORMED, MODULAR, POLYMERIC, VERTEBROPLASTY *(Orthopedics) 87OBL*

Benvenue Medical, Inc. 408-454-9300
3052 Bunker Hill Ln Ste 120, Santa Clara, CA 95054
Kiva VCF Treatment System

CEMENT, BONE, VERTEBROPLASTY, PRE-FORMED, MODULAR *(Orthopedics) 87OBM*

DFine Inc. 866-963-3463
3047 Orchard Pkwy, San Jose, CA 95134
SPACE 360 Delivery System; StabiliT Vertebral Augmentation Sys

Osseon Therapeutics, Inc. 877-567-7366
2330 Circadian Way, Santa Rosa, CA 95407
OsseoPerm 1.0 Bone Cement

CEMENT, DENTAL *(Dental And Oral) 76EMA*

American Dental Products, Inc. 800-846-7120
603 Country Club Dr Ste B, Bensenville, IL 60106
American dental products, root canal sealer, walch's improveed formula.

Bisco, Inc. 847-534-6000
1100 W Irving Park Rd, Schaumburg, IL 60193
Dental adhesive cement.

Chameleon Dental Products, Inc. 913-281-5552
200 N 6th St, Kansas City, KS 66101
No common name listed.

Cooley & Cooley, Ltd. 800-215-4487
8550 Westland West Blvd, Houston, TX 77041
DOC'S BEST ANTIMICROBIAL COPPER CEMENTS retard decay, stimulates secondary dentin, and is biologically and mechanically superior. It can be used with composite restorations, orthodontic bands, and with metal restorations. Laboratory results report Strep mutans, Staph aureus and Lactobacillus paracasei are all killed 100% when exposed to this cement. Toxicology testing reports no toxicity or mutagenicity with any of Doc's Best or COPALITE products.

D.C.A. (Dental Corporation Of America) 800-638-6684
889 S Matlack St, West Chester, PA 19382
$54.95 per unit, variety to choose from, for all.

Den-Mat Holdings, Llc 805-922-8491
2727 Skyway Dr, Santa Maria, CA 93455
No common name listed.

Dent Zar, Inc. 800-444-1241
6362 Hollywood Blvd Ste 214, Los Angeles, CA 90028
Dental cements.

CEMENT, DENTAL *(cont'd)*

Dental Technologies, Inc. 847-677-5500
6901 N Hamlin Ave, Lincolnwood, IL 60712
Zinc phophate dental cement.

Dentalez Group 866-DTE-INFO
101 Lindenwood Dr Ste 225, Valleybrooke Corporate Center Malvern, PA 19355

Dentalez Group, Stardental Division 717-291-1161
1816 Colonial Village Ln, Lancaster, PA 17601
Rc cement non-staining.

Dentsply Canada, Ltd. 800-263-1437
161 Vinyl Ct., Woodbridge, ONT L4L 4A3 Canada

Dshealthcare Inc. 201-871-1232
85 W Forest Ave, Englewood, NJ 07631
Endodontic filling materials and cements.

Essential Dental Systems, Inc. 800-223-5394
89 Leuning St, South Hackensack, NJ 07606

Gc America, Inc. 708-597-0900
3737 W 127th St, Alsip, IL 60803
Reinforced glass ionomer cement.

Glenroe Technologies 800-237-4060
1912 44th Ave E, Bradenton, FL 34203
Various bonding; band cement kits.

Harry J. Bosworth Company 800-323-4352
7227 Hamlin Ave, Skokie, IL 60076
Zinc phosphate cement. ZMENT zinc oxide eugenol temporary cement. MEGABOND crown and bridge resin cement, SUPEREBA cement.

Ivoclar Vivadent, Inc. 800-533-6825
175 Pineview Dr, Amherst, NY 14228
VARIOLINK II, two viscosity, three shades, radiopaque fluoride releasing multi-purpose dental cement, dual cement.

J. Morita Usa, Inc. 888-566-7482
9 Mason, Irvine, CA 92618
BISTITE II DC is the most comprehensive self-etching, dual-cured, all-purpose adhesive resin cement system. The main kit components are the resin cement pastes contained in the 'Super Syringe' and a series of primers used to enhance bonding to various substrates. Bistite II DC is available in three radiopaque shades: Clear, Dentin, and Ivory.

Kerr Corp. 714-516-7400
28200 Wick Rd, Romulus, MI 48174
Temporary cement.

Lancer Orthodontics, Inc. 760-304-2705
253 Pawnee St, San Marcos, CA 92078
Zinc phosphate cement, polycarboxylate cement, glass ionomer cemen.

Lund Dental Mfg. 661-222-7267
3829 Hayvenhurst Dr, Encino, CA 91436
Root canal cement (or) root canal sealer.

Majestic Drug Co., Inc. 845-436-0011
PO Box 490, 4996 Main St., Route 42, S Fallsburg, NY 12779
Dental cement other than zinc oxide-eugenol.

Medental Intl. 760-727-5889
3008 Palm Hill Dr, Vista, CA 92084
Various types.

Medidenta International, Inc. 800-221-0750
3923 62nd St, PO Box 409, Woodside, NY 11377

Mizzy, Inc. Of National Keystone 800-333-3131
616 Hollywood Ave, Cherry Hill, NJ 08002
Flecks Zinc Phosphate cement is used by dentists worldwide. It is completely impervious to oral fluids and retains full cementing strength in the thinnest film.

Moyco Technologies, Inc. 800-331-8837
200 Commerce Dr, Montgomeryville, PA 18936
$15.00 per kit.

Nobel Biocare Usa, Llc 800-579-6515
22715/22725 Savi Ranch Parkway, Yorba Linda, CA 92887
Temporary dental cement.

Novocol, Inc. 303-665-7535
416 S Taylor Ave, Louisville, CO 80027
Zinc phosphate cement, glass ionomer cement, polycarboxylate cement orthodontic.

Oratech, Llc 801-553-4493
475 W 10200 S, South Jordan, UT 84095
Dental cement.

CEMENT, DENTAL *(cont'd)*

Pac-Dent Intl., Inc. 909-839-0888
21078 Commerce Point Dr, Walnut, CA 91789
Type o putty temporary cement.

Parkell, Inc. 800-243-7446
300 Executive Dr, Edgewood, NY 11717
C & B-METABOND adhesive cement that bonds metal to tooth structure. TOTABOND, adhesive cement, easy to use 4-meta-based cement for all adhesive applications.

Pentron Clinical Technologies 203-265-7397
68-70 North Plains Industrial, Road, Wallingford, CT 06492
Cement,dental.

Pentron Laboratory Technologies 203-265-7397
53 N Plains Industrial Rd, Wallingford, CT 06492
Cement, dental.

Plastodent 718-792-3554
2881 Middletown Rd, Bronx, NY 10461

Pulpdent Corp. 800-343-4342
80 Oakland St, Watertown, MA 02472
Dental resin cement.

Rite-Dent Manufacturing Corp. 305-693-8626
3750 E 10th Ct, Hialeah, FL 33013
Various types of dental cement.

Roth Drug Co. 312-733-1478
669 West Ohio St., --, Chestnut Street, IL 60610
Dental cement, zinc oxide-eugenol (zoe).

Shofu Dental Corporation 800-827-4638
1225 Stone Dr, San Marcos, CA 92078
MONOCEM, GLASIONOMER, CX-PLUS, HY-BOND POLYCARBOXYLATE, HY-BOND POLYCARBOXYLATE TEMPORARY CEMENT, HY-BOND ZINC OXIDE EUGENOL TEMPORARY, HY-BOND ZINC PHOSPHATE

Sterngold 800-243-9942
23 Frank Mossberg Dr, PO Box 2967, Attleboro, MA 02703
Tempolock NE - Temporary Cement Automix Non-Eugenol, zinc oxide. Remains flexible under the temporary for easy removal without damage to the tooth or adjacent tooth or tissue.

Temrex Corp. 516-868-6221
112 Albany Ave, P.o. Box 182, Freeport, NY 11520
Temporary dental cement.

Ultradent Products, Inc. 801-553-4586
505 W 10200 S, South Jordan, UT 84095
Oxygen barrier solution.

Water Pik, Inc. 970-221-6129
1730 E Prospect Rd, Fort Collins, CO 80525
Dental cements.

Westside Packaging, Llc. 909-570-3508
1700 S Baker Ave Ste A, Ontario, CA 91761
Dental cement.

CEMENT, EAR, NOSE AND THROAT *(Ear/Nose/Throat) 77NEA*

Biomet Microfixation Inc. 800-874-7711
1520 Tradeport Dr, Jacksonville, FL 32218
Ear nose and throat cement.

CEMENT, HYDROXYAPATITE *(Surgery) 79MGN*

Synthes (Usa) - Development Center 719-481-5300
1230 Wilson Dr, West Chester, PA 19380
Carbonated apatite cement.

Zimmer Dental, Inc. 800-854-7019
1900 Aston Ave, Carlsbad, CA 92008
$30.00/gram for CALCITITE 2040 and 4060 hydroxylapatite (HA) particles for alveolar-ridge augmentation and filling periodontal lesions.

CEMENT, ORTHOPEDIC (BONE) *(Orthopedics) 87QIW*

Dentsply Canada, Ltd. 800-263-1437
161 Vinyl Ct., Woodbridge, ONT L4L 4A3 Canada

Stryker Spine 866-457-7463
2 Pearl Ct, Allendale, NJ 07401

Zimmer Holdings, Inc. 800-613-6131
1800 W Center St, PO Box 708, Warsaw, IN 46580

CEMENT, STOMAL APPLIANCE, OSTOMY
(Gastro/Urology) 78EZR

Biomed Laboratories, Inc. 972-282-8008
11910 Shiloh Rd Ste 142, Dallas, TX 75228

Hollister, Inc. 847-680-2849
366 Draft Ave, Stuarts Draft, VA 24477

CEMENT, STOMAL APPLIANCE, OSTOMY *(cont'd)*

Ldb Medical, Inc. 800-243-2554
2909 Langford Rd Ste B500, Norcross, GA 30071
LAPIDES.

Old 97 Co. 813-247-6677
2306 N 35th St, Tampa, FL 33605
Stomal appliance cement.

Smith & Nephew, Inc. 800-876-1261
11775 Starkey Rd, Largo, FL 33773
SKIN-BOND and SKIN-HESIVE cements.

Torbot Group, Inc. 800-545-4254
1367 Elmwood Ave, Cranston, RI 02910

Xennovate Medical Llc 765-939-2037
1080 University Blvd, Richmond, IN 47374
Ostomy adhesive.

CENTRIFUGE, BLOOD BANK, DIAGNOSTIC *(Hematology) 81KSO*

Beckman Coulter, Inc. 800-742-2345
250 S Kraemer Blvd, PO Box 8000, Brea, CA 92821

Micro Typing Systems, Inc. 908-218-8177
1295 SW 29th Ave, Pompano Beach, FL 33069
Centrifuge.

Novosci Corp. 281-363-4949
2828 N Crescentridge Dr, The Woodlands, TX 77381

Ortho-Clinical Diagnostics, Inc. 800-828-6316
513 Technology Blvd, Rochester, NY 14626
Blood bank test system.

Pro Scientific Inc. 800-584-3776
99 Willenbrock Rd, Oxford, CT 06478

Thermo Fisher Scientific (Asheville) Llc 828-658-4400
275 Aiken Rd, Asheville, NC 28804

Thermo Fisher Scientific - Laboratory Equipment Division Headquarters 800-662-7477
450 Fortune Blvd, Milford, MA 01757

CENTRIFUGE, CELL WASHING *(Hematology) 81JQC*

Biomet, Inc. 574-267-6639
56 E Bell Dr, PO Box 587, Warsaw, IN 46582
Platelet separation kits.

Cardiogenesis Corp. 800-238-2205
11 Musick, Irvine, CA 92618
General purpose centrifuge for clinical use. - CELLERATOR PLATELET

Depuy Spine, Inc. 800-227-6633
325 Paramount Dr, Raynham, MA 02767
Centrifuges (micro, ultra, refrigerated) for clinical use.

Ericomp, Inc. 800-541-8471
10211 Pacific Mesa Blvd Ste 411, San Diego, CA 92121

Forsan Mfg. 201-391-4100
30 Craig Rd, Montvale, NJ 07645
Tabletop centrifuge.

Haemonetics Corp. 781-848-7100
400 Wood Rd, P.O.Box 9114, Braintree, MA 02184
Centrifugal red cell washing system.

Harvest Technologies, Corp. 508-732-7500
40 Grissom Rd Ste 100, Plymouth, MA 02360
General purpose centrifuge for laboratory use,hat kit.

Iris Sample Processing 800-782-8774
60 Glacier Dr, Westwood, MA 02090
Various models of general purpose centrifuges and accessories.

Kendro Laboratory Products 800-252-7100
308 Ridgefield Ct, Asheville, NC 28806

Medical Sales & Service Group 888-357-6520
10 Woodchester Dr, Acton, MA 01720

Sakura Finetek U.S.A., Inc. 800-725-8723
1750 W 214th St, Torrance, CA 90501
$6,500 for CYTO-TEK centrifuge.

Sarstedt, Inc. 800-257-5101
PO Box 468, 1025, St. James Church Road, Newton, NC 28658
Micro, Ultra, Refrigerated.

Thermo Fisher Scientific (Asheville) Llc 828-658-4400
275 Aiken Rd, Asheville, NC 28804

Thermo Fisher Scientific - Laboratory Equipment Division Headquarters 800-662-7477
450 Fortune Blvd, Milford, MA 01757

CENTRIFUGE, CELL WASHING *(cont'd)*

Vulcon Technologies 816-966-1212
718 Main St, Grandview, MO 64030
Clinical centrifuge.

CENTRIFUGE, CELL WASHING, AUTOMATED, IMMUNO-HEMATOLOGY *(Hematology) 81KSN*

Haemonetics Corp. 781-848-7100
400 Wood Rd, P.O.Box 9114, Braintree, MA 02184
Centrifugal red cell washing system.

Helmer, Inc. 800-743-5637
15425 Herriman Blvd, Noblesville, IN 46060
Automated Cell Washing System

Ortho-Clinical Diagnostics, Inc. 800-828-6316
513 Technology Blvd, Rochester, NY 14626
Cell washing system.

Thermo Fisher Scientific - Laboratory Equipment Division Headquarters 800-662-7477
450 Fortune Blvd, Milford, MA 01757

CENTRIFUGE, CONTINUOUS FLOW *(Chemistry) 75UKI*

Alfa Laval Inc 866-253-2528
955 Mearns Rd, Warminster, PA 18974

Beckman Coulter, Inc. 800-742-2345
250 S Kraemer Blvd, PO Box 8000, Brea, CA 92821

Haemonetics Corp. 800-225-5242
400 Wood Rd, P.O. Box 9114, Braintree, MA 02184
(MICRO, ULTRA, REFRIGERATED) FOR CLINICAL USE

Thermo Fisher Scientific - Laboratory Equipment Division Headquarters 800-662-7477
450 Fortune Blvd, Milford, MA 01757

CENTRIFUGE, EXPLOSION-PROOF *(Chemistry) 75UKJ*

Alfa Laval Inc 866-253-2528
955 Mearns Rd, Warminster, PA 18974

Thermo Fisher Scientific - Laboratory Equipment Division Headquarters 800-662-7477
450 Fortune Blvd, Milford, MA 01757

CENTRIFUGE, FLOOR *(Pathology) 88QJA*

Beckman Coulter, Inc. 800-635-3497
740 W 83rd St, Hialeah, FL 33014

Beckman Coulter, Inc. 800-742-2345
250 S Kraemer Blvd, PO Box 8000, Brea, CA 92821

Global Focus (G.F.M.D. Ltd.) 800-527-2320
2280 Springlake Rd Ste 106, Dallas, TX 75234
SILENCER centrifuge.

Kendro Laboratory Products 800-252-7100
308 Ridgefield Ct, Asheville, NC 28806

Pro Scientific Inc. 800-584-3776
99 Willenbrock Rd, Oxford, CT 06478
Hettich has a range of floor/underbench centrifuges including the Rotanta 46 RC (capacity 4x750ml), Rotanta 46 RSC Robotic (capacity 4x750ml)and the Rotixa 50S (capacity 4x1000ml).

Thermo Fisher Scientific - Laboratory Equipment Division Headquarters 800-662-7477
450 Fortune Blvd, Milford, MA 01757
Centrifuges, benchtop and floor models.

CENTRIFUGE, GENERAL (OVER 5,000 RPM) *(Toxicology) 91DOT*

Beckman Coulter, Inc. 800-635-3497
740 W 83rd St, Hialeah, FL 33014

Beckman Coulter, Inc. 800-742-2345
250 S Kraemer Blvd, PO Box 8000, Brea, CA 92821

Kendro Laboratory Products 800-252-7100
308 Ridgefield Ct, Asheville, NC 28806

Medical Sales & Service Group 888-357-6520
10 Woodchester Dr, Acton, MA 01720

Pro Scientific Inc. 800-584-3776
99 Willenbrock Rd, Oxford, CT 06478
The complete range of Hettich centrifuges from micro to macro, from tabletop to floor standing are available to meet your needs.

Separation Technology Inc 800-777-6668
1096 Rainer Dr, Altamonte Springs, FL 32714
PlasmaPrep Centrifuge provides STAT plasma/serum separation in 2 minutes or platelet-rich plasma in 30 seconds. Additional 3-minute spin cycle. 6-place rotor. Uses 2-, 3-, 5-, 7-, and 10-mL collection tubes. Automatic out-of-balance shutdown.

CENTRIFUGE, GENERAL (OVER 5,000 RPM) *(cont'd)*

Statspin, Inc. 800-782-8774
60 Glacier Dr, Westwood, MA 02090
15,000 rpm STATSPIN MP for rapid plasma prep; 120-second hematocrits; lipemia clearing with LIPOCLEAR; total of 6 application-specific cycles.

Thermo Fisher Scientific - Laboratory Equipment Division Headquarters 800-662-7477
450 Fortune Blvd, Milford, MA 01757

CENTRIFUGE, GENERAL (UP TO 5,000 RPM) *(Pathology) 88KDR*

Alfa Laval Inc 866-253-2528
955 Mearns Rd, Warminster, PA 18974

Appropriate Technical Resources, Inc. 800-827-5931
9157 Whiskey Bottom Rd, PO Box 460, Laurel, MD 20723

Beckman Coulter, Inc. 800-742-2345
250 S Kraemer Blvd, PO Box 8000, Brea, CA 92821

Cygnus Inc. 973-523-0668
510 E 41st St, Paterson, NJ 07504

Helmer, Inc. 800-743-5637
15425 Herriman Blvd, Noblesville, IN 46060
Complete Line of Centrifuges

Kendro Laboratory Products 800-252-7100
308 Ridgefield Ct, Asheville, NC 28806

Lw Scientific 800-726-7345
865 Marathon Pkwy, Lawrenceville, GA 30046
The new Straight 8 series of horizontal swing-out centrifuges meets the demands for low-cost, high-performance, straight-line separations in clinics and labs. Higher g-forces and a compact gel line eliminates respins and re-mixing and improves lab efficiency. With variable speed control, the Straight 8 series will also spin other fluids such as urine, semen, and fecal floatations, and the digital tachometer will ensure samples are spun at the correct g-forces.

Medical Sales & Service Group 888-357-6520
10 Woodchester Dr, Acton, MA 01720

Pro Scientific Inc. 800-584-3776
99 Willenbrock Rd, Oxford, CT 06478
The complete range of Hettich centrifuges from micro to macro, from tabletop to floor standing are available to meet your needs.

Statspin, Inc. 800-782-8774
60 Glacier Dr, Westwood, MA 02090
STATSPIN EXPRESS 2. Primary Tube Centrifuge produces platelet-poor plasma in two minutes. Accepts standard 5-mL blood tubes.

Thermo Fisher Scientific - Laboratory Equipment Division Headquarters 800-662-7477
450 Fortune Blvd, Milford, MA 01757

Ward's Natural Science Establishment, Inc. 800-962-2660
PO Box 92912, 5100 W. Henrietta Rd., Rochester, NY 14692

CENTRIFUGE, HEMATOCRIT *(Hematology) 81GKG*

Bd Diagnostic Systems 800-675-0908
7 Loveton Cir, Sparks, MD 21152

Beckman Coulter, Inc. 800-742-2345
250 S Kraemer Blvd, PO Box 8000, Brea, CA 92821

Iris Sample Processing 800-782-8774
60 Glacier Dr, Westwood, MA 02090
Centrifuge and accessories.

Lw Scientific 800-726-7345
865 Marathon Pkwy, Lawrenceville, GA 30046
Models include the M-24 24-place microhematocrit centrifuge and the M-24-Combo, a combination microhematocrit and test-tube centrifuge.

Plaza Medical, Inc. 877-695-4441
9780 E Girard Ave, Denver, CO 80231
$795.00 per unit.

Pro Scientific Inc. 800-584-3776
99 Willenbrock Rd, Oxford, CT 06478
Hematocrit determination with standard capillaries is carried out in the Haematokrit 20 or Mikro 20, with the segmented 24-place rotor. Every capillary has its own segment or chamber. The lid of the rotor is evaluation disc and cover in one. Another rotor model taking 20 capillaries for quantitative buffy coat analysis is also available.

Thermo Fisher Scientific - Laboratory Equipment Division Headquarters 800-662-7477
450 Fortune Blvd, Milford, MA 01757

CENTRIFUGE, MICROHEMATOCRIT *(Hematology) 81QJB*

Beckman Coulter, Inc. 800-742-2345
250 S Kraemer Blvd, PO Box 8000, Brea, CA 92821

Brinkmann Instruments (Canada) Ltd. 800-263-8715
6670 Campobello Rd., Mississauga, ONT L5N 2L8 Canada

Pro Scientific Inc. 800-584-3776
99 Willenbrock Rd, Oxford, CT 06478
Hematocrit determination with standard capillaries is carried out in the Haematokrit 20 or Mikro 20, with the segmented 24-place rotor. Every capillary has its own segment or chamber. The lid of the rotor is evaluation disc and cover in one. Another rotor model taking 20 capillaries for quantitative buffy coat analysis is also available.

Separation Technology Inc 800-777-6668
1096 Rainer Dr, Altamonte Springs, FL 32714
HemataSTAT provides a quantitative hematocrit in 60 seconds. Built-in digital tube reader. Built-in tachometer. Low cost per test. Quiet. Spins up to 6 samples at a time. Optional battery pack for field use. Disposable tube holders in case of sealant blowout. Gasket seal for user protection from aerosols. Displays in 5 languages.

Statspin, Inc. 800-782-8774
60 Glacier Dr, Westwood, MA 02090
CRITSPIN uHCT 120-second microhematocrit centrifuge, sample sizes: less than 10 microliters, volume not critical.

Thermo Fisher Scientific - Laboratory Equipment Division Headquarters 800-662-7477
450 Fortune Blvd, Milford, MA 01757

United Products & Instruments, Inc. 800-588-9776
182 Ridge Rd Ste E, Dayton, NJ 08810
Unico® Model C-MH30 is made of formed metal and has a baked paint application that is acid and reagent resistant. A safety switch built into the handle assembly disconnects the power to the motor whenever the latch is lifted. The hematocrit tray is made of plastic composite material backed by an aluminum shell for durability and lighter weight. The brushed motor is mounted on rubber mounts to provide quite running and less vibration. Visit us at www.unico1.com for more information on this and other lab instruments from UNICO

CENTRIFUGE, MICROSEDIMENTATION *(Hematology) 81GHK*

Brinkmann Instruments (Canada) Ltd. 800-263-8715
6670 Campobello Rd., Mississauga, ONT L5N 2L8 Canada

Thermo Fisher Scientific - Laboratory Equipment Division Headquarters 800-662-7477
450 Fortune Blvd, Milford, MA 01757

CENTRIFUGE, REFRIGERATED *(Pathology) 88QJC*

Alfa Laval Inc 866-253-2528
955 Mearns Rd, Warminster, PA 18974

Beckman Coulter, Inc. 800-742-2345
250 S Kraemer Blvd, PO Box 8000, Brea, CA 92821

Global Focus (G.F.M.D. Ltd.) 800-527-2320
2280 Springlake Rd Ste 106, Dallas, TX 75234
SILENCER centrifuge. Also, nonrefrigerated.

Kendro Laboratory Products 800-252-7100
308 Ridgefield Ct, Asheville, NC 28806

Pro Scientific Inc. 800-584-3776
99 Willenbrock Rd, Oxford, CT 06478
Hettich has a full range of refrigerated centrifuge, including the Mikro 22R (capacity 60x1.5/2ml and 6x50ml), Universal 32R (capacity 4x100ml, Rotina 35R (capacity 4x100ml), Rotina 46R (capacity 4x650ml), Rotanta 46R (capacity 4x750ml)and the Rotixa 50RS (capacity 4x1000ml).

Thermo Fisher Scientific - Laboratory Equipment Division Headquarters 800-662-7477
450 Fortune Blvd, Milford, MA 01757

CENTRIFUGE, TABLETOP *(Pathology) 88QJD*

Beckman Coulter, Inc. 800-635-3497
740 W 83rd St, Hialeah, FL 33014

Beckman Coulter, Inc. 800-742-2345
250 S Kraemer Blvd, PO Box 8000, Brea, CA 92821

Global Focus (G.F.M.D. Ltd.) 800-527-2320
2280 Springlake Rd Ste 106, Dallas, TX 75234
SILENCER centrifuge.

Kendro Laboratory Products 800-252-7100
308 Ridgefield Ct, Asheville, NC 28806

CENTRIFUGE, TABLETOP *(cont'd)*

Lw Scientific 800-726-7345
865 Marathon Pkwy, Lawrenceville, GA 30046
The Ultra tabletop centrifuge models include the U8F-fixed speed, U8V-variable speed, U8S-selectable speed, and U8T with digital tachometer. The Combo V24 centrifuge accepts different rotors for hematocrits, test tubes, and microtubes.

Medical Sales & Service Group 888-357-6520
10 Woodchester Dr, Acton, MA 01720

Pro Scientific Inc. 800-584-3776
99 Willenbrock Rd, Oxford, CT 06478
There is a wide range of Hettich tabletop centrifuges (some with optional refrigeration) available from the; EBA 20 (capacity 8x15ml), EBA 21 (capacity 6x50ml, Haematokrit 20 (24 capillaries), Mikro 20 (capacity 30x.2ml), Mikro 22 (capacity 60x1.5/2ml), Rotofix 32 (capacity 4x100ml), Universal 32 (capacity 4x100ml), Rotina 35 (capacity 4x100ml), Rotina 46 (capacity 4x650ml) and the Rotanta 46 (capacity 4x750ml).

Separation Technology Inc 800-777-6668
1096 Rainer Dr, Altamonte Springs, FL 32714
Micro-12 microcentrifuge has variable speed to 10,000 rpm/7,176 X g. Accommodates twelve 1.5-, 0.5-, 0.4-, and 0.2-mL tubes. Use for quick spin downs, microfiltration, and small-volume blood separations. Quiet, cool running.

Thermo Fisher Scientific - Laboratory Equipment Division Headquarters 800-662-7477
450 Fortune Blvd, Milford, MA 01757

Thermo Savant 800-634-8886
100 Colin Dr, Holbrook, NY 11741
Low cost refrigerated microcentrifuge (SPEEDFUGE) is compact, extremely quiet. Benchtop centrifuge accommodates centrifugal filtration/concentration devices and standard tubes.

Ubs Instruments Corporation 818-710-1195
7745 Alabama Ave Ste 7, Canoga Park, CA 91304
Mobile and desktop centrifuges for physicians and medical examiners.

United Products & Instruments, Inc. 800-588-9776
182 Ridge Rd Ste E, Dayton, NJ 08810
UNICO is proud to introduce powerful and economical new benchtop centrifuges, the PowerSpin Series. The UNICO PowerSpin LX spins at 4000 RPM, insur ing a clean, more complete separation of cellular components thus yielding a superior serum or plasma specimen. The PowerSpin Series entrifuges are extremely quiet for a better working environment. All PowerSpin models feature maintenance-free brushless motors and have a safety lid latch, timer, on/ off switch as well as other features that are normally only found on units costing much more. For more information on this and other instruments from UNICO please visit us at www.unico1.com

CEPHALOMETER *(Dental And Oral) 76EAG*

Barton Matthew, Inc. 734-420-2326
11251 N Ridge Rd, Plymouth, MI 48170
Wall mounted, low cost, cephalostat for exisitng dental operatories.

Margraf Dental Manufacturing, Inc. 800-762-2641
611 Harper Ave, Jenkintown, PA 19046
Cephalometric system.

Wehmer Corporation 800-323-0229
1151 N Main St, Lombard, IL 60148
4 models available - wall mounted units start at $1,650; counterbalanced stand units start at $3,850- X-ray equipment is not included. $3,100 for mobile cephalometer; $995.00 for electric cephalometry chair.

CERAMICS, TRIPHOS./HYDROXYAPATITE, CA. (NON-LOAD BEARING) *(Orthopedics) 87LMN*

Gyrus Ent L.L.C., Sub. Of Gyrus Acmi, Inc. 508-804-2739
2925 Appling Rd, Bartlett, TN 38133
Various types and sizes of hydroxypatite blocks.

CERCLAGE, FIXATION *(Orthopedics) 87JDQ*

Abbott Spine, Inc. 847-937-6100
12708 Riata Vista Cir Ste B-100, Austin, TX 78727
Metallic bone fixaton appliance or cable.

Acumed Llc 503-627-9957
5885 NW Cornelius Pass Rd, Hillsboro, OR 97124
Cerlage,fixation (wire & cable).

Arthrex, Inc. 239-643-5553
1370 Creekside Blvd, Naples, FL 34108
Cerclage kit for orthopedic uses.

CERCLAGE, FIXATION *(cont'd)*

Biomet, Inc. 574-267-6639
56 E Bell Dr, PO Box 587, Warsaw, IN 46582
Parham band.

Pioneer Surgical Technology 800-557-9909
375 River Park Cir, Marquette, MI 49855

Stryker Spine 866-457-7463
2 Pearl Ct, Allendale, NJ 07401

Synthes (Usa) 610-719-5000
35 Airport Rd, Horseheads, NY 14845
Various types and sizes of cerclage wires.

Warsaw Orthopedic, Inc. 901-396-3133
2500 Silveus Xing, Warsaw, IN 46582
Cable devices-sterile and non-sterile.

Zimmer Holdings, Inc. 800-613-6131
1800 W Center St, PO Box 708, Warsaw, IN 46580

CHAIR, ADJUSTABLE, MECHANICAL *(Physical Med) 89INN*

Activeaid, Inc. 800-533-5330
101 Activeaid Rd, Redwood Falls, MN 56283
Carechair pediatric reclining commode.

American Massage Products, Inc. 716-934-2648
341 Central Ave, Silver Creek, NY 14136
Heat and massage reclining chair - electrical; ac-powered.

Arjo, Inc. 800-323-1245
50 Gary Ave Ste A, Roselle, IL 60172

Biofit Engineered Products 800-597-0246
PO Box 109, Waterville, OH 43566
BIOFIT, ergonomic chairs for anesthesiologists, O.R. nurses, and surgeons (BT, BE, EE series). 25 models. Chairs with ergonomic backrests, backrest tilt controls, and pneumatic seat-height adjustments.

Care Products Inc. 757-224-0177
10701 N Ware Rd, McAllen, TX 78504
Various models of mechanical adjustable chairs.

Chattanooga Group 800-592-7329
4717 Adams Rd, Hixson, TN 37343
For cervical traction.

Community Products, Llc 845-658-7723
2032 Route 213, Rifton, NY 12471
Bath chair, chair, commode.

Community Products, Llc 845-658-7723
Platte Clove Rd., Elka Park, NY 12427

Daystar Manufacturing, Incorporated 620-342-4440
3701 W 6th Ave, Emporia, KS 66801
Folding chair with pneumatically adjustable seat height.

Ergogenesis, Llc 800-364-5299
1 Bodybilt Pl, Navasota, TX 77868
Ergonomic chair.

Gillette Children's Specialty Healthcare 612-229-3805
200 University Ave E, Saint Paul, MN 55101
Sitting support orthosis.

Global Surgical Corp. 314-861-3388
3610 Tree Court Industrial Blvd, Saint Louis, MO 63122
H-chair.

Healthpostures, Llc 320-864-4359
2725 12th St E, Glencoe, MN 55336
Adjustable angle support chair.

Hill-Rom Holdings, Inc. 800-445-3730
1069 State Road 46 E, Batesville, IN 47006

Hill-Rom, Inc. 812-934-7777
4115 Dorchester Rd Unit 600, North Charleston, SC 29405
Chair (various).

Intarsia Ltd. 203-355-1357
14 Martha Ln, Gaylordsville, CT 06755
Insert, tot chair, totchair ii.

Invincible Office Furniture Co. 800-558-4417
PO Box 1117, Manitowoc, WI 54221

Kaye Products, Inc. 919-732-6444
535 Dimmocks Mill Rd, Hillsborough, NC 27278
Posture control system to add to adjustable bench to maintain alignment of pelvis and lower extremities to improve sitting posture. Also, adjustable, mechanical bolster, corner, and other chairs.

Ki-Add Specialized Support Technology, Inc. 920-468-8100
6500 Avalon Blvd, Los Angeles, CA 90003
Patient chairs with accesories.

CHAIR, ADJUSTABLE, MECHANICAL *(cont'd)*

L.P.A. Medical, Inc. 888-845-6447
460 Desrochers, Ste. 150D, Vanier, QUEBE G1M 1C2 Canada
Optimum Posturo-Pedic positioning chair, Series 1000.

La-Z-Boy Incorporated 734-242-1444
1284 N Telegraph Rd, Monroe, MI 48162
La-z-boy.

Laszlo Corp. 314-830-3222
2573 Millvalley Dr, Florissant, MO 63031
Attachment for wheeled chair.

Leland Manufacturing Llc 812-367-1761
1300 N Broad St, Leland, Leland, MS 38756

Made Rite Rocker Inc. 203-723-5600
44 Gorman St, Naugatuck, CT 06770
Made rite chair.

Mjm International Corporation 956-781-5000
2003 N Veterans Blvd Ste 10, San Juan, TX 78589
Various models of mechanical adjustable chairs.

Physiomedics Manufacturing, Llc 952-201-1463
15320 Minnetonka Blvd Ste 104, Minnetonka, MN 55345
Adjustable mechanical chair.

Quantum Medical Imaging, Llc 631-567-5800
2002 Orville Dr N Ste B, Ronkonkoma, NY 11779
Positioning chair.

Rifton Equipment 800-571-8198
PO Box 260, Rifton, NY 12471
Adjustable chairs, corner sitter, advancement chair, therapeutic seating, and accessible desk.

The Anthros Medical Group 785-544-6592
807 E Spring St, Highland, KS 66035
Tilt in space chair.

Tumble Forms, Inc. 262-387-8720
1013 Barker Rd, Dolgeville, NY 13329
Multiple.

Vms Rehab Systems, Inc. 800-731-8482
2487 Kaladar Ave., Unit 106, Ottawa K1V 8B9 Canada
Alda chair

CHAIR, BATH *(General) 80QJF*

Activeaid, Inc. 800-533-5330
101 Activeaid Rd, Redwood Falls, MN 56283
The Tubby II folding bath bench provides a reversible and foldable chair for tub use. It is padded for comfort and based on an all-steel frame for strength and stability.

Allman Products 800-223-6889
21101 Itasca St, Chatsworth, CA 91311
Bath benches.

Alsons Corp. 800-421-0001
3010 Mechanic Rd, P.O. Box 282, Hillsdale, MI 49242

Arjo, Inc. 800-323-1245
50 Gary Ave Ste A, Roselle, IL 60172

Columbia Medical Manufacturing Llc 800-454-6612
13577 Larwin Cir, Santa Fe Springs, CA 90670
Columbia Medical SureTrans Omni and Elite Reclining Transfer Systems are multi-functional transfer systems that provide positioning, slide over the tub for use in the bath and can be used as a roll-in shower chair. The Omni can also be used as a commode or toileting seat.

Convaquip Industries, Inc. 800-637-8436
4834 Derrick Dr, PO Box 3417, Abilene, TX 79601
Bariatric; weight certified to 650 lb. Also Tub Transfer Bench, Bariatric, weight certified to 850 lb.

Flaghouse, Inc. 800-793-7900
601 US Highway 46 W, Hasbrouck Heights, NJ 07604

Home Aid Products 888-823-7605
111 Esna Park Dr., Unit 9, Markham, ONT L3R-1H2 Canada
Bath safety seats, various heights and models. Transfer benches with padded or blow-molded seats.

Invacare Corporation 800-333-6900
1 Invacare Way, Elyria, OH 44035
INVACARE.

Invacare Supply Group, An Invacare Co. 800-225-4792
75 October Hill Rd, Holliston, MA 01746
Carry full line of bath safety products from: Invacare, Rubbermaid, & TFI.

Maddak Inc. 800-443-4926
661 State Route 23, Wayne, NJ 07470

CHAIR, BATH *(cont'd)*

Parsons A.D.L. Inc. 800-263-1281
R.R. #2, 1986 Sideroad 15, Tottenham, ONT L0G 1W0 Canada
A variety of bath chairs of various heights, bath boards, bath lifts and other bathing accessories

Rifton Equipment 800-571-8198
PO Box 260, Rifton, NY 12471
3 sizes of bath chair with option of soft fabric or nylon fabric. Tub stand or shower stand available.

Sunrise Medical 800-333-4000
7477 Dry Creek Pkwy, Longmont, CO 80503

TFI Healthcare 800-526-0178
600 W Wythe St, Petersburg, VA 23803
Bath bench: Model #4325 without back, Model #4310 with back; also, heavy duty bath bench Model #4328/1 without back, maximum weight 500 lbs.

Tuffcare 800-367-6160
3999 E La Palma Ave, Anaheim, CA 92807

Wenzelite Rehab Supplies, Llc 800-706-9255
220 36th St, 99 Seaview Blvd, Brooklyn, NY 11232
The DOLPHIN BATH CHAIR features an aluminum frame covered in a removable mesh fabric, adjustable positioning belts and headrest and an angle adjustable seat and back. A height adjustable base is available. The OTTER BATH CHAIR features a plastic frame, height adjustable legs, positioning & leg straps and head cushions. The seat and back are angle adjustable. A height adjustable Tub Stand is available.

Whitehall Manufacturing 800-782-7706
15125 Proctor Ave, City Of Industry, CA 91746

CHAIR, BIRTHING *(Obstetrics/Gyn) 85QJG*

Bryton Corp. 800-567-9500
4310 Guion Rd, Indianapolis, IN 46254
Birthing Chairs new, preowned & remanufactured, replacement mattresses, mattress Comfi-Toppers, etc

Lic Care 800-323-5232
2935A Northeast Pkwy, Atlanta, GA 30360

CHAIR, BLOOD DONOR *(General) 80FML*

American Massage Products, Inc. 716-934-2648
341 Central Ave, Silver Creek, NY 14136
Massage, adjustable electric bed.

Brandt Industries, Inc. 800-221-8031
4461 Bronx Blvd, Bronx, NY 10470
20700 and 20701: with and without drawers.

Custom Comfort Medtek 800-749-0933
3939 Forsyth Rd Ste A, Winter Park, FL 32792
Custom blood-donor chairs chairs come in different heights, widths, and colors (18 to choose from) and are available in reclining, hydraulic, foldable, or stackable models.

Dacor Manufacturing Co., Inc. 618-939-8700
8718 Hanover Industrial Dr, Columbia, IL 62236

Major Lab. Manufacturing 800-598-2621
4408 N Sewell Ave, Oklahoma City, OK 73118
Specimen drawing, 7 models - $416.00 to $557.00 each.

Mobile Designs, Inc. 530-244-1050
4650 Caterpillar Rd, Redding, CA 96003
Blood donor chair.

Pisces Productions, Inc. 707-829-1496
380 Morris St Ste A, Sebastopol, CA 95472
Donor table.

S&W By Hausmann 888-428-7626
130 Union St, Northvale, NJ 07647

Winco, Inc. 800-237-3377
5516 SW 1st Ln, Ocala, FL 34474
Chairs.

CHAIR, BLOOD DRAWING *(General) 80WZB*

Biodex Medical Systems, Inc. 800-224-6339
20 Ramsey Rd, Shirley, NY 11967

Covidien Lp 508-261-8000
15 Hampshire St, Mansfield, MA 02048

Custom Comfort Medtek 800-749-0933
3939 Forsyth Rd Ste A, Winter Park, FL 32792
Custom blood-donor chairs chairs come in different heights, widths, and colors (18 to choose from) and are available in reclining, hydraulic, foldable, or stackable models.

CHAIR, BLOOD DRAWING *(cont'd)*

Enochs Examining Room Furniture, Inc. 800-428-2305
PO Box 50559, Indianapolis, IN 46250
$698.00 per unit (standard).

Labconco Corp. 800-821-5525
8811 Prospect Ave, Kansas City, MO 64132
Three models available ó Single Chair, Single Chair with Side Cabinet or Double Chair with Cabinet in between.

Mayo Medical, S.A. De C.V. 800-715-3872
Edison 1141 Nte., Col. Talleres, Monterrey N.L. 64480 Mexico

Schueler & Company, Inc. 516-487-1500
PO Box 528, Stratford, CT 06615

United Metal Fabricators, Inc. 800-638-5322
1316 Eisenhower Blvd, Johnstown, PA 15904
Blood drawing chair with or without drawer.

CHAIR, DENTAL *(Dental And Oral) 76QJH*

Alliance H. Inc Dentech Equipment 360-988-7080
901 W Front St, Sumas, WA 98295
Swivel, remote infrared foot control, Trendelenbourg position, 12 designer color, 5-year warranty.

American Biomed Instruments, Inc. 718-235-8900
11 Wyona St, Brooklyn, NY 11207

Beaverstate Dental, Inc. 800-237-2303
115 S Elliott Rd, Newberg, OR 97132

Dansereau Health Products, Inc. 800-423-5657
250 E Harrison St, Corona, CA 92879
$1,795.00 for CALIFORNIAN chair. $2,195.00 for NEW AM2 - CHAIR AMERICA.

Dentalez Group 866-DTE-INFO
101 Lindenwood Dr Ste 225, Valleybrooke Corporate Center Malvern, PA 19355

Dentsply Canada, Ltd. 800-263-1437
161 Vinyl Ct., Woodbridge, ONT L4L 4A3 Canada

Dexta Corporation 800-733-3982
962 Kaiser Rd, Napa, CA 94558
Orthodontic and other dental patient chairs.

Dntlworks Equipment Corporation 800-847-0694
7300 S Tucson Way, Centennial, CO 80112
Six models of portable patient chairs are available. Two chairs have a foot-pump-type hydraulic base, and four are scissors-leg based. Select from Supreme, Basic, UltraLite, or ProLite PDC models depending on your needs. Chair weights range from 68 lb down to 29 lb.

Forest Dental Products Inc 800-423-3535
6200 NE Campus Ct, Hillsboro, OR 97124

Galaxy Medical Manufacturing Co. 800-876-4599
5411 Sheila St, Commerce, CA 90040
Dental examination x-ray chairs.

Health Science Products, Inc. 800-237-5794
1489 Hueytown Rd, Hueytown, AL 35023
INTEGRA ergonomically designed for patient comfort and for the proper chairside body position, posture and direct vision of the dentist and the assistant.

J. Morita Usa, Inc. 888-566-7482
9 Mason, Irvine, CA 92618
SPACELINE FEEL 21 patient support and delivery system is developed to prevent unnecessary musculoskeletal stress during daily practice. The bio-mechanically derived design meets the highest standards of ergonomics. This helps to reduce back, neck, shoulder, arm, and hand ailments, which impair both clinicians' health and the potential to achieve peak performance. The effortless access to instruments improves the operator's productivity. With one light directed to the mandible and the other to the maxilla, the touchless fixed twin lights are intended to eliminate any need to adjust the lights while reducing cross-contamination.

Link Ergonomics Corp. 800-424-5465
902 E 4th St, Joplin, MO 64801
LINK dental stools for dentist and assistant.

Mastercraft Dental Co. Of Texas 972-775-8757
880 Eastgate Rd, P.O. Box 882, Midlothian, TX 76065
Orthodontic chair w/power back.

Midmark Corporation 800-643-6275
60 Vista Dr, P.O. Box 286, Versailles, OH 45380

Mobile Dental Equipment Corp.(M-Dec) 425-747-5424
13300 SE 30th St Ste 101, Bellevue, WA 98005
Portable, lightweight, dental patient chair. $1395.

CHAIR, DENTAL *(cont'd)*

Pelton & Crane Co., 704-588-2126
11727 Fruehauf Dr, Charlotte, NC 28273
SPIRIT 3000 ,SPIRIT 2000 and SPIRIT 1500.

Planmeca U.S.A. Inc 630-529-2300
100 Gary Ave Ste A, Roselle, IL 60172
PLANMECA Dental Chair

Royal Dental Manufacturing, Inc. 425-743-0988
12414 Highway 99, Everett, WA 98204
$5,090.00 for Model R16; $3,490.00 for Model GP2; $2,050.00 for Model OR2; $2,820.00 for Model OR2S; $1,700.00 for Model OR2M; $6,250.00 for Signet Model 2230, $5,190.00 for Signet Model 2210;$6,990.00 for Domain Model 2250,hydraulic; $6,390.00 for Domain Model 2240, electro-mechanical.

Schueler & Company, Inc. 516-487-1500
PO Box 528, Stratford, CT 06615

Sds (Summit Dental Systems) 800-275-3368
3560 NW 53rd Ct, Fort Lauderdale, FL 33309

CHAIR, DENTAL (WITH UNIT) *(Dental And Oral) 76KLC*

A-Dec, Inc. 800-547-1883
2601 Crestview Dr, Newberg, OR 97132
A-dec dental chair.

Boyd Industries, Inc.
12900 44th St N, Clearwater, FL 33762
Various dental chairs without units.

Craftmaster Contour Equipment, Inc. 817-568-9260
6900 South Fwy Ste B9, Ft Worth, TX 76134
Contour ii chair and deanna chair on power base.

Dansereau Health Products, Inc. 800-423-5657
250 E Harrison St, Corona, CA 92879
CLINIC SERIES - $3,695.00 to $3,995.00. CHAIR AMERICA SERIES - $3,895.00 to $4,495.00. CALIFORNIA ORTHODONTIC SERIES - $2,995.00 to $3,995.00.

Dentalez Of Alabama 251-937-6781
2500 S US Highway 31, Bay Minette, AL 36507
Chair, dental.

Engle Dental Systems, Inc. 503-359-9390
4115 24th Ave Ste A, Forest Grove, OR 97116
The Sequoia dental chair is a hydraulically driven chair featuring five user-programmable positions, roughly 17 in. of vertical lift, 360× rotation, thin back with lumbar support, and an adjustable double-articulating headrest.

Forest Dental Products Inc 800-423-3535
6200 NE Campus Ct, Hillsboro, OR 97124

Kavo Dental Manufacturing Inc 202-828-0850
901 W Oakton St, Des Plaines, IL 60018
Various models of dental chairs and accessories.

Midmark Corporation 800-643-6275
60 Vista Dr, P.O. Box 286, Versailles, OH 45380

Pelton & Crane 704-588-2126
11727 Fruehauf Dr, Charlotte, NC 28273
Dental chairs and accessories.

Pelton & Crane Co., 704-588-2126
11727 Fruehauf Dr, Charlotte, NC 28273
SPIRIT 1500 AND SPIRIT 2000.

Planmeca U.S.A. Inc 630-529-2300
100 Gary Ave Ste A, Roselle, IL 60172
Compact dental units

Sds (Summit Dental Systems) 800-275-3368
3560 NW 53rd Ct, Fort Lauderdale, FL 33309

CHAIR, DENTAL, WITHOUT OPERATIVE UNIT
(Dental And Oral) 76NRU

Klean N Konstant Dental Water Company, Llc 205-422-3904
2204 Longleaf Blvd, Vestavia, AL 35243
Dental unit waterline cleanser.

United Medical Enterprises 757-224-0177
4049 Allen Station Rd, Augusta, GA 30906
Dental chair head rest cover.

CHAIR, DIALYSIS (WITH SCALE) *(Gastro/Urology) 78WQV*

Scale-Tronix, Inc. 800-873-2001
200 E Post Rd, White Plains, NY 10601
Under-chair dialysis scale with electronic scale; $2,495 for single station, $4,495, for twin station. Chair not included.

CHAIR, DIALYSIS, POWERED (WITHOUT SCALE)
(Gastro/Urology) 78FKS

G.E.M. Water Systems, Int'L., Llc 800-755-1707
6351 Orangethorpe Ave, Buena Park, CA 90620

CHAIR, DIALYSIS, UNPOWERED (WITHOUT SCALE)
(Gastro/Urology) 78FIA

Diasol, Inc. 800-366-0546
13212 Raymer St, North Hollywood, CA 91605
Dialysis chair. 33, 35, or 37 in., with two side tables and casters, Trendelenburg position. Removable arm for easy transfer of wheelchair-bound patients. Heat and massage options available. Daisy--Protected Butterfly (19-256A) protected fistula needle. 8-mm pre- and post-pump bloodlines.

G.E.M. Water Systems, Int'L., Llc 800-755-1707
6351 Orangethorpe Ave, Buena Park, CA 90620

Lee Medical International, Inc. 800-433-8950
612 Distributors Row, Harahan, LA 70123
Lumex chairs.

CHAIR, EXAMINATION AND TREATMENT *(General) 80FRK*

Brandt Industries, Inc. 800-221-8031
4461 Bronx Blvd, Bronx, NY 10470
23730: ent chair, general use. Treatment chairs. 23500 and 23110: mammography. 23030: other models.

Dansereau Health Products, Inc. 800-423-5657
250 E Harrison St, Corona, CA 92879
AMERICA Series: America 1 Op $3,895.00, America 2 Op $4,495.00, America 3 Op $4,295.00 and the America 4 Op $4,295.00

Dexta Corporation 800-733-3982
962 Kaiser Rd, Napa, CA 94558
$4,695 for multi-purpose chair unit.

Global Surgical Corp. 314-861-3388
3610 Tree Court Industrial Blvd, Saint Louis, MO 63122
Straight- back chair.

HAAG-STREIT USA, INC. 800-787-5426
3535 Kings Mills Rd, Mason, OH 45040
$4,985 to $1,195 for chair.

Jedmed Instruments Co. 314-845-3770
5416 Jedmed Ct, Saint Louis, MO 63129

Living Earth Crafts 800-358-8292
3210 Executive Rdg, Vista, CA 92081
SOMACHAIR, is a massage and examination chair.

Mayo Medical, S.A. De C.V. 800-715-3872
Edison 1141 Nte., Col. Talleres, Monterrey N.L. 64480 Mexico
Chaisse lounge.

Md International, Inc. 305-669-9003
11300 NW 41st St, Doral, FL 33178

Medical Technology Industries, Inc. 800-924-4655
3555 W 1500 S, Salt Lake City, UT 84104
Exam/treatment chairs.

Midmark Corporation 800-643-6275
60 Vista Dr, P.O. Box 286, Versailles, OH 45380

Pibbs Inc., P.S. 718-445-8046
133-15 32nd Ave., Flushing, NY 11354-4008

Profex Medical Products 800-325-0196
2224 E Person Ave, Memphis, TN 38114

Stille-Sonesta, Inc. 800-665-1614
1610 S Interstate 35E Ste 203, Carrollton, TX 75006

Stretchair Patient Transfer Systems, Inc, 800-237-1162
8110 Ulmerton Rd, Largo, FL 33771
PORTAZAM, portable/collapsible lightweight multi-functional exam chair. Designed specially for OB-GYN/Ultrasound.

Stryker Medical 800-869-0770
3800 E Centre Ave, Portage, MI 49002

Topcon Medical Systems, Inc. 800-223-1130
37 W Century Rd, Paramus, NJ 07652
Five ophthalmic chairs: $1,690.00, $1,990.00, $4,390.00, $5,390.00, and $5,790.00.

United Metal Fabricators, Inc. 800-638-5322
1316 Eisenhower Blvd, Johnstown, PA 15904
Adjustable height, head rest and reclining back to horizontal position. Industrial, ENT, podiatric, health service, examination and treatment chair. Also, manually or electro-hydraulically adjustable.

Wy'East Medical Corp. 503-657-3101
16700 SE 120th Ave, PO Box 1625, Clackamas, OR 97015
TC-300 Treatment Chair.

CHAIR, FLOTATION THERAPY *(General) 80QJI*
Pyramid Industries, Llc 888-343-3352
3911 Schaad Rd Unit 102, Knoxville, TN 37921
ACTIV-AIR BATTERY OPERATED ALTERNATING PRESSURE CHAIR CUSHION. Rechargeable battery lasts a minimum of 10 hours.

CHAIR, GERIATRIC *(General) 80FRJ*
A.R.C. Distributors 800-296-8724
PO Box 599, Centreville, MD 21617
INVACARE Traditional Three Position Recliner-exceptional comfort, durability & PRICE!! Recliner features upright sitting, elevated leg or full recline. Available in 6 colors.

Ac Healthcare Supply, Inc. 905-448-4706
11651 230th St, Cambria Heights, NY 11411
Medical chair and table.

Adden Furniture, Inc. 800-625-3876
26 Jackson St, Lowell, MA 01852

Basic American Medical Products 800-849-6664
2935A Northeast Pkwy, Atlanta, GA 30360

Broda Enterprises Inc. 800-668-0637
385 Phillip St., Waterloo, ONT N2L 5R8 Canada
BRODA SEATING.

Care Products Inc. 757-224-0177
10701 N Ware Rd, McAllen, TX 78504
Geriatric chair.

Colonial Scientific Ltd. 902-468-1811
201 Brownlow Ave., Unit 52, Dartmouth, NS B3B-1W2 Canada

Falcon Products, Inc. 800-873-3252
10650 Gateway Blvd, Saint Louis, MO 63132

Healthline Medical Products, Inc. 407-656-0704
1065 E Story Rd, Oakland, FL 34787

Invacare Corporation 800-333-6900
1 Invacare Way, Elyria, OH 44035
INVACARE.

Mjm International Corporation 956-781-5000
2003 N Veterans Blvd Ste 10, San Juan, TX 78589
Multiple positional geriatric chairs.

Newschoff Chairs, Inc. 800-203-8916
909 N.E. St., Sheboygan, WI 53081

Paoli, Inc. 800-457-7415
PO Box 30, Paoli, IN 47454

Radix Corp. 204-697-2349
#2-572 South Fifth St., Pembina, ND 58271
QUIESCENCE, HERITAGE designed for ease of entry and exit, open-flo seat design for incontinent patients.

Shelby-Williams Industries 800-873-3252
5303 E Morris Blvd, Morristown, TN 37813

Thompson Contract Inc. 631-589-7337
41 Keyland Ct, Bohemia, NY 11716

Thyssenkrupp Access Corp. 800-925-3100
4001 E 138th St, Grandview, MO 64030

Uplift Technologies, Inc. 800-387-0896
125-11 Morris Dr., Dartmouth, NS B3B 1M2 Canada
Geriatric chair

Winco, Inc. 800-237-3377
5516 SW 1st Ln, Ocala, FL 34474
Chairs.

Youngs, Inc. 800-523-5454
55 E Cherry Ln, Souderton, PA 18964

CHAIR, GERIATRIC, WHEELED *(General) 80FRM*
A.R.C. Distributors 800-296-8724
PO Box 599, Centreville, MD 21617
INVACARE Traditional Three Position Recliner-exceptional comfort, durability, and price. Recliner features upright sitting, elevated leg or full recline. Available in 6 colors.

Alan's Wheelchairs & Repairs 800-693-4344
109 S Harbor Blvd Ste B, Fullerton, CA 92832

Broda Enterprises Inc. 800-668-0637
385 Phillip St., Waterloo, ONT N2L 5R8 Canada
BRODA SEATING Fully reclining chairs, semi-reclining chairs, and tilt-in space chairs.

L.P.A. Medical, Inc. 888-845-6447
460 Desrochers, Ste. 150D, Vanier, QUEBE G1M 1C2 Canada
OPTIMUM Posturo-Pedic positioning chair, Series 1000.

CHAIR, GERIATRIC, WHEELED *(cont'd)*
Total Care 800-334-3802
PO Box 1661, Rockville, MD 20849

CHAIR, INFANT TREATMENT *(General) 80UDI*
Custom Comfort 800-749-0933
PO Box 4779, Winter Park, FL 32793
Infant Phlebotomy Station comes in three styles of infant phlebotomy stations including wall mounted and free standing.

CHAIR, NEUROSURGICAL *(Cns/Neurology) 84HBN*
Crist Instrument Co., Inc. 301-393-8615
111 W 1st St, Hagerstown, MD 21740
Customized Primate Chairs for Brain Mapping, Neurological, Vision, Audio & Behavioral Studies. Models available for Awake subjects placed in MRI apparatus.

CHAIR, OPERATIVE *(Dental And Oral) 76EFG*
Dentalez Group 866-DTE-INFO
101 Lindenwood Dr Ste 225, Valleybrooke Corporate Center
Malvern, PA 19355

Midmark Corporation 800-643-6275
60 Vista Dr, P.O. Box 286, Versailles, OH 45380

3m Unitek 800-634-5300
2724 Peck Rd, Monrovia, CA 91016

CHAIR, OPHTHALMIC, AC-POWERED *(Ophthalmology) 86HME*
Burton Co., R.H. 800-848-0410
3965 Brookham Dr, Grove City, OH 43123
$4,295.00 for Burton 2201 AC powered chair and stand unit. Ophthalmic AC-powered chair and stand, $5,195.00 for Burton XL3303.

Dexta Corporation 800-733-3982
962 Kaiser Rd, Napa, CA 94558
$4,695 for multi-purpose chair unit, $6,995 for powered ophthalmic surgery table.

HAAG-STREIT USA, INC. 800-787-5426
3535 Kings Mills Rd, Mason, OH 45040
$4,395 & $4,985 for motorized ophthalmic chairs.

Marco Ophthalmic, Inc. 800-874-5274
11825 Central Pkwy, Jacksonville, FL 32224
4 models - $5,150.00 for electric recline; $4,995.00 for tilt recline; and $40955.00 and $3,895.00 for manual recline. (List prices)

Topcon Medical Systems, Inc. 800-223-1130
37 W Century Rd, Paramus, NJ 07652
Four ophthalmic chairs: $1,690.00, $4,390.00, $5,390.00, and $5,790.

Western Ophthalmics Corporation 800-426-9938
19019 36th Ave W Ste G, Lynnwood, WA 98036

Woodlyn, Inc. 800-331-7389
2920 Malmo Dr, Ophthalmic Instruments and Equipment
Arlington Heights, IL 60005
Model 4000. Fully motorized by a foot petal or by the Millennium Instrument Stand. Adjusts from full-upright to prone position. Auto return, full-range rotation 320 degrees. Wheel-chair accessible. Call for current prices.

CHAIR, OPHTHALMIC, MANUAL *(Ophthalmology) 86HMD*
HAAG-STREIT USA, INC. 800-787-5426
3535 Kings Mills Rd, Mason, OH 45040
$2,495, $3,195 and $3,595.

Link Ergonomics Corp. 800-424-5465
902 E 4th St, Joplin, MO 64801
LINK ophthalmology chairs for examination and operative treatment.

Topcon Medical Systems, Inc. 800-223-1130
37 W Century Rd, Paramus, NJ 07652
Manual exam chair: $1,990.00. Adjustable stools: $195.00, $295.00, $395.00 and $495.00.

CHAIR, OTHER *(General) 80QJO*
A.R.C. Distributors 800-296-8724
PO Box 599, Centreville, MD 21617
Bariatric products: Bariatric Wheelchairs, Stretchers, Commodes, Walkers, and Patient Lifts. Available in 350lb to 1000lb capacities.

Adden Furniture, Inc. 800-625-3876
26 Jackson St, Lowell, MA 01852

Arjo, Inc. 800-323-1245
50 Gary Ave Ste A, Roselle, IL 60172

Atd-American Co. 800-523-2300
135 Greenwood Ave, Wyncote, PA 19095

CHAIR, OTHER *(cont'd)*

Back Support Systems 800-669-2225
67684 San Andreas St, Desert Hot Springs, CA 92240
ROLLITURE $349.00 orthopedic chair comes in 5 styles.

Bed-Check Corporation 800-523-7956
307 E Brady St, Tulsa, OK 74120
CHAIR-CHECK II, monitoring systems include battery powered, rechargable portable control units with an audible alarm and pressure-sensitive Sensormat pads.

Bevco Ergonomic Seating 800-864-2991
2246 W Bluemound Rd Ste A, Waukesha, WI 53186
BEVCO model 6003 office chair. Pneumatic height adjustment, tilting seat and back, waterfall front seat, optional ergonomic adjustable arms, casters, lumbar back support. 12-year guarantee, lifetime on pneumatic cylinder. BEVCO 7000CR and 7000E series ergonomic chairs and stools for cleanroom and ESD applications. BEVCO 4000CR/ 4000ECR class 100 cleanroom and ESD cleanroom chairs (16) models for contamination control and state control.

Brandrud Furniture, Inc. 253-838-6500
1502 20th St NW, Auburn, WA 98001
Sleeper chairs, sofas, gliders, recliner/treatment chairs, patient chairs, hip chairs, multiple seating units for lobbies/waiting areas.

Brandt Industries, Inc. 800-221-8031
4461 Bronx Blvd, Bronx, NY 10470
23410: chair/table. Hydrotherapy chairs.

Brewer Company, The 888-873-9371
N88W13901 Main St, Menomonee Falls, WI 53051
#1200: Side Chair with Arms, #1250: Side Chair without Arms

Broda Enterprises Inc. 800-668-0637
385 Phillip St., Waterloo, ONT N2L 5R8 Canada
BRODA SEATING Glider rockers.

Champion Manufacturing, Llc. 800-998-5018
2601 Industrial Pkwy, Elkhart, IN 46516
Sleeper chair for patient room use in pediatrics; critical care patients' rooms.

Columbia Medical Manufacturing Llc 800-454-6612
13577 Larwin Cir, Santa Fe Springs, CA 90670
Columbia Medical Contour AquaLift. The Columbia Medical Contour AquaLift bathlifter is a fully portable, easy to store, lightweight bath lifter ideal for use at home or in long term care facilities. The Contour AquaLift presents a perfect solution for people who have difficulty getting in and out of the bath. Powered by a low voltage battery for safety, the AquaLift can lift up to 325 lbs. Pediatric version available.

Country Craft Furniture, Inc. 800-569-1968
5318 Railroad Ave, Flowery Branch, GA 30542

Custom Comfort 800-749-0933
PO Box 4779, Winter Park, FL 32793
MULTI-MED: donor chair, four different styles available with features that include adjustable-height arm rests, storage accessories and pneumatic reclining mechanism; recliner chair, multi-purpose that can be used in almost any department, adjustablearms increase versatility. DRAW-MED phlebotomy chairs that are available with fully adjustable arm rests, over seven styles including chairs that are extra wide and extra tall. Also available, Ulti-med, three different styles of chairs capable of reclining. Ideal for blood banks or labs. now introducing the 'Versa-Med' series reclying chair. The chair has three versatile positions: upright, recline, and full recline. It is equipped with fully adjustable padded arm rests that move back with the chair when reclined. The 25' seat hight provides the technician and patient comfortable sitting and working hight.

Dansereau Health Products, Inc. 800-423-5657
250 E Harrison St, Corona, CA 92879
Stools for assistants and doctors; X-ray chairs.

Fleetwood Group, Incorporated 800-257-6390
PO Box 1259, Holland, MI 49422
Padded recovery lounge with detachable headrest.

Garaventa (Canada) Ltd. 800-663-6556
7505 - 134A St., Surrey, BC V3W-7B3 Canada
$2,195 for EVACU-TRAC emergency evacuation chair.

Gendron, Inc. 800-537-2521
400 E Lugbill Rd, Archbold, OH 43502
SUPER WIDE Wheel chairs extrawide 20-30 in. seat width, folding. Bariatric wheelchairs, all styles, for weight capacities of 350-800 pounds.

Gunnell, Inc. 800-551-0055
8440 State Rd, Millington, MI 48746
Kidster, Rehab TNT, Multi-adjustable chair (MAC), recline and mobility (RAM), and simplex seating.

CHAIR, OTHER *(cont'd)*

HAAG-STREIT USA, INC. 800-787-5426
3535 Kings Mills Rd, Mason, OH 45040
$1,195 for laser examination chair.

Hard Manufacturing Co. 800-873-4273
230 Grider St, Buffalo, NY 14215
$152 for Model E7520 side-chair with no arms; also, $237 for Model E7530 high-back easy chair with arms.

Hill-Rom Holdings, Inc. 800-445-3730
1069 State Road 46 E, Batesville, IN 47006
Sleepers' chairs & chairs for visitors in waiting rooms.

Innovative Products Unlimited, Inc. 800-833-2826
2120 Industrial Dr, Niles, MI 49120
$300.00 per transfer chair, and $145 - $175 per commode chair.

L.P.A. Medical, Inc. 888-845-6447
460 Desrochers, Ste. 150D, Vanier, QUEBE G1M 1C2 Canada
THERA-GLIDE Safety Gliders help prevent falls with a patented automatic-locking system that prevents rocking while entering or exiting the chair. Once safely seated, the lock disengages, permitting the user to experience a soothing gliding motion. When exiting the THERA-GLIDE, the lock automatically engages again for a steady, safe egress. Ideal for LDRP, Geriatric, and Dimentia applications.

Leisure-Lift, Inc. 800-255-0285
1800 Merriam Ln, Kansas City, KS 66106

Link Ergonomics Corp. 800-424-5465
902 E 4th St, Joplin, MO 64801
LINK task chairs for secretarial and business area.

Med-Lift & Mobility, Inc. 800-748-9438
310 S. Madison, Calhoun City, MS 38916
MR. COMFORT Multi-directional massage chair with rollers.

Mission X-Ray 800-676-8718
45459 Industrial Pllace, Suite 1, Fremont, CA 94538-6450
X-ray turntable chair.

Mxe, Inc. 800-252-1801
12107 Jefferson Blvd, Culver City, CA 90230
MXE Deluxe Hydraulic Mammography Chair, reclining and non-reclining mammography chairs. MXE's Ergo Chair for Technologists.

Nk Medical Products Inc. 800-274-2742
10123 Main St, PO Box 627, Clarence, NY 14031
3-Position Medical Recliners, Patient Seating, Bariatric Seating

Paoli, Inc. 800-457-7415
PO Box 30, Paoli, IN 47454

Radix Corp. 204-697-2349
#2-572 South Fifth St., Pembina, ND 58271
Fully upholstered seating.

Rand-Scot Inc. 800-467-7967
401 Linden Center Dr, Fort Collins, CO 80524
BBD Wheelchair Cushion: Bye-Bye Decubiti, rubber air-filled cushion.

Rockaway Chairs 800-256-6601
111 Alexander Rd Apt 11, West Monroe, LA 71291
Physician's waiting room furniture, styled without cushions, seams or welting and high arms to allow patients to get in and out of easily; also, Queen Anne style dining room furniture, beds and bedroom furniture, wood rockers and porch furniture.

S & B Robertson Research And Developments, Inc. 7057995537
R.R. #1, The Glen, Omemee, ONT K0L-2W0 Canada
The RIC Powered Elevating Office Chair. This chair provides independent access to a standard desk or table. It raises the chair seat to the user's standing level and lowers the person to the standard desk or table height.

Sauder Manufacturing Co. 800-537-1530
930 W Barre Rd, Archbold, OH 43502
Patient rooms, dining, and lobby chairs. Special Edition Series, chairs designed for very large people up to 750 pounds. Three styles available.

Shelby-Williams Industries 800-873-3252
5303 E Morris Blvd, Morristown, TN 37813
Health care seating.

Shepherd Caster Corporation 800-253-0868
203 Kerth St, Saint Joseph, MI 49085
Chair bases, IV poles and chairs, stools.

Stille-Sonesta, Inc. 800-665-1614
1610 S Interstate 35E Ste 203, Carrollton, TX 75006

CHAIR, OTHER *(cont'd)*

Thompson Contract Inc. 631-589-7337
41 Keyland Ct, Bohemia, NY 11716
Cafeteria, office and reception area chairs. Patient room chair.

Wehmer Corporation 800-323-0229
1151 N Main St, Lombard, IL 60148
$895 for each electric powered cephalometric chair.

CHAIR, PEDIATRIC *(General) 80QJJ*

Clarke Health Care Products, Inc. 888-347-4537
1003 International Dr, Oakdale, PA 15071
Dukki pediatric shower/commode chair, BugEe pediatric seating mobile push system, Corzo stroller.

Gunnell, Inc. 800-551-0055
8440 State Rd, Millington, MI 48746
KIDSTER pediatric chair.

Invacare Corporation 800-333-6900
1 Invacare Way, Elyria, OH 44035
INVACARE Comet, jr., Orbit, MVP jr., Solara jr., Spree, 9000 Jymni wheelchairs.

Kaye Products, Inc. 919-732-6444
535 Dimmocks Mill Rd, Hillsborough, NC 27278
Adaptive chairs with V-shaped back or bolster seat or adjustable height, all with removable trays, abductors, for children.

Newschoff Chairs, Inc. 800-203-8916
909 N.E. St., Sheboygan, WI 53081

Octostop Inc. 450-978-9805
1675 Saint Elzear, west, Laval, QUE H7L-3N6 Canada
$1115.00.

Rifton Equipment 800-571-8198
PO Box 260, Rifton, NY 12471
Adjustable chairs, corner sitter, Rifton Advancement chair, therapeutic seating, and accessible desk.

Snug Seat, Inc. 800-336-7684
12801 E Independence Blvd, PO Box 1739, Matthews, NC 28105
The WOMBAT seating system is a multifunctioning positioning chair for children who require sitting support and stabilization. Our high-Low bases allow the seat to raise to desk height and lower to floor height, allowing the child to interact with peers or work at a computer.

Thompson Contract Inc. 631-589-7337
41 Keyland Ct, Bohemia, NY 11716

Wenzelite Rehab Supplies, Llc 800-706-9255
220 36th St, 99 Seaview Blvd, Brooklyn, NY 11232
MSS TILT & RECLINE, pediatric positioning system for severely involved. Available on high or low frame with many adjustments. Standard accessories include tray, lateral supports, foot rest and adjustable headrest. It tilts & reclines up to 45 degrees. SEAT2GO pediatric lightweight padded positioning system for children up to 75 pounds. It can be used on the floor or at the table. It features a double strap trunk support and fastening straps to secure it to any chair. It can be used as an insert in a stroller. It only weighs 8 lbs and you can take it with you wherever you go. The FIRST CLASS SCHOOL CHAIR is a height and depth adjustable seat with armrests and pelvic belt. Optional accessories include a trunk harness, abductor, lateral supports, tray, footrest, headrest and wedges, hip guides, anti-tippers, leg extensions and a mobility base.

Youngs, Inc. 800-523-5454
55 E Cherry Ln, Souderton, PA 18964

CHAIR, PODIATRIC *(Orthopedics) 87QJK*

Md International, Inc. 305-669-9003
11300 NW 41st St, Doral, FL 33178

Midmark Corporation 800-643-6275
60 Vista Dr, P.O. Box 286, Versailles, OH 45380

CHAIR, POSITION, ELECTRIC *(Physical Med) 89INO*

Alc, Inc. 262-502-4665
N114W19049 Clinton Dr, Germantown, WI 53022
Lift chair.

Berkline/Benchcraft Llc 423-585-1517
1 Berkline Dr, Morristown, TN 37813
Lift chair.

Dream Inventors Design Llc 208-882-3082
4805 Robinson Park Rd, Moscow, ID 83843
Electric positioning chair.

Franklin Corp. 662-456-4286
600 Franklin Dr, P.o. Box 569, Houston, MS 38851
Various types of lift chairs.

CHAIR, POSITION, ELECTRIC *(cont'd)*

Invacare Corporation 800-333-6900
1 Invacare Way, Elyria, OH 44035
INVACARE

Leisure-Lift, Inc. 800-255-0285
1800 Merriam Ln, Kansas City, KS 66106

Nor-Am Patient Care Products, Inc. 800-387-7103
2388 Speers Rd., Oakville, ONT L6L 5M2 Canada
Dolphin chair lift

Posture Dynamics, Inc. 732-278-2081
415 Jarob Ct, Point Pleasant Boro, NJ 08742
Biophysiometer is a computer aided positioning chair, which helps to balance the patient's spine by using the Pelvis as a fulcrum.

Stille-Sonesta, Inc. 800-665-1614
1610 S Interstate 35E Ste 203, Carrollton, TX 75006

Two Rivers, Llc 423-626-4990
3199 Hwy. 25 E North, Tazewell, TN 37879
Lift chair.

Ultrassage, Inc. 514-344-1083
5680 Rue Pare, Mont-Royal, QUEBE H4P 2M2 Canada
Massage furniture.

CHAIR, POSTURE, FOR CARDIAC AND PULMONARY TREATMENT *(Anesthesiology) 73BYN*

Camtec 410-228-1156
1959 Church Creek Rd, Cambridge, MD 21613
Chair cardiac.

Neutral Posture, Inc. 979-778-0502
3904 N Texas Ave, Bryan, TX 77803
Ergonomic.

Stille-Sonesta, Inc. 800-665-1614
1610 S Interstate 35E Ste 203, Carrollton, TX 75006

CHAIR, REHABILITATION *(General) 80QJL*

Good Sports 412-731-3032
1701 Monongahela Ave, Pittsburgh, PA 15218
Rehabilitation equipment by Bailey Manufacturing.

Invacare Corporation 800-333-6900
1 Invacare Way, Elyria, OH 44035
INVACARE.

Paoli, Inc. 800-457-7415
PO Box 30, Paoli, IN 47454

CHAIR, ROTATING *(Cns/Neurology) 84WHW*

Micromedical Technologies, Inc. 800-334-4154
10 Kemp Dr, Chatham, IL 62629
SYSTEM 2000 Chair with zero backlash drive system, 60ft/lbs. torque, accelerates 200lb-subject to 300 deg./sec.2., +/- 0.5% velocity accuracy. Provides rotational stimuli for assessment of the vestibular ocular reflex (vor). Enhancements: infrared video camera, laser projector, optokinetic drum and enclosure.

Quadromed Inc. 800-363-0192
5776 Thimens Ave., St-Laurent, QUE H4R 2K9 Canada

CHAIR, SEAT LIFTING (STANDING AID) *(General) 80UMP*

Alsons Corp. 800-421-0001
3010 Mechanic Rd, P.O. Box 282, Hillsdale, MI 49242

Altimate Medical, Inc. 800-342-8968
PO Box 180, 262 West 1st St., Morton, MN 56270
EASYSTAND Evolv's natural lifting action offers comfortable support from sitting to standing. Designed to give the support needed for proper standing position. The EASYSTAND MAGICIAN and EasyStand Magician-ei (Early Intervention), and the EasyStand Evolv Youth are seating/standing systems for kids to use during the school day EASYSTAND Evolv Glider combines therapeutic standing with leg and arm movement to create the ultimate standing experience. The EasyStand StrapStand lifts the user directly out of their wheelchair. The EASYSTAND Mobile option allows users to self propel while standing.

Arjo, Inc. 800-323-1245
50 Gary Ave Ste A, Roselle, IL 60172

Basic American Medical Products 800-849-6664
2935A Northeast Pkwy, Atlanta, GA 30360

Ergodyne 800-225-8238
1021 Bandana Blvd E Ste 220, Saint Paul, MN 55108
Lateral patient transfer device eliminates risk of back injury, increased comfort, increased productivity.

CHAIR, SEAT LIFTING (STANDING AID) *(cont'd)*

Golden Technologies, Inc. 800-624-6374
401 Bridge St, Old Forge, PA 18518
Golden Technologies offers 29 different models of lift and recline chairs to fit most customers needs, including the Relaxer with MaxiComfort, featuring zero gravity-like positioning for the utmost in comfort.

L.P.A. Medical, Inc. 888-845-6447
460 Desrochers, Ste. 150D, Vanier, QUEBE G1M 1C2 Canada
Optima Lift Chairs are made for today's busy healthcare facilities. Removable chaise cushions and moisture-impermeable fabrics make the Optima Lift Chair easy to clean and disinfect. Swivel wheels for moving and a compact wall-hugger design lets it fit where ordinary reclining lift-chairs won't . A collection of Crypton and leatherette fabrics compliment any décor. And if you prefer to select your own fabric, we do COM (customer's own material).

Med-Lift & Mobility, Inc. 800-748-9438
310 S. Madison, Calhoun City, MS 38916

Pride Mobility Products Corp. 800-800-8586
182 Susquehanna Ave, Exeter, PA 18643

Rand-Scot Inc. 800-467-7967
401 Linden Center Dr, Fort Collins, CO 80524
Personal standing frame for a user with upper body strength.

Wheelchair Sales And Service Co., Inc. 877-736-0376
315 Main St, West Springfield, MA 01089
Golden Technologies, Pride Mobility.

CHAIR, SHOWER *(General) 80QJM*

A.R.C. Distributors 800-296-8724
PO Box 599, Centreville, MD 21617
INVACARE Class Shower Chair has blow molded design, drain holes and handles on seat, fixed and adjustable height available. Non-marring, non-slip rubber tips, with or without back. Wheelchairs of Kansas Shower-Commode Chair -swing away & removable arms & back, 600lb capacity.

Access Mobility, Inc. 800-336-1147
5240 Elmwood Ave, Indianapolis, IN 46203

Activeaid, Inc. 800-533-5330
101 Activeaid Rd, Redwood Falls, MN 56283
Traum-Aid reclining shower wheelchair for the spinal cord injured. Also available shower commode.

Alimed, Inc. 800-225-2610
297 High St, Dedham, MA 02026

Alsons Corp. 800-421-0001
3010 Mechanic Rd, P.O. Box 282, Hillsdale, MI 49242

Aqua Glass Corporation 800-632-0911
320 Industrial Park Rd, Adamsville, TN 38310
Wheelchair Shower, a wheelchair can wheel directly into the shower.

Arjo, Inc. 800-323-1245
50 Gary Ave Ste A, Roselle, IL 60172
Patient shower cabinet with adjustable lift hygiene chair, toilet function, water and disinfectant spray.

Clarke Health Care Products, Inc. 888-347-4537
1003 International Dr, Oakdale, PA 15071
Aquatec, Aquatec, OceanVIP Tilt shower chair. stainless-steel shower/commode chair, Aquatec OCean stainless steel shower/commode chair.OceanSP self propelled chair

Convaquip Industries, Inc. 800-637-8436
4834 Derrick Dr, PO Box 3417, Abilene, TX 79601
Bariatric Wheeled Transport Shower Chairs. Weight certified from 650 lb. to 750 lbs.

Duralife, Inc. 800-443-5433
195 Phillips Park Dr, Williamsport, PA 17702

Elcoma Metal Fabricating Canada 705-526-9636
878 William St., P.O. Box 685, Midland, ONT L4R-4P4 Canada
Shower seat and other assistive devices. All colors, configurations, lengths and diameters.

Independent Care Products, Inc. 800-695-8151
PO Box 6258, Abilene, TX 79608
The radial shower swing arm will accommodate a person from the chair to the shower. It can be used over a tub as well as in the shower entry. This system has safety locking features for easy accessibility as well as 360 degree rotation on the support arm and 360 degree rotation on the chair assembly. This is a stationary mounting system. Now Available for Bariatric Individuals.

Innovative Products Unlimited, Inc. 800-833-2826
2120 Industrial Dr, Niles, MI 49120
$180.00 each.

CHAIR, SHOWER *(cont'd)*

Invacare Corporation 800-333-6900
1 Invacare Way, Elyria, OH 44035
INVACARE Mariner Rehab Shower Commode Chair, I-Fit Shower Chair, CareGuard Shower Chair.

Larkotex Company 800-972-3037
1002 Olive St, Texarkana, TX 75501

Newschoff Chairs, Inc. 800-203-8916
909 N.E. St., Sheboygan, WI 53081

O&M Enterprise 847-258-4515
641 Chelmsford Ln, Elk Grove Village, IL 60007
CHAIR SHOWER

R. D. Equipment, Inc. 508-362-7498
230 Percival Dr, West Barnstable, MA 02668

Rifton Equipment 800-571-8198
PO Box 260, Rifton, NY 12471
Shower chair - 3 sizes of bath chair fit this mobile shower stand with locking casters

Total Care 800-334-3802
PO Box 1661, Rockville, MD 20849

Tub Master Lc 800-833-0260
413 Virginia Dr, Orlando, FL 32803
Shower & Tub Seats

Tuffcare 800-367-6160
3999 E La Palma Ave, Anaheim, CA 92807

Wheelchairs Of Kansas 800-537-6454
204 W 2nd St, Ellis, KS 67637
FOLDING SHOWER CHAIR is portable and easily folds for the bariatric showering needs; It is constructed with a heavy-duty, stainless steel frame and our signature double x-brace design for support; The anti-tip base is stable and secure for a bariatric individual; Special reinforced seating; Extra large non-marring rubber caps; 600 lb. weight capacity. TUB TRANSFER BENCH offers versatility for the design of any home; Multiple styles of benches are available, such as with a commode seat and/or a detachable back bar, depending upon the individual needs; It is constructed of a heavy-duty, stainless steel frame and an anti-tip base for durablity and strength; detachable back is reversible for either side; Water resistant, anti-bacterial padded seat; Baked, powder-coat finish to resist fading and chipping; 600 lb. weight capacity.

CHAIR, SITZ BATH *(General) 80QJN*

Arjo Canada, Inc. 800-665-4831
1575 South Gateway Rd., Unit C, Mississauga, ONT L4W-5J1 Canada

Tuffcare 800-367-6160
3999 E La Palma Ave, Anaheim, CA 92807

CHAIR, SURGICAL, AC-POWERED *(Surgery) 79GBB*

Blue Horizon Medical 321-217-2717
3129 Ginger Cir, Orlando, FL 32826
Hand control.

Champion Mfg. Inc. 800-998-5018
2601 Industrial Pkwy, Elkhart, IN 46516
Power recliner.

Dexta Corporation 800-733-3982
962 Kaiser Rd, Napa, CA 94558
$5495.

Elmed, Inc. 630-543-2792
60 W Fay Ave, Addison, IL 60101

Md International, Inc. 305-669-9003
11300 NW 41st St, Doral, FL 33178

Midmark Corporation 800-643-6275
60 Vista Dr, P.O. Box 286, Versailles, OH 45380

Stille-Sonesta, Inc. 800-665-1614
1610 S Interstate 35E Ste 203, Carrollton, TX 75006

Transmotion Medical Inc. 866-860-8447
1441 Wolf Creek Trail, Sharon Center, OH 44274
'various models of operating chairs'.

CHAIR, SURGICAL, NON-ELECTRICAL *(Surgery) 79FZK*

Alimed, Inc. 800-225-2610
297 High St, Dedham, MA 02026

Biofit Engineered Products 800-597-0246
PO Box 109, Waterville, OH 43566
BIOFIT BT series ergonomic chair - 7 models. Chair with ergonomic backrest with tilt, concave seat, adjustable seat height, chrome-plated metal parts, and dual-wheel polyurethane casters.

CHAIR, WITH CASTERS *(Physical Med) 89INM*

Arjo, Inc. 800-323-1245
50 Gary Ave Ste A, Roselle, IL 60172
Fully submersible poolchair to assist disabled swimmers into and out of the water providing total mobility throught the pool area.

Bergeron Health Care 800-371-2778
15 S 2nd St, Dolgeville, NY 13329
Various models of postioning device for people with physical disabilities.

Bodypoint, Inc. 800-547-5716
558 1st Ave S Ste 300, Seattle, WA 98104
Monkey, Pediatric Sitter for children 9 months to 5 years.

Care Products Inc. 757-224-0177
10701 N Ware Rd, McAllen, TX 78504
Various models of chairs with casters.

Evermed Corp. 714-777-9997
4999 E La Palma Ave, Anaheim, CA 92807
Evermed.

Flocast Llc. 315-429-8407
15 S 2nd St, Dolgeville, NY 13329
Various models of postioning device for people with physical disabilities.

Global Surgical Corp. 314-861-3388
3610 Tree Court Industrial Blvd, Saint Louis, MO 63122
Stool.

Healthline Medical Products, Inc. 407-656-0704
1065 E Story Rd, Oakland, FL 34787

L.P.A. Medical, Inc. 888-845-6447
460 Desrochers, Ste. 150D, Vanier, QUEBE G1M 1C2 Canada
OPTIMUM Posturo-Pedic positioning chair, Series 1000.

Larkotex Company 800-972-3037
1002 Olive St, Texarkana, TX 75501

Laszlo Corp. 314-830-3222
2573 Millvalley Dr, Florissant, MO 63031
Attachment for wheeled chair.

Maddak Inc. 800-443-4926
661 State Route 23, Wayne, NJ 07470
ABLEWARE.

Mathison Industries, Inc. 775-284-1020
220 Coney Island Dr, Sparks, NV 89431
Operator's stools.

May Corp.
103 E. Espelee Street, Grygla, MN 56727
Various types of geri chairs and accessories.

Medical Depot 516-998-4600
99 Seaview Blvd, Port Washington, NY 11050
Chairs.

Mjm International Corporation 956-781-5000
2003 N Veterans Blvd Ste 10, San Juan, TX 78589
Various models of shower chairs with casters.

Movingpeople.Net Canada, Inc. 416-739-8333
500 Norfinch Dr, Downsview M3N 1Y4 Canada
Mechanical chair with casters for home and work use

Penner Manufacturing Inc 800-732-0717
102 Grant St, PO Box 523, Aurora, NE 68818
Transfer chair.

Sunrise Machine And Tool, Inc. 218-847-3386
1380 Legion Rd, Detroit Lakes, MN 56501
Wheel chair.

Sunrise Medical Hhg Inc 303-218-4505
7128 Ambassador Rd, Baltimore, MD 21244
Dependent pediatric stroller style wheelchair.

Triaid, Inc. 301-759-3525
637 N Centre St, Cumberland, MD 21502
Theraplay stool.

Tumble Forms, Inc. 262-387-8720
1013 Barker Rd, Dolgeville, NY 13329
Multiple.

Winco, Inc. 800-237-3377
5516 SW 1st Ln, Ocala, FL 34474
Patient transfer chair.

CHAIR/TABLE, MEDICAL *(General) 80KMN*

Champion Manufacturing, Llc. 800-998-5018
2601 Industrial Pkwy, Elkhart, IN 46516
Heavy duty recliners and recliner-transporters for dialysis, chemotherapy and physical therapy, outpatient recovery.

Champion Mfg. Inc. 800-998-5018
2601 Industrial Pkwy, Elkhart, IN 46516
Relciner-transporter chair.

Clinton Industries, Inc 717-848-3519
1140 Edison St, York, PA 17403
Various medical chairs and tables.

Custom Comfort 800-749-0933
PO Box 4779, Winter Park, FL 32793
Custom Comfort's Exam Tables are built for comfort and to last. Our 8010 exam table features heavy-duty steel legs. All corners and joints of the table are reinforced with steel brackets that prevent unnecessary stress on critical areas. The tabletop is padded with high-density foam and is upholstered using medical grade seamless vinyl for easy cleaning and available in eighteen colors. You can also choose from three different styles of storage features that allow various combinations to maximize your storage needs. The 8020 series exam tables have all the same features as the 8010 series but are constructed of high quality 1 1/4 in. plywood laminated with our WilsonArt platinum color formica.

Hill-Rom, Inc. 812-934-7777
4115 Dorchester Rd Unit 600, North Charleston, SC 29405
Patient chairs, overbed tables and accessories.

Indigenous Peoples Technology And Education Center 352-465-4545
10575 SW 147th Cir, Dunnellon, FL 34432
Portable chair.

LIFTnWALK LP 972-837-4615
PO Box 742855, Dallas, TX 75374
BUDDY SAFETY ROLLER SEAT, removable seat. BUDDY SEAT.

Lloyd Table Co. 319-455-2110
102 W Main St # 122, Lisbon, IA 52253
Various types and models Of examining and therapy tables.

Mayo Medical, S.A. De C.V. 800-715-3872
Edison 1141 Nte., Col. Talleres, Monterrey N.L. 64480 Mexico

Medical Depot 516-998-4600
99 Seaview Blvd, Port Washington, NY 11050
Chair tables, wheeled.

Mobile Designs, Inc. 530-244-1050
4650 Caterpillar Rd, Redding, CA 96003
Table.

O&M Enterprise 847-258-4515
641 Chelmsford Ln, Elk Grove Village, IL 60007
Chair Examination

Oakworks, Inc. 800-558-8850
923 E Wellspring Rd, New Freedom, PA 17349
Medical treatment table.

P.B. Connections, Inc. 412-825-6095
341 Marguerite Ave, Wilmerding, PA 15148
Support chair.

Stille-Sonesta, Inc. 800-665-1614
1610 S Interstate 35E Ste 203, Carrollton, TX 75006

Tumble Forms, Inc. 262-387-8720
1013 Barker Rd, Dolgeville, NY 13329
Multiple.

Wal-Star, Inc. 434-685-1094
696 Inman Rd, Danville, VA 24541
Chair and table, medical.

CHAMBER, ACOUSTIC, TESTING *(Ear/Nose/Throat) 77EWC*

Eckel Industries Of Canada Limited 800-563-3574
15 Allison Ave., P.O. Box 776, Morrisburg, ONT K0C 1X0 Canada
AB-Series - single person audiometric screening booths; CL-Series - single-wall audiometric rooms for the hearing aid specialists, audiologists, doctors offices & clinics; G-Series - clinical series of audiometric single-wall, double-wall, multi-room suites for diagnostics and research in hospitals and research facilities.

Industrial Acoustics Co., Inc. 718-931-8000
1160 Commerce Ave, Bronx, NY 10462
3 single room models - $3250 for MINI SERIES 250 $5150 for 400-A; $14250 for 1201-A with double walls. 4 double room models - $18400 for 402-A-CT; $32000 for 1202-A-CT with double walls; $27300 for 1402-A-CT and $27700 for 1602-A-CT.

CHAMBER, ACOUSTIC, TESTING *(cont'd)*

Kelleher Medical, Inc. 804-378-9956
3049 St Marys Way, Powhatan, VA 23139

Medi 800-947-6334
4814 E 2nd St, Benicia, CA 94510
Audiometers-(diagnostic, Industrial, High frequency, Pediatric)

Starkey Laboratories, Inc. 800-328-8602
6700 Washington Ave S, Eden Prairie, MN 55344
$8,950 for hearing science lab.

Tremetrics 800-825-0121
7625 Golden Triangle Dr, Eden Prairie, MN 55344
$3,100 for AR901, single room, single wall model. Weighs 765 lbs. OSCAR 7, Electro-Acoustic Ear & Sound Level Monitor, bioacoustic calibrator and monitor for ambient noise levels in acoustic enclosures. Pauses hearing test if noise levels are exceeded. $1,250.00.

Tsi Medical Ltd. 800-661-7263
47 Athabascan Ave., Unit 105, Sherwood Park, AB T8A-4H3 Canada

CHAMBER, ANAEROBIC *(Microbiology) 83VDW*

Almore International, Inc. 503-643-6633
PO Box 25214, Portland, OR 97298
Anaerobic jar (VACU-QUIK). $215.00 to $355.00.

Coy Laboratory Products, Inc. 734-475-2200
14500 Coy Dr, Grass Lake, MI 49240
Environmental chambers.

CHAMBER, CONSTANT TEMPERATURE (ENVIRONMENTAL) *(Microbiology) 83UFT*

Biocold Environmental 636-349-0300
239 Seebold Spur, Fenton, MO 63026
Stability test chambers for testing medical devices (controlling humidity, temperature, light, etc.)

Cincinnati Sub-Zero Products, Inc., Medical Division 800-989-7373
12011 Mosteller Rd, Cincinnati, OH 45241

Cmt, Inc. 800-659-9140
PO Box 297, Hamilton, MA 01936

Environmental Growth Chambers 800-321-6854
510 Washington St, Chagrin Falls, OH 44022
neg. 20, +4C, +37C or variable temp. environmental chambers.

Fts Systems 800-824-0400
PO Box 158, 3538 Main Street,, Stone Ridge, NY 12484

Harris Environmental Systems, Inc. 888-771-4200
11 Connector Rd, Andover, MA 01810
Environmental rooms, cold and warm rooms, dry rooms, and test chambers.

Hotpack 800-523-3608
10940 Dutton Rd, Philadelphia, PA 19154

Kendro Laboratory Products 800-252-7100
308 Ridgefield Ct, Asheville, NC 28806
$4,000 to $20,000 ea.

Percival Scientific Inc. 800-695-2743
505 Research Dr, Perry, IA 50220
Constant temperature and humidity chamber and microbiology incubator: bioassays research and development culture growth.

Powers Scientific, Inc. 800-998-0500
PO Box 268, Pipersville, PA 18947
Also stability and walk-in chambers.

Singleton Corp. 888-456-0643
3280 W 67th Pl, Cleveland, OH 44102

So-Low Environmental Equipment 513-772-9410
10310 Spartan Dr, Cincinnati, OH 45215

Thermal Product Solutions 800-586-2473
2121 Reach Rd, Williamsport, PA 17701

Thermal Product Solutions 800-216-7725
2121 Reach Rd, Williamsport, PA 17701

CHAMBER, DECOMPRESSION, ABDOMINAL *(Obstetrics/Gyn) 85HEE*

Avid Medical 800-886-0584
9000 Westmont Dr, Stonehouse Commerce Park, Toano, VA 23168
Cervical anesthesia needle for administration of local anesthesia prior to biopsy or other surgical procedure.

Biocompatibles Inc. 877-783-5463
115 Hurley Rd Bldg 3, Oxford, CT 06478
Intercervical block needle.

CHAMBER, DECOMPRESSION, ABDOMINAL *(cont'd)*

Kelsar, S.A. 508-261-8000
Blvd. Insurgentes, Libriamento a La, Tijuana 22450 Mexico
Paracervical/pudendal trays w/wo drugs

CHAMBER, ENVIRONMENTAL, PLATELET STORAGE *(Hematology) 81KSH*

Associated Environmental Systems 978-772-0022
31 Willow Rd, Ayer, MA 01432
Test.

Caron Products And Services, Inc. 800-648-3042
PO Box 715, Marietta, OH 45750
With refrigeration and humidification options and a wide variety of applications, these 30 cubic foot chambers have all stainless steel interiors and microprocessor controls.

Helmer, Inc. 800-743-5637
15425 Herriman Blvd, Noblesville, IN 46060
Platelet Storage Incubators and Agitators

Thermo Fisher Scientific (Asheville) Llc 740-373-4763
Millcreek Rd., Marietta, OH 45750
Various models of platelet incubators.

CHAMBER, FREEZING *(Chemistry) 75VFW*

Environmental Growth Chambers 800-321-6854
510 Washington St, Chagrin Falls, OH 44022
Negative 20C storage or working cold rooms.

CHAMBER, HYPERBARIC *(Anesthesiology) 73CBF*

Cantylight 716-625-4227
6100 Donner Rd, Lockport, NY 14094

Hyperbaric Technologies, Inc. 619-336-2022
3224 Hoover Ave, National City, CA 91950
Various models of hyperbaric systems.

Hypertec, Inc. 800-218-3588
301B E Main St, Olney, TX 76374
New & Remanufactured Hyperbaric chambers.

Marine Dynamics Corp. 951-699-4299
6475 E. Pch, #412, Long Beach, CA 90803
Hyperbaric chambers/decompression chambers.

Perry Baromedical Corp. 800-741-4376
3660 Interstate Park Way, Riviera Beach, FL 33404
SIGMA 34, SIGMA PLUS, SIGMA II & SIGMA MP, Hyberbaric systems. $129,900.00 to $169,900 for monoplace hyperbaric chambers, $325,000.00 for dual place hyperbaric chambers, $575,000.00 and up, depending on size, for custom multiplace hyperbaric chambers. SIGMA 34, monoplace hyperbaric system, a more spacious patient environment that allows patient to recline at a more comfortable level.

Reimers Systems, Inc. 877-734-6377
8210 Cinder Bed Rd Ste D, Lorton, VA 22079
Monoplace and multiplace hyperbaric chambers and environmental control systems.

Sechrist Industries, Inc. 800-732-4747
4225 E La Palma Ave, Anaheim, CA 92807

CHAMBER, HYPERBARIC OXYGEN *(Physical Med) 89IQD*

Environmental Tectonics Corp. 215-355-9100
125 James Way, Southampton, PA 18966

Tampa Hyperbaric Enterprise 813-391-9473
10104 Lake Cove Ln, Tampa, FL 33618
Multiplace Hyperbaric Chamber - six person hyperbaric chamber with (or without) mobile trailer.

CHAMBER, HYPOBARIC *(General) 80UKU*

Cantylight 716-625-4227
6100 Donner Rd, Lockport, NY 14094

CHAMBER, ISOLATION, PATIENT CARE *(General) 80FRR*

Clean Air Technology, Inc. 800 459 6320
41105 Capital Dr, Canton, MI 48187
Personnel Isolation Containment Modules, self contained, modular, single bed, negative air pressure, HEPA filtered with or without entry airlock, clear flexible or clear ascrylic sidewalls.

Crist Instrument Co., Inc. 301-393-8615
111 W 1st St, Hagerstown, MD 21740
Individual testing set-up chamber for primates to perform behavioral, vision, audio, and similar tasking acitivities. Customized options are available.

Peace Medical, Inc. 973-672-2120
50 S Center St Ste 11, Orange, NJ 07050
Isolation chamber.

CHAMBER, ISOLATION, PATIENT TRANSPORT *(General) 80LGN*

Clean Air Technology, Inc. 800 459 6320
41105 Capital Dr, Canton, MI 48187
Personnel Isolation Transport Stretcher, (PICM), for single person containment while transporting, negative air pressure, battery powered HEPA filtered stretcher environment, zippered openings on side and glove ports, battery charger, lightweight, optional fold up stretcher cart with wheels.

Isovac Products Llc • 630-679-1740
1306 Enterprise Dr Ste C, Romeoville, IL 60446
Hepa-filtered patient isolation unit.

CHAMBER, OXYGEN, TOPICAL, EXTREMITY *(Surgery) 79KPJ*

Advanced Hyperbaric Technologies, Inc. 800-327-4325
124 Colts Neck Rd, Farmingdale, NJ 07727
Topical sacral hyperbaric oxygen chamber.

Numotech, Inc. 818-772-1579
9420 Reseda Blvd Ste 504, Northridge, CA 91324
Numobag kit.

Sparton Medical Systems 440-878-4630
22740 Lunn Rd, Strongsville, OH 44149
Topical oxygen bandage.

CHAMBER, SLIDE CULTURE *(Pathology) 88KIY*

Erie Scientific 603-431-8410
20 Post Rd, Portsmouth Park, Newington, NH 03801
Various.

Thermo Fisher Scientific (Rochester) 585-899-7600
75 Panorama Creek Dr, Panorama, NY 14625
Various.

Wescor, Inc. 800-453-2725
459 S Main St, Logan, UT 84321
SLIDEPRO-I5, slide incubator for fixing specimens to the slide. Temperature adjustable from 40 degrees C to 100 degrees C. Sells for $575.00.

CHANGER, CASSETTE, RADIOGRAPHIC *(Radiology) 90IXT*

Fujifilm Medical Systems Usa, Inc. 800-431-1850
419 West Ave, Stamford, CT 06902

CHANGER, RADIOGRAPHIC FILM/CASSETTE *(Radiology) 90KPX*

Agfa Corporation 877-777-2432
PO Box 19048, 10 South Academy Street, Greenville, SC 29602

Ge Medical Systems, Llc 262-548-2355
3000 N Grandview Blvd, W-417, Waukesha, WI 53188
Changex chest changer.

Multi Imager Service, Inc 800-400-4549
13865 Magnolia Ave Bldg C, Chino, CA 91710
AGFA-Kodak-Imation-3M-Sterling-DuPont Laser imagers. Buy, sell, service, trade, lease. Also Dry Laser Imagers and Printers, PACS, DICOM, Digital Storage, Film Handling, Magazines, Cassettes & supplies.

CHANGER, TUBE, ENDOTRACHEAL *(Anesthesiology) 73LNZ*

Armstrong Medical Industries, Inc. 800-323-4220
575 Knightsbridge Pkwy, Lincolnshire, IL 60069

Instrumentation Industries, Inc. 800-633-8577
2990 Industrial Blvd, Bethel Park, PA 15102
Endotracheal tube changer.

Neotech Products, Inc. 800-966-0500
27822 Fremont Ct, Valencia, CA 91355
NEOBAR: Endotracheal Tube Holder for neonates, infants and pediatric patients. Unique one piece ET tube holder in which no tape ever contacts skin of neonate.

CHARGER, BATTERY *(General) 80WJM*

Access Battery Inc. 800-654-9845
12104 W Carmen Ave, Division of Alpha Source, Inc. Milwaukee, WI 53225
Battery chargers for communications, cellular, computer, camcorder and medical devices.

Aiv, Inc. (Formerly American Iv) 800-990-2911
7485 Shipley Ave, Harmans, MD 21077
AC Adapters (power sources and battery chargers) for leading ambulatory and portable infusion pumps.

Anton/Bauer - Custom Power Systems 800-422-3473
14 Progress Dr, Shelton, CT 06484
Custom and standard batteries, chargers, and power supplies for high-power, critical-use applications.

CHARGER, BATTERY *(cont'd)*

Japlar Group, Inc. 800-486-8658
4500 Alpine Ave, Cincinnati, OH 45242

Lester Electrical Of Nebraska, Inc. 402-477-8988
625 W A St, Lincoln, NE 68522
LESTRONIC II fully automatic wheelchair battery charger, 24 volt, 8 amp with fully automated shut-off. Dual-mode charger model, SCR controlled, designed to charge sealed or conventional batteries. Lester POWER CUBE for charging sealed, no-maintenance batteries up to 35 amps, hour rated, 24 volt, 5 amps with 12-hour positive shutoff.

Mk Battery 800-372-9253
1645 S Sinclair St, Anaheim, CA 92806
MK Battery has a complete line of premium quality battery chargers for all of your charging needs. Products include a 12V, 6 Amp charger and 24V, 8 Amp chargers.

Nica-Power Battery Corp. 800-565-6422
5155 Spectrum Way, Mississauga, ON L4W 5A1 Canada

Rayovac 800-331-4522
601 Rayovac Drive, Madison, WI 53744-4960
I-C3 15-minute-rechargeable NiMH Cells and chargers. AA & AAA NiMH 2000 mAh.

Tungstone Power Inc 800-232-3557
623 Main St, Woburn, MA 01801

W&W Manufacturing Co. 800-221-0732
800 S Broadway, Hicksville, NY 11801
MASTERCHARGER 6 six station charger for nickel cadmium and nickel-metal hydride batteries. Capable of charging six batteries of different voltage and capacities simultaneously.
MASTERCHARGER Ia - single unit rapid charger that charges nickel cadmium & nickel-metal hydride batteries.

CHART, ANATOMICAL TRAINING *(General) 80UKS*

Alimed, Inc. 800-225-2610
297 High St, Dedham, MA 02026

Armstrong Medical Industries, Inc. 800-323-4220
575 Knightsbridge Pkwy, Lincolnshire, IL 60069

Galloway Plastics, Inc. 847-615-8900
940 W North Shore Dr, Lake Bluff, IL 60044

Hager Worldwide, Inc. 800-328-2335
13322 Byrd Dr, Odessa, FL 33556

Helena Laboratories 409-842-3714
PO Box 752, Beaumont, TX 77704
Educational wall charts.

Kilgore International, Inc. 800-892-9999
36 W Pearl St, Coldwater, MI 49036

Lafayette Instrument Company 800-428-7545
PO Box 5729, 3700 Sagamore Pkwy,, Lafayette, IN 47903
Teaching labs: human physiology chart recorders.

Medco Supply Company 800-556-3326
500 Fillmore Ave, Tonawanda, NY 14150
Flip charts 11'x14', Desktop charts 11'x14', 20'x26': Rigid lamination, flexible lamination, or heavy paper.

Medical Plastics Laboratory, Inc. 800-433-5539
226 FM 116, Industrial Air Park, PO Box 38, Gatesville, TX 76528
Anatomical Charts available for Systems of the Body, Organs, Structures and Diseases & Disorders. Laminated (rigid & light) charts are 20' wide and 26' high, have metal eyelets in each top corner for convenient wall hanging and are markable (write-on, wipe-off). Charts are also available in soft cover book (11' x 14'), grouped as Systems & Structures and Diseases & Disorders. 3-D Raised Relief Charts are also available.

Sound Feelings 818-757-0600
18375 Ventura Blvd # 8000, Tarzana, CA 91356
Richman Body-Type Classification Method wall poster illustrates 45 different body types. Used to validate inherent physical variety and redefine the 'perfect' body.

CHART, VISUAL ACUITY *(Ophthalmology) 86HOX*

Allegheny Plastics, Inc. 412-776-0100
1224 Freedom Rd, Cranberry Township, PA 16066
Corneal rust ring remover-eye spud.

Ama Optics, Inc. 305-538-4124
314 W San Marino Dr, Miami Beach, FL 33139
Potential acuity tester.

George Tiemann & Co. 800-843-6266
25 Plant Ave, Hauppauge, NY 11788

CHART, VISUAL ACUITY *(cont'd)*

Good-Lite Co. 800-362-3860
865 Muirfield Dr, Bartlett, IL 60133
Cabinets, charts & accessories. Also, new model; a visual acuity screener for schools that with extensive R&D has been brought into the computer age with a new computer color, cleaner lines and improved switch.

Mast/Keystone View 800-806-6569
2200 Dickerson Rd, Reno, NV 89503

Medworks Instruments 800-323-9790
PO Box 581, Chatham, IL 62629
$5.50 per 10 units.

National Optronics 434-295-9126
100 Avon St, Charlottesville, VA 22902
Vision tester.

Richmond Products, Inc. 505-275-2406
4400 Silver Ave SE, Albuquerque, NM 87108
Hematocrit control.

Science 20/20, Inc. 760-753-7928
681 Encinitas Blvd Ste 302, Encinitas, CA 92024
Visual-acuity chart software.

Vestibular Technologies, Llc 307-637-5711
205 County Road 128a, Suite 200, Cheyenne, WY 82007-1831
Various models of visual acuity charts.

Vision Assessment Corp. 847-239-5889
2675 Coyle Ave, Elk Grove Village, IL 60007
Vectographic projector slide, projector slide.

Western Ophthalmics Corporation 800-426-9938
19019 36th Ave W Ste G, Lynnwood, WA 98036

William Lembeck, Inc. 718-263-3134
54 Continental Ave, Forest Hills, NY 11375
Potential vision test.

CHECK VALVE, RETROGRADE FLOW (IN-LINE) *(General) 80MJF*

B. Braun Oem Division, B. Braun Medical Inc. 866-8-BBRAUN
824 12th Ave, Bethlehem, PA 18018
The ULTRASITE positive displacement IV system from the OEM Division of B. Braun Medical Inc. features a needle-free design ideal for the intermittent injection, aspiration or infusion of fluids.

Halkey-Roberts Corp. 800-303-4384
2700 Halkey Roberts Pl N, Saint Petersburg, FL 33716

Np Medical, Inc. 978-368-4514
101 Union St, Clinton, MA 01510

Spirax Sarco, Inc. 800-575-0394
1150 Northpoint Blvd, Blythewood, SC 29016

Vernay Laboratories, Inc. 800-666-5227
120 E South College St, Yellow Springs, OH 45387

CHEMICAL, FILM PROCESSOR *(Radiology) 90VGU*

Holmes Dental Corp. 800-322-5577
50 S Penn St, Hatboro, PA 19040
QYK FIX.

Image Marketing Corp. 800-466-7032
1636 N 24th St, PO Box 30935, Mesa, AZ 85213
FILM QUICK-CT Automatic black and white film developer for retinal angiography and specular microscopy.

Medlink Imaging, Inc. 800-456-7800
200 Clearbrook Rd, Elmsford, NY 10523

Simon & Company Inc., H.R. 800-638-9460
3515 Marmenco Ct, Baltimore, MD 21230
2- and 3-part developer and fixer.

Solutek Corp. 800-403-0770
94 Shirley St, Roxbury, MA 02119

Ti-Ba Enterprises, Inc. 585-247-1212
25 Hytec Cir, Rochester, NY 14606
Ti-Ba sell new and remanufactured Kodak and Konica Minolta Medical X-ray film processors.

White Mountain Imaging 603-648-2124
1617 Battle St, Webster, NH 03303
X-ray processing chemicals and X-ray chemical mixer.

Xma (X-Ray Marketing Associates, Inc.) 800-325-8880
1205 W Lakeview Ct, Windham Lakes Business Park
Romeoville, IL 60446

CHEMICAL, HEPARIN COATING *(Cardiovascular) 74LIS*

Polysciences, Inc. 800-523-2575
400 Valley Rd, Warrington, PA 18976
Tridodecylmethylammonium heparinate (TDMAC-Heparin).

CHEST, DRY ICE *(General) 80VDK*

Tegrant Corporation, Thermosafe Brands 847-398-0110
3930 N Ventura Dr Ste 450, Arlington Heights, IL 60004

Thermosafe Brands 847-398-0110
3930 N Ventura Dr Ste 450, Arlington Heights, IL 60004
Dry ice chests, also dry ice block makers.

CHILLING UNIT *(Physical Med) 89IMF*

Aqua Products Company, Inc. 800-849-4264
14301 C R Koon Hwy, Newberry, SC 29108
York Stlye Medical Chilers in 1.5 to 20 tons are designed for your MRI, liner accelerators, lab, lasers, electron microscopes, pet scans, and sterilizers. Also Aqua Starr Spot Cooling, cools workstations - per ton - using a high pressure fan coil and 44 degrees Fahrenheit chilled water - this is a permanent installation. Hydro Star Chillers: Some York Medical Chillers are available is a dual circuit with 100% back-up designer for MRIs and liner accelerators.

Chattanooga Group 800-592-7329
4717 Adams Rd, Hixson, TN 37343
COLPAC. Freezer.

Cryopak Industries, Inc. 800-667-2532
1055 Derwent Way, Delta, BC V3M 5R4 Canada
ICE-PAK® Rigid plastic bottle is used in coolers, keeps food cold and fresh. MICROBAN® anti-microbial protection built into plastic to inhibit growth of common household bacteria, fungi, mold, mildew and odors.

Imi Cornelius, Inc. 800-551-4423
500 Regency Dr, Glendale Heights, IL 60139
Refrigerated liquid chillers.

Isocomforter, Inc. 877-277-0367
3531 SW Corporate Pkwy, Palm City, FL 34990
Portable cold-therapy system.

Polar Products, Inc. 800-763-8423
540 S Main St Ste 951, Akron, OH 44311
Kool Max Body Cooling Systems: We have a complete line of lightweight, cost effective body cooling solutions. Our cooling vests and systems are used by Haz Mat teams, the military, and people with multiple sclerosis, in industrial applications and many other fields. Our best-selling vest is the Kool Max Vest, a cotton vest with ten insulated pockets to insert ten Kool Max ice packs into (which are included.) The vest is light at five lbs., adjustable to fit most sizes and can easily be worn under clothing.

Polyscience, Division Of Preston Industries Inc. 800-229-7569
6600 W Touhy Ave, Niles, IL 60714
PolyScience 5000 and 6000 Series Recirculating Chillers feature adjustable temperature, pressure, and flow rate alarms which alert the user instantly to problems ó such as blocked cooling lines or overload conditions ó which could damage equipment or compromise precision. They're ideal for magnetic resonance imaging systems and other imaging equipment that require precise temperature control and dependable heat removal. These high-performance chillers are capable of maintaining process temperatures from -10× to up to +70×C with ±0.1×C stability and are available with ° to 1 HP compressors.

CHISEL (OSTEOTOME) *(Surgery) 79KDG*

Ascent Healthcare Solutions 480-763-5300
10232 S 51st St, Phoenix, AZ 85044
Chisel.

Biomet Microfixation Inc. 800-874-7711
1520 Tradeport Dr, Jacksonville, FL 32218
Various types of chisels.

Biomet, Inc. 574-267-6639
56 E Bell Dr, PO Box 587, Warsaw, IN 46582
Various types of chisel (osteotome).

E.A. Beck & Co. 949-645-4072
657 W 19th St Ste E, P O Box 10857, Costa Mesa, CA 92627
Chisel.

Holmed Corporation 508-238-3351
40 Norfolk Ave, South Easton, MA 02375

Kmedic 800-955-0559
190 Veterans Dr, Northvale, NJ 07647

Medtronic Sofamor Danek Instrument Manufacturing 901-396-3133
7375 Adrianne Pl, Bartlett, TN 38133
Multiple (chisels & osteotomes).

Medtronic Sofamor Danek Usa, Inc. 901-396-3133
4340 Swinnea Rd, Memphis, TN 38118
Multiple (chisels & osteotomes).

CHISEL (OSTEOTOME) *(cont'd)*

Micro-Aire Surgical Instruments, Inc. 800-722-0822
1641 Edlich Dr, Charlottesville, VA 22911
Femoral canal cement removal tools.

Tuzik Boston 800-886-6363
104 Longwater Dr, Assinippi Park, Norwell, MA 02061

Warsaw Orthopedic, Inc. 901-396-3133
2500 Silveus Xing, Warsaw, IN 46582
Multiple (chisels & osteotomes).

CHISEL, BONE, SURGICAL *(Dental And Oral) 76EML*

Aesculap Implant Systems Inc. 1-800-234-9179
3773 Corporate Pkwy, Center Valley, PA 18034

Arnold Tuber Industries 716-648-3363
97 Main St, Hamburg, NY 14075
Chisel, bone, surgical, dental hand instruments.

Bausch & Lomb Surgical 636-255-5051
3365 Tree Court Ind Blvd, Saint Louis, MO 63122

Biomet Microfixation Inc. 800-874-7711
1520 Tradeport Dr, Jacksonville, FL 32218
Various types of chisels.

Coltene/Whaledent Inc. 330-916-8858
235 Ascot Pkwy, Cuyahoga Falls, OH 44223
Explorer.

Dental Usa, Inc. 815-363-8003
5005 McCullom Lake Rd, McHenry, IL 60050
Chisel.

E.A. Beck & Co. 949-645-4072
657 W 19th St Ste E, P O Box 10857, Costa Mesa, CA 92627
Bone chisel.

Elmed, Inc. 630-543-2792
60 W Fay Ave, Addison, IL 60101

George Tiemann & Co. 800-843-6266
25 Plant Ave, Hauppauge, NY 11788

H & H Co. 909-390-0373
4435 E Airport Dr Ste 108, Ontario, CA 91761
Chisel, bone, all types.

Hu-Friedy Manufacturing Co., Inc. 800-483-7433
3232 N Rockwell St, Chicago, IL 60618
$18.70 to $35.25 each, 36 types.

I.E.D., Inc. 231-728-9154
1938 Sanford St, Muskegon, MI 49441
Osteotomes.

Kmedic 800-955-0559
190 Veterans Dr, Northvale, NJ 07647

Lenox-Maclaren Surgical Corp. 720-890-9660
657 S Taylor Ave Ste A, Colorado Technology Center
Louisville, CO 80027
Chisel, bone surgical / all different.

Miltex Inc. 800-645-8000
589 Davies Dr, York, PA 17402

Nordent Manufacturing, Inc. 800-966-7336
610 Bonnie Ln, Elk Grove Village, IL 60007
$32.50 per unit (standard).

Pac-Dent Intl., Inc. 909-839-0888
21078 Commerce Point Dr, Walnut, CA 91789
Various types of chisel.

Premier Dental Products Co. 888-670-6100
1710 Romano Dr, PO Box 4500, Plymouth Meeting, PA 19462

Suter Dental Manufacturing Company, Inc. 800-368-8376
632 Cedar St, Chico, CA 95928

Tuzik Boston 800-886-6363
104 Longwater Dr, Assinippi Park, Norwell, MA 02061

Zimmer Holdings, Inc. 800-613-6131
1800 W Center St, PO Box 708, Warsaw, IN 46580

CHISEL, MASTOID *(Ear/Nose/Throat) 77JYD*

Bausch & Lomb Surgical 636-255-5051
3365 Tree Court Ind Blvd, Saint Louis, MO 63122

Clinimed, Incorporated 877-CLINIMED
303 Markus Ct, Sandy Brae Industrial Park, Newark, DE 19713

Tuzik Boston 800-886-6363
104 Longwater Dr, Assinippi Park, Norwell, MA 02061

CHISEL, MIDDLE EAR *(Ear/Nose/Throat) 77JYE*

Aesculap Implant Systems Inc. 1-800-234-9179
3773 Corporate Pkwy, Center Valley, PA 18034

CHISEL, MIDDLE EAR *(cont'd)*

Bausch & Lomb Surgical 636-255-5051
3365 Tree Court Ind Blvd, Saint Louis, MO 63122

Clinimed, Incorporated 877-CLINIMED
303 Markus Ct, Sandy Brae Industrial Park, Newark, DE 19713

Jedmed Instruments Co. 314-845-3770
5416 Jedmed Ct, Saint Louis, MO 63129

Koros Usa, Inc. 805-529-0825
610 Flinn Ave, Moorpark, CA 93021
Endoscopic or thoracoscopic forceps.

Tuzik Boston 800-886-6363
104 Longwater Dr, Assinippi Park, Norwell, MA 02061

CHISEL, NASAL *(Ear/Nose/Throat) 77KAN*

Bausch & Lomb Surgical 636-255-5051
3365 Tree Court Ind Blvd, Saint Louis, MO 63122

Biomet Microfixation Inc. 800-874-7711
1520 Tradeport Dr, Jacksonville, FL 32218
Various types of chisels.

Clinimed, Incorporated 877-CLINIMED
303 Markus Ct, Sandy Brae Industrial Park, Newark, DE 19713

Gyrus Ent L.L.C., Sub. Of Gyrus Acmi, Inc. 508-804-2739
2925 Appling Rd, Bartlett, TN 38133
Various.

Miltex Inc. 800-645-8000
589 Davies Dr, York, PA 17402

Tuzik Boston 800-886-6363
104 Longwater Dr, Assinippi Park, Norwell, MA 02061

CHISEL, ORTHOPEDIC *(Orthopedics) 87QJU*

Fehling Surgical Instruments 800-FEHLING
509 Broadstone Ln NW, Acworth, GA 30101

Holmed Corporation 508-238-3351
40 Norfolk Ave, South Easton, MA 02375

Zimmer Holdings, Inc. 800-613-6131
1800 W Center St, PO Box 708, Warsaw, IN 46580

CHISEL, OSTEOTOME, SURGICAL *(Dental And Oral) 76EMM*

Biomet Microfixation Inc. 800-874-7711
1520 Tradeport Dr, Jacksonville, FL 32218
Various types of chisels.

H & H Co. 909-390-0373
4435 E Airport Dr Ste 108, Ontario, CA 91761
Chisel, osteotome, all types.

Hu-Friedy Manufacturing Co., Inc. 800-483-7433
3232 N Rockwell St, Chicago, IL 60618
$39.00 to $134.00 each, 29 types.

Kmedic 800-955-0559
190 Veterans Dr, Northvale, NJ 07647

Oratronics, Inc. 212-986-0050
405 Lexington Ave, New York, NY 10174
Osteotome implant depth penetrator.

Pac-Dent Intl., Inc. 909-839-0888
21078 Commerce Point Dr, Walnut, CA 91789
Various types of chisel.

Princeton Medical Group, Inc. 800-875-0869
1189 Royal Links Dr, Mt Pleasant, SC 29466

Renick Ent., Inc. 561-863-4183
1211 W 13th St, Riviera Beach, FL 33404
Ostetomes and surgical kits

Salvin Dental Specialties, Inc. 800-535-6566
3450 Latrobe Dr, Charlotte, NC 28211
Various types of chisels and osteotomes.

Tuzik Boston 800-886-6363
104 Longwater Dr, Assinippi Park, Norwell, MA 02061

CHISEL, SURGICAL, MANUAL *(Surgery) 79FZO*

Advanced Spine Technology, Inc. 415-241-2400
457 Mariposa St, San Francisco, CA 94107
Chisel.

Bausch & Lomb Surgical 636-255-5051
3365 Tree Court Ind Blvd, Saint Louis, MO 63122

Biomet Microfixation Inc. 800-874-7711
1520 Tradeport Dr, Jacksonville, FL 32218
Various types of chisels.

Biomet, Inc. 574-267-6639
56 E Bell Dr, PO Box 587, Warsaw, IN 46582
Various types of chisel.

CHISEL, SURGICAL, MANUAL *(cont'd)*

Dental Usa, Inc. 815-363-8003
5005 McCullom Lake Rd, McHenry, IL 60050
Dental surgical chisel.

Kmedic 800-955-0559
190 Veterans Dr, Northvale, NJ 07647

Medisiss 866-866-7477
2747 SW 6th St, Redmond, OR 97756
Various chisel,surgical,manual,sterile.

Putnam Precision Products 845-278-2141
3859 Danbury Rd, Brewster, NY 10509

Sterilmed, Inc. 763-488-3400
11400 73rd Ave N Ste 100, Maple Grove, MN 55369
Chisel.

Tuzik Boston 800-886-6363
104 Longwater Dr, Assinippi Park, Norwell, MA 02061

Zimmer Holdings, Inc. 800-613-6131
1800 W Center St, PO Box 708, Warsaw, IN 46580

Zimmer Spine, Inc. 800-655-2614
7375 Bush Lake Rd, Minneapolis, MN 55439
Manual surgical chisel.

CHLAMYDIA TRACHOMATIS *(Microbiology) 83MGM*

Akers Biosciences, Inc. 800-451-8378
201 Grove Rd, West Deptford, NJ 08086
HEALTHTEST.

Chembio Diagnostic Systems, Inc. 631-924-1135
3661 Horseblock Rd, Medford, NY 11763
Immunochromatographic assay for the visual detection of chlamydia antigen.

Gen-Probe, Inc. 800-523-5001
10210 Genetic Center Dr, San Diego, CA 92121
PACE Specimen Collection Kits for Endocervical Specimens - for collection and transport of endocervical specimens to be used with either PACE 2 System or the AMPLIFIED CHLAMYDIA TRACHOMATIS assays. PACE Specimens Collection Kits for Urethral and Conjunctival Specimens - for collection and transport of male urethral and conjunctival AMPLIFIED CHLAMYDIA TRACHOMATIS assays. PACE Specimens Collection Kits for Urethral and Conjunctival Specimens - for collection and transport of male urethral and conjunctival specimens to be used with either the PACE 2 System or the AMPLIFIED CHLAMYDIA TRACHOMATIS Assay. PACE Specimens Collection Kits for Endocervical Specimens - for collection and transport of endocervical specimens to be used with either the PACE 2 System or the AMPLIFIED CHLAMYDIA TRACHOMATIS Assay. Swab Specimen Preparation Kit - processing kit used to prepare endocervical and male urethral swab specimens for testing in the GEN-PROBE AMPLIFIED CHLAMYDIA TRACHOMATIS Assay. PACE 2 Chlamydia Trachomatis Probe Competition Assay - supplemental test to verify non-specific signal in endocervical and male urethral swab specimens that test positive in the PACE 2 System assays for Chlamydia trachomatis. PACE 2 System for Chlamydia Trachomatis - for direct detection of Chlamydia trachomatis from endocervical, male urethral, and conjuctival swab specimens.

CHLAMYDIA, DNA REAGENTS *(Microbiology) 83LSK*

Ameritek Usa, Inc. 425-379-2580
125 130th St SE Ste 200, Everett, WA 98208
Chlamydia test kit.

Bio-Medical Products Corp. 800-543-7427
10 Halstead Rd, Mendham, NJ 07945
Chlamydia screening test kit. Immunochromatographic 20 minute test. Rapid chlamydia test, 10 minutes. $8.00 per test.

Prodesse, Inc. 888-589-6974
W229N1870 Westwood Dr, Waukesha, WI 53186
Pneumoplex® - Multiplex PCR Reagents for simultaneous detection and differentiation of Mycoplasma pneumoniae, Legionella pneumophila, Legionella micdadei, Chlamydophila pneumoniae, and Bordetella pertussis - Research Use Only

Qiagen Gaithersburg, Inc. 800-344-3631
1201 Clopper Rd, Gaithersburg, MD 20878
Reagents for the detection of chlamydia trachomatis (ct) dna.

Thermo Biostar, Inc. 800-637-3717
331 S 104th St, Louisville, CO 80027
100% specific, with results in 19 minutes. Test and treat in a single office visit.

CHLORIDIMETER *(Gastro/Urology) 78QJW*

Labconco Corp. 800-821-5525
8811 Prospect Ave, Kansas City, MO 64132
A columteric titrator used to quantitatively measure sodium chloride ion content in clinical samples such as urine, serum and biological extracts.

CHOLEDOCHOSCOPE, FLEXIBLE OR RIGID *(Gastro/Urology) 78FBN*

Gyrus Acmi, Inc. 508-804-2739
300 Stillwater P.o.box 1971, Stamford, CT 06902
Choledochoscope.

Karl Storz Endoscopy-America Inc. 800-421-0837
600 Corporate Pointe, Culver City, CA 90230
Flexible 7.5 Fr. and 15.5 Fr. outside diameters. Passive two-way deflection system.

Machida, Inc. 914-365-0600
40 Ramland Rd S, Orangeburg, NY 10962
No common name listed.

Mahe International Inc. 800-294-7946
468 Craighead St, Nashville, TN 37204

Olympus America, Inc. 800-645-8160
3500 Corporate Pkwy, PO Box 610, Center Valley, PA 18034
Flexible choledochoscope.

Pentax Medical Company 800-431-5880
102 Chestnut Ridge Rd, Montvale, NJ 07645
$16,170.00 for flexible choledocho-cysto-nephroscope with a distal tip diameter of 4.8mm, and a channel size of 2.2mm; fully immersible.

Pentax Southern Region Service Center 201-571-2300
8934 Kirby Dr, Houston, TX 77054
Choledochoscope.

Pentax West Coast Service Center 800-431-5880
10410 Pioneer Blvd Ste 2, Santa Fe Springs, CA 90670
Pentax choledochoscope.

Richard Wolf Medical Instruments Corp. 800-323-9653
353 Corporate Woods Pkwy, Vernon Hills, IL 60061

CHOLEDOCHOSCOPE, MINI-DIAMETER (5MM OR LESS) *(Gastro/Urology) 78WZV*

Olympus America, Inc. 800-645-8160
3500 Corporate Pkwy, PO Box 610, Center Valley, PA 18034

CHOLINESTERASE, ANTIGEN, ANTISERUM, CONTROL *(Toxicology) 91DCQ*

Creative Laboratory Products, Inc. 317-293-2991
6420 Guion Rd, Indianapolis, IN 46268

CHROMATOGRAPHIC BACTERIAL IDENTIFICATION *(Microbiology) 83JSQ*

Biolog, Inc. 800-284-4949
21124 Cabot Blvd, Hayward, CA 94545

Microcheck, Inc. 877-934-3284
142 Gould Road, Northfield, VT 05663
$40.00 to $90.00 ea. for ID and comparative analysis. Identifies over 1,500 species of yeast, mycobacteria, fungi and actinomycetes. 96 hour turnaround standard. 48 hour STAT turnaround.

Midi, Inc. 302-737-4297
125 Sandy Dr, Newark, DE 19713
Sherlock microbial identification system.

CHROMATOGRAPHIC BARBITURATE IDENTIFICATION (THIN LAYER) *(Toxicology) 91DKX*

Pochemco, Inc. 413-536-2900
724 Main St, Holyoke, MA 01040
Iodoplatinate for non-volatile organic substances; mercuric sulfate.

CHROMATOGRAPHIC DERIVATIVE, TOTAL LIPIDS *(Chemistry) 75CFB*

Ameritek Usa, Inc. 425-379-2580
125 130th St SE Ste 200, Everett, WA 98208
Dengue test kit.

Matreya Llc 800-342-3595
168 Tressler St, Pleasant Gap, PA 16823
Various l-lecithin/sphingomyelin solutions.

CHROMATOGRAPHIC SEPARATION, CPK ISOENZYMES *(Chemistry) 75JHT*

Biomerieux Inc. 800-682-2666
100 Rodolphe St, Durham, NC 27712

CHROMATOGRAPHIC SEPARATION, CPK ISOENZYMES *(cont'd)*

Health Chem Diagnostics Llc 954-979-3845
3341 W McNab Rd, Pompano Beach, FL 33069
Chromatographic separation, cpk isoenzymes.

Nano-Ditech Corporation 609-409-0700
7 Clarke Dr, Cranbury, NJ 08512
Chromatographic separation, cpk isoenzymes.

CHROMATOGRAPHIC SEPARATION, LECITHIN-SPHINGOMYELIN RATIO *(Chemistry) 75JHG*

Helena Laboratories 409-842-3714
PO Box 752, Beaumont, TX 77704

Sita Associates 630-968-3727
720 Williamsburg Ct, Oak Brook, IL 60523
Lecithin-sphingomyelin standards.

CHROMATOGRAPHIC, CYSTINE *(Chemistry) 75JLD*

Mission Pharmacal Co. 210-696-8400
10999 W Interstate 10 Ste 1000, San Antonio, TX 78230
UROCYSTIN Qualitative screening test for urine cystine concentration.

CHROMATOGRAPHIC, PHOSPHOLIPIDS *(Chemistry) 75JNT*

Health Chem Diagnostics Llc 954-979-3845
3341 W McNab Rd, Pompano Beach, FL 33069
Chromatographic, phospholipids.

CHROMATOGRAPHIC/FLUOROMETRIC METHOD, CATECHOLAMINES *(Chemistry) 75CHQ*

Basi (Bioanalytical Systems, Inc.) 800-845-4246
2701 Kent Ave, West Lafayette, IN 47906
Electrochemical in vitro diagnostic kits for catecholamines, urinary metanephrines, and plasma homocysteine.

Bio-Rad Laboratories Inc., Clinical Systems Div. 800-224-6723
4000 Alfred Nobel Dr, Hercules, CA 94547
Various.

Bio-Rad Laboratories, Life Science Group 800-424-6723
2000 Alfred Nobel Dr, Hercules, CA 94547

CHROMATOGRAPHY (GAS), CLINICAL USE *(Toxicology) 91KZQ*

Celsis Laboratory Group 800-523-5227
165 Fieldcrest Ave, Edison, NJ 08837

Puregas 800-521-5351
226 Commerce St Unit A, Broomfield, CO 80020

Varian Scientific Instruments 925-939-2400
2700 Mitchell Dr, Walnut Creek, CA 94598
Automated gas chromatography system.

CHROMATOGRAPHY (LIQUID, GEL), CLINICAL USE *(Toxicology) 91KZR*

Varian Scientific Instruments 925-939-2400
2700 Mitchell Dr, Walnut Creek, CA 94598
Automated liquid chromatography system.

CHROMATOGRAPHY EQUIPMENT, GAS *(Chemistry) 75QJY*

Agilent Technologies, Inc. 877-424-4536
5301 Stevens Creek Blvd, Santa Clara, CA 95051

Antek Instruments, Inc. 281-580-0339
300 Bammel Westfield Rd, Houston, TX 77090
Nitrogen-specific GC detector and sulfur chemiluminescent detector.

Buck Scientific, Inc. 800-562-5566
58 Fort Point St, Norwalk, CT 06855
Buck 910/310 gas chromatographs (GC). Mainframe and oven GCs with the following detectors: TCD, FID, ECD, HID, NPD, PID, FPD, or any combination, most accessories.

Cobert Associates, Inc. 800-972-4766
2302 Weldon Pkwy, Saint Louis, MO 63146

Gow-Mac Instrument Co. 610-954-9000
277 Brodhead Rd, Bethlehem, PA 18017
Six models starting at $4,600 using either thermal conductivity detectors, flame ionization detectors, or discharge ionization detectors; temperature programming available. Also, binary gas analyzers, total hydrocarbon analyzers, aromatic hydrocarbon analyzers, gas-leak detectors, moisture-in-gases analyzers.

Puregas 800-521-5351
226 Commerce St Unit A, Broomfield, CO 80020

Tremetrics 800-825-0121
7625 Golden Triangle Dr, Eden Prairie, MN 55344
$15,000 for microprocessor-controlled system with 2 detector mounts, backlit vacuum fluorescent display, keypad memory.

CHROMATOGRAPHY EQUIPMENT, ION EXCHANGE *(Toxicology) 91DJY*

Beckman Coulter, Inc. 800-742-2345
250 S Kraemer Blvd, PO Box 8000, Brea, CA 92821

Bio-Rad Laboratories, Life Science Group 800-424-6723
2000 Alfred Nobel Dr, Hercules, CA 94547
Modular and integrated systems, classical columns, resins.

Image Molding, Inc. 800-525-1875
4525 Kingston St, Denver, CO 80239
Solid phase extraction columns and custom filtration columns. Also, empty columns.

Polymer Laboratories, Now A Part Of Varian, Inc. 800-767-3963
160 Old Farm Rd, Amherst Fields Research Park, Amherst, MA 01002

Varian Inc 650-424-5078
25200 Commercentre Dr, Lake Forest, CA 92630
Solid phase extraction columns & plates.

CHROMATOGRAPHY EQUIPMENT, LIQUID *(Chemistry) 75QJZ*

Agilent Technologies, Inc. 877-424-4536
5301 Stevens Creek Blvd, Santa Clara, CA 95051

Basi (Bioanalytical Systems, Inc.) 800-845-4246
2701 Kent Ave, West Lafayette, IN 47906
$6,000 to $45,000 for electrochemical, fluorescent, and UV/VIS detection systems; manual and automated chromatographs with data-acquisition software.

Beckman Coulter, Inc. 800-742-2345
250 S Kraemer Blvd, PO Box 8000, Brea, CA 92821

Bio-Rad Laboratories, Life Science Group 800-424-6723
2000 Alfred Nobel Dr, Hercules, CA 94547
Analyzers & systems for protein, carbohydrate, organic acid & base.

Cobert Associates, Inc. 800-972-4766
2302 Weldon Pkwy, Saint Louis, MO 63146

Esa, Inc. 800-959-5095
22 Alpha Rd, Chelmsford, MA 01824

Jasco, Inc. 800-333-5272
8649 Commerce Dr, Easton, MD 21601
$9,500.00 per unit (standard).

Kontes Glass Co. 888-546-2531
1022 Spruce St, Vineland, NJ 08360

Nest Group Inc., The 800-347-6378
45 Valley Rd, Southborough, MA 01772
SPRITE, PICCOLO, and CAPELLINI, small volume LC-MS capillary columns for RPC, HILIC or Ion Exchange

Polymer Laboratories, Now A Part Of Varian, Inc. 800-767-3963
160 Old Farm Rd, Amherst Fields Research Park, Amherst, MA 01002

Waters Corp. 800-252-4752
34 Maple St, Milford, MA 01757
$9850-$23,425 for preparative-type systems.

Whatman Inc. 732-885-6529
800 Centennial Ave Bldg 1, Piscataway, NJ 08854

CHROMATOGRAPHY EQUIPMENT, PAPER *(Chemistry) 75QKA*

Beckman Coulter, Inc. 800-742-2345
250 S Kraemer Blvd, PO Box 8000, Brea, CA 92821

Kontes Glass Co. 888-546-2531
1022 Spruce St, Vineland, NJ 08360

Schleicher & Schuell, Inc. 800-245-4024
10 Optical Ave, PO Box 2012, Keene, NH 03431

Varian Sample Preparation Products 800-421-2825
24201 Frampton Ave, Harbor City, CA 90710

Whatman Inc. 732-885-6529
800 Centennial Ave Bldg 1, Piscataway, NJ 08854

CHROMATOGRAPHY EQUIPMENT, THIN LAYER *(Toxicology) 91DPA*

Camag Scientific, Inc. 800-334-3909
515 Cornelius Harnett Dr, Wilmington, NC 28401
Products for sample application, development, etc.

Cobert Associates, Inc. 800-972-4766
2302 Weldon Pkwy, Saint Louis, MO 63146

Farrand Optical Components & Instruments, Div. Of Ruhle Co. 914-287-4035
99 Wall St, Valhalla, NY 10595
Tlc plate scanner.

Helena Laboratories 409-842-3714
PO Box 752, Beaumont, TX 77704

CHROMATOGRAPHY EQUIPMENT, THIN LAYER *(cont'd)*

Kontes Glass Co. 888-546-2531
1022 Spruce St, Vineland, NJ 08360
$7,250 per unit, fiber-optic multimedia scanner.

Varian Inc 650-424-5078
25200 Commercentre Dr, Lake Forest, CA 92630
Chromatographic system, tlc, drug testing.

Whatman Inc. 732-885-6529
800 Centennial Ave Bldg 1, Piscataway, NJ 08854

CHROMATOGRAPHY, LIQUID, PERFORMANCE, HIGH
(Toxicology) 91MAS

Antek Instruments, Inc. 281-580-0339
300 Bammel Westfield Rd, Houston, TX 77090
Nitrogen specific HPLC detector.

Beckman Coulter, Inc. 800-742-2345
250 S Kraemer Blvd, PO Box 8000, Brea, CA 92821

Bio-Rad Laboratories, Life Science Group 800-424-6723
2000 Alfred Nobel Dr, Hercules, CA 94547
$60-$100 for resins; $75-$2000 for packed columns; $30-$75 for equipment (columns, holders, filtration materials); $550 for sample injector; $900 for strip chart recorder; $4,500 for UV monitor. $35,000 per system.

Celsis Laboratory Group 800-523-5227
165 Fieldcrest Ave, Edison, NJ 08837
Anti-inflammatory analyses, steroid analyses, preservative analyses and pharmaceutical analyses.

Chiral Technologies, Inc. 800-6-Chiral
800 N 5 Points Rd, West Chester, PA 19380
DAICEL chiral columns, method for preparing and analyzing enantiomers in quantities ranging from milligrams and grams to kilograms.

Cobert Associates, Inc. 800-972-4766
2302 Weldon Pkwy, Saint Louis, MO 63146

Eprogen, Inc. 800-556-4272
8205 S Cass Ave Ste 106, Darien, IL 60561
Columns, HPLC (a complete line).

GP Instruments 888-215-6855
11130 Kingston Pike Ste 1200, Knoxville, TN 37934
HPLC autosamplers featuring micro-titer plates, 128-vial tray, priority sampling, optional refrigeration, multiple injections per vial, and more. HPLC pumps also available.

Hitachi High Technologies America, Inc. 800-548-9001
3100 N 1st St, San Jose, CA 95134
The Hitachi LaChrom Elite HPLC system is a reliability-proven high-accuracy high-performance chromatography equipment.

Honeywell Burdick & Jackson 800-368-0050
1953 Harvey St, Muskegon, MI 49442

Jasco, Inc. 800-333-5272
8649 Commerce Dr, Easton, MD 21601
Systems range from $9000 to $40000.

Medical Sales & Service Group 888-357-6520
10 Woodchester Dr, Acton, MA 01720

Myco Instrumentation Source, Inc. 425-228-4239
PO Box 354, Renton, WA 98057

Polymer Laboratories, Now A Part Of Varian, Inc. 800-767-3963
160 Old Farm Rd, Amherst Fields Research Park, Amherst, MA 01002
HPLC detectors. Polymeric reversed phase columns & media. POLYMERIC PLRP-S 300A, reversed phase columns & media for peptides & proteins.

Regis Technologies, Inc. 800-323-8144
8210 Austin Ave, Morton Grove, IL 60053

Richard Scientific, Inc. 800-840-3030
285 Bel Marin Keys Blvd Ste M, Novato, CA 94949
Sedex ELS universal/mass detector for HPLC, GPC, SFC and CCC. Rheos solvent delivery system for micro HPLC, LC-MS.

Spectron Corp. 425-827-9317
934 S Burlington Blvd # 603, Burlington, WA 98233
Reconditioned equipment.

Thermo Fisher Scientific 800-437-2999
PO Box 712099, Cincinnati, OH 45271

Waters Corp. 800-252-4752
34 Maple St, Milford, MA 01757
4 models, $8,895-$12,795, single and dual detector, isocratic and gradient types; fixed or variable wave length UV/visible absorbance detection. Special purpose system available (mino acid analyzers).

CHROMATOGRAPHY, THIN LAYER, TRICYCLIC ANTIDEPRESSANT DRUGS *(Toxicology) 91MLK*

Amedica Biotech, Inc. 510-785-5980
28301 Industrial Blvd Ste K, Hayward, CA 94545
Drug screen tricyclic antidepressant test.

Biosite Incorporated 888-246-7483
9975 Summers Ridge Rd, San Diego, CA 92121
Fluorescence immunoassay for detection of drugs of abuse in urine.

Branan Medical Corp. 949-598-7166
140 Technology Dr Ste 400, Irvine, CA 92618
Immunochromatographical test (qualitative determination of tca in human urine).

Express Diagnostics Int'L, Inc. 507-526-3951
1550 Industrial Dr, Blue Earth, MN 56013
Drugs of abuse screening test.

CHROME ALUM HEMATOXYLIN *(Pathology) 88ICI*

Sci Gen, Inc. 310-324-6576
333 E Gardena Blvd, Gardena, CA 90248
FDA: Medical Device Manufacturing and packaging. Focus on Histology, Cytology, Analytical and General purpose Reagents, Chemistry, and Sterling and Disinfecting agents.

CHRONAXIMETER, PHYSICAL MEDICINE *(Physical Med) 89IKP*

R.J. Lindquist Co. 213-382-1268
2419 James M Wood Blvd, Los Angeles, CA 90006
Various models - stimulator - chronaximeter.

CINEANGIOGRAPH (CARDIAC CATHETERIZATION)
(Radiology) 90QKB

Heartlab, Inc. 800-959-3205
1 Crosswind Dr, Westerly, RI 02891

King's Medical 330-653-3968
1894 Georgetown Rd, Hudson, OH 44236

M & I Medical Sales, Inc. 305-663-6444
4711 SW 72nd Ave, Miami, FL 33155

Stallion Technologies, Inc. 315-476-4330
1201 E Fayette St, Syracuse, NY 13210

CIRCUIT, BREATHING (W CONNECTOR, ADAPTER, Y PIECE)
(Anesthesiology) 73CAI

Alero, Inc. 951-273-7890
1550 Consumer Cir, Corona, CA 92880
Breathing circuits.

Anesthesia Associates, Inc. 760-744-6561
460 Enterprise St, San Marcos, CA 92078
Large variety of configurations available in both Latex Free and traditional Latex. Many selections of masks, elbows, adapters, inserts, pop-offs, inlets, sampling and sensing ports, tubing styles and lengths, bags and scavenging options.

Cardinal Health 207, Inc. 610-862-0800
1100 Bird Center Dr, Palm Springs, CA 92262
Adult/pediatric/infant reusable breathing circuit.

Customed, Inc. 787-801-0101
Calle Igualdad #7, Fajardo, PR 00738
Anesthesia custom circuit hospital de la concepcion 900-178.

Eastmed Enterprises, Inc. 856-797-0131
11 Brandywine Dr, Marlton, NJ 08053
Guedel and Berman airways.

Instrumentation Industries, Inc. 800-633-8577
2990 Industrial Blvd, Bethel Park, PA 15102
Adapter, tube, tracheal, swivel adapters for endotube/trach tube. Adapter Y, swivel Y, and slip-proof Y.

Intersurgical Inc. 315-451-2900
417 Electronics Pkwy, Liverpool, NY 13088

Lampac International Ltd. 636-797-3659
230 N Lake Dr, Hillsboro, MO 63050

Medi-Part,Inc. 847-639-2584
5844 N Rice Lake Rd, P.o. Box 276, Mercer, WI 54547
Various types of breathing circuits.

Medical Mfg., Inc. 415-282-5580
1290 Sanchez St # 2, San Francisco, CA 94114
Various anesthesia respiratory breathing circuit pack kit.

Medline Industries, Inc. 800-633-5886
1 Medline Pl, Mundelein, IL 60060

Optimize Mfg. Co. 520-287-4605
Apdo Postal 205-A,, Parque Industrial San Ramon
Nogales, Sonora Mexico
An-trol ii anesthesia circle system

CIRCUIT, BREATHING (W CONNECTOR, ADAPTER, Y PIECE) *(cont'd)*

Promedic, Inc. 239-498-2155
3460 Pointe Creek Ct Apt 102, Bonita Springs, FL 34134

ReNu Medical Inc. 877-252-1110
9800 Evergreen Way, Everett, WA 98204
MULTIPLE MODELS; REPROCESSED CIRCUIT BREATHING

Respironics Colorado 800-345-6443
12301 Grant St Unit 190, Thornton, CO 80241
Various prices and styles of ventilator breathing circuits.

Romed, Llc 562-438-8904
4224 E Massachusetts St, Long Beach, CA 90814
Cushioned protection for oxygen tubing.

Seven Harvest Intl. Import & Export 765-456-3584
108 N Dixon Rd, Kokomo, IN 46901
Swivel; oxygen breathing connector.

Smiths Medical Asd Inc. 800-258-5361
10 Bowman Dr, Keene, NH 03431
Various types of anesthesia breathing circuits.

Thompson Engineering 858-748-5677
11472 Tree Hollow Ln, San Diego, CA 92128
Various nasal cannulas, oxygen tubing, flow control valve.

Ventlab Corp. 336-753-5000
155 Boyce Dr, Mocksville, NC 27028
Curcuit, breathing, ventilator.

CIRCUIT, BREATHING, VENTILATOR *(Anesthesiology) 73QEL*

Anesthesia Associates, Inc. 760-744-6561
460 Enterprise St, San Marcos, CA 92078
Large variety of configurations available in both Latex Free and traditional Latex. Many selections of masks, elbows, adapters, inserts, pop-offs, inlets, sampling and sensing ports, tubing styles and lengths, bags and scavenging options.

Bio-Med Devices, Inc. 800-224-6633
61 Soundview Rd, Guilford, CT 06437
Ventilator circuits and test lungs, for home care and hospital ventilators and CPAP systems.

Bunnell Incorporated 800-800-4358
436 Lawndale Dr, Salt Lake City, UT 84115
Bunnell jet ventilator humidifier breathing circuit.

Clearmedical, Inc. 425-883-1522
14150 NE 20th St Ste F1, Bellevue, WA 98007
Systems and services for reprocessing anesthesia and respiratory circuits and related equipment.

Instrumentation Industries, Inc. 800-633-8577
2990 Industrial Blvd, Bethel Park, PA 15102

Intersurgical Inc. 315-451-2900
417 Electronics Pkwy, Liverpool, NY 13088

Repex Medical Products, Inc. 305-740-0133
5240 SW 64th Ave, Miami, FL 33155

CIRCULATOR, BREATHING CIRCUIT *(Anesthesiology) 73CAG*

Medline Industries, Inc. 800-633-5886
1 Medline Pl, Mundelein, IL 60060

Smiths Medical Asd, Inc. 847-793-0135
330 Corporate Woods Pkwy, Vernon Hills, IL 60061
Ippb breathing circuits, (with manifold) + nebulizers.

CIRCULATOR, WATER BATH *(Chemistry) 75SFW*

Brinkmann Instruments (Canada) Ltd. 800-263-8715
6670 Campobello Rd., Mississauga, ONT L5N 2L8 Canada

Brinkmann Instruments, Inc. 800-645-3050
PO Box 1019, Westbury, NY 11590

Caron Products And Services, Inc. 800-648-3042
PO Box 715, Marietta, OH 45750
Refrigerated bath/circulator available with wide temperature ranges and external circulation pumping ability.

Cole-Parmer Instrument Inc. 800-323-4340
625 E Bunker Ct, Vernon Hills, IL 60061

Polyscience, Division Of Preston Industries Inc. 800-229-7569
6600 W Touhy Ave, Niles, IL 60714
Programmable Model 9112. This top-of-the-line model features a wide temperature range and time/temperature programmability. Programs can be set directly from the front panel with the aid of the Select/Set knob and multi-language display, or from a PC using the RS-232 interface. LabView™ drivers and Excel® macros offer even greater programming and data logging convenience. Remote probe capability plus 5-speed pressure/ suction (duplex) pump further enhance the capabilities of the Model 9112.

CIRCULATOR, WATER BATH *(cont'd)*

Pro Scientific Inc. 800-584-3776
99 Willenbrock Rd, Oxford, CT 06478
The 45U Memmert water bath, from 10-100 degrees Celsius is a circulating water bath with the following standard features;high grade stainless steel, microprocessor PID control, integral self-diagnostics, digital timer, digital temperature display, overtemperature protection and corrosion proof large-area heating system on three sides of the working space ensuring optimum temperature uniformity.

Thermo Fisher Scientific 877-843-7668
81 Wyman St, Waltham, MA 02451

CIRCULATORY ASSIST UNIT, CARDIAC *(Cardiovascular) 74QKD*

Abiomed, Inc. 800-422-8666
22 Cherry Hill Dr, Danvers, MA 01923
Bi-ventricular cardiac-assist unit driven with pneumatic pump and disposable blood pumps.

Biomation 888-667-2324
335 Perth St., P.O. Box 156, Almonte, ON K0A 1A0 Canada
Circulator Boot end-diastolic pneumatic compression system for arterial and venous insufficiency

Rozinn By Scottcare Corporation 800-243-9412
4791 W 150th St, Cleveland, OH 44135
NICORE External Counterpulsation (ECP) provides new revenue while benefiting over 80% of patients. Intelligent technologies deliver effective therapy and seamlessly integrate with IT systems, track outcomes and improve efficiency.

Scottcare Corporation 800-243-9412
4791 W 150th St, Cleveland, OH 44135
NICORE Advantage opens the door to new revenue opportunities while addressing today's demanding clinical environment. ScottCare designed the NICORE Advantage External Counterpulsation (ECP) system to deliver effective therapy and seamlessly integrate with information technology systems, track patient outcomes and improve efficiency for clinicians. External Counterpulsation (ECP) provides an opportunity to treat and improve the quality of life for ino optionî angina and heart failure patients who are refractory to medications and those who are non-surgical candidates. Clinical studies have demonstrated that ECP therapy benefits more than 80% of patients treated, with significant improvement in relief of the symptoms, increased functional capacity, and reduced dependence on medication.

CIRCULATORY ASSIST UNIT, INTRA-AORTIC BALLOON *(Cardiovascular) 74QKE*

Datascope Cardiac Assist Div. 800-777-4222
15 Law Dr, Fairfield, NJ 07004
Intra-aortic balloon pumps.

Datascope Corp. 800-288-2121
14 Philips Pkwy, Montvale, NJ 07645
System 95 Intra-Aortic Balloon Pump System 97e with Cardio Sync Software. Intra-aortic balloon pump with monitor, pacemaker rejection, ESU and transport capability.

CIRCULATORY ASSIST UNIT, LEFT VENTRICULAR *(Cardiovascular) 74DSQ*

Cardiac Assist, Inc. 412-963-7770
240 Alpha Dr, Pittsburgh, PA 15238
Ab-180 css.

Medtronic Cardiovascular Surgery, The Heart Valve Div. 800-328-2518
1851 E Deere Ave, Santa Ana, CA 92705
Various sizes of apical left ventricle connectors.

Medtronic Heart Valves 800-227-3191
8299 Central Ave NE, Spring Lake Park, MN 55432
Various sizes.

Micromed Technology, Inc. 713-838-9210
8965 Interchange Dr, Houston, TX 77054
Left ventricular assist device.

Peter Schiff Enterprise 931-537-6505
4900 Forrest Hill Rd, Cookeville, TN 38506
Various sizes of mechanical ventricular assist cups.

Syncardia Systems, Inc. 866-771-9437
1992 E Silverlake Rd, Tucson, AZ 85713
Total artificial heart.

Whalen Biomedical Incorporated 617-868-4433
11 Miller St, Somerville, MA 02143
The EPAD is a valveless, pneumatically driven cardiac assist device for providing short term right or left ventricular support.

CIRCULATORY ASSIST UNIT, LEFT VENTRICULAR *(cont'd)*

World Heart Inc. 801-355-6255
7799 Pardee Ln, Oakland, CA 94621
Novacor N100 left ventricular assist system.

World Heart Inc. 888-843-5827
4750 Wiley Post Way Ste 120, Salt Lake City, UT 84116
HeartQuest(TM) VAD is a centrifugal, magnetically levitated, magnetically driven, implantable assist device. It is durable, small, and has a full range of hemodynamic output.(This device is currently under development and has not recieved clearance from any regulatory agency; this description is provided for informational purposes only.)

CLAMP AND CUTTER, UMBILICAL *(Obstetrics/Gyn) 85NBZ*

Busse Hospital Disposables, Inc. 631-435-4711
75 Arkay Dr, Hauppauge, NY 11788
Umbilical cord clamp & clamp.

CLAMP, AORTA *(Cardiovascular) 74QKI*

Clinimed, Incorporated 877-CLINIMED
303 Markus Ct, Sandy Brae Industrial Park, Newark, DE 19713

Codman & Shurtleff, Inc 800-225-0460
325 Paramount Dr, Raynham, MA 02767

Fehling Surgical Instruments 800-FEHLING
509 Broadstone Ln NW, Acworth, GA 30101

Miltex Inc. 800-645-8000
589 Davies Dr, York, PA 17402

Princeton Medical Group, Inc. 800-875-0869
1189 Royal Links Dr, Mt Pleasant, SC 29466

CLAMP, BONE *(Orthopedics) 87HXD*

Biomet Microfixation Inc. 800-874-7711
1520 Tradeport Dr, Jacksonville, FL 32218
Various types of clamps.

Biomet, Inc. 574-267-6639
56 E Bell Dr, PO Box 587, Warsaw, IN 46582
Various types of clamp.

Cardinal Health, Snowden Pencer Products 847-689-8410
5175 S Royal Atlanta Dr, Tucker, GA 30084
Various styles of clamps.

Kmedic 800-955-0559
190 Veterans Dr, Northvale, NJ 07647

Medtronic Sofamor Danek Instrument Manufacturing 901-396-3133
7375 Adrianne Pl, Bartlett, TN 38133
Multiple (orthopedic clamps).

Medtronic Sofamor Danek Usa, Inc. 901-396-3133
4340 Swinnea Rd, Memphis, TN 38118
Multiple (orthopedic clamps).

Nobel Biocare Usa, Llc 800-579-6515
22715/22725 Savi Ranch Parkway, Yorba Linda, CA 92887
Surgical instrument.

Pos-T-Vac, Inc. 800-279-7434
1701 N 14th Ave, P.O. Box 1436, Dodge City, KS 67801
The clamp.

Qfc Plastics, Inc. 817-649-7400
728 111th St, Arlington, TX 76011
Clamp.

Sta-Sof Breast Compressor-Clamp 310-470-8798
10571 Wyton Dr, Los Angeles, CA 90024
Breast compressor clamp.

Symmetry Medical Usa, Inc. 574-267-8700
486 W 350 N, Warsaw, IN 46582
Manual surgical instrument for general use.

Terumo Cardiovascular Systems (Tcvs) 800-283-7866
28 Howe St, Ashland, MA 01721
Clamp.

Tuzik Boston 800-886-6363
104 Longwater Dr, Assinippi Park, Norwell, MA 02061

Warsaw Orthopedic, Inc. 901-396-3133
2500 Silveus Xing, Warsaw, IN 46582
Multiple (orthopedic clamps).

Zimmer Holdings, Inc. 800-613-6131
1800 W Center St, PO Box 708, Warsaw, IN 46580

CLAMP, BRONCHUS *(Ear/Nose/Throat) 77QKJ*

Clinimed, Incorporated 877-CLINIMED
303 Markus Ct, Sandy Brae Industrial Park, Newark, DE 19713

CLAMP, BRONCHUS *(cont'd)*

Miltex Inc. 800-645-8000
589 Davies Dr, York, PA 17402

CLAMP, BULLDOG *(Surgery) 79QKK*

Miltex Inc. 800-645-8000
589 Davies Dr, York, PA 17402

Novare Surgical Systems, Inc. 408-873-3161
10440 Bubb Rd Ste A, Cupertino, CA 95014

Roboz Surgical Instrument Co., Inc. 800-424-2984
PO Box 10710, Gaithersburg, MD 20898

Scanlan International, Inc. 800-328-9458
1 Scanlan Plz, Saint Paul, MN 55107
Disposable bulldog clamps and shunt clamp.

Sterion, Incorporated 800-328-7958
13828 Lincoln St NE, Ham Lake, MN 55304
Silicone covered, parallel clamping jaws provide equal occluding pressure while minimizing vessel trauma.

CLAMP, CANNULA *(Gastro/Urology) 78FKC*

Bausch & Lomb Surgical 636-255-5051
3365 Tree Court Ind Blvd, Saint Louis, MO 63122

Lifemed Of California 800-543-3633
1216 S Allec St, Anaheim, CA 92805

Medical Innovations International Inc. 507-289-0761
6256 34th Ave NW, Rochester, MN 55901
Rochester Reusable Cannula Clamp™.

Sorin Group Usa 800-289-5759
14401 W 65th Way, Arvada, CO 80004

CLAMP, CAROTID ARTERY *(Cns/Neurology) 84HCE*

Biomet Microfixation Inc. 800-874-7711
1520 Tradeport Dr, Jacksonville, FL 32218
Various types of clamps.

Depuy-Raynham, A Div. Of Depuy Orthopaedics 800-451-2006
325 Paramount Dr, Raynham, MA 02767
Various.

Kmedic 800-955-0559
190 Veterans Dr, Northvale, NJ 07647

Tuzik Boston 800-886-6363
104 Longwater Dr, Assinippi Park, Norwell, MA 02061

CLAMP, CIRCUMCISION *(Obstetrics/Gyn) 85HFX*

Allied Healthcare Products, Inc. 800-444-3954
1720 Sublette Ave, Saint Louis, MO 63110

Busse Hospital Disposables, Inc. 631-435-4711
75 Arkay Dr, Hauppauge, NY 11788
Circumcision tray.

Generic Medical Device, Inc. 253-853-3594
5727 Baker Way NW Ste 201, Gig Harbor, WA 98332
Circumcision clamp.

Princeton Medical Group, Inc. 800-875-0869
1189 Royal Links Dr, Mt Pleasant, SC 29466

Surgical Implant Generation Network (Sign) 509-371-1107
451 Hills St, Richland, WA 99354
Wrench.

Tri-State Hospital Supply Corp. 800-248-4058
301 Catrell Dr, PO Box 170, Howell, MI 48843
Gomco style.

CLAMP, DIALYSIS ARM *(Gastro/Urology) 78NOO*

Snow Products, Inc. 847-381-5222
27W996 Industrial Ave Ste 6, Lake Barrington, IL 60010
Dialysis arm clamp.

CLAMP, EYELID, OPHTHALMIC *(Ophthalmology) 86HOD*

Aero Contact Lens, Inc. 269-345-3202
2958 Business One Dr, Kalamazoo, MI 49048
No common name listed.

B. Graczyk, Inc. 269-782-2100
27826 Burmax Park, Dowagiac, MI 49047
Various types of clamps.

Bausch & Lomb Surgical 636-255-5051
3365 Tree Court Ind Blvd, Saint Louis, MO 63122

Fortrad Eye Instruments Corp. 973-543-2371
8 Franklin Rd, Mendham, NJ 07945

George Tiemann & Co. 800-843-6266
25 Plant Ave, Hauppauge, NY 11788

CLAMP, EYELID, OPHTHALMIC *(cont'd)*

Katena Products, Inc. 800-225-1195
4 Stewart Ct, Denville, NJ 07834

CLAMP, FIXATION, CHOLANGIOGRAPHY *(Surgery) 79WZW*

Boss Instruments, Ltd. 800-210-2677
395 Reas Ford Rd Ste 120, Earlysville, VA 22936

Cook Inc. 800-457-4500
PO Box 489, Bloomington, IN 47402

Elmed, Inc. 630-543-2792
60 W Fay Ave, Addison, IL 60101

Princeton Medical Group, Inc. 800-875-0869
1189 Royal Links Dr, Mt Pleasant, SC 29466

CLAMP, HEMODIALYSIS UNIT BLOOD LINE *(Gastro/Urology) 78UCO*

Dravon Medical, Inc. 503-656-6600
11465 SE Highway 212, PO Box 69, Clackamas, OR 97015
Disposable hemostat A-clamp.

Molded Products Inc. 800-435-8957
1112 Chatburn Ave, Harlan, IA 51537
Tube-occluding forceps.

CLAMP, HEMORRHOIDAL *(Gastro/Urology) 78QKL*

Codman & Shurtleff, Inc 800-225-0460
325 Paramount Dr, Raynham, MA 02767

CLAMP, INTESTINAL *(Gastro/Urology) 78QKM*

Codman & Shurtleff, Inc 800-225-0460
325 Paramount Dr, Raynham, MA 02767

Princeton Medical Group, Inc. 800-875-0869
1189 Royal Links Dr, Mt Pleasant, SC 29466

CLAMP, LAPAROSCOPY *(Surgery) 79WZX*

Boss Instruments, Ltd. 800-210-2677
395 Reas Ford Rd Ste 120, Earlysville, VA 22936

Elmed, Inc. 630-543-2792
60 W Fay Ave, Addison, IL 60101

Ethicon Endo-Surgery, Inc. 800-USE-ENDO
4545 Creek Rd, Cincinnati, OH 45242
10mm thoracic, Glassman clamp, 10mm modified Allis clamp.

Mediflex Surgical Products 800-879-7575
250 Gibbs Rd, Islandia, NY 11749

CLAMP, LINE *(Gastro/Urology) 78FKK*

Directmed, Inc. 516-656-3377
150 Pratt Oval, Glen Cove, NY 11542

Rush Medical 401-461-9132
18 Gallup Ave, Cranston, RI 02910
Line or tube clamp.

Sorin Group Usa 800-289-5759
14401 W 65th Way, Arvada, CO 80004

CLAMP, MUSCLE, OPHTHALMIC *(Ophthalmology) 86HOB*

B. Graczyk, Inc. 269-782-2100
27826 Burmax Park, Dowagiac, MI 49047
Various types of clamps.

Bausch & Lomb Surgical 636-255-5051
3365 Tree Court Ind Blvd, Saint Louis, MO 63122

Katena Products, Inc. 800-225-1195
4 Stewart Ct, Denville, NJ 07834

Princeton Medical Group, Inc. 800-875-0869
1189 Royal Links Dr, Mt Pleasant, SC 29466

CLAMP, NON-ELECTRICAL *(Gastro/Urology) 78FFN*

George Tiemann & Co. 800-843-6266
25 Plant Ave, Hauppauge, NY 11788

Molded Products Inc. 800-435-8957
1112 Chatburn Ave, Harlan, IA 51537
Fistula pressure clamp.

CLAMP, OSSICLE HOLDING *(Ear/Nose/Throat) 77JYF*

Bausch & Lomb Surgical 636-255-5051
3365 Tree Court Ind Blvd, Saint Louis, MO 63122

CLAMP, OTHER *(Surgery) 79QKR*

Adelberg Laboratories Inc. 818-784-1141
16821 Oak View Dr, Encino, CA 91436
Offers a newly introduced Model IV Precision V-Clamp for infusion sets that is very attractively priced and delivers a minimal flow-rate deviation, which is superior to most others. Model IV is superior to licensed technology by Abbott Laboratories and Baxter Labotatories. Other design elements include improved tug resistance and ease of adjustment. High-pressure shutoff is built in.

Benlan Inc. 905-829-5004
2760 Brighton Rd., Oakville, ONT L6H 5T4 Canada
Sheet clamps for drainage bags.

Birkova Products 888-567-4502
809 4th St, Gothenburg, NE 69138
Surgical table clamping devices, siderail clamps, Clark sockets, etc.

Bryton Corp. 800-567-9500
4310 Guion Rd, Indianapolis, IN 46254
Wide range of clamping devices for all types of surgical tables.

Dma Med-Chem Corporation 800-362-1833
49 Watermill Ln, Great Neck, NY 11021
Compression clamp and disc system for cardiac cath lab.

Dravon Medical, Inc. 503-656-6600
11465 SE Highway 212, PO Box 69, Clackamas, OR 97015
Disposable towel and sponge clamp.

Health Supply Company Inc., The 770-452-0090
2902 Marlin Cir, Atlanta, GA 30341
LIL MAC accessory clamp, spring loaded to ensure proper stability and placement designed to fit US & European tables.

I.E.D., Inc. 231-728-9154
1938 Sanford St, Muskegon, MI 49441
Clamp for heart valve surgery.

Mission X-Ray 800-676-8718
45459 Industrial Pllace, Suite 1, Fremont, CA 94538-6450
Headclamps.

Mizuho Osi 800-777-4674
30031 Ahern Ave, Union City, CA 94587
Traction clamp.

Novare Surgical Systems, Inc. 408-873-3161
10440 Bubb Rd Ste A, Cupertino, CA 95014
Cygnet flexible shaft clamp for MIS procedures

Pryor Products 800-854-2280
1819 Peacock Blvd, Oceanside, CA 92056
Both standard and custom c-clamp products are available.

Ross Disposable Products 800-649-6526
401 Traders Blvd E, Unit 10, Mississauga, ON L4Z 2H8 Canada
Multi-purpose clamps.

Troemner Llc 800-352-7705
201 Wolf Dr, PO Box 87, West Deptford, NJ 08086
3-prong, 2-prong, large variety of specialty clamps

CLAMP, PATENT DUCTUS *(Surgery) 79QKN*

Codman & Shurtleff, Inc 800-225-0460
325 Paramount Dr, Raynham, MA 02767

CLAMP, PENILE *(Gastro/Urology) 78FHA*

Aesculap Implant Systems Inc. 1-800-234-9179
3773 Corporate Pkwy, Center Valley, PA 18034

C. R. Bard, Inc., Bard Urological Div. 888-367-2273
13183 Harland Dr NE, Covington, GA 30014

Greenwald Surgical Co., Inc. 219-962-1604
2688 Dekalb St, Gary, IN 46405
Incontinence clamps/ meatus clamps.

Gt Urological, Llc 612-379-3578
1313 5th St SE, Minneapolis, MN 55414
Penile clamp.

Gyrx, Llc 904-641-2599
10302 Deerwood Park Blvd Ste 209, Jacksonville, FL 32256
Urological clamp for males.

Richard Wolf Medical Instruments Corp. 800-323-9653
353 Corporate Woods Pkwy, Vernon Hills, IL 60061

Tuzik Boston 800-886-6363
104 Longwater Dr, Assinippi Park, Norwell, MA 02061

CLAMP, PERIPHERAL VASCULAR *(Cardiovascular) 74QKO*

Clinimed, Incorporated 877-CLINIMED
303 Markus Ct, Sandy Brae Industrial Park, Newark, DE 19713

Codman & Shurtleff, Inc 800-225-0460
325 Paramount Dr, Raynham, MA 02767

CLAMP, PERIPHERAL VASCULAR *(cont'd)*

Fehling Surgical Instruments 800-FEHLING
509 Broadstone Ln NW, Acworth, GA 30101

Scanlan International, Inc. 800-328-9458
1 Scanlan Plz, Saint Paul, MN 55107

CLAMP, RUBBER DAM *(Dental And Oral) 76EEF*

Coltene/Whaledent Inc. 330-916-8858
235 Ascot Pkwy, Cuyahoga Falls, OH 44223
Rubber dam clamp.

Hager Worldwide, Inc. 800-328-2335
13322 Byrd Dr, Odessa, FL 33556
FIT

Heraeus Kulzer, Inc., Dental Products Division 574-299-6662
4315 S Lafayette Blvd, South Bend, IN 46614
Rubber dam clamp.

Hu-Friedy Manufacturing Co., Inc. 800-483-7433
3232 N Rockwell St, Chicago, IL 60618
$9.15 each, 42 types.

Miltex Dental Technologies, Inc. 516-576-6022
589 Davies Dr, York, PA 17402
Rubber dam clamps.

Ultradent Products, Inc. 801-553-4586
505 W 10200 S, South Jordan, UT 84095
Rubber dam & accessories.

CLAMP, SKULL *(Cns/Neurology) 84QKQ*

Schaerer Mayfield Usa 800-755-6381
4900 Charlemar Dr, Cincinnati, OH 45227
MAYFIELD brand of skull clamps and cranial stabilization products.

CLAMP, SURGICAL, GENERAL & PLASTIC SURGERY *(Surgery) 79GDJ*

Argon Medical Devices Inc. 903-675-9321
1445 Flat Creek Rd, Athens, TX 75751
Vessel clude.

B & H Medical Products, Inc. 520-296-5544
8925 E Golf Links Rd, Tucson, AZ 85730
Manual, external clamp for dialysis only.

Bausch & Lomb Surgical 636-255-5051
3365 Tree Court Ind Blvd, Saint Louis, MO 63122

Biomet Microfixation Inc. 800-874-7711
1520 Tradeport Dr, Jacksonville, FL 32218
Various types of clamps.

Biomet, Inc. 574-267-6639
56 E Bell Dr, PO Box 587, Warsaw, IN 46582
Various types of chisel for general and plastic surgery.

Bryton Corp. 800-567-9500
4310 Guion Rd, Indianapolis, IN 46254
Wide range of clamps for surgical tables, orthopedic tables and urology tables.

Cascade Life Solutions, Llc 616-977-2505
3710 Sysco Ct SE, Grand Rapids, MI 49512
Tourniquet kit with snare.

Chase Medical, Lp 972-783-0644
1876 Firman Dr, Richardson, TX 75081
Various models of tourniquet kit (sterile/non sterile).

Civco Medical Instruments Co., Inc. 319-656-4447
102 1st St S, Kalona, IA 52247
General purpose clamp.

Edwards Lifesciences Technology Sarl 949-250-2500
State Rd. 402 N.km 1.4, Anasco, PR 00610-1577
Various surgical clips and clamps.

Health Supply Company Inc., The 770-452-0090
2902 Marlin Cir, Atlanta, GA 30341
Midkiff GEOSTATIC Clamp. Principles of geostasis employed. Low in profile. Each clamping function independent and silent. Helpful in lithotomy positioning.

International Hospital Supply Co. 800-398-9450
6914 Canby Ave Ste 105, Reseda, CA 91335

Kmedic 800-955-0559
190 Veterans Dr, Northvale, NJ 07647

Mediflex Surgical Products 800-879-7575
250 Gibbs Rd, Islandia, NY 11749
Adjustable ratcheting clamp conforms to any size liver for hepatic surgery.

CLAMP, SURGICAL, GENERAL & PLASTIC SURGERY *(cont'd)*

Micrins Surgical Instruments, Inc. 800-833-3380
28438 N Ballard Dr, Lake Forest, IL 60045

Princeton Medical Group, Inc. 800-875-0869
1189 Royal Links Dr, Mt Pleasant, SC 29466

Qfc Plastics, Inc. 817-649-7400
728 111th St, Arlington, TX 76011
Clamp.

Rhein Medical, Inc. 800-637-4346
5460 Beaumont Center Blvd Ste 500, Suite 500, Tampa, FL 33634

Scanlan International, Inc. 800-328-9458
1 Scanlan Plz, Saint Paul, MN 55107

Solos Endoscopy 800-388-6445
65 Sprague St # B, Boston/dedham Commerce Park, Boston, MA 02136
Manual surgical instruments for general use.

Surge Medical Solutions, Llc. 616-977-2516
3710 Sysco Ct SE, Grand Rapids, MI 49512
Tourniquet kit with snare.

Terumo Cardiovascular Systems (Tcvs) 800-283-7866
28 Howe St, Ashland, MA 01721
Surgery accessories.

Tools For Surgery, Llc 631-444-4448
1339 Stony Brook Rd, Stony Brook, NY 11790
Intestinal occluding clamp.

Tuzik Boston 800-886-6363
104 Longwater Dr, Assinippi Park, Norwell, MA 02061

Ussc Puerto Rico, Inc. 203-845-1000
Building 911-67, Sabanetas Industrial Park, Ponce, PR 00731
Clamp.

Zimmer Spine, Inc. 800-655-2614
7375 Bush Lake Rd, Minneapolis, MN 55439
Surgical clamp.

CLAMP, TUBING *(General) 80WUF*

Carolina Biological Supply Co. 800-334-5551
2700 York Rd, Burlington, NC 27215

Clinimed, Incorporated 877-CLINIMED
303 Markus Ct, Sandy Brae Industrial Park, Newark, DE 19713

Directmed, Inc. 516-656-3377
150 Pratt Oval, Glen Cove, NY 11542

Halkey-Roberts Corp. 800-303-4384
2700 Halkey Roberts Pl N, Saint Petersburg, FL 33716
Mechanical, adjustable ratchet-type, shutoff-type, and manually operated tube clamps.

Hospira 800-441-4100
268 E 4th St, Ashland, OH 44805
Roller and slide clamp.

Medical Plastic Devices (Mpd), Inc. 866-633-9835
161 Oneida Dr., Pointe Claire, QUE H9R 1A9 Canada

Smiths Medical Asd, Inc. 800-848-1757
6250 Shier Rings Rd, Dublin, OH 43016

Speedy Products Co. 800-388-2001
225 Cash St, Jacksonville, TX 75766
SPEEDY CLAMP; Nylon hose clamp.

Z-Man Corporation 616-281-6108
1359 Pickett St SE, Kentwood, MI 49508
Easy Open Pinch Clamp

CLAMP, TUBING, BLOOD, AUTOMATIC *(Gastro/Urology) 78FIG*

Biomet Microfixation Inc. 800-874-7711
1520 Tradeport Dr, Jacksonville, FL 32218
Various types of clamps.

Dravon Medical, Inc. 503-656-6600
11465 SE Highway 212, PO Box 69, Clackamas, OR 97015
Disposable tube occluding forcep.

Rocky Mountain Research, Inc. 801-359-6060
825 N 300 W Ste 500, Salt Lake City, UT 84103
Various types of automatic tubing clamps.

Sorin Group Usa 800-289-5759
14401 W 65th Way, Arvada, CO 80004

CLAMP, UMBILICAL *(Obstetrics/Gyn) 85HFW*

Directmed, Inc. 516-656-3377
150 Pratt Oval, Glen Cove, NY 11542
HOSPITAL'S UMBILICAL CLAMP sterile/non-sterile non-reopening chord clamp.

CLAMP, UMBILICAL *(cont'd)*

Miltex Inc. 800-645-8000
589 Davies Dr, York, PA 17402

Precision Dynamics Corp. 800-772-1122
13880 Del Sur St, San Fernando, CA 91340
SECURLINE umbilical cord clamp provides a safe and easy method for sealing the umbilical cord. Features a dual gripping surface to hold cord clamp securely while stabilizing.

Ross Disposable Products 800-649-6526
401 Traders Blvd E, Unit 10, Mississauga, ON L4Z 2H8 Canada

Specialty Medical Products Co. 801-295-6023
3063 S Davis Blvd, Bountiful, UT 84010
Umbilical cord clamp.

CLAMP, UTERINE *(Obstetrics/Gyn) 85HGC*

Biomet Microfixation Inc. 800-874-7711
1520 Tradeport Dr, Jacksonville, FL 32218
Various types of clamps.

International Hospital Supply Co. 800-398-9450
6914 Canby Ave Ste 105, Reseda, CA 91335

Tuzik Boston 800-886-6363
104 Longwater Dr, Assinippi Park, Norwell, MA 02061

CLAMP, VASCULAR *(Cardiovascular) 74DXC*

Aesculap Implant Systems Inc. 1-800-234-9179
3773 Corporate Pkwy, Center Valley, PA 18034

Argon Medical Devices Inc. 903-675-9321
1445 Flat Creek Rd, Athens, TX 75751
Vessel loops.

Biomet Microfixation Inc. 800-874-7711
1520 Tradeport Dr, Jacksonville, FL 32218
Various types of clamps.

Boston Scientific Corp. 408-935-3400
150 Baytech Dr, San Jose, CA 95134
Coronary shunt.

Cardiva Medical, Inc. 650-964-8900
2585 Leghorn St, Mountain View, CA 94043
Various models of sterile vascular closure systems.

Clinimed, Incorporated 877-CLINIMED
303 Markus Ct, Sandy Brae Industrial Park, Newark, DE 19713

Codman & Shurtleff, Inc 800-225-0460
325 Paramount Dr, Raynham, MA 02767

Edwards Lifesciences Research Medical 949-250-2500
6864 Cottonwood St, Midvale, UT 84047
Vascular clamp.

Edwards Lifesciences Technology Sarl 949-250-2500
State Rd. 402 N.km 1.4, Anasco, PR 00610-1577
Vascular clamp.

Edwards Lifesciences, Llc. 800-424-3278
1 Edwards Way, Irvine, CA 92614

Fehling Surgical Instruments 800-FEHLING
509 Broadstone Ln NW, Acworth, GA 30101

International Hospital Supply Co. 800-398-9450
6914 Canby Ave Ste 105, Reseda, CA 91335

Interventional Hemostasis Products, Inc. 503-638-9743
1815 NW 169th Pl Ste 6030, Beaverton, OR 97006
Vascular clamp,pressure disc,mobile clamp,hand held.

Kelsar, S.A. 508-261-8000
Blvd. Insurgentes, Libriamento a La, Tijuana 22450 Mexico
Silcone vascular tapes, vascular tourniquets/kits (various)

Maquet Cardiovascular LLC 888-880-2874
45 Barbour Pond Dr, Wayne, NJ 07470

Marine Polymer Technologies, Inc. 888-666-2560
461 Boston St Unit B5, Topsfield, MA 01983
Clamp, vascular.

Mcpherson Enterprises, Inc. 813-931-4201
3851 62nd Ave N Ste A, Pinellas Park, FL 33781
Carotid shunt.

Miltex Inc. 800-645-8000
589 Davies Dr, York, PA 17402

Neomend, Inc. 949-916-1630
9272 Jeronimo Rd Ste 119, Irvine, CA 92618
Sterile vascular pressure cuff.

Novare Surgical Systems, Inc. 408-873-3161
10440 Bubb Rd Ste A, Cupertino, CA 95014
Various.

CLAMP, VASCULAR *(cont'd)*

Novosci Corp. 281-363-4949
2828 N Crescentridge Dr, The Woodlands, TX 77381

Princeton Medical Group, Inc. 800-875-0869
1189 Royal Links Dr, Mt Pleasant, SC 29466

Prosurge Instruments, Inc. 866-832-7874
199 Laidlaw Ave, Jersey City, NJ 07306

Scanlan International, Inc. 800-328-9458
1 Scanlan Plz, Saint Paul, MN 55107

Synovis Life Technologies, Inc 800-255-4018
2575 University Ave W, Saint Paul, MN 55114
Flo-Rester; Flo-Thru

Synovis Surgical Innovations 800-255-4018
2575 University Ave W, Saint Paul, MN 55114
FLO-RESTER Internal Vessel Occluder, a vascular occluder used in cardiac bypass and peripheral vascular surgery. FLO-THRU Intraluminal Shunt for use in coronary artery or peripheral-vascular procedures to shunt blood at the anastomotic site while allowing blood to flow distal to the anastomosis.

Tuzik Boston 800-886-6363
104 Longwater Dr, Assinippi Park, Norwell, MA 02061

Tz Medical Inc. 800-944-0187
7272 SW Durham Rd Ste 800, Portland, OR 97224
Clamp and disks.

Vascular Solutions, Inc. 763-656-4300
5025 Cheshire Ln N, Plymouth, MN 55446
Vascular clamp accessory.

Voss Medical Products 210-650-3124
4235 Centergate St, San Antonio, TX 78217
Coronary clamp.

CLAMP, VASCULAR, REPROCESSED *(Cardiovascular) 74NMF*

Sterilmed, Inc. 763-488-3400
11400 73rd Ave N Ste 100, Maple Grove, MN 55369
Femoral compression device.

CLAMP, WIRE, ORTHODONTIC *(Dental And Oral) 76ECN*

Acme-Monaco Corp. 860-224-1349
75 Winchell Rd, New Britain, CT 06052

Biomet Microfixation Inc. 800-874-7711
1520 Tradeport Dr, Jacksonville, FL 32218
Various types of clamps.

Forestadent Usa 314-878-5985
2315 Weldon Pkwy, Saint Louis, MO 63146
Orthodontic wire clamp.

G & H Wire Co. 800-526-1026
2165 Earlywood Dr, Franklin, IN 46131

H & H Co. 909-390-0373
4435 E Airport Dr Ste 108, Ontario, CA 91761
Clamp, wire.

Highland Metals, Inc. 800-368-6484
419 Perrymont Ave, San Jose, CA 95125
Ligature wire, retainer wire.

Inman Orthodontic Laboratories, Inc. 954-340-8477
9381 W Sample Rd, Coral Springs, FL 33065
Coil spring compressing component.

Ortho Organizers, Inc. 760-448-8730
1822 Aston Ave, Carlsbad, CA 92008
Molar rotator.

Pyramid Orthodontics 800-752-8884
4328 Redwood Hwy Ste 100, San Rafael, CA 94903

3m Unitek 800-634-5300
2724 Peck Rd, Monrovia, CA 91016

CLASP, PREFORMED *(Dental And Oral) 76EHP*

Cdm Dental 541-928-4444
812 Water Ave NE, Albany, OR 97321
Aesthetic Perfection Acetal Resin

Forestadent Usa 314-878-5985
2315 Weldon Pkwy, Saint Louis, MO 63146
Preformed clasp.

G & H Wire Co. 800-526-1026
2165 Earlywood Dr, Franklin, IN 46131

CLASP, WIRE *(Dental And Oral) 76EJW*

G & H Wire Co. 800-526-1026
2165 Earlywood Dr, Franklin, IN 46131

CLASP, WIRE *(cont'd)*

Inman Orthodontic Laboratories, Inc. 954-340-8477
9381 W Sample Rd, Coral Springs, FL 33065
Clasp, wire.

CLASSIFIER, PROGNOSTIC, RECURRENCE RISK ASSESSMENT, RNA GENE EXPRESSION, BREAST CANCER *(Immunology) 82NYI*

Agendia Inc. 888-321-2732
22 Morgan, Irvine, CA 92618
MAMMAPRINT

CLEANER, BEDPAN (STERILIZER) *(General) 80QKS*

American Autoclave Co. 800 421 5161
7819 Riverside Rd E, Sumner, WA 98390
Automatic and manual, flushes and sterilizes.

Getinge Usa, Inc. 800-475-9040
1777 E Henrietta Rd, Rochester, NY 14623
GETINGE

Independent Solutions, Inc. 847-498-0500
900 Skokie Blvd Ste 118, Northbrook, IL 60062
SEMCO floor mounted or surfaced wall mounted or flush wall mounted.

Sloan Valve Co. 800-9VA-LVE9
10500 Seymour Ave, Franklin Park, IL 60131
Bed Pan Washers.

Unit Chemical Corp. 800-879-8648
7360 Commercial Way, Henderson, NV 89011
ODOR-X Disinfectant

CLEANER, DENTURE *(Dental And Oral) 76EFT*

Accupac, Inc. 215-256-7011
1501 Industrial Blvd., Mainland, PA 19451
Denture cleanser.

Align Technology, Inc. 408-470-1000
881 Martin Ave, Santa Clara, CA 95050
Cleanser,denture,over the counter.

Block Drug Co., Inc. 973-889-2578
2149 Harbor Ave., Memphis, TN 38113
Various.

Cascade Dental Products Co. 541-386-2012
924 12th St, Hood River, OR 97031
Denture cleanser.

Centurion Medical Products Corp. 517-545-1135
3310 S Main St, Salisbury, NC 28147

Deseret Laboratories Inc. 435-628-8786
1414 E 3850 S, Saint George, UT 84790
Types of denture cleansers.

Groupe Novalab Inc. 819-474-2580
2350 Rue Power, Drummondville J2C 7Z4 Canada
Cleanser, denture, otc

Harry J. Bosworth Company 800-323-4352
7227 Hamlin Ave, Skokie, IL 60076
Powder denture cleaner.

Mid-Continental Dental Supply Co., Ltd. 204-888-5031
242 Alboro St, Headingley R4J 1A4 Canada
Denture cleanser

Moyco Technologies, Inc. 800-331-8837
200 Commerce Dr, Montgomeryville, PA 18936
Moycodent plastic teeth cleaner. $5.00 per vial.

Pfizer Pharmaceuticals Ltd 212-573-7291
Km 1.9 Rte. 689, Vega Baja, PR 00694-0786
Denture cleanser tablets.

Protech Professional Products, Inc. 561-493-9818
2900 Commerce Park Dr Ste 10, Boynton Beach, FL 33426
Denture cleaner.

Regent Labs, Inc. 954-426-4403
700 W Hillsboro Blvd Ste 2-206, Deerfield Bch, FL 33441
Denture cleanser.

Smile Brite Distributing Llc 585-248-9260
5 Boughton Ave, Pittsford, NY 14534
Orthodontic and denture cleaner.

Tri-State Hospital Supply Corp. 517-545-1135
3173 E 43rd St, Yuma, AZ 85365

Winn-Sol Products 414-231-2031
1853 Delaware St, Oshkosh, WI 54902
Miradent.

CLEANER, DENTURE, MECHANICAL *(Dental And Oral) 76JER*

Align Technology, Inc. 408-470-1000
881 Martin Ave, Santa Clara, CA 95050
Mechanical cleaner.

Alldente Intl., Inc. 416-944-0086
600-94 Cumberland St, Toronto M5R 1A3 Canada
Mechanical denture cleaner

Den-Mat Holdings, Llc 805-922-8491
2727 Skyway Dr, Santa Maria, CA 93455
No common name listed.

Nanzee Dental Products 717-792-9795
2916 Robin Rd, York, PA 17404
Clean dent.

Pfizer Pharmaceuticals Ltd 212-573-7291
Km 1.9 Rte. 689, Vega Baja, PR 00694-0786
Efferdent,2-layer efferdent and efferdent plus tablets.

Smile Brite Distributing Llc 585-248-9260
5 Boughton Ave, Pittsford, NY 14534
Sonic cleaner unit.

3m Espe Dental Products 651-733-7767
2501 Otis Corley Dr, Bentonville, AR 72712
Tango Tongue Cleaner

CLEANER, ELECTROSURGICAL TIP *(Surgery) 79UMT*

Amd-Ritmed, Inc. 800-445-0340
295 Firetower Road, Tonawanda, NY 14150

Xodus Medical, Inc. 800-963-8776
702 Prominence Dr, Westmoreland Business & Research Park
New Kensington, PA 15068
Cautery Tip Cleanear

CLEANER, FORCEPS, BIOPSY *(Cardiovascular) 74WTL*

Prosurge Instruments, Inc. 866-832-7874
199 Laidlaw Ave, Jersey City, NJ 07306

Scholten Surgical Instruments, Inc. 209-365-1393
170 Commerce St Ste 101, Lodi, CA 95240
Endomyocardial biopsy forceps cleaning device, portable syringe operated unit, $135.00

CLEANER, LENS, CONTACT *(Ophthalmology) 86LPN*

Allergan 800-366-6554
2525 Dupont Dr, Irvine, CA 92612

Allergan Sales, Llc 714-246-4388
8301 Mars Dr, Waco, TX 76712
Contact lens products.

Bausch & Lomb Inc., Greenville Solutions Plant 585-338-6000
8507 Pelham Rd, Greenville, SC 29615
Various types of contact lens solutions.

Bausch & Lomb Pharmaceutical, Inc. 800-227-1427
8500 Hidden River Pkwy, Tampa, FL 33637
Contact lens cleaner.

Bausch & Lomb, Vision Care 800-553-5340
1400 Goodman St N, Rochester, NY 14609
RENU, SENSITIVE EYES and BAUSCH & LOMB.

Ciba Vision Corporation 800-875-3001
11460 Johns Creek Pkwy, Duluth, GA 30097

Edmund Industrial Optics 800-363-1992
101 E Gloucester Pike, Barrington, NJ 08007

Irenda Corp. 323-770-4222
14131 Avalon Blvd, Los Angeles, CA 90061
250mg salt tablets.

Kc Pharmaceuticals, Inc. 909-598-9499
3201 Producer Way, Pomona, CA 91768
Also eye care solutions.

Lens Dynamics, Inc. 303-237-6927
14998 W 6th Ave Ste 830, Golden, CO 80401
Polish.

Lobob Laboratories, Inc. 800-83-LOBOB
1440 Atteberry Ln, San Jose, CA 95131
LOBOB hard contact lens cleaner; Optimum by LOBOB cleaning, disinfecting, storage solution for RGP lenses. Optimum by LOBOB Gas permeable wetting/rewetting solution. SOF/PRO multi-purpose solution for cleaning, disinfecting, and storage of soft lenses.

Mcneil-Ppc, Inc. 908-874-1402
100 Jefferson Rd, Parsippany, NJ 07054
Lubricating-rewetting eye drops.

CLEANER, LENS, CONTACT *(cont'd)*

Nomax, Inc. 314-961-2500
40 N Rock Hill Rd, Saint Louis, MO 63119
Various salt & effervescent enzyme tablets.

Questech International, Inc. 800-966-5367
3810 Gunn Hwy, Tampa, FL 33618
Automatic contact lens cleaner for all lenses. For consumer use.

Shamir Usa, Inc. 818-889-6292
29800 Agoura Rd Ste 102, Agoura Hills, CA 91301
lens, material, coating

The Lifestyle Co. Inc. 800-622-0777
1800 State Route 34 Ste 401, Wall Township, NJ 07719
PuriLens Ultra PF-- sterile, unpreserved saline

CLEANER, MEDICAL DEVICE *(General) 80MDZ*

Case Medical, Inc. 888-227-2273
65 Railroad Ave, Ridgefield, NJ 07657
clean all surgical instruments

Clinical Diagnostic Solutions, Inc. 954-791-1773
1800 NW 65th Ave, Plantation, FL 33313
Detergent reagent.

Contec, Inc. 800-289-5762
525 Locust Grv, Spartanburg, SC 29303
PROSAT(R) Sterile(TM) wipers have been sterilized using an E-Beam radiation process and are validated sterile per the AAMI/ISO 11137 Method 1 Guidelines. The presaturated wipers are packaged in a resealable pouch with a tamper evident label.

Friedheim Tool Company 619-474-3600
1433 Roosevelt Ave, National City, CA 91950
Steam jet & vapor cleaner.

Gibbons Surgical Corp. 800-959-1989
1112 Jensen Dr Ste 101, Virginia Beach, VA 23451
TRIPLE ENZYMATIC CLEANER AND CART WASH CONTAIN PROTEASE, AMYLASE AND LIPASE ENZYMES TO BREAK DOWN PROTEINS, CARBOHYDRATES/STARCHES AND FATS ON REUSABLE SURGICAL INSTRUMENTS. PRODUCTS HAVE A NEUTRAL PH, AND CONTAIN A DETERGENT AND ANTICORROSIVE AGENT. PRODUCT LINE ALSO INCLUDES INSTRUMENT LUBRICANT.

Health Care Logistics, Inc. 800-848-1633
450 Town St, PO Box 25, Circleville, OH 43113
Medical clean up kits.

Heraeus Kulzer, Inc., Dental Products Division 574-299-6662
4315 S Lafayette Blvd, South Bend, IN 46614
General purpose enzymatic cleaner.

Intersect Systems, Inc. 360-577-1062
1152 3rd Avenue, Suite D & E, Longview, WA 98632
Wash Concentrate and Probe Rinse for Beckman Synchron CX4,5 and 7

Ultra Tec Manufacturing, Inc. 877-542-0609
1025 E Chestnut Ave, Santa Ana, CA 92701
ULTRAPOL 1200 medical and optical device polisher for grinding and polishing endoscopes, microlens and laser fiber components.

Veridien Corp. 800-345-5444
7600 Bryan Dairy Rd Ste F, Largo, FL 33777
VIRAGUARD, disinfectant/cleaner. Organic, non-toxic (OSHA 29 CFR 1910 1200), non-aqueous and biodegradable (OECD guidelines 302B) intermediate surface disinfectant/cleaner and instrument presoak.

CLEANER, NEEDLE *(General) 80QKU*

Hamilton Company 800-648-5950
4990 Energy Way, Reno, NV 89502

CLEANER, SYRINGE *(General) 80QKV*

Hamilton Company 800-648-5950
4990 Energy Way, Reno, NV 89502

CLEANER, ULTRASONIC, DENTAL LABORATORY
(Dental And Oral) 76ECA

Denplus Inc. 800-344-4424
205 - 1221 Labadie, Longueuil, QUE J4N 1E2 Canada

Esma, Inc. 800-276-2466
450 Taft Dr, South Holland, IL 60473
Automatic Ultrasonic Instument Washer. Clean/Rinse/Dry in a single tank using preprogrammed cycles similar to that of a dishwasher.

Hu-Friedy Manufacturing Co., Inc. 800-483-7433
3232 N Rockwell St, Chicago, IL 60618
Ultrasonic detergent, ultrasonic presoak and ultrasonic inserts.

CLEANER, ULTRASONIC, DENTAL LABORATORY *(cont'd)*

Midmark Corporation 800-643-6275
60 Vista Dr, P.O. Box 286, Versailles, OH 45380

Misonix, Inc. 800-694-9612
1938 New Hwy, Farmingdale, NY 11735

Motloid Company 800-662-5021
300 N Elizabeth St, Chicago, IL 60607
Ultrasonic cleaners.

CLEANER, ULTRASONIC, MEDICAL INSTRUMENT
(General) 80FLG

Action Llc 757-491-4175
1112 Jensen Dr Ste 103, Virginia Beach, VA 23451
Triple enzymatic cleaning solutions for use with ultrasonic cleaners.

American Eagle Instruments, Inc. 406-549-7451
6575 Butler Creek Rd, Missoula, MT 59808
Ultrasonic cleaning solution.

B. Graczyk, Inc. 269-782-2100
27826 Burmax Park, Dowagiac, MI 49047
Various sizes of cleaner.

Barnstead International 412-490-8425
2555 Kerper Blvd, Dubuque, IA 52001
Various ultrasonic cleaners.

Blue Wave Ultrasonics 800-373-0144
960 S Rolff St, Davenport, IA 52802
Wash, rinse and dry ultrasonic medical model deluxe ultrasonic cleaning consoles, matching console rinsers, matching console dryer, tabletop ultrasonic cleaners. All cleaners include magnetostrictive transducers backed by an unconditional lifetime warranty.

Brain Power, Inc. 800-327-2250
4470 SW 74th Ave, Miami, FL 33155
Designed for cleaning surgical instruments and small tools. Available in units with capacities ranging from 1 pint to 7 gallons.

Branson Ultrasonics Corp. 203-796-2235
41 Eagle Rd, P.o. Box 1961, Danbury, CT 06810
Ultrasonic benchtop cleaner.

Buxton Medical Equipment Corp. 631-957-4500
1178 Route 109, Lindenhurst, NY 11757
$18,000 to $350 for all models.

Caig Laboratories, Inc. 800-224-4123
12200 Thatcher Ct, Poway, CA 92064
CAIG DeoxIT and DeoxIT Gold clean and lubricate all contacts and connectors. They minimize electrical resistance thus reducing energy consumption and improving equipment performance.

Cetylite Industries, Inc. 856-665-6111
9051 River Rd, Pennsauken, NJ 08110
General purpose ultrasonic cleaner concentrate.

Cole-Parmer Instrument Inc. 800-323-4340
625 E Bunker Ct, Vernon Hills, IL 60061

Colonial Scientific Ltd. 902-468-1811
201 Brownlow Ave., Unit 52, Dartmouth, NS B3B-1W2 Canada

Coltene/Whaledent Inc. 330-916-8858
235 Ascot Pkwy, Cuyahoga Falls, OH 44223
Ultrasonic cleaner system.

Custom Ultrasonics, Inc. 215-364-1477
144 Railroad Dr, Hartsville, PA 18974
Thorough cleaning, rinsing, and lubricating of rigid surgical instruments through computer-driven process. Features two independently operated processing chambers.

Daztech, Inc. 215-669-3102
424 Broad St, Perkasie, PA 18944
Custom ultrasonics.

Dencraft 800-328-9729
PO Box 57, Moorestown, NJ 08057
Many models available for ultrasonic cleaning.

Dentronix, Inc. 800-523-5944
235 Ascot Pkwy, Cuyahoga Falls, OH 44223
$1,495.00 per unit. Designed for optimum cleaning of orthodontic instruments, and includes a plier rack stand for ease of use.

Dentsply Canada, Ltd. 800-263-1437
161 Vinyl Ct., Woodbridge, ONT L4L 4A3 Canada

Dgh Technology, Inc. 800-722-3883
110 Summit Dr Ste B, Exton, PA 19341
MINIMAX instrument cleanser for surgical diamond tools and hand-held instrumentation.

CLEANER, ULTRASONIC, MEDICAL INSTRUMENT *(cont'd)*

Dshealthcare Inc. 201-871-1232
85 W Forest Ave, Englewood, NJ 07631
Pro.sonic.

Encompas Unlimited, Inc. 800-825-7701
PO Box 516, Tallevast, FL 34270
For all surgical instruments and endoscopic accessories, 4 sizes - $868 for 3-3/8 qt unit, $1,449 for 11 qt unit, $2,449 for 5-1/2 gallon.

Enzyme Solutions, Inc. 260-497-0851
7601 Honeywell Dr, Fort Wayne, IN 46825
Enzymatic cleaner.

Esma, Inc. 800-276-2466
450 Taft Dr, South Holland, IL 60473
Automated Ultrasonic -cleaning/rinsing/drying - washers and 3 chambered - cleaning/rinsing/drying systems for ultrasonic cleaning of instruments.

Forward Technology 320-286-2578
260 Jenks Ave SW, Cokato, MN 55321
Aqueous, alcohol, high-pressure spray, and ultrasonic technologies to replace CFC and other solvent-cleaning methods.

Getinge Usa, Inc. 800-475-9040
1777 E Henrietta Rd, Rochester, NY 14623
GETINGE.

Harry J. Bosworth Company 800-323-4352
7227 Hamlin Ave, Skokie, IL 60076
VIGILANCE.

L&R Manufacturing Co. 201-991-5330
577 Elm St, PO Box 607, Kearny, NJ 07032
ULTRA DOSE General Purpose Cleaner Powder is a single-dose super concentrated powder for the cleaning of medical instruments and for use in an ultrasonic cleaning machine. SWEEP ZONE ultrasonic cleaning machine with Sweep Zone technology. Alters cleaning +/-2 khZ in the tank. Includes pulse width modulation, long power output and the 'smart circuit'.

Md International, Inc. 305-669-9003
11300 NW 41st St, Doral, FL 33178

Medical Technologies Co. 800-280-3220
1728 W Park Center Dr Ste A, Fenton, MO 63026

Mettler Electronics Corp. 800-854-9305
1333 S Claudina St, Anaheim, CA 92805
CAVITATOR: Five models - $605.00 for ME 2.1, $625.00 for ME 4.6, $1,175.00 for ME 11, $1,650.00 for ME 5.5, and $4,915.00 for ME 18 18.

Misonix, Inc. 800-694-9612
1938 New Hwy, Farmingdale, NY 11735
With or without temperature control.

Northeastern Sonics 800-243-2452
130 Lenox Ave Ste 23, Stamford, CT 06906

Novozymes Biologicals, Inc. 540-389-9361
111 Kessler Mill Rd, Salem, VA 24153
Ultrasonic medical instrument cleaner.

Pemaco, Inc. 314-231-3399
2030 S 3rd St, Saint Louis, MO 63104
Ultrasonic cleaner.

Pentax Medical Company 800-431-5880
102 Chestnut Ridge Rd, Montvale, NJ 07645
$1,108.00 to $1,322.00 for an ultrasonic cleaning machine available with or without a heater.

Ramco Equipment 908-687-6700
32 Montgomery St, Hillside, NJ 07205

Stoelting 800-558-5807
502 Highway 67, Kiel, WI 53042

Tuttnauer Usa Co. Ltd. 800-624-5836
25 Power Dr, Hauppauge, NY 11788
Stainless steel tank equipped with sixty minute timer. Durable vinyl clad steel housing. All units equipped with a drain. Optional heater available. Models: CSU1(0.8 gal capacity), CSU3(3 gal capacity).

Tuzik Boston 800-886-6363
104 Longwater Dr, Assinippi Park, Norwell, MA 02061

U.S. Medical Systems, Inc. 512-347-8800
3160 Bee Caves Rd Ste 300C, Austin, TX 78746
Multipurpose medical instrument cleaner.

Ulmer Pharmacal Co. 800-848-5637
PO Box 408, 1614 Industry Ave., Park Rapids, MN 56470
KLER-RO LIQUID $4.64 per 1000 ml.

CLEANER, ULTRASONIC, MEDICAL INSTRUMENT *(cont'd)*

Ultra Clean Systems, Inc. 877-935-6624
12700 Dupont Cir, Tampa, FL 33626
Cannulated Instrument Cleaner cleans cannulated and standard surgical instruments - Countertop Model 1100. Model 1500 series floor model ultrasonic cleaner for cannulated and regular surgical instruments - floor model. Standard Tabletop ultrasonic cleaner for non-cannulated surgical instruments. Ranges from .5 gal to 5.0 gal.

Ultradent Products, Inc. 801-553-4586
505 W 10200 S, South Jordan, UT 84095
Ultrasonic medical instrument cleaner.

United Biotech 866-753-5700
1421 Main St, Rahway, NJ 07065
Ultrasonic medical instrument cleaner.

Y.I. Ventures, Llc 314-344-0010
2260 Wendt St, Algonquin, IL 60102
Ultrasonic solution: non-ionic & biodegradable.

Young Colorado, Llc. 800-325-1881
13705 Shoreline Ct E, Earth City, MO 63045
Ultrasonic cleaner for medical instruments.

CLEANROOM EQUIPMENT *(General) 80VAA*

Advance Tabco 800-645-3166
200 Heartland Blvd, Edgewood, NY 11717
Furniture.

Advanced Input Systems 800-444-5923
600 W Wilbur Ave, Coeur D Alene, ID 83815
MEDIGENIC Cleanable keyboard and mouse with cleaning alert.

Aes Clean Technology, Inc. 888-237-2532
422 Stump Rd, Montgomeryville, PA 18936
AES specializes in the design/build of cGMP Cleanrooms and is the exclusive manufacturer and distributor of the MSS Pharma Wall and Walk-On Ceiling System. Products feature laminar flow modules, ContainAire' weigh/dispense booths, air showers, modular cleanrooms, turnkey HVAC systems, process services and third-party certification/validation services.

Air Control, Inc. 252-492-2300
237 Raleigh Rd, Henderson, NC 27536
MICROVOID.

Airex, Inc. 425-222-3665
13704 SE 17th St, Bellevue, WA 98005
M100 and E100 HEPA/ULPA mobile, self-contained air contamination control systems for industry and medicine. Attachable enclosures for positive or negative pressurized applications.

Bio-Safe America Corp. 800-767-4284
3250 S Susan St Ste B, Sterilaire Medical Division
Santa Ana, CA 92704
Surgery rooms and patient isolation rooms.

Camfil Farr 800-300-3277
2121 E Paulhan St, Rancho Dominguez, CA 90220
FB series fluid seal and GB series gasket seal bag-in/bag-out containment systems; versatile systems for containment of hazardous materials.

Clean Air Technology, Inc. 800 459 6320
41105 Capital Dr, Canton, MI 48187
Turnkey design and build firm specializing in Class 1 to Class 100,000 modular cleanrooms for the medical, pharmaceutical, electronic, semiconductor and aerospace industries. Provides design, construction, start-up, testing and operational services. Also, aseptic fill and containment module.

Cleanroom Systems 800-825-3268
7000 Performance Dr, Syracuse, NY 13212
HEPAIR, self-contained HVAC systems for cleanrooms half ton to 22 ton capacities.

Climet Instruments Co. 909-793-2788
1320 W Colton Ave, Redlands, CA 92374
Airborne particle counters and cleanroom equipment.

Cole-Parmer Instrument Inc. 800-323-4340
625 E Bunker Ct, Vernon Hills, IL 60061
Cleansphere benchtop mini-cleanroom.

Contamination Control Products 877-553-2676
1 3rd Ave # 578, Neptune, NJ 07753
Air showers, laminar flow workstations and HEPA filter modules.

Deltatrak, Inc. 800-962-6776
PO Box 398, Pleasanton, CA 94566
Analytical/monitoring equipment.

CLEANROOM EQUIPMENT *(cont'd)*

Harris Environmental Systems, Inc. 888-771-4200
11 Connector Rd, Andover, MA 01810
Cleanrooms.

Hemco Corp. 816-796-2900
111 S Powell Rd, Independence, MO 64056
Portable cleanroom with vertical laminar airflow supplied through a pressurized plenum and ceiling-mounted HEPA filters.

Hydrofera Llc 866-861-7548
322 Main St, Willimantic, CT 06226
Polyvinyl alcohol (PVA) foam products. SAUFERA bacteriostatic PVA foam.

La Calhene 320-358-4713
1325 S Field Ave, PO Box 567, Rush City, MN 55069
Portable cleanrooms.

Lacey Manufacturing Co. 203-336-0121
1146 Barnum Ave, PO Box 5156, Bridgeport, CT 06610

Liberty Industries, Inc. 800-828-5656
133 Commerce St, East Berlin, CT 06023

Lm Air Technology, Inc. 866-381-8200
1467 Pinewood St, Cleanroom & Lab Equipment - Mfger Rahway, NJ 07065
Portable laminar downflow rooms; Class 100,000 to Class 10 clean environment, works on ambient or ducted air. Options include anti-static grid or bar, ULPA filters or stainless-steel frame.

Micro Care Corp. 800-638-0125
595 John Downey Dr, New Britain, CT 06051
Vertrel® specialty solvents and carrying agents. Micro Care is the North American distributor of these unique DuPont solvents. Nonflammable, ozone-safe, non-toxic and easy to handle, these cleaners are ideal for use in medical applications. They easily remove light oils, grease, inks and inorganic contamination. Unlike water-based cleaners, the Vertrel products will not support biological growth and are compatible with sterilization processes. They offer easy handling, evaporate quickly, and leave no residues on parts or surfaces. Solvency can be tailored to your specific application with a variety of additives, and the products also can be mixed with lubricants to deliver smooth, effortless movement of plastic, metal, ceramic or glass pieces/tools/scapels etc.

Morrison Medical 800-438-6677
3735 Paragon Dr, Columbus, OH 43228
Clean up system I and II, infection control kits for cleaning messes. One time use for spill control.

Nypro Inc. 978-365-9721
101 Union St, Clinton, MA 01510
Cleanroom manufacturing for precision injection molding & device assembly.

Plastic And Metal Center, Inc. 949-770-8230
23162 La Cadena Dr, Laguna Hills, CA 92653
CLEAR PLEX I or stainless steel garment dispensers and environmental chambers custom made or stock.

Purified Micro Environments, Div. Of Germfree Laboratories 800-888-5357
11 Aviator Way, Ormond Beach, FL 32174
Modular cleanrooms. All stainless steel frame modular cleanrooms. Class 100,000 up to Class 10.

Qrp, Inc. 800-832-3882
3925 N Runway Dr, PO Box 28802, Tucson, AZ 85705
Gloves & Fingercots for cleanrooms, ESD, thermal protection, chemical protection, dry box gloves, and general purpose applications.

Spirig Advanced Technologies, Inc. 413-788-6191
144 Oakland St, Springfield, MA 01108
PTS MATS cleanroom mats.

Surgical Technologies, Inc. 800-777-9987
292 E Lafayette Frontage Rd, Saint Paul, MN 55107

Taylor Wharton 800-898-2657
4075 Hamilton Blvd, Theodore, AL 36582
Containment for liquid gases.

Telemed Systems Inc. 800-481-6718
8 Kane Industrial Dr, Hudson, MA 01749
Scope channel cleaning, reusable & disposable available.

The Evercare Company 800-435-6223
3440 Preston Ridge Rd Ste 650, Alpharetta, GA 30005
$18.64 for adhesive floor roller/needle finder with 40 layers of disposable tape (8in. x 20ft.) and plastic extension handle. Picks up bacteria-laden particulates and lost needles from critical area floor.

CLEANROOM EQUIPMENT *(cont'd)*

Uniclean Cleanroom Garment Services 877-544-4432
8 Hixon Pl, A UNIFIRST CO., Maplewood, NJ 07040
Garment service.

CLEANSER, ROOT CANAL *(Dental And Oral) 76KJJ*

Acadental 913-384-7390
5830 Woodson Rd Ste 3, Mission, KS 66202
Edta syringe.

Den-Mat Holdings, Llc 805-922-8491
2727 Skyway Dr, Santa Maria, CA 93455
Cavity cleanser.

Jordco, Inc. 800-752-2812
595 NW 167th Ave, Beaverton, OR 97006
Root canal lubricating gel

Medical Products Laboratories, Inc. 215-677-2700
9990 Global Rd, Philadelphia, PA 19115
Cleanser, root canal.

Miltex Dental Technologies, Inc. 516-576-6022
589 Davies Dr, York, PA 17402
Various solutions for cleaning and drying the root canal.

Oratech, Llc 801-553-4493
475 W 10200 S, South Jordan, UT 84095
Root canal cleanser.

Ultradent Products, Inc. 801-553-4586
505 W 10200 S, South Jordan, UT 84095
Chelating agent.

CLEARING AGENT *(Pathology) 88KEM*

Alpha-Tec Systems, Inc. 800-221-6058
12019 NE 99th St Ste 1780, Vancouver, WA 98682
Clearing agent.

American Mastertech Scientific, Inc. 209-368-4031
1330 Thurman St, Lodi, CA 95240
Clearing agents.

Amresco Inc. 800-366-1313
30175 Solon Industrial Pkwy, Solon, OH 44139
HISTOCHOICE is a safe and effective clearing agent for histology. It is nontoxic, noncarcinogenic, nonflammable and virtually odorless.

Anatech, Ltd. 800-262-8324
1020 Harts Lake Rd, Battle Creek, MI 49037
PRO-PAR CLEARANT; xylene free clearing agent.

E K Industries, Inc. 877-EKI-CHEM
1403 Herkimer St, Joliet, IL 60432
Limonene.

Hemo-De, Inc. 817-379-7328
2000 Whitley Rd Ste H, Keller, TX 76248
Clearing agent, chemical reagent.

Sci Gen, Inc. 310-324-6576
333 E Gardena Blvd, Gardena, CA 90248
FDA: Medical Device Manufacturing and packaging. Focus on Histology, Cytology, Analytical and General purpose Reagents, Chemistry, and Sterling and Disinfecting agents.

Statspin, Inc. 800-782-8774
60 Glacier Dr, Westwood, MA 02090
LIPOCLEAR's lipemic plasma clearing reagent in prefilled micro-tubes.

Vegamed, Inc. 787-807-0392
39 Calle Las Flores, Edificio Multifabril #5, Vega Baja, PR 00693
Bru-water.

CLEARING OIL *(Pathology) 88IJZ*

Sci Gen, Inc. 310-324-6576
333 E Gardena Blvd, Gardena, CA 90248
FDA: Medical Device Manufacturing and packaging. Focus on Histology, Cytology, Analytical and General purpose Reagents, Chemistry, and Sterling and Disinfecting agents.

U S Biotex Corp. 606-652-4700
RR 1 Box 62, Webbville, KY 41180
Oil, clearing.

CLIMBER, CURB, WHEELCHAIR *(Physical Med) 89IMN*

Patterson Medical Supply, Inc. 262-387-8720
W68N158 Evergreen Blvd, Cedarburg, WI 53012
Roylan wheelchair foot support.

CLIP, ANEURYSM (INTRACRANIAL) *(Cns/Neurology) 84HCH*

Aesculap Implant Systems Inc. 1-800-234-9179
3773 Corporate Pkwy, Center Valley, PA 18034
Yasangil aneurysm clips for permanent or temporary occlusion.

Cardinal Health, Snowden Pencer Products 847-689-8410
5175 S Royal Atlanta Dr, Tucker, GA 30084
Various types and sizes of aneurysm clips.

Codman & Shurtleff, Inc 800-225-0460
325 Paramount Dr, Raynham, MA 02767

Mizuho America Inc. 800-699-2547
133 Brimbal Ave, Beverly, MA 01915
SUGITA clips for clipping brain aneurysms.

Nmt Medical, Inc. 617-737-0930
27-43 Wormwood St, Boston, MA 02210
Aneurysm clip.

Scanlan International, Inc. 800-328-9458
1 Scanlan Plz, Saint Paul, MN 55107

CLIP, BANDAGE *(General) 80QLD*

Jero Medical Equipment & Supplies, Inc. 800-457-0644
1701 W 13th St, Chicago, IL 60608

CLIP, HEMOSTATIC *(Surgery) 79MCH*

Cook Endoscopy 336-744-0157
4900 Bethania Station Rd # &, 5951 Grassy Creek Blvd. Winston Salem, NC 27105
Endoscopic clipping device.

Elmed, Inc. 630-543-2792
60 W Fay Ave, Addison, IL 60101

Ethicon Endo-Surgery, Inc. 877-384-4266
3801 University Blvd SE, Albuquerque, NM 87106
Sterile and nonsterile ligating clips.

CLIP, IMPLANTABLE *(Surgery) 79FZP*

Abbott Vascular Inc. 800-227-9902
400 Saginaw Dr, Redwood City, CA 94063
Implantable clip.

Aesculap Implant Systems Inc. 1-800-234-9179
3773 Corporate Pkwy, Center Valley, PA 18034

Biomet, Inc. 574-267-6639
56 E Bell Dr, PO Box 587, Warsaw, IN 46582
Various types of implantable clips, radiographic markers.

Cardica, Inc. 888-544-7194
900 Saginaw Dr, Redwood City, CA 94063
Implantable clip & delivery system.

Devicor Medical Products Inc. 262-857-9300
10505 Corporate Dr Ste 207, Pleasant Prairie, WI 53158
14G CorMARK Biopsy Site Identifier; Caris Site Marker

Ethicon Endo-Surgery, Inc. 877-384-4266
3801 University Blvd SE, Albuquerque, NM 87106
Various types of sterile and non-sterile ligating clips and appliers.

Gyrx, Llc 904-641-2599
10302 Deerwood Park Blvd Ste 209, Jacksonville, FL 32256
Implantable clip.

Kelsar, S.A. 508-261-8000
Blvd. Insurgentes, Libriamento a La, Tijuana 22450 Mexico
Ligating clip

Senorx, Inc. 949-362-4800
11 Columbia, Aliso Viejo, CA 92656
Biopsy site marker.

St. Jude Medical Atrial Fibrillation 800.748.7335
6500 Wedgwood Rd N, Maple Grove, MN 55311
Implantable clip and delivery system.

Ussc Puerto Rico, Inc. 203-845-1000
Building 911-67, Sabanetas Industrial Park, Ponce, PR 00731
Multiple.

CLIP, IMPLANTABLE, MALLEABLE *(Cns/Neurology) 84HBP*

Depuy-Raynham, A Div. Of Depuy Orthopaedics 800-451-2006
325 Paramount Dr, Raynham, MA 02767
Various implanted malleable clips.

CLIP, INSTRUMENT *(Surgery) 79QLF*

Arosurgical Instruments Corp. 800-776-1751
537 Newport Center Dr Ste 101, Newport Beach, CA 92660
BEARtm micro vessel clamps. For veins and arteries from 0.2mm Dia. to 5.0mm Dia. CALL FOR FREE SAMPLES.

Bolt Bethel, Llc 763-434-5900
23530 University Avenue Ext NW, PO Box 135, Bethel, MN 55005

CLIP, INSTRUMENT *(cont'd)*

Putnam Precision Products 845-278-2141
3859 Danbury Rd, Brewster, NY 10509

CLIP, INSTRUMENT, FORMING/CUTTING *(Cns/Neurology) 84HBS*

Busse Hospital Disposables, Inc. 631-435-4711
75 Arkay Dr, Hauppauge, NY 11788
Sterile/non-sterile skin staple removers.

CLIP, IRIS RETRACTOR *(Ophthalmology) 86HOC*

Bausch & Lomb Surgical 636-255-5051
3365 Tree Court Ind Blvd, Saint Louis, MO 63122

Eagle Vision, Inc. 800-222-7584
8500 Wolf Lake Dr Ste 110, Memphis, TN 38133
Graether pupil expander, 1 size.

Genesee Biomedical, Inc. 800-786-4890
1308 S Jason St, Denver, CO 80223
INTRA-ART Coronary Artery Retraction Clip. Improves approach and access to the coronary arteries by simply retracting the fat layer.

Howard Instruments, Inc. 205-553-4453
4749 Appletree Ln, Tuscaloosa, AL 35405

J. Barot & Assoc. 321-383-7574
1125 White Dr, P.o. Box 5293, Titusville, FL 32780
Clip, iris retractor.

Jedmed Instruments Co. 314-845-3770
5416 Jedmed Ct, Saint Louis, MO 63129

Microvision, Inc. 603-474-5566
34 Folly Mill Rd, Seabrook, NH 03874
Iris retractor.

Milvella Limited 952-746-1369
12100 Singletree Ln, Eden Prairie, MN 55344
Sterile pupil dilator.

Surgical Instrument Manufacturers, Inc. 800-521-2985
1650 Headland Dr, Fenton, MO 63026

CLIP, LENS, TRIAL, OPHTHALMIC *(Ophthalmology) 86HPB*

Gulden Ophthalmics 800-659-2250
225 Cadwalader Ave, Elkins Park, PA 19027

CLIP, LIGATURE *(Surgery) 79SJG*

Ethicon Endo-Surgery, Inc. 800-USE-ENDO
4545 Creek Rd, Cincinnati, OH 45242
LIGACLIP cartridge clips, tantalum: 6 and 20 (SM), 6 and 20 (med), 6 (med/lg) and 6 (lg); ligating clips 6 (med) and (lg), titanium; extra clips, 13 1/2in. (lg), 11 1/2in. (med), 9 3/8in. (sm) and (med), appliers, 20 count. ABSOLOK small, medium, medium/large and large absorbable, ligating clips, 10. Cartridge base clips for (sm), (med), (med/lg) and (lg), reuseable. Cartridge extra clips: 6(sm), (med), (med/lg) and (lg), 20 (sm) and (med), stainless steel; 6 and 20 (sm) titanium. Single clip appliers: 10mm shaft (m/l) and (l), reuseable. Multiple clip applier, ligate and divide, 12mm. Also, clip remover, 10in. reuseable.

Teleflex Medical 800-334-9751
2917 Weck Drive, Research Triangle Park, NC 27709
HEM-O-LOK ligating clip system, polymer non-absorbable locking clips for vessel ligation.

CLIP, NOSE *(Anesthesiology) 73BXJ*

A-M Systems, Inc. 800-426-1306
131 Business Park Loop, Sequim, WA 98382
Available with Foam or Rubber Pads. Sold 100 per package. $31.80 per package

Amici, Inc. 610-948-7100
518 Vincent St, Spring City, PA 19475

Creative Biomedics, Inc. 949-366-2300
924 Calle Negocio Ste A, San Clemente, CA 92673
Nose Clip

Directmed, Inc. 516-656-3377
150 Pratt Oval, Glen Cove, NY 11542

Hans Rudolph, Inc. 816-363-5522
7200 Wyandotte St, Kansas City, MO 64114
Nose clip.

Instrumentation Industries, Inc. 800-633-8577
2990 Industrial Blvd, Bethel Park, PA 15102

Mercury Medical 800-237-6418
11300 49th St N, Clearwater, FL 33762

Niagara Pharmaceuticals Div. 905-690-6277
60 Innovation Dr., Flamborough, ONT L9H-7P3 Canada
HEALTH SAVER no. 143 for plastic nose clips with head straps.

CLIP, NOSE *(cont'd)*
Sdi Diagnostics, Inc. 800-678-5782
10 Hampden Dr, South Easton, MA 02375
THE KLIP noseclip for PRT is a disposable, one-piece, snug-fitting noseclip for PFT tests.
Seven Harvest Intl. Import & Export 765-456-3584
108 N Dixon Rd, Kokomo, IN 46901
Nose clips.
Sunmed Healthcare 727-531-7266
12393 Belcher Rd S Ste 460, Largo, FL 33773
Vacumed 800-235-3333
4538 Westinghouse St, Ventura, CA 93003

CLIP, OTHER *(Surgery) 79QLK*
Alto Development Corp. 732-938-2266
5206 Asbury Rd, Wall Township, NJ 07727
Connector clips, Raney clips.
Directmed, Inc. 516-656-3377
150 Pratt Oval, Glen Cove, NY 11542
Howard Instruments, Inc. 205-553-4453
4749 Appletree Ln, Tuscaloosa, AL 35405
CLOSEMATE Clip System and CLOSEMATE Remover, Clips that have only minimal penetration to reduce patient pain during surgery
Taut, Inc. 800-231-8288
2571 Kaneville Ct, Geneva, IL 60134
TAUT Safety Klip is designed not to restrict draining fluids, to assure easy insertion of the drain through the Klip, to facilitate fast and easy advancement of the drain postoperatively, and to maximize patient comfort.
Zimmer Orthopaedic Surgical Products 800-321-5533
PO Box 10, 200 West Ohio Ave., Dover, OH 44622

CLIP, REMOVABLE (SKIN) *(Surgery) 79FZQ*
Codman & Shurtleff, Inc 800-225-0460
325 Paramount Dr, Raynham, MA 02767
Depuy-Raynham, A Div. Of Depuy Orthopaedics 800-451-2006
325 Paramount Dr, Raynham, MA 02767
Various.
Mikron Precision, Inc. 310-515-6221
1558 W 139th St Ste C, Gardena, CA 90249
Wound clip.
Propper Manufacturing Co., Inc. 800-832-4300
3604 Skillman Ave, Long Island City, NY 11101
Tuzik Boston 800-886-6363
104 Longwater Dr, Assinippi Park, Norwell, MA 02061
Warsaw Orthopedic, Inc. 901-396-3133
2500 Silveus Xing, Warsaw, IN 46582
Skin closure clips.

CLIP, SCALP *(Cns/Neurology) 84HBO*
Acra Cut, Inc. 978-263-0250
989 Main St, Acton, MA 01720
Scalp clips.
Codman & Shurtleff, Inc 800-225-0460
325 Paramount Dr, Raynham, MA 02767
Medtronic Neurosurgery 800-468-9710
125 Cremona Dr, Goleta, CA 93117
Kit, clip gun.
Teleflex Medical 800-334-9751
2917 Weck Drive, Research Triangle Park, NC 27709
RANEY clips.
Zimmer Holdings, Inc. 800-613-6131
1800 W Center St, PO Box 708, Warsaw, IN 46580

CLIP, SUTURE *(Surgery) 79QLH*
Fortrad Eye Instruments Corp. 973-543-2371
8 Franklin Rd, Mendham, NJ 07945
Miltex Inc. 800-645-8000
589 Davies Dr, York, PA 17402
Roboz Surgical Instrument Co., Inc. 800-424-2984
PO Box 10710, Gaithersburg, MD 20898

CLIP, TANTALUM, OPHTHALMIC *(Ophthalmology) 86HQW*
University Of Washington 206-616-5130
T281 Health Science, Seattle, WA 98195
Tantalum implant gun.

CLIP, TOWEL *(Surgery) 79QLI*
Codman & Shurtleff, Inc 800-225-0460
325 Paramount Dr, Raynham, MA 02767

CLIP, TOWEL *(cont'd)*
Elmed, Inc. 630-543-2792
60 W Fay Ave, Addison, IL 60101
Miltex Inc. 800-645-8000
589 Davies Dr, York, PA 17402
Moyco Technologies, Inc. 800-331-8837
200 Commerce Dr, Montgomeryville, PA 18936
Plaza Towel Holder, Inc. 877-874-8394
PO Box 4737, Wichita, KS 67204
Towel holders, coat racks and hat racks.
Toolmex Corporation 800-992-4766
1075 Worcester St, Natick, MA 01760
Whitehall Manufacturing 800-782-7706
15125 Proctor Ave, City Of Industry, CA 91746
Towel drying racks.

CLIP, TUBAL OCCLUSION *(Obstetrics/Gyn) 85HGB*
Biomet Microfixation Inc. 800-874-7711
1520 Tradeport Dr, Jacksonville, FL 32218
Various types of clamps.
Richard Wolf Medical Instruments Corp. 800-323-9653
353 Corporate Woods Pkwy, Vernon Hills, IL 60061
Hulka Clips.

CLIP, VAS DEFERENS *(Surgery) 79NJC*
Gyrx, Llc 904-641-2599
10302 Deerwood Park Blvd Ste 209, Jacksonville, FL 32256
Implantable clip.

CLIP, VASCULAR *(Cardiovascular) 74DSS*
Aesculap Implant Systems Inc. 1-800-234-9179
3773 Corporate Pkwy, Center Valley, PA 18034
Biomet Microfixation Inc. 800-874-7711
1520 Tradeport Dr, Jacksonville, FL 32218
Various types of clips.
Covidien Lp 508-261-8000
15 Hampshire St, Mansfield, MA 02048
Fehling Surgical Instruments 800-FEHLING
509 Broadstone Ln NW, Acworth, GA 30101
Lemaitre Vascular, Inc. 781-221-2266
63 2nd Ave, Burlington, MA 01803
The AnastoClip® VCS® Vessel Closure System provides rapid and precise vascular anastomosis. AnastoClip creates an interrupted anastomosis, or vessel attachment site, that is designed to expand and contract as the vessel pulses, which is believed to improve the durability of the attachment.

CLIP, VENA CAVA *(Cardiovascular) 74DST*
Aesculap Implant Systems Inc. 1-800-234-9179
3773 Corporate Pkwy, Center Valley, PA 18034
Fehling Surgical Instruments 800-FEHLING
509 Broadstone Ln NW, Acworth, GA 30101

CLIP, WOUND *(Surgery) 79QLJ*
Codman & Shurtleff, Inc 800-225-0460
325 Paramount Dr, Raynham, MA 02767
Roboz Surgical Instrument Co., Inc. 800-424-2984
PO Box 10710, Gaithersburg, MD 20898

CLIPPER, HAIR *(General) 80QLB*
Homedics Inc. 800-333-8282
3000 N Pontiac Trl, Commerce Township, MI 48390

CLIPPER, NAIL *(General) 80QLC*
Amson Products 718-435-3728
1401 42nd St, Brooklyn, NY 11219
Jero Medical Equipment & Supplies, Inc. 800-457-0644
1701 W 13th St, Chicago, IL 60608
Premier Medical Products 888-PREMUSA
1710 Romano Dr, Plymouth Meeting, PA 19462

CLOCK, ELAPSED TIME *(General) 80QLL*
Bender, Inc. 800-356-4266
700 Fox Chase, Highlands Corp. Center, Coatesville, PA 19320
ZT 1490 Clock and/or elapsed time indicator using 3/4 inch or 2 1/2 inch red LED display. Maintains time without power. All voltages and frequencies. Code Blue input.
Chrono-Log Corp. 800-247-6665
2 W Park Rd, Havertown, PA 19083
Crest Healthcare Supply 800-328-8908
195 3rd St, Dassel, MN 55325

CLOCK, ELAPSED TIME *(cont'd)*

Independent Solutions, Inc. 847-498-0500
900 Skokie Blvd Ste 118, Northbrook, IL 60062
Bender digital or analog, surface or recess wall mounted, local or remote control, synchronous or non-synchronous.

Meylan Corporation 888-769-9667
543 Valley Rd, Upper Montclair, NJ 07043
$90.00 to $110.00 for elapsed time meters; $100.00 to $390.00 for mechanical or electric interval timers.

Novel Products, Inc. 800-323-5143
PO Box 408, Rockton, IL 61072
Reaction time tester: Calibrated Lexan dropsticks.

Rauland-Borg Corp. 800-752-7725
3450 Oakton St, Skokie, IL 60076
Digital master program clocks, digital and analog secondary clocks.

Symmetricom Timing, Test & Measurement 800-544-0233
34 Tozer Rd, Beverly, MA 01915
Standards, frequency, hydrogen, rubidium, cesium and quartz; for use in applications where precise time and frequency control are required. Oscillators, oven controlled, crystal; timing devices end distribution. RD-05, RD-1, RD-2 Remote Time Display. ND-2, ND-4 Network Time Display.

CLOSURE, OTHER *(General) 80WSY*

Atrion Medical Products, Inc. 800-343-9334
1426 Curt Francis Rd NW, Arab, AL 35016
Bottle closure, dispensing tips for pharmaceuticals.

Bausch & Stroebel Machine Company, Inc. 866-512-2637
112 Nod Rd Ste 17, Clinton, CT 06413
Packaging machine.

Bio Plas, Inc. 415-472-3777
4340 Redwood Hwy Ste A15, San Rafael, CA 94903
Safety caps for re-capping blood collection tubes; 4 sizes, 7 colors, non-aerosoling.

Covidien Lp 508-261-8000
15 Hampshire St, Mansfield, MA 02048
Wound closure devices.

Halkey-Roberts Corp. 800-303-4384
2700 Halkey Roberts Pl N, Saint Petersburg, FL 33716
Closures for drainage, enema, and enteral-feeding bags.

CLOTHING, PROTECTIVE *(General) 80WMY*

Argus-Hazco 800-332-0435
6501 Centerville Business Pkwy, Dayton, OH 45459
Personal protective clothing.

Atd-American Co. 800-523-2300
135 Greenwood Ave, Wyncote, PA 19095

Cleanwear Products Ltd. 416-438-4831
54 Crockford Rd., Toronto, ON M1R-3C3 Canada
Chemo-safe and infectious diseases protection kits, Tyvek isolation gowns.

Clopay Plastic Products Company 800-282-2260
8585 Duke Blvd, Mason, OH 45040

Designs For Comfort, Inc. 800-443-9226
PO Box 671044, Marietta, GA 30066
HEADLINER Rail Roader Hat brim for protection from the sun for women bald from chemotherapy.

Fabrite Laminating Corp. 973-777-1406
70 Passaic St, Wood Ridge, NJ 07075

Health-Pak, Inc. 315-724-8370
2005 Beechgrove Pl, Utica, NY 13501
OSHA Protective Wear Kits.

Hipsavers, Inc. 800-358-4477
7 Hubbard St, Canton, MA 02021
Hip Protective Underwear. Polycotton underwear with thin super-shock absorbent pads sewn in to cover the hip bone.

Jero Medical Equipment & Supplies, Inc. 800-457-0644
1701 W 13th St, Chicago, IL 60608
Disposable Coveralls, Disposable Trouser, Disposable Lab Coats, Disposable Bibs, Aprons

Kappler Protective Apparel & Fabrics 800-600-4019
115 Grimes Dr, Guntersville, AL 35976

Lohmann & Rauscher, Inc. 800-279-3863
6001 SW 6th Ave Ste 101, Topeka, KS 66615
High Visibility Saftey Apparel

CLOTHING, PROTECTIVE *(cont'd)*

Newtex Industries, Inc. 585-924-9135
8050 Victor Mendon Rd, Victor, NY 14564
150 Series Approach, 750 Series Proximity, 2000 Series Fire Entry suits. Suits for approach, proximity and fire entry applications. Also available, kiln suits.

Precept Medical Products, Inc. 800-438-5827
PO Box 2400, 370 Airport Road/, Arden, NC 28704

San-I-Pak,Pacific Inc. 800-875-7264
23535 S Bird Rd, Tracy, CA 95304
Hazardous Material Suits are disposable suits and can be used for handling all manner of hazardous materials.

Servicios Paraclinicios S.A. 83-33-8400
Madero No. 3330 Pte., Monterrey N.L. 64020 Mexico

Skil-Care Corp. 800-431-2972
29 Wells Ave, Yonkers, NY 10701
Fireproof apron for smokers.

Sleep Sauna, Inc. 800-229-5210
608 13th Ave, Council Bluffs, IA 51501
$60.00 for nylon occlusive suit for dermatological use. $13.00 for nylon foot covers for occlusion.

Standard Textile 800-999-0400
1 Knollcrest Dr, Cincinnati, OH 45237

Western Medical, Ltd. 800-628-8276
214 Carnegie Ctr Ste 100, Princeton, NJ 08540
GLEN-SLEEVE II cotton and Lycra sleeves for arms and lower legs, protects against tears and abrasions. Heel and elbow protectors, HIP ARMOR hip protection girdle, also with pads.

CLOTHING, PROTECTIVE, SUN *(Surgery) 79MIW*

Wetmore Assoc., Inc. 425-303-9520
2815 Wetmore Ave, Everett, WA 98201
Solumbra.

White Knight Healthcare 800-851-4431
Calle 16, Number 780, Agua Prieta, Sonora Mexico
Various types of protective clothing

CO-OXIMETER *(Hematology) 81VHJ*

Thermo Fisher Scientific Inc. 781-622-1000
81 Wyman St, Waltham, MA 02451
CO-oximetry control.

COAGULATOR, CULDOSCOPIC *(Obstetrics/Gyn) 85HFI*

Solos Endoscopy 800-388-6445
65 Sprague St # B, Boston/dedham Commerce Park, Boston, MA 02136
Gynecologic laparoscope & accessories.

COAGULATOR, HYSTEROSCOPIC (WITH ACCESSORIES) *(Obstetrics/Gyn) 85HFH*

Elmed, Inc. 630-543-2792
60 W Fay Ave, Addison, IL 60101

Richard Wolf Medical Instruments Corp. 800-323-9653
353 Corporate Woods Pkwy, Vernon Hills, IL 60061

Wisap America 800-233-8448
8231 Melrose Dr, Lenexa, KS 66214

COAGULATOR, LAPAROSCOPIC, UNIPOLAR *(Obstetrics/Gyn) 85HFG*

Cameron-Miller, Inc. 800-621-0142
5410 W Roosevelt Rd, Road #241, Chicago, IL 60644

Elmed, Inc. 630-543-2792
60 W Fay Ave, Addison, IL 60101

Instrumed Oem 800-368-1301
2801 S Vallejo St, Englewood, CO 80110

Lican Medical Products Ltd. 519-737-1142
5120 Halford Dr., Windsor, ON N9A 6J3 Canada

Md International, Inc. 305-669-9003
11300 NW 41st St, Doral, FL 33178

Richard Wolf Medical Instruments Corp. 800-323-9653
353 Corporate Woods Pkwy, Vernon Hills, IL 60061

Smith & Nephew, Inc., Endoscopy Division 800-343-8386
150 Minuteman Rd, Andover, MA 01810

Synectic Medical Product Development 203-877-8488
60 Commerce Park, Milford, CT 06460

Transamerican Technologies International 800-322-7373
2246 Camino Ramon, San Ramon, CA 94583
ACCU-SURG '3 in 1' instrument for suction, irrigation and electrosurgery.

COAGULATOR/CUTTER, ENDOSCOPIC, BIPOLAR
(Obstetrics/Gyn) 85HIN

Aesculap Implant Systems Inc. 1-800-234-9179
3773 Corporate Pkwy, Center Valley, PA 18034

Biomet Microfixation Inc. 800-874-7711
1520 Tradeport Dr, Jacksonville, FL 32218
Coagulator-cutter, endoscopic, bipolar.

Ellman International, Inc. 800-835-5355
3333 Royal Ave, Rockville Centre, NY 11572

Elmed, Inc. 630-543-2792
60 W Fay Ave, Addison, IL 60101

Greenwald Surgical Co., Inc. 219-962-1604
2688 Dekalb St, Gary, IN 46405
Biterminal cervical electrodes; handles; cords and plugs.

Gyrus Medical Inc., Sub. Of Gyrus Acmi, Inc. 508-804-2739
6655 Wedgwood Rd N Ste 160, Maple Grove, MN 55311
Endoscopic bicoag coagulating forceps.

Gyrus Medical, Inc. 800-852-9361
6655 Wedgwood Rd N Ste 105, Maple Grove, MN 55311
Bipolar cutting and coagulation device in three shapes: J hook, C hook, high-angle top; 33-cm length, 5-cm diameter.

Integral Design Inc. 781-740-2036
52 Burr Rd, Hingham, MA 02043

Karl Storz Endoscopy-America Inc. 800-421-0837
600 Corporate Pointe, Culver City, CA 90230
Including accessories.

Kirwan Surgical Products, Inc. 888-547-9267
180 Enterprise Dr, PO Box 427, Marshfield, MA 02050
Disposable and reusable bipolar pencils.

Mahe International Inc. 800-294-7946
468 Craighead St, Nashville, TN 37204

Md International, Inc. 305-669-9003
11300 NW 41st St, Doral, FL 33178

Richard Wolf Medical Instruments Corp. 800-323-9653
353 Corporate Woods Pkwy, Vernon Hills, IL 60061

Surgical Instrument Manufacturers, Inc. 800-521-2985
1650 Headland Dr, Fenton, MO 63026

Synectic Medical Product Development 203-877-8488
60 Commerce Park, Milford, CT 06460

Wisap America 800-233-8448
8231 Melrose Dr, Lenexa, KS 66214

COAGULATOR/CUTTER, ENDOSCOPIC, UNIPOLAR
(Obstetrics/Gyn) 85KNF

Aesculap Implant Systems Inc. 1-800-234-9179
3773 Corporate Pkwy, Center Valley, PA 18034

Cameron-Miller, Inc. 800-621-0142
5410 W Roosevelt Rd, Road #241, Chicago, IL 60644

East Coast Surgical Inc. 717-361-0400
64 Pheasant Ct, Elizabethtown, PA 17022
Endoscopic cautery-cutting electrodes, monopolar electrodes.

Elmed, Inc. 630-543-2792
60 W Fay Ave, Addison, IL 60101

Instrumed Oem 800-368-1301
2801 S Vallejo St, Englewood, CO 80110

J. Jamner Surgical Instruments, Inc 800-431-1123
9 Skyline Dr, Hawthorne, NY 10532

Karl Storz Endoscopy-America Inc. 800-421-0837
600 Corporate Pointe, Culver City, CA 90230

Md International, Inc. 305-669-9003
11300 NW 41st St, Doral, FL 33178

Richard Wolf Medical Instruments Corp. 800-323-9653
353 Corporate Woods Pkwy, Vernon Hills, IL 60061

Smith & Nephew, Inc., Endoscopy Division 800-343-8386
150 Minuteman Rd, Andover, MA 01810

Synectic Medical Product Development 203-877-8488
60 Commerce Park, Milford, CT 06460

Transamerican Technologies International 800-322-7373
2246 Camino Ramon, San Ramon, CA 94583
ACCU-SURG '3 in 1' instrument for suction, irrigation and electrosurgery.

Wisap America 800-233-8448
8231 Melrose Dr, Lenexa, KS 66214

COAT, LABORATORY *(General) 80VKC*

Alimed, Inc. 800-225-2610
297 High St, Dedham, MA 02026

Atd-American Co. 800-523-2300
135 Greenwood Ave, Wyncote, PA 19095

Border Opportunity Saver Systems, Inc. 830-775-0992
10 Finegan Rd, Del Rio, TX 78840
Disposable lab coats.

Carolina Biological Supply Co. 800-334-5551
2700 York Rd, Burlington, NC 27215

Clean Esd Products, Inc. 510-257-5080
48340 Milmont Dr, Fremont, CA 94538
#PG501 barrier gowns priced at $76.25/case, 50/case. One size fits all.

Cms Worldwide, Inc. 800-426-4633
30011 Ivy Glenn Dr Ste 215, Laguna Niguel, CA 92677
Impervious labcoat - White, with side & breast pocket.

General Econopak, Inc. 888-871-8568
1725 N 6th St, Philadelphia, PA 19122
GEPCO lab coats, smocks and scrub attire for O.R.

Global Healthcare 800-601-3880
1495 Hembree Rd Ste 700, Roswell, GA 30076
Impervious and regular lab coats.

Health-Pak, Inc. 315-724-8370
2005 Beechgrove Pl, Utica, NY 13501
Disposable, nonwoven coverall.

Kappler Protective Apparel & Fabrics 800-600-4019
115 Grimes Dr, Guntersville, AL 35976

Maytex Corp. 800-462-9839
23521 Foley St, Hayward, CA 94545
Professional, disposable lab jacket with knit cuffs and collar, 5 snaps, 3 pockets.

Mydent International 800-275-0020
80 Suffolk Ct, Hauppauge, NY 11788
Protective Apparel: DEFEND Lab Coats/Gowns; Non-woven poly disposable clothing for personal protection.

Pfb Inter-Apparel Corp. 800-828-7629
1930 Harrison St Ste 304, Hollywood, FL 33020

Precept Medical Products, Inc. 800-438-5827
PO Box 2400, 370 Airport Road/, Arden, NC 28704

Tronex Healthcare Industries 800-833-1181
2 Cranberry Rd, One Tronex Centre, Parsippany, NJ 07054
Nonwoven PPSB material for comfort, breathability, and protection. Several styles offered in fluid resistant or PE-coated fluid impervious styles, different lengths, knotched or knitted collars, w/or w/out pockets, knitted or elastic cuffs. Four to five plastic snaps for front closure. Offers protection from fluid exposure. White, Blue.

COATING, DENTURE HYDROPHILIC, RESIN
(Dental And Oral) 76EBE

Global Dental Products 516-221-8844
PO Box 537, Bellmore, NY 11710
TUBULITEC anti-bacterial primer. Seals dentinal tubules.

COATING, FILLING MATERIAL, RESIN *(Dental And Oral) 76EBD*

Bisco, Inc. 847-534-6000
1100 W Irving Park Rd, Schaumburg, IL 60193
Various types of coating and filling material.

Centrix, Inc. 800-235-5862
770 River Rd, Shelton, CT 06484

Den-Mat Holdings, Llc 805-922-8491
2727 Skyway Dr, Santa Maria, CA 93455
No common name listed.

Dent Zar, Inc. 800-444-1241
6362 Hollywood Blvd Ste 214, Los Angeles, CA 90028
Filling resins coating.

Dental Technologies, Inc. 847-677-5500
6901 N Hamlin Ave, Lincolnwood, IL 60712
Core form material composite.

Dentalez Group 866-DTE-INFO
101 Lindenwood Dr Ste 225, Valleybrooke Corporate Center
Malvern, PA 19355

Drm Research Laboratories, Inc. 203-488-5555
29 Business Park Dr, Branford, CT 06405
Dental composite filling material.

COATING, FILLING MATERIAL, RESIN *(cont'd)*

Foremost Dental Llc. 201-894-5500
242 S Dean St, Englewood, NJ 07631
Resin coating.

Ivoclar Vivadent, Inc. 800-533-6825
175 Pineview Dr, Amherst, NY 14228

Lang Dental Manufacturing Co., Inc. 800-222-5264
175 Messner Dr, Wheeling, IL 60090
Ortho jet clear and wide orthodontic resins in a variety of sizes and colors.

Scientific Pharmaceuticals, Inc. 800-634-3047
3221 Producer Way, Pomona, CA 91768
$150.00 for 30-g kit with accessories.

Zenith/Dmg Brand 800-662-6383
242 S Dean St, Division of Foremost Dental LLC, Englewood, NJ 07631

COIL, MAGNETIC RESONANCE, SPECIALTY *(Radiology) 90MOS*

Advanced Imaging Research, Inc. 216-426-1461
4700 Lakeside Ave E Ste 400, Cleveland, OH 44114
Mri coils.

Confirma, Inc. 877-811-2356
11040 Main St Ste 100, Bellevue, WA 98004
Access Breast Coil is an eight channel, dual-purpose coil design for breast MRI

Ge Medical Systems, Llc 262-312-7117
3200 N Grandview Blvd, Waukesha, WI 53188
Mr coils (accessory), magnetic resonance giagnostic device.

Intermagnetics General Corporation 800-657-0891
PO Box 461, 450 Old Niskayuna Road, Latham, NY 12110
Peripheral Vascular Coil is designed for magnetic-resonance imaging of the lower extremities using MR angiography protocols.

Invivo 800-331-3220
12501 Research Pkwy, Orlando, FL 32826
Multiple

Magna-Lab, Inc. 516-393-5874
6800 Jericho Tpke Ste 120W, Syosset, NY 11791
Magnetic resonance device.

Micromri, Inc. 267-212-1119
1429 Walnut St Ste 1102, Philadelphia, PA 19102

Midwest Rf, Llc 262-367-8254
535 Norton Dr, PO Box 350, Hartland, WI 53029
MRI quadrature and phased-array surface coils.

Mr Instruments, Inc. 952-746-1435
5610 Rowland Rd Ste 145, Minnetonka, MN 55343
Head coil.

Neocoil, Llc 262-347-1250
N27 W23910a Paul Rd., Pewaukee, WI 53072
Magnetic resonance speciality coil.

Surgi-Vision, Inc. 301-527-2000
20 Firstfield Rd Ste 200, Gaithersburg, MD 20878
EE MR coil.

Usa Instruments, Inc. 330-562-1000
1515 Danner Dr, Aurora, OH 44202
Magnetic resonance imaging coil (various types).

COLLAGEN, HEMOSTATIC, MICROSURGICAL
(Cns/Neurology) 84MFQ

Datascope Interventional Products Division 800-225-5827
1300 MacArthur Blvd, Mahwah, NJ 07430

COLLAGEN, PLATELET AGGREGATION AND ADHESION
(Hematology) 81GHX

Kensey Nash Corporation 484-713-2100
735 Pennsylvania Dr, Exton, PA 19341
Variety of collagen based products, insoluble collagen powders and soluble collagen. Extensive biocompatibility testing and certifications.

Nano Mask Inc. 888-656-3697
175 Cassia Way Ste A115, Henderson, NV 89014
Superstat - Enhanced hemostatic collagen

COLLAR, CERVICAL NECK *(Orthopedics) 87QLP*

Alex Orthopedic, Inc. 800-544-2539
PO Box 201442, Arlington, TX 76006

Alimed, Inc. 800-225-2610
297 High St, Dedham, MA 02026

Armstrong Medical Industries, Inc. 800-323-4220
575 Knightsbridge Pkwy, Lincolnshire, IL 60069

COLLAR, CERVICAL NECK *(cont'd)*

Corflex, Inc. 800-426-7353
669 E Industrial Park Dr, Manchester, NH 03109

Dalco International, Inc. 888-354-5515
8433 Glazebrook Ave, Richmond, VA 23228

Dixie Ems Supply 800-347-3494
385 Union Ave, Brooklyn, NY 11211
$85.00 per 10 (med).

Ferno-Washington, Inc. 800-733-3766
70 Weil Way, Wilmington, OH 45177

Fla Orthopedics, Inc. 800-327-4110
2881 Corporate Way, Miramar, FL 33025

Florida Manufacturing Corp. 800-447-2372
501 Beville Rd, South Daytona, FL 32119

Formedica Ltd. 800-361-9671
1481 Rue Begin, St Laurent, QUE H4R 1V8 Canada
$60.00 per 10 (med).

Frank Stubbs Co., Inc 800-223-1713
2100 Eastman Ave Ste B, Oxnard, CA 93030

Freeman Manufacturing Company 800-253-2091
900 W Chicago Rd, PO Box J, Sturgis, MI 49091

Hermell Products, Inc. 800-233-2342
9 Britton Dr, PO Box 7345, Bloomfield, CT 06002
Four-way cervical quick-collar.

Ita-Med Co. 888-9IT-AMED
310 Littlefield Ave, South San Francisco, CA 94080
Foam extra-firm Philadelphia, adult and pediatric.

J. T. Posey Co. 800-447-6739
5635 Peck Rd, Arcadia, CA 91006

Jobri Llc 800-432-2225
520 N Division St, Konawa, OK 74849
MOR-LOC, E-Z FIT.

Larkotex Company 800-972-3037
1002 Olive St, Texarkana, TX 75501

Lohmann & Rauscher, Inc. 800-279-3863
6001 SW 6th Ave Ste 101, Topeka, KS 66615

Medical Specialties, Inc. 800-582-4040
4600 Lebanon Rd, Mint Hill, NC 28227

Morrison Medical 800-438-6677
3735 Paragon Dr, Columbus, OH 43228
Universal custom collars, preemie sizes, plus S, M, L & XL, wide or narrow.

O&M Enterprise 847-258-4515
641 Chelmsford Ln, Elk Grove Village, IL 60007
COLLAR CERIVAL ALL TYPES SIZE

Ortholine 800-243-3351
13 Chapel St, Norwalk, CT 06850
Serpentine Foam 2.0 to 4.5 in. Universal & Sized. Rigid Philadelphia Collars, Miami J, Acute Care, Thoracic Extention & Occian Long Term Collar Back.

Ossur Americas 800-257-8440
1414 Metropolitan Ave, West Deptford, NJ 08066
Miami Occian Collar Back with IntuiTech viscoelastic foam.

Paramedical Distributors 800-245-3278
2020 Grand Blvd, Kansas City, MO 64108

Rogers Foam Corp. 714-538-3033
808 W Nicolas Ave, Orange, CA 92868

Roloke 800-533-8212
127 W Hazel St, Inglewood, CA 90302
Patented. ABM multi-positional neck collar. The head and neck can be supported in a choice of rotated positions to better protect nerves and joints.

Roloke Company 800-533-8212
127 W Hazel St, Inglewood, CA 90302
Multi-positional neck collar. User can place head and neck in a choice of positions and rotation.

Scott Specialties, Inc./Cmo Inc./Ginny Inc. 800-255-7136
512 M St, Belleville, KS 66935

Seattle Systems 360-697-5656
26296 12 Trees Ln NW Bldg 1, Poulsbo, WA 98370

Slawner Ltd., J. 514-731-3378
5713 Cote Des Neiges Rd., Montreal, QUE H3S 1Y7 Canada

Southwest Technologies, Inc. 800-247-9951
1746 E Levee St, North Kansas City, MO 64116

COLLAR, CERVICAL NECK *(cont'd)*

St. John Companies 800-435-4242
25167 Anza Dr, PO Box 800460, Santa Clarita, CA 91355
A size to fit every throat. High quality thyroid collar and other protective apparel.

Star Medical Systems 800-626-3006
8301 Torresdale Ave Ste 13, Philadelphia, PA 19136
Pillows, cervical - large selection of cervical pillows for the neck and back. Support, for the back - many back supports to cater to all patient's injuries. Manufacturer of about 40 different types of products with aluminum stays & without.

Surgical Appliance Industries 800-888-0458
3960 Rosslyn Dr, Cincinnati, OH 45209

Tetra Medical Supply Corp. 800-621-4041
6364 W Gross Point Rd, Niles, IL 60714

Total Care 800-334-3802
PO Box 1661, Rockville, MD 20849

Truform Orthotics & Prosthetics 800-888-0458
3960 Rosslyn Dr, Cincinnati, OH 45209

U.S. Orthotics, Inc. 800-825-5228
8605 Palm River Rd, Tampa, FL 33619
Soft foam neck collars.

Zimmer Holdings, Inc. 800-613-6131
1800 W Center St, PO Box 708, Warsaw, IN 46580

Zimmer Orthopaedic Surgical Products 800-321-5533
PO Box 10, 200 West Ohio Ave., Dover, OH 44622

COLLAR, EXTRICATION *(General) 80WMR*

Ambu, Inc. 800-262-8462
6740 Baymeadow Dr, Glen Burnie, MD 21060
PERFIT, PERFIT ACE

Armstrong Medical Industries, Inc. 800-323-4220
575 Knightsbridge Pkwy, Lincolnshire, IL 60069

Ossur Americas 800-257-8440
1414 Metropolitan Ave, West Deptford, NJ 08066
NecLoc and NecLoc Kids Extrication Collars

COLLAR, ICE *(General) 80QLR*

Hospital Marketing Svcs. Company, Inc. 800-786-5094
162 Great Hill Rd./ Ind. Park, Naugatuck, CT 06770
COL-PRESS instant ice pack - 4in. x 11in., cat. no. 6400, 24/case.

Tetra Medical Supply Corp. 800-621-4041
6364 W Gross Point Rd, Niles, IL 60714

COLLECTOR, BLOOD, VACUUM-ASSISTED *(Hematology) 81KST*

Baxter Healthcare S.A. 847-948-2000
Rd. 721, Km. 0.3, Aibonito, PR 00609
Sterile access device for blood collection.

Bio-Plexus, Inc. 800-223-0010
129 Reservoir Rd, Vernon, CT 06066

Daxor Corporation 865-425-0555
107 Meco Ln, Oak Ridge, TN 37830
Blood collection system.

Habley Medical Technology Corp. 800-729-1994
15721 Bernardo Heights Pkwy Ste B-30, San Diego, CA 92128
Safety blood-collection devices with indefinite shelf life.

Lynn Peavey Co. 913-888-0600
14865 W 105th St, Lenexa, KS 66215
Peavey blood alcohol kit.

COLLECTOR, FRACTION *(Chemistry) 75QLS*

Tudor Scientific Glass Co., Inc. 800-336-4666
555 Edgefield Rd, Belvedere, SC 29841
Gas and liquid.

COLLECTOR, OSTOMY *(Gastro/Urology) 78EXB*

Coloplast Manufacturing Us, Llc 800-533-0464
1840 W Oak Pkwy, Marietta, GA 30062
One and two-piece ostomy pouches with skin barrier.

Hollister, Inc. 847-680-2849
366 Draft Ave, Stuarts Draft, VA 24477

Invacare Supply Group, An Invacare Co. 800-225-4792
75 October Hill Rd, Holliston, MA 01746
Carry full lines of ostomy appliances & pouches from: Hollistor, Covatec, Coloplast, Genairex, Bard & Cymed.

Kem Ent., Inc. 888-562-8802
PO Box 6342, Grand Rapids, MI 49516
Accessory to ostomy collector/air release vent.

COLLECTOR, OSTOMY *(cont'd)*

Ldb Medical, Inc. 800-243-2554
2909 Langford Rd Ste B500, Norcross, GA 30071
LAPIDES.

Metro Medical Supply Wholesale 800-768-2002
200 Cumberland Bnd, Nashville, TN 37228

North American Latex Corp. 812-268-6608
49 Industrial Park Dr, Sullivan, IN 47882
Collector, latex.

Torbot Group, Inc. 800-545-4254
1367 Elmwood Ave, Cranston, RI 02910

X-O Corporation 214-388-5590
8311 Eastpoint Dr Ste 100, Dallas, TX 75227
X-o odor neutralizer/ x-o plus odor neutralizer.

COLLECTOR, SPECIMEN *(Microbiology) 83LIO*

Ability Building Center, Inc. 507-281-6262
1911 14th St NW, P.O. Box 6938, Rochester, MN 55901
PROTOCULT fecal collection device, disposable.

Andwin Scientific 800-497-3113
6636 Variel Ave, Woodland Hills, CA 91303
Safetex Chlamydia trachomatis specimen collection kit.

Bagco 800-533-1931
1650 Airport Rd NW Ste 104, Kennesaw, GA 30144
Two-compartment TEARZONE zipper bag , the safest specimen transport available. This non-perforated TEARZONE give access to the enclosed specimen by either zipping open or tearing the bag open at the tear zone, all packed in tissue-style soft packed dispenser bags.

Becton, Dickinson & Co. 308-872-6811
150 S 1st Ave, Broken Bow, NE 68822
Various (list attached).

Becton, Dickinson & Co., (Bd) Preanalytical System 201-847-6280
1575 Airport Rd, Sumter, SC 29153
Various (list attached).

Bio-Rad Laboratories, Inc. 425-881-8300
14620 NE North Woodinville Way, Way, Suite 200 Woodinville, WA 98072
Various specimen collection kits.

Busse Hospital Disposables, Inc. 631-435-4711
75 Arkay Dr, Hauppauge, NY 11788
Specimen collector.

Chematics, Inc. 574-834-4080
Hwy. 13 South, North Webster, IN 46555
Collection of plasma with filter paper.

Custom Bottle/Lerman Container 800-315-6681
10 Great Hill Rd, Naugatuck, CT 06770

Lps Industries, Inc. 800-275-4577
10 Caesar Pl, Moonachie, NJ 07074
LOC-TOP reclosable polyethylene bags, biohazard/OSHA standard.

Medela, Inc. 800-435-8316
1101 Corporate Dr, McHenry, IL 60050
Specimen cup for collection of tissue samples for use with Medela aspirators.

Meridian Bioscience, Inc. 800-696-0739
3471 River Hills Dr, Cincinnati, OH 45244
Materials necessary for collecting and transporting conjunctival and male and female urethral specimens to be tested for Chlamydia.

Neo Medical Inc. 888-450-3334
42514 Albrae St, Fremont, CA 94538
Entero test capsule.

Sanderson-Macleod, Inc. 866-522-3481
1199 S Main St, P.O. Box 50, Palmer, MA 01069

COLLECTOR, SPUTUM *(Anesthesiology) 73QLT*

Covidien Lp 508-261-8000
15 Hampshire St, Mansfield, MA 02048

Orasure Technologies, Inc. 610-882-1820
1745 Eaton Ave, Bethlehem, PA 18018
Non sputum; oral fluid. Collector of Mucosal Transudate: ORA-SURE oral specimen collection device for HIV-1 antibody testing.

Starplex Scientific Inc. 800-665-0954
50A Steinway Blvd., Etobicoke, ONT M9W 6Y3 Canada
5ml, 10ml & 30ml vials.

COLLECTOR, SWEAT *(Chemistry) 75VCX*

Pacific Biometrics, Inc. 949-455-9724
25651 Atlantic Ocean Dr Ste A1, El Toro, CA 92630
OSTEOPATCH system combines a transdermal sweat collection device with proprietary assays for the detection of biochemical markers of bone loss in sweat and a proprietary method for laboratory analysis.

Ultracell Medical Technologies, Inc. 877-SPO-NGE1
183 Providence New London Tpke, North Stonington, CT 06359
ULTRACELL P.V.A. headband.

Wescor, Inc. 800-453-2725
459 S Main St, Logan, UT 84321
Priced at $1,995.00 for sweat stimulation and collection of error-free sweat samples for cystic fibrosis laboratory diagnosis.

COLLECTOR, URINE *(Gastro/Urology) 78KNX*

Allen Medical Systems, Inc. 800-433-5774
1 Post Office Sq, Acton, MA 01720
Urine collector and accessories

Bio-Medical Products Corp. 800-543-7427
10 Halstead Rd, Mendham, NJ 07945
Urine vacuum tube.

C. R. Bard, Inc., Bard Urological Div. 888-367-2273
13183 Harland Dr NE, Covington, GA 30014

Caring Hands, Inc. 208-691-9524
4347 N Alderbrook Dr, Dalton Gdns, ID 83815
Urine collection, non-invasive/Travelmate. Non-invasive female urinary device, winner of the 2001 Medical Device Excellence Awards in the over-the-counter category.

Cleveland Medical Devices, Inc. 877-253-8363
4415 Euclid Ave, Cleveland, OH 44103
LIBERTY VALVE, urinary leg-bag drainage system for power wheelchair users with a patented 2-switch mechanism that can be easily used without finger/hand movement.

Coloplast Manufacturing Us, Llc 612-302-4992
1185 Willow Lake Blvd, Vadnais Heights, MN 55110
Sterile female urine specimen catheter.

Covidien Lp 508-261-8000
15 Hampshire St, Mansfield, MA 02048

Global Healthcare 800-601-3880
1495 Hembree Rd Ste 700, Roswell, GA 30076
Rectalgular, Pear shaped, economic type and pediatric.

Imed Technology, Inc. 972-732-7333
17408 Tamaron Dr, Dallas, TX 75287
Bedside uring drain bags - sterile.

Jaisons International, Inc. 203-261-1653
22 Bittersweet Ln, Trumbull, CT 06611
Catheters.

Kelsar, S.A. 508-261-8000
Blvd. Insurgentes, Libriamento a La, Tijuana 22450 Mexico
Urinary drainage brags

Ldb Medical, Inc. 800-243-2554
2909 Langford Rd Ste B500, Norcross, GA 30071
LAPIDES.

Medtronic Blood Management 612-514-4000
18501 E Plaza Dr, Parker, CO 80134
Closed urinary drainage system.

Reach Global Industries, Inc. (Reachgood) 888-518-8389
8 Corporate Park Ste 300, Irvine, CA 92606
Various.

Rochester Medical Corp. 800-615-2364
1 Rochester Medical Dr NW, Stewartville, MN 55976
Leg bags, extension tubing, lg. holders.

Terumo Cardiovascular Systems (Tcvs) 800-283-7866
28 Howe St, Ashland, MA 01721
Urinary drainagebag.

Vygon Corp. 800-544-4907
2495 General Armistead Ave, Norristown, PA 19403

COLLECTOR, URINE, DISPOSABLE *(Gastro/Urology) 78FFH*

Coloplast Manufacturing Us, Llc 800-533-0464
1840 W Oak Pkwy, Marietta, GA 30062
CONVEEN thigh and calf urinary leg bags for use with catheters and CONVEEN urinary, pocket shaped urinary drip collector for male urinary dribbling incontinence.

Cook Urological, Inc. 800-457-4500
1100 W Morgan St, P.O. Box 227, Spencer, IN 47460

COLLECTOR, URINE, DISPOSABLE *(cont'd)*

Covidien Lp 508-261-8000
15 Hampshire St, Mansfield, MA 02048

Farmatap S.A. De C.V.
117 Alfonso Esparza Oteo, Mexico Df 01020 Mexico
No common name listed

Image Molding, Inc. 800-525-1875
4525 Kingston St, Denver, CO 80239
Case of 500.

Medi Inc 800-225-8634
75 York Ave, P.O. Box 302, Randolph, MA 02368

Precision Dynamics Corp. 800-772-1122
13880 Del Sur St, San Fernando, CA 91340

Rocket Medical Plc. 800-707-7625
150 Recreation Park Dr Ste 3, Hingham, MA 02043

Ross Disposable Products 800-649-6526
401 Traders Blvd E, Unit 10, Mississauga, ON L4Z 2H8 Canada

Starplex Scientific Inc. 800-665-0954
50A Steinway Blvd., Etobicoke, ONT M9W 6Y3 Canada

COLLECTOR, URINE, POWERED, NON INDWELLING CATHETER *(Gastro/Urology) 78NZU*

Omni Measurement Systems, Inc. 802-865-5223
1150 Airport Dr, South Burlington, VT 05403
Automatic bladder relief device.

Progressive Operations, Inc. 314-570-5153
8455 Wabash Ave, Saint Louis, MO 63134
Urine collector.

COLLIMATOR, RADIOGRAPHIC, AUTOMATIC *(Radiology) 90IZW*

Control-X Medical, Inc. 800-777-9729
1755 Atlas St, Columbus, OH 43228

Ge Medical Systems, Llc 262-548-2355
3000 N Grandview Blvd, W-417, Waukesha, WI 53188
Beam limiting device - collimator.

Margraf Dental Manufacturing, Inc. 800-762-2641
611 Harper Ave, Jenkintown, PA 19046
Podiatry collimator.

Progeny, Inc. 847-415-9800
675 Heathrow Dr, Lincolnshire, IL 60069
Collimators, various types.

Xma (X-Ray Marketing Associates, Inc.) 800-325-8880
1205 W Lakeview Ct, Windham Lakes Business Park
Romeoville, IL 60446

COLLIMATOR, RADIOGRAPHIC, MANUAL *(Radiology) 90IZX*

Americomp, Inc. 800-458-1782
2901 W Lawrence Ave, Chicago, IL 60625

Amrad 888-772-6723
2901 W Lawrence Ave, Chicago, IL 60625

Control-X Medical, Inc. 800-777-9729
1755 Atlas St, Columbus, OH 43228

Marconi Medical Systems 800-323-0550
595 Miner Rd, Cleveland, OH 44143

Progeny, Inc. 847-415-9800
675 Heathrow Dr, Lincolnshire, IL 60069
Collimators, various types.

Xma (X-Ray Marketing Associates, Inc.) 800-325-8880
1205 W Lakeview Ct, Windham Lakes Business Park
Romeoville, IL 60446

COLLIMATOR, THERAPEUTIC X-RAY, HIGH VOLTAGE *(Radiology) 90IYK*

Varian Medical Systems 800-544-4636
3100 Hansen Way, Palo Alto, CA 94304
The Millennium 120-leaf multileaf collimator.

COLLIMATOR, THERAPEUTIC X-RAY, ORTHOVOLTAGE *(Radiology) 90IYI*

Sun Nuclear Corp. 321-259-6862
425 Pineda Ct Ste A, Melbourne, FL 32940
In-vivo dosimetry system.

COLLIMATOR, X-RAY *(Dental And Oral) 76EHB*

Margraf Dental Manufacturing, Inc. 800-762-2641
611 Harper Ave, Jenkintown, PA 19046
Periapical and cephalometric.

COLLIMATOR, X-RAY *(cont'd)*

Wehmer Corporation 800-323-0229
1151 N Main St, Lombard, IL 60148
Accurate X-ray beam alignment plus protection from stray radiation, $295.

COLLODION *(Pathology) 88IAW*

Mavidon Medical Products 800-654-0385
1820 2nd Ave N, Lake Worth, FL 33461
Collodian.

Scholle Chemical Corp. 404-761-0604
2300 W Point Ave, Atlanta, GA 30337
Various types of collodion.

The Electrode Store 360-829-0400
PO Box 188, Enumclaw, WA 98022
$4.00 per tube. $55.00 per pint.

COLONOSCOPE, GASTRO-UROLOGY *(Gastro/Urology) 78FDF*

Avantis Medical Systems, Inc. 408-733-1901
263 Santa Ana Ct, Sunnyvale, CA 94085
Endoscope.

Neoguide Systems, Inc. 408-321-8844
2712 Orchard Pkwy, San Jose, CA 95134
Neoguide endoscopy system and accessories.

Olympus America, Inc. 800-645-8160
3500 Corporate Pkwy, PO Box 610, Center Valley, PA 18034

Pentax Medical Company 800-431-5880
102 Chestnut Ridge Rd, Montvale, NJ 07645
$15,540.00 for several models of fiberoptic colonoscopes with insertion tube diameters of 12.8mm and a channel size of 3.8mm, including a two channel and pediatric model. $25,410.00 to $26,775.00 for video colonoscopes with built-in CCD at insertion tube. Various models with insertion tube diameters (11.6 to 12.8mm) and channel sizes (2.8 to 4.2mm). All fully immersible. EC-3400 Series ideal for pediatric use. Several available with zoom magnification.

Pentax Southern Region Service Center 201-571-2300
8934 Kirby Dr, Houston, TX 77054
Colonoscope.

Pentax West Coast Service Center 800-431-5880
10410 Pioneer Blvd Ste 2, Santa Fe Springs, CA 90670
Pentax colonoscope.

Spirus Medical, Inc. 781-297-7220
1063 Turnpike St, PO Box 258, Stoughton, MA 02072
Endo-Ease Advantage; Endo-Ease Vista

Stryker Gi 866-672-5757
1420 Lakeside Pkwy Ste 110, Flower Mound, TX 75028
Colonoscope, gastro-urology.

COLONOSCOPE, GENERAL & PLASTIC SURGERY
(Surgery) 79FTJ

Dma Med-Chem Corporation 800-362-1833
49 Watermill Ln, Great Neck, NY 11021

COLORIMETER, GENERAL USE *(Chemistry) 75JJQ*

Alt Bioscience,Llc 859-231-3061
235 Bolivar St, Lexington, KY 40508
Colorimeter.

Artel, Inc. 207-854-0860
25 Bradley Dr, Westbrook, ME 04092
Various types of photometers.

Awareness Technology, Inc. 722-283-6540
1935 SW Martin Hwy, Palm City, FL 34990
$2,600 to $4,800 per colorimeter, depending on model. Other custom optical laboratory instrumentation available.

Barnstead International 412-490-8425
2555 Kerper Blvd, Dubuque, IA 52001
Various spectrophotometers.

Bayer Healthcare Llc 914-524-2955
555 White Plains Rd Fl 5, Tarrytown, NY 10591
Spectrophotometer.

Bayer Healthcare, Llc 574-256-3430
430 S Beiger St, Mishawaka, IN 46544
Spectrophotometer.

Beckman Coulter, Inc. 800-742-2345
250 S Kraemer Blvd, PO Box 8000, Brea, CA 92821

Bio-Rad Laboratories, Inc. 425-881-8300
6565 185th Ave NE, Redmond, WA 98052
Eia reader.

COLORIMETER, GENERAL USE *(cont'd)*

Biosite Incorporated 888-246-7483
9975 Summers Ridge Rd, San Diego, CA 92121
Fluorometer for clinical use.

Biotek Instruments, Inc. 802-655-4040
100 Tigan St, Highland Park, Winooski, VT 05404
Various models of manual and automated eia readers.

Bioveris Corporation 301-869-9800
16020 Industrial Dr, Gaithersburg, MD 20877
Detection system.

Brinkmann Instruments (Canada) Ltd. 800-263-8715
6670 Campobello Rd., Mississauga, ONT L5N 2L8 Canada
General and fiber optic probe colorimeters.

Brinkmann Instruments, Inc. 800-645-3050
PO Box 1019, Westbury, NY 11590

Clinical Data Inc 800-937-5449
1 Gateway Ctr Ste 702, Newton, MA 02458
Laboratory instrumentation.

Continental Hydrodyne Systems, Inc. 800-543-9283
1025 Mary Laidley Dr, Covington, KY 41017
EZ-CHECK, Colorimeter used for water analysis with patent pending. Curve fit and technology.

Coral Biotechnology 760-727-8224
110 Bosstick Blvd, San Marcos, CA 92069
Luminometer.

Dynex Technologies, Inc. 800-288-2354
14340 Sullyfield Cir, Chantilly, VA 20151
Microplate reader,luminometer.

Exocell, Inc. 800-234-3962
1880 John F Kennedy Blvd Ste 200, Philadelphia, PA 19103
Handheld device for measurement of analytes by calorimetry.

Hunter Associates Lab., Inc. 703-471-6870
11491 Sunset Hills Rd, Reston, VA 20190
These instruments measure the reflected or transmitted color of a wide range of pharmaceutical products. Use them to measure the reflected color of tablets, caplets, capsules and dip strips or to measure the color of clear liquid such as increasing yellowness with drug aging.

Hyperion, Inc. 305-238-3020
14100 SW 136th St, Miami, FL 33186
$965.00-$9,000.00.

Integrity Products, Inc. 816-965-0308
12910 7th St, Grandview, MO 64030
Valve insert replacement part for chemistry analyzer.

Koehler Instrument Co., Inc. 800-878-9070
1595 Sycamore Ave, Bohemia, NY 11716
Measures the following 16 color scales: US Pharmacopeia scale (USP 21); European Pharmacopoeia; Iodine Color; Hazen Color (APHA Color, Pt/Co Color); Gardner Color; Lovibond®; Klett Color; Hess-Ives Color; Yellowness Index; CIE-L, a*, b* Values; CIE-L*, a*, b* Difference; Hunter Lab Values; Chromaticity Coordinates; Tristimulus Values; Saybolt Color (ASTM D156, ISO 2049, NF M 07-003); and Mineral Oil Color (ASTM D1500, NF M 60-104).*

Lamotte Co. 800-344-3100
802 Washington Ave, PO Box 329, Chestertown, MD 21620
Portable, direct reading chlorine, fluorine, pH colorimeters for drinking, swimming pool and other water testing (fully portable). EPA accepted methods.

Lifescan, Inc. 800-227-8862
1000 Gibraltar Dr, Milpitas, CA 95035
Whole blood glucose meter (reflectance photometer).

Medtox Diagnostics, Inc. 800-334-1116
1640 Nova Ln, Burlington, NC 27215
Colorimeter.

COLORIMETER, GENERAL USE *(cont'd)*

Nutech Molding Corporation 1-800-423-5278
PO Box 840, 2024 Broad St,, Pocomoke City, MD 21851
These photometric colorimeters use specific light filters to give readings on a unique KlettTM scale. The readings are directly proportional to the concentration or optical density of a solution, in accordance with Beers Law. Two matched photocells and a suspension galvanometer give the instrument a broad range of measurement making it light and ambient temperature independent. A fully compensated and carefully balanced electrical circuit provides accuracy and consistency in readings while using simple and rugged equipment. The precision galvanometer has an illuminated logarithmic scale, graduated from 1 to 1000 KlettTM and the scale is graduated in units proportional to the optical density. Repeatability is ±.33% of the full scale. Two units are available. The Industrial Model accepts rectangular solution cells, which can be used in either of two directions. Measurements can then be taken at depths of 10mm, 20mm, or 40mm. A reduction plate is available to minimize solution depth to 2.5mm. An adapter is available which permits the use of test tubes. The Clinical Model uses standard 14.25 x 125mm test tubes. Calibrated or uncalibrated tubes are available. In addition, micro test tubes can be used for samples as small as 2.5 ml. Both models are supplied with the two most commonly used filters, blue for 400-450nm and green for 520-580nm. Additional filters are available to permit measurements over the complete visual range. Each unit has detailed instructions, standards and guides for a wide range of tests.

Orbeco Analytical Systems, Inc. 800-922-5242
185 Marine St, Farmingdale, NY 11735
$895.00, 7 filters calibrated for 94 water tests. Portable, direct-reading.

Ortho-Clinical Diagnostics, Inc. 800-828-6316
513 Technology Blvd, Rochester, NY 14626
Spectrophotometer.

Photo Research, Inc. 818-341-5151
9731 Topanga Canyon Pl, Chatsworth, CA 91311
SPECTRA COLORIMETER $10,500 per unit (standard). PR 650

Qiagen Gaithersburg, Inc. 800-344-3631
1201 Clopper Rd, Gaithersburg, MD 20878
Microplate luminometer; dcr-1 luminometer.

Qualigen, Inc. 760-918-9165
2042 Corte Del Nogal, Carlsbad, CA 92011
Photometer for clinical use.

Teco Diagnostics 714-693-7788
1268 N Lakeview Ave, Anaheim, CA 92807
Spectrophotometer-for clinical use.

Terumo Medical Corporation 800-283-7866
950 Elkton Blvd, P.O.Box 605, Elkton, MD 21921
Colorimeter/spectrophotometer.

Turner Biosystems, Inc. 408-636-2414
645 N Mary Ave, Sunnyvale, CA 94085
Luminometer.

COLORIMETRIC METHOD, CPK OR ISOENZYMES
(Chemistry) 75JHY

Abbott Diagnostics Intl, Biotechnology Ltd 787-846-3500
Road #2 KM. 58.0 , PO Box 278, Cruce Davila, Barceloneta, PR 00617
Assay for detection of creatine kinase.

Biosite Incorporated 888-246-7483
9975 Summers Ridge Rd, San Diego, CA 92121
Fluorescencei immunoassay for ck-mb, troponin i and myoglobin.

Dade Behring, Inc. 800-948-3233
1717 Deerfield Rd, Deerfield, IL 60015

Health Chem Diagnostics Llc 954-979-3845
3341 W McNab Rd, Pompano Beach, FL 33069
Colorimetric method, cpk or isoenzymes.

Myers-Stevens Group, Inc. 903-566-6696
2931 Vail Ave, Commerce, CA 90040
Eia test for the quantitation of cpk-mb.

COLORIMETRIC METHOD, GAMMA-GLUTAMYL TRANSPEPTIDASE *(Chemistry) 75JPZ*

Abbott Diagnostics Div. 626-440-0700
820 Mission St, South Pasadena, CA 91030
Various assays for detection of ggtp.

Beckman Coulter, Inc. 800-635-3497
740 W 83rd St, Hialeah, FL 33014
$0.18 per test.

COLORIMETRIC METHOD, GAMMA-GLUTAMYL TRANSPEPTIDASE *(cont'd)*

Dade Behring, Inc. 800-948-3233
1717 Deerfield Rd, Deerfield, IL 60015

Genzyme Corp. 800-325-2436
160 Christian St, Oxford, CT 06478
Carboxy Substrate, kinetic, IFCC, GPNA.

Intersect Systems, Inc. 360-577-1062
1152 3rd Avenue, Suite D & E, Longview, WA 98632
Colorimetric, gamma glutamyltransferase, Liquid Stable GGT.

Raichem, Division Of Hemagen Diagnostics, Inc. 800-438-6100
8225 Mercury Ct, San Diego, CA 92111
Gamma-GT reagent.

Sterling Diagnostics, Inc. 800-637-2661
36645 Metro Ct, Sterling Heights, MI 48312
L-gamma glutamylnitroanilide/glycylglycine.

COLORIMETRIC METHOD, LIPOPROTEINS *(Chemistry) 75JHM*

Hemagen Diagnostics, Inc. 800-436-2436
9033 Red Branch Rd, Columbia, MD 21045
Various high-density lipoprotein cholesterol methods.

Jas Diagnostics, Inc. 305-418-2320
7220 NW 58th St, Miami, FL 33166
Ldl cholesterol.

Sterling Diagnostics, Inc. 800-637-2661
36645 Metro Ct, Sterling Heights, MI 48312
High density lipoprotein (hdl) cholesterol.

Vital Diagnostics Inc. 714-672-3553
1075 W Lambert Rd Ste D, Brea, CA 92821
Hdl-cholesterol precipitating reagent.

COLORIMETRIC METHOD, TRIGLYCERIDES *(Chemistry) 75JGY*

Amresco Inc. 800-366-1313
30175 Solon Industrial Pkwy, Solon, OH 44139
Hitachi, RA technicon manual and automated systems.

Bayer Healthcare Llc 914-524-2955
555 White Plains Rd Fl 5, Tarrytown, NY 10591
Test for triglycerides in plasma or serum.

Beckman Coulter, Inc. 800-635-3497
740 W 83rd St, Hialeah, FL 33014
$0.17 per test.

Biomerieux Inc. 800-682-2666
100 Rodolphe St, Durham, NC 27712

Caldon Bioscience, Inc. 909-628-9944
2100 S Reservoir St, Pomona, CA 91766
Triglyceride reagent.

Caldon Biotech, Inc. 757-224-0177
2251 Rutherford Rd, Carlsbad, CA 92008
Triglyceride reagent.

Dade Behring, Inc. 800-948-3233
1717 Deerfield Rd, Deerfield, IL 60015

Diagnostic Specialties 732-549-4011
4 Leonard St, Metuchen, NJ 08840
$238.00 per 100-test kit.

Genzyme Corp. 800-325-2436
160 Christian St, Oxford, CT 06478
GPO, enzymatic, endpoint.

Harvey, R.J. Instrument Corp. 201-664-1380
123 Patterson St, Hillsdale, NJ 07642

Polymer Technology Systems, Inc. 317-870-5610
7736 Zionsville Rd, Indianapolis, IN 46268
Triglycirides test.

Raichem, Division Of Hemagen Diagnostics, Inc. 800-438-6100
8225 Mercury Ct, San Diego, CA 92111

COLORIMETRIC, OCCULT BLOOD IN URINE *(Hematology) 81JIO*

Arkray Factory Usa, Inc. 952-646-3168
5182 W 76th St, Minneapolis, MN 55439
Urine test strips.

Bayer Healthcare Llc 914-524-2955
555 White Plains Rd Fl 5, Tarrytown, NY 10591
Test for ph, protein, glucose, ketone, bilirubin & blood in urine.

Bayer Healthcare, Llc 574-256-3430
430 S Beiger St, Mishawaka, IN 46544
Test for ph, protein, glucose, ketone, bilirubin & blood in urine.

COLORIMETRIC, XYLOSE *(Chemistry) 75JOC*

Genova Diagnostics 828-253-0621
63 Zillicoa St, Asheville, NC 28801
Intestinal permeability test system.

Nerl Diagnostics Llc. 401-824-2046
14 Almeida Ave, East Providence, RI 02914
D-xylose.

COLORIMETRY, ACETAMINOPHEN *(Toxicology) 91LDP*

Biosite Incorporated 888-246-7483
9975 Summers Ridge Rd, San Diego, CA 92121
Fluorescence immunoassay for detection of drugs of abuse in urine.

Carolina Liquid Chemistries Corp. 800-471-7272
510 W Central Ave Ste C, Brea, CA 92821
Acetaminophen reagent.

Genzyme Corp. 800-325-2436
160 Christian St, Oxford, CT 06478
Enzymatic rate. Enzymatic endpoint.

Stanbio Laboratory, Inc. 830-249-0772
1261 N Main St, Boerne, TX 78006
ACETAZYME $121.00 for 40 acetazyme test kits containing lypohilized enzyme reagent, enzyme diluent, color reagent 1 and 2, acetaminophen standard 1 (1.0 mmol/l) and 2 (2.0 mmol/l).

COLORIMETRY, CHOLINESTERASE *(Toxicology) 91DIH*

Eqm Research, Inc. 513-661-0560
3638 Glenmore Ave, Cheviot, OH 45211
Cholinesterase test system.

Teco Diagnostics 714-693-7788
1268 N Lakeview Ave, Anaheim, CA 92807
Cholinesterase.

COLORIMETRY, CRESOL RED, CARBON-DIOXIDE *(Chemistry) 75CIL*

Health Chem Diagnostics Llc 954-979-3845
3341 W McNab Rd, Pompano Beach, FL 33069
Cresol red colorimetry, carbon-dioxide.

COLORIMETRY, SALICYLATE *(Toxicology) 91DKJ*

Genzyme Corp. 800-325-2436
160 Christian St, Oxford, CT 06478
Enzymatic, endpoint.

Sterling Diagnostics, Inc. 800-637-2661
36645 Metro Ct, Sterling Heights, MI 48312
Salicylate reagent set.

COLOSTOMY APPLIANCE, DISPOSABLE *(Gastro/Urology) 78EZS*

Coloplast Manufacturing Us, Llc 800-533-0464
1840 W Oak Pkwy, Marietta, GA 30062
COLOPLAST, ASSURA one-or two- piece pouches and flanges; transparent or opaque; open or closed.

Cook Urological, Inc. 800-457-4500
1100 W Morgan St, P.O. Box 227, Spencer, IN 47460

Marlen Manufacturing & Development Co. 216-292-7060
5150 Richmond Rd, Bedford, OH 44146
Ileostomy, urostomy and colostomy appliances. ULTRA one-piece colostomy (disposable with adhesive skin barrier).

Smith & Nephew, Inc. 800-876-1261
11775 Starkey Rd, Largo, FL 33773
Fecal incontinence collection bag; also, BANISH II liquid ostomy appliance deodorant and ODO-WAY ostomy appliance deodorant in pill form.

Torbot Group, Inc. 800-545-4254
1367 Elmwood Ave, Cranston, RI 02910

3m Co. 888-364-3577
3M Center, Saint Paul, MN 55144
3M STOMASEAL ADHESIVE DIS

3m Company 651-733-4365
601 22nd Ave S, Brookings, SD 57006

COLPOSCOPE *(Obstetrics/Gyn) 85HEX*

Air Techniques, Inc. 800-247-8324
1295 Walt Whitman Rd, Melville, NY 11747
Medscope

Carl Zeiss Surgical, Inc. 800-442-4020
1 Zeiss Dr, Thornwood, NY 10594

Codman & Shurtleff, Inc 800-225-0460
325 Paramount Dr, Raynham, MA 02767

COLPOSCOPE *(cont'd)*

Coopersurgical, Inc. 800-243-2974
95 Corporate Dr, Trumbull, CT 06611
114 models, priced from $2,745 to $19,395. With or without lasers.

Elmed, Inc. 630-543-2792
60 W Fay Ave, Addison, IL 60101

Gyrus Acmi, Inc. 508-804-2739
93 N Pleasant St, Norwalk, OH 44857
Colposcope (and colpomicroscope).

Hill-Med, Inc. 305-594-7474
7217 NW 46th St, Miami, FL 33166
Additional products: microscope, Halter, cryosurgery, stress test.

Intermed Group, Inc. 561-586-3667
3550 23rd Ave S Ste 1, Lake Worth, FL 33461
Colposcope; video colposcope; video zoom colposcope.

Jedmed Instruments Co. 314-845-3770
5416 Jedmed Ct, Saint Louis, MO 63129

Leica Microsystems (Canada) Inc. 800-205-3422
400 - 111 Granton Drive, Richmond Hill, ONT L4B 1L5 Canada

Mahe International Inc. 800-294-7946
468 Craighead St, Nashville, TN 37204

Md International, Inc. 305-669-9003
11300 NW 41st St, Doral, FL 33178

Medgyn Products, Inc. 800-451-9667
328 Eisenhower Ln N, Lombard, IL 60148
Binocular colposcope model AL-102 with interchangeable eyepieces (10, 13.5 & 18x magnification) and built-in green filter to view blood vessels in detail. Colposcope AL-104. 5 step magnification with fiber-optic light source and Nikon optics beam splitter for documentation.

R Medical Supply 800-882-7578
620 Valley Forge Rd Ste F, Hillsborough, NC 27278
5 separate models, each with numerous options.

Richard Wolf Medical Instruments Corp. 800-323-9653
353 Corporate Woods Pkwy, Vernon Hills, IL 60061

Seiler Precision Microscopes, Div. Of Seiler Instrument Co. 800-489-2282
170 E Kirkham Ave, Saint Louis, MO 63119
900 SERIES COLPOSCOPES - Model 935, 955 and 965Z colposcopes with dual-port power supply, video and digital video accessories.

Superior Medical Limited 800-268-7944
520 Champagne Dr., Toronto, ONT M3J 2T9 Canada

Techman Int'L Corp. 508-248-2900
242 Sturbridge Rd, Charlton, MA 01507
Colposcope (and colpomicroscope).

Wallach Surgical Devices, Inc. 800-243-2463
235 Edison Rd, Orange, CT 06477
$5615.00 for ZOOMSCOPE colposcope 4-20x; $5015.00 for ZOOMSTAR center post-scope.$4720 is for Tristar Triple Magnification Colopscope $7870.00 is for Tristar with Video Camera.

Western Scientific Co., Inc. 877-489-3726
4104 24th St # 183, San Francisco, CA 94114

COLUMN, ADSORPTION, LIPID *(Cardiovascular) 74WTP*

Croll Reynolds Company, Inc. 908-232-4200
751 Central Ave, PO Box 668, Westfield, NJ 07090
Carbon adsorption equipment. Regenerative and non-regenerative activated-carbon adsorption equipment and systems for highly efficient removal of volatile organic compounds and odors.

Kaneka Pharma America Llc 800-526-3522
546 5th Ave Fl 21, New York, NY 10036
LIPOSORBER LA-15 System utilizes two columns containing dextran sulfate cellulose as an adsorbent which removes selectively apolipoprotein-B containing particles (LDL, VLDL, Lp(a)) from plasma.

COLUMN, ADSORPTION, LIPOPROTEIN, LOW DENSITY *(General) 80LXW*

Kaneka Pharma America Llc 800-526-3522
546 5th Ave Fl 21, New York, NY 10036
LIPOSORBER LA-15 System utilizes two columns containing dextran sulfate cellulose as an adsorbent which removes selectively apolipoprotein-B containing particles (LDL, VLDL, Lp(a)) from plasma.

COLUMN, CHROMATOGRAPHY *(Chemistry) 75QJX*

Bdh, Inc. 800-268-0310
350 Evans Ave., Toronto, ONT M8Z 1K5 Canada
Reagents & Stains.

Beckman Coulter, Inc. 800-742-2345
250 S Kraemer Blvd, PO Box 8000, Brea, CA 92821

Berghof/America 800-544-5004
3773 NW 126th Ave Bldg 1, Coral Springs, FL 33065
Pure PTFE chromatography columns with PTFE tube with push-in PTFE stopcock and with PTFE perforated support disk.

Bio-Rad Laboratories, Life Science Group 800-424-6723
2000 Alfred Nobel Dr, Hercules, CA 94547

Biochemical Diagnostics, Inc. 800-223-4835
180 Heartland Blvd, Edgewood, NY 11717
Extraction columns for GC/MS sample preparation.

Chiral Technologies, Inc. 800-6-Chiral
800 N 5 Points Rd, West Chester, PA 19380
DAICEL.

Eprogen, Inc. 800-556-4272
8205 S Cass Ave Ste 106, Darien, IL 60561
Porous and non-porous HPLC columns for reversed phase, ion exange, size exclusion, and hydrophobic interaction chromatography.

Hamilton Company 800-648-5950
4990 Energy Way, Reno, NV 89502

Kontes Glass Co. 888-546-2531
1022 Spruce St, Vineland, NJ 08360

PerkinElmer 800-762-4000
940 Winter St, Waltham, MA 02451
Empty and prefilled columns.

Polymer Laboratories, Now A Part Of Varian, Inc. 800-767-3963
160 Old Farm Rd, Amherst Fields Research Park, Amherst, MA 01002
PLgel, PLgel 20UM MIXED-A, PLgel 10UM MIXED-B, PLgel 5UM MIXED-C, PLgel 5UM MIXED-D, PLgel 3UM MIXED-E, PLgel 50A TO 10A, PLgel MiniMIX, PLgel Olexis, PL aquagel-OH, PlusPore, PL Rapide, PolarGel-M, PolarGel-L, PL Polymer Calibrants, PL Polymer Standards, EasiCal, EasiVial. High performance and fully characterized calibrants for GPC/SEC. PL Hi-Plex resin-based for the analysis of carbohydrates, saccharides, alcohols and organic acids.

United Chemical Technologies, Inc. 800-385-3153
2731 Bartram Rd, Bristol, PA 19007
CLEAN SCREEN bonded-phase extraction columns or solid-phase extraction columns for forensic and clinical application in sample preparation. CLEAN-UP bonded phase or solid-phase extraction columns for use by analytical chemists and pharmaceutical analysts in sample preparation.

Varian Sample Preparation Products 800-421-2825
24201 Frampton Ave, Harbor City, CA 90710
Extraction columns (solid phase extraction), sample preparation.

Waters Corp. 800-252-4752
34 Maple St, Milford, MA 01757
Gel and liquid chromatography columns and accessories.

Whatman Inc. 732-885-6529
800 Centennial Ave Bldg 1, Piscataway, NJ 08854
HPLC column.

COLUMN, CHROMATOGRAPHY, HYDROXYPROLINE *(Chemistry) 75JMM*

Quidel Corp. 858-552-1100
2981 Copper Rd, Santa Clara, CA 95051
Enzyme immunoassay for deoxypyridinium.

Rockland Immunochemicals, Inc. 800-656-ROCK
PO Box 326, Gilbertsville, PA 19525
Affinity column.

COLUMN, ION EXCHANGE WITH COLORIMETRY, DELTA-AMINOLEVULINIC *(Chemistry) 75JKL*

Bio-Rad Laboratories Inc., Clinical Systems Div. 800-224-6723
4000 Alfred Nobel Dr, Hercules, CA 94547
Ala test method.

Image Molding, Inc. 800-525-1875
4525 Kingston St, Denver, CO 80239
Columns only.

COLUMN, LIFE SUPPORT (ELECTRICAL/GAS) *(General) 80UMS*

Aga Linde Healthcare P.R. Inc. 787-622-7900
PO Box 363868, GPO Box 364727, San Juan, PR 00936
General.

COLUMN, LIFE SUPPORT (ELECTRICAL/GAS) *(cont'd)*

Allied Healthcare Products, Inc. 800-444-3954
1720 Sublette Ave, Saint Louis, MO 63110

Berchtold Corp. 800-243-5135
1950 Hanahan Rd, Charleston, SC 29406
TELETOM suspended medical gas delivery system.

Independent Solutions, Inc. 847-498-0500
900 Skokie Blvd Ste 118, Northbrook, IL 60062
Class 1, free-standing or ceiling suspended, plastic laminate or stainless steel. U.L. listed. Fired, manually retractable or pneumatically retractable.

COLUMN, LIQUID CHROMATOGRAPHY *(Toxicology) 91DPM*

Alltech Associates, Inc. 847-282-2090
17434 Mojave St, Hesperia, CA 92345

Beckman Coulter, Inc. 800-742-2345
250 S Kraemer Blvd, PO Box 8000, Brea, CA 92821

Chromatography Sciences Co. (Csc) 800-668-4752
5750 Vanden Abeele, St-Laurent, QUE H4S 1R9 Canada
CSC-SIL. CSC-VITESSE - 5 c.m. column for test HPLC. $195.

Dionex Corp. 408-737-0700
1228 Titan Way, P.O. Box 3603, Sunnyvale, CA 94085

Harvard Apparatus, Inc. 800-272-2775
84 October Hill Rd, Holliston, MA 01746

Jordi Associates, Flp 508-966-1301
4 Mill St, Bellingham, MA 02019
Also available, Jordi Hydroxylated DVB columns. Analytical and preparative. Reverse phase and normal phase columns. Bulk packing material. Jordi 'J-Clean' SPE Cartridges - analytical and prep cleanup, extract phenols & acidic pesticides. Also for nucleic acid preparations & polar drug metal. Jordi Bullet Columns - RP & NP Bullet, Sulfonated Polar Pac SCX Bullet, PolarPac Way Aqueous Bullet, C18 Bullet, Glucose Bullet, RP Hydroxylated Bullet.

Melcor Technologies, Inc. 408-247-0350
1030 E El Camino Real # 435, Sunnyvale, CA 94087
BIOSPHER polymer methacrylate HPLC sorbents and packed columns. Silica HPLC sorbents and packed columns.

Polylc Inc. 410-992-5400
9151 Rumsey Rd Ste 180, Columbia, MD 21045

Polymer Laboratories, Now A Part Of Varian, Inc. 800-767-3963
160 Old Farm Rd, Amherst Fields Research Park, Amherst, MA 01002

Thermo Fisher Scientific 800-437-2999
PO Box 712099, Cincinnati, OH 45271

Trans-Genomic 888-233-9283
12325 Emmet St, Omaha, NE 68164

Varian, Inc. 800-926-3000
3120 Hansen Way, Palo Alto, CA 94304

Waters Corp. 800-252-4752
34 Maple St, Milford, MA 01757

COMMODE (TOILET) *(General) 80QLV*

Access Mobility, Inc. 800-336-1147
5240 Elmwood Ave, Indianapolis, IN 46203

Activeaid, Inc. 800-533-5330
101 Activeaid Rd, Redwood Falls, MN 56283
Jon-A-Chair pediatric commode bath chair.

Basic American Medical Products 800-849-6664
2935A Northeast Pkwy, Atlanta, GA 30360

Bio-Medic Health Services, Inc. 800-525-0072
5041B Benois Rd Bldg B, Roanoke, VA 24018

Clarke Health Care Products, Inc. 888-347-4537
1003 International Dr, Oakdale, PA 15071
Toilevator raised toilet platform.raises entire toilet from floor 3 inches, includes all hardware and pipe extensions.

Colonial Scientific Ltd. 902-468-1811
201 Brownlow Ave., Unit 52, Dartmouth, NS B3B-1W2 Canada

Columbia Medical Manufacturing Llc 800-454-6612
13577 Larwin Cir, Santa Fe Springs, CA 90670
Columbia Medical Positioning Commodes can be used freestanding or fit over any toilet. The orthopedic-contoured backs include support belts and harness for extra support. Lo and Hi-Back options are available.

Convaquip Industries, Inc. 800-637-8436
4834 Derrick Dr, PO Box 3417, Abilene, TX 79601
Bariatric Bedside Commodes. Weight certified to 850 lb.to 1500 lbs., depending on item.

COMMODE (TOILET) *(cont'd)*

Duralife, Inc. 800-443-5433
195 Phillips Park Dr, Williamsport, PA 17702
3 in 1 commode.

Gendron, Inc. 800-537-2521
400 E Lugbill Rd, Archbold, OH 43502
$467.00 for obese commode with 700lb. capacity.

Invacare Canada 800-668-5324
5970 Chedworth Way, Mississauga, ONT L5R 3T9 Canada

Invacare Corporation 800-333-6900
1 Invacare Way, Elyria, OH 44035
INVACARE All-In-One Aluminum Commode, All-In-One Steel Commode, Bariatric Commode, Heavy-Duty Commode, Drop-Arm Commode.

Larkotex Company 800-972-3037
1002 Olive St, Texarkana, TX 75501

Rest Assured Inc. 800-852-7378
4006 S 21st St, PO Box 163, Phoenix, AZ 85040
Commode Comfort Support System, bathroom aid that assures complete privacy for its user without sacrificing safety and security.

Rifton Equipment 800-571-8198
PO Box 260, Rifton, NY 12471
Commode for handicapped, multiple accessories - for use with toilet or pan, 3 sizes, fully adjustable.

S & B Robertson Research And Developments, Inc. 7057995537
R.R. #1, The Glen, Omemee, ONT K0L-2W0 Canada
VALETTE water-powered elevating toilet seat. Raises the standard height toilet seat to the user's standing level and lowers the user to the level of the bowl. With a reverse motion, the unit returns the user to a standing position.

Sunrise Medical 800-333-4000
7477 Dry Creek Pkwy, Longmont, CO 80503

TFI Healthcare 800-526-0178
600 W Wythe St, Petersburg, VA 23803
Model #DME21/2 low back model; also, Model #DME23/2 2 in I commode/bath bench, maximum weight 450 lbs.; extra wide model 3240/1 holds maximum weight 700 lbs.

Tuffcare 800-367-6160
3999 E La Palma Ave, Anaheim, CA 92807

Wheelchairs Of Kansas 800-537-6454
204 W 2nd St, Ellis, KS 67637
SHOWER COMMODE CHAIR is designed to be used as a 3-in-1 unit, as a bedside commode, over the toilet or in the shower; Constructed of heav-duty stainless steel, the rigid frame is designed for bariatric individuals; Detachable & swingaway armrest; Anti-bacterial, fluid resistant & detachable back; Swingaway footrests; Locking front casters; 600 lb. weight capacity. BARI-COMMODE is a bedside commode designed for bariatric individuals; The heavy-duty stainless steel construction has a rigid frame; Fixed or height adjustable legs with non-marring rubber caps; Water resistant, anti-bacterial padded seat; Detachable back bar; 600 lb. & 1000 lb. weight capacity.

Whitehall Manufacturing 800-782-7706
15125 Proctor Ave, City Of Industry, CA 91746
Concealed toilet units with cabinet swing-out/lightweight hinged toilet cover/hinged toilet cabinet, floor mount or fixed position divided up into Singette, Swivette, Stylette, Modulette, or Versalette Series; 1.6 gpf (gallons per flush).

COMMODE SEAT *(General) 80QLU*

A.R.C. Distributors 800-296-8724
PO Box 599, Centreville, MD 21617
INVACARE All In One, Stationary, Safeguard and Extra Wide commodes with a wide variety of features providing comfort, stability and easy adjustability. All In One Commode can be used as a toilet safety frame, a raised toilet seat, or as a stationary commode. Stationary Commode is designed for bedside use. Safeguard Commode is designed for use as a raised toilet seat or a toilet safety frame. Extra Wide Commode is designed for bedside use. Its extra large seat makes it more comfortable. Its weight limit is 450 lbs. Wheelchairs of Kansas Commode Chair -drop arm & removable back, 600lb & 1000lb. capacities.

Alimed, Inc. 800-225-2610
297 High St, Dedham, MA 02026

American Bantex Corp. 800-633-4839
1815 Rollins Rd, Burlingame, CA 94010

Home Aid Products 888-823-7605
111 Esna Park Dr., Unit 9, Markham, ONT L3R-1H2 Canada
Bariatric wheeled transport shower chair and commode. Adjustable-height pediatric commode.

COMMODE SEAT *(cont'd)*

Invacare Corporation 800-333-6900
1 Invacare Way, Elyria, OH 44035
INVACARE.

Maddak Inc. 800-443-4926
661 State Route 23, Wayne, NJ 07470
TALL-ETTE/LOCK-IN-EL elevated toilet seats.

Medegen Medical Products, Llc 800-233-1987
209 Medegen Drive, Gallaway, TN 38036-0228
ROOM-MATES.

Rifton Equipment 800-571-8198
PO Box 260, Rifton, NY 12471
Potty chair, multiple accessories - for use with toilet or pan, 3 sizes, fully adjustable.

Sani-Med, A Division Of Sanderson Plumbing Products, Inc. 800-647-1042
PO Box 1367, Columbus, MS 39703
Usage for home health care, institutional, residential and commercial.

Sanitor Manufacturing Co. 800-379-5314
1221 W Centre Ave, Portage, MI 49024
NEAT SEAT Disposable toilet seat covers & dispensers.

Sunrise Medical 800-333-4000
7477 Dry Creek Pkwy, Longmont, CO 80503

TFI Healthcare 800-526-0178
600 W Wythe St, Petersburg, VA 23803
Raised toilet seat and safety frame commode, Model #DME 22/2 3 in 1 in. commode with removable back; also Model #5411/1 in. adjustable 5 bracket universal blow molded raised toilet seat.

Toto Kiki Usa, Inc. 888-295-8134
1155 Southern Rd, Morrow, GA 30260
ZOE, computerized wash/dry toilet seat. CHLOE, computerized bidet toilet seat. PORTABLE WASH LE, handheld portable bidet device.

Tuffcare 800-367-6160
3999 E La Palma Ave, Anaheim, CA 92807

COMMUNICATION EQUIPMENT *(General) 80VBO*

Aiphone Corporation 425-455-0510
1700 130th Ave NE, Bellevue, WA 98005
Intercom systems. Color Video Sentry provides security and the convenience of being able to both hear and see in color who's at the door before answering it.

Assistive Technology, Inc. 800-793-9227
333 Elm St Ste 115, Dedham, MA 02026
Mercury Windows XP-Based Augmentative and Alternative Communication Device. Mercury SE dedicated, speech-generating device.

Callconnect Communications, Inc. 800-733-2255
5720 Flatiron Pkwy, Washington, DC 20301
Hospital telecommunicaion system. Also, hospital answering telephone.

Crest Healthcare Supply 800-328-8908
195 3rd St, Dassel, MN 55325
Doctors' in-out register system. Pillow speakers.

David Clark Company, Inc. 800-900-3434
360 Franklin St, Worcester, MA 01604
intercoms for emergency vehicles

Dukane Communication Systems 519-748-5352
461 Manitou Dr., Kitchener, ON N2C 1L5 Canada
3200; MCS350; STARCall Plus; ProCare.

Dynavox Systems Inc. 866-396-2869
2100 Wharton St Ste 400, Pittsburgh, PA 15203
DYNA VOX 3100, augmentatine communication device with a dynamic touch screen, 'concept-tagged' searchable vocabulary, word prediction MD on board environmental control unit. DYNA MITE 3100, small, lightweight augmentative communication device with a dynamic touch screen, 'concept-tagged' searchable vocabulary, word prediction MD on board environmental control unit.

Ericsson, Inc. 434-528-7000
100 Mountain View Dr, Lynchburg, VA 24502
Mobile radios, hand-held radios; talk-back paging system, trunked radio systems for 800 and 900 MHz frequencies, and coded transmission guarded systems.

Ge Medical Systems Information Technologies 800-643-6439
8200 W Tower Ave, Milwaukee, WI 53223
IMPACT.wf system is the first automatic alarm-notification system that displays an ECG waveform on a wireless receiver, allowing caregivers to make informed decisions without checking a monitor.

COMMUNICATION EQUIPMENT *(cont'd)*

Jeron Electronic Systems, Inc. 800-621-1903
1743 W Rosehill Dr # 55, Chicago, IL 60660
Provider® nurse call system requires no IP address or PC to operate. It fully integrates with common mobile communication tools and can be configured on site. Provider is the only true Cat-5 wired system, offering 5 distinct, user-friendly master consoles and a 5-year warranty.

July Soft 800-350-7693
610 E Knox Dr, Tucson, AZ 85705
REMINDERPRO Appointment Confirmation System calls patients to remind them of appointments or needed services, in the voice of a familiar staff member. LABRETRIEVER Provides a 24-hour lab test results patient hotline for confidential routine lab test results.

Micronova Technology, Inc. 615-662-1304
914 Harpeth Valley Pl, Nashville, TN 37221

Ofs, Specialty Photonics Division 888-438-9936
55 Darling Dr, Avon, CT 06001
HCS, ULTRASIL, ALL SILICA Low or High OH, With or Without PYROCOAT - Complete line of USP Class VI, non-toxic, biocompatible, and sterilizable fibers for uses in laser power delivery and medical sensors, fiber, cable, and assemblies. Also available for factory automation data links, industrial sensors, radiation analysis, laser welding and cutting, illumination, etc.

Optelecom-Nkf, Inc 800-293-4237
12920 Cloverleaf Center Dr, Germantown, MD 20874
Fiber-optic communication systems (video, audio, and data transmitters and receivers).

Passy-Muir Inc. 800-634-5397
4521 Campus Dr, Irvine, CA 92612
Passy-Muir™ closed-position 'no leak' Tracheostomy & Ventilator Swallowing and Speaking valves (PMVs.) The only swallowing & speaking valves that are interchangeable for use on or off the ventilator (with the exception of the PMV™ 2020 for metal trach tubes.) Independent research has shown that the closed position PMV improves swallowing, reduces aspiration, facilitates secretion management, and reduces weaning and decannulation time. Reimbursable by Medicare, Medicaid, MediCal, and CCS.

Prentke Romich Company 800-262-1984
1022 Heyl Rd, Wooster, OH 44691
Pathfinder Plus speech synthesis and digitalized speech; alternative keyboard to most computers. Direct or indirect keyboard selection technique available. Combination static keyboard and touch screen; portable. SpringBoard Plus digitized speech, versatile and easy to implement; portable. Vantage Plus speech synthesis and digitalized speech via touch screen. Direct or indirect keyboard selection technique available. Portable. Vanguard Plus speech synthesis and digitalized speech via touch screen. Direct or indirect keyboard selection technique available. Portable.

Rauland-Borg Corp. 800-752-7725
3450 Oakton St, Skokie, IL 60076
Hands free duplex intercoms, flush or desk mounted.

Rf Technologies 800-669-9946
3125 N 126th St, Brookfield, WI 53005
Voice alarm annunciator.

Spectralink Corporation 800-676-5465
5755 Central Ave, Boulder, CO 80301
SpectraLink's Link Wireless Telephone Systems provide healthcare staff with lightweight wireless handsets that make and receive telephone calls anywhere in the facility with no service charges or usage fees. In addition, these handsets seamlessly integrate with many third-party messaging applications such as nurse call systems and other patient monitoriing systems.

Sunrise Medical 800-333-4000
7477 Dry Creek Pkwy, Longmont, CO 80503

Talk-A-Phone Co. 773-539-1100
5013 N Kedzie Ave, Chicago, IL 60625
Intercom systems.

Tash International Inc. 800-463-5685
91 Station St., Unit 1, Ajax, ONT L1S 3H2 Canada
Communication aids.

Trademark Medical Llc 800-325-9044
449 Soverign Ct, St. Louis, MO 63011
SILENT SPEAKER - communication system for patients unable to speak.

COMMUNICATION EQUIPMENT *(cont'd)*

Ultrascope 800-677-2673
2401 Distribution St, Charlotte, NC 28203
SPEAKER BOARD: $10.00 each, simplifies communication for non-English speaking or those who can't speak; flexible 8 x 11 in. board with pen where appropriate word/words can be circled or underlined in English and foreign language interpretation is given. Models for English, English/Spanish and English/International, where any language may be added.

Ultratec, Inc. 800-482-2424
450 Science Dr, Madison, WI 53711
Compact/C portable TYY with full-size keyboard, two-line LCD display, 32k memory, long-lasting batteries, digital cell phone compatible, and acoustic use. MINICOM IV TTY, SUPERCOM 4400 TTY non-printers. Also, PayPhone TTY and PayPhone ITY ST, designed for use with a public telephone.

Visicomm Industries 866-221-3131
911A Milwaukee Ave, Burlington, WI 53105
Personnel and message waiting call systems, signalling system; each with three LEDs (green, red, amber); one cable, low voltage, site-to-site, any number per site.

COMMUNICATION SYSTEM, EMERGENCY ALERT, PERSONAL

(General) 80VFG

Actall Corp. 800-598-1745
3925 Monaco Pkwy Unit D, Denver, CO 80207
Crisis controllers. Computer security. PALS 9000 Personal Alert Locating System is an indoor-outdoor tracking location integration system. Also PALS 9000 L2L, personal alarm 'location to location' - indoor - outdoor wireless tracking fully supervised system.

Aiphone Corporation 425-455-0510
1700 130th Ave NE, Bellevue, WA 98005

Alpha Communications 800-666-4800
42 Central Dr, Farmingdale, NY 11735
AlphaSure™ PC based emergency call/ door monitor/ check-in/ facility management systems. AlphaSure™ can be customized to fit all notification needs. AlphaSure™ monitors and reports on patients, residents, doors, elevators, plant systems.

American Medical Alert Corp. 800-286-2622
3265 Lawson Blvd, Oceanside, NY 11572
VOICECARE for two-way communication with EMTs; Model 800, tabletop personal emergency response system; Model 1000, flush-mounted personal emergency response system.

Crest Healthcare Supply 800-328-8908
195 3rd St, Dassel, MN 55325

Edwards Signaling & Security Systems 800-336-4206
41 Woodford Ave, Plainville, CT 06062
Call for assistance signaling products. Phone page. Strobe.

Heritage Medcall 800-396-6157
202 E Virginia Ave, Tampa, FL 33603
Visual Nurse Call system, Wired and Wireless Emergency Call systems, Office flow and Patient Tracking system

Pioneer Medical Systems 800-234-0683
3408 Howell St Ste D, Duluth, GA 30096
Alzheimer's wandering persons system. Personal emergency response system.

Rf Technologies 800-669-9946
3125 N 126th St, Brookfield, WI 53005
Code Alert, Quick Response emergency response system.

Ring Communications, Inc. 516-585-7464
57 Trade Zone Dr, Ronkonkoma, NY 11779
Internal Communications System with Annuciation for OR's, ER's, and general administration. Small-department-size systems, or for the entire facility. Feature rich. Can be used in elevator, parking garages, and stairwells; ADA compliant.

Senior Technologies 800-824-2996
PO Box 80238, 1620 N 20th Circle, Lincoln, NE 68501
ARIAL Wireless Communication System.

Tel-Tron Technologies Corporation 904-255-1921
220 Fentress Blvd, Daytona Beach, FL 32114
Smoke warning.

Ultratec, Inc. 800-482-2424
450 Science Dr, Madison, WI 53711

COMMUNICATION SYSTEM, NON-POWERED

(Physical Med) 89ILP

Champion America 800-521-7000
PO Box 3092, Branford, CT 06405
Braille/Tactile directional signs.

COMMUNICATION SYSTEM, NON-POWERED *(cont'd)*

Civco Medical Instruments Co., Inc. 319-656-4447
102 1st St S, Kalona, IA 52247
Various types of foot switch holders.

Insiphil (Us) Llc 408-616-8700
650 Vaqueros Ave Ste F, Sunnyvale, CA 94085

Vidatak, Llc 734-477-6942
9080 Santa Monica Blvd Ste 103, Los Angeles, CA 90069
Dry-erase communication board,device,aid/augmentative.

COMMUNICATION SYSTEM, POWERED *(Physical Med) 89ILQ*

Aionex, Inc. 615-851-4477
104 Space Park N, Goodlettsville, TN 37072

Assisted Access-Nfss, Inc. 800-950-9655
822 Preston Ct, Lake Villa, IL 60046
Various equipment and devices for the hearing impaired.

Boost Technology, Llc 415-334-8246
1601 Ocean Ave, San Francisco, CA 94112
Accessory to speech generating device.

Control Bionics 202-257-7090
333 N Broad St, Fairborn, OH 45324

Curbell Electronics Inc. 716-667-3377
20 Centre Dr, Orchard Park, NY 14127
Pillow speakers, call cords, adaptors, and jumpers.

Gn Resound Corporation 800-582-4327
Seaport Center, 220 Saginaw Drive, Redwood City, CA 94063-4725

Hill-Rom Manufacturing, Inc. 800-445-3730
1225 Crescent Green Dr., Suite 200, Cary, NC 27511
Nurse communication system.

Honeywell Hommed, Llc 888-353-5440
3400 Intertech Dr Ste 200, Brookfield, WI 53045
Home vital signs monitor.

Insiphil (Us) Llc 408-616-8700
650 Vaqueros Ave Ste F, Sunnyvale, CA 94085

Lingraphicare America, Inc. 888-274-2742
15 Spring St Fl 2, Princeton, NJ 08542
Speech-generating device (sometines called AAC or Augmentative Communication Device).

Logovox Systems, Inc. 925-253-8303
128 Diablo View Dr, Orinda, CA 94563
Logovox, logobox.

Neural Signals,Inc. 770-220-9964
3688 Clearview Ave Ste 110, Atlanta, GA 30340
Speech generating device.

Scotty Technology Of The Americas, Inc. 910-395-6100
6714 Netherlands Dr, Wilmington, NC 28405
Telehome care system with electronic stethoscope.

Stat-Chek Company 800-248-6618
PO Box 9636, Bend, OR 97708
Between doctors and nurses.

Varitronics, Inc. 800-345-1244
620 Park Way, Broomall, PA 19008
Doctor nurse call systems. Non-verbal interoffice communication systems.

COMMUNICATION SYSTEM, ROOM STATUS *(General) 80THE*

Alpha Communications 800-666-4800
42 Central Dr, Farmingdale, NY 11735
AlphaStatus - Customizable Room Status systems for Doctor's Offices, Surgical Suites, Public facilities.

Callcare 800-345-9414
1370 Arcadia Rd, Lancaster, PA 17601
Complete or add-on audio and visual signaling used in haelathcare facilities.

Crest Healthcare Supply 800-328-8908
195 3rd St, Dassel, MN 55325
Visible/audible system with up to 10 indicators. Pillow speakers.

Kelkom Systems 800-985-3556
418 MacArthur Ave, Redwood City, CA 94063
Staff Vector light message communication system for combination doctor/nurse follower, room status, and emergency call.

Rf Technologies 800-669-9946
3125 N 126th St, Brookfield, WI 53005
Wanderer monitoring system prevents patients or residents from wandering into unsafe areas. For Alzheimer's and other forms of dementia.

COMPACTOR, FIXED *(General) 80TBJ*

Caddy Corporation 856-467-4222
509 Sharptown Road, Bridgeport, NJ 08014-0345

S&G Enterprises, Inc. 800-233-3721
N115W19000 Edison Dr, Germantown, WI 53022
RAM FLAT 8 models--compaction force 12,200 to 85,000 lb.; 5-to 55-gal. volume; weighing 550 to 3700 lb. Models are designed for compaction within 55 gallon drums, drum crushers to crush drums down to 4-6 inches, or dual-use machines that can perform both functions.

COMPLEMENT *(Immunology) 82KTQ*

Cedarlane Laboratories Ltd. 800-268-5058
5516 8th Line R.R. 2, Hornby, ONT L0P 1E0 Canada
Complement - standard rabbit complement HLA-ABC, Low-Tox H-HLA-DR. Low-Tox-M (mouse) and custom batches (+ guinea pig complements.) Lympholyte isolation of viable mouse, rat or rabbit and human lymphocytes. Anti-sera for tissue typing, positive control serum, anti-human, B-cell anti-serum.

Rockland Immunochemicals, Inc. 800-656-ROCK
PO Box 326, Gilbertsville, PA 19525

COMPLEXONE, CRESOLPHTHALEIN, CALCIUM *(Chemistry) 75CIC*

Beckman Coulter, Inc. 800-635-3497
740 W 83rd St, Hialeah, FL 33014
$0.06 per test.

Biomerieux Inc. 800-682-2666
100 Rodolphe St, Durham, NC 27712

Caldon Bioscience, Inc. 909-628-9944
2100 S Reservoir St, Pomona, CA 91766
Calcium.

Caldon Biotech, Inc. 757-224-0177
2251 Rutherford Rd, Carlsbad, CA 92008
Calcium.

Carolina Liquid Chemistries Corp. 800-471-7272
510 W Central Ave Ste C, Brea, CA 92821
Ca.

Diagnostic Specialties 732-549-4011
4 Leonard St, Metuchen, NJ 08840
$106.00 per 100g.

Genchem, Inc. 714-529-1616
510 W Central Ave Ste D, Brea, CA 92821
Calcium reagent.

Health Chem Diagnostics Llc 954-979-3845
3341 W McNab Rd, Pompano Beach, FL 33069
Cresolphthalein complexone, calcium.

Hemagen Diagnostics, Inc. 800-436-2436
9033 Red Branch Rd, Columbia, MD 21045
Various calcium methods.

Jas Diagnostics, Inc. 305-418-2320
7220 NW 58th St, Miami, FL 33166
Calcium (cpc).

Sandare Intl., Inc. 972-293-7440
910 Kck Way, Cedar Hill, TX 75104
Calcium cresolphthalein complexone.

Sterling Diagnostics, Inc. 800-637-2661
36645 Metro Ct, Sterling Heights, MI 48312
Calicum reagent set.

Teco Diagnostics 714-693-7788
1268 N Lakeview Ave, Anaheim, CA 92807
Calcium.

Vital Diagnostics Inc. 714-672-3553
1075 W Lambert Rd Ste D, Brea, CA 92821
Various total calcium reagents.

COMPONENT, CAST *(Orthopedics) 87LGF*

Ac Healthcare Supply, Inc. 905-448-4706
11651 230th St, Cambria Heights, NY 11411
Cast component.

Bionix Development Corp. 800-551-7096
5154 Enterprise Blvd, Toledo, OH 43612
Various vacuum bag and low melt plastic cast supports.

Debusk Orthopedic Casting (Doc) 865-362-2334
420 Straight Creek Rd Ste 1, New Tazewell, TN 37825
Various types of plasters.

COMPONENT, CAST *(cont'd)*

Dj Orthopedics De Mexico, S.A. De C.V. 690-727-1280
Blvd., Delagacion La Presa, Tijuana 22397 Mexico
Cast component

Dj Orthopedics De Mexico, S.A. De C.V. 690-727-1280
Ave. Venustiano Carranza 6802, Castillo, Tijuana 22100 Mexico
Cast component

Dm Systems, Inc. 800-254-5438
1316 Sherman Ave, Evanston, IL 60201
CASTWEDGE™ CAST ADJUSTER is utilized to hold open a uni-or bi-valved cast for control of swelling. It also enhances standard open wedging techniques. The CastWedge™ comes in five different sizes for greater flexibility in treatment (10mm, 15mm, 20mm, 25mm, 30mm). The CastWedge™ is notched in such a way as to keep it in place after the realignment is complete. Made of an impact resistant, radiolucent material, the CastWedge™ will not interfere with the X-rays of a casted fracture.

International Hospital Supply Co. 800-398-9450
6914 Canby Ave Ste 105, Reseda, CA 91335
Cast-removal instrument and supplies.

Just Packaging Inc. 908-753-6700
450 Oak Tree Ave, South Plainfield, NJ 07080
Various types cast components.

Medline Manufacturing And Services Llc 847-837-2759
1 Medline Pl, Mundelein, IL 60060
Under cast padding.

Ossur Americas 949-268-3155
742 Pancho Rd, Camarillo, CA 93012

Pedinol Pharmacal, Inc. 800-733-4665
30 Banfi Plz N, Farmingdale, NY 11735

Protectair Inc. 800-235-7932
59 Eisenhower Ln S, Lombard, IL 60148
Casting accessories.

Smith & Nephew, Mexico Inc. 901-396-2121
San Francisco Cuautlalpan #101, Naucalpan, Edo. De Mexico Mexico
Various

Sukol Scientific, Inc. 305-468-0085
8311 NW 68th St, Miami, FL 33166
Component cast.

W.L. Gore & Associates,Inc 928-526-3030
1505 North Fourth St., Flagstaff, AZ 86004
Cast liner.

COMPONENT, CERAMIC *(General) 80VFE*

Alceram Tech Inc 516-849-3666
57 2nd St, Ronkonkoma, NY 11779
Industrial ceramics, sapphire components, and bio-ceramics including stabilized Zinconia and aluminum oxide. Zinconia oxide - FDA Approved for implants.

Berghof/America 800-544-5004
3773 NW 126th Ave Bldg 1, Coral Springs, FL 33065
Chemware PTFE watch glasses. Can be used as a beaker cover.

Bolt Bethel, Llc 763-434-5900
23530 University Avenue Ext NW, PO Box 135, Bethel, MN 55005

Dynamics Research Corp. 800-522-4321
60 Frontage Rd, Andover, MA 01810

Morgan Advance Ceramics 800-433-0638
26 Madison Rd, Fairfield, NJ 07004

Tp Orthodontics, Inc. 800-348-8856
100 Center Plz, La Porte, IN 46350
Orthodontic bracket.

Vee Gee Scientific, Inc. 800-423-8842
13600 NE 126th Pl Ste A, Kirkland, WA 98034
Glassware.

COMPONENT, CERAMIC *(cont'd)*

Zimmer Dental, Inc. 800-854-7019
1900 Aston Ave, Carlsbad, CA 92008
PureForm ceramic components are designed for cemented restorations. They closely resemble the shapes and shade of natural teeth, providing esthetic outcomes for dental implant patients and less preparation time and cost for the dental laboratory. PureForm components are comprised of a new ceramic material a blend of Aluminum Oxide and Zirconia that is stronger than pure alumina products and easier to prepare than pure Zirconia products. Shading of the ceramic is done in the manufacturing process, resulting in consistent color close to that of natural teeth. PureForm components are sold as two separate pieces: metal core abutments that are specific to the internal hexagon with friction-fit and Spline® dental implant connections and diameters, and ceramic copings sized according to average tooth shapes. These nearly natural shapes reduce the time usually required of the dental laboratory technician to pare down the ceramic to a desired shape and size. The ceramic coping serves as the foundation for the porcelain applied by the laboratory to create the final restoration. No additional ceramic crown or wax-up is necessary. The dental laboratory can use the PureForm plastic try-in kit to determine the appropriate PureForm ceramic coping. PureForm copings are available in six configurations designed according to four basic tooth shapes. Each ceramic coping flares to 4.5mm and will fit any of the core abutments. Core abutments are offered in 0.5mm or 1.5mm cuff heights for optimal esthetics in areas of low gingival margins or thin tissue.

3m Unitek 800-634-5300
2724 Peck Rd, Monrovia, CA 91016
Ceramic bracket.

COMPONENT, ELECTRICAL *(General) 80WKG*

Adit/Electron Tubes 800-521-8382
100 Forge Way Ste F, Rockaway, NJ 07866
High-voltage power supplies. Also, photo multiplier tubes.

Altech Corporation 908-806-9400
35 Royal Rd, Flemington, NJ 08822
Electric wire terminals connector; foot-operated switch control.

Berchtold Corp. 800-243-5135
1950 Hanahan Rd, Charleston, SC 29406

Bhk, Inc. 909-983-2973
1480 N Claremont Blvd, Claremont, CA 91711
Standard and custom power supplies (A/C and D/C) for light-source applications.

Crest Healthcare Supply 800-328-8908
195 3rd St, Dassel, MN 55325
Bulbs and fuses.

Dan Kar Corporation 800-942-5542
PO Box 279, 192 New Boston St C, Wilmington, MA 01887
Low- and high-voltage power supplies.

Evolution Medical Products, Inc. 877-223-3999
74 Eastwood Dr, Deerfield, IL 60015
CORD CADDY medical cord storage and retrieval system for organizing and managing monitor leads, cables and high pressure hoses used with monitors, anesthesia machines and ventilators.

Industrial Specialities Manufacturing, Inc. 800-781-8487
2741 W Oxford Ave Unit 6, Englewood, CO 80110
FILTERTREK filtration line.

Kloehn Co., Ltd. 800-358-4342
10000 Banburry Cross Dr, Las Vegas, NV 89144
Syringe drive modules and intellect valve modules.

Linak U.S. Inc. 502-253-5595
2200 Stanley Gault Pkwy, Louisville, KY 40223
24 VDC electrical linear actuator systems for articulation of beds.

Marinco Specialty Wiring Devices 800-767-8541
2655 Napa Valley Corporate Dr, Napa, CA 94558
Available in 15 & 20 amp hospital grade electrical wiring devices using the exculsive PERMA-LOCK terminal & featuring the exclusive MAG-VU window for fast inspection. Also available, 15 amp 125 volt right angle hospital grade electrical wiring device using PERMA-LOCK terminals.

Merit Cables, Inc. 877-637-4848
830 N Poinsettia St, Santa Ana, CA 92701
Cable and leadwire products for medical monitoring systems.

Minnesota Wire & Cable Co. 800-258-6922
1835 Energy Park Dr, Saint Paul, MN 55108
Full project management for all electrical interconnection programs.

COMPONENT, ELECTRICAL *(cont'd)*

Motloid Company 800-662-5021
300 N Elizabeth St, Chicago, IL 60607
Electrical soldering equipment and supplies. Tin plater, electric.

R. B. Annis Instruments, Inc. 317-637-9282
1101 N Delaware St, Indianapolis, IN 46202
HELMHOLTZ COIL - magnetic field standards.

Reheat Co., Inc. 800-373-4328
10 School St, Danvers, MA 01923
Heaters, controllers, timers.

Star Case Manufacturing Co., Inc. 800-822-7827
648 Superior Ave, Munster, IN 46321
Mechanical and electrical component lift devices.

Supertex, Inc. 800-222-9883
1235 Bordeaux Dr, Sunnyvale, CA 94089
Supertex designs, develops, manufactures and markets semiconductor high voltage interface solutions by integrating high performance low voltage complementary metal oxide semiconductor (CMOS) process and high voltage double-diffused metal oxide semiconductor (DMOS) process into one chip. Supertex is a publicly held mixed signal semiconductor manufacturer, focused in high voltage interface products for use in the telecommunication, networking system, flat panel display, medical and industrial electronic industries.

Theragenics Corp. 770-271-0233
5203 Bristol Industrial Way, Buford, GA 30518
THERASEED, Palladium 103 isotope. Also available, radioactive palladium titanium isotope seeds.

COMPONENT, ELECTRONIC *(General) 80VAF*

Aci Medical, Inc. 800-667-9451
1857 Diamond St, San Marcos, CA 92078
Electronic assemblies.

Aventric Technologies 800-228-3343
1551 E Lincoln Ave Ste 166, Madison Heights, MI 48071
Sony Medical: VCRs, printers, monitors, sales and repair service; print media, parts and supplies

B-Tec Solutions Inc. 215-785-2400
913 Cedar Ave, Croydon, PA 19021

B. Braun Oem Division, B. Braun Medical Inc. 866-8-BBRAUN
824 12th Ave, Bethlehem, PA 18018

Caton Connector Corp. 877-522-2866
26 Wapping Rd, Kingston, MA 02364

Connor-Winfield Corp. 630-851-4722
2111 Comprehensive Dr, Aurora, IL 60505

Crest Healthcare Supply 800-328-8908
195 3rd St, Dassel, MN 55325
Healthcare TV system components: TV receivers and wired remote jumper cables. Signal system components and sound system components.

Crist Instrument Co., Inc. 301-393-8615
111 W 1st St, Hagerstown, MD 21740
Commutators to resolve small animal movements into rotational direction and capture brain-wave data with minimal noise transmission.

Current Controls, Inc. 585-593-1544
353 S Brooklyn Ave, Wellsville, NY 14895

Dynamics Research Corp. 800-522-4321
60 Frontage Rd, Andover, MA 01810

Electronic Industries Alliance 703-907-7500
2500 Wilson Blvd, Arlington, VA 22201

Halbar North, Inc. 650-349-4700
3 37th Ave, San Mateo, CA 94403
computer grade electrolytic, aluminum electrolytic, film, filters, machining svcs., engineering and value added assembly, transformers, chokes, pulse, isolation, LAN, high frequency, permanent magnet motors, gear motors, tach generators, precision, rotary, linear, and modular encoders, etc.

Hamamatsu Corp. 800-524-0504
360 Foothill Rd, Bridgewater, NJ 08807
Photomultipliers, photodiodes, image intensifiers, image converter, and related products. Imaging systems, video microscopy systems, light sources.

Itm Partners, Ltd. 210-651-9066
5925 Corridor Pkwy, Schertz, TX 78154
Parts for x-ray equipment.

Microcision Llc 800-264-3811
5805 Keystone St, Philadelphia, PA 19135

COMPONENT, ELECTRONIC *(cont'd)*

Minnesota Wire & Cable Co. 800-258-6922
1835 Energy Park Dr, Saint Paul, MN 55108
Full project management for all electrical interconnection programs.

National Graphic Supply 800-223-7130
226 N Allen St, Albany, NY 12206
Full line supplier of photographic supplies, equipment and electronics.

Peripheral Dynamics Inc. 800-253-0253
5150 Campus Dr, Plymouth Meeting, PA 19462
Video and diagnostic instruments.

Purdy Electronics Corp. 408-523-8201
720 Palomar Ave, Sunnyvale, CA 94085
Fan, Interoptic, and Interswitch, and Interfan

Rf Industries, Inc. 800-233-1728
7610 Miramar Rd, San Diego, CA 92126
Our RF Neulink division provides telemtery tansmitters and recieivers in VHF, UHF and 900 MHz frequency bands. Our RF Connectors division designs and manufactures coaxial connectors including BNC, TNC, N, UHF, MINI-UHF, MB, SMA, SMB, MCX cable connectors. Our product line also includes cable assemblies, crimp tool kits and universal adapter kits. Also available are cable assemblies made with RG-58/U coaxial cable. Custom cables and lengths also available.

Sensors, Inc. 734-429-2100
6812 State Rd, Saline, MI 48176
OEM - module, CO2.

Sensym Ict 800-573-6796
1804 McCarthy Blvd, Milpitas, CA 95035
The model 1865 force/pressure sensor is designed for use in infusion pumps. Base price in volume is $32.00.

Sr Instruments, Inc. 800-654-6360
600 Young St, Tonawanda, NY 14150

Thales Components Corporation 973-812-9000
40G Commerce Way, PO Box 540, Totowa, NJ 07512
Tetrode power grid tubes,X-ray image amplifier tubes, therapy microwave tubes, radiation therapy microwave tubes, charged coupled devices, solid state X-ray detectors.

Two Technologies Inc. 215-441-5305
419 Sargon Way, Horsham, PA 19044
Handheld computer and handheld terminals.

Ultratec, Inc. 800-482-2424
450 Science Dr, Madison, WI 53711
COMPACT/C TTY and SUPERCOM 4400 TTY non-printing keyboards.

Vectron International 717-486-6060
100 Watts St, Mount Holly Springs, PA 17065
Quartz crystals and oscillators.

X P Power 978-287-7200
305 Foster St, Littleton, MA 01460
Medical switching AC/DC power supply consists of the open-frame series 24-, 40-, 65-, 110-, 130-, and 200-W single- and multi-output switching power supplies. Desktop supplies include 30-, 50-, 90-, 110-, and 130-W, and are single- and multiple-output external switching power supplies. Four power platforms in our Modular Series range from 150 to 450 W.

COMPONENT, EXERCISE *(Physical Med) 89IOD*

Advanced Therapy Products, Inc. 800-548-4550
PO Box 3420, Glen Allen, VA 23058
Work cube.

Balance Systems, Inc. 1-888-274-5444
1644 Plaza Way Ste 317, Walla Walla, WA 99362
FLEXTEND-AC Grip-free Upper Extremity Exercise System including over 50 theraputic exercises.

Bioflex Medical Magnetics, Inc. 954-565-8500
3370 NE 5th Ave, Oakland Park, FL 33334
Medical Magnetic Braces, Supports, foot care, Jewelry and Sleep Products

Bird & Cronin, Inc. 651-683-1111
1200 Trapp Rd, Saint Paul, MN 55121
Physical therapy weights.

Breg, Inc., An Orthofix Company 800-897-BREG
2611 Commerce Way, Vista, CA 92081
Ankle, shoulder, knee, back therapy kits.

Circular Traction Supply, Inc. 800-247-6535
7602 Talbert Ave Ste 9, Huntington Beach, CA 92648
Exercise weight belt.

COMPONENT, EXERCISE *(cont'd)*

Cuff Toughener 601-853-3966
103 Weldon Dr, Madison, MS 39110
Rotator cuff rehabilitative device.

Cybex International, Inc. 508-533-4300
10 Trotter Dr, Medway, MA 02053

Discount Dme 714-630-9590
1265 N Grove St Ste A, Anaheim, CA 92806
Resistive band therapy , exercise bands & tubing.

Dj Orthopedics De Mexico, S.A. De C.V. 690-727-1280
Blvd., Delagacion La Presa, Tijuana 22397 Mexico
Cpm pads

Dj Orthopedics De Mexico, S.A. De C.V. 690-727-1280
Ave. Venustiano Carranza 6802, Castillo, Tijuana 22100 Mexico
Cpm pads

Doctors Orders 866-356-0771
731 Construction Ct Ste B, Zeeland, MI 49464
Pressure feedback ball.

Erigon 361-387-8276
1301 Dakota St, Robstown, TX 78380
Exercise component.

Grav-Trac 813-932-8710
6040 Country Club Rd, Wesley Chapel, FL 33544
Hanging bar for back pain relief.

Home Stretch Products, Inc. 847-816-1852
536 McKinley Ave, Libertyville, IL 60048
Lower extremity tissue stretching device.

Ideal Products 800-321-5490
1287 County Road 623, Broseley, MO 63932
BACK AT YA Rebounder - Medicine ball exercise partner with adjustable angle for a variety of plyometric exercises. Also available, Mobile Storage Rack. PVC pipe storage rack for large therapy exercise balls.

Instrumentation Industries, Inc. 800-633-8577
2990 Industrial Blvd, Bethel Park, PA 15102
Inspiratory, variable resistance.

J.S. Associates 813-975-4354
8403 Ridgebrook Cir, Odessa, FL 33556
Bolster, exercise/massage.

Kenad Sg Medical, Inc. 800-825-0606
2692 Huntley Dr, Memphis, TN 38132
Various exerciser components.

Lifeline Usa 800-553-6633
3201 Syene Rd, Madison, WI 53713
Tuf-Nex.

Little Shepherd Industries 870-453-4874
316 River Run Lane, Flippin, AR 72634
Game and exercise board.

Maribelle Manufacturing Inc. 888-655-3459
9520 Natasha Place, Sidney, BC V8L-4P9 Canada
Exercise assist system, portable frames & clamps footwear.

Medical Depot 516-998-4600
99 Seaview Blvd, Port Washington, NY 11050
Exercise pulley.

Nautilus, Inc. 360-859-2900
16400 SE Nautilus Dr, Vancouver, WA 98683
Full line of variable resistance strength training machines, including single station, multi-station and rehabilitation machines. These machines include four-bar linkage, range limiters and other safety-oriented features for safe and productive training.

Novel Products, Inc. 800-323-5143
PO Box 408, Rockton, IL 61072
Cross crawl exerciser.

Pediatric Intensive Therapy, Inc. 786-543-8165
18639 SW 107th Ave, Cutler Bay, FL 33157
Exercise cage, exercise cage unit.

Profex Medical Products 800-325-0196
2224 E Person Ave, Memphis, TN 38114

Pyraback.Com 713-859-7568
10339 Belfast Rd, La Porte, TX 77571
Back exercise device.

Ralston Group 334-875-2298
656 Lake Lanier Rd, Selma, AL 36701
Weights used to strengthen male and female pelvic floor muscles.

COMPONENT, EXERCISE *(cont'd)*

Richardson Products, Inc. 888-928-7297
9408 Gulfstream Rd, Frankfort, IL 60423
Exercise devices.

Rk Froom & Co., Inc. 310-327-5125
903 Cunningham Ln S, Salem, OR 97302
Arm support.

The Hygenic Corp. 800-321-2135
1245 Home Ave, Akron, OH 44310
Soft weights, various weights, various colors.

The Pettibon System 888-774-6258
2118 Jackson Hwy, Chehalis, WA 98532
Head weight,hip weight,shoulder weight,weight bar/bag.

Thera-Tronics, Inc. 800-267-6211
623 Mamaroneck Ave, Mamaroneck, NY 10543
Multi-weight station and weight station.

Therafin Corporation 800-843-7234
19747 Wolf Rd, Mokena, IL 60448
Various exercise aids.

Thompson Medical Specialties 800-777-4949
3404 Library Ln, Saint Louis Park, MN 55426

Top Shelf Manufacturing, Llc 209-834-8185
1851 Paradise Rd Ste B, Tracy, CA 95304
Cpm pads.

Truform Orthotics & Prosthetics 800-888-0458
3960 Rosslyn Dr, Cincinnati, OH 45209

Vision Quest Industries, Inc. 800-266-6969
18011 Mitchell S, Irvine, CA 92614
Various types of excise kits.

COMPONENT, METAL, OTHER *(General) 80WOS*

Alsons Corp. 800-421-0001
3010 Mechanic Rd, P.O. Box 282, Hillsdale, MI 49242
Shower heads.

American Coil Spring Co. 231-726-4021
1041 E Keating Ave, Muskegon, MI 49442
Custom production of precision cold-formed metal products: coiled springs including compression, extension, torsion, double torsion, and garter; flat springs; constant force springs; wire forms; and small stampings.

American Micro Products, Inc. 800-479-2193
4288 Armstrong Blvd, Batavia, OH 45103
Manufacture and assembly of precision engineered medical devices as a contract manufacturer. Full prototyping and process development available. Materials include all types of titanium, stainless steel, aluminum, precious metals and super alloys.

Bolt Bethel, Llc 763-434-5900
23530 University Avenue Ext NW, PO Box 135, Bethel, MN 55005

Cadence Science Inc. 888-717-7677
1979 Marcus Ave Ste 215, New Hyde Park, NY 11042
Custom products fabricated from such metals as stainless steel, brass, aluminum, titanium and platinum via precision cutting, tip reducing, bending, flaring, EDM and specialty machining.

Deringer-Ney, Inc. 860-242-2281
2 Douglas St, Ney Industrial Park, Bloomfield, CT 06002
Fine Wire and Films

Engineers Express, Inc. 800-255-8823
7 Industrial Park Rd, Medway, MA 02053

Fecom Corporation 800-292-3362
12 Stults Rd Ste 103, Dayton, NJ 08810
Heat Sinks: Extruded, Stamped, CPU Coolers, Extrusion Profiles, Bonded Fin & Assembled Fin, Custom Design, Assembly, and Accessories

Grace Manufacturing, Inc. 479-968-5455
614 Sr 247, Russellville, AR 72802

Greatbatch Inc 716-759-5600
10000 Wehrle Dr, Clarence, NY 14031

Hart Enterprises, Inc. 616-887-0400
400 Apple Jack Ct, Sparta, MI 49345

Imetra, Inc. 914-592-2800
200 Clearbrook Rd, Elmsford, NY 10523
Precision components of ruby, sapphire & ceramics for instrumentation and analytical equipment.

Ispg, Inc. 860-355-8511
517 Litchfield Rd, New Milford, CT 06776
Tubular stainless steel products

COMPONENT, METAL, OTHER *(cont'd)*

Lyons Tool And Die Company 800-422-9363
185 Research Pkwy, Meriden, CT 06450
Rapid prototyping. Production of medical devices in class 10,000 clean rooms. Medical knives and scissors. Precision metal stamping. Engineering services.

Microcision Llc 800-264-3811
5805 Keystone St, Philadelphia, PA 19135
Stainless-steel catheter connectors.

Mission X-Ray 800-676-8718
45459 Industrial Pllace, Suite 1, Fremont, CA 94538-6450
Framework for chiropractic x-ray equipment.

Nanomaterials, Inc. 401-433-7022
9 Preston Dr, Barrington, RI 02806
Nano-sized metal particles.

Okay Industries, Inc. 860-225-8707
200 Ellis St, P.O. Box 2470, New Britain, CT 06051

Patient Instrumentation Corp. 610-799-4436
4117 Route 309, Schnecksville, PA 18078
Linde, Air Products, Foregger and Melco Medical gas outlet parts.

Penn United Technology, Inc. 724-352-1507
799 N Pike Rd, Cabot, PA 16023
Designing and building metal-stamping disposable components.

Phillips Plastics Corp. 877-508-0252
1201 Hanley Rd, Hudson, WI 54016
Metal Injection Molding

Precision Medical Products, Inc. 717-335-3700
44 Denver Rd, PO Box 300, Denver, PA 17517

Putnam Precision Products 845-278-2141
3859 Danbury Rd, Brewster, NY 10509
Custom made components.

R. B. Annis Instruments, Inc. 317-637-9282
1101 N Delaware St, Indianapolis, IN 46202
Production-type bulk erasers for magnetic tape, floppy discs, and steel parts.

Revtek Industries, Llc 503-659-1650
4288 SE International Way, Portland, OR 97222
Precision machined medical & dental components.

Rms Company 763-783-5074
8600 Evergreen Blvd NW, Minneapolis, MN 55433
Titanium, platinum, stainless-steel, other medical grade metals / polymers used for surgical implants/ devices and orthopedic instrumentation.

Safe-T-Rack Systems, Inc. 800-344-0619
4325 Dominguez Rd Ste A, Rocklin, CA 95677

Specialized Medical Devices, Llc 800-463-1874
300 Running Pump Rd, Lancaster, PA 17603

Stewart Efi, Lcc 800-678-7931
630 Central Park Ave, Yonkers, NY 10704

Tegra Medical Inc. 508-541-4200
9 Forge Pkwy, Franklin, MA 02038

Tfx Medical Oem 800-548-6600
50 Plantation Dr, Jaffrey, NH 03452

Troy Manufacturing Co. 440-834-8262
17090 Rapids Rd, PO Box 448, Burton, OH 44021
Non-implant used for wound-drainage kits.

Vita Needle Company 781-444-1780
919 Great Plain Ave, Needham, MA 02492

West Pharmaceutical Services, Inc. 800-231-3000
101 Gordon Dr, Franklin Ctr, PA 19341
Pharmaceutical seals for high-speed filling operations.

Wilkinson Company, Inc. 208-777-8332
590 S Clearwater Loop Ste C, Post Falls, ID 83854
High purity precious metals and alloys in stamped forms, rings and other shapes.

COMPONENT, OPTICAL *(General) 80SHS*

Cadmet, Inc. 800-543-7282
155 Planebrook Rd, P.O. Box 24, Malvern, PA 19355

Dynamics Research Corp. 800-522-4321
60 Frontage Rd, Andover, MA 01810

Edmund Industrial Optics 800-363-1992
101 E Gloucester Pike, Barrington, NJ 08007

COMPONENT, OPTICAL *(cont'd)*

International Crystal Laboratories 973-478-8944
11 Erie St, Garfield, NJ 07026
Optical Crystal. REAL CRYSTAL, IR Sample Card. An IR sample Card with a non-absorbing crystal sample substrate, replaces 3M IR cards.

Klarmann Rulings, Inc. 800-252-2401
480 Charles Bancroft Hwy, Litchfield, NH 03052
Reticles and stage micrometers.

Lighthouse Imaging Corp. 207-253-5350
477 Congress St, Portland, ME 04101

Nanoptics, Inc. 352-378-6620
3014 NE 21st Way, Gainesville, FL 32609
Supplier of ultra bright plastic optical fiber for illumination and POF image bundles

Newport Franklin, Inc. 800-598-6783
8 Forge Pkwy, Franklin, MA 02038

Photon Technology International, Inc. 609-894-4420
300 Birmingham Road, Birmingham, NJ 08011-0272
Optical Building Blocks; Consists of light sources, monochromators, detectors, and lasers for spectroscopic experiment.

Schott North America, Inc. 315-255-2791
62 Columbus St, Auburn, NY 13021
SCHOTT manufactures and supplies fiberoptic and LED illumination solutions for machine vision, industrial OEM, microscopy, forensic and medical applications. Our product catalog features photos, drawings, and technical specifications for more than 400 standard products, from light sources to backlights, ringlights, bundles, goosenecks, lightlines, halogen light sources, and a variety of accessories. Please visit www.us.schott.com/fiberoptics to request our product catalog or literature.

COMPONENT, OTHER *(General) 80WXA*

A.R.C. Distributors 800-296-8724
PO Box 599, Centreville, MD 21617
POLECAT IV transport system for wheelchair and stretcher patients. POLECAT facilitates moving patients using infusion pumps mounted on portable (wheeled) IV poles. Forms a single unit for improved safety and productivity.

Accu-Glass Llc 800-325-4796
10765 Trenton Ave, Saint Louis, MO 63132
Precision glass flow restrictors for infusion devices/flush devices. Precision glass tubing for thermometers, fiber optics, ampules and more.

Apex Medical Technologies, Inc. 800-345-3208
10064 Mesa Ridge Ct Ste 202, San Diego, CA 92121
Specializing in thin-film dip molding of synthetic elastomer materials. Materials range from thermoplastic polyurethanes to synthetic polyisoprene latex and can be incorporated to customer requirements into products or components from catheter balloons to probe covers. Capabilities include prototype product development through contract production manufacturing.

AstraZeneca Pharmaceuticals LP 302-886-3000
PO Box 15437, 1800 Concord Pike, Wilmington, DE 19850
Visible and UV light curable adhesives for assembly of medical products. Photocurable adhesives are formulated for bonding, tacking, sealing, encapsulating and potting applications.

Bak Electronics, Inc. 800-894-6000
PO Box 623, Mount Airy, MD 21771
Discrimination systems. Post generators. Stimulus isolators.

Chamberlin Rubber Company, Inc. 585-427-7780
3333 Brighton Henrietta Town Line Rd, PO Box 22700
Rochester, NY 14623

Cte Chem Tec Equipment Co. 800-222-2177
234 SW 12th Ave, Deerfield Beach, FL 33442
Hardware including gages and meters.

Deringer-Ney, Inc. 860-242-2281
2 Douglas St, Ney Industrial Park, Bloomfield, CT 06002
Custom Alloys

Directmed, Inc. 516-656-3377
150 Pratt Oval, Glen Cove, NY 11542

Ear Technology Corp. 800-327-8547
207 E Myrtle Ave, PO Box 1516, Johnson City, TN 37601
DRY & STORE: device for drying, conditioning, and sanitizing hearing aids.

Engineers Express, Inc. 800-255-8823
7 Industrial Park Rd, Medway, MA 02053

COMPONENT, OTHER *(cont'd)*

Ernst Flow Industries 800-992-2843
116 Main St, Farmingdale, NJ 07727
Manufacturer of level gages, sight flow indicators, sight windows, flow monitors, gage glass and gaskets.

Ezy-Ramp Co. 800-835-8513
4502 N Armenia Ave, Tampa, FL 33603
Disposal of durable medical equipment, consumable supples.

Hoover Precision Products, Inc 906-632-7310
1390 Industrial Park Dr, Sault S Marie, MI 49783
Diagnostic kit components.

In Vivo Metric 707-433-2949
PO Box 397, Healdsburg, CA 95448
Pressure-sensitive components.

Invivo 800-331-3220
12501 Research Pkwy, Orlando, FL 32826
Plug-in devices for MRI platforms for head, neck, wrist, knee, breast and more.

Leedal, Inc. 847-498-0111
3453 Commercial Ave, Northbrook, IL 60062
Stainless steel tanks and waterjackets; thermostatic water controls; water filters.

Lyons Tool And Die Company 800-422-9363
185 Research Pkwy, Meriden, CT 06450
Rapid prototyping. Production of medical devices in class 10,000 clean rooms. Medical knives and scissors. Precision metal stamping. Engineering services.

Macdee, Inc. 734-475-9165
13800 Luick Dr, Chelsea, MI 48118
Components for diagnostic equipment.

Master Bond, Inc. 201-343-8983
154 Hobart St, Hackensack, NJ 07601
Anaerobic, conductive, cyanoacrylate/methacrylate, epoxy and hot-melt adhesives.

Med Labs Inc. 800-968-2486
28 Vereda Cordillera, Goleta, CA 93117
BITE-OR-PUFF: Pneumatic switch for nurse call or control of computers, toys, games, buzzers and other low power devices. Operated by bite, puff, or squeeze- $73.00.

Medcovers, Inc 800-948-8917
500 W Goldsboro St, Kenly, NC 27542
Replacement headgear for CPAP units.

Medela, Inc. 800-435-8316
1101 Corporate Dr, McHenry, IL 60050
SUPPLEMENTAL NURSING SYSTEM (SNS) - a breastfeeding assistance kit for adoptive and nursing mothers.

Medrad, Inc. 800-633-7231
100 Global View Dr, Warrendale, PA 15086
Surface coils for MR. Direct, OEM and private label distribution.

Micronova 888-816-4876
3431 Lomita Blvd, Torrance, CA 90505
Cleanroom tape.

Minnesota Wire & Cable Co. 800-258-6922
1835 Energy Park Dr, Saint Paul, MN 55108
Full project management for electrical interconnection programs.

Nanomaterials, Inc. 401-433-7022
9 Preston Dr, Barrington, RI 02806
Aluminum oxide and aluminum powder. Nano-sized ceramic and composite particles.

Newport Glass Works, Ltd. 714-484-8100
PO Box 127, Stanton, CA 90680
Quartz, fused silica, optical glass blanks, Pyrex blanks, laser protection eyewear glass blanks, etc.

Phillips Plastics Corp. 877-508-0252
1201 Hanley Rd, Hudson, WI 54016
Medical device design, engineering, and assembly services.

Plitek, L.L.C 800-966-1250
69 Rawls Rd, Des Plaines, IL 60018
Pressure sensitive adhesives, films, wovens, non-wovens, filtered-PTFE, adhesive coatings. Product Ideas: Filters, Wound care, Drug Delivery applications, Skin contact approved materials, FDA approved products, surgical drapes, ostomy care, hydrogel products, skin tape.

Rms Company 763-783-5074
8600 Evergreen Blvd NW, Minneapolis, MN 55433
Precision machined components for use in implantable and instrumentation devices.

COMPONENT, OTHER *(cont'd)*

S&G Enterprises, Inc. 800-233-3721
N115W19000 Edison Dr, Germantown, WI 53022
PAK-MORE disk developed to be used with 55-gal drum compactors. This disposable device locks into the drum to prevent the springback of the compacted material, increase compaction ratios, and decrease disposal costs.

Selco Products Company 800-257-3526
605 S East St, Anaheim, CA 92805
Control knobs of all different colors and sizes; push-on, collet, and slider knobs, control knob accessories, push buttons for switches.

Sensidyne, Inc. 800-451-9444
16333 Bay Vista Dr, Clearwater, FL 33760
High-efficiency micro air pumps for diverse applications.

Shared Systems, Inc. 888-474-2733
PO Box 211587, 3961 Columbia Rd, Augusta, GA 30917
Non-serum based blocking buffers.

Sr Instruments, Inc. 800-654-6360
600 Young St, Tonawanda, NY 14150

Tailored Label Products, Inc. 800-727-1344
W165N5731 Ridgewood Dr, Menomonee Falls, WI 53051

Tmp Technologies, Inc. 716-895-6100
1200 Northland Ave, Buffalo, NY 14215
Other.

Transamerican Technologies International 800-322-7373
2246 Camino Ramon, San Ramon, CA 94583
Adapters to connect video cameras and digital cameras to microscopes, colposcopes and ophthalmic slit lamps.

Trelleborg Sealing Solutions 800-466-1727
510 Burbank St, Broomfield, CO 80020
Spring-energized seals and rotary PTFE lip seals.

Tyco Healthcare Group Lp 800-445-5025
2 Ludlow Park Dr, Chicopee, MA 01022
Conductive and hydrogel adhesives and finished device fabrication. Specializing in skin contact products.

Vernay Laboratories, Inc. 800-666-5227
120 E South College St, Yellow Springs, OH 45387

West Pharmaceutical Services, Inc. 800-231-3000
101 Gordon Dr, Franklin Ctr, PA 19341
Medical device components and assemblies made from elastomers, metal and plastic.

Whatman Inc. 732-885-6529
800 Centennial Ave Bldg 1, Piscataway, NJ 08854
Vacu-Guard. Vacuum pump protector.

Young Innovations, Inc. 800-325-1881
13705 Shoreline Ct E, Earth City, MO 63045
Metal and disposable prophyangles.

COMPONENT, PAPER *(General) 80WSM*

British Marketing Enterprises, Inc. 800-358-8220
1825 Bush St, San Francisco, CA 94109
Specifically, disposables, or paper goods.

Perfecseal 877-828-7501
PO Box 2968, 3500 North Main St., Oshkosh, WI 54903

Pm Company 800-327-4359
1500 Kemper Meadow Dr, Cincinnati, OH 45240
Printer papers offer superior images giving crisp, legible readouts for accurate analysis and dianosis for virtually all types of medical/laboratory printer applications, including vision/ear screens, blood testing & lab charting.

Sandt Products, Inc. 800-441-8764
1275 Loop Rd, Lancaster, PA 17601
Paper for recorder or measuring devices. 2 to 8 1/2 in wide rolls of fanfold paper. Thermal or bond impact printers.

Suppleyes, Inc. 800-727-3725
4890 Hammond Industrial Dr Ste A, Cumming, GA 30041
Thermal paper for optometry.

Tailored Label Products, Inc. 800-727-1344
W165N5731 Ridgewood Dr, Menomonee Falls, WI 53051

COMPONENT, PLASTIC *(General) 80VAE*

Achilles Usa, Inc. 425-353-7000
1407 80th St SW, Everett, WA 98203
Flexible PVC film and sheeting in Class I to VI formulations, for medical ID tags and bands, blood bags, medical waste bags, etc.

Aci Medical, Inc. 800-667-9451
1857 Diamond St, San Marcos, CA 92078

COMPONENT, PLASTIC *(cont'd)*

Bruin Plastics Co. 800-556-7764
61 Joslin Rd, Glendale, RI 02826

C&J Industries, Inc. 814-724-4950
760 Water St, Meadville, PA 16335

Cadco Dental Products 800-833-8267
600 E Hueneme Rd, Oxnard, CA 93033
Paper/plastic self-sealing autoclave pouches.

Cal Bionics, Inc. 415-892-1892
1777 Indian Valley Rd, Novato, CA 94947
HYDROFILCON (METHAFILCON A) plastics for contact lenses.

Coeur Inc., Sheboygan 800-874-4240
3411 Behrens Pkwy, Sheboygan, WI 53081

Delstar Technologies Inc 512-447-7000
220 E Saint Elmo Rd, Austin, TX 78745
Plastic netting for use as support/separation for membrane.

Deringer-Ney, Inc. 860-242-2281
2 Douglas St, Ney Industrial Park, Bloomfield, CT 06002
Precision Insert Molded Components

Directmed, Inc. 516-656-3377
150 Pratt Oval, Glen Cove, NY 11542

Drummond Scientific Co. 800-523-7480
500 Park Way # 700, Broomall, PA 19008
Plastic and glass diagnostic kits.

Dux Dental 800-833-8267
600 E Hueneme Rd, Oxnard, CA 93033
Paper/plastic self-sealing autoclave pouches.

Genesis Manufacturing, Inc. 317-485-7887
720 E Broadway St, Fortville, IN 46040
Contract Radio-Frequency (RF) Welding. From development to manufacturing and packaging.

Genpore, A Division Of General Polymeric Corp. 800-654-4391
1136 Morgantown Rd, Reading, PA 19607
Custom porous polymers

Globe Medical Tech, Inc. 713-365-9595
1766 W Sam Houston Pkwy N, Houston, TX 77043
Plastic components for IV sets, blood sets, vein sets, and other medical disposables.

Gvs Filter Technology Inc. 317-471-3700
5353 W 79th St, Indianapolis, IN 46268
Y-sites, male luer locks with or without caps and with or without rotating hub, needle access ports for bags, female luer lock to tube connectors, and many other small components. All non-latex.

Gw Plastics, Inc. 802-234-9941
239 Pleasant St, Bethel, VT 05032
Close tolerance engineered resins.

Hart Enterprises, Inc. 616-887-0400
400 Apple Jack Ct, Sparta, MI 49345

Hoover Precision Products, Inc 906-632-7310
1390 Industrial Park Dr, Sault S Marie, MI 49783
Molding and subassemblies

Kindt Collins Co. 800-321-3170
12651 Elmwood Ave, Cleveland, OH 44111
Bristles for toothbrushes.

Lemans Industries Corp. 800-289-5667
79 Express St, Plainview, NY 11803
Disposable plastic covers for wheelchairs, mattress bags.

Lifemed Of California 800-543-3633
1216 S Allec St, Anaheim, CA 92805

Lucomed Inc. 800-633-7877
45 Kulick Rd, Fairfield, NJ 07004

Medical Plastic Devices (Mpd), Inc. 866-633-9835
161 Oneida Dr., Pointe Claire, QUE H9R 1A9 Canada

Minnesota Rubber & Qmr Plastics 952-927-1400
1100 Xenium Ln N, Minneapolis, MN 55441
Custom molding of rubber & plastic components.

MOS Plastics Inc. 408-944-9407
2308 Zanker Rd, San Jose, CA 95131

Motloid Company 800-662-5021
300 N Elizabeth St, Chicago, IL 60607
PLASTIPAC & PLASTICLEAR Plastic separating sheets and workpans.

Moyco Technologies, Inc. 800-331-8837
200 Commerce Dr, Montgomeryville, PA 18936
Nipper.

COMPONENT, PLASTIC *(cont'd)*

Nanoptics, Inc. 352-378-6620
3014 NE 21st Way, Gainesville, FL 32609
Supplier of ultra bright plastic optical fiber for illumination and POF image bundles

Nypro Inc. 978-365-9721
101 Union St, Clinton, MA 01510
Precision injection molding & cleanroom assembly.

Plitek, L.L.C 800-966-1250
69 Rawls Rd, Des Plaines, IL 60018
Film Extrusion: EVA, APET, Cyclo-Olefin Copolymers and Polymers(Optically clear film with Master drug file), HDPE, LDPE.

Precision Medical Products, Inc. 717-335-3700
44 Denver Rd, PO Box 300, Denver, PA 17517

Putnam Precision Products 845-278-2141
3859 Danbury Rd, Brewster, NY 10509
Teflon, Vesoel, Lexan, Kelf, Tefcel, Polypropylene.

R.C.A. Rubber Company, The 800-321-2340
1833 E Market St, P.O. Box 9240, Akron, OH 44305
Stair treads - rubber and vinyl.

Sabin Corporation 800-264-4510
PO Box 788, PO Box 788, Bloomington, IN 47402
Medical plastics.

Saint-Gobain Performance Plastics/Clearwater 800-541-6880
4451 110th Ave N, Clearwater, FL 33762

Tak Systems 800-333-9631
14 Kendrick Rd Ste 5, Wareham, MA 02571
49.99 for 1-lb. container of Hydroplastic low-temperature thermoformable plastic that softens in hot water for custom medical and dental applications.

Tfx Medical Oem 800-548-6600
50 Plantation Dr, Jaffrey, NH 03452

The Tech Group 480-281-4500
14677 N 74th St, Scottsdale, AZ 85260
Customer specified injection molding, mold construction and medical device assembly.

Trax Cleanroom Products 800-520-8729
3352 Swetzer Rd, P.O. Box 2089, Loomis, CA 95650
Vinyl curtains for use as airflow shields, softwall panels, and strip curtains.

Trelleborg Sealing Solutions 800-466-1727
510 Burbank St, Broomfield, CO 80020
Polymeric roller-element bearings, plain, thrust and flange bearings and bearing materials.

Unilab, Inc. 9058559093
2355 Royal Windsor Dr., Unit 3, Mississauga, ON L5M-5R5 Canada
Plastic laminate counter tops.

United Laboratory Plastics 800-722-2499
PO Box 8585, 1724A Westpark Ctr., Saint Louis, MO 63126
Disposable laboratory plastics, pipet tips, microcentrifuge tubes, gloves, pipettors, lab refrigerators and freezers, timers.

Vernay Laboratories, Inc. 800-666-5227
120 E South College St, Yellow Springs, OH 45387

West Pharmaceutical Services, Inc. 800-231-3000
101 Gordon Dr, Franklin Ctr, PA 19341
Custom manufacturing of plastic components for drug delivery systems and devices.

COMPONENT, RUBBER *(General) 80VAL*

California Medical Innovations 800-229-5871
873 E Arrow Hwy, Pomona, CA 91767
Custom manufactured neoprene, plastisol, and natural latex rubber devices.

Calley & Currier Co. 800-762-5500
1 Greenleaf Woods Dr Unit 202, Portsmouth, NH 03801
Rubber crutch grips, with or without handles.

Chamberlin Rubber Company, Inc. 585-427-7780
3333 Brighton Henrietta Town Line Rd, PO Box 22700
Rochester, NY 14623

Csi International, Inc. 303-795-8273
4301 S Federal Blvd Ste 116, Englewood, CO 80110

Hi-Tech Rubber, Inc. 800-924-4832
3191 E La Palma Ave, Anaheim, CA 92806
Molded silicone rubber.

Hospira 800-441-4100
268 E 4th St, Ashland, OH 44805
Custom-molded shapes.

COMPONENT, RUBBER *(cont'd)*

Kent Elastomer Products, Inc. 800-331-4762
1500 Saint Clair Ave, PO Box 668, Kent, OH 44240

Lifemed Of California 800-543-3633
1216 S Allec St, Anaheim, CA 92805

Minnesota Rubber & Qmr Plastics 952-927-1400
1100 Xenium Ln N, Minneapolis, MN 55441
Custom molding of rubber & plastic components.

Moyco Technologies, Inc. 800-331-8837
200 Commerce Dr, Montgomeryville, PA 18936
Silicone-rubber stops are sterilizable at temperatures up to 450 degrees Fahrenheit and are used to record canal working measurement.

Plasticoid Co., The 410-398-2800
249 W High St, Elkton, MD 21921

R.C.A. Rubber Company, The 800-321-2340
1833 E Market St, P.O. Box 9240, Akron, OH 44305
Stair treads - rubber and vinyl.

Vernay Laboratories, Inc. 800-666-5227
120 E South College St, Yellow Springs, OH 45387

West Pharmaceutical Services, Inc. 800-231-3000
101 Gordon Dr, Franklin Ctr, PA 19341
Custom manufacturing of rubber components for drug delivery systems and devices.

COMPONENT, SILICONE *(General) 80VAM*

Allergan 800-624-4261
71 S Los Carneros Rd, Goleta, CA 93117
Solid silicone blocks.

Csi International, Inc. 303-795-8273
4301 S Federal Blvd Ste 116, Englewood, CO 80110

Degania Silicone, Inc. 401-333-8199
1226 Mendon Rd, Cumberland, RI 02864
Silicone vessel loops that are sterile packaged under private label.

Excel Medical Products, Llc 810-714-4775
3145 Copper Ave, Fenton, MI 48430
Excel Medical Products is an FDA-Registered, ISO and GMP compliant contract manufacturer specializing in medical components and devices. Excel Medical Products offers the following services and capabilities: Class 100,000 clean room manufacturing and assembly, thermoplastic and elastomer injection molding, LSR (liquid silicone rubber) injection molding, compression molding, insert molding, custom assembly, custom kitting, pouch sealing, tray sealing, and pad printing. Additional capabilities included adhesive, solvent and UV bonding, tipping, flaring, skiving and micro drilling. We also offers product development, process development and mold design services. Excel Medical Products provides custom solutions from conception to completion.

Helix Medical, Inc. 800-266-4421
1110 Mark Ave, Carpinteria, CA 93013

Hi-Tech Rubber, Inc. 800-924-4832
3191 E La Palma Ave, Anaheim, CA 92806

Lifemed Of California 800-543-3633
1216 S Allec St, Anaheim, CA 92805

Master Bond, Inc. 201-343-8983
154 Hobart St, Hackensack, NJ 07601
Adhesives.

Moyco Technologies, Inc. 800-331-8837
200 Commerce Dr, Montgomeryville, PA 18936
Silicone-rubber stops are sterilizable at temperatures up to 450 degrees Fahrenheit and are used to record canal working measurement.

Plasticoid Co., The 410-398-2800
249 W High St, Elkton, MD 21921

Smiths Medical Asd 800-424-8662
5700 W 23rd Ave, Gary, IN 46406
Custom and stock; pilot balloons; cuffs; plugs and luers.

Specialty Manufacturing, Inc. 800-269-6204
2210 Midland Rd, Saginaw, MI 48603
Silicone balloon.

United Chemical Technologies, Inc. 800-385-3153
2731 Bartram Rd, Bristol, PA 19007
Specialty silanes, silicone fluids, and silicone elastomers.

Vernay Laboratories, Inc. 800-666-5227
120 E South College St, Yellow Springs, OH 45387

COMPONENT, SILICONE *(cont'd)*

West Pharmaceutical Services, Inc. 800-231-3000
101 Gordon Dr, Franklin Ctr, PA 19341
Injection molding of silicone and thermoplastic elastomers.

COMPONENT, TRACTION, INVASIVE *(Orthopedics) 87JEC*

Acumed Llc 503-627-9957
5885 NW Cornelius Pass Rd, Hillsboro, OR 97124
Small bone fixator.

Ascent Healthcare Solutions 480-763-5300
10232 S 51st St, Phoenix, AZ 85044
External fixation device.

Autogenesis, Inc. 410-665-2017
8700 Old Harford Rd, Baltimore, MD 21234
AUTOMATOR 2000, Autogenesis' Automator 2000 is a programmable, motorized divice used for limb lengthening and deformity correction. The device is compatible with most manufacturers' unilateral and circular fixators. Automator 2000 performs distraction according to the physician's prescription continuously throughout the day. Research indicates the frequent distractions in small increments can promote superior new bone and soft tissue regeneration.

Biomet, Inc. 574-267-6639
56 E Bell Dr, PO Box 587, Warsaw, IN 46582
Various types of skeletal traction.

Depuy Orthopaedics, Inc. 800-473-3789
700 Orthopaedic Dr, P.O. Box 988, Warsaw, IN 46582
Various types of invasive traction components.

Precision Medical Devices, Inc. 717-795-9480
5020 Ritter Rd Ste 211, Mechanicsburg, PA 17055
Tibial retractor.

Synthes (Usa) 610-719-5000
35 Airport Rd, Horseheads, NY 14845
Various types and sizes of invasive traction components.

Zimmer Holdings, Inc. 800-613-6131
1800 W Center St, PO Box 708, Warsaw, IN 46580

COMPONENT, TRACTION, NON-INVASIVE *(Orthopedics) 87KQZ*

Arthrex, Inc. 239-643-5553
1370 Creekside Blvd, Naples, FL 34108
Various.

Bray Corporation 760-345-6689
14149 Calle Contesa, Victorville, CA 92392
Vertebral distraction pump (v.d.p.).

Care Rehab And Orthopaedic Products, Inc. 703-448-9644
3930 Horseshoe Bend Rd, Keysville, VA 23947
Cervical traction device.

Cimex Medical Innovations, Llc 985-871-0802
72385 Industry Park Rd, Covington, LA 70435
Shoulder trac.

Dm Systems, Inc. 800-254-5438
1316 Sherman Ave, Evanston, IL 60201
HEELIFT® TRACTION BOOT provides the same heel pressure relief and added benefits of the existing Heelift® products while preventing fracture pain with up to ten pounds of straight skin traction. The Velcro® traction straps can be removed for continued relief in a post surgical setting.

Ossur Americas 949-268-3155
742 Pancho Rd, Camarillo, CA 93012

Rycor Medical, Inc. 800-227-9267
2053 Atwater Dr, North Port, FL 34288
RYCOR Finger Traps mesh fabric gripping device to apply traction on upper extremities.

Sam Medical Products 503-639-5474
4909 South Coast Hwy., #245, Newport, OR 97365
Pelvic sling, circumferential sacroiliac sling orthosis.

Smith & Nephew Inc., Endoscopy Div. 978-749-1000
76 S Meridian Ave, Oklahoma City, OK 73107
Non-invasive traction component.

The Saunders Group 800-445-9836
4250 Norex Dr, Chaska, MN 55318
Traction device.

Vmg Medical, Inc. 540-337-1996
542 Walnut Hills Rd, Staunton, VA 24401
Traction belt, harness.

COMPONENT, WHEELCHAIR *(Physical Med) 89KNN*

Accessible Designs, Inc. 210-341-0008
401 Isom Rd Ste 520, San Antonio, TX 78216
Wheelchair disc brake/lock system with two piece hub design.

American Track Roadsters, Inc. 303-986-9300
3535 S Kipling St Unit A, Lakewood, CO 80235
Various models of wheelchair armrests / legrests / positioning pads.

Aquila Corporation 608-782-0031
1309 Norplex Dr Ste 6, La Crosse, WI 54601
Wheelchair cushion.

Body Tech 1 Nw 866-315-0640
10727 47th Pl W, Mukilteo, WA 98275
Components, wheelchair.

C & D Technologies Inc., Dynasty Div. 215-619-2700
900 E Keefe Ave, Milwaukee, WI 53212
Wheelchair battery.

Caspian Designs, Inc. 310-396-5258
2632 Lincoln Blvd, Santa Monica, CA 90405
Wheelchair component.

Cortical Systematics Llc. 877-468-5383
5324 E 18th St, Tucson, AZ 85711
Modular wheelchair propulsion system.

Crest Healthcare Supply 800-328-8908
195 3rd St, Dassel, MN 55325
Wheelchair parts.

Fortress Scientifique Du Quebec Ltee. 418-847-5225
2160 Rue De Celles, Quebec G2C 1X8 Canada
Various controllers,seating systems,power bases and other components for wheelch

Gerber Chair Mates, Inc. 814-269-9531
1171 Ringling Ave, Johnstown, PA 15902
$310.00-$345.00 SWING-AWAY amputee stump support attaches to front rigging of the wheelchair, has horizontal adjustment for varied stump length, vertical adjustment for cushion thickness and swing-away action for ease in transfer.

Invacare Corporation 800-333-6900
1 Invacare Way, Elyria, OH 44035
INVACARE.

Kenda American Airless 800-248-4737
7120 Americana Pkwy, Reynoldsburg, OH 43068
Airless inner tubes for wheelchair tires, airless tires for wheelchairs, SUPERLITE combination caster wheel tire & bearing, standard pneumatic wheelchair tires (all sizes), INNTERTHANES for 3 & 4 wheel carts; also available, pneumatic tires and inner tires for all sizes.

Magic Wheels, Inc. 206-282-0760
3837 13th Ave W Ste 104, Seattle, WA 98119
2-speed manual wheelchair.

Mrc Industries Inc. 516-328-6900
85 Denton Ave, New Hyde Park, NY 11040
Various types of cushions.

Nova Health Products, Llc 843-673-0702
1138 Annelle Dr, Florence, SC 29505
Various components for wheelchairs.

Sunrise Medical Hhg Inc 303-218-4505
6724 Preston Ave # 1, Livermore, CA 94551

Sunrise Medical Hhg Inc 303-218-4505
2615 W Casino Rd # 2B, Everett, WA 98204

Sunrise Medical Hhg Inc 303-218-4505
2842 N Business Park Ave, Fresno, CA 93727

Tuffcare 800-367-6160
3999 E La Palma Ave, Anaheim, CA 92807

210 Innovations, Llc
34 Taugwonk Spur Rd Unit 10, Stonington, CT 06378
Various types of wheelchair components.

COMPOUND, RESINOUS, COMPOSITE *(Dental And Oral) 76VLQ*

Danville Materials 800-827-7940
3420 Fostoria Way Ste A200, San Ramon, CA 94583
Starflow & Accolade flowable composites. High compressive strength, excellent esthetics.

Essential Dental Systems, Inc. 800-223-5394
89 Leuning St, South Hackensack, NJ 07606

George Taub Products & Fusion Co., Inc. 800-828-2634
277 New York Ave, Jersey City, NJ 07307
DE-TAK 15cc Liquid in self dispensing bottle, use it to prevent composite resin from sticking to placement instruments.

COMPOUND, RESINOUS, COMPOSITE *(cont'd)*

Purified Protein, Inc. 866-339-6589
3443 Tripp Ct, San Diego, CA 92121
Calcium phosphate and other compounds contracted for.

Vident 800-828-3839
3150 E Birch St, Brea, CA 92821
3D-Direct universal composite in 3D-Master shades.

COMPRESS, COLD *(General) 80QLW*

Armstrong Medical Industries, Inc. 800-323-4220
575 Knightsbridge Pkwy, Lincolnshire, IL 60069

Balance Systems, Inc. 1-888-274-5444
1644 Plaza Way Ste 317, Walla Walla, WA 99362
Self-cooling compression wrap.

Bruder Healthcare Company 888-827-8337
3150 Engineering Pkwy, Alpharetta, GA 30004
Conforming, Soothing Cold Packs, Assorted Shapes and Sizes

Certified Safety Manufacturing 800-854-7474
1400 Chestnut Ave, Kansas City, MO 64127
CERTI-COOL.

Cincinnati Sub-Zero Products, Inc., Medical Division 800-989-7373
12011 Mosteller Rd, Cincinnati, OH 45241
Cold therapy systems for post-surgical applications help to reduce edema and promote faster rehabilitation. Products include CSZ's Electri-Cool II and Portable Cold Therapy Unit. Temperature Therapy pads are available in a variety of configurations for many applications.

Cryopak Industries, Inc. 800-667-2532
1055 Derwent Way, Delta, BC V3M 5R4 Canada
Flexible when frozen, freezer safe, reusable, nontoxic. Available in different sizes.

Dura-Kold Corp. 800-541-7199
3525 S Purdue St, Oklahoma City, OK 73179
Reusable compression ice wraps for in- and out-patient orthopedic surgical procedures and rehabilitation, providing up to 2 hours of cold compression.

Larkotex Company 800-972-3037
1002 Olive St, Texarkana, TX 75501
Extra wide commode, constructed of 1' heavy-gauge steel with solid welds and a white epoxy finish. 850 pound test capacity, seat width is 24', seat height is 19'.

Ludlow Technological Products 800-445-5025
2 Ludlow Park Dr, Chicopee, MA 01022
Hot and cold comnpress products.

Micro-Aire Surgical Instruments, Inc. 800-722-0822
1641 Edlich Dr, Charlottesville, VA 22911

Ortholine 800-243-3351
13 Chapel St, Norwalk, CT 06850
Trulife Cold Therapy Systems. Micro cool thermoelectric device. Cold Therapy Coolers and special design blankets. ACTIVE-ICE cold therapy products.

Precision Therapeutics, Inc. 800-544-0076
8400 E Prentice Ave Ste 700, Greenwood Village, CO 80111
$9.00 to $4.25 for SOFT PACK, hot or cold compress, reusable, various sizes; also available, from $2.19 for SOFT ICE, hot or cold compress, reusable, various sizes.

Romaine, Inc. D.B.A. Koldcare 800-294-7101
2026 Sterling Ave, Elkhart, IN 46516
KOLD COMPRESS Freezable, flexible cold pads for use on neck and lumbar area. Comes in two sizes, 4' x 9' and 9' x 13'. Product is non-toxic and reusable up to 3 years.

COMPRESS, GAUZE *(General) 80QLX*

Certified Safety Manufacturing 800-854-7474
1400 Chestnut Ave, Kansas City, MO 64127

Protector Canada Inc. 800-268-6594
1111 Flint Rd., Unit 23, Toronto, ON M3J 3C7 Canada

COMPRESS, MOIST HEAT *(Physical Med) 89QLY*

Armstrong Medical Industries, Inc. 800-323-4220
575 Knightsbridge Pkwy, Lincolnshire, IL 60069

Medi Inc 800-225-8634
75 York Ave, P.O. Box 302, Randolph, MA 02368
Reusable unit.

Micro-Aire Surgical Instruments, Inc. 800-722-0822
1641 Edlich Dr, Charlottesville, VA 22911

COMPRESS, MOIST HEAT *(cont'd)*

Polar Products, Inc. 800-763-8423
540 S Main St Ste 951, Akron, OH 44311
Professional quality moist heat wraps that use non-organic, no-odor therapeutic beads to collect moisture from humidity in the air. These beads will never break down or become rancid as wraps using barley or other organic fill can.

COMPRESSION INSTRUMENT *(Orthopedics) 87HWN*

Abbott Spine, Inc. 847-937-6100
12708 Riata Vista Cir Ste B-100, Austin, TX 78727
Compression instrument.

Aci Medical, Inc. 800-667-9451
1857 Diamond St, San Marcos, CA 92078
ArtAssist(R) increases arterial blood flow by applying intermittent pneumatic compression to the foot, ankle and calf. This therapeutic device helps patients with peripheral arterial disease including non-surgical candidates, diabetic and non-diabetic arterial ulcers, intermittent claudication and rest pain.

Aircast Llc 800-321-9549
1430 Decision St, Vista, CA 92081
Cyro/Cuff cold and compression system.

Alimed, Inc. 800-225-2610
297 High St, Dedham, MA 02026

Bio Compression Systems, Inc. 800-888-0908
120 W Commercial Ave, Moonachie, NJ 07074
SEQUENTIAL CIRCULATOR lymphedema pumps, cold compression pumps for edema and gradient compression pumps.

Biodermis Corp. 800-322-3729
6000 S Eastern Ave Ste 9D, Las Vegas, NV 89119
EPIFOAM Post Operative Compression Foam Device; post-operative compress foam device after lipectomy procedures.

Biomet, Inc. 574-267-6639
56 E Bell Dr, PO Box 587, Warsaw, IN 46582
Compression device.

Circulator Boot Corp. 610-240-9980
72 Pennsylvania Ave, Malvern, PA 19355
Plastic double-walled leg bags, rigid boot (3 sizes). Canvas legging. Compression instrument. Task specific ECG monitor. All components function together as circulatory assist, limb circulatory assist and/or as venous assist/lymph return unit.

DJO Inc. 800-336-6569
1430 Decision St, Vista, CA 92081

Interventional Spine, Inc. 800-497-0484
13700 Alton Pkwy Ste 160, Irvine, CA 92618
Various types of compression instruments.

K2m, Inc. 866-526-4171
751 Miller Dr SE Ste F1, Leesburg, VA 20175
Compressor.

Lenox-Maclaren Surgical Corp. 720-890-9660
657 S Taylor Ave Ste A, Colorado Technology Center
Louisville, CO 80027
Instrument, compression (pliers).

Luckman Corporation 215-659-1664
1930 Old York Rd, Abington, PA 19001
T-BOLT III dental air compressors.

Medtronic Sofamor Danek Instrument Manufacturing 901-396-3133
7375 Adrianne Pl, Bartlett, TN 38133
Plate and screw compression devices.

Medtronic Sofamor Danek Usa, Inc. 901-396-3133
4340 Swinnea Rd, Memphis, TN 38118
Plate and screw compression devices.

Richardson Products, Inc. 888-928-7297
9408 Gulfstream Rd, Frankfort, IL 60423
Volumeter.

Warsaw Orthopedic, Inc. 901-396-3133
2500 Silveus Xing, Warsaw, IN 46582
Plate and screw compression devices.

Zimmer Holdings, Inc. 800-613-6131
1800 W Center St, PO Box 708, Warsaw, IN 46580

Zimmer Spine, Inc. 800-655-2614
7375 Bush Lake Rd, Minneapolis, MN 55439
Compression instrument.

Zimmer Trabecular Metal Technology 800-613-6131
10 Pomeroy Rd, Parsippany, NJ 07054
Patella clamp.

COMPRESSION UNIT, INTERMITTENT (ANTI-EMBOLISM PUMP)
(Cardiovascular) 74QLZ

Brotherston Homecare Inc., Pxi Div. 800-695-9729
1388 Bridgewater Rd, Bensalem, PA 19020
Pneumatic compression paddle, priced $225.00.

Chattanooga Group 800-592-7329
4717 Adams Rd, Hixson, TN 37343
PRESSION single chamber and sequential.

Freeman Manufacturing Company 800-253-2091
900 W Chicago Rd, PO Box J, Sturgis, MI 49091
Sixteen inflatable polyurethane garments are available.

Huntleigh Healthcare Llc. 800-223-1218
40 Christopher Way, Eatontown, NJ 07724
4 models: $410.00 (homecare), $630.00 (sequential), $750.00 (anti-embolism) and $2,900 (hospital).

COMPRESSOR, AIR, PORTABLE *(Anesthesiology) 73BTI*

Air Techniques, Inc. 800-247-8324
1295 Walt Whitman Rd, Melville, NY 11747
AIRDENT II air abrasion unit.

Allied Healthcare Products, Inc. 800-444-3954
1720 Sublette Ave, Saint Louis, MO 63110
Medical.

Bvs, Inc. 877-877-4821
949 Poplar Road, Honey Brook, PA 19344-0250
Diaphragm air compressors with electronic unloader and solid-state control to prevent motor burn-out from overload.

Cardinal Health 207, Inc. 610-862-0800
1100 Bird Center Dr, Palm Springs, CA 92262
Portable air compressor.

Dansereau Health Products, Inc. 800-423-5657
250 E Harrison St, Corona, CA 92879
Dental air compressor, DHP Precision 101 priced at $1,895.00. DHP Precision 202 at $2,995.00

Dntlworks Equipment Corporation 800-847-0694
7300 S Tucson Way, Centennial, CO 80112
Three models of portable dental compressors with air reservoirs are available. These powerful, oil-free units are clean, quiet and efficient. Combine them with any of our portable delivery units.

Emepe International, Inc. 813-994-9690
18108 Sugar Brooke Dr, Tampa, FL 33647
Large, for pipeline system, and portable, for hospital respiratory therapy. Also, smaller units for homecare (nebulizer).

Enviro Guard, Inc. 800-438-1152
201 Shannon Oaks Cir Ste 115, Cary, NC 27511

Frank Scholz X-Ray Corp. 508-586-8308
244 Liberty St, Brockton, MA 02301
$570.00 per unit (standard).

Hamilton Medical, Inc. 800-426-6331
4990 Energy Way, Reno, NV 89502
VENTILAIR II compressor, air, purrable.

Invacare Corporation 800-333-6900
1 Invacare Way, Elyria, OH 44035
INVACARE Aspirator 50 PSI Compressor.

Jun-Air Usa,Inc. 800-458-6247
1350 Abbott Ct, Buffalo Grove, IL 60089
For ophthalmologic use.

Mada, Inc. 800-526-6370
625 Washington Ave, Carlstadt, NJ 07072

Med Systems 800-345-9061
2631 Ariane Dr, San Diego, CA 92117
Model 2580 air compressor drives Model 2500 air percussor in home applications.

Medical Industries America Inc. 800-759-3038
2636 289th Pl, Adel, IA 50003
MAXI Priced from $360.00; for continuous 50 P.S.I. use.

Medsonic U.S.A., Inc. 716-565-1700
8865 Sheridan Dr, Clarence, NY 14031
WHISPER aerosol compressor.

Pegasus Research Corp. 877-632-0255
3505 Cadillac Ave Ste G5, Costa Mesa, CA 92626
Nebulizer/humidifier heater.

Phipps & Bird, Inc. 800-955-7621
1519 Summit Ave, Richmond, VA 23230
40 psi; fully adjustable; 14 lb weight.

COMPRESSOR, AIR, PORTABLE *(cont'd)*

Precision Medical, Inc. 800-272-7285
300 Held Dr, Northampton, PA 18067
50 psi, 14 lpm.

Repex Medical Products, Inc. 305-740-0133
5240 SW 64th Ave, Miami, FL 33155
Medical Air COmpressor

The Electrode Store 360-829-0400
PO Box 188, Enumclaw, WA 98022
$250.00-$475.00.

Thomas Products Division 920-457-4891
3524 Washington Ave, Sheboygan, WI 53081

COMPRESSOR, CARDIAC, EXTERNAL *(Cardiovascular) 74DRM*

Advanced Circulatory Systems, Inc. 952-947-9590
7615 Golden Triangle Dr Ste A, Eden Prairie, MN 55344
Compression-de-compression cpr.

Huntleigh Healthcare Llc. 800-223-1218
40 Christopher Way, Eatontown, NJ 07724

Zoll Circulation 800-321-4277
249 Humboldt Ct, Sunnyvale, CA 94089
Automatic mechanical chest compressor.

COMPRESSOR, EXTERNAL, CARDIAC, POWERED
(General) 80FQI

Brunswick Laboratories 800-362-3482
50 Commerce Way, Norton, MA 02766
Chest compressions and lung ventilations. Displaced manual CPR. LSL (Life Support Litter) - Transport device with capability of conducting CPR during transport.

Dencraft 800-328-9729
PO Box 57, Moorestown, NJ 08057
A/R

COMPRESSOR, ORBITAL *(Ophthalmology) 86HOA*

Abinitio Holdings, Inc. 813-891-1889
5303 E Longboat Blvd, Tampa, FL 33615
Band eye (tm).

COMPUTER AND SOFTWARE, MEDICAL *(General) 80LNX*

Alaska Native Tribal Health Consortium 907-729-1900
4000 Ambassador Dr, Anchorage, AK 99508
Computers and software, medical.

Allscripts-Misys Healthcare Solutions 919-847-8102
222 Merchandise Mart Plz Ste 2024, Chicago, IL 60654
Software and hardware to manage appointment scheduling, patient billing, claims processing, collections, computerized patient records and EDI.

American Medical Software 800-423-8836
PO Box 236, Edwardsville, IL 62025
Our HIPAA-ready AMS Practice Management PLUS System includes the Medical Management System for billing with electronic claims filing, integrated Electronic Medical Records System, Appointment Scheduling Module, and Handheld Pocket PC Module.

Ampronix, Inc. 800-400-7972
15 Whatney, Irvine, CA 92618
Ampronix carries a full line-up of Medical grade monitors. CRT based displays from 8'-24' diag, featuring landscape & portrait models from Barco, Sony, Chromomaxx, DataRay, Modalixx, Medvix, Clinton and others.

Analytic Bio-Chemistries Laboratory 757-224-0177
1680 Loretta Ave Ste D, Feasterville Trevose, PA 19053
3.5 inch floppy disk.

Antek Healthware, Inc. 800-359-0911
228 Business Center Dr, Reisterstown, MD 21136
LabDAQ, laboratory information system. LabDAQ LIS is a fully integrated Windows application. It is a PC based system for physician office labs, hospital and reference labs. DAQreporter provides physicians with lab and other testing results through a secure Internet port. DAQbilling Practice Management System is a complete system with integrated scheduling, billing and electronic claim submission, financial management (complete A/R) tools and a rules data base.

Areeda Assoc., Ltd. 323-653-5515
1160 Glen Arbor Ave, Los Angeles, CA 90041
Seemor.

Avreo, Inc. 800-354-0680
450 Azalea Road, Charleston, SC 29406
Picture Archiving and Communication system.

COMPUTER AND SOFTWARE, MEDICAL *(cont'd)*

Biomedix Inc. 877-854-0012
4215 White Bear Pkwy, Saint Paul, MN 55110
Custom Lab is a reporting, accreditation, and laboratory management package for non-invasive vascular exams. Features include auto-generated interpretations; ICD9 and CPT coding; Data export to ICAVL Accreditation Software; and Business development graphics.

Clinicomp Intl. 800-350-8202
9655 Towne Centre Dr, San Diego, CA 92121
Clinician Documentation System with EMR

Csam, Inc. 563-359-7917
1890 14th St, Bettendorf, IA 52722
Urea kinetic modeling software.

Curlin Medical, Inc. 714-893-2200
15751 Graham St, Huntington Beach, CA 92649
Software interface.

Dome Imaging Systems, Inc. 866-752-6271
400 5th Ave, Waltham, MA 02451
Planar--a global leader in medical display solutions--offers the Invitium, a revolutionary point-of-care workstation. The Invitium provides a unique level of patient safety and comfort, as well as ease of use for hospital staff. It meets the stringent UL 2601 and IEC 60601 certifications, ensuring a level of safety greater than that provided by most standard electronic equipment. Portable and compact, the Invitium offers truly superior system flexibility. Both the Tk7 workstation and the Tn4 thin client models consist of a computer and a flat-panel monitor, all neatly packaged in a soft-white form factor that blends in with clinical environments. The computer and monitor can be mounted on desk stands, mobile carts, arm mounts, or wall mounts for flexibility and optimal use of limited space. The computer's rugged exterior withstands impact, and its fluid-resistant enclosure protects the system from spills and leaks, in compliance with the IPX1 standard. The enclosure material is also designed to withstand cleaning with hospital-grade disinfectants. The monitor is a 15-inch, color active-matrix liquid-crystal display (AMLCD). It includes an acrylic overlay for protection from punctures or scratches, and can also include an optional touchscreen. The Invitium provides a substantial variety of ports for connecting peripheral devices. It can provide wireless or 10/100-base-T Ethernet connectivity. It also supports sound through speakers and amplifiers that are built into the monitor. The entire system can be powered by either a single power supply or an optional battery system.

Draeger Medical Systems, Inc. 215-660-2626
16 Electronics Ave, Danvers, MA 01923
Multiple.

Etreby Computer Company, Inc. 800-843-7988
2145 W La Palma Ave, Anaheim, CA 92801
APOTHECARE-2000 Pharmaceutical Care Software. Therapy assessment and clinical information and documentation software. Disease managment protocols and pharmacist care plans assist in setting therapeutic goals, intervention, and outcome monitoring.

Healthmark, Inc. 971-236-9171
8440 SE Sunnybrook Blvd Ste 210, Clackamas, OR 97015
Computers and software, medical.

Impac Medical Systems, Inc. 888-464-6722
100 W Evelyn Ave, Mountain View, CA 94041
PowerPath, Anatomic Pathology System ---IntelliLab, Laboratory Information System ---Cancer Registry Systems

Imsi, Integrated Modular Systems Inc. 800-220-9729
2500 W Township Line Rd, PO Box 616, Havertown, PA 19083
Teleradiology, PACS, RIS, Mini-RIS, DICOM and HL7 Interfaces, Mammo-Tracking, Voice Recognition, Remote Transcription, etc...

Infosys, Inc. 800-978-4636
1821 Walden Office Sq Ste 350, Schaumburg, IL 60173
Practice/clinic; rehabilitation rural health. Medsys practice medical management Windows-based software offers integrated scheduling, billing, A/R report, managed care and electronic claims. Single-user systems start at $3000, including training & support. Also available, Rehabilitation and Physical Therapy and Nursing Homes and Assisted Living Software.

July Soft 800-350-7693
610 E Knox Dr, Tucson, AZ 85705
REMINDERPRO Appointment Confirmation System calls patients to remind them of appointments or needed services, in the voice of a familiar staff member.

COMPUTER AND SOFTWARE, MEDICAL *(cont'd)*

Laborie Medical Technologies Inc. 888-522-6743
6415 Northwest Dr., Units 7-14, Mississauga, ONT L4V-1X1 Canada
DELPHIS OFFICE: Office urodynamics system, Delphis Portable, portable urodynamics system. DOLPHIN: Dolphin patient management software.

Matrox Electronic Systems, Ltd. 800-804-6243
1055 St. Regis Blvd., Dorval, QUE H9P 2T4 Canada
Cost-effective high-performance hardware and software for developing machine vision, image analysis, and medical imaging applications.

Medical Soft, Inc. 937-293-2575
1800 Southwood Ln W, Dayton, OH 45419
Obstetric ultrasound software.

Medinotes Corporation 877-633-6683
1025 Ashworth Rd Ste 222, West Des Moines, IA 50265
Practice Panorama is an advanced tool for filtering medical data from the Charting Plus EMR system. This software can print multi-variable queries or export the data to Word, Excel, Access, or Crystal Reports.

Mindways Software, Inc. 512-912-0871
3001 S Lamar Blvd Ste 302, Austin, TX 78704
Medical computers and software.

MOS Plastics Inc. 408-944-9407
2308 Zanker Rd, San Jose, CA 95131

Neurotron Medical 609-896-3444
800 Silvia St, Ewing, NJ 08628
Computer software, medical data storage & management.

Nihon Kohden America, Inc. 800-325-0283
90 Icon, Foothill Ranch, CA 92610
Our family of products includes instrumentation for Epilepsy Monitoring, Electroencephalography, Ambulatory Recording for EEG/PSG, Polysomnography, Portable EEG/PSG, ICU/OR Monitoring, Electromyography and Evoked Potentials.

Nuclear Cardiology Systems, Inc. 303-541-0044
5660 Airport Blvd Ste 101, Boulder, CO 80301
Nuclear medicine spect computer.

Ortivus 800-537-3927
2324 Sweet Parkway Rd, PO Box 276, Decorah, IA 52101
EMS:Sweet-Billing, Sweet-Field Data, Sweet-CAD, Sweet-Online 'subscription' Billing. PUBLIC SAFETY:AVeL-CAD, AVeL-BASE, AVeL-MobiCAD, AVeL-RadioGATE

Radiology Information Systems, Inc. 703-713-3313
43676 Trade Center Pl Ste 100, Dulles, VA 20166
Ris scan view system.

Rahd Ocology Products / Electronic Services Mart, Inc. 314-524-0103
500 Airport Rd, Saint Louis, MO 63135
Radiation therapy treatment planning system.

Scientific Imaging, Inc. 303-681-9402
97 Slate Lane, Mt. Crested Butte, CO 81225
Nuclear medicine computer.

Spacelabs Medical Inc. 800-522-7212
5150 220th Ave SE, Issaquah, WA 98029
Various medical computer and software applications.

Surgical Information Systems, Inc. 678-507-1610
11605 Haynes Bridge Rd Ste 200, Alpharetta, GA 30009
Surgical information system.

Syntermed, Inc. 404-814-5277
3340 Peachtree Rd NE, Tower Place Ctr., Suite 1800
Atlanta, GA 30326
SPECT and PET studies.

COMPUTER AND SOFTWARE, MEDICAL *(cont'd)*

Thought Technology Ltd. 800-361-3651
2180 Belgrave Ave., Montreal, QUE H4A 2L8 Canada
ProComp Infiniti™ with BioGraph®Infiniti Software is a powerful clinical tool, designed in conjunction with some of the leading clinicians in the field. The system comes packaged with the Legacy and Multimodality Suites providing you with a variety of options for your client, with just one database. With this 8-channel system you can record EEG, EKG, EMG, Temperature, Skin Conductance, Heart Rate/Blood Volume Pulse, Respiration and Voltage, providing you with the most complete view of your client’s physiology. The system offers a variety of screens with an array of animations and audio feedbacks that you can change on the fly. The highly integrated system’s new features are high-speed channels, automatic sensor recognition, impedance checking and compact flash memory. The ability to switch between five screens during a session provides your client with the ultimate training experience. Powerful new audio features include split midi tracks, which allow your client’s brain to control a virtual orchestra instrument by instrument. EEG Coherence, video, event counters, discrete feedback and reward animations, and powerful trend reports are all part of the infinite ways you can evaluate and train your patients.*

Translite 281-240-3111
8410 Highway 90A, Sugar Land, TX 77478
Skin examination microscope.

Triple G Systems Group, Inc. 905-305-0041
600-3100 Steeles Ave E, Markham L3R 8T3 Canada
Laboratory information system

Vital Images,Inc. 800-231-0607
5850 Opus Pkwy Ste 300, Minnetonka, MN 55343
Vitrea 2 is advanced clinical software that allows clinicians to view CT and MR image data in 2D and 3D. The software allows for advanced diagnosis, less-invasive screening and improved treatment planning.

Vna Systems, Inc. 404-264-0160
1414 Epping Forest Dr NE, Atlanta, GA 30319
Computer cardiac catheterization laboratory (optical correlator).

Wr Medical Electronics Co. 800-321-6387
123 2nd St N, Stillwater, MN 55082
WR Test Works: Neurological Testing Management Software. Operating software for peripheral sensory and autonomic nervous-system characterization.

COMPUTER AND SOFTWARE, MEDICAL, OPHTHALMIC USE
(Ophthalmology) 86LQB

Carl Zeiss Meditec Inc. 877-486-7473
5160 Hacienda Dr, Dublin, CA 94568
HUMPHREY ATLAS CORNEAL TOPOGRAPHY SYSTEM WITH MASTERVUE SOFTWARE with a small, 12x18 in. footprint, 8,000 datapoints, a powerful computer, and superior central and peripheral coverage, the highly accurate, affordable and portable ATLAS is the right fit for every office. Hardware features include ethernet and modem for LAN compatibility and exam transfer. Optional software includes Advanced Refractive Diagnostics, PRK Simulated Ablation, and Healing Trend Display as well as MASTERFIT Contact Lens Fitting Module.

Lc Technologies, Inc. 800-393-4293
1483 Chain Bridge Rd Ste 104, McLean, VA 22101
Eyegaze communication system.

Topcon Medical Systems, Inc. 800-223-1130
37 W Century Rd, Paramus, NJ 07652
Diagnostic software: $600.00 for color-mapping software; a family of IMAGEnet products including IMAGEnet Professional, IMAGEnet Lite, IMAGEnet EZ Lite, and Auto Mosaic for multi-field imaging (please call for current pricing).

COMPUTER EQUIPMENT *(General) 80VAX*

Actall Corp. 800-598-1745
3925 Monaco Pkwy Unit D, Denver, CO 80207
THEFT ALERT II, Computer security - wireless and fully supervised. Crisis Controller, security system software, wireless.

American Medical Software 800-423-8836
PO Box 236, Edwardsville, IL 62025
IBM or compatible computers available to turnkey with medical software.

Amrel / American Reliance, Inc. 800-654-9838
11801 Goldring Rd, Arcadia, CA 91006
Rugged mobile computers including notebook and tablet PCs

COMPUTER EQUIPMENT *(cont'd)*

Analogic Corporation 978-326-4000
8 Centennial Dr, Peabody, MA 01960
Data acquisition boards.

Ansoft Corp. 412-261-3200
225 W Station Square Dr Ste 200, Pittsburgh, PA 15219

Anthro Corporation 800-325-3841
10450 SW Manhasset Dr, Tualatin, OR 97062
Specifically, computer furniture.

Biocomp Research Institute 800-246-3526
6542 Hayes Dr, Los Angeles, CA 90048
$11,995.00 for Biocomp 4 channel system includes computer system with VGA monitor, enhanced keyboard, 5 1/4 in. floppy, 3 1/2 in. floppy, 30 megabyte hard disk, dot matrix printer; $18,990.00 for Biocomp 8 channel system with VGA monitor, enhanced keyboard, 5 1/4 in. floppy, 3 1/2 in. floppy, 30 megabyte hard disk, dot matrix printer. Computer upgrades available.

Biofeedback Instrument Corp. 212-222-5665
255 W 98th St Apt 3D, New York, NY 10025
$3,000 for computerized biofeedback system, $4,000 for computerized muscle scanner EMG, Resp, Temp, SCL, HR. Also, Procomp Infiniti 8 channel computerized biofeedback system, $5700, Heart Tracker - $395.00, HeartScanner - $1495; $6,000 for Orion/Perry incontinence computerized system. $3,000 for Myotrac 3g incontinence system. Mindset QEEG/neuromap - $2195-16ch; $2995 - 24Ch.

Buxco Research Systems 910-794-6980
219 Station Rd Ste 202, Wilmington, NC 28405
Data loggers, scrolling monitors, extended analysis.

Datascope Corp. 800-288-2121
14 Philips Pkwy, Montvale, NJ 07645
Central station monitoring system including dual trace recorder, mouse, keyboard, central processing unit, flat panel or CRT display. Optional features: 1 hour, 24 hour or 72 hour disclosures, arrhythmia detection and CIS/HIS interface. Also available is Visa II, a central station monitoring system including dual trace, recorder, mouse, keyboard, central processing unit, arrhythmia detection, flat panel or CRT display. Optional features: 24 hour disclosure, paging, networking, remote view station, vital access, T-link, and ST segment analysis.

Delta Products Corp. 510-668-5100
4405 Cushing Pkwy, Fremont, CA 94538
Data storage and accessories. Chip inductors, resister networks.

Digital Dynamics, Inc. 800-765-1288
5 Victor Sq, Scotts Valley, CA 95066
K-Series K6 Industrial PC, ruggedized PC for harsh environments.

Ekeg Electronics Co. Ltd. 604-857-0828
PO Box 46199, Stn. D, Vancouver, BC V6J 5G5 Canada
Expanded computer keyboard and mouse for persons with severe motor disabilities.

Epix, Inc. 847-465-1818
381 Lexington Dr, Buffalo Grove, IL 60089
PC-computer compatible imaging boards with extensive image capture, processing, and display capabilities. Commonly used in CT, MRI, and ultrasound imaging.

Fleetwood Group, Incorporated 800-257-6390
PO Box 1259, Holland, MI 49422
$400 to $500 for wheelchair accessible computer workstations. Computer tables also available.

Flo Healthcare 877-356-4040
5801 Goshen Springs Rd Ste A, Norcross, GA 30071

Humanware 800-722-3393
175 Mason Cir, Concord, CA 94520
Kurzweil text-to-speech scanning systems include KURZWEIL 1000 full-function reading system for the blind.

Imsi, Integrated Modular Systems Inc. 800-220-9729
2500 W Township Line Rd, PO Box 616, Havertown, PA 19083
MED WEBGATE, Internet accessible radiology information system.

Insiphil (Us) Llc 408-616-8700
650 Vaqueros Ave Ste F, Sunnyvale, CA 94085
Computer equipment for sight impaired people (blind), incl. talking unit.

COMPUTER EQUIPMENT *(cont'd)*

Kaypentax 800-289-5297
2 Bridgewater Ln, Lincoln Park, NJ 07035
VISI-PITCH IV, Model 3950 is an integrated, hardware and software PC-based system that provides simple, innovative real-time displays of important speech/voice parameters for visual feedback and the ability to make quantitative measurements to track therapy progress. Swallowing Workstation, Model 7200, is a unique combination of diverse technologies integrated into a powerful modular system to assist clinicians in performing exams and monitoring, in real time, of the swallowing process.

Kem Medical Products Corp. 800-553-0330
75 Price Pkwy, Farmingdale, NY 11735
Sterile Processing Microsystems is a bar code driven microcomputer system for tracking surgical instruments, labor productivity, etc.

Lionville Systems, Inc. 800-523-7114
501 Gunnard Carlson Dr, Coatesville, PA 19320
iCarts Support Mobile Computing and Bar Code Charting Systems. The ergonomically designed iCart combines the security features of a medication cart with the timesaving efficiency of bedside computingÓ

Medical Marketplace 760-242-4171
18737 US Highway 18 Ste 5A, Apple Valley, CA 92307
Mobile MRI, CT and Nuclear Medicine equipment, as well as Ultrasound systems, and numerous other diagnostic imaging equipment solutions.

Mercury Computer Systems, Inc. 978-256-1300
201 Riverneck Rd, Chelmsford, MA 01824

Modulus Data Systems, Inc. 888-663-8547
386 Main St Ste 200, Redwood City, CA 94063
UROCOMP CYTOCOMP $1,295 for urine microscopy terminal and $1,395 for cytology terminal. MODULUS LIS $100,000.00 to $800,000.00 DIFFCOUNT III $529.00 to $649.00 per unit (standard). COMP-U-DIFF $1,250.00 to $649.00 per unit (standard). DIFFCOUNT III $529.00 to $649.00 per unit (standard). UROCOCOMP $1,395.00 to $1,895.00 for urinalysis or cytology workstation.

Polar Electro Inc. 1-800-227-1314
1111 Marcus Ave Ste M15, New Hyde Park, NY 11042

Quality Systems, Inc. 800-888-7955
18111 Von Karman Ave Ste 600, Irvine, CA 92612

Ramco Innovations/ Sunx Sensors 800-280-6933
PO Box 65310, 1207 Maple Street, West Des Moines, IA 50265
Data acquisition and handling systems.

Scc Soft Computer 800-763-8352
5400 Tech Data Dr, Clearwater, FL 33760
SOFTA/R, Offers advanced features to meet the specific billing requirements of a clinical environment. Automated online features include medical necessity checking, bundling and unbundling, payor defined and 72 hour rule billing.

Smead Manufacturing Co. 1-88-USE-SMEAD
600 Smead Blvd, Hastings, MN 55033
SMEADLINK Records Management Software System, Imaging.

Swisslog Translogic Corporation 800-525-1841
10825 E 47th Ave, Denver, CO 80239
Computer control, hardware and software package for computerized pneumatic tube system.

Tash International Inc. 800-463-5685
91 Station St., Unit 1, Ajax, ONT L1S 3H2 Canada
$150 to $700 for computer keyboard emulators; $375 to $900 for expanded keyboards.

Tegrant Corporation, Protexic Brands 800-289-9966
800 5th Ave, P.O. Box 448, New Brighton, PA 15066
Fasteners for securing component parts.

Tekscan, Inc. 800-248-3669
307 W 1st St, South Boston, MA 02127

U.F.I. 805-772-1203
545 Main St Ste C2, Morro Bay, CA 93442
$550.00 for SLIC 8000.

White Systems, Inc. 800-275-1442
30 Boright Ave, Kenilworth, NJ 07033
Software file storage units and tracking devices.

COMPUTER SOFTWARE *(General) 80VBH*

Academy Savant 800-472-8268
PO Box 3670, Fullerton, CA 92834
Computer-based training for the lab, including chromatography; spectroscopy; general lab techniques and safety; fundamentals of atomic absorbtion spectrometry; fundamentals of inductively coupled plasma spectrometry; mass spectrometry fundamentals (includes computer software, video, and manual); SpectraBook, Volumes 1 & 2 (software teaches principles of interpretation for IR, H NMR, Mass Spec, and 13C NMR (PC/Windows or Macintosh)); introduction to gas chromatography; Introduccion A La Cromatografia De Gases (Spanish/English bilingual edition. Fundamentals of Gas Chromatography/Mass Spectrometry includes resolution optimization, column types, inlet systems for packed and capillary columns, enrichment techniques, interfaces, ionization modes, mass filters, data acquisition, and qualitative and quantitative analysis. HPLC Training Pro Series: HPLC interactive training and troubleshooting software modules include Introduction, Method Development, Equipment, Troubleshooting, Separation Modes, Calculations Assistant and Identification, Quantification Techniques of HPLC, and Introduction To LC/MS. Software teaches the combined techniques of liquid chromatography and mass spectrometry: HPLC separation modes and equipment; MS inlets, and ionization modes. Runs under Windows on PC.

Accu-Med Services 800-777-9141
300 Techne Center Dr, Milford, OH 45150
Marketing software. Windows software to cost a prospective resident prior to admission, prepare MDS, care plans progress. Contact manager to market programs and follow-ups with discharge planners. Therapy management system for rehabilitation workflow and information.

Achieve Healthcare Technologies 800-869-1322
7690 Golden Triangle Dr, Eden Prairie, MN 55344
Clinical and financial software and IT services for the long-term care industry.

Activant Solutions Inc. 800-776-7438
19 W College Ave, Yardley, PA 19067
Medical distribution software.

Advanced American Biotechnology (Aab) 714-870-0290
1166 E Valencia Dr Unit 6C, Fullerton, CA 92831
$2,865 for DNA programs (Apple & IBM); also, $995 for 1-D and 2-D analysis program software to re-analyze any 1-D and 2-D separation, $995 for 3-D reconstruction program software to stack CAT, NMR images.

Aesculap Implant Systems Inc. 1-800-234-9179
3773 Corporate Pkwy, Center Valley, PA 18034
INSTA-COUNT computerized program for management of surgical instrumentation.

Algor, Inc. 800-48-ALGOR
150 Beta Dr, Pittsburgh, PA 15238
Algor Design and Finite Element Analysis Software offers a range of FEA capabilities including Mechanical Event Simulation, linear and nonlinear stress, vibration and natural frequencies, heat transfer, electrostatics, fluid flow, piping design and composite materials. Algor's Mechanical Event Simulation family of products realistically simulates motion and flexing in mechanical events of an FEA model, eliminating the need to input a force and computes and shows resulting stresses on the computer model at each instant in time. Algor's InCAD family helps egineers create more reliable products in less time by providing seamless interoperability between CAD and Algor's full range of modeling, FEA and Mechanical Event Simulation software products. Algor's PIPEPAK provides piping design, analysis, visualization, and reporting.

Allscripts-Misys Healthcare Solutions 919-847-8102
222 Merchandise Mart Plz Ste 2024, Chicago, IL 60654
Integrated medical-software packages.

American Orthodontics Corp. 800-558-7687
1714 Cambridge Ave, Sheboygan, WI 53081
PHOTO-EZE, orthodontic software.

Arrhythmia Research Technology, Inc. 978-345-0181
25 Sawyer Passway, Fitchburg, MA 01420
PREDICTOR 7 software: signal-averaging electrocardiography software; sophisticated, high-resolution, comprehensive acquisition and analysis workstation.

Aspyra, Inc. 800-437-9000
26115 Mureau Rd Ste A, Calabasas, CA 91302

COMPUTER SOFTWARE *(cont'd)*

Base4 877-246-2424
601-6299 Airport Rd, Mississauga, ON L4V 1N3 Canada
On-site information systems management, customized programming and specialized products. PHARMATRIX, and integrated solution to aid in scientific discovery and development and to facilitate virtual collaboration and knowledge management. ALLIANCE MANAGER, manages alliances through a secure, third party. Complete audit version control for managing intelectual property.

Baxa Corporation 800-567-2292
9540 S Maroon Circle, Suite 400, Englewood, CO 80112
ABACUS TPN Calculation Software complements Baxa hardware for a complete state-of-the-art system for automated sterile compounding.

Beckman Coulter, Inc. 800-742-2345
250 S Kraemer Blvd, PO Box 8000, Brea, CA 92821

Berkeley Nucleonics Corp. 800-234-7858
2955 Kerner Blvd, San Rafael, CA 94901
DOSE RATE v.2 software package allows users to detect peak dose rates, average dose rates and store results. This new utility requires three seconds to perform acquisition, analysis, identification and software algorithm optimization. Users can review full dose rate calculations and isotope specific calculations simultaneously in real time. Also including model 6899 for field printing of MCA reports using battery-powered systems. This is the first MCA to offer users the ability to print without the need of a computer.

Bio-Optics, Inc. 503-493-8000
1525 NE 41st Ave, Portland, OR 97232
BAMBI and THUMPER For assessing the health of corneas for diagnosis and transplantation by shape and size of cells and cell loss by computerized morphometric analysis system.

Bioclinica, Inc. 800-748-9032
826 Newtown Yardley Rd Ste 101, Newtown, PA 18940
Image processing software.

Biocomp Research Institute 800-246-3526
6542 Hayes Dr, Los Angeles, CA 90048
$11,995.00 for Biocomp 4 channel system includes computer system with VGA monitor, enhanced keyboard, 5 1/4 in. floppy, 3 1/2 in. floppy, 30 megabyte hard disk, dot matrix printer; $18,990.00 for Biocomp 8 channel system with VGA monitor, enhanced keyboard, 5 1/4 in. floppy, 3 1/2 in. floppy, 30 megabyte hard disk, dot matrix printer. Computer upgrades available.

Bose Corporation - Electroforce Systems Group 800-273-0437
10250 Valley View Rd Ste 113, Eden Prairie, MN 55344
WinTest® Control Software & Software Updates, an intuitive design allows quick test set-ups and the flexible hardware & software platform allows for multiple axis, sensors & virtually any chamber control configuration. WinTest® Version 4.0 software, to be released in the late summer 2007, includes 4 major user and test performance features to enhance your laboratory's productivity.

Bradley Company, A Sub. Of Xerox Corporation 216-292-7220
4829 Galaxy Pkwy, Cleveland, OH 44128
Inventory software automates response time to orders. Features include ordering picktickets, receipt tracking and on-line catalogue. Priced from $65K. Purchasing software tracks regular and blanket purchase orders on-line. Priced from $45K. Forms Management software for complete thorough forms specifications, state verification, security levels, reporting for physical and electronic forms. Priced from 25K. Demand Print software; enterprise-side application automates orders to form's job ticket and image and then routes it electronically to networked publishing system. Priced from $50K. Spectrum Plus software streamlines the production and distribution process for traditional documents, print on demand items, electronic forms and other supplies. Modules include web-based requisitioning, inventory control, purchasing, print on demand, kit management, job tracking, forms management.

Buxco Research Systems 910-794-6980
219 Station Rd Ste 202, Wilmington, NC 28405
Acquisition system tissue and cardio-pulmonary mechanics.

California Scientific 800-284-8112
4005 Seaport Blvd, West Sacramento, CA 95691
BrainMaker for designing, building, training, testing, and running neural networks. Artificial neural networks use a simplified version of the brain's architecture to duplicate many of the brain's most useful abilities, such as pattern recognition, trend analysis, and generalized learning from any set of data. Fact files may be logically connected together to create very large databases. $195 for BrainMaker and $795 for BrainMaker Professional software.

COMPUTER SOFTWARE *(cont'd)*

Captiva Software Corporation 800-783-3378
601 Oakmont Ln Ste 200, Westmont, IL 60559
CODELINK contains all ICD-9-CM, CPT, and HCPCS codes; CODELINK PLUS contains Medicare regulations; and CODELINK PROFESSIONAL contains Medicare and usual-, customary-, and reasonable-fee information.

Cedaron Medical, Inc. 800-424-1007
PO Box 2100, Davis, CA 95617
Treatment Outcomes Software. Computer outcomes products for specialty medicines. Certified vendor for ACC and STS. Specialties include orthopaedics, cardiology, thoracic surgery, oncology, diabetes, stroke, rehab, etc.

Cerner Corp. 866-221-8877
2800 Rockcreek Pkwy, Kansas City, MO 64117
Cerner offers more than 60 solutions that span the healthcare continuum, from broad personal health records and electronic medical records to department-specific solutions (laboratory, radiology, etc.).

Chemsw, Inc. 800-536-0404
4771 Mangels Blvd, Fairfield, CA 94534
Software for environmental, water chemistry, chromatography, and biochemistry.

Clinical Reference Systems 800-237-8401
335 Interlocken Pkwy, Broomfield, CO 80021
Patient education software.

Compsee, Inc. 800-628-3888
400 N Main St, PO Box 1209, Mount Gilead, NC 27306
Bar code tracking software used in conjunction with a portable terminal for remote collection of item numbers via scanning of bar code labels.

Computers Unlimited 406-255-9500
2407 Montana Ave, Billings, MT 59101
Providing completely integrated TIMS software, managing every aspect of your business. From DMERC-certified processing to distribution sales, offering superior software, hardware, programming, training, and 24-hour customer service.

Computrition, Inc. 800-222-4488
19808 Nordhoff Pl, Chatsworth, CA 91311
Computrition offers completely integrated foodservice and nutrition care management software systems for the healthcare industry. Features include ingredient, recipe, & menu management and complete diet office automation, including automatic correction of patient menus for allergies, dislikes, diet order restrictions, and meal patterns.

Current Medicine Group Llc 800-427-1796
400 Market St Ste 700, Philadelphia, PA 19106
Database software.

Database, Inc. 919-493-6969
3100 Tower Blvd Ste 304, Durham, NC 27707
TLS - The Laboratory System. $50,000+ for clinical laboratory software system.

Db Consultants, Inc 610-847-5065
198 Tabor Rd, PO Box 580, Ottsville, PA 18942
AS/PC is a powerful, versatile, integrated medical billing, practice management, and patient information software system. It includes HIPAA-compliant electronic claims submission. More than 15,000 healthcare professionals rely on AS/PC daily for quality care.

Dicon, Inc. 800-426-0493
2355 S 1070 W, Salt Lake City, UT 84119
$3,000 for Fieldview analysis software. $4,000 for advanced Fieldview analysis software. Interactive CD-ROM, Pathways to Interpretation takes the mystery out of interpretation of visual fields.

Digisonics, Inc. 713-529-7979
3701 Kirby Dr Ste 930, Houston, TX 77098
Analysis of fetal growth, echocardiology, carotid/vascular ultasound, cardiac cath, pelvic ultrasound and infertility.

COMPUTER SOFTWARE *(cont'd)*

Dps, Inc. 800-654-4689
3685 Priority Way South Dr Ste 100, Indianapolis, IN 46240
DPS EXTEND utilizes the advanced capabilities of the IBM I-series to integrate sales order processing through inventory management/purchasing and all financial functions. K3S-REPLENISH, an inventory management software solution that features demand forcasting, seasonal profile and trending analysis, integrated alternate source buying, overstock and transfer functions, and multiple 'what if' simulators. DPS FLASH, e.business solution that helps you merge existing business processes and legacy systems with Web technology to provide on-line catalogs, order entry, order tracking and delivery status, on-line customer support, product availability checks, and more. DP5 BLAST, an e-business application written in Java that allows for bi-directional flow of information between your company headquarters and its affiliate offices, partners, or stores. Communication is secure and real-time, providing the ideal environment for 'e-collaboration'. DPS ZAP, a bar code or warehouse management system that streamlines every aspect of your warehouse operation, reducing many of the costs associated with warehousing. DPS ZAP provides real-time tools for tracking warehouse activities.

Drg International, Inc. 800-321-1167
1167 US Highway 22, Mountainside, NJ 07092
MEDIARC, computer software Holter; patient data archivization of ECG data.

Duxbury Systems, Inc. 978-692-3000
270 Littleton Rd Ste 6, Westford, MA 01886
Duxbury System's DBT is the standard for braille translator word-processing software. DBT has versions for Windows XP, Windows 95, Windows 98, Windows NT, Macintosh, and UNIX. This simple-looking software does the hard work of translating and formatting your print document into braille. Handles over 30 braille languages.

Endovia Medical, Inc. 781-255-1888
150 Kerry Pl, Norwood, MA 02062
Unique set of laparoscopic instruments that combine a robotic telemanipulator and artificial intelligence software to increase a surgeon's dexterity and transmit a sense of touch to the surgeon's hand.

Epic Systems Corp. 608-271-9000
1979 Milky Way, Verona, WI 53593
Epiccare ambulatory electronic medical record--comprehensive care-delivery tool with demonstrated return-on-investment benefits that provide proactive decision support, time-saving documentation tools, and streamlined workflows. Modular Epiccare inpatient electronic medical record facilitates data storage and retrieval in an acute-care workflow and streamlines the tasks which doctors and nurses perform every day. Epiccare Home Health automates home-care and hospice activities with remote access to important patient information and streamlined patient documentation. Nurse Call Center/Nurse Triage improves an organization's ability to triage calls by providing real-time access to valuable patient data. Epicweb light electronic medical record can be quickly and inexpensively installed to reduce costs by reducing chart pulls, eliminating redundant tests, and managing risk. Mychart empowers patients by providing them secure access to their records across all providers in an organization. Epiclink helps connect and enhance the relationships between an organization and providers at affiliated organizations.

Ericomp, Inc. 800-541-8471
10211 Pacific Mesa Blvd Ste 411, San Diego, CA 92121

Esha Research 503-585-6242
4747 Skyline Rd S Ste 100, Salem, OR 97306
The FOOD PROCESSOR nutrient analysis software generates an analysis of nutrition and fitness information for diets, menus, recipes and nutrient goals. Software shows diet excesses and deficiencies with personalized recommendations based on client's age, weight, sex, height and activity level. Call 1-800-659-3742 (ESHA) for free demo disk or download from http://www.esha.com

Etg Genesys Sales And Support 800-522-6331
2935 Crockett St, Fort Worth, TX 76107
GENESYS, computerized/software for lab information management.

Etreby Computer Company, Inc. 800-843-7988
2145 W La Palma Ave, Anaheim, CA 92801
ETREBY SYSTEM-2000 Pharmacy Management System is a retail pharmacy dispersing, billing, accounts receivable and telecommunications software.

Evergreen Research, Inc. 303-526-7402
433 Park Point Dr Ste 140, Golden, CO 80401

COMPUTER SOFTWARE *(cont'd)*

Fluke Biomedical 800-648-7952
6920 Seaway Blvd, Everett, WA 98203
Biomedical equipment management program and software for bar code printers;

Freedom Data Systems, Inc. 800-932-9000
228 Maple St Fl 1, Manchester, NH 03103
Pharmacy computer software and hardware.

Ge Medical Systems Information Technologies 800-643-6439
8200 W Tower Ave, Milwaukee, WI 53223

Gene Logic 800-436-3564
50 W Watkins Mill Rd, Gaithersburg, MD 20878
Software for compiling and evaluating databases of gene expression products.

Health Care Software, Inc. (Hcs) 800-524-1038
PO Box 2430, Farmingdale, NJ 07727
INTERACTANT fully integrated financial and clinical information systems exclusively for the healthcare industry.

Heartlab, Inc. 800-959-3205
1 Crosswind Dr, Westerly, RI 02891
The Agfa Heartlab Cardiovascular solution provides enterprise storage management and reporting for multiple modalities, long term archiving, web based access for anytime-anywhere access to information, and bi-directional electronic communication between clinical and hospital information systems.

Hex Laboratory Systems 800-729-2085
1042B N El Camino Real Ste 308, Encinitas, CA 92024
LAB/HEX is a fully integrated, multi-site, multi-tasking LIS. Ideal for independent laboratories, hospitals, clinics, veterinary and research. LAB/HEX automates all laboratory departments, including microbiology, cytology and pathology. Flexible and user-definable for Molecular Diagnostics, Cytogenetics and other specialty labs. Features include Cash Management, Electronic Claims, Remote Ordering, Faxing, Printing and Inquiry. VET/HEX is a full featured veterinary information system. LABCENTRAL is a Web-based order entry and result inquiry for medical laboratories and their providers. LABCENTRAL can be used with any LIS.

Hokanson Inc., D.E. 800-999-8251
12840 NE 21st Pl, Bellevue, WA 98005
NIVP3 Computer program (software) collects data from Hokanson instruments. Produces finished patient reports with Doppler and plethysmographic waveforms.

Horizon Healthcare Technologies 800-477-5827
PO Box 27809, Saint Louis, MO 63146
MasterSeries software includes CareMaster (medical records), AccountMaster (billing), BusinessMaster Financial Series, BusinessMaster Employee Management Series, and Small Business Option for smaller facilities.

Howard Medical Company 800-443-1444
1690 N Elston Ave, Chicago, IL 60642
$35,000.00 for complete bar code inventory control system incl. computer equipment, par level restocking, patient charge, and general stores inventory.

Idx Systems Corporation 802-862-1022
1400 Shelburne Rd, South Burlington, VT 05403
Markets software and hardware products, operating systems, communication and installation services, and training to group practices, clinics, managed care organizations, faculty practice plans, imaging centers, hospitals and integrated delivery networks.

Image Analysis, Inc. 800-548-4849
1380 Burkesville St, Columbia, KY 42728
QCT systems for bone mineral density analysis or for QCT lung nodule system; both include automated CT/PC software, simultaneous scan calibration phantom with multiple CaHA densities and quality control torso phantom. Options include dicom systems, 3-D analysis, DXAVIEW projection measurement of spine and hip, and CT calibrated coronary calcium analysis.

Imaging Associates, Inc. 800-821-3230
11110 Westlake Dr, Charlotte, NC 28273
IMAGE QUEST communication software for radilogy, cardiology, endosurgery and pathology.

Imsi, Integrated Modular Systems Inc. 800-220-9729
2500 W Township Line Rd, PO Box 616, Havertown, PA 19083
RIS, PACS, Teleradiology, Mammography Tracking, HL7 and DICOM Interfaces, Voice Recognition, Transcription, etc...

Indec Systems, Inc. 408-986-1600
2210 Martin Ave, Santa Clara, CA 95050
ECHOPLAQUE 2.5, TapeMeasure.

COMPUTER SOFTWARE *(cont'd)*

Infometrix, Inc. 425-402-1450
10634 E Riverside Dr Ste 250, Bothell, WA 98011
PIROUETTE, pattern recognition software that can be used for bacterial identification and predicting disease states.

Information Data Management, Inc. 800-249-4276
9701 W Higgins Rd Ste 500, Rosemont, IL 60018
IDM SURROUND: Surround is an open laboratory system that collects test results from multiple sources and performs applicable decision making. The system collates the data based on client requirements and has multiple transfer options to meet client needs. Surround provides the ability to review the status of all testing at any time. IDM Embarc is a stand alone sample management module that communicates with Surround and NGI to track information on required tests as well as tracks shipping information.

Instromedix, A Card Guard Co. 800-633-3361
10255 W Higgins Rd Ste 100, Rosemont, IL 60018
EKG software and cardiac-monitoring system for transtelephonic and on-site pacemaker recording and reporting.

Integrated Software Design, Inc. 800-600-2242
171 Forbes Blvd Ste 3000, Mansfield, MA 02048
On-Tap allows you to add bar codes to documents printed from Windows, UNIX or VMS application software.

J&S Medical Associates 800-229-6000
35 Tripp St Ste 1, Framingham, MA 01702
LABTRAK L.I.S. information software interfaced to many of the leading hematology & chemistry instruments sold that collates all patient & QL info. & regulatory info. required under CLIA.

Jbm Service Limited 800-663-2280
1405 Menu Road, Westbank, BC V4T-2R9 Canada
RMS Equipment Management software provides complete database to manage equipment, parts, people and vendors.

Kelleher Medical, Inc. 804-378-9956
3049 St Marys Way, Powhatan, VA 23139
DR. SPEECH is video imaging software which allows simultaneous real time video imaging, fundamental frequency, EGG tracing, voice assessment, therapy, training and documentation.

Kettler International 757-427-2400
PO Box 2747, 1355 London Bridge Rd, Virginia Beach, VA 23450
Ergo Concept training software for use with Kettler ergometers. CD-ROM, interface cable 9-pole SUB-D, cable w/ 15-pole SUB-d socket and +/- buttons. Computer-assisted monitoring and assessment of training, resident load profiles for every performance standard, freely programmable courses, training animation, and computer simulation.

Labtronics, Inc. 519-767-1061
546 Governors Rd, Guelph, ONT N1K-1E3 Canada
PC-compatible software for laboratory information systems. Pipette calibration software.

Lds Life Science (Formerly Gould Instrument Systems Inc.) 216-328-7000
5525 Cloverleaf Pkwy, Valley View, OH 44125
Data aquisition system: Software application for smooth muscle research.

Life Care Technologies, Inc. 800-671-0580
4710 Eisenhower Blvd Ste A10, Tampa, FL 33634
LifeCare PIN (Perinatal Information Network) Mother/Baby perinatal information system. Surviellance, archiving, multidepartmental charting.

Linseis, Inc. 800-732-6733
PO Box 666, Princeton Junction, NJ 08550
Computer-based measurement and evaluation software package for thermoanalytical equipment consisting of keyboard, computer, graphical monitor and printer.

Logic Product Development 612-672-9495
411 Washington Ave N Ste 101, Minneapolis, MN 55401
Experienced electrical engineers and computer scientists compose Logic's systems and software team, which specializes in designing, coding, and integrating software with embedded and distributed hardware systems. The software team's experience with networking and communication protocols compliments the electrical engineering team's hardware experience, and has resulted in the design and development of complex distributed and net-based information systems. The software team has also leveraged its embedded experience into higher-level web and Windows based systems that control or use embedded and/or remote access devices.

COMPUTER SOFTWARE *(cont'd)*

Logical Technology, Inc. 800-266-7591
6907 N Knoxville Ave, Peoria, IL 61614
HAZMIN is an integrated set of environmental software modules providing comprehensive MSDS and environmental management, a database of regulated chemicals, and a material review system. The MSDS Management Module software is the cornerstone of a solid Hazard Communication Program for a facility or corporation. MSDS management software offers Right-To-Know compliance coupled with superior MSDS data management. The Regulated Substance Database (RegSub™) Module is the premier List-of-Lists. The List-of-Lists documents employee exposure risks and regulatory impact of hazardous chemicals. The Environmental Reporting Module allows complete chemical inventory tracking and environmental reporting for Tier II, Form R Thresholds and Releases, VOC emissions and more. The Environmental Reporting Module comes in two configurations: CHEMInventory™ and the full Environmental Reporting Module. The Material Process Control Module documents the approved usage and storage of hazardous materials (i.e. MSDS(s)) at a specific location and augments the MSDS with facility-specific training.

Lumedx Corp. 800-966-0669
110 110th Ave NE, Bellevue, WA 98004
Package of tools and services to help medical institutions enhance quality of patient care, reduce costs, streamline workflow, increase patient volume, and grow revenue.

Mckesson General Medical 800-446-3008
8741 Landmark Rd, Richmond, VA 23228

Medical Graphics Corporation 800-950-5597
350 Oak Grove Pkwy, Saint Paul, MN 55127
BREEZEEX cardiopulmonary exercise testing software for use with CPX/D and CARDIO2 Systems.

Medical Manager Health Systems, Inc. 800-222-7701
516 Clyde Ave, Mountain View, CA 94043
THE MEDICAL MANAGER SOFTWARE has over 25,000 installations and offers Practice management, office management, collections, electronic claims, managed care, lab interface, clinical and financial information, voice recognition interface, EDI interface, and quality care guidelines, electronic medical records, and claims adjudiction.

Medical Systems Ltd. 310-445-8590
11444 W Olympic Blvd, Los Angeles, CA 90064
Marketing information systems software.

Medinotes Corporation 877-633-6683
1025 Ashworth Rd Ste 222, West Des Moines, IA 50265
CHARTING PLUS, an innovative and effective electronic medical record system for busy ambulatory care clinics in a variety of specialties (Cardiology, Dermatology, Internal Medicine, Neurology, OB-GYN, Ophthalmology, Optometry, Orthopaedics, Podiatry, Primary Care, Rheumatology, and Urology).

Mediware Information Systems, Inc. 800-255-0026
11711 W 79th St, Lenexa, KS 66214

Meta Health Technology Inc. 800-334-6840
330 7th Ave, New York, NY 10001
Meta Health Technology Inc. develops, markets and supports healthcare software that operates in Windows PC and client/server environments used on site by healthcare facilities, from hospitals to physician groups and HMOs. The software solution automates the Health Information department with modules for chart abstracting, chart tracking, deficiency analysis, release of information imaging, and electronic signature.

Micromedex, Inc. 303-486-6400
6200 S Syracuse Way Ste 300, Greenwood Village, CO 80111
Various databases available. POISINDEX system toxicology database for identification and management of commercial, industrial, pharmaceutical, zoologic, and botanic substances; DRUGDEX system drug information database, which includes evaluations and consults of investigational, foreign, FDA-approved, and OTC drugs; DISEASEDEX General Medicine provides inpatient disease information, from diagnosis to teatment options accessable in a matter of seconds. DISEASEDEX Emergency Medicine referenced clinical database that presents data for the practice of acute-care medicine; and TOMES (Toxicology, Occupational Medicine & Environmental Series) system for information on clinical effects and workplace standards of industrial chemicals. The Healthcare Series compilation of databases is also available, as is SAFETY DEX, a tool for managing healthcare MSDS.

COMPUTER SOFTWARE *(cont'd)*

Molecular Devices 610-873-5610
402 Boot Rd, Downingtown, PA 19335
Meta Series Imaging Systems (MetaMorph and MetaFluor) for biological imaging, acquisition and analysis for common applications such as multi-dimensional imaging, 3D deconvolution, 3D reconstruction, colocalization & brightness measurements, morphometry, motion analysis, ratio imaging, time lapse and more.

Noraxon Usa, Inc. 800-364-8985
13430 N Scottsdale Rd Ste 104, Scottsdale, AZ 85254
Variety of software packages available, from data acquistion with or without video synchronization to our full featured software, MyoResearch XP Master Edition. It features all analysis, reports and applications and editor mode to create user defined setups with video capturing capabilities included.

Ocg Technology, Inc. 914-576-8457
56 Harrison St, New Rochelle, NY 10801
Accounts receivable management software. Medical billing.

Ortivus 800-537-3927
2324 Sweet Parkway Rd, PO Box 276, Decorah, IA 52101
EMS:Sweet-Billing, Sweet-Field Data, Sweet-CAD, Sweet-Online 'subscription' Billing. PUBLIC SAFETY:AVeL-CAD, AVeL-BASE, AVeL-MobiCAD, AVeL-RadioGATE

Pentax Medical Company 800-431-5880
102 Chestnut Ridge Rd, Montvale, NJ 07645
ENDOPRO - This basic software system is an indispensable computer software tool that allows complete management of all your endoscopic data and information. Acting as the hub from which all user applications are accessed, endoPRO allows your staff to manage scheduling, patient flow, and data & image management throughout the facility. Other highlights include completely customizable inferfaces, automatic data collection, image review and reporting, Q/A queries, ad hoc reports and networking capabilities. Call for quote. DOC-U-SCRIBE - An add-on module of endoPRO, this cost-effective software offers an alternative to dictation, allowing the endoscopist to generate quick and easy procedure reports with annotated images. Doc-U-Scribe utilizes customizable templates that combine physician input with information entered by other staff members that interact with the patient throughout the procedure. This collaborative approach to reporting reduces redundancy and minimizes errors while increasing overall efficiency. Call for quote. MOTION PICTURE STUDIO (MPS) - An add-on module of endoPRO that enables real-time, full-motion video recording during a procedure, and allows users to create and edit still images from video. Video segments can be indexed and catalogued in a database from quick retrieval. MPS is available in Standalone, Networked and Mobile options. Call for quote. NURSING NOTES - An add-on module to endoPRO that permits paperless documentation and real-time entering of nurses notes during all phases of patient care. Using this software, the nursing staff can combine their notes during all phases of the procedure into an electronic document which can be shared with physician notes and/or other users. Call for quote.

Perimed, Inc. 877-374-3589
6785 Wallings Rd Ste 2C-2D, North Royalton, OH 44133
$2,500 for PERISOFT software package.

Photo Research, Inc. 818-341-5151
9731 Topanga Canyon Pl, Chatsworth, CA 91311
for Spectrometers - color - graphic

Physicians Practice Management 800-252-6635
320 W 8th St Ste 218, Bloomington, IN 47404
Integrated medical-software packages.

Powerway, Inc. 800-964-9004
429 N Pennsylvania St Ste 400, Indianapolis, IN 46204
Powerway SUITE 2000 software improves enterprise collaboration and performance through creation, control, and sharing of documents, data and knowledge.

Prentke Romich Company 800-262-1984
1022 Heyl Rd, Wooster, OH 44691
WiVik 3.0 provides access to any application in the latest Windows operating systems.Resizable keyboards, macros for persons with poor pointing skills or low vision.

Psyche Systems 800-345-1514
321 Fortune Blvd, Milford, MA 01757
Developing/marketing turnkey clinical laboratory data processing systems, (Digital Corp. hardware) and other vendors for PC clients.

Quality Systems, Inc. 800-888-7955
18111 Von Karman Ave Ste 600, Irvine, CA 92612
QSI SYSTEM & NEXTGEN. Packages for dental and medical group practices. Electronic medical record systems.

COMPUTER SOFTWARE *(cont'd)*

Qualityworx, Inc. 877-825-4379
11 Valley Rd, Kinnelon, NJ 07405
Customized software validation and FDA QSR compliance solutions for safety-critical software design, development, and test applications. QualityWare assesses software development/test process compliance, and develops/implements appropriate corrective actions to establish/regain compliance that include: developing policies, developing validation plans, creating.executing test protocols, and conducting training.

Radcal Corp. 800-423-7169
426 W Duarte Rd, Monrovia, CA 91016
XLPRO is a Microsoft EXCEL add-in that provides drop-down menu control of all 9000 series functions and automatic data capture directly into spreadsheets of your own design. Example templates are also provided and they are fully customized to meet your changing needs. Computer requirements: spare serial port and ability to run EXCEL 4,5,6 or 7.

Radiographic Digital Imaging, Inc. 310-921-9559
20406 Earl St, Torrance, CA 90503
Xscan provides the complete teleradiology software solution, incorporating scanner interface, patient file management, image manipulation and communications elements, all perfectly matched to your Cobrascan x-ray digitizer.

Radiometer America, Inc. 800-736-0600
810 Sharon Dr, Westlake, OH 44145
pH/blood-gas patient results, calilbration and quality-control data management. RADIANCE data-management software system.

Respironics Georgia, Inc. 724-387-4559
175 Chastain Meadows Ct NW, Kennesaw, GA 30144
ALICE & NIGHTWATCH for sleep testing.

Rice Lake Weighing Systems 800-472-6703
230 W Coleman St, Rice Lake, WI 54868
Software for high accuracy piece counting, percentage determination, mass unit conversion, statistical programs and more.

Rms Instruments 905-677-5533
6877-1 Goreway Dr., Mississauga, ONT L4V 1L9 Canada
High speed, high resolution thermal printer.

Rockland Technimed Limited Rtl 845-426-1136
3 Larissa Ct, Airmont, NY 10952
Integrated medical-software packages.

Roper Scientific, Inc. 800-874-9789
3440 E Britannia Dr, Tucson, AZ 85706
WINSPEC Software package for spectroscopy systems.

Scc Soft Computer 800-763-8352
5400 Tech Data Dr, Clearwater, FL 33760
SCC is a leading developer and supplier of clinical information systems for hospitals and independent laboratories specializing in multisite environments. SCC's modules include SoftLab, SoftMic, SoftBank, SoftPath, SoftDonor, SoftRad and SoftA/R, SoftRx, SoftWeb for Physicians and SoftETC for education, training and competency.

Soltec Corp. 800-423-2344
12977 Arroyo St, San Fernando, CA 91340

Sony Electronics, Inc., Medical Systems Div. 800-686-7669
1 Sony Dr, Park Ridge, NJ 07656
Clinical software.

SourceMedical 866-245-8093
100 Grandview Pl Ste 400, Birmingham, AL 35243

Supertech, Inc. 800-654-1054
PO Box 186, Elkhart, IN 46515
$450.00, Radiographic technique computer disk: Print your own technique charts with SUPERTECH software penetrometer and master film.

Swisslog Translogic Corporation 800-525-1841
10825 E 47th Ave, Denver, CO 80239
Matrix software component for computerized pneumatic tube system.

Symyx Technologies, Inc. 408-764-2000
1263 E Arques Ave, Sunnyvale, CA 94085
The Xenobiotic Metabolism structure-searchable database contains known metabolic transformations for chemical compounds, generally drugs.

Systec Computer Associates, Inc. 631-473-5620
28 N Country Rd, Mount Sinai, NY 11766
LIFETEC blood-bank systems. LIFETEC N.T., a Windows-based program for use with blood-bank systems.

COMPUTER SOFTWARE *(cont'd)*

Tcs Scientific Corp. 215-862-3910
6467 Stoney Hill Rd, New Hope, PA 18938
HAS-101 for Hemox Analyzer, HAS-200 USB version.

Tecan U.S., Inc. 800-338-3226
4022 Stirrup Creek Dr Ste 310, Durham, NC 27703
MICROPLATE-data processing software, GEMINI-pipetting software for life science applications, FACTS-flexible assay computer and task scheduler, LOGIC-flexible sample oriented software for diagnostic applications and MAGELLAN.

Telecation 800-584-9964
7112 W Jefferson Ave Ste 307, Lakewood, CO 80235
Aspen and Aspen Enterprise are 32-bit client/server LIMS that provide sample and QC tracking, data import and export, workload management, flexible report generation, Internet awareness and much more. Both systems help facilities comply with the key guidelines of the Good Automated Laboratory Practices and NELAC. Modules for instrument maintenance and calibration, chemical and supply inventory, statistical quality control, barcoding, industrial pretreatment, water and wastewater management are available. Instrument interfacing with barcode supported.

Thermo Spectra-Tech 800-243-9186
2 Research Dr, PO Box 869, Shelton, CT 06484
Complete Windows-based software tailored specifically for microspectroscopy and dedicated for IRUS infrared microanalysis system. Foundation Series, sample-handling accessories utilize a single common base module, the 'foundation,' which mounts in your spectrometer's sampling compartment. IR Cards for transmission analyzes, disposable cards, available in polyethylene and polytetrafluoroethylene. Two centered sampling positions, which gives the ability to run two samples on each card. Useful for qualitative IR transmission analysis of organic liquids, materials soluble in organic solvents, semi-solids and pastes.

Tremetrics 800-825-0121
7625 Golden Triangle Dr, Eden Prairie, MN 55344
FOSHM Safety & Health software for Windows 95, 98 and NT. Comprehensive database management for employee health records, job status, work restrictions with reporting functions for OSHA and state requirements.

U.F.I. 805-772-1203
545 Main St Ste C2, Morro Bay, CA 93442

Unetixs Vascular, Inc. 800-486-3849
115 Airport St, North Kingstown, RI 02852
AUTOSEQUENCE software for MULTILAB 2LHSTI and 2CP automated vascular testing workstation.

Vitalworks 800-278-0037
239 Ethan Allen Hwy, Ridgefield, CT 06877
Integrated medical-software package for billing, accounts receivable, appointment scheduling, transcription, managed care, electronic claim procsssing/remittance, collection, and recall.

3m Health Information Systems 800-367-2447
575 Murray Blvd, Murray, UT 84123

COMPUTER SOFTWARE, HOME HEALTHCARE

(General) 80WVJ

Apothacare 800-736-8456
PO Box 2226, Everett, WA 98213
Pharmacist's Companion Series brings it all together, everything you need to practice consulting pharmacy and pharmaceutical care. Designed by pharmacists for pharmacists to use in nursing homes, board & care homes, hospitals and individual consultations.

Etreby Computer Company, Inc. 800-843-7988
2145 W La Palma Ave, Anaheim, CA 92801
Home-infusion software featuring easy-to-use TPN, IVPB, and home healthcare database-management and formulation program.

Infosys, Inc. 800-978-4636
1821 Walden Office Sq Ste 350, Schaumburg, IL 60173
Windows-based home health/nursing home software modules includes caregiver and patient scheduling, billing, AR, electronic claims, oasis data collection and analysis, clinical and patient records. Starts at $3,000, training and support available.

Omnisys, Inc. 800-448-6891
2824 Terrell Rd Ste 602, Greenville, TX 75402

COMPUTER SOFTWARE, HOSPITAL/NURSING MANAGEMENT

(General) 80WSJ

Accu-Med Services 800-777-9141
300 Techne Center Dr, Milford, OH 45150
Software for long-term care facilities featuring residential billing, electronic billing, accounts receivable/payable, general ledger, etc.

COMPUTER SOFTWARE, HOSPITAL/NURSING MANAGEMENT
(cont'd)

Cirius Group Inc. 925-685-9300
140 Gregory Ln Ste 240, Pleasant Hill, CA 94523

Dps, Inc. 800-654-4689
3685 Priority Way South Dr Ste 100, Indianapolis, IN 46240
DPS EXTEND utilizes the advanced capabilities of the IBM AS/400 to integrate sales order processing through inventory management/purchasing and all financial functions. K3S-REPLENISH, an inventory management software solution that features demand forcasting, seasonal profile and trending analysis, integrated alternate source buying, overstock and transfer functions, and multiple 'what if' simulators.

Drg International, Inc. 800-321-1167
1167 US Highway 22, Mountainside, NJ 07092
MEDIARC DIGI-GRAPH, system offers solutions for clinical applications to archive images from X-ray devices, angiographies, ultrasound scanners, video-endoscopies and microscopies in real-time mode. System can be configured with any Windows-based software.

Ge Medical Systems Information Technologies 800-643-6439
8200 W Tower Ave, Milwaukee, WI 53223
Windows NT platform.

Health Care Software, Inc. (Hcs) 800-524-1038
PO Box 2430, Farmingdale, NJ 07727
INTERACTANT fully integrated financial and clinical information systems exclusively for the healthcare industry.

Horizon Healthcare Technologies 800-477-5827
PO Box 27809, Saint Louis, MO 63146
Horizon.

Idx Systems Corporation 802-862-1022
1400 Shelburne Rd, South Burlington, VT 05403
Markets software and hardware products, operating systems, communication and installation services, and training to group practices, clinics, managed care organizations, faculty practice plans, imaging centers, laboratories, hospitals and multi-entity organizations.

Impac Medical Systems, Inc. 888-464-6722
100 W Evelyn Ave, Mountain View, CA 94041
Practice management aplications for radiation and medical oncology.

Life Care Technologies, Inc. 800-671-0580
4710 Eisenhower Blvd Ste A10, Tampa, FL 33634
LifeCare PIN (Perinatal Information Network) Mother/Baby perinatal information system. Surviellance, archiving, multidepartmental charting.

Medcare Products, Inc. 800-695-4479
151 Cliff Rd E Ste 40, Burnsville, MN 55337
Patient Transfer Education

Melyx Corporation 888-886-3599
21830 Industrial Blvd, Rogers, MN 55374
We have an innovative and comprehensive range of affordable software applications for facilities of all types and sizes. Our computer software is flexible and accommodates small, medium and large facilities, as well as multi-facility companies. Our various types of clinical and financial software include admissions and MDS, care plans, accounts receivable, accounts payable, general ledger, and payroll. Our business management software includes a purchase order inventory system, a fixed assets system and a report generator.

Pentax Medical Company 800-431-5880
102 Chestnut Ridge Rd, Montvale, NJ 07645
NURSING NOTES - An add-on module to endoPRO that permits paperless documentation and real-time entering of nurses notes during all phases of patient care. Using this software, the nursing staff can combine their notes during all phases of the procedure into an electronic document which can be shared with physician notes and/or other users. Call for quote. ENDOPRO - This basic software system is an indispensable computer software tool that allows complete management of all your endoscopic data and information. Acting as the hub from which all user applications are accessed, endoPRO allows your staff to manage scheduling, patient flow, and data & image management throughout the facility. Other highlights include completely customizable inferfaces, automatic data collection, image review and reporting, Q/A queries, ad hoc reports and networking capabilities. Call for quote. DOC-U-SCRIBE - An add-on module of endoPRO, this cost-effective software offers an alternative to dictation, allowing the endoscopist to generate quick and easy procedure reports with annotated images. Doc-U-Scribe utilizes customizable templates that combine physician input with information entered by other staff members that interact with the patient throughout the procedure. This collaborative approach to reporting reduces redundancy and minimizes errors while increasing overall efficiency. Call for quote. MOTION PICTURE STUDIO (MPS) - An add-on module of endoPRO that enables real-time, full-motion video recording during a procedure, and allows users to create and edit still images from video. Video segments can be indexed and catalogued in a database from quick retrieval. MPS is available in Standalone, Networked and Mobile options. Call for quote.

Rauland-Borg Corp. 800-752-7725
3450 Oakton St, Skokie, IL 60076
TRACER System for location of hospital personnel and equipment. ID tags attached to clothing or equipment transmit position to sensors and RESPONDER IV Nurse Call System. Management software HL7 version interfaces to hospital's ADT system. RESPONDER NET for a networked PC interface that makes RESPONDER IV Nurse Call System information available on any networked PC. Staff assignments, patient/staff information, staff sign-on, and bed status are all available on networked PC's.

Rlisys Practice Solutions, Inc. 800-447-2205
1 Aloha Ln, Peoria, IL 61615
Medical Practice Management Software for Ophthalmologists, Optometrists, and Opticians. Electronic Claims; Patient Recalls; Inventory; EDI. EMR interface.

Scc Soft Computer 800-763-8352
5400 Tech Data Dr, Clearwater, FL 33760
SoftRad® SCC's latest Radiology Information System (RIS)developed for modern radiology environments, offering rules-based scheduling/conflict checking, patient tracking, automated report distribution! PACS/HIS interfacing and Web-viewing of signed reports/laboratory results also available!

Surgical Safety Products, Inc. 800-953-7889
2018 Oak Ter Ste 400, Sarasota, FL 34231
OASIS, network of touch screen terminals located in hospitals used for training healthcare workers and the management/reporting of accidental exposures to blood pathogens.

Televox Software, Inc. 800-644-4266
1110 Montlimar Dr Ste 700, Mobile, AL 36609
HOUSECALLS automatically reminds and confirms upcoming appointments. LABCALLS allows patients 24-7 secure access to lab test results via phone or web. VOX ON-HOLD is a customized on-hold program that markets elective services and information.. TeleVox's WEB DESIGN team designs and hosts custom websites.

Wallace Computer Services, Inc 800-782-4892
2275 Cabot Dr, Lisle, IL 60532
Bar code applications.

COMPUTER SOFTWARE, INDUSTRIAL *(General) 80WSN*

Ocg Technology, Inc. 914-576-8457
56 Harrison St, New Rochelle, NY 10801
Prime Care Patient Management System. Patient centered interactive computer program that automates the production and documentation of a complete medical record of the patient/physician encoutner; prints prescription, cross checks for drug interactions, prints educational material for patients concerning medications, disease management and course treatment and provides the physician with extensive reference material.

COMPUTER, AUDIOMETRY *(Ear/Nose/Throat) 77WQJ*

Intelligent Hearing Systems, Corp. 800-447-9783
6860 SW 81st St, Miami, FL 33143
IVRA, automated behavioral hearing evaluation. VVRA, video-based automated behavioral hearing evaluation.

Micro Audiometrics Corp. 800-729-9509
655 Keller Rd, Murphy, NC 28906
$1,995.00 for MICROLAB computerized audiometer. $300.00 for talkover option.

COMPUTER, BAR CODE *(General) 80VFR*

Activant Solutions Inc. 800-776-7438
19 W College Ave, Yardley, PA 19067
Warehouse management.

Avery Dennison Corporation 626-304-2000
150 N Orange Grove Blvd, Pasadena, CA 91103
PRESIDAX bar code printer and label system.

Gdm Electronic And Medical 408-945-4100
2070 Ringwood Ave, San Jose, CA 95131

Integrated Software Design, Inc. 800-600-2242
171 Forbes Blvd Ste 3000, Mansfield, MA 02048
enLabel is a compliance labeling web portal from which you can print all of your compliance labels on any printer. enLabel makes it easy to produce labels that are fully compliant with FDA, OSHA and other standards.

Tailored Label Products, Inc. 800-727-1344
W165N5731 Ridgewood Dr, Menomonee Falls, WI 53051
Complete systems, thermal transfer printer, ribbon & labels. UL recognized & CSA approved.

COMPUTER, BLOOD PRESSURE *(Cardiovascular) 74DSK*

Cardinal Healthcare 209, Inc. 610-862-0800
5225 Verona Rd, Fitchburg, WI 53711
Lab 9000.

Computerized Screening, Inc. (Csi) 800-533-9230
9550 Gateway Dr, Reno, NV 89521
Computerized vital-signs monitors with non-invasive testing and full telehealth. Supports electronic health records.

Draeger Medical Systems, Inc. 215-660-2626
16 Electronics Ave, Danvers, MA 01923
Multiple infinity systems.

Ge Medical Systems Information Technologies 800-643-6439
8200 W Tower Ave, Milwaukee, WI 53223

Invivo Corporation 425-487-7000
12601 Research Pkwy, Orlando, FL 32826
Invasive blood-pressure montitor.

COMPUTER, BRAIN MAPPING *(Cns/Neurology) 84VKG*

Biofeedback Instrument Corp. 212-222-5665
255 W 98th St Apt 3D, New York, NY 10025
Mindset; computerized (16 channel simultaneous EEG) client system, $2195; 24 channel $2995). Neuroguide neuromap analysis and normative database - $2995. Used Cadwell and other systems.

COMPUTER, CARDIAC CATHETERIZATION LABORATORY
(Cardiovascular) 74QMA

Cardiac Services, Inc. 800-722-5742
618 Grassmere Park Dr., Ste. 17, Nashville, TN 37211
Mobile catheterization labs.

Heartlab, Inc. 800-959-3205
1 Crosswind Dr, Westerly, RI 02891
The Agfa Heartlab Cardiovascular solution provides enterprise storage management and reporting for multiple modalities, long term archiving, web based access for anytime-anywhere access to information, and bi-directional electronic communication between clinical and hospital information systems.

Infimed, Inc. 315-453-4545
121 Metropolitan Park Dr, Liverpool, NY 13088
PlatinumOne Cardiac and ComboLab are digital image acquisition systems that offer more clinically advanced features for higher productivity and better patient care. New features include LVA & QCA, customizable doctor's preferences & thumbnail display.

Mennen Medical Corp. 800-223-2201
2540 Metropolitan Dr, Trevose, PA 19053
HORIZON SE, HORIZON LITE, HORIZON COMPACT cath-lab information systems. Features: angiographic imaging, data analysis, shunt determination, cardiac output, flows, resistances, quantitative coronary artery analysis, report generation, 40 hemodynamic channels and full disclosure.

COMPUTER, CARDIAC CATHETERIZATION LABORATORY
(cont'd)

Mikron Digital Imaging, Inc. 800-925-3905
30425 8 Mile Rd, Livonia, MI 48152
Shimadzu: full line Omega cath/electrophysio catheterization labs.

Sanders Data Systems, Llc 650-857-0455
3980 Bibbits Dr, Palo Alto, CA 94303
ViewPlus cardiac DICOM image viewing software, QCAPlus coronary artery quantitiation software, QLVAPlus left ventricular analysis software

Scimage, Inc. 866-724-6243
4916 El Camino Real Ste 200, Los Altos, CA 94022
Cardiology Image and Information Management Solution (CIIMS)

COMPUTER, CHEMISTRY ANALYZER *(Chemistry) 75JQP*

Abbott Point Of Care Inc. 609-443-9300
104 Windsor Center Dr, East Windsor, NJ 08520
Central data station.

Agilent Technologies, Inc. 877-424-4536
5301 Stevens Creek Blvd, Santa Clara, CA 95051

American Medical Diagnostics, Inc. 703-938-6500
4031 University Dr Ste 200, Fairfax, VA 22030
Distributed, computer-based network for collaborative diagnostics between medica.

Arkray Factory Usa, Inc. 952-646-3168
5182 W 76th St, Minneapolis, MN 55439
Diabetes data management software.

B & C Biotech 951-894-6650
24910 Washington Ave Ste 204, Murrieta, CA 92562
Smart hormone management.

Beckman Coulter, Inc. 800-635-3497
740 W 83rd St, Hialeah, FL 33014
DACOS system.

Beckman Coulter, Inc. 800-742-2345
250 S Kraemer Blvd, PO Box 8000, Brea, CA 92821

Cardinal Health 303, Inc. 571-521-8907
12120 Sunset Hills Rd Fl 3, Reston, VA 20190
Wireless care collect.

Cardiocom LLC 888-243-8881
7980 Century Blvd, Chanhassen, MN 55317
Dataprocessing module.

Cerner Corporation Innovation Campus 816-201-1368
10234 Marion Park Dr, Kansas City, MO 64137

Data Innovations, Inc. 802-658-2850
120 Kimball Ave Ste 100, South Burlington, VT 05403
Laboratory instrument interface.

De Novo Software 213-384-7000
3250 Wilshire Blvd Ste 803, Los Angeles, CA 90010
Flow cytometry data analysis software.

Draeger Medical Systems, Inc. 215-660-2626
16 Electronics Ave, Danvers, MA 01923
Calculator/data processing module for clinical use.

Global Care Quest 949-330-7450
65 Enterprise Ste 350, Aliso Viejo, CA 92656
Medical dashboard.

Hycor Biomedical, Inc. 800-382-2527
7272 Chapman Ave, Garden Grove, CA 92841
Treatment set calculation software.

Integramed America, Inc. 914-253-8000
2 Manhattanville Rd, Purchase, NY 10577
Artworks stats.

Iris Diagnostics 800-776-4747
9172 Eton Ave, Chatsworth, CA 91311
Serial data protocol converter.

Lexicor Medical Technology, Inc. 706-447-1074
2840 Wilderness Pl Ste E, Boulder, CO 80301
Laboratory information mgmt. system software.

Medical Automation Systems 434-971-7953
2000 Holiday Dr Ste 500, Charlottesville, VA 22901
Data management systems.

Medical Decisions Network 434-971-7953
2000 Holiday Dr Ste 200, Charlottesville, VA 22901
Mdn-cgs insulin dosing calculator,icutracker,mdn-nbi national benchmarking initi.

COMPUTER, CHEMISTRY ANALYZER *(cont'd)*

Monogen, Inc. 847-573-6700
3630 Burwood Dr, Waukegan, IL 60085
Calculator data processor module for clinical use.

Monterey Medical Solutions, Inc. 831-210-5514
455 Canyon Del Rey Blvd Ste 411, Monterey, CA 93940
Tpn calculating software.

Opti Medical Systems Inc. 770-510-4444
235 Hembree Park Dr, Roswell, GA 30076
Calculator/data processing module for clinical use.

Pds Health, Inc. 800-440-2417
112 Intracoastal Pointe Dr, Jupiter, FL 33477
Central data transfer station,diabetes data management software.

Pointone Systems, Llc 414-771-1802
10437 W Innovation Dr, Milwaukee, WI 53226

Precision Systems, Inc. 508-655-7010
16 Tech Cir, Natick, MA 01760
ANALETTE, P.C. computer-controlled robotic spectrophotometer with diode array-holographic gratings, bar code and full chemistry capabilities.

Standing Stone, Inc. 203-227-8710
49 Richmondville Ave, Westport, CT 06880
Coagclinic.

Sunquest Information Systems, Inc 520-570-2347
250 S Williams Blvd, Tucson, AZ 85711

Thermo - Industrial Hygiene Division 508-520-0430
27 Forge Pkwy, Franklin, MA 02038
ICP and EDXRF techniques for elemental analysis.

Vertex International, Inc. 540-989-6945
7429 Fort Mason Dr, Roanoke, VA 24018
Computer database software.

Waters Corp. 800-252-4752
34 Maple St, Milford, MA 01757
Data control workstations (LC, GC, IC), networking systems.

COMPUTER, CLINICAL LABORATORY *(Chemistry) 75QMB*

Beckman Coulter, Inc. 800-742-2345
250 S Kraemer Blvd, PO Box 8000, Brea, CA 92821

Dawning Technologies, Inc. 800-332-0499
6140 Mid Metro Dr Ste 5, Fort Myers, FL 33966
Complete interface solutions including the JavaLin interface, capable of establishing an HL7 or ASTM compliant interface to any host system, properly mapped and encrypted. Options include a new robust Enhanced Microbiology Interface capability. Dawning's JResultNet Clinical Router Software is a complete interface engine that can manage a population of remote device connections and any number of host-system connections. JResultNet includes a large number of optional features that can be added as plug-in modules, including a Downtime ID Module, a Broadcast Manager Module, a Bio-Rad QC Connection Module, a Rules Module, an Automatic Backup System Module, and others. These systems can be integrated into any LIS environment or with an LAS.

Indec Systems, Inc. 408-986-1600
2210 Martin Ave, Santa Clara, CA 95050
IVUS PLUS.

Labfusions 909-592-8131
437 S Cataract Ave Ste 5, San Dimas, CA 91773
Software.

Life Care Technologies, Inc. 800-671-0580
4710 Eisenhower Blvd Ste A10, Tampa, FL 33634
PERFORMANCE PHARMACY SYSTEM.

Medical Information Technology, Inc. (Meditech) 781-821-3000
Meditech Circle, Westwood, MA 02090
Software for data collection, microbiology specimen mgt. cytology, pathology, infection control, blood bank, and outpatient services management.

Modulus Data Systems, Inc. 888-663-8547
386 Main St Ste 200, Redwood City, CA 94063
MODULUS LIS $100,000.00 to $800,000.00.

Psyche Systems 800-345-1514
321 Fortune Blvd, Milford, MA 01757
$100,000 - $400,000 for Labweb system.

COMPUTER, CLINICAL LABORATORY *(cont'd)*

Scc Soft Computer 800-763-8352
5400 Tech Data Dr, Clearwater, FL 33760
SoftLab, SCC's flagship LIS solution, is at the center of SCC's suite of laboratory information systems. With stand-alone or integrated modules that include SoftMic® for Microbiology and SoftPath® for Anatomic Pathology, the SoftLab suite provides quantifiable improvements in workflow efficiency and cost-per-test reductions in a wide variety of clinical laboratory environments. With features such as medical necessity checking, incorporated outreach functionality, point-of-care testing integration, web enabled, specimen tracking and parallel processing, SoftLab establishes itself as the de facto standard LIS for the industry.

Scientific Software, Inc. 519-767-1061
546 Governors Rd., Guelph, ONT N1K-1E3 Canada
Chromatography acquisition hardware.

COMPUTER, DIAGNOSTIC, PRE-PROGRAMMED, SINGLE-FUNCTION *(Cardiovascular) 74DXG*

Advanced Mechanical Technology, Inc. (Amti) 800-422-AMTI
176 Waltham St, Watertown, MA 02472

Arrow International, Inc. 800-523-8446
2 Berry Dr, Mount Holly, NJ 08060
Balloon therma-type catheter.

Bayer Healthcare Llc 914-524-2955
555 White Plains Rd Fl 5, Tarrytown, NY 10591
Data management systems.

Bayer Healthcare, Llc 574-256-3430
430 S Beiger St, Mishawaka, IN 46544
Data management systems.

Ge Medical Systems Information Technologies 800-643-6439
8200 W Tower Ave, Milwaukee, WI 53223

Hemo Sapiens, Inc. 928-202-4453
325 Lookout Dr, Sedona, AZ 86351
Noninvasive cardiac output.

Hospira, Inc. 877-946-7747
755 Jarvis Dr, Morgan Hill, CA 95037

Icu Medical (Ut), Inc 949-366-2183
4455 Atherton Dr, Salt Lake City, UT 84123
Thermodilution cardiac output computer.

COMPUTER, DIAGNOSTIC, PROGRAMMABLE *(Cardiovascular) 74DQK*

Advanced Biosensor, Inc. 803-407-3044
400 Arbor Lake Dr Ste B450, Columbia, SC 29223
Holter analysis program.

Agfa Healthcare Corp. 864-421-1815
1 Crosswind Dr, Westerly, RI 02891
Ecg management system.

Boston Scientific-Neurovascular 510-440-7700
47900 Bayside Pkwy, Fremont, CA 94538
Real time position management rpm system.

Cambridge Heart, Inc. 888-CAM-WAVE
100 Ames Pond Dr Ste 100, Tewksbury, MA 01876
HearTwave II MTWA System

Catheffects, Llc. 916-677-1790
1100 Melody Ln, Roseville, CA 95678
Electrophysiology mapping system.

Critical Care Systems, Inc. 954-989-4400
5000 Hollywood Blvd, Hollywood, FL 33021
Automated critical care data management system.

Draeger Medical Systems, Inc. 215-660-2626
16 Electronics Ave, Danvers, MA 01923
Programmable diagnostic computer.

Ep Medsystems, Inc. 609-753-8533
575 N Route 73 Bldg D, West Berlin, NJ 08091
Ep workstation, computerized electrophysiology workstation.

Ge Medical Systems Information Technologies 800-643-6439
8200 W Tower Ave, Milwaukee, WI 53223
MAC LAB computerized cardiac Cath Lab; physiological monitoring and measuring system; MUSE cardiology management system.

Hemo Sapiens, Inc. 928-202-4453
325 Lookout Dr, Sedona, AZ 86351
Non-invasive hemodynamic monitoring & management system.

COMPUTER, DIAGNOSTIC, PROGRAMMABLE *(cont'd)*

Imsi, Integrated Modular Systems Inc. 800-220-9729
2500 W Township Line Rd, PO Box 616, Havertown, PA 19083
RADIN Cardiology Imaging Software. Win2K platform. Windows PCs. Easy Integration. Full Functionality and Tools. Cost Effective Licensing.

International Technidyne Corporation 732-548-5700
8 Olsen Ave, Edison, NJ 08820
Diagnostic computer.

Medical Imaging Applications, Llc 319-358-1529
832 Forest Hill Dr, Coralville, IA 52241
Vascular analysis tools.

Medical Information Technology, Inc. (Meditech) 781-821-3000
Meditech Circle, Westwood, MA 02090
Software for nursing inquiry, medical records, pharmacy, admissions, accounting, & materials mgt. Handheld point of care computer.

Medicomp, Inc. 800-23-HEART
7845 Ellis Rd, Melbourne, FL 32904
Full disclosure with total beat annotations, superimposition, editing.

Medtronic Ep Systems 763-514-4000
8299 Central Ave NE, Spring Lake Park, Minneapolis, MN 55432
Cardiac mapping system.

Micro Bio-Physic Laboratory, Inc. 626-451-6813
5917 Oak Ave # 357, Temple City, CA 91780
Progammable diagnostic system.

New Product Development, Inc. 315-434-9000
6700 Old Collamer Rd, East Syracuse, NY 13057
Holter system/aecg system.

Non-Invasive Monitoring Systems, Inc. 305-575-4200
4400 Biscayne Blvd, Miami, FL 33137
Respitrace pt, respievents, respievents, version 4.2.

Northeast Monitoring, Inc. 866-346-5837
2 Clock Tower Pl Ste 555, Maynard, MA 01754
Holter and Event Software

Premier Heart, Llc. 516-883-3383
14 Vanderventer Ave Ste 138, Port Washington, NY 11050
Computerized ekg analysis system.

Spacelabs Medical Inc. 800-522-7212
5150 220th Ave SE, Issaquah, WA 98029
Holter analyzer software.

St. Jude Medical Atrial Fibrillation (Endocardial Solutions) 800-374-8038
1350 Energy Ln Ste 110, Saint Paul, MN 55108
Cardiac mapping system.

Unicom 800-556-2828
6 Blackstone Valley Pl Ste 402, Lincoln, RI 02865
HI-IQ 2.5 is the premiere quality assurance & inventory management database that helps you to manage track and analyze your interventional radiology patient records, encounters & inventory. HI-IQ is the only application that gives you the ability to link individual patient encounters to inventory usage, allowing in-depth procedural and cost data analysis of one encounter or a group of encounters.

Witt Biomedical Corporation 800-669-1328
305 North Dr, Melbourne, FL 32934
CALYSTO SERIES IV Physiological Monitoring System; a Windows based hemodynamic monitoring equipment for cardiac cath labs; full hemodynamic analysis. Complete relational database and multiple software packages included.

COMPUTER, ECG INTERPRETATION (ARRHYTHMIA)
(Cardiovascular) 74QMC

Midmark Diagnostics Group 800-624-8950
3300 Fujita St, Torrance, CA 90505
The IQmark Digital ECG is a compact, portable device that easily connects to a Windows computer. It features full interpretations, pediatrics to adults, using the Telemed® Analysis algorithm; 12-channel monitoring, storage, review and serial comparison; lead-off detection; local or network database, archive and e-mail capabilities; reports printed on plain paper; and a weight of less than 11 oz., with no moving parts.

Mortara Instrument, Inc. 800-231-7437
7865 N 86th St, Milwaukee, WI 53224
Tabletop noninvasive microprocessor ECG device to identify patients at risk of sudden death syndrome. Also available, LCD display to preview ECG data prior to printing.

COMPUTER, HEMATOLOGY ANALYZER *(Hematology) 81JWS*

Beckman Coulter, Inc. 800-635-3497
740 W 83rd St, Hialeah, FL 33014
ACCUCOMP computers and data terminals available for different models of Coulter cell counters.

Horiba Abx 888-903-5001
34 Bunsen, Irvine, CA 92618

COMPUTER, IMAGE, ENDOSCOPIC *(General) 80WLE*

Ge Healthcare Technologies Surgery Navigation 800-708-3856
439 S Union St, Lawrence, MA 01843
CT and MRI data used to construct a 3-D computer image to aid the surgeon with navigation in difficult-to-visualize areas.

Immersion Medical 800-929-4709
55 W Watkins Mill Rd, Gaithersburg, MD 20878
Medical simulators for teaching purposes. Interventional radiology simulator, bronchoscopy simulator, vascular access simulator, volume visualization software.

Imsi, Integrated Modular Systems Inc. 800-220-9729
2500 W Township Line Rd, PO Box 616, Havertown, PA 19083
RADIN Endoscopy Imaging, PACS viewing, Teleradiology, etc...

Koaman International 909-983-4888
656 E D St, Ontario, CA 91764
Fluorescein in situ hybridization; comparative genome hybridization.

Pentax Medical Company 800-431-5880
102 Chestnut Ridge Rd, Montvale, NJ 07645
ENDOPRO - This basic software system is an indispensable computer software tool that allows complete management of all your endoscopic data and information. Acting as the hub from which all user applications are accessed, endoPRO allows your staff to manage scheduling, patient flow, and data & image management throughout the facility. Other highlights include completely customizable interfaces, automatic data collection, image review and reporting, Q/A queries, ad hoc reports and networking capabilities. Call for quote. DOC-U-SCRIBE - An add-on module of endoPRO, this cost-effective software offers an alternative to dictation, allowing the endoscopist to generate quick and easy procedure reports with annotated images. Doc-U-Scribe utilizes customizable templates that combine physician input with information entered by other staff members that interact with the patient throughout the procedure. This collaborative approach to reporting reduces redundancy and minimizes errors while increasing overall efficiency. Call for quote. MOTION PICTURE STUDIO (MPS) - An add-on module of endoPRO that enables real-time, full-motion video recording during a procedure, and allows users to create and edit still images from video. Video segments can be indexed and catalogued in a database from quick retrieval. MPS is available in Standalone, Networked and Mobile options. Call for quote. NURSING NOTES - An add-on module to endoPRO that permits paperless documentation and real-time entering of nurses notes during all phases of patient care. Using this software, the nursing staff can combine their notes during all phases of the procedure into an electronic document which can be shared with physician notes and/or other users. Call for quote.

COMPUTER, IMAGING, PRESURGERY *(Surgery) 79WIY*

Carl Zeiss Surgical, Inc. 800-442-4020
1 Zeiss Dr, Thornwood, NY 10594
STN image-guided surgery is for surgical planning and intra-operative tool navigation using encoded instruments and/or surgical microscope.

Imsi, Integrated Modular Systems Inc. 800-220-9729
2500 W Township Line Rd, PO Box 616, Havertown, PA 19083
Complete Diagnostic Image Viewing. Full Functionality. All modalities. Very Cost Effective Licensing. Standard computers and hardware utilized.

Merge Healthcare 877-741-5369
6737 W Washington St Ste 2250, Milwaukee, WI 53214
Diagnostic imaging interface equipment.

COMPUTER, NUCLEAR MEDICINE *(Radiology) 90QMD*

Aaeon Electronics, Inc. 888-223-6687
3 Crown Plz, Hazlet, NJ 07730
GENE-8310 is a single board computer with high resolution graphics in a very small space and with lower power requirements.

Analogic Corporation 978-326-4000
8 Centennial Dr, Peabody, MA 01960
High-performance imaging workstation.

Capintec, Inc. 800-631-3826
6 Arrow Rd, Ramsey, NJ 07446

COMPUTER, NUCLEAR MEDICINE *(cont'd)*

Diagnostix Plus, Inc. 516-536-2670
100 N Village Ave Ste 33, Rockville Centre, NY 11570
Remanufactured, upgraded new and used nuclear medicine computers.

Indec Systems, Inc. 408-986-1600
2210 Martin Ave, Santa Clara, CA 95050

Marconi Medical Systems 800-323-0550
595 Miner Rd, Cleveland, OH 44143

Mushield Company, Inc., The 888-669-3539
9 Ricker Ave, Londonderry, NH 03053
GB ENCLOSURE MRI monitor enclosure. Eliminates EMI interference up to 30 gauss. Custom and off-the-shelf designs.

Optimed Technologies, Inc. 973-575-9911
20 New Dutch Ln, Fairfield, NJ 07004
Automated clinical reports, Image storage and retrieval, Image distribution (WEB) etc. DICOM viewers

COMPUTER, OXYGEN-UPTAKE *(Anesthesiology) 73BZL*

Aei Technologies Inc. 630-548-3545
300 William Pitt Way, Pittsburgh, PA 15238
Oxygen uptake system.

Korr Medical Technologies, Inc. 801-483-2080
2463 S 3850 W Ste 200, Salt Lake City, UT 84120
Indirect calorimeter.

Microlife Usa, Inc. 888-314-2599
424 Skinner Blvd Apt C, Dunedin, FL 34698
Medgem

Piranha Plastics, Llc. 408-855-9650
3531 Thomas Rd, Santa Clara, CA 95054
Medgem.

Waters Medical Systems, Llc 205-612-5221
2112 15th St NW, Rochester, MN 55901
Oxygen consumption computer.

COMPUTER, PATIENT DATA MANAGEMENT *(General) 80VHN*

Accu-Med Services 800-777-9141
300 Techne Center Dr, Milford, OH 45150
Web based software for providing your QM picture on demand. At a glance you can identify residents at risk of triggering a QM, allowing you to be pro-active.

American Medical Software 800-423-8836
PO Box 236, Edwardsville, IL 62025
Electronic Medical Records Software for Paperless Patient Charts, Prescription Writing, Reminders, and much more.

Bd Diagnostic Systems 800-675-0908
7 Loveton Cir, Sparks, MD 21152

Bio-Medical Instruments, Inc. 800-521-4640
2387 E 8 Mile Rd, Warren, MI 48091

Biofeedback Instrument Corp. 212-222-5665
255 W 98th St Apt 3D, New York, NY 10025
Dedicated 8 channel biofeedback computer model Procomp/Infiniti: $5,700 with Temp, EMG, SCL feedback monitor display modalities. JJ C2 12 channel biofeedback computerized system w/ EEG, EMG TEMP, GSR, RESP, HR for $3,195.

C&S Research Corporation 800-545-8460
625 Clark Ave Ste 21B, King Of Prussia, PA 19406
The Medical Management System is a complete medical practice management system that is customized to fit the requirements of each individual practice.

Captiva Software Corporation 800-783-3378
601 Oakmont Ln Ste 200, Westmont, IL 60559
CLAIMS EDITOR medical claims editing software performs coding, clinical, and Medicare edits. Physicians Fee Reports provide listings of the usual, customary, and reasonable (UCR) fees for the 30th, 50th, 65th, 80th, and 95th percentiles.

Cardiac Science Corp. 800-777-1777
500 Burdick Pkwy, Deerfield, WI 53531
Pyramis

Database, Inc. 919-493-6969
3100 Tower Blvd Ste 304, Durham, NC 27707
TMR - The Medical Record. $25,000 and up for multi-user, patient medical management and practice management system.

Datacard Group 800-621-6972
11111 Bren Rd W, Minnetonka, MN 55343
Patient ID card magnetic-stripe card readers, patient-ID-card imprinters, smart card and smart-card readers.

COMPUTER, PATIENT DATA MANAGEMENT *(cont'd)*

Idx Systems Corporation 802-862-1022
1400 Shelburne Rd, South Burlington, VT 05403
IDXTENDR is a relational, scaleable product line that leverages advanced client-server architecture and web-based technology to facilitate the flow of patient data in healthcare settings. IDXTENDR provides a relational solution designed to grow as your organization grows and comes packaged to meet your specific site requirements whether you are a group practice, MSO, hospital, or integrated delivery network (IDN).

Imsi, Integrated Modular Systems Inc. 800-220-9729
2500 W Township Line Rd, PO Box 616, Havertown, PA 19083
IDOM, Imaging department operations management system - registration, patient history, scheduling, transcription, management reports and interfaces. Medical records department systems and mammography tracking systems also available. CARE TRACK, Unix/Windows based software used for patient follow-up and care tracking system. SCHED STAT, patient scheduling system utilizing an HL7 engine and robotic terminal asst. INTEGRATED IMAGE, Image distribution and management system.

Information Data Management, Inc. 800-249-4276
9701 W Higgins Rd Ste 500, Rosemont, IL 60018
ACCUTRAK, a UNIX-based on-line tracking system for all customer contacts including complaints, non-complaints and product revision requests. Developed to meet SMDA requirements, it records customer contact information, logs the resolution or action taken in response to the call, provides documented logs and generates management reports to analyze customer contacts. IDM Select Series For Blood Centers, includes the Donor Management Information System (DMIS) that provides advanced features in Donor Registration, Deferral Management, HLA. DMIS also includes Red Cell Antigen Matching, Ad Hoc Management Report Capabilities and User Administration. IDM INTOUCH, a donor recruiting system which uses the latest in X-Windows technology to provide an advanced environment for creating targeted recruitment lists, donor scheduling and project management and analysis. IDM Plasma Center Management System, PCMS is designed to maximize staff productivity, assist with regulatory compliance, optimize donor resource management and provide management analyses to continually improve center operations.

Information Health Network 800-443-0613
PO Box 23056, Lansing, MI 48909
Medical records software for orthopedic, neurosurgery, OB/GYN, urology, cardiovascular, ENT, ophthalmic and general surgery physicians. Software can be run over the Internet. Interactive video for patient information data collection.

Life Care Technologies, Inc. 800-671-0580
4710 Eisenhower Blvd Ste A10, Tampa, FL 33634
LifeCare PIN (Perinatal Information Network) Mother/Baby perinatal information system. Surviellance, archiving, multidepartmental charting. E-MAR electronic medication administration record.

Md International, Inc. 305-669-9003
11300 NW 41st St, Doral, FL 33178

Medical Information Technology, Inc. (Meditech) 781-821-3000
Meditech Circle, Westwood, MA 02090
Software for nurse station communications, nursing care management, admissions data capture and retrieval, and results entry and inquiry from virtually all departments.

Mediware Information Systems, Inc. 800-255-0026
11711 W 79th St, Lenexa, KS 66214
Hemocare data management system for total blood bank management; also available, Surgiware provides scheduling, case cart management, intraoperative logging and user-defined reporting for OR system. An Digimedics for hospital pharmacies.

Newbold Corporation 800-552-3282
450 Weaver St, Rocky Mount, VA 24151
ADDRESSOGRAPH 2000 Series electric Healthcare imprinters and supplies.

Optimed Technologies, Inc. 973-575-9911
20 New Dutch Ln, Fairfield, NJ 07004
Patient data storage and retrieval. Automated Clinical report generation. WEB Serversolutions for access to patient data (Imaging and reports)

COMPUTER, PATIENT DATA MANAGEMENT *(cont'd)*

Pentax Medical Company 800-431-5880
102 Chestnut Ridge Rd, Montvale, NJ 07645
ENDOPRO - This basic software system is an indispensable computer software tool that allows complete management of all your endoscopic data and information. Acting as the hub from which all user applications are accessed, endoPRO allows your staff to manage scheduling, patient flow, and data & image management throughout the facility. Other highlights include completely customizable inerfaces, automatic data collection, image review and reporting, Q/A queries, ad hoc reports and networking capabilities. Call for quote. DOC-U-SCRIBE - An add-on module of endoPRO, this cost-effective software offers an alternative to dictation, allowing the endoscopist to generate quick and easy procedure reports with annotated images. Doc-U-Scribe utilizes customizable templates that combine physician input with information entered by other staff members that interact with the patient throughout the procedure. This collaborative approach to reporting reduces redundancy and minimizes errors while increasing overall efficiency. Call for quote. MOTION PICTURE STUDIO (MPS) - An add-on module of endoPRO that enables real-time, full-motion video recording during a procedure, and allows users to create and edit still images from video. Video segments can be indexed and catalogued in a database from quick retrieval. MPS is available in Standalone, Networked and Mobile options. Call for quote. NURSING NOTES - An add-on module to endoPRO that permits paperless documentation and real-time entering of nurses notes during all phases of patient care. Using this software, the nursing staff can combine their notes during all phases of the procedure into an electronic document which can be shared with physician notes and/or other users. Call for quote.

Per-Se Technologies 877-737-3773
1145 Sanctuary Pkwy Ste 200, Alpharetta, GA 30009
ORSOS comprehensive surgical-management information system including scheduling, inventory control, management reporting, perioperative charting, remote scheduling, and personnel scheduling. ONE-CALL enterprise-wide patient scheduling. ANSOS nurse staffing and management. ONE-STAFF enterprise-wide staff scheduling and management. BUSINESS1 enterprise-wide patient financial-management system. MedAxxis physician practice management system.

Radiometer America, Inc. 800-736-0600
810 Sharon Dr, Westlake, OH 44145
RADIANCE data-management software system.

Scc Soft Computer 800-763-8352
5400 Tech Data Dr, Clearwater, FL 33760
SoftWeb™ is a web-enabled Physician Order Entry and Reporting application providing quick access to pertinent patient data obtained from various information systems. Allows Order Entry from Physician Office and Queries by various search criteria, with graphical results and data displayed. A valuable decision support tool for providing innovative and robust outreach solution to physician office from hospital lab or reference lab.

Sorin Group Usa 800-289-5759
14401 W 65th Way, Arvada, CO 80004

Sunrise Medical 800-333-4000
7477 Dry Creek Pkwy, Longmont, CO 80503

Thought Technology Ltd. 800-361-3651
2180 Belgrave Ave., Montreal, QUE H4A 2L8 Canada
MYOTRAC 3G provides clinicians with graphical displays either in the unit alone or connected to a PC, to analyze and monitor pelvic floor muscle activity for the treatment of incontinence, and other urology problems. Built-in memory allows practitioners to record and download session data to a PC. MYOTRAC 3G can analyze muscle strength, fatigue, latency to contract and relaxation. The unit has a full range of statistical capabilities. MYOTRAC 3, a highly sensitive dual-channel sEMG unit, enables clinicians to customize patient assessment and training regiments for incontinence. It can be connected to any window compatible PC for easy real-time monitoring or data analysis with our continence software.

Timemed Labeling Systems, Inc. 800-323-4840
144 Tower Dr, Burr Ridge, IL 60527
Computer labeling systems and label printers.

Turbo-Doc Emr 800-977-4868
771 Buschmann Rd Ste G, Paradise, CA 95969
Electronic Medical Record Software

Veritech Corporation 413-525-3368
168 Denslow Rd, East Longmeadow, MA 01028
Multimedia patient education system & software for orthopedic surgeons. An in-office system that explains total implant procedures, provides implied consent, FS 36, and includes take home video.

COMPUTER, PATIENT DATA MANAGEMENT *(cont'd)*

Vitalcom, Inc. 800-888-0077
15222 Del Amo Ave, Tustin, CA 92780
VCOM clinical information system to acquire, interpret, and distribute real-time patient data throughout a healthcare facility or IHDN.

COMPUTER, PATIENT MONITOR *(Anesthesiology) 73QME*

Axon Systems, Inc. 800-888-2966
400 Oser Ave Ste 2200, Hauppauge, NY 11788
Neurological workstation. Simultaneous, 32 channel, multimodality EEP/EP/EMG monitoring for OR/ICU applications. Built-in transcranial MEP stimulator. Trend all parameters with event alarms. Review and print reports while monitoring. Dual video input for microscope and camera. Import and display vital signs. Multiple site remote monitoring via network, internet or modem. Portable and fixed location platforms.

Bio-Feedback Systems, Inc. 303-444-1411
2736 47th St, Boulder, CO 80301
$2,245 for interface to IBM P.C. includes software.

Bio-Logic Systems Corp. 800-323-8326
1 Bio Logic Plz, Mundelein, IL 60060
BRAINATLAS, CEEGRAPH - microcomputer based systems which perform diagnostic monitoring of EEG and evoked response.

Datascope Corp. 800-288-2121
14 Philips Pkwy, Montvale, NJ 07645
DATATRAC anesthesia record keeping system.

Ge Medical Systems Information Technologies 800-643-6439
8200 W Tower Ave, Milwaukee, WI 53223
Bedside or bedside network to PC interface program which permits PC computer to be interfaced to the bedside monitor or the Marquette monitoring network directly for the collection of monitored parameters and data. Information can then be manipulated to suit the users' needs. Product is provided with a data services manual providing information regarding programming and applications.

Mennen Medical Corp. 800-223-2201
2540 Metropolitan Dr, Trevose, PA 19053
ENVOY patient monitor 8 trace color display, up to 32 parameters, 24 'smart' modules, including ECG, RESP, APNEA, Invasive BP, non-invasiveBP, EtCO2, SpO2, cardiac output, dual temp, data management, printer options.

Nihon Kohden America, Inc. 800-325-0283
90 Icon, Foothill Ranch, CA 92610

Oridion Medical Inc. 888-674-3466
140 Towne& Country Drive, SuiteB, Danville, CA 94526
Multi-parameter patient monitoring systems/measuring stations.

Thought Technology Ltd. 800-361-3651
2180 Belgrave Ave., Montreal, QUE H4A 2L8 Canada
FlexComp Infiniti™ is a computerized physiological monitoring system that can monitor up to 10 sensors (or 40, when used with 4 encoders) of EMG, EKG, EEG, HR/BVP, temperature, skin conductance, respiration, goniometer and force sense adaptor. It will even allow you to read the analog output from a third-party device, using our Voltage Isolator. The FlexComp Infiniti™ has been designed for the power user who requires 2048 s/s and /or will be doing research. The FlexComp™ Infiniti’s power is brought to life with the BioGraph®Infiniti Software. Currently the system includes the Multimodality and Legacy Suites. The high-speed channel capabilities will be fully realized with the Developer Tools and custom suites, coming in 2004. This modular design facilitates the conservation of your computer disk space by using the software/suite that best suits your needs for each application. The FlexComp Infiniti™ is a total monitoring system, ideal for all power users, clinicians and researchers alike, which allows you to customize the application to better fulfill your needs.*

COMPUTER, PULMONARY FUNCTION DATA
(Anesthesiology) 73BZC

Cardinal Health 207, Inc. 610-862-0800
1100 Bird Center Dr, Palm Springs, CA 92262
Wireless portable ergospirometry system.

Cardinal Health 207, Inc. 800-231-2466
22745 Savi Ranch Pkwy, Yorba Linda, CA 92887
$5,000-$43,000 for screening system & full PFT lab.

Go-Mi, Inc. 415-453-3409
740 Fawn Dr, San Anselmo, CA 94960
Lung function testing.

Hans Rudolph, Inc. 816-363-5522
7200 Wyandotte St, Kansas City, MO 64114
Directional control valve for respiratory circuits.

COMPUTER, PULMONARY FUNCTION DATA *(cont'd)*

Lds Life Science (Formerly Gould Instrument Systems Inc.) 216-328-7000
5525 Cloverleaf Pkwy, Valley View, OH 44125
Data acquisition system: Software application for cardio-pulmonary research.

Medical Graphics Corporation 800-950-5597
350 Oak Grove Pkwy, Saint Paul, MN 55127
CPF-S/D disposable flow sensor with pneumotachograph flow-measuring spirometer. IBM compatable desk-top computer. Software library.

Parvo Medics, Inc. 801-942-7796
6526 S State St Ste 202, Murray, UT 84107
Truemax 2400.

Respironics California, Inc. 724-387-4559
2271 Cosmos Ct, Carlsbad, CA 92011
Pulmonary function data monitor/calculator.

Respironics Novametrix, Llc. 724-387-4559
5 Technology Dr, Wallingford, CT 06492
Pulmonary function data monitor/calculator.

Telefelx Medical 919-544-8000
900 W University Dr, Arlington Heights, IL 60004
Calculator, pulmonary function data.

Treymed, Inc. 262-820-1294
N56W24790 N Corporate Cir Ste C, Sussex, WI 53089
Respiratory mechanics monitor.

Vacumed 800-235-3333
4538 Westinghouse St, Ventura, CA 93003
Pulmonary metabolic measurement system for O2 uptake, CO2 production, and RQ.

Vitalograph, Inc. 800-255-6626
13310 W 99th St, Lenexa, KS 66215
SPIROTRAC III software for lung function testing$995.00

COMPUTER, PULMONARY FUNCTION INTERPRETATOR (DIAGNOSTIC) *(Anesthesiology) 73BZM*

Medical Graphics Corporation 800-950-5597
350 Oak Grove Pkwy, Saint Paul, MN 55127
MGC desktop diagnostic/CATH system to measure oxygen uptake and calculate cardiac output (Q-Direct Fick) IBM compatible system includes computer, respiratory/flow module with physiologic waveform analyzer, gfas exchange module incl. rapid response oxygen and carbon dioxide analyzers, and MGC Cath-Diret Fick cardiac output software. Also: breath-by-breath analysis of 40 metabolic parameters with CAD/NET graphics computer, O2 analyzer, CO2 analyzer, ECG monitor/recorder, waveform analyzer & flow module.

Midmark Diagnostics Group 800-624-8950
3300 Fujita St, Torrance, CA 90505
The IQmark Digital Spirometer has met or exceeded the requirements of the ATS. All standard spirometry measurements are available including FEV6, as recommended by the NLHEP. Standard features on this computer-based spirometer include full-loop, FVC, SVC, MVV, and pre/post BD tests; local or network database storage; trending software; and archive and e-mail capabilities. It is lightweight, weighing only 10 oz., and has no moving parts.

Stethographics, Inc. 508-320-2841
1153 Centre St Ste 4381, Jamaica Plain, MA 02130
Pulmonary function interpretor.

COMPUTER, PULMONARY FUNCTION LABORATORY
(Anesthesiology) 73QMF

Jones Medical Instrument Co. 800-323-7336
200 Windsor Dr, Oak Brook, IL 60523
$3,450.00 per unit (standard).

Medical Graphics Corporation 800-950-5597
350 Oak Grove Pkwy, Saint Paul, MN 55127
PF/X and CPX/MAX with disposable flow sensor. IBM compatible modular 160bit desk-top computer, software library, networking capabilities, breath by breath N2 FRC w/o bags & DLCO. Desktop diagnostic CPX cardiopulmonary exercise testing system, CCM critical care management system, CPF-S clinical pulmonary function system-spirometry equipment, all with breath-by-breath gas exchange data acquisition, calculation and real-time display of flow, oxygen & CO2 physiologic waveform.

COMPUTER, PULMONARY FUNCTION, PREDICTED VALUES
(Anesthesiology) 73BTY

Cardinal Health 207, Inc. 610-862-0800
1100 Bird Center Dr, Palm Springs, CA 92262
Metabolic computer,handheld spirometer to test lung function.

Midmark Diagnostics Group 800-624-8950
3300 Fujita St, Torrance, CA 90505
The IQmark Digital Spirometer has met or exceeded the requirements of the ATS. All standard spirometry measurements are available including FEV6, as recommended by the NLHEP. Standard features on this computer-based spirometer include full-loop, FVC, SVC, MVV, and pre/post BD tests; local or network database storage; trending software; and archive and e-mail capabilities. It is lightweight, weighing only 10 oz., and has no moving parts.

COMPUTER, RADIOGRAPHIC DATA *(Radiology) 90WKA*

Capintec, Inc. 800-631-3826
6 Arrow Rd, Ramsey, NJ 07446

Carl Zeiss Meditec Inc. 877-486-7473
5160 Hacienda Dr, Dublin, CA 94568
A/B Scan's responsive technology makes examinations faster and more accurate. The quad imaging feature offers four different scans to view simultaneously, allowing comparison of real-time serial imagery on-screen and easier identification of complex pathology. On-screen icons help screens guide the operator in managing the system.

Multi Imager Service, Inc 800-400-4549
13865 Magnolia Ave Bldg C, Chino, CA 91710
Founded in 1983, Multi Imager specializes in diagnostic-quality film imaging and digital imaging technologies, including film-based video imagers, wet-film-based laser imagers, dry-film imagers, digital acquisition/storage and transmission devices, computed radiography, PACS, and more. Multi Imager provides technical support and training, parts supply, and sales of new as well as refurbished equipment used with a broad range of modalities, including CT, MRI, ultrasound, nuclear medicine, and others.

Openmed Technologies Corporation 877-717-6215
256 W Cummings Park, Woburn, MA 01801
OpenMed Manager, 'always available' PACS image archive that obsoletes the delayed availability associated with older architectures with image pre-fetch requirements

Supertech, Inc. 800-654-1054
PO Box 186, Elkhart, IN 46515
SUPERTECH permits you to create your own technique charts, custom to your equipment.

Ti-Ba Enterprises, Inc. 585-247-1212
25 Hytec Cir, Rochester, NY 14606
Ti-Ba sells all the computed radiography (CR) products by Konica Minolta Medical Imaging and Radlink

Varian Medical Systems 800-544-4636
3100 Hansen Way, Palo Alto, CA 94304
ARIA Oncology Information management system, with modules for surgical, medical, and radiation oncology. Includes a comprehensive oncology-specific electronic medical record (EMR). Optional local area network system with remote data entry workstations, simulator workstation. Built using industry standard communication protocols and an open architecture design, ARIA provides virtually unlimited enterprise-wide connectivity.

Vitalworks 800-278-0037
239 Ethan Allen Hwy, Ridgefield, CT 06877
RadConnect RIS radiology-information system is for appointment scheduling, transcription, film tracking, mammography tracking, marketing module, ACR reporting--all fully integrated with filmless radiology, billing, and more.

COMPUTER, RADIOGRAPHIC IMAGE ANALYSIS

(Radiology) 90UFD

Advanced American Biotechnology (Aab) 714-870-0290
1166 E Valencia Dr Unit 6C, Fullerton, CA 92831
$9,995 for video camera image analyzer (Apple computer); also, $5,995 for ELISA reader (end point and kinetics) video imaging system and software, $7,995 for DNA sequence reader-editor video imaging system; $22,995 for confocal video imaging and microscopy video imaging system (macro and microscopic). Image Analyzer: Color or monchrome CCD video camera, frame grabber, image analysis for morphology, FISH Fluorescent in Situ Hybridization...B/W system IA...$4,995 color system...$6,995. Particle Size-Shape Analyzer: Macroscopic and microscopic, CCD video camera, grabber, software, Automatic or manual, 9 parameters of sorting. Size range 0.1-2,000um...$7,995. DNA Sequence Reading Analysis Program: Un-distort, automatic-manual sequence reading, read complement, gel match, sequence search, complement, Fingerprinting...$995. RFLP, PCR, RAPD Analysis Program: Quantify, Reads MW, comparison report of all peaks in all lanes, dendrogram analysis, gel match & % similarity. Process negative or positive image. Non-linear background correction. Brightness-contrast...$1,495. Dots-ELISA (Microtiterplate) Analysis Program: Read standard 96 wells, part of, or 360. Images acquired by any scanner. Automatic or manual of straight or tilted image. Standard curve. % confidence...$495. Grid, High density dot blots analysis program: Read up to 150,000 spots for human genome, DNA fingerprinting, send, as all s contrast-brightness & pallete...$1,495. Karyotyping analysis program: Automatic sorting and re-mapping of chromosomes in metaphase according to length or p:q ratio. Human, Plants, animals, birds & insect...$1,495. Chromosomes analysis & FISH: Multicolor or B/W analysis of metaphase or microscopic images. Measurement of distance, radius, curve, angular. Fitlers, arihemtic operations, morphology, statistical & correlation analysis...$2,850. 1D Main (One-dimensional) analysis program: for electophoresis & TLC. Quantify (1D, 2D, PCR, RFLP, DNA & TLC). Read MW, Compare, Overlay, fingerprint, % similarity, 2D analysis, user-defined report, comparison report, image analysis, send, annotate. Undistort, global background correction, brightness-contrast, color palette. Windows or MAC...$495. 1D Advanced & Dendograms + 1D Main analysis programs: Compare many lanes, add, subtract, average, different maps, graphs and tables. Window or MAC...$1,995. Biotech pkgA Analysis Programs: 1D, 2D, DNA sequence, PCR-RFLP-RAPD, automatic fingerprinting, main and advanced s. Dots-ELISA, dynamic comparison. Windows or MAC...$2,850. Biotech pkgB analysis programs: Do-it-all 14 s: 1D, 2D, DNA sequence, PCR-RFLP-RAPD, main and advanced s. Dots-ELISA, colony count, dendograms, image analysis, chromosomes analysis, karyotyping, dynamic comparison, Windows or MAC...$5,500. 2D Main & Advanced (Two-Dimensional) analysis programs: Quantify few or all spots, Read MW & IEP. Compare 2 or many gel, add, subtract, average, overlay. Windows or MAC...$1,995. Gel Documentation and Analysis: FL-IM-II: 0.0003 lux low-light CCD video camera, frame grabber, lens, UV filter, metal dark room, UV & white light transilluminator & 1D main...$7,995. Inexpensive Gel Documentation & Analysis: IM-0, 0.03 lux CCD video camera, UV filter, frame grabber, lens, dark room cone & 1D main...$3,995.

Agfa Corp. 800-581-2432
100 Challenger Rd, Ridgefield Park, NJ 07660

Analogic Corporation 978-326-4000
8 Centennial Dr, Peabody, MA 01960
Data Acquisition (DAS) for computer tomography; spectrometers, gradient coil amplifiers, RF power amplifier sub-systems for magnetic resonance images; image processors for med. applications; full & front-end sub-systems & transducers for ultrasound imaging; AP400 and AP500 series array processors; cardiac digital imaging system for cardiovascular X-ray diagnosis and interventions.

COMPUTER, RADIOGRAPHIC IMAGE ANALYSIS *(cont'd)*

Dome Imaging Systems, Inc. 866-752-6271
400 5th Ave, Waltham, MA 02451
Planar--a global leader in medical displays--offers the DOME CX family of flat panels, specifically designed to provide high-quality, high-resolution displays for the medical-imaging market. The DOME CX family consists of the C2, C3, C5, and C5i flat-panel displays. These displays provide exceptional benefits, with technology and lifecycle cost advantages that are unique to all-digital flat-panel display systems. Offering excellent viewing angles and superior image crispness, the CX flat panels can display up to 3061 distinct shades of gray--significantly more than alternative flat panels and the highest level of displayable gray shades on the market today. All CX flat panels use an active-matrix liquid-crystal display (AMLCD) panel that produces crisp, clear, and consistent display. They generate much lower electro-magnetic emissions and heat, and consume much less power than traditional CRT displays, providing users with an energy-efficient and cost-effective product. As a significant advantage in space-constrained healthcare environments, the compact, lightweight CX displays take up little desk space, operate in portrait or landscape mode, and can be wall mounted. The CX displays are designed to provide quality-controlled, high-resolution display. They are fully DICOM calibrated and use exclusive RightLight technology to automatically monitor display luminance and maintain DICOM conformance. Through the DOME CXtra software, they offer unprecedented ease of use, reliability, and quality assurance. CXtra provides access to display-system information through local and remote interfaces. Users and administrators have access to calibration state, luminance levels, hours of backlight operation, panel temperature, serial numbers, and firmware-revision levels.

Elekta, Inc. 800-535-7355
4775 Peachtree Industrial Blvd, Building 300, Suite 300
Norcross, GA 30092
Radiosurgery.

Faxitron X-Ray, Llc 888-465-9729
225 Larkin Dr Ste 1, Wheeling, IL 60090
Faxitron digital radiography system. The Faxitron Model DX-50 functions as a direct digital, cabinet x-ray imaging system when combined with a desktop computer dedicated controller and high-resolution monitor. The system is the result of five years of digital camera experience and special x-ray tube design.

Fujifilm Medical Systems Usa, Inc. 800-431-1850
419 West Ave, Stamford, CT 06902

Image Analysis, Inc. 800-548-4849
1380 Burkesville St, Columbia, KY 42728
Bone density using standard CT scanner.

Imsi, Integrated Modular Systems Inc. 800-220-9729
2500 W Township Line Rd, PO Box 616, Havertown, PA 19083
RADIN. Full functionality. Tele-Rad and PACS viewing. Cost Effective Licensing. Standard software and hardware components.

Indec Systems, Inc. 408-986-1600
2210 Martin Ave, Santa Clara, CA 95050

Medlink Imaging, Inc. 800-456-7800
200 Clearbrook Rd, Elmsford, NY 10523

Nds Surgical Imaging, Inc. 866-637-5237
5750 Hellyer Ave, San Jose, CA 95138
Diagnostic and Review quality monochrome flat panels. 510K certified use for Digital Mammography.

Openmed Technologies Corporation 877-717-6215
256 W Cummings Park, Woburn, MA 01801
OpenMed Radiology diagnostic workstation

Rockland Technimed Limited Rtl 845-426-1136
3 Larissa Ct, Airmont, NY 10952
Software and workstation for image analysis and 3 D Recon of injury zone

Scimage, Inc. 866-724-6243
4916 El Camino Real Ste 200, Los Altos, CA 94022
PACS Workstation

Stallion Technologies, Inc. 315-476-4330
1201 E Fayette St, Syracuse, NY 13210

COMPUTER, STRESS EXERCISE *(Cardiovascular) 74QMG*

Cardiac Science Corp. 800-777-1777
500 Burdick Pkwy, Deerfield, WI 53531
Quest and ExTOL

Cardinal Health 207, Inc. 800-231-2466
22745 Savi Ranch Pkwy, Yorba Linda, CA 92887
$15,000 for ECG stress system incl. ST analysis.

COMPUTER, STRESS EXERCISE *(cont'd)*

Cybex International, Inc. 800-667-6544
10 Trotter Dr, Medway, MA 02053

Ge Medical Systems Information Technologies 800-643-6439
8200 W Tower Ave, Milwaukee, WI 53223
Complete system with arrythmia documentation, interpretation, final report, 3-16 leads, resting ECG analysis, storage, etc. Several models available.

Hillusa Corp. 305-594-7474
7215 NW 46th St, Miami, FL 33166

Md International, Inc. 305-669-9003
11300 NW 41st St, Doral, FL 33178

Medical Graphics Corporation 800-950-5597
350 Oak Grove Pkwy, Saint Paul, MN 55127
CARDIO-2 Breath-by-breath analysis of 60 metabolic parameters with CAD/NET graphics computer, disposable flow monitor O2 analyzer, CO2 analyzer, ECG monitor/recorder, waveform analyzer & flow module.

Mortara Instrument, Inc. 800-231-7437
7865 N 86th St, Milwaukee, WI 53224
PC-based color stress test system provides ST levels for current and reference data on-screen in ST profile bargraph.

Tsi Medical Ltd. 800-661-7263
47 Athabascan Ave., Unit 105, Sherwood Park, AB T8A-4H3 Canada

COMPUTER, ULTRASOUND *(Radiology) 90VHG*

Circadian Systems 800-669-7001
8099 Savage Way, Valley Springs, CA 95252
SCAN-MATE II ultrasound--lightweight, portable, battery-operated system that allows safe, real-time imaging for in-office, mobile unit, ER, clinic, hospital, at-home or nursing-home use. SCAN-MATE is highly useful for initial or general diagnosis, pain or trauma assessment, serial tracking of emerging conditions. Additionally, initial screening is accomplished without delays and the added expense of hospital scheduling. Also available, Medison 2000 and 4500 Ultrasound Systems are compact mobile imaging units for private practice or hospital usage, offering exceptional image resolution.

Complete System Diagnostics, Inc. 800-722-4273
1170 N Lincoln St Ste 108, Dixon, CA 95620
Ultrasound Systems

Davis Medical Electronics, Inc. 800-422-3547
2441 Cades Way Ste 200, Vista, CA 92081
Hewlett Packard cardiographs, stress systems, and ultrasound. Quinton stress systems and zymed holter.

Gwb International, Ltd. 888-436-4826
PO Box 370, 76 Prospect Street, Marshfield Hills, MA 02051
High frequency ultrasound for skin research. DUB, Digital Ultrasound Imaging System, a high resolution ultrasound for dermatology.

Imaging Associates, Inc. 800-821-3230
11110 Westlake Dr, Charlotte, NC 28273

Imsi, Integrated Modular Systems Inc. 800-220-9729
2500 W Township Line Rd, PO Box 616, Havertown, PA 19083
RADIN Imaging. Full funcionality. Tele-Rad and PACS Viewing. DICOM. Standard software (MS) and hardware components.

Indec Systems, Inc. 408-986-1600
2210 Martin Ave, Santa Clara, CA 95050

Meza Medical Equipment 888-308-7116
108 W Nakoma St, San Antonio, TX 78216

CONCENTRATE, DIALYSIS, HEMODIALYSIS (LIQUID OR POWDER) *(Gastro/Urology) 78KPO*

Advanced Renal Technologies, Inc. 425-453-8777
40 Lake Bellevue Dr Ste 100, Suite 100, Bellevue, WA 98005
Acid concentrate for hemodialysis.

Century Pharmaceuticals, Inc. 317-849-4210
10377 Hague Rd, Indianapolis, IN 46256
Various dialysate concentrates for hempdialysis.

Clariant 704-331-7000
4000 Monroe Rd, Charlotte, NC 28205
Color concentrates.

Clinical Pharmacies, Inc. 800-669-6973
21622 Surveyor Cir # 8-C, Huntington Beach, CA 92646
Hemodialysis concentrates. Dialysate concentrate for hemodialysis.

Di-Chem Concentrate, Inc. 763-422-8311
509 Fishing Creek Rd, Lewisberry, PA 17339
Dialysate concentrate.

CONCENTRATE, DIALYSIS, HEMODIALYSIS (LIQUID OR POWDER) *(cont'd)*

Di-Chem, Inc. 763-422-8311
12297 Ensign Ave N, Champlin, MN 55316
Dialysate additives(liquid or powder).

Dialysis Solutions Inc. 905-669-3832
380 Elgin Mills Rd E, Richmond Hill L4C 5H2 Canada
Sterile bicarbontae renal dialysis concentrate

Diasol, Inc. 800-366-0546
13212 Raymer St, North Hollywood, CA 91605
Dialysate acid concentrate and sodium bicarbonate powder and liquid. Custom formulations; additives.

Nxstage Medical, Inc. 866-697-8243
439 S Union St Fl 5, Lawrence, MA 01843
Premixed dialysate.

Rismed Oncology Systems 256-534-6993
2494 Washington St NW, Huntsville, AL 35811
Liquid concentrate, Acid and BiCarbonate, also in powder.

Rockwell Medical Technologies, Inc. 800-449-3353
30142 S Wixom Rd, Wixom, MI 48393
Hemodialysis concentrate solutions and powders.

Rockwell Medical Technologies, Inc. 248-960-9009
604 High Tech Ct, Greer, SC 29650
Various.

Sorb Technology, Inc. 405-682-1993
3631 SW 54th St, Oklahoma City, OK 73119
Dialysate concentrates, powdered.

CONCENTRATOR, CLINICAL SAMPLE *(Chemistry) 75JJH*

Alpha-Tec Systems, Inc. 800-221-6058
12019 NE 99th St Ste 1780, Vancouver, WA 98682
Formalin-ethyl acetate concentrator.

Cds Analytical, Inc. 800-541-6593
465 Limestone Rd, Oxford, PA 19363

Millipore Corporation 877-246-2247
290 Concord Rd, Billerica, MA 01821
30; AMERICON ULTRA; CENTRIFREE; CENTRIPREP; MINICON; MINIPLUS; 000 NMWL; 000 NMWL); CENTRICON; IMMERSIBLE MOLECULAR SE; IMMERSIBLE MOLECULAR SEPARATOR; ULTRAFREE CL; ULTRAFREE CL (30

Pml Microbiologicals 800-628-7014
27120 SW 95th Ave, Wilsonville, OR 97070

Roche Molecular Systems, Inc. 925-730-8110
4300 Hacienda Dr, Pleasanton, CA 94588
Sample preparation for nucleic acid testing.

Spectrum Laboratories, Inc. 800-634-3300
18617 S Broadwick St, Rancho Dominguez, CA 90220
Disposable/Reusable: Membrane conc. systems, 1.0 - 10ml; Hollow Fiber conc. System, up to 800ml.

Zymark Corporation 508-435-9500
68 Elm St, Hopkinton, MA 01748
Models available to evaporate samples $5,900.00 up to 500 ml.

CONCENTRATOR, OXYGEN *(Anesthesiology) 73RJM*

Airsep Corp. 800-874-0202
401 Creekside Dr, Amherst, NY 14228
FORLIFE 5 lpm oxygen concentrator. NEWLIFE 5 lpm oxygen concentrator.

Allied Healthcare Products, Inc. 800-444-3954
1720 Sublette Ave, Saint Louis, MO 63110

American Biomed Instruments, Inc. 718-235-8900
11 Wyona St, Brooklyn, NY 11207

Invacare Corporation 800-333-6900
1 Invacare Way, Elyria, OH 44035
INVACARE Platinum XL oxygen concentrator (IRC5LX, IRC5LX02), INVACARE HomeFill II Complete Home Oxygen System.

Metro Medical Supply Wholesale 800-768-2002
200 Cumberland Bnd, Nashville, TN 37228

Nidek Medical Products Inc. 800-822-9255
3949 Valley East Industrial Dr, Birmingham, AL 35217
MARK 5 oxygen concentrator - 5 liters.

Respironics Colorado 800-345-6443
12301 Grant St Unit 190, Thornton, CO 80241
Travel DC operated and AC stationary. 6 liter, 13 PSI, performance of 93 + - 3% oxygen concentration at .5 to 5 LPM. $3,250.00.

CONCENTRATOR, OXYGEN *(cont'd)*

Respironics Georgia, Inc. 724-387-4559
175 Chastain Meadows Ct NW, Kennesaw, GA 30144
MILLENNIUM 3 & 5 L oxygen concentrator with optional oxygen indicator.

Sunrise Medical 800-333-4000
7477 Dry Creek Pkwy, Longmont, CO 80503

CONDENSER, AMALGAM AND FOIL, OPERATIVE
(Dental And Oral) 76EKG

Buffalo Dental Mfg. Co., Inc. 516-496-7200
159 Lafayette Dr, Syosset, NY 11791
Mallet, plugging, condenser amalgam & gold foil.

Dentalez Group 866-DTE-INFO
101 Lindenwood Dr Ste 225, Valleybrooke Corporate Center
Malvern, PA 19355

H & H Co. 909-390-0373
4435 E Airport Dr Ste 108, Ontario, CA 91761
Condenser.

Hu-Friedy Manufacturing Co., Inc. 800-483-7433
3232 N Rockwell St, Chicago, IL 60618
$20.55 to $22.10 each, 33 types.

Micro-Dent Inc. 866-526-1166
379 Hollow Hill Rd, Wauconda, IL 60084
Condenser.

Nordent Manufacturing, Inc. 800-966-7336
610 Bonnie Ln, Elk Grove Village, IL 60007
$15.75 per unit (standard).

Premier Dental Products Co. 888-670-6100
1710 Romano Dr, PO Box 4500, Plymouth Meeting, PA 19462

Sci-Dent, Inc. 800-323-4145
210 Dowdle St Ste 2, Algonquin, IL 60102

Suter Dental Manufacturing Company, Inc. 800-368-8376
632 Cedar St, Chico, CA 95928

Water Pik, Inc. 970-221-6129
1730 E Prospect Rd, Fort Collins, CO 80525
Mechanical amalgam condenser.

Wykle Research, Inc. 775-887-7500
2222 College Pkwy, Carson City, NV 89706
Amalgam condenser.

CONDENSER, HEAT AND MOISTURE (ARTIFICIAL NOSE)
(Anesthesiology) 73BYD

Amerivac Usa Inc. 908-486-5200
1207 Pennsylvania Ave, Linden, NJ 07036
Various types of artificial nose.

Ballard Medical Products 770-587-7835
12050 Lone Peak Pkwy, Draper, UT 84020
Ballard flex.

Intersurgical Inc. 315-451-2900
417 Electronics Pkwy, Liverpool, NY 13088
HYDRO-TRACH T, HYDRO-THERM, FILTA-THERM, CLEAR-THERM.

Medicomp 763-389-4473
12535 316th Ave, Princeton, MN 55371
Heat moisture exchanger/artificial nose.

Pall Corporation 800-645-6532
25 Harbor Park Dr, Port Washington, NY 11050
Various.

Pall Lifesciences Puerto Rico Llc 516-801-9064
Carr. 194, Km. O.4, Fajardo, PR 00738
Various.

Smiths Medical Asd Inc. 800-258-5361
10 Bowman Dr, Keene, NH 03431
Heat and moisture exchanger.

Sunmed Usa Llc. 310-531-8222
841 Apollo St Ste 334, El Segundo, CA 90245

Synergetics Usa, Inc. 800-600-0565
3845 Corporate Centre Dr, O Fallon, MO 63368
Condenser.

Ventlab Corp. 336-753-5000
155 Boyce Dr, Mocksville, NC 27028
Artificial nose, heat & moisture exchanger.

CONDENSER, MICROSCOPE *(Pathology) 88KEI*

Western Scientific Co., Inc. 877-489-3726
4104 24th St # 183, San Francisco, CA 94114

CONDITIONER, SIGNAL, PHYSIOLOGICAL
(Cns/Neurology) 84GWK

Bio-Feedback Systems, Inc. 303-444-1411
2736 47th St, Boulder, CO 80301

Grass Technologies, An Astro-Med, Inc. Product Gro 401-828-4002
53 Airport Park Drive, Rockland, MA 02370
Electrode selector.

Nellcor Puritan Bennett (Melville) Ltd. 613-238-1840
700-141 Laurier Ave W, Ottawa K1P 5J3 Canada
Sleep eeg software

Nihon Kohden America, Inc. 800-325-0283
90 Icon, Foothill Ranch, CA 92610

Nite Train'R 503-626-8833
9735 SW Sunshine Ct Ste 100, Beaverton, OR 97005
Enuresis conditioning device.

Soltec Corp. 800-423-2344
12977 Arroyo St, San Fernando, CA 91340

CONDOM *(Obstetrics/Gyn) 85HIS*

Actavis Mid Atlantic Llc 973-889-6960
1877 Kawai Rd, Lincolnton, NC 28092
Personal lubricant.

Alatech Healthcare, Llc. 334-886-9337
595 E Lawrence Harris Hwy, Slocomb, AL 36375
Various types and sizes of rubber contraceptive condoms.

Ansell Healthcare, Inc. 800-952-9916
200 Schulz Dr, Red Bank, NJ 07701

Apex Medical Technologies, Inc. 800-345-3208
10064 Mesa Ridge Ct Ste 202, San Diego, CA 92121
MALE-FACTORPAK and HY-GENE seminal-fluid-collection condom.

Biofilm, Inc. 800-848-5900
3225 Executive Rdg, Vista, CA 92081

Church & Dwight Co., Inc. 609-279-7715
1851 Touchstone Rd, Colonial Heights, VA 23834
Latex condoms.

Conquest Condoms Llc 305-279-0089
9020 SW 83rd St, Miami, FL 33173
Condoms.

Cyprus Personal Care Products, Inc. 415-771-0333
2269 Chestnut St # 237, San Francisco, CA 94123
Condoms.

Female Health Company, The 800-884-1601
515 N State St Ste 2250, Suite 2225, Chicago, IL 60654
FC female condom is the first and only device under a woman's control, designed to prevent the spread of AIDS, other sexually transmitted diseases, as well as unintended pregnancy.

Hospital Specialty Company 800-321-9832
500 Memorial Dr, Nicholasville, KY 40356

Imaging Associates, Inc. 800-821-3230
11110 Westlake Dr, Charlotte, NC 28273

J&J Healthcare Products Div Mcneil-Ppc, Inc 866-565-2229
199 Grandview Rd, Skillman, NJ 08558

Line One Laboratories Inc. 818-886-2288
21230 Lassen St, Chatsworth, CA 91311
Condoms (various types).

Lmr International, Inc. 334-687-4610
1600 State Docks Rd, Eufaula, AL 36027
Condoms.

Manexim Multicorp, Ltd. 416-955-0737
62 Harrington Cres, Willowdale M2M 2Y5 Canada
Condom (contraceptive)

Medi-Hut Co., Inc. 800-882-0139
1935 Swarthmore Ave, Lakewood, NJ 08701

Neo Medical Inc. 888-450-3334
42514 Albrae St, Fremont, CA 94538
Nonspermicidaal seminal collection condom.

Oceans Seven Int'L. 502-634-3221
6620 Escondido St, Hughes Airport Center, Las Vegas, NV 89119
Latex condom.

Okamoto U.S.A., Inc. 800-283-7546
18 King St, Stratford, CT 06615
Latex condoms. Beyond Seven Studded, textured latex condom for enhanced stimulation.

CONDOM *(cont'd)*

San-Mar Laboratories, Inc. 914-592-3130
4 Warehouse Ln, Elmsford, NY 10523
Lubricating jelly.

Scientimed Corp. 510-763-5405
4109 Balfour Ave, Oakland, CA 94610
Condom.

The Female Health Co. 312-595-9123
515 N State St, St. #2225, Chicago, IL 60654

Trigg Laboratories, Inc. 757-224-0177
28650 Braxton Ave, Valencia, CA 91355
Wet light.

CONDOM WITH NONOXYNOL-9 *(Obstetrics/Gyn) 85LTZ*

Church & Dwight Co., Inc. 609-279-7715
1851 Touchstone Rd, Colonial Heights, VA 23834
Condom.

Cyprus Personal Care Products, Inc. 415-771-0333
2269 Chestnut St # 237, San Francisco, CA 94123
Condoms with nonoxynol-9.

Jaisons International, Inc. 203-261-1653
22 Bittersweet Ln, Trumbull, CT 06611
SHARE.

Lmr International, Inc. 334-687-4610
1600 State Docks Rd, Eufaula, AL 36027
Condoms.

CONDOM, NON-LATEX *(Obstetrics/Gyn) 85MOL*

Church & Dwight Co., Inc. 609-279-7715
1851 Touchstone Rd, Colonial Heights, VA 23834
Condom non-laxtex.

Gammadirect Medical Division 847-267-5929
PO Box 383, Lake Forest, IL 60045
Aukuflex polyurethane condom for seminal collection.

CONDUIT, VALVED, PULMONIC *(Cardiovascular) 74MWH*

Medtronic Cardiovascular Surgery, The Heart Valve Div. 800-328-2518
1851 E Deere Ave, Santa Ana, CA 92705
Pulmonary valved conduit.

CONE, RADIOGRAPHIC *(Radiology) 90IZT*

Margraf Dental Manufacturing, Inc. 800-762-2641
611 Harper Ave, Jenkintown, PA 19046
Periapical x-ray and TMJ x-ray equipment.

CONE, RADIOGRAPHIC, LEAD-LINED *(Dental And Oral) 76EAH*

Margraf Dental Manufacturing, Inc. 800-762-2641
611 Harper Ave, Jenkintown, PA 19046
Cone (PID's) for all x-ray units. Manufactured in various lengths for specific techniques.

CONFORMER, OPHTHALMIC *(Ophthalmology) 86HQN*

Advanced Ocular Prosthetics Inc. 412-787-7277
1111 Oakdale Rd Ste 5, Oakdale, PA 15071
Ophthalmic conformer.

Austin Ocular Prosthetics Center, Llc 512-452-3100
711 W 38th St Ste G1A, Austin, TX 78705

B. Graczyk, Inc. 269-782-2100
27826 Burmax Park, Dowagiac, MI 49047
Various types & sizes of conformers.

Center For Ocular Reconstruction 301-652-9282
4833 Rugby Ave Fl 4, Bethesda, MD 20814

Danz Inc. 973-783-2955
460 Bloomfield Ave Ste 302, Montclair, NJ 07042

Gulden Ophthalmics 800-659-2250
225 Cadwalader Ave, Elkins Park, PA 19027

Henthorn Ocular Prosthetics 316-688-5235
744 S Hillside St, Wichita, KS 67211
Conformer, ophthalmic.

Jardon Eye Prosthetics, Inc. 248-424-8560
15920 W 12 Mile Rd, Southfield, MI 48076
Silicone and lucite conformer.

John J. Kelley Associates Ltd. 215-567-1377
1528 Walnut St Ste 1801, Mid City East, PA 19102
Various conformers and post-operative drains.

Kolberg Ocular Products, Inc. 858-695-2021
9663 Tierra Grande St Ste 201, San Diego, CA 92126
Ophthalmic conformer.

CONFORMER, OPHTHALMIC *(cont'd)*

Miller Artificial Eye Laboratory, Inc. 419-474-3939
3030 W Sylvania Ave Ste 13, Toledo, OH 43613
Ophthalmic conformer.

Ocular Concepts Llc. 503-699-7700
4035 Mercantile Dr Ste 208, Lake Oswego, OR 97035
Conformer.

Oculo Plastik Inc. 888-381-3292
200 Sauve West, Montreal, QUE H3L-1Y9 Canada
Acrylic conformers: triangular in five radii (14, 16, 18, 18/20 & 22mm) and in three sizes (S, M, L). Also, the new-allen universal conformer.

Randal Minor Ocular Prosthetics Inc. 813-949-2500
1628 Dale Mabry Hwy Ste 110, Lutz, FL 33548
Ophthalmic conformer.

Richard Danz And Sons, Inc. 212-697-5722
104 E 40th St, New York, NY 10016
Post-op conformer.

Soper Brothers & Associates 713-521-1263
1213 Hermann Dr Ste 320, Houston, TX 77004
Ophthalmic conformer.

Southwest Artificial Eyes, Inc. 210-737-3937
PO Box 100636, San Antonio, TX 78201
Conformer.

Technical Products, Inc. 800-226-8434
805 Marathon Pkwy Ste 150, Lawrenceville, GA 30046
Silicone, solid and perforated.

Thompson Ocular Prosthetics, Inc. 210-223-3754
4118 McCullough Ave Ste 16, San Antonio, TX 78212
Ocular conformer.

Total Molding Services, Inc. 215-538-9613
354 East Broad St., Trumbauersville, PA 18970
Small, Medium, & Large Conformers.

Turntine Ocular Prosthetics, Inc 913-962-6299
6342 Long Ave Ste H, Lenexa, KS 66216
Ophthalmic conformer.

Western Ophthalmics Corporation 800-426-9938
19019 36th Ave W Ste G, Lynnwood, WA 98036

CONFORMER, OPHTHALMIC, BIOLOGICAL TISSUE *(Ophthalmology) 86NQB*

Bio-Tissue, Inc. 305-412-0098
7000 SW 97th Ave Ste 211, Miami, FL 33173
Ophthalmic conformer with amniotic membrane.

CONNECTOR, AIRWAY (EXTENSION) *(Anesthesiology) 73BZA*

Allied Healthcare Products, Inc. 800-444-3954
1720 Sublette Ave, Saint Louis, MO 63110

Amerivac Usa Inc. 908-486-5200
1207 Pennsylvania Ave, Linden, NJ 07036
Various types of oxygen swivel connectors.

Ballard Medical Products 770-587-7835
12050 Lone Peak Pkwy, Draper, UT 84020
Metered dose inhaler adapter.

Beevers Manufacturing, Inc. 800-818-4025
14670 Baker Creek Rd, McMinnville, OR 97128
For the pediatric tracheostoma patient not continuously ventilated. Protects exposed trach tube opening from accidental occlusion by bedding, dressings, clothing, 'fat little chin,' etc.

Dhd Healthcare Corporation 800-847-8000
PO Box 6, One Madison Street, Wampsville, NY 13163
ULTRASET, VENTLOK, and DURALIFE. CIRCUVENT.

Instrumentation Industries, Inc. 800-633-8577
2990 Industrial Blvd, Bethel Park, PA 15102

Intersurgical Inc. 315-451-2900
417 Electronics Pkwy, Liverpool, NY 13088
SUPERSET, MICROMOUNT. Also, accessory kit for monitoring nitric oxide .

Invivo Corporation 425-487-7000
12601 Research Pkwy, Orlando, FL 32826
Airway connector for side-stream co2.

Mercury Medical 800-237-6418
11300 49th St N, Clearwater, FL 33762

Mergenet Medical Inc. 888-925-2526
6601 Lyons Rd Ste B1-B4, Coconut Creek, FL 33073
Trach-Assist

CONNECTOR, AIRWAY (EXTENSION) *(cont'd)*

Phase Ii Medical Mfg., Inc. 603-332-8900
88 Airport Dr Ste 100, Rochester, NH 03867
Double swivel adaptor for bronchoscopy.

Primary Medical Co., Inc. 727-520-1920
6541 44th St N Ste 6003, Pinellas Park, FL 33781
Flex tube, various lengths.

Smiths Medical Asd Inc. 800-258-5361
10 Bowman Dr, Keene, NH 03431
Various types of tracheostomy connectors and accessories.

Smiths Medical Asd, Inc. 610-578-9600
9255 Customhouse Plz Ste N, San Diego, CA 92154
Airway intubation set with accessories (sterile and non-sterile).

Woodhead L.P. 847-272-7990
3411 Woodhead Dr, Northbrook, IL 60062
Hospital grade connectors and plugs.

CONNECTOR, CATHETER *(Surgery) 79GCD*

Becton Dickinson Infusion Therapy Systems, Inc. 888-237-2762
9450 S State St, Sandy, UT 84070

Benlan Inc. 905-829-5004
2760 Brighton Rd., Oakville, ONT L6H 5T4 Canada

Boston Scientific Corporation 508-652-5578
780 Brookside Dr, Spencer, IN 47460

C. R. Bard, Inc., Bard Urological Div. 888-367-2273
13183 Harland Dr NE, Covington, GA 30014

Cadence Science Inc. 888-717-7677
1979 Marcus Ave Ste 215, New Hyde Park, NY 11042

Covidien Lp 508-261-8000
15 Hampshire St, Mansfield, MA 02048

Dynamics Research Corp. 800-522-4321
60 Frontage Rd, Andover, MA 01810

Globalmed Inc. 613-394-9844
155 N. Murray St., Trenton, ONT K8V-5R5 Canada
Catheter mounts and patient connections.

Intravascular Incorporated 800-917-3234
3600 Burwood Dr, Waukegan, IL 60085
FloStar Needleless Connector - patented 'dual-valve' needle free connector for use on venous or arterial lines with luer lock or luer slip in intravenous therapy. Available stand alone or on extension sets.

Kck Industries 888-800-1967
14941 Calvert St, Van Nuys, CA 91411

Kelsar, S.A. 508-261-8000
Blvd. Insurgentes, Libriamento a La, Tijuana 22450 Mexico
Catheter connectors (various)

Medline Manufacturing And Services Llc 847-837-2759
1 Medline Pl, Mundelein, IL 60060
Catheter connectors.

Medovations, Inc. 800-558-6408
102 E Keefe Ave, Milwaukee, WI 53212

Microcision Llc 800-264-3811
5805 Keystone St, Philadelphia, PA 19135

Rgi Medical Manufacturing Inc. 352-378-3633
2321 NW 66th Ct Ste W4, Gainesville, FL 32653
Coiled extension, connecting tube, catheter connector.

Vygon Corp. 800-544-4907
2495 General Armistead Ave, Norristown, PA 19403

CONNECTOR, HYDROCEPHALIC *(Cns/Neurology) 84UAS*

Microcision Llc 800-264-3811
5805 Keystone St, Philadelphia, PA 19135

CONNECTOR, SHUNT *(Gastro/Urology) 78FJQ*

Apothecary Products, Inc. 800-328-2742
11750 12th Ave S, Burnsville, MN 55337

Lifemed Of California 800-543-3633
1216 S Allec St, Anaheim, CA 92805

Microcision Llc 800-264-3811
5805 Keystone St, Philadelphia, PA 19135
CSF (cerebral spinal fluid) shunt parts.

CONNECTOR, SUCTION/IRRIGATION *(Surgery) 79SIP*

Covidien Lp 508-261-8000
15 Hampshire St, Mansfield, MA 02048

Medovations, Inc. 800-558-6408
102 E Keefe Ave, Milwaukee, WI 53212

CONNECTOR, SUCTION/IRRIGATION *(cont'd)*

Moldpro, Inc. 603-721-6286
36 Denman Thompson Hwy, Swanzey, NH 03446
Suction Tubing Connectors (bulk, non-sterile)

CONNECTOR, TUBING, BLOOD *(Cardiovascular) 74WJY*

Astro Seal, Inc. 951-787-6670
827 Palmyrita Ave Ste B, Riverside, CA 92507
Implantable hemetic feedthrough.

Brevet, Inc. 949-474-7000
16661 Jamboree Rd, Irvine, CA 92606
Disposable connector, sterilization trays, perfusion adapters, luer nuts available.

Excel Medical Products, Llc 810-714-4775
3145 Copper Ave, Fenton, MI 48430
Excel-6 and Excel-9 precision y-connector with Touhy-Borst adapter hemostasis valve

Gish Biomedical, Inc. 800-938-0531
22942 Arroyo Vis, Rancho Santa Margarita, CA 92688
Y-type polycarbonate connectors, packaged sterile and non-sterile.

Medi Inc 800-225-8634
75 York Ave, P.O. Box 302, Randolph, MA 02368

Molded Products Inc. 800-435-8957
1112 Chatburn Ave, Harlan, IA 51537
Recirculation sets.

Sorin Group Usa 800-289-5759
14401 W 65th Way, Arvada, CO 80004

CONNECTOR, TUBING, BLOOD, INFUSION, T-TYPE *(Gastro/Urology) 78FKB*

Erika De Reynosa, S.A. De C.V. 781-402-9068
Brecha E99 Sur; Parque, Industrial Reynos, Bldg. Ii Cd, Reynosa, Tamps Mexico
Heparin t connector

Lifemed Of California 800-543-3633
1216 S Allec St, Anaheim, CA 92805

Novosci Corp. 281-363-4949
2828 N Crescentridge Dr, The Woodlands, TX 77381

Np Medical, Inc. 978-368-4514
101 Union St, Clinton, MA 01510

Stryker Puerto Rico, Ltd. 939-307-2500
Hwy. 3, Km. 131.2, Las Guasimas Ind. Park, Arroyo, PR 00714
Y connector.

Vygon Corp. 800-544-4907
2495 General Armistead Ave, Norristown, PA 19403

CONNECTOR, TUBING, DIALYSATE *(Gastro/Urology) 78FKY*

Castle Pines Medical, Inc. 303-442-4514
14883 E Hinsdale Ave Ste 2, Centennial, CO 80112
Pump segment rinse lines and t connector.

Directmed, Inc. 516-656-3377
150 Pratt Oval, Glen Cove, NY 11542

Filtrona Extrusion, Inc./Pexcor Medical Products Div. 800-755-7528
764 S Athol Rd, P.O. Box 659, Athol, MA 01331

CONNECTOR, URETERAL CATHETER *(Gastro/Urology) 78EYK*

Boston Scientific Corporation 508-652-5578
780 Brookside Dr, Spencer, IN 47460

CONSERVER, OXYGEN *(Anesthesiology) 73NFB*

Essex Cryogenics Of Missouri, Inc. 314-832-8077
8007 Chivvis Dr, Saint Louis, MO 63123
Escort, escort conserver.

Inovo, Inc. 239-643-6577
2975 Horseshoe Dr S Ste 600, Naples, FL 34104
Oxygen conserver.

Medical Electronic Devices, Inc. 310-618-0306
2807 Oregon Ct Ste D6, Torrance, CA 90503
Oxygen conserver.

Superior Products, Inc. 216-651-9400
3786 Ridge Rd, Cleveland, OH 44144
Oxygen conserver.

The Respiratory Group 314-659-4311
4150 Carr Lane Ct, Saint Louis, MO 63119
Liquid oxygen conserving device.

CONSOLE, HEART-LUNG MACHINE, CARDIOPULMONARY BYPASS *(Cardiovascular) 74DTQ*

Cardiovention, Inc. 408-873-3400
19200 Stevens Creek Blvd Ste 200, Cupertino, CA 95014
Carriovention powerbase tm console.

National Welders 919-544-3772
630 United Dr, Durham, NC 27713
Lung diffusion gases.

Sorin Group Usa 800-289-5759
14401 W 65th Way, Arvada, CO 80004

Terumo Cardiovascular Systems, Corp 800-521-2818
6200 Jackson Rd, Ann Arbor, MI 48103
Heart Lung Machine modular, integrated console & computerized.

CONSOLE, PATIENT SERVICE *(General) 80RKA*

Allied Healthcare Products, Inc. 800-444-3954
1720 Sublette Ave, Saint Louis, MO 63110

Hill-Rom Holdings, Inc. 800-445-3730
1069 State Road 46 E, Batesville, IN 47006

Independent Solutions, Inc. 847-498-0500
900 Skokie Blvd Ste 118, Northbrook, IL 60062
Class 1 flush, semi-flush and surface wall mounted; single-tier and multi-tier; all aluminum construction. UL listed.

Vista Lighting 800-576-2135
1805 Pittsburgh Ave, Erie, PA 16502

CONTAINER, CRYOBIOLOGICAL STORAGE *(Microbiology) 83VFX*

American Fluoroseal Corp. 800-360-1050
431 E Diamond Ave Ste A, Gaithersburg, MD 20877
KryoSure FEP (Teflon) tissue culture bags for cryopreservation of cells, tissues,and reagents. Cryogenic storage. From 2 ml to 18 liter. Priced from $12 to $103.

CONTAINER, EMBEDDING *(Pathology) 88KER*

Globe Scientific, Inc. 800-394-4562
610 Winters Ave, Paramus, NJ 07652
Embedding cassettes.

Richard-Allan Scientific 269-544-5628
4481 Campus Dr, Kalamazoo, MI 49008
Various.

Sci Gen, Inc. 310-324-6576
333 E Gardena Blvd, Gardena, CA 90248
FDA: Medical Device Manufacturing and packaging. Focus on Histology, Cytology, Analytical and General purpose Reagents, Chemistry, and Sterling and Disinfecting agents.

Simport Plastics Ltd. 450-464-1723
2588 Bernard-Pilon, Beloeil, QUE J3G 4S5 Canada

Surgipath Medical Industries, Inc. 800-225-3035
PO Box 528, 5205 Route 12, Richmond, IL 60071

CONTAINER, EVACUATED *(General) 80TBL*

Baxter Healthcare Corporation, Global Drug Delivery 888-229-0001
25212 W Il Route 120, Round Lake, IL 60073
Evacuated glass containers.

Sterion, Incorporated 800-328-7958
13828 Lincoln St NE, Ham Lake, MN 55304
Surgidyne Closed System for Wound Drainage of active and passive wounds.

The Metrix Co. 800-752-3148
4400 Chavenelle Rd, Dubuque, IA 52002

CONTAINER, FROZEN DONOR TISSUE STORAGE *(General) 80LPZ*

Charter Medical, Ltd. 336-768-6447
3948 Westpoint Blvd Ste A, Winston Salem, NC 27103
Blood freezing bags.

Hydro-Med Products, Inc. 214-350-5100
3400 Royalty Row, Irving, TX 75062
Container, frozen donor tissue storage.

Instant Systems, Inc. 800-340-4029
883 Norfolk Sq, Norfolk, VA 23502
Various types of sterile and non-sterile cryoloc containers.

Stericon, Inc. 708-865-8790
2315 Gardner Rd, Broadview, IL 60155
Cryogenically durable plastic bags.

Tegrant Corporation, Thermosafe Brands 847-398-0110
3930 N Ventura Dr Ste 450, Arlington Heights, IL 60004
Diagnostic Specimen Shippers

CONTAINER, IV *(General) 80KPE*

Advance Medical Designs, Inc. 800-221-3679
1241 Atlanta Industrial Dr, Marietta, GA 30066

App Pharmaceuticals, Llc 847-330-3953
1501 E Woodfield Rd Ste 300E, Schaumburg, IL 60173
Tamper evident seal.

Avail Medical Products 858-635-2206
5950 Nancy Ridge Dr Ste 500, San Diego, CA 92121
Vitalmix plus empty i.v. container.

B. Braun Oem Division, B. Braun Medical Inc. 866-8-BBRAUN
824 12th Ave, Bethlehem, PA 18018
Dual-chambered container to store both drug and diluent.

B. Braun Of Puerto Rico, Inc. 610-691-5400
215.7 Insular Rd., Sabana Grande, PR 00637
Various types of sterile iv mixing containers/bags and accessories.

Baxter Healthcare Corporation Nutrition 888-229-0001
1 Baxter Pkwy, Deerfield, IL 60015
QUICK MIX Container.

Baxter Healthcare Corporation, Global Drug Delivery 888-229-0001
25212 W Il Route 120, Round Lake, IL 60073
Large and small volume parenterals, premix medications, VIAFLEX containers, evacuated glass containers.

Baxter Healthcare S.A. 847-948-2000
Rd. 721, Km. 0.3, Aibonito, PR 00609
Various sterile empty solution containers.

Custom Tape Company 651-228-7044
6270 Claude Way, Inver Grove Heights, MN 55076
Tamper evident seal.

Deuteronomy Management Services,Inc. 850-897-3321
1439 Live Oak St Ste A, Niceville, FL 32578
Decanting device.

Entracare, Llc 913-451-2234
11315 Strang Line Rd, Lenexa, KS 66215
Mix container with attached transfer set.

Health Care Logistics, Inc. 800-848-1633
450 Town St, PO Box 25, Circleville, OH 43113
Various.

Hospira Inc. 877-946-7747
275 N Field Dr, Lake Forest, IL 60045
Multiple

Jorgensen Laboratories 970-669-2500
1450 Van Buren Ave, Loveland, CO 80538

Lucomed Inc. 800-633-7877
45 Kulick Rd, Fairfield, NJ 07004

Medi-Dose, Inc. 800-523-8966
70 Industrial Dr, Ivyland, PA 18974

Millipore Corporation 877-246-2247
290 Concord Rd, Billerica, MA 01821
Intravenous solution bags.

Plasco, Inc. 847-662-4400
Carretera Presta La Amistad, Km.19, Acuna, Coahila Mexico
Empty solution transfer container for total parenteral nutrition

The Metrix Co. 800-752-3148
4400 Chavenelle Rd, Dubuque, IA 52002
SECURE Total parenteral nutrition bags, 250ml. through 4000ml. (available in plastic also).

Tulox Plastics Corp. 800-234-1118
PO Box 984, 401 S. Miller Ave., Marion, IN 46952
Calibrated cylinders used as I. V. chambers.

Walkmed Infusion Llc 303-420-9569
4080 Youngfield St, Wheat Ridge, CO 80033
Various types of sterile reservoir bags.

West Pharmaceutical Services, Inc. 800-231-3000
101 Gordon Dr, Franklin Ctr, PA 19341
Pharmaceutical containers.

CONTAINER, LIQUID NITROGEN *(Anesthesiology) 73VFY*

Premier Medical Products 888-PREMUSA
1710 Romano Dr, Plymouth Meeting, PA 19462

CONTAINER, LIQUID OXYGEN *(Anesthesiology) 73VFZ*

Caire, Inc. 800-482-2473
1800 Sandy Plains Industrial Parkway, Suite 316, Marietta, GA 30066
LIBERATOR, LO-LOSS, Liquid oxygen reservoir.

CONTAINER, LIQUID OXYGEN *(cont'd)*

Cryofab, Inc. 800-426-2186
540 N Michigan Ave, Kenilworth, NJ 07033
Liquid-oxygen accessories.

CONTAINER, MEDICATION, GRADUATED LIQUID
(General) 80KYW

Apothecary Products, Inc. 800-328-2742
11750 12th Ave S, Burnsville, MN 55337

Baxa Corporation 800-567-2292
9540 S Maroon Circle, Suite 400, Englewood, CO 80112
KWIK-VIAL. Unit dose container with labeling. Tamper-evident.

Centurion Medical Products Corp. 517-545-1135
3310 S Main St, Salisbury, NC 28147

Medi-Dose, Inc. 800-523-8966
70 Industrial Dr, Ivyland, PA 18974

Mps Acacia 800-486-6677
785 Challenger St, Brea, CA 92821

Tecan U.S., Inc. 800-338-3226
4022 Stirrup Creek Dr Ste 310, Durham, NC 27703
GENESIS Automated Pipetter automated liquid handling system.

Tri-State Hospital Supply Corp. 517-545-1135
3173 E 43rd St, Yuma, AZ 85365

Ware Medics Glass Works, Inc. 845-429-6950
PO Box 368, Garnerville, NY 10923
Pharmaceutical graduates.

CONTAINER, MEDICATION, HOME-USE *(General) 80WPQ*

Carex Health Brands 800-526-8051
921 E Amidon St, PO Box 2526, Sioux Falls, SD 57104
7-day pill organizer, medium and large, helps organize a week's dosage of pills. It features raised, embossed letters and braille for the sight-impaired; Mediplanner and Mediplanner II has 28 compartments allowing for medications to be dispensed up to 4 times per day for an entire week. The Medi/Chest is comprised of 7 day planners in an organizer tray. The day planners can be removed for convenience when traveling.

Health Enterprises 800-633-4243
90 George Leven Dr, North Attleboro, MA 02760
Pill organizer.

Niagara Pharmaceuticals Div. 905-690-6277
60 Innovation Dr., Flamborough, ONT L9H-7P3 Canada
HEALTH SAVER no. 137 plastic pill boxes with live hinge.

Optelec U.S., Inc. 800-828-1056
3030 Enterprise Ct Ste C, Vista, CA 92081

Pioneer Medical Systems 800-234-0683
3408 Howell St Ste D, Duluth, GA 30096
Pill dispenser. Lets elderly know when to take medicine.

CONTAINER, SHARPES *(General) 80MMK*

Bd Medical 760-631-6520
4665 North Ave, Oceanside, CA 92056
Sharps container.

Bemis Mfg. Co. 920-467-5206
Hwy. Pp West, Sheboygan Falls, WI 53085
Sharps container.

Healer Products, Llc 914-663-6300
427 Commerce Ln Ste 1, West Berlin, NJ 08091
Sharps container.

Intermex Trading & Supports Sa De Cv. 52-553-58953
Rio Neva 33 Col.cuauthemoc, Mexico City Of, Df Mexico
Medical waste disposal containers

Kimchuk, Inc. 203-790-7800
Corporate Drive, Danbury, CT 06810-4130
Demolizer #47 one-gallon point of generation sharps container.

Medical Action Industries, Inc. 800-645-7042
25 Heywood Rd, Arden, NC 28704
Needle counters.

O&M Enterprise 847-258-4515
641 Chelmsford Ln, Elk Grove Village, IL 60007
CONTAINER-SHARPES

Oxus Environmental, Llc 207-487-5300
264 Industrial Park St, Pittsfield, ME 04967
Segrimed single deposit container,sterisharp 3 gallon rsdc.

Pro-Western Plastics Ltd. 780-459-4491
30 Riel Dr., P.O. Box 261, St. Albert, ALB T8N-1N3 Canada

CONTAINER, SHARPES *(cont'd)*

Rd Industries, Inc. 800-759-7090
11811 Calhoun Rd, Omaha, NE 68152
Sharps container.

Safetec Of America, Inc. 800-456-7077
887 Kensington Ave, Buffalo, NY 14215
PERSONAL SHARPS SYSTEM includes everything you need to dispose of sharps, after a single use: containers, labels, and 2 gram Red Z Zafety Pac.

Stericycle 847-367-5910
28161 N Keith Dr, Lake Forest, IL 60045
Biobox Traptop (Various Sizes)

Sterilogic Waste Systems, Inc. 315-455-5600
6691 Pickard Dr, Syracuse, NY 13211
Reusable sharps container.

Stik Stoppers, Inc. 541-726-7869
3777 Douglas Dr, Springfield, OR 97478
Sharps container.

Wcm Waste & Compliance Management, Inc. 760-930-9101
6054 Corte Del Cedro, Carlsbad, CA 92011
Srs 800, sms 2400, srs 2400, sms 4000, sms 10000.

CONTAINER, SLIDE MAILER *(Microbiology) 83TDB*

C & A Scientific Co. Inc. 703-330-1413
7241 Gabe Ct, Manassas, VA 20109
PREMIERE Cardboard slides mailer, single & double.

Thermosafe Brands 847-398-0110
3930 N Ventura Dr Ste 450, Arlington Heights, IL 60004

CONTAINER, SPECIMEN MAILER AND STORAGE
(Pathology) 88KDT

Alpha-Tec Systems, Inc. 800-221-6058
12019 NE 99th St Ste 1780, Vancouver, WA 98682
Transport container.

Bio-Medical Products Corp. 800-543-7427
10 Halstead Rd, Mendham, NJ 07945
$105.00 per case of 12ml stabilized urinalysis, screw-cap, transport tubes, eliminating need for refrigeration (500 per case); $108.50 per case of stabilized urine culture transport tubes (500 per case).

C & A Scientific Co. Inc. 703-330-1413
7241 Gabe Ct, Manassas, VA 20109
PREMIERE Cardboard slides mailer, single, double, 4 place & 20capacity folder. Plastic slide mailers, single & double & 5 piece capacity.

Copan Diagnostics, Inc. 800-216-4016
26055 Jefferson Ave, Murrieta, CA 92562
Swabs.

Doxtech, Llc. 503-641-1865
10025 SW Allen Blvd, Beaverton, OR 97005
Security kits for collection/shipping for urine drug testing and evidence specimens.

Evolution Diagnostic Laboratory, Inc. 800-932-8908
475 Highway 70 Fl 2, Lakewood, NJ 08701
Semen collection container.

Exakt Technologies, Inc. 800-866-7172
7002 Broadway Ext, Oklahoma City, OK 73116
EXAKT-PAK packaging for transporting diagnostic specimens, infectious substances, retrieved medical devices, blood, and blood products. Certified to meet the D.O.T and I.A.T.A. regulations for Class 6.2. Custom designs available.

Heritage Labs Intl., Llc 913-764-1045
1111 West Old 56 Hwy., Olathe, KS 66061
Various.

Hycor Biomedical, Inc. 800-382-2527
7272 Chapman Ave, Garden Grove, CA 92841
Centrifuge tube cap.

Image Molding, Inc. 800-525-1875
4525 Kingston St, Denver, CO 80239
Case of 500.

Meridian Bioscience, Inc. 800-696-0739
3471 River Hills Dr, Cincinnati, OH 45244
PARA-PAK CLEAN For the routine collection, transportation and examination of stool specimens for intestinal parasites.

Rayson Co. Inc., W.R. 800-526-1526
720 S Dickerson St, Burgaw, NC 28425
Disposable medical specimen slide holders.

CONTAINER, SPECIMEN MAILER AND STORAGE *(cont'd)*

Richard-Allan Scientific 269-544-5628
4481 Campus Dr, Kalamazoo, MI 49008
Various specimen mailers & storage containers.

Sarstedt, Inc. 800-257-5101
PO Box 468, 1025, St. James Church Road, Newton, NC 28658

Simport Plastics Ltd. 450-464-1723
2588 Bernard-Pilon, Beloeil, QUE J3G 4S5 Canada

Sonoco 513-874-7655
4633 Dues Dr, Cincinnati, OH 45246
Affordable United Nations Class 6.2 Certified shippers for transport and mail of infectious substances and diagnostic specimens. Paper outer container with metal bottom and metal screwcap top. Aluminum screwcap inner container. Fill in blank labeled box included. Other paper-based cans and tubes, all types and sizes.

Statlab Medical Products, Inc. 800-442-3573
106 Hillside Dr, Lewisville, TX 75057
1 and 2 slide mailer, 20 slide folders, ziplock bags with pouch.

Tegrant Corporation, Thermosafe Brands 847-398-0110
3930 N Ventura Dr Ste 450, Arlington Heights, IL 60004
Cryonegic Shipper for clinical trials acts as a storage and transport system (all in one).

Terumo Cardiovascular Systems (Tcvs) 800-283-7866
28 Howe St, Ashland, MA 01721
Bodily fluid waste container.

Thermosafe Brands 847-398-0110
3930 N Ventura Dr Ste 450, Arlington Heights, IL 60004
Blood tube mailers.

Tip, Inc. 314-729-2969
2 Muirfield Ln, PO Box 410208, Saint Louis, MO 63141
Breast specimen compressor and container. SM 59 dimension 5.0 x 9.0 cms. LG 11 dimension 9.0 x 11.5 cms. CO75 core breast specimen container is 7.5 cm diameter

Vonco Products, Inc. 800-323-9077
201 Park Ave, Lake Villa, IL 60046
Tamper-evident specimen transport bags.

CONTAINER, SPECIMEN MAILER AND STORAGE, NON-STERILE *(Pathology) 88NNK*

Celera Corporation 510-749-4219
1401 Harbor Bay Pkwy, Alameda, CA 94502

Mortech Manufacturing Company 757-224-0177
411 N Aerojet Dr, Azusa, CA 91702

Varian Inc 650-424-5078
25200 Commercentre Dr, Lake Forest, CA 92630
Specimen container.

CONTAINER, SPECIMEN MAILER AND STORAGE, TEMPERATURE CONTROL *(Pathology) 88KDW*

Access Business Group Llc 616-787-4964
7575 E Fulton St, Ada, MI 49355
Genetic test specimen mailer.

Babytooth Technologies, Llc. 802-226-7300
2468 Route 103, Proctorsville, VT 05153
Hyopthermic transport systems.

Becton Dickinson And Company 800-284-6845
1 Becton Dr, Franklin Lakes, NJ 07417
Culture swabs; MULTIPLE; VACUTAINER BRAND SP

Celera Corporation 510-749-4219
1401 Harbor Bay Pkwy, Alameda, CA 94502

Covidien Lp 508-261-8000
15 Hampshire St, Mansfield, MA 02048

Exakt Technologies, Inc. 800-866-7172
7002 Broadway Ext, Oklahoma City, OK 73116
EXAKT-PAK insulated packaging for transporting diagnostic specimens, infectious substances, retrieved medical devices, blood, and blood products. Certified to meet the D.O.T and I.A.T.A. regulations for Class 6.2. Custom designs available.

Heritage Labs Intl., Llc 913-764-1045
1111 West Old 56 Hwy., Olathe, KS 66061
Various.

Packaging Products Corp. 800-225-0484
198 Herman Melville Blvd, New Bedford, MA 02740
ARCTIC BOX insulated shipping containers, cut sheet.

Sarstedt, Inc. 800-257-5101
PO Box 468, 1025, St. James Church Road, Newton, NC 28658

CONTAINER, SPECIMEN MAILER AND STORAGE, TEMPERATURE CONTROL *(cont'd)*

Sci Gen, Inc. 310-324-6576
333 E Gardena Blvd, Gardena, CA 90248
FDA: Medical Device Manufacturing and packaging. Focus on Histology, Cytology, Analytical and General purpose Reagents, Chemistry, and Sterling and Disinfecting agents.

Thermosafe Brands 847-398-0110
3930 N Ventura Dr Ste 450, Arlington Heights, IL 60004

Ussc Puerto Rico, Inc. 203-845-1000
Building 911-67, Sabanetas Industrial Park, Ponce, PR 00731
Endoscopic tissue specimen collection device.

CONTAINER, SPECIMEN MAILER AND STORAGE, TEMPERATURE CONTROLLED, NON-STERILE *(Pathology) 88NNL*

Capitol Vial 334-887-8311
2039 McMillan St, Auburn, AL 36832
Urine drug screen collection kit.

CONTAINER, SPECIMEN, ALL TYPES *(General) 80FMH*

Ampac Flexibles 952-693-2475
5305 Parkdale Dr, Minneapolis, MN 55416

Apex Medical Technologies, Inc. 800-345-3208
10064 Mesa Ridge Ct Ste 202, San Diego, CA 92121
HY-GENE (TM) SEMINAL FLUID COLLECTI; MALE FACTOR PAK (; PAK (

Beekley Corp. 860-583-4700
150 Dolphin Rd, Bristol, CT 06010
Accugrid/coretainer.

Berghof/America 800-544-5004
3773 NW 126th Ave Bldg 1, Coral Springs, FL 33065
Various Teflon bottles, jars and transfer containers available.

C & A Scientific Co. Inc. 703-330-1413
7241 Gabe Ct, Manassas, VA 20109
PREMIERE Specimen bags, 6x9 biohazard printing zip-lock, leak proof.

C. R. Bard, Inc., Bard Urological Div. 888-367-2273
13183 Harland Dr NE, Covington, GA 30014

Centurion Medical Products Corp. 517-545-1135
3310 S Main St, Salisbury, NC 28147

Covidien Lp 508-261-8000
15 Hampshire St, Mansfield, MA 02048

Culture Kits, Inc. 888-680-6853
14 Prentice St, PO Box 748, Norwich, NY 13815

Customs Hospital Products, Inc 800-426-2780
6336 SE 107th Ave, Portland, OR 97266
Container, specimen non-sterile, plastic.

Diagnostics For The Real World, Ltd. 408-773-1511
840 Del Rey Ave, Sunnyvale, CA 94085

Doxtech, Llc. 503-641-1865
10025 SW Allen Blvd, Beaverton, OR 97005
Tamperproof and leakproof specimen container for urine drug testing and evidence storage.

E-Z-Em, Inc. 516-333-8230
750 Summa Ave, Westbury, NY 11590
Specimen containers.

Encompas Unlimited, Inc. 800-825-7701
PO Box 516, Tallevast, FL 34270
$74.50 for acrylic specimen caddy, holds 6 specimen vials in a safe and organized fashion.

Freund Container 800-363-9822
4200 Commerce Ct Ste 206, Corporate Center II, Lisle, IL 60532

Garren Scientific, Inc. 800-342-3725
15916 Blythe St Unit A, Van Nuys, CA 91406
Garren Graduated Drug Testing 60cc. Bottle for use in toxicology and methadone treatment.

Globe Scientific, Inc. 800-394-4562
610 Winters Ave, Paramus, NJ 07652
Sterile and non-sterile for storage and transport; also, fecal sample container.

Health Care Logistics, Inc. 800-848-1633
450 Town St, PO Box 25, Circleville, OH 43113
Specimen transporter.

Huhtamaki Consumer Packaging, Inc. 913-583-3025
100 State St, Fulton, NY 13069
Specimen containers or cups.

CONTAINER, SPECIMEN, ALL TYPES *(cont'd)*

Icu Medical (Ut), Inc 949-366-2183
4455 Atherton Dr, Salt Lake City, UT 84123
Collection arthroscopy oraspecimen trap.

Jero Medical Equipment & Supplies, Inc. 800-457-0644
1701 W 13th St, Chicago, IL 60608

Kentron Health Care, Inc. 615-384-0573
3604 Kelton Jackson Rd, P.o. Box 120, Springfield, TN 37172
Specimen container, sterile.

Lsl Industries, Inc. 888-225-5575
5535 N Wolcott Ave, Chicago, IL 60640
$18.00 per 100 sterile specimen cups.

Mckesson General Medical 800-446-3008
8741 Landmark Rd, Richmond, VA 23228

Medchannel Llc 617-314-9861
1241 Adams St Apt 110, Dorchester Center, MA 02124
Tissue bag.

Medegen Medical Products, Llc 800-233-1987
209 Medegen Drive, Gallaway, TN 38036-0228
LAB-CHOICE 24-hour specimen containers, graduated, 3000mL, amber colored.

Medi Inc 800-225-8634
75 York Ave, P.O. Box 302, Randolph, MA 02368

Medi-Dose, Inc. 800-523-8966
70 Industrial Dr, Ivyland, PA 18974
Tamper-evident bottles and caps, seals and locks.

Medical Action Industries, Inc. 800-645-7042
25 Heywood Rd, Arden, NC 28704
Cup.

Medline Industries, Inc. 800-633-5886
1 Medline Pl, Mundelein, IL 60060

Medtronic Spine Llc 877-690-5353
1221 Crossman Ave, Sunnyvale, CA 94089
Sterile specimen container for transport and storage.

Monogen, Inc. 847-573-6700
3630 Burwood Dr, Waukegan, IL 60085
Monoprep, sample collection vials.

O&M Enterprise 847-258-4515
641 Chelmsford Ln, Elk Grove Village, IL 60007
CONTAINER-SPECIMEN

Parter Medical Products 800-666-8282
17015 Kingsview Ave, Carson, CA 90746
Specimen-collection container.

Polar Plastic Ltd. 514-331-0207
4210 Thimens Blvd., St. Laurent, QUE H4R 2B9 Canada
POLAR RX. Graduated 6oz urine cup etched PRTD 10oz graduated cup PRTD 4oz specimen screw cup.

Profex Medical Products 800-325-0196
2224 E Person Ave, Memphis, TN 38114

Quintron Instrument Company 800-542-4448
3712 W Pierce St, Milwaukee, WI 53215
Gas impermeable bags ranging from 60 cc to 1500 liters.

Rd Plastics Company, Inc. 615-781-0007
4825 Trousdale Dr Ste 203, Nashville, TN 37220
Specimen bag transport.

Samco Scientific Corporation 800-522-3359
1050 Arroyo St, San Fernando, CA 91340
POWER Leak resistant designed, cap and vial system sterile, non-sterile. Five sizes available 90/48, 90/53, 120ml/53mm, 60ml/48, 40ml/48mm.

Simport Plastics Ltd. 450-464-1723
2588 Bernard-Pilon, Beloeil, QUE J3G 4S5 Canada

Sonoco 513-874-7655
4633 Dues Dr, Cincinnati, OH 45246
Affordable United Nations Class 6.2 Certified shippers for transport and mail of infectious substances and diagnostic specimens. Paper outer container with metal bottom and metal screwcap top. Aluminum screwcap inner container. Fill in the blank labeled box included. Other paper-based cans and tubes, all types and sizes.

Starplex Scientific Corp. 423-479-4108
705 Industrial Dr SW, Cleveland, TN 37311

Starplex Scientific Inc. 800-665-0954
50A Steinway Blvd., Etobicoke, ONT M9W 6Y3 Canada
HISTOPLEX Histology specimen storage and transport container with leak-resistant caps.

CONTAINER, SPECIMEN, ALL TYPES *(cont'd)*

Statlab Medical Products, Inc. 800-442-3573
106 Hillside Dr, Lewisville, TX 75057
From 1/2 oz. to 165 oz.

Stedim Biosystems, Inc. 800-914-6644
1910 Mark Ct, Concord, CA 94520
FLEXBOY Flexible carboy system for bio-pharmaceutical processing with a wide selection of components and fittings for your individual needs. Sizes 50 ml-50l. FLEXEL 3D system, integrated, modular system for storage, containment and shipment of large volume sterile fluids. Reusable tank with single use bag. FLEXEL 3D bag, single web laminated high barrier film optimized in a 3D configuration. For use in-house or with the FLEXEL 3D system.

Surgipath Medical Industries, Inc. 800-225-3035
PO Box 528, 5205 Route 12, Richmond, IL 60071

Tagg Industries L.L.C. 800-548-3514
23210 Del Lago Dr, Laguna Hills, CA 92653
Insulated traditional specimen lockbox available with extra-long, heavy-duty strap to hang from most office doors. Available in size 14in. x 10-3/4in. x 7in.; Dual-door specimen lockbox may be positioned at top or sides of door. Available in two sizes.

Tegrant Corporation, Thermosafe Brands 847-398-0110
3930 N Ventura Dr Ste 450, Arlington Heights, IL 60004

Terriss-Consolidated Industries 800-342-1611
807 Summerfield Ave, Asbury Park, NJ 07712
Stainless steel containers.

Thermosafe Brands 847-398-0110
3930 N Ventura Dr Ste 450, Arlington Heights, IL 60004

Tri-State Hospital Supply Corp. 517-545-1135
3173 E 43rd St, Yuma, AZ 85365

Viscot Medical, Llc 800-221-0658
32 West St, PO Box 351, East Hanover, NJ 07936
Natural and red sharps containers in 1.5 and 2.5 gallons with metal locking wall cabinets. 24 hour specimen collection containers.

CONTAINER, SPECIMEN, LAPAROSCOPIC *(Surgery) 79WYS*

Encompas Unlimited, Inc. 800-825-7701
PO Box 516, Tallevast, FL 34270

CONTAINER, SPECIMEN, NON-STERILE *(General) 80NNI*

Capitol Vial 334-887-8311
2039 McMillan St, Auburn, AL 36832
Various specimen containers.

Kentron Health Care, Inc. 615-384-0573
3604 Kelton Jackson Rd, P.o. Box 120, Springfield, TN 37172
Specimen container.

Monogen, Inc. 847-573-6700
3630 Burwood Dr, Waukegan, IL 60085
Specimen transport and storage container (prefilled) accessories empty vials bul.

Qfc Plastics, Inc. 817-649-7400
728 111th St, Arlington, TX 76011
Bowl.

Rd Plastics Company, Inc. 615-781-0007
4825 Trousdale Dr Ste 203, Nashville, TN 37220
Multiple/sample bags.

Richard-Allan Scientific 269-544-5628
4481 Campus Dr, Kalamazoo, MI 49008
Various specimen mailers & storage containers.

Starplex Scientific Corp. 423-479-4108
705 Industrial Dr SW, Cleveland, TN 37311

Statsure Diagnostic Systems, Inc. 508-872-2625
1881 Worcester Rd, Framingham, MA 01701

CONTAINER, SPECIMEN, URINE, DRUGS OF ABUSE, OVER THE COUNTER *(Chemistry) 75MPQ*

Ac Healthcare Supply, Inc. 905-448-4706
11651 230th St, Cambria Heights, NY 11411
Otc test sample collection systems.

Apex Plastics 660-258-7283
570 Main St, Brookfield, MO 64628

Phamatech Inc. 858-643-5555
10151 Barnes Canyon Rd, San Diego, CA 92121
Otc collection kit for drug of abuse testing.

CONTAINER, STERILIZATION (TRAY) *(General) 80RVS*

Advanced Medical Innovations, Inc. 888-367-2641
9410 De Soto Ave Ste J, Chatsworth, CA 91311
SECURE-IT-Y, instrument counting organization & handling system; D&C gynecological instrument tray, various specialty instrument stringers.

Akorn, Inc. 800-535-7155
2500 Millbrook Dr, Buffalo Grove, IL 60089
Sterilization tray with silicone mat for diamond knives, titanium and other instruments.

Alimed, Inc. 800-225-2610
297 High St, Dedham, MA 02026

Anspach Effort, Inc. 800-327-6887
4500 Riverside Dr, Palm Beach Gardens, FL 33410
Sterilization/storage cases.

Bausch & Lomb Surgical 636-255-5051
3365 Tree Court Ind Blvd, Saint Louis, MO 63122

Case Medical, Inc. 888-227-2273
65 Railroad Ave, Ridgefield, NJ 07657
Design and manufacturing of aluminum, stainless steel and high impact plastic cases and trays. Orthopedic, dental, general surgery, endoscopy.

Codman & Shurtleff, Inc 800-225-0460
325 Paramount Dr, Raynham, MA 02767

Encompas Unlimited, Inc. 800-825-7701
PO Box 516, Tallevast, FL 34270
$325.00 gas autoclaving tray for flexible endoscopes.

Greatbatch Medical 716-759-5600
3735 N Arlington Ave, Indianapolis, IN 46218
Aluminum, stainless steel plastic case and tray systems for specific and generic purposes (dental and medical); ultrasonic cleaner baskets and trays; sterilizer cases and trays.

Ivry 305-448-9858
216 Catalonia Ave Ste 106, Coral Gables, FL 33134

Johnson & Johnson Medical Division Of Ethicon, Inc. 800-423-4018
2500 E Arbrook Blvd, Arlington, TX 76014

Katena Products, Inc. 800-225-1195
4 Stewart Ct, Denville, NJ 07834

Kls-Martin L.P. 800-625-1557
11239-1 St. John`s Industrial, Parkway South
Jacksonville, FL 32250
MARTIN Container.

Kmi Surgical Ltd. 800-528-2900
110 Hopewell Rd, Laird Professional Building, Downingtown, PA 19335
Microsurgical instrument sterilization trays.

Medegen Medical Products, Llc 800-233-1987
209 Medegen Drive, Gallaway, TN 38036-0228
MED-ASSIST Stainless steel.

Medin Corporation 800-922-0476
90 Dayton Ave, Bldg. 16 C, Passaic, NJ 07055

Micromedics 800-624-5662
1270 Eagan Industrial Rd, Saint Paul, MN 55121
Instru-Safe systems keep surgical instruments organized in sets and protect the instruments during transportation, storage, and sterile processing...saving time in surgery and reducing instrument damage.

Miltex Inc. 800-645-8000
589 Davies Dr, York, PA 17402
Sterlization Container

Nalge Nunc International 800-625-4327
75 Panorama Creek Dr, Rochester, NY 14625
NALGENE rectangular and round configurations. Spill-resistant pipet and instrument sterilizing pan.

Palmero Health Care 800-344-6424
120 Goodwin Pl, Stratford, CT 06615
Cold sterilization holding tray.

Phelan Manufacturing Corp. 800-328-2358
2523 Minnehaha Ave, Minneapolis, MN 55404

Placon Corporation 800-541-1535
6096 McKee Rd, Fitchburg, WI 53719
Thermoformed specialty medical device trays for implants, vascular devices, catheters, ampoules, and surgical kits

Polar Ware Co. 800-237-3655
2806 N 15th St, Sheboygan, WI 53083
Medical perforated sterilization trays, many sizes available. Solid instrument trays and sterilization units also available.

CONTAINER, STERILIZATION (TRAY) *(cont'd)*

Pst 413-447-8051
1520 East St, Pittsfield, MA 01201

Rhein Medical, Inc. 800-637-4346
5460 Beaumont Center Blvd Ste 500, Suite 500, Tampa, FL 33634
Sterilization trays for micro instruments.

Richard Wolf Medical Instruments Corp. 800-323-9653
353 Corporate Woods Pkwy, Vernon Hills, IL 60061

Riley Medical, Inc. 800-245-3300
27 Wrights Lndg, Auburn, ME 04210
FLASHPAK sterilization trays.

San-I-Pak,Pacific Inc. 800-875-7264
23535 S Bird Rd, Tracy, CA 95304
#1 Sterilization bags - #2 Autoclave - #3 Decontamination - #4 Polypropylene bags. Polypropylene bags used for the treatment of infectious waste in steam sterilizers. Bags to fit in instrument, retort, HiVac, tube or cart sterilization.

Scanlan International, Inc. 800-328-9458
1 Scanlan Plz, Saint Paul, MN 55107
VIP system, sterilization tray systems (plastic and metal).

Schueler & Company, Inc. 516-487-1500
PO Box 528, Stratford, CT 06615

Simpex Medical, Inc. 800-851-9753
401 E Prospect Ave, Mount Prospect, IL 60056

Smith & Nephew, Inc., Endoscopy Division 800-343-8386
130 Forbes Blvd, Mansfield, MA 02048

Stephens Instruments, Inc. 800-354-7848
2500 Sandersville Rd, Lexington, KY 40511
$220.00 per unit (standard).

Stryker Spine 866-457-7463
2 Pearl Ct, Allendale, NJ 07401

United Dental Manufacturers, Inc. 918-878-0450
PO Box 700874, Tulsa, OK 74170
Mini Box 2000, Basic Box 2000, Semi Box 2000.

CONTAINER, SURGICAL INSTRUMENT *(Surgery) 79VEE*

Case Design Corp. 800-847-4176
333 School Ln, Telford, PA 18969

Case Medical, Inc. 888-227-2273
65 Railroad Ave, Ridgefield, NJ 07657
Design and manufacturing of aluminum, stainless steel and high impact plastic cases and trays.

Elmed, Inc. 630-543-2792
60 W Fay Ave, Addison, IL 60101
Full- and half-size containers, $270 to $495, three inner tray sizes, stackable, color coded.

Fortrad Eye Instruments Corp. 973-543-2371
8 Franklin Rd, Mendham, NJ 07945

Geen Healthcare Inc. 800-565-4336
931 Progress Ave. Ste.13, Scarborough, ONT M1G 3V5 Canada
POLARWARE - medical blue plastic and steel containers. i.e. bowls, basins, instrument holders, etc.

Greatbatch Medical 716-759-5600
3735 N Arlington Ave, Indianapolis, IN 46218
Aluminum, stainless steel and plastic containers. Orthopedic and sterilization.

Healthmark Industries 800-521-6224
22522 E 9 Mile Rd, Saint Clair Shores, MI 48080
11 models of lightweight 3-part container systems for safety collecting, soaking, transporting and processing contaminated instruments and sharps.

Johnson & Johnson Medical Division Of Ethicon, Inc. 800-423-4018
2500 E Arbrook Blvd, Arlington, TX 76014

Medline Industries, Inc. 800-633-5886
1 Medline Pl, Mundelein, IL 60060
TASKITS solid aluminum instrument container systems with solid lids and bottoms to prevent instrument damage. Two-valve system allows sterilization without disposable filters.

Paragon Medical, Inc. 800-225-6975
8 Matchett Dr, Pierceton, IN 46562
Surgical instrument delivery system. Custom and standard reusable sterilization containers for organizing and protecting instruments and instrument sets during transport, sterilization and storage.

CONTAINER, SURGICAL INSTRUMENT *(cont'd)*

Star Case Manufacturing Co., Inc. 800-822-7827
648 Superior Ave, Munster, IN 46321
Specialized cases and containers for all surgical related instruments and devices.

Surgical Tools, Inc. 800-774-2040
1106 Monroe St, Bedford, VA 24523

Tray-Pak Corporation 888-926-1777
PO Box 14804, Tuckerton Road & Reading Crest Avenue Reading, PA 19612
Thermoformed trays, custom made for surgical kits.

Western Case, Inc. 877-593-2182
14351 Chambers Rd, Tustin, CA 92780
Instrument cases.

CONTAINER, TRANSPORT, KIDNEY *(Gastro/Urology) 78KDK*

Thermosafe Brands 847-398-0110
3930 N Ventura Dr Ste 450, Arlington Heights, IL 60004

CONTAINER, URINE SPECIMEN *(General) 80SEE*

Bio-Medical Products Corp. 800-543-7427
10 Halstead Rd, Mendham, NJ 07945
$105.00 per case of 12ml stabilized urinalysis, screw-cap, transport tubes, eliminating need for refrigeration (500 per case); $95.00 per case of 90ml stabilized urine transport containers (400 per case); $108.50 per case of stabilized urine culture transport tubes (500 per case). 40 ml, 60 ml, 90 ml, 120 ml and also sterile 120 ml screw cap containers.

Cargille Laboratories 973-239-6633
55 Commerce Rd, Cedar Grove, NJ 07009
STABILUR and CULT-UR urinary sediment/chemistry specimen three-day room temperature stabilizer tablets. Four sizes STABILUR tablets for urine volumes from 5 to 56 cc. Three sizes CULT-UR tablets for urine volumes of 5, 10, and 56 cc. Bottles of 1,000 and 10,000 are approximately $0.06 to $0.09 per tablet depending on size of tablet, bottle, and bottles ordered.

Chagrin Safety Supply, Inc. 800-227-0468
8227 Washington St # 1, Chagrin Falls, OH 44023

Covidien Lp 508-261-8000
15 Hampshire St, Mansfield, MA 02048

Helena Plastics 800-227-1727
3700 Lakeville Hwy Ste 200, Petaluma, CA 94954

Image Molding, Inc. 800-525-1875
4525 Kingston St, Denver, CO 80239
Case of 1000 tubes and caps.

Mckesson General Medical 800-446-3008
8741 Landmark Rd, Richmond, VA 23228

Medegen Medical Products, Llc 800-233-1987
209 Medegen Drive, Gallaway, TN 38036-0228
UROLEX Translucent, disposable containers with screw cap. ClikSeal Container Specimen is translucent with blue cover, very leak resistant. Available in sterile or non-sterile packaging. CLIKSEAL very leak resistant, great for pneumatic tube systems, 3 or 4oz container available, sterile or nonsterile packing.

Medi Inc 800-225-8634
75 York Ave, P.O. Box 302, Randolph, MA 02368

Profex Medical Products 800-325-0196
2224 E Person Ave, Memphis, TN 38114

Ross Disposable Products 800-649-6526
401 Traders Blvd E, Unit 10, Mississauga, ON L4Z 2H8 Canada

Samco Scientific Corporation 800-522-3359
1050 Arroyo St, San Fernando, CA 91340
24-hour urine specimen container, 3000ml, 2500ml, and 3500ml for 24-hour collection of urine specimen.

Simport Plastics Ltd. 450-464-1723
2588 Bernard-Pilon, Beloeil, QUE J3G 4S5 Canada

Starplex Scientific Inc. 800-665-0954
50A Steinway Blvd., Etobicoke, ONT M9W 6Y3 Canada
LEAKBUSTERS Leakproof plastic urine container, available in a variety of sizes and materials.

Thermosafe Brands 847-398-0110
3930 N Ventura Dr Ste 450, Arlington Heights, IL 60004

CONTINUOUS POSITIVE AIRWAY PRESSURE UNIT (CPAP, CPPB) *(Anesthesiology) 73QMH*

Ambu, Inc. 800-262-8462
6740 Baymeadow Dr, Glen Burnie, MD 21060

CONTINUOUS POSITIVE AIRWAY PRESSURE UNIT (CPAP, CPPB) *(cont'd)*

Beevers Manufacturing, Inc. 800-818-4025
14670 Baker Creek Rd, McMinnville, OR 97128
In combination with your existing infant NCPAP prongs, Cannulaide improves the pressure seal and helps reduce skin irritation.

Cardinal Health 207, Inc. 800-231-2466
22745 Savi Ranch Pkwy, Yorba Linda, CA 92887
Infant flow system provides a ventilatory support strategy that eases spontaneous respiration while simultaneously restoring the infant's functional residual capacity to reduce the work of breathing.

Hamilton Medical, Inc. 800-426-6331
4990 Energy Way, Reno, NV 89502
ARABELLA - NCPAP system. Mixing gas monitor with nasal prongs.

Invacare Corporation 800-333-6900
1 Invacare Way, Elyria, OH 44035
Polaris EX CPAP, Polaris EX Heated Humidifier

Medcovers, Inc 800-948-8917
500 W Goldsboro St, Kenly, NC 27542
Replacement headgear for CPAP units.

Respironics Colorado 800-345-6443
12301 Grant St Unit 190, Thornton, CO 80241
$1,260.00 - delivers CPAP with ramp, 3- to 18-cm H2O.

Respironics Georgia, Inc. 724-387-4559
175 Chastain Meadows Ct NW, Kennesaw, GA 30144
TRANQUILITY quest & TRANQUILITY plus CPAP systems provide various options for the treatment of obstructive sleep apnea syndrome.

Sleepnet Corporation 800-742-3646
5 Merrill Industrial Dr, Hampton, NH 03842
IQ, Phantom, and MiniMe nasal masks and Mojo SleepMask full face mask for CPAP therapy. Masks feature flexible shells; soft, contoured gel cushions; embedded bendable ring for a comfortable, compliant fit. Latex free and hypoallergenic.

Sunrise Medical 800-333-4000
7477 Dry Creek Pkwy, Longmont, CO 80503

Vacumed 800-235-3333
4538 Westinghouse St, Ventura, CA 93003
Nasal CPAP generator; also available, nasal CPAP masks and accessories.

Vitaid Ltd. 800-267-9301
300 International Dr, Williamsville, NY 14221
Boussignac CPAP - single use

CONTINUOUS, VENTILATOR, HOME USE
(Anesthesiology) 73NOU

Respironics California, Inc. 724-387-4559
2271 Cosmos Ct, Carlsbad, CA 92011
Ventilator.

CONTOURING, INSTRUMENT, MATRIX, OPERATIVE
(Dental And Oral) 76EKF

Addent, Inc. 203-778-0200
43 Miry Brook Rd, Danbury, CT 06810
The Trimax Composite Instrument provides a better way to create posterior composite restorations. Improved polymerization of deep restorations as well as tight anatomically correct contact areas are only two of the Trimax instruments' many benefits. By combining the inherent advantages of optically clear disposable micro light guides that are shaped to fit different size teeth and an ergonomically correct triangular instrument handle, the Trimax instrument makes ideal posterior composite placement easy, fast and accurate.

Almore International, Inc. 503-643-6633
PO Box 25214, Portland, OR 97298
$77.50 per unit (standard).

C.E.J. Dental Products Inc. 949-493-2449
32332 Camino Capistrano Ste 101, San Juan Capistrano, CA 92675
Contouring instrument, multiple sizes and shapes.

Envision Dental Solutions 208-529-4321
2515 Channing Way, Idaho Falls, ID 83404
Contact forcep, contact maker, matrix contouring forcep.

CONTRACEPTIVE CERVICAL CAP *(Obstetrics/Gyn) 85LLQ*

Femcap Incorporated 858-792-2624
14058 Mira Montana Dr, Del Mar, CA 92014
Cervical cap-barrier contraceptive device.

Yama, Inc. 908-206-8706
650 Liberty Ave, Union, NJ 07083
Diaphragm / cervical cap.

PRODUCT DIRECTORY

CONTRACT ASSEMBLY *(General) 80WVW*

Advanced Polymers, Inc. 603-327-0600
29 Northwestern Dr, Salem, NH 03079
Extrusion of polymeric tubing, heat shrink tubing, balloon fabrication and other processing and catheter prototyping.

Altron, Inc. 763-427-7735
6700 Bunker Lake Blvd NW, Ramsey, MN 55303
Custom electronics assembly.

Antibodies, Inc. 800-824-8540
PO Box 1560, Davis, CA 95617
ISO13485, CGMP, small- and medium-run contract manufacturing and assembly of reagents and diagnostic kits.

Armm, Inc. 714-848-8190
17744 Sampson Ln, Huntington Beach, CA 92647
Tubing sets, filter assemblies with fittings, ultrasonic welding services, packaging services, electromechanical devices.

Avail Medical Products, Inc. 866-552-2112
201 Main St, 1600 Wells Fargo Tower, Fort Worth, TX 76102
Full-service outsource design and manufacturing for sterile, single-use medical devices. From initial product concept through finished goods, fulfillment and distribution. Design, process development and validation, manufacturing, injection molding, packaging, sterilization services management, manufacturing transfer.

B. Braun Oem Division, B. Braun Medical Inc. 866-8-BBRAUN
824 12th Ave, Bethlehem, PA 18018

Brady Corporation 800-541-1686
6555 W Good Hope Rd, PO Box 571, Milwaukee, WI 53223
Contract assembly and packaging, including leadwire insertion, pouch packaging, and full lot traceability.

Catheter Research, Inc. (Cri) 317-872-0074
5610 W 82nd St, Indianapolis, IN 46278
Contract assembly and packaging, product development and re-design, sourcing, centerless grinding, 510(k) preparation, Class 100,000 cleanroom available.

Coeur Inc., Sheboygan 800-874-4240
3411 Behrens Pkwy, Sheboygan, WI 53081

Command Medical Products, Inc. 386-672-8116
15 Signal Ave, Ormond Beach, FL 32174
A full range of assembly services, including UV bonding, solvent bonding, tipping, eye punching, silk screening, pad printing, impulse sealing, and kit packing.

Controltek, Inc. 360-896-9375
3905 NE 112th Ave, Vancouver, WA 98682
Circuit assembly, cables, box build, test services.

Csi Holdings 615-452-9633
170 Commerce Way, Gallatin, TN 37066

Deringer-Ney, Inc. 860-242-2281
2 Douglas St, Ney Industrial Park, Bloomfield, CT 06002
Contract Assembly and Manufacturing

Dravon Medical, Inc. 503-656-6600
11465 SE Highway 212, PO Box 69, Clackamas, OR 97015
OEM contract assembly and packaging.

Enova Medical Technologies 866-773-0539
1839 Buerkle Rd, Saint Paul, MN 55110
Class 10000 cleanroom available. Automated and manual systems.

Enpath Medical, Inc. 800-559-2613
2300 Berkshire Ln N, Minneapolis, MN 55441
Cleanroom assembly of stimulation leads, catheters, implants, introducers, and pacing accessory kits. Assembly using laser welding.

Evergreen Research, Inc. 303-526-7402
433 Park Point Dr Ste 140, Golden, CO 80401

Gdm Electronic And Medical 408-945-4100
2070 Ringwood Ave, San Jose, CA 95131

Globe Medical Tech, Inc. 713-365-9595
1766 W Sam Houston Pkwy N, Houston, TX 77043
Manufacturing and assembling of medical disposables such as IV sets, vein sets, burettes, blood sets, syringes, etc. at our Class 100,000 cleanroom facility to meet your private-labeling needs and specifications.

Gw Plastics, Inc. 802-234-9941
239 Pleasant St, Bethel, VT 05032
Class 10,000 assembly, automatic. Automatic & manual assembly.

CONTRACT ASSEMBLY *(cont'd)*

Harmac Medical Products, Inc. 716-897-4500
2201 Bailey Ave, Buffalo, NY 14211
Contract manufacturer of custom disposable medical devices offering assembly, solvent bonding, heat sealing, packaging, and sterilization services. OEM and private-labeled products. Class 100,000 cleanrooms.

Innovative Surgical Products, Inc. 714-836-4474
2761 Walnut Ave, Tustin, CA 92780
Complete assemblies or sub-assemblies; contract packaging of trays, pouches, kits etc. and ETO or radiation sterilization services.

Intersurgical Inc. 315-451-2900
417 Electronics Pkwy, Liverpool, NY 13088

Ipax, Inc. 303-975-2444
2622 S Zuni St, Englewood, CO 80110
Custom assembly.

J-Pac, Llc 603-692-9955
25 Centre Rd, Somersworth, NH 03878
Cleanroom assembly of sterile, disposable medical devices utilizing core competencies that include RF and ultrasonic cutting and welding, vacuum and pressure forming, proprietary cutting and edge treatment of implantable textiles, heat sealing and welding, and design and development of customized automation and tooling.

Lifemed Of California 800-543-3633
1216 S Allec St, Anaheim, CA 92805
Lifemed contract assembly and manufacturing services.

Lucomed Inc. 800-633-7877
45 Kulick Rd, Fairfield, NJ 07004

Lyons Tool And Die Company 800-422-9363
185 Research Pkwy, Meriden, CT 06450
Rapid prototyping. Production of medical devices in class 10,000 clean rooms. Medical knives and scissors. Precision metal stamping. Engineering services.

M&C Specialties Co. 800-441-6996
90 James Way, Southampton, PA 18966

Mack Molding Co. 802-375-2511
608 Warm Brook Rd, Arlington, VT 05250
Custom injection molding and assembly of plastic parts.

Metronix 813-972-1212
12421 N Florida Ave Ste D201, Tampa, FL 33612
Life Saving Prouducts,Wheelchairs, Patient Room Furniture, Reclining chairs,Manikins for safety, training aids for emergency , medical and rescue personnel

Millipore Corporation 877-246-2247
290 Concord Rd, Billerica, MA 01821
Contract sterile fill of fluids.

Novosci Corp. 281-363-4949
2828 N Crescentridge Dr, The Woodlands, TX 77381

Oliver Medical 800-253-3893
445 6th St NW, Grand Rapids, MI 49504
Design and Assembly

Pacon Manufacturing Corporation 732-357-8020
400 Pierce St # B, Somerset, NJ 08873
Custom assembly kit.

Pepin Manufacturing, Inc. 800-291-6505
1875 S Highway 61, Lake City, MN 55041
Automated or hand.

Phillips Plastics Corp. 877-508-0252
1201 Hanley Rd, Hudson, WI 54016

Precision Medical Products, Inc. 717-335-3700
44 Denver Rd, PO Box 300, Denver, PA 17517

Quality Bioresources, Inc. 888-674-7224
1015 N Austin St, Seguin, TX 78155

Rahd Oncology Products 800-844-0103
10762 Indian Head Industrial Blvd, Saint Louis, MO 63132
Provides service for the oncology industry.

Rms Company 763-783-5074
8600 Evergreen Blvd NW, Minneapolis, MN 55433
Contract assembly, packaging, labeling in Class 100,000 clean room.

Specialteam Medical Services, Inc. 714-694-0348
22445 La Palma Ave Ste F, Yorba Linda, CA 92887

Surgical Technologies, Inc. 800-777-9987
292 E Lafayette Frontage Rd, Saint Paul, MN 55107
Assembly, packaging and sterilization services. Located in St. Paul, MN, and a European facility in Amsterdam, the Netherlands.

Tailored Label Products, Inc. 800-727-1344
W165N5731 Ridgewood Dr, Menomonee Falls, WI 53051

CONTRACT ASSEMBLY *(cont'd)*

The Tech Group 480-281-4500
14677 N 74th St, Scottsdale, AZ 85260
Clean rooms, sonic welding, solvent bonding, decorating and packaging capabilities.

Tmp Technologies, Inc. 716-895-6100
1200 Northland Ave, Buffalo, NY 14215
General.

CONTRACT LABORATORY *(General) 80VAB*

Andersen Products, Inc., 800-523-1276
3202 Caroline Dr, Health Science Park, Haw River, NC 27258
Sterilization validation services.

Axiom Analytical, Inc. 949-757-9300
1451 Edinger Ave Ste A, Tustin, CA 92780
Sampling systems providing rapid inspection of incoming materials, surface analysis of polymers, analysis of multiple sample streams and rapid waste water analysis.

B. Braun Oem Division, B. Braun Medical Inc. 866-8-BBRAUN
824 12th Ave, Bethlehem, PA 18018

Bachem Bioscience, Inc. 800-634-3183
3700 Horizon Dr, King Of Prussia, PA 19406
Custom syntheses of products of customer's choice (amino acid derivatives, peptides, proteins, enzyme substracts and inhibitors, organic chemicals) are performed, also in industrial quantities, according to GMP requirements. All custom inquiries are treated with absolute discretion and confidentiality.

Basi (Bioanalytical Systems, Inc.) 800-845-4246
2701 Kent Ave, West Lafayette, IN 47906
Contract analytical laboratory services for the pharmaceutical industry.

Bd Lee Laboratories 800-732-9150
1475 Athens Hwy, Grayson, GA 30017
Custom fermentation; custom polyclonal antisera.

Currie Medical Specialties, Inc. 800-669-3521
730 Los Angeles Ave, Monrovia, CA 91016

Dynatec Scientific Labs, Inc. 915-849-1322
11940 Golden Gate Rd, El Paso, TX 79936
Ethylene oxide, steam and radiation support services.

Idexx Laboratories, Inc. 800-548-6733
1 Idexx Dr, Westbrook, ME 04092

Interstate Blood Bank, Inc. 800-258-9557
5700 Pleasant View Rd, Memphis, TN 38134
Blood bank laboratory services, incl. sampling and testing for clinical trials.

J&S Medical Associates 800-229-6000
35 Tripp St Ste 1, Framingham, MA 01702
$1,000-$5,000 for full service hematology contract, $5,000-$8,000 for full service contract Beckman Astra. $7,000 Olympus demand. Service Bio Chem Atal 6000, AVL, MLA 700,800, Coulter and Sequoia Turner, Roche Mira, Beckman CX 3.

Lab Corp Of America 800-833-3984
1904 Alexander Drive, Durham, NC 27709-2652

Lab Corp. 800-222-7566
430 S Spring St, Burlington, NC 27215

Microcheck, Inc. 877-934-3284
142 Gould Road, Northfield, VT 05663
$40.00 to $90.00 ea. for ID and comparative analysis. Identifies over 1,500 species of yeast, mycobacteria, fungi and actinomycetes. 96 hour turnaround standard. 48 hour STAT turnaround.

Osteotech, Inc. 800-537-9842
51 James Way, Eatontown, NJ 07724
Bone and tissue processing.

Pro Science, Inc., Glass Shop Div. 800-267-1616
92 Railside Rd., Toronto, ONT M3A 1A3 Canada
Custom laboratory glassware and apparatus. Borosilicate or quartz glass.

Psychemedics Corp. 800-628-8073
125 Nagog Park Ste 200, Acton, MA 01720
Historical substance-abuse tests using hair samples; price depends on volume.

Quantachrome 800-989-2476
1900 Corporate Dr, Boynton Beach, FL 33426
Complete fine particle characterization.

Quest Diagnostics, Inc. 800-222-0446
3 Giralda Farms, Madison, NJ 07940

CONTRACT LABORATORY *(cont'd)*

Specialty Laboratories, Inc. 800-421-7110
27027 Tourney Rd, Valencia, CA 91355
Clinical reference laboratory.

Sterigenics International, Inc. 800-472-4508
2015 Spring Rd Ste 650, Oak Brook, IL 60523
Laboratory services include contract testing, contract research and product development using pilot EO and steam sterilization vessels. BIER vessel. Protocol and validation services.

Sts Duotek, Inc 800-836-4850
370 Summit Point Dr, Henrietta, NY 14467
Non-routine and routine, in vivo and in vitro biocompatibility/toxicology evaluations, vivarium, USP microbiology testing, sterility testing, microbial limits and bioburden testing, antibiotic assay studies, package integrity/shelf-life, disinfectant ocular products, microbiology testing. Also, gas chromatography, HPLC, UV/Visible spectrophotometry, particle counts and size analysis, and other analytical chemistry testing methods.

Trace Laboratories-East 410-584-9099
5 N Park Dr, Hunt Valley, MD 21030
Full service laboratory specializing in chemical, electrical, mechanical, environmental, thermal,and metallographical studies,failure analysis, and contamination/material identification. The company emphasizes technical expertise and dedication to customer service. It is ISO 9001:2000,ISO 17025, and A2LA accredited and is a certificated UL Agency.

Truett Labs 626-334-5106
798 N Coney Ave, Azusa, CA 91702
Only manufacturing.

CONTRACT MANUFACTURING *(General) 80VAC*

Accellent El Paso 915-771-9112
31 Butterfield Trail Blvd Ste C, El Paso, TX 79906
Broad variety of medical devices

Acme-Monaco Corp. 860-224-1349
75 Winchell Rd, New Britain, CT 06052
Custom, medical use guidewires for OEM. Special guidewire design, prototype development and fabrication available.

Advanced Biomedical Devices, Inc. (Abd, Inc.) 978-470-1177
Dundee Park, Bldg. 17, Andover, MA 01810
Contract engineering and design.

Advanced Polymers, Inc. 603-327-0600
29 Northwestern Dr, Salem, NH 03079
Full-service polymer manufacturing, extrusion polymers and other processing and prototyping.

Alceram Tech Inc 516-849-3666
57 2nd St, Ronkonkoma, NY 11779

Alsons Corp. 800-421-0001
3010 Mechanic Rd, P.O. Box 282, Hillsdale, MI 49242
Shower heads.

American Fluoroseal Corp. 800-360-1050
431 E Diamond Ave Ste A, Gaithersburg, MD 20877
FEP (Teflon) tissue culture bags for cryogenics, cell culture and reagent storage.

Amici, Inc. 610-948-7100
518 Vincent St, Spring City, PA 19475
Private label breathing devices manufacturing. Also, DRY-ALL moisture indicating dessicant. Adapters in various sizes.

Andersen Products, Inc., 800-523-1276
3202 Caroline Dr, Health Science Park, Haw River, NC 27258
Contract manufacturing, packaging, and sterilization of disposable medical devices.

Antibodies, Inc. 800-824-8540
PO Box 1560, Davis, CA 95617
ISO9001, cGMP, small and medium-run contract manufacturing and assembly of reagents and diagnostic kits.

Apex Medical Technologies, Inc. 800-345-3208
10064 Mesa Ridge Ct Ste 202, San Diego, CA 92121
Specializing in thin-film dip molding of synthetic elastomer materials. Materials range from thermoplastic polyurethanes to synthetic polyisoprene latex and can be incorporated to customer requirements into products or components from catheter balloons to probe covers. Capabilities include prototype product development through contract production manufacturing.

Apw Eder Industries, Inc. 414-761-0400
2250 W South Branch Blvd, Oak Creek, WI 53154
Circuit boards and microprocessors.

CONTRACT MANUFACTURING *(cont'd)*

Arlon Engineered Coated Products 800-232-7181
6110 Rittiman Rd, San Antonio, TX 78218
Pressure-sensitive tapes and films; custom laminating.

Armm, Inc. 714-848-8190
17744 Sampson Ln, Huntington Beach, CA 92647
Full service manufacture of disposable medical devices.

Associated Design And Manufacturing Co. 800-837-8257
8245 Backlick Rd Ste K, Lorton, VA 22079

Astro Seal, Inc. 951-787-6670
827 Palmyrita Ave Ste B, Riverside, CA 92507
Medical connectors for: heart pacers, cochlear implants, cardiac and respiratory monitors, exploratory probes, and remote analyzing devices.

Atc Technologies, Inc. 781-939-0725
30B Upton Dr, Wilmington, MA 01887
OEM full service including assemblies and packaging.

Atrion Medical Products, Inc. 800-343-9334
1426 Curt Francis Rd NW, Arab, AL 35016

Avail Medical Products, Inc. 866-552-2112
201 Main St, 1600 Wells Fargo Tower, Fort Worth, TX 76102
Full-service outsource design and manufacturing for sterile, single-use medical devices. From initial product concept through finished goods, fulfillment and distribution. Design, process development and validation, manufacturing, injection molding, packaging, sterilization services management, manufacturing transfer.

Avery Dennison Corporation 626-304-2000
150 N Orange Grove Blvd, Pasadena, CA 91103
Contract manufacturing for disposable medical devices.

B-Tec Solutions Inc. 215-785-2400
913 Cedar Ave, Croydon, PA 19021

B. Braun Oem Division, B. Braun Medical Inc. 866-8-BBRAUN
824 12th Ave, Bethlehem, PA 18018
The OEM Division of B. Braun Medical Inc. offers a complete range of contract services throughout the medical product life cycle, including design and prototyping, manufacturing, packaging, sterilization, quality control and regulatory guidance.

Bausch & Lomb, Inc. 813-724-6600
21 N Park Place Blvd, Clearwater, FL 33759
Manufacturer of ophthalmic lenses.

Beckman Coulter, Inc. 800-742-2345
250 S Kraemer Blvd, PO Box 8000, Brea, CA 92821

Benchmark Electronics, Inc. 409-849-6550
3600 Technology Dr., Angleton, TX 77515
Printed circuit board assemblies.

Benchmark Electronics, Inc. 507-452-8932
4065 Theurer Blvd, Winona, MN 55987
Electronic printed circuit board assemblies (PCBA), electronic final system assembly (box build, system integration), FDA Manufacturer of Record.

Benlan Inc. 905-829-5004
2760 Brighton Rd., Oakville, ONT L6H 5T4 Canada
P.V.C. Medical Tubing, Clamps, Sheets; Extrusions, Injection Moldings.

Bio Breeders, Inc. 617-926-5278
116 Temperton Parkway, Watertown, MA 02472

Bio Med Sciences, Inc. 800-257-4566
7584 Morris Ct Ste 218, Allentown, PA 18106
Breathable hydrophobic membrane.

Biolitec, Inc. 800-934-2377
515 Shaker Rd, East Longmeadow, MA 01028
Manufacturer of sterile OEM fiber optic laser delivery systems (25 to 100 watts), PCS hard clad and all-silica optical fiber (248nm to 2.1 microns). Jackets include nylon, polyimide, and Teflon.

Bioserv Corporation 858-450-3123
5340 Eastgate Mall, San Diego, CA 92121
Contract services for diagnostic test kits, powder and liquid filling, lyophilization, and packaging. Certified Class 100,000 to Class 100 rooms for medical device and pharmaceutical manufacturing.

Biosig Instruments, Inc. 800-463-5470
PO Box 860, Champlain, NY 12919
SENSORS For measurement of any fitness parameters.

CONTRACT MANUFACTURING *(cont'd)*

Bolt Bethel, Llc 763-434-5900
23530 University Avenue Ext NW, PO Box 135, Bethel, MN 55005
Bolt Bethel, LLC is a precision contract manufacturer specializing in the production of intricate and complex medical instruments, devices, and components. Utilizing the latest techniques, the company produces surgical instruments, infusion ports, orthopedic implants, surgical staplers, endoscopic and arthroscopic components, and electrosurgical equipment, as well as a wide variety of various medical components. Instruments, devices, and components are manufactured from stainless steel, titanium, cobalt chrome, nitinol, and plastic, as well as exotic materials. Major capabilities include CNC turning and milling, CNC Swiss turning, grinding, lapping, honing, EDM, and light assembly. Typical finishes are from 4-16 micro inches and tolerances are held as close as 0.000011 of an inch.

Bpsp Co. (Medical Z Corp.) 800-368-7478
6800 Alamo Downs Pkwy, San Antonio, TX 78238
Manufacturer of customized pressure garments.

Brady Corporation 800-541-1686
6555 W Good Hope Rd, PO Box 571, Milwaukee, WI 53223
OEM contract manufacturing of medical devices, electrodes, transdermal patches, diagnostic components. Full-service development assistance, from prototypes through automated manufacturing.

Brady Precision Converting, Llc 214-275-9595
1801 Big Town Blvd Ste 100, Mesquite, TX 75149
Diecutting, laminating, printing and packaging of medical devices. Precision converters.

Burton Medical Products, Inc. 800-444-9909
21100 Lassen St, Chatsworth, CA 91311
Lamps, lights, illuminators etc.

C&J Industries, Inc. 814-724-4950
760 Water St, Meadville, PA 16335

Cadence Science Inc. 888-717-7677
1979 Marcus Ave Ste 215, New Hyde Park, NY 11042
Needle assemblies, cannulas, tubing and fittings.

Capintec, Inc. 800-631-3826
6 Arrow Rd, Ramsey, NJ 07446
Wipe test counter; hot cells.

Carley Lamps 310-325-8474
1502 W 228th St, Torrance, CA 90501
Custom-made hi-intensity sub-miniature lamps, vacuum or gas filled, halogen and reflectors.

Carver Inc. 260-563-7577
1569 Morris St, Wabash, IN 46992
Designer and manufacturer of custom presses and accessories, including hydraulic presses from 12 to 100 tons pressure.

Casco Manufacturing Solutions, Inc. 800-843-1339
3107 Spring Grove Ave, Cincinnati, OH 45225
Specializing in radio requency sealing and ultrasonic bonding as well as traditional cut and sew operations.

Catheter Research, Inc. (Cri) 317-872-0074
5610 W 82nd St, Indianapolis, IN 46278
Contract assembly and packaging, product development and re-design, sourcing, centerless grinding, 510(k) preparation, Class 100,000 cleanroom available.

Clarke Manufacturing, Inc. 414-444-7003
3000 W Clarke St, Milwaukee, WI 53210
Contract manufacturing bone screws and orthopedic instrumentation.

Clinimed, Incorporated 877-CLINIMED
303 Markus Ct, Sandy Brae Industrial Park, Newark, DE 19713

Coeur Inc., Sheboygan 800-874-4240
3411 Behrens Pkwy, Sheboygan, WI 53081
Medical tubing and custom medical device assembly.

Command Medical Products, Inc. 386-672-8116
15 Signal Ave, Ormond Beach, FL 32174
RF welding of bags, extrusion of medical tubing, assembly and packaging of custom disposable medical devices.

Controltek, Inc. 360-896-9375
3905 NE 112th Ave, Vancouver, WA 98682

Csi Holdings 615-452-9633
170 Commerce Way, Gallatin, TN 37066

Currie Medical Specialties, Inc. 800-669-3521
730 Los Angeles Ave, Monrovia, CA 91016

Dacor Manufacturing Co., Inc. 618-939-8700
8718 Hanover Industrial Dr, Columbia, IL 62236

CONTRACT MANUFACTURING *(cont'd)*

Dade Behring, Inc. 800-948-3233
1717 Deerfield Rd, Deerfield, IL 60015
OEM sensors and modules.

Degania Silicone, Inc. 401-333-8199
1226 Mendon Rd, Cumberland, RI 02864
Silicone rubber medical devices and catheters that are sold under the private label of its customers.

Dicon, Inc. 800-426-0493
2355 S 1070 W, Salt Lake City, UT 84119

Disetronic Sterile Products 800-280-7801
124 Heritage Ave, Portsmouth, NH 03801
Catheters, infusion devices and extension sets.

Dravon Medical, Inc. 503-656-6600
11465 SE Highway 212, PO Box 69, Clackamas, OR 97015
Custom vinyl bags; from drainage to blood handling.

Dynamics Research Corp. 800-522-4321
60 Frontage Rd, Andover, MA 01810
Metal fabrication.

Edmund Industrial Optics 800-363-1992
101 E Gloucester Pike, Barrington, NJ 08007
Custom microscopes.

Elcoma Metal Fabricating Canada 705-526-9636
878 William St., P.O. Box 685, Midland, ONT L4R-4P4 Canada
Custom tubular fabricating to FDA specification. Custom design, color and materials.

Engineered Assemblies Corporation 201-288-4477
380 North St, Teterboro, NJ 07608
Battery design, manufacturing and distribution service for high and low volume manufacturing for Medical, Telecommunication and security equipments.

Enova Medical Technologies 866-773-0539
1839 Buerkle Rd, Saint Paul, MN 55110
Automated and semi-automated custom designed systems. Contract Medical Device Design, ISO 13485 Certified.

Enpath Medical, Inc. 800-559-2613
2300 Berkshire Ln N, Minneapolis, MN 55441
Catheter, introducer, stimulation leads, pacing accessory kits, delivery systems, implant tools, precision laser processing including welding and ablation.

Esco Medical Instruments, Inc. 800-970-3726
21 William Penn Dr, Stony Brook, NY 11790
Micromachining of medical components and assembly of medical instruments.

Excel Medical Products, Llc 810-714-4775
3145 Copper Ave, Fenton, MI 48430
Excel Medical Products is an FDA-Registered, ISO and GMP compliant contract manufacturer specializing in medical components and devices. Excel Medical Products offers the following services and capabilities: Class 100,000 clean room manufacturing and assembly, thermoplastic and elastomer injection molding, LSR (liquid silicone rubber) injection molding, insert molding, custom assembly, custom kitting, pouch sealing, tray sealing, and pad printing. Additional capabilities included adhesive, solvent and UV bonding, tipping, flaring, skiving and micro drilling. We also offers product development, process development and mold design services. Excel Medical Products provides custom solutions from conception to completion.

Filtrona Extrusion, Inc./Pexcor Medical Products Div. 800-755-7528
764 S Athol Rd, P.O. Box 659, Athol, MA 01331

Foothills Industries, Inc. 828-652-4088
300 Rockwell Dr, Marion, NC 28752
Sub-contract.

Forest Dental Products Inc 800-423-3535
6200 NE Campus Ct, Hillsboro, OR 97124

Forward Technology 320-286-2578
260 Jenks Ave SW, Cokato, MN 55321
Plastic-bonding equipment, spin welders, hot-plate welders, leak testers, thermostaking equipment, ultrasonic welders, and vibration welders.

Freund Container 800-363-9822
4200 Commerce Ct Ste 206, Corporate Center II, Lisle, IL 60532
Plastic, metal and glass containers.

Galloway Plastics, Inc. 847-615-8900
940 W North Shore Dr, Lake Bluff, IL 60044
Custom anatomical models.

CONTRACT MANUFACTURING *(cont'd)*

Gdm Electronic And Medical 408-945-4100
2070 Ringwood Ave, San Jose, CA 95131

Genesis Manufacturing, Inc. 317-485-7887
720 E Broadway St, Fortville, IN 46040
Contract Radio-Frequency (RF) Welding. From development to manufacturing and packaging.

Gerstner & Sons Inc. 937-228-1662
20 Gerstner Way, Dayton, OH 45402
Custom wood instrument cases. Custom wood presentation cases. Wood display chests and cases.

Gettig Pharmaceutical Instrument Co., Div Of Gettig Technologies Inc. 814-422-8892
1 Streamside Pl. W., Spring Mills, PA 16875-0085
Injection molded devices for various pharmaceutical applications.

Globe Medical Tech, Inc. 713-365-9595
1766 W Sam Houston Pkwy N, Houston, TX 77043
Can meet your private-label needs and specifications at our Class 100,000 cleanroom facility for medical disposables including IV sets, small vein sets, burettes, blood sets, syringes and needles, etc.

Guild Optical Associates, Inc. 603-889-6247
11 Columbia Dr, Amherst, NH 03031
Custom sapphire lenses, windows, mirrors and other optical components. Window sizes from 1mm diameter; lenses from 8mm with any combination of plano, concave or convex configurations. We produce these parts with precision dimensional tolerances and superior fit and finishes

Harmac Medical Products, Inc. 716-897-4500
2201 Bailey Ave, Buffalo, NY 14211
Full-service contract manufacturer of custom disposable medical devices. Class 100,000 cleanrooms. Services include: assembly, RF-welding, solvent bonding, packaging, sterilization, product engineering, insert molding, and injection molding.

Hart Enterprises, Inc. 616-887-0400
400 Apple Jack Ct, Sparta, MI 49345
Special-application needles and custom medical devices.

Heatron, Inc. 913-651-4420
3000 Wilson Ave, Leavenworth, KS 66048
Custom heating element manufacturing.

Helix Medical, Inc. 800-266-4421
1110 Mark Ave, Carpinteria, CA 93013

Hi-Tech Rubber, Inc. 800-924-4832
3191 E La Palma Ave, Anaheim, CA 92806

Hi-Tronics Designs, Inc. 973-347-4865
999 Willow Grove St, Hackettstown, NJ 07840
Contract manufacturing and design of implantable and external arrhythmia monitors, cardiovascular stimulators, bone growth stimulators and neurologic stimulators and ventricle assist devices.

Holmed Corporation 508-238-3351
40 Norfolk Ave, South Easton, MA 02375

Hydrofera Llc 866-861-7548
322 Main St, Willimantic, CT 06226

I.W. Tremont Co. 973-427-3800
79 4th Ave, Hawthorne, NJ 07506
Filter products and absorbent media.

Innova Corp. 860-242-3210
68 E Dudley Town Rd, Bloomfield, CT 06002
Electrodes, dressings and other die cut, laminated P.S.A. disposable products.

Innovative Surgical Products, Inc. 714-836-4474
2761 Walnut Ave, Tustin, CA 92780
Assembly, packaging, sealing, labeling and sterilization according to customer specifications.

Instrument Technology, Inc. 413-562-3606
33 Airport Rd, Westfield, MA 01085

Ironwood Industries, Inc. 847-362-8681
115 S Bradley Rd, Libertyville, IL 60048
Plastics assembly and packaging, ultrasonic welding, thermal insertion/staking, adhesive bonding, transfer printing and surface treatment.

Ispg, Inc. 860-355-8511
517 Litchfield Rd, New Milford, CT 06776
Stainless-steel tubing, blunts, cutoffs, custom-ground cannulae; huber cannulae standard and custom glass syringes. Special needles.

CONTRACT MANUFACTURING *(cont'd)*

J-Pac, Llc 603-692-9955
25 Centre Rd, Somersworth, NH 03878
J-PAC manufactures products supporting the medical device and diagnostic market segments. Custom tooling and automation are developed as needed to meet client manufacturing requirements. Sterile, disposable medical device assembly and packaging are a specialty.

Kapco (Kent Adhesive Products Co.) 800-791-8964
1000 Cherry St, Kent, OH 44240

Kawasumi Laboratories America, Inc. 800-529-2786
4723 Oak Fair Blvd, Tampa, FL 33610

Kent Elastomer Products, Inc. 800-331-4762
1500 Saint Clair Ave, PO Box 668, Kent, OH 44240
Custom manufacturing of a wide variety of tubing materials in a broad array of materials, sizes, colors and lengths.

Kenyon Industries, Inc. 973-962-4844
235 Margaret King Ave, Ringwood, NJ 07456
Specializing in disposables including medical and dental instruments, dental examination kits and medical patient care kits and trays.

Konigsberg Instruments, Inc. 626-449-0016
2000 E Foothill Blvd, Pasadena, CA 91107
Qualified (FDA, CE/MDD) Medical Manufacturing Services

Lacey Manufacturing Co. 203-336-0121
1146 Barnum Ave, PO Box 5156, Bridgeport, CT 06610
Disposable medical products.

Lake Region Manufacturing, Inc. 952-448-5111
340 Lake Hazeltine Dr, Chaska, MN 55318
Lead tips & other pacing lead machined parts; coils, springs, wires and phaco tips.

Lifecore Biomedical, Inc. 952-368-4300
3515 Lyman Blvd, Chaska, MN 55318
Contract aseptic fill of liquids into syringes or vials. Specializing in difficult-to-fill (viscous) formulations. Development validation and scale-up services related to aseptic manufacturing are available.

Lifemed Of California 800-543-3633
1216 S Allec St, Anaheim, CA 92805
Lifemed contract assembly and manufacturing services.

Lyons Tool And Die Company 800-422-9363
185 Research Pkwy, Meriden, CT 06450
Rapid prototyping. Production of medical devices in class 10,000 clean rooms. Medical knives and scissors. Precision metal stamping. Engineering services.

M&C Specialties Co. 800-441-6996
90 James Way, Southampton, PA 18966
Medical tapes, die cutting, lamination and printing of pressure sensitive tapes.

Medegen 800-520-7999
930 S Wanamaker Ave, Ontario, CA 91761
Mold fabrication, I.V. components, luer-lock connectors, custom medical molding (plastic).

Medegen Medical Products, Llc 800-233-1987
209 Medegen Drive, Gallaway, TN 38036-0228
Injection molding & blow molding plastics, stainless steel forming.

Medical Concepts Development 800-345-0644
2500 Ventura Dr, Saint Paul, MN 55125
Wide-web converting of thin films, non-wovens and soft metal roll goods.

Medical Plastic Devices (Mpd), Inc. 866-633-9835
161 Oneida Dr., Pointe Claire, QUE H9R 1A9 Canada

Meditron Inc D.B.A. Medcare Usa 800-243-2442
3435 Montee Gagnon, Terrebonne, QUEBE J6Y-1J4 Canada

Medovations, Inc. 800-558-6408
102 E Keefe Ave, Milwaukee, WI 53212

Metronix 813-972-1212
12421 N Florida Ave Ste D201, Tampa, FL 33612
Patient care furniture, various monitors, morgue and pathology equipment.

Mettler-Toledo, Inc. 800-METTLER
1900 Polaris Pkwy, Columbus, OH 43240
Reaction carolorimeter; density meters; thermal analysis instruments.

Microcision Llc 800-264-3811
5805 Keystone St, Philadelphia, PA 19135
Close-tolerance machining (0.0002) of medical implants and device parts. Fine hand deburring.

Microsurgical Laboratories 713-723-6900
11333 Chimney Rock Rd Ste 120, Houston, TX 77035

CONTRACT MANUFACTURING *(cont'd)*

Microtek Medical, Inc 800-936-9248
512 N Lehmberg Rd, Columbus, MS 39702
Equipment covers, specialty patient drapes, endoscope instrument accessories, wound drainage.

Minnesota Wire & Cable Co. 800-258-6922
1835 Energy Park Dr, Saint Paul, MN 55108

Moll Industries, Inc. 972-663-6900
13455 Noel Rd Ste 1310, Dallas, TX 75240

Mycoscience, Inc. 860-684-0030
25 Village Hill Rd, Willington, CT 06279
Includes contract R&D/diagnostics and contract laboratory services.

National Medical Products 800-940-6262
9775 Mining Dr Ste 104, Jacksonville, FL 32257
Medical positioning products. Orthopedic, general, physical therapy.

Navion Biomedical Corp. 781-341-8058
312 Tosca Dr, Stoughton, MA 02072

Nemcomed 800-255-4576
801 Industrial Dr, Hicksville, OH 43526
Contract machines.

Nortech Systems Incorporated 952-345-2244
1120 Wayzata Blvd E Ste 201, Wayzata, MN 55391

Nova Biomedical 800-458-5813
200 Prospect St, Waltham, MA 02453
Contract manufacturing of medical products and diagnostic analyzers.

Nuell, Inc. 800-829-7694
PO Box 55, 312 East Van Buren St., Leesburg, IN 46538
Contract manufacturing of orthopedic devices.

Numed Canada, Inc. 613-936-2592
45, Second Street West, Cornwall, ONT K6J 1G3 Canada

Nypro Inc. 978-365-9721
101 Union St, Clinton, MA 01510
Custom medical device and component manufacturing.

Ophtec Usa, Inc. 561-989-8767
6421 Congress Ave Ste 112, Boca Raton, FL 33487
Ophthalmology products.

Optometrics Llc 978-772-1700
8 Nemco Way, Stony Brook Ind. Pk., Ayer, MA 01432
Optical components and instruments, Including Diffraction Gratings, Monochromators and Modules, Interference Filters, Laser Optics & Products, Wire Grid Polarizers.

Orchid Unique 989-746-0780
6688 Dixie Hwy, Bridgeport, MI 48722
Reamers. Saw blades, stainless steel and carbide burs, drills, routers, rasps and special cutting assemblies.

Otto Bock Heathcare 800-328-4058
2 Carlson Pkwy N Ste 100, Minneapolis, MN 55447
Orthopedic seating system.

Pall Corporation 800-521-1520
600 S Wagner Rd, Ann Arbor, MI 48103
Custom filtration products for OEM applications; solid phase supports for immunodiagnostic test kits.

Pentagon Co., The 800-414-8888
17130 Devonshire St Ste 101, Northridge, CA 91325

Pepin Manufacturing, Inc. 800-291-6505
1875 S Highway 61, Lake City, MN 55041
Precision die cutting, slitting, laminating, island placement, coating, inflatable products, membrane switches, wound-care products, TENS electrodes, transdermal products, and diagnostic test kits.

Performance Systematix Inc 616-949-9090
5569 33rd St SE, Grand Rapids, MI 49512
Custom filters: In-house engineering, design & manufacturing capabilities.

Pgm 585-458-4300
1305 Emerson St, Rochester, NY 14606
Specializing in close-tolerance critical components. Full-service organization, offering CAD/CAM, modeling, in-house tooling, stampings, CNC multiaxis turning, milling, grinding, precision deburring and assembly. Sheetmetal, paint, welding.

Phillips Plastics Corp. 877-508-0252
1201 Hanley Rd, Hudson, WI 54016

CONTRACT MANUFACTURING *(cont'd)*

Phytron, Inc. 800-96P-HYTR
600 Blair Park Rd Ste 220, Williston, VT 05495
Stepper motors, 2-phase with diameters ranging from 19 to 125 mm, with a resolution of up to 500 full steps per revolution. All can be rated for vacuum, cryogenic and high temperature environments. Stepper motor controls, high efficient power stage for 2-phase stepper motors. Also available, positioning systems including translation, rotational, goniometers and linear actuators for high precision positioning.

Plexus Corp 425-482-1300
20001 N Creek Pkwy, Bothell, WA 98011
Service organization to respond to issues facing today's competitive medical electronics industry, including providing design resources for new product development, enhancing existing products to provide logical extensions, supporting product manufacturing requirements, contributing expertise to non-electronic related companies, and entering into partnerships with start-up companies.

Plexus Corp. 877-733-5919
55 Jewelers Park Dr, PO Box 156, Neenah, WI 54956
Electronic manufacturing services (EMS).

Plitek, L.L.C 800-966-1250
69 Rawls Rd, Des Plaines, IL 60018
High-technology fabricated film and plastic products. Prototyping services to help during product development with NO tooling charge. Three Clean room manfucaturing facilities available.

Point Medical Corp. 219-663-1775
891 E Summit St, Crown Point, IN 46307
Subassembly, assembly, catheters, other. Convert from latex. Implant grade.

Precision Medical Products, Inc. 717-335-3700
44 Denver Rd, PO Box 300, Denver, PA 17517
Insert molding, plastic joining, swaging, wire forming, micro machining, polishing/tumbling, plastic extrusion, metal stamping, metal joining, coining, injection molding, pointing, micro grooving, plastic tipping & forming, grinding & honing, metal tipping & forming, hypodermic needle manufacturing and component assembly services, manufacturing bifurcated vaccinating needle for smallpox vaccination.

Precision Optics Corp. 800-447-2812
22 E Broadway, Gardner, MA 01440
Advanced lens design, optical system design, structural design and analysis, prototype production and evaluation, optics testing, and high-volume optical system manufacture; video endocouplers, endoscopes and fiberoptic eyepieces.

Princeton Case Co., Inc. 908-687-1750
667 Lehigh Ave, Union, NJ 07083
Custom carrying cases with customized foam inserts.

Progressive Dynamics Medical, Inc. 269-781-4241
507 Industrial Rd, Marshall, MI 49068
Electrical & mechanical components.

Putnam Precision Products 845-278-2141
3859 Danbury Rd, Brewster, NY 10509
Mechanical sub assemblies, components.

Radix Corp. 204-697-2349
#2-572 South Fifth St., Pembina, ND 58271
Casegoods for the healthcare market built/matched to the customer's requirements.

Renick Ent., Inc. 561-863-4183
1211 W 13th St, Riviera Beach, FL 33404
medical device and surgical device manufacturing

Richards Micro-Tool, Inc. 508-746-6900
250 Nicks Road,, Plymouth, MA 02360-2800

Rms Company 763-783-5074
8600 Evergreen Blvd NW, Minneapolis, MN 55433
Contract manufacturing.

Rose Technologies Company 616-233-3000
1440 Front Ave NW, Grand Rapids, MI 49504

Roskamp Champion 800-366-2563
2975 Airline Cir, Waterloo, IA 50703

S4j Manufacturing Services, Inc. 888-S4J-LUER
2685 NE 9th Ave, Cape Coral, FL 33909
Contract manufacturing and designing of tubing connectors.

Saes Memry 203-739-1100
3 Berkshire Blvd, Bethel, CT 06801

Sanderson-Macleod, Inc. 866-522-3481
1199 S Main St, P.O. Box 50, Palmer, MA 01069
Contract manufacture of brushes.

CONTRACT MANUFACTURING *(cont'd)*

Shippert Medical Technologies Corp. 800-888-8663
6248 S Troy Cir Ste A, Centennial, CO 80111
PVA foam packing products.

Shore Medical, Inc. 714-628-9785
1050 N Batavia St Ste C, Orange, CA 92867

Sigma-Aldrich Corp. 800-521-8956
3050 Spruce St, Saint Louis, MO 63103
Chemical Contract Manufacturing.

Smi 920-876-3361
Industrial Park, 544 Sohn Drive, Elkhart Lake, WI 53020
Diagnostic strips and wound care products.

Smiths Medical Asd 800-424-8662
5700 W 23rd Ave, Gary, IN 46406
Silicone extrusion and molding; silicone catheter and cannula assembly, printing and packaging; device design and development.

Sparton Electronics Florida, Inc. 800-824-0682
5612 Johnson Lake Rd, De Leon Springs, FL 32130
Surface-mount technology, printed circuit boards, and final assembly and test of complex products.

Specialized Medical Devices, Llc 800-463-1874
300 Running Pump Rd, Lancaster, PA 17603
Design, development of precision components.

Specialteam Medical Services, Inc. 714-694-0348
22445 La Palma Ave Ste F, Yorba Linda, CA 92887

Spectra Medical Devices, Inc. 866-938-8649
4C Henshaw St, Woburn, MA 01801
Specializing in custom sets.

Sr Instruments, Inc. 800-654-6360
600 Young St, Tonawanda, NY 14150

Stewart Efi, Lcc 800-678-7931
630 Central Park Ave, Yonkers, NY 10704

Sunlite Plastics, Inc. 262-253-0600
W194N11340 McCormick Dr, Germantown, WI 53022
Full service, FDA-approved contract manufacturer for medical industry. Complete range of service available from extrusion to sterilization.

Sunmedica 530-229-1600
1661 Zachi Way, Redding, CA 96003
Compressive, supportive, tapeless dressing to secure sterile dressing, with pockets for cold therapy modalities post operatively/post injury. Designed for the hip, knee & shoulder. ORTHOPLUG is a canal plug, cement restrictor.

Surgical Technologies, Inc. 800-777-9987
292 E Lafayette Frontage Rd, Saint Paul, MN 55107

Symmetry Medical, Inc. 574-268-2252
3724 N State Road 15, Warsaw, IN 46582

Tailored Label Products, Inc. 800-727-1344
W165N5731 Ridgewood Dr, Menomonee Falls, WI 53051
Custom manufacturing of disposable pressure sensitive medical products; printed, die cut and laminated.

Tapemark 800-535-1998
1685 Marthaler Ln, West St Paul, MN 55118
Disposable medical products laminated, printed, die-cut, pouched.

Tecomet, A Subsidiary Of Viasys Healthcare Inc. 978-658-3379
115 Eames St, Wilmington, MA 01887
Medical components including orthopedic implants, heart pumps, maxillofacial mesh.

Tegra Medical Inc. 508-541-4200
9 Forge Pkwy, Franklin, MA 02038

The Metrix Co. 800-752-3148
4400 Chavenelle Rd, Dubuque, IA 52002
Custom manufacturer of medical devices, specializing in RF sealing, assembly and packaging of bags and tube sets.

The Tech Group 480-281-4500
14677 N 74th St, Scottsdale, AZ 85260
Customer specified injection molding, mold construction and medical device assembly.

Tmp Technologies, Inc. 716-895-6100
1200 Northland Ave, Buffalo, NY 14215

Transylvania Vocational Services 828-884-3195
11 Mountain Industrial Dr, PO Box 1115, Brevard, NC 28712

Tua Systems, Inc. 321-453-3200
3645 N Courtenay Pkwy, Merritt Island, FL 32953
Contract coating including hydrophobic, hydrophilic, anti-clotting and anti-microbial coatings.

CONTRACT MANUFACTURING *(cont'd)*

Tyco Healthcare Group Lp 800-445-5025
2 Ludlow Park Dr, Chicopee, MA 01022
Polymer formulations, hydrogels and polymeric components for biomedical devices.

Ufp Technologies, Inc. 630-543-2855
1235 W National Ave, Addison, IL 60101
Impregnated foams for patches and bandages, filters, gaskets and operating table pads. Specialty foam parts.

United Chemical Technologies, Inc. 800-385-3153
2731 Bartram Rd, Bristol, PA 19007
Specialty silanes, silicone fluids, and silicone elastomers.

Valley Products Co. 800-451-8874
PO Box 187, York New Salem, PA 17371
Cotton, polyester, nylon and orthopedic webbing (TAPEPAX). Labels, cords and fasteners. Labels printed and woven sewed in. Custom printing on twill tape.

Vernay Laboratories, Inc. 800-666-5227
120 E South College St, Yellow Springs, OH 45387

Vital Concepts, Inc. 800-984-2300
4334 Brockton Dr SE Ste F, Grand Rapids, MI 49512

Weiss Aug Co., Inc. 973-887-7600
220 Merry Ln, PO Box 520, East Hanover, NJ 07936
Miniature precision metal stampings, precision thermoplastic injection molding, insert molding, and custom assembly of components, utilizing strong product development team.

Zibra Corp. 800-758-8773
640 American Legion Hwy, Westport, MA 02790

Zyloware Corporation 800-765-3700
1136 46th Rd, Long Island City, NY 11101
Contract manufacturer of eyeglasses frames and sunglasses.

Zymogenetics 206-442-6600
1201 Eastlake Ave E, Seattle, WA 98102
Enzyme and insulin manufacturer.

CONTRACT MANUFACTURING, PHARMACEUTICALS/CHEMICALS *(General) 80WXH*

Amresco Inc. 800-366-1313
30175 Solon Industrial Pkwy, Solon, OH 44139
Manufacturer of clinical diagnostic and research chemicals and pharmaceutical intermediates.

Bachem Bioscience, Inc. 800-634-3183
3700 Horizon Dr, King Of Prussia, PA 19406
Supplier of bulk peptide pharmaceuticals with unique capabilities in large-scale synthesis and purification.

Bell-More Labs, Inc. 410-239-7554
4030 Gill Ave, Hampstead, MD 21074

Bristol-Myers Group Company 800-332-2056
PO Box 4500, Princeton, NJ 08543
Cardiovascular, oncology therapy, anti-infectives.

Caledon Laboratories Ltd. 877-cal-edon
40 Armstrong Ave., Georgetown, ONT L7G 4R9 Canada
Wide range of Lab chemicals.

Chattem, Inc. 800-366-6077
1715 W 38th St, Chattanooga, TN 37409
Gold Bond lotions, anti-itch powders and creams. Pamprin PMS treatment. Flexall 454, Icy Hot, Capzasin, Aspercreme topical analgesic. Benzodent dental product for sores on gums. Herpecin-l lip balm for cold sores. Bull Frog Sunscreens. pHisoderm acne products. Selsun Blue antidandruff shampoo and conditioner.

Cis-Us, Inc. 800-221-7554
10 Deangelo Dr, Bedford, MA 01730
MAA, MDP, DTPA, sulfur colloid, pyrophosphate, LDO.

Citra Anticoagulants, Inc. 800-299-3411
55 Messina Dr, Braintree, MA 02184

Cytosol Ophthalmics, Inc. 800-234-5166
PO Box 1408, 1325 William White Place, NE, Lenoir, NC 28645
Contract manufacturing of medical devices and liquid pharmaceuticals.

Dpt Laboratories, Ltd. 866-225-5378
4040 Broadway St Ste 401, San Antonio, TX 78209

Gdm Electronic And Medical 408-945-4100
2070 Ringwood Ave, San Jose, CA 95131

Global Pharmaeuticals: A Division Of Impax Labs Inc. 800-296-9227
3735 Castor Ave, Philadelphia, PA 19124

CONTRACT MANUFACTURING, PHARMACEUTICALS/CHEMICALS *(cont'd)*

Inamco International Corp. 800-724-4003
801 Montrose Ave, South Plainfield, NJ 07080
MEDICOS

King Pharmaceuticals, Inc. 800-525-8466
501 5th St, Bristol, TN 37620

Lockett Medical Corp. 401-421-6599
3 Richmond Sq, Providence, RI 02906

Medicos Laboratories, Inc. (Mdt) 800-724-4003
801 Montrose Ave, South Plainfield, NJ 07080

Meridian Life Science, Inc. 800-327-6299
5171 Wilfong Rd, Memphis, TN 38134
cGMP Production of recombinants in insect or E. Coli cells.

Regeneron Pharmaceuticals, Inc. 914-345-7400
777 Old Saw Mill River Rd, Tarrytown, NY 10591
In Clinical Trials for Cancer and Age Related Macular Degeneration (VEGF Trap); Rheumatoid Arthritis (IL-1 Trap); Astham/Allergy (IL-4/13/ Trap); Obesity (AXOKINE); and on going preclinical research and development.

Regis Technologies, Inc. 800-323-8144
8210 Austin Ave, Morton Grove, IL 60053
Pharmaceuticals/chemicals, custom synthesis under G.M.P. conditions.

Reliable Biopharmeceutical 314-429-7700
1945 Walton Rd, Saint Louis, MO 63114

Solvay Pharmaceuticals 800-241-1643
901 Sawyer Rd, Marietta, GA 30062

Tapemark 800-535-1998
1685 Marthaler Ln, West St Paul, MN 55118
Contract manufacturing with expertise in soluble film for drug delivery, both Rx and OTC. Delivery of active via topical wipes, patches, transdermal, hydrogels.

Technical Marketing, Inc. 954-370-0855
1776 N Pine Island Rd Ste 306, Plantation, FL 33322
Generic pharmaceuticals.

UCB Inc. 770-970-7500
1950 Lake Park Dr SE, Smyrna, GA 30080

CONTRACT MANUFACTURING, PRODUCT, DISPOSABLE
(General) 80WLY

Advance Medical Designs, Inc. 800-221-3679
1241 Atlanta Industrial Dr, Marietta, GA 30066
Private labeling for equipment manufacturers.

Allergan 800-366-6554
2525 Dupont Dr, Irvine, CA 92612
Disposable products for cataract surgery.

Ambiderm, S.A. De C.V. 800-800-8008
Carr. A Bosques De San Isidro 1136, Col. Bosques De San Isidro
Zapopan, Jalisco 45147 Mexico
AMBERDERM disposable medical clothing manufactured with fabric made by Dupont composed of 45% of dacron polyester and 55% wood pulp.

Andersen Products, Inc., 800-523-1276
3202 Caroline Dr, Health Science Park, Haw River, NC 27258
Contract manufacturing, packaging, and EO sterilization of disposable medical devices.

Armm, Inc. 714-848-8190
17744 Sampson Ln, Huntington Beach, CA 92647
Full service manufacture of disposable medical devices.

Avail Medical Products, Inc. 866-552-2112
201 Main St, 1600 Wells Fargo Tower, Fort Worth, TX 76102
Full-service outsource design and manufacturing for sterile, single-use medical devices. From initial product concept through finished goods, fulfillment and distribution. Design, process development and validation, manufacturing, injection molding, packaging, sterilization services management, manufacturing transfer.

Battery Specialties 800-854-5759
3530 Cadillac Ave, Costa Mesa, CA 92626
Assembly of battery packs.

Bio Med Sciences, Inc. 800-257-4566
7584 Morris Ct Ste 218, Allentown, PA 18106
Breathable hydrophobic membrane.

CONTRACT MANUFACTURING, PRODUCT, DISPOSABLE
(cont'd)

Biolitec, Inc. 800-934-2377
515 Shaker Rd, East Longmeadow, MA 01028
Manufacture disposable fiber optic laser delivery systems (25 to 100 watts). Manufactured to customer specifications (248nm to 2.1 micron). All products are for single use and sterilized.

Biomedical Polymers, Inc. 800-253-3684
42 Linus Allain Ave, Gardner, MA 01440
Medical product.

Bioteque America, Inc. 800-889-9008
340 E Maple Ave Ste 204A, Langhorne, PA 19047
Disposable ob/gyn products; pessaries.

Brady Corporation 800-541-1686
6555 W Good Hope Rd, PO Box 571, Milwaukee, WI 53223
OEM custom contract manufacturing of disposable electrodes, tapes and patches, cleanroom assembly and contract sterilization services.

Brady Precision Converting, Llc 214-275-9595
1801 Big Town Blvd Ste 100, Mesquite, TX 75149
Rotary and flat-bed die cutting of medical adhesives, non-wovens, foam, films, etc. to meet exact specifications.

California Medical Innovations 800-229-5871
873 E Arrow Hwy, Pomona, CA 91767
Latex products.

Catheter Research, Inc. (Cri) 317-872-0074
5610 W 82nd St, Indianapolis, IN 46278
Contract assembly and packaging, product development and re-design, sourcing, centerless grinding, 510(k) preparation, Class 100,000 cleanroom available.

Colby Manufacturing Corp. 800-969-3718
1016 Branagan Dr, Tullytown, PA 19007
Contract manufacturing of disposable products.

Command Medical Products, Inc. 386-672-8116
15 Signal Ave, Ormond Beach, FL 32174
Plastic medical disposables of all varieties.

Csi Holdings 615-452-9633
170 Commerce Way, Gallatin, TN 37066

Dhd Healthcare Corporation 800-847-8000
PO Box 6, One Madison Street, Wampsville, NY 13163
Custom manufacturing of complete medical devices.

Directmed, Inc. 516-656-3377
150 Pratt Oval, Glen Cove, NY 11542
Contract manufacturing, product, disposable.

Enpath Medical, Inc. 800-559-2613
2300 Berkshire Ln N, Minneapolis, MN 55441
Catheter, introducer, dilator, pacing accessory kits, delivery systems, implant tool, stimulation leads, precision laser processing.

Evergreen Research, Inc. 303-526-7402
433 Park Point Dr Ste 140, Golden, CO 80401

Frantz Medical Development Ltd. 440-255-1155
7740 Metric Dr, Mentor, OH 44060

Gdm Electronic And Medical 408-945-4100
2070 Ringwood Ave, San Jose, CA 95131

Genesis Manufacturing, Inc. 317-485-7887
720 E Broadway St, Fortville, IN 46040
Contract Radio-Frequency (RF) Welding. From development to manufacturing and packaging.

Grand Rapids Foam Technologies 877-GET-GRFT
2788 Remico St SW, Wyoming, MI 49519

Harmac Medical Products, Inc. 716-897-4500
2201 Bailey Ave, Buffalo, NY 14211
Full-service contract manufacturer of custom plastic medical disposables. Wide range of products including: custom bags and sets, needle assemblies, infusion disposables, Huber needle sets, custom catheters, pressure lines, medical subassemblies, and components. Offering product design and development, assembly, heat sealing, RF-welding, insert/injection molding, packaging, and sterilization. ISO 9001 and EN 46001 certified.

Hospital Marketing Svcs. Company, Inc. 800-786-5094
162 Great Hill Rd./ Ind. Park, Naugatuck, CT 06770

Intersurgical Inc. 315-451-2900
417 Electronics Pkwy, Liverpool, NY 13088

CONTRACT MANUFACTURING, PRODUCT, DISPOSABLE
(cont'd)

J-Pac, Llc 603-692-9955
25 Centre Rd, Somersworth, NH 03878
Cleanroom manufacturing, packaging, and contract sterilization of sterile, disposable medical devices in the cardiovascular, orthopedics, urology, general surgery, and ObGyn market segments, among others. J-PAC supports all stages of development and ongoing manufacturing.

Jero Medical Equipment & Supplies, Inc. 800-457-0644
1701 W 13th St, Chicago, IL 60608
Wearing apparels.

Lifemed Of California 800-543-3633
1216 S Allec St, Anaheim, CA 92805
Lifemed contract assembly and manufacturing services.

Lucomed Inc. 800-633-7877
45 Kulick Rd, Fairfield, NJ 07004
Customized manufacturer of hemodialysis blood tubing, CAPD-CCPD CAVH-CVVH sets, OEM components, IV and blood administration sets, and EVA bags.

Lyons Tool And Die Company 800-422-9363
185 Research Pkwy, Meriden, CT 06450
Rapid prototyping. Production of medical devices in class 10,000 clean rooms. Medical knives and scissors. Precision metal stamping. Engineering services.

M&C Specialties Co. 800-441-6996
90 James Way, Southampton, PA 18966

Medical Concepts Development 800-345-0644
2500 Ventura Dr, Saint Paul, MN 55125
Surgical drapes, pouches, adhesive films, non-wovens, and soft-metals.

Medical Products, Inc. 800-638-0489
511 E Walnut St, PO Box 207, Ripley, MS 38663
Medical supplies.

Medovations, Inc. 800-558-6408
102 E Keefe Ave, Milwaukee, WI 53212

Medtech Group Inc., The 800-348-2759
6 Century Ln, South Plainfield, NJ 07080
Medical device assembly. Medical products manufacturing: ultrasonic welding/solvent bonding/manual assembly, product printing, packaging and sterilization, surgical staple manufacturing.

Minnesota Wire & Cable Co. 800-258-6922
1835 Energy Park Dr, Saint Paul, MN 55108
Specialize in unique custom wire and cable assemblies.

Precision Medical Products, Inc. 717-335-3700
44 Denver Rd, PO Box 300, Denver, PA 17517

Sontec Instruments Inc. 303-790-9411
7248 S Tucson Way, Centennial, CO 80112
See Sontec Instruments, Inc.

Specialteam Medical Services, Inc. 714-694-0348
22445 La Palma Ave Ste F, Yorba Linda, CA 92887

Tailored Label Products, Inc. 800-727-1344
W165N5731 Ridgewood Dr, Menomonee Falls, WI 53051

Tapemark 800-535-1998
1685 Marthaler Ln, West St Paul, MN 55118
Contract manufacturing for laminated and/or die cut products for applications such as wound care, in heat-seal or cold-seal pouch. Strong expertise in adhesives.

Tegra Medical Inc. 508-541-4200
9 Forge Pkwy, Franklin, MA 02038

Tmp Technologies, Inc. 716-895-6100
1200 Northland Ave, Buffalo, NY 14215
General.

Valmark, Inc. 613-822-3107
P.O. Box 190, Gloucester, ONT K1X-1A4 Canada
Premium quality Autoclave Bags for the collection and disposal of biohazardoud materials. Extra strong and durable, seamless side construction, user friendly, instructions in English, French, and Spanish. 4 sizes.

Vital Concepts, Inc. 800-984-2300
4334 Brockton Dr SE Ste F, Grand Rapids, MI 49512

Vonco Products, Inc. 800-323-9077
201 Park Ave, Lake Villa, IL 60046
Custom plastic bags.

CONTRACT MANUFACTURING, PRODUCT, DISPOSABLE *(cont'd)*

Zirc Company 800-328-3899
3918 State Highway 55 SE, Buffalo, MN 55313
Dispos-a-Screens and Saliva Ejector Screens, Dispos-a-Bowl disposable alginate mixing bowl.

CONTRACT MANUFACTURING, PRODUCT, DURABLE *(General) 80WLX*

Alimed, Inc. 800-225-2610
297 High St, Dedham, MA 02026
High-density charcoal-gray polyfoam custom positioners available either uncovered or covered with black conductive vinyl.

Alsons Corp. 800-421-0001
3010 Mechanic Rd, P.O. Box 282, Hillsdale, MI 49242
Hand showers.

Applied Medical Technology, Inc. 800-869-7382
8000 Katherine Blvd, Brecksville, OH 44141
Enteral-feeding gastro-intestinal and urology devices, silicone molding, assembly.

Bay Corporation 888-835-3800
867 Canterbury Rd, Westlake, OH 44145
Medical fittings, connections, tubing, hoses, male/female quick connect couplers; all for use in anesthesia, resuscitation and respiratory care.

Berghof/America 800-544-5004
3773 NW 126th Ave Bldg 1, Coral Springs, FL 33065
Custom fabrication of Teflon products.

Clinimed, Incorporated 877-CLINIMED
303 Markus Ct, Sandy Brae Industrial Park, Newark, DE 19713

Colby Manufacturing Corp. 800-969-3718
1016 Branagan Dr, Tullytown, PA 19007
Contract and OEM manufacturing of durable medical devices.

Controltek, Inc. 360-896-9375
3905 NE 112th Ave, Vancouver, WA 98682
Electronic systems.

Dentsply Canada, Ltd. 800-263-1437
161 Vinyl Ct., Woodbridge, ONT L4L 4A3 Canada

Evergreen Research, Inc. 303-526-7402
433 Park Point Dr Ste 140, Golden, CO 80401

Gdm Electronic And Medical 408-945-4100
2070 Ringwood Ave, San Jose, CA 95131

Light Age Inc. 732-563-0600
500 Apgar Dr, Somerset, NJ 08873
OEM laser source for dermatology manufactured to customer specifications.

Lyons Tool And Die Company 800-422-9363
185 Research Pkwy, Meriden, CT 06450
Rapid prototyping. Production of medical devices in class 10,000 clean rooms. Medical knives and scissors. Precision metal stamping. Engineering services.

Micro-Aire Surgical Instruments, Inc. 800-722-0822
1641 Edlich Dr, Charlottesville, VA 22911
Development and prototyping to full OEM production of new products.

Plexus Corp 425-482-1300
20001 N Creek Pkwy, Bothell, WA 98011
Service organization to respond to issues facing today's competitive medical electronics industry, including providing design resources for new product development, enhancing existing products to provide logical extensions, supporting product manufacturing requirements, contributing expertise to non-electronic related companies, and entering into partnerships with start-up companies.

Precision Medical Products, Inc. 717-335-3700
44 Denver Rd, PO Box 300, Denver, PA 17517

Progressive Dental Supply/Progressive Orthodontics Seminars 800-443-3106
1701 E Edinger Ave Ste C1, Santa Ana, CA 92705
Nickel titanium separating spring.

Rycor Medical, Inc. 800-227-9267
2053 Atwater Dr, North Port, FL 34288
Custom hospital equipment.

S4j Manufacturing Services, Inc. 888-S4J-LUER
2685 NE 9th Ave, Cape Coral, FL 33909
Contract manufacturing and designing of tubing connectors.

CONTRACT MANUFACTURING, PRODUCT, DURABLE *(cont'd)*

Sparton Electronics Florida, Inc. 800-824-0682
5612 Johnson Lake Rd, De Leon Springs, FL 32130
Noninvasive electronic products; complex therapeutic and diagnostic equipment.

CONTRACT MANUFACTURING, REAGENT *(General) 80WLH*

Amresco Inc. 800-366-1313
30175 Solon Industrial Pkwy, Solon, OH 44139
Manufacturer of clinical diagnostic and research chemicals and pharmaceutical intermediates.

Antibodies, Inc. 800-824-8540
PO Box 1560, Davis, CA 95617
Contract reagent manufacturing and packaging. Contract antisera production, purification, labeling and packaging.

Bell-More Labs, Inc. 410-239-7554
4030 Gill Ave, Hampstead, MD 21074

Dpt Laboratories, Ltd. 866-225-5378
4040 Broadway St Ste 401, San Antonio, TX 78209

Genzyme Diagnostics 800-999-6578
115 Summit Dr, Exton, PA 19341
Diagnostic clinical chemistries.

International Immunology Corp. 800-843-2853
PO Box 972, Murrieta, CA 92564
Goat antiserum, goat antibodies and Human Calibrator/Controls etc.

Irvine Scientific 800-437-5706
2511 Daimler St, Santa Ana, CA 92705
Amniostat-FLM & Mycotrim RS & GU diagnostic test kits.

Pointe Scientific, Inc. 800-445-9853
5449 Research Dr, Canton, MI 48188
A complete line of diagnostic chemistry reagents.

Polymer Laboratories, Now A Part Of Varian, Inc. 800-767-3963
160 Old Farm Rd, Amherst Fields Research Park, Amherst, MA 01002
We endeavor to offer the widest possible range of materials from stock, however, we recognize that some customers may wish to purchase something different. We regularly enter into custom or contract manufacture projects with our clients.

Quality Bioresources, Inc. 888-674-7224
1015 N Austin St, Seguin, TX 78155
OEM filling and lyophilization

Reliable Biopharmeceutical 314-429-7700
1945 Walton Rd, Saint Louis, MO 63114

Shared Systems, Inc. 888-474-2733
PO Box 211587, 3961 Columbia Rd, Augusta, GA 30917

Tapemark 800-535-1998
1685 Marthaler Ln, West St Paul, MN 55118
Combination reagent/device products such as test strips

CONTRACT PACKAGING *(General) 80VAO*

Advanced Biomedical Devices, Inc. (Abd, Inc.) 978-470-1177
Dundee Park, Bldg. 17, Andover, MA 01810

Andersen Products, Inc., 800-523-1276
3202 Caroline Dr, Health Science Park, Haw River, NC 27258
Contract manufacturing, packaging, and EO sterilization of disposable medical devices.

Arc/Otsego 607-432-8595
35 Academy St, PO Box 490, Oneonta, NY 13820
Packaging of medical disposables; repackaging and relabeling.

Armm, Inc. 714-848-8190
17744 Sampson Ln, Huntington Beach, CA 92647
Pouches and blister sealing; bulk; implants.

Atrion Medical Products, Inc. 800-343-9334
1426 Curt Francis Rd NW, Arab, AL 35016

Avail Medical Products, Inc. 866-552-2112
201 Main St, 1600 Wells Fargo Tower, Fort Worth, TX 76102
Full-service outsource design and manufacturing for sterile, single-use medical devices. From initial product concept through finished goods, fulfillment and distribution. Design, process development and validation, manufacturing, injection molding, packaging, sterilization services management, manufacturing transfer.

B. Braun Oem Division, B. Braun Medical Inc. 866-8-BBRAUN
824 12th Ave, Bethlehem, PA 18018

Bioseal 800-441-7325
167 W Orangethorpe Ave, Placentia, CA 92870
Repackaging of OR disposables & gauze cotton balls.

CONTRACT PACKAGING *(cont'd)*

Bioserv Corporation 858-450-3123
5340 Eastgate Mall, San Diego, CA 92121
Contract services for complete EIA kit manufacture, device assembly, bulk formulation, powder and liquid filling, lyophilization, and packaging.

Biosure, Inc. 800-345-2267
12301 Loma Rica Dr Unit G, Grass Valley, CA 95945

Brady Precision Converting, Llc 214-275-9595
1801 Big Town Blvd Ste 100, Mesquite, TX 75149
Form-Fill-Seal packaging. Fully validated.

C&J Industries, Inc. 814-724-4950
760 Water St, Meadville, PA 16335

Care Line, Inc. 800-251-1157
2210 Lake Rd, Greenbrier, TN 37073
Stocking distributor of a complete line of patient care products. Products available in bulk and prepicked custom trays. In house printing services available. OEM contract packing and fulfillment services.

Catheter Research, Inc. (Cri) 317-872-0074
5610 W 82nd St, Indianapolis, IN 46278
Contract assembly and packaging, product development and re-design, sourcing, centerless grinding, 510(k) preparation, Class 100,000 cleanroom available.

Command Medical Products, Inc. 386-672-8116
15 Signal Ave, Ormond Beach, FL 32174
Kit packing, blister sealing, pouch and bag packaging.

Cytyc Corporation 603-668-7688
2 E Perimeter Rd, Londonderry, NH 03053
Liquid and powder filling, tray packaging, and pouch processing, form, fill and seal.

Disetronic Sterile Products 800-280-7801
124 Heritage Ave, Portsmouth, NH 03801

Dpt Laboratories, Ltd. 866-225-5378
4040 Broadway St Ste 401, San Antonio, TX 78209

Dravon Medical, Inc. 503-656-6600
11465 SE Highway 212, PO Box 69, Clackamas, OR 97015
OEM contract assembly and packaging.

Enova Medical Technologies 866-773-0539
1839 Buerkle Rd, Saint Paul, MN 55110
Form, fill and seal; RF; Blister; Povelt sealing.

Excel Medical Products, Llc 810-714-4775
3145 Copper Ave, Fenton, MI 48430
Excel Medical Products is an FDA-Registered, ISO and GMP compliant contract manufacturer specializing in medical components and devices. Excel Medical Products offers contract packaging and the following services and capabilities: Class 100,000 clean room manufacturing and assembly, thermoplastic and elastomer injection molding, LSR (liquid silicone rubber) injection molding, insert molding, custom assembly, custom kitting, pouch sealing, tray sealing, and pad printing. Additional capabilities included adhesive, solvent and UV bonding, tipping, flaring, skiving and micro drilling. We also offers product development, process development and mold design services. Excel Medical Products provides custom solutions from conception to completion.

Gdm Electronic And Medical 408-945-4100
2070 Ringwood Ave, San Jose, CA 95131
Contract manufacturing and service. Quick turn, small or large production runs - kit assembly, packaging & labeling, bar coding.

Harmac Medical Products, Inc. 716-897-4500
2201 Bailey Ave, Buffalo, NY 14211
Contract manufacturer offering assembly, packaging, and sterilization services. Custom labeling and printing; heat-sealed paper pouches and polyethylene bags.

Hospital Marketing Svcs. Company, Inc. 800-786-5094
162 Great Hill Rd./ Ind. Park, Naugatuck, CT 06770

Innovative Surgical Products, Inc. 714-836-4474
2761 Walnut Ave, Tustin, CA 92780
Complete assemblies or sub-assemblies; contract packaging of trays, pouches, kits etc. and ETO or radiation sterilization services.

J-Pac, Llc 603-692-9955
25 Centre Rd, Somersworth, NH 03878
J-PAC supports the medical, pharmaceutical, and veterinary markets. Services include package design, prototyping, and validation; packaging process development and validation; and qualification of subsequent sterilization processes. Thermoformed tray put-ups are a specialty, with numerous active dock-to-stock programs. J-PAC packages products that are consigned, as well as products that are fabricated in-house.

CONTRACT PACKAGING *(cont'd)*

Lacey Manufacturing Co. 203-336-0121
1146 Barnum Ave, PO Box 5156, Bridgeport, CT 06610

Lifemed Of California 800-543-3633
1216 S Allec St, Anaheim, CA 92805
Contract packaging, Lifemed contract packaging services.

Lyons Tool And Die Company 800-422-9363
185 Research Pkwy, Meriden, CT 06450
Rapid prototyping. Production of medical devices in class 10,000 clean rooms. Medical knives and scissors. Precision metal stamping. Engineering services.

Medical Packaging Inc. 800-257-5282
470 Route 31 N, PO Box 500, Ringoes, NJ 08551
Selective repackaging for unit-dose dispensing, clinical studies, physicians samples, prescriptions, and compliance packages.

Medical Sterile Products, Inc. 800-292-2887
Road 413 Km. 0.2 BO. Ensenada, Rincon, PR 00743

Meditron Inc D.B.A. Medcare Usa 800-243-2442
3435 Montee Gagnon, Terrebonne, QUEBE J6Y-1J4 Canada

Novosci Corp. 281-363-4949
2828 N Crescentridge Dr, The Woodlands, TX 77381

Pacon Manufacturing Corporation 732-357-8020
400 Pierce St # B, Somerset, NJ 08873
Flow Wrap; FF&S; papers, films, foils

Pl Medical Co., Llc. 800-874-0120
321 Ellis St, New Britain, CT 06051

Plastic And Metal Center, Inc. 949-770-8230
23162 La Cadena Dr, Laguna Hills, CA 92653
Vacuum formed short run trays to specs specializing in design and development of the mold. Assembly equipment also available.

Precision Medical Products, Inc. 717-335-3700
44 Denver Rd, PO Box 300, Denver, PA 17517

Protection Products, Inc. 800-869-6818
PO Box 59367, Homewood, AL 35259

Quality Bioresources, Inc. 888-674-7224
1015 N Austin St, Seguin, TX 78155

Sharp Corporation 800-892-6197
23 Carland Rd, Conshohocken, PA 19428
Packaging of pharmaceuticals, personal care products and health and beauty aids.

Specialteam Medical Services, Inc. 714-694-0348
22445 La Palma Ave Ste F, Yorba Linda, CA 92887

Sts Duotek, Inc 800-836-4850
370 Summit Point Dr, Henrietta, NY 14467
Contract packaging, assembly, testing, and sterilization services. Assembly and packaging include pouching, form, fill, seal, tray, and lid and kit assembly for the medical device industry.

Tapemark 800-535-1998
1685 Marthaler Ln, West St Paul, MN 55118
Packaging individual product into heat-seal or cold-seal pouches, primary boxes. Also, single-use or dose Snap!® packaging contains your cream, gel, paste, or lotion and opens easily with one hand.

Tray-Pak Corporation 888-926-1777
PO Box 14804, Tuckerton Road & Reading Crest Avenue
Reading, PA 19612

Unette Corporation 973-328-6800
88 N Main St, Wharton, NJ 07885
Contract packaging of liquid products: bottle filling, tube filling and foil pouch packaging.

Windstone Medical Packaging, Inc. 800-637-7056
1602 4th Ave N, Billings, MT 59101

CONTRACT R&D, DIAGNOSTICS *(General) 80VAN*

Advanced Biotechnologies, Inc. 800-426-0764
9108 Guilford Rd, Rivers Park II, Columbia, MD 21046
Antisera, virus and monoclonal antibodies.

Akers Biosciences, Inc. 800-451-8378
201 Grove Rd, West Deptford, NJ 08086

Amgen Inc. 800-28-AMGEN
1 Amgen Center Dr, Thousand Oaks, CA 91320
Vaccine research and development.

Amresco Inc. 800-366-1313
30175 Solon Industrial Pkwy, Solon, OH 44139
Manufacturer of clinical diagnostic and research chemicals and pharmaceutical intermediates.

CONTRACT R&D, DIAGNOSTICS *(cont'd)*

Antibodies, Inc. 800-824-8540
PO Box 1560, Davis, CA 95617
ISO9001, cGMP, small and medium-run contract manufacturing of diagnostic kits.

Atrion Medical Products, Inc. 800-343-9334
1426 Curt Francis Rd NW, Arab, AL 35016

Bio-Clin, Inc. 314-647-3244
5977 S.W. Avenue, St. Louis, MO 63139
ELISA diagnostics.

Biomedical Technologies, Inc. 781-344-9942
378 Page St, Stoughton, MA 02072
Custom radioiodination, antiserum production, protein purification.

Biozyme Laboratories International Ltd. 800-423-8199
9939 Hibert St Ste 101, San Diego, CA 92131
Diagnostic enzymes and biochemicals for clinical chemistry.

Casco Manufacturing Solutions, Inc. 800-843-1339
3107 Spring Grove Ave, Cincinnati, OH 45225

Celsis Laboratory Group 800-523-5227
165 Fieldcrest Ave, Edison, NJ 08837
Contract testing facility providing analytical services in the areas of analytical chemistry, microbiology, toxicology, and method development and validation.

Cmt, Inc. 800-659-9140
PO Box 297, Hamilton, MA 01936
More than 15 years of experience in medical device research, design and development, specializing in mechanical and fluid management products.

Covance Laboratories ,Inc 800-742-8378
3301 Kinsman Blvd, Madison, WI 53704
Mammalian & genetic toxicology; analytical support, immuno and clinical chemistry, surgery.

Dpt Laboratories, Ltd. 866-225-5378
4040 Broadway St Ste 401, San Antonio, TX 78209

Evergreen Research, Inc. 303-526-7402
433 Park Point Dr Ste 140, Golden, CO 80401

Gilead Sciences 650-574-3000
333 Lakeside Dr, Foster City, CA 94404
Liposome drug delivery systems.

Gillette Environmental Health And Safety 781-292-8101
37 A St, Needham, MA 02494

H&W Technology, Llc. 585-218-0385
PO Box 20281, Rochester, NY 14602
H & W represents SMP GmbH, a leading German laboratory specializing in cleaning and sterilization validation. H & W is also a representatve of EBRO datalogging solutions, providing wired and wireless temperature, humidity and pressure datalogging for a variety of applications.

Habley Medical Technology Corp. 800-729-1994
15721 Bernardo Heights Pkwy Ste B-30, San Diego, CA 92128
Artificial urinary sphincter, in development. Safety syringes, safety blood-collection devices, safety scalpels, safety I.V. devices, and toplicators are also available to custom design any medically related device. Habley has been issued over 450 U.S. patents.

Innovation Genesis, Llc 617-234-0070
1 Canal Park, Cambridge, MA 02141
Technology and product strategy, design and development for medical device companies. Experience with devices ranging from home health care, diagnostics, imaging, surgical tools and procedures, and cardiology to advanced ER and OR systems.

Intracel Corporation 301-668-8400
93 Monocacy Blvd Ste A8, Frederick, MD 21701
Diagnostic assay is for quantitation of lipoprotein(a)[lp(a)] in human plasma or serum. Also for qualitative measurement of fibrin/fibrinogren degradation products (FDP) in human urine.

Medipoint, Inc. 800-445-0525
72 E 2nd St, Mineola, NY 11501
Goldenrod Animal Lancets for drawing Blood from mice in research.

Merlin's Medical Supply 800-639-9322
699 Mobil Ave, Camarillo, CA 93010

Mycoscience, Inc. 860-684-0030
25 Village Hill Rd, Willington, CT 06279
Includes contract manufacturing and contract laboratory services.

Numed Canada, Inc. 613-936-2592
45, Second Street West, Cornwall, ONT K6J 1G3 Canada

CONTRACT R&D, DIAGNOSTICS *(cont'd)*

Oncogene Research Products 800-854-3417
10394 Pacific Center Ct, San Diego, CA 92121
Biological research with antibodies and peptides.

Product Investigations, Inc. 610-825-5855
151 E 10th Ave, Conshohocken, PA 19428
Medical/clinical research service (R&D).

Prometic Biotherapeutics, Inc. 301-917-6320
9800 Medical Center Dr Ste C110, Rockville, MD 20850

Quality Bioresources, Inc. 888-674-7224
1015 N Austin St, Seguin, TX 78155
OEM filling and lyophilization

Roper Scientific, Inc. 800-874-9789
3440 E Britannia Dr, Tucson, AZ 85706
Digital electronic camera systems.

Shore Medical, Inc. 714-628-9785
1050 N Batavia St Ste C, Orange, CA 92867

Spectral Diagnostics Inc. 888-426-4264
135-2 The West Mall, Toronto, ON M9C 1C2 Canada
Cardiac STATUS CK-MB/Myoglobin Point of Care Test Kit. Rapid format device to detect elevated levels of CK-MB and/or Myoglobin in whole blood, plasma, or serum. Aids in the diagnosis of acute myocardial infarction. Cardiac STATUS Troponin I Point of Care Test Kit. Rapid format device to detect elevated levels of Troponin I in whole blood, plasma, or serum. Aids in the diagnosis of chest pain.

STI Optronics, Inc. 425-827-0460
2755 Northup Way, Bellevue, WA 98004

Sts Duotek, Inc 800-836-4850
370 Summit Point Dr, Henrietta, NY 14467

Synectic Medical Product Development 203-877-8488
60 Commerce Park, Milford, CT 06460
Medical/surgical product development, consulting, and trouble-shooting services available. Experienced in mechanical engineering, industrial design, materials application, medical product manufacturing, tooling, and quality control. Special consideration given to ergonomics and aesthetic factors. We bring together medical practitioners, industrial designers, engineers, and marketing groups; our methods reduce time to market, develop and design products, and enhance productivity during and after the development process.

Tegra Medical Inc. 508-541-4200
9 Forge Pkwy, Franklin, MA 02038
Prototyping services.

Trinity Biotech, Inc. 716-483-3851
2823 Girts Rd, Jamestown, NY 14701
Diagnostics manufacturer, including infectious disease and auto-immune disease ELISAs.

UCB Inc. 770-970-7500
1950 Lake Park Dr SE, Smyrna, GA 30080
Research on pharmaceutical drug delivery enhancement via the skin. Also, research on targeting specific brain sites with pharmaceutica.

Varian Vacuum Products 800-882-7426
121 Hartwell Ave, Lexington, MA 02421
Leak detection equipment with superior sensitivity capable of detecting 1x10 to the -10 power atm-cc/sec. HELITEST portable leak detector unit. Very compact and easy to use with visual and audio leak settings.

Viacirq, Inc. 724-745-2362
Division of ThermaSolutions, Inc., 400 SouthPOinte Blvd, Plaza 1, Suite #23
Canonsburg, PA 15317
ThermoChem HT System is fully integrated system specifically designed for delivering Intraperitoneal Hyperthermia.

Wi Inc 303-762-1693
96 Inverness Dr E Ste N, Englewood, CO 80112
Contract product development of blood diagnostic devices

CONTRACT R&D, EQUIPMENT *(General) 80WUH*

Applied Medical Technology, Inc. 800-869-7382
8000 Katherine Blvd, Brecksville, OH 44141
Polymer and molding technology of silicones and plastics.

ARRK Product Development Group 800-735-2775
8880 Rehco Rd, San Diego, CA 92121
Complete rapid product development services include rapid prototyping, CAD/CAM and CNC machining, vacu-pressure moldings and castings, QuickCast and aluminum castings, fabrication and rapid tooling. Aluminum and steel injection.

CONTRACT R&D, EQUIPMENT *(cont'd)*

Astro Seal, Inc. 951-787-6670
827 Palmyrita Ave Ste B, Riverside, CA 92507

B-Tec Solutions Inc. 215-785-2400
913 Cedar Ave, Croydon, PA 19021

Cmt, Inc. 800-659-9140
PO Box 297, Hamilton, MA 01936
Research, design and development of diagnostic and therapeutic devices. 15+ years experience in the medical field applying mechanical and electrical engineering from technology assessment to production.

Colby Manufacturing Corp. 800-969-3718
1016 Branagan Dr, Tullytown, PA 19007
Contract R&D of medical devices, including surgical instruments.

Crist Instrument Co., Inc. 301-393-8615
111 W 1st St, Hagerstown, MD 21740
Reward Delivery Systems for Primate testing. Both liquid and semi-liquid state devices available.

Evans Group, Inc., The 973-616-1400
230 W Parkway Unit 7-1, Pompton Plains, NJ 07444
Concept to Prototype including design and testing. Prototype to Production including Business Development, Engineering and Quality Assurance.

Evergreen Research, Inc. 303-526-7402
433 Park Point Dr Ste 140, Golden, CO 80401

Filtrona Extrusion, Inc./Pexcor Medical Products Div. 800-755-7528
764 S Athol Rd, P.O. Box 659, Athol, MA 01331

Frantz Medical Development Ltd. 440-255-1155
7740 Metric Dr, Mentor, OH 44060

Gillette Environmental Health And Safety 781-292-8101
37 A St, Needham, MA 02494

Hayes Medical, Inc. 800-240-0500
1115 Windfield Way Ste 100, El Dorado Hills, CA 95762

Hema Metrics Inc. 800-546-5463
695 N Kays Dr, Kaysville, UT 84037
CRITLINE absolute hematocrit and blood volume monitor capable of continuous real-time, noninvasive diagnostic monitoring of HCT, change in blood volume, saturation.

Hi-Tronics Designs, Inc. 973-347-4865
999 Willow Grove St, Hackettstown, NJ 07840
Contract design and prototype for various external and implantable medical devices. Medical grade software development and qualification, custom integrated circuit design.

Indec Systems, Inc. 408-986-1600
2210 Martin Ave, Santa Clara, CA 95050
FOUNDATION 2000.

Innovation Genesis, Llc 617-234-0070
1 Canal Park, Cambridge, MA 02141
Technology and product strategy, design and development for medical device companies. Experience with devices ranging from home health care, diagnostics, imaging, surgical tools and procedures, and cardiology to advanced ER and OR systems.

Kensey Nash Corporation 484-713-2100
735 Pennsylvania Dr, Exton, PA 19341
Rapid design and development of resorbable biomaterial-based medical products. Large well equipped development laboratories with analytical, chemical and mechanical test capabilities. Class 100,000 cleanroom, injection molding, and assembly of collagen and absorbable polymer devices. Product applications include cardiovascular, orthopedic, wound repair, and surgical specialties.

Konigsberg Instruments, Inc. 626-449-0016
2000 E Foothill Blvd, Pasadena, CA 91107
Qualified (FDA, CE/MDD) Medical Device Design and Quality Services

Leander Health Technologies/Healthcare Division 800-635-8188
1525 Vivian Ct, Port Orchard, WA 98367
Chiropractic equipment.

Medegen 800-520-7999
930 S Wanamaker Ave, Ontario, CA 91761
Product designing.

Micromanipulator Co., Inc., The 800-972-4032
1555 Forrest Way, Carson City, NV 89706
Products and accessories to aid in embryo recovery, grading, splitting, injection, micromanipulation and photomicrography.

Microsurgical Laboratories 713-723-6900
11333 Chimney Rock Rd Ste 120, Houston, TX 77035

CONTRACT R&D, EQUIPMENT *(cont'd)*

Nanoptics, Inc. 352-378-6620
3014 NE 21st Way, Gainesville, FL 32609
Contract R&D can be done using POF image bundles, GRIN lenses and illuminator fiber combinations

Nemcomed 800-255-4576
801 Industrial Dr, Hicksville, OH 43526
Contract R & D for medical devices - Orthopedic instrumentation

Nova Biomedical 800-458-5813
200 Prospect St, Waltham, MA 02453
Optical and electrochemical diagnostic technologies for blood-chemistry and immunoassay applications.

Okay Industries, Inc. 860-225-8707
200 Ellis St, P.O. Box 2470, New Britain, CT 06051

Optelecom-Nkf, Inc 800-293-4237
12920 Cloverleaf Center Dr, Germantown, MD 20874
Fiber optics for lasers and communications systems.

Plexus Corp 425-482-1300
20001 N Creek Pkwy, Bothell, WA 98011
Service organization to respond to issues facing today's competitive medical electronics industry, including providing design resources for new product development, enhancing existing products to provide logical extensions, supporting product manufacturing requirements, contributing expertise to non-electronic related companies, and entering into partnerships with start-up companies.

S & B Robertson Research And Developments, Inc. 7057995537
R.R. #1, The Glen, Omemee, ONT K0L-2W0 Canada

Saes Memry 203-739-1100
3 Berkshire Blvd, Bethel, CT 06801

Sagentia Inc 410-654-0090
11403 Cronhill Dr Ste B, Owings Mills, MD 21117
Contract engineering.

Smith Group 800-227-3008
225 Bush St Fl 11, San Francisco, CA 94104

Sparton Electronics Florida, Inc. 800-824-0682
5612 Johnson Lake Rd, De Leon Springs, FL 32130

Spectrum Laboratories, Inc. 800-634-3300
18617 S Broadwick St, Rancho Dominguez, CA 90220
Hollow fiber device development. Ability to develop hollow fiber devices and manufacture them on OEM, private label or third-party basis.

Sr Instruments, Inc. 800-654-6360
600 Young St, Tonawanda, NY 14150

Stratagene 800-424-5444
11011 N Torrey Pines Rd, La Jolla, CA 92037
Biotechnical R&D.

Tmp Technologies, Inc. 716-895-6100
1200 Northland Ave, Buffalo, NY 14215
General.

Triangle Biomedical Sciences, Inc. 919-384-9393
3014 Croasdaile Dr, Durham, NC 27705
Medical device development.

Wi Inc 303-762-1693
96 Inverness Dr E Ste N, Englewood, CO 80112
Contract development of hardware and disposable devices

CONTRACT STERILIZATION *(General) 80VAD*

Andersen Products, Inc., 800-523-1276
3202 Caroline Dr, Health Science Park, Haw River, NC 27258
Ethylene oxide sterilization of medical devices, specializing in small- to medium-size lots.

Armm, Inc. 714-848-8190
17744 Sampson Ln, Huntington Beach, CA 92647
Validations also performed.

Cytosol Ophthalmics, Inc. 800-234-5166
PO Box 1408, 1325 William White Place, NE, Lenoir, NC 28645
Contract steam sterilization.

Dravon Medical, Inc. 503-656-6600
11465 SE Highway 212, PO Box 69, Clackamas, OR 97015
OEM sterilization 100% (ETO). Small loads.

Dumex Medical Surgical Products Ltd. 800-463-9613
104 Shorting Rd., Scarborough, ONT M1S 3S4 Canada

Enova Medical Technologies 866-773-0539
1839 Buerkle Rd, Saint Paul, MN 55110
In house ETO chambers. EN550 Certified

CONTRACT STERILIZATION *(cont'd)*

Hospira — 800-441-4100
268 E 4th St, Ashland, OH 44805
Gamma--medical products only.

Innovative Surgical Products, Inc. — 714-836-4474
2761 Walnut Ave, Tustin, CA 92780
Complete assemblies or sub-assemblies; contract packaging of trays, pouches, kits etc. and ETO or radiation sterilization services.

Iotron Technologies, Inc. — 604-945-8838
1425 Kebet Way, Port Coquitlam, BC V3C 6L3 Canada
Electron Beam Sterilization to disposable medical product manufacturers. The facility utilizes a 10 MeV-60kW accelerator to provide maximum penetration, tight dose tolerance capabilities and high through-put. Warehouse & distribution capabilities, dosemitry lab, R & D co-operative agreement.

J-Pac, Llc — 603-692-9955
25 Centre Rd, Somersworth, NH 03878
J-PAC offers total supply-chain management for your sterile, disposable medical device, including all forms of sterilization through strategic partners. J-PAC routinely provides sterile medical product via dock-to-stock programs that include EtO and gamma sterilization.

Lemco Enterprises, Inc. — 580-226-7808
3204 Hale Rd, Ardmore, OK 73401

Medtronic Dlp — 616-643-5200
620 Watson St SW, Grand Rapids, MI 49504

Midwest Sterilization Corp. — 573-243-8456
1204 Lenco Ave, Jackson, MO 63755
Contract sterilization in 160,000 sq.ft. facility in Jackson, Missouri and 175,000 sq.ft. facility in Laredo, Texas. 100% ETO and nitrogen purge.

Parter Medical Products — 800-666-8282
17015 Kingsview Ave, Carson, CA 90746

Specialteam Medical Services, Inc. — 714-694-0348
22445 La Palma Ave Ste F, Yorba Linda, CA 92887

Sterigenics International, Inc. — 800-472-4508
2015 Spring Rd Ste 650, Oak Brook, IL 60523
FDA registered. ISO 9002 certified. 40 facilities worldwide. Provider of contract gamma, ethylene oxide and electron beam sterilization services to include assistance with material evaluation, process conversion, validation, quality assurance, quarterly dose audit maintenance, turnaround reduction and sterilization cost efficiencies. Sterigenics' worldwide network of irradiation and Ethylene oxide facilities offer medical device manufacturers fast, flexible, precision processing for any size production lot. Guaranteed processing, conversion assistance and other customized services are available.

Sterilization Services — 404-344-8423
6005 Boat Rock Blvd SW, Atlanta, GA 30336
Ethylene oxide.

Sterilization Services Of Tennessee, Inc. — 901-947-2217
2396 Florida St, Memphis, TN 38109
Ethylene Oxide.

Sterilization Services Of Virginia, Inc. — 804-236-1652
5674 Eastport Blvd, Richmond, VA 23231
Ethylene oxide.

Sterimark/Etigam — 419-868-1800
1031 Calle Trepadora #D, Toledo, OH 43635-2796
Sterilization throughput indicators.

Steris Isomedix Services — 973-887-2754
9 Apollo Dr, Whippany, NJ 07981
Contract ethylene oxide sterilization services at plants in MA, TX SC & CA. Contract gamma sterilization services at 11 plants in NY, NJ, MA, OH, IL, SC, UT, TX, PR and Ontario. Also, manufacturing validation service of drug, device, food and other manufacturing operations. Electron beam service in IL.

Sts Duotek, Inc — 800-836-4850
370 Summit Point Dr, Henrietta, NY 14467
Ethylene-oxide and steam sterilization of medical devices.

Surgical Technologies, Inc. — 800-777-9987
292 E Lafayette Frontage Rd, Saint Paul, MN 55107
Full service assembly, packaging and sterilization services.

Windstone Medical Packaging, Inc. — 800-637-7056
1602 4th Ave N, Billings, MT 59101

CONTRACTOR, SURGICAL *(Surgery) 79FZR*

Biomet, Inc. — 574-267-6639
56 E Bell Dr, PO Box 587, Warsaw, IN 46582
Various types and styles of rib contractors.

CONTRAST ENHANCEMENT UNIT, MICROSCOPE
(Microbiology) 83RGS

Micromanipulator Co., Inc., The — 800-972-4032
1555 Forrest Way, Carson City, NV 89706
Products and accessories to aid in embryo recovery, grading, splitting, injection, micromanipulation and photomicrography.

Modulation Optics, Inc. — 516-609-000
40 Garvies Point Rd, Glen Cove, NY 11542
Objectives and condensers for hoffman modulation contrast microscopy.

Western Scientific Co., Inc. — 877-489-3726
4104 24th St # 183, San Francisco, CA 94114

CONTROL MATERIAL, BLOOD CIRCULATING EPITHELIAL CANCER CELL *(Hematology) 81NRS*

Veridex, Llc — 877-837-4339
1001 US Highway Route 202 N., Raritan, NJ 08869
Circulating tumor cell control kit.

CONTROL SYSTEM, CATHETER, STEERABLE
(Cardiovascular) 74DXX

Intraluminal Therapeutics, Inc. — 800-513-4458
6354 Corte Del Abeto Ste A, Carlsbad, CA 92011
Steerable catheter control system.

Stereotaxis, Inc. — 866-646-2346
4320 Forest Park Ave Ste 100, Saint Louis, MO 63108
Various models of catheter control systems.

CONTROL SYSTEM, ENERGY *(General) 80VBT*

Maxwell Technologies Power Systems — 877-511-4324
9244 Balboa Ave, San Diego, CA 92123
MEDI-ISO 50- to 500-kVA isolation transformers, UL544. All voltages and configurations for medical applications.

Vicon Industries Inc. — 800-645-9116
89 Arkay Dr, Hauppauge, NY 11788
NOVA 1500, V1422, V1466, V1300 and V1344 control and switching systems. Microprocessor-based control systems designed to control any size CCTV installation. Includes ProTech graphic command and control module.

CONTROL, ALCOHOL *(Toxicology) 91DKC*

Aalto Scientific Ltd. — 760-431-7922
1959 Kellogg Ave, Carlsbad, CA 92008
Ammonia, ethanol controls.

Clinical Controls International — 805-528-4039
1236 Los Osos Valley Rd Ste T, Los Osos, CA 93402
Serum alcohol control.

CONTROL, ANALYTE (ASSAYED AND UNASSAYED)
(Chemistry) 75JJX

Aalto Scientific Ltd. — 760-431-7922
1959 Kellogg Ave, Carlsbad, CA 92008
In vitro diagnostic controls/calibrators, made with human/animal base. Single specified analyte controls.

Abbott Point Of Care Inc. — 609-443-9300
104 Windsor Center Dr, East Windsor, NJ 08520
Various cardiac marker controls.

Acrometrix — 707-746-8888
6058 Egret Ct, Benicia, CA 94510
Negative hbv dna,hiv-1 rna,hcv rna controls unassayed.

Analytical Control Systems, Inc. — 317-841-0458
9058 Technology Dr, Fishers, IN 46038
LDH, LD/CK & CKMB ENZYME CONTROLS

Arkray Factory Usa, Inc. — 952-646-3168
5182 W 76th St, Minneapolis, MN 55439
Blood glucose control solution.

Arkray Usa — 800-818-8877
5198 W 76th St, Edina, MN 55439
Assure 3, ASSURE II, ASSURE, SUPREME II, QUICKTEK, Advance Intuition, and Advance Micro-draw CONTROL SOLUTION-Control solution is used to validate the performance of the corresponding blood glucose monitoring system . It has a known range of glucose.

Bayer Healthcare Llc — 914-524-2955
555 White Plains Rd Fl 5, Tarrytown, NY 10591
Control materials.

Bayer Healthcare, Llc — 574-256-3430
430 S Beiger St, Mishawaka, IN 46544
Control materials.

CONTROL, ANALYTE (ASSAYED AND UNASSAYED) *(cont'd)*

Bbi Diagnostics, A Division Of Seracare Life Scien 508-244-6428
375 West St, West Bridgewater, MA 02379
Accurun r 150 hsv igg positive control.

Biocell Laboratories, Inc. 800-222-8382
2001 E University Dr, Rancho Dominguez, CA 90220
Serum, urine, spinal fluid.

Biomerieux Inc. 800-682-2666
100 Rodolphe St, Durham, NC 27712

Bionostics, Inc. 978-772-7070
7 Jackson Rd, Devens, MA 01434
Rna medical multi-meter glucose calibration verification control.

Biosite Incorporated 888-246-7483
9975 Summers Ridge Rd, San Diego, CA 92121
Quality control material assayed & unassayed.

Carolina Liquid Chemistries Corp. 800-471-7272
510 W Central Ave Ste C, Brea, CA 92821
Homocysteine controls.

Chembio Diagnostic Systems, Inc. 631-924-1135
3661 Horseblock Rd, Medford, NY 11763
Hcg controls.

Clinical Controls International 805-528-4039
1236 Los Osos Valley Rd Ste T, Los Osos, CA 93402
Various types of analyte controls: whole blood glucose control.

Dade Behring, Inc. 800-948-3233
1717 Deerfield Rd, Deerfield, IL 60015

Diagnostic Devices Inc. 704-285-6400
9300 Harris Corners Pkwy Ste 450, Charlotte, NC 28269
Quality control material (assayed and unassayed).

Diagnostic Hybrids, Inc. 740-589-3300
1055 E State St Ste 100, Athens, OH 45701
Various types of single analyte controls.

Diasorin Inc 800-328-1482
1951 Northwestern Ave S, PO Box 285, Stillwater, MN 55082

Diazyme Laboratories 858-455-4761
12889 Gregg Ct, Poway, CA 92064
Homocysteine enzymatic assay.

Genzyme Diagnostics 617-252-7500
6659 Top Gun St, San Diego, CA 92121
Assayed & unassayed controls.

Health Chem Diagnostics Llc 954-979-3845
3341 W McNab Rd, Pompano Beach, FL 33069
Single (specified) analyte controls (assayed and unassayed).

Helena Laboratories 409-842-3714
PO Box 752, Beaumont, TX 77704

Hycor Biomedical, Inc. 800-382-2527
7272 Chapman Ave, Garden Grove, CA 92841
Serum protein control.

Jas Diagnostics, Inc. 305-418-2320
7220 NW 58th St, Miami, FL 33166
Fructosamine.

Lifescan, Inc. 800-227-8862
1000 Gibraltar Dr, Milpitas, CA 95035
Glucose control solution.

More Diagnostics, Inc. 800-758-0978
PO Box 6714, Los Osos, CA 93412
Cyclosporine C2 Control, multi-level, whole-blood, assayed.

Nipro Diagnostics, Inc. 1-800-342-7226
2400 NW 55th Ct, Fort Lauderdale, FL 33309
High glucose control, low glucose control.

Qualigen, Inc. 760-918-9165
2042 Corte Del Nogal, Carlsbad, CA 92011
Quality controls.

Raichem, Division Of Hemagen Diagnostics, Inc. 800-438-6100
8225 Mercury Ct, San Diego, CA 92111
RAI-TROL single analyte Fructosamine controls, Serum I and II.

Sorrento Biochemical, Inc. 858-259-0717
3443 Tripp Ct, San Diego, CA 92121
Glucose control.

Synergent Biochem, Inc. 562-809-3389
12026 Centralia Rd Ste G, Hawaiian Gardens, CA 90716
HDL/LDL lipid calibrator & controls.

CONTROL, ANALYTE (ASSAYED AND UNASSAYED) *(cont'd)*

Third Wave Technologies, Inc. 888-898-2357
502 S Rosa Rd, Madison, WI 53719
Invader assay controls.

CONTROL, ANTISERUM, ANTIGEN, ACTIVATOR, C3, COMPLEMENT *(Immunology) 82DAC*

Kent Laboratories, Inc. 360-398-8641
777 Jorgensen Pl, Bellingham, WA 98226
C-3 (BIC/BIA) radial immunodiffusion kit (INACTIVATOR).

CONTROL, BLOOD GAS *(Chemistry) 75JJS*

Air Liquide America Corporation, Cambridge Div. 800-638-1197
821 Chesapeake Dr, Cambridge, MD 21613
$65.00 to $85.00 for disposable cylinders.

Air Liquide Healthcare America Corporation 713-402-2152
8428 Market Street Rd, Houston, TX 77029
Blood gas calibration mixtures.

Bionostics, Inc. 978-772-7070
7 Jackson Rd, Devens, MA 01434
Blood gas controls with electrolytes and glucose.

Dade Behring, Inc. 800-948-3233
1717 Deerfield Rd, Deerfield, IL 60015

Health Chem Diagnostics Llc 954-979-3845
3341 W McNab Rd, Pompano Beach, FL 33069
Controls for blood-gases, (assayed and unassayed).

Nova Biomedical 800-458-5813
200 Prospect St, Waltham, MA 02453
Assayed for pH, PCO2, PO2, Na, K, ionized Ca, ionized magnesium, BUN, Cl and glucose.

Radiometer America, Inc. 800-736-0600
810 Sharon Dr, Westlake, OH 44145
QUALICHECK aqueous- and fluorocarbon-based controls.

Rna Medical, A Division Of Bionostics, Inc. 800-533-6162
7 Jackson Rd, Devens, MA 01434
QC products for all major brands of blood gas/critical blood analytes instruments. Blood-gas calibration verification controls.

Thermo Fisher Scientific Inc. 781-622-1000
81 Wyman St, Waltham, MA 02451

CONTROL, CELL COUNTER, NORMAL AND ABNORMAL *(Hematology) 81JCN*

Beckman Coulter, Inc. 800-635-3497
740 W 83rd St, Hialeah, FL 33014
Low, normal and high levels with and without platelets.

Bio-Rad, Diagnostics Group 800-854-6737
9500 Jeronimo Rd, Irvine, CA 92618

Fertility Solutions, Inc. 800-959-7656
13000 Shaker Blvd, Cleveland, OH 44120
Sperm count material.

Hycor Biomedical, Inc. 800-382-2527
7272 Chapman Ave, Garden Grove, CA 92841
Hematology cbc control.

R & D Systems, Inc. 1-800-343-7475
614 McKinley Pl NE, Minneapolis, MN 55413
Impedance and laser controls.

CONTROL, COAGULATION, PLASMA *(Hematology) 81GGN*

Abbott Point Of Care Inc. 609-443-9300
104 Windsor Center Dr, East Windsor, NJ 08520
Various coagulation controls.

American Diagnostica, Inc. 888-234-4435
500 West Ave, Stamford, CT 06902
DIMERTEST monoclonal fdp latex & EIA kits. Factor-deficient plasma tests, IMUBIND t-PA, PAI-1, & u-PA ELISA kits.

Analytical Control Systems, Inc. 317-841-0458
9058 Technology Dr, Fishers, IN 46038
Plasma Coagulation Controls available in human & animal plasma configurations. For quality control of APTT and PT systems. Excellent precision within range and very long stability (2 years refrigerated and unreconstituted.) Plasma Coagulation INR controls available in low, moderate and high INR values.

Bio/Data Corp. 215-441-4000
155 Gibraltar Rd, Horsham, PA 19044
Coagulation control plasma.

Biomerieux Inc. 800-682-2666
100 Rodolphe St, Durham, NC 27712
VERIFY LEVEL 1-normal contol. VERIFY LEVEL 2 and 3-abnormal controls.

CONTROL, COAGULATION, PLASMA *(cont'd)*

Biosite Incorporated 888-246-7483
9975 Summers Ridge Rd, San Diego, CA 92121
Single analyte control - d-dimer.

Dade Behring, Inc. 800-948-3233
1717 Deerfield Rd, Deerfield, IL 60015

Diagnostica Stago, Inc. 800-222-COAG
5 Century Dr, Parsippany, NJ 07054

Fisher Diagnostics 877-722-4366
11515 Vanstory Dr Ste 125, Huntersville, NC 28078
Coagulation reference plasma: normal, abnormal.

Health Chem Diagnostics Llc 954-979-3845
3341 W McNab Rd, Pompano Beach, FL 33069
Plasma, coagulation control.

Helena Laboratories 409-842-3714
PO Box 752, Beaumont, TX 77704

International Technidyne Corp. 800-631-5945
23 Nevsky St, Edison, NJ 08820

International Technidyne Corporation 732-548-5700
8 Olsen Ave, Edison, NJ 08820
Quality control reagents.

Medtronic Blood Management 612-514-4000
18501 E Plaza Dr, Parker, CO 80134
Calcium chloride.

Precision Biologic, Inc. 800-267-2796
900 Windmill Rd., Ste. 100, Dartmouth, NS B3B 1P7 Canada
CRYOCHECK coagulation calibration and control plasmas.

Wortham Laboratories Inc 423-296-0090
6340 Bonny Oaks Dr, Chattanooga, TN 37416
Heparin control plasma.

CONTROL, COOMBS *(Hematology) 81UJQ*

Biomerieux Inc. 800-682-2666
100 Rodolphe St, Durham, NC 27712
Coombs control cells.

Dade Behring, Inc. 800-948-3233
1717 Deerfield Rd, Deerfield, IL 60015

CONTROL, DRUG MIXTURE *(Toxicology) 91DIF*

Aalto Scientific Ltd. 760-431-7922
1959 Kellogg Ave, Carlsbad, CA 92008
Serum protein control.

Bayer Healthcare, Llc 574-256-3430
430 S Beiger St, Mishawaka, IN 46544
Control materials.

Bio Diagnostic Intl. 562-691-7850
1300 Pioneer St Ste C-, Brea, CA 92821
Serum anticonvulsants controls.

Biosite Incorporated 888-246-7483
9975 Summers Ridge Rd, San Diego, CA 92121
Drug mixture controls- amp, mamp, bar, bzo, coc, opi, pcp, thc and tca.

Clinical Controls International 805-528-4039
1236 Los Osos Valley Rd Ste T, Los Osos, CA 93402
No common name listed.

Health Chem Diagnostics Llc 954-979-3845
3341 W McNab Rd, Pompano Beach, FL 33069
Drug mixture control materials.

Hycor Biomedical, Inc. 800-382-2527
7272 Chapman Ave, Garden Grove, CA 92841
Therapeutic drug control (tdc).

Kaulson Laboratories, Inc. 973-226-9494
693 Bloomfield Ave, West Caldwell, NJ 07006
Drug screen control (qualitative).

Synergent Biochem, Inc. 562-809-3389
12026 Centralia Rd Ste G, Hawaiian Gardens, CA 90716
Liquid urine drugs of abuse control.

The Quality Assurance Service Corp. 706-863-6536
310 Commerce Dr, Martinez, GA 30907
Qac controls.

CONTROL, DRUG SPECIFIC *(Toxicology) 91LAS*

Clinical Controls International 805-528-4039
1236 Los Osos Valley Rd Ste T, Los Osos, CA 93402
Whole blood cyclosporin a control.

CONTROL, DRUG SPECIFIC *(cont'd)*

Lin-Zhi International, Inc. 408-732-3856
687 N Pastoria Ave, Sunnyvale, CA 94085
Phencyclidine controls, opiate controls, cocaince controls & amphetaimines cntrl.

Microgenics Corporation 800-232-3342
46360 Fremont Blvd, Fremont, CA 94538

Opus Diagnostics, Inc. 877-944-1777
1 Parker Plz, Fort Lee, NJ 07024
Innofluor Topiramate; Teicoplanin control set.

CONTROL, ELECTROLYTE (ASSAYED AND UNASSAYED)
(Chemistry) 75JJR

Aalto Scientific Ltd. 760-431-7922
1959 Kellogg Ave, Carlsbad, CA 92008

Beckman Coulter, Inc. 800-742-2345
250 S Kraemer Blvd, PO Box 8000, Brea, CA 92821

Biocell Laboratories, Inc. 800-222-8382
2001 E University Dr, Rancho Dominguez, CA 90220
Serum, urine, spinal fluid.

Bionostics, Inc. 978-772-7070
7 Jackson Rd, Devens, MA 01434
Ise electrolyte control.

Health Chem Diagnostics Llc 954-979-3845
3341 W McNab Rd, Pompano Beach, FL 33069
Electrolyte controls (assayed and unassayed).

Nova Biomedical 800-458-5813
200 Prospect St, Waltham, MA 02453
Assayed for electrolytes, ionized Ca, ionized magnesium, pH, glucose, creatinine, BUN, total protein, and osmolality.

Radiometer America, Inc. 800-736-0600
810 Sharon Dr, Westlake, OH 44145
QUALICHECK.

Rna Medical, A Division Of Bionostics, Inc. 800-533-6162
7 Jackson Rd, Devens, MA 01434

Thermo Fisher Scientific Inc. 781-622-1000
81 Wyman St, Waltham, MA 02451
Measured parameters: NA, K, Ca, Cl, Li, Glucose, Blood Gas.

CONTROL, ENZYME (ASSAYED AND UNASSAYED)
(Chemistry) 75JJT

Aalto Scientific Ltd. 760-431-7922
1959 Kellogg Ave, Carlsbad, CA 92008
Aalto Sci. LDH Isoenzyme Control

Beckman Coulter, Inc. 800-635-3497
740 W 83rd St, Hialeah, FL 33014
2 levels available.

Biocell Laboratories, Inc. 800-222-8382
2001 E University Dr, Rancho Dominguez, CA 90220
Serum, urine.

Clinical Controls International 805-528-4039
1236 Los Osos Valley Rd Ste T, Los Osos, CA 93402
Various types of enzyme controls: ckmb/ld-1 immunohibition control.

Dade Behring, Inc. 800-948-3233
1717 Deerfield Rd, Deerfield, IL 60015

Health Chem Diagnostics Llc 954-979-3845
3341 W McNab Rd, Pompano Beach, FL 33069
Enzyme controls (assayed and unassayed).

Helena Laboratories 409-842-3714
PO Box 752, Beaumont, TX 77704

Myers-Stevens Group, Inc. 903-566-6696
2931 Vail Ave, Commerce, CA 90040
Cpk enzyme controls.

Quantimetrix Corporation 800-624-8380
2005 Manhattan Beach Blvd, Redondo Beach, CA 90278
Sweat control for cystic fibrosis testing. Three-level control with simulated sweat matrix to be used to control sweat analysis for chloride, sodium, conductivity, and osmolality.

Verichem Laboratories, Inc. 401-461-0180
90 Narragansett Ave, Providence, RI 02907
No common name listed.

Worthington Biochemical Corp. 800-445-9603
730 Vassar Ave, Lakewood, NJ 08701

CONTROL, FOOT DRIVING, AUTOMOBILE, MECHANICAL *(Physical Med) 89KHZ*

Drive-Master Co., Inc. 973-808-9709
37 Daniel Rd, Fairfield, NJ 07004

Forward Motions, Inc. 877-364-8267
214 Valley St, Dayton, OH 45404

Handicaps, Inc. 800-782-4335
4335 S Santa Fe Dr, Englewood, CO 80110
$185.00 for left foot gas pedal, and $60.00 for park brake extension.

CONTROL, HAND DRIVING, AUTOMOBILE, MECHANICAL *(Physical Med) 89IPQ*

Complete Mobility Systems Inc. 800-788-7479
1915 County Road C W, Roseville, MN 55113
Wide range of devices enabling persons with varying disabilities to operate their vehicles.

Drive-Master Co., Inc. 973-808-9709
37 Daniel Rd, Fairfield, NJ 07004
Ultra-Lite XL push-pull mechanical hand control. Low-effort steering. No-effort steering. Low-effort brake. No-effort brake. Backup steering system. Backup brake system. Horizontal steering unit.

Driving Aids Development Corporation 800-767-6435
9417 Delancey Dr, Vienna, VA 22182
Mechanical/vacuum assisted hand driving control.

Forward Motions, Inc. 877-364-8267
214 Valley St, Dayton, OH 45404

Handicaps, Inc. 800-782-4335
4335 S Santa Fe Dr, Englewood, CO 80110
SUPERGRADE 4, $585.00 for hand driving controls, and $26.00 for steering devices (para). $420.00 for hand brake/clutch (only), and $320.00 for portable hand controls. Portable Hand Control - Temporary use only, $320.00. Comes in carrying case for people who fly and rent vehicles often, or persons who want to drive someone else's vehicle on a temporary basis.

Monmouth Equipment & Service Co. Inc. 732-919-1444
5105 Rts. 33/34, Farmingdale, NJ 07727
Monmouth vans.

Palmer Industries 800-847-1304
PO Box 5707, Endicott, NY 13763
PALMER Handcycle for Children. Handpedal cycles for children.

CONTROL, HEAVY METALS *(Toxicology) 91DIE*

Kaulson Laboratories, Inc. 973-226-9494
693 Bloomfield Ave, West Caldwell, NJ 07006
Blood & urine heavy metal controls.

Utak Laboratories, Inc. 800-235-3442
25020 Avenue Tibbitts, Valencia, CA 91355
Whole blood lead controls are offered in four separate blood lead decision levels classified as background, mild toxicity and moderate toxicity elevated ranges. Assayed for blood lead by graphite furnace atomic absorption spectrophotometry and anode stripping voltammetry.

CONTROL, HEMOGLOBIN *(Hematology) 81GGM*

Chembio Diagnostic Systems, Inc. 631-924-1135
3661 Horseblock Rd, Medford, NY 11763
Sickling hemoglobin controls.

Cone Bioproducts 830-379-0197
1012 N Austin St, Seguin, TX 78155
Hemoglobin a1c linearity set.

Dade Behring, Inc. 800-948-3233
1717 Deerfield Rd, Deerfield, IL 60015

Hycor Biomedical, Inc. 800-382-2527
7272 Chapman Ave, Garden Grove, CA 92841
Hemoglobin control.

PerkinElmer 800-762-4000
940 Winter St, Waltham, MA 02451

Rna Medical, A Division Of Bionostics, Inc. 800-533-6162
7 Jackson Rd, Devens, MA 01434
Hemoglobin controls for the Hemocue Analyzers

Sandare Intl., Inc. 972-293-7440
910 Kck Way, Cedar Hill, TX 75104
Hemoglogin controls.

Stanbio Laboratory, Inc. 830-249-0772
1261 N Main St, Boerne, TX 78006
$42.00 for 3 x 2ml tri-level hemoglobin control set with abnormal low, normal and abnormal high control.

CONTROL, HEMOGLOBIN *(cont'd)*

Thermo Fisher Scientific Inc. 781-622-1000
81 Wyman St, Waltham, MA 02451

CONTROL, HEMOGLOBIN, ABNORMAL *(Hematology) 81JCM*

Diagnostic Technology, Inc. 631-582-4949
175 Commerce Dr Ste L, Hauppauge, NY 11788
Sickle cell hemaglobin control for testing presence of hemoglobin s.

Helena Laboratories 409-842-3714
PO Box 752, Beaumont, TX 77704

Nichols Institute Diagnostics 949-940-7200
1311 Calle Batido, San Clemente, CA 92673
Human chronic gonadotropin immunoassay system.

PerkinElmer 800-762-4000
940 Winter St, Waltham, MA 02451

CONTROL, MULTI ANALYTE, ALL KINDS (ASSAYED AND UNASSAYED) *(Chemistry) 75JJY*

Aalto Scientific Ltd. 760-431-7922
1959 Kellogg Ave, Carlsbad, CA 92008
Human based control.

Abbott Point Of Care Inc. 609-443-9300
104 Windsor Center Dr, East Windsor, NJ 08520
Various control solutions.

Acrometrix 707-746-8888
6058 Egret Ct, Benicia, CA 94510
All kinds of multi-analyte controls.

Air Liquide Healthcare America Corporation 713-402-2152
8428 Market Street Rd, Houston, TX 77029
Lung diffusion calibration mixtures.

Analytical Control Systems, Inc. 317-841-0458
9058 Technology Dr, Fishers, IN 46038
HDL controls, HDL and LDL controls, lipoprotein electrophoresis controls, total lipid controls, Apo(A) and Apo(B) controls, Lp(a) controls, and cardiolipid controls are available. CPK controls, alkaline phosphatase controls, electrophoretic total-protein controls, zero calibrators, and ACE controls available.

Awareness Technology, Inc. 722-283-6540
1935 SW Martin Hwy, Palm City, FL 34990
Instrument performance check sets for photometers and microplate readers.

Bbi Diagnostics, A Division Of Seracare Life Scien 508-244-6428
375 West St, West Bridgewater, MA 02379
Accurn 155 anti-treponema (suphilis) positive control.

Beckman Coulter, Inc. 800-635-3497
740 W 83rd St, Hialeah, FL 33014
2 levels (chemistry); low, normal & high level (hematology).

Beckman Coulter, Inc. 800-742-2345
250 S Kraemer Blvd, PO Box 8000, Brea, CA 92821

Bio-Rad Laboratories 800-866-0305
12945 Alcosta Blvd, San Ramon, CA 94583
Virotrol quality-assurance reagents for use with viral-testing procedures including HIV, hepatitis, rubella, and herpes virus assays.

Bio-Rad Laboratories, Diagnostic Group 800-224-6723
524 Stone Rd Ste A, Benicia, CA 94510
Chemistry controls, multi analyte.

Bio-Rad, Diagnostics Group 800-854-6737
9500 Jeronimo Rd, Irvine, CA 92618
Spec. Controls: IA, TDM, tumor marker, hemoglobin, anemia, spinal fluid, chemistry, pediatric, toxicology, immunology, urine, blood gas, whole blood, isoenzyme, drug free serum, and endocrine, hematology, cardiac marker, diabetes, alcohol, urine metals, molecules bioloy & autoimmune.

Biocell Laboratories, Inc. 800-222-8382
2001 E University Dr, Rancho Dominguez, CA 90220
Lipid, APO A-1, APO-B, spinal-fluid control, urine, serum.

Biomerieux Inc. 800-682-2666
100 Rodolphe St, Durham, NC 27712

Bionostics, Inc. 978-772-7070
7 Jackson Rd, Devens, MA 01434
Multiple.

Bioprocessing, Inc. 207-615-0571
1045 Riverside St, Portland, ME 04103
Tumor marker proteins and antibodies, cell culture services

CONTROL, MULTI ANALYTE, ALL KINDS (ASSAYED AND UNASSAYED) *(cont'd)*

Bioresource Technology, Inc. 954-792-5222
11924 Miramar Pkwy, Flamingo Park Of Commerce, Miramar, FL 33025
Quality control, assayed material.

Biosite Incorporated 888-246-7483
9975 Summers Ridge Rd, San Diego, CA 92121
Various.

Carolina Liquid Chemistries Corp. 800-471-7272
510 W Central Ave Ste C, Brea, CA 92821
Chemistry controls.

Clinical Controls International 805-528-4039
1236 Los Osos Valley Rd Ste T, Los Osos, CA 93402
Varios types of: liquid ckbm/ld-1 immunoinhibition control.

Cliniqa Corporation 800-728-9558
774 N Twin Oaks Valley Rd Ste C, San Marcos, CA 92069
For cardiac, thyroid, tumor markers, serum proteins, and immunology controls and calibrators. ImmuTROL hs CRP Control, a three-level true liquid high-sensitivity CRP control suitable for use with reagent kits measuring very low levels of CRP, including tests for MCI prognostication and neonatal testing. ImmuTROL Tumor Marker Control, a 14-constituent human serum based TLC (true liquid control). Product comes as a three-level finished kit or can be manufactured to spec on an OEM basis.

Compass Bioscience 626-359-9645
1850 Evergreen St, Duarte, CA 91010
Quality control material (assayed & unassayed).

Dade Behring, Inc. 800-948-3233
1717 Deerfield Rd, Deerfield, IL 60015

Diagnostic Hybrids, Inc. 740-589-3300
1055 E State St Ste 100, Athens, OH 45701
Various types of multi-analyte controls.

Health Chem Diagnostics Llc 954-979-3845
3341 W McNab Rd, Pompano Beach, FL 33069
Multi-analyte controls, all kinds (assayed and unassayed).

Helena Laboratories 409-842-3714
PO Box 752, Beaumont, TX 77704

Hemagen Diagnostics, Inc. 800-436-2436
9033 Red Branch Rd, Columbia, MD 21045
Various enzyme verifiers and chemistry controls.

Jas Diagnostics, Inc. 305-418-2320
7220 NW 58th St, Miami, FL 33166
Level i & ii controls (multi analyte).

Maine Standards Company, Llc 800-377-9684
765 Roosevelt Trl Ste 9A, Windham, ME 04062
Various unassayed quality control materials.

More Diagnostics, Inc. 800-758-0978
PO Box 6714, Los Osos, CA 93412
Tac/CsA, Immunosuppressant Control, multi-level whole blood control containing cyclosporine and tacrolimus, assayed. Rap/Tac/CSA, Immunosuppressant Control, multi-level, whole-blood, containing sirolimus (rapamycin,)cyclosporine and tacrolimus, assayed. CARDIAC MARKERS CONTROL, multi-level serum control containing troponin, CKMB and myoglobin, assayed and hsCRP, unassayed.

Opti Medical Systems Inc. 770-510-4444
235 Hembree Park Dr, Roswell, GA 30076
Chemistry controls.

Osmetech, Inc. 800-373-6767
757 S Raymond Ave, Pasadena, CA 91105
Chemistry controls.

Polymer Technology Systems, Inc. 317-870-5610
7736 Zionsville Rd, Indianapolis, IN 46268
Multi-analyte chemistry controls.

Quantimetrix Corporation 800-624-8380
2005 Manhattan Beach Blvd, Redondo Beach, CA 90278
Ammonia/alcohol, urine chemistry, urine drugs-of-abuse screen control, bilirubin, spinal fluid, and microalbumin. Dip and spin combinition dipsticks/microscopics control. Spinalscopics spinal-fluid cell-count control.

Scantibodies Laboratory, Inc. 619-258-9300
9336 Abraham Way, Santee, CA 92071
Serum control.

Synergent Biochem, Inc. 562-809-3389
12026 Centralia Rd Ste G, Hawaiian Gardens, CA 90716
Liquid lipid control.

CONTROL, MULTI ANALYTE, ALL KINDS (ASSAYED AND UNASSAYED) *(cont'd)*

Teco Diagnostics 714-693-7788
1268 N Lakeview Ave, Anaheim, CA 92807
Multi-analyte controls, all kinds (assayed and unassayed).

Tripath Imaging, Inc. 919-206-7140
780 Plantation Dr, Burlington, NC 27215
Cell line control.

Vital Diagnostics Inc. 714-672-3553
1075 W Lambert Rd Ste D, Brea, CA 92821
Various linearity standards and assayed controls.

CONTROL, PLASMA, ABNORMAL *(Hematology) 81GGC*

Corgenix Medical Corporation 800-729-5661
11575 Main St, Broomfield, CO 80020
REAADS COAGULATION CONTROL 2

Dade Behring, Inc. 800-948-3233
1717 Deerfield Rd, Deerfield, IL 60015

Health Chem Diagnostics Llc 954-979-3845
3341 W McNab Rd, Pompano Beach, FL 33069
Control, plasma, abnormal.

Helena Laboratories 409-842-3714
PO Box 752, Beaumont, TX 77704

Life Therapeutics Inc. 404-300-5000
780 Park North Blvd Ste 100, Clarkston, GA 30021
La plasma.

Precision Biologic, Inc. 800-267-2796
900 Windmill Rd., Ste. 100, Dartmouth, NS B3B 1P7 Canada
CRYOCHECK ABNORMAL 1 REFERENCE CONTROL, CRYOCHECK ABNORMAL 2 REFERENCE CONTROL and CRYOCHECK ABNORMAL 1 CONTROL, CRYOCHECK ABNORMAL 2 CONTROL

Wortham Laboratories Inc 423-296-0090
6340 Bonny Oaks Dr, Chattanooga, TN 37416
Abnormal coagulation control.

CONTROL, PLATELET *(Hematology) 81GJP*

Bio-Rad Laboratories, Diagnostic Group 800-224-6723
524 Stone Rd Ste A, Benicia, CA 94510
Platelet control.

Dade Behring, Inc. 800-948-3233
1717 Deerfield Rd, Deerfield, IL 60015

Diagnostic Technology, Inc. 631-582-4949
175 Commerce Dr Ste L, Hauppauge, NY 11788
Platelet control.

R & D Systems, Inc. 1-800-343-7475
614 McKinley Pl NE, Minneapolis, MN 55413

CONTROL, URINALYSIS (ASSAYED AND UNASSAYED) *(Chemistry) 75JJW*

Arkray Usa 800-818-8877
5198 W 76th St, Edina, MN 55439
DIASCREEN LIQUID CONTROLS-Positive and negative controls help complywith quality assurance testing standards, no measuring or mixing required. Convenient and ready to use.

Bayer Healthcare Llc 914-524-2955
555 White Plains Rd Fl 5, Tarrytown, NY 10591
Urinalysis controls.

Bayer Healthcare, Llc 574-256-3430
430 S Beiger St, Mishawaka, IN 46544
Urinalysis controls.

Bio-Rad Laboratories, Diagnostic Group 800-224-6723
524 Stone Rd Ste A, Benicia, CA 94510
Urinalysis dipstick & microscopic controls.

Bio-Rad, Diagnostics Group 800-854-6737
9500 Jeronimo Rd, Irvine, CA 92618
For quantitative and qualitative (dipstick) urine analysis of level I and level II.

Biocell Laboratories, Inc. 800-222-8382
2001 E University Dr, Rancho Dominguez, CA 90220

Compass Bioscience 626-359-9645
1850 Evergreen St, Duarte, CA 91010
Quality control materials (assayed & unassayed).

Cst Technologies, Inc. 800-448-4407
55 Northern Blvd Ste 200, Great Neck, NY 11021
URISUB, $55.00 per liter - urine substitute for urine controls.

CONTROL, URINALYSIS (ASSAYED AND UNASSAYED) *(cont'd)*

Elsohly Labs, Inc. 662-236-2609
5 Industrial Park Dr, Oxford, MS 38655
Various types of laboratory urine controls.

Health Chem Diagnostics Llc 954-979-3845
3341 W McNab Rd, Pompano Beach, FL 33069
Urinalysis controls (assayed and unassayed).

Hycor Biomedical, Inc. 800-382-2527
7272 Chapman Ave, Garden Grove, CA 92841
Urinalysis controls.

Image Molding, Inc. 800-525-1875
4525 Kingston St, Denver, CO 80239
Standardized microscopic urinalysis system.

Iris Diagnostics 800-776-4747
9172 Eton Ave, Chatsworth, CA 91311
Normal/abnormal level specific gravity control.

Iris International, Inc. 800-776-4747
9162 Eton Ave, Chatsworth, CA 91311
IRISPEC CA/CB includes two part, reactive urine chemistry control.

Kenlor Industries, Inc. 714-647-0770
1560 E Edinger Ave Ste A1, Santa Ana, CA 92705
Liquid urine control.

Myers-Stevens Group, Inc. 903-566-6696
2931 Vail Ave, Commerce, CA 90040
Controls for routine urinalysis.

Quantimetrix Corporation 800-624-8380
2005 Manhattan Beach Blvd, Redondo Beach, CA 90278
DIPPER urine dipstick control, DROPPER urine dipstick control, DROPPER PLUS point-of-care urine dipstick control.

Research Triangle Institute
3040 Cornwallis Rd., Research Triangle Park, NC 27709
Urine pt samples, urine qc samples.

Roche Diagnostics 800-361-2070
201 Armand-Frappier Blvd., Laval, QUE H7V 4A2 Canada
CHEMSTRIP retail prices are approximately $8-10 CDN per package of test strips. MICRAL, retail price is $86.60 per package of tests.

Uridynamics, Inc. 317-915-7896
6786 Hawthorn Park Dr, Indianapolis, IN 46220
Urinary ph, urinary specific gravity, urinary quality control material.

Valley Biomedical Products/Ser., Inc. 540-868-0800
121 Industrial Dr, Winchester, VA 22602
Dental curing light.

CONTROLLER, FOOT, HANDPIECE AND CORD
(Dental And Oral) 76EBW

A-Dec, Inc. 800-547-1883
2601 Crestview Dr, Newberg, OR 97132
Electric handpiece.

Aesculap Implant Systems Inc. 1-800-234-9179
3773 Corporate Pkwy, Center Valley, PA 18034

Dentalez Group 866-DTE-INFO
101 Lindenwood Dr Ste 225, Valleybrooke Corporate Center
Malvern, PA 19355

Dentalez Group, Stardental Division 717-291-1161
1816 Colonial Village Ln, Lancaster, PA 17601
X-ray machine, dental.

Md International, Inc. 305-669-9003
11300 NW 41st St, Doral, FL 33178

Obtura Spartan 800-344-1321
13729 Shoreline Ct E, Earth City, MO 63045
Portable dental systems.

Osada, Inc. 800-426-7232
8436 W 3rd St Ste 695, Los Angeles, CA 90048
XL030/VSFP/LHP6-L5M-MCC6 also EXL-40R/VSFP/LHP8-L8M-MC. XL 230/MVFP/LHP6-L5M-MCC6, EXL-M40/MYFP/LHP12-L12M-MC12. OSADA XL-230: Low-speed/high-torque portable electric handpieces with variable speed foot pedal, magnetic sensors and laboratory or chainside handpiece assembly. OSADA EXL-M40: Brushless micromotor handpiece system for laboratory complete with MVFP foot pedal and LHP12 brushless handpiece assembly up to 40,000mm (RPM).

Zimmer Holdings, Inc. 800-613-6131
1800 W Center St, PO Box 708, Warsaw, IN 46580

CONTROLLER, GAS, CARDIOPULMONARY BYPASS
(Cardiovascular) 74DTX

Terumo Cardiovascular Systems, Corp 800-521-2818
6200 Jackson Rd, Ann Arbor, MI 48103

CONTROLLER, INFUSION *(Cardiovascular) 74QMI*

Directmed, Inc. 516-656-3377
150 Pratt Oval, Glen Cove, NY 11542
GEMINI FLOW, infusion set with two attached drip chambers to allow access to two different bags: one chamber is 20 drop, the second is 60 drop.

Microsurgical Technology, Inc. 425-556-0544
PO Box 2679, Redmond, WA 98073

CONTROLLER, INFUSION, INTRAVENOUS
(Cardiovascular) 74QMJ

B. Braun Oem Division, B. Braun Medical Inc. 866-8-BBRAUN
824 12th Ave, Bethlehem, PA 18018

Habley Medical Technology Corp. 800-729-1994
15721 Bernardo Heights Pkwy Ste B-30, San Diego, CA 92128
Patented new infusion delivery devices and controllers.

The Smartpill Corporation 800-644-4162
847 Main St, Buffalo, NY 14203

CONTROLLER, INJECTOR, ANGIOGRAPHIC
(Cardiovascular) 74DQF

Hospira, Inc. 877-946-7747
1776 Centennial Dr, McPherson, KS 67460
Cartridge actuator (plastic).

CONTROLLER, OXYGEN (BLENDER) *(Anesthesiology) 73QMK*

Bio-Med Devices, Inc. 800-224-6633
61 Soundview Rd, Guilford, CT 06437
$700 for air oxygen blender - $800 for MRI version. Several models: hi-lo-flo, lo-flo, hi-flo, 2 3/4 lbs. in weight.

CONTROLLER, PH *(Chemistry) 75UHE*

Analytical Measurements, Inc. 800-635-5580
100 Hoffman Pl, Hillside, NJ 07205
$610.00 each.

Cole-Parmer Instrument Inc. 800-323-4340
625 E Bunker Ct, Vernon Hills, IL 60061

Omega Engineering, Inc. 800-848-4286
1 Omega Dr, Stamford, CT 06907
Microprocessor-based pH controller featuring manual or automatic temperature compensation and 0.01 pH resolution. 1/8 DIN panel size with standard analog output.

CONTROLLER, PUMP SPEED, CARDIOPULMONARY BYPASS
(Cardiovascular) 74DWA

Minnetronix Inc. 888-301-1025
1635 Energy Park Dr, Saint Paul, MN 55108
Tandem Heart Escort Controller, Levitronix Centrimag Primary Consol

Terumo Cardiovascular Systems, Corp 800-521-2818
6200 Jackson Rd, Ann Arbor, MI 48103

CONTROLLER, SUCTION, INTRACARDIAC, CARDIOPULMONARY BYPASS *(Cardiovascular) 74DWD*

Terumo Cardiovascular Systems (Tcvs) 800-283-7866
28 Howe St, Ashland, MA 01721
Suction control.

CONTROLLER, TEMPERATURE, CARDIOPULMONARY BYPASS *(Cardiovascular) 74DWC*

Alpha Omega Mfg. Inc. 936-687-4993
PO Box 387, 110 Main Street, Grapeland, TX 75844
Heater-cooler.

Alsius Corp. 949-453-0150
15770 Laguna Canyon Rd Ste 150, Irvine, CA 92618
Heat exchange system.

Cincinnati Sub-Zero Products, Inc., Medical Division 800-989-7373
12011 Mosteller Rd, Cincinnati, OH 45241
Hemotherm dual-reservoir cooler/heater provides precise blood temperature control during cardiac by-pass surgery without need for ice.

Md International, Inc. 305-669-9003
11300 NW 41st St, Doral, FL 33178

Terumo Cardiovascular Systems, Corp 800-521-2818
6200 Jackson Rd, Ann Arbor, MI 48103

CONTROLLER, TEMPERATURE, HUMIDIFIER *(General) 80QML*

Clean Air Technology, Inc. 800 459 6320
41105 Capital Dr, Canton, MI 48187
Cleanroom temperature and humidity control systems for new construction, upgrades. Control systems for FDA data logging for validatable facilities.

Cleanroom Systems 800-825-3268
7000 Performance Dr, Syracuse, NY 13212
ADVANCAIR, self-contained custom built HVAC systems for tight temperature and humidity control.

Cmt, Inc. 800-659-9140
PO Box 297, Hamilton, MA 01936

Oven Industries, Inc. 1-877-766-6836
207 Hempt Rd, Mechanicsburg, PA 17050

Taga Medical Technologies 800-651-9490
34675 Melinz Pkwy Ste 105, Eastlake, OH 44095
CPAP humidification device for home care.

CONTROLLER, TEMPERATURE, OTHER *(General) 80QMM*

Burling Instruments, Inc. 973-635-9481
16 River Rd, Chatham, NJ 07928
Solid State temperature controller.

Cmt, Inc. 800-659-9140
PO Box 297, Hamilton, MA 01936

Eurotherm Inc. 703-443-0000
741F Miller Dr SE, Leesburg, VA 20175
Range of 1/32, 1/16, 1/8 and 1/4 temperature and process controllers, indicators, programmers and alarms.

Everest Interscience, Inc. 800-422-4342
1891 N Oracle Rd, Tucson, AZ 85705

Lake Shore Cryotronics, Inc. 614-891-2243
575 McCorkle Blvd, Westerville, OH 43082
Temperature sensors, temperature controllers and temperature transmitters.

Luwa Lepco 713-461-1131
1750 Stebbins Dr, Houston, TX 77043
Central plant air conditioning. All types of large scale chilled water, hot water, steam, and low dewpoint systems. Also laminar flow ceilings; specialty dual grid cleanroom ceiling that produces absolute uniform airflow. Gas fuel based air conditioning systems. Membrane Diffusion is a laminar flow and flush grid ceiling system that provides the best laminarity available in class 1 thru class 100,000 cleanrooms.

Movincool/Denso Sales California, Inc. 800-264-9573
3900 Via Oro Ave, Long Beach, CA 90810
Portable air conditioning unit for primary, supplementary or emergency cooling anywhere it's needed in the hospital, pharmacy or laboratory. Eight models offer selection of cooling capacity from 10,000 to 60,000 Btu/hr. OFFICE PRO 60 Portable air conditioner, cools overheating computer or telecom equipment in minutes. The Office Pro 60 provides 60,000 Btu/hr of cooling and operates on 230V power. It is designed to keep electronics operating by air-conditioning down to 65 degrees F. The Office Pro 60 features a programmable digital controller for automatic operation even after hours and weekends and a two-speed fan to control airflow. With the MovinCool portable air conditioner there's no costly installation necessary. You simply wheel the unit where you need it, plug it in and it goes to work. Instantly! Suggested price is $9,995.00

Oven Industries, Inc. 1-877-766-6836
207 Hempt Rd, Mechanicsburg, PA 17050
Temperature controller/alarm units.

Psg Controls, Inc. 800-523-2558
1225 Tunnel Rd, Perkasie, PA 18944

Tcp Reliable, Inc. 888-TCP-3393
551 Raritan Center Pkwy, Edison, NJ 08837
TCP Reliable is a manufacturer of insulated shipping containers, phase change materials and temperature monitoring devices. TCP provides all the packaging materials and services to ship temperature sensitive products. Our ISTA Certified laboratory tests new and existing packaging configurations to ensure the packaging materials maintain the products specified temperature range.

United Electric Controls Co. 617-926-1000
180 Dexter Ave, P.O. Box 9143, Watertown, MA 02472
Electro-mechanical temperature controllers and indicators, temp. switches and thermostats, temperature recorders, circular charts. Also, One Series electronic pressure and temp. switch is the first instrument of its kind with on-board diagnostics. This completely self-contained field device provides monitoring functions traditionally performed separately by transmitters, switches and guages.

CONTROLLER, TEMPERATURE, PROGRAMMABLE *(Chemistry) 75VGA*

Cmt, Inc. 800-659-9140
PO Box 297, Hamilton, MA 01936

Reheat Co., Inc. 800-373-4328
10 School St, Danvers, MA 01923
Temperature controls, programable RS232/RS485.

CONVEYOR, GUIDED VEHICLE *(General) 80TGS*

Bruno Independent Living Aids, Inc. 800-882-8183
1780 Executive Dr, Oconomowoc, WI 53066

Swisslog Translogic Corporation 800-525-1841
10825 E 47th Ave, Denver, CO 80239
Documents/Materials, X-Rays.

CONVEYOR, TRAY *(General) 80TFG*

Adamation, Inc. 800-225-3075
87 Adams St, PO Box 95037, Newton, MA 02458
Soiled tray and tray makeup conveyors.

Bausch & Stroebel Machine Company, Inc. 866-512-2637
112 Nod Rd Ste 17, Clinton, CT 06413

Caddy Corporation 856-467-4222
509 Sharptown Road, Bridgeport, NJ 08014-0345
Soiled tray conveyors for dishware and trays - hospital tray makeup conveyors.

Servolift/Eastern Corp. 800-727-3786
266 Hancock St, Dorchester, MA 02125

CORD, ELECTRIC, ENDOSCOPE *(Gastro/Urology) 78FFZ*

Boehm Surgical Instrument Corp. 716-436-6584
966 Chili Ave, Rochester, NY 14611
Cord, electric for endoscope.

Bryan Corp. 800-343-7711
4 Plympton St, Woburn, MA 01801
Unipolar, bipolar and high frequency connecting cords.

Electro Surgical Instrument Co., Inc. 888-464-2784
37 Centennial St, Rochester, NY 14611
Conducting cord.

Elmed, Inc. 630-543-2792
60 W Fay Ave, Addison, IL 60101

Ethicon Endo-Surgery, Inc. 800-USE-ENDO
4545 Creek Rd, Cincinnati, OH 45242
ENDOPATH bovie pin and banana plug to 90 degrees NJ jack; bovie pin to straight jack, electrosurgery.

Kirwan Surgical Products, Inc. 888-547-9267
180 Enterprise Dr, PO Box 427, Marshfield, MA 02050
Monopolar endoscopic cords.

CORD, ELECTRIC, INSTRUMENT, SURGICAL, TRANSURETHRAL *(Gastro/Urology) 78FBJ*

Greenwald Surgical Co., Inc. 219-962-1604
2688 Dekalb St, Gary, IN 46405
Various types of active machine cords for resectoscopes.

CORD, RETRACTION *(Dental And Oral) 76MVL*

Medical Products Laboratories, Inc. 215-677-2700
9990 Global Rd, Philadelphia, PA 19115
Cord, retraction with & without hemostatic agent.

Pascal Co., Inc. 425-602-3633
2929 Northup Way, Bellevue, WA 98004
Retraction cord.

Ultradent Products, Inc. 801-553-4586
505 W 10200 S, South Jordan, UT 84095
Retraction cord.

CORKSCREW *(Orthopedics) 87HWI*

Biomet, Inc. 574-267-6639
56 E Bell Dr, PO Box 587, Warsaw, IN 46582
Femoral head remover.

Zimmer Holdings, Inc. 800-613-6131
1800 W Center St, PO Box 708, Warsaw, IN 46580

Zimmer Trabecular Metal Technology 800-613-6131
10 Pomeroy Rd, Parsippany, NJ 07054
Acetabular insert remover.

CORSET *(Orthopedics) 87QMN*

Baron Medical Supply 888-702-2766
709 Grand St, Brooklyn, NY 11211
Lumbar sacral and abdominal corsets.

CORSET *(cont'd)*

Freeman Manufacturing Company 800-253-2091
900 W Chicago Rd, PO Box J, Sturgis, MI 49091

Larkotex Company 800-972-3037
1002 Olive St, Texarkana, TX 75501

Paramedical Distributors 800-245-3278
2020 Grand Blvd, Kansas City, MO 64108

Slawner Ltd., J. 514-731-3378
5713 Cote Des Neiges Rd., Montreal, QUE H3S 1Y7 Canada

Truform Orthotics & Prosthetics 800-888-0458
3960 Rosslyn Dr, Cincinnati, OH 45209

CORYNEBACTERIUM DIPHTHERIAE, VIRULENCE STRIP *(Microbiology) 83KFI*

Bd Diagnostic Systems 800-675-0908
7 Loveton Cir, Sparks, MD 21152

COTTON, ROLL *(Dental And Oral) 76EFN*

Barnhardt Mfg. Co. 704-376-0380
1100 Hawthorne Ln, Charlotte, NC 28205
Various sizes of sterile and non sterile cotton rolls.

Carolina Absorbent Cotton Co. 800-277-0377
1100 Hawthorne Ln, Charlotte, NC 28205

Chagrin Safety Supply, Inc. 800-227-0468
8227 Washington St # 1, Chagrin Falls, OH 44023

Customs Hospital Products, Inc 800-426-2780
6336 SE 107th Ave, Portland, OR 97266
Multiple, non-sterile.

Degasa, S.A. De C.V. 525-5-483 31
Prolongacion Canal De, Miramontes #3775 Col. Ex-Hacienda San Juan Del. Tlalpan Mexico
Protec cotton, roll;protec cotton balls

Kentron Health Care, Inc. 615-384-0573
3604 Kelton Jackson Rd, P.o. Box 120, Springfield, TN 37172
Cotton roll.

Mydent International 800-275-0020
80 Suffolk Ct, Hauppauge, NY 11788
DEFEND Dental Rolls non-sterile (100% cotton) non-cellulose size #2).

Omnia, Inc. 863-619-8100
3125 Drane Field Rd Ste 29, Lakeland, FL 33811
Cotton rolls.

Palmero Health Care 800-344-6424
120 Goodwin Pl, Stratford, CT 06615
Cotton roll holders.

Starkey Glencoe 952-947-4734
2915 10th St E, Glencoe, MN 55336
Oto-block.

Tidi Products, Llc 920-751-4380
570 Enterprise Dr, Neenah, WI 54956
Cotton roll, dental.

COUCH, RADIATION THERAPY, POWERED *(Radiology) 90JAI*

Best Nomos Corp. 800-70-NOMOS
1 Best Dr, Pittsburgh, PA 15202
The Nomos CRANE; powered radiation therapy patient support assembly.

Composiflex, Inc. 800-673-2544
8100 Hawthorne Dr, Erie, PA 16509
Low x-ray absorption, high strength carbon fiber couch tops.

Elekta, Inc. 800-535-7355
4775 Peachtree Industrial Blvd, Building 300, Suite 300 Norcross, GA 30092
Radiation therapy positioning systems.

Medtec 800-842-8688
1401 8th St SE, PO Box 320, Orange City, IA 51041
The nomos crane II.

Neutron Products, Inc. 301-349-5001
22301 Mount Ephraim Rd, Dickerson, MD 20842

COULOMETRIC METHOD, CARBON-DIOXIDE *(Chemistry) 75CHS*

Abbott Diagnostics Div. 626-440-0700
820 Mission St, South Pasadena, CA 91030
Carbon dioxide.

COUNTER, CELL *(Microbiology) 83QMQ*

American Bantex Corp. 800-633-4839
1815 Rollins Rd, Burlingame, CA 94010

COUNTER, CELL *(cont'd)*

Beckman Coulter, Inc. 800-635-3497
740 W 83rd St, Hialeah, FL 33014
Complete series of models with 1 to 18 parameters; from $4,495 to $152,000.

Climet Instruments Co. 909-793-2788
1320 W Colton Ave, Redlands, CA 92374
$7,500.00 per unit (standard).

Drew Scientific, Inc. 800-433-0945
4230 Shilling Way, Dallas, TX 75237

Fisher Healthcare 800-766-7000
9999 Veterans Memorial Dr, Houston, TX 77038

Humagen Fertility Diagnostics, Inc. 800-937-3210
2400 Hunters Way, Charlottesville, VA 22911
$90.00 for Counting Chambers disposable cell counting chambers (50 chambers).

Immunicon Corporation 215-830-0777
3401 Masons Mill Rd Ste 100, Huntingdon Valley, PA 19006
The CellTracks Analyzer II is a semi-automated fluorescence microscope taht is designed for rare cell analysis, including circultating tumor cells and circulating endothelial cells.

Lw Scientific 800-726-7345
865 Marathon Pkwy, Lawrenceville, GA 30046
5-key or 8-key differential counters.

Medical Sales & Service Group 888-357-6520
10 Woodchester Dr, Acton, MA 01720

Modulus Data Systems, Inc. 888-663-8547
386 Main St Ste 200, Redwood City, CA 94063
DIFFCOUNT III $529.00 to $649.00 per unit (standard).

Myco Instrumentation Source, Inc. 425-228-4239
PO Box 354, Renton, WA 98057

New Brunswick Scientific Co., Inc. 800-631-5417
PO Box 4005, Edison, NJ 08818
NucleoCounter (R) automated mammalian cell counting device. Uses patented fluorescence technology to accurately count mammalian cells, without regard to cell size or morphology. Eliminates time-consuming manual evaluation, as well as errors caused by operator subjectivity.

Orbeco Analytical Systems, Inc. 800-922-5242
185 Marine St, Farmingdale, NY 11735
$85.00 per unit (standard) improved double Neubauer ruling.

Spectrex Corp. 800-822-3940
3580 Haven Ave, Redwood City, CA 94063
$16,000 for laser particle counter.

Spectron Corp. 425-827-9317
934 S Burlington Blvd # 603, Burlington, WA 98233
Reconditioned equipment.

COUNTER, CELL OR PARTICLE, AUTOMATED *(Hematology) 81GKL*

Adit/Electron Tubes 800-521-8382
100 Forge Way Ste F, Rockaway, NJ 07866

Alicia Diagnostics, Inc. 407-365-8498
1274 Alafaya Trl, Oviedo, FL 32765
Cbc complete bloodcell count equipment.

Bd Biosciences 408-954-6307
2350 Qume Dr, San Jose, CA 95131
Flow cytometer.

Beckman Coulter, Inc. 800-526-3821
11800 SW 147th Ave, Miami, FL 33196
Automated cell counter.

Beckman Coulter, Inc. 800-635-3497
740 W 83rd St, Hialeah, FL 33014
Uses conductivity technique; 105 specimens/hr. throughput.

Cell Science Systems, Ltd. Corp. 954-426-2304
1239 E Newport Center Dr Ste 101, Deerfield Beach, FL 33442
Hematology particle counter.

Diagnostic Technology, Inc. 631-582-4949
175 Commerce Dr Ste L, Hauppauge, NY 11788
Cbc hematology analyzer.

Drew Scientific, Inc. 800-433-0945
4230 Shilling Way, Dallas, TX 75237
Semi-automated red and white blood cell and platelet counter which also measures hemoglobin indices.

Hamilton Thorne Biosciences 978-921-2050
181 Elliott St, 100 Cummings Center-suite 465e, Beverly, MA 01915
Sperm cell analyzer.

COUNTER, CELL OR PARTICLE, AUTOMATED *(cont'd)*

Horiba Abx 888-903-5001
34 Bunsen, Irvine, CA 92618
Automated cell counter.

Iris Diagnostics 800-776-4747
9172 Eton Ave, Chatsworth, CA 91311
Body fluids analyzer.

Minitube Of America, Inc 608-845-1502
419 Venture Ct, Verona, WI 53593
Computer automated cell and particle counter.

Sunshine Instruments 800-343-1199
2200 Michener St, Philadelphia, PA 19115

COUNTER, CELL, DIFFERENTIAL CLASSIFIER, AUTOMATED
(Hematology) 81GKZ

Abbott Diagnostics Div. 847-937-7988
1921 Hurd Dr, Irving, TX 75038
Automated differential cell classifier system.

Alicia Diagnostics, Inc. 407-365-8498
1274 Alafaya Trl, Oviedo, FL 32765
Cbc diff complete bloodcell count equipment with differential.

Bd Biosciences 408-954-6307
2350 Qume Dr, San Jose, CA 95131
Nucleic acid dye.

Beckman Coulter, Inc. 800-526-3821
11800 SW 147th Ave, Miami, FL 33196
Differential cell counters, automated, antibodies and accessories.

Cytek Development, Inc. 510-657-0102
4059 Clipper Ct, Fremont, CA 94538
Facscan,facscalibur.

Drew Scientific, Inc. 800-433-0945
4230 Shilling Way, Dallas, TX 75237

Guava Technologies, Inc. 866-448-2827
25801 Industrial Blvd, Hayward, CA 94545
Various models of personal cell analysis machines.

Horiba Abx 888-903-5001
34 Bunsen, Irvine, CA 92618
Automated differential cell counter.

Modulus Data Systems, Inc. 888-663-8547
386 Main St Ste 200, Redwood City, CA 94063
COMP-U-DIFF $1,250.00 per unit (standard).

Pointcare Technologies Inc. 508-281-6925
181 Cedar Hill St, Marlborough, MA 01752
Flowcare analyzer.

Qbc Diagnostics, Inc. 814-342-6205
200 Shadylane Dr, Philipsburg, PA 16866
Automated differential cell counter.

COUNTER, COLONY *(Microbiology) 83QMR*

Advanced American Biotechnology (Aab) 714-870-0290
1166 E Valencia Dr Unit 6C, Fullerton, CA 92831
Sorting: Video camera, lens, stand, transilluminator and software with background correction, automatic or manual, user-defined sorting dark, faint or translucent, size area, perimeter, circularity, for microbial and tissue culture, cell count Ames test, microscope attachment...$7,995.

American Bantex Corp. 800-633-4839
1815 Rollins Rd, Burlingame, CA 94010

Orbeco Analytical Systems, Inc. 800-922-5242
185 Marine St, Farmingdale, NY 11735
$580.00 per unit (standard) Quebec type.

Ultra-Lum, Inc. 800-809-6559
1480 N Claremont Blvd, Claremont, CA 91711
Omega Series or Gel Explorer Series Imaging Systems.

Ward's Natural Science Establishment, Inc. 800-962-2660
PO Box 92912, 5100 W. Henrietta Rd., Rochester, NY 14692

COUNTER, DIFFERENTIAL HAND TALLY *(Hematology) 81GKM*

Meylan Corporation 888-769-9667
543 Valley Rd, Upper Montclair, NJ 07043
$82.00 to $1280.00 for electromechanical & electronic counters.

Modulus Data Systems, Inc. 888-663-8547
386 Main St Ste 200, Redwood City, CA 94063
DIFFCOUNT III $529.00 to $649.00 per unit (standard).

COUNTER, DIFFERENTIAL HAND TALLY *(cont'd)*

United Products & Instruments, Inc. 800-588-9776
182 Ridge Rd Ste E, Dayton, NJ 08810
Manual differential counters have been used for decades in the clinical laboratory. Each unit is sold with a WBC maturation series picto-strip just above the key windows. Unico® offers the two most popular counters: 5 key with total window, and 8 key with total window. Visit us at www.unico1.com for more information on this and other laboratory instruments from UNICO

COUNTER, GAMMA, GENERAL USE *(Toxicology) 91DNR*

Biodex Medical Systems, Inc. 800-224-6339
20 Ramsey Rd, Shirley, NY 11967

Bioscan, Inc. 800-255-7226
4590 MacArthur Blvd NW, Washington, DC 20007

Capintec, Inc. 800-631-3826
6 Arrow Rd, Ramsey, NJ 07446

Dosimeter Division Of Arrow Tech Inc 800-322-8258
5 Eastmans Rd, Parsippany, NJ 07054

Laboratory Technologies, Inc. 800-542-1123
43 W 900 Rte. 64, Maple Park, IL 60151
Single well gamma counter with full RIA software.

Medical Sales & Service Group 888-357-6520
10 Woodchester Dr, Acton, MA 01720

Mgm Instruments 800-551-1415
925 Sherman Ave, Hamden, CT 06514
$7,200 for ISOCOMP I single-well gamma counter with data reduction, on-board printer, and RS232 port.

Myco Instrumentation Source, Inc. 425-228-4239
PO Box 354, Renton, WA 98057

Spectron Corp. 425-827-9317
934 S Burlington Blvd # 603, Burlington, WA 98233
Reconditioned equipment.

Titertek Instruments, Inc. 256-859-8600
330 Wynn Dr NW, Huntsville, AL 35805

COUNTER, GAMMA, RADIOIMMUNOASSAY (MANUAL)
(Toxicology) 91DNM

Capintec, Inc. 800-631-3826
6 Arrow Rd, Ramsey, NJ 07446

COUNTER, NEEDLE *(Surgery) 79QMT*

Advanced Medical Innovations, Inc. 888-367-2641
9410 De Soto Ave Ste J, Chatsworth, CA 91311
Sharps Safety Station Needle Counter boxes featuring one handed recapping and exchanging for hypodermic needles in surgery and anesthesia; most user friendly blade remover; Counting device for needles including scalpel blades; Scalpel holder; featuring the AUTO-LOCK closure mechnism keeps sharps safely inside, but opens easily for recount.

Anchor Products Company 800-323-5134
52 W Official Rd, Addison, IL 60101
$157.40 for case of 40, and $203.00 for case of 80.

COUNTER, PILL *(General) 80VDQ*

Nova Packaging Systems 978-537-8534
7 New Lancaster Rd, Leominster, MA 01453
SWIFT COUNT tablet & capsule counter.

COUNTER, PLATELET, AUTOMATED *(Hematology) 81GKX*

Beckman Coulter, Inc. 800-635-3497
740 W 83rd St, Hialeah, FL 33014
2 semi-automated models; using conductivity technique. Model T660 adds platelets to automated 5 parameter analysis (WBC, RBC, HGB, MCV and platelets).

COUNTER, PLATELET, MANUAL *(Hematology) 81GLG*

Beckman Coulter, Inc. 800-526-3821
11800 SW 147th Ave, Miami, FL 33196
Manual blood cell counting device.

Cambridge Diagnostic Products, Inc. 800-525-6262
6880 NW 17th Ave, Fort Lauderdale, FL 33309
$38.00 for 4-oz CAMCO Platecount.

Pochemco, Inc. 413-536-2900
724 Main St, Holyoke, MA 01040
Rees-ecker diluting fluid.

Ricca Chemical Company Llc 817-461-5601
1490 Lammers Pike, Batesville, IN 47006

Ricca Chemical Company, Llc 817-461-5601
448 W Fork Dr, Arlington, TX 76012
Rees and ecker blood diluting fluid.

COUNTER, RADIATION *(Radiology) 90RNU*

Alimed, Inc. 800-225-2610
297 High St, Dedham, MA 02026
Wipe-test counter designed to meet NRC requirements for determining surface radioactive-contamination levels.

Canberra Industries 800-243-3955
800 Research Pkwy, Meriden, CT 06450

Capintec, Inc. 800-631-3826
6 Arrow Rd, Ramsey, NJ 07446

Dosimeter Division Of Arrow Tech Inc 800-322-8258
5 Eastmans Rd, Parsippany, NJ 07054
$400-$1,000 per unit, miniature and full size, digital and analog models. Miniature units available with GM or scintillation probes.

Johnson & Associates Inc., Wm. B. 304-645-6568
200 AEI Dr., Lewisburg, WV 24902
22 models, portables, survey meters, geiger, & counting room units - $295 to $2,250 each.

Lnd, Inc. 516-678-6141
3230 Lawson Blvd, Oceanside, NY 11572
Full line, $32 to $3,000 per unit; x-ray and position sensitive proportional counters; beam monitors; alpha, beta, gamma GM detectors.

Ludlum Measurements, Inc. 800-622-0828
501 Oak St, Sweetwater, TX 79556
$485.00 to $6,575.00 per unit; micro R, portal, alarm, and recording models; beta/gamma hand & shoe model; Geiger Mueller probes. Alpha, beta, gamma and neutron detectors, shielded well counters.

Marconi Medical Systems 800-323-0550
595 Miner Rd, Cleveland, OH 44143

Micrad, Inc. 865-690-6389
312 Trossachs Ln, Knoxville, TN 37922

Ortec - (Advanced Measurement Technology) 800-251-9750
801 S Illinois Ave, Oak Ridge, TN 37830

Owens Scientific Inc. 281-394-2311
23230 Sandsage Ln, Katy, TX 77494

S.E. International, Inc. 800-293-5759
436 Farm Rd, PO Box 39, Summertown, TN 38483
8 models available from $279.00 to $685.00 for handheld ionizing radiation detectors.

COUNTER, SCINTILLATION *(Chemistry) 75QMU*

Beckman Coulter, Inc. 800-742-2345
250 S Kraemer Blvd, PO Box 8000, Brea, CA 92821

Canberra Industries 800-243-3955
800 Research Pkwy, Meriden, CT 06450

Capintec, Inc. 800-631-3826
6 Arrow Rd, Ramsey, NJ 07446

Johnson & Associates Inc., Wm. B. 304-645-6568
200 AEI Dr., Lewisburg, WV 24902
Scintillation probes, $295 to $625, connect to $325 meter.

Ludlum Measurements, Inc. 800-622-0828
501 Oak St, Sweetwater, TX 79556
$350.00 to $630.00 for alpha, beta, gamma and neutron detectors, $1,110.00 for shielded well scintillators.

Marconi Medical Systems 800-323-0550
595 Miner Rd, Cleveland, OH 44143

Soltec Corp. 800-423-2344
12977 Arroyo St, San Fernando, CA 91340

COUNTER, SCINTILLATION, LIQUID, TOXICOLOGY *(Toxicology) 91DNY*

Adit/Electron Tubes 800-521-8382
100 Forge Way Ste F, Rockaway, NJ 07866

Beckman Coulter, Inc. 800-742-2345
250 S Kraemer Blvd, PO Box 8000, Brea, CA 92821

Ludlum Measurements, Inc. 800-622-0828
501 Oak St, Sweetwater, TX 79556

COUNTER, SPONGE, SURGICAL *(Surgery) 79LWH*

Advanced Medical Innovations, Inc. 888-367-2641
9410 De Soto Ave Ste J, Chatsworth, CA 91311
SPONGECHECK - 2 bagging systems with a stainless steel adjustable height kick bucket with blood catch basin. Suture Packet Organizers and Counters, organizes by size in a compact slotted foam with adhesive backing. 10 & 20 packet capacity sizes available for minor and major services.

COUNTER, SPONGE, SURGICAL *(cont'd)*

Amd-Ritmed, Inc. 800-445-0340
295 Firetower Road, Tonawanda, NY 14150
Sponge Count & Disposal System. 5 count panels and hardware.

Clearcount Medical Solutions, Inc. 412-931-7233
101 Bellevue Rd Ste 203, Pittsburgh, PA 15229
Surgical sponge counter.

Diamond Edge Co. 727-586-2927
928 W Bay Dr, Largo, FL 33770
Surgical blade cleaning sponge.

Medical Action Industries, Inc. 800-645-7042
25 Heywood Rd, Arden, NC 28704
Sponge counter glove.

Rf Surgical Systems Inc. Technical Center 760-994-8198
9740 Appaloosa Rd Ste 150, San Diego, CA 92131
Scanning system.

Sms Technologies, Inc. 858-587-6900
9877 Waples St, San Diego, CA 92121
Scanning system.

Surgicount Medical, Inc. 951-587-6201
43460 Ridge Park Dr Ste 140, Temecula, CA 92590
Surgical sponge scale.

Xodus Medical, Inc. 800-963-8776
702 Prominence Dr, Westmoreland Business & Research Park
New Kensington, PA 15068
Sponge Counter Bags

COUNTER, SURGICAL INSTRUMENT *(Surgery) 79VDL*

Advanced Medical Innovations, Inc. 888-367-2641
9410 De Soto Ave Ste J, Chatsworth, CA 91311
SECURE-IT-Y, instrument rack system that protects and controls the finger-ringed surgical instrument during processing and during the surgical procedure. Also, adjustable instrument organizer, which replaces a rolled towel on the Mayo and the back table. Available reusable/autoclavable as well as disposable in various sizes for the Mayo and the back table; lint free. No time wasted in stringing instruments and rolling towels.

COUNTER, URINE PARTICLE *(Pathology) 88LKM*

Iris Diagnostics 800-776-4747
9172 Eton Ave, Chatsworth, CA 91311
Automated urinalysis system.

COUNTERSINK *(Orthopedics) 87HWW*

Ascent Healthcare Solutions 480-763-5300
10232 S 51st St, Phoenix, AZ 85044
Countersink.

Biomet, Inc. 574-267-6639
56 E Bell Dr, PO Box 587, Warsaw, IN 46582
Bone screw countersink.

Interventional Spine, Inc. 800-497-0484
13700 Alton Pkwy Ste 160, Irvine, CA 92618
Various types of countersinks.

Kmedic 800-955-0559
190 Veterans Dr, Northvale, NJ 07647

Medtronic Sofamor Danek Instrument Manufacturing 901-396-3133
7375 Adrianne Pl, Bartlett, TN 38133
Countersink.

Medtronic Sofamor Danek Usa, Inc. 901-396-3133
4340 Swinnea Rd, Memphis, TN 38118
Countersink.

Small Bone Innovations, Inc. 215-428-1791
1380 S Pennsylvania Ave, Morrisville, PA 19067
Countersink.

Warsaw Orthopedic, Inc. 901-396-3133
2500 Silveus Xing, Warsaw, IN 46582
Countersink.

Zimmer Holdings, Inc. 800-613-6131
1800 W Center St, PO Box 708, Warsaw, IN 46580

Zimmer Trabecular Metal Technology 800-613-6131
10 Pomeroy Rd, Parsippany, NJ 07054
Countersink tamp.

COUPLER, OPTICAL, LAPAROSCOPIC *(General) 80SHM*
Precision Optics Corp. 800-447-2812
22 E Broadway, Gardner, MA 01440
Custom-made versatile interface between camera and endoscope, couple to almost any camera. Also, custom fiberoptic eyepieces for direct view or coupling to a camera.
Wisap America 800-233-8448
8231 Melrose Dr, Lenexa, KS 66214

COVER, ARM BOARD *(General) 80QMX*
Bryton Corp. 800-567-9500
4310 Guion Rd, Indianapolis, IN 46254
Arm board pads & covers for all types of surgical tables.
General Econopak, Inc. 888-871-8568
1725 N 6th St, Philadelphia, PA 19122
Jms Converters Inc Dba Sabee Products & Stanford Prof Prod 215-396-3302
67 Buck Rd Ste B7, Huntingdon Valley, PA 19006
Disposable armboard cover.
Precision Dynamics Corp. 800-772-1122
13880 Del Sur St, San Fernando, CA 91340
Profex Medical Products 800-325-0196
2224 E Person Ave, Memphis, TN 38114

COVER, BARRIER, PROTECTIVE *(General) 80MMP*
Alimed, Inc. 800-225-2610
297 High St, Dedham, MA 02026
Deuteronomy Management Services,Inc. 850-897-3321
1439 Live Oak St Ste A, Niceville, FL 32578
Equipment covers.
Intl. Medsurg Connection, Inc. 847-619-9926
935 N Plum Grove Rd Ste V, Schaumburg, IL 60173
Bandbags, domebags, setup covers, cassette covers.
Jero Medical Equipment & Supplies, Inc. 800-457-0644
1701 W 13th St, Chicago, IL 60608
Medsep Corp., A Subsidiary Of Pall Corp. 516-484-5400
1630 W Industrial Park St, Covina, CA 91722
Needle protection/sample tube device.
Mydent International 800-275-0020
80 Suffolk Ct, Hauppauge, NY 11788
Barrier Film: DEFEND Barrier Film; Adhesive film size 4' x 6' to cover light handles, tubing, and other items to be protected.
Protek Medical Products, Inc. 319-545-7100
4125 Westcor Ct, Coralville, IA 52241
Various.
Sanax Protective Products, Inc. 800-379-9929
236 Upland Ave, Newton Highlands, MA 02461
Span Packaging Services Llc. 864-627-4155
4611A Dairy Dr, Greenville, SC 29607
Allkare barrier wipe.
Wrapped In Comfort 877-205-0901
15760 Via Sonata, San Lorenzo, CA 94580
Phototherapy light drape.

COVER, BEDPAN *(General) 80QMY*
Lac-Mac Ltd. 800-461-0001
425 Rectory St., London, ONT N5W 3W5 Canada
Ross Disposable Products 800-649-6526
401 Traders Blvd E, Unit 10, Mississauga, ON L4Z 2H8 Canada

COVER, BEDRAIL *(General) 80VFA*
Genesis Manufacturing, Inc. 317-485-7887
720 E Broadway St, Fortville, IN 46040
Contract Radio-Frequency (RF) Welding. From development to manufacturing and packaging.
Hos-Pillow Corp. 800-468-7874
1011 Campus Dr, Mundelein, IL 60060
Bed rail pads.
Profex Medical Products 800-325-0196
2224 E Person Ave, Memphis, TN 38114
Skil-Care Corp. 800-431-2972
29 Wells Ave, Yonkers, NY 10701

COVER, BIOPSY FORCEPS *(Gastro/Urology) 78FFF*
Koros Usa, Inc. 805-529-0825
610 Flinn Ave, Moorpark, CA 93021
Grasper, cup forceps, curette.
Prosurge Instruments, Inc. 866-832-7874
199 Laidlaw Ave, Jersey City, NJ 07306

COVER, BIOPSY FORCEPS *(cont'd)*
Stryker Gi 866-672-5757
1420 Lakeside Pkwy Ste 110, Flower Mound, TX 75028
Gastroenterology, urology biopsy instrument.

COVER, BURR HOLE (CRANIAL) *(Cns/Neurology) 84GXR*
Bioplate, Inc. 310-815-2100
3643 Lenawee Ave, Los Angeles, CA 90016
Burr hole cover.
Codman & Shurtleff, Inc 800-225-0460
325 Paramount Dr, Raynham, MA 02767
Integra Lifesciences Of Ohio 800-654-2873
4900 Charlemar Dr Bldg A, Cincinnati, OH 45227
Burr hole covers.
Integra Neurosciences Pr 800-654-2873
Road 402 North, Km 1.2, Anasco, PR 00610
Todd burr-hole button.
Kls-Martin L.P. 800-625-1557
11239-1 St. John`s Industrial, Parkway South
Jacksonville, FL 32250
Medtronic Image-Guided Neurologics, Inc. 800-707-0933
2290 W Eau Gallie Blvd, Melbourne, FL 32935
Burr hole cover.
Medtronic Neurosurgery 800-468-9710
125 Cremona Dr, Goleta, CA 93117
Invisx cranial fixation locks, invisx cranial fixation tools reusable & disposab.
Synthes (Usa) 610-719-5000
35 Airport Rd, Horseheads, NY 14845
Various types and sizes of burr hole covers.
W.L. Gore & Associates,Inc 928-526-3030
1505 North Fourth St., Flagstaff, AZ 86004
Burr hole cover.

COVER, CAMERA *(Surgery) 79TBN*
Advance Medical Designs, Inc. 800-221-3679
1241 Atlanta Industrial Dr, Marietta, GA 30066
Closed Camera Drape allows user to change out scopes during procedures while maintaining sterility.
Alimed, Inc. 800-225-2610
297 High St, Dedham, MA 02026
Microtek Medical, Inc 800-936-9248
512 N Lehmberg Rd, Columbus, MS 39702
All styles camera drapes.
Preferred Medical Products 800-441-1161
PO Box 100, Ducktown, TN 37326
Tapco Medical, Inc. 818-225-5376
23981 Craftsman Rd, Calabasas, CA 91302
Wisap America 800-233-8448
8231 Melrose Dr, Lenexa, KS 66214

COVER, CART *(General) 80WKB*
Atlantic Medco, Inc. 800-203-8444
166 Bloomfield Ave, Verona, NJ 07044
Bussard & Son Inc., R.D. 800-252-2692
415 25th Ave SW, Albany, OR 97322
Covers for linen carts, supply carts, laundry hampers plus custom manufactured covers and CART TOPPER systems.
Crest Healthcare Supply 800-328-8908
195 3rd St, Dassel, MN 55325
Exchange Cart Accessories 800-823-1490
1 Commerce Dr, Freeburg, IL 62243
General Econopak, Inc. 888-871-8568
1725 N 6th St, Philadelphia, PA 19122
OR/SPD supply cart covers (all sizes custom made to order).
Healthmark Industries 800-521-6224
22522 E 9 Mile Rd, Saint Clair Shores, MI 48080
$20 to 75 per roll of 50 disposable cart covers for case carts. Also, reusable.
Herculite Products, Inc. 800-772-0036
PO Box 435, Emigsville, PA 17318
Hos-Pillow Corp. 800-468-7874
1011 Campus Dr, Mundelein, IL 60060
All sizes of cart covers for food, medicine and linen; available in nylon and Staph-check.
Intermetro Industries Corp. 800-441-2714
651 N Washington St, Wilkes Barre, PA 18705
METRO cart covers for METRO shelves and carts.

COVER, CART *(cont'd)*

Iron Duck, A Div. Of Fleming Industries, Inc. 800-669-6900
20 Veterans Dr, Chicopee, MA 01022
Supply and linen cart covers in many fabrics, used to conform with JCAH standards.

Jero Medical Equipment & Supplies, Inc. 800-457-0644
1701 W 13th St, Chicago, IL 60608

Profex Medical Products 800-325-0196
2224 E Person Ave, Memphis, TN 38114

Tecni-Quip 800-826-1245
960 Crossroads Blvd, PO Box 2050, Seguin, TX 78155
TECNI-QUIP Durable cart covers in staph check material Velcro or zipper closures. Manufactured for any size or brand of cart.

Trax Cleanroom Products 800-520-8729
3352 Swetzer Rd, P.O. Box 2089, Loomis, CA 95650
Made from flexible vinyl or polyurethane.

Windquest 800-562-4257
3311 Windquest Dr, Holland, MI 49424

COVER, CAST *(General) 80KIA*

Alimed, Inc. 800-225-2610
297 High St, Dedham, MA 02026

Alphaprotech, Inc. 229-242-1931
1287 W Fairway Dr, Nogales, AZ 85621

Carolina Narrow Fabric Co. 336-631-3000
1100 Patterson Ave, Winston Salem, NC 27101
Cover for orthopaedic cast.

Mlw Inc. 970-434-2222
510 Fruitvale Ct Ste C, Grand Junction, CO 81504
Cast protector.

Orthomed Products, Inc. 800-338-8512
12150 Charles Dr Unit 5, Grass Valley, CA 95945
AQUASHIELD Reusable Orthopedic Cast Cover protects casts, bandages and skin from water damage during showering, bathing and swimming. Leg models incorporate the SKIDSAFE non-slip sole that provides traction on slippery floors. Made from elastic polyurethane; forms comfortable, watertight seal without straps or buckles; ready-to-use arm and leg sizes for children and adults.

Patterson Medical Supply, Inc. 262-387-8720
W68N158 Evergreen Blvd, Cedarburg, WI 53012
Cast gards.

Trademark Medical Llc 800-325-9044
449 Soverign Ct, St. Louis, MO 63011
SHOWER SAFE Cast and bandage protectors, waterproof for shower and bath.

W. L. Gore & Associates, Inc. 800-437-8181
PO Box 2400, Flagstaff, AZ 86003
BANDAGE COVER; COCOON CAST

W.L. Gore & Associates,Inc 928-526-3030
1505 North Fourth St., Flagstaff, AZ 86004
Cocoon cast & bandage cover.

COVER, CLAMP *(Surgery) 79TBO*

Axiom Medical, Inc. 800-221-8569
19320 Van Ness Ave, Torrance, CA 90501
Soft silicone instrument jaw covers in various sizes: snap-clamp.

Scanlan International, Inc. 800-328-9458
1 Scanlan Plz, Saint Paul, MN 55107
SOFT GRIP and SURG-I-PAW clamp covers.

Sterion, Incorporated 800-328-7958
13828 Lincoln St NE, Ham Lake, MN 55304
Silicone and radiopaque fabric instrument covers. Sterile and non-sterile.

COVER, FILM, X-RAY *(Radiology) 90WZJ*

Alimed, Inc. 800-225-2610
297 High St, Dedham, MA 02026
PROTEX-RAY see-through covers for handling and transporting x-ray cassettes.

Flow X-Ray Corporation 800-356-9729
100 W Industry Ct, Deer Park, NY 11729

Laminex, Inc. 800-438-8850
9900 Brookford St, Charlotte, NC 28273
Laminating film, equipment (I.D. supplies).

St. John Companies 800-435-4242
25167 Anza Dr, PO Box 800460, Santa Clarita, CA 91355
Disposable cassette covers eliminate risk of contamination with heavy duty clear polyethylene plastic. Three sizes available.

COVER, FILM, X-RAY *(cont'd)*

Uniflex Inc., Medical Packaging Division 800-223-0564
383 W John St, Hicksville, NY 11801
PROTEX-RAY Radiolucent disposable cassette covers protect cassettes from contamination. Four sizes to fit all cassettes.

COVER, HEAD, SURGICAL *(Surgery) 79RXN*

Adex Medical, Inc. 800-873-4776
6101 Quail Valley Ct, Riverside, CA 92507
Nurses Cap, 21', 24', White & Blue

Angelica Image Apparel 800-222-3112
700 Rosedale Ave, Saint Louis, MO 63112

Atd-American Co. 800-523-2300
135 Greenwood Ave, Wyncote, PA 19095

Cellucap Manufacturing Co. 800-523-3814
4626 N 15th St, Philadelphia, PA 19140
Beard restraints.

Global Concepts, Ltd. 818-363-7195
19464 Eagle Ridge Ln, Northridge, CA 91326

Johnson & Johnson Medical Division Of Ethicon, Inc. 800-423-4018
2500 E Arbrook Blvd, Arlington, TX 76014

Kerr Group 800-524-3577
1400 Holcomb Bridge Rd, Roswell, GA 30076

Lac-Mac Ltd. 800-461-0001
425 Rectory St., London, ONT N5W 3W5 Canada

New York Hospital Disposables, Inc. 718-384-1620
101 Richardson St, Brooklyn, NY 11211

Omnical, Inc. 818-837-7531
557 Jessie St, San Fernando, CA 91340
Nurses' and surgeons' caps.

Sanax Protective Products, Inc. 800-379-9929
236 Upland Ave, Newton Highlands, MA 02461

Tronex Healthcare Industries 800-833-1181
2 Cranberry Rd, One Tronex Centre, Parsippany, NJ 07054
Bouffant cap in breathable, fluid resistant polypropylene spunbond for nurses or patients features a durable elastic band. Sizes 21' and 24' in White or Soft Blue. Flat packed 100 caps per box, five boxes per carton allows for neat, single piece dispensing.

COVER, HEEL STIRRUP *(Orthopedics) 87QMZ*

Principle Business Enterprises, Inc. 800-467-3224
PO Box 129, Dunbridge, OH 43414
STIRRUP-MATES disposable foam covers for OB/GYN stirrups for patient comfort and hygiene.

COVER, LAPAROSCOPE *(Surgery) 79WZL*

Elmed, Inc. 630-543-2792
60 W Fay Ave, Addison, IL 60101

COVER, LAUNDRY HAMPER *(General) 80TCK*

Bruin Plastics Co. 800-556-7764
61 Joslin Rd, Glendale, RI 02826

General Econopak, Inc. 888-871-8568
1725 N 6th St, Philadelphia, PA 19122
All sizes.

Herculite Products, Inc. 800-772-0036
PO Box 435, Emigsville, PA 17318

Hos-Pillow Corp. 800-468-7874
1011 Campus Dr, Mundelein, IL 60060
Anti-bacterial covers for linen, food and medication carts.

Imperial Fastener Co., Inc. 954-782-7130
1400 SW 8th St, Pompano Beach, FL 33069
Linen cart covers - custom made to fabric, size, color, type of closure etc.

Medline Industries, Inc. 800-633-5886
1 Medline Pl, Mundelein, IL 60060

Steele Canvas Basket Co., Inc. 800-541-8929
201 Williams St, Chelsea, MA 02150

COVER, LIMB *(Physical Med) 89IPM*

Abc Health Solutions Llc 720-962-5412
14008 SE 238th Ln, Kent, WA 98042
Various models of limb covers.

Breg, Inc., An Orthofix Company 800-897-BREG
2611 Commerce Way, Vista, CA 92081
Limb cover.

COVER, LIMB *(cont'd)*

Brown Medical Industries 800-843-4395
1300 Lundberg Dr W, Spirit Lake, IA 51360
SEAL-TIGHT is a waterproof cast protector, available in 21 sizes.

Centurion Medical Products Corp. 517-545-1135
3310 S Main St, Salisbury, NC 28147

Circulator Boot Corp. 610-240-9980
72 Pennsylvania Ave, Malvern, PA 19355

Debusk Orthopedic Casting (Doc) 865-362-2334
420 Straight Creek Rd Ste 1, New Tazewell, TN 37825
Non-sterile stockinette.

Dj Orthopedics De Mexico, S.A. De C.V. 690-727-1280
Blvd., Delagacion La Presa, Tijuana 22397 Mexico
Limb wraps

Dj Orthopedics De Mexico, S.A. De C.V. 690-727-1280
Ave. Venustiano Carranza 6802, Castillo, Tijuana 22100 Mexico
Limb wraps

Endolite North America, Ltd. 937-291-3636
105 Westpark Rd, Centerville, OH 45459
Prosthetic limb cover.

Farabloc Development Corp. 604-941-8201
211-3030 Lincoln Ave, Coquitlam V3B 6B4 Canada
Farabloc limb cover

Foot Levelers, Inc. 540-345-0008
518 Pocahontas Ave NE, P.o. Box 12611, Roanoke, VA 24012
Fas scan (foot analysis system).

Hipsavers, Inc. 800-358-4477
7 Hubbard St, Canton, MA 02021

Juzo 800-222-4999
PO Box 1088, 80 Chart Road, Cuyahoga Falls, OH 44223
Elastic support stump shrinker and suspension sleeves.

Prostep Manufacturing, Inc. 225-751-2100
9542 Brookline Ave Ste A, Baton Rouge, LA 70809
The 'Prostep CastSox' is the only patented product of its kind on the market today. The 'Prostep CastSox' covers the exposed toes of a patient wearing an ankle, foot or leg cast or bandage. The fabric repels moisture away from the skin to keep the toes clean and dry. Available in camouflage patterned fabric and 8 cast matching colors. Also available in two different styles. The 'Standard CastSox' for anytime, anywhere and the 'Lined CastSox' for colder climates or just for that extra coverage sometimes needed. The 'Prostep CastSox' is a great wardrobe accessory for home, school or work.

Protex Medical Products, Inc. 318-397-5465
913 Wood St, West Monroe, LA 71291
Limb cover.

Rx Textiles, Inc. 704-283-9787
3107 Chamber Dr, Monroe, NC 28110
Liners.

Tamarack Habilitation Technologies, Inc. 763-795-0057
1670 94th Ln NE, Blaine, MN 55449
Self-adhesive material for friction management.

Tri-State Hospital Supply Corp. 517-545-1135
3173 E 43rd St, Yuma, AZ 85365

Trulife, Inc. 360-697-5656
26296 12 Trees Ln NW, Poulsbo, WA 98370
Limb cover.

Vq Orthocare
1390 Decision St Ste A, Vista, CA 92081
Prosthetic and orthotic accessory.

COVER, MATTRESS *(General) 80FMW*

A.M.G. Medical, Inc. 888-396-1213
8505 Dalton Rd., Montreal, QUE H4T-IV5 Canada

Achilles Usa, Inc. 425-353-7000
1407 80th St SW, Everett, WA 98203

Allman Products 800-223-6889
21101 Itasca St, Chatsworth, CA 91311

American Health Systems 800-234-6655
PO Box 26688, Greenville, SC 29616
ULTRAFORM; Therapeutic Replacement Cover for Mattresses.

Anatomic Concepts, Inc. 951-549-6800
1691 N Delilah St, Corona, CA 92879
Mattress overlay, unpowered, foam.

COVER, MATTRESS *(cont'd)*

Asi Medical Equipment, Ltd. 800-527-0443
1735 N Interstate 35E, Carrollton, TX 75006
Alternating pressure dual-layer overlay. Provides massaging therapy to enhance circulation and blood flow.

Atd-American Co. 800-523-2300
135 Greenwood Ave, Wyncote, PA 19095

Barjan Mfg., Ltd. 631-420-5588
28 Baiting Place Rd, Farmingdale, NY 11735
Bed pan.

Basic American Medical Products 800-849-6664
2935A Northeast Pkwy, Atlanta, GA 30360

Best Manufacturing Group Llc 800-843-3233
1633 Broadway Fl 18, New York, NY 10019
Vinyls, cloth, zippered, fitted, ties.

Bruin Plastics Co. 800-556-7764
61 Joslin Rd, Glendale, RI 02826

Casco Manufacturing Solutions, Inc. 800-843-1339
3107 Spring Grove Ave, Cincinnati, OH 45225
C-MATT brand mattress covers and replacement covers for healthcare and insituional surfaces.

Civco Medical Instruments Co., Inc. 319-656-4447
102 1st St S, Kalona, IA 52247
Uni/cover.

Comfort Care Products Corp. 803-321-0020
258 Industrial Park Rd, Newberry, SC 29108

Crest Healthcare Supply 800-328-8908
195 3rd St, Dassel, MN 55325

Derby Industries 757-224-0177
24350 State Road 23, South Bend, IN 46614
Mattress cover.

Dowling Textiles 770-957-3981
615 Macon Rd, McDonough, GA 30253
Various types of mattress covers.

Eirsan Care Inc. 201-880-8615
624 Monroe St Apt 2A, Hoboken, NJ 07030
Mattress & pillow cover.

Foam Craft 714-459-9971
2441 Cypress Way, Fullerton, CA 92831

G. Hirsch And Co., Inc. 650-692-8770
870 Mahler Rd, Burlingame, CA 94010
Waterproof sheeting.

Grant Airmass Corporation 800-243-5237
126 Chestnut Hill Rd, PO Box 3456, Stamford, CT 06903

Hawaii Medical, Llc 781-826-5565
750 Corporate Park Dr, Pembroke, MA 02359

Herculite Products, Inc. 800-772-0036
PO Box 435, Emigsville, PA 17318
SURE-CHEK FUSION Fabrics; these healthcare fabrics complement pressure management mattresses, pads, and cushions. The protective polymer membrane & highly stretchable fabric work together to offer protection and comfort.

Hill-Rom Manufacturing, Inc. 800-638-2546
4349 Corporate Rd, Charleston, SC 29405

Hos-Pillow Corp. 800-468-7874
1011 Campus Dr, Mundelein, IL 60060
$5.14 to $9.15 per unit (flat, with anchor band or fitted).

Huntleigh Healthcare Llc. 800-223-1218
40 Christopher Way, Eatontown, NJ 07724

J. Lamb, Inc. A Division Of The Strongwater Group 888-379-6453
250 Moonachie Ave, Moonachie, NJ 07074
Allergy-relief beddding; zippered mattress encasing.

Joerns Healthcare, Inc. 715-341-3600
1032 N Fourth St, Baldwyn, MS 38824
Various.

Kentron Health Care, Inc. 615-384-0573
3604 Kelton Jackson Rd, P.o. Box 120, Springfield, TN 37172
Hospital mattress.

Kreg Medical, Inc. 312-275-7002
2240 W Walnut St, Chicago, IL 60612
Mattress cover.

Lakeland De Mexico S.A. De C.V. 516-981-9700
Rancho La Soledad Lote No. 2, Fracc. Poniente C.p. Celaya, Guajuato Mexico
Mattress cover

COVER, MATTRESS *(cont'd)*

Medcovers, Inc 800-948-8917
500 W Goldsboro St, Kenly, NC 27542

Medical Depot 516-998-4600
99 Seaview Blvd, Port Washington, NY 11050
Mattress.

Mes, Inc. 800-423-2215
1968 E US Highway 90, Seguin, TX 78155
Part#0127 is a standard hospital mattress dust cover, 50 per roll; Part#0129 is a bariatric mattress dust cover, also 50 per roll

North America Mattress Corp. 503-655-6163
10768 SE Highway 212, Clackamas, OR 97015
Mattress.

Postcraft Co. 800-528-4844
625 W Rillito St, Tucson, AZ 85705
Synthetic mattress and pillow covers.

Precision Fabrics Group, Inc. 888-733-5759
301 E Meadowview Rd, Greensboro, NC 27406
Various types of pristine encasements.

Precision Fabrics Group, Inc. 888-733-5759
323 Virginia Ave., Vinton, VA 24179
Various types of pristine encasements.

Primo, Inc. 770-486-7394
417 Dividend Dr Ste B, Peachtree City, GA 30269
Cover, mattress (medical purposes).

Priva (Usa), Inc. 516-255-1736
96 Atlantic Ave, Lynbrook, NY 11563
Mattress covers for medical purposes.

Richardson Products, Inc. 888-928-7297
9408 Gulfstream Rd, Frankfort, IL 60423
Cover.

Riegel Consumer Products Div. 800-845-2232
PO Box E, 51 Riegel Road, Johnston, SC 29832
Mattress pads.

Rogers Foam Corporation 617-623-3010
609 Boone Trail Road, Clinchport, VA 24244

Roho Group, The 800-851-3449
100 N Florida Ave, Belleville, IL 62221
PRODIGY Mattress overlay is designed for individuals who are at risk from breakdown and/or have a stage I or II ischemic ulcer. The non-powered, multi-zoned, adjustable mattress overlay has interconnected air cells.

Sca Personal Care, North America 270-796-9300
7030 Louisville Rd, Bowling Green, KY 42101
Incontinence under pads.

Stryker Medical 800-869-0770
3800 E Centre Ave, Portage, MI 49002

Supracor, Inc. 800-787-7226
2050 Corporate Ct, San Jose, CA 95131
Cover, mattress products.

Tempur-Medical, Inc. 888-255-3302
1713 Jaggie Fox Way, Lexington, KY 40511
Tempur-Med PU Cover

Truform Orthotics & Prosthetics 800-888-0458
3960 Rosslyn Dr, Cincinnati, OH 45209

Val Med 800-242-5355
3700 Desire Pkwy, Ace Bayou Group, New Orleans, LA 70126

Western Textile Productos De Mexico S.De R.L. Dec. 314-225-9400
Francisco Murguia #514 Nte., M.muzquiz, Coahuila Mexico
Various

928735 Ontario, Ltd. 905-660-1030
8-24 Viceroy Rd, Concord L4K 2L9 Canada
Waterproof & dust-mite proof mattress & pillow protectors which reduce allergens

COVER, MATTRESS, CONDUCTIVE *(General) 80QNA*

Bruin Plastics Co. 800-556-7764
61 Joslin Rd, Glendale, RI 02826

Bryton Corp. 800-567-9500
4310 Guion Rd, Indianapolis, IN 46254
Conductive mattresses, pads & covers for surgical tables, orthopedic tables, obstetrical tables, urology tables & stretchers.

Casco Manufacturing Solutions, Inc. 800-843-1339
3107 Spring Grove Ave, Cincinnati, OH 45225

COVER, MATTRESS, CONDUCTIVE *(cont'd)*

Herculite Products, Inc. 800-772-0036
PO Box 435, Emigsville, PA 17318

Profex Medical Products 800-325-0196
2224 E Person Ave, Memphis, TN 38114

Trax Cleanroom Products 800-520-8729
3352 Swetzer Rd, P.O. Box 2089, Loomis, CA 95650
Available in blue/black. or green/black.

Waterloo Bedding Co. Ltd. 800-203-4293
141 Weber St. S, Waterloo, ONT N2J 2A9 Canada

COVER, MATTRESS, WATERPROOF *(General) 80QNB*

Allman Products 800-223-6889
21101 Itasca St, Chatsworth, CA 91311
Vinyl mattress cover.

Atd-American Co. 800-523-2300
135 Greenwood Ave, Wyncote, PA 19095

Best Manufacturing Group Llc 800-843-3233
1633 Broadway Fl 18, New York, NY 10019

Bruin Plastics Co. 800-556-7764
61 Joslin Rd, Glendale, RI 02826

Casco Manufacturing Solutions, Inc. 800-843-1339
3107 Spring Grove Ave, Cincinnati, OH 45225
C-MATT brand, patented RF-welded seam technology, mattress cover and replacement covers for C-MATT Prevention mattress and standard healthcare mattresses.

General Econopak, Inc. 888-871-8568
1725 N 6th St, Philadelphia, PA 19122
Vinyl mattress covers.

Genesis Manufacturing, Inc. 317-485-7887
720 E Broadway St, Fortville, IN 46040
Contract Radio-Frequency (RF) Welding. From development to manufacturing and packaging.

Herculite Products, Inc. 800-772-0036
PO Box 435, Emigsville, PA 17318

Hos-Pillow Corp. 800-468-7874
1011 Campus Dr, Mundelein, IL 60060
$3.35 per piece of waterproof mattress underpad.

Medline Industries, Inc. 800-633-5886
1 Medline Pl, Mundelein, IL 60060

Mes, Inc. 800-423-2215
1968 E US Highway 90, Seguin, TX 78155
Vinyl Zippered Mattress Protectors in two sizes: Part#6063 is for standard hospital mattresses and part#6065 is for bariatric mattresses

Postcraft Co. 800-528-4844
625 W Rillito St, Tucson, AZ 85705
Vinyl mattress and pillow covers (waterproof).

Precision Dynamics Corp. 800-772-1122
13880 Del Sur St, San Fernando, CA 91340

Profex Medical Products 800-325-0196
2224 E Person Ave, Memphis, TN 38114

Ross Disposable Products 800-649-6526
401 Traders Blvd E, Unit 10, Mississauga, ON L4Z 2H8 Canada

The Neurological Research And Development Group 800-327-6759
115 Rotary Dr, West Hazleton, PA 18202

Waterloo Bedding Co. Ltd. 800-203-4293
141 Weber St. S, Waterloo, ONT N2J 2A9 Canada

COVER, MICROSCOPE *(Microbiology) 83QNC*

Microtek Medical, Inc 800-936-9248
512 N Lehmberg Rd, Columbus, MS 39702
Styles to fit all microscope brands.

Western Scientific Co., Inc. 877-489-3726
4104 24th St # 183, San Francisco, CA 94114

COVER, OTHER *(General) 80WHO*

Advance Medical Designs, Inc. 800-221-3679
1241 Atlanta Industrial Dr, Marietta, GA 30066
C-ARM KOVERS, MICRO-KOVERS, LIGHT HANDLE KOVERS, CAMERA KOVERS, microscope drapes, C-ARM drapes, video camera/laser drapes; equipment drapes for the operating room (sterile disposables). Disposable light-handle covers for O.R. lights.

Construction Specialties Inc. 800-233-8493
6696 Route. 405, Muncy, PA 17756
Wall covering.

COVER, OTHER *(cont'd)*

Dazian Fabrics,Llc. 877-232-9426
124 Enterprise Ave S, PO Box 2121, Secaucus, NJ 07094
Geriatric upholstery fabric.

Diestco Manufacturing Corp. 800-795-2392
PO Box 6504, Chico, CA 95927
WEATHERBEE, scooter/wheelchair cover protects your vehicle when being stored or transported. WEATHERMUFF, hand and controls' shield protects your scooter, tiller or power chair joystick. WEATHERCHAPS, lap, leg and feet covers provide waterproof protection for lower body.

General Econopak, Inc. 888-871-8568
1725 N 6th St, Philadelphia, PA 19122
Multi-use/disposable oxygen tank covers. Patient jacket and shirts, hats, hoods, beard covers, and adult blankets, shoe covers, SPD cart and truck covers, shelf and tray liners, window and closet curtains.

Hos-Pillow Corp. 800-468-7874
1011 Campus Dr, Mundelein, IL 60060
Pillow protectors - reusable as well as disposable.

Jaece Industries, Inc. 716-694-2811
908 Niagara Falls Blvd, North Tonawanda, NY 14120
Absorbent liners: protect benchtops, floors, and carts with this highly absorbent cover. Backing is waterproof and resistant to most chemicals.

Lemans Industries Corp. 800-289-5667
79 Express St, Plainview, NY 11803
Disposable Plastic Covers for ventillators , all sizes of durable medical equipment and split-spring hospital beds. Also, clear and buff colored covers available for J.C.A.H.O accreditation.

Medical Action Industries, Inc 800-645-7042
500 Express Dr S, Brentwood, NY 11717
Dust cover.

Memcath Technologies Llc 651-450-7400
1777 Oakdale Ave, Saint Paul, MN 55118
PTFE Endoscope covers with clarified PTFE tips & side access chanels

Mes, Inc. 800-423-2215
1968 E US Highway 90, Seguin, TX 78155
Clear Plastic Equipment covers on rolls or flat in a box, also padded covers for transport

Microtek Medical, Inc 800-936-9248
512 N Lehmberg Rd, Columbus, MS 39702
Extensive line of Microtek equipment covers for OR, radiology, cardiac cath lab.

Neotech Products, Inc. 800-966-0500
27822 Fremont Ct, Valencia, CA 91355
NEOSMILE: Temperature Probe Cover holds temp probe securely to patient with skin friendly hydrocolloid.

Omnical, Inc. 818-837-7531
557 Jessie St, San Fernando, CA 91340
Beard covers.

Pacon Manufacturing Corporation 732-357-8020
400 Pierce St # B, Somerset, NJ 08873
Custom drapes.

Palmero Health Care 800-344-6424
120 Goodwin Pl, Stratford, CT 06615
Disposable dental paper tray covers.

Parker Laboratories, Inc. 800-631-8888
286 Eldridge Rd, Fairfield, NJ 07004
Disposable, latex-free probe/transducer cover pregelled with Aquasonic 100 Ultrasound Transmission Gel.

Polyzen, Inc. 919-319-9599
1041 Classic Rd, Apex, NC 27539
BARRIER SLEEVE products to prevent contagious viral transmission. Light transparent clear-scope or probe covers for UV/laser ultrasound probe cover. Polyurethane instrument covers/sheaths.

Precision Dynamics Corp. 800-772-1122
13880 Del Sur St, San Fernando, CA 91340

Preferred Medical Products 800-441-1161
PO Box 100, Ducktown, TN 37326
Offered in sterile and nonsterile. Also custom items available.

Progressive Dynamics Medical, Inc. 269-781-4241
507 Industrial Rd, Marshall, MI 49068
SOFT-FLEX Warming covers.

COVER, OTHER *(cont'd)*

Sonoco-Stancap Division 770-476-9088
3150 Clinton Ct, Norcross, GA 30071
STANCAP, disposable glass cover paper, can be printed in 6 colors.

Sterion, Incorporated 800-328-7958
13828 Lincoln St NE, Ham Lake, MN 55304
Covers for Stienmann pins and k-wires. Three sizes fits all 11 pins. Also, instrument guards (covers) and endoscope guards (covers).

Trademark Medical Llc 800-325-9044
449 Soverign Ct, St. Louis, MO 63011
Arm shield for protection of patient during surgery.

Uniflex Inc., Medical Packaging Division 800-223-0564
383 W John St, Hicksville, NY 11801
PROTEX-RAY clear film disposable cassette covers.

Whatman Inc. 732-885-6529
800 Centennial Ave Bldg 1, Piscataway, NJ 08854
Benchkote/Benchkote Plus. Lab benchtop protective covering.

COVER, PROBE, TRANSDUCER *(Surgery) 79WHN*

Emt Medical Co., Inc. 800-473-5333
PO Box 294, Poulsbo, WA 98370

Kentec Medical Inc. 800-825-5996
17871 Fitch, Irvine, CA 92614
ACCUTEMP Probe Covers, infant. Insulated temperature probe covers.

Omni Medical Supply Inc. 800-860-6664
4153 Pioneer Dr, Commerce Township, MI 48390

Preferred Medical Products 800-441-1161
PO Box 100, Ducktown, TN 37326

COVER, SEAT, TOILET, SANITARY *(General) 80WHM*

Columbia Medical Manufacturing Llc 800-454-6612
13577 Larwin Cir, Santa Fe Springs, CA 90670
Columbia Medical SecureSeat Toilet Supports feature orthopedic contoured backs to support upper body and torso. Lo and Hi-Back options are available. Fits all toilets.

Hygolet Usa 800-494-6538
349 SE 2nd Ave, Deerfield Beach, FL 33441
HYGOLET Toilet seat. Automatically provides users with a clean hygienic toilet seat. No more paper seat covers. Keeps restrooms and toilet seats cleaner.

Jero Medical Equipment & Supplies, Inc. 800-457-0644
1701 W 13th St, Chicago, IL 60608

Sanitor Manufacturing Co. 800-379-5314
1221 W Centre Ave, Portage, MI 49024
NEAT SEAT Disposable toilet seat covers and dispensers.

Variety Ability Systems Inc. 800-891-4514
2 Kelvin Ave., Unit 3, Toronto, ONT M4C-5C8 Canada
Aquanant, Toileting System - Supports children in a forward-leaning posture that promotes relaxation and helps them to function on the toilet.

COVER, SHOE, CONDUCTIVE *(General) 80QNE*

Cms Worldwide, Inc. 800-426-4633
30011 Ivy Glenn Dr Ste 215, Laguna Niguel, CA 92677
Spun-bonded shoe covers. Polypropylene blue. Non-skid available. 150 pairs per carton.

General Econopak, Inc. 888-871-8568
1725 N 6th St, Philadelphia, PA 19122

Kerr Group 800-524-3577
1400 Holcomb Bridge Rd, Roswell, GA 30076

Lac-Mac Ltd. 800-461-0001
425 Rectory St., London, ONT N5W 3W5 Canada

COVER, SHOE, CONDUCTIVE *(cont'd)*

Medline Industries, Inc. 800-633-5886
1 Medline Pl, Mundelein, IL 60060

O&M Enterprise 847-258-4515
641 Chelmsford Ln, Elk Grove Village, IL 60007
COVER SHOE CONDUCTIVE/NON CONDUCTIVE

Pharaoh Trading Company 866-929-4913
9701 Brookpark Rd, Knollwood Plaza, Suite 241, Cleveland, OH 44129

Precept Medical Products, Inc. 800-438-5827
PO Box 2400, 370 Airport Road/, Arden, NC 28704

Tronex Healthcare Industries 800-833-1181
2 Cranberry Rd, One Tronex Centre, Parsippany, NJ 07054
Fluid resistant, breathable, PPSB Blue nonskid shoe cover with white, non skid, zzz marking. Flexible elastic closure, one size fits all. Size 16 x 7 cm. 100 shoe covers per box, three boxes per carton.

COVER, SHOE, NON-CONDUCTIVE *(General) 80QNF*

Atd-American Co. 800-523-2300
135 Greenwood Ave, Wyncote, PA 19095

General Econopak, Inc. 888-871-8568
1725 N 6th St, Philadelphia, PA 19122

Janin Group, Inc. 800-323-5389
14A Stonehill Rd, Oswego, IL 60543
PEDIDRY Waterproof boot.

Kerr Group 800-524-3577
1400 Holcomb Bridge Rd, Roswell, GA 30076

Medline Industries, Inc. 800-633-5886
1 Medline Pl, Mundelein, IL 60060

Ross Disposable Products 800-649-6526
401 Traders Blvd E, Unit 10, Mississauga, ON L4Z 2H8 Canada

COVER, SHOE, OPERATING ROOM *(Surgery) 79FXP*

Adex Medical, Inc. 800-873-4776
6101 Quail Valley Ct, Riverside, CA 92507
Shoe Cover Non-Skid, Universal, Blue

Alphaprotech, Inc. 229-242-1931
1287 W Fairway Dr, Nogales, AZ 85621

Alphaprotech, Inc. 520-281-0127
2224 Cypress St, Valdosta, GA 31601

Busse Hospital Disposables, Inc. 631-435-4711
75 Arkay Dr, Hauppauge, NY 11788
Multiple.

Cellucap Manufacturing Co. 800-523-3814
4626 N 15th St, Philadelphia, PA 19140

Civco Medical Instruments Co., Inc. 319-656-4447
102 1st St S, Kalona, IA 52247
No common name listed.

Clean Esd Products, Inc. 510-257-5080
48340 Milmont Dr, Fremont, CA 94538
#804, Regular shoe cover priced at $8.00/bag, 100pcs/bag.

Cleanwear Products Ltd. 416-438-4831
54 Crockford Rd., Toronto, ON M1R-3C3 Canada
Disposable shoe covers.

Cypress Medical Products 800-334-3646
1202 S. Rte. 31, McHenry, IL 60050
Regular and non-skid shoe covers.

Darco International, Inc. 800-999-8866
810 Memorial Blvd, Huntington, WV 25701
Post-operative shoe cover.

Depuy Orthopaedics, Inc. 800-473-3789
700 Orthopaedic Dr, P.O. Box 988, Warsaw, IN 46582
Various types of operating-room shoe covers.

General Econopak, Inc. 888-871-8568
1725 N 6th St, Philadelphia, PA 19122
Disposable shoe covers.

Global Concepts, Ltd. 818-363-7195
19464 Eagle Ridge Ln, Northridge, CA 91326

Global Healthcare 800-601-3880
1495 Hembree Rd Ste 700, Roswell, GA 30076
Regular and non-skid shoe covers.

Health-Pak, Inc. 315-724-8370
2005 Beechgrove Pl, Utica, NY 13501
Nonwoven poly spunbonded.

In Disposables Inc. 800-269-4568
PO Box 528, Stratford, CT 06615
Non-skid, fluid resistant - color blue, packed 150 pair/cs.

COVER, SHOE, OPERATING ROOM *(cont'd)*

Janin Group, Inc. 800-323-5389
14A Stonehill Rd, Oswego, IL 60543
PEDIDRY Waterproof shoe cover.

Kappler Protective Apparel & Fabrics 800-600-4019
115 Grimes Dr, Guntersville, AL 35976

Kentron Health Care, Inc. 615-384-0573
3604 Kelton Jackson Rd, P.o. Box 120, Springfield, TN 37172
Shoe covers.

Lakeland De Mexico S.A. De C.V. 516-981-9700
Rancho La Soledad Lote No. 2, Fracc. Poniente C.p. Celaya, Guajuato Mexico
Shoe cover

Maquilas Teta-Kawi, S.A. De C.V. 413-593-6400
Carretera Internacional, Km 1969, Enpalme, Sonora Mexico
Shoe cover

Maytex Corp. 800-462-9839
23521 Foley St, Hayward, CA 94545
Non-skid, fluid-resistant.

Medical Action Industries, Inc. 800-645-7042
25 Heywood Rd, Arden, NC 28704
Shoe cover.

New York Hospital Disposables, Inc. 718-384-1620
101 Richardson St, Brooklyn, NY 11211

North Safety Products 401-943-4400
1101 B Calle Neutron, Parque Industrial Maran, Mexicali, B.c. Mexico
Shoe covers

Omnical, Inc. 818-837-7531
557 Jessie St, San Fernando, CA 91340

Pfb Inter-Apparel Corp. 800-828-7629
1930 Harrison St Ste 304, Hollywood, FL 33020

Sanax Protective Products, Inc. 800-379-9929
236 Upland Ave, Newton Highlands, MA 02461

Scientimed Corp. 510-763-5405
4109 Balfour Ave, Oakland, CA 94610
Shoecovers.

Sloan Corp. 402-597-5700
13316 A St, Omaha, NE 68144
Knee high.

Sri Surgical 813-891-9550
6801 Longe St, Stockton, CA 95206
Shoe cover.

Sri Surgical 813-891-9550
7086 Industrial Row Dr, Mason, OH 45040

Sri Surgical 813-891-9550
1416 Dogwood Way, Mebane, NC 27302

Sri Surgical 813-891-9550
2595 Custer Rd Ste B, Salt Lake City, UT 84104

Sri Surgical 813-891-9550
6675 Business Pkwy Ste A, Elkridge, MD 21075

Sri Surgical 813-891-9550
12950 Executive Dr, Sugar Land, TX 77478

Sri Surgical 813-891-9550
6024 Century Oaks Dr, Chattanooga, TN 37416

Sri Surgical 813-891-9550
1441 Patton Pl Ste 139, Carrollton, TX 75007

Sri Surgical 813-891-9550
2240 E Artesia Blvd, Long Beach, CA 90805

Sri Surgical Express Inc. 813-891-9550
4501 Acline Dr E Ste 170, Tampa, FL 33605

Tidi Products, Llc 920-751-4380
570 Enterprise Dr, Neenah, WI 54956
Shoe cover.

Toolmex Corporation 800-992-4766
1075 Worcester St, Natick, MA 01760

U-Ten Corporation 630-289-8058
1286 Humbracht Cir, Bartlett, IL 60103
Shoe covers.

Web-Tex, Inc. 888-633-2723
5445 De Gaspe Ave., Ste. 702, Montreal, QC H2T 3B2 Canada

White Knight Healthcare 800-851-4431
Calle 16, Number 780, Agua Prieta, Sonora Mexico
Cover, shoe, operating-room

COVER, STOOL *(General) 80QNG*

Bryton Corp. 800-567-9500
4310 Guion Rd, Indianapolis, IN 46254
Covers for surgical stools, conductive or non-conductive.

Profex Medical Products 800-325-0196
2224 E Person Ave, Memphis, TN 38114

COVER, THERMOMETER *(General) 80QND*

American Diagnostic Corporation (Adc) 800-232-2670
55 Commerce Dr, Hauppauge, NY 11788
Disposable sheaths for mercury in glass, and stick digital thermometers

Her-Mar, Inc. 800-327-8209
8550 NW 30th Ter, Doral, FL 33122
$7.00 per 100 (standard).

O&M Enterprise 847-258-4515
641 Chelmsford Ln, Elk Grove Village, IL 60007
COVER-PROBE THERMOMETER

Ross Disposable Products 800-649-6526
401 Traders Blvd E, Unit 10, Mississauga, ON L4Z 2H8 Canada

COVER, TIP, PROBE, CAUTERIZATION *(Surgery) 79WWP*

Megadyne Medical Products, Inc. 800-747-6110
11506 S State St, Draper, UT 84020
E-Z CLEAN, disposable, non-stick cautery tips, blades, needles, MicroFine needles, and laparoscopic electrodes. ALL-IN-ONE, laparoscopic suction/irrigation/cautery pencil & electrodes. MEGA Tip and Indicator Shaft laparoscopic electrodes. LEEP electrodes and standard electrosurgical pencils.

COVERSLIP, MICROSCOPE SLIDE *(Pathology) 88KES*

C & A Scientific Co. Inc. 703-330-1413
7241 Gabe Ct, Manassas, VA 20109
PREMIERE Microscope cover glass in assorted sizes and thickness. PREMIERE Microscope Slide Storage Box plastic storage box-holds 25 microscope slides. PREMIERE Canvas Carrying Case microscope carrying case.

Cadence Science Inc. 888-717-7677
1979 Marcus Ave Ste 215, New Hyde Park, NY 11042
20 types, #1 or #2, square or rect.

Carolina Biological Supply Co. 800-334-5551
2700 York Rd, Burlington, NC 27215

Corning Inc., Science Products Division 800-492-1110
45 Nagog Park, Acton, MA 01720

Erie Scientific 603-431-8410
20 Post Rd, Portsmouth Park, Newington, NH 03801
Microscope slide coverslip.

Hacker Instruments And Industries Inc. 800-442-2537
1132 Kincaid Bridge Rd, PO Box 1176, Winnsboro, SC 29180
HCM4000 state-of-the-art automated coverslipper. Unique dispensing system delivers mountant bubble free. Suitable for cytology and histology. Slide carrier interfaces with most automated stainers

Hampton Research 800-452-3899
34 Journey, Aliso Viejo, CA 92656

Image Molding, Inc. 800-525-1875
4525 Kingston St, Denver, CO 80239

Kimble Glass, Inc. 888-546-2531
537 Crystal Ave, Vineland, NJ 08360
KIMBLE.

Leica Microsystems (Canada) Inc. 800-205-3422
400 - 111 Granton Drive, Richmond Hill, ONT L4B 1L5 Canada
LEICA, CV 5000 Robotic coverslipper with a throughput rate of up to 500 slides/hr.

Leica Microsystems Inc. 800-248-0123
2345 Waukegan Rd, Bannockburn, IL 60015
CV5030 coverslipper with throughput rate of 500 slides per hour.

Mccrone Microscopes & Accessories 800-622-8122
850 Pasquinelli Dr, Westmont, IL 60559
Various laboratory supplies including particle, fiber, and paint pigment slide reference sets; slides; coverslips; microtools.

One Lambda, Inc. 800-822-8824
21001 Kittridge St, Canoga Park, CA 91303
Insta-seal cover, fluoro seal cover.

Propper Manufacturing Co., Inc. 800-832-4300
3604 Skillman Ave, Long Island City, NY 11101

Rayson Co. Inc., W.R. 800-526-1526
720 S Dickerson St, Burgaw, NC 28425
Disposable plastic coverslips.

COVERSLIP, MICROSCOPE SLIDE *(cont'd)*

Statlab Medical Products, Inc. 800-442-3573
106 Hillside Dr, Lewisville, TX 75057
ANAPATH microscope slide coverslip available in various sizes and packaged with desiccant.

Surgipath Medical Industries, Inc. 800-225-3035
PO Box 528, 5205 Route 12, Richmond, IL 60071
Automatic Coverslipper

Thermo Fisher Scientific (Rochester) 585-899-7600
75 Panorama Creek Dr, Panorama, NY 14625
Microscope slide coverslip.

Ware Medics Glass Works, Inc. 845-429-6950
PO Box 368, Garnerville, NY 10923

3m Hutchinson 320-234-2000
905 Adams St SE, Hutchinson, MN 55350
Slides and coverslips.

CRADLE, PATIENT, RADIOGRAPHIC *(Radiology) 90KXH*

Composiflex, Inc. 800-673-2544
8100 Hawthorne Dr, Erie, PA 16509
Low absorption, high strength carbon fiber cradles.

Forest Imaging, Inc 619-218-6460
5288 Eastgate Mall, San Diego, CA 92121
Weight bearing table/cradle.

Oakworks, Inc. 800-558-8850
923 E Wellspring Rd, New Freedom, PA 17349
Spinal Imaging Platform for cervical flexion/extension. Promotes patient stability during procedures while providing comfortable access to specific regions.

Radscan Medical Equipment, Inc. 623-580-0556
23620 N 20th Dr Ste 16, Phoenix, AZ 85085

Vermont Composites, Inc. 802-442-9964
25 Performance Dr, Bennington, VT 05201
Low absorption carbon cradles.

CRIMPER, PIN *(Orthopedics) 87HXQ*

Biomet, Inc. 574-267-6639
56 E Bell Dr, PO Box 587, Warsaw, IN 46582
Dee fixation clamp.

Medtronic Sofamor Danek Instrument Manufacturing 901-396-3133
7375 Adrianne Pl, Bartlett, TN 38133
Various tension crimper.

Medtronic Sofamor Danek Usa, Inc. 901-396-3133
4340 Swinnea Rd, Memphis, TN 38118
Various tension crimper.

Warsaw Orthopedic, Inc. 901-396-3133
2500 Silveus Xing, Warsaw, IN 46582
Various tension crimper.

Zimmer Holdings, Inc. 800-613-6131
1800 W Center St, PO Box 708, Warsaw, IN 46580

CRIMPER, WIRE, ENT *(Ear/Nose/Throat) 77JXT*

Aesculap Implant Systems Inc. 1-800-234-9179
3773 Corporate Pkwy, Center Valley, PA 18034

Bausch & Lomb Surgical 636-255-5051
3365 Tree Court Ind Blvd, Saint Louis, MO 63122

Clinimed, Incorporated 877-CLINIMED
303 Markus Ct, Sandy Brae Industrial Park, Newark, DE 19713

CROWN AND BRIDGE, TEMPORARY, RESIN *(Dental And Oral) 76EBG*

American Tooth Industries 800-235-4639
1200 Stellar Dr, Oxnard, CA 93033
JUSTI.

Artisan Dental Laboratory 800-222-6721
2532 SE Hawthorne Blvd, Portland, OR 97214

Astron Dental Corporation 847-726-8787
815 Oakwood Rd Ste G, Lake Zurich, IL 60047
Vinyl crown & bridge resin.

Cdm Dental 541-928-4444
812 Water Ave NE, Albany, OR 97321
Poly-Carb

Cmp Industries Llc 800-888-5868
413 N Pearl St, Albany, NY 12207
$49.90 per unit (standard).

CROWN AND BRIDGE, TEMPORARY, RESIN *(cont'd)*

Coltene/Whaledent Inc. 330-916-8858
235 Ascot Pkwy, Cuyahoga Falls, OH 44223
Temporary crown & bridge material.

Danville Materials 800-827-7940
3420 Fostoria Way Ste A200, San Ramon, CA 94583
Temporary crown and bridge composite.

Den-Mat Holdings, Llc 805-922-8491
2727 Skyway Dr, Santa Maria, CA 93455
No common name listed.

Dental Technologies, Inc. 847-677-5500
6901 N Hamlin Ave, Lincolnwood, IL 60712
Temporary crown and bridge material.

Direct Crown, Llc 888-910-4490
895 Country Club Rd Ste B100, Eugene, OR 97401
Temporary/provisional.

Drm Research Laboratories, Inc. 203-488-5555
29 Business Park Dr, Branford, CT 06405
Crown & bridge dental composite material.

Dshealthcare Inc. 201-871-1232
85 W Forest Ave, Englewood, NJ 07631
Temporary crown and bridge material.

Ellman International, Inc. 800-835-5355
3333 Royal Ave, Rockville Centre, NY 11572

Gc America, Inc. 708-597-0900
3737 W 127th St, Alsip, IL 60803
Temporary crown & bridge resin.

Harry J. Bosworth Company 800-323-4352
7227 Hamlin Ave, Skokie, IL 60076
TRIM, TRIM II, ULTRATRIM, TRIMPLUS, TRIMVW.

Hennessy Dental Laboratory 800-694-6862
3709 Interstate Park Rd S, Riviera Beach, FL 33404

Ivoclar Vivadent, Inc. 800-533-6825
175 Pineview Dr, Amherst, NY 14228
SYSTEMP.C&B

Kay See Dental Mfg. Co. 816-842-2817
124 Missouri Ave, Kansas City, MO 64106
Temporary crown & bridge material.

Kerr Corp. 949-255-8766
1717 W Collins Ave, Orange, CA 92867
Crown and bridge, temporary, resin.

Motloid Company 800-662-5021
300 N Elizabeth St, Chicago, IL 60607
COLDPAC & LITEPAC Acrylic temporary crown and bridge.

Newtech Dental Laboratories 866-635-5227
1141 Smile Ln, Lansdale, PA 19446
Dental prosthetics.

Pac-Dent Intl., Inc. 909-839-0888
21078 Commerce Point Dr, Walnut, CA 91789
Crown and bridge material.

Parkell, Inc. 800-243-7446
300 Executive Dr, Edgewood, NY 11717
SNAP introductory kit. SMARTEMP, automix provisional c&b material, extrude form an automix impression gun. 1/1 mix ratio self-curve composite.

Pentron Clinical Technologies 203-265-7397
68-70 North Plains Industrial, Road, Wallingford, CT 06492
Crown & bridge temporary, resin.

Pentron Laboratory Technologies 203-265-7397
53 N Plains Industrial Rd, Wallingford, CT 06492
Crown and bridge,temporary,resin.

Plastodent 718-792-3554
2881 Middletown Rd, Bronx, NY 10461

Reliance Dental Mfg., Co. 708-597-6694
5805 W 117th Pl, Alsip, IL 60803
Various types of plastics and acrylics.

Sterngold 800-243-9942
23 Frank Mossberg Dr, PO Box 2967, Attleboro, MA 02703
InstaTemp Max - Bis-Acryl Composite for Temporary Crowns, Bridges, Inlays, Onlays and Attachment Pick-up.

Temrex Corp. 516-868-6221
112 Albany Ave, P.o. Box 182, Freeport, NY 11520
Temporary non-eugenol cement.

CROWN AND BRIDGE, TEMPORARY, RESIN *(cont'd)*

Water Pik, Inc. 970-221-6129
1730 E Prospect Rd, Fort Collins, CO 80525
Temporary crown and bridge resin.

Westside Packaging, Llc. 909-570-3508
1700 S Baker Ave Ste A, Ontario, CA 91761
Temporary crown & bridge resin.

CROWN, PREFORMED *(Dental And Oral) 76ELZ*

Adar International Inc. 404-457-7510
3350 Riverwood Pkwy SE Ste 1900, Atlanta, GA 30339
Crown.

American Dental Center Of Provo 801-375-8200
777 N 500 W Ste 201B, Provo, UT 84601
Pfm crown, pfm bridge.

American Diversified Dental Systems 800-637-2330
22991 La Cadena Dr, Laguna Hills, CA 92653
Insta-Tray Crown Stablizer

Americus Form & Function 440-237-0200
12316 York Rd, North Royalton, OH 44133
Crown.

Artisan Dental Laboratory 800-222-6721
2532 SE Hawthorne Blvd, Portland, OR 97214

Artistic Dental Lab, Incorporated 757-224-0177
1500 Crescent Dr Ste 204, Carrollton, TX 75006
Crown.

Aurum Ceramic Dental Laboratories Llp 403-228-5199
1320 N Howard St, Spokane, WA 99201
Dental prosthesis.

Bonita Dental Lab 239-495-3368
10915 Bonita Beach Rd SE Ste 1152, Bonita Springs, FL 34135
Various.

Den-Mat Holdings, Llc 805-922-8491
2727 Skyway Dr, Santa Maria, CA 93455
No common name listed.

Denart Aesthetic Design, S.F. 415-392-2233
450 Sutter St Rm 1215, San Francisco, CA 94108
Dental gold / metal crowns.

Dentsply Canada, Ltd. 800-263-1437
161 Vinyl Ct., Woodbridge, ONT L4L 4A3 Canada

Elgar Dental Products, Inc. 702-699-5655
3374 Racquet St, Las Vegas, NV 89121
Temporary preformed crown.

Harry J. Bosworth Company 800-323-4352
7227 Hamlin Ave, Skokie, IL 60076
B-crowns, Molar B-crowns.

Hennessy Dental Laboratory 800-694-6862
3709 Interstate Park Rd S, Riviera Beach, FL 33404

Intergrated Dental Solutions, Inc. 858-643-1143
6195 Cornerstone Ct E Ste 108, San Diego, CA 92121
Crown & bridge.

Mason Dental Midwest, Inc. 734-525-1070
12752 Stark Rd, Livonia, MI 48150
Crowns.

Mayclin Dental Studio, Inc. 952-926-1809
7505 Highway 7 Ste 100, Saint Louis Park, MN 55426
Various type of temporary crowns.

Pentron Clinical Technologies 203-265-7397
68-70 North Plains Industrial, Road, Wallingford, CT 06492
Core build-up caps.

Pentron Laboratory Technologies 203-265-7397
53 N Plains Industrial Rd, Wallingford, CT 06492
Preformed crown.

Princeton Laboratory Services, Llc 732-738-8108
340 Mac Ln, Keasbey, NJ 08832
Dental crown.

Rite-Dent Manufacturing Corp. 305-693-8626
3750 E 10th Ct, Hialeah, FL 33013
Various types of polycarbonate crown.

White Bite, Inc. 502-222-2647
5006 Hickory Hill Dr, La Grange, KY 40031
White pedo crown.

3m Espe Dental Products 949-863-1360
2111 McGaw Ave, Irvine, CA 92614
$139.25, $207.50, $177.85, $200.85, $131.85, $268.35, $171.15, $254.35, $243.15, $335.35, and $357.75 per unit.

CRUSHER, PILL *(General) 80QNK*

American Medical Industries 605-428-5501
330 E 3rd St Ste 2, Dell Rapids, SD 57022
EZ-SWALLOW pill crusher. Also available as combination pill crusher/pill splitter. EZ-SWALLOW combination unit. Pill crusher, pill splitter, and storage in one unit.

Geritrex Corp. 800-736-3437
144 E Kingsbridge Rd, Mount Vernon, NY 10550
Metal base.

International Crystal Laboratories 973-478-8944
11 Erie St, Garfield, NJ 07026
E-Z PRESS, laboratory press, low/weight lab press for pressing tablets and KBr pellets.

Medi-Dose, Inc. 800-523-8966
70 Industrial Dr, Ivyland, PA 18974

Ocelco, Inc. 800-328-5343
1111 Industrial Park Rd SW, Brainerd, MN 56401

Ross Disposable Products 800-649-6526
401 Traders Blvd E, Unit 10, Mississauga, ON L4Z 2H8 Canada

Trademark Medical Llc 800-325-9044
449 Soverign Ct, St. Louis, MO 63011
MOBEL 100 durable crusher.

CRUSHER, SYRINGE *(General) 80QNL*

Franklin Miller Inc 800-932-0599
60 Okner Pkwy, Livingston, NJ 07039

CRUSHER, VIAL, LABORATORY *(General) 80WPN*

S&G Enterprises, Inc. 800-233-3721
N115W19000 Edison Dr, Germantown, WI 53022
The VYLEATER® is designed for the bulk collection of liquids from glass and plastic vials. It destroys glass, plastic, Thinprep®, histology, urine & scintillation vials and recovers the liquid contents. Waste vials are processed through a shredder and the residue rinsed away before safely depositing the liquid into one container and the destroyed vials into a separate container. Applications include the draining of vials used in urinalysis, cytology and environmental testing and the secure destruction of pharmaceutical products with and expired shelf life or failed QA standards. The VYLEATER® reduces disposal costs and exposure of hazardous materials by technicians.

Ware Medics Glass Works, Inc. 845-429-6950
PO Box 368, Garnerville, NY 10923
Mortars and pestles.

CRUTCH *(Physical Med) 89IPR*

A&A Orthopedics, Incorporated 757-224-0177
12250 SW 129th Ct Bldg 1, Miami, FL 33186
Wood & aluminum crutch.

Access Mobility, Inc. 800-336-1147
5240 Elmwood Ave, Indianapolis, IN 46203

Adtech Systems Research, Inc 937-426-3329
1342 N Fairfield Rd, Beavercreek, OH 45432
Forearm crutch.

Alex Orthopedic, Inc. 800-544-2539
PO Box 201442, Arlington, TX 76006

Alimed, Inc. 800-225-2610
297 High St, Dedham, MA 02026

American Innovations, Inc. 800-223-3913
123 N Main St, Dublin, PA 18917
Accessories, crutches.

Bio-Medic Health Services, Inc. 800-525-0072
5041B Benois Rd Bldg B, Roanoke, VA 24018

Biomet, Inc. 574-267-6639
56 E Bell Dr, PO Box 587, Warsaw, IN 46582
Various types of crutch.

Calley & Currier Co. 800-762-5500
1 Greenleaf Woods Dr Unit 202, Portsmouth, NH 03801
Five sizes, with or without accessories.

Convaquip Industries, Inc. 800-637-8436
4834 Derrick Dr, PO Box 3417, Abilene, TX 79601
Bariatric Crutches weight certified to 700 lbs.

Cypress Medical Products 800-334-3646
1202 S. Rte. 31, McHenry, IL 60050
UNA-BODY push-button aluminum crutches, in Youth (4ft., 6in. to 5ft., 2in.), Medium (5ft., 2in. to 5ft., 10in.) and Tall (5ft., 10in. to 6ft., 6in.).

DJO Inc. 800-336-6569
1430 Decision St, Vista, CA 92081

CRUTCH *(cont'd)*

Dynatronics Corp. Chattanooga Operations 801-568-7000
6607 Mountain View Rd, Ooltewah, TN 37363
Various types of aluminum crutches.

G. Hirsch And Co., Inc. 650-692-8770
870 Mahler Rd, Burlingame, CA 94010
Various types of crutches.

Gendron, Inc. 800-537-2521
400 E Lugbill Rd, Archbold, OH 43502
$27.00 per pair.

Invacare Corporation 800-333-6900
1 Invacare Way, Elyria, OH 44035
INVACARE Quick-Adjust Crutches, Quick-Change Crutches, Bariatric Crutches, Forearm Crutches

Kaye Products, Inc. 919-732-6444
535 Dimmocks Mill Rd, Hillsborough, NC 27278
Adjustable handgrip, full forearm cuff, metal back, front with Velcro closure. For children 1 year to adult, 7 sizes available.

Keen Mobility Company 503-285-9090
6500 NE Halsey St Ste B, Portland, OR 97213

Lamico, Inc. 920-231-1672
474 Marion Rd, Oshkosh, WI 54901
Wooden crutch.

Larkotex Company 800-972-3037
1002 Olive St, Texarkana, TX 75501

Lofstrand Co. 800-221-0142
3435 Collins Pl, Flushing, NY 11354
Fore-arm crutch, 20 different styles. $60 per pair--also, with pushbutton under the arm crutch, $30 per pair.

Medical Depot 516-998-4600
99 Seaview Blvd, Port Washington, NY 11050
Crutches.

Medline Industries, Inc. 800-633-5886
1 Medline Pl, Mundelein, IL 60060

Mobility Concepts, L.L.C. 660-668-3918
16999 Boyer Ave, Cole Camp, MO 65325
Canadan crutch, forearm crutch.

Ortho-Med, Inc. 800-547-5571
3208 SE 13th Ave, Portland, OR 97202

Orthotic Mobility Systems, Inc. 301-949-2444
10421 Metropolitan Ave, Kensington, MD 20895
Crutch.

Ossur Americas 949-268-3155
742 Pancho Rd, Camarillo, CA 93012

Paramedical Distributors 800-245-3278
2020 Grand Blvd, Kansas City, MO 64108
Wood and/or aluminum crutches and tips.

Parsons A.D.L. Inc. 800-263-1281
R.R. #2, 1986 Sideroad 15, Tottenham, ONT L0G 1W0 Canada
Forearm crutches with orthopaedic grips, very light weight and strong.

Patterson Medical Supply, Inc. 262-387-8720
W68N158 Evergreen Blvd, Cedarburg, WI 53012
Crutch.

Perfect Care 718-805-7800
8927 126th St, Richmond Hill, NY 11418
Crutch.

Productos Rubbermaid, Sociedad Anonima De Capital 540-542-8363
Kmi-Ote, Carretera Cadereyta-Allende
Cadereyta Jimenez 67450 Mexico
Various

Profex Medical Products 800-325-0196
2224 E Person Ave, Memphis, TN 38114

Truform Orthotics & Prosthetics 800-888-0458
3960 Rosslyn Dr, Cincinnati, OH 45209

Tuffcare 800-367-6160
3999 E La Palma Ave, Anaheim, CA 92807

Wheelchairs Of Kansas 800-537-6454
204 W 2nd St, Ellis, KS 67637
Bariatric CRUTCHES in multiple lengths; Constructed of heavy-duty steel that is designed specifically for bariatric needs; Height adjustable in 1' increments; Extra large rubber caps for stability; Soft, cushioned hand grips and underarm pads; 500 lb. weight capacity.

CRUTCH, PTOSIS *(Ophthalmology) 86HJZ*

Fci Ophthalmics 800-932-4202
64 Schoosett St, Pembroke, MA 02359
Ptosis Sling Set (silicone); Ptose-Up (ePTFE) for frontalis suspension.

CRYOPHTHALMIC UNIT *(Ophthalmology) 86HPS*

Keeler Instruments Inc. 800-523-5620
456 Park Way, Broomall, PA 19008
$2,650 for CTU model with accessories. N20/CO2 - CRYOMASTER CONSOLE $4,950 w/accessories. N20/CO2 probes $1,995.

Md International, Inc. 305-669-9003
11300 NW 41st St, Doral, FL 33178

Mira, Inc. 508-278-7877
414 Quaker Hwy, Uxbridge, MA 01569
Cryo.

Wallach Surgical Devices, Inc. 800-243-2463
235 Edison Rd, Orange, CT 06477
$1045 for non-AC-powered cryosurgical unit, $2,640.00 for console unit.

CRYOSURGICAL UNIT *(Surgery) 79GEH*

Alcon Research, Ltd. 800-862-5266
6201 South Fwy, Fort Worth, TX 76134

Cryogen, Inc. 858-450-7400
10700 Bren Rd W, Minnetonka, MN 55343
Cryosurgical system & accessories.

Cryosurgery, Inc. 800-729-1624
5829 Old Harding Rd, Nashville, TN 37205
VERRUCA-FREEZE cryosurgery system: hassle-free, non-hazmat, self-contained unit, portable and lightweight. Kit includes a 162ml canister, 6 transparent limiting cones, instruction book, instructional CD, sample pack of CRYOBUDS, insulator and practice media. 80ml Kit also available.

Dermatologic Lab & Supply, Inc. 800-831-6273
608 13th Ave, Council Bluffs, IA 51501
Delasco FrigiSpray liquid nitrogen apparatus for cryosurgery

Dma Med-Chem Corporation 800-362-1833
49 Watermill Ln, Great Neck, NY 11021

Elmed, Inc. 630-543-2792
60 W Fay Ave, Addison, IL 60101
N20/C02 units--two stand-alone ($850) and four console ($985 to $1,845); 75 psi to -80 deg C.

Healthtronics Inc. 888-252-6575
9825 Spectrum Dr Bldg B, Austin, TX 78717
Accessories

Hill-Med, Inc. 305-594-7474
7217 NW 46th St, Miami, FL 33166

Md International, Inc. 305-669-9003
11300 NW 41st St, Doral, FL 33178

Orasure Technologies, Inc. 800-869-3538
220 E 1st St, Bethlehem, PA 18015
HISTOFREEZER cryosurgical wart treatment.

Pds Manufacturing, Inc. 817-329-2701
577 Commerce St Ste A, Southlake, TX 76092
Cryosurgical device.

Premier Medical Products 888-PREMUSA
1710 Romano Dr, Plymouth Meeting, PA 19462
Nitrospray Plus - Liquid Nitrogen (N2) based cryosurgical unit.

Sanarus Medical, Inc. 925-460-5730
4696 Willow Rd, Pleasanton, CA 94588
Visica treatment system.

Schering-Plough Healthcare Products, Inc. 862-245-5115
4207 Michigan Avenue Rd NE, Cleveland, TN 37323
Cryosurgical unit and accessories.

Scott-Gross Co., Inc. 859-231-0225
664 Magnolia Ave, Lexington, KY 40505
Various.

Southland Cryogenics, Inc. 800-872-2796
8350 Mosley Rd, Houston, TX 77075
CRYOGUN, Cryosurgical device using liquid nitrogen to attain results. Available in 2 sizes. A variety of tips available.

Wallach Surgical Devices, Inc. 800-243-2463
235 Edison Rd, Orange, CT 06477
$1045 for non-AC-powered cryosurgical unit. $8,245.00 for cryosurgical PAINBLOCKER unit.

CRYOSURGICAL UNIT, GYNECOLOGIC *(Obstetrics/Gyn) 85HGJ*

Coopersurgical, Inc. 800-243-2974
95 Corporate Dr, Trumbull, CT 06611
$1,545 for complete system with 4 tips, gas cylinder, mobile cart, and carrying case.

Dma Med-Chem Corporation 800-362-1833
49 Watermill Ln, Great Neck, NY 11021

Md International, Inc. 305-669-9003
11300 NW 41st St, Doral, FL 33178

R Medical Supply 800-882-7578
620 Valley Forge Rd Ste F, Hillsborough, NC 27278

Wallach Surgical Devices, Inc. 800-243-2463
235 Edison Rd, Orange, CT 06477
$1045 for non-AC-powered cryosurgical unit.

CRYOSURGICAL, UNIT, UROLOGY *(Surgery) 79FAZ*

Central Welder's Supply, Inc. 800-728-2068
127D Lee Rd, Watsonville, CA 95076
Liquid nitrogen N.F.

CRYOTHERAPY, UNIT, OPHTHALMIC *(Ophthalmology) 86HQA*

Keeler Instruments Inc. 800-523-5620
456 Park Way, Broomall, PA 19008

Mira, Inc. 508-278-7877
414 Quaker Hwy, Uxbridge, MA 01569
Ophthalmic trichiasis probe.

CRYPTOSPORIDIUM SPP. *(Microbiology) 83MHJ*

Biosite Incorporated 888-246-7483
9975 Summers Ridge Rd, San Diego, CA 92121
Visual immunoassay for detection of crytosporidium,giardia,entamoeba histolytica.

Ivd Research, Inc. 760-929-7744
5909 Sea Lion Pl Ste D, Carlsbad, CA 92010
Cryptosporidium stool antigen elisa.

Meridian Bioscience, Inc. 800-696-0739
3471 River Hills Dr, Cincinnati, OH 45244
A direct immunofluorescent procedure for the simultaneous detection of Cryptosporidium oocysts and Giardia cysts in stool.

CRYSTAL VIOLET *(Hematology) 81GGD*

Bd Diagnostic Systems 800-675-0908
7 Loveton Cir, Sparks, MD 21152

Medical Chemical Corp. 800-424-9394
19430 Van Ness Ave, Torrance, CA 90501
$13.50 per 500mL.

Rocky Mountain Reagents,Inc. 303-762-0800
3207 W Hampden Ave, Englewood, CO 80110

CUFF, BLOOD PRESSURE *(Cardiovascular) 74DXQ*

A&D Medical 800-726-7099
1756 Automation Pkwy, San Jose, CA 95131
$16.95 for UA-279 (small cuff); $16.95 for UA-280 (adult cuff); and $27.95 for UA-281 (adult large).

Advanced Medical Instruments, Inc. 918-250-0566
3061 W Albany St, Broken Arrow, OK 74012
Neonatal blood pressure cuff.

Alimed, Inc. 800-225-2610
297 High St, Dedham, MA 02026

Anesthesia Associates, Inc. 760-744-6561
460 Enterprise St, San Marcos, CA 92078
Large variety of sizes from premature to conical extreme obese. Multiple options for number of tubes and end connectors. Various material selections available.

Armstrong Medical Industries, Inc. 800-323-4220
575 Knightsbridge Pkwy, Lincolnshire, IL 60069

Ascent Healthcare Solutions 480-763-5300
10232 S 51st St, Phoenix, AZ 85044
Tourniquet cuffs.

Biomet, Inc. 574-267-6639
56 E Bell Dr, PO Box 587, Warsaw, IN 46582
Various types of sterile and non-sterile inflation cuffs.

Bowen Medical Services, Inc. 386-362-1345
709 Industrial Ave SW, Live Oak, FL 32064
Cover for blood pressure cuffs.

Carolina Medical, Inc. 800-334-4531
157 Industrial Dr, King, NC 27021
Full range of segmental air cuffs from 2 to 22cm in width. Volumetric cuffs for plethysmographic results in ml/dl available.

CUFF, BLOOD PRESSURE *(cont'd)*

Cas Medical Systems, Inc. 800-227-4414
44 E Industrial Rd, Branford, CT 06405
Neonatal and adult blood-pressure cuffs.

Creative Health Products, Inc. 800-742-4478
5148 Saddle Ridge Rd, Plymouth, MI 48170
AMERICAN DIAGNOSTIC, Nylon Cuff and Bladder for child, adult, large adult and thigh sizes with one or two tube. Child 2 tube $12.50, Adult 2 tube $14.40, Large Adult 2 tube $20.50, Thigh 2 tube $26.90. Adult 1 tube $14.40, Large Adult 1 tube $20.50 from CHP.

David Scott Company 800-804-0333
59 Fountain St, Framingham, MA 01702

Demetech Corp. 888-324-2447
3530 NW 115th Ave, Doral, FL 33178
Manual blood pressure kit, aneroid sphygmomanometer.

Edmund Industrial Optics 800-363-1992
101 E Gloucester Pike, Barrington, NJ 08007

Elmed, Inc. 630-543-2792
60 W Fay Ave, Addison, IL 60101

Ethox International 800-521-1022
251 Seneca St, Buffalo, NY 14204
Blood pressure cuff sterile & non-sterile.

Frontier Medical Products, Inc. 800-367-6828
140 S Park St, Port Washington, WI 53074

Ge Medical Systems Information Technologies 800-558-5544
4502 Woodland Corporate Blvd, Tampa, FL 33614
CRITIKON and DURA-CUF, SOFT CUF, CLASSIC CUF.

Generic Medical, Inc. 678-879-1000
4064 Nine McFarland Dr Ste D, Alpharetta, GA 30004
Blood pressure cuff.

Genesis Manufacturing, Inc. 317-485-7887
720 E Broadway St, Fortville, IN 46040
Contract Radio-Frequency (RF) Welding. From development to manufacturing and packaging.

Health Care Logistics, Inc. 800-848-1633
450 Town St, PO Box 25, Circleville, OH 43113
Disposable surgi-cuff / BP cuff.

Her-Mar, Inc. 800-327-8209
8550 NW 30th Ter, Doral, FL 33122
$25.00 each.

Hokanson Inc., D.E. 800-999-8251
12840 NE 21st Pl, Bellevue, WA 98005
Specialty vascular cuffs are available in 11 sizes from 1.6 to 22 cm, straight segmental, digit and contour; digit cuffs are also available in a disposable variety.

Icu Medical (Ut), Inc 949-366-2183
4455 Atherton Dr, Salt Lake City, UT 84123
Various sizes and configurations of sterile monitoring kits.

Invivo Corporation 425-487-7000
12601 Research Pkwy, Orlando, FL 32826
Neonatal blood pressure cuffs (disposable).

Johnson & Johnson Medical Division Of Ethicon, Inc. 800-423-4018
2500 E Arbrook Blvd, Arlington, TX 76014
Disposable.

Kck Industries 888-800-1967
14941 Calvert St, Van Nuys, CA 91411

Kentron Health Care, Inc. 615-384-0573
3604 Kelton Jackson Rd, P.o. Box 120, Springfield, TN 37172
Aneroid sphygmomanometer.

Kerma Medical Products, Inc. 757-398-8400
400 Port Centre Pkwy, Portsmouth, VA 23704
Blood pressure unit.

Kerr Group 800-524-3577
1400 Holcomb Bridge Rd, Roswell, GA 30076

Lampac International Ltd. 636-797-3659
230 N Lake Dr, Hillsboro, MO 63050
Cuff, blood pressure - digital manual inflate, autodeflate and autoinflate.

Md International, Inc. 305-669-9003
11300 NW 41st St, Doral, FL 33178

Meddex, S.A. 5-581-8022
Calz. Ermita Iztapalapa, #855,, Col. Sta. Isabel Industrial Cd. Mexico, D.f. Mexico
Aneroid sphygmanometer

CUFF, BLOOD PRESSURE *(cont'd)*

Medical Accessories, Inc. 800-275-1624
92 Youngs Rd, Trenton, NJ 08619
Box of 10 disposable cuffs (Velcro) for use with DINAMAP and single tube monitors.

Medworks Instruments 800-323-9790
PO Box 581, Chatham, IL 62629
$13.50 per unit thigh, adult.

Nova Health Systems, Inc. 800-225-NOVA
1001 Broad St, Utica, NY 13501
Disposable, neonatal blood-pressure cuffs.

Pedia Pals, Llc 888-733-4272
965 Highway 169 N, Plymouth, MN 55441
Benjamin Bear Blood Pressure Cuff, Bulb and Kit.

Pioneer Center For Human Services 815-344-1230
4001 W Dayton St, McHenry, IL 60050
Blood pressure cuff.

Primary Medical Co., Inc. 727-520-1920
6541 44th St N Ste 6003, Pinellas Park, FL 33781
Blood-pressure cuff, various sizes.

Propper Manufacturing Co., Inc. 800-832-4300
3604 Skillman Ave, Long Island City, NY 11101

Schueler & Company, Inc. 516-487-1500
PO Box 528, Stratford, CT 06615

Sharn, Inc. 800-325-3671
4517 George Rd Ste 200, Tampa, FL 33634

Smi 920-876-3361
Industrial Park, 544 Sohn Drive, Elkhart Lake, WI 53020

Statcorp, Inc. 800-992-0014
14476 Duval Pl W Ste 303, Jacksonville, FL 32218
Disposable blood pressure cuffs. Cuffs avavilable in double bladder, in both double and single hose, full bladder design. Personal cuff. Disposable blood pressure cuffs. Available in double or single tube, soft fabric, reusable; 8 sizes; neonatal.

Sunbeam Products, Inc. 561-912-4100
2381 NW Executive Center Dr, Boca Raton, FL 33431
Blood pressure cuff.

Technicuff Corp. 800-276-2833
2525 Industrial St, Leesburg, FL 34748
Cuff, blood-pressure.

Trimline Medical Products Corp. 800-526-3538
34 Columbia Rd, Branchburg, NJ 08876
PRE-GAGED cuff has clearly visible guides to determine proper cuff sizes; also includes antimicrobial treatment to protect against bacterial growth and mildew. Also available, neonatal, infant, disposable, extended use and bladderless cuffs and latex-free inflation systems.

Tuzik Boston 800-886-6363
104 Longwater Dr, Assinippi Park, Norwell, MA 02061

Vasamed 800-695-2737
7615 Golden Triangle Dr Ste C, Eden Prairie, MN 55344
LASERDOPP skin perfusion pressure measurement system.

W.A. Baum Co., Inc. 888-281-6061
620 Oak St, Copiague, NY 11726
Aneroid blood pressure cuffs.

Welch Allyn, Inc. 800-535-6663
4341 State Street Rd, Skaneateles Falls, NY 13153

Zefon International 800-282-0073
5350 SW 1st Ln, Ocala, FL 34474
Disposable blood pressure cuffs in a large range of sizes and material choices available for distribution or OEM.

CUFF, INFLATION *(General) 80FLZ*

Clinimed, Incorporated 877-CLINIMED
303 Markus Ct, Sandy Brae Industrial Park, Newark, DE 19713

Fluke Biomedical 800-648-7952
6920 Seaway Blvd, Everett, WA 98203
Automated cuff inflation for NIBP monitor testing.

Genesis Manufacturing, Inc. 317-485-7887
720 E Broadway St, Fortville, IN 46040
Contract Radio-Frequency (RF) Welding. From development to manufacturing and packaging.

Tuzik Boston 800-886-6363
104 Longwater Dr, Assinippi Park, Norwell, MA 02061

CUFF, NERVE *(Cns/Neurology) 84JXI*

Axogen Inc. 888-296-4361
13859 Progress Blvd Ste 100, Alachua, FL 32615
AxoGuard Nerve Connector; AxoGuard Nerve Protector

Biomet, Inc. 574-267-6639
56 E Bell Dr, PO Box 587, Warsaw, IN 46582
Nerve pin, nerve approximator.

Collagen Matrix, Inc. 201-405-1477
509 Commerce St, Franklin Lakes, NJ 07417
Collagen nerve cuff.

Salumedica, L.L.C. 404-589-1727
4451 Atlanta Rd SE Ste 138, Smyrna, GA 30080
Salumedica(tm) nerve cuff.

Synovis Micro Companies Alliance, Inc. 651-603-3700
439 Industrial Ln, Birmingham, AL 35211
Nerve cuff, woven polyglycolic acid tube.

CUFF, PUSHER, WHEELCHAIR *(Physical Med) 89INC*

Alimed, Inc. 800-225-2610
297 High St, Dedham, MA 02026

CUFF, TRACHEAL TUBE, INFLATABLE *(Anesthesiology) 73BSK*

Anesthesia Associates, Inc. 760-744-6561
460 Enterprise St, San Marcos, CA 92078
Cuff Pressure Monitor, ET Tube, w/ Max Hold Gauge -40 to +80 cmH2O. LuerM fitting. PN 00-198

Bausch & Lomb Surgical 636-255-5051
3365 Tree Court Ind Blvd, Saint Louis, MO 63122

Schueler & Company, Inc. 516-487-1500
PO Box 528, Stratford, CT 06615

CUFF, TRACHEOSTOMY TUBE *(Ear/Nose/Throat) 77JOH*

Apdyne Medical Company 800-457-6853
1049 S Vine St, Denver, CO 80209
HYGIENA TRACHE cuffed tracheostomy tube with an auxiliary independent airway for speaking or suctioning.

Bausch & Lomb Surgical 636-255-5051
3365 Tree Court Ind Blvd, Saint Louis, MO 63122

Dale Medical Products, Inc. 800-343-3980
7 Cross St, Plainville, MA 02762
Tracheostomy Tube Holder #240 fits most. #242 fits neonate to infant. Endotracheal Tube Holder #245 fits most adults, #246 fits infants & pediatrics

Kelsar, S.A. 508-261-8000
Blvd. Insurgentes, Libriamento a La, Tijuana 22450 Mexico
Tracheostomy tubes and care set/kits and accessories

Luminaud, Inc. 800-255-3408
8688 Tyler Blvd, Mentor, OH 44060
Assorted laryngectomy filters. Price ranging from $3.75 - $18.00.

Smiths Medical Asd 800-424-8662
5700 W 23rd Ave, Gary, IN 46406
AIRE-CUF, FOME-CUF & TTS (tight-to-shaft).

CULDOSCOPE *(Obstetrics/Gyn) 85HEW*

Gyrus Acmi, Inc. 508-804-2739
93 N Pleasant St, Norwalk, OH 44857
Various sizes and kinds of culdoscopes and accessories.

Gyrus Acmi, Inc. 508-804-2739
300 Stillwater P.o.box 1971, Stamford, CT 06902
Various sizes and kinds of culdoscopes and accessories.

Karl Storz Endoscopy-America Inc. 800-421-0837
600 Corporate Pointe, Culver City, CA 90230

Mahe International Inc. 800-294-7946
468 Craighead St, Nashville, TN 37204

Richard Wolf Medical Instruments Corp. 800-323-9653
353 Corporate Woods Pkwy, Vernon Hills, IL 60061

CULTURE MEDIA, AMINO ACID ASSAY *(Microbiology) 83JRZ*

Alpha Biosciences, Inc. 877-825-7428
3651 Clipper Mill Rd, Baltimore, MD 21211
Various types of microbiolgical assay culture media.

Bd Diagnostic Systems 800-675-0908
7 Loveton Cir, Sparks, MD 21152

CULTURE MEDIA, ANAEROBIC TRANSPORT *(Microbiology) 83JSL*

Oxoid, Inc. 800-567-8378
800 Proctor Ave, Ogdensburg, NY 13669
Dehydrated.

CULTURE MEDIA, ANAEROBIC TRANSPORT *(cont'd)*

Remel 800-255-6730
12076 Santa Fe Dr, Lenexa, KS 66215

CULTURE MEDIA, ANTIBIOTIC ASSAY *(Microbiology) 83JSA*

Bd Diagnostic Systems 800-675-0908
7 Loveton Cir, Sparks, MD 21152

Oxoid, Inc. 800-567-8378
800 Proctor Ave, Ogdensburg, NY 13669
Dehydrated.

Pedinol Pharmacal, Inc. 800-733-4665
30 Banfi Plz N, Farmingdale, NY 11735

CULTURE MEDIA, ANTIMICROBIAL SUSCEPTIBILITY TEST *(Microbiology) 83JSO*

Bd Diagnostic Systems 800-675-0908
7 Loveton Cir, Sparks, MD 21152

Biomerieux Industry 800-634-7656
595 Anglum Rd, Hazelwood, MO 63042

Culture Kits, Inc. 888-680-6853
14 Prentice St, PO Box 748, Norwich, NY 13815
Mueller-Hinton.

Emd Chemicals Inc. 800-222-0342
480 S Democrat Rd, Gibbstown, NJ 08027

Hardy Diagnostics 800-226-2222
1430 W McCoy Ln, Santa Maria, CA 93455
Various culture media for disk diffusion susceptibilty testing of microorganisms.

Trek Diagnostic Systems, Inc. 608-8373788
210 Business Park Dr, Sun Prairie, WI 53590
Various culture media for antimicrobial susceptibility test.

Zeus Scientific, Inc. 800-286-2111
PO Box 38, Raritan, NJ 08869

CULTURE MEDIA, ENRICHED *(Microbiology) 83KZI*

Acumedia Manufacturers, Inc. 800-783-3212
620 Lesher Pl, Lansing, MI 48912
More than 250 different formulas available, along with custom products.

Alpha Biosciences, Inc. 877-825-7428
3651 Clipper Mill Rd, Baltimore, MD 21211
Various types of enriched culture media.

Bd Diagnostic Systems 800-675-0908
7 Loveton Cir, Sparks, MD 21152

Becton Dickinson And Co. 656-860-1553
2801 Industrial Dr, Monona, WI 53713
Various.

Biocell Laboratories, Inc. 800-222-8382
2001 E University Dr, Rancho Dominguez, CA 90220
Tissue-culture sera.

Biomed Diagnostics, Inc. 541-830-3000
1388 Antelope Rd, White City, OR 97503
InPouch TV test Kit for Trichomonas vaginalis. Used for inoculation, transportation, incubation, reading in a single thatis not opened after specimen is introduced in it. Test kits can be stored at room temperature until ready to be used.

Culture Kits, Inc. 888-680-6853
14 Prentice St, PO Box 748, Norwich, NY 13815
URI-THREE urine culture. URI-TWO two media (C. L. E. D./ MacConkey II) urine culture.

Healthlink 904-996-7758
3611 St Johns Bluff Rd S Ste 1, Jacksonville, FL 32224
Culture media.

Incell Corporation, Llc 210-877-0100
12734 Cimarron Path, San Antonio, TX 78249
L broth.

Oxyrase, Inc. 419-589-8800
175 Illinois Ave S, Mansfield, OH 44905
Anaerobic blood agar plates.

CULTURE MEDIA, FOR ISOLATION OF PATHOGENIC NEISSERIA *(Microbiology) 83JTY*

Bd Diagnostic Systems 800-675-0908
7 Loveton Cir, Sparks, MD 21152

Biomerieux Industry 800-634-7656
595 Anglum Rd, Hazelwood, MO 63042

CULTURE MEDIA, FOR ISOLATION OF PATHOGENIC NEISSERIA *(cont'd)*

Culture Kits, Inc. 888-680-6853
14 Prentice St, PO Box 748, Norwich, NY 13815
GONI-KIT for isolation of pathogenic neisseria.

Gibson Laboratories, Inc. 859-254-9500
1040 Manchester St, Lexington, KY 40508
Thayer-martin selective agar with trimethoprim.

Hardy Diagnostics 800-226-2222
1430 W McCoy Ln, Santa Maria, CA 93455
Various selective media for the isolation of Neisseria gonorrhea from clinical specimens.

Healthlink 904-996-7758
3611 St Johns Bluff Rd S Ste 1, Jacksonville, FL 32224
Gc media.

Northeast Laboratory Services, Inc. 800-244-8378
227 China Rd, Winslow, ME 04901
Prepared microbiological culture media.

Oxoid, Inc. 800-567-8378
800 Proctor Ave, Ogdensburg, NY 13669
Dehydrated.

Pml Microbiologicals 800-628-7014
27120 SW 95th Ave, Wilsonville, OR 97070

Remel 800-255-6730
12076 Santa Fe Dr, Lenexa, KS 66215

Smith River Biologicals 276-930-2369
9388 Charity Hwy, Ferrum, VA 24088
Various types of culture media for the isolation of pathogenic neisseria.

CULTURE MEDIA, GENERAL NUTRIENT BROTH
(Microbiology) 83JSC

Advanced Biotechnologies, Inc. 800-426-0764
9108 Guilford Rd, Rivers Park II, Columbia, MD 21046

Anaerobe Systems 408-782-7557
15906 Concord Cir, Morgan Hill, CA 95037
Lombard-dowell (ld) medium with glucose.

Bd Diagnostic Systems 800-675-0908
7 Loveton Cir, Sparks, MD 21152

Biocell Laboratories, Inc. 800-222-8382
2001 E University Dr, Rancho Dominguez, CA 90220

Biomerieux Industry 800-634-7656
595 Anglum Rd, Hazelwood, MO 63042

Carolina Biological Supply Co. 800-334-5551
2700 York Rd, Burlington, NC 27215

Hardy Diagnostics 800-226-2222
1430 W McCoy Ln, Santa Maria, CA 93455
Various culture media for cultivation of non-fastidious micro-organisms.

Healthlink 904-996-7758
3611 St Johns Bluff Rd S Ste 1, Jacksonville, FL 32224
Broth media.

Ml Lifesciences 949-699-3800
17 Hammond Ste 408, Irvine, CA 92618

Northeast Laboratory Services, Inc. 800-244-8378
227 China Rd, Winslow, ME 04901
Prepared microbiological culture media.

Oxoid, Inc. 800-567-8378
800 Proctor Ave, Ogdensburg, NY 13669
Dehydrated.

Pml Microbiologicals 800-628-7014
27120 SW 95th Ave, Wilsonville, OR 97070

Q.I. Medical, Inc. 800-837-8361
440 Lower Grass Valley Rd Ste C, Nevada City, CA 95959

Qiagen Gaithersburg, Inc. 800-344-3631
1201 Clopper Rd, Gaithersburg, MD 20878
Pipettor, microplate handler, incubator.

Remel 800-255-6730
12076 Santa Fe Dr, Lenexa, KS 66215

Remel Atlanta, Div. Of Remel, Inc. 800-255-6730
2797 Peterson Pl, Norcross, GA 30071

Smith River Biologicals 276-930-2369
9388 Charity Hwy, Ferrum, VA 24088
Various types of general nutrient broth culture media.

CULTURE MEDIA, MUELLER HINTON AGAR BROTH
(Microbiology) 83JTZ

Bd Diagnostic Systems 800-675-0908
7 Loveton Cir, Sparks, MD 21152

Carolina Biological Supply Co. 800-334-5551
2700 York Rd, Burlington, NC 27215

Culture Kits, Inc. 888-680-6853
14 Prentice St, PO Box 748, Norwich, NY 13815
URINE DUO urine culture and drug sensitivity test.

Gibson Laboratories, Inc. 859-254-9500
1040 Manchester St, Lexington, KY 40508
Mueller hinton agar.

Healthlink 904-996-7758
3611 St Johns Bluff Rd S Ste 1, Jacksonville, FL 32224
Mueller hinton agar.

Northeast Laboratory Services, Inc. 800-244-8378
227 China Rd, Winslow, ME 04901
Prepared microbiological culture media.

Pml Microbiologicals 800-628-7014
27120 SW 95th Ave, Wilsonville, OR 97070

Remel 800-255-6730
12076 Santa Fe Dr, Lenexa, KS 66215

Smith River Biologicals 276-930-2369
9388 Charity Hwy, Ferrum, VA 24088
Various types of antimicrobial susceptibility test agars.

Trek Diagnostic Systems, Inc. 608-8373788
210 Business Park Dr, Sun Prairie, WI 53590
Various.

CULTURE MEDIA, MULTIPLE BIOCHEMICAL TEST
(Microbiology) 83JSE

Anaerobe Systems 408-782-7557
15906 Concord Cir, Morgan Hill, CA 95037
Carbohydrate fermentation media.

Bd Diagnostic Systems 800-675-0908
7 Loveton Cir, Sparks, MD 21152

Biomerieux Industry 800-634-7656
595 Anglum Rd, Hazelwood, MO 63042

Hardy Diagnostics 800-226-2222
1430 W McCoy Ln, Santa Maria, CA 93455
Various culture media for testing biochemical response of clinical and environmental isolates to various substrates.

Microbiological Specialties 602-867-7323
3311 E Charter Oak Rd, Phoenix, AZ 85032
Enzyme-ase i tubes.

Northeast Laboratory Services, Inc. 800-244-8378
227 China Rd, Winslow, ME 04901
Prepared microbiological culture media.

Oxoid, Inc. 800-567-8378
800 Proctor Ave, Ogdensburg, NY 13669
Dehydrated.

Pml Microbiologicals 800-628-7014
27120 SW 95th Ave, Wilsonville, OR 97070

Remel 800-255-6730
12076 Santa Fe Dr, Lenexa, KS 66215

Smith River Biologicals 276-930-2369
9388 Charity Hwy, Ferrum, VA 24088
Various types of multiple biochemical test culture media.

Usb Corporation 800-321-9322
26111 Miles Rd, Cleveland, OH 44128
Research biochemical.

CULTURE MEDIA, NON-PROPAGATING TRANSPORT
(Microbiology) 83JSM

Alpha Biosciences, Inc. 877-825-7428
3651 Clipper Mill Rd, Baltimore, MD 21211
Various types of multipurpose transport mediums.

Bd Diagnostic Systems 800-675-0908
7 Loveton Cir, Sparks, MD 21152

Hardy Diagnostics 800-226-2222
1430 W McCoy Ln, Santa Maria, CA 93455
CMV transport for use in transporting specimens for culture of viruses, chlamydiae and mycoplasma.

Hobbs Medical, Inc. 860-684-5875
8 Spring St, Stafford Springs, CT 06076
Saccomanno solution.

CULTURE MEDIA, NON-PROPAGATING TRANSPORT *(cont'd)*

Medical Packaging Corporation 800-792-0600
941 Avenida Acaso, Camarillo, CA 93012
SNAPSWAB & CULTURE-PAK Culture Collection and Transport System. Ready to use, disposable, sterile, culture collection device for use in the collection, preservation, and transport of clinical specimens to the laboratory for bacteriological analysis. Available in single or dual. Rayon swab with modified Stuarts, Amies or Cary-Blair media.

Mml Diagnostics Packaging, Inc. 800-826-7186
1625 NW Sundial Rd, P.O. Box 458, Troutdale, OR 97060
Culture transport tubes. Parasitology Specimen Transport. Bacteriology Specimen Transport.

Pml Microbiologicals 800-628-7014
27120 SW 95th Ave, Wilsonville, OR 97070

Remel 800-255-6730
12076 Santa Fe Dr, Lenexa, KS 66215

Smith River Biologicals 276-930-2369
9388 Charity Hwy, Ferrum, VA 24088
Various types of non-propagating transport culture media.

CULTURE MEDIA, NON-SELECTIVE AND DIFFERENTIAL
(Microbiology) 83JSH

Alpha Biosciences, Inc. 877-825-7428
3651 Clipper Mill Rd, Baltimore, MD 21211
Various types of differential culture media.

Anaerobe Systems 408-782-7557
15906 Concord Cir, Morgan Hill, CA 95037
Lombard-dowell (ld) starch agar.

Bd Diagnostic Systems 800-675-0908
7 Loveton Cir, Sparks, MD 21152

Becton Dickinson And Co. 656-860-1553
2801 Industrial Dr, Monona, WI 53713
Various bbl non-selective and differential culture media.

Culture Kits, Inc. 888-680-6853
14 Prentice St, PO Box 748, Norwich, NY 13815
URINE DUO urine culture and drug sensitivity test; URI KIT urine screening kit; URI-THREE urine culture. 2 Media Urine culture and transport mechanism.

Gibson Laboratories, Inc. 859-254-9500
1040 Manchester St, Lexington, KY 40508
Corn meal agar deeps.

Healthlink 904-996-7758
3611 St Johns Bluff Rd S Ste 1, Jacksonville, FL 32224
Blood agar.

Northeast Laboratory Services, Inc. 800-244-8378
227 China Rd, Winslow, ME 04901
Prepared microbiological culture media.

Oral Biotech 541-928-4445
812 Water Ave NE, Albany, OR 97321

Oxoid, Inc. 800-567-8378
800 Proctor Ave, Ogdensburg, NY 13669
Dehydrated.

Pml Microbiologicals 800-628-7014
27120 SW 95th Ave, Wilsonville, OR 97070

Remel 800-255-6730
12076 Santa Fe Dr, Lenexa, KS 66215

Smith River Biologicals 276-930-2369
9388 Charity Hwy, Ferrum, VA 24088
Various types of non-selective and differential culture media.

CULTURE MEDIA, NON-SELECTIVE AND NON-DIFFERENTIAL
(Microbiology) 83JSG

Alpha Biosciences, Inc. 877-825-7428
3651 Clipper Mill Rd, Baltimore, MD 21211
Various types of multipurpose culture mediums.

Anaerobe Systems 408-782-7557
15906 Concord Cir, Morgan Hill, CA 95037
Chopped meat glucose starch (cmgs) medium.

Bd Diagnostic Systems 800-675-0908
7 Loveton Cir, Sparks, MD 21152

Becton Dickinson And Co. 656-860-1553
2801 Industrial Dr, Monona, WI 53713
Various bbl non-selective and non-differential culture media.

CULTURE MEDIA, NON-SELECTIVE AND NON-DIFFERENTIAL
(cont'd)

Biolab Co. 809-787-5746
Ave. Teniente Nelson Martinez,, N-59 Alturas De Flamboyan
Bayamon, PR 00959
Bacterial culture media.

Biomerieux Industry 800-634-7656
595 Anglum Rd, Hazelwood, MO 63042
Dehydrated culture media.

Biosource International Incorporated, Rockville Div. 800-242-0607
1106 Taft St, Rockville, MD 20850
Various types of sterile and non-sterile multipurpose culture medium.

Gibson Laboratories, Inc. 859-254-9500
1040 Manchester St, Lexington, KY 40508
1.5% agar plate.

Healthlink 904-996-7758
3611 St Johns Bluff Rd S Ste 1, Jacksonville, FL 32224
Culture media, non-selective and non-differential (various types).

Key Scientific Products 325-773-3918
1113 E Reynolds St, Stamford, TX 79553
Dehyrated or tableted culture media to be used in isolation and identification.

Ml Lifesciences 949-699-3800
17 Hammond Ste 408, Irvine, CA 92618

Northeast Laboratory Services, Inc. 800-244-8378
227 China Rd, Winslow, ME 04901
Prepared microbiological culture media.

Oxoid, Inc. 800-567-8378
800 Proctor Ave, Ogdensburg, NY 13669
Dehydrated.

Oxyrase, Inc. 419-589-8800
175 Illinois Ave S, Mansfield, OH 44905
Anaerobic blood agar plates.

Pierce Bac-T, Inc.
367A County Road D W, New Brighton, MN 55112
Sheep blood agar.

Pml Microbiologicals 800-628-7014
27120 SW 95th Ave, Wilsonville, OR 97070

Remel 800-255-6730
12076 Santa Fe Dr, Lenexa, KS 66215

Smith River Biologicals 276-930-2369
9388 Charity Hwy, Ferrum, VA 24088
Various types of non-selective and non-differential culture media.

Trek Diagnostic Systems, Inc. 608-8373788
210 Business Park Dr, Sun Prairie, WI 53590
Various.

CULTURE MEDIA, PROPAGATING TRANSPORT
(Microbiology) 83JSN

Bd Diagnostic Systems 800-675-0908
7 Loveton Cir, Sparks, MD 21152

Smith River Biologicals 276-930-2369
9388 Charity Hwy, Ferrum, VA 24088
Various types of propagating transport culture media.

CULTURE MEDIA, SELECTIVE AND DIFFERENTIAL
(Microbiology) 83JSI

Advanced Biotechnologies, Inc. 800-426-0764
9108 Guilford Rd, Rivers Park II, Columbia, MD 21046

Atcc 800-638-6597
10801 University Blvd, PO Box 1549, Manassas, VA 20110
$20.00 for UNIPLUS cultures with its appropriate growth medium. $20.00 for PRECEPTROL cultures; popular rapid ID and antibiotic susceptibility control, testing, assay and teaching strains. Animal and plant viruses, microorganisms, algae, bacteria, fungi, protozoa, yeasts, chlamydiae, rickettsiae, cell lines and recombinant DNA materials. Biological cultures for quality control.

Bd Diagnostic Systems 800-675-0908
7 Loveton Cir, Sparks, MD 21152

Becton Dickinson And Co. 656-860-1553
2801 Industrial Dr, Monona, WI 53713
Culture media.

Biomed Diagnostics, Inc. 541-830-3000
1388 Antelope Rd, White City, OR 97503
Dermatophyte test medium.

CULTURE MEDIA, SELECTIVE AND DIFFERENTIAL *(cont'd)*

Culture Kits, Inc. 888-680-6853
14 Prentice St, PO Box 748, Norwich, NY 13815
STREP-KIT selective media strep; URI-THREE urine culture; STAPH-KIT staphylococcus aureus test kit; CANDI-KIT candida albicans test kit.

Gibson Laboratories, Inc. 859-254-9500
1040 Manchester St, Lexington, KY 40508
Tergitol agar h with ttc.

Hardy Diagnostics 800-226-2222
1430 W McCoy Ln, Santa Maria, CA 93455
Various culture media for the selective isolation and differentation of micro-organisms from clinical specimens.

Healthlink 904-996-7758
3611 St Johns Bluff Rd S Ste 1, Jacksonville, FL 32224
Selective media.

Impact Diagnostic International 909-621-5118
748 E Bonita Ave Ste 211, Pomona, CA 91767
Various type of microbiological media, culture media, selective and differential.

Ivoclar Vivadent, Inc. 800-533-6825
175 Pineview Dr, Amherst, NY 14228
CRT BACTERIA

Key Scientific Products 325-773-3918
1113 E Reynolds St, Stamford, TX 79553
Multiple-media for use in isolating and indentifying organisms.

Ml Lifesciences 949-699-3800
17 Hammond Ste 408, Irvine, CA 92618

Oral Biotech 541-928-4445
812 Water Ave NE, Albany, OR 97321

Oxoid, Inc. 800-567-8378
800 Proctor Ave, Ogdensburg, NY 13669
Dehydrated.

Pml Microbiologicals 800-628-7014
27120 SW 95th Ave, Wilsonville, OR 97070

Remel 800-255-6730
12076 Santa Fe Dr, Lenexa, KS 66215

Sabhi, Inc. 601-956-3169
1303 Riverwood Dr, Jackson, MS 39211
Various types of culture media (selective and differential).

Smith River Biologicals 276-930-2369
9388 Charity Hwy, Ferrum, VA 24088
Various types of selective and differential culture media.

CULTURE MEDIA, SELECTIVE AND NON-DIFFERENTIAL
(Microbiology) 83JSJ

Acuderm Inc. 800-327-0015
5370 NW 35th Ter Ste 106, Fort Lauderdale, FL 33309
Fungal culture media.

Alpha Biosciences, Inc. 877-825-7428
3651 Clipper Mill Rd, Baltimore, MD 21211
Various types of selective culture media.

Anaerobe Systems 408-782-7557
15906 Concord Cir, Morgan Hill, CA 95037
Campylobacter selective medium.

Bd Diagnostic Systems 800-675-0908
7 Loveton Cir, Sparks, MD 21152

Becton Dickinson And Co. 656-860-1553
2801 Industrial Dr, Monona, WI 53713
Various bbl selective and non-differential culture media.

Culture Kits, Inc. 888-680-6853
14 Prentice St, PO Box 748, Norwich, NY 13815
DERM-KIT dermathophyte test kit.

Gibson Laboratories, Inc. 859-254-9500
1040 Manchester St, Lexington, KY 40508
Columbia cna.

Healthlink 904-996-7758
3611 St Johns Bluff Rd S Ste 1, Jacksonville, FL 32224
Multiple.

Northeast Laboratory Services, Inc. 800-244-8378
227 China Rd, Winslow, ME 04901
Prepared microbiological culture media.

Oxoid, Inc. 800-567-8378
800 Proctor Ave, Ogdensburg, NY 13669
Dehydrated.

CULTURE MEDIA, SELECTIVE AND NON-DIFFERENTIAL *(cont'd)*

Oxyrase, Inc. 419-589-8800
175 Illinois Ave S, Mansfield, OH 44905
Various types of kanamycin,vancomycin laced blood agar plates.

Pml Microbiologicals 800-628-7014
27120 SW 95th Ave, Wilsonville, OR 97070

Remel 800-255-6730
12076 Santa Fe Dr, Lenexa, KS 66215

Smith River Biologicals 276-930-2369
9388 Charity Hwy, Ferrum, VA 24088
Various types of selective and non-differential culture media.

CULTURE MEDIA, SELECTIVE BROTH *(Microbiology) 83JSD*

Bd Diagnostic Systems 800-675-0908
7 Loveton Cir, Sparks, MD 21152

Biomerieux Industry 800-634-7656
595 Anglum Rd, Hazelwood, MO 63042

Gibson Laboratories, Inc. 859-254-9500
1040 Manchester St, Lexington, KY 40508
Brain heart infusion with 6.5% nacl.

Healthlink 904-996-7758
3611 St Johns Bluff Rd S Ste 1, Jacksonville, FL 32224
Gn broth.

Northeast Laboratory Services, Inc. 800-244-8378
227 China Rd, Winslow, ME 04901
Prepared microbiological culture media.

Oxoid, Inc. 800-567-8378
800 Proctor Ave, Ogdensburg, NY 13669
Dehydrated.

Pml Microbiologicals 800-628-7014
27120 SW 95th Ave, Wilsonville, OR 97070

Remel 800-255-6730
12076 Santa Fe Dr, Lenexa, KS 66215

Smith River Biologicals 276-930-2369
9388 Charity Hwy, Ferrum, VA 24088
Various types of selective broth culture media.

CULTURE MEDIA, SINGLE BIOCHEMICAL TEST
(Microbiology) 83JSF

Anaerobe Systems 408-782-7557
15906 Concord Cir, Morgan Hill, CA 95037
Lombard-dowell (ld) glucose agar.

Bd Diagnostic Systems 800-675-0908
7 Loveton Cir, Sparks, MD 21152

Biomerieux Industry 800-634-7656
595 Anglum Rd, Hazelwood, MO 63042

Gibson Laboratories, Inc. 859-254-9500
1040 Manchester St, Lexington, KY 40508
Cystine tryptic agar with dulcitol.

Microbiological Specialties 602-867-7323
3311 E Charter Oak Rd, Phoenix, AZ 85032
Various media and test (litmus milk).

Northeast Laboratory Services, Inc. 800-244-8378
227 China Rd, Winslow, ME 04901
Prepared microbiological culture media.

Pml Microbiologicals 800-628-7014
27120 SW 95th Ave, Wilsonville, OR 97070

Remel 800-255-6730
12076 Santa Fe Dr, Lenexa, KS 66215

Smith River Biologicals 276-930-2369
9388 Charity Hwy, Ferrum, VA 24088
Various types of single biochemical test culture media.

CULTURE MEDIA, SUPPLEMENTS *(Microbiology) 83JSK*

Advanced Biotechnologies, Inc. 800-426-0764
9108 Guilford Rd, Rivers Park II, Columbia, MD 21046

Bd Diagnostic Systems 800-675-0908
7 Loveton Cir, Sparks, MD 21152

Bd Lee Laboratories 800-732-9150
1475 Athens Hwy, Grayson, GA 30017
Bacterial enrichments.

Becton Dickinson And Co. 656-860-1553
2801 Industrial Dr, Monona, WI 53713
Various bbl media supplements.

Biocell Laboratories, Inc. 800-222-8382
2001 E University Dr, Rancho Dominguez, CA 90220
Fetal, neonate, and cadet bovine sera.

CULTURE MEDIA, SUPPLEMENTS *(cont'd)*

Hardy Diagnostics 800-226-2222
1430 W McCoy Ln, Santa Maria, CA 93455
Various culture media for the cultivation of fastidious micro-organisms.

Incell Corporation, Llc 210-877-0100
12734 Cimarron Path, San Antonio, TX 78249
Supplement mix.

Northeast Laboratory Services, Inc. 800-244-8378
227 China Rd, Winslow, ME 04901
Prepared microbiological culture media.

Pml Microbiologicals 800-628-7014
27120 SW 95th Ave, Wilsonville, OR 97070

Remel 800-255-6730
12076 Santa Fe Dr, Lenexa, KS 66215

CULTURE MEDIA, SYNTHETIC CELL AND TISSUE *(Pathology) 88KIT*

Diagnostic Hybrids, Inc. 740-589-3300
1055 E State St Ste 100, Athens, OH 45701
Tissue culture media.

Hyclone Laboratories, Inc. 435-792-8000
925 W 1800 S, Logan, UT 84321
Various (serum-free).

Incell Corporation, Llc 210-877-0100
12734 Cimarron Path, San Antonio, TX 78249
M3 family of media.

Lonza Walkersville, Inc. 201-316-9200
8830 Biggs Ford Rd, Walkersville, MD 21793
Serum-free media.

Mediatech, Inc. 800-235-5476
13884 Park Center Rd, Herndon, VA 20171

Millipore Corporation 877-246-2247
290 Concord Rd, Billerica, MA 01821
Tissue culture containers.

Nova-Tech, Inc. 308-381-8841
1982 E Citation Way, Central Ne. Regional Airport
Grand Island, NE 68801
Animal and human sera.

Oral Health Products, Inc. 918-622-9412
6847 E 40th St, Tulsa, OK 74145
Poh disclosing wafers.

Safc Biosciences, Inc. 913-469-5580
320 Swamp Bridge Rd, Denver, PA 17517
Various.

Safc Biosciences, Inc. 913-469-5580
13804 W 107th St, Lenexa, KS 66215

Scytek Laboratories, Inc. 435-755-9848
205 S 600 W, Logan, UT 84321
Media and components, synthetic cell and tissue culture.

Sigma-Aldrich Manufacturing, Llc. 913-469-5580
3506 S Broadway, Saint Louis, MO 63118
Various synthetic cell and tissue cultures.

Terumo Medical Corporation 800-283-7866
950 Elkton Blvd, P.O.Box 605, Elkton, MD 21921
Terumo sensibead eia progesterone kit.

CULTURE MEDIA, VITAMIN ASSAY *(Microbiology) 83JSB*

Bd Diagnostic Systems 800-675-0908
7 Loveton Cir, Sparks, MD 21152

CULTURED ANIMAL AND HUMAN CELLS *(Pathology) 88KIR*

Abbott Molecular, Inc. 847-937-6100
1300 E Touhy Ave, Des Plaines, IL 60018
Quality control slides.

Diagnostic Hybrids, Inc. 740-589-3300
1055 E State St Ste 100, Athens, OH 45701
Various.

Lampire Biological Laboratories 215-795-2838
PO Box 270, Pipersville, PA 18947
Defibrinated sheep blood, sterile; animal blood in Alsever's, sheep/horse/bovine, defibrinated horse blood; sterile, washed sheep red blood cells, 10%; goose blood/chicken blood/rabbit blood and guinea pig blood.

Powell Products, Inc. 800-840-9205
4940 Northpark Dr, Colorado Springs, CO 80918
Sterile individually packaged DNA collection swabs

CULTURED ANIMAL AND HUMAN CELLS *(cont'd)*

Qc Sciences 866-709-0523
4851 Lake Brook Dr, Glen Allen, VA 23060
Qcs control slides.

Tripath Imaging, Inc. 919-206-7140
780 Plantation Dr, Burlington, NC 27215
Tissue and cell line controls.

Ventana Medical Systems, Inc. 800-227-2155
1910 E Innovation Park Dr, Oro Valley, AZ 85755
Various tissue and cell line control slides.

CUP, DENTURE *(Dental And Oral) 76QNT*

Denplus Inc. 800-344-4424
205 - 1221 Labadie, Longueuil, QUE J4N 1E2 Canada

Hager Worldwide, Inc. 800-328-2335
13322 Byrd Dr, Odessa, FL 33556
DENTO BOX (denture box).

Lang Dental Manufacturing Co., Inc. 800-222-5264
175 Messner Dr, Wheeling, IL 60090
Denture duplicator flasks for fabricating temporary or duplicate dentures in 45 minutes. Priced at $88.00.

Lsl Industries, Inc. 888-225-5575
5535 N Wolcott Ave, Chicago, IL 60640
$31.50 per case of 250 denture containers.

Maddak Inc. 800-443-4926
661 State Route 23, Wayne, NJ 07470
ABLEWARE.

Medegen Medical Products, Llc 800-233-1987
209 Medegen Drive, Gallaway, TN 38036-0228
ROOM-MATES Disposable, sterilizable, plastic.

Moyco Technologies, Inc. 800-331-8837
200 Commerce Dr, Montgomeryville, PA 18936

Polar Plastic Ltd. 514-331-0207
4210 Thimens Blvd., St. Laurent, QUE H4R 2B9 Canada
POLAR RX. Blue PPR embossed lid ID loose fit lid.

Ross Disposable Products 800-649-6526
401 Traders Blvd E, Unit 10, Mississauga, ON L4Z 2H8 Canada

CUP, EYE *(Ophthalmology) 86LXQ*

Afassco, Inc. 800-441-6774
2244 Park Pl Ste C, Minden, NV 89423
Plastic eye cups.

Healer Products, Llc 914-663-6300
427 Commerce Ln Ste 1, West Berlin, NJ 08091
Cup, eye.

Maddak Inc. 800-443-4926
661 State Route 23, Wayne, NJ 07470
ABLEWARE.

Oculo Plastik Inc. 888-381-3292
200 Sauve West, Montreal, QUE H3L-1Y9 Canada
Red rubber ophthalmic suction cups for prostheses and protective shield removal.

Ware Medics Glass Works, Inc. 845-429-6950
PO Box 368, Garnerville, NY 10923
Eye wash cups.

CUP, GERIATRIC FEEDING *(General) 80QNV*

Medegen Medical Products, Llc 800-233-1987
209 Medegen Drive, Gallaway, TN 38036-0228
ROOM-MATES Sterilizable plastic.

CUP, MEDICINE *(General) 80QNW*

Crosstex International 800-223-2497
10 Ranick Rd, Hauppauge, NY 11788
Plastic or paper cups.

Crosstex International Ltd., W. Region 800-707-2737
14059 Stage Rd, Santa Fe Springs, CA 90670
Plastic or paper cups.

Crosstex International,Inc. 888-276-7783
10 Ranick Rd, Hauppauge, NY 11788
CROSSTEX Plastic or paper cups.

Cypress Medical Products 800-334-3646
1202 S. Rte. 31, McHenry, IL 60050
Polypropylene, graduated, 1oz. medicine cups.

Medegen Medical Products, Llc 800-233-1987
209 Medegen Drive, Gallaway, TN 38036-0228
ROOM-MATES Disposable and stainless steel.

CUP, MEDICINE *(cont'd)*

Medi-Dose, Inc. 800-523-8966
70 Industrial Dr, Ivyland, PA 18974

Oak Ridge Products 888-650-7444
211 Berg St, Algonquin, IL 60102
One ounce graduated, polypropylene.

Polar Plastic Ltd. 514-331-0207
4210 Thimens Blvd., St. Laurent, QUE H4R 2B9 Canada
POLAR RX. 1oz PPR 7.5cc/ml 2.5cc/ml markings.

Polar Ware Co. 800-237-3655
2806 N 15th St, Sheboygan, WI 53083
Stainless steel, reusable plastic.

Poly Scientific R&D Corp. 800-645-5825
70 Cleveland Ave, Bay Shore, NY 11706
Pre-filled cups in various sizes. Wide-mouth cups also available.

Profex Medical Products 800-325-0196
2224 E Person Ave, Memphis, TN 38114

Ross Disposable Products 800-649-6526
401 Traders Blvd E, Unit 10, Mississauga, ON L4Z 2H8 Canada

Ware Medics Glass Works, Inc. 845-429-6950
PO Box 368, Garnerville, NY 10923
Medicine glasses with or without lip.

CUP, PROPHYLAXIS *(Dental And Oral) 76EHK*

Abrasive Technology, Inc. 740-548-4100
8400 Green Meadows Dr N, Lewis Center, OH 43035
Accessory to oral cavity abrasive polishing agent.

Allpro, Inc. 423-587-2199
6930 W 116th Ave Ste 10, P.o. Box 733, Broomfield, CO 80020
Prophy cup (screw type, snap-on and latch mandrel styles).

Anderson Moulds, Inc. 209-943-1145
3131 E Anita St, Stockton, CA 95205
Single use prophylaxis angle.

Bradrock Industries, Inc. 757-224-0177
75 Bradrock Dr, Des Plaines, IL 60018
Dental prophy, angle prophy.

Buffalo Dental Mfg. Co., Inc. 516-496-7200
159 Lafayette Dr, Syosset, NY 11791
Prophylaxis cup.

Dental Resources 717-866-7571
52 King St, Myerstown, PA 17067
Prophy cups.

Denticator International, Inc. 800-325-1881
13705 Shoreline Ct E, Earth City, MO 63045
$22.00 for 144 units (various sizes); $54.95 per 164 pcs. of disposable Prophy angles incl. Prophy cups.

Floss & Go, Inc. 310-394-6700
1112 Montana Ave Ste D, Santa Monica, CA 90403
Prophy paste.

Miltex Dental Technologies, Inc. 516-576-6022
589 Davies Dr, York, PA 17402
Prophy cups.

Pac-Dent Intl., Inc. 909-839-0888
21078 Commerce Point Dr, Walnut, CA 91789
Prophy cup.

Preventive Technologies, Inc. 704-849-2416
1150 Crews Rd Ste H, Matthews, NC 28105
Disposable prophy angle.

Ultradent Products, Inc. 801-553-4586
505 W 10200 S, South Jordan, UT 84095
Prophylaxis cups.

Water Pik, Inc. 970-221-6129
1730 E Prospect Rd, Fort Collins, CO 80525
Various models.

Young Innovations, Inc. 800-325-1881
13705 Shoreline Ct E, Earth City, MO 63045

3m Espe Dental Products 651-733-7767
2501 Otis Corley Dr, Bentonville, AR 72712
Singles Disposable Prophy Angles

CURETTE *(Orthopedics) 87HTF*

Abbott Spine, Inc. 847-937-6100
12708 Riata Vista Cir Ste B-100, Austin, TX 78727
Curette.

CURETTE *(cont'd)*

Biomet Microfixation Inc. 800-874-7711
1520 Tradeport Dr, Jacksonville, FL 32218
Curette.

Biomet, Inc. 574-267-6639
56 E Bell Dr, PO Box 587, Warsaw, IN 46582
Orthopedic curettes.

Carl Heyer, Inc. 800-284-5550
1872 Bellmore Ave, North Bellmore, NY 11710

Dental Usa, Inc. 815-363-8003
5005 McCullom Lake Rd, McHenry, IL 60050
Dental curette.

Depuy Spine, Inc. 800-227-6633
325 Paramount Dr, Raynham, MA 02767
Various types/sizes of curettes.

Dermatologic Lab & Supply, Inc. 800-831-6273
608 13th Ave, Council Bluffs, IA 51501
Surgical curette.

DJO Inc. 800-336-6569
1430 Decision St, Vista, CA 92081

Fehling Surgical Instruments 800-FEHLING
509 Broadstone Ln NW, Acworth, GA 30101

Fortrad Eye Instruments Corp. 973-543-2371
8 Franklin Rd, Mendham, NJ 07945

George Tiemann & Co. 800-843-6266
25 Plant Ave, Hauppauge, NY 11788

Health Supply Company Inc., The 770-452-0090
2902 Marlin Cir, Atlanta, GA 30341
ENDOCYTE (disposable) non-suction curette, obtains comprehensive sample of endometrial tissue for histological examination.

Holmed Corporation 508-238-3351
40 Norfolk Ave, South Easton, MA 02375

Invuity, Inc. 760-744-4447
334 Via Vera Cruz Ste 255, San Marcos, CA 92078
Curette.

Invuity, Inc. 415-655-2100
39 Stillman St, San Francisco, CA 94107

Kmedic 800-955-0559
190 Veterans Dr, Northvale, NJ 07647

Marina Medical Instruments, Inc. 800-697-1119
955 Shotgun Rd, Sunrise, FL 33326
Various.

Medgyn Products, Inc. 800-451-9667
328 Eisenhower Ln N, Lombard, IL 60148
ENDOSAMPLER, disposable curette for sampling the uterine endometrium.

Medtronic Sofamor Danek Instrument Manufacturing 901-396-3133
7375 Adrianne Pl, Bartlett, TN 38133
Multiple (orthopedic curettes).

Medtronic Sofamor Danek Usa, Inc. 901-396-3133
4340 Swinnea Rd, Memphis, TN 38118
Multiple (orthopedic curettes).

Milex Products, Inc. 800-621-1278
4311 N Normandy Ave, Chicago, IL 60634
$156.20 per box of 25 EXPLORA curettes (3-mm o.d. and 4-mm o.d.).

Pappas Surgical Instruments, Llc 508-429-1049
7 October Hill Rd, Holliston, MA 01746
Various types of curettes.

Precision Medical Manufacturing Corporation 866-633-4626
852 Seton Ct, Wheeling, IL 60090
Brun Bone Curettes,set of nine most used sizes, made of stainless steel with hollow handles tha are hard to bend or come apart from shank of curette.

Spine Wave, Inc. 203-944-9494
2 Enterprise Dr Ste 302, Shelton, CT 06484
Ring curette.

Symmetry Medical Usa, Inc. 574-267-8700
486 W 350 N, Warsaw, IN 46582
Manual surgical instrument for general use.

Symmetry Tnco 888-447-6661
15 Colebrook Blvd, Whitman, MA 02382

CURETTE *(cont'd)*

Trans American Medical / Tamsco Instruments 708-430-7777
7633 W 100th Pl, Bridgeview, IL 60455
Gynecological.

Tuzik Boston 800-886-6363
104 Longwater Dr, Assinippi Park, Norwell, MA 02061

Ussc Puerto Rico, Inc. 203-845-1000
Building 911-67, Sabanetas Industrial Park, Ponce, PR 00731
Surgical curette.

Warsaw Orthopedic, Inc. 901-396-3133
2500 Silveus Xing, Warsaw, IN 46582
Multiple (orthopedic curettes).

Whitney Products, Inc. 800-338-4237
6153 W Mulford St Ste C, Niles, IL 60714
WHITNEY; small blue plastic curette used to remove excess bone cement before implanting prosthetic hip or knee joints. Sterile and disposable. WHITNEY LARGE CURETTE; large yellow plastic curette used to remove excess bone cement before implanting prosthetic hip or knee joints. WHITNEY SCULPS FORK; black plastic sculps tool to remove large amounts of excess bone cement in hip and knee surgeries.

Zimmer Holdings, Inc. 800-613-6131
1800 W Center St, PO Box 708, Warsaw, IN 46580

Zimmer Spine, Inc. 800-655-2614
7375 Bush Lake Rd, Minneapolis, MN 55439
Curette.

CURETTE, ADENOID *(Ear/Nose/Throat) 77KBJ*

Aesculap Implant Systems Inc. 1-800-234-9179
3773 Corporate Pkwy, Center Valley, PA 18034

Bausch & Lomb Surgical 636-255-5051
3365 Tree Court Ind Blvd, Saint Louis, MO 63122

Biomet Microfixation Inc. 800-874-7711
1520 Tradeport Dr, Jacksonville, FL 32218
Curette, adenoid.

Clinimed, Incorporated 877-CLINIMED
303 Markus Ct, Sandy Brae Industrial Park, Newark, DE 19713

Toolmex Corporation 800-992-4766
1075 Worcester St, Natick, MA 01760

Tuzik Boston 800-886-6363
104 Longwater Dr, Assinippi Park, Norwell, MA 02061

CURETTE, BIOPSY, BRONCHOSCOPE (NON-RIGID)
(Anesthesiology) 73BST

Hcmi, Inc. 773-588-2444
2146 E Pythian St, Springfield, MO 65802
Flexion-distraction table.

International Hospital Supply Co. 800-398-9450
6914 Canby Ave Ste 105, Reseda, CA 91335

Tuzik Boston 800-886-6363
104 Longwater Dr, Assinippi Park, Norwell, MA 02061

CURETTE, BIOPSY, BRONCHOSCOPE (RIGID)
(Anesthesiology) 73JEL

Biomet Microfixation Inc. 800-874-7711
1520 Tradeport Dr, Jacksonville, FL 32218
Curette, biopsy, bronchoscope (rigid).

Tuzik Boston 800-886-6363
104 Longwater Dr, Assinippi Park, Norwell, MA 02061

CURETTE, EAR *(Ear/Nose/Throat) 77JYG*

Aesculap Implant Systems Inc. 1-800-234-9179
3773 Corporate Pkwy, Center Valley, PA 18034

Bausch & Lomb Surgical 636-255-5051
3365 Tree Court Ind Blvd, Saint Louis, MO 63122

Biomet Microfixation Inc. 800-874-7711
1520 Tradeport Dr, Jacksonville, FL 32218
Ear curette.

Bionix Development Corp. 800-551-7096
5154 Enterprise Blvd, Toledo, OH 43612
Various types of disposable ear curettes.

Clinimed, Incorporated 877-CLINIMED
303 Markus Ct, Sandy Brae Industrial Park, Newark, DE 19713

Ear Technology Corp. 800-327-8547
207 E Myrtle Ave, PO Box 1516, Johnson City, TN 37601

CURETTE, EAR *(cont'd)*

Fray Products Corp. 800-288-6580
2495 Main St, Buffalo, NY 14214
Disposable, flexible, available in four sizes, economical, safe, and effective.

George Tiemann & Co. 800-843-6266
25 Plant Ave, Hauppauge, NY 11788

Health Care Logistics, Inc. 800-848-1633
450 Town St, PO Box 25, Circleville, OH 43113
Various sizes and types of non-sterile disposable ear curettes.

Karetech, Llc 415-824-3769
3573 22nd St, San Francisco, CA 94114
Ear wax remover.

Kmedic 800-955-0559
190 Veterans Dr, Northvale, NJ 07647

Miltex Inc. 800-645-8000
589 Davies Dr, York, PA 17402
Disposable 19-320 Green ring tip, 19-321 White loop tip, 19-322 Blue small spoon tip, 19-323 Yellow large spoon tip.

Omni Medical Supply Inc. 800-860-6664
4153 Pioneer Dr, Commerce Township, MI 48390

Premier Medical Products 888-PREMUSA
1710 Romano Dr, Plymouth Meeting, PA 19462
Disposable Double-Ended Ear Curette in 3 different styles.

Princeton Medical Group, Inc. 800-875-0869
1189 Royal Links Dr, Mt Pleasant, SC 29466

Shoney Scientific, Inc. 262-970-0170
West 223 North 720 Saratoga Drive,, Suite 120, Waukesha, WI 53186
Ear curette.

Surgical Instrument Manufacturers, Inc. 800-521-2985
1650 Headland Dr, Fenton, MO 63026

Trans American Medical / Tamsco Instruments 708-430-7777
7633 W 100th Pl, Bridgeview, IL 60455

Tuzik Boston 800-886-6363
104 Longwater Dr, Assinippi Park, Norwell, MA 02061

CURETTE, ENDODONTIC *(Dental And Oral) 76EKT*

Acteon Inc. 800-289-6367
124 Gaither Dr Ste 140, Mount Laurel, NJ 08054

Aesculap Implant Systems Inc. 1-800-234-9179
3773 Corporate Pkwy, Center Valley, PA 18034

Biolase Technology, Inc. 888-424-6527
4 Cromwell, Irvine, CA 92618

Biomet Microfixation Inc. 800-874-7711
1520 Tradeport Dr, Jacksonville, FL 32218
Curette, endodontic.

Dental Usa, Inc. 815-363-8003
5005 McCullom Lake Rd, McHenry, IL 60050
Curette.

Miltex Dental Technologies, Inc. 516-576-6022
589 Davies Dr, York, PA 17402
Various endodontic curettes.

Pac-Dent Intl., Inc. 909-839-0888
21078 Commerce Point Dr, Walnut, CA 91789
Various types of curettes.

Premier Dental Products Co. 888-670-6100
1710 Romano Dr, PO Box 4500, Plymouth Meeting, PA 19462

CURETTE, ETHMOID *(Ear/Nose/Throat) 77KAO*

Aesculap Implant Systems Inc. 1-800-234-9179
3773 Corporate Pkwy, Center Valley, PA 18034

Clinimed, Incorporated 877-CLINIMED
303 Markus Ct, Sandy Brae Industrial Park, Newark, DE 19713

CURETTE, NASAL *(Ear/Nose/Throat) 77KAP*

Aesculap Implant Systems Inc. 1-800-234-9179
3773 Corporate Pkwy, Center Valley, PA 18034

Arlington Scientific, Inc. Asi 800-654-0146
1840 N Technology Dr, Springville, UT 84663
The Rhino-probe Curette is a sterile, disposable nasal mucosal collection device designed to collect the optimum specimen with little or no discomfort to the patient. Rhino-probe provides consistent and uniform mucosal samples with 100 to 1000 times more cells than any other method. Cells do not adhere to the device and no degranulation or distortion is seen after staining. Samples obtained can help determine cellular immunological response. Call us for more information.

CURETTE, NASAL *(cont'd)*

Bausch & Lomb Surgical 636-255-5051
3365 Tree Court Ind Blvd, Saint Louis, MO 63122

Biomet Microfixation Inc. 800-874-7711
1520 Tradeport Dr, Jacksonville, FL 32218
Curette, nasal.

Invotec Intl. 800-998-8580
6833 Phillips Industrial Blvd, Jacksonville, FL 32256
Curette nasal.

Kmedic 800-955-0559
190 Veterans Dr, Northvale, NJ 07647

Surgical Instrument Manufacturers, Inc. 800-521-2985
1650 Headland Dr, Fenton, MO 63026

CURETTE, OPERATIVE *(Dental And Oral) 76EKE*

Aesculap Implant Systems Inc. 1-800-234-9179
3773 Corporate Pkwy, Center Valley, PA 18034

Dental Usa, Inc. 815-363-8003
5005 McCullom Lake Rd, McHenry, IL 60050
Curette.

H & H Co. 909-390-0373
4435 E Airport Dr Ste 108, Ontario, CA 91761
Curette, sinus or bone.

Hu-Friedy Manufacturing Co., Inc. 800-483-7433
3232 N Rockwell St, Chicago, IL 60618

Pac-Dent Intl., Inc. 909-839-0888
21078 Commerce Point Dr, Walnut, CA 91789
Various types of curettes.

Premier Dental Products Co. 888-670-6100
1710 Romano Dr, PO Box 4500, Plymouth Meeting, PA 19462

Ultradent Products, Inc. 801-553-4586
505 W 10200 S, South Jordan, UT 84095
Enamel hatchet.

CURETTE, OPHTHALMIC *(Ophthalmology) 86HNZ*

Accutome, Inc. 610-889-0200
3222 Phoenixville Pike, Malvern, PA 19355
Various ophthalmic curette.

B. Graczyk, Inc. 269-782-2100
27826 Burmax Park, Dowagiac, MI 49047
Various types & sizes of curettes.

Bausch & Lomb Surgical 636-255-5051
3365 Tree Court Ind Blvd, Saint Louis, MO 63122

Demetech Corp. 888-324-2447
3530 NW 115th Ave, Doral, FL 33178
Opthalmic curette.

Eye Care And Cure 800-486-6169
4646 S Overland Dr, Tucson, AZ 85714
Curette.

Fortrad Eye Instruments Corp. 973-543-2371
8 Franklin Rd, Mendham, NJ 07945

Katena Products, Inc. 800-225-1195
4 Stewart Ct, Denville, NJ 07834

Rhein Medical, Inc. 800-637-4346
5460 Beaumont Center Blvd Ste 500, Suite 500, Tampa, FL 33634

Total Titanium, Inc. 618-473-2429
140 East Monroe St., Hecker, IL 62248
Various types of ophthalmic curettes.

CURETTE, PERIODONTIC *(Dental And Oral) 76EMS*

Aesculap Implant Systems Inc. 1-800-234-9179
3773 Corporate Pkwy, Center Valley, PA 18034

American Eagle Instruments, Inc. 406-549-7451
6575 Butler Creek Rd, Missoula, MT 59808
Various sizes & styles of periodontic instruments.

Arnold Tuber Industries 716-648-3363
97 Main St, Hamburg, NY 14075
Curette, periodontic, dental hand instruments.

Biomet Microfixation Inc. 800-874-7711
1520 Tradeport Dr, Jacksonville, FL 32218
Curette, periodontic.

Dental Usa, Inc. 815-363-8003
5005 McCullom Lake Rd, McHenry, IL 60050
Curette.

Dentalez Group 866-DTE-INFO
101 Lindenwood Dr Ste 225, Valleybrooke Corporate Center
Malvern, PA 19355

CURETTE, PERIODONTIC *(cont'd)*

Dentalez Group, Stardental Division 717-291-1161
1816 Colonial Village Ln, Lancaster, PA 17601
Rc cement non-staining.

H & H Co. 909-390-0373
4435 E Airport Dr Ste 108, Ontario, CA 91761
Curette, periodontic.

Hu-Friedy Manufacturing Co., Inc. 800-483-7433
3232 N Rockwell St, Chicago, IL 60618
$24.60 to $30.00 each, 160 types.

Micro-Dent Inc. 866-526-1166
379 Hollow Hill Rd, Wauconda, IL 60084
Curette, periodontic.

Nordent Manufacturing, Inc. 800-966-7336
610 Bonnie Ln, Elk Grove Village, IL 60007
$19.50 per unit (standard).

Pac-Dent Intl., Inc. 909-839-0888
21078 Commerce Point Dr, Walnut, CA 91789
Various types of curettes.

Pdt, Inc. 406-626-4153
12201 Moccasin Ct, Missoula, MT 59808
Various.

Premier Dental Products Co. 888-670-6100
1710 Romano Dr, PO Box 4500, Plymouth Meeting, PA 19462

Salvin Dental Specialties, Inc. 800-535-6566
3450 Latrobe Dr, Charlotte, NC 28211
Various types of periodontal curettes.

Sci-Dent, Inc. 800-323-4145
210 Dowdle St Ste 2, Algonquin, IL 60102

Suter Dental Manufacturing Company, Inc. 800-368-8376
632 Cedar St, Chico, CA 95928

Wykle Research, Inc. 775-887-7500
2222 College Pkwy, Carson City, NV 89706
Periodontic curette.

CURETTE, SUCTION, ENDOMETRIAL *(Obstetrics/Gyn) 85HHK*

Apple Medical Corp. 508-357-2700
28 Lord Rd Ste 135, Marlborough, MA 01752
One-touch.

Femsuite, Llc 415-561-2565
220 Halleck St Ste 120B, San Francisco, CA 94129
Endometrial suction curette.

Marina Medical Instruments, Inc. 800-697-1119
955 Shotgun Rd, Sunrise, FL 33326
Various.

Medical Systems, Inc. 800-441-1973
30 Winter Sport Ln, PO Box 966, Williston, VT 05495
Endometrial sampling device.

Milex Products, Inc. 800-621-1278
4311 N Normandy Ave, Chicago, IL 60634
$15.00 per unit (standard) with tis-u-trap; $232.50 per box of 50 of endometrial pipet curettes.

Ob Specialties, Inc. 800-325-6644
1799 Northwood Ct, Oakland, CA 94611

Premier Medical Products 888-PREMUSA
1710 Romano Dr, Plymouth Meeting, PA 19462

R Medical Supply 800-882-7578
620 Valley Forge Rd Ste F, Hillsborough, NC 27278

Rocket Medical Plc. 800-707-7625
150 Recreation Park Dr Ste 3, Hingham, MA 02043

Select Medical Systems 800-441-1973
30 Winter Sport Ln, PO Box 966, Williston, VT 05495
SELECTCELLS STANDARD Endometrial Sampling Device, 3.1mm diameter. SELECTCELLS MINI Endometrial Sampling Device, 1.9mm small-diameter.

Tuzik Boston 800-886-6363
104 Longwater Dr, Assinippi Park, Norwell, MA 02061

CURETTE, SURGICAL *(Surgery) 79FZS*

Acuderm Inc. 800-327-0015
5370 NW 35th Ter Ste 106, Fort Lauderdale, FL 33309
Disposable dermal curette.

Aesculap Implant Systems Inc. 1-800-234-9179
3773 Corporate Pkwy, Center Valley, PA 18034

Ascent Healthcare Solutions 480-763-5300
10232 S 51st St, Phoenix, AZ 85044
Curette.

CURETTE, SURGICAL *(cont'd)*

Bausch & Lomb Surgical 636-255-5051
3365 Tree Court Ind Blvd, Saint Louis, MO 63122

Cardinal Health, Snowden Pencer Products 847-689-8410
5175 S Royal Atlanta Dr, Tucker, GA 30084
Various types of currettes.

Codman & Shurtleff, Inc 800-225-0460
325 Paramount Dr, Raynham, MA 02767

E-Global Medical Equipment, L.L.C. 866-422-1845
2f 500 Lincoln St., Allston, MA 02134
Curette, surgical, general use.

Elmed, Inc. 630-543-2792
60 W Fay Ave, Addison, IL 60101

George Tiemann & Co. 800-843-6266
25 Plant Ave, Hauppauge, NY 11788

In'Tech Medical, Incorporated 757-224-0177
2851 Lamb Pl Ste 15, Memphis, TN 38118
Curette.

Katena Products, Inc. 800-225-1195
4 Stewart Ct, Denville, NJ 07834

Koros Usa, Inc. 805-529-0825
610 Flinn Ave, Moorpark, CA 93021
Grasper, cup forceps, curette.

Lenox-Maclaren Surgical Corp. 720-890-9660
657 S Taylor Ave Ste A, Colorado Technology Center
Louisville, CO 80027
Curette, surgical / all different.

Medtronic, Inc. 800-633-8766
710 Medtronic Pkwy, Minneapolis, MN 55432
Kyphon Express

Princeton Medical Group, Inc. 800-875-0869
1189 Royal Links Dr, Mt Pleasant, SC 29466

Roboz Surgical Instrument Co., Inc. 800-424-2984
PO Box 10710, Gaithersburg, MD 20898

Zimmer Holdings, Inc. 800-613-6131
1800 W Center St, PO Box 708, Warsaw, IN 46580

Zimmer Trabecular Metal Technology 800-613-6131
10 Pomeroy Rd, Parsippany, NJ 07054
Ring curette, straight.

CURETTE, SURGICAL, DENTAL *(Dental And Oral) 76EMK*

Aesculap Implant Systems Inc. 1-800-234-9179
3773 Corporate Pkwy, Center Valley, PA 18034

Arnold Tuber Industries 716-648-3363
97 Main St, Hamburg, NY 14075
Curette, surgical, dental, dental hand instruments.

Biomet Microfixation Inc. 800-874-7711
1520 Tradeport Dr, Jacksonville, FL 32218
Curette, surgical dental.

Dental Usa, Inc. 815-363-8003
5005 McCullom Lake Rd, McHenry, IL 60050
Curette.

Hu-Friedy Manufacturing Co., Inc. 800-483-7433
3232 N Rockwell St, Chicago, IL 60618
$28.80 to $43.65 each, 18 types.

Kmedic 800-955-0559
190 Veterans Dr, Northvale, NJ 07647

Nordent Manufacturing, Inc. 800-966-7336
610 Bonnie Ln, Elk Grove Village, IL 60007
$29.50 per unit (standard).

Pac-Dent Intl., Inc. 909-839-0888
21078 Commerce Point Dr, Walnut, CA 91789
Various types of curettes.

Premier Dental Products Co. 888-670-6100
1710 Romano Dr, PO Box 4500, Plymouth Meeting, PA 19462

Salvin Dental Specialties, Inc. 800-535-6566
3450 Latrobe Dr, Charlotte, NC 28211
Various types of curettes.

Sci-Dent, Inc. 800-323-4145
210 Dowdle St Ste 2, Algonquin, IL 60102

Toolmex Corporation 800-992-4766
1075 Worcester St, Natick, MA 01760

CURETTE, UTERINE *(Obstetrics/Gyn) 85HCY*

Allied Healthcare Products, Inc. 800-444-3954
1720 Sublette Ave, Saint Louis, MO 63110

CURETTE, UTERINE *(cont'd)*

Biomet Microfixation Inc. 800-874-7711
1520 Tradeport Dr, Jacksonville, FL 32218
Curette, uterine.

British Marketing Enterprises, Inc. 800-358-8220
1825 Bush St, San Francisco, CA 94109
Full listing is curette laminaria.

Busse Hospital Disposables, Inc. 631-435-4711
75 Arkay Dr, Hauppauge, NY 11788
Various sizes of sterite, straight or curved curettes.

Coopersurgical, Inc. 800-243-2974
95 Corporate Dr, Trumbull, CT 06611
23 models, priced from $55 to $90.

Femsuite, Llc 415-561-2565
220 Halleck St Ste 120B, San Francisco, CA 94129
Endocervical curette.

Gyrus Acmi, Inc. 508-804-2739
93 N Pleasant St, Norwalk, OH 44857
Curette, urterine.

Health Supply Company Inc., The 770-452-0090
2902 Marlin Cir, Atlanta, GA 30341
ENDOCYTE (disposable) non-suction curette, obtains comprehensive sample of endometrial tissue for histological examination.

Karl Storz Endoscopy-America Inc. 800-421-0837
600 Corporate Pointe, Culver City, CA 90230

Kmedic 800-955-0559
190 Veterans Dr, Northvale, NJ 07647

Marina Medical Instruments, Inc. 800-697-1119
955 Shotgun Rd, Sunrise, FL 33326
Various.

Medgyn Products, Inc. 800-451-9667
328 Eisenhower Ln N, Lombard, IL 60148
Disposable - Flex & Rigid sizes 4mm-16mm.

Milex Products, Inc. 800-621-1278
4311 N Normandy Ave, Chicago, IL 60634
$156.20 per box of 25 endometrial explora curettes.

Miltex Inc. 800-645-8000
589 Davies Dr, York, PA 17402

Premier Medical Products 888-PREMUSA
1710 Romano Dr, Plymouth Meeting, PA 19462

Princeton Medical Group, Inc. 800-875-0869
1189 Royal Links Dr, Mt Pleasant, SC 29466

R Medical Supply 800-882-7578
620 Valley Forge Rd Ste F, Hillsborough, NC 27278

Rms Medical Products 800-624-9600
24 Carpenter Rd, Chester, NY 10918
The Curette, minimizes patient discomfort. Round tip allows for safer insertion. Sharp cutting edge assures adequate tissue sample. Centimeter markings permit a uterine length measurement. Malleable shaft conforms to the shape of the uterus. Curette available in 2mm and 3mm sizes to accommodate post- and premenopausal uteri.

Rocket Medical Plc. 800-707-7625
150 Recreation Park Dr Ste 3, Hingham, MA 02043

Thomas Medical Inc. 800-556-0349
5610 West 82 2nd Street, Indianpolis, IN 46278

Toolmex Corporation 800-992-4766
1075 Worcester St, Natick, MA 01760

Tuzik Boston 800-886-6363
104 Longwater Dr, Assinippi Park, Norwell, MA 02061

CURING UNIT, ACRYLIC *(Dental And Oral) 76VEH*

Concepts International, Inc. 800-627-9729
224 E Main St, Summerton, SC 29148
Curing Light Shield--hand-held flat and curved curing light shield and tipshield for curing guns.

CURING UNIT, ACRYLIC *(cont'd)*

Kinetic Instruments, Inc. 800-233-2346
17 Berkshire Blvd, Bethel, CT 06801
The SunliteLAZER High Intensity curing and handpiece illumination system combines LED light curing technology with fiberoptic handpiece illumination. The power supply has two independent variable output circuits that support any brand dental handpiece, even two different brand handpieces on the same dental unit. The third circuit supports an LED curing light that is integrated with the dental unit ie.- stores on the dental hanger and operates with the dental unit foot control. The LED curing light provides heat-free, noise-free blue light at precisely the 470-nm range required to cure CQ initiated composites at 2.5mm thickness in 5 seconds. Sunlite fiber optic illumination systems are also available without the curing light circuitry in 2 circuit and 3 circuit variable output models. The TransCure Portable LED curing light and transilluminator is a battery-operated design that can provide 1000 cures on a single recharge, with transillumination capability. The device offers both noise-free, heat-free blue LED light for restorative curing and white LED light for visual transillumination procedures indicating fractures, caries, and obliterated canals.

Lang Dental Manufacturing Co., Inc. 800-222-5264
175 Messner Dr, Wheeling, IL 60090
AQUAPRES pressure curing vessels priced at $195.00.

Lemoy International, Inc. 847-427-0840
95 King St, Elk Grove Village, IL 60007
INITIATOR 150 watts of Xenon power, 100% American made and made to order.

Sterngold 800-243-9942
23 Frank Mossberg Dr, PO Box 2967, Attleboro, MA 02703
Stern-Tech Light Box - A light-polymerization unit using the combination of UVA and blue light universal field operation.

CURRENT LIMITER, PATIENT LEADS *(Cardiovascular) 74QNX*

Rf Industries, Inc. 800-233-1728
7610 Miramar Rd, San Diego, CA 92126
Our Bioconnect division provides cable and lead wires for connecting an individual to a machine, including ECG snap leads, ECG patient cables, resting ECG cables, apnea cables and leads, DIN safety systems, and pressure-monitoring products.

CURTAIN, CUBICLE *(General) 80QNY*

Atd-American Co. 800-523-2300
135 Greenwood Ave, Wyncote, PA 19095

Best Manufacturing Group Llc 800-843-3233
1633 Broadway Fl 18, New York, NY 10019
Fire retardent.

Bruin Plastics Co. 800-556-7764
61 Joslin Rd, Glendale, RI 02826

Colonial Scientific Ltd. 902-468-1811
201 Brownlow Ave., Unit 52, Dartmouth, NS B3B-1W2 Canada
Cubicle curtains, and track

Covoc Corp. 800-725-3266
1194 E Valencia Dr, Fullerton, CA 92831
Cubicle curtains and cubicle track.

Crest Healthcare Supply 800-328-8908
195 3rd St, Dassel, MN 55325

Dazian Fabrics,Llc. 877-232-9426
124 Enterprise Ave S, PO Box 2121, Secaucus, NJ 07094
Curtains and draperies.

Fablok Mills, Inc. 908-464-1950
140 Spring St, New Providence, NJ 07974
Cubicle curtain mesh. Mesh bags.

General Econopak, Inc. 888-871-8568
1725 N 6th St, Philadelphia, PA 19122
Disposable/multi-use, standard size 90 x 140 inch. All other sizes custom made to order.

Herculite Products, Inc. 800-772-0036
PO Box 435, Emigsville, PA 17318

Imperial Fastener Co., Inc. 954-782-7130
1400 SW 8th St, Pompano Beach, FL 33069
All items are custom made. Breakaway style cubical curtains and window draperies.

Independent Solutions, Inc. 847-498-0500
900 Skokie Blvd Ste 118, Northbrook, IL 60062
ARNCO Flame-retardant; with or w/o nylon mesh tops.

Medline Industries, Inc. 800-633-5886
1 Medline Pl, Mundelein, IL 60060

CURTAIN, CUBICLE *(cont'd)*

Postcraft Co. 800-528-4844
625 W Rillito St, Tucson, AZ 85705
Vinyl and mesh cubicle curtains.

Salsbury Industries 800-640-4341
1010 E 62nd St, Los Angeles, CA 90001

Standard Textile 800-999-0400
1 Knollcrest Dr, Cincinnati, OH 45237

Trax Cleanroom Products 800-520-8729
3352 Swetzer Rd, P.O. Box 2089, Loomis, CA 95650
Available in clear, translucent, or colored materials.

Waterloo Bedding Co. Ltd. 800-203-4293
141 Weber St. S, Waterloo, ONT N2J 2A9 Canada

Webb Manufacturing Co. 800-932-2634
1241 Carpenter St, Philadelphia, PA 19147

CURTAIN, PROTECTIVE, RADIOGRAPHIC *(Radiology) 90IWQ*

Aadco Medical, Inc. 800-225-9014
2279 VT Route 66, Randolph, VT 05060
X-ray protective drape.

Bar-Ray Products, Inc. 800-359-6115
95 Monarch St, Littlestown, PA 17340

Lite Tech, Inc. 610-650-8690
975 Madison Ave, Norristown, PA 19403
X-ray machine shields & curtains.

Shielding International, Inc. 800-292-2247
PO Box Z, 2150 NW Andrews Drive, Madras, OR 97741
Custom curtains; coated lead vinyl sheeting; blockers.

Trans American Medical, Inc. 801-796-7335
965 W 325 N, Lindon, UT 84042
Radiographic curtain.

CURTAIN, SHOWER *(General) 80TBP*

Atd-American Co. 800-523-2300
135 Greenwood Ave, Wyncote, PA 19095

Bruin Plastics Co. 800-556-7764
61 Joslin Rd, Glendale, RI 02826

Covoc Corp. 800-725-3266
1194 E Valencia Dr, Fullerton, CA 92831
Vinyl shower curtains, nylon shower curtains, decorative fabric shower curtains.

Herculite Products, Inc. 800-772-0036
PO Box 435, Emigsville, PA 17318

Hos-Pillow Corp. 800-468-7874
1011 Campus Dr, Mundelein, IL 60060
Vinyl shower curtain. All sizes.

Imperial Fastener Co., Inc. 954-782-7130
1400 SW 8th St, Pompano Beach, FL 33069
Curtains - fabric, size, color custom made.

Independent Solutions, Inc. 847-498-0500
900 Skokie Blvd Ste 118, Northbrook, IL 60062
Flame retardant, antibacterial, antimicrobial, mildewproof.

Postcraft Co. 800-528-4844
625 W Rillito St, Tucson, AZ 85705
Vinyl and nylon shower curtains. Deluxe Nylon Shower Curtain, white and champagne color, flame retardant, bacteria and mildew resistant, metal grommets, reversed bottom hem, machine washable. Sizes in 3'x6', 4'x6', and 6'x6' plus custom sizes.

Waterloo Bedding Co. Ltd. 800-203-4293
141 Weber St. S, Waterloo, ONT N2J 2A9 Canada

Webb Manufacturing Co. 800-932-2634
1241 Carpenter St, Philadelphia, PA 19147

CUSHION, DENTURE, OTC *(Dental And Oral) 76EHS*

K. W. Griffen Co. 203-846-1923
100 Pearl St, Norwalk, CT 06850
Denture cushions.

CUSHION, EARPHONE (FOR AUDIOMETRIC TESTING) *(Ear/Nose/Throat) 77ETT*

Audiology Products 877-218-6358
126 N Wenatchee Ave, c/o Pak It Rite, Wenatchee, WA 98801
Disposable audiometer earphone cushion cover.

Grason & Associates, Llc 603-899-3089
71 Conifer Rd, P.o. Box 289, Rindge, NH 03461
Accessory to audometers & auditory.

CUSHION, FLOTATION *(Physical Med) 89KIC*

Action Products, Inc. 800-228-7763
954 Sweeney Dr, Hagerstown, MD 21740
Low maintenance cushions for aid in the prevention of decubitus ulcers. Wide range of standard sizes available as well as custom sizes. Price range - $89 to $249 on standard items.

Alternative Products 904-378-9081
5351 Ramona Blvd Ste 7, Jacksonville, FL 32205
Wheelchair cushion.

Amf Support Surfaces, Inc. 951-549-6800
1691 N Delilah St, Corona, CA 92879
Flotation cushion.

Crown Mfg. Co. 905-545-2546
53 Gibson Ave, Hamilton L8L 6J7 Canada
Orthopaedic back cushions

E-Global Medical Equipment, L.L.C. 866-422-1845
2f 500 Lincoln St., Allston, MA 02134
Cushion, floatation.

Federal Foam Technologies, Inc. 715-490-7788
312 Industrial Rd, Ellsworth, WI 54011
Wheelchair cushion.

Grant Airmass Corporation 800-243-5237
126 Chestnut Hill Rd, PO Box 3456, Stamford, CT 06903
Powered flotation cushion.

Health Ent., Inc. 508-695-0727
90 George Leven Dr, North Attleboro, MA 02760
Flotation cushion.

Huntleigh Healthcare Llc. 800-223-1218
40 Christopher Way, Eatontown, NJ 07724
Various

Hydro-Med Products, Inc. 214-350-5100
3400 Royalty Row, Irving, TX 75062
Cushion, flotation.

Keen Mobility Company 503-285-9090
6500 NE Halsey St Ste B, Portland, OR 97213

Kinetic Concepts, Inc. 800-275-4524
8023 Vantage Dr, San Antonio, TX 78230
Flotation cushion.

Leeder Group, Inc. 305-436-5030
8508 NW 66th St, Miami, FL 33166
Gel foam flotation cushions.

Medisearch P.R., Inc. 787-864-0684
Machete Industrial Center, Guayama, PR 00784
Seat cushion.

Numotech, Inc. 818-772-1579
9420 Reseda Blvd Ste 504, Northridge, CA 91324
Pneumatic compression seat.

Paramount Manufacturing 503-612-8442
10360 SW Spokane Ct, Tualatin, OR 97062
Convoluted foam (eggcrate) mattress for beds and wheelchairs.

Roho Group, The 800-851-3449
100 N Florida Ave, Belleville, IL 62221
DRY FLOATATION products. Exclusive distributor of the ROHO DRY FLOATATION product line. Wheelchair cushion, accessories and mattresses.

Skedco, Inc. 503-639-2119
16420 SW 72nd Ave, PO Box 230487, Portland, OR 97224
Flotation system for rescue stretcher for SKED and basket stretcher.

Southwest Technologies, Inc. 800-247-9951
1746 E Levee St, North Kansas City, MO 64116
Gel cushion.

Sundance Enterprises, Inc. 317-831-6447
236 E Washington St, Po. Box 146, Mooresville, IN 46158
Various types of flaircair.

Tele-Made Disposables, Inc. 888-822-4299
3215 Huffman Eastgate Rd, Huffman, TX 77336
Gel mattress overlay.

Tss Foam Industries Corp. 716-538-2321
2770 Caledonia Leroy Rd, Caledonia, NY 14423
Gel cushion.

Tuffcare 800-367-6160
3999 E La Palma Ave, Anaheim, CA 92807

Wcw,Inc 518-686-0725
1 Mechanic St, Hoosick Falls, NY 12090
Cushion, flotation.

CUSHION, FLOTATION, THERAPEUTIC *(Physical Med) 89MOC*

Dallas Trim Industries Corp. 972-278-3598
2511 National Dr, Garland, TX 75041
No-sorz plus.

Leeder Group, Inc. 305-436-5030
8508 NW 66th St, Miami, FL 33166
Wheelchair cushion air pressure reducing.

Ongoing Care Solutions, Inc. 800-375-0207
6545 44th St N Ste 4007, Pinellas Park, FL 33781
Pressure reducing wheel chair cushion.

Tuffcare 800-367-6160
3999 E La Palma Ave, Anaheim, CA 92807

CUSHION, FOOT *(Orthopedics) 87QNZ*

Aetna Foot Products/Div. Of Aetna Felt Corporation 800-390-3668
2401 W Emaus Ave, Allentown, PA 18103
COMFOOT Brand and SCOTT FOOT CARE pre-cut foot pads.

Aetrex Worldwide, Inc 800-526-2739
414 Alfred Ave, Teaneck, NJ 07666
ANTI-SHOX, foot supports absorb shock and treat the discomfort of heel pain, arch strain and ball of foot ailments.

Alimed, Inc. 800-225-2610
297 High St, Dedham, MA 02026

Allman Products 800-223-6889
21101 Itasca St, Chatsworth, CA 91311

Bauerfeind Usa, Inc. 800-423-3405
55 Chastain Rd NW Ste 112, Kennesaw, GA 30144
VISCOPED S, full-length viscoelastic insole to relieve foot and joint pain.

Care Apparel Industries 800-326-6262
12709 91st Ave, Richmond Hill, NY 11418
For edema and diabetic foot conditions. Slippers for thoses with edema or diabetic condition.

Ehob, Inc. 800-899-5553
250 N Belmont Ave, Indianapolis, IN 46222
FOOT WAFFLE Air Cushion.

Emerald Medical Products Corp. 206-781-9450
2405 NW Market St Ste 305, Seattle, WA 98107
Cushions for Orthopedic Surgery (TIBIAL NAILING PILLOW and HENLEY'S INCLINE PILLOW)

Fabrite Laminating Corp. 973-777-1406
70 Passaic St, Wood Ridge, NJ 07075

Grand Rapids Foam Technologies 877-GET-GRFT
2788 Remico St SW, Wyoming, MI 49519

Hapad, Inc. 800-544-2723
5301 Enterprise Blvd, Bethel Park, PA 15102
100% natural wool felt orthopaedic foot products and sports replacement insoles for quick and effective treatment of common, painful foot complaints.

J. T. Posey Co. 800-447-6739
5635 Peck Rd, Arcadia, CA 91006

Langer, Inc. 800-645-5520
450 Commack Rd, Deer Park, NY 11729

Paramedical Distributors 800-245-3278
2020 Grand Blvd, Kansas City, MO 64108
Insoles, heel cushions, pads, materials, etc.

Pedifix, Inc. 800-424-5561
310 Guinea Rd, Brewster, NY 10509

Serum International Inc. 800-361-7726
4400 Autoroute Chomeoey, Laval, QUE H7R-6E9 Canada

Span-America Medical Systems, Inc. 800-888-6752
70 Commerce Ctr, Greenville, SC 29615
Foot drop stops and cast elevators.

Spenco Medical Corp. 254-772-6000
PO Box 2501, Waco, TX 76702
SPENCO® gel cushion insole.

CUSHION, OTHER *(General) 80QOD*

Alex Orthopedic, Inc. 800-544-2539
PO Box 201442, Arlington, TX 76006
Bed wedge.

Allman Products 800-223-6889
21101 Itasca St, Chatsworth, CA 91311
Sheepskin crutch cushion; foam wedge cushions, orthopedic cushions.

CUSHION, OTHER *(cont'd)*

Armstrong Medical Industries, Inc. 800-323-4220
575 Knightsbridge Pkwy, Lincolnshire, IL 60069
CPR kneeling pads.

Bryton Corp. 800-567-9500
4310 Guion Rd, Indianapolis, IN 46254
Cushions and pads for surgical, orthopedic, urology, obstetrical and surgical table accessories such as leg holders and knee rests.

Chamberlin Rubber Company, Inc. 585-427-7780
3333 Brighton Henrietta Town Line Rd, PO Box 22700
Rochester, NY 14623

Chestnut Ridge Foam, Inc. 800-234-2734
PO Box 781, Latrobe, PA 15650
CR SAFGUARD (flame-resistant) cushioning for x-ray pads & stretcher mattresses, bedrail pads, positioning devices, and seat cushioning

Comfort Care Products Corp. 803-321-0020
258 Industrial Park Rd, Newberry, SC 29108
Overlay pads.

Core Products International, Inc. 800-365-3047
808 Prospect Ave, Osceola, WI 54020
Inflatable backrest, adjust the level of support with the squeeze of a handle, deluxe foam-laminated cover for comfort, and 60' positioning belt.

Crest Healthcare Supply 800-328-8908
195 3rd St, Dassel, MN 55325
Bed pads.

Fabrite Laminating Corp. 973-777-1406
70 Passaic St, Wood Ridge, NJ 07075
reusable bed pad

Genesis Manufacturing, Inc. 317-485-7887
720 E Broadway St, Fortville, IN 46040
Contract Radio-Frequency (RF) Welding. From development to manufacturing and packaging.

Grand Rapids Foam Technologies 877-GET-GRFT
2788 Remico St SW, Wyoming, MI 49519
Facial Support, Gourney, Seating, Examination

Hermell Products, Inc. 800-233-2342
9 Britton Dr, PO Box 7345, Bloomfield, CT 06002
Foam slant bed wedge.

Homedics Inc. 800-333-8282
3000 N Pontiac Trl, Commerce Township, MI 48390
Inflatable travel pillows, seat bottoms, massage cushions and pillows.

Invacare Corporation 800-333-6900
1 Invacare Way, Elyria, OH 44035
KSS, ContourU, Shape Sensor, INVACARE, Infinity, Essential, PinDot, AirFlo, Silhouette, Personal Seat VF, Ulti-Mate, FloGel, ViscoFoam.

Langer, Inc. 800-645-5520
450 Commack Rd, Deer Park, NY 11729

Lohmann & Rauscher, Inc. 800-279-3863
6001 SW 6th Ave Ste 101, Topeka, KS 66615

Mccarty's Sacro-Ease Llc 800-635-3557
3329 Industrial Ave S, Coeur D Alene, ID 83815
MCBACK support.

Profex Medical Products 800-325-0196
2224 E Person Ave, Memphis, TN 38114

Regency Product International 800-845-7931
4732 E 26th St, Vernon, CA 90058
Available in any style.

Roho Group, The 800-851-3449
100 N Florida Ave, Belleville, IL 62221
MOSAIC cushion provides a functional and stable environment for clients at risk for or who have a history of skin breakdown. The cushion has interconnected air cells and the cover is washable, reusable and moisture-resistant.

Roloke Company 800-533-8212
127 W Hazel St, Inglewood, CA 90302
Good'n Bed nulti-positional bed wedge.

Southwest Technologies, Inc. 800-247-9951
1746 E Levee St, North Kansas City, MO 64116
Foot/elbow gel cushion.

Tetra Medical Supply Corp. 800-621-4041
6364 W Gross Point Rd, Niles, IL 60714

CUSHION, OTHER *(cont'd)*

Tri-State Hospital Supply Corp. 800-248-4058
301 Catrell Dr, PO Box 170, Howell, MI 48843
HUBGUARD adhesive cushions in several configurations and sizes for anchoring I.V. catheters.

CUSHION, RING, FOAM RUBBER *(General) 80QOA*

Chamberlin Rubber Company, Inc. 585-427-7780
3333 Brighton Henrietta Town Line Rd, PO Box 22700
Rochester, NY 14623

Grand Rapids Foam Technologies 877-GET-GRFT
2788 Remico St SW, Wyoming, MI 49519

Hermell Products, Inc. 800-233-2342
9 Britton Dr, PO Box 7345, Bloomfield, CT 06002
Foam convoluted invalid ring.

Invacare Corporation 800-333-6900
1 Invacare Way, Elyria, OH 44035
INVACARE.

Lundy Medical Product, Llc 480-473-7330
9376 E Bahia Dr Ste D101, Scottsdale, AZ 85260
Vinyl covered foam. Head rest disposable/reusable. Item no. 1008.

Sunrise Medical 800-333-4000
7477 Dry Creek Pkwy, Longmont, CO 80503

Tailored Label Products, Inc. 800-727-1344
W165N5731 Ridgewood Dr, Menomonee Falls, WI 53051

CUSHION, RING, INFLATABLE *(General) 80QOB*

Addto, Inc. 773-278-0294
816 N Kostner Ave, Chicago, IL 60651

Alimed, Inc. 800-225-2610
297 High St, Dedham, MA 02026
Inflatable, soft plastic barium ring for lower G.I. exam.

Hermell Products, Inc. 800-233-2342
9 Britton Dr, PO Box 7345, Bloomfield, CT 06002
Inflatable invalid ring.

Medical Devices International, Div. Of Plasco, Inc. 800-438-7634
512 N Lehmberg Rd, Columbus, MS 39702
Inflatable ring cushion, double wall construction, 17x15 in.

Ross Disposable Products 800-649-6526
401 Traders Blvd E, Unit 10, Mississauga, ON L4Z 2H8 Canada

CUSHION, STOOL *(General) 80QOC*

Brandt Industries, Inc. 800-221-8031
4461 Bronx Blvd, Bronx, NY 10470
Revolving stools, pneumatic stools, hydraulic stools, ergonomic task stool.

Bryton Corp. 800-567-9500
4310 Guion Rd, Indianapolis, IN 46254
Surgery stools, & replacement cushions, conductive & non-conductive.

Grand Rapids Foam Technologies 877-GET-GRFT
2788 Remico St SW, Wyoming, MI 49519

Profex Medical Products 800-325-0196
2224 E Person Ave, Memphis, TN 38114

Shamrock Medical, Inc. 503-233-5055
3620 SE Powell Blvd, Portland, OR 97202
Lumbar, hip and cervical cushions.

CUSHION, TABLE, SURGICAL *(Surgery) 79LWG*

Aadco Medical, Inc. 800-225-9014
2279 VT Route 66, Randolph, VT 05060
Replacement surgical table pads.

Bryton Corp. 800-567-9500
4310 Guion Rd, Indianapolis, IN 46254
Cushions and pads for all types of surgical, orthopedic, urology, and obstetrical tables.

Burlington Medical Supplies, Inc. 800-221-3466
3 Elmhurst St, PO Box 3194, Newport News, VA 23603

E-Global Medical Equipment, L.L.C. 866-422-1845
2f 500 Lincoln St., Allston, MA 02134
Surgical table cushion.

Grand Rapids Foam Technologies 877-GET-GRFT
2788 Remico St SW, Wyoming, MI 49519

Polymer Concepts, Inc. 877-820-3163
7561 Tyler Blvd Ste 8, Mentor, OH 44060
Various models of surgical table pads.

Royal Converting, Inc. 865-938-7828
1615 Highway 33 S, New Tazewell, TN 37825

CUSHION, WHEELCHAIR (PAD) *(Physical Med) 89IMP*

Action Products, Inc. 800-228-7763
954 Sweeney Dr, Hagerstown, MD 21740
XACT contour cushion and TWISTER Light cushion. Positioning cushions for wheelchair users in high risk of skin breakdown. Price range - $389 to 509 on standard sizes.

Activeaid, Inc. 800-533-5330
101 Activeaid Rd, Redwood Falls, MN 56283

Airerx Healthcare, Llc 615-244-3327
1843 Air Lane Dr, Nashville, TN 37210
Wheelchair cushion.

Alex Orthopedic, Inc. 800-544-2539
PO Box 201442, Arlington, TX 76006

Alimed, Inc. 800-225-2610
297 High St, Dedham, MA 02026

Alliance Prosthetics & Orthotics, Inc. 562-921-0353
14535 Valley View Ave Ste U, Santa Fe Spgs, CA 90670
Custom molded wheelchair seat & back inserts.

Allman Products 800-223-6889
21101 Itasca St, Chatsworth, CA 91311

Alternative Products 904-378-9081
5351 Ramona Blvd Ste 7, Jacksonville, FL 32205
Contour positioning cushion.

American Health Systems 800-234-6655
PO Box 26688, Greenville, SC 29616
ULTRAFORM; manufactures a standard 4' cushion, Low-Profile 2.5' cushion for the more active patient, a Wedge Cushion for positioning and pressure relief. Custom sizes available.

Anatomic Concepts, Inc. 951-549-6800
1691 N Delilah St, Corona, CA 92879
Wheelchair pad/cushion.

Aspen Seating, Llc 303-781-1633
4211 S Natches Ct Ste G, Sheridan, CO 80110
Wheelchair cushion.

Blue Earth, Inc. 518-237-5585
31 Ontario St, 2nd Floor - Front, Cohoes, NY 12047
Wheelchair cushion.

Broda Enterprises Inc. 800-668-0637
385 Phillip St., Waterloo, ONT N2L 5R8 Canada
BRODA SEATING.

Cfi Medical Solutions (Contour Fabricators, Inc.) 810-750-5300
14241 N Fenton Rd, Fenton, MI 48430

Chestnut Ridge Foam, Inc. 800-234-2734
PO Box 781, Latrobe, PA 15650
*TRIFLEX dual memory foam cushion. Two layers of high quality "memory foam". Descending increase in firmness to maximize pressure reduction benefits. Base support cushioning avoids "bottoming out". Top covering is a fluid-resistant four-way stretch fabric with a polyurethane coating. Base Covering: Durable no-slip vinyl. Heavy duty zippered cover * Also available without a zipper*

Comfort Care Products Corp. 803-321-0020
258 Industrial Park Rd, Newberry, SC 29108
NOVEX cover is antimicrobial, flame retardant ticking; foam wedged cushion, with gel insert.

Confortaire Inc 662-842-2966
2133 S Veterans Blvd, Tupelo, MS 38804
Cushion, wheelchair.

Creative Foam Medical Systems 800-446-4644
405 Industrial Dr, Bremen, IN 46506
Various types of coated foam cushions.

Dallas Trim Industries Corp. 972-278-3598
2511 National Dr, Garland, TX 75041
Wheelchair cushion.

David Scott Company 800-804-0333
59 Fountain St, Framingham, MA 01702
Available in BLUE DIAMOND gel and gel/foam.

Doh,Ddsd,Csb 505-841-5287
1000 Main St NW, P.o. Box 1269, Los Lunas, NM 87031
Custom molded seating systems.

Dynamic Systems, Inc. 828-683-3523
235 Sunlight Dr, Leicester, NC 28748
Orthopedic viscoelastic cushion material: SunMate, Pudgee, Laminar, and Liquid SunMate FIPS (foam-in-place seating).

E-Global Medical Equipment, L.L.C. 866-422-1845
2f 500 Lincoln St., Allston, MA 02134
Wheelchair seat & back cushions, inserts.

CUSHION, WHEELCHAIR (PAD) *(cont'd)*

Easy Seat Llc 877-327-9732
2361 S 1560 W Ste 200, Woods Cross, UT 84087
Wheel chair cushion.

Essential Medical Supply, Inc. 800-826-8423
6420 Hazeltine National Dr, Orlando, FL 32822
REHAB 1.

Freedom Designs, Inc. 800-331-8551
2241 N Madera Rd, Simi Valley, CA 93065

Genesis Manufacturing, Inc. 317-485-7887
720 E Broadway St, Fortville, IN 46040
Contract Radio-Frequency (RF) Welding. From development to manufacturing and packaging.

Global One Medical, Inc. 561-842-7727
3707 Interstate Park Rd S, Riviera Beach, FL 33404
Floatation cushion: wheelchair cushion: anti-decubitus cushion.

Grand Rapids Foam Technologies 877-GET-GRFT
2788 Remico St SW, Wyoming, MI 49519

Grant Airmass Corporation 800-243-5237
126 Chestnut Hill Rd, PO Box 3456, Stamford, CT 06903
Alternating pressure-relief seat pad.

Hermell Products, Inc. 800-233-2342
9 Britton Dr, PO Box 7345, Bloomfield, CT 06002
Urethane foam, latex, convoluted and gel cushions.

Huntleigh Healthcare Llc. 800-223-1218
40 Christopher Way, Eatontown, NJ 07724
$170.00 for alternating pressure seat cushion.

Intarsia Ltd. 203-355-1357
14 Martha Ln, Gaylordsville, CT 06755
Solid seat insert, drop seat, cushion contoured seat.

Invacare Canada 800-668-5324
5970 Chedworth Way, Mississauga, ONT L5R 3T9 Canada

Invacare Corporation 800-333-6900
1 Invacare Way, Elyria, OH 44035
INVACARE.

J. T. Posey Co. 800-447-6739
5635 Peck Rd, Arcadia, CA 91006

Keen Mobility Company 503-285-9090
6500 NE Halsey St Ste B, Portland, OR 97213

Kees Goebel Medical Specialties, Inc. 800-354-0445
9663 Glades Dr, Hamilton, OH 45011
$45.00 to $105.00 for TEMPERFOAM wheelchair cushion.

Marken International, Inc. 800-564-9248
W231N2811 Roundy Cir E Ste 100, Pewaukee, WI 53072
Seat cushion, pressure equalization and/or positioning.

Medi-Dyne Healthcare Products, L.L.C. 800-810-1740
1812 Industrial Blvd, Colleyville, TX 76034
AllorGel Cushion lightweight cushion combines viscoelastic gel with high density polyfoam for maximum comfort and pressure reduction. Ideal for wheelchair patients, drivers, pilots and stadium seats. Helps eliminate pressure ulcers.

Medical Depot 516-998-4600
99 Seaview Blvd, Port Washington, NY 11050
Wheelchair.

Next Generation Co. 800-598-4303
41740 Enterprise Cir N Ste 108, Temecula, CA 92590
Cushion, wheelchair.

Parsons A.D.L. Inc. 800-263-1281
R.R. #2, 1986 Sideroad 15, Tottenham, ONT L0G 1W0 Canada
Foam comfort cushions, wedges, optional hard bases, with stretch knit covers or Bucktex breathable waterproof covers.

Patterson Medical Supply, Inc. 262-387-8720
W68N158 Evergreen Blvd, Cedarburg, WI 53012
Thera-flo fluid floatation cushion (water or gel filled).

Polymer Concepts, Inc. 877-820-3163
7561 Tyler Blvd Ste 8, Mentor, OH 44060
Various models of wheelchair cushions.

Profex Medical Products 800-325-0196
2224 E Person Ave, Memphis, TN 38114

Regency Product International 800-845-7931
4732 E 26th St, Vernon, CA 90058
Available in 3 styles.

Royal Converting, Inc. 865-938-7828
1615 Highway 33 S, New Tazewell, TN 37825

Saginaw Medical Service, Inc. 989-793-4444
3960 Tittabawassee Rd, Saginaw, MI 48604

CUSHION, WHEELCHAIR (PAD) *(cont'd)*

Scott Specialties, Inc. 785-527-5627
1827 Meadowlark Rd, Clay Center, KS 67432
Various types of wheelchair cushions.

Scott Specialties, Inc. 785-527-5627
1820 E 7th St, Concordia, KS 66901

Sheepskin Ranch, Inc. 800-366-9950
3408 Indale Rd, Fort Worth, TX 76116
$55.00 for SOFSHEEP lamb or sheepskin seating pad.

Silipos Inc. 800-229-4404
704 Williams Road, Niagara Falls, NY 14304

Simon & Simon Mobility Services 210-614-1414
9207 Huebner Rd, San Antonio, TX 78240
Simon & simon medical equipment co., inc.

Skil-Care Corp. 800-431-2972
29 Wells Ave, Yonkers, NY 10701
Drop Seat lowers seat of standard folding wheelchair 4', comes complete with selection of various cushions. Bariatric cushions.

Slide Free Llc 601-213-3758
22 Lake Eddins 163815, Pachuta, MS 39347
Wheelchair pad.

Southwest Technologies, Inc. 800-247-9951
1746 E Levee St, North Kansas City, MO 64116
Gel cushion for wheelchairs.

Span-America Medical Systems, Inc. 800-888-6752
70 Commerce Ctr, Greenville, SC 29615
GEL-T, GEOMATT, and PRT (pressure-relieving therapy), wheelchair cushions.

Spenco Medical Corp. 254-772-6000
PO Box 2501, Waco, TX 76702
Seat padding, made from SILICORE® padding fibers.

Star Cushion Products, Inc. 618-539-7070
5 Commerce Dr, Freeburg, IL 62243
Wheelchair cushion.

Sunnyrec Corp. 310-638-4368
20505 Belshaw Ave, Carson, CA 90746
Hexcare-deluxe.

Sunrise Medical 800-333-4000
7477 Dry Creek Pkwy, Longmont, CO 80503
Positioning accessories for wheelchairs; cushion for pressure relief whenuser is out of wheelchair (straps to body).

Sunrise Medical Hhg Inc 303-218-4505
7128 Ambassador Rd, Baltimore, MD 21244
Various sizes and shapes of wheelchair cushions and inerts.

Sunrise Medical Hhg Inc 303-218-4505
2010 E Spruce Cir, Olathe, KS 66062
Wheelchair cushion.

Sunrise Medical Hhg Inc 303-218-4505
6724 Preston Ave # 1, Livermore, CA 94551

Sunrise Medical Hhg Inc 303-218-4505
2615 W Casino Rd # 2B, Everett, WA 98204

Sunrise Medical Hhg Inc 303-218-4505
2842 N Business Park Ave, Fresno, CA 93727

Supracor, Inc. 800-787-7226
2050 Corporate Ct, San Jose, CA 95131
Various sizes/configurations to make cushions, wheelchair.

Synergy Rehab Technologies, Inc. 407-344-8440
2440 Smith St Ste E, Kissimmee, FL 34744
Various models of wheelchair cushions.

Tele-Made Disposables, Inc. 888-822-4299
3215 Huffman Eastgate Rd, Huffman, TX 77336
Wheelchair cushion.

Tempur-Medical, Inc. 888-255-3302
1713 Jaggie Fox Way, Lexington, KY 40511
Tempur-Med Wheelchair Cushion, ViscoRide Wheelchair Cuhsion.

Tex-Tenn Corp. 800-251-3027
108 Kwickway Ln # 118, PO Box 8219, Gray, TN 37615
Polyester fabric pads. Special polyester pad with corrugated rubberized coating: High pile polyester pad fabric with corrugated rubberized coating.

Therafin Corporation 800-843-7234
19747 Wolf Rd, Mokena, IL 60448
Various shapes and sizes of wheelchair cushion and inserts.

Thompson Medical Specialties 800-777-4949
3404 Library Ln, Saint Louis Park, MN 55426

CUSHION, WHEELCHAIR (PAD) *(cont'd)*

Tuffcare 800-367-6160
3999 E La Palma Ave, Anaheim, CA 92807

Ufp Technologies, Inc. 630-543-2855
1235 W National Ave, Addison, IL 60101
Custom manufacturer of convoluted cushion pads, standard convoluted bed and wheelchair pads, impregnated foams for patches and bandages, filters & operating table pads.

Ultimex Corp. 727-403-3090
6250 42nd St N Ste 30, Pinellas Park, FL 33781
Wheelchair seat cushion, back supports, attachable arm rests, arm trays.

Variety Ability Systems Inc. 800-891-4514
2 Kelvin Ave., Unit 3, Toronto, ONT M4C-5C8 Canada
Kidsert™ is a simple, lightweight cushion that can be added to children's products such as strollers and high chairs. It has unique features to provide extra comfort and support for young children.

Ventura Enterprises 317-745-2989
35 Lawton Ave, Danville, IN 46122

Vitacare Medical Products Inc. 800-263-9068
331 Bowes Rd., Concorrd, ONT L4K-1J2 Canada

CUSP, GOLD AND STAINLESS STEEL *(Dental And Oral) 76ELO*

Intergrated Dental Solutions, Inc. 858-643-1143
6195 Cornerstone Ct E Ste 108, San Diego, CA 92121
Crown & bridge with metal occlusal surface.

CUSPIDOR *(Dental And Oral) 76QOE*

Beaverstate Dental, Inc. 800-237-2303
115 S Elliott Rd, Newberg, OR 97132

Forest Dental Products Inc 800-423-3535
6200 NE Campus Ct, Hillsboro, OR 97124

Midmark Corporation 800-643-6275
60 Vista Dr, P.O. Box 286, Versailles, OH 45380

Sds (Summit Dental Systems) 800-275-3368
3560 NW 53rd Ct, Fort Lauderdale, FL 33309

CUSTOM PROSTHESIS *(Orthopedics) 87WLZ*

Allergan 800-624-4261
71 S Los Carneros Rd, Goleta, CA 93117
Malar prosthesis.

Freeman Manufacturing Company 800-253-2091
900 W Chicago Rd, PO Box J, Sturgis, MI 49091
Orthotic soft goods.

Maramed Orthopedic Systems 800-327-5830
2480 W 82nd St, No. 8, Hialeah, FL 33016

Otto Bock Heathcare 800-328-4058
2 Carlson Pkwy N Ste 100, Minneapolis, MN 55447
Prosthetic and orthotic componentry.

Slawner Ltd., J. 514-731-3378
5713 Cote Des Neiges Rd., Montreal, QUE H3S 1Y7 Canada
Custom manufacturing of orthotics, prosthetics, orthopedic shoes etc.

CUTTER, BONE, ULTRASONIC *(Cns/Neurology) 84JXJ*

Holmed Corporation 508-238-3351
40 Norfolk Ave, South Easton, MA 02375

Misonix, Inc. 800-694-9612
1938 New Hwy, Farmingdale, NY 11735
BC-20 & BC-40 Ultrasonic (Hard Tissue) Bone Cutter for orthopedic, neuro-, cranio- and maxillofacial surgery.

CUTTER, CAST *(Orthopedics) 87QGZ*

Alimed, Inc. 800-225-2610
297 High St, Dedham, MA 02026

Bsn Medical, Inc 800-552-1157
5825 Carnegie Blvd, Charlotte, NC 28209
AMERICAN ORTHOPAEDIC™ CAST CUTTER is specially designed for rugged use - the perfect tool for power and endurance. Internally lubriacated for longer service. Switch is designed and placed so that it will not break if dropped. Hex drive provides 6 blade rotations.

Paramedical Distributors 800-245-3278
2020 Grand Blvd, Kansas City, MO 64108

Slawner Ltd., J. 514-731-3378
5713 Cote Des Neiges Rd., Montreal, QUE H3S 1Y7 Canada

Stryker Corp. 800-726-2725
2825 Airview Blvd, Portage, MI 49002

Zimmer Orthopaedic Surgical Products 800-321-5533
PO Box 10, 200 West Ohio Ave., Dover, OH 44622

CUTTER, CAST, AC-POWERED *(Orthopedics) 87LGH*

Alimed, Inc. 800-225-2610
297 High St, Dedham, MA 02026

Bsn Medical, Inc. 800-552-1157
100 Beiersdorf Drive, Rutherford College, NC 28671
Various.

Debusk Orthopedic Casting (Doc) 865-362-2334
420 Straight Creek Rd Ste 1, New Tazewell, TN 37825
Powered cast saw.

Elite Medical Equipment 719-659-7926
5470 Kates Dr, Colorado Springs, CO 80919
Cast cutter.

Her-Mar, Inc. 800-327-8209
8550 NW 30th Ter, Doral, FL 33122

CUTTER, DOWEL *(Cns/Neurology) 84GZQ*

Osteotech, Inc. 800-537-9842
51 James Way, Eatontown, NJ 07724
Threaded cortial bone dowel.

CUTTER, LINEAR, LAPAROSCOPIC *(Surgery) 79SIM*

Ethicon Endo-Surgery, Inc. 800-USE-ENDO
4545 Creek Rd, Cincinnati, OH 45242
ENDOPATH 60mm endoscopic linear cutter. ENDOPATH EZ35 35mm endoscopic linear cutter.

Okay Industries, Inc. 860-225-8707
200 Ellis St, P.O. Box 2470, New Britain, CT 06051

CUTTER, OPERATIVE *(Dental And Oral) 76EKD*

Aesculap Implant Systems Inc. 1-800-234-9179
3773 Corporate Pkwy, Center Valley, PA 18034

Axis Dental 800-355-5063
800 W Sandy Lake Rd Ste 100, Coppell, TX 75019

Biomet, Inc. 574-267-6639
56 E Bell Dr, PO Box 587, Warsaw, IN 46582
Instrument, manual, surgical.

Carl Heyer, Inc. 800-284-5550
1872 Bellmore Ave, North Bellmore, NY 11710

Dental Usa, Inc. 815-363-8003
5005 McCullom Lake Rd, McHenry, IL 60050
Various types of instruments.

Hu-Friedy Manufacturing Co., Inc. 800-483-7433
3232 N Rockwell St, Chicago, IL 60618

Kmedic 800-955-0559
190 Veterans Dr, Northvale, NJ 07647

Nordent Manufacturing, Inc. 800-966-7336
610 Bonnie Ln, Elk Grove Village, IL 60007
$16.75 per unit (standard).

Premier Dental Products Co. 888-670-6100
1710 Romano Dr, PO Box 4500, Plymouth Meeting, PA 19462

Sds De Mexico, S.A. De C.V. 714-516-7484
Circuito Sur 31, Parque Industrial Nelson, Mexicali 21395 Mexico
Operative cutting instrument

Suter Dental Manufacturing Company, Inc. 800-368-8376
632 Cedar St, Chico, CA 95928

CUTTER, ORTHOPEDIC *(Orthopedics) 87HTZ*

Arthrex, Inc. 239-643-5553
1370 Creekside Blvd, Naples, FL 34108
Percutaneous knot cutter.

Biomet, Inc. 574-267-6639
56 E Bell Dr, PO Box 587, Warsaw, IN 46582
Various types of pin cutting instruments.

Depuy Spine, Inc. 800-227-6633
325 Paramount Dr, Raynham, MA 02767
Rod cutter.

Holmed Corporation 508-238-3351
40 Norfolk Ave, South Easton, MA 02375

Integral Design Inc. 781-740-2036
52 Burr Rd, Hingham, MA 02043

Karl Storz Endoscopy-America Inc. 800-421-0837
600 Corporate Pointe, Culver City, CA 90230
For arthroscopy use.

Kmedic 800-955-0559
190 Veterans Dr, Northvale, NJ 07647

Mahe International Inc. 800-294-7946
468 Craighead St, Nashville, TN 37204

CUTTER, ORTHOPEDIC *(cont'd)*

Medtronic Sofamor Danek Instrument Manufacturing 901-396-3133
7375 Adrianne Pl, Bartlett, TN 38133
Various rongeurs.

Medtronic Sofamor Danek Usa, Inc. 901-396-3133
4340 Swinnea Rd, Memphis, TN 38118
Various rongeurs.

Micrins Surgical Instruments, Inc. 800-833-3380
28438 N Ballard Dr, Lake Forest, IL 60045

Optimal Healthcare Products 800-364-8574
11444 W Olympic Blvd Ste 900, Los Angeles, CA 90064

Smith & Nephew, Inc., Endoscopy Division 800-343-8386
150 Minuteman Rd, Andover, MA 01810
Disposable arthroscopic blades.

Smith & Nephew, Inc., Endoscopy Division 800-343-8386
130 Forbes Blvd, Mansfield, MA 02048

Symmetry Tnco 888-447-6661
15 Colebrook Blvd, Whitman, MA 02382

Warsaw Orthopedic, Inc. 901-396-3133
2500 Silveus Xing, Warsaw, IN 46582
Various rongeurs.

Zimmer Holdings, Inc. 800-613-6131
1800 W Center St, PO Box 708, Warsaw, IN 46580

Zimmer Spine, Inc. 800-655-2614
7375 Bush Lake Rd, Minneapolis, MN 55439
Orthopedic cutting instrument.

Zimmer Trabecular Metal Technology 800-613-6131
10 Pomeroy Rd, Parsippany, NJ 07054
13mn shaver.

CUTTER, PILL *(General) 80WTB*

American Medical Industries 605-428-5501
330 E 3rd St Ste 2, Dell Rapids, SD 57022
EZ-SWALLOW Pill Splitter. Also available in a combination pill crusher/pill spliter. EZ-SWALLOW combination unit. Pill crusher, pill splitter, and storage in one unit.

Health Enterprises 800-633-4243
90 George Leven Dr, North Attleboro, MA 02760
PS-12 PILLSPLITTER splits hard to swallow pills.

Trademark Medical Llc 800-325-9044
449 Soverign Ct, St. Louis, MO 63011
EZ SWALLOW combo splitter/crusher

CUTTER, RING *(General) 80FNS*

Becton Dickinson And Co. 866-906-8080
411 Waverley Oaks Rd, Waltham, MA 02452

Biomet, Inc. 574-267-6639
56 E Bell Dr, PO Box 587, Warsaw, IN 46582
Ring cutting saw.

Clinimed, Incorporated 877-CLINIMED
303 Markus Ct, Sandy Brae Industrial Park, Newark, DE 19713

Dermatologic Lab & Supply, Inc. 800-831-6273
608 13th Ave, Council Bluffs, IA 51501
Ring cutter.

Dixie Ems Supply 800-347-3494
385 Union Ave, Brooklyn, NY 11211
$24.00 per unit (standard).

Elmed, Inc. 630-543-2792
60 W Fay Ave, Addison, IL 60101

General Scientific Safety Equipment Co. 800-523-0166
2553 E Somerset St Fl 1, Philadelphia, PA 19134

Kentron Health Care, Inc. 615-384-0573
3604 Kelton Jackson Rd, P.o. Box 120, Springfield, TN 37172
Ring cutter.

Kmedic 800-955-0559
190 Veterans Dr, Northvale, NJ 07647

M .W. Mooney & Co., Inc. 800-230-5770
415 Williamson Way Ste 9, Ashland, OR 97520
GEM battery-powered ring cutter for emergency care.

Normed 800-288-8200
PO Box 3644, Seattle, WA 98124
Ring cutter.

Rockford Medical & Safety Co. 800-435-9451
2420 Harrison Ave, PO Box 5646, Rockford, IL 61108

CUTTER, RING *(cont'd)*

Trans American Medical / Tamsco Instruments 708-430-7777
7633 W 100th Pl, Bridgeview, IL 60455
Floor & medium grade surgical stainless steel.

Triboro Supplies Inc 800-369-7546
994 Grand Blvd, Deer Park, NY 11729

Tuzik Boston 800-886-6363
104 Longwater Dr, Assinippi Park, Norwell, MA 02061

CUTTER, SKIN GRAFT *(Surgery) 79RTO*

Zimmer Orthopaedic Surgical Products 800-321-5533
PO Box 10, 200 West Ohio Ave., Dover, OH 44622

CUTTER, SKIN GRAFT, EXPANDED MESH *(Surgery) 79RTP*

TI Tate Mfg, Inc. 765-452-8283
1500 N Webster St, Kokomo, IN 46901

Zimmer Orthopaedic Surgical Products 800-321-5533
PO Box 10, 200 West Ohio Ave., Dover, OH 44622

CUTTER, SURGICAL *(Surgery) 79FZT*

Biomet Microfixation Inc. 800-874-7711
1520 Tradeport Dr, Jacksonville, FL 32218
Surgical cutter.

Boston Medical Products, Inc. 800-433-2674
117 Flanders Rd, Westborough, MA 01581
Stainless steel Montgomery tracheal fenestrator, in sizes 4, 6, 8 and 10.

Cincinnati Surgical Company 800-544-3100
11256 Cornell Park Dr, Cincinnati, OH 45242

Depuy Mitek, A Johnson & Johnson Company 800-451-2006
50 Scotland Blvd, Bridgewater, MA 02324
Suture cutter.

Ethicon Endo-Surgery, Inc. 800-USE-ENDO
4545 Creek Rd, Cincinnati, OH 45242
PROXIMATE linear cutter: thin tissue 55mm; 55mm and 75mm thick tissue with lock-out, 4-row with no-knife; 60mm regular, 4-row, with no knife; 60mm regular, 4-row with knife, lock-out; 30mm regular, 6-row, with knife; linear cutter reload, 55mm for TLC55 and TL455, blue and TCT55 and T4T55, green. Linear cutter reload: 30mm regular tissue, ELC35 and EL45; 60mm, regular tissue, titanium for ELC60, EL460, ETC60 and ET460; 60mm, 4 row, thick tissue.

Hospira, Inc. 877-946-7747
755 Jarvis Dr, Morgan Hill, CA 95037
$3,600.00 for heated-blade electronic surgical system.

Medisiss 866-866-7477
2747 SW 6th St, Redmond, OR 97756
Various cutters,surgical,sterile.

Okay Industries, Inc. 860-225-8707
200 Ellis St, P.O. Box 2470, New Britain, CT 06051

Precision Surgical Intl., Inc. 800-776-8493
PO Box 726, Noblesville, IN 46061
Various styles and sizes of surgical cutters.

Stryker Puerto Rico, Ltd. 939-307-2500
Hwy. 3, Km. 131.2, Las Guasimas Ind. Park, Arroyo, PR 00714
Arthoscopic shavers and cutters.

Symmetry Medical Usa, Inc. 574-267-8700
486 W 350 N, Warsaw, IN 46582
Manual surgical instrument for general use.

Zimmer Spine, Inc. 800-655-2614
7375 Bush Lake Rd, Minneapolis, MN 55439
Surgical cutter.

CUTTER, SUTURE *(Surgery) 79UEN*

Cincinnati Surgical Company 800-544-3100
11256 Cornell Park Dr, Cincinnati, OH 45242

CUTTER, SYRINGE AND NEEDLE *(General) 80QOG*

Franklin Miller Inc 800-932-0599
60 Okner Pkwy, Livingston, NJ 07039

CUTTER, VITREOUS ASPIRATION, AC-POWERED *(Ophthalmology) 86HQE*

Allergan 800-366-6554
2525 Dupont Dr, Irvine, CA 92612
BKS-1000 refractive unit allowing partial removal of cornea and cutting without freezing tissue previously.

Bausch & Lomb Surgical 636-255-5051
3365 Tree Court Ind Blvd, Saint Louis, MO 63122

Elmed, Inc. 630-543-2792
60 W Fay Ave, Addison, IL 60101

CUTTER, VITREOUS ASPIRATION, AC-POWERED *(cont'd)*

H.S. International Co., Inc. 800-811-0072
5040 Commercial Cir Ste A, Concord, CA 94520
Pneumatic, anterior and posterior, 20, 23, 25 gauge. Also infusion sleeves available, along with disposable soft tip needles (20 gauge).

Imonti And Associates Inc., M. 949-248-1058
25707 Compass Way, San Juan Capistrano, CA 92675
Pro-Vit Anterior/posterior guillotine vitreous cutter. Disposable. For pneumatic systems available from 18 psi to 30 psi. PRO-VIT single use or reusable irrigation sleeve for PRO-VIT vitreous cutter. PRO-VIT, pneumatic, guillotine vitrectomy cutter single use and reusable.

Medical Instrumentation Development Labs 800-929-5227
557 McCormick St, San Leandro, CA 94577
Supra-Vit and Vitamate. Vit Enhancer. AVE. Vitreous Cutters, up to 2500 cuts per minute.

Microvision, Inc. 603-474-5566
34 Folly Mill Rd, Seabrook, NH 03874
Vitrectomy probe.

Microworld Medical Instruments, Inc. 510-534-7401
4640 Malat St, Oakland, CA 94601
20- and 25-ga pneumatic vitrectomy cutters.

Peregrine Surgical, Ltd. 215-348-0456
51 Britain Dr, Doylestown, PA 18901
Ophthalmic guillotine cutter.

Promex Technologies, Llc 317-736-0128
3049 Hudson St, Franklin, IN 46131
Automated vitrectomy device.

Synergetics Usa, Inc. 800-600-0565
3845 Corporate Centre Dr, O Fallon, MO 63368
Vitreous aspiration and cutting instrument.

Syntec, Inc. 636-566-6500
733 Mansion Rd, Winfield, MO 63389
Vitrectomy device.

Visioncare Devices, Inc. 530-243-5047
1246 Redwood Blvd, Redding, CA 96003
Vitrectomy cutter and accessories.

CUTTER, VITREOUS INFUSION SUCTION *(Ophthalmology) 86QOH*

Alcon Research, Ltd. 800-862-5266
6201 South Fwy, Fort Worth, TX 76134

Bausch & Lomb Surgical 636-255-5051
3365 Tree Court Ind Blvd, Saint Louis, MO 63122

CUTTER, WIRE AND PIN *(Orthopedics) 87HXZ*

Biomet Microfixation Inc. 800-874-7711
1520 Tradeport Dr, Jacksonville, FL 32218
Various types of cutters.

Biomet, Inc. 574-267-6639
56 E Bell Dr, PO Box 587, Warsaw, IN 46582
Various types of wire cutters.

Depuy Spine, Inc. 800-227-6633
325 Paramount Dr, Raynham, MA 02767
Screw/bolt cutter.

Depuy-Raynham, A Div. Of Depuy Orthopaedics 800-451-2006
325 Paramount Dr, Raynham, MA 02767
Various types of orthopedic wire cutters.

Holmed Corporation 508-238-3351
40 Norfolk Ave, South Easton, MA 02375

Interventional Spine, Inc. 800-497-0484
13700 Alton Pkwy Ste 160, Irvine, CA 92618
Various types of wire cutters.

K2m, Inc. 866-526-4171
751 Miller Dr SE Ste F1, Leesburg, VA 20175
Cutter.

Key Surgical, Inc. 800-541-7995
8101 Wallace Rd Ste 100, Eden Prairie, MN 55344
Wire and bolt cutters.

Kmedic 800-955-0559
190 Veterans Dr, Northvale, NJ 07647
Ranging in size from 10in., 16in., and 22in., stainless steel, end-cutting pliers cut wire up to 7mm.

Koros Usa, Inc. 805-529-0825
610 Flinn Ave, Moorpark, CA 93021
Wire cutter.

CUTTER, WIRE AND PIN *(cont'd)*

Medtronic Sofamor Danek Instrument Manufacturing — 901-396-3133
7375 Adrianne Pl, Bartlett, TN 38133
Various types of orthopedic wire cutters.

Medtronic Sofamor Danek Usa, Inc. — 901-396-3133
4340 Swinnea Rd, Memphis, TN 38118
Various types of orthopedic wire cutters.

Schleuniger, Inc. — 877-902-1470
87 Colin Dr, Manchester, NH 03103
Programmable cutting machine for wire, tubing, flat ribbon, and fiberoptic cable.

Simpex Medical, Inc. — 800-851-9753
401 E Prospect Ave, Mount Prospect, IL 60056

Small Bone Innovations, Inc. — 215-428-1791
1380 S Pennsylvania Ave, Morrisville, PA 19067
Orthopedic manual surgical instrument.

Stryker Corp. — 800-726-2725
2825 Airview Blvd, Portage, MI 49002

Stryker Spine — 866-457-7463
2 Pearl Ct, Allendale, NJ 07401

Symmetry Medical Usa, Inc. — 574-267-8700
486 W 350 N, Warsaw, IN 46582
Orthopedic manual surgical instrument.

Toolmex Corporation — 800-992-4766
1075 Worcester St, Natick, MA 01760
Wire, pin, cutters.

Tuzik Boston — 800-886-6363
104 Longwater Dr, Assinippi Park, Norwell, MA 02061

Warsaw Orthopedic, Inc. — 901-396-3133
2500 Silveus Xing, Warsaw, IN 46582
Various types of orthopedic wire cutters.

Westcon Orthopedics, Inc. — 800-382-4975
4 Craig Rd, Neshanic Station, NJ 08853
Pin, capping device, external.

Zimmer Holdings, Inc. — 800-613-6131
1800 W Center St, PO Box 708, Warsaw, IN 46580

Zimmer Trabecular Metal Technology — 800-613-6131
10 Pomeroy Rd, Parsippany, NJ 07054
Cutter.

CUTTER, X-RAY FILM *(Radiology) 90TFP*

Schueler & Company, Inc. — 516-487-1500
PO Box 528, Stratford, CT 06615

CUVETTE, SPECTROPHOTOMETER *(Chemistry) 75TBQ*

Beckman Coulter, Inc. — 800-742-2345
250 S Kraemer Blvd, PO Box 8000, Brea, CA 92821

Bio Plas, Inc. — 415-472-3777
4340 Redwood Hwy Ste A15, San Rafael, CA 94903
Disposable cuvettes for spectrophotometers and clinical analyzers with low background absorbance, for UV and visible use.

Biomerieux Inc. — 800-682-2666
100 Rodolphe St, Durham, NC 27712

Buck Scientific, Inc. — 800-562-5566
58 Fort Point St, Norwalk, CT 06855
LIGHT PATH OPTICAL All standard cuvettes.

Globe Scientific, Inc. — 800-394-4562
610 Winters Ave, Paramus, NJ 07652
Macro, semi-micro, and UV types.

Laboratory Environment Support Systems, Inc. — 800-621-6404
7755 E Evans Rd, Scottsdale, AZ 85260
L.E.S.S. INC. makes laboratory plastic reusable. Your laboratory saves up to 50% on disposable plastic and enhances the environment.

CUVETTE, THERMOSTATED *(Chemistry) 75JRI*

Laboratory Environment Support Systems, Inc. — 800-621-6404
7755 E Evans Rd, Scottsdale, AZ 85260
L.E.S.S. INC. makes laboratory plastic reusable. Your laboratory saves up to 50% on disposable plastic and enhances the environment.

CYANOMETHEMOGLOBIN *(Hematology) 81GKK*

Medical Chemical Corp. — 800-424-9394
19430 Van Ness Ave, Torrance, CA 90501
$24.50 per unit.

CYLINDER, CARBON-DIOXIDE *(Surgery) 79QUA*

Aga Linde Healthcare P.R. Inc. — 787-622-7900
PO Box 363868, GPO Box 364727, San Juan, PR 00936
Surgery.

CYLINDER, COMPRESSED GAS, WITH VALVE *(Anesthesiology) 73ECX*

Aga Linde Healthcare P.R. Inc. — 787-622-7900
PO Box 363868, GPO Box 364727, San Juan, PR 00936
Anesth/Pul Med.

Catalina Cylinders — 714-890-0999
7300 Anaconda Ave, Garden Grove, CA 92841

Emepe International, Inc. — 813-994-9690
18108 Sugar Brooke Dr, Tampa, FL 33647
Cylinders, aluminum or steel, large or small. Valves and fittings. Transfillers.

Erie Medical — 800-932-2293
10225 82nd Ave, Lakeview Corporate Park, Pleasant Prairie, WI 53158
Portable unit, systems supplied in both soft shoulder bag or hard blow-molded carrying cases.

Flotec, Inc. — 800-401-1723
7625 W New York St, Indianapolis, IN 46214
Medical gas cylinder regulators and wall mounted flow meters available for all medical gases & gas blends. True flow restrictor technology. Not gravity sensitive. MRI Compatible & Safe.

Life Corporation — 800-700-0202
1776 N Water St, Milwaukee, WI 53202
LIFE, OxygenPac Portable emergency oxygen units, clear cover and wall-mounted, off/on lever control, resuscitation mask with one-way valve for hygiene, 6lpm 90min. supply, refillable. Also available 6 & 12 lpm NORM & HIGH, 0-25 lpm variable, and demand-valve for 100% oxygen resuscitation. GSA Federal Supply Schedule.

Mada, Inc. — 800-526-6370
625 Washington Ave, Carlstadt, NJ 07072

Oxia U.S. Ltd. — 262-369-1978
665 Industrial Ct Unit B, Hartland, WI 53029
Cylinder, canister.

Safe-T-Rack Systems, Inc. — 800-344-0619
4325 Dominguez Rd Ste A, Rocklin, CA 95677
Compressed gas cylinder restraint and storage system for either interior or exterior use.

U O Equipment Co. — 800-231-6372
5863 W 34th St, Houston, TX 77092

CYLINDER, GAS (EMPTY) *(Anesthesiology) 73KGA*

Air Liquide America Corporation — 800-820-2522
2700 Post Oak Blvd Ste 1800, Houston, TX 77056
Blood gas calibrators. Gas cylinder stands and holders.

Airpot Corporation — 800-848-7681
35 Lois St, Norwalk, CT 06851

Catalina Cylinders — 714-890-0999
7300 Anaconda Ave, Garden Grove, CA 92841

Hy-Mark Cylinders, Inc. — 757-245-7331
305 E St, Hampton, VA 23661
Cylinder, gas (empty) / aluminum medical oxygen cylinder.

Life Corporation — 800-700-0202
1776 N Water St, Milwaukee, WI 53202
LIFE OxygenPac and LIFE O2 SoftPac emergency oxygen units with cylinders, complete.

Linweld Inc. — 402-323-8450
9920 Deer Park Rd, Waverly, NE 68462

Respiratory Science Industries Ltd — 516-561-6161
1325 M St, Elmont, NY 11003
Refill small oxygen cylinders from large oxygen cylinders.

Special Gas Services Inc — 919-621-0980
PO Box 727, Mount Laurel, NJ 08054

CYLINDER, OXYGEN *(Anesthesiology) 73VFF*

Aga Linde Healthcare P.R. Inc. — 787-622-7900
PO Box 363868, GPO Box 364727, San Juan, PR 00936
Anesth/Pul Med.

All-Can Medical, Inc. — 905-677-1302
7575 Kimbel St., Mississauga, ONT L5S 1C8 Canada

Allied Healthcare Products, Inc. — 800-444-3954
1720 Sublette Ave, Saint Louis, MO 63110
Medical gas piping systems.

Armstrong Medical Industries, Inc. — 800-323-4220
575 Knightsbridge Pkwy, Lincolnshire, IL 60069

CYLINDER, OXYGEN *(cont'd)*

Catalina Cylinders 714-890-0999
7300 Anaconda Ave, Garden Grove, CA 92841

Chad Therapeutics, Inc. 800-423-8870
21622 Plummer St, Chatsworth, CA 91311
Oxygen transfilling system.

Contemporary Products, Inc. 800-424-2444
530 Riverside Industrial Pkwy, Portland, ME 04103

Erie Medical 800-932-2293
10225 82nd Ave, Lakeview Corporate Park, Pleasant Prairie, WI 53158
See Canister, Oxygen.

Life Corporation 800-700-0202
1776 N Water St, Milwaukee, WI 53202
LIFE, OxygenPac Portable emergency oxygen units, clear cover and wall-mounted, off/on lever control, resuscitation mask with one-way valve for hygiene, 6lpm 90min. supply, refillable. Also available 6 & 12 lpm NORM & HIGH, 0-25 lpm variable, and demand-valve for 100% oxygen resuscitation. GSA Federal Supply Schedule.

Luxfer Gas Cylinders 800-764-0366
3016 Kansas Ave, Riverside, CA 92507
Ultra-lightweight carbon-composite medical oxygen cylinders & lightweight all-aluminum medical oxygen cylinders.

U O Equipment Co. 800-231-6372
5863 W 34th St, Houston, TX 77092

CYSTIC FIBROSIS SYSTEM *(Gastro/Urology) 78QOI*

Axcan Pharma Inc. 800-950-8085
22 Inverness Center Pkwy, Birmingham, AL 35242
Mucus clearance device for cystic fibrosis(K940986)

Wescor, Inc. 800-453-2725
459 S Main St, Logan, UT 84321
Priced at $1,995.00 for the Macroduct sweat stimulation and collection system for error-free sweat samples for analysis in the Sweat-Chek sweat conductivity analyzer for $ 1,395.00 for the laboratory diagnosis of cystic fibrosis. Cystic Fibrosis System: Nanoduct Neonatal Sweat Analysis System (4,195.00), an integrated system for inducing and analyzing sweat for in situ laboratory diagnosis of cystic fibrosis requiring only three microliters of sweat for analysis along with the Nanoduct Patient Simulator for running CAP survey samples.

CYSTOMETER, ELECTRICAL RECORDING
(Gastro/Urology) 78EXQ

Ashlar Holdings, Llc 573-785-8766
1908 Greenwood Dr Ste B, Poplar Bluff, MO 63901

Richard Wolf Medical Instruments Corp. 800-323-9653
353 Corporate Woods Pkwy, Vernon Hills, IL 60061

CYSTOMETRIC GAS (CARBON-DIOXIDE) OR HYDRAULIC DEVICE *(Gastro/Urology) 78FAP*

Medtronic Neuromodulation 763-514-4000
710 Medtronic Pkwy, Minneapolis, MN 55432
Various types of cystometric gas (carbon-dioxide) on hydraulic devices.

CYSTOSCOPE *(Gastro/Urology) 78FAJ*

Advanced Endoscopy Devices, Inc. 818-227-2720
22134 Sherman Way, Canoga Park, CA 91303
Compatible to any manufacturer's sheaths.

Artes Medical Inc. 888-278-3345
5870 Pacific Center Blvd, San Diego, CA 92121
Various types of cystoscopes,diagnostic.

Boehm Surgical Instrument Corp. 716-436-6584
966 Chili Ave, Rochester, NY 14611
Cystoscope diagnostic.

Cortek Endoscopy, Inc. 847-526-2266
260 Jamie Ln Ste D, Wauconda, IL 60084
Gastroenterology.

Electro Surgical Instrument Co., Inc. 888-464-2784
37 Centennial St, Rochester, NY 14611
Kelly cystoscopes.

Global Endoscopy, Inc. 888-434-3398
914 Estes Ct, Schaumburg, IL 60193
Cystoscope.

Gyrus Acmi, Inc. 508-804-2739
93 N Pleasant St, Norwalk, OH 44857
Endoscopes and accessories.

Gyrus Acmi, Inc. 508-804-2739
300 Stillwater P.o.box 1971, Stamford, CT 06902
Cystoscope, diagnostic.

CYSTOSCOPE *(cont'd)*

Karl Storz Endoscopy-America Inc. 800-421-0837
600 Corporate Pointe, Culver City, CA 90230
Standard flexible and rigid cystoscopes. Rigid 4 mm cystoscopes available in a range of viewing angles. Flexible 15.5 Fr. cystoscopes provide an intuitive deflection mechanism. Filter kit available for photodynamic diagnosis (PDD).

Mahe International Inc. 800-294-7946
468 Craighead St, Nashville, TN 37204

Medifix, Inc 847-965-1898
8727 Narragansett Ave, Morton Grove, IL 60053
Cystoscopes.

Medivision Endoscopy 800-349-5367
1210 N Jefferson St, Anaheim, CA 92807
Independent service center specializing in rigid endoscope repairs and sales. Quality Control Department on premises. Provide customized maintenance reports to customers and distributors. Conduct technical training seminars and in-service programs. Manufacturer of new endoscopes.

Olympus America, Inc. 800-645-8160
3500 Corporate Pkwy, PO Box 610, Center Valley, PA 18034

Pentax Medical Company 800-431-5880
102 Chestnut Ridge Rd, Montvale, NJ 07645
$10,080.00 for fiber cystoscope with distal tip diameter of 4.8mm and channel size 2.2mm. $19,320.00 for color video cystoscope with CCD chip and a distal tip of 5.3mm and a channel size of 2.0mm; all fully immersable.

Pentax Southern Region Service Center 201-571-2300
8934 Kirby Dr, Houston, TX 77054
Cystoscope.

Pentax West Coast Service Center 800-431-5880
10410 Pioneer Blvd Ste 2, Santa Fe Springs, CA 90670
Pentax cystoscope.

Rei Rotolux Enterprises, Inc. 888-773-7611
4145 North Service Rd, Ste. 200, Burlington, ON L7L 6A3 Canada
2.7mm and 4mm are available, all are autoclavable. Custom configurations are available.

Richard Wolf Medical Instruments Corp. 800-323-9653
353 Corporate Woods Pkwy, Vernon Hills, IL 60061

Suneva Medical, Inc. 858-550-9999
5870 Pacific Center Blvd, San Diego, CA 92121
UROSCOPE

CYSTOTOME, OPHTHALMIC *(Ophthalmology) 86HNY*

Alcon Manufacturing, Ltd. 817-551-6813
714 Columbia Ave, Sinking Spring, PA 19608
Various types andmodels of ophthalmic cystotomes.

Becton Dickinson And Co. 866-906-8080
411 Waverley Oaks Rd, Waltham, MA 02452

Eagle Laboratories 800-782-6534
10201 Trademark St Ste A, Rancho Cucamonga, CA 91730

Hurricane Medical 941-751-0588
5315 Lena Rd, Bradenton, FL 34211
Ophthalmic cystotome.

Katena Products, Inc. 800-225-1195
4 Stewart Ct, Denville, NJ 07834

Kmi Surgical Ltd. 800-528-2900
110 Hopewell Rd, Laird Professional Building, Downingtown, PA 19335
Disposable unit.

Medone Surgical, Inc. 941-359-3129
670 Tallevast Rd, Sarasota, FL 34243
Various.

Micromachining Technologies, Inc. 314-785-6800
2345 Millpark Dr Ste A, Maryland Heights, MO 63043
Disposable anterior capsulotomy cystotome.

Microsurgical Technology, Inc. 425-556-0544
PO Box 2679, Redmond, WA 98073

Miltex Inc. 800-645-8000
589 Davies Dr, York, PA 17402

Oasis Medical, Inc. 800-528-9786
514 S Vermont Ave, Glendora, CA 91741

Rhein Medical, Inc. 800-637-4346
5460 Beaumont Center Blvd Ste 500, Suite 500, Tampa, FL 33634
Disposable and reusable ophthalmic instruments.

CYSTOURETHROSCOPE *(Gastro/Urology) 78FBO*

Gyrus Acmi, Inc. 508-804-2739
93 N Pleasant St, Norwalk, OH 44857
Various cystourethroscopes.

Gyrus Acmi, Inc. 508-804-2739
300 Stillwater P.o.box 1971, Stamford, CT 06902
Various cystourethroscopes.

Karl Storz Endoscopy-America Inc. 800-421-0837
600 Corporate Pointe, Culver City, CA 90230
Rigid and flexible versions available.

Mahe International Inc. 800-294-7946
468 Craighead St, Nashville, TN 37204

Olympus America, Inc. 800-645-8160
3500 Corporate Pkwy, PO Box 610, Center Valley, PA 18034

Richard Wolf Medical Instruments Corp. 800-323-9653
353 Corporate Woods Pkwy, Vernon Hills, IL 60061

Vision-Sciences, Inc. 800-874-9975
40 Ramland Rd S Ste 1, Orangeburg, NY 10962
Flexible Cystoscope and EndoSheath System

CYTOCENTRIFUGE *(Pathology) 88IFB*

Cytyc Surgical Products 800-442-9892
250 Campus Dr, Marlborough, MA 01752
Cytocentrifyge.

Iris Sample Processing 800-782-8774
60 Glacier Dr, Westwood, MA 02090
Cytocentrifuge and accessories.

Monogen, Inc. 847-573-6700
3630 Burwood Dr, Waukegan, IL 60085
Cytopreparation device and accessories.

Pro Scientific Inc. 800-584-3776
99 Willenbrock Rd, Oxford, CT 06478
The easy to handle Cyto Chambers allow no contamination, volumes up to 8ml, sediments of different sizes and up to 8 sediments per slide. The various accessories include one or two funnel chambers, slide carriers, filter cards and Cyto angle chambers. The Hettich Cyto System does not require a dedicated unit and may be utilized with any of Hettich's benchtop centrifuges.

Statspin, Inc. 800-782-8774
60 Glacier Dr, Westwood, MA 02090
CYTOFUGE compact, low-cost, versitile cytocentrifuge.

Thermo Fisher Scientific - Laboratory Equipment Division Headquarters 800-662-7477
450 Fortune Blvd, Milford, MA 01757

Tripath Imaging, Inc. 919-206-7140
780 Plantation Dr, Burlington, NC 27215
Centrifuge.

Wescor, Inc. 800-453-2725
459 S Main St, Logan, UT 84321
CYTOPRO; $5,795.00 Model 7620 Cytocentrifuge with 9 stored programs, 8 sample chamber capacity for easy-to-use cell deposition on microscope slides; sealed rotor.

CYTOKERATINS *(Immunology) 82LYE*

Cell Marque Corp. 916-746-8977
6600 Sierra College Blvd, Rocklin, CA 95677
Cytokeratin (polyclonal).

CYTOMEGALOVIRUS, DNA REAGENTS *(Microbiology) 83LSO*

Prodesse, Inc. 888-589-6974
W229N1870 Westwood Dr, Waukesha, WI 53186
Herpes Mplex(TM) Multiplex PCR Reagents for simultaneous detection of HSV-1, HSV-2, CMV, EBV, VZV and HHV-6 - Research Use Only

Qiagen Gaithersburg, Inc. 800-344-3631
1201 Clopper Rd, Gaithersburg, MD 20878
Cmv dna assay.

United Biotech, Inc. 650-961-2910
211 S Whisman Rd Ste E, Mountain View, CA 94041
ELISA detecting Cytomegalovirus IgG and Cytomegalovirus IgM

DAM, DENTAL *(Dental And Oral) 76QOK*

Cardent International, Inc. 866-764-6832
1568 NW 89th Ct, Doral, FL 33172

Dentalez Group 866-DTE-INFO
101 Lindenwood Dr Ste 225, Valleybrooke Corporate Center
Malvern, PA 19355

DAM, DENTAL *(cont'd)*

Gammadirect Medical Division 847-267-5929
PO Box 383, Lake Forest, IL 60045
DamEZ intra-oral dental dam allows for quick placement and dry operating field.

DAM, RUBBER *(Dental And Oral) 76EIE*

Apex Medical Technologies, Inc. 800-345-3208
10064 Mesa Ridge Ct Ste 202, San Diego, CA 92121
Synthetic Polyisoprene Rubber Dam, free of latex proteins and rubber accelerators

Cao Group, Inc. 801-256-9282
4628 Skyhawk Dr, West Jordan, UT 84084
Tissue isolation gel.

Cdm Dental 541-928-4444
812 Water Ave NE, Albany, OR 97321
Power block.

Coltene/Whaledent Inc. 330-916-8858
235 Ascot Pkwy, Cuyahoga Falls, OH 44223
Dental dam.

Cooley & Cooley, Ltd. 800-215-4487
8550 Westland West Blvd, Houston, TX 77041
VALUE DAM- a latex rubber dam material. Heavy non-tear thickness in mint 6 x 6 inch size.

Den-Mat Holdings, Llc 805-922-8491
2727 Skyway Dr, Santa Maria, CA 93455
Paint-on rubber dam kits containing paint-on rubber dam.

Dental Technologies, Inc. 847-677-5500
6901 N Hamlin Ave, Lincolnwood, IL 60712
Gingival dam.

Heraeus Kulzer, Inc., Dental Products Division 574-299-6662
4315 S Lafayette Blvd, South Bend, IN 46614
Ivory rubber dam.

Innovate Medical, L.L.C. 423-854-9694
225 White Top Rd. Ext., Bluff City, TN 37618
Rubber dental dam.

Manufacturera Dental Continental 523-633-8329
2113 Calle Indust Del Plastico, 269 Fracc Zapopan Indust Norte
Zapopan, Jalisco Mexico
Rubber dam

Moyco Technologies, Inc. 800-331-8837
200 Commerce Dr, Montgomeryville, PA 18936

Novocol, Inc. 303-665-7535
416 S Taylor Ave, Louisville, CO 80027
Isolation material, dam material, spacer material.

Oraceutical Llc 413-528-5070
815 Pleasant St, Lee, MA 01238
Barrier material.

Pentron Clinical Technologies 203-265-7397
68-70 North Plains Industrial, Road, Wallingford, CT 06492
Rubber dam and accessories.

Rite-Dent Manufacturing Corp. 305-693-8626
3750 E 10th Ct, Hialeah, FL 33013
Various types of rubber dams.

Spectrum Dental Llc. 310-845-8345
8554 Hayden Pl, Culver City, CA 90232
Soft tissue isolation system.

The Hygenic Corp. 800-321-2135
1245 Home Ave, Akron, OH 44310
Dental dam.

Ultradent Products, Inc. 801-553-4586
505 W 10200 S, South Jordan, UT 84095
Rubber dam caulking material.

Zirc Company 800-328-3899
3918 State Highway 55 SE, Buffalo, MN 55313
INSTI-DAM Rubber Dam; built-in flexible frame, prepunched hole. Radiographs may be taken.

DECALCIFIER DEVICE, ELECTROLYTIC *(Pathology) 88KDZ*

Ethox International 800-521-1022
251 Seneca St, Buffalo, NY 14204
Infuser bag.

DECALCIFIER SOLUTION, ELECTROLYTIC *(Pathology) 88IFF*

Sci Gen, Inc. 310-324-6576
333 E Gardena Blvd, Gardena, CA 90248
FDA: Medical Device Manufacturing and packaging. Focus on Histology, Cytology, Analytical and General purpose Reagents, Chemistry, and Sterling and Disinfecting agents.

DECONTAMINATION KIT *(Surgery) 79MAC*

Burch Manufacturing Co., Inc. 515-573-4136
618 1st Ave N, Fort Dodge, IA 50501
DB-85 collapsible decontamination booth. Use it where even hazardous chemicals are located.In hospitals, factories or any hazardous materials incident. Steel framework assembles in minutes. Includes carrying case for easy transport. 6 ft high x 4 ft wide x 4 ft deep. Weights 68 lb.

Caltech Industries, Inc. 800-234-7700
2420 Schuette Rd, Midland, MI 48642
Biohazard spill kit containing bleach or non-bleach disinfectant (all inclusive) to efficiently and safely decontaminate surfaces relative to bloodborne pathogens and other human body fluids.

Centurion Medical Products Corp. 517-545-1135
3310 S Main St, Salisbury, NC 28147

Laboratory Technologies, Inc. 800-542-1123
43 W 900 Rte. 64, Maple Park, IL 60151

North Safety Products 401-943-4400
1101 B Calle Neutron, Parque Industrial Maran, Mexicali, B.c. Mexico
Bloodborne pathogen protection kit

Tri-State Hospital Supply Corp. 517-545-1135
3173 E 43rd St, Yuma, AZ 85365

U.S. Army Pine Bluff Arsenal 870-540-3622
10020 Kabrich Cir, Pine Bluff, AR 71602
Decontamination kit, skin.

DEFIBRILLATOR, AUTOMATIC IMPLANTABLE CARDIOVERTER, WITH CARDIAC RESYNCHRONIZATION
(Cardiovascular) 74NIK

Medtronic Puerto Rico Operations Co., Juncos 763-514-4000
Road 31, Km. 24, Hm 4, Ceiba Norte Industrial Park, Juncos, PR 00777
Icd with cardiac resynchronization.

DEFIBRILLATOR, AUTOMATIC, EXTERNAL, FOR OUT-OF-HOSPITAL USE *(Cardiovascular) 74NPN*

Concord Medical Products 978-857-5884
72 Bristers Hill Rd, Concord, MA 01742
External defibrillator.

DEFIBRILLATOR, BATTERY-POWERED *(Cardiovascular) 74QOR*

Ardus Medical, Inc. 800-878-1388
11297 Grooms Rd, Cincinnati, OH 45242

Commercial/Medical Electronics, Inc. 800-324-4844
1519 S Lewis Ave, Tulsa, OK 74104

St. Jude Medical, Inc. 800-328-9634
1 Saint Jude Medical Dr, Saint Paul, MN 55117
Fortify implantable cardioverter defibrillator

Superior Medical Limited 800-268-7944
520 Champagne Dr., Toronto, ONT M3J 2T9 Canada

Welch Allyn Protocol, Inc. 800-462-0777
2 Corporate Dr Ste 110, Long Grove, IL 60047
MRL PIC, portable intensive care system. MRL LifeQuest AED, automatic external defibrillator.

Zoll Medical Corp. 800-348-9011
269 Mill Rd, Chelmsford, MA 01824
$5995 for ZOLL D-900 defibrillator. Simple, easy to use inexpensive defibrillation in non-critical areas of the hospital.

DEFIBRILLATOR, BATTERY-POWERED, HIGH ENERGY
(Cardiovascular) 74DRK

Ge Medical Systems Information Technologies 800-643-6439
8200 W Tower Ave, Milwaukee, WI 53223
Defibrillator, DC-powered including paddles; multiple models.

Ge Medical Systems, Llc 262-548-2355
3000 N Grandview Blvd, W-417, Waukesha, WI 53188
D.c. befibrillator.

DEFIBRILLATOR, BATTERY-POWERED, LOW ENERGY
(Cardiovascular) 74LDD

Ballard Medical Products 770-587-7835
12050 Lone Peak Pkwy, Draper, UT 84020
Dc-defibrillator, low-energy, (including paddles).

DEFIBRILLATOR, BATTERY-POWERED, LOW ENERGY *(cont'd)*

Kimball Electronics Tampa 813-814-8114
13750 Reptron Blvd, Tampa, FL 33626
Defibrillator.

Physio-Control, Inc. 800-442-1142
11811 Willows Rd NE, Redmond, WA 98052
LIFEPAK 20 Defibrillator / Monitor. The 20 is highly intuitive to use, and adapts to various patient environments. It skillfully combines an AED function for the infrequent BLS-trained responder, with manual capability so that ALS trained clinicians can quickly and easily deliver advanced diagnostic and therapeutic care.

Tz Medical Inc. 800-944-0187
7272 SW Durham Rd Ste 800, Portland, OR 97224
Defibrillator adapters.

Welch Allyn Protocol, Inc. 800-462-0777
2 Corporate Dr Ste 110, Long Grove, IL 60047
PIC Portable Intensive Care System. ECG monitor, defibrillator, external pacer, NIBP, SPO2, IBP, CO2 - $15,000.

DEFIBRILLATOR, EXTERNAL, AUTOMATIC
(Cardiovascular) 74MKJ

Ansen Corporation 315-393-3573
100 Chimney Point Dr, Ogdensburg, NY 13669
Automatic external defibrillator.

Banyan International Corp. 800-351-4530
PO Box 1779, 2118 E. Interstate 20, Abilene, TX 79604
Philips FR2 and Onsite AEDs; Medtronic LifePak 500 AED; Zoll AED Plus.

Cardiac Science Corp. 800-777-1777
500 Burdick Pkwy, Deerfield, WI 53531
CardioVive AED.

Cardiac Science Corporation (Ca) 888-274-3342
25351 Commercentre Dr Ste 250, Lake Forest, CA 92630
The POWERHEART AED G3 line offers the layperson the latest in public-access defibrillation, with professional models for ACLS trained, providing continuous monitoring during and after cardiac arrest as well as protecting a victim against the reoccurence of a cardiac arrhythmia post-resuscitation. Newest models include the POWERHEART AED G3, POWERHEART AED G3 PRO and the POWERHEART AED G3 AUTOMATIC. POWERHEART CRM bedside cardiac monitor/defibrillator/external pacer is designed for in-hospital use. Continuously monitors, detects, and treats patients at risk of life-threatening ventricular arrhythmias, with little or no human intervention.

Defibtech Llc 866-333-4248
741 Boston Post Rd Ste 201, Guilford, CT 06437
Semi-automatic external defibrillator.

Devon Medical 800-571-3135
1100 1st Ave Ste 100, King Of Prussia, PA 19406

Heartsine Technologies, Inc. 866-478-7463
121 Friends Ln Ste 400, Newtown, PA 18940
Automatic external defibrillators.

Md International, Inc. 305-669-9003
11300 NW 41st St, Doral, FL 33178

O&M Enterprise 847-258-4515
641 Chelmsford Ln, Elk Grove Village, IL 60007
DEFIBRILLATOR

Physio-Control, Inc. 800-442-1142
11811 Willows Rd NE, Redmond, WA 98052
LIFEPAK 300 automatic advisory defibrillator. FIRST MEDIC semi-automatic defilbullators (i.e., FIRST MEDIC or 710 defibullators). LIFEPAK II defibrillator/pacemaker. Mates to LIFEPAK II diagnostic cardiac monitor. LIFEPAK 500 automated external defibrillator, 7 pounds, very simple to operate. Automated defibrillator intended for use by targeted responders (security personnel, police and other responding to cardiac arrest victims.)

Tsi Medical Ltd. 800-661-7263
47 Athabascan Ave., Unit 105, Sherwood Park, AB T8A-4H3 Canada

Welch Allyn Protocol Inc. 800-289-2500
8500 SW Creekside Pl, Beaverton, OR 97008
Defibrillator, automatic, external.

Welch Allyn Protocol, Inc. 800-462-0777
2 Corporate Dr Ste 110, Long Grove, IL 60047
AED 10 defibrillator.

DEFIBRILLATOR, IMPLANTABLE, AUTOMATIC
(Cardiovascular) 74LWS

Arizona Device Manufacturing 763-505-0874
2350 W Medtronic Way, Tempe, AZ 85281
Implantable cardioverter defibrillator.

Biotronik, Inc. 503-635-3594
6024 Jean Rd, Lake Oswego, OR 97035
VARIOUS MODELS OF CRT-DS

Cardiac Pacemakers, Inc. 800-227-3422
4100 Hamline Ave N, P.O. Box 64079, Saint Paul, MN 55112
AICD automatic, implantable cardioverter defibrillator.

Ela Medical, Inc. 800-352-6466
2950 Xenium Ln N, Plymouth, MN 55441
Alto 2 is a dual-chamber rate responsive ICD with a unique PARAD/PARAD+ al;gorithm allowing pacing in the slow VT zone

Maquet Puerto Rico Inc. 408-635-3900
No. 12, Rd. #698, Dorado, PR 00646
Various models of aicds.

Medtronic Puerto Rico Operations Co., Juncos 763-514-4000
Road 31, Km. 24, Hm 4, Ceiba Norte Industrial Park, Juncos, PR 00777
Implantable cardioverter defibrillator.

Medtronic Puerto Rico Operations Co.,Med Rel 763-514-4000
Road 909, Km. 0.4., Barrio Mariana, Humacao, PR 00792
Implantable cardioverter defibrillator.

Medtronic, Inc. 800-633-8766
710 Medtronic Pkwy, Minneapolis, MN 55432
JEWEL, JEWEL CD, JEWEL PCD, PCD.

DEFIBRILLATOR, LINE-POWERED *(Cardiovascular) 74QOS*

Cardiac Science Corp. 800-777-1777
500 Burdick Pkwy, Deerfield, WI 53531
DC200

New Life Systems, Inc. 954-972-4600
PO Box 8767, Coral Springs, FL 33075
AC/DC powered defibrillator with printer.

Welch Allyn Protocol, Inc. 800-462-0777
2 Corporate Dr Ste 110, Long Grove, IL 60047
MRL LITE, ECG, defibrillator, optional AED.

World Medical Equipment, Inc. 800-827-3747
3915 152nd St NE, Marysville, WA 98271

Zoll Medical Corp. 800-348-9011
269 Mill Rd, Chelmsford, MA 01824

DEFIBRILLATOR/MONITOR, BATTERY-POWERED
(Cardiovascular) 74QOO

Biomedics, Inc. 949-458-1998
23322 Peralta Dr Ste 11, Laguna Hills, CA 92653

Datascope Corp. 800-288-2121
14 Philips Pkwy, Montvale, NJ 07645
PASSPORT defibrillator multi-parameter monitor/defibrillator.

Md International, Inc. 305-669-9003
11300 NW 41st St, Doral, FL 33178

Physio-Control, Inc. 800-442-1142
11811 Willows Rd NE, Redmond, WA 98052
LIFEPAK 9 (9A, 9B) defibullator/monitor. LIFEPAK 10 defibrillator/monitor. LIFEPAK 12 series defibrillator/monitor. ECG, 12-lead SP02, external pacing and defibrillation (AED or manual).

Welch Allyn Protocol, Inc. 800-462-0777
2 Corporate Dr Ste 110, Long Grove, IL 60047
PIC system.

World Medical Equipment, Inc. 800-827-3747
3915 152nd St NE, Marysville, WA 98271

Zoll Medical Corp. 800-348-9011
269 Mill Rd, Chelmsford, MA 01824
$ 8,500 for ZOLL PD1200 defibrillator/monitor/non-invasive temporary pacemaker. Defibrillation, pacing and monitoring via one set of disposable skin electrodes. Advisory Defibrilator/Monitor. PD/D 2000 an AC Battery operated combined AED/ALS unit for hospitals with external pacing, internal/external electrodes, pacing. Also available, Automated defibrillator/monitor 1700 AC/Battery operated combined AED/ALS unit for hospitals with external pacing.

DEFIBRILLATOR/MONITOR, LINE-POWERED
(Cardiovascular) 74QOP

Biomedics, Inc. 949-458-1998
23322 Peralta Dr Ste 11, Laguna Hills, CA 92653

Md International, Inc. 305-669-9003
11300 NW 41st St, Doral, FL 33178

DEFIBRILLATOR/MONITOR, LINE-POWERED *(cont'd)*

New Life Systems, Inc. 954-972-4600
PO Box 8767, Coral Springs, FL 33075
AC/DC powered defibrillator with printer.

DEFOAMER, CARDIOPULMONARY BYPASS
(Cardiovascular) 74DTP

Cardiovention, Inc. 408-873-3400
19200 Stevens Creek Blvd Ste 200, Cupertino, CA 95014
Defoamer.

Terumo Cardiovascular Systems, Corp 800-521-2818
6200 Jackson Rd, Ann Arbor, MI 48103

DEFROSTER, DRUG, FROZEN *(General) 80SHJ*

Mmi Of Mississippi, Inc. 800-448-5918
PO Box 488, Crystal Springs, MS 39059

DEGREASER, SKIN, SURGICAL *(Surgery) 79KOY*

Mavidon Medical Products 800-654-0385
1820 2nd Ave N, Lake Worth, FL 33461
Lemonprep, skin prep.

Miller-Stephenson Chemical Company, Inc. 800-992-2424
George Washington Highway, Danbury, CT 06810-7378

DEHUMIDIFIER *(General) 80WUX*

Bry-Air, Inc. 877-379-2479
10793 State Rt. 37 W., Sunbury, OH 43074
Built to prevent mold condensation on injection molding machines up to 1000 tn.

Harris Environmental Systems, Inc. 888-771-4200
11 Connector Rd, Andover, MA 01810
Custom dehumidification.

DELIVERY SYSTEM, ALLERGEN AND VACCINE *(General) 80LDH*

Alkaline Corp. 732-531-7830
20 Meridian Rd Ste 9, Eatontown, NJ 07724
Allergy prick test needle.

Bio Plas, Inc. 415-472-3777
4340 Redwood Hwy Ste A15, San Rafael, CA 94903
ASTRAL Inoculation System--1- and 10-uL inoculation loop system; streaking needles; Clone-Piks.

Hill Top Research Corp 513-831-3114
PO Box 138, 6088 Main & Mill Streets, Miamiville, OH 45147
Hill top chamber r.

Hollister-Stier Laboratories, Llc 800-992-1120
3525 N Regal St, Spokane, WA 99207
QUINTEST and QUINTIP skin test devices (sterile)for allergy testing.

Insource, Inc. 800-366-3829
PO Box 9, Bastian, VA 24314
Injectable vaccines and Medical Supply

Panatrex, Inc. 714-630-5582
1648 Sierra Madre Cir, Placentia, CA 92870
Skin prick test.

Q.T.I. Corp. 760-723-9825
879 Del Valle Dr, Fallbrook, CA 92028
Allergy skin test device-sterile.

DELIVERY SYSTEM, PNEUMATIC TUBE *(General) 80TDT*

Air Link International 800-388-8237
1189 N Grove St Ste A, Anaheim, CA 92806
Used to transport and/or convey pharmacy products and lab specimens throughout hospitals.

Filtrona Extrusion, Inc./Pexcor Medical Products Div. 800-755-7528
764 S Athol Rd, P.O. Box 659, Athol, MA 01331

Swisslog Translogic Corporation 800-525-1841
10825 E 47th Ave, Denver, CO 80239
Specimens, records, and pharmaceuticals. ECO SEAL sealed carriers.

DEMAGNETIZER *(General) 80WIS*

R. B. Annis Instruments, Inc. 317-637-9282
1101 N Delaware St, Indianapolis, IN 46202
For surgical tools and steel components, from small to medium units to those large enough to walk through.

Walker Ldj Scientific, Inc. 800-962-4638
10 Rockdale St, Worcester, MA 01606

DEMINERALIZER *(Chemistry) 75QOU*

Medro Systems, Inc. 972-542-8200
416 Industrial Blvd, McKinney, TX 75069
Dual column and mixed bed.

Thermo Fisher Scientific Inc. 563-556-2241
2555 Kerper Blvd, Dubuque, IA 52001

DENSITOMETER *(Cardiovascular) 74DXM*

Advanced American Biotechnology (Aab) 714-870-0290
1166 E Valencia Dr Unit 6C, Fullerton, CA 92831
$15,995 for microdensitometry station with 1-D or 2-D laser scanner, video densitometer and programs. $36,500 for full microdensitometry station with laser and video densitometers and microscope, IBM 386, 80Mb hard disk, color printer and program. Imaging densitometer (flatbed scanner): Reflectance transmission, 1cmx1cm - 35cmx45cm sample size, 42 um resolution, 0-3 OD, wet or dry gels and stained samples & software...R-500s...$3,995 TR-500...$9,995.

Alimed, Inc. 800-225-2610
297 High St, Dedham, MA 02026

Beckman Coulter, Inc. 800-742-2345
250 S Kraemer Blvd, PO Box 8000, Brea, CA 92821

Caprock Developments Inc. 800-222-0325
475 Speedwell Ave, PO Box 95, Morris Plains, NJ 07950

Civco Medical Instruments Co., Inc. 319-656-4447
102 1st St S, Kalona, IA 52247
Densitometer.

Helena Laboratories 409-842-3714
PO Box 752, Beaumont, TX 77704

Petrolab Company 518-783-5133
874 Albany Shaker Rd, Latham, NY 12110
Pellet press.

X-Rite, Inc. 888-826-3044
4300 44th St SE, Grand Rapids, MI 49512
$775.00 for battery-operated unit with .02D accuracy; $1,100.00 for regular unit with 1-, 2-, and 3-mm apertures and 0 to 5D range. Both models for B/W film.

DENSITOMETER, BONE, DUAL PHOTON *(Radiology) 90WRK*

Coopersurgical, Inc. 800-243-2974
95 Corporate Dr, Trumbull, CT 06611

Xma (X-Ray Marketing Associates, Inc.) 800-325-8880
1205 W Lakeview Ct, Windham Lakes Business Park
Romeoville, IL 60446

DENSITOMETER, BONE, SINGLE PHOTON *(Radiology) 90KGI*

Alara Inc. 800-410-2525
47505 Seabridge Dr, Fremont, CA 94538
Bone mineral densitometer.

Bone Density Measurement International, Llc 301-631-0008
550 Highland St Ste 303, Frederick, MD 21701
Qct bone mineral analysis software.

Compumed, Inc. 800-421-3395
5777 W Century Blvd Ste 360, Los Angeles, CA 90045
Osteogram (radiographic absorptiometry).

Ge Medical Systems Ultrasound And Primary Care Dia 608-826-7050
726 Heartland Trl, Madison, WI 53717
Bone densitometers.

Hologic, Inc. 800-343-9729
35 Crosby Dr, Bedford, MA 01730

Lone Oak Medical Technologies 267-221-0661
3805 Old Easton Rd, Doylestown, PA 18902
Bone mineral densitometer.

Mindways Software, Inc. 512-912-0871
3001 S Lamar Blvd Ste 302, Austin, TX 78704
Hip qct bmd.

Xma (X-Ray Marketing Associates, Inc.) 800-325-8880
1205 W Lakeview Ct, Windham Lakes Business Park
Romeoville, IL 60446

DENSITOMETER, LABORATORY *(Chemistry) 75UKK*

Advanced American Biotechnology (Aab) 714-870-0290
1166 E Valencia Dr Unit 6C, Fullerton, CA 92831
5 models Soft Laser Scanning Densitometers - $5,950 for std unit; $8,950 for UV unit; $15,990 for std 2-D unit; $18,990 for UV 2-D unit; $28,995 for laser DNA sequencing densitometer $4,995 for video densitometer for ELISA reading and AIDS with blots reading capabilities.

DENSITOMETER, LABORATORY *(cont'd)*

Beckman Coulter, Inc. 800-742-2345
250 S Kraemer Blvd, PO Box 8000, Brea, CA 92821

Bio-Rad Laboratories, Life Science Group 800-424-6723
2000 Alfred Nobel Dr, Hercules, CA 94547
Model GS-670 imaging densitometer offers rapid graphical imaging and quantitation capabilities for a wide range of sample types and sizes.

Blake Industries, Inc. 908-233-7240
660 Jerusalem Rd, Scotch Plains, NJ 07076

Camag Scientific, Inc. 800-334-3909
515 Cornelius Harnett Dr, Wilmington, NC 28401

Helena Laboratories 409-842-3714
PO Box 752, Beaumont, TX 77704
$16,275 for CliniScan 1260 electrophoresis densitometer with programmable microprocessor and reflectance, fluorescent, visible, UV scanning. $27,900 for EDC 1376 for densitometer with greater automation.

Kontes Glass Co. 888-546-2531
1022 Spruce St, Vineland, NJ 08360

Mettler-Toledo, Inc. 800-METTLER
1900 Polaris Pkwy, Columbus, OH 43240
Three density/specific gravity models measure, automatically calculate, display and print three, four or five-place density-related values.

Sebia Electrophoresis 800-835-6497
400-1705 Corporate Drive, Norcross, GA 30093

DENSITOMETER, RADIOGRAPHIC *(Radiology) 90VGD*

Advanced American Biotechnology (Aab) 714-870-0290
1166 E Valencia Dr Unit 6C, Fullerton, CA 92831
Imager, 0.0003 lux video densitometer, safe alternative to radioactive labeling and more sensitive.

Alimed, Inc. 800-225-2610
297 High St, Dedham, MA 02026
Quickly and automatically measures the optical density of film. In less than a minute, it can read and calculate a complete set of control-strip data.

Health Care Exports, Inc. 800-847-0173
5701 NW 74th Ave, Miami, FL 33166
Bone densitometers, refurbished.

Image Analysis, Inc. 800-548-4849
1380 Burkesville St, Columbia, KY 42728

Owens Scientific Inc. 281-394-2311
23230 Sandsage Ln, Katy, TX 77494

S&S Technology 281-815-1300
10625 Telge Rd, Houston, TX 77095

Supertech, Inc. 800-654-1054
PO Box 186, Elkhart, IN 46515
Nuclear Associates and ESECO products available

Xma (X-Ray Marketing Associates, Inc.) 800-325-8880
1205 W Lakeview Ct, Windham Lakes Business Park
Romeoville, IL 60446

DENSITOMETER, RADIOGRAPHY, DIGITAL, QUANTITATIVE *(Radiology) 90WIR*

Alimed, Inc. 800-225-2610
297 High St, Dedham, MA 02026
Quickly measures the optical density of film. Designed to measure diffuse transmission density per American National Standards Institute.

Image Analysis, Inc. 800-548-4849
1380 Burkesville St, Columbia, KY 42728

Osteometer Meditech, Inc. 866-421-7762
12515 Chadron Ave, Hawthorne, CA 90250

Telos Medical Equipment (Austin & Assoc., Inc.) 800-934-3029
1109 Sturbridge Rd, Fallston, MD 21047
TELOS stress device for quantitative ligament evaluation of the ankle, knee, elbow, wrist, and shoulder pre- and post-treatment.

DENSITOMETER/SCANNER (INTEGRATING, REFLECTANCE, TLC, RADIO) *(Chemistry) 75JQT*

Abbott Diagnostics Div. 847-937-7988
1921 Hurd Dr, Irving, TX 75038
Reflectance analyzer.

DENSITOMETER/SCANNER (INTEGRATING, REFLECTANCE, TLC, RADIO) *(cont'd)*

Advanced American Biotechnology (Aab) 714-870-0290
1166 E Valencia Dr Unit 6C, Fullerton, CA 92831
Video densitometer II for reading electrophoresis, TLC and image analysis. Flat bed scanner and program for electrophoresis TLC and image analysis.

Helena Laboratories 409-842-3714
PO Box 752, Beaumont, TX 77704

Kontes Glass Co. 888-546-2531
1022 Spruce St, Vineland, NJ 08360
$7,250.00 per unit (standard).

Myers-Stevens Group, Inc. 903-566-6696
2931 Vail Ave, Commerce, CA 90040
Reflectometer used in the quantitation of eia assays.

PerkinElmer 800-762-4000
940 Winter St, Waltham, MA 02451

Sebia Electrophoresis 800-835-6497
400-1705 Corporate Drive, Norcross, GA 30093

DENTAL CEMENT W/OUT ZINC-OXIDE EUGENOL AS AN ULCER COVERING FOR PAIN RELIEF *(Dental And Oral) 76MZW*

Kleen Test Products Corporation 262-284-6600
216 12th St NE, Strasburg, OH 44680
Z-octyl cyanocrylate.

Rite-Dent Manufacturing Corp. 305-693-8626
3750 E 10th Ct, Hialeah, FL 33013
Various types of cement w/o zinc-oxide eugenol.

DENTAL LABORATORY EQUIPMENT *(Dental And Oral) 76WOJ*

American Biomed Instruments, Inc. 718-235-8900
11 Wyona St, Brooklyn, NY 11207
Dental X-Ray Equipment, dental chairs and supplies.

American Diversified Dental Systems 800-637-2330
22991 La Cadena Dr, Laguna Hills, CA 92653
The Spray Opaque System, Complete. Everything supplied except air supply.

Ami Dental, Inc. 800-969-0405
9000 Southwest Fwy Ste 328, Houston, TX 77074
Dental supplies and equipment.

Attachments International, Inc. 800-999-3003
824 Cowan Rd, Burlingame, CA 94010
Instrument attachments and implant components.

Belmed, Inc. 888-723-5893
887 Delta Rd, Red Lion, PA 17356
Dental Equipment - Analgesia systems and accessories, anesthesia equipment and accessories, and oxygen units and accessories

Conger Dental Supply, Inc. 800-255-3983
302 Rosedale Ln, Bristol, TN 37620

Danville Materials 800-827-7940
3420 Fostoria Way Ste A200, San Ramon, CA 94583
PREP START Dental air abrasion unit, countertop air abrasion cavity preparation system for use with all composite resin and pit and fissure restorations.

Denplus Inc. 800-344-4424
205 - 1221 Labadie, Longueuil, QUE J4N 1E2 Canada

Dentalaire Products 800-866-6881
17150 Newhope St Ste 407, Fountain Valley, CA 92708
Silent compressors, dental handpiece parts, verinary dental equipment.

Dentsply Canada, Ltd. 800-263-1437
161 Vinyl Ct., Woodbridge, ONT L4L 4A3 Canada

Forest Dental Products Inc 800-423-3535
6200 NE Campus Ct, Hillsboro, OR 97124

George Taub Products & Fusion Co., Inc. 800-828-2634
277 New York Ave, Jersey City, NJ 07307
Dental laboratory material: TRU-FIT Die spacer, MINUTE STAIN tooth shade resin stains, GLAZE glazes, thinners, brushes, INSTA-GLAZE porcelain polishing material, and FUSION porcelain repair primer. Stereo Microscope available in 8 or 16 power optics. Heavy weighted base, with goose neck stand allows optics to rotate 360 degrees. Does not require electricity, only ambient light. Great for technician or QC viewing. Protective glass shield prevents dust from entering optics from below. Optics made by Olympus.

Hager Worldwide, Inc. 800-328-2335
13322 Byrd Dr, Odessa, FL 33556

DENTAL LABORATORY EQUIPMENT *(cont'd)*

Handler Manufacturing Co. 800-274-2635
612 North Ave E, Westfield, NJ 07090
Full line of dental lab equipment.

Harry J. Bosworth Company 800-323-4352
7227 Hamlin Ave, Skokie, IL 60076
Pressure pot, laboratory burs, neocryl orthodontic acrylics.

Jordco, Inc. 800-752-2812
595 NW 167th Ave, Beaverton, OR 97006
Disposable acrylic polishing wheel

Mds Products, Inc. 800-637-2330
22991 La Cadena Dr, Laguna Hills, CA 92653
The Spray Opaque System, Everything you need except the air supply.

Menlo Tool Co., Inc. 810-756-6010
22760 Dequindre Rd, Warren, MI 48091

Pall Medical 888-676-7255
600 S Wagner Rd, Ann Arbor, MI 48103

Sterngold 800-243-9942
23 Frank Mossberg Dr, PO Box 2967, Attleboro, MA 02703
Blasters, model pinning and torches.

Tekscan, Inc. 800-248-3669
307 W 1st St, South Boston, MA 02127
T-SCAN II computerized occlusal analysis renders a dynamic on-screen analysis of medial/lateral, anterior/posterior balance.

Vida Medica, S.A. De C.V. 5-557-4346
Calle 6 No. 376 Col. Francisco I. Madero, Mexico D.F. 11480 Mexico

Wecom, Inc. 800-628-4115
20 Warrick Ave, Glassboro, NJ 08028
Dental Laboratory Workbox with 1/8 thk Plexiglass Cardshield with internal storage. Military NSN: 6520-00-514-2394. Made to Spec Mil-W-45059, .025 thk Type 304 Stainless Steel with rolled safety edges. Measures 7.25 X 8.50 x 4.75 Hi; stackable and Autoclave safe.WECOM INC Part Number 1526-501. User reference: Case Pan, Dental

Wells Dental, Inc. 800-233-0521
PO Box 106, 5860 Flynn Creek Road, Comptche, CA 95427
Complete engine units, high speed spindles, gold/chrome finishing machines, laboratory handpieces and super quick chucks.

DENTIFRICE *(Dental And Oral) 76QPA*

Amson Products 718-435-3728
1401 42nd St, Brooklyn, NY 11219
1.5 oz to 2.75 oz.

Donovan Industries 800-334-4404
13401 McCormick Dr, Tampa, FL 33626
Cornstarch and talc powder, emery boards, toothpaste, deodorant, manicure sticks, shaving cream, razors, shower caps.

New World Imports 800-329-1903
160 Athens Way, Nashville, TN 37228
Disposable toothbrushes, FRESHMINT toothpaste.

Sonoco-Stancap Division 770-476-9088
3150 Clinton Ct, Norcross, GA 30071
Toothbrush caddy, can be printed in 6 colors.

DENTURE, GOLD *(Dental And Oral) 76ELN*

Hennessy Dental Laboratory 800-694-6862
3709 Interstate Park Rd S, Riviera Beach, FL 33404

Hong Kong Dental Lab 415-330-9099
9 Silliman St Ste C, San Francisco, CA 94134
Denture.

Masel Co., Inc. 800-423-8227
2701 Bartram Rd, Bristol, PA 19007

DENTURE, PLASTIC, TEETH *(Dental And Oral) 76ELM*

A Plus Dental Lab 215-996-4177
1700 Horizon Dr, --suite 104, Chalfont, PA 18914
Full denture, pl denture, temporary crowns.

American Dental Center Of Provo 801-375-8200
777 N 500 W Ste 201B, Provo, UT 84601
Denture, partial denture.

American Dental Designs Inc. 215-643-3232
1116 Horsham Rd, North Wales, PA 19454
Dentures plastic teeth.

American Tooth Industries 800-235-4639
1200 Stellar Dr, Oxnard, CA 93033
JUSTI BLEND.

DENTURE, PLASTIC, TEETH *(cont'd)*

Choices Technologies 425-765-9400
21730 176th Ave SE, Kent, WA 98042
Acrylic denture teeth.

D. Sign Dental Lab, Inc. 757-224-0177
690 W Fremont Ave Ste 9C, Sunnyvale, CA 94087
Plastic dentures.

Dentsply Canada, Ltd. 800-263-1437
161 Vinyl Ct., Woodbridge, ONT L4L 4A3 Canada

Global Dentech Inc. 215-654-1237
1116 Horsham Rd, North Wales, PA 19454
Crown, bridge and denture.

Hermanson Dental 800-328-9648
1055 Highway 36 E, Saint Paul, MN 55109

Hong Kong Dental Lab 415-330-9099
9 Silliman St Ste C, San Francisco, CA 94134
Denture.

Ivoclar Vivadent, Inc. 800-533-6825
175 Pineview Dr, Amherst, NY 14228
ANTARIS/POSTARIS, SR VIVODENT PE, SR ORTHOTYP PE, SR ORTHOPLANE/SR ORTHOLINGUAL, SR ORTHOSIT PE.

Kerr Corp. 714-516-7400
28200 Wick Rd, Romulus, MI 48174
Denture material.

Lisadent Corp. 516-822-9393
35 Broadway, Hicksville, NY 11801

Univac Dental Company 800-523-2559
113 Park Dr, PO Box 447, Montgomeryville, PA 18936
Acrylic Teeth.

Valplast Intl. Corp. 718-361-7440
3430 31st St, Long Island City, NY 11106
Denture teeth.

Vident 800-828-3839
3150 E Birch St, Brea, CA 92821

DENTURE, PREFORMED *(Dental And Oral) 76EKO*

Artisan Dental Laboratory 800-222-6721
2532 SE Hawthorne Blvd, Portland, OR 97214

Dental Procedures, Inc. L.L.C. 973-267-6195
9 Baer Ct, Morristown, NJ 07960
Preformed denture kit.

Hennessy Dental Laboratory 800-694-6862
3709 Interstate Park Rd S, Riviera Beach, FL 33404

Hermanson Dental 800-328-9648
1055 Highway 36 E, Saint Paul, MN 55109

Ivoclar Vivadent, Inc. 800-533-6825
175 Pineview Dr, Amherst, NY 14228

Vident 800-828-3839
3150 E Birch St, Brea, CA 92821
VITAPAN and Physiodens denture teeth, including Lingoform for lingualized occlusion technique

DEPRESSOR, ORBITAL *(Ophthalmology) 86HNX*

Accutome, Inc. 610-889-0200
3222 Phoenixville Pike, Malvern, PA 19355
Depressors.

Bausch & Lomb Surgical 636-255-5051
3365 Tree Court Ind Blvd, Saint Louis, MO 63122

Fortrad Eye Instruments Corp. 973-543-2371
8 Franklin Rd, Mendham, NJ 07945

Stephens Instruments, Inc. 800-354-7848
2500 Sandersville Rd, Lexington, KY 40511
$21.00 each.

DEPRESSOR, TONGUE *(General) 80FMA*

Adex Medical, Inc. 800-873-4776
6101 Quail Valley Ct, Riverside, CA 92507
Tongue Depressor Wood

Aesculap Implant Systems Inc. 1-800-234-9179
3773 Corporate Pkwy, Center Valley, PA 18034

Biomet Microfixation Inc. 800-874-7711
1520 Tradeport Dr, Jacksonville, FL 32218
Tongue depressor.

Bovie Medical Corp. 800-537-2790
5115 Ulmerton Rd, Clearwater, FL 33760
Attaches to penlight.

DEPRESSOR, TONGUE *(cont'd)*

Chagrin Safety Supply, Inc. 800-227-0468
8227 Washington St # 1, Chagrin Falls, OH 44023

Citmed 251-866-5519
18601 S Main St, Citronelle, AL 36522
Infant, junior, senior tongue depressor, sterile/non-sterile.

Clinimed, Incorporated 877-CLINIMED
303 Markus Ct, Sandy Brae Industrial Park, Newark, DE 19713

Codman & Shurtleff, Inc 800-225-0460
325 Paramount Dr, Raynham, MA 02767

Directmed, Inc. 516-656-3377
150 Pratt Oval, Glen Cove, NY 11542

E.A. Beck & Co. 949-645-4072
657 W 19th St Ste E, P O Box 10857, Costa Mesa, CA 92627
Tongue depressor.

Electro Surgical Instrument Co., Inc. 888-464-2784
37 Centennial St, Rochester, NY 14611
Various types styles and sizes of lighted tongue depressors.

Elma Medtec Products Inc. 204-348-7164
Po Box 160, Elma R0E 0Z0 Canada
Depressor, tongue

First Aid Bandage Co., Inc. 888-813-8214
3 State Pier Rd, New London, CT 06320
Flex-o-Blade multi-purpose tongue blades.

Glenroe Technologies 800-237-4060
1912 44th Ave E, Bradenton, FL 34203
Orthodontic tongue block.

H. A. Stiles Co. 800-447-8537
170 Forest St, Westbrook, ME 04092
Depressor wood tongue.

Healer Products, Llc 914-663-6300
427 Commerce Ln Ste 1, West Berlin, NJ 08091
Tongue depressor.

Inter-Med, Inc. 877-418-4782
2200 Northwestern Ave, Racine, WI 53404
Tongue depressor or tongueblade.

Kentron Health Care, Inc. 615-384-0573
3604 Kelton Jackson Rd, P.o. Box 120, Springfield, TN 37172
Tongue depressor.

Md Products, Llc 843-971-2684
506 Hickory Cv, Mt Pleasant, SC 29464
Tongue depressor.

Miltex Inc. 800-645-8000
589 Davies Dr, York, PA 17402

North Safety Products 401-943-4400
1101 B Calle Neutron, Parque Industrial Maran, Mexicali, B.c. Mexico
Depressor, tongue

Oak Ridge Products 888-650-7444
211 Berg St, Algonquin, IL 60102
TONGUE BLADES, senior and junior sized, sterile and non-sterile.

Pharaoh Trading Company 866-929-4913
9701 Brookpark Rd, Knollwood Plaza, Suite 241, Cleveland, OH 44129

Puritan Medical Products Company Llc 800-321-2313
31 School St., Guilford, ME 04443-0149

Richardson Products, Inc. 888-928-7297
9408 Gulfstream Rd, Frankfort, IL 60423
Tongue depressor.

Schueler & Company, Inc. 516-487-1500
PO Box 528, Stratford, CT 06615

Solon Manufacturing Co. 800-341-6640
338 Madison Ave Ste 7, Skowhegan, ME 04976
Assorted packs, sterile, non-sterile and flavored, 4 1/2, 5 1/2, and 6 in.

Welch Allyn, Inc. 800-535-6663
4341 State Street Rd, Skaneateles Falls, NY 13153

DEPRESSOR, TONGUE, DENTAL *(Dental And Oral) 76EJC*

Puritan Medical Products Company Llc 800-321-2313
31 School St., Guilford, ME 04443-0149

Schueler & Company, Inc. 516-487-1500
PO Box 528, Stratford, CT 06615

DEPRESSOR, TONGUE, ENT, METAL *(Ear/Nose/Throat) 77KBL*

Aesculap Implant Systems Inc. 1-800-234-9179
3773 Corporate Pkwy, Center Valley, PA 18034
Metal tongue.

DEPRESSOR, TONGUE, ENT, METAL *(cont'd)*

Clinimed, Incorporated 877-CLINIMED
303 Markus Ct, Sandy Brae Industrial Park, Newark, DE 19713

DEPRESSOR, TONGUE, ENT, WOOD *(Ear/Nose/Throat) 77EWF*

Amsino International, Inc. 800-MD-AMSINO
855 Towne Center Dr, Pomona, CA 91767
AMSINO white birch, non-sterile wood tongue depressors. Available in three sizes: senior, junior, and infant. Items AS019, AS020, and AS022.

C & A Scientific Co. Inc. 703-330-1413
7241 Gabe Ct, Manassas, VA 20109
PREMIERE Wood, smooth, clean in senior & junior sizes.

Puritan Medical Products Company Llc 800-321-2313
31 School St., Guilford, ME 04443-0149

Solon Manufacturing Co. 800-341-6640
338 Madison Ave Ste 7, Skowhegan, ME 04976
4-1/2-, 5-1/2-, and 6-in. white birch wood, smooth finish. Available in sterile or non-sterile. Assorted packs.

DERMABRASION UNIT *(Surgery) 79QPC*

Aesthetic Technologies, Inc. 303-469-0965
14828 W 6th Ave Ste 9B, Golden, CO 80401
Parisian Peel 'Encore' microdermabrasion and dermaphoresis system combines microdermabrasion and ultrasound technologies in the 'Parisian Phoresis' treatment. Dead skin is removed via microdermabrasion; then, ultrasound drives in topicals.

Altair Instruments, Inc. 805-388-8503
330 Wood Rd Ste J, Camarillo, CA 93010
Diamondtome, Micro-Dermabrador, skin rejuvenation instrument.

Excelladerm Corp. 877-969-7546
300065 Comercio, Rancho Santa Margarita, CA 92688
Dermabrasion Equipment and Skin Rejuevenation Systems.

Innovative Med Inc. 877-779-9492
4 Autry Ste B, Irvine, CA 92618
IMI offers a variety of Microdermabrasion systems and accessories. The lightweight (14 lbs) and portable Portapeel 1050, which uses the disposable crystal capsule system making for a very hasslefree and time saving microdermabraison system. A range of Esthetician and Physician models available.

Medical Device Resource Corporation 800-633-8423
23392 Connecticut St, Hayward, CA 94545
Dermabrasion and dermapigmentation equipment.

New Laser Science, Inc. 858-487-5880
PO Box 27210, San Diego, CA 92198
Microdermabrator -EURO PEEL - dermabrasion machine used to perform micro-dermabrasion for skin resurfacing.

Schumann Inc., A. 978-369-6782
167 Hayward Mill Rd, Concord, MA 01742
$5,980.00 for Derma-3 high speed (60,000 RPM) unit, without freezing; weighs 31lb.; 4 handpiece styles; chuck one: 3.5mm.

DERMATOME *(Surgery) 79GFD*

Aesculap Implant Systems Inc. 1-800-234-9179
3773 Corporate Pkwy, Center Valley, PA 18034

Biomet, Inc. 574-267-6639
56 E Bell Dr, PO Box 587, Warsaw, IN 46582
Dermatome blade.

Dadson Mfg. Corp. 816-847-2388
1109 NW Valley Ridge Dr, Blue Springs, MO 64029
Dermatome.

Dermamed Intl, Inc. 610-358-4447
394 Parkmount Rd., Lenni, PA 19052
Micro dermabrasion.

Edge Systems Corporation 800-603-4996
2277 Redondo Ave, Signal Hill, CA 90755
Dermabrasion system.

Genesis Biosystems, Inc. 888-577-7335
1500 Eagle Ct, Lewisville, TX 75057
Various models of microdermabrador(s).

Havel's Inc. 800-638-4770
3726 Lonsdale St, Cincinnati, OH 45227

Med-Aesthetic Solutions, Inc. 505-341-2577
6808 Academy Parkway East NE, Bldg. A Suite 1
Albuquerque, NM 87109
Microdermabrasion.

Micro Current Technology, Inc. 206-778-5717
2244 1st Ave S, Seattle, WA 98134
Various models of micro-dermabrasion.

DERMATOME *(cont'd)*

Zimmer Holdings, Inc. 800-613-6131
1800 W Center St, PO Box 708, Warsaw, IN 46580

Zimmer Orthopaedic Surgical Products 800-321-5533
PO Box 10, 200 West Ohio Ave., Dover, OH 44622
Dermatome skin cutter.

DESICCATOR *(Chemistry) 75QPE*

Boekel Scientific 800-336-6929
855 Pennsylvania Blvd, Feasterville Trevose, PA 19053
variou sizes and types of lab cabinet desiccators

Carolina Biological Supply Co. 800-334-5551
2700 York Rd, Burlington, NC 27215

Cole-Parmer Instrument Inc. 800-323-4340
625 E Bunker Ct, Vernon Hills, IL 60061

Energy Beam Sciences, Inc. 800-992-9037
29 Kripes Rd Ste B, East Granby, CT 06026

Gilson Company, Inc. 800-444-1508
PO Box 200, Lewis Center, OH 43035

Labconco Corp. 800-821-5525
8811 Prospect Ave, Kansas City, MO 64132
A molded fiberglass cabinet having one cubic foot of interior space that provides a low humidity environment for the storage of moisture-sensitive materials including thin layer chromatography plates, halide salt cells for IR spectrophotometers and chemical standards.

Laminar Flow, Inc. 800-553-FLOW
102 Richard Rd, PO Box 2427, Warminster, PA 18974
Acrylic storage box 1, 2 or 3 doors available. Fixed or adjustable shelves, antistatic also available.

Multisorb Technologies, Inc. 800-445-9890
325 Harlem Rd, Buffalo, NY 14224
Desiccants and oxygen absorbers for various applications.

Nalge Nunc International 800-625-4327
75 Panorama Creek Dr, Rochester, NY 14625
NALGENE durable polycarbonate desiccators with and without stopcock.

Nutech Molding Corporation 1-800-423-5278
PO Box 840, 2024 Broad St,, Pocomoke City, MD 21851

Structure Probe, Inc., Spi Supplies 800-2424-SPI
569 E Gay St, PO Box 656, West Chester, PA 19380

W.A. Hammond Drierite Co. 937-376-2927
138 Dayton Ave, P.O. Box 460, Xenia, OH 45385
Drierite desiccant.

DETECTOR, AIR BUBBLE *(Gastro/Urology) 78FJF*

Biomerieux Inc. 800-682-2666
100 Rodolphe St, Durham, NC 27712

Md International, Inc. 305-669-9003
11300 NW 41st St, Doral, FL 33178

Parks Medical Electronics, Inc. 503-649-7007
PO Box 5669, Aloha, OR 97006
PARKS $995.00 for Model 915-BL.

Total Molding Services, Inc. 215-538-9613
354 East Broad St., Trumbauersville, PA 18970
Small-bore Y connector.

DETECTOR, ARRHYTHMIA ALARM *(Cardiovascular) 74DSI*

Cardiac Telecom Corporation 800-355-2594
212 Outlet Way Ste 1, Greensburg, PA 15601
HEARTLink II powers the Telemetry@Home real-time, home-based cardiac surveillance system/service.

CardioNet 888-312-BEAT
227 Washington St Ste 300, Conshohocken, PA 19428

Criticare Systems, Inc. 262-798-5361
20925 Crossroads Cir, Waukesha, WI 53186
Non-invasive vital signs monitor.

Draeger Medical Systems, Inc. 215-660-2626
16 Electronics Ave, Danvers, MA 01923
Various models of patient monitors.

Fukuda Denshi Usa, Inc. 800-365-6668
17725 NE 65th St Ste C, Redmond, WA 98052
Various.

Invivo Corporation 425-487-7000
12601 Research Pkwy, Orlando, FL 32826
Various types of arrhythmia detectors and alarm monitors.

DETECTOR, ARRHYTHMIA ALARM *(cont'd)*

Medicomp, Inc. 800-23-HEART
7845 Ellis Rd, Melbourne, FL 32904
Epicardia 4000 Holter monitoring system

Mennen Medical Corp. 800-223-2201
2540 Metropolitan Dr, Trevose, PA 19053
ENVOY patient monitor with 5- or 12-lead ECG module. ENSEMBLE CENTRAL STATION, 1-12 patient central station, Windows-type user interface, for Envoy, Horizon XL monitors, and Horizon 4200 telemetry.

Spacelabs Healthcare 800-522-7025
5150 220th Ave SE, Issaquah, WA 98029
Ultraview Digital Telemetry, Ultraview SL monitors, 90496; 91496; Command Modules, PCMS recorders

Spacelabs Medical Inc. 800-522-7212
5150 220th Ave SE, Issaquah, WA 98029
Various ecg/arrhythmia monitors and accessories.

Welch Allyn Protocol Inc. 800-289-2500
8500 SW Creekside Pl, Beaverton, OR 97008
Arrhythmia detector.

DETECTOR, BETA/GAMMA *(Chemistry) 75JJJ*

Ballard Medical Products 770-587-7835
12050 Lone Peak Pkwy, Draper, UT 84020
Counter (beta, gamma) for clinical use.

Biodex Medical Systems, Inc. 800-224-6339
20 Ramsey Rd, Shirley, NY 11967

Capintec, Inc. 800-631-3826
6 Arrow Rd, Ramsey, NJ 07446

Daxor Corporation 865-425-0555
107 Meco Ln, Oak Ridge, TN 37830
Gamma counter.

Dosimeter Division Of Arrow Tech Inc 800-322-8258
5 Eastmans Rd, Parsippany, NJ 07054

In/Us Systems, Inc. 800-875-4687
5809 N 50th St, Tampa, FL 33610
B-RAM and G-RAM beta/gamma detectors; GC-RAM beta detector. On-line radioactivity detector for HPLC and GC.

Johnson & Associates Inc., Wm. B. 304-645-6568
200 AEI Dr., Lewisburg, WV 24902
22 models, portables, survey meters, geiger, & counting room units - $125 to $2,495 each.

Lnd, Inc. 516-678-6141
3230 Lawson Blvd, Oceanside, NY 11572

Marconi Medical Systems 800-323-0550
595 Miner Rd, Cleveland, OH 44143

Owens Scientific Inc. 281-394-2311
23230 Sandsage Ln, Katy, TX 77494

Reflex Industries, Inc. 619-562-1821
9530 Pathway St Ste 105, Santee, CA 92071
I-125 or co-57 reference sources.

DETECTOR, BLOOD FLOW, ULTRASONIC (DOPPLER)
(Cardiovascular) 74ULR

Biomedix Inc. 877-854-0012
4215 White Bear Pkwy, Saint Paul, MN 55110
Portable Vascular Laboratory (PVL) - priced from $10,500 for the standard PVL, this portable device can come complete with printer, cart/carry case, laptop & all necessary accessories for non-invasive testing.

Blatek, Inc. 814-231-2085
2820 E College Ave Ste F, State College, PA 16801

Cone Instruments, Inc. 800-321-6964
5201 Naiman Pkwy, Solon, OH 44139

Hokanson Inc., D.E. 800-999-8251
12840 NE 21st Pl, Bellevue, WA 98005
Hokanson vascular Dopplers are all continuous wave bidirectional models, available in multiple sizes and configurations. Pocket Dopplers are available as stand-alone devices, and with a real-time chart recorder. Computerized complete vascular system (CVS4) also includes plethysmographs for peripheral vascular blood flow exams. Portable and tabletop instruments are also available.

Huntleigh Healthcare Llc. 800-223-1218
40 Christopher Way, Eatontown, NJ 07724
3 portable Dopplers - $550.00, $750.00 or $850.00.

Md International, Inc. 305-669-9003
11300 NW 41st St, Doral, FL 33178

DETECTOR, BLOOD FLOW, ULTRASONIC (DOPPLER) *(cont'd)*

Millar Instruments, Inc. 800.669.2343
6001 Gulf Fwy Ste A, Houston, TX 77023
Blood velocity Doppler catheter (incl. 20MHz Doppler crystal) measuring coronary blood flow directions and changes.

Parks Medical Electronics, Inc. 503-649-7007
PO Box 5669, Aloha, OR 97006
PARKS Tabletop models: $595 for #811-B, 3 lbs., $795 for #810-A, 8 lbs., $650 for #811-BL, 3.5 lbs., $650 for #811-BTS, 3 lbs., $650 for #812, 3 lbs.; also, two pocket models - $395 for #840 $540 for #841-A.

Vascular Technology Incorporated 800-550-0856
12 Murphy Dr, Nashua, NH 03062
VTI intraoperative surgical Doppler.

Vmed Technology, Inc. (Formerly Ems Products, Inc.) 425-497-9149
16149 Redmond Way # 108, Redmond, WA 98052
ULTRASCOPE Blood flow and fetal.

DETECTOR, BLOOD LEAKAGE *(Gastro/Urology) 78FJD*

Serim Research Corp. 574-264-3440
3506 Reedy Dr, Elkhart, IN 46514
Test for blood in dialysate fluid.

DETECTOR, BUBBLE, CARDIOPULMONARY BYPASS
(Cardiovascular) 74KRL

Luna Innovations Incorporated 540-769-8400
1 Riverside Cir Ste 400, Roanoke, VA 24016
EDAC QUANTIFIER

Terumo Cardiovascular Systems (Tcvs) 800-283-7866
28 Howe St, Ashland, MA 01721
Bubble trap.

Terumo Cardiovascular Systems, Corp 800-521-2818
6200 Jackson Rd, Ann Arbor, MI 48103

DETECTOR, CARIES *(Dental And Oral) 76LFC*

Addent, Inc. 203-778-0200
43 Miry Brook Rd, Danbury, CT 06810
The MicroluxTM transilluminator provides a focused beam of cool white light for use in clinical diagnosis of caries, calculus, crown fractures and root canal orifice. The light is powered by a high intensity light emitting diode (LED) and transmitted through a focused glass fiber optic element. By using the technique of fiber optic transillumination, the scope of oral diagnosis can be greatly improved without the introduction of additional x-rays

American Dental Products, Inc. 800-846-7120
603 Country Club Dr Ste B, Bensenville, IL 60106
Caries detector plus.

Danville Materials 800-827-7940
3420 Fostoria Way Ste A200, San Ramon, CA 94583
Caries Finder Red & Green is licensed under the only researched and proven formula.

Gresco Products, Inc. 800-527-3250
13391 Murphy Rd, P.o. Box 865, Stafford, TX 77477
Caries detector.

Novocol, Inc. 303-665-7535
416 S Taylor Ave, Louisville, CO 80027
Caries detector, caries indicator.

Oratech, Llc 801-553-4493
475 W 10200 S, South Jordan, UT 84095
Caries detection device.

Ultradent Products, Inc. 801-553-4586
505 W 10200 S, South Jordan, UT 84095
Caries indicator.

DETECTOR, CENTROMERE *(Pathology) 88IJW*

Antibodies, Inc. 800-824-8540
PO Box 1560, Davis, CA 95617
Anti-Human Centromere antiserum

DETECTOR, DEEP VEIN THROMBOSIS *(Cardiovascular) 74QOM*

Huntleigh Healthcare Llc. 800-223-1218
40 Christopher Way, Eatontown, NJ 07724

DETECTOR, ELECTROCHEMICAL, CHROMATOGRAPHY, LIQUID *(Toxicology) 91LEQ*

Basi (Bioanalytical Systems, Inc.) 800-845-4246
2701 Kent Ave, West Lafayette, IN 47906
LC-3C, LC-4C; BAS 200B, electrochemical detectors and pulsed amperometric detectors.

DETECTOR, ELECTROCHEMICAL, CHROMATOGRAPHY, LIQUID *(cont'd)*

Esa, Inc. 800-959-5095
22 Alpha Rd, Chelmsford, MA 01824

Texas Photonics, Inc. 972-412-7111
3213 Main St, Rowlett, TX 75088

DETECTOR, ELECTROSTATIC VOLTAGE *(General) 80QTQ*

Julie Industries, Inc 978-276-0820
PO Box 153, North Reading, MA 01864

Monroe Electronics, Inc. 800-821-6001
100 Housel Ave, Lyndonville, NY 14098

DETECTOR, ETHYLENE-OXIDE LEAKAGE *(General) 80UMV*

American Gas & Chemical Co., Ltd. 800-288-3647
220 Pegasus Ave, Northvale, NJ 07647
$740.00 for wall-mounted toxic gas monitor to detect ethylene oxide.

Andersen Products, Inc., 800-523-1276
3202 Caroline Dr, Health Science Park, Haw River, NC 27258

Interscan Corp. 800-458-6153
21700 Nordhoff St, P.O. Box 2496, Chatsworth, CA 91311
$1,990.00 ea. for portable survey units, and $2750.00 and up for fixed systems. Full data acquisition/archiving/reporting system available.

DETECTOR, HEMODIALYSIS UNIT AIR BUBBLE-FOAM *(Gastro/Urology) 78QZV*

Medisystems Corporation 800-369-6334
439 S Union St Fl 5, Lawrence, MA 01843
Hemodialysis kits.

DETECTOR, HIS BUNDLE *(Cardiovascular) 74RAD*

Seecor, Inc. 972-288-3278
844 Dalworth Dr Ste 6, Mesquite, TX 75149
$6,686.00 per unit (standard); CARDIO-PROBE-HIS bundle detection and conduction mapping.

DETECTOR, LEAKAGE, MEDICAL GAS *(General) 80WPI*

Enmet Corp. 734-761-1270
PO Box 979, Ann Arbor, MI 48106
Toxic gas detectors.

Forward Technology 320-286-2578
260 Jenks Ave SW, Cokato, MN 55321
Pressure-decay leak testers to check for presence of leaks in critical medical components.

Himmelstein & Co., S. 800-632-7873
2490 Pembroke Ave, Hoffman Estates, IL 60169
Automatic, pressure decay leak test system.

Lifegas Llc 866-543-3427
1500 Indian Trail Lilburn Rd, Norcross, GA 30093
Medical Specialty Gases: LifeGas supplies a full line of gases for therapy, calibration, biological culture growth and various blood and pulmonary function testing. The range of medical gases and mixtures encompasses both in vivo (drug) and in vitro (device) applications. Use FDA's Compressed Medical Gases Guidelines.

Mercury Medical 800-237-6418
11300 49th St N, Clearwater, FL 33762
STAT CO2 end tidal CO2 detector. A colorimetric end tidal CO2 detector for verification of proper ET tube placement.

Patient Instrumentation Corp. 610-799-4436
4117 Route 309, Schnecksville, PA 18078
Testing of medical and laboratory gas systems.

Sensidyne, Inc. 800-451-9444
16333 Bay Vista Dr, Clearwater, FL 33760
SENSALERT stationary gas-detection system.

Sunshine Instruments 800-343-1199
2200 Michener St, Philadelphia, PA 19115

U.E. Systems, Inc. 800-223-1325
14 Hayes St, Elmsford, NY 10523
Oxygen/nitrous oxide leak detector electric emission detector, bearing monitor. ULTRAPROBE 10,000 Digital Ultrasonic inspection system.

DETECTOR, METAL, MAGNETIC *(Ophthalmology) 86RGN*

R. B. Annis Instruments, Inc. 317-637-9282
1101 N Delaware St, Indianapolis, IN 46202
$84.00 for 2-Gauss unit (8 ranges available); magnetic field. Helmholtz type magnetic-field standards. (See Magnetometer.)

DETECTOR, MICROWAVE LEAKAGE *(General) 80RGX*

Cober Electronics, Inc. 203-855-8755
151 Woodward Ave, Norwalk, CT 06854
Test systems.

Narda Safety Test Solutions 631-231-1700
435 Moreland Rd, Hauppauge, NY 11788
Checks microwave oven leakage to CDRH specifications.

Simpson Electric Co. 715-588-3311
520 Simpson Ave, PO Box 99, Lac Du Flambeau, WI 54538
Model 380-2. $643.55 per unit (standard).

DETECTOR, RADIOISOTOPE *(Radiology) 90WQO*

Berkeley Nucleonics Corp. 800-234-7858
2955 Kerner Blvd, San Rafael, CA 94901
Radiation isotope identifier. SAM Model 935 surveillance and measurement real-time isotope identifier, using gamma and neutron detectors and an MCA.

In/Us Systems, Inc. 800-875-4687
5809 N 50th St, Tampa, FL 33610
Radioisotope detectors for HPLC, GC, B-RAM, G-RAM, & GC-RAM.

DETECTOR, STRAIN *(General) 80RWM*

Alderon Biosciences, Inc. 919-544-8220
2810 Meridian Pkwy Ste 152, Durham, NC 27713
Molecular Detection for PCR products

Lds Life Science (Formerly Gould Instrument Systems Inc.) 216-328-7000
5525 Cloverleaf Pkwy, Valley View, OH 44125

DETECTOR, ULTRAVIOLET *(Dental And Oral) 76EAQ*

Eit, Inc. 703-478-0700
108 Carpenter Dr, Sterling, VA 20164
SPOTCURE, UVICURE PLUS, UV POWER PUCK, MICROCURE, POWERMAP & MAP PLUS Ultraviolet detectors. SPOTCURE UV intensity meter determines the efficiency in watts/cm2 of UV spot curing systems. UVICURE PLUS is a UV integrating radiometer which provides total dosage in joules/cm2 and peak UV intensity in watts/cm2 of one UV wavelength. UV POWER PUCK is the same as UVICURE PLUS except the dosage and peak UV intensity are given for four UV wavelengths. POWERMAP & MAP PLUS are UV temperature and intensity profiling systems.

Solar Light Co. 215-517-8700
100 E Glenside Ave, Glenside, PA 19038
UV radiometer.

Texas Photonics, Inc. 972-412-7111
3213 Main St, Rowlett, TX 75088

DETECTOR/REMOVER, LICE *(General) 80LJL*

American Comb Corp. 973-523-6551
22 Kentucky Ave, Paterson, NJ 07503
Lice comb.

Apothecary Products, Inc. 800-328-2742
11750 12th Ave S, Burnsville, MN 55337
Includes comb.

Block Drug Co., Inc. 973-889-2578
2149 Harbor Ave., Memphis, TN 38113
Lice comb.

Cfl Industries, Inc. 732-299-8790
331 Toledo St, Sebastian, FL 32958
Spray device for tick removal.

Del Pharmaceuticals, Inc. 516-844-2020
1830 Carver Dr, Rocky Point, NC 28457
Lice comb.

Health Ent., Inc. 508-695-0727
90 George Leven Dr, North Attleboro, MA 02760
Medicomb, acumed.

Health Enterprises 800-633-4243
90 George Leven Dr, North Attleboro, MA 02760
MEDI COMB Lice Comb.

Icp Medical 314-429-1000
10486 Baur Blvd, Saint Louis, MO 63132
Lice removal kit.

Kiel Laboratories, Inc. 770-534-0079
2225 Centennial Dr, Gainesville, GA 30504
Klout (tm) complete head lice treatment kit.

Larada Sciences Inc. 801-533-5423
350 W 800 N Ste 203, Salt Lake City, UT 84103
LouseBuster

DETECTOR/REMOVER, LICE *(cont'd)*

Qualis Group Llc 515-243-3000
4600 Park Ave, Des Moines, IA 50321
Lice egg remover gel, combo kit, solution kit, lice comb-3 pack, metal lice comb.

Safe Solutions, Inc. 616-677-2850
2530 Hayes St, Marne, MI 49435
Lice comb and shampoo kit.

DETERGENT *(Hematology) 81JCB*

Advanced Medical Science & Technology, Llc 410-628-1856
1 Stonegate Ct, Cockeysville, MD 21030
Manually liquid based cytology preparation system.

Beckman Coulter, Inc. 800-635-3497
740 W 83rd St, Hialeah, FL 33014

Bio-Rad Laboratories, Diagnostic Group 800-224-6723
524 Stone Rd Ste A, Benicia, CA 94510
Detergents/cleaning agents.

Carochem, Inc. 919-682-5121
744 E Markham Ave # 15699, Durham, NC 27701
Powdered blend for surgical instrument cleaning.

Chester Labs, Inc. 800-354-9709
1900 Section Rd, Cincinnati, OH 45237
ORGANISOL, hospital ware detergent.

Diagnostic Technology, Inc. 631-582-4949
175 Commerce Dr Ste L, Hauppauge, NY 11788
Isotonic detergent cleaner.

Germiphene Corp. 519-759-7100
1379 Colborne St. E, Brantford, ONT N3T-5M1 Canada
Enzymtic detergent

Haemo-Sol, Inc. 800-821-5676
7301 York Rd, Baltimore, MD 21204

Micro-Scientific Industries, Inc. 888-253-2536
1225 Carnegie St Ste 101, Rolling Meadows, IL 60008
For use in all areas of the healthcare facility where cross contamination is a concern. 3-minute contact time kills 100% of bacteria, viruses, mycobacteria and fungion surfaces.

Micronova 888-816-4876
3431 Lomita Blvd, Torrance, CA 90505

Stanbio Laboratory, Inc. 830-249-0772
1261 N Main St, Boerne, TX 78006
$21.50 for 1,000 ml, $51.00 for 3,800ml, BIO-CLEAN. $25.00 for 1,000ml, BIO-CLEAN II.

Ultra Clean Systems, Inc. 877-935-6624
12700 Dupont Cir, Tampa, FL 33626
Ultra Wash concentrated detergent for ultrasonic cleaners and automatic washers.

DEVICE, ABLATION, THERMAL, ENDOMETRIAL
(Obstetrics/Gyn) 85MNB

Cytyc Surgical Products 800-442-9892
250 Campus Dr, Marlborough, MA 01752
Impedance controlled endometrial ablation system.

DEVICE, ABLATION, THERMAL, ULTRASONIC
(Gastro/Urology) 78MIK

Focus Surgery, Inc. 317-541-1580
3940 Pendleton Way, Indianapolis, IN 46226
Image Guided High Intensity Focused Ultrasound (HIFU)Therapy

Urologix, Inc. 800-475-1403
14405 21st Ave N, Minneapolis, MN 55447

DEVICE, ANALYSIS, ANTERIOR SEGMENT
(Ophthalmology) 86MXK

Clarity Medical Systems 925-463-7984
5775 W Las Positas Blvd Ste 200, Pleasanton, CA 94588
Ac powered slitlamp biomicroscope.

Nidek, Inc. 510-226-5700
47651 Westinghouse Dr, Fremont, CA 94539
Ac-powered slitlamp biomicroscope.

DEVICE, ANASTOMOSIS, BIOFRAGMENTABLE *(Surgery) 79SIW*

Covidien Lp 508-261-8000
15 Hampshire St, Mansfield, MA 02048

DEVICE, ANASTOMOTIC, MICROVASCULAR
(Cardiovascular) 74MVR

Novare Surgical Systems, Inc. 408-873-3161
10440 Bubb Rd Ste A, Cupertino, CA 95014
Enclose Cardiac Anastomotic Assist Device. Eliminates need for partial occlusion clamp during CABG procedures.

Synovis Micro Companies Alliance, Inc. 651-603-3700
439 Industrial Ln, Birmingham, AL 35211
Microvascular anastomotic device.

DEVICE, ANTI-SNORING *(Ear/Nose/Throat) 77LRK*

Airway Management Inc. 214-369-0978
6116 N Central Expy Ste 605, Dallas, TX 75206
Various models of anti-snoring devices.

Aztec Orthodontic Laboratory, Inc. 520-744-1588
7750 N Red Wing Cir, Tucson, AZ 85741
Tap ii,t,oasys.

Biotemps Dental Laboratory 949-440-2683
2181 Dupont Dr, Irvine, CA 92612
Snoring device.

Dental Prosthetic Services, Inc. 319-393-1990
1150 Old Marion Rd NE, Cedar Rapids, IA 52402
Dental devices for snoring & sleep apnea.

Dental Systems Group 315-732-3151
601 State St, Utica, NY 13502
Intra oral device for snoring and sleep apnea.

Dream Systems, L.L.C. 650-369-9227
6 Malory Ct, Redwood City, CA 94061
Dental device for snoring and obstructive sleep apnea.

Dresch/Tolson Dental Lab 952-345-6300
4024 N Holland Sylvania Rd, Toledo, OH 43623
Anti-snoring device.

E. Benson Hood Laboratories, Inc. 800-942-5227
575 Washington St, Pembroke, MA 02359
QUIET NIGHT, silicone device dilates the nasal valve.

Frantz Design, Inc. 512-451-3311
3202 Oakmont Blvd, Austin, TX 78703
Various.

Heumann & Associates Dental Lab 952-541-9622
520 SE 5th St, Topeka, KS 66607
Anti-snoring device.

Lantz Dental Prosthetics, Inc. 419-866-1515
6490 Wheatstone Ct, Maumee, OH 43537
Elastic mandibular advancement (ema) appliance.

Netwal Dental Laboratory 608-782-1724
115 5th Ave S Ste 307, La Crosse, WI 54601
Intraoral device for sleep apnea.

Nose Breathe 808-949-8876
2065 S King St Ste 304, Honolulu, HI 96826
Nose breathe mouthpiece for heavy snorer.

Orthodontic Technologies, Inc. 713-861-0033
5524 Cornish St, Houston, TX 77007
Dental device for snoring and sleep apnea.

Ottawa Dental Laboratory, Ltd 815-434-0655
1304 Starfire Dr, Ottawa, IL 61350
Snoring appliance.

Precise Plastics 814-474-5504
7700 Middle Rd, Fairview, PA 16415
Intra-oral mandibular repositioner.

Precision Dental Laboratories, Inc. 701-280-9089
6 Broadway N Ste 200, Fargo, ND 58102
Mild to moderate sleep apnea and snoring device.

Pro-Tex International, Inc. 209-545-1691
5038 Salida Blvd, Salida, CA 95368
Snore guard, anti-snoring device.

Professional Dental Laboratory Corporation
1400 W Indiana Ave, P.o. Box 877, Elkhart, IN 46516
Dental devices for snoring and sleep apnea.

Restore Medical Inc. 866-869-7237
2800 Patton Rd, Saint Paul, MN 55113
Palatal implant system.

Somnomed Inc. 940-381-5200
3537 Teasley Ln, Denton, TX 76210
Mandibular advancement device.

DEVICE, ANTI-SNORING *(cont'd)*

Town & Country Dental Studios 516-868-8641
275 S Main St, Freeport, NY 11520
Sleep apnea appliance, anti-snoring appliance.

DEVICE, ANTI-TIP, WHEELCHAIR *(Physical Med) 89IMR*

Alimed, Inc. 800-225-2610
297 High St, Dedham, MA 02026

Care Products Inc. 757-224-0177
10701 N Ware Rd, McAllen, TX 78504
Shower/commode chair.

Mjm International Corporation 956-781-5000
2003 N Veterans Blvd Ste 10, San Juan, TX 78589
Self propelled aquatic chair, wheelchair.

Sunrise Medical Hhg Inc 303-218-4505
2842 N Business Park Ave, Fresno, CA 93727

Tuffcare 800-367-6160
3999 E La Palma Ave, Anaheim, CA 92807

DEVICE, ASSIST, CPR *(Anesthesiology) 73LYM*

American Diagnostic Corporation (Adc) 800-232-2670
55 Commerce Dr, Hauppauge, NY 11788
CPR Valve mask

Armstrong Medical Industries, Inc. 800-323-4220
575 Knightsbridge Pkwy, Lincolnshire, IL 60069
Complete CPR training system includes adult, child and infant apparatus.

Certified Safety Manufacturing 800-854-7474
1400 Chestnut Ave, Kansas City, MO 64127
CPROTECTOR.

Eagle Health Supplies, Inc. 800-755-8999
535 W Walnut Ave, Orange, CA 92868
CPR mouth barrier.

Guppie Ent., Inc. 541-548-0748
9251 SW Geneva View Rd, Crooked River Ranch, OR 97760
Barrier device used during cpr.

K. W. Griffen Co. 203-846-1923
100 Pearl St, Norwalk, CT 06850
Cpr kit.

Medical Action Industries, Inc. 800-645-7042
25 Heywood Rd, Arden, NC 28704
Cpr device.

Medical Safety Systems Inc. 888-803-9303
230 White Pond Dr, Akron, OH 44313

Mtm Health Products Ltd. 800-263-8253
2349 Fairview St., Burlington, ONT L7R 2E3 Canada
CPR LANDMARC an assistive device that attaches to the landmark position on the chest to make chest compressions during CPR easier and more accurate. MTM SHIELD for emergency CPR, faceshield-type emergency resuscitator with one-way valve and soft faceshield. Positive one-way valve with patient exhaust port, prevents direct mouth to mouth contact with patient, disposable.

North Safety Products 401-943-4400
1101 B Calle Neutron, Parque Industrial Maran, Mexicali, B.c. Mexico
Rescue breather

Plasco, Inc. 847-662-4400
Carretera Presta La Amistad, Km.19, Acuna, Coahila Mexico
Mouth to mouth resuscitation kit

Rondex Products, Inc. 815-226-0452
PO Box 1829, Rockford, IL 61110
Model 2230 CPR RESCUE KIT; mask, valve, mouthpiece. CPR ISO-SHIELD has two valves located in the bite block, grips below shield barrier allows the operator to place and remove the barrier without touching the top side. This reduces the risk of spreading contamination to the opertor's mouth side of the barrier. Model 9140 & 91402 CPR POCKET RESCUE MASK, mask with valve folds down into plastic pocket case. Double valves placed in valve mouthpiece increases operator safety.

Vector Firstaid, Inc. 800-999-4423
316 N Corona Ave, Ontario, CA 91764

Vitaid Ltd. 800-267-9301
300 International Dr, Williamsville, NY 14221
Boussignac CPR Tube - continuous insufflation

DEVICE, ASSISTIVE LISTENING *(Ear/Nose/Throat) 77LZI*

Doc's Proplugs, Inc. 800-521-2982
719 Swift St Ste 100, Santa Cruz, CA 95060
Earmold/Adapter called Doc's Protune used to secure budstyle earphones securely in the ear for ALD and Walkman.

DEVICE, ASSISTIVE LISTENING *(cont'd)*

Sennheiser Electronic Corp. 877-736-6434
1 Enterprise Dr, Old Lyme, CT 06371
SENNHEISER, Direct Ear SET 250:personal infrared assistive listening system. SENNHEISER, Mikroport 2013-PLL personal FM system to assist hearing impaired. SENNHEISER, SI1015INT, rack mountable, half rack, two channel transmitter. SENNHEISER, SZI1029-24, emitter with operating voltage of 24V DC. SENNHEISER SZI1029 Emitter with operating voltage of 120 VAC. SP230, two channel, portable transmitter/emitter. SI30/ SZI30, Two channel, medium area, modulator and emitter. DIRECT EAR, set 100 TV listening system, compatible with many performance theaters using infrared systems operating at 95 kHz.

DEVICE, BIOPSY, PERCUTANEOUS *(Surgery) 79MJG*

Angiotech 800-424-6779
241 W Palatine Rd, Wheeling, IL 60090
SPRITACRE closed-tip atraumatic spinal needle for local and regional anesthesia. Bone-marrow needle for biopsy, aspiration, and bone-marrow harvesting.

Beekley Corp. 860-583-4700
150 Dolphin Rd, Bristol, CT 06010
Foam device for eliminating negative stroke margin.

Gammadirect Medical Division 847-267-5929
PO Box 383, Lake Forest, IL 60045
AukuProbe Bone Biopsy Needle is specifically designed for iliac crest biopsy.

Havel's Inc. 800-638-4770
3726 Lonsdale St, Cincinnati, OH 45227

Interventional Spine, Inc. 800-497-0484
13700 Alton Pkwy Ste 160, Irvine, CA 92618
Biopsy needle.

Medtronic Spine Llc 877-690-5353
1221 Crossman Ave, Sunnyvale, CA 94089
Biopsy needle.

Osseon Therapeutics, Inc. 877-567-7366
2330 Circadian Way, Santa Rosa, CA 95407

DEVICE, CLOSURE, PUNCTURE, HEMOSTATIC *(Cardiovascular) 74WYE*

Datascope Interventional Products Division 800-225-5827
1300 MacArthur Blvd, Mahwah, NJ 07430
VASOSEAL VHD and needle depth indicator kit for use with VASOSEAL VHD. VASOSEAL ES, extra vascular arterial sealing, utilizes unique temporary arterial locator system that better locates femoral artery. One size fits 5 to 8 french sheath sizes.

Kensey Nash Corporation 484-713-2100
735 Pennsylvania Dr, Exton, PA 19341
ANGIOSEAL developed to seal femoral artery punctures post-catheterization. Holder of approximately 25 U.S. and worldwide patents covering the closure of punctures in tissue.

Mcdalt Medical Corp. 800-841-5774
2225 Prestonwood Dr Ste 100-A, Arlington, TX 76012
Scion Sci-Pro, the dstal protection device. Radius medical snare device with Micro-Snares for cath labs, interventional radiology, et al.

Ranfac Corp. 800-2RANFAC
30 Doherty Ave, Avon Industrial Park, Avon, MA 02322
The Puncture Closure Device is efficient with its one hand operation and enables the surgeon to rapidly close multiple trocar sites securely and safely in a single device. The Puncture Closure Devise is used to tack up hernia mesh prior to final placement, to ligate abdominal wall bleeding and for percutaneous suturing. With a 14-gauge outside diameter, the Puncture Closure Device accommodates any size suture and any size trocar.

DEVICE, COMMUNICATIONS, IMAGES, OPHTHALMIC *(Ophthalmology) 86NFG*

Clarity Medical Systems 925-463-7984
5775 W Las Positas Blvd Ste 200, Pleasanton, CA 94588
Medical image communications device.

Image Technology Laboratories, Inc. 845-338-3366
602 Enterprise Dr, Kingston, NY 12401
Ris/pacs.

Inoveon Corp. 405-271-9025
800 Research Pkwy Ste 370, Oklahoma City, OK 73104
Diabetic retinopathy photography device.

Joslin Diabetes Center 617-226-5808
1 Joslin Pl, Boston, MA 02215
Medical image communications device.

DEVICE, COMMUNICATIONS, IMAGES, OPHTHALMIC *(cont'd)*

Smith & Nephew Inc., Endoscopy Div. 978-749-1000
76 S Meridian Ave, Oklahoma City, OK 73107
Software, integration broker, hl7.

Tc Imaging Solutions 757-224-0177
2432 Cheyenne Trl, Traverse City, MI 49684
Medical image communications device.

DEVICE, CONDITIONING, AVERSION *(Cns/Neurology) 84HCB*

Hq, Inc. 941-721-7588
210 9th Street Dr W # 208-210, Palmetto, FL 34221
Self injurious behavior inhibiting system.

The Judge Rotenberg Educational Center, Inc. 781-828-2202
240 Turnpike St, Canton, MA 02021
Graduated electronic decelerator.

DEVICE, CORONARY SAPHENOUS VEIN BYPASS GRAFT, TEMPORARY, FOR EMBOLIZATION PROTECTION
(Cardiovascular) 74NFA

Abbott Vascular, Vascular Solutions 800-227-9902
26531 Ynez Rd, Temecula, CA 92591
Embolic protection device.

Ev3 Inc. 800-716-6700
4600 Nathan Ln N, Plymouth, MN 55442
Embolic protection device.

Lumen Biomedical, Inc. 763-577-9600
14505 21st Ave N Ste 212, Plymouth, MN 55447
Percutaneous catheter.

Medtronic Vascular 707-525-0111
3576 Unocal Pl, Santa Rosa, CA 95403
Distal protection system

DEVICE, CYSTOMETRIC, HYDRAULIC *(Gastro/Urology) 78FEN*

C. R. Bard, Inc., Bard Urological Div. 888-367-2273
13183 Harland Dr NE, Covington, GA 30014

Medan Inc. 541-231-4141
131 NW 4th St Ste 395, Corvallis, OR 97330
Urodynamic device.

Medtronic Neuromodulation 763-514-4000
710 Medtronic Pkwy, Minneapolis, MN 55432
Various types of cystometric, hydraulic devices.

Myo/Kinetic Systems, Inc. 414-255-1005
North 84 West 13562 Leon Rd., Menomonee Falls, WI 53051
Urodynamic equipment.

Unisensor Usa, Inc. 603-926-5200
1 Park Ave Ste 6, Hampton, NH 03842
Urodynamics measurement system.

Wolfe Tory Medical, Inc. 801-281-3000
79 W 4500 S Ste 18, Salt Lake City, UT 84107
Cystometric tubing and infusion set.

DEVICE, DERMAL REPLACEMENT *(Surgery) 79MDD*

Integra Lifesciences Corporation 800-654-2873
105 Morgan Ln, Plainsboro, NJ 08536
INTEGRA Artificial Skin Regeneration Template is a biosynthetic implantable wound couver, indicated for the postexcisional treatment of life-threatening full-thickness or deep partial-thickness thermal injury. It is the first artificial skin that regenerates dermal tissue to receive approval to market by the US Food and Drug Administration(FDA).

DEVICE, DIAGNOSTIC, NON-PHYSIOLOGICAL
(Cns/Neurology) 84MHM

Quadromed Inc. 800-363-0192
5776 Thimens Ave., St-Laurent, QUE H4R 2K9 Canada

DEVICE, DYSFUNCTION, ERECTILE *(Gastro/Urology) 78LST*

Bio-Feedback Systems, Inc. 303-444-1411
2736 47th St, Boulder, CO 80301

Life-Tech, Inc. 281-491-6600
4235 Greenbriar Dr, Stafford, TX 77477
Cavropump and PC system for cavernosometry

Timm Medical Technologies, Inc. 800-966-2796
6585 City West Pkwy, Eden Prairie, MN 55344
ESTEEM Manual System, ESTEEM Battery System, ERECAID CLASSIC, vacuum erection devices.

DEVICE, DYSFUNCTION, ERECTILE *(cont'd)*

Vivus, Inc. 650-934-5200
1172 Castro St, Mountain View, CA 94040
MUSE non-injectable delivery system for alprostadil. Is indicated for the treatment of erectile dysfunction. MUSE is a non-injectable, transurethral drug delivery system consisting of a prefilled plastic applicator containing a urethral suppository of alprostadil.

DEVICE, EMBOLIZATION, ARTIFICIAL *(Cns/Neurology) 84HCG*

Biocure, Inc. 678-966-3400
2975 Gateway Dr Ste 100, Norcross, GA 30071
Embolic agent sterile.

Biosphere Medical, Inc. 781-681-7900
1050 Hingham St, Rockland, MA 02370
Embolization device.

Boston Scientific-Neurovascular 510-440-7700
47900 Bayside Pkwy, Fremont, CA 94538
Spheres or emboli.

Cordis Neurovascular, Inc. 800-327-7714
14201 NW 60th Ave, Miami Lakes, FL 33014
Embolization device.

Edwards Lifesciences, Llc. 800-424-3278
1 Edwards Way, Irvine, CA 92614
Side-branch-occlusion system.

Ev3 Neurovascular 800-716-6700
9775 Toledo Way, Irvine, CA 92618
Neurovascular embolization device.

Ivalon, Inc. 800-948-2566
1015 Cordova St, San Diego, CA 92107
Ivalon PVA Embolization Particles for permanent therapeutic occlusion and preoperative occlusion of arteriovenous malformations (AVMs) and hypervascular tumors.

Maquet Cardiovascular LLC 888-880-2874
45 Barbour Pond Dr, Wayne, NJ 07470
NEUROVASCULAR - CONTOUR

Microvention, Inc. 949-461-3314
75 Columbia, Aliso Viejo, CA 92656
Embolization coil.

Micrus Corporation 408-830-5900
610 Palomar Ave, Sunnyvale, CA 94085
MicroCoils and microcatheters for use in embolization of cerebral aneurysms.

Micrus Endovascular Corporation 888-550-4120
821 Fox Ln, San Jose, CA 95131
Catheter system for delivery of embolic coil systems.

Surgica Corporation 800-979-5090
PO Box 723, Pollock Pines, CA 95726
PVA foam embolization particles.

DEVICE, ENGORGEMENT, CLITORAL *(Obstetrics/Gyn) 85NBV*

Nu Gyn, Inc 763-398-0108
1633 County Highway 10 Ste 15, Spring Lake Park, MN 55432
Eros-clitoral therapy device.

DEVICE, FERTILITY, CONTRACEPTIVE, DIAGNOSTIC
(Obstetrics/Gyn) 85MEE

Monarch Art Plastics, Llc. 856-235-5151
3838 Church Rd, Mount Laurel, NJ 08054
Gestational calculator

Pheromone Science Corp. 416-861-9854
443 King St. E, Toronto, ONT M5A-1L5 Canada
FDA Approved Indications for Use: Fertilite-OVI (PSCFertility Monitor) is an over-the-counter ('OTC') in vitro diagnostic ('IVD') device intended for use by women as an aid in conception, by measuring hormone-induced changes in the composition of the perspiration on the skin during the menstrual cycle. Properly used, it gives more notice for conceiving and is not invasive. It is NOT to be used for contraception. FERTILIT...: a small, non-invasive device in the form of a wristwatch, which is comfortably worn for six continuous hours each day from early in the menstrual cycle (starting on days 1 - 3) until FERTILIT... announces (typically on day 8 - 12 of the cycle) that ovulation will occur in four days. FERTILIT... employs a disposable biosensor that extradermally measures chloride ions from the skin surface of the skin. The biosensor is filled with a gel that is gradually depleted over time (the sensor itself has a lifespan of one month and will be sold as a consumable). The watch like device incorporates an interactive microprocessor that runs proprietary software algorithms to analyze the ion changes. The proprietary algorithms reliably enables FERTILIT... to provide its four-day advance notice of ovulation. As the chloride ion surge peaks, the device informs the user that ithe

fertility window has opened, which commences the four-day countdown to ovulation. The FERTILIT... watch displays the fertility status of the user as non-fertile (NF), fertile (FT), ovulating (OV) or less fertile (LF). FT is indicated for the four days prior to ovulation since intercourse during any of these days can reasonably result in conception. OV is indicated for two days, comprising the predicted day of the LH surge, and an additional day to account for the 0-24 hours required for the actual time of egg release (ovulation). Results can be viewed at any time on the LCD screen of the watch, and/or the user can be alerted of her fertility status via optional audio signals. An optional accessory coupled with the appropriate software allows the results to be viewed as a computer-generated graphical printout which can be sent to medical professionals via a data transmission upload unit (base and cable) or via a modem unit uploading the data through telephone lines.

DEVICE, FLUSH, VASCULAR ACCESS *(General) 80NGT*

Excelsior Medical Corp. 732-776-7525
1933 Heck Ave, Neptune, NJ 07753
Pre-filled flush syringe.

DEVICE, GERMICIDAL, ULTRAVIOLET *(General) 80MKB*

Ultra-Lum, Inc. 800-809-6559
1480 N Claremont Blvd, Claremont, CA 91711
Midsize and Large Ultraviolet Crosslinker Systems.

DEVICE, HEMOSTASIS, VASCULAR *(Cardiovascular) 74MGB*

Abbott Vascular Inc. 800-227-9902
400 Saginaw Dr, Redwood City, CA 94063
Suture-mediated closure device.

Avd 503-223-2333
2326 NW Everett St, Portland, OR 97210

Datascope Corp. 800-288-2121
14 Philips Pkwy, Montvale, NJ 07645
VASOSEAL.

Datascope Interventional Products Division 800-225-5827
1300 MacArthur Blvd, Mahwah, NJ 07430
Vasoseal Low Profile hemostasis device is a downsized VHD device available in sizes 1to 5. Vasoseal Elite hemostasis device features Datascope's proprietary sponge collagen.

Ensure Medical, Inc. 408-745-7610
762 San Aleso Ave, Sunnyvale, CA 94085
Vascular hemostasis device.

Excel Medical Products, Llc 810-714-4775
3145 Copper Ave, Fenton, MI 48430
The Excel-6 and Excel-9 are high-pressure precision y-connectors, with Touhy-Borst adapter, commonly used in angioplasty and stent procedures. They can be provided individual or bulk, sterile or non-sterile. The Excel-6 (.083 in. - 6 Fr.) and Excel-9 (.120 in. - 9 Fr.) hemostasis valves incorporate a unique flow adjustment design for better control, as well as an increased angle for ease of use and maximum patient comfort.

Medtronic Perfusion Systems 800-328-3320
7611 Northland Dr N, Brooklyn Park, MN 55428
Management system.

Scion Cardio-Vascular, Inc. 305-259-8880
14256 SW 119th Ave, Miami, FL 33186
CLO-SUR PLUS P.A.D. Antimicrobial Barrier Topical Hemostasis Dressing 10/box

St. Jude Medical, Puerto Rico, B.V. 787-746-1111
Lot 20, Caguas West Industrial Park, Caguas, PR 00726-0998
Vascular puncture closure device.

Vascular Solutions, Inc. 888-240-6001
6464 Sycamore Ct N, Maple Grove, MN 55369
Vascular hemostasis device.

Vascular Solutions, Inc. 763-656-4300
5025 Cheshire Ln N, Plymouth, MN 55446
Vascular hemostasis device.

Whalen Biomedical Incorporated 617-868-4433
11 Miller St, Somerville, MA 02143
A fibrin-based hemostatic agent/tissue adhesive for intra-operative or topical use.

DEVICE, HYPERTHERMIA (BLANKET, PLUMBING & HEAT EXCHANGER) *(Cardiovascular) 74BTE*

Adroit Medical Systems, Inc. 800-267-6077
1146 Carding Machine Rd, Loudon, TN 37774
Soft-Air convective warming systems. Nine types of blankets: Adult, Pediatric, Neonate, Upper Body, Lower Body, Torso, Warming Tube, Full Body Sugical Access and Lower Body Surgical Access.

DEVICE, INCONTINENCE, FECAL *(Gastro/Urology) 78WLL*

California Medical Innovations 800-229-5871
873 E Arrow Hwy, Pomona, CA 91767

Dumex Medical Surgical Products Ltd. 800-463-9613
104 Shorting Rd., Scarborough, ONT M1S 3S4 Canada
Abdominal Pads - unique, super-absorbant, unsurpassed quality for your peace of mind.

Revelation L.L.C. 800-510-5012
PO Box 486, 437 Howard Ave, Bridgeport, CT 06601
Prostate Pants, Reusable Briefs: Stops leakage of prostate conditions

Smith & Nephew, Inc. 800-876-1261
11775 Starkey Rd, Largo, FL 33773
Fecal incontinence collection bag; also, BANISH II liquid ostomy appliance deodorant and ODO-WAY ostomy appliance deodorant in pill form.

DEVICE, INCONTINENCE, FECAL, IMPLANTED *(Gastro/Urology) 78MIP*

Uroplasty, Inc. 952-426-6140
5420 Feltl Rd, Minnetonka, MN 55343

DEVICE, INCONTINENCE, MECHANICAL/HYDRAULIC *(Gastro/Urology) 78EZY*

Kay See Dental Mfg. Co. 816-842-2817
124 Missouri Ave, Kansas City, MO 64106
Diaphragm wax.

Neurodyne Medical Corp. 800-963-8633
186 Alewife Brook Pkwy, Cambridge, MA 02138
IA-250 allows any NeuroDyne EMG instrument to be used with standard vaginal and rectal EMG sensors for muscle reeducation.

Park Surgical Co., Inc. 800-633-7878
5001 New Utrecht Ave, Brooklyn, NY 11219
MALE BAG Male incontinence device.

Uromedica, Inc. 763-694-9880
1840 Berkshire Ln N, Plymouth, MN 55441
Implantable balloon occlusion device.

DEVICE, INCONTINENCE, OCCLUSION, URETHRAL *(Gastro/Urology) 78MNG*

Apple Medical Corp. 508-357-2700
28 Lord Rd Ste 135, Marlborough, MA 01752
Incontinence device.

Cook Biotech, Incorporated 888-299-4224
1425 Innovation Pl, West Lafayette, IN 47906
Urethral Sling & pelvic floor repair

Praxis, Llc. 508-400-3969
1110 Washington St, Holliston, MA 01746
Urethral bulker.

Smiths Medical Asd 800-424-8662
5700 W 23rd Ave, Gary, IN 46406
On-Command male incontinence catheter. Intraurethral urological catheter for management of urinary dysfunction with patient activated magnetic valve.

Solace Therapeutics, Inc 760-431-0153
5865 Avenida Encinas Ste 142B, Carlsbad, CA 92008
Female urinary incontinence device.

Uromend, Llc 540-980-0886
1321 Hopkins Dr, Pulaski, VA 24301
Penile or urethral incontinence clamp.

DEVICE, INCONTINENCE, PASTE-ON *(Gastro/Urology) 78EXI*

Bioderm, Inc. 800-373-7006
12320 73rd Ct, Largo, FL 33773
External male incontinence.

Care Electronics, Inc. 303-444-2273
4700 Sterling Dr Ste D, Boulder, CO 80301
WET SENSE; silent monitoring system that alerts staff to change wet bedding, garments.

DEVICE, INCONTINENCE, UROSHEATH TYPE, NON-STERILE *(Gastro/Urology) 78NNX*

Coloplast Manufacturing Us, Llc 612-302-4992
1185 Willow Lake Blvd, Vadnais Heights, MN 55110
Male external catheter.

Hollister, Inc. 847-680-2849
366 Draft Ave, Stuarts Draft, VA 24477

DEVICE, INFLATION, MIDDLE EAR *(Ear/Nose/Throat) 77MJV*

American Medical Industries 605-428-5501
330 E 3rd St Ste 2, Dell Rapids, SD 57022
Home Care Ear Exam Kit aids the home consumer in the early detection and monitoring of ear ailments. The kit includes a high-intensity exam light, four various-sized speculums, and a fully illustrated guidebook with actual color photographs and explanations.

Micromedics 800-624-5662
1270 Eagan Industrial Rd, Saint Paul, MN 55121
The new EarPopper™ is designed to treat otitis media by non-invasively aerating the middle ear. This simple and safe device can be used in the office or at home. NIH sponsored clinical studies have shown that the EarPopper™ can eliminate the need for vent tube surgery in a significant number of cases.

DEVICE, JAW TRACKING, FOR DIAGNOSIS OF TMJ/MPD DISORDERS *(Dental And Oral) 76NFR*

Water Pik, Inc. 970-221-6129
1730 E Prospect Rd, Fort Collins, CO 80525
Jaw tracking device.

DEVICE, JAW TRACKING, FOR MONITORING JAW POSITIONS
(Dental And Oral) 76NFS

Bio-Research Associates, Inc. 414-357-7525
9275 N 49th St Ste 150, Brown Deer, WI 53223
Mandibular movement recorder.

Whip Mix Corp. 502-637-1451
1730 E Prospect Rd Ste 101, Fort Collins, CO 80525

DEVICE, LIMITING, BEAM, DIAGNOSTIC, X-RAY
(Radiology) 90KPW

Ar Custom Medical Products, Ltd. 516-242-7501
19 W Industry Ct Ste A, Deer Park, NY 11729
Ad-1 beam limiting device.

Dentalez Group, Stardental Division 717-291-1161
1816 Colonial Village Ln, Lancaster, PA 17601
Rectangular position indicating device.

Radcal Corp. 800-423-7169
426 W Duarte Rd, Monrovia, CA 91016
Non-invasive and invasive KVP meters, for single phase to high frequency x-ray machines.

DEVICE, LIMITING, BEAM, TELETHERAPY *(Radiology) 90KQA*

Neutron Products, Inc. 301-349-5001
22301 Mount Ephraim Rd, Dickerson, MD 20842

DEVICE, LIMITING, BEAM, TELETHERAPY, RADIONUCLIDE
(Radiology) 90IWD

Marconi Medical Systems 800-323-0550
595 Miner Rd, Cleveland, OH 44143

Neutron Products, Inc. 301-349-5001
22301 Mount Ephraim Rd, Dickerson, MD 20842

DEVICE, LOCKING, CLAMP, INSTESTINAL
(Gastro/Urology) 78FFR

Aesculap Implant Systems Inc. 1-800-234-9179
3773 Corporate Pkwy, Center Valley, PA 18034

Tuzik Boston 800-886-6363
104 Longwater Dr, Assinippi Park, Norwell, MA 02061

DEVICE, MEASUREMENT, POTENTIAL, SKIN
(Cns/Neurology) 84HCJ

Barefoot Medical 760-967-8225
1902 Calle Buena Ventura, Oceanside, CA 92056
BAREFOOT, transparent, flexible and disposable dermal ulcer measuring device available in 7 cm and 10 cm sizes, boxed and padded.

Caldwell, Justiss & Co., Inc. 800-643-4343
622 W Sycamore St, P.O. Box 520, Fayetteville, AR 72703
$450.00 SKYNDEX SYSTEM I body fat electronic calculator; measures percent body fat using three different formulas, LCD display.

General Assembly Corporation 877-GACNC4U
140 Industrial Park Way, West Jefferson, NC 28694

Solarius Development Inc. 800-731-1220
550 E Weddell Dr Ste 3, Sunnyvale, CA 94089
DERMAPROFILE, laser-based non-contact Skin Measurement System permits skin surface changes to be objectively measured to determine changes of skin with treatment of cosmetics, creams, cleansers and soaps, etc.

DEVICE, MEASUREMENT, POTENTIAL, SKIN *(cont'd)*

U.F.I. 805-772-1203
545 Main St Ste C2, Morro Bay, CA 93442
$655.00 for Model 2701.

DEVICE, MEASUREMENT, VELOCITY, CONDUCTION, NERVE
(Cns/Neurology) 84JXE

Ad-Tech Medical Instrument Corp. 800-776-1555
1901 William St, Racine, WI 53404
Spinal Electrode for motor evoked potential monitoring during spinal surgery.

Cadwell Laboratories 800-245-3001
909 N Kellogg St, Kennewick, WA 99336
SIERRA II EMG/EP. CENTRAL EEG/EMG/EP.

Medtronic Neuromodulation 763-514-4000
710 Medtronic Pkwy, Minneapolis, MN 55432
Neuro-urodynamics suite.

Minisun, Llc 559-439-4600
935 E Mill Creek Dr, Fresno, CA 93720
Revolutionary device for physical activity assessment, energy expenditure measurement, functional assessment, and behavior monitoring

Neoprobe Corporation 800-793-0079
425 Metro Pl N Ste 300, Dublin, OH 43017
Quantix/ND for the real-time noninvasive measurement of CBF in the ICA

Neumed Inc. 800-367-1238
800 Silvia St, Ewing, NJ 08628
Brevio NCS-Monitor: Accurate diagnosis of Carpal Tunnel Syndrome and other peripheral neuropathies. Automatically evaluates Sensory, Motor, and F-wave responses of the median and ulnar nerves using a single non-invasive Neuro-sensor.

Neurometrix, Inc. 888-786-7287
62 4th Ave, Waltham, MA 02451
Nerve conduction monitoring system.

Neurotron Medical 609-896-3444
800 Silvia St, Ewing, NJ 08628
Nerve conduction monitor.

Phipps & Bird, Inc. 800-955-7621
1519 Summit Ave, Richmond, VA 23230
Nerve conduction chamber for student education.

Scientific Imaging, Llc 770-926-3060
9878 Main St Ste 125, Woodstock, GA 30188
Electromyograph.

DEVICE, NEEDLE DESTRUCTION *(General) 80MTV*

Safeguard Medical Technologies, Llc 330-547-2166
14200 Ellsworth Rd, Berlin Center, OH 44401
Insulin needle destruction device.

DEVICE, OCCLUSION, CARDIAC, TRANSCATHETER
(Cardiovascular) 74MLV

Aga Medical Corporation. 888-546-4407
5050 Nathan Ln N, Plymouth, MN 55442
AMPLATZER PFO Occluder-- The PFO Occluder is indicated for transcatheter closure of Patent Foramen Ovale. On October 31, 2006, the AMPLATZER PFO Occluder trnsferred from HDE status to IDE use under the PFO Access Registry. The device is also in clinical study in the PREMUIM and RESPECT Trials under IDE from the FDA in the United States. The device is CE marked for sale in EU countries, and has approval for sale in many countries worlwide.AMPLATZER Septal Occluder-- The Septal Occluder is indicated for transcatheter closure of Artial Septal Defect in the secundum position or from fenestrated Fontab procedure. The Occluder is a self-expandable device made from a Nitinol wire mesh that expands to close the defect. Polyester fabric is sewn into the occluder with polyester thread. The fabric provides as surface for thrombosis and tissue ingrowth that closes the communication. The Septal Occluder has CE mark and FDA approval for sale in the U.S.

Cardia Inc. 651-691-4100
2900 Lone Oak Pkwy Ste 130, Eagan, MN 55121
Intrasept, pfo closure device.

Nmt Medical, Inc. 617-737-0930
27-43 Wormwood St, Boston, MA 02210
Cardioseal.

W. L. Gore & Associates, Inc. 800-437-8181
PO Box 2400, Flagstaff, AZ 86003
SEPTAL OCCLUDER

DEVICE, OCCLUSION, CARDIAC, TRANSCATHETER *(cont'd)*

W.L. Gore & Associates,Inc 928-526-3030
1505 North Fourth St., Flagstaff, AZ 86004
Septal occluder.

DEVICE, OTOACOUSTIC *(Ear/Nose/Throat) 77MLJ*

Audiphone Hearing Instruments 800-721-9611
3333 Kingman St Ste 205, Metairie, LA 70006
OTODYNAMICS, LTD ILO 92, IL088 Otoacoustic emission units.

Bio-Logic Systems Corp. 800-323-8326
1 Bio Logic Plz, Mundelein, IL 60060
Distortion Product (DPOAE) and Transient (TEOAE) otoacoustic emission test system. AUDX DPOAE and/or TEOAE system performs tests without connection to a computer. Scout Sport (DPOAE and/or TEOAE) provides otoacoustic emissions testing via interface to a notebook computer.

Tsi Medical Ltd. 800-661-7263
47 Athabascan Ave., Unit 105, Sherwood Park, AB T8A-4H3 Canada

DEVICE, PASTE-ON FOR INCONTINENCE, NON-STERILE *(Gastro/Urology) 78NOA*

Hollister, Inc. 847-680-2849
366 Draft Ave, Stuarts Draft, VA 24477

DEVICE, PERIPHERAL ELECTROMAG. FIELD TO AID WOUND HEALING *(Surgery) 79MBQ*

Rodale Electronics, Inc. 631-231-0044
20 Oser Ave, Hauppauge, NY 11788
Wound healing device.

DEVICE, POSITIVE PRESSURE BREATHING, INTERMITTENT *(Anesthesiology) 73NHJ*

Ps Solutions, Inc. 972-548-8080
411 Interchange St, McKinney, TX 75071
Noncontinuous ventilator.

DEVICE, REMOVAL, PACEMAKER ELECTRODE, PERCUTANEOUS *(Cardiovascular) 74MFA*

Cook Vascular, Incorporated 800-457-4500
1186 Montgomery Ln, Vandergrift, PA 15690
LIBERATOR Locking Stylet - Universal locking stylet used during the removal of transvenous cardiac leads. Packaged individually.

Spectranetics Corp. 800-633-0960
9965 Federal Dr, Colorado Springs, CO 80921
Laser-assisted pacemaker lead removal device. Laser sheath designed to thread over an implanted pacing lead and ablate through scar tissue, thereby aiding in the extraction of the pacing lead.

DEVICE, REPOSITIONING, JAW *(Dental And Oral) 76LQZ*

Dreamwrx Dental Laboratory 949-448-9985
1911 Colorado Blvd, Los Angeles, CA 90041
Intraoral device for snoring and obstructive sleep apnea.

Dresch/Tolson Dental Lab 952-345-6300
4024 N Holland Sylvania Rd, Toledo, OH 43623
Adjustable pm positioner, pm positioner.

Heumann & Associates Dental Lab 952-541-9622
520 SE 5th St, Topeka, KS 66607
Adjustable pm positioner, pm positioner.

Inventive Resources, Inc. 209-545-1691
5038 Salida Blvd, Salida, CA 95368
Bite guard, night guard, bite plate.

Jumar Corp. 928-442-0038
329 N Alarcon St, Prescott, AZ 86301
Dental splint.

National Dentex Corp 508-907-7800
2 Vision Dr Ste 3, Natick, MA 01760
Snoring intraoral device.

Nti-Tss, Inc. 574-258-5963
2303 Blue Smoke Trl, Mishawaka, IN 46544
Jaw repositioning device.

Pro-Tex International, Inc. 209-545-1691
5038 Salida Blvd, Salida, CA 95368
Bite guard,night guard,bite plate.

Talon Acrylics, Inc. 888-433-2551
850 NE 102nd Ave, Portland, OR 97220
'TALON' Thermoplastic Acrylic Elastomer is used in fabrication of TMJ/D Splints, Night Guards, Repositioning Stints, Sleep Apnea Anti-Snore Appliances.

DEVICE, RETRIEVAL, PERCUTANEOUS *(Cardiovascular) 74MMX*

Ev3 Inc. 800-716-6700
9600 54th Ave N, Plymouth, MN 55442
Retrieval device (various models).

Ev3 Inc. 800-716-6700
4600 Nathan Ln N, Plymouth, MN 55442
Retrieval device (various models).

Idev Technologies, Inc. 866-806-4338
253 Medical Center Blvd, Webster, TX 77598
Texan or snare.

DEVICE, SEMEN ANALYSIS *(Obstetrics/Gyn) 85MNA*

Biocoat, Inc. 215-734-0888
211 Witmer Rd, Horsham, PA 19044
Hydrophilic lubricious coatings.

Embryotech Laboratories, Inc. 800-673-7500
323 Andover St, Wilmington, MA 01887

Humagen Fertility Diagnostics, Inc. 800-937-3210
2400 Hunters Way, Charlottesville, VA 22911
$15.00 for disposable manual semen analysis kit.

Irvine Scientific 800-437-5706
2511 Daimler St, Santa Ana, CA 92705

Promega Corp. 800-356-9526
2800 Woods Hollow Rd, Fitchburg, WI 53711

Select Medical Systems 800-441-1973
30 Winter Sport Ln, PO Box 966, Williston, VT 05495
Sperm Select System sperm preparation kit. Convenient in-office kit for intrauterine insemination.

Wisconsin Pharmacal Co. Llc 800-558-6614
PO Box 198, Jackson, WI 53037
Home test kit- Sperm count

Zander Medical Supplies, Inc. / Zander Ivf, Inc. 800-820-3029
755 8th Ct Ste 4, Vero Beach, FL 32962
Zander Spermometer for easy reading of sperm concentration, MSC1 Migration-Sedimentation chamber for separation of motile sperm.

DEVICE, SPINAL VERTEBRAL BODY REPLACEMENT *(Orthopedics) 87MQP*

Abbott Spine, Inc. 847-937-6100
12708 Riata Vista Cir Ste B-100, Austin, TX 78727
Vertebral body replacement.

Alphatec Spine, Inc. 760-494-6769
5818 El Camino Real, Carlsbad, CA 92008
Vetebral body replacement device.

Amedica Corporation 801-839-3500
1885 W 2100 S, Salt Lake City, UT 84119
Valeo Spacer System

Atlas Spine Inc. 561-741-1108
1555 Jupiter Park Dr Ste 4, Jupiter, FL 33458
Vertebral body replacement.

Depuy Spine, Inc. 800-227-6633
325 Paramount Dr, Raynham, MA 02767
Stackable cage.

Implex Corp. 800-613-6131
1800 W Center St, Warsaw, IN 46580

Ionics Medical Corp. 910-428-9726
248 Bird Haven Lane, Ether, NC 27247-0179
Vertically-expandable vertebral-body replacement prosthesis, various sizes.

K2m, Inc. 866-526-4171
751 Miller Dr SE Ste F1, Leesburg, VA 20175
Vertebral body replacement device.

Lanx Inc. 303-443-7500
390 Interlocken Cres, Broomfield, CO 80021
Vbr system.

Nuvasive, Inc. 800-475-9131
7475 Lusk Blvd, San Diego, CA 92121
Vertebral body replacement device.

Orthovita, Inc. 610-640-1775
77 Great Valley Pkwy, Malvern, PA 19355
Various sizes of vertebral body replacement, vbr devices.

Rkl Technologies, Inc. 951-738-8000
245 Citation Cir, Corona, CA 92880
Vertebral body replacement.

Rsb Spine Llc. 866-241-2104
2530 Superior Ave E Ste 703, Cleveland, OH 44114
Interplate vbr system.

DEVICE, SPINAL VERTEBRAL BODY REPLACEMENT *(cont'd)*

Spinal Elements, Inc. 760-607-0121
2744 Loker Ave W Ste 100, Carlsbad, CA 92010
Vertebral body replacement.

Spine Wave, Inc. 203-944-9494
2 Enterprise Dr Ste 302, Shelton, CT 06484
Vertebral body replacement device.

Spineworks Medical Inc. 408-986-8950
1735 N 1st St Ste 245, San Jose, CA 95112

Titan Spine Llc. 1-866-822-7800
6140 W Executive Dr Ste A, Mequon, WI 53092
ENDOSKELETON TA VERTE

Us Spine Inc. 561-367-7463
3600 Fau Blvd Ste 101, Boca Raton, FL 33431
Titanium mesh.

Vertiflex (Tm), Incorporated 1-866-268-6486
1351 Calle Avanzado, San Clemente, CA 92673
Octane

Warsaw Orthopedic, Inc. 901-396-3133
2500 Silveus Xing, Warsaw, IN 46582
Interbody fixator.

Zimmer Trabecular Metal Technology 800-613-6131
10 Pomeroy Rd, Parsippany, NJ 07054
Hedrocel vertebral body replacement.

DEVICE, STABILIZER, HEART *(Cardiovascular) 74MWS*

Ascent Healthcare Solutions 480-763-5300
10232 S 51st St, Phoenix, AZ 85044
Heart stabilizer.

Bioventrix 925-830-1000
12647 Alcosta Blvd Ste 400, San Ramon, CA 94583
Ventricular sizing mandrel.

Boston Scientific Corp. 408-935-3400
150 Baytech Dr, San Jose, CA 95134
Cardiac access device.

Genesee Biomedical, Inc. 800-786-4890
1308 S Jason St, Denver, CO 80223

Maquet Puerto Rico Inc. 408-635-3900
No. 12, Rd. #698, Dorado, PR 00646
Cardiac off pump surgical stabilizer.

DEVICE, STORAGE, IMAGE, DIGITAL *(Radiology) 90LMB*

Acuo Technologies 651-730-4110
7200 Hudson Blvd N Ste 230, Oakdale, MN 55128
Acuomed.

Agfa Corporation 877-777-2432
PO Box 19048, 10 South Academy Street, Greenville, SC 29602

Agfa Healthcare Corp. 864-421-1815
580 Gotham Pkwy, Carlstadt, NJ 07072
Archive.

Agfa Healthcare Corp. 864-421-1815
1 Crosswind Dr, Westerly, RI 02891
Xa capture system.

Aspyra, Inc. 904-854-2107
8649 Baypine Rd, Jacksonville, FL 32256
Clinical image management system.

Avnet, Inc. 480-643-2000
3201 East Harbor, Phoenix, AZ 85034
Same.

Black Diamond Video, Inc. 215-348-3896
1151 Harbor Bay Pkwy Ste 208, Alameda, CA 94502
Dvi processor.

Candelis, Inc. 949-798-8101
18821 Bardeen Ave, Irvine, CA 92612

Canon U.S.A., Inc. 949-932-3100
15975 Alton Pkwy, Irvine, CA 92618
Various models.

Compu Tech Inc 407-788-6353
407 Wekiva Springs Rd Ste 347, Longwood, FL 32779
TIMS image acqusition and viewing software

Datafirst Corp. 800-634-8504
5124 Departure Dr, Raleigh, NC 27616
Data Archive Systems

Datcard Systems Inc 949-932-1300
7 Goodyear, Irvine, CA 92618
Cd burner.

DEVICE, STORAGE, IMAGE, DIGITAL *(cont'd)*

Dejarnette Research Systems 410-583-0680
401 Washington Ave Ste 1010, Towson, MD 21204
Image archive (digital).

Efotoxpress Inc. 510-979-9100
46560 Fremont Blvd Ste 115, Fremont, CA 94538
Pass.

Emageon Inc. 262-369-3379
1200 Corporate Dr Ste 200, Birmingham, AL 35242
Digital image storage device.

Empiric Systems, Llc 866-367-4742
3800 Paramount Pkwy Ste 130, Morrisville, NC 27560
Various medical image storage functions used in conjunction with a radiology inf.

Erad/Image Medical Corp. 864-234-7430
9 Pilgrim Rd Ste 312, Greenville, SC 29607
Medical image storage device.

Fastec Medical Systems 866-463-3633
802 Whitewater Dr, Fullerton, CA 92833
Automatic dicom cd burner.

Fotofinder Systems, Inc. 443-283-3865
9693 Gerwig Ln Ste S, Columbia, MD 21046
Digital camera and image storage system.

Ge Healthcare It 847-277-5000
540 W Northwest Hwy, Barrington, IL 60010
Medical image storage devices.

Genesis Digital Imaging, Inc. 888-436-3444
12921 W Washington Blvd, Los Angeles, CA 90066

Healthline Medical Imaging 704-655-0447
705 Northeast Dr Ste 17, Davidson, NC 28036
Medical image communications device.

Hewlett-Packard Company 408-472-2702
20555 State Highway 249, Houston, TX 77070
Medical image storage device.

Imageflow Inc. 408-569-3860
730 Bantry Ct, Sunnyvale, CA 94087
Medical image management device.

Imaging Archive International, Llc. 770-565-6166
5966 Exeter Cir, Norcross, GA 30071
Image archive storage device.

Imsi, Integrated Modular Systems Inc. 800-220-9729
2500 W Township Line Rd, PO Box 616, Havertown, PA 19083
TeleRadiology and PACS Viewing with Internet Explorer 5.0 or higher on Standard PCs. All DICOM Modalities may be used.

Invoke Imaging, Inc. 630-271-8111
1250 Palmer St, Downers Grove, IL 60516
Various pacs archive devices.

Iquire, Llc 845-277-1846
2 Fallsview Ln, Brewster, NY 10509
Image capture device.

Medical Data Technologies, Inc. 866-643-7424
1421 Oakfield Dr, Brandon, FL 33511
Directrad.

Medical Digital Developers Llc 508-393-3100
767 Lexington Ave Rm 505, New York, NY 10065
Endoscopic image storage device.

Medicor Imaging, Div. Of Lead Technologies Inc. 704-227-2642
1201 Greenwood Clfs Ste 400, Charlotte, NC 28204
Medical image storage device.

Medstrat, Inc. 630-960-8700
1901 Butterfield Rd Ste 600, Downers Grove, IL 60515
Various models of storage devices.

Meta Fusion, Inc. 408-345-0500
15209 Blue Gum Ct, Saratoga, CA 95070
Medical image store.

Mitsui / Mam-A 719-262-2430
10045 Federal Dr, Colorado Springs, CO 80908
Duplicator.

Mpacs, Llc. 608-827-7111
7601 Ganser Way, Madison, WI 53719
Pacs, picture archiving and communications systems.

Neurostar Solutions, Inc. 404-575-4222
75 5th St NW Ste 206, Atlanta, GA 30308
Archive system.

DEVICE, STORAGE, IMAGE, DIGITAL *(cont'd)*

Openmed Technologies Corporation 877-717-6215
256 W Cummings Park, Woburn, MA 01801
OpenMed Manager, multi-media medical image archive and distribution management system

Penrad Technologies, Inc. 763-475-3388
10580 Wayzata Blvd Ste 200, Hopkins, MN 55305
Film scanning software.

Pentax Southern Region Service Center 201-571-2300
8934 Kirby Dr, Houston, TX 77054
Image management system.

Pentax West Coast Service Center 800-431-5880
10410 Pioneer Blvd Ste 2, Santa Fe Springs, CA 90670
Pentax image management systems.

Practiceworks Systems, Llc. 800-944-6365
1765 the Exchange SE, Atlanta, GA 30339
Image storage software for digital dental radiographs.

Provation Medical, Inc. 612-313-1564
800 Washington Ave N Ste 400, Minneapolis, MN 55401
Medical procedure documentation and coding compliance software.

Rorke Data, Incorporated 757-224-0177
7626 Golden Triangle Dr, Eden Prairie, MN 55344
Data archiving system.

Smith & Nephew Inc., Endoscopy Div. 978-749-1000
76 S Meridian Ave, Oklahoma City, OK 73107
Medical image storage device.

Smith Companies Dental Products 800-336-3263
4368 Enterprise St, Fremont, CA 94538
ScanRite Dental Film Scanner. In less than 10 seconds, digitizes #0-, 1-, and 2-size dental film. Use to make diagnostic quality prints, e-mail or view enlarged.

Sorna Corporation 651-406-9900
2020 Silver Bell Rd Ste 17, Eagan, MN 55122
Cd burner system.

Stryker Imaging 888-795-4624
1410 Lakeside Pkwy Ste 600, Flower Mound, TX 75028
Digital image storage device.

Technofrolics 617-441-8870
11 Miller St, Somerville, MA 02143
Digital video recorder (dvr) & playback,perusal system.

Televere Systems 800-385-9593
1611 Center Ave, Janesville, WI 53546
Radiological digital image storage.

Teramedica, Inc. 414-908-7713
10400 W Innovation Dr Ste 200, Milwaukee, WI 53226
Digital image storage and retrivial system.

Thinking Systems Corporation 727-217-0909
750 94th Ave N Ste 211, Saint Petersburg, FL 33702
Image server.

Vision Systems Group, A Division Of Viking Systems 508-366-3668
134 Flanders Rd, Westborough, MA 01581
Digital image storage devices.

DEVICE, STORAGE, IMAGES, OPHTHALMIC
(Ophthalmology) 86NFF

Canon U.S.A., Inc. 949-932-3100
15975 Alton Pkwy, Irvine, CA 92618
Various models.

Clarity Medical Systems 925-463-7984
5775 W Las Positas Blvd Ste 200, Pleasanton, CA 94588
Medical image storage.

Connected Medical Systems Llc 662-455-4523
2005 Highway 82 W, Greenwood, MS 38930
Medical digital imaging system.

Nidek, Inc. 510-226-5700
47651 Westinghouse Dr, Fremont, CA 94539
Medical image storage device.

DEVICE, SUTURING, ENDOSCOPIC *(Surgery) 79MFJ*

Endogastric Solutions, Inc. 425-307-9226
8210 154th Ave NE, Redmond, WA 98052
Endoscopic suture device.

Mediflex Surgical Products 800-879-7575
250 Gibbs Rd, Islandia, NY 11749

Wisap America 800-233-8448
8231 Melrose Dr, Lenexa, KS 66214

DEVICE, SUTURING, STAPLING, GRAFT, AORTIC
(Surgery) 79NCA

Cardica, Inc. 888-544-7194
900 Saginaw Dr, Redwood City, CA 94063
Aortic anastomotic system.

DEVICE, TRANSURETHRAL, FOR CONTROLLED URINATION
(Gastro/Urology) 78MXU

Rochester Medical Corp. 800-615-2364
1 Rochester Medical Dr NW, Stewartville, MN 55976
Urethral insert.

DEVICE, ULTRASOUND, SINUS *(Ear/Nose/Throat) 77LWI*

E. Benson Hood Laboratories, Inc. 800-942-5227
575 Washington St, Pembroke, MA 02359
Czaja-McCaffrey Stent Introducer, Introducing Tracheobronchoscopy: a device used to directly visualize the endolarynx, subgloths, trachea, and proximal bronchial airways.

Ultracell Medical Technologies, Inc. 877-SPO-NGE1
183 Providence New London Tpke, North Stonington, CT 06359
ULTRACELL Nasal-sinus packing. Various sizes of sinus packing made of P.V.A. sponge. Used to pack the middle turbinate, preventing lateralizing by gentle pressure on the mucosa during post-op period.

DI (O-HYDROXYPHENYLIMINE) ETHANE, CALCIUM
(Chemistry) 75CHZ

Mid-Delta Home Health & Hospice 800-543-9055
405 N Hayden St, Belzoni, MS 39038
Monofilaments for Diabetic Sensory Testing

DIACETYL-MONOXIME, UREA NITROGEN *(Chemistry) 75CDW*

Diagnostic Specialties 732-549-4011
4 Leonard St, Metuchen, NJ 08840
$39.50 per 1000ml.

Health Chem Diagnostics Llc 954-979-3845
3341 W McNab Rd, Pompano Beach, FL 33069
Diacetyl-monoxime, urea nitrogen.

Stanbio Laboratory, Inc. 830-249-0772
1261 N Main St, Boerne, TX 78006
$80.00 for 250 urea nitrogen test sets with color reagent, acid reagent, and standards (25, 50 and 75mg/dl). $41.00 for 4 x 50ml enzymatic urea nitrogen test kits with enzyme and color reagent, and standard (25mg/dl). $42.00 for 20 x 6.5ml UV-rate urea nitrogen test kits with reagent and standard (30mg/dl).

DIALYSATE DELIVERY SYSTEM, CENTRAL MULTIPLE PATIENT
(Gastro/Urology) 78FKQ

Alden Medical Llc 413-747-9717
360 Cold Spring Ave, West Springfield, MA 01089
Diacide.

Rismed Oncology Systems 256-534-6993
2494 Washington St NW, Huntsville, AL 35811
Dialysate delivery systems, sigle and multi stations

DIALYSATE DELIVERY SYSTEM, PERITONEAL, SEMI-AUTOMATIC *(Gastro/Urology) 78KPF*

Baxter Healthcare Corp., Renal Division 847-948-2000
7511 114th Ave, Largo, FL 33773
Renal therapy clinical data management software.

DIALYSATE DELIVERY SYSTEM, SINGLE PATIENT
(Gastro/Urology) 78FKP

B. Braun Medical Inc., Renal Therapies Div. 800-854-6851
824 12th Ave, Bethlehem, PA 18018

Baxter Healthcare Corp., Renal Division 847-948-2000
7511 114th Ave, Largo, FL 33773
Sps single patient system.

Chf Solutions, Inc. 763-463-4600
7601 Northland Dr N Ste 170, Brooklyn Center, MN 55428
Chf systems 100.

G.E.M. Water Systems, Int'L., Llc 800-755-1707
6351 Orangethorpe Ave, Buena Park, CA 90620
Sodium bicarbonate mixing & delivery system, mixes and monitors sodium bicarbonate solution and delivers it to the dialysis patients.

Integrated Biomedical Technology, Inc. 574-264-0025
2931 Moose Trl, Elkhart, IN 46514
Watercheck 2 reagent strip, chloramine test strips.

Nxstage Medical, Inc. 866-697-8243
439 S Union St Fl 5, Lawrence, MA 01843
Hemodialysis accessory.

DIALYSATE DELIVERY SYSTEM, SORBENT REGENERATED
(Gastro/Urology) 78FKT

Sorb Technology, Inc. 405-682-1993
3631 SW 54th St, Oklahoma City, OK 73119
Sorbent cartridges.

DIALYSIS UNIT TEST EQUIPMENT *(Gastro/Urology) 78QPJ*

Mesa Laboratories, Inc. 800-992-6372
12100 W 6th Ave, Lakewood, CO 80228
DIGITAL METERS FOR TESTING CONDUCTIVITY, TEMPERATURE, pH, AND PRESSURE FOR THE VERIFICATION AND CALIBRATION OF DIALYSIS DELIVERY SYSTEMS.

Precision Systems, Inc. 508-655-7010
16 Tech Cir, Natick, MA 01760
Osmometers.

DIALYZER *(Chemistry) 75JQQ*

Harvard Apparatus, Inc. 800-272-2775
84 October Hill Rd, Holliston, MA 01746
96-Well Equilibrium Dialyzer is suitable for many applications including protein and protein-drug binding assays, receptor binding assays, ligand binding assays and protein-protein and protein-DNA interactions.

DIALYZER REPROCESSING SYSTEM *(Gastro/Urology) 78LIF*

Alden Medical Llc 413-747-9717
360 Cold Spring Ave, West Springfield, MA 01089
Formasure.

G.E.M. Water Systems, Int'L., Llc 800-755-1707
6351 Orangethorpe Ave, Buena Park, CA 90620
Manual Dialyzer Reprocessing System, reprocesses artificial kidneys by cleaning, testing, and disinfecting so they can be used many times on the same patient.

Integrated Biomedical Technology, Inc. 574-264-0025
2931 Moose Trl, Elkhart, IN 46514
Peracetic acid test strips.

Mesa Laboratories, Inc. 800-992-6372
12100 W 6th Ave, Lakewood, CO 80228
RDM DATA MANAGEMENT SYSTEM FOR DIALYZER REPROCESSING.

Molded Products Inc. 800-435-8957
1112 Chatburn Ave, Harlan, IA 51537
Disposable storage cap.

Serim Research Corp. 574-264-3440
3506 Reedy Dr, Elkhart, IN 46514
Test for levels of glutaraldehyde potency in high level disinfec.

Sparton Medical Systems 440-878-4630
22740 Lunn Rd, Strongsville, OH 44149
Dialyzer reprocessing system.

DIALYZER, CAPILLARY, HOLLOW FIBER (HEMODIALYSIS)
(Gastro/Urology) 78FJI

Baxter Healthcare Corporation, Renal 888-229-0001
1620 S Waukegan Rd, Waukegan, IL 60085
CA dialyzers.

Castle Pines Medical, Inc. 303-442-4514
14883 E Hinsdale Ave Ste 2, Centennial, CO 80112
Dialyzer blood port cap and dialyzer port cap.

Interpore Cross International 800-722-4489
181 Technology Dr, Irvine, CA 92618
Ultraconcentrator manifold with extension set. Graft delivery syringe. Disposable system for intraoperative collection of autologous growth factors.

Medisystems Corporation 800-369-6334
439 S Union St Fl 5, Lawrence, MA 01843

Rismed Oncology Systems 256-534-6993
2494 Washington St NW, Huntsville, AL 35811
Dialyzers, regular and hiflux

Spectrum Laboratories, Inc. 800-634-3300
18617 S Broadwick St, Rancho Dominguez, CA 90220
ZYMAX Microporous Hollow Fiber Bioreactors. Have microporous membranes which allow proteins to exit the extracapillary space. Reduces feed-back inhibition. CELLFLO, KROSFLO and MINIKROS supplied non-pyrogenic, with low bioburden and no preservatives. Priced to be disposable.

DIALYZER, HIGH PERMEABILITY *(Gastro/Urology) 78KDI*

Baxter Healthcare Corp., Renal Division 847-948-2000
7511 114th Ave, Largo, FL 33773
Dialyzer.

DIALYZER, HIGH PERMEABILITY *(cont'd)*

Baxter Healthcare Corporation, Renal 888-229-0001
1620 S Waukegan Rd, Waukegan, IL 60085
CA Cellulose acetate. Cellulose triacetate. CF Capillary flow. Hollow fiber.

Chf Solutions, Inc. 763-463-4600
7601 Northland Dr N Ste 170, Brooklyn Center, MN 55428
System 100; s-100 ultrafiltration console, uf 500 set, venous access catheters,.

Nephros, Inc. 201-343-5202
41 Grand Ave, River Edge, NJ 07661
Various

Nxstage Medical, Inc. 866-697-8243
439 S Union St Fl 5, Lawrence, MA 01843
Hemofiltration system and accessories.

Terumo Cardiovascular Systems (Tcvs) 800-283-7866
28 Howe St, Ashland, MA 01721
Hemoconcentrators.

DIALYZER, LABORATORY *(Chemistry) 75UFV*

Nest Group Inc., The 800-347-6378
45 Valley Rd, Southborough, MA 01772
HARVARD APPARATUS 96-Well DispoEquilibrium dialysers; small volume (10-250 µl) dialysis plates for buffer exchange or protein binding studies.

Spectrum Laboratories, Inc. 800-634-3300
18617 S Broadwick St, Rancho Dominguez, CA 90220
For equilibrium, flow, stirring flow and water dialyses; capacities: 1-50 ml. $44.00 to $56.00.

DIALYZER, PARALLEL FLOW (HEMODIALYSIS)
(Gastro/Urology) 78FJG

Medisystems Corporation 800-369-6334
439 S Union St Fl 5, Lawrence, MA 01843

DIAPER, ADULT *(General) 80QPL*

Allman Products 800-223-6889
21101 Itasca St, Chatsworth, CA 91311

American Associated Companies, Inc. 800-849-7060
120 Carnegie Pl Ste 202, Fayetteville, GA 30214

Arc Home Health Products 800-278-8595
PO Box 615, Oneonta, NY 13820

Atd-American Co. 800-523-2300
135 Greenwood Ave, Wyncote, PA 19095

Best Manufacturing Group Llc 800-843-3233
1633 Broadway Fl 18, New York, NY 10019
Contoured pin and pinless, snaps.

Bio-Medic Health Services, Inc. 800-525-0072
5041B Benois Rd Bldg B, Roanoke, VA 24018

Comfort Touch 888-8BR-IEFS
PO Box 630104, Miami, FL 33163

Duraline Medical Products, Inc. 800-654-3376
324 Werner St, P.O. Box 67, Leipsic, OH 45856

East Atlantic Trading/Triangle Healthcare Inc. 800-243-4635
76 National Rd, Edison, NJ 08817

Fabrite Laminating Corp. 973-777-1406
70 Passaic St, Wood Ridge, NJ 07075
reusable diaper

Feather-Soft Disposable Hospital Products, Inc. 303-470-0200
P.O. Box 360470, Highlands Ranch, CO 80163-0470
Disposable.

Freestyle Medical Supplies, Inc. 800-841-5330
336 Green Rd, Stoney Creek, ON L8E 2B2 Canada
Adult Swim Diaper unisex design. Lightweight 100% nylon outer won't weigh swimmer down. Dries quickly gusseted legs ensures any solid waist stays inside. Adjustable waist. Available small, medium and large.

Gallimore Healthcare Inc. 800-387-0208
#23A Railside Rd., Toronto, ONT M3A-1B2 Canada

Geri-Care Products 201-440-0409
250 Moonachie Ave, Moonachie, NJ 07074
Reusable Incontinence Diapers & Briefs

Hospital Specialty Company 800-321-9832
500 Memorial Dr, Nicholasville, KY 40356

Howard Medical Company 800-443-1444
1690 N Elston Ave, Chicago, IL 60642
$44/case (72/count) for disposable diapers for sizes youth thru XXlarge.

DIAPER, ADULT *(cont'd)*

Humanicare International, Inc. 800-631-5270
9 Elkins Rd, East Brunswick, NJ 08816
DIGNITY PLUS premium adult disposable briefs. Five sizes available. DIGNITY adult disposable briefs 4 sizes.

Invacare Supply Group, An Invacare Co. 800-225-4792
75 October Hill Rd, Holliston, MA 01746
Carry full lines of adult incontinence products from: Invacare, SCA, First Quality, Kimberly-Clark & Kendall.

Lew Jan Textile 800-899-0531
366 Veterans Memorial Hwy Ste 4, Commack, NY 11725

Paperpak 800-428-8363
545 W Terrace Dr, San Dimas, CA 91773
New line of ATTENDS adult briefs with and without waistband. CONFIDENCE Trim Fit adult briefs and wingfold designs available.

Principle Business Enterprises, Inc. 800-467-3224
PO Box 129, Dunbridge, OH 43414
TRANQUILITY SLIMLINE disposable briefs for heavy incontinence. Disposable.

DIAPER, PEDIATRIC *(General) 80QPM*

Atd-American Co. 800-523-2300
135 Greenwood Ave, Wyncote, PA 19095

Best Manufacturing Group Llc 800-843-3233
1633 Broadway Fl 18, New York, NY 10019
Gauze and birdseye cotton, squared and prefolds.

Children's Medical Ventures, Inc. 800-345-6443
191 Wyngate Dr, Monroeville, PA 15146
WEE PEE DIAPER premature size.

Crosswell International Corporation 305-648-0777
101 Madeira Ave, Coral Gables, FL 33134

Dma Med-Chem Corporation 800-362-1833
49 Watermill Ln, Great Neck, NY 11021
WEE-PEE

Duraline Medical Products, Inc. 800-654-3376
324 Werner St, P.O. Box 67, Leipsic, OH 45856

Feather-Soft Disposable Hospital Products, Inc. 303-470-0200
P.O. Box 360470, Highlands Ranch, CO 80163-0470

Freestyle Medical Supplies, Inc. 800-841-5330
336 Green Rd, Stoney Creek, ON L8E 2B2 Canada
KOOSHIES Hospital Diapers - baby diapers designed specifically for use in hospitals and institutions. Available in four sizes fitting preemies (2-4lbs.) to toddlers (23-45lbs.).

Hospital Specialty Company 800-321-9832
500 Memorial Dr, Nicholasville, KY 40356

Howard Medical Company 800-443-1444
1690 N Elston Ave, Chicago, IL 60642
size 1 thru 6, extra absorbent, cloth like backing, velcro closure, channel insert, polymer with fitted leg and waist

Kerr Group 800-524-3577
1400 Holcomb Bridge Rd, Roswell, GA 30076

R. Sabee Company 920-882-7350
1718 W 8th St, Appleton, WI 54914

DIAPHRAGM, CONTRACEPTIVE *(Obstetrics/Gyn) 85HDW*

Milex Products, Inc. 800-621-1278
4311 N Normandy Ave, Chicago, IL 60634
WIDESEAL DIAPHRAGM at $37.50 to $25 per unit.

Ortho-Mcneil-Janssen Pharmaceuticals, Inc. 800-526-7736
1000 US Highway 202, Raritan, NJ 08869

Yama, Inc. 908-206-8706
650 Liberty Ave, Union, NJ 07083
Vaginal contraceptive device.

DIASTASE *(Pathology) 88IBC*

American Mastertech Scientific, Inc. 209-368-4031
1330 Thurman St, Lodi, CA 95240
Multiple.

Ventana Medical Systems, Inc. 800-227-2155
1910 E Innovation Park Dr, Oro Valley, AZ 85755
Diastase.

DIATHERMY, SHORTWAVE *(Physical Med) 89IMJ*

Amrex Electrotherapy Equipment 800-221-9069
641 E Walnut St, Carson, CA 90746

Coventina Healthcare Enterprises, Inc. 412-915-6442
1297 Royal Park Blvd, South Park, PA 15129
Short-wave diathermy.

DIATHERMY, SHORTWAVE *(cont'd)*

Elmed, Inc. 630-543-2792
60 W Fay Ave, Addison, IL 60101

Md International, Inc. 305-669-9003
11300 NW 41st St, Doral, FL 33178

Mettler Electronics Corp. 800-854-9305
1333 S Claudina St, Anaheim, CA 92805
*AUTO*THERM: Starting at $4,495.00 for mobile Auto*Therm 390 with maximum output of 100 watts, continuous or pulsed. $14,995 for Auto*Therm 395 continuous and pulsed diathermy, with a set of plate applicators and a inductive drum applicator. A variety of other applicators available.*

R.J. Lindquist Co. 213-382-1268
2419 James M Wood Blvd, Los Angeles, CA 90006
Shortwave diathermy.

Zimmer Medizinsystems 800-327-3576
25 Mauchly Ste 300, Irvine, CA 92618
High frequency electromagnetic fields, inductive field method, patented spiral electrode, pulsed and continuous options.

DIATHERMY, SHORTWAVE, PULSED *(Physical Med) 89ILX*

Adm Tronics Unlimited, Inc. 201-767-6040
224 Pegasus Ave, Northvale, NJ 07647
SOFPULSE - electrotherapeutic device for the reduction of pain and edema in post-operative soft tissue.

Innovamed, Inc. 801-885-9085
13524 Oakridge Dr, Alpine, UT 84004
Pulse electromagnetic field stimulator.

DIATHERMY, ULTRASONIC (PHYSICAL THERAPY) *(Physical Med) 89IMI*

Amrex Electrotherapy Equipment 800-221-9069
641 E Walnut St, Carson, CA 90746
SYNCHROSONIC U/50 portable. U/20 portable.

Cardinal Health, Snowden Pencer Products 847-689-8410
5175 S Royal Atlanta Dr, Tucker, GA 30084
Therapeutic deep heat device.

Chattanooga Group 800-592-7329
4717 Adams Rd, Hixson, TN 37343
INTELECT ultrasound and electrotherapy products.

Dynatronics Corp. 800-874-6251
7030 Park Centre Dr, Salt Lake City, UT 84121
DYNATRON 150:Mult: frequency capability, watertight sound heads in 4 sizes.

Elmed, Inc. 630-543-2792
60 W Fay Ave, Addison, IL 60101
$1,375 for model 6175 with one transducer, 20-W maximum intensity. 0-30 minute timer, optional electrical stimulator. Tabletop model, weighs 28 lb.

Fibra-Sonics, A Division Of Misonix, Inc. 631-694-9555
1938 New Hwy, Farmingdale, NY 11735
Ultra sound physical therapy device.

Kesner C.R. 630-232-8118
2520 Kaneville Ct, Geneva, IL 60134
Electrically powered. Also available: combination units - muscle stimulator and therapeutic ultrasound, electrically powered.

Kmi Kolster Methods, Inc. 909-737-5476
3185 Palisades Dr, Corona, CA 92880
External ultrasound.

Md International, Inc. 305-669-9003
11300 NW 41st St, Doral, FL 33178

Med-Fit Systems, Inc. 800-831-7665
3553 Rosa Way, Fallbrook, CA 92028

Mettler Electronics Corp. 800-854-9305
1333 S Claudina St, Anaheim, CA 92805
SONICATOR: $1,500 or Sonicator 740 with a 5 cmð dual frequency applicator, optional 1 and 10 cmð applicators available, weighs 4 lbs.; $1,410.00 for Sonicator 716 with one transducer, 20 watt maximum output, 1-20 minute timer; portable style, wall mount optional, weighs 7lbs. Also available, $1,410.00 for smaller treatment areas, Sonicator 715, (5cmð head) with 10 watt max. output. $1,750.00 for Sonicator 730 1 and 3 MH2 with three of four applicators, 10 cmð, 5cmð, 1 cmð.

Rich-Mar Corporation 800-762-4665
PO Box 879, 15499 E 590 Rd, Inola, OK 74036
$3499 for the AutoSound 5.6 - Automatic Hands-Free Ultrasound. $1799.00 for Therasound 3.5, $1599.00 for Therasound 3.4, $1299.00 for Therasound 3.1.

DIATHERMY, ULTRASONIC (PHYSICAL THERAPY) *(cont'd)*

Shantel Medical Supply 888-577-5688
5600 Peck Rd, Arcadia, CA 91006
Ultrsonic treatment device, handheld.

Thera-Tronics, Inc. 800-267-6211
623 Mamaroneck Ave, Mamaroneck, NY 10543

DIAZO (COLORIMETRIC), NITRITE (URINARY, NON-QUANTITATIVE) *(Chemistry) 75JMT*

Arkray Factory Usa, Inc. 952-646-3168
5182 W 76th St, Minneapolis, MN 55439
Urine test strips.

Bayer Healthcare Llc 914-524-2955
555 White Plains Rd Fl 5, Tarrytown, NY 10591
Test for nitrite and leukocytes in urine.

DIAZO, P-NITROANILINE/VANILLIN, VANILMANDELIC ACID *(Chemistry) 75CDF*

Bio-Analysis, Inc. 310-828-7423
1701 Berkeley St, Santa Monica, CA 90404
Hva,vma.

Bio-Rad Laboratories Inc., Clinical Systems Div. 800-224-6723
4000 Alfred Nobel Dr, Hercules, CA 94547
Various.

Biochemical Diagnostics, Inc. 800-223-4835
180 Heartland Blvd, Edgewood, NY 11717

Key Instruments 215-357-6488
250 Andrews Rd, Trevose, PA 19053
Flowmeter.

DIAZONIUM COLORIMETRY, UROBILINOGEN (URINARY, NON-QUANT.) *(Chemistry) 75CDM*

Arkray Factory Usa, Inc. 952-646-3168
5182 W 76th St, Minneapolis, MN 55439
Urine test strips.

Bayer Healthcare Llc 914-524-2955
555 White Plains Rd Fl 5, Tarrytown, NY 10591
Test for uroilnogen in urine.

Bayer Healthcare, Llc 574-256-3430
430 S Beiger St, Mishawaka, IN 46544
Test for uroilnogen in urine.

Lifeline Medical, Inc. 800-452-4566
22 Shelter Rock Ln, Danbury, CT 06810
Urinary chemistry strips.

Ricca Chemical Company Llc 817-461-5601
1490 Lammers Pike, Batesville, IN 47006

Ricca Chemical Company, Llc 817-461-5601
448 W Fork Dr, Arlington, TX 76012
Ehrlich aldehyde.

DIE, WIRE BENDING, ENT *(Ear/Nose/Throat) 77JXW*

Bausch & Lomb Surgical 636-255-5051
3365 Tree Court Ind Blvd, Saint Louis, MO 63122

Clinimed, Incorporated 877-CLINIMED
303 Markus Ct, Sandy Brae Industrial Park, Newark, DE 19713

Gyrus Ent L.L.C., Sub. Of Gyrus Acmi, Inc. 508-804-2739
2925 Appling Rd, Bartlett, TN 38133
Various types and sizes of ent wire bending dies.

DIFFERENTIAL RATE KINETIC METHOD, CPK OR ISOENZYMES *(Chemistry) 75JHS*

Caldon Biotech, Inc. 757-224-0177
2251 Rutherford Rd, Carlsbad, CA 92008
Creatine kinase.

Health Chem Diagnostics Llc 954-979-3845
3341 W McNab Rd, Pompano Beach, FL 33069
Differential rate kinetic method, cpk or isoenzymes.

Sterling Diagnostics, Inc. 800-637-2661
36645 Metro Ct, Sterling Heights, MI 48312
Cpk reagent set (colorimetric).

Teco Diagnostics 714-693-7788
1268 N Lakeview Ave, Anaheim, CA 92807
Cratine kinase (ck-mb).

DIFFRACTOMETER, X-RAY *(Chemistry) 75QPO*

Blake Industries, Inc. 908-233-7240
660 Jerusalem Rd, Scotch Plains, NJ 07076

DIFFRACTOMETER, X-RAY *(cont'd)*

Lnd, Inc. 516-678-6141
3230 Lawson Blvd, Oceanside, NY 11572

Myco Instrumentation Source, Inc. 425-228-4239
PO Box 354, Renton, WA 98057

Spectron Corp. 425-827-9317
934 S Burlington Blvd # 603, Burlington, WA 98233
Reconditioned equipment.

DIGITAL IMAGE, STORAGE AND COMMUNICATIONS, NON-DIAGNOSTIC, LABORATORY INFORMATION SYSTEM *(Chemistry) 75NVV*

Ann Arbor Digital Devices 734-834-5156
699 Skynob Dr, Ann Arbor, MI 48105

Sunquest Information Systems, Inc 520-570-2347
250 S Williams Blvd, Tucson, AZ 85711

DILATOR, BLUNT *(Surgery) 79WZY*

Boss Instruments, Ltd. 800-210-2677
395 Reas Ford Rd Ste 120, Earlysville, VA 22936

Coopersurgical, Inc. 800-243-2974
95 Corporate Dr, Trumbull, CT 06611

Elmed, Inc. 630-543-2792
60 W Fay Ave, Addison, IL 60101

Fehling Surgical Instruments 800-FEHLING
509 Broadstone Ln NW, Acworth, GA 30101

Richard Wolf Medical Instruments Corp. 800-323-9653
353 Corporate Woods Pkwy, Vernon Hills, IL 60061

Wisap America 800-233-8448
8231 Melrose Dr, Lenexa, KS 66214

DILATOR, CATHETER *(Surgery) 79GCC*

Boston Scientific Corporation 508-652-5578
780 Brookside Dr, Spencer, IN 47460

Boston Scientific Corporation 800-225-2732
1 Boston Scientific Pl, Natick, MA 01760

Cook Endoscopy 336-744-0157
4900 Bethania Station Rd # &, 5951 Grassy Creek Blvd. Winston Salem, NC 27105
Various types of biliary and pancreatic dilation catheters.

Tfx Medical Oem 800-548-6600
50 Plantation Dr, Jaffrey, NH 03452

DILATOR, CATHETER, URETERAL *(Gastro/Urology) 78EZN*

Aesculap Implant Systems Inc. 1-800-234-9179
3773 Corporate Pkwy, Center Valley, PA 18034

Boston Scientific Corporation 800-225-2732
1 Boston Scientific Pl, Natick, MA 01760

C. R. Bard, Inc., Bard Urological Div. 888-367-2273
13183 Harland Dr NE, Covington, GA 30014

Cook Urological, Inc. 800-457-4500
1100 W Morgan St, P.O. Box 227, Spencer, IN 47460

Onset Medical Corporation 949-716-1100
13900 Alton Pkwy Ste 120, Irvine, CA 92618
Sterile catheter for access during nephrostomy procedures.

DILATOR, CERVICAL, EXPANDABLE *(Obstetrics/Gyn) 85HDN*

Coopersurgical, Inc. 800-243-2974
95 Corporate Dr, Trumbull, CT 06611

R Medical Supply 800-882-7578
620 Valley Forge Rd Ste F, Hillsborough, NC 27278

DILATOR, CERVICAL, FIXED SIZE *(Obstetrics/Gyn) 85HDQ*

Berkeley Medevices, Inc. 800-227-2388
1330 S 51st St, Richmond, CA 94804
Denniston dilators.

Ipas 919-967-7052
PO Box 5027, Chapel Hill, NC 27514
Denniston Dilators.

Marina Medical Instruments, Inc. 800-697-1119
955 Shotgun Rd, Sunrise, FL 33326
Various.

Rocket Medical Plc. 800-707-7625
150 Recreation Park Dr Ste 3, Hingham, MA 02043

Shoney Scientific, Inc. 262-970-0170
West 223 North 720 Saratoga Drive,, Suite 120, Waukesha, WI 53186
Reusable and disposable os dilators.

DILATOR, CERVICAL, HYGROSCOPIC-LAMINARIA
(Obstetrics/Gyn) 85HDY

Berkeley Medevices, Inc. 800-227-2388
1330 S 51st St, Richmond, CA 94804
Laminaria tent.

Medgyn Products, Inc. 800-451-9667
328 Eisenhower Ln N, Lombard, IL 60148
Sizes: 2, 3, 4, 5, 6, 8, and 10mm.

Milex Products, Inc. 800-621-1278
4311 N Normandy Ave, Chicago, IL 60634
DILATERIA at $105.60 per dozen (standard).

R Medical Supply 800-882-7578
620 Valley Forge Rd Ste F, Hillsborough, NC 27278
Japanese and Norwegian brands available.

DILATOR, COMMON DUCT *(Gastro/Urology) 78QPR*

Codman & Shurtleff, Inc 800-225-0460
325 Paramount Dr, Raynham, MA 02767

DILATOR, ESOPHAGEAL *(Gastro/Urology) 78KNQ*

Cook Endoscopy 336-744-0157
4900 Bethania Station Rd # &, 5951 Grassy Creek Blvd.
Winston Salem, NC 27105
Esophageal/biliary dilator.

Medovations, Inc. 800-558-6408
102 E Keefe Ave, Milwaukee, WI 53212
WEIGHTRIGHT mercury free bougies. Maloney and Hurst styles. SAFEGUIDE endoscopic wire-guided dilator.

Safestitch Medical Inc. 305-575-4145
4400 Biscayne Blvd Ste 760, Miami, FL 33137

DILATOR, ESOPHAGEAL (METAL OLIVE) GASTRO-UROLOGY
(Gastro/Urology) 78EZM

Precision Medical Manufacturing Corporation 866-633-4626
852 Seton Ct, Wheeling, IL 60090

DILATOR, ESOPHAGEAL, ENT *(Ear/Nose/Throat) 77KCF*

Cook Endoscopy 336-744-0157
4900 Bethania Station Rd # &, 5951 Grassy Creek Blvd.
Winston Salem, NC 27105
Esophageal baloon dilators.

Medovations, Inc. 800-558-6408
102 E Keefe Ave, Milwaukee, WI 53212

DILATOR, EXPANSIVE IRIS (ACCESSORY)
(Ophthalmology) 86MMC

Fci Ophthalmics 800-932-4202
64 Schoosett St, Pembroke, MA 02359
Morcher Pupil Dilator

Western Ophthalmics Corporation 800-426-9938
19019 36th Ave W Ste G, Lynnwood, WA 98036

DILATOR, FASCIA, UMBILICAL *(Surgery) 79WZZ*

Automated Medical Products Corp. 800-832-4567
PO Box 2508, Edison, NJ 08818
DEEP SURTURE MIS Fascial structuring device.

Richard Wolf Medical Instruments Corp. 800-323-9653
353 Corporate Woods Pkwy, Vernon Hills, IL 60061

Wisap America 800-233-8448
8231 Melrose Dr, Lenexa, KS 66214

DILATOR, LACRIMAL *(Ophthalmology) 86HNW*

Accutome, Inc. 610-889-0200
3222 Phoenixville Pike, Malvern, PA 19355
Dilators.

Bausch & Lomb Surgical 636-255-5051
3365 Tree Court Ind Blvd, Saint Louis, MO 63122

Biomet Microfixation Inc. 800-874-7711
1520 Tradeport Dr, Jacksonville, FL 32218
Various types of dilators.

Eagle Vision, Inc. 800-222-7584
8500 Wolf Lake Dr Ste 110, Memphis, TN 38133
Coroneo Punctal Gauge, a complete gauging/dilating system in one instrument in increments from 0.5mm up to 1.0mm diameters. Takes the place of multiple instrument gauge sets.

Eye Care And Cure 800-486-6169
4646 S Overland Dr, Tucson, AZ 85714
Dilator.

Fortrad Eye Instruments Corp. 973-543-2371
8 Franklin Rd, Mendham, NJ 07945

DILATOR, LACRIMAL *(cont'd)*

George Tiemann & Co. 800-843-6266
25 Plant Ave, Hauppauge, NY 11788

Jedmed Instruments Co. 314-845-3770
5416 Jedmed Ct, Saint Louis, MO 63129

Katena Products, Inc. 800-225-1195
4 Stewart Ct, Denville, NJ 07834

Stephens Instruments, Inc. 800-354-7848
2500 Sandersville Rd, Lexington, KY 40511
$12.00 per unit (standard).

Surgical Instrument Manufacturers, Inc. 800-521-2985
1650 Headland Dr, Fenton, MO 63026

Total Titanium, Inc. 618-473-2429
140 East Monroe St., Hecker, IL 62248
Various types of lachrimal dilators.

Walsh Medical Devices Inc. 800-449-7615
1200 South Service Rd W, Unit 3, Oakville, ONT L6L 5T7 Canada
Lacrimal intubation set

Western Ophthalmics Corporation 800-426-9938
19019 36th Ave W Ste G, Lynnwood, WA 98036

DILATOR, NASAL *(Ear/Nose/Throat) 77LWF*

Biomet Microfixation Inc. 800-874-7711
1520 Tradeport Dr, Jacksonville, FL 32218
Various types of dilators.

Boyd Associates Inc. 330-854-5433
465 Trelake Dr, Canal Fulton, OH 44614
Nasal dilator.

Breathe With Eez Corp. 800-826-7077
PO Box 37, Albertson, NY 11507
Therapeutic nasal dilator.

Bwell Inc. 865-982-2184
1723 Saint Ives Blvd, Alcoa, TN 37701
Nasal dilator.

Cns, Inc. 800-441-0417
7615 Smetana Ln, Eden Prairie, MN 55344
Breathe Right nasal strips.

E-Global Medical Equipment, L.L.C. 866-422-1845
2f 500 Lincoln St., Allston, MA 02134
Dilator for general surgical use.

Incredible Scents, Inc. 516-676-7500
1009 Glen Cove Ave, Glen Head, NY 11545

Pureline Oralcare, Inc. 831-662-9500
804 Estates Dr, Aptos, CA 95003
Anti-snoring device.

Santa Barbara Medco, Inc. 651-452-1977
1270 Eagan Industrial Rd, Eagan, MN 55121
Nasal dilator.

Schering-Plough Healthcare Products, Inc. 862-245-5115
4207 Michigan Avenue Rd NE, Cleveland, TN 37323
Nasal strips.

Silver Eagle Labs Inc. 650-522-9700
204 W Spear St, Carson City, NV 89703
Nasal dilator.

Ventus Medical, Inc. 650-632-4160
1301 Shoreway Rd Ste 340, Belmont, CA 94002

Woodleaf Corporation 949-675-2121
1700 W Oceanfront Apt D, Newport Beach, CA 92663
Nasal dialator.

DILATOR, OTHER *(Surgery) 79QPW*

Arosurgical Instruments Corp. 800-776-1751
537 Newport Center Dr Ste 101, Newport Beach, CA 92660
Vessel DILATORS for microsurgery, 12 to 18cm, STR, CVD & ANGL. 0.2mm to 0.5mm tips. Titanium or Stainless Steel.

Carl Heyer, Inc. 800-284-5550
1872 Bellmore Ave, North Bellmore, NY 11710

Encompas Unlimited, Inc. 800-825-7701
PO Box 516, Tallevast, FL 34270
Dilator storage tray, $475.00. Protects 11 dilators.

Medgyn Products, Inc. 800-451-9667
328 Eisenhower Ln N, Lombard, IL 60148
Pratt dilators.

Tfx Medical Oem 800-548-6600
50 Plantation Dr, Jaffrey, NH 03452
Split sheath/dilator and dilator/sheath assemblies.

DILATOR, PORT, LAPAROSCOPIC *(Surgery) 79SIN*

Dma Med-Chem Corporation 800-362-1833
49 Watermill Ln, Great Neck, NY 11021
Balloons.

Wisap America 800-233-8448
8231 Melrose Dr, Lenexa, KS 66214

DILATOR, RECTAL *(Gastro/Urology) 78FFP*

Aesculap Implant Systems Inc. 1-800-234-9179
3773 Corporate Pkwy, Center Valley, PA 18034

Milex Products, Inc. 800-621-1278
4311 N Normandy Ave, Chicago, IL 60634
Vaginal and rectal dilator. Available in sets of 4/$135.00.

Specialty Surgical Products, Inc. 406-961-0102
1131 US Highway 93 N, Victor, MT 59875
Pediatric anal dilator.

Tools For Surgery, Llc 631-444-4448
1339 Stony Brook Rd, Stony Brook, NY 11790
Anal dilators.

DILATOR, TRACHEAL *(Ear/Nose/Throat) 77KCG*

Aesculap Implant Systems Inc. 1-800-234-9179
3773 Corporate Pkwy, Center Valley, PA 18034

Clinimed, Incorporated 877-CLINIMED
303 Markus Ct, Sandy Brae Industrial Park, Newark, DE 19713

Codman & Shurtleff, Inc 800-225-0460
325 Paramount Dr, Raynham, MA 02767

Tuzik Boston 800-886-6363
104 Longwater Dr, Assinippi Park, Norwell, MA 02061

DILATOR, URETHRAL *(Gastro/Urology) 78KOE*

Biomet Microfixation Inc. 800-874-7711
1520 Tradeport Dr, Jacksonville, FL 32218
Various types of dilators.

C. R. Bard, Inc., Bard Urological Div. 888-367-2273
13183 Harland Dr NE, Covington, GA 30014

Cook Urological, Inc. 800-457-4500
1100 W Morgan St, P.O. Box 227, Spencer, IN 47460

DILATOR, URETHRAL, MECHANICAL *(Gastro/Urology) 78FAH*

Aesculap Implant Systems Inc. 1-800-234-9179
3773 Corporate Pkwy, Center Valley, PA 18034

Miltex Inc. 800-645-8000
589 Davies Dr, York, PA 17402

Richard Wolf Medical Instruments Corp. 800-323-9653
353 Corporate Woods Pkwy, Vernon Hills, IL 60061

DILATOR, UTERINE *(Obstetrics/Gyn) 85QPV*

Codman & Shurtleff, Inc 800-225-0460
325 Paramount Dr, Raynham, MA 02767

Miltex Inc. 800-645-8000
589 Davies Dr, York, PA 17402

Premier Medical Products 888-PREMUSA
1710 Romano Dr, Plymouth Meeting, PA 19462

Princeton Medical Group, Inc. 800-875-0869
1189 Royal Links Dr, Mt Pleasant, SC 29466

R Medical Supply 800-882-7578
620 Valley Forge Rd Ste F, Hillsborough, NC 27278

DILATOR, VAGINAL *(Obstetrics/Gyn) 85HDX*

Advanced Medical Innovations, Inc. 888-367-2641
9410 De Soto Ave Ste J, Chatsworth, CA 91311
A complete line of German S.S. quality Women's Health Instruments: Stainless Steel; Insulated Instruments for Electrosurgical Procedures; Disposable Specula. SAF-T-VIEW, Ob-Gyn 4-bladed vaginal expanders for ideal cervix exposure for diagnostic & surgical procedures. INSTRU-HOLD, instrument holder, an attachment to the 4-bladed expander line to hold an instrument which keeps the cervix under traction, and freeing the surgeon's hand. Also sells under the WHOLE-IN-ONE trademark. Another international line of 4 bladed speculum is featured under the name Universal 2&4 Bladed speculum. This is a one handed simple design with enhanced comfort for the patient. Comes in all sizes including X-large.

Biomet Microfixation Inc. 800-874-7711
1520 Tradeport Dr, Jacksonville, FL 32218
Various types of dilators.

Kmedic 800-955-0559
190 Veterans Dr, Northvale, NJ 07647

DILATOR, VAGINAL *(cont'd)*

Milex Products, Inc. 800-621-1278
4311 N Normandy Ave, Chicago, IL 60634
VAGINAL-HYMENAL at $135.00 for set of 4.

R Medical Supply 800-882-7578
620 Valley Forge Rd Ste F, Hillsborough, NC 27278

Syracuse Medical Devices, Inc. 315-449-0657
214 Hurlburt Rd, Syracuse, NY 13224
Applied to minimize shrinkage of vagina during and/or after irradiation or surgery. White polyethylene, six inches long, four diameters.

Tuzik Boston 800-886-6363
104 Longwater Dr, Assinippi Park, Norwell, MA 02061

Ware Medics Glass Works, Inc. 845-429-6950
PO Box 368, Garnerville, NY 10923

DILATOR, VASCULAR *(Cardiovascular) 74QPQ*

Becton Dickinson Infusion Therapy Systems, Inc. 888-237-2762
9450 S State St, Sandy, UT 84070

Endovascular Instruments, Inc. 360-750-1150
2501 SE Columbia Way Ste 150, Vancouver, WA 98661

Fehling Surgical Instruments 800-FEHLING
509 Broadstone Ln NW, Acworth, GA 30101

Princeton Medical Group, Inc. 800-875-0869
1189 Royal Links Dr, Mt Pleasant, SC 29466

Scanlan International, Inc. 800-328-9458
1 Scanlan Plz, Saint Paul, MN 55107
Vascular tunneler.

DILATOR, VESSEL *(Gastro/Urology) 78FKA*

Vygon Corp. 800-544-4907
2495 General Armistead Ave, Norristown, PA 19403

DILATOR, VESSEL, PERCUTANEOUS CATHETERIZATION *(Cardiovascular) 74DRE*

Argon Medical Devices Inc. 903-675-9321
1445 Flat Creek Rd, Athens, TX 75751
Introducer kit; vessel dilator.

Becton Dickinson Infusion Therapy Systems, Inc. 888-237-2762
9450 S State St, Sandy, UT 84070

Cook Inc. 800-457-4500
PO Box 489, Bloomington, IN 47402

Cook Vascular, Incorporated 800-457-4500
1186 Montgomery Ln, Vandergrift, PA 15690
PERFECTA Electrosurgical dissection sheath - an RF-powered sheath designed to locally dissect and dilate tissue surrounding cardiac leads. A device used in lead-extraction procedures. RF-energy-powered dilator sheath for use during the removal of transvenous cardiac leads. NEEDLE'S EYE Snare - Specialized nitinol snare used in retrieving cardiac leads and other catheters. Provided with or without 16 French femoral sheath set.

Datascope Corp., Cardiac Assist Division 201-307-5400
1300 MacArthur Blvd, Mahwah, NJ 07430
Vessel dilator.

Enpath Medical, Inc. 800-559-2613
2300 Berkshire Ln N, Minneapolis, MN 55441

Ev3 Neurovascular 800-716-6700
9775 Toledo Way, Irvine, CA 92618
Introducer sheath.

Galt Medical Corp. 800-639-2800
2220 Merritt Dr, Garland, TX 75041
Various types of sterile and non sterile dilators.

Maquet Puerto Rico Inc. 408-635-3900
No. 12, Rd. #698, Dorado, PR 00646
Various.

Merit Medical Systems, Inc. 801-253-1600
1111 S Velasco St, Angleton, TX 77515
Various.

Navilyst Medical 800-833-9973
100 Boston Scientific Way, Marlborough, MA 01752
Various types of sterile dilators and dilator kits.

Tfx Medical Oem 800-548-6600
50 Plantation Dr, Jaffrey, NH 03452

Thomas Medical Products, Inc. 866-446-3003
65 Great Valley Pkwy, Malvern, PA 19355
Dilator.

Vnus Medical Technologies, Inc. 888-797-8346
5799 Fontanoso Way, San Jose, CA 95138
Multiple, dilator, introducer sheath, needle and guide wire.

DILATOR, VESSEL, SURGICAL *(Cardiovascular) 74DWP*

Aesculap Implant Systems Inc. 1-800-234-9179
3773 Corporate Pkwy, Center Valley, PA 18034

Biomet Microfixation Inc. 800-874-7711
1520 Tradeport Dr, Jacksonville, FL 32218
Various types of dilators.

Clinimed, Incorporated 877-CLINIMED
303 Markus Ct, Sandy Brae Industrial Park, Newark, DE 19713

Depuy-Raynham, A Div. Of Depuy Orthopaedics 800-451-2006
325 Paramount Dr, Raynham, MA 02767
Various surgical dilators.

Eriem Surgical 800-833-3380
28438 N Ballard Dr, Lake Forest, IL 60045

Fehling Surgical Instruments 800-FEHLING
509 Broadstone Ln NW, Acworth, GA 30101

Micrins Surgical Instruments, Inc. 800-833-3380
28438 N Ballard Dr, Lake Forest, IL 60045

Neo Medical Inc. 888-450-3334
42514 Albrae St, Fremont, CA 94538
Subcutaneous catheter passer.

Synovis Life Technologies, Inc 800-255-4018
2575 University Ave W, Saint Paul, MN 55114
Intravascular Probe; Vascular Probe

Synovis Surgical Innovations 800-255-4018
2575 University Ave W, Saint Paul, MN 55114
The VASCULAR PROBE, an intravascular probe for coronary and peripheral vascular surgery.

Terumo Cardiovascular Systems (Tcvs) 800-283-7866
28 Howe St, Ashland, MA 01721
Pediatric insulation pad.

Terumo Cardiovascular Systems, Corp 800-521-2818
6200 Jackson Rd, Ann Arbor, MI 48103

DILUENT, BLOOD CELL *(Hematology) 81GIF*

American Red Cross Diagnostic Manufacturing Divisi 202-303-5640
9319 Gaither Rd, Gaithersburg, MD 20877
Bovine albumin 3%.

Beckman Coulter, Inc. 800-635-3497
740 W 83rd St, Hialeah, FL 33014
ISOTON II and ISOTON III.

Bio-Rad Laboratories, Diagnostic Group 800-224-6723
524 Stone Rd Ste A, Benicia, CA 94510
Blood cell diluent.

Biosure, Inc. 800-345-2267
12301 Loma Rica Dr Unit G, Grass Valley, CA 95945
BioSure Sheath Solution, 8X concentrate save on shipping costs. For use on flow cytometry instruments and blood analyzers.

Cst Technologies, Inc. 800-448-4407
55 Northern Blvd Ste 200, Great Neck, NY 11021
$190.00 per liter for PRO-DIL: protein diluent. CTRLSUB $95.00 per liter, synthetic control base. SERADIL $195.00 per liter, serum diluent.

Diagnostic Technology, Inc. 631-582-4949
175 Commerce Dr Ste L, Hauppauge, NY 11788
Isotonic blood cell diluent.

E K Industries, Inc. 877-EKI-CHEM
1403 Herkimer St, Joliet, IL 60432
Various saline solutions.

Edge Medical Imaging, Inc. 703-919-4732
6003 Woodlake Ln, Alexandria, VA 22315
Blood cell diluent.

Health Chem Diagnostics Llc 954-979-3845
3341 W McNab Rd, Pompano Beach, FL 33069
Diluent, blood cell.

Horiba Abx 888-903-5001
34 Bunsen, Irvine, CA 92618
Liquid reagent used to suspend blood cells for counting.

Iris Diagnostics 800-776-4747
9172 Eton Ave, Chatsworth, CA 91311
Blood cell diluent.

Nerl Diagnostics Llc. 401-824-2046
14 Almeida Ave, East Providence, RI 02914
Blood cell dilutants.

DILUENT, BLOOD CELL *(cont'd)*

Ortho-Clinical Diagnostics, Inc. 800-828-6316
513 Technology Blvd, Rochester, NY 14626
Saline diluent.

Rocky Mountain Reagents,Inc. 303-762-0800
3207 W Hampden Ave, Englewood, CO 80110

Sterling Diagnostics, Inc. 800-637-2661
36645 Metro Ct, Sterling Heights, MI 48312

Sysmex Reagents America, Inc. 847-996-4512
10716 Reagan St, Los Alamitos, CA 90720
Various types.

Valley Biomedical Products/Ser., Inc. 540-868-0800
121 Industrial Dr, Winchester, VA 22602
Dental curing light.

Vegamed, Inc. 787-807-0392
39 Calle Las Flores, Edificio Multifabril #5, Vega Baja, PR 00693
Isotonic diluent.

DILUTER *(Chemistry) 75QPX*

Air Techniques International 410-363-9696
11403 Cronridge Dr, Owings Mills, MD 21117

Beckman Coulter, Inc. 800-635-3497
740 W 83rd St, Hialeah, FL 33014
DDIII prepares 1:500 and 1:50,000 dilutions.

Beckman Coulter, Inc. 800-742-2345
250 S Kraemer Blvd, PO Box 8000, Brea, CA 92821

Covidien Lp 508-261-8000
15 Hampshire St, Mansfield, MA 02048

Hamilton Company 800-648-5950
4990 Energy Way, Reno, NV 89502

Kloehn Co., Ltd. 800-358-4342
10000 Banburry Cross Dr, Las Vegas, NV 89144
Syringe drive diluters/dispensers (pumps).

Thermo Fisher Scientific 800-345-0206
22 Friars Dr, Hudson, NH 03051
Dilutor dispensers.

Zymark Corporation 508-435-9500
68 Elm St, Hopkinton, MA 01748

DILUTER, BLOOD CELL, AUTOMATED *(Hematology) 81GKH*

Bd Biosciences 408-954-6307
2350 Qume Dr, San Jose, CA 95131
Sample processor.

Beckman Coulter, Inc. 800-526-3821
11800 SW 147th Ave, Miami, FL 33196
Automated blood cell diluting apparatus.

Beckman Coulter, Inc. 800-635-3497
740 W 83rd St, Hialeah, FL 33014
DDIII prepares 1:500 and 1:50,000 dilutions.

Fisher Healthcare 800-766-7000
9999 Veterans Memorial Dr, Houston, TX 77038

Sparton Medical Systems 440-878-4630
22740 Lunn Rd, Strongsville, OH 44149
Automated blood cell diluting apparatus.

DISC, STRIP AND REAGENT, MICROORGANISM DIFFERENTIATION *(Microbiology) 83JTO*

Alpha Scientific Medical, Inc. 909-802-7000
1751 Yeager Ave, La Verne, CA 91750

Bayer Healthcare Llc 914-524-2955
555 White Plains Rd Fl 5, Tarrytown, NY 10591
Three way test for bacteriuria in urine.

Bayer Healthcare, Llc 574-256-3430
430 S Beiger St, Mishawaka, IN 46544
Three way test for bacteriuria in urine.

Bd Diagnostic Systems 800-675-0908
7 Loveton Cir, Sparks, MD 21152

Biomerieux Industry 800-634-7656
595 Anglum Rd, Hazelwood, MO 63042
Micro-organisms - lyophilized.

Emd Chemicals Inc. 800-222-0342
480 S Democrat Rd, Gibbstown, NJ 08027
HEMACOLOR stain set 3 x 16oz.

Exmoor Plastics Inc. 317-244-1014
304 Gasoline Aly, Indianapolis, IN 46222
SHAH silicone discs and strips for splinting tympanum and for lining wounds before dressing. Sterile, from $3.20 each.

DISC, STRIP AND REAGENT, MICROORGANISM DIFFERENTIATION *(cont'd)*

Hardy Diagnostics — 800-226-2222
1430 W McCoy Ln, Santa Maria, CA 93455
Various reagents and rapid identification kits for the differentiation and identification of microorganisms.

Health Chem Diagnostics Llc — 954-979-3845
3341 W McNab Rd, Pompano Beach, FL 33069
Discs, strips and reagents, microorganism differentiation.

Key Scientific Products — 325-773-3918
1113 E Reynolds St, Stamford, TX 79553
Buffered substrates for use in identifying microorganisms through biochemical re.

Medi-Tech Holdings, Inc. — 714-841-8603
15209 Springdale St, Huntington Beach, CA 92649
Various types of free radical test.

Nerl Diagnostics Llc. — 401-824-2046
14 Almeida Ave, East Providence, RI 02914
Visispot kits, kit for the differential id of enterococcus.

Pml Microbiologicals — 800-628-7014
27120 SW 95th Ave, Wilsonville, OR 97070

Remel — 800-255-6730
12076 Santa Fe Dr, Lenexa, KS 66215

Remel Atlanta, Div. Of Remel, Inc. — 800-255-6730
2797 Peterson Pl, Norcross, GA 30071
Staphylochrome reagent for identification of clumping factor in staphylolcocci; oxichrome reagent.

DISC, SUSCEPTIBILITY, ANTIMICROBIAL *(Microbiology) 83JTN*

Bd Diagnostic Systems — 800-675-0908
7 Loveton Cir, Sparks, MD 21152

Eli Lilly And Co. — 317-276-4000
Lilly Corporate Ctr, Drop Code 2622, Indianapolis, IN 46285
Discs for testing susceptibility to nebciin 10mcg.

DISCRIMINATOR, TWO-POINT *(Cns/Neurology) 84GWI*

Cybernetic Research Laboratories, Inc. — 520-571-8065
3562 E 42nd Stra, Tucson, AZ 85713
Two-point discriminator.

Medworks Instruments — 800-323-9790
PO Box 581, Chatham, IL 62629
$9.90 per unit (standard).

Patterson Medical Supply, Inc. — 262-387-8720
W68N158 Evergreen Blvd, Cedarburg, WI 53012
Touch discriminator.

DISH, PETRI *(Chemistry) 75QPY*

Bd Diagnostic Systems — 800-675-0908
7 Loveton Cir, Sparks, MD 21152

Berghof/America — 800-544-5004
3773 NW 126th Ave Bldg 1, Coral Springs, FL 33065
PFA, stackable Petri dish with dish serving as its own cover, or PTFE, rigid construction Petri dish. Four types of evaporating dishes also available.

Carolina Biological Supply Co. — 800-334-5551
2700 York Rd, Burlington, NC 27215

Edmund Industrial Optics — 800-363-1992
101 E Gloucester Pike, Barrington, NJ 08007

Nalge Nunc International — 800-625-4327
75 Panorama Creek Dr, Rochester, NY 14625
NALGENE disposable polstyrene and reusable polymethlypentene and polycarbonate dishes.

Nutech Molding Corporation — 1-800-423-5278
PO Box 840, 2024 Broad St,, Pocomoke City, MD 21851

Parter Medical Products — 800-666-8282
17015 Kingsview Ave, Carson, CA 90746
Various types & sizes, call for quotation.

Phoenix Biomedical Products, Inc. — 9056708299
7085 Tomken Rd., Mississauga, ONT L5S-1R7 Canada
STARdish sterile, plastic petri dish available in different sizes.

Polar Plastic Ltd. — 514-331-0207
4210 Thimens Blvd., St. Laurent, QUE H4R 2B9 Canada
POLAR RX. semi-stacking, non-stacking-15x150 marbec dish with pull pocket.

Simport Plastics Ltd. — 450-464-1723
2588 Bernard-Pilon, Beloeil, QUE J3G 4S5 Canada

DISH, PETRI *(cont'd)*

Valmark, Inc. — 613-822-3107
P.O. Box 190, Gloucester, ONT K1X-1A4 Canada
ULTRA-DISH Easy hand opening and closing edges of tops and bottoms. 100 percent sterility guaranteed, consistently flat bottoms, manual or machine use.

Ware Medics Glass Works, Inc. — 845-429-6950
PO Box 368, Garnerville, NY 10923

DISH, TISSUE CULTURE *(Pathology) 88KIZ*

Bd Biosciences Discovery Labware — 978-901-7431
1 Becton Cir, Durham, NC 27712
Various sizes, styles & models of sterile, non-sterile disposable tissue culture.

Eye Care And Cure — 800-486-6169
4646 S Overland Dr, Tucson, AZ 85714
Petri dish.

Qiagen Gaithersburg, Inc. — 800-344-3631
1201 Clopper Rd, Gaithersburg, MD 20878
Pipettor, microplate handler, incubator.

Sarstedt, Inc. — 800-257-5101
PO Box 468, 1025, St. James Church Road, Newton, NC 28658

Simport Plastics Ltd. — 450-464-1723
2588 Bernard-Pilon, Beloeil, QUE J3G 4S5 Canada

Thermo Fisher Scientific (Rochester) — 585-899-7600
75 Panorama Creek Dr, Panorama, NY 14625
Various tissue culture dishes.

DISINFECTOR, LIQUID *(General) 80QPZ*

AmSan — 800-327-3528
1930 Energy Park Dr Ste 260, Saint Paul, MN 55108

Beaumont Products, Inc. — 800-451-7096
1560 Big Shanty Dr NW, Kennesaw, GA 30144
CITRUS II, germicidal deodorizing cleaner. Broad spectrum, antimicrobial surface cleaner. Mild, non-alcohol formula. Cleans, deodorizes and disinfects surfaces, equipment and non-critical instruments leaving a plesant citrus fragrance. CITRUS II Antibacterial Soap kills germs. Has moisturizers and a light citrus fragrance.

Betco Corp. — 800-462-3826
1001 Brown Ave, Toledo, OH 43607

Brulin & Co. Inc. — 800-776-7149
2920 Drive A.J. Brown Avenue, Indianapolis, IN 46205
Disinfectant used against HIV-1 (Human Immunodificiency Virus). Maxima 128 is effective against Hepatitis B and HIV.

Caltech Industries, Inc. — 800-234-7700
2420 Schuette Rd, Midland, MI 48642
CITRACE disinfectant spray, RTU. Pressurized spray germicide for disinfecting surfaces and deodorizing air. OSHA acceptable for bloodborne pathogens. Now kills HBV. CITREX hospital spray disinfectant. Pressurized spray disinfectant kills TB, HIV. OSHA acceptable for bloodborne pathogens. DISPATCH cleaner disinfectant spray, RTU. Cleaner disinfectant with bleach, fast acting, non-pressured spray for cleaning and disinfecting in one step. New 30 Second TB claim. OSHA acceptable for bloodborne pathogens. PRECISE foam cleaner disinfectant spray. Hospital foam disinfectant, pressurized spray for cleaning and disinfecting in one step. New HBV and HCV claims. OSHA acceptable for bloodborne pathogens. PRECISE QTB Hospital Cleaner Disinfectant, liquid OSHA acceptable for bloodborne pathogens. New HBC, HCV claims.

Canberra Corp. — 419-841-6616
3610 N Holland Sylvania Rd, Toledo, OH 43615

Carochem, Inc. — 919-682-5121
744 E Markham Ave # 15699, Durham, NC 27701
Hospital disinfectant for disinfection of inanimate objects and floors.

Carroll Co. — 800-527-5722
2900 W Kingsley Rd, Garland, TX 75041

Crosstex International — 800-223-2497
10 Ranick Rd, Hauppauge, NY 11788
SANITEX PLUS Surface spray disinfectant and cleaner.

Dentronix, Inc. — 800-523-5944
235 Ascot Pkwy, Cuyahoga Falls, OH 44223
ULTRACARE Disinfectant Cleaner Concentrate kills HIV-1, HBV and HBC plus an additional 129 organisms. Safe for all surfaces, and odor-free, Ultracare is proven effective in the presence of 98% organic soil, and cleans and disinfects in one step. Economical and easy to use.

Essential Industries Inc. — 800-551-9679
PO Box 12, 28391 Essential Road, Merton, WI 53056

DISINFECTOR, LIQUID *(cont'd)*

Ferno-Washington, Inc. 800-733-3766
70 Weil Way, Wilmington, OH 45177
Designed to kill the tuberculocidal bacteria. Removes blood or other organic matter from vinyl surfaces, and disinfects whirlpools, tubs, stretchers, mattresses and more.

Genlabs 800-882-5227
5568 Schaefer Ave, Chino, CA 91710
Janitorial Supplies

Ivry 305-448-9858
216 Catalonia Ave Ste 106, Coral Gables, FL 33134
Odor/stain eradicator for home and hospital use.

Johnson & Johnson Medical Division Of Ethicon, Inc. 800-423-4018
2500 E Arbrook Blvd, Arlington, TX 76014

Johnsondiversey, Inc. 262-631-4001
8310 16th St, P.O. Box 902, Sturtevant, WI 53177

Jvs Solutions 800-325-3303
1200 Switzer Ave, Saint Louis, MO 63147

KIK Custom Products 800-479-6603
1 W Hegeler Ln, Danville, IL 61832

Lee Medical International, Inc. 800-433-8950
612 Distributors Row, Harahan, LA 70123
Diacide dialysis disinfectant.

Mada, Inc. 800-526-6370
625 Washington Ave, Carlstadt, NJ 07072

Mckesson General Medical 800-446-3008
8741 Landmark Rd, Richmond, VA 23228
Povidone-iodine solution.

Medical Chemical Corp. 800-424-9394
19430 Van Ness Ave, Torrance, CA 90501
WAVICIDE-06 disinfectant - $4.00/qt, $9.00/gal. WAVICIDE-01 disinfectant - $5.17/qt, $18.00/gal.

Micro-Scientific Industries, Inc. 888-253-2536
1225 Carnegie St Ste 101, Rolling Meadows, IL 60008

Noble Pine Products Co. 800-359-4913
PO Box 41, Centuck Station, Yonkers, NY 10710
STERIFAB disinfectant.

Orthodontic Supply & Equipment Co., Inc. 800-638-4003
7851 Airpark Rd Ste 202, Gaithersburg, MD 20879
Cold sterilization solution.

Palmero Health Care 800-344-6424
120 Goodwin Pl, Stratford, CT 06615
DISCIDE ULTRA disinfecting spray. Kills HIV, Herpes and Adenovirus in one minute.

Pharmacal Research Labs. Inc. 800-243-5350
PO Box 369, Naugatuck, CT 06770
Laboratory animal care.

Pharmaceutical Innovations, Inc. 973-242-2900
897 Frelinghuysen Ave, Newark, NJ 07114
T-SPRAY - Ultrasound disinfectant detergent. Designed to clean and disinfect all ultrasound probes and transducers after each use between patients. Available in 250ml bottles @$6.75 each 12/bottles per box. T-SPRAY II - For cleaning and disinfecting mammography compressor plates, cassettes, ultrasound probes and transducers. Available in 250ml bottles @ $6.75 each 12/bottles per box. M-SPRAY 2000 - 21st century disinfectant mammography cleaner. For cleaning and disinfecting mammography components which come in contact with body tissue. Available in 250ml bottles @ $6.75 each 12/bottles per box.

Ppr Direct, Inc. 800-526-3668
74 20th St, Brooklyn, NY 11232
PRO CLEARZ anti-fungal liquid.

Preserve International 800-995-1607
PO Box 17003, Reno, NV 89511
ADVANTAGE 128 - phenolic; triple phenolic. ADVANTAGE 256 - triple phenolic.

Professional Disposables International, Inc. 800-999-6423
2 Nice Pak Park, Orangeburg, NY 10962
SANI-CLOTH Hard surface disinfect and anti-microbial hand wipes.

DISINFECTOR, LIQUID *(cont'd)*

Safetec Of America, Inc. 800-456-7077
887 Kensington Ave, Buffalo, NY 14215
SANIZIDE PLUS and BIOZIDE help you comply with OSHA Bloodborne Pathogens Standard. Ready-to-use, broad spectrum, hospital grade, hard surface disinfectants/deodorizers. Both are EPA registered. SANIZIDE PLUS is tuberculocidal and virucidal -- kills HIV, HBV, and HCV! Dual quaternary ammonium compound is alcohol-free and non-flammable. Packaging: 2-, 16-, or 32-oz spray bottles, or 1-gallon refill. BIOZIDE is a tuberculocidal, virucidal, phenolic formula. Safe on surfaces that will not be harmed by alcohol. Packaging: single-use pouch with a heavy-duty dry 8 x 8-in. wipe, in 2-, 4-, or 16-oz spray bottles, or 1-gallon refill.

Spartan Chemical Company, Inc. 800-537-8990
1110 Spartan Dr, Maumee, OH 43537

Stepan Co. 800-745-7837
22 W Frontage Rd, Northfield, IL 60093

Steris Corporation 800-884-9550
5960 Heisley Rd, Mentor, OH 44060
Products for both high-risk and routine skin disinfection.

Surco Products 800-556-0111
292 Alpha Dr, RIDC Industrial Park, Pittsburgh, PA 15238
Air fresheners, deodorizers, odor neutralizers.

Ulmer Pharmacal Co. 800-848-5637
PO Box 408, 1614 Industry Ave., Park Rapids, MN 56470
PHENEEN $3.33 per 1000 ml.

Ultra Clean Systems, Inc. 877-935-6624
12700 Dupont Cir, Tampa, FL 33626
Ultra Cleanzyme triple enzymatic solution for ultrasonic cleaners. Also for presoaking.

Unit Chemical Corp. 800-879-8648
7360 Commercial Way, Henderson, NV 89011
Liquid disinfectant & detergent.

West Penetone Corp 800-631-1652
700 Gotham Pkwy, Carlstadt, NJ 07072

Youngs, Inc. 800-523-5454
55 E Cherry Ln, Souderton, PA 18964

DISINFECTOR, MEDICAL DEVICE *(General) 80MEC*

Clariant Corporation 800-548-6902
625 East Catawba Ave., Charlotte, NC 28210

Steris Corporation 814-452-3100
2424 W 23rd St, Erie, PA 16506
Washer disinfector.

Unit Chemical Corp. 800-879-8648
7360 Commercial Way, Henderson, NV 89011
Both Liquid & Dry Forms of Disinfectant

Vision Pro Llc 800-892-3937
4309 I 49 S Service Rd, Opelousas, LA 70570
Device cleaner.

DISINFECTOR, PASTEURIZATION *(General) 80QQA*

Cenorin 800-426-1042
6324 S 199th Pl Ste 107, Kent, WA 98032
HLD Systems medical device cleaning and high level disinfection systems, assuring safety through full immersion pasteurization technology. Our systems provide you with the process control and complete assurance that reprocessed devices will be clean, bacteria and viral free, and safe for the next patient use use.

DISINTEGRATOR, BIOLOGICAL CELL *(Microbiology) 83UFW*

Carver Inc. 260-563-7577
1569 Morris St, Wabash, IN 46992

Parr Instrument Co. 800-872-7720
211 53rd St, Moline, IL 61265

Thermo Spectronic 800-654-9955
820 Linden Ave, Rochester, NY 14625
Non-disruptive FRENCH pressure cell disintegrator.

Virtis, An Sp Industries Company 800-431-8232
815 Route 208, Gardiner, NY 12525
Ultrasonic, Virsonic cell disrupter.

DISK, ABRASIVE *(Dental And Oral) 76EHJ*

Abrasive Technology, Inc. 740-548-4100
8400 Green Meadows Dr N, Lewis Center, OH 43035
Various types of abrasive disks.

Aesculap Implant Systems Inc. 1-800-234-9179
3773 Corporate Pkwy, Center Valley, PA 18034

DISK, ABRASIVE *(cont'd)*

Align Technology, Inc. 408-470-1000
881 Martin Ave, Santa Clara, CA 95050
Disk,abrasive.

American Diversified Dental Systems 800-637-2330
22991 La Cadena Dr, Laguna Hills, CA 92653
Perla-Dia Grinding Discs.

Buffalo Dental Mfg. Co., Inc. 516-496-7200
159 Lafayette Dr, Syosset, NY 11791
Abrasive points & stones.

Dedeco Intl., Inc. 845-887-4840
11617 Route 97, Long Eddy, NY 12760
Various types of abrasive disks.

Den-Mat Holdings, Llc 805-922-8491
2727 Skyway Dr, Santa Maria, CA 93455
No common name listed.

Ec Moore Company, Inc 800-331-3548
13325 Leonard St, Dearborn, MI 48126

G & H Wire Co. 800-526-1026
2165 Earlywood Dr, Franklin, IN 46131

Heraeus Kulzer, Inc., Dental Products Division 574-299-6662
4315 S Lafayette Blvd, South Bend, IN 46614
Polishing wheel.

Ivoclar Vivadent, Inc. 800-533-6825
175 Pineview Dr, Amherst, NY 14228
Astropol.

Kerr Corp. 714-516-7400
28200 Wick Rd, Romulus, MI 48174
Abrasive disc.

Mds Products, Inc. 800-637-2330
22991 La Cadena Dr, Laguna Hills, CA 92653
ADDS-IT Super-Cuts, Cut Off Disks, Box of 100.

Miltex Dental Technologies, Inc. 516-576-6022
589 Davies Dr, York, PA 17402
Various abrasive disks.

Mizzy, Inc. Of National Keystone 800-333-3131
616 Hollywood Ave, Cherry Hill, NJ 08002
Use our wide variety of Keystone mounted and unmounted stones, discs, points and rubber wheels for many cutting and finishing applications in the dental laboratory

Moyco Technologies, Inc. 800-331-8837
200 Commerce Dr, Montgomeryville, PA 18936
$8.00 per pack of 400 paper abrasive disks.

Pentron Clinical Technologies 203-265-7397
68-70 North Plains Industrial, Road, Wallingford, CT 06492
Abrasive device and accessories.

Shofu Dental Corporation 800-827-4638
1225 Stone Dr, San Marcos, CA 92078
SUPER-SNAPS

Ultradent Products, Inc. 801-553-4586
505 W 10200 S, South Jordan, UT 84095
Abrasive disks.

3m Espe Dental Products 949-863-1360
2111 McGaw Ave, Irvine, CA 92614
$26.00, $17.40 and $22.90/refills per unit.

DISK, PINHOLE, OPHTHALMIC *(Ophthalmology) 86HKH*

Gulden Ophthalmics 800-659-2250
225 Cadwalader Ave, Elkins Park, PA 19027

Western Ophthalmics Corporation 800-426-9938
19019 36th Ave W Ste G, Lynnwood, WA 98036

DISLODGER, STONE, BASKET, URETERAL, METAL *(Gastro/Urology) 78FFL*

Annex Medical, Inc. 952-942-7576
6018 Blue Circle Dr, Minnetonka, MN 55343
3.0 or smaller with flat wire or helical baskets.

Boston Scientific Corporation 508-652-5578
780 Brookside Dr, Spencer, IN 47460

C. R. Bard, Inc., Bard Urological Div. 888-367-2273
13183 Harland Dr NE, Covington, GA 30014

Cook Endoscopy 336-744-0157
4900 Bethania Station Rd # &, 5951 Grassy Creek Blvd. Winston Salem, NC 27105
Stone extraction basket.

Cook Urological, Inc. 800-457-4500
1100 W Morgan St, P.O. Box 227, Spencer, IN 47460

DISLODGER, STONE, BASKET, URETERAL, METAL *(cont'd)*

Greenwald Surgical Co., Inc. 219-962-1604
2688 Dekalb St, Gary, IN 46405
Various types of ureteral stone dislodgers.

Hobbs Medical, Inc. 860-684-5875
8 Spring St, Stafford Springs, CT 06076
Stone wire retrieval baskets.

Percutaneous Systems, Incorporated 650-493-4200
3260 Hillview Ave Ste 100, Palo Alto, CA 94304
Accordion.

Sterilmed, Inc. 763-488-3400
11400 73rd Ave N Ste 100, Maple Grove, MN 55369
Reprocessed stone retrieval basket.

DISLODGER, STONE, BASKET, URETERAL, METAL, REPROCESSED *(Gastro/Urology) 78NQU*

Sterilmed, Inc. 763-488-3400
11400 73rd Ave N Ste 100, Maple Grove, MN 55369
Stone retrieval basket.

DISLODGER, STONE, FLEXIBLE *(Gastro/Urology) 78FGO*

Annex Medical, Inc. 952-942-7576
6018 Blue Circle Dr, Minnetonka, MN 55343
3.0 or smaller with flat wire or helical baskets.

Boston Scientific Corporation 508-652-5578
780 Brookside Dr, Spencer, IN 47460

Boston Scientific Corporation 800-225-2732
1 Boston Scientific Pl, Natick, MA 01760

Cook Urological, Inc. 800-457-4500
1100 W Morgan St, P.O. Box 227, Spencer, IN 47460

Gyrus Acmi, Inc. 508-804-2739
93 N Pleasant St, Norwalk, OH 44857
Dislodger, stone, flexible.

DISLODGER, STORE, BILIARY *(Gastro/Urology) 78LQR*

Ballard Medical Products 770-587-7835
12050 Lone Peak Pkwy, Draper, UT 84020
Biliary stone extractor.

Boston Scientific Corporation 800-225-2732
1 Boston Scientific Pl, Natick, MA 01760

DISPENSER, CEMENT *(Orthopedics) 87KIH*

Abbott Spine, Inc. 847-937-6100
12708 Riata Vista Cir Ste B-100, Austin, TX 78727
Cement dispenser.

Advanced Biomaterial Systems, Inc. 973-635-9040
100 Passaic Ave, Chatham, NJ 07928
Bone cement mixer and dispenser.

Codman & Shurtleff, Inc 800-225-0460
325 Paramount Dr, Raynham, MA 02767

Depuy Orthopaedics, Inc. 800-473-3789
700 Orthopaedic Dr, P.O. Box 988, Warsaw, IN 46582
Various types of cement dispensers.

Depuy-Raynham, A Div. Of Depuy Orthopaedics 800-451-2006
325 Paramount Dr, Raynham, MA 02767
Various types of cement dispensers.

DFine Inc. 866-963-3463
3047 Orchard Pkwy, San Jose, CA 95134
SPACE 360 Delivery System; StabiliT Vertebral Augmentation Sys

Integra Lifesciences Corp. 609-275-0500
311 Enterprise Dr, Plainsboro, NJ 08536
Bone cement delivery system.

Medtronic Puerto Rico Operations Co.,Med Rel 763-514-4000
Road 909, Km. 0.4., Barrio Mariana, Humacao, PR 00792
Dispenser, cement.

Medtronic Sofamor Danek Usa, Inc. 901-396-3133
4340 Swinnea Rd, Memphis, TN 38118
Dispenser, cement.

Medtronic Spine Llc 877-690-5353
1221 Crossman Ave, Sunnyvale, CA 94089
Various.

Orthovita, Inc. 610-640-1775
77 Great Valley Pkwy, Malvern, PA 19355
Cement dispenser.

Osseon Therapeutics, Inc. 877-567-7366
2330 Circadian Way, Santa Rosa, CA 95407
OsseoFlex 1.0 Steerable Needle

DISPENSER, CEMENT *(cont'd)*

Precision Medical Devices, Inc. 717-795-9480
5020 Ritter Rd Ste 211, Mechanicsburg, PA 17055
Bone cement gun, nozzle and restrictor plug.

Skeletal Kinetics, Llc 408-366-5000
10201 Bubb Rd, Cupertino, CA 95014
Syringe.

Spine Wave, Inc. 203-944-9494
2 Enterprise Dr Ste 302, Shelton, CT 06484
Various types of cement dispensers and accessories.

Spineworks Medical Inc. 408-986-8950
1735 N 1st St Ste 245, San Jose, CA 95112

Stryker Puerto Rico, Ltd. 939-307-2500
Hwy. 3, Km. 131.2, Las Guasimas Ind. Park, Arroyo, PR 00714
Cement dispenser and various sterile accessories.

Synthes (Usa) - Development Center 719-481-5300
1230 Wilson Dr, West Chester, PA 19380
Cement dispenser.

Warsaw Orthopedic, Inc. 901-396-3133
2500 Silveus Xing, Warsaw, IN 46582
Dispenser, cement.

DISPENSER, DISC, SENSITIVITY, ANTIBIOTIC
(Microbiology) 83VCS

Bd Diagnostic Systems 800-675-0908
7 Loveton Cir, Sparks, MD 21152

Culture Kits, Inc. 888-680-6853
14 Prentice St, PO Box 748, Norwich, NY 13815
Ampicillin, augmentin, carbenicillin, cefamandole, cefoxitin, cephalothin, chloramphenicol, cinoxacin, clindamycin, colistin, doxycycline, erythromycin, gentamicin, methanamine mandelate, nafcillin, nalidixic acid, nitrofurantoin, penicillin, piperacillin, sulfonamide, tetracycline, trimeth/sulfa, trimethoprim, tobramycin and vancomycin.

DISPENSER, FLUID *(General) 80TGU*

B. Braun Oem Division, B. Braun Medical Inc. 866-8-BBRAUN
824 12th Ave, Bethlehem, PA 18018

Baxa Corporation 800-567-2292
9540 S Maroon Circle, Suite 400, Englewood, CO 80112
EXACTA-MED, oral liquid and ointment dispensers.

Beckman Coulter, Inc. 800-742-2345
250 S Kraemer Blvd, PO Box 8000, Brea, CA 92821

Cadence Science Inc. 888-717-7677
1979 Marcus Ave Ste 215, New Hyde Park, NY 11042

Ems Pacific, Inc. 800-575-5093
4480 Enterprise St Ste D, Fremont, CA 94538
Pre-settable, adjustable shot range fluid-dispensing system; from 0.005 mL to 12.5 mL in different model of piston pumps; selections of pump models to handle variety of viscous fluid from 1,000 cps to 150,000 cps; pump cylinder and piston available in metal and non-metal wetted parts; selections of valve type: valve or valveless; in pneumatic or motorized configuration.

Encynova 303-465-4800
557 Burbank St Unit C, Broomfield, CO 80020
The Travcyl fluid motion system provides digital control of fluid for precision dispensing of volumes from single microliters to 1.2 liters per minute with +- 0.1% accuracy.

Engineers Express, Inc. 800-255-8823
7 Industrial Park Rd, Medway, MA 02053

Garren Scientific, Inc. 800-342-3725
15916 Blythe St Unit A, Van Nuys, CA 91406
GARREN EZ DISPENSER bleach and water dispenser.

H & S Manufacturing, Inc. 800-827-3091
727 E Broadway, Williston, ND 58801
NEW-AID & HEP-AID disposable kits for cleanup of body fluids.

Hamilton Company 800-648-5950
4990 Energy Way, Reno, NV 89502

Highland Labs, Inc. 508-429-2918
42 Pope Rd # B, Holliston, MA 01746
Soap and fluid dispensers with stainless steel stands, hand or thigh operated.

Medi-Dose, Inc. 800-523-8966
70 Industrial Dr, Ivyland, PA 18974

Nalge Nunc International 800-625-4327
75 Panorama Creek Dr, Rochester, NY 14625
NALGENE precise and variable volume dispensers for fast, easy dispensing of bases, aqueous solutions and alcohols.

DISPENSER, FLUID *(cont'd)*

National Instrument Co., Inc. 800-526-1301
4119 Fordleigh Rd, Baltimore, MD 21215

Q.I. Medical, Inc. 800-837-8361
440 Lower Grass Valley Rd Ste C, Nevada City, CA 95959
SAFE-FIL Dispenser, fluid, needleless vial adaptors.

Safe-Tec Clinical Products, Inc. 800-356-6033
142 Railroad Dr, Ivyland, PA 18974
SAFEPETTE Harvesting Dispenser provides the means to safely and conveniently expel controlled droplet amounts of serum on plasma from the SAFECAP capillary tube.

Stedim Biosystems, Inc. 800-914-6644
1910 Mark Ct, Concord, CA 94520
Stedim 100 Autoclavable Drug Delivery Bags, the alternative to PVC for autoclavable I.V. drug delivery bags. Manufactured from polypropylene, Stedim 100 offers high-quality packaging with a broad range of compatibilities and low extractables.

Taylor 800-255-0626
PO Box 410, Rockton, IL 61072
Surgical Slush Unit for freezing saline

Tricontinent 800-937-4738
12555 Loma Rica Dr, Grass Valley, CA 95945

Varian Sample Preparation Products 800-421-2825
24201 Frampton Ave, Harbor City, CA 90710

DISPENSER, ICE *(General) 80TBU*

Follett Corp. 800-523-9361
801 Church Ln, Easton, PA 18040
Ice dispensers for on-floor patient care. Ice production of 400 pounds per day. Storage capacities from 25-90 pounds. SENSORSAFE ice dispenser for patient care using infra-red sensing to actuate dispensing.

Hoshizaki America, Inc. 800-438-6087
618 Highway 74 S, Peachtree City, GA 30269
Cubelet iemaker/dispensers. Designed for dependability, the stainless-steel exterior provides long life and easy maintenance. Easy-to-chew, dry Cubelet ice is produced and stored in a sanitary built-in storage bin, with selectable continuous or portion-controlled ice dispensing. DCM Cubelet icemaker/dispensers dispense ice and/or water; air-cooled models have removable, cleanable air filters for more efficient operation and dependable performance.

Imi Cornelius, Inc. 800-551-4423
500 Regency Dr, Glendale Heights, IL 60139

Marvel Scientific 800-962-2521
233 Industrial Pkwy, PO Box 997, Richmond, IN 47374
Compact and built for light commercial use; daily ice production from 15lb/24hr to 51lb/24hr.

U-Line Corporation 800-779-2547
8900 N 55th St, PO Box 245040, Milwaukee, WI 53223
Ice maker.

DISPENSER, LIQUID, LABORATORY *(Chemistry) 75VCT*

Beckman Coulter, Inc. 800-742-2345
250 S Kraemer Blvd, PO Box 8000, Brea, CA 92821

Berghof/America 800-544-5004
3773 NW 126th Ave Bldg 1, Coral Springs, FL 33065
Teflon safety reagent dispensers and PTFE dropper bottles.

Brinkmann Instruments, Inc. 800-645-3050
PO Box 1019, Westbury, NY 11590

Ems Pacific, Inc. 800-575-5093
4480 Enterprise St Ste D, Fremont, CA 94538
Pre-settable, adjustable shot range fluid-dispensing system; from 0.005 mL to 12.5 mL in different model of piston pumps; selections of pump models to handle variety of viscous fluid from 1,000 cps to 150,000 cps; pump cylinder and piston available in metal and non-metal wetted parts; selections of valve type: valve or valveless; in pneumatic or motorized configuration.

Nalge Nunc International 800-625-4327
75 Panorama Creek Dr, Rochester, NY 14625
NALGENE precise and variable volume dispensers for fast, easy dispensing of bases, aqueous solutions and alcohols.

Nutech Molding Corporation 1-800-423-5278
PO Box 840, 2024 Broad St,, Pocomoke City, MD 21851

DISPENSER, LIQUID, UNIT-DOSE *(General) 80VDP*

Baxa Corporation 800-567-2292
9540 S Maroon Circle, Suite 400, Englewood, CO 80112
EXACTA-MED, oral liquid and ointment dispensers.

DISPENSER, LIQUID, UNIT-DOSE *(cont'd)*

Liquid Control 330-494-1313
8400 Port Jackson Ave NW, North Canton, OH 44720
single component dispenser with shot size capabilities from 0.0002 cc's to 2.5000 cc's. use with silicones, epoxies, urethanes, and other materials.

Medi-Dose, Inc. 800-523-8966
70 Industrial Dr, Ivyland, PA 18974

Medical Packaging Inc. 800-257-5282
470 Route 31 N, PO Box 500, Ringoes, NJ 08551
Unit-dose filling machine for injectable syringes, and oral pediatric syringes;unit dose cups.

Nova Packaging Systems 978-537-8534
7 New Lancaster Rd, Leominster, MA 01453

Safetec Of America, Inc. 800-456-7077
887 Kensington Ave, Buffalo, NY 14215
ANTISEPTIC BIO-HAND CLEANER (a.b.h.c) kills 99.99% of most germs in as little as 15 seconds, without soap and water! Contains 66.5% Ethyl Alcohol and aloe vera to add moisture to skin. Available in Fresh or Citrus Scents. SANIWASH handwash contains PCMX for antimicrobial action and aloe vera to help moisturize hands when washing.

DISPENSER, MEDICATION, LIQUID *(General) 80KYX*

Apothecary Products, Inc. 800-328-2742
11750 12th Ave S, Burnsville, MN 55337
EZY-DOSE, Compakt Oral Syringe is a tubular liquid medication delivery device.

B. Braun Medical, Inc. 610-596-2536
901 Marcon Blvd, Allentown, PA 18109

B. Braun Of Puerto Rico, Inc. 610-691-5400
215.7 Insular Rd., Sabana Grande, PR 00637
Liquid medication dispenser, pharmacy.

Carex Health Brands 800-526-8051
921 E Amidon St, PO Box 2526, Sioux Falls, SD 57104
Measures in increments up to 2 teaspoons (10 cc) and comes with a filler tube which simplifies the task of drawing medicine from bottles.

Centurion Medical Products Corp. 517-545-1135
3310 S Main St, Salisbury, NC 28147

Covidien Lp 508-261-8000
15 Hampshire St, Mansfield, MA 02048
MONOJECT oral medication syringes, clear for routine medications and amber for light-senstive medications.

Dorel Design & Development Center 781-364-3542
25 Forbes Blvd, Foxboro, MA 02035

Health Care Logistics, Inc. 800-848-1633
450 Town St, PO Box 25, Circleville, OH 43113
Various.

Inter-Med, Inc. 877-418-4782
2200 Northwestern Ave, Racine, WI 53404
Liquid medication syringe.

Kentron Health Care, Inc. 615-384-0573
3604 Kelton Jackson Rd, P.o. Box 120, Springfield, TN 37172
Medicine cup.

Levine Health Products 800-426-6763
21101 NE 108th St, Redmond, WA 98053
Glass amber Boston round bottles with glass pippettes or lids

Medco Supply Company 800-556-3326
500 Fillmore Ave, Tonawanda, NY 14150
Oral medications including pain relief, ibuprofen, aspirin, antacid, allergy, cold, flu, sinus relief, sore throat and cough.

Medical Instill Technologies, Inc. 860-350-1900
201 Housatonic Ave, New Milford, CT 06776
Drug administration device.

Medline Manufacturing And Services Llc 847-837-2759
1 Medline Pl, Mundelein, IL 60060
Medicine cups.

Medtronic Spine Llc 877-690-5353
1221 Crossman Ave, Sunnyvale, CA 94089
Various types of sterile syringes.

Monroe Mfg., Inc. 318-338-3172
3030 Aurora Ave, 2nd Fl., Monroe, LA 71201
Medinurser medidropper medispoon.

Mps Acacia 800-486-6677
785 Challenger St, Brea, CA 92821

DISPENSER, MEDICATION, LIQUID *(cont'd)*

Munchkin, Inc. 800-247-2223
16689 Schoenborn St, North Hills, CA 91343
Various.

Norwood Promotional Products, Inc. 651-388-1298
5151 Moundview Dr, Red Wing, MN 55066

Paramark Corporation 443-436-9400
2605 Lord Baltimore Dr Ste H, Baltimore, MD 21244
Medicine dropper.

Sharn, Inc. 800-325-3671
4517 George Rd Ste 200, Tampa, FL 33634
NUMIMED Pacifier for dispencing liquid medicine and vitamins. NUMINOSE pacifier for inhaling decongestant.

Tri-State Hospital Supply Corp. 517-545-1135
3173 E 43rd St, Yuma, AZ 85365

Welcon, Inc. 800-877-0923
7409 Pebble Dr, Fort Worth, TX 76118
Feeding syringes.

DISPENSER, MERCURY AND/OR ALLOY *(Dental And Oral) 76EHE*

Dentalez Group 866-DTE-INFO
101 Lindenwood Dr Ste 225, Valleybrooke Corporate Center
Malvern, PA 19355

Dentsply Canada, Ltd. 800-263-1437
161 Vinyl Ct., Woodbridge, ONT L4L 4A3 Canada

Harry J. Bosworth Company 800-323-4352
7227 Hamlin Ave, Skokie, IL 60076
CROWN mercury dispenser.

Kerr Corp. 714-516-7400
28200 Wick Rd, Romulus, MI 48174
Mercury and alloy dispenser.

Wykle Research, Inc. 775-887-7500
2222 College Pkwy, Carson City, NV 89706
Tablet and mercury dispenser.

DISPENSER, MICROBIOLOGY MEDIA *(Microbiology) 83JTB*

Beckman Coulter, Inc. 800-742-2345
250 S Kraemer Blvd, PO Box 8000, Brea, CA 92821

Ika-Works, Inc. 800-733-3037
2635 Northchase Pkwy SE, Wilmington, NC 28405
Disperser/homogenizer designed for samples as small as a tenth of a milliliter. Handheld low-voltage drive weighs sixteen ounces.

DISPENSER, NARCOTIC *(General) 80QQC*

Baxa Corporation 800-567-2292
9540 S Maroon Circle, Suite 400, Englewood, CO 80112
KWIK-VIAL, pharmacy vial (tamper evident). EXACTA-MED, oral dispenser.

Brandt Industries, Inc. 800-221-8031
4461 Bronx Blvd, Bronx, NY 10470
Narcotics safes.

Life Care Technologies, Inc. 800-671-0580
4710 Eisenhower Blvd Ste A10, Tampa, FL 33634
MEDSERV & E-MAR automated dispensing & electronic mar. MedServ

DISPENSER, OTHER *(General) 80WJO*

Ak, Ltd. 503-669-0986
18412 NE Halsey St, Portland, OR 97230
Protective glove dispenser or bootie/bouffant/glove dispenser.

Alpha Scientific Corporation 800-242-5989
293 Great Valley Pkwy, Malvern, PA 19355
DIFF-SAFE Blood dispenser for hematology labs. SEG-SAFE is a segment processor for blood banks.

American Medical Alert Corp. 800-286-2622
3265 Lawson Blvd, Oceanside, NY 11572
MED-TIME electronic medication reminder and dispensing system.

American Medical Industries 605-428-5501
330 E 3rd St Ste 2, Dell Rapids, SD 57022
PILBOX Classic offers 7-day, one-button dispensing for up to four times a day. Mini PILBOX 7-day and Micro PILBOX single-day offer slide-open tablet dispensing for up to three times per day.

Atrion Medical Products, Inc. 800-343-9334
1426 Curt Francis Rd NW, Arab, AL 35016
Bottle closure, dispensing tips for pharmaceuticals.

Baxa Corporation 800-567-2292
9540 S Maroon Circle, Suite 400, Englewood, CO 80112
Specialty dispensers for topical and vaginal applications to prevent wrong-route errors.

DISPENSER, OTHER *(cont'd)*

Bowman Manufacturing Company, Inc. 360-435-5005
17301 51st Ave NE, Arlington, WA 98223
Full line of Dispensers for glove boxes, face masks, bandages, bio-hazard bags, bouffant caps, safety glasses, ear plugs, shoe covers, hair nets, and wipers(both premoistened and dry) provide for Medical, Dental, Food Service, and Industrial markets.

Brevis Corp. 800-383-3377
225 W 2855 S, Salt Lake City, UT 84115
Glove, mask and gown dispenser.

Brinkmann Instruments (Canada) Ltd. 800-263-8715
6670 Campobello Rd., Mississauga, ONT L5N 2L8 Canada

Cms Worldwide, Inc. 800-426-4633
30011 Ivy Glenn Dr Ste 215, Laguna Niguel, CA 92677
Metal dispensers, coated, for gloves, masks and other applications. Enamel coated. Imprint available.

Compumed, Inc. 800-722-4417
PO Box 339, Meeteetse, WY 82433
COMPUMED Computerized medication management system.

Covidien Lp 508-261-8000
15 Hampshire St, Mansfield, MA 02048

Ems Pacific, Inc. 800-575-5093
4480 Enterprise St Ste D, Fremont, CA 94538
Pre-settable, adjustable shot range fluid-dispensing system; from 0.005 mL to 12.5 mL in different model of piston pumps; selections of pump models to handle variety of viscous fluid from 1,000 cps to 150,000 cps; pump cylinder and piston available in metal and non-metal wetted parts; selections of valve type: valve or valveless; in pneumatic or motorized configuration.

Liquid Control 330-494-1313
8400 Port Jackson Ave NW, North Canton, OH 44720
POSIRATIO; two, three and other plural component meter mix, and dispense systems for use with silicones, epoxies, and other materials. POSIMETER; system for metering, mixing, and injecting two and three component silicones into the screw or mold of a molding press. POSIDOT; meter, mix and dispense system for two component silicones, epoxies, and other materials in shot sizes from 0.005 and 05.0 cc's.

National Instrument Llc 866-258-1914
4119 Fordleigh Rd, Baltimore, MD 21215
Metering systems consist of piston fillers, peristaltic pumps, rotary pumps, Ivek Pumps, among others.

One Lambda, Inc. 800-822-8824
21001 Kittridge St, Canoga Park, CA 91303
LAMBDA JET III cell dispenser and LAMBDA DOT III reagent dispenser.

Pinnacle Products, Inc. 800-878-3902
21401 Hemlock Ave, Lakeville, MN 55044
PINNACLE GLOVE DISPENSER.

Safetec Of America, Inc. 800-456-7077
887 Kensington Ave, Buffalo, NY 14215
ANTISEPTIC BIO-HAND CLEANER (a.b.h.c) kills 99.99% of most germs in as little as 15 seconds, without soap and water! Contains 66.5% Ethyl Alcohol and aloe vera to add moisture to skin. Available in original Fresh or Citrus Scents.

Thermo Fisher Scientific 800-345-0206
22 Friars Dr, Hudson, NH 03051
Robotic dispensing system.

Thermo Fisher Scientific Inc. 563-556-2241
2555 Kerper Blvd, Dubuque, IA 52001

DISPENSER, PARAFFIN *(Pathology) 88IDW*

Barnstead International 412-490-8425
2555 Kerper Blvd, Dubuque, IA 52001
Tissue embedding center.

Glenroe Technologies 800-237-4060
1912 44th Ave E, Bradenton, FL 34203
Orthodontic archwire markers.

Hacker Instruments And Industries Inc. 800-442-2537
1132 Kincaid Bridge Rd, PO Box 1176, Winnsboro, SC 29180
PD-2.0. Three-gallon capacity. Engineered for safety and lasting dependability.

Sci Gen, Inc. 310-324-6576
333 E Gardena Blvd, Gardena, CA 90248
FDA: Medical Device Manufacturing and packaging. Focus on Histology, Cytology, Analytical and General purpose Reagents, Chemistry, and Sterling and Disinfecting agents.

DISPENSER, PIPETTE *(Chemistry) 75WVX*

Ashton Pumpmatic, Inc. 800-395-1012
858 Distribution Dr, Dayton, OH 45434
PUMPMATIC pipette/liquid-handling system. 1-, 5-, and 10-ml sterile and non-sterile.

Intersciences Inc. 800-661-6431
169 Idema Rd., Markham, ONT L3R 1A9 Canada

Mg Scientific, Inc. 800-343-8338
8500 107th St, Pleasant Prairie, WI 53158

Nutech Molding Corporation 1-800-423-5278
PO Box 840, 2024 Broad St,, Pocomoke City, MD 21851

Standard Instrumentation, Div. Preiser Scientific 800-624-8285
94 Oliver St, Saint Albans, WV 25177

Tudor Scientific Glass Co., Inc. 800-336-4666
555 Edgefield Rd, Belvedere, SC 29841

DISPENSER, SLIDE *(Chemistry) 75QQD*

Nutech Molding Corporation 1-800-423-5278
PO Box 840, 2024 Broad St,, Pocomoke City, MD 21851

DISPENSER, SOAP *(General) 80TBV*

American Specialties, Inc. 914-476-9000
441 Saw Mill River Rd, Yonkers, NY 10701

Bobrick Washroom Equipment, Inc. 818-764-1000
11611 Hart St, North Hollywood, CA 91605

Chester Labs, Inc. 800-354-9709
1900 Section Rd, Cincinnati, OH 45237
PROVUE, manual dispensing system featuring a unique 3MP - pump that gives a precise dosage of 1ml.

Concepts International, Inc. 800-627-9729
224 E Main St, Summerton, SC 29148
Automatic soap dispenser; hands-free, infrared activated.

Gojo Industries, Inc 800-321-9647
1 Gojo Plz Ste 500, Akron, OH 44311
PROVON, PURELL, DERMAPRO.

Highland Labs, Inc. 508-429-2918
42 Pope Rd # B, Holliston, MA 01746
Soap and fluid dispensers with stainless steel stands. Foot operated. Model 488 Antimicrobial Soap/Solution Dispenser allows use of disabled hand operated dispensers in a completely 'hands-free way'.

K W Griffen Company 800-424-5556
100 Pearl St, Norwalk, CT 06850
Anti-microbial.

Questech International, Inc. 800-966-5367
3810 Gunn Hwy, Tampa, FL 33618
Hygeia Touchfree Soap Dispenser uses an infrared, motion-activated mechanism to automatically dispense liquid soap without hand contact. .

Safetec Of America, Inc. 800-456-7077
887 Kensington Ave, Buffalo, NY 14215
SANIWASH handwash contains PCMX for antimicrobial action and aloe vera to help moisturize hands when washing. Available in many other packaging options, as well as the 800 ml. wallmount dispenser.

Silverstone Packaging, Inc.-Your One Stop Supplier 800-413-1108
1401 Lakeland Ave, Bohemia, NY 11716

Spartan Chemical Company, Inc. 800-537-8990
1110 Spartan Dr, Maumee, OH 43537

DISPENSER, SOLID MEDICATION *(Physical Med) 89NXB*

Burggraf Industries 202-789-2111
899 Highway 70, Gallaway, TN 38036

Honeywell Hommed, Llc 888-353-5440
3400 Intertech Dr Ste 200, Brookfield, WI 53045
Medication reminder.

Lifetechniques Inc., Medsignals Corp. Div. 210-222-2067
217 Alamo Plz Ste 200, San Antonio, TX 78205
Solid medication dispenser.

DISPENSER, SYRINGE AND NEEDLE *(General) 80WSB*

Engineers Express, Inc. 800-255-8823
7 Industrial Park Rd, Medway, MA 02053

Kloehn Co., Ltd. 800-358-4342
10000 Banburry Cross Dr, Las Vegas, NV 89144
Syringe drive diluters/dispensers (pumps).

Medi-Dose, Inc. 800-523-8966
70 Industrial Dr, Ivyland, PA 18974

DISPENSER, THORASCOPIC *(Cardiovascular) 74SIZ*

Karl Storz Endoscopy-America Inc. 800-421-0837
600 Corporate Pointe, Culver City, CA 90230
Video-assisted instruments for thoracoscopic procedures; rib spreaders, scissors, graspers, dissectors, retractors, clip appliers.

DISPENSER, TISSUE, TOILET *(General) 80WIW*

Royce Rolls Ringer Co. 800-253-9638
PO Box 1831, 16 Riverview Terrace, Grand Rapids, MI 49501
Four different models of one to four roll dispensers.

DISPENSER, TOWEL *(General) 80WIX*

Palmero Health Care 800-344-6424
120 Goodwin Pl, Stratford, CT 06615
DISCIDE disinfecting towelettes. Kills HIV, Herpes and Adenovirus in one minute. Foil packets and canisters.

Safetec Of America, Inc. 800-456-7077
887 Kensington Ave, Buffalo, NY 14215
Personal Antimicrobial Wipes by Safetec (p.a.w.s.) remove soil from hands and kill 99.99% of most germs in as little as 15 seconds. 5' x 8' towelettes are formulated with PCMX and SD Alcohol, plus aloe vera to help moisturize the skin. Packaged as individually-wrapped, pre-moistened towelettes, or in pull-out, 50-count and 160-count dispenser tubs. Available in original Fresh or Citrus Scents.

DISPLAY, CATHODE-RAY TUBE *(Cardiovascular) 74DXJ*

Draeger Medical Systems, Inc. 215-660-2626
16 Electronics Ave, Danvers, MA 01923
Multiple.

Fukuda Denshi Usa, Inc. 800-365-6668
17725 NE 65th St Ste C, Redmond, WA 98052
Display, cathode-ray tube, medical.

Grass Technologies, An Astro-Med, Inc. Product Gro 401-828-4002
53 Airport Park Drive, Rockland, MA 02370
Crt signal display.

Mushield Company, Inc., The 888-669-3539
9 Ricker Ave, Londonderry, NH 03053
Custom CRT shielding to eliminate electro-magnetic interference.

Spacelabs Medical Inc. 800-522-7212
5150 220th Ave SE, Issaquah, WA 98029
Patient monitors and accessories.

DISRUPTER, CELL *(Microbiology) 83VFS*

Scientific Industries, Inc. 888-850-6208
70 Orville Dr, Bohemia, NY 11716

DISSECTOR, SURGICAL, GENERAL & PLASTIC SURGERY *(Surgery) 79GDI*

American White Cross - Houston 609-514-4744
15200 North Fwy, Houston, TX 77090
Round stick sponges, flat stick.

Atricure, Inc. 888.347.6403
6217 Centre Park Dr, West Chester, OH 45069
Surgical dissector.

Bausch & Lomb Surgical 636-255-5051
3365 Tree Court Ind Blvd, Saint Louis, MO 63122

Biomet Microfixation Inc. 800-874-7711
1520 Tradeport Dr, Jacksonville, FL 32218
Various types of dissectors.

Boston Scientific - Marina Bay Customer Fulfillment Center 617-689-6000
500 Commander Shea Blvd, Quincy, MA 02171
Various.

Cardinal Health, Snowden Pencer Products 847-689-8410
5175 S Royal Atlanta Dr, Tucker, GA 30084
Various styles of general and plastic surgery surgical dissectors.

Carwild Corp. 860-442-4914
3 State Pier Rd, New London, CT 06320
Endoscopic and dissection sticks.

Coapt Systems, Inc. 650-461-7600
1820 Embarcadero Rd, Palo Alto, CA 94303
Dissector.

Codman & Shurtleff, Inc 800-225-0460
325 Paramount Dr, Raynham, MA 02767

Evera Medical, Inc. 650-287-2884
353 Vintage Park Dr Ste F, Foster City, CA 94404
Dissector.

DISSECTOR, SURGICAL, GENERAL & PLASTIC SURGERY *(cont'd)*

First Aid Bandage Co., Inc. 888-813-8214
3 State Pier Rd, New London, CT 06320
Kittner, Peanut, and Cherry dissectors. USP cotton woven, nonwoven, and polyester dissectors for tissue dissection. Also available for endoscopic use.

George Tiemann & Co. 800-843-6266
25 Plant Ave, Hauppauge, NY 11788

Gyrus Medical, Inc. 800-852-9361
6655 Wedgwood Rd N Ste 105, Maple Grove, MN 55311
Bipolar dissector/grasper used for laparoscopy.

Invuity, Inc. 760-744-4447
334 Via Vera Cruz Ste 255, San Marcos, CA 92078
Dissector.

Invuity, Inc. 415-655-2100
39 Stillman St, San Francisco, CA 94107

Karl Storz Endoscopy-America Inc. 800-421-0837
600 Corporate Pointe, Culver City, CA 90230
For various reconstructive and therapeutic endoscopy procedures.

Kmi Kolster Methods, Inc. 909-737-5476
3185 Palisades Dr, Corona, CA 92880
Dissectors.

Lican Medical Products Ltd. 519-737-1142
5120 Halford Dr., Windsor, ON N9A 6J3 Canada
Laparoscopic unipolar dissectors.

Mcneil Healthcare, Inc. 203-932-6263
481 Elm St, West Haven, CT 06516
Cherry sponge,peanut sponge,kittner sponge,stick sponge.

Medtronic Spine Llc 877-690-5353
1221 Crossman Ave, Sunnyvale, CA 94089
Various.

Micrins Surgical Instruments, Inc. 800-833-3380
28438 N Ballard Dr, Lake Forest, IL 60045

Scanlan International, Inc. 800-328-9458
1 Scanlan Plz, Saint Paul, MN 55107
LOFTUS carotid erdarterectomy set and endarterectomy dissector.

Smith & Nephew, Inc., Endoscopy Division 800-343-8386
150 Minuteman Rd, Andover, MA 01810

Sterilmed, Inc. 763-488-3400
11400 73rd Ave N Ste 100, Maple Grove, MN 55369
Dissector.

Ussc Puerto Rico, Inc. 203-845-1000
Building 911-67, Sabanetas Industrial Park, Ponce, PR 00731
Surgical dissector.

Warsaw Orthopedic, Inc. 901-396-3133
2500 Silveus Xing, Warsaw, IN 46582
Various dissectors.

Wells Johnson Co. 800-528-1597
8000 S Kolb Rd, Tucson, AZ 85756

Zimmer Holdings, Inc. 800-613-6131
1800 W Center St, PO Box 708, Warsaw, IN 46580

DISSECTOR, TONSIL *(Ear/Nose/Throat) 77KBM*

American White Cross - Houston 609-514-4744
15200 North Fwy, Houston, TX 77090
Tonsil sponge.

Biomet Microfixation Inc. 800-874-7711
1520 Tradeport Dr, Jacksonville, FL 32218
Various types of dissectors.

Clinimed, Incorporated 877-CLINIMED
303 Markus Ct, Sandy Brae Industrial Park, Newark, DE 19713

George Tiemann & Co. 800-843-6266
25 Plant Ave, Hauppauge, NY 11788

Mcneil Healthcare, Inc. 203-932-6263
481 Elm St, West Haven, CT 06516
Tonsil sponge.

Prosurge Instruments, Inc. 866-832-7874
199 Laidlaw Ave, Jersey City, NJ 07306

DISTILLING UNIT *(Chemistry) 75QQF*

Brinkmann Instruments (Canada) Ltd. 800-263-8715
6670 Campobello Rd., Mississauga, ONT L5N 2L8 Canada
Distilling unit with titration. Adds all reagents to a closed system for accuracy and safety. Records sample data and results with a built-in printer.

DISTILLING UNIT *(cont'd)*

Consolidated Stills & Sterilizers 617-782-6072
76 Ashford St, Boston, MA 02134
$400 to $30,000 per unit (standard).

Kontes Glass Co. 888-546-2531
1022 Spruce St, Vineland, NJ 08360
$3,816.40 per unit (standard).

Labconco Corp. 800-821-5525
8811 Prospect Ave, Kansas City, MO 64132

Thermo Fisher Scientific Inc. 563-556-2241
2555 Kerper Blvd, Dubuque, IA 52001

Tuttnauer Usa Co. Ltd. 800-624-5836
25 Power Dr, Hauppauge, NY 11788
Provides pure water. Removes up to 99% of most tap water contaminants. Four models: 9000 (1 gallon), 7000 (4 gallon), 7000-8 (8 gallon) & 7000-12 (12 gallon).

DISTILLING UNIT, MOLECULAR *(Chemistry) 75UFX*

Kontes Glass Co. 888-546-2531
1022 Spruce St, Vineland, NJ 08360

Scientific Glass & Instruments, Inc. 877-682-1481
PO Box 6, Houston, TX 77001

DISTOMETER *(Ophthalmology) 86HMM*

Western Ophthalmics Corporation 800-426-9938
19019 36th Ave W Ste G, Lynnwood, WA 98036

DNA DEVICE, HEPATITIS B, VIRAL *(Microbiology) 83MKT*

Qiagen Gaithersburg, Inc. 800-344-3631
1201 Clopper Rd, Gaithersburg, MD 20878
Digene hbv dna assay.

DNA-PROBE, CHROMOSOME, HUMAN *(Hematology) 81MAO*

Abbott Molecular, Inc. 847-937-6100
1300 E Touhy Ave, Des Plaines, IL 60018
Fluorescence in situ hybridication (fish) reagents-asr ivd.

Genetic Testing Institute 262-754-1000
20925 Crossroads Cir Ste 200, Waukesha, WI 53186
Platelet antigen typing kit.

Koaman International 909-983-4888
656 E D St, Ontario, CA 91764

DNA-PROBE, GARDNERELLA VAGINALIS *(Microbiology) 83MJM*

Quidel Corp. 858-552-1100
2981 Copper Rd, Santa Clara, CA 95051
Vaginal fluid test for the detection of gardnerella vaginalis.

DNA-PROBE, HER/NEU *(Immunology) 82MMM*

Cortex Biochem, Inc. 800-888-7713
1933 Davis St Ste 321, San Leandro, CA 94577
MagaZorb nucleic-acid isolation (RNA/DNA); magnetic particles; magnetic separators.

DNA-PROBE, NUCLEIC ACID AMPLIFICATION, CHLAMYDIA *(Microbiology) 83MKZ*

Abbott Molecular, Inc. 847-937-6100
1300 E Touhy Ave, Des Plaines, IL 60018
Pcr ct assay.

Bd Diagnostic Systems 800-675-0908
7 Loveton Cir, Sparks, MD 21152

Gen-Probe, Inc. 800-523-5001
10210 Genetic Center Dr, San Diego, CA 92121
GASDirect Test - DNA probe assay which uses nucleic acid hybridization for the qualitative detection of Group A Streptococcal rRNA as an aid in the diagnosis of Group A Streptococcal pharyngitis from throat swabs. AMPLIFIED CHLAMYDIA TRACHOMATIS (AMP CT) Assay - direct target-amplified nucleic acid probe test for the qualitative detection of Chlamydia trachomatis nucleic acids in endovervical and male urethral swab specimens and in femal and male urine specimens. APTIMA Combo 2 Assay - direct target amplified nucleic acid probe test for the qualitative detection and differentiation of Chlamydia trachomatis and Neisseria gonorrhoea in endocervical and male urethral swab specimens and in male and female urine specimens.

Roche Molecular Systems, Inc. 925-730-8110
4300 Hacienda Dr, Pleasanton, CA 94588
Various chlamydia thrachomatis tests, chlamydia serological reagents.

DNA-PROBE, REAGENT *(Microbiology) 83MBT*

Affymetrix, Inc. 888-DNA-CHIP
3420 Central Expy, Santa Clara, CA 95051

DNA-PROBE, REAGENT *(cont'd)*

Qiagen Gaithersburg, Inc. 800-344-3631
1201 Clopper Rd, Gaithersburg, MD 20878
Multiple.

DOME, PRESSURE TRANSDUCER *(General) 80QQH*

Hospira, Inc. 877-946-7747
755 Jarvis Dr, Morgan Hill, CA 95037

Smiths Medical Asd, Inc. 800-848-1757
6250 Shier Rings Rd, Dublin, OH 43016

DOPPLER, BLOOD FLOW, TRANSCRANIAL *(Cardiovascular) 74WSD*

Md International, Inc. 305-669-9003
11300 NW 41st St, Doral, FL 33178

Multigon Industries, Inc. 800-289-6858
1 Odell Plz, Yonkers, NY 10701

Neoprobe Corporation 800-793-0079
425 Metro Pl N Ste 300, Dublin, OH 43017
Quantix/OR for the intraoperative measurement of blood flow volume based upon the simultaneous measurement of velocity and blood vessel diameter

New Life Systems, Inc. 954-972-4600
PO Box 8767, Coral Springs, FL 33075
Peripheral vascular Doppler.

Perimed, Inc. 877-374-3589
6785 Wallings Rd Ste 2C-2D, North Royalton, OH 44133
PERIFLUX 5000; PF5000 Laser Doppler/Transcutaneous System; measures blood flow, transcutaneous oxygen and carbon dioxide. The multi-channel system can hold any combination of 4 modules.

Spencer Technologies 800-684-0586
701 16th Ave, Seattle, WA 98122
Ease of use makes the Transcranial Doppler practical for a wider range of health professionals.

DOPPLER, FLOW MAPPING *(Radiology) 90VHA*

Mizuho America Inc. 800-699-2547
133 Brimbal Ave, Beverly, MA 01915
Mizuho Surgical Doppler for intraoperative evaluation of blood flow.

Unetixs Vascular, Inc. 800-486-3849
115 Airport St, North Kingstown, RI 02852

DOSIMETER, ETHYLENE-OXIDE *(General) 80VDZ*

Andersen Products, Inc., 800-523-1276
3202 Caroline Dr, Health Science Park, Haw River, NC 27258
DOSIMETER Chemical Integrator for use with ANDERSEN gas-sterilization systems.

Assay Technology Inc 800-833-1258
1252 Quarry Ln, Pleasanton, CA 94566
Sampling media (HBr-treated charcoal) analyzed by GC/ECD. Monitor for 15 minutes to 12 hours. Box of 5 monitors

Enviro Guard, Inc. 800-438-1152
201 Shannon Oaks Cir Ste 115, Cary, NC 27511

DOSIMETER, NITROUS-OXIDE *(Anesthesiology) 73VEA*

Assay Technology Inc 800-833-1258
1252 Quarry Ln, Pleasanton, CA 94566
Sampling media (molecular sieve) analyzed by GC/ECD. Sample for 15 minutes to 8 hours. Box of 5 monitors

Enviro Guard, Inc. 800-438-1152
201 Shannon Oaks Cir Ste 115, Cary, NC 27511

Nspire Health, Inc 800-574-7374
1830 Lefthand Cir, Longmont, CO 80501
Non-nitrous oxide. KOKO Dosimeter automated, stand-alone dosimeter used to deliver reproducible, variable doses of an aerosol for challenge testing, diagnosis and therapy.

DOSIMETER, RADIATION *(Radiology) 90QQI*

Biodex Medical Systems, Inc. 800-224-6339
20 Ramsey Rd, Shirley, NY 11967

Capintec, Inc. 800-631-3826
6 Arrow Rd, Ramsey, NJ 07446

Dosimeter Division Of Arrow Tech Inc 800-322-8258
5 Eastmans Rd, Parsippany, NJ 07054
$125.00 for direct reading pencil type unit with ion chambers. Also, low energy dosimeters, standard type dosimeters, line or battery operated dosimeter chargers, dosimeter viewer-chargers, and dosimeter accessories (end caps, logbooks, clips, clip removers, etc.).

DOSIMETER, RADIATION *(cont'd)*

Landauer, Inc. 800-323-8830
2 Science Rd, Glenwood, IL 60425
Personnel radiation dosimeters to measure x-ray, beta, gamma radiation and neutrons. NVLAP accredited, full range of reports, ALARA aids; interactive computer system, dosimetry management PC software. CBT Radiation Safety Training and related services. Low-level gamma radiation dosimeter, down to 1/10 millirem. Comprehensive diagnostic evaluation backed by over 50 years experience.

Lnd, Inc. 516-678-6141
3230 Lawson Blvd, Oceanside, NY 11572

Mirion Technologies 925-543-0800
3000 Executive Pkwy Ste 222, Bishop Ranch 8, San Ramon, CA 94583
Film badges, TLD badges, neutron badges, x-ray badges, personnel radiation monitoring badges, dosimeters.

Owens Scientific Inc. 281-394-2311
23230 Sandsage Ln, Katy, TX 77494

Rocket Medical Plc. 800-707-7625
150 Recreation Park Dr Ste 3, Hingham, MA 02043
Cardiac drain.

S.E. International, Inc. 800-293-5759
436 Farm Rd, PO Box 39, Summertown, TN 38483
Direct reading and electronic dosimeters

Schueler & Company, Inc. 516-487-1500
PO Box 528, Stratford, CT 06615

Simpson Electric Co. 715-588-3311
520 Simpson Ave, PO Box 99, Lac Du Flambeau, WI 54538
Model 897. Used for audiometric testing. $751.70 for dosimeter system, noise.

DOUCHE, VAGINAL *(Obstetrics/Gyn) 85HED*

Hospira 800-441-4100
268 E 4th St, Ashland, OH 44805

Medline Industries, Inc. 800-633-5886
1 Medline Pl, Mundelein, IL 60060

Medline Manufacturing And Services Llc 847-837-2759
1 Medline Pl, Mundelein, IL 60060
Vaginal irrigators,sterile.

DRAIN, NASOBILIARY *(Gastro/Urology) 78QAN*

Redi-Tech Medical Products,Llc 800-824-1793
529 Front St Ste 125, Berea, OH 44017

DRAIN, PENROSE *(Gastro/Urology) 78QQL*

Covidien Lp 508-261-8000
15 Hampshire St, Mansfield, MA 02048

Taut, Inc. 800-231-8288
2571 Kaneville Ct, Geneva, IL 60134
Non-latex elastomer drains with internal longitudinal ribs to prevent occlusion. External 1 inch increments to control postoperative advancement, ten sizes available.

DRAIN, SUCTION, CLOSED *(Surgery) 79QCL*

Andersen Products, Inc., 800-523-1276
3202 Caroline Dr, Health Science Park, Haw River, NC 27258
SHIRLEY wound-drainage system, bi-lumen, radio-opaque, for continuous self-regulated suction.

Armm, Inc. 714-848-8190
17744 Sampson Ln, Huntington Beach, CA 92647
MedDrain silicone closed wound drains.

Aspen Surgical 800-328-7958
6945 Southbelt Dr SE, Caledonia, MI 49316
S-Vac Fluted Channel Drains or S-Vac Perforated Drains for post-surgical wound drainage

Axiom Medical, Inc. 800-221-8569
19320 Van Ness Ave, Torrance, CA 90501
Self-contained, portable, single and Bilumen

Bemis Mfg. Co. 800-558-7651
300 Mill St, Sheboygan Falls, WI 53085
QUICK-DRAIN and VAC-U-PORT Confined Liquid Infectious Waste Management Systems. Closed systems that drains suction canister contents directly into sanitary sewer system.

Degania Silicone, Inc. 401-333-8199
1226 Mendon Rd, Cumberland, RI 02864
Silicone round and flat drains and 100cc evacuators that are sterile packaged under private label.

Dielectrics, Inc. 800-472-7286
300 Burnett Rd, Chicopee, MA 01020

DRAIN, SUCTION, CLOSED *(cont'd)*

Hanson Medical, Inc. 800-771-2215
825 Riverside Ave Ste 2, Paso Robles, CA 93446
Drain, suction, facial; drain, suction, seroma, hematoma; drain, suction, flat; drain, suction, round.

DRAIN, SUMP *(Gastro/Urology) 78QQM*

Andersen Products, Inc., 800-523-1276
3202 Caroline Dr, Health Science Park, Haw River, NC 27258
ANDERSEN nasogastric tube with or without stylet, double-lumen, radio-opaque with anti-reflux filter.

Armm, Inc. 714-848-8190
17744 Sampson Ln, Huntington Beach, CA 92647
MedDrain line of Silicone Sump Drains. Mediastinal, double and mono sump, filtered.

Axiom Medical, Inc. 800-221-8569
19320 Van Ness Ave, Torrance, CA 90501
Large variety of sizes, styles in silicone, coated silicone.

Covidien Lp 508-261-8000
15 Hampshire St, Mansfield, MA 02048

Medovations, Inc. 800-558-6408
102 E Keefe Ave, Milwaukee, WI 53212
Gastric sump tube.

Novosci Corp. 281-363-4949
2828 N Crescentridge Dr, The Woodlands, TX 77381
Sump sets.

Vygon Corp. 800-544-4907
2495 General Armistead Ave, Norristown, PA 19403

DRAIN, T *(Gastro/Urology) 78QQN*

Zimmer Holdings, Inc. 800-613-6131
1800 W Center St, PO Box 708, Warsaw, IN 46580

DRAIN, TEE (WATER TRAP) *(Anesthesiology) 73BYH*

Ballard Medical Products 770-587-7835
12050 Lone Peak Pkwy, Draper, UT 84020
Water trap.

Blue Sky Medical Group Incorporated 727-392-1261
5924 Balfour Ct Ste 102, Carlsbad, CA 92008
Moisture sensor.

Directmed, Inc. 516-656-3377
150 Pratt Oval, Glen Cove, NY 11542

Instrumentation Industries, Inc. 800-633-8577
2990 Industrial Blvd, Bethel Park, PA 15102

Intersurgical Inc. 315-451-2900
417 Electronics Pkwy, Liverpool, NY 13088

Smith & Nephew, Inc. 800-876-1261
970 Lake Carillon Dr Ste 110, Saint Petersburg, FL 33716
AQUALERT

Smiths Medical Asd Inc. 800-258-5361
10 Bowman Dr, Keene, NH 03431
Various types of water traps.

Smiths Medical Asd, Inc. 847-793-0135
330 Corporate Woods Pkwy, Vernon Hills, IL 60061
Water trap.

Thayer Medical Corp. 520-790-5393
4575 S Palo Verde Rd Ste 337, Tucson, AZ 85714
Valved tee adapter.

DRAIN, THORACIC (CHEST) *(Anesthesiology) 73QQO*

Armm, Inc. 714-848-8190
17744 Sampson Ln, Huntington Beach, CA 92647
MedDrain silicone thoracic silicone drains.

Atrium Medical Corp. 800-528-7486
5 Wentworth Dr, Hudson, NH 03051
ATRIUM family of water-seal chest-drain systems, including single, dual, infant, pediatric, and autotransfusion water-seal chest-drainage systems. Both water-controlled and dry-suction systems available.

Axiom Medical, Inc. 800-221-8569
19320 Van Ness Ave, Torrance, CA 90501
Coated silicone 8Fr-40Fr, PVC.

California Medical Laboratories, Inc. 714-556-7365
1570 Sunland Ln, Costa Mesa, CA 92626

Covidien Lp 508-261-8000
15 Hampshire St, Mansfield, MA 02048

DRAIN, THORACIC (CHEST) *(cont'd)*

Degania Silicone, Inc. 401-333-8199
1226 Mendon Rd, Cumberland, RI 02864
Silicone chest drains with ROP stripe.

Filtrona Extrusion, Inc./Pexcor Medical Products Div. 800-755-7528
764 S Athol Rd, P.O. Box 659, Athol, MA 01331

Medovations, Inc. 800-558-6408
102 E Keefe Ave, Milwaukee, WI 53212

Rocket Medical Plc. 800-707-7625
150 Recreation Park Dr Ste 3, Hingham, MA 02043

Smiths Medical Asd 800-424-8662
5700 W 23rd Ave, Gary, IN 46406
Thoracic catheter with PLEUR-A-GUIDES for children and adults.

Uresil, Llc 800-538-7374
5418 Touhy Ave, Skokie, IL 60077
TRU-CLOSE Pneumothorax kit. Thoracic vent procedure tray for pneumothorax.

Utah Medical Products, Inc. 800-533-4984
7043 Cottonwood St, Midvale, UT 84047
THORA-CATH silicone chest drainage catheter sold with trocar. For use with hemo or pneumothorax.

Vygon Corp. 800-544-4907
2495 General Armistead Ave, Norristown, PA 19403

DRAIN, THORACIC, WATER SEAL *(Anesthesiology) 73CCS*

Allied Healthcare Products, Inc. 800-444-3954
1720 Sublette Ave, Saint Louis, MO 63110

Atrium Medical Corp. 800-528-7486
5 Wentworth Dr, Hudson, NH 03051
ATRIUM family of water-seal chest-drain systems, including single, dual, infant, pediatric, and auto-transfusion water-seal chest drainage systems. Both water-controlled and dry-suction systems available.

Covidien Lp 508-261-8000
15 Hampshire St, Mansfield, MA 02048

Gish Biomedical, Inc. 800-938-0531
22942 Arroyo Vis, Rancho Santa Margarita, CA 92688
Reservoir with integrated water seal/manometer.

Medela, Inc. 800-435-8316
1101 Corporate Dr, McHenry, IL 60050
Disposable canister with integrated water seal for thoracic drainage.

Medi Inc 800-225-8634
75 York Ave, P.O. Box 302, Randolph, MA 02368

Ohio Medical Corp. 800-662-5822
1111 Lakeside Dr, Gurnee, IL 60031
Reusable sealed thoracic manometer with separate manometer and underwater seal chambers with precision needle value for bubble regulation.

DRAINAGE SYSTEM, URINE, CLOSED *(Gastro/Urology) 78EYZ*

Bioderm, Inc. 800-373-7006
12320 73rd Ct, Largo, FL 33773
Tubeholder.

Centurion Medical Products Corp. 517-545-1135
3310 S Main St, Salisbury, NC 28147

Covidien Lp 508-261-8000
15 Hampshire St, Mansfield, MA 02048

Dj Orthopedics De Mexico, S.A. De C.V. 690-727-1280
Blvd., Delagacion La Presa, Tijuana 22397 Mexico
Catheter strap

Dj Orthopedics De Mexico, S.A. De C.V. 690-727-1280
Ave. Venustiano Carranza 6802, Castillo, Tijuana 22100 Mexico
Catheter strap

Farmatap S.A. De C.V.
117 Alfonso Esparza Oteo, Mexico Df 01020 Mexico
No common name listed

Kelsar, S.A. 508-261-8000
Blvd. Insurgentes, Libriamento a La, Tijuana 22450 Mexico
Combination kit and accessories

Key / Sun Medical Services, Inc. 847-546-4795
5483 N Northwest Hwy, Chicago, IL 60630
Trademarked 'poly-gel' closed drainage systems with patented liqsorb anti-microbial polymer pouch designed to safely and effectively reduce UTI.

DRAINAGE SYSTEM, URINE, CLOSED *(cont'd)*

Lsl Industries, Inc. 888-225-5575
5535 N Wolcott Ave, Chicago, IL 60640
$59.50 per case of 10 (Model #1616 & 1618).

Medline Industries, Inc. 800-633-5886
1 Medline Pl, Mundelein, IL 60060

Medline Manufacturing And Services Llc 847-837-2759
1 Medline Pl, Mundelein, IL 60060
Drainage bags,sterile.

Mentor Corp. 800-525-0245
201 Mentor Dr, Santa Barbara, CA 93111
Six urine drainage bags for a variety of uses.

Reach Global Industries, Inc. (Reachgood) 888-518-8389
8 Corporate Park Ste 300, Irvine, CA 92606
Various types of sterile and non-sterile urine collection bags.

Tri-State Hospital Supply Corp. 517-545-1135
3173 E 43rd St, Yuma, AZ 85365

Vygon Corp. 800-544-4907
2495 General Armistead Ave, Norristown, PA 19403

DRAINAGE UNIT, URINARY *(General) 80SED*

Covidien Lp 508-261-8000
15 Hampshire St, Mansfield, MA 02048

Eastman Medical Products Inc. 800-373-4410
2000 Powell St Ste 1540, Emeryville, CA 94608
PATHO-SORB Urinary Drainage System; PATHO-SORB Leg Bag System. Anionic polyacrylamide-absorbent polymer in drainage system solidifies liquid urine and reduces migration of bacteria into catheter site and bladder, thereby greatly reducing UTI's.

Invacare Supply Group, An Invacare Co. 800-225-4792
75 October Hill Rd, Holliston, MA 01746
Carry full lines of urologicals from: Invacare, Bard, Coloplast, Kendall, Mentor, Hollister, Rochester, Rusch.

Lsl Industries, Inc. 888-225-5575
5535 N Wolcott Ave, Chicago, IL 60640
$49.90 per case of 20 urinary drainage bags with antireflux bag and latex sampling port. $35.90 per case of 20 standard drainage bags.

Medi Inc 800-225-8634
75 York Ave, P.O. Box 302, Randolph, MA 02368

Medical Devices International, Div. Of Plasco, Inc. 800-438-7634
512 N Lehmberg Rd, Columbus, MS 39702
6 models: urinary drainage units with hook hanger, center entry; 2000 mL.

Mentor Corp. 800-525-0245
201 Mentor Dr, Santa Barbara, CA 93111

Smith & Nephew, Inc. 800-876-1261
11775 Starkey Rd, Largo, FL 33773
FEATHER-LITE soft urinary pouches.

Urocare Products, Inc. 800-423-4441
2735 Melbourne Ave, Pomona, CA 91767
Quick drain valve.

Zimmer Holdings, Inc. 800-613-6131
1800 W Center St, PO Box 708, Warsaw, IN 46580

DRAPE, ADHESIVE, AEROSOL *(Surgery) 79KGT*

Ferndale Laboratories, Inc. 248-548-0900
780 W 8 Mile Rd, Detroit, MI 48220
Mastisol.

Lifescience Plus, Inc. 650-565-8172
473 Sapena Ct Ste 7, Santa Clara, CA 95054
Drape.

M&C Specialties Co. 800-441-6996
90 James Way, Southampton, PA 18966
Non-aerosol.

DRAPE, INCISION, SURGICAL *(Surgery) 79WVZ*

Foothills Industries, Inc. 828-652-4088
300 Rockwell Dr, Marion, NC 28752

Johnson & Johnson Medical Division Of Ethicon, Inc. 800-423-4018
2500 E Arbrook Blvd, Arlington, TX 76014

DRAPE, MICROSCOPE, OPHTHALMIC *(Ophthalmology) 86HMW*

Foothills Industries, Inc. 828-652-4088
300 Rockwell Dr, Marion, NC 28752

Gyrus Ent L.L.C., Sub. Of Gyrus Acmi, Inc. 508-804-2739
2925 Appling Rd, Bartlett, TN 38133
Various.

DRAPE, MICROSCOPE, OPHTHALMIC *(cont'd)*

Mti-Medical Technique, Inc. 800-426-9053
8060 E Research Ct, Tucson, AZ 85710
Drapes, microscopes, and equipment covers and all specialty barriers for c-arms, both standard and mini types.

DRAPE, PATIENT, OPHTHALMIC *(Ophthalmology) 86HMT*

Atd-American Co. 800-523-2300
135 Greenwood Ave, Wyncote, PA 19095

Foothills Industries, Inc. 828-652-4088
300 Rockwell Dr, Marion, NC 28752

Gyrus Ent L.L.C., Sub. Of Gyrus Acmi, Inc. 508-804-2739
2925 Appling Rd, Bartlett, TN 38133
Occular occluder.

Haywood Vocational Opportunities 828-456-4455
56 Scates St, Waynesville, NC 28786
Various sizes and types of drapes.

Howard Instruments, Inc. 205-553-4453
4749 Appletree Ln, Tuscaloosa, AL 35405

Jedmed Instruments Co. 314-845-3770
5416 Jedmed Ct, Saint Louis, MO 63129

Johnson & Johnson Medical Division Of Ethicon, Inc. 800-423-4018
2500 E Arbrook Blvd, Arlington, TX 76014

Keeler Instruments Inc. 800-523-5620
456 Park Way, Broomall, PA 19008
$32.00 per pkg. of 24 ea. disposable drape supports (min. order 4 pkgs.).

Kerr Group 800-524-3577
1400 Holcomb Bridge Rd, Roswell, GA 30076
Nonwoven disposable.

Medical Concepts Development 800-345-0644
2500 Ventura Dr, Saint Paul, MN 55125
Soft, low-glare plastic, aggressive adhesive, and lint-free poly release liners.

Solos Endoscopy 800-388-6445
65 Sprague St # B, Boston/dedham Commerce Park, Boston, MA 02136
Surgical drape & drape accessories.

Trident Medical Products 800-647-4448
1201 Summit Ave, Fort Worth, TX 76102
Trident Face Drape Support. Relieves patient anxiety and claustrophobia during surgery by elevating drape away from face.

DRAPE, PURE LATEX SHEET, WITH SELF-RETAINING FINGER COT *(Gastro/Urology) 78EYX*

Visioncare Devices, Inc. 530-243-5047
1246 Redwood Blvd, Redding, CA 96003
Probe covers.

DRAPE, SURGICAL *(Surgery) 79KKX*

Abbott Associates 203-878-2370
620 West Ave, Milford, CT 06461
Drapes and towels.

Advance Medical Designs, Inc. 800-221-3679
1241 Atlanta Industrial Dr, Marietta, GA 30066

Allergan 800-624-4261
71 S Los Carneros Rd, Goleta, CA 93117
Non-magnetic surgical instrument drape.

Angelica Image Apparel 800-222-3112
700 Rosedale Ave, Saint Louis, MO 63112

Angiosystems, Inc. 800-441-4256
7 Hopkins Pl., Ducktown, TN 37326
RADPAD radiation protection drapes. Surgical drapes incorporating RADPAD shields to protect against scatter radiation. Drapes for angiograms, dialysis access declotting, biventricular pacing, vertebroplasty, tipps, CT scan, pediatric collimation, neonatal collimation, and gonadal protection. Also offered are femoral angio drapes, angio window drapes, eye drapes, biopsy drapes, brachial drapes, subfemoral drapes, and specialty drapes.

Atd-American Co. 800-523-2300
135 Greenwood Ave, Wyncote, PA 19095

Avail Medical Products, Inc. 858-635-2206
1225 N. 28th Avenue, Suite 500, Dallas, TX 75261
Instrument pad.

Bard Shannon Limited 908-277-8000
San Geronimo Industrial Park, Lot # 1, Road # 3, Km 79.7
Humacao, PR 00791
Meditract,laparoscopic product.

DRAPE, SURGICAL *(cont'd)*

Biomet, Inc. 574-267-6639
56 E Bell Dr, PO Box 587, Warsaw, IN 46582
Various types of surgical drapes.

Boyd Converting Co., Inc. 800-262-2242
PO Box 287, South Lee, MA 01260
Surgical drape.

Busse Hospital Disposables, Inc. 631-435-4711
75 Arkay Dr, Hauppauge, NY 11788
Sterile,non-sterile,fenestrated,non-fenestrated,adhesive strips/patches,various.

Centurion Medical Products Corp. 517-545-1135
3310 S Main St, Salisbury, NC 28147

Clopay Plastic Products Company 800-282-2260
8585 Duke Blvd, Mason, OH 45040

Crown Health Care Laundry Services, Inc. 850-438-7578
3805 Highway 41 North, Selma, AL 36701
Textile packs.

Customed, Inc. 787-801-0101
Calle Igualdad #7, Fajardo, PR 00738
Fanfold drape.

Davol Inc., Sub. C.R. Bard, Inc. 800-556-6275
100 Crossings Blvd, Warwick, RI 02886
Adjustable wound protector/retractor.

Depuy Orthopaedics, Inc. 800-473-3789
700 Orthopaedic Dr, P.O. Box 988, Warsaw, IN 46582
Various types of surgical drapes.

Foothills Industries, Inc. 828-652-4088
300 Rockwell Dr, Marion, NC 28752

Galia Textil S.A. De C.V. 246-1-6-066
Lote 3 Manzana 4, Parque Industrial, Tlaxcala Mexico
O.r. towels

Global Healthcare 800-601-3880
1495 Hembree Rd Ste 700, Roswell, GA 30076
Sterile Drapes and Packs

Greenco Industries, Inc. 608-328-8311
1601 4th Ave W, Monroe, WI 53566
Fenistrated surgical towel/drape.

Gyrus Ent L.L.C., Sub. Of Gyrus Acmi, Inc. 508-804-2739
2925 Appling Rd, Bartlett, TN 38133
Various.

Hydro-Med Products, Inc. 214-350-5100
3400 Royalty Row, Irving, TX 75062
Drape, surgical.

Imalux Corporation 216-502-0755
11000 Cedar Ave Ste 250, Cleveland, OH 44106
Sheath.

Innova Corp. 860-242-3210
68 E Dudley Town Rd, Bloomfield, CT 06002

Intl. Medsurg Connection, Inc. 847-619-9926
935 N Plum Grove Rd Ste V, Schaumburg, IL 60173
Towels.

Kerma Medical Products, Inc. 757-398-8400
400 Port Centre Pkwy, Portsmouth, VA 23704
Or towels.

Lakeland De Mexico S.A. De C.V. 516-981-9700
Rancho La Soledad Lote No. 2, Fracc. Poniente C.p.
Celaya, Guajuato Mexico
Surgical drape and drape accessories

Maquilas Teta-Kawi, S.A. De C.V. 413-593-6400
Carretera Internacional, Km 1969, Enpalme, Sonora Mexico
Various

Mckesson General Medical 800-446-3008
8741 Landmark Rd, Richmond, VA 23228
Minor procedure drapes.

Medical Concepts Development 800-345-0644
2500 Ventura Dr, Saint Paul, MN 55125
A complete line of soft, low-glare plastic, non-woven and fluid collection disposable surgical drapes. ACTI-Gard Anitmicrobial Incise Drapes: Iodine base antimicrobial agent within ACTI-Gard.

Microtek Medical, Inc 800-936-9248
512 N Lehmberg Rd, Columbus, MS 39702
Specialty surgical drapes for orthopedics, arthroscopy, neuro, obstetrics, ophthalmology. Full line of incise, aperture and utility drapes, including anti-microbial.

DRAPE, SURGICAL *(cont'd)*

Minrad, Inc. 716-855-1068
50 Cobham Dr, Orchard Park, NY 14127
Sterile surgical drape.

Odyssey Medical, Inc. 901-383-7777
5828 Shelby Oaks Dr, Memphis, TN 38134
Surgical drape.

Pacon Manufacturing Corporation 732-357-8020
400 Pierce St # B, Somerset, NJ 08873
Fenestrated, non-fenestrated, polylined custom drapes.

Protek Medical Products, Inc. 319-545-7100
4125 Westcor Ct, Coralville, IA 52241
Various.

Qsum Biopsy Disposables Llc 720-304-2135
6539 Stearns Ave, Boulder, CO 80303
Non-sterile stereotactic procedure equipment draping.

Rx Textiles, Inc. 704-283-9787
3107 Chamber Dr, Monroe, NC 28110
Surgical drape.

Savoy Medical Supply 631-234-7003
745 Calebs Path, Hauppauge, NY 11788

Spectra Medical Devices, Inc. 866-938-8649
4C Henshaw St, Woburn, MA 01801

Sri Surgical 813-891-9550
6801 Longe St, Stockton, CA 95206
Surgical drape and drape accessories.

Standard Textile 800-999-0400
1 Knollcrest Dr, Cincinnati, OH 45237

Standard Textile Co., Inc. 888-999-0400
PO Box 371805, Cincinnati, OH 45222
Fenestrated and non-fenestrated drapes.

Sterilmed, Inc. 763-488-3400
11400 73rd Ave N Ste 100, Maple Grove, MN 55369
Surgcal drape.

Sterimed, Inc. 770-387-0771
10 River Ct., Cartersville, GA 30120
Surgical drape.

Terumo Cardiovascular Systems (Tcvs) 800-283-7866
28 Howe St, Ashland, MA 01721
Surgical drape.

Tri-State Hospital Supply Corp. 517-545-1135
3173 E 43rd St, Yuma, AZ 85365

Vnus Medical Technologies, Inc. 888-797-8346
5799 Fontanoso Way, San Jose, CA 95138
Drapes,barrier,sterile patient ready.

Vygon Corp. 800-544-4907
2495 General Armistead Ave, Norristown, PA 19403

Wave Form Systems, Inc. 800-332-8749
7737 SW Nimbus Ave, Beaverton, OR 97008

Webster Enterprises Of Jackson County, Inc. 828-586-8981
140 Little Savannah Rd, Sylva, NC 28779
Disposable surgical drapes.

White Knight Healthcare 800-851-4431
Calle 16, Number 780, Agua Prieta, Sonora Mexico
Various types of sterile and non-sterile drapes

3m Company 651-733-4365
601 22nd Ave S, Brookings, SD 57006

DRAPE, SURGICAL INSTRUMENT, MAGNETIC *(Surgery) 79WQC*

Advanced Medical Innovations, Inc. 888-367-2641
9410 De Soto Ave Ste J, Chatsworth, CA 91311
Reusable (Autoclavable) Instrument Magnetic Drape with Unique Reinforcement (special fabric between the layers of silicone for long lasting performance) for safety, security and durability. Disposable magnetic drapes are also available.

Xodus Medical, Inc. 800-963-8776
702 Prominence Dr, Westmoreland Business & Research Park
New Kensington, PA 15068
Saf-T Pass Transfer Drape

DRAPE, SURGICAL, DISPOSABLE *(Surgery) 79FZJ*

Advance Medical Designs, Inc. 800-221-3679
1241 Atlanta Industrial Dr, Marietta, GA 30066
Glass Lens Microscope Drapes, Probe Covers.

Alcon Research, Ltd. 800-862-5266
6201 South Fwy, Fort Worth, TX 76134

DRAPE, SURGICAL, DISPOSABLE *(cont'd)*

Atd-American Co. 800-523-2300
135 Greenwood Ave, Wyncote, PA 19095

Biomet, Inc. 574-267-6639
56 E Bell Dr, PO Box 587, Warsaw, IN 46582
Various types of surgical drapes.

Carl Zeiss Surgical, Inc. 800-442-4020
1 Zeiss Dr, Thornwood, NY 10594
OPMI.

Cfi Medical Solutions (Contour Fabricators, Inc.) 810-750-5300
14241 N Fenton Rd, Fenton, MI 48430

Foothills Industries, Inc. 828-652-4088
300 Rockwell Dr, Marion, NC 28752

General Econopak, Inc. 888-871-8568
1725 N 6th St, Philadelphia, PA 19122
All sizes, sterile and non-sterile.

Innova Corp. 860-242-3210
68 E Dudley Town Rd, Bloomfield, CT 06002

Janin Group, Inc. 800-323-5389
14A Stonehill Rd, Oswego, IL 60543
Waterproof foot switch control drape.

Jms Converters Inc Dba Sabee Products & Stanford Prof Prod 215-396-3302
67 Buck Rd Ste B7, Huntingdon Valley, PA 19006

Johnson & Johnson Medical Division Of Ethicon, Inc. 800-423-4018
2500 E Arbrook Blvd, Arlington, TX 76014

Kerr Group 800-524-3577
1400 Holcomb Bridge Rd, Roswell, GA 30076

Medical Concepts Development 800-345-0644
2500 Ventura Dr, Saint Paul, MN 55125
A complete list of plastic, non-woven and fluid collection surgical drapes; latex free, and ACTI-Gard Antimicrobial Incise Drapes.

Mylan Technologies, Inc. 800-532-5226
110 Lake St, Saint Albans, VT 05478
High moisture vapor permeable, USP Class VI urethane and Hytrel co-polyester films along with adhesive coated.

Nds Surgical Imaging, Inc. 866-637-5237
5750 Hellyer Ave, San Jose, CA 95138
Barrier protection products for touchscreen applications

Pacon Manufacturing Corporation 732-357-8020
400 Pierce St # B, Somerset, NJ 08873
Film, tissue/poly, non-woven.

Precept Medical Products, Inc. 800-438-5827
PO Box 2400, 370 Airport Road/, Arden, NC 28704
Expanding line for coronary & peripheral cath labs

Preferred Medical Products 800-441-1161
PO Box 100, Ducktown, TN 37326

Psc Medical, Inc. 888-986-4276
4930 W Nassau St # 284, Tampa, FL 33607
Manufacturer of a variety of disposable drapes/covers for use on Zeiss, Leica and Moeller microscopes, C-arms, Mini C-arm covers (Fluoroscan, OEC), laser-camera covers, banded bags. PSC also has the ability to customize products for its customers.

Ross Disposable Products 800-649-6526
401 Traders Blvd E, Unit 10, Mississauga, ON L4Z 2H8 Canada

Smith & Nephew Inc. 800-463-7439
2100 52nd Ave., Lachine, QUE H8T 2Y5 Canada

Spectrum Laboratories, Inc. 800-634-3300
18617 S Broadwick St, Rancho Dominguez, CA 90220

U-Ten Corporation 630-289-8058
1286 Humbracht Cir, Bartlett, IL 60103
MAYO STAND COVER

Viscot Medical, Llc 800-221-0658
32 West St, PO Box 351, East Hanover, NJ 07936
Emergency drape - 18x26in. with 2-3/4in. fenestration or nonfenestrated. 24x36in. with 4in. fenestration or nonfenestrated with and without adhesive patches. Plastic drapes, and non-woven drapes in various sizes.

Xodus Medical, Inc. 800-963-8776
702 Prominence Dr, Westmoreland Business & Research Park
New Kensington, PA 15068
Sharps Saf-T Zone

DRAPE, SURGICAL, ENT *(Ear/Nose/Throat) 77ERY*

Atd-American Co. 800-523-2300
135 Greenwood Ave, Wyncote, PA 19095

DRAPE, SURGICAL, ENT *(cont'd)*

Gyrus Ent L.L.C., Sub. Of Gyrus Acmi, Inc. 508-804-2739
2925 Appling Rd, Bartlett, TN 38133
Various types and sizes of ent surgical drapes.

Invotec Intl. 800-998-8580
6833 Phillips Industrial Blvd, Jacksonville, FL 32256
Endoscopy camera drape.

Johnson & Johnson Medical Division Of Ethicon, Inc. 800-423-4018
2500 E Arbrook Blvd, Arlington, TX 76014

Kerr Group 800-524-3577
1400 Holcomb Bridge Rd, Roswell, GA 30076
Nonwoven disposable.

Medical Concepts Development 800-345-0644
2500 Ventura Dr, Saint Paul, MN 55125
Unique, standard and custom styles available.

Mylan Technologies, Inc. 800-532-5226
110 Lake St, Saint Albans, VT 05478
High moisture vapor permeable, USP Class VI urethane and Hytrel co-polyester films along with adhesive coated.

Oto-Med, Inc. 800-433-7703
1090 Empire Dr, Lake Havasu City, AZ 86404
Otology Surgery Drape & Neurotology Surgery Drape: Effective fluid and infection control drapes.

The Sewing Source, Inc. 919-478-3900
802 E Nash St, Spring Hope, NC 27882
Drape, surgical ent.

White Knight Healthcare 800-851-4431
Calle 16, Number 780, Agua Prieta, Sonora Mexico
Various types of sterile & non-sterile drapes

DRAPE, SURGICAL, REUSABLE *(Surgery) 79QQQ*

Atd-American Co. 800-523-2300
135 Greenwood Ave, Wyncote, PA 19095

Best Manufacturing Group Llc 800-843-3233
1633 Broadway Fl 18, New York, NY 10019
Custom made to specs.

Carl Zeiss Surgical, Inc. 800-442-4020
1 Zeiss Dr, Thornwood, NY 10594

Graham Medical Products/Div. Of Little Rapids Corp 866-429-1408
2273 Larsen Rd, Green Bay, WI 54303

Johnson & Johnson Medical Division Of Ethicon, Inc. 800-423-4018
2500 E Arbrook Blvd, Arlington, TX 76014

Lac-Mac Ltd. 800-461-0001
425 Rectory St., London, ONT N5W 3W5 Canada

Medline Industries, Inc. 800-633-5886
1 Medline Pl, Mundelein, IL 60060

Palmero Health Care 800-344-6424
120 Goodwin Pl, Stratford, CT 06615

Xodus Medical, Inc. 800-963-8776
702 Prominence Dr, Westmoreland Business & Research Park New Kensington, PA 15068
Saf-T Pass Reusable Transfer Drape

DRAPE, UROLOGICAL, DISPOSABLE *(Gastro/Urology) 78EYY*

Foothills Industries, Inc. 828-652-4088
300 Rockwell Dr, Marion, NC 28752

Kerr Group 800-524-3577
1400 Holcomb Bridge Rd, Roswell, GA 30076

Mylan Technologies, Inc. 800-532-5226
110 Lake St, Saint Albans, VT 05478
High moisture vapor permeable, USP Class VI urethane and Hytrel co-polyester films along with adhesive coated.

White Knight Healthcare 800-851-4431
Calle 16, Number 780, Agua Prieta, Sonora Mexico
Various types of protective clothing

DRESS, SCRUB, DISPOSABLE *(Surgery) 79RRV*

Adenna Inc. 888-323-3662
11932 Baker Pl, Santa Fe Springs, CA 90670
Latex free, disposable medical gown.

Atd-American Co. 800-523-2300
135 Greenwood Ave, Wyncote, PA 19095

DRESS, SCRUB, DISPOSABLE *(cont'd)*

General Econopak, Inc. 888-871-8568
1725 N 6th St, Philadelphia, PA 19122
All sizes.

Global Healthcare 800-601-3880
1495 Hembree Rd Ste 700, Roswell, GA 30076
All sizes.

Health-Pak, Inc. 315-724-8370
2005 Beechgrove Pl, Utica, NY 13501

Mylan Technologies, Inc. 800-532-5226
110 Lake St, Saint Albans, VT 05478
High moisture vapor permeable yet biologically occlusive extrusion laminates of non-woven fabrics and the MEDIFILM series of USP Class VI elastomeric films in bulk rolls.

New York Hospital Disposables, Inc. 718-384-1620
101 Richardson St, Brooklyn, NY 11211

Precept Medical Products, Inc. 800-438-5827
PO Box 2400, 370 Airport Road/, Arden, NC 28704

DRESS, SCRUB, REUSABLE *(Surgery) 79RRW*

Angelica Image Apparel 800-222-3112
700 Rosedale Ave, Saint Louis, MO 63112

Best Manufacturing Group Llc 800-843-3233
1633 Broadway Fl 18, New York, NY 10019
BEST Mfg. Inc.

Medline Industries, Inc. 800-633-5886
1 Medline Pl, Mundelein, IL 60060

DRESS, SURGICAL *(Surgery) 79FYE*

Angelica Image Apparel 800-222-3112
700 Rosedale Ave, Saint Louis, MO 63112

Berkley Medical Resources, Inc. 412-438-3000
49 Virginia Ave, Uniontown, PA 15401
Face mask.

Biomed Resource, Inc. 310-323-3888
3388 Rosewood Ave, Los Angeles, CA 90066
Jumpsuit, coverall, lab coat.

Clopay Plastic Products Company 800-282-2260
8585 Duke Blvd, Mason, OH 45040

Depuy Orthopaedics, Inc. 800-473-3789
700 Orthopaedic Dr, P.O. Box 988, Warsaw, IN 46582
Various types of surgical dresses.

Dowling Textiles 770-957-3981
615 Macon Rd, McDonough, GA 30253
Various types of surgical dresses.

Global Concepts, Ltd. 818-363-7195
19464 Eagle Ridge Ln, Northridge, CA 91326

Mylan Technologies, Inc. 800-532-5226
110 Lake St, Saint Albans, VT 05478
High moisture vapor permeable yet biologically occlusive extrusion laminates of non-woven fabrics and the MEDIFILM series of USP Class VI elastomeric films in bulk rolls.

The Sewing Source, Inc. 919-478-3900
802 E Nash St, Spring Hope, NC 27882
Dress, scrub.

White Knight Healthcare 800-851-4431
Calle 16, Number 780, Agua Prieta, Sonora Mexico
Scrub dress

DRESSING, AEROSOL *(General) 80QQT*

Mylan Pharmaceuticals Inc 888-523-7835
Research Triangle Pa, Morgantown, NC 27709
PRODERM emollient spray dressing.

Statlab Medical Products, Inc. 800-442-3573
106 Hillside Dr, Lewisville, TX 75057
STATFREEZE Freeze Spray, environmentally friendly aerosol used for firming tissue blocks.

DRESSING, BURN, PORCINE *(Surgery) 79KGN*

Arthrex, Inc. 239-643-5553
1370 Creekside Blvd, Naples, FL 34108
Collagen dowel.

Brennen Medical, Llc 651-429-7413
1290 Hammond Rd, Saint Paul, MN 55110
Biosynthetic (porcine skin) wound dressing.

Collagen Matrix, Inc. 201-405-1477
509 Commerce St, Franklin Lakes, NJ 07417
Collagen topical wound dressing.

DRESSING, BURN, PORCINE *(cont'd)*

Pegasus Biologics, Inc. 949-585-9430
10 Pasteur Ste 150, Irvine, CA 92618
Wound dressing.

Tei Biosciences Inc. 617-268-1616
7 Elkins St, Boston, MA 02127
Wound, dressing.

DRESSING, FOAM *(General) 80QQV*

Carrington Laboratories, Inc. 800-527-5216
2001 W Walnut Hill Ln, Irving, TX 75038
CARRASMART foam for the management of moisture in wounds. The self-adhesive, hydrophilic foam dressing helps to balance the moisture in the wound through a combination of absorptive and evaporative properties.

Coloplast Manufacturing Us, Llc 800-533-0464
1840 W Oak Pkwy, Marietta, GA 30062
BIATIN adhesive or non-adhesive super-absorbent foam dressings for wound management. Adhesive includes hydrocolloid border.

Ferris Mfg Corp. 800-765-9636
16 W300 83rd St., Burr Ridge, IL 60527-5848
PolyMem Wound Care Dressings, The Pink Dressing. A unique patented formula in 28 sizes and configurations include, non-adhesives, Island Dressings, Strips, Cavity Fillers, Calcium Alginates, Super Thick and Silver dressings

Gentell 800-840-9041
3600 Boundbrook Ave, Trevose, PA 19053
GENTELL LO-PROFILE PLUS FOAM DRESSINGS are waterproof, absorbent foam with an island design. Its dense sturdy structure provides the wound with protection from external threats and its porous texture is highly absorbent. A non-abrasive adhesive border affixes the dressing and creates a water-resistant bacterial barrier in which the wound can heal. GENTELL LO-PROFILE FOAM DRESSINGS are available in 4'x4' and 6'x6' sizes.

Innova Corp. 860-242-3210
68 E Dudley Town Rd, Bloomfield, CT 06002

Mpm Medical, Inc. 800-232-5512
2301 Crown Ct, Irving, TX 75038
MPM's Foam Dressing Bordered & Non-Bordered. A unique specialty foam that quickly absorbs large amounts of fluid. This foam has a waterproof top layer. It is available in many sizes including a fenestrated tube site dressing.

Mylan Pharmaceuticals Inc 888-523-7835
Research Triangle Pa, Morgantown, NC 27709
FLEXZAN; Dressing for non- to lightly draining wounds.

Mylan Technologies, Inc. 800-532-5226
110 Lake St, Saint Albans, VT 05478
MEDIFILM, series of USP Class VI extruded Hytrel co-polyester, urethane and Pebax high moisture vapor films, available with hypoallergenic acrylic or hydrocolloid adhesive systems, laminated to synergistic absorbent foams and available in rolls.

Packaging Alternatives Corp. 714-662-0277
1685 Toronto Way, Costa Mesa, CA 92626

Smith & Nephew, Inc. 800-876-1261
11775 Starkey Rd, Largo, FL 33773
Allevyn hydrophilic polyurethane foam with Opsite film waterproof backing layer and I.V. prep. antiseptic, protective dressings.

Tailored Label Products, Inc. 800-727-1344
W165N5731 Ridgewood Dr, Menomonee Falls, WI 53051

DRESSING, GEL *(General) 80WKJ*

Alimed, Inc. 800-225-2610
297 High St, Dedham, MA 02026

Brady Corporation 800-541-1686
6555 W Good Hope Rd, PO Box 571, Milwaukee, WI 53223
Manufacturing of hydrogel dressings to customer specifications for wound care, drug delivery and cosmetic applications.

Brady Precision Converting, Llc 214-275-9595
1801 Big Town Blvd Ste 100, Mesquite, TX 75149
Hydrogel dressings that can be formulated with ingredients to meet specific wound healing requirements.

Carrington Laboratories, Inc. 800-527-5216
2001 W Walnut Hill Ln, Irving, TX 75038
$5.65 for 3.5 oz CARRINGTON moisture barrier cream, $6.00 for 4 oz. CARRADERM moisturizing cream. $14.50 for 3 oz. CARRASYN hydrogel wound dressing. $14.99 for 16 oz. of CARRAKLENZ; $6.65 for 6 oz. of same.

DRESSING, GEL *(cont'd)*

Coloplast Manufacturing Us, Llc 800-533-0464
1840 W Oak Pkwy, Marietta, GA 30062
PURILON, WOUND'DRES sterile or non-sterile hydrogel for absorption and hydration.

Covidien Lp 508-261-8000
15 Hampshire St, Mansfield, MA 02048
INTERPAN wound dressing gel is designed for extended wear, adherence provides a moist wound bed, can be removed without trauma to the wound.

Donell 800-324-7455
1801 Taylor Ave, Louisville, KY 40213
K-Derm Gel is a topical Vitamin K gel, it has a mild gel formula which is helpful in rosacea, as well as bruises and broken capillaries; may help fade spider veins.

Gentell 800-840-9041
3600 Boundbrook Ave, Trevose, PA 19053
GENTELL Hydrogel; is an aloe barbadensis, aloe vera based hydrating wound gel that protects the wound bed and enhances the moist environment essential to the healing process. Aloe is rich in the complex carbohydrate characterized as poly dispersed B-(1,4)-linked acetylated mannin. Aloe is also a source of mono and poly saccharides, amino acids, glycoproteins, vitamins and enzymes. GENTELL HYDROGEL is available in 4oz tube and 8 oz spray bottle.

Innova Corp. 860-242-3210
68 E Dudley Town Rd, Bloomfield, CT 06002
Hydrogels, wounds and burn.

Johnson & Johnson Medical Division Of Ethicon, Inc. 800-423-4018
2500 E Arbrook Blvd, Arlington, TX 76014

Katecho, Inc. 515-244-1212
4020 Gannett Ave, Des Moines, IA 50321
Conductive adhesive hydrogels for patient monitoring and stimulation. EEG, EKG, Pacing, Defibrillation, Cardioversion.

Lohmann & Rauscher, Inc. 800-279-3863
6001 SW 6th Ave Ste 101, Topeka, KS 66615

M&C Specialties Co. 800-441-6996
90 James Way, Southampton, PA 18966

Mpm Medical, Inc. 800-232-5512
2301 Crown Ct, Irving, TX 75038
MPM REPEL Wound Dressing is a waterproof composite dressing that can be used on moderate to heavily draining wounds including those that are infected. MPM Multi Layered Dressing, is a non-waterproof composite dressing that is also highly absorbtive designed to be used on moderate to heavily draining wounds. MPM Excel Hydrocolloid is a transparent occlusive dressing. The transparency allows the clinician to view the progress or non-progress of the wound without removal thereby reducing trauma to the wound and allowing the clinician to make treatment judgements. The MPM Hydrocolloid absorbs exudate and is designed to stay on for five to seven days. It is available in various sizes including those specifically designed for the sacrum. MPM's ExcelGel is an amorphous hydrogel dressing composed of aloe vera and glycerin to moisturize the wound bed to create a natural moist wound healing environment. MPM's ExcelGel can be used for the management of pressure ulcers, stage II - IV, stasis ulcers, first and second degree burns. It is available in 3 oz. and 1 oz. tubes. MPM's CoolMagic Gel Sheet is a solid hydrogel composed of 90% water and 10% polyethelene. It is designed to be used on cuts, burns, abrasions, vascular ulcers, diabetic ulcers, pressure ulcers and radiation reactions. This product is naturally cooling, soothing and excellent for reducing the pain from burns and skin reactions due to radiation. The gel sheets are available in four sizes including a fenestrated tube site dressing. MPM manufactures hydrogel saturated gauze pads in four sizes. These pads are referred to as MPM GelPads. They are indicated for use in packing wounds. These gelpads help establish a moist wound environment and by packing the wound causes the wound to heal from the bottom up.

Mylan Technologies, Inc. 800-532-5226
110 Lake St, Saint Albans, VT 05478
MEDIFILM, series of USP Class VI extruded Hytrel co-polyester, urethane and Pebax high moisture vapor films, available with hypoallergenic acrylic or hydrocolloid adhesive systems, laminated to synergistic absorbent foams and available in rolls.

Pharmaceutical Innovations, Inc. 973-242-2900
897 Frelinghuysen Ave, Newark, NJ 07114
EVRON GEL - Breast self-examination lubricant. Improves the quality of the examination by reducing friction between the breast tissue and the fingers. 6 - 10ml packets per unit/$5.95 each.

DRESSING, GEL *(cont'd)*

Safetec Of America, Inc. 800-456-7077
887 Kensington Ave, Buffalo, NY 14215
Safetec Burn Gel and Burn Spray are recommended for the quick, soothing pain relief of minor burns. Packaging: single-use 1/8 oz. pouch, 2 oz. spray, 4 oz. spray, or 4 oz. flip-top bottle.

Smith & Nephew, Inc. 800-876-1261
11775 Starkey Rd, Largo, FL 33773
Intrasite interactive hydrogel dressing for debriding, desloughing and absorbing.

Southwest Technologies, Inc. 800-247-9951
1746 E Levee St, North Kansas City, MO 64116
ELASTO-GEL(Tm) PLUS (with tape) & also must have hyphin ELASTO-GEL (Tm) (without tape), Toe-Aid (Tm) and Comfort Aid,Toe and wound gel dressing.

Tyco Healthcare Group Lp 800-445-5025
2 Ludlow Park Dr, Chicopee, MA 01022
Hydrogel dressings for wound care.

Weaver & Company 303-366-1804
565 Nucla Way Ste B, Aurora, CO 80011
Medical gels and pastes.

DRESSING, GERMICIDAL *(General) 80QQW*

Acrymed, Inc. 503-624-9830
9560 SW Nimbus Ave, Beaverton, OR 97008
SilvaSorb Silver Antimicrobial Dressings, line of advanced moist, hydrophilic dressings; many sizes and formats. SilvaSorb Site dressings now available for infection control of percutaneous devices.

Mylan Technologies, Inc. 800-532-5226
110 Lake St, Saint Albans, VT 05478
MEDIFILM, series of USP Class VI extruded Hytrel co-polyester, urethane and Pebax high moisture vapor films, available with hypoallergenic acrylic or hydrocolloid adhesive systems, laminated to synergistic absorbent foams and available in either rolls or converted, packaged dressings - incl. IV site dressings.

DRESSING, LAYER, CHARCOAL *(General) 80WSE*

Smith & Nephew, Inc. 800-876-1261
11775 Starkey Rd, Largo, FL 33773
Carbonet dressing with activated charcoal layer, non-adherent wound contact layer and absorbent fleece for the management of draining, malodorous wounds.

DRESSING, NON-ADHERENT *(General) 80QQX*

Albahealth Llc 800-262-2404
425 N Gateway Ave, Rockwood, TN 37854
ALBAHEALTH Petrolatum or Zerform.

Astellas Pharma Us, Inc. 800-888-7704
3 Parkway N, Deerfield, IL 60015
Hercon Laboratories' transparent dressing.

Covidien Lp 508-261-8000
15 Hampshire St, Mansfield, MA 02048
XEROFLO sterile gauze dressing, non-adhering permeable dressing consisting of fine mesh, absorbent gauze impregnated with a water-in-oil emulsion containing bismuth-tribromopherate.

Csi Holdings 615-452-9633
170 Commerce Way, Gallatin, TN 37066

Delstar Technologies, Inc. 800-521-6713
601 Industrial Rd, Middletown, DE 19709
DELNET nonwoven fabric, nonadherent facings, porous, non-stick net for use on wound and burn care products. DEL PORE meltblown nonwoven fabric provides precise uniformity, breathability and controlled porosity for demanding applications such as face masks and surgical drapes and gowns.

Derma Sciences 609-514-4744
214 Carnegie Ctr Ste 300, Princeton, NJ 08540
DERMAGRAN zinc-saline wet dressings for the management of venous statis ulcers, skin ulcerations, pressure sores, minor thermal burns, lacerations, cuts and abrasions.

Dukal Corporation 800-243-0741
5 Plant Ave, Hauppauge, NY 11788

Gentell 800-840-9041
3600 Boundbrook Ave, Trevose, PA 19053
GENTELL COMFORTELL is a Composite WOund Dressing with four distinct layers. This dressing combines an excellent absorbent layer with a selectively permeable barrier that allows the wound to breathe while keeping contaminates out. A special spunlace tape border holds the dressing securely in place while the waterproof backing can be wiped off when soiled. GENTELL COMFORTELL is available in 4'x4' and 6'x6' sizes.

DRESSING, NON-ADHERENT *(cont'd)*

Innova Corp. 860-242-3210
68 E Dudley Town Rd, Bloomfield, CT 06002

Johnson & Johnson Medical Division Of Ethicon, Inc. 800-423-4018
2500 E Arbrook Blvd, Arlington, TX 76014

Lohmann & Rauscher, Inc. 800-279-3863
6001 SW 6th Ave Ste 101, Topeka, KS 66615

Medi-Tech International Corp. 800-333-0109
26 Court St, Brooklyn, NY 11242
SPAND-GEL hydrogel absorption dressing for dermal ulcers - wound contaminant absorbent & moisturizing to enhance tissue granulation in stage I, II, III & IV. Gel sheets to maintain moist environment for treatment of burns and donor site skin grafts.

Pacon Manufacturing Corporation 732-357-8020
400 Pierce St # B, Somerset, NJ 08873
Custom and stock.

Shippert Medical Technologies Corp. 800-888-8663
6248 S Troy Cir Ste A, Centennial, CO 80111
Derma Net, Stretch-Net, Aquagauze.

Smith & Nephew Inc. 800-463-7439
2100 52nd Ave., Lachine, QUE H8T 2Y5 Canada

Smith & Nephew, Inc. 800-876-1261
11775 Starkey Rd, Largo, FL 33773
Transite exudate transfer film.

Winfield Laboratories 800-527-4616
PO Box 832297, Richardson, TX 75083
N-TERFACE, break-away wound dressing, highly absorbant, nonoccursive, burn/wound dressing with releasably attached wound contact layer. 5 sizes available.

Wisap America 800-233-8448
8231 Melrose Dr, Lenexa, KS 66214

DRESSING, OTHER *(General) 80FRO*

Abbott Vascular Inc. 800-227-9902
400 Saginaw Dr, Redwood City, CA 94063
Wound dressing.

Acrymed, Inc. 503-624-9830
9560 SW Nimbus Ave, Beaverton, OR 97008
ACRYDERM Advanced Wound Dressing composed of sheet hydrogel available in five sizes.

Aegis Medical 203-838-9081
10 Wall St, Norwalk, CT 06850
Wound care dressings.

Albahealth Llc 800-262-2404
425 N Gateway Ave, Rockwood, TN 37854
ALBAHEALTH Wet dressings (distilled water & saline).

American White Cross - Houston 609-514-4744
15200 North Fwy, Houston, TX 77090
Topical hemostatic spray.

Anacapa Technologies, Inc. 909-394-7795
301 E Arrow Hwy Ste 106, San Dimas, CA 91773
Hydrogel dressing.

Angiosystems, Inc. 800-441-4256
7 Hopkins Pl., Ducktown, TN 37326
Arnold-King pressure dressing.

Argentum Medical Llc 708-927-9398
424 Stamp Creek Rd Ste F, Salem, SC 29676
Sterile wound dressing.

Becton Dickinson Infusion Therapy Systems, Inc. 888-237-2762
9450 S State St, Sandy, UT 84070
Transparent dressings.

Belcher Pharmaceuticals, Inc. 727-544-8866
12393 Belcher Rd S Ste 420, Largo, FL 33773
Dressing, wound & burn, hydrogel with drug or biologic.

Bioseal 800-441-7325
167 W Orangethorpe Ave, Placentia, CA 92870
Sterile dressings.

Birchwood Laboratories, Inc. 800-328-6156
7900 Fuller Rd, Eden Prairie, MN 55344
ARD (anoperineal dressing), 12 boxes and ARD (mild anal leakage) 24 dressings/box 12 boxes/case

Brecon Knitting Mills, Inc. 800-841-2821
PO Box 478, Talladega, AL 35161
Interface for brace stump shrinker.

DRESSING, OTHER *(cont'd)*

Brennen Medical, Llc 651-429-7413
1290 Hammond Rd, Saint Paul, MN 55110
Topical wound dressing.

Bsn-Jobst 704-554-9933
5825 Carnegie Blvd, Charlotte, NC 28209
Hydrocolloid dressing.

Busse Hospital Disposables, Inc. 631-435-4711
75 Arkay Dr, Hauppauge, NY 11788
Various.

Cenorin 800-426-1042
6324 S 199th Pl Ste 107, Kent, WA 98032
Aqua Guard self-adhesive, latex-free moisture barriers protect wound dressings and vascular devices while showering.

Coloplast Manufacturing Us, Llc 800-533-0464
1840 W Oak Pkwy, Marietta, GA 30062
COMFEEL PLUS Ulcer - absorbent dermal ulcer dressing and COLOPLAST skin barrier protection for skin around stomas and draining wounds.

Cook Biotech, Incorporated 888-299-4224
1425 Innovation Pl, West Lafayette, IN 47906
Wound and Burn

Covidien Lp 508-261-8000
15 Hampshire St, Mansfield, MA 02048
Hydrocolloid and composite.

Crosslink-D, Inc 203-318-8270
3480 Industrial Blvd Ste 105, West Sacramento, CA 95691
Liquid bandage.

Dale Medical Products, Inc. 800-343-3980
7 Cross St, Plainville, MA 02762
Nasal Dressing Support #600.

Delstar Technologies, Inc. 800-521-6713
601 Industrial Rd, Middletown, DE 19709
DELNET coverstock, perforated film for use as a facing material on feminine hygiene and incontinence products.

Derma Sciences 609-514-4744
214 Carnegie Ctr Ste 300, Princeton, NJ 08540
DERMAGRAN hydrophilic wound dressing with impregnated gauze pad.

Dr. Len's Medical Products Llc 678-908-8180
412 Atwood Rd, Erdenheim, PA 19038
Abrams all-in-one with silver abrams foam dressing 4x4, 4x8 and 4x11 with silver.

Dukal Corporation 800-243-0741
5 Plant Ave, Hauppauge, NY 11788
SiteLine transparent film dressing.

Dumex Medical Surgical Products Ltd. 800-463-9613
104 Shorting Rd., Scarborough, ONT M1S 3S4 Canada
Self-adhesive dressing covering - permeable, non-woven, hypoallergenic, cross-elastic flexibility and radiotranslucent. Algicell: Calcium Alginate Wound dressing, sterile dressing to absorb large amounts of wound drainage. Foam Dressing Adhesive: hydrophilic wound dressing. Absorbs-a-Salt: Wet dressing, khydrophilic wound dressing. Dumex Iodoform Packing Strips, for packing wounds.

Durden Enterprises 800-554-5673
1317 4th Ave, P.O. Box 909, Auburn, GA 30011
100W & 200W Wedge Pressure Dressing - 2 sizes, wedge pressure dressings, convenient, eliminates need for sandbag, completely self-contained.

Dynarex Corp. 888-356-2739
10 Glenshaw St, Orangeburg, NY 10962
DYNAREX surgical dressings available in peel down envelopes and tray packaging.

Ferndale Laboratories, Inc. 248-548-0900
780 W 8 Mile Rd, Detroit, MI 48220
Wound and skin emulsion.

General Econopak, Inc. 888-871-8568
1725 N 6th St, Philadelphia, PA 19122
Burn-dressing pad, non-medicated, lintfree, sterile.

DRESSING, OTHER *(cont'd)*

Gentell 800-840-9041
3600 Boundbrook Ave, Trevose, PA 19053
GENTELL CALCIUM ALGINATE DRESSINGS are a comfortable, advanced fiber structured alginate, with a highly absorbent capacity. These advanced alginate dressings are used to absorb, collect and cotain exudate while providing a moist healing environment. These dressings are applied in a dry form. A reaction between the calcium in the dressing and the sodium in the wound exudate results in a chemical exchange that creates a gel like substance. GENTELL CALCIUM ALGINATE is available in 2'x2', 4'x4' and 12' Rope.

H & H Co. 909-390-0373
4435 E Airport Dr Ste 108, Ontario, CA 91761
Gauze dressing.

Hartmann-Conco Inc. 800-243-2294
481 Lakeshore Pkwy, Rock Hill, SC 29730
Contex LF reinforced 'latex-free' bandage, used for compression and support.

Healer Products, Llc 914-663-6300
427 Commerce Ln Ste 1, West Berlin, NJ 08091
Multiple bandages.

Hemcon Medical Technologies, Inc. 877-247-0196
10575 SW Cascade Ave Ste 130, Portland, OR 97223

Hercon Laboratories Corp. 717-764-1191
101 Sinking Springs Ln., Emigsville, PA 17318
Transdermal drug delivery systems

Imonti And Associates Inc., M. 949-248-1058
25707 Compass Way, San Juan Capistrano, CA 92675
$99.50/case of ten sterile units, Catalog #12-1 Gentle Care surgical dressing, used in areola and nipple reconstruction.

Innova Corp. 860-242-3210
68 E Dudley Town Rd, Bloomfield, CT 06002
Foam, burn, gel, non adherent, wound, breathable, universal and permeable. Also available, hydrocolloid wound dressings in full size or island dressings.

Integra Neurosciences Pr 800-654-2873
Road 402 North, Km 1.2, Anasco, PR 00610
Sterile antimicrobial dressing.

Invacare Supply Group, An Invacare Co. 800-225-4792
75 October Hill Rd, Holliston, MA 01746
Carry full lines of all General & Speciality wound care from: Invacare, 3M, J&J, AMD, & Kendall.

Johnson & Johnson Medical Division Of Ethicon, Inc. 800-423-4018
2500 E Arbrook Blvd, Arlington, TX 76014

K W Griffen Company 800-424-5556
100 Pearl St, Norwalk, CT 06850

K. W. Griffen Co. 203-846-1923
100 Pearl St, Norwalk, CT 06850
Wound & blister dresseing (non-adhering dressing).

Kelsar, S.A. 508-261-8000
Blvd. Insurgentes, Libriamento a La, Tijuana 22450 Mexico
Owens surgical dressings

Kerma Medical Products, Inc. 757-398-8400
400 Port Centre Pkwy, Portsmouth, VA 23704
Various sizes dressing, sterille non-adherent pads.

Kli Corp. 317-846-7452
1119 3rd Ave SW, Carmel, IN 46032
Entertainer's Secret, a spray for dry sore throat and hoarse voice, is formulated to resemble natural secretions. Sodium carboxymethylcellulose, aloe vera gel and glycerin - each a proxy for a naturally secreted type of mucus (globular, strand and sheet) - are blended into a buffered, aqueous hypertonic solution. Unlike some other sore throat remedies, it does not contain numbing anesthetics, alcohol, antiseptics, analgesics, antihistamines, decongestants, anti-inflammatory agents or any other 'medicinal' ingredient that can produce unwanted side effects. The honey-apple flavor imparts a pleasant mellow taste. Entertainer's Secret is packaged in a two ounce (60 ml) polyethylene bottle which fits conveniently into pocket or purse and has a built-in locking mechanism so it won't leak or spill. Each bottle delivers about 85 sprays. There are 12 bottles per carton with four cartons (48 bottles) per shipper case. Individuls may order directly: Two bottles are $15.00 (US) and six bottles are $35.00 (US). Bulk prices available on request.

Lexamed 419-693-5307
705 Front St, Northwood, OH 43605
Sterile dressing.

DRESSING, OTHER *(cont'd)*

Lohmann & Rauscher, Inc. 800-279-3863
6001 SW 6th Ave Ste 101, Topeka, KS 66615

Marel Corporation 203-934-8187
5 Saw Mill Rd, West Haven, CT 06516
Burn dressing, burn compress, ABD (combine) pad.

Marine Polymer Technologies, Inc. 888-666-2560
461 Boston St Unit B5, Topsfield, MA 01983
Dressing, wound, drug.

Matrx 716-662-6650
145 Mid County Dr, Orchard Park, NY 14127
Dressing.

Mcneil Healthcare, Inc. 203-932-6263
481 Elm St, West Haven, CT 06516
Burn compress,burn gauze pads,custom burn dressings,non adherent burn pads.

Medi-Tech International Corp. 800-333-0109
26 Court St, Brooklyn, NY 11242
SPAND-GEL - primary hydrogel wound absorption dressing filler for dermal ulcers - wound contaminant absorbent & moisturizing to enhance tissue granulation in stages I-IV. Gel sheets to maintain moist environment for treatment of burns and donor site skin grafts.

Medical Action Industries, Inc. 800-645-7042
25 Heywood Rd, Arden, NC 28704
Wound dressing.

Mpm Medical, Inc. 800-232-5512
2301 Crown Ct, Irving, TX 75038
MPM's calcium alginate absorptive dressing is called EXCELGINATE. ExcelGinate is a highly absorptive dressing designed to be used in heavily draining wounds. The fibers are tightly woven to maintain the product's integrity upon removal. This product does not melt in the wound. It is indicated for pressure ulcers, trauma wounds, donor sites, diabetic ulcers and arterial venous ulcers. The ExcelGinate is available in five sizes including a 6' and 12' rope.

Mylan Technologies, Inc. 800-532-5226
110 Lake St, Saint Albans, VT 05478
Complete family of extruded, custom adhesive coated Hytrel co-polyester, urethane and Pebax high moisture vapor permeable, occlusive films available in roll form or converted, packaged dressings - incl. for IV sites.

O&M Enterprise 847-258-4515
641 Chelmsford Ln, Elk Grove Village, IL 60007
DRESSING NONADHERENT/HYDRO

Omiderm Ltd. 415-753-9989
1 Oakwood Blvd Ste 50, Hollywood, FL 33020
Dressing.

Patterson Medical Supply, Inc. 262-387-8720
W68N158 Evergreen Blvd, Cedarburg, WI 53012
Dressing.

Protector Canada Inc. 800-268-6594
1111 Flint Rd., Unit 23, Toronto, ON M3J 3C7 Canada
Sterile pressure dressing. Adhesive dressings, vinyl and stretch fabric.

Sca Personal Care, North America 270-796-9300
7030 Louisville Rd, Bowling Green, KY 42101
Wound dressing, various sizes, sterile and nonsterile.

Select Fabricators, Inc. 585-393-0650
5310 North St Bldg 5, Canandaigua, NY 14424
Sterile wound dressing.

Shippert Medical Technologies Corp. 800-888-8663
6248 S Troy Cir Ste A, Centennial, CO 80111

Silipos Inc. 800-229-4404
704 Williams Road, Niagara Falls, NY 14304

Smith & Nephew Inc. 800-463-7439
2100 52nd Ave., Lachine, QUE H8T 2Y5 Canada

Smith & Nephew, Inc. 800-876-1261
11775 Starkey Rd, Largo, FL 33773

Smith & Nephew, Inc. 800-876-1261
970 Lake Carillon Dr Ste 110, Saint Petersburg, FL 33716
WOUND AND BURN, HYDROGEL W/DRUG AND/OR BIOLOGIC - SOLOSITE GEL

Southwest Technologies, Inc. 800-247-9951
1746 E Levee St, North Kansas City, MO 64116
Hydrolyzed collagen in four deliveries: powder, amorphous gel, sheet gel and lotion

Swiss American Products, Inc. 800-633-8872
2055 Luna Rd Ste 126, Carrollton, TX 75006
Wound dressing.

Tagg Industries L.L.C. 800-548-3514
23210 Del Lago Dr, Laguna Hills, CA 92653
CASTBLAST, an aerosol that is specifically formulated to relieve itching and odor that is caused by wearing a cast.

The Hymed Group Corp. 610-865-9876
1890 Bucknell Dr, Bethlehem, PA 18015
Polysulfated glycosaminoglycan (PSGAG)-CHONDROPROTEC, and sodium hyaluronate (HA)- HYCOAT, available sterile in vials.

Tri-State Hospital Supply Corp. 800-248-4058
301 Catrell Dr, PO Box 170, Howell, MI 48843
Catheter site dressings: SITEGUARD MVP transparent dressing with high moisture-vapor transmission rate, SORBAVIEW 2000 absorbent window, and VERSADERM fabric border dressing.

Udl Laboratories, Inc. 281-240-1000
12720 Dairy Ashford Rd, Sugar Land, TX 77478
Topical wound dressing.

Vascular Solutions, Inc. 763-656-4300
5025 Cheshire Ln N, Plymouth, MN 55446
Topical hemostat.

Vygon Corp. 800-544-4907
2495 General Armistead Ave, Norristown, PA 19403
Transparent dressings.

Western Medical, Ltd. 800-628-8276
214 Carnegie Ctr Ste 100, Princeton, NJ 08540
COPRESS, Cohesive Dressing, used to retain or in compression - bandages that stick to themselves, not to the skin.

Z-Medica Corporation 203-294-0000
4 Fairfield Blvd, Wallingford, CT 06492
QUIKCLOT COMBAT GAUZE; QUIKCLOT EMERGENCY DRESSING; QUIKCLOT eX; QUIKCLOT HEMOSTATIC FORMULA

Zens Manufacturing, Inc.. 414-372-7060
2435 N Martin Luther King Dr, PO Drawer 12504, Milwaukee, WI 53212
Tublar gauze bandage, non sterile, nat stock no 6510-00-200. Many medical textile products.

DRESSING, PERIODONTAL *(Dental And Oral) 76TBW*

The Hymed Group Corp. 610-865-9876
1890 Bucknell Dr, Bethlehem, PA 18015
Type I collagen for oral wounds -hyCURE ORAL gel. The only product of its kind for denture sores, ulcers, surgical wounds, burns, extraction sites, and traumatic wounds.

DRESSING, PERMEABLE, MOISTURE *(General) 80WKL*

Brady Precision Converting, Llc 214-275-9595
1801 Big Town Blvd Ste 100, Mesquite, TX 75149
Thin film breathable dressings made to customer specifications.

Innova Corp. 860-242-3210
68 E Dudley Town Rd, Bloomfield, CT 06002

Johnson & Johnson Medical Division Of Ethicon, Inc. 800-423-4018
2500 E Arbrook Blvd, Arlington, TX 76014

Kerr Group 800-524-3577
1400 Holcomb Bridge Rd, Roswell, GA 30076

Lohmann & Rauscher, Inc. 800-279-3863
6001 SW 6th Ave Ste 101, Topeka, KS 66615

Mylan Technologies, Inc. 800-532-5226
110 Lake St, Saint Albans, VT 05478
MEDIFILM, series of USP Class VI extruded Hytrel co-polyester, urethane and Pebax high moisture vapor films, available with hypoallergenic acrylic or hydrocolloid adhesive systems, laminated to synergistic absorbent foams and available in either rolls or converted, packaged dressings.

Scapa Medical 310-419-0567
540 N Oak St, Inglewood, CA 90302
Air and moisture-vapor permeable, transparent high MVTR polyurethane dressing, 510(k) approved, available for private labeling.

Smith & Nephew, Inc. 800-876-1261
11775 Starkey Rd, Largo, FL 33773
Opsite transparent adhesive wound and IV dressing.

Vygon Corp. 800-544-4907
2495 General Armistead Ave, Norristown, PA 19403
Transparent dressing (vapor permeable).

DRESSING, ROLLER GAUZE *(General) 80QQZ*

Covidien Lp 508-261-8000
15 Hampshire St, Mansfield, MA 02048
INTERSORB roll stretch gauze, 6-ply wide mesh, 1005 cotton gauze roll, 4 1/2 in. x 4 1/3 yards. Available sterile (individual package) and non-sterile (bulk). Cost-effective.

Kck Industries 888-800-1967
14941 Calvert St, Van Nuys, CA 91411
Wound-care dressings.

DRESSING, SKIN GRAFT, DONOR SITE *(General) 80QRA*

Coloplast Manufacturing Us, Llc 800-533-0464
1840 W Oak Pkwy, Marietta, GA 30062
COMFEEL PLUS hydrocolloid dressings for Stages I-IV and leg ulcers, skin tears, donor sites.

Lifecell Corp. 800-367-5737
1 Millennium Way, Branchburg, NJ 08876
ALLODERM Biological skin replacement (for wounds).

Medi-Tech International Corp. 800-333-0109
26 Court St, Brooklyn, NY 11242
SPAND-GEL gel sheets to maintain moist enviroment for treatment of burns and donor site skin grafts.

Winfield Laboratories 800-527-4616
PO Box 832297, Richardson, TX 75083
N-TERFACE, break-away wound dressing, nonadherent, absorbant, patent-pending releasable wound contact layer. 5 sizes available.

Wisap America 800-233-8448
8231 Melrose Dr, Lenexa, KS 66214

DRESSING, TRACHEOSTOMY TUBE *(Ear/Nose/Throat) 77QRB*

Surgic Aid, Inc. 800-338-5213
37 Crystal Ave # 287, Derry, NH 03038

DRESSING, UNIVERSAL *(General) 80QRC*

Carrington Laboratories, Inc. 800-527-5216
2001 W Walnut Hill Ln, Irving, TX 75038

Coloplast Manufacturing Us, Llc 800-533-0464
1840 W Oak Pkwy, Marietta, GA 30062
COMFEEL PLUS Ulcer Care System - absorbent dermal ulcer dressing and COLOPLAST skin barrier protection for skin around stomas and draining wounds.

Covidien Lp 508-261-8000
15 Hampshire St, Mansfield, MA 02048

Dixie Ems Supply 800-347-3494
385 Union Ave, Brooklyn, NY 11211
$207.00 per 100 (med).

Dukal Corporation 800-243-0741
5 Plant Ave, Hauppauge, NY 11788

Innova Corp. 860-242-3210
68 E Dudley Town Rd, Bloomfield, CT 06002

Johnson & Johnson Medical Division Of Ethicon, Inc. 800-423-4018
2500 E Arbrook Blvd, Arlington, TX 76014

Lohmann & Rauscher, Inc. 800-279-3863
6001 SW 6th Ave Ste 101, Topeka, KS 66615

Medi-Tech International Corp. 800-333-0109
26 Court St, Brooklyn, NY 11242
Open netted tubular elastic dressing retainer and gel dressings.

Medikmark Inc. 800-424-8520
3600 Burwood Dr, Waukegan, IL 60085
Central line reinsertion trays. Chloraprep.

Mylan Pharmaceuticals Inc 888-523-7835
Research Triangle Pa, Morgantown, NC 27709
SORBSAN calcium alginate topical wound dressing and BIOBRANE temporary burn wound dressing.

Orange-Sol Medical Products, Inc. 800-877-7771
1400 N Fiesta Blvd Ste 100, Gilbert, AZ 85233

Rockford Medical & Safety Co. 800-435-9451
2420 Harrison Ave, PO Box 5646, Rockford, IL 61108

Smith & Nephew, Inc. 800-876-1261
970 Lake Carillon Dr Ste 110, Saint Petersburg, FL 33716
WOUND, DRUG - Exu-Dry

Web-Tex, Inc. 888-633-2723
5445 De Gaspe Ave., Ste. 702, Montreal, QC H2T 3B2 Canada
Surgical.

Western Medical, Ltd. 800-628-8276
214 Carnegie Ctr Ste 100, Princeton, NJ 08540

DRESSING, UNIVERSAL *(cont'd)*

Winfield Laboratories 800-527-4616
PO Box 832297, Richardson, TX 75083

DRESSING, WOUND AND BURN, HYDROGEL *(Surgery) 79MGQ*

Acrymed, Inc. 503-624-9830
9560 SW Nimbus Ave, Beaverton, OR 97008
ACRYDERM STRANDS Absorbent Dressing. Highly absorbent wound-cavity filler for heavily draining wound.

Afassco, Inc. 800-441-6774
2244 Park Pl Ste C, Minden, NV 89423
Aqua Skin - unique hydrogel dressing.

Balance Systems, Inc. 1-888-274-5444
1644 Plaza Way Ste 317, Walla Walla, WA 99362
COLDFLEX sterile burn dressing.

Brennen Medical, Llc 651-429-7413
1290 Hammond Rd, Saint Paul, MN 55110
Beta glucan gel.

Burnfree Products Division 888-909-2876
9382 S 670 W, Sandy, UT 84070
First aid dressings in various sizes, sterile product, for application immediately on burns, wounds prior to seeking medical treatment.

Cobe Chemical Co. 562-942-2426
8616 Slauson Ave, Pico Rivera, CA 90660
Glycerin with hyaluronic acid and fibronectin gel.

Concept Health, Llc 215-364-3600
3600 Boundbrook Ave, Trevose, PA 19053
Hydrogel.

Corium International, Inc. 616-656-4563
4558 50th St SE, Grand Rapids, MI 49512
Sterile antimicrobial wound dressing.

Curapharm, Inc. 619-449-7388
10054 Prospect Ave Ste F, Santee, CA 92071
Phytacare alginate hydrogel dressing.

Dumex Medical Surgical Products Ltd. 800-463-9613
104 Shorting Rd., Scarborough, ONT M1S 3S4 Canada
Dumex pak-Its cotton guaze packing impregnated with hydrogel, for packing wounds. Sterile Hydrogel, wound management.

Hartmann-Conco Inc. 800-243-2294
481 Lakeshore Pkwy, Rock Hill, SC 29730
Aquacare wet therapy wound dressing that delivers 24-hour solution for activity rinsing chronic wounds. Aquacare Plus wet therapy wound dressing with water-repellent layer that delivers 24-hour solution for actively rinsing chronic wounds. Aquaclear hydrogel sterile dressing available in non-adhesive and adhesive presentations. Sorbalgon calcium-alginate dressings in two sizes, plus a 12-in. ribbon. Cosmopore soft absorbent gauze dressing with adhesive border. Permacol, a vapor-permeable, hydrocolloid dressing available in five sizes.

Healer Products, Llc 914-663-6300
427 Commerce Ln Ste 1, West Berlin, NJ 08091
Water gel dressing.

Hemcon Medical Technologies, Inc. 877-247-0196
10575 SW Cascade Ave Ste 130, Portland, OR 97223

Innova Corp. 860-242-3210
68 E Dudley Town Rd, Bloomfield, CT 06002

K. W. Griffen Co. 203-846-1923
100 Pearl St, Norwalk, CT 06850
Burn relief dressing.

Lohmann & Rauscher, Inc. 800-279-3863
6001 SW 6th Ave Ste 101, Topeka, KS 66615

Mcmerlin Dental Products, Lp 972-602-3746
1610 W Polo Rd, Grand Prairie, TX 75052
Hydrogel oral wound dressing.

Medi-Tech International Corp. 800-333-0109
26 Court St, Brooklyn, NY 11242
SPAND-GEL Specialty sheets.

Mpm Medical, Inc. 800-232-5512
2301 Crown Ct, Irving, TX 75038

Nbs Medical Products Inc. 888-800-8192
257 Livingston Ave, New Brunswick, NJ 08901
Wound and burn care products, including hydrogels and hydrocolloids and products for treating ulcers, lacerations, and puncture wounds.

Sage Pharmaceuticals, Inc. 318-635-1594
5408 Interstate Dr, Shreveport, LA 71109

DRESSING, WOUND AND BURN, HYDROGEL *(cont'd)*

Swiss American Products, Inc. 800-633-8872
2055 Luna Rd Ste 126, Carrollton, TX 75006
Eutra gel (also marketed as elta gel).

The Hymed Group Corp. 610-865-9876
1890 Bucknell Dr, Bethlehem, PA 18015
CellerateRX - 60% collagen for a variety of wounds, forms a film when left to air dry, reduces pain at the wound site, reduces the chance of scarring.

DRESSING, WOUND AND BURN, INTERACTIVE
(Surgery) 79MGR

Acrymed, Inc. 503-624-9830
9560 SW Nimbus Ave, Beaverton, OR 97008
SilvaSorb Gel, silver antimicrobial wound and burn hydrogel dressing

Advanced Biohealing Inc. 858-754-3863
10933 N Torrey Pines Rd Ste 200, La Jolla, CA 92037
Human fibroblast-derived dermal,temporary skin substitute.

Invitrx, Inc. 877-468-4879
23322 Madero Ste J, Mission Viejo, CA 92691
Autologous cultured skin graft.

DRESSING, WOUND AND BURN, OCCLUSIVE *(Surgery) 79MGP*

Allied Healthcare Products, Inc. 800-444-3954
1720 Sublette Ave, Saint Louis, MO 63110

Bio Med Sciences, Inc. 800-257-4566
7584 Morris Ct Ste 218, Allentown, PA 18106
SILON-TSR temporary skin replacement for advanced woundcare, including laser resurfacing. SILON-DUAL DRESS is a single dressing with two different functions. One side consists of an open-celled hydrophilic foam; the other side consists of SILON-TSR semioccusive film. The SILON (colored blue) is perforated to allow exudate to wick away from the wound.

Brecon Knitting Mills, Inc. 800-841-2821
PO Box 478, Talladega, AL 35161

Certified Safety Manufacturing 800-854-7474
1400 Chestnut Ave, Kansas City, MO 64127
Certi-Burn Dressing

Cook Urological, Inc. 800-457-4500
1100 W Morgan St, P.O. Box 227, Spencer, IN 47460
Oasis.

Covidien Lp 508-261-8000
15 Hampshire St, Mansfield, MA 02048
OWENS surgical dressing.

Dukal Corporation 800-243-0741
5 Plant Ave, Hauppauge, NY 11788

Dumex Medical Surgical Products Ltd. 800-463-9613
104 Shorting Rd., Scarborough, ONT M1S 3S4 Canada
DUPRESS Dumex Pak-its 'Absorbs-a-Salt' cotton guaze packing: for packing wounds. Self Adhesive Foam Island Dressing: occlusive wound dressing. Hydrocolloid Thin Dressing: occlusive wound dressing. Film dressing: occlusive wound dressing.

Euromed, Inc. 845-359-4039
25 Corporate Dr, Orangeburg, NY 10962
Wound dressings for chronic, acute, post op,indications. Central and peripheral line hydrocolloid dressings.Consumer OTC bandages for minor abrasions, blisters,burns and facial blemishes. Hydrocolloid Roll Goods.

Genzyme Corp. 800-232-7546
64 Sidney St, Cambridge, MA 02139
Dressing used in burn treatment.

Geritrex Corp. 800-736-3437
144 E Kingsbridge Rd, Mount Vernon, NY 10550
Hydrophor gauze, 3 x 8 or 8 x 8-in.

Green Field Medical Sourcing, Inc. 512-894-3002
14141 W Highway 290 Ste 410, Austin, TX 78737
Occlusive chest wound dressing.

Healer Products, Llc 914-663-6300
427 Commerce Ln Ste 1, West Berlin, NJ 08091
Wound dressing.

Innova Corp. 860-242-3210
68 E Dudley Town Rd, Bloomfield, CT 06002

Innovative Wound Management, Llc 440-461-1295
29001 Cedar Rd Ste 325, Cleveland, OH 44124
Wound dressing or bandage.

Johnson & Johnson Medical Division Of Ethicon, Inc. 800-423-4018
2500 E Arbrook Blvd, Arlington, TX 76014

DRESSING, WOUND AND BURN, OCCLUSIVE *(cont'd)*

Lohmann & Rauscher, Inc. 800-279-3863
6001 SW 6th Ave Ste 101, Topeka, KS 66615

M&C Specialties Co. 800-441-6996
90 James Way, Southampton, PA 18966

Medi-Tech International Corp. 800-333-0109
26 Court St, Brooklyn, NY 11242
Non-occlusive SPAND-GEL gel sheets to maintain moist enviroment for treatment of burns and donor site skin grafts.

Medix Pharmaceuticals Americas, Inc. 888-242-3463
12505 Starkey Rd Ste M, Largo, FL 33773
Biafine WDE (wound-dressing emulsion) for all types of partial/full-thickness wounds, first/second-degree burns and general dry-skin conditions. Biafine RE (radiodermatitis emulsion) for all types of radiation dermatitis (redness, erythema, dry and moist desquamations) and general dry-skin conditions (PPE/hand-foot syndrome).

Mylan Pharmaceuticals Inc 888-523-7835
Research Triangle Pa, Morgantown, NC 27709
HYDROCOL is a hydrocolloid wound dressing.

Mylan Technologies, Inc. 800-532-5226
110 Lake St, Saint Albans, VT 05478
MEDIFILM, series of USP Class VI extruded Hytrel co-polyester, urethane and Pebax high moisture vapor films, available with hypoallergenic acrylic or hydrocolloid adhesive systems, laminated to synergistic absorbent foams and available in rolls.

Romaine, Inc. D.B.A. Koldcare 800-294-7101
2026 Sterling Ave, Elkhart, IN 46516
KOOLABURN comes in a variety of sizes from a 2' x 2' pad to a 50' x 72' fire blanket. Gelled water is imbedded in polyester dressings and cools by evaporation. Gel is not wet or messy and has a 5 year shelf life. For use on 1st & 2nd degree burns.

Scapa Medical 310-419-0567
540 N Oak St, Inglewood, CA 90302

Southwest Technologies, Inc. 800-247-9951
1746 E Levee St, North Kansas City, MO 64116
Elasto-Gel semi-occlusive dressings.

Spenco Medical Corp. 254-772-6000
PO Box 2501, Waco, TX 76702
2ND SKIN® Moist Burn Pad.

Surgic Aid, Inc. 800-338-5213
37 Crystal Ave # 287, Derry, NH 03038

The Hymed Group Corp. 610-865-9876
1890 Bucknell Dr, Bethlehem, PA 18015
Medical hydrolysate of type I collagen: CellerateRX powder and gel for a variety of wounds...helps reduce the chance of scarring, acts as a tissue adhesive, reduces pain at the wound site.

W.L. Gore & Associates,Inc 928-526-3030
1505 North Fourth St., Flagstaff, AZ 86004
Wound & burn dressing.

Water-Jel Technologies 800-275-3433
50 Broad St, Carlstadt, NJ 07072
COOL-JEL: burn cream available in unit dose (3.5 grams) or 4 oz. size. BURN-JEL: burn cream with lidocaine available in unit dose (3.5 grams) or 4 oz. size.

Winfield Laboratories 800-527-4616
PO Box 832297, Richardson, TX 75083
N-TERFACE, 5 sizes available. Break-away wound dressing.

Zimmer Holdings, Inc. 800-613-6131
1800 W Center St, PO Box 708, Warsaw, IN 46580

DRESSING, WOUND AND BURN, OCCLUSIVE, HEATED
(Surgery) 79MSA

Integrity Medical Devices Inc 609-567-8175
360 Fairview Ave, Hammonton, NJ 08037
Occlusive burn and wound dressing.

DRESSING, WOUND, HYDROGEL W/OUT DRUG AND/OR BIOLOGIC *(Surgery) 79NAE*

Adelphia Medical Inc. 410-742-7104
1525 Edgemore Ave Ste 1, Salisbury, MD 21801

Ameriderm Laboratories, Ltd. 973-279-5100
13 Kentucky Ave, Paterson, NJ 07503
Hydrogel non sterile.

Corium International, Inc. 616-656-4563
4558 50th St SE, Grand Rapids, MI 49512
Sterile wound dressing.

DRESSING, WOUND, HYDROGEL W/OUT DRUG AND/OR BIOLOGIC *(cont'd)*

Global Biomedics Corporation 800-473-1122
11005 Indian Trl Ste 102, Dallas, TX 75229
Hydrogel dressing.

Global Health Products, Inc 757-224-0177
1099 Jay St Ste E, Rochester, NY 14611
Notear.

Integrity Medical Devices Inc 609-567-8175
360 Fairview Ave, Hammonton, NJ 08037
Hydrogel dressing.

Royal Converting, Inc. 865-938-7828
1615 Highway 33 S, New Tazewell, TN 37825

Soluble Systems, Llc 757-877-8899
2520 58th St, Hampton, VA 23661

DRESSING, WOUND, HYDROPHILIC *(Surgery) 79NAC*

Adelphia Medical Inc. 410-742-7104
1525 Edgemore Ave Ste 1, Salisbury, MD 21801

American White Cross - Houston 609-514-4744
15200 North Fwy, Houston, TX 77090
Hydophilic wound dressing.

Biolife, Llc 800-722-7559
1235 Tallevast Rd, Sarasota, FL 34243
Hydrophilic wound dressing.

Brady Precision Converting, Llc 214-275-9595
1801 Big Town Blvd Ste 100, Mesquite, TX 75149
A variety of absorbent dressings made for OEM's with foams and other absorbent materials.

Dr. Len's Medical Products Llc 678-908-8180
412 Atwood Rd, Erdenheim, PA 19038
Abrams all-in-one.

Hollister, Inc. 847-680-2849
366 Draft Ave, Stuarts Draft, VA 24477

Integrity Medical Devices Inc 609-567-8175
360 Fairview Ave, Hammonton, NJ 08037
Hydrophilic wound dressing.

Kentron Health Care, Inc. 615-384-0573
3604 Kelton Jackson Rd, P.o. Box 120, Springfield, TN 37172
Wound dressings.

Marine Polymer Technologies, Inc. 888-666-2560
461 Boston St Unit B5, Topsfield, MA 01983
Hydrophilic wound dressing.

Royal Converting, Inc. 865-938-7828
1615 Highway 33 S, New Tazewell, TN 37825

Rynel, Inc. 207-882-0200
11 Twin Rivers Dr, Wiscasset, ME 04578
Hydrophilic polyurethane dressing.

3m Company 651-733-4365
601 22nd Ave S, Brookings, SD 57006

DRESSING, WOUND, OCCLUSIVE *(Surgery) 79NAD*

Aso Corporation 941-379-0300
300 Sarasota Center Blvd, Sarasota, FL 34240
Hydrocolloid, Scar Treatment

Blue Sky Medical Group Incorporated 727-392-1261
5924 Balfour Ct Ste 102, Carlsbad, CA 92008
Npwt transparent adhesive dressing.

Brady Precision Converting, Llc 214-275-9595
1801 Big Town Blvd Ste 100, Mesquite, TX 75149
Sterile composite dressings made to customer specifications.

Corium International, Inc. 616-656-4563
4558 50th St SE, Grand Rapids, MI 49512
Various sizes of transparent film dressings.

Dr. Len's Medical Products Llc 678-908-8180
412 Atwood Rd, Erdenheim, PA 19038
Abrams surgical dressing.

Gelsmart Llc 973-884-8995
30 Leslie Ct Ste B-202, Whippany, NJ 07981
Gel, wound dressing.

Global Health Products, Inc 757-224-0177
1099 Jay St Ste E, Rochester, NY 14611
Defend - defend-plus - medifoam - retare.

Health Ent., Inc. 508-695-0727
90 George Leven Dr, North Attleboro, MA 02760
Occlusive wound dressing.

DRESSING, WOUND, OCCLUSIVE *(cont'd)*

Hollister, Inc. 847-680-2849
366 Draft Ave, Stuarts Draft, VA 24477

Innovative Wound Management, Llc 440-461-1295
29001 Cedar Rd Ste 325, Cleveland, OH 44124
Occlusive wound dressing.

Integra Lifesciences Corp. 609-275-0500
311 Enterprise Dr, Plainsboro, NJ 08536
Transparent dressing.

Integrity Medical Devices Inc 609-567-8175
360 Fairview Ave, Hammonton, NJ 08037
Non-adhering dressing.

Polygell Llc. 973-884-8995
30 Leslie Ct, Whippany, NJ 07981
Gel, wound dressing.

Royal Converting, Inc. 865-938-7828
1615 Highway 33 S, New Tazewell, TN 37825

3m Company 651-733-4365
601 22nd Ave S, Brookings, SD 57006

DRILL, BONE *(Orthopedics) 87QRE*

Biolectron, Inc. 800-524-0677
25 Commerce Dr, Allendale, NJ 07401
CURVTEK pneumatic drill and cartridge system to create curved tunnels in bone for soft tissue reattachment.

International Hospital Supply Co. 800-398-9450
6914 Canby Ave Ste 105, Reseda, CA 91335

Kls-Martin L.P. 800-625-1557
11239-1 St. John`s Industrial, Parkway South
Jacksonville, FL 32250
Bone drills.

Micro-Aire Surgical Instruments, Inc. 800-722-0822
1641 Edlich Dr, Charlottesville, VA 22911

Miltex Inc. 800-645-8000
589 Davies Dr, York, PA 17402

Minnesota Bramstedt Surgical, Inc. 800-456-5052
1835 Energy Park Dr, Saint Paul, MN 55108
The Woodpecker - a total hip broaching system.

Richards Micro-Tool, Inc. 508-746-6900
250 Nicks Road,, Plymouth, MA 02360-2800

Simpex Medical, Inc. 800-851-9753
401 E Prospect Ave, Mount Prospect, IL 60056

Smith & Nephew, Inc., Endoscopy Division 800-343-8386
150 Minuteman Rd, Andover, MA 01810
Battery operated.

Stryker Corp. 800-726-2725
2825 Airview Blvd, Portage, MI 49002

Stryker Spine 866-457-7463
2 Pearl Ct, Allendale, NJ 07401

Tegra Medical Inc. 508-541-4200
9 Forge Pkwy, Franklin, MA 02038

Vilex, Inc. 800-872-4911
345 Old Curry Hollow Rd, Pittsburgh, PA 15236

DRILL, BONE, POWERED *(Dental And Oral) 76DZI*

Aesculap Implant Systems Inc. 1-800-234-9179
3773 Corporate Pkwy, Center Valley, PA 18034

Altair Instruments, Inc. 805-388-8503
330 Wood Rd Ste J, Camarillo, CA 93010

Biomet Microfixation Inc. 800-874-7711
1520 Tradeport Dr, Jacksonville, FL 32218
Various types of drills.

Jedmed Instruments Co. 314-845-3770
5416 Jedmed Ct, Saint Louis, MO 63129

Nobel Biocare Usa, Llc 800-579-6515
22715/22725 Savi Ranch Parkway, Yorba Linda, CA 92887
Surgical drill, amorphous diamond-like coated drill.

Oratronics, Inc. 212-986-0050
405 Lexington Ave, New York, NY 10174
Abutment kit (bone spiral).

Osada, Inc. 800-426-7232
8436 W 3rd St Ste 695, Los Angeles, CA 90048
PEDO30W/SH29S-LVS-MCS8. Saw attachment handpieces to Pedo 30W/LVS: SSH, SOH & SRH. OSADA saw handpieces: attachments to E-coupler LVS, SSH (sagittal), SOH (oscillating) and SRH (reciprocating).

DRILL, CANNULATED *(Orthopedics) 87QRF*

Stryker Spine 866-457-7463
2 Pearl Ct, Allendale, NJ 07401

Zimmer Holdings, Inc. 800-613-6131
1800 W Center St, PO Box 708, Warsaw, IN 46580
5-12mm with Trinkle fitting.

DRILL, CRANIAL *(Cns/Neurology) 84QRG*

Aesculap Implant Systems Inc. 1-800-234-9179
3773 Corporate Pkwy, Center Valley, PA 18034
ELAN-E electric cable-connected cranial drill; 18,000 max RPM. Standard perforator hit, craniotome, burr and twist bits. Weighs 19 oz. Borchardt chuck included.

Codman & Shurtleff, Inc 800-225-0460
325 Paramount Dr, Raynham, MA 02767
3 models - $1,750 for model 20,000; 20,000 max RPM; wght. 20 oz. $1,350 for AIR DRILL; 100,000 max RPM; wght. 5 oz; $1,850 for UNITIZED 1000; 1,000 max RPM; wght 28 oz. All models with pneumatic power, nitrogen gas.

Integrated Surgical Systems 530-792-2600
1850 Research Park Dr, Davis, CA 95618
NeuroMate system is currently designed to perform stereotactic functional Neurosurgeries such as tumor biopsy, Parkinson's disease and Epilepsy electrode implantation, Neuroendoscopy, etc.

Kirwan Surgical Products, Inc. 888-547-9267
180 Enterprise Dr, PO Box 427, Marshfield, MA 02050
Disposable wire pass drills and cranio blades.

Richards Micro-Tool, Inc. 508-746-6900
250 Nicks Road,, Plymouth, MA 02360-2800

Stryker Spine 866-457-7463
2 Pearl Ct, Allendale, NJ 07401

DRILL, DENTAL, INTRAORAL *(Dental And Oral) 76DZA*

Abrasive Technology, Inc. 740-548-4100
8400 Green Meadows Dr N, Lewis Center, OH 43035
Intraoral, dental drills.

Aesculap Implant Systems Inc. 1-800-234-9179
3773 Corporate Pkwy, Center Valley, PA 18034

Align Technology, Inc. 408-470-1000
881 Martin Ave, Santa Clara, CA 95050
Drill,dental,intraoral.

Arnold Tuber Industries 716-648-3363
97 Main St, Hamburg, NY 14075
Intraoral dental drill.

Biomet 3i 800-342-5454
4555 Riverside Dr, Palm Beach Gardens, FL 33410
Various including the OSSEOCISION® Surgical Drill System

Biomet Microfixation Inc. 800-874-7711
1520 Tradeport Dr, Jacksonville, FL 32218
Various types of drills.

Bisco, Inc. 847-534-6000
1100 W Irving Park Rd, Schaumburg, IL 60193
Root canal drill, various types.

Citizens Development Center 214-637-2911
8800 Ambassador Row, Dallas, TX 75247
Burr and drill set.

Coltene/Whaledent Inc. 330-916-8858
235 Ascot Pkwy, Cuyahoga Falls, OH 44223
Dental drill.

D&S Dental, Llc 423-928-1299
3111 Hanover Rd, Johnson City, TN 37604
Rotary files.

Dentalez Group 866-DTE-INFO
101 Lindenwood Dr Ste 225, Valleybrooke Corporate Center Malvern, PA 19355

Dentalez Group, Stardental Division 717-291-1161
1816 Colonial Village Ln, Lancaster, PA 17601
Intra oral device for snoring and sleep apnea.

H & H Co. 909-390-0373
4435 E Airport Dr Ste 108, Ontario, CA 91761
Drill, dental, intraoral.

Kavo Dental Corp. 800-323-8029
340 East Route 22, Lake Zurich, IL 60047

Miltex Dental Technologies, Inc. 516-576-6022
589 Davies Dr, York, PA 17402
Various types of intraoral drills.

DRILL, DENTAL, INTRAORAL *(cont'd)*

O Company 800-228-0477
600 Paisano St NE, Albuquerque, NM 87123
Tri-spade drill anti-chatter.

Oco Inc. 800-228-0477
600 Paisano St NE Ste A, Albuquerque, NM 87123
Dental drill.

Osada, Inc. 800-426-7232
8436 W 3rd St Ste 695, Los Angeles, CA 90048
XL-30W/FS/SH28S-LVS-MCC6. XL-30W/VSFP/SH, LVSA-MCC8.

Palisades Dental, Llc 201-569-0050
111 Cedar Ln, Englewood, NJ 07631
Dental drill.

Precision Dental Int, Inc. 818-992-1888
21361 Deering Ct, Canoga Park, CA 91304
Dental drill.

Renick Ent., Inc. 561-863-4183
1211 W 13th St, Riviera Beach, FL 33404
3 flute vibration free drills.

Spring Health Products, Inc. 800-800-1680
705 General Washington Ave Ste 701, Norristown, PA 19403
High-speed drills.

DRILL, INTRAMEDULLARY *(Cns/Neurology) 84QRI*

Zimmer Holdings, Inc. 800-613-6131
1800 W Center St, PO Box 708, Warsaw, IN 46580

DRILL, MANUAL (WITH BURR, TREPHINE & ACCESSORIES) *(Cns/Neurology) 84HBG*

Bausch & Lomb Surgical 636-255-5051
3365 Tree Court Ind Blvd, Saint Louis, MO 63122

Biomet Microfixation Inc. 800-874-7711
1520 Tradeport Dr, Jacksonville, FL 32218
Various types of drills.

George Tiemann & Co. 800-843-6266
25 Plant Ave, Hauppauge, NY 11788

Medtronic Neurosurgery 800-468-9710
125 Cremona Dr, Goleta, CA 93117
Ventriculostomy kit, cranial hand drill kit.

Mpp Hand Drill Company Llc. 715-294-3400
807 Prospect Ave, Osceola, WI 54020
Manual drill, hand drill.

Rsb Spine Llc. 866-241-2104
2530 Superior Ave E Ste 703, Cleveland, OH 44114
Various drills, burrs, trephines.

DRILL, MIDDLE EAR SURGERY *(Ear/Nose/Throat) 77QRJ*

Acumed Instruments Corp. 800-234-5045
5286 Evanwood Ave, Oak Park, CA 91377

Jedmed Instruments Co. 314-845-3770
5416 Jedmed Ct, Saint Louis, MO 63129

Micro-Aire Surgical Instruments, Inc. 800-722-0822
1641 Edlich Dr, Charlottesville, VA 22911
Otologic drill.

DRILL, ORAL SURGERY *(Dental And Oral) 76QRK*

Bvr Aero Precision Corporation 815-874-2471
3358 N Publishers Dr # 60, Rockford, IL 61109

Embo-Optics, Llc. 887-885-6400
100 Cummings Ctr # 326B, Beverly, MA 01915
Portable IV illuminator with lighted monitoring feature aids medical personnel in assuring that all IV solutions and medications are infusing properly and at the correct infusion rate. Greatly enhance patient safety in aiding to prevent any adverse events during infusion.

Fc Industries Inc. 937-275-8700
4900 Webster St, Dayton, OH 45414

Medidenta International, Inc. 800-221-0750
3923 62nd St, PO Box 409, Woodside, NY 11377

Micro-Aire Surgical Instruments, Inc. 800-722-0822
1641 Edlich Dr, Charlottesville, VA 22911

Osada, Inc. 800-426-7232
8436 W 3rd St Ste 695, Los Angeles, CA 90048
PEDO-30W/SH26SP-LVSA-MCS8. (XL S30 oral surgery - implant.) XLS30/FS/CS031+CH67IC-LVSA-MCC8 with irrigation pump.

DRILL, PERFORATOR *(Cns/Neurology) 84QRL*

Codman & Shurtleff, Inc 800-225-0460
325 Paramount Dr, Raynham, MA 02767

DRILL, PERFORATOR *(cont'd)*

Miltex Inc. 800-645-8000
589 Davies Dr, York, PA 17402

DRILL, POWERED COMPOUND (WITH BURR, TREPHINE & ACCESSORIES) *(Cns/Neurology) 84HBF*

Acra Cut, Inc. 978-263-0250
989 Main St, Acton, MA 01720
Cranial perforator, disposable & resuable.

Bausch & Lomb Surgical 636-255-5051
3365 Tree Court Ind Blvd, Saint Louis, MO 63122

Codman & Shurtleff, Inc 800-225-0460
325 Paramount Dr, Raynham, MA 02767

DRILL, SURGICAL, ENT (ELECTRIC OR PNEUMATIC) *(Ear/Nose/Throat) 77ERL*

Clinimed, Incorporated 877-CLINIMED
303 Markus Ct, Sandy Brae Industrial Park, Newark, DE 19713

Gyrus Ent L.L.C., Sub. Of Gyrus Acmi, Inc. 508-804-2739
2925 Appling Rd, Bartlett, TN 38133
Various types of ent surgical drills.

H&H Instruments
4950 Crescent Technical Ct, St Augustine, FL 32086
Hhi electric rotary drill.

Jedmed Instruments Co. 314-845-3770
5416 Jedmed Ct, Saint Louis, MO 63129

Karl Storz Endoscopy-America Inc. 800-421-0837
600 Corporate Pointe, Culver City, CA 90230

Mednet Locator, Inc. 800-754-5070
7000 Shadow Oaks Dr, Memphis, TN 38125
Microdrill.

Medtronic Powered Surgical Solutions 800-643-2773
4620 N Beach St, Haltom City, TX 76137
Various models of motors.

Promex Technologies, Llc 317-736-0128
3049 Hudson St, Franklin, IN 46131
Promex ent tissue removal system.

Warsaw Orthopedic, Inc. 901-396-3133
2500 Silveus Xing, Warsaw, IN 46582
Drill.

DRILLS, BURRS, TREPHINES AND ACCESSORIES (MANUAL), REPROCESSED *(Cns/Neurology) 84NLO*

Ascent Healthcare Solutions 480-763-5300
10232 S 51st St, Phoenix, AZ 85044
Drills,burrs,trephines & accessories(manual).

DRINK, GLUCOSE TOLERANCE *(Chemistry) 75MRV*

Vegamed, Inc. 787-807-0392
39 Calle Las Flores, Edificio Multifabril #5, Vega Baja, PR 00693
Bru-glucola 100.

Vineland Syrup Inc. 856-691-5772
723 S East Blvd, Vineland, NJ 08360
Glucose tolerance drink.

DRIVER, BAND, ORTHODONTIC *(Dental And Oral) 76ECT*

G & H Wire Co. 800-526-1026
2165 Earlywood Dr, Franklin, IN 46131

Glenroe Technologies 800-237-4060
1912 44th Ave E, Bradenton, FL 34203
Elastomeric ligature ties.

Lancer Orthodontics, Inc. 760-304-2705
253 Pawnee St, San Marcos, CA 92078
Driver, band, orthodontic.

Premier Dental Products Co. 888-670-6100
1710 Romano Dr, PO Box 4500, Plymouth Meeting, PA 19462

DRIVER, BONE STAPLE *(Orthopedics) 87QRO*

Stryker Spine 866-457-7463
2 Pearl Ct, Allendale, NJ 07401

Telos Medical Equipment (Austin & Assoc., Inc.) 800-934-3029
1109 Sturbridge Rd, Fallston, MD 21047
MEMODYN STAPLE, Compression staples for bone fixation of arthrodesis fusion and osteotomy surgeries of the foot, ankle, and hand.

Zimmer Holdings, Inc. 800-613-6131
1800 W Center St, PO Box 708, Warsaw, IN 46580

DRIVER, BONE STAPLE, POWERED *(Orthopedics) 87HXJ*

Medisiss 866-866-7477
2747 SW 6th St, Redmond, OR 97756
Various staple drivers,sterile.

DRIVER, PROSTHESIS *(Orthopedics) 87HWR*

Biomet, Inc. 574-267-6639
56 E Bell Dr, PO Box 587, Warsaw, IN 46582
Various types of prosthesis driver.

Bioquest 480-350-9944
2211 W 1st St Ste 106, Tempe, AZ 85281
Knee driver.

Boston Scientific Corporation 508-652-5578
780 Brookside Dr, Spencer, IN 47460

Centinel Spine Inc. 952-885-0500
505 Park Ave Fl 14, New York, NY 10022
STALIF C Inserter

DJO Inc. 800-336-6569
1430 Decision St, Vista, CA 92081

Motion Control, Inc. 888-696-2767
2401 S 1070 W Ste B, Salt Lake City, UT 84119
Utah ServoPro System.

Nemcomed 800-255-4576
801 Industrial Dr, Hicksville, OH 43526
New version control Hip Stem Inserter and Universal Hip Stem Extractor.

Stryker Spine 866-457-7463
2 Pearl Ct, Allendale, NJ 07401

Warsaw Orthopedic, Inc. 901-396-3133
2500 Silveus Xing, Warsaw, IN 46582
Various types of prosthesis drivers.

Zimmer Holdings, Inc. 800-613-6131
1800 W Center St, PO Box 708, Warsaw, IN 46580

Zimmer Trabecular Metal Technology 800-613-6131
10 Pomeroy Rd, Parsippany, NJ 07054
Hip stem bullet nose impactor.

DRIVER, SURGICAL, PIN *(Surgery) 79GFC*

Abbott Spine, Inc. 847-937-6100
12708 Riata Vista Cir Ste B-100, Austin, TX 78727
Torque limiter.

Biomet, Inc. 574-267-6639
56 E Bell Dr, PO Box 587, Warsaw, IN 46582
Various types of drivers for surgical pins.

Depuy Spine, Inc. 800-227-6633
325 Paramount Dr, Raynham, MA 02767
Pin driver.

Kmedic 800-955-0559
190 Veterans Dr, Northvale, NJ 07647

Rush-Berivon, Inc. 800-251-7874
1010 19th St, P.O. Box 1851, Meridian, MS 39301
$225.00/per 6mm or 5mm units); for 3mm, 2mm, or 1.6mm units.

Stryker Spine 866-457-7463
2 Pearl Ct, Allendale, NJ 07401

Symmetry Medical Usa, Inc. 574-267-8700
486 W 350 N, Warsaw, IN 46582
Surgical instrument motors and accessories-attachments.

Vilex, Inc. 931-474-7550
111 Moffitt St, McMinnville, TN 37110

Zimmer Holdings, Inc. 800-613-6131
1800 W Center St, PO Box 708, Warsaw, IN 46580

DRIVER, WIRE *(Orthopedics) 87SGD*

Kmedic 800-955-0559
190 Veterans Dr, Northvale, NJ 07647

Micro-Aire Surgical Instruments, Inc. 800-722-0822
1641 Edlich Dr, Charlottesville, VA 22911

Stryker Corp. 800-726-2725
2825 Airview Blvd, Portage, MI 49002

Vilex, Inc. 800-872-4911
345 Old Curry Hollow Rd, Pittsburgh, PA 15236

Westcon Orthopedics, Inc. 800-382-4975
4 Craig Rd, Neshanic Station, NJ 08853
S&S 15, Battery operated, disposable driver for orthopedic wires, sterile.

DRIVER, WIRE, AND BONE DRILL, MANUAL
(Dental And Oral) 76DZJ

Aesculap Implant Systems Inc. 1-800-234-9179
3773 Corporate Pkwy, Center Valley, PA 18034

Biomet Microfixation Inc. 800-874-7711
1520 Tradeport Dr, Jacksonville, FL 32218
Various types of drills.

Kmedic 800-955-0559
190 Veterans Dr, Northvale, NJ 07647

DRIVER/EXTRACTOR, BONE NAIL/PIN *(Orthopedics) 87QRM*

Holmed Corporation 508-238-3351
40 Norfolk Ave, South Easton, MA 02375

Miltex Inc. 800-645-8000
589 Davies Dr, York, PA 17402
Autoclavable stainless steel pin pullers.

Minnesota Bramstedt Surgical, Inc. 800-456-5052
1835 Energy Park Dr, Saint Paul, MN 55108
The Woodpecker - total hip broaching device also used for extraction of intramedullary nails.

Stryker Spine 866-457-7463
2 Pearl Ct, Allendale, NJ 07401

Westcon Orthopedics, Inc. 800-382-4975
4 Craig Rd, Neshanic Station, NJ 08853
Cap, pin, external. Disposable wire driver, S&S 15, battery operated, disposable driver for orthopedic wires, sterile.

Zimmer Holdings, Inc. 800-613-6131
1800 W Center St, PO Box 708, Warsaw, IN 46580

DRIVER/EXTRACTOR, BONE PLATE *(Orthopedics) 87QRN*

Holmed Corporation 508-238-3351
40 Norfolk Ave, South Easton, MA 02375

Zimmer Holdings, Inc. 800-613-6131
1800 W Center St, PO Box 708, Warsaw, IN 46580

DROPPER, EAR *(Ear/Nose/Throat) 77KCM*

Src Medical, Inc. 781-826-9100
263 Winter St, Hanover, MA 02339
Various droppers, ent.

DROPPER, EYE *(Ophthalmology) 86QRP*

Kc Pharmaceuticals, Inc. 909-598-9499
3201 Producer Way, Pomona, CA 91768

Medi Inc 800-225-8634
75 York Ave, P.O. Box 302, Randolph, MA 02368

Mps Acacia 800-486-6677
785 Challenger St, Brea, CA 92821

Owen Mumford Usa, Inc. 800-421-6936
1755 W Oak Commons Ct Ste A, Marietta, GA 30062

Profex Medical Products 800-325-0196
2224 E Person Ave, Memphis, TN 38114

The Hymed Group Corp. 610-865-9876
1890 Bucknell Dr, Bethlehem, PA 18015
Collasate Opthalmic Drops for corneal wound healing, and lubrication.

DROPPER, MEDICINE *(General) 80QRQ*

Apothecary Products, Inc. 800-328-2742
11750 12th Ave S, Burnsville, MN 55337

Carex Health Brands 800-526-8051
921 E Amidon St, PO Box 2526, Sioux Falls, SD 57104
Ideal for administering medicine to children, as it dispenses medication at the back of the mouth beyond the taste buds. It is calibrated in 1-tsp and 55-cc increments.

Health Enterprises 800-633-4243
90 George Leven Dr, North Attleboro, MA 02760

Medi Inc 800-225-8634
75 York Ave, P.O. Box 302, Randolph, MA 02368

Plasticoid Co., The 410-398-2800
249 W High St, Elkton, MD 21921
Dropper assemblies complete dropper assemblies with plastic/glass pipette with/without caps in various sizes, including custom made.

Profex Medical Products 800-325-0196
2224 E Person Ave, Memphis, TN 38114

Ross Disposable Products 800-649-6526
401 Traders Blvd E, Unit 10, Mississauga, ON L4Z 2H8 Canada

Ware Medics Glass Works, Inc. 845-429-6950
PO Box 368, Garnerville, NY 10923

DROPPER, NOSE *(Ear/Nose/Throat) 77QRR*

Medi Inc 800-225-8634
75 York Ave, P.O. Box 302, Randolph, MA 02368

Pennsylvania Glass Products Co. 412-621-2853
430 N Craig St, Pittsburgh, PA 15213
Precision.

DRUG METABOLIZING ENZYME GENOTYPING SYSTEMS
(Toxicology) 91NTI

Roche Molecular Systems, Inc. 925-730-8110
4300 Hacienda Dr, Pleasanton, CA 94588
Cytochrome p450 cyp2c19 test, cytochrome p450 cyp2d6 test.

Third Wave Technologies, Inc. 888-898-2357
502 S Rosa Rd, Madison, WI 53719
In vitro diagnostic molecular test.

DRUM, EYE KNIFE TEST *(Ophthalmology) 86HMS*

Bausch & Lomb Surgical 636-255-5051
3365 Tree Court Ind Blvd, Saint Louis, MO 63122

Surgistar Inc. 800-995-7086
2310 La Mirada Dr, Vista, CA 92081
Specialty needles and cannulas for ophthalmology and ENT

DRUM, OPTICOKINETIC *(Ophthalmology) 86HOW*

Gn Otometrics North America 800-289-2150
125 Commerce Dr, Schaumburg, IL 60173
Optokinetic stimulator.

Western Ophthalmics Corporation 800-426-9938
19019 36th Ave W Ste G, Lynnwood, WA 98036

Western Systems Research, Inc. 626-578-7363
127 N Madison Ave Ste 24, Pasadena, CA 91101
Okn drum.

DRYER, FILM, RADIOGRAPHIC *(Dental And Oral) 76EGW*

Carr Corporation 800-952-2398
1547 11th St, Santa Monica, CA 90401

Ge Medical Systems, Llc 262-548-2355
3000 N Grandview Blvd, W-417, Waukesha, WI 53188
Dryer for x-ray film.

S&S Technology 281-815-1300
10625 Telge Rd, Houston, TX 77095

Schueler & Company, Inc. 516-487-1500
PO Box 528, Stratford, CT 06615

DRYER, LABWARE *(Chemistry) 75TBY*

Bry-Air, Inc. 877-379-2479
10793 State Rt. 37 W., Sunbury, OH 43074
Resin dryer.

Industrial Specialities Manufacturing, Inc. 800-781-8487
2741 W Oxford Ave Unit 6, Englewood, CO 80110

Mcgill Airpressure Corp. 614-829-1200
1777 Refugee Rd, Columbus, OH 43207
Vacuum drying systems.

Nutech Molding Corporation 1-800-423-5278
PO Box 840, 2024 Broad St,, Pocomoke City, MD 21851

Reheat Co., Inc. 800-373-4328
10 School St, Danvers, MA 01923

DRYER, RESPIRATORY/ANESTHESIA EQUIPMENT
(General) 80WPV

Allied Healthcare Products, Inc. 800-444-3954
1720 Sublette Ave, Saint Louis, MO 63110
Air dryer.

Cenorin 800-426-1042
6324 S 199th Pl Ste 107, Kent, WA 98032
ThermaSure custom configured drying cabinets reduce the risk of water or airborne contamination after reprocessing, or may be used as a drying station prior to sterilization.

Draeger Safety, Inc. 800-922-5518
101 Technology Dr, Pittsburgh, PA 15275
Respiratory protection equipment.

Industrial Specialities Manufacturing, Inc. 800-781-8487
2741 W Oxford Ave Unit 6, Englewood, CO 80110

Olympic Medical Corp. 206-767-3500
5900 1st Ave S, Seattle, WA 98108

Perma Pure Llc 800-337-3762
8 Executive Dr, Toms River, NJ 08755
Breath dryer, Nafion tubing.

DRYER, RESPIRATORY/ANESTHESIA EQUIPMENT *(cont'd)*

Taga Medical Technologies 800-651-9490
34675 Melinz Pkwy Ste 105, Eastlake, OH 44095

DRYING UNIT *(Chemistry) 75JRJ*

American Dryer, Inc. 800-485-7003
12932 Farmington Rd, Livonia, MI 48150
$244.00 for heated air dryer for hands or hair.

Bayer Healthcare Llc 914-524-2955
555 White Plains Rd Fl 5, Tarrytown, NY 10591
Slide dryer.

Denton Vacuum, Inc. 856-439-9100
1259 N Church St, Moorestown, NJ 08057
$1,650 for DCP-1 critical point dryer.

Pedinol Pharmacal, Inc. 800-733-4665
30 Banfi Plz N, Farmingdale, NY 11735
Formalyde-10 spray; Lazerformalyde solution, and roll-on, Pedi-Boro Soak Paks, Pedi-Dri and Pedi-Pro topical powder, and Breezee Mist foot powder.

Thermo Savant 800-634-8886
100 Colin Dr, Holbrook, NY 11741
SPEEDGEL Compact, integrated, no-maintenance gel dryer with integral, oil-free, vacuum pump. Large drying surface accommodates sequencing or smaller gels.

DUAL CHAMBER, ANTI-TACHYCARDIA, PULSE GENERATOR
(Cardiovascular) 74LWY

St. Jude Medical Cardiac Rhythm Management Div. 800-777-2237
15900 Valley View Ct, Sylmar, CA 91342

DUAL CHAMBER, IMPLANTABLE PULSE GENERATOR
(Cardiovascular) 74LWP

Boston Scientific Corp. 612-582-7448
6645 185th Ave NE, Redmond, WA 98052
Pulse generator, DDD.

Medtronic Puerto Rico Operations Co., Juncos 763-514-4000
Road 31, Km. 24, Hm 4, Ceiba Norte Industrial Park, Juncos, PR 00777
Pulse generator,dual chamber.

DUODENOSCOPE, ESOPHAGO/GASTRO *(Gastro/Urology) 78FDT*

Olympus America, Inc. 800-645-8160
3500 Corporate Pkwy, PO Box 610, Center Valley, PA 18034

Pentax Medical Company 800-431-5880
102 Chestnut Ridge Rd, Montvale, NJ 07645
$19,425.00 for fiberoptic duodenoscope with insertion tube diameter of 11.3mm and a channel size of 4.2mm. $28,140.00 to $31,710.00 for several video duodenoscopes. Color CCD endoscope with insertion tube diameter range of 7.4mm to 12.1mm and channel size of 2.2mm to 4.8mm diameter; suitable for therapeutic and diagnostic procedures. All fully immersible.

Pentax Southern Region Service Center 201-571-2300
8934 Kirby Dr, Houston, TX 77054
Duodenoscope.

Pentax West Coast Service Center 800-431-5880
10410 Pioneer Blvd Ste 2, Santa Fe Springs, CA 90670
Pentax duodenoscope.

DUPLICATOR, X-RAY FILM *(Radiology) 90TFQ*

AMD Technologies Inc. 800-423-3535
218 Bronwood Ave, Los Angeles, CA 90049

Bidwell Industrial Group, Inc., Blu-Ray Division 860-343-5353
2055 S Main St, Middletown, CT 06457
Compact portable radiograph duplicator.

Marconi Medical Systems 800-323-0550
595 Miner Rd, Cleveland, OH 44143

Schueler & Company, Inc. 516-487-1500
PO Box 528, Stratford, CT 06615

Spectronics Corporation 800-274-8888
956 Brush Hollow Rd, Westbury, NY 11590
SPECTROLINE Hand-held X-ray film duplicator.

Techno-Aide, Inc. 800-251-2629
7117 Centennial Blvd, Nashville, TN 37209

Wolf X-Ray Corporation 800-356-9729
100 W Industry Ct, Deer Park, NY 11729
Makes quick copies of all sizes; medical film.

Xma (X-Ray Marketing Associates, Inc.) 800-325-8880
1205 W Lakeview Ct, Windham Lakes Business Park
Romeoville, IL 60446

DURA-SUBSTITUTE *(Cns/Neurology) 84GXQ*

Bridger Biomed, Inc. 908-277-8000
2430 N 7th Ave, Bozeman, MT 59715
Dura substitute, sterile.

Collagen Matrix, Inc. 201-405-1477
509 Commerce St, Franklin Lakes, NJ 07417
Dura subsitute.

Cook Biotech, Incorporated 888-299-4224
1425 Innovation Pl, West Lafayette, IN 47906
Dural Substitute

Pegasus Biologics, Inc. 949-585-9430
10 Pasteur Ste 150, Irvine, CA 92618
Dura substitute.

Shelhigh, Inc. 908-206-8706
650 Liberty Ave, Union, NJ 07083
Dura substitute.

Synovis Life Technologies, Inc 800-255-4018
2575 University Ave W, Saint Paul, MN 55114
Dura-Guard

Synovis Surgical Innovations 800-255-4018
2575 University Ave W, Saint Paul, MN 55114
DURA-GUARD Dural Repair Patch, a processed bovine pericardial patch for use as a dural substitute for the closure of dura mater during neurosurgery.

W.L. Gore & Associates,Inc 928-526-3030
1505 North Fourth St., Flagstaff, AZ 86004
Dura substitute.

DUSTING POWDER, SURGICAL *(Surgery) 79KGP*

Grain Processing Corporation 800-448-4472
1600 Oregon St, Muscatine, IA 52761
Absorbable dusting powder.

National Starch & Chemical Co. 317-656-2227
1001 Bedford Rd, North Kansas City, MO 64116
Surgical dusting powder.

Premier Brands Of America, Inc. 914-667-6200
120 Pearl St, Mount Vernon, NY 10550
Various foot powders.

DYE-BINDING, ALBUMIN, BROMCRESOL, GREEN
(Chemistry) 75CIX

Abbott Diagnostics Div. 626-440-0700
820 Mission St, South Pasadena, CA 91030
Albumin bcg.

Beckman Coulter, Inc. 800-635-3497
740 W 83rd St, Hialeah, FL 33014
$0.045 per test.

Biomerieux Inc. 800-682-2666
100 Rodolphe St, Durham, NC 27712

Caldon Bioscience, Inc. 909-628-9944
2100 S Reservoir St, Pomona, CA 91766
Albumin.

Caldon Biotech, Inc. 757-224-0177
2251 Rutherford Rd, Carlsbad, CA 92008
Albumin.

Carolina Liquid Chemistries Corp. 800-471-7272
510 W Central Ave Ste C, Brea, CA 92821
Albumin or alb.

Genchem, Inc. 714-529-1616
510 W Central Ave Ste D, Brea, CA 92821
Albumin reagent.

Health Chem Diagnostics Llc 954-979-3845
3341 W McNab Rd, Pompano Beach, FL 33069
Bromcresol green dye-binding, albumin.

Jas Diagnostics, Inc. 305-418-2320
7220 NW 58th St, Miami, FL 33166
Albumin.

Medical Chemical Corp. 800-424-9394
19430 Van Ness Ave, Torrance, CA 90501
$22.00 per unit.

Stanbio Laboratory, Inc. 830-249-0772
1261 N Main St, Boerne, TX 78006
$31.50 for 500ml with albumin standard (3ml).

Sterling Diagnostics, Inc. 800-637-2661
36645 Metro Ct, Sterling Heights, MI 48312
Albumin (bcg) reagent set.

DYE-BINDING, ALBUMIN, BROMCRESOL, GREEN *(cont'd)*

Teco Diagnostics 714-693-7788
1268 N Lakeview Ave, Anaheim, CA 92807
Albumin.

Vital Diagnostics Inc. 714-672-3553
1075 W Lambert Rd Ste D, Brea, CA 92821
Various albumin reagents.

DYE-BINDING, ALBUMIN, BROMCRESOL, PURPLE
(Chemistry) 75CJW

Abbott Diagnostics Div. 626-440-0700
820 Mission St, South Pasadena, CA 91030
Albumin bcp.

Carolina Liquid Chemistries Corp. 800-471-7272
510 W Central Ave Ste C, Brea, CA 92821
Albumin reagent.

Intersect Systems, Inc. 360-577-1062
1152 3rd Avenue, Suite D & E, Longview, WA 98632

DYNAMOMETER, AC-POWERED *(Orthopedics) 87LBB*

Ametek 727-536-7831
8600 Somerset Dr, Largo, FL 33773
Isometric strength dynamometer.

Cybernetic Research Laboratories, Inc. 520-571-8065
3562 E 42nd Stra, Tucson, AZ 85713
Ac powered dynamometer.

JTECH Medical 800-985-8324
470 West Longdale Dr., Suite G, Salt Lake City, UT 84115

Kada Research, Inc. 281-385-9951
21218 Kingsland Blvd, Katy, TX 77450
Force measurement device.

Mekanika, Inc. 561-417-7244
3998 Fau Blvd Ste 210, Boca Raton, FL 33431
Spinal stiffness gauge.

DYNAMOMETER, GRIP-STRENGTH (SQUEEZE)
(Anesthesiology) 73BSH

Alimed, Inc. 800-225-2610
297 High St, Dedham, MA 02026

Creative Health Products, Inc. 800-742-4478
5148 Saddle Ridge Rd, Plymouth, MI 48170
$191.00 for CHP analog unit, and $233.00 for CHP digital unit.

Dynatronics Corp. 800-874-6251
7030 Park Centre Dr, Salt Lake City, UT 84121

Elmed, Inc. 630-543-2792
60 W Fay Ave, Addison, IL 60101

Lafayette Instrument Company 800-428-7545
PO Box 5729, 3700 Sagamore Pkwy,, Lafayette, IN 47903
Lafayette Model #78010, JAMAR Model #J00105.

DYNAMOMETER, NON-POWERED *(Orthopedics) 87HRW*

Ametek 727-536-7831
8600 Somerset Dr, Largo, FL 33773
Dmg250, eg250-m muscle strength dynamometer.

Christy Manufacturing Corp. 925-462-7982
1228 Quarry Ln Ste F, Pleasanton, CA 94566
Bulb dynamometer.

Iopi Northwest Company, Llc 425-333-5721
5901 Tolt River Rd NE, Carnation, WA 98014
Tongue strengh measuring device.

JTECH Medical 800-985-8324
470 West Longdale Dr., Suite G, Salt Lake City, UT 84115
Pressure Stimulus Device. Commander Algometer measures pressure applied by examiner to elicit a response for pain tolerance, pain threshold and trigger point tenderness.

Richardson Products, Inc. 888-928-7297
9408 Gulfstream Rd, Frankfort, IL 60423
Dynamometer.

Slawner Ltd., J. 514-731-3378
5713 Cote Des Neiges Rd., Montreal, QUE H3S 1Y7 Canada

Tuzik Boston 800-886-6363
104 Longwater Dr, Assinippi Park, Norwell, MA 02061

Zimmer Trabecular Metal Technology 800-613-6131
10 Pomeroy Rd, Parsippany, NJ 07054
Cks patella peg stop drill.

DYNAMOMETER, OTHER *(Cns/Neurology) 84GWH*

Advanced Mechanical Technology, Inc. (Amti) 800-422-AMTI
176 Waltham St, Watertown, MA 02472

DYNAMOMETER, PHYSICAL MEDICINE, ELECTRONIC
(Physical Med) 89IKG

Bte Technologies, Inc. 800-331-8845
7455 New Ridge Rd Ste L, Hanover, MD 21076
PrimusRS -Isometric, Isotonic, Isokinetic, Eccentric, CPM, Task Simulation, Hand Therapy, Lifting Evaluations, Sports Medicine. Simulator II- Isometric, Isotonic, Task Simulation, Hand Therapy, Geriatrics, Lifting Evaluations.

Cybex International, Inc. 800-667-6544
10 Trotter Dr, Medway, MA 02053
$41,990 for CYBEX 350; $38,990 for CYBEX 330; $29,990 for CYBEX 325 systems for extremity testing, exercise and rehabilitation.

EAR IRRIGATION KIT *(General) 80OGQ*

Centurion Medical Products Corp. 517-545-1135
3310 S Main St, Salisbury, NC 28147

Tri-State Hospital Supply Corp. 517-545-1135
3173 E 43rd St, Yuma, AZ 85365

ECHOCARDIOGRAPH (ULTRASONIC SCANNER)
(Cardiovascular) 74DXK

Analogic Corporation 978-326-4000
8 Centennial Dr, Peabody, MA 01960
Transesophageal echocardiography - single plane probe or bi-plane probe.

Biosound Esaote, Inc. 800-428-4374
8000 Castleway Dr, Indianapolis, IN 46250
MyLab 30CV, MyLab 50, CARIS PLUS, MEGAS ES, TECHNOS MPX

Imacor Llc. 516-393-0970
50 Charles Lindbergh Blvd Ste 200, Uniondale, NY 11553
ImaCor Zura Imaging System; ImaCor Zura TEE system; Zura

Jaco Medical Equipment Inc. 858-278-7743
4848 Ronson Ct Ste E, San Diego, CA 92111

Nasiff Assoc., Inc. 315-676-2346
841 County Route 37 # 1, Central Square, NY 13036
Electrocardiograph, patient leads.

New Life Systems, Inc. 954-972-4600
PO Box 8767, Coral Springs, FL 33075

Pyramid Medical Llc 800-764-1154
10940 Portal Dr, Los Alamitos, CA 90720
Refurbished Ultrasound from all leading Mfr.'s. 'Save thousands, ... without Compromise!' Warranty included.

Universal Ultrasound 800-842-0607
299 Adams St, Bedford Hills, NY 10507
SHIMADZU ultrasound, BIOSOUND ultrasound, Mindray Ultrasound MEDISON ultrasound.

EIA, BLASTOMYCES DERMATITIDIS *(Microbiology) 83MJL*

Gen-Probe, Inc. 800-523-5001
10210 Genetic Center Dr, San Diego, CA 92121
AccuProbe BLASTOMYCES DERMATITIDIS Culture Identification Test - For the identification of Blastomyces dermatitidis isolated from culture.

EJECTOR, SALIVA *(Ear/Nose/Throat) 77QSD*

Chagrin Safety Supply, Inc. 800-227-0468
8227 Washington St # 1, Chagrin Falls, OH 44023

Covidien Lp 508-261-8000
15 Hampshire St, Mansfield, MA 02048

Crosstex International 800-223-2497
10 Ranick Rd, Hauppauge, NY 11788

Crosstex International Ltd., W. Region 800-707-2737
14059 Stage Rd, Santa Fe Springs, CA 90670

Crosstex International,Inc. 888-276-7783
10 Ranick Rd, Hauppauge, NY 11788
CROSSTEX.

Pelton & Crane Co., 704-588-2126
11727 Fruehauf Dr, Charlotte, NC 28273

ELASTOMER, OTHER *(General) 80WWD*

Advansource Biomaterials Corp. 978-657-0075
229 Andover St, Wilmington, MA 01887
CHRONOFLEX AL ether-free, biodurable aliphatic thermoplastic polyurethane elastomers. CHRONOFLEX AR aromatic, solution-grade biodurable segmented polyurethane elastomers. CHRONO FLEX C ether free, biodurable aromatic thermoplastic polyurethane elastomer. CHRONOPRENE extremely soft, rubbery thermoplastic elastomer. CHRONOTHANE aromatic thermoplastic polyurethane elastomers. HYDROTHANE aliphatic, hydrophilic thermoplastic polyurethane elastomeric hydrogels. POLYBLEND aromatic, polyurethane hybrid elastoplastic mixtures. POLYWELD two-component reactive cast elastomer for potting/encapsulating.

Chamberlin Rubber Company, Inc. 585-427-7780
3333 Brighton Henrietta Town Line Rd, PO Box 22700
Rochester, NY 14623

Diamond Polymers, Inc. 888-437-4674
1353 Exeter Rd, Akron, OH 44306
ABS, PP, PE, SAN, PS, PC.

Saint-Gobain Performance Plastics/Clearwater 800-541-6880
4451 110th Ave N, Clearwater, FL 33762
C-FLEX thermoplastic elastomer USPVI Approved.

Tmp Technologies, Inc. 716-895-6100
1200 Northland Ave, Buffalo, NY 14215
General.

Tpv Manufacturingÿ 978-425-8940
2 Shaker Rd Unit A101, Shirley, MA 01464
Thermoplastic elastomers (TPEs) and thermoplastic vulcanizates (TPVs).

Vernay Laboratories, Inc. 800-666-5227
120 E South College St, Yellow Springs, OH 45387

ELASTOMER, SILICONE (SCAR MANAGEMENT) *(Surgery) 79MDA*

Allied Biomedical 800-276-1322
PO Box 392, Ventura, CA 93002
CIMEOSIL - Cimeosil Scar Gel, Cimeosil Laser Gel, Cimeosil Gel Sheeting. Silicone based medical device for treatment of keloids and hypertrophic scars. Laser gel used for erythema after laser resurfacing, chemical peel, etc.

Bio Med Sciences, Inc. 800-257-4566
7584 Morris Ct Ste 218, Allentown, PA 18106
SILON-SES silicone elastomer sheeting combines one-sided adherence and durability for effective, comfortable scar management. SILON-TEX silicone bonded textile combines silicone with a soft and pliable fabric for pressure garments to treat scars. SILON-STS Silicone Thermoplastic splinting combines silicone with a rigid splinting material for transparent facemasks.

Biodermis Corp. 702-260-4466
6000 South Eastern, Sutie 9d, Las Vegas, NV 89119
Silicone gel sheeting.

Biodermis Corp. 800-322-3729
6000 S Eastern Ave Ste 9D, Las Vegas, NV 89119
Gel sheeting.

Blaine Labs, Inc. 800-307-8818
11037 Lockport Pl, Santa Fe Springs, CA 90670
Silicone for scar management.

Brennen Medical, Llc 651-429-7413
1290 Hammond Rd, Saint Paul, MN 55110
Silicone elastomer gel sheeting.

Christy Manufacturing Corp. 925-462-7982
1228 Quarry Ln Ste F, Pleasanton, CA 94566
Elastomer.

Donell 800-324-7455
1801 Taylor Ave, Louisville, KY 40213

Hanson Medical, Inc. 800-771-2215
825 Riverside Ave Ste 2, Paso Robles, CA 93446
Silicone scar gel.

Jenline Industries, Inc. 734-451-0020
92 Blackburn Ctr, Gloucester, MA 01930
Elastomer, silicone, for scar management.

Jmm Distributing, Inc 360-308-9841
10332 Central Valley Rd NE, Poulsbo, WA 98370
Scar less generation iii topical gel.

Lyne Laboratories, Inc. 508-583-8700
10 Burke Dr, Brockton, MA 02301
Silicone gel.

ELASTOMER, SILICONE (SCAR MANAGEMENT) *(cont'd)*

Nearly Me Technologies, Inc. 800-887-3370
3630 South I 35, Suite A, Waco, TX 76702-1475
Silicone gel sheets.

Patterson Medical Supply, Inc. 262-387-8720
W68N158 Evergreen Blvd, Cedarburg, WI 53012
Various types of elastomer putty, foam and gel.

Pillar Surgical, Inc. 800-367-0445
PO Box 8141, La Jolla, CA 92038
Various.

Polygell Llc. 973-884-8995
30 Leslie Ct, Whippany, NJ 07981
Silicone gel sheets-lined and unlined.

Rejuveness Pharamceuticals, Inc. 518-584-5017
125 High Rock Ave, Saratoga Springs, NY 12866
Polydimethyl siloxane sheet.

Spectrum Designs Medical, Inc. 800-239-6399
6387 Rose Ln Ste B, Carpinteria, CA 93013
Spectragel for keloid scars.

Torbot Group Inc., Jobskin Division 800-207-1074
653 Miami St, Toledo, OH 43605
Burn compression garments.

ELASTOMER, SILICONE BLOCK *(Surgery) 79MIB*

Aesthetic And Reconstructive Technologies, Inc. 775-853-6800
3545 Airway Dr Ste 106, Reno, NV 89511
Silicone carving block.

Allied Biomedical 800-276-1322
PO Box 392, Ventura, CA 93002
Multiple durometers/colors available: custom service: AlliedSil implant grade sheeting - long term and short term implantable available in non-reinforced and reinforced.

Bentec Medical, Inc. 757-224-0177
1380 E Beamer St, Woodland, CA 95776
Silcone sheeting.

Hanson Medical, Inc. 800-771-2215
825 Riverside Ave Ste 2, Paso Robles, CA 93446
Silicone elastomer sheeting implant grade.

Pillar Surgical, Inc. 800-367-0445
PO Box 8141, La Jolla, CA 92038
Various.

Spectrum Designs Medical, Inc. 800-239-6399
6387 Rose Ln Ste B, Carpinteria, CA 93013
Calf and gluteal implants, sterile. Preformed-contour silicone carving blocks (Block I and Block VI implants) used to enhance the calf and buttock areas in both men and women.

ELASTOMER, SILICONE RUBBER *(General) 80QSE*

Alimed, Inc. 800-225-2610
297 High St, Dedham, MA 02026

Allergan 800-624-4261
71 S Los Carneros Rd, Goleta, CA 93117

Chamberlin Rubber Company, Inc. 585-427-7780
3333 Brighton Henrietta Town Line Rd, PO Box 22700
Rochester, NY 14623

United Chemical Technologies, Inc. 800-385-3153
2731 Bartram Rd, Bristol, PA 19007
Specialty silanes, silicone fluids, and silicone elastomers.

Vernay Laboratories, Inc. 800-666-5227
120 E South College St, Yellow Springs, OH 45387

ELECTRO-OCULOGRAPH *(Ophthalmology) 86QTM*

Lkc Technologies, Inc. 800-638-7055
2 Professional Dr Ste 222, Gaithersburg, MD 20879
UTAS-E3000mf and EPIC-4000.

ELECTROCARDIOGRAPH, AMBULATORY (WITH ANALYSIS ALGORITHM) *(Cardiovascular) 74MLO*

CardioNet 888-312-BEAT
227 Washington St Ste 300, Conshohocken, PA 19428

eCardio Diagnostics 888-747-1442
1717 N Sam Houston Pkwy W, Houston, TX 77038
eVolution

Md International, Inc. 305-669-9003
11300 NW 41st St, Doral, FL 33178

ELECTROCARDIOGRAPH, AMBULATORY (WITH ANALYSIS ALGORITHM) *(cont'd)*

Medicomp, Inc. 800-23-HEART
7845 Ellis Rd, Melbourne, FL 32904
CardioPAL SAVI - Auto capture Event monitor that analyzes rate, rhythm, morphology, and p-wave abnormalities for the detection of both symptomatic and asymptomatic events.

Memtec Corp. 603-893-8080
68 Stiles Rd Ste D, Salem, NH 03079
Holter recorder model 700.

Rozinn By Scottcare Corporation 800-243-9412
4791 W 150th St, Cleveland, OH 44135
Rozinn's Holter for Windows+ analysis systems can be configured for any Holter application. They feature arrhythmia morphology templating, multi-level editing, superimposition, and page-mode scanning. All systems are based on Intel Microprocessors running the latest Microsoft Windows® OS.

ELECTROCARDIOGRAPH, AMBULATORY(WITHOUT ANALYSIS) *(Cardiovascular) 74MWJ*

Advanced Biosensor, Inc. 803-407-3044
400 Arbor Lake Dr Ste B450, Columbia, SC 29223
Holter recorder.

Braemar, Inc. 800-328-2719
1285 Corporate Center Dr Ste 150, Eagan, MN 55121

Datrix 760-480-8874
340 State Pl, Escondido, CA 92029
Various.

eCardio Diagnostics 888-747-1442
1717 N Sam Houston Pkwy W, Houston, TX 77038
eTrigger; eTrigger Plus

Inovise Medical, Inc. 503-431-3800
10565 SW Nimbus Ave Ste 100, Portland, OR 97223
Cardiovise ecg interpretative software.

Spacelabs Medical Inc. 800-522-7212
5150 220th Ave SE, Issaquah, WA 98029
Holter recorder.

ELECTROCARDIOGRAPH, INTERPRETIVE

(Cardiovascular) 74UER

Eresearchtechnology Inc. 215-972-0420
1818 Market St Ste 1000, Philadelphia, PA 19103

Ge Medical Systems Information Technologies 800-643-6439
8200 W Tower Ave, Milwaukee, WI 53223
12- or 15-lead electrocardiograph, portable or line-operated with 6 to 15 channels. Available options include signal-averaged ECG for late potential analysis, pacemaker evaluation, vectorcardiography, Holter and modem telephone for remote transmission. Transmitting ECG carts. Several models available.

M & I Medical Sales, Inc. 305-663-6444
4711 SW 72nd Ave, Miami, FL 33155

Meza Medical Equipment 888-308-7116
108 W Nakoma St, San Antonio, TX 78216

Midmark Diagnostics Group 800-624-8950
3300 Fujita St, Torrance, CA 90505
The IQmark Digital ECG is a compact, portable device that easily connects to a Windows computer. It features full interpretations, pediatrics to adults, using the Telemed® Analysis algorithm; 12-channel monitoring, storage, review and serial comparison; lead-off detection; local or network database, archive, and e-mail capabilities; reports printed on plain paper; and a weight of less than 11 oz., with no moving parts.

Mortara Instrument, Inc. 800-231-7437
7865 N 86th St, Milwaukee, WI 53224
ELI 100, ELI 200 models available with simultaneous 12-lead acquisition with sampling rate of 500 s/second. Portable, battery or AC power and user-selectable ID formats.

Omni Medical Supply Inc. 800-860-6664
4153 Pioneer Dr, Commerce Township, MI 48390

Qrs Diagnostic, Llc 800-465-8408
14755 27th Ave N, Plymouth, MN 55447
Universal ECG Electrocardiograph, works with Windows 98/ME/2000/XP; 12-lead with optional narrative interpretation; portable device with real-time ECG data; variety of reporting capabilities.

Tsi Medical Ltd. 800-661-7263
47 Athabascan Ave., Unit 105, Sherwood Park, AB T8A-4H3 Canada

ELECTROCARDIOGRAPH, MULTI-CHANNEL

(Cardiovascular) 74QSJ

Cardiac Science Corp. 800-777-1777
500 Burdick Pkwy, Deerfield, WI 53531
Eclipse 850i, Eclipse Plus, and Universal ECG Atria 3000.

Carolina Biological Supply Co. 800-334-5551
2700 York Rd, Burlington, NC 27215

Circadian Systems 800-669-7001
8099 Savage Way, Valley Springs, CA 95252
Automated, portable, one-touch operation, automatic sensitivity, automated stylus positioning, battery or line operated, LCD display, thermal hot-dot printing simultaneous acquisition.

Dh Biomedical, Inc. 800-600-8791
1712 9th St W, Bradenton, FL 34205
Cardiovit AT-10 plus, manufactured by Schiller.

Elmed, Inc. 630-543-2792
60 W Fay Ave, Addison, IL 60101

Galix Biomedical Instrumentation, Inc. 305-534-5905
2555 Collins Ave Ste C-5, Miami Beach, FL 33140
HIGH PERFORMANCE COMPUTERIZED ECG: 10 seconds of virtually artifact-free ECG data acquired simultaneously from all 12 leads. Digital filters for increased accuracy; Line, Muscle, Baseline Drift. Unique patient cable; only 5 low cost, fully shielded, 2-lead cables connected to the data acquisition box. Smallest fully isolated data acquisition box connected to the USB port of any PC; no batteries needed. Easy integration to an unlimited database. Complete ECG and report can be transmitted over internet to another PC

Ge Medical Systems Information Technologies 800-643-6439
8200 W Tower Ave, Milwaukee, WI 53223
12-lead electrocardiograph with interpretation, portable or line-operated with 6 to 12 channels. Available options include signal-averaged ECG for late potential analysis, pacemaker evaluation, vectorcardiography, Holter analysis, modem and cellular telephone for remote transmission.

Md International, Inc. 305-669-9003
11300 NW 41st St, Doral, FL 33178

Midmark Diagnostics Group 800-624-8950
3300 Fujita St, Torrance, CA 90505
The IQmark Digital ECG is a compact, portable device that easily connects to a Windows computer. It features full interpretations, pediatrics to adults, using the Telemed® Analysis algorithm; 12-channel monitoring, storage, review and serial comparison; lead-off detection; local or network database, archive and e-mail capabilities; reports printed on plain paper; and a weight of less then 11 oz., with no moving parts.

Mortara Instrument, Inc. 800-231-7437
7865 N 86th St, Milwaukee, WI 53224
High resolution ECG's, 3-4 channels with interpretation, battery powered.

New Life Systems, Inc. 954-972-4600
PO Box 8767, Coral Springs, FL 33075
ECG with or w/o analyzer.

Nihon Kohden America, Inc. 800-325-0283
90 Icon, Foothill Ranch, CA 92610

Pulse Biomedical Inc. 610-666-5510
1305 Catfish Ln, Norristown, PA 19403
QRS-Card

Ubs Instruments Corporation 818-710-1195
7745 Alabama Ave Ste 7, Canoga Park, CA 91304
Single- and multi-channel ECG units with or without interpretations.

ELECTROCARDIOGRAPH, SINGLE CHANNEL

(Cardiovascular) 74DPS

Accusync Medical Research Corp. 203-877-1610
132 Research Dr, Milford, CT 06460
Egg synchronizer.

Active Corporation 207-326-9100
PO Box 1000, 15 Main Street, Castine, ME 04421
Cardiac monitor.

Agfa Healthcare Corp. 864-421-1815
1 Crosswind Dr, Westerly, RI 02891
Ecg management system.

Biotek Instruments, Inc. 802-655-4040
100 Tigan St, Highland Park, Winooski, VT 05404
Electrocardiograph monitor and machine analyzer.

ELECTROCARDIOGRAPH, SINGLE CHANNEL *(cont'd)*

Cambridge Heart, Inc. 888-CAM-WAVE
100 Ames Pond Dr Ste 100, Tewksbury, MA 01876
Electrocardiograph.

Cardiac Science Corp. 800-777-1777
500 Burdick Pkwy, Deerfield, WI 53531
EK10 and Elite II

Cardinal Healthcare 209, Inc. 610-862-0800
5225 Verona Rd, Fitchburg, WI 53711
Lab.

Cardiomag Imaging, Inc. 518-381-1000
450 Duane Ave, Schenectady, NY 12304
Magnetocardiograph.

Cardiosoft, L.P. 713-623-4009
1776 Yorktown St Ste LL30, Houston, TX 77056
Electrocardiograph.

Compumed, Inc. 800-421-3395
5777 W Century Blvd Ste 360, Los Angeles, CA 90045
Electrocardiograph.

Diagnostic Monitoring Software 775-589-6049
PO Box 3109, 292 Kingsbury Grade, #32, Stateline, NV 89449
Electrocardiograph monitor; electrocardiograph.

Elmed, Inc. 630-543-2792
60 W Fay Ave, Addison, IL 60101
Two models--$1,545 for CARDIOLINE ETA L/O with manual lead selection, heated-stylus recording method; weighs 11 lb. $1,475 for ETA 150 with manual lead selection, automatic lead marker; weighs 7 lb.

Fukuda Denshi Usa, Inc. 800-365-6668
17725 NE 65th St Ste C, Redmond, WA 98052
Electrocardiograph.

Ge Medical Systems Information Technologies 800-643-6439
8200 W Tower Ave, Milwaukee, WI 53223

Her-Mar, Inc. 800-327-8209
8550 NW 30th Ter, Doral, FL 33122
$1,500.00 each.

Hillusa Corp. 305-594-7474
7215 NW 46th St, Miami, FL 33166

Inovise Medical, Inc. 503-431-3800
10565 SW Nimbus Ave Ste 100, Portland, OR 97223
Electrocardiograph phonocardiograph.

Instromedix, A Card Guard Co. 800-633-3361
10255 W Higgins Rd Ste 100, Rosemont, IL 60018

Integrated Medical Devices, Inc. 888-486-6900
549 Electronics Pkwy, Liverpool, NY 13088
Transtelephonic Cardiac Event Recorders

Intelwave, Llc 732-738-8800
1090 King Georges Post Rd Ste 1004, Edison, NJ 08837
Ecg monitor heart rate variability system.

Jabil Global Services 502-240-1000
11201 Electron Dr, Louisville, KY 40299
Electrograph.

Jayza Corp. 305-477-1136
7215 NW 41st St Ste A, Miami, FL 33166

Md International, Inc. 305-669-9003
11300 NW 41st St, Doral, FL 33178

Monarch Art Plastics, Llc. 856-235-5151
3838 Church Rd, Mount Laurel, NJ 08054
Ekg ruler.

Monebo Technologies, Inc. 512-732-0235
1800 Barton Creek Blvd, Austin, TX 78735
Patient monitor.

Nasiff Assoc., Inc. 315-676-2346
841 County Route 37 # 1, Central Square, NY 13036
Electrocardiograph,patient leads.

New Life Systems, Inc. 954-972-4600
PO Box 8767, Coral Springs, FL 33075
Portable or non-portable, with or w/o analyzer.

Nihon Kohden America, Inc. 800-325-0283
90 Icon, Foothill Ranch, CA 92610

Omni Medical Supply Inc. 800-860-6664
4153 Pioneer Dr, Commerce Township, MI 48390

Q-Med, Inc. 732-544-5544
100 Metro Park S., 3rd Fl., South Amboy, NJ 08878
EKG, Interp 1000-Interpretative electrocardiograph.

ELECTROCAUTERY UNIT, BATTERY-POWERED
(Surgery) 79QSK

Alcon Research, Ltd. 800-862-5266
6201 South Fwy, Fort Worth, TX 76134

Bovie Medical Corp. 800-537-2790
5115 Ulmerton Rd, Clearwater, FL 33760

Hospira, Inc. 877-946-7747
755 Jarvis Dr, Morgan Hill, CA 95037
$350.00 for heated-blade unit.

Mectra Labs, Inc. 800-323-3968
PO Box 350, Two Quality Way, Bloomfield, IN 47424
ELECTRO LAVAGE.

Shippert Medical Technologies Corp. 800-888-8663
6248 S Troy Cir Ste A, Centennial, CO 80111
HOTSY CAUTERY, high-temperature surgical cauteries, disposable, sterile fine tip and loop tip. Also, distributor of Aaron electrocautery products.

ELECTROCAUTERY UNIT, ENDOSCOPIC *(Obstetrics/Gyn) 85HIM*

Elmed, Inc. 630-543-2792
60 W Fay Ave, Addison, IL 60101

George Tiemann & Co. 800-843-6266
25 Plant Ave, Hauppauge, NY 11788

Md International, Inc. 305-669-9003
11300 NW 41st St, Doral, FL 33178

Repro-Med Systems, Inc. 845-469-2042
24 Carpenter Rd, Chester, NY 10918

Richard Wolf Medical Instruments Corp. 800-323-9653
353 Corporate Woods Pkwy, Vernon Hills, IL 60061

Total Molding Services, Inc. 215-538-9613
354 East Broad St., Trumbauersville, PA 18970

ELECTROCAUTERY UNIT, GYNECOLOGIC
(Obstetrics/Gyn) 85HGI

Apple Medical Corp. 508-357-2700
28 Lord Rd Ste 135, Marlborough, MA 01752
Electrocautery and accessories.

Bovie Medical Corp. 800-537-2790
5115 Ulmerton Rd, Clearwater, FL 33760

Greenwald Surgical Co., Inc. 219-962-1604
2688 Dekalb St, Gary, IN 46405
Bovie conization.

Rms Medical Products 800-624-9600
24 Carpenter Rd, Chester, NY 10918
GYNECO thermal cautery system.

Rotburg Instruments Of America Inc. 954-331-8046
1560 Sawgrass Corporate Pkwy Fl 4, Sunrise, FL 33323
Various types of sterile and non-sterile gynecologic electrocautery electordes a.

Surgrx, Inc. 877-7-SURGRX
101 Saginaw Dr, Redwood City, CA 94063
Electrosurgical open and laparoscopic instruments.

Tino, S.A. De C.V. 800-024-77-55
Hospital #631, Guadalajara, JALIS 44200 Mexico

ELECTROCAUTERY UNIT, LINE-POWERED *(Surgery) 79QSL*

Biomedics, Inc. 949-458-1998
23322 Peralta Dr Ste 11, Laguna Hills, CA 92653

Elmed, Inc. 630-543-2792
60 W Fay Ave, Addison, IL 60101

Her-Mar, Inc. 800-327-8209
8550 NW 30th Ter, Doral, FL 33122
$1,950.00 each.

Hospira, Inc. 877-946-7747
755 Jarvis Dr, Morgan Hill, CA 95037
$2,950 for model 150, heated mechanical scapel type with digital temp display, pencil grip. Weighs 9.5 lbs. Temperature range 110deg. to 270deg. C.

Integra Radionics 800-466-6814
22 Terry Ave, Burlington, MA 01803

Jayza Corp. 305-477-1136
7215 NW 41st St Ste A, Miami, FL 33166

Jedmed Instruments Co. 314-845-3770
5416 Jedmed Ct, Saint Louis, MO 63129

Md International, Inc. 305-669-9003
11300 NW 41st St, Doral, FL 33178

ELECTROCAUTERY UNIT, LINE-POWERED *(cont'd)*

World Medical Equipment, Inc. 800-827-3747
3915 152nd St NE, Marysville, WA 98271

ELECTROCONVULSIVE THERAPY UNIT (ELECTROSHOCK)
(Cns/Neurology) 84GXC

Mecta Corporation 503-612-6780
19799 SW 95th Ave, Suite B, Bldg. D, Tualatin, OR 97062
MECTA SPECTRUM 5000 and 4000 ECT devices--the company's fourth-generation products--continue to provide the latest technological advances and patient standard of care, while offering increased clinical safety and efficacy. The new .3 msec Ultrabrief Parameters have been shown to sharply reduce cognitive side effects in patients. The 5000 devices offer up to six channels of monitoring ECG, EEG, and optical motion sensing. They also offer the patented EEG Data Analysis, under exclusive license from Duke University. Also available, with or without a personal computer, is Remote Monitoring Software with data logging and printing capabilities for Windows 95, 98 and NT. Add RMSManager, the industry's only ECT database and record-management system for easy analysis and organization of your ECT data. Both software packages are available for the 5000 models. All four models have the CUL classification, UL classification, and CE certification, ISO 9001, and are licensed by Health Canada and other government agencies, allowing them to be marketed worldwide.

Somatics, Llc 847-234-6761
910 Sherwood Dr Ste 23, Lake Bluff, IL 60044
E.c.t. machine.

ELECTRODE, ABLATION, TISSUE, CONDUCTION, PERCUTANEOUS *(Cardiovascular) 74LPB*

Boston Scientific-Neurovascular 510-440-7700
47900 Bayside Pkwy, Fremont, CA 94538
Radio frequency generator.

Cardima, Inc. 888-354-0300
47266 Benicia St, Fremont, CA 94538
Various electrode ablation catheters.

Cryocor, Inc. 858-909-2213
9717 Pacific Heights Blvd, San Diego, CA 92121
Cardiac ablation system.

Ep Technologies, Inc. 888-272-1001
2710 Orchard Pkwy, San Jose, CA 95134
Cardiac ablation system.

Medtronic Ep Systems 763-514-4000
8299 Central Ave NE, Spring Lake Park, Minneapolis, MN 55432
Cardiac ablation system.

Medtronic Puerto Rico Operations Co., Villalba 763-514-4000
PO Box 6001, Rd. 149, Km. 56.3, Villalba, PR 00766
Cardiac ablation system.

Sterilmed, Inc. 763-488-3400
11400 73rd Ave N Ste 100, Maple Grove, MN 55369
Ablation catheter.

ELECTRODE, BIOPOTENTIAL, SURFACE, COMPOSITE
(Physical Med) 89IKA

In Vivo Metric 707-433-2949
PO Box 397, Healdsburg, CA 95448
Reusable Ag-AgCl electrodes for clear and stable recordings of skin biopotentials. Features include 1mm thick Ag-AgCl sensor element, low offset and low noise. Priced $15-$25.

Integral Design Inc. 781-740-2036
52 Burr Rd, Hingham, MA 02043

Oxford Instruments 800-438-8322
300 Baker Ave Ste 150, Concord, MA 01742
TECA NCS 2000 disposable surface electrodes.

Reade Advanced Materials 401-433-7000
PO Box 15039, Riverside, RI 02915
READE - high-purity composite fabrications made to customer specification for medical applications.

ELECTRODE, BIOPOTENTIAL, SURFACE, METALLIC
(Physical Med) 89IKB

Electro-Cap International, Inc. 800-527-2193
1011 W Lexington Rd, PO Box 87, Eaton, OH 45320

The Electrode Store 360-829-0400
PO Box 188, Enumclaw, WA 98022
160 types: to $28.00.

U.F.I. 805-772-1203
545 Main St Ste C2, Morro Bay, CA 93442
$19.00 for Model 1081 SNP Biode.

ELECTRODE, BLOOD GAS, CARBON-DIOXIDE
(Anesthesiology) 73QSO

Radiometer America, Inc. 800-736-0600
810 Sharon Dr, Westlake, OH 44145

Thermo Fisher Scientific Inc. 781-622-1000
81 Wyman St, Waltham, MA 02451

ELECTRODE, BLOOD GAS, OXYGEN *(Anesthesiology) 73QSP*

Radiometer America, Inc. 800-736-0600
810 Sharon Dr, Westlake, OH 44145

Thermo Fisher Scientific Inc. 781-622-1000
81 Wyman St, Waltham, MA 02451

ELECTRODE, BLOOD PH *(Chemistry) 75CHL*

Abbott Point Of Care Inc. 609-443-9300
104 Windsor Center Dr, East Windsor, NJ 08520
Blood gases test.

General Air Service And Supply 303-892-7003
6330 Colorado Blvd, Commerce City, CO 80022
Clinical blood gases.

National Welders 919-544-3772
630 United Dr, Durham, NC 27713
Blood gases.

Opti Medical Systems Inc. 770-510-4444
235 Hembree Park Dr, Roswell, GA 30076
Automated blood gas/ electrolyte analyzer.

Osmetech, Inc. 800-373-6767
757 S Raymond Ave, Pasadena, CA 91105
Automated blood gas/ electrolyte analyzer.

Polar Cryogenics, Inc. 503-239-5252
2734 SE Raymond St, Portland, OR 97202
Blood-gas mixture & lung diffusion mixture.

Radiometer America, Inc. 800-736-0600
810 Sharon Dr, Westlake, OH 44145

Respironics California, Inc. 724-387-4559
2271 Cosmos Ct, Carlsbad, CA 92011
End tidal co2 monitor.

Respironics Novametrix, Llc. 724-387-4559
5 Technology Dr, Wallingford, CT 06492
End tidal co2 monitor.

Thermo Fisher Scientific Inc. 781-622-1000
81 Wyman St, Waltham, MA 02451

Vital Diagnostics Inc. 714-672-3553
1075 W Lambert Rd Ste D, Brea, CA 92821
Various reagents for the measurement of bicarbonate.

ELECTRODE, CATHETER TIP *(Cardiovascular) 74QSQ*

Dynamics Research Corp. 800-522-4321
60 Frontage Rd, Andover, MA 01810

ELECTRODE, CLIP, FETAL SCALP (AND APPLICATOR)
(Obstetrics/Gyn) 85HIQ

Rocket Medical Plc. 800-707-7625
150 Recreation Park Dr Ste 3, Hingham, MA 02043

ELECTRODE, CORNEAL *(Ophthalmology) 86HLZ*

Cardinal Healthcare 209, Inc. 610-862-0800
5225 Verona Rd, Fitchburg, WI 53711
Erg-jet electrode.

Hansen Ophthalmic Development Lab 319-338-1285
745 Avalon Pl, Coralville, IA 52241
Electrode for electroretinography.

ELECTRODE, CORTICAL *(Cns/Neurology) 84GYC*

Ad-Tech Medical Instrument Corp. 800-776-1555
1901 William St, Racine, WI 53404
Wyler subdural strips and grids.

Cardinal Healthcare 209, Inc. 610-862-0800
5225 Verona Rd, Fitchburg, WI 53711
Electrode, cortical.

Grass Technologies, An Astro-Med, Inc. Product Gro 401-828-4002
53 Airport Park Drive, Rockland, MA 02370
Cortical electrode.

Pmt Corp. 800-626-5463
1500 Park Rd, Chanhassen, MN 55317

ELECTRODE, CUTANEOUS *(Cns/Neurology) 84GXY*

Ambu A/S 457-225-2210
6740 Baymeadow Dr, Glen Burnie, MD 21060
Tens electrode,surface electrode.

Ambu, Inc. 800-262-8462
6740 Baymeadow Dr, Glen Burnie, MD 21060

Avazzia, Inc. 214-575-2820
13154 Coit Rd Ste 200, Dallas, TX 75240
Electrode pads, ear clips. flex, roller and chest electrodes.

Bio-Logic Systems Corp. 800-323-8326
1 Bio Logic Plz, Mundelein, IL 60060

Bio-Research Associates, Inc. 414-357-7525
9275 N 49th St Ste 150, Brown Deer, WI 53223
Emg electrode.

Bioflex, Inc. 614-236-8079
3055 Templeton Rd, Columbus, OH 43209
Stimulation garments such as pants, trousers, arm sleeves, belts etc.

Biomed Products Llc. 916-852-8620
11300 Sanders Dr Ste 26, Rancho Cordova, CA 95742
Biopotential skin electrode.

Cadwell Laboratories 800-245-3001
909 N Kellogg St, Kennewick, WA 99336
CADWELL safe electrodes.

Cardinal Healthcare 209, Inc. 610-862-0800
5225 Verona Rd, Fitchburg, WI 53711
Surface electrodes.

Dermawave, Llc 561-784-0599
15693 83rd Ln N, Loxahatchee, FL 33470
Cutaneous electrodes.

Docxs Biomedical Products And Accessories 707-462-2351
564 S Dora St Ste A-1, Ukiah, CA 95482
Biopoteutial skin electrodes, probes, sensors and reference electrodes.

Fisher Scientific Co., Llc. 201-703-3131
1 Reagent Ln, Fair Lawn, NJ 07410
Gill hematoxylin stain.

Grass Technologies, An Astro-Med, Inc. Product Gro 401-828-4002
53 Airport Park Drive, Rockland, MA 02370
Surface electrode.

Hospira Sedation, Inc. 877-946-7747
5 Billerica Ave, 101 Billerica Avenue, North Billerica, MA 01862
Various.

Hydrodot, Inc. 978-399-0206
238 Littleton Rd Ste 202, Westford, MA 01886
Eeg electrode.

Invivo Corporation 425-487-7000
12601 Research Pkwy, Orlando, FL 32826
Ecg electode.

Lead-Lok, Inc. 208-263-5071
500 Airport Way, Sandpoint, ID 83864
Reusable tens-nmes electrode.

Medi-Source, Inc. 740-524-0358
7719 State Route 656, Sunbury, OH 43074
Stimulation electrodes for tens and nmes.

Medtronic Neuromodulation 763-514-4000
710 Medtronic Pkwy, Minneapolis, MN 55432
Surface electrode.

Microstim Technology, Inc. 772-283-0408
1849 SW Crane Creek Ave, Palm City, FL 34990
Neurology- cutaneous tens electrode.

Naimco, Inc. 423-648-7730
4120 S Creek Rd, Chattanooga, TN 37406
Neurostimulation electrodes.

Neumed Inc. 800-367-1238
800 Silvia St, Ewing, NJ 08628
TheraKnit Garment Electrodes: Glove, sock, elbow sleeve, and knee sleeve for electrotherapy treatment to reduce edema and associated pain. Use with TENS, HVPC, Microcurrent, etc. Available in different sizes.

Neurotron Medical 609-896-3444
800 Silvia St, Ewing, NJ 08628
Electrode, cutaneous for tens.

ELECTRODE, CUTANEOUS *(cont'd)*

Newwave Medical Llc 888-513-9283
1239 Durham Rd, Whitewright, TX 75491
Various.

Nuvasive, Inc. 800-475-9131
7475 Lusk Blvd, San Diego, CA 92121
Emg surface electrodes.

Patterson Medical Supply, Inc. 262-387-8720
W68N158 Evergreen Blvd, Cedarburg, WI 53012
Various types of metallic electrodes.

Respironics California, Inc. 724-387-4559
2271 Cosmos Ct, Carlsbad, CA 92011
Transcutaneous co2/o2 electrode.

Respironics Novametrix, Llc. 724-387-4559
5 Technology Dr, Wallingford, CT 06492
Transcutaneous co2/o2 electrode.

Rhythmlink International, LLC 866-633-3754
1140 First St. South, Columbia, SC 29209
RHYTHMLINK DISC ELECTRODES; RLI CUTANEOUS DISPOSABLE ELECTRODE

Rochester Electro Medical, Inc. 813-963-2933
4212 Cypress Gulch Dr, Lutz, FL 33559
Eeg, emg, and evoked potential electrodes and clips.

Rs Medical 800-683-0353
14001 S.E. First St., Vancouver, WA 98684
RS-FBG Full Back Conductive Garment; RS-LB Low Back Conductive Garment

Selective Med Components, Inc. 740-397-7838
564 Harcourt Rd, Mount Vernon, OH 43050
Electrodes for tens and nmes.

Smiths Medical Asd, Inc. 610-578-9600
9255 Customhouse Plz Ste N, San Diego, CA 92154
Temperature monitor with sensors.

Vision Quest Industries, Inc. 800-266-6969
18011 Mitchell S, Irvine, CA 92614
Cutaneous electrodes.

ELECTRODE, CYSTOSCOPIC *(Gastro/Urology) 78QSR*

Karl Storz Endoscopy-America Inc. 800-421-0837
600 Corporate Pointe, Culver City, CA 90230
Flexible electrodes in a range of shapes.

Mahe International Inc. 800-294-7946
468 Craighead St, Nashville, TN 37204

ELECTRODE, DEFIBRILLATOR *(Cardiovascular) 74QSS*

Katecho, Inc. 515-244-1212
4020 Gannett Ave, Des Moines, IA 50321
External disposable defibrillation and pacing electrodes.

Medtronic, Inc. 800-633-8766
710 Medtronic Pkwy, Minneapolis, MN 55432
TRANSVENE PCD.

Physio-Control, Inc. 800-442-1142
11811 Willows Rd NE, Redmond, WA 98052
QUIK-COMBO Pacing/defibrillation/ECG electrodes. Disposable adhesive, single application electrodes for delivery of noninvasive pacing therapy, defibrillation and/or ECG monitoring.

Tyco Healthcare Group Lp 800-445-5025
2 Ludlow Park Dr, Chicopee, MA 01022

ELECTRODE, DEPTH *(Cns/Neurology) 84GZL*

Ad-Tech Medical Instrument Corp. 800-776-1555
1901 William St, Racine, WI 53404
Spencer probe depth electrode. Spinal Electrode for motor evoked potential monitoring during spinal surgery.

Cardinal Healthcare 209, Inc. 610-862-0800
5225 Verona Rd, Fitchburg, WI 53711
Micro guide.

Cyberkinetics Neurotechnology Systems, Inc. 508-549-9981
100 Foxboro Blvd Ste 240, Foxborough, MA 02035
Depth electrode.

Fhc, Inc 800-326-2905
1201 Main St, Bowdoin, ME 04287
microTargeting® Electrodes

Pmt Corp. 800-626-5463
1500 Park Rd, Chanhassen, MN 55317

ELECTRODE, ECG, HAND-HELD *(Cardiovascular) 74WPX*

Cw Medical, Inc. 909-591-5220
5595 Daniels St Ste E, Chino, CA 91710
Digital TENS: a compact electric stimulator great for the nerves of the body. This device gives a transcutaneous effect for the acupuncture points and site of pain for the human body. Product features compact for better portability,LCD display & digital operation more accurate for prescription, ergonomic design, large buttons for easy operation,6 different stimulation modes,maximum output-200Hz for severe intense pain, intensity adjustable to 9,and preset 10 minute timer. Easy to use as well as long lasting.

ELECTRODE, ECG, RADIOLUCENT *(Cardiovascular) 74WLP*

Cas Medical Systems, Inc. 800-227-4414
44 E Industrial Rd, Branford, CT 06405
Solid gel, radiotranslucent ECG electrodes, prewired.

Taylor Industries, Inc. 800-339-1361
2706 Industrial Dr, Jefferson City, MO 65109

Tyco Healthcare Group Lp 800-445-5025
2 Ludlow Park Dr, Chicopee, MA 01022

ELECTRODE, ELECTRO-OCULOGRAPH *(Ophthalmology) 86QSX*

Integral Design Inc. 781-740-2036
52 Burr Rd, Hingham, MA 02043

ELECTRODE, ELECTROCARDIOGRAPH *(Cardiovascular) 74DRX*

Affinity Medical Technologies Llc 949-477-9495
1732 Reynolds Ave, Irvine, CA 92614
Patient cable.

Ambu A/S 457-225-2210
6740 Baymeadow Dr, Glen Burnie, MD 21060
Ecg electrode.

Ballard Medical Products 770-587-7835
12050 Lone Peak Pkwy, Draper, UT 84020
Disposable ecg monitoring electrodes.

Bio-Detek, Inc. 800-225-1310
525 Narragansett Park Dr, Pawtucket, RI 02861

Cambridge Heart, Inc. 888-CAM-WAVE
100 Ames Pond Dr Ste 100, Tewksbury, MA 01876
Ecg electrode.

Cardiac Science Corp. 800-777-1777
500 Burdick Pkwy, Deerfield, WI 53531
Blue Max, CardioSens, and Heartline

Cardio Command, Inc. 800-231-6370
4920 W Cypress St Ste 110, Tampa, FL 33607
TAPSYSTEM cardiac stimulator. Transesophageal atrial pacing (TAP) and P-wave amplification using TAPSCOPE, esophageal stethoscope; TAPCATH four-F catheter.

Cas Medical Systems, Inc. 800-227-4414
44 E Industrial Rd, Branford, CT 06405
Neonatal ECG electrode, prewired.

Dma Med-Chem Corporation 800-362-1833
49 Watermill Ln, Great Neck, NY 11021

Don Tay Industries 262-789-9102
2383 S 162nd St, New Berlin, WI 53151
Ekg electrode.

Elmed, Inc. 630-543-2792
60 W Fay Ave, Addison, IL 60101

Ge Medical Systems Information Technologies 800-643-6439
8200 W Tower Ave, Milwaukee, WI 53223
Full line of adult and infant monitoring and diagnostic electrodes.

Gereonics, Inc. 949-929-9319
25501 Aria Dr, Mission Viejo, CA 92692
Skin electrodes.

Inovise Medical, Inc. 503-431-3800
10565 SW Nimbus Ave Ste 100, Portland, OR 97223
Ecg sensor w/heartsound microphone.

Instromedix, A Card Guard Co. 800-633-3361
10255 W Higgins Rd Ste 100, Rosemont, IL 60018

Kentron Health Care, Inc. 615-384-0573
3604 Kelton Jackson Rd, P.o. Box 120, Springfield, TN 37172
Electrocardiograph electrodes.

Lead-Lok, Inc. 208-263-5071
500 Airport Way, Sandpoint, ID 83864
Disposable electrode-solid & wet get, snap & pre-wire.

ELECTRODE, ELECTROCARDIOGRAPH *(cont'd)*

Ludlow Technological Products 800-445-5025
2 Ludlow Park Dr, Chicopee, MA 01022
Pre-gelled cardiac monitoring electrodes; also available, SOFT-E neonatal/pediatric electrodes.

Md International, Inc. 305-669-9003
11300 NW 41st St, Doral, FL 33178

Med-Dyne 502-429-4140
2775 S Floyd St, Louisville, KY 40209

Medtronic Inc, Paceart 763-514-4000
4265 Lexington Ave N, Arden Hills, MN 55126
Wrist electrodes.

Micron Products, Inc. 800-370-5500
25 Sawyer Passway, Fitchburg, MA 01420
ECG electrodes.

Multi Biosensors, Inc. 915-581-9684
4944 Vista Grande Cir, El Paso, TX 79922
Various sizes and shapes of disposable electrodes.

New Life Systems, Inc. 954-972-4600
PO Box 8767, Coral Springs, FL 33075

Nikomed U.S.A., Inc. 800-355-6456
2000 Pioneer Rd, Huntingdon Valley, PA 19006
Monitoring ecg electrodes.

Omni Medical Supply Inc. 800-860-6664
4153 Pioneer Dr, Commerce Township, MI 48390
Disposable, foam construction for use in holter and stress testing applications.

Physio-Control, Inc. 800-442-1142
11811 Willows Rd NE, Redmond, WA 98052
LIFEPATCH ECG electrodes (Ag/AgCl, disposable). QUIK-COMBO pacing/defibrillation/ECG electrodes. Disposable adhesive, single application electrodes for delivery of noninvasive pacing therapy, defibrillation and/or ECG monitoring.

Quality Rapid Service Mounts, Inc. 800-418-8342
8617 Eagle Point Blvd, Lake Elmo, MN 55042

R & D Medical Products, Inc. 949-472-9346
20492 Crescent Bay Dr Ste 106, Lake Forest, CA 92630
EKG electrode.

Select Engineering, Inc. 800-971-4500
260 Lunenburg St, Fitchburg, MA 01420
Disposable, molded, plastic, Silver/silver chloride coated snap and eyelet sensors for ECG (EKG), EEG and EMG electrodes. SELECT RADIO TRANSLUCENT, (X-Ray Transparent) one piece, two piece and prewired styles of snap and eyelet sensors for ECG electrodes.

Taylor Industries, Inc. 800-339-1361
2706 Industrial Dr, Jefferson City, MO 65109
Monitoring electrode.

The Pandah Co. 336-993-4579
408 Drayton Park Dr, Kernersville, NC 27284
Ekg electrodes.

Tsi Medical Ltd. 800-661-7263
47 Athabascan Ave., Unit 105, Sherwood Park, AB T8A-4H3 Canada

Tyco Healthcare Group Lp 800-445-5025
2 Ludlow Park Dr, Chicopee, MA 01022

U.F.I. 805-772-1203
545 Main St Ste C2, Morro Bay, CA 93442
$19.00 each.

Ubs Instruments Corporation 818-710-1195
7745 Alabama Ave Ste 7, Canoga Park, CA 91304
Disposable electrodes for ECG/EKG and Holter monitoring uses.

Vermed, Inc. 802-463-9976
9 Lovell Dr, Bellows Falls, VT 05101
Ver - med.

3m Co. 888-364-3577
3M Center, Saint Paul, MN 55144
3M RED DOT ELECTRODES

ELECTRODE, ELECTROCARDIOGRAPH, LONG-TERM *(Cardiovascular) 74WOW*

Taylor Industries, Inc. 800-339-1361
2706 Industrial Dr, Jefferson City, MO 65109

ELECTRODE, ELECTROCARDIOGRAPH, MULTI-FUNCTION *(Cardiovascular) 74MLN*

Ballard Medical Products 770-587-7835
12050 Lone Peak Pkwy, Draper, UT 84020
Disposable,multi-function electrodes.

ELECTRODE, ELECTROCARDIOGRAPH, MULTI-FUNCTION
(cont'd)

Ludlow Technological Products 800-445-5025
2 Ludlow Park Dr, Chicopee, MA 01022
QUANTUM EDGE Multi-Function Defibrillation Electrodes.

Taylor Industries, Inc. 800-339-1361
2706 Industrial Dr, Jefferson City, MO 65109

ELECTRODE, ELECTROENCEPHALOGRAPHIC
(Cns/Neurology) 84QSU

Electro-Cap International, Inc. 800-527-2193
1011 W Lexington Rd, PO Box 87, Eaton, OH 45320

Integral Design Inc. 781-740-2036
52 Burr Rd, Hingham, MA 02043

Oxford Instruments 800-438-8322
300 Baker Ave Ste 150, Concord, MA 01742
Re-usable TECA Gold Cup & silver/silver chloride reusable surface electrodes for EEG/EP studies.

Pmt Corp. 800-626-5463
1500 Park Rd, Chanhassen, MN 55317

Rhythmlink International, LLC 866-633-3754
1140 First St. South, Columbia, SC 29209
Disposable EEG Cup Electrodes, Reusable EEG Cup Electrodes

The Electrode Store 360-829-0400
PO Box 188, Enumclaw, WA 98022
$55.00 for set/10 surface electrodes. $28.00 for set/10 presterilized disposable needle electrodes.

ELECTRODE, ELECTROMYOGRAPHIC *(Cns/Neurology) 84QSV*

Bio-Medical Instruments, Inc. 800-521-4640
2387 E 8 Mile Rd, Warren, MI 48091

Chalgren Enterprises, Inc. 408-847-3994
380 Tomkins Ct, Gilroy, CA 95020
CHALGREN reusable and disposable needle, disc and ring electrodes.

Integral Design Inc. 781-740-2036
52 Burr Rd, Hingham, MA 02043

Laborie Medical Technologies Inc. 888-522-6743
6415 Northwest Dr., Units 7-14, Mississauga, ONT L4V-1X1 Canada
EMG Patch electrodes designed for a secure fit and excellent contact. Priced at $16.50.

Neurodyne Medical Corp. 800-963-8633
186 Alewife Brook Pkwy, Cambridge, MA 02138
Variety of non-gelled and pre-gelled electrodes for surface EMG applications, including both foam and stretchable backing.

Oxford Instruments 800-438-8322
300 Baker Ave Ste 150, Concord, MA 01742
TECA Monopolar Needle, Concentric Needle, NCS 2000 disposable EMG electrodes, MyoJect needle.

The Electrode Store 360-829-0400
PO Box 188, Enumclaw, WA 98022
Protectrode; $200.00 per 25 disposable concentric needles, $107 to $150 for presterilized disposable monopolar needles. From $5 for shielded or unshielded harness.

U.F.I. 805-772-1203
545 Main St Ste C2, Morro Bay, CA 93442
$19.00 each.

ELECTRODE, ELECTRONYSTAGMOGRAPHIC
(Ophthalmology) 86QSW

Gn Otometrics 800-289-2150
125 Commerce Dr, Schaumburg, IL 60173
$30.00 each for reusable, $30.00 for 48 disposable units.

ELECTRODE, ELECTROSURGERY, LAPAROSCOPIC
(Surgery) 79SII

Atc Technologies, Inc. 781-939-0725
30B Upton Dr, Wilmington, MA 01887

Boss Instruments, Ltd. 800-210-2677
395 Reas Ford Rd Ste 120, Earlysville, VA 22936

Cameron-Miller, Inc. 800-621-0142
5410 W Roosevelt Rd, Road #241, Chicago, IL 60644

Ellman International, Inc. 800-835-5355
3333 Royal Ave, Rockville Centre, NY 11572

Encision Inc. 303-444-2600
6797 Winchester Cir, Boulder, CO 80301
AEM laparoscopic electrosurgical electrodes with AEM technology built in to eliminate stray energy due to insulation failure or capacitive coupling.

ELECTRODE, ELECTROSURGERY, LAPAROSCOPIC *(cont'd)*

Ethicon Endo-Surgery, Inc. 800-USE-ENDO
4545 Creek Rd, Cincinnati, OH 45242

Gibbons Surgical Corp. 800-959-1989
1112 Jensen Dr Ste 101, Virginia Beach, VA 23451

Md International, Inc. 305-669-9003
11300 NW 41st St, Doral, FL 33178

Mediflex Surgical Products 800-879-7575
250 Gibbs Rd, Islandia, NY 11749

Olsen Medical 800-297-6344
3001 W Kentucky St, Louisville, KY 40211
Available with Standard Hook, J Hook, L Hook, Hockeystick and Spatula Tip styles. All styles available with pen, cable and/or hex connectors

Transamerican Technologies International 800-322-7373
2246 Camino Ramon, San Ramon, CA 94583
ACCU-SURG '3 in 1' instrument for suction, irrigation and electrosurgery.

Valleylab 800-255-8522
5920 Longbow Dr, Boulder, CO 80301
Pencil grip laparoscopic handset. Selection of retractable electrode tip configurations.

Wisap America 800-233-8448
8231 Melrose Dr, Lenexa, KS 66214

ELECTRODE, ELECTROSURGICAL, ACTIVE (BLADE)
(Surgery) 79FAS

Cameron-Miller, Inc. 800-621-0142
5410 W Roosevelt Rd, Road #241, Chicago, IL 60644

Cardiomed Supplies Inc. 800-387-9757
5 Gormley Industrial Ave., P.O. Box 575
Gormley, ONT L0H 1 Canada
Various configurations to cut, excise and coagulate tissue.

Dermatologic Lab & Supply, Inc. 800-831-6273
608 13th Ave, Council Bluffs, IA 51501
Electrolite Disposable spherical tip Electrosurgical Electrodes (patented)

Elmed, Inc. 630-543-2792
60 W Fay Ave, Addison, IL 60101

Greenwald Surgical Co., Inc. 219-962-1604
2688 Dekalb St, Gary, IN 46405
Various types of cystoscope, and resectoscope cutting, coagulating, and fulgurat.

Gyrus Acmi, Inc. 508-804-2739
93 N Pleasant St, Norwalk, OH 44857
Electrode, electrosurgical, active, urological.

Gyrus Acmi, Inc. 508-804-2739
300 Stillwater P.o.box 1971, Stamford, CT 06902
Various sizes and kinds urological active electrosurgical electrodes.

Incisiontech 800-213-7809
9 Technology Dr, Staunton, VA 24401

Instrumed Oem 800-368-1301
2801 S Vallejo St, Englewood, CO 80110
Electrosurgical blades, balls, needles and loops.

Karl Storz Endoscopy-America Inc. 800-421-0837
600 Corporate Pointe, Culver City, CA 90230

Mahe International Inc. 800-294-7946
468 Craighead St, Nashville, TN 37204

Md International, Inc. 305-669-9003
11300 NW 41st St, Doral, FL 33178

New England Medical Corp. 845-778-4200
2274 Albany Post Rd, Walden, NY 12586
Cervical Large Loop Excision Electrode.

Ob Specialties, Inc. 800-325-6644
1799 Northwood Ct, Oakland, CA 94611

Olsen Medical 800-297-6344
3001 W Kentucky St, Louisville, KY 40211
Full line of reusable and single use electrodes, including blade, needle and ball. available in lengths from 2 3/4' to 6' (selected styles up to 10')

Richard Wolf Medical Instruments Corp. 800-323-9653
353 Corporate Woods Pkwy, Vernon Hills, IL 60061

Utah Medical Products, Inc. 800-533-4984
7043 Cottonwood St, Midvale, UT 84047
EPITOME® Scalpel and OPTI-MICRO™ microdissecction needle electrosurgical electrodes for precise dissection and improved healing properties compared to standard electrosurgical electrodes.

ELECTRODE, ELECTROSURGICAL, ACTIVE (BLADE) *(cont'd)*

Valleylab 800-255-8522
5920 Longbow Dr, Boulder, CO 80301
EDGE™ coated electrodes. Single use electrosurgical pencils. Choice of handswitch or footswitch activation.

ELECTRODE, ELECTROSURGICAL, ACTIVE, FOOT CONTROLLED *(Surgery) 79UEB*

Bausch & Lomb Surgical 636-255-5051
3365 Tree Court Ind Blvd, Saint Louis, MO 63122

Cameron-Miller, Inc. 800-621-0142
5410 W Roosevelt Rd, Road #241, Chicago, IL 60644

Durden Enterprises 800-554-5673
1317 4th Ave, P.O. Box 909, Auburn, GA 30011

Elmed, Inc. 630-543-2792
60 W Fay Ave, Addison, IL 60101

Md International, Inc. 305-669-9003
11300 NW 41st St, Doral, FL 33178

Olsen Medical 800-297-6344
3001 W Kentucky St, Louisville, KY 40211
Reusable and single use Foot Controlled handpieces

Omnitech Systems, Inc. 866-266-9490
450 Campbell St Ste 2, Valparaiso, IN 46385
Resectoscope Electrodes (TURP). Patented coagulating/vaporizing tips.

Richard Wolf Medical Instruments Corp. 800-323-9653
353 Corporate Woods Pkwy, Vernon Hills, IL 60061

Sigma Products Ltd. 845-778-4200
2274 Albany Post Rd, Walden, NY 12586
CONEFOR Cone Biopsy $20.

ELECTRODE, ELECTROSURGICAL, ACTIVE, UROLOGICAL, REPROCESSED *(Gastro/Urology) 78NLW*

Sterilmed, Inc. 763-488-3400
11400 73rd Ave N Ste 100, Maple Grove, MN 55369
Reprocessed endoscopic electrodes.

ELECTRODE, ELECTROSURGICAL, RETURN (GROUND, DISPERSIVE) *(Surgery) 79JOS*

Apple Medical Corp. 508-357-2700
28 Lord Rd Ste 135, Marlborough, MA 01752
Ball electrode.

Bovie Medical Corp. 800-537-2790
5115 Ulmerton Rd, Clearwater, FL 33760

Cameron-Miller, Inc. 800-621-0142
5410 W Roosevelt Rd, Road #241, Chicago, IL 60644

Cardinal Health, Snowden Pencer Products 847-689-8410
5175 S Royal Atlanta Dr, Tucker, GA 30084
Electrosurgical cutting and coagulating device and accessories.

Elmed, Inc. 630-543-2792
60 W Fay Ave, Addison, IL 60101

Hantel Technologies 510-487-1561
721 Sandoval Way, Hayward, CA 94544
Electrodes.

Innova Corp. 860-242-3210
68 E Dudley Town Rd, Bloomfield, CT 06002
OEM custom design and manufacture.

Karl Storz Endoscopy-America Inc. 800-421-0837
600 Corporate Pointe, Culver City, CA 90230
Full line of vaporization electrodes for prostate therapy.

Lmi Lightwave Medical Industries Ltd. 604-275-3400
250-13155 Delf Pl, Richmond, BC V6V 2A2 Canada
Optoelectric electrosurgical pencil

Md International, Inc. 305-669-9003
11300 NW 41st St, Doral, FL 33178

Megadyne Medical Products, Inc. 800-747-6110
11506 S State St, Draper, UT 84020
MEGA Soft is a unique, patented, patient return electrode that guards against burns, eliminate adhesives and shaving of patients. They are environmentally friendly and cost effective.

Neomend, Inc. 949-916-1630
9272 Jeronimo Rd Ste 119, Irvine, CA 92618
Sterile loop electrode, electrosurgical device.

Omnitech Systems, Inc. 866-266-9490
450 Campbell St Ste 2, Valparaiso, IN 46385
Resectoscope cutting loop electrode.

Pmt Corp. 800-626-5463
1500 Park Rd, Chanhassen, MN 55317

ELECTRODE, ELECTROSURGICAL, RETURN (GROUND, DISPERSIVE) *(cont'd)*

Respiratory Diagnostics, Inc. 425-881-8300
47987 Fremont Blvd, Fremont, CA 94538
Catheter eletrode.

Robert Joseph Craig Sa De Cv 905-5600803
Blvd De Santa Monica 106-204, Jardines De, Tlalnepantla Mexico
Disposable foam electrode

Rotburg Instruments Of America Inc. 954-331-8046
1560 Sawgrass Corporate Pkwy Fl 4, Sunrise, FL 33323
Various types of sterile and non-sterile electrosurgical electrodes.

Sigma Products Ltd. 845-778-4200
2274 Albany Post Rd, Walden, NY 12586
NEW ENGLAND MEDICAL LLETZ Electrodes $9-$12.

Smi 920-876-3361
Industrial Park, 544 Sohn Drive, Elkhart Lake, WI 53020

Sterilmed, Inc. 763-488-3400
11400 73rd Ave N Ste 100, Maple Grove, MN 55369
Reprocessed electrosurgical electrode.

Teleflex Medical 800-334-9751
2917 Weck Drive, Research Triangle Park, NC 27709

Transamerican Technologies International 800-322-7373
2246 Camino Ramon, San Ramon, CA 94583
ACCU-SURG, Bipolar Laparoscopic Electrodes. Surgical tools for cutting and coagulation used primarily for laparoscopic GYN and general surgery procedures.

Unimed Surgical Products, Inc. 727-546-1900
10401 Belcher Rd S, Largo, FL 33777
Electrosurgical electrodes for cutting & coagulation.

Valley Forge Scientific Corp. 610-666-7500
136 Green Tree Road, Suite 100, Oaks, PA 19456
Bipolar dual tip electrode used for bipolar cutting and/or coagulation during bipolar electrosurgical procedure.

Valleylab 800-255-8522
5920 Longbow Dr, Boulder, CO 80301
Single-use standard and REM PolyHesive™ II patient return electrodes.

ELECTRODE, ESOPHAGEAL *(Gastro/Urology) 78QSY*

Cardio Command, Inc. 800-231-6370
4920 W Cypress St Ste 110, Tampa, FL 33607
TAPSCOPE, esophageal stethoscope; TAPCATH Five-French catheter.

Microelectrodes, Inc. 603-668-0692
40 Harvey Rd, Bedford, NH 03110
$360, Esophageal pH

ELECTRODE, FETAL SCALP *(Obstetrics/Gyn) 85QSZ*

Medical Accessories, Inc. 800-275-1624
92 Youngs Rd, Trenton, NJ 08619
ECG single spiral fetal monitoring electrode.

Ob Specialties, Inc. 800-325-6644
1799 Northwood Ct, Oakland, CA 94611

Tyco Healthcare Group Lp 800-445-5025
2 Ludlow Park Dr, Chicopee, MA 01022

ELECTRODE, FLEXIBLE SUCTION COAGULATOR *(Gastro/Urology) 78FEH*

Cameron-Miller, Inc. 800-621-0142
5410 W Roosevelt Rd, Road #241, Chicago, IL 60644

ELECTRODE, GEL *(Cardiovascular) 74WOV*

Alimed, Inc. 800-225-2610
297 High St, Dedham, MA 02026

Bpsp Co. (Medical Z Corp.) 800-368-7478
6800 Alamo Downs Pkwy, San Antonio, TX 78238

Cas Medical Systems, Inc. 800-227-4414
44 E Industrial Rd, Branford, CT 06405
Neonatal ECG electrodes, prewired.

Innova Corp. 860-242-3210
68 E Dudley Town Rd, Bloomfield, CT 06002
NexGel, Hydrogel-Adhesive Gel, conductive adhesive gels for electrode use, attaching devices to the body, use in neonatal applications.

Ludlow Technological Products 800-445-5025
2 Ludlow Park Dr, Chicopee, MA 01022
Pregelled cardiac monitoring electrodes.

Med-Dyne 502-429-4140
2775 S Floyd St, Louisville, KY 40209

ELECTRODE, GEL *(cont'd)*

Neotech Products, Inc. 800-966-0500
27822 Fremont Ct, Valencia, CA 91355
NEOLEAD:Hydrocolloid/Hydrogel Neonatal Electrode. Does not fall off infants prematurely. This is the first true innovation in electrodes in years!

Parker Laboratories, Inc. 800-631-8888
286 Eldridge Rd, Fairfield, NJ 07004
SIGNASPRAY, electrode & skin prep. solution.

Romaine, Inc. D.B.A. Koldcare 800-294-7101
2026 Sterling Ave, Elkhart, IN 46516
T.E.N.S. Link gelled water electrode for transcutaneous nerve stimulation. 2' x 48' and 3 x 72' wraps.

Smi 920-876-3361
Industrial Park, 544 Sohn Drive, Elkhart Lake, WI 53020

Taylor Industries, Inc. 800-339-1361
2706 Industrial Dr, Jefferson City, MO 65109

Tyco Healthcare Group Lp 800-445-5025
2 Ludlow Park Dr, Chicopee, MA 01022
Hydrogels for medical electrodes, cardiovascular and muscle stimulation. Component of finished device production.

ELECTRODE, HOLTER *(Cardiovascular) 74WOU*

Electro Medical Equipment Co., Inc. 800-423-2926
12015 Industriplex Blvd, Baton Rouge, LA 70809

Taylor Industries, Inc. 800-339-1361
2706 Industrial Dr, Jefferson City, MO 65109

Tyco Healthcare Group Lp 800-445-5025
2 Ludlow Park Dr, Chicopee, MA 01022

ELECTRODE, ION SELECTIVE (NON-SPECIFIED) *(Chemistry) 75JJP*

Baltimore Laboratories, Inc. 203-445-8423
887 Main St, Monroe, CT 06468
Electro chemical analyzer.

Brinkmann Instruments, Inc. 800-645-3050
PO Box 1019, Westbury, NY 11590

Health Science Products, Llc 757-224-0177
1010 S Beeline Hwy, Payson, AZ 85541
Electrochemical analyzer.

Medica Corp. 800-777-5983
5 Oak Park Dr, Bedford, MA 01730
pH.

Orion Research, Inc. 800-225-1480
166 Cummings Ctr, Beverly, MA 01915
ORION $281 for epoxy body REDOX combination electrode.

Thermo Fisher Scientific Inc. 781-622-1000
81 Wyman St, Waltham, MA 02451

Von London Phonix Co 713-772-6666
6103 Glenmont Dr, Houston, TX 77081

ELECTRODE, ION SPECIFIC, CALCIUM *(Chemistry) 75JFP*

Abbott Point Of Care Inc. 609-443-9300
104 Windsor Center Dr, East Windsor, NJ 08520
Ionized calcium test.

Medica Corp. 800-777-5983
5 Oak Park Dr, Bedford, MA 01730

Opti Medical Systems Inc. 770-510-4444
235 Hembree Park Dr, Roswell, GA 30076
Automated blood gas/electrolyte analyzer.

Orion Research, Inc. 800-225-1480
166 Cummings Ctr, Beverly, MA 01915
ORION $507 for liquid membrane PVC body unit w/ 2 sensors.

Osmetech, Inc. 800-373-6767
757 S Raymond Ave, Pasadena, CA 91105
Automated blood gas/electrolyte analyzer.

Thermo Fisher Scientific Inc. 781-622-1000
81 Wyman St, Waltham, MA 02451
Standard and custom.

ELECTRODE, ION SPECIFIC, CHLORIDE *(Chemistry) 75CGZ*

Abbott Point Of Care Inc. 609-443-9300
104 Windsor Center Dr, East Windsor, NJ 08520
Chloride.

Medica Corp. 800-777-5983
5 Oak Park Dr, Bedford, MA 01730

ELECTRODE, ION SPECIFIC, CHLORIDE *(cont'd)*

Opti Medical Systems Inc. 770-510-4444
235 Hembree Park Dr, Roswell, GA 30076
Automated blood gas/ electrolyte analyzer.

Orion Research, Inc. 800-225-1480
166 Cummings Ctr, Beverly, MA 01915
ORION 2 models - $298 for half cell and $508 for combination.

Osmetech, Inc. 800-373-6767
757 S Raymond Ave, Pasadena, CA 91105
Automated blood gas/ electrolyte analyzer.

Synermed Intl., Inc. 317-896-1565
17408 Tiller Ct Ste 1900, Westfield, IN 46074
Ise reagents, chloride.

Thermo Fisher Scientific Inc. 781-622-1000
81 Wyman St, Waltham, MA 02451
Standard and custom.

Vital Diagnostics Inc. 714-672-3553
1075 W Lambert Rd Ste D, Brea, CA 92821
Various reagents for the measurement of chloride.

ELECTRODE, ION SPECIFIC, POTASSIUM *(Chemistry) 75CEM*

Abbott Point Of Care Inc. 609-443-9300
104 Windsor Center Dr, East Windsor, NJ 08520
Potassium test.

Health Chem Diagnostics Llc 954-979-3845
3341 W McNab Rd, Pompano Beach, FL 33069
Electrode, ion specific, potassium.

Jas Diagnostics, Inc. 305-418-2320
7220 NW 58th St, Miami, FL 33166
Ise diluent, internal reference and standard.

Medica Corp. 800-777-5983
5 Oak Park Dr, Bedford, MA 01730

Opti Medical Systems Inc. 770-510-4444
235 Hembree Park Dr, Roswell, GA 30076
Automated blood gas/electrolyte analyzer.

Orion Research, Inc. 800-225-1480
166 Cummings Ctr, Beverly, MA 01915
ORION $542 for liquid membrane PVC body unit w/ 2 sensors.

Osmetech, Inc. 800-373-6767
757 S Raymond Ave, Pasadena, CA 91105
Automated blood gas/electrolyte analyzer.

Synermed Intl., Inc. 317-896-1565
17408 Tiller Ct Ste 1900, Westfield, IN 46074
Ise reagents, potassium.

Thermo Fisher Scientific Inc. 781-622-1000
81 Wyman St, Waltham, MA 02451
Standard and custom.

Vital Diagnostics Inc. 714-672-3553
1075 W Lambert Rd Ste D, Brea, CA 92821
Various reagents and an electrode for the measurement of potassium.

ELECTRODE, ION SPECIFIC, SODIUM *(Chemistry) 75JGS*

Abbott Point Of Care Inc. 609-443-9300
104 Windsor Center Dr, East Windsor, NJ 08520
Sodium test.

Alfa Wassermann, Inc. 800-220-4488
4 Henderson Dr, West Caldwell, NJ 07006
Potassium, chloride.

Carolina Liquid Chemistries Corp. 800-471-7272
510 W Central Ave Ste C, Brea, CA 92821
Electrolyte reference fluid.

Genchem, Inc. 714-529-1616
510 W Central Ave Ste D, Brea, CA 92821
Ise reference reagent,buffer.

Harvey, R.J. Instrument Corp. 201-664-1380
123 Patterson St, Hillsdale, NJ 07642

Health Chem Diagnostics Llc 954-979-3845
3341 W McNab Rd, Pompano Beach, FL 33069
Electrode, ion specific, sodium.

Jas Diagnostics, Inc. 305-418-2320
7220 NW 58th St, Miami, FL 33166
Ise diluent, internal reference and standard.

Medica Corp. 800-777-5983
5 Oak Park Dr, Bedford, MA 01730

ELECTRODE, ION SPECIFIC, SODIUM *(cont'd)*

Opti Medical Systems Inc. 770-510-4444
235 Hembree Park Dr, Roswell, GA 30076
Automated blood gas/ electrolyte analyzer.

Orion Research, Inc. 800-225-1480
166 Cummings Ctr, Beverly, MA 01915
ORION 2 models - $315 for ROSS half cell epoxy and $390 for ROSS combination glass.

Osmetech, Inc. 800-373-6767
757 S Raymond Ave, Pasadena, CA 91105
Automated blood gas/ electrolyte analyzer.

Synermed Intl., Inc. 317-896-1565
17408 Tiller Ct Ste 1900, Westfield, IN 46074
Ise reagents, sodium.

Teco Diagnostics 714-693-7788
1268 N Lakeview Ave, Anaheim, CA 92807
Ise reagent set for cx system.

Thermo Fisher Scientific Inc. 781-622-1000
81 Wyman St, Waltham, MA 02451
Standard and custom.

Vital Diagnostics Inc. 714-672-3553
1075 W Lambert Rd Ste D, Brea, CA 92821
Various reagents for the measurment of sodium.

ELECTRODE, ION SPECIFIC, UREA NITROGEN

(Chemistry) 75CDS

Abbott Point Of Care Inc. 609-443-9300
104 Windsor Center Dr, East Windsor, NJ 08520
Bun test.

Genchem, Inc. 714-529-1616
510 W Central Ave Ste D, Brea, CA 92821
Bun3.

Opti Medical Systems Inc. 770-510-4444
235 Hembree Park Dr, Roswell, GA 30076
Automated blood gas-electrolyte analyzer.

Orion Research, Inc. 800-225-1480
166 Cummings Ctr, Beverly, MA 01915
ORION 1 model (ammonia) - $455 for gas sensory, epoxy body.

Vital Diagnostics Inc. 714-672-3553
1075 W Lambert Rd Ste D, Brea, CA 92821
Various urea/urea nitrogen reagents.

ELECTRODE, LABORATORY PH *(Chemistry) 75UHF*

Analytical Measurements, Inc. 800-635-5580
100 Hoffman Pl, Hillside, NJ 07205
$60.00 each.

Beckman Coulter, Inc. 800-742-2345
250 S Kraemer Blvd, PO Box 8000, Brea, CA 92821

Brinkmann Instruments (Canada) Ltd. 800-263-8715
6670 Campobello Rd., Mississauga, ONT L5N 2L8 Canada

Brinkmann Instruments, Inc. 800-645-3050
PO Box 1019, Westbury, NY 11590

Cole-Parmer Instrument Inc. 800-323-4340
625 E Bunker Ct, Vernon Hills, IL 60061

Extech Instruments Corp. 781-890-7440
285 Bear Hill Rd, Waltham, MA 02451
Priced from $45.00.

Microelectrodes, Inc. 603-668-0692
40 Harvey Rd, Bedford, NH 03110
$225.00 each.

Omega Engineering, Inc. 800-848-4286
1 Omega Dr, Stamford, CT 06907
Gel-filled electrodes have a clear, epoxy-body construction measuring the entire pH range from 0 to 14 pH units at 0 to 100 degrees C.

Orion Research, Inc. 800-225-1480
166 Cummings Ctr, Beverly, MA 01915
ORION Various models, including ROSS performance, routine ph half cell, reference half cell, combination glass-body, & gel filled electrodes - from $79 to $349 each.

Sensorex Corp. 714-895-4344
11751 Markon Dr, Garden Grove, CA 92841
Prices start at $45.

Von London Phonix Co 713-772-6666
6103 Glenmont Dr, Houston, TX 77081

ELECTRODE, METALLIC WITH SOFT PAD COVERING

(Physical Med) 89IKS

Tetra Medical Supply Corp. 800-621-4041
6364 W Gross Point Rd, Niles, IL 60714
Several styles and sizes, all self-adhering and reusable.

ELECTRODE, MYOCARDIAL *(Cardiovascular) 74QTA*

Ela Medical, Inc. 800-352-6466
2950 Xenium Ln N, Plymouth, MN 55441

Ge Industrial, Sensing 800-833-9438
1100 Technology Park Dr, Billerica, MA 01821

ELECTRODE, NASOPHARYNGEAL *(Cns/Neurology) 84GZK*

Cardinal Healthcare 209, Inc. 610-862-0800
5225 Verona Rd, Fitchburg, WI 53711
Nasopharyngeal electrode.

Grass Technologies, An Astro-Med, Inc. Product Gro 401-828-4002
53 Airport Park Drive, Rockland, MA 02370
Nasopharyngeal electrode.

Rochester Electro Medical, Inc. 813-963-2933
4212 Cypress Gulch Dr, Lutz, FL 33559
Nasopharyngeal electrodes.

ELECTRODE, NEEDLE *(Cns/Neurology) 84GXZ*

Ambu A/S 457-225-2210
6740 Baymeadow Dr, Glen Burnie, MD 21060
Monopolar needle electrode.

Ambu, Inc. 800-262-8462
6740 Baymeadow Dr, Glen Burnie, MD 21060
Monopolar, Conecntric, Subdermal and Inoject Needles Electrodes

Argon Medical Devices Inc. 903-675-9321
1445 Flat Creek Rd, Athens, TX 75751
Electrode needle.

Cadwell Laboratories 800-245-3001
909 N Kellogg St, Kennewick, WA 99336
CADWELL safe electrodes.

Cardinal Healthcare 209, Inc. 610-862-0800
5225 Verona Rd, Fitchburg, WI 53711
Multiple.

Grass Technologies, An Astro-Med, Inc. Product Gro 401-828-4002
53 Airport Park Drive, Rockland, MA 02370
Needle electrode.

Gyrus Medical, Inc. 800-852-9361
6655 Wedgwood Rd N Ste 105, Maple Grove, MN 55311
BILAP single-wire bipolar needle electrode used for cutting in laparoscopic procedures.

Incisiontech 800-213-7809
9 Technology Dr, Staunton, VA 24401

Isurgical 847-949-9744
26625 N Countryside Lake Dr, Mundelein, IL 60060
Isurg sterile subdermal needle electrodes (for single use only).

Jari Electrode Supply 800-745-1934
380 Tomkins Ct, Gilroy, CA 95020
For use in electrophysiological monitoring and testing.

K. W. Griffen Co. 203-846-1923
100 Pearl St, Norwalk, CT 06850
Disposable needle electrode for single use only.

Medtronic Neuromodulation 763-514-4000
710 Medtronic Pkwy, Minneapolis, MN 55432
Needle electrode.

Oxford Instruments 800-438-8322
300 Baker Ave Ste 150, Concord, MA 01742
TECA Monopolar Needle & Concentric Needle disposable electrodes, MyoJect needle.

Quadromed Inc. 800-363-0192
5776 Thimens Ave., St-Laurent, QUE H4R 2K9 Canada

Rhythmlink International, LLC 866-633-3754
1140 First St. South, Columbia, SC 29209
RHYTHMLINK INTL. SUBD

Rochester Electro Medical, Inc. 813-963-2933
4212 Cypress Gulch Dr, Lutz, FL 33559
Subdermal needles and sphenoidal electrodes.

Singer Medical Products Inc., Md Systems Div. 630-860-6500
3800 Buckner St, El Paso, TX 79925
Needle electrode.

ELECTRODE, NEEDLE *(cont'd)*

The Electrode Store 360-829-0400
PO Box 188, Enumclaw, WA 98022
Protectrode; $200.00 per 25 disposable concentric needles; $150.00 per 50 disposable monopolar needles. From $32.00 for set/10 EEG electrode (stainless steel).

ELECTRODE, NEEDLE, ANESTHESIOLOGY
(Cns/Neurology) 84BWR

Diros Technology, Inc. 905-415-3440
232 Hood Road, Markham, ON L3R 3K8 Canada
OWL Needle Kits

Quadromed Inc. 800-363-0192
5776 Thimens Ave., St-Laurent, QUE H4R 2K9 Canada

ELECTRODE, NEEDLE, DIAGNOSTIC ELECTROMYOGRAPH
(Physical Med) 89IKT

Ambu A/S 457-225-2210
6740 Baymeadow Dr, Glen Burnie, MD 21060
Needle electrode.

Cardinal Healthcare 209, Inc. 610-862-0800
5225 Verona Rd, Fitchburg, WI 53711
Multiple.

Medtronic Neuromodulation 763-514-4000
710 Medtronic Pkwy, Minneapolis, MN 55432
Needle electrode.

Oxford Instruments 800-438-8322
300 Baker Ave Ste 150, Concord, MA 01742
TECA Monopolar Needle & Concentric Needle disposable electrodes, MyoJect needle.

Rhythmlink International, LLC 866-633-3754
1140 First St. South, Columbia, SC 29209
RLI Concentric Needle, Monopolar Needle

Rochester Electro Medical, Inc. 813-963-2933
4212 Cypress Gulch Dr, Lutz, FL 33559
Reference/ground needles, monopolar needles and nerve block needles.

The Electrode Store 360-829-0400
PO Box 188, Enumclaw, WA 98022
Protectrode; From $107.00 per package for disposable monopolar needle electrodes, $200.00 per 25 disposable concentric needles.

ELECTRODE, NEUROLOGICAL *(Cns/Neurology) 84QTB*

Ad-Tech Medical Instrument Corp. 800-776-1555
1901 William St, Racine, WI 53404
Sphenoidal, epidural peg, custom foramen ovale electrodes.

Canadian Medical Products, Ltd. 800-267-0572
850 Tapscott Rd., Unit 21, Scarborough, ONT M1X-1N4 Canada

Compex Technologies, Inc. 866-676-6489
1811 Old Highway 8 NW, New Brighton, MN 55112
Complete line of reusable and disposable sterile and non-sterile electrodes (made in U.S.A.).

Electro-Cap International, Inc. 800-527-2193
1011 W Lexington Rd, PO Box 87, Eaton, OH 45320

Integral Design Inc. 781-740-2036
52 Burr Rd, Hingham, MA 02043

Medical Science Products, Inc. 800-456-1971
517 Elm Ridge Ave, P.O. Box 381, Canal Fulton, OH 44614
GLO-TRODES: Reusable pigtail electrode in Day-glo colors and in 5 sizes.

Rhodes Medical Instruments, Inc. 805-684-1099
PO Box 133, Summerland, CA 93067
Research - specials.

The Electrode Store 360-829-0400
PO Box 188, Enumclaw, WA 98022

ELECTRODE, NEUROMUSCULAR STIMULATOR
(Cns/Neurology) 84QTC

American Imex 800-521-8286
16520 Aston, Irvine, CA 92606
DERMATRODE - TENS and muscle stimulator electrodes. Silver-silver chloride conductive liner. High heat/high humidity applications. Superior silver electrodes. Conductive sheet of silver, improved current dispersions & lower impedature, hypoallergenic conductive gel.

ELECTRODE, NEUROMUSCULAR STIMULATOR *(cont'd)*

Axelgaard Manufacturing Company, Ltd. 760-728-3430
520 Industrial Way, Fallbrook, CA 92028
Neurostimulation electrodes made in the USA. All PALS electrodes utilize the patented stainless steel fabric increasing conformity and comfort.

Bloomex International, Inc. 201-703-9799
295 Molnar Dr, Elmwood Park, NJ 07407

Compex Technologies, Inc. 866-676-6489
1811 Old Highway 8 NW, New Brighton, MN 55112
Complete line of reusable and disposable sterile and non-sterile electrodes (made in U.S.A.).

Empi, Inc. 800-328-2536
599 Cardigan Rd, Saint Paul, MN 55126
SUE electrodes for TENS & NMS applications.

Innova Corp. 860-242-3210
68 E Dudley Town Rd, Bloomfield, CT 06002

Katecho, Inc. 515-244-1212
4020 Gannett Ave, Des Moines, IA 50321

Life-Tech, Inc. 281-491-6600
4235 Greenbriar Dr, Stafford, TX 77477
Stimitrode disposable surface electrodes for peripheral nerve stimulation

Mylon-Tech Health Technologies Inc. 613-728-1667
301 Moodie Dr., Ste. 205, Ottawa, ON K2H 9C4 Canada
Wide range of different electrode types for all NMES devices.

Tyco Healthcare Group Lp 800-445-5025
2 Ludlow Park Dr, Chicopee, MA 01022

Zimmer Medizinsystems 800-327-3576
25 Mauchly Ste 300, Irvine, CA 92618
Hygienic single use, multi-function, self-adhesive electrodes. Available in different sizes and shapes. Cost effective, OSHA safe.

ELECTRODE, OTHER *(General) 80QTI*

Ad-Tech Medical Instrument Corp. 800-776-1555
1901 William St, Racine, WI 53404
Cueva Nerve Monitoring Electrode for intraoperative monitoring during skull base surgery.

American Catheter Corp. 800-345-6714
13047 S Highway 475, Ocala, FL 34480

Aspect Medical Systems, Inc. 617-559-7000
141 Needham St, Newton, MA 02464
ZIPPREP Self-prepping, low impedance disposable electrodes.

Axon Systems, Inc. 800-888-2966
400 Oser Ave Ste 2200, Hauppauge, NY 11788
Complete line of neurological testing accessories, including electrodes, probes and electrode application materials, for neurological monitoring.

Bak Electronics, Inc. 800-894-6000
PO Box 623, Mount Airy, MD 21771
Electrode activation system.

Bloomex International, Inc. 201-703-9799
295 Molnar Dr, Elmwood Park, NJ 07407
CARBONFLEX electrodes & MEDFLEX wire lead system.

Bovie Medical Corp. 800-537-2790
5115 Ulmerton Rd, Clearwater, FL 33760
Blades, balls, needles, and loop and square electrodes.

Brady Corporation 800-541-1686
6555 W Good Hope Rd, PO Box 571, Milwaukee, WI 53223
OEM contract manufacturing of disposable electrodes, for applications including monitoring, TENS, drug delivery, ECG, transdermal, muscle stimulation, diagnostics, defibrillation and grounding.

Cadmet, Inc. 800-543-7282
155 Planebrook Rd, P.O. Box 24, Malvern, PA 19355

Comfort Technologies, Inc. 800-321-7846
381 Mountain Blvd, Watchung, NJ 07069
COMPATCH electrodes and accessories.

Compex Technologies, Inc. 866-676-6489
1811 Old Highway 8 NW, New Brighton, MN 55112
Complete line of reusable and disposable sterile and non-sterile electrodes (made in U.S.A.).

Coopersurgical, Inc. 800-243-2974
95 Corporate Dr, Trumbull, CT 06611
$15.00 each for disposable electrodes for Letz procedure (sold in boxes of 5/box). 16 different sets, $28 each for reusable electrodes for Letz procedure.

ELECTRODE, OTHER *(cont'd)*

Danlee Medical Products, Inc. 800-433-7797
6075 E Molloy Rd Bldg 5, Syracuse, NY 13211
E-CLIP LEADSTABILIZER attaches to any electrode to eliminate the use of adhesive tapes used to secure leadwires during Holter, stress, and telemetry. Maximizes patient comfort, eliminates cleaning leadwires and may reduce motion induced artifact. Also available, CLIPTRODE ELECTRODE, same as above only the E-CLIP is preattached to a quality Holter/Stress electrode manufactured exclusively for Danlee.

Dma Med-Chem Corporation 800-362-1833
49 Watermill Ln, Great Neck, NY 11021

Electro-Cap International, Inc. 800-527-2193
1011 W Lexington Rd, PO Box 87, Eaton, OH 45320

Electro-Med Health Industries 800-232-3644
PO Box 610484, Miami, FL 33261
Disposable and reusable electrodes; carbon electrodes. Accessories for electro-therapeutic devices.

Harvard Apparatus, Inc. 800-272-2775
84 October Hill Rd, Holliston, MA 01746
Electroporation Generators and Specialty Electrodes. ECM 830 Square Wave Generator, ECM 630 Exponential Decay Wave Generator, ECM 399 Basic Exponential Decay Wave Generator, ECM 2001 Electrofusion Generator and a large selection of Specialty Electrodes including the Genepaddles, Genetrodes, Tweezertrodes and Caliper Electrodes

Innova Corp. 860-242-3210
68 E Dudley Town Rd, Bloomfield, CT 06002
OEM custom design and manufacture.

Integra Radionics 800-466-6814
22 Terry Ave, Burlington, MA 01803

Integral Design Inc. 781-740-2036
52 Burr Rd, Hingham, MA 02043

Iomed, Inc. 800-621-3347
2441 S 3850 W Ste A, Salt Lake City, UT 84120
TRANSQ iontophoresis electrode. Drug delivery electrode.

Katecho, Inc. 515-244-1212
4020 Gannett Ave, Des Moines, IA 50321
External disposable pacing and defibrillation electrodes.

Kirwan Surgical Products, Inc. 888-547-9267
180 Enterprise Dr, PO Box 427, Marshfield, MA 02050
Mono- and bi-polar endoscopic electrodes.

Life-Tech, Inc. 281-491-6600
4235 Greenbriar Dr, Stafford, TX 77477

Lynn Medical 888-596-6633
764 Denison Ct, Bloomfield Hills, MI 48302
CARBOCONE radiotranslucent electrode.

Medica Corp. 800-777-5983
5 Oak Park Dr, Bedford, MA 01730
Electrode, ion specific, lithium.

Medical Accessories, Inc. 800-275-1624
92 Youngs Rd, Trenton, NJ 08619
ECG single spiral fetal monitoring electrode.

Megadyne Medical Products, Inc. 800-747-6110
11506 S State St, Draper, UT 84020
E-Z CLEAN, laparoscopic electrodes. MEGA TIP & INDICATOR SHAFT, resposable laparascopic electrode which combines the benefits of the E-Z CLEAN non-stick coating and the safety of the patented Indicator Shaft at an economical price.

Neotech Products, Inc. 800-966-0500
27822 Fremont Ct, Valencia, CA 91355
NEOLEAD:Hydrocolloid/Hydrogel Neonatal Electrode. The first neonatal electrode that does not fall off prematurely.

Olsen Medical 800-297-6344
3001 W Kentucky St, Louisville, KY 40211
MIDAS TOUCH - monoplar electrodes.

Premier Medical Products 888-PREMUSA
1710 Romano Dr, Plymouth Meeting, PA 19462
TruCone Rotational Cone Biopsy Electrode to obtain precise cervical cone biopsies.

Prizm Medical, Inc. 770-622-0933
PO Box 40, Oakwood, GA 30566
Electro-Mesh and Silver-Thera electrodes

Rich-Mar Corporation 800-762-4665
PO Box 879, 15499 E 590 Rd, Inola, OK 74036
Self-adhesive electrodes. Easy and safe self-adhesive electrodes available in different sizes. Multiple uses and OSHA safe.

ELECTRODE, OTHER *(cont'd)*

Thermo Fisher Scientific Inc. 781-622-1000
81 Wyman St, Waltham, MA 02451
Standard and custom lithium electrodes.

Thomas Medical Inc. 800-556-0349
5610 West 82 2nd Street, Indianpolis, IN 46278
Electrodes, loop and acccessories.

Tyco Healthcare Group Lp 800-445-5025
2 Ludlow Park Dr, Chicopee, MA 01022

Utah Medical Products, Inc. 800-533-4984
7043 Cottonwood St, Midvale, UT 84047
UtahLoop® and UtahBall® electrodes with exclusive SAFE-T-GAUGE for depth control for treatment of cervical dysplasias.

Zimmer Medizinsystems 800-327-3576
25 Mauchly Ste 300, Irvine, CA 92618
Hygienic single use, multi-function, self-adhesive electrodes. Available in different sizes and shapes. Cost effective, OSHA safe.

Zoll Medical Corp. 800-348-9011
269 Mill Rd, Chelmsford, MA 01824
Multi-function electrode. Multiple therapy electrodes allowing quick and easy switching between defibrillation and pacing. Preconnected, pediatric.

ELECTRODE, PACEMAKER, EXTERNAL *(Cardiovascular) 74QTD*

Biotronik, Inc. 503-635-3594
6024 Jean Rd, Lake Oswego, OR 97035
VARIOUS MODELS OF STERO

Cardio Command, Inc. 800-231-6370
4920 W Cypress St Ste 110, Tampa, FL 33607
TAPSYSTEM cardiac stimulator. Transesophageal atrial pacing (TAP) and P-wave amplification using TAPSCOPE, esophageal stethoscope; TAPCATH four-F catheter.

Covidien Lp 508-261-8000
15 Hampshire St, Mansfield, MA 02048
FLEXON stainless steel unit.

Katecho, Inc. 515-244-1212
4020 Gannett Ave, Des Moines, IA 50321

Tyco Healthcare Group Lp 800-445-5025
2 Ludlow Park Dr, Chicopee, MA 01022

ELECTRODE, PACEMAKER, TEMPORARY
(Cardiovascular) 74LDF

Edwards Lifesciences Technology Sarl 949-250-2500
State Rd. 402 N.km 1.4, Anasco, PR 00610-1577
Electrode, pacemaker, temporary.

Ethicon, Llc. 908-218-2887
Rd. 183, Km. 8.3,, Industrial Area Hato, San Lorenzo, PR 00754
Sterile temporary pacing wire.

Medtronic Heart Valves 800-227-3191
8299 Central Ave NE, Spring Lake Park, MN 55432
Various models.

Oscor, Inc. 800-726-7267
3816 Desoto Blvd, Palm Harbor, FL 34683
Temporary pacing lead.

Teleflex Medical 800-334-9751
2917 Weck Drive, Research Triangle Park, NC 27709
Cardiac pacing wire.

ELECTRODE, PH *(Gastro/Urology) 78FFT*

Analytical Measurements, Inc. 800-635-5580
100 Hoffman Pl, Hillside, NJ 07205
2 models - $60.00 and up.

Arizona Device Manufacturing 763-505-0874
2350 W Medtronic Way, Tempe, AZ 85281
Various types of ph electrodes (stomach).

Beckman Coulter, Inc. 800-742-2345
250 S Kraemer Blvd, PO Box 8000, Brea, CA 92821

Cole-Parmer Instrument Inc. 800-323-4340
625 E Bunker Ct, Vernon Hills, IL 60061

Corning Inc., Science Products Division 800-492-1110
45 Nagog Park, Acton, MA 01720

Filterspun 800-432-0108
624 N Fairfield St, Amarillo, TX 79107

Heidelberg Medical, Inc. 706-745-9698
627 Gainesville Hwy Ste B, Blairsville, GA 30512
Heidelberg ph capsule.

ELECTRODE, PH *(cont'd)*

Konigsberg Instruments, Inc. 626-449-0016
2000 E Foothill Blvd, Pasadena, CA 91107
Pure Antimony pH sensors for ambulatory monitoring. Reusable Probes may be 3.25 mm diameter pH only with 1 to 8 elements, or pH elements may be incorporated into 4 mm dia and 4.65 mm dia GI Motility Probes.

Medtronic Neuromodulation 763-514-4000
710 Medtronic Pkwy, Minneapolis, MN 55432
Various types of ph electrodes (stomach).

Microelectrodes, Inc. 603-668-0692
40 Harvey Rd, Bedford, NH 03110
$360

Omega Engineering, Inc. 800-848-4286
1 Omega Dr, Stamford, CT 06907
ALPHA high-accuracy pH electrodes feature a special internal design which allows rapid, stable readings even during large temperature shifts.

Orbeco Analytical Systems, Inc. 800-922-5242
185 Marine St, Farmingdale, NY 11735
$52.00 each (standard) polymer sealed combination.

Orion Research, Inc. 800-225-1480
166 Cummings Ctr, Beverly, MA 01915
ORION 30 models, including ROSS performance, routine pH half cell, reference half cell, combination glass-body, & gel filled electrodes - from $79 to $349 each.

Sandhill Scientific, Inc. 800-468-4556
9150 Commerce Center Cir Ste 500, Highlands Ranch, CO 80129

Von London Phonix Co 713-772-6666
6103 Glenmont Dr, Houston, TX 77081

Zinetics Medical, Inc. 800-648-4070
1050 E South Temple, Salt Lake City, UT 84102
Enteral feeding tube with pH level electrode/sensor at the tip.

ELECTRODE, SPECIFIC ION *(Chemistry) 75UFY*

Beckman Coulter, Inc. 800-742-2345
250 S Kraemer Blvd, PO Box 8000, Brea, CA 92821
ENDURAGLAS, FAST GLASS, FUTURA, MICROPORE, PERMA-FILL, PERMA-PROBE or STAR pH electrodes.

Brinkmann Instruments (Canada) Ltd. 800-263-8715
6670 Campobello Rd., Mississauga, ONT L5N 2L8 Canada

Dade Behring, Inc. 800-948-3233
1717 Deerfield Rd, Deerfield, IL 60015

Microelectrodes, Inc. 603-668-0692
40 Harvey Rd, Bedford, NH 03110
$140.00 and up each.

Orion Research, Inc. 800-225-1480
166 Cummings Ctr, Beverly, MA 01915
ORION 29 types - $215 to $728 each, including Ag, BF, Br, Ca, Cd, Cl, ClO, CN, CO2, Cu, F, Fisher, Hardness, I, K, Na, NH, NO, O2, Pb, & SCN.

ELECTRODE, SURFACE *(Anesthesiology) 73BWY*

Dymedix Corporation 888-212-1100
5985 Rice Creek Pkwy Ste 201, Shoreview, MN 55126
Dual EMG snap-ons for leg or intercostal; Triple pre-wired EMG/EOG with color-coded wiring; Pre-distanced 3-in-1 Chin electrode patch.

Integral Design Inc. 781-740-2036
52 Burr Rd, Hingham, MA 02043

Jari Electrode Supply 800-745-1934
380 Tomkins Ct, Gilroy, CA 95020
For use in electrophysiological monitoring and testing.

U.F.I. 805-772-1203
545 Main St Ste C2, Morro Bay, CA 93442
$19.00 for Model 1081 SNP Biode.

ELECTRODE, SWEAT TEST *(Chemistry) 75QTF*

Tyco Healthcare Group Lp 800-445-5025
2 Ludlow Park Dr, Chicopee, MA 01022

ELECTRODE, TENS *(Cns/Neurology) 84WHU*

Alimed, Inc. 800-225-2610
297 High St, Dedham, MA 02026

Ambu, Inc. 800-262-8462
6740 Baymeadow Dr, Glen Burnie, MD 21060

Arizona Dme--Durable Medical Equipment, Inc. 888-665-2568
PO Box 15413, Scottsdale, AZ 85267
CPM(S), Bracing C Custom, Post-Op., etc.

ELECTRODE, TENS *(cont'd)*

Axelgaard Manufacturing Company, Ltd. 760-728-3430
520 Industrial Way, Fallbrook, CA 92028
PALS PLATINUM neurostimulation electrodes with knitted stainless steel fabric. VALUTRODE. Neurostimulation electrodes, carbon film based.

Biomedical Life Systems, Inc. 800-726-8367
2448 Cades Way, Vista, CA 92081

Innova Corp. 860-242-3210
68 E Dudley Town Rd, Bloomfield, CT 06002

Katecho, Inc. 515-244-1212
4020 Gannett Ave, Des Moines, IA 50321

Medical Science Products, Inc. 800-456-1971
517 Elm Ridge Ave, P.O. Box 381, Canal Fulton, OH 44614
THE SOFT HEART (2.5in. heart-shape), THE CONDUCTOR (2x2.75in. rectangle), and THE SOFT SPOT (2in. round) disposable, breathable and bathable TENS electrodes designed for multiple day use with solid gel polymer conductor and center ridge PIN connector. POLYSTIM II (thin profile) reusable TENS electrodes. Sizes: 1.1/4in., 2in., or 3in. round, 2x3.5in. or 2x2in. and 3.5x7in. paravertebral. Both types with center Pin connection, Pin or Snap configuration, synthetic conductive polymer with flesh colored cloth.

Mylon-Tech Health Technologies Inc. 613-728-1667
301 Moodie Dr., Ste. 205, Ottawa, ON K2H 9C4 Canada
Excellent variety of different self-adhering electrodes.

Neumed Inc. 800-367-1238
800 Silvia St, Ewing, NJ 08628
TheraKnit Wrap Electrodes: Self-adhering conductive wrap for electrotherapy treatment to reduce edema and associated pain. Use with TENS, HVPC, Microcurrent, etc. Available in beige, blue, and red.

Pepin Manufacturing, Inc. 800-291-6505
1875 S Highway 61, Lake City, MN 55041
Manufacturer of TENS and EMS for all FES applications.

Pharmaceutical Innovations, Inc. 973-242-2900
897 Frelinghuysen Ave, Newark, NJ 07114
Spray. $4.95 250ml ELECTRO MIST electrolyte spray for muscle stimulation.

Smi 920-876-3361
Industrial Park, 544 Sohn Drive, Elkhart Lake, WI 53020

Tailored Label Products, Inc. 800-727-1344
W165N5731 Ridgewood Dr, Menomonee Falls, WI 53051

Zimmer Medizinsystems 800-327-3576
25 Mauchly Ste 300, Irvine, CA 92618
Hygienic single use, multi-function, self-adhesive electrodes. Available in different sizes and shapes. Cost effective, OSHA safe.

ELECTRODE, TRANSCUTANEOUS, CARBON-DIOXIDE *(Anesthesiology) 73QTG*

Radiometer America, Inc. 800-736-0600
810 Sharon Dr, Westlake, OH 44145
Combined tcPCO-2/tcPO-2 electrode.

Respironics, Inc 800-345-6443
1010 Murry Ridge Ln, Murrysville, PA 15668
$950.00 per unit.

ELECTRODE, TRANSCUTANEOUS, OXYGEN *(Anesthesiology) 73QTH*

Radiometer America, Inc. 800-736-0600
810 Sharon Dr, Westlake, OH 44145
Combined tcPCO-2/tcPO-2 electrode.

Respironics, Inc 800-345-6443
1010 Murry Ridge Ln, Murrysville, PA 15668
$950.00 per unit.

ELECTROENCEPHALOGRAPH *(Cns/Neurology) 84GWQ*

Aspect Medical Systems, Inc. 617-559-7000
1 Upland Rd, Norwood, MA 02062
Electroencephalograph.

Aspect Medical Systems, Inc. 617-559-7000
141 Needham St, Newton, MA 02464
A-1000 EEG Monitor 4-Channel EEG brain monitor with the bispectral index.

Bio-Feedback Systems, Inc. 303-444-1411
2736 47th St, Boulder, CO 80301
$1,450 for ALPHA/THETA and $2,195 for TWILIGHT LEARNING, EEG biofeedback equipment. $2,245 for 1 channel hardware & software to interface to PC compatible.

ELECTROENCEPHALOGRAPH *(cont'd)*

Bio-Logic Systems Corp. 800-323-8326
1 Bio Logic Plz, Mundelein, IL 60060
CEEGRAPH, family of digital EEG instruments offer a wide range of products; from kits & portable instruments to laboratory based & reader stations.

Burke L. Mays And Associates, Inc. 615-791-6247
315 Springhouse Cir, Franklin, TN 37067
Electroencephalograph system.

Cadwell Laboratories 800-245-3001
909 N Kellogg St, Kennewick, WA 99336
CADWELL EASY II all 24 or 32 channels. Full digital EEG system with optional polysomnography, digital video & analysis packages. Includes photo stimulator, power supply, floor stand and software.

Cardinal Healthcare 209, Inc. 610-862-0800
5225 Verona Rd, Fitchburg, WI 53711
Video eeg.

Cleveland Medical Devices, Inc. 877-253-8363
4415 Euclid Ave, Cleveland, OH 44103
CRYSTAL-EEG Model 10 is a mobile, intermediate range, wireless EEG system consisting of a transmitter, receiver assembly, software, patient accessories and PC operator interface.

Compumedics Usa, Ltd. 915-225-0303
7850 Paseo Del Norte, El Paso, TX 79912
Electroencephalograph.

Computational Diagnostics, Inc. 412-681-9990
5001 Baum Blvd Ste 426, Pittsburgh, PA 15213
Neurophysiological monitoring system.

Cyberkinetics Neurotechnology Systems, Inc. 508-549-9981
100 Foxboro Blvd Ste 240, Foxborough, MA 02035
Electroencephalograph.

Draeger Medical Systems, Inc. 215-660-2626
16 Electronics Ave, Danvers, MA 01923
Monitor.

Electrical Geodesics, Inc. 541-687-7962
2979 Chad Dr, Eugene, OR 97408
Various models of eeg system equipment.

Electrical Geodesics, Incorporated 541-687-7962
1600 Millrace Dr Ste 307, Eugene, OR 97403
Geodesic EEG System 300 (32, 64,128, 256 electrodes - cart or portable). Geodesic EEG Systems 140 and 120 (32 channels. Appropriate for routine clinical EEG, LTM, video EEG and research applications. Suitable for pediatric and adult populations.

Electro-Cap International, Inc. 800-527-2193
1011 W Lexington Rd, PO Box 87, Eaton, OH 45320

Grass Technologies, An Astro-Med, Inc. Product Gro 401-828-4002
53 Airport Park Drive, Rockland, MA 02370
Home to office portable eeg recorder.

Hydrodot, Inc. 978-399-0206
238 Littleton Rd Ste 202, Westford, MA 01886
Eeg headpiece.

I.M.A. Electronics, Inc. 352-378-7551
6614 NW 26th Ter, Gainesville, FL 32653
Electroencephalograph.

Individual Monitoring Systems, Inc. 410-296-7723
1055 Taylor Ave Ste 300, Baltimore, MD 21286
Actitrac.

La Mont Medical, Inc. 888-452-6688
555 Donofrio Dr, Madison, WI 53719
LA MONT DIGITAL Acquisition Devices including computer interface cards, Programmable EEG and SLEEP amplifiers (PRO AMPS), jackboxes, cables . LA MONT VANGARD SYSTEMS (V Series) for LTM (long Term Epilepsy Monitoring), Routine EEG (REEG) and SLEEP (PSG). LA MONT NCI SYSTEMS (N Series) Service.

Lds Life Science (Formerly Gould Instrument Systems Inc.) 216-328-7000
5525 Cloverleaf Pkwy, Valley View, OH 44125

Lexicor Medical Technology, Inc. 706-447-1074
2840 Wilderness Pl Ste E, Boulder, CO 80301
Elecroencephalograph.

Manufacturing Technology, Inc. 850-664-6070
70 Ready Ave NW, Fort Walton Beach, FL 32548
Activity monitor.

Neurocybernetics, Inc. 516-482-9001
21601 Vanowen St Ste 100, Canoga Park, CA 91303
Eeg signal spectrum analyzer & monitoring data acquisition system.

Nihon Kohden America, Inc. 800-325-0283
90 Icon, Foothill Ranch, CA 92610

Spacelabs Medical Inc. 800-522-7212
5150 220th Ave SE, Issaquah, WA 98029
Various electroencephalograph modules and accessories.

Vsm Medtech (Formerly Ctf Systems) 604-472-2300
9 Burbidge Street, Coquitlam, BC V3K 7B2 Canada
Magnetoencephalograph: biomagnetometer

4-D Neuroimaging 858-453-6300
9727 Pacific Heights Blvd, San Diego, CA 92121
Magnetic encephalograph.

ELECTROFOCUSING EQUIPMENT *(Chemistry) 75UFZ*

Bio-Rad Laboratories, Life Science Group 800-424-6723
2000 Alfred Nobel Dr, Hercules, CA 94547
Complete systems including cells and kits.

Mettler-Toledo Process Analytical, Inc. 800-352-8763
299 Washington St, Woburn, MA 01801
Flat surface pH sensors.

PerkinElmer 800-762-4000
940 Winter St, Waltham, MA 02451
Unit for IEF with the ISOSCAN, general purpose PC-based densitometer.

ELECTROGLOTTOGRAPH *(Ear/Nose/Throat) 77KLX*

U.F.I. 805-772-1203
545 Main St Ste C2, Morro Bay, CA 93442
$525.00 for Model 2991.

ELECTROLYSIS EQUIPMENT, OTHER *(General) 80WPK*

Eel Electronics Mfg. Co. 910-944-4780
160 S May St Apt 2, Southern Pines, NC 28387
Super Phaser Gold non-invasive permanent hair removal Class 1 medical device

ELECTROLYSIS UNIT, OPHTHALMIC *(Ophthalmology) 86HRO*

Biomet, Inc. 574-267-6639
56 E Bell Dr, PO Box 587, Warsaw, IN 46582
Various types of hemostat.

ELECTROMYOGRAPH, DIAGNOSTIC *(Physical Med) 89IKN*

B & L Engineering 714-505-9492
3002 Dow Ave Ste 416, Tustin, CA 92780
Active surface emg electrode.

Bio-Research Associates, Inc. 414-357-7525
9275 N 49th St Ste 150, Brown Deer, WI 53223
Electromyograph, 8 channel.

Cadwell Laboratories 800-245-3001
909 N Kellogg St, Kennewick, WA 99336
CADWELL SIERRA II EMG/EP. All protocols 2 or 4 channel. Cadwell Cascade 8 or 16 channels. All protocals including surgical monitoring CADWELL CENTRAL EMG/EP/EEG.

Cardinal Healthcare 209, Inc. 610-862-0800
5225 Verona Rd, Fitchburg, WI 53711
Electroneurodiagnostic system (ep/emg).

Compumedics Usa, Ltd. 915-225-0303
7850 Paseo Del Norte, El Paso, TX 79912
Emg/ep system.

Delsys, Inc. 617-236-0599
650 Beacon St Fl 6, Boston, MA 02215
Emg system.

Electronic Mfg. Co. 813-855-4068
13440 Wright Cir, Tampa, FL 33626
Semg, surface electromyography.

Excel Tech. Ltd. 905-829-5300
2568 Bristol Cir, Oakville L6H 5S1 Canada
Various

Medtronic Sofamor Danek Usa, Inc. 901-396-3133
4340 Swinnea Rd, Memphis, TN 38118
Monopolar stimulating instrumentation.

Minnetronix Inc. 888-301-1025
1635 Energy Park Dr, Saint Paul, MN 55108
CERSR Electromyography System

ELECTROMYOGRAPH, DIAGNOSTIC *(cont'd)*

Neurocom International, Inc. 503-653-2144
9570 SE Lawnfield Rd, Clackamas, OR 97015
Electromyogram, surface.

Omnia Technology An Optimation Company 585-321-2300
2550 Gray Falls Dr Ste 207, Houston, TX 77077
Diagnostic electromyograph.

Oxford Instruments 800-438-8322
300 Baker Ave Ste 150, Concord, MA 01742
TECA Synergy 2, 5, 10 channel, diagnostic electromyographs with multiple features.

Spinematrix, Inc. 330-665-6780
202 Montrose West Ave Ste 360, Copley, OH 44321
Surface electromyography (semg) diagnostic device.

ELECTRONYSTAGMOGRAPH (ENG) *(Ophthalmology) 86QTL*

Gn Otometrics 800-289-2150
125 Commerce Dr, Schaumburg, IL 60173
$19,900.00 for computer based electronystagmograph with analysis and permanent storage capability. CHARTR VNG videonystagmograph eye movement recorder for diagnosis of balance disorders is available for $26,500.00.

Micromedical Technologies, Inc. 800-334-4154
10 Kemp Dr, Chatham, IL 62629
Meta 4 computerized ENG system with 4-channel programmable EOG amplifier for recording both horizontal and vertical eye movement; quadlight calibration bar, PC compatible computer with two disk drives, monitor and laserjet printer. Also, VORTEQ focus auto-rotational test hard- and software plus VORTEQ tuning fork transducer. Also, computerized electronystagmograph (ENG), FOCUS 2-channel computerized ENG with programmable EOG amplifier for recording eye movements. PC compatible computer, color graphics display, laser printer, and quad lightbar. Nystagmus, caloric, and ocular motor testing available. Visual Eyes infrared video ENG allows simultaneous subjective observation of eye movements and objective collection and analysis of eye movement waveforms during vestibular testing and rehabilitation.

Western Ophthalmics Corporation 800-426-9938
19019 36th Ave W Ste G, Lynnwood, WA 98036

ELECTROPHORESIS EQUIPMENT, CELLULOSE ACETATE MEMBRANE *(Chemistry) 75UEO*

Camag Scientific, Inc. 800-334-3909
515 Cornelius Harnett Dr, Wilmington, NC 28401

Helena Laboratories 409-842-3714
PO Box 752, Beaumont, TX 77704

Olympus America, Inc. 800-645-8160
3500 Corporate Pkwy, PO Box 610, Center Valley, PA 18034

ELECTROPHORESIS EQUIPMENT, GEL *(Chemistry) 75UGG*

Beckman Coulter, Inc. 800-742-2345
250 S Kraemer Blvd, PO Box 8000, Brea, CA 92821

Bio-Rad Laboratories, Life Science Group 800-424-6723
2000 Alfred Nobel Dr, Hercules, CA 94547
$875-$1,600 for slabs; $950 for 1-slab DNA sequencer, 33 cm x 40 cm; $380 for gradient maker, 100 ml mix chambers, 100 ml reservoir; $800 for slab dryer; $750 for constant voltage/current/power.

Cbs Scientific Co., Inc. 800-243-4959
PO Box 856, Del Mar, CA 92014

Crescent Chemical Co., Inc. 800-877-3225
2 Oval Dr, Islandia, NY 11749
All products necessary for SDS or IEF electrophoresis.

Helena Laboratories 409-842-3714
PO Box 752, Beaumont, TX 77704

Idea Scientific Co. 800-433-2535
PO Box 13210, Minneapolis, MN 55414
$250.00 for 10x15 cm chameleon Submarine Agarose Gel electorphoresis equipment. $290.00 for Genie Western blot apparatus for 15x15 cm gels.

Intersciences Inc. 800-661-6431
169 Idema Rd., Markham, ONT L3R 1A9 Canada
GELCLONE Horizontal gel electrophoresis boxes.

Nutech Molding Corporation 1-800-423-5278
PO Box 840, 2024 Broad St,, Pocomoke City, MD 21851

PerkinElmer 800-762-4000
940 Winter St, Waltham, MA 02451

Sebia Electrophoresis 800-835-6497
400-1705 Corporate Drive, Norcross, GA 30093

ELECTROPHORESIS EQUIPMENT, GEL *(cont'd)*

Ultra-Lum, Inc. 800-809-6559
1480 N Claremont Blvd, Claremont, CA 91711
Ultracam Series, Gel Explorer Series, or Omega Series of Gel Documentation Systems.

Uvp, Llc 800-452-6788
2066 W 11th St, Upland, CA 91786
GDS Electrophoresis gel documentation system.

ELECTROPHORESIS EQUIPMENT, LIQUID *(Chemistry) 75JJN*

Beckman Coulter, Inc. 800-742-2345
250 S Kraemer Blvd, PO Box 8000, Brea, CA 92821

Lonza Rockland, Inc. 207-594-3400
191 Thomaston St, Rockland, ME 04841
Various sizes of seakem, seaplaque, isogel agarose powders,gelbond f.

Princeton Separations, Inc. 732-431-3338
100 Commerce Ave, Freehold, NJ 07728
Accessories for electrophonetic determinations.

ELECTROPHORESIS EQUIPMENT, THIN-LAYER *(Chemistry) 75UIU*

Uvp, Llc 800-452-6788
2066 W 11th St, Upland, CA 91786
Ultraviolet transilluminators and UV lamps.

ELECTROPHORESIS INSTRUMENTATION *(Immunology) 82JZS*

Beckman Coulter, Inc. 800-742-2345
250 S Kraemer Blvd, PO Box 8000, Brea, CA 92821

Bio-Rad Laboratories, Life Science Group 800-424-6723
2000 Alfred Nobel Dr, Hercules, CA 94547
Affinity purified antibodies.

Helena Laboratories 409-842-3714
PO Box 752, Beaumont, TX 77704
Immunoelectrophoresis; immunofixation electrophoresis.

Idea Scientific Co. 800-433-2535
PO Box 13210, Minneapolis, MN 55414
$200.00 for SURF-BLOT Western blot strip analysis system. $180.00 for MINI-GENIE complete Western blot apparatus for 10x12cm gels.

Olympus America, Inc. 800-645-8160
3500 Corporate Pkwy, PO Box 610, Center Valley, PA 18034

Sebia Electrophoresis 800-835-6497
400-1705 Corporate Drive, Norcross, GA 30093

Wepco Products, Inc 775-772-5910
1930 Gilly Ln, Concord, CA 94518
Semi-dry electrophoresis blotting devices.

ELECTROPHORETIC SEPARATION, ALKALINE PHOSPHATASE ISOENZYMES *(Chemistry) 75CIN*

Dade Behring, Inc. 800-948-3233
1717 Deerfield Rd, Deerfield, IL 60015

Health Chem Diagnostics Llc 954-979-3845
3341 W McNab Rd, Pompano Beach, FL 33069
Electrophoretic separation, alkaline phosphatase isoenzymes.

Helena Laboratories 409-842-3714
PO Box 752, Beaumont, TX 77704

PerkinElmer 800-762-4000
940 Winter St, Waltham, MA 02451

Quantimetrix Corporation 800-624-8380
2005 Manhattan Beach Blvd, Redondo Beach, CA 90278

Sebia Electrophoresis 800-835-6497
400-1705 Corporate Drive, Norcross, GA 30093

ELECTROPHORETIC SEPARATION, LIPOPROTEINS *(Chemistry) 75JHO*

Beckman Coulter, Inc. 800-742-2345
250 S Kraemer Blvd, PO Box 8000, Brea, CA 92821

Berkeley Heartlab, Inc. 510-263-4033
960 Atlantic Ave Ste 100, Alameda, CA 94501
Hdl,ldl subfraction test.

Berkeley Nucleonics Corp. 800-234-7858
2955 Kerner Blvd, San Rafael, CA 94901
SAM935 from Berkeley Nucleonics offers users the fastest, most accurate nuclear detection available.

Helena Laboratories 409-842-3714
PO Box 752, Beaumont, TX 77704

ELECTROPHORETIC SEPARATION, LIPOPROTEINS *(cont'd)*

Quantimetrix Corporation 800-624-8380
2005 Manhattan Beach Blvd, Redondo Beach, CA 90278
LIPOPRINT LDL or LIPOPRINT HDL systems - simple polyacrylamide gel electrophoresis system for separation of various subfractions of LDL and HDL.

Sebia Electrophoresis 800-835-6497
400-1705 Corporate Drive, Norcross, GA 30093

ELECTROPHORETIC, GLUCOSE-6-PHOSPHATE DEHYDROGENASE *(Hematology) 81JLM*

Helena Laboratories 409-842-3714
PO Box 752, Beaumont, TX 77704

ELECTROPHORETIC, LACTATE DEHYDROGENASE ISOENZYMES *(Chemistry) 75CFE*

Biomerieux Inc. 800-682-2666
100 Rodolphe St, Durham, NC 27712

Creative Laboratory Products, Inc. 317-293-2991
6420 Guion Rd, Indianapolis, IN 46268

Dade Behring, Inc. 800-948-3233
1717 Deerfield Rd, Deerfield, IL 60015

Health Chem Diagnostics Llc 954-979-3845
3341 W McNab Rd, Pompano Beach, FL 33069
Electrophoretic, lactate dehydrogenase isoenzymes.

Helena Laboratories 409-842-3714
PO Box 752, Beaumont, TX 77704
Also, CPK or isoenzymes.

Sebia Electrophoresis 800-835-6497
400-1705 Corporate Drive, Norcross, GA 30093

ELECTROPHORETIC, PROTEIN FRACTIONATION
(Chemistry) 75CEF

Budenheim Usa, Inc 800-645-3044
245 Newtown Rd Ste 305, Plainview, NY 11803

Helena Laboratories 409-842-3714
PO Box 752, Beaumont, TX 77704
Electrophoretic, High Res. Protein.

Princeton Separations, Inc. 732-431-3338
100 Commerce Ave, Freehold, NJ 07728
Reagents for qualitative or quantitative analysis of human protein.

Sebia Electrophoresis 800-835-6497
400-1705 Corporate Drive, Norcross, GA 30093

ELECTRORETINOGRAPH (ERG) *(Ophthalmology) 86QTN*

Lkc Technologies, Inc. 800-638-7055
2 Professional Dr Ste 222, Gaithersburg, MD 20879
UTAS-E3000mf and EPIC-4000. Standard and optional multi-focal ERG capability is available on both the UTAS-E3000mf as well as the EPIC 4000.

ELECTRORHEOGRAPH *(General) 80TBZ*

Spacelabs Healthcare 800-522-7025
5150 220th Ave SE, Issaquah, WA 98029
CardioExpress

U.F.I. 805-772-1203
545 Main St Ste C2, Morro Bay, CA 93442
$6,250.00 for Model 2994.

ELECTROSURGICAL EQUIPMENT, GENERAL PURPOSE
(Surgery) 79UCP

Ams Innovative Center-San Jose 800-356-7600
3070 Orchard Dr, San Jose, CA 95134

Buffalo Filter, A Division Of Medtek Devices Inc. 800-343-2324
595 Commerce Dr, Amherst, NY 14228
Full line of smoke evacuation systems for use with electrosurgical units to capture smoke plume generated from all procedures, including tubing, in-line filters, adapters for connection to ESU pencils, remote switch activators.

Cameron-Miller, Inc. 800-621-0142
5410 W Roosevelt Rd, Road #241, Chicago, IL 60644

Coopersurgical, Inc. 800-243-2974
95 Corporate Dr, Trumbull, CT 06611

Ellman International, Inc. 800-835-5355
3333 Royal Ave, Rockville Centre, NY 11572

Elmed, Inc. 630-543-2792
60 W Fay Ave, Addison, IL 60101

ELECTROSURGICAL EQUIPMENT, GENERAL PURPOSE *(cont'd)*

Encision Inc. 303-444-2600
6797 Winchester Cir, Boulder, CO 80301
AEM EM-2 system monitor dynamicaly monitors electrosurgical instruments during surgery. Deactivates generator if a problem arises due to insulation failure or capacitive coupling.

Ethicon Endo-Surgery, Inc. 800-USE-ENDO
4545 Creek Rd, Cincinnati, OH 45242

Florida Life Systems 727-321-9554
3446 5th Ave N, Saint Petersburg, FL 33713

Gyrus Medical, Inc. 800-852-9361
6655 Wedgwood Rd N Ste 105, Maple Grove, MN 55311
PK Bipolar generator incorporates PK technology for use in endourology, laparoscopic, and open procedures. Featuring vapor-pulsed coagulation for improved tissue management. Also offering effective bipolar cutting modalities.

Innovasive Devices, Inc. 800-435-6001
734 Forest St, Marlborough, MA 01752

International Hospital Supply Co. 800-398-9450
6914 Canby Ave Ste 105, Reseda, CA 91335

J. Jamner Surgical Instruments, Inc 800-431-1123
9 Skyline Dr, Hawthorne, NY 10532

M & I Medical Sales, Inc. 305-663-6444
4711 SW 72nd Ave, Miami, FL 33155

Mark Medical Manufacturing, Inc. 610-269-4420
530 Brandywine Ave, Downingtown, PA 19335
Monopolar and bipolar forceps and nonconductive instruments in titanium or stainless steel.

Md International, Inc. 305-669-9003
11300 NW 41st St, Doral, FL 33178

Medgyn Products, Inc. 800-451-9667
328 Eisenhower Ln N, Lombard, IL 60148

Olsen Medical 800-297-6344
3001 W Kentucky St, Louisville, KY 40211
Bipolar and Monopolar Forceps, and Electrodes.

Olympus America, Inc. 800-645-8160
3500 Corporate Pkwy, PO Box 610, Center Valley, PA 18034

Premier Medical Products 888-PREMUSA
1710 Romano Dr, Plymouth Meeting, PA 19462

Richard Wolf Medical Instruments Corp. 800-323-9653
353 Corporate Woods Pkwy, Vernon Hills, IL 60061

Shippert Medical Technologies Corp. 800-888-8663
6248 S Troy Cir Ste A, Centennial, CO 80111
Generators, electrodes, cauteries. All Aaron electrosurgical products.

Solta Medical, Inc. 877-782-2286
25881 Industrial Blvd, Hayward, CA 94545
electrosurgical, cutting & coagulation & accessories

Superior Medical Limited 800-268-7944
520 Champagne Dr., Toronto, ONT M3J 2T9 Canada

Thomas Medical Inc. 800-556-0349
5610 West 82 2nd Street, Indianpolis, IN 46278

Valleylab 800-255-8522
5920 Longbow Dr, Boulder, CO 80301
Full family of generators: FORCE FX™, FORCE EZ™ electrosurgical geneators with Instant Response™ technology; SURGISTAT™ II, office-based system. Full line electrosurgical accessories.

Wallach Surgical Devices, Inc. 800-243-2463
235 Edison Rd, Orange, CT 06477

ELECTROSURGICAL EQUIPMENT, SPECIAL PURPOSE
(Surgery) 79UCQ

Cameron-Miller, Inc. 800-621-0142
5410 W Roosevelt Rd, Road #241, Chicago, IL 60644

Florida Life Systems 727-321-9554
3446 5th Ave N, Saint Petersburg, FL 33713

Gyrus Medical, Inc. 800-852-9361
6655 Wedgwood Rd N Ste 105, Maple Grove, MN 55311
PK Generator designed for use in endourology, laparoscopic, and open procedures.

Mahe International Inc. 800-294-7946
468 Craighead St, Nashville, TN 37204

Md International, Inc. 305-669-9003
11300 NW 41st St, Doral, FL 33178

Olsen Medical 800-297-6344
3001 W Kentucky St, Louisville, KY 40211
Bipolar and Monopolar Forceps and Electrodes

ELECTROSURGICAL EQUIPMENT, SPECIAL PURPOSE *(cont'd)*

R Medical Supply 800-882-7578
620 Valley Forge Rd Ste F, Hillsborough, NC 27278
OB/GYN excision procedures.

Utah Medical Products, Inc. 800-533-4984
7043 Cottonwood St, Midvale, UT 84047
FINESSE and FINESSE II electrosurgical generator and integrated smoke evacuation systems for loop excision procedures.

Valley Forge Scientific Corp. 610-666-7500
136 Green Tree Road, Suite 100, Oaks, PA 19456
Bipolar Electrosurgical Coagulator - Low powered generator used with electrode instruments for surgical coagulation in microsurgical procedures.

Valleylab 800-255-8522
5920 Longbow Dr, Boulder, CO 80301
FORCE FX™, electrosurgical equipment for cardiothoracic and urologic procedures.

ELECTROSURGICAL UNIT, ANESTHESIOLOGY ACCESSORIES
(Surgery) 79BWA

Intermed Group, Inc. 561-586-3667
3550 23rd Ave S Ste 1, Lake Worth, FL 33461
Intermed es-5000 electrosurgical unit.

Micrins Surgical Instruments, Inc. 800-833-3380
28438 N Ballard Dr, Lake Forest, IL 60045

Reznik Instrument, Inc. 847-673-3444
7337 Lawndale Ave, Skokie, IL 60076
Electrosurgical unit.

ELECTROSURGICAL UNIT, CARDIOVASCULAR
(Cardiovascular) 74DWG

Cameron-Miller, Inc. 800-621-0142
5410 W Roosevelt Rd, Road #241, Chicago, IL 60644

Valleylab 800-255-8522
5920 Longbow Dr, Boulder, CO 80301
FORCE FX™, for demanding cardiovascular procedures.

ELECTROSURGICAL UNIT, CUTTING & COAGULATION DEVICE
(Surgery) 79GEI

Accellent Inc. 866-899-1392
100 Fordham Rd, Wilmington, MA 01887

Aesculap Implant Systems Inc. 1-800-234-9179
3773 Corporate Pkwy, Center Valley, PA 18034

Alto Development Corp. 732-938-2266
5206 Asbury Rd, Wall Township, NJ 07727
Electrosurgical knives.

American Biosurgical 770-416-1992
1850 Beaver Ridge Cir Ste B, Norcross, GA 30071
AB Monopolar Cable/Cord; AB Bipolar Cable/Cord

Apple Medical Corp. 508-357-2700
28 Lord Rd Ste 135, Marlborough, MA 01752
Bipolar electrocautery inserts.

Applied Surgical, Llc 205-259-2050
300 Riverchase Pkwy E, Birmingham, AL 35244
Foot switch & smoke evacuator.

Aragon Surgical Inc. 650-543-3100
1810 Embarcadero Rd Ste B, Palo Alto, CA 94303
Electrosurgical device.

Argon Medical Devices Inc. 903-675-9321
1445 Flat Creek Rd, Athens, TX 75751
Electrosurgical pencil.

Arthrex Manufacturing 239-643-5553
1958 Trade Center Way, Naples, FL 34109
Electrosurgical devices.

Arthrex, Inc. 239-643-5553
1370 Creekside Blvd, Naples, FL 34108
Various cutting and coagulating electrosurgical devices.

Ascent Healthcare Solutions 480-763-5300
10232 S 51st St, Phoenix, AZ 85044
Linear cutter & coagulator, bipolar cords, somnoplasty system.

Asthmatx, Inc. 1-877-810-6060
888 Ross Dr Ste 100, Sunnyvale, CA 94089
Catherter.

Atek Medical 800-253-1540
620 Watson St SW, Grand Rapids, MI 49504
Electrosurgical knife cleaner, electrocautery knife blade, electrosurgical.

ELECTROSURGICAL UNIT, CUTTING & COAGULATION DEVICE *(cont'd)*

Atricure, Inc. 888.347.6403
6217 Centre Park Dr, West Chester, OH 45069
Electrosurgical coagulation device.

Ballard Medical Products 770-587-7835
12050 Lone Peak Pkwy, Draper, UT 84020
Active cord.

Barrx Medical, Incorporated 888-662-2779
540 Oakmead Pkwy, Sunnyvale, CA 94085
Electrosurgical unit and accessories.

Biomet, Inc. 574-267-6639
56 E Bell Dr, PO Box 587, Warsaw, IN 46582
Various types of cautery devices.

Biosearch Medical Products, Inc. 908-722-5000
35 Industrial Pkwy, Branchburg, NJ 08876
Biopolar hemostatic probe.

Boston Scientific Corp. 408-935-3400
150 Baytech Dr, San Jose, CA 95134
Biopolar scissors.

Bovie Medical Corp. 800-537-2790
5115 Ulmerton Rd, Clearwater, FL 33760
Aaron Laparoscopic is a stainless steel laparoscopic electrode: 32 cm L hook, J hook, blade, ball, needle, curved & spatula. Aaron 800 is a 30 watt high frequency desiccator for dermatologic and plastic surgery. Aaron 1200 is a 120 watt electrosurgical generator for small office procedures including cut, blend, coag, fulguration and bipolar settings. Aaron 1250 electrosurgical unit, cutting and coagulating device, 120 watt electrosurgical unit for office/surgi-center procedures, uses standard 3-prong two button pencil or foot control with pad sensing. Aaron 2100unit, cutting and coagulating device, 200 watt electrosurgical generator for surgi-center or hospital has 9 blend settings, tissue sensing and pad sensing.

Cameron-Miller, Inc. 800-621-0142
5410 W Roosevelt Rd, Road #241, Chicago, IL 60644

Cardinal Health, Snowden Pencer Products 847-689-8410
5175 S Royal Atlanta Dr, Tucker, GA 30084
Various styles of electrocautery laparoscopic instruments.

Cook Endoscopy 336-744-0157
4900 Bethania Station Rd # &, 5951 Grassy Creek Blvd. Winston Salem, NC 27105
Various types of papillotomes/sphincterotomes.

Coopersurgical, Inc. 800-243-2974
95 Corporate Dr, Trumbull, CT 06611
$3,995 for electrosurgical generator.

Cosman Company, Inc. 781-272-6561
76 Cambridge St, Burlington, MA 01803
Electrosurgical coagulator with sterile & non sterile accessories.

Davol Inc., Sub. C.R. Bard, Inc. 800-556-6275
100 Crossings Blvd, Warwick, RI 02886
Laparoscopic bipolar,unipolar electrosurgical tips.

Depuy Mitek, A Johnson & Johnson Company 800-451-2006
50 Scotland Blvd, Bridgewater, MA 02324
Electorsurgical scissor & handle; electrosurgical cutting & coagulation systems.

Depuy-Raynham, A Div. Of Depuy Orthopaedics 800-451-2006
325 Paramount Dr, Raynham, MA 02767
Various electrosurgical cutting & coagulation devices and accessories.

Durden Enterprises 800-554-5673
1317 4th Ave, P.O. Box 909, Auburn, GA 30011
Electrosurgical unit with foot control and optional suction control.

Ep Technologies, Inc. 888-272-1001
2710 Orchard Pkwy, San Jose, CA 95134
Electrosugical.

Ethicon Endo-Surgery, Inc. 877-384-4266
3801 University Blvd SE, Albuquerque, NM 87106
Various types of sterile electrosurgical devices and accesories.

Greenwald Surgical Co., Inc. 219-962-1604
2688 Dekalb St, Gary, IN 46405
Electrosurgical cutting and coagulation instruments - various types.

Gyrus Acmi, Inc. 508-804-2739
93 N Pleasant St, Norwalk, OH 44857
Device, electrosurgical cutting & coagulation & accessories.

ELECTROSURGICAL UNIT, CUTTING & COAGULATION DEVICE *(cont'd)*

Gyrus Acmi, Inc. 508-804-2739
300 Stillwater P.o.box 1971, Stamford, CT 06902
Various kinds and sizes, sterile and non-sterile.

Gyrus Ent L.L.C., Sub. Of Gyrus Acmi, Inc. 508-804-2739
2925 Appling Rd, Bartlett, TN 38133
Electro surgical generator and accessories.

Gyrus Medical Inc., Sub. Of Gyrus Acmi, Inc. 508-804-2739
6655 Wedgwood Rd N Ste 160, Maple Grove, MN 55311
Sterile & nonsterile endoscope electrosurgical instrumentation & accessories.

Gyrus Medical, Inc. 800-852-9361
6655 Wedgwood Rd N Ste 105, Maple Grove, MN 55311
BILAP bipolar laparoscopic cutting and coagulation electrosurgical device with irrigation and aspiration. Single-patient use.

Halt Medical Inc. 925-634-7943
131 Sand Creek Rd Ste B, Brentwood, CA 94513
Halt 2000 RF Ablation System; Tulip 1000

Hemostatix Medical Technologies, Llc 901-261-0012
8400 Wolf Lake Dr Ste 109, Bartlett, TN 38133
Thermal scalpel system; esu scalpel system; hemostatic surgical system.

Hill-Med, Inc. 305-594-7474
7217 NW 46th St, Miami, FL 33166

I.C. Medical, Inc. 623-780-0700
2002 W Quail Ave, Phoenix, AZ 85027
Various types of electrosurgical accessories.

Innervision Inc. 901-682-0417
6258 E Shady Grove Rd, Memphis, TN 38120

Integral Design Inc. 781-740-2036
52 Burr Rd, Hingham, MA 02043

Intuitive Surgical, Inc. 888-409-4774
1266 Kifer Rd, Sunnyvale, CA 94086
Various electrosurgical cutting & coagulation & accessories.

J. Jamner Surgical Instruments, Inc 800-431-1123
9 Skyline Dr, Hawthorne, NY 10532

Karl Storz Endoscopy-America Inc. 800-421-0837
600 Corporate Pointe, Culver City, CA 90230
Includes various accessories.

Kirwan Surgical Products, Inc. 888-547-9267
180 Enterprise Dr, PO Box 427, Marshfield, MA 02050
Disposable and reusable monopolar suction coagulators.

Lmi Lightwave Medical Industries Ltd. 604-275-3400
250-13155 Delf Pl, Richmond, BC V6V 2A2 Canada
Various

Maquet Puerto Rico Inc. 408-635-3900
No. 12, Rd. #698, Dorado, PR 00646
Cutting devices.

Mark Medical Manufacturing, Inc. 610-269-4420
530 Brandywine Ave, Downingtown, PA 19335
Monopolar and bipolar forceps and nonconductive instruments in titanium or stainless steel.

Md International, Inc. 305-669-9003
11300 NW 41st St, Doral, FL 33178

Medelec Industries 888-522-6452
6800 Bird Rd, Miami, FL 33155
Electrosurgical pen.

Medical Action Industries, Inc. 800-645-7042
25 Heywood Rd, Arden, NC 28704
Cautery tip cleaners.

Medisiss 866-866-7477
2747 SW 6th St, Redmond, OR 97756
Various electrosurgical cutting and coagulation and accessories,sterile.

Medsphere International, Inc 510-656-8232
48531 Warm Springs Blvd Ste 417, Fremont, CA 94539
Electrosurgical electrodes.

Medtronic Neuromodulation 763-514-4000
710 Medtronic Pkwy, Minneapolis, MN 55432
Various models of cartridge kits.

Medtronic Puerto Rico Operations Co., Villalba 763-514-4000
PO Box 6001, Rd. 149, Km. 56.3, Villalba, PR 00766
Various models of cartridge kits.

ELECTROSURGICAL UNIT, CUTTING & COAGULATION DEVICE *(cont'd)*

Medtronic Sofamor Danek Instrument Manufacturing 901-396-3133
7375 Adrianne Pl, Bartlett, TN 38133
Various electrosurgical accessories.

Medtronic Sofamor Danek Usa, Inc. 901-396-3133
4340 Swinnea Rd, Memphis, TN 38118
Various electrosurgical accessories.

Megadyne Medical Products, Inc. 800-747-6110
11506 S State St, Draper, UT 84020
The Mega Power electrosurgical generator is simple on the outside and advanced on the inside. The E-Z Pen reusable electrosurgical pencils incorporate a counting mechanism and lock-out device that prevents use of the product beyond its safe product life. This provides clinicians with a safe, economical product. Disposable electrosurgical pencils with or without holster, button and rocker switch configurations.

Microline Pentax, Inc. 978-922-9810
800 Cummings Ctr Ste 157X, Beverly, MA 01915
'3 mm selec-tip' laparoscopic scissors.

Minnetronix Inc. 888-301-1025
1635 Energy Park Dr, Saint Paul, MN 55108
EN BLOC BIOPSY SYSTEM

nContact Surgical, Inc. 919-466-9810
1001 Aviation Pkwy Ste 400, Morrisville, NC 27560
Electrosurgical device and accessories.

Neomedix Corp. 949-258-8355
15042 Parkway Loop Ste A, Tustin, CA 92780
Electro surgical bipolar handpiece.

New Deantronics, Ltd. 925-280-8388
1990 N California Blvd Ste 1040, Walnut Creek, CA 94596
Device, electrosurgical, cutting and coagulation and accessories.

Novasys Medical, Inc. 510-226-4060
39684 Eureka Dr, Newark, CA 94560
Electro surgical device.

Pcn, Inc. 508-880-7140
125 John Hancock Rd, Taunton, MA 02780
Coagulation device.

Premier Medical Products 888-PREMUSA
1710 Romano Dr, Plymouth Meeting, PA 19462
Model 2001e Electrosurgical Unit, 120 watts MAXIMUM power output. Five distinct operating modes: cut, blend, coagulation, fulguration, and bipolar.

Quantum Interconnect, Inc. 817-231-1400
3400 Northern Cross Blvd, Fort Worth, TX 76137
Monopolar electrosurgical cable.

Respiratory Diagnostics, Inc. 425-881-8300
47987 Fremont Blvd, Fremont, CA 94538
Various.

Rhytec Incorporated 781-474-9832
130 Turner St Bldg 2, South Waltham, MA 02453
Electrosurgical generator and accessories.

Rontron Engineering, Inc. 203-488-5020
131 Commercial Pkwy, Branford, CT 06405
Electrosurgical genertor.

Rotburg Instruments Of America Inc. 954-331-8046
1560 Sawgrass Corporate Pkwy Fl 4, Sunrise, FL 33323
Various types of sterile and non-sterile electrosurgical pencils, electrodes, co.

Rubicor Medical, Inc. 650-587-3446
600 Chesapeake Dr, Redwood City, CA 94063
Sterile biopsy device & non-sterle accessories.

Salient Surgical Technologies Inc. 800-354-2808
180 International Dr, Portsmouth, NH 03801
BIPOLAR DEVICES; BIPOLAR PUMP GENERATOR; TISSUELINK MONOPOLAR

Senorx, Inc. 949-362-4800
11 Columbia, Aliso Viejo, CA 92656
Electrosurigal unit & accessories, non-sterile , sterile.

Silverglide Surgical Technologies 303-444-1970
5398 Manhattan Cir Ste 120, Boulder, CO 80303
Replacement electrosurgical electrode tip.

Smith & Nephew Inc., Endoscopy Div. 978-749-1000
76 S Meridian Ave, Oklahoma City, OK 73107
Electrosurgical generator.

ELECTROSURGICAL UNIT, CUTTING & COAGULATION DEVICE *(cont'd)*

Solos Endoscopy 800-388-6445
65 Sprague St # B, Boston/dedham Commerce Park, Boston, MA 02136
Electrosurgical cutting & coagulation device & accessories.

Source One Technologies 408-376-3400
120 Knowles Dr, Los Gatos, CA 95032
Electrosurgical device and accessories.

Spinus, Llc 603-758-1444
8 Merrill Industrial Dr, Hampton, NH 03842
Electrosurgical electrode.

Starion Instruments 800-782-7466
775 Palomar Ave, Sunnyvale, CA 94085
Various.

Std Med, Inc. 781-828-4400
75 Mill St, PO Box 420, Stoughton, MA 02072
Suction irrigation unit with electrosurgical tip.

Stellartech Research Corp. 408-331-3000
1346 Bordeaux Dr, Sunnyvale, CA 94089
Electrosurgical cutting device.

Sterilmed, Inc. 763-488-3400
11400 73rd Ave N Ste 100, Maple Grove, MN 55369
Arthroscopic electrode probes.

Stryker Puerto Rico, Ltd. 939-307-2500
Hwy. 3, Km. 131.2, Las Guasimas Ind. Park, Arroyo, PR 00714
Radio frequency ablation system.

Surgrx, Inc. 877-7-SURGRX
101 Saginaw Dr, Redwood City, CA 94063
Electrosurgical open and laparoscopic instruments.

Synergetics Usa, Inc. 800-600-0565
3845 Corporate Centre Dr, O Fallon, MO 63368
Various.

Teleflex Medical 800-334-9751
2917 Weck Drive, Research Triangle Park, NC 27709
And accessories.

Thermage, Inc. 510-782-2286
25881 Industrial Blvd, Hayward, CA 94545
Electrosurgical unit & accessories.

Thermosurgery Technologies, Inc. 602-264-7300
2901 W Indian School Rd, Phoenix, AZ 85017
ThermoMed 1.8 (Localized current field (lcf) radio frequency (rf) instrument.)

Tyco Electronics/Precision Interconnect 503-673-5027
10025 SW Freeman Dr, Wilsonville, OR 97070
Electrosurgical cables.

Ussc Puerto Rico, Inc. 203-845-1000
Building 911-67, Sabanetas Industrial Park, Ponce, PR 00731
Multiple.

Valley Forge Scientific Corp. 610-666-7500
136 Green Tree Road, Suite 100, Oaks, PA 19456
Generator used with electrode hand-held instrument for surgical bipolar. Irrigation system used to provide sterile water or saline irrigation during surgical procedures. Bipolar electrosurgical coagulator/cutting system. High power electrosurgical generator used with electrode hand-held and laparoscopic instruments for surgical bipolar cutting and/or coagulation.

Vnus Medical Technologies, Inc. 888-797-8346
5799 Fontanoso Way, San Jose, CA 95138
Bipolar electrosurgical instrument.

Warsaw Orthopedic, Inc. 901-396-3133
2500 Silveus Xing, Warsaw, IN 46582
Various electrosurgical accessories.

Xenotec Ltd. 949-640-4053
511 Hazel Dr, Corona Del Mar, CA 92625
Units are available with hand or foot controls and with line or battery power. Monopolar and bipolar lectrodes are reusable or disposable.

ELECTROSURGICAL UNIT, DENTAL *(Dental And Oral) 76EKZ*

Coltene/Whaledent Inc. 330-916-8858
235 Ascot Pkwy, Cuyahoga Falls, OH 44223
Dental electrosurge.

Dencraft 800-328-9729
PO Box 57, Moorestown, NJ 08057

Dentalez Group 866-DTE-INFO
101 Lindenwood Dr Ste 225, Valleybrooke Corporate Center
Malvern, PA 19355

ELECTROSURGICAL UNIT, DENTAL *(cont'd)*

Dentsply Canada, Ltd. 800-263-1437
161 Vinyl Ct., Woodbridge, ONT L4L 4A3 Canada

Ellman International, Inc. 800-835-5355
3333 Royal Ave, Rockville Centre, NY 11572
Dental and medical.

Lemoy International, Inc. 847-427-0840
95 King St, Elk Grove Village, IL 60007
AUTOSURG Electrocautery unit for dentists/physicians/veterinarians 100% American made and made to order.

Macan Engineering Company 302-645-8068
21 Shay Ln, P.O. BOX 166 Milton, Milton, DE 19968
$975.00 per unit (standard), Model MC-4. $1250.00 for RadioSurge model.

ELECTROSURGICAL UNIT, GASTROENTEROLOGY

(Gastro/Urology) 78FAR

Accellent El Paso 915-771-9112
31 Butterfield Trail Blvd Ste C, El Paso, TX 79906
BPH Microwave Catheter

Cameron-Miller, Inc. 800-621-0142
5410 W Roosevelt Rd, Road #241, Chicago, IL 60644

Gyrus Medical, Inc. 800-852-9361
6655 Wedgwood Rd N Ste 105, Maple Grove, MN 55311
Bipolar coagulation therapeutic system; water bottle for irrigation.

Hobbs Medical, Inc. 860-684-5875
8 Spring St, Stafford Springs, CT 06076
Polypectomy snare.

Valleylab 800-255-8522
5920 Longbow Dr, Boulder, CO 80301
FORCE FX™ electrosurgical generator.

ELECTROSURGICAL UNIT, GENERAL PURPOSE (ESU)

(Surgery) 79QTV

American Bio-Medical Service Corporation (Abmsc) 800-755-9055
631 W Covina Blvd, Sales,Service and Refurbishing Center
San Dimas, CA 91773

Biomedics, Inc. 949-458-1998
23322 Peralta Dr Ste 11, Laguna Hills, CA 92653

Cameron-Miller, Inc. 800-621-0142
5410 W Roosevelt Rd, Road #241, Chicago, IL 60644

D.R.E., Inc. 800-462-8195
1800 Williamson Ct, Louisville, KY 40223
DRE's ASG series are the latest electrosurgical generators with fully digital implementation. This digital technology offers a completely innovative dimension to electrosurgery for use in today's modern OR and surgical outpatient center. Monopolar and bipolar functions satisfy all surgical demands with maximum safety and a user-friendly interface.

Dermatologic Lab & Supply, Inc. 800-831-6273
608 13th Ave, Council Bluffs, IA 51501
Delasco Electricator in-office coagulation unit (45 watts)

Elmed, Inc. 630-543-2792
60 W Fay Ave, Addison, IL 60101
Twelve tabletop models for varied applications and microsurgery. Available with fiber-optic light source and gas insufflator.

Gyrus Medical, Inc. 800-852-9361
6655 Wedgwood Rd N Ste 105, Maple Grove, MN 55311
Monopolar/bipolar electrosurgical generators for laparoscopic and endoscopic use. Output: bipolar cut, coag, and blend waveforms.

Integral Design Inc. 781-740-2036
52 Burr Rd, Hingham, MA 02043

Kirwan Surgical Products, Inc. 888-547-9267
180 Enterprise Dr, PO Box 427, Marshfield, MA 02050
Solid state bipolar generator.

Koaman International 909-983-4888
656 E D St, Ontario, CA 91764

Macan Engineering Company 302-645-8068
21 Shay Ln, P.O. BOX 166 Milton, Milton, DE 19968
$850.00 for Model MC-6 per unit (standard). Small surgical electrosurgical unit $950.00 for Model MD-9.

Md International, Inc. 305-669-9003
11300 NW 41st St, Doral, FL 33178

Olympus America, Inc. 800-645-8160
3500 Corporate Pkwy, PO Box 610, Center Valley, PA 18034

ELECTROSURGICAL UNIT, GENERAL PURPOSE (ESU) *(cont'd)*

Parkell, Inc. 800-243-7446
300 Executive Dr, Edgewood, NY 11717
SENSIMATIC

Richard Wolf Medical Instruments Corp. 800-323-9653
353 Corporate Woods Pkwy, Vernon Hills, IL 60061

Rontron Engineering, Inc. 203-488-5020
131 Commercial Pkwy, Branford, CT 06405
High-isolation generator, 100-W, battery powered.

Valleylab 800-255-8522
5920 Longbow Dr, Boulder, CO 80301
Full family of generators: FORCE FX™, FORCE EZ™ electrosurgical geneators with Instant Response™ technology; SURGISTAT™ II, office-based system; Force™ 1C and Force™ 2 general purpose generators.

Wallach Surgical Devices, Inc. 800-243-2463
235 Edison Rd, Orange, CT 06477
$3545.00 for electrosurgical unit with starter kit.

Whittemore Enterprises, Inc. 800-999-2452
11149 Arrow Rte, Rancho Cucamonga, CA 91730

ELECTROSURGICAL UNIT, NEUROLOGICAL
(Cns/Neurology) 84HAM

Accellent El Paso 915-771-9112
31 Butterfield Trail Blvd Ste C, El Paso, TX 79906
Bipolar electrocautery sets

Compass International, Inc. 800-933-2143
1815 14th St NW, Rochester, MN 55901
Compass mono-polar coagulation probe and bi-polar forceps. Instruments for neurosurgery.

D.B.I. America Corp. 813-909-9005
254 Crystal Grove Blvd, Lutz, FL 33548
Electrosurgical unit.

Nikomed U.S.A., Inc. 800-355-6456
2000 Pioneer Rd, Huntingdon Valley, PA 19006
Grounding pad or dispersive pad.

ELECTROSURGICAL, CUTTING & COAGULATION ACCESSORIES, LAPAROSCOPIC & ENDOSCOPIC, REPROCESSED *(Surgery) 79NUJ*

Aubrey Group 949-581-0188
6 Cromwell Ste 100, Irvine, CA 92618

ELECTROSURGICAL, RADIO FREQUENCY, REFRACTIVE CORRECTION *(Ophthalmology) 86MWD*

Refractec, Inc. 949-784-2600
5 Jenner Ste 150, Irvine, CA 92618
Decdrosurgical device.

ELECTROSURGICAL, UNIT, GASTROENTEROLOGY
(Gastro/Urology) 78KNS

Ballard Medical Products 770-587-7835
12050 Lone Peak Pkwy, Draper, UT 84020
Papillotomes.

Boston Scientific Corporation 800-225-2732
1 Boston Scientific Pl, Natick, MA 01760

Bovie Medical Corp. 800-537-2790
5115 Ulmerton Rd, Clearwater, FL 33760

Cook Endoscopy 336-744-0157
4900 Bethania Station Rd # &, 5951 Grassy Creek Blvd. Winston Salem, NC 27105
Papillotomes.

Gyrus Acmi, Inc. 508-804-2739
93 N Pleasant St, Norwalk, OH 44857
Unit, electrosurgical, endoscopic (with or without accessories).

Medtronic Neuromodulation 763-514-4000
710 Medtronic Pkwy, Minneapolis, MN 55432
Various.

Ultroid, Llc And Ultroid Technologies, Incorporated 727-865-1929
405 Central Ave Ste 100, Saint Petersburg, FL 33701
Hemorrhoid management system.

ELECTROTHERAPEUTIC UNIT *(General) 80QTW*

Chattanooga Group 800-592-7329
4717 Adams Rd, Hixson, TN 37343
INTELECT ultrasound, stimulator and combo models.

ELECTROTHERAPEUTIC UNIT *(cont'd)*

Diapulse Corporation Of America 800-536-6636
475 Northern Blvd, Great Neck, NY 11021
DIAPULSE non-thermal electromagnetic therapy unit for non-invasive postoperative edema and pain treatment in superficial soft tissues. 65 microseconds pulse duration, 80-600 pulses/sec. pulse frequency, and 27.12MHz high frequency.

Orthofix Inc. 800-535-4492
1720 Bray Central Dr, McKinney, TX 75069
Portable, battery-powered pulsed electromagnetic fields for treatment of recalcitrant bone fractures.

Prizm Medical, Inc. 770-622-0933
PO Box 40, Oakwood, GA 30566
Micro-Z and Micro-Z Mini stimulators

Zimmer Medizinsystems 800-327-3576
25 Mauchly Ste 300, Irvine, CA 92618
Low and medium frequency currents, modular construction, automatic surging and switch off, LED display for all functions, color options.

ELEVATOR, ADSON *(Surgery) 79QTX*

Codman & Shurtleff, Inc 800-225-0460
325 Paramount Dr, Raynham, MA 02767

Fehling Surgical Instruments 800-FEHLING
509 Broadstone Ln NW, Acworth, GA 30101

ELEVATOR, ENT *(Ear/Nose/Throat) 77KAD*

Aesculap Implant Systems Inc. 1-800-234-9179
3773 Corporate Pkwy, Center Valley, PA 18034

Bausch & Lomb Surgical 636-255-5051
3365 Tree Court Ind Blvd, Saint Louis, MO 63122

Biomet Microfixation Inc. 800-874-7711
1520 Tradeport Dr, Jacksonville, FL 32218
Various types of elevators.

Clinimed, Incorporated 877-CLINIMED
303 Markus Ct, Sandy Brae Industrial Park, Newark, DE 19713

George Tiemann & Co. 800-843-6266
25 Plant Ave, Hauppauge, NY 11788

Tuzik Boston 800-886-6363
104 Longwater Dr, Assinippi Park, Norwell, MA 02061

ELEVATOR, NEUROSURGICAL *(Cns/Neurology) 84QTY*

Codman & Shurtleff, Inc 800-225-0460
325 Paramount Dr, Raynham, MA 02767

Zimmer Holdings, Inc. 800-613-6131
1800 W Center St, PO Box 708, Warsaw, IN 46580

ELEVATOR, ORTHOPEDIC *(Orthopedics) 87HTE*

Codman & Shurtleff, Inc 800-225-0460
325 Paramount Dr, Raynham, MA 02767

Depuy Spine, Inc. 800-227-6633
325 Paramount Dr, Raynham, MA 02767
Various sizes/styles of elevators.

Equip For Independence, Inc. 800-216-4881
333 Mamaroneck Ave Ste 383, White Plains, NY 10605

George Tiemann & Co. 800-843-6266
25 Plant Ave, Hauppauge, NY 11788

Holmed Corporation 508-238-3351
40 Norfolk Ave, South Easton, MA 02375

In'Tech Medical, Incorporated 757-224-0177
2851 Lamb Pl Ste 15, Memphis, TN 38118
Elevator.

Kmedic 800-955-0559
190 Veterans Dr, Northvale, NJ 07647

Medtronic Sofamor Danek Instrument Manufacturing 901-396-3133
7375 Adrianne Pl, Bartlett, TN 38133
Multiple elevators, orthopedic.

Medtronic Sofamor Danek Usa, Inc. 901-396-3133
4340 Swinnea Rd, Memphis, TN 38118
Multiple elevators, orthopedic.

Musculoskeletal Transplant Foundation 732-661-0202
1232 Mid Valley Dr, Jessup, PA 18434

Warsaw Orthopedic, Inc. 901-396-3133
2500 Silveus Xing, Warsaw, IN 46582
Multiple elevators, orthopedic.

Zimmer Holdings, Inc. 800-613-6131
1800 W Center St, PO Box 708, Warsaw, IN 46580

ELEVATOR, ORTHOPEDIC *(cont'd)*

Zimmer Spine, Inc. 800-655-2614
7375 Bush Lake Rd, Minneapolis, MN 55439
Elevator.

ELEVATOR, OTHER *(General) 80QTZ*

Inclinator Co. Of America 800-343-9007
601 Gibson Blvd, Harrisburg, PA 17104
ELEVETTE home elevators and accessibility lifts. SPECTRALIFT, industry's only fiberglass wheelchair lift with travel to 57'.

National Medical Products 800-940-6262
9775 Mining Dr Ste 104, Jacksonville, FL 32257
2000 In-Bed Arm Cast Elevator: 16 x 13 1/2 x 12 for post-op or casted arm. 505 In-Bed Arm Elevator: for post-op or casted arm, also excellent for IV elevation. Available for pediatrics. 706 Bedside Leg Elevator: Bedsize width, elevates the heels and malleoli, prevention of pressure sores. Used in orthopedics, wound care, general nursing for in-bed patients, trauma and diabetic patients.

Rf Technologies 800-669-9946
3125 N 126th St, Brookfield, WI 53005
Deactivation option.

Swisslog Translogic Corporation 800-525-1841
10825 E 47th Ave, Denver, CO 80239
Material handling. Also available Matrix, Pneumatic Tube System Software.

Thyssenkrupp Access Corp. 800-925-3100
4001 E 138th St, Grandview, MO 64030
Elevators for residential use and public access buildings like churches and schools. Signet features a customized cab for new construction and the Rise is a pitless elevator and is designed for existing construction

ELEVATOR, SURGICAL, DENTAL *(Dental And Oral) 76EMJ*

Aesculap Implant Systems Inc. 1-800-234-9179
3773 Corporate Pkwy, Center Valley, PA 18034

Arnold Tuber Industries 716-648-3363
97 Main St, Hamburg, NY 14075
Elevator, surgical, dental, dental hand instruments.

Biomet Microfixation Inc. 800-874-7711
1520 Tradeport Dr, Jacksonville, FL 32218
Various types of elevators.

Dental Usa, Inc. 815-363-8003
5005 McCullom Lake Rd, McHenry, IL 60050
Surgical elevator.

E.A. Beck & Co. 949-645-4072
657 W 19th St Ste E, P O Box 10857, Costa Mesa, CA 92627
Elevator.

H & H Co. 909-390-0373
4435 E Airport Dr Ste 108, Ontario, CA 91761
Elevator, all types.

Hu-Friedy Manufacturing Co., Inc. 800-483-7433
3232 N Rockwell St, Chicago, IL 60618
$50.70 each, 70 types.

Js Dental Mfg., Inc. 800-284-3368
196 N Salem Rd, Ridgefield, CT 06877
Luxator,(the original) elevator.

Micro-Dent Inc. 866-526-1166
379 Hollow Hill Rd, Wauconda, IL 60084
Elevator, dental.

Nordent Manufacturing, Inc. 800-966-7336
610 Bonnie Ln, Elk Grove Village, IL 60007
$39.50 per unit (standard).

Oratronics, Inc. 212-986-0050
405 Lexington Ave, New York, NY 10174
Periosteal elevator.

Pac-Dent Intl., Inc. 909-839-0888
21078 Commerce Point Dr, Walnut, CA 91789
Various types of elevator.

Premier Dental Products Co. 888-670-6100
1710 Romano Dr, PO Box 4500, Plymouth Meeting, PA 19462

Symmetry Medical Usa, Inc. 574-267-8700
486 W 350 N, Warsaw, IN 46582
Dental hand instrument.

Trans American Medical / Tamsco Instruments 708-430-7777
7633 W 100th Pl, Bridgeview, IL 60455

Tuzik Boston 800-886-6363
104 Longwater Dr, Assinippi Park, Norwell, MA 02061

ELEVATOR, SURGICAL, GENERAL & PLASTIC SURGERY *(Surgery) 79GEG*

Bausch & Lomb Surgical 636-255-5051
3365 Tree Court Ind Blvd, Saint Louis, MO 63122

Biomet Microfixation Inc. 800-874-7711
1520 Tradeport Dr, Jacksonville, FL 32218
Various types of elevators.

Biomet, Inc. 574-267-6639
56 E Bell Dr, PO Box 587, Warsaw, IN 46582
Various types of elevator.

Cardinal Health, Snowden Pencer Products 847-689-8410
5175 S Royal Atlanta Dr, Tucker, GA 30084
Various types of elevators.

Codman & Shurtleff, Inc 800-225-0460
325 Paramount Dr, Raynham, MA 02767

Depuy Mitek, A Johnson & Johnson Company 800-451-2006
50 Scotland Blvd, Bridgewater, MA 02324
Elevator.

Dermatologic Lab & Supply, Inc. 800-831-6273
608 13th Ave, Council Bluffs, IA 51501
Elevator.

George Tiemann & Co. 800-843-6266
25 Plant Ave, Hauppauge, NY 11788

Invuity, Inc. 760-744-4447
334 Via Vera Cruz Ste 255, San Marcos, CA 92078
Surgical elevator.

Invuity, Inc. 415-655-2100
39 Stillman St, San Francisco, CA 94107

Kmedic 800-955-0559
190 Veterans Dr, Northvale, NJ 07647

Lenox-Maclaren Surgical Corp. 720-890-9660
657 S Taylor Ave Ste A, Colorado Technology Center
Louisville, CO 80027
Elevator, surgical / all different.

Mcpherson Enterprises, Inc. 813-931-4201
3851 62nd Ave N Ste A, Pinellas Park, FL 33781
Abdominal lift.

Mediflex Surgical Products 800-879-7575
250 Gibbs Rd, Islandia, NY 11749
Surgical elevator, abdominal wall system, stainless steel, economically priced.

Micrins Surgical Instruments, Inc. 800-833-3380
28438 N Ballard Dr, Lake Forest, IL 60045

Salvin Dental Specialties, Inc. 800-535-6566
3450 Latrobe Dr, Charlotte, NC 28211
Various types of surgical elevators.

Small Bone Innovations, Inc. 215-428-1791
1380 S Pennsylvania Ave, Morrisville, PA 19067
Elevator, surgical, general & plastic surgery.

Surgical Instrument Manufacturers, Inc. 800-521-2985
1650 Headland Dr, Fenton, MO 63026

Symmetry Medical Usa, Inc. 574-267-8700
486 W 350 N, Warsaw, IN 46582
Manual surgical instrument for general use.

Tuzik Boston 800-886-6363
104 Longwater Dr, Assinippi Park, Norwell, MA 02061

Ussc Puerto Rico, Inc. 203-845-1000
Building 911-67, Sabanetas Industrial Park, Ponce, PR 00731
Surgical rib elevator.

Wells Johnson Co. 800-528-1597
8000 S Kolb Rd, Tucson, AZ 85756

Zimmer Holdings, Inc. 800-613-6131
1800 W Center St, PO Box 708, Warsaw, IN 46580

ELEVATOR, UTERINE *(Obstetrics/Gyn) 85HDP*

Clinical Innovations, Inc. 888-268-6222
747 W 4170 S, Murray, UT 84123
ClearView Uterine Manipulator

Miltex Inc. 800-645-8000
589 Davies Dr, York, PA 17402

Thomas Medical Inc. 800-556-0349
5610 West 82 2nd Street, Indianpolis, IN 46278

ELEVATOR, WHEELCHAIR *(Physical Med) 89ING*

Garaventa (Canada) Ltd. 800-663-6556
7505 - 134A St., Surrey, BC V3W-7B3 Canada
$12,000 to $35,000 for GARAVENTA STAIR-LIFT.

The National Wheel-O-Vator Co., Inc. 800-551-9095
509 W Front St, Roanoke, IL 61561
Vertical and inclined platform lifting device.

Thyssenkrupp Access Corp. 800-925-3100
4001 E 138th St, Grandview, MO 64030
Stairway lifts and wheelchair lifts for both residential and commercial applications.

EMBOLIZATION DEVICE *(Cardiovascular) 74KRD*

Biocure, Inc. 678-966-3400
2975 Gateway Dr Ste 100, Norcross, GA 30071
Artificial embolization device.

Boston Scientific Corporation 800-225-2732
1 Boston Scientific Pl, Natick, MA 01760
CRAGG FX infusion wires, standard occlusion balloon catheters, Glidecath hydrophilic coated catheters.

Closure Medical 888-257-7633
5250 Greens Dairy Rd, Raleigh, NC 27616
AVACRYL; n-Butyl cyanoacrylate for treatment of arteriovenous malformations within the central nervous system (clinical research and/or compassionate usage.

Concentric Medical, Inc. 650-938-2100
301 E Evelyn Ave, Mountain View, CA 94041
Embolization particles.

Cordis Neurovascular, Inc. 800-327-7714
14201 NW 60th Ave, Miami Lakes, FL 33014
Detachable coil.

Ivalon, Inc. 800-948-2566
1015 Cordova St, San Diego, CA 92107
Ivalon PVA Embolization Particles for permanent therapeutic occlusion and preoperative occlusion of arteriovenous malformations (AVMs) and hypervascular tumors.

EMERGENCY RESPONSE SAFETY KIT *(Surgery) 79OKI*

Legend Aerospace, Inc. 305-883-8804
8300 NW South River Dr, Medley, FL 33166

EMULSION, OIL, (TITRIMETRIC), LIPASE *(Chemistry) 75CFG*

Sterling Diagnostics, Inc. 800-637-2661
36645 Metro Ct, Sterling Heights, MI 48312

EMULSION, OLIVE OIL (TURBIDIMETRIC), LIPASE *(Chemistry) 75CET*

Teco Diagnostics 714-693-7788
1268 N Lakeview Ave, Anaheim, CA 92807
Lipase reagent set (colipase method).

ENCAPSULATOR, FLUID *(General) 80WUM*

Armstrong Medical Industries, Inc. 800-323-4220
575 Knightsbridge Pkwy, Lincolnshire, IL 60069

Cdc Products Corp. 800-636-7363
1801 Falmouth Ave, New Hyde Park, NY 11040
Emergency clean-up powder for liquid and semi-liquid accidents; emergency clean-up kits and personal protection kits for blood and body fluid spills. Liquid enzyme used in drains, septic tanks, floors, tables. Cannot come in touch with food

Colby Manufacturing Corp. 800-969-3718
1016 Branagan Dr, Tullytown, PA 19007
ViraSorb Super Solidifier works faster and stays solid. ViraSorb penetrates canister contents to gel infectious blood and body fluids faster than other solidifiers. Once gelled, the contents will not crystallize or become slippery and will remain solid throughout the disposal process to guard against spills or leaks. Choose from single-use or multi-use bottles or dissolvable pouches. One dissolvable pouch can solidify up to 500 cc of fluid and can be conveniently pre-loaded before a procedure for a closed system. Since ViraSorb is glutaraldehyde-free, chlorine-free and phenol-free, it provides a cost-effective, safety conscious means of disposal that can be incinerated.

H & S Manufacturing, Inc. 800-827-3091
727 E Broadway, Williston, ND 58801
SPRINGTIME Cleanup absorbents.

Inotech Biosystems International, Inc. 800-635-4070
15713 Crabbs Branch Way Ste 110, Rockville, MD 20855
Instrument that encapsulates cells and other biologicals in polymer microbeads (100- to 1000-um diameter).

ENCAPSULATOR, FLUID *(cont'd)*

Microtek Medical, Inc 800-936-9248
512 N Lehmberg Rd, Columbus, MS 39702
LTS Liquid Treatment System line of encapsulators and solidifiers.

Safetec Of America, Inc. 800-456-7077
887 Kensington Ave, Buffalo, NY 14215
RED Z, YELLOW Z and GREEN Z encapsulate and solidify blood and body fluids, and help prevent leaks and spills from suction canisters. Makes clean-up and disposal of body fluid spills easier. One ounce solidifies and encapsulates 1 liter of fluid. Available in single-use pouches, shaker top and needlenose bottles, as well as bulk sizes. YELLOW Z deodorizes as it solidifies, and GREEN Z is incinerator-friendly. ACID LOCK neutralizes and solidifies low pH fluid (acidic) spills. ALKY neutralizes and solidifies high pH fluid (alkaline) spills. PETRO LOCK absorbs petroleum-based spill. Convenient Spill Kits also available.

Spartan Chemical Company, Inc. 800-537-8990
1110 Spartan Dr, Maumee, OH 43537
STERIPHENE II disinfectant deodorant. Aerosol and ready-to-use. Also, PD-64 Phenolic Disinfectant (and cleaner). All meet OSHA Bloodborne Pathogen Standard for cleanup of blood/body fluid spills.

ENCLOSURE, BACTERIOLOGICAL SAFETY *(Chemistry) 75UHT*

Kewaunee Scientific Corp. 704-873-7202
2700 W Front St, PO Box 1842, Statesville, NC 28677

Labconco Corp. 800-821-5525
8811 Prospect Ave, Kansas City, MO 64132

Nuaire, Inc. 800-328-3352
2100 Fernbrook Ln N, Plymouth, MN 55447
Laminar air-flow safety cabinets.

Purified Micro Environments, Div. Of Germfree Laboratories 800-888-5357
11 Aviator Way, Ormond Beach, FL 32174

ENDODONTIC INSTRUMENT *(Dental And Oral) 76QUC*

Acteon Inc. 800-289-6367
124 Gaither Dr Ste 140, Mount Laurel, NJ 08054

Almore International, Inc. 503-643-6633
PO Box 25214, Portland, OR 97298
$29.95 per Endo-Ring.

Biolase Technology, Inc. 888-424-6527
4 Cromwell, Irvine, CA 92618

Dentalez Group 866-DTE-INFO
101 Lindenwood Dr Ste 225, Valleybrooke Corporate Center
Malvern, PA 19355

J. Morita Usa, Inc. 888-566-7482
9 Mason, Irvine, CA 92618
DENTAPORT ZX, new to J. Morita's well-recognized endodontic product line, is a low-speed endodontic handpiece with a large LCD display. Easy to read, Root ZX-like screen allows the clinician to better visualize the file movement during the instrumentation. The Dentaport ZX offers 3 automatic safety functions - Auto Start / Stop, Auto Apical Reverse and Auto Torque Reverse, 8-speed setting up to 400 rpm, and 11 torque setting selection. Proven Root ZX technology combined with low-speed endodontic handpiece delivers extreme accuracy and reliability.

Jordco, Inc. 800-752-2812
595 NW 167th Ave, Beaverton, OR 97006
Endoring, endodontic hand held file holding device including the hand held Endoring and the bulk file storage case the Endoring FileCaddy

Medidenta International, Inc. 800-221-0750
3923 62nd St, PO Box 409, Woodside, NY 11377

Moyco Technologies, Inc. 800-331-8837
200 Commerce Dr, Montgomeryville, PA 18936

Osada, Inc. 800-426-7232
8436 W 3rd St Ste 695, Los Angeles, CA 90048
ENDEX and ENDEX PLUS Electronic apex sensor; ENAC: OE505ultrasonic endodontic system.

Parkell, Inc. 800-243-7446
300 Executive Dr, Edgewood, NY 11717
Thermique Gutta Percha Thermal Condenser

ENDOILLUMINATOR *(Ophthalmology) 86MPA*

Alcon Manufacturing, Ltd. 817-551-6813
714 Columbia Ave, Sinking Spring, PA 19608
Ophthalmic light guide.

Iscience Interventional 650-421-2700
4055 Campbell Ave, Menlo Park, CA 94025
Iscience fiberoptic illuminator.

ENDOILLUMINATOR *(cont'd)*

Peregrine Surgical, Ltd. 215-348-0456
51 Britain Dr, Doylestown, PA 18901
Bausch & lomb light pipe, 25 ga.

Romc, Inc. 508-829-4602
37 Kris Alan Dr, Holden, MA 01520

Synergetics Usa, Inc. 800-600-0565
3845 Corporate Centre Dr, O Fallon, MO 63368
Various.

ENDOILLUMINATOR, REPROCESSED *(Ophthalmology) 86NKZ*

Sterilmed, Inc. 763-488-3400
11400 73rd Ave N Ste 100, Maple Grove, MN 55369
Light pipes.

ENDOSCOPE *(Gastro/Urology) 78KOG*

Advanced Endoscopy Devices, Inc. 818-227-2720
22134 Sherman Way, Canoga Park, CA 91303
Endoscopes and instruments available for gynecology, urology, arthroscopy, laparoscopy, hysteroscopy, etc. Repair of forceps, sheaths, work elements, cannulas, etc.

Aesculap Implant Systems Inc. 1-800-234-9179
3773 Corporate Pkwy, Center Valley, PA 18034
Accesories are also available.

Armstrong Medical Industries, Inc. 800-323-4220
575 Knightsbridge Pkwy, Lincolnshire, IL 60069
SCOPESAFE locking fiber optic scope storage cabinet, can be wall or cart mounted.

Avail Medical Products, Inc. 858-635-2206
1225 N. 28th Avenue, Suite 500, Dallas, TX 75261
Endoscopic anti-fog kit.

Avantis Medical Systems, Inc. 408-733-1901
263 Santa Ana Ct, Sunnyvale, CA 94085
Endoscope.

Aztec Medical Products, Inc. 800-223-3859
106 Ingram Rd, Williamsburg, VA 23188
EndoCaddy stores and protects your valuable endoscopes. Endocaddy includes bracket, tube, vapor lid(s) and mounting hardware.

Ballard Medical Products 770-587-7835
12050 Lone Peak Pkwy, Draper, UT 84020
Guidewire.

Bard Shannon Limited 908-277-8000
San Geronimo Industrial Park, Lot # 1, Road # 3, Km 79.7
Humacao, PR 00791
Reusable & disposable cartridges.

Boston Scientific - Marina Bay Customer Fulfillment Center 617-689-6000
500 Commander Shea Blvd, Quincy, MA 02171
Various types of biopsy forceps.

Boston Scientific Corporation 508-652-5578
8600 NW 41st St, Doral, FL 33166

Boston Scientific Corporation 800-225-2732
1 Boston Scientific Pl, Natick, MA 01760

Byrne Medical, Inc. 800-490-9869
2021 Airport Rd, Conroe, TX 77301
Sterile water bottle adapter. EndoGator Water System and EndoGator Irrigation Channel Tubing for Endoscope Irrigation

C. R. Bard, Inc., Bard Urological Div. 888-367-2273
13183 Harland Dr NE, Covington, GA 30014

Candela Corp. 800-733-8550
530 Boston Post Rd, Wayland, MA 01778

Carbon Medical Technologies, Inc. 877-277-1788
1290 Hammond Rd, Saint Paul, MN 55110
Various types of injection needle and cannula.

Cardinal Health, Snowden Pencer Products 847-689-8410
5175 S Royal Atlanta Dr, Tucker, GA 30084
Endoscope,endoscopic instruments and or accessories.

Carl Zeiss Surgical, Inc. 800-442-4020
1 Zeiss Dr, Thornwood, NY 10594

Clarus Medical, Llc. 763-525-8400
1000 Boone Ave N Ste 300, Minneapolis, MN 55427
Fluid irrigation pump.

Cook Endoscopy 336-744-0157
4900 Bethania Station Rd # &, 5951 Grassy Creek Blvd.
Winston Salem, NC 27105
Sullivan variable stiffness cable.

ENDOSCOPE *(cont'd)*

Corpak Medsystems, Inc. 800-323-6305
100 Chaddick Dr, Wheeling, IL 60090
Endoscope catheter placement forceps.

Davol Inc., Sub. C.R. Bard, Inc. 800-556-6275
100 Crossings Blvd, Warwick, RI 02886
Overtube, guidewire, retrieval forceps, suturing, staple removal instrument.

Dixon Medical Inc 770-457-0602
3710 Longview Dr, Atlanta, GA 30341

Endochoice Inc. 888-682-3636
11810 Wills Rd Ste 100, Alpharetta, GA 30009
Blox

Endogastric Solutions, Inc. 425-307-9226
8210 154th Ave NE, Redmond, WA 98052
StomaphyX

Endoscopy Support Services, Inc. 800-349-3636
3 Fallsview Ln, Brewster, NY 10509

Ethicon Endo-Surgery, Inc. 877-384-4266
3801 University Blvd SE, Albuquerque, NM 87106
Various types of sterile surgical staplers and accessories.

Fort Wayne Metals Research Prod. Corp. 260-747-4154
9609 Ardmore Ave, Fort Wayne, IN 46809
Various grades, properties, shapes of precision wire, including strands and cables.

Gi Supply 800-451-5797
200 Grandview Ave, Camp Hill, PA 17011
Spot Endoscopic Marker - biocompatible, non-pyrogenic suspension for marking or 'tattooing' the GI tract.

Gyrus Acmi, Inc. 508-804-2739
93 N Pleasant St, Norwalk, OH 44857
Endoscope and/or accessories.

Gyrus Acmi, Inc. 508-804-2739
300 Stillwater P.o.box 1971, Stamford, CT 06902
Endoscope and/or accessories.

Gyrus Ent L.L.C., Sub. Of Gyrus Acmi, Inc. 508-804-2739
2925 Appling Rd, Bartlett, TN 38133
Various.

Innervision Inc. 901-682-0417
6258 E Shady Grove Rd, Memphis, TN 38120

Instratek, Inc. 281-890-8020
210 Spring Hill Dr Ste 130, Spring, TX 77386

Instrument Technology, Inc. 413-562-3606
33 Airport Rd, Westfield, MA 01085
Micro, rigid, flexible and video endoscopes.

International Hospital Supply Co. 800-398-9450
6914 Canby Ave Ste 105, Reseda, CA 91335

Isee 3d, Inc. 514-908-2233
100-4 Car Westmount, Westmount H3Z 2S6 Canada
Stereoscopic video imaging system for use with endoscopic equipment

Island Biosurgical, Llc 425-251-3455
18 Meadow Ln, Mercer Island, WA 98040
FISTULA SCOPE bladder endoscope for closing fistules. URETHRA PORT is a urethral access system used in conjunction with fistula scope.

Karl Storz Endoscopy-America Inc. 800-421-0837
600 Corporate Pointe, Culver City, CA 90230
Rigid or flexible versions for adult and pediatric laparoscopy, thoracoscopy, urology, ENT, plastic surgery, neuroendoscopy, cardiovascular surgery, anesthesia, spinal surgery, maxillofacial and oral surgery, and gynecology applications.

Kmi Kolster Methods, Inc. 909-737-5476
3185 Palisades Dr, Corona, CA 92880
Endoscope.

Lsi Solutions Inc. 585-869-6641
7796 Victor Mendon Rd, Victor, NY 14564
Various endoscopes and/or endoscope accessories.

Mahe International Inc. 800-294-7946
468 Craighead St, Nashville, TN 37204

Matlock Endoscopic Repairs, Sales, And Service, Inc. 800-394-9822
4320 Kenilwood Dr Ste 107, Nashville, TN 37204

ENDOSCOPE *(cont'd)*

Medifix, Inc 847-965-1898
8727 Narragansett Ave, Morton Grove, IL 60053
Arthroscope, cystoscope, laparoscope, op-laparoscore and accessories.

Mediflex Surgical Products 800-879-7575
250 Gibbs Rd, Islandia, NY 11749

Medtronic Neuromodulation 763-514-4000
710 Medtronic Pkwy, Minneapolis, MN 55432
Endoscope system.

N-Tech Endoscopy, Inc. 480-348-7861
14255 N 79th St Ste 3, Scottsdale, AZ 85260
Artroscope, cystoscope, laparoscope/double & sinlge pancture.

Nanoptics, Inc. 352-378-6620
3014 NE 21st Way, Gainesville, FL 32609
Tracheal intubation fiberscope.

Navilyst Medical 800-833-9973
100 Boston Scientific Way, Marlborough, MA 01752
Torque device.

Ndo Surgical, Inc. 877-337-8887
125 High St Ste 7, Mansfield, MA 02048
Endoscope and accessories.

New Life Systems, Inc. 954-972-4600
PO Box 8767, Coral Springs, FL 33075
All types of endoscopes.

Newport Optical Laboratories, Inc. 714-484-3200
10564C Fern Ave, Stanton, CA 90680

Northgate Technologies Inc. 800-348-0424
600 Church Rd, Elgin, IL 60123
Continuous flow, fluid management system for endoscpoic, irrigation and distention in urology, gynecology, and arthroscopy.

Nuvo, Inc. 814-899-4220
5368 Kuhl Rd., Corry, PA 16407
Monitor system.

Olympus America, Inc. 800-645-8160
3500 Corporate Pkwy, PO Box 610, Center Valley, PA 18034

Optim Incorporated 800-225-7486
64 Technology Park Rd, Sturbridge, MA 01566
ENT, urological, neurological, upper GI, gynecological. Prices range from $3,000 to $10,000.

Pentax Southern Region Service Center 201-571-2300
8934 Kirby Dr, Houston, TX 77054
Endoscope accessories.

Pentax West Coast Service Center 800-431-5880
10410 Pioneer Blvd Ste 2, Santa Fe Springs, CA 90670
Pentax endoscope accessories.

Precision Optics Corp. 800-447-2812
22 E Broadway, Gardner, MA 01440
Precision optics POC-11 laparoscope features outstanding brightness, sharpness and clarity throughout the entire field of view. Also available: an endoscope measuring 425 mm long, 10 mm diam.

Romc, Inc. 508-829-4602
37 Kris Alan Dr, Holden, MA 01520

Scican 800-667-7733
1440 Don Mills Rd., Toronto, ON M3B 3P9 Canada
SCICAN Endoscopes--a wide range of scopes available.

Smith & Nephew Inc., Endoscopy Div. 978-749-1000
76 S Meridian Ave, Oklahoma City, OK 73107
Cameras and accessories.

Solos Endoscopy 800-388-6445
65 Sprague St # B, Boston/dedham Commerce Park, Boston, MA 02136
Endoscope and accessories.

Spirus Medical, Inc. 781-297-7220
1063 Turnpike St, PO Box 258, Stoughton, MA 02072
Endo-Ease Discovery SB, Endo-Ease Advantage; Endo-Ease Vista

Sterilmed, Inc. 763-488-3400
11400 73rd Ave N Ste 100, Maple Grove, MN 55369
Snares/retrieval baskets.

Stryker Gi 866-672-5757
1420 Lakeside Pkwy Ste 110, Flower Mound, TX 75028
Colonoscope, gastro-urology.

Stryker Puerto Rico, Ltd. 939-307-2500
Hwy. 3, Km. 131.2, Las Guasimas Ind. Park, Arroyo, PR 00714
Insufflator tubing w/ filter.

ENDOSCOPE *(cont'd)*

Transamerican Technologies International 800-322-7373
2246 Camino Ramon, San Ramon, CA 94583
ACCU-BEAM, Endoscopic Video Adapter. Universal adapter for rigid and flexible endoscopes.

Usgi Medical 949-369-3890
1140 Calle Cordillera, San Clemente, CA 92673
Overtube.

Ussc Puerto Rico, Inc. 203-845-1000
Building 911-67, Sabanetas Industrial Park, Ponce, PR 00731
Endoscope and/or accessories.

Vision Systems Group, A Division Of Viking Systems 508-366-3668
134 Flanders Rd, Westborough, MA 01581
Various endoscopic cameras and accessories to endoscopes.

W.L. Gore & Associates,Inc 928-526-3030
1505 North Fourth St., Flagstaff, AZ 86004
Gore laparoscopic suture passer.

Welch Allyn, Inc. 800-535-6663
4341 State Street Rd, Skaneateles Falls, NY 13153

Whittemore Enterprises, Inc. 800-999-2452
11149 Arrow Rte, Rancho Cucamonga, CA 91730

Zibra Corp. 800-758-8773
640 American Legion Hwy, Westport, MA 02790

Zutron Medical Llc 816-225-3172
1911 Broadway St, Kansas City, MO 64108
Stiffening wire, stiffening device.

ENDOSCOPE AND ACCESSORIES, AC-POWERED

(Surgery) 79GCP

Ams Innovative Center-San Jose 800-356-7600
3070 Orchard Dr, San Jose, CA 95134

Codman & Shurtleff, Inc 800-225-0460
325 Paramount Dr, Raynham, MA 02767

Deknatel Snowden-Pencer 800-367-7874
5175 S Royal Atlanta Dr, Tucker, GA 30084

J. Jamner Surgical Instruments, Inc 800-431-1123
9 Skyline Dr, Hawthorne, NY 10532

Karl Storz Endoscopy-America Inc. 800-421-0837
600 Corporate Pointe, Culver City, CA 90230

Mahe International Inc. 800-294-7946
468 Craighead St, Nashville, TN 37204

Nbs Medical Products Inc. 888-800-8192
257 Livingston Ave, New Brunswick, NJ 08901
Endoscope accessories, including accessories for insufflation, suction/irrigation, and smoke evacuation.

O'Ryan Industries, Inc. 800-426-4311
12711 NE 95th St, PO Box 1736, Vancouver, WA 98682
Light source.

Sony Electronics, Inc., Medical Systems Div. 800-686-7669
1 Sony Dr, Park Ridge, NJ 07656

Welch Allyn, Inc. 800-535-6663
4341 State Street Rd, Skaneateles Falls, NY 13153

ENDOSCOPE AND ACCESSORIES, BATTERY-POWERED

(Surgery) 79GCS

Karl Storz Endoscopy-America Inc. 800-421-0837
600 Corporate Pointe, Culver City, CA 90230

Mahe International Inc. 800-294-7946
468 Craighead St, Nashville, TN 37204

Utah Medical Products, Inc. 800-533-4984
7043 Cottonwood St, Midvale, UT 84047
Endoscope accessory bulb irrigator - CMI Pathfinder Plus Bulb Irrigator attaches to endoscope and gives physician total control of continuous or pulsatile irrigation during delicate endoscopic procedures.

ENDOSCOPE, DIRECT VISION *(Surgery) 79GCR*

Bryan Corp. 800-343-7711
4 Plympton St, Woburn, MA 01801
5mm/10mm 0degrees.

Instrument Technology, Inc. 413-562-3606
33 Airport Rd, Westfield, MA 01085
Micro, rigid, flexible and video endoscopes.

Karl Storz Endoscopy-America Inc. 800-421-0837
600 Corporate Pointe, Culver City, CA 90230

ENDOSCOPE, DIRECT VISION *(cont'd)*

Mahe International Inc. 800-294-7946
468 Craighead St, Nashville, TN 37204

Richard Wolf Medical Instruments Corp. 800-323-9653
353 Corporate Woods Pkwy, Vernon Hills, IL 60061

Smith & Nephew, Inc., Endoscopy Division 800-343-8386
150 Minuteman Rd, Andover, MA 01810

Wisap America 800-233-8448
8231 Melrose Dr, Lenexa, KS 66214

ENDOSCOPE, ELECTRONIC (VIDEOENDOSCOPE)
(Surgery) 79VKP

Boss Instruments, Ltd. 800-210-2677
395 Reas Ford Rd Ste 120, Earlysville, VA 22936

Calmaquip Engineering Corp. 305-592-4510
7240 NW 12th St, Miami, FL 33126

Instrument Technology, Inc. 413-562-3606
33 Airport Rd, Westfield, MA 01085
Micro, rigid, flexible and video endoscopes.

Richard Wolf Medical Instruments Corp. 800-323-9653
353 Corporate Woods Pkwy, Vernon Hills, IL 60061

Smith & Nephew, Inc., Endoscopy Division 800-343-8386
150 Minuteman Rd, Andover, MA 01810

Welch Allyn, Inc. 800-535-6663
4341 State Street Rd, Skaneateles Falls, NY 13153

ENDOSCOPE, FETAL BLOOD SAMPLING
(Obstetrics/Gyn) 85HGK

Rocket Medical Plc. 800-707-7625
150 Recreation Park Dr Ste 3, Hingham, MA 02043

Romc, Inc. 508-829-4602
37 Kris Alan Dr, Holden, MA 01520

ENDOSCOPE, FIBEROPTIC *(Surgery) 79GDB*

Biomet, Inc. 574-267-6639
56 E Bell Dr, PO Box 587, Warsaw, IN 46582
Fiber optic endoscope.

Clarus Medical, Llc. 763-525-8400
1000 Boone Ave N Ste 300, Minneapolis, MN 55427
Light cable.

Electro Surgical Instrument Co., Inc. 888-464-2784
37 Centennial St, Rochester, NY 14611
Various types, styles and sizes of fiber optic endoscopes.

Insitu Technologies, Inc. 651-389-1017
5810 Blackshire Path, Inver Grove Heights, MN 55076
Endoscope.

Instrument Technology, Inc. 413-562-3606
33 Airport Rd, Westfield, MA 01085
Micro, rigid, flexible and video endoscopes.

Md International, Inc. 305-669-9003
11300 NW 41st St, Doral, FL 33178

Olympus America, Inc. 800-645-8160
3500 Corporate Pkwy, PO Box 610, Center Valley, PA 18034

Pentax Medical Company 800-431-5880
102 Chestnut Ridge Rd, Montvale, NJ 07645
Upper G.I., duodeno, choledocho-nephro, and lower G.I. fiberscopes.

Precision Optics Corp. 800-447-2812
22 E Broadway, Gardner, MA 01440
Fiber scopes to diameters as small as 0.5mm. We can produce micro lenses to sizes as small as 0.2mm in diameter using our proprietary micro-precision™ technology with the quality of ground lenses approaching the cost of gradient index (GRIN) lenses

Romc, Inc. 508-829-4602
37 Kris Alan Dr, Holden, MA 01520

Welch Allyn, Inc. 800-535-6663
4341 State Street Rd, Skaneateles Falls, NY 13153

ENDOSCOPE, FLEXIBLE *(Gastro/Urology) 78GCQ*

Clarus Medical, Llc. 763-525-8400
1000 Boone Ave N Ste 300, Minneapolis, MN 55427
Endoscope.

Convergent Laser Technologies 800-848-8200
1660 S Loop Rd, Alameda, CA 94502
Flexible endoscopes with high quality viewing optics and advanced fused fiber technology. Also available with portable light source for more convenient use in office and clinics.

Endoscopy Support Services, Inc. 800-349-3636
3 Fallsview Ln, Brewster, NY 10509

ENDOSCOPE, FLEXIBLE *(cont'd)*

Hmb Endoscopy Products 800-659-5743
3746 SW 30th Ave, Fort Lauderdale, FL 33312
Gastroscopes, Colonoscopes, Sigmoidoscopes, Choledocoscopes, Bronchoscopes,Cystoscopes, Rhinolaryngoscopes, Duodenoscopes, Laparoscopes, Arthroscopes, Sinusscopes, Resectoscopes, Hysteroscopes.

Instrument Technology, Inc. 413-562-3606
33 Airport Rd, Westfield, MA 01085
Micro, rigid, flexible and video endoscopes.

Lsvp International, Inc. 866-969-0100
4692 El Camino Real Unit 126, Los Altos, CA 94022
insertion tubes and other repair accessories

Matlock Endoscopic Repairs, Sales, And Service, Inc. 800-394-9822
4320 Kenilwood Dr Ste 107, Nashville, TN 37204

Medi-Globe Corporation 800-966-1431
110 W Orion St Ste 136, Tempe, AZ 85283
Flexible endoscopy accessories.

Metron Optics, Inc. 858-755-4477
PO Box 690, 813 Academy Drive, Solana Beach, CA 92075
METRON OPTICS, 3D video endoscopes.

Mobile Instrument Service And Repair, Inc. 800-722-3675
333 Water Ave, Bellefontaine, OH 43311
Repair/refurbishment of all makes and models.

Richard Wolf Medical Instruments Corp. 800-323-9653
353 Corporate Woods Pkwy, Vernon Hills, IL 60061

Welch Allyn, Inc. 800-535-6663
4341 State Street Rd, Skaneateles Falls, NY 13153

ENDOSCOPE, NEUROLOGICAL *(Cns/Neurology) 84GWG*

Aesculap Implant Systems Inc. 1-800-234-9179
3773 Corporate Pkwy, Center Valley, PA 18034

Clarus Medical, Llc. 763-525-8400
1000 Boone Ave N Ste 300, Minneapolis, MN 55427
Endoscope.

Codman & Shurtleff, Inc 800-225-0460
325 Paramount Dr, Raynham, MA 02767

Karl Storz Endoscopy-America Inc. 800-421-0837
600 Corporate Pointe, Culver City, CA 90230
Full line of diagnostic and operative models in various sizes for pediatric to adult use.

Koros Usa, Inc. 805-529-0825
610 Flinn Ave, Moorpark, CA 93021
Videoscope.

Medtronic Neurosurgery 800-468-9710
125 Cremona Dr, Goleta, CA 93117
Neurological endoscopes.

Optim Incorporated 800-225-7486
64 Technology Park Rd, Sturbridge, MA 01566

Richard Wolf Medical Instruments Corp. 800-323-9653
353 Corporate Woods Pkwy, Vernon Hills, IL 60061

Romc, Inc. 508-829-4602
37 Kris Alan Dr, Holden, MA 01520

Warsaw Orthopedic, Inc. 901-396-3133
2500 Silveus Xing, Warsaw, IN 46582
Various scopes.

Zimmer Spine 508-643-0983
23 W Bacon St, Plainville, MA 02762
ENDIUS Spine Endoscopy System endoscope and camera for posterior spine procedures.

ENDOSCOPE, OPHTHALMIC *(Gastro/Urology) 78KYH*

Endo Optiks, Inc. 800-756-3636
39 Sycamore Ave, Little Silver, NJ 07739
Laser microendoscopes under 1mm for ophthalmic and otolaryngology.

Ophthalmic Technologies, Inc. 416-631-9123
12-37 Kodiak Cres, Downsview M3J 3E5 Canada
Ophthalmic endoscope

ENDOSCOPE, RIGID *(Surgery) 79GCM*

Advanced Endoscopy Devices, Inc. 818-227-2720
22134 Sherman Way, Canoga Park, CA 91303
Capability to manufacture any size, diameter, or angle of view.

Ams Innovative Center-San Jose 800-356-7600
3070 Orchard Dr, San Jose, CA 95134

PRODUCT DIRECTORY

ENDOSCOPE, RIGID *(cont'd)*

Bryan Corp. 800-343-7711
4 Plympton St, Woburn, MA 01801
5mm/10mm 0,30,70 degrees.

Cameron-Miller, Inc. 800-621-0142
5410 W Roosevelt Rd, Road #241, Chicago, IL 60644

Elmed, Inc. 630-543-2792
60 W Fay Ave, Addison, IL 60101

Endoscopy Support Services, Inc. 800-349-3636
3 Fallsview Ln, Brewster, NY 10509

Gyrus Ent L.L.C., Sub. Of Gyrus Acmi, Inc. 508-804-2739
2925 Appling Rd, Bartlett, TN 38133
Regid endoscope.

Instrument Technology, Inc. 413-562-3606
33 Airport Rd, Westfield, MA 01085
Micro, rigid, flexible and video endoscopes.

Karl Storz Endoscopy-America Inc. 800-421-0837
600 Corporate Pointe, Culver City, CA 90230
For adult and pediatric laparoscopy, thoracoscopy, urology, ENT, plastic surgery, neuroendoscopy, cardiovascular surgery, anesthesia, spinal surgery, maxillofacial and oral surgery, and gynecology applications.

Mahe International Inc. 800-294-7946
468 Craighead St, Nashville, TN 37204

Md International, Inc. 305-669-9003
11300 NW 41st St, Doral, FL 33178

Medivision Endoscopy 800-349-5367
1210 N Jefferson St, Anaheim, CA 92807
Independent service center specializing in rigid endoscope repairs and sales. Quality Control Department on premises. Provide customized maintenance reports to customers and distributors. Conduct technical training seminars and in-service programs. Manufacturer of new endoscopes.

Metron Optics, Inc. 858-755-4477
PO Box 690, 813 Academy Drive, Solana Beach, CA 92075
METRON OPTICS, 3D video endoscopes.

Mobile Instrument Service And Repair, Inc. 800-722-3675
333 Water Ave, Bellefontaine, OH 43311
Repair/refurbishment of all makes and models.

Princeton Medical Group, Inc. 800-875-0869
1189 Royal Links Dr, Mt Pleasant, SC 29466

Richard Wolf Medical Instruments Corp. 800-323-9653
353 Corporate Woods Pkwy, Vernon Hills, IL 60061

Smith & Nephew, Inc., Endoscopy Division 800-343-8386
150 Minuteman Rd, Andover, MA 01810

Sohniks Endoscopy, Inc. 651-452-4059
930 Blue Gentian Rd Ste 1400, Eagan, MN 55121
Various types of rigidendoscopes.

Welch Allyn, Inc. 800-535-6663
4341 State Street Rd, Skaneateles Falls, NY 13153

ENDOSCOPE, TRANSCERVICAL (AMNIOSCOPE)
(Obstetrics/Gyn) 85HEZ

Mahe International Inc. 800-294-7946
468 Craighead St, Nashville, TN 37204

Richard Wolf Medical Instruments Corp. 800-323-9653
353 Corporate Woods Pkwy, Vernon Hills, IL 60061

ENDOSCOPIC SUTURE/PLICATION SYSTEM, GASTROESOPHAGEAL REFLUX DISEASE (GERD)
(Gastro/Urology) 78ODE

Endogastric Solutions, Inc. 425-307-9226
8210 154th Ave NE, Redmond, WA 98052
EsophyX

ENDOSCOPIC TISSUE APPROXIMATION DEVICE
(Gastro/Urology) 78OCW

Apollo Endosurgery, Inc. 877-ENDO-130
7000 Bee Caves Rd Ste 350, Austin, TX 78746
Overstitch Tissue Approximation

Endogastric Solutions, Inc. 425-307-9226
8210 154th Ave NE, Redmond, WA 98052
StomaphyX Plus/ Titan

ENT DRUG APPLICATOR *(Ear/Nose/Throat) 77LRD*

Aeris Therapeutics, Inc. 781-937-0110
10K Gill St, Woburn, MA 01801
Dual lumen catheter,administration device.

ENT DRUG APPLICATOR *(cont'd)*

Ballard Medical Products 770-587-7835
12050 Lone Peak Pkwy, Draper, UT 84020
Mdi actuator.

Bionix Development Corp. 800-551-7096
5154 Enterprise Blvd, Toledo, OH 43612
Portable/ tabletop ear irrigation system.

Customed, Inc. 787-801-0101
Calle Igualdad #7, Fajardo, PR 00738
Sterile surgical tray.

ENT MANUAL SURGICAL INSTRUMENT *(Ear/Nose/Throat) 77LRC*

Acclarent, Inc. 877-775-2789
1525B Obrien Dr, Menlo Park, CA 94025
Various types of balloon catheters and inflation devices.

Boss Instruments, Ltd. 800-210-2677
395 Reas Ford Rd Ste 120, Earlysville, VA 22936

Cardinal Health, Snowden Pencer Products 847-689-8410
5175 S Royal Atlanta Dr, Tucker, GA 30084
Various types of cartilage punches.

Exmoor Plastics Inc. 317-244-1014
304 Gasoline Aly, Indianapolis, IN 46222
EXMOOR Suction clearance kit, procedure pack for toilet of the external ear canal.

Gyrus Ent L.L.C., Sub. Of Gyrus Acmi, Inc. 508-804-2739
2925 Appling Rd, Bartlett, TN 38133
Various.

International Hospital Supply Co. 800-398-9450
6914 Canby Ave Ste 105, Reseda, CA 91335

Jedmed Instruments Co. 314-845-3770
5416 Jedmed Ct, Saint Louis, MO 63129

Magnum Medical 800-336-9710
3265 N Nevada St, Chandler, AZ 85225

Micrins Surgical Instruments, Inc. 800-833-3380
28438 N Ballard Dr, Lake Forest, IL 60045

Solos Endoscopy 800-388-6445
65 Sprague St # B, Boston/dedham Commerce Park, Boston, MA 02136
Various manual surgical instruments.

Surgical Laser Technologies, Inc. 800-366-4758
147 Keystone Dr, Montgomeryville, PA 18936

Symmetry Tnco 888-447-6661
15 Colebrook Blvd, Whitman, MA 02382
ENT manual surgical instruments: various punches, curettes, probes (w/ & w/out suction capabilty).

ENTEROSCOPE *(Gastro/Urology) 78FDA*

Pentax Medical Company 800-431-5880
102 Chestnut Ridge Rd, Montvale, NJ 07645
$34,650.00 to $34,755.00 for small bowel enteroscope with insertion tube diameters 11.6mm to 11.7mm and channel size 3.5mm to 3.8mm; forward water jet; fully immersible.

ENTRANCE, X-RAY DARKROOMS *(Radiology) 90VGS*

Xma (X-Ray Marketing Associates, Inc.) 800-325-8880
1205 W Lakeview Ct, Windham Lakes Business Park
Romeoville, IL 60446

ENVELOPE, FILM, X-RAY *(Radiology) 90WZI*

Alimed, Inc. 800-225-2610
297 High St, Dedham, MA 02026

Opco Laboratory, Inc. 978-345-2522
704 River St, Fitchburg, MA 01420
Thin film optical coatings.

Pl Medical Co., Llc. 800-874-0120
321 Ellis St, New Britain, CT 06051
X-ray filling envelopes.

St. John Companies 800-435-4242
25167 Anza Dr, PO Box 800460, Santa Clarita, CA 91355
Over 15 different varieties of film filing envelopes and category jackets.

Xma (X-Ray Marketing Associates, Inc.) 800-325-8880
1205 W Lakeview Ct, Windham Lakes Business Park
Romeoville, IL 60446

ENVIRONMENTAL CONTROL SYSTEM, POWERED
(Physical Med) 89IQA

Aes Clean Technology, Inc. 888-237-2532
422 Stump Rd, Montgomeryville, PA 18936

ENVIRONMENTAL CONTROL SYSTEM, POWERED *(cont'd)*

Aionex, Inc. 615-851-4477
104 Space Park N, Goodlettsville, TN 37072

Alarm Electronics Mfg. Co. Inc. 828-632-3365
44 All Healing Springs Rd, Taylorsville, NC 28681
Communication aid.

Anguil Environmental Systems, Inc. 800-488-0230
8855 N 55th St, Milwaukee, WI 53223
Design and construction of cost-effective air pollution control systems in standard and custom sizes of 100-200,000 SCFM. Complete environmental systems meet regulatory requirements worldwide.

Control Bionics 202-257-7090
333 N Broad St, Fairborn, OH 45324

Croll Reynolds Company, Inc. 908-232-4200
751 Central Ave, PO Box 668, Westfield, NJ 07090
Ethylene oxide cleanup systems for sterilizers. EtO scrubber system consists of packed towers, reaction tank, valves and pumps, and acid catalyst. Alternate compact design utilizing injection-bubbler technique.

Ekeg Electronics Co. Ltd. 604-857-0828
PO Box 46199, Stn. D, Vancouver, BC V6J 5G5 Canada
Expanded computer keyboard and mouse for persons with severe motor disabilities.

Health Watch Personal Response Systems 561-994-6699
6400 Park of Commerce Blvd Ste 1A, Boca Raton, FL 33487
Personal emergency response system.

Hill-Rom, Inc. 812-934-7777
4115 Dorchester Rd Unit 600, North Charleston, SC 29405
Environmental control system.

Interact Plus 800-944-8002
2225 Drake Ave SW Ste 2, Huntsville, AL 35805
Environmental control unit.

Kinetic Concepts, Inc. 800-275-4524
8023 Vantage Dr, San Antonio, TX 78230
Powered environmental control.

Lab Safety Supply, Inc. 800-356-0783
401 S Wright Rd, Janesville, WI 53546

Quartet Technology, Inc. 978-649-4328
87 Progress Ave, Tyngsboro, MA 01879
The Simplicity Series Environmental Control Unit (ECU) allows someone with a physical disability to control their

Tash International Inc. 800-463-5685
91 Station St., Unit 1, Ajax, ONT L1S 3H2 Canada
$40 to $800 for environmental controls.

Tektone Sound & Signal Manufacturing, Inc. 828-524-9967
277 Industrial Park Rd, Franklin, NC 28734
Various nurse call systems.

Weitbrecht Communications, Inc. 800-233-9130
926 Colorado Ave, Santa Monica, CA 90401
Alerting, paging, and signaling devices for the deaf and hard of hearing.

ENVIRONMENTAL CONTROL SYSTEM, POWERED, REMOTE
(Physical Med) 89ILR

Quartet Technology, Inc. 978-649-4328
87 Progress Ave, Tyngsboro, MA 01879
The Simplicity Series Environmental Control Unit (ECU) allows someone with a physical disability to control their home, hospital, or work environment. By a simple voice command or activating a switch a user can control their built-in telephone, nurse call, electric bed, thermostat, doors, lights, TV, computer and more. Go mobile with your Simplicity ECU from your wheelchair with our radio remote package.

ENZYMATIC (U.V.), PYRUVIC ACID *(Chemistry) 75JLT*

Calbiotech, Inc. 619-660-6162
10461 Austin Dr Ste G, Spring Valley, CA 91978
Mitochondrial antibody (ma) elisa.

ENZYMATIC ESTERASE-OXIDASE, CHOLESTEROL
(Chemistry) 75CHH

Abbott Diagnostics Div. 626-440-0700
820 Mission St, South Pasadena, CA 91030
Cholesterol.

Accuech, Llc 760-599-6555
2641 La Mirada Dr, Vista, CA 92081
Cholesterol test.

ENZYMATIC ESTERASE-OXIDASE, CHOLESTEROL *(cont'd)*

Amresco Inc. 800-366-1313
30175 Solon Industrial Pkwy, Solon, OH 44139
Liquid Direct HDL Cholesterol Kit used for qunatitative determination of high density lipoprotein cholesterol in serum. This automated two reagent test is the fastest fully automatable liquid direct HDL method available and has been validated for hospital reference and physician office labs.

Beckman Coulter, Inc. 800-635-3497
740 W 83rd St, Hialeah, FL 33014
$0.14 per test.

Beckman Coulter, Inc. 800-742-2345
250 S Kraemer Blvd, PO Box 8000, Brea, CA 92821

Biomerieux Inc. 800-682-2666
100 Rodolphe St, Durham, NC 27712

Caldon Bioscience, Inc. 909-628-9944
2100 S Reservoir St, Pomona, CA 91766
Cholesterol.

Caldon Biotech, Inc. 757-224-0177
2251 Rutherford Rd, Carlsbad, CA 92008
Cholesterol.

Carolina Liquid Chemistries Corp. 800-471-7272
510 W Central Ave Ste C, Brea, CA 92821
Cholesterol or chol.

Chematics, Inc. 574-834-4080
Hwy. 13 South, North Webster, IN 46555
Solid phase determination of total cholesterol, enzymatic esterase-oxdase.

Diagnostic Specialties 732-549-4011
4 Leonard St, Metuchen, NJ 08840
Cholesterol reagent kit. CE/CO Enzymated cholesterol reagents.

Genchem, Inc. 714-529-1616
510 W Central Ave Ste D, Brea, CA 92821
Cholesterol reagent.

Genzyme Corp. 800-325-2436
160 Christian St, Oxford, CT 06478
Cholesterol assay kit, enzymatic 505nm.

Harvey, R.J. Instrument Corp. 201-664-1380
123 Patterson St, Hillsdale, NJ 07642
Cholesterol enzymatic lipase-oxidase.

Health Chem Diagnostics Llc 954-979-3845
3341 W McNab Rd, Pompano Beach, FL 33069
Enzymatic esterase--oxidase, cholesterol.

Hemagen Diagnostics, Inc. 800-436-2436
9033 Red Branch Rd, Columbia, MD 21045
Various cholesterol methods.

Intersect Systems, Inc. 360-577-1062
1152 3rd Avenue, Suite D & E, Longview, WA 98632
Enzymatic esterase-oxidase cholesterol, Enzymatic Cholesterol.

Jas Diagnostics, Inc. 305-418-2320
7220 NW 58th St, Miami, FL 33166
Cholesterol.

Polymer Technology Systems, Inc. 317-870-5610
7736 Zionsville Rd, Indianapolis, IN 46268
Bioscanner plus and lipid panel test strips.

St. Paul Biotech 714-903-1000
11555 Monarch St, Garden Grove, CA 92841
Total cholesterol test.

Stanbio Life Sciences, Division Of Stanbio Laboratory 830-249-0772
25235 Leer Dr, Elkhart, IN 46514

Sterling Diagnostics, Inc. 800-637-2661
36645 Metro Ct, Sterling Heights, MI 48312
Cholesterol reagent set.

Synermed Intl., Inc. 317-896-1565
17408 Tiller Ct Ste 1900, Westfield, IN 46074
Cholesterol reagent kit & hdl cholesterol reagent kit.

Teco Diagnostics 714-693-7788
1268 N Lakeview Ave, Anaheim, CA 92807
Cholesterol liquid reagent.

Vital Diagnostics Inc. 714-672-3553
1075 W Lambert Rd Ste D, Brea, CA 92821
Various total cholesterol reagents.

ENZYMATIC METHOD, AMMONIA *(Chemistry) 75JIF*

Abbott Diagnostics Div. 626-440-0700
820 Mission St, South Pasadena, CA 91030
Ammonia.

Carolina Liquid Chemistries Corp. 800-471-7272
510 W Central Ave Ste C, Brea, CA 92821
Ammonia reagent.

Genzyme Corp. 800-325-2436
160 Christian St, Oxford, CT 06478
Ammonia, endpoint. Enzymatic, rate.

Raichem, Division Of Hemagen Diagnostics, Inc. 800-438-6100
8225 Mercury Ct, San Diego, CA 92111
Ammonia Reagent (Test System).

Teco Diagnostics 714-693-7788
1268 N Lakeview Ave, Anaheim, CA 92807
Ammonia.

ENZYMATIC METHOD, BILIRUBIN *(Chemistry) 75JFM*

Hemagen Diagnostics, Inc. 800-436-2436
9033 Red Branch Rd, Columbia, MD 21045
Analyst total bilirubin.

ENZYMATIC METHOD, BLOOD, OCCCULT, FECAL *(Chemistry) 75TGO*

Biomerica, Inc. 800-854-3002
17571 Von Karman Ave, Irvine, CA 92614
#1000 occult blood in stool test. EZ DETECT, fecal occult test without diet restrictions & stool handling.

Cambridge Diagnostic Products, Inc. 800-525-6262
6880 NW 17th Ave, Fort Lauderdale, FL 33309
CAMCO Pak Guaiac: $56.00 for 100; $160.00 for 300; $380.00 for 1,000. Developer 10's-$55.00.Control 10's-$55.00.

Fujirebio Diagnostics, Inc. (Fdi) 877-861-7246
201 Great Valley Pkwy, Malvern, PA 19355
HEMP-SP immunochemical/agglutination method test for detection of hemoglobin in feces; performed on microplates.

Helena Laboratories 409-842-3714
PO Box 752, Beaumont, TX 77704

ENZYMATIC METHOD, BLOOD, OCCULT, URINARY *(Chemistry) 75JIP*

Bayer Healthcare Llc 914-524-2955
555 White Plains Rd Fl 5, Tarrytown, NY 10591
Test for occult blood in urine.

Bayer Healthcare, Llc 574-256-3430
430 S Beiger St, Mishawaka, IN 46544
Multiple.

Cambridge Diagnostic Products, Inc. 800-525-6262
6880 NW 17th Ave, Fort Lauderdale, FL 33309
$40.00 for 100 guaiac tablets and 100 filter paper squares.

ENZYMATIC METHOD, CREATININE *(Chemistry) 75JFY*

Bayer Healthcare Llc 914-524-2955
555 White Plains Rd Fl 5, Tarrytown, NY 10591
Test for leukocytes,nitrite,blood,ph,creatinine,sg,ketone,protein low/high,.

Bayer Healthcare, Llc 574-256-3430
430 S Beiger St, Mishawaka, IN 46544
Test for leukocytes,nitrite,blood,ph,creatinine,sg,ketone,protein low/high,.

Hemagen Diagnostics, Inc. 800-436-2436
9033 Red Branch Rd, Columbia, MD 21045
Analyst creatinine.

Polymer Technology Systems, Inc. 317-870-5610
7736 Zionsville Rd, Indianapolis, IN 46268
Creatinine test.

ENZYMATIC METHOD, GALACTOSE *(Chemistry) 75JIA*

Astoria-Pacific,Inc. 800-536-3111
PO Box 830, Clackamas, OR 97015
For determining galactose content in infant blood serum.

Neo-Genesis, A Division Of Natus 503-657-8000
15140 SE 82nd Dr Ste 270, Clackamas, OR 97015
Galactose test system.

ENZYMATIC METHOD, GLUCOSE (URINARY, NON-QUANTITATIVE) *(Chemistry) 75JIL*

Ameritek Usa, Inc. 425-379-2580
125 130th St SE Ste 200, Everett, WA 98208
Urinalysis strips.

ENZYMATIC METHOD, GLUCOSE (URINARY, NON-QUANTITATIVE) *(cont'd)*

Arkray Factory Usa, Inc. 952-646-3168
5182 W 76th St, Minneapolis, MN 55439
Urine test strips.

Bayer Healthcare Llc 914-524-2955
555 White Plains Rd Fl 5, Tarrytown, NY 10591
Test for glucose in urine.

Bayer Healthcare, Llc 574-256-3430
430 S Beiger St, Mishawaka, IN 46544
Multiple.

Iris Diagnostics 800-776-4747
9172 Eton Ave, Chatsworth, CA 91311
Semi-automated urine chemistry analyzer.

Neo Pharm Inc. 714-226-0070
10532 Walker St Ste B, Cypress, CA 90630
Urinary glucose (non-quantitative) test system.

Stanbio Laboratory, Inc. 830-249-0772
1261 N Main St, Boerne, TX 78006
$42.00 for 250ml enzymatic glucose test set with liquid reagent and 100mg/dl standard.

Teco Diagnostics 714-693-7788
1268 N Lakeview Ave, Anaheim, CA 92807
Urine reagent strips.

ENZYMATIC METHOD, LACTIC ACID *(Chemistry) 75KHP*

Abbott Diagnostics Div. 626-440-0700
820 Mission St, South Pasadena, CA 91030
Various.

Abbott Point Of Care Inc. 609-443-9300
104 Windsor Center Dr, East Windsor, NJ 08520
Lactate test.

ENZYMATIC METHOD, TROPONIN SUBUNIT *(Chemistry) 75MMI*

Abbott Point Of Care Inc. 609-443-9300
104 Windsor Center Dr, East Windsor, NJ 08520
Cardiac troponin i test.

Access Bio Incorporate 732-297-2222
2033 Rt. 130 Unit H, Monmouth Junction, NJ 08852
Cardiac myoglobin/ckmb/troponin i rapid test.

Ameritek Usa, Inc. 425-379-2580
125 130th St SE Ste 200, Everett, WA 98208
Troponin i test kit.

Bio-Medical Products Corp. 800-543-7427
10 Halstead Rd, Mendham, NJ 07945
Rapid serum troponin I test, 15 minutes. $8.00 per test.

Biocheck, Inc. 650-573-1968
323 Vintage Park Dr, Foster City, CA 94404
Troponin i eia test kit.

Chembio Diagnostic Systems, Inc. 631-924-1135
3661 Horseblock Rd, Medford, NY 11763
Immunochromatographic assay for visual detection of troponin i antigen.

Lusys Laboratories Inc. 858-546-0902
10054 Mesa Ridge Ct Ste 118, San Diego, CA 92121
For determination of troponin i in serum.

Nano-Ditech Corporation 609-409-0700
7 Clarke Dr, Cranbury, NJ 08512
Immunoassay method tropin subunit.

ENZYMATIC, CARBON-DIOXIDE *(Chemistry) 75KHS*

Genzyme Corp. 800-325-2436
160 Christian St, Oxford, CT 06478
Carbon dioxide assay kit. Enzymatic, endpoint.

Intersect Systems, Inc. 360-577-1062
1152 3rd Avenue, Suite D & E, Longview, WA 98632
Enzymatic carbon dioxide, Single Vial CO2. Also available Enzymatic carbon dioxide Dual Vial CO2.

Jas Diagnostics, Inc. 305-418-2320
7220 NW 58th St, Miami, FL 33166
Carbon dioxide.

Raichem, Division Of Hemagen Diagnostics, Inc. 800-438-6100
8225 Mercury Ct, San Diego, CA 92111
Carbon dioxide (Co2) reagent, test system, enzymatic.

Synermed Intl., Inc. 317-896-1565
17408 Tiller Ct Ste 1900, Westfield, IN 46074
Enzymatic co2 reagent kit.

ENZYMATIC, CARBON-DIOXIDE *(cont'd)*

Teco Diagnostics 714-693-7788
1268 N Lakeview Ave, Anaheim, CA 92807
Carbon dioxide.

ENZYME IMMUNOASSAY, AMPHETAMINE *(Toxicology) 91DKZ*

Acro Biotech Llc. 909-466-6892
9500 7th St Ste M, Rancho Cucamonga, CA 91730
Point of care rapid test.

Alfa Scientific Designs, Inc. 877-204-5071
13200 Gregg St, Poway, CA 92064
Various.

Amedica Biotech, Inc. 510-785-5980
28301 Industrial Blvd Ste K, Hayward, CA 94545
Drug screen amphetamine test.

Ameditech, Inc. 858-535-1968
10340 Camino Santa Fe Ste F, San Diego, CA 92121
Multi-drug amphetamine etc. test system.

American Bio Medica Corp. 800-227-1243
122 Smith Rd, Kinderhook, NY 12106
One step lateral flow immunoassay.

American Bio Medica Corp. 856-241-2320
603 Heron Dr Ste 3, Logan Township, NJ 08085
One step lateral flow immunoassay.

Biosite Incorporated 888-246-7483
9975 Summers Ridge Rd, San Diego, CA 92121
Fluorescence immunoassay for detection of drugs of abuse in urine.

Branan Medical Corp. 949-598-7166
140 Technology Dr Ste 400, Irvine, CA 92618
Immunochromatographical test for qualitative determination of amphetamines.

Carolina Liquid Chemistries Corp. 800-471-7272
510 W Central Ave Ste C, Brea, CA 92821
Amphetamine reagent.

Express Diagnostics Int'L, Inc. 507-526-3951
1550 Industrial Dr, Blue Earth, MN 56013
Drugs of abuse screening test.

Germaine Laboratories, Inc. 210-692-4192
4139 Gardendale St Ste 101, San Antonio, TX 78229
Various types, amphetamines tests.

Innovacon, Inc. 858-535-2030
4106 Sorrento Valley Blvd, San Diego, CA 92121
Amphetamine drug of abuse test.

Jant Pharmacal Corp. 800-676-5565
16255 Ventura Blvd Ste 505, Encino, CA 91436
Test to detect amphetamine in human urine.

Lin-Zhi International, Inc. 408-732-3856
687 N Pastoria Ave, Sunnyvale, CA 94085
Homogeneous enzyme immunoassay for the determination of amphetamines lvl in urin.

Medtox Diagnostics Inc. 800-334-1116
1238 Anthony Rd, Burlington, NC 27215
EZ-SCREEN competitive enzyme immunoassay screening test for amphetamines and metabolites.

Medtox Diagnostics, Inc. 800-334-1116
1640 Nova Ln, Burlington, NC 27215
Immunochromatographic assay for amphetamines (amp).

Microgenics Corporation 800-232-3342
46360 Fremont Blvd, Fremont, CA 94538

Myers-Stevens Group, Inc. 903-566-6696
2931 Vail Ave, Commerce, CA 90040
Eia test for the detection of amphetamines.

Pan Probe Biotech, Inc. 858-689-9936
7396 Trade St, San Diego, CA 92121
Determination of amphetamine in human urine.

QuantRx Biomedical Corp. 503-252-9565
5920 NE 112th Ave, Portland, OR 97220
ACCUSTEP DOA SINGLE AND

Rapid Diagnostics, Div. Of Mp Biomedicals, Llc 800-888-7008
1429 Rollins Rd, Burlingame, CA 94010
Rapid Amphetamine test.

St. Paul Biotech 714-903-1000
11555 Monarch St, Garden Grove, CA 92841
Amphetamine test.

ENZYME IMMUNOASSAY, AMPHETAMINE *(cont'd)*

Teco Diagnostics 714-693-7788
1268 N Lakeview Ave, Anaheim, CA 92807
One step amphetamine card test.

Ucp Biosciences, Inc. 408-392-0064
1445 Koll Cir Ste 111, San Jose, CA 95112
Amphetamine test system.

Varian Inc 650-424-5078
25200 Commercentre Dr, Lake Forest, CA 92630
Drug testing devices.

W.H.P.M., Inc. 978-927-3808
9662 Telstar Ave, El Monte, CA 91731
Drug of abuse screening.

ENZYME IMMUNOASSAY, BARBITURATE *(Toxicology) 91DIS*

Abbott Diagnostics Div. 626-440-0700
820 Mission St, South Pasadena, CA 91030
Barbiturates.

Abbott Laboratories 800-223-2064
100 Abbott Park Rd, Abbott Park, IL 60064
TDX BARBITURATES II ASSAY

Amedica Biotech, Inc. 510-785-5980
28301 Industrial Blvd Ste K, Hayward, CA 94545
Drug screen barbiturates test.

American Bio Medica Corp. 800-227-1243
122 Smith Rd, Kinderhook, NY 12106
One step lateral flow immunoassay.

American Bio Medica Corp. 856-241-2320
603 Heron Dr Ste 3, Logan Township, NJ 08085
One step lateral flow immunoassay.

Biosite Incorporated 888-246-7483
9975 Summers Ridge Rd, San Diego, CA 92121
Fluorescence immunoassay for detection of drugs of abuse in urine.

Branan Medical Corp. 949-598-7166
140 Technology Dr Ste 400, Irvine, CA 92618
Immunochromatographical test for the qualitative determination of barbiturates.

Carolina Liquid Chemistries Corp. 800-471-7272
510 W Central Ave Ste C, Brea, CA 92821
Barbiturate reagent.

Express Diagnostics Int'L, Inc. 507-526-3951
1550 Industrial Dr, Blue Earth, MN 56013
Drugs of abuse screening test.

Germaine Laboratories, Inc. 210-692-4192
4139 Gardendale St Ste 101, San Antonio, TX 78229
Various types, barbiturate.

Innovacon, Inc. 858-535-2030
4106 Sorrento Valley Blvd, San Diego, CA 92121
Barbiturates drug of abuse.

Medtox Diagnostics Inc. 800-334-1116
1238 Anthony Rd, Burlington, NC 27215
EZ-SCREEN competitive enzyme immunoassay screening test for barbiturates and metabolites.

Medtox Diagnostics, Inc. 800-334-1116
1640 Nova Ln, Burlington, NC 27215
Immunochromatographic assay for barbiturates (bar).

Microgenics Corporation 800-232-3342
46360 Fremont Blvd, Fremont, CA 94538

Pan Probe Biotech, Inc. 858-689-9936
7396 Trade St, San Diego, CA 92121
Determination of barbiturate in human urine.

Phamatech Inc. 858-643-5555
10151 Barnes Canyon Rd, San Diego, CA 92121
Lateral flow immunoassay for barbiturates.

QuantRx Biomedical Corp. 503-252-9565
5920 NE 112th Ave, Portland, OR 97220
ACCUSTEP DOA SINGLE AND

Rapid Diagnostics, Div. Of Mp Biomedicals, Llc 800-888-7008
1429 Rollins Rd, Burlingame, CA 94010
Rapid Barbiturate test.

St. Paul Biotech 714-903-1000
11555 Monarch St, Garden Grove, CA 92841
Barbiturate test.

Ucp Biosciences, Inc. 408-392-0064
1445 Koll Cir Ste 111, San Jose, CA 95112
Barbiturate test system.

ENZYME IMMUNOASSAY, BARBITURATE *(cont'd)*

Varian Inc 650-424-5078
25200 Commercentre Dr, Lake Forest, CA 92630
Drug testing devices.

Victorch Meditek, Inc. 858-530-9191
7313 Carroll Rd Ste A-B, San Diego, CA 92121
One step multiple drugs of abuse assays.

ENZYME IMMUNOASSAY, BENZODIAZEPINE *(Toxicology) 91JXM*

Abbott Diagnostics Div. 626-440-0700
820 Mission St, South Pasadena, CA 91030
Benzodiazepine.

Abbott Diagnostics Intl, Biotechnology Ltd 787-846-3500
Road #2 KM. 58.0 , PO Box 278, Cruce Davila, Barceloneta, PR 00617
Various.

Acro Biotech Llc. 909-466-6892
9500 7th St Ste M, Rancho Cucamonga, CA 91730
Point of care rapid test.

Amedica Biotech, Inc. 510-785-5980
28301 Industrial Blvd Ste K, Hayward, CA 94545
Drug screen benzodiazepines test.

American Bio Medica Corp. 800-227-1243
122 Smith Rd, Kinderhook, NY 12106
One step lateral flow immunoassay.

American Bio Medica Corp. 856-241-2320
603 Heron Dr Ste 3, Logan Township, NJ 08085
One step lateral flow immunoassay.

Biosite Incorporated 888-246-7483
9975 Summers Ridge Rd, San Diego, CA 92121
Fluorescence immunoassay for detection of drugs of abuse in urine.

Branan Medical Corp. 949-598-7166
140 Technology Dr Ste 400, Irvine, CA 92618
Immunochromatographical test (qualitative derтermination bzo human urine).

Carolina Liquid Chemistries Corp. 800-471-7272
510 W Central Ave Ste C, Brea, CA 92821
Benzodiazepine reagent.

Express Diagnostics Int'L, Inc. 507-526-3951
1550 Industrial Dr, Blue Earth, MN 56013
Drugs of abuse screening test.

Germaine Laboratories, Inc. 210-692-4192
4139 Gardendale St Ste 101, San Antonio, TX 78229
Various types, benzodiazipine.

Innovacon, Inc. 858-535-2030
4106 Sorrento Valley Blvd, San Diego, CA 92121
Benzodiazepine test.

Jant Pharmacal Corp. 800-676-5565
16255 Ventura Blvd Ste 505, Encino, CA 91436
Test to detect benzodiazepines in human urine.

Medtox Diagnostics, Inc. 800-334-1116
1640 Nova Ln, Burlington, NC 27215
Immunochromatographic assay for benzodiazipines (bzo).

Microgenics Corporation 800-232-3342
46360 Fremont Blvd, Fremont, CA 94538

Nubenco Ent., Inc. 800-633-1322
1 Kalisa Way Ste 207, Paramus, NJ 07652
Benzodiazepines test kit.

Pan Probe Biotech, Inc. 858-689-9936
7396 Trade St, San Diego, CA 92121
Determination of benzodiazepine in human urine.

Phamatech Inc. 858-643-5555
10151 Barnes Canyon Rd, San Diego, CA 92121
Lateral flow immunoassay for benzodiazepines.

QuantRx Biomedical Corp. 503-252-9565
5920 NE 112th Ave, Portland, OR 97220
ACCUSTEP DOA SINGLE AND

Rapid Diagnostics, Div. Of Mp Biomedicals, Llc 800-888-7008
1429 Rollins Rd, Burlingame, CA 94010
Rapid Benzodiazepine test.

Sun Biomedical Laboratories, Inc. 888-440-8388
604 Vpr Center, 1001 Lower Landing Road, Blackwood, NJ 08012
Benzodiazepines test--drug-screening urine test.

Ucp Biosciences, Inc. 408-392-0064
1445 Koll Cir Ste 111, San Jose, CA 95112
Benzodiazepine test system.

ENZYME IMMUNOASSAY, BENZODIAZEPINE *(cont'd)*

Varian Inc 650-424-5078
25200 Commercentre Dr, Lake Forest, CA 92630
Drug testing devices.

ENZYME IMMUNOASSAY, CANNABINOIDS *(Toxicology) 91LDJ*

Abbott Diagnostics Div. 626-440-0700
820 Mission St, South Pasadena, CA 91030
Cannabinoids.

Acro Biotech Llc. 909-466-6892
9500 7th St Ste M, Rancho Cucamonga, CA 91730
Point of care rapid test.

Alfa Scientific Designs, Inc. 877-204-5071
13200 Gregg St, Poway, CA 92064
Various.

Amedica Biotech, Inc. 510-785-5980
28301 Industrial Blvd Ste K, Hayward, CA 94545
Drug screen thc test.

Ameditech, Inc. 858-535-1968
10340 Camino Santa Fe Ste F, San Diego, CA 92121
Various.

American Bio Medica Corp. 800-227-1243
122 Smith Rd, Kinderhook, NY 12106
One step lateral flow immunoassay.

American Bio Medica Corp. 856-241-2320
603 Heron Dr Ste 3, Logan Township, NJ 08085
One step lateral flow immunoassay.

Biosite Incorporated 888-246-7483
9975 Summers Ridge Rd, San Diego, CA 92121
Fluorescence immunoassay for detection of drugs of abuse in urine.

Branan Medical Corp. 949-598-7166
140 Technology Dr Ste 400, Irvine, CA 92618
Various.

Carolina Liquid Chemistries Corp. 800-471-7272
510 W Central Ave Ste C, Brea, CA 92821
Cannabinoid reagent.

Escreen, Inc. 800-881-0722
2205 W Parkside Ln, Phoenix, AZ 85027
Escreen drugs of abuse screening system.

Express Diagnostics Int'L, Inc. 507-526-3951
1550 Industrial Dr, Blue Earth, MN 56013
Drugs of abuse screening test.

Germaine Laboratories, Inc. 210-692-4192
4139 Gardendale St Ste 101, San Antonio, TX 78229
Various types, cannabinoids & thc.

Innovacon, Inc. 858-535-2030
4106 Sorrento Valley Blvd, San Diego, CA 92121
Thc drug of abuse test.

Jant Pharmacal Corp. 800-676-5565
16255 Ventura Blvd Ste 505, Encino, CA 91436
Test to detect THC in human urine.

Lin-Zhi International, Inc. 408-732-3856
687 N Pastoria Ave, Sunnyvale, CA 94085
Homogeneous enzyme immunoassay for the determination of cannabinoids in urine.

Medtox Diagnostics Inc. 800-334-1116
1238 Anthony Rd, Burlington, NC 27215
EZ-SCREEN competitive cannabinoid/cocaine/opiates enyzme immunoassay screening test for cannabinoid/cocaine/opiates and metabolites.

Myers-Stevens Group, Inc. 903-566-6696
2931 Vail Ave, Commerce, CA 90040
Test for the detection of cannabinoids.

Nano-Ditech Corporation 609-409-0700
7 Clarke Dr, Cranbury, NJ 08512
Enzyme immunoassay, cannabinoids.

Nubenco Ent., Inc. 800-633-1322
1 Kalisa Way Ste 207, Paramus, NJ 07652
Cannabinoid (thc) test kit.

Pan Probe Biotech, Inc. 858-689-9936
7396 Trade St, San Diego, CA 92121
Determination of marijuana (thc) in human urine.

Phamatech Inc. 858-643-5555
10151 Barnes Canyon Rd, San Diego, CA 92121
Thc rapid test.

ENZYME IMMUNOASSAY, CANNABINOIDS *(cont'd)*

QuantRx Biomedical Corp. 503-252-9565
5920 NE 112th Ave, Portland, OR 97220
ACCUSTEP DOA SINGLE AND

Rapid Diagnostics, Div. Of Mp Biomedicals, Llc 800-888-7008
1429 Rollins Rd, Burlingame, CA 94010
Rapid THC test

St. Paul Biotech 714-903-1000
11555 Monarch St, Garden Grove, CA 92841
Marijuana test.

Sun Biomedical Laboratories, Inc. 888-440-8388
604 Vpr Center, 1001 Lower Landing Road, Blackwood, NJ 08012
Thc/co combo test--drug-screening urine test.

Teco Diagnostics 714-693-7788
1268 N Lakeview Ave, Anaheim, CA 92807
Onestep marijuana card test.

Ucp Biosciences, Inc. 408-392-0064
1445 Koll Cir Ste 111, San Jose, CA 95112
Cannabinoid test system.

Varian Inc 650-424-5078
25200 Commercentre Dr, Lake Forest, CA 92630
Drug testing devices.

ENZYME IMMUNOASSAY, CARBAMAZEPINE *(Toxicology) 91KLT*

Abbott Diagnostics Div. 626-440-0700
820 Mission St, South Pasadena, CA 91030
Various assays for detection of carbamazepine.

Abbott Diagnostics Intl, Biotechnology Ltd 787-846-3500
Road #2 KM. 58.0 , PO Box 278, Cruce Davila, Barceloneta, PR 00617
Various assays for detection of carbamazepine.

Beckman Coulter, Inc. 800-742-2345
250 S Kraemer Blvd, PO Box 8000, Brea, CA 92821

Microgenics Corporation 800-232-3342
46360 Fremont Blvd, Fremont, CA 94538

Opus Diagnostics, Inc. 877-944-1777
1 Parker Plz, Fort Lee, NJ 07024
Innofluor carbamazipine reagent set.

ENZYME IMMUNOASSAY, COCAINE *(Toxicology) 91JXO*

Biosite Incorporated 888-246-7483
9975 Summers Ridge Rd, San Diego, CA 92121
Fluorescence immunoassay for detection of drugs of abuse ini urine.

Medtox Diagnostics Inc. 800-334-1116
1238 Anthony Rd, Burlington, NC 27215
EZ-SCREEN multiple enyzme immunoassay screening test for cannabinoid/cocaine and metabolites.

Teco Diagnostics 714-693-7788
1268 N Lakeview Ave, Anaheim, CA 92807
Onestep cocaine/benzoyl/ergonine card test.

ENZYME IMMUNOASSAY, COCAINE AND COCAINE METABOLITES *(Toxicology) 91DIO*

Abbott Diagnostics Div. 626-440-0700
820 Mission St, South Pasadena, CA 91030
Cocaine.

Acro Biotech Llc. 909-466-6892
9500 7th St Ste M, Rancho Cucamonga, CA 91730
Point of care rapid test.

Alfa Scientific Designs, Inc. 877-204-5071
13200 Gregg St, Poway, CA 92064
Various.

Amedica Biotech, Inc. 510-785-5980
28301 Industrial Blvd Ste K, Hayward, CA 94545
Drug screen cocaine test.

Ameditech, Inc. 858-535-1968
10340 Camino Santa Fe Ste F, San Diego, CA 92121
Various.

American Bio Medica Corp. 800-227-1243
122 Smith Rd, Kinderhook, NY 12106
One-step lateral flow immuno assay.

American Bio Medica Corp. 856-241-2320
603 Heron Dr Ste 3, Logan Township, NJ 08085
One-step lateral flow immuno assay.

Ameritek Usa, Inc. 425-379-2580
125 130th St SE Ste 200, Everett, WA 98208
Cocaine test kit.

ENZYME IMMUNOASSAY, COCAINE AND COCAINE METABOLITES *(cont'd)*

Biosite Incorporated 888-246-7483
9975 Summers Ridge Rd, San Diego, CA 92121
Visual immunoassay for detection of drugs of abuse in urine.

Branan Medical Corp. 949-598-7166
140 Technology Dr Ste 400, Irvine, CA 92618
Various.

Carolina Liquid Chemistries Corp. 800-471-7272
510 W Central Ave Ste C, Brea, CA 92821
Cocaine reagent.

Escreen, Inc. 800-881-0722
2205 W Parkside Ln, Phoenix, AZ 85027
Escreen drugs of abuse screening system.

Express Diagnostics Int'L, Inc. 507-526-3951
1550 Industrial Dr, Blue Earth, MN 56013
Drugs of abuse screening test.

Germaine Laboratories, Inc. 210-692-4192
4139 Gardendale St Ste 101, San Antonio, TX 78229
Various types, cocaine tests.

Innovacon, Inc. 858-535-2030
4106 Sorrento Valley Blvd, San Diego, CA 92121
Cocaine drug of abuse test.

Lin-Zhi International, Inc. 408-732-3856
687 N Pastoria Ave, Sunnyvale, CA 94085
Homogeneous enzyme immunoassay for the determination of benzoylecgonine in urine.

Medtox Diagnostics Inc. 800-334-1116
1238 Anthony Rd, Burlington, NC 27215
EZ-SCREEN enzyme immunoassay screening test for cocaine and cocaine metabolites.

Medtox Diagnostics, Inc. 800-334-1116
1640 Nova Ln, Burlington, NC 27215
Immunochromatographic assay for cocaine (coc).

Nano-Ditech Corporation 609-409-0700
7 Clarke Dr, Cranbury, NJ 08512
Enzyme immunoassay, cocaine and cocaine metabolites.

Neo Pharm Inc. 714-226-0070
10532 Walker St Ste B, Cypress, CA 90630
Cocaine and cocaine metabolites test system.

Nubenco Ent., Inc. 800-633-1322
1 Kalisa Way Ste 207, Paramus, NJ 07652
Cocaine test kit.

QuantRx Biomedical Corp. 503-252-9565
5920 NE 112th Ave, Portland, OR 97220
ACCUSTEP DOA SINGLE AND

Rapid Diagnostics, Div. Of Mp Biomedicals, Llc 800-888-7008
1429 Rollins Rd, Burlingame, CA 94010
Rapid cocaine test

St. Paul Biotech 714-903-1000
11555 Monarch St, Garden Grove, CA 92841
Cocaine test.

Varian Inc 650-424-5078
25200 Commercentre Dr, Lake Forest, CA 92630
Drug testing devices.

W.H.P.M., Inc. 978-927-3808
9662 Telstar Ave, El Monte, CA 91731
Drug of abuse screening.

ENZYME IMMUNOASSAY, DIGITOXIN *(Toxicology) 91LFM*

Dade Behring, Inc. 800-948-3233
1717 Deerfield Rd, Deerfield, IL 60015

Microgenics Corporation 800-232-3342
46360 Fremont Blvd, Fremont, CA 94538

Opus Diagnostics, Inc. 877-944-1777
1 Parker Plz, Fort Lee, NJ 07024
Innofluor digitoxin reagent set.

ENZYME IMMUNOASSAY, DIGOXIN *(Toxicology) 91KXT*

Abbott Diagnostics Intl, Biotechnology Ltd 787-846-3500
Road #2 KM. 58.0 , PO Box 278, Cruce Davila, Barceloneta, PR 00617
Digoxin.

Alfa Wassermann, Inc. 800-220-4488
4 Henderson Dr, West Caldwell, NJ 07006
Thyroxine (T4), T uptake.

ENZYME IMMUNOASSAY, DIGOXIN *(cont'd)*

Microgenics Corporation 800-232-3342
46360 Fremont Blvd, Fremont, CA 94538
No pretreatment digoxin assay.

Myers-Stevens Group, Inc. 903-566-6696
2931 Vail Ave, Commerce, CA 90040
Eia test for the quantitation of digoxin.

ENZYME IMMUNOASSAY, DIPHENYLHYDANTOIN
(Toxicology) 91DIP

Abbott Diagnostics Div. 626-440-0700
820 Mission St, South Pasadena, CA 91030
Phenytoin.

Microgenics Corporation 800-232-3342
46360 Fremont Blvd, Fremont, CA 94538

ENZYME IMMUNOASSAY, ETHOSUXIMIDE *(Toxicology) 91DLF*

Bayer Healthcare, Llc 574-256-3430
430 S Beiger St, Mishawaka, IN 46544
Test for ethosuximide in serum or plasma.

ENZYME IMMUNOASSAY, FETAL FIBRONECTIN
(Chemistry) 75LKV

Cytyc Corporation 888-773-8376
1240 Elko Dr, Sunnyvale, CA 94089
Thi system.

Cytyc Surgical Products 800-442-9892
250 Campus Dr, Marlborough, MA 01752
Tli iq system.

ENZYME IMMUNOASSAY, GENTAMICIN *(Toxicology) 91LCD*

Microgenics Corporation 800-232-3342
46360 Fremont Blvd, Fremont, CA 94538

ENZYME IMMUNOASSAY, METHADONE *(Toxicology) 91DJR*

Abbott Diagnostics Div. 626-440-0700
820 Mission St, South Pasadena, CA 91030
Methadone.

Abbott Laboratories 800-223-2064
100 Abbott Park Rd, Abbott Park, IL 60064
Various

Amedica Biotech, Inc. 510-785-5980
28301 Industrial Blvd Ste K, Hayward, CA 94545
Drug screen methadone test.

American Bio Medica Corp. 800-227-1243
122 Smith Rd, Kinderhook, NY 12106
One step lateral flow immunoassay.

American Bio Medica Corp. 856-241-2320
603 Heron Dr Ste 3, Logan Township, NJ 08085
Methadone test system.

Biosite Incorporated 888-246-7483
9975 Summers Ridge Rd, San Diego, CA 92121
Visual immunoassay for detection of drugs of abuse in urine.

Branan Medical Corp. 949-598-7166
140 Technology Dr Ste 400, Irvine, CA 92618
Immunochromatographical test (qualitative determination of methadone in urine).

Carolina Liquid Chemistries Corp. 800-471-7272
510 W Central Ave Ste C, Brea, CA 92821
Methadone reagent.

Express Diagnostics Int'L, Inc. 507-526-3951
1550 Industrial Dr, Blue Earth, MN 56013
Drugs of abuse screening test.

Germaine Laboratories, Inc. 210-692-4192
4139 Gardendale St Ste 101, San Antonio, TX 78229
Various types, methadone.

Innovacon, Inc. 858-535-2030
4106 Sorrento Valley Blvd, San Diego, CA 92121
Methadone drug of abuse.

Jant Pharmacal Corp. 800-676-5565
16255 Ventura Blvd Ste 505, Encino, CA 91436
Test to detect methadone in human urine.

Lin-Zhi International, Inc. 408-732-3856
687 N Pastoria Ave, Sunnyvale, CA 94085
Homoglnlous enzyme immunoassay for the determination of methadone in urine.

Medtox Diagnostics, Inc. 800-334-1116
1640 Nova Ln, Burlington, NC 27215
Immunochromatographic assay for methadone (mtd).

ENZYME IMMUNOASSAY, METHADONE *(cont'd)*

Microgenics Corporation 800-232-3342
46360 Fremont Blvd, Fremont, CA 94538

Pan Probe Biotech, Inc. 858-689-9936
7396 Trade St, San Diego, CA 92121
Determination of methadone in human urine.

Phamatech Inc. 858-643-5555
10151 Barnes Canyon Rd, San Diego, CA 92121
Lateral flow immunoassay for methadone.

QuantRx Biomedical Corp. 503-252-9565
5920 NE 112th Ave, Portland, OR 97220
ACCUSTEP DOA SINGLE AND

Rapid Diagnostics, Div. Of Mp Biomedicals, Llc 800-888-7008
1429 Rollins Rd, Burlingame, CA 94010
Rapid Methadone test.

St. Paul Biotech 714-903-1000
11555 Monarch St, Garden Grove, CA 92841
Methadone test.

Ucp Biosciences, Inc. 408-392-0064
1445 Koll Cir Ste 111, San Jose, CA 95112
Methadone test system.

ENZYME IMMUNOASSAY, N-ACETYLPROCAINAMIDE
(Toxicology) 91LAN

Bayer Healthcare, Llc 574-256-3430
430 S Beiger St, Mishawaka, IN 46544
Test for napa [n-acetylprocainamide] test kit.

Microgenics Corporation 800-232-3342
46360 Fremont Blvd, Fremont, CA 94538

ENZYME IMMUNOASSAY, NON-RADIOLABELED, TOTAL THYROXINE *(Chemistry) 75KLI*

Abbott Diagnostics Intl, Biotechnology Ltd 787-846-3500
Road #2 KM. 58.0 , PO Box 278, Cruce Davila, Barceloneta, PR 00617
Fluorescence polarization immunoassay (fpia) for the quantitavive determination.

Biocheck, Inc. 650-573-1968
323 Vintage Park Dr, Foster City, CA 94404
Total thyroxine eia test kit.

Biotecx Laboratories, Inc. 800-535-6286
15225 Gulf Hwy, #F106, Houston, TX 77034

Chemux Bioscience, Inc. 650-872-1800
50 S Linden Ave Ste 7, South San Francisco, CA 94080
Total thyroxine(t4) enzyme immunoassay kits.

Hemagen Diagnostics, Inc. 800-436-2436
9033 Red Branch Rd, Columbia, MD 21045
Various thyroxine methods.

Microgenics Corporation 800-232-3342
46360 Fremont Blvd, Fremont, CA 94538

Myers-Stevens Group, Inc. 903-566-6696
2931 Vail Ave, Commerce, CA 90040
Eia test for the quantitation of thyroxin.

Neo-Genesis, A Division Of Natus 503-657-8000
15140 SE 82nd Dr Ste 270, Clackamas, OR 97015
Total thyroxine test system.

Repromedix Corp. 781-937-8893
86 Cummings Park, Woburn, MA 01801
Reprobead t4 enyme immuno assay reagent kit.

Teco Diagnostics 714-693-7788
1268 N Lakeview Ave, Anaheim, CA 92807
T4 (total thyroxine) eia microtiter assay.

ENZYME IMMUNOASSAY, OPIATES *(Toxicology) 91DJG*

Abbott Diagnostics Div. 626-440-0700
820 Mission St, South Pasadena, CA 91030
Opiates.

Abbott Laboratories 800-223-2064
100 Abbott Park Rd, Abbott Park, IL 60064
AXSYM OPIATES

Acro Biotech Llc. 909-466-6892
9500 7th St Ste M, Rancho Cucamonga, CA 91730
Point of care rapid test.

Alfa Scientific Designs, Inc. 877-204-5071
13200 Gregg St, Poway, CA 92064
Various.

ENZYME IMMUNOASSAY, OPIATES *(cont'd)*

Amedica Biotech, Inc. 510-785-5980
28301 Industrial Blvd Ste K, Hayward, CA 94545
Drug screen oxycodone test.

Ameditech, Inc. 858-535-1968
10340 Camino Santa Fe Ste F, San Diego, CA 92121
Various.

American Bio Medica Corp. 800-227-1243
122 Smith Rd, Kinderhook, NY 12106
One step lateral flow immunoassay.

American Bio Medica Corp. 856-241-2320
603 Heron Dr Ste 3, Logan Township, NJ 08085
One step lateral flow immunoassay.

Biosite Incorporated 888-246-7483
9975 Summers Ridge Rd, San Diego, CA 92121
Fluorescence immunoassay for detection of drugs of abuse in urine.

Branan Medical Corp. 949-598-7166
140 Technology Dr Ste 400, Irvine, CA 92618
Immunochromatographical test for the qualitative derternination of morphine.

Carolina Liquid Chemistries Corp. 800-471-7272
510 W Central Ave Ste C, Brea, CA 92821
Opiate reagent.

Escreen, Inc. 800-881-0722
2205 W Parkside Ln, Phoenix, AZ 85027
Escreen drugs of abuse screening system.

Express Diagnostics Int'L, Inc. 507-526-3951
1550 Industrial Dr, Blue Earth, MN 56013
Drugs of abuse screening test.

Germaine Laboratories, Inc. 210-692-4192
4139 Gardendale St Ste 101, San Antonio, TX 78229
Various types, opiates tests.

Innovacon, Inc. 858-535-2030
4106 Sorrento Valley Blvd, San Diego, CA 92121
Opiates drug of abuse test.

Lin-Zhi International, Inc. 408-732-3856
687 N Pastoria Ave, Sunnyvale, CA 94085
Homgeneous enzyme immunoassay for the determination of opiates level in urine.

Medtox Diagnostics Inc. 800-334-1116
1238 Anthony Rd, Burlington, NC 27215
EZ-SCREEN competitive enyzme immunoassay screening test for opiates and metabolites.

Medtox Diagnostics, Inc. 800-334-1116
1640 Nova Ln, Burlington, NC 27215
Immunochromatographic assay for opiates (opi).

Myers-Stevens Group, Inc. 903-566-6696
2931 Vail Ave, Commerce, CA 90040
Eia test for the detection of opiates.

Nano-Ditech Corporation 609-409-0700
7 Clarke Dr, Cranbury, NJ 08512
Enzyme immunoassay, opiates.

Neo Pharm Inc. 714-226-0070
10532 Walker St Ste B, Cypress, CA 90630
Opiates test system.

Nubenco Ent., Inc. 800-633-1322
1 Kalisa Way Ste 207, Paramus, NJ 07652
Morphine/opiates/heroin test kit.

Pan Probe Biotech, Inc. 858-689-9936
7396 Trade St, San Diego, CA 92121
Determination of opiates (morphine) in human urine.

Phamatech Inc. 858-643-5555
10151 Barnes Canyon Rd, San Diego, CA 92121
Oxycodone rapid test; opiate rapid test.

Psychemedics Corp. 800-628-8073
125 Nagog Park Ste 200, Acton, MA 01720

Psychmedics Corp. 978-206-8220
125 Nagog Park, Acton, MA 01720
RADIOIMMUNOASSAY

Rapid Diagnostics, Div. Of Mp Biomedicals, Llc 800-888-7008
1429 Rollins Rd, Burlingame, CA 94010
Rapid opiate test

Ucp Biosciences, Inc. 408-392-0064
1445 Koll Cir Ste 111, San Jose, CA 95112
Opiates test system.

ENZYME IMMUNOASSAY, OPIATES *(cont'd)*

Varian Inc 650-424-5078
25200 Commercentre Dr, Lake Forest, CA 92630
Drug testing devices.

W.H.P.M., Inc. 978-927-3808
9662 Telstar Ave, El Monte, CA 91731
Drug of abuse screening.

ENZYME IMMUNOASSAY, OTHER *(Chemistry) 75VKK*

American Diagnostica, Inc. 888-234-4435
500 West Ave, Stamford, CT 06902
DIMERTEST monoclonal fdp latex & EIA kits for plasma; ACTIBIND t-PA + u-PA ELISA kits.

Beckman Coulter, Inc. 800-742-2345
250 S Kraemer Blvd, PO Box 8000, Brea, CA 92821

Biomedical Technologies, Inc. 781-344-9942
378 Page St, Stoughton, MA 02072
$540 per 2500-tube Involucrin ELISA kit. $380 per kit; 96-well plate. Intact Osteocalcin ELISA Kit. $310 per 96-well Human Fibronectin ELISA Kit. CYCLIC AMP EIA kit, $295/kit of 2 x 96 wells. catalog no. BT-730. CYCLIC GMP EIA KIT, $295/kit of 2 x 96 wells, catalog no. BT-740. Rat Osteocalcin EIA Kit, $350/kit of 1 x 96 wells, catalog no. BT-490. Mouse Osteocalcin EIA Kit (BT-470), $370/kit (1 x 96 wells).

Biomerica, Inc. 800-854-3002
17571 Von Karman Ave, Irvine, CA 92614
Candida IgG, IgM, IgA; Helicobacter pylori IgG, IgM, IgA; also available, #7018 ultrasensitive TSH ELISA test; GAP H. pylori IgG.

Biotecx Laboratories, Inc. 800-535-6286
15225 Gulf Hwy, #F106, Houston, TX 77034
Enzyme immunoassay for TotalThyroxine, TotalTiliodothylonine, and control. OPTICOAT T3 and OPTICOAT TSH.

Diagnostica Stago, Inc. 800-222-COAG
5 Century Dr, Parsippany, NJ 07054

Diagnostics Biochem Canada Inc. 519-681-8731
1020 Hargrieve Rd., London, ONT N6E 1P5 Canada
ELISA Human Chorionic Gonadotropin - $79.00 for 100 assay tubes. ELISA Human Growth Hormone - $79.00 for 100 assay tubes. ELISA Thyroid Stimulating Hormone - $79.00 for 100 assay tubes.

Drg International, Inc. 800-321-1167
1167 US Highway 22, Mountainside, NJ 07092
Microtiter plate-ELISA: C-Peptide, 17-OH Progesterone, thyroids and hormones. Tumor markers, infectious diseases, progesterone, estradiol and cortisol-saliva det'n., etc.

Genzyme 800-332-1042
500 Kendall St, Cambridge, MA 02142

Immco Diagnostics, Inc. 800-537-8378
60 Pineview Dr, Buffalo, NY 14228
IMMUGEL, IMMULISA anti-ENA RNP, Sm, SS-A/RO, SS-B/LA; Anti-DS DNA and anti-gliadin, RF, histone enzyme immunoassays. IMMURLOT, Western blot for ANA; IMMULISA, ELISA for TPO and Tg. ELISAs for the detection of thyroglobulin and thyroperoxidate.

Immuno-Mycologics, Inc. 800-654-3639
PO Box 1151, Norman, OK 73070
Candida enzyme immunoassay (CEIA) test system; also, YXP systemic fungal medium kit for isolation and culture of systemic fungi.

Kronus, Inc. 800-822-6999
12554 W Bridger St Ste 108, Boise, ID 83713
Autoimmune disease diagnostic kits/autoantibody detection kits. Thyroid peroxidase (TPO) Ab EIA tests and thyroglobulin Ab EIA tests for Hashimoto's disease. META-Tg, Serum Thyroglobulin EIA Test Kit; Enzyme immunoassay for the measurement of thyroglobulin in serum.

Lifesign 800-526-2125
71 Veronica Ave, Somerset, NJ 08873
STATUS STREPA $105.00 per kit of 30 tests. $293.00 per kit of 90 tests. UNISTEP MONO.

Microgenics Corporation 800-232-3342
46360 Fremont Blvd, Fremont, CA 94538
Cortisol enzyme immunoassay; non-isotopic total T3 assay; and non-isotopic vitamin B12 and folate assays. Tobramycin & ferritin.

Neometrics, A Division Of Natus 800-645-3616
150 Motor Pkwy Ste 203, Hauppauge, NY 11788
Accuwell T4, neonatal blood spot T4

ENZYME IMMUNOASSAY, OTHER *(cont'd)*

Nuclin Diagnostics, Inc. 847-498-5210
3322 Commercial Ave, Northbrook, IL 60062
Enzyme activity assays. New products include the COLORIPASE CL-700, a stat colorimetric test for determining pancreatic lipase levels in serum and plasma.

Orasure Technologies, Inc. 800-869-3538
220 E 1st St, Bethlehem, PA 18015
Serum/sweat/urine/saliva tests for detection of various therapeutic drugs and drugs of abuse; homogeneous and microplate. Q.E.D. saliva alcohol test.

Oxis International, Inc. 800-547-3686
468 N Camden Dr Fl 2, Beverly Hills, CA 90210
ACCUFLUOR FPIA analyzer for TDM.

Pierce Biotechnology 800-487-4885
30 Commerce Way, Woburn, MA 01801
Human, mouse, rat and pig cytokine ELISA kits; human and mouse chemokine ELISA kits; human and mouse cell surface marker ELISA kits; human apoptosis marker ELISA kits; and matched pairs for cytokine measurement.

Ramco Laboratories, Inc. 281-313-1200
4100 Greenbriar Dr Ste 200, Stafford, TX 77477
Ferritin enzyme immunoassay; Von Willebrand factor enzyme immunoassay; transferrin receptor enzyme immunoassay

Rockland Immunochemicals, Inc. 800-656-ROCK
PO Box 326, Gilbertsville, PA 19525
Substrate enzyme.

Salimetrics, Llc 800-790-2258
101 Innovation Blvd Ste 302, State College, PA 16803
Alpha-Amylase Kinetic Reaction Kit - Androstenedione EIA Kit -

Surmodics, Inc. 866-SURMODX
9924 W 74th St, Eden Prairie, MN 55344
STABILCOAT immunoassay stabilizer effectively protects protein components that need to be dried and stored long term. STABILZYME conjugate stabilizers extend the shelf life of horseradish peroxidose and alkaline phosphatase conjugates in solution. STABILGUARD biomolecule stabilizer is an animal-protein-free immunoassay stabilizer.

ENZYME IMMUNOASSAY, PHENCYCLIDINE *(Toxicology) 91LCM*

Abbott Diagnostics Div. 626-440-0700
820 Mission St, South Pasadena, CA 91030
Pcp.

Acro Biotech Llc. 909-466-6892
9500 7th St Ste M, Rancho Cucamonga, CA 91730
Point of care rapid test.

Amedica Biotech, Inc. 510-785-5980
28301 Industrial Blvd Ste K, Hayward, CA 94545
Drug screen pcp test.

Ameditech, Inc. 858-535-1968
10340 Camino Santa Fe Ste F, San Diego, CA 92121
Various.

American Bio Medica Corp. 800-227-1243
122 Smith Rd, Kinderhook, NY 12106
One step lateral flow immunoassay.

American Bio Medica Corp. 856-241-2320
603 Heron Dr Ste 3, Logan Township, NJ 08085
One step lateral flow immunoassay.

Biosite Incorporated 888-246-7483
9975 Summers Ridge Rd, San Diego, CA 92121
Fluorescence immunoassay for detection of drugs of abuse in urine.

Branan Medical Corp. 949-598-7166
140 Technology Dr Ste 400, Irvine, CA 92618
Immunochromatographical test for qualitative determination of pcp in humam urine.

Carolina Liquid Chemistries Corp. 800-471-7272
510 W Central Ave Ste C, Brea, CA 92821
Phencyclidine reagent.

Dade Behring, Inc. • 800-948-3233
1717 Deerfield Rd, Deerfield, IL 60015

Escreen, Inc. 800-881-0722
2205 W Parkside Ln, Phoenix, AZ 85027
Escreen drugs of abuse screening system.

Express Diagnostics Int'L, Inc. 507-526-3951
1550 Industrial Dr, Blue Earth, MN 56013
Drugs of abuse screening test.

ENZYME IMMUNOASSAY, PHENCYCLIDINE *(cont'd)*

Germaine Laboratories, Inc. 210-692-4192
4139 Gardendale St Ste 101, San Antonio, TX 78229
Various types, phencyclidine tests.

Innovacon, Inc. 858-535-2030
4106 Sorrento Valley Blvd, San Diego, CA 92121
Pcp drug of abuse test.

Jant Pharmacal Corp. 800-676-5565
16255 Ventura Blvd Ste 505, Encino, CA 91436
Test to detect phencyclidine in human urine.

Lin-Zhi International, Inc. 408-732-3856
687 N Pastoria Ave, Sunnyvale, CA 94085
Homogeneous enzyme immunoassay for the determination of phencyclidin in urine.

Lusys Laboratories Inc. 858-546-0902
10054 Mesa Ridge Ct Ste 118, San Diego, CA 92121
Enzyme immunoassay for amp, bzd, coc, opi, thc.

Medtox Diagnostics Inc. 800-334-1116
1238 Anthony Rd, Burlington, NC 27215
EZ-SCREEN competitive enzyme immunoassay screening test for PCP and PCP metabolites.

Medtox Diagnostics, Inc. 800-334-1116
1640 Nova Ln, Burlington, NC 27215
Immunochromatographic assay for phencyclidine (pcp).

Microgenics Corporation 800-232-3342
46360 Fremont Blvd, Fremont, CA 94538

Nano-Ditech Corporation 609-409-0700
7 Clarke Dr, Cranbury, NJ 08512
Enzyme immunoassay, phencyclidine.

Pan Probe Biotech, Inc. 858-689-9936
7396 Trade St, San Diego, CA 92121
Determination of phencyclidine in human urine.

Phamatech Inc. 858-643-5555
10151 Barnes Canyon Rd, San Diego, CA 92121
Pcp rapid test.

QuantRx Biomedical Corp. 503-252-9565
5920 NE 112th Ave, Portland, OR 97220
ACCUSTEP DOA SINGLE AND

Rapid Diagnostics, Div. Of Mp Biomedicals, Llc 800-888-7008
1429 Rollins Rd, Burlingame, CA 94010
Rapid PCP test

Ucp Biosciences, Inc. 408-392-0064
1445 Koll Cir Ste 111, San Jose, CA 95112
Phecyclidine test system.

Varian Inc 650-424-5078
25200 Commercentre Dr, Lake Forest, CA 92630
Drug testing devices.

W.H.P.M., Inc. 978-927-3808
9662 Telstar Ave, El Monte, CA 91731
Drug of abuse screening.

ENZYME IMMUNOASSAY, PHENOBARBITAL *(Toxicology) 91DLZ*

Abbott Diagnostics Div. 626-440-0700
820 Mission St, South Pasadena, CA 91030
Assay for the detection of phenobarbital.

Microgenics Corporation 800-232-3342
46360 Fremont Blvd, Fremont, CA 94538

ENZYME IMMUNOASSAY, PRIMIDONE *(Toxicology) 91DJD*

Abbott Laboratories 800-223-2064
100 Abbott Park Rd, Abbott Park, IL 60064
TDX PRIMIDONE

Bayer Healthcare, Llc 574-256-3430
430 S Beiger St, Mishawaka, IN 46544
Test for primidone in serum or plasma.

ENZYME IMMUNOASSAY, PROCAINAMIDE *(Toxicology) 91LAR*

Bayer Healthcare, Llc 574-256-3430
430 S Beiger St, Mishawaka, IN 46544
Test for procainamide in serum or plasma.

ENZYME IMMUNOASSAY, PROPOXYPHENE *(Toxicology) 91JXN*

Abbott Diagnostics Div. 626-440-0700
820 Mission St, South Pasadena, CA 91030
Propoxyphene.

Amedica Biotech, Inc. 510-785-5980
28301 Industrial Blvd Ste K, Hayward, CA 94545
Drug test propoxyphene test.

ENZYME IMMUNOASSAY, PROPOXYPHENE *(cont'd)*

American Bio Medica Corp. 856-241-2320
603 Heron Dr Ste 3, Logan Township, NJ 08085
Propoxyphene test system.

Biosite Incorporated 888-246-7483
9975 Summers Ridge Rd, San Diego, CA 92121
Visual immunoassay for detection of drugs of abuse in urine.

Carolina Liquid Chemistries Corp. 800-471-7272
510 W Central Ave Ste C, Brea, CA 92821
Propoxyphene reagent.

Express Diagnostics Int'L, Inc. 507-526-3951
1550 Industrial Dr, Blue Earth, MN 56013
Drugs of abuse screening test.

Germaine Laboratories, Inc. 210-692-4192
4139 Gardendale St Ste 101, San Antonio, TX 78229
Propoxyphene.

Innovacon, Inc. 858-535-2030
4106 Sorrento Valley Blvd, San Diego, CA 92121
Propoxyphene drug of abuse test.

Lin-Zhi International, Inc. 408-732-3856
687 N Pastoria Ave, Sunnyvale, CA 94085
Homogeneous enzyme immunoassay for the determination of propoxyphene in urine.

Medtox Diagnostics, Inc. 800-334-1116
1640 Nova Ln, Burlington, NC 27215
Immunochromatographic assay for propoxyphene and norpropoxyphene (pbx).

Rapid Diagnostics, Div. Of Mp Biomedicals, Llc 800-888-7008
1429 Rollins Rd, Burlingame, CA 94010
Rapid Propoxyphene test.

Ucp Biosciences, Inc. 408-392-0064
1445 Koll Cir Ste 111, San Jose, CA 95112
Propoxyphene test system.

ENZYME IMMUNOASSAY, QUINIDINE *(Toxicology) 91LBZ*

Opus Diagnostics, Inc. 877-944-1777
1 Parker Plz, Fort Lee, NJ 07024
Innofluor quinidine reagent set.

Oxis International, Inc. 800-547-3686
468 N Camden Dr Fl 2, Beverly Hills, CA 90210
Fluorescence polarization immunoassay, 100 test kit.

ENZYME IMMUNOASSAY, THEOPHYLLINE *(Toxicology) 91KLS*

Abbott Diagnostics Div. 626-440-0700
820 Mission St, South Pasadena, CA 91030
Theophylline.

Accuech, Llc 760-599-6555
2641 La Mirada Dr, Vista, CA 92081
Theophylline test.

Microgenics Corporation 800-232-3342
46360 Fremont Blvd, Fremont, CA 94538

ENZYME IMMUNOASSAY, VALPROIC ACID *(Toxicology) 91LEG*

Bayer Healthcare, Llc 574-256-3430
430 S Beiger St, Mishawaka, IN 46544
Test for valproic acid in serum or plasma.

Microgenics Corporation 800-232-3342
46360 Fremont Blvd, Fremont, CA 94538

Opus Diagnostics, Inc. 877-944-1777
1 Parker Plz, Fort Lee, NJ 07024
Innofluor valporic acid reagent set.

Oxis International, Inc. 800-547-3686
468 N Camden Dr Fl 2, Beverly Hills, CA 90210
Fluorescence polarization immunoassay, 100 test kit.

ENZYME LINKED IMMUNOABSORBENT ASSAY, CHLAMYDIA GROUP *(Microbiology) 83LJC*

Diagnostic Automation/ Cortez Diagnostics Inc,. 818-591-3030
23961 Craftsman Rd Ste D/E/F, Calabasas, CA 91302
Enzyme linked immunoabsorbent assay (chlamydiae group).

Meridian Bioscience, Inc. 800-696-0739
3471 River Hills Dr, Cincinnati, OH 45244
Enzyme immunoassay for the detection of Chlamydia in specimens and cell culture.

Princeton Biomeditech Corp. 732-274-1000
4242 US Highway 1, Monmouth Junction, NJ 08852
BioSign Chlamydia trachomatis direct antigen detection test.

ENZYME LINKED IMMUNOABSORBENT ASSAY, CHLAMYDIA GROUP *(cont'd)*

St. Paul Biotech 714-903-1000
11555 Monarch St, Garden Grove, CA 92841
Chlamydia test.

Wampole Laboratories 800-257-9525
2 Research Way, Princeton, NJ 08540

ENZYME LINKED IMMUNOABSORBENT ASSAY, COCCIDIOIDES IMMITIS *(Microbiology) 83MIY*

Focus Diagnostics, Inc. 714-220-1900
10703 Progress Way, Cypress, CA 90630
Coccidioides immitis serological reagents.

Meridian Bioscience, Inc. 800-696-0739
3471 River Hills Dr, Cincinnati, OH 45244
Enzyme immunoassay for detection of antibodies to Coccidioides immitis in serum.

United Biotech, Inc. 650-961-2910
211 S Whisman Rd Ste E, Mountain View, CA 94041
ELISA for detecting: Herpes I IgG, Herpes I IgM, Herpes II IgG, Herpes II IgM

ENZYME LINKED IMMUNOABSORBENT ASSAY, CYTOMEGALOVIRUS *(Microbiology) 83LFZ*

Akers Biosciences, Inc. 800-451-8378
201 Grove Rd, West Deptford, NJ 08086
HEALTHTEST for CMV.

Bd Diagnostic Systems 800-675-0908
7 Loveton Cir, Sparks, MD 21152

Biocheck, Inc. 650-573-1968
323 Vintage Park Dr, Foster City, CA 94404
Cytomegalovirus igg eia test kit.

Diamedix Corp. 800-327-4565
2140 N Miami Ave, Miami, FL 33127
Is-CMV IgG catalog #720-320 and Is-CMV IgM Capture catalog #720-330.

Quest Intl., Inc. 305-592-6991
8127 NW 29th St, Doral, FL 33122
Anti-cmv igg serological reagents, elisa.

United Biotech, Inc. 650-961-2910
211 S Whisman Rd Ste E, Mountain View, CA 94041
ELISA for detecting CMV IgG.

Zeus Scientific, Inc. 800-286-2111
PO Box 38, Raritan, NJ 08869
96 IgG tests or IgM tests.

ENZYME LINKED IMMUNOABSORBENT ASSAY, HERPES SIMPLEX VIRUS *(Microbiology) 83LGC*

Biocheck, Inc. 650-573-1968
323 Vintage Park Dr, Foster City, CA 94404
Herpes simplex virus-1 igm eia test kit.

Diamedix Corp. 800-327-4565
2140 N Miami Ave, Miami, FL 33127
Is-HSV 1 and 2 IgG catalog #720-340 and Is-HSV 1 and 2 IgM catalog #720-350.

Focus Diagnostics, Inc. 714-220-1900
10703 Progress Way, Cypress, CA 90630
Various.

Meridian Bioscience, Inc. 800-696-0739
3471 River Hills Dr, Cincinnati, OH 45244
Enzyme immunoassay for detection of HSV in direct specimens and culture.

Quest Intl., Inc. 305-592-6991
8127 NW 29th St, Doral, FL 33122
Herpes simplex virus (hsv) serological reagents.

Wampole Laboratories 800-257-9525
2 Research Way, Princeton, NJ 08540

Zeus Scientific, Inc. 800-286-2111
PO Box 38, Raritan, NJ 08869
96 IgG or IgM determinations for HSV-1 or HSV-2.

ENZYME LINKED IMMUNOABSORBENT ASSAY, HISTOPLASMA CAPSULATUM *(Microbiology) 83MIZ*

Focus Diagnostics, Inc. 714-220-1900
10703 Progress Way, Cypress, CA 90630
Histoplasma capsulatum serological reagents.

ENZYME LINKED IMMUNOABSORBENT ASSAY, MUMPS VIRUS
(Microbiology) 83LJY

Calbiotech, Inc. 619-660-6162
10461 Austin Dr Ste G, Spring Valley, CA 91978
Mumps igg elisa.

Diamedix Corp. 800-327-4565
2140 N Miami Ave, Miami, FL 33127
Is-Mumps IgG Catalog# 720-540

Quest Intl., Inc. 305-592-6991
8127 NW 29th St, Doral, FL 33122
Anti-mumps virus, serological reagents, elisa.

Wampole Laboratories 800-257-9525
2 Research Way, Princeton, NJ 08540

Zeus Scientific, Inc. 800-286-2111
PO Box 38, Raritan, NJ 08869
Mumps 96 tests ELISA IgG only.

ENZYME LINKED IMMUNOABSORBENT ASSAY, MYCOPLASMA SPP. *(Microbiology) 83LJZ*

Calbiotech, Inc. 619-660-6162
10461 Austin Dr Ste G, Spring Valley, CA 91978
Mycoplasma pneumonia igg elisa.

Innominata dba GENBIO 800-288-4368
15222 Avenue of Science Ste A, San Diego, CA 92128
Various.

Meridian Bioscience, Inc. 800-696-0739
3471 River Hills Dr, Cincinnati, OH 45244
Enzyme immunoassay for the detection of IgM antibodies to Mycoplasma pneumoniae in serum.

Wampole Laboratories 800-257-9525
2 Research Way, Princeton, NJ 08540

Zeus Scientific, Inc. 800-286-2111
PO Box 38, Raritan, NJ 08869
Mycoplasma 96 tests ELISA IgG only. Mycoplasma 96 tests ELISA IgM only.

ENZYME LINKED IMMUNOABSORBENT ASSAY, NEISSERIA GONORRHOEAE *(Microbiology) 83LIR*

St. Paul Biotech 714-903-1000
11555 Monarch St, Garden Grove, CA 92841
Gonorrhea test.

ENZYME LINKED IMMUNOABSORBENT ASSAY, RESP. SYNCYTIAL VIRUS *(Microbiology) 83MCE*

Chembio Diagnostic Systems, Inc. 631-924-1135
3661 Horseblock Rd, Medford, NY 11763
Rapid immunochromatographic test for detection of rsv in human respiratory sampl.

Meridian Bioscience, Inc. 800-696-0739
3471 River Hills Dr, Cincinnati, OH 45244
Enzyme immunoassay for detection of RSV in nasopharangeal specimens.

ENZYME LINKED IMMUNOABSORBENT ASSAY, ROTAVIRUS
(Microbiology) 83LIQ

Biomol Research Labs 800-942-0430
5120 Butler Pike, Plymouth Meeting, PA 19462

Chembio Diagnostic Systems, Inc. 631-924-1135
3661 Horseblock Rd, Medford, NY 11763
Immunochromatographic assay for visual detection of rotavirus antigen.

Ivd Research, Inc. 760-929-7744
5909 Sea Lion Pl Ste D, Carlsbad, CA 92010
Rotavirus stool antigen elisa.

Meridian Bioscience, Inc. 800-696-0739
3471 River Hills Dr, Cincinnati, OH 45244
Enzyme immunoassay for the detection of Rotavirus in stool.

ENZYME LINKED IMMUNOABSORBENT ASSAY, RUBELLA
(Microbiology) 83LFX

American Laboratory Products Co. 800-592-5726
26 Keewaydin Dr Ste G, Salem, NH 03079

Ameritek Usa, Inc. 425-379-2580
125 130th St SE Ste 200, Everett, WA 98208
Rubella test kit.

Biocheck, Inc. 650-573-1968
323 Vintage Park Dr, Foster City, CA 94404
Rubella igg eia test kit.

ENZYME LINKED IMMUNOABSORBENT ASSAY, RUBELLA
(cont'd)

Diamedix Corp. 800-327-4565
2140 N Miami Ave, Miami, FL 33127
Is-Rubella IgG catalog #720-360 and Is-Rubella IgM capture catalog #720-370.

Innominata dba GENBIO 800-288-4368
15222 Avenue of Science Ste A, San Diego, CA 92128
Enzyme linked dot blot immunoassay, for antibody to rubella virus.

Quest Intl., Inc. 305-592-6991
8127 NW 29th St, Doral, FL 33122
Rubella igm serological reagents, elisa.

Virotech International, Inc. 301-924-8000
12 Meem Ave Ste C, Gaithersburg, MD 20877
Rubella.

Wampole Laboratories 800-257-9525
2 Research Way, Princeton, NJ 08540

Zeus Scientific, Inc. 800-286-2111
PO Box 38, Raritan, NJ 08869
96 IgG tests and IgM tests.

ENZYME LINKED IMMUNOABSORBENT ASSAY, RUBEOLA
(Microbiology) 83LJB

Calbiotech, Inc. 619-660-6162
10461 Austin Dr Ste G, Spring Valley, CA 91978
Measles (rubcola) igg elisa.

Diamedix Corp. 800-327-4565
2140 N Miami Ave, Miami, FL 33127
Is-Measles (Rubeola)-IgG, catalog #720-520.

Quest Intl., Inc. 305-592-6991
8127 NW 29th St, Doral, FL 33122
Anti-rubella serological reagents ,elisa.

Wampole Laboratories 800-257-9525
2 Research Way, Princeton, NJ 08540

Zeus Scientific, Inc. 800-286-2111
PO Box 38, Raritan, NJ 08869
Measles/Rubeola 96 tests ELISA IgG only.

ENZYME LINKED IMMUNOABSORBENT ASSAY, T. CRUZI
(Microbiology) 83MIU

Chembio Diagnostic Systems, Inc. 631-924-1135
3661 Horseblock Rd, Medford, NY 11763
Immunochromatographic assay for visual detection of antibodies to t.cruzi.

ENZYME LINKED IMMUNOABSORBENT ASSAY, TOXOPLASMA GONDII *(Microbiology) 83LGD*

Biocheck, Inc. 650-573-1968
323 Vintage Park Dr, Foster City, CA 94404
Toxoplasma igm eia test kit.

Diamedix Corp. 800-327-4565
2140 N Miami Ave, Miami, FL 33127
Is-ToxoG catalog #720-300 and Is-ToxoM capture catalog #720-310.

Quest Intl., Inc. 305-592-6991
8127 NW 29th St, Doral, FL 33122
Toxoplasma igg serological reagents.

United Biotech, Inc. 650-961-2910
211 S Whisman Rd Ste E, Mountain View, CA 94041
ELISA detecting: Toxo IgG, Toxo IgM

Virotech International, Inc. 301-924-8000
12 Meem Ave Ste C, Gaithersburg, MD 20877
Toxo.

Zeus Scientific, Inc. 800-286-2111
PO Box 38, Raritan, NJ 08869
IgG tests and IgM tests.

ENZYME LINKED IMMUNOABSORBENT ASSAY, TREPONEMA PALLIDUM *(Microbiology) 83LIP*

Bio-Rad Laboratories, Inc. 425-881-8300
14620 NE North Woodinville Way, Way, Suite 200
Woodinville, WA 98072
Multi-analyte detection system syphilis igg.

Diamedix Corp. 800-327-4565
2140 N Miami Ave, Miami, FL 33127
TREP-CHEK™ anti-Treponemal EIA kit Catalog# 720-100

Immunoscience, Inc. 925-460-8111
7066 Commerce Cir Ste D, Pleasanton, CA 94588
Various.

ENZYME LINKED IMMUNOABSORBENT ASSAY, TREPONEMA PALLIDUM *(cont'd)*

Innominata dba GENBIO 800-288-4368
15222 Avenue of Science Ste A, San Diego, CA 92128
Enzyme - linked immunoassay - for borrelia antibodies.

Quest Intl., Inc. 305-592-6991
8127 NW 29th St, Doral, FL 33122
Syphilis igg antibody.

Wampole Laboratories 800-257-9525
2 Research Way, Princeton, NJ 08540

ENZYME LINKED IMMUNOABSORBENT ASSAY, TRICHINELLA SPIRALIS *(Microbiology) 83MDT*

Ivd Research, Inc. 760-929-7744
5909 Sea Lion Pl Ste D, Carlsbad, CA 92010
Trichinella serum elisa.

ENZYME LINKED IMMUNOABSORBENT ASSAY, VARICELLA-ZOSTER *(Microbiology) 83LFY*

Diamedix Corp. 800-327-4565
2140 N Miami Ave, Miami, FL 33127
Is-VZV-IgG, catalog #720-380.

Quest Intl., Inc. 305-592-6991
8127 NW 29th St, Doral, FL 33122
Anti-vzv igg serological reagents, elisa.

Zeus Scientific, Inc. 800-286-2111
PO Box 38, Raritan, NJ 08869
Varicella zoster 96 tests ELISA IgG only.

ENZYME, CELL (ERYTHROCYTIC AND LEUKOCYTIC) *(Hematology) 81JBE*

Biomol Research Labs 800-942-0430
5120 Butler Pike, Plymouth Meeting, PA 19462

Promega Corp. 800-356-9526
2800 Woods Hollow Rd, Fitchburg, WI 53711

ENZYME-LINKED IMMUNOSORBENT ASSAY, HERPES SIMPLEX VIRUS, HSV-1 *(Microbiology) 83MXJ*

Virotech International, Inc. 301-924-8000
12 Meem Ave Ste C, Gaithersburg, MD 20877
Hsv-1.

ENZYME-LINKED IMMUNOSORBENT ASSAY, HERPES SIMPLEX VIRUS, HSV-2 *(Microbiology) 83MYF*

United Biotech, Inc. 650-961-2910
211 S Whisman Rd Ste E, Mountain View, CA 94041
ELISA for detecting: Herpes I IgG, Herpes I IgM, Herpes II, IgG, Herpes II IgM

Virotech International, Inc. 301-924-8000
12 Meem Ave Ste C, Gaithersburg, MD 20877
Hsv-2.

EPILATOR, HIGH-FREQUENCY, NEEDLE-TYPE *(Surgery) 79KCW*

Clareblend, Inc. 800-334-7126
3555 Airway Dr Ste 307, Reno, NV 89511
Various types of needles epilgtors.

Cti Medical Equipment, Inc. 856-424-0503
1910 Marlton Pike E Ste 10, Cherry Hill, NJ 08003
Medi-blend.

Elmed, Inc. 630-543-2792
60 W Fay Ave, Addison, IL 60101

Gentronics 800-950-3265
8721 Santa Monica Blvd # 210, Los Angeles, CA 90069
Electrolysis epilator, hair removal.

Instantron 401-433-6800
3712 Pawtucket Ave, Riverside, RI 02915
Hair removal.

L.P. Systems Corp. 718-805-6926
11608 Myrtle Ave Ste 330, Richmond Hill, NY 11418
Epilator, high frequency, needle-type.

Michael D. Warren Services Ltd. 905-455-1915
211-338 Queen St E, Brampton L6V 1C4 Canada
Sofblend t-80

Precision Electrolysis Needles, Inc. 401-246-1155
166 Bay Spring Ave, Barrington, RI 02806
Epilator high frequency.

R. A. Fischer Co. 800-525-3467
8751 White Oak Ave, Northridge, CA 91325
Shortwave epilator.

EPILATOR, HIGH-FREQUENCY, NEEDLE-TYPE *(cont'd)*

R.A. Fischer Company 800-525-3467
8751 White Oak Ave, Northridge, CA 91325
$1249 for standard unit.

Skin Deep, Inc. 215-728-1035
1926 Cottman Ave, Philadelphia, PA 19111
Multiple needle galvanic epilator.

EPILATOR, HIGH-FREQUENCY, TWEEZER TYPE *(Surgery) 79KCX*

American Hair Removal System, Inc. 800-446-2477
42320 County Road 653, Paw Paw, MI 49079
Tweezer electrolysis-galvanic epilator.

Burke Medical, Llc 727-532-8333
2310 Tall Pines Dr Ste 210, Largo, FL 33771
Carol's secret.

Camda Corp. 213-381-0888
3435 Wilshire Blvd Ste 990, Los Angeles, CA 90010
Epilator, high frequency, tweezer type.

Divine Skin Solutions, Inc. 888-404-7777
11951 Metropolitan Ave, Suite G4, Kew Gardens, NY 11415
Tweezer type electroysis device.

EPSTEIN-BARR VIRUS, DNA REAGENTS *(Microbiology) 83LSF*

Prodesse, Inc. 888-589-6974
W229N1870 Westwood Dr, Waukesha, WI 53186
Herpes Mplex™ - Multiplex PCR Reagents for simultaneous detection of HSV-1, HSV-2, CMV, EBV, VZV and HHV-6 - Research Use Only

EPSTEIN-BARR VIRUS, OTHER *(Microbiology) 83LSE*

Bio-Rad Laboratories, Inc. 425-881-8300
14620 NE North Woodinville Way, Way, Suite 200
Woodinville, WA 98072
Various multi-analyte detection system ebv kits.

Diasorin Inc 800-328-1482
1951 Northwestern Ave S, PO Box 285, Stillwater, MN 55082

Fuller Laboratories 714-525-7660
1135 E Truslow Ave, Fullerton, CA 92831
Ebv vca and ebv ea.

Innominata dba GENBIO 800-288-4368
15222 Avenue of Science Ste A, San Diego, CA 92128
Various.

Quest Intl., Inc. 305-592-6991
8127 NW 29th St, Doral, FL 33122
Anti-eb vca igg serological reagents, elisa.

Zeus Scientific, Inc. 800-286-2111
PO Box 38, Raritan, NJ 08869
EBV-VCA 96 tests ELISA IgM only.

EQUIPMENT, ANALYSIS, PHOTOCHEMICAL *(Chemistry) 75UHG*

Aura Industries, Inc. 800-551-2872
545 8th Ave Rm 5W, New York, NY 10018
PHRED Reactors.

EQUIPMENT, APHERESIS *(Hematology) 81VJC*

Biomerieux Inc. 800-682-2666
100 Rodolphe St, Durham, NC 27712

Caridianbct Inc. 800-525-2623
10810 W Collins Ave, Lakewood, CO 80215
COBE Spectra Apheresis System.

Fenwal Inc. 800-766-1077
3 Corporate Dr, Lake Zurich, IL 60047
AUTOPHERESIS-C System. Plasmapheresis instrument console and support stand for the collection of source plasma and plasma by membrane filtration.

Kaneka Pharma America Llc 800-526-3522
546 5th Ave Fl 21, New York, NY 10036
LIPOSORBER LA-15 System utilizes two columns containing dextran sulfate cellulose as an adsorbent which removes selectively apolipoprotein-B containing particles (LDL, VLDL, Lp(a)) from plasma.

Medtronic Perfusion Systems 800-328-3320
7611 Northland Dr N, Brooklyn Park, MN 55428
Apheresis kits for competitive machines.

EQUIPMENT, BANK, BLOOD, CRYOGENIC (LIQUID NITROGEN)
(Hematology) 81QNO

Bio Plas, Inc. 415-472-3777
4340 Redwood Hwy Ste A15, San Rafael, CA 94903
Cryogenic tubes.

Biohit Inc. 800-922-0784
PO Box 308, 3535 Rte. 66, Bldg. 4, Neptune, NJ 07754

Cryofab, Inc. 800-426-2186
540 N Michigan Ave, Kenilworth, NJ 07033

Ts Scientific 800-258-2796
PO Box 198, Perkasie, PA 18944
$8,000 for standard unit.

EQUIPMENT, BUILDING SECURITY *(General) 80WRQ*

American Medical Alert Corp. 800-286-2622
3265 Lawson Blvd, Oceanside, NY 11572
SILENT PARTNER 2000, personal and environmental interactive security-monitoring system for retail and 24-hour facilities.

Atd-American Co. 800-523-2300
135 Greenwood Ave, Wyncote, PA 19095
Safety and protective security items such as metal detectors, security mirrors, etc.

Dictator U.S., Inc. 877-366-7439
3939 Royal Dr NW Ste 214, Kennesaw, GA 30144
DICTATOR smoke detectors, electric magnets, door closers, door hardware, gas springs, and hydraulic dampers. Also available, DICTAMAT, electric door operators for sliding doors and hingedoors.

Knox Company 800-552-5669
1601 W Deer Valley Rd, Phoenix, AZ 85027
SENTRALOK key capture system holds master key to KNOX-BOX, securely and safely. Heavy duty padlocks, key switches.

Minatronics Corp. 412-488-6435
1 Trimont Ln Apt 850C, Pittsburgh, PA 15211
Fiber Optic Zones of protection can be added to 'Card Access' or 'HVAC' systems

Secure Care Products, Inc. 800-451-7917
39 Chenell Dr, Concord, NH 03301
To provide security for exits and meets safety code 101.

EQUIPMENT, CLEANING, AIR *(General) 80FRF*

Abatement Technologies, Inc. 800-634-9091
605 Satellite Blvd NW Ste 300, Suwanee, GA 30024
HEPA-CARE Air Purification Systems

Air Quality Engineering, Inc. 800-328-0787
7140 Northland Dr N, Minneapolis, MN 55428
Air cleaners available for various room sizes and applications. PM 400 Air Cleaner. Portable HEPA air cleaner with activated carbon. XJ 1000 HEPA filter unit for negative pressure isolation rooms.

Austin Air Systems Limited 716-856-3700
500 Elk St, Buffalo, NY 14210
Healthmate air purifier.

Battle Creek Equipment Co. 800-253-0854
307 Jackson St W, Battle Creek, MI 49037
Air purification system, certified to remove airborne smoke, dust and pollen. $77.00 to $294.00.

Bio-Rad Laboratories, Inc. 425-881-8300
6565 185th Ave NE, Redmond, WA 98052
No common name listed.

Biological Controls Inc. 800-224-9768
749 Hope Rd Ste A, Tinton Falls, NJ 07724
Various types of air purification devices.

Caframo Ltd. 800-567-3556
RR#2 Airport Rd., Wiarton, ONT N0H 2T0 Canada
Fans & heaters.

Clean Air Engineering 800-627-0033
500 W Wood St, Palatine, IL 60067

Clean Air Technology, Inc. 800 459 6320
41105 Capital Dr, Canton, MI 48187
Recirculating air handlers for HEPA filter cleanroom systems.

Controlled Environment Equipment Corp. 800-569-5444
59 Sanford Dr Ste 32, Gorham, ME 04038
Cleanline Sticky Roller- Poly or Foam

Hmi Industries, Inc. 440-846-7873
13325 Darice Pkwy Unit A, Strongsville, OH 44149
Defender.

EQUIPMENT, CLEANING, AIR *(cont'd)*

Masterquest International 315-298-2904
801 Hammond St Ste 200, Coppell, TX 75019
Air cleaner.

Medair, Inc. 800-325-7780
PO Box 635, East Bridgewater, MA 02333
Air-filtration equipment for isolation-room applications. Wall, ceiling, in-line, and portable systems available.

Micro Air Air Cleaners By Metal-Fab 800-835-2830
PO Box 1138, Wichita, KS 67201

Novosci Corp. 281-363-4949
2828 N Crescentridge Dr, The Woodlands, TX 77381
SURGIFRESH and PLUME-INATOR multi-stage and mini air-enhancement systems for laser surgery and electrosurgery.

Patient Instrumentation Corp. 610-799-4436
4117 Route 309, Schnecksville, PA 18078
Cleaning of contaminated medical air and other gas systems.

Premier Medical Products 888-PREMUSA
1710 Romano Dr, Plymouth Meeting, PA 19462
Evacuator/air filtration system and dust extractor for use in any surgical setting whether for laser or electrosurgical procedures.

R&Da Co. 508-747-5803
37 Dwight Ave, Plymouth, MA 02360
ElectroStatic air cleaners, antipollution and anti-odors and anti-airborne-agents.

Sterling Fluid Systems (Usa) 716-773-6450
303 Industrial Dr, Grand Island, NY 14072
Air compressor. Oilless engineered systems for medical breathing air.

Tapcon, Inc. 800-247-3587
521 Sheperd Street, Garland, TX 75042
Several models - from 250 CFM to 20,000 CFM.

United Air Specialists, Inc. 800-252-4647
4440 Creek Rd, Cincinnati, OH 45242

EQUIPMENT, CONTROL, POLLUTION *(General) 80WLA*

Advanced Air Technologies, Inc. 800-295-6583
300 Sleeseman Dr, Corunna, MI 48817

Air Quality Engineering, Inc. 800-328-0787
7140 Northland Dr N, Minneapolis, MN 55428
Air cleaning equipment available for removal of particulate and gaseous contaminants.

Andersen Products, Inc., 800-523-1276
3202 Caroline Dr, Health Science Park, Haw River, NC 27258
Disposer for use with ANDERSEN ethylene-oxide-gas sterilization systems.

Anguil Environmental Systems, Inc. 800-488-0230
8855 N 55th St, Milwaukee, WI 53223
Design and construction of cost-effective air pollution control systems in standard and custom sizes of 100-200,000 SCFM. Complete environmental systems meet regulatory requirements worldwide.

Ars Enterprises 800-735-9277
12900 Lakeland Rd, Santa Fe Springs, CA 90670
EO emission control device.

Bemco, Inc. 805-583-4970
2255 Union Pl, Simi Valley, CA 93065
Environmental testing equipment.

Bvs, Inc. 877-877-4821
949 Poplar Road, Honey Brook, PA 19344-0250
Automatic samplers for water pollution surveillance and control. Non-vacuum for accuracy. All BVS automatic samplers utilize the flooded-suction concept of operation as recommended by the ASTM.

Contamination Control Products 877-553-2676
1 3rd Ave # 578, Neptune, NJ 07753
HEPA filter modules.

Imtek Environmental Corp. 770-667-8621
PO Box 2066, Alpharetta, GA 30023

Misonix, Inc. 800-694-9612
1938 New Hwy, Farmingdale, NY 11735
Air pollution control equipment, scrubbers.

Nucon International, Inc. 800-992-5192
7000 Huntley Rd, Columbus, OH 43229
BRAYCYCLE and BRAYSORB, solvent vapor recovery systems based on the Brayton Cycle technology. They provide clean solvents with no secondary waste created, allowing for direct reuse.

EQUIPMENT, CONTROL, POLLUTION *(cont'd)*

R&Da Co. 508-747-5803
37 Dwight Ave, Plymouth, MA 02360
ElectroStatic anti-pollution precipitators, anti-odors, anti-airborne-agents.

San-I-Pak,Pacific Inc. 800-875-7264
23535 S Bird Rd, Tracy, CA 95304
INFECTIOUS WASTE BUCKETS, are plastic buckets used for storage of dirty, soiled lab glasses and infectious waste.

Veco, S.A. De C.V. 55-688-3566
Pirineos No. 263, Col. General Anaya, Mexico D.F., BENIT 03100 Mexico

EQUIPMENT, CRYOTHERAPY *(Physical Med) 89WOK*

Corflex, Inc. 800-426-7353
669 E Industrial Park Dr, Manchester, NH 03109
CRYOTHERM cold/hot compression wraps anatomically designed for the entire body.

Origen Biomedical, Inc. 512-474-7278
4020 S Industrial Dr Ste 160, Austin, TX 78744
Cryopreservation Solutions

Zimmer Medizinsystems 800-327-3576
25 Mauchly Ste 300, Irvine, CA 92618
CRYO 5 ice wind cryotherapy unit. Ice wind therapy is the latest innovation in cryotherapy. For pain relief and inflammation reduction for 1-3 hours following a 30 sec. to 3 min. treatment.

EQUIPMENT, DEVICE COATING, PROTECTIVE *(General) 80SHH*

Equipment Technology Conveyance 408-496-0686
2320 Walsh Ave Ste D, Santa Clara, CA 95051
Inspection: microscopes.

Implant Sciences Corp. 781-246-0700
107 Audubon Rd Ste 5, Wakefield, MA 01880
Ion implantation and coating services for the biomedical and dental industries, including surface modification by ion implantation, radiopaque coatings, antimicrobial coatings and graded-interface ceramic coatings.

Newport Glass Works, Ltd. 714-484-8100
PO Box 127, Stanton, CA 90680
Laser protective wear.

Pharmaceutical Innovations, Inc. 973-242-2900
897 Frelinghuysen Ave, Newark, NJ 07114
Ultra/Phonic Scanning Pads are for ultrasound scanning of Neonates. Ultra/Phonic Fontanelle Scanning Pads help protect the baby's delicate skin and skull, as removing normal ultrasound gel may damage the skin when removing. They are easy, convenient and fast to use. After examination, lift off baby's head and throw away. There is no clean up.

Spire Corp. 800-510-4815
1 Patriots Park, Bedford, MA 01730

Surmodics, Inc. 866-SURMODX
9924 W 74th St, Eden Prairie, MN 55344

Vergason Technology, Inc. 607-589-4429
166 State Route 224, Van Etten, NY 14889
A world leader in rapid cycle metalizing equipment. Since 1989, VTI's products have led the way for the synchronous manufacture of molded and metalized parts with quality yields never before possible. To achieve the best total solution, VTI can tailor the coatings and processes using a variety of metals, in-chamber base and top coatings, and thermal, sputtering or cathodic arc coating techniques. Medical, decorative, aerospace & defense, automotive & consumer lighting, electronic shielding applications are a few of the markets that VTI's equipment group serves.

EQUIPMENT, EXTRUDING/MOLDING *(General) 80VAJ*

Crest Healthcare Supply 800-328-8908
195 3rd St, Dassel, MN 55325
Wall protection.

Nypro Inc. 978-365-9721
101 Union St, Clinton, MA 01510
State-of-the-art precision injection molding.

Point Medical Corp. 219-663-1775
891 E Summit St, Crown Point, IN 46307
Multi-lumen. Custom extrusion. Tight tolerance.

EQUIPMENT, FILTERING, AIR, ETO *(General) 80WYN*

Abatement Technologies, Inc. 800-634-9091
605 Satellite Blvd NW Ste 300, Suwanee, GA 30024
HEPA-AIRE Portable Air Scrubbers

Fumex Inc. 800-432-7550
1150 Cobb International Pl NW Ste D, Kennesaw, GA 30152

EQUIPMENT, FILTERING, AIR, ETO *(cont'd)*

Lm Air Technology, Inc. 866-381-8200
1467 Pinewood St, Cleanroom & Lab Equipment - Mfger
Rahway, NJ 07065
HEPA & ULPA filtered equipment including Laminar flow

The Kahn Companies 860-529-8643
885 Wells Rd, Wethersfield, CT 06109
Compressed air and gas dehydrators/dryers. Equipment to remove moisture and contamintants from compressed air and gases.

EQUIPMENT, IMMUNOELECTROPHORESIS, ROCKET *(Immunology) 82JZX*

Bio-Rad Laboratories, Life Science Group 800-424-6723
2000 Alfred Nobel Dr, Hercules, CA 94547

Helena Laboratories 409-842-3714
PO Box 752, Beaumont, TX 77704
Laurell rocket electrophoresis for vWF:AG (F. VIII R:Ag), Protein C, and Protein S (free and bound).

Sebia Electrophoresis 800-835-6497
400-1705 Corporate Drive, Norcross, GA 30093

EQUIPMENT, IN VITRO FERTILIZATION/EMBRYO TRANSFER *(Obstetrics/Gyn) 85VIK*

Basi (Bioanalytical Systems, Inc.) 800-845-4246
2701 Kent Ave, West Lafayette, IN 47906

Embryotech Laboratories, Inc. 800-673-7500
323 Andover St, Wilmington, MA 01887
Cryopreserved mouse embryos.

Genx International 888-GEN-XNOW
393 Soundview Rd, Guilford, CT 06437

Rocket Medical Plc. 800-707-7625
150 Recreation Park Dr Ste 3, Hingham, MA 02043

EQUIPMENT, LABORATORY, GEN. PURPOSE (SPECIFIC MEDICAL USE) *(Chemistry) 75LXG*

Abbott Diagnostics Div. 847-937-7988
1921 Hurd Dr, Irving, TX 75038
Temperature cycling instrument.

Act-Aeromed Copan Technologies Llc. 951-549-8793
85 Commerce St, Glastonbury, CT 06033
Disposable transfer pipettes.

Alt Bioscience,Llc 859-231-3061
235 Bolivar St, Lexington, KY 40508
Vial.

Anton Paar Usa 800-722-7556
10215 Timber Ridge Dr, Ashland, VA 23005
$1,700.00-$25,000.00 Density/Specific gravity meters with accuracies from +/- 0.001 gm/cc to +/-0.0000015 gm/cc.

Applied Test Systems, Inc. 800-441-0215
154 Eastbrook Ln, Butler, PA 16002
Lab-test furnaces and ovens to specifications in a wide variety of sizes and temperatures.

Asi Instruments, Inc. 800-531-1105
12900 E 10 Mile Rd, Warren, MI 48089

Aviaradx, Inc. 877-886-6739
11025 Roselle St Ste 200, San Diego, CA 92121
Various types of general purpose laboratory equipment.

Baxter Healthcare Corp., Renal Division 847-948-2000
7511 114th Ave, Largo, FL 33773
Various types of sterile transfer and adapter sets and accessories.

Bd Biosciences 408-954-6307
2350 Qume Dr, San Jose, CA 95131
Laboratory equipment.

Beckman Coulter, Inc. 800-526-3821
11800 SW 147th Ave, Miami, FL 33196
General purpose laboratory equipment labeled or promoted for a specific medicale.

Biocare Medical, Llc 925-603-8003
4040 Pike Ln, Concord, CA 94520
General purpose laboratory equipment, labeled or promoted for a specific use.

EQUIPMENT, LABORATORY, GEN. PURPOSE (SPECIFIC MEDICAL USE) *(cont'd)*

Biogenex Laboratories 800-421-4149
4600 Norris Canyon Rd, San Ramon, CA 94583
OPTIMAX; Equipment, Test, Immunohistology: automated immunostainer and complete system of optimized antibodies and detection reagents. BIOGENEX i6000 automated immunohistostaining system that simultaneously performs IHC, ISH, special stains, and H&E. BIOGENEX i1000 automated antigen retrieval system for high-throughput antigen retrieval, Dewax, and H&E. BIOGENEX iVision Digital Image Analysis System for quantification, detection, and archiving of stained tissue images.

Bose Corporation - Electroforce Systems Group 800-273-0437
10250 Valley View Rd Ste 113, Eden Prairie, MN 55344
Test systems for medical device durability, graft, orthopedic and tissue, materials characterization, rheology, viscoelastic testing. ELECTROFORCE Stent/Graft Series Test Instruments, 3200, 3300 & 3500 Series Test Instruments and our TestBench Series; high performance testing equipment which utilizes a proprietary electro-dynamic linear actuator technology developed by BOSE Corporation.

Brinkmann Instruments (Canada) Ltd. 800-263-8715
6670 Campobello Rd., Mississauga, ONT L5N 2L8 Canada
Grinding mill model ZM-1 for small batches of material from 3 grams up to 100 grams. Also, recirculating chillers with cooling capacity of 15,000 watts.

Brinkmann Instruments, Inc. 800-645-3050
PO Box 1019, Westbury, NY 11590

Caligor 800-472-4346
846 Pelham Pkwy, Pelham, NY 10803
Most medical supplies, including medical and surgical supplies for physicians' offices.

Calmaquip Engineering Corp. 305-592-4510
7240 NW 12th St, Miami, FL 33126

Carclo Technical Plastics - Export 724-539-1833
6009 Enterprise Dr, Export, PA 15632
Various types of evaporation covers.

Carver Inc. 260-563-7577
1569 Morris St, Wabash, IN 46992
Compact pellet press for KBr pellet pressing, compound and formula testing, fluid extractions, etc. Also, bench model automatic compression presses with microprocessor based control of pressure, ramping capabilities.

Celera Corporation 510-749-4219
1401 Harbor Bay Pkwy, Alameda, CA 94502
Accessory,general-purpose software.

Copan Diagnostics, Inc. 800-216-4016
26055 Jefferson Ave, Murrieta, CA 92562
Microbiology inoculation loops and needles.

Cytyc Surgical Products 800-442-9892
250 Campus Dr, Marlborough, MA 01752
General purpose laboratory equipment labeled or promoted for a specific medical.

Daxor Corporation 865-425-0555
107 Meco Ln, Oak Ridge, TN 37830
General purpose lab equipment.

Depuy Spine, Inc. 800-227-6633
325 Paramount Dr, Raynham, MA 02767
Labware.

Dynex Technologies, Inc. 800-288-2354
14340 Sullyfield Cir, Chantilly, VA 20151
Plate washer.

Express Systems And Parts Network Inc 330-995-4350
325 Harris Dr, Aurora, OH 44202

Gentra Systems, Inc. 763-543-0678
13355 10th Ave N Ste 120, Minneapolis, MN 55441
Automated nucleic acid purification instrument.

Hampton Research 800-452-3899
34 Journey, Aliso Viejo, CA 92656

Hudson Control Group, Inc. 973-376-7400
10 Stern Ave, Springfield, NJ 07081
Automated punch for dried blood spots.

Ika-Works, Inc. 800-733-3037
2635 Northchase Pkwy SE, Wilmington, NC 28405
Analytical mills designed to reduce dry, hard and brittle materials such as bone, teeth, coal, coke, limestone and soil for analytical evaluation.

EQUIPMENT, LABORATORY, GEN. PURPOSE (SPECIFIC MEDICAL USE) *(cont'd)*

International Hospital Supply Co. 800-398-9450
6914 Canby Ave Ste 105, Reseda, CA 91335

J & H Berge, Inc. 800-684-1234
4111 S Clinton Ave, South Plainfield, NJ 07080

Lab-Interlink, Inc. 705-860-1220
8950 J St, Omaha, NE 68127
Various.

Lcr-Hallcrest--Florida 847-998-8580
6705 Parke East Blvd Unit A, Tampa, FL 33610
Liquid crystal urine specimen thermometer.

Mccrone Microscopes & Accessories 800-622-8122
850 Pasquinelli Dr, Westmont, IL 60559
Includes polarized light, inverted and general light, fluorescence, and stereo microscopes; digital imaging; heating and freezing stages.

Nanogen, Inc. 877-626-6436
10398 Pacific Center Ct, San Diego, CA 92121
General purpose laboratory equipment.

Nsk America Corporation 800-585-4675
700 Cooper Ct Ste B, Schaumburg, IL 60173
Laboratory equipment, electric and air.

Nutech Molding Corporation 1-800-423-5278
PO Box 840, 2024 Broad St,, Pocomoke City, MD 21851

Portable Medical Laboratories, Inc. 858-755-7385
544 S Nardo Ave, Solana Beach, CA 92075
Portable medical laboratory (laboratory in a suitcase).

Promega Corp. 800-356-9526
2800 Woods Hollow Rd, Fitchburg, WI 53711

Sarstedt, Inc. 800-257-5101
PO Box 468, 1025, St. James Church Road, Newton, NC 28658

Teco Diagnostics 714-693-7788
1268 N Lakeview Ave, Anaheim, CA 92807
Laboratory equipment.

Thermo Fisher Scientific (Rochester) 585-899-7600
75 Panorama Creek Dr, Panorama, NY 14625
Various.

Tomtec 877-866-8323
1000 Sherman Ave, Hamden, CT 06514

Troemner Llc 800-352-7705
201 Wolf Dr, PO Box 87, West Deptford, NJ 08086

Turner Biosystems, Inc. 408-636-2414
645 N Mary Ave, Sunnyvale, CA 94085
Luminometer,multi-functional.

United Laboratory Plastics 800-722-2499
PO Box 8585, 1724A Westpark Ctr., Saint Louis, MO 63126
Rockers, shakers, balances, minicentrifuges and other lab equipment.

Vida Medica, S.A. De C.V. 5-557-4346
Calle 6 No. 376 Col. Francisco I. Madero, Mexico D.F. 11480 Mexico

EQUIPMENT, MANAGEMENT, PAIN, RADIOFREQUENCY, NON-INVASIVE *(General) 80WYB*

Bard Access Systems, Inc. 800-545-0890
605 N 5600 W, Salt Lake City, UT 84116
Portable, battery powered ultrasound scanners.

Biofreeze Performance Health, Inc. 800-246-3733
1245 Home Ave, Akron, OH 44310

EQUIPMENT, MARKING, ELECTROCHEMICAL *(General) 80WXQ*

R&Da Co. 508-747-5803
37 Dwight Ave, Plymouth, MA 02360
Technology to debur machined parts; also eliminate micro burrs on sharp edges, such as on needles and cutting tools.

EQUIPMENT, MOLDING *(General) 80WXE*

Aetrex Worldwide, Inc 800-526-2739
414 Alfred Ave, Teaneck, NJ 07666
VAC PRESS, equipment that is used to form and finish foot orthotics. FOAMART, foot impression system and APEX foot imprinter, used to evaluate foot conditions and make custom foot orthotics.

EQUIPMENT, MOLDING *(cont'd)*

Altman Mfg. Co, Inc. 630-963-0031
1990 Ohio St, Lisle, IL 60532
Deflashing equipment for molded rubber products. RSOM secondary equipment for injection molded rubber products. Die trimming equipment to produce trimmed rubber products. Dies - Shear type - to deflash, punch and trim. Coverting Equipment for Blood bags, sonic welding, assembly, and general automation equipment. Conveying systems, packaging, and cleaning systems.

Carver Inc. 260-563-7577
1569 Morris St, Wabash, IN 46992
Auto Series Presses, automatic benchtop molding presses. Electric presses

Globe Medical Tech, Inc. 713-365-9595
1766 W Sam Houston Pkwy N, Houston, TX 77043
Injection Molding: mold design, sample and production molds for components of medical devices.

EQUIPMENT, SCREENING, SCOLIOSIS *(Orthopedics) 87WRR*

Mizuho Osi 800-777-4674
30031 Ahern Ave, Union City, CA 94587

EQUIPMENT, SHAVING, DISC, SPINAL *(Orthopedics) 87WYA*

Blackstone Medical, Inc. 888-298-5400
90 Brookdale Dr, Springfield, MA 01104

LinkBio Corp. 800-932-0616
300 Round Hill Dr, Rockaway, NJ 07866
Instruments for spinal surgery.

Medtronic Sofamor Danek Usa, Inc 901-399-2346
1800 Pyramid Pl, Memphis, TN 38132
Spinal Orthopedics.

Zimmer Spine 508-643-0983
23 W Bacon St, Plainville, MA 02762
MDS, Micro Debrider System, a powered shaver system with suction and irrigation, side-cutting, blunt-tipped blades for the removal of nucleus tissue from disc.

EQUIPMENT, SUCTION/IRRIGATION, LAPAROSCOPIC *(Surgery) 79WYP*

American Catheter Corp. 800-345-6714
13047 S Highway 475, Ocala, FL 34480
Suction-irrigation electrode probes.

Bryan Corp. 800-343-7711
4 Plympton St, Woburn, MA 01801
5mm/10mm 33cm length with trumpet valve.

Elmed, Inc. 630-543-2792
60 W Fay Ave, Addison, IL 60101

Ethicon Endo-Surgery, Inc. 800-USE-ENDO
4545 Creek Rd, Cincinnati, OH 45242

Exmoor Plastics Inc. 317-244-1014
304 Gasoline Aly, Indianapolis, IN 46222
Range of single use stainless steel or plastic suction equipment including single use myringotome, priced from $4.25.

Genicon 800-936-1020
6869 Stapoint Ct Ste 114, Winter Park, FL 32792
Disposable Laparoscopic Suction Irrigation Products

Md International, Inc. 305-669-9003
11300 NW 41st St, Doral, FL 33178

Megadyne Medical Products, Inc. 800-747-6110
11506 S State St, Draper, UT 84020
ALL-IN-ONE, laparoscopic suction/irrigation/electrocautery hand control unit and electrodes.

Olsen Medical 800-297-6344
3001 W Kentucky St, Louisville, KY 40211
Foot activated suction tubes.

Richard Wolf Medical Instruments Corp. 800-323-9653
353 Corporate Woods Pkwy, Vernon Hills, IL 60061

Smiths Medical Asd, Inc. 800-553-8351
160 Weymouth St, Rockland, MA 02370
Normothermic irrigating system 1129 with power pole for high flow irrigating.

Surgicorp, Inc. 727-934-5000
40347 US Highway 19 N Ste 121, Tarpon Springs, FL 34689
SURGIN, trumpet valves with and without probes, filtered insufflation tubing.

Synectic Medical Product Development 203-877-8488
60 Commerce Park, Milford, CT 06460

EQUIPMENT, SUCTION/IRRIGATION, LAPAROSCOPIC *(cont'd)*

Valleylab 800-255-8522
5920 Longbow Dr, Boulder, CO 80301
Laparoscopic suction/irrigation/coagulator/cutter. Pencil grip handset; retractable electrodes.

Wisap America 800-233-8448
8231 Melrose Dr, Lenexa, KS 66214

EQUIPMENT, SUCTION/IRRIGATION/ELECTROCAUTERY, LAPAROSCOPIC *(Surgery) 79SJK*

Olsen Medical 800-297-6344
3001 W Kentucky St, Louisville, KY 40211
Irrigating bipolar forceps. Suction tubes.

Topcon Canada Inc. 800-361-3515
110 Provencher Ave., Boisbriand, QUE J7G-1N1 Canada

EQUIPMENT, TEST, WESTERN BLOT *(Microbiology) 83WKS*

Advanced American Biotechnology (Aab) 714-870-0290
1166 E Valencia Dr Unit 6C, Fullerton, CA 92831
Profile reader.

Calypte Biomedical Corporation 877-CALYPTE
16290 SW Upper Boones Ferry Rd, Portland, OR 97224
Cambridge Biotech HIV-1 Western blot kit for the detection and confirmation of HIV-1 antibodies in urine and serum.

Fisher Healthcare 800-766-7000
9999 Veterans Memorial Dr, Houston, TX 77038

Immunetics, Inc. 800-227-4765
27 Drydock Ave Ste 6, Boston, MA 02210
Miniblotter multichannel Western blot incubation unit; incubation system with disposable cassettes and kit for detecting human anibodies to Taenia solium.

Orasure Technologies, Inc. 610-882-1820
1745 Eaton Ave, Bethlehem, PA 18018
EPI-BLOT: Western blot HIV-I confirmatory test.

Tecan U.S., Inc. 800-338-3226
4022 Stirrup Creek Dr Ste 310, Durham, NC 27703
Profiblot.

Ultra-Lum, Inc. 800-809-6559
1480 N Claremont Blvd, Claremont, CA 91711
Omega and Gel Explorer Series Imaging Systems.

EQUIPMENT, THERAPY, APNEA *(Anesthesiology) 73WLD*

E. Benson Hood Laboratories, Inc. 800-942-5227
575 Washington St, Pembroke, MA 02359
Eccovison Acoustic Pharyngometer, screen for sleep apnea.

Omni Medical Supply Inc. 800-860-6664
4153 Pioneer Dr, Commerce Township, MI 48390

Respan Prod. Inc. 800-267-4063
8 Erinville Dr., Erin, ONT N0B 1T0 Canada
Disposable respiratory products.

EQUIPMENT, THERAPY, HANDICAPPED/PHYSICAL *(Physical Med) 89WPB*

Abilitations 800-850-8602
PO Box 922668, Norcross, GA 30010
Industries leading solutions based product catalog for children with special needs. Product mix includes movement, positioning, sensory integration, adapted play, aquatics and more.

Aqua Glass Corporation 800-632-0911
320 Industrial Park Rd, Adamsville, TN 38310
All aqua-glass SPECIAL CARE bathing fixtures and products for the physically handicapped come with MICROBAN antibacterial protection that hinders the growth of odor and stain that cause mold and mildew. Aqua-glass bathing fixtures are thus easier to keep clean.

Arjo, Inc. 800-323-1245
50 Gary Ave Ste A, Roselle, IL 60172
See-through pool for hydrotherapy with multiple patients.

EQUIPMENT, THERAPY, HANDICAPPED/PHYSICAL *(cont'd)*

Balance Systems, Inc. 1-888-274-5444
1644 Plaza Way Ste 317, Walla Walla, WA 99362
The Carpal Management System™ (CMS) uniquely combines two clinical and patented technologies that make your computer fit the work you do and makes you more fit to work. The Carpal Management System™ comprises of the Virtually Hands Free™ Mousing System, which is Quill Mouse™, the first patented Grip-Less™ mouse, and the Nib™ software, and in addition the unique and patented FLEXTEND® Orthotic Exercise Glove that rehabilitates most forms of RSI affecting the fingers, hands, wrists, forearms and elbows. The software will remind you of exercise breaks for the FLEXTEND® Orthotic glove(s) along with tracking your exercise routine and progress. Perfect for Home or Office!! Registed under GSA Section 508 of the Rehabilitation Act.

Bergeron Health Care 800-371-2778
15 S 2nd St, Dolgeville, NY 13329
Special Tomato Soft Touch Therapy Rolls and Wedges

Bertec Corporation 877-237-8320
6171 Huntley Rd Ste J, Columbus, OH 43229
Balance and gait training and rehabilitation tools, appropriate for physical therapy. Includes posturography biofeedback balance training protocols and instrumented force measuring treadmills.

Biomation 888-667-2324
335 Perth St., P.O. Box 156, Almonte, ON K0A 1A0 Canada
Distribute physical therapy and psychotherapy equipment including biofeedback, muscle testing, electrical stimulation and psychotherapy.

Bloomex International, Inc. 201-703-9799
295 Molnar Dr, Elmwood Park, NJ 07407

Bte Technologies, Inc. 800-331-8845
7455 New Ridge Rd Ste L, Hanover, MD 21076
PrimusRS- Isometric, Isotonic, Isokinetic, Eccentric, CPM, Task Simulation, Hand Therapy, Lifting Evaluations, Sports Medicine. Simulator II- Isometric, Isotonic, Task Simulation, Hand Therapy, Geriatrics, Lifting Evaluations.

Cardon Rehabilitation Products Inc 800-944-7868
908 Niagara Falls Blvd, Wurlitzer Industrial Park
North Tonawanda, NY 14120
Therapeutic exercise equipment including bilateral pulleys, bench and lateral pulleys.

Commercial/Medical Electronics, Inc. 800-324-4844
1519 S Lewis Ave, Tulsa, OK 74104
Physical therapy equipment.

Enduro Medical Technology, Inc. 860-289-2299
310 Nutmeg Rd S Unit C5, South Windsor, CT 06074
SAM-Y by Enduro, youth model secure ambulation module developed under license with NASA for youth gait training and standing therapy. For use at home and in school.

Essential Medical Supply, Inc. 800-826-8423
6420 Hazeltine National Dr, Orlando, FL 32822
ENDURANCE, FEATHERLIGHT, ROLL EASY, BLAZER.

Flaghouse, Inc. 800-793-7900
601 US Highway 46 W, Hasbrouck Heights, NJ 07604

Kees Goebel Medical Specialties, Inc. 800-354-0445
9663 Glades Dr, Hamilton, OH 45011
Physical therapy products.

Lifeline Usa 800-553-6633
3201 Syene Rd, Madison, WI 53713
Skit rehab kit.

Living Earth Crafts 800-358-8292
3210 Executive Rdg, Vista, CA 92081
Treatment tables: portable, hydraulic and electric models from $339.00 to $1,895.00. 5-year warranty, custom models available.

Magister Corporation 800-396-3130
310 Sylvan St, Chattanooga, TN 37405

Maribelle Manufacturing Inc. 888-655-3459
9520 Natasha Place, Sidney, BC V8L-4P9 Canada
Exercise assist equipment to fit babies up to extra large adults. For MERRY MUSCLES Model F, designed for severely disabled children up to 35 lbs. MARIBELLE EXERCISE ASSIST SYSTEM (MEAS): For #456, for weights of approximately 30-65 lbs; $425.00 for #789, which adjusts to persons 60-100+ lbs; for #JP, for the tall and slim person; for #RA, for the medium adult range; and $750.00 for #XL, which is made to ' measure only - the cost includes custom design in this ' size only; other custom-designed units (within the closest size range) are subject to a $70.00 surcharge over the regular price.

EQUIPMENT, THERAPY, HANDICAPPED/PHYSICAL *(cont'd)*

Med-Fit Systems, Inc. 800-831-7665
3553 Rosa Way, Fallbrook, CA 92028
ACCESStrainer- patented wheelchair exercise device features over 20 different exercises

Meddev Corporation 800-543-2789
730 N Pastoria Ave, Sunnyvale, CA 94085

Nautilus, Inc. 360-859-2900
16400 SE Nautilus Dr, Vancouver, WA 98683

North Coast Medical, Inc. 800-821-9319
18305 Sutter Blvd, Morgan Hill, CA 95037

Parsons A.D.L. Inc. 800-263-1281
R.R. #2, 1986 Sideroad 15, Tottenham, ONT L0G 1W0 Canada
Occupational and physiotherapy supplies.

Pre Pak Products, Inc. 800-544-7257
4055 Oceanside Blvd Ste L, Oceanside, CA 92056
HOME RANGER, over the door pulley for shoulder rehabilitation. Three models to choose from; HOME RANGER ORIGINAL-$14.50 each-has molded rubber handles and a web door-strap, HOME RANGER 92 -$21.00 each-has assisted grip handles and a stainless steel door bracket, HOME RANGER 93-$17.50 each-has assisted grip handles and a web door-strap. Quantity discounts available on all three models. FLEX RANGER, stretch cable with pulley. A multi-use exercise device that covers all stages of rehab - from passive range of motion through resistive, weight bearing exercise. $25.00 each. Quantity discounts available.

Prime Engineering 800-827-8263
4202 W Sierra Madre Ave, Fresno, CA 93722
Standing frames, Prone Stander, standing tables/frames. Multi-position standers.

RDL Supply 214-630-3965
11240 Gemini Ln, Dallas, TX 75229
POWER DOOR openers open interior and exterior doors with push of a button. PFSB swing clear hinges remove doors from inside of frames to increase opening size.

Rifton Equipment 800-571-8198
PO Box 260, Rifton, NY 12471
Adjustable chairs, gait trainers, tricycles with safety features, prone standers, supine standers, dynamic standers, bath chairs, commodes, and other equipment for the disabled.

Scifit 800-278-3933
5151 S 110th East Ave, Tulsa, OK 74146
Power Trainers and PRO2 All Body Exercisers - rehabilitation and fitness equipment for non-impact, aerobic conditioning.

Stairmaster Health And Fitness Products 800-628-8458
1886 Prairie Way, Superior, CO 80027
Exercise equipment, physical therapy equipment.

Stand-N-Go, Inc. 218-739-5252
19051 County Highway 1, Fergus Falls, MN 56537
Stand-N-Go; a mobile standing aid for paraplegics with an attached work station.

Tagg Industries L.L.C. 800-548-3514
23210 Del Lago Dr, Laguna Hills, CA 92653
ACTION ARM, therapeutic aid develops skilled motor movement, increases control and coordination, increases muscular strength and improves accuracy for the arm and shoulder.

Thera-Tronics, Inc. 800-267-6211
623 Mamaroneck Ave, Mamaroneck, NY 10543
Rehab. supplies.

EQUIPMENT, TRACTION, POWERED *(Physical Med) 89ITH*

Advanced Back Technologies, Inc. 631-231-0076
89 Cabot Ct Ste F, Hauppauge, NY 11788
Powered traction device / powered decompression table.

Alimed, Inc. 800-225-2610
297 High St, Dedham, MA 02026

Arizona Dme--Durable Medical Equipment, Inc. 888-665-2568
PO Box 15413, Scottsdale, AZ 85267
CPM(S), Bracing C custom, Post-Op., etc.

Axiom Worldwide, Inc. 813-969-2414
9423 Corporate Lake Dr, Tampa, FL 33634
Various.

Bray Corporation 760-345-6689
14149 Calle Contesa, Victorville, CA 92392
Vertebral distraction pump (v.d.p.).

Cert Health Sciences, Llc 866-990-4444
7036 Golden Ring Rd, Baltimore, MD 21237
Spinemed therapeutic table.

EQUIPMENT, TRACTION, POWERED *(cont'd)*

Chattanooga Group 800-592-7329
4717 Adams Rd, Hixson, TN 37343
TX and TRITON traction table.

Erp Group Professional Products Ltd. 800-361-3537
3232 Autoroute Laval W., Laval, QC H7T 2H6 Canada
Akron traction units and tables.

Lordex, Inc. 281-395-9512
32357 Morton Rd Bldg 3, Brookshire, TX 77423
Lumbar decompression traction machine.

North American Medical Corp (Nam) 770-541-0012
1649 Sands Pl SE Ste A, Marietta, GA 30067
Chiropractic spinal decompression equipment, Medical rehabilitation devices for spinal dysfunction, Electrical modalities and related diagnostic equipment.

North American Medical Corporation 770-541-0012
1649 Sands Pl SE Ste A, Marietta, GA 30067

Spinerx Technology 713-983-9979
6100 Brittmoore Rd Ste S, Houston, TX 77041
Equipment, traction, powered.

Vat-Tech, Inc. 705-687-8717
684 Muskoka Rd N, Gravenhurst P1P 1E7 Canada
Vax-d therapeutic table

Vax-D Medical Technologies Llc 813-343-5000
310 Mears Blvd, Oldsmar, FL 34677
VAX-D Therapy Table.

EQUIPMENT, ULTRASOUND, DOPPLER, EVALUATION, FETAL
(Obstetrics/Gyn) 85LQT

American Biomed Instruments, Inc. 718-235-8900
11 Wyona St, Brooklyn, NY 11207

Hokanson Inc., D.E. 800-999-8251
12840 NE 21st Pl, Bellevue, WA 98005
The OB1 Obstetrical Doppler has a large display of Fetal Heart Rate, detachable waterproof transducer, rechargeable NiCad batteries and carries the Hokanson 5 year warranty.

Imaging Associates, Inc. 800-821-3230
11110 Westlake Dr, Charlotte, NC 28273

Medison America, Inc. 800-829-SONO
11075 Knott Ave Ste C, Cypress, CA 90630

Pyramid Medical Llc 800-764-1154
10940 Portal Dr, Los Alamitos, CA 90720
New PMI 764 and 800 portable ultrasound, 24 month warranty starting from $9500.00 New 3-D System which can be added to your present ultrasound. This will give you all the advantages of 3-D rendering and multi-plane imaging.

Sonosite, Inc. 888-482-9449
21919 30th Dr SE, Bothell, WA 98021
The SonoSite TITAN(TM) is a hand-carried mobile ultrasound system uniquely combining high performance and usability in a lightweight rugged package. The TITAN system offers the high-resolution image quality, features and functionality of a cart-based system while maintaining the flexibility and speed of a grab-and-go solution. The system was designed to be the most intuitive and easy to use ultrasound system available today.

Vmed Technology, Inc. (Formerly Ems Products, Inc.) 425-497-9149
16149 Redmond Way # 108, Redmond, WA 98052
Obstetrical Dopplers for fetal detection as early as eight weeks.

EQUIPMENT, ULTRASOUND, INTRAVASCULAR, 3-DIMENSIONAL *(Cardiovascular) 74WYD*

Imaging Associates, Inc. 800-821-3230
11110 Westlake Dr, Charlotte, NC 28273

EQUIPMENT/ACCESSORIES, LASER, LAPAROSCOPY
(Surgery) 79SIV

Ams Innovative Center-San Jose 800-356-7600
3070 Orchard Dr, San Jose, CA 95134
ADD side-firing laser energy delivery system for broad range of surgical laser applications including ablation, vaporization and coagulation of prostatic tissue.

Buffalo Filter, A Division Of Medtek Devices Inc. 800-343-2324
595 Commerce Dr, Amherst, NY 14228
Accessories for laser, ESU, laparoscopic procedures, tubing, surgical masks, in-line filters, etc.

Olsen Medical 800-297-6344
3001 W Kentucky St, Louisville, KY 40211
Laser safety products: Patient Eye Shields,

EQUIPMENT/ACCESSORIES, LASER, LAPAROSCOPY *(cont'd)*

Reliant Technologies, Inc. 650-473-0200
260 Sheridan Ave Ste 300, Palo Alto, CA 94306

EQUIPMENT/SERVICE, QUALITY CONTROL *(General) 80WQM*

Aerosol Monitoring & Analysis, Inc. 410-684-3327
1331 Ashton Rd Ste A, P.O. Box 646, Hanover, MD 21076
Environmental consulting, health and safety, lab surveys fume hood testing, safety audits, indoor air quality.

Ar Worldwide 800-933-8181
160 Schoolhouse Rd, Souderton, PA 18964
RF Amplifiers, 1 - 50,000 watts, dc to 1 GHz; Microwave Amplifiers, 1 - 2000 watts, .8 to 40 GHz; Antennas, 1 - 15,000 watts, 10 kHz to 40 GHz; Transient Generators from EM Test; Precompliance test systems; Accessories and software; and Vision Series modules.

Ats Laboratories, Inc. 203-579-2700
404 Knowlton St, Bridgeport, CT 06608
Clinical quality assurance phantom for hospital quality assurance programs; full range available; also, phantom lithotripter for clinical teaching and quality assurance purposes; also, endoscopic phantom utilized for evaluating endoscopic imaging systems.

Bioreliance 800-553-5372
14920 Broschart Rd, Rockville, MD 20850
GLP-compliant toxicological testing services offered worldwide. In-depth knowledge of U.S. and international regulations and range of genetic, in vitro and in vivo testing protocols assure complete confidential support for regulatory submissions and nonregulatory safety assessments.

Bomem Inc. 800-858-FTIR
585 Charest Blvd. East, Suite 300, Quebec City, QUE G1K-9H4 Canada
Infrared spectrometer with .002cm resolution for QC applications.

Brown & Sharpe Inc. 800-343-7933
250 Circuit Dr, North Kingstown, RI 02852
Measuring/Inspection Equipment

Bryton Corp. 800-567-9500
4310 Guion Rd, Indianapolis, IN 46254
Service, used equipment. Complete service as well as extensive scheduled maintenance programs for all types of surgical, orthopedic, urological, obstetrical, and major examination tables and surgical lights.

Celsis Laboratory Group 800-523-5227
165 Fieldcrest Ave, Edison, NJ 08837
Testing facility specializing in chemistry, microbiology, sterility testing, sterilization cycle validation, and toxicology including in vitro and in vivo procedures, ISO-10993/FDA Matrix.

Dpt Laboratories, Ltd. 866-225-5378
4040 Broadway St Ste 401, San Antonio, TX 78209

Fumex Inc. 800-432-7550
1150 Cobb International Pl NW Ste D, Kennesaw, GA 30152

Hayes Medical, Inc. 800-240-0500
1115 Windfield Way Ste 100, El Dorado Hills, CA 95762

Lacey Manufacturing Co. 203-336-0121
1146 Barnum Ave, PO Box 5156, Bridgeport, CT 06610

Luwa Lepco 713-461-1131
1750 Stebbins Dr, Houston, TX 77043

Microstat Laboratories, Inc. 877-204-2007
PO Box 115, Dover, MN 55929
Enumeration and identification of particulate matter in pharmaceutical products and medical devices.

Milliken & Company, Anticon Products 800-762-3472
201 Lukken Industrial Dr W # M-836, Lagrange, GA 30240
Cleanroom consumables. Included is cleanroom laundered, lint free wipers and mops. Wipers can be pre-saturated with various cleaning solutions.

Millipore Corporation 800-MILLIPORE
80 Ashby Rd, Bedford, MA 01730
Admixture Quality Control System: Confirms the microbial quality of admixtures.

Novosci Corp. 281-363-4949
2828 N Crescentridge Dr, The Woodlands, TX 77381

Photo Research, Inc. 818-341-5151
9731 Topanga Canyon Pl, Chatsworth, CA 91311
Standards, Calibration and Measurement for lighting industries.

Sonoco Crellin, Inc. 518-392-2000
87 Center St, Chatham, NY 12037
Cleanroom and clean areas available.

EQUIPMENT/SERVICE, QUALITY CONTROL *(cont'd)*

Stellar Technologies, Inc. 888-566-9094
9200 Xylon Ave N Ste 100, Brooklyn Park, MN 55445
Stellar Technologies, Inc. specializes in assisting design and manufacture of implantable assemblies and medical components. Providing Rapid Response for design development, silicone molding, insert overmolding, multiaxis machining, laser machining, marking and welding, wire winding and forming, micro machining and cleanroom assembly.

ERASER, DENTAL STAIN *(Dental And Oral) 76MAU*

Deepak Products, Inc. 305-482-9669
5220 NW 72nd Ave Ste 15, Miami, FL 33166
Bleaching systems.

Pac-Dent Intl., Inc. 909-839-0888
21078 Commerce Point Dr, Walnut, CA 91789
Dental tooth whitening gel.

Twist2it, Inc. 877-PRO-PHYS
3930A 62nd St, Flushing, NY 11377

ERGOMETER, BICYCLE *(Cardiovascular) 74QUN*

Cybex International, Inc. 800-667-6544
10 Trotter Dr, Medway, MA 02053
$1,590 for FITRON with continuous hydraulic braking system. Adjustable seats and handlebars. Optional toe clips on pedals. Also, metabolic systems The Bike, computerized cycle ergometer, $2,590.

Elmed, Inc. 630-543-2792
60 W Fay Ave, Addison, IL 60101

Equilibrated Bio Systems, Inc. 800-327-9490
22 Lawrence Ave Ste LL2, Smithtown, NY 11787

Tsi Medical Ltd. 800-661-7263
47 Athabascan Ave., Unit 105, Sherwood Park, AB T8A-4H3 Canada

ERGOMETER, OTHER *(Anesthesiology) 73QUO*

Concept Ii, Inc. 800-245-5676
105 Industrial Park Dr, Morrisville, VT 05661
CONCEPT II, $725, idoor rower.

Cybex International, Inc. 800-667-6544
10 Trotter Dr, Medway, MA 02053
$2,390 for UBE upper body rehab. and exercise ergometer. $3,890 for computerized Met 100.

ERGOMETER, TREADMILL *(Cardiovascular) 74BYQ*

Cybex International, Inc. 800-667-6544
10 Trotter Dr, Medway, MA 02053
TrackMaster treadmills from $3,390.

Galix Biomedical Instrumentation, Inc. 305-534-5905
2555 Collins Ave Ste C-5, Miami Beach, FL 33140
HIGH PERFORMANCE STRESS TEST SYSTEM: User friendly programmable features like protocols, printing formats, comments, screens, etc. The software controls any RS-232 compatible treadmill or bicycle. With a Windows platform and USB port connection, the computer and printer compatibility is limitless. Hundreds of reports can be stored on a PC database and/or transmitted via Internet.

Hillusa Corp. 305-594-7474
7215 NW 46th St, Miami, FL 33166

Kistler Instrument Corp. 716-691-5100
75 John Glenn Dr, Amherst, NY 14228
GAITWAY instrumented force-meausuring treadmill for assesment and bio-feedback of clinical gait.

Rehamed Intl. Llc. 800-577-4424
522 W Mowry Dr, Homestead, FL 33030
Upper body ergometer that is inclusive for people in wheelchairs

Tsi Medical Ltd. 800-661-7263
47 Athabascan Ave., Unit 105, Sherwood Park, AB T8A-4H3 Canada

ERISOPHAKE *(Ophthalmology) 86HNT*

Bausch & Lomb Surgical 636-255-5051
3365 Tree Court Ind Blvd, Saint Louis, MO 63122

ESOPHAGOSCOPE (FLEXIBLE OR RIGID)
(Ear/Nose/Throat) 77EOX

Boehm Surgical Instrument Corp. 716-436-6584
966 Chili Ave, Rochester, NY 14611
Esophagoscope.

Clinimed, Incorporated 877-CLINIMED
303 Markus Ct, Sandy Brae Industrial Park, Newark, DE 19713

ESOPHAGOSCOPE (FLEXIBLE OR RIGID) *(cont'd)*

Electro Surgical Instrument Co., Inc. 888-464-2784
37 Centennial St, Rochester, NY 14611
Various types, styles and sizes of fiberoptic esophagoscopes.

Karl Storz Endoscopy-America Inc. 800-421-0837
600 Corporate Pointe, Culver City, CA 90230
Adult and pediatric systems.

Mahe International Inc. 800-294-7946
468 Craighead St, Nashville, TN 37204

Olympus America, Inc. 800-645-8160
3500 Corporate Pkwy, PO Box 610, Center Valley, PA 18034

Richard Wolf Medical Instruments Corp. 800-323-9653
353 Corporate Woods Pkwy, Vernon Hills, IL 60061

Tsi Medical Ltd. 800-661-7263
47 Athabascan Ave., Unit 105, Sherwood Park, AB T8A-4H3 Canada

ESOPHAGOSCOPE, GENERAL & PLASTIC SURGERY
(Gastro/Urology) 78GCL

Pentax Southern Region Service Center 201-571-2300
8934 Kirby Dr, Houston, TX 77054
Esophagoscope.

Pentax West Coast Service Center 800-431-5880
10410 Pioneer Blvd Ste 2, Santa Fe Springs, CA 90670
Pentax esophagoscope.

ESTERASE *(Pathology) 88JCH*

Boston Scientific Corporation 508-652-5578
780 Brookside Dr, Spencer, IN 47460

ESTHESIOMETER *(Cns/Neurology) 84GXB*

Christy Manufacturing Corp. 925-462-7982
1228 Quarry Ln Ste F, Pleasanton, CA 94566
Aesthesiometer.

Lafayette Instrument Company 800-428-7545
PO Box 5729, 3700 Sagamore Pkwy,, Lafayette, IN 47903
2-point Model #16011, 3-point Model #16012.

Medical Monofilament Manufacturing 508-746-7877
116 Long Pond Rd, Plymouth, MA 02360
Esthesiometer.

National Hansen's Disease Programs 225-756-3740
1770 Physicians Park Dr, Baton Rouge, LA 70816
Filament.

Patterson Medical Supply, Inc. 262-387-8720
W68N158 Evergreen Blvd, Cedarburg, WI 53012
Esthesiometer.

Timely Neuropathy Testing, Llc 225-638-5343
9553 Island Rd, Ventress, LA 70783
Mono filament sensory (touch) test.

ESTROGEN RECEPTOR ASSAY KIT *(Chemistry) 75LPJ*

Dako North America, Inc 805-566-6655
6392 Via Real, Carpinteria, CA 93013

EUTHYSCOPE, AC-POWERED *(Ophthalmology) 86HMK*

Cadence Science Inc. 888-717-7677
1979 Marcus Ave Ste 215, New Hyde Park, NY 11042

EVACUATOR, BLADDER, MANUALLY OPERATED
(Gastro/Urology) 78FFD

Boston Scientific Corporation 508-652-5578
780 Brookside Dr, Spencer, IN 47460

C. R. Bard, Inc., Bard Urological Div. 888-367-2273
13183 Harland Dr NE, Covington, GA 30014

EVACUATOR, FLUID *(Gastro/Urology) 78FHF*

Boston Scientific Corporation 508-652-5578
780 Brookside Dr, Spencer, IN 47460

EVACUATOR, FUME *(Chemistry) 75QXU*

Bedcolab Ltd. 800-461-6414
2305 Francis Hughes, Laval, QUE H7S 1N5 Canada

Berchtold Corp. 800-243-5135
1950 Hanahan Rd, Charleston, SC 29406
Smoke Evacuator is an option for Teletom Power Booms. It provides filter and vacuum to remove smoke from various surgical procedures utilizing laser and electrosurgery.

Fox Manufacturing, Inc. 928-634-5897
PO Box 309, Cottonwood, AZ 86326
Fume Exhaust Systems for atomic absorption and atomic emission instruments.

EVACUATOR, FUME *(cont'd)*

Fumex Inc. 800-432-7550
1150 Cobb International Pl NW Ste D, Kennesaw, GA 30152

Zimmer Holdings, Inc. 800-613-6131
1800 W Center St, PO Box 708, Warsaw, IN 46580

EVACUATOR, GASTRO-UROLOGY *(Gastro/Urology) 78KQT*

Boston Scientific Corporation 508-652-5578
780 Brookside Dr, Spencer, IN 47460

C. R. Bard, Inc., Bard Urological Div. 888-367-2273
13183 Harland Dr NE, Covington, GA 30014

Civco Medical Instruments Co., Inc. 319-656-4447
102 1st St S, Kalona, IA 52247
Evacuator.

Gri Medical Products, Inc. 800-291-9425
4937 E Red Range Way, Cave Creek, AZ 85331
Intussusception air reduction system, bulb w/ gauge and tubing kits.

Gyrus Acmi, Inc. 508-804-2739
93 N Pleasant St, Norwalk, OH 44857
Evacuator, gastro-urology.

Medovations, Inc. 800-558-6408
102 E Keefe Ave, Milwaukee, WI 53212

EVACUATOR, ORAL CAVITY *(Dental And Oral) 76EHZ*

Coltene/Whaledent Inc. 330-916-8858
235 Ascot Pkwy, Cuyahoga Falls, OH 44223
Evacuation system.

Cpac Equipment, Inc. 800-333-9729
2364 Leicester Road, Leicester, NY 14481-0175

Dental Components, Inc. 503-538-8343
305 N Springbrook Rd, Newberg, OR 97132
Vacuum valves.

Dental Innovators, Inc. 877-921-3919
1642 N Mockingbird Pl, Orange, CA 92867

Dentalez Group 866-DTE-INFO
101 Lindenwood Dr Ste 225, Valleybrooke Corporate Center
Malvern, PA 19355

Dentalez Of Alabama 251-937-6781
2500 S US Highway 31, Bay Minette, AL 36507
Evacuator, oral cavity.

Dentsply Canada, Ltd. 800-263-1437
161 Vinyl Ct., Woodbridge, ONT L4L 4A3 Canada

Dntlworks Equipment Corporation 800-847-0694
7300 S Tucson Way, Centennial, CO 80112
Portable and mobile units have adjustable strength, high and low volume evacuation features. PortaVac is easily carried to remote sites, while the Mobile Vacuum Unit rolls smoothly between operatories.

Hager Worldwide, Inc. 800-328-2335
13322 Byrd Dr, Odessa, FL 33556
MIRASUCTO, PELLOTTE, MIRASUC, SUGITIP, & CHIRU TIP, POLYMATIC, MIRASUC 3P, CHIRUSUC.

Hygo Plastic, Inc. 414-375-4011
1376 Cheyenne Ave, Grafton, WI 53024
Hve tips.

Inter-Med, Inc. 877-418-4782
2200 Northwestern Ave, Racine, WI 53404
Oral evacuation tube.

Lorvic Corp. 800-325-1881
13705 Shoreline Ct E, Earth City, MO 63045
Various types and models of aspirators and evacuators.

Matrx By Midmark 800-847-1000
145 Mid County Dr, Orchard Park, NY 14127

Pac-Dent Intl., Inc. 909-839-0888
21078 Commerce Point Dr, Walnut, CA 91789
Surgical aspirator tips.

Pascal Co., Inc. 425-602-3633
2929 Northup Way, Bellevue, WA 98004
Oral evacuator tip.

Pelton & Crane Co., 704-588-2126
11727 Fruehauf Dr, Charlotte, NC 28273

Plastek Industries, Inc. 336-271-3210
880 Huffman St, Greensboro, NC 27405
Plastic oral evacuator tip, disposable.

Ramvac Dental Products Inc 800-572-6822
3100 1st Ave, Spearfish, SD 57783

EVACUATOR, ORAL CAVITY *(cont'd)*

Salvin Dental Specialties, Inc. 800-535-6566
3450 Latrobe Dr, Charlotte, NC 28211
Various types of oral evacuators and accessories.

Sds (Summit Dental Systems) 800-275-3368
3560 NW 53rd Ct, Fort Lauderdale, FL 33309

Small Beginnings Inc. 760-949-7707
17525 Alder St Ste 28, Hesperia, CA 92345
Oral cavity evacuator.

Team Technologies Molding 630-937-0380
1300 Nagel Blvd, Batavia, IL 60510
Oral care suction device.

EVACUATOR, VAPOR, CEMENT MONOMER
(Orthopedics) 87JDY

Biomet, Inc. 574-267-6639
56 E Bell Dr, PO Box 587, Warsaw, IN 46582
Cementation system.

Depuy Orthopaedics, Inc. 800-473-3789
700 Orthopaedic Dr, P.O. Box 988, Warsaw, IN 46582
Various types of cement monomer vapor evacuators.

Niche Medical, Inc. 800-633-1055
55 Access Rd, Warwick, RI 02886
Evacuation & containment system.

Stryker Puerto Rico, Ltd. 939-307-2500
Hwy. 3, Km. 131.2, Las Guasimas Ind. Park, Arroyo, PR 00714
Cement monomer evacuator.

Zimmer Holdings, Inc. 800-613-6131
1800 W Center St, PO Box 708, Warsaw, IN 46580

EVAPORATOR *(Chemistry) 75JRK*

Brinkmann Instruments (Canada) Ltd. 800-263-8715
6670 Campobello Rd., Mississauga, ONT L5N 2L8 Canada

Brinkmann Instruments, Inc. 800-645-3050
PO Box 1019, Westbury, NY 11590

Cole-Parmer Instrument Inc. 800-323-4340
625 E Bunker Ct, Vernon Hills, IL 60061

Denton Vacuum, Inc. 856-439-9100
1259 N Church St, Moorestown, NJ 08057
$12,000 for DV502A high vacuum carbon coater; $4,900 for DESK II gold sputter coater.

Glas-Col , Llc 800-452-7265
711 Hulman St, PO Box 2128, Terre Haute, IN 47802

Kontes Glass Co. 888-546-2531
1022 Spruce St, Vineland, NJ 08360

Labconco Corp. 800-821-5525
8811 Prospect Ave, Kansas City, MO 64132
Vortex evaporators (RAPIDVAP) and Multi-Sample Concentrators (CENTRIVAP).

Organomation Associates, Inc. 978-838-7300
266 River Rd W, Berlin, MA 01503
N-EVAP, MULTIVAP, MICROVAP 10 models of nitrogen evaporators, from 12 to 100 positions. S-EVAP solvent evaporaters for KD or round flasks, waste solvent collection standard on all units.

Thermo Savant 800-634-8886
100 Colin Dr, Holbrook, NY 11741
SPEEDVAC Component integrated and automated systems for sample drying and concentration. Large and small capacity. Evaporates from any type of vessel.

EVOKED POTENTIAL UNIT, AUDIOMETRIC
(Cns/Neurology) 84VDA

Bio-Logic Systems Corp. 800-323-8326
1 Bio Logic Plz, Mundelein, IL 60060
NAVIGATOR PRO - microcomputer based systems which perform all AUDITORY EVOKED POTENTIALS, bone conduction, ECOG, P-300, 40Hz ERP, Master Auditory Steady State Response (MASTER, ASSR), Stacked ABR, Cochlear Hydrops (CHAMP), VEMP's, ENoG (external unit) and BioMap.

Intelligent Hearing Systems, Corp. 800-447-9783
6860 SW 81st St, Miami, FL 33143
SMART-EP: full featured auditory evoked potential system. SMART SCREENER: automated newborn hearing screener.

EVOKED RESPONSE UNIT *(Cns/Neurology) 84QUT*

Bio-Logic Systems Corp. 800-323-8326
1 Bio Logic Plz, Mundelein, IL 60060
NAVIGATOR PRO - microcomputer based systems which perform all modalities of AUDITORY EVOKED POTENTIALS (AEP), bone conduction, ECOG, P-300, 40Hz ERP, Multiple Auditory Steady State Response (MASTER, ASSR), Stacked ABR, Cochlear Hydrops (CHAMP), VEMP's, ENoG (external unit) and BioMap.

Cadwell Laboratories 800-245-3001
909 N Kellogg St, Kennewick, WA 99336
CADWELL SIERRA II EMG/EP does all protocals. CADWELL CASCADE EMG/EP. CADWELL CENTRAL EEG/EMG/EP. SIERRA II (2-4 ch) EMG/EP, Windows 98/xP/2000.

Lkc Technologies, Inc. 800-638-7055
2 Professional Dr Ste 222, Gaithersburg, MD 20879
The UTAS-E3000mf and the EPIC 4000 offers both VEP and Sweep VEP capability. The EPIC 4000 offers VEP and Sweep VEP in a cost and space efficient standalone system.

Md International, Inc. 305-669-9003
11300 NW 41st St, Doral, FL 33178

Nihon Kohden America, Inc. 800-325-0283
90 Icon, Foothill Ranch, CA 92610

Tsi Medical Ltd. 800-661-7263
47 Athabascan Ave., Unit 105, Sherwood Park, AB T8A-4H3 Canada

EVOKED RESPONSE UNIT, AUDITORY *(Ear/Nose/Throat) 77ETZ*

Bio-Logic Systems Corp. 800-323-8326
1 Bio Logic Plz, Mundelein, IL 60060
NAVIGATOR PRO - electrodiagnostic system complete with laptop computer and printer which performs AEP with optional two amplifier channels, bone conduction, ECOG, P-300, 40Hz ERP, digital filtering, graphmaster, MASTER (ASSR, Steady State EP), Stacked ABR, Cochlear Hydrops (CHAMP), Screening ABR (ABAER), Screening and diagnostic OAE (DP and TE); SCOUT SPORT performs diagnostic DPOAE and/or TEOAE - must be interfaced to a notebook computer to perform and VEMP's, ENoG (external unit) and BioMap.

Intelligent Hearing Systems, Corp. 800-447-9783
6860 SW 81st St, Miami, FL 33143
SMART-EP, SMART SCREENER, SMARTEP-ASSR

Natus Medical Inc. 800-255-3901
1501 Industrial Rd, San Carlos, CA 94070
The ALGO Newborn Hearing Screener uses patented AABR technology, providing an accurate, objective and cost-effective method of screening all newborns for hearing loss before hospital discharge.

EXAMINATION DEVICE, AC-POWERED *(General) 80KZF*

Aadco Medical, Inc. 800-225-9014
2279 VT Route 66, Randolph, VT 05060
Examination light.

Advanced Motion Measurement, Llc 602-263-8657
1202 E Maryland Ave Ste 1J, Phoenix, AZ 85014
Spine motion analyzer.

Burton Medical Products, Inc. 800-444-9909
21100 Lassen St, Chatsworth, CA 91311

Cameron-Miller, Inc. 800-621-0142
5410 W Roosevelt Rd, Road #241, Chicago, IL 60644

Global Surgical Corp. 314-861-3388
3610 Tree Court Industrial Blvd, Saint Louis, MO 63122
Halogen console lightsource.

Hill-Rom, Inc. 812-934-7777
4115 Dorchester Rd Unit 600, North Charleston, SC 29405
Various.

Jedmed Instruments Co. 314-845-3770
5416 Jedmed Ct, Saint Louis, MO 63129

Lic Care 800-323-5232
2935A Northeast Pkwy, Atlanta, GA 30360

Lucid, Inc. 585-239-9800
2320 Brighton Henrietta Town Line Rd, Rochester, NY 14623
Vivascope 1500.

Maquet, Inc. 843-552-8652
7371 Spartan Blvd E, N Charleston, SC 29418
Various models of ac-powered medical examination lights.

Medical Depot 516-998-4600
99 Seaview Blvd, Port Washington, NY 11050
Examination lamp.

Welch Allyn, Inc. 800-535-6663
4341 State Street Rd, Skaneateles Falls, NY 13153

EXCAVATOR, DENTAL, OPERATIVE *(Dental And Oral) 76EKC*

Aesculap Implant Systems Inc. 1-800-234-9179
3773 Corporate Pkwy, Center Valley, PA 18034

Biomet Microfixation Inc. 800-874-7711
1520 Tradeport Dr, Jacksonville, FL 32218
Excavator, dental, operative.

Cameron-Miller, Inc. 800-621-0142
5410 W Roosevelt Rd, Road #241, Chicago, IL 60644

Dental Usa, Inc. 815-363-8003
5005 McCullom Lake Rd, McHenry, IL 60050
Excavator.

Dentalez Group 866-DTE-INFO
101 Lindenwood Dr Ste 225, Valleybrooke Corporate Center Malvern, PA 19355

Dentalez Group, Stardental Division 717-291-1161
1816 Colonial Village Ln, Lancaster, PA 17601
Explorer, operative.

E.A. Beck & Co. 949-645-4072
657 W 19th St Ste E, P O Box 10857, Costa Mesa, CA 92627
Spoon or excavator.

Frank J. May, Inc. 215-923-3165
256 S 11th St, Philadelphia, PA 19107
Various types of dental hand inst.

Hu-Friedy Manufacturing Co., Inc. 800-483-7433
3232 N Rockwell St, Chicago, IL 60618
$21.00 to 22.85, 25 types.

Micro-Dent Inc. 866-526-1166
379 Hollow Hill Rd, Wauconda, IL 60084
Excavators.

Miltex Dental Technologies, Inc. 516-576-6022
589 Davies Dr, York, PA 17402
Various dental excavators.

Nordent Manufacturing, Inc. 800-966-7336
610 Bonnie Ln, Elk Grove Village, IL 60007
$17.50 per unit (standard).

Pac-Dent Intl., Inc. 909-839-0888
21078 Commerce Point Dr, Walnut, CA 91789
Various types of excavator.

Premier Dental Products Co. 888-670-6100
1710 Romano Dr, PO Box 4500, Plymouth Meeting, PA 19462

Sci-Dent, Inc. 800-323-4145
210 Dowdle St Ste 2, Algonquin, IL 60102

Suter Dental Manufacturing Company, Inc. 800-368-8376
632 Cedar St, Chico, CA 95928

Ultradent Products, Inc. 801-553-4586
505 W 10200 S, South Jordan, UT 84095
Excavator.

EXCAVATOR, EAR *(Ear/Nose/Throat) 77JYH*

Aesculap Implant Systems Inc. 1-800-234-9179
3773 Corporate Pkwy, Center Valley, PA 18034

EXERCISE STAIR *(Physical Med) 89QUU*

Alimed, Inc. 800-225-2610
297 High St, Dedham, MA 02026

Cybex International, Inc. 508-533-4300
10 Trotter Dr, Medway, MA 02053

Hausmann Industries, Inc. 888-428-7626
130 Union St, Northvale, NJ 07647
6 models - $1,175 to $1,985.

Hoggan Health Industries, Inc. 800-678-7888
8020 S 1300 W, West Jordan, UT 84088
SPRINT STEP electronic display stair climber.

Life Fitness 800-735-3867
10601 Belmont Ave, Franklin Park, IL 60131

Nautilus, Inc. 360-859-2900
16400 SE Nautilus Dr, Vancouver, WA 98683
StairMaster climber products

Thera-Tronics, Inc. 800-267-6211
623 Mamaroneck Ave, Mamaroneck, NY 10543

EXERCISER, ARM *(Physical Med) 89QUV*

Creative Health Products, Inc. 800-742-4478
5148 Saddle Ridge Rd, Plymouth, MI 48170
HUDSON UBE Ergometer, portable table top upper body ergometer with pulse monitor $489.00 for CHP. MONARK Arm Ergometer rehab trainer table top model $1189.00.

EXERCISER, ARM *(cont'd)*

Elginex Corporation 800-279-3762
270 Eisenhower Ln N Unit 4-A, Lombard, IL 60148
$810 to $2,354 for wall pulley systems.

Hausmann Industries, Inc. 888-428-7626
130 Union St, Northvale, NJ 07647
Exercise pulley weight sets - $44.50 to $965.00 ea.

Hoggan Health Industries, Inc. 800-678-7888
8020 S 1300 W, West Jordan, UT 84088
Sprint Upper Body Ergometer provides cardiovascular exercise and upper-body conditioning. Adjustable crank arms provide foward or backward motion, wheel chair accessible, self-contained.

Optp 888-819-0121
3800 Annapolis Ln N Ste 165, PO Box 47009, Minneapolis, MN 55447
B.O.I.N.G., oscillating flexible exercise rod for shoulder and arm.

EXERCISER, BICYCLE *(Physical Med) 89QUW*

Alimed, Inc. 800-225-2610
297 High St, Dedham, MA 02026

Battle Creek Equipment Co. 800-253-0854
307 Jackson St W, Battle Creek, MI 49037
HEALTH BIKE, welded frame and shipped set-up. $229.00 PULSESTAR, adjustable resistance, UPS shippable. $249.00

Champion Manufacturing, Llc. 800-998-5018
2601 Industrial Pkwy, Elkhart, IN 46516

Creative Health Products, Inc. 800-742-4478
5148 Saddle Ridge Rd, Plymouth, MI 48170
MONARK ergometer bikes, Professional Model 828E $1198.00; weight ergometer Model 874E $1388.75. CATEYE ergometer bikes and recumbents, Models EC-3200 $655.00, EC-1600 $1487.00, EC-3500 $969.00, EC-3700 $1759.00, EC-C400 $1110.00, EC-C400R $1529.00, EC-UB200 $2225.00 from CHP.

Cybex International, Inc. 508-533-4300
10 Trotter Dr, Medway, MA 02053
Exercycle

Dedicated Distribution 800-325-8367
640 Miami Ave, Kansas City, KS 66105

Elmed, Inc. 630-543-2792
60 W Fay Ave, Addison, IL 60101

Hoggan Health Industries, Inc. 800-678-7888
8020 S 1300 W, West Jordan, UT 84088
SPRINT recumbent bikes features eddy current resistance system, self-powered, easy to use, walk through feature provides easy entry and exit.

Kettler International 757-427-2400
PO Box 2747, 1355 London Bridge Rd, Virginia Beach, VA 23450
Ergometer SX1, semi-recumbent, stationary exercise bike (suitable for therapeutic training in accordance with DIN EN 957-1/5, class A). Training computer - power in watts (25-400), energy consumption in kilojoules, distance covered, speed, pulse rate, recovery pulse raye, 10 resident training programs, PC interface. Electromagnetic eddy-current brake. Also Ergometer AX1, upright, stationary bike (same in accordance as the SX1, class A), and almost all the same features as the SX1.

Life Fitness 800-735-3867
10601 Belmont Ave, Franklin Park, IL 60131
Lifecycle.

Med-Fit Systems, Inc. 800-831-7665
3553 Rosa Way, Fallbrook, CA 92028

Nautilus, Inc. 360-859-2900
16400 SE Nautilus Dr, Vancouver, WA 98683
Musculoskeletal and rehabilitation exercisers for medical therapy and home-use; also available. Products from Schwinn Fitness, StairMaster, and Nautilus.

Thera-Tronics, Inc. 800-267-6211
623 Mamaroneck Ave, Mamaroneck, NY 10543

Vacumed 800-235-3333
4538 Westinghouse St, Ventura, CA 93003

EXERCISER, CHEST *(Physical Med) 89QUX*

Alimed, Inc. 800-225-2610
297 High St, Dedham, MA 02026

Cybex International, Inc. 800-667-6544
10 Trotter Dr, Medway, MA 02053
Trunk extension/Flexion (TEF) testing & rehab unit, $43,990.

Elginex Corporation 800-279-3762
270 Eisenhower Ln N Unit 4-A, Lombard, IL 60148
$810 to $2,354 for wall pulley systems.

EXERCISER, CHEST *(cont'd)*

Fitness Plus, Inc. 888-778-4019
PO Box 516, Valley City, ND 58072

Hausmann Industries, Inc. 888-428-7626
130 Union St, Northvale, NJ 07647
$467.00 per unit (standard).

Med-Fit Systems, Inc. 800-831-7665
3553 Rosa Way, Fallbrook, CA 92028

Nautilus, Inc. 360-859-2900
16400 SE Nautilus Dr, Vancouver, WA 98683
$500 for abduction/lower back exercise machine for home-use. Musculoskeletal and rehabilitation exercisers for medical therapy and home-use.

EXERCISER, FINGER, POWERED *(Physical Med) 89JFA*

Jace Systems 800-800-4276
2 Pin Oak Ln Ste 200, Cherry Hill, NJ 08003
The JACE hand CPM, at 10.5 oz is the lightest on the market. Allowing for full 0-260 degrees of motion and full isolated MCP joint motion, 0-90 degrees. With Features including a Warm-up mode- gently and gradually progresses to the full range of programmed motion, and Dynamic Tension mode- converts CPM to low-load prolonged stress to the tissues while reading tissue resistance and automatically adjusting range of motion.

Kinetic Muscles, Inc. 480-557-0448
2103 E Cedar St Ste 3, Tempe, AZ 85281
Neuromuscular therapy device.

Meddev Corporation 800-543-2789
730 N Pastoria Ave, Sunnyvale, CA 94085
THUMBHELPER and FINGERHELPER are progressive resistive force exercisers for exercising individual fingers and thumb.

Orthologic Canada 602-286-5520
901 Dillingham Rd, Pickering L1W 2Y5 Canada
Various types

Zimmer Holdings, Inc. 800-613-6131
1800 W Center St, PO Box 708, Warsaw, IN 46580

EXERCISER, HAND *(Physical Med) 89QUY*

Alimed, Inc. 800-225-2610
297 High St, Dedham, MA 02026

Ball Dynamics International, Llc 800-752-2255
14215 Mead St, Longmont, CO 80504

Bte Technologies, Inc. 800-331-8845
7455 New Ridge Rd Ste L, Hanover, MD 21076
PrimusRS- Isometric, Isotonic, Isokinetic, Eccentric, CPM, Task Simulation, Hand Therapy, Lifting Evaluations, Sports Medicine. Simulator II- Isometric, Isotonic, Task Simulation, Hand Therapy, Geriatrics, Lifting Evaluations.

Cfi Medical Solutions (Contour Fabricators, Inc.) 810-750-5300
14241 N Fenton Rd, Fenton, MI 48430

Creative Health Products, Inc. 800-742-4478
5148 Saddle Ridge Rd, Plymouth, MI 48170
GRIP MASTER Hand and Finger Exercisers, 5 lb, 7 lb or 9 lb per finger $ 11.50 each from CHP.

George C. Bishop Company 800-476-7374
PO Box 684, Horsham, PA 19044
$5.60 per unit (2oz standard) for BISHOP'S PUTTY.

J. T. Posey Co. 800-447-6739
5635 Peck Rd, Arcadia, CA 91006

Maddak Inc. 800-443-4926
661 State Route 23, Wayne, NJ 07470
ABLEWARE.

Magister Corporation 800-396-3130
310 Sylvan St, Chattanooga, TN 37405
Eggsercizer Hand Exercise for finger, hand and forearm rehabiliation; 4 resistances

Meddev Corporation 800-543-2789
730 N Pastoria Ave, Sunnyvale, CA 94085
HANDHELPER: progressive resistive rubberband hand exerciser. ISO HANDHELPER: progressive resisitve forcehand exerciser. SOFT TOUCH: kit using three densities of foam to offer graded levels of exercise progression. THE ULTIMATE HAND HELPER, progressive resistive rubberband hand exerciser curved for varied muscle interaction.

Southwest Technologies, Inc. 800-247-9951
1746 E Levee St, North Kansas City, MO 64116
Cloth covered gel hand exerciser.

EXERCISER, ISOROBIC *(Physical Med) 89SGS*

Fitness Motivation Institute Of America, Inc. 800-538-7790
26685 Sussex Hwy Ste A, Seaford, DE 19973
$299.95 for isorobic exerciser unit with video instructions.

Nautilus, Inc. 360-859-2900
16400 SE Nautilus Dr, Vancouver, WA 98683
Musculoskeletal and rehabilitation exercisers for medical therapy and home-use.

EXERCISER, LEG AND ANKLE *(Physical Med) 89QUZ*

Alimed, Inc. 800-225-2610
297 High St, Dedham, MA 02026

Cfi Medical Solutions (Contour Fabricators, Inc.) 810-750-5300
14241 N Fenton Rd, Fenton, MI 48430

Colonial Scientific Ltd. 902-468-1811
201 Brownlow Ave., Unit 52, Dartmouth, NS B3B-1W2 Canada
Medical weights for rehabilitaion.

Cybex International, Inc. 800-667-6544
10 Trotter Dr, Medway, MA 02053
$3,390.00 for leg and knee exerciser ORTHOTRON KT1.

Dm Systems, Inc. 800-254-5438
1316 Sherman Ave, Evanston, IL 60201
ANKLETOUGH® REHAB SYSTEM is a progressive resistive strengthening program for the prevention or post injury treatment of ankle sprains or fractures. The AnkleTough® straps are available as a set of four progressive resistance strengths or as an 8-pack (same strength) available in each of the 4 resistive tensions. We have improved patient compliance with an exercise instruction guide and resistive straps easily carried in purse or pocket.

Elginex Corporation 800-279-3762
270 Eisenhower Ln N Unit 4-A, Lombard, IL 60148
$550.00 for standard unit; Foot exerciser $25.00 for ARCHXERCISER.

Fitness Plus, Inc. 888-778-4019
PO Box 516, Valley City, ND 58072

Hausmann Industries, Inc. 888-428-7626
130 Union St, Northvale, NJ 07647
Weight belts - 1/2 to 20 lb. - $6.85 to $40.25 ea.

Optp 888-819-0121
3800 Annapolis Ln N Ste 165, PO Box 47009, Minneapolis, MN 55447
ROCK balance platform for ankle rehabilitation.

Pre Pak Products, Inc. 800-544-7257
4055 Oceanside Blvd Ste L, Oceanside, CA 92056
ANKLE WEIGHT BAG, progressive, resistive exercise device for strengthening lower extremity; $15.25 each, quantity discounts available.

Rand-Scot Inc. 800-467-7967
401 Linden Center Dr, Fort Collins, CO 80524
Saratoga Cycle: Exerciser, leg and ankle; Saratoga Cycle, Colorado Sport cycle, adjustable height cycle table, adjustable table for Monark Rehabtrainer and Spirit Cycles for arm and leg use.

Zimmer Holdings, Inc. 800-613-6131
1800 W Center St, PO Box 708, Warsaw, IN 46580

EXERCISER, MEASURING *(Physical Med) 89ISD*

Biodex Medical Systems, Inc. 800-224-6339
20 Ramsey Rd, Shirley, NY 11967
Upper Body Cycle, BioStep Semi-Recumbent Elliptical Trainer and RTM Treadmill.

Breg, Inc., An Orthofix Company 800-897-BREG
2611 Commerce Way, Vista, CA 92081
Balance board.

Bte Technologies, Inc. 800-331-8845
7455 New Ridge Rd Ste L, Hanover, MD 21076
PrimusRS- Comprehensive system for functional evaluation and rehabilitation; EvalTech- Comprehensive Functional Capacity Evaluation and Post Offer of Employment Testing system; MCU- Multi-Cervical Unit measures the three planes of motion of the cervical spine and provides resistive exercises for strengthening.

Creative Health Products, Inc. 800-742-4478
5148 Saddle Ridge Rd, Plymouth, MI 48170
BACK, LEG & CHEST STRENGTH TESTER, $323.50.00 for CHP Analog unit, $ 465.00 for CHP Digital unit

Cybex International, Inc. 800-667-6544
10 Trotter Dr, Medway, MA 02053
$52,900 for trunk extension flexion testing & rehab. system; $38,900 for torso rotation testing & rehab. system: $42,700 for lifting capability screening & training system; $25,990 for LiftTask Lifting capability and training unit.

EXERCISER, MEASURING *(cont'd)*

Fitness Motivation Institute Of America, Inc. 800-538-7790
26685 Sussex Hwy Ste A, Seaford, DE 19973
$1,895.00 for digital strength meter.

Lifeline Usa 800-553-6633
3201 Syene Rd, Madison, WI 53713
Multi-use shoulder pulley with door attachment, add-on attachment, and metal door bracket.

Nautilus, Inc. 360-859-2900
16400 SE Nautilus Dr, Vancouver, WA 98683
Musculoskeletal and rehabilitation exercisers for medical therapy and home-use.

Performance Health Technologies 800-722-4749
427 River View Plz, Trenton, NJ 08611
Core:Tx for Stroke Survivors assists with neuromuscular reeducation, by tracking and measuring range of motion in real-time as patient performs exercises.

EXERCISER, NON-MEASURING *(Physical Med) 89ION*

Advanced Circulatory Systems, Inc. 952-947-9590
7615 Golden Triangle Dr Ste A, Eden Prairie, MN 55344
Respiratory muscle trainer.

Ameret Llc 913-888-5248
9025 Rosehill Rd, Lenexa, KS 66215
Exerciser.

Apec, Inc. 800-746-8421
2740 N 49th St Apt 6, Lincoln, NE 68504
Tibialis anterior muscle exerciser.

Backproject Corporation 408-280-7500
341 N Montgomery St, San Jose, CA 95110

Backstrong International Llc. 714-671-1150
710 N Brea Blvd Ste G, Brea, CA 92821
Variable angle roman chair.

Ball Dynamics International, Llc 800-752-2255
14215 Mead St, Longmont, CO 80504

Battle Creek Equipment Co. 800-253-0854
307 Jackson St W, Battle Creek, MI 49037
PEDLAR, Light workout exerciser, $49.95.

Biomet Microfixation Inc. 800-874-7711
1520 Tradeport Dr, Jacksonville, FL 32218
Hand-operated jaw exerciser.

Breg, Inc., An Orthofix Company 800-897-BREG
2611 Commerce Way, Vista, CA 92081
Balance execiser.

Christy Manufacturing Corp. 925-462-7982
1228 Quarry Ln Ste F, Pleasanton, CA 94566
Active exerciser.

Columbia-Inland Corporation 503-657-6676
415 17th St Ste 2, Oregon City, OR 97045
Therapeutic mobility device.

Community Products, Llc 845-658-7723
2032 Route 213, Rifton, NY 12471
Tricycle.

Depuy Orthopaedics, Inc. 800-473-3789
700 Orthopaedic Dr, P.O. Box 988, Warsaw, IN 46582
Various types of non-measuring exercisers.

Dj Orthopedics De Mexico, S.A. De C.V. 690-727-1280
Blvd., Delagacion La Presa, Tijuana 22397 Mexico
Cpm pads

Dj Orthopedics De Mexico, S.A. De C.V. 690-727-1280
Ave. Venustiano Carranza 6802, Castillo, Tijuana 22100 Mexico
Cpm pads

DJO Inc. 800-336-6569
1430 Decision St, Vista, CA 92081
Digi-Flex exerciser system.

Dynatronics Corp. Chattanooga Operations 801-568-7000
6607 Mountain View Rd, Ooltewah, TN 37363
Overdoor pulley.

Elginex Corporation 800-279-3762
270 Eisenhower Ln N Unit 4-A, Lombard, IL 60148
$810 to $2,354 for wall pulley systems.

Empi 651-415-9000
Clear Lake Industrial Park, Clear Lake, SD 57226
Knee exercise orthosis.

EXERCISER, NON-MEASURING *(cont'd)*

Engineering Marketing Assoc. Dba Impulse Training Systems 800-964-2362
PO Box 2312, 339 Millard Farmer Industrial Blvd, Newnan, GA 30264
Inertial Exercise Training

Et Training Systems, Llc 313-864-1317
3494 Cambridge Ave, Detroit, MI 48221
Resistance trainer exerciser.

Evolve Projects, Llc 330-253-5060
75 E Market St, Attn: Matthew A. Heinle, Akron, OH 44308

Fitness Plus, Inc. 888-778-4019
PO Box 516, Valley City, ND 58072
WEIGHT STACK.

Foot Levelers, Inc. 540-345-0008
518 Pocahontas Ave NE, P.o. Box 12611, Roanoke, VA 24012
Exerciser.

Freedom Concepts, Inc. 800-661-9915
45117 RPO Regent, Winnipeg, MB R2C 5C7 Canada
Alternative mobility aid.

Function Technologies, Inc. 517-702-0912
805 N Jenison Ave, Lansing, MI 48915
The health well.

Gesturetek Health-Gesturetek Inc 408-216-8087
530 Lakeside Dr Ste 280, Sunnyvale, CA 94085

Gull Works Mfg. Llc 801-423-2812
685 E 600 S, Salem, UT 84653
Therapeutic tricycle.

Harmonizer
448 Silver Oaks Dr Apt 5, Kent, OH 44240
Exercise platform.

Hausmann Industries, Inc. 888-428-7626
130 Union St, Northvale, NJ 07647

Health Equipment Manufacturers, Inc. 269-962-6181
702 S Reed Rd, Fremont, IN 46737
Exceriser.

Kneebourne Therapeutic, Llc 317-776-2770
15299 Stony Creek Way, Noblesville, IN 46060
Nonmeasuring exerciser.

Lordex, Inc. 281-395-9512
32357 Morton Rd Bldg 3, Brookshire, TX 77423
Exercise equipment.

M.W. Sales And Service, Inc. 830-303-2508
2549 Odaniel Rd, Seguin, TX 78155
Weighted or pressure devices.

Maddak Inc. 800-443-4926
661 State Route 23, Wayne, NJ 07470
ABLEWARE.

Miles Ahead Products 615-834-0195
3137 Glencliff Rd, Nashville, TN 37211
Passive stretching device lower leg and foot.

Nautilus, Inc. 360-859-2900
16400 SE Nautilus Dr, Vancouver, WA 98683
Musculoskeletal and rehabilitation exercisers for medical therapy and home-use.

Nesar Systems, Inc. 724-827-8172
420 Ashwood Rd, Darlington, PA 16115
Shoulder rehabilitation device.

Nu-Back 262-695-1660
140 Sussex St, Pewaukee, WI 53072
Fit-back.

Olympic Sport, Inc. 914-347-4737
500 Executive Blvd, Elmsford, NY 10523
Hand strengthening glove.

Oral-Tx, Llc 580-832-3058
121 S Market St, Cordell, OK 73632
Facial exerciser.

Patterson Medical Supply, Inc. 262-387-8720
W68N158 Evergreen Blvd, Cedarburg, WI 53012
Various types of excerise equipment (barbellskickboards,paddles, mats).

Posturizer, Inc.
89 Lincoln Ave, Mastic Beach, NY 11951
Postural realignment exercise device.

EXERCISER, NON-MEASURING *(cont'd)*

Powerlung, Inc. 713-465-1180
10690 Shadow Wood Dr Ste 100, Houston, TX 77043
Respiratory muscle strength training device.

Pre Pak Products, Inc. 800-544-7257
4055 Oceanside Blvd Ste L, Oceanside, CA 92056
THE ROPE, $13.50 each, quantity discounts. A simple stretching device to be used as an excercise and rehab regimen. Helps create flexible muscles and joints, allowing the body to move through a pain-free range of motion. Comes complete with web-strap, custom braided rope & rubber handles. THE ROLLER, $13.50 each, a highly effective device for treatment of soft tissue and musculo-skeletal problems: trigger points, myofascial adhesions, forward head syndrome, excessive kyphosis,occipital/axis contractures. Made of solid, tree-farmed hardwood and will not become distorted or deteriorate over time.

Quadriciser Corporation 865-689-5003
6624 Central Avenue Pike, Knoxville, TN 37912
Cpm device (continuous passive motion) device.

Ram Plus, Llc 435-781-1646
983 N 2175 W, Vernal, UT 84078
Exerciser, non-measuring.

Rehab Innovations, Inc. 402-445-4335
8727 Ames Ave, Omaha, NE 68134
Therapeutic exercise equipment class i.

Rehabilitation Technical Components, Corp. 919-732-1705
3913 Devonwood Rd, Hillsborough, NC 27278
Finger flexon glove.

Richardson Products, Inc. 888-928-7297
9408 Gulfstream Rd, Frankfort, IL 60423
Exercise equipment.

Shuttle Systems By Contemporary Design Co. 800-334-5633
10005 Mt. Baker Hwy., Glacier, WA 98244-5089
The Shuttle Miniclinic by Contemporary Design is a three foot long 20 pound portable leg press for safe, controlled, graduated lower-extremity exercise leading to faster safer healing and recovery from knee and hip surgery such as total hip replacements, total knee replacement, ACL repairs and stroke recovery patterning.

Smc Medical Manufacturing Division 715-247-3500
360 Reed St, Somerset, WI 54025
Back stretching product.

Tangle, Inc. 650-616-7900
439C Eccles Ave, South San Francisco, CA 94080
Non-measuring exerciser.

Team America Health & Fitness, Inc 800-642-5419
675 Racquet Club Ln, Thousand Oaks, CA 91360
EGX for EXER-GENIE standard unit; prices range from $69.95-$149.95. THE TRAINER rehab and training systems using variable isokinetic resistance device, portable, price range: $95.00-$199.95 (rope friction device). THE TRAINER Skate Belt, skating rehab and strength/skill development using variable resistance, adjustable harness, for ice skating or rollerblading. THE TRAINER Fit For Sport, variable rope friction system to aid in static, dynamic, functional muscle, joint and movement rehab and strength development. EXER-GENIE EXERCISER/THE TRAINER, variable-resistance rope friction device, employing variable isokinetic, isometric, and isotonic movements, $199-$299. THE TRAINER EXER-GENIE Rehab and Training System, speed development system, 120-ft. rope friction used for walking, jogging, or running rehab and speed developments. Indoor or out.

The Hygenic Corp. 800-321-2135
1245 Home Ave, Akron, OH 44310
Hand exerciser.

The Pettibon System 888-774-6258
2118 Jackson Hwy, Chehalis, WA 98532
Wobble chair,various non measuring exercise equipment,fulcrum exercise program.

The Saunders Group 800-445-9836
4250 Norex Dr, Chaska, MN 55318
Various types of exercisers with handles.

Therafin Corporation 800-843-7234
19747 Wolf Rd, Mokena, IL 60448
Various exercise aids.

Therapeutic Dimensions, Inc. 509-323-9275
319 W Hastings Rd, Po Box 28307, Spokane, WA 99218
Resistive hand exerciser.

EXERCISER, NON-MEASURING *(cont'd)*

Total Molding Services, Inc. 215-538-9613
354 East Broad St., Trumbauersville, PA 18970
Therabite jaw-motion rehab system.

Total Motion, Inc. 281-386-8747
19606 Piney Place Ct, Houston, TX 77094
Exerciser.

Tri W-G Group 800-437-8011
215 12th Ave NE, PO Box 905, Valley City, ND 58072
FITNESS PLUS Weight stack units for rehab.

Tumble Forms, Inc. 262-387-8720
1013 Barker Rd, Dolgeville, NY 13329
Multiple.

Viscolas, Inc. 800-548-2694
8801 Consolidated Dr, Soddy Daisy, TN 37379
Hand exerciser.

EXERCISER, OTHER *(Physical Med) 89QVE*

American Imex 800-521-8286
16520 Aston, Irvine, CA 92606
PFX2- Pelvic floor exerciser.

Aplix, Inc. 704-588-1920
12300 Steele Creek Rd, Charlotte, NC 28273

Athena Feminine Technologies, Inc 866-308-4436
179 Moraga Way, Orinda, CA 94563
The Athena Pelvic Muscle Trainer is a cordless productthat is inserted like a tampon and is controlled by a remote control. The PMT automatically stimulates the pelvic floor muscles to do Kegel exercises. It has a 15-minute cycle and then shuts off automatically. The intensity of the contractions is easily controlled. Clinical studies prove that the Athena PMT is safe and effective. The Athena Pelvic Muscle Trainer is FDA approved and Medicare reimbursable. It will be available by prescription.

Cfi Medical Solutions (Contour Fabricators, Inc.) 810-750-5300
14241 N Fenton Rd, Fenton, MI 48430

Columbia Medical Manufacturing Llc 800-454-6612
13577 Larwin Cir, Santa Fe Springs, CA 90670
TheraGait Training System for Facilities and Personal Use. The Columbia Medical TheraGait meets the rehabilitation needs of many patients. Combined with its unique ambulation support system for added safety and comfort, the TheraGait makes rehabilitation therapy easier and safer for both the patient and caregiver.

Cybex International, Inc. 800-667-6544
10 Trotter Dr, Medway, MA 02053
$1,495 and up for variable resistance weight exercise and rehab. unit; $7,625 for KINETRON II lower limb exercise and training model.

Dm Systems, Inc. 800-254-5438
1316 Sherman Ave, Evanston, IL 60201
ADJUSTICIZER™ EXERCISE SYSTEM is a totally adjustable bungee cord strengthening device. It is the only such device that can be adjusted for both length and tension. It also comes with a 64-page exercise manual so that anyone can strengthen all muscle groups conveniently. The Adjusticizer™ is a six-ounce total body workout!

Engineering Marketing Assoc. Dba Impulse Training Systems 800-964-2362
PO Box 2312, 339 Millard Farmer Industrial Blvd, Newnan, GA 30264
High Performance Inertial Exercise Trainer

Equipment Shop, Inc. 800-525-7681
PO Box 33, Bedford, MA 01730
Tricycle accessories. Back support, upright handlebars, foot pedal attachments and pommel for positioning on a tricycle for the physically challenged. $125.35 a set.

Fitness Plus, Inc. 888-778-4019
PO Box 516, Valley City, ND 58072
Abdominal, back, cervical and multi-hip exercisers.

Heart Rate, Inc. 800-237-2271
3190 Airport Loop Dr, Costa Mesa, CA 92626
$1,895 to $4,995for VERSA CLIMBER Total Body exercise machine.

Hoggan Health Industries, Inc. 800-678-7888
8020 S 1300 W, West Jordan, UT 84088
CAMSTAR selectorized variable resistance single station exercising equipment; SPRINT CIRCUIT 15 piece resistance training circuit; cast plate, rubber plated, chrome and stainless dumbbells; beauty bells, SPRINT CROSS TRAINER elliptical.

I-Rep, Inc. 800-828-0852
508 Chaney St Ste B, Lake Elsinore, CA 92530
Exercise equipment.

EXERCISER, OTHER *(cont'd)*

Jace Systems 800-800-4276
2 Pin Oak Ln Ste 200, Cherry Hill, NJ 08003
The JACE Toe CPM is the ONLY device specifically designed to assist with rehabilitation of the toe joints. The JACE Toe CPM has a Handheld Controller with easy to set parameters:Range of motion 0 to 90 degrees extension and 0 to 60 degrees flexion, adjustable speed and pause with optional muscle stim capability.

Kettler International 757-427-2400
PO Box 2747, 1355 London Bridge Rd, Virginia Beach, VA 23450
Medic Sport, back trainer with height and angle adjustment and comfortable kneeling position designed to avoid excessive strain to the spinal column.

Lafayette Instrument Company 800-428-7545
PO Box 5729, 3700 Sagamore Pkwy,, Lafayette, IN 47903
Fitness-evaluation equipment, FIT-KIT, Model 01180, Canadian standards test.

Life Fitness 800-735-3867
10601 Belmont Ave, Franklin Park, IL 60131
Elliptical trainer.

Magister Corporation 800-396-3130
310 Sylvan St, Chattanooga, TN 37405
REP Band latex-free exercise bands and tubing

Medx Corporation 800-876-6339
1401 NE 77th St, Ocala, FL 34479
Lumbar extension and cervical extension. Designed for muscle testing and rehabilitation.

Noram Solutions 800-387-7103
PO Box 543, Lewiston, NY 14092
(SABA) rehabilitation equipment as used in medical exercise therapy (MET). TARGET Balance Trainer with visual & audio feedback.

Ooltewah Manufacturing 800-251-6040x25
5722 Main St, P.O. Box 587, Ooltewah, TN 37363
Therapeutic weights.

Ppr Direct, Inc. 800-526-3668
74 20th St, Brooklyn, NY 11232
SuperKegel incontinence exerciser.

Pre Pak Products, Inc. 800-544-7257
4055 Oceanside Blvd Ste L, Oceanside, CA 92056
WEB-SLIDE EXERCISE RAIL SYSTEM. This home exercise and rehab training station is an in-clinic system containing everything the clinician needs to quickly and effectively teach patients exercises they can perform at home. $548.50 includes: 3 Exercise Rails, a Storage Rack to hold 16 pieces of exercise equipment, a 14 piece inventory of assorted exercise devices, a 2' x 3' Product Wall Poster, and 5 'Tear-Off' Sheet Exercise Pads for each of the 5 exercise devices in the system. Components also sold separately.

True Fitness 800-426-6570
865 Hoff Rd, St Peters, MO 63366
TRUE ELLIPTICAL, full commercial elliptical cross trainer with standard-contact heart rate. TRUE UPRIGHT, upright stationary bike with a commercial 3-year warranty. RECUMBENT - 750R, recumbent stationary bike - full commercial - 3-year parts and labor warranty. TNT 2000 - True Natural Trainer, arm powered treadmill - full commercial use - 3-years parts and labor warranty.

Universal Gym Equipment 800-843-3906
PO Box 1296, PO Box 1270, West Point, MS 39773
CENTURION weight training equipment; SPARTAN and MAXIMUS compact weight training equipment; POWER CIRCUIT powder coated weight equipment. PROFLEX Flexibility system.

EXERCISER, PASSIVE, MEASURING *(Physical Med) 89ISC*

Ormed Corporation 800-440-2784
599 Cardigan Rd, Saint Paul, MN 55126
ARTROMOT and K3 continuous passive motion device (CPM) for the knee, ARTROMOT K4 CPM for the knee and hip joint, ARTROMOT S2 CPM for the shoulder, ARTROMOT SB CPM for shoulder attachment to bed, ARTROMOT SP2 CPM for the ankle and ARTROMOT E CPM for elbow. ARTROMOT S2Pro anatomically correct shoulder CPM.

EXERCISER, PASSIVE, NON-MEASURING (CPM MACHINE)
(Physical Med) 89IOO

Action Products, Inc. 800-228-7763
954 Sweeney Dr, Hagerstown, MD 21740
Hand exercises for hot/cold therapy. It will never fully compress or lose its shape. Builds hand, wrist, and arm strength.

EXERCISER, PASSIVE, NON-MEASURING (CPM MACHINE) *(cont'd)*

Capstone Therapeutics 800-937-5520
1275 W Washington St, Tempe, AZ 85281
LEGASUS CPM continuous passive motion therapy for total knee replacements, ligament reconstruction, and repairs. WAVEFLEX CFT continuous passive motion therapy for the hand. Also model CPM 9000AT continuous passive motion therapy for the ankle, and ORTHOMOTION continuous passive motion therapy for the shoulder.

Chattanooga Group 800-592-7329
4717 Adams Rd, Hixson, TN 37343
OPTIFLEX and OPTIFLEX-S cont. passive motion devices. Allows hyperextention (-10 deg) to full knee-flexion, (120 deg). OPTIFLEX-T Trolley, OPTI-LIFT, bedmount and storage rack accessories.

Dedicated Distribution 800-325-8367
640 Miami Ave, Kansas City, KS 66105
Continuous passive motion machines.

Empi, Inc. 800-328-2536
599 Cardigan Rd, Saint Paul, MN 55126
Continuous motion therapy system CM-100 with or without neuromuscular stimulator.

Jace Systems 800-800-4276
2 Pin Oak Ln Ste 200, Cherry Hill, NJ 08003
The JACE Knee CPM is the Ultimate in patient comfort, convenience and portability...built to withstand the rigors of hospital and home use. The JACE Knee CPM has a Handheld Controller with easy to set parameters:Range of motion -3 to 120 degrees, adjustable speeds and pause and optional muscle stim capability. The JACE CPM also has a Warm-Up mode which gently and gradually progresses to the full range of programmed motion.

Orthomotion Inc. 800-387-5139
901 Dillingham Rd., Pickering, ONT L1W 2Y5 Canada
Lower limb and knee continuous motion with multifunctional controller, lightweight, quiet. Range 10 to 135 degee, fold up ease to storage, transport equipment.

Reha Partner Inc. 866-282-4558
530 Means St NW Ste 120, Atlanta, GA 30318
The CHALLENGER bikes and trycycles are available as 16' and 20'. They have a low frame for easy straddling and they are adjustable to grow. Direct drive or forward driven/backward freewheeling are available. I wide range of available options makes sure the CHALLENGER bike will fit to the needs of your child.

Select Medical Products, Inc. 800-276-7237
6531 47th St N, Pinellas Park, FL 33781
Continuous passive motion knee, hand, elbow, toe, & shoulder devices.

EXERCISER, POWERED *(Anesthesiology) 73BXB*

B2 Imports, Llc 918-557-5729
12807 E 90th St N, Owasso, OK 74055
Powered exercise equipment.

Bio-Gate Usa, Inc. 714-670-2771
6800 Orangethorpe Ave Ste E, Buena Park, CA 90620
Gait rehabilitation equipment.

Breg, Inc., An Orthofix Company 800-897-BREG
2611 Commerce Way, Vista, CA 92081
Shoulder continuous passive motion device.

Care Rehab And Orthopaedic Products, Inc. 703-448-9644
3930 Horseshoe Bend Rd, Keysville, VA 23947
Powered exercise equipment.

Conray, Inc. 623-465-7881
1950 E Watkins St Ste 110, Phoenix, AZ 85034
Water tread mill.

Discount Dme 714-630-9590
1265 N Grove St Ste A, Anaheim, CA 92806
Cpm device.

Endless Pools, Inc. 800-233-0741
200 E Dutton Mill Rd, Aston, PA 19014
Endless pool.

In Home Products, Inc. 800-810-8475
12015 Shiloh Rd Ste 158-B, Dallas, TX 75228
IN HOME PT MACHINE: designed for Paraplegics, Quadriplegics, Stroke Victims, and the elderly. Simple to use, no transferring out of wheelchair.Enhanced digital controls.

Interactive Motion Technologies, Inc. 617-497-6330
37 Spinelli Pl, Cambridge, MA 02138
Powered robotic exerciser.

EXERCISER, POWERED *(cont'd)*

Juvent Inc. 732-748-8866
300 Atrium Dr, Somerset, NJ 08873
Exerciser, powered.

Mckelor Technologies, Ltd. 800-273-5233
6312 Seeds Rd, Grove City, OH 43123
Continuous passive motion (CPM) devices.

Md Systems, Inc. 614-818-3000
5805 Chandler Ct, Westerville, OH 43082
Hand dynamometer.

Medical Graphics Corporation 800-950-5597
350 Oak Grove Pkwy, Saint Paul, MN 55127
CPE 2000/CARDIO-KEY compute- controlled work rate, electr. braked.

Nespa Enterprises, Inc. 888-479-4677
2800 Richter Ave Ste C, Oroville, CA 95966
Therapy pools.

Non-Invasive Monitoring Systems, Inc. 305-575-4200
4400 Biscayne Blvd, Miami, FL 33137
Acceleration platform.

Orbital Enterprises Llc 440-349-5100
6850 Cochran Rd, Solon, OH 44139
Continuous passive motion device.

Orthologic Canada 602-286-5520
901 Dillingham Rd, Pickering L1W 2Y5 Canada
Various types

Ozark Systems Manufacturing, Llc. 479-524-9778
501 N Lincoln St, Siloam Springs, AR 72761
Motorized bicycle exercise trainer (mbet).

Pneumex, Inc. 800-447-5792
2605 N Boyer Ave, Sandpoint, ID 83864
Unweight system.

Rehabtek Llc 847-853-8380
2510 Wilmette Ave, Wilmette, IL 60091
Continuous passive and active motion device.

Restorative Therapies Inc. 800-609-9166
907 S Lakewood Ave, Baltimore, MD 21224

Seca Corp. 800-542-7322
1352 Charwood Rd Ste E, Hanover, MD 21076
Three models available of cardiotest ergometer cycles and special order items.

Shapemaster Usa, Inc. 918-585-2377
823 S Detroit Ave Ste 410, Tulsa, OK 74120
Power assisted exercise machines.

T.C. Dynamics, Inc. 248-706-2021
5235 Greer Rd, West Bloomfield, MI 48324
'multiple', backpro cpm and backpro cpm lx.

Therapease Innovation, Llc 435-671-0886
32 N 1025 E, Lindon, UT 84042
Continuous passive motion device.

Value Tool Site Location 352-481-2659
10250 NE 130th Ave, Fort Mc Coy, FL 32134

Vision Quest Industries, Inc. 800-266-6969
18011 Mitchell S, Irvine, CA 92614
Continuous passive motion powered exercise equipment.

EXERCISER, RESPIRATORY *(Anesthesiology) 73QVA*

Covidien Lp 508-261-8000
15 Hampshire St, Mansfield, MA 02048

Creative Health Products, Inc. 800-742-4478
5148 Saddle Ridge Rd, Plymouth, MI 48170
POWERbreathe; strengthens inspiratory muscles, available in 3 models- wellness, fitness, sports peformance, $74.95 each for CHP unit

Medi Inc 800-225-8634
75 York Ave, P.O. Box 302, Randolph, MA 02368

Respironics New Jersey, Inc. 800-804-3443
5 Woodhollow Rd, Parsippany, NJ 07054
THRESHOLD, PFLEX, $9.95 for PFLEX variable resistance inspiratory muscle trainer. THRESHOLD, $24.95 variable resistance inspiratory muscle trainer.

EXERCISER, SHOULDER *(Physical Med) 89QVB*

Alimed, Inc. 800-225-2610
297 High St, Dedham, MA 02026

EXERCISER, SHOULDER *(cont'd)*

Bte Technologies, Inc. 800-331-8845
7455 New Ridge Rd Ste L, Hanover, MD 21076
PrimusRS- Isometric, Isotonic, Isokinetic, Eccentric, CPM, Task Simulation, Hand Therapy, Lifting Evaluations, Sports Medicine. Simulator II- Isometric, Isotonic, Task Simulation, Hand Therapy, Geriatrics, Lifting Evaluations.

Elginex Corporation 800-279-3762
270 Eisenhower Ln N Unit 4-A, Lombard, IL 60148
$810 to $2,354 for wall pulley systems.

Fitness Plus, Inc. 888-778-4019
PO Box 516, Valley City, ND 58072

Hausmann Industries, Inc. 888-428-7626
130 Union St, Northvale, NJ 07647
$467.00 per unit (standard).

EXERCISER, TRAPEZE *(Physical Med) 89QVC*

Zimmer Holdings, Inc. 800-613-6131
1800 W Center St, PO Box 708, Warsaw, IN 46580

EXERCISER, WRIST *(Physical Med) 89VLC*

Alimed, Inc. 800-225-2610
297 High St, Dedham, MA 02026

Balance Systems, Inc. 1-888-274-5444
1644 Plaza Way Ste 317, Walla Walla, WA 99362
FLEXTEND orthotic glove for the prevention and rehabilitation of carpal-tunnel syndrome and other repetitive-strain injuries.

Elginex Corporation 800-279-3762
270 Eisenhower Ln N Unit 4-A, Lombard, IL 60148
$810 to $2,354 for wall pulley systems. $6.60 and up for therapeutic weight cuffs weighing 1/4lb. to 20lbs., sold individually or in institutional sets; variable weight sets available in 5, 10, 15 & 20lb. sizes.

I-Rep, Inc. 800-828-0852
508 Chaney St Ste B, Lake Elsinore, CA 92530

Lifeline Usa 800-553-6633
3201 Syene Rd, Madison, WI 53713
Ankle and wrist attachment kit.

EXHAUST SYSTEM, SURGICAL *(Surgery) 79FYD*

Acuderm Inc. 800-327-0015
5370 NW 35th Ter Ste 106, Fort Lauderdale, FL 33309
Surgical smoke evacuator.

Biomet, Inc. 574-267-6639
56 E Bell Dr, PO Box 587, Warsaw, IN 46582
Various surgical exhaust apparatus.

Buffalo Filter, A Division Of Medtek Devices Inc. 800-343-2324
595 Commerce Dr, Amherst, NY 14228
LAPEVAC

Corpak Medsystems, Inc. 800-323-6305
100 Chaddick Dr, Wheeling, IL 60090
Smoke filtration systems-various sterile and non sterile.

Depuy Orthopaedics, Inc. 800-473-3789
700 Orthopaedic Dr, P.O. Box 988, Warsaw, IN 46582
Apparatus, exhaust, surgical (various types).

Dermatologic Lab & Supply, Inc. 800-831-6273
608 13th Ave, Council Bluffs, IA 51501
Saft-Evac Smoke Evacuator to remove plume from in-office electrosurgery procedures

Edge Systems Corporation 800-603-4996
2277 Redondo Ave, Signal Hill, CA 90755
Smoke evacuator.

I.C. Medical, Inc. 623-780-0700
2002 W Quail Ave, Phoenix, AZ 85027
Various types of smoke evacuators & sterile & non- sterile accessories.

Medtek Devices, Inc. 716-835-7000
595 Commerce Dr, 155 Pineview Dr., Amherst, NY 14228
Various smoke evacuators & filters.

Niche Medical, Inc. 800-633-1055
55 Access Rd, Warwick, RI 02886
SmartVac Smoke Evacuation System is ultra quiet, powerful, user friendly with a low cost per procedure. It safely collects hazardous surgical smoke/plume direct from the operative site.

Recto Molded Products Inc., Quinn Healthcare Products 513-871-5544
4425 Appleton St, Cincinnati, OH 45209
Laser smoke evacuator or filtrator.

EXHAUST SYSTEM, SURGICAL *(cont'd)*

Surgimedics 800-840-9906
2950 Mechanic St, Lake City, PA 16423
Surgifresh mini plume inator purevac.

Vision Pro Llc 800-892-3937
4309 I 49 S Service Rd, Opelousas, LA 70570
Handheld fixation device with plume evacuation, irrigation, aspiration and air d.

EXOENZYME, MULTIPLE, STREPTOCOCCAL
(Microbiology) 83GTP

Biomerieux Inc. 800-682-2666
100 Rodolphe St, Durham, NC 27712

E-Y Laboratories, Inc. 800-821-0044
107 N Amphlett Blvd, San Mateo, CA 94401
Exoenzymes.

Luminex Corp. 888-219-8020
12212 Technology Blvd, Austin, TX 78727
xMAP

EXOPHTHALMOMETER *(Ophthalmology) 86HLS*

Eagle Vision, Inc. 800-222-7584
8500 Wolf Lake Dr Ste 110, Memphis, TN 38133

Gulden Ophthalmics 800-659-2250
225 Cadwalader Ave, Elkins Park, PA 19027

Western Ophthalmics Corporation 800-426-9938
19019 36th Ave W Ste G, Lynnwood, WA 98036

Woodlyn, Inc. 800-331-7389
2920 Malmo Dr, Ophthalmic Instruments and Equipment
Arlington Heights, IL 60005
Model 43300. The Woodlyn Prism Exophthalmometer is designed for accuracy and simplicity in the measurements of the exophthalmos. Call for current prices.

EXPANDER, SKIN, INFLATABLE *(Surgery) 79LCJ*

Allergan 800-624-4261
71 S Los Carneros Rd, Goleta, CA 93117
Tissue expander.

Brava, Llc 305-856-4242
2601 S Bayshore Dr Ste 725, Coconut Grove, FL 33133
Breast enhancement and shaping system.

Pmt Corp. 800-626-5463
1500 Park Rd, Chanhassen, MN 55317

Specialty Surgical Products, Inc. 406-961-0102
1131 US Highway 93 N, Victor, MT 59875
Various types of tissue expanders.

Stryker Puerto Rico, Ltd. 939-307-2500
Hwy. 3, Km. 131.2, Las Guasimas Ind. Park, Arroyo, PR 00714
Compartment syndrome pressure monitor system.

EXPANDER, SURGICAL, SKIN GRAFT *(Surgery) 79FZW*

Biomet Microfixation Inc. 800-874-7711
1520 Tradeport Dr, Jacksonville, FL 32218
Expander, surgical, skin graft.

Brennen Medical, Llc 651-429-7413
1290 Hammond Rd, Saint Paul, MN 55110
Skin graft mesher.

Lenox-Maclaren Surgical Corp. 720-890-9660
657 S Taylor Ave Ste A, Colorado Technology Center
Louisville, CO 80027
Graft surgical.

Pmt Corp. 800-626-5463
1500 Park Rd, Chanhassen, MN 55317

Zimmer Holdings, Inc. 800-613-6131
1800 W Center St, PO Box 708, Warsaw, IN 46580

Zimmer Orthopaedic Surgical Products 800-321-5533
PO Box 10, 200 West Ohio Ave., Dover, OH 44622

EXPANDER, TISSUE, ORBITAL *(Ophthalmology) 86NFM*

Innovia Llc 305-378-2651
12415 SW 136th Ave Ste 3, Miami, FL 33186
Orbital tissue expander.

EXPLORER, OPERATIVE *(Dental And Oral) 76EKB*

Biomet Microfixation Inc. 800-874-7711
1520 Tradeport Dr, Jacksonville, FL 32218
Explorer, operative.

Dental Usa, Inc. 815-363-8003
5005 McCullom Lake Rd, McHenry, IL 60050
Explorer.

EXPLORER, OPERATIVE *(cont'd)*

Dentalez Group 866-DTE-INFO
101 Lindenwood Dr Ste 225, Valleybrooke Corporate Center Malvern, PA 19355

Dentalez Group, Stardental Division 717-291-1161
1816 Colonial Village Ln, Lancaster, PA 17601
Explorer, operative.

Dentlight Inc. 972-889-8857
1411 E Campbell Rd Ste 500, Richardson, TX 75081
Dental explorer.

E.A. Beck & Co. 949-645-4072
657 W 19th St Ste E, P O Box 10857, Costa Mesa, CA 92627
Explorer.

H & H Co. 909-390-0373
4435 E Airport Dr Ste 108, Ontario, CA 91761
Explorer, all types.

Hartzell & Son, G. 800-950-2206
2372 Stanwell Cir, Concord, CA 94520

Hu-Friedy Manufacturing Co., Inc. 800-483-7433
3232 N Rockwell St, Chicago, IL 60618
$9.60 to $13.65 for single-end; $9.60 to $17.20 for double-end, 16 types.

Micro-Dent Inc. 866-526-1166
379 Hollow Hill Rd, Wauconda, IL 60084
Explorer.

Miltex Dental Technologies, Inc. 516-576-6022
589 Davies Dr, York, PA 17402
Various single and doubled-ended endodontic explorers.

Nordent Manufacturing, Inc. 800-966-7336
610 Bonnie Ln, Elk Grove Village, IL 60007
$10.50 per unit (standard).

Pdt, Inc. 406-626-4153
12201 Moccasin Ct, Missoula, MT 59808
Various.

Premier Dental Products Co. 888-670-6100
1710 Romano Dr, PO Box 4500, Plymouth Meeting, PA 19462

Sci-Dent, Inc. 800-323-4145
210 Dowdle St Ste 2, Algonquin, IL 60102

Suter Dental Manufacturing Company, Inc. 800-368-8376
632 Cedar St, Chico, CA 95928

U.S.A. Delta.Inc 305-557-1435
7830 W 28th Ave Apt 213, Hialeah, FL 33018
Explorer operatives.

Ultradent Products, Inc. 801-553-4586
505 W 10200 S, South Jordan, UT 84095
Explorer.

Wykle Research, Inc. 775-887-7500
2222 College Pkwy, Carson City, NV 89706
Operative explorer.

EXPRESSOR *(Ophthalmology) 86HNS*

Fortrad Eye Instruments Corp. 973-543-2371
8 Franklin Rd, Mendham, NJ 07945

George Tiemann & Co. 800-843-6266
25 Plant Ave, Hauppauge, NY 11788

EXPRESSOR, LENS LOOP *(Ophthalmology) 86RES*

Fortrad Eye Instruments Corp. 973-543-2371
8 Franklin Rd, Mendham, NJ 07945

EXTERNAL MANDIBULAR FIXATOR AND/OR DISTRACTOR
(Dental And Oral) 76MQN

Biomet Microfixation Inc. 800-874-7711
1520 Tradeport Dr, Jacksonville, FL 32218
Distraction devices.

Orthonetx, Inc. 877-370-0477
2301 W 205th St Ste 102, Torrance, CA 90501
Distraction device, dental bone plate.

EXTRACORPOREAL PHOTOPHERESIS SYSTEM
(Gastro/Urology) 78LNR

Therakos, Inc., A Johnson & Johnson Company 877-865-6850
437 Creamery Way, Exton, PA 19341
Photopheresis procedural kit. UVAR instrument for performing photopheresis.

EXTRACTABLE ANTINUCLEAR ANTIBODY (RNP/SM), ANTIGEN/CONTROL *(Immunology) 82LLL*

American Laboratory Products Co. 800-592-5726
26 Keewaydin Dr Ste G, Salem, NH 03079
Qualitative screen for anti-SS-A, SS-B, Sm, RNP/Sm, Jo-1 and Scl-70. Individual semi-quantitative assays also available.

Bio-Rad Laboratories Inc., Clinical Systems Div. 800-224-6723
4000 Alfred Nobel Dr, Hercules, CA 94547
Eia ena test kits.

Corgenix Medical Corporation 800-729-5661
11575 Main St, Broomfield, CO 80020
REAADS Anti-Jo-1

Hycor Biomedical, Inc. 800-382-2527
7272 Chapman Ave, Garden Grove, CA 92841
Autoimmune diagnostic kits.

Innominata dba GENBIO 800-288-4368
15222 Avenue of Science Ste A, San Diego, CA 92128
Enzyme - linked immunoassay - for ssa/b antibodies.

Micro Detect, Inc. 714-832-8234
2852 Walnut Ave Ste H1, Tustin, CA 92780
Mdi sm test.

Quest Intl., Inc. 305-592-6991
8127 NW 29th St, Doral, FL 33122
Anti-sb serological reagents, elisa.

Zeus Scientific, Inc. 800-286-2111
PO Box 38, Raritan, NJ 08869
Poly-ENA for detection of antibodies to RNP, Sm, SSA(Ro) & SSB.

EXTRACTION/CHROMATOGRAPHY, NINHYDRIN, HYDROXYPROLINE *(Chemistry) 75JMN*

Aura Industries, Inc. 800-551-2872
545 8th Ave Rm 5W, New York, NY 10018
SPEEDMAN Solid phase extraction disc manifold.

Tudor Scientific Glass Co., Inc. 800-336-4666
555 Edgefield Rd, Belvedere, SC 29841

EXTRACTOR, CATARACT *(Ophthalmology) 86QHF*

Allergan 800-366-6554
2525 Dupont Dr, Irvine, CA 92612
PRESTIGE advanced cataract extraction system.

Bausch & Lomb Surgical 636-255-5051
3365 Tree Court Ind Blvd, Saint Louis, MO 63122

Biomedics, Inc. 949-458-1998
23322 Peralta Dr Ste 11, Laguna Hills, CA 92653
Phaco-Emulsifiers, Vitrectomy units (Alcon & Storz).

Eagle Laboratories 800-782-6534
10201 Trademark St Ste A, Rancho Cucamonga, CA 91730

EXTRACTOR, METAL, MAGNETIC *(Surgery) 79QVF*

Adept-Med International, Inc. 800-222-8445
665 Pleasant Valley Rd, Diamond Springs, CA 95619
MAGNATREVE magnetic floor sweep for hands-free collection of sharps and other ferrous metals.

Alcon Research, Ltd. 800-862-5266
6201 South Fwy, Fort Worth, TX 76134

EXTRACTOR, NAIL *(Orthopedics) 87HWB*

Advanced Bio-Surfaces, Inc. 952-912-5400
5909 Baker Rd Ste 550, Minnetonka, MN 55345
Extractor.

Biomet, Inc. 574-267-6639
56 E Bell Dr, PO Box 587, Warsaw, IN 46582
Various types of orthopedic extractor.

Depuy Mitek, A Johnson & Johnson Company 800-451-2006
50 Scotland Blvd, Bridgewater, MA 02324
Various types of removal tools.

Design Standards Corp. 603-826-7744
Ceda Industrial Park, Charlestown, NH 03603
Surgical staple extractor, laparoscopic.

Interventional Spine, Inc. 800-497-0484
13700 Alton Pkwy Ste 160, Irvine, CA 92618
Various types of extractors.

K2m, Inc. 866-526-4171
751 Miller Dr SE Ste F1, Leesburg, VA 20175
Extractor.

Kmedic 800-955-0559
190 Veterans Dr, Northvale, NJ 07647

EXTRACTOR, NAIL *(cont'd)*

Medtronic Sofamor Danek Instrument Manufacturing — 901-396-3133
7375 Adrianne Pl, Bartlett, TN 38133
Multiple (driver-extractors).

Medtronic Sofamor Danek Usa, Inc. — 901-396-3133
4340 Swinnea Rd, Memphis, TN 38118
Multiple (driver-extractors).

Minnesota Bramstedt Surgical, Inc. — 800-456-5052
1835 Energy Park Dr, Saint Paul, MN 55108
The Woodpecker - total hip broaching device also used for extraction of intramedullary nails.

Nobel Biocare Usa, Llc — 800-579-6515
22715/22725 Savi Ranch Parkway, Yorba Linda, CA 92887
Surgical instrument.

Oratronics, Inc. — 212-986-0050
405 Lexington Ave, New York, NY 10174
Implant remover.

Rush-Berivon, Inc. — 800-251-7874
1010 19th St, P.O. Box 1851, Meridian, MS 39301
1 model (for 2-6mm pins) - $484.00. With 3 interchangeable heads - additional heads available at $48.00 each.

Shukla Medical — 732-474-1762
151 Old New Brunswick Rd, Piscataway, NJ 08854

Spine Wave, Inc. — 203-944-9494
2 Enterprise Dr Ste 302, Shelton, CT 06484
Pin puller.

Stryker Spine — 866-457-7463
2 Pearl Ct, Allendale, NJ 07401

Surgical Implant Generation Network (Sign) — 509-371-1107
451 Hills St, Richland, WA 99354
Extractor.

Warsaw Orthopedic, Inc. — 901-396-3133
2500 Silveus Xing, Warsaw, IN 46582
Multiple (driver-extractors).

Zimmer Holdings, Inc. — 800-613-6131
1800 W Center St, PO Box 708, Warsaw, IN 46580

Zimmer Spine, Inc. — 800-655-2614
7375 Bush Lake Rd, Minneapolis, MN 55439
Extractor.

Zimmer Trabecular Metal Technology — 800-613-6131
10 Pomeroy Rd, Parsippany, NJ 07054
Slide hammer.

EXTRACTOR, PLASMA *(Hematology) 81QVG*

Applied Biosystems — 800-345-5724
850 Lincoln Centre Dr, Foster City, CA 94404
$42,000 for model 3404A DNA/RNA extractor, $20,500 for model 152A DNA/RNA separation system.

Biomerieux Inc. — 800-682-2666
100 Rodolphe St, Durham, NC 27712

Inotech Biosystems International, Inc. — 800-635-4070
15713 Crabbs Branch Way Ste 110, Rockville, MD 20855
Heparin adsorbent. Heparin removal from plasma.

Organomation Associates, Inc. — 978-838-7300
266 River Rd W, Berlin, MA 01503
ROT-X-TRACT Liquid-solid or liquid-liquid, extractors hold 5 to 10 samples.

EXTRACTOR, VACUUM, FETAL *(Obstetrics/Gyn) 85HDB*

Clinical Innovations, Inc. — 888-268-6222
747 W 4170 S, Murray, UT 84123
Kiwi Vacuum Delivery System is a unit designed for complete control without an assistant. Palm Pump is a safe vacuum system that fits in hand.

Koaman International — 909-983-4888
656 E D St, Ontario, CA 91764

Ob Scientific, Inc. — 262-532-8200
N112W18741 Mequon Rd, Germantown, WI 53022
Fetal vacuum extractor cup.

Ob Specialties, Inc. — 800-325-6644
1799 Northwood Ct, Oakland, CA 94611
MITYVAC Vacuum Delivery System; MYSTIC One-Piece Unit

Pristech Products, Inc — 800-432-8722
6952 Fairgrounds Pkwy, PO Box 680728, San Antonio, TX 78238
MITY VAC vacuum extraction device for use in labor and delivery of infants. Cup for use with vacuum extraction device.

EXTRACTOR, VACUUM, FETAL *(cont'd)*

Utah Medical Products, Inc. — 800-533-4984
7043 Cottonwood St, Midvale, UT 84047
CMI Vacuum Delivery System equipment is used for assisting delivery of the infant's head in vaginal or Caesarean procedures, instead of forceps. Equipment consists of sterile cup, tube & fluid trap sets usually used with a hand operated vacuum pump which can be steam sterilized. Also available is an educational video which demonstrates how to use this CMI equipment correctly. Note: CMI sterile vacuum cup, tube & fluid trap sets can also be used with an electric vacuum pump, if desired.

EXTRICATION EQUIPMENT *(General) 80TCA*

Armstrong Medical Industries, Inc. — 800-323-4220
575 Knightsbridge Pkwy, Lincolnshire, IL 60069

Dixie Ems Supply — 800-347-3494
385 Union Ave, Brooklyn, NY 11211
$189.00 per unit (standard).

Hermell Products, Inc. — 800-233-2342
9 Britton Dr, PO Box 7345, Bloomfield, CT 06002
Extricating collars (1 & 2 piece).

Rapid Deployment Products — 877-433-7569
157 Railroad Dr, Ivyland, PA 18974
PRO-LITE Speedboard - short extrication board.

EYE, ARTIFICIAL, CUSTOM *(Ophthalmology) 86HQI*

Jardon Eye Prosthetics, Inc. — 248-424-8560
15920 W 12 Mile Rd, Southfield, MI 48076

Legrand Assoc. — 800-523-4314
313 S 17th St, Philadelphia, PA 19103
Custom artificial eyes (occular prosthetics).

EYE, ARTIFICIAL, NON-CUSTOM *(Ophthalmology) 86HQH*

Advanced Ocular Prosthetics Inc. — 412-787-7277
1111 Oakdale Rd Ste 5, Oakdale, PA 15071
Artificial eye.

Albuquerque Eye Prosthetics, Inc. — 505-884-2927
4117 Montgomery Blvd NE, Albuquerque, NM 87109
Eye, artificial, non-custom.

Anderson Eye Prosthetics — 801-262-6711
164 E 5900 S # 101-B, Murray, UT 84107
Prosthetic eye.

Austin Ocular Prosthetics Center, Llc — 512-452-3100
711 W 38th St Ste G1A, Austin, TX 78705

Bruce Cook, Prosthetics — 314-567-7585
2821 N Ballas Rd Ste 215, Saint Louis, MO 63131
Custom artificial eye.

Carole Lewis Stolpe' B.C.O. — 310-271-8801
435 N Bedford Dr Ste 411, Beverly Hills, CA 90210
Prosthetic eyes.

Carolina Eye Prosthetics, Inc. — 336-228-7877
420 Maple Ave, Burlington, NC 27215
Custom fitted plastic ocular prosthesis.

Center For Ocular Prosthetics, Llc. — 503-229-8490
2525 NW Lovejoy St Ste 306, Portland, OR 97210
Prosthetic or artificial eye.

Center For Ocular Reconstruction — 301-652-9282
4833 Rugby Ave Fl 4, Bethesda, MD 20814

Dallas Eye Prosthetics — 214-739-5355
8226 Douglas Ave Ste 415, Dallas, TX 75225
Custom ocular prosthesis.

Daniel T Acosta — 619-235-8950
635 C St Apt 502, San Diego, CA 92101
Custom ocular prosthetics.

Dean B. Scott, Ocularist — 847-965-4455
5225 Old Orchard Rd Ste 27B, Skokie, IL 60077
Eye prosthesis.

Dean B. Scott, Ocularist — 847-965-4455
1901 S Osprey Ave, Sarasota, FL 34239
Eye prosthesis.

Dean B. Scott, Ocularist — 847-965-4455
4101 Evans Ave, Fort Myers, FL 33901
Eye prosthesis.

Dean B. Scott, Ocularist — 847-965-4455
1319 Butterfield Rd Ste 524, Downers Grove, IL 60515
Eye prosthesis.

EYE, ARTIFICIAL, NON-CUSTOM *(cont'd)*

Department Of Veterans Affairs Medical Center 503-220-8262
3710 SW US Veterans Hospital Rd, Portland, OR 97239
Artificial eye.

Doss K. Tannehill - Ocularist 808-738-5300
752 17th Ave, Honolulu, HI 96816
Custom ocular prosthesis.

Erickson Labs Northwest 425-823-1861
12911 120th Ave NE Ste C10, Kirkland, WA 98034
Artificial eye.

Eye Prosthetics Of Utah, Inc. 801-942-1600
7050 Highland Dr Ste 220, Salt Lake City, UT 84121
Eye, artificial, custom.

Eye Prosthetics Of Wisconsin, Inc. 262-363-1528
4781 Hayes Rd, Madison, WI 53704
Artificial eye.

Eye Restoration Clinic 866-364-6544
4606 S Garnett Rd Ste 302, Tulsa, OK 74146
Custom artificial eyes.

Fort Worth Eye Prosthetics, Inc. 817-429-8086
1350 S Main St Ste 2450, Fort Worth, TX 76104
Custom ocular prosthesis.

Frank Tanaka, Ocularist, Inc. 813-978-1142
3000 E Fletcher Ave Ste 310, Tampa, FL 33613
Artificial eye.

Glenn Reams, Ocularist 800-426-8995
221 NW McNary Ct, Lees Summit, MO 64086
Artificial eye.

Glenn Reams, Ocularist 800-426-8995
1020 W Buena Vista Rd, Evansville, IN 47710
Artificial eye.

Glenn Reams, Ocularist 800-426-8995
610 S Floyd St, Louisville, KY 40202
Artificial eye.

Glenn Reams, Ocularist 800-426-8995
2845 Farrell Cres, Owensboro, KY 42303
Artificial eye.

Henthorn Ocular Prosthetics 316-688-5235
744 S Hillside St, Wichita, KS 67211
Eye, artificial, non-custom.

Intermountain Ocular Prosthetics, Inc. 208-378-8200
2995 N Cole Rd Ste 115, Boise, ID 83704
Eye, artificial, non-custom.

June R.R. Nichols, Ocularist Ltd. 847-803-5050
1767 E Oakton St, Des Plaines, IL 60018
Artificial eye.

L.J. Greiner & Sons, Inc. 973-977-9441
63 Danforth Ave # 69, Paterson, NJ 07501
Custom made Artificial eye.

Maloney's Custom Ocular Prosthetics, Inc. 503-675-1320
4035 Mercantile Dr Ste 208, Lake Oswego, OR 97035
Various types of custom plastic artificial eyes.

Miller Artificial Eye Laboratory, Inc. 419-474-3939
3030 W Sylvania Ave Ste 13, Toledo, OH 43613
Artificial eye.

Ocu-Labs, Inc. 952-854-6702
7851 Metro Pkwy Ste 225, Bloomington, MN 55425
Prosthesis, eye, internal.

Ocular Prosthetics, Inc. 323-462-6004
321 N Larchmont Blvd Ste 711, Los Angeles, CA 90004

Rocky Mountain Anaplastology, Inc. 303-973-8482
3405 S Yarrow St Unit C, Lakewood, CO 80227
Artificial eyes (custom made).

S.P. Artificial Eye Co. 270-665-5515
374 Broadway, La Center, KY 42056
Artificial eye (plastic).

S.W. Florida Prosthetic Clinic 239-936-0033
13691 Metro Pkwy Ste 100, Fort Myers, FL 33912
Eye prosthesis.

Sng Prosthetic Eye Institute 561-391-7099
6018 SW 18th St Ste C2, Boca Raton, FL 33433
Sng prosthetic eye ins.

Soper Brothers & Associates 713-521-1263
1213 Hermann Dr Ste 320, Houston, TX 77004
Non-custom artificial eye.

EYE, ARTIFICIAL, NON-CUSTOM *(cont'd)*

Southwest Artificial Eyes, Inc. 210-737-3937
PO Box 100636, San Antonio, TX 78201
Artificial eye.

Steven R. Young Ocularist, Inc. 510-836-2123
411 30th St Ste 512, Oakland, CA 94609
Eye, artificial, custom.

The Eye Concern, Inc. 480-962-5841
1450 S Dobson Rd Ste A206, Mesa, AZ 85202
Artificial eye, ocular prosthesis.

Thomas Ocular Prosthetics Labs, Inc. 901-753-4724
1900 Kirby Pkwy Ste 102, Germantown, TN 38138
Prosthesis, eye, internal.

Thompson Ocular Prosthetics, Inc. 210-223-3754
4118 McCullough Ave Ste 16, San Antonio, TX 78212
Ocular prosthesis/artificial eye.

Tomas L. Ortega 956-630-2887
San Borja 1361, Mexico City Mexico
Artificial eye

Turntine Ocular Prosthetics, Inc 913-962-6299
6342 Long Ave Ste H, Lenexa, KS 66216
Artificial eye.

EYEGLASSES *(Ophthalmology) 86QVI*

Aura Lens Products, Inc. 800-281-2872
51 8th St N, PO Box 763, St. Cloud,, Sauk Rapids, MN 56379

Briggs Corporation 800-247-2343
PO Box 1698, 7300 Westown Pkwy., Des Moines, IA 50306

Burlington Medical Supplies, Inc. 800-221-3466
3 Elmhurst St, PO Box 3194, Newport News, VA 23603
Lead glasses.

Davis Lead Apron, Inc. 800-483-3979
4560 W 34th St, PO Box 924585, Houston, TX 77092
Eyeglasses for Radiology Protection

Dispensers Optical Service Corp. 800-626-4545
1815 Plantside Dr, Louisville, KY 40299
Military optical lenses, eyewear, and goggles

General Scientific Safety Equipment Co. 800-523-0166
2553 E Somerset St Fl 1, Philadelphia, PA 19134

H.L. Bouton Co., Inc. 800-426-1881
PO Box 840, Buzzards Bay, MA 02532
Disposable.

Lesco Optical 520-323-1538
4444 E Grant Rd, Tucson, AZ 85712

Novosci Corp. 281-363-4949
2828 N Crescentridge Dr, The Woodlands, TX 77381

Oxy-View, Inc. 877-699-8439
109 Inverness Dr E Ste C, Englewood, CO 80112
Oxy-View oxygen-therapy eyewear. Eyeglass frames used in the delivery of oxygen to oxygen-dependent patients.

Safilo Usa 800-631-1188
801 Jefferson Rd, Parsippany, NJ 07054
Opthalmic eyewear. Also available GUCCI, RALPH LAUREN, CHRISTIAN DIOR, NINE WEST and FOSSIL eyewear.

Schott Glass Technologies, Inc. 570-457-7485
400 York Ave, Duryea, PA 18642
Various types from basic clear to tint crown glasses.

Sellstrom Manufacturing Co. 800-323-7402
1 Sellstrom Dr, Palatine, IL 60067
20/20 eyewear - clear polycarbonate lenses.

Soderberg Optical, Inc. 800-755-5655
230 Eva St, Saint Paul, MN 55107

Transtracheal Systems, Inc. 800-527-2667
109 Inverness Dr E Ste C, Englewood, CO 80112
The OxyView eyeglass frame is designed to deliver up to 5 liters per minute of oxygen to patients who require continuous supplemental oxygen. Oxygen patients who also must wear glasses or hearing aids will appreciate the comfort of the OxyView frame, since it eliminates the nasal cannula tubing over the ears. Of European design, these frames are lightweight, stylish, and likely to improve compliance with oxygen therapy when the patient is out in public. There are 5 different frame designs, and each is available in two gold-tone colors or black. Patients may have their eyecare professional fit different types of prescription or non-prescription lenses such as bifocal, sunglasses, etc.

EYEGLASSES, SAFETY *(Ophthalmology) 86TCB*

Aearo Company 800-678-4163
5457 W 79th St, Indianapolis, IN 46268
SPLASHMASTER protective prescription eyewear with single vision or progressive power multifocal lenses. Anti-fog coating provides visual clarity in high humidity and temperature changes.

Alimed, Inc. 800-225-2610
297 High St, Dedham, MA 02026
COMBO SHIELD combines full eye protection with a surgical face mask. COMBO-C is a traditional elastic headband-style cone mask. COMBO-CE is the same as COMBO-C except it has adjustable, elastic earloops. MEDS seal out potentially harmful splashes of blood and other bodily fluids. ADD-A-MASK attaches directly to the face mask to help guard against splashes to the eyes. 1/2 COVERALL fits over glasses and is adjustable. COVERALL is full-face protection.

Aura Lens Products, Inc. 800-281-2872
51 8th St N, PO Box 763, St. Cloud,, Sauk Rapids, MN 56379
Standard safety glasses, prescription and non-prescription; also, X-ray laser and glassblowers shielding eyeglasses, prescription and nonprescription.

Branford Laboratories 843-832-8004
PO Box 51000, Summerville, SC 29485
Lead glasses.

Burkhart Roentgen Intl. Inc. 800-USA-XRAY
5201 8th Ave S, Gulfport, FL 33707
Lead glass spectacles and goggles with or w/o prescription lenses as well as full wrap-around protection.

Co/Op Optical Vision Designs 866-733-2667
2424 E 8 Mile Rd, E. of Dequindre, Detroit, MI 48234

Concepts International, Inc. 800-627-9729
224 E Main St, Summerton, SC 29148
Colorful safety wear, 12 colors, distortion-free, hard-coated polycarbonate lenses; comes with case and cord; curing light glasses.

Crosstex International,Inc. 888-276-7783
10 Ranick Rd, Hauppauge, NY 11788
IC EYEWEAR, protective safety eyewear utilizing face mask support system incorporates small hooks on temple to allow you to comfortably attach ear loop masks.

H.L. Bouton Co., Inc. 800-426-1881
PO Box 840, Buzzards Bay, MA 02532
UFO Series, stylish safety spectacles.

Hager Worldwide, Inc. 800-328-2335
13322 Byrd Dr, Odessa, FL 33556
UVEX (anti scratch, anti fog, anti glare, ultra violet coating).

Infab Corp. 805-987-5255
3651 Via Pescador, Camarillo, CA 93012
Radiographic protective. New LOWER PRICES effective June 1, 2003!

Intec Industries, Inc. 205-251-5600
2024 12th Ave N, Birmingham, AL 35234
Disposable.

Lase-R Shield, A Bacou-Dalloz Company 800-288-1164
7011 Prospect Pl NE, Albuquerque, NM 87110
Priced from $19.00; complete line of safety eyeglasses for visitor or staff.

Medco Supply Company 800-556-3326
500 Fillmore Ave, Tonawanda, NY 14150
Large selection.

Medical Safety Systems Inc. 888-803-9303
230 White Pond Dr, Akron, OH 44313

Novosci Corp. 281-363-4949
2828 N Crescentridge Dr, The Woodlands, TX 77381
COLORGUARD Laser safety eyeglasses, multiple wavelengths, glass or polycarbonate in spectacles, goggles, shields for laser protection. Splash shields in thin polycarbonate for splash protection only.

Pulse Medical Inc. 800-342-5973
4131 SW 47th Ave Ste 1404, Davie, FL 33314
Lead, radiographic glasses with a large selection of style and comfort.

Rochester Optical Mfg. Company 585-254-0022
1260 Lyell Ave, Rochester, NY 14606

Rockford Medical & Safety Co. 800-435-9451
2420 Harrison Ave, PO Box 5646, Rockford, IL 61108

Schott Glass Technologies, Inc. 570-457-7485
400 York Ave, Duryea, PA 18642

EYEGLASSES, SAFETY *(cont'd)*

Schueler & Company, Inc. 516-487-1500
PO Box 528, Stratford, CT 06615

Surgical Safety Products, Inc. 800-953-7889
2018 Oak Ter Ste 400, Sarasota, FL 34231
MEDI-SPECS RX ultra-lightweight prescription glasses. Glasses are pre-manufactured with corrective lenses that include 85-90% of the most common prescriptions used. They can be custom fit, have bifocal capability and feature OSHA-recommended side shields now required for the operating room.

Trademark Medical Llc 800-325-9044
449 Soverign Ct, St. Louis, MO 63011
FACE-FIT splashguard protective cover goggles, also available as Anti-Fogging model. Also, spectacles and face shield.

Western Ophthalmics Corporation 800-426-9938
19019 36th Ave W Ste G, Lynnwood, WA 98036

Zee Medical, Inc. 800-841-8417
22 Corporate Park, Irvine, CA 92606

EYEPIECE, LENS, NON-PRESCRIPTION, ENDOSCOPIC
(Gastro/Urology) 78FEI

Access Optics Llc 918-294-1234
2001 N Willow Ave, Broken Arrow, OK 74012
Endoscope camera coupler(s).

Mahe International Inc. 800-294-7946
468 Craighead St, Nashville, TN 37204

EYEPIECE, LENS, PRESCRIPTION, ENDOSCOPIC
(Gastro/Urology) 78FDZ

Duffens Optical 800-432-2475
400 SE Quincy St, Topeka, KS 66603
Opthalmic eyeware.

Mahe International Inc. 800-294-7946
468 Craighead St, Nashville, TN 37204

FACE BOW *(Dental And Oral) 76KCR*

Almore International, Inc. 503-643-6633
PO Box 25214, Portland, OR 97298
$125.00 (standard).

Classone Orthodontics, Inc. 806-799-0608
5064 50th St, Lubbock, TX 79414
Various types of facebows.

Ivoclar Vivadent, Inc. 800-533-6825
175 Pineview Dr, Amherst, NY 14228
UNIVERSAL TRANSFERBOW SYSTEM

Lancer Orthodontics, Inc. 760-304-2705
253 Pawnee St, San Marcos, CA 92078
Various types of face bows.

Masel Co., Inc. 800-423-8227
2701 Bartram Rd, Bristol, PA 19007

Ortho Organizers, Inc. 760-448-8730
1822 Aston Ave, Carlsbad, CA 92008
Various types of facebows.

Oscar, Inc. 317-849-2618
11793 Technology Ln, Fishers, IN 46038
Face bows - various sizes and kinds.

Panadent Corp. 800-368-9777
22573 Barton Rd, Grand Terrace, CA 92313
The PANA-MOUNT Face Bow features wrench or wrenchless detachable bite-fork assemblies which allows the face-bow to be used for multiple patients without having to mount casts immediately. It has a standard 22mm nasion relator as well as an orbital pointer. Comfortable ear pieces and foam nasion pad increase patient comfort. The face-bow can be used as an average axis ear-bow as well as a true transverse axis bow (in conjunction with the Axis Mounting System and Axi-Path Recorder).

Water Pik, Inc. 970-221-6129
1730 E Prospect Rd, Fort Collins, CO 80525
Various models of facebows and springbow.

Whip Mix Corp. 502-637-1451
1730 E Prospect Rd Ste 101, Fort Collins, CO 80525

Whip-Mix Corporation 800-626-5651
361 Farmington Ave, PO Box 17183, Louisville, KY 40209

3m Unitek 800-634-5300
2724 Peck Rd, Monrovia, CA 91016

FACIAL FRACTURE APPLIANCE, EXTERNAL *(Surgery) 79FYI*

Biomet Microfixation Inc. 800-874-7711
1520 Tradeport Dr, Jacksonville, FL 32218
Various types of external facial fracture appliances (prosthesis).

FACIAL TISSUE *(General) 80QVK*

Chagrin Safety Supply, Inc. 800-227-0468
8227 Washington St # 1, Chagrin Falls, OH 44023

Crosstex International Ltd., W. Region 800-707-2737
14059 Stage Rd, Santa Fe Springs, CA 90670

Crosstex International,Inc. 888-276-7783
10 Ranick Rd, Hauppauge, NY 11788
CROSSTEX.

Jero Medical Equipment & Supplies, Inc. 800-457-0644
1701 W 13th St, Chicago, IL 60608

Kerr Group 800-524-3577
1400 Holcomb Bridge Rd, Roswell, GA 30076

Niagara Pharmaceuticals Div. 905-690-6277
60 Innovation Dr., Flamborough, ONT L9H-7P3 Canada
LENS SAVER all-purpose, low-lint tissue; 4.5 x 8.3 inches, 300 sheets per box with 60 per case.

Paperpak 800-428-8363
545 W Terrace Dr, San Dimas, CA 91773
TISSUE PAK 50 sheets per box, 200 boxes per case. The product code is T-584.

FACILITY, EQUIPMENT, MEDICAL, MOBILE *(General) 80WUC*

Bond Caster And Wheel Corporation 800-233-2663
230 S Penn St, PO Box 339, Manheim, PA 17545
Tripod Dolly for excellent manuverability and access to tight places. Custom carts for manufacturing equipment and machines and end user equipment and instruments are produced in a variety of materials.

Calmaquip Engineering Corp. 305-592-4510
7240 NW 12th St, Miami, FL 33126
Mobile hospitals.

Choice Medical Systems, Inc. 727-347-8833
1426 Pasadena Ave S, South Pasadena, FL 33707
Reconditioned ultrasound,thermal printers, VCRs, monitors, Gel and Thermal Paper supplies.

Colonial Scientific Ltd. 902-468-1811
201 Brownlow Ave., Unit 52, Dartmouth, NS B3B-1W2 Canada
High density mobile shelving systems for medical records.

Dornier Medtech America 800-367-6437
1155 Roberts Blvd NW, Kennesaw, GA 30144
Mobile lithotriptor systems, urology imaging systems, orthopedic shock wave device systems, medical and aesthetic lasers.

Duke Diagnostic Resale 516-496-3503
257 Cold Spring Rd, Syosset, NY 11791
Pre owned.

Electrolux Home Products - North America 877-435-3287
250 Bobby Jones Expy, PO Box 212378, Augusta, GA 30907
Major appliances.

Ge Medical Systems Information Technologies 800-558-5544
4502 Woodland Corporate Blvd, Tampa, FL 33614
4 & 8 patient central station system that connects up to 8 DINAMAP & DINAMAP PLUS monitors via hardwire or wireless network.

Medical Coaches, Inc. 607-432-1333
399 County Highway 58, P.O. Box 129, Oneonta, NY 13820
Mobile magnetic resonance imaging (MRI) trailers to house Siemens and Philips MRI systems. Trailers to house Siemens, Philips, Hitachi, and GE positron emission tomography (PET) and positron emission tomography/computed tomography (PET/CT) systems. Mobile mutiphasic medical, medical diagnostic treatment, x-ray mammography, CT units and TV broadcast/production units in trailer and self-propelled versions.

Mobile Medical International Corporation 800-748-2322
2176 Portland St Ste 4, PO Box 672, Saint Johnsbury, VT 05819
Mobile Surgery Units providing the only U.S. healthcare compliant, state-licensable, & Medicare certified mobile operating room solution; pre-op/recovery area and 400 sq ft OR with adjacent clean and soiled utility rooms; integrated systems for nurse call, medical gas, plumbing, electrical, intrusion alarm, fire alarm, communications and fire suppression; redundant systems for power, communicatiosn and plumbing. Mobile Breast Care Center is a mobile facility designed to screen, diagnose, and educate women on breast care. Unit is self contained and includes ultrasound stereotactic biopsy and multi-function workstations.

FACILITY, EQUIPMENT, MEDICAL, MOBILE *(cont'd)*

Oshkosh Specialty Vehicles 800-596-aksv
16745 Lathrop Ave, Harvey, IL 60426
Mobile MRI, PET/CT, PET, CT, Cath labs, digital mammograpy and medical clinic units, mobile field hospital systems, and relocatable medical buildings.

Progressive Medical International 800-764-0636
2460 Ash St, Vista, CA 92081
Medical and hospital equipment. Emergency care, rescue and safety products.

Quad Med 800-933-7334
PO Box 550773, 11210 Philips Ind. Blvd. E., Suite 10
Jacksonville, FL 32255
Emergency medical supplies and equipment. Pedi-Immobilizer, Grip-ET, Pad-Pro. Featuring Kimberly-Clark, Kendall, ConMed, Ferno, Rusch products and many more.

Ultron Systems, Inc. 805-529-1485
5105 Maureen Ln, Moorpark, CA 93021
Processing for semiconductors. Also, Ionizing Air Pencil, neutralizes static on small parts and devices. Pencil sized for fine point-of use applications.

FASTENER, CRANIOPLASTY PLATE *(Cns/Neurology) 84HBW*

Biomet, Inc. 574-267-6639
56 E Bell Dr, PO Box 587, Warsaw, IN 46582
Poly-l-lactric acid/ polyglycolic acid microplate.

FASTENER, FIXATION, BIODEGRADABLE, HARD TISSUE
(Orthopedics) 87MBJ

Depuy Orthopaedics, Inc. 800-473-3789
700 Orthopaedic Dr, P.O. Box 988, Warsaw, IN 46582
Various types of biodegradable hard tissue fixation fasteners.

Depuy-Raynham, A Div. Of Depuy Orthopaedics 800-451-2006
325 Paramount Dr, Raynham, MA 02767
Various types of biodegradable hard tissue fixation fasteners.

FASTENER, FIXATION, BIODEGRADABLE, SOFT TISSUE
(Orthopedics) 87MAI

Arthrex, Inc. 239-643-5553
1370 Creekside Blvd, Naples, FL 34108
Various sterile bioabsorbable suture anchors.

Biomet, Inc. 574-267-6639
56 E Bell Dr, PO Box 587, Warsaw, IN 46582
Various types of lactosorb sterile & non-sterile.

Coapt Systems, Inc. 650-461-7600
1820 Embarcadero Rd, Palo Alto, CA 94303
Brow lift device & installation kit.

Depuy Mitek, A Johnson & Johnson Company 800-451-2006
50 Scotland Blvd, Bridgewater, MA 02324
Fastner, fixation, biodegradable soft tissue.

Ethicon, Inc. 800-4-ETHICON
Route 22 West, Somerville, NJ 08876

Karl Storz Endoscopy-America Inc. 800-421-0837
600 Corporate Pointe, Culver City, CA 90230

Macropore Biosurgery, Inc. 858-458-0900
6740 Top Gun St, San Diego, CA 92121
Bone screws and tacks.

Mar-Lee Companies 978-534-8305
190 Authority Dr, Fitchburg, MA 01420
Same.

Scandius Biomedical, Inc. 978-486-4088
11A Beaver Brook Rd, Littleton, MA 01460
Sterile soft tissue fixation devices and instrumentation.

Tornier Inc. 978-232-9997
100 Cummings Ctr Ste 444C, Beverly, MA 01915
Bio-absorbable bone anchor.

Ussc Puerto Rico, Inc. 203-845-1000
Building 911-67, Sabanetas Industrial Park, Ponce, PR 00731
Bioberadable fastners.

FASTENER, FIXATION, NON-BIODEGRADABLE, SOFT TISSUE
(Orthopedics) 87MBI

Anulex Technologies, Inc 877-326-8539
5600 Rowland Rd Ste 280, Minnetonka, MN 55343
Rimclose Bone Anchor

Arthrex Manufacturing 239-643-5553
1958 Trade Center Way, Naples, FL 34109
Screw,fastener.

FASTENER, FIXATION, NON-BIODEGRADABLE, SOFT TISSUE *(cont'd)*

Arthrex, Inc. 239-643-5553
1370 Creekside Blvd, Naples, FL 34108
Bone screws.

Biomet, Inc. 574-267-6639
56 E Bell Dr, PO Box 587, Warsaw, IN 46582
Harpoon suture anchor.

Bonutti Research, Inc. 217-342-3412
2600 S Raney St, Effingham, IL 62401
Various.

Boston Scientific - Marina Bay Customer Fulfillment Center 617-689-6000
500 Commander Shea Blvd, Quincy, MA 02171
Bone anchor system.

Depuy Mitek, A Johnson & Johnson Company 800-451-2006
50 Scotland Blvd, Bridgewater, MA 02324
Fastener, fixation, non-biodegradable, soft tissue.

Depuy Orthopaedics, Inc. 800-473-3789
700 Orthopaedic Dr, P.O. Box 988, Warsaw, IN 46582
Fastener, fixation, nondegradable, soft tissue (various types).

Depuy-Raynham, A Div. Of Depuy Orthopaedics 800-451-2006
325 Paramount Dr, Raynham, MA 02767
Various types of nondegradable soft tissue fixation fasteners.

Ethicon, Inc. 800-4-ETHICON
Route 22 West, Somerville, NJ 08876

Innovasive Devices, Inc. 800-435-6001
734 Forest St, Marlborough, MA 01752

Scandius Biomedical, Inc. 978-486-4088
11A Beaver Brook Rd, Littleton, MA 01460
Sterile soft tissue fixation devices and instrumentation.

Tornier Inc. 978-232-9997
100 Cummings Ctr Ste 444C, Beverly, MA 01915
Suture applicator.

Zimmer Holdings, Inc. 800-613-6131
1800 W Center St, PO Box 708, Warsaw, IN 46580
Soft tissue attachment anchor.

Zimmer Trabecular Metal Technology 800-613-6131
10 Pomeroy Rd, Parsippany, NJ 07054
Implex screw and washer.

FC, ANTIGEN, ANTISERUM, CONTROL *(Immunology) 82DBN*

Antibodies, Inc. 800-824-8540
PO Box 1560, Davis, CA 95617

Dako North America, Inc 805-566-6655
6392 Via Real, Carpinteria, CA 93013

FC, FITC, ANTIGEN, ANTISERUM, CONTROL *(Immunology) 82DBK*

Antibodies, Inc. 800-824-8540
PO Box 1560, Davis, CA 95617

Dako North America, Inc 805-566-6655
6392 Via Real, Carpinteria, CA 93013

FC, RHODAMINE, ANTIGEN, ANTISERUM, CONTROL *(Immunology) 82DBH*

Alerchek, Inc. 877-282-9542
203 Anderson St, Portland, ME 04101
FLIPSCREEN SPECIFIC E ASSAY KIT

FELT *(Surgery) 79UKN*

Aetna Foot Products/Div. Of Aetna Felt Corporation 800-390-3668
2401 W Emaus Ave, Allentown, PA 18103
COMFOOT Brand and SCOTT FOOT CARE pre-cut pads, rolls and sheets in various thicknesses.

National Nonwovens 800-333-3469
PO Box 150, Easthampton, MA 01027
Podiatric felt.

FERMENTATION EQUIPMENT *(Microbiology) 83UGA*

Appropriate Technical Resources, Inc. 800-827-5931
9157 Whiskey Bottom Rd, PO Box 460, Laurel, MD 20723

Bioscience Contract Production Corp. 410-563-9200
5901 E Lombard St, Baltimore, MD 21224

Mettler-Toledo Process Analytical, Inc. 800-352-8763
299 Washington St, Woburn, MA 01801
Sensors - pH, O2, redox, CO2,.

FERMENTATION EQUIPMENT *(cont'd)*

New Brunswick Scientific Co., Inc. 800-631-5417
PO Box 4005, Edison, NJ 08818
Full line of research through production fermentors and bioreactors for submerged culture of bacteria, yeast, mammalian, animal, insect or plant culture. Available with interchangeable autoclavable vessels, or as sterilizable-in-place systems. BioFlo (R) 110 research fermentors available in conveniently pre-packaged kits for fermentation or cell culture.

Virtis, An Sp Industries Company 800-431-8232
815 Route 208, Gardiner, NY 12525
1- to 2-liter laboratory and omni-culture benchtop fermenters.

FERRIC CHLORIDE, PHENYLKETONES (URINARY, NON-QUANTITATIVE) *(Chemistry) 75JGK*

Rocky Mountain Reagents,Inc. 303-762-0800
3207 W Hampden Ave, Englewood, CO 80110

FERROZINE (COLORIMETRIC) IRON BINDING CAPACITY *(Chemistry) 75JMO*

Abbott Diagnostics Div. 626-440-0700
820 Mission St, South Pasadena, CA 91030
Iron binding capacity assays.

Carolina Liquid Chemistries Corp. 800-471-7272
510 W Central Ave Ste C, Brea, CA 92821
Unsaturated iron binding capacity reagent.

Genzyme Corp. 800-325-2436
160 Christian St, Oxford, CT 06478
Unsaturated iron binding capacity, endpoint, 595nm.

Health Chem Diagnostics Llc 954-979-3845
3341 W McNab Rd, Pompano Beach, FL 33069
Ferrozine (colorimetric) iron binding capacity.

Jas Diagnostics, Inc. 305-418-2320
7220 NW 58th St, Miami, FL 33166
Iron (uibc).

Sandare Intl., Inc. 972-293-7440
910 Kck Way, Cedar Hill, TX 75104
No common name listed.

Sterling Diagnostics, Inc. 800-637-2661
36645 Metro Ct, Sterling Heights, MI 48312
Ferrozine colorimetric iron and iron binding reagent set.

Synermed Intl., Inc. 317-896-1565
17408 Tiller Ct Ste 1900, Westfield, IN 46074
Uibc reagent kit.

Teco Diagnostics 714-693-7788
1268 N Lakeview Ave, Anaheim, CA 92807
Iron/total iron binding capacity (iron/tibc).

Vital Diagnostics Inc. 714-672-3553
1075 W Lambert Rd Ste D, Brea, CA 92821
Iron binding capacity sample pretreatment kit.

FERTILITY DIAGNOSTIC DEVICE *(Obstetrics/Gyn) 85LHD*

Biosense Corporation 215-348-2977
450 East St, Doylestown, PA 18901
Fertility monitor proceptive.

Embryotech Laboratories, Inc. 800-673-7500
323 Andover St, Wilmington, MA 01887

Neo Medical Inc. 888-450-3334
42514 Albrae St, Fremont, CA 94538
Seminal collection device.

Ovusoft, Llc. 757-722-0991
120 W Queens Way Ste 202, Hampton, VA 23669
Tcoyf fertility software.

FETAL DOPPLER ULTRASOUND *(Obstetrics/Gyn) 85LXE*

Huntleigh Healthcare Llc. 800-223-1218
40 Christopher Way, Eatontown, NJ 07724
FETAL DOPPLEX II, D920 AUDIO DOPPLEX, D900 MINI DOPPLEX, MULTI DOPPLEX II.

FIBER, ABSORBENT *(General) 80FRL*

A Plus International, Inc 909-591-5168
5138 Eucalyptus Ave, Chino, CA 91710
Operating room towels.

Abbott Associates 203-878-2370
620 West Ave, Milford, CT 06461
Non-adherent dressings, wing sponges, paint sticks.

Adelphia Medical Inc. 410-742-7104
1525 Edgemore Ave Ste 1, Salisbury, MD 21801

FIBER, ABSORBENT *(cont'd)*

American Fiber & Finishing, Inc. 800-522-2438
PO Box 2488, Albemarle, NC 28002
Sterile Cotton Balls

Barnhardt Mfg. Co. 704-376-0380
1100 Hawthorne Ln, Charlotte, NC 28205
Various sizes and packages of absorbent fiber.

Bioseal 800-441-7325
167 W Orangethorpe Ave, Placentia, CA 92870
Sterile cotton & rayon balls, pads, squares.

Bowers Medical Supply Co. 800-663-0047
3691 Viking Way, Unit 11, Richmond, BC V6V 2J6 Canada
Pressure bandage large and small

Brennen Medical, Llc 651-429-7413
1290 Hammond Rd, Saint Paul, MN 55110
Sterile isotonic saline solution.

Carolina Absorbent Cotton 704-405-4002
4969 Energy Way, Reno, NV 89502

Centurion Medical Products Corp. 517-545-1135
3310 S Main St, Salisbury, NC 28147

Confection Medicale D.R. Inc. 514-252-5553
200-4220 Rue De Rouen, Montreal H1V 3T2 Canada
Various types

Customs Hospital Products, Inc 800-426-2780
6336 SE 107th Ave, Portland, OR 97266
'balls' multiple non-sterile.

Dukal Corporation 800-243-0741
5 Plant Ave, Hauppauge, NY 11788

International Technidyne Corporation 732-548-5700
8 Olsen Ave, Edison, NJ 08820
Blotting paper.

K. W. Griffen Co. 203-846-1923
100 Pearl St, Norwalk, CT 06850
Absorbent cotton.

Marine Polymer Technologies, Inc. 888-666-2560
461 Boston St Unit B5, Topsfield, MA 01983
Medical absorbent pad.

North Safety Products 401-943-4400
1101 B Calle Neutron, Parque Industrial Maran, Mexicali, B.c. Mexico
Various sizes

Omnia, Inc. 863-619-8100
3125 Drane Field Rd Ste 29, Lakeland, FL 33811
Cotton header roll.

Respond Industries, Inc. 1-800-523-8999
9500 Woodend Rd, Edwardsville, KS 66111
Various sizes and styles of gauze pads.

Safetec Of America, Inc. 800-456-7077
887 Kensington Ave, Buffalo, NY 14215
ZORB sheets are tissue-based papers impregnated withsuper absorbent polymers. SUPER BARRIER ZORBS have an added poly backing for protection against fluid penetration. ZAFETY PACS are an ideal absorbent for specimen transport -- a single-use pac of solidifier encased in a porous, non-woven material, allowing the solidifier and fluid to mix.

Sentinel Consumer Products, Inc. 440-974-8144
7750 Tyler Blvd, Mentor, OH 44060

Standard Textile Augusta, Inc. 513-761-9255
1701 Goodrich St, Augusta, GA 30904
Various sizes of surgical towels.

Suburban Adult Services, Inc. 716-496-5551
441 Indian Church Rd, West Seneca, NY 14224
Eye patch kit, sterile.

Suburban Adult Services, Inc. 716-496-5551
118 King St, East Aurora, NY 14052

Tidi Products, Llc 920-751-4380
570 Enterprise Dr, Neenah, WI 54956
Trauma dressing- various sizes and types sterile and non-sterile-roll type absor.

Tillotson Healthcare Corp. 888-335-7500
10 Glenshaw St, Orangeburg, NY 10962
SUPER FLUFF, sterile and non-sterile, high absorbency dressing bandages. Features a crinkle weave pattern for superior wicking action. SENSI WRAP, sterile and non-sterile, self-adherent; USP Type VIII gauze bandages. Features a two ply Duo Cling bandage for non-constricting stretch and flex qualities with mild compression.

FIBER, ABSORBENT *(cont'd)*

Tri-State Hospital Supply Corp. 517-545-1135
3173 E 43rd St, Yuma, AZ 85365

U-Ten Corporation 630-289-8058
1286 Humbracht Cir, Bartlett, IL 60103
Operating room towels.

3m Company 651-733-4365
601 22nd Ave S, Brookings, SD 57006

FIBEROPTIC LIGHT SOURCE & CARRIER

(Ear/Nose/Throat) 77EQH

Biomet Microfixation Inc. 800-874-7711
1520 Tradeport Dr, Jacksonville, FL 32218
Source, carrier, fiberoptic light.

Bulbworks, Inc. 800-334-2852
80 N Dell Ave Unit 5, Kenvil, NJ 07847
Replacement Lamps For All Types Of Fiberoptic Equipment

Chiu Technical Corp. 631-544-0606
252 Indian Head Rd, Kings Park, NY 11754
$248.00 for FO 150-115.

Clinimed, Incorporated 877-CLINIMED
303 Markus Ct, Sandy Brae Industrial Park, Newark, DE 19713

Codman & Shurtleff, Inc 800-225-0460
325 Paramount Dr, Raynham, MA 02767

Electro Surgical Instrument Co., Inc. 888-464-2784
37 Centennial St, Rochester, NY 14611
Various fiber optic lighting systems, light sources, cables,and adaptors.

Elmed, Inc. 630-543-2792
60 W Fay Ave, Addison, IL 60101

Fiberoptic Components, Llc 978-422-0422
2 Spratt Tech. Way, Sterling, MA 01564
Fiber optic light guide.

Gyrus Ent L.L.C., Sub. Of Gyrus Acmi, Inc. 508-804-2739
2925 Appling Rd, Bartlett, TN 38133
Various types and sizes of fiberoptic light carrier scources.

Health Care Logistics, Inc. 800-848-1633
450 Town St, PO Box 25, Circleville, OH 43113
Battery operated penlight handles for laryngscopes blades.

Integra Luxtec, Inc. 800-325-8966
99 Hartwell St, West Boylston, MA 01583

Invuity, Inc. 760-744-4447
334 Via Vera Cruz Ste 255, San Marcos, CA 92078
Fiberoptic cables.

Invuity, Inc. 415-655-2100
39 Stillman St, San Francisco, CA 94107

Jedmed Instruments Co. 314-845-3770
5416 Jedmed Ct, Saint Louis, MO 63129

Karl Storz Endoscopy-America Inc. 800-421-0837
600 Corporate Pointe, Culver City, CA 90230

Kelleher Medical, Inc. 804-378-9956
3049 St Marys Way, Powhatan, VA 23139

Linos Photonics, Inc 800-334-5678
459 Fortune Blvd, Milford, MA 01757
Laser light sources.

Mahe International Inc. 800-294-7946
468 Craighead St, Nashville, TN 37204

Peregrine Surgical, Ltd. 215-348-0456
51 Britain Dr, Doylestown, PA 18901
Various disposable fiber optic probes (cords w/handpieces).

Progressive Dynamics Medical, Inc. 269-781-4241
507 Industrial Rd, Marshall, MI 49068
150 watt halogen light source.

Schott North America, Inc. 315-255-2791
62 Columbus St, Auburn, NY 13021
SCHOTT manufactures and supplies fiberoptic and LED illumination solutions for machine vision, industrial OEM, microscopy, forensic, and medical applications. Our product catalog features photos, drawings, and technical specifications for more than 400 standard products, from light sources to backlights, ringlights, bundles, goosenecks, lightlines, halogen light sources, and a variety of accessories. Please visit www.us.schott.com/fiberoptics to request our product catalog or literature.

Scope Technology, Inc. 860-963-1141
1 Vision Rd, Pomfret, CT 06258
Medical light guide.

FIBEROPTIC LIGHT SOURCE & CARRIER *(cont'd)*

Sunoptic Technologies 877-677-2832
6018 Bowdendale Ave, Jacksonville, FL 32216
Fiberoptic cables, all types, sizes and lengths, standard or custom, autoclavable. Several models of solid state high intensity universal fiberoptic lightsources, 150W, 300W, and xenon types available. UL and CSA listed. Custom work and prototypes of fiberoptic cables.

Techman Int'L Corp. 508-248-2900
242 Sturbridge Rd, Charlton, MA 01507
Fiberoptic cable.

Tsi Medical Ltd. 800-661-7263
47 Athabascan Ave., Unit 105, Sherwood Park, AB T8A-4H3 Canada

FIBRILLATOR *(Cardiovascular) 74QVT*

Seecor, Inc. 972-288-3278
844 Dalworth Dr Ste 6, Mesquite, TX 75149
AC and battery powered units; Model 2039 - AC fibrillator.

FIBRILLATOR, AC-POWERED *(Cardiovascular) 74LIW*

Peter Schiff Enterprise 931-537-6505
4900 Forrest Hill Rd, Cookeville, TN 38506
Battery operated ac cardiac fibrilliator.

Seecor, Inc. 972-288-3278
844 Dalworth Dr Ste 6, Mesquite, TX 75149

FIBRIN MONOMER PARACOAGULATION *(Hematology) 81JBN*

Biomerieux Inc. 800-682-2666
100 Rodolphe St, Durham, NC 27712

Diagnostica Stago, Inc. 800-222-COAG
5 Century Dr, Parsippany, NJ 07054

FIBRIN SPLIT PRODUCTS *(Hematology) 81GHH*

Access Bio Incorporate 732-297-2222
2033 Rt. 130 Unit H, Monmouth Junction, NJ 08852
D-dimer test.

Biosite Incorporated 888-246-7483
9975 Summers Ridge Rd, San Diego, CA 92121
Fluorescence immunoassay for d-dimer.

Fisher Diagnostics 877-722-4366
11515 Vanstory Dr Ste 125, Huntersville, NC 28078

R2 Diagnostics, Inc. 574-288-4377
1801 Commerce Dr, South Bend, IN 46628
Dimtek d-dimerfibrotek fdp.

FIBROMETER *(Hematology) 81GIE*

Bd Diagnostic Systems 800-675-0908
7 Loveton Cir, Sparks, MD 21152

FILE *(Orthopedics) 87HTP*

Biomet Microfixation Inc. 800-874-7711
1520 Tradeport Dr, Jacksonville, FL 32218
Various types of files.

Biomet, Inc. 574-267-6639
56 E Bell Dr, PO Box 587, Warsaw, IN 46582
Orthopedic bone file.

Carr Corporation 800-952-2398
1547 11th St, Santa Monica, CA 90401
X-ray film files.

Elmed, Inc. 630-543-2792
60 W Fay Ave, Addison, IL 60101

Integral Design Inc. 781-740-2036
52 Burr Rd, Hingham, MA 02043

Kmedic 800-955-0559
190 Veterans Dr, Northvale, NJ 07647

Zimmer Trabecular Metal Technology 800-613-6131
10 Pomeroy Rd, Parsippany, NJ 07054
Bone file.

FILE, BONE, SURGICAL *(Dental And Oral) 76EMI*

Aesculap Implant Systems Inc. 1-800-234-9179
3773 Corporate Pkwy, Center Valley, PA 18034

Biomet Microfixation Inc. 800-874-7711
1520 Tradeport Dr, Jacksonville, FL 32218
Various types of files.

Deknatel Snowden-Pencer 800-367-7874
5175 S Royal Atlanta Dr, Tucker, GA 30084

Dental Usa, Inc. 815-363-8003
5005 McCullom Lake Rd, McHenry, IL 60050
File.

FILE, BONE, SURGICAL *(cont'd)*

E.A. Beck & Co. 949-645-4072
657 W 19th St Ste E, P O Box 10857, Costa Mesa, CA 92627
Bone file.

Elmed, Inc. 630-543-2792
60 W Fay Ave, Addison, IL 60101

H & H Co. 909-390-0373
4435 E Airport Dr Ste 108, Ontario, CA 91761
File, bone, all types.

Hu-Friedy Manufacturing Co., Inc. 800-483-7433
3232 N Rockwell St, Chicago, IL 60618
$53.55 each, 11 types.

Kmedic 800-955-0559
190 Veterans Dr, Northvale, NJ 07647

Miltex Inc. 800-645-8000
589 Davies Dr, York, PA 17402

Nordent Manufacturing, Inc. 800-966-7336
610 Bonnie Ln, Elk Grove Village, IL 60007
$52.50 per unit (standard).

Premier Dental Products Co. 888-670-6100
1710 Romano Dr, PO Box 4500, Plymouth Meeting, PA 19462

Salvin Dental Specialties, Inc. 800-535-6566
3450 Latrobe Dr, Charlotte, NC 28211
Various types of bone files.

Symmetry Medical Usa, Inc. 574-267-8700
486 W 350 N, Warsaw, IN 46582
Dental hand instrument.

FILE, CALLOUS *(Surgery) 79QVU*

Alimed, Inc. 800-225-2610
297 High St, Dedham, MA 02026

FILE, MARGIN FINISHING, OPERATIVE *(Dental And Oral) 76EKA*

Aesculap Implant Systems Inc. 1-800-234-9179
3773 Corporate Pkwy, Center Valley, PA 18034

Dental Usa, Inc. 815-363-8003
5005 McCullom Lake Rd, McHenry, IL 60050
File.

Hu-Friedy Manufacturing Co., Inc. 800-483-7433
3232 N Rockwell St, Chicago, IL 60618
$28.70 each, 3 types.

Micro-Dent Inc. 866-526-1166
379 Hollow Hill Rd, Wauconda, IL 60084
Knife.

Premier Dental Products Co. 888-670-6100
1710 Romano Dr, PO Box 4500, Plymouth Meeting, PA 19462

Suter Dental Manufacturing Company, Inc. 800-368-8376
632 Cedar St, Chico, CA 95928

FILE, PERIODONTIC *(Dental And Oral) 76EMR*

Biomet Microfixation Inc. 800-874-7711
1520 Tradeport Dr, Jacksonville, FL 32218
Various types of files.

Dental Usa, Inc. 815-363-8003
5005 McCullom Lake Rd, McHenry, IL 60050
File.

E.A. Beck & Co. 949-645-4072
657 W 19th St Ste E, P O Box 10857, Costa Mesa, CA 92627
File.

H & H Co. 909-390-0373
4435 E Airport Dr Ste 108, Ontario, CA 91761
File, periodontic.

Hu-Friedy Manufacturing Co., Inc. 800-483-7433
3232 N Rockwell St, Chicago, IL 60618
$32.95 each, 16 types.

Nordent Manufacturing, Inc. 800-966-7336
610 Bonnie Ln, Elk Grove Village, IL 60007
$38.50 to $28.50 each in various sizes.

Suter Dental Manufacturing Company, Inc. 800-368-8376
632 Cedar St, Chico, CA 95928

Zoll Dental 800-239-2904
7450 N Natchez Ave, Niles, IL 60714
Root planing files.

FILE, PULP CANAL, ENDODONTIC *(Dental And Oral) 76EKS*

D&S Dental, Llc 423-928-1299
3111 Hanover Rd, Johnson City, TN 37604
Hand files, endodontic.

FILE, PULP CANAL, ENDODONTIC *(cont'd)*

Dental Usa, Inc. 815-363-8003
5005 McCullom Lake Rd, McHenry, IL 60050
File.

Dentalez Group 866-DTE-INFO
101 Lindenwood Dr Ste 225, Valleybrooke Corporate Center
Malvern, PA 19355

International Plastics, Llc 262-781-2270
4965 N. Campbell Dr., Menomonee Falls, WI 53051
Rotary endodontic file.

Js Dental Mfg., Inc. 800-284-3368
196 N Salem Rd, Ridgefield, CT 06877
S-file, engine s-file.

Kerr Corp. 714-516-7400
28200 Wick Rd, Romulus, MI 48174
Pulp canal file.

Maximum Dental, Inc. 631-245-2176
600 Meadowlands Pkwy Ste 269, Secaucus, NJ 07094

Miltex Dental Technologies, Inc. 516-576-6022
589 Davies Dr, York, PA 17402
Various engine-driven endodontic instruments.

Moyco Technologies, Inc. 800-331-8837
200 Commerce Dr, Montgomeryville, PA 18936
FLEX-R, ONYX-R, ONYX-H, K-FILES & HEDSTROM.

Plastic Endo, Llc 866-752-3636
318 W Half Day Rd # 247, Buffalo Grove, IL 60089
Dental hand instrument.

Pulpdent Corp. 800-343-4342
80 Oakland St, Watertown, MA 02472
17% EDTA solution.

Special Products, Inc. 800-538-6836
2540 Greenwood Dr, Kissimmee, FL 34744
File system.

Ultradent Products, Inc. 801-553-4586
505 W 10200 S, South Jordan, UT 84095
Disinfecting solution.

United Dental Manufacturers, Inc. 918-878-0450
PO Box 700874, Tulsa, OK 74170
K-file, Hedstroem file.

United Dental Mfg., Inc. 717-845-7511
608 Rolling Hills Dr, Johnson City, TN 37604
Various.

FILE, SURGICAL, GENERAL & PLASTIC SURGERY
(Surgery) 79GEO

Bausch & Lomb Surgical 636-255-5051
3365 Tree Court Ind Blvd, Saint Louis, MO 63122

Biomet Microfixation Inc. 800-874-7711
1520 Tradeport Dr, Jacksonville, FL 32218
Various types of files.

Deknatel Snowden-Pencer 800-367-7874
5175 S Royal Atlanta Dr, Tucker, GA 30084
Nasal bone file.

Kmedic 800-955-0559
190 Veterans Dr, Northvale, NJ 07647

Symmetry Medical Usa, Inc. 574-267-8700
486 W 350 N, Warsaw, IN 46582
Manual surgical instrument for general use.

FILIFORM, WITH FILIFORM FOLLOWER *(Gastro/Urology) 78FBW*

Cook Urological, Inc. 800-457-4500
1100 W Morgan St, P.O. Box 227, Spencer, IN 47460

FILLER, BONE CEMENT (FOR VERTEBROPLASTY)
(Orthopedics) 87NDN

Advanced Biomaterial Systems, Inc. 973-635-9040
100 Passaic Ave, Chatham, NJ 07928
Pmma.

Medtronic Sofamor Danek Usa, Inc. 901-396-3133
4340 Swinnea Rd, Memphis, TN 38118
Cement, bone, vertebroplasty.

Medtronic Spine Llc 877-690-5353
1221 Crossman Ave, Sunnyvale, CA 94089
Sterile polymethylmethacrylate, pmma, bone cement.

Stryker Puerto Rico, Ltd. 939-307-2500
Hwy. 3, Km. 131.2, Las Guasimas Ind. Park, Arroyo, PR 00714
Pmma bone cement.

FILLER, BONE VOID, MEDICATED *(Orthopedics) 87MVB*

Bacterin International Inc. 406-388-0480
664 Cruiser Ln, Belgrade, MT 59714
OsteoSelect DBM Putty

FILLER, BONE VOID, NON-OSTEOINDUCTION
(Physical Med) 89MBS

Medtronic Sofamor Danek Usa, Inc. 901-396-3133
4340 Swinnea Rd, Memphis, TN 38118
Synthetic bone substitute.

FILLER, BONE VOID, OSTEOINDUCTION *(Physical Med) 89MBP*

Berkeley Advanced Biomaterials, Inc. 510-883-0500
901 Grayson St Unit 101, Berkeley, CA 94710
Sterile bone void fillers include synthetic bone grafts and human DBM putty, dough, and strips.

FILLER, BOVINE PROTEIN MIXTURE, BONE MORPHOGENETIC PROTEINS, COLLAGEN SCAFFOLD, OSTEOINDUCTION
(Physical Med) 89MPY

Stryker Biotech 508-416-5200
35 South St, Hopkinton, MA 01748
Bone morphogentic protein combination device. - OP-1 Implant, OP-1 Putty

Stryker Biotech 603-298-3000
9 Technology Dr, West Lebanon, NH 03784
Bone morphogentic protein combination device.

FILLER, CALCIUM SULFATE PREFORMED PELLETS
(Orthopedics) 87MQV

Arthrex, Inc. 239-643-5553
1370 Creekside Blvd, Naples, FL 34108
Bone substitute.

Biomet, Inc. 574-267-6639
56 E Bell Dr, PO Box 587, Warsaw, IN 46582
Various types of bone graft substitute.

Biostructures, Llc 949-553-1743
3700 Campus Dr Ste 204, Newport Beach, CA 92660
Filler,bone void, calcium compound.

Collagen Matrix, Inc. 201-405-1477
509 Commerce St, Franklin Lakes, NJ 07417
Filer,bone void, calciun compound.

Depuy Spine, Inc. 800-227-6633
365 Ravendale Dr, Mountain View, CA 94043
Bone graft substiture.

Depuy Spine, Inc. 800-227-6633
325 Paramount Dr, Raynham, MA 02767
B-tricalcium phosphate.

Medtronic Sofamor Danek Usa, Inc. 901-396-3133
4340 Swinnea Rd, Memphis, TN 38118
Bone, void filler.

Musculoskeletal Transplant Foundation 800-433-6576
125 May St Ste 300, Edison Corp Ctr, Edison, NJ 08837
Bone void filler containing human demineralized bone matrix.

Nanotherapeutics, Inc. 386-462-9663
13859 Progress Blvd Ste 300, Alachua, FL 32615
Bone void filler, bone graft substitute.

Novabone Products, Llc 386-462-7660
13709 Progress Blvd Ste 33, Alachua, FL 32615
NovaBone - Synthetic Bone Void Filler;

Nuvasive, Inc. 800-475-9131
7475 Lusk Blvd, San Diego, CA 92121
Bone void filler.

Orthovita, Inc. 610-640-1775
77 Great Valley Pkwy, Malvern, PA 19355
Various sizes and shapes of sterile bone graft material.

RTI Biologics Inc. 877-343-6832
11621 Research Cir, Alachua, FL 32615
Filler, bone void, calcium compound.

Skeletal Kinetics, Llc 408-366-5000
10201 Bubb Rd, Cupertino, CA 95014
Bone void filler.

Spinecraft Llc 708-531-9700
2215 Enterprise Dr, Westchester, IL 60154
Bone void filler.

Synthes (Usa) - Development Center 719-481-5300
1230 Wilson Dr, West Chester, PA 19380
Bone void filler.

FILLER, CALCIUM SULFATE PREFORMED PELLETS *(cont'd)*

Therics, Llc 330-475-8600
1800 Triplett Blvd, Akron, OH 44306
Bone void fillers.

Wright Medical Group, Inc. 800-238-7117
5677 Airline Rd, Arlington, TN 38002

FILLER, RECOMBINANT HUMAN BONE MORPHOGENETIC PROTEIN, COLLAGEN SCAFFOLD WITH METAL PROSTHESIS, OSTEOINDUCTION *(Orthopedics) 87NEK*

Medtronic Sofamor Danek Usa, Inc. 901-396-3133
4340 Swinnea Rd, Memphis, TN 38118
Collagen sponge.

FILLING, INSTRUMENT PLASTIC, DENTAL
(Dental And Oral) 76EIY

Denbur, Inc. 630-969-6865
433 Plaza Dr Ste 4, Westmont, IL 60559
Tooth fracture locator.

Dental Usa, Inc. 815-363-8003
5005 McCullom Lake Rd, McHenry, IL 60050
Various types of instruments.

Dentalez Group 866-DTE-INFO
101 Lindenwood Dr Ste 225, Valleybrooke Corporate Center
Malvern, PA 19355

Dentsply Canada, Ltd. 800-263-1437
161 Vinyl Ct., Woodbridge, ONT L4L 4A3 Canada

E.A. Beck & Co. 949-645-4072
657 W 19th St Ste E, P O Box 10857, Costa Mesa, CA 92627
Plastic filling instrument.

Garrison Dental Solutions 616-842-2244
110 Dewitt Ln, Spring Lake, MI 49456
Composite instruments.

Glenroe Technologies 800-237-4060
1912 44th Ave E, Bradenton, FL 34203
Cement spatula.

Hager Worldwide, Inc. 800-328-2335
13322 Byrd Dr, Odessa, FL 33556
MIRAFILL.

Hartzell & Son, G. 800-950-2206
2372 Stanwell Cir, Concord, CA 94520

Hu-Friedy Manufacturing Co., Inc. 800-483-7433
3232 N Rockwell St, Chicago, IL 60618
$22.80 to $26.45 each.

Nordent Manufacturing, Inc. 800-966-7336
610 Bonnie Ln, Elk Grove Village, IL 60007
$18.00 per unit (standard).

Premier Dental Products Co. 888-670-6100
1710 Romano Dr, PO Box 4500, Plymouth Meeting, PA 19462

Sci-Dent, Inc. 800-323-4145
210 Dowdle St Ste 2, Algonquin, IL 60102

Suter Dental Manufacturing Company, Inc. 800-368-8376
632 Cedar St, Chico, CA 95928

Trans American Medical / Tamsco Instruments 708-430-7777
7633 W 100th Pl, Bridgeview, IL 60455
Medium grade surgical stainless steel.

Ultradent Products, Inc. 801-553-4586
505 W 10200 S, South Jordan, UT 84095
Composite packer.

United Dental Manufacturers, Inc. 918-878-0450
PO Box 700874, Tulsa, OK 74170

United Dental Mfg., Inc. 717-845-7511
608 Rolling Hills Dr, Johnson City, TN 37604
Dental plastic filling instruments.

Young O/S Llc 800-325-1881
1663 Fenton Business Park Ct, Fenton, MO 63026
Heated gutta purcha system.

3m Espe Dental Products 949-863-1360
2111 McGaw Ave, Irvine, CA 92614
From $69.95 to $165.50 per unit.

FILM, X-RAY *(Radiology) 90EAL*

Agfa Corp. 800-581-2432
100 Challenger Rd, Ridgefield Park, NJ 07660
X-ray film and CURIX automated daylight film center.

FILM, X-RAY *(cont'd)*

Burkhart Roentgen Intl. Inc. 800-USA-XRAY
5201 8th Ave S, Gulfport, FL 33707
Blue and green sensitive in stock, all sizes.

Chemplex Industries, Inc. 800-424-3675
2820 SW 42nd Ave, Palm City, FL 34990

Flow X-Ray Corporation 800-356-9729
100 W Industry Ct, Deer Park, NY 11729
All types of x-ray film medical and dental x-ray film

Gammadirect Medical Division 847-267-5929
PO Box 383, Lake Forest, IL 60045
Beta-Elk Laser digitizer is user friendly and allows for efficient film management-DICOM compatible. Filed film can be accessed from home.

I.B.F. Corporation 800-423-3456
44 Plauderville Ave, Garfield, NJ 07026
RXB (blue) and RXG (green) standard, MM single emulsion and DUP-X duplicating x-ray film; also, MSF blue half speed x-ray film.

Kodak Canada Inc., Health Imaging Division 800-295-5526
3500 Eglinton Ave. W., Toronto, ONT M6M 1V3 Canada

Marconi Medical Systems 800-323-0550
595 Miner Rd, Cleveland, OH 44143

Medlink Imaging, Inc. 800-456-7800
200 Clearbrook Rd, Elmsford, NY 10523
Blue sensitive, orthochromatic, CRT. 1/2 speed Blue-Duplicating.

Pl Medical Co., Llc. 800-874-0120
321 Ellis St, New Britain, CT 06051
Blue high speed, 1/2 speed, green sensitive.

Polyzen, Inc. 919-319-9599
1041 Classic Rd, Apex, NC 27539
Radiology barrier films.

Schueler & Company, Inc. 516-487-1500
PO Box 528, Stratford, CT 06615

Simon & Company Inc., H.R. 800-638-9460
3515 Marmenco Ct, Baltimore, MD 21230

St. John Companies 800-435-4242
25167 Anza Dr, PO Box 800460, Santa Clarita, CA 91355
Top quality x-ray film at competitive prices.

Ti-Ba Enterprises, Inc. 585-247-1212
25 Hytec Cir, Rochester, NY 14606
Medical X-ray Film. Please call us for your price on Physicians Choice Medical X-ray Film from Konica Minolta.

White Mountain Imaging 603-648-2124
1617 Battle St, Webster, NH 03303
FUJI/WMI X-RAY FILM

Wolf X-Ray Corporation 800-356-9729
100 W Industry Ct, Deer Park, NY 11729
Blue and green sensitive film in all popular sizes.

Xma (X-Ray Marketing Associates, Inc.) 800-325-8880
1205 W Lakeview Ct, Windham Lakes Business Park
Romeoville, IL 60446

FILM, X-RAY, DENTAL, EXTRAORAL *(Dental And Oral) 76EHC*

Agfa Corporation 877-777-2432
PO Box 19048, 10 South Academy Street, Greenville, SC 29602

D.C.A. (Dental Corporation Of America) 800-638-6684
889 S Matlack St, West Chester, PA 19382
$54.00per 100 and $23.75 per pad (100 sheets) of x-ray tracing paper.

G & H Wire Co. 800-526-1026
2165 Earlywood Dr, Franklin, IN 46131

Goetze Dental 800-692-0804
3939 NE 33rd Ter, Kansas City, MO 64117

Orthodontic Supply & Equipment Co., Inc. 800-638-4003
7851 Airpark Rd Ste 202, Gaithersburg, MD 20879

Schueler & Company, Inc. 516-487-1500
PO Box 528, Stratford, CT 06615

Sirona Dental Systems Llc 800-659-5977
4835 Sirona Dr Ste 100, Charlotte, NC 28273

3m Espe Dental Products 949-863-1360
2111 McGaw Ave, Irvine, CA 92614
$113.40 for panoramic x-ray film.

FILM, X-RAY, DENTAL, INTRAORAL *(Dental And Oral) 76EAO*

Goetze Dental 800-692-0804
3939 NE 33rd Ter, Kansas City, MO 64117

FILM, X-RAY, DENTAL, INTRAORAL *(cont'd)*

Marconi Medical Systems 800-323-0550
595 Miner Rd, Cleveland, OH 44143

Minimax Company 800-292-2620
100 W Industry Ct, Deer Park, NY 11729
Periapical, children size, bitewings.

Orthodontic Supply & Equipment Co., Inc. 800-638-4003
7851 Airpark Rd Ste 202, Gaithersburg, MD 20879

Schueler & Company, Inc. 516-487-1500
PO Box 528, Stratford, CT 06615

Wolf X-Ray Corporation 800-356-9729
100 W Industry Ct, Deer Park, NY 11729

FILM, X-RAY, SPECIAL PURPOSE *(Radiology) 90IWZ*

Agfa Corporation 877-777-2432
PO Box 19048, 10 South Academy Street, Greenville, SC 29602

Agfa Healthcare Corp. 864-421-1815
1636 Bushy Park Rd, Goose Creek, SC 29445

Carestream Health, Inc. 888-777-2072
150 Verona St, Rochester, NY 14608
Various types of duplicating, extraoral and introral film.

Codonics 800-444-1198
17991 Englewood Dr, Middleburg Heights, OH 44130
Codonics DirectVista Film offers superior diagnostic quality available in 14'x17', 11'x14' and 8'x10'. All film sizes print on the Horizon Multi-media Imager product line.

Fr Chemical 603-648-2194
524 S Columbus Ave, Mount Vernon, NY 10550
X-ray processing solutions.

Fujifilm Manufacturing Usa, Inc. 864-223-2888
103 Spray Shed Rd, Greenwood, SC 29649
X-ray film.

Hayes Manufacturing Services, Inc. 408-496-1816
3330 Victor Ct, Santa Clara, CA 95054

Holorad Llc 801-983-6075
2929 S Main St, Salt Lake City, UT 84115
Holographic medical imaging film.

Medlink Imaging, Inc. 800-456-7800
200 Clearbrook Rd, Elmsford, NY 10523

Xma (X-Ray Marketing Associates, Inc.) 800-325-8880
1205 W Lakeview Ct, Windham Lakes Business Park
Romeoville, IL 60446

FILTER PAPER *(Chemistry) 75QVV*

Enzo Biochem, Inc. 212-583-0100
527 Madison Ave, New York, NY 10022
Glass fiber filters, discs or sheets.

Great Lakes Filters/Filpaco Industries 517-639-8470
301 Arch Ave, Hillsdale, MI 49242
Single source distributor of filtration products.

Pall Corporation 800-521-1520
600 S Wagner Rd, Ann Arbor, MI 48103

Schleicher & Schuell, Inc. 800-245-4024
10 Optical Ave, PO Box 2012, Keene, NH 03431

Terriss-Consolidated Industries 800-342-1611
807 Summerfield Ave, Asbury Park, NJ 07712

The Hilliard Corporation 607-733-7121
100 W 4th St, Elmira, NY 14901

Whatman Inc. 732-885-6529
800 Centennial Ave Bldg 1, Piscataway, NJ 08854

FILTER, AIR *(General) 80QVW*

Air Quality Engineering, Inc. 800-328-0787
7140 Northland Dr N, Minneapolis, MN 55428
SMOKEMASTER electrostatic precipitator. MIRACLE AIR media air cleaners. Both available for various room sizes and applications. XJ 1000 HEPA filter unit for negative pressure isolation rooms.

Airguard 800-999-3458
3807 Bishop Ln, Louisville, KY 40218
VARI-KLEAN, gas phase adsorption carbon filter.

Airistar Technologies, L.L.C. 800-755-8006
2330 Ernie Krueger Cir, Waukegan, IL 60087
Portable air-purification systems that use Airistar's advanced six-step Hexaflow purification process featuring superior HEPA filtration, the next generation of HEPA technology.

Atlantic Ultraviolet Corp. 631-273-0500
375 Marcus Blvd, Hauppauge, NY 11788
SANITAIRE Portable room air sterilizers.

FILTER, AIR *(cont'd)*

Bio-Safe America Corp. 800-767-4284
3250 S Susan St Ste B, Sterilaire Medical Division
Santa Ana, CA 92704
HEPA.uhpa

Camfil Farr 800-300-3277
2121 E Paulhan St, Rancho Dominguez, CA 90220
Cleanroom air filtration systems and HEPA air filters.

Clean Air Technology, Inc. 800 459 6320
41105 Capital Dr, Canton, MI 48187
HEPA filters, pre-filters, BAG IN-BAG OUT filter systems and HEPA filter systems for modular cleanrooms, soft wall cleanrooms, containment modules, Bio-Hazard level P2 and P3 negative air pressure laboratories.

Cloud 9 630-595-5000
777 N Edgewood Ave, Wood Dale, IL 60191

Esa, Inc. 800-959-5095
22 Alpha Rd, Chelmsford, MA 01824
Air filter analyses.

Filterspun 800-432-0108
624 N Fairfield St, Amarillo, TX 79107
Filter, liquid.

Filtertek Inc. 800-248-2461
11411 Price Rd, Hebron, IL 60034
Filter elements (parts).

Fts Systems 800-824-0400
PO Box 158, 3538 Main Street,, Stone Ridge, NY 12484
Recirculating coolers for cost-effective cooling/heat removal. System provides a clean circulating medium at a constant temperature.

Genx International 888-GEN-XNOW
393 Soundview Rd, Guilford, CT 06437

Great Lakes Filters/Filpaco Industries 517-639-8470
301 Arch Ave, Hillsdale, MI 49242
Single source distributor of filtration products.

Gvs Filter Technology Inc. 317-471-3700
5353 W 79th St, Indianapolis, IN 46268
Hydrophobic vents (all radiation stable) for catheters, IV sets, bags, canisters, and other types of systems that require venting or isolation from the environment. Some have integral caps, some do not. All available on an OEM basis.

Industrial Specialities Manufacturing, Inc. 800-781-8487
2741 W Oxford Ave Unit 6, Englewood, CO 80110

La Calhene 320-358-4713
1325 S Field Ave, PO Box 567, Rush City, MN 55069

Liberty Industries, Inc. 800-828-5656
133 Commerce St, East Berlin, CT 06023

Lm Air Technology, Inc. 866-381-8200
1467 Pinewood St, Cleanroom & Lab Equipment - Mfger
Rahway, NJ 07065
LO-PRO T-grid filter blower module, 24 x 48 x 9 profile, with replaceable HEPA filter. Less than 62 dBA at 70 FPM 50 lbs. Operates on less than 2 amps. Two-year warranty.

Lydall, Inc. 860-646-1233
1 Colonial Rd, Manchester, CT 06042
Filtration media for air, liquids and diagnostic devices. Glass papers for laboratory analyses.

Mars Air Doors 800-421-1266
14716 S Broadway St, Gardena, CA 90248
Clean air filters.

Mectra Labs, Inc. 800-323-3968
PO Box 350, Two Quality Way, Bloomfield, IN 47424
Hydrophobic insufflation filter, 0.1mm particulate air filter, hydrophobic media with 10' attached tubing.

Medi-Dose, Inc. 800-523-8966
70 Industrial Dr, Ivyland, PA 18974

Millipore Corporation 800-MILLIPORE
80 Ashby Rd, Bedford, MA 01730

Niche Medical, Inc. 800-633-1055
55 Access Rd, Warwick, RI 02886
Full line of competitive filters for many of the smoke evacuation units on the market today as well as inline filters.

Novosci Corp. 281-363-4949
2828 N Crescentridge Dr, The Woodlands, TX 77381

Pall Corporation 800-521-1520
600 S Wagner Rd, Ann Arbor, MI 48103

FILTER, AIR *(cont'd)*

Performance Systematix Inc 616-949-9090
5569 33rd St SE, Grand Rapids, MI 49512
Air vent filters for particle/bacteria removal. Hydrophobic filter media allows free air passage while blocking liquids.

Permatron Corp. 800-882-8012
1180 Pratt Blvd, Elk Grove Village, IL 60007

Porvair Filtration Group Inc 803-327-5008
454 Anderson Rd S, BTC 514, Rock Hill, SC 29730

Purified Micro Environments, Div. Of Germfree Laboratories 800-888-5357
11 Aviator Way, Ormond Beach, FL 32174
Portable fume/particulate filtration. Small, portable carbon filtered air filtration unit.

Schleicher & Schuell, Inc. 800-245-4024
10 Optical Ave, PO Box 2012, Keene, NH 03431

Smiths Medical Asd, Inc. 800-848-1757
6250 Shier Rings Rd, Dublin, OH 43016

Trion, Inc. 800-884-0002
101 McNeill Rd, Sanford, NC 27330

United Air Specialists, Inc. 800-252-4647
4440 Creek Rd, Cincinnati, OH 45242

Veco, S.A. De C.V. 55-688-3566
Pirineos No. 263, Col. General Anaya, Mexico D.F., BENIT 03100 Mexico
Environmental engineering.

Vital Concepts, Inc. 800-984-2300
4334 Brockton Dr SE Ste F, Grand Rapids, MI 49512
37 and 50 mm insufflation filters for insufflation procedures with 2in., 6in., 2ft., 6ft., and 12ft. tubing.

FILTER, ASPIRATOR *(Surgery) 79WIF*

Armm, Inc. 714-848-8190
17744 Sampson Ln, Huntington Beach, CA 92647
0.2 micron, hydrophobic, high flow.

Medela, Inc. 800-435-8316
1101 Corporate Dr, McHenry, IL 60050
Odor, overflow and bacteria filters for use with Medela aspirators.

Schueler & Company, Inc. 516-487-1500
PO Box 528, Stratford, CT 06615

FILTER, BACTERIAL, BREATHING CIRCUIT
(Anesthesiology) 73CAH

A-M Systems, Inc. 800-426-1306
131 Business Park Loop, Sequim, WA 98382
3 types- mainflow low pressure filter; nebulizer higher pressure unit (both autoclavable)

Accent Plastics 951-273-7777
1925 Elise Cir, Corona, CA 92879
Microgard.

Airex, Inc. 425-222-3665
13704 SE 17th St, Bellevue, WA 98005
M100 mobile self-contained ultra-clean air delivery system with attachable, quick setup and easily accessible pos/neg patient isolation chamber.

Alliance Tech Medical, Inc. 661-588-5102
5305 Mission Cir, Granbury, TX 76049
Pulmonary function filter.

Allied Healthcare Products, Inc. 800-444-3954
1720 Sublette Ave, Saint Louis, MO 63110

Amici, Inc. 610-948-7100
518 Vincent St, Spring City, PA 19475
Bacteria/virus filter.

Arc Medical, Inc. 800-950-ARC1
4296 Cowan Rd, Tucker, GA 30084
HepaStatic,circuitGuard, circuit protection system, a unitized constructed filter for safe reuse of anesthesia breathing circuits. FilterFlo.

Ballard Medical Products 770-587-7835
12050 Lone Peak Pkwy, Draper, UT 84020
Filter, bacterial, breathing-circuit.

Camfil Farr 800-300-3277
2121 E Paulhan St, Rancho Dominguez, CA 90220

Creative Biomedics, Inc. 949-366-2300
924 Calle Negocio Ste A, San Clemente, CA 92673
Clear Advantage Filter

FILTER, BACTERIAL, BREATHING CIRCUIT *(cont'd)*

Directmed, Inc. 516-656-3377
150 Pratt Oval, Glen Cove, NY 11542
Bacterial/Viral filter - air filter for breathing circuits.

Enternet Medical, Inc. 888-887-6638
1676 Village Grn, Crofton, MD 21114
Various types of bacteria filters.

Globalmed Inc. 613-394-9844
155 N. Murray St., Trenton, ONT K8V-5R5 Canada
150- and 200-g bacterial/viral filters.

Intersurgical Inc. 315-451-2900
417 Electronics Pkwy, Liverpool, NY 13088
FILTA-GUARD, CLEAR-GUARD, FILTA-THERM, CLEAR-THERM.

Jostra Bentley, Inc. 302-454-9959
Rd. 402 N. Km 1.4, Industrial Park, Anasco, PR 00610-1577
Biologic gas line filter.

Kaz, Inc. 518-828-0450
1 Vapor Trl, Hudson, NY 12534
Air cleaner, filters.

Medicomp 763-389-4473
12535 316th Ave, Princeton, MN 55371
No common name listed.

Medline Industries, Inc. 800-633-5886
1 Medline Pl, Mundelein, IL 60060

Millipore Corporation 800-MILLIPORE
80 Ashby Rd, Bedford, MA 01730

Nano Mask Inc. 888-656-3697
175 Cassia Way Ste A115, Henderson, NV 89014
2H Breathing System Filter

Nspire Health, Inc 800-574-7374
1830 Lefthand Cir, Longmont, CO 80501
KOKOMoe PFT Filter; pulmonary function/spirometry. One-piece is disposable and can be used for spirometry and full lung volume testing.

Pall Corporation 800-645-6532
25 Harbor Park Dr, Port Washington, NY 11050
Various.

Pall Corporation 800-521-1520
600 S Wagner Rd, Ann Arbor, MI 48103

Pall Lifesciences Puerto Rico Llc 516-801-9064
Carr. 194, Km. O.4, Fajardo, PR 00738
Breathing circuit filter.

Porous Media Corp. 651-653-2000
1350 Hammond Rd, Saint Paul, MN 55110
Breathing circuit filter.

Promedic, Inc. 239-498-2155
3460 Pointe Creek Ct Apt 102, Bonita Springs, FL 34134

Smiths Medical Asd Inc. 800-258-5361
10 Bowman Dr, Keene, NH 03431
Breathing filter.

Smiths Medical Asd, Inc. 847-793-0135
330 Corporate Woods Pkwy, Vernon Hills, IL 60061
Bacterial filter.

Smiths Medical Asd, Inc. 800-848-1757
6250 Shier Rings Rd, Dublin, OH 43016

Spirometrics Medical Equipment Co., Llc 207-657-6700
22 Shaker Rd, Gray, ME 04039
Particulant hydrophobic filter.

Terumo Cardiovascular Systems (Tcvs) 800-283-7866
28 Howe St, Ashland, MA 01721
Gas filter.

Vacumed 800-235-3333
4538 Westinghouse St, Ventura, CA 93003
5 sizes available.

Ventlab Corp. 336-753-5000
155 Boyce Dr, Mocksville, NC 27028
Filter, bacterial, breathing circuit.

Vitalograph, Inc. 800-255-6626
13310 W 99th St, Lenexa, KS 66215
Bacterial/viral filter. Combined filter and mouthpiece in one unit. Complies with international standards for low back-pressure. Re-useable adaptors available. Box of 50 $80.00.

FILTER, BACTERIOLOGICAL, LABORATORY *(Chemistry) 75UGC*

Airguard 800-999-3458
3807 Bishop Ln, Louisville, KY 40218

FILTER, BACTERIOLOGICAL, LABORATORY *(cont'd)*

Camfil Farr 800-300-3277
2121 E Paulhan St, Rancho Dominguez, CA 90220
Cleanroom air filtration systems and HEPA air filters.

Corning Inc., Science Products Division 800-492-1110
45 Nagog Park, Acton, MA 01720
Rapid bacterial enumeration kit.

Ge Infrastructure Water & Process Technologies 877-522-7867
5951 Clearwater Dr, Minnetonka, MN 55343

Millipore Corporation 800-MILLIPORE
80 Ashby Rd, Bedford, MA 01730
MILLIDISK, MILLEX, MILLIPAK and ADDI-CHEK filters.

Pall Corporation 800-521-1520
600 S Wagner Rd, Ann Arbor, MI 48103

Q.I. Medical, Inc. 800-837-8361
440 Lower Grass Valley Rd Ste C, Nevada City, CA 95959

Schleicher & Schuell, Inc. 800-245-4024
10 Optical Ave, PO Box 2012, Keene, NH 03431

Sdi Diagnostics, Inc. 800-678-5782
10 Hampden Dr, South Easton, MA 02375
Bacterial/viral filter for pulmonary function testing.

The Hilliard Corporation 607-733-7121
100 W 4th St, Elmira, NY 14901

Thermo Fisher Scientific Inc. 563-556-2241
2555 Kerper Blvd, Dubuque, IA 52001

Whatman Inc. 732-885-6529
800 Centennial Ave Bldg 1, Piscataway, NJ 08854

FILTER, BLOOD, CARDIOPULMONARY BYPASS, ARTERIAL LINE *(Cardiovascular) 74DTM*

Edwards Lifesciences Research Medical 949-250-2500
6864 Cottonwood St, Midvale, UT 84047
Arterial filter.

Gish Biomedical, Inc. 800-938-0531
22942 Arroyo Vis, Rancho Santa Margarita, CA 92688
Arterial filter with or without integral bypass in 25- and 40-micron size.

Jostra Bentley, Inc. 302-454-9959
Rd. 402 N. Km 1.4, Industrial Park, Anasco, PR 00610-1577
Arterial filter.

Medicalcv, Inc. 800-328-2060
9725 S Robert Trl, Inver Grove Heights, MN 55077
INTERFACE.

Medtronic Blood Management 612-514-4000
18501 E Plaza Dr, Parker, CO 80134
Arterial filter.

Medtronic Perfusion Systems 800-328-3320
7611 Northland Dr N, Brooklyn Park, MN 55428
AIRSTAR arterial blood filter. Custom perfusion tubing packs.

Millipore Corporation 800-MILLIPORE
80 Ashby Rd, Bedford, MA 01730

Novosci Corp. 281-363-4949
2828 N Crescentridge Dr, The Woodlands, TX 77381

Pall Corporation 800-645-6532
25 Harbor Park Dr, Port Washington, NY 11050
Multiple.

Pall Corporation 800-521-1520
600 S Wagner Rd, Ann Arbor, MI 48103

Pall Lifesciences Puerto Rico Llc 516-801-9064
Carr. 194, Km. O.4, Fajardo, PR 00738
Multiple.

Sorin Group Usa 800-289-5759
14401 W 65th Way, Arvada, CO 80004

Terumo Cardiovascular Systems (Tcvs) 800-283-7866
125 Blue Ball Rd, Elkton, MD 21921
Arterial filter.

Terumo Cardiovascular Systems (Tcvs) 800-283-7866
28 Howe St, Ashland, MA 01721
Arterial filter.

FILTER, BLOOD, CARDIOTOMY SUCTION LINE, CARDIOPULMONARY *(Cardiovascular) 74JOD*

Gish Biomedical, Inc. 800-938-0531
22942 Arroyo Vis, Rancho Santa Margarita, CA 92688
Reservoir with integrated water seal/manometer.

FILTER, BLOOD, CARDIOTOMY SUCTION LINE, CARDIOPULMONARY *(cont'd)*

Medicalcv, Inc. 800-328-2060
9725 S Robert Trl, Inver Grove Heights, MN 55077
INTERFACE.

Millipore Corporation 800-MILLIPORE
80 Ashby Rd, Bedford, MA 01730

Pall Corporation 800-645-6532
25 Harbor Park Dr, Port Washington, NY 11050
Various.

Pall Corporation 800-521-1520
600 S Wagner Rd, Ann Arbor, MI 48103

Pall Lifesciences Puerto Rico Llc 516-801-9064
Carr. 194, Km. O.4, Fajardo, PR 00738
Various.

Sorin Group Usa 800-289-5759
14401 W 65th Way, Arvada, CO 80004

Terumo Cardiovascular Systems (Tcvs) 800-283-7866
28 Howe St, Ashland, MA 01721
Cardiotomy filter/reservoir.

Terumo Cardiovascular Systems, Corp 800-521-2818
6200 Jackson Rd, Ann Arbor, MI 48103
Reservoir cardiotomy with filter and defoamer.

Vitalcor, Inc. 800-874-8358
100 Chestnut Ave, Westmont, IL 60559
Cardiotomy.

FILTER, BLOOD, DIALYSIS *(Gastro/Urology) 78FKJ*

Apheresis Technologies, Inc. 800-749-9284
PO Box 2081, Palm Harbor, FL 34682
Plasma separator.

Gvs Filter Technology Inc. 317-471-3700
5353 W 79th St, Indianapolis, IN 46268
We offer many different types of transducer protectors, both gas permeable and non-permeable. Some with built-in reservoirs for blood collection, and some standard 25mm housings. All bacterial and viral retentive. Many different connector configurations.

Haemonetics Corp. 781-848-7100
400 Wood Rd, P.O.Box 9114, Braintree, MA 02184
Microaggregate filter.

Millipore Corporation 800-MILLIPORE
80 Ashby Rd, Bedford, MA 01730

Porex Corporation 800-241-0195
500 Bohannon Rd, Fairburn, GA 30213
INSTRUMENT SPECIFIC removes fibrin and gel separation particulates.

Serim Research Corp. 574-264-3440
3506 Reedy Dr, Elkhart, IN 46514
Test for levels of residual chlorine in rinse water.

FILTER, CELL COLLECTION, TISSUE PROCESSING *(Pathology) 88KET*

Corning Inc., Science Products Division 800-492-1110
45 Nagog Park, Acton, MA 01720

Corning, Inc. 607-433-3100
275 River St, Oneonta, NY 13820
Various vessels for cell and tissue culture.

Cytyc Surgical Products 800-442-9892
250 Campus Dr, Marlborough, MA 01752
Tissue processing equipment.

Millipore Corporation 800-MILLIPORE
80 Ashby Rd, Bedford, MA 01730

Monogen, Inc. 847-573-6700
3630 Burwood Dr, Waukegan, IL 60085
Various monoprep capsule, monoprep demo kit, slide preparation kit,starter kit.

Nalge Nunc International 800-625-4327
75 Panorama Creek Dr, Rochester, NY 14625
NALGENE analytical filter units and funnels. Single use sterile and reusable styles.

Tripath Imaging, Inc. 919-206-7140
780 Plantation Dr, Burlington, NC 27215
Tissue processing reagents.

FILTER, CONDUCTION, ANESTHESIA *(Anesthesiology) 73BSN*

Millipore Corporation 800-MILLIPORE
80 Ashby Rd, Bedford, MA 01730

FILTER, CONDUCTION, ANESTHESIA *(cont'd)*

Pall Corporation 800-521-1520
600 S Wagner Rd, Ann Arbor, MI 48103

Sdi Diagnostics, Inc. 800-678-5782
10 Hampden Dr, South Easton, MA 02375

Vacumed 800-235-3333
4538 Westinghouse St, Ventura, CA 93003

FILTER, GAS *(Anesthesiology) 73QVX*

Armm, Inc. 714-848-8190
17744 Sampson Ln, Huntington Beach, CA 92647
SuperFlow filters for insufflation. With and without tubing.

Filtertek Inc. 800-248-2461
11411 Price Rd, Hebron, IL 60034
Filter elements (parts).

Gish Biomedical, Inc. 800-938-0531
22942 Arroyo Vis, Rancho Santa Margarita, CA 92688
Extracorporeal-gas-line filter.

Mectra Labs, Inc. 800-323-3968
PO Box 350, Two Quality Way, Bloomfield, IN 47424
CO2 PATIENT FILTER, Insufflation filter, filters CO2 during insufflation, completely disposable, tubing included, adapts to all major brands of insufflators.

Millipore Corporation 800-MILLIPORE
80 Ashby Rd, Bedford, MA 01730
MILLEX LS, MILLEX FH.

Novosci Corp. 281-363-4949
2828 N Crescentridge Dr, The Woodlands, TX 77381

Pall Corporation 800-521-1520
600 S Wagner Rd, Ann Arbor, MI 48103
INTERVENE MAX-FLOW Gas Filter features high airflow rates and low back-pressure to maximize performances in sufflation, oxygen (concentration), vacuum protection, and ventilation applications.

Porvair Filtration Group Inc 803-327-5008
454 Anderson Rd S, BTC 514, Rock Hill, SC 29730

Spectrum Laboratories, Inc. 800-634-3300
18617 S Broadwick St, Rancho Dominguez, CA 90220
MEDIAKAP high-surface-area, compact filtration modules. Hollow-fiber filters for gas, media, and reagent sterilization. Also available on OEM or private-label basis.

FILTER, INFUSION LINE *(General) 80FPB*

B. Braun Medical, Inc. 610-596-2536
901 Marcon Blvd, Allentown, PA 18109
MULTIPLE

B. Braun Of Puerto Rico, Inc. 610-691-5400
215.7 Insular Rd., Sabana Grande, PR 00637
Infusion line filter.

Baxa Corporation 800-567-2292
9540 S Maroon Circle, Suite 400, Englewood, CO 80112
SUPOR CAPSULE, large-volume filter designed to batch filter 50 to 100 liters of non-cellular pharmaceutical solutions.

Benlan Inc. 905-829-5004
2760 Brighton Rd., Oakville, ONT L6H 5T4 Canada

Entracare, Llc 913-451-2234
11315 Strang Line Rd, Lenexa, KS 66215
Extension and filter sets, macro and micro, sterile.

Gvs Filter Technology Inc. 317-471-3700
5353 W 79th St, Indianapolis, IN 46268
GVS offers a new Hi-Flo IV filter, available on an OEM basis, 0.2µm, 1.2µm (other pore sizes avaialbel). Four vents for Speedflow Adult filter, two vents for Speedflow Kids configuration, and new innovative Speedflow Baby will be available late this year.

Hospira Inc. 877-946-7747
275 N Field Dr, Lake Forest, IL 60045
MULTIPLE, MICROFILTER

Jostra Bentley, Inc. 302-454-9959
Rd. 402 N. Km 1.4, Industrial Park, Anasco, PR 00610-1577
Blood infusion line.

Medi-Dose, Inc. 800-523-8966
70 Industrial Dr, Ivyland, PA 18974

Millipore Corporation 800-MILLIPORE
80 Ashby Rd, Bedford, MA 01730
IVEX, IV-EXPRESS, IV-EXPRESS PEDI, NUTRIVEX, MICROVEX.

Mps Acacia 800-486-6677
785 Challenger St, Brea, CA 92821

FILTER, INFUSION LINE *(cont'd)*

Pall Corporation 800-645-6532
25 Harbor Park Dr, Port Washington, NY 11050
Various.

Pall Corporation 800-521-1520
600 S Wagner Rd, Ann Arbor, MI 48103

Pall Lifesciences Puerto Rico Llc 516-801-9064
Carr. 194, Km. O.4, Fajardo, PR 00738
Various.

FILTER, INTRAVASCULAR, CARDIOVASCULAR
(Cardiovascular) 74DTK

Millipore Corporation 800-MILLIPORE
80 Ashby Rd, Bedford, MA 01730

Navilyst Medical 800-833-9973
100 Boston Scientific Way, Marlborough, MA 01752
Various sterile vascular access devices.

Nmt Medical, Inc. 617-737-0930
27-43 Wormwood St, Boston, MA 02210
Various models of sterile vena cava filters.

FILTER, INTRAVENOUS TUBING *(General) 80QVY*

B. Braun Oem Division, B. Braun Medical Inc. 866-8-BBRAUN
824 12th Ave, Bethlehem, PA 18018

Benlan Inc. 905-829-5004
2760 Brighton Rd., Oakville, ONT L6H 5T4 Canada

Churchill Medical Systems, Inc. 800-468-0585
935 Horsham Rd Ste M, Horsham, PA 19044
IV filter kit.

Directmed, Inc. 516-656-3377
150 Pratt Oval, Glen Cove, NY 11542

Ge Infrastructure Water & Process Technologies 877-522-7867
5951 Clearwater Dr, Minnetonka, MN 55343

Gvs Filter Technology Inc. 317-471-3700
5353 W 79th St, Indianapolis, IN 46268
GVS offers a new Hi-Flo IV filter, available on an OEM basis. 0.2µm and 1.2µm pore sizes (other pore sizes available). Four vents for Speedflow Adult filter, two vents for Speedflow Kids, and new innovative Speedflow Baby is now available.

Medi-Dose, Inc. 800-523-8966
70 Industrial Dr, Ivyland, PA 18974

Millipore Corporation 800-MILLIPORE
80 Ashby Rd, Bedford, MA 01730
MICROVEX in-line filter for neonatal and outpatient ambulatory IV therapies.

Mps Acacia 800-486-6677
785 Challenger St, Brea, CA 92821

Pall Corporation 800-521-1520
600 S Wagner Rd, Ann Arbor, MI 48103

Smiths Medical Asd, Inc. 800-848-1757
6250 Shier Rings Rd, Dublin, OH 43016

The Metrix Co. 800-752-3148
4400 Chavenelle Rd, Dubuque, IA 52002

FILTER, KIDNEY STONE *(Gastro/Urology) 78QVZ*

Gerson Co. Inc., Louis M. 800-225-8623
15 Sproat St, Middleboro, MA 02346
Hygenic filters with nylon tip and sides for easy detection of Calculi. Used in arthroscopies and general purpose liquid filtration.

Ross Disposable Products 800-649-6526
401 Traders Blvd E, Unit 10, Mississauga, ON L4Z 2H8 Canada

FILTER, LENS *(Ophthalmology) 86WXB*

Barr Associates, Inc. 978-692-7513
2 Lyberty Way, Westford, MA 01886
Design development and manufacturing of precision optical filters in wavelengths from 0.1 through 30.0 microns.

Glass Fab, Inc. 585-262-4000
257 Ormond St, PO Box 31880, Rochester, NY 14605

Newport Franklin, Inc. 800-598-6783
8 Forge Pkwy, Franklin, MA 02038
Optical filters and components; also available, interference filters including fluorescence filter sets. Also, fluorescent filter sets.

Newport Glass Works, Ltd. 714-484-8100
PO Box 127, Stanton, CA 90680
Colored filter glass.

FILTER, LENS *(cont'd)*

Princeton Instruments - Acton 978-263-3584
15 Discovery Way, Acton, MA 01720
Optical filters (UV-VIS-NIR).

FILTER, MEMBRANE *(Chemistry) 75UGD*

Alfa Laval Inc 866-253-2528
955 Mearns Rd, Warminster, PA 18974

Berghof/America 800-544-5004
3773 NW 126th Ave Bldg 1, Coral Springs, FL 33065
Chemically inert, non-contaminating, non-flammable Teflon filter membranes. Non-adhesive, non-clogging, high retention efficiency, self gasketing, and heat sealable.

Bio-Rad Laboratories, Life Science Group 800-424-6723
2000 Alfred Nobel Dr, Hercules, CA 94547

Corning Inc., Science Products Division 800-492-1110
45 Nagog Park, Acton, MA 01720
Disposable membrane filter unit.

Filtertek Inc. 800-248-2461
11411 Price Rd, Hebron, IL 60034
Filter elements (parts).

Ge Infrastructure Water & Process Technologies 877-522-7867
5951 Clearwater Dr, Minnetonka, MN 55343

Lydall, Inc. 860-646-1233
1 Colonial Rd, Manchester, CT 06042
Filtration media for air, liquids and diagnostic devices. Glass papers for laboratory analyses.

Millipore Corporation 800-MILLIPORE
80 Ashby Rd, Bedford, MA 01730
DURAPORE, MF (nitrocellulose), Millipore Express (PES), UPE, Polypropylene, and Hi-Flow Capillary Flow.

Nalge Nunc International 800-625-4327
75 Panorama Creek Dr, Rochester, NY 14625
NALGENE nylon cellulose nitrate, certified water quality cellulose nitrate and cellulose acetate membrane.

Pall Corporation 800-521-1520
600 S Wagner Rd, Ann Arbor, MI 48103

Porvair Filtration Group Inc 803-327-5008
454 Anderson Rd S, BTC 514, Rock Hill, SC 29730

Schleicher & Schuell, Inc. 800-245-4024
10 Optical Ave, PO Box 2012, Keene, NH 03431
Nitrocellulose, cellulose acetate, nylon, regenerated cellulose, PVDF.

Spectrum Laboratories, Inc. 800-634-3300
18617 S Broadwick St, Rancho Dominguez, CA 90220
Macroporous: nylon, flourocarbon, PP, PE, SS. Molecularporous UF: Types C and F (MWCOs 500-1,000,000) $57.00 to $140.00/10.

Thermo Fisher Scientific Inc. 563-556-2241
2555 Kerper Blvd, Dubuque, IA 52001

Thermo Oriel 800-715-393
150 Long Beach Blvd, Stratford, CT 06615

Whatman Inc. 732-885-6529
800 Centennial Ave Bldg 1, Piscataway, NJ 08854

FILTER, PRE-BYPASS, CARDIOPULMONARY BYPASS *(Cardiovascular) 74KRJ*

Gish Biomedical, Inc. 800-938-0531
22942 Arroyo Vis, Rancho Santa Margarita, CA 92688

Medicalcv, Inc. 800-328-2060
9725 S Robert Trl, Inver Grove Heights, MN 55077
INTERFACE.

Medtronic Perfusion Systems 800-854-3570
7611 Northland Dr N, Brooklyn Park, MN 55428

Pall Corporation 800-645-6532
25 Harbor Park Dr, Port Washington, NY 11050
Various.

Pall Lifesciences Puerto Rico Llc 516-801-9064
Carr. 194, Km. O.4, Fajardo, PR 00738
Various.

Porous Media Corp. 651-653-2000
1350 Hammond Rd, Saint Paul, MN 55110
Cardiopulmonary pre-bypass filter.

Terumo Cardiovascular Systems (Tcvs) 800-283-7866
28 Howe St, Ashland, MA 01721
Prebypass filter.

FILTER, RADIOGRAPHIC *(Radiology) 90VGF*

Alimed, Inc. 800-225-2610
297 High St, Dedham, MA 02026

FILTER, RADIOGRAPHIC *(cont'd)*

Delta Products Corp. 510-668-5100
4405 Cushing Pkwy, Fremont, CA 94538
Medical EMI/RFI filters.

Octostop Inc. 450-978-9805
1675 Saint Elzear, west, Laval, QUE H7L-3N6 Canada
$240.00 for THE BOOMERANG, filter for x-ray of the shoulder, etc. $225.00 for the INGOT filter for x-ray of the hip, etc. Prism, $146.00. Gentle slope, $118.00. Ridges $1850.00.

St. John Companies 800-435-4242
25167 Anza Dr, PO Box 800460, Santa Clarita, CA 91355
Soft texture filters which improve diagnostic capabilities through increased detail at lower costs and less radiation exposure to patient.

Supertech, Inc. 800-654-1054
PO Box 186, Elkhart, IN 46515
X-Ray Clear-Pb filters.

Xma (X-Ray Marketing Associates, Inc.) 800-325-8880
1205 W Lakeview Ct, Windham Lakes Business Park
Romeoville, IL 60446

FILTER, STEAM *(General) 80QWC*

Spirax Sarco, Inc. 800-575-0394
1150 Northpoint Blvd, Blythewood, SC 29016

FILTER, SYRINGE *(General) 80QWD*

Baxa Corporation 800-567-2292
9540 S Maroon Circle, Suite 400, Englewood, CO 80112
SUPOR syringe filter, connects to syringe for filtering of passing fluid. 32- and 25-mm filter available in 0.2-, 0.45-, 0.8-, 1.2-, and 5.0-micron configurations.

Filtertek Inc. 800-248-2461
11411 Price Rd, Hebron, IL 60034

Ge Infrastructure Water & Process Technologies 877-522-7867
5951 Clearwater Dr, Minnetonka, MN 55343

Millipore Corporation 800-MILLIPORE
80 Ashby Rd, Bedford, MA 01730
MILLEX.

Nalge Nunc International 800-625-4327
75 Panorama Creek Dr, Rochester, NY 14625
NALGENE with 7-, 13-, 25-, or 50mm diameter membrane. Cellulose acetate, nylon, PTFE and surfactant-free cellulose acetate membranes. 0.2-, 0.45-, 0.8-um pore sizes.

Porvair Filtration Group Inc 803-327-5008
454 Anderson Rd S, BTC 514, Rock Hill, SC 29730

Schleicher & Schuell, Inc. 800-245-4024
10 Optical Ave, PO Box 2012, Keene, NH 03431
SPARTAN, UNIFLO, CENTREX.

Spectrum Laboratories, Inc. 800-634-3300
18617 S Broadwick St, Rancho Dominguez, CA 90220
DYNAGARD syringe filters. Thin and narrow-shaped syringe filters for hard to reach places. Compact shape is ideal for epidural procedure kits. Available on an OEM or private label basis.

Whatman Inc. 732-885-6529
800 Centennial Ave Bldg 1, Piscataway, NJ 08854
13mm syringe filter.

FILTER, VENA CAVA *(Cardiovascular) 74QWE*

Boston Scientific Corporation 800-225-2732
1 Boston Scientific Pl, Natick, MA 01760

Cook Inc. 800-457-4500
PO Box 489, Bloomington, IN 47402

M & I Medical Sales, Inc. 305-663-6444
4711 SW 72nd Ave, Miami, FL 33155

Millipore Corporation 800-MILLIPORE
80 Ashby Rd, Bedford, MA 01730

FILTER, VENTILATOR *(Anesthesiology) 73QWF*

A-M Systems, Inc. 800-426-1306
131 Business Park Loop, Sequim, WA 98382

Intersurgical Inc. 315-451-2900
417 Electronics Pkwy, Liverpool, NY 13088
FILTA-GUARD, FILTA-THERM, CLEAR-GUARD, CLEAR-THERM.

Millipore Corporation 800-MILLIPORE
80 Ashby Rd, Bedford, MA 01730

Pall Corporation 800-521-1520
600 S Wagner Rd, Ann Arbor, MI 48103

Perma Pure Llc 800-337-3762
8 Executive Dr, Toms River, NJ 08755

FINDER, VEIN *(General) 80SER*
Liquid Crystal Resources, L.L.C. 800-527-1419
1820 Pickwick Ln, Glenview, IL 60026
Liquid crystal.

FINGER COT *(General) 80LZB*
Afassco, Inc. 800-441-6774
2244 Park Pl Ste C, Minden, NV 89423
Alimed, Inc. 800-225-2610
297 High St, Dedham, MA 02026
Arthrex, Inc. 239-643-5553
1370 Creekside Blvd, Naples, FL 34108
Finger cot.
Corflex, Inc. 800-426-7353
669 E Industrial Park Dr, Manchester, NH 03109
General Scientific Safety Equipment Co. 800-523-0166
2553 E Somerset St Fl 1, Philadelphia, PA 19134
Healer Products, Llc 914-663-6300
427 Commerce Ln Ste 1, West Berlin, NJ 08091
Finger cot.
Hospira 800-441-4100
268 E 4th St, Ashland, OH 44805
Non-latex rubber formula, custom shapes available.
Inland Specialties, Inc. 800-741-0022
7655 Matoaka Rd, Sarasota, FL 34243
Available in extra-small, small, medium and large.
Liberty Industries, Inc. 800-828-5656
133 Commerce St, East Berlin, CT 06023
Profex Medical Products 800-325-0196
2224 E Person Ave, Memphis, TN 38114
Ross Disposable Products 800-649-6526
401 Traders Blvd E, Unit 10, Mississauga, ON L4Z 2H8 Canada
Zimmer Holdings, Inc. 800-613-6131
1800 W Center St, PO Box 708, Warsaw, IN 46580

FIRST AID KIT WITHOUT DRUG *(Surgery) 79OHO*
Legend Aerospace, Inc. 305-883-8804
8300 NW South River Dr, Medley, FL 33166

FITTING, LUER *(General) 80QWK*
Anesthesia Associates, Inc. 760-744-6561
460 Enterprise St, San Marcos, CA 92078
Available in Standard and Luer-Lock varieties, in both Male and Female, or as sets. Chrome Plated Brass or Aluminum.
B. Braun Oem Division, B. Braun Medical Inc. 866-8-BBRAUN
824 12th Ave, Bethlehem, PA 18018
Cadence Science Inc. 888-717-7677
1979 Marcus Ave Ste 215, New Hyde Park, NY 11042
Churchill Medical Systems, Inc. 800-468-0585
935 Horsham Rd Ste M, Horsham, PA 19044
Luer lock adapters, male and female luer lock caps, rotating male luer lock.
Directmed, Inc. 516-656-3377
150 Pratt Oval, Glen Cove, NY 11542
Engineers Express, Inc. 800-255-8823
7 Industrial Park Rd, Medway, MA 02053
Halkey-Roberts Corp. 800-303-4384
2700 Halkey Roberts Pl N, Saint Petersburg, FL 33716
Luer syringe check valves.
Hamilton Company 800-648-5950
4990 Energy Way, Reno, NV 89502
Hospira 800-441-4100
268 E 4th St, Ashland, OH 44805
Medical components for IV delivery.
Intersurgical Inc. 315-451-2900
417 Electronics Pkwy, Liverpool, NY 13088
Medegen 800-520-7999
930 S Wanamaker Ave, Ontario, CA 91761
Precision-molded luer adaptors for OEMs.
Medi-Dose, Inc. 800-523-8966
70 Industrial Dr, Ivyland, PA 18974
Medical Plastic Devices (Mpd), Inc. 866-633-9835
161 Oneida Dr., Pointe Claire, QUE H9R 1A9 Canada
Microcision Llc 800-264-3811
5805 Keystone St, Philadelphia, PA 19135
Mps Acacia 800-486-6677
785 Challenger St, Brea, CA 92821

FITTING, LUER *(cont'd)*
Novosci Corp. 281-363-4949
2828 N Crescentridge Dr, The Woodlands, TX 77381
Richard Wolf Medical Instruments Corp. 800-323-9653
353 Corporate Woods Pkwy, Vernon Hills, IL 60061
S4j Manufacturing Services, Inc. 888-S4J-LUER
2685 NE 9th Ave, Cape Coral, FL 33909
Luer taper medical connectors, adaptors & stopcocks, reusable.
Smiths Medical Asd, Inc. 800-848-1757
6250 Shier Rings Rd, Dublin, OH 43016
Spectra Medical Devices, Inc. 866-938-8649
4C Henshaw St, Woburn, MA 01801
Plastic and metal available, all configurations. Short lead time and attractive pricing.
Vita Needle Company 781-444-1780
919 Great Plain Ave, Needham, MA 02492
Stock and custom short runs, male and female luer lock, luerslip, threaded, hose barbs.
Vygon Corp. 800-544-4907
2495 General Armistead Ave, Norristown, PA 19403

FITTING, OTHER *(General) 80QWJ*
B. Braun Oem Division, B. Braun Medical Inc. 866-8-BBRAUN
824 12th Ave, Bethlehem, PA 18018
Bay Corporation 888-835-3800
867 Canterbury Rd, Westlake, OH 44145
Medical fittings, connections, tubing, hoses, male/female quick connect couplers; all for use in anesthesia, resuscitation and respiratory care.
Chamberlin Rubber Company, Inc. 585-427-7780
3333 Brighton Henrietta Town Line Rd, PO Box 22700
Rochester, NY 14623
Gaskets, Seals, Strips, Pads, Sheet Rubber (Silicone, Neoprene, Viton, EPDM, etc), Sponge, Foam, Extrusions, Molded Parts, 3M Adhesives, Slit Tape, Tubing, Custom Hose Assemblies, Hose Clamps, Couplings and Fittings, Flexible Ducting and Matting (Cleanroom and Anti Fatigue). Our Gaskets and Hose Assemblies are made and shipped Factory Direct! 'Tell us what you need and we will give you what you want'. We serve our customers as 'Kings' with old fashioned Hard Work, Honesty and Integrity!
Engineers Express, Inc. 800-255-8823
7 Industrial Park Rd, Medway, MA 02053
Industrial Specialities Manufacturing, Inc. 800-781-8487
2741 W Oxford Ave Unit 6, Englewood, CO 80110
Intersurgical Inc. 315-451-2900
417 Electronics Pkwy, Liverpool, NY 13088
Kloehn Co., Ltd. 800-358-4342
10000 Banburry Cross Dr, Las Vegas, NV 89144
Fittings and connectors for the direct mounting of various sizes of Teflon type tubing.
Medical Fittings 800-331-2685
300 Held Dr, Northampton, PA 18067
Medical Plastic Devices (Mpd), Inc. 866-633-9835
161 Oneida Dr., Pointe Claire, QUE H9R 1A9 Canada
Mercury Medical 800-237-6418
11300 49th St N, Clearwater, FL 33762
Saint-Gobain Performance Plastics--Akron 800-798-1554
2664 Gilchrist Rd, Akron, OH 44305
TYGOPURE, sanitary fittings available in PVDF, Polypropylene and Polysufone. Seamless and tapered fluid path, one piece construction for low pressure applications.

FITTING, QUICK CONNECT (GAS CONNECTOR) *(General) 80QWL*
Aga Linde Healthcare P.R. Inc. 787-622-7900
PO Box 363868, GPO Box 364727, San Juan, PR 00936
General.
Allied Healthcare Products, Inc. 800-444-3954
1720 Sublette Ave, Saint Louis, MO 63110
Armstrong Medical Industries, Inc. 800-323-4220
575 Knightsbridge Pkwy, Lincolnshire, IL 60069
Schrader.
Dhd Healthcare Corporation 800-847-8000
PO Box 6, One Madison Street, Wampsville, NY 13163
VENTLOK.
Engineers Express, Inc. 800-255-8823
7 Industrial Park Rd, Medway, MA 02053

FITTING, QUICK CONNECT (GAS CONNECTOR) *(cont'd)*

Medical Fittings 800-331-2685
300 Held Dr, Northampton, PA 18067

Precision Medical, Inc. 800-272-7285
300 Held Dr, Northampton, PA 18067

S4j Manufacturing Services, Inc. 888-S4J-LUER
2685 NE 9th Ave, Cape Coral, FL 33909

Woodhead L.P. 847-272-7990
3411 Woodhead Dr, Northbrook, IL 60062

FIXATION APPLIANCE, MULTIPLE COMPONENT

(Orthopedics) 87KTT

Alphatec Spine, Inc. 760-494-6769
5818 El Camino Real, Carlsbad, CA 92008
Alphatec external fixation system.

Ascent Healthcare Solutions 480-763-5300
10232 S 51st St, Phoenix, AZ 85044
External fixation device.

Biomet, Inc. 574-267-6639
56 E Bell Dr, PO Box 587, Warsaw, IN 46582
Various types of external wrist plates.

Bolt Bethel, Llc 763-434-5900
23530 University Avenue Ext NW, PO Box 135, Bethel, MN 55005

Depuy Mitek, Inc. 800-451-2006
325 Paramount Dr, Raynham, MA 02767

Depuy Orthopaedics, Inc. 800-473-3789
700 Orthopaedic Dr, P.O. Box 988, Warsaw, IN 46582
Various types.

Depuy-Raynham, A Div. Of Depuy Orthopaedics 800-451-2006
325 Paramount Dr, Raynham, MA 02767
Various types.

Millennium Medical Technologies, Inc. 505-988-7595
460 Saint Michaels Dr Ste 901, Santa Fe, NM 87505
External wrist fixator.

Nutek Orthopaedics, Llc 954-779-1400
301 S.w. 7th St., Ft. Lauderdale, FL 33301
Wrist plate.

Orthofix Inc. 800-535-4492
1720 Bray Central Dr, McKinney, TX 75069
Correction of length or deformity; Internal fracture fixation - Hip

Orthonetx, Inc. 877-370-0477
2301 W 205th St Ste 102, Torrance, CA 90501
Distraction device femur.

R&R Medical, Inc. 877-776-9972
2225 Park Place Dr., Slatington, PA 18080
Single/multiple component metallic bone fixation appliances and accessories.

Rigid Fx Orthopedics, Incorporated 512-443-7770
3601 S Congress Ave Ste B400, Austin, TX 78704
Wrist fixator.

Small Bone Innovations, Inc. 215-428-1791
1380 S Pennsylvania Ave, Morrisville, PA 19067
Single/multiple component metallic bone fixation appliances and accessories.

Sterilmed, Inc. 763-488-3400
11400 73rd Ave N Ste 100, Maple Grove, MN 55369
Appliance, fixation.

Stryker Spine 866-457-7463
2 Pearl Ct, Allendale, NJ 07401

Synthes (Usa) 610-719-5000
35 Airport Rd, Horseheads, NY 14845
Various types and sizes of multiple component fixation devices.

Truform Orthotics & Prosthetics 800-888-0458
3960 Rosslyn Dr, Cincinnati, OH 45209
Prefabricated orthopedic appliances and supports.

Warsaw Orthopedic, Inc. 901-396-3133
2500 Silveus Xing, Warsaw, IN 46582
Screwdrivers, wrenches, taps, guide pins, etc.

Zimmer Manufacturing B.V. 800-613-6131
Route 1, Km. 123.4, Bldg. 1, Turpeaux Industrial Park
Mercedita, PR 00715
Various.

FIXATION APPLIANCE, SINGLE COMPONENT

(Orthopedics) 87KTW

Ascent Healthcare Solutions 480-763-5300
10232 S 51st St, Phoenix, AZ 85044
External fixation device.

Depuy Orthopaedics, Inc. 800-473-3789
700 Orthopaedic Dr, P.O. Box 988, Warsaw, IN 46582
Various types of single component fixation appliances, nail/blade/plate comb.

Synthes (Usa) 610-719-5000
35 Airport Rd, Horseheads, NY 14845
Various types and sizes of single component fixation devices.

Truform Orthotics & Prosthetics 800-888-0458
3960 Rosslyn Dr, Cincinnati, OH 45209
Prefabricated orthopedic appliances and supports.

Warsaw Orthopedic, Inc. 901-396-3133
2500 Silveus Xing, Warsaw, IN 46582
Plate.

FIXATION DEVICE, AC-POWERED, OPHTHALMIC

(Ophthalmology) 86HPL

Hansen Ophthalmic Development Lab 319-338-1285
745 Avalon Pl, Coralville, IA 52241
A distant fixation device for children.

Ophthalmic Intl. 480-837-6165
16857 E Saguaro Blvd, Fountain Hills, AZ 85268
Pneumatic Trabeculoplasty Device.

Western Ophthalmics Corporation 800-426-9938
19019 36th Ave W Ste G, Lynnwood, WA 98036

FIXATION DEVICE, BATTERY-POWERED, OPHTHALMIC

(Ophthalmology) 86HKJ

Western Ophthalmics Corporation 800-426-9938
19019 36th Ave W Ste G, Lynnwood, WA 98036

FIXATION DEVICE, EXTRA-CRANIAL (HEAD FRAME)

(Orthopedics) 87VKH

Crist Instrument Co., Inc. 301-393-8615
111 W 1st St, Hagerstown, MD 21740
MRI stereotaxic frames for macaques and baboons permits these animal subjects to be placed in MRIs. New models for small animals; mice, rats, etc. Will customize to fit your equipment.

Elekta Inc. 800-535-7355
4775 Peachtree Industrial Blvd, Bldg. 300, Suite 300
Norcross, GA 30092
Leksell Gamma Knife.

George Tiemann & Co. 800-843-6266
25 Plant Ave, Hauppauge, NY 11788

Keeler Instruments Inc. 800-523-5620
456 Park Way, Broomall, PA 19008
SPECTRA Indirect Ophthalmoscope. The Spectra is a durable indirect with key beams and filters incorporated. This instrument can be utilized either on a frame or headband and is easily interchangeable $1,564. The Spectra features a 6 watt xenon type bulb.

Quatro Composites 858-513-4300
13250 Gregg St Ste A1, Poway, CA 92064

Spencer Technologies 800-684-0586
701 16th Ave, Seattle, WA 98122
MARC 600 Transcranial Doppler Probe. Head-fixation device for unilateral or bilateral monitoring.

FIXATION DEVICE, JAW FRACTURE *(Orthopedics) 87TCT*

Ebi, Llc 800-526-2579
100 Interpace Pkwy, Parsippany, NJ 07054
External unilateral fixation EBI XFIX Dynafix system for fracture management and reconstruction.

George Tiemann & Co. 800-843-6266
25 Plant Ave, Hauppauge, NY 11788

Lifecore Biomedical, Inc. 952-368-4300
3515 Lyman Blvd, Chaska, MN 55318
TEFGEN Barrier Membranes are to restore defective jawbone.

Unisplint Corp. 770-271-0646
4485 Commerce Dr Ste 106, Buford, GA 30518
$25.00 per unit (standard).

FIXATION DEVICE, SPINAL (EXTERNAL) *(Orthopedics) 87UAP*

Capstone Therapeutics 800-937-5520
1275 W Washington St, Tempe, AZ 85281
OrthoFrame, external fixation device designed for ease of application and maximum versatility.

Ebi, Llc 800-526-2579
100 Interpace Pkwy, Parsippany, NJ 07054
SPINE LINK

Encore Medical Corporation 800-456-8696
9800 Metric Blvd, Austin, TX 78758
ISOBAR, ISOLOCK,SECUPLATE, CC CAGES - a family of products that includes cervical plates, pedicle screws, rods, hooks, and interbody fusion devices.

Microcision Llc 800-264-3811
5805 Keystone St, Philadelphia, PA 19135

Orthofix Inc. 800-535-4492
1720 Bray Central Dr, McKinney, TX 75069
External fixation systems.

FIXATION DEVICE, TRACHEAL TUBE *(Anesthesiology) 73CBH*

Allegiance Group, Inc. 805-569-1694
4025 Lago Dr, Santa Barbara, CA 93110
Prepare lock.

Ambu A/S 457-225-2210
6740 Baymeadow Dr, Glen Burnie, MD 21060
Endotracheal tube holder.

Applied Medical Technology, Inc. 800-869-7382
8000 Katherine Blvd, Brecksville, OH 44141

Biomedix, Inc. 800-627-2765
3895 W Vernal Pike, Bloomington, IN 47404
ENDOGRIP. Endotracheal Tube Holder features a simple two-piece construction that promotes quick applications, strength and the easy repositioning of the tube from side to side. This design requires no tape, buttons, snaps or pins.

Biomet Microfixation Inc. 800-874-7711
1520 Tradeport Dr, Jacksonville, FL 32218
Cotten-lorenz laryngeal prosthesis.

Bioseal 800-441-7325
167 W Orangethorpe Ave, Placentia, CA 92870
Sterile trach type.

Ergomed, Inc. 210-377-2217
5426 Billington Dr, San Antonio, TX 78230
Tracheal tube securing devices.

Health Care Logistics, Inc. 800-848-1633
450 Town St, PO Box 25, Circleville, OH 43113
Securement devices for endotracheal and tracheostomy tube.

Hollister, Inc. 847-680-2849
366 Draft Ave, Stuarts Draft, VA 24477

Insight Medical Products, Llc 561-742-3650
710 NE 7th St Apt 403, Boynton Beach, FL 33435
Endotracheal tube holder.

Intersurgical Inc. 315-451-2900
417 Electronics Pkwy, Liverpool, NY 13088
SECUR-ET, endotracheal tube fixation device.

Lifestream Medical Corporation 407-529-9920
12024 Green Emerald Ct, Orlando, FL 32837
Trach chain.

Marpac Inc. 800-334-6413
8436 Washington Pl NE, Albuquerque, NM 87113
ET Adhesive Tape quickly secures an endotracheal tube with out the trouble of tearing tape. No assembly required, ET Adhesive Tape makes your job easier. Soft cotton/foam neckband and choice of Silk or Cloth tape assure patient comfort. Individually wrapped for immediate use. Work quickly and efficiently! Sold in boxes of 25 or 100.

Mes, Inc. 800-423-2215
1968 E US Highway 90, Seguin, TX 78155
Part#9101 Endotracheal Tube Holder with elastic strap is completely latex free

Precision Medical, Inc. 800-272-7285
300 Held Dr, Northampton, PA 18067

Ventlab Corp. 336-753-5000
155 Boyce Dr, Mocksville, NC 27028
Fixation device tracheal tube.

Ximedix, Inc. 800-999-6349
4829 Northpark Dr, Colorado Springs, CO 80918
Endotracheal tube stabiliztion system; tube holder.

FIXATIVE, ACID CONTAINING *(Pathology) 88LDW*

American Mastertech Scientific, Inc. 209-368-4031
1330 Thurman St, Lodi, CA 95240
Multiple.

Ricca Chemical Company Llc 888-467-4222
1841 Broad St, Pocomoke City, MD 21851
Various

Ricca Chemical Company Llc 817-461-5601
1490 Lammers Pike, Batesville, IN 47006

Ricca Chemical Company, Llc 817-461-5601
448 W Fork Dr, Arlington, TX 76012
Various.

Richard-Allan Scientific 269-544-5628
4481 Campus Dr, Kalamazoo, MI 49008
Multiple.

Sci Gen, Inc. 310-324-6576
333 E Gardena Blvd, Gardena, CA 90248
FDA: Medical Device Manufacturing and packaging. Focus on Histology, Cytology, Analytical and General purpose Reagents, Chemistry, and Sterling and Disinfecting agents.

Ventana Medical Systems, Inc. 800-227-2155
1910 E Innovation Park Dr, Oro Valley, AZ 85755
Fixative.

Zeus Scientific, Inc. 800-286-2111
PO Box 38, Raritan, NJ 08869
Tissue fixative and wash solution; 12 x 10 ml tissue fixative, 4 x 120 ml wash solution.

FIXATIVE, ALCOHOL CONTAINING *(Pathology) 88LDZ*

American Mastertech Scientific, Inc. 209-368-4031
1330 Thurman St, Lodi, CA 95240
Multiple types of alcohol containing fixative.

American Spraytech, L.L.C. 908-725-6060
205 Meister Ave, Branchburg, NJ 08876
Cytology fixative spray.

Anatech, Ltd. 800-262-8324
1020 Harts Lake Rd, Battle Creek, MI 49037
Zinc Formalin: unbuffered zinc formalin fixative; Z-FIX: buffered zinc formalin fixative; PREFER Fixative, formalin free fixative. All available in gallon, 5 gallon drum and prefill sizes

Cambridge Diagnostic Products, Inc. 800-525-6262
6880 NW 17th Ave, Fort Lauderdale, FL 33309
CAMCO Stain Pak 3-16 oz bottles; Fixative, Solution I and Solution II $70.00. Fixative Solution-1 Gallon-$70.00. Solution I [red]-1 Gallon-$128.00. Solution II [blue]-1 Gallon-$133.00.

Lgm International Inc. 410-472-9930
3030 Venture Ln Ste 106, Melbourne, FL 32934
Fixative, alcohol containing.

Medical Packaging Corporation 800-792-0600
941 Avenida Acaso, Camarillo, CA 93012
Cytology fixative; combines 95% ethyl alcohol & 2.5% carbowax; 1-oz and 4-oz bottles packed 100/cs and 40/case. Also available: acetone and methanol fixatives.

Monogen, Inc. 847-573-6700
3630 Burwood Dr, Waukegan, IL 60085
Various: monofix, monolex, monosol.

Ricca Chemical Company Llc 888-467-4222
1841 Broad St, Pocomoke City, MD 21851
Various

Ricca Chemical Company Llc 817-461-5601
1490 Lammers Pike, Batesville, IN 47006

Ricca Chemical Company, Llc 817-461-5601
448 W Fork Dr, Arlington, TX 76012
Various.

Richard-Allan Scientific 269-544-5628
4481 Campus Dr, Kalamazoo, MI 49008
Fix-rite.

Sci Gen, Inc. 310-324-6576
333 E Gardena Blvd, Gardena, CA 90248
FDA: Medical Device Manufacturing and packaging. Focus on Histology, Cytology, Analytical and General purpose Reagents, Chemistry, and Sterling and Disinfecting agents.

Spectra-Tint 585-546-8050
250 Cumberland St Ste 228, Rochester, NY 14605
Formal dehyde-free compound histology fixative.

FIXATIVE, ALCOHOL CONTAINING *(cont'd)*

Tripath Imaging, Inc. 919-206-7140
780 Plantation Dr, Burlington, NC 27215
Fixative solutions.

FIXATIVE, FORMALIN CONTAINING *(Pathology) 88LDY*

American Mastertech Scientific, Inc. 209-368-4031
1330 Thurman St, Lodi, CA 95240
Multiple types of formalin containing fixative.

Meridian Bioscience, Inc. 800-696-0739
3471 River Hills Dr, Cincinnati, OH 45244
PARA-PAK FORMALIN and MF For the routine collection, transportation, preservation and examination of stool specimens for intestinal parasites.

Michclone Associates, Inc. 248-583-1150
1197 Rochester Rd Ste L, Troy, MI 48083
10% neutral buffered formalin.

Richard-Allan Scientific 269-544-5628
4481 Campus Dr, Kalamazoo, MI 49008
Formalin containing fixatives.

Sci Gen, Inc. 310-324-6576
333 E Gardena Blvd, Gardena, CA 90248
FDA: Medical Device Manufacturing and packaging. Focus on Histology, Cytology, Analytical and General purpose Reagents, Chemistry, and Sterling and Disinfecting agents.

Scytek Laboratories, Inc. 435-755-9848
205 S 600 W, Logan, UT 84321
Fixative, formalin-containing.

Spectra-Tint 585-546-8050
250 Cumberland St Ste 228, Rochester, NY 14605
Compound histology fixative for biopsies.

Statlab Medical Products, Inc. 800-442-3573
106 Hillside Dr, Lewisville, TX 75057
ANAPATH.

U S Biotex Corp. 606-652-4700
RR 1 Box 62, Webbville, KY 41180
10% non-buffered formalin.

FIXATIVE, METALLIC CONTAINING *(Pathology) 88LDX*

Alpha-Tec Systems, Inc. 800-221-6058
12019 NE 99th St Ste 1780, Vancouver, WA 98682
Schaudin's fixative.

American Mastertech Scientific, Inc. 209-368-4031
1330 Thurman St, Lodi, CA 95240
Multiple types of metallic containing fixative.

Meridian Bioscience, Inc. 800-696-0739
3471 River Hills Dr, Cincinnati, OH 45244
Para-Pak LV-PVA, Co-PVA, Zn-PVA For the routine collection, transportation, preservation and examination of stool specimens for intestinal parasites with or without mercury.

Michclone Associates, Inc. 248-583-1150
1197 Rochester Rd Ste L, Troy, MI 48083
B-5 fixative.

Ricca Chemical Company Llc 888-467-4222
1841 Broad St, Pocomoke City, MD 21851
Various

Ricca Chemical Company Llc 817-461-5601
1490 Lammers Pike, Batesville, IN 47006

Ricca Chemical Company, Llc 817-461-5601
448 W Fork Dr, Arlington, TX 76012
B-5 fixative.

Sci Gen, Inc. 310-324-6576
333 E Gardena Blvd, Gardena, CA 90248
FDA: Medical Device Manufacturing and packaging. Focus on Histology, Cytology, Analytical and General purpose Reagents, Chemistry, and Sterling and Disinfecting agents.

FLAME PHOTOMETER, PESTICIDES (DEDICATED INSTRUMENTS) *(Toxicology) 91DMM*

Medical Sales & Service Group 888-357-6520
10 Woodchester Dr, Acton, MA 01720

FLASK, DEWAR *(Chemistry) 75QPH*

Cole-Parmer Instrument Inc. 800-323-4340
625 E Bunker Ct, Vernon Hills, IL 60061

International Cryogenics, Inc. 800-886-2796
4040 Championship Dr, Indianapolis, IN 46268

FLASK, DEWAR *(cont'd)*

Nalge Nunc International 800-625-4327
75 Panorama Creek Dr, Rochester, NY 14625
NALGENE double wall polyethylene construction with insulating foam. Sizes from 1 to 10 liters.

Southland Cryogenics, Inc. 800-872-2796
8350 Mosley Rd, Houston, TX 77075
Dewar, Liquid Nitrogen: insulated containers for storage of liquid nitrogen to be used in cryosurgery; available in 10 sizes.

United Silica Products, Inc. 973-209-8854
3 Park Dr, Franklin, NJ 07416

FLASK, SPINNER *(Pathology) 88KJD*

Berghof/America 800-544-5004
3773 NW 126th Ave Bldg 1, Coral Springs, FL 33065
Teflon Erlenmeyer flasks and round bottom flasks.

FLASK, TISSUE CULTURE *(Pathology) 88KJA*

Corning Inc., Life Sciences 207-985-5310
2 Alfred Rd, Kennebunk, ME 04043
Flasks, cluster plates, porous substrates for misc. cell culture applications.

Ethox International 800-521-1022
251 Seneca St, Buffalo, NY 14204
Tissue culture-various size sterile.

Sarstedt, Inc. 800-257-5101
PO Box 468, 1025, St. James Church Road, Newton, NC 28658

Thermo Fisher Scientific (Rochester) 585-899-7600
75 Panorama Creek Dr, Panorama, NY 14625
Various sizes and configurations of tissue culture flasks.

FLOOR MAT *(General) 80TCC*

Ace Hose & Rubber Company 888-223-4673
1333 S Jefferson St, Chicago, IL 60607
Chemical resistant lab mat; also, anti-fatigue standing mats for laboratories.

Aegis Floorsystems 972-788-2233
14286 Gillis Rd, Dallas, TX 75244
Floor safety surface. Safety service.

Alimed, Inc. 800-225-2610
297 High St, Dedham, MA 02026

Atd-American Co. 800-523-2300
135 Greenwood Ave, Wyncote, PA 19095

Colby Manufacturing Corp. 800-969-3718
1016 Branagan Dr, Tullytown, PA 19007
SURGISAFE absorbent floor pads are an effective method of containing and controlling blood and body fluids on the floor generated during fluid intensive procedures. Available with or without fluid-barrier backing in various sizes and absorption efficacies.

Construction Specialties Inc. 800-233-8493
6696 Route. 405, Muncy, PA 17756

Crown Mats 800-628-5463
2100 Commerce Dr, Fremont, OH 43420

Durable Corporation 877-938-7225
75 N Pleasant St, Norwalk, OH 44857
Grand Stand smooth rubber surface with sponge rubber base. Anti-fatigue mat. Tread Grid vinyl runner with gripper surface. SPECTRA-DELUXE Olefin Pile on vinyl carpet mat. Also available, SUPERDEKS 100% recycled PVC top banded to resilient sponge base. Excellent anti-slip/anti-fatigue mat.

Magister Corporation 800-396-3130
310 Sylvan St, Chattanooga, TN 37405
AIREX professional mats for physical therapy and exercise are available in many different sizes and colors.

Markel Industries, Inc. 860-646-5303
PO Box 1388, 135A Sheldon Road, Manchester, CT 06045
Disposable adhesive entrance mats.

National Nonwovens 800-333-3469
PO Box 150, Easthampton, MA 01027
Superabsorbent floor pads.

Pawling Corp., Architectural Prod. Div. 800-431-3456
32 Nelson Hill Rd, PO Box 200, Wassaic, NY 12592
Entrance and lobby mats, anti-fatigue mats, gratings, and roll-up mats.

R.C.A. Rubber Company, The 800-321-2340
1833 E Market St, P.O. Box 9240, Akron, OH 44305

FLOOR MAT *(cont'd)*

Tapeswitch Corporation 800-234-8273
100 Schmitt Blvd, Farmingdale, NY 11735
Pressure sensitive mats detect patient or personnel movement.

FLOOR MAT, ANTIBACTERIAL *(General) 80QWM*

Ace Hose & Rubber Company 888-223-4673
1333 S Jefferson St, Chicago, IL 60607
Chemical resistant lab mats.

Atd-American Co. 800-523-2300
135 Greenwood Ave, Wyncote, PA 19095
Bath mat

Chamberlin Rubber Company, Inc. 585-427-7780
3333 Brighton Henrietta Town Line Rd, PO Box 22700
Rochester, NY 14623

Controlled Environment Equipment Corp. 800-569-5444
59 Sanford Dr Ste 32, Gorham, ME 04038
$59/case (120 sheets, 18in.x45in.), $85/case (120 sheets, 26in.x45in.).

Lab Safety Supply, Inc. 800-356-0783
401 S Wright Rd, Janesville, WI 53546

Liberty Industries, Inc. 800-828-5656
133 Commerce St, East Berlin, CT 06023
Tacky mats

National Nonwovens 800-333-3469
PO Box 150, Easthampton, MA 01027
Superabsorbent floor pads.

FLOORING *(General) 80VBC*

Aegis Floorsystems 972-788-2233
14286 Gillis Rd, Dallas, TX 75244
TUB SAFE, slip resistant surface treatment for porcelain tubs and shower stalls. FRICTION, flooring coating quarry tile, concrete/terrazzoand ceramic tile

Dur-A-Flex, Inc. 800-253-3539
95 Goodwin St, East Hartford, CT 06108
Epoxy, urethane and MMA flooring/resurfacing materials.

R.C.A. Rubber Company, The 800-321-2340
1833 E Market St, P.O. Box 9240, Akron, OH 44305
Flooring - rubber - tile and sheet.

Regupol America 800-537-8737
33 Keystone Dr, Lebanon, PA 17042
Resillient flooring for use in physical therapy facilities.

FLOSS, DENTAL *(Dental And Oral) 76JES*

Ait Dental, Inc. 800-762-1765
1226 International Dr, Eau Claire, WI 54701

Almore International, Inc. 503-643-6633
PO Box 25214, Portland, OR 97298
Ultimate Flosser Hand Held Flosser

Alsco Industries, Inc. 508-347-1199
174 Charlton Rd, Po Box 1168, Sturbridge, MA 01566

Amden Corp. 949-581-9988
2533 N Carson St, Carson City, NV 89706
Sonifloss.

American White Cross - Houston 609-514-4744
15200 North Fwy, Houston, TX 77090
Dental floss.

Ams Industries 510-667-0673
14680 Doolittle Dr, San Leandro, CA 94577
Dental floss case.

Apc Industries 323-255-7101
3030 Fletcher Dr, Glassell, CA 90065

Bergman Oral Care 909-627-3651
13745 Seminole Dr, Chino, CA 91710
Flossbrite.

C & A Scientific Co. Inc. 703-330-1413
7241 Gabe Ct, Manassas, VA 20109
PREMIERE Disposable dental floss/toothpicks.

Coats American, Inc. 704-329-5800
Rt. 64 West, Hendersonville, NC 27739
Dental floss.

Cowan Plastics, Llc 401-351-1400
610 Manton Ave, Providence, RI 02909
Disposable flosser.

Den-Mat Holdings, Llc 805-922-8491
2727 Skyway Dr, Santa Maria, CA 93455
No common name listed.

FLOSS, DENTAL *(cont'd)*

Dentek Oral Care, Inc. 865-983-1300
307 Excellence Way, Maryville, TN 37801
Floss threader.

Du-More, Inc. 425-489-6088
1751 S 1st St, Rogers, AR 72756

Gudebrod, Inc. 877-249-2211
274 Shoemaker Rd, Pottstown, PA 19464
Dental floss and dental tape.

Hager Worldwide, Inc. 800-328-2335
13322 Byrd Dr, Odessa, FL 33556
MIRA FLOSS floss holder.

J&J Healthcare Products Div Mcneil-Ppc, Inc 866-565-2229
199 Grandview Rd, Skillman, NJ 08558

L.A.K. Enterprises, Inc. 800-824-3112
423 Broadway Ste 501, Millbrae, CA 94030
Dental floss holder and threader.

Lactona Corporation 215-692-9000
1669 School Rd, P.o. Box 428, Hatfield, PA 19440

Locin Industries Ltd. 800-663-8270
#200-18 Gostick Pk., North Vancouver, BC V7M- 3G Canada
LAZY FLOSS dental floss & KIDS FLOSS $49.95/M.

Loops, L.L.C. 360-366-3009
PO Box 2936, Ferndale, WA 98248
Floss loops dental floss.

Norwood Promotional Products, Inc. 651-388-1298
5151 Moundview Dr, Red Wing, MN 55066
Dental floss.

Novamin Technology Inc. 386-418-1551
13859 Progress Blvd Ste 600, Alachua, FL 32615
Dental floss; floss.

Nysarc, Columbia County Chapter, Inc. 518-672-4451
PO Box 2, Mellenville, NY 12544
Dental floss.

Oral Health Products, Inc. 918-622-9412
6847 E 40th St, Tulsa, OK 74145
Poh dental floss.

Oramaax Dental Products,Inc. 516-771-8514
216 N Main St Ste A1, Freeport, NY 11520
Dental floss.

Quden Inc. 450-243-6101
8 Maple, Cp 510, Knowlton J0E 1V0 Canada
Dental floss

Ranir, Llc 616-698-8880
4701 E Paris Ave SE, Grand Rapids, MI 49512

Ruthal Industries Ltd. 800-445-6640
1 Industrial Ave., Mahwah, NJ 07430-2113

Staino, Llc 845-887-5746
11617 State Route 97, Long Eddy, NY 12760
Types of dental floss.

Sunstar Butler 800-J BUTLER
4635 W Foster Ave, Chicago, IL 60630

Team Technologies, Inc. 423-587-2199
5949 Commerce Blvd, Morristown, TN 37814
Dental floss.

Tecstar Mfg. Company 262-255-5790
W190N11701 Moldmakers Way, Germantown, WI 53022
Brytonpick (dental floss-pick).

Ultradent Products, Inc. 801-553-4586
505 W 10200 S, South Jordan, UT 84095
Retraction cord.

W.L. Gore & Associates,Inc 928-526-3030
1505 North Fourth St., Flagstaff, AZ 86004
Dental floss.

Whitehill Manufacturing, Inc. 281-240-8782
12701 Executive Dr Ste 614, Meadows Place, TX 77477
Dental floss.

Young Innovations Llc Dba Plak Smacker 800-558-6684
755 Trademark Cir, Corona, CA 92879
Floss-o-matic.

FLOWMETER, BACK-PRESSURE COMPENSATED, THORPE TUBE *(Anesthesiology) 73CAX*

Allied Healthcare Products, Inc. 800-444-3954
1720 Sublette Ave, Saint Louis, MO 63110

FLOWMETER, BACK-PRESSURE COMPENSATED, THORPE TUBE *(cont'd)*

Blue White Industries, Inc. 714-893-8529
14931 Chestnut St, Westminster, CA 92683

Concoa 800-225-0473
1501 Harpers Rd, Virginia Beach, VA 23454
805 Series flowmeters.

Harris Products Group 800-241-0804
2345 Murphy Blvd, Gainesville, GA 30504
Harris Calorific.

Life Corporation 800-700-0202
1776 N Water St, Milwaukee, WI 53202
LIFE Flowmeters.

Ohmeda Medical 800-345-2700
8880 Gorman Rd, Laurel, MD 20723
Oxygen flowmeter.

Precision Medical, Inc. 800-272-7285
300 Held Dr, Northampton, PA 18067

Superior Products, Inc. 216-651-9400
3786 Ridge Rd, Cleveland, OH 44144
Flowmeter, medical gas flowmeter.

FLOWMETER, BLOOD, INTRAVENOUS *(Cardiovascular) 74DPW*

Arrow International, Inc. 800-523-8446
9 Plymouth St, Everett, MA 02149
Hemosonic 100 non-invasive transesophageal hemodynamic monitor.

Cardinal Healthcare 209, Inc. 610-862-0800
5225 Verona Rd, Fitchburg, WI 53711
Vascular probe.

Carolina Medical, Inc. 800-334-4531
157 Industrial Dr, King, NC 27021
$6,900.00 for FM501D electromagnetic flowmeter for research use. $7,595.00 for FM701D CLINIFLOW II for operating room use.

Escalon Trek Medical 800-433-8197
2440 S 179th St, New Berlin, WI 53146
Doppler vascular access monitor.

Hemedex Incorporated 866-HEMEDEX
222 3rd St Ste T123, Cambridge, MA 02142
Tissue perfusion monitoring system

Huntleigh Healthcare Llc. 800-223-1218
40 Christopher Way, Eatontown, NJ 07724
Vascular Assist - a handheld vascular assessment unit incorporating color spectrum analysis.

Koven Technology, Inc. 800-521-8342
12125 Woodcrest Executive Dr Ste 320, Saint Louis, MO 63141
Dopplers - , Model ES-1000SPM SMARTDOP®, Model DVM-4300T, Model HD-307, Model ES-100VX MINIDOPPLER®, Model ES-100X MINIDOP®, BIDOP® 3, SMARTDOP® 45, SMARTDOP® 20, SMARTDOP® 30, SMARTDOP® 50 Frequency Analyzer Doppler, Model ES-101EX-8 EchoSounder™; SMART-V-LINK Vascular Software

Terumo Cardiovascular Systems, Corp 800-521-2818
6200 Jackson Rd, Ann Arbor, MI 48103

Volcano Corporation 800-228-4728
3661 Valley Centre Dr Ste 200, San Diego, CA 92130
Doppler, instrument monitor.

FLOWMETER, BLOOD, OTHER *(Cardiovascular) 74WSR*

Millar Instruments, Inc. 800.669.2343
6001 Gulf Fwy Ste A, Houston, TX 77023
20MHz pulsed Doppler velocimeter for use with Doppler catheter to measure coronary blood flow velocity.

Neoprobe Corporation 800-793-0079
425 Metro Pl N Ste 300, Dublin, OH 43017
Flowguard; Quantix

Pmt Corp. 800-626-5463
1500 Park Rd, Chanhassen, MN 55317
TempTrac monitors blood flow in revascularized tissue, such as replanted digits, limbs, and free flaps. 4-channel LED readout and audible/visual alarm system.

Transonic Systems Inc. 800-353-3569
34 Dutch Mill Rd, Warren Road Business Park, Ithaca, NY 14850
TRANSONIC Flowmeter HT300 - series Transit-time ultrasonic blood volume flow monitors for intraoperative use during cardiac, transplant, vascular and neuro-surgery. BLF21, BLF21A, BLF21D Laser Doppler monitor to track blood flow in skin and other tissue surfaces during and after plastic and reconstructive surgery, cardiac and transplant surgery.

FLOWMETER, BLOOD, OTHER *(cont'd)*

Vasamed 800-695-2737
7615 Golden Triangle Dr Ste C, Eden Prairie, MN 55344
LASERFLO for laser Doppler perfusion monitor for continuous tissue blood flow measurements.

FLOWMETER, BLOOD, ULTRASONIC *(Gastro/Urology) 78QWP*

Parks Medical Electronics, Inc. 503-649-7007
PO Box 5669, Aloha, OR 97006
PARKS Five tabletop models: $1,300 for #806-CB, weighs 8 lbs., rechargeable; $1,500 for #909, 7.5 lbs., $3,445 for #1050-C, 17 lbs., rechargeable; $3,750 for #1052-C 17 lbs., rechargeable.

Verathon Inc. 800-331-2313
21222 30th Dr SE Ste 120, Bothell, WA 98021
VERSADOPP 5, 10, and 1000 economical, portable 5- and 10-MHz Doppler device for vascular disease assessment, deep venous occlusion detection, arterial-flow comparative studies, systolic pressure measurement, and other peripheral vascular exams. VERSADOPP 1000 is a bi-directional system that includes exam protocols, waveform display, 5- and 10-MHz Doppler probes, chart recorder, and external speaker.

FLOWMETER, DIALYSATE *(Gastro/Urology) 78FIS*

Cte Chem Tec Equipment Co. 800-222-2177
234 SW 12th Ave, Deerfield Beach, FL 33442
LPH flow switch maintains flow at designated set points and emits an electrical signal when fow parameters deviate from the norm. MAO flow meter monitors flow and continually emits a signal which describes the liquid flow rates of media.

FLOWMETER, GAS (OXYGEN), CALIBRATED *(Anesthesiology) 73BXY*

Aalborg Instruments & Controls, Inc. 800-866-3837
20 Corporate Dr, Orangeburg, NY 10962
Mass Flow Instrumentation, V.A. Rotameters Values

Aga Linde Healthcare P.R. Inc. 787-622-7900
PO Box 363868, GPO Box 364727, San Juan, PR 00936
Anesth/Pul Med.

Air Products And Chemicals, Inc. 800-654-4567
7201 Hamilton Blvd, Allentown, PA 18195

Allied Healthcare Products, Inc. 800-444-3954
1720 Sublette Ave, Saint Louis, MO 63110

Blue White Industries, Inc. 714-893-8529
14931 Chestnut St, Westminster, CA 92683

Cole-Parmer Instrument Inc. 800-323-4340
625 E Bunker Ct, Vernon Hills, IL 60061
Hand-held gas mass flowmeter measures flow of air, nitrogen, hydrogen, helium, carbon dioxide, and argon.

Datex-Ohmeda Inc. 608-221-1551
3030 Ohmeda Dr, Madison, WI 53718
Calibration flowmeter.

Dey, L.P. 800-755-5560
2751 Napa Valley Corporate Dr, Napa, CA 94558
ASTECH peak-flow meter is durable and has an enclosed indicator and permanent mouthpiece. Its full range scale accommodates both adults and children. The color zone allows personalized zone-based asthma management.

Dixie Ems Supply 800-347-3494
385 Union Ave, Brooklyn, NY 11211
$42.00 per unit (standard).

Emepe International, Inc. 813-994-9690
18108 Sugar Brooke Dr, Tampa, FL 33647
Oxygen and air flowmeter. Different flow ranges. With or withour power-take-off. Single or duplexes; also, custom assembled.

Erie Medical 800-932-2293
10225 82nd Ave, Lakeview Corporate Park, Pleasant Prairie, WI 53158
Back-pressure compensated flowmeter on piston-style regulator in 0-8 and 0-15 liter/min flow models.

Farley Inc., W.T. 800-327-5397
931 Via Alondra, Camarillo, CA 93012
Dual scale 0-5 and 5-15 LPM, dual tapered flow tube provides finer low flow accuracy; Model #3-700, $32.00.

Flotec, Inc. 800-401-1723
7625 W New York St, Indianapolis, IN 46214
Twelve-position flow rotor dial settings. True flow restricor technology. Available for all medical gases & gas blends as well as all inlet connections. Not gravity sensitive. MRI Compatible & Safe.

Kontes Glass Co. 888-546-2531
1022 Spruce St, Vineland, NJ 08360

FLOWMETER, GAS (OXYGEN), CALIBRATED *(cont'd)*

Life Corporation 800-700-0202
1776 N Water St, Milwaukee, WI 53202
LIFE Flowmeters.

Mada, Inc. 800-526-6370
625 Washington Ave, Carlstadt, NJ 07072

Michigan Instruments, Inc. 800-530-9939
4717 Talon Ct SE, Grand Rapids, MI 49512
The FlowAnalyser™ PF-300, a ventilator tester, measures bi-directional flow, pressure, temperature, humidity and O2 concentration. The unique feature of choosing the measuring mode between 'Adult-', 'Pediatric-' and 'High Frequency ventilation' proves the FlowAnalyser™ to be the ideal calibration tool for all ventilators, anesthesia machines and spirometers. It integrates a very simple and intuitive multilingual user interface, with its FlowLab™ software adding a wide range of graphical analysis capability.

Respironics California, Inc. 724-387-4559
2271 Cosmos Ct, Carlsbad, CA 92011
Transcutaneous monitor gas calibrator, o2/co2.

Respironics Novametrix, Llc. 724-387-4559
5 Technology Dr, Wallingford, CT 06492
Transcutaneous monitor gas calibrator, o2/co2.

Spiracle Technology 714-418-1091
16520 Harbor Blvd Ste D, Fountain Valley, CA 92708
Flow control valve.

Sun-Med 800-433-2797
12393 Belcher Rd S Ste 450, Largo, FL 33773

Terumo Cardiovascular Systems, Corp 800-521-2818
6200 Jackson Rd, Ann Arbor, MI 48103

Tri-Tech Medical, Inc. 800-253-8692
35401 Avon Commerce Pkwy, Avon, OH 44011
Various.

U O Equipment Co. 800-231-6372
5863 W 34th St, Houston, TX 77092

FLOWMETER, GAS, NON-BACK-PRESSURE COMPENSATED, BOURDON GAUGE *(Anesthesiology) 73CCN*

Life Corporation 800-700-0202
1776 N Water St, Milwaukee, WI 53202
LIFE Flowmeters.

FLOWMETER, METER, CEREBRAL BLOOD, XENON CLEARANCE *(Cns/Neurology) 84UEW*

Diversified Diagnostic Products, Inc. 281-955-5323
11603 Windfern Rd, Houston, TX 77064
$129,000.00 for XECT SYSTEM 2 stable Xenon/CT for quantitative cerebral blood flow determination. XECT SYSTEM 2 is high resolution, quantitative cerebral blood flow measuring device used in conjuncion with CT scanners.

FLOWMETER, PULMONARY FUNCTION *(Anesthesiology) 73VHT*

Dhd Healthcare Corporation 800-847-8000
PO Box 6, One Madison Street, Wampsville, NY 13163
asmaPlan Peak Flowmeter

Mada, Inc. 800-526-6370
625 Washington Ave, Carlstadt, NJ 07072
Peak flowmeter, adult and pediatric.

Validyne Engineering Sales Corp. 800-423-5851
8626 Wilbur Ave, Northridge, CA 91324
MP45 Pressure Transducer for use with Pneumatachs.

FLOWMETER, URINE, DISPOSABLE *(Gastro/Urology) 78FFG*

C. R. Bard, Inc., Bard Urological Div. 888-367-2273
13183 Harland Dr NE, Covington, GA 30014

Medispec Ltd. - Usa 888-663-3477
20410 Observation Dr Ste 102, Germantown, MD 20876
UROSPEC, device for measuring urine flow rates.

W.O.M. World Of Medicine Usa, Inc. 888-469-4378
4531 36th St, Orlando, FL 32811
Uropower UL201, (ULTRACOMPACT 9500 automatic flowmeter)

FLUID, BOUIN'S *(Pathology) 88IGN*

American Mastertech Scientific, Inc. 209-368-4031
1330 Thurman St, Lodi, CA 95240
Multiple types of bouin's fluid.

E K Industries, Inc. 877-EKI-CHEM
1403 Herkimer St, Joliet, IL 60432
Bouin's fluid.

FLUID, BOUIN'S *(cont'd)*

Hydrol Chemical Co. 610-622-3603
520 Commerce Dr, Yeadon, PA 19050
Bouins solution.

Labchem, Inc. 412-826-5230
200 William Pitt Way, Pittsburgh, PA 15238
Bouin's fluid, tissue fixative (lc11790).

Medical Chemical Corp. 800-424-9394
19430 Van Ness Ave, Torrance, CA 90501
$17.00 per 500mL, $40.00 per gal., $85.00 per 2.5 gal.

Poly Scientific R&D Corp. 800-645-5825
70 Cleveland Ave, Bay Shore, NY 11706

Polysciences, Inc. 800-523-2575
400 Valley Rd, Warrington, PA 18976

Ricca Chemical Company Llc 817-461-5601
1490 Lammers Pike, Batesville, IN 47006

Ricca Chemical Company, Llc 817-461-5601
448 W Fork Dr, Arlington, TX 76012
Bouin's fluid.

Rowley Biochemical Institute 978-739-4883
10 Electronics Ave, Danvers Industrial Park, Danvers, MA 01923

Sci Gen, Inc. 310-324-6576
333 E Gardena Blvd, Gardena, CA 90248
FDA: Medical Device Manufacturing and packaging. Focus on Histology, Cytology, Analytical and General purpose Reagents, Chemistry, and Sterling and Disinfecting agents.

FLUID, INTRAOCULAR *(Ophthalmology) 86LWL*

Cima Technology, Inc. 724-733-2627
3253 Old Frankstown Rd Ste C, Pittsburgh, PA 15239
Hydroxypropylmethylcellulose visco-surgical device; sodium hyaluronate visco-sur.

Fluoromed, L.P.
2350 Double Creek Dr, Round Rock, TX 78664
Fluoromed apf-215m.

Oasis Medical, Inc. 800-528-9786
514 S Vermont Ave, Glendora, CA 91741
VISCO SHIELD HPMC Viscoelastic for Export Only.

Peregrine Surgical, Ltd. 215-348-0456
51 Britain Dr, Doylestown, PA 18901
Tubing set.

FLUID, MANUAL CELL DILUTING *(Hematology) 81JCG*

J&S Medical Associates 800-229-6000
35 Tripp St Ste 1, Framingham, MA 01702
$18.00 for 20 liters of J & S blood cell dilutent. $65.00 for J & S T Pack.

FLUID, RED CELL DILUTING *(Hematology) 81GJN*

E K Industries, Inc. 877-EKI-CHEM
1403 Herkimer St, Joliet, IL 60432
Hayem diluting fluid.

Harvey, R.J. Instrument Corp. 201-664-1380
123 Patterson St, Hillsdale, NJ 07642

Ortho-Clinical Diagnostics, Inc. 800-828-6316
513 Technology Blvd, Rochester, NY 14626
Saline diluent for red cells.

Ricca Chemical Company Llc 817-461-5601
1490 Lammers Pike, Batesville, IN 47006

Ricca Chemical Company, Llc 817-461-5601
448 W Fork Dr, Arlington, TX 76012
Hayem diluting fluid.

Rocky Mountain Reagents,Inc. 303-762-0800
3207 W Hampden Ave, Englewood, CO 80110

FLUID, RED CELL LYSING *(Hematology) 81GGK*

Bd Biosciences 408-954-6307
2350 Qume Dr, San Jose, CA 95131
Red cell lysing products.

Beckman Coulter, Inc. 800-635-3497
740 W 83rd St, Hialeah, FL 33014
ZAPOGLOBIN, LYSE 5 III DIFF, LYSE 5 II, LYSE 5 III.

Bio-Rad Laboratories, Diagnostic Group 800-224-6723
524 Stone Rd Ste A, Benicia, CA 94510
Lysing fluid.

Clinical Diagnostic Solutions, Inc. 954-791-1773
1800 NW 65th Ave, Plantation, FL 33313
Hemoglobin/lyse reagent.

FLUID, RED CELL LYSING *(cont'd)*

Diagnostic Technology, Inc. 631-582-4949
175 Commerce Dr Ste L, Hauppauge, NY 11788
Rbc lysing reagent.

Health Chem Diagnostics Llc 954-979-3845
3341 W McNab Rd, Pompano Beach, FL 33069
Products, red-cell lysing products.

Horiba Abx 888-903-5001
34 Bunsen, Irvine, CA 92618
Liquid reagent used to treat white and red cells.

Iris Diagnostics 800-776-4747
9172 Eton Ave, Chatsworth, CA 91311
Red-cell lysing reagent.

J&S Medical Associates 800-229-6000
35 Tripp St Ste 1, Framingham, MA 01702
$120.00 for 4 liters of J & S lysing reagent.

Sterling Diagnostics, Inc. 800-637-2661
36645 Metro Ct, Sterling Heights, MI 48312

Sysmex Reagents America, Inc. 847-996-4512
10716 Reagan St, Los Alamitos, CA 90720
Various types.

Vegamed, Inc. 787-807-0392
39 Calle Las Flores, Edificio Multifabril #5, Vega Baja, PR 00693
Lysing reagent.

FLUID, WHITE CELL DILUTING *(Hematology) 81GGJ*

E K Industries, Inc. 877-EKI-CHEM
1403 Herkimer St, Joliet, IL 60432
Various solutions of acetic acid.

Pochemco, Inc. 413-536-2900
724 Main St, Holyoke, MA 01040
Acetic acid, 3% & 5%.

Ricca Chemical Company Llc 817-461-5601
1490 Lammers Pike, Batesville, IN 47006

Ricca Chemical Company, Llc 817-461-5601
448 W Fork Dr, Arlington, TX 76012
Turk blood diluting fluid.

Rocky Mountain Reagents,Inc. 303-762-0800
3207 W Hampden Ave, Englewood, CO 80110

FLUIDIC, PHACOEMULSIFICATION/FRAGMENTATION
(Ophthalmology) 86MUS

Biomedics, Inc. 949-458-1998
23322 Peralta Dr Ste 11, Laguna Hills, CA 92653

Nidek, Inc. 510-226-5700
47651 Westinghouse Dr, Fremont, CA 94539
Phacofragmentation system.

Phaco Solutions, Inc. 209-536-9707
19395 Village Dr, Sonora, CA 95370
Multiple types of phacoemulsification handpieces.

FLUIDIZED THERAPY, UNIT, DRY HEAT *(Physical Med) 89LBG*

Adroit Medical Systems, Inc. 800-267-6077
1146 Carding Machine Rd, Loudon, TN 37774
Digital Heat Therapy Pump with real time temperature display. Soft-Temp pads are the only kind made from polyurethene (a soft, flexible rubber-like material that will not pinch off when folded).

FLUIDOTHERAPY UNIT *(Physical Med) 89LSB*

Colonial Scientific Ltd. 902-468-1811
201 Brownlow Ave., Unit 52, Dartmouth, NS B3B-1W2 Canada
Heat modality.

Thermo Electric Company 800-523-2002
1193 McDermott Dr, West Chester, PA 19380
Fluido-therapy.

FLUORESCENCE POLARIZATION IMMUNOASSAY, CARBAMAZEPINE *(Toxicology) 91LGI*

Oxis International, Inc. 800-547-3686
468 N Camden Dr Fl 2, Beverly Hills, CA 90210
100 test kit.

FLUORESCENCE POLARIZATION IMMUNOASSAY, DIPHENYLHYDANTOIN *(Toxicology) 91LGR*

Abbott Diagnostics Intl, Biotechnology Ltd 787-846-3500
Road #2 KM. 58.0 , PO Box 278, Cruce Davila, Barceloneta, PR 00617
Various assays for detection of phenytoin.

Opus Diagnostics, Inc. 877-944-1777
1 Parker Plz, Fort Lee, NJ 07024
Innofluor phenytoin reagent set.

FLUORESCENCE POLARIZATION IMMUNOASSAY, DIPHENYLHYDANTOIN *(cont'd)*

Oxis International, Inc. 800-547-3686
468 N Camden Dr Fl 2, Beverly Hills, CA 90210
100 test kit.

FLUORESCENCE POLARIZATION IMMUNOASSAY, PHENOBARBITAL *(Toxicology) 91LGQ*

Abbott Diagnostics Intl, Biotechnology Ltd 787-846-3500
Road #2 KM. 58.0 , PO Box 278, Cruce Davila, Barceloneta, PR 00617
Various assays for detection of phenobarbital.

Opus Diagnostics, Inc. 877-944-1777
1 Parker Plz, Fort Lee, NJ 07024
Innofluor phenobarbital reagent set.

Oxis International, Inc. 800-547-3686
468 N Camden Dr Fl 2, Beverly Hills, CA 90210
100 test kit.

FLUORESCENCE POLARIZATION IMMUNOASSAY, THEOPHYLLINE *(Toxicology) 91LGS*

Abbott Diagnostics Intl, Biotechnology Ltd 787-846-3500
Road #2 KM. 58.0 , PO Box 278, Cruce Davila, Barceloneta, PR 00617
Various assays for detection of theophylline.

Opus Diagnostics, Inc. 877-944-1777
1 Parker Plz, Fort Lee, NJ 07024
Innofluor theophylline reagent set.

Oxis International, Inc. 800-547-3686
468 N Camden Dr Fl 2, Beverly Hills, CA 90210
100 test kit.

FLUORESCENCE POLARIZATION IMMUNOASSAY, TOBRAMYCIN *(Toxicology) 91LFW*

Abbott Laboratories 800-223-2064
100 Abbott Park Rd, Abbott Park, IL 60064
TDX/TDXFLX & TDXFLX THEOPHYLLINE MO

Opus Diagnostics, Inc. 877-944-1777
1 Parker Plz, Fort Lee, NJ 07024
Innofluor tobramycin reagent set.

Oxis International, Inc. 800-547-3686
468 N Camden Dr Fl 2, Beverly Hills, CA 90210
Tobramycin, vancomycin, gentamicin, quinidine, phenytoin and digoxin test kits.

FLUORESCENCE POLARIZATION, IMMUNOASSAY, CYCLOSPORINE *(Chemistry) 75MGU*

Abbott Diagnostics Intl, Biotechnology Ltd 787-846-3500
Road #2 KM. 58.0 , PO Box 278, Cruce Davila, Barceloneta, PR 00617
Fluorescence polarization immunoassay to quantitate cyclosporine in human whole.

FLUORESCENT IMMUNOASSAY GENTAMICIN
(Toxicology) 91LCQ

Oxis International, Inc. 800-547-3686
468 N Camden Dr Fl 2, Beverly Hills, CA 90210
Fluorescence polarization immunoassay 100 test kit.

FLUORESCENT IMMUNOASSAY, DIPHENYLHYDANTOIN
(Toxicology) 91LES

Dade Behring, Inc. 800-948-3233
1717 Deerfield Rd, Deerfield, IL 60015

FLUORESCENT IMMUNOASSAY, PRIMIDONE
(Toxicology) 91LFT

Dade Behring, Inc. 800-948-3233
1717 Deerfield Rd, Deerfield, IL 60015

FLUORESCENT IMMUNOASSAY, TOBRAMYCIN
(Toxicology) 91LCR

Bayer Healthcare, Llc 574-256-3430
430 S Beiger St, Mishawaka, IN 46544
Test for tobramycin in serum or plasma.

FLUORESCENT PROC. (QUAL.), GALACTOSE-1-PHOSPHATE URIDYL *(Chemistry) 75KQP*

Astoria-Pacific,Inc. 800-536-3111
PO Box 830, Clackamas, OR 97015
For determination of galactose-1-phosphate uridyl trasnferase activity in w.blod.

Bio-Rad Laboratories Inc., Clinical Systems Div. 800-224-6723
4000 Alfred Nobel Dr, Hercules, CA 94547
Coda galt assay.

FLUOROMETER *(Immunology) 82JZT*

Access Genetics 952-942-0671
7550 Market Place Dr, Eden Prairie, MN 55344
Software that processes analytical instrument output signals.

Dynex Technologies, Inc. 800-288-2354
14340 Sullyfield Cir, Chantilly, VA 20151
Fluorometer.

Farrand Optical Components & Instruments, Div. Of Ruhle Co. 914-287-4035
99 Wall St, Valhalla, NY 10595
Filter and grating fluorometers. Polarization fluorometers. HPLC fluorometers. Dual Emission Real-time fluorometers. OEM Fluorescence detectors.

Hitachi High Technologies America, Inc. 800-548-9001
3100 N 1st St, San Jose, CA 95134
Offering two models of fluorescence spectrophotometers, the F-2500 and F-7000 with a wide range of accessories.

Horiba Jobin Yvon Inc 866-JOBINYVON
3880 Park Ave, Edison, NJ 08820
Spectrofluorometer-the most sensitive systems available for application from protein unfolding to energy transfer and even pharmaceutical screening. Research lifetime systems to routine analytical push-button operation are presented. New Microwell Plate Reader expands the applications of SPEX Spectrofluorometers. SPEX FLUOROMAX-3, the world's most sensitive spectrofluorometer is now smaller and even more sensitive. Experiments are automated for trouble-free operation.

Medicos Laboratories, Inc. (Mdt) 800-724-4003
801 Montrose Ave, South Plainfield, NJ 07080

Myco Instrumentation Source, Inc. 425-228-4239
PO Box 354, Renton, WA 98057

Olis: On-Line Instrument Systems, Inc. 800-852-3504
130 Conway Dr Ste A, Bogart, GA 30622

Spectron Corp. 425-827-9317
934 S Burlington Blvd # 603, Burlington, WA 98233
Reconditioned equipment.

Standard Instrumentation, Div. Preiser Scientific 800-624-8285
94 Oliver St, Saint Albans, WV 25177

Tecan U.S., Inc. 800-338-3226
4022 Stirrup Creek Dr Ste 310, Durham, NC 27703
Spectra Fluor, Spectra Fluor Plus, Safire, Polarion, Ultra.

Thermo Spectronic 800-654-9955
820 Linden Ave, Rochester, NY 14625
High-performance spectrofluorometer.

Turner Designs 877-316-8049
845 W Maude Ave, Sunnyvale, CA 94085

Xiril 302-655-7035
91 Lukens Dr Ste A, New Castle, DE 19720
Microplate luminescence (luminometer).

FLUOROMETER, CHEMISTRY *(Chemistry) 75KHO*

Abbott Diagnostics Div. 847-937-7988
1921 Hurd Dr, Irving, TX 75038
Drug monitoring and immune fluorometric system.

Abbott Diagnostics Intl, Biotechnology Ltd 787-846-3500
Road #2 KM. 58.0 , PO Box 278, Cruce Davila, Barceloneta, PR 00617
Drug monitoring and immunofluorometric system (automated fluorescence polarizati).

Barnstead International 412-490-8425
2555 Kerper Blvd, Dubuque, IA 52001
Fluorometer.

Biosite Incorporated 888-246-7483
9975 Summers Ridge Rd, San Diego, CA 92121
Triage meter.

Biotek Instruments, Inc. 802-655-4040
100 Tigan St, Highland Park, Winooski, VT 05404
Microplate fluorometer/plate reader.

Diamond Diagnostics, Inc. 508-429-0450
333 Fiske St, Holliston, MA 01746

Luminex Corp. 888-219-8020
12212 Technology Blvd, Austin, TX 78727
Fluorometer or fluorescence measurement instrument.

Matech 818-991-8500
31304 Via Colinas Ste 102, Westlake Village, CA 91362
Fluorescent reference standard.

FLUOROMETER, CHEMISTRY *(cont'd)*

Ortho-Clinical Diagnostics, Inc. 908-218-8177
Route 202, Raritan, NJ 08869
Immunodiagnostic analyzer.

Ortho-Clinical Diagnostics, Inc. 585-453-3768
1000 Lee Rd, Rochester, NY 14606
Immunodiagnostic analyzer.

Ortho-Clinical Diagnostics, Inc. 585-453-3768
100 Indigo Creek Dr, Rochester, NY 14626
VITROS ECI IMMUNOD; VITROS ECI IMMUNODIAGNOSTIC SYSTEM; VITROS ECiQ Immunodiagnostic System

Turner Designs 877-316-8049
845 W Maude Ave, Sunnyvale, CA 94085

FLUOROMETER, TOXICOLOGY *(Toxicology) 91DPR*

Aviv Biomedical, Inc. 732-370-1300
750 Vassar Ave, Lakewood, NJ 08701
Lead-poisoning screening.

Dade Behring, Inc. 800-948-3233
1717 Deerfield Rd, Deerfield, IL 60015
STRATUS immunoassay system (fluorometric).

Thermo Spectronic 800-654-9955
820 Linden Ave, Rochester, NY 14625
High-performance spectrofluorometer.

FLUOROMETRIC MEASUREMENT, PORPHYRINS *(Chemistry) 75JKJ*

Bio-Rad Laboratories, Life Science Group 800-424-6723
2000 Alfred Nobel Dr, Hercules, CA 94547

Frontier Scientific, Inc., 453-753-1901
PO Box 31, Logan, UT 84323
$68.89 per kit (12 vials) PFS-9 protoporphyrin fluorescence standard; $33.30 per kit - (12 vials) CFS-3 coproporphyrin fluorescence standard; $38.30 per kit - (12 vials) UFS-1 uroporphyrin fluorescence standard. Full line or research porphyrins and bile pigments.

Kaulson Laboratories, Inc. 973-226-9494
693 Bloomfield Ave, West Caldwell, NJ 07006
Protoporphyrin.

FLUOROMETRIC METHOD, CPK OR ISOENZYMES *(Chemistry) 75JHX*

Biosite Incorporated 888-246-7483
9975 Summers Ridge Rd, San Diego, CA 92121
Fluorescence immunoassay for ckmb,tropinin i and myoglobin.

Helena Laboratories 409-842-3714
PO Box 752, Beaumont, TX 77704

FLUOROMETRY, MORPHINE *(Toxicology) 91DJJ*

Branan Medical Corp. 949-598-7166
140 Technology Dr Ste 400, Irvine, CA 92618
Fluorometry, morphine.

Jant Pharmacal Corp. 800-676-5565
16255 Ventura Blvd Ste 505, Encino, CA 91436
Test to detect morphine in human urine.

Teco Diagnostics 714-693-7788
1268 N Lakeview Ave, Anaheim, CA 92807
Onestep morphine card test.

FLUOROPHOTOMETER *(Chemistry) 75VEC*

Bean Products 800-726-8365
1500 S Western Ave Ste 4BN, Chicago, IL 60608

FLUSHING DEVICE, AUTOMATIC *(Anesthesiology) 73KFY*

Hospira, Inc. 877-946-7747
755 Jarvis Dr, Morgan Hill, CA 95037

Smiths Medical Asd, Inc. 800-848-1757
6250 Shier Rings Rd, Dublin, OH 43016

FLUXMETER *(General) 80TCE*

R. B. Annis Instruments, Inc. 317-637-9282
1101 N Delaware St, Indianapolis, IN 46202
$73.00 to $190.00 for hand-held unit; ranges from 0.5 to 400 Gauss. (See Magnetometer.)

FOAM, PLASTIC *(General) 80WVT*

Aetna Foot Products/Div. Of Aetna Felt Corporation 800-390-3668
2401 W Emaus Ave, Allentown, PA 18103
COMFOOT Brand and SCOTT FOOT CARE non-plastic pre-cut pads, rolls and sheets in various thicknesses.

FOAM, PLASTIC *(cont'd)*

Crest Foam Industries 201-807-0809
100 Carol Pl, Moonachie, NJ 07074
Environmentally friendly and extraordinarily versatile material that can be fabricated into virtually any configuration, and used in thousands of different products and applications.

Crown Mats 800-628-5463
2100 Commerce Dr, Fremont, OH 43420
Foam products.

Grand Rapids Foam Technologies 877-GET-GRFT
2788 Remico St SW, Wyoming, MI 49519

Placon Corporation 800-541-1535
6096 McKee Rd, Fitchburg, WI 53719
Thermoformed specialty medical device trays for implants, vascular devices, catheters, ampoules, and surgical kits.

Porex Corporation 800-241-0195
500 Bohannon Rd, Fairburn, GA 30213
Rigid POREX porous plastics in standard products and custom molded shapes.

Regupol America 800-537-8737
33 Keystone Dr, Lebanon, PA 17042

Tailored Label Products, Inc. 800-727-1344
W165N5731 Ridgewood Dr, Menomonee Falls, WI 53051

FOIL, DENTAL *(Dental And Oral) 76QOX*

Almore International, Inc. 503-643-6633
PO Box 25214, Portland, OR 97298
$14.95 for Shimstock occlusion foil.

Ivoclar Vivadent, Inc. 800-533-6825
175 Pineview Dr, Amherst, NY 14228
MAT FOIL Mat gold with a thin overlay of gold foil covering the surfaces. It has been developed for ease of handling and superior cavity adaptibility.

FOIL, OPHTHALMIC *(Ophthalmology) 86UAY*

Reade Advanced Materials 401-433-7000
PO Box 15039, Riverside, RI 02915
READE - high-purity metal foils and wires for medical applications, manufactured to customer specifications.

FOLDERS AND INJECTORS, INTRAOCULAR LENS (IOL)
(Ophthalmology) 86MSS

Eyekon Medical, Inc 800-633-9248
2451 Enterprise Rd, Clearwater, FL 33763

Staar Surgical Co. 800-292-7902
1911 Walker Ave, Monrovia, CA 91016
MicroSTAAR Injector System (TF/PF)

Tekia, Inc. 949-699-1300
17 Hammond Ste 414, Irvine, CA 92618
Tek-Clear Accommodative IOL, Kelman Duet Phakic IOL and 3-piece foldable silicone, hydrophilic IOLs.

FOODSERVICE PRODUCT/EQUIPMENT *(General) 80VAV*

Accu Scan Instruments, Inc. 800-822-1344
5098 Trabue Rd, Columbus, OH 43228
Monitor drinking/feeding behavior.

Adamation, Inc. 800-225-3075
87 Adams St, PO Box 95037, Newton, MA 02458
Dishwashing machines and food waste disposal units.

Aladdin Synergetics, Inc. 800-888-8018
250 E Main St, Hendersonville, TN 37075
All types of patient meal delivery trays, componenets and covers are offered for pellet, insulated trays, and trays pertaining to cook/chill systems.

Caddy Corporation 856-467-4222
509 Sharptown Road, Bridgeport, NJ 08014-0345
Self-leveling equipment (dish dispenser/storage), utility distribution system, banquet dish storage carts.

Carter-Hoffmann 800-323-9793
1551 McCormick Blvd, Mundelein, IL 60060
Tray make-up support equipment.

Central Paper Products Company 800-339-4065
PO Box 4480, Manchester, NH 03108
Cups, plates and napkins.

Cres Cor 877-273-7267
5925 Heisley Rd, Mentor, OH 44060
Heated cabinets, utility cabinets, racks, banquet cabinets, dish dollies, Roast-N-Hold convection ovens, and more.

FOODSERVICE PRODUCT/EQUIPMENT *(cont'd)*

Edlund Co. 800-772-2126
159 Industrial Pkwy, Burlington, VT 05401

Electro-Steam Generator Corp. 888-783-2624
1000 Bernard St, Alexandria, VA 22314
Steam generator.

Fawn Vendors, Inc. 800-548-1982
8040 University Blvd, Des Moines, IA 50325
Medical Supply Vending Machine will vend samples, gloves, etc., that are used in hospitals, doctor's office and medical centers. Full line of automatic vending equipment. Including cold drink and snack vending equipment.

Imi Cornelius, Inc. 800-551-4423
500 Regency Dr, Glendale Heights, IL 60139
Ice and beverage dispensers.

Intermetro Industries Corp. 800-441-2714
651 N Washington St, Wilkes Barre, PA 18705
METRO dish dollies; heated cabinets, cooler shelving, SS prep tables, ice carts.

International Hospital Supply Co. 800-398-9450
6914 Canby Ave Ste 105, Reseda, CA 91335

Jones-Zylon Company 800-848-8160
305 N Center St, West Lafayette, OH 43845
Autoclavable and disposable hospital bedside plastics.

Kold-Draft 800-840-9577
1525 E Lake Rd, Erie, PA 16511
Ice makers, ice bins, ice crushers and ice dispensers.

Leedal, Inc. 847-498-0111
3453 Commercial Ave, Northbrook, IL 60062
Stainless steel sinks.

Medegen Medical Products, Llc 800-233-1987
209 Medegen Drive, Gallaway, TN 38036-0228
ROOM-MATES Disposable, sterilizable plastic & stainless steel water pitchers and tumblers.

Medirex Systems Ltd. 800-387-9848
P.O. Box 40 Station F, Toronto, ONT M4Y 2L4 Canada
Hospital menus and healthcare placemats.

Multi Marketing & Manufacturing, Inc. 303-794-5955
PO Box 1070, 5401 Prince Street, Littleton, CO 80160
UN-SKRU $8.95 plus $3.00 s/h screw top opener for 1/2in to 5in size tops; to be mounted underneath the cabinet; available in white and brown to match kitchen and workshop cabinets.

Piper Products, Inc. 800-492-3431
300 S 84th Ave, Wausau, WI 54401

Polder, Inc. 800-431-2133
8 Slater St, Port Chester, NY 10573
$15.00 for POLDER 1 gram diet scale, #934-90.

Royal Paper Products, Inc. 800-666-6655
PO Box 151, Coatesville, PA 19320
Bouffant Caps, Hairnets, Disposable Aprons,Beard Protectors, Scouring Pads, Sponges

Science Products 800-888-7400
1043 Lancaster Ave, Berwyn, PA 19312
DIGI-VOICE Speech modified scale for the visually impaired. DIGI-VOICE Talking Foodservice Thermometer.

Sonoco-Stancap Division 770-476-9088
3150 Clinton Ct, Norcross, GA 30071
STANCAP sanitary paperboard covers for food-service trays and glasses in 45 sizes. STANCOASTER paperboards, various sizes.

Taylor 800-255-0626
PO Box 410, Rockton, IL 61072
Manufacturer of equipment for carbonated and non-carbonated slush beverages, shake, soft serve, frozen yogurt, custard, smoothie dispensing freezers and grills.

Testo, Inc. 800-227-0729
40 White Lake Rd, Sparta, NJ 07871
MAGNUM food-service thermometer.

Thermosafe Brands 847-398-0110
3930 N Ventura Dr Ste 450, Arlington Heights, IL 60004

Westlund Engineering, Inc. 727-572-4343
12400 44th St N, Clearwater, FL 33762
Placers for food trays, lids and domes

Wilbur Curtis Company 800-421-6150
6913 W Acco St, Montebello, CA 90640
Coffee brewing systems, coffee urns & brewers, decanter and ice tea dispensers.

FOODSERVICE PRODUCT/EQUIPMENT *(cont'd)*

Youngs, Inc. 800-523-5454
55 E Cherry Ln, Souderton, PA 18964

FOOTREST, WHEELCHAIR *(Physical Med) 89IMM*

Alimed, Inc. 800-225-2610
297 High St, Dedham, MA 02026

Gendron, Inc. 800-537-2521
400 E Lugbill Rd, Archbold, OH 43502
$76.00 pair.

Invacare Corporation 800-333-6900
1 Invacare Way, Elyria, OH 44035
INVACARE.

Kareco International, Inc. 800-8KA-RECO
299 Rte. 22 E., Green Brook, NJ 08812-1714

Miller's Adaptive Technologies 800-837-4544
2023 Romig Rd, Akron, OH 44320
A wide range of foot supports including one and two piece foot cradles-A dynamic articulating footrest hanger.

Sunrise Medical Hhg Inc 303-218-4505
2842 N Business Park Ave, Fresno, CA 93727

Tuffcare 800-367-6160
3999 E La Palma Ave, Anaheim, CA 92807

FOOTSTOOL *(General) 80OWV*

Brandt Industries, Inc. 800-221-8031
4461 Bronx Blvd, Bronx, NY 10470
Footstools, handrail.

Brewer Company, The 888-873-9371
N88W13901 Main St, Menomonee Falls, WI 53051
#11001: Pneumatic Exam Stool with chrome base(available with back and footring), #1010: Spin Lift Exam Stool with chrome base(available with back), #22500: Pneumatic Exam Stool with plastic base (available with back), #22400: Spin Lift Exam Stool with plastic base (available with back), #21435: Ergonomic Task Chair (available with back and arms), #21340: Foot Operated Stool (available with back), #21520B/#21521B: Laboratory Stool

Clinimed, Incorporated 877-CLINIMED
303 Markus Ct, Sandy Brae Industrial Park, Newark, DE 19713

Convaquip Industries, Inc. 800-637-8436
4834 Derrick Dr, PO Box 3417, Abilene, TX 79601
Bariatric Footstool - Capacity 1000 lbs.

Custom Comfort Medtek 800-749-0933
3939 Forsyth Rd Ste A, Winter Park, FL 32792
Chrome-plated foot stool comes with an 11 x 14-in. platform and optional 34-in. handrail.

Pedigo Products 360-695-3500
4000 SE Columbia Way, Vancouver, WA 98661
Stacking or non-stacking, chrome or stainless steel, various sizes.

FOOTSTOOL, CONDUCTIVE *(General) 80QWU*

Mayo Medical, S.A. De C.V. 800-715-3872
Edison 1141 Nte., Col. Talleres, Monterrey N.L. 64480 Mexico
Stainless steel, revolving and adjustable.

Phelan Manufacturing Corp. 800-328-2358
2523 Minnehaha Ave, Minneapolis, MN 55404
$75.00 for add-a-unit step stand.

FOOTSTOOL, NON-CONDUCTIVE *(General) 80QWV*

Brandt Industries, Inc. 800-221-8031
4461 Bronx Blvd, Bronx, NY 10470
$48.00 for footstool 1600Z.

Brewer Company, The 888-873-9371
N88W13901 Main St, Menomonee Falls, WI 53051
#11200: Step Stool; #11220: Step Stool with Handrail

Hausmann Industries, Inc. 888-428-7626
130 Union St, Northvale, NJ 07647
$49.75 per unit (standard).

Larkotex Company 800-972-3037
1002 Olive St, Texarkana, TX 75501

O&M Enterprise 847-258-4515
641 Chelmsford Ln, Elk Grove Village, IL 60007
FOOT STOOLS CONDUCTIVE/NON CONDUCTIVE

Schueler & Company, Inc. 516-487-1500
PO Box 528, Stratford, CT 06615

FOOTSTOOL, OPERATING ROOM *(Surgery) 79FZL*

Blickman 800-247-5070
39 Robinson Rd, Lodi, NJ 07644
Stacking footstools designed for surgery suites, diagnostic centers and outpatient facilities.

United Metal Fabricators, Inc. 800-638-5322
1316 Eisenhower Blvd, Johnstown, PA 15904
All stainless steel construction with conductive rubber non-skid tread and foot tips. (Also chrome- plated available).

FORCEPS *(Orthopedics) 87HTD*

Abbott Spine, Inc. 847-937-6100
12708 Riata Vista Cir Ste B-100, Austin, TX 78727
Forceps.

American Surgical Instrument Corp. 800-628-2879
26 Plaza Dr, Westmont, IL 60559
Foldable and implantation forceps.

Arista Surgical Supply Co. Inc. 800-223-1984
297 High St, Dedham, MA 02026
All types.

Arthrex California, Inc. 239-643-5553
20509 Earlgate St, Walnut, CA 91789
Grasper/forceps.

Biomet Microfixation Inc. 800-874-7711
1520 Tradeport Dr, Jacksonville, FL 32218
Various types of forceps.

Biomet Sports Medicine, Inc 800-348-9500
56 E Bell Dr, Warsaw, IN 46582
Hand instruments.

Biomet, Inc. 574-267-6639
56 E Bell Dr, PO Box 587, Warsaw, IN 46582
Various types of orthopedic forceps.

Boss Instruments, Ltd. 800-210-2677
395 Reas Ford Rd Ste 120, Earlysville, VA 22936
Ophthalmic; vascular/cardiovascular; ENT, plastic surgery; neurosurgical, orthopedic, micro surgery, general surgery.

Busse Hospital Disposables, Inc. 631-435-4711
75 Arkay Dr, Hauppauge, NY 11788
Sterile/non-sterile, plastic disposable forceps.

Carl Heyer, Inc. 800-284-5550
1872 Bellmore Ave, North Bellmore, NY 11710

Conformis, Inc. 781-860-5111
2 4th Ave, Burlington, MA 01803
Forceps.

Cook Endoscopy 336-744-0157
4900 Bethania Station Rd # &, 5951 Grassy Creek Blvd. Winston Salem, NC 27105
Various grasping and retrieval forceps, soehendra stent retriever.

Deknatel Snowden-Pencer 800-367-7874
5175 S Royal Atlanta Dr, Tucker, GA 30084

Denovo Dental, Inc. 800-854-7949
5130 Commerce Dr, Baldwin Park, CA 91706

Dental Usa, Inc. 815-363-8003
5005 McCullom Lake Rd, McHenry, IL 60050
Dental forceps.

Depuy Spine, Inc. 800-227-6633
325 Paramount Dr, Raynham, MA 02767
Forceps.

Dermatologic Lab & Supply, Inc. 800-831-6273
608 13th Ave, Council Bluffs, IA 51501
Surgical forceps.

DJO Inc. 800-336-6569
1430 Decision St, Vista, CA 92081

Endoscopy Support Services, Inc. 800-349-3636
3 Fallsview Ln, Brewster, NY 10509

Fehling Surgical Instruments 800-FEHLING
509 Broadstone Ln NW, Acworth, GA 30101

Fortrad Eye Instruments Corp. 973-543-2371
8 Franklin Rd, Mendham, NJ 07945

George Tiemann & Co. 800-843-6266
25 Plant Ave, Hauppauge, NY 11788
Orthopedic forceps and instruments for mandibular joint surgery.

H & H Co. 909-390-0373
4435 E Airport Dr Ste 108, Ontario, CA 91761
Forceps, surgical, all types.

FORCEPS *(cont'd)*

Harvard Apparatus, Inc. 800-272-2775
84 October Hill Rd, Holliston, MA 01746

Healer Products, Llc 914-663-6300
427 Commerce Ln Ste 1, West Berlin, NJ 08091
Forceps, tweezers.

Health Care Logistics, Inc. 800-848-1633
450 Town St, PO Box 25, Circleville, OH 43113
Various types of forceps.

J. Jamner Surgical Instruments, Inc 800-431-1123
9 Skyline Dr, Hawthorne, NY 10532

K. W. Griffen Co. 203-846-1923
100 Pearl St, Norwalk, CT 06850
Forceps.

Karl Storz Endoscopy-America Inc. 800-421-0837
600 Corporate Pointe, Culver City, CA 90230

Kentron Health Care, Inc. 615-384-0573
3604 Kelton Jackson Rd, P.o. Box 120, Springfield, TN 37172
Forceps.

Kenyon Industries, Inc. 973-962-4844
235 Margaret King Ave, Ringwood, NJ 07456
Disposable.

King Tool, Inc. 800-587-9445
5350 Love Ln, Bozeman, MT 59718
Meniscal suture grabbers.

Kirwan Surgical Products, Inc. 888-547-9267
180 Enterprise Dr, PO Box 427, Marshfield, MA 02050
Bipolar electrosurgical forceps. Non-stick bipolar forceps.

Kmedic 800-955-0559
190 Veterans Dr, Northvale, NJ 07647

Lican Medical Products Ltd. 519-737-1142
5120 Halford Dr., Windsor, ON N9A 6J3 Canada
Arthroscopy forceps: blunt, scoop, grasper, scissors and miniature types; also available, thoracic forceps.

Mahe International Inc. 800-294-7946
468 Craighead St, Nashville, TN 37204

Marina Medical Instruments, Inc. 800-697-1119
955 Shotgun Rd, Sunrise, FL 33326
Various.

Medtronic Puerto Rico Operations Co.,Med Rel 763-514-4000
Road 909, Km. 0.4., Barrio Mariana, Humacao, PR 00792
Various forceps.

Medtronic Sofamor Danek Instrument Manufacturing 901-396-3133
7375 Adrianne Pl, Bartlett, TN 38133
Multiple forceps.

Medtronic Sofamor Danek Usa, Inc. 901-396-3133
4340 Swinnea Rd, Memphis, TN 38118
Multiple forceps.

Medtronic Spine Llc 877-690-5353
1221 Crossman Ave, Sunnyvale, CA 94089
Sterile tweezers.

Musculoskeletal Transplant Foundation 732-661-0202
1232 Mid Valley Dr, Jessup, PA 18434

Odyssey Medical, Inc. 901-383-7777
5828 Shelby Oaks Dr, Memphis, TN 38134
Forceps.

Princeton Medical Group, Inc. 800-875-0869
1189 Royal Links Dr, Mt Pleasant, SC 29466

Prosurge Instruments, Inc. 866-832-7874
199 Laidlaw Ave, Jersey City, NJ 07306

Qfc Plastics, Inc. 817-649-7400
728 111th St, Arlington, TX 76011
Forceps.

Razoraid Incorporated 410-585-1395
7301 Park Heights Ave Apt 207, Baltimore, MD 21208
Razoraid-a ingrown hair extricator.

Ross Disposable Products 800-649-6526
401 Traders Blvd E, Unit 10, Mississauga, ON L4Z 2H8 Canada

Salvin Dental Specialties, Inc. 800-535-6566
3450 Latrobe Dr, Charlotte, NC 28211
Various types of forceps.

Sca Personal Care, North America 270-796-9300
7030 Louisville Rd, Bowling Green, KY 42101
Forceps, disposable.

FORCEPS *(cont'd)*

Scanlan International, Inc. 800-328-9458
1 Scanlan Plz, Saint Paul, MN 55107

Small Bone Innovations, Inc. 215-428-1791
1380 S Pennsylvania Ave, Morrisville, PA 19067
Forceps.

Smith & Nephew, Inc., Endoscopy Division 800-343-8386
150 Minuteman Rd, Andover, MA 01810

Smith & Nephew, Inc., Endoscopy Division 800-343-8386
130 Forbes Blvd, Mansfield, MA 02048

Spine Wave, Inc. 203-944-9494
2 Enterprise Dr Ste 302, Shelton, CT 06484
Forceps.

Standard Instrumentation, Div. Preiser Scientific 800-624-8285
94 Oliver St, Saint Albans, WV 25177

Stern Inc., Walter 516-883-9100
68 Sintsink Dr E, P.O. Box 571, Port Washington, NY 11050
Surgical and laboratory stainless steel scissors, forceps, tweezers.

Stryker Spine 866-457-7463
2 Pearl Ct, Allendale, NJ 07401

Symmetry Medical Usa, Inc. 574-267-8700
486 W 350 N, Warsaw, IN 46582
Manual surgical instrument for general use.

Symmetry Tnco 888-447-6561
15 Colebrook Blvd, Whitman, MA 02382
Endoscopic forceps.

Synovis Micro Companies Alliance, Inc. 651-603-3700
439 Industrial Ln, Birmingham, AL 35211
Forcep.

Trans American Medical / Tamsco Instruments 708-430-7777
7633 W 100th Pl, Bridgeview, IL 60455
Floor & medium grade surgical stainless steel.

Triboro Supplies Inc 800-369-7546
994 Grand Blvd, Deer Park, NY 11729

Tuzik Boston 800-886-6363
104 Longwater Dr, Assinippi Park, Norwell, MA 02061

Warsaw Orthopedic, Inc. 901-396-3133
2500 Silveus Xing, Warsaw, IN 46582
Multiple forceps.

Wexler Surgical Supplies 800-414-1076
11333 Chimney Rock Rd Ste 110, Houston, TX 77035

Zimmer Holdings, Inc. 800-613-6131
1800 W Center St, PO Box 708, Warsaw, IN 46580

Zimmer Spine 508-643-0983
23 W Bacon St, Plainville, MA 02762
FLEXTIP steerable rongeurs for discectomy.

FORCEPS, ARTICULATION PAPER *(Dental And Oral) 76EFK*

Aesculap Implant Systems Inc. 1-800-234-9179
3773 Corporate Pkwy, Center Valley, PA 18034

Almore International, Inc. 503-643-6633
PO Box 25214, Portland, OR 97298
$10.00 to $98.50 per unit (standard).

Buffalo Dental Mfg. Co., Inc. 516-496-7200
159 Lafayette Dr, Syosset, NY 11791
Articulator forceps.

Dental Usa, Inc. 815-363-8003
5005 McCullom Lake Rd, McHenry, IL 60050
Forceps.

E.A. Beck & Co. 949-645-4072
657 W 19th St Ste E, P O Box 10857, Costa Mesa, CA 92627
Miller forcep.

Hu-Friedy Manufacturing Co., Inc. 800-483-7433
3232 N Rockwell St, Chicago, IL 60618
$21.35 each.

Miltex Dental Technologies, Inc. 516-576-6022
589 Davies Dr, York, PA 17402
Miller-type articulating paper forceps.

Pascal Co., Inc. 425-602-3633
2929 Northup Way, Bellevue, WA 98004
Articulation forceps.

Premier Dental Products Co. 888-670-6100
1710 Romano Dr, PO Box 4500, Plymouth Meeting, PA 19462

Prosurge Instruments, Inc. 866-832-7874
199 Laidlaw Ave, Jersey City, NJ 07306

FORCEPS, ARTICULATION PAPER *(cont'd)*

Pulpdent Corp. 800-343-4342
80 Oakland St, Watertown, MA 02472
No common name listed.

FORCEPS, BIOPSY *(Surgery) 79SIR*

American Catheter Corp. 800-345-6714
13047 S Highway 475, Ocala, FL 34480

Atc Technologies, Inc. 781-939-0725
30B Upton Dr, Wilmington, MA 01887

Boston Scientific - Maple Grove 800-553-5878
1 Scimed Pl, Maple Grove, MN 55311

Cook Inc. 800-457-4500
PO Box 489, Bloomington, IN 47402

Endo-Therapeutics, Inc. 888-294-2377
15251 Roosevelt Blvd Ste 204, Clearwater, FL 33760

Mahe International Inc. 800-294-7946
468 Craighead St, Nashville, TN 37204

Medi-Globe Corporation 800-966-1431
110 W Orion St Ste 136, Tempe, AZ 85283
Electric and Non-Electric Flexible Endoscopic Procedures

Okay Industries, Inc. 860-225-8707
200 Ellis St, P.O. Box 2470, New Britain, CT 06051

Prosurge Instruments, Inc. 866-832-7874
199 Laidlaw Ave, Jersey City, NJ 07306

Rocket Medical Plc. 800-707-7625
150 Recreation Park Dr Ste 3, Hingham, MA 02043

Telemed Systems Inc. 800-481-6718
8 Kane Industrial Dr, Hudson, MA 01749

United States Endoscopy Group 800-769-8226
5976 Heisley Rd, Mentor, OH 44060
Disposable 2-3mm biopsy forceps; hot and cold biopsy forceps. Reusable biopsy forceps.

Wisap America 800-233-8448
8231 Melrose Dr, Lenexa, KS 66214

FORCEPS, BIOPSY, BRONCHOSCOPE (NON-RIGID)
(Anesthesiology) 73BWH

American Surgical Instrument Corp. 800-628-2879
26 Plaza Dr, Westmont, IL 60559

Ballard Medical Products 770-587-7835
12050 Lone Peak Pkwy, Draper, UT 84020
Reuseable biopsy forceps.

Cook Endoscopy 336-744-0157
4900 Bethania Station Rd # &, 5951 Grassy Creek Blvd.
Winston Salem, NC 27105
Flexible biopsy forceps.

International Hospital Supply Co. 800-398-9450
6914 Canby Ave Ste 105, Reseda, CA 91335

Lsvp International, Inc. 866-969-0100
4692 El Camino Real Unit 126, Los Altos, CA 94022
Quality reusable instruments available for $199 and under.

Mahe International Inc. 800-294-7946
468 Craighead St, Nashville, TN 37204

Surgi-Aid Endoscopics, Inc. 480-988-0916
3553 E Wildhorse Dr, Gilbert, AZ 85297
Biopsy forceps, non-rigid.

Tuzik Boston 800-886-6363
104 Longwater Dr, Assinippi Park, Norwell, MA 02061

FORCEPS, BIOPSY, BRONCHOSCOPE (RIGID)
(Anesthesiology) 73JEK

Aesculap Implant Systems Inc. 1-800-234-9179
3773 Corporate Pkwy, Center Valley, PA 18034

American Catheter Corp. 800-345-6714
13047 S Highway 475, Ocala, FL 34480

Biomet Microfixation Inc. 800-874-7711
1520 Tradeport Dr, Jacksonville, FL 32218
Various types of forceps.

International Hospital Supply Co. 800-398-9450
6914 Canby Ave Ste 105, Reseda, CA 91335

Karl Storz Endoscopy-America Inc. 800-421-0837
600 Corporate Pointe, Culver City, CA 90230
Various styles.

Mahe International Inc. 800-294-7946
468 Craighead St, Nashville, TN 37204

FORCEPS, BIOPSY, BRONCHOSCOPE (RIGID) *(cont'd)*

Prosurge Instruments, Inc. 866-832-7874
199 Laidlaw Ave, Jersey City, NJ 07306

Surgi-Aid Endoscopics, Inc. 480-988-0916
3553 E Wildhorse Dr, Gilbert, AZ 85297
Biopsy forcep, rigid.

Tuzik Boston 800-886-6363
104 Longwater Dr, Assinippi Park, Norwell, MA 02061

FORCEPS, BIOPSY, ELECTRIC *(Gastro/Urology) 78KGE*

Apollo Endosurgery, Inc. 877-ENDO-130
7000 Bee Caves Rd Ste 350, Austin, TX 78746
Endoscopic Monopolar Scissors

Ballard Medical Products 770-587-7835
12050 Lone Peak Pkwy, Draper, UT 84020
Disposable, coagulating, biopsy forceps.

Cook Endoscopy 336-744-0157
4900 Bethania Station Rd # &, 5951 Grassy Creek Blvd.
Winston Salem, NC 27105
Hot biopsy forceps.

Esco Medical Instruments, Inc. 800-970-3726
21 William Penn Dr, Stony Brook, NY 11790

Karl Storz Endoscopy-America Inc. 800-421-0837
600 Corporate Pointe, Culver City, CA 90230

Lsvp International, Inc. 866-969-0100
4692 El Camino Real Unit 126, Los Altos, CA 94022
Quality reusable instruments available for $199 and under.

Preiser Scientific, Inc. 800-624-8285
94 Oliver St, P.O. Box 1330, Saint Albans, WV 25177
Motorized forceps (Microgrippers).

FORCEPS, BIOPSY, ELECTRIC, REPROCESSED
(Gastro/Urology) 78NLU

Medisiss 866-866-7477
2747 SW 6th St, Redmond, OR 97756
Various reprocessed electric biopsy forceps, sterile.

Sterilmed, Inc. 763-488-3400
11400 73rd Ave N Ste 100, Maple Grove, MN 55369
Biopsy forceps, hot.

FORCEPS, BIOPSY, GYNECOLOGICAL *(Obstetrics/Gyn) 85HFB*

Ac Healthcare Supply, Inc. 905-448-4706
11651 230th St, Cambria Heights, NY 11411
Obstetric-gynecologic specialized manual instrument.

Aesculap Implant Systems Inc. 1-800-234-9179
3773 Corporate Pkwy, Center Valley, PA 18034

Apple Medical Corp. 508-357-2700
28 Lord Rd Ste 135, Marlborough, MA 01752
Biopsy instrument.

Berkeley Medevices, Inc. 800-227-2388
1330 S 51st St, Richmond, CA 94804

Biomet Microfixation Inc. 800-874-7711
1520 Tradeport Dr, Jacksonville, FL 32218
Various types of forceps.

Codman & Shurtleff, Inc 800-225-0460
325 Paramount Dr, Raynham, MA 02767

Elmed, Inc. 630-543-2792
60 W Fay Ave, Addison, IL 60101

Karl Storz Endoscopy-America Inc. 800-421-0837
600 Corporate Pointe, Culver City, CA 90230

Lican Medical Products Ltd. 519-737-1142
5120 Halford Dr., Windsor, ON N9A 6J3 Canada

Lsvp International, Inc. 866-969-0100
4692 El Camino Real Unit 126, Los Altos, CA 94022
Quality reusable instruments available for $199 and under.

Marina Medical Instruments, Inc. 800-697-1119
955 Shotgun Rd, Sunrise, FL 33326
Various.

Miltex Inc. 800-645-8000
589 Davies Dr, York, PA 17402

Premier Medical Products 888-PREMUSA
1710 Romano Dr, Plymouth Meeting, PA 19462

Princeton Medical Group, Inc. 800-875-0869
1189 Royal Links Dr, Mt Pleasant, SC 29466

Prosurge Instruments, Inc. 866-832-7874
199 Laidlaw Ave, Jersey City, NJ 07306

FORCEPS, BIOPSY, GYNECOLOGICAL *(cont'd)*

R Medical Supply 800-882-7578
620 Valley Forge Rd Ste F, Hillsborough, NC 27278

Richard Wolf Medical Instruments Corp. 800-323-9653
353 Corporate Woods Pkwy, Vernon Hills, IL 60061

Rocket Medical Plc. 800-707-7625
150 Recreation Park Dr Ste 3, Hingham, MA 02043

Tuzik Boston 800-886-6363
104 Longwater Dr, Assinippi Park, Norwell, MA 02061

FORCEPS, BIOPSY, NON-ELECTRIC *(Gastro/Urology) 78FCL*

Accellent El Paso 915-771-9112
31 Butterfield Trail Blvd Ste C, El Paso, TX 79906
Endoscopic biopsy forceps

Aesculap Implant Systems Inc. 1-800-234-9179
3773 Corporate Pkwy, Center Valley, PA 18034

Annex Medical, Inc. 952-942-7576
6018 Blue Circle Dr, Minnetonka, MN 55343
3.0 Fr. flexible cup biopsy forceps (disposable).

Ballard Medical Products 770-587-7835
12050 Lone Peak Pkwy, Draper, UT 84020
Various types of non-electric biopsy forceps.

Boston Scientific Corporation 508-652-5578
8600 NW 41st St, Doral, FL 33166

Cameron-Miller, Inc. 800-621-0142
5410 W Roosevelt Rd, Road #241, Chicago, IL 60644

Cook Endoscopy 336-744-0157
4900 Bethania Station Rd # &, 5951 Grassy Creek Blvd.
Winston Salem, NC 27105
Various grasping & retrieval forceps, stent retriever.

Endochoice Inc. 888-682-3636
11810 Wills Rd Ste 100, Alpharetta, GA 30009

Esco Medical Instruments, Inc. 800-970-3726
21 William Penn Dr, Stony Brook, NY 11790

Gibbons Surgical Corp. 800-959-1989
1112 Jensen Dr Ste 101, Virginia Beach, VA 23451

Gyrus Acmi, Inc. 508-804-2739
93 N Pleasant St, Norwalk, OH 44857
Forceps, biopsy, nonelectric.

Lsvp International, Inc. 866-969-0100
4692 El Camino Real Unit 126, Los Altos, CA 94022
Quality reusable instruments available for $199 and under.

Medi-Globe Corporation 800-966-1431
110 W Orion St Ste 136, Tempe, AZ 85283
Biopsy forceps and foreign body retrievers.

Medical Engineering Laboratory, Inc. 704-487-0166
108 W Warren St Ste 207, Shelby, NC 28150
Biopsy forceps.

Primed Instruments, Inc. 877-565-0565
1080 Tristar Dr., Unit 14, Mississauga, ONTAR L5T 1P1 Canada
Reusable and Disposable Biopsy Forceps.

Princeton Medical Group, Inc. 800-875-0869
1189 Royal Links Dr, Mt Pleasant, SC 29466

Prosurge Instruments, Inc. 866-832-7874
199 Laidlaw Ave, Jersey City, NJ 07306

Rotburg Instruments Of America Inc. 954-331-8046
1560 Sawgrass Corporate Pkwy Fl 4, Sunrise, FL 33323
Various types of sterile and non-sterile gastroenterology-urology biopsy forceps.

Spectrascience, Inc. 858-847-0200
11568 Sorrento Valley Rd Ste 11, San Diego, CA 92121
Biopsy forceps, sterile, accessory to an endoscope.

Sterilmed, Inc. 763-488-3400
11400 73rd Ave N Ste 100, Maple Grove, MN 55369
Biopsy forceps.

Surgi-Aid Endoscopics, Inc. 480-988-0916
3553 E Wildhorse Dr, Gilbert, AZ 85297
Biopsy forceps, non-electric.

Tuzik Boston 800-886-6363
104 Longwater Dr, Assinippi Park, Norwell, MA 02061

FORCEPS, BIOPSY, NON-ELECTRIC, REPROCESSED *(Gastro/Urology) 78NON*

Medisiss 866-866-7477
2747 SW 6th St, Redmond, OR 97756
Various reprocessed non-electric biopsy forceps sterile.

FORCEPS, DISCONNECT *(Gastro/Urology) 78FJR*

Aesculap Implant Systems Inc. 1-800-234-9179
3773 Corporate Pkwy, Center Valley, PA 18034

FORCEPS, DRESSING *(Surgery) 79QWW*

Bausch & Lomb Surgical 636-255-5051
3365 Tree Court Ind Blvd, Saint Louis, MO 63122

Codman & Shurtleff, Inc 800-225-0460
325 Paramount Dr, Raynham, MA 02767

Directmed, Inc. 516-656-3377
150 Pratt Oval, Glen Cove, NY 11542

Elmed, Inc. 630-543-2792
60 W Fay Ave, Addison, IL 60101

Fine Surgical Instrument, Inc. 800-851-5155
741 Peninsula Blvd, Hempstead, NY 11550

Fortrad Eye Instruments Corp. 973-543-2371
8 Franklin Rd, Mendham, NJ 07945

Integral Design Inc. 781-740-2036
52 Burr Rd, Hingham, MA 02043

Katena Products, Inc. 800-225-1195
4 Stewart Ct, Denville, NJ 07834

Kirwan Surgical Products, Inc. 888-547-9267
180 Enterprise Dr, PO Box 427, Marshfield, MA 02050

Kmedic 800-955-0559
190 Veterans Dr, Northvale, NJ 07647

Kta, Instruments, Inc. 888-830-9KTA
3051 Brighton-Third St., 1st Fl., Brooklyn, NY 11235

Medworks Instruments 800-323-9790
PO Box 581, Chatham, IL 62629
$.90 per unit (5-1/2in).

Mine Safety Appliances Company 866-MSA-1001
121 Gamma Dr, Pittsburgh, PA 15238

Princeton Medical Group, Inc. 800-875-0869
1189 Royal Links Dr, Mt Pleasant, SC 29466

Prosurge Instruments, Inc. 866-832-7874
199 Laidlaw Ave, Jersey City, NJ 07306

Roboz Surgical Instrument Co., Inc. 800-424-2984
PO Box 10710, Gaithersburg, MD 20898

Rocket Medical Plc. 800-707-7625
150 Recreation Park Dr Ste 3, Hingham, MA 02043

Toolmex Corporation 800-992-4766
1075 Worcester St, Natick, MA 01760

Zimmer Holdings, Inc. 800-613-6131
1800 W Center St, PO Box 708, Warsaw, IN 46580

FORCEPS, DRESSING, DENTAL *(Dental And Oral) 76EFL*

Aesculap Implant Systems Inc. 1-800-234-9179
3773 Corporate Pkwy, Center Valley, PA 18034

Biomet Microfixation Inc. 800-874-7711
1520 Tradeport Dr, Jacksonville, FL 32218
Various types of forceps.

Dental Usa, Inc. 815-363-8003
5005 McCullom Lake Rd, McHenry, IL 60050
Forceps.

Dentalez Group 866-DTE-INFO
101 Lindenwood Dr Ste 225, Valleybrooke Corporate Center
Malvern, PA 19355

E.A. Beck & Co. 949-645-4072
657 W 19th St Ste E, P O Box 10857, Costa Mesa, CA 92627
Dressing forcep.

Grobet File Co. 800-847-4188
1912 Whitney Rd, Cheyenne, WY 82007
Forceps; dental pliers.

H & H Co. 909-390-0373
4435 E Airport Dr Ste 108, Ontario, CA 91761
Forceps, dressing, cotton.

Holmes Dental Corp. 800-322-5577
50 S Penn St, Hatboro, PA 19040

Micro-Vac, Inc. 800-729-1020
5905 E 5th St, Tucson, AZ 85711
Sterilization products

Miltex Dental Technologies, Inc. 516-576-6022
589 Davies Dr, York, PA 17402
Various dental dressing forceps.

Prosurge Instruments, Inc. 866-832-7874
199 Laidlaw Ave, Jersey City, NJ 07306

FORCEPS, DRESSING, DENTAL *(cont'd)*

Tuzik Boston 800-886-6363
104 Longwater Dr, Assinippi Park, Norwell, MA 02061

FORCEPS, ELECTROSURGICAL *(Surgery) 79QWX*

Cameron-Miller, Inc. 800-621-0142
5410 W Roosevelt Rd, Road #241, Chicago, IL 60644

Codman & Shurtleff, Inc 800-225-0460
325 Paramount Dr, Raynham, MA 02767

Dermatologic Lab & Supply, Inc. 800-831-6273
608 13th Ave, Council Bluffs, IA 51501
Delasco Bipolar Electrosurgery Forceps (McPherson, Adson, Semkin, Cushing, Gerald)

Elmed, Inc. 630-543-2792
60 W Fay Ave, Addison, IL 60101

Gyrus Medical, Inc. 800-852-9361
6655 Wedgwood Rd N Ste 105, Maple Grove, MN 55311
BICOAG bipolar forceps for laparoscopic procedures; 33- and 45-cm lengths available, marco and micro jaw. Also available, BICOAG bipolar cutting forceps. Bipolar electrosurgical forceps with transection capabilites.

Integral Design Inc. 781-740-2036
52 Burr Rd, Hingham, MA 02043

Jedmed Instruments Co. 314-845-3770
5416 Jedmed Ct, Saint Louis, MO 63129

Karl Storz Endoscopy-America Inc. 800-421-0837
600 Corporate Pointe, Culver City, CA 90230

Kirwan Surgical Products, Inc. 888-547-9267
180 Enterprise Dr, PO Box 427, Marshfield, MA 02050
Complete line of bipolar coagulating forceps, including titanium, and disposable electrosurgical bipolar coagulating forceps.

Mahe International Inc. 800-294-7946
468 Craighead St, Nashville, TN 37204

Olsen Medical 800-297-6344
3001 W Kentucky St, Louisville, KY 40211

Richard Wolf Medical Instruments Corp. 800-323-9653
353 Corporate Woods Pkwy, Vernon Hills, IL 60061

Valleylab 800-255-8522
5920 Longbow Dr, Boulder, CO 80301
Monopolar and non-stick bipolar forceps, handswitch or footswitch activated.

FORCEPS, ENDOSCOPIC *(Gastro/Urology) 78QWY*

Advanced Endoscopy Devices, Inc. 818-227-2720
22134 Sherman Way, Canoga Park, CA 91303
KWIK-KLEEN, arthroscopic procedures luer port for quick internal shaft cleaning.

Ams Innovative Center-San Jose 800-356-7600
3070 Orchard Dr, San Jose, CA 95134

Atc Technologies, Inc. 781-939-0725
30B Upton Dr, Wilmington, MA 01887

Bryan Corp. 800-343-7711
4 Plympton St, Woburn, MA 01801
5mm/10mm 33cm length, insulated and non insulated, various styles.

Deknatel Snowden-Pencer 800-367-7874
5175 S Royal Atlanta Dr, Tucker, GA 30084

Elmed, Inc. 630-543-2792
60 W Fay Ave, Addison, IL 60101

Ethicon Endo-Surgery, Inc. 800-USE-ENDO
4545 Creek Rd, Cincinnati, OH 45242
Bipolar endoscopic forceps.

Frantz Medical Development Ltd. 440-255-1155
7740 Metric Dr, Mentor, OH 44060

Gyrus Medical, Inc. 800-852-9361
6655 Wedgwood Rd N Ste 105, Maple Grove, MN 55311

J. Jamner Surgical Instruments, Inc 800-431-1123
9 Skyline Dr, Hawthorne, NY 10532

Karl Storz Endoscopy-America Inc. 800-421-0837
600 Corporate Pointe, Culver City, CA 90230

Kirwan Surgical Products, Inc. 888-547-9267
180 Enterprise Dr, PO Box 427, Marshfield, MA 02050
Mono- and bi-polar endoscopic forceps.

Lsvp International, Inc. 866-969-0100
4692 El Camino Real Unit 126, Los Altos, CA 94022
Quality reusable instruments available for $199 and under.

Mahe International Inc. 800-294-7946
468 Craighead St, Nashville, TN 37204

FORCEPS, ENDOSCOPIC *(cont'd)*

Md International, Inc. 305-669-9003
11300 NW 41st St, Doral, FL 33178

Olympus America, Inc. 800-645-8160
3500 Corporate Pkwy, PO Box 610, Center Valley, PA 18034

Pentax Medical Company 800-431-5880
102 Chestnut Ridge Rd, Montvale, NJ 07645
Complete line of fully autoclavable forceps (fenestrated, spiked, grasping, extra large cups, crocodile, and window) for use with all types of endoscopes. Also available are single use biopsy forceps and shears.

Prosurge Instruments, Inc. 866-832-7874
199 Laidlaw Ave, Jersey City, NJ 07306

Richard Wolf Medical Instruments Corp. 800-323-9653
353 Corporate Woods Pkwy, Vernon Hills, IL 60061

Smith & Nephew, Inc., Endoscopy Division 800-343-8386
150 Minuteman Rd, Andover, MA 01810

Synectic Medical Product Development 203-877-8488
60 Commerce Park, Milford, CT 06460

FORCEPS, ENT *(Ear/Nose/Throat) 77KAE*

Aesculap Implant Systems Inc. 1-800-234-9179
3773 Corporate Pkwy, Center Valley, PA 18034

Bausch & Lomb Surgical 636-255-5051
3365 Tree Court Ind Blvd, Saint Louis, MO 63122

Biomet Microfixation Inc. 800-874-7711
1520 Tradeport Dr, Jacksonville, FL 32218
Various types of forceps.

Clinimed, Incorporated 877-CLINIMED
303 Markus Ct, Sandy Brae Industrial Park, Newark, DE 19713

Invotec Intl. 800-998-8580
6833 Phillips Industrial Blvd, Jacksonville, FL 32256
Forceps nasal.

Karl Storz Endoscopy-America Inc. 800-421-0837
600 Corporate Pointe, Culver City, CA 90230
Adult and pediatric versions.

Micrins Surgical Instruments, Inc. 800-833-3380
28438 N Ballard Dr, Lake Forest, IL 60045

Prosurge Instruments, Inc. 866-832-7874
199 Laidlaw Ave, Jersey City, NJ 07306

Solos Endoscopy 800-388-6445
65 Sprague St # B, Boston/dedham Commerce Park, Boston, MA 02136
Forceps,ent.

Tuzik Boston 800-886-6363
104 Longwater Dr, Assinippi Park, Norwell, MA 02061

FORCEPS, EPILATION *(Surgery) 79QWZ*

Jedmed Instruments Co. 314-845-3770
5416 Jedmed Ct, Saint Louis, MO 63129

Katena Products, Inc. 800-225-1195
4 Stewart Ct, Denville, NJ 07834

FORCEPS, FIXATION *(Surgery) 79QXA*

Elmed, Inc. 630-543-2792
60 W Fay Ave, Addison, IL 60101

George Tiemann & Co. 800-843-6266
25 Plant Ave, Hauppauge, NY 11788

Katena Products, Inc. 800-225-1195
4 Stewart Ct, Denville, NJ 07834

Miltex Inc. 800-645-8000
589 Davies Dr, York, PA 17402

FORCEPS, GALLBLADDER (BILIARY DUCT) *(Gastro/Urology) 78QXB*

Codman & Shurtleff, Inc 800-225-0460
325 Paramount Dr, Raynham, MA 02767

Elmed, Inc. 630-543-2792
60 W Fay Ave, Addison, IL 60101

Mahe International Inc. 800-294-7946
468 Craighead St, Nashville, TN 37204

Princeton Medical Group, Inc. 800-875-0869
1189 Royal Links Dr, Mt Pleasant, SC 29466

FORCEPS, GENERAL & PLASTIC SURGERY *(Surgery) 79GEN*

Aesculap Implant Systems Inc. 1-800-234-9179
3773 Corporate Pkwy, Center Valley, PA 18034

FORCEPS, GENERAL & PLASTIC SURGERY *(cont'd)*

Anesthesia Associates, Inc. 760-744-6561
460 Enterprise St, San Marcos, CA 92078
Magill Forceps in 3 sizes. Special Aillon Tube Bender for difficult nasotracheal intubation. Stainless Steel.

Arosurgical Instruments Corp. 800-776-1751
537 Newport Center Dr Ste 101, Newport Beach, CA 92660
AROSforceps for MICRO & PLASTIC surgery. 8 to 23cm, STR, CVD & ANGL, Jeweler's micro fcps, Titanium, Stainless Steel, DIAMOND DUSTED tips, with tying platforms, 0.1mm to 3.0mm tips.

Bausch & Lomb Surgical 636-255-5051
3365 Tree Court Ind Blvd, Saint Louis, MO 63122

Biomet Microfixation Inc. 800-874-7711
1520 Tradeport Dr, Jacksonville, FL 32218
Various types of forceps.

Biomet, Inc. 574-267-6639
56 E Bell Dr, PO Box 587, Warsaw, IN 46582
Various types of forceps.

Bionix Development Corp. 800-551-7096
5154 Enterprise Blvd, Toledo, OH 43612
Various.

Cardinal Health, Snowden Pencer Products 847-689-8410
5175 S Royal Atlanta Dr, Tucker, GA 30084
Various types of forceps.

Centurion Medical Products Corp. 517-545-1135
3310 S Main St, Salisbury, NC 28147

Codman & Shurtleff, Inc 800-225-0460
325 Paramount Dr, Raynham, MA 02767

Depuy-Raynham, A Div. Of Depuy Orthopaedics 800-451-2006
325 Paramount Dr, Raynham, MA 02767
Various types of forceps.

Electro Surgical Instrument Co., Inc. 888-464-2784
37 Centennial St, Rochester, NY 14611
Various types, styles and sizes of forceps for grasping manipulating and biopsy.

George Tiemann & Co. 800-843-6266
25 Plant Ave, Hauppauge, NY 11788

Grobet File Co. 800-847-4188
1912 Whitney Rd, Cheyenne, WY 82007
Dissecting forceps, tweezers.

Gyrus Acmi, Inc. 508-804-2739
93 N Pleasant St, Norwalk, OH 44857
Various sizes and kinds of forceps.

Gyrus Medical, Inc. 800-852-9361
6655 Wedgwood Rd N Ste 105, Maple Grove, MN 55311
PK CUTTING FORCEPS utilize bipolar electrosurgical energy to dissect, coagulate, grasp, and cut tissue during laparoscopic surgery.

Health Care Logistics, Inc. 800-848-1633
450 Town St, PO Box 25, Circleville, OH 43113
Various sizes of disposable sterile wound forceps.

Incisive Surgical, Inc. 877-246-7672
14405 21st Ave N Ste 130, Plymouth, MN 55447
INSORB|1 Single User Forceps

Integral Design Inc. 781-740-2036
52 Burr Rd, Hingham, MA 02043

International Hospital Supply Co. 800-398-9450
6914 Canby Ave Ste 105, Reseda, CA 91335

Invuity, Inc. 760-744-4447
334 Via Vera Cruz Ste 255, San Marcos, CA 92078
Forceps.

Invuity, Inc. 415-655-2100
39 Stillman St, San Francisco, CA 94107

J. Jamner Surgical Instruments, Inc 800-431-1123
9 Skyline Dr, Hawthorne, NY 10532

Kirwan Surgical Products, Inc. 888-547-9267
180 Enterprise Dr, PO Box 427, Marshfield, MA 02050

Kmedic 800-955-0559
190 Veterans Dr, Northvale, NJ 07647

Koros Usa, Inc. 805-529-0825
610 Flinn Ave, Moorpark, CA 93021
Vascular forceps.

Laschal Surgical, Inc. 914-949-8577
4 Baltusrol Dr, Purchase, NY 10577
Pressure controlled forceps.

FORCEPS, GENERAL & PLASTIC SURGERY *(cont'd)*

Medisiss 866-866-7477
2747 SW 6th St, Redmond, OR 97756
Various forceps,sterile.

Micrins Surgical Instruments, Inc. 800-833-3380
28438 N Ballard Dr, Lake Forest, IL 60045

Molded Products Inc. 800-435-8957
1112 Chatburn Ave, Harlan, IA 51537
Disposable forcep.

Neogen Corporation 800-234-5333
620 Lesher Pl, Lansing, MI 48912
For veterinary use only.

Normed 800-288-8200
PO Box 3644, Seattle, WA 98124
Various types and sizes of general medical forceps.

Olsen Medical 800-297-6344
3001 W Kentucky St, Louisville, KY 40211
Full line of Bipolar and Monopolar Forceps

Precision Surgical Intl., Inc. 800-776-8493
PO Box 726, Noblesville, IN 46061
Various forceps.

Princeton Medical Group, Inc. 800-875-0369
1189 Royal Links Dr, Mt Pleasant, SC 29466
TITANIUM & S/S MICROSURGICAL INSTRUMENTS

Prosurge Instruments, Inc. 866-832-7374
199 Laidlaw Ave, Jersey City, NJ 07306

Rhein Medical, Inc. 800-637-4346
5460 Beaumont Center Blvd Ste 500, Suite 500, Tampa, FL 33634

Schueler & Company, Inc. 516-487-1500
PO Box 528, Stratford, CT 06615

Small Bone Innovations, Inc. 215-428-1791
1380 S Pennsylvania Ave, Morrisville, PA 19067
Forceps, general & plastic surgery.

Solos Endoscopy 800-388-6445
65 Sprague St # B, Boston/dedham Commerce Park, Boston, MA 02136
Manual surgical instruments for general use.

Sporicidin International 800-424-3733
121 Congressional Ln, Rockville, MD 20852
Sporicidin Antimicrobial Lotion Soap is categorized by FDA as a surgical scrub and healthcare personnel handwash. It kills 99.9% of gram-positive and gram-negative pathogens tested, yet is gentle enough for routine daily handwashing. Pleasant scent.

Tri-State Hospital Supply Corp. 517-545-1135
3173 E 43rd St, Yuma, AZ 85365

Tuzik Boston 800-886-6363
104 Longwater Dr, Assinippi Park, Norwell, MA 02061

Vnus Medical Technologies, Inc. 888-797-8346
5799 Fontanoso Way, San Jose, CA 95138
Forcep, mosquito.

W.L. Gore & Associates,Inc 928-526-3030
1505 North Fourth St., Flagstaff, AZ 86004
Forcep.

FORCEPS, GRASPING, ATRAUMATIC *(Surgery) 79QKT*

Ams Innovative Center-San Jose 800-356-7600
3070 Orchard Dr, San Jose, CA 95134

Boss Instruments, Ltd. 800-210-2677
395 Reas Ford Rd Ste 120, Earlysville, VA 22936

Bryan Corp. 800-343-7711
4 Plympton St, Woburn, MA 01801
5mm/10mm 33cm length, insulated and non insulated, various styles.

Elmed, Inc. 630-543-2792
60 W Fay Ave, Addison, IL 60101

Ethicon Endo-Surgery, Inc. 800-USE-ENDO
4545 Creek Rd, Cincinnati, OH 45242
ENDOPATH 10mm thoracic, disposable, right-angle; also, 10mm thoracic curved disposable Kelly forceps. Instrument grasper, short with ratchet handle and unipolar cautery, 5mm. Blunt grasper, 5mm with handle, ratchet handle, with tooth and handle and with tooth and ratch, reuseable. Allis and Babcock graspers, 10mm, bowel, disposable.

Fehling Surgical Instruments 800-FEHLING
509 Broadstone Ln NW, Acworth, GA 30101

Md International, Inc. 305-669-9003
11300 NW 41st St, Doral, FL 33178

Mediflex Surgical Products 800-879-7575
250 Gibbs Rd, Islandia, NY 11749

FORCEPS, GRASPING, ATRAUMATIC *(cont'd)*

Princeton Medical Group, Inc. 800-875-0869
1189 Royal Links Dr, Mt Pleasant, SC 29466
TITANIUM & S/S INSTRUMENTS

Prosurge Instruments, Inc. 866-832-7874
199 Laidlaw Ave, Jersey City, NJ 07306

Richard Wolf Medical Instruments Corp. 800-323-9653
353 Corporate Woods Pkwy, Vernon Hills, IL 60061

Smith & Nephew, Inc., Endoscopy Division 800-343-8386
150 Minuteman Rd, Andover, MA 01810

Synectic Medical Product Development 203-877-8488
60 Commerce Park, Milford, CT 06460

FORCEPS, GRASPING, FLEXIBLE ENDOSCOPIC
(Gastro/Urology) 78QXC

Advanced Endoscopy Devices, Inc. 818-227-2720
22134 Sherman Way, Canoga Park, CA 91303
Forceps, endoscopic: instruments for urology/gyn, general surgery, arthroscopy, bronc-eso-ent.

Cathguide, Division Of Scilogy Corp. 305-269-0500
9135 Fontainebleau Blvd Apt 5, Miami, FL 33172

Cook Urological, Inc. 800-457-4500
1100 W Morgan St, P.O. Box 227, Spencer, IN 47460

Deknatel Snowden-Pencer 800-367-7874
5175 S Royal Atlanta Dr, Tucker, GA 30084

Elmed, Inc. 630-543-2792
60 W Fay Ave, Addison, IL 60101

Karl Storz Endoscopy-America Inc. 800-421-0837
600 Corporate Pointe, Culver City, CA 90230

Lsvp International, Inc. 866-969-0100
4692 El Camino Real Unit 126, Los Altos, CA 94022
Quality reusable instruments available for $199 and under.

Mahe International Inc. 800-294-7946
468 Craighead St, Nashville, TN 37204

Richard Wolf Medical Instruments Corp. 800-323-9653
353 Corporate Woods Pkwy, Vernon Hills, IL 60061

Synectic Medical Product Development 203-877-8488
60 Commerce Park, Milford, CT 06460

Wisap America 800-233-8448
8231 Melrose Dr, Lenexa, KS 66214

FORCEPS, GRASPING, TRAUMATIC *(Surgery) 79QLE*

Ams Innovative Center-San Jose 800-356-7600
3070 Orchard Dr, San Jose, CA 95134

Bryan Corp. 800-343-7711
4 Plympton St, Woburn, MA 01801
5mm/10mm 33cm length, insulated and non insulated, various styles.

Elmed, Inc. 630-543-2792
60 W Fay Ave, Addison, IL 60101

Md International, Inc. 305-669-9003
11300 NW 41st St, Doral, FL 33178

Mediflex Surgical Products 800-879-7575
250 Gibbs Rd, Islandia, NY 11749

Prosurge Instruments, Inc. 866-832-7874
199 Laidlaw Ave, Jersey City, NJ 07306

Richard Wolf Medical Instruments Corp. 800-323-9653
353 Corporate Woods Pkwy, Vernon Hills, IL 60061

Smith & Nephew, Inc., Endoscopy Division 800-343-8386
150 Minuteman Rd, Andover, MA 01810

Synectic Medical Product Development 203-877-8488
60 Commerce Park, Milford, CT 06460

FORCEPS, HEMOSTATIC *(Surgery) 79QXD*

Bausch & Lomb Surgical 636-255-5051
3365 Tree Court Ind Blvd, Saint Louis, MO 63122

Codman & Shurtleff, Inc 800-225-0460
325 Paramount Dr, Raynham, MA 02767

Dixie Ems Supply 800-347-3494
385 Union Ave, Brooklyn, NY 11211
$5.60 per unit (3-1/2in).

Elmed, Inc. 630-543-2792
60 W Fay Ave, Addison, IL 60101

Fehling Surgical Instruments 800-FEHLING
509 Broadstone Ln NW, Acworth, GA 30101

Fine Surgical Instrument, Inc. 800-851-5155
741 Peninsula Blvd, Hempstead, NY 11550

FORCEPS, HEMOSTATIC *(cont'd)*

Fortrad Eye Instruments Corp. 973-543-2371
8 Franklin Rd, Mendham, NJ 07945

J. Jamner Surgical Instruments, Inc 800-431-1123
9 Skyline Dr, Hawthorne, NY 10532

Jedmed Instruments Co. 314-845-3770
5416 Jedmed Ct, Saint Louis, MO 63129

Katena Products, Inc. 800-225-1195
4 Stewart Ct, Denville, NJ 07834

Kmedic 800-955-0559
190 Veterans Dr, Northvale, NJ 07647

Kta, Instruments, Inc. 888-830-9KTA
3051 Brighton-Third St., 1st Fl., Brooklyn, NY 11235

Lican Medical Products Ltd. 519-737-1142
5120 Halford Dr., Windsor, ON N9A 6J3 Canada

Medworks Instruments 800-323-9790
PO Box 581, Chatham, IL 62629
$1.30 per unit (3-1/2in to 5-1/2 in).

Nordent Manufacturing, Inc. 800-966-7336
610 Bonnie Ln, Elk Grove Village, IL 60007
$30.00 per unit (standard).

Prestige Medical Corporation 800-762-3333
8600 Wilbur Ave, Northridge, CA 91324
Hemostatic and tungsten forceps.

Princeton Medical Group, Inc. 800-875-0869
1189 Royal Links Dr, Mt Pleasant, SC 29466

Prosurge Instruments, Inc. 866-832-7874
199 Laidlaw Ave, Jersey City, NJ 07306

Roboz Surgical Instrument Co., Inc. 800-424-2984
PO Box 10710, Gaithersburg, MD 20898

Rocket Medical Plc. 800-707-7625
150 Recreation Park Dr Ste 3, Hingham, MA 02043

Scanlan International, Inc. 800-328-9458
1 Scanlan Plz, Saint Paul, MN 55107

Toolmex Corporation 800-992-4766
1075 Worcester St, Natick, MA 01760

Trans American Medical 800-626-9232
7633 W 100th Pl, Bridgeview, IL 60455
KELLY 5.5 in. straight and curved, satin or polished. MOSQUITO 5 in. straight and curved, satin or polished. U.S. made.

Zimmer Holdings, Inc. 800-613-6131
1800 W Center St, PO Box 708, Warsaw, IN 46580

FORCEPS, INTESTINAL (CLAMPS) *(Gastro/Urology) 78QXE*

Codman & Shurtleff, Inc 800-225-0460
325 Paramount Dr, Raynham, MA 02767

Elmed, Inc. 630-543-2792
60 W Fay Ave, Addison, IL 60101

Fine Surgical Instrument, Inc. 800-851-5155
741 Peninsula Blvd, Hempstead, NY 11550

Kta, Instruments, Inc. 888-830-9KTA
3051 Brighton-Third St., 1st Fl., Brooklyn, NY 11235

Prosurge Instruments, Inc. 866-832-7874
199 Laidlaw Ave, Jersey City, NJ 07306

FORCEPS, LAPAROSCOPY, BIPOLAR, ELECTROSURGICAL
(Surgery) 79SJX

Genicon 800-936-1020
6869 Stapoint Ct Ste 114, Winter Park, FL 32792
Bipolar Electrosurgical Instrumentation for Laparoscopic Surgery. Products are available in 5mm diameter and 33cm and 45cm products.

Gyrus Medical, Inc. 800-852-9361
6655 Wedgwood Rd N Ste 105, Maple Grove, MN 55311

Okay Industries, Inc. 860-225-8707
200 Ellis St, P.O. Box 2470, New Britain, CT 06051

FORCEPS, LAPAROSCOPY, ELECTROSURGICAL
(Surgery) 79WZD

Gyrus Medical, Inc. 800-852-9361
6655 Wedgwood Rd N Ste 105, Maple Grove, MN 55311
BICOAG bipolar laparoscopic cutting forceps. Intended for laparoscopic and other MIS procedures; available in a variety of micro- or maxi-jaw configurations.

Mediflex Surgical Products 800-879-7575
250 Gibbs Rd, Islandia, NY 11749

FORCEPS, LUNG *(Surgery) 79QXF*

Ethicon Endo-Surgery, Inc. 800-USE-ENDO
4545 Creek Rd, Cincinnati, OH 45242
ENDOPATH 10mm disposable thoracic forceps.

Miltex Inc. 800-645-8000
589 Davies Dr, York, PA 17402

Richard Wolf Medical Instruments Corp. 800-323-9653
353 Corporate Woods Pkwy, Vernon Hills, IL 60061

FORCEPS, OBSTETRICAL *(Obstetrics/Gyn) 85HDA*

Aesculap Implant Systems Inc. 1-800-234-9179
3773 Corporate Pkwy, Center Valley, PA 18034

Biomet Microfixation Inc. 800-874-7711
1520 Tradeport Dr, Jacksonville, FL 32218
Various types of forceps.

Codman & Shurtleff, Inc 800-225-0460
325 Paramount Dr, Raynham, MA 02767

Cook Ob/Gyn 800-541-5591
1100 W Morgan St, Spencer, IN 47460

Cook Urological, Inc. 800-457-4500
1100 W Morgan St, P.O. Box 227, Spencer, IN 47460

Elmed, Inc. 630-543-2792
60 W Fay Ave, Addison, IL 60101

George Tiemann & Co. 800-843-6266
25 Plant Ave, Hauppauge, NY 11788

Kmedic 800-955-0559
190 Veterans Dr, Northvale, NJ 07647

Miltex Inc. 800-645-8000
589 Davies Dr, York, PA 17402

Prosurge Instruments, Inc. 866-832-7874
199 Laidlaw Ave, Jersey City, NJ 07306

Rocket Medical Plc. 800-707-7625
150 Recreation Park Dr Ste 3, Hingham, MA 02043

Solos Endoscopy 800-388-6445
65 Sprague St # B, Boston/dedham Commerce Park, Boston, MA 02136
Forceps,obstetrical.

Toolmex Corporation 800-992-4766
1075 Worcester St, Natick, MA 01760

Tuzik Boston 800-886-6363
104 Longwater Dr, Assinippi Park, Norwell, MA 02061

FORCEPS, OPHTHALMIC *(Ophthalmology) 86HNR*

Accutome, Inc. 610-889-0200
3222 Phoenixville Pike, Malvern, PA 19355
Forceps.

Addition Technology, Inc. 847-297-8419
155 Moffett Park Dr Ste B-1, Sunnyvale, CA 94089

Akorn, Inc. 800-535-7155
2500 Millbrook Dr, Buffalo Grove, IL 60089
Titanium and stainless steel corneal/tissue, tying, fixation, lens implanting and capsulorhexis forceps.

Alcon Manufacturing, Ltd. 817-551-6813
714 Columbia Ave, Sinking Spring, PA 19608
Various sizes & types of ophthalmic forceps.

American Surgical Instrument Corp. 800-628-2879
26 Plaza Dr, Westmont, IL 60559
Lens holding forceps with 0.2mm peg to fit into manipulation hole of lens.

B. Graczyk, Inc. 269-782-2100
27826 Burmax Park, Dowagiac, MI 49047
Various types of forceps.

Back-Mueller, Inc. 314-531-6640
2700 Clark Ave, Saint Louis, MO 63103
Various type of forceps.

Bausch & Lomb Surgical 636-255-5051
3365 Tree Court Ind Blvd, Saint Louis, MO 63122

Capital Instruments, Ltd. 425-271-3756
6210 Lake Washington Blvd SE, Bellevue, WA 98006
Various types.

Demetech Corp. 888-324-2447
3530 NW 115th Ave, Doral, FL 33178
Ophthalmic forceps.

Diamond Edge Co. 727-586-2927
928 W Bay Dr, Largo, FL 33770
Forceps.

FORCEPS, OPHTHALMIC *(cont'd)*

Dutch Ophthalmic Usa, Inc. 800-753-8824
10 Continental Dr Bldg 1, Exeter, NH 03833
Various models of forceps.

Eagle Vision, Inc. 800-222-7584
8500 Wolf Lake Dr Ste 110, Memphis, TN 38133
Various forceps.

Elmed, Inc. 630-543-2792
60 W Fay Ave, Addison, IL 60101

Eye Care And Cure 800-486-6169
4646 S Overland Dr, Tucson, AZ 85714
Forceps.

Fischer Surgical Inc. 314-303-7753
1343 Pine Dr, Arnold, MO 63010
Various types of ophthalmic forceps.

Fortrad Eye Instruments Corp. 973-543-2371
8 Franklin Rd, Mendham, NJ 07945

Glaukos Corp. 949-367-9600
26051 Merit Cir Ste 103, Laguna Hills, CA 92653
Various types of sterile & non-sterile ophthalmic forceps.

Gyrus Ent L.L.C., Sub. Of Gyrus Acmi, Inc. 508-804-2739
2925 Appling Rd, Bartlett, TN 38133
Various.

Hai Laboratories, Inc. 781-862-9384
320 Massachusetts Ave, Lexington, MA 02420
Ophthalmic forceps - various types.

Harvey Precision Instruments 707-793-2300
217 Fairway Rd, Cape Haze, FL 33947
Various ophthalmic forceps.

International Hospital Supply Co. 800-398-9450
6914 Canby Ave Ste 105, Reseda, CA 91335

J. Jamner Surgical Instruments, Inc 800-431-1123
9 Skyline Dr, Hawthorne, NY 10532

Jedmed Instruments Co. 314-845-3770
5416 Jedmed Ct, Saint Louis, MO 63129
Micro needle forceps for grasping of anterior or posterior capsules, secondary membranes, and various vitreous strands and for intravitreal cutting in combination with a second instrument; no sutures required, forceps protruding from tip of 24-gauge needle.

Katena Products, Inc. 800-225-1195
4 Stewart Ct, Denville, NJ 07834

Keeler Instruments Inc. 800-523-5620
456 Park Way, Broomall, PA 19008
$208. to $287. for Hoskin instruments.

Kmedic 800-955-0559
190 Veterans Dr, Northvale, NJ 07647

Krause Surgical Instrument Corp. 314-842-0327
5544 Robert Wood Dr, Saint Louis, MO 63128
Ophthalmic forceps.

Labtician Ophthalmics, Inc. 800-265-8391
2140 Winston Park Dr., Unit 6, Oakville, ONTAR L6H 5V5 Canada
Frederick sleeve forceps.

Medone Surgical, Inc. 941-359-3129
670 Tallevast Rd, Sarasota, FL 34243
Various types of micro forceps.

Micro-Select Instruments, Inc. 636-273-5227
165 Duckworth St, Saint Clair, MO 63077
Forceps.

Prosurge Instruments, Inc. 866-832-7874
199 Laidlaw Ave, Jersey City, NJ 07306

Rhein Medical, Inc. 800-637-4346
5460 Beaumont Center Blvd Ste 500, Suite 500, Tampa, FL 33634
Kershner forceps, Utrata capsulorhexis forceps, tying, lens insertion, fixation, lens folding.

Rhein Mfg., Inc. 314-997-1775
2269 Grissom Dr, Saint Louis, MO 63146
Various sizes and types of ophthalmic surgical forceps.

Stephens Instruments, Inc. 800-354-7848
2500 Sandersville Rd, Lexington, KY 40511
$35.00 per unit (standard).

Surgical Eye Enterprise 636-282-2800
1763 Engle Dr, Arnold, MO 63010
Various.

Surgical Instrument Manufacturers, Inc. 800-521-2985
1650 Headland Dr, Fenton, MO 63026

FORCEPS, OPHTHALMIC *(cont'd)*

Synergetics Usa, Inc. 800-600-0565
3845 Corporate Centre Dr, O Fallon, MO 63368
Forceps.

Total Titanium, Inc. 618-473-2429
140 East Monroe St., Hecker, IL 62248
Various types of ophthalmic forceps.

Western Ophthalmics Corporation 800-426-9938
19019 36th Ave W Ste G, Lynnwood, WA 98036

FORCEPS, RONGEUR, SURGICAL *(Dental And Oral) 76EMH*

Aesculap Implant Systems Inc. 1-800-234-9179
3773 Corporate Pkwy, Center Valley, PA 18034

Arnold Tuber Industries 716-648-3363
97 Main St, Hamburg, NY 14075
Forceps, rongeur, surgical, dental hand instruments.

Biomet Microfixation Inc. 800-874-7711
1520 Tradeport Dr, Jacksonville, FL 32218
Various types of forceps.

Dental Usa, Inc. 815-363-8003
5005 McCullom Lake Rd, McHenry, IL 60050
Forceps.

E.A. Beck & Co. 949-645-4072
657 W 19th St Ste E, P O Box 10857, Costa Mesa, CA 92627
Ronguer.

Elmed, Inc. 630-543-2792
60 W Fay Ave, Addison, IL 60101

H & H Co. 909-390-0373
4435 E Airport Dr Ste 108, Ontario, CA 91761
Rongeur, dental.

Hu-Friedy Manufacturing Co., Inc. 800-483-7433
3232 N Rockwell St, Chicago, IL 60618
$213.20 to $236.65, 17 types.

Kmedic 800-955-0559
190 Veterans Dr, Northvale, NJ 07647

Oratronics, Inc. 212-986-0050
405 Lexington Ave, New York, NY 10174
Bone rongeurs.

Premier Dental Products Co. 888-670-6100
1710 Romano Dr, PO Box 4500, Plymouth Meeting, PA 19462

Prosurge Instruments, Inc. 866-832-7874
199 Laidlaw Ave, Jersey City, NJ 07306

Salvin Dental Specialties, Inc. 800-535-6566
3450 Latrobe Dr, Charlotte, NC 28211
Various types of rongeurs and accessories.

Symmetry Medical Usa, Inc. 574-267-8700
486 W 350 N, Warsaw, IN 46582
Dental hand instrument.

Tuzik Boston 800-886-6363
104 Longwater Dr, Assinippi Park, Norwell, MA 02061

FORCEPS, RUBBER DAM CLAMP *(Dental And Oral) 76EJG*

Coltene/Whaledent Inc. 330-916-8858
235 Ascot Pkwy, Cuyahoga Falls, OH 44223
Rubber dam clamp forceps.

Dental Usa, Inc. 815-363-8003
5005 McCullom Lake Rd, McHenry, IL 60050
Forceps, rubber dam clamps.

Hager Worldwide, Inc. 800-328-2335
13322 Byrd Dr, Odessa, FL 33556
FIT.

Heraeus Kulzer, Inc., Dental Products Division 574-299-6662
4315 S Lafayette Blvd, South Bend, IN 46614
Rubber dam forceps.

Miltex Dental Technologies, Inc. 516-576-6022
589 Davies Dr, York, PA 17402
Various rubber dam clamp forceps.

Moyco Technologies, Inc. 800-331-8837
200 Commerce Dr, Montgomeryville, PA 18936

Premier Dental Products Co. 888-670-6100
1710 Romano Dr, PO Box 4500, Plymouth Meeting, PA 19462

Prosurge Instruments, Inc. 866-832-7874
199 Laidlaw Ave, Jersey City, NJ 07306

FORCEPS, SPECIMEN *(Gastro/Urology) 78QXG*

Richard Wolf Medical Instruments Corp. 800-323-9653
353 Corporate Woods Pkwy, Vernon Hills, IL 60061

FORCEPS, SPONGE *(Surgery) 79QXH*

Codman & Shurtleff, Inc 800-225-0460
325 Paramount Dr, Raynham, MA 02767

Directmed, Inc. 516-656-3377
150 Pratt Oval, Glen Cove, NY 11542

Elmed, Inc. 630-543-2792
60 W Fay Ave, Addison, IL 60101

Kmedic 800-955-0559
190 Veterans Dr, Northvale, NJ 07647

Princeton Medical Group, Inc. 800-875-0869
1189 Royal Links Dr, Mt Pleasant, SC 29466

Prosurge Instruments, Inc. 866-832-7874
199 Laidlaw Ave, Jersey City, NJ 07306

Richard Wolf Medical Instruments Corp. 800-323-9653
353 Corporate Woods Pkwy, Vernon Hills, IL 60061

Rocket Medical Plc. 800-707-7625
150 Recreation Park Dr Ste 3, Hingham, MA 02043

Zimmer Holdings, Inc. 800-613-6131
1800 W Center St, PO Box 708, Warsaw, IN 46580

FORCEPS, STERILIZER TRANSFER *(General) 80QXI*

Clinimed, Incorporated 877-CLINIMED
303 Markus Ct, Sandy Brae Industrial Park, Newark, DE 19713

Sterigenics International, Inc. 800-472-4508
2015 Spring Rd Ste 650, Oak Brook, IL 60523
Providing overnight re-useable instrument sterilization services for hospitals, surgical centers, labs and research facilities in four markets (Los Angeles, Chicago, Atlanta and Salt Lake City. This service meets AAMI, ISO and JCAHO standards for sterilization compliance, assisting the healthcare and research facility to reduce its in-house sterilization que, in a cost and time effective manner.

FORCEPS, STONE MANIPULATION *(Gastro/Urology) 78QXJ*

Codman & Shurtleff, Inc 800-225-0460
325 Paramount Dr, Raynham, MA 02767

Cook Urological, Inc. 800-457-4500
1100 W Morgan St, P.O. Box 227, Spencer, IN 47460

Elmed, Inc. 630-543-2792
60 W Fay Ave, Addison, IL 60101

Karl Storz Endoscopy-America Inc. 800-421-0837
600 Corporate Pointe, Culver City, CA 90230

Mahe International Inc. 800-294-7946
468 Craighead St, Nashville, TN 37204

Miltex Inc. 800-645-8000
589 Davies Dr, York, PA 17402

Richard Wolf Medical Instruments Corp. 800-323-9653
353 Corporate Woods Pkwy, Vernon Hills, IL 60061

FORCEPS, SUCTION *(Surgery) 79QXK*

Codman & Shurtleff, Inc 800-225-0460
325 Paramount Dr, Raynham, MA 02767

Integral Design Inc. 781-740-2036
52 Burr Rd, Hingham, MA 02043

Kirwan Surgical Products, Inc. 888-547-9267
180 Enterprise Dr, PO Box 427, Marshfield, MA 02050

Scanlan International, Inc. 800-328-9458
1 Scanlan Plz, Saint Paul, MN 55107

FORCEPS, SURGICAL, GYNECOLOGICAL
(Obstetrics/Gyn) 85HCZ

Biomet Microfixation Inc. 800-874-7711
1520 Tradeport Dr, Jacksonville, FL 32218
Various types of forceps.

Elmed, Inc. 630-543-2792
60 W Fay Ave, Addison, IL 60101

International Hospital Supply Co. 800-398-9450
6914 Canby Ave Ste 105, Reseda, CA 91335

Kmedic 800-955-0559
190 Veterans Dr, Northvale, NJ 07647

Lican Medical Products Ltd. 519-737-1142
5120 Halford Dr., Windsor, ON N9A 6J3 Canada
Laparoscopic forceps.

Marina Medical Instruments, Inc. 800-697-1119
955 Shotgun Rd, Sunrise, FL 33326
Various.

Princeton Medical Group, Inc. 800-875-0869
1189 Royal Links Dr, Mt Pleasant, SC 29466

FORCEPS, SURGICAL, GYNECOLOGICAL *(cont'd)*

Prosurge Instruments, Inc. 866-832-7874
199 Laidlaw Ave, Jersey City, NJ 07306

Reznik Instrument, Inc. 847-673-3444
7337 Lawndale Ave, Skokie, IL 60076
Forceps.

Rocket Medical Plc. 800-707-7625
150 Recreation Park Dr Ste 3, Hingham, MA 02043

Toolmex Corporation 800-992-4766
1075 Worcester St, Natick, MA 01760

Triboro Supplies Inc 800-369-7546
994 Grand Blvd, Deer Park, NY 11729

Tuzik Boston 800-886-6363
104 Longwater Dr, Assinippi Park, Norwell, MA 02061

FORCEPS, TISSUE *(Surgery) 79QXL*

Bausch & Lomb Surgical 636-255-5051
3365 Tree Court Ind Blvd, Saint Louis, MO 63122

Codman & Shurtleff, Inc 800-225-0460
325 Paramount Dr, Raynham, MA 02767

Deknatel Snowden-Pencer 800-367-7874
5175 S Royal Atlanta Dr, Tucker, GA 30084

Elmed, Inc. 630-543-2792
60 W Fay Ave, Addison, IL 60101

Ethicon Endo-Surgery, Inc. 800-USE-ENDO
4545 Creek Rd, Cincinnati, OH 45242
ENDOPATH 10mm thoracic, disposable.

Fortrad Eye Instruments Corp. 973-543-2371
8 Franklin Rd, Mendham, NJ 07945

Integral Design Inc. 781-740-2036
52 Burr Rd, Hingham, MA 02043

J. Jamner Surgical Instruments, Inc 800-431-1123
9 Skyline Dr, Hawthorne, NY 10532

Jedmed Instruments Co. 314-845-3770
5416 Jedmed Ct, Saint Louis, MO 63129

Katena Products, Inc. 800-225-1195
4 Stewart Ct, Denville, NJ 07834

Kirwan Surgical Products, Inc. 888-547-9267
180 Enterprise Dr, PO Box 427, Marshfield, MA 02050

Kmedic 800-955-0559
190 Veterans Dr, Northvale, NJ 07647

Medcare Technologies 800-388-6235
850 Saint Paul St, Rochester, NY 14605
Disposable, bulk, non-sterile.

Medworks Instruments 800-323-9790
PO Box 581, Chatham, IL 62629
$1.00 per unit (5-1/2in, 1 x 2th).

Miltex Inc. 800-645-8000
589 Davies Dr, York, PA 17402

Nordent Manufacturing, Inc. 800-966-7336
610 Bonnie Ln, Elk Grove Village, IL 60007
$28.50 per unit (5-1/2in, 1 x 2th).

Olsen Medical 800-297-6344
3001 W Kentucky St, Louisville, KY 40211
Full line of tissue forceps

Prosurge Instruments, Inc. 866-832-7874
199 Laidlaw Ave, Jersey City, NJ 07306

Rhein Medical, Inc. 800-637-4346
5460 Beaumont Center Blvd Ste 500, Suite 500, Tampa, FL 33634

Rocket Medical Plc. 800-707-7625
150 Recreation Park Dr Ste 3, Hingham, MA 02043

Scanlan International, Inc. 800-328-9458
1 Scanlan Plz, Saint Paul, MN 55107

Toolmex Corporation 800-992-4766
1075 Worcester St, Natick, MA 01760

Zimmer Holdings, Inc. 800-613-6131
1800 W Center St, PO Box 708, Warsaw, IN 46580

FORCEPS, TONSIL *(Ear/Nose/Throat) 77QXM*

Clinimed, Incorporated 877-CLINIMED
303 Markus Ct, Sandy Brae Industrial Park, Newark, DE 19713

Elmed, Inc. 630-543-2792
60 W Fay Ave, Addison, IL 60101

Integral Design Inc. 781-740-2036
52 Burr Rd, Hingham, MA 02043

FORCEPS, TONSIL *(cont'd)*

Kirwan Surgical Products, Inc. 888-547-9267
180 Enterprise Dr, PO Box 427, Marshfield, MA 02050

FORCEPS, TOOTH EXTRACTOR, SURGICAL
(Dental And Oral) 76EMG

Aesculap Implant Systems Inc. 1-800-234-9179
3773 Corporate Pkwy, Center Valley, PA 18034

Arnold Tuber Industries 716-648-3363
97 Main St, Hamburg, NY 14075
Forceps, tooth extractor, surgical, dental hand instruments.

Biomet Microfixation Inc. 800-874-7711
1520 Tradeport Dr, Jacksonville, FL 32218
Various types of forceps.

Brasseler Usa - Komet Medical 800-535-6638
1 Brasseler Blvd, Savannah, GA 31419

Dental Usa, Inc. 815-363-8003
5005 McCullom Lake Rd, McHenry, IL 60050
Forceps.

E.A. Beck & Co. 949-645-4072
657 W 19th St Ste E, P O Box 10857, Costa Mesa, CA 92627
Forcep.

H & H Co. 909-390-0373
4435 E Airport Dr Ste 108, Ontario, CA 91761
Tooth extractor.

Hu-Friedy Manufacturing Co., Inc. 800-483-7433
3232 N Rockwell St, Chicago, IL 60618
$118.60 to $184.60 each, 35 types.

Long And Rossi Products 303-233-9581
895 Field St, Lakewood, CO 80215
Tooth extractor.

Miltex Inc. 800-645-8000
589 Davies Dr, York, PA 17402
Root Tip Carbide Beak extracting forceps. DEF845/TC delicate 7 1/4' lower root tip, DEF849/TC delicate 7 1/2' upper root tip, DEF849S/TC delicate 6 1/2' peclo upper root tip, DEF859/TC delicate 5 3/8' lower root tip. Pedoclontic extracting forceps. DEFA upper molar 4 3/4', DEFB lower root 4 1/4', DEFC lower molar universal 4 1/4', DEFE upper front 4 1/2', DEFF upper root 4 1/2', DEFH pedoupper & lower 4 1/2'.

Nordent Manufacturing, Inc. 800-966-7336
610 Bonnie Ln, Elk Grove Village, IL 60007
$105.00 per unit (standard).

Premier Dental Products Co. 888-670-6100
1710 Romano Dr, PO Box 4500, Plymouth Meeting, PA 19462

Prosurge Instruments, Inc. 866-832-7874
199 Laidlaw Ave, Jersey City, NJ 07306

Pulpdent Corp. 800-343-4342
80 Oakland St, Watertown, MA 02472
No common name listed.

Salvin Dental Specialties, Inc. 800-535-6566
3450 Latrobe Dr, Charlotte, NC 28211
Various types of extraction forceps.

FORCEPS, TUBE INTRODUCTION *(Anesthesiology) 73BWB*

Aesculap Implant Systems Inc. 1-800-234-9179
3773 Corporate Pkwy, Center Valley, PA 18034

Eastmed Enterprises, Inc. 856-797-0131
11 Brandywine Dr, Marlton, NJ 08053
Various sizes of magill forceps.

Mercury Medical 800-237-6418
11300 49th St N, Clearwater, FL 33762

Primary Medical Co., Inc. 727-520-1920
6541 44th St N Ste 6003, Pinellas Park, FL 33781
Forceps, tube introduction, various sizes.

Tuzik Boston 800-886-6363
104 Longwater Dr, Assinippi Park, Norwell, MA 02061

FORCEPS, UTILITY *(Surgery) 79QXN*

Codman & Shurtleff, Inc 800-225-0460
325 Paramount Dr, Raynham, MA 02767

Elmed, Inc. 630-543-2792
60 W Fay Ave, Addison, IL 60101

George Tiemann & Co. 800-843-6266
25 Plant Ave, Hauppauge, NY 11788

Katena Products, Inc. 800-225-1195
4 Stewart Ct, Denville, NJ 07834

FORCEPS, UTILITY *(cont'd)*

Mine Safety Appliances Company 866-MSA-1001
121 Gamma Dr, Pittsburgh, PA 15238

Prosurge Instruments, Inc. 866-832-7874
199 Laidlaw Ave, Jersey City, NJ 07306

Zimmer Holdings, Inc. 800-613-6131
1800 W Center St, PO Box 708, Warsaw, IN 46580

FORCEPS, WIRE CLOSURE, ENT *(Ear/Nose/Throat) 77JXX*

Aesculap Implant Systems Inc. 1-800-234-9179
3773 Corporate Pkwy, Center Valley, PA 18034

Bausch & Lomb Surgical 636-255-5051
3365 Tree Court Ind Blvd, Saint Louis, MO 63122

Biomet Microfixation Inc. 800-874-7711
1520 Tradeport Dr, Jacksonville, FL 32218
Various types of forceps.

Clinimed, Incorporated 877-CLINIMED
303 Markus Ct, Sandy Brae Industrial Park, Newark, DE 19713

Gyrus Ent L.L.C., Sub. Of Gyrus Acmi, Inc. 508-804-2739
2925 Appling Rd, Bartlett, TN 38133
Various types and sizes of ent wire closure forceps.

Prosurge Instruments, Inc. 866-832-7874
199 Laidlaw Ave, Jersey City, NJ 07306

FORCEPS, WIRE HOLDING *(Orthopedics) 87HYA*

Biomet, Inc. 574-267-6639
56 E Bell Dr, PO Box 587, Warsaw, IN 46582
Various types of wire holding forceps.

J. Jamner Surgical Instruments, Inc 800-431-1123
9 Skyline Dr, Hawthorne, NY 10532

Kls-Martin L.P. 800-625-1557
11239-1 St. John`s Industrial, Parkway South
Jacksonville, FL 32250
Wire twisting forceps.

Kmedic 800-955-0559
190 Veterans Dr, Northvale, NJ 07647

Prosurge Instruments, Inc. 866-832-7874
199 Laidlaw Ave, Jersey City, NJ 07306

Smith & Nephew, Inc., Endoscopy Division 800-343-8386
130 Forbes Blvd, Mansfield, MA 02048

Stryker Spine 866-457-7463
2 Pearl Ct, Allendale, NJ 07401

Toolmex Corporation 800-992-4766
1075 Worcester St, Natick, MA 01760

Zimmer Holdings, Inc. 800-613-6131
1800 W Center St, PO Box 708, Warsaw, IN 46580

FORK *(Orthopedics) 87HXE*

K2m, Inc. 866-526-4171
751 Miller Dr SE Ste F1, Leesburg, VA 20175
Fork.

Medtronic Sofamor Danek Usa, Inc. 901-396-3133
4340 Swinnea Rd, Memphis, TN 38118
Fork, fork hammer.

R. D. Equipment, Inc. 508-362-7498
230 Percival Dr, West Barnstable, MA 02668
Right angle folding fork.

Warsaw Orthopedic, Inc. 901-396-3133
2500 Silveus Xing, Warsaw, IN 46582
Fork, fork hammer.

Zimmer Trabecular Metal Technology 800-613-6131
10 Pomeroy Rd, Parsippany, NJ 07054
Hip retractor.

FORK, TUNING *(Cns/Neurology) 84GWX*

Biomet Microfixation Inc. 800-874-7711
1520 Tradeport Dr, Jacksonville, FL 32218
Fork, tuning.

Kmedic 800-955-0559
190 Veterans Dr, Northvale, NJ 07647

Medworks Instruments 800-323-9790
PO Box 581, Chatham, IL 62629
1024 to 64 frequencies, professional.

Miltex Inc. 800-645-8000
589 Davies Dr, York, PA 17402

Phipps & Bird, Inc. 800-955-7621
1519 Summit Ave, Richmond, VA 23230

FORK, TUNING, ENT *(Ear/Nose/Throat) 77ETQ*

Aesculap Implant Systems Inc. 1-800-234-9179
3773 Corporate Pkwy, Center Valley, PA 18034

Clinimed, Incorporated 877-CLINIMED
303 Markus Ct, Sandy Brae Industrial Park, Newark, DE 19713

Hal-Hen Company, Inc. 800-242-5436
180 Atlantic Ave, Garden City Park, NY 11040
Complete set of turning revaks; $135.00 per unit (standard).

Jedmed Instruments Co. 314-845-3770
5416 Jedmed Ct, Saint Louis, MO 63129

Princeton Medical Group, Inc. 800-875-0869
1189 Royal Links Dr, Mt Pleasant, SC 29466

Riverbank Laboratories 630-232-2207
2613 Kaneville Ct, PO Box 110, Geneva, IL 60134

FORMALDEHYDE (FORMALIN, FORMOL) *(Pathology) 88IGG*

Advanced Chemical Sensors Inc. 561-338-3116
3201 N Dixie Hwy Ste 3, Boca Raton, FL 33431
Electronic instruments and monitoring badges. Electronic instruments provide real time measurement and alarm with data logging capability. Monitoring badges provide a written record from an independent laboratory.

American Mastertech Scientific, Inc. 209-368-4031
1330 Thurman St, Lodi, CA 95240
Multiple.

Anatech, Ltd. 800-262-8324
1020 Harts Lake Rd, Battle Creek, MI 49037
Formalin containing fixative Z-5 is a B5 replacement fixative.Sold as an one quart concentrate to make 820 ml of fixative.

B/R Instrument Corp. 800-922-9206
9119 Centreville Rd, Easton, MD 21601
PUREFORM 2100, Formalin Recycling System, recycles formalin from tissue processor and surgical specimens. Formalin can be re-used in the same process. Accessories available.

E K Industries, Inc. 877-EKI-CHEM
1403 Herkimer St, Joliet, IL 60432
Formaldehyde.

Fisher Scientific Co., Llc. 201-703-3131
1 Reagent Ln, Fair Lawn, NJ 07410
Formalin fixative & 405 formaldehyde fixative.

Hydrol Chemical Co. 610-622-3603
520 Commerce Dr, Yeadon, PA 19050
Formaldehyde (formalin, formol).

Kem Medical Products Corp. 800-553-0330
75 Price Pkwy, Farmingdale, NY 11735

Lamotte Co. 800-344-3100
802 Washington Ave, PO Box 329, Chestertown, MD 21620
Formaldehyde samplers and analyzer, dialysis use.

Medical Chemical Corp. 800-424-9394
19430 Van Ness Ave, Torrance, CA 90501
$20.00 per 4000mL.

Pochemco, Inc. 413-536-2900
724 Main St, Holyoke, MA 01040
Formaldehyde.

Poly Scientific R&D Corp. 800-645-5825
70 Cleveland Ave, Bay Shore, NY 11706

Polysciences, Inc. 800-523-2575
400 Valley Rd, Warrington, PA 18976
Methanol free and 10% methanol free.

Proper Chem Ltd. 631-420-8000
280 Smith St, Farmingdale, NY 11735

Ricca Chemical Company Llc 817-461-5601
1490 Lammers Pike, Batesville, IN 47006

Ricca Chemical Company, Llc 817-461-5601
448 W Fork Dr, Arlington, TX 76012
Formaldehyde solution.

Rocky Mountain Reagents,Inc. 303-762-0800
3207 W Hampden Ave, Englewood, CO 80110

Sci Gen, Inc. 310-324-6576
333 E Gardena Blvd, Gardena, CA 90248
FDA: Medical Device Manufacturing and packaging. Focus on Histology, Cytology, Analytical and General purpose Reagents, Chemistry, and Sterling and Disinfecting agents.

Wessels And Associates 248-547-7177
131 Cambridge Blvd, Pleasant Ridge, MI 48069
10% neutral buffered formalin.

FORMALIN, NEUTRAL BUFFERED *(Pathology) 88IFP*

American Mastertech Scientific, Inc. 209-368-4031
1330 Thurman St, Lodi, CA 95240
Multiple.

Anatech, Ltd. 800-262-8324
1020 Harts Lake Rd, Battle Creek, MI 49037
NBF;5 gallon drum of standard 10% neutral buffered formalin; CB FORMALIN is concentrate form of NBF, sold in one gallon units, addition of water makes standard NBF.

Diagnostic Technology, Inc. 631-582-4949
175 Commerce Dr Ste L, Hauppauge, NY 11788
10% v/v neutralized formalin.

E K Industries, Inc. 877-EKI-CHEM
1403 Herkimer St, Joliet, IL 60432
Neutral buffered formalin carson millonig formulation & fixative.

Fisher Scientific Co., Llc. 201-703-3131
1 Reagent Ln, Fair Lawn, NJ 07410
Buffered formalin (10% buffered formalin phosphate).

Hydrol Chemical Co. 610-622-3603
520 Commerce Dr, Yeadon, PA 19050
Buffered formalin.

Meridian Bioscience, Inc. 800-696-0739
3471 River Hills Dr, Cincinnati, OH 45244
$210.00 per case of formalin and polyvinyl alcohol.

National Nonwovens 800-333-3469
PO Box 150, Easthampton, MA 01027
Formaldehyde neutralizer pads, used for grossing tissue in formalin to neutralize vapors.

Pochemco, Inc. 413-536-2900
724 Main St, Holyoke, MA 01040
Formalin concentrate; formalin, neutral buffered.

Poly Scientific R&D Corp. 800-645-5825
70 Cleveland Ave, Bay Shore, NY 11706
10% buffered formalin or any dilution.

Polysciences, Inc. 800-523-2575
400 Valley Rd, Warrington, PA 18976
10% buffered neutral formalin.

Ricca Chemical Company Llc 817-461-5601
1490 Lammers Pike, Batesville, IN 47006

Ricca Chemical Company, Llc 817-461-5601
448 W Fork Dr, Arlington, TX 76012
Various.

Richard-Allan Scientific 269-544-5628
4481 Campus Dr, Kalamazoo, MI 49008
Multiple.

Rocky Mountain Reagents,Inc. 303-762-0800
3207 W Hampden Ave, Englewood, CO 80110

Sci Gen, Inc. 310-324-6576
333 E Gardena Blvd, Gardena, CA 90248
FDA: Medical Device Manufacturing and packaging. Focus on Histology, Cytology, Analytical and General purpose Reagents, Chemistry, and Sterling and Disinfecting agents.

Scytek Laboratories, Inc. 435-755-9848
205 S 600 W, Logan, UT 84321
Formalin, neutral buffered.

Spectra-Tint 585-546-8050
250 Cumberland St Ste 228, Rochester, NY 14605
Forma-fix i.

Statlab Medical Products, Inc. 800-442-3573
106 Hillside Dr, Lewisville, TX 75057
ANAPATH 10% Neutral and Carson-Milldnig's formalin, and pre-buffered formalin concentrate, plus pre-filled vials available, also 20%.

Surgipath Medical Industries, Inc. 800-225-3035
PO Box 528, 5205 Route 12, Richmond, IL 60071

U S Biotex Corp. 606-652-4700
RR 1 Box 62, Webbville, KY 41180
Formalin, neutral buffered.

Wessels And Associates 248-547-7177
131 Cambridge Blvd, Pleasant Ridge, MI 48069
Formalin.

FORMALIN-SALINE *(Pathology) 88IGC*

Pochemco, Inc. 413-536-2900
724 Main St, Holyoke, MA 01040
Formalin saline.

FORMALIN-SALINE *(cont'd)*

Rocky Mountain Reagents,Inc. 303-762-0800
3207 W Hampden Ave, Englewood, CO 80110

FORMS, MEDICAL AND PATIENT *(General) 80QXP*

Hessler Forms & Labels 800-346-1304
106 Susan Dr Ste 1, Elkins Park, PA 19027
Custom forms made: CMNs & HCFAs.

Lionville Systems, Inc. 800-523-7114
501 Gunnard Carlson Dr, Coatesville, PA 19320
Medication records, patient profiles, doctor's order forms; plastic flip-top and paperboard med boxes; and record files.

Medirex Systems Ltd. 800-387-9848
P.O. Box 40 Station F, Toronto, ONT M4Y 2L4 Canada
Medical forms and patient menus.

Newbold Corporation 800-552-3282
450 Weaver St, Rocky Mount, VA 24151
PatientWorks, An E-forms software solution. Addressograph Healthcare introduces its newest product for patient forms automation.

St. John Companies 800-435-4242
25167 Anza Dr, PO Box 800460, Santa Clarita, CA 91355
HCFA-1500 available in continuous, later-printable and faxable formats, for UB-92 (HCFA-1450); meets all of HCFA's latest printing standards for Medicare and Medical claims.

FORNIXSCOPE *(Ophthalmology) 86HKG*

Ocular Innovations, Inc. 813-645-2355
1121 Lewis Ave, Sarasota, FL 34237
Eye lid retractor.

FOUNTAIN, EYE WASH *(Chemistry) 75TCG*

Afassco, Inc. 800-441-6774
2244 Park Pl Ste C, Minden, NV 89423
Emergency Eye Wash Station.

Concepts International, Inc. 800-627-9729
224 E Main St, Summerton, SC 29148
Emergency eye-wash station.

Haws Corporation 775-359-4712
1455 Kleppe Ln, Sparks, NV 89431

Hemco Corp. 816-796-2900
111 S Powell Rd, Independence, MO 64056

Lab Safety Supply, Inc. 800-356-0783
401 S Wright Rd, Janesville, WI 53546

Medical Safety Systems Inc. 888-803-9303
230 White Pond Dr, Akron, OH 44313
Eye wash station.

Nevin Laboratories, Inc 800-544-5337
5000 S Halsted St, Chicago, IL 60609
Emergency eyewash station. Faucet mounted on existing sink or deck mounted.

Niagara Pharmaceuticals Div. 905-690-6277
60 Innovation Dr., Flamborough, ONT L9H-7P3 Canada
HEALTH SAVER self-contained eye wash station additive and conditioner for portable units. Used as a bactericide, algicide and fungicide.

Nutech Molding Corporation 1-800-423-5278
PO Box 840, 2024 Broad St,, Pocomoke City, MD 21851

Rockford Medical & Safety Co. 800-435-9451
2420 Harrison Ave, PO Box 5646, Rockford, IL 61108
Emergency eye shower.

Vector Firstaid, Inc. 800-999-4423
316 N Corona Ave, Ontario, CA 91764
1/2 oz. 32 oz bottles of all sizes. Sterile clear bottles of all sizes.

FRAME, RUBBER DAM *(Dental And Oral) 76EJE*

Coltene/Whaledent Inc. 330-916-8858
235 Ascot Pkwy, Cuyahoga Falls, OH 44223
Rubber dam frame.

Dentalez Group 866-DTE-INFO
101 Lindenwood Dr Ste 225, Valleybrooke Corporate Center
Malvern, PA 19355

Dentalez Group, Stardental Division 717-291-1161
1816 Colonial Village Ln, Lancaster, PA 17601
Unit, operative dental.

Hager Worldwide, Inc. 800-328-2335
13322 Byrd Dr, Odessa, FL 33556
FIT, PLAST FRAME.

FRAME, RUBBER DAM *(cont'd)*

Manufacturera Dental Continental 523-633-8329
2113 Calle Indust Del Plastico, 269 Fracc Zapopan Indust Norte
Zapopan, Jalisco Mexico
Rubber dam frame

Miltex Dental Technologies, Inc. 516-576-6022
589 Davies Dr, York, PA 17402
Rubber dam frame.

Moyco Technologies, Inc. 800-331-8837
200 Commerce Dr, Montgomeryville, PA 18936

Pac-Dent Intl., Inc. 909-839-0888
21078 Commerce Point Dr, Walnut, CA 91789
Various sizes and types of rubber dam holders.

Pulpdent Corp. 800-343-4342
80 Oakland St, Watertown, MA 02472
Rubber dam frame.

Young Innovations, Inc. 800-325-1881
13705 Shoreline Ct E, Earth City, MO 63045

FRAME, SPECTACLE (EYEGLASSES) *(Ophthalmology) 86HQZ*

Alpha Optics, Llc. 212-431-9190
5408 46th St, Maspeth, NY 11378
Various.

Ao Eyewear, Inc. 508-764-3214
529 Ashland Ave Ste 3, P.o. Box 1064, Southbridge, MA 01550
Sunglass frames.

Artcraft New York 800-828-8288
57 Goodway Dr S, Rochester, NY 14623
Prescription-Quality Safety and Dress Frames

Atlantic Optical Co., Inc. 800-423-5175
20801 Nordhoff St, Chatsworth, CA 91311

Avada Eyewear Inc. 800-844-2034
5605 Florida Mining Blvd S Bldg 200, Suite 210, Jacksonville, FL 32257
AVADA EYEWEAR INC. LINES ARE AS FOLLOWS: KAMANARI, OLIMPIC, RARE FORM, PURE & SIMPLE, INVISION

Barrier Eyewear 561-317-5324
840 13th St Ste 31, Lake Park, FL 33403
Frame for eyeglass.

Centennial Optical Ltd. 416-739-8539
158 Norfinch Dr., Downsview, ONTAR M3N 1X6 Canada
Various.

Co/Op Optical Vision Designs 866-733-2667
2424 E 8 Mile Rd, E. of Dequindre, Detroit, MI 48234

Colors In Optics Ltd. 866-465-2656
366 5th Ave Rm 1003, New York, NY 10001

Criss Optical Manufacturing Co., Inc. 800-835-2023
3628 S West St, Wichita, KS 67217

Dispensers Optical Service Corp. 800-626-4545
1815 Plantside Dr, Louisville, KY 40299
Ballistic and laser protective eyewear.

Diversified Ophthalmics, Inc. 800-626-2281
250 McCullough St, Cincinnati, OH 45226

Embassy Creations, Inc. 800-367-3341
122 Manton Ave # L4, Providence, RI 02909
Eyeglass cases.

Euro-Frames, Inc. 800-422-2773
2985 Glendale Blvd, Los Angeles, CA 90039
CLUB L.A.

European Eyewear Corp. 941-322-6771
630 Myakka Rd, Sarasota, FL 34240
Various.

Fine & Particular Ey 914-834-4358
2001 Palmer Ave Ste 103, Larchmont, NY 10538

Focal Point Opticians 510-923-0568
2638 Ashby Ave, Berkeley, CA 94705
A clipon that can hold a prescription lens.

I Connection 914-834-4358
2001 Palmer Ave Ste 103, Larchmont, NY 10538

Incite International, Inc. 816-220-7533
2749 NW Hunter Dr, Blue Springs, MO 64015

Kentek Corporation 603-435-7201
1 Elm St, Pittsfield, NH 03263
Eyewear frames without lenses.

L'Amy, Inc. 800-USA-LAMY
37 Danbury Rd, Wilton, CT 06897

FRAME, SPECTACLE (EYEGLASSES) *(cont'd)*

Lehrer Brillenperfektion Werks, Inc. 818-407-1890
3908 N 5th St, North Las Vegas, NV 89032
Frame, spectacle.

Lenscrafters, Inc. 770-305-7352
9926 International Blvd, Cincinnati, OH 45246
Spectacle frames.

Marcolin Usa 888-627-2654
7543 E Tierra Buena Ln, Scottsdale, AZ 85260

Minima Timon Lunetterie, Inc. 888-661-0404
614 Av. Champagneur, Outremont H2V 3P6 Canada
Minima

Ockiobel, Inc. 305-261-6144
777 NW 72nd Ave Ste 2K20, Miami, FL 33126
Eyeglasses.

Optical Shop Of Aspen 800-647-2345
25 Brookline, Aliso Viejo, CA 92656
Including Matsuda, Hiero, Chrome Hearts, and Kieselstein-Cord jewelry style eyewear. Sterling silver and electro plated gold accents available from the Kieselstein-Cord line. HIERO, high end ophthalmic and sunglass frames. Metal, plastic and titanium frames are available. Clayton-Franklin, retro styled eyewear. Old and new design collide to produce a contemporary masterpiece. Metal and plastic frames are available. Each frame comes in clear or sunglass; sunglass frames come with polarized lenses. CHROME HEARTS: Designer frame incorporating chrome accents into frame design.

Optical Suppliers, Inc. 808-486-2933
99-1253 Halawa Valley St, Aiea, HI 96701
Eyeglasses.

Paris Miki, Inc. 425-883-2464
2863 152nd Ave NE, Redmond, WA 98052

Parmelee Industries, Inc. 800-821-5218
8101 Lenexa Dr, Lenexa, KS 66214
Complete prescription eyewear for safety, computer user as well as streetwear eyewear.

Philadelphia Vision Center 215-568-0700
1100 Market St, Philadelphia, PA 19107
Spectacle frames.

Randolph Engineering, Inc. 781-961-6070
26 Thomas Patten Dr, Randolph, MA 02368
Spectacle frames.

Revolution Eyewear, Inc. 310-777-8399
997 Flower Glen St, Simi Valley, CA 93065
Eyeglass frame.

Rochester Optical Mfg. Company 585-254-0022
1260 Lyell Ave, Rochester, NY 14606
Spectacle frame.

Solo Bambini 650-340-1773
729 Occidental Ave, San Mateo, CA 94402
Spectacle frames.

Spectrum Optical 323-931-4349
6154 W 6th St, Los Angeles, CA 90048
Frames.

Sperian Eye & Face Protection Inc. 401-232-1200
10 Thurber Blvd, Smithfield, RI 02917
Spectacle frames.

Styloptic Intl., S.A. De C.V. 301-242-2330
274 Playa Villa Del Mar, Mexico City Mexico
Frame

Surgin Surgical Instrumentation, Inc. (Surgin Inc.) 714-832-6300
37 Shield, Irvine, CA 92618
Accessories to phacoemulsification systems.

The Optical Shop 405-514-0903
1111 S Eastern Ave, Oklahoma City, OK 73129
Metal optical frame.

U.S. Vision Optical, Inc. 856-228-1000
5 Harmon Dr, Blackwood, NJ 08012
Optical frames.

United Syntek Corp. 888-665-2326
3557 Denver Dr, Denver, NC 28037
Eyewear.

Zyloware Corporation 800-765-3700
1136 46th Rd, Long Island City, NY 11101
Contract manufacturer of frames.

FRAME, TRACTION *(Orthopedics) 87QXQ*

Florida Manufacturing Corp. 800-447-2372
501 Beville Rd, South Daytona, FL 32119

Freeman Manufacturing Company 800-253-2091
900 W Chicago Rd, PO Box J, Sturgis, MI 49091

Inland Specialties, Inc. 800-741-0022
7655 Matoaka Rd, Sarasota, FL 34243
Traction overdoor.

Invacare Corporation 800-333-6900
1 Invacare Way, Elyria, OH 44035
INVACARE.

Lossing Orthopedic 800-328-5216
PO Box 6224, Minneapolis, MN 55406
Lumbar frame; cervical frame.

Mizuho Osi 800-777-4674
30031 Ahern Ave, Union City, CA 94587
FULL LINE, MULTIPLE FRAME TYPES

Zimmer Holdings, Inc. 800-613-6131
1800 W Center St, PO Box 708, Warsaw, IN 46580

Zimmer Orthopaedic Surgical Products 800-321-5533
PO Box 10, 200 West Ohio Ave., Dover, OH 44622
ZIMCODE.

FRAME, TRIAL, OPHTHALMIC *(Ophthalmology) 86HPA*

Avi-Advanced Visual Instruments Inc. 212-262-7878
321 W 44th St Ste 902, New York, NY 10036
Ophthalmic trial lens frame, universal lens holder.

Eye Care And Cure 800-486-6169
4646 S Overland Dr, Tucson, AZ 85714
Trial frame.

Gulden Ophthalmics 800-659-2250
225 Cadwalader Ave, Elkins Park, PA 19027

Reichert, Inc. 888-849-8955
3362 Walden Ave, Depew, NY 14043
Used with trial lens set to aid in refractive error diagnosis.

Topcon Medical Systems, Inc. 800-223-1130
37 W Century Rd, Paramus, NJ 07652
$200.00

Western Ophthalmics Corporation 800-426-9938
19019 36th Ave W Ste G, Lynnwood, WA 98036

Woodlyn, Inc. 800-331-7389
2920 Malmo Dr, Ophthalmic Instruments and Equipment
Arlington Heights, IL 60005
Model 26000. The Woodlyn Lightweight Trial Frame has a wide range of adjustments including 48 to 80 mm P.D. adjustment, variable horizontal, and vertical bridge movements, and a free rocking saddle bridge for comfortable nose fit. Call for current prices.

FRAME, TURNING *(Orthopedics) 87QXR*

Stryker Medical 800-869-0770
3800 E Centre Ave, Portage, MI 49002

FREEZE DRYING EQUIPMENT *(Chemistry) 75UGF*

Appropriate Technical Resources, Inc. 800-827-5931
9157 Whiskey Bottom Rd, PO Box 460, Laurel, MD 20723
Heto's FD 2.5 bench top freeze dryer. Large 12 liter condenser at -55 degrees C, high cooling capacity, and multi-purpose performance.

Fts Systems 800-824-0400
PO Box 158, 3538 Main Street,, Stone Ridge, NY 12484

Labconco Corp. 800-821-5525
8811 Prospect Ave, Kansas City, MO 64132
FREEZONE Freeze Dry Systems in capacities from 1 liter to 18 liter, including the NEW The FreeZone Triad offers it all for lypholization....stopping tray dryer and sample freeze drying with four sample valves on the left side. Samples for both types of freeze drying can be run at once.

Virtis, An Sp Industries Company 800-431-8232
815 Route 208, Gardiner, NY 12525
2- to 35-liter ice condenser capacity. Freezemobile research freeze dryers. 'K' Series BenchTop freeze dryers. AdVantage freeze dryer.

Ward's Natural Science Establishment, Inc. 800-962-2660
PO Box 92912, 5100 W. Henrietta Rd., Rochester, NY 14692

FREEZER, BLOOD CELL *(Hematology) 81KSP*

Thermo Fisher Scientific (Asheville) Llc 740-373-4763
Millcreek Rd., Marietta, OH 45750
Various models of blast freezers.

FREEZER, BLOOD STORAGE *(Hematology) 81KSE*

Action Africa - Artique Refrigeration 520-762-9293
16335 S Houghton Rd # 115, Corona De Tucson, AZ 85641
Blood storage refrigerator.

Bally Refrigerated Boxes, Inc. 800-24-BALLY
135 Little Nine Rd, Morehead City, NC 28557

Barnstead International 412-490-8425
2555 Kerper Blvd, Dubuque, IA 52001
Various blood storage refrigerator thermometers.

Case In Point 801-647-5437
3917 Viewcrest Dr, Salt Lake City, UT 84124
Portable temperature control case for pharmaceuticals.

Environmental Growth Chambers 800-321-6854
510 Washington St, Chagrin Falls, OH 44022
Negative 20C storage or working cold lab rooms

Harris Environmental Systems, Inc. 888-771-4200
11 Connector Rd, Andover, MA 01810

Helmer, Inc. 800-743-5637
15425 Herriman Blvd, Noblesville, IN 46060
Plasma Freezers

Kendro Laboratory Products 800-252-7100
308 Ridgefield Ct, Asheville, NC 28806
$4,000 to $13,000 ea.

Mgr Equipment Corp. 516-239-3030
22 Gates Ave, Inwood, NY 11096
Blood bank, refrigerator, mechanical, biological.

Nor-Lake Inc., Nor-Lake Scientific 715-386-2323
Second & Elm St., Hudson, WI 54016
Refigerator, freezer, blood storage.

Rtf Mfg. Co. Llc. 800-836-0744
793 Route 66, Hudson, NY 12534
Rtf mfg.

So-Low Environmental Equipment 513-772-9410
10310 Spartan Dr, Cincinnati, OH 45215

Thermo Fisher Scientific (Asheville) Llc 740-373-4763
Millcreek Rd., Marietta, OH 45750
Various models of blood storage refrigerators.

Thermo Fisher Scientific (Asheville) Llc 828-658-4400
275 Aiken Rd, Asheville, NC 28804

Thermogenesis Corp. 800-783-8357
2711 Citrus Rd, Rancho Cordova, CA 95742
THERMOGENESIS, Ultrarapid freezer. Available in 2 sizes

FREEZER, BONE *(Orthopedics) 87TCH*

Kendro Laboratory Products 800-252-7100
308 Ridgefield Ct, Asheville, NC 28806

FREEZER, LABORATORY, BIOLOGICAL *(Chemistry) 75UKL*

Environmental Growth Chambers 800-321-6854
510 Washington St, Chagrin Falls, OH 44022
Negatvie 20C storage or working cold lab rooms

Helmer, Inc. 800-743-5637
15425 Herriman Blvd, Noblesville, IN 46060
Laboratory Freezers

Kendro Laboratory Products 800-252-7100
308 Ridgefield Ct, Asheville, NC 28806
$4,000 to $13,000 ea.

New Brunswick Scientific Co., Inc. 800-631-5417
PO Box 4005, Edison, NJ 08818
Line of nine upright and chest ultra-low temperature (-85oC) freezers, available with inventory racking, autodiallers, CO2 and LN2 controller back-up, data logging software, chart recorders and more. Space-saving VIP freezers utilize vacuum insulation panel technology to provide up to 30% more storage capacity than freezers of equal size. Personal-sized model also available for use on or under the bench, providing the ultimate in convenience and sample security.

So-Low Environmental Equipment 513-772-9410
10310 Spartan Dr, Cincinnati, OH 45215

FREEZER, LABORATORY, GENERAL PURPOSE *(Chemistry) 75JRM*

Bally Refrigerated Boxes, Inc. 800-24-BALLY
135 Little Nine Rd, Morehead City, NC 28557

Barnstead International 412-490-8425
2555 Kerper Blvd, Dubuque, IA 52001
Various freezers.

FREEZER, LABORATORY, GENERAL PURPOSE *(cont'd)*

Environmental Growth Chambers 800-321-6854
510 Washington St, Chagrin Falls, OH 44022
Negative 20C storage or cold working lab rooms

Kendro Laboratory Products 800-252-7100
308 Ridgefield Ct, Asheville, NC 28806

Marvel Scientific 800-962-2521
233 Industrial Pkwy, PO Box 997, Richmond, IN 47374
15AF tabletop freezer. 1.5-cu-ft, -20 degrees, may be built-in or free standing, requires zero clearance from top sides. 4.5 cu ft to 29 cu ft. Commercial and utility freezers are also available, including hazard-location and flammable-material models.

Mfg One, Llc 703-437-9838
3900 Skyhawk Dr, Chantilly, VA 20151
Surgical slush machine.

Nor-Lake Inc., Nor-Lake Scientific 715-386-2323
Second & Elm St., Hudson, WI 54016
Multiple.

So-Low Environmental Equipment 513-772-9410
10310 Spartan Dr, Cincinnati, OH 45215

Standard Instrumentation, Div. Preiser Scientific 800-624-8285
94 Oliver St, Saint Albans, WV 25177

Virtis, An Sp Industries Company 800-431-8232
815 Route 208, Gardiner, NY 12525
35-cu-ft. unit. Genesis, Ultra, VirTual and Benchmark pilot and production lyophilizers.

Whitehall Manufacturing 800-782-7706
15125 Proctor Ave, City Of Industry, CA 91746
Single or 12-pack, re-usable Glazier-Packs are gelfilled, utilized with cold therapy treatment.

FREEZER, LABORATORY, ULTRA-LOW TEMPERATURE
(Chemistry) 75UKM

Kendro Laboratory Products 800-252-7100
308 Ridgefield Ct, Asheville, NC 28806
$4,000 to $13,000 ea.

New Brunswick Scientific Co., Inc. 800-631-5417
PO Box 4005, Edison, NJ 08818
Line of nine upright and chest models for storing samples at -85oC. Available with inventory racking, autodiallers, CO2 and LN2 controller back-up, data logging software, chart recorders and more. Space-saving VIP models utilize vacuum insulation panel technology to provide up to 30% more storage capacity than freezers of equal size. Personal-sized model also available for use on or under the bench, providing the ultimate in convenience and sample security.

Nuaire, Inc. 800-328-3352
2100 Fernbrook Ln N, Plymouth, MN 55447

So-Low Environmental Equipment 513-772-9410
10310 Spartan Dr, Cincinnati, OH 45215

FUCHSIN, BASIC *(Pathology) 88KKW*

American Mastertech Scientific, Inc. 209-368-4031
1330 Thurman St, Lodi, CA 95240
Multiple.

Richard-Allan Scientific 269-544-5628
4481 Campus Dr, Kalamazoo, MI 49008
Basic fuchsin.

FULL FIELD DIGITAL, SYSTEM, X-RAY, MAMMOGRAPHIC
(Radiology) 90MUE

Lorad, A Hologic Company 800-321-4659
36 Apple Ridge Rd, Danbury, CT 06810
Full field digital system x-ray mammographic.

FURNACE, PORCELAIN *(Dental And Oral) 76VEJ*

Preiser Scientific, Inc. 800-624-8285
94 Oliver St, P.O. Box 1330, Saint Albans, WV 25177
Furnaces

Thermo Fisher Scientific Inc. 563-556-2241
2555 Kerper Blvd, Dubuque, IA 52001

Vident 800-828-3839
3150 E Birch St, Brea, CA 92821
VITA Vacumat 40T and 4000T furnaces. AGF Automatic glazing furnace for staining and glazing. VITA Inceramat 3 furnace.

Whip-Mix Corporation 800-626-5651
361 Farmington Ave, PO Box 17183, Louisville, KY 40209

FURNITURE, GENERAL *(General) 80VBP*

Adden Furniture, Inc. 800-625-3876
26 Jackson St, Lowell, MA 01852
Furniture for lounges, acute and psychiatric care facilities and offices.

Allsteel Inc. 800-624-9212
2210 2nd Ave, Muscatine, IA 52761
Contemporary and traditional steel and wood desks and chairs; lateral and vertical steel and wood files; systems furniture.

American Seating 616-732-6600
401 American Seating Ctr NW, Grand Rapids, MI 49504
Framework lab furniture system integrates the benefits of both traditional fixed and modular benchwork.

Atd-American Co. 800-523-2300
135 Greenwood Ave, Wyncote, PA 19095
Office, lobby and conference room furniture. Cafeteria, library and training room furniture.

Bevco Ergonomic Seating 800-864-2991
2246 W Bluemound Rd Ste A, Waukesha, WI 53186
Laboratory and office chairs and stools, hat and coat racks, hangers (chairs from $66.00, quantity discounts available). Class 10 cleanroom and ESD/cleanroom seating. BEVCO 7000 CR series is 16 models for cleanroom and ESD/cleanroom applications-class 10 certified. BEVCO 5000CR/ECR series, class 10 cleanroom, ESD cleanroom seating. 16 models for static and contamination control.

Bibbero Systems, Inc. 800-242-2376
1300 N McDowell Blvd, Petaluma, CA 94954
Wood Mallet Office Furniture, Tennsco high density filing cabinet systems.

Brandrud Furniture, Inc. 253-838-6500
1502 20th St NW, Auburn, WA 98001
All office seating: wood frame upholstered products, conference and occasional tables.

Buckstaff Co. 800-755-5890
1127 S Main St, Oshkosh, WI 54902
Convalescent chairs, lounges, cafeteria and library furniture. Bariatrics seating

Budget Buddy Company, Inc. 800-208-3375
PO Box 590, Belton, MO 64012
Charting desk and folding wall desk $129.95-269.95 each.

Century Woodworking Corp. 330-753-2024
846 Coventry Rd, Barberton, OH 44203
Medical wall desk, nurse supply station, radiology wardrobe cabinet; call for brochures.

Enochs Examining Room Furniture, Inc. 800-428-2305
PO Box 50559, Indianapolis, IN 46250
Examining room furniture.

ERG International 800-446-1186
361 Bernoulli Cir, Oxnard, CA 93030
Seating and tables for every department of the medical facility including lobbies, waiting areas, patient rooms, admitting/administration, lecture hall, dining/cafeteria, etc.

Fleetwood Group, Incorporated 800-257-6390
PO Box 1259, Holland, MI 49422
$470 for book or magazine display cabinets, $240 for book cases (48x42x18). Also, wireless response system.

Genie Scientific, Inc. 800-545-8816
17430 Mount Cliffwood Cir, Fountain Valley, CA 92708
New and reconditioned laboratory furniture.

Grosfillex, Inc. 800-233-3186
230 Old West Penn Ave, Robesonia, PA 19551
Indoor/outdoor furniture.

Hale Manufacturing Co., F.E. 800-USE-HALE
120 Benson Pl, PO Box 186, Frankfort, NY 13340
Bookcases (wooden).

Hausmann Industries, Inc. 888-428-7626
130 Union St, Northvale, NJ 07647
Examining room furniture.

Haworth, Inc. 800-426-8562
1 Haworth Ctr, Holland, MI 49423

Health Care Furnishings, Inc. 800-648-5744
63 Pebble Beach Dr, Little Rock, AR 72212
Furniture, interior design.

Henry Schein, Inc. 631-843-5500
135 Duryea Rd, Melville, NY 11747
Dental operatory equipment. Schein Crusader.

FURNITURE, GENERAL *(cont'd)*

International Hospital Supply Co. 800-398-9450
6914 Canby Ave Ste 105, Reseda, CA 91335
Disposable, x-ray film, vacutainers.

L.P.A. Medical, Inc. 888-845-6447
460 Desrochers, Ste. 150D, Vanier, QUEBE G1M 1C2 Canada
Thera-Glide safety glider.

Lista International Corp. 800-722-3020
106 Lowland St, Holliston, MA 01746
Tool and parts storage cabinets, modular drawer storage cabinets, mobile drawer/shelf/cabinet work centers, overhead cabinets, workbenches, Storage Wall(R) systems (combination of drawers, shelves and roll-out trays).

Midmark Corporation 800-643-6275
60 Vista Dr, P.O. Box 286, Versailles, OH 45380
Examining room furniture.

Nevin Laboratories, Inc 800-544-5337
5000 S Halsted St, Chicago, IL 60609
Examining room furniture.

Newschoff Chairs, Inc. 800-203-8916
909 N.E. St., Sheboygan, WI 53081

Ortoprocess Mr. 57688118
Av. Del Taller #351 Col. Alvaro Obregon, Mexico D.F. 15990 Mexico
Includes wheel chairs and walking auxilary.

Penco Products Inc. 800-562-1000
PO Box 378, 99 Brower Ave., Oaks, PA 19456
Personnel lockers.

Rockaway Chairs 800-256-6601
111 Alexander Rd Apt 11, West Monroe, LA 71291
Padded sleeper benches, sofas, loveseats, chairs. Also, observation systems, and folding doors, accordian doors, and movable walls. Also, Alzheimer's facility furniture - hopsital room sleeper bench with seamless seats, solid oak frame, available in any stain in 60' or 72' lengths.

Shelby-Williams Industries 800-873-3252
5303 E Morris Blvd, Morristown, TN 37813
Function room furniture.

Shure Manufacturing Corp. 800-227-4873
1901 W Main St, Washington, MO 63090
Laboratory and pharmacy furniture.

Space Tables, Inc. 800-328-2580
11511 95th Ave N, Maple Grove, MN 55369
Adjustable tables for nursing homes.

Stackbin Corporation 800-333-1603
29 Powder Hill Rd, Lincoln, RI 02865
Workbenches, workstations, desks and adjustable workstation stool.

Techno-Aide, Inc. 800-251-2629
7117 Centennial Blvd, Nashville, TN 37209
Ergonomic Furniture: ht. adj.

Thermo Scientific Hamilton 920-794-6800
1316 18th St, Two Rivers, WI 54241

Thompson Contract Inc. 631-589-7337
41 Keyland Ct, Bohemia, NY 11716

Tri-State Surgical Supply & Equipment 800-424-5227
409 Hoyt St, Brooklyn, NY 11231
Medical supplies, furniture, equipment. Wheelchairs, beds, recliners, walkers, mattresses, syringes, solutions, bandages, etc.

Unilab, Inc. 9058559093
2355 Royal Windsor Dr., Unit 3, Mississauga, ON L5M-5R5 Canada
Modular, mobile, and free standing laboratory furniture. Also available are plastic laminate, epoxy resin and stainless steel counter tops.

United Metal Fabricators, Inc. 800-638-5322
1316 Eisenhower Blvd, Johnstown, PA 15904
Examining room furniture.

FURNITURE, PATIENT ROOM *(General) 80TCJ*

Adden Furniture, Inc. 800-625-3876
26 Jackson St, Lowell, MA 01852

American Of Martinsville 276-632-2061
128 E Church St, Martinsville, VA 24112

Atd-American Co. 800-523-2300
135 Greenwood Ave, Wyncote, PA 19095

Basic American Medical Products 800-849-6664
2935A Northeast Pkwy, Atlanta, GA 30360

Basic American Metal Products 800-365-2338
336 Trowbridge Dr, PO Box 907, Fond Du Lac, WI 54937

FURNITURE, PATIENT ROOM *(cont'd)*

Buckstaff Co. 800-755-5890
1127 S Main St, Oshkosh, WI 54902

Budget Buddy Company, Inc. 800-208-3375
PO Box 590, Belton, MO 64012
Charting products and folding wall desk $129.95-265.95 each.

Calmaquip Engineering Corp. 305-592-4510
7240 NW 12th St, Miami, FL 33126

Clinimed, Incorporated 877-CLINIMED
303 Markus Ct, Sandy Brae Industrial Park, Newark, DE 19713

Colonial Scientific Ltd. 902-468-1811
201 Brownlow Ave., Unit 52, Dartmouth, NS B3B-1W2 Canada
Visitor chairs, overbed telephones, overbed tables.

Country Craft Furniture, Inc. 800-569-1968
5318 Railroad Ave, Flowery Branch, GA 30542

Custom Comfort Medtek 800-749-0933
3939 Forsyth Rd Ste A, Winter Park, FL 32792
A wide selection of patient and lab furniture includes blood-drawing chairs, dialysis chairs, exam tables, cabinets, supply carts, foot stools, IV poles, privacy screens, exam lights, transport chairs, mayo stands, supply organizers, medical stools, mobile workstations, infant phlebotomy stations, wheel-chair phlebotomy arms, and bariatric chairs.

Durfold Corporation 800-345-6349
102 Upton Dr, Jackson, MS 39209
Sleepchairs and sofas.

Hard Manufacturing Co. 800-873-4273
230 Grider St, Buffalo, NY 14215
Chairs, casegoods, overbed tables, cabinets, beds.

Hausmann Industries, Inc. 888-428-7626
130 Union St, Northvale, NJ 07647

Hill-Rom Holdings, Inc. 800-445-3730
1069 State Road 46 E, Batesville, IN 47006

Hospital Systems, Inc. 925-427-7800
750 Garcia Ave, Pittsburg, CA 94565

Kewaunee Scientific Corp. 704-873-7202
2700 W Front St, PO Box 1842, Statesville, NC 28677
Laboratory furniture--casework (wood and steel), fume hoods.

L.P.A. Medical, Inc. 888-845-6447
460 Desrochers, Ste. 150D, Vanier, QUEBE G1M 1C2 Canada
Thera-Glide safety glider.

M.C. Healthcare Products, Inc. 800-268-8671
4658 Ontario St., Beamsville, ONT L0R 1B4 Canada
Dressers for patient rooms with 3 or 4 drawers. Laminate and veneers prestige series.

Mayo Medical, S.A. De C.V. 800-715-3872
Edison 1141 Nte., Col. Talleres, Monterrey N.L. 64480 Mexico

Newschoff Chairs, Inc. 800-203-8916
909 N.E. St., Sheboygan, WI 53081
Patient room and lobby furniture.

Nk Medical Products Inc. 800-274-2742
10123 Main St, PO Box 627, Clarence, NY 14031
Bedside Cabinets, Bed-in-a-Box, Beds, Overbed Tables

Pedicraft, Inc. 800-223-7649
4134 Saint Augustine Rd, Jacksonville, FL 32207
Fold-away beds for visitors, cribs and other furniture.

Radix Corp. 204-697-2349
#2-572 South Fifth St., Pembina, ND 58271
Patient room, lounge/waiting room, armoires, headboards, footboards, and child-size furniture; available in a variety of hardwood and plastic laminates.

Rockaway Chairs 800-256-6601
111 Alexander Rd Apt 11, West Monroe, LA 71291
All wood bedside cabinets-beds, overbed tables.

S&W By Hausmann 888-428-7626
130 Union St, Northvale, NJ 07647

Shelby-Williams Industries 800-873-3252
5303 E Morris Blvd, Morristown, TN 37813
Wall coverings.

Stryker Medical 800-869-0770
3800 E Centre Ave, Portage, MI 49002

Sunrise Medical 800-333-4000
7477 Dry Creek Pkwy, Longmont, CO 80503

Total Care 800-334-3802
PO Box 1661, Rockville, MD 20849

GAG, MOUTH *(Ear/Nose/Throat) 77KBN*

Aesculap Implant Systems Inc. 1-800-234-9179
3773 Corporate Pkwy, Center Valley, PA 18034

Bausch & Lomb Surgical 636-255-5051
3365 Tree Court Ind Blvd, Saint Louis, MO 63122

Biomet Microfixation Inc. 800-874-7711
1520 Tradeport Dr, Jacksonville, FL 32218
Gag, mouth.

Clinimed, Incorporated 877-CLINIMED
303 Markus Ct, Sandy Brae Industrial Park, Newark, DE 19713

Codman & Shurtleff, Inc 800-225-0460
325 Paramount Dr, Raynham, MA 02767

E.A. Beck & Co. 949-645-4072
657 W 19th St Ste E, P O Box 10857, Costa Mesa, CA 92627
Mouth gag.

Electro Surgical Instrument Co., Inc. 888-464-2784
37 Centennial St, Rochester, NY 14611
Various types styles and sizes of mouth gags with fiberoptic light.

Exmoor Plastics Inc. 317-244-1014
304 Gasoline Aly, Indianapolis, IN 46222
Dental protection from the mouth gag or laryngoscope, priced from $6.30 each.

Hu-Friedy Manufacturing Co., Inc. 800-483-7433
3232 N Rockwell St, Chicago, IL 60618
$11.00 to $198.75, 9 types.

Kmedic 800-955-0559
190 Veterans Dr, Northvale, NJ 07647

Miltex Inc. 800-645-8000
589 Davies Dr, York, PA 17402

Toolmex Corporation 800-992-4766
1075 Worcester St, Natick, MA 01760

Trans American Medical / Tamsco Instruments 708-430-7777
7633 W 100th Pl, Bridgeview, IL 60455

GARMENT, PROTECTIVE, FOR INCONTINENCE
(Gastro/Urology) 78EYQ

Ac Healthcare Supply, Inc. 905-448-4706
11651 230th St, Cambria Heights, NY 11411
Protective garment for incontinence.

American Disposables, Inc. 413-967-6201
6 E Main St, Ware, MA 01082
Adult disposable diaper.

Arc Home Health Products 800-278-8595
PO Box 615, Oneonta, NY 13820

Arcus Medical Llc 704-332-3424
2327 Distribution St, Charlotte, NC 28203
Brief and pad for incontinence.

Articulos Higienicos S.A. De C.V. 52-55-58997980
Av. Asoc. Nacional De Industriales 10, Parque Ind. Cuamatla Cuautitlan Izcalli, EDO. 54730 Mexico
Protective disposable adult diapers for incontinence.

Atd-American Co. 800-523-2300
135 Greenwood Ave, Wyncote, PA 19095

Attends Healthcare Products 252-752-1100
2321 Arrow Highway, La Verne, CA 91750
Various incontinent garments.

Attends Healthcare Products 252-752-1100
1029 Old Creek Rd, Greenville, NC 27834

Biomed Resource, Inc. 310-323-3888
3388 Rosewood Ave, Los Angeles, CA 90066
Adult brief,disposable.

Care Apparel Industries 800-326-6262
12709 91st Ave, Richmond Hill, NY 11418
Complete line of clothing for individuals requiring adaptive and incontinent wear.

Central Paper Products Company 800-339-4065
PO Box 4480, Manchester, NH 03108
Procter & Gamble ATTENDS.

Douglas & Harper Mfg. Co., Inc. 912-367-4149
1126 S Main St, Baxley, GA 31513
Incontinent pants and liner.

Duraline Medical Products, Inc. 800-654-3376
324 Werner St, P.O. Box 67, Leipsic, OH 45856

GARMENT, PROTECTIVE, FOR INCONTINENCE *(cont'd)*

Freestyle Medical Supplies, Inc. 800-841-5330
336 Green Rd, Stoney Creek, ON L8E 2B2 Canada
FREESTYLE Maxi Briefs - all-in-one garment for moderate to heavy incontinence or total loss of bladder/bowel control. Available in six sizes: XS-Junior to X-Large. FREESTYLE Mini Briefs - all-in-one garment for light to moderate incontinence or loss of bladder control. Available in two styles, men's and women's; and in three sizes, small, medium, and large. All washable up to 350 times. FREESTYLE Swim Diaper for protection in pools, ideal for nydro therapy-incontinent product.

G. Hirsch And Co., Inc. 650-692-8770
870 Mahler Rd, Burlingame, CA 94010
Various sizes of adult and child disposable briefs and undergarments.

Genuine Care Rehab. Svc., Inc. 405-604-5907
2401 NW 23rd St Ste 17, Oklahoma City, OK 73107
Prosthetic sportswear garment.

Geri-Care Products 201-440-0409
250 Moonachie Ave, Moonachie, NJ 07074
Reusable Adult Incontinence Briefs & Diapers

Gomez Packaging Corp. 973-569-9500
75 Wood St, Paterson, NJ 07524
Diapers.

Gyrx, Llc 904-641-2599
10302 Deerwood Park Blvd Ste 209, Jacksonville, FL 32256
Incontinence garments.

Humanicare International, Inc. 800-631-5270
9 Elkins Rd, East Brunswick, NJ 08816
Reusable DIGNITY w/waterproof pocket $10.95 unisex, (genderized) FREE & ACTIVE $17.95 absorbent garments (genderized)LADY DIGNITY w/waterproof pouch panty; $9.95 each for SIR DIGNITY w/pouch brief; $8.95 for DIGNITY PLUS w/barrier panel Regular brief; and $11.95 DIGNITY men's boxershorts w/waterproof pouch; $7.95 DIGNITY DUCHESS floralpanty w/barrier panel, DIGNITY FREE & ACTIVEBRIEFMATES pads, liners, guards, undergarments, diapers and underpads.

Ideal Brands, Inc. 213-422-8526
1513 Mirasol St, Commerce, CA 90023

Kck Industries 888-800-1967
14941 Calvert St, Van Nuys, CA 91411

Livedo Usa, Inc. 252-237-1373
4925 Livedo Dr, Wilson, NC 27893
Adult diaper.

Presto Absorbent Products, Inc. 715-839-2085
3925 N Hastings Way, Eau Claire, WI 54703
Adult incontinence briefs.

Presto Absorbent Products-Atlanta
1070 Atlanta Industrial Dr, Marietta, GA 30066
Adult incontinence briefs.

Principle Business Ent. 419-352-1551
Pine Lake Industrial Pk., Dunbridge, OH 43414
Adult incontinent diaper, shields & pads.

Principle Business Enterprises, Inc. 800-467-3224
PO Box 129, Dunbridge, OH 43414
TRANQUILITY SLIMLINE Adjustable brief, undergarment for heavy incontinence. Also available in beltless fitted liner.

Quality Packaging Industries Llc 573-334-6700
5830 State Highway V, Jackson, MO 63755
Adult diaper--Femcare products.

Revelation L.L.C. 800-510-5012
PO Box 486, 437 Howard Ave, Bridgeport, CT 06601
BeKleenDri: Underwear and incontinence products that prevent the growth and spread of microbes, bacteria, yeast and fungi in the garments. BeKleenDri Pants and Underwear: stop the growth of infections in the Perineal area by using 'Prevention Cotton' to reduce the Bio Burden. Variations for Regular Briefs, incontinence and disposables.

Salk Inc. 800-343-4497
119 Braintree St Ste 701, 4th Floor, Boston, MA 02134

Sca Personal Care, North America 270-796-9300
7030 Louisville Rd, Bowling Green, KY 42101
Disposable underpads.

Stryker Gi 866-672-5757
1420 Lakeside Pkwy Ste 110, Flower Mound, TX 75028
Disposable undergarment.

Tidi Products, Llc 920-751-4380
570 Enterprise Dr, Neenah, WI 54956
Adult brief/diaper.

GARMENT, PROTECTIVE, FOR INCONTINENCE *(cont'd)*

Truform Orthotics & Prosthetics 800-888-0458
3960 Rosslyn Dr, Cincinnati, OH 45209

Tytex, Inc. 401-762-4100
601 Park East Dr, Highland Industrial Park, Woonsocket, RI 02895
Mesh pants.

Western Textile Productos De Mexico S.De R.L. Dec. 314-225-9400
Francisco Murguia #514 Nte., M.muzquiz, Coahuila Mexico
Various

White Knight Healthcare 800-851-4431
Calle 16, Number 780, Agua Prieta, Sonora Mexico
Various types of protective clothing

GARMENT, STORAGE, PERITONEAL DIALYSIS CATHETER
(Physical Med) 89OAG

Worldtechnological, Llc 423-305-0355
2016 Dodson Ave Ste B, Chattanooga, TN 37406

GAS CHROMATOGRAPH, ALCOHOL (DEDICATED INSTRUMENTS) *(Toxicology) 91DLS*

Cds Analytical, Inc. 800-541-6593
465 Limestone Rd, Oxford, PA 19363

GAS CHROMATOGRAPHY, AMPHETAMINE *(Toxicology) 91DOD*

Ameritek Usa, Inc. 425-379-2580
125 130th St SE Ste 200, Everett, WA 98208
Amphetamine test kit.

GAS CHROMATOGRAPHY, COCAINE *(Toxicology) 91DIN*

Medtox Diagnostics Inc. 800-334-1116
1238 Anthony Rd, Burlington, NC 27215
VERDICT Immunochromatographic screening test for cocaine and cocaine metabolite(benzoylleganial).

GAS CHROMATOGRAPHY, METHAMPHETAMINE
(Toxicology) 91LAF

Abbott Diagnostics Div. 626-440-0700
820 Mission St, South Pasadena, CA 91030
Amphetamine.

Amedica Biotech, Inc. 510-785-5980
28301 Industrial Blvd Ste K, Hayward, CA 94545
Drug screen mdma test.

Ameditech, Inc. 858-535-1968
10340 Camino Santa Fe Ste F, San Diego, CA 92121
Various.

American Bio Medica Corp. 800-227-1243
122 Smith Rd, Kinderhook, NY 12106
One step lateral flow immunoassay.

American Bio Medica Corp. 856-241-2320
603 Heron Dr Ste 3, Logan Township, NJ 08085
One step lateral flow immunoassay.

Ameritek Usa, Inc. 425-379-2580
125 130th St SE Ste 200, Everett, WA 98208
Methamphetamine test kit.

Biosite Incorporated 888-246-7483
9975 Summers Ridge Rd, San Diego, CA 92121
Fluorescence immunoassay for detection of drugs of abuse in urine.

Branan Medical Corp. 949-598-7166
140 Technology Dr Ste 400, Irvine, CA 92618
Immunochromatographical test for the qualitative determination.

Escreen, Inc. 800-881-0722
2205 W Parkside Ln, Phoenix, AZ 85027
Escreen drugs of abuse screening system.

Express Diagnostics Int'L, Inc. 507-526-3951
1550 Industrial Dr, Blue Earth, MN 56013
Drugs of abuse screening test.

Germaine Laboratories, Inc. 210-692-4192
4139 Gardendale St Ste 101, San Antonio, TX 78229
Various types.

Innovacon, Inc. 858-535-2030
4106 Sorrento Valley Blvd, San Diego, CA 92121
Methamphetamine drug of abuse test.

Jant Pharmacal Corp. 800-676-5565
16255 Ventura Blvd Ste 505, Encino, CA 91436
Test to detect methamphetamine in human urine.

GAS CHROMATOGRAPHY, METHAMPHETAMINE *(cont'd)*

Pan Probe Biotech, Inc. 858-689-9936
7396 Trade St, San Diego, CA 92121
Determination of methamphetamine in human urine.

Phamatech Inc. 858-643-5555
10151 Barnes Canyon Rd, San Diego, CA 92121
Methamphetamine rapid test.

QuantRx Biomedical Corp. 503-252-9565
5920 NE 112th Ave, Portland, OR 97220

Rapid Diagnostics, Div. Of Mp Biomedicals, Llc 800-888-7008
1429 Rollins Rd, Burlingame, CA 94010
Rapid methamphetamin test

Teco Diagnostics 714-693-7788
1268 N Lakeview Ave, Anaheim, CA 92807
One step methamphetamine card test.

GAS CHROMATOGRAPHY, MORPHINE *(Toxicology) 91DMY*

Ameritek Usa, Inc. 425-379-2580
125 130th St SE Ste 200, Everett, WA 98208
Morphine test kit.

GAS CHROMATOGRAPHY, OPIATES *(Toxicology) 91DJF*

Medtox Diagnostics Inc. 800-334-1116
1238 Anthony Rd, Burlington, NC 27215
VERDICT Immunochromatographic screening test for opiates and opiates metabolites(morphine and cocaine).

GAS MIXTURES, LABORATORY *(General) 80WPF*

Aga Linde Healthcare P.R. Inc. 787-622-7900
PO Box 363868, GPO Box 364727, San Juan, PR 00936
General.

Air Products And Chemicals, Inc. 800-654-4567
7201 Hamilton Blvd, Allentown, PA 18195

Lenox Laser 800-494-6537
12530 Manor Rd, Glen Arm, MD 21057
Gas mixing systems: accurate and convenient gas mixing system for producing high quality gas mixtures. The system is based on precision flow calibrated orifices.

GAS MIXTURES, MAGNETIC RESONANCE IMAGING
(Radiology) 90WPG

Air Products And Chemicals, Inc. 800-654-4567
7201 Hamilton Blvd, Allentown, PA 18195

GAS MIXTURES, MEDICAL *(General) 80THJ*

Aga Linde Healthcare P.R. Inc. 787-622-7900
PO Box 363868, GPO Box 364727, San Juan, PR 00936
General.

Air Liquide America Corporation, Cambridge Div. 800-638-1197
821 Chesapeake Dr, Cambridge, MD 21613
$65.00 to $80.00 for disposable cylinders, lung diffusion, laser surgical, biological atmospheres gas mixtures.

Air Products And Chemicals, Inc. 800-654-4567
7201 Hamilton Blvd, Allentown, PA 18195

All-Can Medical, Inc. 905-677-1302
7575 Kimbel St., Mississauga, ONT L5S 1C8 Canada

Colonial Scientific Ltd. 902-468-1811
201 Brownlow Ave., Unit 52, Dartmouth, NS B3B-1W2 Canada

GAS MIXTURES, STERILIZATION *(General) 80WPE*

Aga Linde Healthcare P.R. Inc. 787-622-7900
PO Box 363868, GPO Box 364727, San Juan, PR 00936
General.

Lifegas Llc 866-543-3427
1500 Indian Trail Lilburn Rd, Norcross, GA 30093
LifeGas provides sterilization gas and services, including regulatory and in-service training.

GAS, CALIBRATED (SPECIFIED CONCENTRATION)
(Anesthesiology) 73BXK

Agl Welding Supply Co., Inc. 973-478-5000
600 Route 46, Clifton, NJ 07013
Calibration gas.

Air Liquide America Corporation, Cambridge Div. 800-638-1197
821 Chesapeake Dr, Cambridge, MD 21613
$65.00 to $80.00 for disposable cylinders.

Air Liquide America Specialty Gases Llc 713-402-2152
1311 New Savannah Rd, Augusta, GA 30901

Air Liquide Healthcare America Corporation 713-402-2152
12550 Arrow Rte, Etiwanda, CA 91739

GAS, CALIBRATED (SPECIFIED CONCENTRATION) *(cont'd)*

Air Products And Chemicals, Inc. 800-654-4567
7201 Hamilton Blvd, Allentown, PA 18195

Ge Medical Systems Information Technologies 800-643-6439
8200 W Tower Ave, Milwaukee, WI 53223

General Air Service And Supply 303-892-7003
6330 Colorado Blvd, Commerce City, CO 80022
Lung diffusion mixture.

Gospro, Inc. 808-842-2282
2305 Kamehameha Hwy, Honolulu, HI 96819
Lung diffusion gas, blood gas.

Haun Specialty Gases, Inc. 315-463-5769
6481 Ridings Rd, Syracuse, NY 13206
Multiple.

Inweld Corp. 317-248-0651
5353 W Southern Ave, Indianapolis, IN 46241
Blood gas mixtures.

Linde Gas Puerto Rico Inc. 908-771-1669
Carr 869 Km 1 Hm 8s Flamboya, Catano, PR 00962
Aerobic gas mixture.

Linde Gas Usa Llc 216-642-6600
3930 Michigan St, Hammond, IN 46323
Aerobic gas mixture.

Matheson Tri-Gas, Inc. 972-893-5600
8200 Washington St NE, Albuquerque, NM 87113
Blood gas.

Matheson Tri-Gas, Inc. 505-222-0219
2200 Houston Ave, Houston, TX 77007

Mg Industries 610-695-7628
1 Steel Rd E, U.S. Industrial Park, Morrisville, PA 19067
Patient lift.

Middlesex Gases & Technologies, Inc. 617-387-5050
292 2nd St, Everett, MA 02149
Calibration gas.

Nexair, Llc. 901-729-5547
1211 N McLean Blvd, Memphis, TN 38108
Clinical blood gas mixture.

Polar Cryogenics, Inc. 503-239-5252
2734 SE Raymond St, Portland, OR 97202
Calibration gas mixture.

Portland Welding Supply 207-772-3036
40 Madison St, South Portland, ME 04106
Gas, calibration, specified concentration.

Praxair Distribution Inc., Southeast Llc 440-234-1075
403 Zell Dr, Orlando, FL 32824
Clinical blood gas mixtures.

Praxair Distribution, Inc. 440-234-1075
2801 Montopolis Dr, Austin, TX 78741

Praxair Distribution, Inc. 440-234-1075
1930 Loveridge Rd, Pittsburg, CA 94565

Praxair Distribution, Inc. 440-234-1075
9 Judith Ln, Cahokia, IL 62206

Praxair Distribution, Inc. 440-234-1075
19200 Hawthorne Blvd, Torrance, CA 90503

Praxair Distribution, Inc. 440-234-1075
12000 Roosevelt Rd, Hillside, IL 60162

Praxair-Puerto Rico 440-234-1075
Rt. 931 & 189, Gurabo, PR 00778
Clinical blood gas mixtures.

Pulmonox Medical Corporation 888-464-8742
5243-53 Ave, Tofield, ALB T0B 4J0 Canada
Various

Roberts Oxygen Co., Inc. 301-315-9090
17011 Railroad St, Gaithersburg, MD 20877
Lung diffusion gas mixtures.

Scott Specialty Gases 215-766-8861
6141 Easton Road Box 310, Plumsteadville, PA 18949
Various types of gas calibration condcentrates.

Spec Connection Intl Inc. 813-618-0400
34310 State Road 54, Zephyrhills, FL 33543
Lung diffusion.

Specialty Gases Of America, Inc. 419-729-7732
6055 Brent Dr, Toledo, OH 43611
Lung diffusion mixtures, laser mixtures blood gas calibration mixtures.

GAS, CALIBRATED (SPECIFIED CONCENTRATION) *(cont'd)*

Thermo Fisher Scientific Inc. 781-622-1000
81 Wyman St, Waltham, MA 02451

Valley National Gases Wv Llc 724-834-9200
1055 Garden St, Greensburg, PA 15601
Various types of gas.

Welco-Cgi Gas Technologies 440-234-1075
145 Shimersville Rd, Bethlehem, PA 18015
Clinical blood gas mixtures.

GAS, COLLECTING VESSEL *(Anesthesiology) 73KGK*

Centurion Medical Products Corp. 517-545-1135
3310 S Main St, Salisbury, NC 28147

K. W. Griffen Co. 203-846-1923
100 Pearl St, Norwalk, CT 06850
Adhesive bandages.

Quintron Instrument Company 800-542-4448
3712 W Pierce St, Milwaukee, WI 53215
Gas collection devices for neonates, children, and adults.

Smiths Medical Asd Inc. 800-258-5361
10 Bowman Dr, Keene, NH 03431
Various types, lengths, and sizes of tubing and bags used as a part of a gas sca.

Tri-State Hospital Supply Corp. 517-545-1135
3173 E 43rd St, Yuma, AZ 85365

GAS, GLC *(Toxicology) 91DMS*

Mg Industries 610-695-7628
1 Steel Rd E, U.S. Industrial Park, Morrisville, PA 19067
Patient lift.

GAS, LASER GENERATING *(Surgery) 79NXF*

Air Liquide America Specialty Gases Llc 713-402-2152
1311 New Savannah Rd, Augusta, GA 30901

Air Liquide Healthcare America Corporation 713-402-2152
12550 Arrow Rte, Etiwanda, CA 91739

Matheson Tri-Gas, Inc. 505-222-0219
2200 Houston Ave, Houston, TX 77007

GAS, REATTACHMENT PROCEDURE, RETINAL *(Ophthalmology) 86LPO*

Scott Specialty Gases 215-766-8861
6141 Easton Road Box 310, Plumsteadville, PA 18949
Perfluoropropane (c3 f8) gas.

GAS-MACHINE, ANALGESIA *(Anesthesiology) 73ELI*

Accutron, Inc. 800-531-2221
1733 W Parkside Ln, Phoenix, AZ 85027

Dentalez Group 866-DTE-INFO
101 Lindenwood Dr Ste 225, Valleybrooke Corporate Center
Malvern, PA 19355

Matrx By Midmark 800-847-1000
145 Mid County Dr, Orchard Park, NY 14127
Portable and wall mount nitrous oxide/oxygen mixers for the dental industry. Delivery ranges from 30-100% oxygen.

Ohio Medical Corp. 800-662-5822
1111 Lakeside Dr, Gurnee, IL 60031
Healthcair medical gas distribution equipment is a complete line of wall outlets, valves, valve boxes, medical gas alarms and manifolds.

Porter Instrument Division Parker Hannifin Corp 800-457-2001
245 Township Line Rd, Hatfield, PA 19440
$2500 per unit (standard MXR) for dental analgesia use.

GAS-MACHINE, ANESTHESIA *(Anesthesiology) 73BSZ*

Aga Linde Healthcare P.R. Inc. 787-622-7900
PO Box 363868, GPO Box 364727, San Juan, PR 00936
Anesth/ Pul Med.

American Bio-Medical Service Corporation (Abmsc) 800-755-9055
631 W Covina Blvd, Sales,Service and Refurbishing Center
San Dimas, CA 91773

Anesthesia Equipment Supply, Inc. 253-631-8008
24301 Roberts Dr, Black Diamond, WA 98010
Anesthesia gas machine.

Calmaquip Engineering Corp. 305-592-4510
7240 NW 12th St, Miami, FL 33126

Cardinal Medical Specialties, Inc. 502-969-9652
4708 Pinewood Rd, Louisville, KY 40218
Anesthesia gas machine.

GAS-MACHINE, ANESTHESIA *(cont'd)*

D.R.E., Inc. 800-462-8195
1800 Williamson Ct, Louisville, KY 40223
DRE Integra MRI-Compatible Anesthesia Machines, models SP I, SP II, and VSO2. Ranging from the portable, 27 lb, VSO2, to the SP II, a dual-vaporizer free-standing unit.

Datex-Ohmeda (Canada) 800-268-1472
1093 Meyerside Dr., Unit 2, Mississauga, ONT L5T-1J6 Canada

Datex-Ohmeda Inc. 608-221-1551
3030 Ohmeda Dr, Madison, WI 53718
Various anesthesia gas-machine.

Draeger Medical Systems, Inc. 215-660-2626
16 Electronics Ave, Danvers, MA 01923
Gas machine for anesthesia or analgesia.

Engler Engineering Corp. 800-445-8581
1099 E 47th St, Hialeah, FL 33013
A.D.S. 1000 Veterinary positive pressure anesthesia machine/ ventilator. Electronic valve system. Lab mode for small animals and Normal mode for animals upto 150 lbs. $ 3495.00

G. Dundas Co.,Inc. 253-631-8008
24301 Roberts Dr, Black Diamond, WA 98010
Accessories & components for anethesia gas machines.

International Hospital Supply Co. 800-398-9450
6914 Canby Ave Ste 105, Reseda, CA 91335

Matrx 716-662-6650
145 Mid County Dr, Orchard Park, NY 14127
Analgesia gas machine.

Md International, Inc. 305-669-9003
11300 NW 41st St, Doral, FL 33178

Oceanic Medical Products, Inc. 913-874-2000
8005 Shannon Industrial Park, Ln., Atchison, KS 66002
Gas machine,anesthesia.

Safer Sleep Llc 425-861-8262
3322 W End Ave Ste 705, Nashville, TN 37203
Anesthetic safety and automated record keeper system.

Whittemore Enterprises, Inc. 800-999-2452
11149 Arrow Rte, Rancho Cucamonga, CA 91730

World Medical Equipment, Inc. 800-827-3747
3915 152nd St NE, Marysville, WA 98271
Specialize in refurbished anesthesia machines such as North American Drager and Datex-Ohmeda as well as OR tables, lights, autoclaves, monitors, and accessories.

GASTROSCOPE, FLEXIBLE *(Gastro/Urology) 78QYC*

Olympus America, Inc. 800-645-8160
3500 Corporate Pkwy, PO Box 610, Center Valley, PA 18034

Pentax Medical Company 800-431-5880
102 Chestnut Ridge Rd, Montvale, NJ 07645
$15,015.00 to $16,000.00 for several models of therapeutic upper G.I. fiberscopes. Insertion tube diameters range from 4.9mm to 9.8mm and channel sizes from 2.0 to 2.8mm. Some models are available with a forward water jet system, and a special white tip for laser applications. $18,900.00 to $25,200.00 for several models of video gastroscopes with various insertion tube diameters (5.1mm to 12.8mm) and channel sizes (2.0mm to 4.2mm), including a two channel model. All are fully immersible and have a color CCD chip.

GASTROSCOPE, GASTRO-UROLOGY *(Gastro/Urology) 78FDS*

Avantis Medical Systems, Inc. 408-733-1901
263 Santa Ana Ct, Sunnyvale, CA 94085
Endoscope.

Pentax Southern Region Service Center 201-571-2300
8934 Kirby Dr, Houston, TX 77054
Gastroscope.

Pentax West Coast Service Center 800-431-5880
10410 Pioneer Blvd Ste 2, Santa Fe Springs, CA 90670
Pentax gastroscope.

GASTROSCOPE, GENERAL & PLASTIC SURGERY *(Gastro/Urology) 78GCK*

Mahe International Inc. 800-294-7946
468 Craighead St, Nashville, TN 37204

Richard Wolf Medical Instruments Corp. 800-323-9653
353 Corporate Woods Pkwy, Vernon Hills, IL 60061

GASTROSCOPE, RIGID *(Gastro/Urology) 78QYD*

Richard Wolf Medical Instruments Corp. 800-323-9653
353 Corporate Woods Pkwy, Vernon Hills, IL 60061

GAUGE, DEPTH *(Orthopedics) 87HTJ*

Abbott Spine, Inc. 847-937-6100
12708 Riata Vista Cir Ste B-100, Austin, TX 78727
Depth gauge.

Arthrex, Inc. 239-643-5553
1370 Creekside Blvd, Naples, FL 34108
Variuos depth gauges.

Biomet, Inc. 574-267-6639
56 E Bell Dr, PO Box 587, Warsaw, IN 46582
Bone screw depth gauge.

Depuy Mitek, A Johnson & Johnson Company 800-451-2006
50 Scotland Blvd, Bridgewater, MA 02324
Depth guage.

Depuy Orthopaedics, Inc. 800-473-3789
700 Orthopaedic Dr, P.O. Box 988, Warsaw, IN 46582
Various types of depth gauges.

Depuy Spine, Inc. 800-227-6633
325 Paramount Dr, Raynham, MA 02767
Depth gauge.

Depuy-Raynham, A Div. Of Depuy Orthopaedics 800-451-2006
325 Paramount Dr, Raynham, MA 02767
Various types of depth gauges.

Interventional Spine, Inc. 800-497-0484
13700 Alton Pkwy Ste 160, Irvine, CA 92618
Various types of depth gages.

K2m, Inc. 866-526-4171
751 Miller Dr SE Ste F1, Leesburg, VA 20175
Depth gauge.

Kls-Martin L.P. 800-625-1557
11239-1 St. John`s Industrial, Parkway South
Jacksonville, FL 32250

Kmedic 800-955-0559
190 Veterans Dr, Northvale, NJ 07647

Medtronic Sofamor Danek Instrument Manufacturing 901-396-3133
7375 Adrianne Pl, Bartlett, TN 38133
Multiple (depth gauges).

Medtronic Sofamor Danek Usa, Inc. 901-396-3133
4340 Swinnea Rd, Memphis, TN 38118
Multiple (depth gauges).

Musculoskeletal Transplant Foundation 800-433-6576
125 May St Ste 300, Edison Corp Ctr, Edison, NJ 08837
Sbs' trial spacer.

Musculoskeletal Transplant Foundation 732-661-0202
1232 Mid Valley Dr, Jessup, PA 18434

Small Bone Innovations, Inc. 215-428-1791
1380 S Pennsylvania Ave, Morrisville, PA 19067
Depth gauge.

Smith & Nephew, Inc., Endoscopy Division 800-343-8386
130 Forbes Blvd, Mansfield, MA 02048

Stryker Spine 866-457-7463
2 Pearl Ct, Allendale, NJ 07401

Surgical Implant Generation Network (Sign) 509-371-1107
451 Hills St, Richland, WA 99354
Depth gauge.

Symmetry Medical Usa, Inc. 574-267-8700
486 W 350 N, Warsaw, IN 46582
Depth gauge for clinical use.

Warsaw Orthopedic, Inc. 901-396-3133
2500 Silveus Xing, Warsaw, IN 46582
Multiple (depth gauges).

Zimmer Holdings, Inc. 800-613-6131
1800 W Center St, PO Box 708, Warsaw, IN 46580

Zimmer Spine, Inc. 800-655-2614
7375 Bush Lake Rd, Minneapolis, MN 55439
Depth gague.

Zimmer Trabecular Metal Technology 800-613-6131
10 Pomeroy Rd, Parsippany, NJ 07054
Depth gauge.

GAUGE, DEPTH, INSTRUMENT, DENTAL *(Dental And Oral) 76EIL*

Aesculap Implant Systems Inc. 1-800-234-9179
3773 Corporate Pkwy, Center Valley, PA 18034

Align Technology, Inc. 408-470-1000
881 Martin Ave, Santa Clara, CA 95050
Gauge,depth,instrument,dental.

GAUGE, DEPTH, INSTRUMENT, DENTAL *(cont'd)*

Basic Dental Implant Systems, Inc. 505-884-1922
3321 Columbia Dr NE, Albuquerque, NM 87107
Dental depth gauge instrument.

Biomet Microfixation Inc. 800-874-7711
1520 Tradeport Dr, Jacksonville, FL 32218
Gauge, depth, instrument, dental.

Coltene/Whaledent Inc. 330-916-8858
235 Ascot Pkwy, Cuyahoga Falls, OH 44223
Depth gauge.

Dental Usa, Inc. 815-363-8003
5005 McCullom Lake Rd, McHenry, IL 60050
Gauge.

Dentalez Group 866-DTE-INFO
101 Lindenwood Dr Ste 225, Valleybrooke Corporate Center
Malvern, PA 19355

Moyco Technologies, Inc. 800-331-8837
200 Commerce Dr, Montgomeryville, PA 18936

Nobel Biocare Usa, Llc 800-579-6515
22715/22725 Savi Ranch Parkway, Yorba Linda, CA 92887
Surgical or prosthetic instrument.

Oco Inc. 800-228-0477
600 Paisano St NE Ste A, Albuquerque, NM 87123
Depth gauge.

Oratronics, Inc. 212-986-0050
405 Lexington Ave, New York, NY 10174
Channel curette and depth gauge.

Panadent Corp. 800-368-9777
22573 Barton Rd, Grand Terrace, CA 92313
BioEsthetic level gauge is used to help align the average axis face-bow horizontal so the anterior esthetic plane of the teeth can be established correctly on the articulator. The Adjustable Nasion Relator is used in conjunction with the level guage to level the face-bow in the sagittal plane when the patients head is erect. The nasion is calibrated in millimeters from nasion. There is a long and a short extension with each kit which allows the anterior reference pont to be changed in a range from 25mm to 45mm (short: 25-35mm, long: 35-45mm).

Salvin Dental Specialties, Inc. 800-535-6566
3450 Latrobe Dr, Charlotte, NC 28211
Depth gauge.

Suter Dental Manufacturing Company, Inc. 800-368-8376
632 Cedar St, Chico, CA 95928

Symmetry Medical Usa, Inc. 574-267-8700
486 W 350 N, Warsaw, IN 46582
Dental hand instrument.

GAUGE, GAS PRESSURE, CYLINDER/PIPELINE
(Anesthesiology) 73BXH

Aga Linde Healthcare P.R. Inc. 787-622-7900
PO Box 363868, GPO Box 364727, San Juan, PR 00936
Anesth/Pul Med.

Dresser Inc., Dresser Measurement Division 203-426-3115
PO Box 5605, Newtown, CT 06470

Life Corporation 800-700-0202
1776 N Water St, Milwaukee, WI 53202
LIFE Gauges.

Mg Industries 610-695-7628
1 Steel Rd E, U.S. Industrial Park, Morrisville, PA 19067
Patient lift.

Precision Medical, Inc. 800-272-7285
300 Held Dr, Northampton, PA 18067

Tri-Tech Medical, Inc. 800-253-8692
35401 Avon Commerce Pkwy, Avon, OH 44011
Various.

GAUGE, LENS, OPHTHALMIC *(Ophthalmology) 86HLN*

B. Graczyk, Inc. 269-782-2100
27826 Burmax Park, Dowagiac, MI 49047
Various types & sizes of gauges.

Western Ophthalmics Corporation 800-426-9938
19019 36th Ave W Ste G, Lynnwood, WA 98036

GAUGE, MASTOID *(Ear/Nose/Throat) 77JYI*

Bausch & Lomb Surgical 636-255-5051
3365 Tree Court Ind Blvd, Saint Louis, MO 63122

Clinimed, Incorporated 877-CLINIMED
303 Markus Ct, Sandy Brae Industrial Park, Newark, DE 19713

GAUGE, MASTOID *(cont'd)*

Tuzik Boston 800-886-6363
104 Longwater Dr, Assinippi Park, Norwell, MA 02061

GAUGE, MEASURING *(Ear/Nose/Throat) 77JYJ*

Accutome, Inc. 610-889-0200
3222 Phoenixville Pike, Malvern, PA 19355
Block gauge.

Cole-Parmer Instrument Inc. 800-323-4340
625 E Bunker Ct, Vernon Hills, IL 60061
Digital and mechanical force gauges.

Eagle Vision, Inc. 800-222-7584
8500 Wolf Lake Dr Ste 110, Memphis, TN 38133
Coroneo Punctal Gauge, a complete gauging/dilating system in one instrument in increments from 0.5mm up to 1.0mm diameters. Takes the place of multiple instrument gauge sets.

Novel Products, Inc. 800-323-5143
PO Box 408, Rockton, IL 61072
Patient flexibility testing equipment.

Richardson Products, Inc. 888-928-7297
9408 Gulfstream Rd, Frankfort, IL 60423
Measuring device.

Solarius Development Inc. 800-731-1220
550 E Weddell Dr Ste 3, Sunnyvale, CA 94089
LASERSCAN, noncontact measuring system can verify dimensional specifications, such as flatness, step height, roughness, thickness and volume.

Soltec Corp. 800-423-2344
12977 Arroyo St, San Fernando, CA 91340

GAUGE, PRESSURE *(General) 80WVV*

Dickson Co 800-757-3747
930 S Westwood Ave, Addison, IL 60101
Pressure data loggers and chart recorders. Including our PRXA. A microprocessor-based differential pressure recorder designed for use in hospital isolation rooms, HVAC balancing, pressure monitoring and clean room monitoring. Its large digital display and 8' diameter chart deliver easy to read results.

Marsh Bellofram 800-727-5646
8019 Ohio River Blvd., Newell, WV 26050
Low-pressure diaphragm and other pressure gauges.

Noshok, Inc. 440-243-0888
1010 W Bagley Rd, Berea, OH 44017
1 1/2 through 6-inch diameter, 30-inch vacuum up to 30,000 psi. Special 1 1/2 30 Hg to 300 psi angioplasty gauge, luminous dial.

Novosci Corp. 281-363-4949
2828 N Crescentridge Dr, The Woodlands, TX 77381

Soltec Corp. 800-423-2344
12977 Arroyo St, San Fernando, CA 91340

GAUGE, PRESSURE, CORONARY, CARDIOPULMONARY BYPASS *(Cardiovascular) 74DXS*

Atek Medical 800-253-1540
620 Watson St SW, Grand Rapids, MI 49504
Pressure display box, patient transport box, Ecmo pressure box.

Edwards Lifesciences Research Medical 949-250-2500
6864 Cottonwood St, Midvale, UT 84047
Pressure display set.

Noshok, Inc. 440-243-0888
1010 W Bagley Rd, Berea, OH 44017
Compound pressure gauge - lead-free solder - level IV cleanliness.

Terumo Cardiovascular Systems, Corp 800-521-2818
6200 Jackson Rd, Ann Arbor, MI 48103

GAUGE, STRAIN *(General) 80RWN*

Hokanson Inc., D.E. 800-999-8251
12840 NE 21st Pl, Bellevue, WA 98005
Hokanson manufactures strain gauges for use with our strain gauge plethysmographs. Digit sizes range from 4.5 to 11 cm in 0.5 cm increments, and limb gauges can be made up to 50 cm in 2cm increments. Strain gauges available with Mercury or Indium-Gallium.

Soltec Corp. 800-423-2344
12977 Arroyo St, San Fernando, CA 91340
Complete line of strain gauges for 'all' applications. Request catalog.

GAUSSMETER *(General) 80WWL*

Lake Shore Cryotronics, Inc. 614-891-2243
575 McCorkle Blvd, Westerville, OH 43082

GAUSSMETER *(cont'd)*

R. B. Annis Instruments, Inc. 317-637-9282
1101 N Delaware St, Indianapolis, IN 46202
Small, hand-held instruments, accurately calibrated magnetometer.

Walker Ldj Scientific, Inc. 800-962-4638
10 Rockdale St, Worcester, MA 01606
Magnetic measuring instrument - gaussmeters.

GAUZE ROLL *(Surgery) 79QYE*

Aso Corporation 941-379-0300
300 Sarasota Center Blvd, Sarasota, FL 34240

Covidien Lp 508-261-8000
15 Hampshire St, Mansfield, MA 02048
STA-TITE elastic gauze for wrapping, 2-ply cotton, wide mesh gauze, available in 2in., 3in., 4in. and 6in. widths - all 4.5 yards long.

Dermapac, Inc. 203-924-7148
PO Box 852, Shelton, CT 06484
Procedural kits/packs - Custom kits.

Dukal Corporation 800-243-0741
5 Plant Ave, Hauppauge, NY 11788

East Atlantic Trading/Triangle Healthcare Inc. 800-243-4635
76 National Rd, Edison, NJ 08817

GAUZE, ABSORBABLE *(Surgery) 79GEM*

Adex Medical, Inc. 800-873-4776
6101 Quail Valley Ct, Riverside, CA 92507
Cotton Gauze, Steril, Non Steril

Amd-Ritmed, Inc. 800-445-0340
295 Firetower Road, Tonawanda, NY 14150

Carwild Corp. 860-442-4914
3 State Pier Rd, New London, CT 06320

Covidien Lp 508-261-8000
15 Hampshire St, Mansfield, MA 02048
Petrolatum sterile, non-adhering protective dressing consisting of absorbent, fine mesh gauze impregnated with xeroform in a petrolatum blend.

Degasa, S.A. De C.V. 525-5-483 31
Prolongacion Canal De, Miramontes #3775 Col. Ex-Hacienda San Juan Del. Tlalpan Mexico
Gauze

Dumex Medical Surgical Products Ltd. 800-463-9613
104 Shorting Rd., Scarborough, ONT M1S 3S4 Canada

K W Griffen Company 800-424-5556
100 Pearl St, Norwalk, CT 06850

Mydent International 800-275-0020
80 Suffolk Ct, Hauppauge, NY 11788
DEFEND cotton filled 2 in. x 2 in. 8 ply non-sterile.

Vonex Medical Supplies Inc. 888-866-3920
29-601 Magnetic Dr., Toronto M3J 3J2 Canada
Gauze, absorbable

GAUZE, NON-ABSORBABLE, NON-MEDICATED (INTERNAL SPONGE) *(Surgery) 79GEK*

Bioseal 800-441-7325
167 W Orangethorpe Ave, Placentia, CA 92870
Sterile packing gauze.

Carwild Corp. 860-442-4914
3 State Pier Rd, New London, CT 06320

Degasa, S.A. De C.V. 525-5-483 31
Prolongacion Canal De, Miramontes #3775 Col. Ex-Hacienda San Juan Del. Tlalpan Mexico
Protec simple gauze (sterilized)

First Aid Bandage Co., Inc. 888-813-8214
3 State Pier Rd, New London, CT 06320
USP North American cotton, varied sizes, available x-ray and non-x-ray.

Mcneil Healthcare, Inc. 203-932-6263
481 Elm St, West Haven, CT 06516
Lap sponges,x-ray sponges.

GAUZE, NON-ABSORBABLE, X-RAY DETECTABLE (INTERNAL SPONGE) *(Surgery) 79GDY*

Adi Medical Division Of Asia Dynamics (Group) Inc. 877-647-7699
1565 S Shields Dr, Waukegan, IL 60085

American White Cross - Houston 609-514-4744
15200 North Fwy, Houston, TX 77090
Triangle sponges.

GAUZE, NON-ABSORBABLE, X-RAY DETECTABLE (INTERNAL SPONGE) *(cont'd)*

Bioseal 800-441-7325
167 W Orangethorpe Ave, Placentia, CA 92870
Sterile packing gauze.

Carwild Corp. 860-442-4914
3 State Pier Rd, New London, CT 06320

Centurion Medical Products Corp. 517-545-1135
3310 S Main St, Salisbury, NC 28147

Clearcount Medical Solutions, Inc. 412-931-7233
101 Bellevue Rd Ste 203, Pittsburgh, PA 15229
Surgical sponge.

Dukal Corporation 800-243-0741
5 Plant Ave, Hauppauge, NY 11788

First Aid Bandage Co., Inc. 888-813-8214
3 State Pier Rd, New London, CT 06320
USP North American cotton sponges; all sizes, strung and non-strung, latex free.

Johnson & Johnson Medical Division Of Ethicon, Inc. 800-423-4018
2500 E Arbrook Blvd, Arlington, TX 76014

Lifescience Plus, Inc. 650-565-8172
473 Sapena Ct Ste 7, Santa Clara, CA 95054
Gauze sponge.

Marel Corporation 203-934-8187
5 Saw Mill Rd, West Haven, CT 06516
X-ray gauze sponge, packing sponge.

Mcneil Healthcare, Inc. 203-932-6263
481 Elm St, West Haven, CT 06516
X-ray packing,x-ray vag packing.

Medline Industries, Inc. 800-633-5386
1 Medline Pl, Mundelein, IL 60060

Omnia, Inc. 863-619-8100
3125 Drane Field Rd Ste 29, Lakeland, FL 33811
Gauze sponge, multiple brands.

Parker Anderson Llc 888-799-4289
5030 Paradise Rd Ste A214, Las Vegas, NV 89119
Gauze.

Stryker Puerto Rico, Ltd. 939-307-2500
Hwy. 3, Km. 131.2, Las Guasimas Ind. Park, Arroyo, PR 00714
Femoral canal sponge.

Surgic Aid, Inc. 800-338-5213
37 Crystal Ave # 287, Derry, NH 03038

Tri-State Hospital Supply Corp. 517-545-1135
3173 E 43rd St, Yuma, AZ 85365

Ultracell Medical Technologies, Inc. 877-SPO-NGE1
183 Providence New London Tpke, North Stonington, CT 06359
ULTRACELL P.V.A. orthopedic sponges, various sizes. Sponges used in hip, knee and other types of surgery. All sponges are made of P.V.A. sponge.

GAUZE/SPONGE, NONRESORBABLE FOR EXTERNAL USE *(Surgery) 79NAB*

American White Cross - Houston 609-514-4744
15200 North Fwy, Houston, TX 77090
Gauze/sponge, nonresorbable for external use.

Aso Llc 941-379-0300
12120 Esther Lama Dr Ste 112, El Paso, TX 79936
Non-woven pads.

Beacon Promotions, Inc. 507-354-3900
2121 S Bridge St, New Ulm, MN 56073
Various types of sterile and non sterile gauze-sponge-swabs.

Centurion Medical Products Corp. 517-545-1135
3310 S Main St, Salisbury, NC 28147

Crosstex International, Inc. 516-482-9001
621 Hurricane Shoals Rd NW Ste G, Lawrenceville, GA 30046

Customs Hospital Products, Inc 800-426-2780
6336 SE 107th Ave, Portland, OR 97266
Various sizes of gauze.

Elastic Corporation Of America 704-328-5381
455 Highway 70, Columbiana, AL 35051
Various sizes of gauze bandages.

Global Healthcare 800-601-3880
1495 Hembree Rd Ste 700, Roswell, GA 30076
Sterile/Non-sterile

GAUZE/SPONGE, NONRESORBABLE FOR EXTERNAL USE
(cont'd)

Gyrus Ent L.L.C., Sub. Of Gyrus Acmi, Inc. 508-804-2739
2925 Appling Rd, Bartlett, TN 38133
Various.

Healer Products, Llc 914-663-6300
427 Commerce Ln Ste 1, West Berlin, NJ 08091
Sponge gauze.

Health Ent., Inc. 508-695-0727
90 George Leven Dr, North Attleboro, MA 02760
Tubular gauze, tubular stockinette.

Intl. Medsurg Connection, Inc. 847-619-9926
935 N Plum Grove Rd Ste V, Schaumburg, IL 60173
Gauze, various sizes and piles.

K. W. Griffen Co. 203-846-1923
100 Pearl St, Norwalk, CT 06850
Asborbent surgical sponge.

Kentron Health Care, Inc. 615-384-0573
3604 Kelton Jackson Rd, P.o. Box 120, Springfield, TN 37172
Gauze sponges for external use.

Ks Manufacturing, Inc. 508-427-5727
254 Bodwell St Ste E, Avon, MA 02322
Wound dressing, bandage.

Laboratorios Jaloma, S.A. De C.V. 3-617-5010
Aquiles Serdan No. 438, Guadalajara, Jalisco Mexico
Sterile cotton pads

Lifescience Plus, Inc. 650-565-8172
473 Sapena Ct Ste 7, Santa Clara, CA 95054
Gauze, sponge.

Maxpak, Llc 863-682-0123
2808 New Tampa Hwy, Lakeland, FL 33815
Non-woven pads.

Medspring Group, Inc. 801-295-9750
533 W 2600 S Ste 105, Bountiful, UT 84010
Gauze.

Omnia, Inc. 863-619-8100
3125 Drane Field Rd Ste 29, Lakeland, FL 33811
Abd pad/roll.

Pac-Dent Intl., Inc. 909-839-0888
21078 Commerce Point Dr, Walnut, CA 91789
Non-woven sponge.

Parker Anderson Llc 888-799-4289
5030 Paradise Rd Ste A214, Las Vegas, NV 89119
Hemostatic gauze (sterile) non resorbable for external use.

Qfc Plastics, Inc. 817-649-7400
728 111th St, Arlington, TX 76011
Sponge.

Sunmed Usa Llc. 310-531-8222
841 Apollo St Ste 334, El Segundo, CA 90245

Tidi Products, Llc 920-751-4380
570 Enterprise Dr, Neenah, WI 54956
Sponge, external for medical and dental use.

Tri-State Hospital Supply Corp. 517-545-1135
3173 E 43rd St, Yuma, AZ 85365

United Medical Enterprises 757-224-0177
4049 Allen Station Rd, Augusta, GA 30906
Non woven gauze sponges sterile and non sterile for external use.

3d Medical Concepts, Llc 205-987-0935
1061 Morgan Park Rd, Pelham, AL 35124
Sponge.

GEL, ELECTRODE, ELECTROCARDIOGRAPH
(Cardiovascular) 74DYA

Cardiac Science Corp. 800-777-1777
500 Burdick Pkwy, Deerfield, WI 53531

Md International, Inc. 305-669-9003
11300 NW 41st St, Doral, FL 33178

Parker Laboratories, Inc. 800-631-8888
286 Eldridge Rd, Fairfield, NJ 07004
SIGNAPAD, SIGNACREME and TENSIVE, conductive adhesive gel, electrode cream, paste and electrode pads.

Pharmaceutical Innovations, Inc. 973-242-2900
897 Frelinghuysen Ave, Newark, NJ 07114
$2.65 per 250ml LECTRON II TENS, ECG, electrosurgical gel; $4.95 per 250ml SPRAYTRODE conductive ECG spray; $6.45 per 250ml PREPTRODE gentle conductive electrode skin preparation.

GEL, ELECTRODE, ELECTROCARDIOGRAPH *(cont'd)*

Physio-Control, Inc. 800-442-1142
11811 Willows Rd NE, Redmond, WA 98052
DERMAJEO electrode gel.

Taylor Industries, Inc. 800-339-1361
2706 Industrial Dr, Jefferson City, MO 65109

GEL, ELECTRODE, ELECTROSURGICAL *(Surgery) 79JOT*

Innova Corp. 860-242-3210
68 E Dudley Town Rd, Bloomfield, CT 06002

Pharmaceutical Innovations, Inc. 973-242-2900
897 Frelinghuysen Ave, Newark, NJ 07114
$2.65 per 250ml LECTRON II, ECG, electrosurgical gel.

Triad Disposables 800-288-1288
19355 Janacek Ct, Brookfield, WI 53045
Ultrasound gel.

GEL, ELECTRODE, PULP TESTER *(Dental And Oral) 76EAS*

C.E.J. Dental Products Inc. 949-493-2449
32332 Camino Capistrano Ste 101, San Juan Capistrano, CA 92675
Dental conducting gel, multiple, various viscosities and colors.

GEL, ELECTRODE, STIMULATOR *(Cns/Neurology) 84GYB*

Alimed, Inc. 800-225-2610
297 High St, Dedham, MA 02026

Cadwell Laboratories 800-245-3001
909 N Kellogg St, Kennewick, WA 99336
CADWELL safe electrodes.

Docxs Biomedical Products And Accessories 707-462-2351
564 S Dora St Ste A-1, Ukiah, CA 95482
Electrode gel.

E-Z-Em, Inc. 516-333-8230
750 Summa Ave, Westbury, NY 11590
Contact and coupling media ultrasound and accessories.

Grass Technologies, An Astro-Med, Inc. Product Gro 401-828-4002
53 Airport Park Drive, Rockland, MA 02370
Electrode paste (gel).

H.B. Gordon Mfg. Co., Inc. 310-327-5240
751 E Artesia Blvd, Carson, CA 90746
Electrode gel.

Mavidon Medical Products 800-654-0385
1820 2nd Ave N, Lake Worth, FL 33461
Electrode jelly.

Oxford Instruments 800-438-8322
300 Baker Ave Ste 150, Concord, MA 01742
Electrode conductivity gel.

Pharmaceutical Innovations, Inc. 973-242-2900
897 Frelinghuysen Ave, Newark, NJ 07114
$2.65 per 250ml LECTRON II TENS, ECG, electrosurgical gel; $3.00 per 90ml Q.R. (Quick Recovery) defibrillator gel; $4.95 for 250 ml bottle to $49.95 for 4 liter container of ELECTRO-MIST, an electrolyte spray for muscle stimulation.

Rochester Electro Medical, Inc. 813-963-2933
4212 Cypress Gulch Dr, Lutz, FL 33559
Electrode jelly.

3m Company 651-733-4365
601 22nd Ave S, Brookings, SD 57006

GEL, ELECTRODE, TENS *(Physical Med) 89IKC*

Arizona Dme--Durable Medical Equipment, Inc. 888-665-2568
PO Box 15413, Scottsdale, AZ 85267

Electro Therapeutic Devices Inc. 800-268-3834
570 Hood Rd., Ste. 14, Markham, ONT L3R 4G7 Canada

Electro-Cap International, Inc. 800-527-2193
1011 W Lexington Rd, PO Box 87, Eaton, OH 45320

Elmed, Inc. 630-543-2792
60 W Fay Ave, Addison, IL 60101

Gn Otometrics 800-289-2150
125 Commerce Dr, Schaumburg, IL 60173
$6.00 per 8 oz. tube.

Innova Corp. 860-242-3210
68 E Dudley Town Rd, Bloomfield, CT 06002
Gel, electrodes, TENS, electrosurgical, electrocardiograph.

Lumiscope Company, Inc. 800-672-8293
1035 Centennial Ave, Piscataway, NJ 08854

GEL, ELECTRODE, TENS *(cont'd)*

Parker Laboratories, Inc. 800-631-8888
286 Eldridge Rd, Fairfield, NJ 07004
TENSIVE SPECTRA 360.

Pharmaceutical Innovations, Inc. 973-242-2900
897 Frelinghuysen Ave, Newark, NJ 07114
$2.65 per 250ml LECTRON II TENS, ECG, electrosurgical gel; $4.95 per 50g TAC gel electrically conductive adhesive; $5.50 per 15ml PRE TAC conductive TENS skin preparation; $5.75 per 60ml AFTER-TENS care cream; $4.75 per 60ml RES-OFF adhesive residue remover.

Tailored Label Products, Inc. 800-727-1344
W165N5731 Ridgewood Dr, Menomonee Falls, WI 53051

Tetra Medical Supply Corp. 800-621-4041
6364 W Gross Point Rd, Niles, IL 60714
Foam, Cloth, Carbon, round or square. Reusable, self-adhering and flexible.

Weiman Healthcare Solutions 800-837-8140
755 Tri State Pkwy, Gurnee, IL 60031
Conductive, multi-purpose gel for electro-medical procedures; conductive gel for use with ultrasound procedures.

GEL, FILTER *(Chemistry) 75UGB*

Bio-Rad Laboratories, Life Science Group 800-424-6723
2000 Alfred Nobel Dr, Hercules, CA 94547

GEL, SUPPORT *(Immunology) 82JZR*

Allen Medical Systems, Inc. 800-433-5774
1 Post Office Sq, Acton, MA 01720
Protect and pamper your patients with luxurious Allen® Polymer Gel Pads

Epicentre Technologies 800-284-8474
726 Post Rd, Madison, WI 53713
GELASE Jellies. Gel for digestion preparation.

Pharmaceutical Innovations, Inc. 973-242-2900
897 Frelinghuysen Ave, Newark, NJ 07114
Light transmitting gel. Used for laser and pulsed light, depilatory absorbs thermal energy, ultra clear, stays in place and reduces patient complaints.

Qed Bioscience, Inc. 800-929-2114
10919 Technology Pl Ste C, San Diego, CA 92127
Affinity resins for specific plasma and serum protein depletion: removal of human serum albumin, IgG, fibrinogen and transferrin from serum, plasma, CSF, urine.

Somervell Laboratories 254-897-4085
1102A Bluebonnet St, Glen Rose, TX 76043
Ultrasound gel.

GEL, ULTRASONIC COUPLING *(Physical Med) 89QYF*

Biofreeze Performance Health, Inc. 800-246-3733
1245 Home Ave, Akron, OH 44310

Cardiac Science Corp. 800-777-1777
500 Burdick Pkwy, Deerfield, WI 53531

Chester Labs, Inc. 800-354-9709
1900 Section Rd, Cincinnati, OH 45237
LIQUA-SONIC, gel.

Labthermics Technologies 217-351-7722
701 Devonshire Dr, Champaign, IL 61820
SONOTHERM ultrasonic gel.

Parker Laboratories, Inc. 800-631-8888
286 Eldridge Rd, Fairfield, NJ 07004
POLYSONIC, AQUASONIC CLEAR and AQUASONIC 100, ultrasound lotion.

GEL, ULTRASONIC COUPLING *(cont'd)*

Pharmaceutical Innovations, Inc. 973-242-2900
897 Frelinghuysen Ave, Newark, NJ 07114
$2.45 per 250ml GAMMA massage and ultrasound gel; $2.45 per 250ml ULTRA/PHONIC conductivity gel. ULTRA PHONIC FREE, odorless, colorless, free of propylene glycol, glycerin, environmentally and user friendly. $2.45 per 250 ml bottle, $20.75 per 5 ltr. ULTRA PHONIC WHITE, ultrasound transmission medium which is also a cosmetic grade massage lotion. $2.45 per 250ml bottle, $19.95 per 4 ltr.container. ULTRA PHONIC FOCUS - Conforming Gel Pad. Is a solidified gel pad which is used to obtain near field imaging, or for scanning over bony prominent areas. Available in 2 sizes: 1.5 cm x 9 cm = $6.50 each and 2.5 cm x 9 cm = $7.00 each. ULTRA PHONICS SG, stabilized formula resists liquefying from body heat and salts in perspiration remaining uniform throughout the procedure, less is required, cleanup is minimized. $2.45 per 250 ml bottle, $19.25 per 4 ltr. container, $20.75 per 5 ltr. container, and $39.00 per 10 ltr. container. OTHER-SONIC, $1.52 per 250 ml bottle, $13.75 per 5 ltr. container.

GEL, ULTRASONIC TRANSMISSION *(General) 80SDY*

Alimed, Inc. 800-225-2610
297 High St, Dedham, MA 02026

Cone Instruments, Inc. 800-321-6964
5201 Naiman Pkwy, Solon, OH 44139

Coopersurgical, Inc. 800-243-2974
95 Corporate Dr, Trumbull, CT 06611

Ideal Medical Source, Inc. 800-537-0739
2805 East. Oakland Blvd, Suite 352, Fort Lauderdale, FL 33306

Life-Tech, Inc. 281-491-6600
4235 Greenbriar Dr, Stafford, TX 77477

Md International, Inc. 305-669-9003
11300 NW 41st St, Doral, FL 33178

Medical Equipment Specialists, Inc. 800-795-6641
107 Otis St, Northborough, MA 01532
GELISONDE II, ultrasonic coupling medium. 250 ml per bottle; 12 bottles per box. Specially formulated for fetal monitoring.

Medison America, Inc. 800-829-SONO
11075 Knott Ave Ste C, Cypress, CA 90630

Mettler Electronics Corp. 800-854-9305
1333 S Claudina St, Anaheim, CA 92805
$39.00 for SONIGEL 12x9.5 oz tubes, $19.75 for 1x4 liter and $69.50 for 4x4 liter.

Parker Laboratories, Inc. 800-631-8888
286 Eldridge Rd, Fairfield, NJ 07004
AQUASONIC CLEAR, AQUASONIC 100 and AQUAFLEX.

Pharmaceutical Innovations, Inc. 973-242-2900
897 Frelinghuysen Ave, Newark, NJ 07114
$2.45 per 250 ml GAMMA massage and ultrasound gel. $2.45 per 250 ml ULTRA/PHONIC conductivity gel. ULTRA PHONIC FREE, odorless, colorless, free of propylene glycol, glycerin, environmentally and user friendly. $2.45 per 250 ml bottle, $20.75 per 5 ltr. ULTRA PHONIC WHITE, ultrasound transmission medium which is also a cosmetic grade massage lotion. $2.45 per 250 ml bottle, $19.95 per 4 ltr. container. ULTRA PHONIC FOCUS -Conforming Gel Pad. Is a solidified gel pad which is used to obtain near field imaging, or for scanning over bony prominent areas. Available in 2 sizes: 1.5 cm x 9 cm = $6.50 each and 2.5 cm x 9 cm = $7.00 each. ULTRA PHONIC SG, stabilized formula resists liquefying from body heat and salts in perspiration remaining uniform throughout the procedure, less is required, cleanup is minimized. $2.45 per 250 ml bottle, $19.25 per 4 ltr. container, $20.75 per 5 ltr. container, and $39.00 per 10 ltr. container. OTHER-SONIC, $1.52 per 250 ml bottle, $13.75 per 5 ltr. container.

Products Group International, Inc. 800-336-5299
447 Main St., Lyons, CO 80540

Rich-Mar Corporation 800-762-4665
PO Box 879, 15499 E 590 Rd, Inola, OK 74036
Coupling gels and lotions for ultrasound transmission. Both made with natural healing aloe vera.

Schueler & Company, Inc. 516-487-1500
PO Box 528, Stratford, CT 06615

Shimadzu Medical Systems 800-228-1429
20101 S Vermont Ave, Torrance, CA 90502

GEL, ULTRASONIC TRANSMISSION *(cont'd)*

Sonotech Inc. 800-458-4254
774 Marine Dr, Bellingham, WA 98225
CLEAR IMAGE Ultrasound Scanning Gel has acoustic properties which minimize refraction through the skin while optimizing coupling. Clear Image is fragrance- and dye-free, contains no silicones, surfactacts, alcohol, or mineral oil, which can degrade transducers and electrical connectors.(br)(br) CLEAR IMAGE SINGLES prevent cross contamination through 15 or 30 ml unit dose packets containing CLEAR IMAGE scanning gel. (br)(br) LITHOCLEAR and LITHOCLEAR with Aloe present a clear pathway for shockwave acoustics in ESWL lithotripsy with no reflection or scattering due to micro or macro air bubbles.

St. John Companies 800-435-4242
25167 Anza Dr, PO Box 800460, Santa Clarita, CA 91355
SPEE-D-GLIDE ultrasound transmission gel offers exceptional coupling, effectively directing energy ways to the patients tissue. It's water-soluble, non-staining, non-allergenic, non-irritating and bacteriostatic free.

Universal Ultrasound 800-842-0607
299 Adams St, Bedford Hills, NY 10507

GELATIN *(Pathology) 88IEX*

Bd Diagnostic Systems 800-675-0908
7 Loveton Cir, Sparks, MD 21152

Polysciences, Inc. 800-523-2575
400 Valley Rd, Warrington, PA 18976

GELATIN FOR SPECIMEN ADHESION *(Pathology) 88IFZ*

American Mastertech Scientific, Inc. 209-368-4031
1330 Thurman St, Lodi, CA 95240
Multiple.

Spectra-Tint 585-546-8050
250 Cumberland St Ste 228, Rochester, NY 14605
Float-affix.

U S Biotex Corp. 606-652-4700
RR 1 Box 62, Webbville, KY 41180
Gelatin adhesive.

GENERAL HEMATOLOGY REAGENT *(Pathology) 88KQD*

Utak Laboratories, Inc. 800-235-3442
25020 Avenue Tibbitts, Valencia, CA 91355
UTAK Homocysteine Controls are available in four concentration levels. This sulfur containing amino acid has been implicated as an increased risk factor in cardiovascular disease; measurement of the plasma or serum levels has become a tool in diagnosis.

GENERAL MEDICAL DEVICE *(General) 80LDQ*

Astellas Pharma Us, Inc. 800-888-7704
3 Parkway N, Deerfield, IL 60015
Compounding devices: transfer pins, chemo pins, transfer spike vented needles.

Axcan Pharma Inc. 800-950-8085
22 Inverness Center Pkwy, Birmingham, AL 35242
Mucus clearance device for chronic bronchitis and bronchiectasis (K946083).

B. Braun Oem Division, B. Braun Medical Inc. 866-8-BBRAUN
824 12th Ave, Bethlehem, PA 18018

Bio-Medical Service De Mexico, S.A. De C.V. 5-286-7943
Amsterdam #87, Mexico D.F. 06170 Mexico
Including incubators, vacuums, fans.

Calmaquip Engineering Corp. 305-592-4510
7240 NW 12th St, Miami, FL 33126
Incubators, operating rooms, respirators, supplies and tools, central piping and medical gases.

Cowan Plastics, Llc 401-351-1400
610 Manton Ave, Providence, RI 02909

Emerald Medical Products Corp. 206-781-9450
2405 NW Market St Ste 305, Seattle, WA 98107
Custom medical device, manufacturing, and product development.

Globe Medical Tech, Inc. 713-365-9595
1766 W Sam Houston Pkwy N, Houston, TX 77043
Provide turn key solution for disposable medical products. Our services include: patent evaluation, design, FDA application, prototype, injection molding and clean room assembly / manufacturing.

GENERAL MEDICAL DEVICE *(cont'd)*

Globetec Nonwovens 410-287-2207
40 Industrial Rd, North East, MD 21901
MICROSTAT BFE/VFE electrostatic filter media. High-efficiency removal of viral and bacterial contamination in gaseous stream applications. Also available nonwoven and depth filter media engineered materials for removal of particulate (solid or liquids) from fluid (gas or liquid) streams. Soaker Pad: needle felts designed for fluid absoption for many medical applications including incontinence.

Hart Enterprises, Inc. 616-887-0400
400 Apple Jack Ct, Sparta, MI 49345
Custom medical devices.

Huntleigh Healthcare Llc. 800-223-1218
40 Christopher Way, Eatontown, NJ 07724
DOPPLEX locking device to help prevent a Doppler from being misplaced, dropped or stolen.

I-Rep, Inc. 800-828-0852
508 Chaney St Ste B, Lake Elsinore, CA 92530
JOG PATELLA MOBILIZER is a mobilizing device for the patella.

Integrated Orbital Implants, Inc. 800-424-6537
12625 High Bluff Dr Ste 314, San Diego, CA 92130
OK Motility Peg System for integrated implants converts a standard hypodermic needle into a handy drill.

Mclean Medical And Scientific, Inc. 800-777-9987
292 E Lafayette Frontage Rd, Saint Paul, MN 55107
Surgical devices, all materials.

Medi 800-947-6334
4814 E 2nd St, Benicia, CA 94510
Interacoustics EP 15 and EP 25. Brain stem system.

Medicool, Inc. 800-426-3227
20460 Gramercy Pl, Torrance, CA 90501
Insulin cooling unit for traveling diabetics.

Medikmark Inc. 800-424-8520
3600 Burwood Dr, Waukegan, IL 60085
Pain management kits.

Medtronic Sofamor Danek Usa, Inc 901-399-2346
1800 Pyramid Pl, Memphis, TN 38132
Fracture orthopedic internal fixation device.

Mesa Laboratories, Inc. 800-992-6372
12100 W 6th Ave, Lakewood, CO 80228
Data Trace is a self contained instrument for measuring and recording temperature, humidity and pressure.

Mini-Mitter Company, Inc. 800-685-2999
20300 Empire Ave Ste B3, Bend, OR 97701
Mini-Logger is an extremely lightweight, wearable data logger for simultaneous monitoring of temperature and activity along with Inter-Beat Interval for HRV analysis. Alternatively, the unit can be programmed to pick up and record heart rate instead of IBI.

Mono Research Lab Ltd. 716-634-6800
5436 Main St Ste 4, Williamsville, NY 14221
Physical strength measurements.

National Instrument Co., Inc. 800-526-1301
4119 Fordleigh Rd, Baltimore, MD 21215
FILAMATIC filing machines ranges from bench-top filler to one-person production lines. Automatic and semi-automatic liquid filing machines are available in a wide variety of models to fill from micoliters of free-flowing, semi-viscous or vicous products. FILAMATICS monoblocs provide multifunctional capabilities of filing, plugging, stoppering and capping with the touch of a button. CAPAMATIC stoppering machines provide a simple, reliable means of closing containers with standard or lyophilization stoppers and aluminum crimp caps sizes to 30mm. CAPAMATIC screwcapping machines utilize servo torquing - the perfect capping methodology for accurate screwcap applications. The salient features of servo torque control are that it provides extremely accurate application torque due to total speed/dwell profile control, automatic reject feedback, preset control parameters for different caps, optional real time data access. Servo control in combination with our patented extremely low inertia quick-change chuck guarantees the most high-speed application torque available in the industry.

Northern Technologies Intl. Corp. 800-328-2433
6680 N Highway 49, Lino Lakes, MN 55014
Corrosion inhibitor products.

Surgical Tools, Inc. 800-774-2040
1106 Monroe St, Bedford, VA 24523

GENERAL MEDICAL DEVICE *(cont'd)*

Taga Medical Technologies 800-651-9490
34675 Melinz Pkwy Ste 105, Eastlake, OH 44095
Taga Button Enteral Feeding Device is a low profile feeding device for adults and pediatrics.

Timm Medical Technologies, Inc. 800-966-2796
6585 City West Pkwy, Eden Prairie, MN 55344
THERMOFLEX System (Wit prostatic treatment) - administers thermal treatment to the prostate using heated water for the treatment of symptoms due to benign prostatic Hyperplasia (BPH).

Woodward Laboratories, Inc. 800-780-6999
125 Columbia Ste B, Aliso Viejo, CA 92656
Diabetic Basics Antimicrobial Healthy Foot Kit. Provides trio of germ-killing products, foot sanitizer, lotion and powder that help to prevent foot infections for individuals with limited mobility.

GENERAL PURPOSE HEMATOLOGY DEVICE
(Hematology) 81LOQ

Globe Scientific, Inc. 800-394-4562
610 Winters Ave, Paramus, NJ 07652
Disposable needle holder. Fits 13mm and 16mm blood collection tubes and all common needle units. Single-use.

Pioneer Center For Human Services 815-344-1230
4001 W Dayton St, McHenry, IL 60050
Test tube & reaction trays.

GENERAL PURPOSE MICROBIOLOGY DIAGNOSTIC DEVICE
(Microbiology) 83LIB

Abbott Molecular, Inc. 847-937-6100
1300 E Touhy Ave, Des Plaines, IL 60018
Amplification detection system.

Bd Biosciences Discovery Labware 978-901-7431
1 Becton Cir, Durham, NC 27712
Various styles and sizes of sterile and non-sterile disposable assay and immunoa.

Dawning Technologies, Inc. 800-332-0499
6140 Mid Metro Dr Ste 5, Fort Myers, FL 33966
This is a new version of our JavaLin interface designed for use with microbiology instruments. It produces HL7 or ASTM compliant messaging using a new organization of these complex records, reducing the interpretive load on the LIS.

Focus Diagnostics, Inc. 714-220-1900
10703 Progress Way, Cypress, CA 90630
Various parvovirus elisa kits and components.

Healthlink 904-996-7758
3611 St Johns Bluff Rd S Ste 1, Jacksonville, FL 32224
Dip paddle.

J&S Medical Associates 800-229-6000
35 Tripp St Ste 1, Framingham, MA 01702
VISISPOT presumptive visual test for enterococci and strep A, both on the same card.

Metabolic Solutions, Inc. 866-302-1998
460 Amherst St, Nashua, NH 03063
14C erythromycin breath test to measure in vivo CYP3A4 activity

Micromanipulator Co., Inc., The 800-972-4032
1555 Forrest Way, Carson City, NV 89706
Products and accessories to aid in embryo recovery, grading, splitting, injection, micromanipulation and photomicrography.

Virotek, L.L.C. 847-634-4500
900 Asbury Dr, Buffalo Grove, IL 60089
Inoculating loop.

GENERAL USE SURGICAL SCISSORS *(Surgery) 79LRW*

Acuderm Inc. 800-327-0015
5370 NW 35th Ter Ste 106, Fort Lauderdale, FL 33309
Disposable scissors.

Aesculap Implant Systems Inc. 1-800-234-9179
3773 Corporate Pkwy, Center Valley, PA 18034

Arista Surgical Supply Co. Inc. 800-223-1984
297 High St, Dedham, MA 02026

Ascent Healthcare Solutions 480-763-5300
10232 S 51st St, Phoenix, AZ 85044
Scissor tips.

Berring Precision Blades Llc 352-383-8333
9236 Wildwood Ln, Robertsville, MO 63072
General surgical scissors.

GENERAL USE SURGICAL SCISSORS *(cont'd)*

Biomet Microfixation Inc. 800-874-7711
1520 Tradeport Dr, Jacksonville, FL 32218
Various types of scissors.

Cardinal Health, Snowden Pencer Products 847-689-8410
5175 S Royal Atlanta Dr, Tucker, GA 30084
Various styles of scissors for general surgical use.

Carl Heyer, Inc. 800-284-5550
1872 Bellmore Ave, North Bellmore, NY 11710

Centurion Medical Products Corp. 517-545-1135
3310 S Main St, Salisbury, NC 28147

Clauss Tools 800-225-2377
1931 Black Rock Tpke, Fairfield, CT 06825
Dental, veterinarian, paramedic and pathologist shears.

Cook Endoscopy 336-744-0157
4900 Bethania Station Rd # &, 5951 Grassy Creek Blvd. Winston Salem, NC 27105
Scissors, general use, surgical.

Dermatologic Lab & Supply, Inc. 800-831-6273
608 13th Ave, Council Bluffs, IA 51501
Surgical scissors.

Gyrus Acmi, Inc. 508-804-2739
93 N Pleasant St, Norwalk, OH 44857
Scissors, general, surgical.

Gyrus Medical, Inc. 800-852-9361
6655 Wedgwood Rd N Ste 105, Maple Grove, MN 55311
Scissors cut, coagulate, and dissect tissue using the PK bipolar mode during laparscopic surgical prodecures.

Health Care Logistics, Inc. 800-848-1633
450 Town St, PO Box 25, Circleville, OH 43113
Various makes of surgical scissors.

International Hospital Supply Co. 800-398-9450
6914 Canby Ave Ste 105, Reseda, CA 91335

Laschal Surgical, Inc. 914-949-8577
4 Baltusrol Dr, Purchase, NY 10577
Uniband scissors/featherlite scissors.

Marina Medical Instruments, Inc. 800-697-1119
955 Shotgun Rd, Sunrise, FL 33326
Various.

Medisiss 866-866-7477
2747 SW 6th St, Redmond, OR 97756
Various general surgical scissors,sterile.

Micrins Surgical Instruments, Inc. 800-833-3380
28438 N Ballard Dr, Lake Forest, IL 60045

Micro Stamping Corp. 513-573-0085
140 Belmont Dr, Somerset, NJ 08873
Surgical scissors.

Miltex Dental Technologies, Inc. 516-576-6022
589 Davies Dr, York, PA 17402
Various utility scissors.

Normed 800-288-8200
PO Box 3644, Seattle, WA 98124
Various types & sizes of general medical scissors.

Precision Surgical Intl., Inc. 800-776-8493
PO Box 726, Noblesville, IN 46061
Various types of scissors.

Prosurge Instruments, Inc. 866-832-7874
199 Laidlaw Ave, Jersey City, NJ 07306

Rocket Medical Plc. 800-707-7625
150 Recreation Park Dr Ste 3, Hingham, MA 02043

Schueler & Company, Inc. 516-487-1500
PO Box 528, Stratford, CT 06615

Solos Endoscopy 800-388-6445
65 Sprague St # B, Boston/dedham Commerce Park, Boston, MA 02136
Manual surgical instruments for general use.

Symmetry Medical Usa, Inc. 574-267-8700
486 W 350 N, Warsaw, IN 46582
Manual surgical instrument for general use.

Synergetics Usa, Inc. 800-600-0565
3845 Corporate Centre Dr, O Fallon, MO 63368
Various.

Trans American Medical 800-626-9232
7633 W 100th Pl, Bridgeview, IL 60455
Operating and dressing scissors. 5.5 in. sharp/blunt or sharp/sharp; curved or straight; satin or polished. U.S. made.

GENERAL USE SURGICAL SCISSORS *(cont'd)*

Trans American Medical / Tamsco Instruments 708-430-7777
7633 W 100th Pl, Bridgeview, IL 60455
Floor grade surgical stainless steel.

Tri-State Hospital Supply Corp. 517-545-1135
3173 E 43rd St, Yuma, AZ 85365

Triboro Supplies Inc 800-369-7546
994 Grand Blvd, Deer Park, NY 11729

GENERATOR, AEROSOL *(Ear/Nose/Throat) 77QAH*

A&H Products, Inc. 918-835-8081
PO Box 470686, Tulsa, OK 74147

Air Techniques International 410-363-9696
11403 Cronridge Dr, Owings Mills, MD 21117
Model TDA-4BI, 5B, 6C and PSL jet atomizer.

Medical Industries America Inc. 800-759-3038
2636 289th Pl, Adel, IA 50003
AEROMAX Priced from $63.00; for nebulization of medication. SPORT NEB; priced from $49, small, lightweight nebulizer compressor.

Monaghan Medical Corp. 800-833-9653
5 Latour Ave Ste 1600, P.O. Box 2805, Plattsburgh, NY 12901
AeroChamber Plus Valved Holding Chamber: Aerosol delivery system. AeroTrach Plus Valved Holding Chamber: Aerosol delivery system for tracheostomy patient.

San-I-Pak,Pacific Inc. 800-875-7264
23535 S Bird Rd, Tracy, CA 95304
#1 Odor Control - #2 Ozone Generator - #3 Deoderizer. This Generator converts oxygen to ozone,wich oxidizes bacteria that causes odors.Used in garbage compactors, sterlizers and sewage treatment. Air purification for allergies. Waste cans and hampers with integral ozone generator eliminates airborne pathogens and odor. Only for hospital and lab rooms.

Tsi Incorporated 800-874-2811
500 Cardigan Rd, Shoreview, MN 55126
The Vibrating Orifice Aerosol Generator creates uniform, highly monodisperse particles from 1 to 200 micrometers.

GENERATOR, DIAGNOSTIC X-RAY, HIGH VOLTAGE, 3-PHASE *(Radiology) 90VHL*

Advanced Instrument Development, Inc. 800-243-9729
2545 Curtiss St, Downers Grove, IL 60515
Expos-AID; MULTIPLE

Americomp, Inc. 800-458-1782
2901 W Lawrence Ave, Chicago, IL 60625
With anatomical programming.

Amrad 888-772-6723
2901 W Lawrence Ave, Chicago, IL 60625

Control-X Medical, Inc. 800-777-9729
1755 Atlas St, Columbus, OH 43228
Microprocessor controlled.

Gtr Labs, Inc. 888-871-9232
510 Elk St, Gassaway, WV 26624
SMARTGEN, INTELLIGEN, VALUGEN x-ray generators offer affordable prices as a result of using complete software control in a state of the art design. Designed by a team of service engineers for fast and easy installation and calibration.

Medlink Imaging, Inc. 800-456-7800
200 Clearbrook Rd, Elmsford, NY 10523

Shimadzu Medical Systems 800-228-1429
20101 S Vermont Ave, Torrance, CA 90502
2 models, 150 KVp, 800-1250 mA, 80-100 KW ratings, UD1508-30, AUD150G.

Spellman High Voltage Electronics Corp. 631-630-3000
475 Wireless Blvd, Hauppauge, NY 11788

Xma (X-Ray Marketing Associates, Inc.) 800-325-8880
1205 W Lakeview Ct, Windham Lakes Business Park
Romeoville, IL 60446

GENERATOR, DIAGNOSTIC X-RAY, HIGH VOLTAGE, SINGLE PHASE *(Radiology) 90IZO*

Americomp, Inc. 800-458-1782
2901 W Lawrence Ave, Chicago, IL 60625

Amrad 888-772-6723
2901 W Lawrence Ave, Chicago, IL 60625

Ar Custom Medical Products, Ltd. 516-242-7501
19 W Industry Ct Ste A, Deer Park, NY 11729
Mammographic x-ray generator.

GENERATOR, DIAGNOSTIC X-RAY, HIGH VOLTAGE, SINGLE PHASE *(cont'd)*

Bay Shore Medical Equipment Corp. 631-586-1991
235 S Fehr Way, Bay Shore, NY 11706
Multiple.

Control-X Medical, Inc. 800-777-9729
1755 Atlas St, Columbus, OH 43228
Microprocessor controlled.

Custom X-Ray Service, Inc. 602-439-3100
2120 W Encanto Blvd, Phoenix, AZ 85009

Del Medical Systems 800-800-6006
11550 King St, Franklin Park, IL 60131
Computer based radiographic generator; anatomically programmed.

Ge Medical Systems, Llc 262-548-2355
3000 N Grandview Blvd, W-417, Waukesha, WI 53188
Various types of x-ray generators.

Gtr Labs, Inc. 888-871-9232
510 Elk St, Gassaway, WV 26624
SMARTGEN, INTELLIGEN, VALUGEN x-ray generators offer affordable prices as a result of using complete software control in a state of the art design. Designed by a team of service engineers for fast and easy installation and calibration.

Hcmi, Inc. 773-588-2444
2146 E Pythian St, Springfield, MO 65802
X-ray generator and control.

Linear Medical Corporation 303-962-5730
1130 W 124th Ave Ste 400, Westminster, CO 80234
X-ray generator unit.

Medimaging Tecnology, Inc. 800-244-9035
49 Herb Hill Rd, Glen Cove, NY 11542

Quantum Medical Imaging, Llc 631-567-5800
2002 Orville Dr N Ste B, Ronkonkoma, NY 11779
High-voltage x-ray generators.

Raymax Medical Corp. 905-791-3020
20 Strathearn Ave, Unit 3, Brampton, ONT L6T 4P7 Canada
Generator-single phase 360 ma unit

Shimadzu Medical Systems 800-228-1429
20101 S Vermont Ave, Torrance, CA 90502
2 models, 150 kVp, 500 mA, 50 KW ratings, UD150L-30 and UD150LF.

Spellman High Voltage Electronics Corp. 631-630-3000
475 Wireless Blvd, Hauppauge, NY 11788
High-voltage generator

Xma (X-Ray Marketing Associates, Inc.) 800-325-8880
1205 W Lakeview Ct, Windham Lakes Business Park
Romeoville, IL 60446

GENERATOR, ELECTRONIC NOISE (FOR AUDIOMETRIC TESTING) *(Ear/Nose/Throat) 77ETS*

Simpson Electric Co. 715-588-3311
520 Simpson Ave, PO Box 99, Lac Du Flambeau, WI 54538
$715.90 for dosimeter system, noise.

GENERATOR, GAS, MICROBIOLOGY *(Microbiology) 83KZJ*

Air Liquide America Specialty Gases Llc 713-402-2152
1311 New Savannah Rd, Augusta, GA 30901

Bd Diagnostic Systems 800-675-0908
7 Loveton Cir, Sparks, MD 21152

Oxoid, Inc. 800-567-8378
800 Proctor Ave, Ogdensburg, NY 13669
Anaerobic micro-aerophilic, carbon dioxide.

GENERATOR, IONIZED AIR *(Anesthesiology) 73RCO*

Julie Industries, Inc 978-276-0820
PO Box 153, North Reading, MA 01864
Hurricane 300 dual fan, extended range ionizing air blower delivers 300 CFM of ionized air, 115 volt 50/60 hz.

GENERATOR, OXYGEN, PORTABLE *(Anesthesiology) 73CAW*

Carleton Life Support Systems Inc. 563-383-6204
2734 Hickory Grove Rd, Davenport, IA 52804
Oxygen concentrator.

Glenn Medical Systems, Inc. 330-453-1177
511 12th St NE, Canton, OH 44704
Oxygen generator.

Igs Generon Americas 713-937-5200
11985 FM 529 Rd, Houston, TX 77041
Oxygen generator.

GENERATOR, OXYGEN, PORTABLE *(cont'd)*

Inogen, Inc. 805-562-0500
326 Bollay Dr, Goleta, CA 93117
Inogen one oxygen concentrator.

On Site Gas Systems, Inc. 888-748-3429
35 Budney Rd, Newington, CT 06111
Oxygen generator.

Oxair Ltd. 716-298-8288
8320 Quarry Rd, Niagara Falls, NY 14304
Various models of oxygen generators systems.

Oxlife Llc 828-684-7353
141 Twin Springs Rd, Hendersonville, NC 28792
Oxygen concentrator.

Pacific Consolidated Industries, Llc 951-479-0872
12201 Magnolia Ave, Riverside, CA 92503
Deployable oxygen concetration system (doc s).

Sequal Technologies Inc. 800-826-4610
11436 Sorrento Valley Rd, San Diego, CA 92121
Portable oxygen concentrators

Sparton Medical Systems 440-878-4630
22740 Lunn Rd, Strongsville, OH 44149
Portable oxygen generator.

Tennessee Medical Equipment, Inc. 731-635-2119
4637 Highway 19 E, Ripley, TN 38063
Various.

GENERATOR, OZONE *(Anesthesiology) 73RJR*

Bhk, Inc. 909-983-2973
1480 N Claremont Blvd, Claremont, CA 91711
Standard and custom 185-nm generating mercury lamps for efficient generation of ozone in air or water.

Fuller Ultraviolet Corp. 815-469-3301
9416 Gulfstream Rd, Frankfort, IL 60423
$500.00 per unit (standard).

GENERATOR, POWER, ELECTROSURGICAL *(Surgery) 79SHL*

Coopersurgical, Inc. 800-243-2974
95 Corporate Dr, Trumbull, CT 06611
Five output waveforms, three cutting modes, and two coagulating modes. 180-watt maximum cutting power, 90-watt maximum coagulating power.

Ellman International, Inc. 800-835-5355
3333 Royal Ave, Rockville Centre, NY 11572

Gyrus Medical, Inc. 800-852-9361
6655 Wedgwood Rd N Ste 105, Maple Grove, MN 55311

Md International, Inc. 305-669-9003
11300 NW 41st St, Doral, FL 33178

Richard Wolf Medical Instruments Corp. 800-323-9653
353 Corporate Woods Pkwy, Vernon Hills, IL 60061

GENERATOR, PULSATILE FLOW, CARDIOPULMONARY BYPASS *(Cardiovascular) 74JOR*

Jayza Corp. 305-477-1136
7215 NW 41st St Ste A, Miami, FL 33166

Medtronic, Inc. 800-633-8766
710 Medtronic Pkwy, Minneapolis, MN 55432

Terumo Cardiovascular Systems, Corp 800-521-2818
6200 Jackson Rd, Ann Arbor, MI 48103

GENERATOR, RADIOFREQUENCY LESION *(Cns/Neurology) 84GXD*

Angiodynamics, Inc. 510-771-0400
46421 Landing Pkwy, Fremont, CA 94538
The new RITA Model 1500X Generator provides more power than ever before, for larger, faster ablations. It also offers additional numerous independent temperature displays, and a simple, intuitive panel design for ease of use. As always, RITA provides automatic temperature control and micro infusion for more predictable, controllable ablations in a single session. For use in percutaneous, laparoscopic, or open procedures. Compatible with the latest RITA devices - the Starburst XLi, Starburst XL, Starburst Semi-Flex, and Starburst SDE for ablations of up to 7 cm. Ablations have never been easier.

Ballard Medical Products 770-587-7835
12050 Lone Peak Pkwy, Draper, UT 84020
Disposable, dispersive pads.

Diros Technology, Inc. 905-415-3440
232 Hood Road, Markham, ON L3R 3K8 Canada
OWL Universal RF System

GENERATOR, RADIOFREQUENCY LESION *(cont'd)*

Engineering & Research Assoc., Inc. (D.B.A. Sebra) 800-625-5550
100 N Tucson Blvd, Tucson, AZ 85716
RF GENERATOR, high power radio frequency generators for the medical manufacturing industry.

Neurotherm Inc. 978-777-3916
2 De Bush Ave, Middleton, MA 01949
Rf lesion generator system.

Oscor, Inc. 800-726-7267
3816 Desoto Blvd, Palm Harbor, FL 34683
RF generator.

Respiratory Diagnostics, Inc. 425-881-8300
47987 Fremont Blvd, Fremont, CA 94538
Rf generator.

GENERATOR, RADIOGRAPHIC, CAPACITOR DISCHARGE *(Radiology) 90IZR*

Xma (X-Ray Marketing Associates, Inc.) 800-325-8880
1205 W Lakeview Ct, Windham Lakes Business Park
Romeoville, IL 60446

GENETIC ENGINEERING *(Microbiology) 83UGH*

Applied Biosystems 800-345-5724
850 Lincoln Centre Dr, Foster City, CA 94404
DNA sequence analyzers and DNA and RNA separation systems.

Avi Biopharma, Inc. 503-227-0554
4575 SW Research Way Ste 200, Corvallis, OR 97333
Oligonucleotides.

Enzo Biochem, Inc. 212-583-0100
527 Madison Ave, New York, NY 10022
Non-radioactive DNA labeling and detection.

Interferon Sciences, Inc. 888-728-4372
783 Jersey Ave, New Brunswick, NJ 08901
Interferon.

Koaman International 909-983-4888
656 E D St, Ontario, CA 91764

Var-Lac-Oid Chemical Co., Inc. 201-387-0038
13 Foster St, Bergenfield, NJ 07621
Cesium chloride, osmium tetroxide, RNA purified/free of calcium/sodium.

Zeptometrix Corporation 800-274-5487
872 Main St, Buffalo, NY 14202
Recombinant IL-2, RETRO-TEK HTLV-1 P19 ELISA kit, RETRO-TEK HIV-1 P24 Antigen Elisa, SIV P27 Antigen Elisa. MONOBODY anti-P19 to HTLV-1 core protein. All tests for research use only.

GERM-FREE APPARATUS *(Microbiology) 83UGI*

Aramark Clean Room Services 800-759-0102
7650 Grant St., Hinsdale, IL 60521

Technh, Inc 603-424-4404
8 Continental Blvd, PO Box 476, Merrimack, NH 03054

GIARDIA SPP. *(Microbiology) 83MHI*

Antibodies, Inc. 800-824-8540
PO Box 1560, Davis, CA 95617
Giardia lamblia diagnostic test kit for detection from fresh stool samples.

Biosite Incorporated 888-246-7483
9975 Summers Ridge Rd, San Diego, CA 92121
Enzyme immunoassay for detection of giardia lamblia, entamoeba histolyticaldispa.

Genzyme Diagnostics 617-252-7500
6659 Top Gun St, San Diego, CA 92121
Immunoassay for giardia and cryptosporidium antigen.

Ivd Research, Inc. 760-929-7744
5909 Sea Lion Pl Ste D, Carlsbad, CA 92010
Giardia stool antigen elisa.

Wampole Laboratories 800-257-9525
2 Research Way, Princeton, NJ 08540
Enteric disease diagnostic assays.

GLOVE, AUTOPSY *(Pathology) 88QYH*

Cms Worldwide, Inc. 800-426-4633
30011 Ivy Glenn Dr Ste 215, Laguna Niguel, CA 92677
Autopsy gloves, latex; sizes S, M, L, XL. 17 mil. 12 in. or 14 in. cuff length.

GLOVE, AUTOPSY *(cont'd)*

Howard Medical Company 800-443-1444
1690 N Elston Ave, Chicago, IL 60642
sized, hand specific, 10.5 mil in palm, non sterile, 12 inch beaded cuff

Pm Gloves, Inc. 800-788-9486
13808 Magnolia Ave, Chino, CA 91710
Vinyl and latex.

Sterling Rubber Company 519-843-4032
675 Woodside St., Fergus, ONT N1M 2M4 Canada
STERLING 3600 post mortem gloves. Non-sterile latex gloves, extra thick.

GLOVE, OTHER *(General) 80QYK*

Adi Medical Division Of Asia Dynamics (Group) Inc. 877-647-7699
1565 S Shields Dr, Waukegan, IL 60085

American Health Products Corporation 800-828-2964
80 Internationale Blvd Unit A, Glendale Heights, IL 60139
SAFEPREP food service disposable gloves and heavy duty gloves.

Ansell Protective Products 800-800-0444
200 Schulz Dr, Red Bank, NJ 07701
NITRA-TOUCH powder-free disposable nitrile glove.

Armin Poly-Version, Inc. 516-481-7775
564 Warren Blvd, Garden City, NY 11530

Baldur Systems Corporation 800-736-4716
33235 Transit Ave, Union City, CA 94587
Glove, patient examination, latex, powder-free.

Berghof/America 800-544-5004
3773 NW 126th Ave Bldg 1, Coral Springs, FL 33065
Teflon coated laboratory gloves available in 11in. or 24in. sizes.

Best Manufacturing Co. 800-241-0323
579 Edison St, PO Box 8, Menlo, GA 30731
100% Nitrile, low-modulus disposable glove. Contains no natural rubber proteins. Class 1 medical device for examination.

Brain Power, Inc. 800-327-2250
4470 SW 74th Ave, Miami, FL 33155
$54.95 for Safety Gloves #83000, 6 pack--for protection from dyes, acetone, and chemicals. Sheer, liquid-proof stretch vinyl developed specially for the optical industry.

Chagrin Safety Supply, Inc. 800-227-0468
8227 Washington St # 1, Chagrin Falls, OH 44023

Clean Esd Products, Inc. 510-257-5080
48340 Milmont Dr, Fremont, CA 94538
ABSORBIE 100 percent cotton gloves, ABSORBIE nylon glove liner available in partial finger.

Cms Worldwide, Inc. 800-426-4633
30011 Ivy Glenn Dr Ste 215, Laguna Niguel, CA 92677
High-Risk Safety Examination Gloves. Blue, 15 mil thickness, 12 in. cuff, size S, M, L, & XL. Powdered and powder free. NFPA certification. Nitrile exam gloves, blue, 4mil; sizes XS, S, M, L, XL, XXL. Nitrile safety exam gloves, powder-free, blue, 8mil thick, 12 in. cuff length; sizes S, M, L, XL, XXL.

Edmund Industrial Optics 800-363-1992
101 E Gloucester Pike, Barrington, NJ 08007
For the handling optics.

Exelint International Co. 800-940-3935
5840 W Centinela Ave, Los Angeles, CA 90045
Vinyl, latex, procedure (non-sterile).

Gallimore Healthcare Inc. 800-387-0208
#23A Railside Rd., Toronto, ONT M3A-1B2 Canada
Rubber, latex, vinyl, and nitrile gloves.

Gammadirect Medical Division 847-267-5929
PO Box 383, Lake Forest, IL 60045
Promit seamless nylon gloves are ideal as a liner for latex gloves. They are hydroscopic, super comfortable and reuseable.

General Scientific Safety Equipment Co. 800-523-0166
2553 E Somerset St Fl 1, Philadelphia, PA 19134

George Glove Company, Inc. 800-631-4292
301 Greenwood Ave, Midland Park, NJ 07432

Hatch Corporation 800-347-1200
42374 Avenida Alvarado Ste A, Temecula, CA 92590
Large variety of wheelchair gloves, push gloves, padded palm and finger gloves, 1/2-finger mesh back gloves, and more. Edema gloves made of nylon Lycra for support, available in 3/4 or full finger, also Cryo-Pak for the carpal nerve. Quad Push Gloves designed for quadriplegics and wheelchair users. The entire glove surface is a durable non-slip rubber which wears well and increases gripping and breaking.

GLOVE, OTHER *(cont'd)*

Hospira 800-441-4100
268 E 4th St, Ashland, OH 44805
Specialty gloves.

International Hospital Supply Co. 800-398-9450
6914 Canby Ave Ste 105, Reseda, CA 91335
Sterilie, surgeon's, latex-free, vinyl, non-sterilie exam, latex, latex-free vinyl.

Johnson & Johnson Medical Division Of Ethicon, Inc. 800-423-4018
2500 E Arbrook Blvd, Arlington, TX 76014

Lee Medical International, Inc. 800-433-8950
612 Distributors Row, Harahan, LA 70123
Latex, nitrile, vinyl.

Liberty Industries, Inc. 800-828-5656
133 Commerce St, East Berlin, CT 06023
Various styles available.

Lohmann & Rauscher, Inc. 800-279-3863
6001 SW 6th Ave Ste 101, Topeka, KS 66615

Love Imports 800-944-5523
PO Box 759, Grapeland, TX 75844
Very lightly powdered white latex and latex heavy blue safety gloves.

Ludlow Technological Products 800-445-5025
2 Ludlow Park Dr, Chicopee, MA 01022

Medco Supply Company 800-556-3326
500 Fillmore Ave, Tonawanda, NY 14150
Protective gloves. Latex and latex free.

Medikmark Inc. 800-424-8520
3600 Burwood Dr, Waukegan, IL 60085
Fluoroscopic procedure gloves.

Mi-Co Company 516-481-7775
564 Warren Blvd, Garden City, NY 11530
Disposable, copolymer gloves laminated on paper.

Microflex Corporation 800-876-6866
PO Box 32000, 2301 Robb Drive,, Reno, NV 89533
EVOLUTION ONE powder-free laboratory gloves. EVOLUTION ONE gloves are virtually allergen free and can be stretched to as much as 700% of their original size without damage, significantly reducing the risk of stress-related tearing. DIAMOND GRIP powder-free gloves can be used in the hospital, dental clinic, ambulance, and beyond. MICRO ONE is 20% heavier and stronger than other gloves in its class, for greater protection. TECH ONE is the leading choice among dental offices because of its durable and premium grade low modulus latex. POWERGRIP has rugged durability, a textured grip and is affordable. COLOR TOUCH is color-coded by size, has a textured grip, superior sensitivity, and is made of low modulus latex/low powder. ULTRA ONE has high-risk protection, an extra-long reinforced cuff, superior tactile sensitivity, is powder-free and ultra-durable. SAFEGRIP is powder-free, and provides high-risk protection and a micro-rough surface. SYNETRON is powder-free and has tactile sensitivity.

Newtex Industries, Inc. 585-924-9135
8050 Victor Mendon Rd, Victor, NY 14564
ZETEX gloves and mittens; ZETEX PLUS gloves and mittens, high temperature applications (1100-2000 degrees F). Sized 11', 14', and 23'. Special fabrication per customer specifications available. Zetex & Zetex Plus Gloves are now CE Approved

Perfect Fit Glove 800-245-6837
85 Innsbruck Dr, Buffalo, NY 14227

Pharaoh Trading Company 866-929-4913
9701 Brookpark Rd, Knollwood Plaza, Suite 241, Cleveland, OH 44129
Polyethylene gloves.

Pm Gloves, Inc. 800-788-9486
13808 Magnolia Ave, Chino, CA 91710
powder free synthetic gloves.

Polyzen, Inc. 919-319-9599
1041 Classic Rd, Apex, NC 27539
Custom radiopaque gloves for fluoroscopy and X-ray.

Postcraft Co. 800-528-4844
625 W Rillito St, Tucson, AZ 85705
Vinyl all purpose gloves.

Silverstone Packaging, Inc.-Your One Stop Supplier 800-413-1108
1401 Lakeland Ave, Bohemia, NY 11716

Sterling Rubber Company 519-843-4032
675 Woodside St., Fergus, ONT N1M 2M4 Canada
STERLING 2600 lab gloves, non-sterile, latex.

GLOVE, OTHER *(cont'd)*

Washington Trade International, Inc. 800-327-3379
2633 Willamette Dr NE, Lacey, WA 98516
Variety of other Latex, Nitrile, Vinyl, Chloreprene Surgical, or Industrial Gloves.

World Medical Supply Usa., Inc. 800-545-5475
150 Marseille Dr, PRISTINE GLOVES, Maumelle, AR 72113
PRISTINE powder-free sterile surgical gloves for general, microsurgical, and ophthalmic surgery.

GLOVE, PATIENT EXAMINATION *(General) 80FMC*

Adex Medical, Inc. 800-873-4776
6101 Quail Valley Ct, Riverside, CA 92507
Latex, Vinyl, Nitrile, Examination gloves.

Adi Medical Division Of Asia Dynamics (Group) Inc. 877-647-7699
1565 S Shields Dr, Waukegan, IL 60085

American Health Products Corporation 800-828-2964
80 Internationale Blvd Unit A, Glendale Heights, IL 60139
DERMASAFE Powdered and Powder Free Latex examination gloves, Powdered and Powder Free Synthetic examination gloves, Powder Free Nitrile, Specialty (EMS) gloves, customer kits and Private Labels.

Awi Industries (Usa), Inc. 909-597-0808
14502 Central Ave, Chino, CA 91710
Powdered and latex.

Baldur Systems Corporation 800-736-4716
33235 Transit Ave, Union City, CA 94587
BALDUR powder-free nitrile, ambidextrous, non-sterile, textured surface. Comes in 5 sizes: XS, S, M, L, XL. Available 100 pieces per box, 10 boxes per case.

Best Manufacturing Co.(Fayette Division) 706-862-6712
931 2nd Ave SE, Fayette, AL 35555
Disposable nitrile gloves.

Bibbero Systems, Inc. 800-242-2376
1300 N McDowell Blvd, Petaluma, CA 94954
Patient examination gloves available in latex, safety/high risk latex and synthetic latex FREE. Sizes from small to large.

Bio-Flex International, Inc. 800-755-4588
1250 E Hallandale Beach Blvd PH 1, Hallandale Beach, FL 33009
Latex gloves, synthetic gloves.

Carl Heyer, Inc. 800-284-5550
1872 Bellmore Ave, North Bellmore, NY 11710

Central Paper Products Company 800-339-4065
PO Box 4480, Manchester, NH 03108
Latex examination gloves.

Clean Esd Products, Inc. 510-257-5080
48340 Milmont Dr, Fremont, CA 94538
ULTRA-TOUCH 1112, lightly powdered 9-inch gloves. Also, 1401, regular surface, powder-free 9-inch gloves.

Coast Scientific 800-445-1544
1445 Engineer St, Vista, CA 92081
Lightly powdered and powder free Nitrile examination gloves. High Risk latex examination gloves, 12' in length.

Crosstex International 800-223-2497
10 Ranick Rd, Hauppauge, NY 11788
Lightly Powdered & Powderfree

Crosstex International Ltd., W. Region 800-707-2737
14059 Stage Rd, Santa Fe Springs, CA 90670

Crosstex International,Inc. 888-276-7783
10 Ranick Rd, Hauppauge, NY 11788
CLASSIC, OMEGA, LEFT/RIGHT FITTED, ULTIMATE, ULTRAPLUS.

Dash Medical Gloves, Inc. 800-523-2055
10180 S 54th St, Franklin, WI 53132
Powder free gloves.

Davis Lead Apron, Inc. 800-483-3979
4560 W 34th St, PO Box 924585, Houston, TX 77092
Gloves for Radiology Protection

Delta Gloves 800-220-1262
6865 Shiloh Rd E Ste 400, Alpharetta, GA 30005
EZ-CARE, Delta's new powder free stretch vinyl gloves offer users an affordable alternative to latex exam gloves. Delta's CARE FREE NITREX glove continues to provide users with unsurpassed tactile sensitivity and dexterity without compromising fit or feel.

Digitcare Corporation 888-287-2990
2999 Overland Ave Ste 209, Los Angeles, CA 90064

GLOVE, PATIENT EXAMINATION *(cont'd)*

Dixie Ems Supply 800-347-3494
385 Union Ave, Brooklyn, NY 11211
$39.50 per 1000 (latex, med).

Dma Med-Chem Corporation 800-362-1833
49 Watermill Ln, Great Neck, NY 11021

East Atlantic Trading/Triangle Healthcare Inc. 800-243-4635
76 National Rd, Edison, NJ 08817
Triangle Tropics: Latex exam gloves, vinyl exam gloves, nitrile exam gloves, gauze sponges, isolation gown, bouffant caps, mask (pleated earloop and cone).

Eci Medical Technologies, Inc. 800-668-5289
2 Cook Rd., Bridgewater, NS B4V 3W7 Canada
ELASTYREN Synthetic Examination Glove. ELASTYLITE Synthetic Examination Glove. ELASTYPLUS Synthetic Examination Glove, powder-free.

Global Concepts, Ltd. 818-363-7195
19464 Eagle Ridge Ln, Northridge, CA 91326

Healer Products, Llc 914-663-6300
427 Commerce Ln Ste 1, West Berlin, NJ 08091
Nitrile gloves.

Hospital Therapy Products, Inc. 630-766-7101
757 N Central Ave, Wood Dale, IL 60191
Various sizes gloves.

Intermed Supplies 800-766-3131
7115 Belgold St Ste E, Houston, TX 77066
Latex examination gloves.

Invacare Supply Group, An Invacare Co. 800-225-4792
75 October Hill Rd, Holliston, MA 01746
Carry full line of Invacare brand examination gloves.

Johnson & Johnson Medical Division Of Ethicon, Inc. 800-423-4018
2500 E Arbrook Blvd, Arlington, TX 76014

Kern Surgical Supply, Inc. 800-582-3939
2823 Gibson St, Bakersfield, CA 93308

Lab Safety Supply, Inc. 800-356-0783
401 S Wright Rd, Janesville, WI 53546

Life Guard 626-965-1588
18400 San Jose Ave, City Of Industry, CA 91748
Latex Exam Gloves provides best form fit and reduces hand fatigue. Available in powdered and powder free versions.

Love Imports 800-944-5523
PO Box 759, Grapeland, TX 75844
Very lightly powdered vinyl gloves.

Mckesson General Medical 800-446-3008
8741 Landmark Rd, Richmond, VA 23228

Medspring Group, Inc. 801-295-9750
533 W 2600 S Ste 105, Bountiful, UT 84010
Patient examination glove.

Mexpo International, Inc. 800-838-8299
2695B McCone Ave, Hayward, CA 94545
BLOSSOM, DISCOVERY 2020, SUPERGLOVES, and HORIZON: latex, vinyl, and nitrite examination gloves. Patent-pending gloves: BLOSSOM Latex Powder Free with Aloe Vera, BLOSSOM Latex Powder Free with Aloe Vera + Vitamin E, and BLOSSOM Nitrile Powder Free with Aloe Vera.

Miami Medical Equipment & Supply Corp. 305-592-0111
2150 NW 93rd Ave, Doral, FL 33172

Neogen Corporation 800-234-5333
620 Lesher Pl, Lansing, MI 48912
Also make gloves for veterinary use

Nova Health Products, Llc 843-673-0702
1138 Annelle Dr, Florence, SC 29505
Disposable gloves used in patient examination by doctors.

O&M Enterprise 847-258-4515
641 Chelmsford Ln, Elk Grove Village, IL 60007
GLOVES EXAMINATION LATEX/NON LATEX

Omni Medical Supply Inc. 800-860-6664
4153 Pioneer Dr, Commerce Township, MI 48390

Pacifica Gloves 800-635-4430
1709 E Del Amo Blvd, West Coast Distribution, Carson, CA 90746
PACIFICA vinyl, non-sterile latex gloves.

Pm Gloves, Inc. 800-788-9486
13808 Magnolia Ave, Chino, CA 91710
Vinyl and latex gloves, powdered and powder free.

GLOVE, PATIENT EXAMINATION *(cont'd)*

Quantum Labs, Inc. 800-328-8213
452 Northco Dr Ste 180, Minneapolis, MN 55432

Ross Disposable Products 800-649-6526
401 Traders Blvd E, Unit 10, Mississauga, ON L4Z 2H8 Canada

Sanax Protective Products, Inc. 800-379-9929
236 Upland Ave, Newton Highlands, MA 02461

Scientimed Corp. 510-763-5405
4109 Balfour Ave, Oakland, CA 94610
Examination gloves.

Sempermed Corp. 800-366-9545
13900 49th St N, Clearwater, FL 33762
SEMPERCARE powder-free nitrile exam glove.

Shepard Medical Products 800-354-5683
260 E Lies Rd, Carol Stream, IL 60188

Supertex Industrial, S.A. De C.V. 656-65-57
Carretera a Bosques De San, Isidro # 1136, Zapopan, Jalisco Mexico
Patient examination gloves

Technical Marketing, Inc. 954-370-0855
1776 N Pine Island Rd Ste 306, Plantation, FL 33322
2,000 ambidextrous gloves per case; small, medium and large sizes.

Tg Medical Usa Inc. 626-969-7838
165 N Aspan Ave, TG Medical USA Inc., Azusa, CA 91702
Glove, patient examination, latex, vinyl. Available in extra small, small, medium and large.

Tronex Healthcare Industries 800-833-1181
2 Cranberry Rd, One Tronex Centre, Parsippany, NJ 07054
TRONEX The Choice Nitrile gloves are non-sterile, non-latex and powder free. Six mil thick, high resistance to punctures and chemicals. Ultra low modulus, excellent manual dexterity, sensitivity, and comfort. Small to X-large. ASTM standards, FDA 510(k) A.Q.L. = 1.5

Wehmer Corporation 800-323-0229
1151 N Main St, Lombard, IL 60148
$5.95 per box of 100 latex examination gloves. Also powder free latex.

GLOVE, PATIENT EXAMINATION, LATEX *(General) 80LYY*

Adenna Inc. 888-323-3662
11932 Baker Pl, Santa Fe Springs, CA 90670
Powder free, low protein, textured and smooth surfaces, powdered, etc.

Adi Medical Division Of Asia Dynamics (Group) Inc. 877-647-7699
1565 S Shields Dr, Waukegan, IL 60085

Alimed, Inc. 800-225-2610
297 High St, Dedham, MA 02026

Ambiderm, S.A. De C.V. 800-800-8008
Carr. A Bosques De San Isidro 1136, Col. Bosques De San Isidro Zapopan, Jalisco 45147 Mexico
Surgical and exam latex gloves, also available in different colors.

American Bantex Corp. 800-633-4839
1815 Rollins Rd, Burlingame, CA 94010

American Healthcare Products, Inc. 888-784-1888
1068 Westminster Ave, Alhambra, CA 91803
Manufacturer of the UNISEAL line of latex, vinyl, and nitrile gloves. UNISEAL gloves are available in powdered and powder-free versions and are designed in a variety of lengths and thickness to meet the most demanding requirements of any medical professional. UNISEAL PRODERMA, low-protein, hypoallergenic, powdered, latex gloves. UNISEAL SUREGRIP, low-protein, textured powder-free latex gloves. UNISEAL NITRILE, powdered and powder-free synthetic exam gloves. UNISEAL, safety powder-free, 10 MIL, 12-in. cuff, textured latex exam gloves. UNISEAL High-Risk (Blue) powder-free, 15 MIL, 12-in. cuff, textured exam gloves. UNISEAL SUR-G-GLOVE, sterilized surgical gloves. UNISEAL Sensiflex powder-free, low-protein, sterilized surgical gloves.

Ammex Corp. 800-274-7354
18375 Olympic Ave S, Tukwila, WA 98188

Armstrong Medical Industries, Inc. 800-323-4220
575 Knightsbridge Pkwy, Lincolnshire, IL 60069

Associated Production Services, Inc. 215-364-0211
365 Andrews Rd, Trevose, PA 19053
Latex glove.

GLOVE, PATIENT EXAMINATION, LATEX *(cont'd)*

Baldur Systems Corporation 800-736-4716
33235 Transit Ave, Union City, CA 94587
Glove, patient examination, vinyl powder-free BALDUR in 5 sizes, 100% powder-free vinyl, latex free, ambidextrous, non-sterile, smooth surface (x-s,s,m,l,x-l). Available 100 pieces per box, 10 boxes per case.

Bankier Companies, Inc. 847-647-6565
6151 W Gross Point Rd, Niles, IL 60714
Glove, patient examination, latex.

Best Manufacturing Co.(Fayette Division) 706-862-6712
931 2nd Ave SE, Fayette, AL 35555
Various types of non-sterile including nitrile examination gloves.

Bio-Flex International, Inc. 800-755-4588
1250 E Hallandale Beach Blvd PH 1, Hallandale Beach, FL 33009

C & K Manufacturing & Sales 800-821-7795
28825 Ranney Pkwy, Westlake, OH 44145
Latex medical gloves.

Chagrin Safety Supply, Inc. 800-227-0468
8227 Washington St # 1, Chagrin Falls, OH 44023

Cms Worldwide, Inc. 800-426-4633
30011 Ivy Glenn Dr Ste 215, Laguna Niguel, CA 92677
Latex Exam Gloves, powdered and powder free. Sizes XS, S, M, L, XL, XXL. ISO 9002. AQL1.5. CE. OEM and Private Label Specialists.

Coast Scientific 800-445-1544
1445 Engineer St, Vista, CA 92081
Lightly powdered and powder free.

Crosstex International Ltd., W. Region 800-707-2737
14059 Stage Rd, Santa Fe Springs, CA 90670

Cypress Medical Products 800-334-3646
1202 S. Rte. 31, McHenry, IL 60050
Available in small, medium, and large. 100 per box, 10 boxes per case. Powder-free or hypoallergenic latex gloves available in small, medium and large, 100 per box, 10 boxes per case.

Dash Medical Gloves, Inc. 800-523-2055
10180 S 54th St, Franklin, WI 53132

Delta Gloves 800-220-1262
6865 Shiloh Rd E Ste 400, Alpharetta, GA 30005
DELTA's FMT Series Powder Free Latex Exam Glove offers users unsurpassed tactile sensitivity through its unique polymer coating technology.

Demetech Corp. 888-324-2447
3530 NW 115th Ave, Doral, FL 33178
Disposable latex gloves.

Digitcare Corporation 888-287-2990
2999 Overland Ave Ste 209, Los Angeles, CA 90064

Dynarex Corp. 888-356-2739
10 Glenshaw St, Orangeburg, NY 10962
Available in three sizes, ambidextrous with beaded cuff.

East Atlantic Trading/Triangle Healthcare Inc. 800-243-4635
76 National Rd, Edison, NJ 08817

Genlee 650-697-5831
769 Morningside Dr, Millbrae, CA 94030
ARISTA patient exam gloves, vinyl, nitrile, powder and no powder, latex.

Healer Products, Llc 914-663-6300
427 Commerce Ln Ste 1, West Berlin, NJ 08091
Latex gloves.

Health Care Logistics, Inc. 800-848-1633
450 Town St, PO Box 25, Circleville, OH 43113
Various.

Healthco International, Llc 603-255-4200
2000 Cold Spring Rd, Dixville Notch, Dixville, NH 03576
Latex patient medical examination gloves.

In Disposables Inc. 800-269-4568
PO Box 528, Stratford, CT 06615
Malaysian exam gloves, sizes in x-small, small, medium, large, x-large. Very lightly powdered, non-powdered available.

Inamco International Corp. 800-724-4003
801 Montrose Ave, South Plainfield, NJ 07080

Intermed Supplies 800-766-3131
7115 Belgold St Ste E, Houston, TX 77066

Jaisons International, Inc. 203-261-1653
22 Bittersweet Ln, Trumbull, CT 06611
ULTRA Touch.

GLOVE, PATIENT EXAMINATION, LATEX *(cont'd)*

Johnson & Johnson Medical Division Of Ethicon, Inc. 800-423-4018
2500 E Arbrook Blvd, Arlington, TX 76014

Life Guard 626-965-1588
18400 San Jose Ave, City Of Industry, CA 91748
Nitrile Exam Powder & Powder Free Gloves; 100% nitrile gloves provide the superb latex free hand protection.

Lmr International, Inc. 334-687-4610
1600 State Docks Rd, Eufaula, AL 36027

Love Imports 800-944-5523
PO Box 759, Grapeland, TX 75844
Very lightly powdered or powder-free.

Maytex Corp. 800-462-9839
23521 Foley St, Hayward, CA 94545
Synthetic

Medical Action Industries, Inc. 800-645-7042
25 Heywood Rd, Arden, NC 28704
Glove.

Medicos Laboratories, Inc. (Mdt) 800-724-4003
801 Montrose Ave, South Plainfield, NJ 07080

Mi-Co Company 516-481-7775
564 Warren Blvd, Garden City, NY 11530

Microflex Corporation 800-876-6866
PO Box 32000, 2301 Robb Drive,, Reno, NV 89533
A leading provider of latex and synthetic examination gloves.

Midwest Scientific 800-227-9997
280 Vance Rd, Valley Park, MO 63088
Latex exam gloves - $10.95 per box of 100 powderless, $8.95 per box of 100 with light powder.

Mydent International 800-275-0020
80 Suffolk Ct, Hauppauge, NY 11788
DEFEND hypoallergenic, ADA professionally recognized, sizes: xs, s, m, & l. DEFEND powder-free latex exam glove. Chlorinated process removes all powder. Textured finish for sure grip.

Normed 800-288-8200
PO Box 3644, Seattle, WA 98124
Exam gloves, latex.

North Safety Products 401-943-4400
1101 B Calle Neutron, Parque Industrial Maran, Mexicali, B.c. Mexico
Disposable gloves

Norwood Promotional Products, Inc. 651-388-1298
5151 Moundview Dr, Red Wing, MN 55066
Latex gloves.

Pharaoh Trading Company 866-929-4913
9701 Brookpark Rd, Knollwood Plaza, Suite 241, Cleveland, OH 44129

Pm Gloves, Inc. 800-788-9486
13808 Magnolia Ave, Chino, CA 91710
Premium quality latex exam gloves, lightly powdered & powder free.

Raymar Medical Corp. 216-475-8360
16360 Broadway Ave, Cleveland, OH 44137
Latex examination gloves.

Royal Paper Products, Inc. 800-666-6655
PO Box 151, Coatesville, PA 19320
Exam Grade Latex Gloves, lightly powdered & powder free latex, available in small-medium-large-Xlarge.

S.S. White Burs Inc. 800-535-2877
1145 Towbin Ave, Lakewood, NJ 08701
Latex gloves that are disposable with or without powder. Non-sterile, available in XS, S, M, L.

Sempermed Corp. 800-366-9545
13900 49th St N, Clearwater, FL 33762
POLYMED powder-free latex exam glove.

Shinemound Enterprise, Inc. 978-436-9980
17A Sterling Rd, North Billerica, MA 01862

Tg Medical Usa Inc. 626-969-7838
165 N Aspan Ave, TG Medical USA Inc., Azusa, CA 91702
Available in extra-small, small, medium, and large.

GLOVE, PATIENT EXAMINATION, LATEX *(cont'd)*

Tillotson Healthcare Corp. 888-335-7500
10 Glenshaw St, Orangeburg, NY 10962
FORMULA ONE sterile or non-sterile; polymer lined lightly powdered; low modulus; natural rubber latex; patient examination glove made from Allotex enzyme treated natural rubber latex. Contains (10ug per gram of protein. ULTRA CARE/ULTRA CARE 2, non-sterile; powder free polymer lined; low modulus; natural rubber latex; patient examination glove made from Allotex enzyme treated natural latex. Contains (10ug per gram of protein. DENTAL CARE, nonsterile; powder free polymer lined; low modulus; natural rubber latex; patient examination glove made from Allotex enzyme treated natural rubber latex. Contains (10ug per gram of protein. SENSI GRIP, non-sterile; lightly powdered with USP absorbable dusting powder; bisque finish; natural rubber latex; patient examination glove. Contains (200ug per gram of protein. HPI SIZED MEDICAL, non-sterile; powdered with USP absorbable dusting powder; natural rubber latex; patient examination glove. Sized left and right. POWDER FREE PLUS, non-sterile; powder free; non-chlorinated-siliconized; bisque finish; natural rubber latex; patient examination glove. Contains (50ug per gram of protein. ENTRUST, non-sterile; powder free; chlorinated-polymer lined; bisque finish; natural rubber latex; patient examination glove. Contains (50ug per gram of protein. ACCU TOUCH, non-sterile, powder free; non-chlorinated-polymer lined; microtextrured; natural rubber latex; patient examination glove. Contains (50ug per gram of protein. PRESERVE WITH ALOE VERA, non-sterile, powder free; non-chlorinated-polymer lined; aloe vera inner lining; natural rubber latex; patient examination glove. Contains(50ug per gram of protein. ULTRA PRESERVE WITH ALOE VERA, non-sterile, powder free; non-cholrinated-polymer lined; aloe vera inner lining; green colored; natural rubber latex; patient examintaion glove made from Allotex enzyme treated natural rubber latex. No starch added in manufacturing process; particulate content less than 2mg/dm2. SENSI GRIP LTC, non-sterile; lightly powdered with USP absorbable dusting powder; bisque finish; natural rubber latex; patient examination glove. Contains (200ug per gram of protein. SENSI GRIP LTC POWDER FREE, non-sterile; powder free; chlorinated; polymer inner lining and microtextured outer surface; natural rubber latex patient examintaion glove. Contains 200ug per gram of protein. MULTI CARE, non-sterile, powdered or powder free; poly vinyl chloride (PVC) patient examination glove. NEXT GENERATION VINYL, non-sterile, powder free; stretch poly vinyl chloride (PVC) patient examination glove.

Tillotson Rubber Co., Inc. 781-402-1731
59 Waters Ave, Everett, MA 02149
Various types of non-sterile including nitrile examination gloves.

Tradex International 800-456-8370
5300 Tradex Pkwy, Cleveland, OH 44102
Ambitex brand, non sterile, vinyl.

Tronex Healthcare Industries 800-833-1181
2 Cranberry Rd, One Tronex Centre, Parsippany, NJ 07054
TRONEX The Choice, non-sterile ADA certified. Premium quality, USP approved grade of cornstarch. Lightly and evenly powdered. ASTM, FDA 510(k)of 1.5. X-Small - X-Large. Other styles in double chlorinated Powder Free, Textured, Ultra textured, and High Risk.

Washington Trade International, Inc. 800-327-3379
2633 Willamette Dr NE, Lacey, WA 98516
UniSeal, lightly powdered and powder free.

Youngs, Inc. 800-523-5454
55 E Cherry Ln, Souderton, PA 18964

GLOVE, PATIENT EXAMINATION, POLY *(General) 80LZA*

Adex Medical, Inc. 800-873-4776
6101 Quail Valley Ct, Riverside, CA 92507
Powder free, Medical, small, medium & large 100pcs./box, 10 box/case.

Ammex Corp. 800-274-7354
18375 Olympic Ave S, Tukwila, WA 98188
Nitrite gloves--powder free; GlovePlus nitrite powder free; Glove, patient examination, nitrite.

Cms Worldwide, Inc. 800-426-4633
30011 Ivy Glenn Dr Ste 215, Laguna Niguel, CA 92677
Stretch-vinyl/polymer exam gloves, powdered and powder-free. Cream or white color. ISO9002, CE. Sizes XS, S, M, L, XL. OEM and Private Label Specialists.

Gammadirect Medical Division 847-267-5929
PO Box 383, Lake Forest, IL 60045
Aukuflex Exam Gloves, the first commerical polyurethane glove-improved tactile sensitivity.

GLOVE, PATIENT EXAMINATION, POLY *(cont'd)*

Healthco International, Llc 603-255-4200
2000 Cold Spring Rd, Dixville Notch, Dixville, NH 03576
Polymer patient medical examination gloves(powdered/powder free).

John J. Brogan, Inc. 908-859-2300
1161 3rd Ave, Alpha, NJ 08865
Clinical brand.

Normed 800-288-8200
PO Box 3644, Seattle, WA 98124
Exam gloves, vinyl.

Shinemound Enterprise, Inc. 978-436-9980
17A Sterling Rd, North Billerica, MA 01862

Tillotson Healthcare Corp. 888-335-7500
10 Glenshaw St, Orangeburg, NY 10962
PURE ADVANTAGE, non-sterile; hypoallergic; powdered or powder free; thermal responsive nitrile patient examiniation gloves. DUAL ADVANTAGE, non-sterile; hypoallergenic; powder free polymer lining; thermal responsive nitrile patient examination glove. PolyGlide interior for quick and easy donning when hands are wet. SENSI GRIP LTC BLUE NITRILE, nonsterile, powder-free, moisture-resistant nitrile. High degree of tactile sensitivity. TRUE ADVANTAGE, nonsterile, powder-free purple nitrile. Does not contain carbamates, thiurams, or thiazoles. Ultimate in hand-conforming comfort.

GLOVE, PATIENT EXAMINATION, SPECIALTY *(General) 80LZC*

Adenna Inc. 888-323-3662
11932 Baker Pl, Santa Fe Springs, CA 90670
Nitrile, polyurethane, synthetic gloves, textured.

Cypress Medical Products 800-334-3646
1202 S. Rte. 31, McHenry, IL 60050
SYNTRILE PF a powder free, latex free nitrile glove which eliminates the possibility of latex protein allergies. Packed 100/box in small, medium, large and x-large.

Digitcare Corporation 888-287-2990
2999 Overland Ave Ste 209, Los Angeles, CA 90064

F & L Medical Products Co. 724-845-7028
1129 Industrial Park Rd Ste 3, Vandergrift, PA 15690
Attenuating glove.

Hosmer Dorrance Corp. 408-379-5151
561 Division St, Campbell, CA 95008
Cosmetic glove (passive hand).

Hospira 800-441-4100
268 E 4th St, Ashland, OH 44805
Precision-dipped latex specialty gloves.

Marketing International, Inc. 800-447-0173
PO Box 4835, Topeka, KS 66604
Stainless-steel cut-proof glove for pathology.

Pacifica Gloves 800-635-4430
1709 E Del Amo Blvd, West Coast Distribution, Carson, CA 90746
Powder-free, non-sterile latex and non-sterile vinyl exam.

Tronex Healthcare Industries 800-833-1181
2 Cranberry Rd, One Tronex Centre, Parsippany, NJ 07054
Tronex, The Choice non latex Synthetic in powdered and powder free styles. Exceptional softness, comfort; most similar to latex in elasticity and shaped fit. FDA 510K=1.5, ASTM D5250. In Retail 50 packs or 100 packs.

Washington Trade International, Inc. 800-327-3379
2633 Willamette Dr NE, Lacey, WA 98516
UniSeal Flex-Nitrile Glove: Latex Free, Powder-Free

GLOVE, PATIENT EXAMINATION, VINYL *(General) 80LYZ*

Ac Healthcare Supply, Inc. 905-448-4706
11651 230th St, Cambria Heights, NY 11411
Patient examination glove.

Adenna Inc. 888-323-3662
11932 Baker Pl, Santa Fe Springs, CA 90670
Powder-free and powdered PVC, soft-stretch vinyl.

Adi Medical Division Of Asia Dynamics (Group) Inc. 877-647-7699
1565 S Shields Dr, Waukegan, IL 60085

Alimed, Inc. 800-225-2610
297 High St, Dedham, MA 02026

Ammex Corp. 800-274-7354
18375 Olympic Ave S, Tukwila, WA 98188

GLOVE, PATIENT EXAMINATION, VINYL *(cont'd)*

Baldur Systems Corporation 800-736-4716
33235 Transit Ave, Union City, CA 94587
BALDUR in 5 sizes. Prepowdered vinyl ambidextrous, soft and odorless, white color, X-S, S, M, L, X-L sizes available, 100 pcs/box, 10 boxes/case. Also available with chlorinated/coated 100% natrual rubber powder free latex, ambidextrous, non-sterile, smooth surface.

C & K Manufacturing & Sales 800-821-7795
28825 Ranney Pkwy, Westlake, OH 44145
Vinyl medical gloves.

Certol International, Llc 303-799-9401
6120 E 58th Ave, Commerce City, CO 80022
Vinyl examination gloves.

Chagrin Safety Supply, Inc. 800-227-0468
8227 Washington St # 1, Chagrin Falls, OH 44023

Cms Worldwide, Inc. 800-426-4633
30011 Ivy Glenn Dr Ste 215, Laguna Niguel, CA 92677
Vinyl Exam Gloves, powdered and powder free. ISO 9002, CE, sizes XS, S, M, L, and XL. OEM and Private Label Specialists.

Coast Scientific 800-445-1544
1445 Engineer St, Vista, CA 92081
Lightly powdered and powder free.

Cypress Medical Products 800-334-3646
1202 S. Rte. 31, McHenry, IL 60050
Vinyl examination gloves, available in small, medium, large, extra-large, 100 per box, 10 boxes per case. Medium cuffed, 50 per package, 40 packages per case. TRILON 2000 with MC3 preferred polyvinyl chloride exam glove. Special powder free vinyl exam glove with unique ivory color in small, medium, large, and X-large. Packed 100 per box, 10 boxes per case.

Dash Medical Gloves, Inc. 800-523-2055
10180 S 54th St, Franklin, WI 53132

Delta Gloves 800-220-1262
6865 Shiloh Rd E Ste 400, Alpharetta, GA 30005
DELTA's broad selection of vinyl gloves continues to grow with several new products being added. These gloves are available in both powdered and powder free styles.

Dynarex Corp. 888-356-2739
10 Glenshaw St, Orangeburg, NY 10962
Available in three sizes, pre-powdered for donning.

East Atlantic Trading/Triangle Healthcare Inc. 800-243-4635
76 National Rd, Edison, NJ 08817

In Disposables Inc. 800-269-4568
PO Box 528, Stratford, CT 06615
Strong, pre-powdered exam gloves. Sizes in small, medium, large, x-large.

Jaisons International, Inc. 203-261-1653
22 Bittersweet Ln, Trumbull, CT 06611

Life Guard 626-965-1588
18400 San Jose Ave, City Of Industry, CA 91748
Vinyl Exam Gloves are the best alternative for persons with latex allergy problems.

Maytex Corp. 800-462-9839
23521 Foley St, Hayward, CA 94545

Medtrol, Inc. 847-647-6555
7157 N Austin Ave, Niles, IL 60714
Body fluid clean up kit.

Mi-Co Company 516-481-7775
564 Warren Blvd, Garden City, NY 11530

Mydent International 800-275-0020
80 Suffolk Ct, Hauppauge, NY 11788
DEFEND elastic style, lightly powdered. Sizes: s, m, l, & xl.

Oak Technical, Llc 423-587-0690
208 Industrial Blvd, Tullahoma, TN 37388
Vinyl exam gloves.

Pharaoh Trading Company 866-929-4913
9701 Brookpark Rd, Knollwood Plaza, Suite 241, Cleveland, OH 44129

Pm Gloves, Inc. 800-788-9486
13808 Magnolia Ave, Chino, CA 91710

Royal Paper Products, Inc. 800-666-6655
PO Box 151, Coatesville, PA 19320
Exam Grade Vinyl Gloves, small-medium-large-Xlarge, also available in powder free.

Sempermed Corp. 800-366-9545
13900 49th St N, Clearwater, FL 33762
SEMPERCARE powder-free vinyl exam glove.

GLOVE, PATIENT EXAMINATION, VINYL *(cont'd)*

Shinemound Enterprise, Inc. 978-436-9980
17A Sterling Rd, North Billerica, MA 01862

Silverstone Packaging, Inc.-Your One Stop Supplier 800-413-1108
1401 Lakeland Ave, Bohemia, NY 11716

Tradex International 800-456-8370
5300 Tradex Pkwy, Cleveland, OH 44102

Tronex Healthcare Industries 800-833-1181
2 Cranberry Rd, One Tronex Centre, Parsippany, NJ 07054
TRONEX The Choice, non-sterile, non-latex for people with extreme sensitivity to latex. Exceptional quality vinyl with unique memory feature for better fit. S-XLarge. Powdered or powder free. Packaged in 100 or 50 size retail packs. ASTM, FDA 510(k) of 1.5.

GLOVE, PROTECTIVE, RADIOGRAPHIC *(Radiology) 90IWP*

Aadco Medical, Inc. 800-225-9014
2279 VT Route 66, Randolph, VT 05060
X-ray protective gloves.

Bar-Ray Products, Inc. 800-359-6115
95 Monarch St, Littlestown, PA 17340

Best Glove, Inc. 706-862-6712
579 Edison St, Cloudland, GA 30731
Radiation attenuation glove or x-ray protection glove.

Best Manufacturing Co.(Fayette Division) 706-862-6712
931 2nd Ave SE, Fayette, AL 35555
Radiation attenuation gloves.

Boston Scientific Corporation 508-652-5578
780 Brookside Dr, Spencer, IN 47460

Burlington Medical Supplies, Inc. 800-221-3466
3 Elmhurst St, PO Box 3194, Newport News, VA 23603

Carr Corporation 800-952-2398
1547 11th St, Santa Monica, CA 90401

Chagrin Safety Supply, Inc. 800-227-0468
8227 Washington St # 1, Chagrin Falls, OH 44023

Citow Cervical Visualizer Company 646-460-2984
712 S Milwaukee Ave, Libertyville, IL 60048

Gammadirect Medical Division 847-267-5929
PO Box 383, Lake Forest, IL 60045
Promit-Mamo anti-static gloves prevents dust from settling on mamogram film. The gloves are non-latex, hydroscopic and super comfortable.

Infab Corp. 805-987-5255
3651 Via Pescador, Camarillo, CA 93012
.50mm pb standard and .25mm pb for added dexterity.

International Biomedical, Ltd. 512-873-0033
2725 N Main St, Cleburne, TX 76033
Radiation resistant gloves.

Marconi Medical Systems 800-323-0550
595 Miner Rd, Cleveland, OH 44143

Protech Leaded Eyewear 561-627-9769
4087 Burns Rd, Palm Beach Gardens, FL 33410
Radiation filtering gloves and sleeves.

R & R Industries, Inc. 949-361-9238
1000 Calle Cordillera, San Clemente, CA 92673
Lifters gloves.

Schueler & Company, Inc. 516-487-1500
PO Box 528, Stratford, CT 06615

Shielding International, Inc. 800-292-2247
PO Box Z, 2150 NW Andrews Drive, Madras, OR 97741
Seamless lead gloves and mitts, vnyl or leather; Tri-Rad protective gloves; sterile radiation-resistant and radiation-reducing gloves.

Shielding Intl., Inc. 541-475-7211
2150 N.w. Andrews Dr., Madras, OR 97741
Lead glove.

Supertech, Inc. 800-654-1054
PO Box 186, Elkhart, IN 46515
Latex-Free, Radiation Protective Gloves

Tapco Medical, Inc. 818-225-5376
23981 Craftsman Rd, Calabasas, CA 91302
Flouroshield, Lead-free

Wolf X-Ray Corporation 800-356-9729
100 W Industry Ct, Deer Park, NY 11729
12 in. or 15 in., also mittens.

GLOVE, PROTECTIVE, RADIOGRAPHIC *(cont'd)*

Xma (X-Ray Marketing Associates, Inc.) 800-325-8880
1205 W Lakeview Ct, Windham Lakes Business Park
Romeoville, IL 60446

GLOVE, SURGICAL *(General) 80FPI*

Abbott Laboratories 800-223-2064
100 Abbott Park Rd, Abbott Park, IL 60064

Adex Medical, Inc. 800-873-4776
6101 Quail Valley Ct, Riverside, CA 92507
Surgical Latex Glove, Steril, Size 6.5-9.5

Aegis Medical 203-838-9081
10 Wall St, Norwalk, CT 06850
Disposable operating room gloves.

Branford Laboratories 843-832-8004
PO Box 51000, Summerville, SC 29485
L-3 Lead/latex surgical gloves.

C. R. Bard, Inc., Bard Urological Div. 888-367-2273
13183 Harland Dr NE, Covington, GA 30014

Cms Worldwide, Inc. 800-426-4533
30011 Ivy Glenn Dr Ste 215, Laguna Niguel, CA 92677
Surgical gloves, sterile, Latex, powdered; available in sizes 5.5 to 9.0. Four boxes of 50 pair per case.

Dma Med-Chem Corporation 800-362-1833
49 Watermill Ln, Great Neck, NY 11021

Eci Medical Technologies, Inc. 800-668-5289
2 Cook Rd., Bridgewater, NS B4V 3W7 Canada
ELASTYREN Synthetic Surgeons Glove. ELASTYLITE Synthetic Surgeons Glove, ELASTYPLUS Synthetic Surgeons Glove, powder-free.

Genesee Biomedical, Inc. 800-786-4890
1308 S Jason St, Denver, CO 80223
INTRA-ART Cardiac Retraction Glove. Allows the assistant to raise, rotate and retract the heart in circumflex coronary artery surgery.

Global Concepts, Ltd. 818-363-7195
19464 Eagle Ridge Ln, Northridge, CA 91326

Habley Medical Technology Corp. 800-729-1994
15721 Bernardo Heights Pkwy Ste B-30, San Diego, CA 92128
World's first puncture-evident surgical glove.

Howard Medical Company 800-443-1444
1690 N Elston Ave, Chicago, IL 60642
GANTEX Lightly powdered, $.80/pr. Also available, textured, beaded cuff in 9.5 mm thickness: 50 pr/bx, 4bx/cs. Made in the USA.

Jaisons International, Inc. 203-261-1653
22 Bittersweet Ln, Trumbull, CT 06611
ULTRA-TOUCH

Johnson & Johnson Medical Division Of Ethicon, Inc. 800-423-4018
2500 E Arbrook Blvd, Arlington, TX 76014

Lab Safety Supply, Inc. 800-356-0783
401 S Wright Rd, Janesville, WI 53546

Miami Medical Equipment & Supply Corp. 305-592-0111
2150 NW 93rd Ave, Doral, FL 33172

Sempermed Corp. 800-366-9545
13900 49th St N, Clearwater, FL 33762
SEMPERMED SUPREME powder-free latex surgical glove.

Spectra Medical Devices, Inc. 866-938-8649
4C Henshaw St, Woburn, MA 01801

Spring Health Products, Inc. 800-800-1680
705 General Washington Ave Ste 701, Norristown, PA 19403
Non-sterile latex gloves.

Sterling Rubber Company 519-843-4032
675 Woodside St., Fergus, ONT N1M 2M4 Canada
STERLING 1000 sterile, latex gloves.

Technical Marketing, Inc. 954-370-0855
1776 N Pine Island Rd Ste 306, Plantation, FL 33322
Non-sterile, standard sizes, 1,000 gloves per case.

Tg Medical Usa Inc. 626-969-7838
165 N Aspan Ave, TG Medical USA Inc., Azusa, CA 91702
surgical sterile, latex. Available in sizes 6.5, 7.0, 7.5, 8.0, 8.5, 9.0, 9.5.

World Medical Supply Usa., Inc. 800-545-5475
150 Marseille Dr, PRISTINE GLOVES, Maumelle, AR 72113
PRISTINE powder-free sterile surgical gloves for general, microsurgical, and ophthalmic surgery.

GLOVE, SURGICAL, HYPOALLERGENIC *(General) 80QYI*

Armstrong Medical Industries, Inc. 800-323-4220
575 Knightsbridge Pkwy, Lincolnshire, IL 60069

Cms Worldwide, Inc. 800-426-4633
30011 Ivy Glenn Dr Ste 215, Laguna Niguel, CA 92677
Surgical gloves, synthetic, sterile, powder-free. Sizes 5.5-9.0. Four boxes of 50 pair per case.

Digitcare Corporation 888-287-2990
2999 Overland Ave Ste 209, Los Angeles, CA 90064

Dma Med-Chem Corporation 800-362-1833
49 Watermill Ln, Great Neck, NY 11021

Johnson & Johnson Medical Division Of Ethicon, Inc. 800-423-4018
2500 E Arbrook Blvd, Arlington, TX 76014

GLOVE, SURGICAL, PLASTIC SURGERY *(Surgery) 79KGO*

Adi Medical Division Of Asia Dynamics (Group) Inc. 877-647-7699
1565 S Shields Dr, Waukegan, IL 60085

Advanced Chemical Technology, Inc. 863-687-9603
1706 S Combee Rd, Lakeland, FL 33801
Miracle glove gloving cream.

Best Manufacturing Co.(Fayette Division) 706-862-6712
931 2nd Ave SE, Fayette, AL 35555
Disposable surgical gloves.

Biomet, Inc. 574-267-6639
56 E Bell Dr, PO Box 587, Warsaw, IN 46582
Surgical gloves.

Bonded Logistics, Inc. 704-597-9638
PO Box 480203, 5709 North Graham Street, Charlotte, NC 28269
Surgeon's gloves.

Demetech Corp. 888-324-2447
3530 NW 115th Ave, Doral, FL 33178
Disposable surgeon's gloves.

Depuy Orthopaedics, Inc. 800-473-3789
700 Orthopaedic Dr, P.O. Box 988, Warsaw, IN 46582
Various types of surgeon's glove.

DJO Inc. 800-336-6569
1430 Decision St, Vista, CA 92081
Various off-the-shelf gloves in assorted sizes.

Globe Medical Tech, Inc. 713-365-9595
1766 W Sam Houston Pkwy N, Houston, TX 77043
Surgical gloves, available in sizes 6 to 8 1/2.

Grupo Industrial Latex, S.A. De C.V. 011-523-7653
Riveras Del Pilar, Ave. San Jorge 250-A, Chapala 45900 Mexico
Latex surgical gloves

Guantes Quirurgicos, S.A. De C.V. 525-760-5122
366 Henry Ford Ave.,, Deleg. Gustavo A. Madero
Mexico City, D.f. Mexico
Surgeon's gloves

Healthco International, Llc 603-255-4200
2000 Cold Spring Rd, Dixville Notch, Dixville, NH 03576
Polymer and latex surgeon gloves(powdered/powder free)(sterile).

International Biomedical, Ltd. 512-873-0033
2725 N Main St, Cleburne, TX 76033
Radiation attenuating surgical glove (powered free).

Johnson & Johnson Medical Division Of Ethicon, Inc. 800-423-4018
2500 E Arbrook Blvd, Arlington, TX 76014

Scientimed Corp. 510-763-5405
4109 Balfour Ave, Oakland, CA 94610
Surgical gloves.

Tillotson Healthcare Corp. 888-335-7500
10 Glenshaw St, Orangeburg, NY 10962
PURE ADVANTAGE SURGEONS, sterile surgeon sized; hypoallergenic; powdered or powder free; thermal responsive nitrile surgeon gloves. HPI SENSI GRIP SURGEONS, sterile, surgeon sized; bisque finish; powdered with USP absorbable dusting powder; white or brown color natural rubber latex surgeon gloves. Each glove is air inflated, tested for 13 minutes.

World Medical Supply Usa., Inc. 800-545-5475
150 Marseille Dr, PRISTINE GLOVES, Maumelle, AR 72113
PRISTINE powder-free surgical gloves for general, microsurgical, and ophthalmic surgery.

GLOVE, SURGICAL, POWDER-FREE *(Surgery) 79WWN*

Adex Medical, Inc. 800-873-4776
6101 Quail Valley Ct, Riverside, CA 92507
Surgical Latex Glove, Powder-Free Steril, Size 6.5-9.5

Armstrong Medical Industries, Inc. 800-323-4220
575 Knightsbridge Pkwy, Lincolnshire, IL 60069

Chagrin Safety Supply, Inc. 800-227-0468
8227 Washington St # 1, Chagrin Falls, OH 44023

Cms Worldwide, Inc. 800-426-4633
30011 Ivy Glenn Dr Ste 215, Laguna Niguel, CA 92677
Surgical gloves, sterile, Latex, powder-free. Available in sizes 5.5 to 9.0. Four boxes of 50 pair per case.

Dash Medical Gloves, Inc. 800-523-2055
10180 S 54th St, Franklin, WI 53132
Available powdered and unpowdered.

Digitcare Corporation 888-287-2990
2999 Overland Ave Ste 209, Los Angeles, CA 90064

Dma Med-Chem Corporation 800-362-1833
49 Watermill Ln, Great Neck, NY 11021

East Atlantic Trading/Triangle Healthcare Inc. 800-243-4635
76 National Rd, Edison, NJ 08817
Latex and vinyl for exam.

Howard Medical Company 800-443-1444
1690 N Elston Ave, Chicago, IL 60642
GANTEX powder free, low protein, $2.10/pr. Also available powder free, synthetic, carbex $2.50/pr. 50pr/bx, 4 bx/cs. Last glove made in the USA.

Mydent International 800-275-0020
80 Suffolk Ct, Hauppauge, NY 11788
DEFEND hypoallergenic; silicone process, odorless.

Pacifica Gloves 800-635-4430
1709 E Del Amo Blvd, West Coast Distribution, Carson, CA 90746
PACIFICA latex and vinyl models available.

World Medical Supply Usa., Inc. 800-545-5475
150 Marseille Dr, PRISTINE GLOVES, Maumelle, AR 72113
PRISTINE powder-free sterile surgical gloves for general, microsurgical, and ophthalmic surgery.

GLOVE, UTILITY *(General) 80QYJ*

Adex Medical, Inc. 800-873-4776
6101 Quail Valley Ct, Riverside, CA 92507
Industrial For All Applications

Alimed, Inc. 800-225-2610
297 High St, Dedham, MA 02026

Armin Poly-Version, Inc. 516-481-7775
564 Warren Blvd, Garden City, NY 11530

Carolina Biological Supply Co. 800-334-5551
2700 York Rd, Burlington, NC 27215

Cms Worldwide, Inc. 800-426-4633
30011 Ivy Glenn Dr Ste 215, Laguna Niguel, CA 92677
Utility Gloves, flocklined, yellow, 18 mil. thickness. Available in sizes S, M, L, XL. Foodservice, janitorial, Latex, vinyl and nitrile gloves.

Love Imports 800-944-5523
PO Box 759, Grapeland, TX 75844
Very lightly powdered white latex or latex heavy blue safety gloves.

Medical Safety Systems Inc. 888-803-9303
230 White Pond Dr, Akron, OH 44313
Impervious nitrile gloves for working with chemicals such as acids or corrosives or when cleaning instruments.

Pm Gloves, Inc. 800-788-9486
13808 Magnolia Ave, Chino, CA 91710
Vinyl.

Postcraft Co. 800-528-4844
625 W Rillito St, Tucson, AZ 85705
Vinyl, all purpose utility gloves.

Y.I. Ventures, Llc 314-344-0010
2260 Wendt St, Algonquin, IL 60102
Nitrile autoclavable.

GLUCOSE DEHYDROGENASE, GLUCOSE *(Chemistry) 75LFR*

Abbott Diabetes Care Inc. 510-749-5400
1360 S Loop Rd, Alameda, CA 94502
Automated glucose monitor and test strips.

Arkray Factory Usa, Inc. 952-646-3168
5182 W 76th St, Minneapolis, MN 55439
Blood glucose monitoring system.

GLUCOSE DEHYDROGENASE, GLUCOSE *(cont'd)*

Bayer Healthcare Llc 914-524-2955
555 White Plains Rd Fl 5, Tarrytown, NY 10591
Test for blood glucose.

Insulet Corporation 800-591-3455
9 Oak Park Dr, Bedford, MA 01730
Blood glucose monitor.

Roche Diagnostics Corp. 317-521-2834
Marginal Rd., Punto Oro, Industrial Development, Ponce, PR 00731
Glucose test strips.

Sanmina-Sci Usa, Inc. 256-882-4800
13000 Memorial Pkwy SW, Huntsville, AL 35803
Glucose monitoring system.

GLUCOSE-6-PHOSPHATE DEHYDROGENASE (ERYTHROCYTIC), ELECTRO *(Hematology) 81JBM*

Helena Laboratories 409-842-3714
PO Box 752, Beaumont, TX 77704

GLUCOSE-6-PHOSPHATE DEHYDROGENASE (ERYTHROCYTIC), SCREENING *(Hematology) 81JBF*

Health Chem Diagnostics Llc 954-979-3845
3341 W McNab Rd, Pompano Beach, FL 33069
Glucose-6-phosphate dehydrogenase (erythrocytic), screening.

GLUCOSE-6-PHOSPHATE DEHYDROGENASE (ERYTHROCYTIC), SPOT *(Hematology) 81JBG*

Beckman Coulter, Inc. 800-742-2345
250 S Kraemer Blvd, PO Box 8000, Brea, CA 92821

GLUE, SURGICAL TISSUE *(Surgery) 79MFI*

Cryolife, Inc. 800-438-8285
1655 Roberts Blvd NW, Kennesaw, GA 30144
BIOGLUE.

Micromedics 800-624-5662
1270 Eagan Industrial Rd, Saint Paul, MN 55121
FibriJet Delivery Systems offers a controlled delivery of biologic components through dual and single lumen applicator tips. Six syringe sizes and a variety of specialized tips, including micro, endoscopic, flexible catheter, blending and both manual and air assisted spray, you may conveniently apply the appropriate amount of material to a specified site with simple one-handed operation.

GLUTARALDEHYDE (FIXATIVE) *(Pathology) 88IFT*

Advanced Chemical Sensors Inc. 561-338-3116
3201 N Dixie Hwy Ste 3, Boca Raton, FL 33431
Electronic instruments and monitoring badges. Electronic instruments provide real time measurement and alarm with data logging capability. Monitoring badges provide a written record from an independent laboratory.

E K Industries, Inc. 877-EKI-CHEM
1403 Herkimer St, Joliet, IL 60432
Glutaraldehyde.

Hydrol Chemical Co. 610-622-3603
520 Commerce Dr, Yeadon, PA 19050
Glutaraldehyde.

Kem Medical Products Corp. 800-553-0330
75 Price Pkwy, Farmingdale, NY 11735
Glutaraldehyde neutralizer liquid and mats for spills.

Poly Scientific R&D Corp. 800-645-5825
70 Cleveland Ave, Bay Shore, NY 11706

Sci Gen, Inc. 310-324-6576
333 E Gardena Blvd, Gardena, CA 90248
FDA: Medical Device Manufacturing and packaging. Focus on Histology, Cytology, Analytical and General purpose Reagents, Chemistry, and Sterling and Disinfecting agents.

GOGGLES, PROTECTIVE, EYE *(Ophthalmology) 86WHZ*

Adex Medical, Inc. 800-873-4776
6101 Quail Valley Ct, Riverside, CA 92507
Splash Protective Goggles, Antifog, Flexible, Light Weight, Clear.

Alimed, Inc. 800-225-2610
297 High St, Dedham, MA 02026

Armstrong Medical Industries, Inc. 800-323-4220
575 Knightsbridge Pkwy, Lincolnshire, IL 60069

Concepts International, Inc. 800-627-9729
224 E Main St, Summerton, SC 29148
Infection-control goggles.

Dupaco, Inc. 800-546-4550
4144 Avenida De La Plata, Oceanside, CA 92056
OPTIGARD.

GOGGLES, PROTECTIVE, EYE *(cont'd)*

Edmund Industrial Optics 800-363-1992
101 E Gloucester Pike, Barrington, NJ 08007

Elvex Corporation 800-888-6582
13 Trowbridge Dr, Bethel, CT 06801
Laser safety glasses/spectacles/goggles.

Erb Industries Inc. 800-800-6522
1 Safety Way, Woodstock, GA 30188
STING RAYS & PIRANHAS Safety glasses. Boas, Vipers, Commandos & Toraz polycarbonate safety glasses meet Z87.1 ANSI requirements.

H.L. Bouton Co., Inc. 800-426-1881
PO Box 840, Buzzards Bay, MA 02532
Disposable goggles.

Johnson & Johnson Medical Division Of Ethicon, Inc. 800-423-4018
2500 E Arbrook Blvd, Arlington, TX 76014

Lamba Systems 800-231-1332
99 Wales Ave, Tonawanda, NY 14150
The Revolution goggle is a chemical splash/dust/impact goggle. The antifog eyewear is designed for comfort, fit, and protection. A prescription lens insert is available.

Lase-R Shield, A Bacou-Dalloz Company 800-288-1164
7011 Prospect Pl NE, Albuquerque, NM 87110
Extra-large goggles and spectacles for better field of vision.

Leader Industries Inc. 800-847-2001
1280 Nobel, Boucherville, QUE J4B-5H1 Canada

Medical Safety Systems Inc. 888-803-9303
230 White Pond Dr, Akron, OH 44313

Micromedical Technologies, Inc. 800-334-4154
10 Kemp Dr, Chatham, IL 62629
Video Frenzel Goggles: REALEYES and OPTIMEYES PORTABLE permit easy observation and simultaneous video recording of eye movement during balance testing or vestibular rehabilitation.

Mydent International 800-275-0020
80 Suffolk Ct, Hauppauge, NY 11788
DEFEND RayBloc protective glasses provide max. protection from U.V. and blue-light radiation. Clear-Vue protector glasses are made distortion-free.

National Biological Corp. 800-338-5045
1532 Enterprise Pkwy, Twinsburg, OH 44087
Treatment goggles & street glasses.

Newport Optical Laboratories, Inc. 714-484-3200
10564C Fern Ave, Stanton, CA 90680
Laser protective eye wear.

Noir Manufacturing 800-521-9746
10125 Colonial Industrial Dr, South Lyon, MI 48178
Laser shield. Laser protective eyewear.

Oberon Company ,Div Of The Paramount Corp. 800-322-3348
22 Logan St, PO Box 61008, New Bedford, MA 02740
Polycarbonate scratch resistant goggles, available in non-ventilated, perforated or indirect (splash) ventilated frames. Available with side shields. Frames available in a variety of colors.

Rochester Optical Mfg. Company 585-254-0022
1260 Lyell Ave, Rochester, NY 14606

Sanax Protective Products, Inc. 800-379-9929
236 Upland Ave, Newton Highlands, MA 02461

Sellstrom Manufacturing Co. 800-323-7402
1 Sellstrom Dr, Palatine, IL 60067
Lightweight, flexible and fog free, mini sizes also available.

Trademark Medical Llc 800-325-9044
449 Soverign Ct, St. Louis, MO 63011
MED-VUE protective eyewear; protective goggles, glasses and eyeshields from blood and fluid flashback.

Y.I. Ventures, Llc 314-344-0010
2260 Wendt St, Algonquin, IL 60102
Fog free.

GONIOMETER, AC-POWERED *(Orthopedics) 87KQX*

Advanced Motion Measurement, Llc 602-263-8657
1202 E Maryland Ave Ste 1J, Phoenix, AZ 85014
Motion analysis system (3d-dynamic range-of-motion).

Dynatronics Corp. 800-874-6251
7030 Park Centre Dr, Salt Lake City, UT 84121

GONIOMETER, AC-POWERED *(cont'd)*

Fasstech 978-663-2800
76 Treble Cove Rd Ste 3, North Billerica, MA 01862
SPINAL TOUCH Computerized inclinometer for spinal range-of-motion and impairment rating.

Global Services Group 757-220-8282
350 McLaws Cir Ste 2, Williamsburg, VA 23185

JTECH Medical 800-985-8324
470 West Longdale Dr., Suite G, Salt Lake City, UT 84115

Motus Bioengineering Inc. 707-745-4194
133 Carlisle Way, Benicia, CA 94510
Motus movement monitor.

Nk Biotechnical Corp. 612-541-0411
701 Decatur Ave N Ste 111A, Golden Valley, MN 55427
Ac powered goniometer.

Ppi-Time Zero Inc. 973-278-6500
262 Buffalo Ave, Paterson, NJ 07503
Knee positioning and alignment system.

RamÇ-Hart, Inc. 973-448-0305
95 Allen St, PO Box 400, Netcong, NJ 07857
Goniometer contact angle measurement, wetting, surface tension.

GONIOMETER, MECHANICAL *(Physical Med) 89IKQ*

Alimed, Inc. 800-225-2610
297 High St, Dedham, MA 02026

GONIOMETER, NON-POWERED *(Orthopedics) 87KQW*

Acumar Technology 503-292-7137
1314 SW 57th Ave, Portland, OR 97221
Acumar inclinometer.

Alimed, Inc. 800-225-2610
297 High St, Dedham, MA 02026

Biomet Microfixation Inc. 800-874-7711
1520 Tradeport Dr, Jacksonville, FL 32218
Various types of goniometers.

Biomet, Inc. 574-267-6639
56 E Bell Dr, PO Box 587, Warsaw, IN 46582
Various types of goniometer.

Depuy Spine, Inc. 800-227-6633
325 Paramount Dr, Raynham, MA 02767
Goniometer.

Patterson Medical Supply, Inc. 262-387-8720
W68N158 Evergreen Blvd, Cedarburg, WI 53012
Goniometer.

Plasticards, Inc. Dba Rainbow Printing Co. 800-535-1433
3711 Boettler Oaks Dr, Uniontown, OH 44685
Goniometer, nonpowered.

Princeton Medical Group, Inc. 800-875-0869
1189 Royal Links Dr, Mt Pleasant, SC 29466

Richardson Products, Inc. 888-928-7297
9408 Gulfstream Rd, Frankfort, IL 60423
Goniometer.

Slawner Ltd., J. 514-731-3378
5713 Cote Des Neiges Rd., Montreal, QUE H3S 1Y7 Canada

Sport Tech, Inc. 434-982-5752
391 Ridge Lee Dr, Charlottesville, VA 22903
Ligmaster.

The Saunders Group 800-445-9836
4250 Norex Dr, Chaska, MN 55318
Inclinometer.

GONIOMETER, ORTHOPEDIC *(Orthopedics) 87HTI*

Alimed, Inc. 800-225-2610
297 High St, Dedham, MA 02026

Creative Health Products, Inc. 800-742-4478
5148 Saddle Ridge Rd, Plymouth, MI 48170
TRUE-ANGLE, Goniometer, mechanical and orthopedic CHP TRUE-ANGLE goniometer, 12 1/2', 360 deg., 1 deg. increments $14.00 each.

Holmed Corporation 508-238-3351
40 Norfolk Ave, South Easton, MA 02375

Kmedic 800-955-0559
190 Veterans Dr, Northvale, NJ 07647

Lafayette Instrument Company 800-428-7545
PO Box 5729, 3700 Sagamore Pkwy,, Lafayette, IN 47903
Accurate - extendable goniometer, Model #01135

GONIOMETER, ORTHOPEDIC *(cont'd)*

Medworks Instruments 800-323-9790
PO Box 581, Chatham, IL 62629
$9.00 stainless steel 180 degree 8 inch.

Miltex Inc. 800-645-8000
589 Davies Dr, York, PA 17402

Mizuho Osi 800-777-4674
30031 Ahern Ave, Union City, CA 94587

Paramedical Distributors 800-245-3278
2020 Grand Blvd, Kansas City, MO 64108

RamÇ-Hart, Inc. 973-448-0305
95 Allen St, PO Box 400, Netcong, NJ 07857
Contact angle measurement.

Zimmer Holdings, Inc. 800-613-6131
1800 W Center St, PO Box 708, Warsaw, IN 46580

GOUGE, NASAL *(Ear/Nose/Throat) 77KAQ*

Aesculap Implant Systems Inc. 1-800-234-9179
3773 Corporate Pkwy, Center Valley, PA 18034

Biomet Microfixation Inc. 800-874-7711
1520 Tradeport Dr, Jacksonville, FL 32218
Various types of gouges.

Clinimed, Incorporated 877-CLINIMED
303 Markus Ct, Sandy Brae Industrial Park, Newark, DE 19713

Miltex Inc. 800-645-8000
589 Davies Dr, York, PA 17402

Zimmer Holdings, Inc. 800-613-6131
1800 W Center St, PO Box 708, Warsaw, IN 46580

GOUGE, SURGICAL, GENERAL & PLASTIC SURGERY *(Surgery) 79GDH*

Aesculap Implant Systems Inc. 1-800-234-9179
3773 Corporate Pkwy, Center Valley, PA 18034

Ascent Healthcare Solutions 480-763-5300
10232 S 51st St, Phoenix, AZ 85044
Gouge.

Bausch & Lomb Surgical 636-255-5051
3365 Tree Court Ind Blvd, Saint Louis, MO 63122

Biomet Microfixation Inc. 800-874-7711
1520 Tradeport Dr, Jacksonville, FL 32218
Various types of gouges.

DJO Inc. 800-336-6569
1430 Decision St, Vista, CA 92081

George Tiemann & Co. 800-843-6266
25 Plant Ave, Hauppauge, NY 11788

Holmed Corporation 508-238-3351
40 Norfolk Ave, South Easton, MA 02375

Kmedic 800-955-0559
190 Veterans Dr, Northvale, NJ 07647

Lenox-Maclaren Surgical Corp. 720-890-9660
657 S Taylor Ave Ste A, Colorado Technology Center Louisville, CO 80027
Gouge, surgical / all different.

Micro-Aire Surgical Instruments, Inc. 800-722-0822
1641 Edlich Dr, Charlottesville, VA 22911

Tuzik Boston 800-886-6363
104 Longwater Dr, Assinippi Park, Norwell, MA 02061

Warsaw Orthopedic, Inc. 901-396-3133
2500 Silveus Xing, Warsaw, IN 46582
Various gouges.

Zimmer Holdings, Inc. 800-613-6131
1800 W Center St, PO Box 708, Warsaw, IN 46580

GOWN, EXAMINATION *(General) 80FME*

A.G.A. Electronics Corp. 305-592-1860
7209 NW 41st St, Miami, FL 33166
Examination gown.

Adex Medical, Inc. 800-873-4776
6101 Quail Valley Ct, Riverside, CA 92507
Coveralls.

Adi Medical Division Of Asia Dynamics (Group) Inc. 877-647-7699
1565 S Shields Dr, Waukegan, IL 60085

Alphaprotech, Inc. 229-242-1931
1287 W Fairway Dr, Nogales, AZ 85621

Atd-American Co. 800-523-2300
135 Greenwood Ave, Wyncote, PA 19095

GOWN, EXAMINATION *(cont'd)*

Barjan Mfg., Ltd. 631-420-5588
28 Baiting Place Rd, Farmingdale, NY 11735
Exam gowns.

Biomed Resource, Inc. 310-323-3888
3388 Rosewood Ave, Los Angeles, CA 90066
Disposable gown, isolation gown.

Centurion Medical Products Corp. 517-545-1135
3310 S Main St, Salisbury, NC 28147

Chagrin Safety Supply, Inc. 800-227-0468
8227 Washington St # 1, Chagrin Falls, OH 44023

Digitcare Corporation 888-287-2990
2999 Overland Ave Ste 209, Los Angeles, CA 90064

Ekcomed, Llc 314-303-9757
391 Portsmouth Dr, Saint Charles, MO 63303
Exam gown, exam scrubs, warm-up jacket, comfort clothes.

Exami-Gowns, Inc. 800-962-4696
8647 Ridgelys Choice Dr, Baltimore, MD 21236
EXAMI-ROBE is available in a generous 'One Size Fits All', accomodating patients weighing up to 300 pounds. This gown is available in white only, and can be monogrammed for a personal touch. The robe is manufactured with a pocket on the right front side, has a belt permanently attached in the center back, and raglan sleeves 3/4 length. All fabrics used in manufacturing are 20% Cotton and 80% Polyester.

Global Healthcare 800-601-3880
1495 Hembree Rd Ste 700, Roswell, GA 30076
Disposable.

Graham Medical Products/Div. Of Little Rapids Corp 866-429-1408
2273 Larsen Rd, Green Bay, WI 54303
Pediatric or adult - in white or print. Wide variety of materials and sizes; also examination capes available in variety of colors and styles including new extra long breast examination capes.

Health-Pak, Inc. 315-724-8370
2005 Beechgrove Pl, Utica, NY 13501
Extended wear X-ray procedure glued/sewn gowns.

Hpk Industries Llc 315-724-0196
1208 Broad St, Utica, NY 13501
Examination capes, gowns.

Jero Medical Equipment & Supplies, Inc. 800-457-0644
1701 W 13th St, Chicago, IL 60608
Isolation & Procedures.

Jms Converters Inc Dba Sabee Products & Stanford Prof Prod 215-396-3302
67 Buck Rd Ste B7, Huntingdon Valley, PA 19006
Patient Exam Gowns and Capes

Kappler Protective Apparel & Fabrics 800-600-4019
115 Grimes Dr, Guntersville, AL 35976

Lakeland De Mexico S.A. De C.V. 516-981-9700
Rancho La Soledad Lote No. 2, Fracc. Poniente C.p. Celaya, Guajuato Mexico
Examination gown non-sterile

Mckesson General Medical 800-446-3008
8741 Landmark Rd, Richmond, VA 23228

Monchis S.A.De. D.U. 336-292-8877
Bustamente 514 Col., Arboledas, Montemorelos, N.I Mexico
Disposable apparel, protective apparel

R. Sabee Company 920-882-7350
1718 W 8th St, Appleton, WI 54914

Standard Textile Co., Inc. 888-999-0400
PO Box 371805, Cincinnati, OH 45222
Patient apparel, sterile wearing apparel.

The Sewing Source, Inc. 919-478-3900
802 E Nash St, Spring Hope, NC 27882
Gown, examination.

Tidi Products, Llc 920-751-4380
570 Enterprise Dr, Neenah, WI 54956
Disposable exam gown; disposable exam cape.

Tri-State Hospital Supply Corp. 517-545-1135
3173 E 43rd St, Yuma, AZ 85365

GOWN, EXAMINATION *(cont'd)*

Tronex Healthcare Industries 800-833-1181
2 Cranberry Rd, One Tronex Centre, Parsippany, NJ 07054
Non latex PE Gown with Thumbhooks is fluid impervious for protection against bloodborne pathogens. Thumbhooks keep arms protected when worn under gloves. Individually packaged. Sizes in Unisize and X-Large. Blue.

White Knight Healthcare 800-851-4431
Calle 16, Number 780, Agua Prieta, Sonora Mexico
Gown, examination

GOWN, ISOLATION, SURGICAL *(Surgery) 79FYC*

Adi Medical Division Of Asia Dynamics (Group) Inc. 877-647-7699
1565 S Shields Dr, Waukegan, IL 60085

Angelica Image Apparel 800-222-3112
700 Rosedale Ave, Saint Louis, MO 63112

Armstrong Medical Industries, Inc. 800-323-4220
575 Knightsbridge Pkwy, Lincolnshire, IL 60069

Avent S.A. De C.V. 602-748-6900
Camino De Libramiento, Km. 1.5, Nogales, Sonora Mexico
Various types and sized of cover gowns and apparel

Baldur Systems Corporation 800-736-4716
33235 Transit Ave, Union City, CA 94587
Isolation gowns, Full body length, long sleeves, elastic cuff with ties at the neck and waist, repellency resists moisture, one size fits all, yellow color, 50 pcs per case.

Busse Hospital Disposables, Inc. 631-435-4711
75 Arkay Dr, Hauppauge, NY 11788
Isolation gown,sterile & non-sterle.

Chagrin Safety Supply, Inc. 800-227-0468
8227 Washington St # 1, Chagrin Falls, OH 44023

Cypress Medical Products 800-334-3646
1202 S. Rte. 31, McHenry, IL 60050
Disposable, full length, yellow isolation gowns with ties. Unisize, 50 per case.

Dowling Textiles 770-957-3981
615 Macon Rd, McDonough, GA 30253
Isolation gown.

Dynarex Corp. 888-356-2739
10 Glenshaw St, Orangeburg, NY 10962
Fluid resistant, yellow, universal size, full length with ties.

Fabrite Laminating Corp. 973-777-1406
70 Passaic St, Wood Ridge, NJ 07075

General Econopak, Inc. 888-871-8568
1725 N 6th St, Philadelphia, PA 19122
Disposable, sterile and non-sterile.

Global Healthcare 800-601-3880
1495 Hembree Rd Ste 700, Roswell, GA 30076
Disposable, full length.

Graham Medical Products/Div. Of Little Rapids Corp 866-429-1408
2273 Larsen Rd, Green Bay, WI 54303
Elastic-cuff. Waist and neckties attached. Disposable.

Grand Medical Products 800-521-2055
7222 Ertel Ln, Houston, TX 77040

Health-Pak, Inc. 315-724-8370
2005 Beechgrove Pl, Utica, NY 13501
Regular spunbonded and infection control.

Hpk Industries Llc 315-724-0196
1208 Broad St, Utica, NY 13501
Isolation gown cover gown.

In Disposables Inc. 800-269-4568
PO Box 528, Stratford, CT 06615
Spun-bonded polypropylene, sewn edges. Full length with ties at neck and waist. Packaged 50/cs.

Kappler Protective Apparel & Fabrics 800-600-4019
115 Grimes Dr, Guntersville, AL 35976

Kentron Health Care, Inc. 615-384-0573
3604 Kelton Jackson Rd, P.o. Box 120, Springfield, TN 37172
Isolation gown.

Kerr Group 800-524-3577
1400 Holcomb Bridge Rd, Roswell, GA 30076

GOWN, ISOLATION, SURGICAL *(cont'd)*

Lakeland De Mexico S.A. De C.V. 516-981-9700
Rancho La Soledad Lote No. 2, Fracc. Poniente C.p.
Celaya, Guajuato Mexico
Isolation gown

Medical Action Industries, Inc. 800-645-7042
25 Heywood Rd, Arden, NC 28704
Gown.

Medline Industries, Inc. 800-633-5886
1 Medline Pl, Mundelein, IL 60060

Mexpo International, Inc. 800-838-8299
2695B McCone Ave, Hayward, CA 94545
BLOSSOM - Latex-free and knitted Cuffs.

New York Hospital Disposables, Inc. 718-384-1620
101 Richardson St, Brooklyn, NY 11211

Pfb Inter-Apparel Corp. 800-828-7629
1930 Harrison St Ste 304, Hollywood, FL 33020

Pharaoh Trading Company 866-929-4913
9701 Brookpark Rd, Knollwood Plaza, Suite 241, Cleveland, OH 44129

Precept Medical Products, Inc. 800-438-5827
PO Box 2400, 370 Airport Road/, Arden, NC 28704

Ross Disposable Products 800-649-6526
401 Traders Blvd E, Unit 10, Mississauga, ON L4Z 2H8 Canada

Scientimed Corp. 510-763-5405
4109 Balfour Ave, Oakland, CA 94610
Isolation gowns.

The Sewing Source, Inc. 919-478-3900
802 E Nash St, Spring Hope, NC 27882
O.r./surgeons gown.

Tidi Products, Llc 920-751-4380
570 Enterprise Dr, Neenah, WI 54956
Isolation gown, non-sterile.

Tradewinds Rehabilitation Center, Inc. 219-949-4000
5901 W 7th Ave, Gary, IN 46406
Isolation gowns.

Tronex Healthcare Industries 800-833-1181
2 Cranberry Rd, One Tronex Centre, Parsippany, NJ 07054
Fluid resistant, breathable Polypropylene spunbond with latex free elastic or knitted cuffs, waist and neck ties and full back. Styles also offered with PE coating for fluid impervious protection. Fluid resistant, three-ply SMS material also available. Yellow, blue, and white colors; Unisize and X-Large.

White Knight Healthcare 800-851-4431
Calle 16, Number 780, Agua Prieta, Sonora Mexico
Gown, isolation, surgical

GOWN, OPERATING ROOM, DISPOSABLE *(Surgery) 79FPH*

Ability Building Center, Inc. 507-281-6262
1911 14th St NW, P.O. Box 6938, Rochester, MN 55901

Adenna Inc. 888-323-3662
11932 Baker Pl, Santa Fe Springs, CA 90670
Latex free, disposable medical gown.

Aegis Medical 203-838-9081
10 Wall St, Norwalk, CT 06850

Atd-American Co. 800-523-2300
135 Greenwood Ave, Wyncote, PA 19095

Digitcare Corporation 888-287-2990
2999 Overland Ave Ste 209, Los Angeles, CA 90064

International Hospital Supply Co. 800-398-9450
6914 Canby Ave Ste 105, Reseda, CA 91335

Johnson & Johnson Medical Division Of Ethicon, Inc. 800-423-4018
2500 E Arbrook Blvd, Arlington, TX 76014

Kappler Protective Apparel & Fabrics 800-600-4019
115 Grimes Dr, Guntersville, AL 35976

Kerr Group 800-524-3577
1400 Holcomb Bridge Rd, Roswell, GA 30076

Precept Medical Products, Inc. 800-438-5827
PO Box 2400, 370 Airport Road/, Arden, NC 28704
New Excel Surgeon Gown with generous sizing and other features

White Knight Healthcare 800-851-4431
Calle 16, Number 780, Agua Prieta, Sonora Mexico
Various type of sterile and non-sterile gowns

GOWN, OPERATING ROOM, REUSABLE *(Surgery) 79QYN*

Angelica Image Apparel 800-222-3112
700 Rosedale Ave, Saint Louis, MO 63112

GOWN, OPERATING ROOM, REUSABLE *(cont'd)*

Best Manufacturing Group Llc 800-843-3233
1633 Broadway Fl 18, New York, NY 10019
BEST Mfg. Inc.

International Hospital Supply Co. 800-398-9450
6914 Canby Ave Ste 105, Reseda, CA 91335

Mahe International Inc. 800-294-7946
468 Craighead St, Nashville, TN 37204

Medline Industries, Inc. 800-633-5886
1 Medline Pl, Mundelein, IL 60060

Standard Textile 800-999-0400
1 Knollcrest Dr, Cincinnati, OH 45237

Welch Allyn, Inc. 800-535-6663
4341 State Street Rd, Skaneateles Falls, NY 13153

GOWN, OTHER *(General) 80QYQ*

Adex Medical, Inc. 800-873-4776
6101 Quail Valley Ct, Riverside, CA 92507
Cover Alls.

Angelica Image Apparel 800-222-3112
700 Rosedale Ave, Saint Louis, MO 63112

Atd-American Co. 800-523-2300
135 Greenwood Ave, Wyncote, PA 19095

Cleanwear Products Ltd. 416-438-4831
54 Crockford Rd., Toronto, ON M1R-3C3 Canada
TYVEK isolation gowns.

Cms Worldwide, Inc. 800-426-4633
30011 Ivy Glenn Dr Ste 215, Laguna Niguel, CA 92677
Isolation/barrier gowns. White, blue, yellow, green or pink. Impervious. All sizes.

General Econopak, Inc. 888-871-8568
1725 N 6th St, Philadelphia, PA 19122
Disposable waterproof cover gowns, shorts, skirts, jackets, coveralls, and lab coats.

Gi Supply 800-451-5797
200 Grandview Ave, Camp Hill, PA 17011
DEFENZ disposable fluid resistant gown for healthcare provider.

Global Healthcare 800-601-3880
1495 Hembree Rd Ste 700, Roswell, GA 30076
Barrier gowns, isolation, exam gowns.

Kappler Protective Apparel & Fabrics 800-600-4019
115 Grimes Dr, Guntersville, AL 35976

Lac-Mac Ltd. 800-461-0001
425 Rectory St., London, ONT N5W 3W5 Canada

Ludlow Technological Products 800-445-5025
2 Ludlow Park Dr, Chicopee, MA 01022

O&M Enterprise 847-258-4515
641 Chelmsford Ln, Elk Grove Village, IL 60007
GOWN EXAMINATION/PATIENT/SURGICAL

Sanax Protective Products, Inc. 800-379-9929
236 Upland Ave, Newton Highlands, MA 02461
Barrier gowns.

GOWN, PATIENT *(Surgery) 79FYB*

Adi Medical Division Of Asia Dynamics (Group) Inc. 877-647-7699
1565 S Shields Dr, Waukegan, IL 60085

Allman Products 800-223-6889
21101 Itasca St, Chatsworth, CA 91311

American Health Care Apparel Ltd. 800-252-0584
302 Town Center Blvd, Easton, PA 18040
FASHION - adaptive clothing and footwear designed to aid the caregiver in dressing and undressing someone restricted to a wheelchair or bed with ease.

Angelica Image Apparel 800-222-3112
700 Rosedale Ave, Saint Louis, MO 63112

Arizant Healthcare Inc. 800-733-7775
10393 W 70th St, Eden Prairie, MN 55344
BAIR PAWS warming gown offers warming and gowning in one step. The single use, full coverage gown allows patients to control their own temperature.

Atd-American Co. 800-523-2300
135 Greenwood Ave, Wyncote, PA 19095

Biomni Medical Systems, Inc. 801-768-0166
160 S 1350 E, Lehi, UT 84043
Biopsy.

GOWN, PATIENT *(cont'd)*

Care Apparel Industries 800-326-6262
12709 91st Ave, Richmond Hill, NY 11418

Digitcare Corporation 888-287-2990
2999 Overland Ave Ste 209, Los Angeles, CA 90064

Dowling Textiles 770-957-3981
615 Macon Rd, McDonough, GA 30253
Various types of patient gowns.

Encompass Medical 800-826-4490
16415 Addison Rd Ste 660, Addison, TX 75001

Exami-Gowns, Inc. 800-962-4696
8647 Ridgelys Choice Dr, Baltimore, MD 21236
PEDIATRIC GOWN is a slipover the head full-cut style with cap sleeves, especially designed for children ages 6-10 years old. Available in green only.

Freestyle Medical Supplies, Inc. 800-841-5330
336 Green Rd, Stoney Creek, ON L8E 2B2 Canada
100% cotton flannel gowns, one size fits all, available in men's/women's prints, solids overlap in back of gown.

General Econopak, Inc. 888-871-8568
1725 N 6th St, Philadelphia, PA 19122
Disposable adult, adolescent, and pediatric size patient pajamas.

International Hospital Supply Co. 800-398-9450
6914 Canby Ave Ste 105, Reseda, CA 91335

Kennedy Center, Inc. 203-365-8522
2440 Reservoir Ave, Trumbull, CT 06611
No common name listed.

Lakeland De Mexico S.A. De C.V. 516-981-9700
Rancho La Soledad Lote No. 2, Fracc. Poniente C.p. Celaya, Guajuato Mexico
Patient gowns

Mckesson General Medical 800-446-3008
8741 Landmark Rd, Richmond, VA 23228

Scientimed Corp. 510-763-5405
4109 Balfour Ave, Oakland, CA 94610
Patient exam gowns.

Standard Textile Co., Inc. 888-999-0400
PO Box 371805, Cincinnati, OH 45222
Patient apparel.

The Sewing Source, Inc. 919-478-3900
802 E Nash St, Spring Hope, NC 27882
Gown, patient.

White Knight Healthcare 800-851-4431
Calle 16, Number 780, Agua Prieta, Sonora Mexico
Gown, patient

GOWN, PATIENT, DISPOSABLE *(General) 80QYO*

Adenna Inc. 888-323-3662
11932 Baker Pl, Santa Fe Springs, CA 90670
Latex free, disposable medical gown.

Arc/Otsego 607-432-8595
35 Academy St, PO Box 490, Oneonta, NY 13820
Economical disposable gowns and capes to cover patients during exams and x-rays.

Atd-American Co. 800-523-2300
135 Greenwood Ave, Wyncote, PA 19095

Bibbero Systems, Inc. 800-242-2376
1300 N McDowell Blvd, Petaluma, CA 94954
Disposable exam gowns available in adult, adults plus & pediatric sizes. Exam capes also available in adult sizes.

GOWN, PATIENT, DISPOSABLE *(cont'd)*

Dna Products, Llc 800-535-3189
PO Box 306, New York, NY 10032
Mens disposable boxer made of soft polypropylene. Features a convenient fly front, finished leg openings, and elastic waistband. Intended to be worn once and discarded; available in 5 sizes (S-XXL); 3 white individually wrapped boxers per package; $2.25/package; 40 packages per carton (single size). Mens disposable brief made of soft polypropylene. Features a convenient front opening, elastic leg openings, and wide elastic waistband. Intended to be worn once and discarded; available in 5 sizes (S-XXL); 5 white individually wrapped briefs per package; $2.25/package; 40 packages per carton (single size). Womens disposable brief panty made of soft polypropylene w/cotton crotch and elastic waist and leg openings. Intended to be worn once and discarded; available in 5 sizes (S-XXL); 5 white individually wrapped panties per package; $2.25/package; 40 packages per carton (single size). Womens disposable thong panty made of soft polypropylene w/elastic waist and leg openings. Intended to be worn once and discarded; available in 5 sizes (S-XXL); 7 white individually wrapped panties per package; $2.25/package; 40 packages per carton (single size).

General Econopak, Inc. 888-871-8568
1725 N 6th St, Philadelphia, PA 19122
Adult-, adolescent-, and pediatric-sized patient pajamas.

Gi Supply 800-451-5797
200 Grandview Ave, Camp Hill, PA 17011
MOONPANTS disposable patient shorts with rear trap door.

Graham Medical Products/Div. Of Little Rapids Corp 866-429-1408
2273 Larsen Rd, Green Bay, WI 54303
Pediatric or adult - in white or print. Wide variety of materials and sizes; also examination capes available in variety of colors and styles including new extra long breast examination capes.

Howard Medical Company 800-443-1444
1690 N Elston Ave, Chicago, IL 60642
$35.00 (50 per case) disposable infant gowns; blue dexter. $46.00/cs (50 per case) adult isolation gown meets OSHA regulations for blood-borne pathogens.

Jms Converters Inc Dba Sabee Products & Stanford Prof Prod 215-396-3302
67 Buck Rd Ste B7, Huntingdon Valley, PA 19006

Kerr Group 800-524-3577
1400 Holcomb Bridge Rd, Roswell, GA 30076

Pfb Inter-Apparel Corp. 800-828-7629
1930 Harrison St Ste 304, Hollywood, FL 33020

Precept Medical Products, Inc. 800-438-5827
PO Box 2400, 370 Airport Road/, Arden, NC 28704

Ross Disposable Products 800-649-6526
401 Traders Blvd E, Unit 10, Mississauga, ON L4Z 2H8 Canada

Shinemound Enterprise, Inc. 978-436-9980
17A Sterling Rd, North Billerica, MA 01862

Tronex Healthcare Industries 800-833-1181
2 Cranberry Rd, One Tronex Centre, Parsippany, NJ 07054
PPSB material is comfortable, fluid resistant, and breathable. Sleeveless gown in Dark Blue offers discretion and privacy for the patient. ISO 9001 certified factory quality standard.

Washington Trade International, Inc. 800-327-3379
2633 Willamette Dr NE, Lacey, WA 98516
Isolation Gowns - One size fits all. Color variety.

GOWN, PATIENT, REUSABLE *(General) 80QYP*

Angelica Image Apparel 800-222-3112
700 Rosedale Ave, Saint Louis, MO 63112

Atd-American Co. 800-523-2300
135 Greenwood Ave, Wyncote, PA 19095

Best Manufacturing Group Llc 800-843-3233
1633 Broadway Fl 18, New York, NY 10019
Prints colors, ties, snaps, Std. and full overcap.

Carl Zeiss Surgical, Inc. 800-442-4020
1 Zeiss Dr, Thornwood, NY 10594

Essential Medical Supply, Inc. 800-826-8423
6420 Hazeltine National Dr, Orlando, FL 32822

Exami-Gowns, Inc. 800-962-4696
8647 Ridgelys Choice Dr, Baltimore, MD 21236

Graham Medical Products/Div. Of Little Rapids Corp 866-429-1408
2273 Larsen Rd, Green Bay, WI 54303

GOWN, PATIENT, REUSABLE *(cont'd)*

Johnson & Johnson Medical Division Of Ethicon, Inc. — 800-423-4018
2500 E Arbrook Blvd, Arlington, TX 76014

Medline Industries, Inc. — 800-633-5886
1 Medline Pl, Mundelein, IL 60060

Salk Inc. — 800-343-4497
119 Braintree St Ste 701, 4th Floor, Boston, MA 02134
COMFORT COLLECTION.

GOWN, SURGICAL *(Surgery) 79FYA*

American Medical Devices, Inc. — 800-788-9876
287 S Stoddard Ave, San Bernardino, CA 92401
Disposable surgical gowns.

Angelica Image Apparel — 800-222-3112
700 Rosedale Ave, Saint Louis, MO 63112

Atd-American Co. — 800-523-2300
135 Greenwood Ave, Wyncote, PA 19095

Avent S.A. De C.V. — 770-587-8393
Carretera Intl., Salida Norte, Magdalena, Sonora Mexico
Various types & sizes of sterile, surgical gowns

Avent S.A. De C.V. — 602-748-6900
Camino De Libramiento, Km. 1.5, Nogales, Sonora Mexico
Varous types and sizes of sterile, surgical gowns

Biomet, Inc. — 574-267-6639
56 E Bell Dr, PO Box 587, Warsaw, IN 46582
Various types of surgical gowns.

Customed, Inc. — 787-801-0101
Calle Igualdad #7, Fajardo, PR 00738
Surgeon gown.

Depuy Orthopaedics, Inc. — 800-473-3789
700 Orthopaedic Dr, P.O. Box 988, Warsaw, IN 46582
Various types of surgical gowns.

Dowling Textiles — 770-957-3981
615 Macon Rd, McDonough, GA 30253
Various types of nurses gown.

Exami-Gowns, Inc. — 800-962-4696
8647 Ridgelys Choice Dr, Baltimore, MD 21236

General Econopak, Inc. — 888-871-8568
1725 N 6th St, Philadelphia, PA 19122
Disposable, sterile, regular-back, safety shield gown with impervious sleeves and front shield.

Gi Supply — 800-451-5797
200 Grandview Ave, Camp Hill, PA 17011
DEFENZ disposable fluid resistant gown for healthcare provider.

Global Healthcare — 800-601-3880
1495 Hembree Rd Ste 700, Roswell, GA 30076
Disposable, various sizes, sterile

Health-Pak, Inc. — 315-724-8370
2005 Beechgrove Pl, Utica, NY 13501

Industrias Medison, S.A. De C.V. — 800-851-4431
Lote 7 Manzana 3 Parque, Industrial De Cananea,km.5 Carretera a Inuris, Sonora Mexico
Various

Johnson & Johnson Medical Division Of Ethicon, Inc. — 800-423-4018
2500 E Arbrook Blvd, Arlington, TX 76014

Kappler Protective Apparel & Fabrics — 800-600-4019
115 Grimes Dr, Guntersville, AL 35976
PRO/VENT surgical gown, sterile.

Kerr Group — 800-524-3577
1400 Holcomb Bridge Rd, Roswell, GA 30076

Kleen Laundry & Drycleaning Services, Inc. — 603-448-1134
1 Foundry St, Lebanon, NH 03766
Surgeions gown.

Lac-Mac Ltd. — 800-461-0001
425 Rectory St., London, ONT N5W 3W5 Canada
Surgical gown with GORE TEX material.

Lakeland De Mexico S.A. De C.V. — 516-981-9700
Rancho La Soledad Lote No. 2, Fracc. Poniente C.p. Celaya, Guajuato Mexico
Surgical gown

Maquilas Teta-Kawi, S.A. De C.V. — 413-593-6400
Carretera Internacional, Km 1969, Enpalme, Sonora Mexico
Gown, surgical

GOWN, SURGICAL *(cont'd)*

Maytex Corp. — 800-462-9839
23521 Foley St, Hayward, CA 94545
Full-length, long sleeves, fluid-resistant and fluid-impervious gowns available.

North Safety Products — 401-943-4400
1101 B Calle Neutron, Parque Industrial Maran, Mexicali, B.c. Mexico
Protective gown

Rcmex, S.A. De C.V. — 915-598-4072
Av. Profr. Ramon Rivera Lara, Juarez 31857 Mexico
Sterile & non sterile surgical gown , disposable

Scientimed Corp. — 510-763-5405
4109 Balfour Ave, Oakland, CA 94610
Or gowns.

Sloan Corp. — 402-597-5700
13316 A St, Omaha, NE 68144
Smock.

Sri Surgical — 813-891-9550
6801 Longe St, Stockton, CA 95206
Various.

Standard Textile — 800-999-0400
1 Knollcrest Dr, Cincinnati, OH 45237

Standard Textile Co., Inc. — 888-999-0400
PO Box 371805, Cincinnati, OH 45222
Surgical gown, theater gown, O.R. gown.

Sterilmed, Inc. — 763-488-3400
11400 73rd Ave N Ste 100, Maple Grove, MN 55369
Gown.

The Sewing Source, Inc. — 919-478-3900
802 E Nash St, Spring Hope, NC 27882
O.r./surgeons gown.

White Knight Healthcare — 800-851-4431
Calle 16, Number 780, Agua Prieta, Sonora Mexico
Gown, surgical

GRAFT, ARTERIAL, BIOLOGICAL *(Cardiovascular) 74LOW*

Artegraft, Inc. — 800-631-5264
220 N Center Dr, North Brunswick, NJ 08902
ARTEGRAFT 100% collagen matrix for long term patency as an A-V access or peripheral bypass graft.

Cryolife, Inc. — 800-438-8285
1655 Roberts Blvd NW, Kennesaw, GA 30144
CRYOGRAFT and OA GRAFTS. Also CRYOVEIN.

GRAFT, BONE *(Orthopedics) 87QYR*

Etex Corporation — 617-577-7270
38 Sidney St Ste 370, The Clark Bldg., Cambridge, MA 02139
α-BSM is a synthetic, bioresorbable bone substitute material engineered to mimic the chemical composition and crystalline structure of the mineral content of bone. It is easily implanted into the body as a moldable putty or an injectable paste and undergoes endothermically initiated setting at body temperature. This feature gives the surgeons adequate working time and the required flexibility to achieve a complete defect fill and graft containment after implantation. The material is resorbed through the body's natural cellular remodeling process.

Exactech, Inc. — 800-392-2832
2320 NW 66th Ct, Gainesville, FL 32653

Impladent Ltd. — 800-526-9343
19845 Foothill Ave, Hollis, NY 11423
87QYR Graft, Bone Class III. OsteoGen®, a synthetic bioactive resorbable graft (SBRG), is an osteoconductive, non-ceramic pure hydroxylapatite, simulating chemical, structural, and mechanical properties similar to trabecular human bone. OsteoGen® synthetic bone material is used for augmentation and repair of bone defects or sinus augmentation and is effective with dental implants to fill large trabecular spaces for implant osteotomy support and bone bridging. OsteoGen® is a highly crystalline material, comparable to natural human bone, with no a/? tricalcium phosphates, tetracalcium phosphates, amorphous phases, or bone-inhibiting pyrophosphates found in all ceramic hydroxylapatite (CHA).

Interpore Cross International — 800-722-4489
181 Technology Dr, Irvine, CA 92618
PRO OSTEON resorbable bone graft substitute is for bony voids or gaps of the skeletal system. It provides a bone graft substitute that resorbs and is replaced with bone during the healing process.

Lifecore Biomedical, Inc. — 952-368-4300
3515 Lyman Blvd, Chaska, MN 55318
HAPSET: Hydroxylapatite bone-graft substitute.

GRAFT, BONE *(cont'd)*

Osteotech, Inc. 800-537-9842
51 James Way, Eatontown, NJ 07724
Mineralized allograft bone.

University Of Miami Tissue Bank 888-UMTISSUE
1600 NW 10th Ave # R-12, Miami, FL 33136
Bone allografts, dura mater allografts, soft tissue allografts.

Wright Medical Group, Inc. 800-238-7117
5677 Airline Rd, Arlington, TN 38002

Zimmer Dental, Inc. 800-854-7019
1900 Aston Ave, Carlsbad, CA 92008
$30.00/gram for CALCITITE hydroxylapatite (HA) particles for alveolar-ridge augmentation and filling periodontal lesions.

GRAFT, BOVINE *(Surgery) 79QYS*

Artegraft, Inc. 800-631-5264
220 N Center Dr, North Brunswick, NJ 08902
ARTEGRAFT. The original bovine collagen vascular carotid artery graft with 35 years of continuous clinical performance and proven patency. Available in 6 to 8mm outside diameters and 15 to 52cm lengths. Indications for use include A-V access and peripheral bypass distal to the aorta.

Synovis Surgical Innovations 800-255-4018
2575 University Ave W, Saint Paul, MN 55114
The TISSUE-GUARD family of cross-linked bovine pericardium includes: DURA-GUARD Dural Repair Patch, PERI-GUARD Cardiac Patch, SUPPLE PERI-GUARD Cardiac Patch, and VASCU-GUARD Peripheral Vascular Patch. Synovis also manufactures VERITAS Collagen Matrix, a remodelable bovine pericardium material, for treatment of pelvic organ prolapse and stress urinary incontinence, and for soft tissue repairs.

GRAFT, SKIN *(Surgery) 79QYT*

Genzyme Corp. 800-232-7546
64 Sidney St, Cambridge, MA 02139
Cultured autograft.

Lifecell Corp. 800-367-5737
1 Millennium Way, Branchburg, NJ 08876
Cryopreserved Allograft Skin. Donated cadaver skin for temporary coverage of burn wounds.

Organogenesis Inc. 888-432-5232
150 Dan Rd, Canton, MA 02021
APLIGRAF is approved for use in venous leg ulcers and diabetic foot ulcers. It is a skin substitute that is bilayered and composed of living epidermal (keratinocytes) and dermal (fibroblasts) cells.

GRAFT, VASCULAR, BIOLOGICAL *(Cardiovascular) 74MAK*

Artegraft, Inc. 800-631-5264
220 N Center Dr, North Brunswick, NJ 08902
ARTEGRAFT 100% collagen vascular grafts for A-V access and peripheral bypass, available 6 to 8 mm O.D., and 15 to 52 cm lengths.

Bard Peripheral Vascular, Inc. 800-321-4254
1625 W 3rd St, Tempe, AZ 85281

Corvita Corp. 305-599-3100
8210 NW 27th St, Doral, FL 33122

Hancock/Jaffe Laboratories 949-261-2900
2807 McGaw Ave, Irvine, CA 92614
Vascular bioprosthesis.

Organogenesis Inc. 888-432-5232
150 Dan Rd, Canton, MA 02021
Being developed for use in coronary artery bypass procedures; currently in animal studies.

GRAFT, VASCULAR, BIOLOGICAL, HEMODIALYSIS ACCESS
(Gastro/Urology) 78MDQ

Artegraft, Inc. 800-631-5264
220 N Center Dr, North Brunswick, NJ 08902
ARTEGRAFT. 100% collagen matrix permits natural advantages over synthetic vascular grafts when used for A-V access and peripheral bypass. Available 6 to 8mm O.D., 15 to 52cm lengths.

GRAFT, VASCULAR, SYNTHETIC/BIOLOGICAL COMPOSITE
(Cardiovascular) 74MAL

Atrium Medical Corp. 800-528-7486
5 Wentworth Dr, Hudson, NH 03051
Nonbiological/composite. PTFE vascular grafts in a variety of sizes and configurations for peripheral and AV vascular reconstruction.

Corvita Corp. 305-599-3100
8210 NW 27th St, Doral, FL 33122
Under development.

GRAFT, VASCULAR, SYNTHETIC/BIOLOGICAL COMPOSITE *(cont'd)*

Datascope Corp. 800-288-2121
14 Philips Pkwy, Montvale, NJ 07645

Maquet Cardiovascular LLC 888-880-2874
45 Barbour Pond Dr, Wayne, NJ 07470
HEMASHIELD

GRID, AMSLER *(Ophthalmology) 86HOQ*

Keeler Instruments Inc. 800-523-5620
456 Park Way, Broomall, PA 19008
$32 pkg. of 100.

The Peristat Group, Inc. 714-928-8507
3721 Fillmore St, San Francisco, CA 94123
Amsler grid.

GRID, RADIOGRAPHIC *(Radiology) 90IXJ*

Alimed, Inc. 800-225-2610
297 High St, Dedham, MA 02026
Aluminum interspaced grids for diagnostic radiographs free of mottle and grid-line variations.

Americomp, Inc. 800-458-1782
2901 W Lawrence Ave, Chicago, IL 60625

Badge Machine Products, Inc. 585-394-0330
2491 Brickyard Rd, Canandaigua, NY 14424
Radiographic grid.

Bio-Med U.S.A. Inc. 973-278-5222
111 Ellison St, Paterson, NJ 07505
BIO GRID x-ray grid, light-weight aluminum interpaced.

Burkhart Roentgen Intl. Inc. 800-USA-XRAY
5201 8th Ave S, Gulfport, FL 33707
Grid specialists, all types available.

Burlington Medical Supplies, Inc. 800-221-3466
3 Elmhurst St, PO Box 3194, Newport News, VA 23603
Aluminum grids.

Composiflex, Inc. 800-673-2544
8100 Hawthorne Dr, Erie, PA 16509
Carbon fiber Buckey panels.

Mxe, Inc. 800-252-1801
12107 Jefferson Blvd, Culver City, CA 90230
Standard Grids, CR 'Highline' Grids, Decubitus (lines to short dimension) Grids, Specialty Grids. Grid protectors: k-Edge Slip On, Grid Cap, EZ Slide, Encasement, Slimlite Grid Cassette, Standard Grid Cassette.

Navilyst Medical 800-833-9973
100 Boston Scientific Way, Marlborough, MA 01752
A calibrating grid for cine-angiography.

Progeny, Inc. 847-415-9800
675 Heathrow Dr, Lincolnshire, IL 60069
Bucky.

Reina Imaging 815-356-8181
6107 Lou St, Crystal Lake, IL 60014

Soyee Products, Inc. 800-574-4743
459 Thompson Rd, Thompson, CT 06277

Spectronics Corporation 800-274-8888
956 Brush Hollow Rd, Westbury, NY 11590
Mammography, stationary, Bucky, slip-on, drop-on grids & grid cassettes.

Tuzik Boston 800-886-6363
104 Longwater Dr, Assinippi Park, Norwell, MA 02061

Umi Intl. 888-511-8655
2 E Union Ave, PO Box 170, East Rutherford, NJ 07073
X-ray radiography grid, x-ray mammography grid, x-ray digital grid.

Wehmer Corporation 800-323-0229
1151 N Main St, Lombard, IL 60148
$330 for X-ray filter grid.

Wolf X-Ray Corporation 800-356-9729
100 W Industry Ct, Deer Park, NY 11729
Over 100 different types.

Xma (X-Ray Marketing Associates, Inc.) 800-325-8880
1205 W Lakeview Ct, Windham Lakes Business Park
Romeoville, IL 60446

GRINDER, TISSUE *(Pathology) 88LEC*

Exakt Technologies, Inc. 800-866-7172
7002 Broadway Ext, Oklahoma City, OK 73116
Complete system for embedding, cutting, and grinding undecalcified hard and soft tissue with or without biomaterial implants to thickness of 10 microns.

Glas-Col , Llc 800-452-7265
711 Hulman St, PO Box 2128, Terre Haute, IN 47802
Various sizes and pestle types.

Handler Manufacturing Co. 800-274-2635
612 North Ave E, Westfield, NJ 07090
SANI-GRINDER, used to grind and polish orthotic prosthesis; collect dust from this process.

GUARD, DISK *(Dental And Oral) 76EEJ*

Abrasive Technology, Inc. 740-548-4100
8400 Green Meadows Dr N, Lewis Center, OH 43035
Accessory for abrasive disk.

G & H Wire Co. 800-526-1026
2165 Earlywood Dr, Franklin, IN 46131

Total Molding Services, Inc. 215-538-9613
354 East Broad St., Trumbauersville, PA 18970
Custom Fittable Nightguard for person's with teeth grinding problem

GUIDE *(Orthopedics) 87HXH*

Biopro, Inc. 800-252-7707
2929 Lapeer Rd, Port Huron, MI 48060
Accu-Cut Osteotomy Guide System

DJO Inc. 800-336-6569
1430 Decision St, Vista, CA 92081

Holmed Corporation 508-238-3351
40 Norfolk Ave, South Easton, MA 02375

Stryker Spine 866-457-7463
2 Pearl Ct, Allendale, NJ 07401

Zimmer Holdings, Inc. 800-613-6131
1800 W Center St, PO Box 708, Warsaw, IN 46580

GUIDE, CATHETER *(Cardiovascular) 74WTR*

Angiodynamics, Inc. 518-795-1400
14 Plaza Drive, Latham, NY 12110

Boston Scientific Corp. 800-323-6472
5905 Nathan Ln N, Minneapolis, MN 55442
SOFTIP guiding catheter.

Cardio-Nef, S.A. De C.V. 01-800-024-0240
Rio Grijalva 186, Col. Mitras Norte, Monterrey, N.L. 64320 Mexico

Cook Inc. 800-457-4500
PO Box 489, Bloomington, IN 47402

M & I Medical Sales, Inc. 305-663-6444
4711 SW 72nd Ave, Miami, FL 33155

Vernay Laboratories, Inc. 800-666-5227
120 E South College St, Yellow Springs, OH 45387

GUIDE, DEVICE, ULTRASONIC *(General) 80WXY*

Pharmaceutical Innovations, Inc. 973-242-2900
897 Frelinghuysen Ave, Newark, NJ 07114
ULTRA/PHONIC BP - Breast Phantom. For hand/eye coordination practice for ultrasound guided needle biopsy. Reusable, self-healing and acoustically accurate. Ramdomly embedded target structures. $165.00 each.

Phillips Ultrasound 800-982-2011
22100 Bothell Everett Hwy, P.O. Box 3003, Bothell, WA 98021

GUIDE, DRILL *(Orthopedics) 87QZA*

Holmed Corporation 508-238-3351
40 Norfolk Ave, South Easton, MA 02375

Kls-Martin L.P. 800-625-1557
11239-1 St. John`s Industrial, Parkway South
Jacksonville, FL 32250

Stryker Spine 866-457-7463
2 Pearl Ct, Allendale, NJ 07401

Zimmer Holdings, Inc. 800-613-6131
1800 W Center St, PO Box 708, Warsaw, IN 46580
ACL reconstruction, cannulated.

GUIDE, DRILL, LIGAMENT *(Orthopedics) 87LXI*

Arthrex, Inc. 239-643-5553
1370 Creekside Blvd, Naples, FL 34108
Various types of marking hooks.

GUIDE, GIGLI SAW *(Orthopedics) 87QZB*

Princeton Medical Group, Inc. 800-875-0869
1189 Royal Links Dr, Mt Pleasant, SC 29466

Stryker Spine 866-457-7463
2 Pearl Ct, Allendale, NJ 07401

Zimmer Holdings, Inc. 800-613-6131
1800 W Center St, PO Box 708, Warsaw, IN 46580

GUIDE, INTRAOCULAR LENS *(Ophthalmology) 86KYB*

A.M.O. Puerto Rico Manufacturing, Inc 714-247-8656
Rd. 402, Km. 4.2, Anasco, PR 00610
Intraocular lens (iol) insertion systems.

Fortrad Eye Instruments Corp. 973-543-2371
8 Franklin Rd, Mendham, NJ 07945

Hurricane Medical 941-751-0588
5315 Lena Rd, Bradenton, FL 34211
Surgical glide.

Staar Surgical Co. 800-292-7902
1911 Walker Ave, Monrovia, CA 91016
MicroSTAAR Injector System (P1)

GUIDE, NEEDLE *(Surgery) 79TDD*

Katena Products, Inc. 800-225-1195
4 Stewart Ct, Denville, NJ 07834

Rocket Medical Plc. 800-707-7625
150 Recreation Park Dr Ste 3, Hingham, MA 02043

GUIDE, SURGICAL, INSTRUMENT *(Surgery) 79FZX*

Abbott Spine, Inc. 847-937-6100
12708 Riata Vista Cir Ste B-100, Austin, TX 78727
Guide.

Aesculap Implant Systems Inc. 1-800-234-9179
3773 Corporate Pkwy, Center Valley, PA 18034

Atricure, Inc. 888.347.6403
6217 Centre Park Dr, West Chester, OH 45069
Instrument guide.

Beere Precision Medical Instruments, Kmedic, Telef 919-544-8000
5307 95th Ave, Kenosha, WI 53144
Various types of surgical instrument guides.

Biomet Microfixation Inc. 800-874-7711
1520 Tradeport Dr, Jacksonville, FL 32218
Various types of guides.

Biomet, Inc. 574-267-6639
56 E Bell Dr, PO Box 587, Warsaw, IN 46582
Various types of orthopedic guide.

Boston Scientific - Marina Bay Customer Fulfillment Center 617-689-6000
500 Commander Shea Blvd, Quincy, MA 02171
Various.

Boston Scientific Corporation 508-652-5578
780 Brookside Dr, Spencer, IN 47460

Depuy Mitek, A Johnson & Johnson Company 800-451-2006
50 Scotland Blvd, Bridgewater, MA 02324
Guidewires, drill guide.

Depuy Orthopaedics, Inc. 800-473-3789
700 Orthopaedic Dr, P.O. Box 988, Warsaw, IN 46582
Various surgical guides.

Depuy Spine, Inc. 800-227-6633
325 Paramount Dr, Raynham, MA 02767
Orthopaedic guide.

Innovative Medical Products, Inc. 800-467-4944
87 Spring Lane, Plainville Industrial Pk, Plainville, CT 06062
FEMUR FINDER, a surgical instrument to help the surgeon locate the area to be drilled when inserting a femoral nail. Reduces length of surgery. IMP Innovative Medical Products #198GW Spade Tip Reamerwire for use with FEMUR FINDER cost effective wire to drill through piriformis fossa and direct wire straight into intramedullary canal. Requires less time, less disection.

Inrad 800-558-4647
4375 Donkers Ct SE, Kentwood, MI 49512
Ghiatas Beaded Breast Localization Wire, UltraWire One-handed breast localization device, with safety needle, Stiffening cannula.

Interphase Implants, Inc. 248-442-1460
19928 Farmington Rd, Livonia, MI 48152
Drill guide.

GUIDE, SURGICAL, INSTRUMENT *(cont'd)*

Interventional Spine, Inc. 800-497-0484
13700 Alton Pkwy Ste 160, Irvine, CA 92618
Various types of surgical instrument guides.

Medtronic Sofamor Danek Instrument Manufacturing 901-396-3133
7375 Adrianne Pl, Bartlett, TN 38133
Various types of drill guides & guide wires (pins).

Medtronic Sofamor Danek Usa, Inc. 901-396-3133
4340 Swinnea Rd, Memphis, TN 38118
Various types of drill guides & guide wires (pins).

Medtronic Spine Llc 877-690-5353
1221 Crossman Ave, Sunnyvale, CA 94089
Various.

Small Bone Innovations, Inc. 215-428-1791
1380 S Pennsylvania Ave, Morrisville, PA 19067
Manual surgical instrument for general use.

Surgical Implant Generation Network (Sign) 509-371-1107
451 Hills St, Richland, WA 99354
Various sizes and types of drill guides.

Symmetry Medical Usa, Inc. 574-267-8700
486 W 350 N, Warsaw, IN 46582
Instrument guide.

Tl Tate Mfg, Inc. 765-452-8283
1500 N Webster St, Kokomo, IN 46901
Surgical instruments.

W. L. Gore & Associates, Inc. 800-437-8181
PO Box 2400, Flagstaff, AZ 86003
S.A.M. SILICONE SIZER

W.L. Gore & Associates,Inc 928-526-3030
1505 North Fourth St., Flagstaff, AZ 86004
Surgical guide for measuring prosthesis selection.

Warsaw Orthopedic, Inc. 901-396-3133
2500 Silveus Xing, Warsaw, IN 46582
Various types of drill guides & guide wires (pins).

Zimmer Spine, Inc. 800-655-2614
7375 Bush Lake Rd, Minneapolis, MN 55439
Surgical instrument guide.

Zimmer Trabecular Metal Technology 800-613-6131
10 Pomeroy Rd, Parsippany, NJ 07054
Cementless resection guide 14.

GUIDE, SURGICAL, NEEDLE *(Surgery) 79GDF*

Aesculap Implant Systems Inc. 1-800-234-9179
3773 Corporate Pkwy, Center Valley, PA 18034

Allez Medical Applications, Inc. 714-641-2098
2141 S Standard Ave, Santa Ana, CA 92707
Sterile fascia closure kit with suture passer instrument and needle guide.

Argon Medical Devices Inc. 903-675-9321
1445 Flat Creek Rd, Athens, TX 75751
Arterial needle cournand needle & perc needle.

Biomet Microfixation Inc. 800-874-7711
1520 Tradeport Dr, Jacksonville, FL 32218
Various types of guides.

Boston Scientific - Marina Bay Customer Fulfillment Center 617-689-6000
500 Commander Shea Blvd, Quincy, MA 02171
Various.

Boston Scientific Corp. 408-935-3400
150 Baytech Dr, San Jose, CA 95134
Surgical guide needle.

Boston Scientific Corporation 508-652-5578
8600 NW 41st St, Doral, FL 33166

Havel's Inc. 800-638-4770
3726 Lonsdale St, Cincinnati, OH 45227

Health Care Logistics, Inc. 800-848-1633
450 Town St, PO Box 25, Circleville, OH 43113
Various models of needle holders.

Inrad 800-558-4647
4375 Donkers Ct SE, Kentwood, MI 49512
Blunt needle guide.

Kelsar, S.A. 508-261-8000
Blvd. Insurgentes, Libriamento a La, Tijuana 22450 Mexico
Biofragmentable anastomosis ring, purse string suture and accessories

GUIDE, SURGICAL, NEEDLE *(cont'd)*

Medisiss 866-866-7477
2747 SW 6th St, Redmond, OR 97756
Various surgical needle guides,sterile.

Promex Technologies, Llc 317-736-0128
3049 Hudson St, Franklin, IN 46131
Needle guide, breast lesion localization needle.

Sanarus Medical, Inc. 925-460-5730
4696 Willow Rd, Pleasanton, CA 94588
Surgical guide needle.

Suros Surgical Systems, Inc 877-887-8767
6100 Technology Center Dr, Indianapolis, IN 46278
Trocar style/co-axial introducer needle.

Suturtek Incorporated
51 Middlesex St, North Chelmsford, MA 01863
Minimally invasive suturing device.

Tmx Engineering & Manufacturing, Inc. 714-641-5884
2141 S Standard Ave, Santa Ana, CA 92707
Sterile fascia closure kit with suture passer instrument and needle guide.

Vnus Medical Technologies, Inc. 888-797-8346
5799 Fontanoso Way, San Jose, CA 95138
Arterial needle.

GUIDE, WIRE, ANGIOGRAPHIC (AND ACCESSORIES) *(Cns/Neurology) 84HAP*

Acme-Monaco Corp. 860-224-1349
75 Winchell Rd, New Britain, CT 06052

Boston Scientific Corp. 800-323-6472
5905 Nathan Ln N, Minneapolis, MN 55442
ANGIOPORT guidewire catheter introducer.

Diablo Sales & Marketing, Inc. 925-648-1611
PO Box 3219, Danville, CA 94526
Custom design and manufacturing of catheters and specialty guidewires. Guiding catheters; stent delivery and drug delivery systems.

Fort Wayne Metals Research Prod. Corp. 260-747-4154
9609 Ardmore Ave, Fort Wayne, IN 46809
Various grades, properties and shapes of precision wire.

Guidewire Technologies, Inc. 800-894-4399
26 Keewaydin Dr, Salem, NH 03079

Lake Region Manufacturing, Inc. 952-448-5111
340 Lake Hazeltine Dr, Chaska, MN 55318
Stainless steel and PTFE coated guidewires.

Oscor, Inc. 800-726-7267
3816 Desoto Blvd, Palm Harbor, FL 34683
Lead adaptor.

GUIDEWIRE *(Cardiovascular) 74QYZ*

Acme-Monaco Corp. 860-224-1349
75 Winchell Rd, New Britain, CT 06052
.014 through .080, length 20 cm through 400 cm, J radius 1.5 mm to 15 mm.

Boston Scientific - Maple Grove 800-553-5878
1 Scimed Pl, Maple Grove, MN 55311
ENTRE II guidewire and MAGNET exchange device PTCA guidewire system for exchange of over-the-wire PTCA balloon catheters.

C. R. Bard, Inc. 800-367-2273
730 Central Ave, New Providence, NJ 07974
COMMANDER series offers 54 guidewires addressing six performance categories.

Cardio-Nef, S.A. De C.V. 01-800-024-0240
Rio Grijalva 186, Col. Mitras Norte, Monterrey, N.L. 64320 Mexico

Cardiomed Supplies Inc. 800-387-9757
5 Gormley Industrial Ave., P.O. Box 575
Gormley, ONT L0H 1 Canada
Complete range of stainless steel and teflon coated guide wire - with J and soft end for added safety to the patients.

Cook Inc. 800-457-4500
PO Box 489, Bloomington, IN 47402

Cook Urological, Inc. 800-457-4500
1100 W Morgan St, P.O. Box 227, Spencer, IN 47460

Dma Med-Chem Corporation 800-362-1833
49 Watermill Ln, Great Neck, NY 11021

Fort Wayne Metals Research Prod. Corp. 260-747-4154
9609 Ardmore Ave, Fort Wayne, IN 46809
Various grades, properties and shapes of precision wire.

GUIDEWIRE *(cont'd)*

Guidewire Technologies, Inc. 800-894-4399
26 Keewaydin Dr, Salem, NH 03079

Hospira, Inc. 877-946-7747
755 Jarvis Dr, Morgan Hill, CA 95037

Lake Region Manufacturing, Inc. 952-448-5111
340 Lake Hazeltine Dr, Chaska, MN 55318
Steerable and infusion guidewires. Endoscopic and urological guidewires are also available.

M & I Medical Sales, Inc. 305-663-6444
4711 SW 72nd Ave, Miami, FL 33155

Marconi Medical Systems 800-323-0550
595 Miner Rd, Cleveland, OH 44143

Mcdalt Medical Corp. 800-841-5774
2225 Prestonwood Dr Ste 100-A, Arlington, TX 76012
Diagnostic and interventional.

Medi-Globe Corporation 800-966-1431
110 W Orion St Ste 136, Tempe, AZ 85283
Guidewires for endoscopy. Also multi-feature guidewire.

Medovations, Inc. 800-558-6408
102 E Keefe Ave, Milwaukee, WI 53212

St. Jude Medical Atrial Fibrillation 800-328-3873
14901 Deveau Pl, Minnetonka, MN 55345
Double distal guidewires with 3mm J and straight tip (.025, .032, .038 diameter wires available).

Telemed Systems Inc. 800-481-6718
8 Kane Industrial Dr, Hudson, MA 01749

Tfx Medical Oem 800-548-6600
50 Plantation Dr, Jaffrey, NH 03452

Wytech Industries, Inc. 732-396-3900
960 E Hazelwood Ave, Rahway, NJ 07065
Introducer wire.

GUIDEWIRE, CATHETER *(Cardiovascular) 74DQX*

Abbott Vascular, Cardiac Therapies 800-227-9902
26531 Ynez Rd, Mailing P.O. Box 9018, Temecula, CA 92591
Cardiovascular guidewire.

Abbott Vascular, Vascular Solutions 800-227-9902
26531 Ynez Rd, Temecula, CA 92591
Guide wire.

Acme-Monaco Corp. 860-224-1349
75 Winchell Rd, New Britain, CT 06052
.014 through .080, length 20 cm through 400 cm, J radius 1.5 mm to 15 mm.

Advanced Biomedical Devices, Inc. (Abd, Inc.) 978-470-1177
Dundee Park, Bldg. 17, Andover, MA 01810
VariSoft Guide Wire Extension; VariSoft Steerable Guide Wire

Aga Medical Corporation. 888-546-4407
5050 Nathan Ln N, Plymouth, MN 55442
AMPLATZER® Guidewires--AMPLATZER Guidewires are manufactured from stainless steel and are coated with PTFE, offering excellent glide and positioning capabilities. Guidewire length, diameter, core configuration, and tip configuration are all indicated on the product label.

Angiodynamics, Inc. 800-472-5221
1 Horizon Way, Manchester, GA 31816
0.038 in. O.D. by 70cm J/straight double ended guidewire.

Argon Medical Devices Inc. 903-675-9321
1445 Flat Creek Rd, Athens, TX 75751
Sniper guide wire.

Arrow Internacional De Mexico, S.A. De C.V. 610-378-0131
Modulo 1, Circuito 5, Parque Industrias De America
Col. Panamericana, Chihuahua Mexico
Various types and sizes of wire guides

Arrow International, Inc. 800-523-8446
2400 Bernville Rd, Reading, PA 19605
TRUE TORQUE vascular access guidewires.

Avantec Vascular Corp. 408-329-5425
605 W California Ave, Sunnyvale, CA 94086
Guide wire.

B. Braun Medical, Inc. 610-596-2536
901 Marcon Blvd, Allentown, PA 18109
GUIDEWIRES; TORQUE DEVICE; GUIDEWIRE TRAY

Bard Reynosa S.A. De C.V. 908-277-8000
Blvd. Montebello #1, Parque Industrial Colonial
Reynosa, Tamaulipas Mexico
Various

GUIDEWIRE, CATHETER *(cont'd)*

Becton Dickinson Infusion Therapy Systems, Inc. 888-237-2762
9450 S State St, Sandy, UT 84070

Biosphere Medical, Inc. 781-681-7900
1050 Hingham St, Rockland, MA 02370
Guidewire.

Biotronik, Inc. 503-635-3594
6024 Jean Rd, Lake Oswego, OR 97035
Various models of Catheter accessories

Boston Scientific - Maple Grove 800-553-5878
1 Scimed Pl, Maple Grove, MN 55311

Boston Scientific Corp. 800-323-6472
5905 Nathan Ln N, Minneapolis, MN 55442
Guidewires for angiography and angioplasty procedures.

Boston Scientific Corporation 508-652-5578
8600 NW 41st St, Doral, FL 33166

Boston Scientific Corporation 800-225-2732
1 Boston Scientific Pl, Natick, MA 01760

BridgePoint Medical 763-225-8500
2800 Campus Dr Ste 50, Plymouth, MN 55441
Entera; Stingray Guidewire; Stingray Guidewire - Stiff

C. R. Bard, Inc., Bard Urological Div. 888-367-2273
13183 Harland Dr NE, Covington, GA 30014

Cardio-Nef, S.A. De C.V. 01-800-024-0240
Rio Grijalva 186, Col. Mitras Norte, Monterrey, N.L. 64320 Mexico

Cardiomed Supplies Inc. 800-387-9757
5 Gormley Industrial Ave., P.O. Box 575
Gormley, ONT L0H 1 Canada
BOURASSA guidewires for cath lab.

Cathguide, Division Of Scilogy Corp. 305-269-0500
9135 Fontainebleau Blvd Apt 5, Miami, FL 33172
Various sizes of guidewires.

Concentric Medical, Inc. 650-938-2100
301 E Evelyn Ave, Mountain View, CA 94041
Catheter guidewire.

Conceptus, Inc. 650-962-4000
331 E Evelyn Ave, Mountain View, CA 94041

Cook Inc. 800-457-4500
PO Box 489, Bloomington, IN 47402

Cook Urological, Inc. 800-457-4500
1100 W Morgan St, P.O. Box 227, Spencer, IN 47460

Cook Vascular, Incorporated 800-457-4500
1186 Montgomery Ln, Vandergrift, PA 15690
LIBERATOR Locking System - Universal locking stylet used during the removal of transvenous cardiac leads. Packaged individually.

Cordis Neurovascular, Inc. 800-327-7714
14201 NW 60th Ave, Miami Lakes, FL 33014
Guide wire.

Datascope Corp., Cardiac Assist Division 201-307-5400
1300 MacArthur Blvd, Mahwah, NJ 07430
Catheter guide wire.

Ev3 Inc. 800-716-6700
9600 54th Ave N, Plymouth, MN 55442
Guidewires.

Ev3 Inc. 800-716-6700
4600 Nathan Ln N, Plymouth, MN 55442
Guidewires.

Ev3 Neurovascular 800-716-6700
9775 Toledo Way, Irvine, CA 92618
Guidewire.

Flowcardia, Inc. 408-617-0352
745 N Pastoria Ave, Sunnyvale, CA 94085
Guidewire.

Fort Wayne Metals Research Prod. Corp. 260-747-4154
9609 Ardmore Ave, Fort Wayne, IN 46809
Various grades, properties and shapes of precision wire.

Galt Medical Corp. 800-639-2800
2220 Merritt Dr, Garland, TX 75041
Sterile and non-sterile guidewire.

Guidewire Technologies, Inc. 800-894-4399
26 Keewaydin Dr, Salem, NH 03079

Intella Interventional Systems, Inc. 408-737-7121
870 Hermosa Ave, Sunnyvale, CA 94085
Guidewire.

GUIDEWIRE, CATHETER *(cont'd)*

Interventional Technologies, Inc. 858-268-4488
30590 Cochise Cir, Murrieta, CA 92563
Various models of guide wires.

Intraluminal Therapeutics, Inc. 800-513-4458
6354 Corte Del Abeto Ste A, Carlsbad, CA 92011
Safe-Cross Crossing Wire. A guide wire designed to cross total occlusions with Optical Coherance Reflectometetry and Radio Frequency.

Maquet Puerto Rico Inc. 408-635-3900
No. 12, Rd. #698, Dorado, PR 00646
Various.

Medical Device Technologies, Inc. (Md Tech) 800-338-0440
3600 SW 47th Ave, Gainesville, FL 32608
NEOSOFT Drainage Catheters, nephrostomy, biliary, and abscess drainage. SKATER Drainage Catheters, nephrostomy, biliary, and abscess drainage. TCD Drainage Catheters, nephrostomy, biliary, and abscess drainage.

Medtronic Vascular 707-525-0111
3576 Unocal Pl, Santa Rosa, CA 95403
Guide wire, filter wire

Merit Medical Systems, Inc. 801-253-1600
1111 S Velasco St, Angleton, TX 77515
Guidewire.

Merit Medical Systems, Inc. 800-356-3748
1600 Merit Pkwy, South Jordan, UT 84095
Diagnostic guidewires. Hydrophilic guidewires

Micrus Endovascular Corporation 888-550-4120
821 Fox Ln, San Jose, CA 95131
Wire,guide,catheter.

Navilyst Medical 800-833-9973
100 Boston Scientific Way, Marlborough, MA 01752
Various sterile angiographic guidewires and accessories.

Navion Biomedical Corp. 781-341-8058
312 Tosca Dr, Stoughton, MA 02072
MAPWIRE disposable j-tip guidewire with sensor in its tip. Replaces standard guidewire for catheter placement.

Neo Metrics, Inc. 763-559-4440
Fernbrook Lane N, Suite J, Minneapolis, MN 55447
Access guidewire.

Radius Medical Technologies, Inc. 978-263-4466
15 Craig Rd, Acton, MA 01720
Radius 018 Cougar Wire; Radius Cougar Wire

Sonosite, Inc. 888-482-9449
21919 30th Dr SE, Bothell, WA 98021
LumenVu

Stereotaxis, Inc. 866-646-2346
4320 Forest Park Ave Ste 100, Saint Louis, MO 63108
Cardiodrive Catheter Advancement Sy

Tfx Medical Oem 800-548-6600
50 Plantation Dr, Jaffrey, NH 03452

Toray International America Inc. 800-662-1777
140 Cypress Station Dr Ste 210, Houston, TX 77090
TORAYGUIDE used in percutaneous procedures to introduce and position catheters and other interventional devices in the central and peripheral vasculature.

Vnus Medical Technologies, Inc. 888-797-8346
5799 Fontanoso Way, San Jose, CA 95138
Guide wire.

Volcano Corporation 800-228-4728
3661 Valley Centre Dr Ste 200, San Diego, CA 92130
Doppler guide wire.

Wytech Industries, Inc. 732-396-3900
960 E Hazelwood Ave, Rahway, NJ 07065

GUIDEWIRE, CATHETER, RADIOLOGICAL *(Radiology) 90JAJ*

Acme-Monaco Corp. 860-224-1349
75 Winchell Rd, New Britain, CT 06052
.014 through .080, length 20 cm through 400 cm, J radius 1.5 mm to 15 mm.

Cook Inc. 800-457-4500
PO Box 489, Bloomington, IN 47402

Diablo Sales & Marketing, Inc. 925-648-1611
PO Box 3219, Danville, CA 94526
Custom design and manufacturing of catheters and specialty guidewires. Guiding catheters; stent delivery and drug delivery systems.

GUIDEWIRE, CATHETER, RADIOLOGICAL *(cont'd)*

Fort Wayne Metals Research Prod. Corp. 260-747-4154
9609 Ardmore Ave, Fort Wayne, IN 46809
Various grades, properties and shapes of precision wire.

Guidewire Technologies, Inc. 800-894-4399
26 Keewaydin Dr, Salem, NH 03079

Medical Device Technologies, Inc. (Md Tech) 800-338-0440
3600 SW 47th Ave, Gainesville, FL 32608
MD TECH, WORKER.

Tfx Medical Oem 800-548-6600
50 Plantation Dr, Jaffrey, NH 03452

Uresil, Llc 800-538-7374
5418 Touhy Ave, Skokie, IL 60077
Guidewires for percutaneous placement of catheters.

GUIDEWIRE, CATHETER, REPROCESSED
(Cardiovascular) 74NKQ

Insitu Technologies, Inc. 651-389-1017
5810 Blackshire Path, Inver Grove Heights, MN 55076
Ptca guidewires, .014' guidewires.

GUIDEWIRE, CORONARY, TOTAL OCCLUSION
(Cardiovascular) 74NFN

Boston Scientific Corporation 800-225-2732
1 Boston Scientific Pl, Natick, MA 01760
Kinetix Guidewire

GUILLOTINE, TONSIL *(Ear/Nose/Throat) 77KBO*

Aesculap Implant Systems Inc. 1-800-234-9179
3773 Corporate Pkwy, Center Valley, PA 18034

GUTTA PERCHA *(Dental And Oral) 76EKM*

Coltene/Whaledent Inc. 330-916-8858
235 Ascot Pkwy, Cuyahoga Falls, OH 44223
Gutta percha.

Dentalez Group 866-DTE-INFO
101 Lindenwood Dr Ste 225, Valleybrooke Corporate Center
Malvern, PA 19355

Endodent, Inc. 626-359-5715
851 Meridian St, Duarte, CA 91010
Compounded dental gutta percha as per customer requirements. Also available, Points, Gutta Percha.

Future Dental Technologies, Inc. 909-894-4203
26398 Deere Ct Ste 105, Murrieta, CA 92562
Various; gutta-percha heater (accessory).

Js Dental Mfg., Inc. 800-284-3368
196 N Salem Rd, Ridgefield, CT 06877
Gutta percha points.

Kerr Corp. 714-516-7400
28200 Wick Rd, Romulus, MI 48174
Gutta percha.

Maximum Dental, Inc. 631-245-2176
600 Meadowlands Pkwy Ste 269, Secaucus, NJ 07094

Medidenta International, Inc. 800-221-0750
3923 62nd St, PO Box 409, Woodside, NY 11377

Miltex Dental Technologies, Inc. 516-576-6022
589 Davies Dr, York, PA 17402
Various gutta percha points and cones and accessories.

Moyco Technologies, Inc. 800-331-8837
200 Commerce Dr, Montgomeryville, PA 18936

Pentron Clinical Technologies 203-265-7397
68-70 North Plains Industrial, Road, Wallingford, CT 06492
Gutta-percha.

Precise Dental Internacional S.A.C.V. 818-992-5333
925 Parque Cuzin Belenes Norte, Zapopan, Jalisoo Mexico
Gutta-percha points

Rite-Dent Manufacturing Corp. 305-693-8626
3750 E 10th Ct, Hialeah, FL 33013
Various types of gutta percha.

United Dental Manufacturers, Inc. 918-878-0450
PO Box 700874, Tulsa, OK 74170
Gutta-percha points ISO-DIN 13965 plus accessories.

United Dental Mfg., Inc. 717-845-7511
608 Rolling Hills Dr, Johnson City, TN 37604
Gutta percha, endodontic points.

Zenith/Dmg Brand 800-662-6383
242 S Dean St, Division of Foremost Dental LLC, Englewood, NJ 07631

HALTER, HEAD, TRACTION *(Physical Med) 89IRS*

A&A Orthopedics, Incorporated 757-224-0177
12250 SW 129th Ct Bldg 1, Miami, FL 33186
Head halter.

Alimed, Inc. 800-225-2610
297 High St, Dedham, MA 02026

Bird & Cronin, Inc. 651-683-1111
1200 Trapp Rd, Saint Paul, MN 55121
Head halter.

DJO Inc. 800-336-6569
1430 Decision St, Vista, CA 92081

Dynatronics Corp. Chattanooga Operations 801-568-7000
6607 Mountain View Rd, Ooltewah, TN 37363
Head halter, traction.

Florida Manufacturing Corp. 800-447-2372
501 Beville Rd, South Daytona, FL 32119

Freeman Manufacturing Company 800-253-2091
900 W Chicago Rd, PO Box J, Sturgis, MI 49091

Larkotex Company 800-972-3037
1002 Olive St, Texarkana, TX 75501

Lossing Orthopedic 800-328-5216
PO Box 6224, Minneapolis, MN 55406
LOSSING adjustable head cradle is designed for single patient use, has built-in sub-occipital support and extra padding to allow precise yet comfortable positioning; also, LOSSING adjustable head cradle for mobilization gives firm, locking grip to facilitate posterior and rotation releases.

Morrison Medical 800-438-6677
3735 Paragon Dr, Columbus, OH 43228
HEAD VISE II head immobilizer made of water resistant cardboard; folds up for support; disposable - one time use.

Shamrock Medical, Inc. 503-233-5055
3620 SE Powell Blvd, Portland, OR 97202
Unit incl. detachable chin strap.

Surgical Appliance Industries 800-888-0458
3960 Rosslyn Dr, Cincinnati, OH 45209

Warsaw Orthopedic, Inc. 901-396-3133
2500 Silveus Xing, Warsaw, IN 46582
Various types of head halters and cervical traction devices.

HALTER, HEAD, TRACTION, ORTHOPEDIC *(Orthopedics) 87HSS*

Alimed, Inc. 800-225-2610
297 High St, Dedham, MA 02026

American Orthopedic Supply Co., Inc.
37017 State Highway 79, Cleveland, AL 35049
Head halter.

Biomet, Inc. 574-267-6639
56 E Bell Dr, PO Box 587, Warsaw, IN 46582
Various types of halters, head, traction.

Border Opportunity Saver Systems, Inc. 830-775-0992
10 Finegan Rd, Del Rio, TX 78840

Chattanooga Group 800-592-7329
4717 Adams Rd, Hixson, TN 37343
TXA-1 traction accessory package.

Florida Manufacturing Corp. 800-447-2372
501 Beville Rd, South Daytona, FL 32119

Freeman Manufacturing Company 800-253-2091
900 W Chicago Rd, PO Box J, Sturgis, MI 49091

Larkotex Company 800-972-3037
1002 Olive St, Texarkana, TX 75501

Lohmann & Rauscher, Inc. 800-279-3863
6001 SW 6th Ave Ste 101, Topeka, KS 66615

Lossing Orthopedic 800-328-5216
PO Box 6224, Minneapolis, MN 55406
LOSSING adjustable head cradle is designed for single patient use, has built-in sub-occipital support and extra padding to allow precise yet comfortable positioning; also, LOSSING adjustable head cradle for mobilization gives firm, locking grip to facilitate posterior and rotation releases.

Mizuho Osi 800-777-4674
30031 Ahern Ave, Union City, CA 94587
Full line

Paramedical Distributors 800-245-3278
2020 Grand Blvd, Kansas City, MO 64108

Scott Specialties, Inc. 785-527-5627
1827 Meadowlark Rd, Clay Center, KS 67432
Various types of head halters.

HALTER, HEAD, TRACTION, ORTHOPEDIC *(cont'd)*

Scott Specialties, Inc. 785-527-5627
1820 E 7th St, Concordia, KS 66901

Slawner Ltd., J. 514-731-3378
5713 Cote Des Neiges Rd., Montreal, QUE H3S 1Y7 Canada

Tetra Medical Supply Corp. 800-621-4041
6364 W Gross Point Rd, Niles, IL 60714

The Saunders Group 800-445-9836
4250 Norex Dr, Chaska, MN 55318
Head halter.

Vmg Medical, Inc. 540-337-1996
542 Walnut Hills Rd, Staunton, VA 24401
Head halter.

Zimmer Holdings, Inc. 800-613-6131
1800 W Center St, PO Box 708, Warsaw, IN 46580

Zimmer Orthopaedic Surgical Products 800-321-5533
PO Box 10, 200 West Ohio Ave., Dover, OH 44622
ZIMCODE.

HAMMER, NEUROLOGICAL *(Cns/Neurology) 84QZF*

Codman & Shurtleff, Inc 800-225-0460
325 Paramount Dr, Raynham, MA 02767

Elmed, Inc. 630-543-2792
60 W Fay Ave, Addison, IL 60101

Her-Mar, Inc. 800-327-8209
8550 NW 30th Ter, Doral, FL 33122
$6.50 per unit (standard).

Medworks Instruments 800-323-9790
PO Box 581, Chatham, IL 62629
$28.95 for Troemner pattern. Queen square set comes in twelve and 16 inch with nylon handles and soft or extra soft bumpers for $9.50 per set.

Miltex Inc. 800-645-8000
589 Davies Dr, York, PA 17402

HAMMER, PERCUSSION *(Cns/Neurology) 84QZG*

American Diagnostic Corporation (Adc) 800-232-2670
55 Commerce Dr, Hauppauge, NY 11788
Taylor, buck, babinski hammers

Codman & Shurtleff, Inc 800-225-0460
325 Paramount Dr, Raynham, MA 02767

Elmed, Inc. 630-543-2792
60 W Fay Ave, Addison, IL 60101

Her-Mar, Inc. 800-327-8209
8550 NW 30th Ter, Doral, FL 33122
$2.50 per unit (standard).

Medworks Instruments 800-323-9790
PO Box 581, Chatham, IL 62629
$1.30 per unit, Taylor Tomahawk.

Miltex Inc. 800-645-8000
589 Davies Dr, York, PA 17402

Princeton Medical Group, Inc. 800-875-0869
1189 Royal Links Dr, Mt Pleasant, SC 29466

Riverbank Laboratories 630-232-2207
2613 Kaneville Ct, PO Box 110, Geneva, IL 60134

Trans American Medical / Tamsco Instruments 708-430-7777
7633 W 100th Pl, Bridgeview, IL 60455
All types. Diagnostic.

HAMMER, REFLEX, POWERED *(Physical Med) 89IKO*

Biomet Microfixation Inc. 800-874-7711
1520 Tradeport Dr, Jacksonville, FL 32218
Various types of hammers.

HAMMER, SURGICAL *(Surgery) 79FZY*

Biomet Microfixation Inc. 800-874-7711
1520 Tradeport Dr, Jacksonville, FL 32218
Various types of hammers.

Biomet, Inc. 574-267-6639
56 E Bell Dr, PO Box 587, Warsaw, IN 46582
Various types of surgical hammers.

Elmed, Inc. 630-543-2792
60 W Fay Ave, Addison, IL 60101

Interventional Spine, Inc. 800-497-0484
13700 Alton Pkwy Ste 160, Irvine, CA 92618
Hammer.

Kmedic 800-955-0559
190 Veterans Dr, Northvale, NJ 07647

HAMMER, SURGICAL *(cont'd)*

Midshore Industries, Inc. 410-822-8622
29526 Canvasback Dr, Easton, MD 21601
Various types of surgical hammers,custom,orthopaedic

Tuzik Boston 800-886-6363
104 Longwater Dr, Assinippi Park, Norwell, MA 02061

Zimmer Spine, Inc. 800-655-2614
7375 Bush Lake Rd, Minneapolis, MN 55439
Surgical hammer.

HAND INSTRUMENT, CALCULUS REMOVAL
(Dental And Oral) 76ELA

Dental Concepts Llc 800-592-6661
90 N Broadway, Irvington, NY 10533
Orapik

Dentalez Group 866-DTE-INFO
101 Lindenwood Dr Ste 225, Valleybrooke Corporate Center
Malvern, PA 19355

Dentalez Group, Stardental Division 717-291-1161
1816 Colonial Village Ln, Lancaster, PA 17601
Explorer, operative.

Dentek Oral Care, Inc. 865-983-1300
307 Excellence Way, Maryville, TN 37801
Plaque remover.

Hu-Friedy Manufacturing Co., Inc. 800-483-7433
3232 N Rockwell St, Chicago, IL 60618

Nordent Manufacturing, Inc. 800-966-7336
610 Bonnie Ln, Elk Grove Village, IL 60007
$19.00 per unit (standard).

Premier Dental Products Co. 888-670-6100
1710 Romano Dr, PO Box 4500, Plymouth Meeting, PA 19462

HAND, EXTERNAL LIMB COMPONENT, MECHANICAL
(Physical Med) 89IRA

Brown Medical Industries 800-843-4395
1300 Lundberg Dr W, Spirit Lake, IA 51360
WRISTIMER prevents and minimizes carpal tunnel symdrome.
WRISTIMER PM prevents and minimizes carpal tunnel syndrome.

Franklin Prosthetic Covers 610-666-6645
PO Box 313, Oaks, PA 19456
Custom-made multi-layer silicone cosmetic glove.

Hosmer Dorrance Corp. 408-379-5151
561 Division St, Campbell, CA 95008
Various.

HAND, EXTERNAL LIMB COMPONENT, POWERED
(Physical Med) 89IQZ

Starkey Florida 800-327-7939
2200 N Commerce Pkwy, Weston, FL 33326
Myoelectric and switch controlled electric hand systems.

HANDLE, INSTRUMENT, DENTAL *(Dental And Oral) 76EJB*

A. Titan Instruments, Inc. 716-648-9272
97 Main St, Hamburg, NY 14075
Handles sugical.

Acme-Monaco Corp. 860-224-1349
75 Winchell Rd, New Britain, CT 06052

Aesculap Implant Systems Inc. 1-800-234-9179
3773 Corporate Pkwy, Center Valley, PA 18034

Almore International, Inc. 503-643-6633
PO Box 25214, Portland, OR 97298
HYLITE dental handles with removable cone socket tips at each end. $18.45 each.

American Eagle Instruments, Inc. 406-549-7451
6575 Butler Creek Rd, Missoula, MT 59808
Various sizes and styles of instruments.

Beutlich Lp, Pharmaceuticals 800-238-8542
1541 S Shields Dr, Waukegan, IL 60085
HurriView TM Plaque Indicating Swab Applicators

Biomet 3i 800-342-5454
4555 Riverside Dr, Palm Beach Gardens, FL 33410
Various dental hand instruments.

Biomet Microfixation Inc. 800-874-7711
1520 Tradeport Dr, Jacksonville, FL 32218
Handle, instrument, dental.

Classone Orthodontics, Inc. 806-799-0608
5064 50th St, Lubbock, TX 79414
Instruments.

HANDLE, INSTRUMENT, DENTAL *(cont'd)*

Coltene/Whaledent Inc. 330-916-8358
235 Ascot Pkwy, Cuyahoga Falls, OH 44223
Dam punch.

Common Sense Dental Inc. 616-837-1231
12261 Cleveland St Ste D, Nunica, MI 49448
Dental wedge.

Dental Usa, Inc. 815-363-8003
5005 McCullom Lake Rd, McHenry, IL 60050
Various types of handles.

Dentalez Group 866-DTE-INFO
101 Lindenwood Dr Ste 225, Valleybrooke Corporate Center
Malvern, PA 19355

Dentalez Group, Stardental Division 717-291-1161
1816 Colonial Village Ln, Lancaster, PA 17601
Unit, operative dental.

Dentek Oral Care, Inc. 865-983-1300
307 Excellence Way, Maryville, TN 37801
DenTek EVO Flosser Handle

Dentsply Canada, Ltd. 800-263-1437
161 Vinyl Ct., Woodbridge, ONT L4L 4A3 Canada

E-Z Floss 760-325-1888
PO Box 2292, Palm Springs, CA 92263
Dental instrument handle.

Engler Engineering Corp. 800-445-8581
1099 E 47th St, Hialeah, FL 33013
Marathon inserts - K-1, K-2, K-4, K-Petite.

Garrison Dental Solutions 616-842-2244
110 Dewitt Ln, Spring Lake, MI 49456
Interproximal wedges.

Harry J. Bosworth Company 800-323-4352
7227 Hamlin Ave, Skokie, IL 60076
B-CROWN scissors, HYDROX placement tool, super EBA cement spatula.

Hu-Friedy Manufacturing Co., Inc. 800-483-7433
3232 N Rockwell St, Chicago, IL 60618

Icon Llc 501-374-2929
8 Ten Tee Dr, Maumelle, AR 72113
Dental instrument, handle.

Lightspeed Technology, Inc. 210-495-4942
403 E Ramsey Rd Ste 205, San Antonio, TX 78216
Endodontic hand file.

Micro-Dent Inc. 866-526-1166
379 Hollow Hill Rd, Wauconda, IL 60084
Various type of dental hand instruments.

Miltex Dental Technologies, Inc. 516-576-6022
589 Davies Dr, York, PA 17402
Same.

Nobel Biocare Usa, Llc 800-579-6515
22715/22725 Savi Ranch Parkway, Yorba Linda, CA 92887
Surgical or prosthetic instrument.

Nordent Manufacturing, Inc. 800-966-7336
610 Bonnie Ln, Elk Grove Village, IL 60007
$4.50 for mirror handle.

Orthopli Corp.
10061 Sandmeyer Ln, Philadelphia, PA 19116
Various styles.

Pac-Dent Intl., Inc. 909-839-0888
21078 Commerce Point Dr, Walnut, CA 91789
Disposable micro applicator.

Pascal Co., Inc. 425-602-3633
2929 Northup Way, Bellevue, WA 98004
Retraction cord packing instrument.

Pdt, Inc. 406-626-4153
12201 Moccasin Ct, Missoula, MT 59808
Various types of handles.

Premier Dental Products Co. 888-670-6100
1710 Romano Dr, PO Box 4500, Plymouth Meeting, PA 19462

Pru-Dent Mfg. Inc. 847-301-1170
1929 Wright Blvd, Schaumburg, IL 60193
Dental hand instruments.

Suter Dental Manufacturing Company, Inc. 800-368-8376
632 Cedar St, Chico, CA 95928
TRU-LITE Handle.

HANDLE, INSTRUMENT, DENTAL *(cont'd)*

Symmetry Medical Usa, Inc. 574-267-8700
486 W 350 N, Warsaw, IN 46582
Dental hand instrument.

Ultradent Products, Inc. 801-553-4586
505 W 10200 S, South Jordan, UT 84095
Dental calculus detection system.

Wykle Research, Inc. 775-887-7500
2222 College Pkwy, Carson City, NV 89706
Instrument handle.

Young Microbrush Llc 262-375-4011
1376 Cheyenne Ave, Grafton, WI 53024

HANDLE, INSTRUMENT, LAPAROSCOPIC (ELECTROCAUTERY)
(Surgery) 79SIF

Bolt Bethel, Llc 763-434-5900
23530 University Avenue Ext NW, PO Box 135, Bethel, MN 55005

Ethicon Endo-Surgery, Inc. 800-USE-ENDO
4545 Creek Rd, Cincinnati, OH 45242
ENDOPATH, foot and handle control electrosurgery.

Karl Storz Endoscopy-America Inc. 800-421-0837
600 Corporate Pointe, Culver City, CA 90230

Mediflex Surgical Products 800-879-7575
250 Gibbs Rd, Islandia, NY 11749

Princeton Medical Group, Inc. 800-875-0869
1189 Royal Links Dr, Mt Pleasant, SC 29466
LAPAROSCOPIC DISSECTORS & GRASPERS - MINIATURE AND STANDARD SIZES

Putnam Precision Products 845-278-2141
3859 Danbury Rd, Brewster, NY 10509

Valleylab 800-255-8522
5920 Longbow Dr, Boulder, CO 80301
LIGASURE™ Vessel Sealing System bipolar electrosurgical generator and handsets for open and laparoscopic procedures. Designed to permanently seal vessels up to and including 7mm and tissue bundles.

HANDLE, INSTRUMENT, LAPAROSCOPIC (IRRIGATION)
(Surgery) 79SJH

Ethicon Endo-Surgery, Inc. 800-USE-ENDO
4545 Creek Rd, Cincinnati, OH 45242

HANDLE, KNIFE BLADE *(Surgery) 79RDE*

Arista Surgical Supply Co. Inc. 800-223-1984
297 High St, Dedham, MA 02026

Becton Dickinson And Co. 866-906-8080
411 Waverley Oaks Rd, Waltham, MA 02452

Codman & Shurtleff, Inc 800-225-0460
325 Paramount Dr, Raynham, MA 02767

Dgh Technology, Inc. 800-722-3883
110 Summit Dr Ste B, Exton, PA 19341
Instrument made of titanium and stainless steel, diamond blades.

Elmed, Inc. 630-543-2792
60 W Fay Ave, Addison, IL 60101

Fortrad Eye Instruments Corp. 973-543-2371
8 Franklin Rd, Mendham, NJ 07945

Medical Sterile Products, Inc. 800-292-2887
Road 413 Km. 0.2 BO. Ensenada, Rincon, PR 00743
MIS and opthalmology handles.

Propper Manufacturing Co., Inc. 800-832-4300
3604 Skillman Ave, Long Island City, NY 11101

Toolmex Corporation 800-992-4766
1075 Worcester St, Natick, MA 01760

HANDLE, KNIFE, LAPAROSCOPIC *(Surgery) 79QWG*

Prosurge Instruments, Inc. 866-832-7874
199 Laidlaw Ave, Jersey City, NJ 07306

HANDLE, SCALPEL *(Surgery) 79GDZ*

Back-Mueller, Inc. 314-531-6640
2700 Clark Ave, Saint Louis, MO 63103
Various types of knife holders.

Bausch & Lomb Surgical 636-255-5051
3365 Tree Court Ind Blvd, Saint Louis, MO 63122

Bd Caribe, Ltd. 201-847-4298
Rd. 183, Km. 20.3, Las Piedras, PR 00771
Scalpel handle.

HANDLE, SCALPEL *(cont'd)*

Biomet Microfixation Inc. 800-874-7711
1520 Tradeport Dr, Jacksonville, FL 32218
Various types of scalpels.

Brasseler Usa - Komet Medical 800-535-6638
1 Brasseler Blvd, Savannah, GA 31419

C & A Scientific Co. Inc. 703-330-1413
7241 Gabe Ct, Manassas, VA 20109
PREMIERE stainless steel. #3 & #4 sizes.

Carl Heyer, Inc. 800-284-5550
1872 Bellmore Ave, North Bellmore, NY 11710

Cincinnati Surgical Company 800-544-3100
11256 Cornell Park Dr, Cincinnati, OH 45242

Curetteblade, Inc. 866-287-3883
20 Cedar Blvd Ste 410, Pittsburgh, PA 15228
Reusable, stainless steel scalpel blade handles.

Dental Usa, Inc. 815-363-8003
5005 McCullom Lake Rd, McHenry, IL 60050
Dental scalpel handle.

E.A. Beck & Co. 949-645-4072
657 W 19th St Ste E, P O Box 10857, Costa Mesa, CA 92627
Handle.

H & H Co. 909-390-0373
4435 E Airport Dr Ste 108, Ontario, CA 91761
Scalpel handle, all types.

Kmedic 800-955-0559
190 Veterans Dr, Northvale, NJ 07647

Medical Sterile Products, Inc. 800-292-2887
Road 413 Km. 0.2 BO. Ensenada, Rincon, PR 00743
Miniature edged handle, oral-perio handle, arthro handle, podiatry handle, ENT-micro handle.

Medisiss 866-866-7477
2747 SW 6th St, Redmond, OR 97756
Various scalpel handles,sterile.

Medworks Instruments 800-323-9790
PO Box 581, Chatham, IL 62629
$1.00 per unit (#3 or #4).

Miltex Inc. 800-645-8000
589 Davies Dr, York, PA 17402

Normed 800-288-8200
PO Box 3644, Seattle, WA 98124
Scalpel, handle.

Oratronics, Inc. 212-986-0050
405 Lexington Ave, New York, NY 10174
Scalpel handle.

Personna Medical/Div. Of American Safety Razor Co. 800-457-2222
1 Razor Blade Ln, Verona, VA 24482
PERSONNA PLUS Safety Metal Handles in #3, #3L, #4, #4L, and #7 fit PERSONNA PLUS safety cartridges.

Precision Surgical Intl., Inc. 800-776-8493
PO Box 726, Noblesville, IN 46061
Scalel.

Princeton Medical Group, Inc. 800-875-0869
1189 Royal Links Dr, Mt Pleasant, SC 29466

Propper Manufacturing Co., Inc. 800-832-4300
3604 Skillman Ave, Long Island City, NY 11101

Pulpdent Corp. 800-343-4342
80 Oakland St, Watertown, MA 02472
No common name listed.

Roboz Surgical Instrument Co., Inc. 800-424-2984
PO Box 10710, Gaithersburg, MD 20898

Salvin Dental Specialties, Inc. 800-535-6566
3450 Latrobe Dr, Charlotte, NC 28211
Various types of scalpel handles.

Symmetry Medical Usa, Inc. 574-267-8700
486 W 350 N, Warsaw, IN 46582
Manual surgical instrument for general use.

Toolmex Corporation 800-992-4766
1075 Worcester St, Natick, MA 01760

Tuzik Boston 800-886-6363
104 Longwater Dr, Assinippi Park, Norwell, MA 02061

HANDLING UNIT, AUTOMATIC DAYLIGHT X-RAY FILM
(Radiology) 90UFC

Kodak Canada Inc., Health Imaging Division — 800-295-5526
3500 Eglinton Ave. W., Toronto, ONT M6M 1V3 Canada

HANDPIECE (BRACE), DRILL *(Cns/Neurology) 84HBD*

Biomet Microfixation Inc. — 800-874-7711
1520 Tradeport Dr, Jacksonville, FL 32218
Various types of drills.

Cynthia Flores Castrejon — 52-5-780-36-97
Plazuela #24, Mz 12, Lt 8 Casa, 3 Plazas De Aragon
Nezahualcoyotl, EDO. 57139 Mexico
Cranial drill handpiece (brace).

Zimmer Holdings, Inc. — 800-613-6131
1800 W Center St, PO Box 708, Warsaw, IN 46580

HANDPIECE, AIR-POWERED, DENTAL *(Dental And Oral) 76EFB*

A-Dec, Inc. — 800-547-1883
2601 Crestview Dr, Newberg, OR 97132
High speed handpiece.

Alrand, Inc./Boca Dental Supply, Inc. — 800-5004908
3401 N Federal Hwy Ste 203, Boca Raton, FL 33431
Various types.

Athena Technology, Inc. — 314-344-0010
13705 Shoreline Ct E, Earth City, MO 63045
Multiple.

Bien Air Usa, Inc. — 800-433-2636
17880 Sky Park Cir Ste 140, Irvine, CA 92614

Biomet Microfixation Inc. — 800-874-7711
1520 Tradeport Dr, Jacksonville, FL 32218
Various types of drills.

Dencraft — 800-328-9729
PO Box 57, Moorestown, NJ 08057
Dental handpieces and accessories.

Dentalez Group — 866-DTE-INFO
101 Lindenwood Dr Ste 225, Valleybrooke Corporate Center
Malvern, PA 19355

Dentalez Group, Stardental Division — 717-291-1161
1816 Colonial Village Ln, Lancaster, PA 17601
Handpiece, air-powered, dental.

Dp Manufacture Corp. — 305-640-9894
1460 NW 107th Ave Ste H, Doral, FL 33172
Handpiece & accs.

Dynamic Dental Corp. — 954-753-4693
10791 NW 53rd St Ste 102, Sunrise, FL 33351
High & low speed handpiece.

Handpiece Parts & Products, Inc. — 714-997-4331
707 W Angus Ave, Orange, CA 92868
Dental handpiece/accessories.

Kinetic Instruments, Inc. — 800-233-2346
17 Berkshire Blvd, Bethel, CT 06801
VIPER fiberoptic high speed and fiberoptic low speed handpieces have a proven record of reliability and value for over 25 years. The VIPER handpiece line includes the Viper 360, Viper Hi-Torque, Viper-mini, and Viper low speed handpieces. The Quantum is a high-end fiberoptic high speed handpiece with features comparable to the top brand name handpieces at a fraction of the cost to purchase and to repair.

Lares Research — 800-347-3289
295 Lockheed Ave, Chico, CA 95973

Microtech — 714-966-1645
3633 W MacArthur Blvd Ste 410, Santa Ana, CA 92704
Dental handpiece.

Mti Precision Products — 732-905-7440
175 Oberlin Ave N, Lakewood, NJ 08701
Dental air powered handpiece.

Nsk America Corporation — 800-585-4675
700 Cooper Ct Ste B, Schaumburg, IL 60173
High and low speed handpieces.

Obtura Spartan — 800-344-1321
13729 Shoreline Ct E, Earth City, MO 63045
Portable dental systems.

Pac-Dent Intl., Inc. — 909-839-0888
21078 Commerce Point Dr, Walnut, CA 91789
Barrier, sleeve, tray, t-style, tube, curing light, handpiece, x-ray sleeve.

HANDPIECE, AIR-POWERED, DENTAL *(cont'd)*

Palisades Dental, Llc — 201-569-0050
111 Cedar Ln, Englewood, NJ 07631
Dental handpiece.

Prodrive Systems, Inc. — 866-937-8882
812 Commerce Dr., Ogdensburg, NY 13669
Turbine addembly for dental handpiece.

Shofu Dental Corporation — 800-827-4638
1225 Stone Dr, San Marcos, CA 92078
LAB AIR-Z

Twist2it, Inc. — 877-PRO-PHYS
3930A 62nd St, Flushing, NY 11377
Air-powered scaler.

U.S. Medical Systems, Inc. — 512-347-8800
3160 Bee Caves Rd Ste 300C, Austin, TX 78746
Cleaner / lubricant for dental handpieces.

Ultradent Products, Inc. — 801-553-4586
505 W 10200 S, South Jordan, UT 84095
Dental handpiece and motor.

Vector Research & Development — 253-564-5084
6824 19th St W # 230, University Place, WA 98466
Dental handpiece.

3m Unitek — 800-634-5300
2724 Peck Rd, Monrovia, CA 91016

3s L.L.C. — 866-437-2677
9315 Knightsbridge Ct, Tampa, FL 33647
Dental handpiece lubricant.

HANDPIECE, BELT AND/OR GEAR DRIVEN, DENTAL
(Dental And Oral) 76EFA

Aesculap Implant Systems Inc. — 1-800-234-9179
3773 Corporate Pkwy, Center Valley, PA 18034

Central Welder's Supply, Inc. — 800-728-2068
127D Lee Rd, Watsonville, CA 95076
Compressed nitrogen N.F.

Dentalez Group — 866-DTE-INFO
101 Lindenwood Dr Ste 225, Valleybrooke Corporate Center
Malvern, PA 19355

Jaro, Inc. — 610-527-1889
1111 E Lancaster Ave, Bryn Mawr, PA 19010
Tick kit.

Miltex Inc. — 800-645-8000
589 Davies Dr, York, PA 17402

Stryker Corp. — 800-726-2725
2825 Airview Blvd, Portage, MI 49002

HANDPIECE, CONTRA- AND RIGHT-ANGLE ATTACHMENT, DENTAL *(Dental And Oral) 76EGS*

Airtech Industries, Inc. — 540-949-6565
412 Ohio St, Waynesboro, VA 22980
Disposable prophy angle.

Biomet 3i — 800-342-5454
4555 Riverside Dr, Palm Beach Gardens, FL 33410

Biomet Microfixation Inc. — 800-874-7711
1520 Tradeport Dr, Jacksonville, FL 32218
Various types of drills.

Coltene/Whaledent Inc. — 330-916-8858
235 Ascot Pkwy, Cuyahoga Falls, OH 44223
Right angle handpiece and head.

Deepak Products, Inc. — 305-482-9669
5220 NW 72nd Ave Ste 15, Miami, FL 33166
Disposable prophy angles.

Dentalez Group — 866-DTE-INFO
101 Lindenwood Dr Ste 225, Valleybrooke Corporate Center
Malvern, PA 19355

Dentalez Group, Stardental Division — 717-291-1161
1816 Colonial Village Ln, Lancaster, PA 17601
Scissors, surgical tissue, dental.

Denticator International, Inc. — 800-325-1881
13705 Shoreline Ct E, Earth City, MO 63045
$30.00 for sterilizable unit.

Dp Manufacture Corp. — 305-640-9894
1460 NW 107th Ave Ste H, Doral, FL 33172
Air handpiece.

Dynamic Dental Corp. — 954-753-4693
10791 NW 53rd St Ste 102, Sunrise, FL 33351
Handpiece, contra- and right-angle attachment, dental.

HANDPIECE, CONTRA- AND RIGHT-ANGLE ATTACHMENT, DENTAL *(cont'd)*

Kerr Corp. 714-516-7400
28200 Wick Rd, Romulus, MI 48174
Various accessories.

Medidenta International, Inc. 800-221-0750
3923 62nd St, PO Box 409, Woodside, NY 11377

Miltex Dental Technologies, Inc. 516-576-6022
589 Davies Dr, York, PA 17402
Various dental handpieces, kits, and accessories.

Osada, Inc. 800-426-7232
8436 W 3rd St Ste 695, Los Angeles, CA 90048
SH-series straight handpieces. CS-contra shark with CH-contra head.

Pac-Dent Intl., Inc. 909-839-0888
21078 Commerce Point Dr, Walnut, CA 91789
Disposable prophy angle.

Preventive Technologies, Inc. 704-849-2416
1150 Crews Rd Ste H, Matthews, NC 28105
Prophy angle.

Promident Llc 845-634-3997
242 N Main St, New City, NY 10956

Scodenco, Inc. 918-627-6795
7405 E 31st Pl, Tulsa, OK 74145
Attachment system.

Stryker Corp. 800-726-2725
2825 Airview Blvd, Portage, MI 49002

Team Technologies, Inc. 423-587-2199
5949 Commerce Blvd, Morristown, TN 37814
Disposable prophylaxis angle.

Twist2it, Inc. 877-PRO-PHYS
3930A 62nd St, Flushing, NY 11377
Reciprocating 1/4-turn disposable prophy angle.

Water Pik, Inc. 970-221-6129
1730 E Prospect Rd, Fort Collins, CO 80525
Friction grip, latch and prophylaxis angles.

Young Dental Manufacturing Co 1, Llc 800-325-1881
4401 Paredes Line Rd, Brownsville, TX 78526
Prophylaxis angle.

3m Unitek 800-634-5300
2724 Peck Rd, Monrovia, CA 91016

HANDPIECE, DIRECT DRIVE, AC-POWERED
(Dental And Oral) 76EKX

Aesculap Implant Systems Inc. 1-800-234-9179
3773 Corporate Pkwy, Center Valley, PA 18034

Buffalo Dental Mfg. Co., Inc. 516-496-7200
159 Lafayette Dr, Syosset, NY 11791
Abrasive wheels and points, rubberized bonded base.

Dp Manufacture Corp. 305-640-9894
1460 NW 107th Ave Ste H, Doral, FL 33172
Electric micromotor.

H&H Instruments
4950 Crescent Technical Ct, St Augustine, FL 32086
Hhi electrice console.

Osada, Inc. 800-426-7232
8436 W 3rd St Ste 695, Los Angeles, CA 90048
PEDO-30W and XL30-W/SH28S-LVS-MCC6.

3m Unitek 800-634-5300
2724 Peck Rd, Monrovia, CA 91016

HANDPIECE, FIBEROPTIC *(Dental And Oral) 76THM*

Lares Research 800-347-3289
295 Lockheed Ave, Chico, CA 95973

Sunoptic Technologies 877-677-2832
6018 Bowdendale Ave, Jacksonville, FL 32216
Custom high performance fiberoptics, autoclavable, white light transmitting fibers.

HANDPIECE, ROTARY BONE CUTTING *(Dental And Oral) 76KMW*

Ivry 305-448-9858
216 Catalonia Ave Ste 106, Coral Gables, FL 33134
Dental and oral-maxillofacial bone drill.

HANDRIM, WHEELCHAIR *(Physical Med) 89IMO*

Sunrise Medical Hhg Inc 303-218-4505
2842 N Business Park Ave, Fresno, CA 93727

HANGER, INTRAVENOUS *(General) 80RCM*

Baxter Healthcare Corporation, Global Drug Delivery 888-229-0001
25212 W Il Route 120, Round Lake, IL 60073

Brandt Industries, Inc. 800-221-8031
4461 Bronx Blvd, Bronx, NY 10470
$102.50 for IV stand 35700.

Hospira 800-441-4100
268 E 4th St, Ashland, OH 44805
Plastic extension hanger/hook.

Imperial Fastener Co., Inc. 954-782-7130
1400 SW 8th St, Pompano Beach, FL 33069

Independent Solutions, Inc. 847-498-0500
900 Skokie Blvd Ste 118, Northbrook, IL 60062
ARNCO Ceiling mounted stationary hook or removable, pivotting, wall mounted, or I.V. ceiling track mounted, fixed or adjustable height. Conductive or non-conductive.

Medical Skyhook Company 801-262-1471
PO Box 17213, Salt Lake City, UT 84117

Phelan Manufacturing Corp. 800-328-2358
2523 Minnehaha Ave, Minneapolis, MN 55404
$250.00 for ceiling mounted intravenous hanger.

Pryor Products 800-854-2280
1819 Peacock Blvd, Oceanside, CA 92056
A wide variety of ceiling mounted IV hangers are available.

Salsbury Industries 800-640-4341
1010 E 62nd St, Los Angeles, CA 90001

Vygon Corp. 800-544-4907
2495 General Armistead Ave, Norristown, PA 19403
Intravenous accessories.

HANGER, UROLOGIC *(Gastro/Urology) 78SEG*

Phelan Manufacturing Corp. 800-328-2358
2523 Minnehaha Ave, Minneapolis, MN 55404
$585.00 for ceiling mounted urologic hanger.

HANGER, X-RAY TUBE *(Radiology) 90VHK*

Americomp, Inc. 800-458-1782
2901 W Lawrence Ave, Chicago, IL 60625

Amrad 888-772-6723
2901 W Lawrence Ave, Chicago, IL 60625

Marconi Medical Systems 800-323-0550
595 Miner Rd, Cleveland, OH 44143

HARVESTER, CELL *(Microbiology) 83UFS*

Tomtec 877-866-8323
1000 Sherman Ave, Hamden, CT 06514
HARVESTER 96 is a 96 well cell harvester, fully programmable to control all parameters in harvesting. Available for all plate readers.

HDL VIA LDL & VLDL PRECIPITATION, LIPOPROTEINS
(Chemistry) 75KMZ

Genzyme Corp. 800-325-2436
160 Christian St, Oxford, CT 06478
Enzymatic Direct HDL - homogenous.

HEAD REST, NEUROSURGICAL *(Cns/Neurology) 84HBM*

Composites Horizons, Inc. 626-331-0861
1471 W Industrial Park St, Covina, CA 91722
Radiolucent composite headrests for x-ray, CT & nuclear imaging.

Confortaire Inc 662-842-2966
2133 S Veterans Blvd, Tupelo, MS 38804
Neurosurgical headrest.

Depuy Mitek, Inc. 800-451-2006
325 Paramount Dr, Raynham, MA 02767
Anterior and posterior approach halo adapters are fully compatible with the Mayfield neurosurgical headrest system. These adapters provide added patient security during cervical surgery by reducing the risk of unprotected movements of the cervical spine.

Eagle Vision, Inc. 800-222-7584
8500 Wolf Lake Dr Ste 110, Memphis, TN 38133
Surgical headrests and instruments for primary eyecare.

Integra Lifesciences Of Ohio 800-654-2873
4900 Charlemar Dr Bldg A, Cincinnati, OH 45227
Various neurosurgical headrests.

Mizuho America Inc. 800-699-2547
133 Brimbal Ave, Beverly, MA 01915
Head frames to hold head during neurosurgery.

HEAD REST, NEUROSURGICAL *(cont'd)*

Practical Things, Llc. 310-951-6906
3267 E 3300 S Ste 105, Salt Lake City, UT 84109
Neurosurgical headrest.

Schaerer Mayfield Usa 800-755-6381
4900 Charlemar Dr, Cincinnati, OH 45227
MAYFIELD skull clamp and horseshoe headrest system for cranial fixation and stabilization.

HEADGEAR, EXTRAORAL, ORTHODONTIC
(Dental And Oral) 76DZB

American Orthodontics Corp. 800-558-7687
1714 Cambridge Ave, Sheboygan, WI 53081

Barnhart Industries, Inc. 800-325-9973
3690 Highway M, Imperial, MO 63052
Orthodontic headgear.

Classone Orthodontics, Inc. 806-799-0608
5064 50th St, Lubbock, TX 79414
Various types of release modules.

Fairdale Orthodontic Co., Inc. 513-421-2620
312 W 4th St, Cincinnati, OH 45202
Headgear, extraoral orthodontic-neck pads, neck straps.

Forestadent Usa 314-878-5985
2315 Weldon Pkwy, Saint Louis, MO 63146
Extraoral orthodontic headgear.

G & H Wire Co. 800-526-1026
2165 Earlywood Dr, Franklin, IN 46131
Safety release modules.

Lancer Orthodontics, Inc. 760-304-2705
253 Pawnee St, San Marcos, CA 92078
Facebow, headgear.

Masel Co., Inc. 800-423-8227
2701 Bartram Rd, Bristol, PA 19007

Ortho Organizers, Inc. 760-448-8730
1822 Aston Ave, Carlsbad, CA 92008
Orthodontic headgear.

Orthoband Company, Inc. 800-325-9973
3690 Highway M, Imperial, MO 63052

Orthodontic Design And Production, Inc. 760-734-3995
1370 Decision St Ste D, Vista, CA 92081
Orthodontic headgear.

Oscar, Inc. 317-849-2618
11793 Technology Ln, Fishers, IN 46038
Orthodontic headgear products.

Pacific Coast Mfg., Inc. 425-485-8866
15604 163rd Ave NE, Woodinville, WA 98072
Support chair.

Tp Orthodontics, Inc. 800-348-8856
100 Center Plz, La Porte, IN 46350
Facebows, Neckstraps, Safety Release Modules, Headcaps, Revers Pull Headgear.

3m Unitek 800-634-5300
2724 Peck Rd, Monrovia, CA 91016

HEADLAMP, OPERATING, AC-POWERED
(Ophthalmology) 86HPQ

Ams Innovative Center-San Jose 800-356-7600
3070 Orchard Dr, San Jose, CA 95134

Bulbtronics, Inc. 800-624-2852
45 Banfi Plz N, Farmingdale, NY 11735

Med-General Usa Llc 239-597-9967
1045 Collier Center Way Ste 1, Naples, FL 34110
Headlamp, ent.

Mobile Dental Equipment Corp.(M-Dec) 425-747-5424
13300 SE 30th St Ste 101, Bellevue, WA 98005
Operating headlamp.

Qed, Inc. 859-231-0338
750 Enterprise Dr, Lexington, KY 40510
Halogen headlight.

Western Ophthalmics Corporation 800-426-9938
19019 36th Ave W Ste G, Lynnwood, WA 98036

HEADLAMP, OPERATING, BATTERY-OPERATED
(Ophthalmology) 86HPP

Advanced Medical Science & Technology, Llc 410-628-1856
1 Stonegate Ct, Cockeysville, MD 21030
Surgical headlamp.

HEADLAMP, OPERATING, BATTERY-OPERATED *(cont'd)*

Cool View, Llc 865-982-5552
9530 Gladiolus Blossom Ct, Fort Myers, FL 33908
Surgeon's headlamp, battery-operated.

Interplex Medical, Llc 513-248-5120
25 Whitney Dr Ste 114, Milford, OH 45150
Halogen headlight.

Isolux Llc 239-514-7475
1045 Collier Center Way Ste 6, Naples, FL 34110
Led portable headlight.

Meddev Corporation 800-543-2789
730 N Pastoria Ave, Sunnyvale, CA 94085
MULTARRAY HALOGEN SURGICAL HEADLIGHT Headband and reflector assembly with battery pack. Quartz halogen bulb.

Medical Vision Industries, Inc. 800-775-2088
3117 McHenry Ave Ste B, Modesto, CA 95350
Headlamp.

Qed, Inc. 859-231-0338
750 Enterprise Dr, Lexington, KY 40510
Halogen headlight.

Riverpoint Medical 503-517-8001
809 NE 25th Ave, Portland, OR 97232

HEADLIGHT, ENT *(Ear/Nose/Throat) 77KAF*

Bausch & Lomb Surgical 636-255-5051
3365 Tree Court Ind Blvd, Saint Louis, MO 63122

Cameron-Miller, Inc. 800-621-0142
5410 W Roosevelt Rd, Road #241, Chicago, IL 60644

Clinimed, Incorporated 877-CLINIMED
303 Markus Ct, Sandy Brae Industrial Park, Newark, DE 19713

Codman & Shurtleff, Inc 800-225-0460
325 Paramount Dr, Raynham, MA 02767

Elmed, Inc. 630-543-2792
60 W Fay Ave, Addison, IL 60101

General Scientific Corp. 800-959-0153
77 Enterprise Dr, Ann Arbor, MI 48103

Grams Medical Inc 949-548-7337
2443 Norse Ave, Costa Mesa, CA 92627

Integra Luxtec, Inc. 800-325-8966
99 Hartwell St, West Boylston, MA 01583

Jedmed Instruments Co. 314-845-3770
5416 Jedmed Ct, Saint Louis, MO 63129

Karl Storz Endoscopy-America Inc. 800-421-0837
600 Corporate Pointe, Culver City, CA 90230

Mahe International Inc. 800-294-7946
468 Craighead St, Nashville, TN 37204

Md International, Inc. 305-669-9003
11300 NW 41st St, Doral, FL 33178

Richard Wolf Medical Instruments Corp. 800-323-9653
353 Corporate Woods Pkwy, Vernon Hills, IL 60061

Sunoptic Technologies 877-677-2832
6018 Bowdendale Ave, Jacksonville, FL 32216
Coaxial fixed or variable bright white light spot size fiberoptic headlight, including fiberoptic cable, carrying case, two autoclavable joysticks and two garment clips.

Tsi Medical Ltd. 800-661-7263
47 Athabascan Ave., Unit 105, Sherwood Park, AB T8A-4H3 Canada

Welch Allyn, Inc. 800-535-6663
4341 State Street Rd, Skaneateles Falls, NY 13153

HEADLIGHT, FIBEROPTIC FOCUSING *(Gastro/Urology) 78FCT*

Biomet Microfixation Inc. 800-874-7711
1520 Tradeport Dr, Jacksonville, FL 32218
Headlight, fiberoptic focusing.

Cameron-Miller, Inc. 800-621-0142
5410 W Roosevelt Rd, Road #241, Chicago, IL 60644

Codman & Shurtleff, Inc 800-225-0460
325 Paramount Dr, Raynham, MA 02767

Electro Surgical Instrument Co., Inc. 888-464-2784
37 Centennial St, Rochester, NY 14611
Various types, styles and sizes of fiberoptic head lamps.

Fiberoptic Components, Llc 978-422-0422
2 Spratt Tech. Way, Sterling, MA 01564
Fiber optic lightguide.

HEADLIGHT, FIBEROPTIC FOCUSING *(cont'd)*

Integra Luxtec, Inc. 800-325-8966
99 Hartwell St, West Boylston, MA 01583
Miniature fiberoptic headlight.

Kelleher Medical, Inc. 804-378-9956
3049 St Marys Way, Powhatan, VA 23139

Qed, Inc. 859-231-0338
750 Enterprise Dr, Lexington, KY 40510
Various types.

Sunoptic Technologies 877-677-2832
6018 Bowdendale Ave, Jacksonville, FL 32216
Coaxial fixed or variable bright white light headlights, portable or mobile systems. Fixed type and focusing type. Prices include fiberoptic cable and carrying case. Xenon lightsources also available.

Surgical Tools, Inc. 800-774-2040
1106 Monroe St, Bedford, VA 24523

Techman Int'L Corp. 508-248-2900
242 Sturbridge Rd, Charlton, MA 01507
Multiple.

HEADWALL SYSTEM (PATIENT ROOM) *(General) 80RLO*

Allied Healthcare Products, Inc. 800-444-3954
1720 Sublette Ave, Saint Louis, MO 63110
Premanufactured headwall systems.

Gcx Corp. 800-228-2555
3875 Cypress Dr, Petaluma, CA 94954
POLYMOUNT mounting solutions for patient monitors, fluid-delivery mounting systems and other devices for headwall systems.

Hill-Rom Holdings, Inc. 800-445-3730
1069 State Road 46 E, Batesville, IN 47006

Hospital Systems, Inc. 925-427-7800
750 Garcia Ave, Pittsburg, CA 94565
Medical Equipment Rail System

Independent Solutions, Inc. 847-498-0500
900 Skokie Blvd Ste 118, Northbrook, IL 60062
Class 1 Flatwall or horizontal or island or peninsula or ISI cockpit headwalls for ICU, CCU, neonatal stations, renal dialysis stations, burn units, labor, delivery, emergency and recovery rooms, postpartum, OR holding rooms, medical/surgical patient rooms (private or semiprivate rooms), LDR, et al. UL listed.

Post Glover Lifelink 800-287-4123
167 Gap Way, Erlanger, KY 41018
Patient service consoles can be used in every type of patient care facility bringing power, gases, lights and nurse call systems safely to the patient area.

Stryker Medical 800-869-0770
3800 E Centre Ave, Portage, MI 49002

HEARING AID, AIR CONDUCTION, TRANSCUTANEOUS SYSTEM *(Ear/Nose/Throat) 77NIX*

Gyrus Ent L.L.C., Sub. Of Gyrus Acmi, Inc. 508-804-2739
2925 Appling Rd, Bartlett, TN 38133
Hearing system.

Harris Research & Development, Llc. 800-802-2228
528 E 800 N, Orem, UT 84097
Hearing aid.

Intricon Corporation 651-636-9770
1260 Red Fox Rd, Arden Hills, MN 55112
Multiple

Kezar Enterprises, Inc. 541-334-6100
747 Blair Blvd, Eugene, OR 97402
Various types of hearing aids.

Suncoast Laboratories 714-229-9178
6888 Lincoln Ave Ste G, Buena Park, CA 90620
Suncoast.

HEARING AID, DIRECT DRIVE, PARTIALLY IMPLANTED
(Ear/Nose/Throat) 77MPV

Soundtec, Inc. 405-842-5045
2601 NW Expressway Ste 400, Oklahoma City, OK 73112
Semi-implanted hearing system.

HEARING-AID *(Ear/Nose/Throat) 77ESD*

Ace Hearing Laboratory, Llc 479-273-6006
2304 SE 14th St, Bentonville, AR 72712
Hearing aids.

HEARING-AID *(cont'd)*

Affinity Medical Technology, Llc. 763-744-0412
3025 Harbor Ln N Ste 105, Plymouth, MN 55447
Various types of air conduction hearing aids.

All American Mold Laboratories, Inc. 405-677-2700
2120 S I 35 Service Rd, Oklahoma City, OK 73129
Earmold for air-conduction hearing aid.

Alliance Hearing Systems 828-286-9399
431 S Main St Ste 6, Rutherfordton, NC 28139
Hearing aid.

Ambit Corporation 770-534-4150
1636 Oakbrook Industrial Dr., Gainesville, GA 30507
Hearing aids, hearing instruments or hearing devices.

America Hears, Inc. 215-788-0330
806 Beaver St, Bristol, PA 19007
Behind-the-ear air conduction hearing aids; hearing aid conduction system.

American Hearing Laboratory 972-394-4370
3740 N Josey Ln Ste 125, Carrollton, TX 75007
All in the ear hearing aid.

American Hearing Systems Inc. 763-404-1122
8001 E Bloomington Fwy, Bloomington, MN 55420
Various models of digital hearing aids.

Apherma Corp. 408-524-1634
440 N Wolfe Rd, Sunnyvale, CA 94085
Ite (in the ear); itc (in the canal); cic (completely in the canal)； Ison(All in one)

Argosy 800-328-6105
10300 W 70th St, Eden Prairie, MN 55344
Programmable and conventional ITE, ITC & CIC custom instruments, directional/omnidirectional microphone with digital push-button switch. Holds patents on 3-channel circuit series, DMS remote volume control for the CAMEO, CIC & MANHATTAN circuit.

audifon USA Inc. 800-776-0222
403 Chairman Ct Ste 1, P.O. Box 531700, Debary, FL 32713

Audina Hearing Instruments, Inc. 800-223-7700
165 E Wildmere Ave, Longwood, FL 32750

Audio d 207-893-2920
885 Roosevelt Trail, Windham, ME 04062
Hearing aid, behind the ear and in the ear.

Audio Hearing Aid Service 330-364-6637
617 Wabash Ave NW, New Philadelphia, OH 44663
Hearing aid, behind the ear and in the ear.

Audiphone Hearing Instruments 800-721-9611
3333 Kingman St Ste 205, Metairie, LA 70006

Banco Hearing Centers 941-753-3131
1133 Cortez Rd W, Bradenton, FL 34207
Various hearing aids.

Billedeaux Hearing Center, Llc 337-989-4327
4414 Johnston St Ste D, Lafayette, LA 70503
Americare hearing instruments.

Coast Hearing Aid Lab, Llc 228-539-5400
12100 Highway 49 Ste 314, Gulfport, MS 39503
Various models of air condition hearing aids.

Coast Hearing Services 541-265-6273
904 SW Bay St, Newport, OR 97365
Air-conduction hearing-aid.

Crystal Tone Hearing Instruments 515-255-4144
4217 University Ave, Des Moines, IA 50311
In-the-ear hearing aid.

Dakota Hearing Instruments, Inc. 605-487-7661
340 Main St., Lake Andes, SD 57356
Hearing aids.

Diagnostic Group Llc 952-278-4457
7625 Golden Triangle Dr Ste F, Eden Prairie, MN 55344
Various models of hearing aids.

Digital Hearing Aid Center 530-877-3808
6032 Clark Rd Ste C, Paradise, CA 95969
Analyzer.

Digitone Technology, Inc. 847-413-1688
890 E Higgins Rd Ste 158, Schaumburg, IL 60173
Various models of air-conduction hearing aids.

Directional Hearing Aid Service 208-376-9431
6876 W Fairview Ave, Boise, ID 83704
Hearing aid.

HEARING-AID *(cont'd)*

Discovery Hearing Aid Co-Op, Inc. 800-736-9903
4318 Downtowner Loop N Ste K, Mobile, AL 36609
Hearing aids.

Doc's Proplugs, Inc. 800-521-2982
719 Swift St Ste 100, Santa Cruz, CA 95060
Ready to wear earmold for BTE and radios.

Ear Lab 301-790-3300
363 S Cleveland Ave, Hagerstown, MD 21740
Hearing aid.

Ear Tech, Inc. 941-747-8193
3904 9th Ave W, Bradenton, FL 34205
Hearing-aid.

Ear-Tech Of Puerto Rico 787-841-6913
1469 Calle Aloa, Urb. Mercedita, Ponce, PR 00717
Hearing aid, air conduction.

Earcrafters, Inc. 800-688-3277
5000 Nations Crossing Rd Ste 205, Charlotte, NC 28217
Microclear.

Earmold Connection
6538 Ranch View Ln SE, Eyota, MN 55934
Hearing aid.

El Cajon Hearing Aid Center 619-442-5634
761 Arnele Ave, El Cajon, CA 92020
Hearing aids.

Excel Labs 763-391-7413
106 Central Ave Ste B, Osseo, MN 55369
Sound amplifier.

Fenwick Hearing Instruments 503-464-9441
2888 NW Westover Rd, Portland, OR 97210
Fenwick hearing instruments.

Finetone Hearing Instruments 207-893-2920
885 Roosevelt Trl, Windham, ME 04062
Hearing aid-custom in-the-ear.

Fisher Hearing Aid Service 330-627-2002
25 S Lisbon St, Carrollton, OH 44615
Same - hearing aid air conduction.

General Hearing Instruments, Inc. 504-733-3767
175 Brookhollow Espl., Harahan, LA 70123
Air-conduction hearing aid.

Gn Resound 952-769-8000
8001 E Bloomington Fwy, Bloomington, MN 55420
Hearing aid.

Great Lakes Earmold Lab 440-838-1300
750 Ken Mar Industrial Pkwy, Cleveland, OH 44147
Hearing aid, air conduction.

Harc Mercantile Ltd. 800-445-9968
1111 W Centre Ave, Portage, MI 49024

Healthdrive Ag 617-964-6681
25 Needham St, Newton, MA 02461
Hearing aid.

Hear Ear Inc 574-256-0000
3718 Lincolnway E, Mishawaka, IN 46544
Air conduction hearing aids.

Hearing Aid Depot, Inc 661-729-4315
43935 15th St W, Lancaster, CA 93534

Hearing Aid Express 713-666-1704
11888 Marsh Ln Ste 111, Dallas, TX 75234
Various.

Hearing Aid Express 713-666-1704
5201 Bellaire Blvd, Bellaire, TX 77401
Multiple.

Hearing Aid Factory 409-883-3010
105 Camellia Ave, P.o. Box 61, Orange, TX 77630
Air conduction hearing aid.

Hearing Crafters Of America 417-466-4085
708 E Mount Vernon Blvd, Mount Vernon, MO 65712
Custom built hearing aids.

Hearing Improvement 801-392-4310
1961 Washington Blvd., Ogden, UT 84401-0433
In-the-ear hearing aid.

Hearing Tech, Inc. 520-297-7555
7225 N Oracle Rd Ste 111, Tucson, AZ 85704
Hearing aids.

HEARING-AID *(cont'd)*

Hearing Technologies 727-525-7770
6251 44th St N Ste 109, Pinellas Park, FL 33781
Various hearing aids.

Hearing Today Laboratory, Inc. 913-888-6336
11954 W 95th St, Lenexa, KS 66215
Custom in-the-ear hearing aid.

Hearing Today Laboratory, Inc. 913-888-6336
14473 W Center Rd, Omaha, NE 68144
Custom in the ear hearing aid.

Hearmore Co., Inc. 651-771-4019
1445 White Bear Ave N, Saint Paul, MN 55106
Hearing aid.

Hearmore Company Inc. 800-881-4327
75 W Baseline Rd Ste 9, Gilbert, AZ 85233
Hearing-aid, air-conduction.

Hitec Group Intl. 800-288-8303
8160 S Madison St, Burr Ridge, IL 60527
Assistive-listening device for people who are hard of hearing.

Insound Medical Inc. 510-792-4000
39660 Eureka Dr, Newark, CA 94560
Insound xt services system.

Jade Hearing Instruments 248-922-5600
6803 Dixie Hwy Ste 2, Clarkston, MI 48346
Hearing aid.

Kelly Hearing Aid 702-309-3724
150 S Decatur Blvd, Las Vegas, NV 89107
Hearing aids, various sizes and kinds.

Lifestyle Medical Mfg 520-323-0099
6479 E 22nd St, Tucson, AZ 85710
'in -the-ear' hearing aid.

Littlefield Co. 801-485-1441
1441 E 2100 S, Salt Lake City, UT 84105
Hearing-aid.

Lotus Technology, Inc. 704-658-0406
110 Talbert Pointe Dr, Mooresville, NC 28117
Hearing aid.

Magnatone Hearing Aid Corp. 800-789-6543
170 N Cypress Way, Casselberry, FL 32707
MAGNATONE ITE (in the ear) and BTE (Behind the Ear) for all types of hearing losses, ranging from mild to severe. 100% digital, digitally programmable, rechargeable options, prewired form available.

Manan Technologies, Inc. 812-232-5191
905 S 25th St, Terre Haute, IN 47803
Hearing aids.

Micro Hearing Aids 480-895-2153
10440 E Riggs Rd Ste 120, Sun Lakes, AZ 85248
Micro hearing aids.

Micro-Ear Technology, Inc. 952-995-8800
6425 Flying Cloud Dr, Eden Prairie, MN 55344
Hearing aid.

Midwest City Hearing Aid Center 405-732-8682
1401 S Midwest Blvd, Midwest City, OK 73110
Audio enhancer ite, hca c/c class a,b,d, dynamic eq1,2&3.

Minnesota Wire & Cable Co. 800-258-6922
1835 Energy Park Dr, Saint Paul, MN 55108
Hearing-aid wire, vent-plugs, vent wire and battery pills.

Miracle-Ear 877-268-4264
5000 Cheshire Ln N, Minneapolis, MN 55446
4 types - molded within ear/ear canal, glasses, behind ear, or body.

Novasonic 800-843-0133
PO Box 18484, Saint Paul, MN 55118
*Nova*Sonic 2000, 4000, 5000*

Nu-Ear Electronics 952-947-4734
6769 Mesa Ridge Rd Ste 100, San Diego, CA 92121
Various.

Nu-Ear Electronics 800-626-8327
6769 Mesa Ridge Rd Ste 100, San Diego, CA 92121
NU-EAR, SOUNDEX, SOUND SOURCE, MINISCOPIC, and ACUITY hearing aids for external and internal wear, plus accessories.

Oticon, Inc. 800-526-3921
29 Schoolhouse Rd, Somerset, NJ 08873

Park Surgical Co., Inc. 800-633-7878
5001 New Utrecht Ave, Brooklyn, NY 11219

HEARING-AID *(cont'd)*

Phonic Ear, Inc. 800-227-0735
3880 Cypress Dr, Petaluma, CA 94954
EASY LISTENER sound field system provides mild amplification for students with normal hearing and those with minimal to mild hearing loss in the 10- to 25-decibel range. SOLARIS personal hearing system can supplement the performance of hearing aids and cochlear implants, or it can be used alone to achieve clear speech understanding in situations where speaker-to-listener communication may be impacted by distance, background noise or echo. Both direct audio input (DAI) and teleloop options can be used to couple to hearing aids. Just a few of the proven applications for this wireless technology include teacher-to-student instruction, lectures and business meetings, doctor's visits, watching television and talking in the car or around the dinner table.

Portland Hearing Aid Specialists, Inc. 503-261-9309
8505 SE Stark St, Portland, OR 97216
Hearing aid.

Prairie Labs 952-908-7654
637 12th Ave S, Hopkins, MN 55343
Various types of hearing aids.

Precision Laboratories, Inc. 800-327-4792
830 Sunshine Ln, Altamonte Springs, FL 32714
Hearing aid.

Professional Hearing Aid Service 316-942-4992
851 N West St, Wichita, KS 67203
Professional hearing aid service.

Professional Hearing Aid Service 724-548-4801
141 S Jefferson St, Kittanning, PA 16201
In the ear hearing aid.

Quality Hearing 651-770-5282
2115 County Road D E Ste A100, Maplewood, MN 55109
Hearing aids.

R And L Hearing Services 800-444-8920
3005 Niagara Ln N Ste 2, Minneapolis, MN 55447

R.J.S. Acoustic Services, Inc. 800-826-3180
11919 NE Glisan St, Portland, OR 97220
Various types of hearing aids, air conduction.

Remedy Hearing Aids 760-754-8151
2420 Vista Way Ste 112, Oceanside, CA 92054
Custom-made Digital Hearing Aids, Factory Direct.

Retone, Inc. 866-864-3271
4280 Sunrise Rd, Eagan, MN 55122
Glass.

Rexton, Inc. 763-553-0787
5010 Cheshire Ln N Ste 2, Plymouth, MN 55446
Hearing aid.

Robinson Audiology Laboratories 810-754-3511
8033 E 10 Mile Rd Ste 104, Center Line, MI 48015
Same.

Ruhling Enterprises, Inc. 616-364-0090
4598 Plainfield Ave NE, Grand Rapids, MI 49525
Knapp hearing aid.

Scientific Plastics, Inc. 212-967-1199
243 W 30th St, New York, NY 10001
Earmold.

Sebotek Hearing Systems, Llc 918-388-9000
2488 E 81st St Ste 2000, Tulsa, OK 74137

Songbird Hearing, Inc. 732-828-8300
303 George St Ste 307, New Brunswick, NJ 08901
Hearing aid format selector.

Spectrum Hearing Systems, Inc. 704-237-9100
18636 Starcreek Dr Ste E, Cornelius, NC 28031
Hearing aids.

Starkey California 952-947-4734
2536 W Woodland Dr, Anaheim, CA 92801
Hearing aid.

Starkey East 952-947-4734
535 Route 38 Ste 230, Cherry Hill, NJ 08002
Hearing aid.

Starkey Florida 952-947-4734
2200 N Commerce Pkwy, Weston, FL 33326
In-the-ear hearing aid.

Starkey Florida 800-327-7939
2200 N Commerce Pkwy, Weston, FL 33326

HEARING-AID *(cont'd)*

Starkey Laboratories, Inc. 800-328-8602
6700 Washington Ave S, Eden Prairie, MN 55344
Custom ITE and Canal-BTE, eyeglass, body aids.

Starkey Southeast 952-947-4734
5300 Oakbrook Pkwy, Bldg. 100, Suite 130, Norcross, GA 30093
Various.

Starkey Southwest 952-947-4734
3100 Alvin Devane Blvd, Austin, TX 78741
Various.

Telex Communications, Inc.-Hearing Instrument Grp. 800-328-8212
1200 Portland Avenue S, Burnsville, MN 55357
ACUSOUND COMPRESSION, SOPRANO & ACAPELLA, personal FM sound enhacement system for the hearing impaired and for the profoundly deaf. ITE, BTE, & CIC Hearing instruments for hard of hearing individuals.

The Earmold Co., Ltd. 540-389-1642
814 E 8th St, Salem, VA 24153
Hearing aid.

The Hearing Aid Factory, Inc. 407-649-9696
710 W Colonial Dr Ste 101, Orlando, FL 32804
'in the ear' hearing aid.

Trillium Hearing Technologies, Inc. 813-864-2292
13803 W Hillsborough Ave, Tampa, FL 33635
Hearing aids (various types of).

Unitron Hearing 763-744-3300
2300 Berkshire Ln N Ste A, Plymouth, MN 55441
Hearing aid.

Unitron Industries Ltd. 877-492-6244
20 Beasley Dr., Kitchener, ONT N2G 4X1 Canada
Sound F/X fits a wide range of reverse to precipitous hearing losses. Full section of styles, including completely-in-the-canal, custom and behind the ear. Programmable versions allow hearing professionals to customize five adjustable parameters with Unifit fitting software (NOAH-compatible). US80 Super Power Hearing Aid behind-the-ear model designed to fit severe to profound hearing losses. Programmable version features two programs and eight adjestable parameters. Non-programmable model offers extended low frequency emphasis and four adjustable controls. Supported by Unifit fitting software (NOAH-compatible). Complete line of hearing aids from analog to digital, from CIC to BTE.

VARTA Microbattery Inc. 800-468-2782
1311 Mamaroneck Ave Ste 120, White Plains, NY 10605
Power One V 675, V 312, V 13, V 10, V 5 Zinc Air Hearing Aid Batteries. (The Ultimate Power For Hearing).

Vivatone Hearing Systems, Llc 203-341-9100
1 Gorham Is, Westport, CT 06880
Hearing aid.

Vocal Labs 360-736-7123
114 W Pear St, Centralia, WA 98531
Hearing aid.

Zenith Sound Inc. 847-692-5205
960 N Northwest Hwy, Park Ridge, IL 60068

Zenith/Omni Hearing Instruments, Inc. 203-624-9857
111 Park St Ste K, New Haven, CT 06511
Hearing aids.

Zounds, Inc. 480-813-8400
1910 S Stapley Dr Ste 202, Mesa, AZ 85204
Hearing aid and accessories.

Zounds, Inc. 480-258-6013
4405 E Baseline Rd, Phoenix, AZ 85042

HEARING-AID, BONE-CONDUCTION, PERCUTANEOUS
(Ear/Nose/Throat) 77MKE

M-E Manufacturing And Services, Inc. 763-268-4500
5010 Cheshire Ln N, Plymouth, MN 55446
Various types of hearing aids.

HEARING-AID, GROUP, OR AUDITORY TRAINER
(Ear/Nose/Throat) 77EPF

Listen Technologies Corp. 801-233-8992
14912 Heritagecrest Way, Bluffdale, UT 84065
Various.

Z Sound 847-293-5205
6947 W Birchwood Ave, Niles, IL 60714
Z n d.

HEARING-AID, MASTER *(Ear/Nose/Throat) 77KHL*

Jack Jones Hearing Aid Centers, Inc. 800-722-8534
400 S Henderson St, Ft Worth, TX 76104
Jones ca hearing aid.

Statco Hearing Aid Laboratory 501-771-2444
4000 McCain Blvd, North Little Rock, AR 72116
Hearing aid.

HEARING-AID, PLATE, FACE *(Ear/Nose/Throat) 77LRB*

Affinity Medical Technology, Llc. 763-744-0412
3025 Harbor Ln N Ste 105, Plymouth, MN 55447
Various types of prewired hearing aid faceplates.

America Hears, Inc. 215-788-0330
806 Beaver St, Bristol, PA 19007
Various face plate hearing aids.

American Hearing Systems Inc. 763-404-1122
8001 E Bloomington Fwy, Bloomington, MN 55420
Multiple (alpha, image)prolink,quiklink,quiklink d,diglink.

Audina Hearing Instruments, Inc. 800-223-7700
165 E Wildmere Ave, Longwood, FL 32750

Crystal Tone Hearing Instruments 515-255-4144
4217 University Ave, Des Moines, IA 50311
Hearing aid.

House Of Hearing 480-649-9609
4020 E Main St, Mesa, AZ 85205
Various types of hearing aids.

Master Craft Labs 800-233-1413
PO Box 11, Bethel, MN 55005
Master craft laboratories.

Midwest City Hearing Aid Center 405-732-8682
1401 S Midwest Blvd, Midwest City, OK 73110
Audio enhancer in-the-ear (ite), audio enhancer in-the-canal (itc) & audio enhan.

Stephen Tobias Hearing Center 617-770-3395
382 Quincy Ave, Quincy, MA 02169
Faceplate hearing aid.

HEART, ARTIFICIAL *(Cardiovascular) 74LOZ*

Abiomed, Inc. 800-422-8666
22 Cherry Hill Dr, Danvers, MA 01923
Implantable.

HEART-LUNG BYPASS UNIT (CARDIOPULMONARY)
(Cardiovascular) 74QZM

Gish Biomedical, Inc. 800-938-0531
22942 Arroyo Vis, Rancho Santa Margarita, CA 92688
Custom tubing pack.

Terumo Cardiovascular Systems, Corp 800-521-2818
6200 Jackson Rd, Ann Arbor, MI 48103

HEAT EXCHANGER, EXTRACORPOREAL PERFUSION
(Surgery) 79QZP

Heatron, Inc. 913-651-4420
3000 Wilson Ave, Leavenworth, KS 66048

HEAT EXCHANGER, HEART-LUNG BYPASS
(Cardiovascular) 74DTR

Cardiovention, Inc. 408-873-3400
19200 Stevens Creek Blvd Ste 200, Cupertino, CA 95014
Cardiopulmonary bypass heat exchanger.

Heatron, Inc. 913-651-4420
3000 Wilson Ave, Leavenworth, KS 66048

Jostra Bentley, Inc. 302-454-9959
Rd. 402 N. Km 1.4, Industrial Park, Anasco, PR 00610-1577
Heat exchanger.

Medtronic Blood Management 612-514-4000
18501 E Plaza Dr, Parker, CO 80134
Blood heat exchanger.

Medtronic Perfusion Systems 800-854-3570
7611 Northland Dr N, Brooklyn Park, MN 55428

Terumo Cardiovascular Systems (Tcvs) 800-283-7866
125 Blue Ball Rd, Elkton, MD 21921
CPB heat exchanger.

Terumo Cardiovascular Systems (Tcvs) 800-283-7866
28 Howe St, Ashland, MA 01721
Heat exchanger.

Terumo Cardiovascular Systems, Corp 800-521-2818
6200 Jackson Rd, Ann Arbor, MI 48103

HEAT EXCHANGER, HEART-LUNG BYPASS, AC-POWERED
(Cardiovascular) 74QZQ

Heatron, Inc. 913-651-4420
3000 Wilson Ave, Leavenworth, KS 66048

HEAT EXCHANGER, REGIONAL PERFUSION *(Surgery) 79QZR*

Heatron, Inc. 913-651-4420
3000 Wilson Ave, Leavenworth, KS 66048

Lytron, Inc. 781-933-7300
55 Dragon Ct, Woburn, MA 01801
Dielectric oil cooler and aluminum heat exchanger.

HEAT-SEALING DEVICE *(Hematology) 81KSD*

Centron Technologies, Inc. 215-501-0430
10601 Decatur Rd Ste 100, Philadelphia, PA 19154
Genesis tube sealer.

Engineering & Research Assoc., Inc. (D.B.A. Sebra) 800-625-5550
100 N Tucson Blvd, Tucson, AZ 85716
PIRF and RF sealing equipment.

Forward Technology 320-286-2578
260 Jenks Ave SW, Cokato, MN 55321
Hot-plate welders for bonding thermoplastic parts.

Pac-Dent Intl., Inc. 909-839-0888
21078 Commerce Point Dr, Walnut, CA 91789
Heat sealer.

Sarstedt, Inc. 800-257-5101
PO Box 468, 1025, St. James Church Road, Newton, NC 28658

Trudell Medical Marketing Ltd. 800-265-5494
926 Leathorne St., London, ON N5Z-3M5 Canada

HEATER, BREATHING SYSTEM W/WO CONTROLLER
(Anesthesiology) 73BZE

C.F. Electronics, Inc. 307-742-5200
2052 N 3rd St, Laramie, WY 82072
Inhalation system providing warm moist air and/or oxygen.

Smiths Medical Asd Inc. 800-258-536[illegible]
10 Bowman Dr, Keene, NH 03431
Various types of heated breathing systems.

HEATER, ELECTRICAL INSTRUMENT *(General) 80SGQ*

Heatron, Inc. 913-651-4420
3000 Wilson Ave, Leavenworth, KS 66048
Flexible silcone-rubber, etched-silicone, Kapton, etched-mica and cast-in aluminum and bronze heaters.

Minco Products, Inc. 763-571-312[illegible]
7300 Commerce Ln NE, Minneapolis, MN 55432
Flexible THERMOFOIL instrument heaters featuring etched-foil element with chemical-resistant polyimide insulation and full range of temperature controls.

Research, Inc. 952-941-3300
7128 Shady Oak Rd, Eden Prairie, MN 55344
Infrared, high density I/R heater in various sizes.

Wisap America 800-233-8443
8231 Melrose Dr, Lenexa, KS 66214
Warmers--carbon dioxide warmer, fluid warmer, and laparoscope warmer. THERME3 endoscopic warming system warms and maintains the patient's cricial core body temperature as well as significantly reducing laparoscope fogging, saving valuable time in the operating room.

HEATER, HOT PACK *(Physical Med) 89VFJ*

Hospital Marketing Svcs. Company, Inc. 800-786-5094
162 Great Hill Rd./ Ind. Park, Naugatuck, CT 06770
24 per case.

Whitehall Manufacturing 800-782-7706
15125 Proctor Ave, City Of Industry, CA 91746
Hot pack heating unit. Several sizes, stationary and mobile.

Worldwide Products Heat Packs 800-554-6340
7031 N Via De Paesia, Scottsdale, AZ 85258
QuantumHeat Heat pack provides instant portable and reusable heat.

HEATER, IMMERSION *(Microbiology) 83UGJ*

Cole-Parmer Instrument Inc. 800-323-4340
625 E Bunker Ct, Vernon Hills, IL 60061

Corning Inc., Science Products Division 800-492-11[illegible]0
45 Nagog Park, Acton, MA 01720

HEATER, IMMERSION *(cont'd)*

Polyscience, Division Of Preston Industries Inc. 800-229-7569
6600 W Touhy Ave, Niles, IL 60714
The Model 7312 Immersion Circulator provides ambient +5× to 200×C temperature control, ±0.01×C temperature stability, and can be programmed with up to ten time/temperature profiles. It's ideal for applications where gradual or multi-step heating is required.

HEATER, PERINEAL *(Obstetrics/Gyn) 85KND*

Hospital Marketing Svcs. Company, Inc. 800-786-5094
162 Great Hill Rd./ Ind. Park, Naugatuck, CT 06770
Cat. no. 6350 24 per case.

HEATER, PERINEAL, DIRECT CONTACT *(Obstetrics/Gyn) 85HGZ*

Hospital Marketing Svcs. Company, Inc. 800-786-5094
162 Great Hill Rd./ Ind. Park, Naugatuck, CT 06770
Cat. no 6350 Perineal warm pack/24 per case.

HEATER, PERINEAL, RADIANT, NON-CONTACT *(Obstetrics/Gyn) 85HHA*

Ge Medical Systems Information Technologies 800-643-6439
8200 W Tower Ave, Milwaukee, WI 53223

Richard Wolf Medical Instruments Corp. 800-323-9653
353 Corporate Woods Pkwy, Vernon Hills, IL 60061

United Metal Fabricators, Inc. 800-638-5322
1316 Eisenhower Blvd, Johnstown, PA 15904
Incandescant bulb heat source. Equipped with adjustable width knee crutches.

HEATING MANTLE *(Microbiology) 83UGK*

Glas-Col , Llc 800-452-7265
711 Hulman St, PO Box 2128, Terre Haute, IN 47802
Various sizes for various laboratory vessels.

Minco Products, Inc. 763-571-3121
7300 Commerce Ln NE, Minneapolis, MN 55432

Tudor Scientific Glass Co., Inc. 800-336-4666
555 Edgefield Rd, Belvedere, SC 29841

HEATING UNIT, POWERED *(Physical Med) 89IRQ*

Aragona Medical, Inc. 201-664-8822
184 Rivervale Rd, Rivervale, NJ 07675
Radiant Warmer (Thermal Ceiling); 3 models: Ceiling Mounted, Mobile, and Baby Warmer, Require no disposables.

Chattanooga Group 800-592-7329
4717 Adams Rd, Hixson, TN 37343
HYDROCOLLATOR.

Dynatronics Corp. Chattanooga Operations 801-568-7000
6607 Mountain View Rd, Ooltewah, TN 37363
Powered heating unit.

Kennex Development Inc 626-458-0598
533 S Atlantic Blvd Ste 301, Monterey Park, CA 91754
Various types of powered heating units.

Naimco, Inc. 423-648-7730
4120 S Creek Rd, Chattanooga, TN 37406
Medical heating unit.

Radiant Electric Heat Inc. 262-783-1282
N52w 13670 N. Park Dr., Menomonee Falls, WI 53051
16 x 24 portable stainless steel heater.

Roberts & Gordon Canada, Inc. 905-945-5403
76 Main St. West, Unit 10, Grimsby, ON L3M-1R6 Canada
Infrared heating equipment.

Tetra Medical Supply Corp. 800-621-4041
6364 W Gross Point Rd, Niles, IL 60714
Hydrococollator Brand distributor.

HELMET, CRANIAL, FOR PROTECTIVE USE *(Physical Med) 89NDA*

Becker Orthopedic Appliance Co. 248-588-7480
635 Executive Dr, Troy, MI 48083
Protective helmet.

Richardson Products, Inc. 888-928-7297
9408 Gulfstream Rd, Frankfort, IL 60423
Helmet.

HELMET, SURGICAL *(Surgery) 79FXZ*

Corpak Medsystems, Inc. 800-323-6305
100 Chaddick Dr, Wheeling, IL 60090
Surgical helmet systems and face shields.

HELMET, SURGICAL *(cont'd)*

Depuy Orthopaedics, Inc. 800-473-3789
700 Orthopaedic Dr, P.O. Box 988, Warsaw, IN 46582
Various types of surgical helmets.

DJO Inc. 800-336-6569
1430 Decision St, Vista, CA 92081
Various sterile and non-sterile surgical helmets.

Variety Ability Systems Inc. 800-891-4514
2 Kelvin Ave., Unit 3, Toronto, ONT M4C-5C8 Canada
Protective helmet.

HEMACYTOMETER *(Hematology) 81ULS*

Propper Manufacturing Co., Inc. 800-832-4300
3604 Skillman Ave, Long Island City, NY 11101

HEMATOCRIT CONTROL *(Hematology) 81GLK*

Bionostics, Inc. 978-772-7070
7 Jackson Rd, Devens, MA 01434
Hematocrit controls.

Hycor Biomedical, Inc. 800-382-2527
7272 Chapman Ave, Garden Grove, CA 92841
Hematacrit control.

Richmond Diagnostics, Inc. 732-246-2429
100 Jersey Ave Ste 202-A, Bldg. B, New Brunswick, NJ 08901
Hematocrit control.

Separation Technology Inc 800-777-6668
1096 Rainer Dr, Altamonte Springs, FL 32714
HEMATACHEK hematocrit control stored at room temperature with two-year shelf life and 31-day open-vial stability. Available in low-, normal-, and high-assay levels.

HEMATOCRIT TUBE, RACK, SEALER, HOLDER *(Hematology) 81GHY*

Becton Dickinson And Company 800-284-6845
1 Becton Dr, Franklin Lakes, NJ 07417
HOLDER; RACK; SEALER; TUBE; HEMATOCRIT; MULTIPLE; SEAL-EASE TUBE SEALER AND HOLDER

Chase Scientific Glass, Inc. 412-490-8425
234 Cardiff Valley Rd, Rockwood, TN 37854
Multiple.

Covidien Lp 508-261-8000
15 Hampshire St, Mansfield, MA 02048

Dade Behring, Inc. 800-948-3233
1717 Deerfield Rd, Deerfield, IL 60015

Drummond Scientific Co. 800-523-7480
500 Park Way # 700, Broomall, PA 19008
HEMATO-CLAD Mylar wrapped hematocrit tube, with or without heparin, 75mm length.

Iris Sample Processing 800-782-8774
60 Glacier Dr, Westwood, MA 02090
Micro hematocrit tube reader and assoc.products.

Kimble Chase Life Science And Research Products, Llc. 865-717-2635
234 Cardiff Valley Rd, Ozone, TN 37854

Ram Scientific, Inc. 800-535-6734
PO Box 348, Yonkers, NY 10703
100% plastic SAFE-T-FILL(R) Micro Hematocrit Tubes come either heparinized or plain.

Statspin, Inc. 800-782-8774
60 Glacier Dr, Westwood, MA 02090
SAFECRIT 40-mm/75-mm, treated and untreated plastic hematocrit tubes.

Ware Medics Glass Works, Inc. 845-429-6950
PO Box 368, Garnerville, NY 10923

HEMATOCRIT, MANUAL *(Hematology) 81JPI*

Abbott Point Of Care Inc. 609-443-9300
104 Windsor Center Dr, East Windsor, NJ 08520
I-stat system.

Baxter Healthcare Corp., Renal Division 847-948-2000
7511 114th Ave, Largo, FL 33773
Device, hematocrit measuring.

Hema Metrics Inc. 800-546-5463
695 N Kays Dr, Kaysville, UT 84037

Iris Sample Processing 800-782-8774
60 Glacier Dr, Westwood, MA 02090
Hematocrit measuring device and accessories.

HEMATOCRIT, MANUAL *(cont'd)*

Separation Technology Inc 800-777-6668
1096 Rainer Dr, Altamonte Springs, FL 32714
UltraCrit Hematocrit Measurement Device employs ultrasound technology to accurately measure hematocrit (Hect) in whole blood. The initial application is to screen for suitable blood donors by the blood banking industry.

Thermo Fisher Scientific - Laboratory Equipment Division Headquarters 800-662-7477
450 Fortune Blvd, Milford, MA 01757

Vulcon Technologies 816-966-1212
718 Main St, Grandview, MO 64030
Polycarbonate hematocrit reader.

HEMATOLOGY QUALITY CONTROL MIXTURE *(Hematology) 81JPK*

Beckman Coulter, Inc. 800-635-3497
740 W 83rd St, Hialeah, FL 33014

Bio-Rad Laboratories, Diagnostic Group 800-224-6723
524 Stone Rd Ste A, Benicia, CA 94510
Hematology control mixtures for quality control.

Biomerieux Inc. 800-682-2666
100 Rodolphe St, Durham, NC 27712

Bionostics, Inc. 978-772-7070
7 Jackson Rd, Devens, MA 01434
Hemoglobin control.

Clinical Diagnostic Solutions, Inc. 954-791-1773
1800 NW 65th Ave, Plantation, FL 33313
Control for hematology analyqers that perform 5 part diffs.

Dade Behring, Inc. 800-948-3233
1717 Deerfield Rd, Deerfield, IL 60015

Diagnostic Technology, Inc. 631-582-4949
175 Commerce Dr Ste L, Hauppauge, NY 11788
Multi-parameter hematology calibrator for laser/optic instruments.

Horiba Abx 888-903-5001
34 Bunsen, Irvine, CA 92618
Hematology quality control mixture.

Hycor Biomedical, Inc. 800-382-2527
7272 Chapman Ave, Garden Grove, CA 92841
Control for hematology analyzers.

Iris Diagnostics 800-776-4747
9172 Eton Ave, Chatsworth, CA 91311
Controls.

J&S Medical Associates 800-229-6000
35 Tripp St Ste 1, Framingham, MA 01702
Hematology control, Hematrol; whole blood assayed controls used to check performance and validity of blood cell counters.

R & D Systems, Inc. 1-800-343-7475
614 McKinley Pl NE, Minneapolis, MN 55413

Trillium Diagnostics, Llc. 866-364-0028
915 Union St Ste 3, Bangor, ME 04401
FETALtrol is a tri-level assayed, human blood control designed to document and monitor values obtained from test methods used to determine fetal RBCs in maternal blood samples.

Vegamed, Inc. 787-807-0392
39 Calle Las Flores, Edificio Multifabril #5, Vega Baja, PR 00693
Hematology control.

HEMATOXYLIN WEIGERT'S *(Pathology) 88HYO*

American Mastertech Scientific, Inc. 209-368-4031
1330 Thurman St, Lodi, CA 95240
Multiple.

Richard-Allan Scientific 269-544-5628
4481 Campus Dr, Kalamazoo, MI 49008
Alcoholic hematoxylin.

Rowley Biochemical Institute 978-739-4883
10 Electronics Ave, Danvers Industrial Park, Danvers, MA 01923

HEMOCYTOMETER *(Hematology) 81GHO*

Propper Manufacturing Co., Inc. 800-832-4300
3604 Skillman Ave, Long Island City, NY 11101

HEMODIALYSIS UNIT (KIDNEY MACHINE) *(Gastro/Urology) 78RAA*

B. Braun Medical Inc., Renal Therapies Div. 800-854-6851
824 12th Ave, Bethlehem, PA 18018
Dialog+ Hemodialysis System.

HEMODIALYSIS UNIT (KIDNEY MACHINE) *(cont'd)*

Rismed Oncology Systems 256-534-6993
2494 Washington St NW, Huntsville, AL 35811
Hemodialysis machines, fully automated. Flat screen touch screen monitor, triple pump system, etc. A state of the art dialysis system.

HEMOGLOBIN A2 QUANTITATION *(Hematology) 81JPD*

Bio-Rad Laboratories Inc., Clinical Systems Div. 800-224-6723
4000 Alfred Nobel Dr, Hercules, CA 94547
Variant ii b-thal short, or vii bts.

Helena Laboratories 409-842-3714
PO Box 752, Beaumont, TX 77704

Sebia Electrophoresis 800-835-6497
400-1705 Corporate Drive, Norcross, GA 30093

HEMOGLOBIN C (ABNORMAL HEMOGLOBIN VARIANT) *(Hematology) 81MLL*

Sebia Electrophoresis 800-835-6497
400-1705 Corporate Drive, Norcross, GA 30093

HEMOGLOBIN F QUANTITATION *(Hematology) 81JPC*

Jas Diagnostics, Inc. 305-418-2320
7220 NW 58th St, Miami, FL 33166
Hemoglobin control.

Sebia Electrophoresis 800-835-6497
400-1705 Corporate Drive, Norcross, GA 30093

HEMOGLOBIN M *(Hematology) 81JPB*

Michclone Associates, Inc. 248-583-1150
1197 Rochester Rd Ste L, Troy, MI 48083
Sickle heme control.

HEMOGLOBIN S *(Hematology) 81GIQ*

PerkinElmer 800-762-4000
940 Winter St, Waltham, MA 02451

Primus Diagnostics 800-377-4752
4231 E 75th Ter, Kansas City, MO 64132
ultra2 dual-assay HPLC system for the quantitation of HbA1c and Hb Variants utilizes boronate affinity technology for an interference-free A1c result in 2 minutes and features a 4-minute Quick Scan with an abnormal results automatic reflex to a 10-minute High Resolution Program to aid in Hb variant identification.

Sebia Electrophoresis 800-835-6497
400-1705 Corporate Drive, Norcross, GA 30093

HEMOGLOBIN, RESISTANT, ALKALI *(Hematology) 81GHA*

Analytical Control Systems, Inc. 317-841-0458
9058 Technology Dr, Fishers, IN 46038
QUIK-SEP Hemoglobin Alkali Denaturation Assay provides a reagent set for accurate quantitation of adult Hb F in ranges from 2% to 40% by alkali denaturation. Normal and elevated F controls also available.

HEMOGLOBINOMETER *(Hematology) 81GIG*

Beckman Coulter, Inc. 800-635-3497
740 W 83rd St, Hialeah, FL 33014
$2,195 for hemoglobinometer.

Radiometer America, Inc. 800-736-0600
810 Sharon Dr, Westlake, OH 44145
Hemoximeter.

HEMOGLOBINOMETER, AUTOMATED *(Hematology) 81GKR*

International Technidyne Corporation 732-548-5700
8 Olsen Ave, Edison, NJ 08820
Whole blood hemoglobin test system.

Opti Medical Systems Inc. 770-510-4444
235 Hembree Park Dr, Roswell, GA 30076
Automated blood gas/electrolyte analyzer.

Osmetech, Inc. 800-373-6767
757 S Raymond Ave, Pasadena, CA 91105
Automated blood gas/electrolyte analyzer.

Radiometer America, Inc. 800-736-0600
810 Sharon Dr, Westlake, OH 44145
Hemoximeter system measuring seven parameters; 35-mL sample size.

HEMOGLOBINOMETER, ELECTROPHORETIC ANALYSIS SYSTEM *(Hematology) 81JBD*

Carolina Liquid Chemistries Corp. 800-471-7272
510 W Central Ave Ste C, Brea, CA 92821
Hemolyzing solution.

HEMOGLOBINOMETER, ELECTROPHORETIC ANALYSIS SYSTEM *(cont'd)*

PerkinElmer 800-762-4000
940 Winter St, Waltham, MA 02451

HEMOPERFUSION SYSTEM, SORBENT *(Gastro/Urology) 78FLD*

American Health Care Systems, Inc. 504-831-4867
3350 Ridgelake Dr Ste 255, Metairie, LA 70002
Various types and sizes.

HEMORRHOID CUSHION *(Gastro/Urology) 78LRL*

Grand Rapids Foam Technologies 877-GET-GRFT
2788 Remico St SW, Wyoming, MI 49519

Occk, Inc. 800-526-9731
1710 W Schilling Rd, Salina, KS 67401
Hemorrhoid cushion.

HEMOSTAT *(Orthopedics) 87HRQ*

Cardinal Health, Snowden Pencer Products 847-689-8410
5175 S Royal Atlanta Dr, Tucker, GA 30084
Manual surgical instruments.

Dermatologic Lab & Supply, Inc. 800-831-6273
608 13th Ave, Council Bluffs, IA 51501
Surgical hemostat.

Hartzell & Son, G. 800-950-2206
2372 Stanwell Cir, Concord, CA 94520

Johnson & Johnson Medical Division Of Ethicon, Inc. 800-423-4018
2500 E Arbrook Blvd, Arlington, TX 76014
Surgicel fibrillar absorbable.

Kentron Health Care, Inc. 615-384-0573
3604 Kelton Jackson Rd, P.o. Box 120, Springfield, TN 37172
Forceps hemostat.

Kmedic 800-955-0559
190 Veterans Dr, Northvale, NJ 07647

Medchem Products, Inc. 800-451-4716
160 New Boston St, Woburn, MA 01801
Topical AVITENE microfibrillar collagen hemostat including preloaded applicators: syringe AVITENE; NeuroAVITENE and ENT AVITENE. ENDO-AVITENE topical AVITENE microfibrillar collagen hemostat in an endoscopic delivery device.

Micrins Surgical Instruments, Inc. 800-833-3380
28438 N Ballard Dr, Lake Forest, IL 60045

Pocket Nurse Enterprises, Inc. 800-225-1600
200 1st St, Ambridge, PA 15003

Precision Surgical Intl., Inc. 800-776-8493
PO Box 726, Noblesville, IN 46061
Various types of hemostatic forceps.

Prosurge Instruments, Inc. 866-832-7874
199 Laidlaw Ave, Jersey City, NJ 07306

Symmetry Medical Usa, Inc. 574-267-8700
486 W 350 N, Warsaw, IN 46582
Manual surgical instrument for general use.

Trans American Medical / Tamsco Instruments 708-430-7777
7633 W 100th Pl, Bridgeview, IL 60455

Tuzik Boston 800-886-6363
104 Longwater Dr, Assinippi Park, Norwell, MA 02061

Zimmer Holdings, Inc. 800-613-6131
1800 W Center St, PO Box 708, Warsaw, IN 46580

HEMOSTAT, SURGICAL *(Dental And Oral) 76EMD*

Aesculap Implant Systems Inc. 1-800-234-9179
3773 Corporate Pkwy, Center Valley, PA 18034

Biomet Microfixation Inc. 800-874-7711
1520 Tradeport Dr, Jacksonville, FL 32218
Hemostat, surgical.

Buffalo Dental Mfg. Co., Inc. 516-496-7200
159 Lafayette Dr, Syosset, NY 11791
Surgical hemostat.

Coltene/Whaledent Inc. 330-916-8858
235 Ascot Pkwy, Cuyahoga Falls, OH 44223
Hemostat.

Dshealthcare Inc. 201-871-1232
85 W Forest Ave, Englewood, NJ 07631
Topical hemostatic solution.

E.A. Beck & Co. 949-645-4072
657 W 19th St Ste E, P O Box 10857, Costa Mesa, CA 92627
Mosquito or kelly.

HEMOSTAT, SURGICAL *(cont'd)*

Elmed, Inc. 630-543-2792
60 W Fay Ave, Addison, IL 60101

George Tiemann & Co. 800-843-6266
25 Plant Ave, Hauppauge, NY 11788

H & H Co. 909-390-0373
4435 E Airport Dr Ste 108, Ontario, CA 91761
Hemostat, all types.

Hu-Friedy Manufacturing Co., Inc. 800-483-7433
3232 N Rockwell St, Chicago, IL 60618
$52.75 to $78.75, 13 types.

Kmedic 800-955-0559
190 Veterans Dr, Northvale, NJ 07647

Micrins Surgical Instruments, Inc. 800-833-3380
28438 N Ballard Dr, Lake Forest, IL 60045

Miltex Dental Technologies, Inc. 516-576-6022
589 Davies Dr, York, PA 17402
Various hemostats.

Nordent Manufacturing, Inc. 800-966-7336
610 Bonnie Ln, Elk Grove Village, IL 60007
$30.00 per unit (standard).

Oratronics, Inc. 212-986-0050
405 Lexington Ave, New York, NY 10174
Needle holder.

Premier Dental Products Co. 888-670-6100
1710 Romano Dr, PO Box 4500, Plymouth Meeting, PA 19462

Prosurge Instruments, Inc. 866-832-7874
199 Laidlaw Ave, Jersey City, NJ 07306

Pulpdent Corp. 800-343-4342
80 Oakland St, Watertown, MA 02472
No common name listed.

Salvin Dental Specialties, Inc. 800-535-6566
3450 Latrobe Dr, Charlotte, NC 28211
Various types of surgical hemostats.

Scanlan International, Inc. 800-328-9458
1 Scanlan Plz, Saint Paul, MN 55107

Tuzik Boston 800-886-6363
104 Longwater Dr, Assinippi Park, Norwell, MA 02061

Vartex Instrument Corp. 718-486-5050
311 Wallabout St, Brooklyn, NY 11206
Various forceps.

HEPARIN *(Pathology) 88IAZ*

Baxter Healthcare Corporation, Global Drug Delivery 888-229-0001
25212 W Il Route 120, Round Lake, IL 60073
Heparin sodium in 5% dextrose injections.

Fisher Diagnostics 877-722-4366
11515 Vanstory Dr Ste 125, Huntersville, NC 28078
Heparin controls.

HEPATITIS B TEST (B CORE, BE ANTIGEN & ANTIBODY, B CORE IGM) *(Microbiology) 83LOM*

Abbott Laboratories 800-223-2064
100 Abbott Park Rd, Abbott Park, IL 60064
ARCHITECT HBSAG REAGENT KIT; CALIBRATORS, CONTROLS, CONFIRMATORY; CONFIRMATORY MANUAL DILUENT; REAGENT KIT

Abbott Molecular, Inc. 847-937-6100
1300 E Touhy Ave, Des Plaines, IL 60018
In vitro pcr assay quantitation of hbv.

Chembio Diagnostic Systems, Inc. 631-924-1135
3661 Horseblock Rd, Medford, NY 11763
Immunochromatographic assay for visual detection of hepatitis b surface antigen.

Diasorin Inc 800-328-1482
1951 Northwestern Ave S, PO Box 285, Stillwater, MN 55082
ETI-AB-COREK PLUS for the detection of Total Antibodies to Hepatitis B Core Antigen. ETI-CORE-IgMK PLUS for detection of IgM Antibodies to Hepatitis B Core Antigen. ETI-EBK PLUS for the detection of Hepatitis B Antigen and Antibodies to Hepatitis B Antigen.

Hema Diagnostic Systems, Llc 305-867-6123
1666 Kennedy Causeway, Suite 401, North Bay Village, FL 33141
Rapid 1-2-3 hema hepatitis B whole blood test. Available in strip format or in the new rapid 1-2-3 hema housing.

HEPATITIS B TEST (B CORE, BE ANTIGEN & ANTIBODY, B CORE IGM) *(cont'd)*

Immunoscience, Inc. 925-460-8111
7066 Commerce Cir Ste D, Pleasanton, CA 94588
Colloidal gold rapid immunoassay for hepatitis b.

Inamco International Corp. 800-724-4003
801 Montrose Ave, South Plainfield, NJ 07080
MEDICOS.

St. Paul Biotech 714-903-1000
11555 Monarch St, Garden Grove, CA 92841
Hepatitis b test.

United Biotech, Inc. 650-961-2910
211 S Whisman Rd Ste E, Mountain View, CA 94041
ELISA for detecting HbsAg (Hepatitis B Surface Antigen)

HEXOKINASE, GLUCOSE *(Chemistry) 75CFR*

Abbott Diagnostics Div. 626-440-0700
820 Mission St, South Pasadena, CA 91030
Glucose assay reagent.

Bayer Healthcare, Llc 574-256-3430
430 S Beiger St, Mishawaka, IN 46544
Test for blood glucose.

Beckman Coulter, Inc. 800-635-3497
740 W 83rd St, Hialeah, FL 33014
$0.08 per test.

Beckman Coulter, Inc. 800-742-2345
250 S Kraemer Blvd, PO Box 8000, Brea, CA 92821

Caldon Bioscience, Inc. 909-628-9944
2100 S Reservoir St, Pomona, CA 91766
Glucose (hko.

Caldon Biotech, Inc. 757-224-0177
2251 Rutherford Rd, Carlsbad, CA 92008
Clucose (hkO.

Carolina Liquid Chemistries Corp. 800-471-7272
510 W Central Ave Ste C, Brea, CA 92821
Glucose or glu.

Do Not Disturb, Inc. 770-750-0065
5665 Atlanta Hwy # 10, Alpharetta, GA 30004
Heating insert (accessory to home spa products).

Genchem, Inc. 714-529-1616
510 W Central Ave Ste D, Brea, CA 92821
Glucose reagent.

Genzyme Corp. 800-325-2436
160 Christian St, Oxford, CT 06478
Endpoint.

Health Chem Diagnostics Llc 954-979-3845
3341 W McNab Rd, Pompano Beach, FL 33069
Hexokinase, glucose.

Hemagen Diagnostics, Inc. 800-436-2436
9033 Red Branch Rd, Columbia, MD 21045
Various glucose methods.

Intersect Systems, Inc. 360-577-1062
1152 3rd Avenue, Suite D & E, Longview, WA 98632
Hexokinase glucose, Glucose-Hexokinase.

Jas Diagnostics, Inc. 305-418-2320
7220 NW 58th St, Miami, FL 33166
Glucose-hexokinase.

Raichem, Division Of Hemagen Diagnostics, Inc. 800-438-6100
8225 Mercury Ct, San Diego, CA 92111

Sterling Diagnostics, Inc. 800-637-2661
36645 Metro Ct, Sterling Heights, MI 48312
Glucose reagent set (hk-uv).

Teco Diagnostics 714-693-7788
1268 N Lakeview Ave, Anaheim, CA 92807
Glucose (hexoinase) liquid reagent.

Vital Diagnostics Inc. 714-672-3553
1075 W Lambert Rd Ste D, Brea, CA 92821
Various glucose reagents.

HIGH PERFORMANCE LIQUID CHROMATOGRAPHY, CYCLOSPORINE *(Chemistry) 75MGS*

Justrite Manufacturing Co., L.L.C. 800-798-9250
2454 E Dempster St, Des Plaines, IL 60016
Justrite has Quick-Disconnect Safety Disposal Cans that offer a safe and easy way to collect liquid waste. Quick disconnect fittings allow free flow of solvent into container through tubing.

HIGH PERFORMANCE LIQUID CHROMATOGRAPHY, CYCLOSPORINE *(cont'd)*

Tosoh Bioscience Llc 800-366-4875
156 Keystone Dr, Montgomeryville, PA 18936
HPLC columns for clinical and diagnostic analyses, including hemaglobin analysis, cathecholamines, and antidepressants.

HIGH PRESSURE LIQUID CHROMATOGRAPHY, BARBITURATE *(Toxicology) 91KZY*

Beckman Coulter, Inc. 800-742-2345
250 S Kraemer Blvd, PO Box 8000, Brea, CA 92821

HIGH PRESSURE LIQUID CHROMATOGRAPHY, BENZODIAZEPINE *(Toxicology) 91LAA*

Beckman Coulter, Inc. 800-742-2345
250 S Kraemer Blvd, PO Box 8000, Brea, CA 92821

Bio-Rad Laboratories Inc., Clinical Systems Div. 800-224-6723
4000 Alfred Nobel Dr, Hercules, CA 94547
Benzodiazepines/tricyclic antidepressant test system.

HIGH PRESSURE LIQUID CHROMATOGRAPHY, COCAINE & METABOLITES *(Toxicology) 91LAC*

Beckman Coulter, Inc. 800-742-2345
250 S Kraemer Blvd, PO Box 8000, Brea, CA 92821

HIGH PRESSURE LIQUID CHROMATOGRAPHY, CODEINE *(Toxicology) 91LAE*

Beckman Coulter, Inc. 800-742-2345
250 S Kraemer Blvd, PO Box 8000, Brea, CA 92821

HIGH PRESSURE LIQUID CHROMATOGRAPHY, METHAMPHETAMINE *(Toxicology) 91LAG*

Beckman Coulter, Inc. 800-742-2345
250 S Kraemer Blvd, PO Box 8000, Brea, CA 92821

HIGH PRESSURE LIQUID CHROMATOGRAPHY, OPIATES *(Toxicology) 91LAH*

Beckman Coulter, Inc. 800-742-2345
250 S Kraemer Blvd, PO Box 8000, Brea, CA 92821

HIGH PRESSURE LIQUID CHROMATOGRAPHY, PROPOXYPHENE *(Toxicology) 91LAK*

Beckman Coulter, Inc. 800-742-2345
250 S Kraemer Blvd, PO Box 8000, Brea, CA 92821

HIGH PRESSURE LIQUID CHROMATOGRAPHY, QUININE *(Toxicology) 91LAM*

Beckman Coulter, Inc. 800-742-2345
250 S Kraemer Blvd, PO Box 8000, Brea, CA 92821

Biomet Microfixation Inc. 800-874-7711
1520 Tradeport Dr, Jacksonville, FL 32218
Guard, skin, graft.

HIGH PRESSURE LIQUID CHROMATOGRAPHY, TRICYCLIC DRUG *(Toxicology) 91LFI*

Beckman Coulter, Inc. 800-742-2345
250 S Kraemer Blvd, PO Box 8000, Brea, CA 92821

Pan Probe Biotech, Inc. 858-689-9936
7396 Trade St, San Diego, CA 92121
Determination of tricyclic antidepressant in human urine.

Polymer Laboratories, Now A Part Of Varian, Inc. 800-767-3963
160 Old Farm Rd, Amherst Fields Research Park, Amherst, MA 01002
Varian 385-LC and Varian 380-LC Evaporative light scattering detectors. Also for GPC. PL-LC1120 precise reproducible flow for accurate reliable results, on-board diagnostics for dependable operation, and variable piston stroke for minimal variation in pressure and flow. PL-LC1150 Unique proportioning system for accurate solvent composition, low internal volume for sharp reproducible solvent gradients and ease of set-up/Ease of use. PL-LC1200 high sensitivity and excellent linearity, advanced optical system design for improved reliability, and small footprint.

HIP, HEMI-, FEMORAL, METAL BALL *(Orthopedics) 87LZY*

Bio-Technology Usa, Inc. 305-512-3522
6175 NW 167th St Ste G8, Hialeah, FL 33015
Hip endoprosthesis.

Biomet, Inc. 574-267-6639
56 E Bell Dr, PO Box 587, Warsaw, IN 46582
Various types of sterile hip components.

Depuy Orthopaedics, Inc. 800-473-3789
700 Orthopaedic Dr, P.O. Box 988, Warsaw, IN 46582
Prosthesis, hip, hemi-, femoral, metal ball (various types).

HIP, HEMI-, FEMORAL, METAL BALL *(cont'd)*

Endotec, Inc. 973-762-6100
2546 Hansrob Rd, Orlando, FL 32804
Buechel-pappas femoral head.

Millstone Medical Outsourcing 508-679-8384
1565 N Main St Ste 408, Fall River, MA 02720
Multiple and various.

HOE, PERIODONTIC *(Dental And Oral) 76EMQ*

Aesculap Implant Systems Inc. 1-800-234-9179
3773 Corporate Pkwy, Center Valley, PA 18034

Dental Usa, Inc. 815-363-8003
5005 McCullom Lake Rd, McHenry, IL 60050
Hoe.

E.A. Beck & Co. 949-645-4072
657 W 19th St Ste E, P O Box 10857, Costa Mesa, CA 92627
Hoe.

H & H Co. 909-390-0373
4435 E Airport Dr Ste 108, Ontario, CA 91761
Chisel, periodontic.

Hu-Friedy Manufacturing Co., Inc. 800-483-7433
3232 N Rockwell St, Chicago, IL 60618
$18.45 to $24.60, 6 types.

Premier Dental Products Co. 888-670-6100
1710 Romano Dr, PO Box 4500, Plymouth Meeting, PA 19462

Suter Dental Manufacturing Company, Inc. 800-368-8376
632 Cedar St, Chico, CA 95928

HOLDER, CAMERA, SURGICAL *(Surgery) 79FXR*

Mediflex Surgical Products 800-879-7575
250 Gibbs Rd, Islandia, NY 11749
Holding device for laparoscope instruments, liver retractors and laparoscopes. Starting at $1,595.00

HOLDER, CATHETER *(Gastro/Urology) 78EYJ*

Ac Healthcare Supply, Inc. 905-448-4706
11651 230th St, Cambria Heights, NY 11411
Urological catheter and accessories.

Advanced Materials, Inc. 310-537-5444
20211 S Susana Rd, East Rancho Dominguez, CA 90221
Catheter holder.

Aesculap Implant Systems Inc. 1-800-234-9179
3773 Corporate Pkwy, Center Valley, PA 18034

Aplix, Inc. 704-588-1920
12300 Steele Creek Rd, Charlotte, NC 28273

Armstrong Medical Industries, Inc. 800-323-4220
575 Knightsbridge Pkwy, Lincolnshire, IL 60069

Dale Medical Products, Inc. 800-343-3980
7 Cross St, Plainville, MA 02762
Foley Catheter Tube Holder: #316 legband, fits most adults; #330 legband/waistband, fits most adults

Eclipse Medical, Inc. 877-600-0042
12105 SW 129th Ct Ste 104, Miami, FL 33186
Foley catheter holder.

Insight Biodesign Llc 775-250-0267
1065 Waverly Dr, Reno, NV 89519
Urethral catheter holder.

Intermetro Industries Corp. 800-441-2714
651 N Washington St, Wilkes Barre, PA 18705
SUPERERECTA, STARSYS.

Kentron Health Care, Inc. 615-384-0573
3604 Kelton Jackson Rd, P.o. Box 120, Springfield, TN 37172
Catheter holder/legband.

M.C. Johnson Co., Inc. 800-553-8483
2037 J and C Blvd, Naples, FL 34109
CATH-SECURE holds catheters, gastrostomy & wound drainage tubing; CATH-SECURE DUAL TAB anchors various medical tubings sucha as indwelling urinary catheters, EKG leads, subclavian line ports, jejunostomy and wound drainage tubing; NG SECURE - holder for nasogastric tubes, nasal feeding tubes and oxygen cannulas.

Neotech Products, Inc. 800-966-0500
27822 Fremont Ct, Valencia, CA 91355
NEOBRIDGE: Umbilical catheter holder uses skin friendly hydrocolloid to attach to patient.

Skil-Care Corp. 800-431-2972
29 Wells Ave, Yonkers, NY 10701

HOLDER, CATHETER *(cont'd)*

Taylor Medical Products 814-362-2183
200 Saint Francis Dr Apt 114, Bradford, PA 16701
$25.00 per package of 25 Foley catheter holders.

HOLDER, CRUTCH AND CANE, WHEELCHAIR
(Physical Med) 89IMZ

Feiter's Inc 414-355-7575
8700 W Port Ave, Milwaukee, WI 53224
Holder, crutch and cane, wheelchair.

Sunrise Medical Hhg Inc 303-218-4505
2842 N Business Park Ave, Fresno, CA 93727

Therafin Corporation 800-843-7234
19747 Wolf Rd, Mokena, IL 60448
Cane holder.

Wheelchair Carrier, Inc. 800-541-3213
203 Matzinger Rd, Toledo, OH 43612
Wheelchair carriers priced from $199.00; scooter carriers priced from $558.00. Attach to trailer hitch to transport wheelchairs and scooters.

HOLDER, EAR SPECULUM *(Ear/Nose/Throat) 77JYK*

Aesculap Implant Systems Inc. 1-800-234-9179
3773 Corporate Pkwy, Center Valley, PA 18034

Cameron-Miller, Inc. 800-621-0142
5410 W Roosevelt Rd, Road #241, Chicago, IL 60644

Gyrus Ent L.L.C., Sub. Of Gyrus Acmi, Inc. 508-804-2739
2925 Appling Rd, Bartlett, TN 38133
Various types and sizes of ear speculum holders.

Tuzik Boston 800-886-6363
104 Longwater Dr, Assinippi Park, Norwell, MA 02061

HOLDER, ELECTROSURGICAL ELECTRODE *(Surgery) 79QSM*

Elmed, Inc. 630-543-2792
60 W Fay Ave, Addison, IL 60101

Pharmaceutical Innovations, Inc. 973-242-2900
897 Frelinghuysen Ave, Newark, NJ 07114
PREP N' STAY holds electrodes in place for diaphoretic patients. $5.50 for 15ml bottle.

HOLDER, GAS CYLINDER *(Anesthesiology) 73BSM*

Allied Healthcare Products, Inc. 800-444-3954
1720 Sublette Ave, Saint Louis, MO 63110

Farley Inc., W.T. 800-327-5397
931 Via Alondra, Camarillo, CA 93012
$60.00 for oxygen & E cylinder safety holders for wheelchairs, beds, code carts, free standing and wall mounted. $72.00 for MULTI-OX combination oxygen cylinder floor stand, gurney and bed holder; also available, $72.00 for cylinder safety holder for walkers, keeps cylinder safe while allowing patient to move freely.

Life Corporation 800-700-0202
1776 N Water St, Milwaukee, WI 53202
LIFE, OxygenPac Portable emergency oxygen units, clear cover and wall-mounted, off/on lever control, resuscitation mask with one-way valve for hygiene, 6lpm 90min. supply, refillable. Also available 6 & 12 lpm NORM & HIGH, 0-25 lpm variable, and demand-valve for 100% oxygen resuscitation. GSA Federal Supply Schedule.

Matrx By Midmark 800-847-1000
145 Mid County Dr, Orchard Park, NY 14127

Norco 800-657-6672
1125 W Amity Rd, Boise, ID 83705

Special Gas Services Inc 919-621-0980
PO Box 727, Mount Laurel, NJ 08054

Ziamatic Corp. 800-711-FIRE
10 W College Ave, Yardley, PA 19067
QUIC RELEASE gas cylinder brackets is an oxygen tank system with electrical rack to raise or lower medical oxygen cylinder into or out of a compartment.

Zimmer Holdings, Inc. 800-613-6131
1800 W Center St, PO Box 708, Warsaw, IN 46580

HOLDER, GUIDE, CATHETER *(Cardiovascular) 74DQW*

Richard Wolf Medical Instruments Corp. 800-323-9653
353 Corporate Woods Pkwy, Vernon Hills, IL 60061

HOLDER, HEAD, NEUROSURGICAL (SKULL CLAMP)
(Cns/Neurology) 84HBL

Codman & Shurtleff, Inc 800-225-0460
325 Paramount Dr, Raynham, MA 02767

HOLDER, HEAD, NEUROSURGICAL (SKULL CLAMP) *(cont'd)*

Composite Manufacturing, Inc. 949-361-7580
970 Calle Amanecer Ste B, San Clemente, CA 92673
Head holder.

Frank Scholz X-Ray Corp. 508-586-8308
244 Liberty St, Brockton, MA 02301
$538.45 per unit (standard).

Integra Lifesciences Of Ohio 800-654-2873
4900 Charlemar Dr Bldg A, Cincinnati, OH 45227
Various head holders (skull clamps) and accessories.

Medtronic Image-Guided Neurologics, Inc. 800-707-0933
2290 W Eau Gallie Blvd, Melbourne, FL 32935
Head holder.

Mtd, Inc. 908-362-6807
24 Slabtown Creek Rd, Hardwick, NJ 07825

Precision Medical Manufacturing Corporation 866-633-4626
852 Seton Ct, Wheeling, IL 60090
Hemilaminectomy Retractor 6' with two blades, this retractor has a powerful smooth action with self locking rack and pinion. Frame can be also used with thoracic retractor.

Schaerer Mayfield Usa 800-755-6381
4900 Charlemar Dr, Cincinnati, OH 45227
Modified MAYFIELD skull clamp system. MAYFIELD 2000 radiolucent headrest system.

HOLDER, HEAD, RADIOGRAPHIC *(Radiology) 90IWY*

Alimed, Inc. 800-225-2610
297 High St, Dedham, MA 02026
PROTECTA-COAT head and neck supports.

Best Nomos Corp. 800-70-NOMOS
1 Best Dr, Pittsburgh, PA 15202
TALON head fixation and immobilization system.

Bionix Development Corp. 800-551-7096
5154 Enterprise Blvd, Toledo, OH 43612
Various types of head immobilization devices.

Composiflex, Inc. 800-673-2544
8100 Hawthorne Dr, Erie, PA 16509
Low absorption, high strength carbon fiber head holders.

Creative Foam Medical Systems 800-446-4644
405 Industrial Dr, Bremen, IN 46506
Various types of coated foam head support/holders.

Frank Scholz X-Ray Corp. 508-586-8308
244 Liberty St, Brockton, MA 02301
$538.45 per unit (standard).

Larson Medical Products, Inc. 614-235-9100
2844 Banwick Rd, Columbus, OH 43232
Radiographic head holder.

Marconi Medical Systems 800-323-0550
595 Miner Rd, Cleveland, OH 44143

Portal, Inc. 435-753-3598
1350 N 200 W Ste 6, Logan, UT 84341
Patient positioning & weighting accessory to mri, ct & xray.

Rhodes Medical Products Inc. 904-233-0928
1116 Celebrant Dr, Jacksonville, FL 32225
Rhodes mri pillow.

Vermont Composites, Inc. 802-442-9964
25 Performance Dr, Bennington, VT 05201
Low absorption carbon head holder.

HOLDER, HEART VALVE PROSTHESIS *(Cardiovascular) 74DTJ*

Ats Medical, Inc. 949-380-9333
20412 James Bay Cir, Lake Forest, CA 92630

ATS Medical, Inc. 800-399-1381
3905 Annapolis Ln N Ste 105, Minneapolis, MN 55447
Open Pivot Handle; Open Pivot Hex End Rotator; Open Pivot Holder

Edwards Lifesciences, Llc. 800-424-3278
1 Edwards Way, Irvine, CA 92614

Medtronic Cardiovascular Surgery, The Heart Valve Div. 800-328-2518
1851 E Deere Ave, Santa Ana, CA 92705
Holder or collet.

Medtronic Heart Valves 800-227-3191
8299 Central Ave NE, Spring Lake Park, MN 55432
Holder or collet.

HOLDER, INFANT POSITION *(General) 80FRP*

Children's Medical Ventures, Inc. 800-345-6443
191 Wyngate Dr, Monroeville, PA 15146
BENDY BUMPER & SNUGGLE UP, premature infant positioning aids.

Greenco Industries, Inc. 608-328-8311
1601 4th Ave W, Monroe, WI 53566
Soft circumcision restraint.

Joerns Healthcare, Inc. 715-341-3600
1032 N Fourth St, Baldwyn, MS 38824
Pediatric positioner/holder.

Kerma Medical Products, Inc. 757-398-8400
400 Port Centre Pkwy, Portsmouth, VA 23704
Circumcision restraint belts.

Octostop Inc. 450-978-9805
1675 Saint Elzear, west, Laval, QUE H7L-3N6 Canada
$780.00 for Universal OCTOSTOP infant immobilizer (general).

Tucker Designs Limited 800-780-7979
PO Box 641117, Kenner, LA 70064
Sling, priced from $26.00 on up. Available in 9 different sizes. TUCKER SLING - positioning device for infants and toddlers who need to be elevated. This product is for hospital and home use. Specifically designed for GERD.

HOLDER, INSTRUMENT, LAPAROSCOPIC *(Surgery) 79QNR*

Automated Medical Products Corp. 800-832-4567
PO Box 2508, Edison, NJ 08818
IRON INTERN.

Coopersurgical, Inc. 800-243-2974
95 Corporate Dr, Trumbull, CT 06611

Dma Med-Chem Corporation 800-362-1833
49 Watermill Ln, Great Neck, NY 11021

Kronner Medical 800-706-3533
1443 Upper Cleveland Rapids Rd, Roseburg, OR 97471
Kronner Cannula Site Stitcher - used for closing the cannula site wound during laparoscopic surgery.

Mediflex Surgical Products 800-879-7575
250 Gibbs Rd, Islandia, NY 11749

Thompson Surgical Instruments, Inc. 800-227-7543
10170 E Cherry Bend Rd, Traverse City, MI 49684

HOLDER, INTRAVASCULAR CATHETER *(General) 80KMK*

Centurion Medical Products Corp. 517-545-1135
3310 S Main St, Salisbury, NC 28147

Corium International, Inc. 616-656-4563
4558 50th St SE, Grand Rapids, MI 49512
Various sizes of i.v. transparent dressings.

Four Process, Ltd. 636-677-5650
1480 W Lark Industrial Dr, Fenton, MO 63026
I.V. house.

Genesis Medical Products, Inc. 508-876-1063
40 Farm Hill Rd, Wrentham, MA 02093
I.v. armboards.

Health Care Logistics, Inc. 800-848-1633
450 Town St, PO Box 25, Circleville, OH 43113
Various.

I.V. House, Inc. 800-530-0400
7400 Foxmont Dr, Hazelwood, MO 63042
I.V. HOUSE ULTRA DRESSING--intravenous site protector.

K. W. Griffen Co. 203-846-1923
100 Pearl St, Norwalk, CT 06850
Anchor bandage.

Martin-Mars, Inc. 985-438-4402
415 Camellia Dr, Thibodaux, LA 70301
Tube-securing device. LineBacker is a tapeless device that secures the intravenous line in severe and harsh conditions. Ideal for the emergency environment as well as combat conditions.

Medtronic Ep Systems 763-514-4000
8299 Central Ave NE, Spring Lake Park, Minneapolis, MN 55432
Intravascular catheter securement device.

Modern Medical Technology, Inc. 800-474-4911
2308 Cedar Valley Dr, P.O. Box 659, Cedar Bluff, VA 24609
I/v guard.

Nexus Medical, Llc 913-451-2234
11315 Strang Line Rd, Lenexa, KS 66215
Site securement device.

HOLDER, INTRAVASCULAR CATHETER *(cont'd)*

Pedia Pals, Llc 888-733-4272
965 Highway 169 N, Plymouth, MN 55441
I.V. cover or I.V. guard.

R4 Vascular, Inc. 612-770-4038
7550 Meridian Cir N, Meridian Business Center, Suite 150
Maple Grove, MN 55369
Catheter bandage-cover dressing.

Sterion, Incorporated 800-328-7958
13828 Lincoln St NE, Ham Lake, MN 55304
SecureIt Nasal and Catheter Tube Holders to standardize fastening procedures and hold catheters securely in place.

Tri-State Hospital Supply Corp. 517-545-1135
3173 E 43rd St, Yuma, AZ 85365

Venetec International., Inc. 888-685-0565
12555 High Bluff Dr Ste 100, San Diego, CA 92130
Various.

Wv Iv Pro, Inc. 304-366-6151
2104 Locust Ave, Fairmont, WV 26554

Zefon International 800-282-0073
5350 SW 1st Ln, Ocala, FL 34474
Grip-Lok Universal Securement Device secures various tubes to patients. Sizes available to hold tubes from .8mm to 19mm.

3m Company 651-733-4365
601 22nd Ave S, Brookings, SD 57006

HOLDER, KNIFE *(Surgery) 79RDF*

Becton Dickinson And Co. 866-906-8080
411 Waverley Oaks Rd, Waltham, MA 02452

Xodus Medical, Inc. 800-963-8776
702 Prominence Dr, Westmoreland Business & Research Park
New Kensington, PA 15068
Scalpel Holder

HOLDER, LAPAROSCOPE *(Obstetrics/Gyn) 85UEZ*

Automated Medical Products Corp. 800-832-4567
PO Box 2508, Edison, NJ 08818
IRON INTERN.

Elmed, Inc. 630-543-2792
60 W Fay Ave, Addison, IL 60101

Kronner Medical 800-706-3533
1443 Upper Cleveland Rapids Rd, Roseburg, OR 97471

Mediflex Surgical Products 800-879-7575
250 Gibbs Rd, Islandia, NY 11749
Mobile flexible laparscope and laparoscopic instrument positioner/holder with adjustable rigidity for one hand operation. Built in O.R. rail clamp.

Richard Wolf Medical Instruments Corp. 800-323-9653
353 Corporate Woods Pkwy, Vernon Hills, IL 60061

Thompson Surgical Instruments, Inc. 800-227-7543
10170 E Cherry Bend Rd, Traverse City, MI 49684
Endoscope holders.

HOLDER, LEG *(Surgery) 79UFB*

Bryton Corp. 800-567-9500
4310 Guion Rd, Indianapolis, IN 46254
Leg support systems for surgical procedures designed to fit all major surgical tables.

Holmed Corporation 508-238-3351
40 Norfolk Ave, South Easton, MA 02375

Medmetric Corp. 800-995-6066
7542 Trade St, San Diego, CA 92121
Arthroscopic Leg Holder-LH1000, $975.00.

Medrecon, Inc. 877-526-4323
257 South Ave, Garwood, NJ 07027

Rush-Berivon, Inc. 800-251-7874
1010 19th St, P.O. Box 1851, Meridian, MS 39301
RUSH COUNTERSUPPORT, #950 C S, leg holder in emergency room & OR, $241.00.

HOLDER, LEG, ARTHROSCOPY *(Orthopedics) 87THC*

Alimed, Inc. 800-225-2610
297 High St, Dedham, MA 02026

Bryton Corp. 800-567-9500
4310 Guion Rd, Indianapolis, IN 46254

Equip For Independence, Inc. 800-216-4881
333 Mamaroneck Ave Ste 383, White Plains, NY 10605

HOLDER, LEG, ARTHROSCOPY *(cont'd)*

Maramed Orthopedic Systems 800-327-5830
2480 W 82nd St, No. 8, Hialeah, FL 33016
Leg and hand holders.

Medrecon, Inc. 877-526-4323
257 South Ave, Garwood, NJ 07027

Mizuho Osi 800-777-4674
30031 Ahern Ave, Union City, CA 94587

Richard Wolf Medical Instruments Corp. 800-323-9653
353 Corporate Woods Pkwy, Vernon Hills, IL 60061

Smith & Nephew, Inc., Endoscopy Division 800-343-8386
150 Minuteman Rd, Andover, MA 01810

Telos Medical Equipment (Austin & Assoc., Inc.) 800-934-3029
1109 Sturbridge Rd, Fallston, MD 21047
TELOS knee holder for positioning during arthroscopy. CONTEC supports have multiple adjustments with side to side compression control and cushioned insert. Knee can be completely manipulated on ball joint pivot.

HOLDER, MEDICAL CHART *(General) 80RGK*

Alimed, Inc. 800-225-2610
297 High St, Dedham, MA 02026

Armstrong Medical Industries, Inc. 800-323-4220
575 Knightsbridge Pkwy, Lincolnshire, IL 60069

Budget Buddy Company, Inc. 800-208-3375
PO Box 590, Belton, MO 64012
$26.50 for wall mounted holder.

First Healthcare Products 800-854-8304
6125 Lendell Dr, Sanborn, NY 14132
POLY ring binders, medical chart labels, charting forms protection, visible record system incl. tray and pockets, clipboards. Poly and paper chart dividers/indexing. STAT-ALERT signal/communication devices, charting accessories.

Howard Medical Company 800-443-1444
1690 N Elston Ave, Chicago, IL 60642
$13.25 for clear industructable medical chart holder (bed chart) that hangs on end of bed. NEW; 7 vibrant colored plexiglas.

Ideal Medical Source, Inc. 800-537-0739
2805 East. Oakland Blvd, Suite 352, Fort Lauderdale, FL 33306

Mayo Medical, S.A. De C.V. 800-715-3872
Edison 1141 Nte., Col. Talleres, Monterrey N.L. 64480 Mexico

Medi-Dose, Inc. 800-523-8966
70 Industrial Dr, Ivyland, PA 18974

Medirecord Systems 800-561-9791
P.O. Box 6201 Station A, Saint John, NB E2L 4R6 Canada

National Systems Co. 877-672-4278
31B Durward Pl., Waterloo N2J 3Z9 Canada
Patient charts, chart holders, indexes, racks, self-adhesive pockets, etc.

Omnimed, Inc. (Beam Products) 800-257-2326
800 Glen Ave, Moorestown, NJ 08057

Peter Pepper Products, Inc. 800-496-0204
17929 S Susana Rd, PO Box 5769, Compton, CA 90221

Profex Medical Products 800-325-0196
2224 E Person Ave, Memphis, TN 38114

Stat-Chek Company 800-248-6618
PO Box 9636, Bend, OR 97708
STAT-CHEK attaches to chart holder to alert nurse of the doctor's new orders - $11.60 per dozen; also patient ID card holder - $10.75 per dozen.

HOLDER, NEEDLE *(Gastro/Urology) 78FHQ*

Accutome, Inc. 610-889-0200
3222 Phoenixville Pike, Malvern, PA 19355
Needle holders.

Aesculap Implant Systems Inc. 1-800-234-9179
3773 Corporate Pkwy, Center Valley, PA 18034
DUROGRIP dissecting forceps and needle holders.

Akorn, Inc. 800-535-7155
2500 Millbrook Dr, Buffalo Grove, IL 60089
Nordan delicate curved plus The Blue Max titanium, ophthalmic needle holders.

B. Graczyk, Inc. 269-782-2100
27826 Burmax Park, Dowagiac, MI 49047
Various types of needle holders.

Back-Mueller, Inc. 314-531-6640
2700 Clark Ave, Saint Louis, MO 63103
Various types of needle holders.

HOLDER, NEEDLE *(cont'd)*

Bausch & Lomb Surgical 636-255-5051
3365 Tree Court Ind Blvd, Saint Louis, MO 63122

Biomet Microfixation Inc. 800-874-7711
1520 Tradeport Dr, Jacksonville, FL 32218
Various types of needles.

Boss Instruments, Ltd. 800-210-2677
395 Reas Ford Rd Ste 120, Earlysville, VA 22936
Ophthalmic; vascular/cardiovascular; ENT, plastic surgery; neurosurgical, orthopedic, micro surgery, general surgery.

Boston Scientific Corporation 508-652-5578
8600 NW 41st St, Doral, FL 33166

Cardinal Health, Snowden Pencer Products 847-689-8410
5175 S Royal Atlanta Dr, Tucker, GA 30084
Various types of needle holders.

Cook Urological, Inc. 800-457-4500
1100 W Morgan St, P.O. Box 227, Spencer, IN 47460

Deem Precision Products 562-692-5416
4203 Durfee Ave, Pico Rivera, CA 90660
Hypodermic needle destroyer medical device.

Deknatel Snowden-Pencer 800-367-7874
5175 S Royal Atlanta Dr, Tucker, GA 30084
Endoscopic needle holders.

Demetech Corp. 888-324-2447
3530 NW 115th Ave, Doral, FL 33178
Needle holder.

E.A. Beck & Co. 949-645-4072
657 W 19th St Ste E, P O Box 10857, Costa Mesa, CA 92627
Needle holder.

Elmed, Inc. 630-543-2792
60 W Fay Ave, Addison, IL 60101

Fine Surgical Instrument, Inc. 800-851-5155
741 Peninsula Blvd, Hempstead, NY 11550

George Tiemann & Co. 800-843-6266
25 Plant Ave, Hauppauge, NY 11788

Griff Industries, Inc. 800-709-4743
19761 Bahama St, Northridge, CA 91324
Disposable needle and blade counter.

Hager Worldwide, Inc. 800-328-2335
13322 Byrd Dr, Odessa, FL 33556
CAPTOR, CAPTOR DELUXE, CAP TRAP.

Hartzell & Son, G. 800-950-2206
2372 Stanwell Cir, Concord, CA 94520

Karl Storz Endoscopy-America Inc. 800-421-0837
600 Corporate Pointe, Culver City, CA 90230

Katena Products, Inc. 800-225-1195
4 Stewart Ct, Denville, NJ 07834

Kmedic 800-955-0559
190 Veterans Dr, Northvale, NJ 07647

Kmi Kolster Methods, Inc. 909-737-5476
3185 Palisades Dr, Corona, CA 92880
Needle holders.

Koros Usa, Inc. 805-529-0825
610 Flinn Ave, Moorpark, CA 93021
Micro needle holder.

Kta, Instruments, Inc. 888-830-9KTA
3051 Brighton-Third St., 1st Fl., Brooklyn, NY 11235

Marina Medical Instruments, Inc. 800-697-1119
955 Shotgun Rd, Sunrise, FL 33326
Various.

Medical Safety Systems Inc. 888-803-9303
230 White Pond Dr, Akron, OH 44313
Sharps blood collection needle holder.

Minnesota Bramstedt Surgical, Inc. 800-456-5052
1835 Energy Park Dr, Saint Paul, MN 55108
KANT-SLIP jaw inserts for needle holders.

Molded Products Inc. 800-435-8957
1112 Chatburn Ave, Harlan, IA 51537
Needle case.

Precision Surgical Intl., Inc. 800-776-8493
PO Box 726, Noblesville, IN 46061
Various types of needle holders.

Prosurge Instruments, Inc. 866-832-7874
199 Laidlaw Ave, Jersey City, NJ 07306

HOLDER, NEEDLE *(cont'd)*

Pulpdent Corp. 800-343-4342
80 Oakland St, Watertown, MA 02472
No common name listed.

Scanlan International, Inc. 800-328-9458
1 Scanlan Plz, Saint Paul, MN 55107

Symmetry Medical Usa, Inc. 574-267-8700
486 W 350 N, Warsaw, IN 46582
Manual gastroenterology-urology surgical inst. and acces.

Terumo Medical Corporation 800-283-7866
950 Elkton Blvd, P.O.Box 605, Elkton, MD 21921
Needle holder.

Toolmex Corporation 800-992-4766
1075 Worcester St, Natick, MA 01760

Trans American Medical 800-626-9232
7633 W 100th Pl, Bridgeview, IL 60455
WEBSTER, MAYO-HEGOR all types. U.S. made.

Trans American Medical / Tamsco Instruments 708-430-7777
7633 W 100th Pl, Bridgeview, IL 60455
Floor grade surgical stainless steel.

Tuzik Boston 800-886-6363
104 Longwater Dr, Assinippi Park, Norwell, MA 02061

Uroplasty, Inc. 952-426-6140
5420 Feltl Rd, Minnetonka, MN 55343

Vartex Instrument Corp. 718-486-5050
311 Wallabout St, Brooklyn, NY 11206
Various holders.

Warsaw Orthopedic, Inc. 901-396-3133
2500 Silveus Xing, Warsaw, IN 46582
Holder, needle.

Wexler Surgical Supplies 800-414-1076
11333 Chimney Rock Rd Ste 110, Houston, TX 77035

Wisap America 800-233-8448
8231 Melrose Dr, Lenexa, KS 66214

HOLDER, NEEDLE, CURVED, LAPAROSCOPIC *(Surgery) 79QOJ*

Elmed, Inc. 630-543-2792
60 W Fay Ave, Addison, IL 60101

Ethicon Endo-Surgery, Inc. 800-USE-ENDO
4545 Creek Rd, Cincinnati, OH 45242

Smith & Nephew, Inc., Endoscopy Division 800-343-8386
150 Minuteman Rd, Andover, MA 01810

HOLDER, NEEDLE, LAPAROSCOPIC *(Surgery) 79QNU*

Boss Instruments, Ltd. 800-210-2677
395 Reas Ford Rd Ste 120, Earlysville, VA 22936

Elmed, Inc. 630-543-2792
60 W Fay Ave, Addison, IL 60101

Ethicon Endo-Surgery, Inc. 800-USE-ENDO
4545 Creek Rd, Cincinnati, OH 45242
ENDOPATH, 5mm, handle, reuseable.

Md International, Inc. 305-669-9003
11300 NW 41st St, Doral, FL 33178

Princeton Medical Group, Inc. 800-875-0869
1189 Royal Links Dr, Mt Pleasant, SC 29466

Smith & Nephew, Inc., Endoscopy Division 800-343-8386
150 Minuteman Rd, Andover, MA 01810

Synectic Medical Product Development 203-877-8488
60 Commerce Park, Milford, CT 06460

HOLDER, NEEDLE, ORTHOPEDIC *(Orthopedics) 87HXK*

Biomet Microfixation Inc. 800-874-7711
1520 Tradeport Dr, Jacksonville, FL 32218
Various types of needles.

Biomet, Inc. 574-267-6639
56 E Bell Dr, PO Box 587, Warsaw, IN 46582
Various types of needle holders.

Fehling Surgical Instruments 800-FEHLING
509 Broadstone Ln NW, Acworth, GA 30101

Kmedic 800-955-0559
190 Veterans Dr, Northvale, NJ 07647

Medtronic Sofamor Danek Instrument Manufacturing 901-396-3133
7375 Adrianne Pl, Bartlett, TN 38133
Holder, needle.

HOLDER, NEEDLE, ORTHOPEDIC *(cont'd)*

Nordent Manufacturing, Inc. 800-966-7336
610 Bonnie Ln, Elk Grove Village, IL 60007
$110.00 for unit with carbide inserts; $84.50 for s.s.

Salvin Dental Specialties, Inc. 800-535-6566
3450 Latrobe Dr, Charlotte, NC 28211
Various types of needle holders.

Symmetry Medical Usa, Inc. 574-267-8700
486 W 350 N, Warsaw, IN 46582
Orthopedic manual surgical instrument.

Tuzik Boston 800-886-6363
104 Longwater Dr, Assinippi Park, Norwell, MA 02061

Zimmer Holdings, Inc. 800-613-6131
1800 W Center St, PO Box 708, Warsaw, IN 46580

Zimmer Trabecular Metal Technology 800-613-6131
10 Pomeroy Rd, Parsippany, NJ 07054
Stem holder.

HOLDER, NEEDLE, OTHER *(Surgery) 79RHW*

Arosurgical Instruments Corp. 800-776-1751
537 Newport Center Dr Ste 101, Newport Beach, CA 92660
AROS Needle Holders, FUSION WELDED Tungsten Carbide inserts. Gold Handles. We have a wide variety. go to www.arosurgical.com for complete listing.

Bausch & Lomb Surgical 636-255-5051
3365 Tree Court Ind Blvd, Saint Louis, MO 63122

Cameron-Miller, Inc. 800-621-0142
5410 W Roosevelt Rd, Road #241, Chicago, IL 60644

Codman & Shurtleff, Inc 800-225-0460
325 Paramount Dr, Raynham, MA 02767

Covidien Lp 508-261-8000
15 Hampshire St, Mansfield, MA 02048

Deknatel Snowden-Pencer 800-367-7874
5175 S Royal Atlanta Dr, Tucker, GA 30084
DIAMOND-JAW & MICRO DIAMOND-JAW.

Elmed, Inc. 630-543-2792
60 W Fay Ave, Addison, IL 60101

Holmed Corporation 508-238-3351
40 Norfolk Ave, South Easton, MA 02375

Hu-Friedy Manufacturing Co., Inc. 800-483-7433
3232 N Rockwell St, Chicago, IL 60618
$55.00 to $247.00, 37 types. Sutures (dental) .

Invacare Corporation 800-333-6900
1 Invacare Way, Elyria, OH 44035

Medworks Instruments 800-323-9790
PO Box 581, Chatham, IL 62629
$3.50 per unit (5-1/2in).

Miltex Inc. 800-645-8000
589 Davies Dr, York, PA 17402
Abbey needle holder.

Nordent Manufacturing, Inc. 800-966-7336
610 Bonnie Ln, Elk Grove Village, IL 60007
$110.00 for unit with carbide inserts; $58.50 for s.s.

Ortho Development Corp. 800-429-8339
12187 Business Park Dr, Draper, UT 84020

Premier Dental Products Co. 888-670-6100
1710 Romano Dr, PO Box 4500, Plymouth Meeting, PA 19462

Roboz Surgical Instrument Co., Inc. 800-424-2984
PO Box 10710, Gaithersburg, MD 20898

Stephens Instruments, Inc. 800-354-7848
2500 Sandersville Rd, Lexington, KY 40511
$125.00 per unit (5-1/2in).

Toolmex Corporation 800-992-4766
1075 Worcester St, Natick, MA 01760

Xodus Medical, Inc. 800-963-8776
702 Prominence Dr, Westmoreland Business & Research Park
New Kensington, PA 15068
Needle Counters

Zimmer Holdings, Inc. 800-613-6131
1800 W Center St, PO Box 708, Warsaw, IN 46580

HOLDER, RADIOGRAPHIC CASSETTE, WALL-MOUNTED *(Radiology) 90IXY*

Afc Industries, Inc. 718-747-0237
1316 133rd Pl, College Point, NY 11356
Mobile cassette stand.

HOLDER, RADIOGRAPHIC CASSETTE, WALL-MOUNTED *(cont'd)*

Afp Imaging Corp. 800-592-6666
250 Clearbrook Rd, Elmsford, NY 10523

Bay Shore Medical Equipment Corp. 631-586-1991
235 S Fehr Way, Bay Shore, NY 11706
Multiple.

Brotherston Homecare Inc., Pxi Div. 800-695-9729
1388 Bridgewater Rd, Bensalem, PA 19020
Mobile cassette holder, priced $645.00.

Civco Medical Instruments Co., Inc. 319-656-4447
102 1st St S, Kalona, IA 52247
Equipment holder for ultrasound scanners.

Del Medical Systems 800-800-6006
11550 King St, Franklin Park, IL 60131

Frank Scholz X-Ray Corp. 508-586-8308
244 Liberty St, Brockton, MA 02301
$250.00 per unit (standard).

Ge Medical Systems, Llc 262-548-2355
3000 N Grandview Blvd, W-417, Waukesha, WI 53188
Wall mounted cassette holder.

Midwest X-Ray Equipment Co. 630-892-2414
701 W Illinois Ave, Aurora, IL 60506
Various models of buckys.

Poersch Metal Mfg. Co. 773-722-0890
4027 W Kinzie St # 31, Chicago, IL 60624
Cassette holder.

Qsa-Global Inc. 781-272-2000
40 North Ave, Burlington, MA 01803
Holder, radiographic cassette, wall-mounted.

Quantum Medical Imaging, Llc 631-567-5800
2002 Orville Dr N Ste B, Ronkonkoma, NY 11779
Wall-mounted radiographic cassette holder.

S&S Technology 281-815-1300
10625 Telge Rd, Houston, TX 77095

HOLDER, RETRACTOR *(Surgery) 79WRE*

Automated Medical Products Corp. 800-832-4567
PO Box 2508, Edison, NJ 08818
IRON INTERN.

Mediflex Surgical Products 800-879-7575
250 Gibbs Rd, Islandia, NY 11749
Flexarm universal holder/positioner for use with laparoscopic retractors such as liver retractors, etc.

Thompson Surgical Instruments, Inc. 800-227-7543
10170 E Cherry Bend Rd, Traverse City, MI 49684

Ultracell Medical Technologies, Inc. 877-SPO-NGE1
183 Providence New London Tpke, North Stonington, CT 06359
ULTRACELL Retractor covers. Various sizes of retractor covers are made from P.V.A. sponges. Covers are made for all types of surgery.

HOLDER, SHOULDER, ARTHROSCOPY *(Surgery) 79WRY*

Bauerfeind Usa, Inc. 800-423-3405
55 Chastain Rd NW Ste 112, Kennesaw, GA 30144
OMOTRAIN shoulder support with straps.

Smith & Nephew, Inc., Endoscopy Division 800-343-8386
150 Minuteman Rd, Andover, MA 01810

HOLDER, SPECULUM, ENT *(Ear/Nose/Throat) 77KAG*

Aesculap Implant Systems Inc. 1-800-234-9179
3773 Corporate Pkwy, Center Valley, PA 18034

Biomet Microfixation Inc. 800-874-7711
1520 Tradeport Dr, Jacksonville, FL 32218
Various types of speculums.

Prosurge Instruments, Inc. 866-832-7874
199 Laidlaw Ave, Jersey City, NJ 07306

Tuzik Boston 800-886-6363
104 Longwater Dr, Assinippi Park, Norwell, MA 02061

HOLDER, SYRINGE, LEADED *(Radiology) 90IWR*

Biodex Medical Systems, Inc. 800-224-6339
20 Ramsey Rd, Shirley, NY 11967
Complete selection of Pro-Tec Syringe Shields and shielding accessories.

Inrad 800-558-4647
4375 Donkers Ct SE, Kentwood, MI 49512
Aspiration biopsy syringe gun.

HOLDER, SYRINGE, LEADED *(cont'd)*

Sterex Corp. 800-603-5045
4501 126th Ave N, Clearwater, FL 33762
Shield for hypodermic syringe.

HOLDER, THERMOMETER *(General) 80SAI*

Polar Ware Co. 800-237-3655
2806 N 15th St, Sheboygan, WI 53083
Stainless steel.

Profex Medical Products 800-325-0196
2224 E Person Ave, Memphis, TN 38114

HOLDER, TRACHEOSTOMY TUBE *(Anesthesiology) 73SBH*

Dale Medical Products, Inc. 800-343-3980
7 Cross St, Plainville, MA 02762
Tracheostomy tube holder No. 240 fits most. Endotracheal tube holder #245, (neckband, adult). childrens' neckband #246.

Dhd Healthcare Corporation 800-847-8000
PO Box 6, One Madison Street, Wampsville, NY 13163
DHD Tracheostomy Holder

Marpac Inc. 800-334-6413
8436 Washington Pl NE, Albuquerque, NM 87113
Marpac Tracheostomy collars comfortably secure tracheostomy tubes. Composed of a latex free, soft, breathable neckband and easy Velco adjustment tabs. One piece, 'Perfect Fit' collars come in boxes of 25 or 100. Two piece, 'One Size Fits All' collars come in boxes of 10 or 100.

Welcon, Inc. 800-877-0923
7409 Pebble Dr, Fort Worth, TX 76118

HOLDER, TRANSDUCER *(Anesthesiology) 73SBU*

Northeast Medical Systems Corp. 856-910-8111
901 Beechwood Ave, Cherry Hill, NJ 08002
For cardiac and electrophysiology tables.

Sorin Group Usa 800-289-5759
14401 W 65th Way, Arvada, CO 80004

HOLDER, X-RAY FILM *(Dental And Oral) 76EGZ*

Del Medical Systems 800-800-6006
11550 King St, Franklin Park, IL 60131

Flow X-Ray Corporation 800-356-9729
100 W Industry Ct, Deer Park, NY 11729

Ge Medical Systems, Llc 262-548-2355
3000 N Grandview Blvd, W-417, Waukesha, WI 53188
Film mount for small format photospot films.

Hager Worldwide, Inc. 800-328-2335
13322 Byrd Dr, Odessa, FL 33556
EMMINEX (film holder) & SOFTBITE WING FLAPS (soft bite wing tab holder).

Huestis Medical 800-972-9222
68 Buttonwood St, Bristol, RI 02809
FLEXI-HOLDER x-ray film cassette.

K-Stat, L.L.C. 702-262-1044
8665 W Flamingo Rd # 131-356, Las Vegas, NV 89147
Dental x-ray foam cushion pocket.

Marconi Medical Systems 800-323-0550
595 Miner Rd, Cleveland, OH 44143

Margraf Dental Manufacturing, Inc. 800-762-2641
611 Harper Ave, Jenkintown, PA 19046

Medrecon, Inc. 877-526-4323
257 South Ave, Garwood, NJ 07027

Midwest X-Ray Equipment Co. 630-892-2414
701 W Illinois Ave, Aurora, IL 60506
Various models of cassette trays.

Pac-Dent Intl., Inc. 909-839-0888
21078 Commerce Point Dr, Walnut, CA 91789
Plastic film mount.

Peter Pepper Products, Inc. 800-496-0204
17929 S Susana Rd, PO Box 5769, Compton, CA 90221
Decks, training/AV carts, white boards (preattached).

Precision Dental Int, Inc. 818-992-1888
21361 Deering Ct, Canoga Park, CA 91304
Dental x-ray film holder.

Pulpdent Corp. 800-343-4342
80 Oakland St, Watertown, MA 02472
No common name listed.

S&S Technology 281-815-1300
10625 Telge Rd, Houston, TX 77095

HOLDER, X-RAY FILM *(cont'd)*

Schueler & Company, Inc. 516-487-1500
PO Box 528, Stratford, CT 06615

Sds (Summit Dental Systems) 800-275-3368
3560 NW 53rd Ct, Fort Lauderdale, FL 33309

Soyee Products, Inc. 800-574-4743
459 Thompson Rd, Thompson, CT 06277
Cassette.

Star X-Ray Co., Inc. 800-374-2163
63 Ranick Dr S, Amityville, NY 11701

Steri-Shield Products 805-692-4972
336 S Fairview Ave, Goleta, CA 93117
Wingers.

Temrex Corp. 516-868-6221
112 Albany Ave, P.o. Box 182, Freeport, NY 11520
#3 manila coin envelopes 21/2' x 41/4' end open flap.

Wolf X-Ray Corporation 800-356-9729
100 W Industry Ct, Deer Park, NY 11729

HOLDER, X-RAY FILM CASSETTE, VERTICAL *(Radiology) 90VGT*

Americomp, Inc. 800-458-1782
2901 W Lawrence Ave, Chicago, IL 60625

Bio-Med U.S.A. Inc. 973-278-5222
111 Ellison St, Paterson, NJ 07505
BIO CASSETTES film cassettes, aluminum with window.

Marconi Medical Systems 800-323-0550
595 Miner Rd, Cleveland, OH 44143

Mxe, Inc. 800-252-1801
12107 Jefferson Blvd, Culver City, CA 90230
Grid protectors & film cassette holders: K-Edge Slip On made of carbon fiber, Grid Cap, EZ Slide.

Techno-Aide, Inc. 800-251-2629
7117 Centennial Blvd, Nashville, TN 37209

Xma (X-Ray Marketing Associates, Inc.) 800-325-8880
1205 W Lakeview Ct, Windham Lakes Business Park
Romeoville, IL 60446

HOLDER/SCISSORS, NEEDLE, LAPAROSCOPIC *(Surgery) 79QPN*

Elmed, Inc. 630-543-2792
60 W Fay Ave, Addison, IL 60101

Mediflex Surgical Products 800-879-7575
250 Gibbs Rd, Islandia, NY 11749

Prosurge Instruments, Inc. 866-832-7874
199 Laidlaw Ave, Jersey City, NJ 07306

Richard Wolf Medical Instruments Corp. 800-323-9653
353 Corporate Woods Pkwy, Vernon Hills, IL 60061

Smith & Nephew, Inc., Endoscopy Division 800-343-8386
150 Minuteman Rd, Andover, MA 01810

Synectic Medical Product Development 203-877-8488
60 Commerce Park, Milford, CT 06460

HOLLOW MILL SET *(Orthopedics) 87HWL*

Biomet, Inc. 574-267-6639
56 E Bell Dr, PO Box 587, Warsaw, IN 46582
Hollow mill set.

Zimmer Holdings, Inc. 800-613-6131
1800 W Center St, PO Box 708, Warsaw, IN 46580

HOLOGRAPH, FETAL, ACOUSTICAL *(Obstetrics/Gyn) 85HHX*

Advanced Imaging Technologies, Inc. 509-375-3100
2400 Stevens Dr Ste B, Richland, WA 99354
Fetal holograph (acoustical).

HOMOGENIZER, TISSUE *(Microbiology) 83RAE*

Brinkmann Instruments (Canada) Ltd. 800-263-8715
6670 Campobello Rd., Mississauga, ONT L5N 2L8 Canada

Brinkmann Instruments, Inc. 800-645-3050
PO Box 1019, Westbury, NY 11590

Cole-Parmer Instrument Inc. 800-323-4340
625 E Bunker Ct, Vernon Hills, IL 60061
The hand-held TISSUMITE features a 100-W motor with a built-in speed controller having a range of 5000 to 25,000 rpm.

Corning Inc., Science Products Division 800-492-1110
45 Nagog Park, Acton, MA 01720

Eberbach Corp. 800-422-2558
505 S Maple Rd, Ann Arbor, MI 48103

HOMOGENIZER, TISSUE *(cont'd)*

Kontes Glass Co. 888-546-2531
1022 Spruce St, Vineland, NJ 08360

Omni International, Inc. 540-347-5331
PO Box 861455, Vint Hill Farms, VA 20187
OMNI MIXER Homogenizer, high speed, high shear homogenizer mixer offering aerosol sealed chambers with high speed rotor stator or cutting blade attachments. OMNI-TIPS, PCR Tissue Homogenizing Kits, disposable/reusable plastic rotor stator generator probes ideal for sensitive PCR application.

Pro Scientific Inc. 800-584-3776
99 Willenbrock Rd, Oxford, CT 06478
Handheld or post-mounted laboratory homogenizer for samples from .03ml to multi liters. Sealed containers for aerosol containment available.

Scientific Industries, Inc. 888-850-6208
70 Orville Dr, Bohemia, NY 11716

Troemner Llc 800-352-7705
201 Wolf Dr, PO Box 87, West Deptford, NJ 08086
.03ml - 40 liter capacity

Virtis, An Sp Industries Company 800-431-8232
815 Route 208, Gardiner, NY 12525
Open blade-type rotor/stator, Tempest and Cyclone homogenizers.

HOMOPOLYMER, KARAYA AND ETHYLENE-OXIDE
(Dental And Oral) 76KXX

Kleen Laundry & Drycleaning Services, Inc. 603-448-1134
1 Foundry St, Lebanon, NH 03766
Surgical drape.

Sheffield Pharmaceuticals 800-222-1087
170 Broad St, New London, CT 06320
Denture adhesive.

HOOD, CHEMICAL *(Chemistry) 75RAF*

Bedcolab Ltd. 800-461-6414
2305 Francis Hughes, Laval, QUE H7S 1N5 Canada
Standards - balance air. Radioisotop - perchloric acid.

Hemco Corp. 816-796-2900
111 S Powell Rd, Independence, MO 64056
Uniflow walk-in fume hood with 70 in. height and sliding glass upper sash and hinged lower doors.

Labconco Corp. 800-821-5525
8811 Prospect Ave, Kansas City, MO 64132
PROTECTOR Premier fiberglass hoods in 4ft, 5ft, 6ft and 8ft widths. Also available are the Protector XL Hoods which can be custom to almost any width, and Protector XStream Hood which is a low-flow, high performance hood that saves energy.

HOOD, FUME *(Toxicology) 91RAG*

Bedcolab Ltd. 800-461-6414
2305 Francis Hughes, Laval, QUE H7S 1N5 Canada
Standards - balance air. Radioisotop - perchloric acid.

Biodex Medical Systems, Inc. 800-224-6339
20 Ramsey Rd, Shirley, NY 11967

Capintec, Inc. 800-631-3826
6 Arrow Rd, Ramsey, NJ 07446

Cif Furniture Ltd. 905-738-5821
56 Edilcan Dr., Concord, ONT L4K-3S6 Canada

Cole-Parmer Instrument Inc. 800-323-4340
625 E Bunker Ct, Vernon Hills, IL 60061

Hacker Instruments And Industries Inc. 800-442-2537
1132 Kincaid Bridge Rd, PO Box 1176, Winnsboro, SC 29180
Portable, bench-top unit; fumes are drawn down, away from operator; made in USA.

Hemco Corp. 816-796-2900
111 S Powell Rd, Independence, MO 64056
UNIFLOW fiberglass or stainless steel fume and canopy hoods, wall-mounted or ceiling suspended. Side and rear wall panels, exhaust blowers, blower switches, flexible PVC ducting, vaporproof lights and mounting kits available.

Jamestown Metal Products 716-665-5313
178 Blackstone Ave, Jamestown, NY 14701
ISOLATOR Complete line of bench and walk-in chemical fumehoods. With assorted liner materials including stainless steel.

Kewaunee Scientific Corp. 704-873-7202
2700 W Front St, PO Box 1842, Statesville, NC 28677

HOOD, FUME *(cont'd)*

Lab Fabricators Company 888-431-5444
1802 E 47th St, Cleveland, OH 44103
Laboratory fume hoods with the highest performance in safety and energy savings that can be manufactured to accomodate your specific requirements.

Labconco Corp. 800-821-5525
8811 Prospect Ave, Kansas City, MO 64132
PROTECTOR Fume Hoods in 4ft, 5ft, 6ft and 8ft widths.

Laminar Flow, Inc. 800-553-FLOW
102 Richard Rd, PO Box 2427, Warminster, PA 18974

Misonix, Inc. 800-694-9612
1938 New Hwy, Farmingdale, NY 11735
Ductless fume hoods. Economical chemical workstations.

Purified Micro Environments, Div. Of Germfree Laboratories 800-888-5357
11 Aviator Way, Ormond Beach, FL 32174
Custom stainless steel.

Thermo Scientific Hamilton 920-794-6800
1316 18th St, Two Rivers, WI 54241

HOOD, FUME, CHEMICAL *(Chemistry) 75JRN*

Air Control, Inc. 252-492-2300
237 Raleigh Rd, Henderson, NC 27536
MICROVOID Fume hoods, corrosion resistant and chemical process stations.

Brinkmann Instruments, Inc. 800-645-3050
PO Box 1019, Westbury, NY 11590

Fumex Inc. 800-432-7550
1150 Cobb International Pl NW Ste D, Kennesaw, GA 30152

Genie Scientific, Inc. 800-545-8816
17430 Mount Cliffwood Cir, Fountain Valley, CA 92708

Hemco Corp. 816-796-2900
111 S Powell Rd, Independence, MO 64056
UNIFLOW fiberglass or stainless steel fume and canopy hoods, wall-mounted or ceiling suspended. Side and rear wall panels, exhaust blowers, blower switches, flexible PVC ducting, vaporproof lights and mounting kits available.

Lab Fabricators Company 888-431-5444
1802 E 47th St, Cleveland, OH 44103
A variety of conventional exhaust, smooth air flo and auxiliary air fume hoods are available. All hoods can be customized to suit your individual needs.

Microzone Corporation 877-252-7746
86 Harry Douglas Drive, Ottawa, ONT K2S 2C7 Canada

Nuaire, Inc. 800-328-3352
2100 Fernbrook Ln N, Plymouth, MN 55447
Polypropylene fume hoods and trace metal analysis fume hoods.

HOOD, ISOLATION, LAMINAR AIR FLOW *(General) 80RAH*

Aes Clean Technology, Inc. 888-237-2532
422 Stump Rd, Montgomeryville, PA 18936

Air Control, Inc. 252-492-2300
237 Raleigh Rd, Henderson, NC 27536
MICROVOID.

Bio Air Systems Div. 336-299-2885
PO Box 18547, Greensboro, NC 27419
Pricing architecturally dependent.

Bio-Safe America Corp. 800-767-4284
3250 S Susan St Ste B, Sterilaire Medical Division
Santa Ana, CA 92704
Negative air isolation.

Colonial Scientific Ltd. 902-468-1811
201 Brownlow Ave., Unit 52, Dartmouth, NS B3B-1W2 Canada

Labconco Corp. 800-821-5525
8811 Prospect Ave, Kansas City, MO 64132
PURIFIER Delta Series Class II Type A2 and B2 Biological Safety Cabinets.

Laminar Flow, Inc. 800-553-FLOW
102 Richard Rd, PO Box 2427, Warminster, PA 18974
99.99% to .03 micron - custom built also.

Liberty Industries, Inc. 800-828-5656
133 Commerce St, East Berlin, CT 06023
Freestanding model with optional 2 door cabinet, static eliminator. Countertop model with optional base stand. Both available as total exhaust hood or total recirculation hood. Custom units available.

Luwa Lepco 713-461-1131
1750 Stebbins Dr, Houston, TX 77043

HOOD, ISOLATION, LAMINAR AIR FLOW *(cont'd)*

Microzone Corporation 877-252-7746
86 Harry Douglas Drive, Ottawa, ONT K2S 2C7 Canada

Misonix, Inc. 800-694-9612
1938 New Hwy, Farmingdale, NY 11735
Laminar flow hood for medical and DNA applications. The PCR workstation module disinfecting UV light.

Nuaire, Inc. 800-328-3352
2100 Fernbrook Ln N, Plymouth, MN 55447
$4,450 to $7,400 for 3 freestanding models. $2,695 to $4,750 for 2 countertop models. Optional ultraviolet light. Steel frame, stainless steel work area.

Purified Micro Environments, Div. Of Germfree Laboratories 800-888-5357
11 Aviator Way, Ormond Beach, FL 32174

HOOD, MICROBIOLOGICAL *(Microbiology) 83RAI*

Brinkmann Instruments, Inc. 800-645-3050
PO Box 1019, Westbury, NY 11590

Kewaunee Scientific Corp. 704-873-7202
2700 W Front St, PO Box 1842, Statesville, NC 28677

Nuaire, Inc. 800-328-3352
2100 Fernbrook Ln N, Plymouth, MN 55447

Purified Micro Environments, Div. Of Germfree Laboratories 800-888-5357
11 Aviator Way, Ormond Beach, FL 32174

HOOD, OXYGEN, INFANT *(General) 80FOG*

Allied Healthcare Products, Inc. 800-444-3954
1720 Sublette Ave, Saint Louis, MO 63110

Cardinal Health 207, Inc. 610-862-0800
1100 Bird Center Dr, Palm Springs, CA 92262
Infant oxygen hood.

Medicomp 763-389-4473
12535 316th Ave, Princeton, MN 55371
No common name listed.

Nova Health Systems, Inc. 800-225-NOVA
1001 Broad St, Utica, NY 13501

Olympic Medical Corp. 206-767-3500
5900 1st Ave S, Seattle, WA 98108
$129.50 per unit (standard).

Utah Medical Products, Inc. 800-533-4984
7043 Cottonwood St, Midvale, UT 84047
DISPOSA-HOOD in five sizes, single patient use, precise-concentration oxygen delivery system.

HOOD, SURGICAL *(Surgery) 79FXY*

Angelica Image Apparel 800-222-3112
700 Rosedale Ave, Saint Louis, MO 63112

Atd-American Co. 800-523-2300
135 Greenwood Ave, Wyncote, PA 19095

Depuy Orthopaedics, Inc. 800-473-3789
700 Orthopaedic Dr, P.O. Box 988, Warsaw, IN 46582
Various types of surgical hoods.

General Econopak, Inc. 888-871-8568
1725 N 6th St, Philadelphia, PA 19122

Johnson & Johnson Medical Division Of Ethicon, Inc. 800-423-4018
2500 E Arbrook Blvd, Arlington, TX 76014

Maquilas Teta-Kawi, S.A. De C.V. 413-593-6400
Carretera Internacional, Km 1969, Enpalme, Sonora Mexico
Surgical hood

White Knight Healthcare 800-851-4431
Calle 16, Number 780, Agua Prieta, Sonora Mexico
Cover, shoe, operating-room

HOOK, BONE *(Surgery) 79KIK*

Holmed Corporation 508-238-3351
40 Norfolk Ave, South Easton, MA 02375

HOOK, CORDOTOMY *(Ear/Nose/Throat) 77RAJ*

Codman & Shurtleff, Inc 800-225-0460
325 Paramount Dr, Raynham, MA 02767

Elmed, Inc. 630-543-2792
60 W Fay Ave, Addison, IL 60101

HOOK, EXTERNAL LIMB COMPONENT, MECHANICAL *(Physical Med) 89IQX*

Ada Technologies, Inc. 303-874-8276
8100 Shaffer Pkwy Unit 130, Littleton, CO 80127
Terminal device, gripper, hook, split hook.

Hosmer Dorrance Corp. 408-379-5151
561 Division St, Campbell, CA 95008
Variuos models of prosthetic hooks.

HOOK, EXTERNAL LIMB COMPONENT, POWERED *(Physical Med) 89IQW*

Hosmer Dorrance Corp. 408-379-5151
561 Division St, Campbell, CA 95008
Various.

HOOK, FIBROID, GYNECOLOGICAL *(Obstetrics/Gyn) 85HDE*

Biomet Microfixation Inc. 800-874-7711
1520 Tradeport Dr, Jacksonville, FL 32218
Various types of hooks.

HOOK, GASTRO-UROLOGY *(Gastro/Urology) 78FHB*

Aesculap Implant Systems Inc. 1-800-234-9179
3773 Corporate Pkwy, Center Valley, PA 18034

Biomet Microfixation Inc. 800-874-7711
1520 Tradeport Dr, Jacksonville, FL 32218
Various types of hooks.

HOOK, INCUS *(Ear/Nose/Throat) 77RAK*

Bausch & Lomb Surgical 636-255-5051
3365 Tree Court Ind Blvd, Saint Louis, MO 63122

HOOK, IUD REMOVAL *(Obstetrics/Gyn) 85RAL*

Premier Medical Products 888-PREMUSA
1710 Romano Dr, Plymouth Meeting, PA 19462

R Medical Supply 800-882-7578
620 Valley Forge Rd Ste F, Hillsborough, NC 27278

Thomas Medical Inc. 800-556-0349
5610 West 82 2nd Street, Indianpolis, IN 46278

HOOK, MICROSURGICAL EAR *(Ear/Nose/Throat) 77JYL*

Aesculap Implant Systems Inc. 1-800-234-9179
3773 Corporate Pkwy, Center Valley, PA 18034

Bausch & Lomb Surgical 636-255-5051
3365 Tree Court Ind Blvd, Saint Louis, MO 63122

Biomet Microfixation Inc. 800-874-7711
1520 Tradeport Dr, Jacksonville, FL 32218
Various types of hooks.

Clinimed, Incorporated 877-CLINIMED
303 Markus Ct, Sandy Brae Industrial Park, Newark, DE 19713

George Tiemann & Co. 800-843-6266
25 Plant Ave, Hauppauge, NY 11788

HOOK, OPHTHALMIC *(Ophthalmology) 86HNQ*

Accutome, Inc. 610-889-0200
3222 Phoenixville Pike, Malvern, PA 19355
Hooks.

Advanced Vision Science 800-235-5781
5743 Thornwood Dr, Goleta, CA 93117
Sterile, deisposable Iris Retractors

Akorn, Inc. 800-535-7155
2500 Millbrook Dr, Buffalo Grove, IL 60089
Titanium lens spatula nucleus, straight or angled iris hook plus diamond knives and other titanium instruments.

B. Graczyk, Inc. 269-782-2100
27826 Burmax Park, Dowagiac, MI 49047
Various sizes of sterile & non-sterile hooks.

Bausch & Lomb Surgical 636-255-5051
3365 Tree Court Ind Blvd, Saint Louis, MO 63122

Demetech Corp. 888-324-2447
3530 NW 115th Ave, Doral, FL 33178
Ophthalmic hook.

Fischer Surgical Inc. 314-303-7753
1343 Pine Dr, Arnold, MO 63010
Various types of ophthalmic hooks.

Fortrad Eye Instruments Corp. 973-543-2371
8 Franklin Rd, Mendham, NJ 07945

George Tiemann & Co. 800-843-6266
25 Plant Ave, Hauppauge, NY 11788

HOOK, OPHTHALMIC *(cont'd)*

Hai Laboratories, Inc. 781-862-9884
320 Massachusetts Ave, Lexington, MA 02420
Ophthalmic hook - various types.

Harvey Precision Instruments 707-793-2600
217 Fairway Rd, Cape Haze, FL 33947
Ophthalmic hooks, various.

Integral Design Inc. 781-740-2036
52 Burr Rd, Hingham, MA 02043

Katena Products, Inc. 800-225-1195
4 Stewart Ct, Denville, NJ 07834

Lenstec, Inc. 727-571-2272
2870 Scherer Dr N Ste 300, Saint Petersburg, FL 33716

Micro Medical Instruments 314-845-3663
123 Cliff Cave Rd, Saint Louis, MO 63129
Ophthalmic hooks (iris, Muscle).

Psi/Eye-Ko, Inc. 636-447-1010
804 Corporate Centre Dr, O Fallon, MO 63368
Various types of ophthalmic hooks.

Rhein Medical, Inc. 800-637-4346
5460 Beaumont Center Blvd Ste 500, Suite 500, Tampa, FL 33634
Titanium lens manipulation hook, iris hook and other titanium instruments.

Stephens Instruments, Inc. 800-354-7848
2500 Sandersville Rd, Lexington, KY 40511
$25.00 per unit (standard).

Surgical Instrument Manufacturers, Inc. 800-521-2985
1650 Headland Dr, Fenton, MO 63026

Total Titanium, Inc. 618-473-2429
140 East Monroe St., Hecker, IL 62248
Various types of ophthalmic hooks.

HOOK, OTHER *(Surgery) 79RAT*

Carl Heyer, Inc. 800-284-5550
1872 Bellmore Ave, North Bellmore, NY 11710

Deflecto Corp. 800-428-4328
7035 E 86th St, Indianapolis, IN 46250
Complete line of hidden screw mount, decorative and functional hooks. Mount on wall or use with partitions.

Fortrad Eye Instruments Corp. 973-543-2371
8 Franklin Rd, Mendham, NJ 07945

Katena Products, Inc. 800-225-1195
4 Stewart Ct, Denville, NJ 07834

Kmedic 800-955-0559
190 Veterans Dr, Northvale, NJ 07647

Miltex Inc. 800-645-8000
589 Davies Dr, York, PA 17402

Phelan Manufacturing Corp. 800-328-2358
2523 Minnehaha Ave, Minneapolis, MN 55404
$125.00 per dozen of instrument storage hooks.

Whitney Products, Inc. 800-338-4237
6153 W Mulford St Ste C, Niles, IL 60714
HOOKUP; Plastic hook with self adhesive back.

Zimmer Holdings, Inc. 800-613-6131
1800 W Center St, PO Box 708, Warsaw, IN 46580

HOOK, RHINOPLASTIC *(Surgery) 79RAN*

Bausch & Lomb Surgical 636-255-5051
3365 Tree Court Ind Blvd, Saint Louis, MO 63122

Elmed, Inc. 630-543-2792
60 W Fay Ave, Addison, IL 60101

Miltex Inc. 800-645-8000
589 Davies Dr, York, PA 17402

HOOK, SCLERAL FIXATION *(Ophthalmology) 86RAO*

Bausch & Lomb Surgical 636-255-5051
3365 Tree Court Ind Blvd, Saint Louis, MO 63122

Fortrad Eye Instruments Corp. 973-543-2371
8 Franklin Rd, Mendham, NJ 07945

Katena Products, Inc. 800-225-1195
4 Stewart Ct, Denville, NJ 07834

Miltex Inc. 800-645-8000
589 Davies Dr, York, PA 17402

Stephens Instruments, Inc. 800-354-7848
2500 Sandersville Rd, Lexington, KY 40511
$30.00 per unit (standard).

HOOK, SKIN *(Surgery) 79RAP*

Bausch & Lomb Surgical 636-255-5051
3365 Tree Court Ind Blvd, Saint Louis, MO 63122

Codman & Shurtleff, Inc 800-225-0460
325 Paramount Dr, Raynham, MA 02767

Katena Products, Inc. 800-225-1195
4 Stewart Ct, Denville, NJ 07834

Miltex Inc. 800-645-8000
589 Davies Dr, York, PA 17402

Zimmer Holdings, Inc. 800-613-6131
1800 W Center St, PO Box 708, Warsaw, IN 46580

HOOK, STRABISMUS *(Ophthalmology) 86RAQ*

Bausch & Lomb Surgical 636-255-5051
3365 Tree Court Ind Blvd, Saint Louis, MO 63122

Elmed, Inc. 630-543-2792
60 W Fay Ave, Addison, IL 60101

Fortrad Eye Instruments Corp. 973-543-2371
8 Franklin Rd, Mendham, NJ 07945

Katena Products, Inc. 800-225-1195
4 Stewart Ct, Denville, NJ 07834

Miltex Inc. 800-645-8000
589 Davies Dr, York, PA 17402

Stephens Instruments, Inc. 800-354-7848
2500 Sandersville Rd, Lexington, KY 40511
$27.50 per unit (standard).

HOOK, SURGICAL, GENERAL & PLASTIC SURGERY *(Surgery) 79GDG*

Aesculap Implant Systems Inc. 1-800-234-9179
3773 Corporate Pkwy, Center Valley, PA 18034

Ascent Healthcare Solutions 480-763-5300
10232 S 51st St, Phoenix, AZ 85044
Hook.

Bausch & Lomb Surgical 636-255-5051
3365 Tree Court Ind Blvd, Saint Louis, MO 63122

Biomet Microfixation Inc. 800-874-7711
1520 Tradeport Dr, Jacksonville, FL 32218
Various types of hooks.

Biomet, Inc. 574-267-6639
56 E Bell Dr, PO Box 587, Warsaw, IN 46582
Various types of surgical hooks.

Cardinal Health, Snowden Pencer Products 847-689-8410
5175 S Royal Atlanta Dr, Tucker, GA 30084
Various styles of surgical hooks.

Elmed, Inc. 630-543-2792
60 W Fay Ave, Addison, IL 60101

George Tiemann & Co. 800-843-6266
25 Plant Ave, Hauppauge, NY 11788

Kapp Surgical Instrument, Inc. 800-282-5277
4919 Warrensville Center Rd, Cleveland, OH 44128

Kmedic 800-955-0559
190 Veterans Dr, Northvale, NJ 07647

Micrins Surgical Instruments, Inc. 800-833-3380
28438 N Ballard Dr, Lake Forest, IL 60045

Rocket Medical Plc. 800-707-7625
150 Recreation Park Dr Ste 3, Hingham, MA 02043

Surgical Instrument Manufacturers, Inc. 800-521-2985
1650 Headland Dr, Fenton, MO 63026

Symmetry Medical Usa, Inc. 574-267-8700
486 W 350 N, Warsaw, IN 46582
Manual surgical instrument for general use.

Tuzik Boston 800-886-6363
104 Longwater Dr, Assinippi Park, Norwell, MA 02061

Venosan North America, Inc. 800-432-5347
300 Industrial Park Ave, PO Box 1067, Asheboro, NC 27205
VENOSAN Phlebectomy hooks by Mueller, Oesch and Ramelet.

Vnus Medical Technologies, Inc. 888-797-8346
5799 Fontanoso Way, San Jose, CA 95138
Phlebectomy hook.

Warsaw Orthopedic, Inc. 901-396-3133
2500 Silveus Xing, Warsaw, IN 46582
Hook, surgical.

Zimmer Holdings, Inc. 800-613-6131
1800 W Center St, PO Box 708, Warsaw, IN 46580

HOOK, SYMPATHECTOMY *(Cns/Neurology) 84RAR*

Elmed, Inc. 630-543-2792
60 W Fay Ave, Addison, IL 60101

Miltex Inc. 800-645-8000
589 Davies Dr, York, PA 17402

HOOK, TONSIL SUTURING *(Ear/Nose/Throat) 77KBP*

Aesculap Implant Systems Inc. 1-800-234-9179
3773 Corporate Pkwy, Center Valley, PA 18034

Bausch & Lomb Surgical 636-255-5051
3365 Tree Court Ind Blvd, Saint Louis, MO 63122

HOOK, TRACHEAL *(Ear/Nose/Throat) 77RAS*

Bausch & Lomb Surgical 636-255-5051
3365 Tree Court Ind Blvd, Saint Louis, MO 63122

Codman & Shurtleff, Inc 800-225-0460
325 Paramount Dr, Raynham, MA 02767

Elmed, Inc. 630-543-2792
60 W Fay Ave, Addison, IL 60101

Miltex Inc. 800-645-8000
589 Davies Dr, York, PA 17402

HOOK, TRACHEAL, ENT *(Ear/Nose/Throat) 77KCH*

Aesculap Implant Systems Inc. 1-800-234-9179
3773 Corporate Pkwy, Center Valley, PA 18034

Bausch & Lomb Surgical 636-255-5051
3365 Tree Court Ind Blvd, Saint Louis, MO 63122

Tuzik Boston 800-886-6363
104 Longwater Dr, Assinippi Park, Norwell, MA 02061

HOT WATER PASTEURIZATION DEVICE *(General) 80LDS*

Midbrook, Inc. 517-787-3481
2080 Brooklyn Rd, Jackson, MI 49203
Medical washer.

HOUSEKEEPING EQUIPMENT *(General) 80VBI*

Amano Pioneer Eclipse Corp. 800-334-2246
1 Eclipse Rd, PO Box 909, Sparta, NC 28675
Housekeeping and floor care chemicals.

Cdc Products Corp. 800-636-7363
1801 Falmouth Ave, New Hyde Park, NY 11040
Cleaner and deodorizer for trash cans, urinals, dumpsters, cigarette urns; anti-clog for air conditioning/refrigeration units. Carpet cleaning powder, carptet deodorizer.

Central Paper Products Company 800-339-4065
PO Box 4480, Manchester, NH 03108

Continental Manufacturing Co. 800-325-1051
13330 Lakefront Dr, Earth City, MO 63045
Mopping equipment.

Crest Healthcare Supply 800-328-8908
195 3rd St, Dassel, MN 55325

Geerpres 800-253-0373
1780 Harvey St, Muskegon, MI 49442
CHAMP bucket, ULTRA and NAUTILUS wringers, ROYAL KNIGHT and ROYAL PRINCE stainless steel wringers, DYNAMATE mop handle, GRIPIT tool holders. ERGO KNIGHT, ERGO PRINCE and ERGO KING ergonomic wringers. Downpress wringer with ergonomic handle. GPS 2000, a self-contained cleaning system with microfiber mop head.

Hygolet Usa 800-494-6538
349 SE 2nd Ave, Deerfield Beach, FL 33441
HygoFresh Aerosol Dispenser. Metered aerosol air freshener can be adjusted to spray scent in intervals from 5 to 25 minutes on a day/night or 24 hour schedule.

Lamba Systems 800-231-1332
99 Wales Ave, Tonawanda, NY 14150
25in and 36in 4-sided safety/wet floor caution cones and accessories. 25' high bright yellow or lime green floor signs with messages such as, ' WET FLOOR,' ' WATCH YOUR STEP,' ' CAUTION,' etc. It can be bi-lingual, English/Spanish, English/French, etc. Innovative Lockin'Arm on each side displays message, in addition to messages on the 2-sided sign itself, giving the message on all 4 sides.

Morrison Medical 800-438-6677
3735 Paragon Dr, Columbus, OH 43228
Clean-up systems, contains solidifying powder.

HOUSEKEEPING EQUIPMENT *(cont'd)*

Multi Marketing & Manufacturing, Inc. 303-794-5955
PO Box 1070, 5401 Prince Street, Littleton, CO 80160
HAND KEY-PER; $9.95 plus $3.00 s/h. Multi-purpose household opener helps 8 ways; opens bags, envelopes, pop-top cans, medicine jars and aspirin bottles. Internally installed keys makes turning house and car keys easier.

Nss Enterprises, Inc. 419-531-2121
3115 Frenchmens Rd, Toledo, OH 43607
NSS machies for hard floor and carpet care include: CHARGER burnishers, WRANGLER automatic scrubbers; THOROUGHBRED, MAWERICK, MUSTANG and GALAXY floor machines; MANTA, SIDEWINDER and PORTER sweepers; BP RANGER, COLT, and DESIGNER SERIES wet/dry vacuum; PACER vacuum cleaners; PONY, PREDATOR, and STALLION carpet extractors; and pressurewashers.

Perfex Corp. 800-848-8483
32 Case St., Poland, NY 13431
Hygiene brooms, brushes & squeegees for housekeeping. TRUCLEAN PRO is a flat mopping system designed to isolate contaminants. TRUCLEAN SYSTEM II, compact flat mopping system, designed for small area cleaning. TRUCLEAN Disinfection System, designed for disinfecting surgical service areas of hospitals, nursing homes and healthcare facilities.

R&B Wire Products, Inc. 800-634-0555
2902 W Garry Ave, Santa Ana, CA 92704
Wire Shelving Units in 6 sizes with the availablity of solid shel options.

Royce Rolls Ringer Co. 800-253-9638
PO Box 1831, 16 Riverview Terrace, Grand Rapids, MI 49501
Stainless steel.

Sanitor Manufacturing Co. 800-379-5314
1221 W Centre Ave, Portage, MI 49024
Paper hand towels and dispensers plus disposable toilet seat covers and dispensers.

Sloan Valve Co. 800-9VA-LVE9
10500 Seymour Ave, Franklin Park, IL 60131

Sprayway, Inc. 800-332-9000
484 S Vista Ave, Addison, IL 60101
Multi-purpose cleansing sprays.

Tornado Industries 800-822-8367
7401 W Lawrence Ave, Chicago, IL 60706

Tu-Way American Group 800-537-3750
191 Pearl St., Rockford, OH 45882-0306
Industrial and institutional wet mops/dust mops, specialty cleaning tools, carpet bonnets, wax applicators, wallwash systems.

World Dryer Corp. 800-323-0701
5700 McDermott Dr, Berkeley, IL 60163
Dryers.

HOUSING, X-RAY TUBE, DIAGNOSTIC *(Radiology) 90ITY*

Atlas Medical Technologies 909-923-7387
1137 E Philadelphia St, Ontario, CA 91761

Dunlee 800-238-3780
555 N Commerce St, Aurora, IL 60504
X-ray tube housing assembly.

Dunlee-Tubemaster Facility 800-544-9729
2312 Avenue J, Arlington, TX 76006
Tube housing assembly.

Ge Medical Systems, Llc 847-277-5002
4855 W Electric Ave, West Milwaukee, WI 53219
Various models of x-ray tube housing assemblies.

Gemspro, S.A. De C.V. 262-544-3894
Calle B #504 Parque Industrial, Almacetro, Apodaca, N.I. Mexico
Various

K-Alpha X-Ray 630-860-1364
175 Hansen Ct Ste 108, Wood Dale, IL 60191
X-ray tube and assembly.

Marconi Medical Systems 800-323-0550
595 Miner Rd, Cleveland, OH 44143

North American Imaging, Inc. 805-383-2200
924 Via Alondra, Camarillo, CA 93012
Various models of x-ray tube housings.

Varian Medical Systems Interay 800-468-3729
3235 Fortune Dr, North Charleston, SC 29418
Tube housing assembly.

Varian Medical Systems X-Ray Products 800-432-4422
1678 Pioneer Rd, Salt Lake City, UT 84104

HOUSING, X-RAY TUBE, DIAGNOSTIC *(cont'd)*

Virtual Imaging, Inc. 954-428-6191
720 S Powerline Rd Ste E, Deerfield Bch, FL 33442
Various.

5 Star Imaging, Inc. 727-376-0588
11515 Prosperous Dr, Odessa, FL 33556
Diagnostic x-ray tube housing assembly.

HOUSING, X-RAY TUBE, THERAPEUTIC *(Radiology) 90ITZ*

Atlas Medical Technologies 909-923-7887
1137 E Philadelphia St, Ontario, CA 91761

Bionix Development Corp. 800-551-7096
5154 Enterprise Blvd, Toledo, OH 43612
Bionix radiacare intraoperative therapy system.

Varian Medical Systems X-Ray Products 800-432-4422
1678 Pioneer Rd, Salt Lake City, UT 84104

HUMIDIFIER, HEAT/MOISTURE EXCHANGE
(Anesthesiology) 73RAU

Arc Medical, Inc. 800-950-ARC1
4296 Cowan Rd, Tucker, GA 30084
THERMOFLO and THERMOFLO I Heat/moisture exchange. Clinically effective HCH - caring for patients from intubation to extubation. Moisture output)33 mg H2O/L.

Caframo Ltd. 800-567-3556
RR#2 Airport Rd., Wiarton, ONT N0H 2T0 Canada
Caframo H-15 Humidifier, 15. liter capacity.

Enternet Medical, Inc. 888-887-6638
1676 Village Grn, Crofton, MD 21114
HCH with Sputum Baffle

Intersurgical Inc. 315-451-2900
417 Electronics Pkwy, Liverpool, NY 13088
HYDRO-THERM, CLEAR-THERM, FILTA-THERM, HYDRO-TRACH T.

Medline Industries, Inc. 800-633-5886
1 Medline Pl, Mundelein, IL 60060

Repex Medical Products, Inc. 305-740-0133
5240 SW 64th Ave, Miami, FL 33155

HUMIDIFIER, HEATED *(Anesthesiology) 73RAV*

Dhd Healthcare Corporation 800-847-8000
PO Box 6, One Madison Street, Wampsville, NY 13163
Thera-Mist Heated Humidifier

Enternet Medical, Inc. 888-887-6638
1676 Village Grn, Crofton, MD 21114
Thermax

Pegasus Research Corp. 877-632-0255
3505 Cadillac Ave Ste G5, Costa Mesa, CA 92626
For infant incubators and ventilators.

Sunrise Medical 800-333-4000
7477 Dry Creek Pkwy, Longmont, CO 80503

HUMIDIFIER, NON-DIRECT PATIENT INTERFACE (HOME-USE)
(Anesthesiology) 73KFZ

Afton Medical Llc 707-577-0685
3137 Swetzer Rd Ste C, Loomis, CA 95650
Bubble humidifier.

Battle Creek Equipment Co. 800-253-0854
307 Jackson St W, Battle Creek, MI 49037
Evaporative Humidifier, bacteria blocking polymers prevent the growth of bacteria, mold and spores for maintenance free healthy humidification. $77.00 to $105.00.

Dorel Design & Development Center 781-364-3542
25 Forbes Blvd, Foxboro, MA 02035

Kaz Usa, Inc. 518-828-0450
4755 Southpoint Dr, Memphis, TN 38118
Various types of humidifiers.

Kaz, Inc. 518-828-0450
1 Vapor Trl, Hudson, NY 12534
Various types of humidifiers, non-heated.

Smiths Medical Asd, Inc. 847-793-0135
330 Corporate Woods Pkwy, Vernon Hills, IL 60061
Humidifiers & nebulizers, non-filled.

Sunbeam Products, Inc. 561-912-4100
2381 NW Executive Center Dr, Boca Raton, FL 33431
Humidifier, hot steam vaporizer.

HUMIDIFIER, NON-HEATED *(Anesthesiology) 73RAW*

Allied Healthcare Products, Inc. 800-444-3954
1720 Sublette Ave, Saint Louis, MO 63110

Dixie Ems Supply 800-347-3494
385 Union Ave, Brooklyn, NY 11211
$1.69 per unit (standard).

Precision Medical, Inc. 800-272-7285
300 Held Dr, Northampton, PA 18067

Salter Labs 800-235-4203
100 Sycamore Rd, Arvin, CA 93203
Disposable humidifier (dry).

Sunrise Medical 800-333-4000
7477 Dry Creek Pkwy, Longmont, CO 80503

HUMIDIFIER, RESPIRATORY GAS, (DIRECT PATIENT INTERFACE) *(Anesthesiology) 73BTT*

Ballard Medical Products 770-587-7835
12050 Lone Peak Pkwy, Draper, UT 84020
Heated humidifier.

Bergquist Torrington Company 860-489-0489
89 Commercial Blvd, Torrington, CT 06790
Heated humidifier for cpap.

Cardinal Health 207, Inc. 610-862-0800
1100 Bird Center Dr, Palm Springs, CA 92262
Heated humidifier.

Carlsbad International Export, Inc. 760-438-5323
1954 Kellogg Ave, Carlsbad, CA 92008
Humidifier.

Corpak Medsystems, Inc. 800-323-6305
100 Chaddick Dr, Wheeling, IL 60090
Humidifier - various size chambers.

Emepe International, Inc. 813-994-9690
18108 Sugar Brooke Dr, Tampa, FL 33647
Humidifier for oxygen. Reusable and disposable. Oxygen nebulizer. Heater for nebulizer.

Norco 800-657-6672
1125 W Amity Rd, Boise, ID 83705

Pegasus Research Corp. 877-632-0255
3505 Cadillac Ave Ste G5, Costa Mesa, CA 92626
Bubblestick Bubbler Humidifier Utilizes standard 500- and 1000-ml sterile water sources.

Perma Pure Llc 800-337-3762
8 Executive Dr, Toms River, NJ 08755

Porous Media Corp. 651-653-2000
1350 Hammond Rd, Saint Paul, MN 55110
Humidifier.

Precision Medical, Inc. 800-272-7285
300 Held Dr, Northampton, PA 18067

Resmed Corp. 800-424-0737
14040 Danielson St, Poway, CA 92064
Humidifier, passover.

Resmed Inc. 800-424-0737
9001 Spectrum Center Blvd, San Diego, CA 92123
RESMED PASSOVER HUMIDIFIER

Santa Fe Rubber Products, Inc. 562-693-2776
12306 Washington Blvd, Whittier, CA 90606
Innalation & respiration device diaphragms & hose connections.

Smiths Medical Asd Inc. 800-258-5361
10 Bowman Dr, Keene, NH 03431
Various types of humidifiers and sterile and non-sterile access.

Smiths Medical Asd, Inc. 847-793-0135
330 Corporate Woods Pkwy, Vernon Hills, IL 60061
Various sizes of sterile humidifiers and accessories.

Smiths Medical Asd, Inc. 610-578-9600
9255 Customhouse Plz Ste N, San Diego, CA 92154
Humidifier and accessories.

Superior Products, Inc. 216-651-9400
3786 Ridge Rd, Cleveland, OH 44144
Passover humidifier.

Telefelx Medical 919-544-8000
900 W University Dr, Arlington Heights, IL 60004
Various respiratory gas humidfiers, direct patient interfa.

Tennessee Medical Equipment, Inc. 731-635-2119
4637 Highway 19 E, Ripley, TN 38063
Ap-5 medication device nebulizer.

HUMIDIFIER, RESPIRATORY GAS, (DIRECT PATIENT INTERFACE) *(cont'd)*

Vapotherm, Inc. 866-827-6843
198 Log Canoe Cir, Stevensville, MD 21666
Respiratory gas humidifier.

HYALURONIDASE *(Pathology) 88IBD*

E K Industries, Inc. 877-EKI-CHEM
1403 Herkimer St, Joliet, IL 60432
Schiff reagent (fuchsin-suifurous acid Ts).

HYGROMETER (HUMIDITY INDICATOR) *(Anesthesiology) 73RAX*

Abbeon Cal, Inc. 800-922-0977
123 Gray Ave, Santa Barbara, CA 93101
LUFFT, Opus 200/300 Datalogger, records temperature, humidity and/or condition for downloading to a computer; comes with analysis software.

Cmt, Inc. 800-659-9140
PO Box 297, Hamilton, MA 01936

Dickson Co 800-757-3747
930 S Westwood Ave, Addison, IL 60101
Offering chart recorders, hand held indicators and data loggers.

Edgetech 800-276-3729
19 Brigham St Unit 8, Marlborough, MA 01752
Moisture and humidity instruments. Hygrometers, chilled mirror hygrometer standards, DewTrak products, diffusion cell sensors for moisture and humidity measurements in laboratories, commercial industries and process applications.

Extech Instruments Corp. 781-890-7440
285 Bear Hill Rd, Waltham, MA 02451
$149.00 for hygrometer to indicate and measure temperature and humidity.

Linseis, Inc. 800-732-6733
PO Box 666, Princeton Junction, NJ 08550

The Kahn Companies 860-529-8643
885 Wells Rd, Wethersfield, CT 06109
Ceramic, aluminum oxide, and optical models available. For use with gases, including anesthetics. CERMAX portable hygrometer, a rugged, fully self-contained, portable dewpoint-measuring instrument for portable measurements of moisture in air or other compressed gases. Dewpoint range from -100 to +20 degrees Celsius and typical accuracy of +/- 1 degree Celsius. EASIDEW portable hygrometer, a lower-cost, compact, easy-to-use portable hygrometer, dewpoint measurement range from -100 to +20 degrees Celsius, +/- 2 degrees Celsius accuracy, which includes an integral sampling system, 4-20 mA output, rugged NEMA 4 enclosure, rechargeable nickel-cadmium battery, battery charge indicator and a fixed-orifice-port configuration for selection of dewpoint measurement at atmospheric or line pressure. TRANSMET dewpoint transmitter, dewpont transmitter for process-point measurements of moisture in air or other process gases. Dewpoint range from -100 to +20 degrees Celsius and typical accuracy of +/- 1 degree Celsius; analog or digital output. EASIDEW dewpoint transmitter, a low-cost, rugged ceramic dewpoint transmitter that is economical to purchase, install, and maintain, features full dewpoint range from -100 to +20 degrees Celsius, +/-2 degrees Celsius accuracy and linear 4-20 mA output. CERMET II hygrometer, a single-channel system that includes sensor, interconnecting cable and digital display with 4-20mA output, adjustable alarm relays and capability to display moisture measurement in various engineering units. The new OPTIDEW dewpoint and RH transmitter features single-stage or two-stage sensor for a full range of dewpoint measurements from -60 to +90 degrees Celsius, sealed tight sensors for use in condensing environments, dynamic contamination correction for better accuracy and three models to choose from: wall mount with integrated sensor, bench/panel mount with remote sensor, probe mount for flange or duct installation.

HYPERTHERMIA SYSTEM, AUTOMATIC CONTROL *(Radiology) 90LNE*

Medispec Ltd. - Usa 888-663-3477
20410 Observation Dr Ste 102, Germantown, MD 20876
THERMASPEC 1000 for treatment of BPH.

HYPERTHERMIA UNIT, MICROWAVE *(Radiology) 90RAY*

Bsd Medical Corporation 801-972-5555
2188 W 2200 S, Salt Lake City, UT 84119
For treatment of cancer tumors. Models BSD 500, 2000. Price ranges from $53,000 to $600,000.

HYPERTHERMIA UNIT, MICROWAVE *(cont'd)*

Labthermics Technologies 217-351-7722
701 Devonshire Dr, Champaign, IL 61820
MICROTHERM microwave hyperthermia system SONOTHERM ultrasound and INTERTHERM RF interstitial hyperthermia systems. Also: Ultrasound Hyperthermia Unit, SONOTHERM ultrasound hyperthermia system.

HYPO/HYPERTHERMIA BLANKET *(General) 80RAZ*

Adroit Medical Systems, Inc. 800-267-6077
1146 Carding Machine Rd, Loudon, TN 37774
Water circulating heating and cooling blankets for temperature therapy. Adult and pediatric sizes. Can be used with all hypo-hyperthermia machines.

American Woolen Company 305-635-4000
4000 NW 30th Ave, Miami, FL 33142

Arizant Healthcare Inc. 800-733-7775
10393 W 70th St, Eden Prairie, MN 55344
BAIR HUGGER Warming blanket line available in 23 designs, including an outpatient warming model.

Cincinnati Sub-Zero Products, Inc., Medical Division 800-989-7373
12011 Mosteller Rd, Cincinnati, OH 45241
Available in reusable and single patient use adult, pediatric, and O.R. table sizes; provide highest flow rates resulting in high thermal transfer characteristics. Disposable blankets include Maxi-Therm and Maxi-Therm Lite. Reusable Blankets PlastiPad.

Gaymar Industries, Inc. 800-828-7341
10 Centre Dr, Orchard Park, NY 14127
Random flow design allows quick heating/cooling of water circulating blanket. Wide variety of sizes and types available.

Hos-Pillow Corp. 800-468-7874
1011 Campus Dr, Mundelein, IL 60060
Thermal bedspread blankets as well as wool, acrylic, cotton and polyester blankets.

Md International, Inc. 305-669-9003
11300 NW 41st St, Doral, FL 33178

HYPO/HYPERTHERMIA UNIT, MOBILE *(General) 80RBB*

Aragona Medical, Inc. 201-664-8822
184 Rivervale Rd, Rivervale, NJ 07675
Radiant Warmer: Height adjustable mobile thermal ceiling. Requires no disposables.

Cincinnati Sub-Zero Products, Inc., Medical Division 800-989-7373
12011 Mosteller Rd, Cincinnati, OH 45241
NORMO-O-TEMP hyperthermia unit with total body temperature control. BLANKETROL II Hyper-Hypothermia System for warming or cooling total body temperature.

Gaymar Industries, Inc. 800-828-7341
10 Centre Dr, Orchard Park, NY 14127
MEDI-THERM II microprocessor-controlled unit offers rapid heating/cooling of water blankets. User friendly. MED1 TEMP II provides rapid warming of blood/fluids.

Md International, Inc. 305-669-9003
11300 NW 41st St, Doral, FL 33178

Terumo Cardiovascular Systems, Corp 800-521-2818
6200 Jackson Rd, Ann Arbor, MI 48103
2 models with cooler-heater in single unit. TCM computer aided temperature control, monitor and automatic ice generator.

Thermotek Inc. 877-242-3232
1454 Halsey Way, Carrollton, TX 75007
ProThermo PT-7 Heat, Cool, Contrast, Compression. Designed with the help of top sports physicians and trainers, orthopaedic surgeons, and professors of sports medicine and pain management.

HYPOTHERMIA UNIT *(General) 80RBC*

Aragona Medical, Inc. 201-664-8822
184 Rivervale Rd, Rivervale, NJ 07675
Radiant Warmer (Thermal Ceiling); 3 models: Ceiling Mounted, Mobile, and Baby Warmer. Requires no disposables.

Arizant Healthcare Inc. 800-733-7775
10393 W 70th St, Eden Prairie, MN 55344
BAIR HUGGER patient warming unit. Also, total temperature management system.

HYPOTHERMIA UNIT *(cont'd)*

Cincinnati Sub-Zero Products, Inc., Medical Division 800-989-7373
12011 Mosteller Rd, Cincinnati, OH 45241
WARMAIR system for treating hypothermic patients post-surgically and intra-operatively, model #135.

Gaymar Industries, Inc. 800-828-7341
10 Centre Dr, Orchard Park, NY 14127
THERMACARE convective warmed air unit with warming quilts.

Md International, Inc. 305-669-9003
11300 NW 41st St, Doral, FL 33178

Progressive Dynamics Medical, Inc. 269-781-4241
507 Industrial Rd, Marshall, MI 49068
Warm air hypothermia unit.

HYPOTHERMIA UNIT (BLANKET, PLUMBING & HEAT EXCHANGER) *(Anesthesiology) 73BTF*

Adroit Medical Systems, Inc. 800-267-6077
1146 Carding Machine Rd, Loudon, TN 37774
Allon Whole Body Hypo-Hyperthermia Unit with ThermoWrap Heat Exchange Garments (Infant, Pediatric, Adult, Cardiac, Sugical Access)

Progressive Dynamics Medical, Inc. 269-781-4241
507 Industrial Rd, Marshall, MI 49068
LIFE-AIR 1000 hypothermic therapy system, .2 micro filtration for O.R. or PAC-U; disposable, non-woven, spun bound blanket, high degree of flexibility.

HYPOTHERMIC EQUIPMENT *(Microbiology) 83UGN*

Cincinnati Sub-Zero Products, Inc., Medical Division 800-989-7373
12011 Mosteller Rd, Cincinnati, OH 45241

Md International, Inc. 305-669-9003
11300 NW 41st St, Doral, FL 33178

HYSTEROSCOPE *(Obstetrics/Gyn) 85HIH*

Apple Medical Corp. 508-357-2700
28 Lord Rd Ste 135, Marlborough, MA 01752
Illuminator.

Conceptus, Inc. 650-962-4000
331 E Evelyn Ave, Mountain View, CA 94041

Coopersurgical, Inc. 800-243-2974
95 Corporate Dr, Trumbull, CT 06611
$6,295 for flexible fiberoptic hysteroscope; $2,995 for 4-mm, 30-degree rigid hysteroscope; $3,095 for 2.7-mm hysteroscope.

Cortek Endoscopy, Inc. 847-526-2266
260 Jamie Ln Ste D, Wauconda, IL 60084
Gynecology.

Global Endoscopy, Inc. 888-434-3398
914 Estes Ct, Schaumburg, IL 60193
Hysteroscope (and accessories).

Gyrus Acmi, Inc. 508-804-2739
93 N Pleasant St, Norwalk, OH 44857
Hysteroscope (and accessories).

Gyrus Acmi, Inc. 508-804-2739
300 Stillwater P.o.box 1971, Stamford, CT 06902
Hysteroscope (and accessories).

Henke Sass Wolf Of America, Inc. 508-671-9300
135 Schofield Ave, Dudley, MA 01571
(AND ACCESSORIES)

Karl Storz Endoscopy-America Inc. 800-421-0837
600 Corporate Pointe, Culver City, CA 90230
Diagnostic and operative hysteroscopes with rod-lens telescopes for hospital and office hysteroscopies.

Mahe International Inc. 800-294-7946
468 Craighead St, Nashville, TN 37204

Medgyn Products, Inc. 800-451-9667
328 Eisenhower Ln N, Lombard, IL 60148

Minrad, Inc. 716-855-1068
50 Cobham Dr, Orchard Park, NY 14127
Hysteroscope.

Olympus America, Inc. 800-645-8160
3500 Corporate Pkwy, PO Box 610, Center Valley, PA 18034

Rei Rotolux Enterprises, Inc. 888-773-7611
4145 North Service Rd, Ste. 200, Burlington, ON L7L 6A3 Canada
2.7mm and 4mm are available, all autoclavable . Custom configurations are available.

HYSTEROSCOPE *(cont'd)*

Richard Wolf Medical Instruments Corp. 800-323-9653
353 Corporate Woods Pkwy, Vernon Hills, IL 60061

Smith & Nephew, Inc., Endoscopy Division 800-343-8386
150 Minuteman Rd, Andover, MA 01810

Superior Medical Limited 800-268-7944
520 Champagne Dr., Toronto, ONT M3J 2T9 Canada

Wisap America 800-233-8448
8231 Melrose Dr, Lenexa, KS 66214

HYSTEROSCOPY FLUID *(Obstetrics/Gyn) 85LTA*

Hospira, Inc. 877-946-7747
Hwy. 301 North, Rocky Mount, NC 27801
Hysteroscopic fluid.

IDENTIFICATION PANEL, BLOOD CELL *(Hematology) 81UJR*

Dade Behring, Inc. 800-948-3233
1717 Deerfield Rd, Deerfield, IL 60015

Innovative Chemistry, Inc. 781-837-6709
PO Box 578, Marshfield, MA 02050
AUTHENTIKIT - Cell line identification.

IDENTIFICATION, ALERT, MEDICAL *(General) 80UEU*

Apothecary Products, Inc. 800-328-2742
11750 12th Ave S, Burnsville, MN 55337
Emerge Alert and Protect Your Life brands

Bio-Logics Products, Inc. 800-426-7577
PO Box 505, West Jordan, UT 84084
Alert tags for patient ID bands.

Carex Health Brands 800-526-8051
921 E Amidon St, PO Box 2526, Sioux Falls, SD 57104

Instantel Inc. 800-267-9111
309 Legget Dr., Kanata, ON K2K 3A3 Canada
Wandering patient and medical alert system for home use.

Medicalert Foundation International 800-432-5378
2323 Colorado Ave, Turlock, CA 95382
Emergency medical information service. Membership includes personal identification (emblem, bracelet, wallet card) backed by 24 hour Emergency Response Center. $35 initial enrollment which includes stainless steel emblems. $20 annual renewal fee includes free record updates. 1-800-432-5378 for application and membership information.

R&Da Co. 508-747-5803
37 Dwight Ave, Plymouth, MA 02360
MEDSHEET medical record sheet. A two-sided laser printed sheet in code containing 60,000 characters (30 pages), decodable by flatbed scanner and software. By special order only.

Xenotec Ltd. 949-640-4053
511 Hazel Dr, Corona Del Mar, CA 92625
Foot printing system for newborn infants. Completing clean footprinting system to ensure correct identification of child with mother.

IGA, FERRITIN, ANTIGEN, ANTISERUM, CONTROL *(Immunology) 82CZM*

Dako North America, Inc 805-566-6655
6392 Via Real, Carpinteria, CA 93013

Kent Laboratories, Inc. 360-398-8641
777 Jorgensen Pl, Bellingham, WA 98226

IGE, FERRITIN, ANTIGEN, ANTISERUM, CONTROL *(Immunology) 82DFM*

Dako North America, Inc 805-566-6655
6392 Via Real, Carpinteria, CA 93013

Kent Laboratories, Inc. 360-398-8641
777 Jorgensen Pl, Bellingham, WA 98226

IGG (FD FRAGMENT SPECIFIC), ANTIGEN, ANTISERUM, CONTROL *(Immunology) 82DAQ*

Rockland Immunochemicals, Inc. 800-656-ROCK
PO Box 326, Gilbertsville, PA 19525

IGG IMMUNOASSAY REAGENTS *(Immunology) 82KTO*

Ease Labs, Inc. 650-872-7788
338 N Canal St Ste 9, South San Francisco, CA 94080
Protein a-gold conjugate.

IGG, FERRITIN, ANTIGEN, ANTISERUM, CONTROL
(Immunology) 82DGD

Clinical Controls International 805-528-4039
1236 Los Osos Valley Rd Ste T, Los Osos, CA 93402
Ferritin control.

Dako North America, Inc 805-566-6655
6392 Via Real, Carpinteria, CA 93013

Kent Laboratories, Inc. 360-398-8641
777 Jorgensen Pl, Bellingham, WA 98226

Rockland Immunochemicals, Inc. 800-656-ROCK
PO Box 326, Gilbertsville, PA 19525

IGM, FERRITIN, ANTIGEN, ANTISERUM, CONTROL
(Immunology) 82DFL

Dako North America, Inc 805-566-6655
6392 Via Real, Carpinteria, CA 93013

Kent Laboratories, Inc. 360-398-8641
777 Jorgensen Pl, Bellingham, WA 98226

ILLUMINATOR, COLOR VISION PLATE *(Ophthalmology) 86HJD*

Richmond Products, Inc. 505-275-2406
4400 Silver Ave SE, Albuquerque, NM 87108
Hematocrit control.

Western Ophthalmics Corporation 800-426-9938
19019 36th Ave W Ste G, Lynnwood, WA 98036

ILLUMINATOR, FIBEROPTIC (FOR ENDOSCOPE)
(Gastro/Urology) 78FFS

Ams Innovative Center-San Jose 800-356-7600
3070 Orchard Dr, San Jose, CA 95134

Chiu Technical Corp. 631-544-0606
252 Indian Head Rd, Kings Park, NY 11754
$248.00 for FO 150-115.

Codman & Shurtleff, Inc 800-225-0460
325 Paramount Dr, Raynham, MA 02767

Elmed, Inc. 630-543-2792
60 W Fay Ave, Addison, IL 60101

Gyrus Acmi, Inc. 508-804-2739
93 N Pleasant St, Norwalk, OH 44857
Illuminator, fiberoptic, for endoscope.

Isolux Llc 239-514-7475
1045 Collier Center Way Ste 6, Naples, FL 34110
Xenon fiberoptic light source for medical procedures.

Karl Storz Endoscopy-America Inc. 800-421-0837
600 Corporate Pointe, Culver City, CA 90230

Mahe International Inc. 800-294-7946
468 Craighead St, Nashville, TN 37204

Progressive Dynamics Medical, Inc. 269-781-4241
507 Industrial Rd, Marshall, MI 49068
150 watt halogen light source.

Reznik Instrument, Inc. 847-673-3444
7337 Lawndale Ave, Skokie, IL 60076
Fiber-optic light source.

Richard Wolf Medical Instruments Corp. 800-323-9653
353 Corporate Woods Pkwy, Vernon Hills, IL 60061

Smith & Nephew, Inc., Endoscopy Division 800-343-8386
150 Minuteman Rd, Andover, MA 01810

Sunoptic Technologies 877-677-2832
6018 Bowdendale Ave, Jacksonville, FL 32216
Fiberoptic illuminators, high intensity lightsource, several models, UL and CSA listed.

Vision Systems Group, A Division Of Viking Systems 508-366-3668
134 Flanders Rd, Westborough, MA 01581
Vista illuminatio system.

ILLUMINATOR, FIBEROPTIC, SURGICAL FIELD
(Cns/Neurology) 84HBI

Advanced Dental Systems 480-991-4081
5001 E Desert Jewel Dr, Paradise Valley, AZ 85253
Light source for surgery.

Alcon Manufacturing, Ltd. 817-551-6813
714 Columbia Ave, Sinking Spring, PA 19608
Fiber optic light guide.

Chiu Technical Corp. 631-544-0606
252 Indian Head Rd, Kings Park, NY 11754
$248.00 for FO 150-115.

ILLUMINATOR, FIBEROPTIC, SURGICAL FIELD *(cont'd)*

Escalon Trek Medical 800-433-8197
2440 S 179th St, New Berlin, WI 53146
Fiber optic light source system.

Isolux Llc 239-514-7475
1045 Collier Center Way Ste 6, Naples, FL 34110
Xenon fiber optic light source for surgical procedures.

Sunoptic Technologies 877-677-2832
6018 Bowdendale Ave, Jacksonville, FL 32216
Coaxial fixed or variable spot headlight systems with high intensity 150W, 300W, and xenon lightsources, UL and CSA listed.

ILLUMINATOR, NON-REMOTE *(Surgery) 79FTF*

Medical Vision Industries, Inc. 800-775-2088
3117 McHenry Ave Ste B, Modesto, CA 95350
Illuminator.

ILLUMINATOR, RADIOGRAPHIC FILM *(Radiology) 90IXC*

Alimed, Inc. 800-225-2610
297 High St, Dedham, MA 02026
Bright Spot illuminator increases light intensity to facilitate viewing of dense films.

Alkco Lighting Co. 847-451-0700
11500 Melrose Ave, Franklin Park, IL 60131

AMD Technologies Inc. 800-423-3535
218 Bronwood Ave, Los Angeles, CA 90049
9 models and styles. CATELLA digital imaging display.

Americomp, Inc. 800-458-1782
2901 W Lawrence Ave, Chicago, IL 60625

Brandt Industries, Inc. 800-221-8031
4461 Bronx Blvd, Bronx, NY 10470
Single and banked.

Broadwest Corp. 800-232-2948
304 Elati St, Denver, CO 80223
Broadwest's LumiVue™ flat panel illuminators utilize the latest and most effective features currently available in mammography viewing. Through a unique cold cathode fluorescent lamp, LumiVue™ is able to provide a brightness of 8,000 cd/m2 and a useful life several times longer than that of other fluorescent lamps. Furthermore, its backlight technology employs the highest daylight color temperature for improving contrast rendering and providing a uniformity greater than 90%. To complement its cutting-edge technical features, LumiVue™ has an aesthetically pleasing design less than 3î thick with fully masking shutters and a choice of three color types (Ivory, White, Gray). MAMMOMASK illuminators for mammography feature four shutters to mask transmitted light around mammograms, ultrasound, or standard radiographs. Desktop and wall-mounted models are available in eight sizes, with dimmers and high luminance lighting. QUAL'X high-luminance viewboxes utilize four lamps and reflectors per panel to create a uniform light field. Features include a choice of six colors, gravity film grips, adjustable nylon wire and optional dimmers.

Burkhart Roentgen Intl. Inc. 800-USA-XRAY
5201 8th Ave S, Gulfport, FL 33707
Many types available with and without shutters to fit any budget, as well as motorized.

Burton Medical Products, Inc. 800-444-9909
21100 Lassen St, Chatsworth, CA 91311
Single and Double Bank

Cadco Dental Products 800-833-8267
600 E Hueneme Rd, Oxnard, CA 93033

Carr Corporation 800-952-2398
1547 11th St, Santa Monica, CA 90401

Cone Instruments, Inc. 800-321-6964
5201 Naiman Pkwy, Solon, OH 44139

Control Research, Inc. 847-392-4770
1775 Winnetka Cir, Rolling Meadows, IL 60008
Motorized film viewer.

Dentalez Group 866-DTE-INFO
101 Lindenwood Dr Ste 225, Valleybrooke Corporate Center
Malvern, PA 19355

Diversified Diagnostic Products, Inc. 281-955-5323
11603 Windfern Rd, Houston, TX 77064
$20,000 for high frequency, dimming illuminators and motorized film viewers. $16,000 for Mammoviewer - high frequency, dimming and motorized film viewers specifically for mammography.

Dux Dental 800-833-8267
600 E Hueneme Rd, Oxnard, CA 93033

ILLUMINATOR, RADIOGRAPHIC FILM *(cont'd)*

Flow X-Ray Corporation 800-356-9729
100 W Industry Ct, Deer Park, NY 11729
11 different styles, 125 different models (sizes).

Gagne, Inc. 800-800-5954
41 Commercial Dr, Johnson City, NY 13790

Ge Medical Systems, Llc 262-548-2355
3000 N Grandview Blvd, W-417, Waukesha, WI 53188
Various types and models of illuminators.

Holorad Llc 801-983-6075
2929 S Main St, Salt Lake City, UT 84115
Holographic medical imaging lightbox.

Image Marketing Corp. 800-466-7032
1636 N 24th St, PO Box 30935, Mesa, AZ 85213
SLIMLITE 5000 viewboxes 1' thin. sizes up to 14' x 24' for viewing most medical films. SLIMLITE Viewbox, lightbox for reading x-rays or slides, lightweight and only 1/2' thick. Film sizes up to 9' x 12'. It produces bright, even illumination for easy viewing that can be permanent or portable. LP 204 a cost effective flat panel for viewing x-rays up to 8' x 11' in size. MINILITE View Panel, x-ray viewer, portable workstation, Alc & batteries. MICROLITE portable viewerfor single small films up to 2' x 2'.

Independent Solutions, Inc. 847-498-0500
900 Skokie Blvd Ste 118, Northbrook, IL 60062
MAXANT flush wall mounted or surface wall mounted; single or multiple gang, single or multiple tier. U.L. listed.

Inocraft, Inc. 678-985-2926
478 Northdale Rd Ste 706, Lawrenceville, GA 30046
Various.

Jedmed Instruments Co. 314-845-3770
5416 Jedmed Ct, Saint Louis, MO 63129

Leedal, Inc. 847-498-0111
3453 Commercial Ave, Northbrook, IL 60062

Marconi Medical Systems 800-323-0550
595 Miner Rd, Cleveland, OH 44143

Maxant Technologies, Inc. 800-307-4190
7540 N Caldwell Ave, Niles, IL 60714
Techline 200,300 and 400 Series, X-ray illuminators available in two, three, and four lamp lighting configurations. Also, Mammo-Techline mammography view boxes.

Mayo Medical, S.A. De C.V. 800-715-3872
Edison 1141 Nte., Col. Talleres, Monterrey N.L. 64480 Mexico

Obsidian Medical Technology, Inc. 832-767-9606
5108 Corona Covet, Pleasanton, CA 94588
Digital light box.

Pelton & Crane 704-588-2126
11727 Fruehauf Dr, Charlotte, NC 28273
X-ray view box.

Post Glover Lifelink 800-287-4123
167 Gap Way, Erlanger, KY 41018
X-ray film viewer with low power leakage to be used in operating rooms and anywhere purity of power is important.

Pulse Medical Inc. 800-342-5973
4131 SW 47th Ave Ste 1404, Davie, FL 33314
SLIMVIEW x-ray illuminator, portable, battery or 120V AC powered, 2in. thick. Plastic x-ray developing tank, darkroom film bin and x-ray developing hangers also available.

S&S Technology 281-815-1300
10625 Telge Rd, Houston, TX 77095
Largest selection of quality view boxes, including mammo and over 20 models of motorized viewers, plus x-ray filing systems, darkroom cabinets, and much more. $12,000 to $20,000 for motorized unit. High-intensity x-ray illuminator: $616/unit (non-motorized.). Meter for measuring luminance: $275/unit.

Schueler & Company, Inc. 516-487-1500
PO Box 528, Stratford, CT 06615

Star X-Ray Co., Inc. 800-374-2163
63 Ranick Dr S, Amityville, NY 11701
$137.00 for medical single bank illuminator; $263.00 for double bank illuminator; $576.00 for four bank illuminator.

Topcon Medical Systems, Inc. 800-223-1130
37 W Century Rd, Paramus, NJ 07652
Ophthalmic viewer, $950. Hand-held stereo viewer, $219.

Uber Lucas Intl Llc 410-758-3181
11126 Tuckahoe Rd, Denton, MD 21629

ILLUMINATOR, RADIOGRAPHIC FILM *(cont'd)*

Wolf X-Ray Corporation 800-356-9729
100 W Industry Ct, Deer Park, NY 11729
11 different styles, 125 different models (sizes).

Xma (X-Ray Marketing Associates, Inc.) 800-325-8880
1205 W Lakeview Ct, Windham Lakes Business Park
Romeoville, IL 60446

ILLUMINATOR, RADIOGRAPHIC FILM, EXPLOSION-PROOF
(Radiology) 90JAG

Ge Medical Systems, Llc 262-548-2355
3000 N Grandview Blvd, W-417, Waukesha, WI 53188
Explosion-proof radiographi illuminator.

ILLUMINATOR, ULTRAVIOLET *(Dental And Oral) 76EAR*

Ultra-Lum, Inc. 800-809-6559
1480 N Claremont Blvd, Claremont, CA 91711
Midsize and Large Ultraviolet Crosslinker Systems.

IMAGE DIGITIZER *(Radiology) 90LMA*

Agfa Corporation 877-777-2432
PO Box 19048, 10 South Academy Street, Greenville, SC 29602

Agfa Healthcare Corp. 864-421-1815
580 Gotham Pkwy, Carlstadt, NJ 07072
Digitizer.

Agfa Healthcare Corp. 864-421-1815
1 Crosswind Dr, Westerly, RI 02891
Echo capture system.

Brit Systems Inc. 800-230-7227
1909 Hl Line Dr Ste A, Dallas, TX 75207

Canon Development Americas, Inc 949-932-3100
15955 Alton Pkwy, Irvine, CA 92618
Canon Film Scanner 300, a compact, desk-top size film digitizer. It is fast at several sheets per minute with density-controlled scanning.

Dornier Medtech America 800-367-6437
1155 Roberts Blvd NW, Kennesaw, GA 30144
DORNIER OPUS II digital urology imaging system.

Icad Inc. 866-280-2239
98 Spit Brook Rd Ste 100, Nashua, NH 03062
X-ray film digitizer.

Icrco Inc. 310-921-9559
2580 W 237th St, Torrance, CA 90505
Medical image digitizer.

Imsi, Integrated Modular Systems Inc. 800-220-9729
2500 W Township Line Rd, PO Box 616, Havertown, PA 19083
IMSI Film Digitizers. Perfect for getting film images to DICOM. Easy to use, fast, and very cost effective. Integrates easily with Tele-Rad and PACS.

Maxxvision, Llc 1-877-340-6483
2800 Aurora Rd Ste E, Melbourne, FL 32935
iView by MaxxVision (tm) is a remarkable digital image processing system that uses a hand-held digital wand coupled with a powerful image processor that works in real-time. The enhanced mammographic image is viewed on a compact LCD display with its own enhancement features.

Multi Imager Service, Inc 800-400-4549
13865 Magnolia Ave Bldg C, Chino, CA 91710
Founded in 1983, Multi Imager specializes in diagnostic-quality film imaging and digital imaging technologies, including film-based video imagers, wet-film-based laser imagers, dry-film imagers, digital acquisition/storage and transmission devices, computed radiography, PACS, and more. Multi Imager provides technical support and training, parts supply, and sales of new as well as refurbished equipment used with a broad range of modalities, including CT, MRI, ultrasound, nuclear medicine, and others.

Nai Tech Products 866-342-6629
12919 Earhart Ave, Auburn, CA 95602
Dicombox & MDR-Video

Openmed Technologies Corporation 877-717-6215
256 W Cummings Park, Woburn, MA 01801
OpenMed Capture workstation for 'DICOM-izing' radiologic films, documents, etc. for storage and distibution in the PACS archive

Radiographic Digital Imaging, Inc. 310-921-9559
20406 Earl St, Torrance, CA 90503
Cobrascan x-ray digitizer.

Radlink, Inc. 310-643-6900
2400 Marine Ave, Redondo Beach, CA 90278
Laser film digitizer.

IMAGE DIGITIZER *(cont'd)*

Ti-Ba Enterprises, Inc. 585-247-1212
25 Hytec Cir, Rochester, NY 14606
Ti-Ba sells the Laser Pro 16 x-ray film scanner/digitzer.

Titan Corporation/Systems & Imagery Division 800-622-8554
1200 Woody Burke Rd, PO Box 550, Melbourne, FL 32901
IMAGCLEAR radiographic film digitizer.

Topcon Canada Inc. 800-361-3515
110 Provencher Ave., Boisbriand, QUE J7G-1N1 Canada

Vidar Systems Corp. 703-471-7070
365 Herndon Pkwy, Herndon, VA 20170
X-ray film digitizer.

Xma (X-Ray Marketing Associates, Inc.) 800-325-8880
1205 W Lakeview Ct, Windham Lakes Business Park
Romeoville, IL 60446

IMAGE INTENSIFICATION SYSTEM *(Radiology) 90TCP*

Afp Imaging Corp. 800-592-6666
250 Clearbrook Rd, Elmsford, NY 10523

Camp-Ray, Inc. 520-885-6323
2030 N Klondike Dr, Tucson, AZ 85749

Ge Oec Medical Systems Inc. 800-874-7378
384 Wright Brothers Dr, Salt Lake City, UT 84116
SERIES 9600 Mobile Digital Imaging System. For use in orthopedics, vascular, neuro, urology and billiary surgery.

M & I Medical Sales, Inc. 305-663-6444
4711 SW 72nd Ave, Miami, FL 33155

Mikron Digital Imaging, Inc. 800-925-3905
30425 8 Mile Rd, Livonia, MI 48152
Service and installation.

Thales Components Corporation 973-812-9000
40G Commerce Way, PO Box 540, Totowa, NJ 07512
Radiological Imaging Units (RIU) consist of X-ray Image Intensifier + Optics + CCD Camera

Varian Medical Systems X-Ray Products 800-432-4422
1678 Pioneer Rd, Salt Lake City, UT 84104

IMAGE PROCESSING SYSTEM *(Radiology) 90LLZ*

Advanced Image Enhancement, Inc. 508-344-3097
306 Valentine St, Fall River, MA 02720
Aie region of interest image enhancement software.

Agfa Corporation 877-777-2432
PO Box 19048, 10 South Academy Street, Greenville, SC 29602

Agfa Healthcare Corp. 864-421-1815
580 Gotham Pkwy, Carlstadt, NJ 07072
Pacs, workstations.

Agfa Healthcare Corp. 864-421-1815
1 Crosswind Dr, Westerly, RI 02891
Cardiac network,echo capture system.

Alaska Native Tribal Health Consortium 907-729-1900
4000 Ambassador Dr, Anchorage, AK 99508
System, image processing, radiological.

Alimed, Inc. 800-225-2610
297 High St, Dedham, MA 02026

As Software, Inc. 201-541-1900
560 Sylvan Ave, Englewood Cliffs, NJ 07632
Image acquisition, review and reporting system.

Aspyra, Inc. 904-854-2107
8649 Baypine Rd, Jacksonville, FL 32256
Clinical image management system.

Atlas Medical Technologies 909-923-7887
1137 E Philadelphia St, Ontario, CA 91761
Atlas sells systems to process scanned data into a variety of formats. Virtual, 3D, cardiac scoring.

Avnet, Inc. 480-643-2000
3201 East Harbor, Phoenix, AZ 85034
Image management system.

Barco, Inc 678-475-8137
3059 Premiere Pkwy, Duluth, GA 30097
Image display system, medical image workstation.

Cardinal Healthcare 209, Inc. 610-862-0800
5225 Verona Rd, Fitchburg, WI 53711
Navigation system.

Carl Zeiss Surgical, Inc. 800-442-4020
1 Zeiss Dr, Thornwood, NY 10594

IMAGE PROCESSING SYSTEM *(cont'd)*

Chase Medical, Lp 972-783-0644
1876 Firman Dr, Richardson, TX 75081
Cardiac analysis system.

Coactiv Medical Business Solutions 877-262-2848
900 Ethan Allen Hwy, Ridgefield, CT 06877
Picture, archive, and communication system.

Compass International, Inc. 800-933-2143
1815 14th St NW, Rochester, MN 55901
Cygnus-PFS Image-Guided (frameless) surgery system, hardware and planning software. COMPASS Stereotacic Image-Guided (framed) surgery system, hardware and planning software.

Confirma, Inc. 877-811-2356
11040 Main St Ste 100, Bellevue, WA 98004
CADstream, the standard in CAD for MRI, enhances efficiency and workflow of MRI studies by automating data analysis.

Connect Imaging, Inc.
850 W Hind Dr Ste 116, Honolulu, HI 96821
Picture archiving & communications systems.

Connexmd 206-356-4568
800 W Park Ave Ste 3, Port Townsend, WA 98368
Echoconnex communicator.

Cortechs Labs, Inc. 858-459-9702
1020 Prospect St Ste 304, La Jolla, CA 92037
The deep gray system.

Cybermdx, Inc. 401-228-3772
850 Waterman Ave, East Providence, RI 02914
System,image processing,radiological.

Datacube Inc. 978-777-4200
300 Rosewood Dr, Danvers, MA 01923
Max TD target and development systems. 40 MHz pipeline image processor, hardware, and point and click software.

Direct Radiography 302-631-2700
600 Technology Dr, Newark, DE 19702
Directray operator console.

Direx Systems Corp. 339-502-6013
437 Turnpike St, Canton, MA 02021
Image processing unit.

Dome Imaging Systems, Inc. 866-752-6271
400 5th Ave, Waltham, MA 02451
Active-matrix liquid-crystal display panel.

Edda Technology, Inc. 609-919-9889
5 Independence Way Ste 210, Princeton, NJ 08540
Picture archiving and communications system.

Emageon Inc. 262-369-3379
1200 Corporate Dr Ste 200, Birmingham, AL 35242
Picture archive and communications system.

Fernandez Industries, Inc. 978-371-8431
43 Oak Knoll Rd, Carlisle, MA 01741
Pacs station.

Flow X-Ray Corporation 800-356-9729
100 W Industry Ct, Deer Park, NY 11729

Ge Healthcare Integrated It Solutions 877-519-4471
40 Idx Dr, P.O. Box 1070, South Burlington, VT 05403
Picture archiving and communications system.

Ge Healthcare It 847-277-5000
540 W Northwest Hwy, Barrington, IL 60010
Picture archiving and communications system (pacs).

Ge Medical Systems, Llc 262-548-2355
3000 N Grandview Blvd, W-417, Waukesha, WI 53188
Radiological image processing workstation.

Ge Oec Medical Systems 978-552-5200
439 S Union St, Lawrence, MA 01843
Image guided surgical system & sterile/non-sterile accessories.

Ge Oec Medical Systems Inc. 800-874-7378
384 Wright Brothers Dr, Salt Lake City, UT 84116
SERIES 9600 Mobile Digital Imaging System.

Gvi Technology Partners 330-963-4083
1470 Enterprise Pkwy, Twinsburg, OH 44087
Multi-modality registration workstation.

Healthline Medical Imaging 704-655-0447
705 Northeast Dr Ste 17, Davidson, NC 28036
Picture archive communication systems.

Heart Imaging Technologies, Llc 919-384-5044
5003 Southpark Dr Ste 140, Durham, NC 27713
Image management system.

IMAGE PROCESSING SYSTEM *(cont'd)*

Hologic, Inc. 800-343-9729
35 Crosby Dr, Bedford, MA 01730
RADIOLOGICAL

Hologic|r2, Inc 866-243-2533
2585 Augustine Dr, Santa Clara, CA 95054
Medical imaging workstation.

Icad Inc 603-882-5200
245 Main St Ste 620, White Plains, NY 10601
Medical image processing software.

Icad Inc. 866-280-2239
98 Spit Brook Rd Ste 100, Nashua, NH 03062
Second Look Viewer, PrecisionPoint, Spectra/VividLook CADvue

Icardiogram, Incorporated 919-534-2150
333 E Six Forks Rd, Raleigh, NC 27609
Echoencoder.

Icrco Inc. 310-921-9559
2580 W 237th St, Torrance, CA 90505
Medical viewing and scanning software.

Imaging Sciences International, Llc 215-997-5666
1910 N Penn Rd, Hatfield, PA 19440
X-ray software.

Implant Logic Systems, Ltd. 516-295-1121
76 Spruce St, Cedarhurst, NY 11516
Dental implant surgery planning software.

Innovative Medical Solutions, Inc. 414-774-7614
N2462 W Miner Dr, Waupaca, WI 54981
Tele-echocardiography system.

Life Imaging Systems, Inc. 800-298-8664
195 Dufferin Ave, Unit 3, London N6A 1K7 Canada
3d ultrasound acquisition and postprocessing system

Lumedx Corp. 800-966-0669
110 110th Ave NE, Bellevue, WA 98004
Radiological

Marconi Medical Systems 800-323-0550
595 Miner Rd, Cleveland, OH 44143

Medical Manager Research & Development, Llc 386-462-2148
15151 NW 99th St, Alachua, FL 32615
Image scanning & viewing system.

Medical Metrics, Inc. 713-850-7500
4600 Post Oak Place Dr Ste 359, Houston, TX 77027
Image processing system.

Medical Metrx Solutions
12 Commerce Ave, West Lebanon, NH 03784
Image processing software.

Merlin Engineering Works, Inc. 800-227-1980
1888 Embarcadero Rd, Palo Alto, CA 94303
ME-959 UNISCAN digital scan converter. ME-509 DownScan LT provides video scan conversion from 1023-1125/30 (1249/25) to 525/30 (625/30) for standard video. ME-511 DownscanLX provides video scan conversion, SVGA progressive scan signals to 525-625 line standard video.

Mimvista Corp. 216-896-9798
25200 Chagrin Blvd Ste 200, Cleveland, OH 44122
Image processing software.

Mpacs, Llc. 608-827-7111
7601 Ganser Way, Madison, WI 53719
Picture archiving & communications systems.

Mri Cardiac Services, Incorporated 336-831-1908
8 W 3rd St Ste M9, Winston Salem, NC 27101
Workstation for viewing, organizing and analyzing cardiovascular MRI images in real time for immediate diagnosis and reporting.

Multi Imager Service, Inc 800-400-4549
13865 Magnolia Ave Bldg C, Chino, CA 91710
Founded in 1983, Multi Imager specializes in diagnostic-quality film imaging and digital imaging technologies, including film-based video imagers, wet-film-based laser imagers, dry-film imagers, digital acquisition/storage and transmission devices, computed radiography, PACS, and more. Multi Imager provides technical support and training, parts supply, and sales of new as well as refurbished equipment used with a broad range of modalities, including CT, MRI, ultrasound, nuclear medicine, and others.

Nbs Technologies Inc. 800-524-0419
70 Eisenhower Dr, Paramus, NJ 07652
Printers, digitized cameras, software, and ID systems.

IMAGE PROCESSING SYSTEM *(cont'd)*

Neurostar Solutions, Inc. 404-575-4222
75 5th St NW Ste 206, Atlanta, GA 30308
Pacs-picture archiving and communications system.

Obsidian Medical Technology, Inc. 832-767-9606
5108 Corona Covet, Pleasanton, CA 94588
Various types of picture archiving communications systems.

Optical Electronics, Inc. 520-889-8811
4455 S Park Ave Ste 106, Tucson, AZ 85714
Video imaging and processing units.

Pegasus Imaging Corp. 800-875-7009
4001 N Riverside Dr, Tampa, FL 33603
PICTools Medical

Penn Diagnostics 301-279-5958
14 Clemson Ct, Rockville, MD 20850
Medical imaging processing system.

Prism Clinical Imaging, Inc. 414-727-1930
851 S 70th St Ste 103, Milwaukee, WI 53214
Image processing software.

Problem Solving Concepts, Inc. 800-755-2150
8021 Knue Rd Ste 100, Indianapolis, IN 46250
Picture archiving and communications systems.

Resonance Innovations Llc 402-934-2650
10957 Lake Ridge Dr, Omaha, NE 68136
Image enhancement system.

Scimage, Inc. 866-724-6243
4916 El Camino Real Ste 200, Los Altos, CA 94022
Enterprise wide PACS

Segami Corporation 410-381-2311
8325 Guilford Rd Ste B, Columbia, MD 21046
Image processing system.

Shared P.E.T. Imaging, Llc 330-491-0480
4912 Higbee Ave NW, Nw Suite 100, Canton, OH 44718
Clarity pet.

Smith & Nephew Inc., Endoscopy Div. 978-749-1000
76 S Meridian Ave, Oklahoma City, OK 73107
Picture archiving and communications system.

Solos Endoscopy 800-388-6445
65 Sprague St # B, Boston/dedham Commerce Park, Boston, MA 02136
Picture archiving & communications system.

St. Jude Medical Atrial Fibrillation (Endocardial Solutions) 800-374-8038
1350 Energy Ln Ste 110, Saint Paul, MN 55108
Picture archiving and communication system-software.

Stallion Technologies Inc. 315-476-4330
1201 E Fayette St, Syracuse, NY 13210
Image-processing systems.

Stallion Technologies, Inc. 315-476-4330
1201 E Fayette St, Syracuse, NY 13210

Stryker Imaging 888-795-4624
1410 Lakeside Pkwy Ste 600, Flower Mound, TX 75028
Radiological image processing system.

Televere Systems 800-385-9593
1611 Center Ave, Janesville, WI 53546
Pacs.

Terarecon, Inc. 877-354-1100
2955 Campus Dr Ste 325, San Mateo, CA 94403
Image processing server.

Thinking Systems Corporation 727-217-0909
750 94th Ave N Ste 211, Saint Petersburg, FL 33702
Picture archiving and communications system.

Ti-Ba Enterprises, Inc. 585-247-1212
25 Hytec Cir, Rochester, NY 14606
Ti-Ba sells all the computed radiography (CR) products by Konica Minolta Medical Imaging and Radlink.

Titan Corporation/Systems & Imagery Division 800-622-8554
1200 Woody Burke Rd, PO Box 550, Melbourne, FL 32901
Medical imaging workstation.

Toshiba America Medical Systems 800-421-1968
2441 Michelle Dr, Tustin, CA 92780
Model XA-0220A--Efficiency/EPS Plus.

Universal Pacs, Inc. 225-766-9381
127 Albert Hart Dr, Baton Rouge, LA 70808
UniPACS workstation.

IMAGE PROCESSING SYSTEM *(cont'd)*

Uvp, Llc 800-452-6788
2066 W 11th St, Upland, CA 91786
Image acquisition systems. Image acquisition with CCD camera & zoom lens.

Varian Medical Systems, Oncology Systems 800 278-2747
911 Hansen Way, Bldg.3 M/S C-165, Palo Alto, CA 94304
Various types of image processing device.

Vassol, Inc. 312-601-4431
833 W Jackson Blvd Fl 8, Chicago, IL 60607
Mri flow analysis package.

Velopex International. 888-835-6739
105 E 17th St, Saint Cloud, FL 34769

Viatronix, Inc. 631-444-9700
25 Health Sciences Dr Ste 203, Stony Brook, NY 11790
Image processing system.

Virtual Radiologic Corporation 800-737-0610
11995 Singletree Ln Ste 500, Eden Prairie, MN 55344
vRad PACS; vRad Picture and Archiving System

Vision Chips, Inc. 949-362-0565
27671 La Paz Rd, Laguna Niguel, CA 92677
Ultrasound reporting and image archiving system.

Warsaw Orthopedic, Inc. 901-396-3133
2500 Silveus Xing, Warsaw, IN 46582
Imaging system.

Z-Kat, Inc. 954-927-2044
2903 Simms St, Hollywood, FL 33020
Acustar advanced surgical navigation system.

3dsharp, Inc. 412-648-9211
6425 Forward Ave, Pittsburgh, PA 15217
Medical image enhancement system.

IMAGER, X-RAY, ELECTROSTATIC *(Radiology) 90IXK*

Agfa Corporation 877-777-2432
PO Box 19048, 10 South Academy Street, Greenville, SC 29602

Eklin Medical Systems 408-492-0057
1605 Wyatt Dr, Santa Clara, CA 95054
Various models of x-ray systems.

Fujifilm Medical Systems Usa, Inc. 800-431-1850
419 West Ave, Stamford, CT 06902

Radiographic Digital Imaging, Inc. 310-921-9559
20406 Earl St, Torrance, CA 90503
Cobrascan CR-1 filmless X-ray digitizer.

IMAGER, X-RAY, SOLID STATE (FLAT PANEL/DIGITAL) *(Radiology) 90MQB*

Alara Inc. 800-410-2525
47505 Seabridge Dr, Fremont, CA 94538
CRYSTALVIEW T-100; CRYSTALVIEW T-110; CRYSTALVIEW T-SERIES CR SYSTEM

Canon Development Americas, Inc 949-932-3100
15955 Alton Pkwy, Irvine, CA 92618
CXDI-11, Canon X-ray Digital Radiography System, captures and produces digital images in three seconds and six seconds for next exposure, using amorphous silicon sensor.

Direct Radiography 302-631-2700
600 Technology Dr, Newark, DE 19702
Directray.

Dpix, Llc 650-842-9600
3406 Hillview Ave, Palo Alto, CA 94304

Ge Medical Systems, Llc 262-548-2355
3000 N Grandview Blvd, W-417, Waukesha, WI 53188
Various models of digital radiographic imaging systems.

Lakeshore Technologies Inc. 315-699-2975
7536 W Murray Dr, Cicero, NY 13039
Digital image processor.

Medelex, Inc. 408-774-0692
1170 Mountain View Alviso Rd, Sunnyvale, CA 94089
Digital radiography system.

Phoxxor 251-408-0208
5600 Commerce Blvd E # A, Mobile, AL 36619
Digital x-ray image receptor.

Radlink, Inc. 310-643-6900
2400 Marine Ave, Redondo Beach, CA 90278
Computed radiography.

Stallion Technologies, Inc. 315-476-4330
1201 E Fayette St, Syracuse, NY 13210

IMAGER, X-RAY, SOLID STATE (FLAT PANEL/DIGITAL) *(cont'd)*

Stereotaxis, Inc. 866-646-2346
4320 Forest Park Ave Ste 100, Saint Louis, MO 63108
X-ray system.

Thales Components Corporation 973-812-9000
40G Commerce Way, PO Box 540, Totowa, NJ 07512
Trixell family of Pixium flat-panel x-ray detectors for Radiographic or Real-time medical imaging.

Varian Medical Systems 800-544-4636
3100 Hansen Way, Palo Alto, CA 94304
Varian produces the PaxScan(tm) line of amorphous-silicon X-ray image detectors. Each PaxScan digital imager incorporates a flat panel amorphous-silicon sensor array, a command processor, a power supply, and all interconnecting cables.

Vidar Systems Corp. 703-471-7070
365 Herndon Pkwy, Herndon, VA 20170
Digital radiography system.

Virtual Imaging, Inc. 954-428-6191
720 S Powerline Rd Ste E, Deerfield Bch, FL 33442
Image-intensified fluoroscopic x-ray system.

IMMOBILIZER, ANKLE *(Orthopedics) 87RBF*

Alimed, Inc. 800-225-2610
297 High St, Dedham, MA 02026

Cropper Medical, Inc./Bio Skin 800-541-2455
240 E Hersey St Ste 2, Ashland, OR 97520
Trilok Ankle Brace with Footlok strap.

Formedica Ltd. 800-361-9671
1481 Rue Begin, St Laurent, QUE H4R 1V8 Canada
$3.00 per unit (standard).

Humane Restraint Co Inc 800-356-7472
912 Bethel Cir, Waunakee, WI 53597
Various types of ankle and other restraints.

Klm Laboratories, Inc. 800-556-3668
28280 Alta Vista Ave, Valencia, CA 91355
The Richie Brace is a custom-articulated ankle brace.

Medical Specialties, Inc. 800-582-4040
4600 Lebanon Rd, Mint Hill, NC 28227
ASO ankle stabilizer.

Pedifix, Inc. 800-424-5561
310 Guinea Rd, Brewster, NY 10509
Elastic ankle braces.

Protectair Inc. 800-235-7932
59 Eisenhower Ln S, Lombard, IL 60148

Tartan Orthopedics, Ltd. 888-287-1456
10651 Irma Dr Unit C, Northglenn, CO 80233
$18.00 per unit (standard).

Tetra Medical Supply Corp. 800-621-4041
6364 W Gross Point Rd, Niles, IL 60714

Zimmer Holdings, Inc. 800-613-6131
1800 W Center St, PO Box 708, Warsaw, IN 46580

IMMOBILIZER, ARM *(Orthopedics) 87RBG*

Cfi Medical Solutions (Contour Fabricators, Inc.) 810-750-5300
14241 N Fenton Rd, Fenton, MI 48430

Formedica Ltd. 800-361-9671
1481 Rue Begin, St Laurent, QUE H4R 1V8 Canada
$3.00 per unit (standard).

Inland Specialties, Inc. 800-741-0022
7655 Matoaka Rd, Sarasota, FL 34243
Forearm splint, padded or non-padded, in small, medium and large sizes; also available, Colles splint, padded or non-padded, in small, medium and large sizes.

Medical Specialties, Inc. 800-582-4040
4600 Lebanon Rd, Mint Hill, NC 28227
Wrist and forearm splints.

Mizuho Osi 800-777-4674
30031 Ahern Ave, Union City, CA 94587

Ross Disposable Products 800-649-6526
401 Traders Blvd E, Unit 10, Mississauga, ON L4Z 2H8 Canada

Scott Specialties, Inc./Cmo Inc./Ginny Inc. 800-255-7136
512 M St, Belleville, KS 66935

Tetra Medical Supply Corp. 800-621-4041
6364 W Gross Point Rd, Niles, IL 60714

Zimmer Holdings, Inc. 800-613-6131
1800 W Center St, PO Box 708, Warsaw, IN 46580

IMMOBILIZER, ARM *(cont'd)*

Zimmer Orthopaedic Surgical Products 800-321-5533
PO Box 10, 200 West Ohio Ave., Dover, OH 44622

IMMOBILIZER, CERVICAL *(Orthopedics) 87RBH*

Armstrong Medical Industries, Inc. 800-323-4220
575 Knightsbridge Pkwy, Lincolnshire, IL 60069

Bashaw Medical, Inc. 800-499-3857
4909 Mobile Hwy Ste B, Pensacola, FL 32506
BASHAW CID.

Bsn Medical, Inc 800-552-1157
5825 Carnegie Blvd, Charlotte, NC 28209
Variety of cervical collars available.

Depuy Mitek, Inc. 800-451-2006
325 Paramount Dr, Raynham, MA 02767

Formedica Ltd. 800-361-9671
1481 Rue Begin, St Laurent, QUE H4R 1V8 Canada
$6.00 per unit (standard).

Jerome Medical 800-257-8440
305 Harper Dr, Moorestown, NJ 08057
Halo Traction, Tong Traction

Morrison Medical 800-438-6677
3735 Paragon Dr, Columbus, OH 43228
The HEAD VISE reusable, waterproof & economical, or HEAD VISE II cardboard STICK BLOCKS (peel - stick & throwaway). HEAD BLOCKS disposable.

Ossur Americas 800-257-8440
1414 Metropolitan Ave, West Deptford, NJ 08066
Papoose Infant Spinal Immobilizer

Slawner Ltd., J. 514-731-3378
5713 Cote Des Neiges Rd., Montreal, QUE H3S 1Y7 Canada

Tetra Medical Supply Corp. 800-621-4041
6364 W Gross Point Rd, Niles, IL 60714

Zimmer Orthopaedic Surgical Products 800-321-5533
PO Box 10, 200 West Ohio Ave., Dover, OH 44622

IMMOBILIZER, ELBOW *(Orthopedics) 87RBI*

Alimed, Inc. 800-225-2610
297 High St, Dedham, MA 02026
Elbow orthosis.

Formedica Ltd. 800-361-9671
1481 Rue Begin, St Laurent, QUE H4R 1V8 Canada
$3.00 per unit (standard).

Inland Specialties, Inc. 800-741-0022
7655 Matoaka Rd, Sarasota, FL 34243
Posterior elbow splint, padded or non-padded, in small, medium and large sizes

Orthomotion Inc. 800-387-5139
901 Dillingham Rd., Pickering, ONT L1W 2Y5 Canada
E2 elbow CPM (continuous passive motion).

Restorative Care Of America Inc 800-627-1595
12221 33rd St N, Saint Petersburg, FL 33716
Gradually increases joint extension with static progressive settings. Kydex construction. Kodel or ortho-wick liners included.

Seattle Systems 360-697-5656
26296 12 Trees Ln NW Bldg 1, Poulsbo, WA 98370

Swb Elbow Brace, Ltd. 760-564-9853
56059 Winged Foot, La Quinta, CA 92253
Brace designed to limit extension of the elbow joint; allow joint to heal as activity continues; support the elbow joint laterally and be worn during activity.

Tartan Orthopedics, Ltd. 888-287-1456
10651 Irma Dr Unit C, Northglenn, CO 80233
$38.75 per unit (standard).

Tetra Medical Supply Corp. 800-621-4041
6364 W Gross Point Rd, Niles, IL 60714

Zimmer Holdings, Inc. 800-613-6131
1800 W Center St, PO Box 708, Warsaw, IN 46580

Zimmer Orthopaedic Surgical Products 800-321-5533
PO Box 10, 200 West Ohio Ave., Dover, OH 44622

IMMOBILIZER, INFANT (CIRCUMCISION BOARD)
(Orthopedics) 87RBJ

Brotherston Homecare Inc., Pxi Div. 800-695-9729
1388 Bridgewater Rd, Bensalem, PA 19020

Formedica Ltd. 800-361-9671
1481 Rue Begin, St Laurent, QUE H4R 1V8 Canada
$10.00 per unit (standard).

IMMOBILIZER, INFANT (CIRCUMCISION BOARD) *(cont'd)*

Olympic Medical Corp. 206-767-3500
5900 1st Ave S, Seattle, WA 98108
$174.50 per unit.

Schueler & Company, Inc. 516-487-1500
PO Box 528, Stratford, CT 06615

Tetra Medical Supply Corp. 800-621-4041
6364 W Gross Point Rd, Niles, IL 60714

IMMOBILIZER, KNEE *(Orthopedics) 87RBK*

Alimed, Inc. 800-225-2610
297 High St, Dedham, MA 02026

Bsn Medical, Inc 800-552-1157
5825 Carnegie Blvd, Charlotte, NC 28209
Variety of Knee Immobilizers available.

Cfi Medical Solutions (Contour Fabricators, Inc.) 810-750-5300
14241 N Fenton Rd, Fenton, MI 48430

Corflex, Inc. 800-426-7353
669 E Industrial Park Dr, Manchester, NH 03109
CKI, Compression Knee Immobilizer, provides compression, support, and immobilization.

Dalco International, Inc. 888-354-5515
8433 Glazebrook Ave, Richmond, VA 23228

Darco International, Inc. 800-999-8866
810 Memorial Blvd, Huntington, WV 25701

Fla Orthopedics, Inc. 800-327-4110
2881 Corporate Way, Miramar, FL 33025

Formedica Ltd. 800-361-9671
1481 Rue Begin, St Laurent, QUE H4R 1V8 Canada
$20.00 per unit (standard).

Freeman Manufacturing Company 800-253-2091
900 W Chicago Rd, PO Box J, Sturgis, MI 49091

Information Health Network 800-443-0613
PO Box 23056, Lansing, MI 48909
3X10=0 Full Extension Knee device assists patient in achieving full extension after surgery or trauma.

Inland Specialties, Inc. 800-741-0022
7655 Matoaka Rd, Sarasota, FL 34243
Posterior, tibia and fibula splints, padded and non-padded available in sizes small medium and large; posterior patella splints available in knee and femur lengths.

Jobri Llc 800-432-2225
520 N Division St, Konawa, OK 74849
MOR-LOC.

Larkotex Company 800-972-3037
1002 Olive St, Texarkana, TX 75501

Lohmann & Rauscher, Inc. 800-279-3863
6001 SW 6th Ave Ste 101, Topeka, KS 66615

Ortholine 800-243-3351
13 Chapel St, Norwalk, CT 06850
Deluxe, Mid-line & Economy; Universal and Sized. Pediatric(8') to Tall (26')

Osborn Medical Corp. 800-535-5865
100 W Main St N, PO Box 324, Utica, MN 55979
Knee Immobilzer and stump protector for below knee amputation, immediate post-op.

Restorative Care Of America Inc 800-627-1595
12221 33rd St N, Saint Petersburg, FL 33716
Tri-panel design accomodates multiple circumference sizes. Constructed of washable foam liner and aluminum stays. Pediatric to adult sizes.

Royce Medical 800-521-0601
742 Pancho Rd, Camarillo, CA 93012
Orthopaedic supports and braces. Wrist splints, ankle braces, short leg walking casts, back supports, knee immobilizers and knee supports.

Scott Specialties, Inc./Cmo Inc./Ginny Inc. 800-255-7136
512 M St, Belleville, KS 66935

Seattle Systems 360-697-5656
26296 12 Trees Ln NW Bldg 1, Poulsbo, WA 98370

Signal Medical Corporation 800-246-6324
1000 Des Peres Rd Ste 140, Saint Louis, MO 63131
Positioner, including slide block, boot assembly, base plate, and end stop.

Slawner Ltd., J. 514-731-3378
5713 Cote Des Neiges Rd., Montreal, QUE H3S 1Y7 Canada

IMMOBILIZER, KNEE *(cont'd)*

Sroufe Healthcare Products Llc 888-894-4171
PO Box 347, 601 Sroufe St., Ligonier, IN 46767
Canvas, vinyl, foam laminate, and elastic.

Tartan Orthopedics, Ltd. 888-287-1456
10651 Irma Dr Unit C, Northglenn, CO 80233
$14.50 per unit (standard); 15, 30 and 45 deg. angle knee immobilizers; Neoprene knee sleeve, $11.90/unit.

Tetra Medical Supply Corp. 800-621-4041
6364 W Gross Point Rd, Niles, IL 60714

Total Care 800-334-3802
PO Box 1661, Rockville, MD 20849

U.S. Orthotics, Inc. 800-825-5228
8605 Palm River Rd, Tampa, FL 33619
Universal circumference with various heights.

Zimmer Holdings, Inc. 800-613-6131
1800 W Center St, PO Box 708, Warsaw, IN 46580

Zimmer Orthopaedic Surgical Products 800-321-5533
PO Box 10, 200 West Ohio Ave., Dover, OH 44622

IMMOBILIZER, SHOULDER *(Orthopedics) 87RBL*

Alimed, Inc. 800-225-2610
297 High St, Dedham, MA 02026

Baron Medical Supply 888-702-2766
709 Grand St, Brooklyn, NY 11211

Corflex, Inc. 800-426-7353
669 E Industrial Park Dr, Manchester, NH 03109

Darco International, Inc. 800-999-8866
810 Memorial Blvd, Huntington, WV 25701

Formedica Ltd. 800-361-9671
1481 Rue Begin, St Laurent, QUE H4R 1V8 Canada
$12.00 per unit (standard).

Hermell Products, Inc. 800-233-2342
9 Britton Dr, PO Box 7345, Bloomfield, CT 06002

Mizuho Osi 800-777-4674
30031 Ahern Ave, Union City, CA 94587
Shoulder abduction splint (contoured foam).

Omni Life Science, Inc. 800-448-OMNI
1390 Decision St, Vista, CA 92081
Functional Arm Brace for post-surgical immobilization, adjustable flexion/extension and support.

Orthomotion Inc. 800-387-5139
901 Dillingham Rd., Pickering, ONT L1W 2Y5 Canada
Continuous passive motion.

Protectair Inc. 800-235-7932
59 Eisenhower Ln S, Lombard, IL 60148

Scott Specialties, Inc./Cmo Inc./Ginny Inc. 800-255-7136
512 M St, Belleville, KS 66935

Segufix Systems Ltd. 506-328-8636
110 Queen St., Woodstock, NB E7M-2M6 Canada

Tartan Orthopedics, Ltd. 888-287-1456
10651 Irma Dr Unit C, Northglenn, CO 80233
$6.25 per unit (standard).

Tetra Medical Supply Corp. 800-621-4041
6364 W Gross Point Rd, Niles, IL 60714

U.S. Orthotics, Inc. 800-825-5228
8605 Palm River Rd, Tampa, FL 33619
Soft foam supports with Velcro closures.

Zimmer Holdings, Inc. 800-613-6131
1800 W Center St, PO Box 708, Warsaw, IN 46580

Zimmer Orthopaedic Surgical Products 800-321-5533
PO Box 10, 200 West Ohio Ave., Dover, OH 44622

IMMOBILIZER, THERAPY, RADIATION *(Radiology) 90WUB*

Diacor, Inc. 800-342-2679
3191 Valley St Ste 100A, Salt Lake City, UT 84109
$2,100.00 for RADASSIST bilateral immobilization board. Model RAD-1 for lower lung and abdomen simulation & treatment.

Edwin Corp. 1-888-323-3941
425 Hill Dr Apt H, Glendale, CA 91206
Pediatric immobilizer for medical procedures and x-ray examinations.

Smithers Medical Products, Inc. 330-497-0690
4850 Hossler Dr NW, North Canton, OH 44720
Patient immobilization devices for diagnostic & therapeutic radiology. CT, MRI, PET.

IMMOBILIZER, UPPER BODY *(Orthopedics) 87WUW*

Alimed, Inc. 800-225-2610
297 High St, Dedham, MA 02026

Depuy Mitek, Inc. 800-451-2006
325 Paramount Dr, Raynham, MA 02767
HALO system.

O&M Enterprise 847-258-4515
641 Chelmsford Ln, Elk Grove Village, IL 60007
IMMOBILIZER UPPER/LOWER BODY

IMMOBILIZER, WRIST/HAND *(Orthopedics) 87RBM*

Alimed, Inc. 800-225-2610
297 High St, Dedham, MA 02026

Bsn Medical, Inc 800-552-1157
5825 Carnegie Blvd, Charlotte, NC 28209
Variety of wrist splints available.

Cfi Medical Solutions (Contour Fabricators, Inc.) 810-750-5300
14241 N Fenton Rd, Fenton, MI 48430

Corflex, Inc. 800-426-7353
669 E Industrial Park Dr, Manchester, NH 03109
SIGNATURE wrist splints provide immobilization and support for injured or weak wrists.

Darco International, Inc. 800-999-8866
810 Memorial Blvd, Huntington, WV 25701

Fla Orthopedics, Inc. 800-327-4110
2881 Corporate Way, Miramar, FL 33025

Formedica Ltd. 800-361-9671
1481 Rue Begin, St Laurent, QUE H4R 1V8 Canada
$7.00 per unit (standard).

Hand Biomechanics Lab, Inc. 800-522-5778
77 Scripps Dr Ste 104, Sacramento, CA 95825
AGEE WRISTJACK Fracture Reduction System, a fracture reduction system for distal radius fractures. Also, the AGEE DIGIT WIDGET, an external fixation system to reverse PIP flexion contractures of the fingers.

Humane Restraint Co Inc 800-356-7472
912 Bethel Cir, Waunakee, WI 53597
Various types of wrist and other restraints.

Inland Specialties, Inc. 800-741-0022
7655 Matoaka Rd, Sarasota, FL 34243
Forearm splint, Colles splint, Cockup splint, Mason Allen splints, Bar Colles splint, Metacarpal splint, and Palm Metacarpal splint; padded and non-padded; available in small, medium and large sizes.

Maramed Orthopedic Systems 800-327-5830
2480 W 82nd St, No. 8, Hialeah, FL 33016

Medical Specialties, Inc. 800-582-4040
4600 Lebanon Rd, Mint Hill, NC 28227
Beige elastic wrist splint.

Orthomotion Inc. 800-387-5139
901 Dillingham Rd., Pickering, ONT L1W 2Y5 Canada
Continuous passive motion.

Slawner Ltd., J. 514-731-3378
5713 Cote Des Neiges Rd., Montreal, QUE H3S 1Y7 Canada

Tartan Orthopedics, Ltd. 888-287-1456
10651 Irma Dr Unit C, Northglenn, CO 80233
$11.50 per unit (standard) and wrist wrap made of Neoprene; $10.95 for carpal tunnel motion limiting device.

Tetra Medical Supply Corp. 800-621-4041
6364 W Gross Point Rd, Niles, IL 60714

Zimmer Holdings, Inc. 800-613-6131
1800 W Center St, PO Box 708, Warsaw, IN 46580

Zimmer Orthopaedic Surgical Products 800-321-5533
PO Box 10, 200 West Ohio Ave., Dover, OH 44622

IMMUNOASSAY, OTHER *(Toxicology) 91WQE*

American Diagnostica, Inc. 888-234-4435
500 West Ave, Stamford, CT 06902
ACTIBIND; Tissue factor assay and tissue factor pathway inhibitor; ELISA and cytochemistry test kits.

Bangs Laboratories, Inc. 800-387-0672
9025 Technology Dr, Fishers, IN 46038
Cell separation, chemiluminescent and other immunoassays. Magnetic content from 12 to 60%. Size 1-8um.

Beckman Coulter, Inc. 800-742-2345
250 S Kraemer Blvd, PO Box 8000, Brea, CA 92821

IMMUNOASSAY, OTHER *(cont'd)*

Binding Site, Inc., The 800-633-4484
5889 Oberlin Dr Ste 101, San Diego, CA 92121
IgE ELISA; SCD23 ELISA, dsDNA ELISA.

Biomedical Technologies, Inc. 781-344-9942
378 Page St, Stoughton, MA 02072
MID-TACT Osteocalcin ELISA Kit $325.00/kit Sandwich EIA for human osteocalcin. Measures both Intact (I-49) and major N-terminal fragment (I-43). Catalog No. BT-460 (96 well). INTACT Osteocalcin ELISA Kit $385.00 Sandwich EIA for human osteocalcin. Measures only (I-49) Intact osteocalcin. Catalog No. BT-460 (96 well). Human Epidermal Growth Factor (EGF) ELISA Kit measures human EGF from urine directly. Catalog No. BT-720 for $325/kit (96 well).

Biomerica, Inc. 800-854-3002
17571 Von Karman Ave, Irvine, CA 92614
#7010 Isletest-ICA and Isletest-IAA for detection of Islet cell auto-antibodies and insulin auto-antibodies; also, #1052 free alpha subunit RIA skit - double Ab; ALLERQUANT, 90G detection of IgG antibodies to 90 foods.

Biomerieux Inc. 800-682-2666
100 Rodolphe St, Durham, NC 27712
MDA D-DIMER is a homogeneous latex particle based immunoassay (LIA) developed for the quantitative determination of cross-linked fibrin degradation products containing the D-Dimer domain in citrated human plasma.

Diamedix Corp. 800-327-4565
2140 N Miami Ave, Miami, FL 33127
EIA for autoimmune and infectious disease, including: TPO, TG, MPO, PR-3, ANA, DNA, Immune Complex, CH50, Rheumatoid Factor, DNP, anti-SM, SSA, SSB, RNP, Scl-70, Jo-1; B2-Glycoprotein Screen and IgG/IgM; Cardiolipin Screen, IgA and IgG/IgM; Gliadin IgG and IgA, Toxoplasma IgG and IgM; CMV IgG and IgM, Rubella IgG and IgM, Herpes 1 and 2 IgG and IgM, H. pylori, VZV IgG, EBV, Lyme IgM and IgG/IgM, Mycoplasma, Syphilis, and Measles.

Fona Diagnostics International 800-249-4897
855 Matheson Blvd E, Unit 14, Mississauga, ON L4W 4L6 Canada
ELISA test kits.

Fujirebio Diagnostics, Inc. (Fdi) 877-861-7246
201 Great Valley Pkwy, Malvern, PA 19355
SERODIA-AMC particle-agglutination assay for the detection and titration of anti-microsomal antibodies in human serum. SERODIA-ATG particle-agglutination assay for the detection and titration of anti-thyroglobulin antibodies in human serum.

Oxis International, Inc. 800-547-3686
468 N Camden Dr Fl 2, Beverly Hills, CA 90210
Fluorescence polarization immunoassay, amikane, digitoxin, phenytomin, quinadine, and vancomycim.

Raichem, Division Of Hemagen Diagnostics, Inc. 800-438-6100
8225 Mercury Ct, San Diego, CA 92111
SPIA Serum protein immunoassay, turbidimetric end-point method for assay of apolipoprotein A-1 or B read at 340nm, manual or automated procedure, no predilution of components required.

Seradyn, Inc. 800-428-4072
7998 Georgetown Rd Ste 1000, Indianapolis, IN 46268
Giardia ELISA-antigen detection; Cryptosporidium ELISA-antigen detection; ASO latex slide test; CRP latex slide test. Also available, COLOR VUE Seradyn Color Vue E coli. ELISA antigen detection for E coli in stool samples.

Sun Biomedical Laboratories, Inc. 888-440-8388
604 Vpr Center, 1001 Lower Landing Road, Blackwood, NJ 08012
Rapid assay for metabolites of marijuana, cocaine, opiates, methamphetamine, amphetamine, PCP, barbiturates, TCA, benzodiazibens, and methadone in different test configurations.

Wampole Laboratories 800-257-9525
2 Research Way, Princeton, NJ 08540
CMV CAP M, EBNA-1 IgG, Rube CAP M, Toxo IgG, Toxo IgM, Toxo CAP M, Varicella-zoster IgG, Varicella-zoster IgM, Infectious disease ELISA kits available. Autoimmune disease ELISA kits available are Cardiolopin IgG, Cardiolipin IgM, Cardiolipin IgA, Cardiolipin IgG,A,M, MPO, PR-3 Ribosomal P, ENA combined screen, Jo-1, SCI-70, SS-A (Ro), SS-B (La), dsDNA, Histone, and Mitochondria.

IMMUNOCHEMICAL, LYSOZYME (MURAMIDASE)
(Chemistry) 75JMR

Biomedical Technologies, Inc. 781-344-9942
378 Page St, Stoughton, MA 02072
Human Lysozyme EIA Kit (BT-630), $350/kit (96 well).

IMMUNOCHEMICAL, LYSOZYME (MURAMIDASE) *(cont'd)*

Dako North America, Inc 805-566-6655
6392 Via Real, Carpinteria, CA 93013

IMMUNOCHEMICAL, THYROGLOBULIN AUTOANTIBODY
(Immunology) 82JNL

Biomerica, Inc. 800-854-3002
17571 Von Karman Ave, Irvine, CA 92614
#7015 anti-thyroglobulin ELISA test.

Hycor Biomedical, Inc. 800-382-2527
7272 Chapman Ave, Garden Grove, CA 92841
Tg & tpo autoimmune kits.

Nichols Institute Diagnostics 949-940-7200
1311 Calle Batido, San Clemente, CA 92673
Anti-tpo.

IMMUNOCHEMICAL, TRANSFERRIN *(Immunology) 82JNM*

Nichols Institute Diagnostics 949-940-7200
1311 Calle Batido, San Clemente, CA 92673
Stfr.

Ramco Laboratories, Inc. 281-313-1200
4100 Greenbriar Dr Ste 200, Stafford, TX 77477
Transferrin Receptor Assay - enzyme immunoassay for quantifying the level of transferrin receptors in human serum or plasma.

IMMUNODIFFUSION EQUIPMENT (AGAR CUTTER)
(Chemistry) 75RBN

Bio-Rad Laboratories, Life Science Group 800-424-6723
2000 Alfred Nobel Dr, Hercules, CA 94547

Cadence Science Inc. 888-717-7677
1979 Marcus Ave Ste 215, New Hyde Park, NY 11042

Helena Laboratories 409-842-3714
PO Box 752, Beaumont, TX 77704

IMMUNODIFFUSION METHOD, IMMUNOGLOBULINS (G, A, M)
(Chemistry) 75CGM

Biomerieux Inc. 800-682-2666
100 Rodolphe St, Durham, NC 27712

Meridian Bioscience, Inc. 800-696-0739
3471 River Hills Dr, Cincinnati, OH 45244
Fungal Immunodiffusion System for the detection of antibodies to Aspergillus, Coccidioides, Blastomyces and Histoplasma.

IMMUNODIFFUSION, PROTEIN FRACTIONATION
(Chemistry) 75JQK

Kent Laboratories, Inc. 360-398-8641
777 Jorgensen Pl, Bellingham, WA 98226
Apolioprotein A-1 or B radial immunodiffusion kit.

IMMUNOELECTROPHORETIC, IMMUNOGLOBULINS, (G, A, M)
(Chemistry) 75CFF

Beckman Coulter, Inc. 800-742-2345
250 S Kraemer Blvd, PO Box 8000, Brea, CA 92821

Carolina Liquid Chemistries Corp. 800-471-7272
510 W Central Ave Ste C, Brea, CA 92821
Immunoglobulins.

Dako North America, Inc 805-566-6655
6392 Via Real, Carpinteria, CA 93013

Helena Laboratories 409-842-3714
PO Box 752, Beaumont, TX 77704

IMMUNOFLUORESCENCE EQUIPMENT *(Immunology) 82RBO*

Bio-Rad Laboratories, Life Science Group 800-424-6723
2000 Alfred Nobel Dr, Hercules, CA 94547

Labo America, Inc. 510-445-1257
920 Auburn Ct, Fremont, CA 94538

IMMUNOFLUORESCENT ASSAY, T. CRUZI *(Microbiology) 83MIV*

Ivd Research, Inc. 760-929-7744
5909 Sea Lion Pl Ste D, Carlsbad, CA 92010
Trypanosoma cruzi serum elisa.

United Biotech, Inc. 650-961-2910
211 S Whisman Rd Ste E, Mountain View, CA 94041
ELISA for detecting T. Cruzi (Chagas IgG & IgM)

IMMUNOHISTOCHEMICAL REAGENT, ANTIBODY (MONOCLONAL OR POLYCLONAL) TO P63 PROTEIN IN NUCLEUS OF PROSTATIC BASAL CELLS *(Hematology) 81NTR*

Spring Bioscience 510-979-9460
46755 Fremont Blvd, Fremont, CA 94538

IMMUNOHISTOCHEMISTRY ANTIBODY ASSAY, C-KIT
(Hematology) 81NKF

Ventana Medical Systems, Inc. 800-227-2155
1910 E Innovation Park Dr, Oro Valley, AZ 85755
C-kit antibody.

IMMUNOHISTOCHEMISTRY ASSAY, ANTIBODY, ESTROGEN RECEPTOR *(Pathology) 88MYA*

Cell Marque Corp. 916-746-8977
6600 Sierra College Blvd, Rocklin, CA 95677
Various.

Ventana Medical Systems, Inc. 800-227-2155
1910 E Innovation Park Dr, Oro Valley, AZ 85755
Immunohistochemistry antibody assay, estrogen receptor.

IMMUNOHISTOCHEMISTRY ASSAY, ANTIBODY, PROGESTERONE RECEPTOR *(Pathology) 88MXZ*

Cell Marque Corp. 916-746-8977
6600 Sierra College Blvd, Rocklin, CA 95677
Various.

Ventana Medical Systems, Inc. 800-227-2155
1910 E Innovation Park Dr, Oro Valley, AZ 85755
Immunohistochemistry antibody assay, progesterone receptor.

IMMUNOHISTOCHEMISTRY REAGENTS AND KITS
(Pathology) 88NJT

Advanced Medical Science & Technology, Llc 410-628-1856
1 Stonegate Ct, Cockeysville, MD 21030
(cell & tissue)hpv broad spectrum capsid l1 ihc kit.

Biocare Medical, Llc 925-603-8003
4040 Pike Ln, Concord, CA 94520
Immunohistochemistry reagents.

Diagnostic Biosystems 925-484-3350
1020 Serpentine Ln Ste 114, Pleasanton, CA 94566

Lab Vision Corp. 510-991-2800
47777 Warm Springs Blvd, Fremont, CA 94539
Various immunohistochemistry reagents & kits.

Richard-Allan Scientific 269-544-5628
4481 Campus Dr, Kalamazoo, MI 49008
Various immunohistochemistry reagents & kits.

Scytek Laboratories, Inc. 435-755-9848
205 S 600 W, Logan, UT 84321

Tripath Imaging, Inc. 919-206-7140
780 Plantation Dr, Burlington, NC 27215
Ihc reagents and kits.

Ventana Medical Systems, Inc. 800-227-2155
1910 E Innovation Park Dr, Oro Valley, AZ 85755
Various immunohistochemistry reagents & kits.

IMPACTOR *(Orthopedics) 87HWA*

Abbott Spine, Inc. 847-937-6100
12708 Riata Vista Cir Ste B-100, Austin, TX 78727
Impactor.

Biomet, Inc. 574-267-6639
56 E Bell Dr, PO Box 587, Warsaw, IN 46582
Various types of orthopedic impactors.

Centinel Spine Inc. 952-885-0500
505 Park Ave Fl 14, New York, NY 10022
STALIF C Slap Hammer

George Tiemann & Co. 800-843-6266
25 Plant Ave, Hauppauge, NY 11788

Holmed Corporation 508-238-3351
40 Norfolk Ave, South Easton, MA 02375

Kmedic 800-955-0559
190 Veterans Dr, Northvale, NJ 07647

Lenox-Maclaren Surgical Corp. 720-890-9660
657 S Taylor Ave Ste A, Colorado Technology Center
Louisville, CO 80027
Impactor.

Medtronic Sofamor Danek Usa, Inc. 901-396-3133
4340 Swinnea Rd, Memphis, TN 38118
Impactor.

Nobel Biocare Usa, Llc 800-579-6515
22715/22725 Savi Ranch Parkway, Yorba Linda, CA 92887
Surgical instrument.

Orthogenesis, Inc. 530-672-8560
4315 Product Dr # C, Cameron Park, CA 95682
Impactor for placement of various sizes of acetabular cups.

IMPACTOR *(cont'd)*

Small Bone Innovations, Inc. 215-428-1791
1380 S Pennsylvania Ave, Morrisville, PA 19067
Impactor.

Spine Wave, Inc. 203-944-9494
2 Enterprise Dr Ste 302, Shelton, CT 06484
Mallet.

Stryker Spine 866-457-7463
2 Pearl Ct, Allendale, NJ 07401

Warsaw Orthopedic, Inc. 901-396-3133
2500 Silveus Xing, Warsaw, IN 46582
Impactor.

Zimmer Holdings, Inc. 800-613-6131
1800 W Center St, PO Box 708, Warsaw, IN 46580

Zimmer Spine, Inc. 800-655-2614
7375 Bush Lake Rd, Minneapolis, MN 55439
Impactor.

Zimmer Trabecular Metal Technology 800-613-6131
10 Pomeroy Rd, Parsippany, NJ 07054
Bayonet impactor handle.

IMPLANT, ABSORBABLE (SCLERAL BUCKLING METHOD)
(Ophthalmology) 86HQJ

Labtician Ophthalmics, Inc. 800-265-8391
2140 Winston Park Dr., Unit 6, Oakville, ONTAR L6H 5V5 Canada
Labtician retinal implants (for scleral-buckling method).

Mira, Inc. 508-278-7877
414 Quaker Hwy, Uxbridge, MA 01569
Various sizes of sterile and non-sterile implants.

IMPLANT, COCHLEAR *(Ear/Nose/Throat) 77MCM*

Advanced Bionics Corp. 800-678-2575
12740 San Fernando Rd, Sylmar, CA 91342
Cochlear implant.

Cochlear Americas 303-790-9010
400 Inverness Pkwy Ste 400, Englewood, CO 80112
Nucleus Freedom cochlear implant system consisting of the Nucleus Freedom Contour Advance implant, Freedom ear level and bodyworn speech processors.

Jedmed Instruments Co. 314-845-3770
5416 Jedmed Ct, Saint Louis, MO 63129

IMPLANT, COLLAGEN (NON-AESTHETIC USE) *(Surgery) 79LMI*

C. R. Bard, Inc., Bard Urological Div. 888-367-2273
13183 Harland Dr NE, Covington, GA 30014

Lacrimedics, Inc. 360-376-7095
9 Hope Ln, Eastsound, WA 98245
Dissolvable lacrimal plug.

Tipp Machine & Tool, Inc. 937-387-0880
4201 Little York Rd, Dayton, OH 45414

IMPLANT, COLLAGEN, DERMAL (AESTHETIC USE)
(Surgery) 79LMH

Artes Medical Inc. 888-278-3345
5870 Pacific Center Blvd, San Diego, CA 92121
Various types of dermal inplants.

C. R. Bard, Inc., Bard Urological Div. 888-367-2273
13183 Harland Dr NE, Covington, GA 30014

Genzyme Corporation 617-252-7500
1125 Pleasantview Ter, Ridgefield, NJ 07657
Implant, dermal for aesthetic use.

Suneva Medical, Inc. 858-550-9999
5870 Pacific Center Blvd, San Diego, CA 92121
ArteFill; Bellafill

Uroplasty, Inc. 952-426-6140
5420 Feltl Rd, Minnetonka, MN 55343

IMPLANT, CORNEAL *(Ophthalmology) 86LQE*

Addition Technology, Inc. 847-297-8419
950 Lee St Ste 210, Des Plaines, IL 60016
INTACS prescription inserts reshape the cornea reducing nearsightedness and astigmatism associated with Keratoconus to return tolerence to contact lenses and delay or eliminate the need for a cornea transplant. Intacs are also approved to correct mild nearsightedness without permanent removal of corneal tissue in the central optic zone.

Revision Optics 949-707-2740
25651 Atlantic Ocean Dr Ste A1, Lake Forest, CA 92630
Vue+

IMPLANT, ENDOSSEOUS *(Dental And Oral) 76DZE*

Altiva Corp. 866-425-8482
9800 Southern Pine Blvd Ste I, Charlotte, NC 28273
Dental implant.

Astra Tech Inc 617-871-2783
25 1st St, --, Cambridge, MA 02141
Various types of sterile and non-sterile custom abutments and accessories.

Basic Dental Implant Systems, Inc. 505-884-1922
3321 Columbia Dr NE, Albuquerque, NM 87107
Implant kit & tool kit.

Bicon, Llc 800-882-4266
501 Arborway Fl 2, Boston, MA 02130
Bicon.

Biomet 3i 800-342-5454
4555 Riverside Dr, Palm Beach Gardens, FL 33410
Various endosseous implants and abutments including the NanoTite™ Implant,the NanoTite Tapered Implant and the Certain® PREVAIL® Implant with the Certain® QuickSeat Connection®.

Blue Sky Bio, Llc 847-548-8499
888 E Belvidere Rd Ste 212, Grayslake, IL 60030
Dental implant, endosseous, accessories and instruments.

Crystal Medical Technology 205-733-0901
153 Cahaba Valley Pkwy, Pelham, AL 35124
Dental implant.

Danlin Products, Inc. 505-884-1922
3321 Columbia Dr NE, Albuquerque, NM 87107
Design and manufacture custom medical products. GMP approved.

Deringer-Ney, Inc. 860-242-2281
2 Douglas St, Ney Industrial Park, Bloomfield, CT 06002
Dental Implants, Copings and Screws

Diamodent 714-632-3206
2737 E Regal Park Dr, Anaheim, CA 92806
Ucla & universal abutments.

Dio Usa 213-300-7979
3435 Wilshire Blvd Ste 2210, Los Angeles, CA 90010
Implant system.

Duo-Dent Dental Implant Systems Llc. 800-386-3368
340 W Butterfield Rd Ste 2A, Elmhurst, IL 60126
Duo-Dent Surgical-Prosthetic Kit.

Impladent Ltd. 800-526-9343
19845 Foothill Ave, Hollis, NY 11423
76DZE Implant, Endosseous Class III: Impladent Ltd. manufactures the LaminOss® Osteocompressive Immediate-Load Implant System, featuring one- and two-piece implant modalities. Sinusoidal thread design and aggressive surface provide greater horizontal load-bearing areas to maximize bone interface and reduce stresses. Utilizing the science of osteocompression via sequential surgical technique, bone is laminated during insertion, immediately stabilizing the implant and providing your patient immediate function the day of placement. LaminOss® offers 4 implant designs, in 2 diameters and 4 lengths, with removable morse-taper abutments. Each two-piece implant costs $160.00, and one-piece implants are $190.00 each. Straight abutments and angled abutments are available from $60.00-$66.00. The new SuperSplintTM immediate-splinting chairside prosthetic system offers a prefabricated superstructure for time-saving, cost-effective full-lower existing denture restoration the day of implant surgery.

Implant Center Of The Palm Beaches 561-627-5560
824 US Highway 1 Ste 370, North Palm Beach, FL 33408

Imtec, A 3m Company 800-879-9799
2401 N Commerce St, IMTEC Plaza, Ardmore, OK 73401
Mini Dental iplant and traditional implants.

Intra-Lock International 561-447-8282
6560 W Rogers Cir Ste 24, Boca Raton, FL 33487
Dental implant device.

Microcision Llc 800-264-3811
5805 Keystone St, Philadelphia, PA 19135

Nobel Biocare Usa, Llc 800-579-6515
22715/22725 Savi Ranch Parkway, Yorba Linda, CA 92887
Endosseous dental implant, components & accessories.

O Company 800-228-0477
600 Paisano St NE, Albuquerque, NM 87123
Contract manufacturer of dental implant parts. Attachments for endosseous implants also available.

IMPLANT, ENDOSSEOUS *(cont'd)*

Oco Inc. 800-228-0477
600 Paisano St NE Ste A, Albuquerque, NM 87123
Dental implant.

Oratronics, Inc. 212-986-0050
405 Lexington Ave, New York, NY 10174
Implant endosseous.

Ortho Organizers, Inc. 760-448-8730
1822 Aston Ave, Carlsbad, CA 92008
Implant, endosseous, root-form.

Pacific Implant, Inc. 707-764-5602
920 Rio Dell Ave, Rio Dell, CA 95562
Ramus frame implant; single tooth implant; ramus blade.

Quantum Bioengineering, Ltd. 954-474-4707
7951 SW 6th St, Plantation, FL 33324
Dental implant.

Renew Biocare Corp. 415-367-3646
1001 Bayhill Dr Fl 2, San Bruno, CA 94066
Various.

Renick Ent., Inc. 561-863-4183
1211 W 13th St, Riviera Beach, FL 33404
The complete Cal-form dental line: implants, attachments, drills, surgical kits.

Speedent Dental Supplies 800-706-0644
9591 Central Ave, Montclair, CA 91763
Dental abutments & supplies.

Sterngold 800-243-9942
23 Frank Mossberg Dr, PO Box 2967, Attleboro, MA 02703
IMPLA-MED; External hex titanium screw and cylinder forms. ERA Implant

Straumann Manufacturing, Inc. 978-747-2575
60 Minuteman Rd, Andover, MA 01810
Various implants,accessories and instruments for dental implant system.

Titan Implants, Inc. 1-866-439-0470
18 Columbia Ave, Bergenfield, NJ 07621
Titan Compatible Implants,Attachment & Accessories with Noble-Biocare (NBC) implants, ITI implant, Titan Implants Generation-1 (TIG1) exclusive implant design,3i implants(internal and external),Zimmer(interenal and external),Astra implant, Bicon implants, and Friadent, (Internal and Xive TG)

Vident 800-828-3839
3150 E Birch St, Brea, CA 92821
IMPAC. Abutments for implants, implant accessories and tools for use with implant manufacturer's products.

Zimmer Dental, Inc. 800-854-7019
1900 Aston Ave, Carlsbad, CA 92008
Tapered Screw-Vent® dental implants feature the patented Fixture Mount/Transfer and internal hex connection with friction-fit abutments assures a reliable restoration. The tapered body enhances initial stability while allowing placement in even the most challenging locations. The Screw-Vent® dental implant system offers three prosthetic platforms and a wide selection of restorative components for maximum versatility and optimal esthetics. The platforms are 3.5mm, 4.5mm and 5.7mm. Screw-Vent's friction-fit abutments form a virtual 'cold-weld' when assembled with the implant's internal hex, virtually eliminating micromovement, the leading cause of screw loosening. AdVent™ dental implant is the single-stage solution that minimizes chair time and lessens patient trauma. The immediate loading protocol for the edentulous mandible gives patients function and esthetics with as little as one visit. Its tapered design enhances initial stability, and the internal hex connection with friction-fit abutments assures a reliable restoration. Tapered SwissPlus™ is the single-stage implant is packaged with an all-in-one Fixture Mount/Transfer that can be used for insertion, impression taking and as a customized final abutment. The self-tapping flutes eliminate a step in the placement process, while the double lead threads provide faster implant insertion. The tapered body increases initial stability in soft bone, and a narrow diameter platform allows for use in tight interdental spaces.

IMPLANT, ENDOSSEOUS (BONE FILLING AND/OR AUGMENTATION) *(Dental And Oral) 76LYC*

Bioform Medical, Inc. 262-835-3323
4133 Courtney Rd Ste 10, Franksville, WI 53126
Bone filler.

IMPLANT, ENDOSSEOUS (BONE FILLING AND/OR AUGMENTATION) *(cont'd)*

Biomet 3i 800-342-5454
4555 Riverside Dr, Palm Beach Gardens, FL 33410
OsseoGuard® Resorbable Collagen Membrane-The Protection You Need To Grow-- Biogran® Resorbable Synthetic Bone Graft-The Ideal Graft Material Because It Is Effective, Resorbable And Easy-- Safescraper® Cortical Bone Scraper/Collector,The Simple Way To Natural Value-- University of Miami Allograft(DFDBA & FDBA)-The options you want.The results you expect.The safety you demand.--Calcigen(TM)Oral-The Strength You Need For The Stability You Want

Biomet Microfixation Inc. 800-874-7711
1520 Tradeport Dr, Jacksonville, FL 32218
Bone filling augmentation material.

Biomet, Inc. 574-267-6639
56 E Bell Dr, PO Box 587, Warsaw, IN 46582
Bone cement.

Collagen Matrix, Inc. 201-405-1477
509 Commerce St, Franklin Lakes, NJ 07417
Collagen periodontal membrane.

Dentsply Friadent Ceramed 717-849-4229
12860 W Cedar Dr Ste 110, Lakewood, CO 80228
Various types of sterile bone filling augmentation materials.

Gyrus Ent L.L.C., Sub. Of Gyrus Acmi, Inc. 508-804-2739
2925 Appling Rd, Bartlett, TN 38133
Various.

Imtec, A 3m Company 800-879-9799
2401 N Commerce St, IMTEC Plaza, Ardmore, OK 73401
Gore-Tex, regenerative material barriers.

Kerr Corp. 949-255-8766
1717 W Collins Ave, Orange, CA 92867
Synthetic bone grafting material.

Lifecore Biomedical, Inc. 952-368-4300
3515 Lyman Blvd, Chaska, MN 55318
CALFORMA Calcium Sulfate Barrier. CALMATRIX Calcium Sulfate Binder. CAPSET Calcium Sulfate Barrier. TEFGEN Regenerative Membranes.

Luitpold Pharmaceuticals, Inc. 631-924-4000
1 Luitpold Dr, Shirley, NY 11967
Fixation pins.

Medtronic Sofamor Danek Usa, Inc. 901-396-3133
4340 Swinnea Rd, Memphis, TN 38118
Bone void filler material.

Novabone Products, Llc 386-462-7660
13709 Progress Blvd Ste 33, Alachua, FL 32615
Perioglas - Sythetic Bone Graft Particulate;

Oct Usa, Inc.
17 Hammond Ste 411, Irvine, CA 92618
Various models of synthetic bone grafting material.

Osteogenics Biomedical, Inc. 806-796-1923
4620 71st St Bldg 78-79, Lubbock, TX 79424
Resorbable regenerative membrane.

Smith & Nephew, Inc. 800-343-5717
University Business Park, 12500 Network, Suite 112
Andover, MA 01810
Resorbable regenerative membrane.

Steiner Laboratories 808-371-2700
590 Farrington Hwy, #1010 Suite 7, Kapolei, HI 96707
Regen biocement.

Therics, Llc 330-475-8600
1800 Triplett Blvd, Akron, OH 44306
Bone graft substitute hydroxylapatite blocks synthetic bone substitute.

Unicare Biomedical, Inc. 949-643-6707
22971 Triton Way Ste B, Laguna Hills, CA 92653
Unigraft synthetic bioactive glass bone-graft material. Also, Cytoflex expanded PTFE synthetic barrier membrane for use as a space-making barrier in the treatment of periodontal defects.

W.L. Gore & Associates,Inc 928-526-3030
1505 North Fourth St., Flagstaff, AZ 86004
Periodontal material.

W.L. Gore & Associates,Inc 302-738-4880
345 Inverness Dr S, Bldg. A, Ste. 120, Englewood, CO 80112
Regenerative material.

IMPLANT, EYE VALVE *(Ophthalmology) 86KYF*

E. Benson Hood Laboratories, Inc. 800-942-5227
575 Washington St, Pembroke, MA 02359
Krupin eye valve implant in 4 sizes, ultra-smooth surface treatment.

Glaukos Corp. 949-367-9600
26051 Merit Cir Ste 103, Laguna Hills, CA 92653
Glaucoma/aqueous shunt.

John J. Kelley Associates Ltd. 215-567-1377
1528 Walnut St Ste 1801, Mid City East, PA 19102
Orbital floor implant for blowout fractures of the orbit (teflon).

New World Medical, Inc. 800-832-5327
10763 Edison Ct, Rancho Cucamonga, CA 91730
GLAUCOMA DEVICES, GLAUCOMA SHUNTS, GLAUCOMA VALVES, TUBE INSERTERS, FORCEPS, PERICARDIUM AND SCLERAL TISSUE

IMPLANT, FEMALE INCONTINENCE *(Obstetrics/Gyn) 85MCQ*

Smiths Medical Asd 800-424-8662
5700 W 23rd Ave, Gary, IN 46406
On-Command female incontinence catheter. Intraurethral urological catheter for management of urinary outflow dysfunction with patient activated magnetic valve.

IMPLANT, FIXATION DEVICE, CONDYLAR PLATE
(Orthopedics) 87JDP

Biomet Microfixation Inc. 800-874-7711
1520 Tradeport Dr, Jacksonville, FL 32218
Condylar fixation device.

Biomet, Inc. 574-267-6639
56 E Bell Dr, PO Box 587, Warsaw, IN 46582
Various types of condylar blade plates.

C.O.R.E. Tech, Inc. 574-267-5744
542 E 200 N, Warsaw, IN 46582
Contract manufacturing: trauma, spinal, and reconstructive implants and instrumentation.

Kmedic 800-955-0559
190 Veterans Dr, Northvale, NJ 07647

Panadent Corp. 800-368-9777
22573 Barton Rd, Grand Terrace, CA 92313
Condyle Positioner; AXIS Mounting System and Mounting Plate System; and C.P.I. (CONDYLE Position Indicator). Also, AXI-PATH Recorder, and Bite-Tabs and Bite Trays. Visit... www.panadent.com check out our catalog and or help section to learn more about panadent equipment.

Synthes (Usa) 610-719-5000
35 Airport Rd, Horseheads, NY 14845
Various types and sizes of condylar plate fixation devices.

Zimmer Holdings, Inc. 800-613-6131
1800 W Center St, PO Box 708, Warsaw, IN 46580

IMPLANT, FIXATION DEVICE, PROXIMAL FEMORAL
(Orthopedics) 87JDO

Ascension Orthopedics 512-836-5001
8700 Cameron Rd Ste 100, Austin, TX 78754
Implants, Small Joints

Biomet, Inc. 574-267-6639
56 E Bell Dr, PO Box 587, Warsaw, IN 46582
Various types of proximal femoral fixation devices.

Keller Engineering, Inc. 310-326-6291
3203 Kashiwa St, Torrance, CA 90505

Kinetikos Medical, Inc. 800-546-3845
6005 Hidden Valley Rd Ste 180, Carlsbad, CA 92011
M.B.A., The Maxwell-Brancheau Subtalar Arthroereisis Implant, UNIVERSAL2 Total Wrist Implant, KINETIK Great Toe Implant, K2 Hemi Toe Implant, Kompressor Compression Screw, Katalyst Radial Head Implant, Viper Distal Volar Radius Plate with VALT (Variable Angle Locking Technology) Screws.

Kmedic 800-955-0559
190 Veterans Dr, Northvale, NJ 07647

LinkBio Corp. 800-932-0616
300 Round Hill Dr, Rockaway, NJ 07866
Orthopedic implants

Macdee, Inc. 734-475-9165
13800 Luick Dr, Chelsea, MI 48118

Medtronic Puerto Rico Operations Co.,Med Rel 763-514-4000
Road 909, Km. 0.4., Barrio Mariana, Humacao, PR 00792
Multiple (proximal femoral fixation devices, nails, plates, screws, pins).

IMPLANT, FIXATION DEVICE, PROXIMAL FEMORAL *(cont'd)*

Medtronic Sofamor Danek Usa, Inc. 901-396-3133
4340 Swinnea Rd, Memphis, TN 38118
Multiple (proximal femoral fixation devices, nails, plates, screws, pins).

Stryker Spine 866-457-7463
2 Pearl Ct, Allendale, NJ 07401

Synthes (Usa) 610-719-5000
35 Airport Rd, Horseheads, NY 14845
Various types and sizes of proximal femur fixation devices.

Warsaw Orthopedic, Inc. 901-396-3133
2500 Silveus Xing, Warsaw, IN 46582
Multiple (proximal femoral fixation devices, nails, plates, screws, pins).

Zimmer Manufacturing B.V. 800-613-6131
Route 1, Km. 123.4, Bldg. 1, Turpeaux Industrial Park
Mercedita, PR 00715
Various types and sizes of proximal femoral fixation devices.

IMPLANT, FIXATION DEVICE, SPINAL *(Orthopedics) 87JDN*

Advanced Spine Technology, Inc. 415-241-2400
457 Mariposa St, San Francisco, CA 94107
Various.

Biomet, Inc. 574-267-6639
56 E Bell Dr, PO Box 587, Warsaw, IN 46582
Meurig williams plate.

Bolt Bethel, Llc 763-434-5900
23530 University Avenue Ext NW, PO Box 135, Bethel, MN 55005

Depuy Spine, Inc. 800-227-6633
325 Paramount Dr, Raynham, MA 02767
Various spinal hooks, rods, couplers, wires and related instrument.

Depuy-Raynham, A Div. Of Depuy Orthopaedics 800-451-2006
325 Paramount Dr, Raynham, MA 02767
Interlaminar clamps.

Holmed Corporation 508-238-3351
40 Norfolk Ave, South Easton, MA 02375

Interventional Spine, Inc. 800-497-0484
13700 Alton Pkwy Ste 160, Irvine, CA 92618
RENEW Interspinous Allograft Technology

Kapp Surgical Instrument, Inc. 800-282-5277
4919 Warrensville Center Rd, Cleveland, OH 44128

Life Medical Llc 317-840-3816
10424 Snapper Ct, Indianapolis, IN 46256
'Smart' implant with MEMS devices incorporated into the implant that communicate position, motion, pressure, load, and strain.

Microcision Llc 800-264-3811
5805 Keystone St, Philadelphia, PA 19135

Micron Precision Engineering, Inc. 310-874-4963
939 Evening Shade Dr, San Pedro, CA 90731
Intervertebral disc.

Millstone Medical Outsourcing 508-679-8384
1565 N Main St Ste 408, Fall River, MA 02720
Multiple and various.

Osteotech, Inc. 800-537-9842
51 James Way, Eatontown, NJ 07724
VERSALOK implant and instrument system for anterior correction of spinal deformities, spinal fixation brace.

Pioneer Surgical Technology 800-557-9909
375 River Park Cir, Marquette, MI 49855

Rickman Tool, Inc. 574-223-8198
1202 E 4th St, Rochester, IN 46975
Spinal Orthopedic Implants.

V--Operations Management Consulting, 317-570-5830
7350 E 86th St, Indianapolis, IN 46256

Warsaw Orthopedic, Inc. 901-396-3133
2500 Silveus Xing, Warsaw, IN 46582
Various inplant fixation devices, spinal - sterile and non-sterile.

Zimmer Manufacturing B.V. 800-613-6131
Route 1, Km. 123.4, Bldg. 1, Turpeaux Industrial Park
Mercedita, PR 00715
Various types and sizes of spinal fixation devices and accessories.

IMPLANT, JOINT, TEMPOROMANDIBULAR
(Dental And Oral) 76LZD

Biomet Microfixation Inc. 800-874-7711
1520 Tradeport Dr, Jacksonville, FL 32218
Joint, temporomandibular, implant, dental.

IMPLANT, JOINT, TEMPOROMANDIBULAR *(cont'd)*

Tmj Implants, Inc. 800-825-4865
17301 W Colfax Ave Ste 135, Golden, CO 80401
Fossa Eminence Prosthesis.

Tmj Solution, Inc 805-650-3391
1793 Eastman Ave, Ventura, CA 93003
Tmj implant.

IMPLANT, MUSCLE, PECTORALIS *(Surgery) 79MIC*

Aesthetic And Reconstructive Technologies, Inc. 775-853-6800
3545 Airway Dr Ste 106, Reno, NV 89511
Silicone elastomer pectoralis implant.

Allied Biomedical 800-276-1322
PO Box 392, Ventura, CA 93002
POWERFLEX PEC; POWERFLEX PEC II; NOVACKPEC; contoured carving blocks.

Hanson Medical, Inc. 800-771-2215
825 Riverside Ave Ste 2, Paso Robles, CA 93446
Pectoral implant.

Spectrum Designs Medical, Inc. 800-239-6399
6387 Rose Ln Ste B, Carpinteria, CA 93013
Aiache and Novack pectoral implants, sterile. Pectoral implants used in men to enhance the pectoral area.

IMPLANT, ORBITAL, EXTRA-OCULAR *(Ophthalmology) 86HQX*

Fci Ophthalmics 800-932-4202
64 Schoosett St, Pembroke, MA 02359
Scleral buckles for retinal detachment surgery.

Integrated Orbital Implants, Inc. 800-424-6537
12625 High Bluff Dr Ste 314, San Diego, CA 92130
BIO-EYE Hydroxyapatite Orbital Implant for the anophthalmic patient.

John J. Kelley Associates Ltd. 215-567-1377
1528 Walnut St Ste 1801, Mid City East, PA 19102
'winged sled' (non-sterile).

Mira, Inc. 508-278-7877
414 Quaker Hwy, Uxbridge, MA 01569
Eye implants.

Oculo Plastik Inc. 888-381-3292
200 Sauve West, Montreal, QUE H3L-1Y9 Canada
Codere-Durette, acrylic floor of the orbit. Also trianugular solid PTFE implamts.

IMPLANT, RETINAL *(Ophthalmology) 86WJZ*

Fci Ophthalmics 800-932-4202
64 Schoosett St, Pembroke, MA 02359
Scleral buckling components

IMPLANT, SCLERAL *(Ophthalmology) 86WUA*

Allergan 800-366-6554
2525 Dupont Dr, Irvine, CA 92612
KERATO-LENS & KERATO-PATCH corneal implants for treatment of aphakia.

IMPLANT, SUBPERIOSTEAL *(Dental And Oral) 76ELE*

Jardon Eye Prosthetics, Inc. 248-424-8560
15920 W 12 Mile Rd, Southfield, MI 48076

Microcision Llc 800-264-3811
5805 Keystone St, Philadelphia, PA 19135

O Company 800-228-0477
600 Paisano St NE, Albuquerque, NM 87123
Contract manufacturer of dental implant parts.

Oco Inc. 800-228-0477
600 Paisano St NE Ste A, Albuquerque, NM 87123
Subperiosteal implant.

Pentron Laboratory Technologies 203-265-7397
53 N Plains Industrial Rd, Wallingford, CT 06492
Implant, subperiosteal.

IMPLANTABLE RADIO FREQUENCY TRANSPONDER SYSTEM
(General) 80NRV

Digital Angel Corp. 651-554-1574
490 Villuame Ave, South Saint Paul, MN 55075
Implantable radio frequency identificaiton transponder.

IMPLANTED SUBCUTANEOUS SECUREMENT CATHETER
(General) 80OKC

Interrad Medical 763-225-6699
181 Cheshire Ln N Ste 100, Plymouth, MN 55441

IMPOTENCE DEVICE, MECHANICAL/HYDRAULIC *(Gastro/Urology) 78FHW*

Augusta Medical Systems, Llc 800-827-8382
1025 Broad St, Augusta, GA 30901
New Generation of Vacuum Therapy. Manual and battery operated vacuum erection devices for the treatment of erectile dysfunction. Devices to help with the recovery of Radical Prostatectomy surgery.

Bio-Feedback Systems, Inc. 303-444-1411
2736 47th St, Boulder, CO 80301
Electronic penile plethysmograph - $695 each. Special order.

Encore, Inc. 800-221-6603
7696 15th St E, Sarasota, FL 34243

Mission Pharmacal Co. 210-696-8400
10999 W Interstate 10 Ste 1000, San Antonio, TX 78230
VED external vacuum erection device. Available with either hand-operated or battery-operated pump.

INCINERATOR *(General) 80VBK*

Agile Mfg., Inc 800-476-7436
720 Industrial Park Road, Anderson, MO 64831
Professional incinerators, pathological and infectious waste incinerators for sanitary disposal of hospital and laboratory waste. Various models and sizes are available for on-site disposal.

INCUBATOR, AEROBIC *(Microbiology) 83RBW*

Appropriate Technical Resources, Inc. 800-827-5931
9157 Whiskey Bottom Rd, PO Box 460, Laurel, MD 20723

Carolina Biological Supply Co. 800-334-5551
2700 York Rd, Burlington, NC 27215

Environmental Growth Chambers 800-321-6854
510 Washington St, Chagrin Falls, OH 44022
Walk-in incubators and plant growth chambers.

Hotpack 800-523-3608
10940 Dutton Rd, Philadelphia, PA 19154

New Brunswick Scientific Co., Inc. 800-631-5417
PO Box 4005, Edison, NJ 08818
Incubated/refrigerated shakers in a variety of models and sizes, including bench and large-capacity, space-saving floor models. Also CO2 incubators in choice of water-jacketed or air-jacketed designs.

Percival Scientific Inc. 800-695-2743
505 Research Dr, Perry, IA 50220

Powers Scientific, Inc. 800-998-0500
PO Box 268, Pipersville, PA 18947

Pro Scientific Inc. 800-584-3776
99 Willenbrock Rd, Oxford, CT 06478

Q.I. Medical, Inc. 800-837-8361
440 Lower Grass Valley Rd Ste C, Nevada City, CA 95959

Stratagene 800-424-5444
11011 N Torrey Pines Rd, La Jolla, CA 92037
Laboratory incubators.

Thermal Product Solutions 800-216-7725
2121 Reach Rd, Williamsport, PA 17701

INCUBATOR, ANAEROBIC *(Microbiology) 83RBX*

Hotpack 800-523-3608
10940 Dutton Rd, Philadelphia, PA 19154

Pro Scientific Inc. 800-584-3776
99 Willenbrock Rd, Oxford, CT 06478

INCUBATOR, NEONATAL *(General) 80FMZ*

Colonial Scientific Ltd. 902-468-1811
201 Brownlow Ave., Unit 52, Dartmouth, NS B3B-1W2 Canada

Ge Industrial, Sensing 800-833-9438
1100 Technology Park Dr, Billerica, MA 01821

Ohmeda Medical 800-345-2700
8880 Gorman Rd, Laurel, MD 20723
Ohio Care Plus Incubator for warming of premature infants. GIRAFFE OMNIBED, GIRAFFE Incubator.

Wrapped In Comfort 877-205-0901
15760 Via Sonata, San Lorenzo, CA 94580
Incubator cover, accessory to neonatal incubator.

INCUBATOR, NEONATAL TRANSPORT *(General) 80FPL*

International Biomedical, Ltd. 512-873-0033
2725 N Main St, Cleburne, TX 76033
Airborne.

INCUBATOR, TEST TUBE, PORTABLE *(Microbiology) 83RBY*

Lifesign 800-526-2125
71 Veronica Ave, Somerset, NJ 08873
$190 for MTC model III tubes (17 test capacity each).

INCUBATOR, TEST TUBE, STATIONARY *(Microbiology) 83RBZ*

Boekel Scientific 800-336-6929
855 Pennsylvania Blvd, Feasterville Trevose, PA 19053

Hotpack 800-523-3608
10940 Dutton Rd, Philadelphia, PA 19154
Full line of Multi-Mode CO2 incubators.

Lifesign 800-526-2125
71 Veronica Ave, Somerset, NJ 08873
$299 for MTC model LX tubes (60-test capacity each).

Scientific Industries, Inc. 888-850-6208
70 Orville Dr, Bohemia, NY 11716

INCUBATOR/WATER BATH *(Chemistry) 75JRH*

Brinkmann Instruments, Inc. 800-645-3050
PO Box 1019, Westbury, NY 11590

Nuaire, Inc. 800-328-3352
2100 Fernbrook Ln N, Plymouth, MN 55447
CO-2 water jacketed incubator.

INCUBATOR/WATER BATH, MICROBIOLOGY *(Microbiology) 83JTQ*

Abbott Diagnostics Div. 847-937-7988
1921 Hurd Dr, Irving, TX 75038
Dry incubator.

Barnstead International 412-490-8425
2555 Kerper Blvd, Dubuque, IA 52001
Various.

Boekel Scientific 800-336-6929
855 Pennsylvania Blvd, Feasterville Trevose, PA 19053

Brinkmann Instruments (Canada) Ltd. 800-263-8715
6670 Campobello Rd., Mississauga, ONT L5N 2L8 Canada

Cannon Instrument Co. 800-676-6232
PO Box 16, State College, PA 16804
CT-500, priced at $3,360.00 per unit.

Cole-Parmer Instrument Inc. 800-323-4340
625 E Bunker Ct, Vernon Hills, IL 60061

Coy Laboratory Products, Inc. 734-475-2200
14500 Coy Dr, Grass Lake, MI 49240

Ericomp, Inc. 800-541-8471
10211 Pacific Mesa Blvd Ste 411, San Diego, CA 92121

New Brunswick Scientific Co., Inc. 800-631-5417
PO Box 4005, Edison, NJ 08818
NBS Innova (r) and C-Line water bath shakers provide exceptional temperature control for applications in cell culture, hybridization, and staining/destaining cells. Microprocessor-controlled temperature 5 degrees C above ambient (or cooling temperature if using cooling coil) to 80 degrees C.

Ortho-Clinical Diagnostics, Inc. 800-828-6316
513 Technology Blvd, Rochester, NY 14626
Incubator.

Praxair-Puerto Rico 440-234-1075
Rt. 931 & 189, Gurabo, PR 00778
Biological atmosphere.

Sheldon Mfg., Inc. 503-640-3000
300 N 26th Ave, Cornelius, OR 97113
Water bath, incubator.

Thermo Fisher Scientific 877-843-7668
81 Wyman St, Waltham, MA 02451

Thermo Fisher Scientific (Asheville) Llc 740-373-4763
Millcreek Rd., Marietta, OH 45750
Various models of incubators and water baths.

Thermo Fisher Scientific Inc. 563-556-2241
2555 Kerper Blvd, Dubuque, IA 52001

Welco-Cgi Gas Technologies 440-234-1075
145 Shimersville Rd, Bethlehem, PA 18015
Biological atmosphere.

Young Dental Manufacturing Co 1, Llc 800-325-1881
4401 Paredes Line Rd, Brownsville, TX 78526
Incubator.

INDICATOR METHOD, PROTEIN OR ALBUMIN (URINARY, NON-QUANT.) *(Chemistry) 75JIR*

Ameritek Usa, Inc. 425-379-2580
125 130th St SE Ste 200, Everett, WA 98208
Albumin urine test kit.

Arkray Factory Usa, Inc. 952-646-3168
5182 W 76th St, Minneapolis, MN 55439
Urine test strips.

Bayer Healthcare Llc 914-524-2955
555 White Plains Rd Fl 5, Tarrytown, NY 10591
Various.

Bayer Healthcare, Llc 574-256-3430
430 S Beiger St, Mishawaka, IN 46544
Various.

E K Industries, Inc. 877-EKI-CHEM
1403 Herkimer St, Joliet, IL 60432
Sulfosailcylic acid, 3%.

Kamiya Biomedical Company 206-575-8068
12779 Gateway Dr S, Tukwila, WA 98168
Diagnostic immunoturbidimetric assay for urinary microalbumin and calibrators.

Pochemco, Inc. 413-536-2900
724 Main St, Holyoke, MA 01040
Sulfosalicyclic acid.

Synermed Intl., Inc. 317-896-1565
17408 Tiller Ct Ste 1900, Westfield, IN 46074
Albumin test system.

Teco Diagnostics 714-693-7788
1268 N Lakeview Ave, Anaheim, CA 92807
Urine reagent strips.

INDICATOR, BIOLOGICAL, LIQUID CHEMICAL STERIL. PROCESS *(General) 80MRB*

Raven Biological Laboratories, Inc. 800-728-5702
8607 Park Dr, PO Box 27261, Omaha, NE 68127
PROSPORE, a self-contained biological indicator 4ml growth media impregnated w/spores, w/bromocresol purple color indicator. For steam sterilization. PROSPORE 2: same as PROSPORE plus tube containing spore dot and crushable ampule containing growth media.

INDICATOR, PH, DYE (URINARY, NON-QUANTITATIVE) *(Chemistry) 75CEN*

Arkray Factory Usa, Inc. 952-646-3168
5182 W 76th St, Minneapolis, MN 55439
Urine test strips.

Beutlich Lp, Pharmaceuticals 800-238-8542
1541 S Shields Dr, Waukegan, IL 60085
pH Paper

Bristol-Myers Squibb 732-227-7564
2400 W Lloyd Expy, Evansville, IN 47712
Ph paper.

Quidel Corp. 858-552-1100
2981 Copper Rd, Santa Clara, CA 95051
Various types of vaginal fluid test for ph and amines.

INDICATOR, PHYSICAL/CHEMICAL, STORAGE TEMPERATURE *(General) 80OCI*

3m Co. 888-364-3577
3M Center, Saint Paul, MN 55144
3M Comply Liquid Paracetic Cl #1249, 3M Comply Steri-Gage EO Chemical; Integrator 1244A, 1244B, 1244E; MULTIPLE, 3M Comply Thermalog EO Chemical; Ingegrator; MULTIPLE, 3M Comply Thermalog Steam; Integrator - #2134MM; MULTIPLE, 3M Comply Gas Plasma Ind Tape 1228; MULTIPLE, 3M C omply 1248 Gas Plasma Cl; MULTIPLE, 3M Comply Bowie-Dick Lead Free

INDIRECT FLUORESCENT ANTIBODY TEST, ENTAMOEBA HISTOLYTICA *(Microbiology) 83GWD*

Ivd Research, Inc. 760-929-7744
5909 Sea Lion Pl Ste D, Carlsbad, CA 92010
E. histolytica serum elisa.

INDOPHENOL, BERTHELOT, UREA NITROGEN *(Chemistry) 75CDL*

Sterling Diagnostics, Inc. 800-637-2661
36645 Metro Ct, Sterling Heights, MI 48312
Urea nitrogen reagent set.

INFILTRATOR *(Pathology) 88IDQ*

George Tiemann & Co. 800-843-6266
25 Plant Ave, Hauppauge, NY 11788

INFLATOR, CUFF *(General) 80QNQ*

Elmed, Inc. 630-543-2792
60 W Fay Ave, Addison, IL 60101

Hokanson Inc., D.E. 800-999-8251
12840 NE 21st Pl, Bellevue, WA 98005
Specialized vascular cuff inflators are available in three types: rapid inflator/deflator inflates the largest thigh cuff in 0.3 seconds. A battery operated hand-held model has a built in pump and stores up to 12 pressures simultaneously. An aneroid sphygmomanometer is also available. We also have cuff inflator accessories available.

Statcorp, Inc. 800-992-0014
14476 Duval Pl W Ste 303, Jacksonville, FL 32218
UNIFUSOR: Disposable pressure cuff for infusing blood and I.V. fluids, 500 cc and 1000 cc with 300 Torr gauge and removable hand-bulb, which is for use with THE WOODS PUMP.

INFUSER, PRESSURE (BLOOD PUMP) *(General) 80RLQ*

Armstrong Medical Industries, Inc. 800-323-4220
575 Knightsbridge Pkwy, Lincolnshire, IL 60069

David Clark Company, Inc. 800-900-3434
360 Franklin St, Worcester, MA 01604
1/2 and 1 liter sizes

David Scott Company 800-804-0333
59 Fountain St, Framingham, MA 01702

Dma Med-Chem Corporation 800-362-1833
49 Watermill Ln, Great Neck, NY 11021

Smiths Medical Asd, Inc. 800-553-8351
160 Weymouth St, Rockland, MA 02370
Automated pressure infusor for I. V. fluid therapy.

INFUSION PUMP, ENTERAL *(General) 80LZH*

Ardus Medical, Inc. 800-878-1388
11297 Grooms Rd, Cincinnati, OH 45242

Corpak Medsystems, Inc. 800-323-6305
100 Chaddick Dr, Wheeling, IL 60090
Enternal feeding pump.

Entracare, Llc 913-451-2234
11315 Strang Line Rd, Lenexa, KS 66215
Infusion pump, non sterile.

Novartis Nutrition 800-333-3785
1600 Utica Ave S Ste 600, PO Box 370, Minneapolis, MN 55416
Enteral pump with formula delivery and patient hydration modules.

Omni Medical Supply Inc. 800-860-6664
4153 Pioneer Dr, Commerce Township, MI 48390

Ost Medical Inc. 401-737-3774
11 Knight St Bldg F23, Warwick, RI 02886
Enteral feeding pump.

INFUSION PUMP, INSULIN *(General) 80LZG*

Abbott Diabetes Care Inc. 510-749-5400
1360 S Loop Rd, Alameda, CA 94502
Aviator Insulin Pump

Animas Corp. 877-767-7373
200 Lawrence Dr, West Chester, PA 19380
Pump, infusion, insulin.

Disetronic Medical Systems 800-280-7801
11800 Exit 5 Pkwy, Fishers, IN 46037
PANOMAT micro volume infusion pumps, D-PEN mechanical pen for injection of drugs, PENFINE pen needle for use on insulin pens. H-TRON PLUS only two pump system so that patients don't need to go back to MDI if they have a problem with their primary pump. D-TRON world's most advanced insulin pump. DAHedi world's smallest insulin pump.

Insulet Corporation 800-591-3455
9 Oak Park Dr, Bedford, MA 01730
Insulin infusion pump and remote controller.

Medtronic Minimed 800-933-3322
18000 Devonshire St, Northridge, CA 91325
External and implantable models.

Medtronic Puerto Rico Operations Co., Juncos 763-514-4000
Road 31, Km. 24, Hm 4, Ceiba Norte Industrial Park, Juncos, PR 00777
Infusion pump.

INFUSION STAND *(General) 80FOX*

Ac Healthcare Supply, Inc. 905-448-4706
11651 230th St, Cambria Heights, NY 11411
Infusion stand.

Advanced Medical Innovations, Inc. 888-367-2641
9410 De Soto Ave Ste J, Chatsworth, CA 91311
SAF-T-POLE I.V., pole and irrigation tower for arthroscopy, TURP and hysteroscopy. Saves money and the practitioner's back.

Alimed, Inc. 800-225-2610
297 High St, Dedham, MA 02026

Allen Medical Systems, Inc. 800-433-5774
1 Post Office Sq, Acton, MA 01720
Easy Irrigation Tower - Four independently adjustable hooks each safely support up to 10,000cc of fluid. Comfortable, quick-release knobs permit vertical adjustment of hangers from 51⁄2' to 81⁄2'. (167.5 cm x 259 cm) This nurse-friendly design makes it easy for all personnel to operate effortlessly.

American Medical Mfg., Inc. 800-426-6476
9410 De Soto Ave Ste J, Chatsworth, CA 91311
SAF-T-POLE is a specialized I.V. Pole & Irrigation Tower used for Arthroscopy, Hysteroscopy and TURP surgeries where irrigation requirements are high. The Pole utilizes four independent lift channels with an eight-bag capacity. Each channel adjusts from 5-8 feet in height with no interruptions to continuous flow even during bag replacement. It accommodates the use of higher volume, more economical bags. O.R. designed with a wide 27î diameter uniquely inverted and sturdy 5-legged, no stain base with dual casters. Humanly engineered for ONE HANDED operation; PUSH quick-release handle down to lift the bag up, with half the force required compared to regular I.V. Pole due to two to one mechanical advantage. No need for sand bags for stabilization or step stool to change bags. Different models will hold 2 to 8 bags and will depend on your needs, suitable for critical care, intensive care, emergency department, etc.

Armstrong Medical Industries, Inc. 800-323-4220
575 Knightsbridge Pkwy, Lincolnshire, IL 60069

Atd-American Co. 800-523-2300
135 Greenwood Ave, Wyncote, PA 19095

B. Braun Medical, Inc. 610-596-2536
901 Marcon Blvd, Allentown, PA 18109

Blickman 800-247-5070
39 Robinson Rd, Lodi, NJ 07644
Stainless steel and chrome IV Stands with four, five and six leg bases. Five different height adjustment mechanisms- foot-operated, twist lock, friction knob,thumb control, trigger lock.

Brandt Industries, Inc. 800-221-8031
4461 Bronx Blvd, Bronx, NY 10470
IV poles, many varieties.

Brewer Company, The 888-873-9371
N88W13901 Main St, Menomonee Falls, WI 53051
#43408/#43409: 2-Rams Horn Hook and 4-Rams Horn Hook, 6 leg, Heavy Duty Base; #43416/#43417: 2-Rams Horn Hook and 4-Rams Horn Hook, 5 leg, Short Wheel Base; #11300: 2-Rams Horn Hooks 4 leg base; #11350/#11360: 2-Rams Horn Hook and 4-Rams Horn Hook, 5 leg base; #43403/#43406: 2-Rams Horn Hook and 4-Rams Horn Hook, 4 leg heavy base.

Cameron-Miller, Inc. 800-621-0142
5410 W Roosevelt Rd, Road #241, Chicago, IL 60644

Camtec 410-228-1156
1959 Church Creek Rd, Cambridge, MD 21613
Stand infusion, intravenous.

Clinimed, Incorporated 877-CLINIMED
303 Markus Ct, Sandy Brae Industrial Park, Newark, DE 19713

Crest Healthcare Supply 800-328-8908
195 3rd St, Dassel, MN 55325
I.V. stands and accessories.

Ekos Corp. 888-400-3567
11911 N Creek Pkwy S, Bothell, WA 98011
Infusion stand.

Ethicon, Inc. 800-4-ETHICON
Route 22 West, Somerville, NJ 08876

Farley Inc., W.T. 800-327-5397
931 Via Alondra, Camarillo, CA 93012
$50.00 for aluminum I.V. pole for ambulance gurney.

Galaxy Medical Manufacturing Co. 800-876-4599
5411 Sheila St, Commerce, CA 90040

INFUSION STAND *(cont'd)*

Glo Touch Corporation 734-439-8248
3075 Judd Rd, Milan, MI 48160
IV securement device. IV Protector is an FDA - Class 1 excemst infusion set accessory device -(Anchor joint)- disposable for IV line safety so as to avoid strain, disconnection from patient while in transport.

Health Care Logistics, Inc. 800-848-1633
450 Town St, PO Box 25, Circleville, OH 43113
Various.

Hill-Rom Holdings, Inc. 800-445-3730
1069 State Road 46 E, Batesville, IN 47006

Hill-Rom, Inc. 812-934-7777
4115 Dorchester Rd Unit 600, North Charleston, SC 29405
Infusion stands and accessories.

Homak Manufacturing Company Inc. 800-874-6625
1605 Old Route 18 Ste 4-36, Wampum, PA 16157

Hospira Inc. 877-946-7747
275 N Field Dr, Lake Forest, IL 60045
Hospira IV stand

I.V. League Medical 805-988-1010
460 Lombard St, Oxnard, CA 93030
I.v. stand.

Icu Medical (Ut), Inc 949-366-2183
4455 Atherton Dr, Salt Lake City, UT 84123
I.v. stand and accessories.

Imperial Surgical Ltd. 800-661-5432
581 Orly Ave., Dorval, ONT H9P-1G1 Canada
$220 per unit.

Innovative Medical Designs 317-421-0308
130 West Rampart Rd., Shelbyville, IN 46176
Infusion stand.

Iradimed Corporation 407-677-8022
7457 Aloma Ave Ste 201, Winter Park, FL 32792
Infusion pump stand i.v. pole.

Jedmed Instruments Co. 314-845-3770
5416 Jedmed Ct, Saint Louis, MO 63129

Livengood Engineering Inc. 970-493-2569
1112 Oakridge Dr Unit 104, Fort Collins, CO 80525
Cart, walker.

Maquet, Inc. 843-552-8652
7371 Spartan Blvd E, N Charleston, SC 29418
Various models of infusion stands and poles.

Mayo Medical, S.A. De C.V. 800-715-3872
Edison 1141 Nte., Col. Talleres, Monterrey N.L. 64480 Mexico

Medical Depot 516-998-4600
99 Seaview Blvd, Port Washington, NY 11050
Iv pole.

Medved Products, Inc. 651-482-8413
PO Box 120883, Saint Paul, MN 55112
Heavy duty, stainless steel IV poles and accessories.

Mei Corporation 402-339-3300
4907 S 90th St, Omaha, NE 68127
'The Messerli Connection' Adjustable connector for IV poles and adjustable receiver for wheelchairs, beds, and gurneys. Takes 3-5 seconds to make the switch.

Modular Services Company 405-521-9923
109 NE 38th St, Oklahoma City, OK 73105
Infusion pump stands.

O&M Enterprise 847-258-4515
641 Chelmsford Ln, Elk Grove Village, IL 60007
INFUSION STANDS

Omni Medical Supply Inc. 800-860-6664
4153 Pioneer Dr, Commerce Township, MI 48390

Pedigo Products 360-695-3500
4000 SE Columbia Way, Vancouver, WA 98661
Stainless steel or chrome: pump, gravity feed, hand or foot operated.

Phelan Manufacturing Corp. 800-328-2358
2523 Minnehaha Ave, Minneapolis, MN 55404
$190.00 per IV floor stand.

Pryor Products 800-854-2280
1819 Peacock Blvd, Oceanside, CA 92056
A broad and deep variety of standard and custom IV stands are available. These products are designed to work safely and effectively in their intended patinet care areas.

INFUSION STAND *(cont'd)*

Quality Control Corp. 708-887-5400
7315 W Wilson Ave, Harwood Heights, IL 60706
I.v. stand, i.v. pole.

Sharps Compliance Corp. 713-432-0300
9220 Kirby Dr Ste 500, Houston, TX 77054
PitchIt IV Poles are designed to eliminate the frustration of retrieving, cleaning, bagging, and tagging your old IV poles. These innovative poles are cost-effective, portable, collapsible, lightweight, sturdy and easy to use. They can be unfolded in just seconds and their innovative tripod design allows them to be used on any floor or tabletop. No assembly is required; lower shipping costs than traditional IV poles. Aluminum construction allows for ìpitchingî into recycled waste when IV pole is no longer needed.

Steelcraft, Inc. 800-225-7710
115 W Main St, Millbury, MA 01527

INHALER, NASAL *(Ear/Nose/Throat) 77KCO*

Dedicated Distribution 800-325-8367
640 Miami Ave, Kansas City, KS 66105
Aerochambers for metered dose inhalers.

Dey, L.P. 800-755-5560
2751 Napa Valley Corporate Dr, Napa, CA 94558
Complete line of inhaled solutions, including Ipratropium bromide inhalation solution, cromolyn sodium inhalation USP, albuterol sulfate solution, metaproterenol sulfate inhalation solution, sodium chloride solutions (hypotonic, isotonic and hypertonic), and sterile water solutions.

The Tech Group Tempe 480-281-4400
640 S Rockford Dr, Tempe, AZ 85281
Dry powder inhaler (dpi), pulmonary delivery system (pds).

Wolfe Tory Medical, Inc. 801-281-3000
79 W 4500 S Ste 18, Salt Lake City, UT 84107
Wound irrigation syringe.

INHIBITOR, PERIDURAL FIBROSIS (ADHESION BARRIER)
(Physical Med) 89MLQ

Gliatech Medical, Inc. 216-831-3200
27070 Miles Rd, Solon, OH 44139
Adcon-I adhesion control in barrier gel.

INJECTOR & ACCESSORIES, MANIPULATOR, UTERINE
(Obstetrics/Gyn) 85RCF

Clinical Innovations, Inc. 888-268-6222
747 W 4170 S, Murray, UT 84123
CLEARVIEW Uterine Manipulator injector in convenience kit with accessory sound-dilator, syringe and tip spacer. Full retroversion/anteversion capability and physician control.

Conkin Surgical Instruments Ltd. 416-922-9496
18 Coldwater Rd., Toronto, ON M3B-1Y7 Canada
Valtchev uterine mobilizer, with body and interchangeable obturators and cannulas.

Karl Storz Endoscopy-America Inc. 800-421-0837
600 Corporate Pointe, Culver City, CA 90230

Superior Medical Limited 800-268-7944
520 Champagne Dr., Toronto, ONT M3J 2T9 Canada

Thomas Medical Inc. 800-556-0349
5610 West 82 2nd Street, Indianpolis, IN 46278
Uterine manipulator injector: Zinnanti Manipulator, disposable uterine manipulator injector. Easy Seal Injector: to inject fluid or media for HSG and sono procedures. Makes use of the Easy Seal to seal the cervical canal, no balloons in the uterus blocking view.

Utah Medical Products, Inc. 800-533-4984
7043 Cottonwood St, Midvale, UT 84047
LUMIN laparoscopic uterine manipulator.

INJECTOR AND SYRINGE, ANGIOGRAPHIC, BALLOON INFLATION, REPROCESSED *(Cardiovascular) 74NKU*

Angiodynamics, Inc. 518-795-1400
14 Plaza Drive, Latham, NY 12110
High Pressure Connecting Lines

B. Braun Medical, Inc. 610-596-2536
901 Marcon Blvd, Allentown, PA 18109
ANGIOGRAPHIC; INJECTOR AND SYRINGE

Sterilmed, Inc. 763-488-3400
11400 73rd Ave N Ste 100, Maple Grove, MN 55369
Reprocessed balloon inflation device.

INJECTOR, ANGIOGRAPHIC (CARDIAC CATHETERIZATION)
(Cardiovascular) 74DXT

Acist Medical Systems, Inc. 888-667-6648
7905 Fuller Rd, Eden Prairie, MN 55344
Angiographic injection system.

Argon Medical Devices Inc. 903-675-9321
1445 Flat Creek Rd, Athens, TX 75751
Angiographic injector syringe.

Atrion Medical Products, Inc. 800-343-9334
1426 Curt Francis Rd NW, Arab, AL 35016
Inflation devices QL 1006, QL 1455, QL QL1030, QL2015, QL 2540, and QL 6015. Fluid delivery, injection and pressure delivery devices.

C. R. Bard, Inc., Bard Urological Div. 888-367-2273
13183 Harland Dr NE, Covington, GA 30014

Icu Medical (Ut), Inc 949-366-2183
4455 Atherton Dr, Salt Lake City, UT 84123
Various types angiographic syringes.

Marconi Medical Systems 800-323-0550
595 Miner Rd, Cleveland, OH 44143

Medrad, Inc. 800-633-7231
100 Global View Dr, Warrendale, PA 15086
Angiography injector - Medrad Mark V ProVis injection system.

Navilyst Medical 800-833-9973
100 Boston Scientific Way, Marlborough, MA 01752
Various types of angiographic syringe accessories and contrast injection lines.

Nemoto Medical U.S., Inc. 949-863-9395
24992 Del Monte St, Laguna Hills, CA 92653
Contrast injector syringe, parts and accessories.

INJECTOR, CONTRAST MEDIUM, AUTOMATIC
(Radiology) 90IZQ

Coeur, Inc 800-296-5893
704 Cadet Ct, Lebanon, TN 37087

Cook Inc. 800-457-4500
PO Box 489, Bloomington, IN 47402
$1,275 for pneumatic pressure injector, weighs 6 lbs., uses reusable syringes.

Epix Pharmaceuticals, Inc 781-761-7600
4 Maguire Rd, Lexington, MA 02421

INJECTOR, FLUID, NON-ELECTRIC *(General) 80KZE*

Activa Brand Products Inc. 800-991-4464
36 Fourth St., Charlottetown, PEI C1E-2B3 Canada
PRECI-JET 50 needleless insulin injector, pen shaped, weight: 160g, size: 14x2cm, capacity: 50 units U-100 insulin; front tube assembly contains cylinder & piston, distal end accepts nozzle cap & disposable vial holder, handle contains power source & injection trigger button with safety catch. Injector accepts 2 types of insulin with window showing amount of units loaded.

Avant Medical Corp. 858-202-1560
10225 Barnes Canyon Rd Ste A113, San Diego, CA 92121
Needle-free jet injection system.

Bioject Medical Technologies, Inc. 800-683-7221
20245 SW 95th Ave, Tualatin, OR 97062
Vitajet

Felton International, Inc. 913-599-1590
8210 Marshall Dr, Lenexa, KS 66214
Needle-free jet injector.

National Medical Products, Inc. 949-768-1147
57 Parker, Irvine, CA 92618
Jet injector.

Valeritas, Llc 508-845-1177
800 Boston Tpke, Shrewsbury, MA 01545
Fluid injector.

INJECTOR, INDICATOR *(Cardiovascular) 74DXL*

Advanced Biomedical Devices, Inc. (Abd, Inc.) 978-470-1177
Dundee Park, Bldg. 17, Andover, MA 01810
OMP Injector OMP Gas Dispenser

INJECTOR, INSULIN *(Gastro/Urology) 78WRW*

Activa Brand Products Inc. 800-991-4464
36 Fourth St., Charlottetown, PEI C1E-2B3 Canada
ADVANTA JET, ADVANTA JET ES, and GENTLE JET are needle free insulin injectors.

INJECTOR, INSULIN *(cont'd)*

Bioject Medical Technologies, Inc. 800-683-7221
20245 SW 95th Ave, Tualatin, OR 97062
Jet injector for insulin.

Novo Nordisk Canada, Inc. 800-465-4334
2700 Matheson Blvd. East, 3rd Floor, West Tower
Mississauga, ONT L4W 4 Canada
Insulin Delivery Devices and Needles for use with Insulin Delivery Devices (NovoFine)

Owen Mumford Usa, Inc. 800-421-6936
1755 W Oak Commons Ct Ste A, Marietta, GA 30062
UNIFINE PENTIPS, 29 gauge needles designed for use with all insulin pens. They are specially lubricated and are available in orginal 12mm and short 8mm lengths and come in 50 count packages. 30 gauge needles available in short 8mm lengths in boxes of 100.

Palco Labs, Inc. 800-346-4488
8030 Soquel Ave Ste 104, Santa Cruz, CA 95062
INJECT-EASE, makes insulin syringe injections easy and comfortable.

INJECTOR, JET, GAS-POWERED *(Dental And Oral) 76EGQ*

Bioject Medical Technologies, Inc. 800-683-7221
20245 SW 95th Ave, Tualatin, OR 97062
The Bioject Needle-Free Injection Management System; Biojector 2000 injection unit, $1200.00 each; Bioject needle-free disposable syringes, $2.00 each; CO2 power cartridges, $.80 each. Volume discounts available.

Med-E-Jet D. 800-231-4203
8092 Olmway Ave, Olmsted Falls, OH 44138
For giving injections without needles, call for model number & price, 800-231-4203, Fax 440-235-2247. E-mail spetz@columbus.rr.com

INJECTOR, JET, MECHANICAL-POWERED *(Dental And Oral) 76EGM*

Bioject Medical Technologies, Inc. 800-683-7221
20245 SW 95th Ave, Tualatin, OR 97062
Jet injector for insulin and vaccine.

Mada, Inc. 800-526-6370
625 Washington Ave, Carlstadt, NJ 07072
MADALET XL needle-free injection device.

Mizzy, Inc. Of National Keystone 800-333-3131
616 Hollywood Ave, Cherry Hill, NJ 08002
SYRIJET II or III reduces patient apprehension and discomfort, as well as cross contamination issues, with its needleless technique.

INJECTOR, LYMPHANGIOGRAPHIC *(Cns/Neurology) 84RCB*

Cook Inc. 800-457-4500
PO Box 489, Bloomington, IN 47402

INJECTOR, MEDICATION (INOCULATOR) *(General) 80RCC*

Activa Brand Products Inc. 800-991-4464
36 Fourth St., Charlottetown, PEI C1E-2B3 Canada
PRECI-JET 50 needleless insulin injector, pen shaped, weight: 160g, size: 14x2cm, capacity: 50 units U-100 insulin; front tube assembly contains cylinder & piston, distal end accepts nozzle cap & disposable vial holder, handle contains power source & injection trigger button with safety catch. Injector accepts 2 types of insulin with window showing amount of units loaded.

Mada, Inc. 800-526-6370
625 Washington Ave, Carlstadt, NJ 07072
Inoculator using no needles.

Med-E-Jet D. 800-231-4203
8092 Olmway Ave, Olmsted Falls, OH 44138
For giving injections without needles, call for model number & price 800-231-4203, fax 440-235-2247. E-mail spetz@columbus.rr.com

Meridian Medical Technologies 800-638-8093
10240 Old Columbia Rd, Columbia, MD 21046
Automatic unit for insecticide poisoning antidote (atropen), intramuscular injection.

Owen Mumford Usa, Inc. 800-421-6936
1755 W Oak Commons Ct Ste A, Marietta, GA 30062

INJECTOR, PEN *(General) 80NSC*

Microplastics, Inc. 630-513-2900
406 38th Ave, Saint Charles, IL 60174
Insulin Pen

INJECTOR, SAMPLE *(Chemistry) 75UHV*

Bio-Rad Laboratories, Life Science Group 800-424-6723
2000 Alfred Nobel Dr, Hercules, CA 94547

INJECTOR, SAMPLE *(cont'd)*

Cetac Technologies, Inc. 800-369-2822
14306 Industrial Rd, Omaha, NE 68144

GP Instruments 888-215-6855
11130 Kingston Pike Ste 1200, Knoxville, TN 37934
Fixed-loop and variable-loop HPLC autosamplers.

Jasco, Inc. 800-333-5272
8649 Commerce Dr, Easton, MD 21601

Leap Technologies 800-229-8814
PO Box 969, Carrboro, NC 27510

Spectrum Laboratories, Inc. 800-634-3300
18617 S Broadwick St, Rancho Dominguez, CA 90220
HPLC syringe injectors for Rheodyne, Altex and Waters UK6 valve injection system.

INJECTOR, SYRINGE *(General) 80RCD*

Baxa Corporation 800-567-2292
9540 S Maroon Circle, Suite 400, Englewood, CO 80112
PhaSeal Injector, used with syringe, Protector and Connector to create a closed system for handling hazardous drugs.

Cadence Science Inc. 888-717-7677
1979 Marcus Ave Ste 215, New Hyde Park, NY 11042

Hamilton Company 800-648-5950
4990 Energy Way, Reno, NV 89502

Innovative Med Inc. 877-779-9492
4 Autry Ste B, Irvine, CA 92618
Inderm-PSI and Inderm Basic Plus, the latest in mico-injection therapy guns. www.inderm-psi.com

Medrad, Inc. 800-633-7231
100 Global View Dr, Warrendale, PA 15086
For Angio, CT, and MR Medrad injection systems. Syringe Loaders: Spectris MR Syringe Loader and CT Syringe Loader are easy-to-use, convenient syringe loaders for both the MR and CT modalities.

Meridian Medical Technologies 800-638-8093
10240 Old Columbia Rd, Columbia, MD 21046
Automatic unit for insecticide poisoning antidote (atropen), intramuscular injection. TRUJECT auto-injector-front end activated.

Pharmajet 303-526-4278
24797 Foothills Dr N, Golden, CO 80401
Needle free injection device

Vetter Pharma-Turm, Inc. 215-321-6930
1790 Yardley Langhorne Rd, Heston Hall/Carriage House, Suite 203
Yardley, PA 19067

INJECTOR, THERMAL DILUTION *(Cardiovascular) 74RCE*

Advanced Biomedical Devices, Inc. (Abd, Inc.) 978-470-1177
Dundee Park, Bldg. 17, Andover, MA 01810
OMP 372000 CO2 powered injector for thermal dilution

INJECTOR, VERTEBROPLASTY (DOES NOT CONTAIN CEMENT) *(Orthopedics) 87OAR*

Osseon Therapeutics, Inc. 877-567-7366
2330 Circadian Way, Santa Rosa, CA 95407
OsseoFlex 1.0 Steerable Needle

Vidacare Corp. 800-680-4911
4350 Lockhill Selma Rd Ste 150, Shavano Park, TX 78249
On-Control

INSERT, TUBAL OCCLUSION *(Obstetrics/Gyn) 85HHS*

Accellent El Paso 915-771-9112
31 Butterfield Trail Blvd Ste C, El Paso, TX 79906
Essure

Conceptus, Inc. 650-962-4000
331 E Evelyn Ave, Mountain View, CA 94041
Essure System for Permanent Birth Control

Richard Wolf Medical Instruments Corp. 800-323-9653
353 Corporate Woods Pkwy, Vernon Hills, IL 60061

INSERTER, MYRINGOTOMY TUBE *(Ear/Nose/Throat) 77JYM*

Exmoor Plastics Inc. 317-244-1014
304 Gasoline Aly, Indianapolis, IN 46222
EXMOOR Myringotomy kit, procedure pack for myringotomy with or without vent tubes.

Mednet Locator, Inc. 800-754-5070
7000 Shadow Oaks Dr, Memphis, TN 38125
Ventilation tube.

INSERTER, MYRINGOTOMY TUBE *(cont'd)*

Micromedics 800-624-5662
1270 Eagan Industrial Rd, Saint Paul, MN 55121
The T-Tube Inserter is a reusable instrument that facilitates rapid insertion of any length T-Tube.

INSERTER, SACCULOTOMY TACK *(Ear/Nose/Throat) 77JYN*

Kingswood Technology, Inc. 203-386-1839
44 Rachel Dr, Stratford, CT 06615

INSERTER/REMOVER, LENS, CONTACT *(Ophthalmology) 86KYE*

Dmv Corporation 800-522-9465
1024 Military Rd, Zanesville, OH 43701
Hard lens and RGP Inserter/remover and SOFTLENS inserter/remover. Also available, magnifying mirror for lens insertion/removal and Luma Serter luminous lens guide.

Softsert, Inc. 516-887-2056
19 Reunion Rd, Rye Brook, NY 10573
Softsert+plus $42.50/10 pack soft lens remover/applicator... Original Softsert $35.00/10 pack soft lens applicator... Lensvue2 'viewer/applicator' (To identify an inside out lens and apply it correctly) $99.50/10pack...Combo 12-pack (get aquainted pack) 4 of each of the above for those not familiar with our products)$72.50/12pack.

Western Ophthalmics Corporation 800-426-9938
19019 36th Ave W Ste G, Lynnwood, WA 98036

INSOLES, MEDICAL *(General) 80KYS*

Action Products, Inc. 800-228-7763
954 Sweeney Dr, Hagerstown, MD 21740

Alimed, Inc. 800-225-2610
297 High St, Dedham, MA 02026

Brantlin 954-691-6476
1511 NE 40th St, Pompano Beach, FL 33064
Insole.

Chesson Laboratory Associates, Inc. 919-636-5773
603 Ellis Rd, Durham, NC 27703
Insole.

Crown Mats 800-628-5463
2100 Commerce Dr, Fremont, OH 43420

Diapedia, Llc 814-234-0700
200 Innovation Blvd Ste 241, State College, PA 16803
Multiple density insert.

DJO Inc. 800-336-6569
1430 Decision St, Vista, CA 92081

Flat-D Innovations, Inc. 319-447-4840
7531 Berkshire Dr NE, Cedar Rapids, IA 52402
Flat-d, chair pad, premium, overpad-d, disposable.

K-Fit Orthotics Llc 516-293-6400
1464 Old Country Rd, Plainview, NY 11803
K-fit orthotic foot orthotic / arch support.

Klm Laboratories, Inc. 800-556-3668
28280 Alta Vista Ave, Valencia, CA 91355
Custom Orthotics, Prefabricated insoles & shells. System Rx Shells.

Lohmann & Rauscher, Inc. 800-279-3863
6001 SW 6th Ave Ste 101, Topeka, KS 66615

Mark Medical 800-433-3668
1168 Aster Ave Ste C, Sunnyvale, CA 94086
FEATHER STEPS/SDO Custom Fluid Orthotics containing highly viscous silicone for diabetic ulcers and many other foot aliments. Custom made for precise fit. Also available. META PUMPERS ORTHOTICS - fluid orthotics for runners and athletes. Provides biomechanical alignment and more shock absorption while running. Helps alleviate hip and knee pain, anterior tendonitis, arthritis and patellofemoral joint dysfunction.

Medi-Dyne Healthcare Products, L.L.C. 800-810-1740
1812 Industrial Blvd, Colleyville, TX 76034
TULI heel cups, shock absorbers for the feet; helps prevent heel spurs and shin splints.

Optec Specialties, Inc. 770-513-7380
975 Progress Cir, Lawrenceville, GA 30043
Various.

Ossur Americas 949-268-3155
742 Pancho Rd, Camarillo, CA 93012

Paramedical Distributors 800-245-3278
2020 Grand Blvd, Kansas City, MO 64108
Shoe/foot insoles, cushions, pads, materials, etc.

Pedors Shoes 800-750-6729
1349 Old 41 Hwy NW Ste 130, Marietta, GA 30060

INSOLES, MEDICAL *(cont'd)*

Rehabilitation Technical Components, Corp. 919-732-1705
3913 Devonwood Rd, Hillsborough, NC 27278
Foot orthosis.

Schering-Plough Healthcare Products, Inc. 862-245-5115
4207 Michigan Avenue Rd NE, Cleveland, TN 37323
Various.

Step Forward Co. 253-631-0683
11109 SE Kent Kangley Rd, Kent, WA 98030
Arch support.

Truarch, Inc. 618-592-6468
6062 E 800th Ave, Robinson, IL 62454
Various types of orthotics.

Viscolas, Inc. 800-548-2694
8801 Consolidated Dr, Soddy Daisy, TN 37379
Shoe insoles.

INSTRUMENT GUARD *(Surgery) 79LXZ*

Axiom Medical, Inc. 800-221-8569
19320 Van Ness Ave, Torrance, CA 90501
Silicone tip/clamp covers, multiple sizes.

Healthmark Industries 800-521-6224
22522 E 9 Mile Rd, Saint Clair Shores, MI 48080
STERIGARD Tip Protectors, vented, silicone tip protectors for surgical instruments that prevent instruments from sticking to the tip protector.

Hunter Research Laboratories, Inc. 888-764-5463
1541 S Vine St, Denver, CO 80210
Needle recapping aid (disposable needlestick-prevention aid).

Micrins Surgical Instruments, Inc. 800-833-3380
28438 N Ballard Dr, Lake Forest, IL 60045

INSTRUMENT, BENDING (CONTOURING) *(Orthopedics) 87HXP*

Abbott Spine, Inc. 847-937-6100
12708 Riata Vista Cir Ste B-100, Austin, TX 78727
Bender.

Arthronet Medical, Inc. 949-254-3343
520 Broadway Ste 350, Santa Monica, CA 90401
Orthopedic manual instruments, various.

Biomet, Inc. 574-267-6639
56 E Bell Dr, PO Box 587, Warsaw, IN 46582
Various types of benoing instruments.

Depuy Spine, Inc. 800-227-6633
325 Paramount Dr, Raynham, MA 02767
Contouring instrument.

K2m, Inc. 866-526-4171
751 Miller Dr SE Ste F1, Leesburg, VA 20175
Bender.

Kls-Martin L.P. 800-625-1557
11239-1 St. John`s Industrial, Parkway South
Jacksonville, FL 32250
Plate bending tool, bending pliers.

Medtronic Sofamor Danek Instrument Manufacturing 901-396-3133
7375 Adrianne Pl, Bartlett, TN 38133
Various rod benders.

Medtronic Sofamor Danek Usa, Inc. 901-396-3133
4340 Swinnea Rd, Memphis, TN 38118
Various rod benders.

Musculoskeletal Transplant Foundation 732-661-0202
1232 Mid Valley Dr, Jessup, PA 18434

Warsaw Orthopedic, Inc. 901-396-3133
2500 Silveus Xing, Warsaw, IN 46582
Various rod benders.

Zimmer Holdings, Inc. 800-613-6131
1800 W Center St, PO Box 708, Warsaw, IN 46580

Zimmer Spine, Inc. 800-655-2614
7375 Bush Lake Rd, Minneapolis, MN 55439
Bending or conforming instrument.

Zimmer Trabecular Metal Technology 800-613-6131
10 Pomeroy Rd, Parsippany, NJ 07054
Starter femoral shaver, mini plus number 9.

INSTRUMENT, CLIP REMOVAL *(Cns/Neurology) 84HBQ*

Acra Cut, Inc. 978-263-0250
989 Main St, Acton, MA 01720
Clip remover.

INSTRUMENT, CLIP REMOVAL *(cont'd)*

Mikron Precision, Inc. 310-515-6221
1558 W 139th St Ste C, Gardena, CA 90249
Wound clip remover.

Teleflex Medical 800-334-9751
2917 Weck Drive, Research Triangle Park, NC 27709

Trans American Medical / Tamsco Instruments 708-430-7777
7633 W 100th Pl, Bridgeview, IL 60455
Medium grade surgical stainless steel.

Tuzik Boston 800-886-6363
104 Longwater Dr, Assinippi Park, Norwell, MA 02061

INSTRUMENT, DENTAL, MANUAL *(Dental And Oral) 76QOY*

Abiomed, Inc. 800-422-8666
22 Cherry Hill Dr, Danvers, MA 01923
PERIO TEMP (TM)

Almore International, Inc. 503-643-6633
PO Box 25214, Portland, OR 97298
Soft line trimmer used to cut away flesh and tissue conditioners. $195.00 each.

Becton Dickinson And Co. 866-906-8080
411 Waverley Oaks Rd, Waltham, MA 02452

Bien Air Usa, Inc. 800-433-2636
17880 Sky Park Cir Ste 140, Irvine, CA 92614

Cooley & Cooley, Ltd. 800-215-4487
8550 Westland West Blvd, Houston, TX 77041
FORMATILL-a set of five instruments for carving and creating posterior dental anatomy in composite restorations. Saves the dentists valuable chairtime in create perfect contacts,centric stop, line angles and cusps. No more flat posterior anatomy.

Danville Materials 800-827-7940
3420 Fostoria Way Ste A200, San Ramon, CA 94583
Micro dental plating pen.

Dentalez Group 866-DTE-INFO
101 Lindenwood Dr Ste 225, Valleybrooke Corporate Center
Malvern, PA 19355

Dento-Profile Scale Co. 800-936-8610
1010 8th St Ste A, Coronado, CA 92118
Dental supplies. $595.00 for Dento-Profile scale, $28.00 for Sorenson's sore-spot indicator.

Dentsply Canada, Ltd. 800-263-1437
161 Vinyl Ct., Woodbridge, ONT L4L 4A3 Canada

Forest Dental Products Inc 800-423-3535
6200 NE Campus Ct, Hillsboro, OR 97124

Kls-Martin L.P. 800-625-1557
11239-1 St. John`s Industrial, Parkway South
Jacksonville, FL 32250

Luckman Corporation 215-659-1664
1930 Old York Rd, Abington, PA 19001
ENCORE 403 high speed dental handpieces.

Miltex Inc. 800-645-8000
589 Davies Dr, York, PA 17402

Motloid Company 800-662-5021
300 N Elizabeth St, Chicago, IL 60607
Carvers, spatulas.

Prosurge Instruments, Inc. 866-832-7874
199 Laidlaw Ave, Jersey City, NJ 07306

Ruthal Industries Ltd. 800-445-6640
1 Industrial Ave., Mahwah, NJ 07430-2113

Rx Honing Machine Corporation 800-346-6464
1301 E 5th St, Mishawaka, IN 46544
RX Honing Machines: Detailed instrument sharpening manuals with over 60 pictures and illustrations using Rx honing sets. French, French Canadian, and German available.

Superior Dental & Test 800-528-7297
1501 SE Village Green Dr, Port St Lucie, FL 34952

Suter Dental Manufacturing Company, Inc. 800-368-8376
632 Cedar St, Chico, CA 95928

Toolmex Corporation 800-992-4766
1075 Worcester St, Natick, MA 01760
Dental instruments.

INSTRUMENT, DENTAL, MANUAL *(cont'd)*

Zimmer Dental, Inc. 800-854-7019
1900 Aston Ave, Carlsbad, CA 92008
GemLock™ touchless delivery tools are designed for use with the AdVent™, Tapered Screw-Vent®, Screw-Vent® and SwissPlus™ dental implant systems. The tools quickly and simply take the implant and fixture mount from packaging to the osteotomy. GemLock tools are manufactured from surgical grade stainless steel for consistent durability and strength. Using advanced patent-pending technology, the GemLock retaining mechanism utilizes a spring-loaded synthetic ruby bearing for enhanced reliability. The tools engage the internal hexagon of the fixture mount for increased precision, and provide a narrow profile diameter ideal for use in tight interdental spaces. The GemLock interlocking tools system - a retaining wrench (Cat. # RSR), standard and long retaining hex drivers (Cat. #s RH2.5 and RHL2.5, respectively) and a latch-lock retaining hex (Cat. # RHD2.5) - provides a superior tactile experience for the clinician when placing the implants.

INSTRUMENT, DIAMOND, DENTAL *(Dental And Oral) 76DZP*

A & M Instruments, Inc. 770-772-6404
3565 Trotter Dr, Alpharetta, GA 30004
Diamond burs.

Abrasive Technology, Inc. 740-548-4100
8400 Green Meadows Dr N, Lewis Center, OH 43035
Various types of dental diamond instruments.

Aesculap Implant Systems Inc. 1-800-234-9179
3773 Corporate Pkwy, Center Valley, PA 18034

Align Technology, Inc. 408-470-1000
881 Martin Ave, Santa Clara, CA 95050
Interproximal reduction kit.

Axis Dental 800-355-5063
800 W Sandy Lake Rd Ste 100, Coppell, TX 75019
Diamond rotary instruments and discs.

Cadco Dental Products 800-833-8267
600 E Hueneme Rd, Oxnard, CA 93033
Priced from $9.00 each, 35 rotary curettage diamonds.

Cutting Edge Instruments Inc. 330-916-8858
312 River Rd., Bridgewater Corners, VT 05035
Diamond bur.

Dedeco Intl., Inc. 845-887-4840
11617 Route 97, Long Eddy, NY 12760
Various types of dental diamond instruments.

Den-Mat Holdings, Llc 805-922-8491
2727 Skyway Dr, Santa Maria, CA 93455
No common name listed.

Dent Zar, Inc. 800-444-1241
6362 Hollywood Blvd Ste 214, Los Angeles, CA 90028
Dental diamond instrument.

Dentalez Group 866-DTE-INFO
101 Lindenwood Dr Ste 225, Valleybrooke Corporate Center
Malvern, PA 19355

Dentalez Group, Stardental Division 717-291-1161
1816 Colonial Village Ln, Lancaster, PA 17601
Intra oral device for snoring and sleep apnea.

Dentsply Canada, Ltd. 800-263-1437
161 Vinyl Ct., Woodbridge, ONT L4L 4A3 Canada

Dux Dental 800-833-8267
600 E Hueneme Rd, Oxnard, CA 93033
Priced from $9.00 each, 35 rotary curettage diamonds.

Garrison Dental Solutions 616-842-2244
110 Dewitt Ln, Spring Lake, MI 49456
Diamond burrs, diamond instruments.

Lasco Diamond Products 800-621-4726
PO Box 4657, 9950 Canoga Avenue, Unit A-8, Chatsworth, CA 91313
Diamond Gingival Margin Files; Diamond FG, Surgical, and Laboratory Burs; Specialty burs for Porcelain Veneers, Rotary Gingival Curettage, Micron Finishing Diamonds, Depth Cutters, and more.

Miltex Dental Technologies, Inc. 516-576-6022
589 Davies Dr, York, PA 17402
Various dental diamond instruments.

Miltex Inc. 800-645-8000
589 Davies Dr, York, PA 17402

Moyco Technologies, Inc. 800-331-8837
200 Commerce Dr, Montgomeryville, PA 18936

INSTRUMENT, DIAMOND, DENTAL *(cont'd)*

Pentron Clinical Technologies 203-265-7397
68-70 North Plains Industrial, Road, Wallingford, CT 06492
Dental diamond instrument.

Pentron Laboratory Technologies 203-265-7397
53 N Plains Industrial Rd, Wallingford, CT 06492
3-d dental diamonds.

Premier Dental Products Co. 888-670-6100
1710 Romano Dr, PO Box 4500, Plymouth Meeting, PA 19462

Premier Medical Products 888-PREMUSA
1710 Romano Dr, Plymouth Meeting, PA 19462
Non-dental. Podiatric/dermal. PBS Diamond Burs - Diamond rotary instruments.

Repco 800-726-1852
1227 W Magnolia Ave Ste 310, Fort Worth, TX 76104
Diamond points for periodontology, general and cosmetic dentistry. Also, Diamond+PlusTechnologies, microsurgical diamond instruments for large-and small-bone surgical applications. Superior quality diamond burs and discs to integrate with existing power surgical-drill systems.

S.S. White Burs Inc. 800-535-2877
1145 Towbin Ave, Lakewood, NJ 08701
BLACK coarse, finishing and equilibrating diamond instruments and diamonds for composite (natural matrix).

Salvin Dental Specialties, Inc. 800-535-6566
3450 Latrobe Dr, Charlotte, NC 28211
Various types of dental diamond rotary instruments.

Shofu Dental Corporation 800-827-4638
1225 Stone Dr, San Marcos, CA 92078
ROBOT FG POINTS, GINGICURETTAGE, TPE DIAMONDS, HYBRID POINTS, T & F HYBRID POINTS, SUMMADISK, ROBOT CARBIDE FINISHERS, ROBOT CARBIDE CUTTERS

Spectrum Systems, Llc 717-845-5339
465 S Ogontz St, --, York, PA 17403

Spring Health Products, Inc. 800-800-1680
705 General Washington Ave Ste 701, Norristown, PA 19403
Diamond tools for arthroscopic surgery.

Sterngold 800-243-9942
23 Frank Mossberg Dr, PO Box 2967, Attleboro, MA 02703

Ultradent Products, Inc. 801-553-4586
505 W 10200 S, South Jordan, UT 84095
Dental diamond instruments and dental burs.

Westside Packaging, Llc. 909-570-3508
1700 S Baker Ave Ste A, Ontario, CA 91761
Abrasive device to smooth tooth surface.

3m Unitek 800-634-5300
2724 Peck Rd, Monrovia, CA 91016

INSTRUMENT, DIAMOND, DENTAL, REPROCESSED
(Dental And Oral) 76NLD

Ascent Healthcare Solutions 480-763-5300
10232 S 51st St, Phoenix, AZ 85044
Diamond dental instrument.

INSTRUMENT, DISSECTING, LAPAROSCOPIC *(Surgery) 79QQU*

Boss Instruments, Ltd. 800-210-2677
395 Reas Ford Rd Ste 120, Earlysville, VA 22936

Bryan Corp. 800-343-7711
4 Plympton St, Woburn, MA 01801
5mm/33cm spatula, j hook, l hook insulated with trumpet valve.

Elmed, Inc. 630-543-2792
60 W Fay Ave, Addison, IL 60101

Ethicon Endo-Surgery, Inc. 800-USE-ENDO
4545 Creek Rd, Cincinnati, OH 45242
ENDOPATH straight and curved dissector, short with unipolar cautery, 5mm rotating, 5mm with handle, ratchet handle, curved handle and curved ratchet handle, micro. Blunt dissector, 5mm, disposable. Set 5mm, reuseable. Shaft: 5mm blunt grasper also, with tooth; 5mm micro and curved dissector; 5mm extractor; 5mm hook and micro scissors; 5mm needleholder; all reuseable. Tissue manipulator, 5mm endoscopic. 10mm Babcock grasper, 10mm bowel clamp and 10mm Kelly clamp, disposable and curved. Kelly dissector 10mm bowel, disposable, right-angle and cherry blunt dissector, plastic handle, 3 per kit. Scissors, Metzenbaum 10mm with uniolar cautery rotating shaft.

Genicon 800-936-1020
6869 Stapoint Ct Ste 114, Winter Park, FL 32792
Mono Polar Instrumentation

INSTRUMENT, DISSECTING, LAPAROSCOPIC *(cont'd)*

Md International, Inc. 305-669-9003
11300 NW 41st St, Doral, FL 33178

Prosurge Instruments, Inc. 866-832-7874
199 Laidlaw Ave, Jersey City, NJ 07306

Richard Wolf Medical Instruments Corp. 800-323-9653
353 Corporate Woods Pkwy, Vernon Hills, IL 60061

Smith & Nephew, Inc., Endoscopy Division 800-343-8386
150 Minuteman Rd, Andover, MA 01810

Synectic Medical Product Development 203-877-8488
60 Commerce Park, Milford, CT 06460

INSTRUMENT, DISSECTING, MYOMA, LAPAROSCOPIC
(Surgery) 79QQY

Elmed, Inc. 630-543-2792
60 W Fay Ave, Addison, IL 60101

Richard Wolf Medical Instruments Corp. 800-323-9653
353 Corporate Woods Pkwy, Vernon Hills, IL 60061

Wisap America 800-233-8448
8231 Melrose Dr, Lenexa, KS 66214

INSTRUMENT, ELECTROSURGERY, LAPAROSCOPIC
(Surgery) 79SIJ

Bolt Bethel, Llc 763-434-5900
23530 University Avenue Ext NW, PO Box 135, Bethel, MN 55005

Ethicon Endo-Surgery, Inc. 800-USE-ENDO
4545 Creek Rd, Cincinnati, OH 45242

Mahe International Inc. 800-294-7946
468 Craighead St, Nashville, TN 37204

Premier Medical Products 888-PREMUSA
1710 Romano Dr, Plymouth Meeting, PA 19462
Non-laparoscopic. LOOP insulated gynecology instruments.

Surgicorp, Inc. 727-934-5000
40347 US Highway 19 N Ste 121, Tarpon Springs, FL 34689
Endoscopic, ophthalmic and E.N.T. instrumentation imported directly from the manufacturer.

INSTRUMENT, ELECTROSURGICAL, FIELD FOCUSED
(Cns/Neurology) 84MBZ

Ellman International, Inc. 800-835-5355
3333 Royal Ave, Rockville Centre, NY 11572

Encision Inc. 303-444-2600
6797 Winchester Cir, Boulder, CO 80301
AEM laparoscopic electrosurgical instrument with AEM technology built in.

INSTRUMENT, FORMING, MATERIAL, CRANIOPLASTY
(Cns/Neurology) 84HBX

Codman & Shurtleff, Inc 800-225-0460
325 Paramount Dr, Raynham, MA 02767

Hu-Friedy Manufacturing Co., Inc. 800-483-7433
3232 N Rockwell St, Chicago, IL 60618
SATIN STEEL XTS, Composite instrument line; composite placing, shaping, and forming. 22 types priced from $26.45.

INSTRUMENT, IMPLANTATION, SHUNT *(Cns/Neurology) 84GYK*

Codman & Shurtleff, Inc 800-225-0460
325 Paramount Dr, Raynham, MA 02767

Integra Neurosciences Pr 800-654-2873
Road 402 North, Km 1.2, Anasco, PR 00610
Various styles of instruments.

Medtronic Neurosurgery 800-468-9710
125 Cremona Dr, Goleta, CA 93117
Catheter passer instruments.

Microcision Llc 800-264-3811
5805 Keystone St, Philadelphia, PA 19135

INSTRUMENT, KNOT TYING, SUTURE, LAPAROSCOPIC
(Surgery) 79QRS

Apollo Endosurgery, Inc. 877-ENDO-130
7000 Bee Caves Rd Ste 350, Austin, TX 78746
Overstitch Tissue Approximation

Boss Instruments, Ltd. 800-210-2677
395 Reas Ford Rd Ste 120, Earlysville, VA 22936

Coopersurgical, Inc. 800-243-2974
95 Corporate Dr, Trumbull, CT 06611

Elmed, Inc. 630-543-2792
60 W Fay Ave, Addison, IL 60101

INSTRUMENT, KNOT TYING, SUTURE, LAPAROSCOPIC *(cont'd)*

Princeton Medical Group, Inc. 800-875-0869
1189 Royal Links Dr, Mt Pleasant, SC 29466

Ranfac Corp. 800-2RANFAC
30 Doherty Ave, Avon Industrial Park, Avon, MA 02322

Richard Wolf Medical Instruments Corp. 800-323-9653
353 Corporate Woods Pkwy, Vernon Hills, IL 60061

INSTRUMENT, MANUAL, GENERAL SURGICAL *(Surgery) 79MDM*

Abbott Vascular Inc. 800-227-9902
400 Saginaw Dr, Redwood City, CA 94063
Knot tying device.

Aesculap Implant Systems Inc. 1-800-234-9179
3773 Corporate Pkwy, Center Valley, PA 18034

American Eagle Instruments, Inc. 406-549-7451
6575 Butler Creek Rd, Missoula, MT 59808
Various types of manual general surgical instruments.

American Safety Razor Co. 540-248-8000
1 Razor Blade Ln, Verona, VA 24482
Plus safety scalpel system.

Anulex Technologies, Inc 877-326-8539
5600 Rowland Rd Ste 280, Minnetonka, MN 55343
Manual surgical instrument.

Arthrex Manufacturing 239-643-5553
1958 Trade Center Way, Naples, FL 34109
Grasper, forceps.

Arthrex, Inc. 239-643-5553
1370 Creekside Blvd, Naples, FL 34108
Various.

Bard Reynosa S.A. De C.V. 908-277-8000
Blvd. Montebello #1, Parque Industrial Colonial
Reynosa, Tamaulipas Mexico
Various

Bolt Bethel, Llc 763-434-5900
23530 University Avenue Ext NW, PO Box 135, Bethel, MN 55005

Boston Scientific Corporation 508-652-5578
8600 NW 41st St, Doral, FL 33166

Busse Hospital Disposables, Inc. 631-435-4711
75 Arkay Dr, Hauppauge, NY 11788
Sponge/solution bowls.

Cardinal Health, Snowden Pencer Products 847-689-8410
5175 S Royal Atlanta Dr, Tucker, GA 30084
Manual surgical instruments.

Care Wise Medical Products Corp. 888-462-8725
15750 Vineyard Blvd Ste 160, Morgan Hill, CA 95037

Clinical Resolution Laboratory 213-384-0500
14401 Chambers Rd # 200, Tustin, CA 92780
Manually supplementary surgical,medical instrument.

Codman & Shurtleff, Inc 800-225-0460
325 Paramount Dr, Raynham, MA 02767

Cyberonics, Inc. 800-332-1375
100 Cyberonics Blvd, The Cyberonics Building, Houston, TX 77058
VNS THERAPY MODEL 402 TUNNELER

Cytyc Surgical Products 800-442-9892
250 Campus Dr, Marlborough, MA 01752
Manual surgical instrument.

Dentlight Inc. 972-889-8857
1411 E Campbell Rd Ste 500, Richardson, TX 75081
Dental forceps.

Depuy Orthopaedics, Inc. 800-473-3789
700 Orthopaedic Dr, P.O. Box 988, Warsaw, IN 46582
Various types of general surgical manual instruments.

Depuy-Raynham, A Div. Of Depuy Orthopaedics 800-451-2006
325 Paramount Dr, Raynham, MA 02767
Various types of general surgical manual instruments.

Dermatologic Lab & Supply, Inc. 800-831-6273
608 13th Ave, Council Bluffs, IA 51501
Comedone extractor.

Edrich Health Technologies Inc. 973-656-0777
177 Madison Ave Ste 1, Morristown, NJ 07960

Elmed, Inc. 630-543-2792
60 W Fay Ave, Addison, IL 60101

Entellus Medical 866-620-7615
6705 Wedgwood Ct N, Maple Grove, MN 55311
ENT - Entellus Medical FinESS Sinus Treat

INSTRUMENT, MANUAL, GENERAL SURGICAL *(cont'd)*

Ethicon Endo-Surgery, Inc. 877-384-4266
3801 University Blvd SE, Albuquerque, NM 87106
Various types of manual surgical instruments.

Eye Care And Cure 800-486-6169
4646 S Overland Dr, Tucson, AZ 85714
Surgical instruments.

Fehling Surgical Instruments 800-FEHLING
509 Broadstone Ln NW, Acworth, GA 30101

Florida Life Systems 727-321-9554
3446 5th Ave N, Saint Petersburg, FL 33713

Greatbatch Inc 716-759-5600
1771 E 30th St, Cleveland, OH 44114
Biomec instrument holder.

Holmed Corporation 508-238-3351
40 Norfolk Ave, South Easton, MA 02375

Instratek, Inc. 281-890-8020
210 Spring Hill Dr Ste 130, Spring, TX 77386
Surgical instruments for endoscopic surgical techniques and fixation procedures.

International Hospital Supply Co. 800-398-9450
6914 Canby Ave Ste 105, Reseda, CA 91335
OB/GYN, urology, plastic.

Ivry 305-448-9858
216 Catalonia Ave Ste 106, Coral Gables, FL 33134

J. Jamner Surgical Instruments, Inc 800-431-1123
9 Skyline Dr, Hawthorne, NY 10532

Kelsar, S.A. 508-261-8000
Blvd. Insurgentes, Libriamento a La, Tijuana 22450 Mexico
Various handheld instruments

Kentron Health Care, Inc. 615-384-0573
3604 Kelton Jackson Rd, P.o. Box 120, Springfield, TN 37172
Staple remover.

Laprostop, Llc 858-705-3838
1845 Newport Avenue, San Diego, CA 92107
Trocar accessory.

Magnum Medical 800-336-9710
3265 N Nevada St, Chandler, AZ 85225
First aid kit instruments.

Medchannel Llc 617-314-9861
1241 Adams St Apt 110, Dorchester Center, MA 02124
Dissector, ligator, brush, rule, bag.

Medicept, Inc. 508-231-8842
200 Homer Ave, Ashland, MA 01721
Various types of quick connect cannula sets.

Medline Manufacturing And Services Llc 847-837-2759
1 Medline Pl, Mundelein, IL 60060
Instruments,various.

Medone Surgical, Inc. 941-359-3129
670 Tallevast Rd, Sarasota, FL 34243
Various backflush handles.

Medtronic Spine Llc 877-690-5353
1221 Crossman Ave, Sunnyvale, CA 94089
Various types of sterile handles; introducer tool set/osteo introducer system.

Micrins Surgical Instruments, Inc. 800-833-3380
28438 N Ballard Dr, Lake Forest, IL 60045

Micro Medical Instruments 314-845-3663
123 Cliff Cave Rd, Saint Louis, MO 63129
Manual reusable instruments.

Minrad, Inc. 716-855-1068
50 Cobham Dr, Orchard Park, NY 14127
Surgical instruments.

Nanomed Devices, Inc. 518-862-0151
116 Kennewyck Cir, Slingerlands, NY 12159
Hand held instrument.

Omni-Tract Surgical, A Div. Of Minnesota Scientific, Inc. 800-367-8657
4849 White Bear Pkwy, Saint Paul, MN 55110
Omni-Tract Surgical Retractor System - surgical retractor for general use.

Pac-Dent Intl., Inc. 909-839-0888
21078 Commerce Point Dr, Walnut, CA 91789
Dental hand instrument holder.

INSTRUMENT, MANUAL, GENERAL SURGICAL *(cont'd)*

Personna Medical/Div. Of American Safety Razor Co. 800-457-2222
1 Razor Blade Ln, Verona, VA 24482
PERSONNA PLUS Safety Scalpel System, a system using a deidcated and weighted metal handle with a safety blade cartridge. User never has to touch the blade. Available with 5 handle sizes and 5 blade sizes. Also available in disposable with 5 blade sizes.

Pnavel Systems, Inc. 718-645-6304
1502 E 14th St Ste 2, Brooklyn, NY 11230
Surgical instruments, graspers, cannula, cutters.

Rx Honing Machine Corporation 800-346-6464
1301 E 5th St, Mishawaka, IN 46544
RX Honing Machines: Detailed instrument sharpening manuals with over 150 pictures and diagrams of surgical instruments being sharpened with the Rx system II sharpening machine.

Scanlan International, Inc. 800-328-9458
1 Scanlan Plz, Saint Paul, MN 55107

Schueler & Company, Inc. 516-487-1500
PO Box 528, Stratford, CT 06615

Solos Endoscopy 800-388-6445
65 Sprague St # B, Boston/dedham Commerce Park, Boston, MA 02136
Various surgical instruments.

Sontec Instruments Inc. 303-790-9411
7248 S Tucson Way, Centennial, CO 80112

Spine Wave, Inc. 203-944-9494
2 Enterprise Dr Ste 302, Shelton, CT 06484
Various types of handles.

Sri Surgical 813-891-9550
6801 Longe St, Stockton, CA 95206
Various.

Sri Surgical 813-891-9550
7086 Industrial Row Dr, Mason, OH 45040

Sri Surgical 813-891-9550
1416 Dogwood Way, Mebane, NC 27302

Sri Surgical 813-891-9550
2595 Custer Rd Ste B, Salt Lake City, UT 84104

Sri Surgical 813-891-9550
6675 Business Pkwy Ste A, Elkridge, MD 21075

Sri Surgical 813-891-9550
12950 Executive Dr, Sugar Land, TX 77478

Sri Surgical 813-891-9550
6024 Century Oaks Dr, Chattanooga, TN 37416

Sri Surgical 813-891-9550
1441 Patton Pl Ste 139, Carrollton, TX 75007

Sri Surgical 813-891-9550
2240 E Artesia Blvd, Long Beach, CA 90805

Sri Surgical Express Inc. 813-891-9550
4501 Acline Dr E Ste 170, Tampa, FL 33605

Stonhouse Manufacturing 231-548-5630
7693 Barney Rd, Alanson, MI 49706
Fishhook in skin remover.

Stryker Puerto Rico, Ltd. 939-307-2500
Hwy. 3, Km. 131.2, Las Guasimas Ind. Park, Arroyo, PR 00714
Various manual instruments.

Symmetry Medical Usa, Inc 207-786-2775
111 N Clay St, Claypool, IN 46510
Various types of manual surgical instruments.

Symmetry Medical Usa, Inc. 574-267-8700
486 W 350 N, Warsaw, IN 46582
Manual surgical instrument for general use.

Synergetics Usa, Inc. 800-600-0565
3845 Corporate Centre Dr, O Fallon, MO 63368
Scrapper.

Thermo Oriel 800-715-393
150 Long Beach Blvd, Stratford, CT 06615
Instruments for research use and spectroscopic use.

Thompson Surgical Instruments, Inc. 800-227-7543
10170 E Cherry Bend Rd, Traverse City, MI 49684
Table mounted retractor.

Tino, S.A. De C.V. 800-024-77-55
Hospital #631, Guadalajara, JALIS 44200 Mexico

Ussc Puerto Rico, Inc. 203-845-1000
Building 911-67, Sabanetas Industrial Park, Ponce, PR 00731
Surgical grasper.

INSTRUMENT, MANUAL, GENERAL SURGICAL *(cont'd)*

Velco Tool And Die Co. 949-855-6638
20551 Pascal Way, Lake Forest, CA 92630
Instrument used for passing sutures through soft tissue.

West Coast Surgical Llc. 650-728-8095
141 California Ave Ste 101, Half Moon Bay, CA 94019
Curettes,various types of retractors with removable blades.

World Medical Equipment, Inc. 800-827-3747
3915 152nd St NE, Marysville, WA 98271
Specialize in refurbished ECG, NIBP, SAO2, monitors and defibrillators-Datex-Ohmeda, Nellcor, Dinamap, Physio Control, Datascope as well as OR tables, lights, autoclaves, anesthesia machines, and accessories.

310 Llc 904-382-0911
1901 S Harbor City Blvd Ste 600, Melbourne, FL 32901
Instrument storage pack.

INSTRUMENT, MICROSURGICAL *(Cns/Neurology) 84GZX*

Akorn, Inc. 800-535-7155
2500 Millbrook Dr, Buffalo Grove, IL 60089
Titanium and stainless steel microsurgical tissue, tying forceps, needle holders, scissors, etc.

Altair Instruments, Inc. 805-388-8503
330 Wood Rd Ste J, Camarillo, CA 93010

Ami Dental, Inc. 800-969-0405
9000 Southwest Fwy Ste 328, Houston, TX 77074
Medical supplies.

Arosurgical Instruments Corp. 800-776-1751
537 Newport Center Dr Ste 101, Newport Beach, CA 92660
MICROsurgical instruments. Micro spring handle scissors, 8cm to 18cm, STR & CVD. MICRO needle holders, 12 to18cm, STR & CVD titanium and stainless steel, DIAMOND DUSTED JAWS.

Bausch & Lomb Surgical 636-255-5051
3365 Tree Court Ind Blvd, Saint Louis, MO 63122

Boss Instruments, Ltd. 800-210-2677
395 Reas Ford Rd Ste 120, Earlysville, VA 22936
Ophthalmic, vascular/cardiovascular, ENT, plastic surgery, neurosurgical, orthopedic, general surgery.

Cameron-Miller, Inc. 800-621-0142
5410 W Roosevelt Rd, Road #241, Chicago, IL 60644

Codman & Shurtleff, Inc 800-225-0460
325 Paramount Dr, Raynham, MA 02767

Cynthia Flores Castrejon 52-5-780-36-97
Plazuela #24, Mz 12, Lt 8 Casa, 3 Plazas De Aragon
Nezahualcoyotl, EDO. 57139 Mexico
Various.

Deknatel Snowden-Pencer 800-367-7874
5175 S Royal Atlanta Dr, Tucker, GA 30084
Endoscopic instruments, equipment and scissors.

Eagle Laboratories 800-782-6534
10201 Trademark St Ste A, Rancho Cucamonga, CA 91730
Disposable blades and knives for microsurgery.

Elmed, Inc. 630-543-2792
60 W Fay Ave, Addison, IL 60101

Eriem Surgical 800-833-3380
28438 N Ballard Dr, Lake Forest, IL 60045

Fehling Surgical Instruments 800-FEHLING
509 Broadstone Ln NW, Acworth, GA 30101

Fischer Surgical Inc. 314-303-7753
1343 Pine Dr, Arnold, MO 63010
Various types of microsurgical instruments.

Integral Design Inc. 781-740-2036
52 Burr Rd, Hingham, MA 02043

International Hospital Supply Co. 800-398-9450
6914 Canby Ave Ste 105, Reseda, CA 91335
Surgical, specialty, orthopedic, neuro, endoscopic, and dental instruments.

Ivry 305-448-9858
216 Catalonia Ave Ste 106, Coral Gables, FL 33134

Jedmed Instruments Co. 314-845-3770
5416 Jedmed Ct, Saint Louis, MO 63129

Kapp Surgical Instrument, Inc. 800-282-5277
4919 Warrensville Center Rd, Cleveland, OH 44128
General operating-room-grade surgical instruments; also available, custom stainless-steel surgical instruments.

INSTRUMENT, MICROSURGICAL *(cont'd)*

Katena Products, Inc. 800-225-1195
4 Stewart Ct, Denville, NJ 07834
For cataract, glaucoma and other ophthalmic surgical procedures.

Kirwan Surgical Products, Inc. 888-547-9267
180 Enterprise Dr, PO Box 427, Marshfield, MA 02050

Kmedic 800-955-0559
190 Veterans Dr, Northvale, NJ 07647

Kmi Surgical Ltd. 800-528-2900
110 Hopewell Rd, Laird Professional Building, Downingtown, PA 19335

Lfi, Inc-Laser Fare, Inc. 401-231-4400
1 Industrial Dr S, Lan-Rex Industrial Pk., Smithfield, RI 02917

LinkBio Corp. 800-932-0616
300 Round Hill Dr, Rockaway, NJ 07866

Mark Medical Manufacturing, Inc. 610-269-4420
530 Brandywine Ave, Downingtown, PA 19335
Bipolar and monopolar electrosurgical instruments.

Medone Surgical, Inc. 941-359-3129
670 Tallevast Rd, Sarasota, FL 34243
Various styles of neurosurgery instruments.

Medtronic Sofamor Danek Usa, Inc. 901-396-3133
4340 Swinnea Rd, Memphis, TN 38118
Microsurgical, instruments.

Micrins Surgical Instruments, Inc. 800-833-3380
28438 N Ballard Dr, Lake Forest, IL 60045

Micro-Aire Surgical Instruments, Inc. 800-722-0822
1641 Edlich Dr, Charlottesville, VA 22911

Micromanipulator Co., Inc., The 800-972-4032
1555 Forrest Way, Carson City, NV 89706
Products and accessories to aid in embryo recovery, grading, splitting, injection, micromanipulation and photomicrography.

Miltex Inc. 800-645-8000
589 Davies Dr, York, PA 17402

Mizuho America Inc. 800-699-2547
133 Brimbal Ave, Beverly, MA 01915

Ortho Development Corp. 800-429-8339
12187 Business Park Dr, Draper, UT 84020

Ortho-Med, Inc. 800-547-5571
3208 SE 13th Ave, Portland, OR 97202

Pmt Corp. 800-626-5463
1500 Park Rd, Chanhassen, MN 55317
Disposable.

Prosurge Instruments, Inc. 866-832-7874
199 Laidlaw Ave, Jersey City, NJ 07306

Roboz Surgical Instrument Co., Inc. 800-424-2984
PO Box 10710, Gaithersburg, MD 20898
Microdissecting instruments.

Rocket Medical Plc. 800-707-7625
150 Recreation Park Dr Ste 3, Hingham, MA 02043

Rx Honing Machine Corporation 800-346-6464
1301 E 5th St, Mishawaka, IN 46544
RX Honing Machines: Microsurgical instrument Rx system II sharpening machine with surgical set #92701 or hospital set #92801 include 40+ components for sharpening surgical instruments.

Sable Industries 800-890-0251
4751 Oceanside Blvd Ste G, Oceanside, CA 92056
Blades & knives.

Scanlan International, Inc. 800-328-9458
1 Scanlan Plz, Saint Paul, MN 55107

Smith & Nephew, Inc., Endoscopy Division 800-343-8386
150 Minuteman Rd, Andover, MA 01810
Arthroscopy instruments.

Smith & Nephew, Inc., Endoscopy Division 800-343-8386
130 Forbes Blvd, Mansfield, MA 02048

Specialty Surgical Instrumentation, Inc. 800-251-3000
200 River Hills Dr, Nashville, TN 37210

Surgical Instrument Manufacturers, Inc. 800-521-2985
1650 Headland Dr, Fenton, MO 63026

Surgical Laser Technologies, Inc. 800-366-4758
147 Keystone Dr, Montgomeryville, PA 18936
Endoscopic sinus surgery instruments.

Symmetry Tnco 888-447-6661
15 Colebrook Blvd, Whitman, MA 02382
Endoscopic punches, graspers, scissors.

INSTRUMENT, MICROSURGICAL *(cont'd)*

Synergetics Usa, Inc. 800-600-0565
3845 Corporate Centre Dr, O Fallon, MO 63368
Various.

Toolmex Corporation 800-992-4766
1075 Worcester St, Natick, MA 01760

Tuzik Boston 800-886-6363
104 Longwater Dr, Assinippi Park, Norwell, MA 02061

Venosan North America, Inc. 800-432-5347
300 Industrial Park Ave, PO Box 1067, Asheboro, NC 27205
VENOSAN Instruments for vein surgery.

Vital Concepts, Inc. 800-984-2300
4334 Brockton Dr SE Ste F, Grand Rapids, MI 49512
Pro Point, microsurgical blades - ophthalmic knives.

Warsaw Orthopedic, Inc. 901-396-3133
2500 Silveus Xing, Warsaw, IN 46582
Microsurgical, instruments.

INSTRUMENT, NEEDLE HOLDER/KNOT TYING *(Surgery) 79QPS*

Boss Instruments, Ltd. 800-210-2677
395 Reas Ford Rd Ste 120, Earlysville, VA 22936

Coopersurgical, Inc. 800-243-2974
95 Corporate Dr, Trumbull, CT 06611

Elmed, Inc. 630-543-2792
60 W Fay Ave, Addison, IL 60101

Fehling Surgical Instruments 800-FEHLING
509 Broadstone Ln NW, Acworth, GA 30101

Holmed Corporation 508-238-3351
40 Norfolk Ave, South Easton, MA 02375

Richard Wolf Medical Instruments Corp. 800-323-9653
353 Corporate Woods Pkwy, Vernon Hills, IL 60061

Smith & Nephew, Inc., Endoscopy Division 800-343-8386
150 Minuteman Rd, Andover, MA 01810

Synectic Medical Product Development 203-877-8488
60 Commerce Park, Milford, CT 06460

INSTRUMENT, PASSING, LIGATURE, KNOT TYING
(Cns/Neurology) 84HCF

Apple Medical Corp. 508-357-2700
28 Lord Rd Ste 135, Marlborough, MA 01752
Suture snare.

Boston Scientific Corporation 508-652-5578
780 Brookside Dr, Spencer, IN 47460

Depuy Mitek, A Johnson & Johnson Company 800-451-2006
50 Scotland Blvd, Bridgewater, MA 02324
Suture grasper, knot pusher.

E.A. Beck & Co. 949-645-4072
657 W 19th St Ste E, P O Box 10857, Costa Mesa, CA 92627
Trocar; ligature needle.

Integral Design Inc. 781-740-2036
52 Burr Rd, Hingham, MA 02043

Kirwan Surgical Products, Inc. 888-547-9267
180 Enterprise Dr, PO Box 427, Marshfield, MA 02050

Lsi Solutions Inc. 585-869-6641
7796 Victor Mendon Rd, Victor, NY 14564
Instrument, ligature passing and knot tying.

Ranfac Corp. 800-2RANFAC
30 Doherty Ave, Avon Industrial Park, Avon, MA 02322
Laparoscopic knot-pusher ligater enables doctor to tie multiple extracorporeal surgeon knots with added precision.

Scanlan International, Inc. 800-328-9458
1 Scanlan Plz, Saint Paul, MN 55107
CARDIOVASIVE knot slider and CARDIOVASIVE knot pusher.

Sutura, Inc. 714-437-9801
17080 Newhope St, Fountain Valley, CA 92708
Sterile knot pusher.

Suturtek Incorporated
51 Middlesex St, North Chelmsford, MA 01863
Suture,needle.

Ussc Puerto Rico, Inc. 203-845-1000
Building 911-67, Sabanetas Industrial Park, Ponce, PR 00731
Multiple.

INSTRUMENT, PASSING, SUTURE, LAPAROSCOPIC
(Surgery) 79QSH

Advanced Medical Innovations, Inc. 888-367-2641
9410 De Soto Ave Ste J, Chatsworth, CA 91311
Neutray™ Sharps Passing Tray - A iNeutral Zoneî Tray Pat. Pending: Neutray™ Sharps Passing Tray for hands free transfer of sharps during a surgical procedure. This innovative product has been specifically designed to handle many of the different styles of sharps used in today's O.R. It is the ultimate in safety since all sharp instruments have a specific slot or cavity that they can nestle in while they are being passed safely inside the neutral zone. It has a unique instrument pick-up area that protects the practitioner's hands from sharp or contaminated instruments unlike anything else available in the market today. It can handle virtually all sharps in surgery such as : scalpels & blades; needle/needle holders (all sizes); syringes; sharp instruments (like Iris Scissors); K-wires; Trocars and others. Two trays can be interconnected as an option for a one-handed needle exchange system.

Elmed, Inc. 630-543-2792
60 W Fay Ave, Addison, IL 60101

Inlet Medical, Inc. 800-969-0269
10340 Viking Dr Ste 125, Eden Prairie, MN 55344
CARTER-THOMASON needle-point suture passer includes closure of trocar sites following laparoscopic surgery and suture ligation of lacerated inferior epigastric arteries. CARTER-THOMASON INLET Close Sure, PILOT. METRA PS needle-point suture passer, grasper, suture, knot pusher, suture guides. Use includes shortening, round ligaments for uterine suspension. Also available are the FLEVEST procedure kit for shortening round and uterosacral ligaments for uterine prolapse repair and the AVESTA procedure kit for shortening and reinforcing uterosacral ligaments.

Richard Wolf Medical Instruments Corp. 800-323-9653
353 Corporate Woods Pkwy, Vernon Hills, IL 60061

INSTRUMENT, REMOVAL, MYOMA, LAPAROSCOPIC
(Surgery) 79SJP

Karl Storz Endoscopy-America Inc. 800-421-0837
600 Corporate Pointe, Culver City, CA 90230

Wisap America 800-233-8448
8231 Melrose Dr, Lenexa, KS 66214
POWER-DRIVE MORCELLATOR, MOTO-DRIVE CORDLESS MORCELLATOR, HAND-DRIVE and SEMM TISSUE PUNCH.

INSTRUMENT, SURGICAL, POWERED, PNEUMATIC
(Orthopedics) 87HSZ

Anspach Effort, Inc. 800-327-6887
4500 Riverside Dr, Palm Beach Gardens, FL 33410
Black MaxUniversal Instrument System: high speed pneumatic drill system for all facets of orthopedic and neurologic surgery. Capabilities for working in bone, biometals and bioplastics. Black Max Neuro System with same features as the above except used in neurosurgery.

Arthrex, Inc. 239-643-5553
1370 Creekside Blvd, Naples, FL 34108
Harvesting saw.

Biomet, Inc. 574-267-6639
56 E Bell Dr, PO Box 587, Warsaw, IN 46582
Ossotome.

Brasseler Usa - Medical 805-650-5209
4837 McGrath St Ste J, Ventura, CA 93003
Surgical instrument system.

Clarus Medical, Llc. 763-525-8400
1000 Boone Ave N Ste 300, Minneapolis, MN 55427
Instrument, surgical, orthopedic, pneumatic powered & accessory.

Depuy Orthopaedics, Inc. 800-473-3789
700 Orthopaedic Dr, P.O. Box 988, Warsaw, IN 46582
Various types of orthopedic surgical pneumatic instruments/motors-powered/access.

Depuy-Raynham, A Div. Of Depuy Orthopaedics 800-451-2006
325 Paramount Dr, Raynham, MA 02767
Various types of orthopedic surgical pneumatic instruments/motors-powered/access.

Lfi, Inc-Laser Fare, Inc. 401-231-4400
1 Industrial Dr S, Lan-Rex Industrial Pk., Smithfield, RI 02917

Medtronic Powered Surgical Solutions 800-643-2773
4620 N Beach St, Haltom City, TX 76137
Various models of motors/attach.various sterile/non-sterile accessories.

Micro-Aire Surgical Instruments, Inc. 800-722-0822
1641 Edlich Dr, Charlottesville, VA 22911

INSTRUMENT, SURGICAL, POWERED, PNEUMATIC *(cont'd)*

Minnesota Bramstedt Surgical, Inc. 800-456-5052
1835 Energy Park Dr, Saint Paul, MN 55108
The Woodpecker - a total hip broaching device. Manufactured by IMT and exclusively distributed in North America by MBS. Reduces head pressure, optimizes cutting efficiency and minimizes the need for patient restraint. In addition, bone-marrow emboli is decreased and accurate modeling of the medullary space is achieved.

Paragon Medical, Inc. 800-225-6975
8 Matchett Dr, Pierceton, IN 46562

Richard Wolf Medical Instruments Corp. 800-323-9653
353 Corporate Woods Pkwy, Vernon Hills, IL 60061
RIWO arthroscopic shaver system.

Strenumed, Inc. 805-477-1000
1833 Portola Rd Unit K, Ventura, CA 93003
Rechargable battery.

Symmetry Medical Usa, Inc. 574-267-8700
486 W 350 N, Warsaw, IN 46582
Reamers.

Tava Surgical Instruments 805-650-5209
4837 McGrath St Ste J, Ventura, CA 93003
Surgical instrument system.

INSTRUMENT, VOLUME, BLADDER *(Gastro/Urology) 78WYI*

Verathon Inc. 800-331-2313
21222 30th Dr SE Ste 120, Bothell, WA 98021
BLADDERSCAN is a portable ultrasound instrument that measures bladder volume non-invasively. It provides immediate results, reducing patient trauma and discomfort. It also eliminates diagnostic catheterizations, minimizing the risk of urinary tract infections.

INSTRUMENTATION FOR CLINICAL MULTIPLEX TEST SYSTEMS *(Chemistry) 75NSU*

Affymetrix, Inc. 888-DNA-CHIP
3420 Central Expy, Santa Clara, CA 95051
Affymetrix Genechip Microarray Inst

Affymetrix, Inc. 916-376-1309
890 Embarcadero Dr, West Sacramento, CA 95605
Affymetrix scanner, autoloader, fluidics station, gcosdx software, and workstati.

Ambry Genetics 866-262-7943
100 Columbia Ste 200, Aliso Viejo, CA 92656
BeadXpress System

Autogenomics, Incorporated 760-477-2251
2890 Scott St, Vista, CA 92081
Instrumentation for clinical multiplex test systems.

Bio-Rad Laboratories Inc., Clinical Systems Div. 800-224-6723
4000 Alfred Nobel Dr, Hercules, CA 94547
Multi-analyte detection system.

Cambridge Research & Instrumentation (CRi) 800-383-7924
35B Cabot Rd, Woburn, MA 01801
Tissue Arrayer, Automated, precise TMA creation

Illumina, Inc. 1.800.809.4566
9885 Towne Centre Dr, San Diego, CA 92121
BeadXpress System

Luminex Corp. 888-219-8020
12212 Technology Blvd, Austin, TX 78727
Luminex 100; Luminex 100/200; Luminex 200

INSTRUMENTATION, HIGH PRESSURE LIQUID CHROMATOGRAPHY *(Toxicology) 91LDM*

Bio-Rad Laboratories Inc., Clinical Systems Div. 800-224-6723
4000 Alfred Nobel Dr, Hercules, CA 94547
Cdm system.

Polymer Laboratories, Now A Part Of Varian, Inc. 800-767-3963
160 Old Farm Rd, Amherst Fields Research Park, Amherst, MA 01002

INSUFFLATOR, CARBON-DIOXIDE, AUTOMATIC (FOR ENDOSCOPE) *(Gastro/Urology) 78FCX*

Cmt, Inc. 800-659-9140
PO Box 297, Hamilton, MA 01936

Elmed, Inc. 630-543-2792
60 W Fay Ave, Addison, IL 60101

Mahe International Inc. 800-294-7946
468 Craighead St, Nashville, TN 37204

Richard Wolf Medical Instruments Corp. 800-323-9653
353 Corporate Woods Pkwy, Vernon Hills, IL 60061

INSUFFLATOR, CARBON-DIOXIDE, AUTOMATIC (FOR ENDOSCOPE) *(cont'd)*

Smith & Nephew, Inc., Endoscopy Division — 800-343-8386
150 Minuteman Rd, Andover, MA 01810

Wisap America — 800-233-8448
8231 Melrose Dr, Lenexa, KS 66214
10-20-31 L/min gas warming Insufflators.

INSUFFLATOR, CARBON-DIOXIDE, UTEROTUBAL *(Obstetrics/Gyn) 85HES*

Karl Storz Endoscopy-America Inc. — 800-421-0837
600 Corporate Pointe, Culver City, CA 90230

Mahe International Inc. — 800-294-7946
468 Craighead St, Nashville, TN 37204

INSUFFLATOR, HYSTEROSCOPIC *(Obstetrics/Gyn) 85HIG*

Ams Innovative Center-San Jose — 800-356-7600
3070 Orchard Dr, San Jose, CA 95134

Davol Inc., Sub. C.R. Bard, Inc. — 800-556-6275
100 Crossings Blvd, Warwick, RI 02886
Tubing set,remote control,remote control pads.

Deknatel Snowden-Pencer — 800-367-7874
5175 S Royal Atlanta Dr, Tucker, GA 30084

Elmed, Inc. — 630-543-2792
60 W Fay Ave, Addison, IL 60101

Innervision Inc. — 901-682-0417
6258 E Shady Grove Rd, Memphis, TN 38120

Karl Storz Endoscopy-America Inc. — 800-421-0837
600 Corporate Pointe, Culver City, CA 90230
Control and monitor hysteroscopic irrigation.

Richard Wolf Medical Instruments Corp. — 800-323-9653
353 Corporate Woods Pkwy, Vernon Hills, IL 60061

Solos Endoscopy — 800-388-6445
65 Sprague St # B, Boston/dedham Commerce Park, Boston, MA 02136
Hysteroscopic insufflator.

Wisap America — 800-233-8448
8231 Melrose Dr, Lenexa, KS 66214

INSUFFLATOR, LAPAROSCOPIC *(Obstetrics/Gyn) 85HIF*

Adivamed — 703-729-8836
44141 Bristow Cir, Ashburn, VA 20147
Insuffation tubing

Aragon Surgical Inc. — 650-543-3100
1810 Embarcadero Rd Ste B, Palo Alto, CA 94303
Laparoscopic access device.

C&J Industries, Inc. — 814-724-4950
760 Water St, Meadville, PA 16335
Aragon Lapcap

Cardinal Health, Snowden Pencer Products — 847-689-8410
5175 S Royal Atlanta Dr, Tucker, GA 30084
Laparoscopic insufflator.

Cmt, Inc. — 800-659-9140
PO Box 297, Hamilton, MA 01936

Deknatel Snowden-Pencer — 800-367-7874
5175 S Royal Atlanta Dr, Tucker, GA 30084
Computerized insufflator for laparoscopic gynecological surgery.

Elmed, Inc. — 630-543-2792
60 W Fay Ave, Addison, IL 60101
Three models: $985 for PNEUMOMAT with 18-40 mm Hg insulation pressure, 1-2 LPM flow rate; weighs 24 lb. PNEUMOMAT digital electronic insufflator with 8 LPM flow, $5,495.

Geneva Medical Inc. — 630-232-2507
2571 Kaneville Ct, Geneva, IL 60134
Insufflaotion needle.

Genicon — 800-936-1020
6869 Stapoint Ct Ste 114, Winter Park, FL 32792
Laparoscopic Insufflators in 16 liter and 30 liter configurations with gas heating as an option.

Innervision Inc. — 901-682-0417
6258 E Shady Grove Rd, Memphis, TN 38120

Karl Storz Endoscopy-America Inc. — 800-421-0837
600 Corporate Pointe, Culver City, CA 90230

Lexion Medical, Llc. — 651-635-0000
5000 Township Pkwy, Saint Paul, MN 55110
Laparoscopic filter/heater/hydrator insufflation gas conditioner.

Mahe International Inc. — 800-294-7946
468 Craighead St, Nashville, TN 37204

INSUFFLATOR, LAPAROSCOPIC *(cont'd)*

Medtec Applications, Inc. — 630-628-0444
50 W Fay Ave, Addison, IL 60101
Insufflator.

Northgate Technologies Inc. — 800-348-0424
600 Church Rd, Elgin, IL 60123
CO2 Gas Warmer/Humidifier designed to warm and humidify CO2 gas during laparoscopic procedures. A device that when connected to insufflation tubing warms CO2 gas to body temperature. Also, insufflators with warming and humidification, the 7600 series, up to 40 LPM, electronic variable pressure relief, variable alarm, and computer control gas warming and TAP System (a method of direct measurement of abdominal pressure). The Humi-Flow System is designed for use as a means of warming and humidifying CO2 gas used in providing pneumoperitoneum during laparoscopic procedures. The Humi-Flow System is comprised of a stand-alone Controller and a Gas Warmer-Humidifier.

Reznik Instrument, Inc. — 847-673-3444
7337 Lawndale Ave, Skokie, IL 60076
Co2 and n2o insufflator.

Richard Wolf Medical Instruments Corp. — 800-323-9653
353 Corporate Woods Pkwy, Vernon Hills, IL 60061

Smith & Nephew Inc., Endoscopy Div. — 978-749-1000
76 S Meridian Ave, Oklahoma City, OK 73107
Laproscopic insufflator.

Smith & Nephew, Inc., Endoscopy Division — 800-343-8386
150 Minuteman Rd, Andover, MA 01810

Solos Endoscopy — 800-388-6445
65 Sprague St # B, Boston/dedham Commerce Park, Boston, MA 02136
Various models of insufflators.

Stryker Endoscopy — 800-435-0220
5900 Optical Ct, San Jose, CA 95138

Stryker Puerto Rico, Ltd. — 939-307-2500
Hwy. 3, Km. 131.2, Las Guasimas Ind. Park, Arroyo, PR 00714
Insufflator tube set.

Synectic Medical Product Development — 203-877-8488
60 Commerce Park, Milford, CT 06460

INSUFFLATOR, OTHER *(Surgery) 79RCH*

Deknatel Snowden-Pencer — 800-367-7874
5175 S Royal Atlanta Dr, Tucker, GA 30084
Endoscopic insufflator.

Mahe International Inc. — 800-294-7946
468 Craighead St, Nashville, TN 37204

Medical Device Resource Corporation — 800-633-8423
23392 Connecticut St, Hayward, CA 94545
GS9800 High-flow electronic endoscopic insufflator (15 LPM).

Richard Wolf Medical Instruments Corp. — 800-323-9653
353 Corporate Woods Pkwy, Vernon Hills, IL 60061

Smith & Nephew, Inc., Endoscopy Division — 800-343-8386
150 Minuteman Rd, Andover, MA 01810

Wisap America — 800-233-8448
8231 Melrose Dr, Lenexa, KS 66214
10-20-31 L/min warming insufflators.

INTERVERTEBRAL FUSION DEVICE WITH BONE GRAFT, CERVICAL *(Orthopedics) 87ODP*

Amedica Corporation — 801-839-3500
1885 W 2100 S, Salt Lake City, UT 84119
Valeo Spacer

Benvenue Medical, Inc. — 408-454-9300
3052 Bunker Hill Ln Ste 120, Santa Clara, CA 95054
Benvenue IBF Implant System

Binder Biomedical Inc. — 561-981-2682
2385 NW Executive Center Dr, Boca Raton, FL 33431
Newton

Centinel Spine Inc. — 952-885-0500
505 Park Ave Fl 14, New York, NY 10022
STALIF C

INTRAUTERINE DEVICE, CONTRACEPTIVE (IUD) AND INTRODUCER *(Obstetrics/Gyn) 85HDT*

Ortho-Mcneil-Janssen Pharmaceuticals, Inc. — 800-526-7736
1000 US Highway 202, Raritan, NJ 08869

INTRAVASCULAR RADIATION DELIVERY SYSTEM
(Cardiovascular) 74MOU

Best Vascular, Inc. 770-717-0904
4350 International Blvd, Norcross, GA 30093
Various types of vascular brachytherapy systems including sterile catheters and.

Guidant Corporation 408-845-3995
8934 Kirby Dr, Houston, TX 77054
Source delivery unit.

INTRODUCER, CATHETER *(Cardiovascular) 74DYB*

Abbott Vascular Inc. 800-227-9902
400 Saginaw Dr, Redwood City, CA 94063
Various sizes sterile catheter introducer and dilators for percutaneous use.

Abbott Vascular, Cardiac Therapies 800-227-9902
26531 Ynez Rd, Mailing P.O. Box 9018, Temecula, CA 92591
Sterile rotating hemostatic valve or external plastic valve.

Acumen Medical, Inc. 408-530-1810
275 Santa Ana Ct, Sunnyvale, CA 94085
Introducing catheter.

Angiodynamics, Inc. 518-795-1400
14 Plaza Drive, Latham, NY 12110

Angiodynamics, Inc. 800-472-5221
1 Horizon Way, Manchester, GA 31816
Percutaneous introducer kits, sizes from 6 to 16 french.

Argon Medical Devices Inc. 903-675-9321
1445 Flat Creek Rd, Athens, TX 75751
Innervasc access system.

Arrow Internacional De Mexico, S.A. De C.V. 610-378-0131
Modulo 1, Circuito 5, Parque Industrias De America
Col. Panamericana, Chihuahua Mexico
Various

Arrow International, Inc. 800-523-8446
2 Berry Dr, Mount Holly, NJ 08060
Various.

Arrow International, Inc. 800-523-8446
2400 Bernville Rd, Reading, PA 19605
Percutaneous sheath introducer.

Arrow Medical Products, Ltd. 800-387-7819
2300 Bristol Circle Unit 1, Oakville, ONT L6H-5S3 Canada
Percutaneous sheath introducers. Kits and sets available from $25.00.

Atek Medical 800-253-1540
620 Watson St SW, Grand Rapids, MI 49504
Femoral cannula and introducer.

B. Braun Medical, Inc. 610-596-2536
901 Marcon Blvd, Allentown, PA 18109
Intradyne

B. Braun Oem Division, B. Braun Medical Inc. 866-8-BBRAUN
824 12th Ave, Bethlehem, PA 18018

Bard Reynosa S.A. De C.V. 908-277-8000
Blvd. Montebello #1, Parque Industrial Colonial
Reynosa, Tamaulipas Mexico
Various

Becton Dickinson Infusion Therapy Systems, Inc. 888-237-2762
9450 S State St, Sandy, UT 84070

Bipore, Inc. 201-767-1993
31 Industrial Pkwy, Northvale, NJ 07647
ACCUFLEX, sheath introducer. ACCUFLEX Guiding Sheath for Carotids. ACCUFLEX Dialysis Declotting Sheath.

Boston Scientific Corp. 800-323-6472
5905 Nathan Ln N, Minneapolis, MN 55442
ANGIOPORT catheter introducer.

Cardio-Nef, S.A. De C.V. 01-800-024-0240
Rio Grijalva 186, Col. Mitras Norte, Monterrey, N.L. 64320 Mexico

Cardiomed Supplies Inc. 800-387-9757
5 Gormley Industrial Ave., P.O. Box 575
Gormley, ONT L0H 1 Canada
VALVEKIT Complete range of introducer with locking device for introducing balloon catheter.

Cardiovascular Systems, Inc. 877-CSI-0360
651 Campus Dr, Saint Paul, MN 55112
ViperSheath

Clinical Instruments Intl., Inc. 508-764-2200
278 Worcester St, Southbridge, MA 01550
Introducers.

INTRODUCER, CATHETER *(cont'd)*

Cook Inc. 800-457-4500
PO Box 489, Bloomington, IN 47402

Covidien Lp 508-261-8000
15 Hampshire St, Mansfield, MA 02048

Cryocor, Inc. 858-909-2213
9717 Pacific Heights Blvd, San Diego, CA 92121
Sheath introducer kit.

Datascope Corp. 800-288-2121
14 Philips Pkwy, Montvale, NJ 07645
For use with intra-aortic balloon catheters.

Datascope Corp., Cardiac Assist Division 201-307-5400
1300 MacArthur Blvd, Mahwah, NJ 07430
Catheter introducer set.

Diablo Sales & Marketing, Inc. 925-648-1611
PO Box 3219, Danville, CA 94526
Custom design and manufacturing of catheters and specialty guidewires. Guiding catheters; stent delivery and drug delivery systems.

Dma Med-Chem Corporation 800-362-1833
49 Watermill Ln, Great Neck, NY 11021

Edwards Lifesciences Research Medical 949-250-2500
6864 Cottonwood St, Midvale, UT 84047
Introducer.

Edwards Lifesciences Technology Sarl 949-250-2500
State Rd. 402 N.km 1.4, Anasco, PR 00610-1577
Introducer, catheter.

Enpath Medical, Inc. 800-559-2613
2300 Berkshire Ln N, Minneapolis, MN 55441

Ep Technologies, Inc. 888-272-1001
2710 Orchard Pkwy, San Jose, CA 95134
Intracardiac tontroducing sheath and accessories.

Ethicon Endo-Surgery, Inc. 800-USE-ENDO
4545 Creek Rd, Cincinnati, OH 45242
Percutaneous with catheter ECC05.

Ev3 Inc. 800-716-6700
9600 54th Ave N, Plymouth, MN 55442
Y-connector.

Ev3 Inc. 800-716-6700
4600 Nathan Ln N, Plymouth, MN 55442
Y connector.

Flowmedica, Inc. 866-671-9500
46563 Fremont Blvd, Fremont, CA 94538
Catheter introducer.

Galt Medical Corp. 800-639-2800
2220 Merritt Dr, Garland, TX 75041
Various types of sterile & non-sterile tearaway introducer sheaths.

Hospira, Inc. 877-946-7747
755 Jarvis Dr, Morgan Hill, CA 95037

Icu Medical (Ut), Inc 949-366-2183
4455 Atherton Dr, Salt Lake City, UT 84123
Various.

Inrad 800-558-4647
4375 Donkers Ct SE, Kentwood, MI 49512
Various.

Integra Lifesciences Corp. 609-275-0500
311 Enterprise Dr, Plainsboro, NJ 08536
Introducer needle.

Lifemed Of California 800-543-3633
1216 S Allec St, Anaheim, CA 92805

Medtronic Vascular 707-525-0111
3576 Unocal Pl, Santa Rosa, CA 95403

Medtronic, Inc. 800-633-8766
710 Medtronic Pkwy, Minneapolis, MN 55432
SOLO-TRAK.

Memcath Technologies Llc 651-450-7400
1777 Oakdale Ave, Saint Paul, MN 55118

Merit Medical Systems, Inc. 800-356-3748
1600 Merit Pkwy, South Jordan, UT 84095
Blood containment device. Captiva.

Navilyst Medical 800-833-9973
100 Boston Scientific Way, Marlborough, MA 01752
Various types of introducer sheaths and accessories and introducer sheath kits.

INTRODUCER, CATHETER *(cont'd)*

Neo Medical Inc. 888-450-3334
42514 Albrae St, Fremont, CA 94538
Introduceer, catheter.

Nmt Medical, Inc. 617-737-0930
27-43 Wormwood St, Boston, MA 02210
Sheath.

Onset Medical Corporation 949-716-1100
13900 Alton Pkwy Ste 120, Irvine, CA 92618
Sterile catheter for access during endovascular procedures.

Oscor, Inc. 800-726-7267
3816 Desoto Blvd, Palm Harbor, FL 34683
Lead introducer.

Promex Technologies, Llc 317-736-0128
3049 Hudson St, Franklin, IN 46131
Transjugular liver access set.

Specialized Health Products International, Inc. 800-306-3360
585 W 500 S, Bountiful, UT 84010
Majestik angiographic needle incorporates a built-in safety device which reduces the risk of accidental needlestick injuries.

St. Jude Medical Atrial Fibrillation 800-328-3873
14901 Deveau Pl, Minnetonka, MN 55345
Percutaneous introducer kits in sizes from 4 to 16 french; introducers with hemostasis valves venous introducers and peel-away introducers.

St. Jude Medical Cardiac Rhythm Management Div. 800-777-2237
15900 Valley View Ct, Sylmar, CA 91342
Subclavian cardiac pacing lead introducer sets 8-14Fr.

Taut, Inc. 800-231-8288
2571 Kaneville Ct, Geneva, IL 60134
Provides flexibility in strategically positioning the cholangiogram catheter. Models PI-63 & PI-93 available.

Terumo Medical Corporation 800-283-7866
950 Elkton Blvd, P.O.Box 605, Elkton, MD 21921
Catheter introducer.

Tfx Medical Oem 800-548-6600
50 Plantation Dr, Jaffrey, NH 03452

Thomas Medical Products, Inc. 866-446-3003
65 Great Valley Pkwy, Malvern, PA 19355
Various types of sterile percutaneous introducers.

Thoratec Corporation 800-456-1477
6101 Stoneridge Dr, Pleasanton, CA 94588

Vernay Laboratories, Inc. 800-666-5227
120 E South College St, Yellow Springs, OH 45387

Vlv Associates, Inc. 973-428-2884
30C Ridgedale Ave, East Hanover, NJ 07936
Safety Introducer Needle, OTN & Seldinger

Vnus Medical Technologies, Inc. 888-797-8346
5799 Fontanoso Way, San Jose, CA 95138
Catheter introducer.

Vygon Corp. 800-544-4907
2495 General Armistead Ave, Norristown, PA 19403

W.L. Gore & Associates,Inc 928-526-3030
1505 North Fourth St., Flagstaff, AZ 86004
Introducer sheath.

INTRODUCER, SPHERE *(Ophthalmology) 86HNP*

Bausch & Lomb Surgical 636-255-5051
3365 Tree Court Ind Blvd, Saint Louis, MO 63122

Integral Design Inc. 781-740-2036
52 Burr Rd, Hingham, MA 02043

INTRODUCER, SPINAL NEEDLE *(Anesthesiology) 73BWD*

Covidien Lp 508-261-8000
15 Hampshire St, Mansfield, MA 02048

Incisiontech 800-213-7809
9 Technology Dr, Staunton, VA 24401

Ranfac Corp. 800-2RANFAC
30 Doherty Ave, Avon Industrial Park, Avon, MA 02322

Spectra Medical Devices, Inc. 978-657-0889
260H Fordham Rd, Wilmington, MA 01887
needle introducer

Tegra Medical Inc. 508-541-4200
9 Forge Pkwy, Franklin, MA 02038

INTRODUCER, SYRINGE NEEDLE *(General) 80KZH*

Cadence Science Inc. 888-717-7677
1979 Marcus Ave Ste 215, New Hyde Park, NY 11042

Covidien Lp 508-261-8000
15 Hampshire St, Mansfield, MA 02048

Inrad 800-558-4647
4375 Donkers Ct SE, Kentwood, MI 49512
Introducer, syringe needle.

Medtronic Minimed 800-933-3322
18000 Devonshire St, Northridge, CA 91325
SOF-SERTER.

Neo Medical Inc. 888-450-3334
42514 Albrae St, Fremont, CA 94538
Breakaway needle introducer.

Neomend, Inc. 949-916-1630
9272 Jeronimo Rd Ste 119, Irvine, CA 92618
Sterile needle introducer.

Procedure Products, Inc. 360-693-1832
6622 Oakridge Dr, Gladstone, OR 97027
Introducer needles used to introduce guidewire in angiographic procedures.

Tfx Medical Oem 800-548-6600
50 Plantation Dr, Jaffrey, NH 03452

West Pharmaceutical Services Delaware Acquistion, 903-677-5017
1704 Enterprise St, Athens, TX 75751
Auto-injector.

INTRODUCER, T-TUBE *(Gastro/Urology) 78QTO*

Memcath Technologies Llc 651-450-7400
1777 Oakdale Ave, Saint Paul, MN 55118
To facilitate the introduction of catheters and instruments (endoscopes, resectoscopes, cystoscopes, laproscopy, nysteroscopes, etc.) and like the intermittent catheter to take sterile urine samples. Instillation of therapeutic drugs.

INVERSION UNIT *(Orthopedics) 87THB*

Stl International, Inc. / Teeter Hang Ups 253-840-5252
9902 162nd Street Ct E, Puyallup, WA 98375
Inversion tables, racks, and gravity boots.

IODINE (TINCTURE) *(Pathology) 88IAL*

Dynarex Corp. 888-356-2739
10 Glenshaw St, Orangeburg, NY 10962
Available in both prep and scrub solutions, meets USP and FDA standards.

ION ELECTRODE BASED ENZYMATIC, CREATININE *(Chemistry) 75CGL*

Abbott Point Of Care Inc. 609-443-9300
104 Windsor Center Dr, East Windsor, NJ 08520
Creatine test.

ION EXCHANGE RESIN, EHRLICH'S REAGENT, PORPHOBILINOGEN *(Chemistry) 75JNF*

Bio-Rad Laboratories Inc., Clinical Systems Div. 800-224-6723
4000 Alfred Nobel Dr, Hercules, CA 94547
Porphobilinogen test system.

IONTOPHORESIS DEVICE, DENTAL *(Dental And Oral) 76EGJ*

C & S Electronics, Inc. 402-563-3596
2565 16th Ave, Columbus, NE 68601
Sweat test apparatus.

Empi 651-415-9000
Clear Lake Industrial Park, Clear Lake, SD 57226
Device, iontophoresis, other uses.

Erchonia Medical 214-733-5209
2021 Commerce Dr, McKinney, TX 75069
Foot bath.

Naimco, Inc. 423-648-7730
4120 S Creek Rd, Chattanooga, TN 37406
Iontophoresis drug delivery electrodes.

Selective Med Components, Inc. 740-397-7838
564 Harcourt Rd, Mount Vernon, OH 43050
Iontophoresis electrode.

Travanti Pharma Incorporated 651-730-1008
2520 Pilot Knob Rd Ste 100, Mendota Heights, MN 55120
Ionto phoresis device.

IONTOPHORESIS EQUIPMENT *(Chemistry) 75UGQ*

R.A. Fischer Company — 800-525-3467
8751 White Oak Ave, Northridge, CA 91325
$675 for standard unit.

Wescor, Inc. — 800-453-2725
459 S Main St, Logan, UT 84321
$1,995.00 for Model 3700-Sys MACRODUCT system with fail-safe circuitry, controlled rate of change; visual sweat quantitation.

IONTOPHORESIS UNIT (SWEAT RATE) *(Gastro/Urology) 78RCP*

Wescor, Inc. — 800-453-2725
459 S Main St, Logan, UT 84321
Sweat analysis. $1,395.00 for the model 3120 SWEAT-CHEK sweat conductivity analyzer designed to interface with the MACRODUCT sweat collection system for analysis of microliter sweat samples by electrical conductivity.

IONTOPHORESIS UNIT, PHYSICAL MEDICINE *(Physical Med) 89KTB*

General Medical Co. — 800-432-5362
1935 Armacost Ave, Los Angeles, CA 90025
Iontophoretic sweat control devices for hyperhidrotics. $139.95 for pair of DRIONIC sweat control devices for treatment of sweating underarms, hands or feet.

Iomed, Inc. — 800-621-3347
2441 S 3850 W Ste A, Salt Lake City, UT 84120
PHORESOR iontophoresis unit.

Life-Tech, Inc. — 281-491-6600
4235 Greenbriar Dr, Stafford, TX 77477
NeedleBuster and Iontophor - microprocessor controlled applicators with Meditrodes - disposable drug delivery electrodes

Polychrome Medical — 763-585-9328
2700 Freeway Blvd Ste 750, Brooklyn Center, MN 55430
Ontophoretic test kit.

R. A. Fischer Co. — 800-525-3467
8751 White Oak Ave, Northridge, CA 91325
Galvanic unit.

IRON CHLORIDE-WEIGERT *(Pathology) 88HYQ*

American Mastertech Scientific, Inc. — 209-368-4031
1330 Thurman St, Lodi, CA 95240
Multiple.

IRRADIATOR *(Radiology) 90WIB*

Cis-Us, Inc. — 800-221-7554
10 Deangelo Dr, Bedford, MA 01730
IBL-437C. 3.8 liter blood irradiator.

IRRADIATOR, BLOOD TO PREVENT GRAFT VS HOST DISEASE *(Radiology) 90MOT*

J. L. Shepherd And Assoc. — 818-898-2361
1010 Arroyo St, San Fernando, CA 91340
Blood irradiators (various types).

IRRADIATOR, BLOOD, EXTRACORPOREAL *(Gastro/Urology) 78NAX*

Dkl Construction Management, Inc. — 231-947-6450
323 E Welch Ct Ste B, Traverse City, MI 49686
Ultraviolet blood irradiation device.

IRRIGATING SOLUTION, NON-INJECTABLE *(Surgery) 79LWD*

Ballard Medical Products — 770-587-7835
12050 Lone Peak Pkwy, Draper, UT 84020
Saline vials for inhalation therapy.

Baxter Healthcare Corporation, Global Drug Delivery — 888-229-0001
25212 W Il Route 120, Round Lake, IL 60073
Glycine irrigation. Irrigating solution G. TIS-U-SOL solution. Sodium Chloride irrigation solution, Lactated Ringer's solution.

IRRIGATOR, CALORIC *(Ear/Nose/Throat) 77QFS*

Gn Otometrics — 800-289-2150
125 Commerce Dr, Schaumburg, IL 60173
$5,950 per unit.

Life-Tech, Inc. — 281-491-6600
4235 Greenbriar Dr, Stafford, TX 77477
Caligator computer controlled caloric irrigator

Tsi Medical Ltd. — 800-661-7263
47 Athabascan Ave., Unit 105, Sherwood Park, AB T8A-4H3 Canada

IRRIGATOR, COLONIC *(Gastro/Urology) 78KPL*

Clearwater Colon Hydrotherapy, Inc. — 888-869-6191
3145 SW 74th Ter, Ocala, FL 34474
Colonics.

Dotolo Research Corp. — 800-237-8458
2875 Mcl Dr, Pinellas Park, FL 33782

Dotolo Research Western Div. — 623-936-0500
10199 W Van Buren St Ste 10, Tolleson, AZ 85353
Colon hydrotherapy instrument.

Lifestream Purification Systems, Llc — 877-564-3185
2001 S Lamar Blvd Ste G, Austin, TX 78704
Angel of Water CM-1 Surround.

Progressive Medical Systems, Inc. — 602-421-2484
1221 W Warner Rd Ste 103, Tempe, AZ 85284
Ez flow 1, rosebud.

Specialty Health Products, Inc. — 623-582-4950
21636 N 14th Ave Ste A1, Phoenix, AZ 85027
Colon hydro-therapy instrument.

Tiller Mind Body, Inc. — 210-308-8888
10911 West Ave, San Antonio, TX 78213
Lower bowel evacuation system for colon hydrotherapy.

Ultimate Concepts, Inc. — 801-566-3241
5056 Crimson Patch Way, Riverton, UT 84096
Colon irrigation device.

IRRIGATOR, OCULAR SURGERY *(Ophthalmology) 86KYG*

A.M.O. Puerto Rico Manufacturing, Inc — 714-247-8656
Rd. 402, Km. 4.2, Anasco, PR 00610
I/a tubing packs.

Alcon Manufacturing, Ltd. — 817-551-6813
714 Columbia Ave, Sinking Spring, PA 19608
Various models of operating room instrumentation for ocular surgery.

B. Braun Medical, Inc. — 610-596-2536
901 Marcon Blvd, Allentown, PA 18109

Med-Logics, Inc. — 949-582-3891
26061 Merit Cir Ste 102, Laguna Hills, CA 92653
Vacuum tubing.

Microsurgical Technology, Inc. — 425-556-0544
PO Box 2679, Redmond, WA 98073
INTER TIP I/A handpiece and MST unibody I/A handpiece. AERO DX, AERO TI, 20,000 TI Phaco handpieces. Bi-Manual I/A handpieces.

Mortan, Inc. — 800-423-8659
329 E Pine St, Missoula, MT 59802
MORGAN medi-FLOW Lens

Mortech, Llc. — 406-542-7040
323 SW Higgins Ave, Missoula, MT 59803
Ocular irrigation device.

Neomedix Corp. — 949-258-8355
15042 Parkway Loop Ste A, Tustin, CA 92780
Irrigation tubing.

Syntec, Inc. — 636-566-6500
812 N Truman Blvd, Crystal City, MO 63019
Light probe's.

IRRIGATOR, OCULAR, EMERGENCY *(Ophthalmology) 86WKX*

Mortan, Inc. — 800-423-8659
329 E Pine St, Missoula, MT 59802
MORGAN medi-FLOW Lens

IRRIGATOR, ORAL *(Dental And Oral) 76EFS*

Air Force, Inc. — 616-399-8511
933 Butternut Dr, Holland, MI 49424
Air powered oral irrigator.

Ethicare — 954-742-3599
2190 NW 74th Ave, Sunrise, FL 33313
Hydro-flo.

Global Dental Products — 516-221-8844
PO Box 537, Bellmore, NY 11710
TUBULICID PLUS. Endodontic irrigator.

Health & Hygiene, Inc. — 239-403-9919
4406 Exchange Ave Ste 127, Naples, FL 34104
H2 oral irrigator.

Health Solutions Medical Products, Corp. — 310-837-9594
9027 Monte Mar Dr, Los Angeles, CA 90035

IRRIGATOR, ORAL *(cont'd)*

Inter-Med, Inc. 877-418-4782
2200 Northwestern Ave, Racine, WI 53404
Irrigation and evacuation unit.

Luminaud, Inc. 800-255-3408
8688 Tyler Blvd, Mentor, OH 44060
THERMO-STIM Oral motor stimulator for treatment of delayed swallowing reaction.

Osada, Inc. 800-426-7232
8436 W 3rd St Ste 695, Los Angeles, CA 90048
ID-2. XLS-30 implant handpiece w/irrigation dispenser.

Powell Labs 800-210-6549
480 Roe Ave, Elmira, NY 14901
Unit, oral irrigation.

Showerfloss, Inc. 800-723-2300
20930 Persimmon Pl, Estero, FL 33928
Water or shower pic.Attaches to shower.

Stryker Puerto Rico, Ltd. 939-307-2500
Hwy. 3, Km. 131.2, Las Guasimas Ind. Park, Arroyo, PR 00714
Oral irrigator with various sterile and non-sterile accessories.

The Gillette Company 617-421-7000
800 Boylston St, Prudential Tower Bldg. Fl.45, Boston, MA 02199
Dental water jet.

Water Pik, Inc. 970-221-6129
1730 E Prospect Rd, Fort Collins, CO 80525
Various models, and accessories.

IRRIGATOR, OSTOMY *(Gastro/Urology) 78EXD*

Coloplast Manufacturing Us, Llc 800-533-0464
1840 W Oak Pkwy, Marietta, GA 30062
Colostomy irrigation sets with water regulator and thermometer.

Hollister, Inc. 847-680-2849
366 Draft Ave, Stuarts Draft, VA 24477

Invacare Supply Group, An Invacare Co. 800-225-4792
75 October Hill Rd, Holliston, MA 01746
Carry full lines of irrigation systems from: Coloplast, Convatec, Mentor, Hollister.

Marlen Manufacturing & Development Co. 216-292-7060
5150 Richmond Rd, Bedford, OH 44146

Torbot Group, Inc. 800-545-4254
1367 Elmwood Ave, Cranston, RI 02910

IRRIGATOR, PERINEAL *(Gastro/Urology) 78RCX*

Chester Labs, Inc. 800-354-9709
1900 Section Rd, Cincinnati, OH 45237
Perineal bottle.

Dotolo Research Corp. 800-237-8458
2875 Mcl Dr, Pinellas Park, FL 33782

IRRIGATOR, POWERED NASAL *(Ear/Nose/Throat) 77KMA*

Ethicare 954-742-3599
2190 NW 74th Ave, Sunrise, FL 33313
Ethicare nasal irrigator.

Jedmed Instruments Co. 314-845-3770
5416 Jedmed Ct, Saint Louis, MO 63129

Water Pik, Inc. 970-221-6129
1730 E Prospect Rd, Fort Collins, CO 80525
Nasal irrigator.

IRRIGATOR, SINUS *(Ear/Nose/Throat) 77KAR*

Aesculap Implant Systems Inc. 1-800-234-9179
3773 Corporate Pkwy, Center Valley, PA 18034

Bausch & Lomb Surgical 636-255-5051
3365 Tree Court Ind Blvd, Saint Louis, MO 63122

Ethicare 954-742-3599
2190 NW 74th Ave, Sunrise, FL 33313
Sinus irrigator.

H & H Co. 909-390-0373
4435 E Airport Dr Ste 108, Ontario, CA 91761
Irrigator, sinus.

Jedmed Instruments Co. 314-845-3770
5416 Jedmed Ct, Saint Louis, MO 63129

IRRIGATOR, SUCTION *(General) 80RWY*

American Catheter Corp. 800-345-6714
13047 S Highway 475, Ocala, FL 34480

Armm, Inc. 714-848-8190
17744 Sampson Ln, Huntington Beach, CA 92647
EndoSI suction / irrigator with probe and tubing.

IRRIGATOR, SUCTION *(cont'd)*

Clinimed, Incorporated 877-CLINIMED
303 Markus Ct, Sandy Brae Industrial Park, Newark, DE 19713

Jedmed Instruments Co. 314-845-3770
5416 Jedmed Ct, Saint Louis, MO 63129

Mectra Labs, Inc. 800-323-3968
PO Box 350, Two Quality Way, Bloomfield, IN 47424
MASTER LAVAGE, Laparoscopic suction/irrigation probe. 5mm probe featuring thumb controlled rotary valve. Adapts to major irrigation pumps completely leak free/clog free.

Medovations, Inc. 800-558-6408
102 E Keefe Ave, Milwaukee, WI 53212

Rocket Medical Plc. 800-707-7625
150 Recreation Park Dr Ste 3, Hingham, MA 02043

Smith & Nephew, Inc., Endoscopy Division 800-343-8386
150 Minuteman Rd, Andover, MA 01810
Irrigation pump, Intelijet fluid management system.

Stryker Corp. 800-726-2725
2825 Airview Blvd, Portage, MI 49002

Synectic Medical Product Development 203-877-8488
60 Commerce Park, Milford, CT 06460

Valley Forge Scientific Corp. 610-666-7500
136 Green Tree Road, Suite 100, Oaks, PA 19456
Irrigation system used with bipolar generator to provide saline irrigation during electrosurgical procedures.

IRRIGATOR/COAGULATOR/CUTTER, SUCTION, LAPAROSCOPIC *(Surgery) 79SJR*

Genicon 800-936-1020
6869 Stapoint Ct Ste 114, Winter Park, FL 32792

Valleylab 800-255-8522
5920 Longbow Dr, Boulder, CO 80301
Laparoscopic handsets and electrodes.

ISOKINETIC TESTING AND EVALUATION SYSTEM
(Physical Med) 89IKK

Biodex Medical Systems, Inc. 800-224-6339
20 Ramsey Rd, Shirley, NY 11967
SYSTEM 4. Dynamometer controlled rehabilitation and testing with auto-programming, treatment protocols, and real-time hands-on control.

Bte Technologies, Inc. 800-331-8345
7455 New Ridge Rd Ste L, Hanover, MD 21076
PrimusRS- Isometric, Isotonic, Isokinetic, Eccentric, CPM, Task Simulation, Hand Therapy, Lifting Evaluations, Sports Medicine.

Computer Sports Medicine, Inc. 781-297-2034
101 Tosca Dr, Stoughton, MA 02072
Various models of isokinetic testing and evaluation equipment.

Cybex International, Inc. 800-667-6544
10 Trotter Dr, Medway, MA 02053

Dynatronics Corp. 800-874-6251
7030 Park Centre Dr, Salt Lake City, UT 84121
DYNATRON 2000 patient testing and managment system.

Interactive Motion Technologies, Inc. 617-497-6330
37 Spinelli Pl, Cambridge, MA 02138
Robot therapist.

Interactive Performance Monitoring, Inc. (Ipm) 509-334-6363
1230 NE Hickman Ct, Pullman, WA 99163
Ominikinetic.

Lafayette Instrument Company 800-428-7545
PO Box 5729, 3700 Sagamore Pkwy,, Lafayette, IN 47903
Manual Muscle Tester, Model #01163.

Manufacturing Technology, Inc. 850-664-6070
70 Ready Ave NW, Fort Walton Beach, FL 32548
Activity monitor.

Orthocare Innovations, Llc 425-771-0797
6405 218th St SW Ste 100, Mountlake Ter, WA 98043
Stepwatch activity monitor.

Pneumex, Inc. 800-447-5792
2605 N Boyer Ave, Sandpoint, ID 83864
Back chair.

Spinerx Technology 713-983-9979
6100 Brittmoore Rd Ste S, Houston, TX 77041
Lumbar extension machine.

ISOLATION UNIT, SURGICAL *(General) 80FRT*

Lone Star Medical Products, Inc. 800-331-7427
11211 Cash Rd, Stafford, TX 77477
Patient isolation bubble used in surgery to decrease airborne contamination (= &) 0.3 microns/particle) and/or isolate personnel from hazardous surgical environment; bubble is ventilated by a compressor with HEPA filter and includes ports for surgeons hands.

Post Glover Lifelink 800-287-4123
167 Gap Way, Erlanger, KY 41018
Isolated power panels to assure that there is no chance for electrical shock or power failure due to a fault to ground or spilling of liquids.

Suburban Surgical Co., Inc. 800-323-7366
275 12th St, Wheeling, IL 60090
To accomodate animal cages.

ISOTACHOPHORESIS EQUIPMENT *(Chemistry) 75UGR*

Bio-Rad Laboratories, Life Science Group 800-424-6723
2000 Alfred Nobel Dr, Hercules, CA 94547

IV START KIT *(Surgery) 79LRS*

Audina Hearing Instruments, Inc. 800-223-7700
165 E Wildmere Ave, Longwood, FL 32750

Centurion Medical Products Corp. 517-545-1135
3310 S Main St, Salisbury, NC 28147

Cotran Corp. 800-345-4449
574 Park Ave, PO Box 130, Portsmouth, RI 02871

Crest Healthcare Supply 800-328-8908
195 3rd St, Dassel, MN 55325

Customed, Inc. 787-801-0101
Calle Igualdad #7, Fajardo, PR 00738
I.v. prep kit ryder.

Cypress Medical Products 800-334-3646
1202 S. Rte. 31, McHenry, IL 60050
Features include tourniquet, alcohol prep pad, PVP ointment, PVP prep pad or ampule swab, 2x2 gauze sponges, 3/4in. surgical tape and patient ID label. Other components available.

Kawasumi Laboratories America, Inc. 800-529-2786
4723 Oak Fair Blvd, Tampa, FL 33610
Primary gravity IV sets (84-120') for use in oncology centers and ambulatory surgical suite.

Lsl Industries, Inc. 888-225-5575
5535 N Wolcott Ave, Chicago, IL 60640
Various Types & Configurations including Chloraprep. Price Range mostly $50 to $147

Medikmark Inc. 800-424-8520
3600 Burwood Dr, Waukegan, IL 60085
ChloraPrep

Rd Medical Mfg. Inc. 787-716-6363
Road 183, Km 21.6, Las Piedras Industrial Park, Las Piedras, PR 00771
Various types of iv start kits.

Tri-State Hospital Supply Corp. 517-545-1135
3173 E 43rd St, Yuma, AZ 85365

JAR, APPLICATOR *(Surgery) 79RCY*

Polar Ware Co. 800-237-3655
2806 N 15th St, Sheboygan, WI 53083
Stainless steel.

Profex Medical Products 800-325-0196
2224 E Person Ave, Memphis, TN 38114

Terriss-Consolidated Industries 800-342-1611
807 Summerfield Ave, Asbury Park, NJ 07712
Stainless steel.

JAR, BLADE *(Surgery) 79RCZ*

Profex Medical Products 800-325-0196
2224 E Person Ave, Memphis, TN 38114

JAR, DRESSING *(Surgery) 79RDA*

Freund Container 800-363-9822
4200 Commerce Ct Ste 206, Corporate Center II, Lisle, IL 60532

Medegen Medical Products, Llc 800-233-1987
209 Medegen Drive, Gallaway, TN 38036-0228
MED-ASSIST Stainless steel.

Polar Ware Co. 800-237-3655
2806 N 15th St, Sheboygan, WI 53083
Stainless steel.

Ware Medics Glass Works, Inc. 845-429-6950
PO Box 368, Garnerville, NY 10923
Dressing jars; labeled and unlabeled sundry jars.

JAR, FORCEPS *(Surgery) 79RDB*

Medegen Medical Products, Llc 800-233-1987
209 Medegen Drive, Gallaway, TN 38036-0228
MED-ASSIST Sterilizable plastic.

Polar Ware Co. 800-237-3655
2806 N 15th St, Sheboygan, WI 53083
Stainless steel.

Terriss-Consolidated Industries 800-342-1611
807 Summerfield Ave, Asbury Park, NJ 07712
Stainless steel.

JAR, OPERATING ROOM *(Surgery) 79FTE*

Dencraft 800-328-9729
PO Box 57, Moorestown, NJ 08057

JELLY, CONTACT (FOR TRANSURETHRAL SURGICAL INSTRUMENT) *(Gastro/Urology) 78FHY*

K. W. Griffen Co. 203-846-1923
100 Pearl St, Norwalk, CT 06850
Wire spint.

JELLY, LUBRICATING *(General) 80RFL*

Chester Labs, Inc. 800-354-9709
1900 Section Rd, Cincinnati, OH 45237
E-Z Lubricating Jelly. (Bacteriostat: Methylparaben and Propylparaben; Water Soluble/Sterile).

Covidien Lp 508-261-8000
15 Hampshire St, Mansfield, MA 02048
Pure white petroleum jelly.

Fougera 800-645-9833
60 Baylis Rd, PO Box 2006, Melville, NY 11747
Surgilube

Johnson & Johnson Consumer Products, Inc. 800-526-3967
199 Grandview Rd, Skillman, NJ 08558
K-Y brand lubricating jelly.

Johnson & Johnson Medical Division Of Ethicon, Inc. 800-423-4018
2500 E Arbrook Blvd, Arlington, TX 76014

Professional Disposables International, Inc. 800-999-6423
2 Nice Pak Park, Orangeburg, NY 10962
Bacteriostatic lubricating jelly.

Ulmer Pharmacal Co. 800-848-5637
PO Box 408, 1614 Industry Ave., Park Rapids, MN 56470
SURGEL $5.39 per 1000 ml.

Xttrium Laboratories, Inc. 800-587-3721
415 W Pershing Rd, Chicago, IL 60609
LUBRI-GEL lubricating jelly.

JELLY, LUBRICATING, TRANSURETHRAL SURGICAL INSTRUMENT *(Gastro/Urology) 78FHX*

Culture Kits, Inc. 888-680-6853
14 Prentice St, PO Box 748, Norwich, NY 13815
URO-JET lidocaine HCL.

Elamex S.A. De C.V. 52-16-164333
Av. Insurgentes 4145 lote., Cd. Jiarex, Chih Mexico
Various

Schueler & Company, Inc. 516-487-1500
PO Box 528, Stratford, CT 06615

Taro Pharmaceuticals, Inc. 905-791-8276
130 East Dr, Brampton L6T 1C1 Canada
Sterile lubricating jelly

Triad Disposables 800-288-1288
19355 Janacek Ct, Brookfield, WI 53045
Lubricating jelly.

United-Guardian, Inc. 800-645-5566
230 Marcus Blvd, P.O. Box 18050, Hauppauge, NY 11788
Water soluble lubricating jelly, non-drying (bulk); and radiation stable lubricating jelly.

JIG, PISTON CUTTING, ENT *(Ear/Nose/Throat) 77JXY*

Bausch & Lomb Surgical 636-255-5051
3365 Tree Court Ind Blvd, Saint Louis, MO 63122

Gyrus Ent L.L.C., Sub. Of Gyrus Acmi, Inc. 508-804-2739
2925 Appling Rd, Bartlett, TN 38133
Various types and sizes of ent piston cutting jigs.

JOINT, ELBOW, EXTERNAL LIMB COMPONENT, MECHANICAL
(Physical Med) 89IRD

Becker Orthopedic Appliance Co. 248-588-7480
635 Executive Dr, Troy, MI 48083
Various elbow orthoses and orthosis components.

Hosmer Dorrance Corp. 408-379-5151
561 Division St, Campbell, CA 95008
Various.

JOINT, ELBOW, EXTERNAL LIMB COMPONENT, POWERED
(Physical Med) 89IRE

Hosmer Dorrance Corp. 408-379-5151
561 Division St, Campbell, CA 95008
Various.

JOINT, HIP, EXTERNAL BRACE *(Physical Med) 89ITS*

Alimed, Inc. 800-225-2610
297 High St, Dedham, MA 02026

American Orthopedic Supply Co., Inc.
37017 State Highway 79, Cleveland, AL 35049
Thr.

Becker Orthopedic Appliance Co. 248-588-7480
635 Executive Dr, Troy, MI 48083
Various hip orthoses and orthosis components.

Biomet, Inc. 574-267-6639
56 E Bell Dr, PO Box 587, Warsaw, IN 46582
Various types of external hip braces.

Dj Orthopedics De Mexico, S.A. De C.V. 690-727-1280
Blvd., Delagacion La Presa, Tijuana 22397 Mexico
Hip brace

Dj Orthopedics De Mexico, S.A. De C.V. 690-727-1280
Ave. Venustiano Carranza 6802, Castillo, Tijuana 22100 Mexico
Hip brace

Hendricks Orthotic Prosthetic Enterprises, Inc. 407-850-0411
6439 Milner Blvd Ste 6, Orlando, FL 32809
Joint, hip, external brace.

Hosmer Dorrance Corp. 408-379-5151
561 Division St, Campbell, CA 95008
Various.

Liberating Technologies, Inc. 800-437-0024
325 Hopping Brook Rd Ste A, Holliston, MA 01746

Pfs Med, Inc. 541-349-9646
3295 Cross St, Eugene, OR 97402
Pfs with derot. bar, derot. bar.

Pro Orthopedic Devices, Inc. 800-523-5611
2884 E Ganley Rd, Tucson, AZ 85706
PRO Neoprene rubber joint sleeves and supports.

Restorative Medical, Inc. 270-422-5454
332 Broadway St, Brandenburg, KY 40108
Hip-knee orthosis.

Scott Orthotic Labs, Inc. 800-821-5795
1831 E Mulberry St, Fort Collins, CO 80524
Hip abduction orthosis.

Spinal Solutions, Inc. 770-922-2434
1971 Old Covington Rd NE Ste 103, Conyers, GA 30013
Hip joint.

Tiburon Medical Enterprises 909-654-2333
915 Industrial Way, San Jacinto, CA 92582
Various.

U.S. Orthotics, Inc. 800-825-5228
8605 Palm River Rd, Tampa, FL 33619

Zimmer Holdings, Inc. 800-613-6131
1800 W Center St, PO Box 708, Warsaw, IN 46580

JOINT, HIP, EXTERNAL LIMB COMPONENT *(Physical Med) 89ISL*

Endolite North America, Ltd. 937-291-3636
105 Westpark Rd, Centerville, OH 45459
Artificial limb hip joint.

Hosmer Dorrance Corp. 408-379-5151
561 Division St, Campbell, CA 95008
Various.

Ortho Development Corp. 800-429-8339
12187 Business Park Dr, Draper, UT 84020
PRIMALOC Total Hip System; total hip replacement.

Pro Orthopedic Devices, Inc. 800-523-5611
2884 E Ganley Rd, Tucson, AZ 85706
PRO Neoprene rubber joint sleeves and supports.

JOINT, HIP, EXTERNAL LIMB COMPONENT *(cont'd)*

Signal Medical Corporation 800-246-6324
1000 Des Peres Rd Ste 140, Saint Louis, MO 63131
Capello hip positioner complete with gel pad, including 4' positioning board, saftey clamps 9' pegs, 6' pegs, and 46' gel pad.

JOINT, KNEE, EXTERNAL BRACE *(Physical Med) 89ITQ*

A&A Orthopedics, Incorporated 757-224-0177
12250 SW 129th Ct Bldg 1, Miami, FL 33186
Knee brace.

Airway Division Of Surgical Appliance Industries, Inc. 800-888-0458
3960 Rosslyn Dr, Cincinnati, OH 45209

American Orthopedic Supply Co., Inc.
37017 State Highway 79, Cleveland, AL 35049
Knee brace & immobilizer.

Anodyne Therapy, Llc 813-645-2855
13570 Wright Cir, Tampa, FL 33626
External knee brace.

Baiwa, Inc. 888-247-5633
630 Alma Way, Zephyr Cove, NV 89448
Various types of body joint braces.

Bauerfeind Usa, Inc. 800-423-3405
55 Chastain Rd NW Ste 112, Kennesaw, GA 30144
Non-rigid functional knee brace.

Becker Orthopedic Appliance Co. 248-588-7480
635 Executive Dr, Troy, MI 48083
Various knee orthoses and orthosis components.

Benik Corp. 360-692-5601
11871 Silverdale Way NW Ste 107, Silverdale, WA 98383
Knee support, knee sleeve.

Best Orthopedic And Medical Services, Inc. 800-344-5279
2356B Springs Rd NE, Hickory, NC 28601

Biomet, Inc. 574-267-6639
56 E Bell Dr, PO Box 587, Warsaw, IN 46582
Various types of knee braces.

Bledsoe Brace Systems 888-253-3763
2601 Pinewood Dr, Grand Prairie, TX 75051

Breg, Inc., An Orthofix Company 800-897-BREG
2611 Commerce Way, Vista, CA 92081
Knee bracing for sports medicine/osteoarthritis.

Burke Medical, Llc 727-532-8333
2310 Tall Pines Dr Ste 210, Largo, FL 33771
Knee brace.

Core Products International, Inc. 800-365-3047
808 Prospect Ave, Osceola, WI 54020

Corflex, Inc. 800-426-7353
669 E Industrial Park Dr, Manchester, NH 03109
Control Passive Stretch (CPS) is a dynamic knee brace that provides low-load prolonged force that can result in tissue remodeling over time.

Cramer Products, Inc. 800-255-6621
153 W Warren St, Gardner, KS 66030
Patellar knee strap is one size fits all, with molded foam buttress. Helps relieve the pain of chondromalicia and patellar tendinitis.

Dalco International, Inc. 888-354-5515
8433 Glazebrook Ave, Richmond, VA 23228
Functional, sports and rehabilitation braces.

Dj Orthopedics De Mexico, S.A. De C.V. 690-727-1280
Blvd., Delagacion La Presa, Tijuana 22397 Mexico
Knee braces, functional

Dj Orthopedics De Mexico, S.A. De C.V. 690-727-1280
Ave. Venustiano Carranza 6802, Castillo, Tijuana 22100 Mexico
Knee braces, functional

DJO Inc. 800-336-6569
1430 Decision St, Vista, CA 92081
Functional custom and off-the-shelf knee braces. Post surgical/rehabilitation knee brace.

Dynatronics Corp. Chattanooga Operations 801-568-7000
6607 Mountain View Rd, Ooltewah, TN 37363
Joint, knee, external brace.

Elite Orthopaedics, Inc. 800-284-1688
1535 Santa Anita Ave, South El Monte, CA 91733

Evs Sports Protection 800-229-4EVS
2146 E Gladwick St, Rancho Dominguez, CA 90220

JOINT, KNEE, EXTERNAL BRACE *(cont'd)*

Fla Orthopedics, Inc. 800-327-4110
2881 Corporate Way, Miramar, FL 33025

Frank Stubbs Co., Inc 800-223-1713
2100 Eastman Ave Ste B, Oxnard, CA 93030

Freeman Manufacturing Company 800-253-2091
900 W Chicago Rd, PO Box J, Sturgis, MI 49091
Elastic knee brace and protective orthoses with adjustable flexion/extension and neoprene knee support.

Health Ent., Inc. 508-695-0727
90 George Leven Dr, North Attleboro, MA 02760
Knee brace.

Hosmer Dorrance Corp. 408-379-5151
561 Division St, Campbell, CA 95008
Various.

Inland Specialties, Inc. 800-741-0022
7655 Matoaka Rd, Sarasota, FL 34243
Rehab knee brace with 7 1/2 degree increments for extension/flexion available in short and regular sizes; also available in 'knockdown' version

Ita-Med Co. 888-9IT-AMED
310 Littlefield Ave, South San Francisco, CA 94080
Designed to prevent and treat knee injuries.

Jace Systems 800-800-4276
2 Pin Oak Ln Ste 200, Cherry Hill, NJ 08003
The ideal brace for your patient's recovery. The JACE Tri/Brace functions as a CPM Brace, a Post Operative Brace, and a Rehabilitation Brace.

Just Packaging Inc. 908-753-6700
450 Oak Tree Ave, South Plainfield, NJ 07080
External knee joint.

Kenad Sg Medical, Inc. 800-825-0606
2692 Huntley Dr, Memphis, TN 38132
Knee brace.

Kern Surgical Supply, Inc. 800-582-3939
2823 Gibson St, Bakersfield, CA 93308

Lenox Hill Brace / Seattle Systems 360-697-5656
26296 12 Trees Ln NW, Poulsbo, WA 98370
Functional knee braces.

Maramed Orthopedic Systems 800-327-5830
2480 W 82nd St, No. 8, Hialeah, FL 33016

Medi Usa 800-633-6334
6481 Franz Warner Pkwy, Whitsett, NC 27377
Anatomically knitted knee supports with specially shaped circular silicone buttress and/or opposing patella pull straps.

Omni Life Science, Inc. 800-448-OMNI
1390 Decision St, Vista, CA 92081
Rage ready-to-fit knee braces for ligament instability and O.A.

Ortho Innovations, Inc. 507-269-2895
121 23rd Ave SW, Rochester, MN 55902
Joint, external brace.

Orthorx, Inc. 858-457-3545
8929 University Center Ln Ste 200, San Diego, CA 92122
External knee brace.

Orthosource, Inc. 800-649-5525
17374 W Sunset Blvd, Pacific Palisades, CA 90272
Physical medicine.

Orthotic & Prosthetic Lab, Inc. 314-968-8555
748 Marshall Ave, Webster Groves, MO 63119
O&p orthotic knee brace.

Ossur Americas, Inc 800-222-4284
19762 Pauling, Foothill Ranch, CA 92610
Custom, graphite knee braces, with anatomically correct hinges for optimum brace performance. OTS braces and Osteoarthritis knee braces.

Patterson Medical Supply,•Inc. 262-387-8720
W68N158 Evergreen Blvd, Cedarburg, WI 53012
Metal and plastic knee hinges.

Pfs Med, Inc. 541-349-9646
3295 Cross St, Eugene, OR 97402
Pka.

Primo, Inc. 770-486-7394
417 Dividend Dr Ste B, Peachtree City, GA 30269
Knee immobilizer.

JOINT, KNEE, EXTERNAL BRACE *(cont'd)*

Pro Orthopedic Devices, Inc. 800-523-5611
2884 E Ganley Rd, Tucson, AZ 85706
PRO Neoprene rubber joint sleeves and supports.

Protectair Inc. 800-235-7932
59 Eisenhower Ln S, Lombard, IL 60148

Rehabilitation Technical Components, Corp. 919-732-1705
3913 Devonwood Rd, Hillsborough, NC 27278
(tks) Three Way knee stabilizer.

Restorative Medical, Inc. 270-422-5454
332 Broadway St, Brandenburg, KY 40108
Knee orthosis.

Richardson Products, Inc. 888-928-7297
9408 Gulfstream Rd, Frankfort, IL 60423
Knee brace.

Rs Medical 800-683-0353
14001 S.E. First St., Vancouver, WA 98684
OA Solution Knee Brace

Scott Orthotic Labs, Inc. 800-821-5795
1831 E Mulberry St, Fort Collins, CO 80524
Knee orthosis or knee cage.

Scott Specialties, Inc. 785-527-5627
1827 Meadowlark Rd, Clay Center, KS 67432
Various types of knee braces.

Scott Specialties, Inc. 785-527-5627
1820 E 7th St, Concordia, KS 66901

Scott Specialties, Inc./Cmo Inc./Ginny Inc. 800-255-7136
512 M St, Belleville, KS 66935

Tagg Industries L.L.C. 800-548-3514
23210 Del Lago Dr, Laguna Hills, CA 92653
ISODYN, Functional knee brace, off the shelf.

Tartan Orthopedics, Ltd. 888-287-1456
10651 Irma Dr Unit C, Northglenn, CO 80233
$26.75 per unit (med).

Therafirm, A Knit Rite Company 800-562-2701
120 Osage Ave, Kansas City, KS 66105
Tubular knit, one piece, two-way stretch, 8 in. & 11 in. length.

Tiburon Medical Enterprises 909-654-2333
915 Industrial Way, San Jacinto, CA 92582
Various.

Top Shelf Manufacturing, Llc 209-834-8185
1851 Paradise Rd Ste B, Tracy, CA 95304
Various types of knee braces & support.

Trulife, Inc. 360-697-5656
26296 12 Trees Ln NW, Poulsbo, WA 98370
Knee brace or knee orthosis.

U.S. Orthotics, Inc. 800-825-5228
8605 Palm River Rd, Tampa, FL 33619

Unique Sports Products, Inc. 800-554-3707
840 McFarland Pkwy, Alpharetta, GA 30004
Knee Strap--helps reduce cartilage and ligament movement and the resulting pain.

Vq Orthocare
1390 Decision St Ste A, Vista, CA 92081
Limb orthosis.

Warsaw Orthopedic, Inc. 901-396-3133
2500 Silveus Xing, Warsaw, IN 46582
Various knee braces immobilizers.

Zimmer Holdings, Inc. 800-613-6131
1800 W Center St, PO Box 708, Warsaw, IN 46580

JOINT, KNEE, EXTERNAL LIMB COMPONENT

(Physical Med) 89ISY

Aulie Devices, Inc. 541-548-7355
3615 Northwest Way, Redmond, OR 97756
External prosthetic knee.

Bionix Development Corp. 800-551-7096
5154 Enterprise Blvd, Toledo, OH 43612
Various types of external limb components (knee).

Dj Orthopedics De Mexico, S.A. De C.V. 690-727-1280
Blvd., Delagacion La Presa, Tijuana 22397 Mexico
Sleeve

Dj Orthopedics De Mexico, S.A. De C.V. 690-727-1280
Ave. Venustiano Carranza 6802, Castillo, Tijuana 22100 Mexico
Sleeve

JOINT, KNEE, EXTERNAL LIMB COMPONENT *(cont'd)*

Endolite North America, Ltd. 937-291-3636
105 Westpark Rd, Centerville, OH 45459
Prosthetic limb knee joint.

Hosmer Dorrance Corp. 408-379-5151
561 Division St, Campbell, CA 95008
Various models of artificial, external limb knee joints.

Inland Specialties, Inc. 800-741-0022
7655 Matoaka Rd, Sarasota, FL 34243
Knee brace components, machined to customer specifications, aluminum or stainless steel pieces, anodized or powdercoated in a variety of colors

Mauch, Inc. 800-622-8742
3035 Dryden Rd, Moraine, OH 45439
$653.00 and $1043.00 per unit (standard).

Ohio Willow Wood Company 800-848-4930
15441 Scioto Darby Rd, Mount Sterling, OH 43143
Structural components for ankle, foot, knee and thigh prostheses.

Ossur Americas 517-629-8890
910 Burstein Dr, Albion, MI 49224

Otto Bock Healthcare, Lp 763-489-5106
9420 Delegates Dr Ste 100, Orlando, FL 32837
Various types of external knee components/accessories.

Trulife, Inc. 360-697-5656
26296 12 Trees Ln NW, Poulsbo, WA 98370
Various models of prosthetic knees.

JOINT, SHOULDER, EXTERNAL LIMB COMPONENT
(Physical Med) 89IQQ

Benik Corp. 360-692-5601
11871 Silverdale Way NW Ste 107, Silverdale, WA 98383
Shoulder support.

DJO Inc. 800-336-6569
1430 Decision St, Vista, CA 92081
Off-the-shelf shoulder braces and supports.

Hosmer Dorrance Corp. 408-379-5151
561 Division St, Campbell, CA 95008
Axilla pad.

JOINT, WRIST, EXTERNAL LIMB COMPONENT, MECHANICAL
(Physical Med) 89ISZ

Dick Medical Supply, Llc 614-444-2300
630 Marion Rd, Columbus, OH 43207
Limb restraint.

Hosmer Dorrance Corp. 408-379-5151
561 Division St, Campbell, CA 95008
Various.

Lighthouse Industries 219-879-1550
107 Eastwood Rd, Po Box 8905, Michigan City, IN 46360

Patterson Medical Supply, Inc. 262-387-8720
W68N158 Evergreen Blvd, Cedarburg, WI 53012
Wrist hinge.

KAPPA, PEROXIDASE, ANTIGEN, ANTISERUM, CONTROL
(Immunology) 82DFD

Ventana Medical Systems, Inc. 800-227-2155
1910 E Innovation Park Dr, Oro Valley, AZ 85755
Various immunoglobulin immunological test systems.

KERATOME, AC-POWERED *(Ophthalmology) 86HNO*

Back-Mueller, Inc. 314-531-6640
2700 Clark Ave, Saint Louis, MO 63103
Various types of r-k corneal markers.

Bausch & Lomb Surgical 636-255-5051
3365 Tree Court Ind Blvd, Saint Louis, MO 63122

Fortrad Eye Instruments Corp. 973-543-2371
8 Franklin Rd, Mendham, NJ 07945

Frantz Medical Development Ltd. 440-255-1155
7740 Metric Dr, Mentor, OH 44060
Disposable device.

Katena Products, Inc. 800-225-1195
4 Stewart Ct, Denville, NJ 07834
BARRON Micro Keratome for lasik surgery.

Lasersight Technologies, Inc. 630-530-9700
6848 Stapoint Ct, Winter Park, FL 32792
Ultrashaper durable keratome.

KERATOME, AC-POWERED *(cont'd)*

Med-Logics, Inc. 949-582-3891
26061 Merit Cir Ste 102, Laguna Hills, CA 92653
Microkeratame.

Nidek Inc. 800-223-9044
47651 Westinghouse Dr, Fremont, CA 94539
MK-2000 keratome system.

Nidek, Inc. 510-226-5700
47651 Westinghouse Dr, Fremont, CA 94539
Keratome.

Surgin Surgical Instrumentation, Inc. (Surgin Inc.) 714-832-6300
37 Shield, Irvine, CA 92618
Keratome blades.

KERATOME, BATTERY-POWERED *(Ophthalmology) 86HMY*

Industrial & Medical Design, Inc. 818-642-7501
4741 Deseret Dr, Woodland Hills, CA 91364
Microkeratome.

KERATOME, WATER JET *(Ophthalmology) 86MYD*

Advanced Refractive Technologies 949-940-1300
1062 Calle Negocio Ste D, San Clemente, CA 92673
Hydrokeratome.

KERATOMETER *(Ophthalmology) 86UEK*

Akorn, Inc. 800-535-7155
2500 Millbrook Dr, Buffalo Grove, IL 60089
Titanium, cone shaped Maloney hand-held astigmatism keratometer.

Burton Co., R.H. 800-848-0410
3965 Brookham Dr, Grove City, OH 43123
$1,150.00 for Burton 1040 keratometer with circular fluorescent bulb for clear images; auto refractor/keratometer also available. Autorefractor/Keratometer $9,995.00 Burton Bark 8 Autorefkeratometer measuring mechanism which allows for high speed, accurate refractive power and corneal curvature measurements.

Canon Development Americas, Inc 949-932-3100
15955 Alton Pkwy, Irvine, CA 92618
RK-F1 full refractor/keratometer combination model.

Carl Zeiss Meditec Inc. 877-486-7473
5160 Hacienda Dr, Dublin, CA 94568
HUMPHREY AUTOMATIC REFRACTOR/KERATOMETER The Humphrey Automatic Refractor/Keratometer (HARK) Model 599 is the first full-featured combination automatic refractor/keratometer. The HARK allows for immediate patient response on refraction results with visual acuities. The operator control panel can be positioned at either 90 degrees or 180 degrees to meet office space requirements. COMMUNICOM links the HARK to the Humphrey Lens Analyzer for quick and easy comparison of current and new prescriptions.

Marco Ophthalmic, Inc. 800-874-5274
11825 Central Pkwy, Jacksonville, FL 32224
$2,050.00 for manual keratometer model; $15,000.00 for ARK, 900 automatic refractor/keratometer combination system. (List prices)

Topcon Medical Systems, Inc. 800-223-1130
37 W Century Rd, Paramus, NJ 07652
$2,690.00 and $2,790 for ophthalmometer.

Western Ophthalmics Corporation 800-426-9938
19019 36th Ave W Ste G, Lynnwood, WA 98036

Woodlyn, Inc. 800-331-7389
2920 Malmo Dr, Ophthalmic Instruments and Equipment
Arlington Heights, IL 60005
Model 55000. The Woodlyn Keratometer features precision objectives, achromatic prisms, and uniform illumination. Call for current prices.

KERATOPROSTHESIS, NON-CUSTOM *(Ophthalmology) 86HQM*

Addition Technology, Inc. 847-297-8419
950 Lee St Ste 210, Des Plaines, IL 60016
AlphaCor is a flexible, biotrgratable, one-piece artificial cornea (kertoprosthesis) designed to replace scarred or diseased native cornea.

M.E.E.I. Mfg. 941-492-2560
Claes H Dohlman, Md Room 550I, Meei, 5th Floor, Boston, MA 02114
Keratoprosthesis.

KERATOSCOPE, AC-POWERED *(Ophthalmology) 86HLQ*

Eyequip, Div Of Alliance Medical Marketing 800-393-8676
5150 Palm Valley Rd Ste 305, Ponte Vedra Beach, FL 32082
KERATRON and Scout Portable Corneal Topographer, extremely accurate, full featured and easy-to-operate topographer. State-of-the-art true curvature (IROC) maps.

Eyesys Vision, Inc. 281-885-3800
225 Pennbright Dr Ste 100, Houston, TX 77090
Eyesys portable corneal topography system & eyesys desktop corneal topography.

Lasersight Technologies, Inc. 630-530-9700
6848 Stapoint Ct, Winter Park, FL 32792
Astramax.

Nidek Inc. 800-223-9044
47651 Westinghouse Dr, Fremont, CA 94539
Model PKS-3000 photokeratoscope.

Nidek, Inc. 510-226-5700
47651 Westinghouse Dr, Fremont, CA 94539
Ophthalmic refractometer.

Topcon Medical Systems, Inc. 800-223-1130
37 W Century Rd, Paramus, NJ 07652
KR-8000PA auto refractor with corneal topography: $18,490.00. KR-9000PW wavefront analyzer with corneal topography: $39,990.00. Color-mapping software: $600.00.

KINESTHESIOMETER *(Orthopedics) 87TCU*

Myotronics-Noromed, Inc. 206-243-4214
5870 S 194th St, Kent, WA 98032
$21,150.00 for K7 mandibular kinesiograph, used for occlusion testing. Consists of jaw tracker, dental EMG with optional joint sound recorder.

KINETIC METHOD, GAMMA-GLUTAMYL TRANSPEPTIDASE *(Chemistry) 75JQB*

Caldon Bioscience, Inc. 909-628-9944
2100 S Reservoir St, Pomona, CA 91766
Gamma-glutamyl transpeptidase.

Caldon Biotech, Inc. 757-224-0177
2251 Rutherford Rd, Carlsbad, CA 92008
Gct.

Carolina Liquid Chemistries Corp. 800-471-7272
510 W Central Ave Ste C, Brea, CA 92821
Ggt.

Genchem, Inc. 714-529-1616
510 W Central Ave Ste D, Brea, CA 92821
Ggt reagent.

Hemagen Diagnostics, Inc. 800-436-2436
9033 Red Branch Rd, Columbia, MD 21045
Kinetic method, gamma-glutamyl transpeptidase.

Jas Diagnostics, Inc. 305-418-2320
7220 NW 58th St, Miami, FL 33166
Gamma-gt (ggt).

Synermed Intl., Inc. 317-896-1565
17408 Tiller Ct Ste 1900, Westfield, IN 46074
Gamma-glutamyltransferase (ggt) reagent set.

Teco Diagnostics 714-693-7788
1268 N Lakeview Ave, Anaheim, CA 92807
8-gt liquid reagent.

Vital Diagnostics Inc. 714-672-3553
1075 W Lambert Rd Ste D, Brea, CA 92821
Various gamma-glutamyltransferase reagents.

KIT, ACUPUNCTURE *(Anesthesiology) 73QAA*

M.E.D. Servi-Systems Canada Ltd. 800-267-6868
8 Sweetnam Dr., Stittsville, ONT K2S 1G2 Canada

KIT, ADMINISTRATION, BLOOD *(General) 80QDX*

B. Braun Oem Division, B. Braun Medical Inc. 866-8-BBRAUN
824 12th Ave, Bethlehem, PA 18018

Baxter Healthcare Corporporation, Alternate Care And Channel Team 888-229-0001
25212 W Il Route 120, Round Lake, IL 60073
Administration sets. Filters. Recipient sets.

Codan Us Corporation 800-33-CODAN
3511 W Sunflower Ave, Santa Ana, CA 92704
Anesthesia infusion sets.

KIT, ADMINISTRATION, BLOOD *(cont'd)*

Kawasumi Laboratories America, Inc. 800-529-2786
4723 Oak Fair Blvd, Tampa, FL 33610
Therapeutic Phlebotomy Kits

Medi Inc 800-225-8634
75 York Ave, P.O. Box 302, Randolph, MA 02368

The Metrix Co. 800-752-3148
4400 Chavenelle Rd, Dubuque, IA 52002
Custom contract manufacturer.

KIT, ADMINISTRATION, CARDIOPLEGIA SOLUTION *(Cardiovascular) 74UDD*

Gish Biomedical, Inc. 800-938-0531
22942 Arroyo Vis, Rancho Santa Margarita, CA 92688
Blood-mixing set.

Medtronic Perfusion Systems 800-328-3320
7611 Northland Dr N, Brooklyn Park, MN 55428
Custom perfusion/cardioplegia packs.

Novosci Corp. 281-363-4949
2828 N Crescentridge Dr, The Woodlands, TX 77381

Terumo Cardiovascular Systems, Corp 800-521-2818
6200 Jackson Rd, Ann Arbor, MI 48103
Standard and custom kits available with integrated heat exchanger, pressure and temperature monitoring.

KIT, ADMINISTRATION, ENTERAL *(Gastro/Urology) 78QUJ*

Abbott Laboratories 800-624-7677
1033 Kingsmill Pkwy, Columbus, OH 43229
Case of FLEXIFLO top-fill enteral nutrition system with pre-attached FLEXIFLO pump set, incl. roller clamp & 1000ml bag. Same also available for gravity feeding. 24 pcs. of FLEXIFLO pump sets with 40mm screw top, roller clamp and bacteria retentive air filter. 24 pcs. of FLEXIFLO pump sets with piercing pin. 24 pcs. of FLEXIFLO gravity gavage sets; same also available with piercing pin. Same also available in TOPTAINER system and EASY-FEED for FLEXIFLO III and gravity system. For gravity feeding - choice of screw sets, spike sets, and both rigid and flexible bag and sets pre-attached.

Coeur Inc., Sheboygan 800-874-4240
3411 Behrens Pkwy, Sheboygan, WI 53081

Covidien Lp 508-261-8000
15 Hampshire St, Mansfield, MA 02048

Filtrona Extrusion, Inc./Pexcor Medical Products Div. 800-755-7528
764 S Athol Rd, P.O. Box 659, Athol, MA 01331

Invacare Supply Group, An Invacare Co. 800-225-4792
75 October Hill Rd, Holliston, MA 01746
Carry full lines of kits and solutions from: Ross, Mead-Johnson, Nestle.

Kck Industries 888-800-1967
14941 Calvert St, Van Nuys, CA 91411

Novartis Nutrition 800-333-3785
1600 Utica Ave S Ste 600, PO Box 370, Minneapolis, MN 55416
Sets with 1000mL & 500mL preattached semi-rigid containers; with 1000mL vinyl bag; with spike.

Welcon, Inc. 800-877-0923
7409 Pebble Dr, Fort Worth, TX 76118
UI300, Intermittent Feeding Container with pre-attached gravity set.

KIT, ADMINISTRATION, INTRA-ARTERIAL *(General) 80WVF*

B. Braun Oem Division, B. Braun Medical Inc. 866-8-BBRAUN
824 12th Ave, Bethlehem, PA 18018

Spectra Medical Devices, Inc. 866-938-8649
4C Henshaw St, Woburn, MA 01801
Arterial extension sets.

KIT, ADMINISTRATION, INTRAVENOUS *(General) 80FPA*

Abbott Diagnostics Intl, Biotechnology Ltd 787-846-3500
Road #2 KM. 58.0 , PO Box 278, Cruce Davila, Barceloneta, PR 00617
Various sizes of IV administration sets (sterile).

Accellent El Paso 915-771-9112
31 Butterfield Trail Blvd Ste C, El Paso, TX 79906
Complete line of IV administration sets.

American Medical Devices, Inc. 800-788-9876
287 S Stoddard Ave, San Bernardino, CA 92401

Amsino International, Inc. 800-MD-AMSINO
855 Towne Center Dr, Pomona, CA 91767
AMSINO I.V. administration set is available in a variety of spikes, chambers, tubing lengths, and diameters.

KIT, ADMINISTRATION, INTRAVENOUS *(cont'd)*

Argon Medical Devices Inc. 903-675-9321
1445 Flat Creek Rd, Athens, TX 75751
Hyperbaric kit.

Arkray Factory Usa, Inc. 952-646-3168
5182 W 76th St, Minneapolis, MN 55439
Sterile subcutaneous infusion set.

Arrow Internacional De Mexico, S.A. De C.V. 610-378-0131
Modulo 1, Circuito 5, Parque Industrias De America
Col. Panamericana, Chihuahua Mexico
Multiple

Arrow International, Inc. 800-523-8446
2 Berry Dr, Mount Holly, NJ 08060
High flow solution administration set.

B. Braun Oem Division, B. Braun Medical Inc. 866-8-BBRAUN
824 12th Ave, Bethlehem, PA 18018

B. Braun Of Puerto Rico, Inc. 610-691-5400
215.7 Insular Rd., Sabana Grande, PR 00637
Iv administration set.

Bard Reynosa S.A. De C.V. 908-277-8000
Blvd. Montebello #1, Parque Industrial Colonial
Reynosa, Tamaulipas Mexico
Various

Baxter Healthcare Corp., Renal Division 847-948-2000
7511 114th Ave, Largo, FL 33773
Various sterile sets with/without filters.

Baxter Healthcare Corporporation, Alternate Care And Channel Team 888-229-0001
25212 W Il Route 120, Round Lake, IL 60073
Basic solution. Blood sets. Interlink Access System.

Baxter Healthcare S.A. 847-948-2000
Rd. 721, Km. 0.3, Aibonito, PR 00609
Various sterile sets with/without filters.

Becton Dickinson Infusion Therapy Systems, Inc. 888-237-2762
9450 S State St, Sandy, UT 84070
I.V. start kits and accessories.

Becton, Dickinson & Co., (Bd) Preanalytical System 201-847-6280
1575 Airport Rd, Sumter, SC 29153
Infusion sets.

Beech Medical Products, Inc.
2 South Winchester St., West Swanzey, NH 03469
Shielded needle connector assembly.

Benlan Inc. 905-829-5004
2760 Brighton Rd., Oakville, ONT L6H 5T4 Canada

Biomedix, Inc. 800-627-2765
3895 W Vernal Pike, Bloomington, IN 47404
SELEC-3 is a multi-drip I.V. administration set. Choose between a 10, 15, or 60-drop/cc-volume setting without breaking the line. Each set has two 'Y' port connections and a built-in extension set, with a backflow prevention device. Custom sets available upon request.

Block Medical De Mexico S.A. De C.V. 949-206-2700
La Mesa Parque Industrial, Paseo Reforma S/n, Fracc.
Tijuana, Bc Mexico
Iv administration set

Cardinal Health 303,Inc. 858-458-7830
1515 Ivac Way, Creedmoor, NC 27522
Various administration sets & accessories.

Catheter Innovations, Inc. 800-418-2828
3598 W 1820 S, Salt Lake City, UT 84104
Needle-free valved connector and cap.

Centurion Medical Products Corp. 517-545-1135
3310 S Main St, Salisbury, NC 28147

Charter Medical, Ltd. 336-768-6447
3948 Westpoint Blvd Ste A, Winston Salem, NC 27103
Administration transfer and recipient sets.

Clinical Pharmacies, Inc. 800-669-6973
21622 Surveyor Cir # 8-C, Huntington Beach, CA 92646
Administration sets.

Codan Us Corporation 800-33-CODAN
3511 W Sunflower Ave, Santa Ana, CA 92704

Coeur Inc., Sheboygan 800-874-4240
3411 Behrens Pkwy, Sheboygan, WI 53081

Curlin Medical, Inc. 714-893-2200
15751 Graham St, Huntington Beach, CA 92649
Disposable sets.

KIT, ADMINISTRATION, INTRAVENOUS *(cont'd)*

Custom Healthcare Systems, Inc. 804-421-5959
4205 Eubank Rd, Richmond, VA 23231

Deuteronomy Management Services,Inc. 850-897-3321
1439 Live Oak St Ste A, Niceville, FL 32578
Decanting devices.

Directmed, Inc. 516-656-3377
150 Pratt Oval, Glen Cove, NY 11542

Edwards Lifesciences Research Medical 949-250-2500
6864 Cottonwood St, Midvale, UT 84047
Fluid transfer spike, i.v. administration.

Edwards Lifesciences Technology Sarl 949-250-2500
State Rd. 402 N.km 1.4, Anasco, PR 00610-1577
Set, administration, intravascular.

Entracare, Llc 913-451-2234
11315 Strang Line Rd, Lenexa, KS 66215
Extension sets.

Erika De Reynosa, S.A. De C.V. 781-402-9068
Brecha E99 Sur; Parque, Industrial Reynos, Bldg. Ii
Cd, Reynosa, Tamps Mexico
I.v. administration

Evans Medical Inc. 916-939-2451
1529 Terracina Dr, El Dorado Hills, CA 95762
Infusion set (winged).

Excelsior Medical Corp. 732-776-7525
1933 Heck Ave, Neptune, NJ 07753
Microbore extension set.

Exelint International Co. 800-940-3935
5840 W Centinela Ave, Los Angeles, CA 90045
Huber infusion sets. EXEL I.V. Administration Set.

Filtrona Extrusion, Inc./Pexcor Medical Products Div. 800-755-7528
764 S Athol Rd, P.O. Box 659, Athol, MA 01331

Global Healthcare 800-601-3380
1495 Hembree Rd Ste 700, Roswell, GA 30076
Lure lock, luer slip; with/without needle; various sizes;also include injection site and burette

Globe Medical Tech, Inc. 713-365-9595
1766 W Sam Houston Pkwy N, Houston, TX 77043
I.V. administration sets, available with y-injection sites and flashback bulbs.

Haemonetics Corp. 781-848-7100
400 Wood Rd, P.O.Box 9114, Braintree, MA 02184
Intravenous administration kit and components.

Harmac Medical Products, Inc. 716-897-4500
2201 Bailey Ave, Buffalo, NY 14211
OEM and private-labeled infusion disposables, including infusion bags and sets, extension sets, heparin traps, T-connectors, roller clamps, latex-free injection sites, and infusion components.

Hemerus Medical, Llc. 651-635-0070
5000 Township Pkwy, Saint Paul, MN 55110
Various leukocyte reduction filters sets.

Hospira, Inc. 877-946-7747
Hwy. 301 North, Rocky Mount, NC 27801
Various sizes of iv administration sets (sterile).

Hospira, Inc. 877-946-7747
755 Jarvis Dr, Morgan Hill, CA 95037

Icu Medical (Ut), Inc 949-366-2183
4455 Atherton Dr, Salt Lake City, UT 84123
Various.

Icu Medical, Inc. 800-824-7890
951 Calle Amanecer, San Clemente, CA 92673
Intravascular administration set.

Imp Group Ltd. 902-453-2400
400-2651 Dutch Village Rd, Halifax B3L 4T1 Canada
Set, administration, intravascular

Integra Biotechnical Llc 760-597-9878
2755 Dos Aarons Way Ste B, Vista, CA 92081

Iradimed Corporation 407-677-8022
7457 Aloma Ave Ste 201, Winter Park, FL 32792
Infusion pump administration sets.

Jostra Bentley, Inc. 302-454-9959
Rd. 402 N. Km 1.4, Industrial Park, Anasco, PR 00610-1577
Cardioplegia cooling/administration set.

Kawasumi Laboratories America, Inc. 800-529-2786
4723 Oak Fair Blvd, Tampa, FL 33610

KIT, ADMINISTRATION, INTRAVENOUS *(cont'd)*

Kelsar, S.A. 508-261-8000
Blvd. Insurgentes, Libriamento a La, Tijuana 22450 Mexico
Infusion plug w/wo filter needle

Lexamed 419-693-5307
705 Front St, Northwood, OH 43605
Various.

Lifemed Of California 800-543-3633
1216 S Allec St, Anaheim, CA 92805
IV Set, Buret Set, Extension Set; Lifeline IV & Buret Sets; disposable.

Lucomed Inc. 800-633-7877
45 Kulick Rd, Fairfield, NJ 07004

Medi Inc 800-225-8634
75 York Ave, P.O. Box 302, Randolph, MA 02368

Medical Action Industries, Inc. 800-645-7042
25 Heywood Rd, Arden, NC 28704
I.V. line securing device.

Medical Technologies Of Georgia, Inc. 404-394-2478
15151 Prater Dr, Covington, GA 30014
Multi lumen extension set.

Medron, Inc. 801-974-3010
1518 Gladiola St, Salt Lake City, UT 84104
Injection cap.

Medtronic Minimed 800-933-3322
18000 Devonshire St, Northridge, CA 91325

Merit Medical Systems Inc. 804-416-1030
12701 Kingston Ave, Chesterfield, VA 23837

Merit Medical Systems, Inc. 801-253-1600
1111 S Velasco St, Angleton, TX 77515
Various types of angiography kits eg digital subtraction.

Merit Medical Systems, Inc. 800-356-3748
1600 Merit Pkwy, South Jordan, UT 84095
Fluid administration sets.

Myco Medical 800-454-6926
158 Towerview Ct, Cary, NC 27513
Safety blood collection and infusion sets. IV administration sets. Specialty anesthesia trays and kits.

Navilyst Medical 800-833-9973
100 Boston Scientific Way, Marlborough, MA 01752
Fluid delivery sets.

Nexus Medical, Llc 913-451-2234
11315 Strang Line Rd, Lenexa, KS 66215
Various macro and microbore, extension sets, filter sets, sterile.

Nipro Diabetes Systems, Inc. 888-651-7867
3361 Enterprise Way, Miramar, FL 33025
Infusion set.

Np Medical, Inc. 978-368-4514
101 Union St, Clinton, MA 01510
Plastic IV check valves, plastic IV hooks, custom plastic set components.

Omni Medical Supply Inc. 800-860-6664
4153 Pioneer Dr, Commerce Township, MI 48390

Optimal Healthcare Products 800-364-8574
11444 W Olympic Blvd Ste 900, Los Angeles, CA 90064
The edit function seems to be working.

Prizm Medical, Inc. 770-622-0933
3400 Corporate Way Ste I, Duluth, GA 30096
I.V. administration sets, infusion set, I.V. tubing.

Rd Medical Mfg. Inc. 787-716-6363
Road 183, Km 21.6, Las Piedras Industrial Park, Las Piedras, PR 00771
Various sterile sets with and without filters.

Smiths Medical Asd, Inc. 800-848-1757
6250 Shier Rings Rd, Dublin, OH 43016

Specialized Health Products International, Inc. 800-306-3360
585 W 500 S, Bountiful, UT 84010
LiftLoc Safety Infusion Set. LiftLoc is a safety Huber needle designed to reduce the risk of accidental needlesticks by shielding the needle after use. LiftLoc's low profile and small footprint make dressing the site easy.

Terumo Cardiovascular Systems (Tcvs) 800-283-7866
28 Howe St, Ashland, MA 01721
Iv administration set.

Terumo Medical Corporation 800-283-7866
950 Elkton Blvd, P.O.Box 605, Elkton, MD 21921
Intravascular administration set.

KIT, ADMINISTRATION, INTRAVENOUS *(cont'd)*

Tri-State Hospital Supply Corp. 517-545-1135
3173 E 43rd St, Yuma, AZ 85365

Vascular Solutions, Inc. 763-656-4300
5025 Cheshire Ln N, Plymouth, MN 55446
Lidocaine delivery system.

Venetec International., Inc. 888-685-0565
12555 High Bluff Dr Ste 100, San Diego, CA 92130
Various.

Vlv Associates, Inc. 973-428-2884
30C Ridgedale Ave, East Hanover, NJ 07936
Shielded needle connector.

Vygon Corp. 800-544-4907
2495 General Armistead Ave, Norristown, PA 19403
Intravenous accessories.

Walkmed Infusion Llc 303-420-9569
4080 Youngfield St, Wheat Ridge, CO 80033
Various types of sterile infusion tubing sets.

KIT, ADMINISTRATION, OXYGEN *(Anesthesiology) 73RJH*

Life Corporation 800-700-0202
1776 N Water St, Milwaukee, WI 53202
LIFE, OxygenPac Portable emergency oxygen units, clear cover and wall-mounted, off/on lever control, resuscitation mask with one-way valve for hygiene, 6lpm 90min. supply, refillable. Also available 6 & 12 lpm NORM & HIGH, 0-25 lpm variable, and demand-valve for 100% oxygen resuscitation. GSA Federal Supply Schedule.

Mada, Inc. 800-526-6370
625 Washington Ave, Carlstadt, NJ 07072

Mine Safety Appliances Company 866-MSA-1001
121 Gamma Dr, Pittsburgh, PA 15238

U O Equipment Co. 800-231-6372
5863 W 34th St, Houston, TX 77092
Model 10100 fixed flow inhalator, list price $214.00. Can be ordered with CPR mask for oxygen enriched manual resuscitation. Adjustable models available.

KIT, ADMINISTRATION, PARENTERAL *(Gastro/Urology) 78TGJ*

Covidien Lp 508-261-8000
15 Hampshire St, Mansfield, MA 02048

Lucomed Inc. 800-633-7877
45 Kulick Rd, Fairfield, NJ 07004

Welcon, Inc. 800-877-0923
7409 Pebble Dr, Fort Worth, TX 76118

KIT, ADMINISTRATION, PERITONEAL DIALYSIS, DISPOSABLE
(Gastro/Urology) 78KDJ

B. Braun Of Puerto Rico, Inc. 610-691-5400
215.7 Insular Rd., Sabana Grande, PR 00637
Peritoneal dialysis administration set.

Baxter Healthcare Corp., Renal Division 847-948-2000
7511 114th Ave, Largo, FL 33773
Various sterile peritoneal dialysis solution administration sets & transfer sets.

Baxter Healthcare Corporation, Renal 888-229-0001
1620 S Waukegan Rd, Waukegan, IL 60085
CAPD prep kit.

Erika De Reynosa, S.A. De C.V. 781-402-9068
Brecha E99 Sur; Parque, Industrial Reynos, Bldg. Ii
Cd, Reynosa, Tamps Mexico
Various

Hospira, Inc. 877-946-7747
Hwy. 301 North, Rocky Mount, NC 27801
Peritoneal dialysis solution admin. set [sterile].

Lee Medical International, Inc. 800-433-8950
612 Distributors Row, Harahan, LA 70123

Medisystems Corporation 800-369-6334
439 S Union St Fl 5, Lawrence, MA 01843
Peritoneal dialysis disposables.

Millipore Corporation 877-246-2247
290 Concord Rd, Billerica, MA 01821
Peritoneal dialysis bags.

KIT, ADMISSION (PATIENT UTENSIL) *(General) 80RKC*

Atd-American Co. 800-523-2300
135 Greenwood Ave, Wyncote, PA 19095

Idexx Laboratories, Inc. 800-548-6733
1 Idexx Dr, Westbrook, ME 04092
For Leukemia.

KIT, ADMISSION (PATIENT UTENSIL) *(cont'd)*

Jero Medical Equipment & Supplies, Inc. 800-457-0644
1701 W 13th St, Chicago, IL 60608

Jones-Zylon Company 800-848-8160
305 N Center St, West Lafayette, OH 43845

Lsl Industries, Inc. 888-225-5575
5535 N Wolcott Ave, Chicago, IL 60640
$17.00 for 12 kits containing wash basin, emesis basin, tumbler, soap dish.

New World Imports 800-329-1903
160 Athens Way, Nashville, TN 37228
All disposable kit items. Also, emery boards and manicure sticks, nurses' pencils, disposable razors and personal belongings bags available. Also, Freshscent liquid amenities: lotion, shampoo, conditioner, mouthwash, bath gel.

KIT, ANESTHESIA, CAUDAL *(Anesthesiology) 73QAV*

Covidien Lp 508-261-8000
15 Hampshire St, Mansfield, MA 02048

KIT, ANESTHESIA, CONDUCTION *(Anesthesiology) 73CAZ*

Ballard Medical Products 770-587-7835
12050 Lone Peak Pkwy, Draper, UT 84020
Epidural and spinal anesthesia trays; sure snap epidural.

Becton Dickinson And Company 800-284-6845
1 Becton Dr, Franklin Lakes, NJ 07417
Epilor LOR Syringe; Axillary Block Needle

Biocompatibles Inc. 877-783-5463
115 Hurley Rd Bldg 3, Oxford, CT 06478
Various.

Busse Hospital Disposables, Inc. 631-435-4711
75 Arkay Dr, Hauppauge, NY 11788
Regional anesthesia trays.

Havel's Inc. 800-638-4770
3726 Lonsdale St, Cincinnati, OH 45227

Hospira, Inc. 877-946-7747
Hwy. 301 North, Rocky Mount, NC 27801
Various auesthesin kits [sterile.

Integra Lifesciences Corp. 801-886-9505
3395 W 1820 S, Salt Lake City, UT 84104
Anesthesia kit.

Kelsar, S.A. 508-261-8000
Blvd. Insurgentes, Libriamento a La, Tijuana 22450 Mexico
Spinal kits, epidural kits, w/wo drugs (various)

Neo Medical Inc. 888-450-3334
42514 Albrae St, Fremont, CA 94538
Cla kit.

Thomas Medical Products, Inc. 866-446-3003
65 Great Valley Pkwy, Malvern, PA 19355
Various sterile regional anesthesia trays and sets.

KIT, ANESTHESIA, EPIDURAL *(Anesthesiology) 73QAW*

B. Braun Oem Division, B. Braun Medical Inc. 866-8-BBRAUN
824 12th Ave, Bethlehem, PA 18018

Covidien Lp 508-261-8000
15 Hampshire St, Mansfield, MA 02048

Dma Med-Chem Corporation 800-362-1833
49 Watermill Ln, Great Neck, NY 11021

Havel's Inc. 800-638-4770
3726 Lonsdale St, Cincinnati, OH 45227

Norco 800-657-6672
1125 W Amity Rd, Boise, ID 83705

Vygon Corp. 800-544-4907
2495 General Armistead Ave, Norristown, PA 19403

KIT, ANESTHESIA, OTHER *(Anesthesiology) 73QAZ*

Covidien Lp 508-261-8000
15 Hampshire St, Mansfield, MA 02048

Dma Med-Chem Corporation 800-362-1833
49 Watermill Ln, Great Neck, NY 11021
Critical care anesthesia disposables.

KIT, ANESTHESIA, PARACERVICAL *(Obstetrics/Gyn) 85HEH*

Covidien Lp 508-261-8000
15 Hampshire St, Mansfield, MA 02048

KIT, ANESTHESIA, PUDENDAL *(Obstetrics/Gyn) 85HEG*

Covidien Lp 508-261-8000
15 Hampshire St, Mansfield, MA 02048

KIT, ANESTHESIA, PUDENDAL *(cont'd)*

International Medication Systems, Ltd. 800-423-4136
1886 Santa Anita Ave, South El Monte, CA 91733
O.b. needle guide with needle.

Kelsar, S.A. 508-261-8000
Blvd. Insurgentes, Libriamento a La, Tijuana 22450 Mexico
Paracervical/pudendal trays w/wo drugs

KIT, ANESTHESIA, SPINAL *(Anesthesiology) 73QAY*

Covidien Lp 508-261-8000
15 Hampshire St, Mansfield, MA 02048

KIT, ANGIOGRAPHIC, DIGITAL *(Radiology) 90VGB*

Boston Scientific Corporation 800-225-2732
1 Boston Scientific Pl, Natick, MA 01760
FloSwitch, one-hand operated flow controller stopcock and LeVeen inflator for inflation of angioplasty catheters.

Medical Techniques Usa 801-936-4501
125 N 400 W Ste C, North Salt Lake, UT 84054

KIT, ANGIOGRAPHIC, SPECIAL PROCEDURE *(Radiology) 90VGC*

Boston Scientific Corp. 800-323-6472
5905 Nathan Ln N, Minneapolis, MN 55442

Medical Techniques Usa 801-936-4501
125 N 400 W Ste C, North Salt Lake, UT 84054

Mennen Medical Corp. 800-223-2201
2540 Metropolitan Dr, Trevose, PA 19053
HORIZON ANGIO interventional peripheral vascular analysis physiological monitoring system.

KIT, ASSAY, RECEPTOR, PROGESTERONE *(Chemistry) 75LPI*

Dako North America, Inc 805-566-6555
6392 Via Real, Carpinteria, CA 93013

KIT, BARIUM ENEMA, DISPOSABLE *(Gastro/Urology) 78FCD*

Coloplast Manufacturing Us, Llc 612-302-4992
1185 Willow Lake Blvd, Vadnais Heights, MN 55110
Barium enema kit.

E-Z-Em, Inc. 516-333-8230
750 Summa Ave, Westbury, NY 11590
Barium sulfate suspension.

KIT, BIOPSY *(General) 80QDS*

Covidien Lp 508-261-8000
15 Hampshire St, Mansfield, MA 02048

David Scott Company 800-804-0333
59 Fountain St, Framingham, MA 01702

Ipas 919-967-7052
PO Box 5027, Chapel Hill, NC 27514
Endometrial biopsy kit.

Medical Techniques Usa 801-936-4501
125 N 400 W Ste C, North Salt Lake, UT 84054

Medtronic, Inc. 800-633-8766
710 Medtronic Pkwy, Minneapolis, MN 55432
INRAD, OMNIKIT.

Merit Medical Systems Inc. 804-416-1030
12701 Kingston Ave, Chesterfield, VA 23837

Rms Medical Products 800-624-9600
24 Carpenter Rd, Chester, NY 10918
MASTERSON endometrial biopsy system, DiSaia endocervical biopsy system.

KIT, BIOPSY NEEDLE *(Gastro/Urology) 78FCG*

Angiotech 800-424-6779
241 W Palatine Rd, Wheeling, IL 60090
BIO-CUT semiautomated biopsy needle for core tissue biopsy.

Atrion Medical Products, Inc. 800-343-9334
1426 Curt Francis Rd NW, Arab, AL 35016
Biopsy needles and cannulas.

Avid Medical 800-886-0584
9000 Westmont Dr, Stonehouse Commerce Park, Toano, VA 23168
N.I.T. Automatic Cutting Biopsy Needle, for use with powered reusable gun. Also available are manual style biopsy needles.

Ballard Medical Products 770-587-7835
12050 Lone Peak Pkwy, Draper, UT 84020
Set, biopsy needle and needle, gastro-urology.

Bard Reynosa S.A. De C.V. 908-277-8000
Blvd. Montebello #1, Parque Industrial Colonial
Reynosa, Tamaulipas Mexico
Various types of biopsy instruments/needles & needle sets

KIT, BIOPSY NEEDLE *(cont'd)*

Biocompatibles Inc. 877-783-5463
115 Hurley Rd Bldg 3, Oxford, CT 06478
Cutting biopsy needle.

C. R. Bard, Inc., Bard Urological Div. 888-367-2273
13183 Harland Dr NE, Covington, GA 30014

Cook Endoscopy 336-744-0157
4900 Bethania Station Rd # &, 5951 Grassy Creek Blvd. Winston Salem, NC 27105
Biliary and gastric aspiration needles.

Cook Inc. 800-457-4500
PO Box 489, Bloomington, IN 47402

Cook Urological, Inc. 800-457-4500
1100 W Morgan St, P.O. Box 227, Spencer, IN 47460

Envisioneering Medical Technologies 314-429-7367
1982 Innerbelt Business Center Dr, Drive, Overland, MO 63114
Biopsy kit & neddle guide.

Navilyst Medical 800-833-9973
100 Boston Scientific Way, Marlborough, MA 01752
Ptc procedure tray.

Pneumrx Inc 650-625-8910
530 Logue Ave, Mountain View, CA 94043
Sterile and non-sterile kit, needle, biopsy.

Proact, Ltd. 814-231-2158
112 W Foster Ave, State College, PA 16801
Flexible 165 cm Histological biopsy needle for endoscopic applications.

Promex Technologies, Llc 317-736-0128
3049 Hudson St, Franklin, IN 46131
Chiba,franseen,westcott,spinal style aspiration automated single action core bio.

Sterylab Usa, Llc 390-293-5084
2916 N Graham Rd Ste C, Franklin, IN 46131
Biopsy instrument.

KIT, BIOPSY, GASTRO-UROLOGY *(Gastro/Urology) 78FCH*

Busse Hospital Disposables, Inc. 631-435-4711
75 Arkay Dr, Hauppauge, NY 11788
Basic biopsy tray without biopsy needle.

Navilyst Medical 800-833-9973
100 Boston Scientific Way, Marlborough, MA 01752
Universal procedure tray.

KIT, BLOOD COLLECTION, PHLEBOTOMY *(Cardiovascular) 74RKS*

Bio-Plexus, Inc. 800-223-0010
129 Reservoir Rd, Vernon, CT 06066

Engineering & Research Assoc., Inc. (D.B.A. Sebra) 800-625-5550
100 N Tucson Blvd, Tucson, AZ 85716
Blood collection and processing instruments.

Fenwal Inc. 800-766-1077
3 Corporate Dr, Lake Zurich, IL 60047
Autologous.

Kawasumi Laboratories America, Inc. 800-529-2786
4723 Oak Fair Blvd, Tampa, FL 33610
Blood drawing kit - device for therapeutic phlebotomy, 600-ml blood bag (empty), preattached 16G venipunture needle, pinch clamp, 48-inch tubing length.

KIT, BLOOD DONOR *(Hematology) 81QDZ*

The Metrix Co. 800-752-3148
4400 Chavenelle Rd, Dubuque, IA 52002
Custom contract manufacturer.

KIT, BLOOD PRESSURE, CENTRAL VENOUS *(Cardiovascular) 74QIX*

Hospira, Inc. 877-946-7747
755 Jarvis Dr, Morgan Hill, CA 95037

KIT, BLOOD, TRANSFUSION *(General) 80BRZ*

B. Braun Of Puerto Rico, Inc. 610-691-5400
215.7 Insular Rd., Sabana Grande, PR 00637
Blood administration sets.

Baxter Healthcare S.A. 847-948-2000
Rd. 721, Km. 0.3, Aibonito, PR 00609
Transfusion sets.

KIT, BLOOD, TRANSFUSION *(cont'd)*

Charter Medical, Ltd. 336-768-6447
3948 Westpoint Blvd Ste A, Winston Salem, NC 27103
Fluid reservoir and delivery system.

Haemonetics Corp. 800-225-5242
400 Wood Rd, P.O. Box 9114, Braintree, MA 02184
ORTHOPAT system salvages the patient's own blood during and after surgery.

Sorin Group Usa 800-289-5759
14401 W 65th Way, Arvada, CO 80004
BRAT II Kardiothor autologous blood recovery system; Brat-Pak disposable set for autologous transfusion system plus reinfusion bag.

Vygon Corp. 800-544-4907
2495 General Armistead Ave, Norristown, PA 19403

KIT, BOWEL *(Gastro/Urology) 78SIB*

C.B. Fleet Company Inc. 804-528-4000
PO Box 11349, 4615 Murray Place, Lynchburg, VA 24506
FLEET prep kits. 48 basic units; all kits include 4-Bisacodyl Tablets and Fleet Phospho-soda, and either small volume enema, large-volume enema, or suppository.

Ethicon Endo-Surgery, Inc. 800-USE-ENDO
4545 Creek Rd, Cincinnati, OH 45242
ENDOPATH FLEXTRAY bowel tray delivery system.

KIT, BREAST CANCER DETECTION *(Obstetrics/Gyn) 85TGQ*

American Diagnostica, Inc. 888-234-4435
500 West Ave, Stamford, CT 06902
IMUBIND; Breast cancer prognosis. ICA & ELISA

Mammatech Corp. 800-626-2273
930 NW 8th Ave, Gainesville, FL 32601
$225.00 for breast self-exam videocassette with 2 breast models.

KIT, BURN *(General) 80QEU*

Afassco, Inc. 800-441-6774
2244 Park Pl Ste C, Minden, NV 89423
Several burn kits available.

Allied Healthcare Products, Inc. 800-444-3954
1720 Sublette Ave, Saint Louis, MO 63110

Covidien Lp 508-261-8000
15 Hampshire St, Mansfield, MA 02048

General Scientific Safety Equipment Co. 800-523-0166
2553 E Somerset St Fl 1, Philadelphia, PA 19134

O-Two Systems International Inc. 800-387-3405
7575 Kimbel St., Mississauga, ONT L5S 1C8 Canada
BURN RELIEF 'Gelled Water' burn kits and supplies.

Rockford Medical & Safety Co. 800-435-9451
2420 Harrison Ave, PO Box 5646, Rockford, IL 61108

Romaine, Inc. D.B.A. Koldcare 800-294-7101
2026 Sterling Ave, Elkhart, IN 46516
KOOLABURN STERILE BURN KIT Available in two different sizes. Each contain a variety of gelled water burn dressings in a convenient carrying case.

Vector Firstaid, Inc. 800-999-4423
316 N Corona Ave, Ontario, CA 91764
WATERJEL Water based product with Lidocaine to relieve the pain of all types of burns.

Water-Jel Technologies 800-275-3433
50 Broad St, Carlstadt, NJ 07072
Burn Kits for every need - contain water-based, gel-soaked dressings and accessory items to treat all kinds of burns.

Zimmer Holdings, Inc. 800-613-6131
1800 W Center St, PO Box 708, Warsaw, IN 46580

KIT, CATHETER CARE *(General) 80QHG*

B. Braun Oem Division, B. Braun Medical Inc. 866-8-BBRAUN
824 12th Ave, Bethlehem, PA 18018

Covidien Lp 508-261-8000
15 Hampshire St, Mansfield, MA 02048

Ep Medsystems, Inc. 609-753-8533
575 N Route 73 Bldg D, West Berlin, NJ 08091
PROCATH peel-away sheath introducer kits.

Lsl Industries, Inc. 888-225-5575
5535 N Wolcott Ave, Chicago, IL 60640
$37.00 for 50 kits containing 5 rayon balls, PVP solution kit, PVP ointment pkt., 2 gloves, waterproof drape, 4 x 4 gauze sponge, wooden cotton-tipped applicator, 1 tray.

KIT, CATHETER CARE *(cont'd)*

Medi Inc 800-225-8634
75 York Ave, P.O. Box 302, Randolph, MA 02368

Vygon Corp. 800-544-4907
2495 General Armistead Ave, Norristown, PA 19403
Catheter removal kits.

KIT, CATHETERIZATION, CARDIAC *(Cardiovascular) 74QHK*

Excel Medical Products, Llc 810-714-4775
3145 Copper Ave, Fenton, MI 48430
Excel Angyo PTCA Life Kit

Medical Techniques Usa 801-936-4501
125 N 400 W Ste C, North Salt Lake, UT 84054

KIT, CATHETERIZATION, INTRAVENOUS, WINGED
(Cardiovascular) 74QHL

Becton Dickinson Infusion Therapy Systems, Inc. 888-237-2762
9450 S State St, Sandy, UT 84070
Winged infusion sets.

Covidien Lp 508-261-8000
15 Hampshire St, Mansfield, MA 02048

Kawasumi Laboratories America, Inc. 800-529-2786
4723 Oak Fair Blvd, Tampa, FL 33610
Winged small vein infusion sets, safety and standard available

Medisystems Corporation 800-369-6334
439 S Union St Fl 5, Lawrence, MA 01843

Vygon Corp. 800-544-4907
2495 General Armistead Ave, Norristown, PA 19403

KIT, CATHETERIZATION, STERILE URETHRAL
(Gastro/Urology) 78FCM

Biomet Microfixation Inc. 800-874-7711
1520 Tradeport Dr, Jacksonville, FL 32218
Tray, catheterization, sterile urethral, with or without catheter.

C. R. Bard, Inc., Bard Urological Div. 888-367-2273
13183 Harland Dr NE, Covington, GA 30014

Coloplast Manufacturing Us, Llc 612-302-4992
1185 Willow Lake Blvd, Vadnais Heights, MN 55110
Urethral catheterization system.

Continental Medical Laboratories, Inc. 262-534-2787
813 Ela Ave, Waterford, WI 53185
Urethral catheterization kit.

Covidien Lp 508-261-8000
15 Hampshire St, Mansfield, MA 02048

Customed, Inc. 787-801-0101
Calle Igualdad #7, Fajardo, PR 00738
Foley tray 16 fr. (sterile) 900-402.

Kelsar, S.A. 508-261-8000
Blvd. Insurgentes, Libriamento a La, Tijuana 22450 Mexico
Folye catheter trays- all silicone,coated(elastomer latex,premiun teflon)

Life-Tech, Inc. 281-491-6600
4235 Greenbriar Dr, Stafford, TX 77477

Lsl Industries, Inc. 888-225-5575
5535 N Wolcott Ave, Chicago, IL 60640
$32.95 for 20 kits containing 1 package of 3 povidone iodine swabs, 2 gloves, lubricating jelly, waterproof drape, fenestrated drape, specimen container with lid & label, 14-16Fr. urethral catheter, 1100ml tray. Premium wrapped tray also available.

Mckesson General Medical 800-446-3008
8741 Landmark Rd, Richmond, VA 23228

Medline Industries, Inc. 800-633-5886
1 Medline Pl, Mundelein, IL 60060

Medline Manufacturing And Services Llc 847-837-2759
1 Medline Pl, Mundelein, IL 60060
Catheter trays.

Omni Medical Supply Inc. 800-860-6664
4153 Pioneer Dr, Commerce Township, MI 48390

Rochester Medical Corp. 800-615-2364
1 Rochester Medical Dr NW, Stewartville, MN 55976
Various models of catheterization trays.

Welcon, Inc. 800-877-0923
7409 Pebble Dr, Fort Worth, TX 76118

KIT, CATHETERIZATION, URINARY *(Gastro/Urology) 78QHM*

Boston Scientific Corporation 800-225-2732
1 Boston Scientific Pl, Natick, MA 01760
VTC Nephrostomy catheters.

KIT, CATHETERIZATION, URINARY *(cont'd)*

Covidien Lp 508-261-8000
15 Hampshire St, Mansfield, MA 02048

Medi Inc 800-225-8634
75 York Ave, P.O. Box 302, Randolph, MA 02368

Medline Industries, Inc. 800-633-5886
1 Medline Pl, Mundelein, IL 60060

Welcon, Inc. 800-877-0923
7409 Pebble Dr, Fort Worth, TX 76118

Zimmer Holdings, Inc. 800-613-6131
1800 W Center St, PO Box 708, Warsaw, IN 46580

KIT, CHEST DRAINAGE (THORACENTESIS TRAY)
(General) 80QJS

Atrium Medical Corp. 800-528-7486
5 Wentworth Dr, Hudson, NH 03051

Covidien Lp 508-261-8000
15 Hampshire St, Mansfield, MA 02048
TRU-CLOSE thoracic vent procedure tray.

Medi Inc 800-225-8634
75 York Ave, P.O. Box 302, Randolph, MA 02368

Vygon Corp. 800-544-4907
2495 General Armistead Ave, Norristown, PA 19403

KIT, CHOLECYSTECTOMY *(Gastro/Urology) 78SHX*

Elmed, Inc. 630-543-2792
60 W Fay Ave, Addison, IL 60101

Ethicon Endo-Surgery, Inc. 800-USE-ENDO
4545 Creek Rd, Cincinnati, OH 45242
ENDOPATH FLEXTRAY cholecystectomy tray delivery system.

Gibbons Surgical Corp. 800-959-1989
1112 Jensen Dr Ste 101, Virginia Beach, VA 23451

J. Jamner Surgical Instruments, Inc 800-431-1123
9 Skyline Dr, Hawthorne, NY 10532

Karl Storz Endoscopy-America Inc. 800-421-0837
600 Corporate Pointe, Culver City, CA 90230

Primesource Healthcare, Inc. 888-842-6999
3708 E Columbia St Ste 100, Tucson, AZ 85714
Kit, lapcholy.

Taut, Inc. 800-231-8288
2571 Kaneville Ct, Geneva, IL 60134

KIT, CIRCUMCISION, DISPOSABLE TRAY
(Obstetrics/Gyn) 85QKG

American Medical Devices, Inc. 800-788-9876
287 S Stoddard Ave, San Bernardino, CA 92401

KIT, COLLECTION/TRANSFUSION, MARROW, BONE
(General) 80LWE

Biocompatibles Inc. 877-783-5463
115 Hurley Rd Bldg 3, Oxford, CT 06478
Bone marrow biopsy needle.

Biomedical Enterprises, Inc. 800-880-6528
14785 Omicron Dr Ste 205, San Antonio, TX 78245
BONEHOG, Bone and Marrow Collection System, disposable manual surgical instrument used in drilling or collecting viable bone and marrow. EXCALIBUR Bone Grafting System is the powered version.

Custom Medical Products 407-865-7211
3909 E Semoran Blvd Bldg 599, Apopka, FL 32703
Bone marrow tray.

Exmoor Plastics Inc. 317-244-1014
304 Gasoline Aly, Indianapolis, IN 46222
Mofat-Robinson bone plate collector with single-use filters priced at $275.00 complete.

Kelsar, S.A. 508-261-8000
Blvd. Insurgentes, Libriamento a La, Tijuana 22450 Mexico
Bone marrow biopsy/aspiration needle & trays w/&w/o needles

University Of Washington 206-616-5130
T281 Health Science, Seattle, WA 98195
Bone marrow grafting apparatus.

KIT, CORD BLOOD COLLECTION *(Hematology) 81MYK*

Custom Medical Products 407-865-7211
3909 E Semoran Blvd Bldg 599, Apopka, FL 32703
Blood cord collection kit.

KIT, CRICOTHYROTOMY *(Anesthesiology) 73QNJ*

Cook Inc. 800-457-4500
PO Box 489, Bloomington, IN 47402

Instrumentation Industries, Inc. 800-633-8577
2990 Industrial Blvd, Bethel Park, PA 15102

Smiths Medical Asd 800-424-8662
5700 W 23rd Ave, Gary, IN 46406
NU-TRAKE emergency cricothyrotome/tracheotomy device, RE-TRAKE emergency/reintubation device, PEDIA-THOR emergency thoracostomy device for children and NU-THOR model for adults.

KIT, DENTAL PROPHYLAXIS *(Dental And Oral) 76RMM*

Medikmark Inc. 800-424-8520
3600 Burwood Dr, Waukegan, IL 60085

KIT, DENTURE REPAIR, OTC *(Dental And Oral) 76EBO*

Astron Dental Corporation 847-726-8787
815 Oakwood Rd Ste G, Lake Zurich, IL 60047
Denture reline/repair acrylic material.

Dentsply Canada, Ltd. 800-263-1437
161 Vinyl Ct., Woodbridge, ONT L4L 4A3 Canada

KIT, DIALYSIS, SINGLE NEEDLE (CO-AXIAL FLOW) *(Gastro/Urology) 78LBW*

Lee Medical International, Inc. 800-433-8950
612 Distributors Row, Harahan, LA 70123
Custom kit.

KIT, DISC AGAR GEL DIFFUSION, SERUM LEVEL *(Microbiology) 83JTP*

Biomerieux Inc. 800-682-2666
100 Rodolphe St, Durham, NC 27712

KIT, DISPOSABLE PROCEDURE *(Cardiovascular) 74SGT*

Crosstex International 800-223-2497
10 Ranick Rd, Hauppauge, NY 11788
Dental disposables.

Crosstex International Ltd., W. Region 800-707-2737
14059 Stage Rd, Santa Fe Springs, CA 90670
Dental disposables.

Crosstex International,Inc. 888-276-7783
10 Ranick Rd, Hauppauge, NY 11788
CROSSTEX Dental disposables.

Danlee Medical Products, Inc. 800-433-7797
6075 E Molloy Rd Bldg 5, Syracuse, NY 13211
Customized Hook-up kits for Holter/Stress and Event Recording. Can be private labeled. Choose electrodes, batteries, prep supplies, disposable pouches and more to custom design a kit for your specific requirements.

David Scott Company 800-804-0333
59 Fountain St, Framingham, MA 01702

Excel Medical Products, Llc 810-714-4775
3145 Copper Ave, Fenton, MI 48430
PTCA and custom disposable procedure kits.

Mckesson General Medical 800-446-3008
8741 Landmark Rd, Richmond, VA 23228
Non-sterile.

Medical Techniques Usa 801-936-4501
125 N 400 W Ste C, North Salt Lake, UT 84054

Merit Medical Systems Inc. 804-416-1030
12701 Kingston Ave, Chesterfield, VA 23837

KIT, DISSECTING *(Pathology) 88QQE*

Trans American Medical / Tamsco Instruments 708-430-7777
7633 W 100th Pl, Bridgeview, IL 60455

KIT, DNA DETECTION, HUMAN PAPILLOMAVIRUS *(Microbiology) 83MAQ*

Epicentre Technologies 800-284-8474
726 Post Rd, Madison, WI 53713
SEQUITHERM EXCEL DNA Sequencing Kit. MASTERAMP PCR kits & Buccal swab kit products for high yield PCR, including method for collecting human DNA samples without drawing blood.

Qiagen Gaithersburg, Inc. 800-344-3631
1201 Clopper Rd, Gaithersburg, MD 20878
Digene hpv dna assay.

KIT, EARMOLD IMPRESSION *(Ear/Nose/Throat) 77LDG*

All American Mold Laboratories, Inc. 405-677-2700
2120 S I 35 Service Rd, Oklahoma City, OK 73129
Earmold for air-conduction hearing aid.

K & R Products, Inc. 831-426-6061
33170 Central Ave, Union City, CA 94587
Ear plugs/ear molds.

Northeast Resins & Silicones, Llc. 203-272-4931
122 Spring St Ste C1, Southington, CT 06489
Various - earmold impression material(s).

Oticon, Inc. 800-526-3921
29 Schoolhouse Rd, Somerset, NJ 08873
Oticon ear impression material.

Quest Intl., Inc. 305-592-6991
8127 NW 29th St, Doral, FL 33122
Anti-toxoplasma tgm serological reagents, elisa.

Santa Barbara Medco, Inc. 651-452-1977
1270 Eagan Industrial Rd, Eagan, MN 55121
Silicone ear putty.

Starkey Glencoe 952-947-4734
2915 10th St E, Glencoe, MN 55336
Impression kits, precise, x-acto kits.

KIT, EMERGENCY DRUG *(General) 80QUB*

Caligor 800-472-4346
846 Pelham Pkwy, Pelham, NY 10803

KIT, EMERGENCY, ANAPHYLACTIC *(General) 80UDB*

Banyan International Corp. 800-351-4530
PO Box 1779, 2118 E. Interstate 20, Abilene, TX 79604

KIT, EMERGENCY, CARDIOPULMONARY RESUSCITATION *(General) 80UDC*

Ambu, Inc. 800-262-8462
6740 Baymeadow Dr, Glen Burnie, MD 21060
Including suction equipment.

Armstrong Medical Industries, Inc. 800-323-4220
575 Knightsbridge Pkwy, Lincolnshire, IL 60069

Banyan International Corp. 800-351-4530
PO Box 1779, 2118 E. Interstate 20, Abilene, TX 79604
Stat Kit 700...$585.00; Stat Kit 900...$965.00; First Kit...$199.00

Mtm Health Products Ltd. 800-263-8253
2349 Fairview St., Burlington, ONT L7R 2E3 Canada
COMPLETE CRP KIT weatherproof, zipped bag contains one MTM MOUTH TO MASK resusitator. one CPR Landmarc, and one pair of surgical gloves.

Safetec Of America, Inc. 800-456-7077
887 Kensington Ave, Buffalo, NY 14215
EZ CPR RESCUE/PROTECTION KITS allow for safe use of normal CPR techniques, without fear of cross-contamination. Contains PTP II CPR mask, vinyl gloves, Personal Antimicrobial Hand Wipes (paws), and Biohazard Waste Bag. Kits are available in 3 convenient packaging options: nylon pack, poly bag, or clam shell.

Vitalograph, Inc. 800-255-6626
13310 W 99th St, Lenexa, KS 66215
$438.00 to $690.00, resuscitation and suction.

KIT, EMERGENCY, INSECT STING *(General) 80RCG*

Afassco, Inc. 800-441-6774
2244 Park Pl Ste C, Minden, NV 89423

Health Enterprises 800-633-4243
90 George Leven Dr, North Attleboro, MA 02760
BUG SHIELD and ITCH'S GONE Insect Repellent and relief products.

KIT, ENDODONTIC *(Dental And Oral) 76VEI*

Biolase Technology, Inc. 888-424-6527
4 Cromwell, Irvine, CA 92618

Moyco Technologies, Inc. 800-331-8837
200 Commerce Dr, Montgomeryville, PA 18936
Endoscopic equipment.

KIT, ENEMA *(General) 80QUG*

C.B. Fleet Company Inc. 804-528-4000
PO Box 11349, 4615 Murray Place, Lynchburg, VA 24506
FLEET adult ready to use, disposable saline enema.

Chester Labs, Inc. 800-354-9709
1900 Section Rd, Cincinnati, OH 45237
Phosphate enema (Gent-L-Tip), disposable.

KIT, ENEMA *(cont'd)*

Crosswell International Corporation 305-648-0777
101 Madeira Ave, Coral Gables, FL 33134

Lsl Industries, Inc. 888-225-5575
5535 N Wolcott Ave, Chicago, IL 60640
$38.50 to $42.00 for various types of enema sets.

Marconi Medical Systems 800-323-0550
595 Miner Rd, Cleveland, OH 44143
1500cc unit.

Marlen Manufacturing & Development Co. 216-292-7060
5150 Richmond Rd, Bedford, OH 44146

O&M Enterprise 847-258-4515
641 Chelmsford Ln, Elk Grove Village, IL 60007
KIT ENEMA

KIT, ENEMA (FOR CLEANING PURPOSES)
(Gastro/Urology) 78FCE

American Wellness Foundation 713-622-8499
6105 Beverlyhill St Ste 202, Houston, TX 77057
Enema kit.

Carolina Medical Products Co. 252-753-7111
PO Box 147, 8026 Us 264 Alternate, Farmville, NC 27828
Enema kit.

Colon-Ez Llc 936-756-1970
12126 Kimberly Trce, Conroe, TX 77304
Enema kit.

Energy Medicine Center 949-833-8989
20301 SW Acacia St, Newport Beach, CA 92660
Sitting enema/colon cleaner.

Ergounlimited, Inc. 205-591-9977
5401 9th Ave S, Birmingham, AL 35212
Enema board.

Kelsar, S.A. 508-261-8000
Blvd. Insurgentes, Libriamento a La, Tijuana 22450 Mexico
Enema bag sets / enema bucket

Leyshon Miller Industries 740-695-9188
534 N 1st St, Cambridge, OH 43725
Speculum.

Lifestream Purification Systems, Llc 877-564-3185
2001 S Lamar Blvd Ste G, Austin, TX 78704
Portable colon irrigation kit for internal cleansing.

Medline Industries, Inc. 800-633-5886
1 Medline Pl, Mundelein, IL 60060

The Art Of Living Institute 713-621-0366
7815 Fondren Rd, Houston, TX 77074
Enema kit.

Ultimate Concepts, Inc. 801-566-3241
5056 Crimson Patch Way, Riverton, UT 84096
Enema kit.

Ultimate Trends 800-745-3191
1455 E 8125 S, Sandy, UT 84093
Home gravity colenema kit.

KIT, FEEDING, ADULT (ENTERAL) *(General) 80QVM*

Amsino International, Inc. 800-MD-AMSINO
855 Towne Center Dr, Pomona, CA 91767
AMSINO contains 60-cc syringe, piston or bulb, luer tip adaptor, syringe cap. Packaged in zip-lock bag. Item AS006.

Covidien Lp 508-261-8000
15 Hampshire St, Mansfield, MA 02048
KANGAROO sterile, non-sterile enteral feeding pumps, gastrosomy feeding tubes. DUO-TUBE silicone feeding unit with weighted tip.

Filtrona Extrusion, Inc./Pexcor Medical Products Div. 800-755-7528
764 S Athol Rd, P.O. Box 659, Athol, MA 01331

Frantz Medical Development Ltd. 440-255-1155
7740 Metric Dr, Mentor, OH 44060

KIT, FEEDING, PEDIATRIC (ENTERAL) *(General) 80QVN*

Amsino International, Inc. 800-MD-AMSINO
855 Towne Center Dr, Pomona, CA 91767
AMSINO contains 60-cc syringe, piston or bulb, luer tip adaptor, syringe cap. Packaged in zip-lock bag. Item AS006.

Children's Medical Ventures, Inc. 800-345-6443
191 Wyngate Dr, Monroeville, PA 15146
SAFE-T-CARE, enteral only extension-sets.

KIT, FEEDING, PEDIATRIC (ENTERAL) *(cont'd)*

Covidien Lp 508-261-8000
15 Hampshire St, Mansfield, MA 02048

Filtrona Extrusion, Inc./Pexcor Medical Products Div. 800-755-7528
764 S Athol Rd, P.O. Box 659, Athol, MA 01331

Genesis Industries/Maternal Concepts 800-310-5817
130 S Public St, Elmwood, WI 54740
SUCKLE-CUP INFANT FEEDER is an infant feeding cup, used to aid in feeding infants.

Lact-Aid International 866-866-1239
PO Box 1066, Athens, TN 37371
LACT-AID Nursing Trainer system. Breastfeeding-assistance device supplements infant at breast to aid lactation.

Novartis Nutrition 800-333-3785
1600 Utica Ave S Ste 600, PO Box 370, Minneapolis, MN 55416

KIT, FIRST AID *(Surgery) 79LRR*

Adventure Medical Kits 510-261-7414
5555 San Leandro St Fl 1, Oakland, CA 94621
Medical kits.

Afassco, Inc. 800-441-6774
2244 Park Pl Ste C, Minden, NV 89423
Several sizes standard first-aid kits and emergency response kits. also can custom-make to any fill.

Arkon Safety Equipment, Inc. 514-351-8240
10550 Boul Parkway, Anjou H1J 2K4 Canada
Various

Armstrong Medical Industries, Inc. 800-323-4220
575 Knightsbridge Pkwy, Lincolnshire, IL 60069

B. Braun Oem Division, B. Braun Medical Inc. 866-8-BBRAUN
824 12th Ave, Bethlehem, PA 18018
Critical care kits.

Beacon Promotions, Inc. 507-354-3900
2121 S Bridge St, New Ulm, MN 56073
First aid kit.

C.M.S. Industries Ltd. 800-668-8821
1320 Alberta Ave., Saskatoon, SK S7K 1R5 Canada
CPR key rings, first aid kits, and car safety kits.

Caligor 800-472-4346
846 Pelham Pkwy, Pelham, NY 10803

Certified Safety Manufacturing 800-854-7474
1400 Chestnut Ave, Kansas City, MO 64127
Industrial, commercial.

Cook Inc. 800-457-4500
PO Box 489, Bloomington, IN 47402

Cooperative Workshops, Inc. 888-615-6332
1500 Ewing Dr, Sedalia, MO 65301
Various.

Cramer Products, Inc. 800-255-6621
153 W Warren St, Gardner, KS 66030

Dixie Ems Supply 800-347-3494
385 Union Ave, Brooklyn, NY 11211
$180.00 per unit (basic).

Emergency First Aid Products (Usa), Inc. 518-562-9911
53 Area Development Dr Unit B, Plattsburgh, NY 12901
First aid kits.

Erb Industries Inc. 800-800-6522
1 Safety Way, Woodstock, GA 30188
Personal First Aid Kit pouch.

F.A.S.T. First Aid & Survival Technologies Ltd. 604-540-8300
1687 Cliveden Ave, Delta V3M 6V5 Canada
Kit, first aid

Fieldtex Products, Inc. 800-772-4816
3055 Brighton-Henrietta Tl Rd, Rochester, NY 14623
Soft-sided first-aid kits and supplies.

General Scientific Safety Equipment Co. 800-523-0166
2553 E Somerset St Fl 1, Philadelphia, PA 19134

Healer Products, Llc 914-663-6300
427 Commerce Ln Ste 1, West Berlin, NJ 08091
Multiple first aid kits.

Hospital Specialty Company 800-321-9832
500 Memorial Dr, Nicholasville, KY 40356

Hospitales Y Quirofanos S.A. Dec.V. 5-611-8244
Murillo No. 44 Col. Nonoalco, Deleg. B. Juarez, D.F. 03700 Mexico
Wound Care.

KIT, FIRST AID *(cont'd)*

Johnson & Johnson Consumer Products, Inc. 800-526-3967
199 Grandview Rd, Skillman, NJ 08558

Johnson & Johnson Medical Division Of Ethicon, Inc. 800-423-4018
2500 E Arbrook Blvd, Arlington, TX 76014

Kern Surgical Supply, Inc. 800-582-3939
2823 Gibson St, Bakersfield, CA 93308

Lab Safety Supply, Inc. 800-356-0783
401 S Wright Rd, Janesville, WI 53546

Lhb Industries 800-542-3697
10440 Trenton Ave, Saint Louis, MO 63132
First-aid kit.

Marine Medical Intl., Inc. 954-523-1404
1414 S Andrews Ave, Fort Lauderdale, FL 33316
Kit, first aid.

Medco Supply Company 800-556-3326
500 Fillmore Ave, Tonawanda, NY 14150
Custom and Johnson & Johnson.

Medical Safety Systems Inc. 888-803-9303
230 White Pond Dr, Akron, OH 44313

Medipoint, Inc. 800-445-0525
72 E 2nd St, Mineola, NY 11501
SPLINTER-OUT individually wrapped, sterile splinter removers.

Medistat Medical - Hallmark Sales Corporation 888-MED-ISTA
1601 Peach Leaf St, Houston, TX 77039
Manufacturer of complete line for commercial, institutional, government, and consumer use at affordable prices. Other products include splint kits, burn kits, universal refills, blood/pathogen spill kits, sterile medical/surgical kits, and custom kits. Also sells first aid, safety, and medical supplies.

Metronix 813-972-1212
12421 N Florida Ave Ste D201, Tampa, FL 33612
Wound dressing, splint devices and accessories, immobilization and extraction trauma kits and medical bags.

Mine Safety Appliances Company 866-MSA-1001
121 Gamma Dr, Pittsburgh, PA 15238

Normed 800-288-8200
PO Box 3644, Seattle, WA 98124
Various types & sizes of first aid kits.

North Safety Products 401-943-4400
1101 B Calle Neutron, Parque Industrial Maran, Mexicali, B.c. Mexico
1st aid kit

Norwood Promotional Products, Inc. 651-388-1298
5151 Moundview Dr, Red Wing, MN 55066
First aid kit-various types.

Palmero Health Care 800-344-6424
120 Goodwin Pl, Stratford, CT 06615
DISCIDE ULTRA disinfecting towelettes, hospital level, for use in first aid kits.

Plano Molding Co. 800-451-2122
431 E South St, Plano, IL 60545
747M, Plano Jumbo Medical Box. This item is made of high-impact plastic and features front access to 3 large trays w/ bulk storage in the extra deep bottom. The top opens all the way to allow the trays to cantilever for easy access to total contents. Patented locking system prevents gear spillage, even when the box is unlatched. Dimensions: 20.83 ' L x 11.5 ' W x 12.75 ' H

Quick Point Inc. 636-343-9400
1717 Fenpark Dr, Fenton, MO 63026
First aid kit.

Respond Industries, Inc. 1-800-523-8999
9500 Woodend Rd, Edwardsville, KS 66111
Eye & skin flushing kit.

Rockford Medical & Safety Co. 800-435-9451
2420 Harrison Ave, PO Box 5646, Rockford, IL 61108

Safecross First Aid Ltd. 416-665-0050
1111 Alness St, Toronto M3J 2J1 Canada
Various

Sentinel Consumer Products, Inc. 440-974-8144
7750 Tyler Blvd, Mentor, OH 44060

Total Care 800-334-3802
PO Box 1661, Rockville, MD 20849

KIT, FIRST AID *(cont'd)*

Wisconsin Pharmacal Co. Llc 800-558-6614
PO Box 198, Jackson, WI 53037
Line of first aid kits for outdoor/wilderness use. Retail prices from $10 to $500.

Work 'N Leisure Products, Inc. 508-634-0939
455 Fortune Blvd, Milford, MA 01757
Multiple first aid kits.

Zee Medical, Inc. 800-841-8417
22 Corporate Park, Irvine, CA 92606

1st Aid First 800-613-6770
1690 Lake Hill Rd, Deer Lodge, MT 59722
Custom first aid kit design and supply.

KIT, FORENSIC EVIDENCE *(Pathology) 88TCF*

Garren Scientific, Inc. 800-342-3725
15916 Blythe St Unit A, Van Nuys, CA 91406
Premier Pak, Premier Drug Screen Products: On-site drug screen kit for DOA, alcohol, adulteration with lab confirmation.

Lab Corp Of America 800-833-3984
1904 Alexander Drive, Durham, NC 27709-2652

Medical & Clinical Consortium (Mcc) 877-622-8378
13740 Nelson Ave, City Of Industry, CA 91746
Instant Human IgG Test for detection of human blood in crime scenes.

Sirchie Finger Print Laboratories 800-356-7311
100 Hunter Pl, Youngsville, NC 27596
DNA evidence collection kit.

KIT, FORENSIC EVIDENCE, SEXUAL ASSAULT *(Obstetrics/Gyn) 85QXO*

First Aid Bandage Co., Inc. 888-813-8214
3 State Pier Rd, New London, CT 06320
Markit--components and instructions for uniform and scientific collection and preservation of medicolegal evidence in rape cases and sexual abuse.

Sirchie Finger Print Laboratories 800-356-7311
100 Hunter Pl, Youngsville, NC 27596
Blood and urine evidence collection kits.

KIT, GASTROSTOMY, ENDOSCOPIC, PERCUTANEOUS *(Gastro/Urology) 78SJD*

Abbott Laboratories 800-624-7677
1033 Kingsmill Pkwy, Columbus, OH 43229
FLEXIFLO LAP G laparoscopic gastostomy kit.

KIT, GINGIVAL RETRACTION *(Dental And Oral) 76VEG*

Harry J. Bosworth Company 800-323-4352
7227 Hamlin Ave, Skokie, IL 60076

KIT, GONORRHOEAE TEST (MALE USE) *(Microbiology) 83SGO*

Hema Diagnostic Systems, Llc 305-867-6123
1666 Kennedy Causeway, Suite 401, North Bay Village, FL 33141

KIT, HEMODIALYSIS TUBING *(Gastro/Urology) 78QZU*

B. Braun Medical Inc., Renal Therapies Div. 800-854-6851
824 12th Ave, Bethlehem, PA 18018
DiaLines Bloodline Tubing Sets and SAF T Needlefree Bloodline Tubing Sets.

Kawasumi Laboratories America, Inc. 800-529-2786
4723 Oak Fair Blvd, Tampa, FL 33610

Lifemed Of California 800-543-3633
1216 S Allec St, Anaheim, CA 92805

Lucomed Inc. 800-633-7877
45 Kulick Rd, Fairfield, NJ 07004

Medisystems Corporation 800-369-6334
439 S Union St Fl 5, Lawrence, MA 01843

Megamed Corporation 305-665-6876
7432 SW 48th St, Miami, FL 33155

KIT, HERNIORRHAPHY *(Gastro/Urology) 78SHY*

Ethicon Endo-Surgery, Inc. 800-USE-ENDO
4545 Creek Rd, Cincinnati, OH 45242
ENDOPATH FLEXTRAY herniorrhaphy tray delivery system.

KIT, HYSTERECTOMY *(Obstetrics/Gyn) 85SHZ*

Ethicon Endo-Surgery, Inc. 800-USE-ENDO
4545 Creek Rd, Cincinnati, OH 45242
ENDOPATH FLEXTRAY delivery system.

KIT, IDENTIFICATION, ANAEROBIC *(Microbiology) 83JSP*

Air Liquide Healthcare America Corporation 713-402-2152
8428 Market Street Rd, Houston, TX 77029
Biological atmosphere of anaerobic gas mixtures.

Almore International, Inc. 503-643-6633
PO Box 25214, Portland, OR 97298
$215.00 per unit (standard) to $355.00.

Remel Atlanta, Div. Of Remel, Inc. 800-255-6730
2797 Peterson Pl, Norcross, GA 30071
RAPID ANA II has four identification of medically important anaerobic bacteria.

KIT, IDENTIFICATION, DERMATOPHYTE *(Microbiology) 83JSR*

Dms Laboratories, Inc. 800-567-4367
2 Darts Mill Rd, Flemington, NJ 08822
RAPIDVET-D rapid screening system to detect the presence of dermatophytes on dogs, cats, rabbits and horses. 25 tests. Total testing time is 72 hours maximum for negative results.

KIT, IDENTIFICATION, ENTEROBACTERIACEAE *(Microbiology) 83JSS*

Biomerieux Inc. 800-682-2666
100 Rodolphe St, Durham, NC 27712

Meridian Bioscience, Inc. 800-696-0739
3471 River Hills Dr, Cincinnati, OH 45244
MERITEC culture confirmation products.

Remel Atlanta, Div. Of Remel, Inc. 800-255-6730
2797 Peterson Pl, Norcross, GA 30071
RAPID ONE has four identification of oxidase - negative gram - negative rods (eneterobacteriagae) and other bacteria.

KIT, IDENTIFICATION, GLUCOSE (NON-FERMENT) *(Microbiology) 83JSW*

Bd Diagnostic Systems 800-675-0908
7 Loveton Cir, Sparks, MD 21152

Remel Atlanta, Div. Of Remel, Inc. 800-255-6730
2797 Peterson Pl, Norcross, GA 30071
RAPID NF PLUS has four identification of oxidase - positive gram - negative rods (non-fermentors and vibrio).

KIT, IDENTIFICATION, NEISSERIA GONORRHOEAE *(Microbiology) 83JSX*

Culture Kits, Inc. 888-680-6853
14 Prentice St, PO Box 748, Norwich, NY 13815
GONO-GEN II.

E-Y Laboratories, Inc. 800-821-0044
107 N Amphlett Blvd, San Mateo, CA 94401
Neisseria gonorrhoeae identification kit.

Gen-Probe, Inc. 800-523-5001
10210 Genetic Center Dr, San Diego, CA 92121
PACE 2C for Chlamydia Trachomatis and Neisseria Gonorrhea - single-tube assay to screen for the presence of Chlamydia trachomatis and Neisseria gonorrhea from endocervical and male urethral swab specimens. AccuProbe NEISSERIA GONORRHOEAE Culture Identification Test - for the identification of Neisseria gonorrhoeae isolated from culture.

Remel Atlanta, Div. Of Remel, Inc. 800-255-6730
2797 Peterson Pl, Norcross, GA 30071
RAPID NH has two identification of medically important neisseria and four hour identification of haemophilus.

Sierra Molecular Inc. 209-536-0886
21109 Longeway Rd Ste C, Sonora, CA 95370
Genetic transformation test for indentification of n. gonorrhoeae.

Washington Biotechnology, Inc. 206-292-9734
562 1st Ave S Fl 7, Seattle, WA 98104
Culture-confirmation test

KIT, IDENTIFICATION, YEAST *(Microbiology) 83JXB*

Bayer Healthcare Llc 914-524-2955
555 White Plains Rd Fl 5, Tarrytown, NY 10591
Test for candida species in vaginal specimens.

Bayer Healthcare, Llc 574-256-3430
430 S Beiger St, Mishawaka, IN 46544
Test for candida species in vaginal specimens.

Biolog, Inc. 800-284-4949
21124 Cabot Blvd, Hayward, CA 94545
YT MICROPLATE for identification of approximately 250 species of yeast, both clinical and industrial.

KIT, IDENTIFICATION, YEAST *(cont'd)*

Remel Atlanta, Div. Of Remel, Inc. 800-255-6730
2797 Peterson Pl, Norcross, GA 30071
RAPID YEAST PLUS has four four identification of medically yeast and yeast-like organisms.

Wescor, Inc. 800-453-2725
459 S Main St, Logan, UT 84321
The Fungichrom kit allows the identification of the main human pathogenic yeasts notably via the use on chromogenicsubstrates.

KIT, INCISION AND DRAINAGE *(Surgery) 79RBS*

Atrium Medical Corp. 800-528-7486
5 Wentworth Dr, Hudson, NH 03051

Marlen Manufacturing & Development Co. 216-292-7060
5150 Richmond Rd, Bedford, OH 44146

Medistat Medical - Hallmark Sales Corporation 888-MED-ISTA
1601 Peach Leaf St, Houston, TX 77039
Manufacturer of kits including first aid, body fluid spills, burns, emergency, medical, surgical, obstetrical, exams, minor surgery, biopsy, convenience, procedure trays, disposable instruments, sterile kits. Owns manufacturing and validated sterilization facilities. Can make custom or special order kits. Refills, supplies.

Merit Medical Systems Inc. 804-416-1030
12701 Kingston Ave, Chesterfield, VA 23837

Surgimark, Inc. 800-228-1186
2516 W Washington Ave, Yakima, WA 98903

Technical Products, Inc. 800-226-8434
805 Marathon Pkwy Ste 150, Lawrenceville, GA 30046
Slicone incision drains used in hand and finger surgery.

Zimmer Holdings, Inc. 800-613-6131
1800 W Center St, PO Box 708, Warsaw, IN 46580

KIT, INSTRUMENTS AND ACCESSORIES, SURGICAL *(Surgery) 79FTN*

Advanced Medical Innovations, Inc. 888-367-2541
9410 De Soto Ave Ste J, Chatsworth, CA 91311
SAF-T-SCREEN or Anesthesia IV, pole/screen combination to save precious floor space. Easily adjusts to any height during surgery with the EZ lift system.

Bioseal 800-441-7325
167 W Orangethorpe Ave, Placentia, CA 92870
Custom sterile OR put-ups.

Cardiovascular Research, Inc. 813-832-6222
4810 W Gandy Blvd, Tampa, FL 33611
Surgical instruments. Non-skid vascular surgical forceps.

Care Wise Medical Products Corp. 888-462-8725
15750 Vineyard Blvd Ste 160, Morgan Hill, CA 95037

Cloward Instrument Corporation 808-734-3511
3787 Diamond Head Rd, Honolulu, HI 96816
CLOWARD Anterior cervical fusion kit.

Conkin Surgical Instruments Ltd. 416-922-9496
18 Coldwater Rd., Toronto, ON M3B-1Y7 Canada

Custom Medical Products 407-865-7211
3909 E Semoran Blvd Bldg 599, Apopka, FL 32703
Plastic surgery kit.

Deknatel Snowden-Pencer 800-367-7874
5175 S Royal Atlanta Dr, Tucker, GA 30084

J. Jamner Surgical Instruments, Inc 800-431-1123
9 Skyline Dr, Hawthorne, NY 10532

Kapp Surgical Instrument, Inc. 800-282-5277
4919 Warrensville Center Rd, Cleveland, OH 44128

Lipomax Mfg., Inc. 562-623-9364
13055 Tom White Way Ste G, Norwalk, CA 90650
Various types of cannulas.

Medistat Medical - Hallmark Sales Corporation 888-MED-ISTA
1601 Peach Leaf St, Houston, TX 77039
Manufacturer of kits including first aid, body fluid spills, burns, emergency, medical, surgical, obstetrical, exams, minor surgery, biopsy, convenience, procedure trays, disposable instruments, sterile kits. Owns manufacturing and validated sterilization facilities. Can make custom or special order kits. Refills, supplies.

Microsurgical Laboratories 713-723-6900
11333 Chimney Rock Rd Ste 120, Houston, TX 77035

Millstone Medical Outsourcing 508-679-8384
1565 N Main St Ste 408, Fall River, MA 02720
Multiple and various.

KIT, INSTRUMENTS AND ACCESSORIES, SURGICAL *(cont'd)*

Orchid Unique 989-746-0780
6688 Dixie Hwy, Bridgeport, MI 48722
Machined components and surgical instruments.

Osteomed L.P. 800-456-7779
3880 Arapaho Rd, Addison, TX 75001
M4 Rigid Fixation System; comprehensive system of titanium bone plates, screws and instrumentation for use in craniomaxillofacial reconstruction surgery

Repco 800-726-1852
1227 W Magnolia Ave Ste 310, Fort Worth, TX 76104
AccuSurgical.

Royal Surgical Instruments, Co. 309-547-3656
206 N Robinson St, Lewistown, IL 61542

Rx Honing Machine Corporation 800-346-6464
1301 E 5th St, Mishawaka, IN 46544
RX Honing Machines: Honing sets. Surgical instrument sharpening sets with machine components, instructional manuals, and videos designed for specialties including hospital, surgical, dermatology, ophthalmology, and plastic surgery.

Scanlan International, Inc. 800-328-9458
1 Scanlan Plz, Saint Paul, MN 55107

Transamerican Technologies International 800-322-7373
2246 Camino Ramon, San Ramon, CA 94583
ACCU-SURG, endoscopic instruments - fiber director, s/l cannula, electrosurgical probes, stone/clot aspirator, plus custom instruments.

Wexler Surgical Supplies 800-414-1076
11333 Chimney Rock Rd Ste 110, Houston, TX 77035

KIT, INTRAVENOUS EXTENSION TUBING *(General) 80RCK*

B. Braun Oem Division, B. Braun Medical Inc. 866-8-BBRAUN
824 12th Ave, Bethlehem, PA 18018

Baxter Healthcare Corporporation, Alternate Care And Channel Team 888-229-0001
25212 W Il Route 120, Round Lake, IL 60073
Catheter extension sets. Extension sets. MINI-INFUSER syringe pumps and microbore extension sets. Minivolume extension set.

Benlan Inc. 905-829-5004
2760 Brighton Rd., Oakville, ONT L6H 5T4 Canada

Churchill Medical Systems, Inc. 800-468-0585
935 Horsham Rd Ste M, Horsham, PA 19044

Codan Us Corporation 800-33-CODAN
3511 W Sunflower Ave, Santa Ana, CA 92704

Directmed, Inc. 516-656-3377
150 Pratt Oval, Glen Cove, NY 11542

Eagle Laboratories 800-782-6534
10201 Trademark St Ste A, Rancho Cucamonga, CA 91730

Filtrona Extrusion, Inc./Pexcor Medical Products Div. 800-755-7528
764 S Athol Rd, P.O. Box 659, Athol, MA 01331

Harmac Medical Products, Inc. 716-897-4500
2201 Bailey Ave, Buffalo, NY 14211
OEM and private-labeled custom infusion disposable products, including infusion bags and sets, extension sets, heparin traps, T-connectors, latex-free injection sites, and infusion components.

Industrial Specialities Manufacturing, Inc. 800-781-8487
2741 W Oxford Ave Unit 6, Englewood, CO 80110

Integra Biotechnical Llc 760-597-9878
2755 Dos Aarons Way Ste B, Vista, CA 92081

Kawasumi Laboratories America, Inc. 800-529-2786
4723 Oak Fair Blvd, Tampa, FL 33610
Add-on filter extension tubing for use with Taxol, Erbitux and Remicade infusions. Appropriate for both gravity IV and pump administration sets.

Lifemed Of California 800-543-3633
1216 S Allec St, Anaheim, CA 92805
Lifeline Burette Sets.

Medi Inc 800-225-8634
75 York Ave, P.O. Box 302, Randolph, MA 02368

Medisystems Corporation 800-369-6334
439 S Union St Fl 5, Lawrence, MA 01843

Medtronic Minimed 800-933-3322
18000 Devonshire St, Northridge, CA 91325
42in. PVC subcutaneous set or Polyfin (non-PVC) subcutaneous set, 60in. Polyfin IV extension set.

KIT, INTRAVENOUS EXTENSION TUBING *(cont'd)*

Mps Acacia 800-486-6677
785 Challenger St, Brea, CA 92821

Smiths Medical Asd, Inc. 800-848-1757
6250 Shier Rings Rd, Dublin, OH 43016

Spectra Medical Devices, Inc. 866-938-8649
4C Henshaw St, Woburn, MA 01801

Vygon Corp. 800-544-4907
2495 General Armistead Ave, Norristown, PA 19403
I.V. accessories - extension lines (straight and coiled).

3m Co. 888-364-3577
3M Center, Saint Paul, MN 55144

KIT, INTRAVENOUS, ADMINISTRATION, BURET *(General) 80RCI*

Baxter Healthcare Corporporation, Alternate Care And Channel Team 888-229-0001
25212 W Il Route 120, Round Lake, IL 60073
Buretrol Solution Sets.

Codan Us Corporation 800-33-CODAN
3511 W Sunflower Ave, Santa Ana, CA 92704

Globe Medical Tech, Inc. 713-365-9595
1766 W Sam Houston Pkwy N, Houston, TX 77043
Burette (volumetric) I.V. administration sets, 100-ml and 150-ml burette, 60 drops/ml with Y-injection site.

Lifemed Of California 800-543-3633
1216 S Allec St, Anaheim, CA 92805
Lifeline Burette Sets.

Lucomed Inc. 800-633-7877
45 Kulick Rd, Fairfield, NJ 07004

KIT, IRRIGATION, BLADDER *(Gastro/Urology) 78RCR*

Covidien Lp 508-261-8000
15 Hampshire St, Mansfield, MA 02048

Medi Inc 800-225-8634
75 York Ave, P.O. Box 302, Randolph, MA 02368

KIT, IRRIGATION, EAR *(Ear/Nose/Throat) 77RCS*

Ethicare Products 800-253-3599
PO Box 5027, Fort Lauderdale, FL 33310
With adjustable fan spray nozzle.

Medi Inc 800-225-8634
75 York Ave, P.O. Box 302, Randolph, MA 02368

Oto-Med, Inc. 800-433-7703
1090 Empire Dr, Lake Havasu City, AZ 86404
Levine Irrigation-Suction Kit: Completely assembled - offers a consistent easy-to-set-up system. Sterile disposable

KIT, IRRIGATION, EYE *(Ophthalmology) 86RCT*

Allergan 800-366-6554
2525 Dupont Dr, Irvine, CA 92612
From $50 to $110 CooperVision compatible I/A and Phaco disposable kits.

Armstrong Medical Industries, Inc. 800-323-4220
575 Knightsbridge Pkwy, Lincolnshire, IL 60069

Bausch & Lomb Surgical 636-255-5051
3365 Tree Court Ind Blvd, Saint Louis, MO 63122

Medi Inc 800-225-8634
75 York Ave, P.O. Box 302, Randolph, MA 02368

Microsurgical Technology, Inc. 425-556-0544
PO Box 2679, Redmond, WA 98073

Mortan, Inc. 800-423-8659
329 E Pine St, Missoula, MT 59802
MORGAN medi-FLOW Lens 'Irrigation Station Kit'

Stephens Instruments, Inc. 800-354-7848
2500 Sandersville Rd, Lexington, KY 40511

KIT, IRRIGATION, ORAL *(Ear/Nose/Throat) 77TCR*

Ludlow Technological Products 800-445-5025
2 Ludlow Park Dr, Chicopee, MA 01022
Oral care products.

KIT, IRRIGATION, PERINEAL *(Gastro/Urology) 78RCU*

Dotolo Research Corp. 800-237-8458
2875 Mcl Dr, Pinellas Park, FL 33782

Welcon, Inc. 800-877-0923
7409 Pebble Dr, Fort Worth, TX 76118

KIT, IRRIGATION, STERILE *(Gastro/Urology) 78EYN*

Advanced Medical Innovations, Inc. 888-367-2641
9410 De Soto Ave Ste J, Chatsworth, CA 91311
SAF-T-POLE, irrigation tower for arthroscopic hysteroscopies and TURP surgeries.

Amsino International, Inc. 800-MD-AMSINO
855 Towne Center Dr, Pomona, CA 91767
AMSINO contains 60-cc syringe, piston or bulb, 500-ml container, patient I.D. label luer tip adaptor, syringe cap. Items AS126 and AS120.

B. Braun Of Puerto Rico, Inc. 610-691-5400
215.7 Insular Rd., Sabana Grande, PR 00637
Fluid administration set.

Centurion Medical Products Corp. 517-545-1135
3310 S Main St, Salisbury, NC 28147

Covidien Lp 508-261-8000
15 Hampshire St, Mansfield, MA 02048

Customed, Inc. 787-801-0101
Calle Igualdad #7, Fajardo, PR 00738
Sterile irrigation tray with bulb syringe.

Deknatel Snowden-Pencer 800-367-7874
5175 S Royal Atlanta Dr, Tucker, GA 30084
Hydro dissection pump, irrigation pump.

Kelsar, S.A. 508-261-8000
Blvd. Insurgentes, Libriamento a La, Tijuana 22450 Mexico
Irrigation kits w/bulb or piston syringe (various)

Lsl Industries, Inc. 888-225-5575
5535 N Wolcott Ave, Chicago, IL 60640
$26.00 for 20 trays containing 50ml bulb syringe, 500ml graduated container, 1100ml tray, waterproof drape, alcohol wipe, tip protector. $18.75 for same but without wrap. $26.00 for 20 sterile piston irrigation trays - $18.75 for same but without wrap.

Mckesson General Medical 800-446-3008
8741 Landmark Rd, Richmond, VA 23228

Medline Industries, Inc. 800-633-5886
1 Medline Pl, Mundelein, IL 60060

Medline Manufacturing And Services Llc 847-837-2759
1 Medline Pl, Mundelein, IL 60060
Irrigation procedure trays.

Steris Corporation 814-452-3100
2424 W 23rd St, Erie, PA 16506
Irrigation sets.

Stryker Puerto Rico, Ltd. 939-307-2500
Hwy. 3, Km. 131.2, Las Guasimas Ind. Park, Arroyo, PR 00714
Knife.

Terumo Cardiovascular Systems (Tcvs) 800-283-7866
28 Howe St, Ashland, MA 01721
Irrigation tray.

Tri-State Hospital Supply Corp. 517-545-1135
3173 E 43rd St, Yuma, AZ 85365

Welcon, Inc. 800-877-0923
7409 Pebble Dr, Fort Worth, TX 76118

KIT, IRRIGATION, WOUND *(General) 80RCW*

American Medical Industries 605-428-5501
330 E 3rd St Ste 2, Dell Rapids, SD 57022
EZ-IRRIGATOR irrigation syringe.

Covidien Lp 508-261-8000
15 Hampshire St, Mansfield, MA 02048
Wound cleanser.

Medco Supply Company 800-556-3326
500 Fillmore Ave, Tonawanda, NY 14150

Medi Inc 800-225-8634
75 York Ave, P.O. Box 302, Randolph, MA 02368

Welcon, Inc. 800-877-0923
7409 Pebble Dr, Fort Worth, TX 76118

Zerowet, Inc. 800-438-0938
PO Box 4375, Palos Verdes Peninsula, CA 90274
KLENZALAC, a complete system for high-speed, high-volume wound irrigation, for large, dirty, or complex wounds. Includes ZEROWET SPLASHIELD.

Zimmer Holdings, Inc. 800-613-6131
1800 W Center St, PO Box 708, Warsaw, IN 46580

KIT, LABOR AND DELIVERY *(Obstetrics/Gyn) 85MLS*

Armstrong Medical Industries, Inc. 800-323-4220
575 Knightsbridge Pkwy, Lincolnshire, IL 60069

KIT, LABOR AND DELIVERY *(cont'd)*

Bio-Logics Products, Inc. 800-426-7577
PO Box 505, West Jordan, UT 84084
The Placental Triage Kit (PTK). The iPTKî is designed to help improve how placentas are handled in the birthing room. It standardizes placental triage, making it quicker, more efficient and low cost while optimizing documentation and information on placentas not submitted for pathology examination.

Centurion Medical Products Corp. 517-545-1135
3310 S Main St, Salisbury, NC 28147

Medistat Medical - Hallmark Sales Corporation 888-MED-ISTA
1601 Peach Leaf St, Houston, TX 77039
Manufacturer of kits including first aid, body fluid spills, burns, emergency, medical, surgical, obstetrical, exams, minor surgery, biopsy, convenience, procedure trays, disposable instruments, sterile kits. Owns manufacturing and validated sterilization facilities. Can make custom or special order kits. Refills, supplies.

Morrison Medical 800-438-6677
3735 Paragon Dr, Columbus, OH 43228
OB KITS, Kit obstetrical, disposable for birthing and delivery of babies in emergency situations. Available with many various components to meet your expectations or regulations.

Rockford Medical & Safety Co. 800-435-9451
2420 Harrison Ave, PO Box 5646, Rockford, IL 61108

Tri-State Hospital Supply Corp. 517-545-1135
3173 E 43rd St, Yuma, AZ 85365

Utah Medical Products, Inc. 800-533-4984
7043 Cottonwood St, Midvale, UT 84047
CMI Vacuum Delivery System equipment is used for assisting delivery of the infant's head in vaginal or Caesarean procedures, instead of forceps. Equipment consists of sterile cup, tube & fluid trap sets usually used with a hand operated vacuum pump which can be steam sterilized. Also available is an educational video which demonstrates how to use this CMI equipment correctly. Note: CMI sterile vacuum cup, tube & fluid trap sets can also be used with an electric vacuum pump, if desired.

KIT, LAPAROSCOPY *(Gastro/Urology) 78FDE*

Abbott Laboratories 800-624-7677
1033 Kingsmill Pkwy, Columbus, OH 43229
FLEXIFLO Lap G laparoscopic gastrostomy kit. Includes silicone gastrostomy tube with balloon bumper and radiopaque tip.

American Medical Devices, Inc. 800-788-9876
287 S Stoddard Ave, San Bernardino, CA 92401
Laparoscopy tray.

Boston Scientific Corporation 800-225-2732
1 Boston Scientific Pl, Natick, MA 01760

Deknatel Snowden-Pencer 800-367-7874
5175 S Royal Atlanta Dr, Tucker, GA 30084

Dexterity Surgical, Inc. 210-495-8787
12961 Park Central Ste 1300, San Antonio, TX 78216
Suction irrigation systems and instruments. Disposable and reusable accessories.

Elmed, Inc. 630-543-2792
60 W Fay Ave, Addison, IL 60101

Endovia Medical, Inc. 781-255-1888
150 Kerry Pl, Norwood, MA 02062
Unique set of laparoscopic instruments that combine a robotic telemanipulator and artificial intelligence software to increase a surgeon's dexterity and transmit a sense of touch to the surgeon's hand.

Koros Usa, Inc. 805-529-0825
610 Flinn Ave, Moorpark, CA 93021
Videoscope.

Taut, Inc. 800-231-8288
2571 Kaneville Ct, Geneva, IL 60134
Comprehensive Lap CBDE kit. A one-box approach to the treatment of CBD stones: components include the Trifecta dual-lumen balloon and Intraducer and the Titanium4 wire basket. Tools designed specifically for Transcystic Lap CBDE.

KIT, LARYNGEAL INJECTION *(Ear/Nose/Throat) 77KAA*

Bausch & Lomb Surgical 636-255-5051
3365 Tree Court Ind Blvd, Saint Louis, MO 63122

Mel R. Manufacturas 956-655-1380
417 E Coma Ave Ste 534, Hidalgo, TX 78557
general assembly 'kit' subcontarctor

KIT, LUMBAR PUNCTURE *(Cns/Neurology) 84RFM*

Covidien Lp 508-261-8000
15 Hampshire St, Mansfield, MA 02048

Havel's Inc. 800-638-4770
3726 Lonsdale St, Cincinnati, OH 45227

Utah Medical Products, Inc. 800-533-4984
7043 Cottonwood St, Midvale, UT 84047
MYELO-NATE, specialized tray for collection of cerebrospinal fluid (csf). Needles available separately.

KIT, LYMPHANGIOGRAPHIC *(Cns/Neurology) 84RFN*

Cook Inc. 800-457-4500
PO Box 489, Bloomington, IN 47402

KIT, MATERNITY *(Obstetrics/Gyn) 85RGF*

Hospital Marketing Svcs. Company, Inc. 800-786-5094
162 Great Hill Rd./ Ind. Park, Naugatuck, CT 06770
Cat. no 6300-p4, 6300-p6 6packs, w/ mesh pant, 4 packs w/ mesh pant.

Jones-Zylon Company 800-848-8160
305 N Center St, West Lafayette, OH 43845

Medical Techniques Usa 801-936-4501
125 N 400 W Ste C, North Salt Lake, UT 84054

Tri-State Hospital Supply Corp. 800-248-4058
301 Catrell Dr, PO Box 170, Howell, MI 48843

KIT, MENINGITIS DETECTION *(Microbiology) 83TGR*

Bd Diagnostic Systems 800-675-0908
7 Loveton Cir, Sparks, MD 21152

KIT, MID-STREAM COLLECTION *(General) 80RGZ*

Lsl Industries, Inc. 888-225-5575
5535 N Wolcott Ave, Chicago, IL 60640
$20.00 to $28.50 for 50 sterile midstream urine specimen kits containing 120ml container, twist on cap, specimen label, instruction sheet and povidone-iodine USP wipes or 3-in-1 iodophor wipes plus tissues with the deluxe kit. Also available with castile soap or BKC.

Medi Inc 800-225-8634
75 York Ave, P.O. Box 302, Randolph, MA 02368

Rocket Medical Plc. 800-707-7625
150 Recreation Park Dr Ste 3, Hingham, MA 02043

Starplex Scientific Inc. 800-665-0954
50A Steinway Blvd., Etobicoke, ONT M9W 6Y3 Canada

KIT, MYCOBACTERIA IDENTIFICATION *(Microbiology) 83JSY*

Access Bio Incorporate 732-297-2222
2033 Rt. 130 Unit H, Monmouth Junction, NJ 08852
Tuberculosis test.

Bd Diagnostic Systems 800-675-0908
7 Loveton Cir, Sparks, MD 21152
BACTEC 9000B continuous monitoring, non-invasive culturing device for the detection of mycobacteria. Can hold and test up to 240 culture vials at one time. Media available: MYCO/F - Sputa. BACTEC 460TB radiometric culture device for the detection of mycobacteria; identification and susceptibility testing of M. tuberculosis. Media available: 12B, 13A, PZA, NAP and SIRE Drugs. BACTEC MGIT 960 for mycobacteria testing is designed to meet the needs of medium and high volume laboratories with a 960 tube, space saving capacity. The system has continuous as well as safe, efficient, on-board incubation. It is non-radiometric and uses no sharps in the inoculation or testing.

Biomerieux Inc. 800-682-2666
100 Rodolphe St, Durham, NC 27712
MB/BACT Mycobacteria detection.

KIT, MYCOBACTERIA IDENTIFICATION *(cont'd)*

Gen-Probe, Inc. 800-523-5001
10210 Genetic Center Dr, San Diego, CA 92121
AccuProbe Culture Identification Reagent Kit - reagents for mycobacterial- and fungal-culture identification tests. AccuProbe COCCIDIOIDES IMMITIS Culture Identification Test - for the identification of Coccidioides immitis isolated from culture. AccuProbe ENTEROCOCCUS Culture Identification Test - for the identification fo Enterococcus avium, E. casseliflavus, E. durans, E. faecalis, E. faecium, E. gallinarum, E. hirae, E. mundtii, E. pseudoavium, E. malodorous, and E. raffinosus isolated from culture. AccuProbe HAEMOPHILUS INFLUENZAE Culture Identification Test - for the identification of Haemophilus influenzae isolated from culture. AccuProbe HISTOPLASMA CAPSULATUM Culture Identification Test - for the identification of Histoplasma capsulatum isolated from culture. AccuProbe LISTERIA MONOCYTOGENES Culture Identification Test - for the identification of Listeria monocytogenes isolated from culture. AccuProbe STAPHYLOCOCCUS AUREUS Culture Identification Test - for the identification of Staphylococcus aureus isolated from culture. AccuProbe STAPHYLOCOCCUS PNEUMONIAE Culture Identification Test - for the identification of Staphylococcus pneumoniae isolated from culture.

Hema Diagnostic Systems, Llc 305-867-6123
1666 Kennedy Causeway, Suite 401, North Bay Village, FL 33141
Rapid 1-2-3 hema tuberculosis, whole blood test. In strip format or in our new rapid 1-2-3 hema housing.

Immunoscience, Inc. 925-460-8111
7066 Commerce Cir Ste D, Pleasanton, CA 94588
Mycobacterium tuberculosis assay.

KIT, MYELOGRAM *(Cns/Neurology) 84RHN*

Medical Techniques Usa 801-936-4501
125 N 400 W Ste C, North Salt Lake, UT 84054

KIT, PAP SMEAR *(Obstetrics/Gyn) 85RJW*

Andwin Scientific 800-497-3113
6636 Variel Ave, Woodland Hills, CA 91303
SAFETEX NO TOUCH and SAFETEX CLASSIC kits.

Medical Chemical Corp. 800-424-9394
19430 Van Ness Ave, Torrance, CA 90501
$13.50 per 25 units.

Medical Packaging Corporation 800-792-0600
941 Avenida Acaso, Camarillo, CA 93012
8 kits: standard one slide, standard two slide, mailing one slide, and mailing two slide, which all contain 1 or 2 frosted end glass slides, 1 cervical scraper, 1 cotton- tipped applicator, and 1 ampule cytology fixative (95% ethyl alcohol/2.5% carbowax); also cytology brush one slide, cytology brush two slide, mailing cytology brush one slide, and mailing cytology brush two slide, which all contain the above items, except that CYTOSOFT cytology brush replaces cotton-tipped applicator. All packaged 500 kits/case.

Surgipath Medical Industries, Inc. 800-225-3035
PO Box 528, 5205 Route 12, Richmond, IL 60071

Wallach Surgical Devices, Inc. 800-243-2463
235 Edison Rd, Orange, CT 06477

KIT, PELVIC EXAM *(Obstetrics/Gyn) 85MLT*

Centurion Medical Products Corp. 517-545-1135
3310 S Main St, Salisbury, NC 28147

Tri-State Hospital Supply Corp. 517-545-1135
3173 E 43rd St, Yuma, AZ 85365

Tri-State Hospital Supply Corp. 800-248-4058
301 Catrell Dr, PO Box 170, Howell, MI 48843
Centurion(R) Pelvic Exam Trays built to specific procedural needs. Available items include Centurion(R) specula, steel-alloy forceps, plastic forceps, cervical scrapers, specimen slides, CSR wraps rayon-tipped applicators, rayon balls w/ radiopaque thread, sterile gloves, drapes, gauze.

KIT, PERFUSION, KIDNEY, DISPOSABLE *(Gastro/Urology) 78KDL*

Erika De Reynosa, S.A. De C.V. 781-402-9068
Brecha E99 Sur; Parque, Industrial Reynos, Bldg. Ii Cd, Reynosa, Tamps Mexico
Kidney perfusion kit

KIT, PLAQUE DISCLOSING *(Dental And Oral) 76EAW*

Harry J. Bosworth Company 800-323-4352
7227 Hamlin Ave, Skokie, IL 60076

Sunstar Butler 800-J BUTLER
4635 W Foster Ave, Chicago, IL 60630

KIT, PLAQUE DISCLOSING *(cont'd)*

Young Innovations, Inc. 800-325-1881
13705 Shoreline Ct E, Earth City, MO 63045
Disclosing products. 2-tone old plaque stains blue, new plaque stains red.

KIT, PLATELET ASSOCIATED IGG *(Hematology) 81LLG*

Dms Laboratories, Inc. 800-567-4367
2 Darts Mill Rd, Flemington, NJ 08822
CANITEC ELISA assay for the in-vitro determination of allergen-specific IgE and allergen-specific IgG in canine serum and EQUITEC ELISA assay for equine serum. 15 or 32 tests, total testing time of 5 hours.

Genetic Testing Institute 262-754-1000
20925 Crossroads Cir Ste 200, Waukesha, WI 53186
Modified antigen capture elisa for the detection of ig antibodies to ptl glyprtn.

KIT, PREGNANCY TEST *(Obstetrics/Gyn) 85TFV*

Acon Laboratories, Inc. 858-535-2030
10125 Mesa Rim Rd, San Diego, CA 92121
Pregnancy test strips, devices, midstreams

American Bantex Corp. 800-633-4839
1815 Rollins Rd, Burlingame, CA 94010

Bio-Medical Products Corp. 800-543-7427
10 Halstead Rd, Mendham, NJ 07945
Strips, slides and wands. $2.50 for one test package of one-step pregnancy test (2 minute urine/serum test).

Biomerica, Inc. 800-854-3002
17571 Von Karman Ave, Irvine, CA 92614
EZ- hCG, pregnancy test. One step urine. (#1047).

Bremancos Diagnostics Inc. 800-830-2593
6800 Kitimat Rd., Unit 2, Mississauga, ONT L5N-5M1 Canada

Diagnostic Specialties 732-549-4011
4 Leonard St, Metuchen, NJ 08840
$37.50 for PREGNA CERT latex pregnancy kit, 50 tests per kit. $59.00 for PREGNA SURE membrane ELISA pregnancy test kit, 20 tests per kit.

Drg International, Inc. 800-321-1167
1167 US Highway 22, Mountainside, NJ 07092
Home or office use; one step pregnancy test (BEE-SURE).

Immunostics, Inc. 800-722-7505
3505 Sunset Ave, Ocean, NJ 07712

Inamco International Corp. 800-724-4003
801 Montrose Ave, South Plainfield, NJ 07080
MEDICOS.

Inverness Medical Inc. 732-308-3000
569 Halls Mill Rd, Freehold, NJ 07728
INVERNESS MEDICAL.

Lifesign 800-526-2125
71 Veronica Ave, Somerset, NJ 08873
STATUS HCG Urine/serum pregnancy test. $75.00/Box 25, $137.50/Box 50. 25 miv sensitivity.

Miami Medical Equipment & Supply Corp. 305-592-0111
2150 NW 93rd Ave, Doral, FL 33172

Mizuho Usa, Inc. 858-679-0555
12131 Community Rd, Poway, CA 92064

Omni Medical Supply Inc. 800-860-6664
4153 Pioneer Dr, Commerce Township, MI 48390

Princeton Biomeditech Corp. 732-274-1000
4242 US Highway 1, Monmouth Junction, NJ 08852
BioSign HCG, one-step pregnancy test card; BioStrip P, one-step pregnancy test strip; LifeSign 1, one-step home pregnancy test stick.

R Medical Supply 800-882-7578
620 Valley Forge Rd Ste F, Hillsborough, NC 27278
One-step and slide tests.

Sa Scientific, Inc. 800-272-2710
4919 Golden Quail, San Antonio, TX 78240
One-step, dip stick, lateral and midstream formate for serum and urine. Also, PREGNANCY CHECK pregnancy kit for OTC.

Stanbio Laboratory, Inc. 830-249-0772
1261 N Main St, Boerne, TX 78006
$109.00 for 100 QUICKTELL test kits with antibody and latex reagents.

Syntron Bioresearch, Inc. 800-854-6226
2774 Loker Ave W, Carlsbad, CA 92010

KIT, PREGNANCY TEST *(cont'd)*

Wampole Laboratories 800-257-9525
2 Research Way, Princeton, NJ 08540
CLEARVIEW HCG II chromatographic immunoassay, serum/urine, 25mIV hcG/ml.

Xenotec Ltd. 949-640-4053
511 Hazel Dr, Corona Del Mar, CA 92625
Three types of pregnancy tests - strip, pack, and midstream.

KIT, PREGNANCY TEST, OVER THE COUNTER, HCG
(Chemistry) 75LCX

Ac Healthcare Supply, Inc. 905-448-4706
11651 230th St, Cambria Heights, NY 11411
Pregnancy test kit.

Access Bio Incorporate 732-297-2222
2033 Rt. 130 Unit H, Monmouth Junction, NJ 08852
Pregnancy test kit.

Acon Laboratories, Inc. 858-535-2030
10125 Mesa Rim Rd, San Diego, CA 92121

Advanced Diagnostics, Inc. (Adi) 800-724-4003
801 Montrose Ave, South Plainfield, NJ 07080

Ameritek Usa, Inc. 425-379-2580
125 130th St SE Ste 200, Everett, WA 98208
Pregnancy test.

Arlington Scientific, Inc. Asi 800-654-0146
1840 N Technology Dr, Springville, UT 84663
PROPHASE PLUS one step which requires only 4 drops of urine. Results in 5 minutes.

Azog, Inc. 908-213-2900
1011 US Highway 22, Alpha, NJ 08865
Test for pregnancy (hcg) (urine).

Bio-Med U.S.A. Inc. 973-278-5222
111 Ellison St, Paterson, NJ 07505
BIO ACCU HCG serum/urine one-step pregnancy test kit, $1.20 - $1.60 per kit.

Bioscreen Medical Inc. 570-928-7636
Rr I Box 1045a, Mildred, PA 18632
One step serum/urine pregnancy test.

Biotech Atlantic, Inc. 732-389-4789
Industrial Way W Bay F6, Eatontown, NJ 07724
Pregnancy test kit.

Bremancos Diagnostics Inc. 800-830-2593
6800 Kitimat Rd., Unit 2, Mississauga, ONT L5N-5M1 Canada

Elabsupply 714-446-8740
1001 Starbuck St Apt C306, Fullerton, CA 92833
hCG one-step visual pregnancy tests available in Urine or Urine/Serum Card and Dipstick formats.

Eucardio Laboratory, Inc. 760-632-1824
2216 Silver Peak Pl, Encinitas, CA 92024
Hcg pregnancy test.

Genzyme Diagnostics 617-252-7500
6659 Top Gun St, San Diego, CA 92121
Otc pregnancy test kit.

Germaine Laboratories, Inc. 210-692-4192
4139 Gardendale St Ste 101, San Antonio, TX 78229
Various.

Immunostics, Inc. 800-722-7505
3505 Sunset Ave, Ocean, NJ 07712

Innovacon, Inc. 858-535-2030
4106 Sorrento Valley Blvd, San Diego, CA 92121
One step home pregnancy test strip.

Inverness Medical Professional Diagnostics-San Die 858-535-2030
4106 Sorrento Valley Blvd, San Diego, CA 92121
One step home pregnancy test strip.

Jant Pharmacal Corp. 800-676-5565
16255 Ventura Blvd Ste 505, Encino, CA 91436
Solid phase immunochromatographic assay/detection of hcg in urine.

Mizuho Usa, Inc. 858-679-0555
12131 Community Rd, Poway, CA 92064
Both visual and electronic result readout versions.

Myers-Stevens Group, Inc. 903-566-6696
2931 Vail Ave, Commerce, CA 90040
Over the counter pregnancy test.

KIT, PREGNANCY TEST, OVER THE COUNTER, HCG *(cont'd)*

Neo Pharm Inc. 714-226-0070
10532 Walker St Ste B, Cypress, CA 90630
Hcg test system.

Pacific Integrated Mfg., Inc. 619-921-3464
4364 Bonita Rd # 454, Bonita, CA 91902
Pregnancy test.

Phamatech Inc. 858-643-5555
10151 Barnes Canyon Rd, San Diego, CA 92121
Pregnancy test.

Pulse Scientific, Inc. 800-363-7907
5100 S. Service Rd., Unit 18, Burlington, ONT L7L-6A5 Canada
Pregnancy Test in Strips or cards style to detect HCG in utine or serum.

Rapid Diagnostics, Div. Of Mp Biomedicals, Llc 800-888-7008
1429 Rollins Rd, Burlingame, CA 94010
HCG test.

Sa Scientific, Inc. 800-272-2710
4919 Golden Quail, San Antonio, TX 78240

Scantibodies Laboratory, Inc. 619-258-9300
9336 Abraham Way, Santee, CA 92071
Various models of pregnancy test kits.

Sci International Inc. 301-696-8879
5902 Enterprise Ct, Frederick, MD 21703
Invitro pregnancy test.

St. Paul Biotech 714-903-1000
11555 Monarch St, Garden Grove, CA 92841
Pregnancy test.

Sun Biomedical Laboratories, Inc. 888-440-8388
604 Vpr Center, 1001 Lower Landing Road, Blackwood, NJ 08012
Pregnancy test kit.

Teco Diagnostics 714-693-7788
1268 N Lakeview Ave, Anaheim, CA 92807
Direct pregnancy test.

The Reese Pharmaceutical Co. 800-321-7178
10617 Frank Ave, Cleveland, OH 44106
Preferred pregnancy test kit.

Victorch Meditek, Inc. 858-530-9191
7313 Carroll Rd Ste A-B, San Diego, CA 92121
One step hcg urine pregnancy test.

KIT, PREP *(General) 80RLP*

Border Opportunity Saver Systems, Inc. 830-775-0992
10 Finegan Rd, Del Rio, TX 78840
Kit, Shave Prep

Global Healthcare 800-601-3880
1495 Hembree Rd Ste 700, Roswell, GA 30076
Shave Prep Trays

Leap Technologies 800-229-8814
PO Box 969, Carrboro, NC 27510
Prep & load systems.

Lsl Industries, Inc. 888-225-5575
5535 N Wolcott Ave, Chicago, IL 60640
$21.75 per 100 fixed head, disposable razors; $27.50 per case containing, castile soap sponge, waterproof drape, absorbent towel, 2 cotton tip applicators, fixed head razor, single compartment tray. $33.50 for same but with 2 additional gauze sponges, 1 additional wash cloth and double compartment tray.

Mckesson General Medical 800-446-3008
8741 Landmark Rd, Richmond, VA 23228
Iodine preps and scrubs.

Medi Inc 800-225-8634
75 York Ave, P.O. Box 302, Randolph, MA 02368

Medical Techniques Usa 801-936-4501
125 N 400 W Ste C, North Salt Lake, UT 84054

Medline Industries, Inc. 800-633-5886
1 Medline Pl, Mundelein, IL 60060

Merit Medical Systems Inc. 804-416-1030
12701 Kingston Ave, Chesterfield, VA 23837

Ross Disposable Products 800-649-6526
401 Traders Blvd E, Unit 10, Mississauga, ON L4Z 2H8 Canada

The Evercare Company 800-435-6223
3440 Preston Ridge Rd Ste 650, Alpharetta, GA 30005
$10.00 for 100 disposable surgical prep mitts. Each with one adhesive layer to pick up hair and dead skin flakes after shaving procedure.

KIT, PRESSURE MONITORING (AIR/GAS) *(General) 80RLY*

Cardiomed Supplies Inc. 800-387-9757
5 Gormley Industrial Ave., P.O. Box 575
Gormley, ONT L0H 1 Canada
Complete range of re-usable and disposable pressure monitoring products.

Hospira, Inc. 877-946-7747
755 Jarvis Dr, Morgan Hill, CA 95037
25 different standard kits (plus customized kits). Six kits available.

Smiths Medical Asd, Inc. 800-848-1757
6250 Shier Rings Rd, Dublin, OH 43016

Spectra Medical Devices, Inc. 866-938-8649
4C Henshaw St, Woburn, MA 01801

KIT, QUALITY CONTROL *(Microbiology) 83JTR*

American Biomedical, Inc. 918-437-3009
11333 E Pine St Ste 60, Tulsa, OK 74116
Microbiology reagents qualitly control kit.

Armstrong Medical Industries, Inc. 800-323-4220
575 Knightsbridge Pkwy, Lincolnshire, IL 60069
Universal precaution compliance kit for OSHA bloodborne pathogens compliance.

Arrow International, Inc. 800-523-8446
2400 Bernville Rd, Reading, PA 19605
Infection control systems.

Bio-Test Medical, Inc. 412-444-0933
1017 Executive Dr, Gibsonia, PA 15044
Gram check-gram stain control,afb check, acid fast stain control.

Biomerieux Inc. 800-682-2666
100 Rodolphe St, Durham, NC 27712

Copan Diagnostics, Inc. 800-216-4016
26055 Jefferson Ave, Murrieta, CA 92562
Microbial preservation system.

Genzyme Diagnostics 617-252-7500
6659 Top Gun St, San Diego, CA 92121
Giadial - cryptospordium control kit.

Gibson Laboratories, Inc. 859-254-9500
1040 Manchester St, Lexington, KY 40508
Lyophilized microorganisms.

Healthlink 904-996-7758
3611 St Johns Bluff Rd S Ste 1, Jacksonville, FL 32224
Qc kit.

Micro-Bio-Logics.Inc 800-599-2847
217 Osseo Ave N, Saint Cloud, MN 56303

Microbiologics, Inc. 800-599-BUGS
217 Osseo Ave N, Saint Cloud, MN 56303
EPOWER™;EZ-CFU™;EZ-CFU™ ONE STEP;EZ-COMP™ SAMPLES;EZ-FPC™;EZ-PEC™;EZ-SPORE™;KWIK-STIK™;KW IK-STIK™ PLUS;LYFO DISK®

Remel-Lake Charles, Division Of Remel Inc. 800-256-4376
3941 Ryan St, Lake Charles, LA 70605
Quality control kit for culture media.

Shared Systems, Inc. 888-474-2733
PO Box 211587, 3961 Columbia Rd, Augusta, GA 30917
In vitro diagnostic kits including microbiology, serology, HDL cholesterol and infectious disease.

KIT, QUALITY CONTROL, BLOOD BANKING *(Hematology) 81KSF*

Bbi Diagnostics, A Division Of Seracare Life Scien 508-244-6428
375 West St, West Bridgewater, MA 02379
Accurun1 multi-marker negative control.

Ortho-Clinical Diagnostics, Inc. 800-828-6316
513 Technology Blvd, Rochester, NY 14626
Qc system for blood banking reagent.

KIT, REPAIR, PACEMAKER *(Cardiovascular) 74KFJ*

Maquet Puerto Rico Inc. 408-635-3900
No. 12, Rd. #698, Dorado, PR 00646
Various pacemaker accessories.

St. Jude Medical Cardiac Rhythm Management Div. 800-777-2237
15900 Valley View Ct, Sylmar, CA 91342

KIT, RIA, BASIC PROTEIN, MYELIN *(Immunology) 82MEL*

Dako North America, Inc 805-566-6655
6392 Via Real, Carpinteria, CA 93013
Kit to detect HER2 protein onerexpression in breast carcinoma. Kit to detect EGFR protein.

KIT, SAMPLING, ARTERIAL BLOOD *(Anesthesiology) 73CBT*

Argon Medical Devices Inc. 903-675-9321
1445 Flat Creek Rd, Athens, TX 75751
Various.

Covidien Lp 508-261-8000
15 Hampshire St, Mansfield, MA 02048

Customed, Inc. 787-801-0101
Calle Igualdad #7, Fajardo, PR 00738
Blood gas kit with protector.

Edwards Lifesciences Technology Sarl 949-250-2500
State Rd. 402 N.km 1.4, Anasco, PR 00610-1577
Arterial blood sampling kit.

Icu Medical (Ut), Inc 949-366-2183
4455 Atherton Dr, Salt Lake City, UT 84123
Shielded blunt cannula.

International Medication Systems, Ltd. 800-423-4136
1886 Santa Anita Ave, South El Monte, CA 91733
Arterial blood sampler.

Jostra Bentley, Inc. 302-454-9959
Rd. 402 N. Km 1.4, Industrial Park, Anasco, PR 00610-1577
Custom cardiovascular perfusion kits.

Kramer Scientific Laboratory Products Corp. 201-767-8505
50 Maple St, Norwood, NJ 07648
Arterial blood sampling kit.

Opti Medical Systems Inc. 770-510-4444
235 Hembree Park Dr, Roswell, GA 30076
Arterial blood sampling kit.

Radiometer America, Inc. 800-736-0600
810 Sharon Dr, Westlake, OH 44145
PICO arterial-blood samplers.

Rd Medical Mfg. Inc. 787-716-6363
Road 183, Km 21.6, Las Piedras Industrial Park, Las Piedras, PR 00771
Various types of arterial blood gas kits.

KIT, SAMPLING, BLOOD *(General) 80RQG*

Basi (Bioanalytical Systems, Inc.) 800-845-4246
2701 Kent Ave, West Lafayette, IN 47906
CULEX Automated Blood Sampler system for robotic sampling of blood from freely moving animals (most often rats) for research in pharmacokinetics, drug metabolism, and drug safety assessment.

Biosensors International - Usa 949-553-8300
20280 SW Acacia St Ste 300, Newport Beach, CA 92660
BIOPORT 2, closed blood-sampling system, reduces risk of infections and conserves blood loss.

Covidien Lp 508-261-8000
15 Hampshire St, Mansfield, MA 02048

Dade Behring, Inc. 800-948-3233
1717 Deerfield Rd, Deerfield, IL 60015

Esa, Inc. 800-959-5095
22 Alpha Rd, Chelmsford, MA 01824

Fenwal Inc. 800-766-1077
3 Corporate Dr, Lake Zurich, IL 60047
Site couplers.

International Technidyne Corp. 800-631-5945
23 Nevsky St, Edison, NJ 08820
Fingerstick device. Disposable incision making device in three sizes for safe & painless blood sampling from the finger.

Owen Mumford Usa, Inc. 800-421-6936
1755 W Oak Commons Ct Ste A, Marietta, GA 30062

Porex Corporation 800-241-0195
500 Bohannon Rd, Fairburn, GA 30213
FILTER SAMPLER blood serum filters.

Science Products 800-888-7400
1043 Lancaster Ave, Berwyn, PA 19312
SURE DROP is a small, specially coated fixture that fits over the PROFILE & BASIC to direct the blood drop onto the test strip. Use of the device assists in the placement of the blood drop and also helps to control the size of the sample (sufficient but not excessive), reducing the number of failed tests and the amount of blood required for eact test. SURE GUIDE holds SURE STEP strip to guide blood to the center of the strip.

KIT, SAMPLING, BLOOD *(cont'd)*

Terumo Medical Corp. 800-283-7866
2101 Cottontail Ln, Somerset, NJ 08873

KIT, SAMPLING, BLOOD GAS *(General) 80RQH*

Covidien Lp 508-261-8000
15 Hampshire St, Mansfield, MA 02048

Dade Behring, Inc. 800-948-3233
1717 Deerfield Rd, Deerfield, IL 60015

Radiometer America, Inc. 800-736-0600
810 Sharon Dr, Westlake, OH 44145
PICO arterial-blood samplers.

Terumo Medical Corp. 800-283-7866
2101 Cottontail Ln, Somerset, NJ 08873

KIT, SAMPLING, ENDOMETRIAL *(Obstetrics/Gyn) 85RQI*

Berkeley Medevices, Inc. 800-227-2388
1330 S 51st St, Richmond, CA 94804
Endometrial/endocervical tissue sampling kits (VABRA).

Rocket Medical Plc. 800-707-7625
150 Recreation Park Dr Ste 3, Hingham, MA 02043

KIT, SCREENING, STAPHYLOCOCCUS AUREUS *(Microbiology) 83JWX*

Arlington Scientific, Inc. Asi 800-654-0146
1840 N Technology Dr, Springville, UT 84663
The ASI Staphslide Latex Test is a slide agglutination assay for the qualitative detection of coagulase (both clumping factor and protein A) to identify Staphylococcus aureus to the exclusion of other species of staphylococci. This test is for use on pure culture samples suspected of being S. aureus.

Bd Diagnostic Systems 800-675-0908
7 Loveton Cir, Sparks, MD 21152

J&S Medical Associates 800-229-6000
35 Tripp St Ste 1, Framingham, MA 01702
ACCUTEX qualitative and quantitative latex agglutination kits for RF, ASO, SLE, CRP, Mono and Staph.

Nerl Diagnostics Llc. 401-824-2046
14 Almeida Ave, East Providence, RI 02914
Staph latex kits.

Remel 800-255-6730
12076 Santa Fe Dr, Lenexa, KS 66215

Remel Atlanta, Div. Of Remel, Inc. 800-255-6730
2797 Peterson Pl, Norcross, GA 30071
RAPID STR has four hour identification of medically important streptococci, pediococci, and leucocnostoc.

Wescor, Inc. 800-453-2725
459 S Main St, Logan, UT 84321
Identification of Staphylococcus aureus from isolated colonies

KIT, SCREENING, URINE *(Microbiology) 83JXA*

Abbott Molecular, Inc. 847-937-6100
1300 E Touhy Ave, Des Plaines, IL 60018
Sampling, transport and storage device.

Coral Biotechnology 760-727-8224
110 Bosstick Blvd, San Marcos, CA 92069
Utiscreen.

Culture Kits, Inc. 888-680-6853
14 Prentice St, PO Box 748, Norwich, NY 13815
Uri-Kit single media for urine culture and colony count. Plate contains CLED media.Also available are Dip Paddles for urine culture in 2 combinations, EMB/CLED and MacConkey/CLED.

Escreen, Inc. 800-881-0722
2205 W Parkside Ln, Phoenix, AZ 85027
Escreen drugs of abuse screening system.

Gen-Probe, Inc. 800-523-5001
10210 Genetic Center Dr, San Diego, CA 92121
Urine Specimens Preparation Kit - Processing kit used to prepare female and male urine specimens for testing in the GEN-PROBE® AMPLIFIED CHLAMYDIA TRACHOMATIS Assay.

Hycor Biomedical, Inc. 800-382-2527
7272 Chapman Ave, Garden Grove, CA 92841
Urine screening kit.

Izon Business Products, Inc. 800-447-9989
520 W Nyack Rd, West Nyack, NY 10994
Kits manufacturer, urine, blood, etc.

J&S Medical Associates 800-229-6000
35 Tripp St Ste 1, Framingham, MA 01702
SENTRY urine control for all SAMSHA recommended analytes.

KIT, SCREENING, URINE *(cont'd)*

Lifesign 800-526-2125
71 Veronica Ave, Somerset, NJ 08873
URICULT screening kit CLED/EMB (10 tests) $25.00/bx. CLED/MAC (10 tests) $25.00/bx. CLED/Polymyxin/MAC (10 tests) $25.00/bx. CLED/Polymyxin/EMB (10 tests) $25.00/bx.

Lynn Peavey Co. 913-888-0600
14865 W 105th St, Lenexa, KS 66215
Peavey urine testing kit.

Medical & Clinical Consortium (Mcc) 877-622-8378
13740 Nelson Ave, City Of Industry, CA 91746
Instant Urine Adulteration Test, when testing for drugs of abuse.

Medical Chemical Corp. 800-424-9394
19430 Van Ness Ave, Torrance, CA 90501
$11.00 per 100-test kit.

Meridian Bioscience, Inc. 800-696-0739
3471 River Hills Dr, Cincinnati, OH 45244
FILTRACHECK-UTI Screening kit for urinary tract infections.

Oral Biotech 541-928-4445
812 Water Ave NE, Albany, OR 97321

Oxoid, Inc. 800-567-8378
800 Proctor Ave, Ogdensburg, NY 13669

Qualicum Scientific Ltd. 800-344-4652
35 Antares Dr. #2, Nepean, ONT K2E 8B1 Canada
Various types of dipchex

Sirchie Finger Print Laboratories 800-356-7311
100 Hunter Pl, Youngsville, NC 27596

Starplex Scientific Inc. 800-665-0954
50A Steinway Blvd., Etobicoke, ONT M9W 6Y3 Canada
DIP 'N COUNT Dipslide culture media. A variety of media dip paddles for microbiological screening tests.

Teco Diagnostics 714-693-7788
1268 N Lakeview Ave, Anaheim, CA 92807
Urine reagent strip-specific gravity.

Wampole Laboratories 800-257-9525
2 Research Way, Princeton, NJ 08540
UCG Slide.

KIT, SEROLOGICAL, NEGATIVE CONTROL *(Microbiology) 83MJY*

Shared Systems, Inc. 888-474-2733
PO Box 211587, 3961 Columbia Rd, Augusta, GA 30917

KIT, SEROLOGICAL, POSITIVE CONTROL *(Microbiology) 83MJX*

Bbi Diagnostics, A Division Of Seracare Life Scien 508-244-6428
375 West St, West Bridgewater, MA 02379
Accurn 113 hbc igm positive control.

Qed Bioscience, Inc. 800-929-2114
10919 Technology Pl Ste C, San Diego, CA 92127
Serological infectious disease test kits for sale in North America only.

Shared Systems, Inc. 888-474-2733
PO Box 211587, 3961 Columbia Rd, Augusta, GA 30917

KIT, SEX SELECTION *(Obstetrics/Gyn) 85ULY*

Gametrics Ltd. 307-878-4494
426 Lonesome Country Rd, Alzada, MT 59311
$110.00 for one 22 + X/Y procedure (international sales only).

KIT, SHROUD *(Pathology) 88RSZ*

General Econopak, Inc. 888-871-8568
1725 N 6th St, Philadelphia, PA 19122
Mortuary packs, complete with shroud sheet, chinstrap, ties, and inner and outer ID tags.

Ross Disposable Products 800-649-6526
401 Traders Blvd E, Unit 10, Mississauga, ON L4Z 2H8 Canada

Tri-State Hospital Supply Corp. 800-248-4058
301 Catrell Dr, PO Box 170, Howell, MI 48843

KIT, SITZ BATH *(Physical Med) 89HHC*

Lsl Industries, Inc. 888-225-5575
5535 N Wolcott Ave, Chicago, IL 60640
$19.95 for 10 kits.

Medegen Medical Products, Llc 800-233-1987
209 Medegen Drive, Gallaway, TN 38036-0228
ROOM-MATES.

Medline Industries, Inc. 800-633-5886
1 Medline Pl, Mundelein, IL 60060

KIT, SKIN SCRUB *(General) 80TFI*

Custom Healthcare Systems, Inc. 804-421-5959
4205 Eubank Rd, Richmond, VA 23231

Kck Industries 888-800-1967
14941 Calvert St, Van Nuys, CA 91411

KIT, SMEAR, CERVICAL *(Obstetrics/Gyn) 85MCO*

Canadian Medical Brush, Inc. 905-405-1075
11-7686 Kimbel St, Mississauga L5S 1E9 Canada
Pap smear kit cmb-2020

Cytyc Corporation 800-442-9892
445 Simarano Dr, Marlborough, MA 01752
Fluid-based system for preparing cervical cell samples for cancer screening.

Cytyc Surgical Products 800-442-9892
250 Campus Dr, Marlborough, MA 01752
Fluid-based system for preparing cervical cell samples for cancer screening.

Monogen, Inc. 847-573-6700
3630 Burwood Dr, Waukegan, IL 60085
Cervical cytology slide preparation for use on automated processor.

KIT, SNAKE BITE *(General) 80RTX*

Dixie Ems Supply 800-347-3494
385 Union Ave, Brooklyn, NY 11211
$5.20 per unit (standard).

KIT, SNAKE BITE, SUCTION *(General) 80KYP*

Healer Products, Llc 914-663-6300
427 Commerce Ln Ste 1, West Berlin, NJ 08091
Snake-bite kit.

North Safety Products 401-943-4400
1101 B Calle Neutron, Parque Industrial Maran, Mexicali, B.c. Mexico
Snake bite kit

KIT, SUCTION, AIRWAY (TRACHEAL) *(Anesthesiology) 73CBE*

Allied Healthcare Products, Inc. 800-444-3954
1720 Sublette Ave, Saint Louis, MO 63110

Armstrong Medical Industries, Inc. 800-323-4220
575 Knightsbridge Pkwy, Lincolnshire, IL 60069

Covidien Lp 508-261-8000
15 Hampshire St, Mansfield, MA 02048

Neotech Products, Inc. 800-966-0500
27822 Fremont Ct, Valencia, CA 91355
NEOTECH LITTLE SUCKER: Oral-Nasal Suction Device for pediatric and neonatal patients. Soft tip like bulb syringe with finger control. Gentle on nose and mouth of tiny patients. Replace up to three products with one Little Sucker.

Zimmer Holdings, Inc. 800-613-6131
1800 W Center St, PO Box 708, Warsaw, IN 46580

KIT, SUCTIONING, TRACHEOSTOMY AND NASAL *(Surgery) 79LRQ*

Continental Medical Laboratories, Inc. 262-534-2787
813 Ela Ave, Waterford, WI 53185
Tracheostomy cleaning kit/ tracheostomy care kit.

Customed, Inc. 787-801-0101
Calle Igualdad #7, Fajardo, PR 00738
Sterile tracheostomy care kit.

Engineered Medical Systems 317-246-5500
2055 Executive Dr, Indianapolis, IN 46241
Cricothyroidoyomy/tracheostomy kit.

Kentron Health Care, Inc. 615-384-0573
3604 Kelton Jackson Rd, P.o. Box 120, Springfield, TN 37172
Tracheostomy mask.

KIT, SURGICAL (GENERAL) *(Surgery) 79LRO*

Acuderm Inc. 800-327-0015
5370 NW 35th Ter Ste 106, Fort Lauderdale, FL 33309
Suture kit.

Atrion Medical Products, Inc. 800-343-9334
1426 Curt Francis Rd NW, Arab, AL 35016
Pre- and post-op surgical kits and kit boxes/trays. Distribution of surgical kits and drugs.

Ballard Medical Products 770-587-7835
12050 Lone Peak Pkwy, Draper, UT 84020
Paracentesis devices.

Biomet 3i 800-342-5454
4555 Riverside Dr, Palm Beach Gardens, FL 33410

KIT, SURGICAL (GENERAL) *(cont'd)*

Centurion Medical Products Corp. 517-545-1135
3310 S Main St, Salisbury, NC 28147

Custom Medical Products 407-865-7211
3909 E Semoran Blvd Bldg 599, Apopka, FL 32703
Kit, surgical - general.

Customed, Inc. 787-801-0101
Calle Igualdad #7, Fajardo, PR 00738
Various.

Depuy Orthopaedics, Inc. 800-473-3789
700 Orthopaedic Dr, P.O. Box 988, Warsaw, IN 46582
Various types of accessory kits.

Elamex S.A. De C.V. 52-16-164333
Av. Insurgentes 4145 Iote., Cd. Jiarex, Chih Mexico
Various

Hospital Laundry Services - Sterile Recovery Division 847-229-0900
45 W Hintz Rd, Wheeling, IL 60090
Surgical packs - various types of kits.

In-Sight 401-434-1211
750 Narragansett Park Dr, Rumford, RI 02916
No common name listed.

Kentron Health Care, Inc. 615-384-0573
3604 Kelton Jackson Rd, P.o. Box 120, Springfield, TN 37172
Procedure kits and trays.

Lexamed 419-693-5307
705 Front St, Northwood, OH 43605
Sterile eye surgery kit various components per customer specifications.

Mckesson General Medical 800-446-3008
8741 Landmark Rd, Richmond, VA 23228

Mclean Medical And Scientific, Inc. 800-777-9987
292 E Lafayette Frontage Rd, Saint Paul, MN 55107
Surgical instruments, stainless/titanium.

Medical Techniques Usa 801-936-4501
125 N 400 W Ste C, North Salt Lake, UT 84054

Medicorp, Inc. 514-733-1900
5800 Royalmount, Montreal, QUE H4P 1K5 Canada
T3 RIA or EIA kits to measure T#. T4 RIA or EIA kits to measure T4.

Medline Manufacturing And Services Llc 847-837-2759
1 Medline Pl, Mundelein, IL 60060
Convenience kit.

Porex Surgical, Inc. 800-521-7321
15 Dart Rd, Newnan, GA 30265
TLS and SPG Surgical Drainage systems for post operative small wound draining.

Professional Disposables International, Inc. 800-999-6423
2 Nice Pak Park, Orangeburg, NY 10962
Chlorascrub Swab, Swabstick and Maxi-Swabstick

Savoy Medical Supply 631-234-7003
745 Calebs Path, Hauppauge, NY 11788

Sri Surgical 813-891-9550
6801 Longe St, Stockton, CA 95206
Surgical procedure trays various.

Tri-State Hospital Supply Corp. 517-545-1135
3173 E 43rd St, Yuma, AZ 85365

Ussc Puerto Rico, Inc. 203-845-1000
Building 911-67, Sabanetas Industrial Park, Ponce, PR 00731
Laparoscopic kit.

Vnus Medical Technologies, Inc. 888-797-8346
5799 Fontanoso Way, San Jose, CA 95138
Convenience kit.

Washington-Greene County Branch Pennsylvania Assoc 724-228-0770
566 E Maiden St, Washington, PA 15301
Tracheotomy care kit.

White Knight Healthcare 800-851-4431
Calle 16, Number 780, Agua Prieta, Sonora Mexico
Various types of sterile and non sterile packs

Windstone Medical Packaging, Inc. 800-637-7056
1602 4th Ave N, Billings, MT 59101

Xodus Medical, Inc. 800-963-8776
702 Prominence Dr, Westmoreland Business & Research Park
New Kensington, PA 15068
EZ Kits

KIT, SURGICAL INSTRUMENT, DISPOSABLE *(Surgery) 79KDD*

Acuderm Inc. 800-327-0015
5370 NW 35th Ter Ste 106, Fort Lauderdale, FL 33309
Skin biopsy punch kit.

Bioseal 800-441-7325
167 W Orangethorpe Ave, Placentia, CA 92870
Sterile and ready to use.

Centurion Medical Products Corp. 517-545-1135
3310 S Main St, Salisbury, NC 28147

Clinical Pharmacies, Inc. 800-669-6973
21622 Surveyor Cir # 8-C, Huntington Beach, CA 92646
Dialysis on/off kit, shunt declotting tray.

Custom Healthcare Systems, Inc. 804-421-5959
4205 Eubank Rd, Richmond, VA 23231

Cytyc Surgical Products 800-442-9892
250 Campus Dr, Marlborough, MA 01752
Accessory kit.

Dumex Medical Surgical Products Ltd. 800-463-9613
104 Shorting Rd., Scarborough, ONT M1S 3S4 Canada
Surture removal kit; manual surgical instrument

Ethox International 800-521-1022
251 Seneca St, Buffalo, NY 14204
Surgical instrument kit,disposable.

Gi Supply 800-451-5797
200 Grandview Ave, Camp Hill, PA 17011
Surgical instrument kit (with drugs). Large volume paracentesis kit.

Innovasive Devices, Inc. 800-435-600[illegible]
734 Forest St, Marlborough, MA 01752
Suture fastener and grasper.

Inrad 800-558-4647
4375 Donkers Ct SE, Kentwood, MI 49512
Various models.

Lexamed 419-693-5307
705 Front St, Northwood, OH 43605
Instruments, surgical disposible, sterile.

Magnum Medical 800-336-9710
3265 N Nevada St, Chandler, AZ 85225

Medical Action Industries, Inc. 800-645-7042
25 Heywood Rd, Arden, NC 28704
Basin kit.

Medical Techniques Usa 801-936-4501
125 N 400 W Ste C, North Salt Lake, UT 84054

Medistat Medical - Hallmark Sales Corporation 888-MED-ISTA
1601 Peach Leaf St, Houston, TX 77039
Manufacturer of kits including first aid, body fluid spills, burns, emergency, medical, surgical, obstetrical, exams, minor surgery, biopsy, convenience, procedure trays, disposable instruments, sterile kits. Owns manufacturing and validated sterilization facilities. Can make custom or special order kits. Refills, supplies.

Medline Industries, Inc. 800-633-5886
1 Medline Pl, Mundelein, IL 60060

Merit Medical Systems Inc. 804-416-1030
12701 Kingston Ave, Chesterfield, VA 23837

Millstone Medical Outsourcing 508-679-8384
1565 N Main St Ste 408, Fall River, MA 02720
Multiple and various.

Olsen Medical 800-297-6344
3001 W Kentucky St, Louisville, KY 40211
Complete line of bipolar and monopolar forceps packaged in a kit with cord, tip cleaner, and surgi-wipe.

Qsum Biopsy Disposables Llc 720-304-2135
6539 Stearns Ave, Boulder, CO 80303
Sterile breast biopsy-localization tray.

Rd Medical Mfg. Inc. 787-716-6363
Road 183, Km 21.6, Las Piedras Industrial Park, Las Piedras, PR 00771
Various types of sterile trays and kits.

Scanlan International, Inc. 800-328-9458
1 Scanlan Plz, Saint Paul, MN 55107

Staar Surgical Co. 800-292-7902
1911 Walker Ave, Monrovia, CA 91016

Sterling Medical-Products Intl., Inc. 815-537-5303
401 Market St, Prophetstown, IL 61277
Instrument tray.

Sterling Multi-Products, Inc. 815-537-2381
326 W 5th St, Prophetstown, IL 61277
Instrument tray.

KIT, SURGICAL INSTRUMENT, DISPOSABLE *(cont'd)*

Surgical Instrument Manufacturers, Inc. 800-521-2985
1650 Headland Dr, Fenton, MO 63026

Tri-State Hospital Supply Corp. 517-545-1135
3173 E 43rd St, Yuma, AZ 85365

Tri-State Hospital Supply Corp. 800-248-4058
301 Catrell Dr, PO Box 170, Howell, MI 48843

Windstone Medical Packaging, Inc. 800-637-7056
1602 4th Ave N, Billings, MT 59101

KIT, SUTURE REMOVAL *(Surgery) 79MCZ*

Border Opportunity Saver Systems, Inc. 830-775-0992
10 Finegan Rd, Del Rio, TX 78840

Busse Hospital Disposables, Inc. 631-435-4711
75 Arkay Dr, Hauppauge, NY 11788
Suture removal kits,sterile.

Centurion Medical Products Corp. 517-545-1135
3310 S Main St, Salisbury, NC 28147

Customed, Inc. 787-801-0101
Calle Igualdad #7, Fajardo, PR 00738
Sterile suture removal kit.

Cypress Medical Products 800-334-3646
1202 S. Rte. 31, McHenry, IL 60050
Suture removal kits available with metal or plastic Littauer scissors and forceps, and 4x4 gauze sponge.

K. W. Griffen Co. 203-846-1923
100 Pearl St, Norwalk, CT 06850
Staple remover kit.

Kentron Health Care, Inc. 615-384-0573
3604 Kelton Jackson Rd, P.o. Box 120, Springfield, TN 37172
Suture removal kit, sterile.

Lsl Industries, Inc. 888-225-5575
5535 N Wolcott Ave, Chicago, IL 60640
$26.00 for 50 kits.

Medical Action Industries, Inc. 800-645-7042
25 Heywood Rd, Arden, NC 28704
Suture removal kit.

Medistat Medical - Hallmark Sales Corporation 888-MED-ISTA
1601 Peach Leaf St, Houston, TX 77039
Manufacturer of kits including first aid, body fluid spills, burns, emergency, medical, surgical, obstetrical, exams, minor surgery, biopsy, convenience, procedure trays, disposable instruments, sterile kits. Owns manufacturing and validated sterilization facilities. Can make custom or special order kits. Refills, supplies.

Rd Medical Mfg. Inc. 787-716-6363
Road 183, Km 21.6, Las Piedras Industrial Park, Las Piedras, PR 00771
Various types of sterile suture removal kits.

Tri-State Hospital Supply Corp. 517-545-1135
3173 E 43rd St, Yuma, AZ 85365

Washington-Greene County Branch Pennsylvania Assoc 724-228-0770
566 E Maiden St, Washington, PA 15301
Tracheotomy care kit.

KIT, TEST(DONORS), FOR BLOODBORNE PATHOGEN *(Immunology) 82MYZ*

Bbi Diagnostics, A Division Of Seracare Life Scien 508-244-6428
375 West St, West Bridgewater, MA 02379
Accurun 365 west nile virus rna positive quality control.

KIT, TEST, ALPHA-FETOPROTEIN FOR TESTICULAR CANCER *(Immunology) 82LOJ*

Beckman Coulter Inc. 800-231-7970
445 Medical Center Blvd, Webster, TX 77598
AFP ELISA

Biocheck, Inc. 650-573-1968
323 Vintage Park Dr, Foster City, CA 94404
Alpha-fetoprotein eia test kit.

United Biotech, Inc. 650-961-2910
211 S Whisman Rd Ste E, Mountain View, CA 94041
ELISA quantitative detecting Alpha Fetoprotein (alpha FP)

KIT, TEST, COAGGLUTININ *(Hematology) 81MHS*

Lifesign 800-526-2125
71 Veronica Ave, Somerset, NJ 08873
RUBALEX Latex agglutinate test for Rubella antibodies. 10 IU sensitivity. $245/100 tests, $1100/500 tests. Also available for heteropithis antibody associated with infectious mono at $100/50 test kit and H. pylori antibody in serum at $200/24 test kit.

KIT, TEST, MALARIA *(Toxicology) 91NED*

Access Bio Incorporate 732-297-2222
2033 Rt. 130 Unit H, Monmouth Junction, NJ 08852
Malaria test.

Ameritek Usa, Inc. 425-379-2580
125 130th St SE Ste 200, Everett, WA 98208
Malaria test kit.

Merlin Labs, Inc. 760-804-1782
6082 Corte Del Cedro, Carlsbad, CA 92011
Malaria combo test.

St. Paul Biotech 714-903-1000
11555 Monarch St, Garden Grove, CA 92841
Malaria test.

KIT, TEST, MULTIPLE, DRUGS OF ABUSE, OVER THE COUNTER *(Toxicology) 91MVO*

Ameritek Usa, Inc. 425-379-2580
125 130th St SE Ste 200, Everett, WA 98208
Multi-drug of abuse test.

Immunoscience, Inc. 925-460-8111
7066 Commerce Cir Ste D, Pleasanton, CA 94588
Various.

Medical & Clinical Consortium (Mcc) 877-622-8378
13740 Nelson Ave, City Of Industry, CA 91746
**Instant Drugs of Abuse (AMP, BAR, BZO, COC, THC, M-AMP, OPI, PCP, MOR, MTD, MDMA, TCA)Available as singles and combinations from 2--10 drugs of abuse tests. *Instant Swipe Test for Drugs of Abuse (detects residue, on cars, clothing, lockers, etc.)*

Phamatech Inc. 858-643-5555
10151 Barnes Canyon Rd, San Diego, CA 92121
Home drug test, lateral flow immunoassay.

Sun Biomedical Laboratories, Inc. 888-440-8388
604 Vpr Center, 1001 Lower Landing Road, Blackwood, NJ 08012
Multiple drugs-of-abuse rapid test panel for cocaine, opiates, methamphetamine, THC, and PCP.

KIT, TEST, PERIODONTAL, IN VITRO *(Dental And Oral) 76MCL*

Micronics, Inc. 425-895-9197
8463 154th Ave NE Bldg G, Redmond, WA 98052
ABORhCard

KIT, TEST, SALIVA, HIV-1&2 *(Hematology) 81MWB*

Bremancos Diagnostics Inc. 800-830-2593
6800 Kitimat Rd., Unit 2, Mississauga, ONT L5N-5M1 Canada

Chembio Diagnostic Systems, Inc. 631-924-1135
3661 Horseblock Rd, Medford, NY 11763
Immunochromatogrphic assay for detection of antibodies.

Orasure Technologies, Inc. 800-869-3538
220 E 1st St, Bethlehem, PA 18015
OraSure HIV-1 Oral Fluid Collection device.

KIT, TRACHEOSTOMY CARE *(Anesthesiology) 73SBG*

Covidien Lp 508-261-8000
15 Hampshire St, Mansfield, MA 02048

Custom Healthcare Systems, Inc. 804-421-5959
4205 Eubank Rd, Richmond, VA 23231

Lsl Industries, Inc. 888-225-5575
5535 N Wolcott Ave, Chicago, IL 60640
$22.90 per 20 sterile sets containing waterproof drape, absorbent towel, 2 gloves, trach dressing, 2 pipe cleaners, 2 cotton tip applicators, 2 gauze sponges, 1 cleaning brush, 2 twill tapes.

Medikmark Inc. 800-424-8520
3600 Burwood Dr, Waukegan, IL 60085

Welcon, Inc. 800-877-0923
7409 Pebble Dr, Fort Worth, TX 76118

KIT, TRACHEOTOMY *(Anesthesiology) 73SBJ*

Armstrong Medical Industries, Inc. 800-323-4220
575 Knightsbridge Pkwy, Lincolnshire, IL 60069

Bausch & Lomb Surgical 636-255-5051
3365 Tree Court Ind Blvd, Saint Louis, MO 63122

KIT, TRACHEOTOMY *(cont'd)*

Dixie Ems Supply 800-347-3494
385 Union Ave, Brooklyn, NY 11211
$16.95 per unit (standard).

Mahe International Inc. 800-294-7946
468 Craighead St, Nashville, TN 37204

Smiths Medical Asd 800-424-8662
5700 W 23rd Ave, Gary, IN 46406
PEDIA-TRAKE pediatric emergency cricothyrotomy/tracheotomy device.

KIT, TRICHOMONAS SCREENING *(Microbiology) 83JWZ*

Genzyme Diagnostics 617-252-7500
6659 Top Gun St, San Diego, CA 92121
Test system for trichomonas vaginalis.

KIT, TROCAR *(Surgery) 79SIA*

Mectra Labs, Inc. 800-323-3968
PO Box 350, Two Quality Way, Bloomfield, IN 47424
5mm and 10mm single use trocars

KIT, TUBING, BLOOD, ANTI-REGURGITATION *(Gastro/Urology) 78FJK*

Apheresis Technologies, Inc. 800-749-9284
PO Box 2081, Palm Harbor, FL 34682
Tubeset for plasmapheresis.

B. Braun Medical Inc., Renal Therapies Div. 800-854-6851
824 12th Ave, Bethlehem, PA 18018

Sorin Group Usa 800-289-5759
14401 W 65th Way, Arvada, CO 80004

KIT, TUBING, DIALYSIS, PERITONEAL *(Gastro/Urology) 78RKM*

Medisystems Corporation 800-369-6334
439 S Union St Fl 5, Lawrence, MA 01843

Redi-Tech Medical Products,Llc 800-824-1793
529 Front St Ste 125, Berea, OH 44017

Spectrum Laboratories, Inc. 800-634-3300
18617 S Broadwick St, Rancho Dominguez, CA 90220
Cellulose ester dialysis tubing with a wide range of available retention ratings, from 100 Daltons to 100,000 Daltons. Regenerated cellulose dialysis tubing available for organic solvents. Also available, membranes: cellulose (CE), regenerated cellulose (RC) and poly vimclidene (PVD).

KIT, URINARY DRAINAGE COLLECTION *(Gastro/Urology) 78FCN*

Amsino International, Inc. 800-MD-AMSINO
855 Towne Center Dr, Pomona, CA 91767
AMSINO urinary drainage bag available in diamond shape (A5312), pearl shape (A5302), rectangular shape (A5300); all feature an anti-reflux chamber or valve, sterile fluid pathway. Also available, urinary leg bag, available in both a twist-open valve (A5308, A5309) and a push-pull valve (A5306, A5307).

Centurion Medical Products Corp. 517-545-1135
3310 S Main St, Salisbury, NC 28147

Covidien Lp 508-261-8000
15 Hampshire St, Mansfield, MA 02048

Exelint International Co. 800-940-3935
5840 W Centinela Ave, Los Angeles, CA 90045
EXEL Urine Collection Kit/Tube.

Hospira, Inc. 877-946-7747
Hwy. 301 North, Rocky Mount, NC 27801
Foley catheter kit.

Hycor Biomedical, Inc. 800-382-2527
7272 Chapman Ave, Garden Grove, CA 92841
Urine collection kit.

Kelsar, S.A. 508-261-8000
Blvd. Insurgentes, Libriamento a La, Tijuana 22450 Mexico
Universal drainage trays, drain bag w/flo check, flo rite

Kentron Health Care, Inc. 615-384-0573
3604 Kelton Jackson Rd, P.o. Box 120, Springfield, TN 37172
Urinary drainage bag.

Ldb Medical, Inc. 800-243-2554
2909 Langford Rd Ste B500, Norcross, GA 30071
LAPIDES.

Lsl Industries, Inc. 888-225-5575
5535 N Wolcott Ave, Chicago, IL 60640

Marlen Manufacturing & Development Co. 216-292-7060
5150 Richmond Rd, Bedford, OH 44146

KIT, URINARY DRAINAGE COLLECTION *(cont'd)*

Tri-State Hospital Supply Corp. 517-545-1135
3173 E 43rd St, Yuma, AZ 85365

Trinity Sterile, Inc. 410-860-5123
201 Kiley Dr, Salisbury, MD 21801

Utah Medical Products, Inc. 800-533-4984
7043 Cottonwood St, Midvale, UT 84047
Uri-Cath silicone urinary drainage catheter for collection of urine and accurate output measurement, available as part of a set or separately.

KIT, WESTERN BLOT, HIV-1 *(Hematology) 81MVW*

Maxim Biomedical Incorporated 301-251-0800
1500 E Gude Dr Ste A, Rockville, MD 20850
Hiv-1 western blot kit.

KIT, WOUND DRAINAGE *(General) 80VFP*

Andersen Products, Inc., 800-523-1276
3202 Caroline Dr, Health Science Park, Haw River, NC 27258
SHIRLEY wound-drainage systems, bi-lumen, radio-opaque, for continuous self-regulated suction.

Aspen Surgical 800-328-7958
6945 Southbelt Dr SE, Caledonia, MI 49316
3C (Cross Contamination Control) Collection System for Saber and Sceptre manual evacuators and for VariDyne battery powered wound drainage/collection.

Atrium Medical Corp. 800-528-7486
5 Wentworth Dr, Hudson, NH 03051

Axiom Medical, Inc. 800-221-8569
19320 Van Ness Ave, Torrance, CA 90501
Flat and round silicone drains and suction set for small procedures. 150cc, 20cc and 10cc reservoirs. Available with exclusive hydrophilic coating.

Gish Biomedical, Inc. 800-938-0531
22942 Arroyo Vis, Rancho Santa Margarita, CA 92688
Orthopedic wound drain.

Johnson & Johnson Medical Division Of Ethicon, Inc. 800-423-4013
2500 E Arbrook Blvd, Arlington, TX 76014

Kck Industries 888-800-1967
14941 Calvert St, Van Nuys, CA 91411

Marlen Manufacturing & Development Co. 216-292-7060
5150 Richmond Rd, Bedford, OH 44146

Medikmark Inc. 800-424-8520
3600 Burwood Dr, Waukegan, IL 60085

Medtronic Perfusion Systems 800-328-3320
7611 Northland Dr N, Brooklyn Park, MN 55428
Wound drainage blood collection systems are designed for post-operative use.

Smith & Nephew, Inc. 800-876-1261
11775 Starkey Rd, Largo, FL 33773
BONGORT wound drainage pouches.

Taut, Inc. 800-231-8288
2571 Kaneville Ct, Geneva, IL 60134

Zimmer Holdings, Inc. 800-613-6131
1800 W Center St, PO Box 708, Warsaw, IN 46580

Zimmer Orthopaedic Surgical Products 800-321-5533
PO Box 10, 200 West Ohio Ave., Dover, OH 44622
HEMOVAC; Infection control wound drainage system, helps prevent healthcare personnel from coming in contact with wound drainage.

KIT, WOUND DRAINAGE, CLOSED *(Cns/Neurology) 84SGF*

Aspen Surgical 800-328-7958
6945 Southbelt Dr SE, Caledonia, MI 49316
SABER bulb evacuation system with 3C bag for closed system emptying and reactivation.

Axiom Medical, Inc. 800-221-8569
19320 Van Ness Ave, Torrance, CA 90501
Closed wound kits consisting of variety of sizes and shapes of drains with trocars and suction devices.

David Scott Company 800-804-0333
59 Fountain St, Framingham, MA 01702
Abscess drainage kit, a closed system to better comply w/OSHA requirements not to expose personnel to highly contagious infected body fluid.

Zimmer Holdings, Inc. 800-613-6131
1800 W Center St, PO Box 708, Warsaw, IN 46580

KIT, WOUND DRAINAGE, CLOSED *(cont'd)*

Zimmer Orthopaedic Surgical Products 800-321-5533
PO Box 10, 200 West Ohio Ave., Dover, OH 44622
HEMOVAC.

KIT, WOUND DRESSING *(Surgery) 79MCY*

Ac Healthcare Supply, Inc. 905-448-4706
11651 230th St, Cambria Heights, NY 11411
Wound dressing kit.

American Medical Devices, Inc. 800-788-9876
287 S Stoddard Ave, San Bernardino, CA 92401

Bsn-Jobst 704-554-9933
5825 Carnegie Blvd, Charlotte, NC 28209
Venous leg ulcer management kit.

Busse Hospital Disposables, Inc. 631-435-4711
75 Arkay Dr, Hauppauge, NY 11788
Dressing change tray.

Centurion Medical Products Corp. 517-545-1135
3310 S Main St, Salisbury, NC 28147

Continental Medical Laboratories, Inc. 262-534-2787
813 Ela Ave, Waterford, WI 53185
Wound care kit/wound care management kit.

Covidien Lp 508-261-8000
15 Hampshire St, Mansfield, MA 02048

Custom Healthcare Systems, Inc. 804-421-5959
4205 Eubank Rd, Richmond, VA 23231

Customed, Inc. 787-801-0101
Calle Igualdad #7, Fajardo, PR 00738
Sterile t p n.

Cytyc Surgical Products 800-442-9892
250 Campus Dr, Marlborough, MA 01752
Kit, wound dressing.

Haemonetics Corp. 781-848-7100
400 Wood Rd, P.O.Box 9114, Braintree, MA 02184
Wound drain kit.

Johnson & Johnson Medical Division Of Ethicon, Inc. 800-423-4018
2500 E Arbrook Blvd, Arlington, TX 76014

Medi-Tech International Corp. 800-333-0109
26 Court St, Brooklyn, NY 11242
Kit includes SPAND-GEL hydrogel for Stage II through IV dermal ulcers, SPAN-DRESS absobent non-adherent pads, and SPANDAGE instant stretch bandage.

Merit Medical Systems Inc. 804-416-1030
12701 Kingston Ave, Chesterfield, VA 23837

Ormed Corporation 800-440-2784
599 Cardigan Rd, Saint Paul, MN 55126
EPIGARD synthetic skin substitute for temporary coverage used for protecting and conditioning of soft-tissue wounds.

Quadris Medical 507-389-4319
2030 Lookout Dr, North Mankato, MN 56003
Wound dressing kit.

Tmp Technologies, Inc. 716-895-6100
1200 Northland Ave, Buffalo, NY 14215

Tri-State Hospital Supply Corp. 517-545-1135
3173 E 43rd St, Yuma, AZ 85365

Vygon Corp. 800-544-4907
2495 General Armistead Ave, Norristown, PA 19403
Dressing change trays.

Web-Tex, Inc. 888-633-2723
5445 De Gaspe Ave., Ste. 702, Montreal, QC H2T 3B2 Canada

KIT, YEAST SCREENING *(Microbiology) 83JXC*

Bayer Healthcare Llc 914-524-2955
555 White Plains Rd Fl 5, Tarrytown, NY 10591
Culture test for the detection of candida species in vaginal specimens.

Culture Kits, Inc. 888-680-6853
14 Prentice St, PO Box 748, Norwich, NY 13815
CANDI-KIT candida albicans.

KNIFE, AMPUTATION *(Surgery) 79GDN*

Aesculap Implant Systems Inc. 1-800-234-9179
3773 Corporate Pkwy, Center Valley, PA 18034

Biomet, Inc. 574-267-6639
56 E Bell Dr, PO Box 587, Warsaw, IN 46582
Liston amputation knife.

KNIFE, AMPUTATION *(cont'd)*

Elmed, Inc. 630-543-2792
60 W Fay Ave, Addison, IL 60101

Kmedic 800-955-0559
190 Veterans Dr, Northvale, NJ 07647

Miltex Inc. 800-645-8000
589 Davies Dr, York, PA 17402

Tuzik Boston 800-886-6363
104 Longwater Dr, Assinippi Park, Norwell, MA 02061

KNIFE, CATARACT *(Ophthalmology) 86RDH*

Akorn, Inc. 800-535-7155
2500 Millbrook Dr, Buffalo Grove, IL 60089
Adjustable diamond knife for cataract surgery with titanium handle. 3mm and 3.2mm depth adjustable diamond knife for phacoemulsification, and clear cornea.

Bausch & Lomb Surgical 636-255-5051
3365 Tree Court Ind Blvd, Saint Louis, MO 63122

Becton Dickinson And Co. 866-906-8080
411 Waverley Oaks Rd, Waltham, MA 02452

Dgh Technology, Inc. 800-722-3883
110 Summit Dr Ste B, Exton, PA 19341
Instrument made of titanium and stainless-steel; diamond blades.

Elmed, Inc. 630-543-2792
60 W Fay Ave, Addison, IL 60101

Gwb International, Ltd. 888-436-4826
PO Box 370, 76 Prospect Street, Marshfield Hills, MA 02051
HUCO diamond and crystal blades for ophthalmology.

Havel's Inc. 800-638-4770
3726 Lonsdale St, Cincinnati, OH 45227

Kmi Surgical Ltd. 800-528-2900
110 Hopewell Rd, Laird Professional Building, Downingtown, PA 19335
Cataract and radial keratotomy diamond knives.

Oasis Medical, Inc. 800-528-9786
514 S Vermont Ave, Glendora, CA 91741
PREMIER EDGE disposable knives - Stab, Slit, Clear Cornea, Implant, MVR, Round Tunnel and Crescent Tunnel.

Sable Industries 800-890-0251
4751 Oceanside Blvd Ste G, Oceanside, CA 92056

Stephens Instruments, Inc. 800-354-7848
2500 Sandersville Rd, Lexington, KY 40511
$20.00 per unit (standard).

KNIFE, CERVICAL CONE *(Obstetrics/Gyn) 85HDZ*

New England Medical Corp. 845-778-4200
2274 Albany Post Rd, Walden, NY 12586
Cervical Cone Biopsy Electrode.

KNIFE, DERMATOME *(Surgery) 79RDI*

Bausch & Lomb Surgical 636-255-5051
3365 Tree Court Ind Blvd, Saint Louis, MO 63122

KNIFE, DURA HOOK *(Cns/Neurology) 84RDJ*

Codman & Shurtleff, Inc 800-225-0460
325 Paramount Dr, Raynham, MA 02767

KNIFE, EAR *(Ear/Nose/Throat) 77JYO*

Aesculap Implant Systems Inc. 1-800-234-9179
3773 Corporate Pkwy, Center Valley, PA 18034

Bausch & Lomb Surgical 636-255-5051
3365 Tree Court Ind Blvd, Saint Louis, MO 63122

Becton Dickinson And Co. 866-906-8080
411 Waverley Oaks Rd, Waltham, MA 02452

Biomet Microfixation Inc. 800-874-7711
1520 Tradeport Dr, Jacksonville, FL 32218
Various types of knives.

Elmed, Inc. 630-543-2792
60 W Fay Ave, Addison, IL 60101

George Tiemann & Co. 800-843-6266
25 Plant Ave, Hauppauge, NY 11788

Inciontech 800-213-7809
9 Technology Dr, Staunton, VA 24401
Special purpose and custom-made surgical blades.

Jedmed Instruments Co. 314-845-3770
5416 Jedmed Ct, Saint Louis, MO 63129

Medone Surgical, Inc. 941-359-3129
670 Tallevast Rd, Sarasota, FL 34243
Various.

KNIFE, EAR *(cont'd)*

Miltex Inc. 800-645-8000
589 Davies Dr, York, PA 17402

Surgical Instrument Manufacturers, Inc. 800-521-2985
1650 Headland Dr, Fenton, MO 63026

KNIFE, ENT *(Ear/Nose/Throat) 77KTG*

Becton Dickinson And Co. 866-906-8080
411 Waverley Oaks Rd, Waltham, MA 02452

Biomet Microfixation Inc. 800-874-7711
1520 Tradeport Dr, Jacksonville, FL 32218
Various types of knives.

Havel's Inc. 800-638-4770
3726 Lonsdale St, Cincinnati, OH 45227

Incisiontech 800-213-7809
9 Technology Dr, Staunton, VA 24401
Special purpose and custom-made surgical blades.

Walls Precision Instruments, Llc. 541-894-2520
38800 Deer Creek Rd, Baker City, OR 97814
Cdt speculum.

KNIFE, KERATOME *(Ophthalmology) 86RDK*

Bausch & Lomb Surgical 636-255-5051
3365 Tree Court Ind Blvd, Saint Louis, MO 63122

Becton Dickinson And Co. 866-906-8080
411 Waverley Oaks Rd, Waltham, MA 02452

Crescent Mfg. Co. 800-537-1330
1310 Majestic Dr, Fremont, OH 43420
Crescent. Microkaratome. Blades used in Lasic Surgery.

Dgh Technology, Inc. 800-722-3883
110 Summit Dr Ste B, Exton, PA 19341
Instrument made of titanium and stainless steel; diamond blades.

Eagle Laboratories 800-782-6534
10201 Trademark St Ste A, Rancho Cucamonga, CA 91730

Havel's Inc. 800-638-4770
3726 Lonsdale St, Cincinnati, OH 45227

Incisiontech 800-213-7809
9 Technology Dr, Staunton, VA 24401
Special purpose and custom-made surgical blades.

Kmi Surgical Ltd. 800-528-2900
110 Hopewell Rd, Laird Professional Building, Downingtown, PA 19335
Cataract and radial keratotomy diamond knives.

Rhein Medical, Inc. 800-637-4346
5460 Beaumont Center Blvd Ste 500, Suite 500, Tampa, FL 33634

Stephens Instruments, Inc. 800-354-7848
2500 Sandersville Rd, Lexington, KY 40511
$25.00 per unit (standard).

KNIFE, LAPAROSCOPIC *(Surgery) 79QWI*

Incisiontech 800-213-7809
9 Technology Dr, Staunton, VA 24401

Lyons Tool And Die Company 800-422-9363
185 Research Pkwy, Meriden, CT 06450
Rapid prototyping. Production of medical devices in class 10,000 clean rooms. Medical knives and scissors. Precision metal stamping. Engineering services.

Okay Industries, Inc. 860-225-8707
200 Ellis St, P.O. Box 2470, New Britain, CT 06051

Vital Concepts, Inc. 800-984-2300
4334 Brockton Dr SE Ste F, Grand Rapids, MI 49512
Laparoscopic Kittner, Kittner blunt laparoscopic dissector for all laparoscopic, pelvoscopic & endoscopic procedures.

KNIFE, LARYNGEAL *(Ear/Nose/Throat) 77JZY*

Aesculap Implant Systems Inc. 1-800-234-9179
3773 Corporate Pkwy, Center Valley, PA 18034

Bausch & Lomb Surgical 636-255-5051
3365 Tree Court Ind Blvd, Saint Louis, MO 63122

Incisiontech 800-213-7809
9 Technology Dr, Staunton, VA 24401
Special purpose and custom-made surgical blades.

KNIFE, MARGIN FINISHING, OPERATIVE *(Dental And Oral) 76EJZ*

Aesculap Implant Systems Inc. 1-800-234-9179
3773 Corporate Pkwy, Center Valley, PA 18034

Dental Usa, Inc. 815-363-8003
5005 McCullom Lake Rd, McHenry, IL 60050
Various types of knives.

KNIFE, MARGIN FINISHING, OPERATIVE *(cont'd)*

Hu-Friedy Manufacturing Co., Inc. 800-483-7433
3232 N Rockwell St, Chicago, IL 60618
$14.90 each - 6 sizes of margin trimmers.

Premier Dental Products Co. 888-670-6100
1710 Romano Dr, PO Box 4500, Plymouth Meeting, PA 19462

Suter Dental Manufacturing Company, Inc. 800-368-8376
632 Cedar St, Chico, CA 95928

KNIFE, MENISCUS *(Surgery) 79RDL*

Becton Dickinson And Co. 866-906-8080
411 Waverley Oaks Rd, Waltham, MA 02452

Elmed, Inc. 630-543-2792
60 W Fay Ave, Addison, IL 60101

Havel's Inc. 800-638-4770
3726 Lonsdale St, Cincinnati, OH 45227

Incisiontech 800-213-7809
9 Technology Dr, Staunton, VA 24401
Special purpose and custom-made surgical blades.

Miltex Inc. 800-645-8000
589 Davies Dr, York, PA 17402

Smith & Nephew, Inc., Endoscopy Division 800-343-8386
150 Minuteman Rd, Andover, MA 01810

Symmetry Tnco 888-447-6661
15 Colebrook Blvd, Whitman, MA 02382

KNIFE, MICROTOME *(Pathology) 88RDM*

Becton Dickinson And Co. 866-906-8080
411 Waverley Oaks Rd, Waltham, MA 02452

Boeckeler Instruments, Inc. 800-552-2262
4650 S Butterfield Dr, Tucson, AZ 85714
ultramicrotome diamond knives and GKM glass knife maker

Havel's Inc. 800-638-4770
3726 Lonsdale St, Cincinnati, OH 45227

Incisiontech 800-213-7809
9 Technology Dr, Staunton, VA 24401

Personna Medical/Div. Of American Safety Razor Co. 800-457-2222
1 Razor Blade Ln, Verona, VA 24482
Disposable PERSONNA PLUS (.010' & .012') microtome blades in 2 blade sizes (Low Profile .010' and High Profile .012'. PERSONNA PLUS blades feature MICROCOAT technology to provide smooth, clean ribbons. Ergonomically designed dispenser.

KNIFE, MYRINGOTOMY *(Ear/Nose/Throat) 77JYP*

Aesculap Implant Systems Inc. 1-800-234-9179
3773 Corporate Pkwy, Center Valley, PA 18034

Anchor Products Company 800-323-5134
52 W Official Rd, Addison, IL 60101
$170.00 per box of 20.

Bausch & Lomb Surgical 636-255-5051
3365 Tree Court Ind Blvd, Saint Louis, MO 63122

Becton Dickinson And Co. 866-906-8080
411 Waverley Oaks Rd, Waltham, MA 02452

Havel's Inc. 800-638-4770
3726 Lonsdale St, Cincinnati, OH 45227

Incisiontech 800-213-7809
9 Technology Dr, Staunton, VA 24401
Special purpose and custom-made surgical blades.

Mednet Locator, Inc. 800-754-5070
7000 Shadow Oaks Dr, Memphis, TN 38125
Knife.

Medone Surgical, Inc. 941-359-3129
670 Tallevast Rd, Sarasota, FL 34243
Various.

Micromedics 800-624-5662
1270 Eagan Industrial Rd, Saint Paul, MN 55121
Five blade styles with flexible shafts helps achieve a nearly infinite number of angles.

Sable Industries 800-890-0251
4751 Oceanside Blvd Ste G, Oceanside, CA 92056

KNIFE, NASAL *(Ear/Nose/Throat) 77KAS*

Aesculap Implant Systems Inc. 1-800-234-9179
3773 Corporate Pkwy, Center Valley, PA 18034

Bausch & Lomb Surgical 636-255-5051
3365 Tree Court Ind Blvd, Saint Louis, MO 63122

KNIFE, NASAL *(cont'd)*

Biomet Microfixation Inc. 800-874-7711
1520 Tradeport Dr, Jacksonville, FL 32218
Various types of knives.

Incisiontech 800-213-7809
9 Technology Dr, Staunton, VA 24401
Special purpose and custom-made surgical blades.

Invotec Intl. 800-998-8580
6833 Phillips Industrial Blvd, Jacksonville, FL 32256
Knife, nasal.

Medisiss 866-866-7477
2747 SW 6th St, Redmond, OR 97756
Various nasal knives,sterile.

Symmetry Medical Usa, Inc. 574-267-8700
486 W 350 N, Warsaw, IN 46582
Ear,nose, and throat manual surgical instrument.

KNIFE, OPHTHALMIC *(Ophthalmology) 86HNN*

Accutome, Inc. 610-889-0200
3222 Phoenixville Pike, Malvern, PA 19355
Various diamond opthalmic knives.

Akorn, Inc. 800-535-7155
2500 Millbrook Dr, Buffalo Grove, IL 60089
Micrometer diamond knife for precise depth incisions.

Alcon Manufacturing, Ltd. 817-551-6813
714 Columbia Ave, Sinking Spring, PA 19608
Various sizes and types of ophthalmic cutting instruments.

B. Graczyk, Inc. 269-782-2100
27826 Burmax Park, Dowagiac, MI 49047
Various styles types & sizes of sterile & non-sterile knives.

Back-Mueller, Inc. 314-531-6640
2700 Clark Ave, Saint Louis, MO 63103
Various lens cutters.

Bausch & Lomb Surgical 636-255-5051
3365 Tree Court Ind Blvd, Saint Louis, MO 63122

Becton Dickinson And Co. 866-906-8080
411 Waverley Oaks Rd, Waltham, MA 02452

Cytosol Ophthalmics, Inc. 800-234-5166
PO Box 1408, 1325 William White Place, NE, Lenoir, NC 28645
Stainless-steel disposable blades for cataract procedure. Variety of sizes and designs including stab, slit, phaco, trapezoid, mini-crescent.

Dgh Technology, Inc. 800-722-3883
110 Summit Dr Ste B, Exton, PA 19341
Instrument made of titanium and stainless steel; diamond blades.

Diamond Edge Co. 727-586-2927
928 W Bay Dr, Largo, FL 33770
General purpose knife for ocular surgery.

Escalon Trek Medical 800-433-8197
2440 S 179th St, New Berlin, WI 53146
Mvr blade.

Eye Care And Cure 800-486-6169
4646 S Overland Dr, Tucson, AZ 85714
Knife, ophthalmic, manual opthalmic surgical instrument.

Fortrad Eye Instruments Corp. 973-543-2371
8 Franklin Rd, Mendham, NJ 07945

Gyrus Ent L.L.C., Sub. Of Gyrus Acmi, Inc. 508-804-2739
2925 Appling Rd, Bartlett, TN 38133
Various.

Hai Laboratories, Inc. 781-862-9884
320 Massachusetts Ave, Lexington, MA 02420
Ophthalmic knife - various types.

Havel's Inc. 800-638-4770
3726 Lonsdale St, Cincinnati, OH 45227

Hurricane Medical 941-751-0588
5315 Lena Rd, Bradenton, FL 34211
Ophthalmic knife.

Incisiontech 800-213-7809
9 Technology Dr, Staunton, VA 24401
Special purpose and custom-made surgical blades.

International Science And Technology, Lp 800-867-8081
8665 New Trails Dr Ste 100, The Woodlands, TX 77381
Ophthalmic knife.

Katena Products, Inc. 800-225-1195
4 Stewart Ct, Denville, NJ 07834

KNIFE, OPHTHALMIC *(cont'd)*

Kmi Surgical Ltd. 800-528-2900
110 Hopewell Rd, Laird Professional Building, Downingtown, PA 19335

L.A.B. Instruments, Ltd. 775-883-1205
3692 Green Acres Dr, Carson City, NV 89705
Diamond knife.

Liquidmetal Technologies, Inc. 949-206-8000
25800 Commercentre Dr Ste 100, Lake Forest, CA 92630
Ophthalmic knife blade.

Mark Medical Manufacturing, Inc. 610-269-4420
530 Brandywine Ave, Downingtown, PA 19335
Opthalmic surgical instruments.

Mastel Precision, Inc. 800-657-8057
2843 Samco Rd Unit A, Rapid City, SD 57702
Knife, ophthalmic.

Medone Surgical, Inc. 941-359-3129
670 Tallevast Rd, Sarasota, FL 34243
Various.

Oasis Medical, Inc. 800-528-9786
514 S Vermont Ave, Glendora, CA 91741
FEATHER brand ophthalmic scalpels - Incision, Guarded, Tunnel, Clear Cornea Keratomes, Wound Enlargement, MVR.

Psi/Eye-Ko, Inc. 636-447-1010
804 Corporate Centre Dr, O Fallon, MO 63368
Various types of ophthlamic knifes.

Rhein Medical, Inc. 800-637-4346
5460 Beaumont Center Blvd Ste 500, Suite 500, Tampa, FL 33634
Stainless and titanium diamond knife.

Stephens Instruments, Inc. 800-354-7848
2500 Sandersville Rd, Lexington, KY 40511
$15.00 per unit (standard).

Surgical Instrument Manufacturers, Inc. 800-521-2985
1650 Headland Dr, Fenton, MO 63026

Surgistar Inc. 800-995-7086
2310 La Mirada Dr, Vista, CA 92081
Surgical blades and knives, specially for ophthalmic, ENT, cardiovascular procedures.

Total Titanium, Inc. 618-473-2429
140 East Monroe St., Hecker, IL 62248
Various types of ophthalmic knives.

KNIFE, ORTHOPEDIC *(Orthopedics) 87HTS*

Ascent Healthcare Solutions 480-763-5300
10232 S 51st St, Phoenix, AZ 85044
Cartilage knife.

Biomet Microfixation Inc. 800-874-7711
1520 Tradeport Dr, Jacksonville, FL 32218
Various types of knives.

Depuy Mitek, A Johnson & Johnson Company 800-451-2006
50 Scotland Blvd, Bridgewater, MA 02324
Various types of orthopedic knives.

Depuy Spine, Inc. 800-227-6633
325 Paramount Dr, Raynham, MA 02767
Dissector, surgical knife.

Havel's Inc. 800-638-4770
3726 Lonsdale St, Cincinnati, OH 45227

I.T.I., Inc. 406-251-7000
6150 US Highway 93 S, Missoula, MT 59804
Electroencephalograph.

Incisiontech 800-213-7809
9 Technology Dr, Staunton, VA 24401
Special purpose and custom-made surgical blades.

Kmedic 800-955-0559
190 Veterans Dr, Northvale, NJ 07647

Medisiss 866-866-7477
2747 SW 6th St, Redmond, OR 97756
Various orthopedic knives,sterile.

Medtronic Puerto Rico Operations Co.,Med Rel 763-514-4000
Road 909, Km. 0.4., Barrio Mariana, Humacao, PR 00792
Knife, orthopedic.

Smith & Nephew, Inc., Endoscopy Division 800-343-8386
150 Minuteman Rd, Andover, MA 01810

Spinus, Llc 603-758-1444
8 Merrill Industrial Dr, Hampton, NH 03842
Scalpel.

KNIFE, ORTHOPEDIC *(cont'd)*

Symmetry Medical Usa, Inc. 574-267-8700
486 W 350 N, Warsaw, IN 46582
Orthopedic manual surgical instrument.

Symmetry Tnco 888-447-6661
15 Colebrook Blvd, Whitman, MA 02382

Tuzik Boston 800-886-6363
104 Longwater Dr, Assinippi Park, Norwell, MA 02061

Warsaw Orthopedic, Inc. 901-396-3133
2500 Silveus Xing, Warsaw, IN 46582
Various cartilage knives.

Whitney Products, Inc. 800-338-4237
6153 W Mulford St Ste C, Niles, IL 60714
WHITNEY - Green sculps knife for removing excess bone cement before implanting a prosthesis during hip or knee replacement surgery. Handle has thumb indentation to orient tip in hard-to-reach places. Sterile and disposable.

Zimmer Holdings, Inc. 800-613-6131
1800 W Center St, PO Box 708, Warsaw, IN 46580

Zimmer Trabecular Metal Technology 800-613-6131
10 Pomeroy Rd, Parsippany, NJ 07054
Osteotome.

KNIFE, OTHER *(Surgery) 79RDS*

Becton Dickinson And Co. 866-906-8080
411 Waverley Oaks Rd, Waltham, MA 02452

Hospital Marketing Svcs. Company, Inc. 800-786-5094
162 Great Hill Rd./ Ind. Park, Naugatuck, CT 06770
HMS SURGIBLADE - box of 10 pcs. (#10, 11, 15, 20, 21); box of 10 pcs. (#12, 22 or 23).

Incisiontech 800-213-7809
9 Technology Dr, Staunton, VA 24401
Special purpose and custom-made surgical blades.

Katena Products, Inc. 800-225-1195
4 Stewart Ct, Denville, NJ 07834
Diamond and sapphire knives.

Kinetikos Medical, Inc. 800-546-3845
6005 Hidden Valley Rd Ste 180, Carlsbad, CA 92011
SAFEGUARD Mini Carpal Tunnel Release System, disposable, single use knives & reusable stainless steel guide used for carpal tunnel release.

Lyons Tool And Die Company 800-422-9363
185 Research Pkwy, Meriden, CT 06450
Rapid prototyping. Production of medical devices in class 10,000 clean rooms. Medical knives and scissors. Precision metal stamping. Engineering services.

Neogen Corporation 800-234-5333
620 Lesher Pl, Lansing, MI 48912
For veterinary use only.

Surgipath Medical Industries, Inc. 800-225-3035
PO Box 528, 5205 Route 12, Richmond, IL 60071
Disposable dissection knives

Zivic Laboratories 800-422-5227
178 Toll Gate School Road, Zelienople, PA 16063
Rat and mouse brain block slicers are available in plastic or steel construction with coronal or sagittal divisions. They are available in 1mm, 2mm, 3mm divisions. Brass micron punches used for the removal of discrete regions of the brain in 2mm, 1.5mm, 1mm, .75mm, .69mm, .50mm, and .30mm sizes. Custon carved brain slicers of any size are also available.

KNIFE, PERIODONTIC *(Dental And Oral) 76EMO*

Aesculap Implant Systems Inc. 1-800-234-9179
3773 Corporate Pkwy, Center Valley, PA 18034

Arnold Tuber Industries 716-648-3363
97 Main St, Hamburg, NY 14075
Knife, periodontic, dental hand instruments.

Biomet Microfixation Inc. 800-874-7711
1520 Tradeport Dr, Jacksonville, FL 32218
Various types of knives.

Dental Usa, Inc. 815-363-8003
5005 McCullom Lake Rd, McHenry, IL 60050
Various types of knives.

Dentalez Group 866-DTE-INFO
101 Lindenwood Dr Ste 225, Valleybrooke Corporate Center Malvern, PA 19355

KNIFE, PERIODONTIC *(cont'd)*

Dentalez Group, Stardental Division 717-291-1161
1816 Colonial Village Ln, Lancaster, PA 17601
Rc cement non-staining.

E.A. Beck & Co. 949-645-4072
657 W 19th St Ste E, P O Box 10857, Costa Mesa, CA 92627
Knife.

H & H Co. 909-390-0373
4435 E Airport Dr Ste 108, Ontario, CA 91761
Knife, periodontic.

Hu-Friedy Manufacturing Co., Inc. 800-483-7433
3232 N Rockwell St, Chicago, IL 60618
$28.10 to $40.30 each, 17 types.

Nordent Manufacturing, Inc. 800-966-7336
610 Bonnie Ln, Elk Grove Village, IL 60007
$36.50 per unit (standard).

Premier Dental Products Co. 888-670-6100
1710 Romano Dr, PO Box 4500, Plymouth Meeting, PA 19462

Sci-Dent, Inc. 800-323-4145
210 Dowdle St Ste 2, Algonquin, IL 60102
Gingivectomy knife.

KNIFE, PLASTER *(Orthopedics) 87RDO*

Codman & Shurtleff, Inc 800-225-0460
325 Paramount Dr, Raynham, MA 02767

Miltex Inc. 800-645-8000
589 Davies Dr, York, PA 17402

Zimmer Holdings, Inc. 800-613-6131
1800 W Center St, PO Box 708, Warsaw, IN 46580

KNIFE, SCALPEL *(Surgery) 79RDP*

Alcon Research, Ltd. 800-862-5266
6201 South Fwy, Fort Worth, TX 76134

Cincinnati Surgical Company 800-544-3100
11256 Cornell Park Dr, Cincinnati, OH 45242
Disposable scapels and mini-scalpel.

Dgh Technology, Inc. 800-722-3883
110 Summit Dr Ste B, Exton, PA 19341
Instrument made of titanium and stainless steel; diamond blades.

Elmed, Inc. 630-543-2792
60 W Fay Ave, Addison, IL 60101

Hospital Marketing Svcs. Company, Inc. 800-786-5094
162 Great Hill Rd./ Ind. Park, Naugatuck, CT 06770
Cat. 5510, 5511, 5512, 5515, Sterile-5520, 5521, 5522, 5523, sizes 10-23.

Incisiontech 800-213-7809
9 Technology Dr, Staunton, VA 24401

Magnaplan Corp. 800-361-1192
1320 Rte. 9, Champlain, NY 12919-5007
Handles made of nickel-silver alloy. Blades are easily attached with a simple sliding motion. Push-button type handles make blade changing even simpler and faster. Contour blades made of .005 inches stainless steel.

Mark Medical Manufacturing, Inc. 610-269-4420
530 Brandywine Ave, Downingtown, PA 19335
General surgical instruments.

Miltex Inc. 800-645-8000
589 Davies Dr, York, PA 17402

Msi Precision, Specialty Instrument 800-322-4674
1220 Valley Forge Rd Ste 34, Phoenixville, PA 19460

Rhein Medical, Inc. 800-637-4346
5460 Beaumont Center Blvd Ste 500, Suite 500, Tampa, FL 33634

Toolmex Corporation 800-992-4766
1075 Worcester St, Natick, MA 01760

Trans American Medical / Tamsco Instruments 708-430-7777
7633 W 100th Pl, Bridgeview, IL 60455

KNIFE, SKIN GRAFTING *(Surgery) 79RDQ*

Bausch & Lomb Surgical 636-255-5051
3365 Tree Court Ind Blvd, Saint Louis, MO 63122

Miltex Inc. 800-645-8000
589 Davies Dr, York, PA 17402

KNIFE, STERNUM *(Surgery) 79RDR*

Codman & Shurtleff, Inc 800-225-0460
325 Paramount Dr, Raynham, MA 02767

Miltex Inc. 800-645-8000
589 Davies Dr, York, PA 17402

KNIFE, SURGICAL *(Dental And Oral) 76EMF*

Accutome, Inc. 610-889-0200
3222 Phoenixville Pike, Malvern, PA 19355
Surgical knife.

Aesculap Implant Systems Inc. 1-800-234-9179
3773 Corporate Pkwy, Center Valley, PA 18034

Biomet Microfixation Inc. 800-874-7711
1520 Tradeport Dr, Jacksonville, FL 32218
Various types of knives.

Cardinal Health, Snowden Pencer Products 847-689-8410
5175 S Royal Atlanta Dr, Tucker, GA 30084
Various types of knife handles.

Competitive Engineering Inc. 520-746-0270
3371 E Hemisphere Loop, Tucson, AZ 85706
Manual surgical knife.

Dental Usa, Inc. 815-363-8003
5005 McCullom Lake Rd, McHenry, IL 60050
Dental knife.

Dgh Technology, Inc. 800-722-3883
110 Summit Dr Ste B, Exton, PA 19341
Surgical diamond knives: KOI line, freehand and micrometer.

Elmed, Inc. 630-543-2792
60 W Fay Ave, Addison, IL 60101

Gyrus Ent L.L.C., Sub. Of Gyrus Acmi, Inc. 508-804-2739
2925 Appling Rd, Bartlett, TN 38133
Various.

Hospital Marketing Svcs. Company, Inc. 800-786-5094
162 Great Hill Rd./ Ind. Park, Naugatuck, CT 06770
Sterile - cat. 5510 through 5523; Blade sizes #10 through 23; Disposable-10 per box.

Incisiontech 800-213-7809
9 Technology Dr, Staunton, VA 24401
Special purpose and custom-made surgical blades.

Kmi Surgical Ltd. 800-528-2900
110 Hopewell Rd, Laird Professional Building, Downingtown, PA 19335
Disposable.

Lyons Tool And Die Company 800-422-9363
185 Research Pkwy, Meriden, CT 06450
Rapid prototyping. Production of medical devices in class 10,000 clean rooms. Medical knives and scissors. Precision metal stamping. Engineering services.

Marketing International, Inc. 800-447-0173
PO Box 4835, Topeka, KS 66604
Disposable macro-prep autopsy knife, with stainless-steel blade.NOT DENTAL!

Msi Precision, Specialty Instrument 800-322-4674
1220 Valley Forge Rd Ste 34, Phoenixville, PA 19460

Smith & Nephew, Inc., Endoscopy Division 800-343-8386
130 Forbes Blvd, Mansfield, MA 02048

Stryker Puerto Rico, Ltd. 939-307-2500
Hwy. 3, Km. 131.2, Las Guasimas Ind. Park, Arroyo, PR 00714
Knife.

Surgistar Inc. 800-995-7086
2310 La Mirada Dr, Vista, CA 92081
Various specialty surgical blades.

Tuzik Boston 800-886-6363
104 Longwater Dr, Assinippi Park, Norwell, MA 02061

KNIFE, TONSIL *(Ear/Nose/Throat) 77KBQ*

Aesculap Implant Systems Inc. 1-800-234-9179
3773 Corporate Pkwy, Center Valley, PA 18034

Bausch & Lomb Surgical 636-255-5051
3365 Tree Court Ind Blvd, Saint Louis, MO 63122

Becton Dickinson And Co. 866-906-8080
411 Waverley Oaks Rd, Waltham, MA 02452

Biomet Microfixation Inc. 800-874-7711
1520 Tradeport Dr, Jacksonville, FL 32218
Various types of knives.

Electro Surgical Instrument Co., Inc. 888-464-2784
37 Centennial St, Rochester, NY 14611
Various types,styles and sizes of illuminated tonsil knives, dissectors, retract.

Elmed, Inc. 630-543-2792
60 W Fay Ave, Addison, IL 60101

KNIFE, TONSIL *(cont'd)*

Medisiss 866-866-7477
2747 SW 6th St, Redmond, OR 97756
Various tonsil knives,sterile.

Miltex Inc. 800-645-8000
589 Davies Dr, York, PA 17402

Tuzik Boston 800-886-6363
104 Longwater Dr, Assinippi Park, Norwell, MA 02061

L-GLUTAMYLNITROANILIDE/GLYCYLGLYCINE, GGTP *(Chemistry) 75CGG*

Amresco Inc. 800-366-1313
30175 Solon Industrial Pkwy, Solon, OH 44139
Hitachi, technicon RA, SMAC and SMA systems.

L-LEUCYL B-NAPHTHYLAMIDE, LACTIC ACID *(Chemistry) 75JKI*

Dade Behring, Inc. 800-948-3233
1717 Deerfield Rd, Deerfield, IL 60015

LABEL, BAR CODE *(General) 80WNL*

Avery Dennison Corporation 626-304-2000
150 N Orange Grove Blvd, Pasadena, CA 91103
PRESIDAX bar code printer and label system.

Barcodes West, Llc 206-323-8100
1560 1st Ave S, Seattle, WA 98134
Preprint/blank labels and tags, most any size, shape, numbering sequence, material, adhesive, lamination, up to six colors. Also BUI labels.

Bio-Logics Products, Inc. 800-426-7577
PO Box 505, West Jordan, UT 84084
Bar code labels for blood banking.

Integrated Software Design, Inc. 800-600-2242
171 Forbes Blvd Ste 3000, Mansfield, MA 02048
Tattoo ID is fully integrated software for in-house design and production printing of signs, labels and forms. Allows user to include fixed or fill-in text, graphics and bar codes. Receive data from databases. Print on any printer. Compliant with all popular standards.

Kroy, Llc 888-888-5769
3830 Kelley Ave, Cleveland, OH 44114

Lab Safety Supply, Inc. 800-356-0783
401 S Wright Rd, Janesville, WI 53546

Medi-Hut Co., Inc. 800-882-0139
1935 Swarthmore Ave, Lakewood, NJ 08701

Products International Co. 800-521-5123
2320 W Holly St, Phoenix, AZ 85009
EasyID patient label sheets work in a standard laser printer, are sized for patient records and TabBand ID bands, and are punched to fit file folders.

Tailored Label Products, Inc. 800-727-1344
W165N5731 Ridgewood Dr, Menomonee Falls, WI 53051
Pressure sensitive labels (rolls or fanfolded), nameplates, rating plates, bar code lables, UL/CSA labels.

Timemed Labeling Systems, Inc. 800-323-4840
144 Tower Dr, Burr Ridge, IL 60527
Bar code labeling applications; products include blood bank labels and bar code printers.

Wallace Computer Services, Inc 800-782-4892
2275 Cabot Dr, Lisle, IL 60532
Tapes & labels for all healthcare applications.

LABEL, DEVICE *(General) 80QPF*

Aigner Index, Inc. 800-242-3919
218 Mac Arthur Ave, New Windsor, NY 12553
SUPERSCAN Label Holder, self-adhesive, magnetic and Velcro backing available, xtra large (3x5 and 4x6), barcode compatible.

Avery Dennison Corporation 626-304-2000
150 N Orange Grove Blvd, Pasadena, CA 91103
Patient Charge Recovery System (using labels) for hospital inventory, distribution and patient cost control.

Briggs Corporation 800-247-2343
PO Box 1698, 7300 Westown Pkwy., Des Moines, IA 50306

Healthcare Labels, Inc. 800-323-8323
245 Honey Lake Ct, North Barrington, IL 60010
Full catalog of nursing, pharmacy, anesthesia, IV tubing, microscope slide, patient chart, and blank labels; EDP and bar coded labels; piggy back labels.

Medi-Dose, Inc. 800-523-8966
70 Industrial Dr, Ivyland, PA 18974

LABEL, DEVICE *(cont'd)*

Ross Disposable Products 800-649-6526
401 Traders Blvd E, Unit 10, Mississauga, ON L4Z 2H8 Canada

Scanlan International, Inc. 800-328-9458
1 Scanlan Plz, Saint Paul, MN 55107
SURG-I-BAND color coding system for surgical instruments.

Spirig Advanced Technologies, Inc. 413-788-6191
144 Oakland St, Springfield, MA 01108
CELSISTRIPS temperature recording & sterilization temp. labels.

Stat-Chek Company 800-248-6618
PO Box 9636, Bend, OR 97708
$12.45 to $23.20 per doz. for STAT-CHEK Inventory Control Signals.

Sterion, Incorporated 800-328-7958
13828 Lincoln St NE, Ham Lake, MN 55304
Locking labeling tag.

Surgipath Medical Industries, Inc. 800-225-3035
PO Box 528, 5205 Route 12, Richmond, IL 60071

Tailored Label Products, Inc. 800-727-1344
W165N5731 Ridgewood Dr, Menomonee Falls, WI 53051
Pressure sensitive labels (rolls or fanfolded), nameplates, rating plates, bar code lables, UL/CSA labels.

Timemed Labeling Systems, Inc. 800-323-4840
144 Tower Dr, Burr Ridge, IL 60527
Patient charge labeling systems and label printers.

Veriad 800-423-4643
650 Columbia St, Brea, CA 92821
Pressure sensitive labels for all hospital departments.

LABEL/TAG, STERILE *(Surgery) 79LYV*

Busse Hospital Disposables, Inc. 631-435-4711
75 Arkay Dr, Hauppauge, NY 11788
Sterile label.

Centurion Medical Products Corp. 517-545-1135
3310 S Main St, Salisbury, NC 28147

Tailored Label Products, Inc. 800-727-1344
W165N5731 Ridgewood Dr, Menomonee Falls, WI 53051

Tri-State Hospital Supply Corp. 517-545-1135
3173 E 43rd St, Yuma, AZ 85365

LABELER, X-RAY FILM *(Radiology) 90SGK*

Gri Medical Products, Inc. 800-291-9425
4937 E Red Range Way, Cave Creek, AZ 85331
Date label system.

Marconi Medical Systems 800-323-0550
595 Miner Rd, Cleveland, OH 44143

Revelation Industries 800-833-2139
101 E Oak St, Bozeman, MT 59715
MARKER FOOT differentiated adhesive, cleanly adheres x-ray markers to a film cassette or bucky. 100 pre-cut tabs come in a handy dispenser pack. Puts an end to messy tape and glue residues.

S&S Technology 281-815-1300
10625 Telge Rd, Houston, TX 77095

St. John Companies 800-435-4242
25167 Anza Dr, PO Box 800460, Santa Clarita, CA 91355
Labels for medical imaging, radiology, mammography, nuclear medicine, MRI, ultrasound, CT scan and general hospital use. Wristbands, patient identification.

Tabbies, Div. Of Xertrex International, Inc. 630-773-4160
1530 Glenlake Ave, Itasca, IL 60143

Techno-Aide, Inc. 800-251-2629
7117 Centennial Blvd, Nashville, TN 37209

Xma (X-Ray Marketing Associates, Inc.) 800-325-8880
1205 W Lakeview Ct, Windham Lakes Business Park
Romeoville, IL 60446

LABELING EQUIPMENT *(General) 80VAH*

Apple Converting, Inc. 607-337-4474
65 Hale St, Norwich, NY 13815

Astro-Med, Inc. 800-343-4039
600 E Greenwich Ave, West Warwick, RI 02893
Equipment, supplies, and materials.

LABELING EQUIPMENT *(cont'd)*

Avery Dennison Corporation 626-304-2000
150 N Orange Grove Blvd, Pasadena, CA 91103
INTACS imprinting systems with UPC-A, EAN-13, UPC-E, EAN-8, UPC-A with descenders, ISBN, standard code 39 (no check digit), HIBC primary or secondary, European code 39 (no start/stop characters), code 39, Codabar, interleaved 2 of 5, MSI/Plessey and code 128 option. Rated print speed of up to 3in./sec., max. label width: 3.25in., length: 5.in.

Basi (Bioanalytical Systems, Inc.) 800-845-4246
2701 Kent Ave, West Lafayette, IN 47906
Chads for Vials sampling-labeling system. Thin, flexible, pre-numbered tags, printed on waterproof, solvent-resistant material, for labeling sampling vials, one-at-a-time, or up to 192 vials at a time.

Bausch & Stroebel Machine Company, Inc. 866-512-2637
112 Nod Rd Ste 17, Clinton, CT 06413

Biner Ellison 800-741-2341
2685 S Melrose Dr, Vista, CA 92081
Liquid packaging machinery, cappers, labelers, coders, torque testers, conveyors, bottle washers, induction sealers, and tube sealers.

Champion America 800-521-7000
PO Box 3092, Branford, CT 06405
Bar coding equipment and supplies.

Healthcare Labels, Inc. 800-323-8323
245 Honey Lake Ct, North Barrington, IL 60010

Hospira, Inc. 877-946-7747
755 Jarvis Dr, Morgan Hill, CA 95037
Modified to enhance the safety in the use of device.

Intersign Corp. 800-322-8426
2156 Amnicola Hwy, Chattanooga, TN 37406

Kroy, Llc 888-888-5769
3830 Kelley Ave, Cleveland, OH 44114

Lab Safety Supply, Inc. 800-356-0783
401 S Wright Rd, Janesville, WI 53546

Lacey Manufacturing Co. 203-336-0121
1146 Barnum Ave, PO Box 5156, Bridgeport, CT 06610

Medi-Dose, Inc. 800-523-8966
70 Industrial Dr, Ivyland, PA 18974

Medical Packaging Inc. 800-257-5282
470 Route 31 N, PO Box 500, Ringoes, NJ 08551
On-line computerized printing system for strip packaging machinery, bar code capabilities, and pre-printed labels.

Medical Safety Systems Inc. 888-803-9303
230 White Pond Dr, Akron, OH 44313

Mts Medication Technologies 800-671-0508
2003 Gandy Blvd N Ste 800, Saint Petersburg, FL 33702
Packaging supplies & prescription labels.

Nbs Technologies Inc. 800-524-0419
70 Eisenhower Dr, Paramus, NJ 07652
Wristband, card and label printers; also plastic card embossing machines.

Quint Company 215-533-1988
3725 Castor Ave # 26, Philadelphia, PA 19124
Printing plates for unit dose and blister packaging and medical pouches/lidding. Printing plates for Bellmaote, Hapa, Gottscho, and Metronic inline printers.

Tailored Label Products, Inc. 800-727-1344
W165N5731 Ridgewood Dr, Menomonee Falls, WI 53051

Tray-Pak Corporation 888-926-1777
PO Box 14804, Tuckerton Road & Reading Crest Avenue
Reading, PA 19612

LABORATORY EQUIPMENT, OPHTHALMIC
(Ophthalmology) 86WTY

Co/Op Optical Vision Designs 866-733-2667
2424 E 8 Mile Rd, E. of Dequindre, Detroit, MI 48234

LABORATORY EQUIPMENT, OPHTHALMIC *(cont'd)*

Dac International, Inc. 888-373-3027
6390 Rose Ln, Carpinteria, CA 93013
DLL Series III, CNC lens lathes for contact lens and intraocular lens production. 2-Axis OTT, CNC 2-Axis lathe with oscillating tool toric for the production of toric contact and intraocular lenses. 4XC/T, CNC 4-Axis lathe with flycutting, kinematic toric option, for the production of contact and intraocular lenses. DLL SERIES III/4-AXIS OTT LATHE, for production of contact and intraocular lenses, with oscillating tool technology, capable of producing spheres, aspheres, torics, all with complete edge radius. DSS, Spectacle Lens Surfacing System, consists of a surfacing lathe and three cylinder machines, capable of surfacing, firing, and polishing 240 jobs/day with a single operator.

Dispensers Optical Service Corp. 800-626-4545
1815 Plantside Dr, Louisville, KY 40299
Ophthalmic instrumentation.

Dmv Corporation 800-522-9465
1024 Military Rd, Zanesville, OH 43701
STRONGHOLD and TECHNICIAN'S HELPER units for contact lens modification.

Innovative Imaging, Inc. 800-765-7226
9940 Business Park Dr Ste 155, Sacramento, CA 95827
$10,000.00 to $30,000.00 diagnostic ultrasound systems for ophthalmologists. Clear oscilloscope display of macular traction, edema, holes, tumor vascularity, detachments, etc.

Landec Corp. 650-306-1650
3603 Haven Ave, Menlo Park, CA 94025

Micrins Surgical Instruments, Inc. 800-833-3380
28438 N Ballard Dr, Lake Forest, IL 60045

Newport Glass Works, Ltd. 714-484-8100
PO Box 127, Stanton, CA 90680
Quartz, fused silica, optical glass blanks, Pyrex blanks, laser protection eyewear glass blanks, etc.

Newport Optical Laboratories, Inc. 714-484-3200
10564C Fern Ave, Stanton, CA 90680
Lenses (singlet, achromats, etc.), beamsplitters, precision optics used in medical instrumentation (surgical microscope, lasers, etc.), and mirrors. Also provide thin film coatings on glass and ceramic material.

Oasis Medical, Inc. 800-528-9786
514 S Vermont Ave, Glendora, CA 91741
Ophthalmic disk fluid filters.

Pacific Precision Laboratories, Inc. 800-793-0179
20447 Nordhoff St, Chatsworth, CA 91311
Measurement and inspection solutions for high precision applications.

Topcon Medical Systems, Inc. 800-223-1130
37 W Century Rd, Paramus, NJ 07652
Three models of patternless edgers: ULTIMA 5100, ULTIMA 5100SG, and ULTIMA XPRESS (please call for current pricing). Also aspherical lenses, two models, $295 each.

LABWARE, ASSISTED REPRODUCTION *(Obstetrics/Gyn) 85MQK*

Bd Biosciences Discovery Labware 978-901-7431
1 Becton Cir, Durham, NC 27712
Assisted reproduction labware.

Biocoat, Inc. 215-734-0888
211 Witmer Rd, Horsham, PA 19044
PICSI SPERM SELECTION DEVICE

Genesis Instruments, Inc. 715-639-9209
200 Main St., Elmwood, WI 54740
Culture dish (sterile).

Minitube Of America, Inc 608-845-1502
419 Venture Ct, Verona, WI 53593
Tissue/cell culturing device.

LABWARE, BASIC, DISPOSABLE *(Chemistry) 75RDU*

Biohit Inc. 800-922-0784
PO Box 308, 3535 Rte. 66, Bldg. 4, Neptune, NJ 07754

Burrell Scientific, Inc 800-637-6074
2223 5th Ave, Pittsburgh, PA 15219

Cargille Laboratories 973-239-6633
55 Commerce Rd, Cedar Grove, NJ 07009
Beakers in polypropylene or paper.

Carolina Biological Supply Co. 800-334-5551
2700 York Rd, Burlington, NC 27215

Cole-Parmer Instrument Inc. 800-323-4340
625 E Bunker Ct, Vernon Hills, IL 60061

LABWARE, BASIC, DISPOSABLE *(cont'd)*

Corning Inc., Science Products Division 800-492-1110
45 Nagog Park, Acton, MA 01720

Covidien Lp 508-261-8000
15 Hampshire St, Mansfield, MA 02048

Dade Behring, Inc. 800-948-3233
1717 Deerfield Rd, Deerfield, IL 60015

Fisher Healthcare 800-766-7000
9999 Veterans Memorial Dr, Houston, TX 77038

Helena Plastics 800-227-1727
3700 Lakeville Hwy Ste 200, Petaluma, CA 94954

Image Molding, Inc. 800-525-1875
4525 Kingston St, Denver, CO 80239

Kimble Glass, Inc. 888-546-2531
537 Crystal Ave, Vineland, NJ 08360
KIMBLE.

Labcon North America 800-227-1466
3700 Lakeville Hwy Ste 200, Petaluma, CA 94954
Injection molded plastic disposables.

Medi-Dose, Inc. 800-523-8966
70 Industrial Dr, Ivyland, PA 18974

Moldpro, Inc. 603-721-6286
36 Denman Thompson Hwy, Swanzey, NH 03446
Autosampler tubes and cups

Nutech Molding Corporation 1-800-423-5278
PO Box 840, 2024 Broad St,, Pocomoke City, MD 21851

Precision Dynamics Corp. 800-772-1122
13880 Del Sur St, San Fernando, CA 91340
SECURLINE Permanent lab marker.

Quality Scientific Plastics 800-426-9595
1260 Holm Rd, Petaluma, CA 94954

Sanderson-Macleod, Inc. 866-522-3481
1199 S Main St, P.O. Box 50, Palmer, MA 01069
Disposable brushes.

Schleicher & Schuell, Inc. 800-245-4024
10 Optical Ave, PO Box 2012, Keene, NH 03431
ZAPCAP, EXTRACTOR.

Simport Plastics Ltd. 450-464-1723
2588 Bernard-Pilon, Beloeil, QUE J3G 4S5 Canada

Sonoco-Stancap Division 770-476-9088
3150 Clinton Ct, Norcross, GA 30071

Thermosafe Brands 847-398-0110
3930 N Ventura Dr Ste 450, Arlington Heights, IL 60004

LABWARE, BASIC, REUSABLE *(Chemistry) 75RDV*

Beckman Coulter, Inc. 800-742-2345
250 S Kraemer Blvd, PO Box 8000, Brea, CA 92821

Berghof/America 800-544-5004
3773 NW 126th Ave Bldg 1, Coral Springs, FL 33065
Teflon labware.

Burrell Scientific, Inc 800-637-6074
2223 5th Ave, Pittsburgh, PA 15219

Carolina Biological Supply Co. 800-334-5551
2700 York Rd, Burlington, NC 27215

Cata-Mount Glass, Inc. 802-442-5438
309 County St, Bennington, VT 05201

Cole-Parmer Instrument Inc. 800-323-4340
625 E Bunker Ct, Vernon Hills, IL 60061

Corning Inc., Science Products Division 800-492-1110
45 Nagog Park, Acton, MA 01720

Dade Behring, Inc. 800-948-3233
1717 Deerfield Rd, Deerfield, IL 60015

Dan Kar Corporation 800-942-5542
PO Box 279, 192 New Boston St C, Wilmington, MA 01887
Electrophoresis accessories, electrophoresis glass plates, gradient makers & protective plexiglass shielding.

Edmund Industrial Optics 800-363-1992
101 E Gloucester Pike, Barrington, NJ 08007
Labware, lab construction equipment, and lab meters.

Fisher Healthcare 800-766-7000
9999 Veterans Memorial Dr, Houston, TX 77038

Francis L. Freas Glass Works, Inc. 610-828-0430
148 E 9th Ave, Conshohocken, PA 19428

LABWARE, BASIC, REUSABLE *(cont'd)*

Glass Instruments, Inc. 323-681-0011
2285 E Foothill Blvd, Pasadena, CA 91107
Custom & production glassware for medical R&D.

Healthmark Industries 800-521-6224
22522 E 9 Mile Rd, Saint Clair Shores, MI 48080
Autoclavable plastic trays, boxes and bags.

Kimble Glass, Inc. 888-546-2531
537 Crystal Ave, Vineland, NJ 08360
KONTES.

Kontes Glass Co. 888-546-2531
1022 Spruce St, Vineland, NJ 08360

Kreisers Inc. 800-843-7948
2200 W 46th St, Sioux Falls, SD 57105

Metal Techology, Inc. 800-394-9979
173 Queen Ave SE, Albany, OR 97322
Laboratory crucibles, refractory metal crucibles of Zirconium, Inconel, Nickel, Tantalum, Molybdenum, and Vanadium from 5ml to 1500ml sizes available.

Nalge Nunc International 800-625-4327
75 Panorama Creek Dr, Rochester, NY 14625
NALGENE premium quality bottles and containers; graduated ware; centrifuge ware; tubing and connectors; test tube racks, and safety products.

Nutech Molding Corporation 1-800-423-5278
PO Box 840, 2024 Broad St,, Pocomoke City, MD 21851

Profex Medical Products 800-325-0196
2224 E Person Ave, Memphis, TN 38114

Quartz Scientific, Inc. 800-229-2186
819 East St, Fairport Harbor, OH 44077

Regis Technologies, Inc. 800-323-8144
8210 Austin Ave, Morton Grove, IL 60053
Supplies and chemicals for chromatography.

Schleicher & Schuell, Inc. 800-245-4024
10 Optical Ave, PO Box 2012, Keene, NH 03431
ELUTRAP, TURBOBLOTTER, MINIFOLD.

Stern Inc., Walter 516-883-9100
68 Sintsink Dr E, P.O. Box 571, Port Washington, NY 11050
Agate mortars and pestles, pipette fillers, sodalime and borosilicate glass balls, rubber bulbs all sizes.

Thermosafe Brands 847-398-0110
3930 N Ventura Dr Ste 450, Arlington Heights, IL 60004

Ward's Natural Science Establishment, Inc. 800-962-2660
PO Box 92912, 5100 W. Henrietta Rd., Rochester, NY 14692

LABWARE, BLOOD COLLECTION *(Chemistry) 75JKA*

Alpha Scientific Corp. 800-242-5989
287 Great Valley Pkwy, Malvern, PA 19355
Diff-safe blood dispenser.

Bd Medical 760-631-6520
4665 North Ave, Oceanside, CA 92056
Various sizes,types of blood collection tubes and accessories.

Becton, Dickinson & Co. 308-872-6811
150 S 1st Ave, Broken Bow, NE 68822
Various sizes and types of blood collection tubes and accessories.

Becton, Dickinson & Co., (Bd) Preanalytical System 201-847-6280
1575 Airport Rd, Sumter, SC 29153
Various sizes and types of blood collection tubes and accessories.

Bio Plas, Inc. 415-472-3777
4340 Redwood Hwy Ste A15, San Rafael, CA 94903
Safety caps for re-capping blood collection tubes; 4 sizes, 7 colors, non-aerosoling.

Biomerieux Inc. 800-682-2666
100 Rodolphe St, Durham, NC 27712

Bionostics, Inc. 978-772-7070
7 Jackson Rd, Devens, MA 01434
Capillary blood collection tubes.

Breg, Inc., An Orthofix Company 800-897-BREG
2611 Commerce Way, Vista, CA 92081
Disposable joint aspiration/injection convenience kit.

Chase Scientific Glass, Inc. 412-490-8425
234 Cardiff Valley Rd, Rockwood, TN 37854
Various blood collection tubes & vials.

LABWARE, BLOOD COLLECTION *(cont'd)*

Covidien Lp 508-261-8000
15 Hampshire St, Mansfield, MA 02048
MONOJECT blood collection products.

Gbf Graphics, Inc. 800-GBF-TEAM
7300 Niles Center Rd, Skokie, IL 60077

Greiner Bio-One North America, Inc. 410-592-2060
4238 Capital Dr, Monroe, NC 28110
Various types & sizes of sterile blood collection tubes.

Hycor Biomedical, Inc. 800-382-2527
7272 Chapman Ave, Garden Grove, CA 92841
Urine centrifuge tube.

Image Molding, Inc. 800-525-1875
4525 Kingston St, Denver, CO 80239
Case of 1000 serum separators.

Immunetech, Inc. 650-470-7420
888 Oak Grove Ave Ste 4, Menlo Park, CA 94025
Blood collection device - k021698.

International Technidyne Corp. 800-631-5945
23 Nevsky St, Edison, NJ 08820

International Technidyne Corporation 732-548-5700
8 Olsen Ave, Edison, NJ 08820
Blood specimen collection device.

Iris Sample Processing 800-782-8774
60 Glacier Dr, Westwood, MA 02090
Various types of tubes, vials, and serum separators.

Kimble Chase Life Science And Research Products, Llc. 865-717-2635
234 Cardiff Valley Rd, Ozone, TN 37854

Medical Action Industries, Inc. 800-645-7042
25 Heywood Rd, Arden, NC 28704
Tube.

Ortho-Clinical Diagnostics, Inc. 800-828-6316
513 Technology Blvd, Rochester, NY 14626
Automated cell washing centrifuge.

Qbc Diagnostics, Inc. 814-342-6205
200 Shadylane Dr, Philipsburg, PA 16866
Micro hematocrit tubes.

Safe-Tec Clinical Products, Inc. 800-356-6033
142 Railroad Dr, Ivyland, PA 18974
SAFECAP self-sealing Mylar-wrapped capillary tube. SAFECAP contains a vented plug that seals automatically on contact with blood, and if accidental breakage occurs, a triple Mylar oven-wrap minimizes exposures.

Sarstedt, Inc. 800-257-5101
PO Box 468, 1025, St. James Church Road, Newton, NC 28658

Teco Diagnostics 714-693-7788
1268 N Lakeview Ave, Anaheim, CA 92807
Vacu lab plain tube and gel/clot activator.

Terumo Medical Corporation 800-283-7866
950 Elkton Blvd, P.O.Box 605, Elkton, MD 21921
Capillary blood collection tubes.

LACTIC DEHYDROGENASE, ANTIGEN, ANTISERUM, CONTROL
(Immunology) 82DET

Beckman Coulter, Inc. 800-742-2345
250 S Kraemer Blvd, PO Box 8000, Brea, CA 92821

LAMINAR AIR FLOW UNIT *(General) 80FLJ*

Aes Clean Technology, Inc. 888-237-2532
422 Stump Rd, Montgomeryville, PA 18936

Air Control, Inc. 252-492-2300
237 Raleigh Rd, Henderson, NC 27536
MICROVOID.

Bio-Safe America Corp. 800-767-4284
3250 S Susan St Ste B, Sterilaire Medical Division
Santa Ana, CA 92704
Class 100 hepa air or laser surgery rooms. Class 100 patient isolator. Class 1000 burn unit. Class 10 prefabricated pharmacy.

Contamination Control Products 877-553-2676
1 3rd Ave # 578, Neptune, NJ 07753
Workstations.

Equilibrated Bio Systems, Inc. 800-327-9490
22 Lawrence Ave Ste LL2, Smithtown, NY 11787
TurboAire Challenger(TM) cold-air bronchial-provocation device.

LAMINAR AIR FLOW UNIT *(cont'd)*

La Calhene 320-358-4713
1325 S Field Ave, PO Box 567, Rush City, MN 55069

Laminar Flow, Inc. 800-553-FLOW
102 Richard Rd, PO Box 2427, Warminster, PA 18974
Horizontal and vertical laminar air flow units.

Liberty Industries, Inc. 800-828-5656
133 Commerce St, East Berlin, CT 06023
Various styles and sizes available.

Lm Air Technology, Inc. 866-381-8200
1467 Pinewood St, Cleanroom & Lab Equipment - Mfger Rahway, NJ 07065
Vertical & Horizontal Laminar flow - Painted, Stainless Steel, Laminated or Polypropylene construction

Microzone Corporation 877-252-7746
86 Harry Douglas Drive, Ottawa, ONT K2S 2C7 Canada

LAMINAR AIR FLOW UNIT, FIXED (AIR CURTAIN)
(Chemistry) 75RDW

Aes Clean Technology, Inc. 888-237-2532
422 Stump Rd, Montgomeryville, PA 18936

Air Control, Inc. 252-492-2300
237 Raleigh Rd, Henderson, NC 27536
MICROVOID.

Bedcolab Ltd. 800-461-6414
2305 Francis Hughes, Laval, QUE H7S 1N5 Canada

Berner International Corp. 800-245-4455
111 Progress Ave, Shenango Commerce Park, New Castle, PA 16101
Air curtains, heated and unheated.

Bio Air Systems Div. 336-299-2885
PO Box 18547, Greensboro, NC 27419
Pricing architectually dependent.

Camfil Farr 800-300-3277
2121 E Paulhan St, Rancho Dominguez, CA 90220
Filter module for cleanroom.

Labconco Corp. 800-821-5525
8811 Prospect Ave, Kansas City, MO 64132
PURIFIER Class II TYPE A2 AND B2 Biolgical Safety Cabinets also includes Clean Benches with vertical and hortizontal laminar flow.

Laminar Flow, Inc. 800-553-FLOW
102 Richard Rd, PO Box 2427, Warminster, PA 18974
99.99% to .03 micron custom built.

Liberty Industries, Inc. 800-828-5656
133 Commerce St, East Berlin, CT 06023
Standard or custom units available.

Mars Air Doors 800-421-1266
14716 S Broadway St, Gardena, CA 90248
HEPAC air curtains with H.E.P.A. air filters to remove air-borne contaminants. Heated and unheated air curtains. To repel insects, dust and odors, and seal in heated or refrigerated air. Save energy. WINDGUARD heavy duty industrial air curtains. Heated and unheated air curtains. For oversize doorways to save energy usage, repel wind up to 30 MPH and maximize employee comfort and productivity. Also available ARES - Air Replacement Engeneered System.

Nuaire, Inc. 800-328-3352
2100 Fernbrook Ln N, Plymouth, MN 55447

Purified Micro Environments, Div. Of Germfree Laboratories 800-888-5357
11 Aviator Way, Ormond Beach, FL 32174

LAMINAR AIR FLOW UNIT, MOBILE *(Chemistry) 75RDX*

Aes Clean Technology, Inc. 888-237-2532
422 Stump Rd, Montgomeryville, PA 18936

Air Control, Inc. 252-492-2300
237 Raleigh Rd, Henderson, NC 27536
MICROVOID.

Berner International Corp. 800-245-4455
111 Progress Ave, Shenango Commerce Park, New Castle, PA 16101
MAXAIR, universally designed to fit virtually any opening, the 7 1/2' high MAXAIR air door will protect your lowest concession window to your 8' high doorway. Adjustable motor speed, precision built cross-flow fans allow for best seal available today. Low sound levels, available unheated or w/ optional electric, steam and hot water heating coils. Aluminum construction, light weight, will not fade or discolor.

LAMINAR AIR FLOW UNIT, MOBILE *(cont'd)*

Laminar Flow, Inc. 800-553-FLOW
102 Richard Rd, PO Box 2427, Warminster, PA 18974
99.99% to .03 micron - custom built.

Liberty Industries, Inc. 800-828-5656
133 Commerce St, East Berlin, CT 06023
$4K TO 10K per unit (standard). Custom units available.

Purified Micro Environments, Div. Of Germfree Laboratories 800-888-5357
11 Aviator Way, Ormond Beach, FL 32174

LAMP, ENDOSCOPIC, INCANDESCENT *(Surgery) 79FTI*

Bulbtronics, Inc. 800-624-2852
45 Banfi Plz N, Farmingdale, NY 11735

Bulbworks, Inc. 800-334-2852
80 N Dell Ave Unit 5, Kenvil, NJ 07847
Replacement Lamps For All Types Of Endoscope Equipment

Cameron-Miller, Inc. 800-621-0142
5410 W Roosevelt Rd, Road #241, Chicago, IL 60644

Caprock Developments Inc. 800-222-0325
475 Speedwell Ave, PO Box 95, Morris Plains, NJ 07950

Carley Lamps 310-325-8474
1502 W 228th St, Torrance, CA 90501

Electro Surgical Instrument Co., Inc. 888-464-2784
37 Centennial St, Rochester, NY 14611
Miniature and subminiature lamps in various types, styles, sizes and light outpu.

Karl Storz Endoscopy-America Inc. 800-421-0837
600 Corporate Pointe, Culver City, CA 90230

Lamp Technology, Inc. 800-533-7548
1645 Sycamore Ave, Bohemia, NY 11716

Mahe International Inc. 800-294-7946
468 Craighead St, Nashville, TN 37204

Rei Rotolux Enterprises, Inc. 888-773-7611
4145 North Service Rd, Ste. 200, Burlington, ON L7L 6A3 Canada
Halogen light source.

Richard Wolf Medical Instruments Corp. 800-323-9653
353 Corporate Woods Pkwy, Vernon Hills, IL 60061

LAMP, EXAMINATION (LIGHT) *(General) 80RDZ*

Adjustable Fixture Co. 800-558-2628
3726 N Booth St, Milwaukee, WI 53212
NIGHTINGALE TRU-LIGHT, color-correction for minor procedures. 3 year warranty. Sold through medical dealers. NIGHTINGALE, deluxe examination lamps stay cool to the touch. 3 year warranty. Sold through medical dealers. EXAMLIGHT OB/GYN, examination light whiter, brighter light safest, easiest for pelvic exams. Long life halogen cycle bulb, maintenance-free.

Berchtold Corp. 800-243-5135
1950 Hanahan Rd, Charleston, SC 29406

Brandt Industries, Inc. 800-221-8031
4461 Bronx Blvd, Bronx, NY 10470
Exam lamps: mobile, stationary. Incandescent, fluorescent. Halogen. Woods lights. Illuminated magnifiers.

Bulbtronics, Inc. 800-624-2852
45 Banfi Plz N, Farmingdale, NY 11735

Bulbworks, Inc. 800-334-2852
80 N Dell Ave Unit 5, Kenvil, NJ 07847
Replacement Lamps For All Types Of Examination Lights

Burton Medical Products, Inc. 800-444-9909
21100 Lassen St, Chatsworth, CA 91311
Available are NOVA exam light and GLEAMER procedure light.

Cameron-Miller, Inc. 800-621-0142
5410 W Roosevelt Rd, Road #241, Chicago, IL 60644

Cantylight 716-625-4227
6100 Donner Rd, Lockport, NY 14094

Clinimed, Incorporated 877-CLINIMED
303 Markus Ct, Sandy Brae Industrial Park, Newark, DE 19713

Crest Healthcare Supply 800-328-8908
195 3rd St, Dassel, MN 55325

Dazor Manufacturing Corp. 800-345-9103
11721 Dunlap Industrial Dr, Maryland Heights, MO 63043
Medical inspection lamps, desk lamps, etc. can be viewed and m.s.r.p. pricing found at www.dazor.com and our video microscope, the speckFINDER at www.speckfinder.com

Elmed, Inc. 630-543-2792
60 W Fay Ave, Addison, IL 60101

LAMP, EXAMINATION (LIGHT) *(cont'd)*

Florida Life Systems 727-321-9554
3446 5th Ave N, Saint Petersburg, FL 33713

Galaxy Medical Manufacturing Co. 800-876-4599
5411 Sheila St, Commerce, CA 90040

Goodwin Manufacturing, Inc. 800-282-5267
6980 Pikeview Dr, PO Box 5981, Thomasville, NC 27360
$259.95 for Model #1179, $259.95 for mobile Model #1183-CB, other models from $200.00.

Hill-Rom Holdings, Inc. 800-445-3730
1069 State Road 46 E, Batesville, IN 47006

Independent Solutions, Inc. 847-498-0500
900 Skokie Blvd Ste 118, Northbrook, IL 60062
VISTA or BURTON ceiling mounted or track mounted or wall mounted or portable or headwall mounted or console mounted. UL listed.

Jedmed Instruments Co. 314-845-3770
5416 Jedmed Ct, Saint Louis, MO 63129

Kadan Co. Inc., D.A. 800-325-2326
1 Brigadoon Ln, Waxhaw, NC 28173

Lic Care 800-323-5232
2935A Northeast Pkwy, Atlanta, GA 30360

Mayo Medical, S.A. De C.V. 800-715-3872
Edison 1141 Nte., Col. Talleres, Monterrey N.L. 64480 Mexico
Stainless steel and chrome, goose-neck lamp.

Md International, Inc. 305-669-9003
11300 NW 41st St, Doral, FL 33178

Meddev Corporation 800-543-2789
730 N Pastoria Ave, Sunnyvale, CA 94085
MULTARRAY HALOGEN EXAMINATION LIGHT general purpose/minor surgical procedure halogen light incorporates a patented, computer designed array reflector. Available in floorstand, tablemount, and wall-mounting models.

Medical Illumination International 800-831-1222
547 Library St, San Fernando, CA 91340
Centry diagnostic/exam lights, MED-LITE 13 inch reflector; Med-Exam 11 inch reflector; Versalite exam light

Medical Innovations International Inc. 507-289-0761
6256 34th Ave NW, Rochester, MN 55901
Rochester Patient Exam Light™.

Midmark Corporation 800-643-6275
60 Vista Dr, P.O. Box 286, Versailles, OH 45380

Pibbs Inc., P.S. 718-445-8046
133-15 32nd Ave., Flushing, NY 11354-4008

Roldan Products Corp. 866-922-6800
448 Sovereign Ct, Ballwin, MO 63011
$158.00 per unit (standard) and $122.00 for incandescent examination light.

Schueler & Company, Inc. 516-487-1500
PO Box 528, Stratford, CT 06615

Skytron 800-759-8766
5085 Corporate Exchange Blvd SE, Grand Rapids, MI 49512
Wall- or stand-mounted, Model ST9

Spectronics Corporation 800-274-8888
956 Brush Hollow Rd, Westbury, NY 11590

Sunnex, Inc. 800-445-7869
3 Huron Dr, Natick, MA 01760

Swivelier Co., Inc. 845-353-1455
600 Bradley Hill Rd, Blauvelt, NY 10913

Vista Lighting 800-576-2135
1805 Pittsburgh Ave, Erie, PA 16502

Waldmann Lighting 800-634-0007
9 Century Dr, Wheeling, IL 60090
Halux R 35/2 FX dual spot & flood task light. Halux 50 SX with flexible gooseneck arm.

Welch Allyn, Inc. 800-535-6663
4341 State Street Rd, Skaneateles Falls, NY 13153
LS100 Examination Light Features; halogen light (low-voltage); available with bench, wall or mobile stands.

LAMP, EXAMINATION, CEILING MOUNTED (LIGHT) *(General) 80TCY*

Berchtold Corp. 800-243-5135
1950 Hanahan Rd, Charleston, SC 29406

Burton Medical Products, Inc. 800-444-9909
21100 Lassen St, Chatsworth, CA 91311

LAMP, EXAMINATION, CEILING MOUNTED (LIGHT) *(cont'd)*

Cantylight 716-625-4227
6100 Donner Rd, Lockport, NY 14094

Elmed, Inc. 630-543-2792
60 W Fay Ave, Addison, IL 60101

Florida Life Systems 727-321-9554
3446 5th Ave N, Saint Petersburg, FL 33713

Independent Solutions, Inc. 847-498-0500
900 Skokie Blvd Ste 118, Northbrook, IL 60062
BURTON single or multihead; direct ceiling or track mounted. UL listed.

O&M Enterprise 847-258-4515
641 Chelmsford Ln, Elk Grove Village, IL 60007
LAMP EXAMINATION

Schueler & Company, Inc. 516-487-1500
PO Box 528, Stratford, CT 06615

Skytron 800-759-8766
5085 Corporate Exchange Blvd SE, Grand Rapids, MI 49512
Model ST9 4,200 ea fc single or dual lightheads.

Sunnex, Inc. 800-445-7869
3 Huron Dr, Natick, MA 01760

Vista Lighting 800-576-2135
1805 Pittsburgh Ave, Erie, PA 16502

Waldmann Lighting 800-634-0007
9 Century Dr, Wheeling, IL 60090
Halux Eydite 1050 DM with dimmer. Halux 50DM with 2-step switch.

LAMP, FLUORESCEIN, AC-POWERED *(Surgery) 79HJE*

Bulbtronics, Inc. 800-624-2852
45 Banfi Plz N, Farmingdale, NY 11735
Fluorescent lamp.

Welch Allyn, Inc. 800-535-6663
4341 State Street Rd, Skaneateles Falls, NY 13153

LAMP, HEAT *(General) 80FOI*

Bulbtronics, Inc. 800-624-2852
45 Banfi Plz N, Farmingdale, NY 11735

Bulbworks, Inc. 800-334-2852
80 N Dell Ave Unit 5, Kenvil, NJ 07847
Replacement Lamps For All Types Of Heat Lamps

LAMP, INFRARED *(Physical Med) 89ILY*

Amest Corp. 949-766-9692
30394 Esperanza, Rancho Santa Margarita, CA 92688
Ir radiator.

Anodyne Medical Technologies, Inc 340-772-2846
RR 2 Box 9905, Bldg 2, Kingshill, VI 00850
Heat therapy system.

Anodyne Therapy, Llc 813-645-2855
13570 Wright Cir, Tampa, FL 33626
Heat therapy system.

Astron Dental Corporation 847-726-8787
815 Oakwood Rd Ste G, Lake Zurich, IL 60047
Heat lamp unit.

Atlantis Luminescent Products, Llc 318-894-9490
1405 W Pinhook Rd Ste 205, Lafayette, LA 70503
Infrared lamp.

Avicenna Laser Technology, Inc. 561-722-1153
1209 N Flagler Dr, West Palm Beach, FL 33401
Alt infrared laser.

Bhk, Inc. 909-983-2973
1480 N Claremont Blvd, Claremont, CA 91711
Maxir II infrared grey-body source offered with either sapphire or zinc selenide windows.

Brandt Industries, Inc. 800-221-8031
4461 Bronx Blvd, Bronx, NY 10470
Many varieties.

Bulbtronics, Inc. 800-624-2852
45 Banfi Plz N, Farmingdale, NY 11735

Bulbworks, Inc. 800-334-2852
80 N Dell Ave Unit 5, Kenvil, NJ 07847
Replacement Lamps For All Types Of Infrared Equipment

Caprock Developments Inc. 800-222-0325
475 Speedwell Ave, PO Box 95, Morris Plains, NJ 07950
Short and medium wave

Carley Lamps 310-325-8474
1502 W 228th St, Torrance, CA 90501

LAMP, INFRARED *(cont'd)*

Computerized Thermal Imaging Co. 801-776-4700
1719 W 2800 S, Ogden, UT 84401
Infrared lamp.

Curae'Lase Inc. 843-455-7020
2315 Highway 701 S, Loris, SC 29569
Infrared lamp.

Cutera, Inc. 888-4-CUTERA
3240 Bayshore Blvd, Brisbane, CA 94005
Aesthetic.

Diomedics, Inc. 888-972-4699
342 SE 35th St, Keystone Heights, FL 32656
Infrared heat lamp.

Dynatronics Corp. 800-874-6251
7030 Park Centre Dr, Salt Lake City, UT 84121

Eraser Company, Inc. 800-724-0594
123 Oliva Dr, Mattydale, NY 13211
LUXTHERM infrared heating tools provide cleanroom heat for heat-shrink tubing applications and sealing requirements.

Huntington Mechanical Laboratories, Inc. 800-227-8059
1040 La Avenida St, Mountain View, CA 94043

Io Laser, Inc. 407-296-0544
6140 Edgewater Dr Ste B, Orlando, FL 32810
Infrared, laser.

J. H. Emerson Co. 800-252-1414
22 Cottage Park Ave, Cambridge, MA 02140
Heat lamp.

Jenex Corporation 800-496-4682
733 Overlook Dr, Alliance, OH 44601
Thermal therapy for the relief of insect stings and bites.

Kbd, Inc. 859-331-0800
2550 American Ct, Erlanger, KY 41017
Various models and sizes of sunlamps.

Laser Neurotherapy Development Labs, Inc.
5061 N 30th St Ste 105, Colorado Springs, CO 80919
Therapeutic laser system.

Life Without Pain, Llc 954-786-0007
4600 140th Ave N Ste 190, Clearwater, FL 33762
Various types of infrared lamps.

Litecure, Llc 302-709-0408
930 Old Harmony Rd Ste A, Newark, DE 19713
Infrared lamp.

Mettler Electronics Corp. 800-854-9305
1333 S Claudina St, Anaheim, CA 92805
*Low Level Laser Therapy, LLLT, Laser Sys*Stim 540 with 785 nm laser applicator $4,995, optional SLD/LED cluster applicator, $895.*

New Star Lasers, Inc. 916-677-1900
9085 Foothills Blvd, Roseville, CA 95747
Infrared heat lamp.

Photoactif 480-827-1212
7211 E Southern Ave Ste C-110, Mesa, AZ 85209
Led phototherapy.

Quantum Devices, Inc. 608-924-3000
112 E Orbison St, Barneveld, WI 53507
Quantum warp 10 light delivery system.

Research, Inc. 952-941-3300
7128 Shady Oak Rd, Eden Prairie, MN 55344

Rich-Mar Corporation 800-762-4665
PO Box 879, 15499 E 590 Rd, Inola, OK 74036
$1799 for the AutoPrism Light Therapy device

Silver Bay, Llc 941-306-5812
1431 Tallevast Rd, Sarasota, FL 34243
Infrared heat lamp.

Tridien Medical 954-340-0500
4200 NW 120th Ave, Coral Springs, FL 33065
ANODYNE THERAPY SYSTEM

LAMP, LARYNGOSCOPE *(Ear/Nose/Throat) 77SHF*

Bulbworks, Inc. 800-334-2852
80 N Dell Ave Unit 5, Kenvil, NJ 07847
Replacement Lamps For All Types Of Laryngoscopes

LAMP, LARYNGOSCOPE *(cont'd)*

Carley Lamps 310-325-8474
1502 W 228th St, Torrance, CA 90501
Introducing the new Mediflector® brand medical lamp designed and patented by Carley Lamps. Delivering a minimum of 100% greater light output compared to traditional lamps for Fiberoptic layrngoscopes and other hand held diagnostic instruments. By incorporating a miniature reflector that intercepts and refocuses light normally lost by spherical radiation into a precise spot for unparalleled light intensity, uniformity and repeatability - all accomplished with no increase in wattage, heat generation or battery drain.

Sunmed Healthcare 727-531-7266
12393 Belcher Rd S Ste 460, Largo, FL 33773

LAMP, MICROSCOPE *(Pathology) 88KEG*

Bulbtronics, Inc. 800-624-2852
45 Banfi Plz N, Farmingdale, NY 11735

Bulbworks, Inc. 800-334-2852
80 N Dell Ave Unit 5, Kenvil, NJ 07847
Replacement Lamps For All Types Of Microscopes

C & A Scientific Co. Inc. 703-330-1413
7241 Gabe Ct, Manassas, VA 20109
Whole line of monocular & binocular microscopes.

Caprock Developments Inc. 800-222-0325
475 Speedwell Ave, PO Box 95, Morris Plains, NJ 07950
Including halogen, incandescnt, short arc mercury and xenon

Carl Zeiss Surgical, Inc. 800-442-4020
1 Zeiss Dr, Thornwood, NY 10594

Chiu Technical Corp. 631-544-0606
252 Indian Head Rd, Kings Park, NY 11754
$158.00 HG 100DM.

Edmund Industrial Optics 800-363-1992
101 E Gloucester Pike, Barrington, NJ 08007

Lamp Technology, Inc. 800-533-7548
1645 Sycamore Ave, Bohemia, NY 11716

Nikon Instruments Inc. 800-52-Nikon
1300 Walt Whitman Rd, Melville, NY 11747

Olympus America, Inc. 800-645-8160
3500 Corporate Pkwy, PO Box 610, Center Valley, PA 18034

Thermo Oriel 800-715-393
150 Long Beach Blvd, Stratford, CT 06615

Unitron Ltd 631-589-6666
120 Wilbur Pl Ste C, Bohemia, NY 11716

Western Scientific Co., Inc. 877-489-3726
4104 24th St # 183, San Francisco, CA 94114
Complete line of microscope lamps.

LAMP, NON-HEATING, FOR ADJUNCTIVE USE IN PAIN THERAPY *(Physical Med) 89NHN*

A Major Difference, Inc. 303-755-0112
2950 S Jamaica Ct Ste 300, Aurora, CO 80014
Low level laser therapy.

Em-Probe Inc. 360-297-6858
4110 Ne Carver Dr., Port Gamble, WA 98364
Non-heating infrared lamp.

Erchonia Medical 214-733-5209
2021 Commerce Dr, McKinney, TX 75069
Light therapy device.

Medical Laser Systems Inc 203-481-2395
20 Baldwin Dr, Branford, CT 06405
Infrared laser,low level laser therapy device.

Stargate International, Inc. 303-840-8206
10235 S Progress Way Unit 7, Parker, CO 80134
Light therapy system.

LAMP, OPERATING ROOM *(General) 80FQP*

Aculux, Inc. 239-643-8023
4424 Corporate Sq, Naples, FL 34104
Xenon fiberoptic illuminator, headlamp & cables.

Ams Innovative Center-San Jose 800-356-7600
3070 Orchard Dr, San Jose, CA 95134

Berchtold Corp. 800-243-5135
1950 Hanahan Rd, Charleston, SC 29406
Remote-controlled surgical lighthead for positioning from the sterile field. ENDOLITE switches from general surgical lighting to low-level ambient lighting.

LAMP, OPERATING ROOM *(cont'd)*

Bulbman, Inc. 800-648-1163
630 Sunshine Ln, Reno, NV 89502

Bulbtronics, Inc. 800-624-2852
45 Banfi Plz N, Farmingdale, NY 11735

Bulbworks, Inc. 800-334-2852
80 N Dell Ave Unit 5, Kenvil, NJ 07847
Replacement Lamps For All Types Of Operatory Lights

Burton Medical Products, Inc. 800-444-9909
21100 Lassen St, Chatsworth, CA 91311
Available is GENESIS operating light. Genesis Plus and Genie Plus.

International Hospital Supply Co. 800-398-9450
6914 Canby Ave Ste 105, Reseda, CA 91335

Medical Illumination International 800-831-1222
547 Library St, San Fernando, CA 91340
SYSTEM ONE Surgery lights- Models S2 (20'), S1 Satellite(16'), P1 Video Camera, Centurion Excel surgery light; CENTURION 15' minor surgery light.

Waldmann Lighting 800-634-0007
9 Century Dr, Wheeling, IL 60090
Halux 35/2 FX dual spot and flood task light. Halux 50 SX with flexible gooseneck arm. ISIS minor surgery light.

LAMP, OTHER *(General) 80REF*

Adjustable Fixture Co. 800-558-2628
3726 N Booth St, Milwaukee, WI 53212
BRASS N' COLOR, table/floor lighting with DURA-HARP for multi-housing; SPACESAVER, cabinet-mount lamp; NIGHTINGALE, table, floor and wall lamps; POLYLAMP, table lamps; POLYLAST and FIBER-LAST, shades for multi-housing. 5 year warranty. Sold factory direct to user.

American Diagnostic Corporation (Adc) 800-232-2670
55 Commerce Dr, Hauppauge, NY 11788
Replacement lamps for handheld diagnostic instruments

Bhk, Inc. 909-983-2973
1480 N Claremont Blvd, Claremont, CA 91711
Low-pressure mercury lamps, phosphor-coated mercury lamps, mercury grid lamps, zinc and cadmium lamps, rare-gas lamps (argon, neon, krypton, xenon), infrared lamps.

Boekel Scientific 800-336-6929
855 Pennsylvania Blvd, Feasterville Trevose, PA 19053
Alcohol lamp.

Brandt Industries, Inc. 800-221-8031
4461 Bronx Blvd, Bronx, NY 10470
Low-vision lights, Perineal heater.

Bulbtronics, Inc. 800-624-2852
45 Banfi Plz N, Farmingdale, NY 11735
Deuterium and hollow cathode lamps.

Bulbworks, Inc. 800-334-2852
80 N Dell Ave Unit 5, Kenvil, NJ 07847
All Types Of Specialty Lamps, Including Quartz Halogen, Mercury Arc, Xenon, Incandescent, Fluorescent, Metal Halide And Others.

Caprock Developments Inc. 800-222-0325
475 Speedwell Ave, PO Box 95, Morris Plains, NJ 07950
For all specialty applications

Carley Lamps 310-325-8474
1502 W 228th St, Torrance, CA 90501
Hi-intensity sub-miniature lamps, vacuum or gas filled. Direct sales to OEMs, hospitals and distributors. Aluminum reflectors are custom made reflectors to be used with carley lamps to create light sources for laryngoscopes, flashlights, etc.

Cole-Parmer Instrument Inc. 800-323-4340
625 E Bunker Ct, Vernon Hills, IL 60061

Concepts International, Inc. 800-627-9729
224 E Main St, Summerton, SC 29148
Fluorescent safe lights.

Dazor Manufacturing Corp. 800-345-9103
11721 Dunlap Industrial Dr, Maryland Heights, MO 63043
Illuminated magnifiers and video microscope can be viewed at www.dazor.com and at www.speckfinder.com.

Goodwin Manufacturing, Inc. 800-282-5267
6980 Pikeview Dr, PO Box 5981, Thomasville, NC 27360
Floor and table lamps with and without magnification, from $150 to $350.

Hanovia Specialty Lighting Llc 800-229-3666
825 Lehigh Ave, Union, NJ 07083
$500.00 per unit.

LAMP, OTHER *(cont'd)*

Kadan Co. Inc., D.A. 800-325-2326
1 Brigadoon Ln, Waxhaw, NC 28173

Lamp Technology, Inc. 800-533-7548
1645 Sycamore Ave, Bohemia, NY 11716
Microscope, scientific, precision optical, miniature and subminiature lamps from BLV, Chicago Miniature, GE, Illumination Industries, Lamp Technology, Norelco, Osram, Philips, Sylvania, Taunuslicht, Thorn and Tungsram.

Luxo Corporation 800-222-5896
200 Clearbrook Rd, Elmsford, NY 10523

Medical Illumination International 800-831-1222
547 Library St, San Fernando, CA 91340
Centura variable spotlights in wall, floor, single or dual ceiling, as well as in ChuttleTrak mounts, MEDI-SPOT variable spotlights in floor, wall mount, single and dual ceiling mount and flexi/glide ceiling track mounts.

National Biological Corp. 800-338-5045
1532 Enterprise Pkwy, Twinsburg, OH 44087
HANDISOL UVA and/or UVB hand-held phototherapy system.

Roldan Products Corp. 866-922-6800
448 Sovereign Ct, Ballwin, MO 63011
$135 for halogen low voltage lamp and $107 for fluorescent desk lamp. DAZOR 6950 $150.00 Standard halogen low voltage 20W with bulb, 31' flexible arm, magnetic base holds 100 lbs of straight pull on 1' steel, mounts instantly on any steel wall (plate) or equipment.

Second Source, The 800-776-3924
1480 N Claremont Blvd, Claremont, CA 91711
Replacement lamps for a variety of applications including gas chromatographs, atomic absorbtion, HPLC, colorimeters, fluorometers, and more.

Spectronics Corporation 800-274-8888
956 Brush Hollow Rd, Westbury, NY 11590
SPECTROLINE model Q-22 ultraviolet/white light magnifier lamp has a whole spectrum of fluorescence analysis applications, including medical diagnosis, ophthalmology, dermatology, nondestructive testing, quality control and detection of repairs.

Sunnex, Inc. 800-445-7869
3 Huron Dr, Natick, MA 01760
Halogen bed/reading lamps.

Thermo Fisher Scientific Inc. 781-622-1000
81 Wyman St, Waltham, MA 02451
Halogen lamps for BM/Hitachi chemistry analyzers. ALKO halogen lamps for Hitachi are validated for the following instrument models: Hitachi 704, 717, 736, 737, 747, 902, 911, 914, 917.

Ushio America, Inc. 800-838-7446
5440 Cerritos Ave, Cypress, CA 90630
Xenon lamps for fluorescence microscopy. Ceramic xenon and halogen lamps for fiber-optic illuminators. Germicidal (UV-C), blacklight, and blacklight blue (UV-A and UV-B) for sterilization, inspection, and analysis.

Waldmann Lighting 800-634-0007
9 Century Dr, Wheeling, IL 60090
Omnivue Magnifier with dual illumination levels. RLLE-122 ring magnifier. SNE-136 for broad-range illumination.

Ware Medics Glass Works, Inc. 845-429-6950
PO Box 368, Garnerville, NY 10923
Alcohol lamp.

Woodhead L.P. 847-272-7990
3411 Woodhead Dr, Northbrook, IL 60062
Portable hand lamp.

LAMP, SLIDE WARMING *(Pathology) 88IEH*

Barnstead International 412-490-8425
2555 Kerper Blvd, Dubuque, IA 52001
Lamps.

LAMP, SLIT *(Ophthalmology) 86REC*

Allergan 800-366-6554
2525 Dupont Dr, Irvine, CA 92612
Slit lamp attachments: beam sputter, video adapter & tubes.

Biomedics, Inc. 949-458-1998
23322 Peralta Dr Ste 11, Laguna Hills, CA 92653
ZEISS, COHERENT, ETC

Bulbtronics, Inc. 800-624-2852
45 Banfi Plz N, Farmingdale, NY 11735

LAMP, SLIT *(cont'd)*

Burton Co., R.H. 800-848-0410
3965 Brookham Dr, Grove City, OH 43123
Four models available: $2,795.00 for #825, $2,995.00 for #850, $3,850.00 for #2000, and imaging from $5,200.

Caprock Developments Inc. 800-222-0325
475 Speedwell Ave, PO Box 95, Morris Plains, NJ 07950

Carl Zeiss Meditec Inc. 877-486-7473
5160 Hacienda Dr, Dublin, CA 94568
ZEISS SL 120 SLIT LAMP The Zeiss SL 120 Slit Lamp offers improved optical design and optimum opterating parameters. Light efficiency has improved by 20%. Higher resolution facilitates recognition of ocular details while increasing image contrast. A 20-degree tiltable prism eases gonioscopic and fundus examinations. The SL 120 is ideal for video documentation and fluorescein observation.

Carl Zeiss Surgical, Inc. 800-442-4020
1 Zeiss Dr, Thornwood, NY 10594

Iridex Corporation 800-388-4747
1212 Terra Bella Ave, Mountain View, CA 94043
Slit lamp adapters with and without micromanipulators. Available for IR and visible product lines. Multi-fiber and large-spot-size versions also available.

LAMP, SLIT, BIOMICROSCOPE, AC-POWERED *(Ophthalmology) 86HJO*

Bulbtronics, Inc. 800-624-2852
45 Banfi Plz N, Farmingdale, NY 11735

Carl Zeiss Meditec Inc. 877-486-7473
5160 Hacienda Dr, Dublin, CA 94568
Ultrasound Biomicroscope - The Humphrey Ultrasound Biomicroscope is a breakthrough technology that offers an expansive view of the anterior segment of the eye with unmatched clarity and resolution. Proprietary software is icon-based and user-friendly. Output data can be formatted for use in MS-DOS based graphics programs.

Hai Laboratories, Inc. 781-862-9884
320 Massachusetts Ave, Lexington, MA 02420
Slit lamp microscope.

Marco Ophthalmic, Inc. 800-874-5274
11825 Central Pkwy, Jacksonville, FL 32224
7 models priced at $4,595.00, $5,695.00, $5,860.00, $4,250.00, and $7,225.00. (List prices)

Nidek, Inc. 510-226-5700
47651 Westinghouse Dr, Fremont, CA 94539
Slit lamp.

Ocumetrics, Inc. 650-960-3955
2224 Old Middlefield Way Ste C, Mountain View, CA 94043
Ocular fluorophotometer.

Paradigm Medical Industries, Inc. 801-977-8970
2355 S 1070 W, Salt Lake City, UT 84119
Biomicroscope, slit-lamp, ac-powered.

Reichert, Inc. 888-849-8955
3362 Walden Ave, Depew, NY 14043
XCEL Slit Lamp. Reichert offers a full line of XCEL slit lamps with a complete range of styles and features.

Topcon Medical Systems, Inc. 800-223-1130
37 W Century Rd, Paramus, NJ 07652
Six models of slit lamps: $3,490.00 and $6,890.00 for traditional models; $4,990.00, $6,590.00, $8,690.00, and $9,990.00 for digital-ready models. Optional integrated digital camera attachment: $3,290.00.

Visx Incorporated, A Subsidiary Of Amo Inc. 714-247-8656
1328 Kifer Rd, Sunnyvale, CA 94086
Acpowered slit lamp bimicroscope.

Woodlyn, Inc. 800-331-7389
2920 Malmo Dr, Ophthalmic Instruments and Equipment
Arlington Heights, IL 60005
Model HRI. The Woodlyn HR-1 Slit Lamp features high resolution and consistent quality. Halogen illumination, single joystick controlling both horizontal and vertical movements, and a microscope providing a wide field of view. Call for current prices.

LAMP, SUN, INCANDESCENT *(General) 80REB*

Bulbtronics, Inc. 800-624-2852
45 Banfi Plz N, Farmingdale, NY 11735

LAMP, SURGICAL *(Surgery) 79FTD*

Alkco Lighting Co. 847-451-0700
11500 Melrose Ave, Franklin Park, IL 60131
For minor surgical/outpatient procedures.

Berchtold Corp. 800-243-5135
1950 Hanahan Rd, Charleston, SC 29406

Bulbtronics, Inc. 800-624-2852
45 Banfi Plz N, Farmingdale, NY 11735

Burton Medical Products, Inc. 800-444-9909
21100 Lassen St, Chatsworth, CA 91311

Carley Lamps 310-325-8474
1502 W 228th St, Torrance, CA 90501

Elmed, Inc. 630-543-2792
60 W Fay Ave, Addison, IL 60101

Enova Medical Technologies 866-773-0539
1839 Buerkle Rd, Saint Paul, MN 55110
Halo Cordless LED Surgical Headlight. Battery powered with LED bulbs for use in the O/R.

Md International, Inc. 305-669-9003
11300 NW 41st St, Doral, FL 33178

Medical Illumination International 800-831-1222
547 Library St, San Fernando, CA 91340
SYSTEM ONE S2, S1 surgery lights and P1 video camera; Centurion Excel 16' surgery light, and CENTURION 15' minor surgery light

Qed, Inc. 859-231-0338
750 Enterprise Dr, Lexington, KY 40510
Maxenon.

Skytron 800-759-8766
5085 Corporate Exchange Blvd SE, Grand Rapids, MI 49512
Aurora LED Surgical Light avialable in 18 models featuring state-of-the-art Light Emitting Diode technology and color selection of 4000K (Soft White) or 4500K (Bright white) with excellent shadow control. LED Pod life exceeds 10 years of illumination retaining 90% of intensity. single, dual or triple ceiling-mounted lightheads. Aurora LED uses less than 1/2 the energy to power vs. traditional halogen systems. Extremely energy efficient High Intensity, Bright,Focusable and Cool Surgical Lighting for every procedure.

Smith & Nephew Inc. 800-463-7439
2100 52nd Ave., Lachine, QUE H8T 2Y5 Canada

Steris Corporation 800-884-9550
5960 Heisley Rd, Mentor, OH 44060

Stryker Puerto Rico, Ltd. 939-307-2500
Hwy. 3, Km. 131.2, Las Guasimas Ind. Park, Arroyo, PR 00714
Knife.

Welch Allyn, Inc. 800-535-6663
4341 State Street Rd, Skaneateles Falls, NY 13153

Xodus Medical, Inc. 800-963-8776
702 Prominence Dr, Westmoreland Business & Research Park
New Kensington, PA 15068
Light Handle Covers

LAMP, SURGICAL, INCANDESCENT *(Surgery) 79GBC*

Boehm Surgical Instrument Corp. 716-436-6584
966 Chili Ave, Rochester, NY 14611
Lamp surgical incandescent, miniature.

Brandt Industries, Inc. 800-221-8031
4461 Bronx Blvd, Bronx, NY 10470
Minor surgery lights.

Jedmed Instruments Co. 314-845-3770
5416 Jedmed Ct, Saint Louis, MO 63129

Lamp Technology, Inc. 800-533-7548
1645 Sycamore Ave, Bohemia, NY 11716

LAMP, SURGICAL, XENON *(Surgery) 79FTB*

Biomedics, Inc. 949-458-1998
23322 Peralta Dr Ste 11, Laguna Hills, CA 92653

Bulbtronics, Inc. 800-624-2852
45 Banfi Plz N, Farmingdale, NY 11735

Caprock Developments Inc. 800-222-0325
475 Speedwell Ave, PO Box 95, Morris Plains, NJ 07950

Carley Lamps 310-325-8474
1502 W 228th St, Torrance, CA 90501

Chiu Technical Corp. 631-544-0606
252 Indian Head Rd, Kings Park, NY 11754
$1,130.00 X150T.

Endoscopy Support Services, Inc. 800-349-3636
3 Fallsview Ln, Brewster, NY 10509

LAMP, SURGICAL, XENON *(cont'd)*

Lamp Technology, Inc. 800-533-7548
1645 Sycamore Ave, Bohemia, NY 11716

Sunoptic Technologies 877-677-2832
6018 Bowdendale Ave, Jacksonville, FL 32216
High intensity projectors for fiberoptics, several models of Quartz Halogen, Metal Halide, and Xenon lightsources available.

Transamerican Technologies International 800-322-7373
2246 Camino Ramon, San Ramon, CA 94583
ACCU-BEAM Flash Tubes for Carl Zeiss fundus cameras.

Ushio America, Inc. 800-838-7446
5440 Cerritos Ave, Cypress, CA 90630
Xenon and halogen lamps for overhead surgical lights.

LAMP, ULTRAVIOLET (SPECTRUM A) *(General) 80REE*

Bhk, Inc. 909-983-2973
1480 N Claremont Blvd, Claremont, CA 91711

Brevis Corp. 800-383-3377
225 W 2855 S, Salt Lake City, UT 84115
GlitterBug® Handwash Product Line

Bulbtronics, Inc. 800-624-2852
45 Banfi Plz N, Farmingdale, NY 11735

Caprock Developments Inc. 800-222-0325
475 Speedwell Ave, PO Box 95, Morris Plains, NJ 07950

Harry J. Bosworth Company 800-323-4352
7227 Hamlin Ave, Skokie, IL 60076
CURE ALL Light Curing Unit, UVA light curing unit specially designed for custom trays. Cleans easily with a soft cloth and alcohol.

Ultra-Lum, Inc. 800-809-6559
1480 N Claremont Blvd, Claremont, CA 91711
UVA Ultraviolet Lamps.

LAMP, ULTRAVIOLET, GERMICIDAL *(General) 80RED*

Atlantic Ultraviolet Corp. 631-273-0500
375 Marcus Blvd, Hauppauge, NY 11788
STER-L-RAY 11 fixture types, lamp models.

Bhk, Inc. 909-983-2973
1480 N Claremont Blvd, Claremont, CA 91711
Standard and custom 'pencil'-style mercury lamps for a wide range of applications from sterilization to process-thickness applications.

Bulbtronics, Inc. 800-624-2852
45 Banfi Plz N, Farmingdale, NY 11735

Bulbworks, Inc. 800-334-2852
80 N Dell Ave Unit 5, Kenvil, NJ 07847
Replacement Lamps For All Types Of Equipment Using Germicidal Bulbs

Burton Medical Products, Inc. 800-444-9909
21100 Lassen St, Chatsworth, CA 91311
Burten Ultraviolet (Woods) Lamp

Caprock Developments Inc. 800-222-0325
475 Speedwell Ave, PO Box 95, Morris Plains, NJ 07950

Fuller Ultraviolet Corp. 815-469-3301
9416 Gulfstream Rd, Frankfort, IL 60423
$50.00 per unit (standard).

Glass Instruments, Inc. 323-681-0011
2285 E Foothill Blvd, Pasadena, CA 91107
Ozone generating, custom UV lamps for sterilization & ozone generating applications.

Hanovia Specialty Lighting Llc 800-229-3666
825 Lehigh Ave, Union, NJ 07083
$100.00 per unit (standard).

Spectronics Corporation 800-274-8888
956 Brush Hollow Rd, Westbury, NY 11590

Uvp, Llc 800-452-6788
2066 W 11th St, Upland, CA 91786
Shortwave UV lamps are handheld and supplied with stand, 4-, 6-, 8-, and 15-W lamps (15-W lamps can be wall or ceiling mounted).

LAMP, ULTRAVIOLET, PHYSICAL MEDICINE
(Physical Med) 89IOB

Atlantic Ultraviolet Corp. 631-273-0500
375 Marcus Blvd, Hauppauge, NY 11788

Bhk, Inc. 909-983-2973
1480 N Claremont Blvd, Claremont, CA 91711

Brandt Industries, Inc. 800-221-8031
4461 Bronx Blvd, Bronx, NY 10470
Many varieties.

LAMP, ULTRAVIOLET, PHYSICAL MEDICINE *(cont'd)*

Bulbtronics, Inc. 800-624-2852
45 Banfi Plz N, Farmingdale, NY 11735

Burton Medical Products, Inc. 800-444-9909
21100 Lassen St, Chatsworth, CA 91311

Defiance Metal Prod Co. 419-784-5332
21 Seneca St, Defiance, OH 43512
Ultraviolet light source.

Fuller Ultraviolet Corp. 815-469-3301
9416 Gulfstream Rd, Frankfort, IL 60423
From $16.50 to $74.00.

Glass Instruments, Inc. 323-681-0011
2285 E Foothill Blvd, Pasadena, CA 91107
For AA spectroscopy and spectrophotometry.

Hanovia Specialty Lighting Llc 800-229-3666
825 Lehigh Ave, Union, NJ 07083
$1,200.00 per unit (standard).

Kbd, Inc. 859-331-0800
2550 American Ct, Erlanger, KY 41017
Various models of sunlamps.

Minisun, Llc 559-439-4600
935 E Mill Creek Dr, Fresno, CA 93720
Intelligent Device for Energy Expenditure and Activity - IDEEA is a truely breakthrough in physical activity assessment, energy expenditure measurement, functional assessment, and behavior monitoring

National Biological Corp. 800-338-5045
1532 Enterprise Pkwy, Twinsburg, OH 44087
$16.00-$125.00 for UVA, UVB & UVBNB lamps.

Roldan Products Corp. 866-922-6800
448 Sovereign Ct, Ballwin, MO 63011
$181.00 per unit (standard).

Spectronics Corporation 800-274-8888
956 Brush Hollow Rd, Westbury, NY 11590
E, EA-, EB- and Q-Series lamps.

The Daavlin Company 800-322-8546
205 W Bement St, PO Box 626, Bryan, OH 43506

Uvp, Llc 800-452-6788
2066 W 11th St, Upland, CA 91786
365, 302, and 254mm.

Voltarc Technologies, Inc. 203-578-4600
400 Captain Neville Dr, Waterbury, CT 06705
Various types of una tanning lamp. Specialty low and medium fluorescent lamps (i.e. microscope, inspecion, medical treatment, indoor tanning, etc.)

LANCET, BLOOD *(General) 80FMK*

A.M.G. Medical, Inc. 888-396-1213
8505 Dalton Rd., Montreal, QUE H4T-IV5 Canada

Aimsco, Delta Hi-Tech, Inc. 800-378-0909
3762 Secord St, Salt Lake City, UT 84115
Aimsco Ultra Thin Lancets, 28 & 30 gauge. Aimsco Auto Safety lancet 28 gauge.& AIMSCO Adjustable Lancing device.

Alimed, Inc. 800-225-2610
297 High St, Dedham, MA 02026
Autolet Mark II eliminates accidental cross-contamination from capillary blood samples when used with Unilet disposable lancets.

Arkray Factory Usa, Inc. 952-646-3168
5182 W 76th St, Minneapolis, MN 55439
Blood lancet.

Arkray Usa 800-818-8877
5198 W 76th St, Edina, MN 55439
HAEMOLANCE, HAEMOLANCE PLUS, QUICKLANCE & TECHLITE Lancets and SELECT LITE Lancet Holder. HAEMOLANCE, HAEMOLANCE PLUS & QUICKLANCE - single use, disposable lancet with built-in needle protection system, needle retracts automatically to reduce cross-contamination and accidental needle punctures. TECHLITE Lancets fit most devices. Available in 21, 25, and 28 gauge. SELECT LITE, a lancing device for all capillary blood samples. This easy to use lancing device is compatible with TECHLITE and most general purpose lancets and has an adjustable tip for maximum comfort.

Atrion Medical Products, Inc. 800-343-9334
1426 Curt Francis Rd NW, Arab, AL 35016
Lancet device, blood sampling.

Bayer Healthcare, Llc 574-256-3430
430 S Beiger St, Mishawaka, IN 46544
Lancet, blood.

LANCET, BLOOD *(cont'd)*

Bd Caribe, Ltd. 201-847-4298
Rd. 183, Km. 20.3, Las Piedras, PR 00771
Various types and sizes of blood lancets.

Becton Dickinson And Company 800-284-6845
1 Becton Dr, Franklin Lakes, NJ 07417
BLOOD; LANCET; MICRO-FINE LANCETS; MICROLANCE-BLOOD LANCET; MULTIPLE; MULTIPLE LANCETS; NONE NONE

C & A Scientific Co. Inc. 703-330-1413
7241 Gabe Ct, Manassas, VA 20109
PREIMERE Sterile, stainless steel, blood lancet.

Chematics, Inc. 574-834-4080
Hwy. 13 South, North Webster, IN 46555
Body fluid specimen collector.

Covidien Lp 508-261-8000
15 Hampshire St, Mansfield, MA 02048

Facet Technologies, Llc 770-767-8800
101 Liberty Industrial Pkwy, McDonough, GA 30253
Various.

Facet Technologies, Llc 800-526-2387
112 Townpark Dr NW Ste 300, Kennesaw, GA 30144

Global Healthcare 800-601-3880
1495 Hembree Rd Ste 700, Roswell, GA 30076
Blood Lancets

Hawaii Medical, Llc 781-826-5565
750 Corporate Park Dr, Pembroke, MA 02359

Hosuk America Co. 303-750-3829
1583 S Tucson St, Aurora, CO 80012

Htl-Strefa, Inc. 678-921-2692
1950 Spectrum Cir SE Ste 400, Marietta, GA 30067
1) Safety single-use lancets for professional use, and 2) personal lancets for home diagnostics

International Technidyne Corp. 800-631-5945
23 Nevsky St, Edison, NJ 08820

International Technidyne Corporation 732-548-5700
8 Olsen Ave, Edison, NJ 08820
Incision device.

Jayza Corp. 305-477-1136
7215 NW 41st St Ste A, Miami, FL 33166

K W Griffen Company 800-424-5556
100 Pearl St, Norwalk, CT 06850

K. W. Griffen Co. 203-846-1923
100 Pearl St, Norwalk, CT 06850
Lancet.

Kentron Health Care, Inc. 615-384-0573
3604 Kelton Jackson Rd, P.o. Box 120, Springfield, TN 37172
Blood lancet.

Lifescan, Inc. 800-227-8862
1000 Gibraltar Dr, Milpitas, CA 95035
Lancets, sterile.

Medi-Dose, Inc. 800-523-8966
70 Industrial Dr, Ivyland, PA 18974

Medical Plastic Devices (Mpd), Inc. 866-633-9835
161 Oneida Dr., Pointe Claire, QUE H9R 1A9 Canada
23ga Blood Lancet, all sizes. Also available Safety Lanset.

Medicore, Inc. 800-327-8894
2647 W 81st St, Hialeah, FL 33016
Sterile blood lancet.

Medipoint, Inc. 800-445-0525
72 E 2nd St, Mineola, NY 11501
Stainless Steel, Plastic, and Safety Style Blood Lancets for taking finger-tip blood samples.

Norco Medical 386-734-9080
1501 Lexington Ave, Deland, FL 32724
Lancets.

North Safety Products 401-943-4400
1101 B Calle Neutron, Parque Industrial Maran, Mexicali, B.c. Mexico
Lancet

Owen Mumford Usa, Inc. 800-421-6936
1755 W Oak Commons Ct Ste A, Marietta, GA 30062

Palco Labs, Inc. 800-346-4488
8030 Soquel Ave Ste 104, Santa Cruz, CA 95062
AUTO-LANCET finger lancing device, EZ-LETS sterile capillary blood lancets.

LANCET, BLOOD *(cont'd)*

Propper Manufacturing Co., Inc. 800-832-4300
3604 Skillman Ave, Long Island City, NY 11101

Qualitico Dist's, Inc. 813-264-4788
14025 Clubhouse Cir Apt 2503, Tampa, FL 33618
Lancet.

Ross Disposable Products 800-649-6526
401 Traders Blvd E, Unit 10, Mississauga, ON L4Z 2H8 Canada

Sarstedt, Inc. 800-257-5101
PO Box 468, 1025, St. James Church Road, Newton, NC 28658

Virotek, L.L.C. 847-634-4500
900 Asbury Dr, Buffalo Grove, IL 60089
Safety lancet.

LAPAROSCOPE, FLEXIBLE *(Surgery) 79WXI*

Lican Medical Products Ltd. 519-737-1142
5120 Halford Dr., Windsor, ON N9A 6J3 Canada

Welch Allyn, Inc. 800-535-6663
4341 State Street Rd, Skaneateles Falls, NY 13153

LAPAROSCOPE, GENERAL & PLASTIC SURGERY *(Surgery) 79GCJ*

Advanced Endoscopy Devices, Inc. 818-227-2720
22134 Sherman Way, Canoga Park, CA 91303
2- to 10-mm sizes available.

Aesculap Implant Systems Inc. 1-800-234-9179
3773 Corporate Pkwy, Center Valley, PA 18034

Apple Medical Corp. 508-357-2700
28 Lord Rd Ste 135, Marlborough, MA 01752
Stonegrabber.

Applied Medical Technology, Inc. 800-869-7382
8000 Katherine Blvd, Brecksville, OH 44141

Ballard Medical Products 770-587-7835
12050 Lone Peak Pkwy, Draper, UT 84020
Various endoscopic accessories.

Bard Shannon Limited 908-277-8000
San Geronimo Industrial Park, Lot # 1, Road # 3, Km 79.7 Humacao, PR 00791
Precision pass.

Baxter Healthcare Corporation, Medication Delivery 949-851-9066
17511 Armstrong Ave, Irvine, CA 92614
Endoscope applicator.

Biomet Sports Medicine 530-226-5800
6704 Lockheed Dr, Redding, CA 96002
Innervue with various accessories.

Biomet, Inc. 574-267-6639
56 E Bell Dr, PO Box 587, Warsaw, IN 46582
Various types of endoscopes and accessories.

Biovision Technologies, Llc 303-237-9608
221 Corporate Cir Ste H, Golden, CO 80401
Innervue diagnostic scope system.

Boston Scientific - Marina Bay Customer Fulfillment Center 617-689-6000
500 Commander Shea Blvd, Quincy, MA 02171
Stretch vl stents (stent store).

Boston Scientific Corp. 408-935-3400
150 Baytech Dr, San Jose, CA 95134
Dissector,introducer,endoscope,sterilization tray.

Boston Scientific Corporation 800-225-2732
1 Boston Scientific Pl, Natick, MA 01760

Cardinal Health, Snowden Pencer Products 847-689-8410
5175 S Royal Atlanta Dr, Tucker, GA 30084
Various styles of laparascopes, laparoscopic instruments,cannulas trocars,and la.

Cook Endoscopy 336-744-0157
4900 Bethania Station Rd # &, 5951 Grassy Creek Blvd. Winston Salem, NC 27105
Needle guide.

Cortek Endoscopy, Inc. 847-526-2266
260 Jamie Ln Ste D, Wauconda, IL 60084
Gastroenterology.

Davol Inc., Sub. C.R. Bard, Inc. 800-556-6275
100 Crossings Blvd, Warwick, RI 02886
Laparoscopic irrigator and tips.

LAPAROSCOPE, GENERAL & PLASTIC SURGERY *(cont'd)*

Deknatel Snowden-Pencer 800-367-7874
5175 S Royal Atlanta Dr, Tucker, GA 30084

Elmed, Inc. 630-543-2792
60 W Fay Ave, Addison, IL 60101

Ethicon Endo-Surgery, Inc. 877-384-4266
3801 University Blvd SE, Albuquerque, NM 87106
Various types of sterile and non-sterile surgical trocars and convenience kits.

Geneva Medical Inc. 630-232-2507
2571 Kaneville Ct, Geneva, IL 60134
Surgical trocar and accessories.

Genicon 800-936-1020
6869 Stapoint Ct Ste 114, Winter Park, FL 32792
Ridgid Laparoscopes, Autoclavable in 5mm and 10mm Diameters as well as 33cm and 45cm lengths.

Gibbons Surgical Corp. 800-959-1989
1112 Jensen Dr Ste 101, Virginia Beach, VA 23451
Laparoscope and laparoscopic instruments.

Global Endoscopy, Inc. 888-434-3398
914 Estes Ct, Schaumburg, IL 60193
Laparoscope, general and plastic surgery.

Gyrus Acmi, Inc. 508-804-2739
93 N Pleasant St, Norwalk, OH 44857
Laparoscope, general & plastic surgery and accessories.

Gyrus Acmi, Inc. 508-804-2739
300 Stillwater P.o.box 1971, Stamford, CT 06902
Laparoscope, general & plastic surgery and accessories.

Gyrus Ent L.L.C., Sub. Of Gyrus Acmi, Inc. 508-804-2739
2925 Appling Rd, Bartlett, TN 38133
Instrument wipe.

Henke Sass Wolf Of America, Inc. 508-671-9300
135 Schofield Ave, Dudley, MA 01571

I.C. Medical, Inc. 623-780-0700
2002 W Quail Ave, Phoenix, AZ 85027
Various types.

Innervision Inc. 901-682-0417
6258 E Shady Grove Rd, Memphis, TN 38120

Innovasive Devices, Inc. 800-435-6001
734 Forest St, Marlborough, MA 01752

Intuitive Surgical, Inc. 888-409-4774
1266 Kifer Rd, Sunnyvale, CA 94086
Various.

J. Jamner Surgical Instruments, Inc 800-431-1123
9 Skyline Dr, Hawthorne, NY 10532

Karl Storz Endoscopy-America Inc. 800-421-0837
600 Corporate Pointe, Culver City, CA 90230
Full line of both diagnostic and operating models; rod-lens optics; rigid and semi-rigid versions.

Kmedic 800-955-0559
190 Veterans Dr, Northvale, NJ 07647

Lican Medical Products Ltd. 519-737-1142
5120 Halford Dr., Windsor, ON N9A 6J3 Canada

Lsi Solutions Inc. 585-869-6641
7796 Victor Mendon Rd, Victor, NY 14564
Suture placement device and accessories; color video monitor.

Mahe International Inc. 800-294-7946
468 Craighead St, Nashville, TN 37204

Maquet Puerto Rico Inc. 408-635-3900
No. 12, Rd. #698, Dorado, PR 00646
Blunt tip surgical trocar & dissector.

Mark Medical Manufacturing, Inc. 610-269-4420
530 Brandywine Ave, Downingtown, PA 19335
Insulated and non-insulated laparoscopic instruments.

Mclean Medical And Scientific, Inc. 800-777-9987
292 E Lafayette Frontage Rd, Saint Paul, MN 55107

Md International, Inc. 305-669-9003
11300 NW 41st St, Doral, FL 33178

Mediflex Surgical Products 800-879-7575
250 Gibbs Rd, Islandia, NY 11749
Designed for video, 10-mm 0- to 30-degree to 45- degree, economically priced.

Medisiss 866-866-7477
2747 SW 6th St, Redmond, OR 97756
Various laparoscope accessories, reprocessed, sterile.

LAPAROSCOPE, GENERAL & PLASTIC SURGERY *(cont'd)*

Medivision Endoscopy 800-349-5367
1210 N Jefferson St, Anaheim, CA 92807
Independent service center specializing in rigid endoscope repairs and sales. Quality Control Department on premises. Provide customized maintenance reports to customers and distributors. Conduct technical training seminars and in-service programs. Manufacturer of new endoscopes. Personal Video Display, Head mounted video display that allows user to view video signals while simultaneously observing the surgical site.

Medtec Applications, Inc. 630-628-0444
50 W Fay Ave, Addison, IL 60101
Laparoscope.

Microline Pentax, Inc. 978-922-9810
800 Cummings Ctr Ste 157X, Beverly, MA 01915
Clip applier.

Minrad, Inc. 716-855-1068
50 Cobham Dr, Orchard Park, NY 14127
Laparoscope.

Olympus America, Inc. 800-645-8160
3500 Corporate Pkwy, PO Box 610, Center Valley, PA 18034

Pare Surgical, Inc. 303-689-0187
7332 S Alton Way Ste H, Centennial, CO 80112
Endoscopic suture knot tying device using a 5mm reusable Quik-Stitch Handle and Needle driver or Disposable 5mm Quik-Stitch Handle and Needle driver.

Pentax Southern Region Service Center 201-571-2300
8934 Kirby Dr, Houston, TX 77054
Confocal system.

Pentax West Coast Service Center 800-431-5880
10410 Pioneer Blvd Ste 2, Santa Fe Springs, CA 90670
Pentax confocal system.

Precision Optics Corp. 800-447-2812
22 E Broadway, Gardner, MA 01440
Zero-, 3-, and 45-degree laparoscopes provide bright, high-quality imagery.

Rei Rotolux Enterprises, Inc. 888-773-7611
4145 North Service Rd, Ste. 200, Burlington, ON L7L 6A3 Canada
Different diameters are available. All are autoclavable. Custom configurations are available.

Richard Wolf Medical Instruments Corp. 800-323-9653
353 Corporate Woods Pkwy, Vernon Hills, IL 60061

Smith & Nephew Inc., Endoscopy Div. 978-749-1000
76 S Meridian Ave, Oklahoma City, OK 73107
Laproscopic/endoscopic accessory.

Smith & Nephew, Inc., Endoscopy Division 800-343-8386
150 Minuteman Rd, Andover, MA 01810

Smith & Nephew, Inc., Endoscopy Division 800-343-8386
130 Forbes Blvd, Mansfield, MA 02048

Solos Endoscopy 800-388-6445
65 Sprague St # B, Boston/dedham Commerce Park, Boston, MA 02136
Endoscope & accessories.

Stryker Endoscopy 800-435-0220
5900 Optical Ct, San Jose, CA 95138

Stryker Gi 866-672-5757
1420 Lakeside Pkwy Ste 110, Flower Mound, TX 75028
Laproscope, general & plastic surgery.

Surgiquest, Inc. 203-799-2400
12 Cascade Blvd Ste 2B, Orange, CT 06477
Surgical trocar.

Sutura, Inc. 714-437-9801
17080 Newhope St, Fountain Valley, CA 92708
Disposable vascular suturing device.

Telos Medical Equipment (Austin & Assoc., Inc.) 800-934-3029
1109 Sturbridge Rd, Fallston, MD 21047

The Microoptical Corporation 781-326-8111
33 S West Park, Westwood, MA 02090
Critical data viewers, portable monitors, head mounted displays, head up display.

Tulip Medical Products 800-325-6526
PO Box 7368, San Diego, CA 92167
The TULIP LCI 300 integrated endoscopic imaging system. This integrated and miniaturized video imager combines the patented HiLUX lamp devleoped by Welch Allyn with Sony's HyperHAD camera architecture in a superior performance endoscopic imaging system that weighs less than 5 lbs. and is easily affordable.

LAPAROSCOPE, GENERAL & PLASTIC SURGERY *(cont'd)*

Ussc Puerto Rico, Inc. 203-845-1000
Building 911-67, Sabanetas Industrial Park, Ponce, PR 00731
Laparoscope and accessories.

Vision Systems Group, A Division Of Viking Systems 508-366-3668
134 Flanders Rd, Westborough, MA 01581
Head mounted display.

Warsaw Orthopedic, Inc. 901-396-3133
2500 Silveus Xing, Warsaw, IN 46582
Camera.

Welch Allyn, Inc. 800-535-6663
4341 State Street Rd, Skaneateles Falls, NY 13153

Wisap America 800-233-8448
8231 Melrose Dr, Lenexa, KS 66214

LAPAROSCOPE, GENERAL & PLASTIC SURGERY, REPROCESSED *(Gastro/Urology) 78NLM*

Ascent Healthcare Solutions 480-763-5300
10232 S 51st St, Phoenix, AZ 85044
Trocars,lap scissors,graspers,dissectors,clamps,babcocks,cannula sets.

Henke Sass Wolf Of America, Inc. 508-671-9300
135 Schofield Ave, Dudley, MA 01571

Maquet Cardiovascular LLC 888-880-2874
45 Barbour Pond Dr, Wayne, NJ 07470
5MM ENDOSCOPE; 7MM ENDOSCOPE; SHORT PORT BTT; STERILIZATION TRAY; VASOVIEW DISSECTION CANNULA

Sterilmed, Inc. 763-488-3400
11400 73rd Ave N Ste 100, Maple Grove, MN 55369
Laparoscopic instruments.

Surgiquest, Inc. 203-799-2400
12 Cascade Blvd Ste 2B, Orange, CT 06477
AnchorPortTM

LAPAROSCOPE, GYNECOLOGIC *(Obstetrics/Gyn) 85HET*

Aesculap Implant Systems Inc. 1-800-234-9179
3773 Corporate Pkwy, Center Valley, PA 18034

Apple Medical Corp. 508-357-2700
28 Lord Rd Ste 135, Marlborough, MA 01752
Various.

Cardinal Health, Snowden Pencer Products 847-689-8410
5175 S Royal Atlanta Dr, Tucker, GA 30084
Various types of endoscopic light sources.

Clarus Medical, Llc. 763-525-8400
1000 Boone Ave N Ste 300, Minneapolis, MN 55427
Camera/light source.

Cook Ob/Gyn 800-541-5591
1100 W Morgan St, Spencer, IN 47460
Laparoscopic accessories.

Cortek Endoscopy, Inc. 847-526-2266
260 Jamie Ln Ste D, Wauconda, IL 60084
Gynecology/general surgery.

Elmed, Inc. 630-543-2792
60 W Fay Ave, Addison, IL 60101

Endoplus, Inc. 847-325-5660
431 Lexington Dr Ste A, Buffalo Grove, IL 60089
Various.

Ethicon Endo-Surgery, Inc. 877-384-4266
3801 University Blvd SE, Albuquerque, NM 87106
Various types of sterile surgical trocars and convenience kits.

Global Endoscopy, Inc. 888-434-3398
914 Estes Ct, Schaumburg, IL 60193
Laparoscope, gynecologic (and accessories).

Gyrus Acmi, Inc. 508-804-2739
93 N Pleasant St, Norwalk, OH 44857
Laparoscope, gynecologic (and accessories).

Innervision Inc. 901-682-0417
6258 E Shady Grove Rd, Memphis, TN 38120

Karl Storz Endoscopy-America Inc. 800-421-0837
600 Corporate Pointe, Culver City, CA 90230
Diagnostic, operative and laser; rod-lens optics; rigid and semi-rigid versions available.

Laser, Inc. 800-367-5694
27831 Commercial Park Ln, Tomball, TX 77375
Autoclavable.

LAPAROSCOPE, GYNECOLOGIC *(cont'd)*

Lican Medical Products Ltd. 519-737-1142
5120 Halford Dr., Windsor, ON N9A 6J3 Canada

Mahe International Inc. 800-294-7946
468 Craighead St, Nashville, TN 37204

Maquet Puerto Rico Inc. 408-635-3900
No. 12, Rd. #698, Dorado, PR 00646
Dissector.

Md International, Inc. 305-669-9003
11300 NW 41st St, Doral, FL 33178

Medgyn Products, Inc. 800-451-9667
328 Eisenhower Ln N, Lombard, IL 60148

Mediflex Surgical Products 800-879-7575
250 Gibbs Rd, Islandia, NY 11749

Medtec Applications, Inc. 630-628-0444
50 W Fay Ave, Addison, IL 60101
Safety trocar.

Olympus America, Inc. 800-645-8160
3500 Corporate Pkwy, PO Box 610, Center Valley, PA 18034

Reznik Instrument, Inc. 847-673-3444
7337 Lawndale Ave, Skokie, IL 60076
Laparoscopes.

Richard Wolf Medical Instruments Corp. 800-323-9653
353 Corporate Woods Pkwy, Vernon Hills, IL 60061

Smith & Nephew Inc., Endoscopy Div. 978-749-1000
76 S Meridian Ave, Oklahoma City, OK 73107
Laparoscopes.

Smith & Nephew, Inc., Endoscopy Division 800-343-8386
150 Minuteman Rd, Andover, MA 01810

Solos Endoscopy 800-388-6445
65 Sprague St # B, Boston/dedham Commerce Park, Boston, MA 02136
Gynecologic laparoscope & accessories.

Superior Medical Limited 800-268-7944
520 Champagne Dr., Toronto, ONT M3J 2T9 Canada

Usgi Medical 949-369-3890
1140 Calle Cordillera, San Clemente, CA 92673
Sterile grasper.

Ussc Puerto Rico, Inc. 203-845-1000
Building 911-67, Sabanetas Industrial Park, Ponce, PR 00731
Laparsocope and accessories.

Valley Forge Scientific Corp. 610-666-7500
136 Green Tree Road, Suite 100, Oaks, PA 19456
Laparoscopic bipolar pen-loops, and needle-point electrodes used for laparoscopic surgical procedures.

Welch Allyn, Inc. 800-535-6663
4341 State Street Rd, Skaneateles Falls, NY 13153

LAPAROSCOPE, MICROLAPAROSCOPY *(Surgery) 79SJT*

Genicon 800-936-1020
6869 Stapoint Ct Ste 114, Winter Park, FL 32792
3mm Laparoscopic Manual Instrumentaion

Wisap America 800-233-8448
8231 Melrose Dr, Lenexa, KS 66214
POWER-DRIVE laparoscopic morcellator has intercapable blade diameters of 10, 15, 18, and 20 mm. The device is steam sterilizable and reusable. This system combines the THERME-PNEU computer insufflator, which has a flow rate up to 31 L/min, the AQUA PURATOR BIOTHERME, which warms the irrigation solution to body temperature, and the OPTIC THERME laparoscope preheater, which preheats the laparoscope to prevent fogging.

LARYNGOSCOPE *(Ear/Nose/Throat) 77EQN*

Alimed, Inc. 800-225-2610
297 High St, Dedham, MA 02026

American Diagnostic Corporation (Adc) 800-232-2670
55 Commerce Dr, Hauppauge, NY 11788
Standard and Fiber optic Laryngoscopes blades and handles

Anesthesia Associates, Inc. 760-744-6561
460 Enterprise St, San Marcos, CA 92078
Laryngoscope blades and handles available in both conventional and GreenLine FiberOptic (fully GreenSpecification compatible). Standard, Slim, Bantam, Pediatric, Adjustable and Oversize handles available. Blades made in an incredible variety of special shapes and sizes. Includes Articulated Tip Mac's, Reduced Flanges, German Profiles, Oxygen Ports and other specialties, all at reduced prices. Stainless Steel and Chrome Plated Brass.

Armstrong Medical Industries, Inc. 800-323-4220
575 Knightsbridge Pkwy, Lincolnshire, IL 60069

LARYNGOSCOPE *(cont'd)*

Carley Lamps 310-325-8474
1502 W 228th St, Torrance, CA 90501

Dixie Ems Supply 800-347-3494
385 Union Ave, Brooklyn, NY 11211
$73.00 per unit (standard).

International Hospital Supply Co. 800-398-9450
6914 Canby Ave Ste 105, Reseda, CA 91335

Jedmed Instruments Co. 314-845-3770
5416 Jedmed Ct, Saint Louis, MO 63129

Karl Storz Endoscopy-America Inc. 800-421-0837
600 Corporate Pointe, Culver City, CA 90230
Diagnostic and operative units for adult and pediatric applications.

Kelleher Medical, Inc. 804-378-9956
3049 St Marys Way, Powhatan, VA 23139

Kta, Instruments, Inc. 888-830-9KTA
3051 Brighton-Third St., 1st Fl., Brooklyn, NY 11235

Magnum Medical 800-336-9710
3265 N Nevada St, Chandler, AZ 85225

Mahe International Inc. 800-294-7946
468 Craighead St, Nashville, TN 37204

Md International, Inc. 305-669-9003
11300 NW 41st St, Doral, FL 33178

Mercury Medical 800-237-6418
11300 49th St N, Clearwater, FL 33762
Standard and fiber optic; laryngoscope handles available.

North American Medical Products, Inc. 800-488-6267
6 British American Blvd Ste B, Latham, NY 12110
D.L. Scope - Disposable fiberoptic blades and reusable handle. PORTSCOPE III

Novamed, Llc 800-425-3535
4 Westchester Plz, Elmsford, NY 10523
NovaLite Fiber Optic, Standard and MRI-Compatable Laryngoscope Systems provide a whiter, brighter light source to ensure safer intubations -- even within the magnetic resonance (MR) environment. Available in a complete selection of styles and sizes.

Olympus America, Inc. 800-645-8160
3500 Corporate Pkwy, PO Box 610, Center Valley, PA 18034

Pentax Medical Company 800-431-5880
102 Chestnut Ridge Rd, Montvale, NJ 07645
Several models of flexible naso-pharyngo-laryngoscopes, with various distal tip diameters from 2.4mm to 5.5mm, and channel sizes, 1.2mm to 2.0mm. Fully immersible. Call for quote.

Precision Optics Corp. 800-447-2812
22 E Broadway, Gardner, MA 01440

Primary Medical Co., Inc. 727-520-1920
6541 44th St N Ste 6003, Pinellas Park, FL 33781
Various models non-sterile laryngoscope.

Princeton Medical Group, Inc. 800-875-0869
1189 Royal Links Dr, Mt Pleasant, SC 29466

Shippert Medical Technologies Corp. 800-888-8663
6248 S Troy Cir Ste A, Centennial, CO 80111
Rhinolaryngoscope, Welch Allyn.

Sun-Med 800-433-2797
12393 Belcher Rd S Ste 450, Largo, FL 33773
Conventional laryngoscope blades, Macintosh, Miller, and Wisconsin; GreenLine fiber-optic laryngoscope handles; GreenLine fiber-optic standard laryngscopes blades, MacIntosh and Miller. German-profile MacIntosh and Miller.

Sunmed Healthcare 727-531-7266
12393 Belcher Rd S Ste 460, Largo, FL 33773

Trans American Medical / Tamsco Instruments 708-430-7777
7633 W 100th Pl, Bridgeview, IL 60455
Stainless steel fiber-optic.

Triboro Supplies Inc 800-369-7546
994 Grand Blvd, Deer Park, NY 11729

Welch Allyn, Inc. 800-535-6663
4341 State Street Rd, Skaneateles Falls, NY 13153

LARYNGOSCOPE, FLEXIBLE *(Anesthesiology) 73CAL*

Clarus Medical, Llc. 763-525-8400
1000 Boone Ave N Ste 300, Minneapolis, MN 55427
Laryngoscope.

LARYNGOSCOPE, FLEXIBLE *(cont'd)*

Novamed, Llc 800-425-3535
4 Westchester Plz, Elmsford, NY 10523
NOVALITE Fiber Optic Laryngoscope range includes a complete selection of disposable Macintosh and Miller disposable blades. Available in high quality plexi construction with desired firmness for safe intubations.

Olympus America, Inc. 800-645-8160
3500 Corporate Pkwy, PO Box 610, Center Valley, PA 18034

Parker Medical 303-799-1990
7275 S Revere Pkwy Ste 804, Centennial, CO 80112
Portable, self-contained videoscope with detachable, flexible fiberbundle connected to carrying case containing light source, camera, and TV monitor.

Pentax Southern Region Service Center 201-571-2300
8934 Kirby Dr, Houston, TX 77054
Laryngoscope.

Pentax West Coast Service Center 800-431-5880
10410 Pioneer Blvd Ste 2, Santa Fe Springs, CA 90670
Pentax laryngoscope.

Sunmed Healthcare 727-531-7266
12393 Belcher Rd S Ste 460, Largo, FL 33773

Vision-Sciences, Inc. 800-874-9975
40 Ramland Rd S Ste 1, Orangeburg, NY 10962

LARYNGOSCOPE, RIGID *(Anesthesiology) 73CCW*

Achi Corp. 408-321-9581
2168 Ringwood Ave, San Jose, CA 95131
The Wuscope System is a rigid tubular fiberoptic intubating device for airway management.

Alero, Inc. 951-273-7890
1550 Consumer Cir, Corona, CA 92880
Laryngoscopes blades, handles, connectors and adapters.

Astralite Corporation 800-345-7703
PO Box 689, Somerset, CA 95684
Laropharyngeal Fiberoptic Rigid Endoscope - a precision diagnostic periscope for safe examination and diagnosis of the larynx and pharynx.

Carley Lamps 310-325-8474
1502 W 228th St, Torrance, CA 90501

Ccr Medical, Inc. 888-883-7331
967 43rd Ave NE, Saint Petersburg, FL 33703
Laryngoscope handle, rigid various size, accessory.

Clinimed, Incorporated 877-CLINIMED
303 Markus Ct, Sandy Brae Industrial Park, Newark, DE 19713

Dma Med-Chem Corporation 800-362-1833
49 Watermill Ln, Great Neck, NY 11021

Eastmed Enterprises, Inc. 856-797-0131
11 Brandywine Dr, Marlton, NJ 08053
Conventional and fibroptic laryngoscope blades.

Gyrus Acmi, Inc. 508-804-2739
93 N Pleasant St, Norwalk, OH 44857
Bullard laryngoscope.

Gyrus Acmi, Inc. 508-804-2739
300 Stillwater P.o.box 1971, Stamford, CT 06902
Bullard laryngoscope.

Hartwell Medical Corp. 800-633-5900
6352 Corte Del Abeto Ste J, Carlsbad, CA 92011
GRANDVIEW laryngoscope blade, rigid laryngoscope blade with unique curvature, wider blade surface, and patented reflecting lamp for brighter light source. Designed for emergency-care providers. The GRANDVIEW Blade adult size is now available as a disposable unit. Now you have a choice of a durable or a disposable blade. Both are high quality metal blades, not plastic with brilliant light sources.

Henke Sass Wolf Of America, Inc. 508-671-9300
135 Schofield Ave, Dudley, MA 01571

Her-Mar, Inc. 800-327-8209
8550 NW 30th Ter, Doral, FL 33122
$200.00 per set of three blades with handle.

Instrumentation Industries, Inc. 800-633-8577
2990 Industrial Blvd, Bethel Park, PA 15102

International Respiratory Systems, Inc. 845-562-5546
95 Ann St, Newburgh, NY 12550
Larynogscope blade & handle.

LARYNGOSCOPE, RIGID *(cont'd)*

Intubation Plus, Inc. 814-663-4688
1524 Enterprise Rd, Corry, PA 16407
Laryngoscope.

Kelleher Medical, Inc. 804-378-9956
3049 St Marys Way, Powhatan, VA 23139

Kentron Health Care, Inc. 615-384-0573
3604 Kelton Jackson Rd, P.o. Box 120, Springfield, TN 37172
Laryngoscope handles and blades.

Mahe International Inc. 800-294-7946
468 Craighead St, Nashville, TN 37204

Mainline Medical, Inc. 800-366-2084
3250 Peachtree Corners Cir Ste J, Norcross, GA 30092
Disposable Stainless Steel Fiber Optic Sterile Laryngoscope Blades. Works with ALL Manufactures green system fiber optic Laryngoscope handles.

Mercury Medical 800-237-6418
11300 49th St N, Clearwater, FL 33762
UPSHER brand laryngoscopes.

Minrad, Inc. 716-855-1068
50 Cobham Dr, Orchard Park, NY 14127
Intubating laryngoscope.

Novamed, Llc 800-425-3535
4 Westchester Plz, Elmsford, NY 10523
NOVALITE superior illumination Fiber Optic and Standard Laryngoscopes. Available in a complete range of reusable blades including Macintosh, Miller, Wisconsin, Seward, Robertshaw, etc.

Olympus America, Inc. 800-645-8160
3500 Corporate Pkwy, PO Box 610, Center Valley, PA 18034

Pogo, Inc. 507-280-8868
410 1st Ave NW, Rochester, MN 55901
Laryngoscope vacuum sleeve.

Promedic, Inc. 239-498-2155
3460 Pointe Creek Ct Apt 102, Bonita Springs, FL 34134
Specially designed handle.

Richard Wolf Medical Instruments Corp. 800-323-9653
353 Corporate Woods Pkwy, Vernon Hills, IL 60061

Rtech, Inc. 877-783-2446
739 Brandywine Dr, Moorestown, NJ 08057
Various types and sizes of laryngoscope.

Smiths Medical Asd Inc. 800-258-5361
10 Bowman Dr, Keene, NH 03431
Various.

Sun-Med 800-433-2797
12393 Belcher Rd S Ste 450, Largo, FL 33773

Sunmed Healthcare 727-531-7266
12393 Belcher Rd S Ste 460, Largo, FL 33773
GreenLine/D disposable, STERILE, stainless steel, fiber optic laryngoscope blades are the solution to contamination confronting the EMS Field. Available in 4 MacIntosh, 5 Miller, and 2 Robertshaw sizes. Used with any manufacturer's 'Green' system fiber optic handles, including: AMS, Anesthesia Associates, Heine, Propper, Rusch, Sunmed, and Welch Allyn. Individually packaged sterile - 20 per box.

Welch Allyn, Inc. 800-535-6663
4341 State Street Rd, Skaneateles Falls, NY 13153

LARYNGOSCOPE, SURGICAL *(Surgery) 79GCI*

Boehm Surgical Instrument Corp. 716-436-6584
966 Chili Ave, Rochester, NY 14611
Laryngoscope.

Carley Lamps 310-325-8474
1502 W 228th St, Torrance, CA 90501

Electro Surgical Instrument Co., Inc. 888-464-2784
37 Centennial St, Rochester, NY 14611
Various types and sizes of fiberoptic laryngoscopes.

Karl Storz Endoscopy-America Inc. 800-421-0837
600 Corporate Pointe, Culver City, CA 90230
Versions for adult and pediatric applications.

Mahe International Inc. 800-294-7946
468 Craighead St, Nashville, TN 37204

Mercury Medical 800-237-6418
11300 49th St N, Clearwater, FL 33762
2001 FIBERLIGHT Regular laryngoscope, fiber optic laryngoscope and laryngoscope lamp.

Propper Manufacturing Co., Inc. 800-832-4300
3604 Skillman Ave, Long Island City, NY 11101

LARYNGOSTROBOSCOPE *(Ear/Nose/Throat) 77EQL*

Jedmed Instruments Co. 314-845-3770
5416 Jedmed Ct, Saint Louis, MO 63129

Kelleher Medical, Inc. 804-378-9956
3049 St Marys Way, Powhatan, VA 23139

Pentax Southern Region Service Center 201-571-2300
8934 Kirby Dr, Houston, TX 77054
Laryngostroboscope.

Pentax West Coast Service Center 800-431-5880
10410 Pioneer Blvd Ste 2, Santa Fe Springs, CA 90670
Pentax laryngostroscope.

Richard Wolf Medical Instruments Corp. 800-323-9653
353 Corporate Woods Pkwy, Vernon Hills, IL 60061

LARYNX, ARTIFICIAL BATTERY-POWERED
(Ear/Nose/Throat) 77ESE

Cyberbiomed, Llc 561-582-1955
3605 S Ocean Blvd Apt A335, Palm Beach, FL 33480
Artificial larynx.

Drb Technologies, Inc 610-356-4258
3612 Chapel Rd Ste B, Newtown Square, PA 19073
Artificial larynx, electrolarynx.

E. Benson Hood Laboratories, Inc. 800-942-5227
575 Washington St, Pembroke, MA 02359

Griffin Laboratories 800-330-5969
43391 Business Park Dr Ste C5, Temecula, CA 92590
Artificial larynx, electronic.

Justmed, Inc. 503-524-4223
14780 SW Osprey Dr Ste 260, Beaverton, OR 97007
Battery-powered artificial larynx.

Luminaud, Inc. 800-255-3408
8688 Tyler Blvd, Mentor, OH 44060
$425.00 for COOPER-RAND intraoral models (three types for hand mobility problems). $440.00 for DENRICK 3 neck held artificial larynx, used with oral adapter.

Mountain Precision Mfg. Ltd. Co. 208-322-1111
11000 W Executive Dr, Boise, ID 83713
Battery powered artificial larynx.

Park Surgical Co., Inc. 800-633-7878
5001 New Utrecht Ave, Brooklyn, NY 11219
Electronic larynx.

Smiths Medical Asd 800-424-8662
5700 W 23rd Ave, Gary, IN 46406
Electronically hand held electrolarynx which produces auditory vibrations for voice production in laryngectomees.

Ultravoice, Ltd. 800-985-3000
3612 Chapel Rd, Newtown Square, PA 19073
Artificial larynx.

LASER, ANGIOPLASTY, CORONARY *(Cardiovascular) 74LPC*

Cardiogenesis Corp. 800-238-2205
11 Musick, Irvine, CA 92618
Coro.angio.laser; periph.angio.laser; surgical powered laser inst.

Light Age Inc. 732-563-0600
500 Apgar Dr, Somerset, NJ 08873
OEM laser source, manufactured to customer specification.

LASER, ANGIOPLASTY, PERIPHERAL *(Cardiovascular) 74LWX*

Spectrascience, Inc. 858-847-0200
11568 Sorrento Valley Rd Ste 11, San Diego, CA 92121
Peripheral laser angioplasty system.

LASER, ARGON, SURGICAL *(Surgery) 79ULB*

Alcon Research, Ltd. 800-862-5266
6201 South Fwy, Fort Worth, TX 76134

Allergan 800-366-6554
2525 Dupont Dr, Irvine, CA 92612

Biomedics, Inc. 949-458-1998
23322 Peralta Dr Ste 11, Laguna Hills, CA 92653

Md International, Inc. 305-669-9003
11300 NW 41st St, Doral, FL 33178

LASER, CARBON-DIOXIDE, MICROSURGICAL, ENT
(Ear/Nose/Throat) 77EWG

Biomedics, Inc. 949-458-1998
23322 Peralta Dr Ste 11, Laguna Hills, CA 92653

LASER, CARBON-DIOXIDE, SURGICAL *(Surgery) 79UKZ*

Biomedics, Inc. 949-458-1998
23322 Peralta Dr Ste 11, Laguna Hills, CA 92653
Coherent, Sharplan, Surgilase, LEI, etc

Carl Zeiss Surgical, Inc. 800-442-4020
1 Zeiss Dr, Thornwood, NY 10594

Pulse Systems, Inc. 505-662-7599
422 Connie Ave, Los Alamos, NM 87544

Sun Medical, Inc. 800-678-6633
2607 Aero Dr, Grand Prairie, TX 75052
Nidek Unipulse CO2 laser system.

Surgical Laser Technologies, Inc. 800-366-4758
147 Keystone Dr, Montgomeryville, PA 18936

LASER, COMBINATION *(General) 80WQS*

Alcon Research, Ltd. 800-862-5266
6201 South Fwy, Fort Worth, TX 76134

Biolitec, Inc. 800-934-2377
515 Shaker Rd, East Longmeadow, MA 01028
The biolitec 980nm laser is ideal for soft-tissue applications in medical, dental, and veterinary environments. Compact and portable, it allows controlled tissue sculpting and provides a clean, bloodless field for most surgical procedures. Unlike other medical lasers, the biolitec Ceralas D and SmilePro 980 lasers cut optically ó not thermally ó without collateral tissue damage, charring, or inflammation. Because of their unique wavelength, biolitec's 980nm lasers allow precise, one-step cutting and coagulating. No special cooling or maintenance is required. 15, 25, and 50 watt versions available.

Biomedics, Inc. 949-458-1998
23322 Peralta Dr Ste 11, Laguna Hills, CA 92653

Lambda Physik Usa, Inc. 800-EXCIMER
3201 W Commercial Blvd Ste 110, Fort Lauderdale, FL 33309

Light Age Inc. 732-563-0600
500 Apgar Dr, Somerset, NJ 08873
Transmiocardial revascularization, coronary OEM laser source operating at 380 nm, manufacturered to customer's specification.

Linos Photonics, Inc 800-334-5678
459 Fortune Blvd, Milford, MA 01757

Multi Imager Service, Inc 800-400-4549
13865 Magnolia Ave Bldg C, Chino, CA 91710
Founded in 1983, Multi Imager specializes in diagnostic-quality film imaging and digital imaging technologies, including film-based video imagers, wet-film-based laser imagers, dry-film imagers, digital acquisition/storage and transmission devices, computed radiography, PACS, and more. Multi Imager provides technical support and training, parts supply, and sales of new as well as refurbished equipment used with a broad range of modalities, including CT, MRI, ultrasound, nuclear medicine, and others.

Perimed, Inc. 877-374-3589
6785 Wallings Rd Ste 2C-2D, North Royalton, OH 44133
System 5000 measures blood flow and oxygen.

Princeton Instruments - Acton 978-263-3584
15 Discovery Way, Acton, MA 01720
Excimer and UV laser optics and lenses.

Specialty Surgical Instrumentation, Inc. 800-251-3000
200 River Hills Dr, Nashville, TN 37210

Zander Medical Supplies, Inc. / Zander Ivf, Inc. 800-820-3029
755 8th Ct Ste 4, Vero Beach, FL 32962
Zonal drilling laser installed on inverted microscopes; Anti-vibration tables.

LASER, DENTAL *(Dental And Oral) 76LYB*

Biolase Technology, Inc. 888-424-6527
4 Cromwell, Irvine, CA 92618
WATERLASE - hard and soft tissue dental laser. LASERSMILE - in-office teeth whitening laser system.

Continuum, Inc. 888-532-1064
3150 Central Expy, Santa Clara, CA 95051
Continuum Dental Laser Systems. Delight Er:YAG hard-tissue dental laser system for caries removal and cavity preparation. DioDent diode laser soft-tissue laser system for various soft-tissue laser procedures.

Excel Technology, Inc. 631-784-6100
41 Research Way, East Setauket, NY 11733

Lares Research 800-347-3289
295 Lockheed Ave, Chico, CA 95973
POCKETPRO Nd: Yag Soft Tissue Laser

LASER, DENTAL *(cont'd)*

Light Age Inc. 732-563-0600
500 Apgar Dr, Somerset, NJ 08873
OEM pulsed laser source operating at 375nm, high average power, for hard and soft tissue.

Millennium Dental Technologies, Inc. 562-860-2908
10945 South St Ste 104A, Cerritos, CA 90703
Various.

Quatronix 800-289-7707
41 Research Way, East Setauket, NY 11733

LASER, DIODE, LAPAROSCOPY *(Surgery) 79SJO*

Edmund Industrial Optics 800-363-1992
101 E Gloucester Pike, Barrington, NJ 08007

Surgical Laser Technologies, Inc. 800-366-4758
147 Keystone Dr, Montgomeryville, PA 18936

Texas Photonics, Inc. 972-412-7111
3213 Main St, Rowlett, TX 75088

LASER, DYE *(General) 80WQR*

Alcon Research, Ltd. 800-862-5266
6201 South Fwy, Fort Worth, TX 76134

Ams Innovative Center-San Jose 800-356-7600
3070 Orchard Dr, San Jose, CA 95134
Dye laser outputs red light for photodynamic Tx.

Candela Corp. 800-733-8550
530 Boston Post Rd, Wayland, MA 01778
SPTL-1b Vascular Lesion Laser. Priced at $129,500 for dye laser treatment of vascular dermatological lesions, such as spider veins and port wine stains.

Lambda Physik Usa, Inc. 800-EXCIMER
3201 W Commercial Blvd Ste 110, Fort Lauderdale, FL 33309

LASER, EXCIMER, SURGICAL *(Surgery) 79VIC*

Lambda Physik Usa, Inc. 800-EXCIMER
3201 W Commercial Blvd Ste 110, Fort Lauderdale, FL 33309

Olympus America, Inc. 800-645-8160
3500 Corporate Pkwy, PO Box 610, Center Valley, PA 18034

Spectra Gases, Inc. 800-932-0624
3434 US Highway 22, Branchburg, NJ 08876
Excimer laser gases in pre-mixed gas cylinders for worldwide distribution and related equipment for gas handling. Xenon-129, Helium-3, stable isotopic gases for diagnostic evaluation.

Spectranetics Corp. 800-633-0960
9965 Federal Dr, Colorado Springs, CO 80921
CVX-300 xenon chloride gas excimer laser unit. LASER SHEATH use in conjunction with the CVX-300 to assist in removing pacer or ICD leads by ablating scar tissue.

Surgical Laser Technologies, Inc. 800-366-4758
147 Keystone Dr, Montgomeryville, PA 18936

LASER, FLUORESCENCE CARIES DETECTION *(Dental And Oral) 76NBL*

Air Techniques, Inc. 800-247-8324
1295 Walt Whitman Rd, Melville, NY 11747
Spectra

LASER, GASTROENTEROLOGY/UROLOGY *(Gastro/Urology) 78LNK*

Biomedics, Inc. 949-458-1998
23322 Peralta Dr Ste 11, Laguna Hills, CA 92653
Laserscope, Coherent, etc

Industrial Welding Supplies Of Hattiesburg, Inc. 601-545-1800
1924 Byron St, Hattiesburg, MS 39402
Laser gas mixtures.

Wave Form Systems, Inc. 800-332-8749
7737 SW Nimbus Ave, Beaverton, OR 97008
WAVESTONE Holmium laser for urinary stone fragmentation.

LASER, GYNECOLOGIC *(Obstetrics/Gyn) 85HHR*

International Hospital Supply Co. 800-398-9450
6914 Canby Ave Ste 105, Reseda, CA 91335

Medical Energy, Inc. 850-469-1727
225 E Zaragoza St, Pensacola, FL 32502
LIGHT FORCE SERIES: Light Force 1 (20 watts) and Light Force 2 (30 watts) 980nm lasers.

LASER, HEALING, WOUND *(Surgery) 79LXU*

Spectrum Laser & Technologies, Inc 719-264-7632
2270 Garden of the Gods Rd Ste 103, Colorado Springs, CO 80907
Therapeutic laser system.

LASER, LABORATORY *(Chemistry) 75REH*

Advanced American Biotechnology (Aab) 714-870-0290
1166 E Valencia Dr Unit 6C, Fullerton, CA 92831
4 models Soft Laser Scanning Densitometers - $5,950 for std unit; $8,950 for UV unit; $15,990 for std 2-D unit; $18,990 for UV 2-D unit. Laser Densitometry Station 0-4.2 OD linear range. Reflectance-transmission UV fluorescence and white light. High speed; one lane per 2 sec. 2D in 12 minutes. 1D, 2D, DNA, RFLP software. Scanner attachment to scan 35x45cm X-ray film...$14,500.

Coherent, Inc. 800-527-3786
5100 Patrick Henry Dr, Santa Clara, CA 95054

Kavo Dental Corp. 800-323-8029
340 East Route 22, Lake Zurich, IL 60047
KAVO DIAGNODENT: laser fluorescence caries-detection device.

Lambda Physik Usa, Inc. 800-EXCIMER
3201 W Commercial Blvd Ste 110, Fort Lauderdale, FL 33309

Optelecom-Nkf, Inc 800-293-4237
12920 Cloverleaf Center Dr, Germantown, MD 20874
Fiber-optic lasers.

Quatronix 800-289-7707
41 Research Way, East Setauket, NY 11733

LASER, ND:YAG, LAPAROSCOPY *(Surgery) 79QYU*

Biomedics, Inc. 949-458-1998
23322 Peralta Dr Ste 11, Laguna Hills, CA 92653

Surgical Laser Technologies, Inc. 800-366-4758
147 Keystone Dr, Montgomeryville, PA 18936
Add Diode Laser and Co2 Laser and Holmium Laser

LASER, ND:YAG, SURGICAL *(Surgery) 79ULA*

Alcon Research, Ltd. 800-862-5266
6201 South Fwy, Fort Worth, TX 76134

Allergan 800-366-6554
2525 Dupont Dr, Irvine, CA 92612
$30,000 and up.

Biomedics, Inc. 949-458-1998
23322 Peralta Dr Ste 11, Laguna Hills, CA 92653

Carl Zeiss Surgical, Inc. 800-442-4020
1 Zeiss Dr, Thornwood, NY 10594
Dual-wavelength 1440-nm and 1064-nm surgical YAG laser.

Convergent Laser Technologies 800-848-8200
1660 S Loop Rd, Alameda, CA 94502
OPTICA 100 super pulsed Nd:YAG surgical laser system with Fiber Tip Protection System, real time power display, dual joules counters and ambient beam sensors.

Ddc Technologies, Inc. 866-346-3527
313B Atlantic Ave, Oceanside, NY 11572
Nd:YAG laser for Hair Removal

Dornier Medtech America 800-367-6437
1155 Roberts Blvd NW, Kennesaw, GA 30144
The DORNIER D940 DIODE LASER SYSTEM is a laser transmission system for the treatment of spider and varicose veins. Also available, FIBERTOME Nd:YAG laser.

Focus Medical, Llc. 866-633-5273
23 Francis J Clarke Cir, Bethel, CT 06801
NaturaLase 2 Joule Q-switched 2 joule Nd:YAG, Tattoo Removal, Collagen Remodeling, Hair Removal. Also: NaturaLase LP Long Pulse YAG, Hair Removal, Leg Vein, Facial Vascular Collagen Remodeling

Quatronix 800-289-7707
41 Research Way, East Setauket, NY 11733

Surgical Laser Technologies, Inc. 800-366-4758
147 Keystone Dr, Montgomeryville, PA 18936
CONTACT LASER SYSTEM, $55,000-$90,000 for contact laser, $450 for reusable contact laser scalpels, $375-$495 for reusable contact laser probes, $160 for Nd:YAG fiber, $175-$215 for Nd:YAG fiber with handpiece. Nd: YAG lasers, 25-, 40-, 60-, 100-Watt fiber delivery systems for SLT lasers and lasers with SMA-905 connectors.

Telsar Laboratories Inc 800-255-9938
1 Enviro Way Ste 100, Wood River, IL 62095
The SoftLight laser is the only Yag laser approved for hair removal and skin resurfacing using the patented carbon lotion.

Wave Form Systems, Inc. 800-332-8749
7737 SW Nimbus Ave, Beaverton, OR 97008
PROLASE--Nd: YAG surgical laser fiber. Prolase Blue--HolmiumLaser, Surgical fiber.

LASER, NEODYMIUM:YAG, OPHTHALMIC (POST. CAPSULOTOMY) *(Ophthalmology) 86LXS*

Nidek, Inc. 510-226-5700
47651 Westinghouse Dr, Fremont, CA 94539
Nd, yag laser for posterior capsulotomy and peripheral.

LASER, NEODYMIUM:YAG, SURGICAL, GYNECOLOGIC *(Obstetrics/Gyn) 85LLW*

Surgical Laser Technologies, Inc. 800-366-4758
147 Keystone Dr, Montgomeryville, PA 18936

Transamerican Technologies International 800-322-7373
2246 Camino Ramon, San Ramon, CA 94583
ACCU-BEAM, Fiber Optic Handpiece used with Nd:YAG lasers for surgical procedures.

LASER, NEODYMIUM:YAG, SURGICAL, PULMONARY *(Anesthesiology) 73LLO*

Xintec Corp. / Convergent Laser Tech. 510-832-2130
1660 S Loop Rd, Alameda, CA 94502
Nd:yag surgical laser.

LASER, OPHTHALMIC *(Ophthalmology) 86HQF*

Alcon Research, Ltd. 800-862-5266
6201 South Fwy, Fort Worth, TX 76134

Allergan 800-366-6554
2525 Dupont Dr, Irvine, CA 92612

Biolitec, Inc. 800-934-2377
515 Shaker Rd, East Longmeadow, MA 01028
Laser delivery system and 532mm diode laser (3 watt).

Biomedics, Inc. 949-458-1998
23322 Peralta Dr Ste 11, Laguna Hills, CA 92653

Carl Zeiss Surgical, Inc. 800-442-4020
1 Zeiss Dr, Thornwood, NY 10594
YAG ophthalmic laser and argon ophthalmic laser.

Edmund Industrial Optics 800-363-1992
101 E Gloucester Pike, Barrington, NJ 08007
Optics.

Fine Pitch Technologies, Inc., A Solectron Subsidi 408-957-8500
1077 Gibraltar Dr, Milpitas, CA 95035
Various types of ophthalmic lasers.

Iridex Corporation 800-388-4747
1212 Terra Bella Ave, Mountain View, CA 94043
OcuLight line of IR and visible photocoagulators. Extremely portable (both weigh under 18 lb), solid state reliability, no maintenance required, run on standard wall current.

Lumenis Inc. 800-447-0234
3959 W 1820 S, Salt Lake City, UT 84104

Microvision, Inc. 603-474-5566
34 Folly Mill Rd, Seabrook, NH 03874
Laser probe.

Nidek Inc. 800-223-9044
47651 Westinghouse Dr, Fremont, CA 94539
Model YC-1600 Nd:YAG laser;Model ADC-7000 multi-wavelength krypton, red, yellow, green laser; Model DC-3300 diode laser; and Model GYC-1000 DPSS green laser.

Nidek, Inc. 510-226-5700
47651 Westinghouse Dr, Fremont, CA 94539
Laser,ophthalmic.

Ophthalmed Llc 770-777-6613
11660 Alpharetta Hwy Ste 205, Roswell, GA 30076
Laser-illumination-aspiration probe for ophthalmology.

Peregrine Surgical, Ltd. 215-348-0456
51 Britain Dr, Doylestown, PA 18901
20ga or 25ga disposable laser probe.

Quatronix 800-289-7707
41 Research Way, East Setauket, NY 11733

Sterilmed, Inc. 763-488-3400
11400 73rd Ave N Ste 100, Maple Grove, MN 55369
Laser probe.

Welco-Cgi Gas Technologies 440-234-1075
145 Shimersville Rd, Bethlehem, PA 18015
Laser gas mixture.

LASER, SURGICAL *(Surgery) 79GEX*

Adept Medical Concepts 949-635-9238
29816 Avenida De Las Bandera, Rancho Santa Margarita, CA 92688
Various type & size of laser systems.

LASER, SURGICAL *(cont'd)*

Aesthera Corporation 925-737-2100
6634 Owens Dr, Pleasanton, CA 94588
Aip intense pulsed light system.

Air Liquide Healthcare America Corporation 713-402-2152
8428 Market Street Rd, Houston, TX 77029
Laser instrument, surgical, powered.

Allergan 800-366-6554
2525 Dupont Dr, Irvine, CA 92612

American Lasers, Inc. 626-300-9330
300 E Main St, Alhambra, CA 91801
Ruby laser,nd:yag.

American Medical Bio Care, Inc. 800-676-1434
1201 Dove St Ste 520, Newport Beach, CA 92660
Fluorescent Pulsed Light (FPL) system.

Angiodynamics, Inc. 518-795-1400
14 Plaza Drive, Latham, NY 12110
VenaCure Procedure Kits

Biolitec, Inc. 800-934-2377
515 Shaker Rd, East Longmeadow, MA 01028
Laser delivery system and 980mm diode laser 15, 25, or 50 watt. Dermatology (vascular lesions), dentistry (soft tissue oral cavity), ENT, general surgery, urology, and pulmonary. Soft tissue hemostasis, ablation, incision/excision and vaporization. Both pulsed/cw combined in the same laser.

Biomedics, Inc. 949-458-1998
23322 Peralta Dr Ste 11, Laguna Hills, CA 92653

Biotex, Inc. 713-741-0111
8058 El Rio St, Houston, TX 77054
Sterile laser applicators; diode laser systems.

C. R. Bard, Inc., Bard Urological Div. 888-367-2273
13183 Harland Dr NE, Covington, GA 30014

Candela Corp. 800-733-8550
530 Boston Post Rd, Wayland, MA 01778

Cao Group, Inc. 801-256-9282
4628 Skyhawk Dr, West Jordan, UT 84084
Diode laser 810nm.

Clarus Medical, Llc. 763-525-8400
1000 Boone Ave N Ste 300, Minneapolis, MN 55427
Laser fiber.

Clinicon Corp. 760-439-1700
3025 Industry St Ste A, Oceanside, CA 92054
Laser,laser scanner,accessory,surgical co2 laser,laser beam delivery system,inst.

Continuum, Inc. 888-532-1064
3150 Central Expy, Santa Clara, CA 95051
Medlite C6 and Medlite C3 medical laser systems. The Medlite C6 has four wavelength capability (1064 nm, 650 nm, 585 nm, and 532 nm) and is excellent for removing benign pigmented dermal and epidermal lesions and multicolor tattoos. The Multilite Dye Laser Handpiece system option adds the 585 nm and 650 nm capability to the Medlite C6 system. The Medlite is also used for treating vascular lesions and hair removal. The Medlite C6 has up to a 1 Joule output per pulse in the infrared at 1064 nm. The Medlite C3 has up to a 0.5 Joule per pulse output in the infrared at 1064 nm and has two wavelength capability (1064 nm and 532 nm).

Convergent Laser Technologies 800-848-8200
1660 S Loop Rd, Alameda, CA 94502
PROTEGE Er:YAG laser sytem and accessories, a state-of-the-art erbium laser system with many advanced features such as touch screen controls, variable pulse width, and pre-programmed power settings. Especially adapted for laser skin resurfacing and aesthetic surgery. PROTEGE II Erbium Laser System especially designed for aesthetic laser skin resurfacing with many features and options including fluence display, collimated beam, adjustable spot handpiece, variable pulse width and integrated scanner.

Cutera, Inc. 888-4-CUTERA
3240 Bayshore Blvd, Brisbane, CA 94005
Aesthetic.

Cynosure, Inc. 800-886-2966
5 Carlisle Rd, Westford, MA 01886
Multiple

Ddc Technologies, Inc. 866-346-3527
313B Atlantic Ave, Oceanside, NY 11572
Alexandrite laser for hair removal.

Dusa Pharmaceuticals, Inc. 978-657-7500
25 Upton Dr, Wilmington, MA 01887
Laser powered surgical instrument.

LASER, SURGICAL *(cont'd)*

Edge Systems Corporation 800-603-4996
2277 Redondo Ave, Signal Hill, CA 90755
Smoke evacuation tubing & filter.

Equilasers, Inc
3350 Scott Blvd Bldg 5, Santa Clara, CA 95054
Surgical laser.

Erchonia Medical 214-733-5209
2021 Commerce Dr, McKinney, TX 75069
Low level laser.

Ethicon Endo-Surgery, Inc. 877-384-4266
3801 University Blvd SE, Albuquerque, NM 87106
Various types of bipolar forceps, diode laser system and accessories.

Focus Medical, Llc. 866-633-5273
23 Francis J Clarke Cir, Bethel, CT 06801
NaturaLase Erbium Laser Treatment System, Erbium laser treatment for skin resurfacing

General Air Service And Supply 303-892-7003
6330 Colorado Blvd, Commerce City, CO 80022
Laser gas mixtures.

Gospro, Inc. 808-842-2282
2305 Kamehameha Hwy, Honolulu, HI 96819
Laser gas.

Grayson O Company 800-435-1508
6509 Newell Ave., Kannapolis, NC 28081
Melanin enhancer.

I.C. Medical, Inc. 623-780-0700
2002 W Quail Ave, Phoenix, AZ 85027
Various types.

Incisive, Llc. 510-669-9401
3095 Richmond Pkwy Ste 213, Richmond, CA 94806
Nd: yag pulsed laser.

International Biophysics Corp. 512-326-3244
2101 E Saint Elmo Rd Ste 275, Austin, TX 78744
Mediderm laser.

Intralase Corp. 714-247-8200
9701 Jeronimo Rd, Irvine, CA 92618
Laser keratome.

Inweld Corp. 317-248-0651
5353 W Southern Ave, Indianapolis, IN 46241
Laser gas mixtures.

Iridex Corporation 800-388-4747
1212 Terra Bella Ave, Mountain View, CA 94043
Powered

Isee3d, Inc. 514-908-2234
759 Victoria Square, Ste. 200, Montreal, QUE H2Y-2J7 Canada
3-D Imaging for telemedicine,endoscopy.

Lambda Physik Usa, Inc. 800-EXCIMER
3201 W Commercial Blvd Ste 110, Fort Lauderdale, FL 33309
OPTEX excimer laser for scientific and medical applications. The compact OPTEX excimer laser can operate at 193, 248, 308, and 351 nm. Pulse energies range from 8 to 25 mJ, with repetition rates up to 200 Hz. The OPTEX's small size (600 x 300 x 400 mm3), modular design, fiber-optic connections, and NovaTube Technology simplifies operation and maintenance. OPTEX can be used for applications such as laser microsurgery, ophthalmology, spectroscopy, bioanalysis, photochemistry, and material ablation and ionization. (Note: Lambda Physik lasers are suitable components or light sources for integration into finished medical devices marketed for such medical uses.)

Laser Dental Innovations 877-753-5054
745 Dubanski Dr, San Jose, CA 95123
Laser dental handpiece with 90 degree disposable tip.

Laser Engineering, A Div. Of Ssi 800-251-3000
200 River Hills Dr, Nashville, TN 37210
Various types.

Light Age Inc. 732-563-0600
500 Apgar Dr, Somerset, NJ 08873
EPICARE, alexandrite laser, multimode, pulsed, continuous or timed, for removal of unwanted hair. Ta2 ERASER, alexandrite laser for tattoo removal. EPICARE-LP, hair removal laser, manufacturer direct for dermatological lasers.

Lightwave Technologies Llc 602-738-4226
15354 N. 83rd Way St., 102, Scottsdale, AZ 85260
Various models of led photomodulation devices.

LASER, SURGICAL *(cont'd)*

Matheson Tri-Gas, Inc. 972-893-5600
8200 Washington St NE, Albuquerque, NM 87113
Laser gas mixture.

Medical Energy, Inc. 850-469-1727
225 E Zaragoza St, Pensacola, FL 32502
Light Force 1 and Light Force 2 series; 980nm.

Medical Laser Technologies, Llc 512-626-6267
3708 Ebony Hollow Cv, Austin, TX 78739
Erbium laser.

Medtek Devices, Inc. 716-835-7000
595 Commerce Dr, 155 Pineview Dr., Amherst, NY 14228
Accessory to laser equipment-smoke evacuator filters.

Mg Industries 610-695-7628
1 Steel Rd E, U.S. Industrial Park, Morrisville, PA 19067
Laser instrument, surgical, powered.

Minnetronix Inc. 888-301-1025
1635 Energy Park Dr, Saint Paul, MN 55108
Artilaze Surgical Ablation System

New Laser Science, Inc. 858-487-5880
PO Box 27210, San Diego, CA 92198
New and used. VIRIDIS DERMA 532 - KTP Laser - portable for treating vascular and pigmented lesions. DUALIS - Long pulsed ND:YAG hair removal for all skin types. FIDELIS - Long pulsed, erbium laser for wrinkle removal, laser photo rejuvination of skin and for all skin types.

New Star Lasers, Inc. 916-677-1900
9085 Foothills Blvd, Roseville, CA 95747
Surgical laser system.

Nexair, Llc. 901-729-5547
1211 N McLean Blvd, Memphis, TN 38108
Medical mixture-laser gas mixture.

Nidek Inc. 800-223-9044
47651 Westinghouse Dr, Fremont, CA 94539
Model COL-1040 CO2 laser for general surgery and cosmetic applications; Model DS-66 epistar diode laser for hair removal and vascular lesions.

Nidek, Inc. 510-226-5700
47651 Westinghouse Dr, Fremont, CA 94539
General laser surgical instrument.

North Valley Precision Products, Llc 775-829-2566
4750 Turbo Cir, Reno, NV 89502
Photo therapy.

Novalis Medical, Llc 813-645-2855
813 S West Shore Blvd, Tampa, FL 33609
High intensity, multi-wave length light device.

Omniguide, Inc. 888-666-4484
1 Kendall Sq Bldg 100, 3rd Floor, Cambridge, MA 02139
Laser beam delivery system with sterile disposable fiber assemblies.

Ophthalmed Llc 770-777-6613
11660 Alpharetta Hwy Ste 205, Roswell, GA 30076
Laser probes for endo-ocular laser photocoagulation treatments.

Optical Integrity, Inc. 850-233-5512
8317 Front Beach Rd Ste 21, Panama City Beach, FL 32407
General shape laser fiber.

Optimedica Corporation 888-850-1230
3130 Coronado Dr, Santa Clara, CA 95054
Ophthalmic laser.; PASCAL Streamline Photocoagulator; PASCAL Photocoagulator; Laser Indirect Ophthalmoscope

Palomar Medical Technologies 800-725-6627
82 Cambridge St, Burlington, MA 01803
Develops and manufactures proprietary state-of-the-art laser and pulsed light systems used in cosmetic dermatology and esthetic environments. StarLux, MediLux and EsteLux Systems: Pulsed light devices for the removal of hair, pigmented lesions, vascular lesions, and acne. NeoLux System: A pulsed light device for removal of hair and pigmented lesions. Palomar Q-YAG 5: A Q-switched laser used in cosmetic dermatology for the removal of tattoos and pigmented lesions.

Paradigm Lasers, Inc. 509-232-2040
1620 N Mamer Rd Bldg C, Suite 100, Spokane Valley, WA 99216
Dermatological laser system.

Paradigm-Trex, Llc 858-646-5756
10455 Pacific Center Ct, San Diego, CA 92121
Various models of hand held dermal coolers.

LASER, SURGICAL *(cont'd)*

Peerless Injection Molding, Llc. 310-768-8023
14600 S Main St, Gardena, CA 90248
Intense pulsed light system.

Photoactif 480-827-1212
7211 E Southern Ave Ste C-110, Mesa, AZ 85209
Led phototherapy.

Photomedex, Inc. 760-602-3300
2375 Camino Vida Roble Ste B, Carlsbad, CA 92011
Xeci excimer laser.

Photovac Laser Corp., Inc. 614-875-3300
3513 Farm Bank Way, Grove City, OH 43123

Plc Systems Inc. 508-541-8800
10 Forge Pkwy, Franklin, MA 02038
125MM Handpiece, Touch Focus 200MM Handpiece

Polar Cryogenics, Inc. 503-239-5252
2734 SE Raymond St, Portland, OR 97202
Laser gas mixture.

Praxair Distribution Inc., Southeast Llc 440-234-1075
403 Zell Dr, Orlando, FL 32824
Laser gas mixtures.

Praxair-Puerto Rico 440-234-1075
Rt. 931 & 189, Gurabo, PR 00778
Laser gas mixtures.

Quality Contract Manufacturing, Llc 770-965-3300
4362 Thurmon Tanner Rd, Flowery Branch, GA 30542
Led photomodulation device.

Quantel-Usa, Inc. 406-586-0131
601 Haggerty Ln, Bozeman, MT 59715
Pulsed light system.

Quatronix 800-289-7707
41 Research Way, East Setauket, NY 11733

Ra Medical Systems, Inc. 760-804-1648
2270 Camino Vida Roble Ste L, Carlsbad, CA 92011
308nm excimer laser.

Rainbow Electro-Technologies, Inc. 516-933-0327
41 Moss Ln, Jericho, NY 11753
Epilator.

Sandstone Medical Technologies, Llc 205-290-8251
102 Oxmoor Rd Ste 130, Birmingham, AL 35209
Surgical laser.

Sciton, Inc. 888-646-6999
9255 Commercial St., Palo Alto, CA 94303
Medical laser for tissue ablation and coagulation.

Solta Medical, Inc. 877-782-2286
25881 Industrial Blvd, Hayward, CA 94545
Fraxel III; SR Laser System

Spec Connection Intl Inc. 813-618-0400
34310 State Road 54, Zephyrhills, FL 33543
Laser mixture.

Specialty Surgical Instrumentation, Inc. 800-251-3000
200 River Hills Dr, Nashville, TN 37210

Spectrum International, Inc. 925-768-1122
1130 Burnett Ave Ste J, Concord, CA 94520
Surgical soft tissue diode laser.

Sterilmed, Inc. 763-488-3400
11400 73rd Ave N Ste 100, Maple Grove, MN 55369
Laser probe.

Surgical Laser Technologies, Inc. 800-366-4758
147 Keystone Dr, Montgomeryville, PA 18936

Surgilight, Inc. 407-482-4555
23 Alafaya Woods Blvd # 170, Oviedo, FL 32765
Er: yag laser system.

Synergetics Usa, Inc. 800-600-0565
3845 Corporate Centre Dr, O Fallon, MO 63368
Endooto laser probe.

Technology Delivery Systems, Inc. 866-629-4359
340 E Parker Blvd, Suite 240, Baton Rouge, LA 70808
Laser fiber optic.

Telsar Laboratories Inc 800-255-9938
1 Enviro Way Ste 100, Wood River, IL 62095
Sales of pre-owned laser systems.

Telsar Laboratories, Inc. 618-254-5555
1 Enviro Way Ste 100, Wood River, IL 62095
Laser instrument, surgical, powered.

LASER, SURGICAL *(cont'd)*

Theralight, Inc. 760-930-8000
2794 Loker Ave W Ste 105, Carlsbad, CA 92010
Phototherapy system and accessories.

Transamerican Technologies International 800-322-7373
2246 Camino Ramon, San Ramon, CA 94583
ACCU-BEAM, CO2 Laser Accessories. CO2 laser micromanipulator, handpieces and laparoscope couplers.

Tria Beauty, Inc. 925-701-2540
5880 W Las Positas Blvd Ste 52, Pleasanton, CA 94588
Hair removal laser.

Usa Photonics, Inc. 845-348-4900
169 Main St Fl 1, Nyack, NY 10960
Intense pulsed light system.

Vascular Solutions, Inc. 763-656-4300
5025 Cheshire Ln N, Plymouth, MN 55446
Laser instrument, surgical, powered.

Wave Form Systems, Inc. 800-332-8749
7737 SW Nimbus Ave, Beaverton, OR 97008
Mobile laser for on-site use for hair removal, vascular lesions, leg veins, wrinkle treatment, etc.

Welco-Cgi Gas Technologies 440-234-1075
145 Shimersville Rd, Bethlehem, PA 18015
Laser gas mixtures.

Xintec Corp. / Convergent Laser Tech. 510-832-2130
1660 S Loop Rd, Alameda, CA 94502
Holmium yag surgical laser system.

Zap Lasers, Llc 925-930-6777
2621 Pleasant Hill Rd Ste B, Pleasant Hill, CA 94523
Surgical diode laser.

Zeltiq 925-474-2500
4698 Willow Rd, Pleasanton, CA 94588
Zeltiq System

LASER, SURGICAL, HOLMIUM *(Surgery) 79WXW*

Biomedics, Inc. 949-458-1998
23322 Peralta Dr Ste 11, Laguna Hills, CA 92653

Convergent Laser Technologies 800-848-8200
1660 S Loop Rd, Alameda, CA 94502
ODYSSEY 30 watt Holmium YAG surgical laser system with touch screen control and instant on capability. Especially designed for urological applications such as endoscopic fragmentation of stones in kidney.

Ivry 305-448-9858
216 Catalonia Ave Ste 106, Coral Gables, FL 33134
LASER KIT percutaneous endoscopic laser discectomy.

New Laser Science, Inc. 858-487-5880
PO Box 27210, San Diego, CA 92198

Surgical Laser Technologies, Inc. 800-366-4758
147 Keystone Dr, Montgomeryville, PA 18936

Trimedyne, Inc. 800-733-5273
15091 Bake Pkwy, Irvine, CA 92618
Multiple application OMNIPULSE-MAX 80 watt Holmium laser system with double pulse mode, delivering an effective energy per pulse of up to 7 joules. FDA Clearances in the surgical specialties of urology, lithotripsy, orthopedic/spine, arthroscopy, gynecology, otolaryngology (ENT), general surgery, gastroenterology, plastic surgery.

LASER, SYSTEM, PHACOLYSIS *(Ophthalmology) 86MXO*

Paradigm Medical Industries, Inc. 801-977-8970
2355 S 1070 W, Salt Lake City, UT 84119
Photon ocular surgery workstation.

LASER, THERAPEUTIC *(Radiology) 90REI*

Dynatronics Corp. 800-874-6251
7030 Park Centre Dr, Salt Lake City, UT 84121
DYNATRON 1650 helium-neon cold laser.

Erp Group Professional Products Ltd. 800-361-3537
3232 Autoroute Laval W., Laval, QC H7T 2H6 Canada
Biotherapy lasers from Omega.

Fujifilm Medical Systems Usa, Inc. 800-431-1850
419 West Ave, Stamford, CT 06902
DryPix 7000 and DryPix FM-DP L for centralized imaging applications. DryPix 1000 and 3000 for de-centralized imaging applications.

LASER, THERAPEUTIC *(cont'd)*

Medelco Ltd. 800-268-7927
55 Queens Plate Dr., Unit 9, Toronto, ONT M9W 6P2 Canada
OMNIPROBE and NEUROPROBE, low power therapeutic laser for soft tissue repair and wound healing in physical therapy and rehabilitation.

Multiplex Stimulator Ltd. 800-663-8576
2-1750 McLean Ave., Port Coquitlam, BC V3C 1M9 Canada
Low Level Laser therapy products.

LASER, THERAPY, PAIN *(Cns/Neurology) 84LLP*

Mylon-Tech Health Technologies Inc. 613-728-1667
301 Moodie Dr., Ste. 205, Ottawa, ON K2H 9C4 Canada
Portable laser devices for pain control and soft-tissue treatments.

Spectrum Laser & Technologies, Inc 719-264-7632
2270 Garden of the Gods Rd Ste 103, Colorado Springs, CO 80907
Therapeutic laser system.

LAUNDRY EQUIPMENT *(General) 80TCW*

American Dryer Corp. 508-678-9000
88 Currant Rd, Fall River, MA 02720
ADC drying tumblers, 15 to 670 lb., including Cleanroom dryers.

Cissell Manufacturing Company 888-223-2980
PO Box 990, Shepard Street, Ripon, WI 54971
Laundry dryers with 20-, 30-, 50-, 75-, 80-, 110-, 150-, 175-, and 190-lb capacities. Washers with 40-, 60-, and 80-lb capacities. All types of finishing equipment.

Dexter Apache Holdings, Inc. 800-524-2954
2211 W Grimes Ave, Fairfield, IA 52556
DEXTER & CENTURY laundry dryer.

Electro-Steam Generator Corp. 888-783-2624
1000 Bernard St, Alexandria, VA 22314
Steam generator.

Hoyt Corp. 800-343-9411
251 Forge Rd, Westport, MA 02790

Huebsch Sales 800-553-5120
PO Box 990, Shepard Street, Ripon, WI 54971
Laundry washer-extractors and drying tumblers.

Pellerin Milnor Corp. 800-469-8780
PO Box 400, Kenner, LA 70063
Laundry washer-extractors, 35- to 750-lb capacity, continuous-batch washers. Laundry dryers 55- to 450-lb capacity, freestanding or part of continuous-batch system.

R&B Wire Products, Inc. 800-634-0555
2902 W Garry Ave, Santa Ana, CA 92704
Wire Linen Carts are available in 6 sizes an in 4 shelf options and 3 shelf options with handles. Units have the option of including a solid shelf option to meet Title 22 requirements. All carts have covers available for them.

Tecni-Quip 800-826-1245
960 Crossroads Blvd, PO Box 2050, Seguin, TX 78155
CLEAN CYCLE lint filters for use on institutional laundry dryers and on-premises laundries.

Unimac 800-587-5458
PO Box 990, Ripon, WI 54971
UNIMAC offers a full line of washer-extractors in 18-80 lb capacity hard mounts and 18-250 lb soft mounts; as well as manually controlled drying tumblers in 30-170 lb capacities and microprocessor-controlled 50-, 75-, 120-, and 170-lb units. In addition, UNIMAC offers top-load washers, commercial dryers, and stack dryers.

Wascomat Laundry Equipment 800-645-2204
461 Doughty Blvd, Inwood, NY 11096
Laundry dryers, from 30 lb. capacity to 150 lb. capacities.

Washex, Inc. 800-433-0933
5000 Central Fwy, Wichita Falls, TX 76306
Laundry equipment including continuous-batch laundry systems, self-unloading washer/extractors, end-loading washer/extractors, and side-loading washer/extractors.

LAUNDRY HAMPER *(General) 80TCN*

Alimed, Inc. 800-225-2610
297 High St, Dedham, MA 02026
Brewer's swivel casters resist bacteria.

LAUNDRY HAMPER *(cont'd)*

Approved Medical Systems 951-353-2453
7101 Jurupa Ave Ste 4, Riverside, CA 92504
Priced under $70 each, mini wall mount and isolation room hampers. Its a convenient wall mounted fixture, requiring less than 4" of space when folded. System 90, Deluxe System 90 Hamper Stand; Heavy duty tubular frame sturdy hamper stands--meets Icaho and CDC recommendations. Foot-pedal operated.

Atd-American Co. 800-523-2300
135 Greenwood Ave, Wyncote, PA 19095

Brewer Company, The 888-873-9371
N88W13901 Main St, Menomonee Falls, WI 53051
#33334: Tilt-Top Round 18' Hamper, #11410: Square Tilt-Top Hamper; #33330 Round 18' Hamper, #33395: Folding Hamper

Duralife, Inc. 800-443-5433
195 Phillips Park Dr, Williamsport, PA 17702
Polyvinyl chloride laundry hamper.

Hos-Pillow Corp. 800-468-7874
1011 Campus Dr, Mundelein, IL 60060
Bags and stands.

Innovative Products Unlimited, Inc. 800-833-2826
2120 Industrial Dr, Niles, MI 49120
$177.00 for PVC single, double & triple laundry hamper.

Pedigo Products 360-695-3500
4000 SE Columbia Way, Vancouver, WA 98661
With or without foot operated lid, chrome or stainless steel.

R&B Wire Products, Inc. 800-634-0555
2902 W Garry Ave, Santa Ana, CA 92704
Steel tubular hampers with foot pedal and brakes; comes with leakproof bag; single, double or triple versions.

Steele Canvas Basket Co., Inc. 800-541-8929
201 Williams St, Chelsea, MA 02150

United Metal Fabricators, Inc. 800-638-5322
1316 Eisenhower Blvd, Johnstown, PA 15904
Stainless steel or enamel, washable or disposable bag holding, knock-down design with option of manual and/or foot pedal operated lid.

LAVAGE UNIT *(Gastro/Urology) 78REK*

Atrion Medical Products, Inc. 800-343-9334
1426 Curt Francis Rd NW, Arab, AL 35016
GI balloon inflation device, QL4015, QL6010

LAVAGE UNIT, ENT *(Ear/Nose/Throat) 77REM*

Ethicare Products 800-253-3599
PO Box 5027, Fort Lauderdale, FL 33310
Irrigation unit with adjustable fan spray nozzle for ear, throat and nose.

LAVAGE UNIT, SURGICAL *(Surgery) 79REN*

Micro-Aire Surgical Instruments, Inc. 800-722-0822
1641 Edlich Dr, Charlottesville, VA 22911

Stryker Corp. 800-726-2725
2825 Airview Blvd, Portage, MI 49002

LAVAGE UNIT, WATER JET *(General) 80FQH*

Atek Medical 800-253-1540
620 Watson St SW, Grand Rapids, MI 49504
Blower/mister.

Boston Scientific Corp. 408-935-3400
150 Baytech Dr, San Jose, CA 95134
Blower/mister.

Brasseler Usa - Medical 805-650-5209
4837 McGrath St Ste J, Ventura, CA 93003
Pulse lavage.

Chase Medical, Lp 972-783-0644
1876 Firman Dr, Richardson, TX 75081
Anastomosis visualization devices.

Davol Inc., Sub. C.R. Bard, Inc. 800-556-6275
100 Crossings Blvd, Warwick, RI 02886
Lavage,jet.

Edwards Lifesciences Research Medical 949-250-2500
6864 Cottonwood St, Midvale, UT 84047
Visualization wand.

Griswold Tool And Die, Inc. 517-741-7433
PO Box 86, 8500 M-60 East, Union City, MI 49094
Disposable tips for surgilav tubing.

LAVAGE UNIT, WATER JET *(cont'd)*

H.L. Bouton Co., Inc. 800-426-1881
PO Box 840, Buzzards Bay, MA 02532
LAVOPTIK, personal and wall mounted eyewash units and stations.

Hydrocision, Inc. 888-747-7470
22 Linnell Cir Ste 102, Billerica, MA 01821
Hydrosurgical system for soft-tissue management, including traumatic and chronic wound debridement.

Microaire Surgical Instruments, Llc 434-975-8000
1641 Edlich Dr, Charlottesville, VA 22911

Smith & Nephew, Inc. 800-876-1261
970 Lake Carillon Dr Ste 110, Saint Petersburg, FL 33716
VERSAJET SYSTEMS, VersaJet Hydrosurgery System

Stryker Corp. 800-726-2725
2825 Airview Blvd, Portage, MI 49002

Stryker Puerto Rico, Ltd. 939-307-2500
Hwy. 3, Km. 131.2, Las Guasimas Ind. Park, Arroyo, PR 00714
Various models of jet lavage,various sterile and non-sterile accessories.

Tava Surgical Instruments 805-650-5209
4837 McGrath St Ste J, Ventura, CA 93003
Pulse lavage.

LDL & VLDL PRECIPITATION, CHOLESTEROL VIA ESTERASE-OXIDASE *(Chemistry) 75LBS*

Abbott Diagnostics Div. 626-440-0700
820 Mission St, South Pasadena, CA 91030
Direct hdl.

Accuech, Llc 760-599-6555
2641 La Mirada Dr, Vista, CA 92081
Hdl cholesterol test.

Akers Biosciences, Inc. 800-451-8378
201 Grove Rd, West Deptford, NJ 08086
Rapid cholesterol test directly measures total and bad (LDL) cholesterol and, by computation, good cholesterol (HDL).

Caldon Bioscience, Inc. 909-628-9944
2100 S Reservoir St, Pomona, CA 91766
Hdl.

Caldon Biotech, Inc. 757-224-0177
2251 Rutherford Rd, Carlsbad, CA 92008
Hdl.

Genchem, Inc. 714-529-1616
510 W Central Ave Ste D, Brea, CA 92821
Hdlc precipitating reagent.

Jas Diagnostics, Inc. 305-418-2320
7220 NW 58th St, Miami, FL 33166
Hdl cholesterol.

Raichem, Division Of Hemagen Diagnostics, Inc. 800-438-6100
8225 Mercury Ct, San Diego, CA 92111
LDL & VLDL precipitation by dextran sulfate and magnesium sulfate for assay of HDL cholesterol.

Vital Diagnostics Inc. 714-672-3553
1075 W Lambert Rd Ste D, Brea, CA 92821
Various hdl-cholesterol reagents.

LDL & VLDL PRECIPITATION, HDL *(Chemistry) 75LBR*

Bayer Healthcare Llc 914-524-2955
555 White Plains Rd Fl 5, Tarrytown, NY 10591
Test for hdlc in plasma or serum.

Caliper Systems, Inc. 781-687-9222
23 Crosby Dr, Bedford, MA 01730
Unitized 1:1.

Carolina Liquid Chemistries Corp. 800-471-7272
510 W Central Ave Ste C, Brea, CA 92821
Total lipids.

Diagnostic Specialties 732-549-4011
4 Leonard St, Metuchen, NJ 08840
PEG.

Genzyme 800-332-1042
500 Kendall St, Cambridge, MA 02142

Genzyme Corp. 800-325-2436
160 Christian St, Oxford, CT 06478
Direct LDL.

Intersect Systems, Inc. 360-577-1062
1152 3rd Avenue, Suite D & E, Longview, WA 98632

LDL & VLDL PRECIPITATION, HDL *(cont'd)*

Jas Diagnostics, Inc. 305-418-2320
7220 NW 58th St, Miami, FL 33166
Hdl cholesterol ppt.

Polymer Technology Systems, Inc. 317-870-5610
7736 Zionsville Rd, Indianapolis, IN 46268
Hdl cholesterol test strip.

Raichem, Division Of Hemagen Diagnostics, Inc. 800-438-6100
8225 Mercury Ct, San Diego, CA 92111
RAICHEM HDL-cholesterol direct reagent.

Teco Diagnostics 714-693-7788
1268 N Lakeview Ave, Anaheim, CA 92807
Direct hdl/ldl cholesterol calibrator.

LEAD, PACEMAKER (CATHETER) *(Cardiovascular) 74UCH*

Lake Region Manufacturing, Inc. 952-448-5111
340 Lake Hazeltine Dr, Chaska, MN 55318

Medtronic, Inc. 800-633-8766
710 Medtronic Pkwy, Minneapolis, MN 55432
ACTIVITRAX, ACTIVITRAX II, ACTIVITRAX E, CAPSURE, CAPSURE SP, CAPSUREFIX, CAPSURE Z, ELITE, ELITE II, LEGEND, LEGEND ST, LEGEND II, MICRO MINIX, MINIX, MINIX ST, MINUET, SPECTRAX, SPECTRAX S, SPECTRAX SX, SPECTRAX SX-HT, SPECTRAX SXT, SPECTRAX VL, SPECTRAX VM, SYMBOSIS, SYNERGYST, SYNERGYST II, THERA D, THERA DR, THERA PLUS, THERA S, THERA SR.

St. Jude Medical, Inc. 800-328-9634
1 Saint Jude Medical Dr, Saint Paul, MN 55117

Wytech Industries, Inc. 732-396-3900
960 E Hazelwood Ave, Rahway, NJ 07065

LEAD, PACEMAKER, IMPLANTABLE ENDOCARDIAL
(Cardiovascular) 74QIG

Alto Development Corp. 732-938-2266
5206 Asbury Rd, Wall Township, NJ 07727
Temporary cardiac pacing wires and hook-up accessories.

Cardiac Pacemakers, Inc. 800-227-3422
4100 Hamline Ave N, P.O. Box 64079, Saint Paul, MN 55112
AICD leads systems $550.00 per unit (thin porous tined).

Ela Medical, Inc. 800-352-6466
2950 Xenium Ln N, Plymouth, MN 55441
Carbon tipped electrode, STELA models BT45, BT47, UT46, BJ44, BJ45.

Enpath Medical, Inc. 800-559-2613
2300 Berkshire Ln N, Minneapolis, MN 55441
Epicardial and endocardial implantable pacemaker lead.

Lake Region Manufacturing, Inc. 952-448-5111
340 Lake Hazeltine Dr, Chaska, MN 55318

St. Jude Medical Cardiac Rhythm Management Div. 800-777-2237
15900 Valley View Ct, Sylmar, CA 91342
Unipolar and bipolar silicone or polyurethane insulation with activated carbon electrodes, finned or tined fixation; 5mm, 6mm and VS1 connectors. Bipolar silicone extendable/retractable screw-in with VS1 connector.

LEAD, PACEMAKER, IMPLANTABLE MYOCARDIAL
(Cardiovascular) 74DTB

Cardiac Pacemakers, Inc. 800-227-3422
4100 Hamline Ave N, P.O. Box 64079, Saint Paul, MN 55112
AICD leads systems.

Edwards Lifesciences Technology Sarl 949-250-2500
State Rd. 402 N.km 1.4, Anasco, PR 00610-1577
Electrode, pacemaker, permanent.

Ela Medical, Inc. 800-352-6466
2950 Xenium Ln N, Plymouth, MN 55441

Enpath Medical, Inc. 800-559-2613
2300 Berkshire Ln N, Minneapolis, MN 55441

Ethicon, Inc. 800-4-ETHICON
Route 22 West, Somerville, NJ 08876
Temporary pacing wire/6 product codes.

Fort Wayne Metals Research Prod. Corp. 260-747-4154
9609 Ardmore Ave, Fort Wayne, IN 46809
Various implantable grades, properties, and coatings of precision wire for leads, including DFT(R) wire and cable.

Lake Region Manufacturing, Inc. 952-448-5111
340 Lake Hazeltine Dr, Chaska, MN 55318
Electrode pacemaker - permanent and temporary.

LEAD, PACEMAKER, IMPLANTABLE MYOCARDIAL *(cont'd)*

Maquet Puerto Rico Inc. 408-635-3900
No. 12, Rd. #698, Dorado, PR 00646
Various models of implantable leads.

Medtronic Puerto Rico Operations Co., Villalba 763-514-4000
PO Box 6001, Rd. 149, Km. 56.3, Villalba, PR 00766
Temporary & permanent cardiac pacing leads.

Oscor, Inc. 800-726-7267
3816 Desoto Blvd, Palm Harbor, FL 34683
Permanent pacing lead.

Pace Medical, Inc. 781-890-5656
391 Totten Pond Rd, Waltham, MA 02451
Heart wires.

St. Jude Medical Cardiac Rhythm Management Div. 800-777-2237
15900 Valley View Ct, Sylmar, CA 91342
Unipolar, silicone with sutureless screw-in electrode.

LEAD, PACEMAKER, TEMPORARY ENDOCARDIAL
(Cardiovascular) 74UCI

St. Jude Medical Atrial Fibrillation 800-328-3873
14901 Deveau Pl, Minnetonka, MN 55345
Bipolar standard, semi floating and balloon pacing catheters available in sizes from 4 to 7 french.

LEAD, PACEMAKER, TEMPORARY MYOCARDIAL
(Cardiovascular) 74WQA

Scholten Surgical Instruments, Inc. 209-365-1393
170 Commerce St Ste 101, Lodi, CA 95240
Temporary pacemaker ground wire (disposable indifferent lead).

LECTINS/PROTECTINS *(Hematology) 81KSI*

Biomerieux Inc. 800-682-2666
100 Rodolphe St, Durham, NC 27712
Lectins only.

Dako North America, Inc 805-566-6655
6392 Via Real, Carpinteria, CA 93013

Ortho-Clinical Diagnostics, Inc. 800-828-6316
513 Technology Blvd, Rochester, NY 14626
Direct agglulination test for a1 antigen.

Vector Laboratories, Inc. 800-227-6666
30 Ingold Rd, Burlingame, CA 94010
$65.00 for Lectin Kit I & II; $105.00 for Fluorescein Lectin Kit 1,2, & 3; $105.00 for Rhodamine Lectin Kit I & II; $120.00 for Biotinylated lectin kit 1,2, & 3.

LEG REST *(General) 80RER*

Bryton Corp. 800-567-9500
4310 Guion Rd, Indianapolis, IN 46254
Leg support systems for surgical procedures designed to fit all major surgical tables.

Hermell Products, Inc. 800-233-2342
9 Britton Dr, PO Box 7345, Bloomfield, CT 06002

Senecare Enterprises, Inc. 800-442-4577
350 Central Ave Ste A, Bohemia, NY 11716
PRE-LUBRICTED FOOT & HEEL LIFT SKIN SHIELD SYSTEM. CODE#4201S

LEGGING, COMPRESSION, INFLATABLE, SEQUENTIAL
(Cardiovascular) 74WTT

Aci Medical, Inc. 800-667-9451
1857 Diamond St, San Marcos, CA 92078
VENAPULSE rapid inflation and deflation device used in vascular examinations, ultrasonic imaging and plethysmographic studies.

Huntleigh Healthcare Llc. 800-223-1218
40 Christopher Way, Eatontown, NJ 07724
FLOW PRESS full leg, half leg, and full arm. FLOWPLUS gradient segmental.

LEGGING, COMPRESSION, NON-INFLATABLE *(General) 80LLK*

Alimed, Inc. 800-225-2610
297 High St, Dedham, MA 02026

Coloplast Manufacturing Us, Llc 800-533-0464
1840 W Oak Pkwy, Marietta, GA 30062
CIRCAID, CIRCPLUS and THERA-BOOT non-elastic, adjustable, reusable leggings for lower leg venous disorders.

Elastic Therapy, Inc. 800-849-2497
718 Industrial Park Ave, P.O. Box 4068, Asheboro, NC 27205
Firm compression graduated support stockings; medical/surgical compression stockings. All types.

LEGGING, COMPRESSION, NON-INFLATABLE *(cont'd)*

Geen Healthcare Inc. 800-565-4336
931 Progress Ave. Ste.13, Scarborough, ONT M1G 3V5 Canada
GEEN MEDISOX

Lohmann & Rauscher, Inc. 800-279-3863
6001 SW 6th Ave Ste 101, Topeka, KS 66615
epX Products

Paramedical Distributors 800-245-3278
2020 Grand Blvd, Kansas City, MO 64108
THERAFIRM Compression hose; shear support knee highs, shear support thigh high, maternity pantyhose, firm support pantyhose, men's support socks, anti-embolism stockings.

Shippert Medical Technologies Corp. 800-888-8663
6248 S Troy Cir Ste A, Centennial, CO 80111
VERONIQUE compression garments: full-body girdle, abdominal girdle, compression vest facial band, bras, breast wrap, arm sleeves, male abdominal garment, abnominal binder.

Truform Orthotics & Prosthetics 800-888-0458
3960 Rosslyn Dr, Cincinnati, OH 45209
Medical compression hosiery.

LEGIONELLA DIRECT & INDIRECT FLUORESCENT ANTIBODY REGENTS *(Microbiology) 83LHL*

Bio-Rad Laboratories, Inc. 425-881-8300
6565 185th Ave NE, Redmond, WA 98052
Culture confirmation test for legionella pneumophila.

Focus Diagnostics, Inc. 714-220-1900
10703 Progress Way, Cypress, CA 90630
Legionella ifa serological reagents.

Monoclonal Technologies Inc. 888-683-2414
16335 New Bullpen Rd, Alpharetta, GA 30004
Legionella DFA kits; contract hybridoma production; polyclonal antibody production; ELISA substrates.

Zeus Scientific, Inc. 800-286-2111
PO Box 38, Raritan, NJ 08869
Legionella Direct Fluorescence; test system, and Legionella, Indirect Immunofluorescent. Legionella 96 tests ELISA IgG/IgM/IgA. H. pylori 96 tests ELISA IgG only. Lyme Western Blot 32 tests ELISA IgG only. Lyme Western Blot 32 tests ELISA IgM only. EBV-VCA 96 tests ELISA IgG only.

LEGIONELLA DNA REAGENTS *(Microbiology) 83LQH*

Prodesse, Inc. 888-589-6974
W229N1870 Westwood Dr, Waukesha, WI 53186
Pneumoplex® - Multiplex PCR Reagents for simultaneous detection and differentiation of Mycoplasma pneumoniae, Legionella pneumophila, Legionella micdadei, Chlamydophila pneumoniae and Bordetella pertussis - Research Use Only

LEGIONELLA, SPP., ELISA *(Microbiology) 83MJH*

Ivd Research, Inc. 760-929-7744
5909 Sea Lion Pl Ste D, Carlsbad, CA 92010
Legionella pneumophila urine antigen elisa.

Wampole Laboratories 800-257-9525
2 Research Way, Princeton, NJ 08540

Zeus Scientific, Inc. 800-286-2111
PO Box 38, Raritan, NJ 08869

LENS, CAMERA, SURGICAL *(Surgery) 79FXQ*

Genicon 800-936-1020
6869 Stapoint Ct Ste 114, Winter Park, FL 32792
Single and Three Chip Cameras for Endoscopic Surgery

Newport Glass Works, Ltd. 714-484-8100
PO Box 127, Stanton, CA 90680

LENS, CONDENSING, DIAGNOSTIC *(Ophthalmology) 86HJL*

Ion Vision, Inc. 760-450-4548
7933 Paseo Membrillo, Carlsbad, CA 92009
Ophthalmic, anterior and posterior inner eye viewing lenses.

LENS, CONTACT (OTHER MATERIAL) *(Ophthalmology) 86HQD*

Aero Contact Lens, Inc. 269-345-3202
2958 Business One Dr, Kalamazoo, MI 49048
Sterile aspheric progressive add soft contact lens.

American Contact Lens Inc. 858-487-8684
15970 Bemardo Center Drive, San Diego, CA 92127
Gas-permeable contact lenses. Soft contact lenses.

Art Optical Contact Lens, Inc. 800-253-9364
3175 3 Mile Rd NW, PO Box 1848, Grand Rapids, MI 49534
Rigid gas permeable contact lenses.

LENS, CONTACT (OTHER MATERIAL) *(cont'd)*

Bausch & Lomb, Vision Care 800-553-5340
1400 Goodman St N, Rochester, NY 14609
Seequence, seequence2, Medalist, Occasions, Gold Medalist, Toric, Occasions multi-focal, Medalist Toric, B&L 70, 03, 04, P.S.1, OptimaToric, B3, U3, U4.

Bentec Medical, Inc. 757-224-0177
1380 E Beamer St, Woodland, CA 95776
Rigid gas permeable contact lens blank.

Benz Research And Development Corp. 941-758-8256
6447 Parkland Dr, Sarasota, FL 34243
Rigid gas permeable lenses.

Blanchard Contact Lens, Inc. 603-625-1664
8025 S Willow St Bldg 2, Manchester, NH 03103
Rigid gas permeable contact lens.

Ciba Vision 800-875-3001
11460 Johns Creek Pkwy, Duluth, GA 30097

Ciba Vision Corporation 800-875-3001
11460 Johns Creek Pkwy, Duluth, GA 30097

Contex, Inc. 800-626-6839
4505 Van Nuys Blvd, Sherman Oaks, CA 91403
Contex OK E-System contact lens for overnight orthokeratology

Cooper Vision Carribbean 925-460-3600
500 Road 584 Lot 7, Amuelas Industrial Park, Juana Diaz, PR 00795
Soft contact lenses.

Corneal Lens Lab, Inc. 816-455-0500
621 Moorefield Park Dr Ste F, Richmond, VA 23236
Gas permeable contact lenses.

Firestone Optics, Inc. 816-455-0500
3901 E N.e., 33rd. Terr., Kansas City, MO 64117
Gas permeable contact lenses.

G.T. Laboratories, Inc. 847-998-4776
3333 Warrenville Rd Ste 200, Central Park Of Lisle Center
Lisle, IL 60532
Contact lens blanks.

Ideal Optics, Inc. 612-520-6000
2775 Premiere Pkwy Ste 600, Duluth, GA 30097
Gas permeable, rigid contact lenses.

Innovision, Inc. 402-558-3000
3125 S 61st Ave, Omaha, NE 68106
Rigid gas permeable contact lens.

Lens Dynamics, Inc. 303-237-6927
14998 W 6th Ave Ste 830, Golden, CO 80401
Rigid gas permeable-daily wear.

Lens Express, Inc. 800-536-7397
350 SW 12th Ave, Deerfield Beach, FL 33442

Lobob Laboratories, Inc. 800-83-LOBOB
1440 Atteberry Ln, San Jose, CA 95131
LOBOB rigid hard contact lens wetting solution, soaking solution.

Ocu-Ease Optical Products, Inc. 800-521-8984
629 Tennent Ave, Pinole, CA 94564

Optical Polymer Research, Inc. 352-378-1027
5921 NE 38th St, Gainesville, FL 32609
Oxygen permeable contact lens polymers.

Richardson Limited 602-843-6365
11633 N 38th Ave, Phoenix, AZ 85029
Rigid gas permeable contact lens.

Soderberg Optical, Inc. 800-755-5655
230 Eva St, Saint Paul, MN 55107

Staar Surgical Co. 800-292-7902
1911 Walker Ave, Monrovia, CA 91016
Intraocular contact lens;PMMA lenses, elastic silicone, foldable and toric hydrogel lenses.

The Lagado Corp. 303-789-0933
2890 S Tejon St, Englewood, CO 80110
Rigid gas permeable contact lens.

The Lifestyle Gp Company, L.L.C. 888-379-6645
2530 Trail Mate Dr, Sarasota, FL 34243
Rigid gas permeable contact lens.

Unilens Corp., Usa 727-544-2531
10431 72nd St, Largo, FL 33777
Silicone/acrylate rigid gas permeable contact lenses.

Visionary Contact Lens 714-237-1900
2940 E Miraloma Ave, Anaheim, CA 92806
Rigid gas permeable contact lenses for daily wear (clear and tinted).

LENS, CONTACT (OTHER MATERIAL) *(cont'd)*

Vistakon, Inc. 800-874-5278
7500 Centurion Pkwy, Jacksonville, FL 32256
$1,400.00 per 100 units.

X-Cel Contacts 770-622-9235
2775 Premiere Pkwy Ste 600, Duluth, GA 30097
Gas permeable lenses.

X-Cel Contacts 770-622-9235
1120 Sycamore Ave Ste D, Vista, CA 92081
Gas permeable lenses.

LENS, CONTACT(RIGID GAS PERMEABLE)-EXTENDED WEAR
(Ophthalmology) 86MWL

Con-Cise Contact Lens Co. 800-772-3911
14450 Doolittle Dr, PO Box 2198, San Leandro, CA 94577
Oxyflow EW, Oxyflow HDS, Oxyflow 151, Menicon Z EW, Menicon Z CW.

Rochester Optical Mfg. Company 585-254-0022
1260 Lyell Ave, Rochester, NY 14606

X-Cel Contacts 770-622-9235
2775 Premiere Pkwy Ste 600, Duluth, GA 30097
Gas permeable lenses, extended wear.

X-Cel Contacts 770-622-9235
1120 Sycamore Ave Ste D, Vista, CA 92081
Gas permeable lenses, extended wear.

LENS, CONTACT, (DISPOSABLE) *(Ophthalmology) 86MVN*

Cooper Vision Carribbean 925-460-3600
500 Road 584 Lot 7, Amuelas Industrial Park, Juana Diaz, PR 00795
Contact lens.

LENS, CONTACT, BIFOCAL *(Ophthalmology) 86ULH*

Ciba Vision Corporation 800-875-3001
11460 Johns Creek Pkwy, Duluth, GA 30097

Co/Op Optical Vision Designs 866-733-2667
2424 E 8 Mile Rd, E. of Dequindre, Detroit, MI 48234

Con-Cise Contact Lens Co. 800-772-3911
14450 Doolittle Dr, PO Box 2198, San Leandro, CA 94577
Mandell Seamless Bifocal, EZ Bifocal, Natural Vision Bifocal, Vericon Aspheric Bifocal.

LENS, CONTACT, DISPOSABLE *(Ophthalmology) 86WIZ*

Co/Op Optical Vision Designs 866-733-2667
2424 E 8 Mile Rd, E. of Dequindre, Detroit, MI 48234

Coopervision Inc. 716-385-6810
711 North Rd, Scottsville, NY 14546

Vistakon, Inc. 800-874-5278
7500 Centurion Pkwy, Jacksonville, FL 32256
$250 /100 units.

LENS, CONTACT, EXTENDED-WEAR *(Ophthalmology) 86ULD*

Ciba Vision 800-875-3001
11460 Johns Creek Pkwy, Duluth, GA 30097

Co/Op Optical Vision Designs 866-733-2667
2424 E 8 Mile Rd, E. of Dequindre, Detroit, MI 48234

Con-Cise Contact Lens Co. 800-772-3911
14450 Doolittle Dr, PO Box 2198, San Leandro, CA 94577
Oxyflow EW, Oxyflow HDS, Oxyflow 100, Menicon Z EW, Menicon Z CW.

Coopervision Inc. 800-341-2020
10 Faraday, Irvine, CA 92618
Preference 4-Pack, Preference Standard 4-Pack, Preference Toric 4-Pack, Cooper Toric, CooperClear, CooperClear FW, CooperThin, Vantage(Handling Tint), Vantage Accents(Enhancement Tint), Vantage Thin(Clear), Vantage Thin(Handling tint), Vantage Thing Accents(Enhancement tint), Permaflex Naturals, Permaflex UV Naturals, Peralens XL, Permalens, Permalens Mano(Therapeutic), Permalens High Plus(Aphakic), Hydrasoft DW Toric(Astgmatism), Hydrasoft XW Toric, Hydrasoft Sphere, Hydrasoft XW Sphere, Hydrasoft Aphakic Lenses. Preference 4-Pack flexible wear, planned replacement sphere tetrafilcon A, 43% water material, $31.00. Preference Standard 4-Pack Daily wear planned replacement sphere tetrafilcon A, 43% water material, $31.00. Preference Toric 4-Pack daily wear planned replacement toric tetrafilcon A, 43% water material, $65.00. Cooper Toric daily wear, conventional wear Toric tetrafilcon A, 43% water material, $30.00. CooperClear daily wear conventional wear sphere tetrafilcon A, 43% water material, $13.00. CooperClear FW flexible wear, conventional wear sphere tetrafilcon A, 43% water material, $13.00. CooperThin daily wear, conventional wear sphere polymacon, 38% water material, $25.00. Vantage(Handling tint) daily wear conventional wear sphere tetrafilcon A, 43% water material, $21.00. Vantage Accents(Enhancement tint) daily wear conventional wear sphere tetrafilcon A, 43% water material enhancement tint selection, $25.00. Vantage Thin(Clear) flexible wear conventional wear sphere tetrafilcon A, 43% water material, $21.00. Vantage Thin(Handling tint) flexible wear conventional wear sphere tetrafilcon A, 43% water material, $22.00. Vantage Thin Accents(Enhancement tint) flexible wear conventional wear sphere tetrafilcon A, 43% water material enhancement tint selection, $26.00. Permaflex Naturals flexible wear conventional wear sphere surfilcon A, 74% water material, $32.00. Permaflex UV Naturals flexible wear conventional wear sphere vasurfilcon A, 74% water material, $54.00. Permalens XL extended wear conventional wear sphere perfilcon A, 71% water material, $34.00. Permalens extended wear conventional wear sphere perfilcon A, 71% water material, $53.00. Permalens Mano(Therapeutic) extended wear conventional wear sphere perfilcon A, 71% water material therapeutic lens, $80.00. Permalens High Plus(Aphakic) extended wear conventional wear sphere perfilcon A, 71% water material aphakic lens, $80.00. Hydrasoft DW Toric(Astgmatism) daily wear conventional wear custom toric methafilcon B 55% water material, $55-89. Hydrasoft XW Toric flexible wear conventional wear custom toric methafilcon B, 55% water material, $55.00-89.00. Hydrasoft Sphere daily wear conventional wear sphere methafilcon B, 55% water material, Std. parameters $25, Specialty $45, Custom $75. Hydrasoft XW Sphere flexible wear conventional wear sphere methafilcon B, 55% water material, Std. parameters $25, Specialty $ 45, Custom $ 75. Hydrasoft Aphakic daily or flexible wear, conventional wear sphere methafilcon B, 55% water material, $40.00.

Coopervision Inc. 716-385-6810
711 North Rd, Scottsville, NY 14546

Vistakon, Inc. 800-874-5278
7500 Centurion Pkwy, Jacksonville, FL 32256
$1,200 per 100 units; $4,900/100 pcs. of extended wear, toric lenses.

LENS, CONTACT, GAS-PERMEABLE *(Ophthalmology) 86MRC*

Bausch & Lomb Inc., Greenville Solutions Plant 585-338-6000
8507 Pelham Rd, Greenville, SC 29615
Contact lens care products.

C&E Gp Specialists 800-346-2626
1015 Calle Amanecer, San Clemente, CA 92673
Products, contact lens care, rigid gas permeable.

Ciba Vision 800-875-3001
11460 Johns Creek Pkwy, Duluth, GA 30097

Con-Cise Contact Lens Co. 800-772-3911
14450 Doolittle Dr, PO Box 2198, San Leandro, CA 94577
Oxyflow, Pliaflex, Menicon, Mandell Seamless Bifocal, Natural Vision, Gravity Lens, Mandell / Moore Bitoric, EZ Bifocal, Surgilens.

Genzyme Corporation 617-252-7500
1125 Pleasantview Ter, Ridgefield, NJ 07657
Lubricant-wetting,re-wetting drop.

Paragon Vision Sciences, Inc. 800-528-8279
947 E Impala Ave, Mesa, AZ 85204

LENS, CONTACT, HYDROPHILIC *(Ophthalmology) 86TGY*

Ciba Vision 800-875-3001
11460 Johns Creek Pkwy, Duluth, GA 30097
6 models, all made of phemfilcon A: $24.00 each for DuraSoft 3 lite tint spherical flexible wear lens. $54.00 each for DuraSoft OPTIFIT toric flexible wear lens. $21.00 each for DuraSoft 2 LiteTint spherical daily wear lens. $46.00 for DuraSoft 2 OPTIFIT toric daily wear lens. $48.95 each for DuraSoft 3 colors in blue, green, aqua, $48.95 each for DuraSoft 3 colors in blue, green, aqua, hazel, gray and violet. $51.95 for Complements by DuraSoft hazel, gray and violet. $51.95 for Complements by DuraSoft colors.

Ciba Vision Corporation 800-875-3001
11460 Johns Creek Pkwy, Duluth, GA 30097

Diversified Ophthalmics, Inc. 800-626-2281
250 McCullough St, Cincinnati, OH 45226

Kontur Kontact Lens Co., Inc. 800-227-1320
642 Alfred Nobel Dr, Hercules, CA 94547
$15.00 per spherical lens and $37.50 to $85.00 per toric lens; both types consist of 55% water.

Optikem International, Inc. 800-525-1752
2172 S Jason St, Denver, CO 80223

Vistakon, Inc. 800-874-5278
7500 Centurion Pkwy, Jacksonville, FL 32256
$4,700.00 per 100 units.

LENS, CONTACT, POLYMETHYLMETHACRYLATE
(Ophthalmology) 86HPX

Associated Contacts, Inc. 941-921-1200
2036 Bispham Rd, Sarasota, FL 34231
Rigid gas permeable contact lens.

Ciba Vision 800-875-3001
11460 Johns Creek Pkwy, Duluth, GA 30097
$21.00 for DuraSoft 2 LiteTint spherical lens, $20.00 for DuraSoft 2 clear spherical lens, $69.50 for DuraSoft 3 OptiFit colors, $26.00 for AQUAFLEX Superthin Minus, $27.00 for AQUAFLEX Superthin Plus, $24.00 for DuraSoft 3 LiteTint Flexiwear and $23.00 for DuraSoft 3 clear Flexiwear.

Ciba Vision Corporation 800-875-3001
11460 Johns Creek Pkwy, Duluth, GA 30097

Firestone Optics, Inc. 816-455-0500
3901 E N.e., 33rd. Terr., Kansas City, MO 64117
Pmma contact lenses.

Ideal Optics, Inc. 612-520-6000
2775 Premiere Pkwy Ste 600, Duluth, GA 30097
Contact lenses.

Lens Dynamics, Inc. 303-237-6927
14998 W 6th Ave Ste 830, Golden, CO 80401
Glassflex.

The Lagado Corp. 303-789-0933
2890 S Tejon St, Englewood, CO 80110
Hard contact lens.

X-Cel Contacts 770-622-9235
2775 Premiere Pkwy Ste 600, Duluth, GA 30097
Pmma lenses.

X-Cel Contacts 770-622-9235
1120 Sycamore Ave Ste D, Vista, CA 92081
Pmma lenses.

LENS, CONTACT, POLYMETHYLMETHACRYLATE, DIAGNOSTIC *(Ophthalmology) 86HJK*

Avi-Advanced Visual Instruments Inc. 212-262-7878
321 W 44th St Ste 902, New York, NY 10036
Contact laser & diagnostic,gonioscopy & vitrectomy lens,minature indirect contac.

Ideal Optics, Inc. 612-520-6000
2775 Premiere Pkwy Ste 600, Duluth, GA 30097
Contact lens.

Ocular Instruments, Inc. 800-888-6616
2255 116th Ave NE, Bellevue, WA 98004
Hand-held contact lenses for diagnostic procedures, surgical contact lenses and hand-held contact lenses for laser therapy. Also mirrored contact lenses for diagnosing diseases and disorders of the eye.

LENS, CONTACT, TINTED *(Ophthalmology) 86VJN*

Cal Bionics, Inc. 415-892-1892
1777 Indian Valley Rd, Novato, CA 94947

Ciba Vision 800-875-3001
11460 Johns Creek Pkwy, Duluth, GA 30097
Fresh Look Colors, Fresh Look Color Enhancer, Fresh Look with various tints, Durasoft Colors; also Precision IV Gentle Touch.

LENS, FRESNEL, FLEXIBLE, DIAGNOSTIC *(Ophthalmology) 86HJJ*

Awi Industries (Usa), Inc. 909-597-0808
14502 Central Ave, Chino, CA 91710
Plastic optics, lens assembly. Mirrors - specially coated mirrors for laser surgery equipment.

Dynamics Research Corp. 800-522-4321
60 Frontage Rd, Andover, MA 01810

Gn Otometrics North America 800-289-2150
125 Commerce Dr, Schaumburg, IL 60173
Frenzel lenses.

LENS, FUNDUS, HRUBY, DIAGNOSTIC *(Ophthalmology) 86HJI*

Gyrus Ent L.L.C., Sub. Of Gyrus Acmi, Inc. 508-804-2739
2925 Appling Rd, Bartlett, TN 38133
Various.

LENS, INTRAOCULAR *(Ophthalmology) 86HQL*

A.M.O. Puerto Rico Manufacturing, Inc 714-247-8656
Rd. 402, Km. 4.2, Anasco, PR 00610
Intraocular lenses.

Alcon Manufacturing, Ltd. 304-736-5230
6065 Kyle Ln, Huntington, WV 25702

LENS, INTRAOCULAR *(cont'd)*

Allergan 800-366-6554
2525 Dupont Dr, Irvine, CA 92612
From $305 to $405 per unit, available with ultraviolet blocker.

Bausch & Lomb 585-338-6000
1 Bausch and Lomb Pl, Rochester, NY 14604

Bausch & Lomb Surgical 636-255-5051
3365 Tree Court Ind Blvd, Saint Louis, MO 63122

Bausch & Lomb, Inc. 813-724-6600
21 N Park Place Blvd, Clearwater, FL 33759

Benz Research And Development Corp. 941-758-8256
6447 Parkland Dr, Sarasota, FL 34243
Non-sterile intraocular lens for export only.

Ciba Vision Puerto Rico, Inc. 678-415-3638
El Jibaro Industrial Park, Cidra, PR 00739
Posterior chamber intraocular lens.

Cima Technology, Inc. 724-733-2627
3253 Old Frankstown Rd Ste C, Pittsburgh, PA 15239
Aphakic intraocular lens.

Ellis Ophthalmic Technologies, Inc. 718-656-7390
147-39, 175 St.,, Suite #128, Jamaica, NY 11434
Introcular lens.

Eyekon Medical, Inc 800-633-9248
2451 Enterprise Rd, Clearwater, FL 33763
Single piece, multipiece, hydrophilic acrylic.

Eyekon Medical, Inc. 800-633-9248
2451 Enterprise Rd, Clearwater, FL 33763
Intraocular lens.

Eyeonics, Inc. 949-916-9352
10574 Acacia St Ste D1, Rancho Cucamonga, CA 91730
Intraocular lens.

Howard Instruments, Inc. 205-553-4453
4749 Appletree Ln, Tuscaloosa, AL 35405

Medennium, Inc. 949-789-5385
9 Parker Ste 150, Irvine, CA 92618
Intraoculal lens.

Ophtec Usa, Inc. 561-989-8767
6421 Congress Ave Ste 112, Boca Raton, FL 33487
ARTISAN Myopia lens and ARTISAN Hyperopia lens. Phakic implants for the correction of high myopia and hyperopia.

Ophthalmic Innovations Intl., Inc. 909-937-1033
4290 E Brickell St Ste A, Ontario, CA 91761
Intraocular lens.

Staar Surgical Co. 800-292-7902
1911 Walker Ave, Monrovia, CA 91016
PHAKIC, Implantable Collamer Lens

Tekia, Inc. 949-699-1300
17 Hammond Ste 414, Irvine, CA 92618
kelman duet implant; teklens ; teklens II

Thinoptx, Inc. 276-623-2258
15856 Porterfield Hwy, Abingdon, VA 24210
Posterior chamber intraocular lens.

U.S. Iol, Inc. 800-354-7848
2500 Sandersville Rd, Lexington, KY 40511

LENS, INTRAOCULAR, ANTERIOR CHAMBER
(Ophthalmology) 86UBA

Allergan 800-366-6554
2525 Dupont Dr, Irvine, CA 92612
From $360 to $390 for anterior chamber lenses, priced according to model, with or w/o ultraviolet blocker.

LENS, INTRAOCULAR, MULTIFOCAL *(Ophthalmology) 86MFK*

A.M.O. Puerto Rico Manufacturing, Inc 714-247-8656
Rd. 402, Km. 4.2, Anasco, PR 00610
Multifocal intraocular lens.

LENS, INTRAOCULAR, POSTERIOR CHAMBER
(Ophthalmology) 86UBD

Allergan 800-366-6554
2525 Dupont Dr, Irvine, CA 92612
From $325 to $405 for posterior chamber intraocular lenses, priced according to model; ultraviolet blocking, YAG laser compatible and one piece PMMA styles available.

LENS, MADDOX *(Ophthalmology) 86HKR*

Astron International Inc. 239-435-0136
3410 Westview Dr, Naples, FL 34104
Lens, maddox.

Eye Care And Cure 800-486-6169
4646 S Overland Dr, Tucson, AZ 85714
Maddox lens.

Gulden Ophthalmics 800-659-2250
225 Cadwalader Ave, Elkins Park, PA 19027

LENS, OTHER *(Ophthalmology) 86REV*

Allergan 800-366-6554
2525 Dupont Dr, Irvine, CA 92612
Laser contact lens.

Arw Optical Corp. 910-452-7373
6631 Amsterdam Way # B, Wilmington, NC 28405
Cylinder lenses.

Bausch & Lomb 585-338-6000
1 Bausch and Lomb Pl, Rochester, NY 14604

Diversified Ophthalmics, Inc. 800-626-2281
250 McCullough St, Cincinnati, OH 45226

Fortrad Eye Instruments Corp. 973-543-2371
8 Franklin Rd, Mendham, NJ 07945

Gammadirect Medical Division 847-267-5929
PO Box 383, Lake Forest, IL 60045
BetaSpecs-PM, disposable post-mydriasis lens

General Scientific Corp. 800-959-0153
77 Enterprise Dr, Ann Arbor, MI 48103
Also, surgical loupes. Vision enhancement for dentists and surgeons.

H.L. Bouton Co., Inc. 800-426-1881
PO Box 840, Buzzards Bay, MA 02532
LENSCLEAN, antifog liquid cleaners designed for safety eyewear.

La Croix Optical Co. 870-698-1881
PO Box 2556, Batesville, AR 72503
Manufacturer of custom precision optical components, such as lenses, windows, prisms, mirrors and achromats.

Marco Ophthalmic, Inc. 800-874-5274
11825 Central Pkwy, Jacksonville, FL 32224
Replacement sphere, cylinder and prism lenses.

Navitar, Inc. 800-828-6778
200 Commerce Dr, Rochester, NY 14623
Optical equipment lenses.

Opco Laboratory, Inc. 978-345-2522
704 River St, Fitchburg, MA 01420
Custom optical lenses for analytical instruments.

Peter M. Tolliver 585-244-8788
42 Varinna Dr, Rochester, NY 14618
Lateral View Extender Lens Device

The Lifestyle Co. Inc. 800-622-0777
1800 State Route 34 Ste 401, Wall Township, NJ 07719
MV2 Hydrophilic bifocal soft contact lenses - blister packed - frequent replacement lens.

Vicon Industries Inc. 800-645-9116
89 Arkay Dr, Hauppauge, NY 11788
Video surveillance equipment, including cameras, lenses, monitors, etc. VIDEO MULTIPLEXERS - 16 input multiplexers available in simplex or duplex, color or monochrome with telemetry, alarm detection, digital PTZ functions and screen playback.

Volk Optical Inc. 800-345-8655
7893 Enterprise Dr, Mentor, OH 44060
Diagnostic, therapeutic/laser treatment, and surgical ophthalmic lenses and accessories for eyecare/medical purposes.

LENS, SET, TRIAL, OPHTHALMIC *(Ophthalmology) 86HPC*

Eye Care And Cure 800-486-6169
4646 S Overland Dr, Tucson, AZ 85714
Trial lens set.

Marco Ophthalmic, Inc. 800-874-5274
11825 Central Pkwy, Jacksonville, FL 32224
$1190.00 to $2,360.00 for trial lens sets. (List prices)

Newport Glass Works, Ltd. 714-484-8100
PO Box 127, Stanton, CA 90680

Ocular Instruments, Inc. 800-888-6616
2255 116th Ave NE, Bellevue, WA 98004
Indirect ophthalmoscopy lenses.

LENS, SET, TRIAL, OPHTHALMIC *(cont'd)*

Reichert, Inc. 888-849-8955
3362 Walden Ave, Depew, NY 14043
Lens set with carrying case

Richmond Products, Inc. 505-275-2406
4400 Silver Ave SE, Albuquerque, NM 87108
Hematocrit control.

Topcon Medical Systems, Inc. 800-223-1130
37 W Century Rd, Paramus, NJ 07652
Trial lens set: full diameter $1,075.00; corrected curve, $2,550.00.

Woodlyn, Inc. 800-331-7389
2920 Malmo Dr, Ophthalmic Instruments and Equipment
Arlington Heights, IL 60005
Model 27300S. The Woodlyn Trial Lens Set features a complete selection of full-aperature bi-concave and bi-convex lenses. Call for current prices.

LENS, SPECTACLE (PRESCRIPTION), FOR READING DISCOMFORT *(Ophthalmology) 86NJH*

Crystal Computer Lenses 214-773-3457
104 E US Highway 80 Ste 100, Forney, TX 75126
Computer glasses.

Signet Armorlite, Inc. 760-744-4000
1001 Armorlite Dr, San Marcos, CA 92069
Single vision and multifocal spectacle lenses.

Vision Optics Technologies Ltd. 502-671-0735
1816 Production Ct, Louisville, KY 40299
Lens to provide refractive corrections mounted on a frame.

Vivvid International 447-040-4013
800 N Ferncreek Ave, Orlando, FL 32803
Ophthalmic lens.

LENS, SPECTACLE/EYEGLASSES, CUSTOM (PRESCRIPTION) *(Ophthalmology) 86HRA*

Co/Op Optical Vision Designs 866-733-2667
2424 E 8 Mile Rd, E. of Dequindre, Detroit, MI 48234

Dispensers Optical Service Corp. 800-626-4545
1815 Plantside Dr, Louisville, KY 40299
Semi-finished and finished single vision and multi-focal ophthalmic lenses.

Rochester Optical Mfg. Company 585-254-0022
1260 Lyell Ave, Rochester, NY 14606
Prescription lenses

Southern Optical Laboratory, Inc. 800-333-8498
501 Merritt Ave, Nashville, TN 37203

Titmus Optical Inc. 800-446-1802
690 Hp Way, 3811 CorPOrate Drive, Chester, VA 23836
Industrial prescription safety eyewear in metal/plastic, 60+ styles.

LENS, SPECTACLE/EYEGLASSES, NON-CUSTOM *(Ophthalmology) 86HQG*

Alfa Import And Export 905-457-9941
13 Halldorson Trail, Brampton L6W 4M4 Canada
Spectacle lens blanks

American Optical Lens Mex S. De R.L. De C.V. 408-735-1982
Calle 2, Orienta #133,, C.d. Industrial Mesa De Otay, Tijuana, B.c. Mexico
Spectacle lens

Canada Optix, Inc. 905-238-3332
5181 Bradco Blvd, Mississauga L4W 2A6 Canada
Polycarbonate spectacle lens

Carl Zeiss Vision Inc. 707-763-9911
1030 Worldwide Blvd, Hebron, KY 41048
Spectacle lens.

Carl Zeiss Vision-Kentucky 866-289-7652
1050 Worldwide Blvd, Hebron, KY 41048
Spectacle lens.

Co/Op Optical Vision Designs 866-733-2667
2424 E 8 Mile Rd, E. of Dequindre, Detroit, MI 48234

Coeye, Inc. 321-543-2219
2025 W New Haven Ave, West Melbourne, FL 32904
Prescription spectacle lenses.

Cole Vision Coropration 770-305-7352
2465 Joe Field Rd, Dallas, TX 75229
Prescription spectacles.

Cole Vision Corp. 770-305-7352
2150 Bixby Rd, Lockbourne, OH 43137
Prescription specatacles.

LENS, SPECTACLE/EYEGLASSES, NON-CUSTOM *(cont'd)*

Cole Vision Corporation 770-305-7352
9926 International Blvd, Cincinnati, OH 45246
Prescription spectacles.

Cole Vision Corporation 770-305-7352
4435 Anderson Rd, Knoxville, TN 37918
Prescription spectacles.

Cole Vision Corporation 770-305-7352
1887 S 3230 W, Salt Lake City, UT 84104
Prescription spectacles.

Cole Vision Corporation 770-305-7352
5780 E Shelby Dr, Memphis, TN 38141
Prescription spectacles.

Cole Vision Corporation 513-765-6300
820 Southlake Blvd, Richmond, VA 23236
Prescription spectacles.

Collard-Rose Optical Lab 562-698-2286
12402 Philadelphia St, Whittier, CA 90601
Prescription spectacle lenses.

Ctp Coil Inc. 800-933-2645
1801 Howard St Ste D, Elk Grove Village, IL 60007
Uncut unfinished, microscopic, prismatic lenses for binoculars or monocular frame mounting.

Dietz Laboratories, Inc. 800-792-8934
3124 Stuart Dr, Fort Worth, TX 76110

Essilor Industries 011-331-4977
Sabanetas Industrial Park, Mercedita, PR 00715
Various.

European Eyewear Corp. 941-322-6771
630 Myakka Rd, Sarasota, FL 34240
Spectacles, sunglasses.

Habilis, Inc. 203-377-8835
155 Hill St, Milford, CT 06460
Resolution.

I.F. Optical, Inc. 773-761-3323
2812 W Touhy Ave, Chicago, IL 60645
Single vision lens blanks.

Indo Lens Us, Inc. 800-729-1959
224 James St, Bensenville, IL 60106
Prescription spectable lens-various models.

Landon Lens Manufacturing Corp. 212-348-4020
301 E 69th St, New York, NY 10021
Plastic progressive lenses.

Lenscrafters, Inc. 770-305-7352
9926 International Blvd, Cincinnati, OH 45246
Spectacle lens.

Miki, Inc. 808-943-6454
1450 Ala Moana Blvd Ste 1247, Honolulu, HI 96814
Lenses.

National Vision, Inc. 800-637-3597
296 Grayson Hwy, Attn: Legal/C. Mingle, Lawrenceville, GA 30046
Eyeglasses.

Nikon Optical Canada, Inc. 011-813-5600
100-5075 Rue Fullum, Montreal H2H 2K3 Canada
Ophthalmic progressive addiction lens

Oakley, Inc. 800-431-1439
1 Icon, Foothill Ranch, CA 92610
Sunglasses, prescription.

Ophthonix Inc. 760-842-5772
1491 Poinsettia Ave, Vista, CA 92081
Prescription spectacle lens.

Optical Dynamics Corporation 502-671-2020
10100 Bluegrass Pkwy, Louisville, KY 40299
Prescription spectacle lens.

Optical Suppliers, Inc. 808-486-2933
99-1253 Halawa Valley St, Aiea, HI 96701
Eyeglasses.

Optima, Inc. 203-377-8835
111 Research Dr, Stratford, CT 06615

Oracle Lens Mfg. Corp. 401-736-9600
30 Jefferson Park Rd, Warwick, RI 02888
Polycarbonate plastic prescription lenses.

Paris Miki, Inc. 425-883-2464
2863 152nd Ave NE, Redmond, WA 98052

LENS, SPECTACLE/EYEGLASSES, NON-CUSTOM *(cont'd)*

Polyvision Inc. 888-645-7788
875 E Patriot Blvd Ste 201, Reno, NV 89511
Uncut finished single vision spectacle lens.

Precision Optical Products 619-287-4436
4950 Waring Rd Ste 4, San Diego, CA 92120
Custom spectacle lens.

Rochester Optical Mfg. Company 585-254-0022
1260 Lyell Ave, Rochester, NY 14606

Rodenstock North America, Inc. 614-409-2820
2150 Bixby Rd, Lockbourne, OH 43137
Prescription spectacle lens.

Signet Armorlite, Inc. 760-744-4000
1001 Armorlite Dr, San Marcos, CA 92069
Ophthalmic lens.

Sola Custom Coatings, Inc. 858-509-9899
9117 SE Saint Helens St, Street, Clackamas, OR 97015
Spectacle lens.

Specialty Lens Corp. 800-366-1382
3955 Howick St, Salt Lake City, UT 84107
Various types of prescription lens blanks,plastic or glass,clear or polarized.

Sunglass International Llc 888-478-6764
71 Cypress St, Warwick, RI 02888
Prescription sunglasses.

The Optical Shop 405-514-0903
1111 S Eastern Ave, Oklahoma City, OK 73129
Reading glasses for presbyopia & myopia.

Transitions Optical, Inc. 727-545-0400
9251 Belcher Rd, Pinellas Park, FL 33782
Multiple transitions lenses.

Tri-City Optical 727-528-8873
5600 115th Ave N Ste B, Clearwater, FL 33760
Eyeglasses.

Vision Optics Technologies Ltd. 502-671-0735
1816 Production Ct, Louisville, KY 40299
Lens to provide refractive corrections mounted on a frame.

Vision-Ease Lens, Inc. 800-328-3449
7000 Sunwood Dr NW, Ramsey, MN 55303

Vivvid International 447-040-4013
800 N Ferncreek Ave, Orlando, FL 32803
Ophthalmic lens.

X-Cel Optical Co. 800-747-9235
806 S Benton Dr # 420, Sauk Rapids, MN 56379
Various types of opthelmic semi-finished lens blanks.

Younger Mfg. Co. 310-783-1649
2925 California St, Torrance, CA 90503
Lens blank, semi-finished lens.

LENS, SURGICAL, LASER *(Ophthalmology) 86LQJ*

Alceram Tech Inc 516-849-3666
57 2nd St, Ronkonkoma, NY 11779
Wide Range of custom and stock lenses, in various materials.

Ocular Instruments, Inc. 800-888-6616
2255 116th Ave NE, Bellevue, WA 98004
Glass lenses for vitrectomy surgery.

LENSES, SOFT CONTACT, DAILY WEAR *(Ophthalmology) 86LPL*

Adventures In Color Technology 303-271-9644
1800 Jackson St Ste 214, Golden, CO 80401
Tinted daily wear soft contact lens.

Aero Contact Lens, Inc. 269-345-3202
2958 Business One Dr, Kalamazoo, MI 49048
Sterile toric soft contact lens (various).

Bausch & Lomb 585-338-6000
1 Bausch and Lomb Pl, Rochester, NY 14604

Benz Research And Development Corp. 941-758-8256
6447 Parkland Dr, Sarasota, FL 34243
Soft contact lenses.

Biomed Devices Corp. 540-636-7976
1325 Progress Dr, Front Royal, VA 22630
Soft contact lens.

Ciba Vision Puerto Rico, Inc. 678-415-3638
El Jibaro Industrial Park, Cidra, PR 00739
Various models of hydrophilic contact lenses.

LENSES, SOFT CONTACT, DAILY WEAR *(cont'd)*

Cooper Vision Carribbean 925-460-3600
500 Road 584 Lot 7, Amuelas Industrial Park, Juana Diaz, PR 00795
Multiple models of soft contact lenses.

Cooper Vision, Inc. 510-460-3600
1215 Boissevain Ave, Norfolk, VA 23507
Soft (hydrophilic) contact lens for daily wear.

Coopervision 585-421-0100
370 Woodcliff Dr Ste 200, Fairport, NY 14450

Hydrogel Vision Corporation 877-336-2482
7575 Commerce Ct, Sarasota, FL 34243
Soft(hydrophillic)contact lens.

Ideal Optics, Inc. 612-520-6000
2775 Premiere Pkwy Ste 600, Duluth, GA 30097
Various soft lenses.

Johnson & Johnson Vision Care, Inc. 800-843-2020
7500 Centurion Pkwy Ste 100, Jacksonville, FL 32256
Soft (hydrophilic) contact lens.

Metro Optics Of Austin, Ltd. 512-251-2382
15802 Vision Dr, Pflugerville, TX 78660
Metrosoft soft lens.

Specialeyes Llc 813-645-2855
6447 Parkland Dr Ste 2020, Sarasota, FL 34243
Daily wear contact lens.

Unilens Corp., Usa 727-544-2531
10431 72nd St, Largo, FL 33777
Hydrophilic contact lenses.

Unilens Corp., Usa 800-446-2020
10431 72nd St, Largo, FL 33777

United Contact Lens, Inc. 425-743-7343
19111 61st Ave NE Unit 5, Arlington, WA 98223
Ucl-55.

Wavetouch Technologies, Llc 858-924-9283
15970 Bernardo Center Dr, San Diego, CA 92127
Soft daily wear lenses.

Westcon Contact Lens Co. 770-622-9235
611 Eisenhauer St, Grand Junction, CO 81505
Daily wear soft contact lens.

X-Cel Contacts 770-622-9235
2775 Premiere Pkwy Ste 600, Duluth, GA 30097
Softlens.

LENSES, SOFT CONTACT, EXTENDED WEAR
(Ophthalmology) 86LPM

Cooper Vision Carribbean 925-460-3600
500 Road 584 Lot 7, Amuelas Industrial Park, Juana Diaz, PR 00795
Multiple models of soft contact lenses.

Coopervision 585-421-0100
370 Woodcliff Dr Ste 200, Fairport, NY 14450

Johnson & Johnson Vision Care, Inc. 800-843-2020
7500 Centurion Pkwy Ste 100, Jacksonville, FL 32256
Soft (hydrophilic) contact lens.

Lens Dynamics, Inc. 303-237-6927
14998 W 6th Ave Ste 830, Golden, CO 80401
Technicon.

Unilens Corp., Usa 727-544-2531
10431 72nd St, Largo, FL 33777
Hydrophilic contact lenses.

Unilens Corp., Usa 800-446-2020
10431 72nd St, Largo, FL 33777

Wavetouch Technologies, Llc 858-924-9283
15970 Bernardo Center Dr, San Diego, CA 92127
Soft extended wear lenses.

Westcon Contact Lens Co. 770-622-9235
611 Eisenhauer St, Grand Junction, CO 81505
Soft (hydrophilic) contact lens.

LENSOMETER *(Ophthalmology) 86REW*

Carl Zeiss Meditec Inc. 877-486-7473
5160 Hacienda Dr, Dublin, CA 94568
The Humphrey Lens Analyzer, Model 350 and 360 with SPEXAN are so simple to operate that any office staff member can become an expert with minimal training. On-screen help menus guide the user through the neutralization of PAL's, prism lenses, contact lenses, polycarbonate and other high-index material lenses. The LA 360 with SPEXAN, measures the amount of UV radiation that is transmitted through the lens. Humphrey Lens Analyzers for laboratories, Model 370 and Model 380 with SPEXAN, meet the needs of both edging layout and final inspection. The fully automated Lab Lens Analyzers feature single vision blocking capabilities, software with ANSI tolerance check and a reference point measurement for PALs, making layout and quality control faster and more accurate. Because the instrument is so reliable and easy to operate, you do not need to be a lensometry expert. Less experienced personnel can achieve the same accurate, fast results with a significant increase in quality and productivity for improved profitability.

Marco Ophthalmic, Inc. 800-874-5274
11825 Central Pkwy, Jacksonville, FL 32224
Models priced at $1,375.00 and $1,540.00; $3,050.00 for digital model; $5,695.00 for automatic model. (List prices)

LEUKOCYTE ALKALINE PHOSPHATASE *(Hematology) 81GHD*

Bayer Healthcare Llc 914-524-2955
555 White Plains Rd Fl 5, Tarrytown, NY 10591
Test for leukocytes in urine.

Bayer Healthcare, Llc 574-256-3430
430 S Beiger St, Mishawaka, IN 46544
Test for leukocytes in urine.

Biomerieux Inc. 800-682-2666
100 Rodolphe St, Durham, NC 27712

LIFT, BATH, NON-AC-POWERED *(General) 80FSA*

Access Bridges 707-546-7671
610 Nason St, Santa Rosa, CA 95404
Patient lift.

Arjo Canada, Inc. 800-665-4831
1575 South Gateway Rd., Unit C, Mississauga, ONT L4W-5J1 Canaca

Arjo, Inc. 800-323-1245
50 Gary Ave Ste A, Roselle, IL 60172

Bhm Medical, Inc. 800-868-0441
2001 Tanguay, Magog, QC J1X 5Y5 Canada
Patient lifts and accessories; mobile floor lifts and ceiling track (overhead) lifts.

Cameron-Miller, Inc. 800-621-0142
5410 W Roosevelt Rd, Road #241, Chicago, IL 60644

Can-Dan Rehatec Ltd. 9056487522
3-1378 Sandhill Dr., Ancaster, ONT L9G-4V5 Canada
Bath-Support for Children. Made of S/S.

Clark Medical Products, Inc. 800-889-5295
10-5510 Ambler Drive, Mississauga, ONT L4W- 2V1 Canada
Water Powered Bath Lift is a hydraulic lift that raises to tub height and swivels to facilitate transfering. Fabricated of PVC, aluminum and steel. Also available is VALETTE Water Powered Toilet Lift. This hydraulic lift raises a person from toilet bowl to a standing position. Fabricated of steel and aluminum and white powder coated with a 300lb. capacity. Also available is PAPI-LIFT Battery Powered Toilet Lift. This 12 volt actuator type lift has a 300 lb. capacity and folds for storage and travel. Fabricated of steel and white powder coated.

Clarke Health Care Products, Inc. 888-347-4537
1003 International Dr, Oakdale, PA 15071
Aquatec Beluga battery-powered bathlift, includes reclining back supoport, remote control, battery, and charger.Aqautec Available in wide and with side laterals.

Community Products, Llc 845-658-7723
2032 Route 213, Rifton, NY 12471
Patient lift.

Craftsmen/Access Unlimited 607-669-4822
570 Hance Rd, Binghamton, NY 13903
Non-ac-powered patient lift.

Descent Control Systems, Inc. 801-304-9299
8100 S 1300 W Ste D, West Jordan, UT 84088
Non-ac powered patient lift.

Enneking Medical Inc. 816-300-4279
1801 Guinotte Ave, Kansas City, MO 64120
Non-ac-powered patient lifts.

LIFT, BATH, NON-AC-POWERED *(cont'd)*

G. Hirsch And Co., Inc. 650-692-8770
870 Mahler Rd, Burlingame, CA 94010
Various types of patient lifts and accessories.

H2o Ramps And Lifts, Llc 501-825-8838
7010 Greers Ferry Rd, Greers Ferry, AR 72067
Patient lift.

Handicap Helpers, Inc. 540-565-1889
604 W Main St, Appalachia, VA 24216
Lizzie lift.

Huntleigh Healthcare Llc. 800-223-1218
40 Christopher Way, Eatontown, NJ 07724

Laszlo Corp. 314-830-3222
2573 Millvalley Dr, Florissant, MO 63031
A Lift and Transfer automated system with AC-Powered remote control, seatback adjustment from 90 degrees to 180 degrees, a mobile unit that transports indoors and outdoors. Helps reduce Patient and caregiver injuries.

Liftaid Transport Llc 800-951-4243
46908 Liberty Dr, Wixom, MI 48393
The Lift Aid Transport is a portable patient lifting system that can be used by a single caregiver to lift, transfer, weigh and transport a patient up to 600 pounds with ease, comfort and security.

Mastercare Patient Equipment, Inc. 800-798-5867
2071 14th Ave, PO Box 1435, Columbus, NE 68601
Stretcher lift.

Mckesson General Medical 800-446-3008
8741 Landmark Rd, Richmond, VA 23228

Medi-Man Rehabilitation Products, Inc. 800-268-4256
6200A Tomken Rd., Mississauga, ONT L5T-1X7 Canada
MEDI-LIFTER, BREEZE, ATLANTIS, CYPRESS, ASPEN, SATURN, SUMMIT, CRICKET. Foldable lift. Hydraulic and electric patient lifts, with or without electronic scale. Battery powered patient lifts for general transfer, hygiene care. Bath, ceiling.

Medical Depot 516-998-4600
99 Seaview Blvd, Port Washington, NY 11050
Lift.

Mesa, Inc. 210-699-6911
9807 Fredericksburg Rd, San Antonio, TX 78240
Patient lift.

Mobility Research 480-829-1727
444 W Geneva Dr, Tempe, AZ 85282

Mrc Industries Inc. 516-328-6900
85 Denton Ave, New Hyde Park, NY 11040
Various types of slings.

Nor-Am Patient Care Products, Inc. 800-387-7103
2388 Speers Rd., Oakville, ONT L6L 5M2 Canada
Ready lift

Ortho Innovations, Inc. 507-269-2895
121 23rd Ave SW, Rochester, MN 55902
Patient lift, non-ac-powered.

Penner Manufacturing Inc 800-732-0717
102 Grant St, PO Box 523, Aurora, NE 68818
Various.

Porto-Lift Corp. 800-321-1454
PO Box 5, Higgins Lake, MI 48627

Prism Medical Inc. 800-265-0677
1-116 Rayette Rd, Concord L4K 2G3 Canada
Various

Rehamed Intl. Llc. 800-577-4424
522 W Mowry Dr, Homestead, FL 33030
Various.

Robomedica, Inc. 877-762-6633
1 Technology Dr, Bldg. C, Suite C-511, Irvine, CA 92618
Body weight support.

Sunrise Machine And Tool, Inc. 218-847-3386
1380 Legion Rd, Detroit Lakes, MN 56501
Battery powered patient lift.

Take-Along Lifts, Llc 877-667-6515
125 Pumpkin Hill Rd, New Milford, CT 06776
Portable transfer aid.

Target Compaction, Inc. 315-363-3077
510 Lake Rd, Oneida, NY 13421
Various.

LIFT, BATH, NON-AC-POWERED *(cont'd)*

Tr Group, Inc. 800-752-6900
903 Wedel Ln, Glenview, IL 60025
Patient lift.

Trace Medical Equipment, Inc. 800-323-3786
5000 Varsity Dr, Lisle, IL 60532
Case Carts, and monitor carts, wooden

Vigor Therapy Solutions Llc 269-429-0191
4915 Advance Way, Stevensville, MI 49127
Body weight support.

West Coast Automation, Corp. 509-773-5055
1600 S Roosevelt Ave, Goldendale, WA 98620
Lift, patient, non-ac powered.

Whitehall Manufacturing 800-782-7706
15125 Proctor Ave, City Of Industry, CA 91746
Whirlpool raising and lowering device for treatment of upper/lower extremities in the same unit.

LIFT, PATIENT *(General) 80FNG*

Alimed, Inc. 800-225-2610
297 High St, Dedham, MA 02026

Aquatic Access, Inc. 800-323-5438
417 Dorsey Way, Louisville, KY 40223
Full line of water-powered lifts, providing disabled access to in-ground & above-ground pools, spas, therapy tubs, boats and docks. Including heavy-duty, bariatric pool lifts and custom seating.

Arjo Canada, Inc. 800-665-4831
1575 South Gateway Rd., Unit C, Mississauga, ONT L4W-5J1 Canada

Arjo, Inc. 800-323-1245
50 Gary Ave Ste A, Roselle, IL 60172
Patient lifts for bed, bath, shower, pool etc.

Blevins Medical Inc 866-783-3056
207 Broad St, Marion, VA 24354

Clarke Health Care Products, Inc. 888-347-4537
1003 International Dr, Oakdale, PA 15071
Hydraulic bathlifts, Aquatec Major bathlift available with 4 back supports, fixed angle or recline wiht or without adjustable laterals, custom full length.

Colonial Scientific Ltd. 902-468-1811
201 Brownlow Ave., Unit 52, Dartmouth, NS B3B-1W2 Canada

Columbus Mckinnon Corp., Mobility Products Div. 800-888-0985
140 John James Audubon Pkwy, Amherst, NY 14228
Overhead patient lift and transfer system, freestanding or ceiling mount.

Convaquip Industries, Inc. 800-637-8436
4834 Derrick Dr, PO Box 3417, Abilene, TX 79601
Bariatric Portable Patient lifts with 600 lb. and 1000 lb. capacities.

Crest Healthcare Supply 800-328-8908
195 3rd St, Dassel, MN 55325

Drive-Master Co., Inc. 973-808-9709
37 Daniel Rd, Fairfield, NJ 07004
Rotary and hydraulic lifts for physically handicapped person to get in and out of van.

Enneking Medical Inc. 816-300-4279
1801 Guinotte Ave, Kansas City, MO 64120
Ac-powered patient lifts.

Fablok Mills, Inc. 908-464-1950
140 Spring St, New Providence, NJ 07974

Grant Airmass Corporation 800-243-5237
126 Chestnut Hill Rd, PO Box 3456, Stamford, CT 06903
Water operated patient lift.

Help U Lift 702-435-9001
5653 Wheatfield Dr, Las Vegas, NV 89120
Ac-patient lift.

Hill-Rom Manufacturing, Inc. 800-638-2546
4349 Corporate Rd, Charleston, SC 29405
TRANS-LIFT resident sling lift. TRANS-LIFT resident stand assist.

Horcher Lifting Systems, Inc. 800-582-8732
324 Cypress Rd, Ocala, FL 34472
UNILIFT Ceiling-mounted patient lifts. 24 volt battery powered. Custom installed. Easy to use universal slings. Quiet and smooth operation. Also powered patient lift; electric floor model to help patients stand up. Battery operated and adjustable to accommodate patient height.

LIFT, PATIENT *(cont'd)*

Hovertech International 800-471-2776
513 S Clewell St, Fountain Hill, PA 18015
HoverJack Air Patient Lift is designed to lift a patient from floor to stretcher/bed height in a supine position to reduce the risk of injury to caregiver and patient.

I-Beam Walking Machine 248-477-9808
21755 Ruth St, Farmington Hills, MI 48336
Beam walking assist device.

I.E.D., Inc. 231-728-9154
1938 Sanford St, Muskegon, MI 49441

Invacare Corporation 800-333-6900
1 Invacare Way, Elyria, OH 44035
INVACARE.

Laszlo Corp. 314-830-3222
2573 Millvalley Dr, Florissant, MO 63031
An automated lift system that lifts patient from bed and into the lift chair device without physical exertion for the caregiver. Can adjust seat, and seatback from 180 to 90 degrees which aids in preventing pneumonia. Chair can be used as an exam chair for any medical purpose. Patient can be placed back into bed using same system, excellent for home care management.

Liftaid Transport Llc 800-951-4243
46908 Liberty Dr, Wixom, MI 48393
LIFT AID 2000 system. Over head, whole room structure, 12-volt battery-operated. Lifts up to 500 pounds and provides complete access to entire room. Custom cut to room's dimensions. Does not attach to walls, floor or ceiling. True four point lift bar and soft sling.

Liko North America 888-545-6671
122 Grove St, Franklin, MA 02038

Linak U.S. Inc. 502-253-5595
2200 Stanley Gault Pkwy, Louisville, KY 40223

Medcare Products, Inc. 800-695-4479
151 Cliff Rd E Ste 40, Burnsville, MN 55337
Patient lifts and patient stands.

Nk Medical Products Inc. 800-274-2742
10123 Main St, PO Box 627, Clarence, NY 14031
Manual and Powered Patient Lifts

Noram Solutions 800-387-7103
PO Box 543, Lewiston, NY 14092
Ready Stand Ready Lift and Versa lift. A variety of lifters for all lifting situations.

Penner Manufacturing Inc 800-732-0717
102 Grant St, PO Box 523, Aurora, NE 68818
Patient lift.

Porto-Lift Corp. 800-321-1454
PO Box 5, Higgins Lake, MI 48627
$1115.00 for 300lb capacity model with hydraulic lifting mechanism, adjustable base, chrome finish. Optional head/neck brace, bath/commode adapter, and stretcher attachment. PORTO-LIFT 400lb capacity with hydraulic lifting mechanism, adjustable base, chrome finish. Optional head/neck brace, bath/commode adapter and stretcher attachment. PORTO-LIFT 300 lb capacity with hydraulic lifting mechanism, fixed 'C' base, blue epoxy & chrome finish. Optional headneck brace, bath/commode adapter and stretcher attachment. Pediatric models - 150Lb capacity, adjustable or fixed 'C' base, 4 point or 2 point suspension systems, purple or strawberry colors. $479.40 to $629.40.

Rifton Equipment 800-571-8198
PO Box 260, Rifton, NY 12471
With zero-lifting, a single caregiver can transfer adult clients from their wheelchair to an upright standing or mobility device. Additionally, by lifting entirely from above the waist, the Rifton SoloLift offers convenience and dignity for toileting.

Robomedica, Inc. 877-762-6633
1 Technology Dr, Bldg. C, Suite C-511, Irvine, CA 92618
Body weight support.

Sani-Med, A Division Of Sanderson Plumbing Products, Inc. 800-647-1042
PO Box 1367, Columbus, MS 39703

Smart Medical Technology, Inc 630-964-1689
8404 Wilmette Ave Ste B, Darien, IL 60561
Lateral patient transfer system.

Sperian Protection 800-343-3411
900 Douglas Pike, Smithfield, RI 02917

LIFT, PATIENT *(cont'd)*

Sr Instruments, Inc. 800-654-6360
600 Young St, Tonawanda, NY 14150
Weight module for patient lift, converts patient lift into a precision scale system in seconds. 440 lb/200 kg capacity fits HOYER, INVACARE and other lifts employing compatible lift and sling attachments; 9-V battery operation - 3000+ readings. OEM inquiries welcome.

Sunrise Medical 800-333-4000
7477 Dry Creek Pkwy, Longmont, CO 80503

Surehands Lift & Care Systems 800-724-5305
982 Rte. 1, Pine Island, NY 10969
SUREHANDS offers a unique, patented and exclusive range of Lift&Care systems that meet private and institutional needs for individuals with motor disabilities. Includes permanent and portable models for homes, workplaces, and recreational areas. The SUREHANDS Body Support offers easy and secure transfers for both patient and caregiver, and also the opportunity for independent transfers. All lifts are easily maintained and operated with minimum assistance.

The National Wheel-O-Vator Co., Inc. 800-551-9095
509 W Front St, Roanoke, IL 61561
Portable vertical platform lifting device.

Tr Group, Inc. 800-752-6900
903 Wedel Ln, Glenview, IL 60025
Various.

Tuffcare 800-367-6160
3999 E La Palma Ave, Anaheim, CA 92807

Vancare, Inc. 800-694-4525
1515 1st St, Aurora, NE 68818
VANDER-LIFT patient lift, MET/NRTL listed, single staff transfer, machine washable sling, and smooth, electric movement up/down (non-hydraulic).

Vigor Therapy Solutions Llc 269-429-0191
4915 Advance Way, Stevensville, MI 49127
Body weight support.

Wheelchairs Of Kansas 800-537-6454
204 W 2nd St, Ellis, KS 67637
Two types of LIFT & TRANSFER SYSTEM, Heavy duty 1000 lb. capacity lift transfers safely and comfortably. One style uses a track system to guide patient into position; The other style is a standard hoist lift.

LIFT, STAIR CLIMBING *(General) 80TFX*

Bruno Independent Living Aids, Inc. 800-882-8183
1780 Executive Dr, Oconomowoc, WI 53066
BRUNO ELECTRA-RIDE stairway elevator system for straight rail for in-home.

Ferno-Washington, Inc. 800-733-3766
70 Weil Way, Wilmington, OH 45177

Garaventa (Canada) Ltd. 800-663-6556
7505 - 134A St., Surrey, BC V3W-7B3 Canada
$12,000 to $35,000 for GARAVENTA STAIR-LIFT.

Handi-Ramp 800-876-7267
510 North Ave, Libertyville, IL 60048
Seated stair lifts for all stair configurations.

Inclinator Co. Of America 800-343-9007
601 Gibson Blvd, Harrisburg, PA 17104
Stairlift Model SC

Thyssenkrupp Access Corp. 800-925-3100
4001 E 138th St, Grandview, MO 64030
The Stair-Glide and Flow stair lifts are designed to offer solutions for curved or spiral staircases. The Citia available in either an A/C or BOS power system is designed for straight staircases.

LIFT, WHEELCHAIR *(General) 80REY*

A.R.C. Distributors 800-296-8724
PO Box 599, Centreville, MD 21617
Hoyer Patient Lift hydraulic patient lifters. Weight capacity 300lb, 400lb, and 600lb. Invacare Reliant Lift, Reliant 600 Heavy Duty Lift, Reliant Stand-Up Lift, Hydraulic and Battery Powered Lifts.

Amigo Mobility International 800-248-9131
6693 Dixie Hwy, Bridgeport, MI 48722
New Lift-It requires no installation, used with Class II and III hitches. Lift-All-per unit (200-lb), three-wheeled scooter lift.

LIFT, WHEELCHAIR *(cont'd)*

Bruno Independent Living Aids, Inc. 800-882-8183
1780 Executive Dr, Oconomowoc, WI 53066
Car trunk wheelchair lift, car trunk scooter lift, van/mini-van scooter lift (various van models). Wheelchair lifts for manual and motorized wheelchairs. Full power, platform outside bumper scooter and wheelchair lifts for pick-up trucks. Bruno's lift line includes models that will lift up to 400lbs.

Complete Mobility Systems Inc. 800-788-7479
1915 County Road C W, Roseville, MN 55113
Electric wheelchair lifts and power door operators for full size vans and minivans.

Forward Motions, Inc. 877-364-8267
214 Valley St, Dayton, OH 45404
Vertical wheelchair lifts for commercial or residential use. Buildings.

Garaventa (Canada) Ltd. 800-663-6556
7505 - 134A St., Surrey, BC V3W-7B3 Canada
$12,000 to $35,000 for GARAVENTA STAIR-LIFT.

Handi-Cap Aids Company 800-689-0511
730 W Hefner Rd, Oklahoma City, OK 73114
Wheelchair lifts for vehicles, including standard platform lifts and specialty lifts. New and used, already adapted wheelchair-accessible full-size and mini-vans available.

Handi-Ramp 800-876-7267
510 North Ave, Libertyville, IL 60048
Vertical home lifts, 500-lb capacity, with various lifting heights with options for 90-degree exit platform, special gates, etc.

Handicap Unlimited, Inc. 888-371-0095
5640 Summer Ave Ste 3, Memphis, TN 38134

Handicaps, Inc. 800-782-4335
4335 S Santa Fe Dr, Englewood, CO 80110
$4,950 for SUPERARM 2000 (lift for vans), $4,950 for motorhome lifts, and $6,200 for basement motorhome lifts.

Inclinator Co. Of America 800-343-9007
601 Gibson Blvd, Harrisburg, PA 17104
VL to lift wheelchair and passenger up to 12 feet.

Kino Mobility Inc. 4166355873
18 Lepage Crt, Toronto, ON M3J 1Z9 Canada

Ricon Corp. 800-322-2884
7900 Nelson Rd, Panorama City, CA 91402

Silver Star Mobility 800-555-4385
578 Mason Way, Medford, OR 97501
SILVER STAR lift for transporting power and manual wheelchairs and three- or four-wheel scooters. Also available is the SILVER STAR BACKPACKER, an inside lift for picking up scooters and power wheelchairs and placing them in the rear of minivans.

The National Wheel-O-Vator Co., Inc. 800-551-9095
509 W Front St, Roanoke, IL 61561
Vertical and inclined platform lifting device.

Thyssenkrupp Access Corp. 800-925-3100
4001 E 138th St, Grandview, MO 64030
vertical and inclined platform lifts

LIGATOR, ESOPHAGEAL *(Gastro/Urology) 78MND*

Cook Endoscopy 336-744-0157
4900 Bethania Station Rd # &, 5951 Grassy Creek Blvd. Winston Salem, NC 27105
Band ligators.

Ethicon Endo-Surgery, Inc. 877-384-4266
3801 University Blvd SE, Albuquerque, NM 87106
Various types of esophageal ligators.

LIGATOR, HEMORRHOIDAL *(Gastro/Urology) 78FHN*

Aesculap Implant Systems Inc. 1-800-234-9179
3773 Corporate Pkwy, Center Valley, PA 18034

Biocompatibles Inc. 877-783-5463
115 Hurley Rd Bldg 3, Oxford, CT 06478
Aspiration biopsy needles.

Cook Endoscopy 336-744-0157
4900 Bethania Station Rd # &, 5951 Grassy Creek Blvd. Winston Salem, NC 27105
Band ligator.

Ethicon Endo-Surgery, Inc. 877-384-4266
3801 University Blvd SE, Albuquerque, NM 87106
Various types of hemorrhoidal ligators.

Medchannel Llc 617-314-9861
1241 Adams St Apt 110, Dorchester Center, MA 02124
Tissue ligator.

LIGATOR, HEMORRHOIDAL *(cont'd)*

Miltex Inc. 800-645-8000
589 Davies Dr, York, PA 17402

Redfield Corp. 800-678-4472
336 W Passaic St, Rochelle Park, NJ 07662
Infrared Coagulator

Scanlan International, Inc. 800-328-9458
1 Scanlan Plz, Saint Paul, MN 55107
SCANLAN hemorrhoidal ligator.

LIGATURE, LAPAROSCOPIC *(Surgery) 79SIL*

Covidien Lp 508-261-8000
15 Hampshire St, Mansfield, MA 02048

LIGHT SOURCE, ENDOSCOPE, XENON ARC *(Surgery) 79GCT*

Biomet Sports Medicine 530-226-5800
6704 Lockheed Dr, Redding, CA 96002
Light source.

Bulbtronics, Inc. 800-624-2852
45 Banfi Plz N, Farmingdale, NY 11735

Cardinal Health, Snowden Pencer Products 847-689-8410
5175 S Royal Atlanta Dr, Tucker, GA 30084
Various types of xenon arc endoscopic light sources.

Chiu Technical Corp. 631-544-0606
252 Indian Head Rd, Kings Park, NY 11754
$1,130.00 X150T.

Clarus Medical, Llc. 763-525-8400
1000 Boone Ave N Ste 300, Minneapolis, MN 55427
Light source.

Elmed, Inc. 630-543-2792
60 W Fay Ave, Addison, IL 60101

Integra Luxtec, Inc. 800-325-8966
99 Hartwell St, West Boylston, MA 01583
Solid state Xenon light source.

Karl Storz Endoscopy-America Inc. 800-421-0837
600 Corporate Pointe, Culver City, CA 90230
300-Watt version provides illumination with the color temperature of sunlight.

Mahe International Inc. 800-294-7946
468 Craighead St, Nashville, TN 37204

Mediflex Surgical Products 800-879-7575
250 Gibbs Rd, Islandia, NY 11749
Runs cooler, greater reliability, ceramic xenon lamp, guaranteed for 700 hours of operation, economically priced.

Medtec Applications, Inc. 630-628-0444
50 W Fay Ave, Addison, IL 60101
Fiberoptic photographic lightsource.

Pentax Medical Company 800-431-5880
102 Chestnut Ridge Rd, Montvale, NJ 07645
$24,255.00 for EPK-1000 video color processor with 100 watt xenon light source, air pump, and full screen images. $23,730.00 for EPM-3500 video processor with 300 watt xenon light source, air pump, and IR filter.

Pentax Southern Region Service Center 201-571-2300
8934 Kirby Dr, Houston, TX 77054
Light source.

Pentax West Coast Service Center 800-431-5880
10410 Pioneer Blvd Ste 2, Santa Fe Springs, CA 90670
Pentax light source.

Products For Medicine 800-333-3087
1201 E Ball Rd Ste H, Anaheim, CA 92805
300W XENON LIGHT SOURCE

Richard Wolf Medical Instruments Corp. 800-323-9653
353 Corporate Woods Pkwy, Vernon Hills, IL 60061

Smith & Nephew Inc., Endoscopy Div. 978-749-1000
76 S Meridian Ave, Oklahoma City, OK 73107
Enodscopic illunimators, light sources and accessories.

Smith & Nephew, Inc., Endoscopy Division 800-343-8386
150 Minuteman Rd, Andover, MA 01810

Solos Endoscopy 800-388-6445
65 Sprague St # B, Boston/dedham Commerce Park, Boston, MA 02136
Light source, endoscope, xenon arc.

Sunoptic Technologies 877-677-2832
6018 Bowdendale Ave, Jacksonville, FL 32216
High intensity projectors for fiberoptics, several models of Quartz Halogen, Metal Halide, and Xenon lightsources available.

LIGHT SOURCE, ENDOSCOPIC *(Obstetrics/Gyn) 85HIE*

Bulbtronics, Inc. 800-624-2852
45 Banfi Plz N, Farmingdale, NY 11735

Cameron-Miller, Inc. 800-621-0142
5410 W Roosevelt Rd, Road #241, Chicago, IL 60644

General Scientific Corp. 800-959-0153
77 Enterprise Dr, Ann Arbor, MI 48103

Integra Luxtec, Inc. 800-325-8966
99 Hartwell St, West Boylston, MA 01583
Solid state xenon light source.

Karl Storz Endoscopy-America Inc. 800-421-0837
600 Corporate Pointe, Culver City, CA 90230

Mahe International Inc. 800-294-7946
468 Craighead St, Nashville, TN 37204

Medical Illumination International 800-831-1222
547 Library St, San Fernando, CA 91340

Olympus America, Inc. 800-645-8160
3500 Corporate Pkwy, PO Box 610, Center Valley, PA 18034

Progressive Dynamics Medical, Inc. 269-781-4241
507 Industrial Rd, Marshall, MI 49068
150 watt halogen light source.

Richard Wolf Medical Instruments Corp. 800-323-9653
353 Corporate Woods Pkwy, Vernon Hills, IL 60061

Smith & Nephew, Inc., Endoscopy Division 800-343-8386
150 Minuteman Rd, Andover, MA 01810

Sunoptic Technologies 877-677-2832
6018 Bowdendale Ave, Jacksonville, FL 32216
Fiberoptic illuminators, high intensity lightsources, several models, UL and CSA listed.

Welch Allyn, Inc. 800-535-6663
4341 State Street Rd, Skaneateles Falls, NY 13153
SOLARTEC, Source 100 and Source 270 systems.

Wisap America 800-233-8448
8231 Melrose Dr, Lenexa, KS 66214
100-180-300-W digital xenon.

LIGHT SOURCE, FIBEROPTIC, ROUTINE *(Gastro/Urology) 78FCW*

Bulbtronics, Inc. 800-624-2852
45 Banfi Plz N, Farmingdale, NY 11735

Burton Medical Products, Inc. 800-444-9909
21100 Lassen St, Chatsworth, CA 91311

Cameron-Miller, Inc. 800-621-0142
5410 W Roosevelt Rd, Road #241, Chicago, IL 60644
Quartz-halogen low intensity light with 40 hr. lamp life; discrete 4 level illumination adjustment; weighs 13 lbs.

Cantylight 716-625-4227
6100 Donner Rd, Lockport, NY 14094

Carl Zeiss Surgical, Inc. 800-442-4020
1 Zeiss Dr, Thornwood, NY 10594

Chiu Technical Corp. 631-544-0606
252 Indian Head Rd, Kings Park, NY 11754
$248.00 for FO 150-115.

Codman & Shurtleff, Inc 800-225-0460
325 Paramount Dr, Raynham, MA 02767
$450 to $1,995 for 3 models - $1,995 for high intensity, 300 W model with 75 hr. lamp life. $450 or $750 for 2 low intensity lights with 150 W output, 40 hr. lamp life.

Elmed, Inc. 630-543-2792
60 W Fay Ave, Addison, IL 60101

Hmb Endoscopy Products 800-659-5743
3746 SW 30th Ave, Fort Lauderdale, FL 33312
Xenon Light Sources, Halogen Light Sources, Fiberoptic Light Sources.

Integra Luxtec, Inc. 800-325-8966
99 Hartwell St, West Boylston, MA 01583
Solid state Halogen light source.

Jedmed Instruments Co. 314-845-3770
5416 Jedmed Ct, Saint Louis, MO 63129

Karl Storz Endoscopy-America Inc. 800-421-0837
600 Corporate Pointe, Culver City, CA 90230
Full line of both low and high intensity models.

Kavo Dental Corp. 800-323-8029
340 East Route 22, Lake Zurich, IL 60047

Kelsar, S.A. 508-261-8000
Blvd. Insurgentes, Libriamento a La, Tijuana 22450 Mexico
Various

LIGHT SOURCE, FIBEROPTIC, ROUTINE *(cont'd)*

Mahe International Inc. 800-294-7946
468 Craighead St, Nashville, TN 37204

Olympus America, Inc. 800-645-8160
3500 Corporate Pkwy, PO Box 610, Center Valley, PA 18034

Pentax Medical Company 800-431-5880
102 Chestnut Ridge Rd, Montvale, NJ 07645
$510.00 to $1208.00 for three models of Halogen light sources. Call for details. Also several models of portable 'bedside' endoscope light source accessories and several models of replacemnt lamp kits. Call for quote.

Pentax Southern Region Service Center 201-571-2300
8934 Kirby Dr, Houston, TX 77054
Light source.

Pentax West Coast Service Center 800-431-5880
10410 Pioneer Blvd Ste 2, Santa Fe Springs, CA 90670
Pentax light source.

Progressive Dynamics Medical, Inc. 269-781-4241
507 Industrial Rd, Marshall, MI 49068
150 watt halogen light source.

Qed, Inc. 859-231-0338
750 Enterprise Dr, Lexington, KY 40510
Maxillume 250-1, 250-2, minimax.

Rei Rotolux Enterprises, Inc. 888-773-7611
4145 North Service Rd, Ste. 200, Burlington, ON L7L 6A3 Canada
Small diameter probe utilizing fibreoptics to carry light. Used in endoscopy. Different sizes, configurations are availble.

Richard Wolf Medical Instruments Corp. 800-323-9653
353 Corporate Woods Pkwy, Vernon Hills, IL 60061
3 models available.

Rocket Medical Plc. 800-707-7625
150 Recreation Park Dr Ste 3, Hingham, MA 02043

Smith & Nephew, Inc., Endoscopy Division 800-343-8386
150 Minuteman Rd, Andover, MA 01810

Stryker Corp. 800-726-2725
2825 Airview Blvd, Portage, MI 49002

Sunoptic Technologies 877-677-2832
6018 Bowdendale Ave, Jacksonville, FL 32216
Several models available.

Sylvan Corp. 800-628-3836
32 Billott Ave, Irwin, PA 15642
Maxiscan.

Techman Int'L Corp. 508-248-2900
242 Sturbridge Rd, Charlton, MA 01507
Lightsource.

Transamerican Technologies International 800-322-7373
2246 Camino Ramon, San Ramon, CA 94583
ACCU-BEAM, fiberoptic retrofits for operating microscopes. Features include variable light control, interchangeable filters, high intensity output and wide field illumination.

Vision-Sciences, Inc. 800-874-9975
40 Ramland Rd S Ste 1, Orangeburg, NY 10962

LIGHT SOURCE, FLASH *(Chemistry) 75RFC*

Bulbtronics, Inc. 800-624-2852
45 Banfi Plz N, Farmingdale, NY 11735

Endoscopy Support Services, Inc. 800-349-3636
3 Fallsview Ln, Brewster, NY 10509

Jeron Electronic Systems, Inc. 800-621-1903
1743 W Rosehill Dr # 55, Chicago, IL 60660
SPECTRUM 760; room status, staff-patient sequencing, patient call multi-colored light message system aids staff in clinic management.

Karl Storz Endoscopy-America Inc. 800-421-0837
600 Corporate Pointe, Culver City, CA 90230

Mahe International Inc. 800-294-7946
468 Craighead St, Nashville, TN 37204

Pocket Nurse Enterprises, Inc. 800-225-1600
200 1st St, Ambridge, PA 15003

LIGHT SOURCE, INCANDESCENT, DIAGNOSTIC
(Gastro/Urology) 78FCQ

Adva-Lite, Inc. 727-546-5483
7340 Bryan Dairy Rd, Largo, FL 33777
Disposable patient examining flashlight.

Bulbtronics, Inc. 800-624-2852
45 Banfi Plz N, Farmingdale, NY 11735

LIGHT SOURCE, INCANDESCENT, DIAGNOSTIC *(cont'd)*

Lightolier A Genlyte Co. 978-657-7600
45 Industrial Way, Wilmington, MA 01887
Examination light.

United Metal Fabricators, Inc. 800-638-5322
1316 Eisenhower Blvd, Johnstown, PA 15904

LIGHT SOURCE, PHOTOGRAPHIC, FIBEROPTIC
(Gastro/Urology) 78FCR

B. Graczyk, Inc. 269-782-2100
27826 Burmax Park, Dowagiac, MI 49047
Various sizes and shapes of sterile and non-sterile keratome blades.

Bulbtronics, Inc. 800-624-2852
45 Banfi Plz N, Farmingdale, NY 11735

Karl Storz Endoscopy-America Inc. 800-421-0837
600 Corporate Pointe, Culver City, CA 90230

Mahe International Inc. 800-294-7946
468 Craighead St, Nashville, TN 37204

Sunoptic Technologies 877-677-2832
6018 Bowdendale Ave, Jacksonville, FL 32216
Solid state universal turret, dual 150W and 300W, UL and CSA listed.

LIGHT, BILIRUBIN (PHOTOTHERAPY) *(General) 80TCX*

Burton Medical Products, Inc. 800-444-9909
21100 Lassen St, Chatsworth, CA 91311

Natus Medical Inc. 800-255-3901
1501 Industrial Rd, San Carlos, CA 94070
Natus neoBLUE LED Phototherapy is an innovative phototherapy light, incorporating a state-of-the-art blue LED light source for the treatment of newborn jaundice.

Olympic Medical Corp. 206-767-3500
5900 1st Ave S, Seattle, WA 98108
$1,739.50 floorstand with fluorescent bulbs. Halogen model is $1,993.50.

LIGHT, DENTAL *(Dental And Oral) 76RFD*

Alliance H. Inc Dentech Equipment 360-988-7080
901 W Front St, Sumas, WA 98295

Beaverstate Dental, Inc. 800-237-2303
115 S Elliott Rd, Newberg, OR 97132

Bulbtronics, Inc. 800-624-2852
45 Banfi Plz N, Farmingdale, NY 11735

Dencraft 800-328-9729
PO Box 57, Moorestown, NJ 08057

Dentalez Group 866-DTE-INFO
101 Lindenwood Dr Ste 225, Valleybrooke Corporate Center
Malvern, PA 19355

Dntlworks Equipment Corporation 800-847-0694
7300 S Tucson Way, Centennial, CO 80112
The ProBrite series of halogen and fiber-optic portable lights have a variety of mounting options. These lights can be chair-mounted, post-mounted, or mobile floor-standing. Two styles of headband lights add to your choices.

Forest Dental Products Inc 800-423-3535
6200 NE Campus Ct, Hillsboro, OR 97124

Health Science Products, Inc. 800-237-5794
1489 Hueytown Rd, Hueytown, AL 35023
HSP Glows dental light for tooth shading, a high/low intensity for color matching, with flexible arm and head positioning in a manual or hands-free sensor on/off model.

J. Morita Usa, Inc. 888-566-7482
9 Mason, Irvine, CA 92618
JETLITE 4000 PLUS, an upgraded version of Jetlite 4000 with increased power output of 900-1400 mW/cm2 and a built-in digital light intensity meter. It is a microprocessor controlled curing light designed to perform standard curing techniques as well as ramp-up curing techniques. The Jetlite 4000 Plus allows the user to easily select and rotate between standard and ramp-up (quantum cure) at the touch of a button. Standard features include, digital display countdown timer, audible start and stop signals and choice of nine pre-set curing times (10-90 sec.)

Midmark Corporation 800-643-6275
60 Vista Dr, P.O. Box 286, Versailles, OH 45380

Pelton & Crane Co., 704-588-2126
11727 Fruehauf Dr, Charlotte, NC 28273
LIGHT FANTASTIC Unit/Column Mount.

Sds (Summit Dental Systems) 800-275-3368
3560 NW 53rd Ct, Fort Lauderdale, FL 33309

LIGHT, DENTAL *(cont'd)*

Spring Health Products, Inc. 800-800-1680
705 General Washington Ave Ste 701, Norristown, PA 19403
Curing lights that block out UV.

Sunoptic Technologies 877-677-2832
6018 Bowdendale Ave, Jacksonville, FL 32216
Visible light curing and transillumination, fiberoptic light cables, or high intensity probes for curing guns. Surgical headlights: 150W and 300W high intensity lightsources, UL and CSA listed. Replacement light guides available for bonding.

Welch Allyn, Inc. 800-535-6663
4341 State Street Rd, Skaneateles Falls, NY 13153

Zila, Inc. 800-228-5595
701 Centre Ave, Fort Collins, CO 80526
ViziLite Comprehensive Exam Tray; ViziLite Plus

LIGHT, DENTAL, INTRAORAL *(Dental And Oral) 76RFE*

Dntlworks Equipment Corporation 800-847-0694
7300 S Tucson Way, Centennial, CO 80112
Portable halogen light with gooseneck arm, 4 lb. ProBrite series of portable, gooseneck-style halogen lights.

Lares Research 800-347-3289
295 Lockheed Ave, Chico, CA 95973

Pelton & Crane Co., 704-588-2126
11727 Fruehauf Dr, Charlotte, NC 28273

3m Unitek 800-634-5300
2724 Peck Rd, Monrovia, CA 91016
High power, visible orthodontic curring light with built-in meter to cure bonding adhesives.

LIGHT, EXAMINATION, BATTERY-POWERED *(General) 80KYT*

Adva-Lite, Inc. 727-546-5483
7340 Bryan Dairy Rd, Largo, FL 33777
Adva-lite replaceable battery pocket light.

Bionix Development Corp. 800-551-7096
5154 Enterprise Blvd, Toledo, OH 43612
Bionix reddy lite.

Cejay Engineering, Llc 239-498-8923
25080 Goldcrest Dr, Bonita Springs, FL 34134
Multi-use miniature finger light.

Engineered Medical Solutions Co. Llc. 908-213-9001
85 Industrial Rd Bldg B, Phillipsburg, NJ 08865
Battery powered light.

General Scientific Corp. 800-959-0153
77 Enterprise Dr, Ann Arbor, MI 48103

Kentron Health Care, Inc. 615-384-0573
3604 Kelton Jackson Rd, P.o. Box 120, Springfield, TN 37172
Penlights.

Medical Illumination International 800-831-1222
547 Library St, San Fernando, CA 91340
Centurion Excel Emergency battery-back-up light, available in wall mounted, single ceiling mounted or portable models

Medspring Group, Inc. 801-295-9750
533 W 2600 S Ste 105, Bountiful, UT 84010
Battery-powered medical examination light.

Minrad, Inc. 716-855-1068
50 Cobham Dr, Orchard Park, NY 14127
Flashlight.

Perioptix, Inc. 949-366-3333
230 Market Pl, Escondido, CA 92029
Battery powered portable light source.

Promedic, Inc. 239-498-2155
3460 Pointe Creek Ct Apt 102, Bonita Springs, FL 34134
Transillumination vein locator.

Translite 281-240-3111
8410 Highway 90A, Sugar Land, TX 77478
Battery powered exam light.

Welch Allyn, Inc. 800-535-6663
4341 State Street Rd, Skaneateles Falls, NY 13153

Xemax Surgical Products, Inc. 800-257-9470
712 California Blvd, Napa, CA 94559
Battery powered, rechargable light.

3gen, Llc. 949-481-6384
31521 Rancho Viejo Rd Ste 104, San Juan Capistrano, CA 92675
Battery powered exam light.

LIGHT, FIBEROPTIC, DENTAL *(Dental And Oral) 76EAY*

A-Dec, Inc. 800-547-1883
2601 Crestview Dr, Newberg, OR 97132
Dental fiber optic light sovrce.

Den-Mat Holdings, Llc 805-922-8491
2727 Skyway Dr, Santa Maria, CA 93455
Virtuoso light.

Denbur, Inc. 630-969-6865
433 Plaza Dr Ste 4, Westmont, IL 60559
Wand attachment.

Dent Zar, Inc. 800-444-1241
6362 Hollywood Blvd Ste 214, Los Angeles, CA 90028
Fiber optic dental light.

Dentalez Group 866-DTE-INFO
101 Lindenwood Dr Ste 225, Valleybrooke Corporate Center
Malvern, PA 19355

Dp Manufacture Corp. 305-640-9894
1460 NW 107th Ave Ste H, Doral, FL 33172
Fiber optic rod.

Fiberoptic Components, Llc 978-422-0422
2 Spratt Tech. Way, Sterling, MA 01564
Fiber optic light guide.

Fused Fiberoptics L.L.C. 508-765-1652
79 Golf St, Southbridge, MA 01550
Fiber-optic dental-curing-tip light guides.

H & H Co. 909-390-0373
4435 E Airport Dr Ste 108, Ontario, CA 91761
Light, fiber optic, dental.

Insitu Technologies, Inc. 651-389-1017
5810 Blackshire Path, Inver Grove Heights, MN 55076
Fiberscope diagnostic probe.

Lares Research 800-347-3289
295 Lockheed Ave, Chico, CA 95973

Qed, Inc. 859-231-0338
750 Enterprise Dr, Lexington, KY 40510
Dental headlight, fiber optic light.

Salvin Dental Specialties, Inc. 800-535-6566
3450 Latrobe Dr, Charlotte, NC 28211
Various types of dental fiber optic lights and accessories.

Sds (Summit Dental Systems) 800-275-3368
3560 NW 53rd Ct, Fort Lauderdale, FL 33309

Sunoptic Technologies 877-677-2832
6018 Bowdendale Ave, Jacksonville, FL 32216
Visible light curing and transillumination, fiberoptic light cables, or high intensity probes for curing guns. Surgical headlights. Replacement light guides available for bonding. Intra-oral video endoscopes.

LIGHT, HEADBAND, SURGICAL *(Surgery) 79FSR*

Cameron-Miller, Inc. 800-621-0142
5410 W Roosevelt Rd, Road #241, Chicago, IL 60644

Sunoptic Technologies 877-677-2832
6018 Bowdendale Ave, Jacksonville, FL 32216
Coaxial fixed or variable bright white light headlights, portable or mobile systems, UL and CSA listed.

Vitalcor, Inc. 800-874-8358
100 Chestnut Ave, Westmont, IL 60559
Applied Fiberoptics Gemini headlight system.

LIGHT, HIGH INTENSITY *(Radiology) 90VHH*

Burkhart Roentgen Intl. Inc. 800-USA-XRAY
5201 8th Ave S, Gulfport, FL 33707
Heidelberg examination lights: ceiling or wall-mount and floor models, and the new blue line available in: 30, 80, 90 and 120 lux, all configurations.

Caprock Developments Inc. 800-222-0325
475 Speedwell Ave, PO Box 95, Morris Plains, NJ 07950

Roldan Products Corp. 866-922-6800
448 Sovereign Ct, Ballwin, MO 63011
$70 for high intensity table lamp and $62 for compact 13W table lamp.

Sunoptic Technologies 877-677-2832
6018 Bowdendale Ave, Jacksonville, FL 32216
Surgical headlight, shadow free bright white light, coaxial fixed or variable spot diameter 20mm to 80mm, fixed 100mm. Fiberoptic headlight incorporates coated multiple optical system for a very bright white light. Three year warranty, UL and CSA listed. Variable focus headlight with headband, fiberoptic cable, two autoclavable joysticks, two garment clips and carrying case.

LIGHT, OTHER *(General) 80RFG*

Alkco Lighting Co. 847-451-0700
11500 Melrose Ave, Franklin Park, IL 60131
Undercabinet lighting, night lights, dark room safelights, etc.

American Bio-Medical Service Corporation (Abmsc) 800-755-9055
631 W Covina Blvd, Sales,Service and Refurbishing Center
San Dimas, CA 91773
Operating room lights.

Astralite Corporation 800-345-7703
PO Box 689, Somerset, CA 95684
Replacement bulbs, miniature for diagnostic/endoscopic instruments; replacements for Statham, Burton, Astralite, Welch-Allyn.

Bovie Medical Corp. 800-537-2790
5115 Ulmerton Rd, Clearwater, FL 33760
Battery-operated, flexible surgical lights, and lighted intubation stylet.

Brewer Company, The 888-873-9371
N88W13901 Main St, Menomonee Falls, WI 53051
#163002: Procedure Light- Floor, #163001: Procedure Light- Wall, #163003: Procedure Light- Ceiling, #16100- Halogen Exam Light, #15100: Incandescent Exam Light, #11500 Chrome Gooseneck Exam Lamp

Bulbtronics, Inc. 800-624-2852
45 Banfi Plz N, Farmingdale, NY 11735

Bulbworks, Inc. 800-334-2852
80 N Dell Ave Unit 5, Kenvil, NJ 07847
All Types Of Specialty Lamps, Including Quartz Halogen, Mercury Arc, Xenon, Incandescent, Fluorescent, Metal Halide And Others.

Callcare 800-345-9414
1370 Arcadia Rd, Lancaster, PA 17601
Call-lights and systems.

Clean Air Technology, Inc. 800 459 6320
41105 Capital Dr, Canton, MI 48187
Cleanroom sealed lights. Sealed lights for class 1 Div2 hazardous areas. Explosion proof lights.

Colonial Scientific Ltd. 902-468-1811
201 Brownlow Ave., Unit 52, Dartmouth, NS B3B-1W2 Canada
Examination lights, pharmacy fixtures, overbed lights.

Crest Healthcare Supply 800-328-8908
195 3rd St, Dassel, MN 55325
Emergency lighting.

Deknatel Snowden-Pencer 800-367-7874
5175 S Royal Atlanta Dr, Tucker, GA 30084
Video light source.

Flow X-Ray Corporation 800-356-9729
100 W Industry Ct, Deer Park, NY 11729
Darkroom safety lights.

Gagne, Inc. 800-800-5954
41 Commercial Dr, Johnson City, NY 13790
PORTA-TRACE Thinlite, thin-profile lightbox: 3/4' thick, 22 oz., direct AC plug (no AC adapter), bright and even color corrected light.

Innovative Med Inc. 877-779-9492
4 Autry Ste B, Irvine, CA 92618
Our new Multi Wave Light Therapy system is one of the most versatile LED light therapy systems to hit the market. Because of the unique design, we can generate any wavelength that has been demonstrated to be effective from 395 to 920 nm. The Multi Wave Light Therapy system has multiple programs, all working on the basic principle of healing damaged cells; making them healthy again. ONE PAD - FIVE WAVELENGTHS; RED: 630nm, BLUE: 445nm, IR: 870nm, AMBER: 585nm, GREEN: 533nm. With the Multi Wave system there is no need to change pads or components to achieve the various wavelengths.

Lumitex, Inc. 800-969-5483
8443 Dow Cir, Strongsville, OH 44136
Illuminated retractors and bilirubin phototherapy lights. Also Bard Light BG LUMITEX and LightMat by LUMITEX, disposable surgical illumination devices.

Medical Illumination International 800-831-1222
547 Library St, San Fernando, CA 91340
Century 'Woods Light', VERSALITE exam light; Medi-Vue magnifying light

LIGHT, OTHER *(cont'd)*

Physician Engineered Products, Inc. 800-622-6240
103 Smith St, Fryeburg, ME 04037
PEP has introduced an innovative adult bright light,phototherapy device that offers 8000 or 12000 lux of blue-green light in a most convenient, portable unit that clips under the visor of any brimmed hat - allowing the user to perform most daily activities while receiving the standard 1/2 hour of bright light. It is effective against winter blues and for circadian rhythm adjustment to prevent jet lag, work shift change fatigue and sleep phase insomnias.

Rayovac 800-331-4522
601 Rayovac Drive, Madison, WI 53744-4960
Flashlights and penlights.

Roldan Products Corp. 866-922-6800
448 Sovereign Ct, Ballwin, MO 63011
$81.00 per unit.

Schott North America, Inc. 315-255-2791
62 Columbus St, Auburn, NY 13021
SCHOTT manufactures and supplies fiberoptic and LED illumination solutions for machine vision, industrial OEM, microscopy, forensic, and medical applications. Our product catalog features photos, drawings, and technical specifications for more than 400 standard products, from light sources to backlights, ringlights, bundles, goosenecks, lightlines, halogen light sources, and a variety of accessories. Please visit www.us.schott.com/fiberoptics to request our product catalog or literature.

Siltron Emergency Systems 800-874-3392
290 E Prairie St, Crystal Lake, IL 60014
Emergency lighting & exit signs, UPS & inverter systems for lighting.

Star X-Ray Co., Inc. 800-374-2163
63 Ranick Dr S, Amityville, NY 11701
$75.00 for circular darkroom safelight.

Sunbox Company 800-548-3968
19217 Orbit Dr, Gaithersburg, MD 20879
Medical lighting for phototherapy. Also available, Dawn Simulators.

Suppleyes, Inc. 800-727-3725
4890 Hammond Industrial Dr Ste A, Cumming, GA 30041
Instrument light bulbs for optometry.

Vista Lighting 800-576-2135
1805 Pittsburgh Ave, Erie, PA 16502

Welch Allyn, Inc. 800-535-6663
4341 State Street Rd, Skaneateles Falls, NY 13153
SOLARTEC Source 270 high-intensity universal light source that delivers white light. MULTI LINK port allows the SOLARTEC to power all major bundle designs. SOLARTEC Source 100 high-intensity universal light source that delivers white light. The MULTI LINK port allows the SOLARTEC Source 100 to power all major bundle designs.

Wolf X-Ray Corporation 800-356-9729
100 W Industry Ct, Deer Park, NY 11729
Darkroom safety lights.

3m Espe Dental Products 949-863-1360
2111 McGaw Ave, Irvine, CA 92614
$869.25 for curing light.

LIGHT, OVERBED *(General) 80RFF*

Alkco Lighting Co. 847-451-0700
11500 Melrose Ave, Franklin Park, IL 60131
IMPRESSIONS, Versalume, Textra, Horizon, T5, T8, Up-Light, Down-Light, 2 lamp, 3 lamp, 4 lamp.

Allied Healthcare Products, Inc. 800-444-3954
1720 Sublette Ave, Saint Louis, MO 63110

Burton Medical Products, Inc. 800-444-9909
21100 Lassen St, Chatsworth, CA 91311

Crest Healthcare Supply 800-328-8908
195 3rd St, Dassel, MN 55325

Independent Solutions, Inc. 847-498-0500
900 Skokie Blvd Ste 118, Northbrook, IL 60062
VISTA Fluorescent; one, two, three or four tube; 2', 3' or 4'; with many hospital options. U.L. listed.

Roldan Products Corp. 866-922-6800
448 Sovereign Ct, Ballwin, MO 63011
$92.00 per unit (standard).

Swivelier Co., Inc. 845-353-1455
600 Bradley Hill Rd, Blauvelt, NY 10913
Track lighting.

Vista Lighting 800-576-2135
1805 Pittsburgh Ave, Erie, PA 16502

LIGHT, OVERBED *(cont'd)*

Waldmann Lighting 800-634-0007
9 Century Dr, Wheeling, IL 60090
Amadea for flexible and energy efficient four-way lighting, Medicool E with electronic ballast.

LIGHT, SURGICAL HEADLIGHT *(Dental And Oral) 76EBA*

Bausch & Lomb Surgical 636-255-5051
3365 Tree Court Ind Blvd, Saint Louis, MO 63122

Burton Medical Products, Inc. 800-444-9909
21100 Lassen St, Chatsworth, CA 91311
XenaLux Fiberoptic Headlight.

Cameron-Miller, Inc. 800-621-0142
5410 W Roosevelt Rd, Road #241, Chicago, IL 60644

General Scientific Corp. 800-959-0153
77 Enterprise Dr, Ann Arbor, MI 48103

Genesis Biosystems, Inc. 888-577-7335
1500 Eagle Ct, Lewisville, TX 75057
Surgical headlight.

Gyrus Ent L.L.C., Sub. Of Gyrus Acmi, Inc. 508-804-2739
2925 Appling Rd, Bartlett, TN 38133
Headband for headlight.

Integra Luxtec, Inc. 800-325-8966
99 Hartwell St, West Boylston, MA 01583
Miniature fiber optic headlight.

Keeler Instruments Inc. 800-523-5620
456 Park Way, Broomall, PA 19008
Keelite clip-on headlight with single light source, $995.

Kerr Corp. 949-255-8766
3225 Deming Way Ste 190, Middleton, WI 53562
Dental, headlight.

Md International, Inc. 305-669-9003
11300 NW 41st St, Doral, FL 33178

Medical Sales & Service Group 888-357-6520
10 Woodchester Dr, Acton, MA 01720

Medical Technologies Co. 800-280-3220
1728 W Park Center Dr Ste A, Fenton, MO 63026

Qed, Inc. 859-231-0338
750 Enterprise Dr, Lexington, KY 40510
Dental surgical headlight.

Salvin Dental Specialties, Inc. 800-535-6566
3450 Latrobe Dr, Charlotte, NC 28211
Surgical headlamp and accessories.

Sunoptic Technologies 877-677-2832
6018 Bowdendale Ave, Jacksonville, FL 32216
Surgical headlight, shadow free bright white light, coaxial fixed or variable spot diameter, 20mm to 80mm, fixed 100mm, unique adjustment. Fiberoptic headlight incorporates multiple coated optical system for a very bright white light. Three year warranty, UL and CSA listed. All lightsources can be mounted onto mobile floorstand.

Welch Allyn, Inc. 800-535-6663
4341 State Street Rd, Skaneateles Falls, NY 13153

LIGHT, SURGICAL OPERATING, DENTAL *(Dental And Oral) 76EAZ*

A-Dec, Inc. 800-547-1883
2601 Crestview Dr, Newberg, OR 97132
Dental operating light.

Amelife Llc 302-476-2631
702 N West St Ste 101, Wilmington, DE 19801

Boyd Industries, Inc.
12900 44th St N, Clearwater, FL 33762
Various dental operating lights.

Burton Medical Products, Inc. 800-444-9909
21100 Lassen St, Chatsworth, CA 91311
Genesis Plus, Genie Plus Visionary

Dentalez Group 866-DTE-INFO
101 Lindenwood Dr Ste 225, Valleybrooke Corporate Center
Malvern, PA 19355

Dentalez Of Alabama 251-937-6781
2500 S US Highway 31, Bay Minette, AL 36507
Light, dental.

Dentamerica Inc. 626-912-1388
18688 San Jose Ave, City Of Industry, CA 91748
CELUX.

LIGHT, SURGICAL OPERATING, DENTAL *(cont'd)*

Global Surgical Corp. 314-861-3388
3610 Tree Court Industrial Blvd, Saint Louis, MO 63122
Dental light.

H & H Co. 909-390-0373
4435 E Airport Dr Ste 108, Ontario, CA 91761
Light, operating, dental.

Health Science Products, Inc. 800-237-5794
1489 Hueytown Rd, Hueytown, AL 35023
HSP Glows dental light for tooth shading, flexible positioning and a high-low for color matching (same as light above).

Isolux Llc 239-514-7475
1045 Collier Center Way Ste 6, Naples, FL 34110
Xenon fiber optic light source for dental procedures.

Js Dental Mfg., Inc. 800-284-3368
196 N Salem Rd, Ridgefield, CT 06877
Accessory to curing light, light tip.

Kavo Dental Manufacturing Inc 202-828-0850
901 W Oakton St, Des Plaines, IL 60018
Various models of dental operating lights marketed as 'the environment'.

Md Components Inc. 954-565-5328
3560 NW 53rd Ct, Fort Lauderdale, FL 33309
Dental light.

Midmark Corporation 800-643-6275
60 Vista Dr, P.O. Box 286, Versailles, OH 45380

Pelton & Crane 704-588-2126
11727 Fruehauf Dr, Charlotte, NC 28273
Dental light.

Planmeca U.S.A. Inc 630-529-2300
100 Gary Ave Ste A, Roselle, IL 60172
PLANMECA Delight dental light

Proma, Inc. 310-327-0035
730 Kingshill Pl, Carson, CA 90746
Dental light.

Zila Technical, Inc. 602-266-6700
3418 S 48th St Ste 9, Phoenix, AZ 85040
Dental operating light.

LIGHT, SURGICAL, CARRIER *(Surgery) 79FSZ*

Medtronic Puerto Rico Operations Co.,Med Rel 763-514-4000
Road 909, Km. 0.4., Barrio Mariana, Humacao, PR 00792
Surgical lamp.

Medtronic Sofamor Danek Usa, Inc. 901-396-3133
4340 Swinnea Rd, Memphis, TN 38118
Surgical lamp.

Warsaw Orthopedic, Inc. 901-396-3133
2500 Silveus Xing, Warsaw, IN 46582
Surgical lamp.

LIGHT, SURGICAL, CEILING MOUNTED *(Surgery) 79FSY*

Alkco Lighting Co. 847-451-0700
11500 Melrose Ave, Franklin Park, IL 60131
Recessed fluorescent lighting.

Berchtold Corp. 800-243-5135
1950 Hanahan Rd, Charleston, SC 29406

Burkhart Roentgen Intl. Inc. 800-USA-XRAY
5201 8th Ave S, Gulfport, FL 33707
Heidelberg examination lights: ceiling or wall-mount and floor models, and the new blue line available in 30, 80, 90 and 120 lux, all configurations.

Burton Medical Products, Inc. 800-444-9909
21100 Lassen St, Chatsworth, CA 91311
VISIONARY, Genie Plus, Genesis Plus

Computer Optics Inc. 603-889-2116
120 Derry St, Hudson, NH 03051
Various models of surgical lights.

Elmed, Inc. 630-543-2792
60 W Fay Ave, Addison, IL 60101

Kma Remarketing Corp. 814-371-5242
302 Aspen Way, Dubois, PA 15801
Ceiling mounted surgical light.

Maquet, Inc. 843-552-8652
7371 Spartan Blvd E, N Charleston, SC 29418
Surgical and examination lights.

LIGHT, SURGICAL, CEILING MOUNTED *(cont'd)*

Medical Illumination International 800-831-1222
547 Library St, San Fernando, CA 91340
SYSTEM ONE surgery light, available in S1 (20'), S2 (16'), and P1 video camera in Solo, Duo or Trio ceiling mount configurations; Centurion Excel 16' surgery light, Centurion 15' minor surgery light, available in wall, portable, single, dual or combo fixed ceiling mounts, as well as ChuttleTrak ceiling track mountings

Meza Medical Equipment 888-308-7116
108 W Nakoma St, San Antonio, TX 78216

Nuvo, Inc. 814-899-4220
5368 Kuhl Rd., Corry, PA 16407
Surgical light.

Skytron 800-759-8766
5085 Corporate Exchange Blvd SE, Grand Rapids, MI 49512
Eighteen models with quartz halogen type lamps, 6- to 10-in. diameter circular field. 5 to 8 lamps per model. 12,000-39,000 fc. Center-point mounted. STELLAR Series combines fixed and variable focus into one lighthead. 110-degree vertical travel.

Swivelier Co., Inc. 845-353-1455
600 Bradley Hill Rd, Blauvelt, NY 10913
Surgical ambulance light.

World Medical Equipment, Inc. 800-827-3747
3915 152nd St NE, Marysville, WA 98271
Specialize in refurbished OR lights such as AMSCO/Steris, Burton, Skytron, and ALM as well as OR tables, autoclaves, anesthesia machines, monitors, and accessories.

LIGHT, SURGICAL, CONNECTOR *(Surgery) 79FSX*

Connector Contacts 877-463-9029
714 E Edna Pl, Covina, CA 91723
Contact pins, sockets, and connectors.

Sunoptic Technologies 877-677-2832
6018 Bowdendale Ave, Jacksonville, FL 32216
Custom or standard high performance fiberoptic cables and adaptors, all sizes, all types (autoclavable).

LIGHT, SURGICAL, ENDOSCOPIC *(Surgery) 79FSW*

Aculux, Inc. 239-643-8023
4424 Corporate Sq, Naples, FL 34104
Xenalight fiberoptic illuminator, headlamp & cables.

Advanced Endoscopy Devices, Inc. 818-227-2720
22134 Sherman Way, Canoga Park, CA 91303
Fiberoptic light source and carrier. Halogen and xenon light source. Fiberoptic light cable.

General Scientific Corp. 800-959-0153
77 Enterprise Dr, Ann Arbor, MI 48103

Genicon 800-936-1020
6869 Stapoint Ct Ste 114, Winter Park, FL 32792
Lightsources for Endoscopic Surgery

Medical Illumination International 800-831-1222
547 Library St, San Fernando, CA 91340

Richard Wolf Medical Instruments Corp. 800-323-9653
353 Corporate Woods Pkwy, Vernon Hills, IL 60061

Solos Endoscopy 800-388-6445
65 Sprague St # B, Boston/dedham Commerce Park, Boston, MA 02136
Surgical light source.

Sunoptic Technologies 877-677-2832
6018 Bowdendale Ave, Jacksonville, FL 32216
Fiberoptic cables, all types, sizes and lengths, standard or custom, autoclavable. Custom fiberoptic cables and contract manufacturer. Several models of solid state, high intensity universal fiberoptic lightsources, 150W, 300W and xenon types available, UL and CSA listed. (Custom work and prototypes of fiberoptic cables in 10 days). Coaxial fixed or variable bright white light headlights, UL and CSA listed.

Welch Allyn, Inc. 800-535-6663
4341 State Street Rd, Skaneateles Falls, NY 13153

LIGHT, SURGICAL, FIBEROPTIC *(Surgery) 79FST*

Advanced Dental Systems 480-991-4081
5001 E Desert Jewel Dr, Paradise Valley, AZ 85253
Fiber optic light.

Arthrex, Inc. 239-643-5553
1370 Creekside Blvd, Naples, FL 34108
Various types of light cables and illuminator ends.

Bulbtronics, Inc. 800-624-2852
45 Banfi Plz N, Farmingdale, NY 11735

LIGHT, SURGICAL, FIBEROPTIC *(cont'd)*

Cantylight 716-625-4227
6100 Donner Rd, Lockport, NY 14094

Chiu Technical Corp. 631-544-0606
252 Indian Head Rd, Kings Park, NY 11754
$534.00 DLU-150 dual lamp light source, halogen lamp module, $598.00 DLU dual universal lite source with diaph or dimmer.

Dma Med-Chem Corporation 800-362-1833
49 Watermill Ln, Great Neck, NY 11021

Electro Surgical Instrument Co., Inc. 888-464-2784
37 Centennial St, Rochester, NY 14611
Fiber optic focusable light stand in various types, styles and sizes.

Fiberoptics Technology, Inc. 800-433-5248
1 Fiber Rd, Pomfret, CT 06258
Fiberoptics for surgery.

Florida Life Systems 727-321-9554
3446 5th Ave N, Saint Petersburg, FL 33713

Isolux Llc 239-514-7475
1045 Collier Center Way Ste 6, Naples, FL 34110
Isolux america fiber optic surgical headlight.

Karl Storz Endoscopy-America Inc. 800-421-0837
600 Corporate Pointe, Culver City, CA 90230

Med-General Usa Llc 239-597-9967
1045 Collier Center Way Ste 1, Naples, FL 34110
Led illumination.

Mediflex Surgical Products 800-879-7575
250 Gibbs Rd, Islandia, NY 11749
Laparoscopy light guide, 90-degree swivel at scope connection, manually adjustable, iris at scope connection, 10-ft length.

Mednet Locator, Inc. 800-754-5070
7000 Shadow Oaks Dr, Memphis, TN 38125
Fiberoptic light source.

Microvision, Inc. 603-474-5566
34 Folly Mill Rd, Seabrook, NH 03874
Fiber optic endoillumination probe.

Nuvasive, Inc. 800-475-9131
7475 Lusk Blvd, San Diego, CA 92121
Surgical light.

Progressive Dynamics Medical, Inc. 269-781-4241
507 Industrial Rd, Marshall, MI 49068
150 watt halogen light source.

Sds-Surgical Acuity 888-822-8489
3225 Deming Way Ste 120, Middleton, WI 53562
ZEON Illuminator and zeon lumenare fiber-optic lighting.

Solos Endoscopy 800-388-6445
65 Sprague St # B, Boston/dedham Commerce Park, Boston, MA 02136
Surgical lamp.

Sunoptic Technologies 877-677-2832
6018 Bowdendale Ave, Jacksonville, FL 32216
Fiberoptic headlights and cables, standard or custom, fiberoptic lightsources, several models available, UL and CSA listed.

Vitalcor, Inc. 800-874-8358
100 Chestnut Ave, Westmont, IL 60559
Applied Fiberoptics Sunbeam 300-Watt xenon light source.

Welch Allyn, Inc. 800-535-6663
4341 State Street Rd, Skaneateles Falls, NY 13153
SOLARTEC Source 270 high-intensity universl light source that delivers white light. MULTI LINK port allows the SOLARTEC to power all major bundle designs. SOLARTEC Source 100 high-intensity universal light source that delivers white light. The MULTI LINK port allows the SOLARTEC Source 100 to power all major bundle designs.

LIGHT, SURGICAL, FLOOR STANDING *(Surgery) 79FSS*

Berchtold Corp. 800-243-5135
1950 Hanahan Rd, Charleston, SC 29406

Burton Medical Products, Inc. 800-444-9909
21100 Lassen St, Chatsworth, CA 91311
Outpatient II, CoolSpot II

Kma Remarketing Corp. 814-371-5242
302 Aspen Way, Dubois, PA 15801
Floor standing surgical light.

Maquet, Inc. 843-552-8652
7371 Spartan Blvd E, N Charleston, SC 29418
Minor surgical lights.

Meza Medical Equipment 888-308-7116
108 W Nakoma St, San Antonio, TX 78216

LIGHT, SURGICAL, FLOOR STANDING *(cont'd)*

Midmark Corporation 800-643-6275
60 Vista Dr, P.O. Box 286, Versailles, OH 45380
20 in. lighthead with quartz halogen lamp and mobile stand. Includes dimmer control.

Sunnex, Inc. 800-445-7869
3 Huron Dr, Natick, MA 01760
Examination/minor surgery lamp on caster base.

Sunoptic Technologies 877-677-2832
6018 Bowdendale Ave, Jacksonville, FL 32216
180 watt or 300 watt xenon lightsource featuring small size, quiet operation and intense white light output. Entire system includes lightsource, headlight, and floorstand.

LIGHT, SURGICAL, INSTRUMENT *(Surgery) 79FSQ*

International Hospital Supply Co. 800-398-9450
6914 Canby Ave Ste 105, Reseda, CA 91335

Stryker Puerto Rico, Ltd. 939-307-2500
Hwy. 3, Km. 131.2, Las Guasimas Ind. Park, Arroyo, PR 00714
Knife.

Sunoptic Technologies 877-677-2832
6018 Bowdendale Ave, Jacksonville, FL 32216
Custom or standard high performance fiberoptic cables and adaptors, all sizes, all types (autoclavable).

Varitech Medical Devices, Inc. 815-624-6785
319 Dickop St, South Beloit, IL 61080
Low profile birthing room light 18 inch.

Vitalcor, Inc. 800-874-8358
100 Chestnut Ave, Westmont, IL 60559
Applied Fiberoptics lighted retractors.

LIGHT, THERAPY, SEASONAL AFFECTIVE DISORDER (SAD) *(General) 80MIO*

Bio-Brite, Inc. 800-621-5483
4330 E West Hwy Ste 310, Bethesda, MD 20814

Health Light Inc. 800-265-6020
P.O. Box 3899 LCD 4, Hamilton, ONT L8H-7P2 Canada

Mind Alive Inc. 800-661-6463
9008 51 Ave., Edmonton, ALB T6E-5X4 Canada
DAVID PAL - Audio-Visual Entrainment (AVE) device that stimulates and changes brainwaves to help with SAD, depression, anxiety and insomnia. Can also be helpful in chronic pain management, fibromyalgia, and ADD. Very non-intrusive and very easy to use.

Mylon-Tech Health Technologies Inc. 613-728-1667
301 Moodie Dr., Ste. 205, Ottawa, ON K2H 9C4 Canada
Newest, most efficient light systems for treatment of SAD.

Sunnex Biotechnologies 877-778-6639
167 Lombard Ave. #657, Winnipeg, MAN R3B-0V3 Canada
Patented Low Intensity limited spectrum light therapy unit for the treatment of seasonal and non-seasonal depression, and for chronobiological disorders including adaptation to night work and the treatment of sleep disorders.

LIGHT, ULTRAVIOLET, DERMATOLOGIC *(Surgery) 79FTC*

Avex Industries, Ltd.
27 Allen St, Hudson Falls, NY 12839
Phototherapeutix.

Heartland Tanning, Inc. 816-795-1414
4251 NE Port Dr, Lees Summit, MO 64064
Various.

Interlectric Corp. 800-722-2184
1401 Lexington Ave, Warren, PA 16365
Tanning lamps.

International Tanning Technologies 800-832-8267
5225 W 140th St, Brook Park, OH 44142
Light, ultraviolet, dermatological.

National Biological Corp. 800-338-5045
1532 Enterprise Pkwy, Twinsburg, OH 44087
DERMA-WAND, handheld germicidal (UVC) lamp.

The Richmond Light Co. 888-276-0559
2301 Falkirk Dr, Richmond, VA 23236
Home UVB light source.

Theralight, Inc. 760-930-8000
2794 Loker Ave W Ste 105, Carlsbad, CA 92010
Uva/uvb phototherapy system & accessories.

LIGHT, WOOD'S, FLUORESCENCE *(Microbiology) 83GMB*

Equipro Equipment De Beaute 514-324-2226
11005 Rue Masse, Montreal-Nord H1G 4G5 Canada
Skin scanner

Kentron Health Care, Inc. 615-384-0573
3604 Kelton Jackson Rd, P.o. Box 120, Springfield, TN 37172
Uretheral catheter.

LINEN *(General) 80VBF*

Atd-American Co. 800-523-2300
135 Greenwood Ave, Wyncote, PA 19095

Bba Fiberweb Washougal, Inc. 800-772-7771
3720 Grant St, Washougal, WA 98671
Non-woven fabrics in rolls sent to companies that make diapers, feminine hygiene & medical companies.

Clopay Plastic Products Company 800-282-2260
8585 Duke Blvd, Mason, OH 45040
Fabrics meeting requirements of OSHA bloodborne pathogens rule.

Dazian Fabrics,Llc. 877-232-9426
124 Enterprise Ave S, PO Box 2121, Secaucus, NJ 07094
TRAPEZE, 4-way stretch, flame retardent, 120' polyester/lycra jersey. CELTIC CLOTH, 122' flame-retardent heavyweight polyester.

General Econopak, Inc. 888-871-8568
1725 N 6th St, Philadelphia, PA 19122
Pillowcases, bath towels, and hand towels. Linen packs for Stryker Circle and Wedge Frame, burn/isolation linen pack, sterile. GEPCO Sterile O.R. and OB Linen Packs, either standard or made to order. Burn/isolation Linen Packs, sterile, lintfree, non-allergenic (contents include bed sheets, pillowcase, draw-sheet, washcloth, bath towel, and patient gown).

Geri-Care Products 201-440-0409
250 Moonachie Ave, Moonachie, NJ 07074
SIGNATURE is a product line of knitted sheets.

Global Healthcare 800-601-3880
1495 Hembree Rd Ste 700, Roswell, GA 30076
Disposable pillow cases, mattress cover, blanket, and stretcher sheets

Graham Medical Products/Div. Of Little Rapids Corp 866-429-1408
2273 Larsen Rd, Green Bay, WI 54303
Professional Towels; POLYCEL, assorted colors and styles. Disposable.

Health-Pak, Inc. 315-724-8370
2005 Beechgrove Pl, Utica, NY 13501
Poly spunbonded sewn pillowcases.

Hermell Products, Inc. 800-233-2342
9 Britton Dr, PO Box 7345, Bloomfield, CT 06002
Hospital sheets: fitted, flat and pillowcase in polycotton.

Jms Converters Inc Dba Sabee Products & Stanford Prof Prod 215-396-3302
67 Buck Rd Ste B7, Huntingdon Valley, PA 19006
Disposable pillow covers.

Pelton Shepherd Industries 800-258-3423
812B W Luce St, Stockton, CA 95203
Disposable linen covers.

Pharaoh Trading Company 866-929-4913
9701 Brookpark Rd, Knollwood Plaza, Suite 241, Cleveland, OH 44129
Bed linens and terry towels for healthcare.

Riegel Consumer Products Div. 800-845-2232
PO Box E, 51 Riegel Road, Johnston, SC 29832
Table cloths, napkins, place mats. (CARESS, PERMALUX, PARNELL & BEAUTI-DAMASK.)

Standard Textile Co., Inc. 888-999-0400
PO Box 371805, Cincinnati, OH 45222
Linens for all areas of the institution.

LINEN, BED *(General) 80KME*

A Plus International, Inc 909-591-5168
5138 Eucalyptus Ave, Chino, CA 91710
Baby blanket.

Allman Products 800-223-6889
21101 Itasca St, Chatsworth, CA 91311

LINEN, BED *(cont'd)*

American Woolen Company 305-635-4000
4000 NW 30th Ave, Miami, FL 33142
Cotton thermal blankets. AMERICA'S FINEST Thermal blankets 100 % cotton boil-proof hemmed, tumble dry, preshrunk, and vat dyed. SUPERWEAVE High Performance Blanket, (#2500-72), 50% polyester, 50% acrylic, size 72' x 90' Institutional Medical Blanket, Natusilk, 100% silk, size 90' x 90', 90' x 108'.

Atd-American Co. 800-523-2300
135 Greenwood Ave, Wyncote, PA 19095
Full line of sheets and towels.

Attends Healthcare Products 252-752-1100
2321 Arrow Highway, La Verne, CA 91750
Various.

Attends Healthcare Products 252-752-1100
1029 Old Creek Rd, Greenville, NC 27834

Biomed Resource, Inc. 310-323-3888
3388 Rosewood Ave, Los Angeles, CA 90066
Underpad.

Biomet, Inc. 574-267-6639
56 E Bell Dr, PO Box 587, Warsaw, IN 46582
Various types of cervical pillows.

Bradford Medical, Llc 816-584-8100
8350 N Saint Clair Ave Ste 230, Kansas City, MO 64151
Disposable linens.

Busse Hospital Disposables, Inc. 631-435-4711
75 Arkay Dr, Hauppauge, NY 11788
Same.

Centurion Medical Products Corp. 517-545-1135
3310 S Main St, Salisbury, NC 28147

Commerce Facilitators 703-352-3569
3924 Tedrich Blvd, Fairfax, VA 22031
Transfer sheet.

Dna Products, Llc 800-535-3189
PO Box 306, New York, NY 10032
Disposable flat bed sheet made of soft polypropylene. Measures 36'W x 90'L. At 45 grams per square meter (GSM), fabric is lightweight yet durable. Safety overlock stitching around the edges prevents fraying. Intended for single use; 1 white individually wrapped sheet per package; $1.00/package; 100 packages per carton. Disposable pillowcase made of soft polypropylene. Measures 17.75'W x 11.5'L. At 28 grams per square meter (GSM), fabric is lightweight yet durable. Intended for single use; 1 white individually wrapped pillowcase per package; $0.14/package; 150 packages per carton.

Doctor Down, Inc. 406-883-3052
802 1st St E Ste B, Polson, MT 59860
Emergency rescue wrap.

Essential Medical Supply, Inc. 800-826-8423
6420 Hazeltine National Dr, Orlando, FL 32822
Hospital bed linen sets and individual pack items.

General Econopak, Inc. 888-871-8568
1725 N 6th St, Philadelphia, PA 19122
Disposable bed sheets, incontinence sheets, pillow cases, and vinyl mattress covers.

Graham Medical Products/Div. Of Little Rapids Corp 866-429-1408
2273 Larsen Rd, Green Bay, WI 54303
Disposable sheets and pillowcases. Nonwoven and tissue/poly.

Grupo Industrial C&A, S.A. De C.V. 525-562-0660
Circuito Misioneros #26, Cd. Satelite,anucal-Pan,edo Mexico
W.w.leasing bedding pack

Hawaii Medical, Llc 781-826-5565
750 Corporate Park Dr, Pembroke, MA 02359

Hill-Rom, Inc. 812-934-7777
4115 Dorchester Rd Unit 600, North Charleston, SC 29405
Bedding, disposable, medical.

Hos-Pillow Corp. 800-468-7874
1011 Campus Dr, Mundelein, IL 60060
Dr. Scholls Bedding Products, Medibed dustmite proof products, Serta Bedding Products.

Innovative Disposables 908-222-7111
3611 Kennedy Rd, South Plainfield, NJ 07080
Medical disposable bedding.

Inter-Con-Tex Corp. 570-748-3121
935 Bellefonte Ave, Lock Haven, PA 17745
Sheepskin bed pad.

LINEN, BED *(cont'd)*

Jim-Dar Ent. Corp. 913-321-1368
1922 N 18th St, Kansas City, KS 66104
Bed pillows.

Kentron Health Care, Inc. 615-384-0573
3604 Kelton Jackson Rd, P.o. Box 120, Springfield, TN 37172
Stretcher sheets.

Kerma Medical Products, Inc. 757-398-8400
400 Port Centre Pkwy, Portsmouth, VA 23704
Disposable washcloth.

Lakeland De Mexico S.A. De C.V. 516-981-9700
Rancho La Soledad Lote No. 2, Fracc. Poniente C.p. Celaya, Guajuato Mexico
Medical disposable bedding

Mcairlaid's Inc. 540-352-5050
180 Corporate Dr, Rocky Mount, VA 24151

Mip Inc. 800-361-4964
9100 Ray Lawson Blvd., Montreal, QC H1J-1K8 Canada
Specialty knit-fitted linens.

Normed 800-288-8200
PO Box 3644, Seattle, WA 98124
Emergency rescue blanket.

Paper Pak Industries 909-392-1764
One Paper Pak Way, Washington, GA 30673
Medical disposable bedding.

Paperpak 800-428-8363
545 W Terrace Dr, San Dimas, CA 91773

Riegel Consumer Products Div. 800-845-2232
PO Box E, 51 Riegel Road, Johnston, SC 29832
Mattress pads.

Rock Valley Textiles 608-752-6866
111 Avon St, Janesville, WI 53545
Hospital pad-decubitus bedding.

Rockaway Chairs 800-256-6601
111 Alexander Rd Apt 11, West Monroe, LA 71291
Bedspreads for all size beds - cotton/poly front and back.

Small Beginnings Inc. 760-949-7707
17525 Alder St Ste 28, Hesperia, CA 92345
Disposable pillow covers various types.

Standard Textile Co., Inc. 888-999-0400
PO Box 371805, Cincinnati, OH 45222
Reusable bed linens of various styles and weights.

Tidi Products, Llc 920-751-4380
570 Enterprise Dr, Neenah, WI 54956
Examination table sheeting.

Tri-State Hospital Supply Corp. 517-545-1135
3173 E 43rd St, Yuma, AZ 85365

White Knight Healthcare 800-851-4431
Calle 16, Number 780, Agua Prieta, Sonora Mexico
Bedding, disposable, medical

LINER, CAVITY, CALCIUM HYDROXIDE *(Dental And Oral) 76EJK*

Bisco, Inc. 847-534-6000
1100 W Irving Park Rd, Schaumburg, IL 60193
Oxalate dentin densensitizing agent.

Cadco Dental Products 800-833-8267
600 E Hueneme Rd, Oxnard, CA 93033

Coltene/Whaledent Inc. 330-916-8858
235 Ascot Pkwy, Cuyahoga Falls, OH 44223
Calcium hydroxide cavity liner.

Dshealthcare Inc. 201-871-1232
85 W Forest Ave, Englewood, NJ 07631
Calcium hydroxide cavity liner.

Dux Dental 800-833-8267
600 E Hueneme Rd, Oxnard, CA 93033

Ellman International, Inc. 800-835-5355
3333 Royal Ave, Rockville Centre, NY 11572

George Taub Products & Fusion Co., Inc. 800-828-2634
277 New York Ave, Jersey City, NJ 07307
HYDROXYLINE $18.00 per 6cc base white & 12cc thinner; $16.00 per 6cc base and 12cc thinner of calcium hydroxide liner tooth color.

Global Dental Products 516-221-8844
PO Box 537, Bellmore, NY 11710
TUBELITEC cavity liner. Prevents future contraction gaps from forming.

LINER, CAVITY, CALCIUM HYDROXIDE *(cont'd)*

Ivoclar Vivadent, Inc. 800-533-6825
175 Pineview Dr, Amherst, NY 14228
VIVAGLASS LINER

Js Dental Mfg., Inc. 800-284-3368
196 N Salem Rd, Ridgefield, CT 06877
Calcium hydroxide cavity liner.

Kerr Corp. 714-516-7400
28200 Wick Rd, Romulus, MI 48174
Cavity liner.

Lorvic Corp. 800-325-1881
13705 Shoreline Ct E, Earth City, MO 63045
Calcium hydroxide cavity liner.

Oratech, Llc 801-553-4493
475 W 10200 S, South Jordan, UT 84095
Cavity liner.

Pulpdent Corp. 800-343-4342
80 Oakland St, Watertown, MA 02472
Tempcanal - temporary calcium hydroxide root canal treatment.

Rite-Dent Manufacturing Corp. 305-693-8626
3750 E 10th Ct, Hialeah, FL 33013
Various types of calcium hydroxide USP.

Temrex Corp. 516-868-6221
112 Albany Ave, P.o. Box 182, Freeport, NY 11520
Cavity liner and base.

Ultradent Products, Inc. 801-553-4586
505 W 10200 S, South Jordan, UT 84095
Calcium hydroxide.

LINER, GLOVE *(General) 80WYZ*

Alimed, Inc. 800-225-2610
297 High St, Dedham, MA 02026

Cms Worldwide, Inc. 800-426-4633
30011 Ivy Glenn Dr Ste 215, Laguna Niguel, CA 92677
Glove liners; cotton or nylon.

Midwest Scientific 800-227-9997
280 Vance Rd, Valley Park, MO 63088
100% cotton glove liners fit under latex gloves, s-m-l, 3 dozen pairs $23.00.

LINER, KICK BUCKET *(General) 80RDC*

Profex Medical Products 800-325-0196
2224 E Person Ave, Memphis, TN 38114

LINER, LAUNDRY HAMPER *(General) 80TCL*

Approved Medical Systems 951-353-2453
7101 Jurupa Ave Ste 4, Riverside, CA 92504
Color-coded and designed to withstand impact. Is available with disposable or reusable liners.

Atd-American Co. 800-523-2300
135 Greenwood Ave, Wyncote, PA 19095

Brewer Company, The 888-873-9371
N88W13901 Main St, Menomonee Falls, WI 53051
#31331: Rope Style Hamper Bag (18', 21', and 25')

Bussard & Son Inc., R.D. 800-252-2692
415 25th Ave SW, Albany, OR 97322
Laundry basket liners.

Iron Duck, A Div. Of Fleming Industries, Inc. 800-669-6900
20 Veterans Dr, Chicopee, MA 01022
IMPERVAGARD Impervious replacement liners in many fabrics and sizes.

Profex Medical Products 800-325-0196
2224 E Person Ave, Memphis, TN 38114

Steele Canvas Basket Co., Inc. 800-541-8929
201 Williams St, Chelsea, MA 02150

LIPASE HYDROLYSIS/GLYCEROL KINASE ENZYME, TRIGLYCERIDES *(Chemistry) 75CDT*

Abbott Diagnostics Div. 626-440-0700
820 Mission St, South Pasadena, CA 91030
Various.

Carolina Liquid Chemistries Corp. 800-471-7272
510 W Central Ave Ste C, Brea, CA 92821
Trig.

Genzyme Corp. 800-325-2436
160 Christian St, Oxford, CT 06478

LIPASE HYDROLYSIS/GLYCEROL KINASE ENZYME, TRIGLYCERIDES *(cont'd)*

Health Chem Diagnostics Llc 954-979-3845
3341 W McNab Rd, Pompano Beach, FL 33069
Lipase hydrolysis/glycerol kinase enzyme, triglycerides.

Hemagen Diagnostics, Inc. 800-436-2436
9033 Red Branch Rd, Columbia, MD 21045
Various triglyceride methods.

Intersect Systems, Inc. 360-577-1062
1152 3rd Avenue, Suite D & E, Longview, WA 98632
Lipase hydrolysis/glycerol kinase. Triglyceride, Triglyceride-GPO.

Jas Diagnostics, Inc. 305-418-2320
7220 NW 58th St, Miami, FL 33166
Triglycerides.

Raichem, Division Of Hemagen Diagnostics, Inc. 800-438-6100
8225 Mercury Ct, San Diego, CA 92111
Triglycerides.

Sterling Diagnostics, Inc. 800-637-2661
36645 Metro Ct, Sterling Heights, MI 48312
Triglycerides reagent set.

Synermed Intl., Inc. 317-896-1565
17408 Tiller Ct Ste 1900, Westfield, IN 46074
Triglycerides reagent kit.

Teco Diagnostics 714-693-7788
1268 N Lakeview Ave, Anaheim, CA 92807
Triglyceride reagent.

Vital Diagnostics Inc. 714-672-3553
1075 W Lambert Rd Ste D, Brea, CA 92821
Various triglycerides reagents.

LIPASE-ESTERASE, ENZYMATIC, PHOTOMETRIC, LIPASE
(Chemistry) 75CHI

Carolina Liquid Chemistries Corp. 800-471-7272
510 W Central Ave Ste C, Brea, CA 92821
Lipase reagent.

Jas Diagnostics, Inc. 305-418-2320
7220 NW 58th St, Miami, FL 33166
Lipase.

LIPOPROTEIN, HIGH DENSITY, HDL, OVER-THE-COUNTER
(Chemistry) 75NAQ

Polymer Technology Systems, Inc. 317-870-5610
7736 Zionsville Rd, Indianapolis, IN 46268
Hdl cholesterol test.

LIQUID ANTI-INFECTIVES *(General) 80QAB*

Baxter Healthcare Corporation, Global Drug Delivery 888-229-0001
25212 W Il Route 120, Round Lake, IL 60073
Famotidine.

LIQUID CHROMATOGRAPHY, AMPHETAMINE
(Toxicology) 91DNI

Bio-Rad Laboratories Inc., Clinical Systems Div. 800-224-6723
4000 Alfred Nobel Dr, Hercules, CA 94547
Remedi drug profiling system.

LIQUID CHROMATOGRAPHY, MORPHINE *(Toxicology) 91DPK*

St. Paul Biotech 714-903-1000
11555 Monarch St, Garden Grove, CA 92841
Morphine test.

LIQUID CHROMATOGRAPHY, SALICYLATE *(Toxicology) 91DMX*

Welco-Cgi Gas Technologies 440-234-1075
145 Shimersville Rd, Bethlehem, PA 18015
Helium.

LITHOTRIPTOR *(Gastro/Urology) 78UEP*

Karl Storz Endoscopy-America Inc. 800-421-0837
600 Corporate Pointe, Culver City, CA 90230
Extracorporeal shock wave lithotriptor, ultrasound lithotriptor, and single-shot and continuous pneumatic lithotriptor available.

Light Age Inc. 732-563-0600
500 Apgar Dr, Somerset, NJ 08873
OEM pulsed alexandrite laser operating in the red/near infared for stone destruction.

Mahe International Inc. 800-294-7946
468 Craighead St, Nashville, TN 37204

LITHOTRIPTOR, ELECTRO-HYDRAULIC, EXTRACORPOREAL
(Gastro/Urology) 78VKM

Northgate Technologies Inc. 800-348-0424
600 Church Rd, Elgin, IL 60123
AUTOLITH EHL Lithotripter is used for fragmenting Urinary and Biliary Stones, AUTOLITH is a computer controlled EHL generator with various electrodes to choose from, 1.9Fr., 3Fr., 5Fr., 9Fr., and 250 cm long version for biliary applications.

LITHOTRIPTOR, ELECTRO-HYDRAULIC, PERCUTANEOUS
(Gastro/Urology) 78FFK

Gyrus Acmi, Inc. 508-804-2739
93 N Pleasant St, Norwalk, OH 44857
Electrohydraulic lithotripter.

Karl Storz Endoscopy-America Inc. 800-421-0837
600 Corporate Pointe, Culver City, CA 90230

Richard Wolf Medical Instruments Corp. 800-323-9653
353 Corporate Woods Pkwy, Vernon Hills, IL 60061

LITHOTRIPTOR, EXTRACORPOREAL SHOCK-WAVE, UROLOGICAL *(Gastro/Urology) 78LNS*

Direx Systems Corp. 339-502-6013
437 Turnpike St, Canton, MA 02021
Lithotripter.

E.S.W.L. Products, Inc. 847-419-6844
1542 Barclay Blvd, Buffalo Grove, IL 60089
Extracorporeal shockwave litotriptor.

Fmd, Llc 703-880-4642
7200 Telegraph Square Dr Ste E, Lorton, VA 22079
Extracorporeal shock-wave lithotriptor.

Medispec Ltd. - Usa 888-663-3477
20410 Observation Dr Ste 102, Germantown, MD 20876
ECONOLITH/E-2000

Richard Wolf Medical Instruments Corp. 800-323-9653
353 Corporate Woods Pkwy, Vernon Hills, IL 60061

LITHOTRIPTOR, LASER *(Gastro/Urology) 78WSU*

Candela Corp. 800-733-8550
530 Boston Post Rd, Wayland, MA 01778
MDL 3000 LASERTRIPTER. Priced at $159,500 for ureteral and kidney stone removal.

Dynacon, Inc. 573-594-3813
4924 Pike 451, Curryville, MO 63339
Shock wave lithotriptors for kidney stones. Surgical lasers.

Surgical Laser Technologies, Inc. 800-366-4758
147 Keystone Dr, Montgomeryville, PA 18936

LITHOTRIPTOR, MECHANICAL, BILIARY *(Gastro/Urology) 78LQC*

Boston Scientific Corporation 800-225-2732
1 Boston Scientific Pl, Natick, MA 01760

Cook Endoscopy 336-744-0157
4900 Bethania Station Rd # &, 5951 Grassy Creek Blvd. Winston Salem, NC 27105
Soehendra lithotripsy set.

Medi-Globe Corporation 800-966-1431
110 W Orion St Ste 136, Tempe, AZ 85283
Mechanical.

LITHOTRIPTOR, MULTIPURPOSE *(Gastro/Urology) 78WIL*

Dornier Medtech America 800-367-6437
1155 Roberts Blvd NW, Kennesaw, GA 30144
Dornier's Compact line of lithotripters provides extracorporeal shock-wave lithotripsy for treatment of kidney, ureteral, and bile-duct stones.

LITHOTRIPTOR, ULTRASONIC *(Gastro/Urology) 78FEO*

Fibra-Sonics, A Division Of Misonix, Inc. 631-694-9555
1938 New Hwy, Farmingdale, NY 11735
Ultrasonic lithotriptor.

Karl Storz Endoscopy-America Inc. 800-421-0837
600 Corporate Pointe, Culver City, CA 90230

Misonix, Inc. 800-694-9612
1938 New Hwy, Farmingdale, NY 11735
Misonix 2000 Ultrasonic Lithotriptor for urology.

Richard Wolf Medical Instruments Corp. 800-323-9653
353 Corporate Woods Pkwy, Vernon Hills, IL 60061

LOCATOR, APEX, ROOT *(Dental And Oral) 76LQY*

Acteon Inc. 800-289-6367
124 Gaither Dr Ste 140, Mount Laurel, NJ 08054
NEOSONO.

LOCATOR, APEX, ROOT *(cont'd)*

Ellman International, Inc. 800-835-5355
3333 Royal Ave, Rockville Centre, NY 11572

J. Morita Usa, Inc. 888-566-7482
9 Mason, Irvine, CA 92618
ROOT ZX Apex Locator has been independently evaluated with a clinical accuracy rate of 96.2%. The accuracy of the measurement is not affected by the presence or absence of blood, other discharges, or electrolytes. The large color display is easy to read, providing both precision and high contrast. The action of the meter in the display corresponds exactly to the tactile sensation of using the file. Other features include, no zero-adjustment, automatic calibration, battery power indication and automatic power off function.

Miltex Dental Technologies, Inc. 516-576-6022
589 Davies Dr, York, PA 17402
Various apex locators and accessories.

Parkell, Inc. 800-243-7446
300 Executive Dr, Edgewood, NY 11717
All-fluids electronic apex locator.

LOCATOR, BLEEDING, GASTROINTESTINAL, STRING AND TUBE *(Gastro/Urology) 78FFW*

Bionix Development Corp. 800-551-7096
5154 Enterprise Blvd, Toledo, OH 43612
Feeding tube declogger.

Neo Medical Inc. 888-450-3334
42514 Albrae St, Fremont, CA 94538
Gastro intestinal string test.

LOCATOR, CELL, AUTOMATED *(Hematology) 81JOY*

Carl Zeiss Microimaging Ais, Inc 949-425-5700
31 Columbia, Aliso Viejo, CA 92656
Automated cellular imaging system.

Dako Colorado, Inc. 454-485-9500
4850 Innovation Dr, Fort Collins, CO 80525
Automated cell-locating device.

Ikonisys, Inc 203-776-0791
5 Science Park Ste 1000, New Haven, CT 06511
Automated microscope.

LOCATOR, INTRACORPOREAL DEVICE, ULTRASONIC *(Obstetrics/Gyn) 85HHJ*

Medispec Ltd. - Usa 888-663-3477
20410 Observation Dr Ste 102, Germantown, MD 20876
LITHOSPEC portable/electromagnetic lithotripter for treatment of ureteric, bladder, and renal stones.

LOCATOR, MAGNETIC *(Surgery) 79FTZ*

Lucent Medical Systems, Inc. 425-822-3310
811 Kirkland Ave Ste 100, Kirkland, WA 98033
Magnetic 3D location/tracking system for cardiac catheters, gastrointestinal tubes, and other medical devices.

Medchannel Llc 617-314-9861
1241 Adams St Apt 110, Dorchester Center, MA 02124
Cutter.

Medical Action Industries, Inc 800-645-7042
500 Express Dr S, Brentwood, NY 11717
This

LOCATOR, VEIN, LIQUID CRYSTAL *(General) 80KZA*

AccuVein LLC 816-997-9400
40 Goose Hill Rd, Cold Spring Harbor, NY 11724
AV-300

Plexus Electronic Assembly 847-793-4492
2400 Millbrook Dr, Buffalo Grove, IL 60089

LOCK, CATHETER *(General) 80WLM*

Smiths Medical Asd, Inc. 800-848-1757
6250 Shier Rings Rd, Dublin, OH 43016

LOCK, WIRE, AND LIGATURE, INTRAORAL *(Dental And Oral) 76DYX*

Atlanta Orthodontics 800-535-7166
1247 Zonolite Rd NE, Atlanta, GA 30306

Biomet Microfixation Inc. 800-874-7711
1520 Tradeport Dr, Jacksonville, FL 32218
Various types of ligature.

Glenroe Technologies 800-237-4060
1912 44th Ave E, Bradenton, FL 34203
Orthodontic kobayashi ties.

LOCK, WIRE, AND LIGATURE, INTRAORAL *(cont'd)*

Unisplint Corp. 770-271-0646
4485 Commerce Dr Ste 106, Buford, GA 30518
$15.00 per set.

United Precision Technology 716-634-4331
4085 David Rd, Williamsville, NY 14221
Arch bar.

3m Unitek 800-634-5300
2724 Peck Rd, Monrovia, CA 91016

LOOP, ENDARTERECTOMY *(Cardiovascular) 74RFH*

Codman & Shurtleff, Inc 800-225-0460
325 Paramount Dr, Raynham, MA 02767

Endovascular Instruments, Inc. 360-750-1150
2501 SE Columbia Way Ste 150, Vancouver, WA 98661

LOOP, INOCULATING *(Microbiology) 83RFI*

Alfa Aesar, A Johnson Matthey Company 800-343-0660
26 Parkridge Rd, Ward Hill, MA 01835

Bd Diagnostic Systems 800-675-0908
7 Loveton Cir, Sparks, MD 21152

Biohit Inc. 800-922-0784
PO Box 308, 3535 Rte. 66, Bldg. 4, Neptune, NJ 07754

Covidien Lp 508-261-8000
15 Hampshire St, Mansfield, MA 02048

Globe Scientific, Inc. 800-394-4562
610 Winters Ave, Paramus, NJ 07652
Disposable inoculation loops, 1 ul and 10 ul.

Pml Microbiologicals 800-628-7014
27120 SW 95th Ave, Wilsonville, OR 97070

Rocket Medical Plc. 800-707-7625
150 Recreation Park Dr Ste 3, Hingham, MA 02043
Diathermy loop.

S.C.I. Science Center, Inc. 800-345-0774
PO Box 994, Santa Fe, NM 87504
Inoculating loops with handles. Twisted loop inserts are 3 inches in length with closed ends; inoculating needles, loops, holders, disposable loops, needles, colony isolation probes.

Simport Plastics Ltd. 450-464-1723
2588 Bernard-Pilon, Beloeil, QUE J3G 4S5 Canada
INO-LOOP.

LOOP, LENS *(Ophthalmology) 86RET*

Fortrad Eye Instruments Corp. 973-543-2371
8 Franklin Rd, Mendham, NJ 07945

Jedmed Instruments Co. 314-845-3770
5416 Jedmed Ct, Saint Louis, MO 63129

Katena Products, Inc. 800-225-1195
4 Stewart Ct, Denville, NJ 07834

LOOP, VASCULAR *(Cardiovascular) 74RFK*

Axiom Medical, Inc. 800-221-8569
19320 Van Ness Ave, Torrance, CA 90501
Multiple colors and sizes of silicone loops for retraction, identification, occlusion. Also 'snap' covers.

Berkeley Medevices, Inc. 800-227-2388
1330 S 51st St, Richmond, CA 94804

Key Surgical, Inc. 800-541-7995
8101 Wallace Rd Ste 100, Eden Prairie, MN 55344
KEY Vascular Loops - silicone loops used to occlude, retract, or identify veins, arteries, nerves or tendons during surgical procedures. Mini or maxi size. Available in four colors.

Scanlan International, Inc. 800-328-9458
1 Scanlan Plz, Saint Paul, MN 55107
SURG-I-LOOP PLUS with blunt needle. Vessel loops.

Sterion, Incorporated 800-328-7958
13828 Lincoln St NE, Ham Lake, MN 55304
Vascular occlusion, retraction, and identification loops. Four sizes and four colors. Radiopaque medical grade silicone.

LOOP, WIRE *(Ear/Nose/Throat) 77JYQ*

Biomet Microfixation Inc. 800-874-7711
1520 Tradeport Dr, Jacksonville, FL 32218
Various types of wire.

George Tiemann & Co. 800-843-6266
25 Plant Ave, Hauppauge, NY 11788

LOTION, SKIN CARE *(General) 80VLB*

Aesthetic Technologies, Inc. 303-469-0965
14828 W 6th Ave Ste 9B, Golden, CO 80401
Parisian Peel Satin C--lipid-soluable vitamin C antioxidant topical. This solution is a non-ascorbic acid-based topical in 10% and 20% concentrations. Shelf life of 1 year.

Alimed, Inc. 800-225-2610
297 High St, Dedham, MA 02026

AmSan 800-327-3528
1930 Energy Park Dr Ste 260, Saint Paul, MN 55108
Antimicrobial lotion.

Arjo Canada, Inc. 800-665-4831
1575 South Gateway Rd., Unit C, Mississauga, ONT L4W-5J1 Canada

Beiersdorf, Inc. 800-233-2340
187 Danbury Rd, Wilton Corporate Center, Wilton, CT 06897
EUCERIN Original Lotion, Creme; AQUAPHOR Healing Ointment . EUCERIN Calming Creme EUCERIN PLUS cream and lotion.

Calmoseptine, Inc. 800-800-3405
16602 Burke Ln, Huntington Beach, CA 92647
Ointment.

Chattanooga Group 800-592-7329
4717 Adams Rd, Hixson, TN 37343
MYOSSAGE.

Chester Labs, Inc. 800-354-9709
1900 Section Rd, Cincinnati, OH 45237
APRILFRESH, lotion.

Coloplast Manufacturing Us, Llc 800-533-0464
1840 W Oak Pkwy, Marietta, GA 30062
Creams and lotions treat dry, reddened, irritated skin.

Covidien Lp 508-261-8000
15 Hampshire St, Mansfield, MA 02048
CONSTANT CARE cleansing lotion, conditioning cream, moisture barrier salve.

Crosstex International Ltd., W. Region 800-707-2737
14059 Stage Rd, Santa Fe Springs, CA 90670
Antimicrobial soap and skin care lotion.

Deb Sbs, Inc. 704-263-4240
1100 Highway 27, Stanley, NC 28164
SBS-40 medicated skin cream, SBS-41 medicated skin lotion, SBS-44 protective cream (water-based irritants). SBS-46 protective cream (solvent-based irritant). Medicated skin cream in a hygienically sealed cartridge.

Donell 800-324-7455
1801 Taylor Ave, Louisville, KY 40213
Miracle C-Gel - Vitamin C gel for softer, smoother skin, helps repair ultraviolet damage. Lightening gel - gel made with Kojic & Azelaic acid to lighten age spots, sun spots and freckles. A+010 is an antioxidant formula for firmer, smoother skin. This new formulation, with CoEnzyme Q10, a revolutionary new antioxidant, and Vitamin A with firming qualities, combines two of the most desirable anti-aging ingredients in skincare today. Use for firmer, smoother and softer skin. A+Q10 cream combination of vitamin A with firming quality and Q10 coenzyme Q10 antioxidant, anti-aging and wrinkle cream. Acne gel/Acne cleanser alpha beta gel beta hydroxy cleanser to unroof blackheads and control acne flare-ups. Mini Microdermabrasion features magnesium oxide crystals with anit-oxidants and anti-inflammatory ingredients to exfoliate dry skin cells and stimulate collagen elastin production. Super Suncare is a waterproof sunblock featuring Parsol 1789, which provides broad-spectrum protection from ultraviolet rays that are know to damage even the deepest layer of the skin.

Donovan Industries 800-334-4404
13401 McCormick Dr, Tampa, FL 33626
Hand sanitizer, antibacterial liquid and bar soaps, deodorant soaps, skin lotions, perineal-care sprays and ointments, shampoos.

Geen Healthcare Inc. 800-565-4336
931 Progress Ave. Ste.13, Scarborough, ONT M1G 3V5 Canada
Skin cleaner and conditioner.

Geritrex Corp. 800-736-3437
144 E Kingsbridge Rd, Mount Vernon, NY 10550
Hydrocerin moisturizer alleviates chapped and chafed areas. Available as a cream or lotion. The cream comes in 4-oz and 1-lb jars and the lotion in 8- and 16-oz bottles.

Health Enterprises 800-633-4243
90 George Leven Dr, North Attleboro, MA 02760
BODY SHIELD PLUS Bath Oil.

Home Health 800-445-7137
2100 Smithtown Ave, Ronkonkoma, NY 11779

LOTION, SKIN CARE *(cont'd)*

Kck Industries 888-800-1967
14941 Calvert St, Van Nuys, CA 91411

Lantiseptic Division, Summit Industries, Inc. 800-241-6996
PO Box 7329, Marietta, GA 30065
LANTISEPTIC Skin Protectant, a lanolin rich ointment for skin problems associated with incontinence, pressure sores (Stage I, II), and other skin conditions common to nursing-home patients and Diabetics. Available in 5gr-, .5-, 2.5-, 4-, 4.5-, and 14-oz. sizes. Also available is our Lantiseptic Therapeutic Cream and Lantiseptic All-Body Wash.

Lee Medical International, Inc. 800-433-8950
612 Distributors Row, Harahan, LA 70123

Mckesson General Medical 800-446-3008
8741 Landmark Rd, Richmond, VA 23228

Medco Supply Company 800-556-3326
500 Fillmore Ave, Tonawanda, NY 14150
Large selection.

Medela, Inc. 800-435-8316
1101 Corporate Dr, McHenry, IL 60050
PURELAN 100 - 100% USP modified lanolin for soothing sore nipples.

Medi-Tech International Corp. 800-333-0109
26 Court St, Brooklyn, NY 11242
BURNBLOK AFTER CARE LOTION WITH ALOE VERA. Effective treatment for side effects from radiation therapy, 1st & 2nd degree burns, and thermal burns.

Medical Science Products, Inc. 800-456-1971
517 Elm Ridge Ave, P.O. Box 381, Canal Fulton, OH 44614
Aloe vera lotion and aloe vera gel. Vitamin E lotion and massage crème. Glacier rub.

Ortho Dermatologics 310-642-1150
5760 W 96th St, Los Angeles, CA 90045

P. J. Noyes Company, Inc. 800-522-2469
89 Bridge St, Lancaster, NH 03584
SKIN 1ST moisturizing skin cream/lotion, fragrance free, greaseless.

Pedinol Pharmacal, Inc. 800-733-4665
30 Banfi Plz N, Farmingdale, NY 11735
HYDRISINOL creme (4-oz or 1-lb jar) or lotion (8- and 16-oz plastic bottles); LACTINOL-E creme (4-oz size and 8-oz tube); LAZERCREME (2-oz size); UREACIN 10 lotion (8-oz size); UREACIN 20 creme (4-oz size); and PEDI-BATH salts (6-oz size). HYDRISALIC Gel 1 oz, LACTINOL Lotion 12 oz. CITRADERM facial complex with Vitamin C, 0.5 oz.; TI-SCREEN moisturizing sunscreen lotion spf 15, sports sunscreen gel spf 20, moisturizing sunscreen lotion spf 30, parsol 1879, sunscreen spray spf 23.

Pre Pak Products, Inc. 800-544-7257
4055 Oceanside Blvd Ste L, Oceanside, CA 92056
FREE-UP MASSAGE CREAM - Available in scented and unscented - $9.50 each 8 oz jar provides ideal soft tissue massage medium. Does not contain beeswax; hypo-allergenic, bacteriostatic; $14.95 each 16 oz jar, quantity discounts available. COMFORT TOUCH, low heat massage cream; cool on first contact followed by a warm therapeutic heat. Ideal for mild strains, bruises, muscle aches and pains. $9.95 ea. - 8 oz. jar, $15.50 each - 16 oz. jar, quantity discounts available. RED DOT, deep heat sports cream; quick pain relief from deep muscle strains, aches or arthritis. $12.95 each - 8 oz. jar, $18.95 each - 16 oz. jar, quantity discounts available. RELEASE, deep tissue massage cream; ideal for deep myofascial massage, scar and connective tissue mobilization. $8.95 for 2 oz.

Smith & Nephew, Inc. 800-876-1261
11775 Starkey Rd, Largo, FL 33773
Nursing Care skin care products include the No-rinse Nursing Care Personal Cleanser, the Fragrance-free Nursing Care Moisturizing Lotion and the Nursing Care Barrier Ointment.

Steuart Laboratories 877-210-9664
142 S Main St, Mabel, MN 55954
Pain Formula, made from soybean. Foot Cream, tea tree oil.

The Aloe Institute 941-727-0042
5808 42nd St E, Bradenton, FL 34203
Miracle Foot Repair for dry, cracked and itchy feet. Major U.S. brand for troubled feet. Contains 60% whole leaf aloe vera. V-LOE vaginal itch with 70% aloe. Miracle of Aloe, Aloe All Over is a therapeutic hand and body lotion containing 72% aloe, evening primroe oil, chamomile oil and provides unique relief for dry, cracked and itchy skin. Miracle Rub provides quick relief for arthritis and muscle pain. Includes 46% aloe to speed penetration and softer tissue.

LOTION, SKIN CARE *(cont'd)*

Tri-State Surgical Supply & Equipment 800-424-5227
409 Hoyt St, Brooklyn, NY 11231
Skin care lotion for hands and body.

Ulmer Pharmacal Co. 800-848-5637
PO Box 408, 1614 Industry Ave., Park Rapids, MN 56470
LOBANA body lotion $3.25 per 1000 ml.

Winning Solutions, Inc. 800-899-2563
PO Box 5408, Pagosa Springs, CO 81147
Complete line of aloe-vera-based creams and lotions.

LOUPE, BINOCULAR, LOW POWER *(Ophthalmology) 86HJH*

Alimed, Inc. 800-225-2610
297 High St, Dedham, MA 02026

Almore International, Inc. 503-643-6633
PO Box 25214, Portland, OR 97298
$29.50 to $112.50 per unit (standard).

Aztec Medical Products, Inc. 800-223-3859
106 Ingram Rd, Williamsburg, VA 23188
Binocular loupeice used to determine female breast volume.

Ctp Coil Inc. 800-933-2645
1801 Howard St Ste D, Elk Grove Village, IL 60007
Face mounted spectacle binoculars and binocular flip-up clip-on.

Eschenbach Optik Of America, Inc. 800-487-5389
904 Ethan Allen Hwy, Ridgefield, CT 06877

Mahe International Inc. 800-294-7946
468 Craighead St, Nashville, TN 37204

Perioptix, Inc. 949-366-3333
230 Market Pl, Escondido, CA 92029
Various types of low power loupes.

Scanlan International, Inc. 800-328-9458
1 Scanlan Plz, Saint Paul, MN 55107
Magnifying loupes.

Valley Forge Scientific Corp. 610-666-7500
136 Green Tree Road, Suite 100, Oaks, PA 19456
Used to magnify the field during surgical procedures.

LOUPE, DIAGNOSTIC/SURGICAL *(Surgery) 79FSP*

Carl Zeiss Surgical, Inc. 800-442-4020
1 Zeiss Dr, Thornwood, NY 10594

Codman & Shurtleff, Inc 800-225-0460
325 Paramount Dr, Raynham, MA 02767

Concepts International, Inc. 800-627-9729
224 E Main St, Summerton, SC 29148
Full line of magnifiers that attach to glasses or come with headband. Head-band magnifiers with 6000-candle-power head lights.

Edroy Products Co., Inc. 800-233-8803
245 N Midland Ave, PO Box 998, Nyack, NY 10960
PRO-LOUPE: Headband; wire clip; spring-top, $294.00 per unit (standard) brow bar $320.05 per unit (standard) 2x-approx. 16' working distance, 3x-approx. 11' working distance

Elmed, Inc. 630-543-2792
60 W Fay Ave, Addison, IL 60101

Eschenbach Optik Of America, Inc. 800-487-5389
904 Ethan Allen Hwy, Ridgefield, CT 06877

Five Star Manufacturing, Inc. 877-595-7827
163 Samuel Barnet Blvd, New Bedford, MA 02745
Retractor blade.

General Scientific Corp. 800-959-0153
77 Enterprise Dr, Ann Arbor, MI 48103
Advanced vision enhancement for the professional.

Ivry 305-448-9858
216 Catalonia Ave Ste 106, Coral Gables, FL 33134
Microsurgery.

Jedmed Instruments Co. 314-845-3770
5416 Jedmed Ct, Saint Louis, MO 63129

Keeler Instruments Inc. 800-523-5620
456 Park Way, Broomall, PA 19008
Galilean $945. or Prismatic, $1195 to $1495.

Kerr Corp. 949-255-8766
3225 Deming Way Ste 190, Middleton, WI 53562
Diagnostic/surgical loupes.

Quality Aspirators 800-858-2121
1419 Godwin Ln, Duncanville, TX 75116
Q-OPTICS magnification

LOUPE, DIAGNOSTIC/SURGICAL *(cont'd)*

Roldan Products Corp. 866-922-6800
448 Sovereign Ct, Ballwin, MO 63011
$191.00 per unit (standard).

LOWRY (COLORIMETRIC), TOTAL PROTEIN *(Chemistry) 75JGP*

Clin-Chem Mfg. Llc. 800-359-9691
2560 Business Pkwy Ste C, Minden, NV 89423
For determination of protein in urine or cerebrospinal fluid.

Sita Associates 630-968-3727
720 Williamsburg Ct, Oak Brook, IL 60523
Total protein kit.

LUBRICANT, INSTRUMENT *(General) 80TCZ*

Acheson Colloids Company 800-255-1908
1600 Washington Ave, Port Huron, MI 48060

Altana, Inc. 800-231-0206
60 Baylis Rd, Melville, NY 11747
SURGILUBE sterile bacteriostatic lubricant.

Carochem, Inc. 919-682-5121
744 E Markham Ave # 15699, Durham, NC 27701
Special milky emulsion for lubrication of surgical instruments.

Case Medical, Inc. 888-227-2273
65 Railroad Ave, Ridgefield, NJ 07657

Deknatel Snowden-Pencer 800-367-7874
5175 S Royal Atlanta Dr, Tucker, GA 30084
NUTRA-PH ENDO-MILK lubricant intended to lubricate and protect endoscopic surgical instruments. Used after every cleaning with ENDO-CLEAN unit.

L&R Manufacturing Co. 201-991-5330
577 Elm St, PO Box 607, Kearny, NJ 07032
Barrier milk is a corrosion inhibitor/lubricant for use on surgical instruments. Formulated to remove organic build-up while providing a natural corrosion inhibitor.

Micro Care Corp. 800-638-0125
595 John Downey Dr, New Britain, CT 06051
Micro Dispersion Lubricants -- Micro Care packages a variety of high-performance lubricants for use on medical products in dip, wipe and even aerosol applications. Examples: the VDX Dry Lubricant is a nonflammable, no-aroma, nonmigrating aerosol used for precision 'spot' lubrication. Unique in the entire industry, this product is plastic-safe, nonflammable and ozone-safe. Select VDX for the pinpoint lubrication of friction points between plastic, metal, glass or ceramic components. Other lubricants include dips formulated with PTFE and silicones for use in high-volume applications, ranging from 0.5% to 9% concentrations. Fast-drying, nonflammable and ozone-safe, these lubes allow your precision components to move smoothly, without friction.

Micro-Scientific Industries, Inc. 888-253-2536
1225 Carnegie St Ste 101, Rolling Meadows, IL 60008

Miltex Inc. 800-645-8000
589 Davies Dr, York, PA 17402
Pre-mixed pump spray lubricant for surgical instruments.

Xenotec Ltd. 949-640-4053
511 Hazel Dr, Corona Del Mar, CA 92625
Surgilube provides instant, continuous lubricating action for easy, comfortable insertion of catheters, endoscopes, surgical instruments and gloves into body orifices. used for more hospital procedures than any other surgical lubricant.

LUBRICANT, PATIENT *(General) 80KMJ*

Actavis Mid Atlantic Llc 973-889-6960
1877 Kawai Rd, Lincolnton, NC 28092
Lubricating jelly.

Altana, Inc. 800-231-0206
60 Baylis Rd, Melville, NY 11747

Arthrex, Inc. 239-643-5553
1370 Creekside Blvd, Naples, FL 34108
Lubricant.

Biofilm, Inc. 800-848-5900
3225 Executive Rdg, Vista, CA 92081
ASTROGLIDE patient lubricant.

Centurion Medical Products Corp. 517-545-1135
3310 S Main St, Salisbury, NC 28147

Coloplast Manufacturing Us, Llc 612-302-4992
1185 Willow Lake Blvd, Vadnais Heights, MN 55110
Patient lubricant.

J&J Healthcare Products Div Mcneil-Ppc, Inc 866-565-2229
199 Grandview Rd, Skillman, NJ 08558

LUBRICANT, PATIENT *(cont'd)*

Medical Action Industries, Inc. 800-645-7042
25 Heywood Rd, Arden, NC 28704
Lubricant, patient.

Perrigo New York, Inc. 269-686-2916
1700 Bathgate Ave, Bronx, NY 10457
Lubricating jelly.

Pharmaceutical Innovations, Inc. 973-242-2900
897 Frelinghuysen Ave, Newark, NJ 07114
$2.95 per 150ml GENTLE GEL; $21.50 per box of 25 sterile GENTLE GEL.

Professional Disposables International, Inc. 800-999-6423
2 Nice Pak Park, Orangeburg, NY 10962

Qualis Group Llc 515-243-3000
4600 Park Ave, Des Moines, IA 50321
Personal lubricant liquid.

Reach Global Industries, Inc. (Reachgood) 888-518-8389
8 Corporate Park Ste 300, Irvine, CA 92606
Patient lubricant.

Retroactive Bioscience 859-431-4660
1 Moock Rd Ste 3, Wilder, KY 41071
Patient lubricant.

Span Packaging Services Llc. 864-627-4155
4611A Dairy Dr, Greenville, SC 29607
Lubricant jelly.

Spirus Medical, Inc. 781-297-7220
1063 Turnpike St, PO Box 258, Stoughton, MA 02072

Stony Brook, Inc. 563-388-0588
12047 70th Ave, Blue Grass, IA 52726
Sil-ophtho.

The Aloe Institute 941-727-0042
5808 42nd St E, Bradenton, FL 34203
CHAFE-GUARD anti-friction lubricant to prevent chafing. Comes in a convenient 2 oz. stick applicator. $4.95/retail and $1.65/wholesale. PERFECT MATCH vaginal lubrication with 76% aloe.

Tri-State Hospital Supply Corp. 517-545-1135
3173 E 43rd St, Yuma, AZ 85365

LUBRICANT, PATIENT, VAGINAL, LATEX COMPATIBLE *(Obstetrics/Gyn) 85NUC*

Cosmetic Laboratories Of America 708-450-3153
20245 Sunburst St, Chatsworth, CA 91311
Personal lubricant.

Dlc Laboratories, Inc.
7008 Marcelle St, Paramount, CA 90723
Liquid personal lubricant.

LUBRICANT, VAGINAL, PATIENT *(General) 80MMS*

Biofilm, Inc. 800-848-5900
3225 Executive Rdg, Vista, CA 92081
SILKEN SECRET vaginal lubricant and moisturizer for vaginal dryness in a convenient, single use applicator.

Elamex S.A. De C.V. 52-16-164333
Av. Insurgentes 4145 lote., Cd. Jiarex, Chih Mexico
Various

Jason Natural Products Inc., Personal Care Divisio 310-945-4308
8468 Warner Dr, Culver City, CA 90232
Personal lubricant.

Qualis Group Llc 515-243-3000
4600 Park Ave, Des Moines, IA 50321
Personal lubricating gel.

Sheffield Pharmaceuticals 800-222-1087
170 Broad St, New London, CT 06320
Personal lubricant.

Wal-Med, Inc. 877-542-3688
11302 164th St E, Puyallup, WA 98374
FemGlide Gel Lubricant, Water Based, Glycerin Free

LUMINOMETER *(Chemistry) 75WXK*

Gen-Probe, Inc. 800-523-5001
10210 Genetic Center Dr, San Diego, CA 92121
LEADER 450i, LEADER 501i, and LEADER HC+ luminometers for analyzing cheminluminescent assays.

LUMINOMETER *(cont'd)*

Mgm Instruments 800-551-1415
925 Sherman Ave, Hamden, CT 06514
Luminometer with Injector Systems; $6,240 to $7,600 for OPTOCOMP I semiautomatic; $14,160 to $15,520 for OPTOCOMP II 250-sample. All luminometers include built-in printer and data reduction software.

Turner Designs 877-316-8049
845 W Maude Ave, Sunnyvale, CA 94085

Xiril 302-655-7035
91 Lukens Dr Ste A, New Castle, DE 19720
Lucy1 anthos microplate luminometer.

LUNG, MEMBRANE (FOR LONG-TERM RESPIRATORY SUPPORT) *(Anesthesiology) 73BYS*

Bio-Med Devices, Inc. 800-224-6633
61 Soundview Rd, Guilford, CT 06437
Semi-permanent test lung, $10.00.

Medtronic Perfusion Systems 800-854-3570
7611 Northland Dr N, Brooklyn Park, MN 55428

Puritan Bennett Corp. 925-463-4371
2800 Airwest Blvd, Plainfield, IN 46168
Portable liquid oxygen unit & stationary liquid oxygen unit.

M. LYSODEIKTICUS CELLS (SPECTROPHOTOMETRIC), LYSOZYME *(Chemistry) 75JMQ*

Biomerieux Inc. 800-682-2666
100 Rodolphe St, Durham, NC 27712

MAGNET, AC-POWERED *(Ophthalmology) 86HPO*

Bausch & Lomb Surgical 636-255-5051
3365 Tree Court Ind Blvd, Saint Louis, MO 63122

Schumann Inc., A. 978-369-6782
167 Hayward Mill Rd, Concord, MA 01742
$13,450.00 for std Giant Eye Magnet (13,000 Gauss at contact) explosion-proof (142-301Kg wt).

MAGNET, PERMANENT *(Ophthalmology) 86HPN*

B. Graczyk, Inc. 269-782-2100
27826 Burmax Park, Dowagiac, MI 49047
Various types of magnets.

Miltex Inc. 800-645-8000
589 Davies Dr, York, PA 17402

Schumann Inc., A. 978-369-6782
167 Hayward Mill Rd, Concord, MA 01742
$270.00 for permanent handmagnet (13lb carrying power, weighs .85lb); also electric handmagnet (26lb power, weighs 2lb).

Synergetics Usa, Inc. 800-600-0565
3845 Corporate Centre Dr, O Fallon, MO 63368
Magnet.

MAGNET, PERMANENT, MRI (MAGNETIC RESONANCE IMAGING) *(Radiology) 90WRT*

Atlas Medical Technologies 909-923-7887
1137 E Philadelphia St, Ontario, CA 91761

Mushield Company, Inc., The 888-669-3539
9 Ricker Ave, Londonderry, NH 03053
GB ENCLOSURE MRI monitor enclosure. Eliminates EMI interference up to 30 gauss. Custom and off-the-shelf designs.

Supertech, Inc. 800-654-1054
PO Box 186, Elkhart, IN 46515
MRI Accessories - wheelchair, stretcher, carts, IV Poles, lights, mayo stand, oxygen equipment, step stools, tables, hampers, trash cans, transfer board/chair, tools, sharps containers . . . and so much more.

Wang Nmr Inc. 925-443-0212
550 N Canyon Pkwy, Livermore, CA 94551

Webb Manufacturing Co. 800-932-2634
1241 Carpenter St, Philadelphia, PA 19147
POWER SCAN 1000 is an MRI surface-coil holder.

MAGNET, SUPERCONDUCTING, MRI (MAGNETIC RESONANCE IMAGING) *(Radiology) 90VIM*

Atlas Medical Technologies 909-923-7887
1137 E Philadelphia St, Ontario, CA 91761
Late model GE and Marconi MR units are available at resonable prices.

Mushield Company, Inc., The 888-669-3539
9 Ricker Ave, Londonderry, NH 03053
GB ENCLOSURE MRI monitor enclosure. Eliminates EMI interference up to 30 gauss. Custom and off-the-shelf designs.

MAGNET, SUPERCONDUCTING, MRI (MAGNETIC RESONANCE IMAGING) *(cont'd)*

Nonin Medical, Inc. 800-356-8874
13700 1st Ave N, Plymouth, MN 55441
Pulse oximeter with fiber optic sensor for safe monitoring of sedated patients in MRI.

Wang Nmr Inc. 925-443-0212
550 N Canyon Pkwy, Livermore, CA 94551

MAGNET, TEST, PACEMAKER *(Cardiovascular) 74DTG*

Cyberonics, Inc. 800-332-1375
100 Cyberonics Blvd, The Cyberonics Building, Houston, TX 77058
Model 220, Patient Magnet

Instromedix, A Card Guard Co. 800-633-3361
10255 W Higgins Rd Ste 100, Rosemont, IL 60018

Trivirix International Inc. 320-982-8000
925 6th Ave NE, Milaca, MN 56353
Magnet.

MAGNETIC UNIT, THERAPEUTIC *(Physical Med) 89RFO*

Cbs Medical Technologies Inc. 514-582-9098
225 Chemin des Grands Ducs, Piedmont, QUE J0R 1K0 Canada

Homedics Inc. 800-333-8282
3000 N Pontiac Trl, Commerce Township, MI 48390
Magnetic therapy devices.

Magnet Sales & Manufacturing 800-421-6692
11248 Playa Ct, Culver City, CA 90230
Stock and custom magnets and magnet assemblies made to specification. Expert design assistance, including Finite Element Analysis modeling. Applications experience in Faraday rotators, motors, magnetic couplings, magnetic bearings, beam focusing, deposition technologies, magnetic separation and others. Short lead times for both prototype and production. Quality system based on ISO 9002.

R. B. Annis Instruments, Inc. 317-637-9282
1101 N Delaware St, Indianapolis, IN 46202
Standard coils are 3 1/2-, 4 1/2-, 6-, and 10- in. in diameter inside opening. Plus 6 x 14-, 8 x 24-, and 14 x 16-in. opening. AC or DC available. $558.00 per standard 6 in. Continuous unit.

Roloke Company 800-533-8212
127 W Hazel St, Inglewood, CA 90302
Tectonic magnets. Magnetic products for the entire body. Superior depth of penetration and surface-field strength.

MAGNETOMETER *(General) 80RFP*

R. B. Annis Instruments, Inc. 317-637-9282
1101 N Delaware St, Indianapolis, IN 46202
Pocket magnetometers. Small hand-held instruments available with different ranges, from 1/2 to 100 gauss, full-scale both polarity and intensity measurement on unidirectional fields (magnetic).

MAGNIFIER, HAND-HELD, LOW-VISION *(Ophthalmology) 86HJF*

Becton Dickinson And Company 800-284-6845
1 Becton Dr, Franklin Lakes, NJ 07417
MAGNI-GUIDE

Broadwest Corp. 800-232-2948
304 Elati St, Denver, CO 80223
Viewing accessories including classic magnifiers, Mammomag viewers, aspheric dome magnifiers, headlamp magnifiers, bright spots with iris, and technologists' viewers are available.

Caprock Developments Inc. 800-222-0325
475 Speedwell Ave, PO Box 95, Morris Plains, NJ 07950

Concepts International, Inc. 800-627-9729
224 E Main St, Summerton, SC 29148
Galilean magnifiers.

Ctp Coil Inc. 800-933-2645
1801 Howard St Ste D, Elk Grove Village, IL 60007
Various forms of hi-power and standard magnification handheld units in round and rectangular formats for low vision practice and patient use.

E.W. Pike & Company 908-352-0630
501 Pennsylvania Ave # 517, Elizabeth, NJ 07201
FLASH-O-LENS $50.00 for battery powered, $55.00 for electric unit with 5x magnification. $55.00 and $60.00 for 7x magnification. $65.00 for electric reader with 3x magnification. $125.00 for electric reader stand.

Edmund Industrial Optics 800-363-1992
101 E Gloucester Pike, Barrington, NJ 08007

Eschenbach Optik Of America, Inc. 800-487-5389
904 Ethan Allen Hwy, Ridgefield, CT 06877

MAGNIFIER, HAND-HELD, LOW-VISION *(cont'd)*

Eye Care And Cure 800-486-6169
4646 S Overland Dr, Tucson, AZ 85714
Magnifier.

Freedom Scientific Blv Group, Llc. 727-803-8000
11800 31st Ct N, Saint Petersburg, FL 33716
Hand-held magnifier.

MAGNIFIER, OPERATING *(Surgery) 79RFQ*

Alimed, Inc. 800-225-2610
297 High St, Dedham, MA 02026

Edroy Products Co., Inc. 800-233-8803
245 N Midland Ave, PO Box 998, Nyack, NY 10960
MAGNI-FOCUSER Headband vision-aid for close-up, hands free work and precise quality control. $22.50-23.70 per unit (standard), 1.5X, 1.75, 2.00, 2.25, 2.75, 3.5X. MAGNI-FOCUSER with light $77.85-79.05 per unit, 1.5X, 1.75, 2.00, 2.25, 2.75, 3.5X. MAGNI-SPECS Brow bar, nose piece and Zyl temples $38.20 per unit (standard), 1.5X, 1.75, 2.00, 2.25, 2.75, 3.5X.

Eschenbach Optik Of America, Inc. 800-487-5389
904 Ethan Allen Hwy, Ridgefield, CT 06877

MAINTAINER, SPACE PREFORMED, ORTHODONTIC *(Dental And Oral) 76DYT*

Classone Orthodontics, Inc. 806-799-0608
5064 50th St, Lubbock, TX 79414
Various types of rotation and steiner wedges.

Denovo Dental, Inc. 800-854-7949
5130 Commerce Dr, Baldwin Park, CA 91706

3m Unitek 800-634-5300
2724 Peck Rd, Monrovia, CA 91016

MALAR IMPLANT *(Surgery) 79LZK*

Aesthetic And Reconstructive Technologies, Inc. 775-853-6800
3545 Airway Dr Ste 106, Reno, NV 89511
Silicone elastomer malar implant.

Allied Biomedical 800-276-1322
PO Box 392, Ventura, CA 93002

Hanson Medical, Inc. 800-771-2215
825 Riverside Ave Ste 2, Paso Robles, CA 93446
Silicone malar implant.

Implantech Associates, Inc. 800-733-0833
6025 Nicolle St Ste B, Ventura, CA 93003
BINDER Submalar, TERINO Malar Shell, Combined Submalar Shell.

Pillar Surgical, Inc. 800-367-0445
PO Box 8141, La Jolla, CA 92038
Various.

Spectrum Designs Medical, Inc. 800-239-6399
6387 Rose Ln Ste B, Carpinteria, CA 93013
Malar implants, sterile. Designed to enhance the malar (cheek) area in the aging face.

W.L. Gore & Associates,Inc 928-526-3030
1505 North Fourth St., Flagstaff, AZ 86004
Facial reconstruction prothesis.

MALLET, BONE *(Orthopedics) 87HXL*

Abbott Spine, Inc. 847-937-6100
12708 Riata Vista Cir Ste B-100, Austin, TX 78727
Mallet.

Biomet, Inc. 574-267-6639
56 E Bell Dr, PO Box 587, Warsaw, IN 46582
Various types of orthopedic mallets.

Codman & Shurtleff, Inc 800-225-0460
325 Paramount Dr, Raynham, MA 02767

DJO Inc. 800-336-6569
1430 Decision St, Vista, CA 92081

Elmed, Inc. 630-543-2792
60 W Fay Ave, Addison, IL 60101

George Tiemann & Co. 800-843-6266
25 Plant Ave, Hauppauge, NY 11788

H & H Co. 909-390-0373
4435 E Airport Dr Ste 108, Ontario, CA 91761
Mallet, all types.

Holmed Corporation 508-238-3351
40 Norfolk Ave, South Easton, MA 02375

Integral Design Inc. 781-740-2036
52 Burr Rd, Hingham, MA 02043

MALLET, BONE *(cont'd)*

Kirwan Surgical Products, Inc. 888-547-9267
180 Enterprise Dr, PO Box 427, Marshfield, MA 02050

Kmedic 800-955-0559
190 Veterans Dr, Northvale, NJ 07647

Medtronic Sofamor Danek Instrument Manufacturing 901-396-3133
7375 Adrianne Pl, Bartlett, TN 38133
Multiple (surgical mallets).

Medtronic Sofamor Danek Usa, Inc. 901-396-3133
4340 Swinnea Rd, Memphis, TN 38118
Multiple (surgical mallets).

Miltex Inc. 800-645-8000
589 Davies Dr, York, PA 17402

Precision Medical Manufacturing Corporation 866-633-4626
852 Seton Ct, Wheeling, IL 60090
Bone Mallets are designed to incorporate a proper balance and weight with stainless steel construction. All handles are stainless steel and hollow. Some models come with replaceable nylon head prevents from transmitting the shock to patient.

Rush-Berivon, Inc. 800-251-7874
1010 19th St, P.O. Box 1851, Meridian, MS 39301
$158.00 for 16 oz units.

Salvin Dental Specialties, Inc. 800-535-6566
3450 Latrobe Dr, Charlotte, NC 28211
Mallet.

Stryker Spine 866-457-7463
2 Pearl Ct, Allendale, NJ 07401

Tuzik Boston 800-886-6363
104 Longwater Dr, Assinippi Park, Norwell, MA 02061

Warsaw Orthopedic, Inc. 901-396-3133
2500 Silveus Xing, Warsaw, IN 46582
Multiple (surgical mallets).

Zimmer Holdings, Inc. 800-613-6131
1800 W Center St, PO Box 708, Warsaw, IN 46580

MALLET, DENTAL *(Dental And Oral) 76RFR*

Miltex Inc. 800-645-8000
589 Davies Dr, York, PA 17402

MALLET, OTHER *(Surgery) 79RFS*

Princeton Medical Group, Inc. 800-875-0869
1189 Royal Links Dr, Mt Pleasant, SC 29466
ENT/Orthopedics.

MALLET, SURGICAL, GENERAL & PLASTIC SURGERY *(Surgery) 79GFJ*

Bausch & Lomb Surgical 636-255-5051
3365 Tree Court Ind Blvd, Saint Louis, MO 63122

Biomet Microfixation Inc. 800-874-7711
1520 Tradeport Dr, Jacksonville, FL 32218
Mallet, surgical.

E.A. Beck & Co. 949-645-4072
657 W 19th St Ste E, P O Box 10857, Costa Mesa, CA 92627
Mallet.

Kmedic 800-955-0559
190 Veterans Dr, Northvale, NJ 07647

Lenox-Maclaren Surgical Corp. 720-890-9660
657 S Taylor Ave Ste A, Colorado Technology Center
Louisville, CO 80027
Mallett, surgical.

Miltex Dental Technologies, Inc. 516-576-6022
589 Davies Dr, York, PA 17402
Dental surgical mallet and accessories.

Premier Dental Products Co. 888-670-6100
1710 Romano Dr, PO Box 4500, Plymouth Meeting, PA 19462

Symmetry Medical Usa, Inc. 574-267-8700
486 W 350 N, Warsaw, IN 46582
Manual surgical instrument for general use.

Tuzik Boston 800-886-6363
104 Longwater Dr, Assinippi Park, Norwell, MA 02061

MANDREL *(Dental And Oral) 76RFU*

Miltex Inc. 800-645-8000
589 Davies Dr, York, PA 17402

Moyco Technologies, Inc. 800-331-8837
200 Commerce Dr, Montgomeryville, PA 18936
$10.00 per dozen (standard).

MANIFOLD, GAS *(Chemistry) 75RFV*

Aga Linde Healthcare P.R. Inc. 787-622-7900
PO Box 363868, GPO Box 364727, San Juan, PR 00936
Chemistry.

Air Products And Chemicals, Inc. 800-654-4567
7201 Hamilton Blvd, Allentown, PA 18195

Anspach Effort, Inc. 800-327-6887
4500 Riverside Dr, Palm Beach Gardens, FL 33410
Multiple outlet manifolds with or without regulators.

Engineers Express, Inc. 800-255-8823
7 Industrial Park Rd, Medway, MA 02053

Farley Inc., W.T. 800-327-5397
931 Via Alondra, Camarillo, CA 93012
$65.00 for PORCUPINE oxygen manifold with 4 check valved outlets, $160.00 for OXY-MAN oxygen manifold for ambulance gurneys, $200.00 for multi-casualty manifold for EMS, provides oxygen to multiple casualties simutaneously.

M & I Medical Sales, Inc. 305-663-6444
4711 SW 72nd Ave, Miami, FL 33155

S4j Manufacturing Services, Inc. 888-S4J-LUER
2685 NE 9th Ave, Cape Coral, FL 33909

MANIFOLD, LIQUID *(Chemistry) 75RFW*

Cadence Science Inc. 888-717-7677
1979 Marcus Ave Ste 215, New Hyde Park, NY 11042
12 types.

Engineers Express, Inc. 800-255-8823
7 Industrial Park Rd, Medway, MA 02053

Kimble Glass, Inc. 888-546-2531
537 Crystal Ave, Vineland, NJ 08360
Kontes new SPE glassware and manifolds enable the user to get the most from 3M EMPORE extraction disks. The components are designed specifically for use with solid-phase extraction disks to provide the highest possible recoveries from drinking water, surface water, and wastewater samples. SPE manifolds and glassware are offered for both 47- and 90-mm-diam extraction disks.

S4j Manufacturing Services, Inc. 888-S4J-LUER
2685 NE 9th Ave, Cape Coral, FL 33909

Smiths Medical Asd, Inc. 800-848-1757
6250 Shier Rings Rd, Dublin, OH 43016
MEDIFOLD drug administration manifold.

MANOMETER, LABORATORY *(Chemistry) 75UGT*

Cole-Parmer Instrument Inc. 800-323-4340
625 E Bunker Ct, Vernon Hills, IL 60061

Corning Inc., Science Products Division 800-492-1110
45 Nagog Park, Acton, MA 01720

Eberbach Corp. 800-422-2558
505 S Maple Rd, Ann Arbor, MI 48103

Mercury Medical 800-237-6418
11300 49th St N, Clearwater, FL 33762
Disposable, single patient use manometer for use with Mercury brand resuscitators. Mini Stat CO2 infant/pediatric end tidal CO2 detector. Single patient use end-tidal CO2 detector for patients weighing 1-15 kilograms. Stat CO2 meter single patient use combonation manometer and end tidal CO2 detector.

Meriam Process Technologies 216-281-1100
10920 Madison Ave, Cleveland, OH 44102
U-type, Well type, inclined tube manometers, tank gauges, portable digital manometers, Bellows D/P instruments and digital indicating switch, digital flow totalizers, fire pump flowmeters, laminar flow elements, accutube flow elements, orifice plates and flanges, seal pots, indicating fluids, pressure sources, manometer and tank gauge accessories, and meriam scales. Barometer, digital; SMART.

Scientific Glass & Instruments, Inc. 877-682-1481
PO Box 6, Houston, TX 77001

MANOMETER, SPINAL FLUID *(General) 80FMJ*

Busse Hospital Disposables, Inc. 631-435-4711
75 Arkay Dr, Hauppauge, NY 11788
Lumbar puncture tray.

Kelsar, S.A. 508-261-8000
Blvd. Insurgentes, Libriamento a La, Tijuana 22450 Mexico
Lumbar puncture tray

Rocket Medical Plc. 800-707-7625
150 Recreation Park Dr Ste 3, Hingham, MA 02043

Ware Medics Glass Works, Inc. 845-429-6950
PO Box 368, Garnerville, NY 10923

MANUAL, POLICIES *(General) 80WVL*

Biomed Ink 720-493-5199
3411 Westhaven Pl, Littleton, CO 80126
operating procedures; instruction for use; user manuals; online help; web-based training; labeling; package inserts; submissions; beta testing and usability testing; desktop publishing and technical illustrations; document design and style guides; research; single-source publishing.

Medical Safety Systems Inc. 888-803-9303
230 White Pond Dr, Akron, OH 44313

MARKER, CARDIOPULMONARY BYPASS (VEIN MARKER) *(Cardiovascular) 74MAB*

Genesee Biomedical, Inc. 800-786-4890
1308 S Jason St, Denver, CO 80223
ANASTOMARK Coronary Artery Bypass Graft Markers. Shortening and simplifying post-operative angiography for your patient and cardiologist. Three styles available to mark the anastomoses. Clear, unambiguous x-ray images. Quick and easy implantation.

Med-Edge, Inc. 800-360-3682
1843 Pinehurst Dr, Lewisville, NC 27023
Coronary vein graft marker.

MARKER, IDENTIFICATION, SUTURE *(Surgery) 79MAW*

Sterion, Incorporated 800-328-7958
13828 Lincoln St NE, Ham Lake, MN 55304
Suture Aid Bootie, protect, tag and help locate sutures.

MARKER, OCULAR *(Ophthalmology) 86HMR*

Accutome, Inc. 610-889-0200
3222 Phoenixville Pike, Malvern, PA 19355
Various ophthalmic marker.

Addition Technology, Inc. 847-297-8419
155 Moffett Park Dr Ste B-1, Sunnyvale, CA 94089

Mastel Precision, Inc. 800-657-8057
2843 Samco Rd Unit A, Rapid City, SD 57702
Marker, ocular.

Ocusoft, Inc. 281-342-3350
PO Box 429, Richmond, TX 77406
Corneal marking pads, ocular marker.

Refractec, Inc. 949-784-2600
5 Jenner Ste 150, Irvine, CA 92618
Corneal marker.

Total Titanium, Inc. 618-473-2429
140 East Monroe St., Hecker, IL 62248
Various types of ocular markers.

MARKER, OSTIA, AORTO-SAPHENOUS VEIN *(Surgery) 79KPK*

Cook Inc. 800-457-4500
PO Box 489, Bloomington, IN 47402

Scanlan International, Inc. 800-328-9458
1 Scanlan Plz, Saint Paul, MN 55107
AC & radiomark

Voss Medical Products 210-650-3124
4235 Centergate St, San Antonio, TX 78217
Graft marker.

MARKER, PERIODONTIC *(Dental And Oral) 76EMP*

Aesculap Implant Systems Inc. 1-800-234-9179
3773 Corporate Pkwy, Center Valley, PA 18034

Almore International, Inc. 503-643-6633
PO Box 25214, Portland, OR 97298
$12.50 to $35.00 per unit (standard).

Medic Unique 310-698-0739
2962 Mindanao Dr, Costa Mesa, CA 92626
U-marc.

Premier Dental Products Co. 888-670-6100
1710 Romano Dr, PO Box 4500, Plymouth Meeting, PA 19462

MARKER, RADIOGRAPHIC, IMPLANTABLE *(Surgery) 79NEU*

Bioform Medical, Inc. 262-835-3323
4133 Courtney Rd Ste 10, Franksville, WI 53126
Radiological marker.

Biomet Microfixation Inc. 800-874-7711
1520 Tradeport Dr, Jacksonville, FL 32218
Radiographic marker.

Biomet, Inc. 574-267-6639
56 E Bell Dr, PO Box 587, Warsaw, IN 46582
Various types of implantable radiographic markers.

MARKER, RADIOGRAPHIC, IMPLANTABLE *(cont'd)*

Devicor Medical Products Inc. 262-857-9300
10505 Corporate Dr Ste 207, Pleasant Prairie, WI 53158
8 Gauge MicroMARK II Tissue Marker

Ethicon Endo-Surgery, Inc. 877-384-4266
3801 University Blvd SE, Albuquerque, NM 87106
Various types of implantable tissue markers.

Suros Surgical Systems, Inc 877-887-8767
6100 Technology Center Dr, Indianapolis, IN 46278
Biopsy site tissue marker device.

MARKER, SCLERA (OCULAR) *(Ophthalmology) 86HMQ*

Bausch & Lomb Surgical 636-255-5051
3365 Tree Court Ind Blvd, Saint Louis, MO 63122

Hurricane Medical 941-751-0588
5315 Lena Rd, Bradenton, FL 34211
Preinked marking pads.

Micro Medical Instruments 314-845-3663
123 Cliff Cave Rd, Saint Louis, MO 63129
Lens marker.

Peregrine Surgical, Ltd. 215-348-0456
51 Britain Dr, Doylestown, PA 18901
Marker, sclera.

MARKER, SKIN *(Surgery) 79FZZ*

Accu-Line Products, Inc. 800-363-7740
379 Iyannough Rd Rear Bldg, Hyannis, MA 02601
Surgical marking system that combines a fine point and broad point in one marker. Various styles, rulers, and labels available.

Advantage Medical Systems, Inc. 800-810-1262
2876 S Wheeling Way, Aurora, CO 80014
Bull's Eye Surgical Light Aimer: Compatible with virtually every surgical light in existence, eliminates frustration and wasted minutes adjusting lights (laser guided).

Beekley Corp. 860-583-4700
150 Dolphin Rd, Bristol, CT 06010
Beekley spots.

Centurion Medical Products Corp. 517-545-1135
3310 S Main St, Salisbury, NC 28147

Codman & Shurtleff, Inc 800-225-0460
325 Paramount Dr, Raynham, MA 02767

Colby Manufacturing Corp. 800-969-3718
1016 Branagan Dr, Tullytown, PA 19007
VeriSite and SurgiGuard Patient Labeling Systems for surgical site verification and documentation for the prevention of surgical errors.

Depuy-Raynham, A Div. Of Depuy Orthopaedics 800-451-2006
325 Paramount Dr, Raynham, MA 02767
Various.

First Aid Bandage Co., Inc. 888-813-8214
3 State Pier Rd, New London, CT 06320
Surgiscribe.

Griff Industries, Inc. 800-709-4743
19761 Bahama St, Northridge, CA 91324
TRImarker skin marker and TRImarker CS marker. Triangular pen for marking skin and triangular all-purpose CS marker for marking plastic, glass, foam, etc.

Hospital Marketing Svcs. Company, Inc. 800-786-5094
162 Great Hill Rd./ Ind. Park, Naugatuck, CT 06770
HMS SKIN SKRIBE -box of 10 pcs., #6650. (TWIN TIP marker - box of 10 pcs., #6650-T.) box of 50 pcs., #6653.

I.Z.I. Medical Products, Inc. 800-231-1499
7020 Tudsbury Rd, Baltimore, MD 21244
Various.

Liqui-Mark Corp. 631-236-4333
PO Box 18015, Hauppauge, NY 11788
Skin marker.

Olsen Medical 800-297-6344
3001 W Kentucky St, Louisville, KY 40211
DermaMarker Skin Marking Pen, packged pen only, pen and ruler, and pen, ruler and labels.

Oratronics, Inc. 212-986-0050
405 Lexington Ave, New York, NY 10174
Fine-line tissue marker.

Porex Surgical, Inc. 800-521-7321
15 Dart Rd, Newnan, GA 30265
TLS and SQUEEZE-MARK Surgical Markers.

MARKER, SKIN *(cont'd)*

Precision Dynamics Corp. 800-772-1122
13880 Del Sur St, San Fernando, CA 91340
SECURLINE MARKER II Fine-tip, scrub-resistant skin marker.

Sanford, L.P. 800-323-0749
1 Pencil St, Shelbyville, TN 37160
Skin marker.

Scanlan International, Inc. 800-328-9458
1 Scanlan Plz, Saint Paul, MN 55107
SCANLAN surgical skin markers.

St. John Companies 800-435-4242
25167 Anza Dr, PO Box 800460, Santa Clarita, CA 91355
Determine exact locations of lesions and microcalcifications with the help of SPEE-D-MARK. Eliminate chance of nipple shadow being mistaken.

Surgichip, Inc. 561-694-7776
4398 Hickory Dr, Palm Beach Gardens, FL 33418
Skin marker.

Tri-State Hospital Supply Corp. 517-545-1135
3173 E 43rd St, Yuma, AZ 85365

Viscot Medical, Llc 800-221-0658
32 West St, PO Box 351, East Hanover, NJ 07936
Gentian violet ink skin markers; fine, ultra-fine, borad tips 79FZZ Black, red, blue, green ink; bullet tip laboratory markers.

Xodus Medical, Inc. 800-963-8776
702 Prominence Dr, Westmoreland Business & Research Park
New Kensington, PA 15068
Surgical Skin Markers

MARKER, X-RAY *(Radiology) 90RFX*

All-Craft Wellman Products, Inc. 800-340-3899
4839 E 345th St, Willoughby, OH 44094
Custom-made x-Ray markers using lead letters and numbers; solid lead x-Ray letters, sizes 3/32 through 1 inch; radiopaque mammography markers. Radiographic rulers, 115- and 45-cm length acrylic rulers with radiopaque scales. Also available, radiolucent tissue localizer.

Concepts International, Inc. 800-627-9729
224 E Main St, Summerton, SC 29148
ID ONE--ID printer for x-ray film that prints patient's name, date, etc., onto each x-ray film before developing.

Cone Instruments, Inc. 800-321-6964
5201 Naiman Pkwy, Solon, OH 44139

Flow X-Ray Corporation 800-356-9729
100 W Industry Ct, Deer Park, NY 11729
Lead letters and figures.

Hospital Marketing Svcs. Company, Inc. 800-786-5094
162 Great Hill Rd./ Ind. Park, Naugatuck, CT 06770
HMS SKIN SKRIBE - 100 each/bag, product #6880.

Marconi Medical Systems 800-323-0550
595 Miner Rd, Cleveland, OH 44143

Tabbies, Div. Of Xertrex International, Inc. 630-773-4160
1530 Glenlake Ave, Itasca, IL 60143

Tailored Label Products, Inc. 800-727-1344
W165N5731 Ridgewood Dr, Menomonee Falls, WI 53051

Techno-Aide, Inc. 800-251-2629
7117 Centennial Blvd, Nashville, TN 37209

Wolf X-Ray Corporation 800-356-9729
100 W Industry Ct, Deer Park, NY 11729
Lead letters & figures.

X-Rite, Inc. 888-826-3044
4300 44th St SE, Grand Rapids, MI 49512
$26.00 for 50-ft. roll of 3/8in., $35.25 for 50-ft. roll of 3/4in. marking tape.

MASK, ANALGESIA *(Dental And Oral) 76UDX*

American Diversified Dental Systems 800-637-2330
22991 La Cadena Dr, Laguna Hills, CA 92653
N95 Health Care Particulate Respirator. 2300N95 Air-Flow Particulate Respirator.

Mizzy, Inc. Of National Keystone 800-333-3131
616 Hollywood Ave, Cherry Hill, NJ 08002
Our Comfort Cushion disposable Mask and dental analgesia delivery system sets new standards in comfort, convenience, cleanliness and efficiency

MASK, EYE, PHOTOTHERAPY *(Ophthalmology) 86RGA*

J. T. Posey Co. 800-447-6739
5635 Peck Rd, Arcadia, CA 91006

MASK, EYE, PHOTOTHERAPY *(cont'd)*

Olympic Medical Corp. 206-767-3500
5900 1st Ave S, Seattle, WA 98108
$39.95 for 12 units.

MASK, FACE *(General) 80WKE*

Adenna Inc. 888-323-3662
11932 Baker Pl, Santa Fe Springs, CA 90670
4-fold design forms better protective cone shape. Ultra soft inner layer for comfortable wear. Latex free and fiberglass free. PVC concealed nose piece minimizes x-ray reflection. PFE) 99% and BFE) 99%

Adex Medical, Inc. 800-873-4776
6101 Quail Valley Ct, Riverside, CA 92507
Cone Mask, Ear Loop, Soft Nose Bridge, Blue, White, Pink.

Aearo Company 800-678-4163
5457 W 79th St, Indianapolis, IN 46268
TUFFSHIELD face shield with full-impact protection for orthopedic procedures. Ratchet headband and replacement anti-fog shields available.

Alimed, Inc. 800-225-2610
297 High St, Dedham, MA 02026

Allied Healthcare Products, Inc. 800-444-3954
1720 Sublette Ave, Saint Louis, MO 63110

Armstrong Medical Industries, Inc. 800-323-4220
575 Knightsbridge Pkwy, Lincolnshire, IL 60069
Patient face shields and resuscitation masks.

Aura Lens Products, Inc. 800-281-2872
51 8th St N, PO Box 763, St. Cloud,, Sauk Rapids, MN 56379
Face shielding products: splash, bio-hazard, blood pathogen including faceshields, glasses, goggles and visor shield products.

Chagrin Safety Supply, Inc. 800-227-0468
8227 Washington St # 1, Chagrin Falls, OH 44023

Clean Esd Products, Inc. 510-257-5080
48340 Milmont Dr, Fremont, CA 94538
#PS36, $6.00/box of 50. One size fits all.

Cms Worldwide, Inc. 800-426-4633
30011 Ivy Glenn Dr Ste 215, Laguna Niguel, CA 92677
Isolation face mask: cone mask, osha, fluid resistant; pink, white, or blue; 50 per box.

Concepts International, Inc. 800-627-9729
224 E Main St, Summerton, SC 29148
FULL-FACE splatter shield.

Crosstex International 800-223-2497
10 Ranick Rd, Hauppauge, NY 11788
6 Levels of Mask,all latex free

Crosstex International Ltd., W. Region 800-707-2737
14059 Stage Rd, Santa Fe Springs, CA 90670
MASKENOMICS, six levels of protection, eleven varieties.

Crosstex International,Inc. 888-276-7783
10 Ranick Rd, Hauppauge, NY 11788
ISOFLUID, PROCEDURAL, ISOLITE, ULTRA FLUID, ISOLATOR PLUS, CIRCLE OF PROTECTION.

General Econopak, Inc. 888-871-8568
1725 N 6th St, Philadelphia, PA 19122
Non-allergenic, with ties or earloops; also, with or without safety visor.

Gerson Co. Inc., Louis M. 800-225-8623
15 Sproat St, Middleboro, MA 02346
NIOSH approved Particulate masks with or without valves. Also, TB approved.

Global Concepts, Ltd. 818-363-7195
19464 Eagle Ridge Ln, Northridge, CA 91326

In Disposables Inc. 800-269-4568
PO Box 528, Stratford, CT 06615
3-ply non-woven, non-linting material. Fluid resistant, soft elastic loops; packed 50/bx; 12 boxes/cs. Available in blue, green, pink, yellow or white.

Inamco International Corp. 800-724-4003
801 Montrose Ave, South Plainfield, NJ 07080

Intec Industries, Inc. 205-251-5600
2024 12th Ave N, Birmingham, AL 35234

Ivry 305-448-9858
216 Catalonia Ave Ste 106, Coral Gables, FL 33134

Johnson & Johnson Medical Division Of Ethicon, Inc. 800-423-4018
2500 E Arbrook Blvd, Arlington, TX 76014

K Medical 800-478-5633
PO Box 5224, Fort Lauderdale, FL 33310

MASK, FACE *(cont'd)*

Kerr Group 800-524-3577
1400 Holcomb Bridge Rd, Roswell, GA 30076

Key Surgical, Inc. 800-541-7995
8101 Wallace Rd Ste 100, Eden Prairie, MN 55344
Disposable face shields.

Lee Medical International, Inc. 800-433-8950
612 Distributors Row, Harahan, LA 70123
Full face shields.

M.C. Johnson Co., Inc. 800-553-8483
2037 J and C Blvd, Naples, FL 34109
Anti-fog full face shields. Face shields with disposable lens, ear-loop and tie on masks with shields for protection from splashes of body fluids.

Maytex Corp. 800-462-9839
23521 Foley St, Hayward, CA 94545
Cone, ear-loop, tie-on, fiberglass free, anti-fog, latex-free and fluid-resistant.

Med Systems 800-345-9061
2631 Ariane Dr, San Diego, CA 92117
MEDS Series 2100 anatomical and disposable masks for anesthesia or respiratory pressure breathing circuits; fits over N/G intubated and bearded patients. Available in 3 adult sizes. Mask is disposable. Latex free.

Medicos Laboratories, Inc. (Mdt) 800-724-4003
801 Montrose Ave, South Plainfield, NJ 07080

Mexpo International, Inc. 800-838-8299
2695B McCone Ave, Hayward, CA 94545
BLOSSOM - 3-Ply Earloop face mask, latex free and Duckbill 3-Ply Earloop Face Mask.

Mydent International 800-275-0020
80 Suffolk Ct, Hauppauge, NY 11788
DEPEND Cone, form-fit, tie-on, fluid resistant, spartan and pleated face masks.

Nano Mask Inc. 888-656-3697
175 Cassia Way Ste A115, Henderson, NV 89014
NanoMask - Nanotechnology enhanced face mask

Oberon Company ,Div Of The Paramount Corp. 800-322-3348
22 Logan St, PO Box 61008, New Bedford, MA 02740
Clear Polycarbonate, Impact Resistant Faceshield with Antifog coating on inner surface for visibility. For Surgical and laboratory applications

Omnical, Inc. 818-837-7531
557 Jessie St, San Fernando, CA 91340

Onyx Medical Inc./Face-It 800-333-5773
445 Coloma St, Sausalito, CA 94965
Disposable full face shield, full length with flat viewing area; anti-fog coated. Drape Shield is a disposable full face shield with fluid barrier fabric extending below plastic, Velcro-like facteners close fabric under chin to protect against splash.

Pm Gloves, Inc. 800-788-9486
13808 Magnolia Ave, Chino, CA 91710

Rapid Deployment Products 877-433-7569
157 Railroad Dr, Ivyland, PA 18974

Sanax Protective Products, Inc. 800-379-9929
236 Upland Ave, Newton Highlands, MA 02461

Sellstrom Manufacturing Co. 800-323-7402
1 Sellstrom Dr, Palatine, IL 60067
Full face protective with lift-up window.

Shinemound Enterprise, Inc. 978-436-9980
17A Sterling Rd, North Billerica, MA 01862

Silverstone Packaging, Inc.-Your One Stop Supplier 800-413-1108
1401 Lakeland Ave, Bohemia, NY 11716

Splash Shield, Inc. 800-536-6686
52 Dragon Ct, Woburn, MA 01801
Disposable face protection products to protect entire face from splattered blood and other bodily fluids.

Superior Medical Limited 800-268-7944
520 Champagne Dr., Toronto, ONT M3J 2T9 Canada

MASK, FACE *(cont'd)*

Tronex Healthcare Industries 800-833-1181
2 Cranberry Rd, One Tronex Centre, Parsippany, NJ 07054
Breathable three-ply masks with BFE)98%; outer layer PPSB spunbonded, PP melt blown second layer as filter and third layer of PP thermobond. PVC wire to conform to face is fastened ultrasonically at two side edges. Comes in styles with latex free elastic earloops, tie type, and with face shield and earloops. Fluid resistant. Blue.

Ventlab Corporation 800-593-4654
155 Boyce Dr, Mocksville, NC 27028
Anesthesia masks, resuscitation bags-disposable reusable, peak flow meters, spacers for medication delivery.

Vitalograph, Inc. 800-255-6626
13310 W 99th St, Lenexa, KS 66215
$31.00, cuffed, 5 sizes for resuscitators.

Washington Trade International, Inc. 800-327-3379
2633 Willamette Dr NE, Lacey, WA 98516
Resirattor Masks with or without Valve, also Earloop Masks

Water-Jel Technologies 800-275-3433
50 Broad St, Carlstadt, NJ 07072
Burn Mask - pre-cut with eye / nose / mouth slits -- and soaked in a water-based gel. Cools burns fast, relieves pain, prevents contamination and prepares patient for pre-hospital transport

MASK, GAS, ANESTHESIA *(Anesthesiology) 73BSJ*

A-M Systems, Inc. 800-426-1306
131 Business Park Loop, Sequim, WA 98382
Assorted sizes available

Ac Healthcare Supply, Inc. 905-448-4706
11651 230th St, Cambria Heights, NY 11411
Anesthetic gas mask.

Aga Linde Healthcare P.R. Inc. 787-622-7900
PO Box 363868, GPO Box 364727, San Juan, PR 00936
Anesth/ Pul Med.

Ambu A/S 457-225-2210
6740 Baymeadow Dr, Glen Burnie, MD 21060
Disposable face masks,various sizes.

Ambu, Inc. 800-262-8462
6740 Baymeadow Dr, Glen Burnie, MD 21060
AMBU Face Mask consisting of a mask, gas (anesthetic).

Anesthesia Associates, Inc. 760-744-6561
460 Enterprise St, San Marcos, CA 92078
Excellent fitting reusable masks constructed of various materials including durable silicone, neoprene, plastic, and Latex Free. Sizes from very small to very large. Standard versions as well as Patil-Syracuse endoscopic access versions available.

Corpak Medsystems, Inc. 800-323-6305
100 Chaddick Dr, Wheeling, IL 60090
Face mask.

E-Global Medical Equipment, L.L.C. 866-422-1845
2f 500 Lincoln St., Allston, MA 02134
Laryngeal airway, la & laryngeal airway shield, las.

Eastmed Enterprises, Inc. 856-797-0131
11 Brandywine Dr, Marlton, NJ 08053
Reach toothbrush.

Emepe International, Inc. 813-994-9690
18108 Sugar Brooke Dr, Tampa, FL 33647
Mask, tubing, and breathing bags for respiratory care and anesthesia. Disposable patient circuits.

Engineered Medical Systems 317-246-5500
2055 Executive Dr, Indianapolis, IN 46241
Suprglottic airway.

Hans Rudolph, Inc. 816-363-5522
7200 Wyandotte St, Kansas City, MO 64114
Anesthesia face mask,non-conductive,silicone rubber.

International Hospital Supply Co. 800-398-9450
6914 Canby Ave Ste 105, Reseda, CA 91335

International Respiratory Systems, Inc. 845-562-5546
95 Ann St, Newburgh, NY 12550
Face mask, gas anesthesia.

Med Systems 800-345-9061
2631 Ariane Dr, San Diego, CA 92117
MEDS MASK anesthesia gas mask. Mask is disposable. Latex Free.

Medline Industries, Inc. 800-633-5886
1 Medline Pl, Mundelein, IL 60060

MASK, GAS, ANESTHESIA *(cont'd)*

O-Two Systems International Inc. 800-387-3405
7575 Kimbel St., Mississauga, ONT L5S 1C8 Canada
Universal, Resuscitation and anaesthesia 'Everseal Edge' Facemasks in both PVC and silicone. Also sinigle use cuffed facemasks.

ReNu Medical Inc. 877-252-1110
9800 Evergreen Way, Everett, WA 98204
ANESTHETIC; GAS; MULTIPLE MODELS; REPROCESSED MASK

Smiths Medical Asd Inc. 800-258-5361
10 Bowman Dr, Keene, NH 03431
Various types and sizes of anesthetic gas masks.

Sun-Med 800-433-2797
12393 Belcher Rd S Ste 450, Largo, FL 33773

Sunmed Healthcare 727-531-7266
12393 Belcher Rd S Ste 460, Largo, FL 33773

Thayer Medical Corp. 520-790-5393
4575 S Palo Verde Rd Ste 337, Tucson, AZ 85714
Various types of anesthesia face masks.

Unomedical, Inc. 800-634-6003
5701 S Ware Rd Ste 1, McAllen, TX 78503

Ventlab Corp. 336-753-5000
155 Boyce Dr, Mocksville, NC 27028
Mask, face.

MASK, OTHER *(General) 80RGD*

Afassco, Inc. 800-441-6774
2244 Park Pl Ste C, Minden, NV 89423
One-way valve masks.

Amici, Inc. 610-948-7100
518 Vincent St, Spring City, PA 19475
Inflatable, cushion-type rebreathing mask.

Avid Products 888-575-AVID
72 Johnny Cake Hill Rd, Aquidneck Industrial Park, Middletown, RI 02842
AVID soft nylon sleep mask for relaxation in room or during MRI testing.

Cms Worldwide, Inc. 800-426-4633
30011 Ivy Glenn Dr Ste 215, Laguna Niguel, CA 92677
Isolation face mask: ear-loop face mask, 3-ply, osha, fluid resistant; blue or pink; 50 per box.

Gerson Co. Inc., Louis M. 800-225-8623
15 Sproat St, Middleboro, MA 02346

Medical Safety Systems Inc. 888-803-9303
230 White Pond Dr, Akron, OH 44313
HEPA respirators for respiratory protection from TB and organic vapors.

Mine Safety Appliances Company 866-MSA-1001
121 Gamma Dr, Pittsburgh, PA 15238

Norwood Promotional Products, Inc. 651-388-1298
5151 Moundview Dr, Red Wing, MN 55066
CPR Face Shield

Ross Disposable Products 800-649-6526
401 Traders Blvd E, Unit 10, Mississauga, ON L4Z 2H8 Canada

Sunrise Medical 800-333-4000
7477 Dry Creek Pkwy, Longmont, CO 80503

MASK, OXYGEN, AEROSOL ADMINISTRATION
(Anesthesiology) 73BYG

A-M Systems, Inc. 800-426-1306
131 Business Park Loop, Sequim, WA 98382
Assorted sizes available

Ac Healthcare Supply, Inc. 905-448-4706
11651 230th St, Cambria Heights, NY 11411
Oxygen mask.

Afton Medical Llc 707-577-0685
3137 Swetzer Rd Ste C, Loomis, CA 95650
Oxygen masks.

Ambu A/S 457-225-2210
6740 Baymeadow Dr, Glen Burnie, MD 21060
Resusable face mask, transparent, silicone.

Amerivac Usa Inc. 908-486-5200
1207 Pennsylvania Ave, Linden, NJ 07036
Tracheostomy mask.

Corpak Medsystems, Inc. 800-323-6305
100 Chaddick Dr, Wheeling, IL 60090
Blow-by aerosol and/or oxygen delivery system.

MASK, OXYGEN, AEROSOL ADMINISTRATION *(cont'd)*

Dixie Ems Supply 800-347-3494
385 Union Ave, Brooklyn, NY 11211
$128.00 per 100 (med).

E-Global Medical Equipment, L.L.C. 866-422-1845
2f 500 Lincoln St., Allston, MA 02134
Laryngeal airway, la & laryngeal airway shield, las.

Hans Rudolph, Inc. 816-363-5522
7200 Wyandotte St, Kansas City, MO 64114
Nasal mask.

Healer Products, Llc 914-663-6300
427 Commerce Ln Ste 1, West Berlin, NJ 08091
Rescue breather mask, microshield breather mask, cpr ptp valve mask.

Health Care Logistics, Inc. 800-848-1633
450 Town St, PO Box 25, Circleville, OH 43113
Non-sterile disposable pediatric aerosol mask.

Intersurgical Inc. 315-451-2900
417 Electronics Pkwy, Liverpool, NY 13088

Kentron Health Care, Inc. 615-384-0573
3604 Kelton Jackson Rd, P.o. Box 120, Springfield, TN 37172
Oxygen mask.

Kidsmed 800-241-8338
2198 Ogden Ave, Aurora, IL 60504
Mask, oxygen. Pediatric aerosol masks and MDI spacer masks. Nic the Dragon, Bubbles the Fish, Reggie Rabbit and E-for-Elephant.

Lampac International Ltd. 636-797-3659
230 N Lake Dr, Hillsboro, MO 63050

Life Corporation 800-700-0202
1776 N Water St, Milwaukee, WI 53202
LIFE CPR Masks and LIFE CPR Shields.

Mada, Inc. 800-526-6370
625 Washington Ave, Carlstadt, NJ 07072

Matrx 716-662-6650
145 Mid County Dr, Orchard Park, NY 14127
Mask.

Oxia U.S. Ltd. 262-369-1978
665 Industrial Ct Unit B, Hartland, WI 53029
Shroud, lid, cap.

ReNu Medical Inc. 877-252-1110
9800 Evergreen Way, Everett, WA 98204
MULTIPLE MODELS; OXYGEN; REPROCESSED MASK

Respironics California, Inc. 724-387-4559
2271 Cosmos Ct, Carlsbad, CA 92011
Mask.

Respironics Novametrix, Llc. 724-387-4559
5 Technology Dr, Wallingford, CT 06492
Mask.

Smiths Medical Asd Inc. 800-258-5361
10 Bowman Dr, Keene, NH 03431
Various.

Smiths Medical Asd, Inc. 847-793-0135
330 Corporate Woods Pkwy, Vernon Hills, IL 60061
Various types of adult oxygen masks.

Sterilmed, Inc. 763-488-3400
11400 73rd Ave N Ste 100, Maple Grove, MN 55369
Cpap mask.

Tagg Industries L.L.C. 800-548-3514
23210 Del Lago Dr, Laguna Hills, CA 92653
TRISEAL, disposable cushioned face mask with soft pre-filled air cushion for seal and comfort. See-thru for visual monitoring.

Ventlab Corp. 336-753-5000
155 Boyce Dr, Mocksville, NC 27028
Mask, oxygen.

MASK, OXYGEN, LOW CONCENTRATION, VENTURI
(Anesthesiology) 73BYF

Ac Healthcare Supply, Inc. 905-448-4706
11651 230th St, Cambria Heights, NY 11411
Venturi mask.

Afton Medical Llc 707-577-0685
3137 Swetzer Rd Ste C, Loomis, CA 95650
Venturi masks.

Intersurgical Inc. 315-451-2900
417 Electronics Pkwy, Liverpool, NY 13088

MASK, OXYGEN, LOW CONCENTRATION, VENTURI *(cont'd)*

Life Corporation 800-700-0202
1776 N Water St, Milwaukee, WI 53202
LIFE CPR Masks and LIFE CPR Shields.

O-Two Systems International Inc. 800-387-3405
7575 Kimbel St., Mississauga, ONT L5S 1C8 Canada

Pegasus Research Corp. 877-632-0255
3505 Cadillac Ave Ste G5, Costa Mesa, CA 92626
FLO2, adjustable high-flow oxygen diluter. OXY-PEEP, adjustable high-flow oxygen diluter with Peep valve.

ReNu Medical Inc. 877-252-1110
9800 Evergreen Way, Everett, WA 98204
MULTIPLE MODELS; REPROCESSED MASK; VENTURI

Smiths Medical Asd Inc. 800-258-5361
10 Bowman Dr, Keene, NH 03431
Venturi mask.

MASK, OXYGEN, NON-REBREATHING *(Anesthesiology) 73KGB*

Ac Healthcare Supply, Inc. 905-448-4706
11651 230th St, Cambria Heights, NY 11411
Non-breathing mask.

Advanced Circulatory Systems, Inc. 952-947-9590
7615 Golden Triangle Dr Ste A, Eden Prairie, MN 55344
Nonrebreathing mask.

Afton Medical Llc 707-577-0685
3137 Swetzer Rd Ste C, Loomis, CA 95650
Non-rebreathing mask.

Allied Healthcare Products, Inc. 800-444-3954
1720 Sublette Ave, Saint Louis, MO 63110

Ambu A/S 457-225-2210
6740 Baymeadow Dr, Glen Burnie, MD 21060
Mask, oxygen.

Ambu, Inc. 800-262-8462
6740 Baymeadow Dr, Glen Burnie, MD 21060
Ambu Rescue Mask is a mask, oxygen, with a non breathing one way valve & filter.

Bls Systems, Ltd. 905-339-1069
1055 Industry St, Oakville L6J 2X3 Canada
Ambu rescue mask

Cft, Inc./Life Mask 800-331-8844
14602 N Cave Creek Rd Ste B, Phoenix, AZ 85022
With one-way non-rebreathing valve for mouth to mask resuscitation. CPR Life Mask Resuscitator, cushion mask with one-way valve and bacterial and viral filter for mouth to mask resuscitation.

Corpak Medsystems, Inc. 800-323-6305
100 Chaddick Dr, Wheeling, IL 60090
Cpap mask - various sizes.

Dhd Healthcare Corporation 800-847-8000
PO Box 6, One Madison Street, Wampsville, NY 13163
FLO2 Emergency Non-rebreather High Flow O2 System

Hans Rudolph, Inc. 816-363-5522
7200 Wyandotte St, Kansas City, MO 64114
Accessory seal for a face mask.

Intersurgical Inc. 315-451-2900
417 Electronics Pkwy, Liverpool, NY 13088

Kentron Health Care, Inc. 615-384-0573
3604 Kelton Jackson Rd, P.o. Box 120, Springfield, TN 37172
Non-rebreathing mask.

Life Corporation 800-700-0202
1776 N Water St, Milwaukee, WI 53202
LIFE CPR Masks and LIFE CPR Shields.

O-Two Systems International Inc. 800-387-3405
7575 Kimbel St., Mississauga, ONT L5S 1C8 Canada

Plasco, Inc. 847-662-4400
Carretera Presta La Amistad, Km.19, Acuna, Coahila Mexico
Mask

Salter Labs 800-235-4203
100 Sycamore Rd, Arvin, CA 93203

Smiths Medical Asd, Inc. 847-793-0135
330 Corporate Woods Pkwy, Vernon Hills, IL 60061
Non rebreathing mask.

Sunmed Usa Llc. 310-531-8222
841 Apollo St Ste 334, El Segundo, CA 90245

MASK, OXYGEN, OTHER *(General) 80FQG*

Cardinal Health 207, Inc. 800-231-2466
22745 Savi Ranch Pkwy, Yorba Linda, CA 92887
Disposable, High FIO, for brief treatment with high oxygen concentrations greater than 80% at only 8 liters per minute of oxigen flow. 15/unit.

Intersurgical Inc. 315-451-2900
417 Electronics Pkwy, Liverpool, NY 13088

Kck Industries 888-800-1967
14941 Calvert St, Van Nuys, CA 91411
Resuscitation mask.

Life Corporation 800-700-0202
1776 N Water St, Milwaukee, WI 53202
LIFE CPR Masks and LIFE CPR Shields.

Mercury Medical 800-237-6418
11300 49th St N, Clearwater, FL 33762
Disposable masks.

O&M Enterprise 847-258-4515
641 Chelmsford Ln, Elk Grove Village, IL 60007
MASK, OXYGEN, REBREATHING, FACE MASK W/SHIELD

Passy-Muir Inc. 800-634-5397
4521 Campus Dr, Irvine, CA 92612
Passy-Muir™ PMA™ 2000 O2 adapter allows for easy inhalation of supplemental low-flow oxygen and humidity through the Low Profile PMV™ 2000 Series Speaking Valves. The Passy-Muir PMA 2000 O2 Adapter is small, lightweight, clear in color, and clips onto both the PMV 2000 (Clear) and PMV 2001 (Purple™) Swallowing & Speaking Valves. It is easily removed when not in use. Oxygen is delivered in front of the diaphragm of the PMV to avoid complications associated with devices that provide continuous flow behind the diaphragm of a speaking valve such as air trapping, drying of secretions, and possible cilia damage.

Rondex Products, Inc. 815-226-0452
PO Box 1829, Rockford, IL 61110
Oxygen mask, resuscitation mask.

Southmedic Inc. 800-463-7146
50 Alliance Blvd., Barrie, ONT L4M-5K3 Canada
OXYARM - The First Open Oxygen System

MASK, OXYGEN, PARTIAL REBREATHING *(General) 80RFY*

Allied Healthcare Products, Inc. 800-444-3954
1720 Sublette Ave, Saint Louis, MO 63110

Intersurgical Inc. 315-451-2900
417 Electronics Pkwy, Liverpool, NY 13088

Life Corporation 800-700-0202
1776 N Water St, Milwaukee, WI 53202
LIFE CPR Masks and LIFE CPR Shields.

Mada, Inc. 800-526-6370
625 Washington Ave, Carlstadt, NJ 07072

Rockford Medical & Safety Co. 800-435-9451
2420 Harrison Ave, PO Box 5646, Rockford, IL 61108

MASK, OXYGEN, VENTURI *(Anesthesiology) 73FSC*

Circadiance LLC 1-888-825-9640
1060 Corporate Ln, Export, PA 15632
SleepWeaver

MASK, SCAVENGING *(Anesthesiology) 73KHA*

Ac Healthcare Supply, Inc. 905-448-4706
11651 230th St, Cambria Heights, NY 11411
Scavenging mask.

Matrx 716-662-6650
145 Mid County Dr, Orchard Park, NY 14127
Scavenging mask.

ReNu Medical Inc. 877-252-1110
9800 Evergreen Way, Everett, WA 98204
MULTIPLES MODELS; REPROCESSED MASK; SCAVENGING

MASK, SURGICAL *(Surgery) 79FXX*

Adex Medical, Inc. 800-873-4776
6101 Quail Valley Ct, Riverside, CA 92507
Tie On Mask, Blue, White.

Amd-Ritmed, Inc. 800-445-0340
295 Firetower Road, Tonawanda, NY 14150

Atd-American Co. 800-523-2300
135 Greenwood Ave, Wyncote, PA 19095

Barnhardt Mfg. Co. 704-376-0380
1100 Hawthorne Ln, Charlotte, NC 28205
Dental mask.

MASK, SURGICAL *(cont'd)*

Berkley Medical Resources, Inc. 412-438-3000
49 Virginia Ave, Uniontown, PA 15401
Face mask.

Busse Hospital Disposables, Inc. 631-435-4711
75 Arkay Dr, Hauppauge, NY 11788
Isolation mask (non-surgical).

Certol International, Llc 303-799-9401
6120 E 58th Ave, Commerce City, CO 80022
Face mask,pleated,preformed.

Cms Worldwide, Inc. 800-426-4633
30011 Ivy Glenn Dr Ste 215, Laguna Niguel, CA 92677
Surgical tie-on face mask: 3-ply, osha, fluid resistant; blue or green; 50 per box.

Depuy Orthopaedics, Inc. 800-473-3789
700 Orthopaedic Dr, P.O. Box 988, Warsaw, IN 46582
Various types of surgical masks.

Dowling Textiles 770-957-3981
615 Macon Rd, McDonough, GA 30253
Various types of surgical masks.

Gammadirect Medical Division 847-267-5929
PO Box 383, Lake Forest, IL 60045
BetaSpecs disposable eyeshields

Gerson Co. Inc., Louis M. 800-225-8623
15 Sproat St, Middleboro, MA 02346
TB approved 1730, 2735 and 2735S (Small). All have a 160 mm Hg. rating in the Fluid Penetration Resistance Test.

Global Healthcare 800-601-3880
1495 Hembree Rd Ste 700, Roswell, GA 30076
Tie On, Ear Loop, surgical masks with and without eye shield, Cone masks

Hager Worldwide, Inc. 800-328-2335
13322 Byrd Dr, Odessa, FL 33556
GLOBAL (laser mask) & EARLOOP.

Intec Industries, Inc. 205-251-5600
2024 12th Ave N, Birmingham, AL 35234

Johnson & Johnson Medical Division Of Ethicon, Inc. 800-423-4018
2500 E Arbrook Blvd, Arlington, TX 76014

Kentron Health Care, Inc. 615-384-0573
3604 Kelton Jackson Rd, P.o. Box 120, Springfield, TN 37172
Face mask, surgical mask.

Kerma Medical Products, Inc. 757-398-8400
400 Port Centre Pkwy, Portsmouth, VA 23704
Various masks.

Lampac International Ltd. 636-797-3659
230 N Lake Dr, Hillsboro, MO 63050
Available with ties or earloops.

Medical Action Industries, Inc. 800-645-7042
25 Heywood Rd, Arden, NC 28704
Mask.

Medline Industries, Inc. 800-633-5886
1 Medline Pl, Mundelein, IL 60060

Medspring Group, Inc. 801-295-9750
533 W 2600 S Ste 105, Bountiful, UT 84010
Surgical mask.

Medtek Devices, Inc. 716-835-7000
595 Commerce Dr, 155 Pineview Dr., Amherst, NY 14228
Surgical & laser face masks.

Moldex-Metric, Inc. 800-421-0668
10111 Jefferson Blvd, Culver City, CA 90232
N95 Disposable Respirator

New York Hospital Disposables, Inc. 718-384-1620
101 Richardson St, Brooklyn, NY 11211

Niche Medical, Inc. 800-633-1055
55 Access Rd, Warwick, RI 02886
.01 Micron Laser Masks

North Safety Products 401-943-4400
1101 B Calle Neutron, Parque Industrial Maran, Mexicali, B.c. Mexico
Face mask w/eye shield

Pac-Dent Intl., Inc. 909-839-0888
21078 Commerce Point Dr, Walnut, CA 91789
Disposable mask, disposable surgical mask.

Pharaoh Trading Company 866-929-4913
9701 Brookpark Rd, Knollwood Plaza, Suite 241, Cleveland, OH 44129

MASK, SURGICAL *(cont'd)*

Precept Medical Products, Inc. 800-438-5827
PO Box 2400, 370 Airport Road/, Arden, NC 28704
Facemask with protective neck veil

Prestige Ameritech 817-595-1131
7426 Tower St, Richland Hills, TX 76118
Surgical face mask.

Surgimedics 800-840-9906
2950 Mechanic St, Lake City, PA 16423
Various.

Ultradent Products, Inc. 801-553-4586
505 W 10200 S, South Jordan, UT 84095
Surgical apparel.

United Medical Enterprises 757-224-0177
4049 Allen Station Rd, Augusta, GA 30906
Tie on and earloop surgical medical face mask.

Young Colorado, Llc. 800-325-1881
13705 Shoreline Ct E, Earth City, MO 63045
Surgical apparel.

MASK, X-RAY SHIELD *(Radiology) 90VFC*

AMD Technologies Inc. 800-423-3535
218 Bronwood Ave, Los Angeles, CA 90049

MASKER, TINNITUS *(Ear/Nose/Throat) 77KLW*

audifon USA Inc. 800-776-0222
403 Chairman Ct Ste 1, P.O. Box 531700, Debary, FL 32713

Hal-Hen Company, Inc. 800-242-5436
180 Atlantic Ave, Garden City Park, NY 11040

Micro-Ear Technology, Inc. 952-995-8800
6425 Flying Cloud Dr, Eden Prairie, MN 55344
Tinnitus masker.

Neuromonics Inc. 484-821-1260
2810 Emrick Blvd, Bethlehem, PA 18020
Tinnitus masker.

Sound Techniques Systems, Llc 201-271-0700
710 Denbigh Blvd, Newport News, VA 23608
Tinnitus masker.

Starkey East 952-947-4734
535 Route 38 Ste 230, Cherry Hill, NJ 08002
Tinnitus masker.

Starkey Laboratories, Inc. 800-328-8602
6700 Washington Ave S, Eden Prairie, MN 55344

MASS SPECTROMETER, CLINICAL USE *(Toxicology) 91DOP*

AB Sciex 1 877-740-2129
110 Marsh Dr, Foster City, CA 94404
TripleTOF 5600

Absorption Systems 610-280-7300
436 Creamery Way, Exton, PA 19341
LTQ Orbitrap XL Hybrid Fourier Transform

Basi (Bioanalytical Systems, Inc.) 800-845-4246
2701 Kent Ave, West Lafayette, IN 47906
Mass spectrometry, HPLC, GC, TLC, dissolution, robotics.

Extrel Cms 412-963-7530
575 Epsilon Dr, Pittsburgh, PA 15238

Ge Medical Systems Information Technologies 800-643-6439
8200 W Tower Ave, Milwaukee, WI 53223
MGA-1100 medical mass spectrometer capable of simultaneous measurement of 8 gas channels within a dynamic range of 2-135 atomic mass units (AMU). Configurability of the MGA-1100 allows for use in many applications such as pulmonary function, stress testing, anesthesia, ICU/CCU, hyperbaric studies, and veterinary clinics. Completely self-contained and portable. The advantage multiplexed mass-spectrometer system is capable of connecting up to 31 ICU/CCU or operating rooms. Measures and displays inspired and expired concentrations of O2, N2, N2O, CO2, halothane, ethrane, suprane, and forane. The in-room display presents this data along with waveforms of all measured gases. Trend analysis of all stored parameters up to 16 hours. Remote observatory units may be connected with direct blood-gas input available. Hard-copy documentation for permanent record of patient data. RAMS Quadrupole Mass Spectrometer, capable of simultaneous measuring of up to 10 gas channels within a dynamic range of 1-250 AMU. This unit is configurable and allows for use in many applications such as anesthesia, stress testing, pulmonary function, hyperbaric studies, and research applications.

MASS SPECTROMETER, CLINICAL USE *(cont'd)*

Headwall Photonics, Inc. 978-353-4100
601 River St, Fitchburg, MA 01420
Clinical chemistry absorbance (340-700 nm) OEM module.

Hitachi High Technologies America, Inc. 800-548-9001
3100 N 1st St, San Jose, CA 95134
Hitachi's NanoFrontier incorporates Linear Ion Trap technology with TOF detection affording superior sensitivity, mass accuracy, and resolution. The Hitachi IBA (Information Based Acquisition) intelligent MS/MS provides enhanced protein information at reduced analysis time.

Jeol Usa, Inc. 978-536-2270
11 Dearborn Rd, Peabody, MA 01960

Kratos Analytical Inc. 800-935-0213
100 Red Schoolhouse Rd Bldg A, Spring Valley, NY 10977
Mass spectrometer work stations have high speed GC-MS/LC-MS processing.

Mds Sciex 416-675-6777
71 Four Valley Dr, Concord L4K 4V8 Canada
Mass spectrometer

Mds Sciex 905-660-9005
71 Four Valley Dr., Concord, ON L4K 4V8 Canada
Tandem mass spectrometer.

Spectro Analytical Instruments Inc. 800-548-5809
160 Authority Dr, Fitchburg, MA 01420
Available are ICP spectrometers, ICP-MS spectrometers, and X-ray fluorescent spectrometers.

Spectron Corp. 425-827-9317
934 S Burlington Blvd # 603, Burlington, WA 98233
Reconditioned equipment.

Ta Instruments 302-427-4000
109 Lukens Dr, New Castle, DE 19720

Ulvac Technologies, Inc. 800-998-5822
401 Griffin Brook Dr, Methuen, MA 01844

Varian Scientific Instruments 925-939-2400
2700 Mitchell Dr, Walnut Creek, CA 94598
Bench-top gas chromatograph / mass spectrometer.

MASSAGER, POWERED INFLATABLE TUBE
(Physical Med) 89IRP

Advanced Circulatory Systems, Inc. 952-947-9590
7615 Golden Triangle Dr Ste A, Eden Prairie, MN 55344
Circulatory enhancer.

Grimm Scientific Ind., Inc. 800-223-5395
1403 Pike St, PO Box 2143, Marietta, OH 45750
CYROPress $5,900 for sequential cyrocompression units.

Tactile Systems Technology Inc 866-435-3948
1331 Tyler St NE Ste 200, Minneapolis, MN 55413
Patented lymph preparation and drainage pneumatic device for treatment of lymphedema and chronic wound healing.

MASSAGER, THERAPEUTIC *(Physical Med) 89ISA*

A-1 Engineering 951-537-7240
2533 S San Jacinto Ave, Gilman Hot Springs, CA 92583

Aesthetic Innovations, Inc. 615-269-9166
1704A Gale Ln, Nashville, TN 37212
Visage elev'e.

Alimed, Inc. 800-225-2610
297 High St, Dedham, MA 02026
Electric massagers have flexible necks for tough angles.

Alsons Corp. 800-421-0001
3010 Mechanic Rd, P.O. Box 282, Hillsdale, MI 49242
ADA wall bar and hand shower system.

American Massage Products, Inc. 716-934-2648
341 Central Ave, Silver Creek, NY 14136
Heat and massage pad; hand unit.

Ami, Inc. 800-248-4031
1101 Noank Ledyard Rd, Mystic, CT 06355
Aqua PT Pro- The 3 in 1 Therapy System - Dry hydrotherapy, dry heat therapy, and massage therapy - increase circulation, relieve muscular pain & tension, relax muscles without getting undressed or wet! Now includes Body Profiler Control System with solar touch screen control and AVA Relaxation System.

Ark Therapeutic Services, Inc. 803-438-9779
PO Box 340, 862 A Hwy. 1 South, Lugoff, SC 29078
Therapeutic massager.

MASSAGER, THERAPEUTIC *(cont'd)*

Atzen/Universal Companies, Inc. 800-558-5571
18260 Oak Park Dr, Abingdon, VA 24210
Therapeutic massager (Atzen, LymphMed) for the face and body using vacuum pumps and suction cups (3 sizes). Massage by air suction.

Avazzia, Inc. 214-575-2820
13154 Coit Rd Ste 200, Dallas, TX 75240
Therapeutic massager.

B2 Imports, Llc 918-557-5729
12807 E 90th St N, Owasso, OK 74055
Therapeutic massager.

Body Well Design,Llc 866-293-8444
6206 E Trent Ave Ste 1A, Spokane Valley, WA 99212
Vacuum massage machine.

Cell Science Systems, Ltd. Corp. 954-426-2304
1239 E Newport Center Dr Ste 101, Deerfield Beach, FL 33442
Skin rolling machines used for massage.

Chi Institute 949-361-3976
27130A Paseo Espada Ste 1407, San Juan Capistrano, CA 92675

Conair Corp. 203-351-9000
150 Milford Rd, East Windsor, NJ 08520
Massager.

Cosmo Health, Inc. 626-839-9995
2616 Carlton Pl, Rowland Heights, CA 91748
Cosmo Tens (transcutaneous electrical nerve stimulator).

Cynosure, Inc. 800-886-2966
5 Carlisle Rd, Westford, MA 01886
Electric

Decompression Technology International 903-667-3802
1235 County Road 4244, De Kalb, TX 75559
Vactherapy.

Econnectech Llc. 415-810-9436
2434 14th Ave, San Francisco, CA 94116
Various models econnectech acumassager controller, neck care collars, electrodes.

Electro Medica Office 705-878-5894
33 Williams St. North, Lindsay, ONT K9V-3Z9 Canada
$170.00 for SONAFON intra sound massager.

Facemaster Of Beverly Hills, Inc. 818-222-2461
23961 Craftsman Rd Ste I, Calabasas, CA 91302
Facemaster.

Gaia Holistic,Inc 212-799-9711
20 W 64th St Apt 24E, New York, NY 10023
Heat pad.

General Pysiotherapy, Inc. 800-237-1832
13222 Lakefront Dr, Earth City, MO 63045
PROFESSIONAL THERAPEUTIC MASSAGE MACHINES FOR MUSCLE RELAXATION, TRIGGER-POINT THERAPY, SPORTS REHABILITATION, PHYSICAL THERAPY, AIDS CELLULITE REDUCTION, AIDS LYMPHATIC DRAINAGE, AIDS LACTIC ACID MOBILIZATION

Health Keeper 9000 Usa Inc. 213-385-3933
680 Wilshire Pl Ste 405, Los Angeles, CA 90005
Sae ik health keeper 9000.

Homedics Inc. 800-333-8282
3000 N Pontiac Trl, Commerce Township, MI 48390
Many models of therapeutic massagers available.

Jtl Enterprises 800-699-1008
15395 Roosevelt Blvd, Clearwater, FL 33760
AquaMED Dry Hydrotherapy Massage System

Medical Depot 516-998-4600
99 Seaview Blvd, Port Washington, NY 11050
Massager, therapeutic.

Medsonix 702-873-3700
2626 S Rainbow Blvd Ste 109, Las Vegas, NV 89146
Massager.

Micro Current Technology, Inc. 206-778-5717
2244 1st Ave S, Seattle, WA 98134
Various models of electric therapeutic massagers.

Microstim Technology, Inc. 772-283-0408
1849 SW Crane Creek Ave, Palm City, FL 34990
Massager.

Morfam, Inc. 219-259-4581
3002 N Home St, Mishawaka, IN 46545
Electrical hand-held massagers.

MASSAGER, THERAPEUTIC *(cont'd)*

Nutra Luxe Md, Llc 239-561-9699
6835 International Center Blvd Ste 5, Fort Myers, FL 33912
Hand-held massager system kit, hand-held massager.

Oismueller & Partner, Inc. 770-874-1767
1968 Sixes Rd, Canton, GA 30114
Golden spoon-facial care set.

Patterson Medical Supply, Inc. 262-387-8720
W68N158 Evergreen Blvd, Cedarburg, WI 53012
Massagers and vibrators.

Photoclear, Inc. 888-789-3784
8819 Hoskins Rd, Freeport, TX 77541

Pneu-Mobility, Inc. 610-266-8500
944 Marcon Blvd Ste 110, Allentown, PA 18109
Pneu-wave.

R.J. Lindquist Co. 213-382-1268
2419 James M Wood Blvd, Los Angeles, CA 90006
Vibrator.

Salton, Inc. 202-408-9213
1955 W Field Ct, Lake Forest, IL 60045
Various models of massagers.

Sanuwave Inc. 866-581-6843
11680 Great Oaks Way Ste 350, Alpharetta, GA 30022

Sidmar Mfg., Inc. 800-330-7260
31530 125th St NW, Princeton, MN 55371
Dry hydromassage table.

Southpaw Enterprises, Inc. 800-228-1698
PO Box 1047, Dayton, OH 45401
This unique massager is sure to be a necessity for your client's tactile needs. The powerful two-speed motor allows for an oscillating massage at either 4300 or 5700 vibrations per minute. The flexible îpower-springî mounted head allows for 100% of the vibration energy to be applied to the designated area, instead of in your hands. The integral, rechargeable battery is long lasting at 45 minutes of continual use per charge, or for hours of use with the custom DC cord socket.

The Pettibon System 888-774-6258
2118 Jackson Hwy, Chehalis, WA 98532
Tendon muscle ligament stimulator.

Ultrassage, Inc. 514-344-1083
5680 Rue Pare, Mont-Royal, QUEBE H4P 2M2 Canada
Hand massage unit.

United Laboratories And Manufacturing, Llc 703-787-9600
45000 Underwood Ln Ste F, Sterling, VA 20166
Electric hair dryer, brush.

Voyager Medical Corp. 503-223-3881
5550 SW MacAdam Ave Ste 310, Portland, OR 97239
Therapeautic massager.

Wahl Clipper Corp. 815-548-8342
2900 Locust St, Sterling, IL 61081
Massager.

Webbmed Corporation 678-482-1722
615 Emerald Pkwy, Sugar Hill, GA 30518
Massager, therapeutic, electric.

Wunder Tool & Die, Inc. 509-922-6415
17625 E Euclid Ave, Spokane Valley, WA 99216
Acoustic massager.

Zeltiq 925-474-2500
4698 Willow Rd, Pleasanton, CA 94588
Zeltiq System

MASSAGER, THERAPEUTIC, MANUAL *(Physical Med) 89LYG*

Ark Therapeutic Services, Inc. 803-438-9779
PO Box 340, 862 A Hwy. 1 South, Lugoff, SC 29078
Teething ring.

Ball Dynamics International, Llc 800-752-2255
14215 Mead St, Longmont, CO 80504

Cryo Therapy 763-295-5455
20233 167th St NW, Big Lake, MN 55309

Genesen Pan America, Inc. 714-799-1735
7245 Garden Grove Blvd Ste D, Garden Grove, CA 92841
Acutouch / acurepatch.

Joint Venture Development, Inc. 713-501-0075
1628 Beaconshire Rd, Houston, TX 77077
Therapeutic massager.

MASSAGER, THERAPEUTIC, MANUAL *(cont'd)*

Patterson Medical Supply, Inc. 262-387-8720
W68N158 Evergreen Blvd, Cedarburg, WI 53012
Manual massager.

Photoclear, Inc. 888-789-3784
8819 Hoskins Rd, Freeport, TX 77541

Polar Products, Inc. 800-763-8423
540 S Main St Ste 951, Akron, OH 44311
Roller Ice Cryogenic Massage: This new patent pending product combines soothing massage with cold therapy to provide relief from muscle strains, bruises, chronic pain, migraines and more. The stainless steel roller ball rolls freely in all directions and when frozen, will remain cold for up to one hour. Also available in non-rolling point for trigger-point massage.

The Myo Tool Co. 530-272-7306
1020 McCourtney Rd Ste D, Grass Valley, CA 95949
Self massage device.

MATERIAL, ACRYLIC, DENTAL *(Dental And Oral) 76WKF*

Almore International, Inc. 503-643-6633
PO Box 25214, Portland, OR 97298
Debubblizer; Almore surfactant, 8 oz. and 32 oz. sizes, $10.50 and $25.00 respectively.

Denplus Inc. 800-344-4424
205 - 1221 Labadie, Longueuil, QUE J4N 1E2 Canada

Global Dental Products 516-221-8844
PO Box 537, Bellmore, NY 11710
D.T. Temporary Dressing. Unoxygenated calcium hydroxide paste in sterile packets.

Harry J. Bosworth Company 800-323-4352
7227 Hamlin Ave, Skokie, IL 60076
Trim, Trim II, Trim Plus, Trim VW

Heraeus Kulzer, Inc. 800-431-1785
99 Business Park Dr, Armonk, NY 10504
JELDENT, dual technique resin for pour and press pack technique.

Holmes Dental Corp. 800-322-5577
50 S Penn St, Hatboro, PA 19040
QYK SET Quick setting self cure acrylic, QYK SET for making temporary crowns. INTERIM bisacrylic for temporaries (cartride).

Mizzy, Inc. Of National Keystone 800-333-3131
616 Hollywood Ave, Cherry Hill, NJ 08002
Use Sledghammer, Millenium or our new Diamond D 'Ultra' High Impact Denture Acrylic to form new dentures or to repair fractured dentures.

Motloid Company 800-662-5021
300 N Elizabeth St, Chicago, IL 60607
MIRACRYL & MOLDPAC Acrylic resins, self and heat cure.

Plaskolite West Inc. 800-562-8883
2225 E Del Amo Blvd, Compton, CA 90220
Acrylic manufacturing. IOL Materials

Talon Acrylics, Inc. 888-433-2551
850 NE 102nd Ave, Portland, OR 97220
'TALON' Thermoplastic Acrylic Elastomer is used in fabrication of TMJ/D Splints, Night Guards, Repositioing Stints, Sleep Apnea Anti-Snore Appliances, and other appiances as prescribed. 'REVERE' Thermoplastic Acrylics Elastomer is used in fabrication of Liners/Relines for Compete and Partial Dentures, Overdentures/Gaskets.

Yates & Bird And Motloid 800-662-5021
300 N Elizabeth St, Chicago, IL 60607
Coldpac tooth acrylic. Self-cure temporary crown & bridge material.

MATERIAL, CASTING *(Dental And Oral) 76UDT*

Codman & Shurtleff, Inc 800-225-0460
325 Paramount Dr, Raynham, MA 02767

Dentecon, Inc. 800-423-6088
1249 S La Cienega Blvd, Los Angeles, CA 90035
Thermabond partial and ceramic full crown alloys.

Mds Products, Inc. 800-637-2330
22991 La Cadena Dr, Laguna Hills, CA 92653
Fastcast'n Press formula, dental investment, 100-100gm packets.

Ortho-Med, Inc. 800-547-5571
3208 SE 13th Ave, Portland, OR 97202

Royce Medical 800-521-0601
742 Pancho Rd, Camarillo, CA 93012

Sterngold 800-243-9942
23 Frank Mossberg Dr, PO Box 2967, Attleboro, MA 02703

MATERIAL, DENTAL FILLING *(Dental And Oral) 76QOW*

Centrix, Inc. 800-235-5862
770 River Rd, Shelton, CT 06484

Dentalez Group 866-DTE-INFO
101 Lindenwood Dr Ste 225, Valleybrooke Corporate Center
Malvern, PA 19355

Dentsply Canada, Ltd. 800-263-1437
161 Vinyl Ct., Woodbridge, ONT L4L 4A3 Canada

Harry J. Bosworth Company 800-323-4352
7227 Hamlin Ave, Skokie, IL 60076

J. Morita Usa, Inc. 888-566-7482
9 Mason, Irvine, CA 92618
PALFIQUE ESTELITE's uniquely manufactured spherical filler is responsible for the integrity and esthetics of this technologically advanced composite. Palfique Estelite offers the clinician high resistance to abrasion, minimal color change after polymerization and chameleon effect shade matching. Palfique Estelite is available in 14 radiopaque shades including incisal, cervical and two opaque shades. Palfique Estelite LV Flowable is also available in 3 viscosities.

Mizzy, Inc. Of National Keystone 800-333-3131
616 Hollywood Ave, Cherry Hill, NJ 08002
Zoe powder contains zinc oxide and cotton fibers rendering the mix more dense and better suited as a temporary restorative. The fibers reinforce the filling and act to facilitate removal. Zoe liquid contains predominantly eugenol and an additive to accelerate setting

3m Espe Dental Products 949-863-1360
2111 McGaw Ave, Irvine, CA 92614
Tooth colored resin for dental fillings.

MATERIAL, IMPRESSION *(Dental And Oral) 76ELW*

A Plus Dental Lab 215-996-4177
1700 Horizon Dr, --suite 104, Chalfont, PA 18914
Impression material.

Align Technology, Inc. 408-470-1000
881 Martin Ave, Santa Clara, CA 95050
Material, impression.

Aluwax Dental Products Co. 616-895-4385
5260 Edgewater Dr, Allendale, MI 49401
ALUWAX $10.55 to $15.00 per box; bite registration and impression material. Seven different styles available.

American Dental Products, Inc. 800-846-7120
603 Country Club Dr Ste B, Bensenville, IL 60106
Alginate flavoring.

Cadco Dental Products 800-833-8267
600 E Hueneme Rd, Oxnard, CA 93033
$21.10/box for 12 regular tubes of hydrocolloid materials.

D.C.A. (Dental Corporation Of America) 800-638-6684
889 S Matlack St, West Chester, PA 19382
$29.95 per 50 lbs.

Den-Mat Holdings, Llc 805-922-8491
2727 Skyway Dr, Santa Maria, CA 93455
No common name listed.

Denplus Inc. 800-344-4424
205 - 1221 Labadie, Longueuil, QUE J4N 1E2 Canada

Dental Technologies, Inc. 847-677-5500
6901 N Hamlin Ave, Lincolnwood, IL 60712
Polysulfide rubber impression material.

Dentalez Group 866-DTE-INFO
101 Lindenwood Dr Ste 225, Valleybrooke Corporate Center
Malvern, PA 19355

Dentalez Group, Stardental Division 717-291-1161
1816 Colonial Village Ln, Lancaster, PA 17601
Material, dental impression.

Dentsply Canada, Ltd. 800-263-1437
161 Vinyl Ct., Woodbridge, ONT L4L 4A3 Canada

Dshealthcare Inc. 201-871-1232
85 W Forest Ave, Englewood, NJ 07631
Dental impression material.

Dux Dental 800-833-8267
600 E Hueneme Rd, Oxnard, CA 93033
$21.10/box for 12 regular tubes of hydrocolloid materials.

G & H Wire Co. 800-526-1026
2165 Earlywood Dr, Franklin, IN 46131

Gc America, Inc. 708-597-0900
3737 W 127th St, Alsip, IL 60803
Bite registration.

MATERIAL, IMPRESSION *(cont'd)*

Global Dentech Inc. 215-654-1237
1116 Horsham Rd, North Wales, PA 19454
Crown, bridge, model.

Harry J. Bosworth Company 800-323-4352
7227 Hamlin Ave, Skokie, IL 60076
SUPERGEL, SUPERGEL FRESH, SUPER PASTE. Also available, PLASTOPASTE, PLASTOSIL and SILENE, SUPERBITE PASTE, PLASTOGUM and SUPERSIL.

Holmes Dental Corp. 800-322-5577
50 S Penn St, Hatboro, PA 19040
SORE SPOTTER Sore and pressure spotting pastes.

Ivoclar Vivadent, Inc. 800-533-6825
175 Pineview Dr, Amherst, NY 14228
VIRTUAL IMPRESSION SYSTEM VPS impression materials. ACCU-DENT impression system for removable products.

J. Morita Usa, Inc. 888-566-7482
9 Mason, Irvine, CA 92618
PERFECTIM SYSTEMS VPS Impression Materials offer reliable performance and a range of working/setting times to suit any impression procedure. They are also radiopaque. Blue Velvet cures to a hard, plaster-like set to make a precise template for bite registrations or first-step impressions using the H & H cordless impression technique. Flexi-Velvet is a second step companion to Blue Velvet, it captures perfect margins. Other materials include Single Phase Body for one-step/one-material impressions, Final Wash, and Putty.

Kerr Corp. 714-516-7400
28200 Wick Rd, Romulus, MI 48174
Impression material.

Kottler Research Corp. 850-983-0552
2000 Garcon Point Rd, Milton, FL 32583
Material, dental impression.

Lancer Orthodontics, Inc. 760-304-2705
253 Pawnee St, San Marcos, CA 92078
Alginate.

Matech, Inc. 818-367-2472
13000 San Fernando Rd, Sylmar, CA 91342
Kromatica impression material; replica impression material.

Medental Intl. 760-727-5889
3008 Palm Hill Dr, Vista, CA 92084
Various.

Mid-States Laboratories, Inc. 800-247-3669
600 N Saint Francis St, Wichita, KS 67214
$40.75 for ACCU-FORM silicone impression material. $8.00 per dozen of MID-STATES powder/liquid impression material. $8.00 per cartridge of YELLOW STUFF.

Mydent International 800-275-0020
80 Suffolk Ct, Hauppauge, NY 11788
DEFEND Impression Material: Vinyl polysiloxane, all viscosities of impression material. Bite registration (regular and fast set).

Novocol, Inc. 303-665-7535
416 S Taylor Ave, Louisville, CO 80027
Tray adhesive.

Orthodontic Design And Production, Inc. 760-734-3995
1370 Decision St Ste D, Vista, CA 92081
Orthodontic impression material.

Pac-Dent Intl., Inc. 909-839-0888
21078 Commerce Point Dr, Walnut, CA 91789
Various types of impression material.

Parkell, Inc. 800-243-7446
300 Executive Dr, Edgewood, NY 11717
BLU-MOUSSE & CINCH.

Pentron Clinical Technologies 203-265-7397
68-70 North Plains Industrial, Road, Wallingford, CT 06492
Impression material.

Pentron Laboratory Technologies 203-265-7397
53 N Plains Industrial Rd, Wallingford, CT 06492
Impression, material.

Plastodent 718-792-3554
2881 Middletown Rd, Bronx, NY 10461

Preat Corp. 800-232-7732
2976 Long Valley Rd, P.O. Box 1030, Santa Ynez, CA 93460
Playdough used for intraoral impressions.

Pulpdent Corp. 800-343-4342
80 Oakland St, Watertown, MA 02472
Reliner for compound impressions.

MATERIAL, IMPRESSION *(cont'd)*

Rite-Dent Manufacturing Corp. 305-693-8626
3750 E 10th Ct, Hialeah, FL 33013
Varioius types of alginate.

Robert B. Scott Ocularists Of Florida, Inc. 813-977-7676
3500 E Fletcher Ave Ste 509, Tampa, FL 33613
Scleral shades of plastic powder for artificial eyes; moldeye.

Scican 800-667-7733
1440 Don Mills Rd., Toronto, ON M3B 3P9 Canada
Polysil--a superhydrophilic vinyl polysiloxane impression material delivered in automixing dispensing cartridges. Perfectly suited for a variety of impression techniques.

Tak Systems 800-333-9631
14 Kendrick Rd Ste 5, Wareham, MA 02571
Bite Clips are thermalastic pads, pre-set in adjustable frames. Softens to a paste in hot water. Ready in one minute. Turns clear for correct visual placement. Set to firm elastomer. Ideal for bite registrations.

Ultradent Products, Inc. 801-553-4586
505 W 10200 S, South Jordan, UT 84095
Alginate impression material.

Vident 800-828-3839
3150 E Birch St, Brea, CA 92821
Scan White (Dentaco). Optical impression contrast liquid.

Water Pik, Inc. 970-221-6129
1730 E Prospect Rd, Fort Collins, CO 80525
Dental impression material.

Westside Packaging, Llc. 909-570-3508
1700 S Baker Ave Ste A, Ontario, CA 91761
Bite registration,dental impression material.

3m Espe Dental Products 949-863-1360
2111 McGaw Ave, Irvine, CA 92614
$148.65 and $191.35 for impression material; $131.50 for registration material. $38.50 for masking agents.

3m Unitek 800-634-5300
2724 Peck Rd, Monrovia, CA 91016

MATERIAL, IMPRESSION TRAY, RESIN *(Dental And Oral) 76EBH*

Airway Management Inc. 214-369-0978
6116 N Central Expy Ste 605, Dallas, TX 75206
Resin impression tray material.

Buffalo Dental Mfg. Co., Inc. 516-496-7200
159 Lafayette Dr, Syosset, NY 11791
Sheet resin.

Classone Orthodontics, Inc. 806-799-0608
5064 50th St, Lubbock, TX 79414
Various types of impression trays.

Cmp Industries Llc 800-888-5868
413 N Pearl St, Albany, NY 12207
$32.12 per 1000g.

Coltene/Whaledent Inc. 330-916-8858
235 Ascot Pkwy, Cuyahoga Falls, OH 44223
Custom tray material.

Denplus Inc. 800-344-4424
205 - 1221 Labadie, Longueuil, QUE J4N 1E2 Canada

Dental Resources 717-866-7571
52 King St, Myerstown, PA 17067
Vacuum forming material.

Dental Technologies, Inc. 847-677-5500
6901 N Hamlin Ave, Lincolnwood, IL 60712
Impression tray.

Glenroe Technologies 800-237-4060
1912 44th Ave E, Bradenton, FL 34203
Disposable impression tray.

Harry J. Bosworth Company 800-323-4352
7227 Hamlin Ave, Skokie, IL 60076
FASTRAY custom tray material, FASTRAY LC (Light Cure).

Ivoclar Vivadent, Inc. 800-533-6825
175 Pineview Dr, Amherst, NY 14228
ACCU-TRAY, for removable products. LIGHT TRAY, custom tray material.

Kerr Corp. 714-516-7400
28200 Wick Rd, Romulus, MI 48174
Plastic for custom impression tray.

Lang Dental Manufacturing Co., Inc. 800-222-5264
175 Messner Dr, Wheeling, IL 60090
Instant tray mix. JET tray and AURORA custom tray resin in a variety of sizes.

MATERIAL, IMPRESSION TRAY, RESIN *(cont'd)*

Mycone Dental Supply Co. Inc. T/A Keystone Ind-Myerstown 717-866-7571
52 King St, Myerstown, PA 17067
Vacuum forming material.

Pascal Co., Inc. 425-602-3633
2929 Northup Way, Bellevue, WA 98004
Fluoride treatment tray.

Patterson Medical Supply, Inc. 262-387-8720
W68N158 Evergreen Blvd, Cedarburg, WI 53012
Dental tray.

Plastodent 718-792-3554
2881 Middletown Rd, Bronx, NY 10461

Reliance Dental Mfg., Co. 708-597-6694
5805 W 117th Pl, Alsip, IL 60803
Tray material.

Rite-Dent Manufacturing Corp. 305-693-8626
3750 E 10th Ct, Hialeah, FL 33013
Tray acrylic.

Ultradent Products, Inc. 801-553-4586
505 W 10200 S, South Jordan, UT 84095
Resin impression tray material.

Water Pik, Inc. 970-221-6129
1730 E Prospect Rd, Fort Collins, CO 80525
Impression tray adhesive.

3m Unitek 800-634-5300
2724 Peck Rd, Monrovia, CA 91016

MATERIAL, INVESTMENT *(Dental And Oral) 76EGC*

Astron Dental Corporation 847-726-8787
815 Oakwood Rd Ste G, Lake Zurich, IL 60047
Investment chemical.

Dentsply Canada, Ltd. 800-263-1437
161 Vinyl Ct., Woodbridge, ONT L4L 4A3 Canada

General Dental Products, Inc. 888-367-6212
201 Ogden Ave, Ely, NV 89301

Harry J. Bosworth Company 800-323-4352
7227 Hamlin Ave, Skokie, IL 60076

Heraeus Kulzer, Inc. 800-431-1785
99 Business Park Dr, Armonk, NY 10504
Phosphate bonded investment for dental laboratory use in casting dental alloys.

Heraeus Kulzer, Inc., Dental Products Division 574-299-6662
4315 S Lafayette Blvd, South Bend, IN 46614
Material investment.

Ivoclar Vivadent, Inc. 800-533-6825
175 Pineview Dr, Amherst, NY 14228
Sure-Vest.

Somerset Dental Products (Pentron Ceramics, Inc.) 800-496-9600
500 Memorial Dr, Somerset, NJ 08873
Refractor & investment.

Whip-Mix Corporation 800-626-5651
361 Farmington Ave, PO Box 17183, Louisville, KY 40209

MATERIAL, METALLIC-STAINLESS STEEL, TANTALUM, PLATINUM *(Ear/Nose/Throat) 77ESG*

Advance Tabco 800-645-3166
200 Heartland Blvd, Edgewood, NY 11717
Stainless steel carts.

Wilkinson Company, Inc. 208-777-8332
590 S Clearwater Loop Ste C, Post Falls, ID 83854
High purity precious metals and alloys.

MATERIAL, PREPARATION, SKIN *(Hematology) 81KSC*

Enturia, Inc. (Formerly Medi-Flex) 800-523-0502
11400 Tomahawk Creek Pkwy Ste 310, Leawood, KS 66211
MEDI-FLEX now offers our (2% Chlorhexidine in 70% Isopropyl Alcohol) ChloraPrep Frepp for use as a One-Step prepping system. This One-Step procedure cuts down on prep time while reducing the risk of contaminated Blood Cultures by allowing a thorough scrub and delivers bactericidal action to lower skin layers. Blood Culture Prep Kit: Medi-Flex also offers a two-step prepping procedure when preparing the skin for Blood Cultures. Contents: One 70%Isopropyl Alcohol Frepp and one 2% Tincture of Iodine Sepp. FREPP/SEPP Kit : Frepp- Povidone Iodine, 2% Aqueous, SEPP-10% Povidone Iodine.

MATERIAL, PTFE/CARBON, MAXILLOFACIAL *(Surgery) 79KKY*

Kerr Group 800-524-3577
1400 Holcomb Bridge Rd, Roswell, GA 30076

Osteogenics Biomedical, Inc. 806-796-1923
4620 71st St Bldg 78-79, Lubbock, TX 79424
Bone graft extender.

MATERIAL, RAW, PRODUCTION *(General) 80WJB*

Aalto Scientific Ltd. 760-431-7922
1959 Kellogg Ave, Carlsbad, CA 92008
Purified human enzymes and proteins.

Aetrex Worldwide, Inc 800-526-2739
414 Alfred Ave, Teaneck, NJ 07666
Many materials used in the manufacture of orthotics and prosthetics including PLASTAZOTE, CARBOPLAST II, DERMAPLAST, S.T.S., THERMOCORK, ORTHO FELT, REFLEX and THERMOSKY.

Graham Medical Products/Div. Of Little Rapids Corp 866-429-1408
2273 Larsen Rd, Green Bay, WI 54303

Kamiya Biomedical Company 206-575-8068
12779 Gateway Dr S, Tukwila, WA 98168
Enzymes, substrates, antibodies, antigens and other biological products for diagnostics.

Medical Concepts Development 800-345-0644
2500 Ventura Dr, Saint Paul, MN 55125
Materials include single- and double-coated adhesive films, nonwovens, and soft metals. Company specializes in wide-web converting of roll goods.

Mylan Technologies, Inc. 800-532-5226
110 Lake St, Saint Albans, VT 05478
Raw materials for transdermal and synthetic wound dressings, films and laminates.

Pepin Manufacturing, Inc. 800-291-6505
1875 S Highway 61, Lake City, MN 55041
Large selection of various types, including tapes, adhesives, films, laminates, etc.

United Chemical Technologies, Inc. 800-385-3153
2731 Bartram Rd, Bristol, PA 19007
Specialty silanes, silicone fluids, and silicone elastomers.

MATERIAL, RESTORATION, AESTHETIC, EXTERNAL *(Surgery) 79GBI*

3m Espe Dental Products 949-863-1360
2111 McGaw Ave, Irvine, CA 92614
$48.25/refills for posterior restorative.

MATERIAL, TOOTH SHADE, RESIN *(Dental And Oral) 76EBF*

American Dental Products, Inc. 800-846-7120
603 Country Club Dr Ste B, Bensenville, IL 60106
Light cure composite resin sure paste w/fluoride.

American Medical Technologies, Inc. 361-289-1145
5655 Bear Ln, Corpus Christi, TX 78405
PAC (Plasma Arc Curing) LIGHT high speed curing system. This device will cure most composites in 10 seconds or less and many in only 3 seconds. The PAC also effectively activates most power-bleaching formulas, providing for a faster teethnwhitening process.

American Tooth Industries 800-235-4639
1200 Stellar Dr, Oxnard, CA 93033
JUSTI tooth shade guides.

Biomat Sciences, Inc. 866-4-BIOMAT
7210A Corporate Ct, Frederick, MD 21703
Advanced composite for tooth restoration.

Bisco, Inc. 847-534-6000
1100 W Irving Park Rd, Schaumburg, IL 60193
Dental post cement.

Coltene/Whaledent Inc. 330-916-8858
235 Ascot Pkwy, Cuyahoga Falls, OH 44223
Various.

Den-Mat Holdings, Llc 805-922-8491
2727 Skyway Dr, Santa Maria, CA 93455
No common name listed.

Denali R&D Corporation 781-826-9190
134 Old Washington St, Hanover, MA 02339
Core material.

Denmed Technologies, Inc. 866-433-6633
1531 W Orangewood Ave, Orange, CA 92868
Dental curing light and tooth whitening

MATERIAL, TOOTH SHADE, RESIN *(cont'd)*

Dent Zar, Inc. 800-444-1241
6362 Hollywood Blvd Ste 214, Los Angeles, CA 90028
Filling materials.

Dental Technologies, Inc. 847-677-5500
6901 N Hamlin Ave, Lincolnwood, IL 60712
Composite restorative material.

Dentalez Group 866-DTE-INFO
101 Lindenwood Dr Ste 225, Valleybrooke Corporate Center Malvern, PA 19355

Dentsply Canada, Ltd. 800-263-1437
161 Vinyl Ct., Woodbridge, ONT L4L 4A3 Canada

Gc America, Inc. 708-597-0900
3737 W 127th St, Alsip, IL 60803
Composite.

George Taub Products & Fusion Co., Inc. 800-828-2634
277 New York Ave, Jersey City, NJ 07307
Minute Stains, for modifying the shade of acrylic or composite resins. Makes lifeless temporary resins look lifelike.

Harry J. Bosworth Company 800-323-4352
7227 Hamlin Ave, Skokie, IL 60076

Ivoclar Vivadent, Inc. 800-533-6825
175 Pineview Dr, Amherst, NY 14228
HELIOMOLAR - Regular, Flow and Heavy Body. TETRIC CERAM - Regular, Flow and Heavy Body. COMPOGLASS - Compomer-based filling materials.

Kerr Corp. 714-516-7400
28200 Wick Rd, Romulus, MI 48174
Tooth resin.

Kerr Corp. 949-255-8766
1717 W Collins Ave, Orange, CA 92867
Dental composite restorative.

Lang Dental Manufacturing Co., Inc. 800-222-5264
175 Messner Dr, Wheeling, IL 60090
JET tooth shade. SPLINTLINE and BIS-JET temporary crown and bridge materials in a variety of sizes.

Lee Pharmaceuticals 626-442-3141
1434 Santa Anita Ave, El Monte, CA 91733
Adhesive composite tooth restoratives (resin + enamel conditioner).

Medental Intl. 760-727-5889
3008 Palm Hill Dr, Vista, CA 92084
Various.

Novocol, Inc. 303-665-7535
416 S Taylor Ave, Louisville, CO 80027
Composite, restorative material systems.

Oratech, Llc 801-553-4493
475 W 10200 S, South Jordan, UT 84095
Tooth shade resin material.

Pac-Dent Intl., Inc. 909-839-0888
21078 Commerce Point Dr, Walnut, CA 91789
Composite resin.

Pentron Clinical Technologies 203-265-7397
68-70 North Plains Industrial, Road, Wallingford, CT 06492
Tooth shade resin material.

Pentron Laboratory Technologies 203-265-7397
53 N Plains Industrial Rd, Wallingford, CT 06492
Restorative composite.

Plastodent 718-792-3554
2881 Middletown Rd, Bronx, NY 10461

Premier Dental Products Co. 888-670-6100
1710 Romano Dr, PO Box 4500, Plymouth Meeting, PA 19462

Prime Dental Manufacturing, Inc. 773-539-5927
3735 W Belmont Ave, Chicago, IL 60618
Prime-dent composite restorative material.

Protech Professional Products, Inc. 561-493-9818
2900 Commerce Park Dr Ste 10, Boynton Beach, FL 33426
Tooth acrylic.

Rite-Dent Manufacturing Corp. 305-693-8626
3750 E 10th Ct, Hialeah, FL 33013
Various types of dental composite with enamel bonding.

Ultradent Products, Inc. 801-553-4586
505 W 10200 S, South Jordan, UT 84095
Flowable composite/sealent.

MATERIAL, TOOTH SHADE, RESIN *(cont'd)*

Vident 800-828-3839
3150 E Birch St, Brea, CA 92821
VITA 3D-Master, VITA Classical Shade Guide and VITA Easyshade Digital Shade-Taking Device; Lumibond Bonding & Cementation System; Vita Zeta Crown & Bridge Acrylic Veneering System.

Water Pik, Inc. 970-221-6129
1730 E Prospect Rd, Fort Collins, CO 80525
Composite crown build-up material.

Westside Packaging, Llc. 909-570-3508
1700 S Baker Ave Ste A, Ontario, CA 91761
Tooth shade resin material.

3m Espe Dental Products 949-863-1360
2111 McGaw Ave, Irvine, CA 92614

3m Unitek 800-634-5300
2724 Peck Rd, Monrovia, CA 91016

MATERIAL, TRAINING, AUDIOVISUAL *(General) 80VBD*

Air-Tite Products Co., Inc. 800-231-7762
565 Central Dr Ste 101, Virginia Beach, VA 23454
Coastal Communications various training programs to enhance employee awareness: OSHA Bloodborne Pathogen Standard; Infectious Hazardous Waste; Nursing Assessment.

Armstrong Medical Industries, Inc. 800-323-4220
575 Knightsbridge Pkwy, Lincolnshire, IL 60069
Emergency medical training and ACLS videotapes.

Bio-Feedback Systems, Inc. 303-444-1411
2736 47th St, Boulder, CO 80301
$34.95 or $40.00 per set of three cassette relaxation programs. $17.50 per cassette out of 15 titles of self-help programs. Includes both subliminal and supraliminal formats.

Current Medicine Group Llc 800-427-1796
400 Market St Ste 700, Philadelphia, PA 19106
Including bound books and slide atlases.

Eagle Vision, Inc. 800-222-7584
8500 Wolf Lake Dr Ste 110, Memphis, TN 38133
Instructional video CDs for physician and patient, including dry eye education, Graether information, Monostent.

Eschenbach Optik Of America, Inc. 800-487-5389
904 Ethan Allen Hwy, Ridgefield, CT 06877

Health Imaging Corp. 800-468-7874
1011 Campus Dr, Mundelein, IL 60060

Health Learning Systems, Inc. 800-388-1000
402 Interpace Pkwy, Wayne Interchange Plaza II, Parsippany, NJ 07054
SAGES surgical education program.

Ibiom Instruments Ltd. 450-678-5468
6640 Barry St., Brossard, QUE J4Z 1T8 Canada
Video teaching system for radiology and cardiology. $10,365 for video unit TECHNI-LAB I model TL-10; $15,338 for video unit TECHNI-LAB II model TL-10-21; $19,964 for video unit TECHNI-LAB III model TL-10-35; Standard unit consist of video table, external circular lamp, imbedded light box, compact video camera, electronic push-button module for motorized zoom lens, large b&w video monitor/receiver, small b&w video monitor.

Lab Safety Supply, Inc. 800-356-0783
401 S Wright Rd, Janesville, WI 53546

Lemaitre Vascular, Inc. 781-221-2266
63 2nd Ave, Burlington, MA 01803
LEMAITRE IN SITU videotape, audiotape, book, CDrom.

Lifegas Llc 866-543-3427
1500 Indian Trail Lilburn Rd, Norcross, GA 30093
Special Services: LifeGas provides services to support its medical products including OSHA compliance and safety training; up-to-date information on regulatory standards; ongoing technical and clinical expertise; standardized cylinder packaging and labeling; local Hazardous Materials Emergency Response team. CEU programs for healthcare practitioners.

Mammatech Corp. 800-626-2273
930 NW 8th Ave, Gainesville, FL 32601
$350.00 for clinical breast exam videocassette with 3 breast models.

Maramed Orthopedic Systems 800-327-5830
2480 W 82nd St, No. 8, Hialeah, FL 33016

Medcom, Inc. 800-877-1443
6060 Phyllis Dr, Cypress, CA 90630
Audiovisual education programming. Web-based CME/CE courses with learning management system.

MATERIAL, TRAINING, AUDIOVISUAL *(cont'd)*

Medfilms, Inc. 800-535-5593
4910 W Monte Carlo Dr, Tucson, AZ 85745
Including environment of care, operating room safety, and infection control.

Medical Safety Systems Inc. 888-803-9303
230 White Pond Dr, Akron, OH 44313
OSHA compliance training video.

Optp 888-819-0121
3800 Annapolis Ln N Ste 165, PO Box 47009, Minneapolis, MN 55447
Treat Your Own Back videocassette; $54.00 for The Lumbar Spine book, $129..95 for Low Back Exercises poster.

Passy-Muir Inc. 800-634-5397
4521 Campus Dr, Irvine, CA 92612
Educational materials for clinicians working with tracheotomized and ventilator-dependent patients. Materials include the comprehensive Passy-Muir™ one-day continuing-educaton seminar manual and videotape set, Tracheostomy T. O. M.™ teaching model, Toby Tracheasaurus™ & Toby Tote Pediatric Communication Therapy toys, free Resource Guide, free Clinical Inservice Outline, free Clinical Inservice Video or DVD, free Benefits CD-ROM, and free research literature packet on the Passy-Muir Tracheostomy & Ventilator Swallowing and Speaking Valves.

Pritchett & Hull Associates Inc. 800-241-4925
3440 Oakcliff Rd Ste 110, Atlanta, GA 30340
Patient-education materials--books, slides, CD-ROMs, etc.

Sound Feelings 818-757-0600
18375 Ventura Blvd # 8000, Tarzana, CA 91356
Music-medicine as adjunct for specific conditions.

V.I.E.W. Video 800-843-9843
34 E 23rd St, New York, NY 10010
$24.98 for videotape of how exercise can beat arthritis: low impact aerobic exercise is effective in decreasing pain and stiffness; increased self-sufficiency and improved fitness. Nine gentle exercises set to music. Childbirth Part 1- Pregnancy and Pre-natal Period, $29.98 for video tape 78 minutes covering preparing for pregnancy, nutrition, and exercise, and the psychology of pregnancy. By Dr. John Tyson, medical scientist and clinician. Childbirth Part 2 - Delivery and Post-natal Period, $29.98 for videotape 72 minutes covering the hospital, exercise, delivery, and post-natal care. By Dr. John Tyson, medical scientist and clinician.

Veritech Corporation 413-525-3368
168 Denslow Rd, East Longmeadow, MA 01028
Interactive video simulator; Learning Exchange interactive video system; CME/CEU certification capability, interactive sales education meetings.

Wrs Group, Ltd. 800-299-3366
5045 Franklin Ave, Waco, TX 76710
Wall charts, anatomical and patient care models.

MATRIX, DENTAL *(Dental And Oral) 76DZN*

Abrasive Technology, Inc. 740-548-4100
8400 Green Meadows Dr N, Lewis Center, OH 43035
Dental matrix band.

Accor, Inc. 216-381-2951
1375 Yellowstone Rd, Cleveland Heights, OH 44121
Multisize dental matrix.

Arnel Healthcare, Inc. 516-783-1939
1523 Dewey Ave, North Bellmore, NY 11710
Matrix bands.

Arnel, Inc. 516-486-7098
73 High St, Hempstead, NY 11550
Various.

C.E.J. Dental Products Inc. 949-493-2449
32332 Camino Capistrano Ste 101, San Juan Capistrano, CA 92675
Dental matrix, assorted sizes, metal and polymer types.

Den-Mat Holdings, Llc 805-922-8491
2727 Skyway Dr, Santa Maria, CA 93455
No common name listed.

Dental Usa, Inc. 815-363-8003
5005 McCullom Lake Rd, McHenry, IL 60050
Dental matrix.

Dentalez Group 866-DTE-INFO
101 Lindenwood Dr Ste 225, Valleybrooke Corporate Center
Malvern, PA 19355

Dentalez Group, Stardental Division 717-291-1161
1816 Colonial Village Ln, Lancaster, PA 17601
Intra oral device for snoring and sleep apnea.

MATRIX, DENTAL *(cont'd)*

Dentsply Canada, Ltd. 800-263-1437
161 Vinyl Ct., Woodbridge, ONT L4L 4A3 Canada

Diamond Dental, Inc. 770-381-3799
3545 Cruse Rd Ste 203, Lawrenceville, GA 30044
Dental instruments hand-held dental instruments.

Ellman International, Inc. 800-835-5355
3333 Royal Ave, Rockville Centre, NY 11572

H & H Co. 909-390-0373
4435 E Airport Dr Ste 108, Ontario, CA 91761
Instruments, dental hand.

Ivoclar Vivadent, Inc. 800-533-6825
175 Pineview Dr, Amherst, NY 14228

Lorvic Corp. 800-325-1881
13705 Shoreline Ct E, Earth City, MO 63045
Matrix bands.

Miltex Dental Technologies, Inc. 516-576-6022
589 Davies Dr, York, PA 17402
Various dental matrix materials, shells, and bands.

Moyco Technologies, Inc. 800-331-8837
200 Commerce Dr, Montgomeryville, PA 18936

Pascal Co., Inc. 425-602-3633
2929 Northup Way, Bellevue, WA 98004
Dental matrix strips and contours.

Pulpdent Corp. 800-343-4342
80 Oakland St, Watertown, MA 02472
No common name listed.

Rite-Dent Manufacturing Corp. 305-693-8626
3750 E 10th Ct, Hialeah, FL 33013
Various types of matrix bands.

Ultradent Products, Inc. 801-553-4586
505 W 10200 S, South Jordan, UT 84095
Matrix.

Water Pik, Inc. 970-221-6129
1730 E Prospect Rd, Fort Collins, CO 80525
Various instruments and models.

3m Espe Dental Products 949-863-1360
2111 McGaw Ave, Irvine, CA 92614
$23.10 per unit.

MATTRESS, AIR FLOTATION *(General) 80FNM*

Acclaim Medical Manufacturing Llc 856-234-3216
1000 Atlantic Ave Ste 529, Camden, NJ 08104
Millennium series powered support surfaces amm series powered support surfaces.

Aggressive Solutions, Inc. 972-242-2164
1735 N Interstate 35E, Carrollton, TX 75006
Alternating pressure mattress system.

Ambu A/S 457-225-2210
6740 Baymeadow Dr, Glen Burnie, MD 21060
Immobilizing vaccum matters.

Amf Support Surfaces, Inc. 951-549-6800
1691 N Delilah St, Corona, CA 92879
Low air loss mattress.

Asi Medical Equipment, Ltd. 800-527-0443
1735 N Interstate 35E, Carrollton, TX 75006
Mattress replacements for air support therapy.

Bergad Mattress 888-476-8664
747 Eljer Way, Ford City, PA 16226
Isoform mattress.

Dynamedics Corp. 519-433-7474
30 Adelaide St N, Ste. 205, London, ONT N6B 3N5 Canada
Specialty support surface

Encompass Therapeutic Support Systems 818-546-2466
500 N Central Ave Ste 900, Glendale, CA 91203
Alternating pressure mattress system.

Gaymar Industries, Inc. 800-828-7341
10 Centre Dr, Orchard Park, NY 14127
SPR.PLUS, SOF.CARE, SOF.MATT low air-loss mattress overlay. Provides pressure relief and moisture control. SOF.MATT powered low air-loss mattress replacements.

Genadyne Biotechnologies, Inc. 516-487-8787
65 Watermill Ln, Great Neck, NY 11021
Air pump/alternating pressure, air flotation mattress.

MATTRESS, AIR FLOTATION *(cont'd)*

Hill-Rom Manufacturing, Inc. 800-638-2546
4349 Corporate Rd, Charleston, SC 29405
ACUCAIR continuous airflow system.

Hill-Rom, Inc. 812-934-7777
4115 Dorchester Rd Unit 600, North Charleston, SC 29405
Air mattress.

Hovertech International 800-471-2776
513 S Clewell St, Fountain Hill, PA 18015
HOVERMATT Lateral Transfer and Repositioning Air Mattress reduces friction to make transferring a patient 90% easier. There is no weight limit and the HoverMatt is usable in all hospital departments.

Howard Medical Company 800-443-1444
1690 N Elston Ave, Chicago, IL 60642
$80.00 for 3 layered air mattress with air loss detector, and $75 for air pump.

Huntleigh Healthcare Llc. 800-223-1218
40 Christopher Way, Eatontown, NJ 07724
ALPHAXCELL system uses powered air flotation to support the patient on inflating and deflating air cells. Replaces specialty beds in the acute, home or alternate site environments.

James Consolidated, Inc. 800-884-3317
PO Box 3483, 1867 Ygnacio Valley Rd, Walnut Creek, CA 94598
Lateral rotation. Volkner turning system, Volkner Turning System (VTS), James Air.

Kap Medical 951-340-4360
1395 Pico St, Corona, CA 92881
Low air loss mattress system.

Kinetic Concepts, Inc. 800-275-4524
8023 Vantage Dr, San Antonio, TX 78230
Pressure reducing mattress.

Marcon Group, Inc. 800-547-5021
655 Du Bois St Ste D, San Rafael, CA 94901
Alternating pressure air flotation mattress.

Medical Depot 516-998-4600
99 Seaview Blvd, Port Washington, NY 11050
Air flotation mattress.

Medisearch P.R., Inc. 787-864-0684
Machete Industrial Center, Guayama, PR 00784
Alternating pressure reduction pump and pad system.

Mellen Air Manufacturing, Inc. 800-770-6264
2601 E 28th St Ste 307, Signal Hill, CA 90755
Low Air Loss Mattress, Rem Air 777, Rem Air 2000, Rem Air 777XL

Mrc Industries Inc. 516-328-6900
85 Denton Ave, New Hyde Park, NY 11040
Various types of mattresses.

Northwest Bedding Co. 509-244-3000
6102 S Hayford Rd, Spokane, WA 99224
Various orthopedic mattresses.

Nova Health Systems, Inc. 800-225-NOVA
1001 Broad St, Utica, NY 13501

Pyramid Industries, Llc 888-343-3352
3911 Schaad Rd Unit 102, Knoxville, TN 37921
ULTRA-CARE- A product line of alternating pressure and low airloss mattresses, including bariatric and turning mattresses to reduce the risk or treat existing pressure ulcers.

Rogers Foam Corporation 617-623-3010
609 Boone Trail Road, Clinchport, VA 24244

Scott Technology Llc 203-888-2783
1 Jacks Hill Rd, Oxford, CT 06478
Alternating pressure mattress.

Sentech Medical Systems, Inc. 954-340-0500
4200 NW 120th Ave, Coral Springs, FL 33065
Alternating low air loss mastress overlay.

Span-America Medical Systems, Inc. 800-888-6752
70 Commerce Ctr, Greenville, SC 29615
Pressure Guard Turn Select, Pressure Guard CFT, Pressure Guard APM2, PressureGuard Easy Air

Sunflower Medical L.L.C. 888-321-3382
206 Jerrerson, Ellis, KS 67637
Various.

Sunrise Medical 800-333-4000
7477 Dry Creek Pkwy, Longmont, CO 80503

MATTRESS, AIR FLOTATION *(cont'd)*

Tele-Made Disposables, Inc. 888-822-4299
3215 Huffman Eastgate Rd, Huffman, TX 77336
Powered flotation therapy mattress.

Tempur Production Usa, Inc. 276-431-7174
203 Tempur Pedic Dr Ste 102, Duffield, VA 24244
Low air-loss mattress.

Tempur-Medical, Inc. 888-255-3302
1713 Jaggie Fox Way, Lexington, KY 40511
TempurAP, TempurAIR.

Trlby Innovative L.L.C. 860-482-6848
65 New Litchfield St, Torrington, CT 06790
Unisoft.

Wcw,Inc 518-686-0725
1 Mechanic St, Hoosick Falls, NY 12090
Mattress, air flotation, alternating pressure.

Wheelchairs Of Kansas 800-537-6454
204 W 2nd St, Ellis, KS 67637
Low Air Loss Mattress has the option of static or alternating pressure & is a true low air loss system. Capacity of 1000 lbs., comes with a dark blue.

MATTRESS, ALTERNATING PRESSURE (OR PADS)
(Physical Med) 89ILA

Bio Compression Systems, Inc. 800-888-0908
120 W Commercial Ave, Moonachie, NJ 07074

Bodypoint, Inc. 800-547-5716
558 1st Ave S Ste 300, Seattle, WA 98104
Dreama Sleep and Rest Positioning System. Available in single-bed and crib size.

Casco Manufacturing Solutions, Inc. 800-843-1339
3107 Spring Grove Ave, Cincinnati, OH 45225

Essential Medical Supply, Inc. 800-826-8423
6420 Hazeltine National Dr, Orlando, FL 32822
ENDURANCE D9000 Deluxe APP, D8000 Standard APP, D8800 Pad.

Fabrite Laminating Corp. 973-777-1406
70 Passaic St, Wood Ridge, NJ 07075

Gaymar Industries, Inc. 800-828-7341
10 Centre Dr, Orchard Park, NY 14127
PILLO-PUMP, AIRFLO PLUS, alternating pressure therapy, with or without low air-loss. SOF.MATT pressure relieving powered mattress replacements.

Genesis Manufacturing, Inc. 317-485-7887
720 E Broadway St, Fortville, IN 46040
Contract Radio-Frequency (RF) Welding. From development to manufacturing and packaging.

Grant Airmass Corporation 800-243-5237
126 Chestnut Hill Rd, PO Box 3456, Stamford, CT 06903

Huntleigh Healthcare Llc. 800-223-1218
40 Christopher Way, Eatontown, NJ 07724
$285.00 for institutional pump, $198.00 for homecare pump; 2 types of mattress pads (single-patient use) - bubble pad or AIR-O-PAD (ventilated). Also pressure relieving hospital mattress-PG II $360.00. Pressure relieving nursing home mattress-PG I $450.00.

Tex-Tenn Corp. 800-251-3027
108 Kwickway Ln # 118, PO Box 8219, Gray, TN 37615
Decubitus pads, bed pad fabrics.

Tuffcare 800-367-6160
3999 E La Palma Ave, Anaheim, CA 92807

MATTRESS, BED *(General) 80RGG*

Alimed, Inc. 800-225-2610
297 High St, Dedham, MA 02026

American Health Systems 800-234-6655
PO Box 26688, Greenville, SC 29616
ULTRAFORM; mattresses designed for pressure relief and treatment/prevention of pressure ulcers in high risk patients. Products range from Economy Institutional Mattresses up to Multi-Zone Therapeutic Stage 1 and 2 Treatment Mattresses.High denisty foam cores with IST Interface Surface Technology Design.Ultraform ELITE mattress comes standard with SoftCell Heel Zone. Core design has 600 individual polymer cells to move and shift with patient to prevent shearing forces and pressure. All covers are of healthcare fabrics with superior MVTR ratings.

Asi Medical Equipment, Ltd. 800-527-0443
1735 N Interstate 35E, Carrollton, TX 75006

MATTRESS, BED *(cont'd)*

Atd-American Co. 800-523-2300
135 Greenwood Ave, Wyncote, PA 19095

B.G. Industries, Inc. 800-822-8288
8550 Balboa Blvd Ste 214, Northridge, CA 91325
MAXIFLEX, PERMAFLEX. Inner spring mattress.

Back Support Systems 800-669-2225
67684 San Andreas St, Desert Hot Springs, CA 92240
CONFOURM, with memory foam, theraputic cover and overlay for reduction of bed sores and back and neck pain. Memory foam overlay or mattress with magnets is available in six standard sizes.

Basic American Medical Products 800-849-6664
2935A Northeast Pkwy, Atlanta, GA 30360

Bruin Plastics Co. 800-556-7764
61 Joslin Rd, Glendale, RI 02826

Casco Manufacturing Solutions, Inc. 800-843-1339
3107 Spring Grove Ave, Cincinnati, OH 45225
C-MATT brand Sealed and Comfort mattresses.

Chestnut Ridge Foam, Inc. 800-234-2734
PO Box 781, Latrobe, PA 15650
Pressure Reduction Healthcare mattresses manufactured and sold directly to group purchasing organizations or facilities for maximum value. Traditional and fire-resistant mattresses for general healthcare and long-term care facilities.

Colonial Scientific Ltd. 902-468-1811
201 Brownlow Ave., Unit 52, Dartmouth, NS B3B-1W2 Canada

Comfort Care Products Corp. 803-321-0020
258 Industrial Park Rd, Newberry, SC 29108
Pressure-reduction antimicrobial, fire-resistant cover and made from high-resiliency foam treated to be antimicrobial and flame retardant. FLEXI-COMFORT antimicrobial and flame-retardant staph chek ticking. Solid foam core with 1 in. convoluted peaks top and bottom, also treated to be antimicrobial and flame retardant.

Country Craft Furniture, Inc. 800-569-1968
5318 Railroad Ave, Flowery Branch, GA 30542

Crest Healthcare Supply 800-328-8908
195 3rd St, Dassel, MN 55325

Elite Mattress Manufacturing 800-332-5878
4999 Rear Fyler Avenue, St. Louis, MO 63139

Gaymar Industries, Inc. 800-828-7341
10 Centre Dr, Orchard Park, NY 14127
TOP GARD foam pressure reducing mattress replacements. Symmetric.Aire non-powered self-adjusting mattress replacement system.

Hard Manufacturing Co. 800-873-4273
230 Grider St, Buffalo, NY 14215
$58 to $193 for antibacterial mattresses; sizes for infant cribs, youth and adult beds.

Herculite Products, Inc. 800-772-0036
PO Box 435, Emigsville, PA 17318
SURE-CHEK Healthcare fabric with bidirectional stretch developed for pressure management on mattresses, cushions and pads. SURE-CHEK COMFORT is healthcare fabric for use on mattresses, pads and cushions.

Hill-Rom Holdings, Inc. 800-445-3730
1069 State Road 46 E, Batesville, IN 47006

Hill-Rom Manufacturing, Inc. 800-638-2546
4349 Corporate Rd, Charleston, SC 29405

Huntleigh Healthcare Llc. 800-223-1218
40 Christopher Way, Eatontown, NJ 07724
DFS, DFS2, AUTOEXCEL, ALPHA ACTIVE, ALPHACARE, mattress replacement system for the prevention and management of decubitus problems. The system is designed for home use and fits most types of bedframes. It offers ideal pressure relieving characteristics and utilizes the AutoMatt sensor to optimize support pressures.

Invacare Corporation 800-333-6900
1 Invacare Way, Elyria, OH 44035
INVACARE Phomvantage

M.C. Healthcare Products, Inc. 800-268-8671
4658 Ontario St., Beamsville, ONT L0R 1B4 Canada
Pressure Reduction - unique layered design of contoured modular of polyurethane foam; have excellent pressure reduction capability. Pressure Relief - layered high density polyurethane foam are contoured to provide reduction of decubitus, comfort and durability. CONTOUR, ULTIMA, CIRRUS series.

Md International, Inc. 305-669-9003
11300 NW 41st St, Doral, FL 33178

MATTRESS, BED *(cont'd)*

Melrose Mattress, Inc. 800-500-0233
8241 Lankershim Blvd, North Hollywood, CA 91605
Hospital mattresses. Custom sizes and shapes available.

Milwaukee Mattress & Furniture 800-373-1462
423 N 3rd St, Milwaukee, WI 53203
5 types - Flex-Master units designed to hinge from $134.00 to $191.00 each.

Mip Inc. 800-361-4964
9100 Ray Lawson Blvd., Montreal, QC H1J-1K8 Canada
Theraputic mattresses, INTEGRIDERM.

Newschoff Chairs, Inc. 800-203-8916
909 N.E. St., Sheboygan, WI 53081

Nk Medical Products Inc. 800-274-2742
10123 Main St, PO Box 627, Clarence, NY 14031
Foam Mattresses for Cribs, Bassinets and Beds

Pedicraft, Inc. 800-223-7649
4134 Saint Augustine Rd, Jacksonville, FL 32207
PEDI-MATTRESS; $180.00 to $240.00 per unit. Custom sizes available.

Relax-A-Flex, Inc. 912-598-7010
7 Ramshorn Ct., Skidaway Island, Savannah, GA 31411-1327

Roho Group, The 800-851-3449
100 N Florida Ave, Belleville, IL 62221

Sealy Inc. 800-697-3259
1 Office Parkway Rd, Trinity, NC 27370

Span-America Medical Systems, Inc. 800-888-6752
70 Commerce Ctr, Greenville, SC 29615
PRESSURE GUARD and GEO MATTRESS replacement mattresses are available in a wide range of sizes.

Standard Textile 800-999-0400
1 Knollcrest Dr, Cincinnati, OH 45237

Stryker Medical 800-869-0770
3800 E Centre Ave, Portage, MI 49002

Sunrise Medical 800-333-4000
7477 Dry Creek Pkwy, Longmont, CO 80503

The Neurological Research And Development Group 800-327-6759
115 Rotary Dr, West Hazleton, PA 18202
Bed mattresses and stretcher pads.

Val Med 800-242-5355
3700 Desire Pkwy, Ace Bayou Group, New Orleans, LA 70126

Waterloo Bedding Co. Ltd. 800-203-4293
141 Weber St. S, Waterloo, ONT N2J 2A9 Canada

Zimmer Holdings, Inc. 800-613-6131
1800 W Center St, PO Box 708, Warsaw, IN 46580

MATTRESS, IMMOBILIZATION *(General) 80WLB*

Cfi Medical Solutions (Contour Fabricators, Inc.) 810-750-5300
14241 N Fenton Rd, Fenton, MI 48430
Infant immobilizer.

Hartwell Medical Corp. 800-633-5900
6352 Corte Del Abeto Ste J, Carlsbad, CA 92011
The EVAC U SPLINT mattress provides full-body immobilization and transport of patients with possible spinal injuries. Offers the maximum amount of comfort and stabilization. Vacuum mattress conforms to the shape of the patient, eliminating pressure sores due to transport on a hard surface. Used for back, hip, pelvis, and suspected spinal injuries.

MATTRESS, NON-POWERED FLOTATION THERAPY
(Physical Med) 89IKY

Action Products, Inc. 800-228-7763
954 Sweeney Dr, Hagerstown, MD 21740
Reusable in the hospital, long term care facility and homecare markets. Easy to use. Effective protection from decubitus ulcers. Wide range of sizes. Custom sizes available. Price range from $125 to $525.

Advanced Urethane Technologies, Inc. 630-293-0780
1750 Downs Dr, West Chicago, IL 60185
Foam accessories & pads.

Alternative Products 904-378-9081
5351 Ramona Blvd Ste 7, Jacksonville, FL 32205
Static mattress overlay.

Amf Support Surfaces, Inc. 951-549-6800
1691 N Delilah St, Corona, CA 92879
Accumax quantum,nonpowered flotation therapy mattress.

MATTRESS, NON-POWERED FLOTATION THERAPY *(cont'd)*

Anatomic Concepts, Inc. 951-549-6800
1691 N Delilah St, Corona, CA 92879
Operating-room bed; comfort pads; bed pad protective sleeve.

Capital Bedding, Incorporated 757-224-0177
5262 South Raymond Street, Verona, MS 38879
Standard hospital medical mattress.

Confortaire Inc 662-842-2966
2133 S Veterans Blvd, Tupelo, MS 38804
Therapeutic foam mattress, non-powered.

Creative Bedding Technologies, Inc. 815-444-9088
300 Exchange Dr Ste A, Crystal Lake, IL 60014
Gel overlay pad.

Creative Foam Medical Systems 800-446-4644
405 Industrial Dr, Bremen, IN 46506
Various types of coated foam mattress, flotation therapy pads.

Dynamic Systems, Inc. 828-683-3523
235 Sunlight Dr, Leicester, NC 28748

Ehob, Inc. 800-899-5553
250 N Belmont Ave, Indianapolis, IN 46222
WAFFLE brand air cushions management of pressure ulcers. Waffle brand Treatment Overlay, mattress overlay, using static air to treat stage III and IV pressure ulcers. Waffle Mattress Replacement System, mattresss replacement treats stage III, IV pressure ulcers using static air technology.

Federal Foam Technologies, Inc. 715-490-7788
312 Industrial Rd, Ellsworth, WI 54011
Mattress.

Forum Industries Inc. 210-225-9600
1903 Hormel Dr, Kirby, TX 78219

Gaymar Industries, Inc. 800-828-7341
10 Centre Dr, Orchard Park, NY 14127
SOF.CARE static air bed cushion and SOFCARE inflator or monitor. ISOFLEX, non-powered mattress replacement designed to treat and prevent pressure ulcers.

Genadyne Biotechnologies, Inc. 516-487-8787
65 Watermill Ln, Great Neck, NY 11021
Non powered mattress.

Grand Rapids Foam Technologies 877-GET-GRFT
2788 Remico St SW, Wyoming, MI 49519
Hospital mattress.

Hawaii Medical, Llc 781-826-5565
750 Corporate Park Dr, Pembroke, MA 02359

Hill-Rom Manufacturing, Inc. 800-638-2546
4349 Corporate Rd, Charleston, SC 29405
PRIMA prevention mattress series.

Joerns Healthcare, Inc. 715-341-3600
1032 N Fourth St, Baldwyn, MS 38824
Various.

Keen Mobility Company 503-285-9090
6500 NE Halsey St Ste B, Portland, OR 97213

Kinetic Concepts, Inc. 800-275-4524
8023 Vantage Dr, San Antonio, TX 78230
Pressure reducing mattress.

Kreg Medical, Inc. 312-275-7002
2240 W Walnut St, Chicago, IL 60612
Mattress.

Leeder Group, Inc. 305-436-5030
8508 NW 66th St, Miami, FL 33166
Mattress flotation therapy overlay, non powered.

Medical Depot 516-998-4600
99 Seaview Blvd, Port Washington, NY 11050
Flotation mattress.

Medisearch P.R., Inc. 787-864-0684
Machete Industrial Center, Guayama, PR 00784
Staic air mattress and accessories.

Merlo Co., Llc. 800-290-9199
62038 Minnesota Highway 24, PO Box 570, Litchfield, MN 55355
Underquilt.

Mrc Industries Inc. 516-328-6900
85 Denton Ave, New Hyde Park, NY 11040
Various types of mattresses.

Nasa Tech Memory Foam Sleep Systems 727-447-0957
8300 Ulmerton Rd Ste 100, Largo, FL 33771
Multiple density foam mattress.

MATTRESS, NON-POWERED FLOTATION THERAPY *(cont'd)*

Neonatal, Infant, Pediatric, And Adult — 305-267-8885
815 NW 57th Ave Ste 110, Miami, FL 33126
Mattress, non-powered, non-powered flotation therapy mattress.

Ongoing Care Solutions, Inc. — 800-375-0207
6545 44th St N Ste 4007, Pinellas Park, FL 33781
Mattress flotation therapy - non-powered.

Pata Enterprises, Inc. — 603-883-4534
1120 N Mesquite St, San Antonio, TX 78202
Medical recovery positioning system.

Scott Technology Llc — 203-888-2783
1 Jacks Hill Rd, Oxford, CT 06478
Foam therapy pad,foam mattress.

Star Cushion Products, Inc. — 618-539-7070
5 Commerce Dr, Freeburg, IL 62243
Flotation mattress.

Sunco Llc — 901-412-7589
4187 Senator St, Memphis, TN 38118
Foam mattress.

Symphony Medical Products — 877-470-9995
6320 NW 84th Ave, Miami, FL 33166
Powered transport stretcher.

Tempur Production Usa, Inc. — 276-431-7174
203 Tempur Pedic Dr Ste 102, Duffield, VA 24244
Standard hospital mattress.

Tempur Production Usa, Inc. — 276-431-7174
12907 Tempur-Pedic Pkwy NW, Albuquerque, NM 87120

Tempur-Medical, Inc. — 888-255-3302
1713 Jaggie Fox Way, Lexington, KY 40511
Tempur-Med Mattress

Tuffcare — 800-367-6160
3999 E La Palma Ave, Anaheim, CA 92807

Wcw,Inc — 518-686-0725
1 Mechanic St, Hoosick Falls, NY 12090
Mattress, flotation therapy, non-powered.

MATTRESS, OPERATING TABLE *(General) 80RGH*

Bryton Corp. — 800-567-9500
4310 Guion Rd, Indianapolis, IN 46254
Cushions and pads for all makes and models of surgical tables, orthopedic tables, urological tables and obstetrical tables.

Herculite Products, Inc. — 800-772-0036
PO Box 435, Emigsville, PA 17318

Medrecon, Inc. — 877-526-4323
257 South Ave, Garwood, NJ 07027

Profex Medical Products — 800-325-0196
2224 E Person Ave, Memphis, TN 38114

MATTRESS, REDUCTION, PRESSURE *(General) 80WYO*

American Health Systems — 800-234-6655
PO Box 26688, Greenville, SC 29616
UltraForm; Bariatric Mattresses designed to reduce pressures and increase patient comfort. Standard and custom sizes available.

B.G. Industries, Inc. — 800-822-8288
8550 Balboa Blvd Ste 214, Northridge, CA 91325
MAXIFLOAT Die-cut foam pressure relief mattresses for decubitus care. ACCUMAX QUANTUM CONVERTIBLE pressure relief system automatically creates a custom pressure relieving profile in a dynamic system.

Casco Manufacturing Solutions, Inc. — 800-843-1339
3107 Spring Grove Ave, Cincinnati, OH 45225
C-MAtt Prevention mattress for patients and residents at risk of developing pressure ulcers.

Chestnut Ridge Foam, Inc. — 800-234-2734
PO Box 781, Latrobe, PA 15650
A comprehensive offering of the CAREFLEX and BLUECLOUD with ultra soft memory foam, therapeutic healthcare mattresses combine pressure reduction, comfort, durability,economical. Enhanced value because we sell direct to purchasing groups and facilities direct.

Comfort Care Products Corp. — 803-321-0020
258 Industrial Park Rd, Newberry, SC 29108
Features include flame retardancy and complete anti-microbial protection inside and out. VISCO FLEX specialized, zoned pressure reduction support surface. Unique heel section. SUPRA FLEX dual sided bariatric mattress with exclusive foam coil design. 450 lbs. BARIFLEX-EXTEND bariatric mattress, extra wide featuring our exclusive foam coil core, rated to 1000 lbs. EASY COMFORT II PLUS advanced pressure reduction mattress.

MATTRESS, REDUCTION, PRESSURE *(cont'd)*

Hill-Rom Holdings, Inc. — 800-445-3730
1069 State Road 46 E, Batesville, IN 47006

Hill-Rom Manufacturing, Inc. — 800-638-2546
4349 Corporate Rd, Charleston, SC 29405

Milwaukee Mattress & Furniture — 800-373-1462
423 N 3rd St, Milwaukee, WI 53203
From $260.00 to $280.00.

O&M Enterprise — 847-258-4515
641 Chelmsford Ln, Elk Grove Village, IL 60007
MATTRESS BED EGG CRATE

Pyramid Industries, Llc — 888-343-3352
3911 Schaad Rd Unit 102, Knoxville, TN 37921
GEL-LITE includes GEL_LITE III Gel mattress overlays, standard, lightweight and bariatric models, including Gel wheelchair cushions. Wheelchair cushions are available in all standard sizes and custom sizes from pediatric to bariatric.

Sunrise Medical — 800-333-4000
7477 Dry Creek Pkwy, Longmont, CO 80503

The Neurological Research And Development Group — 800-327-6759
115 Rotary Dr, West Hazleton, PA 18202
Pressure Sore Prevention Mattresses including Gel, Visco Elastic Foam , as well as all other types of foam.

MATTRESS, SILICONE, AND CHAIR CUSHION *(General) 80FNI*

Grand Rapids Foam Technologies — 877-GET-GRFT
2788 Remico St SW, Wyoming, MI 49519

Stryker Medical — 800-869-0770
3800 E Centre Ave, Portage, MI 49002

MATTRESS, WATER *(General) 80RGI*

Genesis Manufacturing, Inc. — 317-485-7887
720 E Broadway St, Fortville, IN 46040
Contract Radio-Frequency (RF) Welding. From development to manufacturing and packaging.

Howard Medical Company — 800-443-1444
1690 N Elston Ave, Chicago, IL 60642
$81.00 for standard water mattress; 36 x 60.

Tetra Medical Supply Corp. — 800-621-4041
6364 W Gross Point Rd, Niles, IL 60714

MATTRESS, WATER, TEMPERATURE REGULATED *(General) 80FOH*

Blue Chip Medical Products, Inc. — 800-795-6115
7-11 Suffern Pl Ste 2, Suffern, NY 10901

Children's Medical Ventures, Inc. — 800-345-6443
191 Wyngate Dr, Monroeville, PA 15146
OASIS Baby Warming System, microprocessor controlled heated water mattress.

Medisearch P.R., Inc. — 787-864-0684
Machete Industrial Center, Guayama, PR 00784
Various.

MEASURER, CORNEAL RADIUS *(Ophthalmology) 86HJB*

Fortrad Eye Instruments Corp. — 973-543-2371
8 Franklin Rd, Mendham, NJ 07945

Vision Medical Instruments, Inc. — 440-338-5981
8147 Chagrin Mills Rd, Chagrin Falls, OH 44022
Ultrasonic pachymeter.

MEASURER, LENS RADIUS, OPHTHALMIC *(Ophthalmology) 86HLF*

Burton Co., R.H. — 800-848-0410
3965 Brookham Dr, Grove City, OH 43123
$1,150.00 for Burton 2030 radius gauge with analog.

Capital Instruments, Ltd. — 425-271-3756
6210 Lake Washington Blvd SE, Bellevue, WA 98006
Incision gauge.

MEASURER, LENS, AC-POWERED *(Ophthalmology) 86HLM*

Burton Co., R.H. — 800-848-0410
3965 Brookham Dr, Grove City, OH 43123
$825.00 for BURTON 2020 lensmeter and $925.00 for BURTON 2021 lensmeter with prism compensator.

Eye Care And Cure — 800-486-6169
4646 S Overland Dr, Tucson, AZ 85714
Lensometer.

MEASURER, LENS, AC-POWERED *(cont'd)*

Reichert, Inc. 888-849-8955
3362 Walden Ave, Depew, NY 14043
AL200 Auto Lensometer. AL200 is an automatic lensmeter that measures progressive lenses and lenses with prisms.

Topcon Medical Systems, Inc. 800-223-1130
37 W Century Rd, Paramus, NJ 07652
Six lensometer models. Manual models: $990.00, $1,590.00, and $1,690.00. Computerized models: $3,290.00, $3,690.00 (with built-in printer), and $4,390.00 (with built-in printer & PD attachment).

MEASURER, STEREOPSIS *(Ophthalmology) 86HLC*

Astron International Inc. 239-435-0136
3410 Westview Dr, Naples, FL 34104
Instrument, measuring, stereopsis.

Mast/Keystone View 800-806-6569
2200 Dickerson Rd, Reno, NV 89503
TELEBINOCULAR.

MEDIA, CONTRAST, RADIOLOGIC *(Radiology) 90KTA*

Ge Medical Systems, Llc 262-548-2355
3000 N Grandview Blvd, W-417, Waukesha, WI 53188
Barium sulfate mixture ndc 12505-024-01/02.

Xma (X-Ray Marketing Associates, Inc.) 800-325-8880
1205 W Lakeview Ct, Windham Lakes Business Park
Romeoville, IL 60446

MEDIA, CONTRAST, ULTRASOUND *(Radiology) 90MJS*

Imaging Associates, Inc. 800-821-3230
11110 Westlake Dr, Charlotte, NC 28273

MEDIA, COUPLING, ULTRASOUND *(Radiology) 90MUI*

Truett Labs 626-334-5106
798 N Coney Ave, Azusa, CA 91702

MEDIA, CULTURE, EX VIVO, TISSUE AND CELL *(Gastro/Urology) 78NDS*

Biolife Solutions, Inc. 607-687-4487
171 Front St, Owego, NY 13827
Hypo thermosol, cryostor, gelstor.

MEDIA, FILTER *(General) 80WXR*

Enhanced Filter Company, Inc. 805-642-2079
2159C Palma Dr Ste C, Ventura, CA 93003
ELECTROSTAT and VARIFLO 100% synthetic air filter media; 10 grades ELECTROSTAT, 3 grades VARIFLO, including HEPA and ULPA. Ultrasorb 100% carbon-fiber adsorption cloth.

Genpore, A Division Of General Polymeric Corp. 800-654-4391
1136 Morgantown Rd, Reading, PA 19607
Custom porous plastic filters.

Globetec Nonwovens 410-287-2207
40 Industrial Rd, North East, MD 21901
MICROSTAT BFE/VFE electrostatic filter media. High-efficiency removal of viral and bacterial contamination in gaseous stream applications. Also available are nonwoven and depth filter media engineered materials for the removal of particulate (solid or liquids) from fluid (gas or liquid) streams.

I.W. Tremont Co. 973-427-3800
79 4th Ave, Hawthorne, NJ 07506
Galss micro fiber and laminated micro fiber filters.

Imtek Environmental Corp. 770-667-8621
PO Box 2066, Alpharetta, GA 30023
Waste water.

Nbs Medical Products Inc. 888-800-8192
257 Livingston Ave, New Brunswick, NJ 08901
Medical filters.

Pall Corporation 800-521-1520
600 S Wagner Rd, Ann Arbor, MI 48103
EMFLON PTFE Media uses an advanced lamination technique making it ideal for healthcare and other air-venting applications.

Performance Systematix Inc 616-949-9090
5569 33rd St SE, Grand Rapids, MI 49512
Gas Line Filters, 25mm Filters, EPA Filters, Cambridge Filters, Suction Canister Filters

Porvair Filtration Group Inc 803-327-5008
454 Anderson Rd S, BTC 514, Rock Hill, SC 29730

MEDIA, GASTROENTEROGRAPHIC CONTRAST (BARIUM SULFATE) *(Radiology) 90UJW*

Alimed, Inc. 800-225-2610
297 High St, Dedham, MA 02026

MEDIA, GASTROENTEROGRAPHIC CONTRAST (BARIUM SULFATE) *(cont'd)*

Bryan Corp. 800-343-7711
4 Plympton St, Woburn, MA 01801
Biotrace Sterile Barium Sulfate, 6 grams, USP.

Marconi Medical Systems 800-323-0550
595 Miner Rd, Cleveland, OH 44143

MEDIA, MOUNTING *(Pathology) 88LEB*

American Mastertech Scientific, Inc. 209-368-4031
1330 Thurman St, Lodi, CA 95240
Multiple.

Cargille Laboratories 973-239-6633
55 Commerce Rd, Cedar Grove, NJ 07009
$47.00 per oz. of MELTMOUNT mounting media, nD = 1.539-1.704.

Diagnostic Hybrids, Inc. 740-589-3300
1055 E State St Ste 100, Athens, OH 45701
Mounting medium.

Lgm International Inc. 410-472-9930
3030 Venture Ln Ste 106, Melbourne, FL 32934
Mounting media.

Poly Scientific R&D Corp. 800-645-5825
70 Cleveland Ave, Bay Shore, NY 11706
Poly mount mounting media (xylene or toluene base).

Polysciences, Inc. 800-523-2575
400 Valley Rd, Warrington, PA 18976
CitraMount for use directly from dlimonene based clearants, PolyMount, miscible with toluene and xylene

Sci Gen, Inc. 310-324-6576
333 E Gardena Blvd, Gardena, CA 90248
FDA: Medical Device Manufacturing and packaging. Focus on Histology, Cytology, Analytical and General purpose Reagents, Chemistry, and Sterling and Disinfecting agents.

MEDIA, MOUNTING, WATER SOLUBLE *(Pathology) 88KEQ*

Immco Diagnostics, Inc. 800-537-8378
60 Pineview Dr, Buffalo, NY 14228
IMMUGLO.

Meridian Bioscience, Inc. 800-696-0739
3471 River Hills Dr, Cincinnati, OH 45244

Polysciences, Inc. 800-523-2575
400 Valley Rd, Warrington, PA 18976
Aqua-Poly/Mount, useful for immunofluorescent techniques Crystalline (99.95%), 2% and 4% solutions

Sci Gen, Inc. 310-324-6576
333 E Gardena Blvd, Gardena, CA 90248
FDA: Medical Device Manufacturing and packaging. Focus on Histology, Cytology, Analytical and General purpose Reagents, Chemistry, and Sterling and Disinfecting agents.

Scytek Laboratories, Inc. 435-755-9848
205 S 600 W, Logan, UT 84321
Media, mounting, water soluble.

MEDIA, MYCOPLASMA DETECTION *(Pathology) 88KIX*

Bd Diagnostic Systems 800-675-0908
7 Loveton Cir, Sparks, MD 21152

MEDIA, POTENTIATING *(Hematology) 81KSG*

Genetic Testing Institute 262-754-1000
20925 Crossroads Cir Ste 200, Waukesha, WI 53186
Potentiating solution for in vitro diagnostic use.

Micro Typing Systems, Inc. 908-218-8177
1295 SW 29th Ave, Pompano Beach, FL 33069
Potentiating media.

Ortho-Clinical Diagnostics, Inc. 800-828-6316
513 Technology Blvd, Rochester, NY 14626
Bovine albumin solution.

MEDIA, RADIOGRAPHIC INJECTABLE CONTRAST *(Radiology) 90VGW*

Epix Pharmaceuticals, Inc 781-761-7600
4 Maguire Rd, Lexington, MA 02421
Injectable intravascular MRI contrast agent.

Mckesson General Medical 800-446-3008
8741 Landmark Rd, Richmond, VA 23228

MEDIA, RADIOGRAPHIC INJECTABLE CONTRAST *(cont'd)*

Rockland Technimed Limited Rtl 845-426-1136
3 Larissa Ct, Airmont, NY 10952
Oxy-17 Tissue Viability Imaging Agent as an oxygen uptake marker using a stable non-radioactive isotope of oxygen, naturally occuring. A smart contrast agent formulation, with image processing and MRI sequences and recon workstations.

MEDIA, REPRODUCTIVE *(Obstetrics/Gyn) 85MQL*

Biocoat, Inc. 215-734-0888
211 Witmer Rd, Horsham, PA 19044
PICSI SPERM SELECTION DEVICE

Conception Technologies 858-824-0888
6835 Flanders Dr Ste 500, San Diego, CA 92121
Sperm separation media.

Genx International 888-GEN-XNOW
393 Soundview Rd, Guilford, CT 06437

Minitube Of America, Inc 608-845-1502
419 Venture Ct, Verona, WI 53593
Assisted reproduction media.

Nidacon Canada Inc. 613-260-0886
250-600 Peter Morand Cres, Ottawa K1G 5Z3 Canada
Sperm separation medium

Sage In-Vitro Fertilization Inc. 203-601-5200
1979 Locust St, Pasadena, CA 91107
Reproductive media and supplements.

MEDIA, SUPPORTING *(Chemistry) 75UIO*

Bio-Rad Laboratories, Life Science Group 800-424-6723
2000 Alfred Nobel Dr, Hercules, CA 94547

Peninsula Laboratories, Inc. 800-650-4442
305 Old County Rd, San Carlos, CA 94070

MEDIA, TRANSPORT/STORAGE, ORGAN/TISSUE *(Cardiovascular) 74MFU*

Preservation Solutions, Inc. 262-723-6715
980 Proctor Dr, Elkhorn, WI 53121
Organ transport solution.

MEDIASTINOSCOPE *(Surgery) 79GCH*

Karl Storz Endoscopy-America Inc. 800-421-0837
600 Corporate Pointe, Culver City, CA 90230
Lerut mediastinoscope enables connection of video camera while working under direct vision to facilitate teaching.

Richard Wolf Medical Instruments Corp. 800-323-9653
353 Corporate Woods Pkwy, Vernon Hills, IL 60061

MEDIASTINOSCOPE, ENT *(Ear/Nose/Throat) 77EWY*

Mahe International Inc. 800-294-7946
468 Craighead St, Nashville, TN 37204

Richard Wolf Medical Instruments Corp. 800-323-9653
353 Corporate Woods Pkwy, Vernon Hills, IL 60061

MEDICAL DISINFECTANTS/CLEANERS FOR INSTRUMENTS *(General) 80LRJ*

Acrymed, Inc. 503-624-9830
9560 SW Nimbus Ave, Beaverton, OR 97008
SILVAGARD surface treatment for medical devices. Nanoparticle silver in solution adds biofilm prevention to any finished device.

Advanced Sterilization Products 800-595-0200
33 Technology Dr, Irvine, CA 92618
High-level disinfectants. CIDEX family of products. CIDEX glutaraldehyde, CIDEX PA solutions for high-level disinfection of instrumentation. ENZOL enzymatic cleaners. Enzymatic detergent for cleaning medical instrumentation. CIDEX, is a fast and effective solution that disinfects a wide range of instruments and endoscopes. A (.55%) ortho-phthalaldehyde solution, CIDEX solution is effective at room temperature and has excellent tuberculocidal and high level disinfection capabilities. For over 35 years the CIDEX glutaraldehyde solutions have provided fast and effective solutions for the high level disinfection of medical instrumentation. The new, non-glutaraldehyde CIDEX OPA Solution provides a rapid alternative to glutaraldehyde. It is effective in only 12 minutes at room temperature, requires no activation and has no offensive odor. The product also includes ENZOL Enzymatic Detergent, an enzymatic detergent with a neutral pH that can be used for pre-cleaning and washing medical instrrumentation, CIDEX Solution Test Strips and CIDEX Solution Trays.

Alden Medical Llc 413-747-9717
360 Cold Spring Ave, West Springfield, MA 01089
General purpose disinfectant.

MEDICAL DISINFECTANTS/CLEANERS FOR INSTRUMENTS *(cont'd)*

Antheros Llc 804-353-6464
1403 Mactavish Ave, Richmond, VA 23230
Disinfectant medical device.

B.M. Group 800-561-9818
4860 Rue Mackenzie, Montreal, QUE H3W 1B3 Canada
Disinfecting and sterilizing solutions

Bersa Group, Inc. 954-920-9991
3430 N 29th Ave, Hollywood, FL 33020
General purpose disinfectants.

Biospan Technologies, Inc. 800-730-8980
6540 Meyer Dr, Washington, MO 63090
Disinfectant cleaners (germicidal cleaners).

Central Solutions, Inc. 913-621-6542
401 Funston Rd, Kansas City, KS 66115
Various types of hard surface disinfectant cleaners.

Certol International, Llc 303-799-9401
6120 E 58th Ave, Commerce City, CO 80022
Iodine disinfectant.

Chemlink Laboratories, Llc. 770-499-8008
1590 N Roberts Rd NW Ste 111, Kennesaw, GA 30144
Hospital grade disinfectant.

Db Square, Llc 402-292-2383
101 Hickory Grove Church Rd, Sumrall, MS 39482
Toothbrush sanitizer.

Frio Technologies, Inc. 210-308-5635
500 Sandau Rd Ste 200, San Antonio, TX 78216
Dental waterline cleaner.

Garrison Dental Solutions 616-842-2244
110 Dewitt Ln, Spring Lake, MI 49456
Dental unit waterline treatment, dental unit waterline solution.

Health Care Logistics, Inc. 800-848-1633
450 Town St, PO Box 25, Circleville, OH 43113
Various.

Intercon Chemical Co. 800-325-9218
1100 Central Industrial Dr, Saint Louis, MO 63110
Disinfectants, general purpose.

Johnsondiversey, Inc. 262-631-4101
8311 16th St Bldg 65C, Sturtevant, WI 53177
Various.

Js Dental Mfg., Inc. 800-284-3368
196 N Salem Rd, Ridgefield, CT 06877
Surface disinfectant.

Liquipak Corp. 989-463-5510
2205 Michigan Ave, Alma, MI 48801
Disinfectant.

Morgan-Gallacher, Inc. 562-695-1232
8707 Millergrove Dr, Santa Fe Springs, CA 90670
Sanitizing solution.

Novocol, Inc. 303-665-7535
416 S Taylor Ave, Louisville, CO 80027
Surface disinfectant.

Patterson Medical Supply, Inc. 262-387-3720
W68N158 Evergreen Blvd, Cedarburg, WI 53012
Various types; chlorazene for hydrothreapy, polysonic for ultrsound.

Perfecto Products Mfg., Inc. 404-352-3863
1800 Marietta Blvd NW, Atlanta, GA 30318
Various types of disinfectants.

Perform Manufacturing Incorporated 913-722-1557
1624 S 45th St, Kansas City, KS 66106
Surface disinfecting wipe.

Puricore Inc. 484-321-2700
508 Lapp Rd, Malvern, PA 19355

Span Packaging Services Llc. 864-627-4155
4611A Dairy Dr, Greenville, SC 29607
General purpose disinfectant.

Splenodex Canada Inc. 514-224-1080
109 Ch Des Ormes Rr 121, Sainte-Anne-Des-Lacs J0R 1B0 Canada
Formac for manual system tray/basket (reuse test for 28 days)

Sporicidin International 800-424-3733
121 Congressional Ln, Rockville, MD 20852
Sporicidin offers a complete line of disinfectant products including solutions, sprays, individually wrapped towelettes, and canister towelettes. All Sporicidin disinfectants are FDA cleared, EPA registered, and OSHA compliant. They contain no alcohol.

MEDICAL DISINFECTANTS/CLEANERS FOR INSTRUMENTS *(cont'd)*

Unit Chemical Corp. 800-879-8648
7360 Commercial Way, Henderson, NV 89011
TIMSEN packets or Liquid TIMSEN.

Wexford Labs, Inc. 314-966-4134
325 Leffingwell Ave, Kirkwood, MO 63122
Various hard surface disinfectants.

Young Colorado, Llc. 800-325-1881
13705 Shoreline Ct E, Earth City, MO 63045
General purpose disinfectant.

MEDICAL RADIOGRAPHIC PERSONAL MONITORING DEVICE *(Radiology) 90LWN*

American Telecare, Inc. 800-323-6667
15159 Technology Dr, Eden Prairie, MN 55344
AVIVA system.

MEDIUM, LYMPHOCYTE SEPARATION *(Hematology) 81JCF*

American Red Cross Diagnostic Manufacturing Divisi 202-303-5640
9319 Gaither Rd, Gaithersburg, MD 20877
Lymphocyte separation solution (lss).

Budenheim Usa, Inc 800-645-3044
245 Newtown Rd Ste 305, Plainview, NY 11803

Dendreon Corp. 866-477-6782
3005 1st Ave, Seattle, WA 98121
Various types.

One Lambda, Inc. 800-822-8824
21001 Kittridge St, Canoga Park, CA 91303
Lymphocyte Isolation Reagents. Lympho-Kwik cell isolation reagents and Fluorobeads cell isolation reagents.

Zeptometrix Corporation 800-274-5487
872 Main St, Buffalo, NY 14202
Lymphokines/cytokines (human) for research use only.

MERCURIC CHLORIDE FORMULATIONS FOR TISSUE *(Pathology) 88IFQ*

American Mastertech Scientific, Inc. 209-368-4031
1330 Thurman St, Lodi, CA 95240
Multiple.

Poly Scientific R&D Corp. 800-645-5825
70 Cleveland Ave, Bay Shore, NY 11706

Rocky Mountain Reagents,Inc. 303-762-0800
3207 W Hampden Ave, Englewood, CO 80110

MERCURIC NITRATE AND DIPHENYL CARBAZONE (TITRIMETRIC) *(Chemistry) 75CHK*

Medical Chemical Corp. 800-424-9394
19430 Van Ness Ave, Torrance, CA 90501
$16.00 per 100-test kit.

MERCURY *(Dental And Oral) 76ELY*

Bethlehem Apparatus Co., Inc. 610-838-7034
890 Front St, Hellertown, PA 18055
Mercury recovery and recycling.

Dentalez Group 866-DTE-INFO
101 Lindenwood Dr Ste 225, Valleybrooke Corporate Center
Malvern, PA 19355

Harry J. Bosworth Company 800-323-4352
7227 Hamlin Ave, Skokie, IL 60076

Mexicana De Equipos Dentales, S,A, 523-684-8110
Guillermo Baca 3738, Lomas De Polanco, Guadalajara 44960 Mexico
Mercury dental

Moyco Technologies, Inc. 800-331-8837
200 Commerce Dr, Montgomeryville, PA 18936

Tuzik Boston 800-886-6363
104 Longwater Dr, Assinippi Park, Norwell, MA 02061

MESH, CARDIOVASCULAR (POLYMERIC) *(Cardiovascular) 74UAK*

W. L. Gore & Associates, Inc. 800-437-8181
PO Box 2400, Flagstaff, AZ 86003
Gore Seamguard Staple Line Reinforc

MESH, METAL *(Gastro/Urology) 78EZX*

Biomet Microfixation Inc. 800-874-7711
1520 Tradeport Dr, Jacksonville, FL 32218
Timesh titanium mesh system.

MESH, METAL *(cont'd)*

Macropore Biosurgery, Inc. 858-458-0900
6740 Top Gun St, San Diego, CA 92121
Surgical mesh.

Nuvasive, Inc. 800-475-9131
7475 Lusk Blvd, San Diego, CA 92121
Surgical mesh.

Zimmer Trabecular Metal Technology 800-613-6131
10 Pomeroy Rd, Parsippany, NJ 07054
Hedrocel trabecular metal reconstructive system.

MESH, ORTHOPEDIC (METALLIC) *(Orthopedics) 87UBH*

V--Operations Management Consulting, 317-570-5830
7350 E 86th St, Indianapolis, IN 46256

Zimmer Holdings, Inc. 800-613-6131
1800 W Center St, PO Box 708, Warsaw, IN 46580

MESH, SURGICAL (STEEL GAUZE) *(Surgery) 79FTM*

Brennen Medical, Llc 651-429-7413
1290 Hammond Rd, Saint Paul, MN 55110
Surgical mesh.

Carbon Medical Technologies, Inc. 877-277-1788
1290 Hammond Rd, Saint Paul, MN 55110
Surgical mesh.

Cook Endoscopy 336-744-0157
4900 Bethania Station Rd # &, 5951 Grassy Creek Blvd.
Winston Salem, NC 27105
Soft tissue graft.

Cook Urological, Inc. 800-457-4500
1100 W Morgan St, P.O. Box 227, Spencer, IN 47460
Stratasis & Surgisis.

Cryolife, Inc. 800-438-8285
1655 Roberts Blvd NW, Kennesaw, GA 30144
PROPATCH SOFT TISSUE REPAIR MATRIX

Depuy Orthopaedics, Inc. 800-473-3789
700 Orthopaedic Dr, P.O. Box 988, Warsaw, IN 46582
Various types of surgical mesh.

Ethicon, Inc. 800-4-ETHICON
Route 22 West, Somerville, NJ 08876

Medtronic Neurosurgery 800-468-9710
125 Cremona Dr, Goleta, CA 93117
Metallic bone fixation appliance or surgical mesh.

Pegasus Biologics, Inc. 949-585-9430
10 Pasteur Ste 150, Irvine, CA 92618
Sterile surgical mesh.

Shelhigh, Inc. 908-206-8706
650 Liberty Ave, Union, NJ 07083
Soft tissue repair.

Stryker Spine 866-457-7463
2 Pearl Ct, Allendale, NJ 07401

Synovis Life Technologies, Inc 800-255-4018
2575 University Ave W, Saint Paul, MN 55114
Peri-Guard; Peri-Strips Sleeve; Peri-Strips Strip; Supple Peri-Guard

Synthes (Usa) - Development Center 719-481-5300
1230 Wilson Dr, West Chester, PA 19380
Various types and sizes of surgical mesh.

Tei Biosciences Inc. 617-268-1616
7 Elkins St, Boston, MA 02127
Surgical mesh.

W.L. Gore & Associates,Inc 928-526-3030
1505 North Fourth St., Flagstaff, AZ 86004
Staple line reinforcement material.

Zimmer Holdings, Inc. 800-613-6131
1800 W Center St, PO Box 708, Warsaw, IN 46580

Zimmer Trabecular Metal Technology 800-613-6131
10 Pomeroy Rd, Parsippany, NJ 07054
Hedrocel trabecular metal reconstructive system.

MESH, SURGICAL, POLYMERIC *(Surgery) 79FTL*

Anulex Technologies, Inc 877-326-8539
5600 Rowland Rd Ste 280, Minnetonka, MN 55343
Surgical mesh.

Atrium Medical Corp. 800-528-7486
5 Wentworth Dr, Hudson, NH 03051
SURGICAL MESH--polypropylene hernia mesh in a variety of shapes and sizes for both open and laparoscopic repair of hernias.

MESH, SURGICAL, POLYMERIC *(cont'd)*

Avail Medical Products, Inc. 858-635-2206
1225 N. 28th Avenue, Suite 500, Dallas, TX 75261
Abdominal wound care dressing.

Bard Shannon Limited 908-277-8000
San Geronimo Industrial Park, Lot # 1, Road # 3, Km 79.7 Humacao, PR 00791
Meshes,flats,plugs.

Bentec Medical, Inc. 757-224-0177
1380 E Beamer St, Woodland, CA 95776
Silo bag.

Boston Scientific - Marina Bay Customer Fulfillment Center 617-689-6000
500 Commander Shea Blvd, Quincy, MA 02171
Surgical mesh.

Bridger Biomed, Inc. 908-277-8000
2430 N 7th Ave, Bozeman, MT 59715
Surgical mesh.

Caldera Medical Inc. 866-422-5337
5171 Clareton Dr, Agoura Hills, CA 91301
Desara

Cook Biotech, Incorporated 888-299-4224
1425 Innovation Pl, West Lafayette, IN 47906
Hernia Repair and soft tissue reinforcement

Covidien Lp 508-261-8000
15 Hampshire St, Mansfield, MA 02048
DEXON absorbable polyglycolic acid mesh.

Davol Inc., Sub. C.R. Bard, Inc. 800-556-6275
100 Crossings Blvd, Warwick, RI 02886
Surgical mesh.

Ethicon Endo-Surgery, Inc. 877-384-4266
3801 University Blvd SE, Albuquerque, NM 87106
(sterile, polymeric mesh).

Ethicon Endo-Surgery, Inc. 800-USE-ENDO
4545 Creek Rd, Cincinnati, OH 45242
PROLENE and MERSIENE mesh, available in sizes including 12in. x 12in., 6in. x 6in., 2.5in. x 4.5in.

Ethicon, Inc. 800-4-ETHICON
Route 22 West, Somerville, NJ 08876
Absorbable and non-absorbable mesh available in various sizes.

Ethicon, Llc. 908-218-2887
Rd. 183, Km. 8.3,, Industrial Area Hato, San Lorenzo, PR 00754
Sterile, polymeric, mesh.

Evera Medical, Inc. 650-287-2884
353 Vintage Park Dr Ste F, Foster City, CA 94404
Surgical mesh.

Generic Medical Device, Inc. 253-853-3594
5727 Baker Way NW Ste 201, Gig Harbor, WA 98332
Surgical mesh.

Kelsar, S.A. 508-261-8000
Blvd. Insurgentes, Libriamento a La, Tijuana 22450 Mexico
Mesh (synthetic, absorbable, surgical, knitted)

Kollsut Scientific Corporation 630-290-5746
3286 N 29th Ct, Hollywood, FL 33020
Nonabsorbable propylene surgical mesh.

Macropore Biosurgery, Inc. 858-458-0900
6740 Top Gun St, San Diego, CA 92121
Surgical mesh.

Maquet Cardiovascular LLC 888-880-2874
45 Barbour Pond Dr, Wayne, NJ 07470
Trelex.

Mast Biosurgery Usa Inc. 858-550-8050
6749 Top Gun St Ste 108, San Diego, CA 92121
Surgical mesh.

Minnesota Medical Development, Inc. 763-354-7105
14305 21st Ave N Ste 100, Minneapolis, MN 55447
Sterile surgical mesh devices.

S Jackson Inc. 800-368-5225
PO Box 4487, Alexandria, VA 22303
SUPRAMESH $62.50 for 15x15 cm non-sterile mesh. Two sheets/box.

Shelhigh, Inc. 908-206-8706
650 Liberty Ave, Union, NJ 07083
Rotator cuff.

Specialty Surgical Products, Inc. 406-961-0102
1131 US Highway 93 N, Victor, MT 59875
Ventral wall defect reduction silo.

Synovis Surgical Innovations 800-255-4018
2575 University Ave W, Saint Paul, MN 55114
Non-polymeric. PERISTRIPS DRY (permanent) and PERISTRIPS DRY WITH VERITAS (remodelable) staple line reinforcements. Strips of bovine pericardial tissue designed to reinforce the staple lines during lung resection and bariatric surgical procedures. PERI-STRIPS DRY is also cleared for the occlusion of the left atrial appendage. Other soft tissue deficiencies amenable to repair include defects of the abdominal and thoracic wall.

Synthes (Usa) - Development Center 719-481-5300
1230 Wilson Dr, West Chester, PA 19380
Various types and sizes of polymeric surgical mesh.

Tei Biosciences Inc. 617-268-1616
7 Elkins St, Boston, MA 02127
Soft tissue repair matrix.

TYRX, Inc. 866-908-8979
1 Deerpark Dr Ste G, Monmouth Junction, NJ 08852
Polymeric surgical mesh.

Ussc Puerto Rico, Inc. 203-845-1000
Building 911-67, Sabanetas Industrial Park, Ponce, PR 00731
Multiple.

W.L. Gore & Associates,Inc 928-526-3030
1505 North Fourth St., Flagstaff, AZ 86004
Surgical mesh.

W.L. Gore & Associates,Inc 302-738-4880
345 Inverness Dr S, Bldg. A, Ste. 120, Englewood, CO 80112
Staple line reinforcement material.

METACRYLATE, METHYL, CRANIOPLASTY
(Cns/Neurology) 84GXP

Advanced Biomaterial Systems, Inc. 973-635-9040
100 Passaic Ave, Chatham, NJ 07928
Polymethylmethacrylate, pmma.

Biomet Microfixation Inc. 800-874-7711
1520 Tradeport Dr, Jacksonville, FL 32218
Craniofacial calcium phosphate ceramic bone filler.

Biomet, Inc. 574-267-6639
56 E Bell Dr, PO Box 587, Warsaw, IN 46582
Bone cement.

Codman & Shurtleff, Inc 800-225-0460
325 Paramount Dr, Raynham, MA 02767

Skeletal Kinetics, Llc 408-366-5000
10201 Bubb Rd, Cupertino, CA 95014
Bone void killer.

Synthes (Usa) - Development Center 719-481-5300
1230 Wilson Dr, West Chester, PA 19380
Bone cement.

METAL, BASE *(Dental And Oral) 76EJH*

A Plus Dental Lab 215-996-4177
1700 Horizon Dr, --suite 104, Chalfont, PA 18914
Artificial teeth.

America Green Dent., Mfg. 323-265-7000
3432 E 14th St, Commerce, CA 90023
Dental alloy.

American Dent-All Inc. 877-864-6294
5140 San Fernando Rd, Glendale, CA 91204
Various.

Ceragroup Industries Inc. 954-670-0208
6555 Powerline Rd Ste 211, Ft Lauderdale, FL 33309
Amalgram alloy.

D. Sign Dental Lab, Inc. 757-224-0177
690 W Fremont Ave Ste 9C, Sunnyvale, CA 94087
Metal alloy.

Dentalium Dental Ceramics, Inc. 949-440-2600
4141 MacArthur Blvd, Newport Beach, CA 92660

Etkon Usa, Inc. 978-747-2575
916 113th St Ste A, Arlington, TX 76011

Golden Triangle Dental Laboratory Inc. 972-910-9912
7475 Las Colinas Blvd Ste A, Irving, TX 75063
Crown/bridges, inlay/onlay.

METAL, BASE *(cont'd)*

Hong Kong Dental Lab 415-330-9099
9 Silliman St Ste C, San Francisco, CA 94134
Alloy.

Ivoclar Vivadent, Inc. 800-533-6825
175 Pineview Dr, Amherst, NY 14228
Variety of Predominantly base metal alloys

Jensen Industries, Inc. 203-239-2090
50 Stillman Rd, North Haven, CT 06473
Dental alloys.

Matech, Inc. 818-367-2472
13000 San Fernando Rd, Sylmar, CA 91342
Durabond,ceradium v,ceradium non-precious ceramic alloy.

Metalor Technologies Usa 800-554-5504
255 John L Dietsch Blvd, PO Box 255, North Attleboro, MA 02763
Solder for non-precious dental alloy.

Mountain Medico, Inc. 909-931-0688
600 N Mountain Ave Ste D204, Upland, CA 91786

Nano-Write Corporation 925-606-1388
2021 Las Positas Ct Ste 121, Livermore, CA 94551
Base metal alloy.

Pentron Laboratory Technologies 203-265-7397
53 N Plains Industrial Rd, Wallingford, CT 06492
Cobalt-chrome ceramic alloy (be and ni free).

Recigno Laboratories Inc. 215-659-7755
509 Davisville Rd, Willow Grove, PA 19090
Partial denture frame & metal crown/bridge.

Talladium, Inc. 661-295-0900
27360 Muirfield Ln, Valencia, CA 91355
Dental alloy.

Vident 800-828-3839
3150 E Birch St, Brea, CA 92821
Vident 90 & 95 alloy; Aurix, Vident 500 Alloy.

Weartech Intl., Inc. 562-698-7847
13032 Park St, Santa Fe Springs, CA 90670
Partial denture casting alloy,non-precious porcelain fused to metal dental alloy.

3m Unitek 800-634-5300
2724 Peck Rd, Monrovia, CA 91016

METAL, MEDICAL *(General) 80WUL*

Deringer-Ney, Inc. 860-242-2281
2 Douglas St, Ney Industrial Park, Bloomfield, CT 06002
Precision Metal Components

Glines And Rhodes, Inc. 508-226-2000
189 East St, P.O. Box 2285, Attleboro, MA 02703
Refiners of Platinum, Palladium, Gold, Silver, Rhodium, Iridium, Titanium, Tungsten and Tantalum.

Nanoprobes, Inc. 877-447-6266
95 Horseblock Rd, Yaphank, NY 11980
Nanogold (1.4 nm) and undecagold (0.8 nm) site-specific gold labeling reagents and covalent Fab and IgG antibody conjugates which give improved penetration and superior labeling. Unique Fluoro Nanogold combines fluorescent and gold-labeled Fab immunoprobes. Gold-labeled lipids, silver enhancement and negative stain reagents, and 3-, 5-, 10-, 15-, and 30-nm colloidal gold conjugates. Principal market: life science researchers.

Profiles, Inc. 800-959-3171
7 First St., Palmer Industrial Park, Palmer, MA 01069

Troy Manufacturing Co. 440-834-8262
17090 Rapids Rd, PO Box 448, Burton, OH 44021

METALLIC REDUCTION METHOD, GLUCOSE (URINARY, NON-QUANT.) *(Chemistry) 75JIM*

Bayer Healthcare Llc 914-524-2955
555 White Plains Rd Fl 5, Tarrytown, NY 10591
Test for reducing sugars in urine.

Bayer Healthcare, Llc 574-256-3430
430 S Beiger St, Mishawaka, IN 46544
Test for reducing sugars in urine.

Eli Lilly And Co. 317-276-4000
Lilly Corporate Ctr, Drop Code 2622, Indianapolis, IN 46285
Urinary glucose non-quantitative test system.

Elite Dental Service 954-825-6392
10188 NW 47th St, Sunrise, FL 33351

METER, BACTERIAL CULTURE GROWTH *(Microbiology) 83UFL*

Biolog, Inc. 800-284-4949
21124 Cabot Blvd, Hayward, CA 94545
Culture medium: BUGM (Biolog universal growth medium) used with GN MICROPLATE and GP MICROPLATE.

METER, CONDUCTIVITY *(Chemistry) 75VCU*

Analyticon Instruments Corp. 973-379-6771
99 Morris Ave, P.O. Box 92, Springfield, NJ 07081
Also pH meters.

Bio-Feedback Systems, Inc. 303-444-1411
2736 47th St, Boulder, CO 80301
2 models: $175 & $945.

Brinkmann Instruments, Inc. 800-645-3050
PO Box 1019, Westbury, NY 11590

Caprock Developments Inc. 800-222-0325
475 Speedwell Ave, PO Box 95, Morris Plains, NJ 07950

Extech Instruments Corp. 781-890-7440
285 Bear Hill Rd, Waltham, MA 02451
Priced from $209.00 to measure conductivity from 10 - 19, 990uS.

Kernco Instruments Co., Inc. 800-325-3875
420 Kenazo Ave., El Paso, TX 79928-7338

Myron L Company 760-438-2021
2450 Impala Dr, Carlsbad, CA 92010

Omega Engineering, Inc. 800-848-4286
1 Omega Dr, Stamford, CT 06907
Benchtop and portable conductivity, TDS resistivity meters.

Orion Research, Inc. 800-225-1480
166 Cummings Ctr, Beverly, MA 01915
ORION 7 models $650 to $1,800 research/QC, portable digital conductivity meter.

METER, CONDUCTIVITY, INDUCTION, REMOTE TYPE *(Gastro/Urology) 78FLB*

Erika De Reynosa, S.A. De C.V. 781-402-9068
Brecha E99 Sur; Parque, Industrial Reynos, Bldg. Ii
Cd, Reynosa, Tamps Mexico
Conductivity monitor

METER, CONDUCTIVITY, NON-REMOTE *(Gastro/Urology) 78FIZ*

Biodynamics Corp. 206-526-0205
4554 9th Ave NE Ste 100, Seattle, WA 98105
Body compositin analyzer.

Erika De Reynosa, S.A. De C.V. 781-402-9068
Brecha E99 Sur; Parque, Industrial Reynos, Bldg. Ii
Cd, Reynosa, Tamps Mexico
Conductivity monitor

Myron L Company 760-438-2021
2450 Impala Dr, Carlsbad, CA 92010
Portable water quality meter with cup.

METER, DIALYSATE CONDUCTIVITY *(Gastro/Urology) 78QPI*

Myron L Company 760-438-2021
2450 Impala Dr, Carlsbad, CA 92010
Direct readout handheld unit with 2% accuracy and 11 to 15 millimhos range - salt concentration.

Thermo Fisher Scientific Inc. 563-556-2241
2555 Kerper Blvd, Dubuque, IA 52001

METER, LEAKAGE CURRENT (AMMETER) *(General) 80REQ*

Simpson Electric Co. 715-588-3311
520 Simpson Ave, PO Box 99, Lac Du Flambeau, WI 54538
Model 229-2 $248.75 per unit (standard). Model 228 $479.00.

Starkey Laboratories, Inc. 800-328-8602
6700 Washington Ave S, Eden Prairie, MN 55344
$299.50 for digital drain meter unit.

Woodhead L.P. 847-272-7990
3411 Woodhead Dr, Northbrook, IL 60062

METER, LIGHT, PHOTOMICROGRAPHIC *(Microbiology) 83RFB*

Photo Research, Inc. 818-341-5151
9731 Topanga Canyon Pl, Chatsworth, CA 91311
LITE MATE $2,295.00 per unit (standard).

METER, OXYGEN *(Anesthesiology) 73RJO*

Omega Engineering, Inc. 800-848-4286
1 Omega Dr, Stamford, CT 06907
Benchtop dissolved.

METER, PATIENT HEIGHT *(General) 80WOB*

Alimed, Inc. 800-225-2610
297 High St, Dedham, MA 02026

Ibiom Instruments Ltd. 450-678-5468
6640 Barry St., Brossard, QUE J4Z 1T8 Canada
STADIOMETER Height rod. PEDIATEC. For adult and neonatle.

Olympic Medical Corp. 206-767-3500
5900 1st Ave S, Seattle, WA 98108
Automatic infant length measurer. $1,958.50 for auto length.

Seca Corp. 800-542-7322
1352 Charwood Rd Ste E, Hanover, MD 21076
Stationary or portable, manual and digital operation economical to high tech computer interface option versions and growth related accessories. Also available, nine models of wall mount stadiometers, seven models of tabletop infantometers and three models of scale mount for adult and infant.

METER, PEAK FLOW, SPIROMETRY *(Anesthesiology) 73BZH*

Armstrong Medical Industries, Inc. 800-323-4220
575 Knightsbridge Pkwy, Lincolnshire, IL 60069

Boehringer Laboratories, Inc. 800-642-4945
500 E Washington St, Norristown, PA 19401
Dual-range unit. Portable peak-flow meter allows convenient, accurate bedside analysis of this parameter.

Creative Biomedics, Inc. 949-366-2300
924 Calle Negocio Ste A, San Clemente, CA 92673
The Peak

Dhd Healthcare Corporation 800-847-8000
PO Box 6, One Madison Street, Wampsville, NY 13163
asmaPlan Peak Flowmeter

Futuremed America, Inc. 800-222-6780
15700 Devonshire St, Granada Hills, CA 91344
$150.00 for S100 SPIROPET. $1200 for SPIROPET II.

Intl. Medical, Inc. 952-890-6547
14470 W Burnsville Pkwy, Burnsville, MN 55306
Imi peak flow meter.

Lifewatch Services, Inc. 877-774-9846
10255 W Higgins Rd Ste 100, O'hare International Center II
Rosemont, IL 60018
Spirometry.

Monaghan Medical Corp. 800-833-9653
5 Latour Ave Ste 1600, P.O. Box 2805, Plattsburgh, NY 12901
TRUZONE.

Nspire Health, Inc 800-574-7374
1830 Lefthand Cir, Longmont, CO 80501
A full range of personal diary spirometers, including PiKo-1, KoKoPeak Pro and Accutrax, provide a simplified approach to monitoring FEV1 and PEFR in asthma and COPD patients at home.

Piko Healthcare Products, Inc. 888-737-5656
908 Main St, Louisville, CO 80027
PiKo (peak flow), PiKo-1 (peak flow and FEV1), PiKo-1P (peak flow, FEV1, and diary questions), PiKo-6P (peak flow, FEV1, FEV^, and diary questions), PAMP software. All products are electronic and low cost.

Respironics Georgia, Inc. 724-387-4559
175 Chastain Meadows Ct NW, Kennesaw, GA 30144

Respironics New Jersey, Inc. 800-804-3443
5 Woodhollow Rd, Parsippany, NJ 07054
PERSONAL BEST, ASSESS, ASTHMA CHECK, ASTHMAMENTOR, $23.00 ASSESS Standard Range peak expiratory flow rates from 60 to 880 lpm and ASSESS Low Range $26.00 peak expiratory flow rates from 30 to 390 lpm. $24.50 Personal Best, portable peak flow meter, with Integrated Asthma Management Zone system, flow rates from 60 to 810 lpm, and Personal Best Low Range (50-390 1pm) $26.00. ASTHMA CHECK, Universal Range from 60 to 810 lpm. ASTHMAMENTOR, $24.95 Universal Range from 60 to 180 lpm with Auto Zone Calculator and Asthma Action Plan.

Spirometrics Medical Equipment Co., Llc 207-657-6700
22 Shaker Rd, Gray, ME 04039
Peak flow meter.

Ulster Scientific, Inc. 845-255-2200
83 S Putt Corners Rd, PO Box 819, New Paltz, NY 12561
WhistleWatch

Vacumed 800-235-3333
4538 Westinghouse St, Ventura, CA 93003
Peak flowmeter.

METER, PEAK FLOW, SPIROMETRY *(cont'd)*

Vitalograph, Inc. 800-255-6626
13310 W 99th St, Lenexa, KS 66215
ASMAPLAN+ Peak flow meter assess the severity of asthma. With color zones $14.00. / Without $11.00

Westmed, Inc. 800-975-7987
5580 S Nogales Hwy, Tucson, AZ 85706
MDILOG electronic to be used with Clinical Trials Model MDILOG. MDILOGII, electronic to be used with Tophat adapter system. Peaklog and display software.

METER, PH, BLOOD *(Chemistry) 75JKO*

Radiometer America, Inc. 800-736-0600
810 Sharon Dr, Westlake, OH 44145
BPH5 automatic analyzer for measurement of scalp pH on 35 uL of blood. Standby mode saves consumables. Upgradable to ABL5 blood-gas analyzer.

METER, PH, GENERAL USE *(Toxicology) 91DNB*

Analytical Measurements, Inc. 800-635-5580
100 Hoffman Pl, Hillside, NJ 07205
$250.00 per unit (standard).

Beckman Coulter, Inc. 800-742-2345
250 S Kraemer Blvd, PO Box 8000, Brea, CA 92821

Brinkmann Instruments (Canada) Ltd. 800-263-8715
6670 Campobello Rd., Mississauga, ONT L5N 2L8 Canada

Capital Controls, MicroChem 215-997-4000
3000 Advance Ln, Colmar, PA 18915

Caprock Developments Inc. 800-222-0325
475 Speedwell Ave, PO Box 95, Morris Plains, NJ 07950

Corning Inc., Science Products Division 800-492-1110
45 Nagog Park, Acton, MA 01720

Devar Inc. 800-566-6822
706 Bostwick Ave, Bridgeport, CT 06605

Extech Instruments Corp. 781-890-7440
285 Bear Hill Rd, Waltham, MA 02451
$119.00 for pH meters measure 0 -14.00 range accurate to 0.02pH.

Kendro Laboratory Products 800-252-7100
308 Ridgefield Ct, Asheville, NC 28806

METER, PH, PORTABLE *(Chemistry) 75JQY*

Analytical Measurements, Inc. 800-635-5580
100 Hoffman Pl, Hillside, NJ 07205
5 models - $290.00 to $500.00, solid state.

Beckman Coulter, Inc. 800-742-2345
250 S Kraemer Blvd, PO Box 8000, Brea, CA 92821

Brinkmann Instruments (Canada) Ltd. 800-263-8715
6670 Campobello Rd., Mississauga, ONT L5N 2L8 Canada

Brinkmann Instruments, Inc. 800-645-3050
PO Box 1019, Westbury, NY 11590

Caprock Developments Inc. 800-222-0325
475 Speedwell Ave, PO Box 95, Morris Plains, NJ 07950

Cole-Parmer Instrument Inc. 800-323-4340
625 E Bunker Ct, Vernon Hills, IL 60061

Corning Inc., Science Products Division 800-492-1110
45 Nagog Park, Acton, MA 01720

Extech Instruments Corp. 781-890-7440
285 Bear Hill Rd, Waltham, MA 02451

Kernco Instruments Co., Inc. 800-325-3875
420 Kenazo Ave., El Paso, TX 79928-7338
6 models: $179-$850, analog or digital, accuracy to 0.02 pH.

Lamotte Co. 800-344-3100
802 Washington Ave, PO Box 329, Chestertown, MD 21620
Digital, portable pH meter uses single 9V battery, also a digital, portable pH meter with automatic temperature compensation and microprocessor keypad entry.

Myron L Company 760-438-2021
2450 Impala Dr, Carlsbad, CA 92010
pDS pH/conductivity meter.

Omega Engineering, Inc. 800-848-4286
1 Omega Dr, Stamford, CT 06907
Non-glass pH electrode and digital meter measures pH, mV, and degrees C.

Orbeco Analytical Systems, Inc. 800-922-5242
185 Marine St, Farmingdale, NY 11735
$325.00 per unit (standard).

METER, PH, PORTABLE *(cont'd)*

Orion Research, Inc. 800-225-1480
166 Cummings Ctr, Beverly, MA 01915
ORION 17 models - $230 to $2,095; analog or digital, accuracy up to .001 pH, portable or benchtop models, temperature compensation available.

Precisa Balances Usa Inc. 877-PRE-CISA
540 Powder Springs St Ste 8, Marietta, GA 30064
pH900 meter--user friendly, simple 2-pt calibration; includes KCl, buffers, and case. Free with the purchase of a Precisa semi-micro balance.

Sentron, Inc. 253-851-7881
7117 Stinson Ave Ste C, Gig Harbor, WA 98335

Settler Medical Electronics Inc.
723 Queenston St, Winnipeg R3N 0X8 Canada
No common name listed

Von London Phonix Co 713-772-6666
6103 Glenmont Dr, Houston, TX 77081

METER, SKIN RESISTANCE, AC-POWERED *(Physical Med) 89IKI*

U.F.I. 805-772-1203
545 Main St Ste C2, Morro Bay, CA 93442
$625.00 for Model 2701.

METER, SKIN RESISTANCE, BATTERY-POWERED *(Physical Med) 89IKJ*

Bio-Feedback Systems, Inc. 303-444-1411
2736 47th St, Boulder, CO 80301
2 models: $175 & $945.

Neurodyne Medical Corp. 800-963-8633
186 Alewife Brook Pkwy, Cambridge, MA 02138
CT3 Skin Conductance Adapter is available for T30 and T33 clinical-series temperature monitors.

U.F.I. 805-772-1203
545 Main St Ste C2, Morro Bay, CA 93442
$625.00 for Model 2701.

METER, ULTRASONIC POWER *(General) 80SDX*

Gentec Electro-Optics Inc. 888-543-6832
445 St-Jean-Baptiste, Ste. 160, Quebec, QUE G2E-5N7 Canada

Medsonic U.S.A., Inc. 716-565-1700
8865 Sheridan Dr, Clarence, NY 14031

Netech, Corp. 800-547-6557
110 Toledo St, Farmingdale, NY 11735
Five Models of Ultrasound Watt Meters are offered with different power ranges. While degassed water is the standard coupling medium, one model uses ultrasound gel.

METER, VOLUME, BLOOD *(Hematology) 81JWO*

Buxco Research Systems 910-794-6980
219 Station Rd Ste 202, Wilmington, NC 28405
Flow volume and pressure analyzer.

Daxor Corporation 865-425-0555
107 Meco Ln, Oak Ridge, TN 37830
Blood volume analyzer.

METHYL METACRYLATE *(Cns/Neurology) 84JXH*

Advanced Chemical Sensors Inc. 561-338-3116
3201 N Dixie Hwy Ste 3, Boca Raton, FL 33431
Monitoring badges for a written record from an independent laboratory.

Codman & Shurtleff, Inc 800-225-0460
325 Paramount Dr, Raynham, MA 02767

MICRO-INJECTOR, TRANSPLANT, GENE *(Microbiology) 83WPR*

Micromanipulator Co., Inc., The 800-972-4032
1555 Forrest Way, Carson City, NV 89706
Products and accessories to aid in embryo recovery, grading, splitting, injection, micromanipulation and photomicrography.

MICRODEBRIDER, ENT, HIGH SPEED, SINGLE USE, REPROCESSED *(Ear/Nose/Throat) 77NLY*

Ascent Healthcare Solutions 480-763-5300
10232 S 51st St, Phoenix, AZ 85044
Ent bur, reprocessed.

MICRODENSITOMETRY METHOD, LIPOPROTEINS *(Chemistry) 75JHL*

Beckman Coulter, Inc. 800-742-2345
250 S Kraemer Blvd, PO Box 8000, Brea, CA 92821

MICRODENSITOMETRY METHOD, LIPOPROTEINS *(cont'd)*

Genzyme Diagnostics 617-252-7500
6659 Top Gun St, San Diego, CA 92121
Hcg urine pregnancy test kit.

MICROELECTRODE *(General) 80RGQ*

Bak Electronics, Inc. 800-894-6000
PO Box 623, Mount Airy, MD 21771

Basi (Bioanalytical Systems, Inc.) 800-845-4246
2701 Kent Ave, West Lafayette, IN 47906
mPTE, mAUE microelectrodes for voltammetry.

Beckman Coulter, Inc. 800-742-2345
250 S Kraemer Blvd, PO Box 8000, Brea, CA 92821

Cameron-Miller, Inc. 800-621-0142
5410 W Roosevelt Rd, Road #241, Chicago, IL 60644

Dynamics Research Corp. 800-522-4321
60 Frontage Rd, Andover, MA 01810

Elmed, Inc. 630-543-2792
60 W Fay Ave, Addison, IL 60101

Lazar Research Laboratories, Inc. 800-824-2066
731 N La Brea Ave Ste 5, Los Angeles, CA 90038
380-micron diameter sensor measures pH, cations and anions; Micro PO2 electrode measures dissolved oxygen in small samples.

MICROFILM/MICROFICHE EQUIPMENT *(General) 80VAZ*

White Systems, Inc. 800-275-1442
30 Boright Ave, Kenilworth, NJ 07033
Microfilm and microfiche storage units.

MICROFILTER, BLOOD TRANSFUSION *(Anesthesiology) 73CAK*

Charter Medical, Ltd. 336-768-6447
3948 Westpoint Blvd Ste A, Winston Salem, NC 27103
40 micron filter.

Corning Inc., Science Products Division 800-492-1110
45 Nagog Park, Acton, MA 01720

Davol Inc., Sub. C.R. Bard, Inc. 800-556-6275
100 Crossings Blvd, Warwick, RI 02886
Solcosept filter.

Fenwal Inc. 800-766-1077
3 Corporate Dr, Lake Zurich, IL 60047
Blood filtration products.

Gvs Filter Technology Inc. 317-471-3700
5353 W 79th St, Indianapolis, IN 46268
Tubular screen filters offered with a variety of pore sizes, resins, and dimensional configurations. These screen filters are compatible with many different types of drip chambers and other tubular components. Also available are disc filters of many different mesh sizes and membrane types.

Icu Medical (Ut), Inc 949-366-2183
4455 Atherton Dr, Salt Lake City, UT 84123
Various sterile combinations of blood filters and administration sets.

Medicalcv, Inc. 800-328-2060
9725 S Robert Trl, Inver Grove Heights, MN 55077
INTERFACE.

Medsep Corp., A Subsidiary Of Pall Corp. 516-484-5400
1630 W Industrial Park St, Covina, CA 91722
Various types of sterile leukocyte reduction filter sets.

Pall Corporation 800-645-6532
25 Harbor Park Dr, Port Washington, NY 11050
Various.

Pall Corporation 800-521-1520
600 S Wagner Rd, Ann Arbor, MI 48103

Pall Lifesciences Puerto Rico Llc 516-801-9064
Carr. 194, Km. O.4, Fajardo, PR 00738
Various.

Statcorp, Inc. 800-992-0014
14476 Duval Pl W Ste 303, Jacksonville, FL 32218
20 micron blood filter sets available in straight administration sets; Y-sets and stand-alone sets.

Terumo Cardiovascular Systems (Tcvs) 800-283-7866
28 Howe St, Ashland, MA 01721
Transfusion filter.

Utah Medical Products, Inc. 800-533-4984
7043 Cottonwood St, Midvale, UT 84047
HEMO-NATE, stainless steal filter media assures absolute retention of particulate larger than 18 micron. Available as part of a set or separately.

MICROFILTER, BLOOD TRANSFUSION *(cont'd)*

Whatman Inc. 732-885-6529
800 Centennial Ave Bldg 1, Piscataway, NJ 08854

MICROMANIPULATOR *(General) 80RGR*

Carl Zeiss Surgical, Inc. 800-442-4020
1 Zeiss Dr, Thornwood, NY 10594

Micromanipulator Co., Inc., The 800-972-4032
1555 Forrest Way, Carson City, NV 89706
Products and accessories to aid in embryo recovery, grading, splitting, injection, micromanipulation and photomicrography.

Nikon Instruments Inc. 800-52-Nikon
1300 Walt Whitman Rd, Melville, NY 11747

Transamerican Technologies International 800-322-7373
2246 Camino Ramon, San Ramon, CA 94583
ACCU-BEAM, CO2 Laser micromanipulators.

Zander Medical Supplies, Inc. / Zander Ivf, Inc. 800-820-3029
755 8th Ct Ste 4, Vero Beach, FL 32962
RI-Integra Micromanipulation station for leading brands of Inverted microscopes with 3 heated surfaces, single and double toolholders including embryo biopsy procedures, proprietory method of 'homing' of pipette tips at operation level.

MICROMANIPULATOR, LABORATORY *(Microbiology) 83UGV*

Brinkmann Instruments (Canada) Ltd. 800-263-8715
6670 Campobello Rd., Mississauga, ONT L5N 2L8 Canada

Minitool, Inc. 408-395-1585
634 University Ave, Los Gatos, CA 95032
Mirrors, chisels, knives.

Technical Instruments (Ti) 650-651-3000
1826 Rollins Rd, Burlingame, CA 94010

MICROMANIPULATORS AND MICROINJECTORS, ASSISTED REPRODUCTION *(Obstetrics/Gyn) 85MQJ*

Exfo America Inc. 800-663-3936
3701 W Plano Pkwy Ste 160, Plano, TX 75075
MICROMANIPULATOR, the piezodrill increases yields and improves productivity for advanced reproductive techniques.

Narishige International Usa, Inc. 800-445-7914
1710 Hempstead Tpke, East Meadow, NY 11554
Assisted reproduction micromanipulators and microinjectors.

MICROMETER, MICROSCOPE *(Pathology) 88KEH*

Huntington Mechanical Laboratories, Inc. 800-227-8059
1040 La Avenida St, Mountain View, CA 94043

Trestle Corp. 949-673-1907
199 Technology Dr Ste 105, Irvine, CA 92618
Microscopy system.

Western Scientific Co., Inc. 877-489-3726
4104 24th St # 183, San Francisco, CA 94114
Standard and custom-made micrometers and reticles.

MICROPLATE *(General) 80WOC*

Awareness Technology, Inc. 722-283-6540
1935 SW Martin Hwy, Palm City, FL 34990
$1,200 for Model Stat Fax 2200 microplate shaker/incubator with variable speeds, temperatures and timer; holds two plates.

Bd Diagnostic Systems 800-675-0908
7 Loveton Cir, Sparks, MD 21152

Biolog, Inc. 800-284-4949
21124 Cabot Blvd, Hayward, CA 94545
GN MICROPLATE for biotyping & identifying aerobic gram-negative bacteria, GP MICROPLATE for biotyping and identifying aerobic gram-positive bacteria, ES MICROPLATE for biotyping E. Coli K12 and S. typhimurium LT2 strains.

Corning Inc., Science Products Division 800-492-1110
45 Nagog Park, Acton, MA 01720

Globe Scientific, Inc. 800-394-4562
610 Winters Ave, Paramus, NJ 07652
96-well, U, V, and flat-bottom microplates.

Lenox Laser 800-494-6537
12530 Manor Rd, Glen Arm, MD 21057
This revolutionary product is designed for use with aggressive chemicals, acidic and alkaline solutions and many other practical applications including fluorescence, deep UV exploration, microscopy and DNA and protein analysis at very high temperatures.

MICROPLATE *(cont'd)*

Medtec, Inc. 919-241-1400
PO Box 16578, Chapel Hill, NC 27516
Verify the chamber temperature of your microplate reader with the Temperature Validation Microplate (TVM). Coming soon: catalog number MT05000.

Molecular Devices Corp. 800-635-5577
1311 Orleans Dr, Sunnyvale, CA 94089
SOFTMAX and SOFTMAX PRO; microplate software.

Titertek Instruments, Inc. 256-859-8600
330 Wynn Dr NW, Huntsville, AL 35805

Tomtec 877-866-8323
1000 Sherman Ave, Hamden, CT 06514
24 flat bottom well plate: 15.5mm diam., 17.8mm deep, 1.9cm bottom area per well, 3.5ml brim volume, made of optical polystrene or inert polypropylene, gamma radiation sterilized, with interstices between wells to be filled with water to hold a uniform temperature on all wells. Turning lid 180 degrees provides two levels of ventilation for oxygen transfer.

MICROSCOPE *(Hematology) 81GJY*

Accu-Scope, Inc. 516-759-1000
7 Littleworth Ln, Sea Cliff, NY 11579
Microscopes and accessories; illuminators.

Akorn, Inc. 800-535-7155
2500 Millbrook Dr, Buffalo Grove, IL 60089
Calibrating microscope for inspection of diamond blade and verification of blade extension of micrometer diamond knives (100x magnification).

C & A Scientific Co. Inc. 703-330-1413
7241 Gabe Ct, Manassas, VA 20109
PREMIERE Monocular, binocular and stereo microscopes. Dual view and trinocular head.

Carl Zeiss Surgical, Inc. 800-442-4020
1 Zeiss Dr, Thornwood, NY 10594

Ken-A-Vision Manufacturing Co., Inc. 800-627-1953
5615 Raytown Rd, Raytown, MO 64133
Microprojector. Projecting microscope $725, 150 watts. NEW - X2000 Microprojector MP2, connects directly to LCD/Video Projectors though VGA connection.

Labo America, Inc. 510-445-1257
920 Auburn Ct, Fremont, CA 94538

Leica Microsystems (Canada) Inc. 800-205-3422
400 - 111 Granton Drive, Richmond Hill, ONT L4B 1L5 Canada
LEICA

Leica Microsystems Inc. 800-248-0123
2345 Waukegan Rd, Bannockburn, IL 60015
MZ-Series and StereoZoom S-Series Stereomicroscopes with ergonomic design for a wide range of applications. DM DigitalMicroscope Research compound microscopes with many automated features. A complete line with precision optics for a wide variety of applications.

Lw Scientific 800-726-7345
865 Marathon Pkwy, Lawrenceville, GA 30046
Models include M5 LabScope infinity-plan laboratory microscope, the M2 LabScope for routine clinical use, the Revelation 3 physician-grade achromatic binocular microscope, and the Observer Series educational monocular and binocular microscopes.

Md International, Inc. 305-669-9003
11300 NW 41st St, Doral, FL 33178

Micromanipulator Co., Inc., The 800-972-4032
1555 Forrest Way, Carson City, NV 89706
Products and accessories to aid in embryo recovery, grading, splitting, injection, micromanipulation and photomicrography.

Microscopy/Microscopy Education 413-746-6931
125 Paridon St Ste 102, Springfield, MA 01118

Minitool, Inc. 408-395-1585
634 University Ave, Los Gatos, CA 95032
Tools.

Nikon Canada Inc., Instrument Div. 905-625-9910
1366 Aerowood Dr., Mississauga, ONT L4W-1C1 Canada

Opti-Quip, Inc. 914-928-2254
548 State Route 32 # 469, Highland Mills, NY 10930
microscope accessories

Portable Medical Laboratories, Inc. 858-755-7385
544 S Nardo Ave, Solana Beach, CA 92075

MICROSCOPE *(cont'd)*

Spirig Advanced Technologies, Inc. 413-788-6191
144 Oakland St, Springfield, MA 01108
Illuminated pocket microscope.

Technical Instruments (Ti) 650-651-3000
1826 Rollins Rd, Burlingame, CA 94010
Confocal scanning microscope.

United Products & Instruments, Inc. 800-588-9776
182 Ridge Rd Ste E, Dayton, NJ 08810
Now you candesign your own microscope by starting with theG-400 and adding the ccessories you need fromour extensive accessory list to meet all yourmicroscope needs.Superb optics and newly designedmechanical ystems assure years ofdependable use.The G400 SERIES is ideal for use inmedical, esearch, agricultural and industriallaboratories, anywhere a versatile, cost efficientmicroscope is needed. Visit us at www.unico1.com for more information on a complete microscope line from UNICO

Vee Gee Scientific, Inc. 800-423-8842
13600 NE 126th Pl Ste A, Kirkland, WA 98034
Clinical.

Wallach Surgical Devices, Inc. 800-243-2463
235 Edison Rd, Orange, CT 06477
$5615.00 for general purpose ZOOMSCOPE 4-20x microscope.

Welch Allyn, Inc. 800-535-6663
4341 State Street Rd, Skaneateles Falls, NY 13153

Western Scientific Co., Inc. 877-489-3726
4104 24th St # 183, San Francisco, CA 94114
Complete line of microscopes; video and digital imaging systems.

Western Scientific Co., Inc. 800-48W-ESCO
2112 W Burbank Blvd, Burbank, CA 91506
Student microscope for use in schools.

MICROSCOPE AND MICROSCOPE ACCESSORIES, REPRODUCTION, ASSISTED *(Obstetrics/Gyn) 85MTX*

Azusa Optronics And Manufacturing Inc. 909-659-3011
2409 S Vineyard Ave, Suite B& C, Ontario, CA 91761
Fertility / ovulation tester.

MICROSCOPE, AUTOMATED, IMAGE ANALYSIS, IMMUNOHISTOCHEMISTRY, OPERATOR INTERVENTION, NUCLEAR INTENSITY & PERCENT POSITIVITY
(Hematology) 81NQN

Aperio Technologies Inc. 866-478-4111
1360 Park Center Dr, Vista, CA 92081
ScanScope XT System

Tripath Imaging, Inc. 919-206-7140
780 Plantation Dr, Burlington, NC 27215
Er-pr assay.

MICROSCOPE, AUTOMATED, IMAGE ANALYSIS, OPERATOR INTERVENTION *(Hematology) 81NOT*

Aperio Technologies Inc. 866-478-4111
1360 Park Center Dr, Vista, CA 92081
ScanScope XT System; ScanScope System

Tripath Imaging, Inc. 919-206-7140
780 Plantation Dr, Burlington, NC 27215
Her2-neu assay.

MICROSCOPE, EAR *(Ear/Nose/Throat) 77RGT*

Carl Zeiss Surgical, Inc. 800-442-4020
1 Zeiss Dr, Thornwood, NY 10594

Jedmed Instruments Co. 314-845-3770
5416 Jedmed Ct, Saint Louis, MO 63129

Medicos Laboratories, Inc. (Mdt) 800-724-4003
801 Montrose Ave, South Plainfield, NJ 07080

Olympus America, Inc. 800-645-8160
3500 Corporate Pkwy, PO Box 610, Center Valley, PA 18034

Tsi Medical Ltd. 800-661-7263
47 Athabascan Ave., Unit 105, Sherwood Park, AB T8A-4H3 Canada

World Medical Equipment, Inc. 800-827-3747
3915 152nd St NE, Marysville, WA 98271

MICROSCOPE, FLUORESCENCE/U.V. *(Pathology) 88IBK*

Cambridge Research & Instrumentation (CRi) 800-383-7924
35B Cabot Rd, Woburn, MA 01801
Nuance Multispectral Imaging

Carl Zeiss Surgical, Inc. 800-442-4020
1 Zeiss Dr, Thornwood, NY 10594

Labo America, Inc. 510-445-1257
920 Auburn Ct, Fremont, CA 94538

MICROSCOPE, FLUORESCENCE/U.V. *(cont'd)*

Leica Microsystems (Canada) Inc. 800-205-3422
400 - 111 Granton Drive, Richmond Hill, ONT L4B 1L5 Canada

Nikon Canada Inc., Instrument Div. 905-625-9910
1366 Aerowood Dr., Mississauga, ONT L4W-1C1 Canada

Portable Medical Laboratories, Inc. 858-755-7385
544 S Nardo Ave, Solana Beach, CA 92075
FLUORESLENS objective lens for converting standard compound microscope to fluorescence microscope. ECONOMY FLUORESCENCE MICROSCOPE -Student microscope with Fluoreslens attached.

Standard Instrumentation, Div. Preiser Scientific 800-624-8285
94 Oliver St, Saint Albans, WV 25177

Western Scientific Co., Inc. 877-489-3726
4104 24th St # 183, San Francisco, CA 94114
Upright and inverted fluorescence microscopes.

MICROSCOPE, INTELLIGENT, AUTOMATED
(Hematology) 81WXZ

Leica Microsystems (Canada) Inc. 800-205-3422
400 - 111 Granton Drive, Richmond Hill, ONT L4B 1L5 Canada

Nikon Canada Inc., Instrument Div. 905-625-9910
1366 Aerowood Dr., Mississauga, ONT L4W-1C1 Canada

MICROSCOPE, INVERTED STAGE, TISSUE CULTURE
(Pathology) 88IBL

Accu-Scope, Inc. 516-759-1000
7 Littleworth Ln, Sea Cliff, NY 11579

Carl Zeiss Surgical, Inc. 800-442-4020
1 Zeiss Dr, Thornwood, NY 10594

Labo America, Inc. 510-445-1257
920 Auburn Ct, Fremont, CA 94538

Leica Microsystems (Canada) Inc. 800-205-3422
400 - 111 Granton Drive, Richmond Hill, ONT L4B 1L5 Canada

Nikon Canada Inc., Instrument Div. 905-625-9910
1366 Aerowood Dr., Mississauga, ONT L4W-1C1 Canada

Nikon Instruments Inc. 800-52-Nikon
1300 Walt Whitman Rd, Melville, NY 11747

Standard Instrumentation, Div. Preiser Scientific 800-624-8285
94 Oliver St, Saint Albans, WV 25177

Western Scientific Co., Inc. 877-489-3726
4104 24th St # 183, San Francisco, CA 94114
Inverted microscopes--brightfield, fluorescence, and phase contrast.

MICROSCOPE, LABORATORY, ELECTRON *(Microbiology) 83RGU*

Electron Microscopy Sciences 800-523-5874
321 Morris Rd, Fort Washington, PA 19034
Accessories & supplies only (electron microscopy).

Jeol Usa, Inc. 978-536-2270
11 Dearborn Rd, Peabody, MA 01960
Scanning electron, transmission electron, auger scanning microprobe, electron x-ray microanalyzer.

Myco Instrumentation Source, Inc. 425-228-4239
PO Box 354, Renton, WA 98057

Spectron Corp. 425-827-9317
934 S Burlington Blvd # 603, Burlington, WA 98233
Reconditioned equipment.

MICROSCOPE, LABORATORY, OPTICAL *(Microbiology) 83RGV*

Accu-Scope, Inc. 516-759-1000
7 Littleworth Ln, Sea Cliff, NY 11579

Bay Optical Instruments 415-431-8711
2401 15th St, San Francisco, CA 94114

Carl Zeiss Surgical, Inc. 800-442-4020
1 Zeiss Dr, Thornwood, NY 10594

Carolina Biological Supply Co. 800-334-5551
2700 York Rd, Burlington, NC 27215

Edmund Industrial Optics 800-363-1992
101 E Gloucester Pike, Barrington, NJ 08007
Stereo, biological, plan, achromatic and many other various types.

George Taub Products & Fusion Co., Inc. 800-828-2634
277 New York Ave, Jersey City, NJ 07307
Stereo Microscope with 8 or 16 power optics. Used for dental lab, or QC viewing. Unit is very portable; has weight base with gooseneck stand. Optics swivel 360 degrees. View under ambient light. Does not require electricity making it very useful in the field as well. Optics made by Olympus.

MICROSCOPE, LABORATORY, OPTICAL *(cont'd)*

Ken-A-Vision Manufacturing Co., Inc. 800-627-1953
5615 Raytown Rd, Raytown, MO 64133
Research grade binocular compound microscopes starting as low as $795. Excellent for video microscopy.

Labo America, Inc. 510-445-1257
920 Auburn Ct, Fremont, CA 94538

Leica Microsystems (Canada) Inc. 800-205-3422
400 - 111 Granton Drive, Richmond Hill, ONT L4B 1L5 Canada
LEICA

Leica Microsystems Inc. 800-248-0123
2345 Waukegan Rd, Bannockburn, IL 60015
MZ-Series and StereoZoom S-Series Stereomicroscopes with ergonomic design for a wide range of applications. DM DigitalMicroscope research compound microscopes with many automated features. A complete line with precision optics for a wide variety of applications.

Meiji Techno America 800-832-0060
3010 Olcott St, Santa Clara, CA 95054
Prices start at $954.00.

Micromanipulator Co., Inc., The 800-972-4032
1555 Forrest Way, Carson City, NV 89706
Products and accessories to aid in embryo recovery, grading, splitting, injection, micromanipulation and photomicrography.

Nikon Canada Inc., Instrument Div. 905-625-9910
1366 Aerowood Dr., Mississauga, ONT L4W-1C1 Canada

Nikon Instruments Inc. 800-52-Nikon
1300 Walt Whitman Rd, Melville, NY 11747

Olympus America, Inc. 800-645-8160
3500 Corporate Pkwy, PO Box 610, Center Valley, PA 18034

Technical Instruments (Ti) 650-651-3000
1826 Rollins Rd, Burlingame, CA 94010

Ted Pella, Inc. 800-237-3526
4595 Mountain Lakes Blvd, Redding, CA 96003
BA400 Laboratory microscope with optional fluorescence kit

United Products & Instruments, Inc. 800-588-9776
182 Ridge Rd Ste E, Dayton, NJ 08810
For over a decade, the G300 series microscopes have led the way in quality, durability, and affordability. UNICO is proud to announce the latest addition to its line: the newly designed G350 Series. The new G350 Series has all the features and quality customers have come to expect only now at a new lower price. The two models in this series are G350 featuring a sliding binocular head and the G354 that comes equipped with a Seidentopf binocular head. Monocular and trinocular versions are also available. Visit us at www.unico1.com for more information on a complete microscope line from UNICO.

Unitron Ltd 631-589-6666
120 Wilbur Pl Ste C, Bohemia, NY 11716

Western Scientific Co., Inc. 877-489-3726
4104 24th St # 183, San Francisco, CA 94114
Complete line of microscopes; video and digital imaging systems.

Western Scientific Co., Inc. 800-48W-ESCO
2112 W Burbank Blvd, Burbank, CA 91506

MICROSCOPE, LASER, SCANNING, ACOUSTIC
(Microbiology) 83UEV

Coherent, Inc. 800-527-3786
5100 Patrick Henry Dr, Santa Clara, CA 95054

Nikon Canada Inc., Instrument Div. 905-625-9910
1366 Aerowood Dr., Mississauga, ONT L4W-1C1 Canada

Technical Instruments (Ti) 650-651-3000
1826 Rollins Rd, Burlingame, CA 94010
Confocal scanning microscope.

MICROSCOPE, LIGHT *(Pathology) 88IBJ*

Accu-Scope, Inc. 516-759-1000
7 Littleworth Ln, Sea Cliff, NY 11579

Carolina Biological Supply Co. 800-334-5551
2700 York Rd, Burlington, NC 27215

Diasys Corporation 800-360-2003
21 W Main St, Waterbury, CT 06702
R/S and FE-2 Series Workstations that works in conjunction with any standard microscope to automate the analysis of urine sediment, and fecal concentrates respectively.

Labo America, Inc. 510-445-1257
920 Auburn Ct, Fremont, CA 94538

MICROSCOPE, LIGHT *(cont'd)*

Micromanipulator Co., Inc., The 800-972-4032
1555 Forrest Way, Carson City, NV 89706
Products and accessories to aid in embryo recovery, grading, splitting, injection, micromanipulation and photomicrography.

Nikon Canada Inc., Instrument Div. 905-625-9910
1366 Aerowood Dr., Mississauga, ONT L4W-1C1 Canada

Nikon Instruments Inc. 800-52-Nikon
1300 Walt Whitman Rd, Melville, NY 11747

Richard-Allan Scientific 269-544-5628
4481 Campus Dr, Kalamazoo, MI 49008
Various.

Ted Pella, Inc. 800-237-3526
4595 Mountain Lakes Blvd, Redding, CA 96003
Laboratory and research microscopes, Motic BA series with optinal digital color imaging.

Translite 281-240-3111
8410 Highway 90A, Sugar Land, TX 77478
Skin examination microscope.

United Products & Instruments, Inc. 800-588-9776
182 Ridge Rd Ste E, Dayton, NJ 08810
Our most advanced and versatile compound microscopes are able to perform allthe intricate and varied functions of microscopes costing thousands of dollarsmore. With continuing improvements, and the addition of new high-power accessories, today's H600 SERIES has even greater potential for research,education and medical applications. UNICO's attention to detail and function mean that your H600 SERIES microscopewill give decades of useful service. Visit us at www.unico1.com for more information on complete microscope line from UNICO

Western Scientific Co., Inc. 877-489-3726
4104 24th St # 183, San Francisco, CA 94114
Complete line of microscopes; video and digital imaging systems.

MICROSCOPE, OPERATING, AC-POWERED, OPHTHALMIC
(Ophthalmology) 86HRM

Accutome, Inc. 610-889-0200
3222 Phoenixville Pike, Malvern, PA 19355
Microscope & accessories.

Bausch & Lomb Surgical 636-255-5051
3365 Tree Court Ind Blvd, Saint Louis, MO 63122

Biomedics, Inc. 949-458-1998
23322 Peralta Dr Ste 11, Laguna Hills, CA 92653
Zeiss, Storz, Leica

Carl Zeiss Surgical, Inc. 800-442-4020
1 Zeiss Dr, Thornwood, NY 10594
Features include fiber optic illumination system for red reflex, optimal depth perception, clarity and resolution, and three integrated angles of illumination.

Endure Medical, Inc. 770-888-3755
1455 Ventura Dr, Cumming, GA 30040
Surgical microscope.

Hill-Med, Inc. 305-594-7474
7217 NW 46th St, Miami, FL 33166

Leica Microsystems (Canada) Inc. 800-205-3422
400 - 111 Granton Drive, Richmond Hill, ONT L4B 1L5 Canada

Md International, Inc. 305-669-9003
11300 NW 41st St, Doral, FL 33178

Questar Corp. 800-247-9607
6204 Ingham Rd, New Hope, PA 18938
$5,000 to $55,000 for diagnostic and research non-invasive microscopes with working distances of 6 to 200in.

Topcon Medical Systems, Inc. 800-223-1130
37 W Century Rd, Paramus, NJ 07652
Four models of ophthalmic microscopes: $9,490.00 for office/ambulatory use; hospital-based use: (please call for current pricing).

Wallach Surgical Devices, Inc. 800-243-2463
235 Edison Rd, Orange, CT 06477
$8295.00 for operating microscope with 200m magnification, with power zoom and power focus.

Woodlyn, Inc. 800-331-7389
2920 Malmo Dr, Ophthalmic Instruments and Equipment
Arlington Heights, IL 60005
Woodlyn Model 9809600 operation microscope. Call for current prices.

MICROSCOPE, OPERATING, NON-ELECTRIC, OPHTHALMIC
(Ophthalmology) 86HRB

Avi-Advanced Visual Instruments Inc. 212-262-7878
321 W 44th St Ste 902, New York, NY 10036
Microscope video adapter, stereo image inverter.

World Medical Equipment, Inc. 800-827-3747
3915 152nd St NE, Marysville, WA 98271

MICROSCOPE, PHASE CONTRAST *(Pathology) 88IBM*

Accu-Scope, Inc. 516-759-1000
7 Littleworth Ln, Sea Cliff, NY 11579

Carl Zeiss Surgical, Inc. 800-442-4020
1 Zeiss Dr, Thornwood, NY 10594

Labo America, Inc. 510-445-1257
920 Auburn Ct, Fremont, CA 94538

Lucid, Inc. 585-239-9800
2320 Brighton Henrietta Town Line Rd, Rochester, NY 14623
Confocal microscopes.

Standard Instrumentation, Div. Preiser Scientific 800-624-8285
94 Oliver St, Saint Albans, WV 25177

Ward's Natural Science Establishment, Inc. 800-962-2660
PO Box 92912, 5100 W. Henrietta Rd., Rochester, NY 14692

Western Scientific Co., Inc. 877-489-3726
4104 24th St # 183, San Francisco, CA 94114
Upright and inverted phase-contrast microscopes.

MICROSCOPE, SURGICAL *(Ear/Nose/Throat) 77EPT*

Biomedics, Inc. 949-458-1998
23322 Peralta Dr Ste 11, Laguna Hills, CA 92653

Camsight Co., Inc. 323-259-1900
3380 N San Fernando Rd, Glassell, CA 90065
Camsight digital surgical scope.

Carl Zeiss Meditec Inc. 877-486-7473
5160 Hacienda Dr, Dublin, CA 94568

Carl Zeiss Surgical, Inc. 800-442-4020
1 Zeiss Dr, Thornwood, NY 10594

Dentalez Group 866-DTE-INFO
101 Lindenwood Dr Ste 225, Valleybrooke Corporate Center
Malvern, PA 19355

Global Surgical Corp. 314-861-3388
3610 Tree Court Industrial Blvd, Saint Louis, MO 63122
Storz sugical microscope system.

Jedmed Instruments Co. 314-845-3770
5416 Jedmed Ct, Saint Louis, MO 63129

Leica Microsystems (Canada) Inc. 800-205-3422
400 - 111 Granton Drive, Richmond Hill, ONT L4B 1L5 Canada

Marco Ophthalmic, Inc. 800-874-5274
11825 Central Pkwy, Jacksonville, FL 32224
$8,550.00 for in-office microscope. (List price)

Products For Medicine 800-333-3087
1201 E Ball Rd Ste H, Anaheim, CA 92805
Bulb replacements for light sources.

Richard Wolf Medical Instruments Corp. 800-323-9653
353 Corporate Woods Pkwy, Vernon Hills, IL 60061

Stereoimaging Corporation 978-649-8592
164 Westford Rd Ste 17, Tyngsboro, MA 01879
Zoom microscope.

Techman Int'L Corp. 508-248-2900
242 Sturbridge Rd, Charlton, MA 01507
Microscope.

Tidi Products, Llc 920-751-4380
570 Enterprise Dr, Neenah, WI 54956
Drape for operation microscopes.

Truevision Systems, Incorporated 805-963-9700
114 E Haley St, Santa Barbara, CA 93101
Microsurgery teaching system.

MICROSCOPE, SURGICAL, GENERAL & PLASTIC SURGERY
(Surgery) 79FSO

Biomedics, Inc. 949-458-1998
23322 Peralta Dr Ste 11, Laguna Hills, CA 92653
Zeiss, Storz, Leica, Wild, etc...

Carl Zeiss Surgical, Inc. 800-442-4020
1 Zeiss Dr, Thornwood, NY 10594

Codman & Shurtleff, Inc 800-225-0460
325 Paramount Dr, Raynham, MA 02767

MICROSCOPE, SURGICAL, GENERAL & PLASTIC SURGERY
(cont'd)

Elmed, Inc. 630-543-2792
60 W Fay Ave, Addison, IL 60101

International Hospital Supply Co. 800-398-9450
6914 Canby Ave Ste 105, Reseda, CA 91335
Arthroscopy, laparoscopy, endoscopy.

Jedmed Instruments Co. 314-845-3770
5416 Jedmed Ct, Saint Louis, MO 63129

Leica Microsystems (Canada) Inc. 800-205-3422
400 - 111 Granton Drive, Richmond Hill, ONT L4B 1L5 Canada

Md International, Inc. 305-669-9003
11300 NW 41st St, Doral, FL 33178

Newport Optical Laboratories, Inc. 714-484-3200
10564C Fern Ave, Stanton, CA 90680

Olympus America, Inc. 800-645-8160
3500 Corporate Pkwy, PO Box 610, Center Valley, PA 18034

Richard Wolf Medical Instruments Corp. 800-323-9653
353 Corporate Woods Pkwy, Vernon Hills, IL 60061

Technical Instruments (Ti) 650-651-3000
1826 Rollins Rd, Burlingame, CA 94010

Wallach Surgical Devices, Inc. 800-243-2463
235 Edison Rd, Orange, CT 06477
$5615.00 for operating zoomscope 4-20x microscope.

Whittemore Enterprises, Inc. 800-999-2452
11149 Arrow Rte, Rancho Cucamonga, CA 91730

MICROSCOPE, SURGICAL, NEUROSURGICAL
(Cns/Neurology) 84HBH

Carl Zeiss Surgical, Inc. 800-442-4020
1 Zeiss Dr, Thornwood, NY 10594

Leica Microsystems (Canada) Inc. 800-205-3422
400 - 111 Granton Drive, Richmond Hill, ONT L4B 1L5 Canada

MICROSCOPE, TISSUE CULTURE *(Microbiology) 83VES*

Accu-Scope, Inc. 516-759-1000
7 Littleworth Ln, Sea Cliff, NY 11579

Labo America, Inc. 510-445-1257
920 Auburn Ct, Fremont, CA 94538

Leica Microsystems (Canada) Inc. 800-205-3422
400 - 111 Granton Drive, Richmond Hill, ONT L4B 1L5 Canada

Nikon Canada Inc., Instrument Div. 905-625-9910
1366 Aerowood Dr., Mississauga, ONT L4W-1C1 Canada

Western Scientific Co., Inc. 877-489-3726
4104 24th St # 183, San Francisco, CA 94114
Inverted and upright microscopes--brightfield, fluorescence, and phase contrast.

MICROTITER DILUTING/DISPENSING DEVICE
(Microbiology) 83JTC

Bio-Rad Laboratories, Inc. 425-881-8300
6565 185th Ave NE, Redmond, WA 98052
Handheld microplate washer.

Cadence Science Inc. 888-717-7677
1979 Marcus Ave Ste 215, New Hyde Park, NY 11042

Dynacon Ent. Ltd. 905-672-8828
2nd Fl, 3565 Nashua Dr, Mississauga L4V 1R1 Canada
Inoculab j 80

Dynex Technologies, Inc. 800-288-2354
14340 Sullyfield Cir, Chantilly, VA 20151
Various.

Progroup Instrument Corp. 800-471-1916
4947 Fosterburg Rd, Alton, IL 62002
The WellPro Automated Liquid Handling System (tm) utilizes a 12 channel liquid head and disposable pipette tips to perform serial dilutions, plate to plate transfers, and plate filling from reservoirs. Working volumes range from 5 to 200ul for the standard tips, and 5 to 120ul for filter tips. The unit operates through a convenient hand held controller eliminating the need for another PC to consume valuable bench space.

Tri-Continent Scientific, Inc. 530-274-4240
12555 Loma Rica Dr # 2, Grass Valley, CA 95945
Various.

Tricontinent 800-937-4738
12555 Loma Rica Dr, Grass Valley, CA 95945

MICROTOME, CRYOSTAT *(Pathology) 88IDP*

Bayer Healthcare Llc 914-524-2955
555 White Plains Rd Fl 5, Tarrytown, NY 10591
Microtome-cryostat.

Hacker Instruments And Industries Inc. 800-442-2537
1132 Kincaid Bridge Rd, PO Box 1176, Winnsboro, SC 29180
Hacker-Bright Clinicut; ideal for clinical pathology; rapid, convenient frozen sections; affordable price. Hacker-Bright OTF; dual, parallel refrigeration; consistent quantitative serial sections; whole body & undecalcified bone sectioning.

Kendro Laboratory Products 800-252-7100
308 Ridgefield Ct, Asheville, NC 28806

Medical Sales & Service Group 888-357-6520
10 Woodchester Dr, Acton, MA 01720

Myco Instrumentation Source, Inc. 425-228-4239
PO Box 354, Renton, WA 98057

Sakura Finetek U.S.A., Inc. 800-725-8723
1750 W 214th St, Torrance, CA 90501
TISSUE-TEK CRYO3 microtome/cryostat features patented ozone disinfection.

Spectron Corp. 425-827-9317
934 S Burlington Blvd # 603, Burlington, WA 98233
Reconditioned equipment.

Technical Products International, Inc. 800-729-4421
5918 Evergreen Blvd, Saint Louis, MO 63134
Complete line of cryostats including a self decontaminating cryostat

MICROTOME, FREEZING ATTACHMENT *(Pathology) 88IDN*

Advanced Spine Technology, Inc. 415-241-2400
457 Mariposa St, San Francisco, CA 94107
Chisel.

Boeckeler Instruments, Inc. 800-552-2262
4650 S Butterfield Dr, Tucson, AZ 85714
Cryo units for microtomes and ultramicrotomes

Hacker Industries, Inc. 803-712-6100
1132 Kincaid Bridge Rd, Winnsboro, SC 29180
Freezing attachment.

MICROTOME, ROTARY *(Pathology) 88IDO*

Boeckeler Instruments, Inc. 800-552-2262
4650 S Butterfield Dr, Tucson, AZ 85714
MT-990, MR-2, MR-3 rotary microtomes from RMC Products line

Energy Beam Sciences, Inc. 800-992-9037
29 Kripes Rd Ste B, East Granby, CT 06026
For sectioning of plastic and embedded specimens.

Hacker Industries, Inc. 803-712-6100
1132 Kincaid Bridge Rd, Winnsboro, SC 29180
Hacker rh-950 rotary.

Hacker Instruments And Industries Inc. 800-442-2537
1132 Kincaid Bridge Rd, PO Box 1176, Winnsboro, SC 29180
H/I 100, 200 & 300 series microtomes. From fully manual to fully automate - dependable and user friendly.

Kendro Laboratory Products 800-252-7100
308 Ridgefield Ct, Asheville, NC 28806

Leica Microsystems Inc. 800-248-0123
2345 Waukegan Rd, Bannockburn, IL 60015
RM2255, one of a series of microtomes for routine histology, pathology, research, biological and clinical applications.

Medical Sales & Service Group 888-357-6520
10 Woodchester Dr, Acton, MA 01720

Sakura Finetek U.S.A., Inc. 800-725-8723
1750 W 214th St, Torrance, CA 90501
ACCU-CUT $6,700 for SRM 200 rotary microtome.

Surgipath Medical Industries, Inc. 800-225-3035
PO Box 528, 5205 Route 12, Richmond, IL 60071
Rotary and Semiautomatic

MICROTOME, SLIDING *(Pathology) 88KFL*

Hacker Industries, Inc. 803-712-6100
1132 Kincaid Bridge Rd, Winnsboro, SC 29180
H/i sliding microtome.

Technical Products International, Inc. 800-729-4421
5918 Evergreen Blvd, Saint Louis, MO 63134
The 8000 retracting base sliding microtome offers the ultimate in versatility combined with strength, accuracy, reliability and, not least, safety.

MICROTOME, ULTRA *(Pathology) 88IDM*

Boeckeler Instruments, Inc. 800-552-2262
4650 S Butterfield Dr, Tucson, AZ 85714
PT-X, PT-XL and PT-PC ultramicrotomes from the RMC Products line

Leica Microsystems (Canada) Inc. 800-205-3422
400 - 111 Granton Drive, Richmond Hill, ONT L4B 1L5 Canada
LEICA

Leica Microsystems Inc. 800-248-0123
2345 Waukegan Rd, Bannockburn, IL 60015
EM UC6 Ultracut with FSC cryochamber for the preparation of specimens for electron microscopy.

MICROTOOLS, ASSISTED REPRODUCTION
(Obstetrics/Gyn) 85MQH

Conception Technologies 858-824-0888
6835 Flanders Dr Ste 500, San Diego, CA 92121
Microtools for assisted reproduction.

Cook Ob/Gyn 800-541-5591
1100 W Morgan St, Spencer, IN 47460

Sage In-Vitro Fertilization Inc. 203-601-5200
1979 Locust St, Pasadena, CA 91107
Various.

MIRROR, CORRIDOR SAFETY *(General) 80TGZ*

Crest Healthcare Supply 800-328-8908
195 3rd St, Dassel, MN 55325
Observation and safety mirrors.

K-10 Enterprizes, Inc. 800-531-7496
PO Box 1170, Mission, TX 78573
$34.50 for 1/4 hemisphere (L intersection); $65.50 for 1/2 hemisphere; $126.00 for full hemisphere; $114.50 for convex 36in. x 24in. surveillance mirror. $120 for 18in. dia. polycarbonate bubble window. $130.00 for 2'X4' mirror dome in tile. New Wall-Eye Mirror $69.50

MIRROR, ENDOSCOPIC *(Surgery) 79GCO*

Aesculap Implant Systems Inc. 1-800-234-9179
3773 Corporate Pkwy, Center Valley, PA 18034

Clinical Instruments Intl., Inc. 508-764-2200
278 Worcester St, Southbridge, MA 01550
Introducers.

San Diego Swiss Machining, Inc. 858-571-6636
9177 Aero Dr Ste A, San Diego, CA 92123
Surgical mirror with fiberoptic and video carrier.

Sohniks Endoscopy, Inc. 651-452-4059
930 Blue Gentian Rd Ste 1400, Eagan, MN 55121
Various types of flexible endoscopes.

MIRROR, ENT *(Ear/Nose/Throat) 77KAI*

Aesculap Implant Systems Inc. 1-800-234-9179
3773 Corporate Pkwy, Center Valley, PA 18034

Bausch & Lomb Surgical 636-255-5051
3365 Tree Court Ind Blvd, Saint Louis, MO 63122

Clinimed, Incorporated 877-CLINIMED
303 Markus Ct, Sandy Brae Industrial Park, Newark, DE 19713

Electro Surgical Instrument Co., Inc. 888-464-2784
37 Centennial St, Rochester, NY 14611
Various sizes and types of mirrors for ent, general, endoscopic and plastic surg.

Jedmed Instruments Co. 314-845-3770
5416 Jedmed Ct, Saint Louis, MO 63129

Mahe International Inc. 800-294-7946
468 Craighead St, Nashville, TN 37204

Md International, Inc. 305-669-9003
11300 NW 41st St, Doral, FL 33178

Miltex Dental Technologies, Inc. 516-576-6022
589 Davies Dr, York, PA 17402
Various ear and throat mirrors.

Princeton Medical Group, Inc. 800-875-0869
1189 Royal Links Dr, Mt Pleasant, SC 29466

Welch Allyn, Inc. 800-535-6663
4341 State Street Rd, Skaneateles Falls, NY 13153

MIRROR, GENERAL & PLASTIC SURGERY *(Surgery) 79FTX*

Bausch & Lomb Surgical 636-255-5051
3365 Tree Court Ind Blvd, Saint Louis, MO 63122

Codman & Shurtleff, Inc 800-225-0460
325 Paramount Dr, Raynham, MA 02767

MIRROR, GENERAL & PLASTIC SURGERY *(cont'd)*

Opco Laboratory, Inc. 978-345-2522
704 River St, Fitchburg, MA 01420
Custom optical mirrors for analytical instruments.

Paul Arpin Mfg. 408-263-4974
1347 Highland Ct, Milpitas, CA 95035
Medical mirror kit.

Richardson Products, Inc. 888-928-7297
9408 Gulfstream Rd, Frankfort, IL 60423
Mirror.

MIRROR, HEADBAND, OPHTHALMIC *(Ophthalmology) 86HKF*

Bausch & Lomb Surgical 636-255-5051
3365 Tree Court Ind Blvd, Saint Louis, MO 63122

Jedmed Instruments Co. 314-845-3770
5416 Jedmed Ct, Saint Louis, MO 63129

MIRROR, LARYNGEAL *(Ear/Nose/Throat) 77RHA*

Aesculap Implant Systems Inc. 1-800-234-9179
3773 Corporate Pkwy, Center Valley, PA 18034

Alimed, Inc. 800-225-2610
297 High St, Dedham, MA 02026

Bausch & Lomb Surgical 636-255-5051
3365 Tree Court Ind Blvd, Saint Louis, MO 63122

Elmed, Inc. 630-543-2792
60 W Fay Ave, Addison, IL 60101

Jedmed Instruments Co. 314-845-3770
5416 Jedmed Ct, Saint Louis, MO 63129

Miltex Inc. 800-645-8000
589 Davies Dr, York, PA 17402

Welch Allyn, Inc. 800-535-6663
4341 State Street Rd, Skaneateles Falls, NY 13153

MIRROR, MIDDLE EAR *(Ear/Nose/Throat) 77RHB*

Bausch & Lomb Surgical 636-255-5051
3365 Tree Court Ind Blvd, Saint Louis, MO 63122

MIRROR, MOUTH *(Dental And Oral) 76EAX*

Aesculap Implant Systems Inc. 1-800-234-9179
3773 Corporate Pkwy, Center Valley, PA 18034

Alliance Precision Plastics 585-426-2630
595 Trabold Rd, Rochester, NY 14624

American Eagle Instruments, Inc. 406-549-7451
6575 Butler Creek Rd, Missoula, MT 59808
Various types of mouth mirrors.

Biomet Microfixation Inc. 800-874-7711
1520 Tradeport Dr, Jacksonville, FL 32218
Mirror, mouth.

Cadco Dental Products 800-833-8267
600 E Hueneme Rd, Oxnard, CA 93033

Classone Orthodontics, Inc. 806-799-0608
5064 50th St, Lubbock, TX 79414
Various types of mirrors.

Clive Craig Co. 805-488-1122
600 E Hueneme Rd, Oxnard, CA 93033
Mouth mirror.

Crystalmark Dental Systems, Inc. 818-240-7596
621 Ruberta Ave, Glendale, CA 91201
Mirror, mouth.

Dental Usa, Inc. 815-363-8003
5005 McCullom Lake Rd, McHenry, IL 60050
Various types of mirrors.

Dentalez Group 866-DTE-INFO
101 Lindenwood Dr Ste 225, Valleybrooke Corporate Center
Malvern, PA 19355

Dentalez Group, Stardental Division 717-291-1161
1816 Colonial Village Ln, Lancaster, PA 17601
X-ray machine, dental.

Dentek Oral Care, Inc. 865-983-1300
307 Excellence Way, Maryville, TN 37801
Mouth mirror.

Denticator International, Inc. 800-325-1881
13705 Shoreline Ct E, Earth City, MO 63045
$.48 per unit (standard).

Dux Dental 800-833-8267
600 E Hueneme Rd, Oxnard, CA 93033

MIRROR, MOUTH *(cont'd)*

Evaporated Metal Films Corp. 800-456-7070
239 Cherry St, Ithaca, NY 14850
Various intra-oral photography mirrors.

G & H Wire Co. 800-526-1026
2165 Earlywood Dr, Franklin, IN 46131

H & H Co. 909-390-0373
4435 E Airport Dr Ste 108, Ontario, CA 91761
Mirror, mouth.

Hager Worldwide, Inc. 800-328-2335
13322 Byrd Dr, Odessa, FL 33556
BRILLIANT & DURATANIC (mouth mirrors).

Hu-Friedy Manufacturing Co., Inc. 800-483-7433
3232 N Rockwell St, Chicago, IL 60618
$10.85 to $13.35 for handles; $5.45 to $7.00 for mirrors.

Inter-Med, Inc. 877-418-4782
2200 Northwestern Ave, Racine, WI 53404
Mirror, mouth.

Kerr Corp. 714-516-7400
28200 Wick Rd, Romulus, MI 48174
Various mouth mirrors.

Masel Co., Inc. 800-423-8227
2701 Bartram Rd, Bristol, PA 19007

Metron Optics, Inc. 858-755-4477
PO Box 690, 813 Academy Drive, Solana Beach, CA 92075
Diamond coated MiniMirrors. Ultra small and thin.

Miltex Dental Technologies, Inc. 516-576-6022
589 Davies Dr, York, PA 17402
Various dental mouth mirrors.

Moyco Technologies, Inc. 800-331-8837
200 Commerce Dr, Montgomeryville, PA 18936
Stainless, plastic and chrome.

Mydent International 800-275-0020
80 Suffolk Ct, Hauppauge, NY 11788
DEFEND MirrorLite: Illuminated mouth mirror.

Nordent Manufacturing, Inc. 800-966-7336
610 Bonnie Ln, Elk Grove Village, IL 60007
$3.50 for mirror handle.

Nu-Lite Retractor, Inc. 718-886-3461
400 E 56th St Apt 4D, New York, NY 10022
Dental mirror-retractor /// mirrored dental retractor.

Parkell, Inc. 800-243-7446
300 Executive Dr, Edgewood, NY 11717
20/20 Double-sided mirrors

Precision Dental Int, Inc. 818-992-1888
21361 Deering Ct, Canoga Park, CA 91304
Mouth mirror.

Qed, Inc. 859-231-0338
750 Enterprise Dr, Lexington, KY 40510
Dental mirror.

Richardson Products, Inc. 888-928-7297
9408 Gulfstream Rd, Frankfort, IL 60423
Mouth mirror.

Ruthal Industries Ltd. 800-445-6640
1 Industrial Ave., Mahwah, NJ 07430-2113
FLOXITE dental mirror light uses high magnification for self-examination. Reusable (3.5in. diameter) or disposable, fitting over any 2in. diameter flashlight 115 volt and 60 Hz (AC).

Salvin Dental Specialties, Inc. 800-535-6566
3450 Latrobe Dr, Charlotte, NC 28211
Photo mirror.

San Diego Swiss Machining, Inc. 858-571-6636
9177 Aero Dr Ste A, San Diego, CA 92123
Various.

Sunstar Butler 800-J BUTLER
4635 W Foster Ave, Chicago, IL 60630

Team Technologies, Inc. 423-587-2199
5949 Commerce Blvd, Morristown, TN 37814
Mirror, mouth.

Trans American Medical / Tamsco Instruments 708-430-7777
7633 W 100th Pl, Bridgeview, IL 60455
Disposable and reusable.

Ultradent Products, Inc. 801-553-4586
505 W 10200 S, South Jordan, UT 84095
Mouth mirror.

MIRROR, MOUTH *(cont'd)*

Wykle Research, Inc. 775-887-7500
2222 College Pkwy, Carson City, NV 89706
Mouth mirror.

Zirc Company 800-328-3899
3918 State Highway 55 SE, Buffalo, MN 55313
Plastic, sterilizable.

Zoll Dental 800-239-2904
7450 N Natchez Ave, Niles, IL 60714
Mirrors.

MIRROR, OBSTETRICAL *(Obstetrics/Gyn) 85RHC*

K-10 Enterprizes, Inc. 800-531-7496
PO Box 1170, Mission, TX 78573
$114.50 for 36 x 24in. surveillance mirror.

MIRROR, POSTURE *(Physical Med) 89RHD*

Alimed, Inc. 800-225-2610
297 High St, Dedham, MA 02026

Hausmann Industries, Inc. 888-428-7626
130 Union St, Northvale, NJ 07647
3 models - $275 to $745 each.

Hygiene Specialties, Inc./Andermac, Inc. 800-824-0214
2626 Live Oak Blvd, Yuba City, CA 95991
Portable mirror with 2 sets of arms, for use on the toilet or flat surface. Double sided 5 in. mirror with magnified and life-sized images. Battery operated lights. Self-cath patients and wound therapists highly recommend this product.

S&W By Hausmann 888-428-7626
130 Union St, Northvale, NJ 07647

MIRROR, SPEECH *(Ear/Nose/Throat) 77RHE*

Alimed, Inc. 800-225-2610
297 High St, Dedham, MA 02026

Maddak Inc. 800-443-4926
661 State Route 23, Wayne, NJ 07470
ABLEWARE.

MITT/WASHCLOTH, PATIENT *(General) 80RHF*

Atlantic Mills, Inc. 800-242-7374
1295 Towbin Ave, Lakewood, NJ 08701
Disposable washcloth (boxed & bulk).

General Econopak, Inc. 888-871-8568
1725 N 6th St, Philadelphia, PA 19122
Disposable washcloths, wipers, hand-towels, 4-ply.

Graham Medical Products/Div. Of Little Rapids Corp 866-429-1408
2273 Larsen Rd, Green Bay, WI 54303
Non-woven washcloths with high wet strength.

Health-Pak, Inc. 315-724-8370
2005 Beechgrove Pl, Utica, NY 13501
Non-woven.

Jero Medical Equipment & Supplies, Inc. 800-457-0644
1701 W 13th St, Chicago, IL 60608

Jms Converters Inc Dba Sabee Products & Stanford Prof Prod 215-396-3302
67 Buck Rd Ste B7, Huntingdon Valley, PA 19006
Disposable patient washcloths.

Principle Business Enterprises, Inc. 800-467-3224
PO Box 129, Dunbridge, OH 43414
TRANQUILITY Personal Cleaning Washcloths which are premoistened and disposable.

MIXER, ALGINATE *(Dental And Oral) 76VEF*

Cadco Dental Products 800-833-8267
600 E Hueneme Rd, Oxnard, CA 93033
IDENTIC & KROMAFAZE Alginate is irreversible hydrocolloid used for impression making. Also available in color changing alginate.

Dux Dental 800-833-8267
600 E Hueneme Rd, Oxnard, CA 93033
IDENTIC & KROMAFAZE Alginate is irreversible hydrocolloid used for impression making. Also available in color changing alginate.

Masel Co., Inc. 800-423-8227
2701 Bartram Rd, Bristol, PA 19007

MIXER, BLOOD BANK, DONOR BLOOD *(Hematology) 81RHG*

Engineering & Research Assoc., Inc. (D.B.A. Sebra) 800-625-5550
100 N Tucson Blvd, Tucson, AZ 85716
SEBRA, blood shaker/weight monitor, SEBRA digital blood shaker/flow and weight monitor.

Pall Corporation 800-645-6532
25 Harbor Park Dr, Port Washington, NY 11050
HemoFlow 400

MIXER, BLOOD TUBE *(Hematology) 81GLE*

Beckman Coulter, Inc. 800-635-3497
740 W 83rd St, Hialeah, FL 33014
$275.00 available with M430 system and separate.

Sarstedt, Inc. 800-257-5101
PO Box 468, 1025, St. James Church Road, Newton, NC 28658

MIXER, BREATHING GASES, ANESTHESIA INHALATION *(Anesthesiology) 73BZR*

Cardinal Health 207, Inc. 610-862-0800
1100 Bird Center Dr, Palm Springs, CA 92262
Nasal continuous positive airway pressure (ncpap).

Maxtec, Inc. 800-748-5355
6526 Cottonwood St, Salt Lake City, UT 84107
MaxBlend. Air/Oxygen Blender w/oxygen monitor. 0-30 IPM.

Respironics California, Inc. 724-387-4559
2271 Cosmos Ct, Carlsbad, CA 92011
Transtracheal continous flow gas delivery system.

Sechrist Industries, Inc. 800-732-4747
4225 E La Palma Ave, Anaheim, CA 92807
Oxygen/air mixer.

MIXER, CHEMICAL, FILM, X-RAY *(Radiology) 90WHY*

Simon & Company Inc., H.R. 800-638-9460
3515 Marmenco Ct, Baltimore, MD 21230

MIXER, CLINICAL LABORATORY *(Chemistry) 75RHH*

Baxa Corporation 800-567-2292
9540 S Maroon Circle, Suite 400, Englewood, CO 80112
MICROMACRO, Compounder TPN compounding systems.

Brinkmann Instruments (Canada) Ltd. 800-263-8715
6670 Campobello Rd., Mississauga, ONT L5N 2L8 Canada
Electronic overhead mixers with high, constant-torque ensure reproducible speeds regardless of load.

Burrell Scientific, Inc 800-637-6074
2223 5th Ave, Pittsburgh, PA 15219
WRIST ACTION SHAKER, laboratory shaker with build-up capabilities that duplicates hand/wrist action.

Cole-Parmer Instrument Inc. 800-323-4340
625 E Bunker Ct, Vernon Hills, IL 60061

Dade Behring, Inc. 800-948-3233
1717 Deerfield Rd, Deerfield, IL 60015

Gilson Company, Inc. 800-444-1508
PO Box 200, Lewis Center, OH 43035

Ika-Works, Inc. 800-733-3037
2635 Northchase Pkwy SE, Wilmington, NC 28405
Laboratory mixers and shakers feature compensation systems and electronic speed controls to ensure stability and repeatability.

Jiffy Mixer Co., Inc. 800-560-2903
1691 California Ave, Corona, CA 92881
5 models - 10.5 to 40 in. shaft length; 1 pint to 50/55 gal. capacity fits 1/4 to 3/4 in. power tools.

Microfluidics International Corporation 800-370-5452
30 Ossipee Rd, Newton Upper Falls, MA 02464
MICROFLUIDIZER Fluid mixer.

Nalge Nunc International 800-625-4327
75 Panorama Creek Dr, Rochester, NY 14625
Mixers and assemblies including mixer overhead drives and lower assemblies/shafts and impellers.

Scientific Industries, Inc. 888-850-6208
70 Orville Dr, Bohemia, NY 11716

Troemner Llc 800-352-7705
201 Wolf Dr, PO Box 87, West Deptford, NJ 08086

Whip-Mix Corporation 800-626-5651
361 Farmington Ave, PO Box 17183, Louisville, KY 40209

MIXER/SCALE, BLOOD *(Hematology) 81KSQ*

Baxter Healthcare Corp., Renal Division 847-948-2000
7511 114th Ave, Largo, FL 33773
Various donor chair accessories.

Centron Technologies, Inc. 215-501-0430
10601 Decatur Rd Ste 100, Philadelphia, PA 19154
Genesis blood collection mixer cm735.

Engineering & Research Assoc., Inc. (D.B.A. Sebra) 800-625-5550
100 N Tucson Blvd, Tucson, AZ 85716
SEBRA, blood shaker/weight monitor, SEBRA digital blood shaker/flow and weight monitor.

Sarstedt, Inc. 800-257-5101
PO Box 468, 1025, St. James Church Road, Newton, NC 28658

Vulcon Technologies 816-966-1212
718 Main St, Grandview, MO 64030
Blood rocker.

MIXING EQUIPMENT, CEMENT *(Orthopedics) 87JDZ*

Advanced Biomaterial Systems, Inc. 973-635-9040
100 Passaic Ave, Chatham, NJ 07928
Bone cement mixer and dispenser.

Depuy Orthopaedics, Inc. 800-473-3789
700 Orthopaedic Dr, P.O. Box 988, Warsaw, IN 46582
Various types of cement mixers for clinical use.

DFine Inc. 866-963-3463
3047 Orchard Pkwy, San Jose, CA 95134

Donatelle 651-746-2900
501 County Rd. E-2 Extension, New Brighton, MN 55112

Medtronic Spine Llc 877-690-5353
1221 Crossman Ave, Sunnyvale, CA 94089
Cement mixer.

Pac-Dent Intl., Inc. 909-839-0888
21078 Commerce Point Dr, Walnut, CA 91789
Various mixing bowls.

Precision Medical Devices, Inc. 717-795-9480
5020 Ritter Rd Ste 211, Mechanicsburg, PA 17055
Bone cement mixer.

Stryker Corp. 800-726-2725
2825 Airview Blvd, Portage, MI 49002

Stryker Puerto Rico, Ltd. 939-307-2500
Hwy. 3, Km. 131.2, Las Guasimas Ind. Park, Arroyo, PR 00714
Cement mixers for clinical use.

Stryker Spine 866-457-7463
2 Pearl Ct, Allendale, NJ 07401

Synthes (Usa) - Development Center 719-481-5300
1230 Wilson Dr, West Chester, PA 19380
Cement mixer.

Zimmer Holdings, Inc. 800-613-6131
1800 W Center St, PO Box 708, Warsaw, IN 46580

MIXING SLAB *(Dental And Oral) 76RHI*

Cadco Dental Products 800-833-8267
600 E Hueneme Rd, Oxnard, CA 93033
$245.00 for Alginator, electrical mixer.

Dux Dental 800-833-8267
600 E Hueneme Rd, Oxnard, CA 93033
$245.00 for Alginator, electrical mixer.

Ivoclar Vivadent, Inc. 800-533-6825
175 Pineview Dr, Amherst, NY 14228

Moyco Technologies, Inc. 800-331-8837
200 Commerce Dr, Montgomeryville, PA 18936
$3.15 per 4x2.5 in. unit (standard).

MOBILIZER, ENT *(Ear/Nose/Throat) 77KAJ*

Aesculap Implant Systems Inc. 1-800-234-9179
3773 Corporate Pkwy, Center Valley, PA 18034

MOIST THERAPY PACK *(Physical Med) 89RHK*

Battle Creek Equipment Co. 800-253-0854
307 Jackson St W, Battle Creek, MI 49037
THERMOPHORE, for temporary pain relief; $74.95 per unit (14 x 27 in.), $59.95 per unit (14 x 14 inch), $49.95 per unit (4 x 17 inch). Thermophore muff is rolled for arthritic hands, $49.95.

Bruder Healthcare Company 888-827-8337
3150 Engineering Pkwy, Alpharetta, GA 30004
Microwave Moist Heat Products

MOIST THERAPY PACK *(cont'd)*

Chattanooga Group 800-592-7329
4717 Adams Rd, Hixson, TN 37343
HYDROCOLLATOR HOTPAC and THERATHERM Digital Moist heating pad.

Medi Inc 800-225-8634
75 York Ave, P.O. Box 302, Randolph, MA 02368

Medical Supplies Corporation T/A.Roberts Manufacturing Co., 800-451-9951
4002 Dillon St, Baltimore, MD 21224
$492.00 for 12 petite moist heat therapy pads, 4' x 13'; each $59.95.

Ooltewah Manufacturing 800-251-6040x25
5722 Main St, P.O. Box 587, Ooltewah, TN 37363
EZ ice cold therapy.

Pelton Shepherd Industries 800-258-3423
812B W Luce St, Stockton, CA 95203
7 sizes canvas & bentonite HYDROTHERM Mst Ht Pk & Cvrs 5100 standard size 10 x 12 in. 5102 cervical (neck) size 6 1/2 in. x 21 in. 5104 oversize 15 in. x 24 in. 5106 half-size 5 in. x 12 in. 5114 in. large size 10 x 18 in. 5116 ex-large size 10 in. x 24 in. 5118 in. knee-shoulder size 10 x 20 in. 5110 standard cover 18 in. x 26 in. (open) 5112 cervical (neck) cover 17 in. x 23 in. (open) 5113 (oversize) 49 in. x 18 1/2 in. (open).

Tetra Medical Supply Corp. 800-621-4041
6364 W Gross Point Rd, Niles, IL 60714

MOIST THERAPY PACK CONDITIONER *(Physical Med) 89RHJ*

Passy-Muir Inc. 800-634-5397
4521 Campus Dr, Irvine, CA 92612
Passy-Muir™ PMA™ 2000 O2 adapter allows for easy inhalation of supplemental low-flow oxygen and humidity through the Low Profile PMV™ 2000 Series Speaking Valves. The Passy-Muir PMA 2000 O2 Adapter is small, lightweight, clear in color, and clips onto both the PMV 2000 (Clear) and PMV 2001 (Purple™) Swallowing & Speaking Valves. It is easily removed when not in use. Oxygen is delivered in front of the diaphragm of the PMV to avoid complications associated with devices that provide continuous flow behind the diaphragm of a speaking valve such as air trapping, drying of secretions, and possible cilia damage.

MOLD, MIDDLE EAR *(Ear/Nose/Throat) 77ETC*

Bausch & Lomb Surgical 636-255-5051
3365 Tree Court Ind Blvd, Saint Louis, MO 63122

Emtech Laboratories, Inc. 800-336-5719
PO Box 12900, Roanoke, VA 24022
Ear pieces to be used with behind the ear hearing aids.

Gyrus Ent L.L.C., Sub. Of Gyrus Acmi, Inc. 508-804-2739
2925 Appling Rd, Bartlett, TN 38133
Various types and sizes of middle ear molds.

Mid-States Laboratories, Inc. 800-247-3669
600 N Saint Francis St, Wichita, KS 67214
Custom earmold for hearing aids and other uses. Available in 10 different materials and over 20 styles. Two NASA based materials available - AUDTEX and APOLLO.

Starkey Laboratories, Inc. 800-328-8602
6700 Washington Ave S, Eden Prairie, MN 55344

MOLDING, CUSTOM *(General) 80WNC*

Aci Medical, Inc. 800-667-9451
1857 Diamond St, San Marcos, CA 92078

Affinity Medical Technologies Llc 949-477-9495
1732 Reynolds Ave, Irvine, CA 92614
Design and develop custom medical interconnect systems.

Atrion Medical Products, Inc. 800-343-9334
1426 Curt Francis Rd NW, Arab, AL 35016

B. Braun Oem Division, B. Braun Medical Inc. 866-8-BBRAUN
824 12th Ave, Bethlehem, PA 18018

Benlan Inc. 905-829-5004
2760 Brighton Rd., Oakville, ONT L6H 5T4 Canada
Injection molding.

C&J Industries, Inc. 814-724-4950
760 Water St, Meadville, PA 16335

Command Medical Products, Inc. 386-672-8116
15 Signal Ave, Ormond Beach, FL 32174
Bubble tubing, taper tubing, straight tubing, paratubing and multi-lumen tubing and coextrusion. In-line printing on tubing available.

Csi International, Inc. 303-795-8273
4301 S Federal Blvd Ste 116, Englewood, CO 80110

MOLDING, CUSTOM (cont'd)

Dana Molded Products, Inc. 847-255-2000
6 N Hickory Ave, Arlington Heights, IL 60004

Elcoma Metal Fabricating Canada 705-526-9636
878 William St., P.O. Box 685, Midland, ONT L4R-4P4 Canada
Custom tubular fabricating to FDA specification. Custom design, color and materials.

Engineering & Research Assoc., Inc. (D.B.A. Sebra) 800-625-5550
100 N Tucson Blvd, Tucson, AZ 85716
PIRF, catheter manufacturing equipment.

Greatbatch Medical 716-759-5600
3735 N Arlington Ave, Indianapolis, IN 46218
Plastic custom trays. Vacuum forming 5 axis mills.

Gw Plastics, Inc. 802-234-9941
239 Pleasant St, Bethel, VT 05032
Prototype through production.

Harmac Medical Products, Inc. 716-897-4500
2201 Bailey Ave, Buffalo, NY 14211
Insert and injection molding. Custom contract manufacturer. Class 100,000 cleanrooms.

Hart Enterprises, Inc. 616-887-0400
400 Apple Jack Ct, Sparta, MI 49345
Custom insert and injection molding. Specializing in small parts.

Helix Medical, Inc. 800-266-4421
1110 Mark Ave, Carpinteria, CA 93013
Silicone molding, LIM, transfer, compression.

Hi-Tech Rubber, Inc. 800-924-4832
3191 E La Palma Ave, Anaheim, CA 92806

International Hospital Supply Co. 800-398-9450
6914 Canby Ave Ste 105, Reseda, CA 91335
Custom trays.

Ironwood Industries, Inc. 847-362-8681
115 S Bradley Rd, Libertyville, IL 60048
Full-service custom injection molder of disposable medical products, offering product design and development, custom assembly and all secondary services. Cleanroom molding and cleanroom assembly capabilities.

Medegen 800-520-7999
930 S Wanamaker Ave, Ontario, CA 91761
Cleanroom injection molding.

Medical Plastic Devices (Mpd), Inc. 866-633-9835
161 Oneida Dr., Pointe Claire, QUE H9R 1A9 Canada

Medtech Group Inc., The 800-348-2759
6 Century Ln, South Plainfield, NJ 07080
Plastic injection molding; engineering and design; tool building.

Micor, Inc. 412-487-1113
2855 Oxford Blvd, Allison Park, PA 15101
Injection molding and custom extrusion (LDPE, HDPE, PVC, PV, PP, nylon and radiopaque).

Minnesota Rubber & Qmr Plastics 952-927-1400
1100 Xenium Ln N, Minneapolis, MN 55441

Minnesota Wire & Cable Co. 800-258-6922
1835 Energy Park Dr, Saint Paul, MN 55108
Tool design and fabrication capability on site.

Ots Corp. 800-221-4769
220 Merrimon Ave, Weaverville, NC 28787
POQ infrared ovens, for thermoforming plastic orthotics & prosthetics.

Packaging Plus Llc 714-522-5400
14450 Industry Cir, La Mirada, CA 90638
Design and manufacturing of thermoformed plastic trays and packages.

Phillips Plastics Corp. 877-508-0252
1201 Hanley Rd, Hudson, WI 54016

Plasticoid Co., The 410-398-2800
249 W High St, Elkton, MD 21921

Plastics One, Inc. 540-772-7950
6591 Merriman Rd, Roanoke, VA 24018

Point Medical Corp. 219-663-1775
891 E Summit St, Crown Point, IN 46307
Liquid, top transfer, compression, micro-molding. Class 10,000.

Porex Corporation 800-241-0195
500 Bohannon Rd, Fairburn, GA 30213

MOLDING, CUSTOM (cont'd)

Precision Medical Products, Inc. 717-335-3700
44 Denver Rd, PO Box 300, Denver, PA 17517
Precision injection and insert molding, through affiliated manufacturer.

Saint-Gobain Performance Plastics/Clearwater 800-541-6880
4451 110th Ave N, Clearwater, FL 33762
Injection molding & custom extrusion.

Team Vantage Molding Llc. 651-464-3900
22455 Everton Ave N, Forest Lake, MN 55025
Precision injection molded parts.

Technh, Inc 603-424-4404
8 Continental Blvd, PO Box 476, Merrimack, NH 03054
Full-service ISO 9001-certified contract manufacturer specializing in injection molding and mold making, catering to the medical and electronics markets. Capabilities include engineering resins, product design and development, plastics engineering, assembly, cleanroom molding, decorating, shielding services, and more.

Tegrant Corporation, Protexic Brands 800-289-9966
800 5th Ave, P.O. Box 448, New Brighton, PA 15066
Protective packaging for medical devices

The Tech Group 480-281-4500
14677 N 74th St, Scottsdale, AZ 85260
Customer specified injection molding, mold construction and medical device assembly.

Vernay Laboratories, Inc. 800-666-5227
120 E South College St, Yellow Springs, OH 45387

MOLDING, INJECTION (General) 80WYJ

Avail Medical Products 814-353-0680
270 Rolling Ridge Dr, Bellefonte, PA 16823

Avail Medical Products, Inc. 866-552-2112
201 Main St, 1600 Wells Fargo Tower, Fort Worth, TX 76102
Full-service outsource design and manufacturing for sterile, single-use medical devices. From initial product concept through finished goods, fulfillment and distribution. Design, process development and validation, manufacturing, injection molding, packaging, sterilization services management, manufacturing transfer.

B. Braun Oem Division, B. Braun Medical Inc. 866-8-BBRAUN
824 12th Ave, Bethlehem, PA 18018

Drummond Scientific Co. 800-523-7480
500 Park Way # 700, Broomall, PA 19008

Filtertek Inc. 800-248-2461
11411 Price Rd, Hebron, IL 60034
Filter products.

Frantz Medical Development Ltd. 440-255-1155
7740 Metric Dr, Mentor, OH 44060

Gw Plastics, Inc. 802-234-9941
239 Pleasant St, Bethel, VT 05032
Full-service supplier of precision-injection-molded components. Class 100,000 cleanroom, multiple plant locations.

Harmac Medical Products, Inc. 716-897-4500
2201 Bailey Ave, Buffalo, NY 14211
Custom injection and insert molding. Contract manufacturer and OEM of disposable medical devices. Class 100,000 cleanrooms.

Ironwood Industries, Inc. 847-362-8681
115 S Bradley Rd, Libertyville, IL 60048
Class 100,000 molding, including insert molding and multi-material molding, in an ISO 9002 certified facility.

Lacey Manufacturing Co. 203-336-0121
1146 Barnum Ave, PO Box 5156, Bridgeport, CT 06610

Lucomed Inc. 800-633-7877
45 Kulick Rd, Fairfield, NJ 07004

Mack Molding Co. 802-375-2511
608 Warm Brook Rd, Arlington, VT 05250
Custom injection molding and assembly of plastic parts.

Medegen 800-520-7999
930 S Wanamaker Ave, Ontario, CA 91761

Medical Plastic Devices (Mpd), Inc. 866-633-9835
161 Oneida Dr., Pointe Claire, QUE H9R 1A9 Canada

Medical Sterile Products, Inc. 800-292-2887
Road 413 Km. 0.2 BO. Ensenada, Rincon, PR 00743

Medtech Group Inc., The 800-348-2759
6 Century Ln, South Plainfield, NJ 07080
Precision injection molding, including two-shot and insert molding of medical products.

MOLDING, INJECTION *(cont'd)*

Molded Products Inc. 800-435-8957
1112 Chatburn Ave, Harlan, IA 51537

Phillips Plastics Corp. 877-508-0252
1201 Hanley Rd, Hudson, WI 54016

Sonoco Crellin, Inc. 518-392-2000
87 Center St, Chatham, NY 12037
Filtration products

Technh, Inc 603-424-4404
8 Continental Blvd, PO Box 476, Merrimack, NH 03054
Full-service ISO 9001-certified contract manufacturer specializing in injection molding and mold making, catering to the medical and electronics markets. Capabilities include engineering resins, product design and development, plastics engineering, assembly, cleanroom molding, decorating, shielding services, and more.

The Tech Group 480-281-4500
14677 N 74th St, Scottsdale, AZ 85260
Customer specified injection molding, mold construction and medical device assembly.

Vernay Laboratories, Inc. 800-666-5227
120 E South College St, Yellow Springs, OH 45387

MOLECULAR WEIGHT EQUIPMENT *(Chemistry) 75UGW*

Polymer Laboratories, Now A Part Of Varian, Inc. 800-767-3963
160 Old Farm Rd, Amherst Fields Research Park, Amherst, MA 01002

Scientific Glass & Instruments, Inc. 877-682-1481
PO Box 6, Houston, TX 77001

MOLESKIN *(General) 80RHL*

Aetna Foot Products/Div. Of Aetna Felt Corporation 800-390-3668
2401 W Emaus Ave, Allentown, PA 18103
COMFOOT Brand and SCOTT FOOT CARE pre-cut foot pads, rolls and sheets in various thicknesses.

Omni Medical Supply Inc. 800-860-6664
4153 Pioneer Dr, Commerce Township, MI 48390

MONITOR, AIRWAY PRESSURE (GAUGE/ALARM)
(Anesthesiology) 73CAP

Ambu A/S 457-225-2210
6740 Baymeadow Dr, Glen Burnie, MD 21060
Disposable pressure manometer.

Datex-Ohmeda Inc. 608-221-1551
3030 Ohmeda Dr, Madison, WI 53718
Airway pressure gauge.

Engineered Medical Systems 317-246-5500
2055 Executive Dr, Indianapolis, IN 46241
Pressure manometer-disposable.

Instrumentation Industries, Inc. 800-633-8577
2990 Industrial Blvd, Bethel Park, PA 15102
Airway pressure gauges. Artificial airway cuff pressure.

Respironics Colorado 800-345-6443
12301 Grant St Unit 190, Thornton, CO 80241
$640.00 - monitors pressues on either positive pressure or negative pressure ventilators and respiratory set-ups; programmable alarm parameters; AC/DC.

Respironics Novametrix, Llc. 724-387-4559
5 Technology Dr, Wallingford, CT 06492
Criterion 40,60.

Respironics, Inc 800-345-6443
1010 Murry Ridge Ln, Murrysville, PA 15668
PNEUMOGARD is an airway pressure monitor with continuous display of distending, mean airway pressures and either ventilator rate, I/E positive pressure or duration of positive pressure.

Smiths Medical Asd, Inc. 610-578-9600
9255 Customhouse Plz Ste N, San Diego, CA 92154
Airway pressure monitor.

Spiracle Technology 714-418-1091
16520 Harbor Blvd Ste D, Fountain Valley, CA 92708
Pressure/time gauge.

MONITOR, AIRWAY PRESSURE (INSPIRATORY FORCE)
(Anesthesiology) 73BXR

Boehringer Laboratories, Inc. 800-642-4945
500 E Washington St, Norristown, PA 19401
Minus 60 cm H2O to plus 60 cm H2O units available. A memory pointer captures the highest inspiratory or expiratory pressure.

MONITOR, AIRWAY PRESSURE (INSPIRATORY FORCE) *(cont'd)*

Dhd Healthcare Corporation 800-847-8000
PO Box 6, One Madison Street, Wampsville, NY 13163
NIF-KIT, RESCAL, NIF-TEE.

Instrumentation Industries, Inc. 800-633-8577
2990 Industrial Blvd, Bethel Park, PA 15102
Maximal static inspiratory pressure gauges.

Medi Inc 800-225-8634
75 York Ave, P.O. Box 302, Randolph, MA 02368

MONITOR, AIRWAY PRESSURE, CONTINUOUS
(Anesthesiology) 73RLV

Cardinal Health 207, Inc. 800-231-2466
22745 Savi Ranch Pkwy, Yorba Linda, CA 92887
Continuous positive airway pressure device for the treatment of sleep disorders.

MONITOR, APNEA *(General) 80FLS*

Draeger Medical Systems, Inc. 215-660-2626
16 Electronics Ave, Danvers, MA 01923
Multiple infinity systems.

East River Ventures Lp 212-644-2322
590 Madison Ave, c/o East River Ventures LP, New York, NY 10022
Apnea monitors, respiratory.

Embla Systems, Inc. 716-691-0718
55 Pineview Dr Ste 100, Buffalo, NY 14228
Sleep study, data acquisition software.

Futuremed America, Inc. 800-222-6780
15700 Devonshire St, Granada Hills, CA 91344
$390.00 for C-PAP.

Ge Medical Systems Information Technologies 800-643-6439
8200 W Tower Ave, Milwaukee, WI 53223

Grass Technologies, An Astro-Med, Inc. Product Gro 401-828-4002
53 Airport Park Drive, Rockland, MA 02370
Respiratory effort transducer.

Medical Cables, Inc. 800-314-51111
1365 Logan Ave, Costa Mesa, CA 92626

Mennen Medical Corp. 800-223-2201
2540 Metropolitan Dr, Trevose, PA 19053
ENVOY patient monitor apnea detection is a software feature of the Envoy.

Omni Medical Supply Inc. 800-860-6664
4153 Pioneer Dr, Commerce Township, MI 48390
Rental of equipment.

Pro-Tech Services, Inc. 800-350-5511
4338 Harbour Pointe Blvd SW, Mukilteo, WA 98275
Various.

Respironics Georgia, Inc. 724-387-4559
175 Chastain Meadows Ct NW, Kennesaw, GA 30144
SMARTMONITOR Models of infant monitor for home use, weighing 5lbs. Use impedance pneumography technique.

Sleep Solutions, Inc. 408-255-0808
2450 El Camino Real Ste 101, Palo Alto, CA 94306
Apnea monitor.

MONITOR, BED OCCUPANCY *(General) 80QDB*

Bed-Check Corporation 800-523-7956
307 E Brady St, Tulsa, OK 74120
BED-CHECK II, easy-to-use fall prevention systems include portable control units and pressure-sensitive Sensormat pads for monitoring bed occupancy, adaptable to all nurse call systems. NURSE CALL ADAPTER, Universal 'Y' Adapter nurse call system, universal 'y' adapter. Also available: MODEL VR Bed-Check Model Va, portable bed occupancy monitor, computer programmable, outcome expecting, adaptable to all nurse call systems, for use with the BED-CHECK SENSORMAT or CHAIR-CHECK SENSORMAT.

MONITOR, BED OCCUPANCY *(cont'd)*

Care Electronics, Inc. 303-444-2273
4700 Sterling Dr Ste D, Boulder, CO 80301
Care Mobility Monitor monitors patients in a bed or chair and alerts a caregiver when they attempt to get up. Care Deluxe Mobility Monitor includes five adjustable alarm sounds, nurse-call interface, low battery monitoring, and auto reset as well. Care Deluxe Occupancy System monitors patients in a bed or chair using pressure sensitive pads and cushions. Also includes five adjustable alarm sounds, four delay settings, auto-reset, nurse-call interface, low battery monitoring, LED indicator. PATIENTCARE WANDERER Monitoring System monitors doorways and halls for attempts to exit. The system monitors 50 residents and identifies the wanderer attempting to exit. Adjustable sensitivity and long battery life transmitters are standard. PATIENTCARE 16/64 Wireless Monitoring System provides wireless nurse-call features, door monitoring, pendant 'help' buttons, and Deluxe Occupancy transmitters. System is fully supervised for reliability. WANDERCARE 100 Monitoring System monitors wanderers at home and notifies caregivers when the wanderer leaves the area. Long range tracking (up to one mile) is included. System can also notify others by phone and pager of the emergency.

Intellectual Property, Llc 608-798-0904
8030 Stagecoach Rd, Cross Plains, WI 53528
A device which detects the presence of flesh without requiring direct contact to the patient.

Nocwatch International, Inc./Fallsaver 877-614-5616
PO Box 1367, Crystal Bay, NV 89402
Wireless position monitor which alarms when patient tries to get up unassisted in time for staff to intervene. Works from a patch on the patient's leg so alarms anywhere the patient is -- in bed, in a wheelchair, on the toilet, down the hall. No false alarms. 'Fall prevention' is probably a better category if you can create it.

Nurse Assist ,Inc. 800-649-6800
3400 Northern Cross Blvd, Fort Worth, TX 76137
Bed Exit Monitor Unit - $230.00, package of 10 disposable pads-$240.00.

Rf Technologies 800-669-9946
3125 N 126th St, Brookfield, WI 53005
Bed and chair alarm available.

Senior Technologies 800-824-2996
PO Box 80238, 1620 N 20th Circle, Lincoln, NE 68501
TABS Mobility Monitor is designed to alert caregivers when a person is leaving a bed, chair or room (emergency alert).

Tapeswitch Corporation 800-234-8273
100 Schmitt Blvd, Farmingdale, NY 11735
Pressure sensitive strips detect patient with switch closure.

MONITOR, BED PATIENT *(General) 80KMI*

Aionex, Inc. 615-851-4477
104 Space Park N, Goodlettsville, TN 37072

Aiv, Inc. (Formerly American Iv) 800-990-2911
7485 Shipley Ave, Harmans, MD 21077
Pulse oximeter adapter cables that connect sensors to leading patient monitors.

Alert Care, Inc. 800-826-7444
591 Redwood Hwy Ste 5200, Mill Valley, CA 94941
AMBULARM is used for fall prevention and restraint reduction. It snaps onto a leg band that the patient wears just above the knee. When alarm approaches a near vertical position as in walking, crawling or kneeling, a position sensitive switch triggers an audio alarm alerting the nearest caregiver. To deactivate the alarm it must be unsnapped from the elastic band. It is especially effective at preventing patient falls and reducing restraints for patients not interested in being tethered or using a pad sensor.

Amelife Llc 302-476-2631
702 N West St Ste 101, Wilmington, DE 19801

American Biomed Instruments, Inc. 718-235-8900
11 Wyona St, Brooklyn, NY 11207

Basic American Metal Products 800-365-2338
336 Trowbridge Dr, PO Box 907, Fond Du Lac, WI 54937

Blackhagen Design 727-736-0582
811 Douglas Ave Ste C, Dunedin, FL 34698

MONITOR, BED PATIENT *(cont'd)*

Care Electronics, Inc. 303-444-2273
4700 Sterling Dr Ste D, Boulder, CO 80301
Care Mobility Monitor monitors patients in a bed or chair and alerts a caregiver when they attempt to get up. Care Deluxe Mobility Monitor includes five adjustable alarm sounds, nurse-call interface, low battery monitoring, and auto reset as well. Care Deluxe Occupancy System monitors patients in a bed or chair using pressure sensitive pads and cushions. Also includes five adjustable alarm sounds, four delay settings, auto-reset, nurse-call interface, low battery monitoring, LED indicator. PATIENTCARE WANDERER Monitoring System monitors doorways and halls for attempts to exit. The system monitors 50 residents and identifies the wanderer attempting to exit. Adjustable sensitivity and long battery life transmitters are standard. PATIENTCARE 16/64 Wireless Monitoring System provides wireless nurse-call features, door monitoring, pendant 'help' buttons, and Deluxe Occupancy transmitters. System is fully supervised for reliability. WANDERCARE 100 Monitoring System monitors wanderers at home and notifies caregivers when the wanderer leaves the area. Long range tracking (up to one mile) is included. System can also notify others by phone and pager of the emergency.

Close Call Corp. 630-663-0189
4617 Cumnor Rd, Downers Grove, IL 60515
Close call or patient alarm.

Curbell Electronics Inc. 716-667-3377
20 Centre Dr, Orchard Park, NY 14127
Bed-patient monitor.

Curbell, Inc. Electronics 800-235-7500
7 Cobham Dr, Orchard Park, NY 14127
CARESENSE bed and chair monitoring systems and patient monitoring systems for acute- and long-term-care situations.

D.R.E., Inc. 800-462-8195
1800 Williamson Ct, Louisville, KY 40223
DRE ASM-5000 Multi-Parameter Patient Monitor feaures ECG with Recorder, SaO2, NIBP, Respiration and Temperature on Neonatal to Adult patients. Using technology developed by the industry's leading names, such as Nellcor and Colin, we can offer this combination of advanced features and a lifetime warranty. The high-resolution, 64-color display shows each parameter in a distinct color and can be viewed from an angle. Powered by AC with a 1-hour battery back-up.

Data Medical 800-790-9978
89 Leuning St Ste 2, South Hackensack, NJ 07606
ACCU-HALT detects holes in barrier products. ACU-LAB - Acu Lab Monitor, detects pinholes, hydration in all types of medical and other gloves. Glove Safety Monitor - detects pinholes & permeabilty in cleanroom gloves & glove boxes.

Datascope Corp. 800-288-2121
14 Philips Pkwy, Montvale, NJ 07645
POINT OF VIEW, monitoring in operating rooms and post-anesthesia care units has modules for patient vital signs and anesthesia gas monitoring.

Dome Imaging Systems, Inc. 866-752-6271
400 5th Ave, Waltham, MA 02451
Planar--a global leader in medical displays--offers the VitalScreen family of flat panels, specifically designed to support the delivery of safe, high-quality care in the healthcare environment. These flat-panel displays provide exceptional display quality, patient safety, and fitness for use. The VitalScreen family consists of the VitalScreen CSR and the VitalScreen S. The VitalScreen CSR is the display of choice when configuration management, safety, and durability are the key concerns. It is the model most often used in applications within high-intensity areas, such as operating rooms, trauma units, and emergency rooms. The VitalScreen S is ideal for patient-monitoring applications that require a medically certified display without configuration management or IPX1 certification. From their inception, the VitalScreen flat panels were designed to address the stringent safety standards for patients, practitioners, and visitors in a hospital environment. The products meet the UL2601 and IEC 60601 standards, which define strict guidelines for equipment that can be used in the patient envelope--the 1.5-meter hemisphere surrounding the patient. These certifications ensure a level of patient and caregiver protection far greater than the safety standards of commodity electronic equipment. Offering excellent viewing angles and superior image crispness, the VitalScreen flat panels display most standard resolutions, from standard VGA up to 1024 x 768 pixels (on the 15-inch displays) and 1280 x 1024 pixels (on the 17.4-inch displays). They use an active-matrix liquid-crystal display (AMLCD) panel that produces crisp, clear display with low radiation emission, thereby reducing radiation-related health concerns associated with CRT monitors.

MONITOR, BED PATIENT *(cont'd)*

Hill-Rom Manufacturing, Inc. 800-445-3730
1225 Crescent Green Dr., Suite 200, Cary, NC 27511
Bed-patient monitoring system software.

Invivo Corporation 425-487-7000
12601 Research Pkwy, Orlando, FL 32826
Various telemetry ecg monitors.

Ivy Biomedical Systems, Inc. 800-247-4614
11 Business Park Dr, Branford, CT 06405
IVY BIOMEDICAL SYSTEMS,INC405T SERIES are portable patient monitor features include ECG response,nibp temp ibp etco2 builtin recorder.price range $8000.00-13,000.00

JVC Americas Corp. 973-315-5000
1700 Valley Rd, Wayne, NJ 07470

Ledtronics 800-579-4875
23105 Kashiwa Ct, Torrance, CA 90505

Matamatic Inc. 800-603-4050
230 Westec Dr, Mount Pleasant, PA 15666
Bed sensor.

Medical Depot 516-998-4600
99 Seaview Blvd, Port Washington, NY 11050
Patient movement alarm.

Nocwatch International, Inc. 775-833-4142
288 Village Blvd Ste 5, Incline Village, NV 89451
Patient monitor.

Nurse Assist ,Inc. 800-649-6800
3400 Northern Cross Blvd, Fort Worth, TX 76137
NURSE ASSIST bed exit monitor. Electronic monitor with above mattress, disposable sensor strip. $230 monitor, package of ten disposable pads $240.00.

Pace Tech, Inc. 800-722-3024
510 N Garden Ave, Clearwater, FL 33755
MiniPack 300 series functions offered are ECG, NIBP, temperature, capnography, pulse oximetry and respiration (12 models available). Can be used for all bedside monitoring, transport and other alternate site applications.

Quality Monitor Systems, Inc. 800-743-5747
1950 Victor Pl, Colorado Springs, CO 80915
Sales and service of used patient monitors.

Rg Electronics, Inc. 888-877-5682
100 Spring Creek Dr, Liberty Hill, TX 78642
Versatex restraint free monitor/alarm.

Scj Enterprises, Inc. 516-797-8903
3 Riviera Dr E, Massapequa, NY 11758
Bed monitor.

Secure Care Products, Inc. 800-451-7917
39 Chenell Dr, Concord, NH 03301
Wandering Patient electronic monitoring system. The electronic sensor lets the staff know if the patient leaves the bed. Also sensors to let staff know if patients leaves a chair.

Senior Technologies 800-824-2996
PO Box 80238, 1620 N 20th Circle, Lincoln, NE 68501
TABS mobility monitors. Alert staff when someone leaving a bed, chair, or wheelchair. Can be used to monitor interior doors.

Smiths Medical Pm, Inc. 800-558-2345
N7W22025 Johnson Dr, Waukesha, WI 53186
Advisor Vital Signs Monitor offers 3 or 5 lead ECG, respiration, NIBP, pulse oximetry, 2 temperature/2 invasive pressure, and recorder.

Sterilmed, Inc. 763-488-3400
11400 73rd Ave N Ste 100, Maple Grove, MN 55369
Hospital bed patient monitoring alarm.

Superior Medical Limited 800-268-7944
520 Champagne Dr., Toronto, ONT M3J 2T9 Canada
Philips Medical patient monitoring/cardiac/obstetric.

Tapeswitch Corporation 800-234-8273
100 Schmitt Blvd, Farmingdale, NY 11735
Pressure sensitive strips detect patient with switch closure.

Transilwrap Co., Inc. 847-678-1800
9201 Belmont Ave, Franklin Park, IL 60131
Hospital bed patient monitoring alarm.

210 Innovations, Llc
34 Taugwonk Spur Rd Unit 10, Stonington, CT 06378
Various patient monitors, bed and wheelchair.

MONITOR, BIOLOGICAL (CONTAMINATION TESTING) *(General) 80QDR*

Alderon Biosciences, Inc. 919-544-8220
2810 Meridian Pkwy Ste 152, Durham, NC 27713
Molecular assays for E. coli, pathogens, and threat agents

Bio-Rad Laboratories, Life Science Group 800-424-6723
2000 Alfred Nobel Dr, Hercules, CA 94547
Products for molecular biology.

Climet Instruments Co. 909-793-2788
1320 W Colton Ave, Redlands, CA 92374
$10,000.00 per unit (standard).

Enviro Guard, Inc. 800-438-1152
201 Shannon Oaks Cir Ste 115, Cary, NC 27511

Interscan Corp. 800-458-6153
21700 Nordhoff St, P.O. Box 2496, Chatsworth, CA 91311
Formaldehyde monitor. $1,990.00 ea. for portable survey units, and $2750.00 and up for fixed systems. Full data acquisition/archiving/reporting system available.

Ludlum Measurements, Inc. 800-622-0828
501 Oak St, Sweetwater, TX 79556

Markel Industries, Inc. 860-646-5303
PO Box 1388, 135A Sheldon Road, Manchester, CT 06045

MONITOR, BLOOD FLOW, ULTRASONIC *(Obstetrics/Gyn) 85HEP*

Blatek, Inc. 814-231-2085
2820 E College Ave Ste F, State College, PA 16801

Cardinal Healthcare 209, Inc. 610-862-0800
5225 Verona Rd, Fitchburg, WI 53711
Transcranial doppler system.

Koven Technology, Inc. 800-521-8342
12125 Woodcrest Executive Dr Ste 320, Saint Louis, MO 63141
ES-100VX MINIDOPPler®; BIDOP® 3; ES-101EX-2 Fetal EchoSounder™

Parks Medical Electronics, Inc. 503-649-7007
PO Box 5669, Aloha, OR 97006

Terumo Cardiovascular Systems, Corp 800-521-2818
6200 Jackson Rd, Ann Arbor, MI 48103
Flow sensor for use with centrifugal blood pump.

Vmed Technology, Inc. (Formerly Ems Products, Inc.) 425-497-9149
16149 Redmond Way # 108, Redmond, WA 98052
Blood flow and PPG recorder.

MONITOR, BLOOD GAS, ON-LINE, CARDIOPULMONARY BYPASS *(Cardiovascular) 74DRY*

International Biophysics Corp. 512-326-3244
2101 E Saint Elmo Rd Ste 275, Austin, TX 78744
Monitor, blood-gas, on-line, cardiopulmonary bypass.

Terumo Cardiovascular Systems (Tcvs) 714-258-8001
1311 Valencia Ave, Tustin, CA 92780
Cdi blood parameter monitor.

Terumo Cardiovascular Systems (Tcvs) 800-283-7866
28 Howe St, Ashland, MA 01721
Blood/gas monitor.

Terumo Cardiovascular Systems, Corp 800-521-2818
6200 Jackson Rd, Ann Arbor, MI 48103

MONITOR, BLOOD GAS, OXYGEN *(Anesthesiology) 73QEB*

Dedicated Distribution 800-325-8367
640 Miami Ave, Kansas City, KS 66105

Sensidyne, Inc. 800-451-9444
16333 Bay Vista Dr, Clearwater, FL 33760
Provides continuous direct-monitoring and spot-checking of oxygen delivery devices in respiratory care, anesthesiology, and oxygen therapy applications.

MONITOR, BLOOD GAS, REAL-TIME *(Cardiovascular) 74UMH*

Allegro Biodiesel Corporation 800-949-4762
6245 Bristol Pkwy Ste 263, Culver City, CA 90230
Trend Care continuous blood-gas monitor that continuously monitors blood gases including pH, PCO2, PO2, and temperature.

MONITOR, BLOOD GAS, TRANSCUTANEOUS CARBON-DIOXIDE *(Anesthesiology) 73TAJ*

Radiometer America, Inc. 800-736-0600
810 Sharon Dr, Westlake, OH 44145
TINA performance 1% drift/hr; 50-sec response time. Weighs 6 lb.

MONITOR, BLOOD GAS, TRANSCUTANEOUS OXYGEN
(Anesthesiology) 73QEC

Radiometer America, Inc. 800-736-0600
810 Sharon Dr, Westlake, OH 44145
TINA single-channel tcPO-2 unit with 20-sec response time.

MONITOR, BLOOD GLUCOSE (TEST) *(Gastro/Urology) 78TGM*

Acon Laboratories, Inc. 858-535-2030
10125 Mesa Rim Rd, San Diego, CA 92121

Dedicated Distribution 800-325-8367
640 Miami Ave, Kansas City, KS 66105

Invacare Supply Group, An Invacare Co. 800-225-4792
75 October Hill Rd, Holliston, MA 01746
Carry full lines of meters from: Invacare, Roche, Bayer, Lifescan..

Inverness Medical Inc. 732-308-3000
569 Halls Mill Rd, Freehold, NJ 07728
Electrochemical blood glucose monitoring system.

Kck Industries 888-800-1967
14941 Calvert St, Van Nuys, CA 91411

Lifescan, Inc. 800-227-8862
1000 Gibraltar Dr, Milpitas, CA 95035
ONE TOUCH II and ONE TOUCH BASIC blood glucose monitor. PENLET II finger puncture device.

Quest Star Medical, Inc. 800-525-6718
10180 Viking Dr, Eden Prairie, MN 55344
Focus blood-glucose monitoring system.

Roche Diagnostics 800-361-2070
201 Armand-Frappier Blvd., Laval, QUE H7V 4A2 Canada
ACCU-CHEK, ADVANTAGE, CHEMSTRIP Retail price of monitors range from $50-200 CDN. Retail price of test strips range from $25-58 CDN per package.

Science Products 800-888-7400
1043 Lancaster Ave, Berwyn, PA 19312
LIFESCAN ONE TOUCH PROFILE - Basic & Surestep glucose analyzer for visually impaired. DIGI-VOICE Speech modules for use with ONE TOUCH POFILE, ONE TOUCH BASIC, or SURESTEP: $275, $219, & $199.

MONITOR, BLOOD PRESSURE, FINGER *(Cardiovascular) 74WZC*

Optelec U.S., Inc. 800-828-1056
3030 Enterprise Ct Ste C, Vista, CA 92081
Talking blood pressure monitor.

MONITOR, BLOOD PRESSURE, INDIRECT (ARTERIAL)
(Cardiovascular) 74RLS

A&D Medical 800-726-7099
1756 Automation Pkwy, San Jose, CA 95131
Ambulatory 24-hour monitoring system; TM-2430 meter/recorder for measurement and recording of blood pressure at a variety of preset intervals; TM-2020 prints out data stored in memory of TM-2420. Aneroid blood pressure monitors $29.95, UA-100 home blood pressure kit w/ attached stethoscope $29.95.

Biomedix Inc. 877-854-0012
4215 White Bear Pkwy, Saint Paul, MN 55110
PADnet Lab, a non-invasive device detects blockages in arteries and the quality of blood flow using pulse volume recording and oscillometric segmental blood pressure measurement.The device is lightweight (about six pounds) and portable and includes a laptop computer and color printer on a medical grade cart. The test can be performed in 20 minutes or less. Test results are transferred to vascular specialists via a HIPAA compliant web server and diagnosis and treatment recommendations are returned to the test site within 24 hours.

Buxco Research Systems 910-794-6980
219 Station Rd Ste 202, Wilmington, NC 28405

Datex-Ohmeda (Canada) 800-268-1472
1093 Meyerside Dr., Unit 2, Mississauga, ONT L5T-1J6 Canada

David Scott Company 800-804-0333
59 Fountain St, Framingham, MA 01702

Ela Medical, Inc. 800-352-6466
2950 Xenium Ln N, Plymouth, MN 55441
Agilis is an ambulatory blood pressure using the oscillometric tecnique.

Koaman International 909-983-4888
656 E D St, Ontario, CA 91764

MONITOR, BLOOD PRESSURE, INDIRECT (ARTERIAL) *(cont'd)*

Lumiscope Company, Inc. 800-672-8293
1035 Centennial Ave, Piscataway, NJ 08854
$59.95 for standard unit; $79.95 for unit with audible/visual display, microphone; $199.95 for uP-based, digital display unit with auto zero, memory and recall.

Mennen Medical Corp. 800-223-2201
2540 Metropolitan Dr, Trevose, PA 19053
ENVOY patient monitor.

Rockford Medical & Safety Co. 800-435-9451
2420 Harrison Ave, PO Box 5646, Rockford, IL 61108

Trimline Medical Products Corp. 800-526-3538
34 Columbia Rd, Branchburg, NJ 08876
TRIMLINE Large face aneroid and mercurial sphygmomanometers available as wall, desk or stand models; also cuff containers and inflation systems, all latex -free.

MONITOR, BLOOD PRESSURE, INDIRECT, ANESTHESIOLOGY
(Anesthesiology) 73BXD

Cas Medical Systems, Inc. 800-227-4414
44 E Industrial Rd, Branford, CT 06405
Neonatal and adult non-invasive blood-pressure monitors.

Ge Medical Systems Information Technologies 800-558-5544
4502 Woodland Corporate Blvd, Tampa, FL 33614
Non invasive BP monitors using oscillometric technique. Available with SPO2 and Temp. PRO SERIES non invasive blood pressure monitor available with SPO2 and temp.

Ge Medical Systems Information Technologies 800-643-6439
8200 W Tower Ave, Milwaukee, WI 53223

Industrial & Biomedical Sensors Corp. 781-891-4201
1377 Main St, Waltham, MA 02451
$1,800 for automatic monitor.

Lifeclinic International, Inc. 301-476-9888
4032 Blackburn Ln, Burtonsville, MD 20866
Health Check Center.

Mennen Medical Corp. 800-223-2201
2540 Metropolitan Dr, Trevose, PA 19053
ENVOY patient monitor.

Omni Medical Supply Inc. 800-860-6664
4153 Pioneer Dr, Commerce Township, MI 48390
Sales, service and rental.

Pace Tech, Inc. 800-722-3024
510 N Garden Ave, Clearwater, FL 33755
VITALMAX 800 & MINIPACK 911 series $1995 to $3795. NIBP w/options of temp, respiration and pulse oximetry. Battery operated, upgradable.

Trimline Medical Products Corp. 800-526-3538
34 Columbia Rd, Branchburg, NJ 08876
TRIMLINE Large face aneroid and mercurial sphygmomanometers available as wall, desk or stand models; also cuff containers and inflation systems, all latex-free.

MONITOR, BLOOD PRESSURE, INDIRECT, AUTOMATIC
(Cardiovascular) 74JOE

Cas Medical Systems, Inc. 800-227-4414
44 E Industrial Rd, Branford, CT 06405
Neonatal and adult non-invasive blood-pressure monitor. Also available with pulse oximetry and temperature options.

Circadian Systems 800-669-7001
8099 Savage Way, Valley Springs, CA 95252
Circadian ambulatory blood-pressure monitoring system monitors blood pressure noninvasively over a 24-hour period. System can be programmed. Final report provides readings for systolic, diastolic, MAP, and heart rate. Information is summarized on an hourly basis and all readings are printed for backup. Entire system office-based, designed for nontechnical staff.

MONITOR, BLOOD PRESSURE, INDIRECT, AUTOMATIC *(cont'd)*

Colin Medical Instruments Corp. 800-829-6427
5850 Farinon Dr, San Antonio, TX 78249
PRESS-MATE Prodigy portable vital signs monitor, with features that include NIBP with dynamic linear cuff deflation, large colorful LEDs, patient ID capability and bar code scanning technology (optional), user-designed cuff interval programs (protocols), motion-tolerant Spo2 (optional), 7-second E-Temp (optional), multiple print options, 2-plane display design, 6-hour battery, 400-line list memory, battery charge indicators, and Gold Standard warranty. PRESS-MATE Model 8800 portable vital signs monitor, with NIBP/PR printer complete with accessories; electronic/tympanic temperature and SPO2 oximetry options available. PRESS-MATE Model 8800 FP with NIBP/ PR, electronic temperature deluxe rolling stand, accessories, optional printer, pulse oximetry option. PRESS-MATE Model 8800 MSP with NIBP/PR, integrated typmanic temperature, deluxe rolling stone, accessories, pulse oximetry option, optional printer. PRESS-MATE ADVANTAGE multi-parameter NIBP monitor is portable and includes ECG, respiration, temperature, SpO2 recorder, high-resolution color, and LCD display.

Computerized Screening, Inc. (Csi) 800-533-9230
9550 Gateway Dr, Reno, NV 89521
Computerized vital-signs monitor with full telehealth, patented seated weight, non-invasive testing and electronic health record support.

Creative Health Products, Inc. 800-742-4478
5148 Saddle Ridge Rd, Plymouth, MI 48170
Digital Blood Pressure Units, Automatic Inflation: AMERICAN DIAGNOSTIC $74.90, OMRON $66.90, MABIS $88.90. Extra cuffs and accessories available from CHP.

Datascope Corp. 800-288-2121
14 Philips Pkwy, Montvale, NJ 07645
ACCUTORR Non-invasive blood pressure monitor using oscillometric technique without printer and with printer.

Devon Medical 800-571-3135
1100 1st Ave Ste 100, King Of Prussia, PA 19406
Take the guessing out of blood pressure monitoring. This digital monitor features state-of-the-art technology that automatically determines ideal cuff inflation. Easier and more accurate than conventional monitors, it's a great addition to any medical facility.

Ge Medical Systems Information Technologies 800-558-5544
4502 Woodland Corporate Blvd, Tampa, FL 33614
Non invasive BP monitors using oscillometric technique. Available with SPO2 and Temp.

Ge Medical Systems Information Technologies 800-643-6439
8200 W Tower Ave, Milwaukee, WI 53223
Unit using oscillometric method. Manual or automatic cycles. Displays systolic, diastolic, and mean pressure.

Her-Mar, Inc. 800-327-8209
8550 NW 30th Ter, Doral, FL 33122

Hill-Med, Inc. 305-594-7474
7217 NW 46th St, Miami, FL 33166
Revelation, records 24, 48, 72 hours, pre- and post-medication.

Hillusa Corp. 305-594-7474
7215 NW 46th St, Miami, FL 33166
Ambulatory blood pressure, 24, 48, 72 recording time.

Industrial & Biomedical Sensors Corp. 781-891-4201
1377 Main St, Waltham, MA 02451
$1,800 for automatic unit, measures systolic and diastolic BP, pulse rate, elapsed time. $400 for digital printer unit. Computer interface capability.

Jayza Corp. 305-477-1136
7215 NW 41st St Ste A, Miami, FL 33166

Mennen Medical Corp. 800-223-2201
2540 Metropolitan Dr, Trevose, PA 19053
ENVOY patient monitor 551-130-000 NIBP for Envoy, HORIZON 9000 WS cath-lab information system.

New Life Systems, Inc. 954-972-4600
PO Box 8767, Coral Springs, FL 33075
All types.

MONITOR, BLOOD PRESSURE, INDIRECT, AUTOMATIC *(cont'd)*

Nonin Medical, Inc. 800-356-8874
13700 1st Ave N, Plymouth, MN 55441
AVANT, combination nonivasive blood pressure and pulse oximeter.

Promed Technologies Inc. 877-977-6633
P.O. Box 2070, Richmond Hill, ONT L4E-1A3 Canada

Suntech Medical, Inc. 800-421-8626
507 Airport Blvd Ste 117, Morrisville, NC 27560
Typically worn for 24 hours, the Oscar 2 is a compact, lightweight monitor which provides the cost-effective solution for monitoring the patient's blood pressure outside the clinical environment. Oscar 2 employs the popular oscillometric technique of blood-pressure measurement used in patient monitors and hospitals worldwide. The elegance and simplicity of Oscar 2 provides for the quickest and easiest patient hook-up. Oscar 2 interfaces to SunTech's newest PC software, AccuWin Pro, for monitor programming as well as data editing and graphic report printout.

Welch Allyn Protocol, Inc. 800-462-0777
2 Corporate Dr Ste 110, Long Grove, IL 60047

MONITOR, BLOOD PRESSURE, INDIRECT, SEMI-AUTOMATIC
(Cardiovascular) 74DXN

Advanced Biosensor, Inc. 803-407-3044
400 Arbor Lake Dr Ste B450, Columbia, SC 29223
Ambulatory blood pressure monitors.

Advanced Medical Instruments, Inc. 918-250-0566
3061 W Albany St, Broken Arrow, OK 74012
Non-invasive blood pressure monitor.

Biotek Instruments, Inc. 802-655-4040
100 Tigan St, Highland Park, Winooski, VT 05404
Non-invasive blood pressure monitor tester (nibpmt).

Breconridge Manufacturing Solutions 315-393-8000
120 Chimney Point Dr, Ogdensburg, NY 13669
Health monitoring kit.

Cardinal Health 303,Inc. 858-458-7830
1515 Ivac Way, Creedmoor, NC 27522
Blood pressure machine & accessories.

Cardiocom LLC 888-243-8881
7980 Century Blvd, Chanhassen, MN 55317
Noninvasive blood pressure measurement system.

Carematix Inc. 312-371-3050
120 S Riverside Plz Ste 2100, Chicago, IL 60606
Blood pressure monitor.

Delphi Medical Systems Colorado Corp. 248-813-6819
4300 Rd. 18, Longmont, CO 80504
Monitoring system.

Demetech Corp. 888-324-2447
3530 NW 115th Ave, Doral, FL 33178
Various type of blood pressure monitors/kit (sphygmomanometer, aneroid.

Draeger Medical Systems, Inc. 215-660-2626
16 Electronics Ave, Danvers, MA 01923
Multiple.

Fukuda Denshi Usa, Inc. 800-365-6668
17725 NE 65th St Ste C, Redmond, WA 98052
Non-invasive blood pressure devices.

G H Medical Inc., Division Of Tsj Inc. 612-331-6299
2010 E Hennepin Ave, Minneapolis, MN 55413
Ambulatory blood pressure monitoring systems 942 or 932.

Healer Products, Llc 914-663-6300
427 Commerce Ln Ste 1, West Berlin, NJ 08091
Blood pressure cuff.

Honeywell Hommed, Llc 888-353-5440
3400 Intertech Dr Ste 200, Brookfield, WI 53045
Review station.

MONITOR, BLOOD PRESSURE, INDIRECT, SEMI-AUTOMATIC
(cont'd)

Hypertension Diagnostics, Inc. 888-785-7392
2915 Waters Rd Ste 108, Eagan, MN 55121
HDI offers a family of CardioVascular Profiling Systems (CPSs), all of which are non-invasive and utilize an upper-arm blood pressure cuff and an unique Arterial PulseWave(tm) Sensor as a complete system. Includes printer and pre-printed report forms as follows: (1) the HDI/PulseWave(tm) CR-2000 Research CPS is offered in the U.S. for 'research purposes only' and provides 15 cardiovascular parameters including cardiac output, SVR, and TVI as well as C1-large artery and C2-small artery elasticity indices (that is, arterial compliance). The system carries a CE Mark as a medical device for patient diagnostic use outside the U.S. and is provided in one of 5 languages besides English; (2) the CVProfilor(R) DO-2020 CPS is offered only in the U.S., has been cleared by the FDA (510k #K001948), carries a UL-Listed product label, and generates a CVProfile(tm) report based on the patient's blood-pressure waveform anaysis which includes a brief medical history as recorded, body-mass index (BMI), blood-pressure values including pulse pressure and heart rate, and both C1 and C2 arterial elasticity (or stiffness) parameters; and (3) the CVProfilor(R) MD-3000 CPS is only offered outside the U.S. (has CE Mark) for physicians in practice to use as an aid in the diagnosis, treatment and monitoring of patients with hypertension and other cardiovascular disease (including diabetes and dyslipidemias).

Icu Medical (Ut), Inc 949-366-2183
4455 Atherton Dr, Salt Lake City, UT 84123
Various types of monitoring kits.

Imetrikus, Inc. 760-804-8800
5875 Avenida Encinas, Carlsbad, CA 92008
Data transfer system.

Intercare Dx, Inc. 310-242-5634
6080 Center Dr Ste 640, Los Angeles, CA 90045
Vascular laboratory.

Invivo Corporation 425-487-7000
12601 Research Pkwy, Orlando, FL 32826
Non-indvelling blood-pressure monitor.

Jabil Global Services 502-240-1000
11201 Electron Dr, Louisville, KY 40299
Blood pressure unit.

Jobar Intl., Inc. 310-222-8682
21022 Figueroa St, Carson, CA 90745
Noninvasive blood-pressure monitor; wrist-type, fully automated. One-touch operation.

Koven Technology, Inc. 800-521-8342
12125 Woodcrest Executive Dr Ste 320, Saint Louis, MO 63141
Nissei Model DS-250 Ambulatory Monitoring System - Compact Korotkoff method patient-worn blood pressure measuring and recording system with analysis software.

Lifeclinic International, Ltd. 800-543-2787
511 Creasman Dr, Winchester, TN 37398
Computerized blood pressure, pulse.

Lumiscope Company, Inc. 800-672-8293
1035 Centennial Ave, Piscataway, NJ 08854
$200 for unit using Korotkoff technique, and non-rechargeable batteries, weighing 1.5 lb.

Medport, Llc 978-927-3808
23 Acorn St, Providence, RI 02903
Blood pressure monitor.

Microfit, Inc. 650-969-7296
1077B Independence Ave, Mountain View, CA 94043
Computerized non-invasive blood pressure, heart rate, body weight system.

Nasiff Assoc., Inc. 315-676-2346
841 County Route 37 # 1, Central Square, NY 13036
Cardio-card nibp (non-invasive blood pressure monitor) mgmt system.

Spacelabs Medical Inc. 800-522-7212
5150 220th Ave SE, Issaquah, WA 98029
Ambulatory blood pressure monitors and accessories.

Sunbeam Products, Inc. 561-912-4100
2381 NW Executive Center Dr, Boca Raton, FL 33431
Blood pressure monitor.

Tensys Medical, Inc. 888-722-7800
5825 Oberlin Dr Ste 100, San Diego, CA 92121
Non-invasive blood pressure monitor.

Visual Telecommunications Network, Inc 703-448-C999
2108 Beechgrove Pl, Utica, NY 13501
Non invasive patient home blood pressure monitoring device.

Zoe Medical, Inc. 978-887-1410
460 Boston St, Topsfield, MA 01983
Telemonitoring system.

MONITOR, BLOOD PRESSURE, INDIRECT, SURGERY
(Surgery) 79FYM

Datascope Corp. 800-288-2121
14 Philips Pkwy, Montvale, NJ 07645
Accutorr Plus lightweight, portable NIBP monitor. Optional features: SpO2, temperature, trend, and recorder.

Fluke Biomedical 800-648-7952
6920 Seaway Blvd, Everett, WA 98203
Non-invasive blood-pressure analyzer.

Smiths Medical Pm, Inc. 800-558-2345
N7W22025 Johnson Dr, Waukesha, WI 53186
SERIES 6004 Noninvasive blood pressure unit allows the measurement of systolic, diastolic, mean arterial pressure with optional printer, pulse oximetry, and temperature.

Trimline Medical Products Corp. 800-526-3538
34 Columbia Rd, Branchburg, NJ 08876
TRIMLINE Large face aneroid and mercurial sphygmomanometers, available as wall, desk or stand models; also cuff containers and inflation systems, all latex-free.

MONITOR, BLOOD PRESSURE, INDIRECT, SURGERY, POWERED *(Surgery) 79FYL*

D.R.E., Inc. 800-462-8195
1800 Williamson Ct, Louisville, KY 40223
The DRE Insight 4A measures 3-lead ECG, respiration, NIBP, and SpO2. This monitor can be used with patients from neonate to adult by use of an intuitive interface. Options include 5-lead ECG, 2-channel IP, 2-channel temperature, capnography, printer, and rechargeable battery.

MONITOR, BLOOD PRESSURE, INDIRECT, TRANSDUCER
(Anesthesiology) 73BZZ

Md International, Inc. 305-669-9003
11300 NW 41st St, Doral, FL 33178

Welch Allyn, Inc. 800-535-6663
4341 State Street Rd, Skaneateles Falls, NY 13153

MONITOR, BLOOD PRESSURE, INVASIVE (ARTERIAL)
(Cardiovascular) 74RLR

Datascope Corp. 800-288-2121
14 Philips Pkwy, Montvale, NJ 07645
DUAL TRACE monitor 2200I with printer for invasive and non-invasive monitoring. For non-invasive model 2100 with printer/without printer.

Edmund Industrial Optics 800-363-1992
101 E Gloucester Pike, Barrington, NJ 08007

Ge Medical Systems Information Technologies 800-643-6439
8200 W Tower Ave, Milwaukee, WI 53223
Unit measuring arterial, pulmonary artery, venous, left atrial, or intracranial pressures. Connections for two transducers. Displays systolic, diastolic, and mean pressure with label. PAW measurement program calculates end-expiration wedge. Unit measures arterial, pulmonary artery, venous, and left atrial or intracranial pressure. Connection for one transducer. (Displays and PAW measurements as listed above.) Unit with additional display of two internal or surface temperatures and difference.

Konigsberg Instruments, Inc. 626-449-0016
2000 E Foothill Blvd, Pasadena, CA 91107
Chronically implantable transducer, -150 to 300 mm Hg, various models 2.5 to 7 mm diameter, 20-60 mV output, for animal research only. For studies periods from a few days to several years.

Lds Life Science (Formerly Gould Instrument Systems Inc.) 216-328-7000
5525 Cloverleaf Pkwy, Valley View, OH 44125

Mennen Medical Corp. 800-223-2201
2540 Metropolitan Dr, Trevose, PA 19053
ENVOY patient monitor 551-170-000 dual BP and cardiac output, 551-180-000 dual BP for Envoy patient monitor. HORIZON 9000 WS cath-lab information system.

Pace Tech, Inc. 800-722-3024
510 N Garden Ave, Clearwater, FL 33755

MONITOR, BLOOD PRESSURE, INVASIVE (ARTERIAL) *(cont'd)*

Smiths Medical Asd, Inc. 800-848-1757
6250 Shier Rings Rd, Dublin, OH 43016

Sorin Group Usa 800-289-5759
14401 W 65th Way, Arvada, CO 80004

MONITOR, BLOOD PRESSURE, INVASIVE (ARTERIAL), ANESTHESIA *(Anesthesiology) 73CAA*

Aga Linde Healthcare P.R. Inc. 787-622-7900
PO Box 363868, GPO Box 364727, San Juan, PR 00936
Anesth/Pul Med.

David Scott Company 800-804-0333
59 Fountain St, Framingham, MA 01702

Pace Tech, Inc. 800-722-3024
510 N Garden Ave, Clearwater, FL 33755
VITALMAX 4000, mini-pack 3000/3100, from $8,795.00-$12,795.00.

MONITOR, BLOOD PRESSURE, VENOUS *(Cardiovascular) 74RLX*

Dedicated Distribution 800-325-8367
640 Miami Ave, Kansas City, KS 66105
Digital and manual blood pressure monitors

Konigsberg Instruments, Inc. 626-449-0016
2000 E Foothill Blvd, Pasadena, CA 91107
Chronically implantable transducer, -150 to 300 mm Hg, various models 2.5 to 7 mm diameter, 20-60 mV output, for animal research only. For studies periods from a few days to several years.

Lds Life Science (Formerly Gould Instrument Systems Inc.) 216-328-7000
5525 Cloverleaf Pkwy, Valley View, OH 44125

Mennen Medical Corp. 800-223-2201
2540 Metropolitan Dr, Trevose, PA 19053
HORIZON 9000 WS cath-lab information system + ENVOY patient monitor.

Q-Med, Inc. 732-544-5544
100 Metro Park S., 3rd Fl., South Amboy, NJ 08878
VASOSPECT venous flow analyzer with interpretive report.

MONITOR, BLOOD PRESSURE, VENOUS, CARDIOPULMONARY BYPASS *(Cardiovascular) 74KRK*

B. Braun Oem Division, B. Braun Medical Inc. 866-8-BBRAUN
824 12th Ave, Bethlehem, PA 18018

B. Braun Of Puerto Rico, Inc. 610-691-5400
215.7 Insular Rd., Sabana Grande, PR 00637
Non-powered venous pressure monitor.

MONITOR, BLOOD PRESSURE, VENOUS, CENTRAL *(Surgery) 79FYO*

Smiths Medical Asd, Inc. 800-848-1757
6250 Shier Rings Rd, Dublin, OH 43016

Trudell Medical Marketing Ltd. 800-265-5494
926 Leathorne St., London, ON N5Z-3M5 Canada
Central monitor foe pressure alarms.

MONITOR, CARBON-DIOXIDE, CUTANEOUS *(Anesthesiology) 73LKD*

Draeger Medical Systems, Inc. 215-660-2626
16 Electronics Ave, Danvers, MA 01923
Monitor.

Respironics California, Inc. 724-387-4559
2271 Cosmos Ct, Carlsbad, CA 92011
Transcutaneous monitor.

Respironics Novametrix, Llc. 724-387-4559
5 Technology Dr, Wallingford, CT 06492
Transcutaneous monitor.

MONITOR, CARDIAC (CARDIOTACHOMETER & RATE ALARM) *(Cardiovascular) 74DRT*

Accusync Medical Research Corp. 203-877-1610
132 Research Dr, Milford, CT 06460
Cardiac monitor.

Biotek Instruments, Inc. 802-655-4040
100 Tigan St, Highland Park, Winooski, VT 05404
Multiparameter simulator, (cardiac monitor tester).

Calmaquip Engineering Corp. 305-592-4510
7240 NW 12th St, Miami, FL 33126

Commercial/Medical Electronics, Inc. 800-324-4844
1519 S Lewis Ave, Tulsa, OK 74104

MONITOR, CARDIAC (CARDIOTACHOMETER & RATE ALARM) *(cont'd)*

Criticare Systems, Inc. 262-798-5361
20925 Crossroads Cir, Waukesha, WI 53186
Vital signs monitor (various models).

Draeger Medical Systems, Inc. 215-660-2626
16 Electronics Ave, Danvers, MA 01923
Multiple.

Electronic Design & Research Co., Inc. 502-433-8660
7331 Intermodal Dr, Louisville, KY 40258
Super-High resolution EKG, Cardio-stimulator, low-noise amplifiers, 50/60 Hz comb notch filters

Fukuda Denshi Usa, Inc. 800-365-6668
17725 NE 65th St Ste C, Redmond, WA 98052
Monitor, cardiac (incl. cardiotachometer & rate alarm).

Ge Medical Systems Information Technologies 800-643-6439
8200 W Tower Ave, Milwaukee, WI 53223

Invivo Corporation 425-487-7000
12601 Research Pkwy, Orlando, FL 32826
Ecg monitor; plethsmograph.

Mednet Healthcare Technologies, Inc. 800-606-5511
100 Ludlow Dr, Ewing, NJ 08638
Heartrak Smart, Heartrak Smart AT, Pacetrak Plus, Pacetrak Speaks

Mennen Medical Corp. 800-223-2201
2540 Metropolitan Dr, Trevose, PA 19053
ENVOY patient monitor 551-104-000 includes ECG, resp, and apnea for Envoy patient monitor.

Nasiff Assoc., Inc. 315-676-2346
841 County Route 37 # 1, Central Square, NY 13036
Cardio card holter system.

Physio-Control, Inc. 800-442-1142
11811 Willows Rd NE, Redmond, WA 98052
Lifepak 11 diagnostic cardiac monitor. Interpretive diagnostic 3-channel 12-lead monitor and recorder.

Proteus Biomedical, Inc. 650-632-4031
2600 Bridge Pkwy Ste 101, Redwood City, CA 94065

Sensor Dynamics, Inc. 510-623-1459
4568 Enterprise St, Fremont, CA 94538
Various models of heart rate monitors.

Spacelabs Medical Inc. 800-522-7212
5150 220th Ave SE, Issaquah, WA 98029
Patient monitors and accessories.

The Ansar Group, Inc. 215-922-6088
240 S 8th St, Philadelphia, PA 19107
Respiratory and cardiac spectral frequency signal monitor.

Vitalcom, Inc. 800-888-0077
15222 Del Amo Ave, Tustin, CA 92780

Welch Allyn Protocol Inc. 800-289-2500
8500 SW Creekside Pl, Beaverton, OR 97008
Vital signs monitor; portable cardiac monitor

Zoe Medical, Inc. 978-887-1410
460 Boston St, Topsfield, MA 01983
Patient monitoring system.

MONITOR, CARDIAC OUTPUT, FLOWMETER *(Cardiovascular) 74KFP*

Konigsberg Instruments, Inc. 626-449-0016
2000 E Foothill Blvd, Pasadena, CA 91107
2 Channel Telemetry Flowmeter; Medical Research, Discovery Research, Safety Pharmacology

Respironics, Inc 800-345-6443
1010 Murry Ridge Ln, Murrysville, PA 15668

MONITOR, CARDIAC OUTPUT, IMPEDANCE PLETHYSMOGRAPHY *(Surgery) 79KFR*

Sorba Medical Systems, Inc. 800-SOR-BA13
165 Bishops Way Ste 152, Brookfield, WI 53005
$20,000 (including printer and cart) for CIC-1000 non-invasive cardiac output monitoring system with continuous storage of data and trend analysis graphs for complete hemodynamic status.

U.F.I. 805-772-1203
545 Main St Ste C2, Morro Bay, CA 93442
$6,250 to $10,250 for Model 2994 (1 to 4 channels).

MONITOR, CARDIAC OUTPUT, THERMAL (BALLOON TYPE CATHETER) *(Surgery) 79KFN*

Ge Medical Systems Information Technologies 800-643-6439
8200 W Tower Ave, Milwaukee, WI 53223

MONITOR, CARDIAC OUTPUT, THERMAL (BALLOON TYPE CATHETER) *(cont'd)*

Mennen Medical Corp. 800-223-2201
2540 Metropolitan Dr, Trevose, PA 19053
ENVOY patient monitor 551-107-000 cardiac output or 2 temps for Envoy patient monitor.

MONITOR, CARDIAC OUTPUT, TREND (ARTERIAL PRESSURE PULSE) *(Surgery) 79KFQ*

Ge Medical Systems Information Technologies 800-643-6439
8200 W Tower Ave, Milwaukee, WI 53223

Netech, Corp. 800-547-6557
110 Toledo St, Farmingdale, NY 11735
Several hand held patient simulators are offered. The MicroSim series provides 5 lead ECG with either 10 arrhythmias or one invasive blood pressure and performance waveforms. The MiniSim is a comprehensive 10 lead ECG simulator with 45 arrhythmias, performance waveforms, 2 invasive blood preesures, respiration, and temperature. In addition, Holter, EEG, and Cardiac Output Simulators are available.

MONITOR, CARDIOPULMONARY LEVEL SENSING
(Cardiovascular) 74DTW

Cardiomedics, Inc. 888-849-0200
18872 Bardeen Ave, Irvine, CA 92612
Cardiopulmonary Diagnostic System

Sanmina-Sci Corp. 408-964-3555
2700 N 1st St, San Jose, CA 95134
Level sensor pad.

Terumo Cardiovascular Systems, Corp 800-521-2818
6200 Jackson Rd, Ann Arbor, MI 48103

MONITOR, CEREBRAL FUNCTION *(Cns/Neurology) 84QJE*

Flowtronics, Inc. 602-997-1364
10250 N 19th Ave Ste B, Phoenix, AZ 85021
Priced from $6,450 to $21,500 for cerebral blood flow monitors.

Olympic Medical Corp. 206-767-3500
5900 1st Ave S, Seattle, WA 98108
New Infant Brain Monitor: The Olympic CFM 6000 can be used in the NICU and other acute care departments to continuously monitor an infant's brain activity. Simple to use, the Olympic CFM enables clinical staff to assess the neurological status of the brain, record and detect seizures, monitor the effects of drugs and other therapies on the brain, identify HIE and predict long-term outcome, and determine the need for further neurological examination or transport. The Olympic CFM produces an amplitude-integrated output (aEEG) ó an easy-to-read record of brain activity and abnormalities. Contact Olympic Medical at 1(800)426-0353 or (01)1-206-767-3500, or visit www.OlympicCFM.com.

MONITOR, CONTAMINATION, ENVIRONMENTAL, PERSONAL
(General) 80WIP

Andersen Products, Inc., 800-523-1276
3202 Caroline Dr, Health Science Park, Haw River, NC 27258
AIRSCAN monitoring system for measuring personnel exposure to ethylene oxide; obtain results same day on-site.

Assay Technology Inc 800-833-1258
1252 Quarry Ln, Pleasanton, CA 94566
CHEM CHIP on-site and CHEM EXPRESS mail-in badges for personal exposure to ethylene oxide, formaldehyde, xylene, glutaraldehyde, halogenated anesthetic gases, nitrous oxide, mercury vapor, hydrogen peroxide, acetic acid, ozone, nitrogen dioxide, ethyl-2-cyanoacrylate and over 100 organic vapors.

Cole-Parmer Instrument Inc. 800-323-4340
625 E Bunker Ct, Vernon Hills, IL 60061

Custom Ultrasonics, Inc. 215-364-1477
144 Railroad Dr, Hartsville, PA 18974
SYSTEM 93 glutaraldehyde fume recovery system. Adjunct to system 83/81/80 designed to remove environmental glutaraldehyde vapors to OSHA guidelines.

Enviro Guard, Inc. 800-438-1152
201 Shannon Oaks Cir Ste 115, Cary, NC 27511

Interscan Corp. 800-458-6153
21700 Nordhoff St, P.O. Box 2496, Chatsworth, CA 91311
$1,990.00 ea. for portable survey units, and $2750.00 and up for fixed systems. Full data acquisition/archiving/reporting system available.

Lab Safety Supply, Inc. 800-356-0783
401 S Wright Rd, Janesville, WI 53546

MONITOR, CONTAMINATION, ENVIRONMENTAL, PERSONAL *(cont'd)*

Medical Safety Systems Inc. 888-803-9303
230 White Pond Dr, Akron, OH 44313
Formaldehyde, radiation, mercury vapor, ethylene oxide gas, nitrous oxide, glutaraldahyde and halogenated anesthetic monitoring badges.

Sensidyne, Inc. 800-451-9444
16333 Bay Vista Dr, Clearwater, FL 33760
Detector and dosimeter tubes for visual indication and measurement of over 300 gases and vapors.

MONITOR, ECG *(Cardiovascular) 74QRW*

Biomedical Systems Corp. 800-877-6334
77 Progress Pkwy Bldg 1, Maryland Hts, MO 63043
12 Lead ECG machine that simultaneously acquires all 12 leads in 15 seconds and then analyzes them with a powerful and accurate 12 lead interpretive program. Supplies instantaneous computer interpretation with bedside printout.

Cardiac Telecom Corporation 800-355-2594
212 Outlet Way Ste 1, Greensburg, PA 15601
An automatic event-driven ECG telemetry unit for institutional use.

Cardiomedics, Inc. 888-849-0200
18872 Bardeen Ave, Irvine, CA 92612
Wireless Holter Monitor and Electrode Patches

Colin Medical Instruments Corp. 800-829-6427
5850 Farinon Dr, San Antonio, TX 78249
The portable PRESS-MATE ADVANTAGE multi-parameter NIBP monitor includes ECG (3/5 lead), SpO2, respiration, temperature, recorder, and high-resolution color LCD display.

Commercial/Medical Electronics, Inc. 800-324-4844
1519 S Lewis Ave, Tulsa, OK 74104

Futuremed America, Inc. 800-222-6780
15700 Devonshire St, Granada Hills, CA 91344
3 Ch. EZ-3 from $1,300 to $1,700. 12Ch. P-8000 -POWER from $2,800. 3Ch. PC-Based ECG Interp. Stress 12Ch Stress test system $5,000.

Ge Medical Systems Information Technologies 800-643-6439
8200 W Tower Ave, Milwaukee, WI 53223
Multi-lead ECG transport monitor, TRAM unit with smart lead fail, dual temperature, non-invasive blood-pressure and pulse oximetry. System is AC or battery powered with a LCD display. TRAM module is compatible with the Solar 7000 physiological patient monitor. Also, the Eagle 4000 patient monitor is available with multi-lead ECG, dual-temperature, non-invasive blood pressure, pulse oximetry with or without invasive blood pressures. The unit is battery operated and portable.

I.P.I.-International Products, Inc. 703-237-2774
1929 Poole Ln, McLean, VA 22101

Ivy Biomedical Systems, Inc. 800-247-4614
11 Business Park Dr, Branford, CT 06405
$2,200 for adult/neonate ECG monitor, Model 101. $5,600 for ECG, temperature, direct press, NIBP monitor. $7900 - $9700 for different configurations; monitors for ECG, two pressures, respiration, ox and pulse. Also available, $7900 - $9900 for adult and neonatal monitor, ECG, respirator, NIBP, pulse ox, 2 temperatures and 2 pressures.

J.M. Baragano Biomedical P.M. And Consulting, Inc. 787-722-4007
808 Ave Fernandez Juncos, San Juan, PR 00907
Flexible monitoring equipment for physiological monitoring in ICU, ER, OR, and other areas within healthcare facilities.

Lechnologies Research, Inc.. 866-321-2342
N64W24801 Main St Ste 107, Sussex, WI 53089
Introducing AfibAlert™, the newest tool for the diagnosis of transient atrial fibrillation. The patented AfibAlert™ is a revolutionary new way of detecting whether the heart is beating normally or is in chaotic atrial fibrillation (AF). Designed for home use, the AfibAlert™ allows the patient to test their heart rhythm on a daily basis, or as often as they wish. Physicians and patients can work together to detect transient atrial fibrillation recurrences for the first time. Stored data can be transmitted via telephone or uploaded to a secure web site for physician review. The AfibAlert™ is available with a physician's prescription.

Md International, Inc. 305-669-9003
11300 NW 41st St, Doral, FL 33178
Holter analyzer system and software with digital recorder.

Med-Dyne 502-429-4140
2775 S Floyd St, Louisville, KY 40209

MONITOR, ECG *(cont'd)*

Mennen Medical Corp. 800-223-2201
2540 Metropolitan Dr, Trevose, PA 19053
ENVOY patient monitor with C51-104-000 5 lead ECG module or with C51-112-000 12 lead ECG module.

Meza Medical Equipment 888-308-7116
108 W Nakoma St, San Antonio, TX 78216

Mortara Instrument, Inc. 800-231-7437
7865 N 86th St, Milwaukee, WI 53224
Non-interpretive single channel, AC/DC, 3 - 4 channel electrocardiograph with printout format. Interpretive version also available.

Nihon Kohden America, Inc. 800-325-0283
90 Icon, Foothill Ranch, CA 92610

Omni Medical Supply Inc. 800-860-6664
4153 Pioneer Dr, Commerce Township, MI 48390

Polar Electro Inc. 1-800-227-1314
1111 Marcus Ave Ste M15, New Hyde Park, NY 11042
Wireless ECG heart rate monitors and accessories.

Rf Industries, Inc. • 800-233-1728
7610 Miramar Rd, San Diego, CA 92126
Our Bioconnect division offers our new 'Pinch Lead' or 'Grabber' patient-monitoring connecting wires.

Scottcare Corporation 800-243-9412
4791 W 150th St, Cleveland, OH 44135
TeleRehab Advantage, an ECG monitoring and practice management system designed specifically for cardiopulmonary rehabilitation professionals. TeleRehab is a computer-based telemetry (in-hospital), and transtelephonic (at-home/satellite location) cardiopulmonary rehabilitation monitoring system that includes comprehensive and integrated data management, report generation, and Outcomes software. Telemetry channels can be combined with transtelephonic (remote location)channels on the same CPU. Includes archiving and report generating. System is networkable and expandable.

Smiths Medical Pm, Inc. 800-558-2345
N7W22025 Johnson Dr, Waukesha, WI 53186
Autocorr Plus, Pulse oximeter/ECG monitor, with 3 or 5 led ECG, pace detect/reject, digital oximetry with SAC (serial autocorrelation) technology, and respiration. A high resolution electroluminescent screen display provides two user configuration traces.

Superior Medical Limited 800-268-7944
520 Champagne Dr., Toronto, ONT M3J 2T9 Canada

Welch Allyn Protocol, Inc. 800-462-0777
2 Corporate Dr Ste 110, Long Grove, IL 60047
MRL LITE.

Zoll Medical Corp. 800-348-9011
269 Mill Rd, Chelmsford, MA 01824
AC/battery operated transport defibrillator/monitor. $8,945 for Zoll PD1400 defibrillator/ monitor/ non-invasive/ temporarypacemaker, lightweight. Defibrillate, pace, and monitor through two electrodes.

MONITOR, ECG, AMBULATORY, REAL-TIME

(Cardiovascular) 74TGX

Cadwell Laboratories 800-245-3001
909 N Kellogg St, Kennewick, WA 99336
CADWELL Easy ambulatory EEG/ECG 32 channel digital recorder, up to 48 hours.

Cardiac Care Units, Inc. 818-592-6004
7745 Alabama Ave, Canoga Park, CA 91304
CCU COMPAS simultaneous 3-channel, microprocessor based, ambulatory cardiac monitoring system with continuous ECG analysis and ST measurement in real time. The system detects, diagnoses, signals and digitally records silent and symptomatic arrhythmias plus ischemic changes and is capable of providing over 75 six second diagnostic ECG strips. COMPAS system generates hard copy report with tabular summaries, bar graphs, and selected event strips. Comprehensive data on arrhythmias, ST segment alterations, heart rates, and total beats. System requires no console. Heart rate variability calculations. Full-disclosure, narrative summary.

Colin Medical Instruments Corp. 800-829-6427
5850 Farinon Dr, San Antonio, TX 78249
ABPM-630 Ambulatory NIBP/PR monitor. Provides 24-hour measurements at user-selected intervals. CO2 driven for quiet readings during business or sleep. Stored information can be analyzed via AA-200 or computer software.

MONITOR, ECG, AMBULATORY, REAL-TIME *(cont'd)*

Ge Medical Systems Information Technologies 800-643-6439
8200 W Tower Ave, Milwaukee, WI 53223
Solid-state recorder acquires 24 hours of two-channel ECG data and analyzes it in real time. Tape recorder model can be used as either a two- or three-channel recorder for up to 48 hours recording.

Ivy Biomedical Systems, Inc. 800-247-4614
11 Business Park Dr, Branford, CT 06405
$3100 - $5950 for neonatal/adult transport monitors displaying ECG, respiration, temperature, pressure, Ox and pulse.

Omni Medical Supply Inc. 800-860-6664
4153 Pioneer Dr, Commerce Township, MI 48390

Q-Med, Inc. 732-544-5544
100 Metro Park S., 3rd Fl., South Amboy, NJ 08878
MONITOR ONE computerized ambulatory long term ECG.

Ubs Instruments Corporation 818-710-1195
7745 Alabama Ave Ste 7, Canoga Park, CA 91304
COMPAS XM Holter Monitor, a real-time miroprocessor based cardiac monitoring system with continuous ECG analysis and ST measurements. Prints 24 hour monitoring reports with 84 sample ECG strips, HRV calculations and Time Domain Parameters. Weighs only 13 oz.

Vitalog, Inc 650-366-8676
643 Bair Island Rd Ste 212, Redwood City, CA 94063
Internet-based Sleep Diagnostic products and services; Positive Airway Pressure Therapy Monitoring system. Ambulatory monitor.

Zoetek Medical Sales & Service, Inc. 800-388-6223
668 Phillips Rd, Victor, NY 14564
Stress Test Systems, Holter Recorders, EKG monitors, etc. Exclusive dealer for Schiller America throughout the Northeastern US.

MONITOR, ECG, ANESTHESIA *(Anesthesiology) 73BRS*

Aga Linde Healthcare P.R. Inc. 787-622-7900
PO Box 363868, GPO Box 364727, San Juan, PR 00936
Anesth/Pul Med.

Aspect Medical Systems, Inc. 617-559-7000
141 Needham St, Newton, MA 02464
A-2000 Monitor.

Mennen Medical Corp. 800-223-2201
2540 Metropolitan Dr, Trevose, PA 19053
ENVOY patient monitor.

Mortara Instrument, Inc. 800-231-7437
7865 N 86th St, Milwaukee, WI 53224
12 lead monitor for ischemic changes during anesthesia.

Pace Tech, Inc. 800-722-3024
510 N Garden Ave, Clearwater, FL 33755
VITALMAX 4000-B configurated or modular $6,495-$12,795. ECG with NIBP, temp., resp., and pulse oximeter. EL display optional invasive pressures.

MONITOR, ECG, ARRHYTHMIA *(Cardiovascular) 74QRX*

eCardio Diagnostics 888-747-1442
1717 N Sam Houston Pkwy W, Houston, TX 77038

Ge Medical Systems Information Technologies 800-643-6439
8200 W Tower Ave, Milwaukee, WI 53223
SOLAR 7000 is a monochrome or color, 8-trace patient monitoring device with network compatibility. System is capable of monitoring ECG, invasive and non-invasive blood pressure, pulse oximetry, SVO2, end-tidal CO2, as well as anesthetic agent analysis through the SAM module. SOLAR 7000 is entirely software configured, offering upgradability via network or direct PC connection. User interface for the system is consistent to trim-knob control for ease of operation. Also available, EAGLE 4000 with ECG, dual temperature, cardiac output, 2 invasive blood pressure, non-invasive blood pressure, and pulse oximetry. Five-trace monochrome or color flat-panel display; system offers battery as well as AC operation. Trim-knob control, user-interface is identical to that found on the SOLAR 7000.

Instromedix, A Card Guard Co. 800-633-3361
10255 W Higgins Rd Ste 100, Rosemont, IL 60018

Lechnologies Research, Inc.. 866-321-2342
N64W24801 Main St Ste 107, Sussex, WI 53089
30-day pre-symptom memory loop recorder with 16 minutes memory.

Life Sensing Instrument Company, Inc. 800-624-2732
329 W Lincoln St, Tullahoma, TN 37388

Medtronic, Inc. 800-633-8766
710 Medtronic Pkwy, Minneapolis, MN 55432

MONITOR, ECG, ARRHYTHMIA *(cont'd)*

Mennen Medical Corp. 800-223-2201
2540 Metropolitan Dr, Trevose, PA 19053
ENVOY patient monitor.

Pinnacle Technology Group, Inc. 800-345-5123
7076 Schnipke Dr, Ottawa Lake, MI 49267
ADI-10 (Arrhythmia Display Interface) is a device that allows you to display any arrhythmia from any simulator onto a TV screen or video projection system. $1035

MONITOR, ECG, SURGERY *(Surgery) 79FYW*

Mortara Instrument, Inc. 800-231-7437
7865 N 86th St, Milwaukee, WI 53224
12 lead monitor for ischemic changes during surgery.

Welch Allyn, Inc. 800-535-6663
4341 State Street Rd, Skaneateles Falls, NY 13153
Electrocardiograph system.

MONITOR, EEG *(Cns/Neurology) 84BRR*

Aga Linde Healthcare P.R. Inc. 787-622-7900
PO Box 363868, GPO Box 364727, San Juan, PR 00936
Neurology.

American Biomed Instruments, Inc. 718-235-8900
11 Wyona St, Brooklyn, NY 11207

Aspect Medical Systems, Inc. 617-559-7000
141 Needham St, Newton, MA 02464
A-1050 EEG Monitor 1 or channel EEG brain monitor with the bispectral index. BIS 1-2000 EEG monitor, status, trend and numeric displays, compact, lightweight and porable.

Bio-Feedback Systems, Inc. 303-444-1411
2736 47th St, Boulder, CO 80301
$1,450 for alpha & theta biofeedback monitor, $2,195 for twilight learning (theta actuated). $2,245 for 1 channel hardware & software to interface to PC compatible.

Bio-Logic Systems Corp. 800-323-8326
1 Bio Logic Plz, Mundelein, IL 60060
BRAIN ATLAS, CEEGRAPH- microcomputer based systems which perform intraoperative monitoring of EEG.

Bio-Medical Instruments, Inc. 800-521-4640
2387 E 8 Mile Rd, Warren, MI 48091
EEG Neurofeedback monitor battery powered. Compuerized 1 - 24 channel.

Cadwell Laboratories 800-245-3001
909 N Kellogg St, Kennewick, WA 99336
CADWELL EEG monitoring system, 32-channel EASY II.

Mennen Medical Corp. 800-223-2201
2540 Metropolitan Dr, Trevose, PA 19053
ENVOY patient monitor.

Sleepmed Incorporated 800-334-5085
200 Corporate Pl Ste 5-B, Peabody, MA 01960
DigiTrace 2700 Plus recorders provide 24 channels and 3 auxiliary channels with on-line automatic seizure and spike analysis. DigiTrace recorders are noted for high quality, low artifact tracings.

Sterogene Bioseparations, Inc. 800-535-2284
5922 Farnsworth Ct, Carlsbad, CA 92008
Computerized, 2-channel and 16-channel, brain-mapping system.

MONITOR, EEG, SURGERY *(Surgery) 79FYX*

Axon Systems, Inc. 800-888-2966
400 Oser Ave Ste 2200, Hauppauge, NY 11788
Neurological workstation. Simultaneous, 32, 16 or 8 channel, multimodality EEP/EP/EMG monitoring for OR/ICU applications. Quantified EEG - Spectral edge, CSA, DSA, CDSA displays. absloute and relative power, burst supppression index. Trend all parameters with event alarms. Review and print reports while monitoring. Import and display vital signs. Multiple site remote monitoring via network, internet or modem. Portable and fixed location platforms.

Bio-Logic Systems Corp. 800-323-8326
1 Bio Logic Plz, Mundelein, IL 60060
BRAIN ATLAS, CEEGRAPH- microcomputer based systems which perform intraoperative monitoring of EEG.

MONITOR, EMG *(Anesthesiology) 73CAB*

Axon Systems, Inc. 800-888-2966
400 Oser Ave Ste 2200, Hauppauge, NY 11788
Comprehensive cranial, nerve root and motor nerve monitoring with eight or sixteen channels of spontaneous or evoked EMG activity. Signal-triggered tones and audible EMG provide identification and assessment of nerve function.

MONITOR, EMG *(cont'd)*

Bio-Medical Instruments, Inc. 800-521-4640
2387 E 8 Mile Rd, Warren, MI 48091

Cadwell Laboratories 800-245-3001
909 N Kellogg St, Kennewick, WA 99336
Cadwell Cascade 8-16 channel EMG/EP console. High performance Laptop based portable system with auto report generation. Provides multi-modality monitoring with display of EMG, SEP, ABR, VEP, triggeved EMG, and MEP activity, interleaving for testing all extremities at the same time, with compressed spectral array, Sentry for automatically sequencing through 8 separate EP protocoles, 16 channel triggered EMG, and remote monitoring via network, internet, intranet.

MONITOR, ESOPHAGEAL MOTILITY, AND TUBE *(Gastro/Urology) 78KLA*

Medtronic Neuromodulation 763-514-4000
710 Medtronic Pkwy, Minneapolis, MN 55432
Various types of esophageal motility catheters.

Narco Bio-Systems 800-433-5615
8508 Cross Park Dr, Austin, TX 78754
Esophageal, anorectal, bilalry and small bowel recording systems. Up to 11 channels with time and event. Automated data analysis.

Sandhill Scientific, Inc. 800-468-4556
9150 Commerce Center Cir Ste 500, Highlands Ranch, CO 80129
InSIGHT EFT system with combined impedance-manometry for esophageal function testing (EFT). The InSIGHT EFT system assesses both bolus transit and muscular function in a single concurrent test. InSIGHT is also available for esophageal, anorectal and biliary manometry.

MONITOR, ESOPHAGEAL PRESSURE *(Gastro/Urology) 78RLU*

Konigsberg Instruments, Inc. 626-449-0016
2000 E Foothill Blvd, Pasadena, CA 91107
Multi-function Motility Catheters. Pressure manometers with one to six solide state pressure sensors, directional and circumferential types, for rapid sphincter tonus and smooth muscle response-coordination assessment. Manometry probes may also include multiple pH elements, EMG electrodes and impedance circuit electrodes, as well as a variety of air and fluid passages and outlets.

MONITOR, EYE MOVEMENT *(Ophthalmology) 86HLL*

Applied Science Laboratories 781-275-4000
175 Middlesex Tpke, Bedford, MA 01730
Product line includes systems from $7,000 to $100,000. The Model 501 Eye Tracking System employs digital signal processors to achieve faster and more precise image analysis and accepts high speed camera inputs.

Bausch & Lomb Surgical 636-255-5051
3365 Tree Court Ind Blvd, Saint Louis, MO 63122

Konigsberg Instruments, Inc. 626-449-0016
2000 E Foothill Blvd, Pasadena, CA 91107
Medical Research, Discovery Research, Safety Pharmacology, Special systems for Biocontainment Levels 2, 3 and 4.

Micromedical Technologies, Inc. 800-334-4154
10 Kemp Dr, Chatham, IL 62629
VISUALEYES VIDEO ENG is for observing and recording eye movements. It allows simultaneous subjective observation of eye movements and objective collection and analysis of waveforms during vestibular testing and rehabilitation.

Nidek Inc. 800-223-9044
47651 Westinghouse Dr, Fremont, CA 94539
Model EAS-100 anterior-segment eye-analyzing system. Model CF-3 confocal microscope.

Sensomotoric Instruments, Inc. 888-SMI-USA1
97 Chapel St, Needham, MA 02492
Binocular Eye Tracking with Horizontal, Vertical, & Torsional measurement. Easy to use windows based SW. Ideal for Clinical Vestibular, Ophthalmic, and Oculomotor Research.

MONITOR, EYE MOVEMENT, DIAGNOSTIC *(Ophthalmology) 86HMC*

Microguide, Inc. 630-964-3368
1635 Plum Ct, Downers Grove, IL 60515
Infrared eye-movement monitor.

MONITOR, EYE MOVEMENT, DIAGNOSTIC *(cont'd)*

Pharmaceutical Innovations, Inc. 973-242-2900
897 Frelinghuysen Ave, Newark, NJ 07114
Ultra/Phonic Ophthalmic Scanning pads is a solid ultrasound gel used for ultrasound of the eye. They eliminate the use of regular ultrasound gel, which is difficult to remove from the eyelid and gets into the patient's causing pain. A pad is placed on the closed eyelid; no other gel or liquid is needed. The pad adds cushioning to help protect the eye. After completion of examination, lift the pad off and throw away. There is no clean up.

MONITOR, FERTILITY *(Obstetrics/Gyn) 85VDI*

Zetek, Inc. 800-367-2837
876 Ventura St, Aurora, CO 80011
CUE fertility monitor predicts ovulation 6 days in advance based on hormonal changes from oral/vaginal measurements.

MONITOR, FETAL *(Obstetrics/Gyn) 85QVQ*

Beckman Coulter, Inc. 800-742-2345
250 S Kraemer Blvd, PO Box 8000, Brea, CA 92821

Ge Medical Systems Information Technologies 800-643-6439
8200 W Tower Ave, Milwaukee, WI 53223

Superior Medical Limited 800-268-7944
520 Champagne Dr., Toronto, ONT M3J 2T9 Canada

Xodus Medical, Inc. 800-963-8776
702 Prominence Dr, Westmoreland Business & Research Park
New Kensington, PA 15068
Labor & Delivery Belts and Straps

MONITOR, FETAL DOPPLER ULTRASOUND
(Obstetrics/Gyn) 85MAA

Coopersurgical, Inc. 800-243-2974
95 Corporate Dr, Trumbull, CT 06611
$595 for Doppler model with speaker, LM-120.

Her-Mar, Inc. 800-327-8209
8550 NW 30th Ter, Doral, FL 33122
$850.00 per unit (2Mhz).

Huntleigh Healthcare Llc. 800-223-1218
40 Christopher Way, Eatontown, NJ 07724
3 portable Dopplers - $495.00, $675.00 or $850.00.

Md International, Inc. 305-669-9003
11300 NW 41st St, Doral, FL 33178

Medgyn Products, Inc. 800-451-9667
328 Eisenhower Ln N, Lombard, IL 60148
Ultrasonic mini-doppler unit with three interchangeable probes (2.25, 5 and 8.2MHz) to measure deep or superficial arterial and venous blood flow, blood pressure and pulse rate plus to detect occlusions and location of patient vessels etc.

Ob Specialties, Inc. 800-325-6644
1799 Northwood Ct, Oakland, CA 94611
Summit,Imex,Medisonic Dopplers.

Parks Medical Electronics, Inc. 503-649-7007
PO Box 5669, Aloha, OR 97006

Philips Medical Systems 949-450-0014
1590 Scenic Ave, Costa Mesa, CA 92626

R Medical Supply 800-882-7578
620 Valley Forge Rd Ste F, Hillsborough, NC 27278

MONITOR, FETAL, CARDIAC *(Obstetrics/Gyn) 85KXN*

Medical Cables, Inc. 800-314-51111
1365 Logan Ave, Costa Mesa, CA 92626

MONITOR, FETAL, ULTRASONIC *(Obstetrics/Gyn) 85KNG*

Cardinal Healthcare 209, Inc. 610-862-0800
5225 Verona Rd, Fitchburg, WI 53711
Dop-tone ii.

Cas Medical Systems, Inc. 800-227-4414
44 E Industrial Rd, Branford, CT 06405
FETALGARD Lite antepartum fetal monitor. Avail. with NIBP.

Cone Instruments, Inc. 800-321-6964
5201 Naiman Pkwy, Solon, OH 44139

Huntleigh Healthcare Llc. 800-223-1218
40 Christopher Way, Eatontown, NJ 07724

Summit Doppler Systems, Inc. 800-554-5090
4620 Technology Dr Ste 100, Golden, CO 80403
Handheld fetal/vascular doppler.

The Newman Group, Llc 847-283-9177
42 Sherwood Ter Ste 2, Lake Bluff, IL 60044
Handheld fetal-vascular doppler.

MONITOR, FETAL, ULTRASONIC, HEART RATE
(Obstetrics/Gyn) 85HEL

Cardinal Healthcare 209, Inc. 610-862-0800
5225 Verona Rd, Fitchburg, WI 53711
Lab monitor ultrasound.

Huntleigh Healthcare Llc. 800-223-1218
40 Christopher Way, Eatontown, NJ 07724

MONITOR, FETAL, ULTRASONIC, HEART SOUND
(Obstetrics/Gyn) 85HEK

Analogic Corporation 978-326-4000
8 Centennial Dr, Peabody, MA 01960
FETALGARD 3000 and FETALGARD Lite antepartum fetal monitor.

Cardinal Healthcare 209, Inc. 610-862-0800
5225 Verona Rd, Fitchburg, WI 53711
Monitor.

MONITOR, GAS, ATMOSPHERIC, ENVIRONMENTAL
(General) 80QUM

American Gas & Chemical Co., Ltd. 800-288-3647
220 Pegasus Ave, Northvale, NJ 07647
$740.00 for wall-mounted toxic gas monitor, designed to detect ethylene oxide.

Andersen Products, Inc., 800-523-1276
3202 Caroline Dr, Health Science Park, Haw River, NC 27258
Ethylene oxide personal- and area-monitoring equipment.

Climet Instruments Co. 909-793-2788
1320 W Colton Ave, Redlands, CA 92374
$12,000.00 per unit (standard).

Enviro Guard, Inc. 800-438-1152
201 Shannon Oaks Cir Ste 115, Cary, NC 27511

Interscan Corp. 800-458-6153
21700 Nordhoff St, P.O. Box 2496, Chatsworth, CA 91311
$1,990.00 ea. for portable survey units, and $2750.00 and up for fixed systems. Full data acquisition/archiving/reporting system available.

Lab Safety Supply, Inc. 800-356-0783
401 S Wright Rd, Janesville, WI 53546

Landauer, Inc. 800-323-8830
2 Science Rd, Glenwood, IL 60425
RADTRAK Radon monitoring equipment.

Nevin Laboratories, Inc 800-544-5337
5000 S Halsted St, Chicago, IL 60609
Vapor monitors for measuring nitrous oxide, formaldehyde, glutaraldehyde in the workplace.

Sensors, Inc. 734-429-2100
6812 State Rd, Saline, MI 48176
Measures Carbon Monoxide (CO), Acetylene (C2H2), Methane (CH4) to 3,000 PPM. Module multi-gas pulmonary function.

MONITOR, HEART RATE, OTHER *(Cardiovascular) 74QZO*

Alere Medical, Inc. 775-829-8885
595 Double Eagle Ct Ste 1000, Reno, NV 89521
Alere Medical is a privately held medical technology and services company and leader in the development of phone and Internet-based cardiac patient monitoring systems. Alere's suite of products establishes remote connectivity and communication between patients, their physicians, family members and care managers. Currently in use in 29 states, the Alere Heart Monitoring Program system enables patients with congestive heart failure to have their condition assessed daily, using the patented DayLink monitor, to avoid a crisis such as emergency care or hospitalization. The Alere Heart Monitoring Program improves patient outcomes, reduces provider costs and enriches overall care. Founded in 1996, Alere Medical is based in Reno, NV. For more information about Alere, visit www.alere.com.

Brytech Inc. 613-731-5800
600 Peter Morand Crescent, Suite 240, Ottawa, ONT K1G-5Z3 Canada
HCM

Datascope Corp. 800-288-2121
14 Philips Pkwy, Montvale, NJ 07645
Expert modular high-end vital signals monitor featuring touch-screen display 6 traces, 6 IBP's, NIBP, SpO2, ST segment analysis, arrhythmia, 2 temperatures, CO, hemodynamics and CO2. Also available MR Monitor full featured vital signs monitor with ECG, NIBP, SpO2, temperature, recorder and complete gas analysis that can be placed in the magnet room. Optional features: remote display. Also available Passport portable multiparameter monitor featuring ECG, respiration, NIBP, SpO2, and temperature. Optional features: IBP and recorder.

MONITOR, HEART RATE, OTHER *(cont'd)*

Elmed, Inc. 630-543-2792
60 W Fay Ave, Addison, IL 60101

Florida Life Systems 727-321-9554
3446 5th Ave N, Saint Petersburg, FL 33713
Vital signs monitors.

Genesee Biomedical, Inc. 800-786-4890
1308 S Jason St, Denver, CO 80223
Myocardial Needle Temperature Sensor, myocardial needles of 4 different lentghs used to measure TAG temperature of the heart.

Heart Rate, Inc. 800-237-2271
3190 Airport Loop Dr, Costa Mesa, CA 92626
$295 for 1-2-3-Heartrate Monitor; exercise monitor using NASA ECG capacitive sensors and polar compatible heart beat transmitters. Five models ranging from $295 to $365.

Lds Life Science (Formerly Gould Instrument Systems Inc.) 216-328-7000
5525 Cloverleaf Pkwy, Valley View, OH 44125

Neogen Corporation 800-234-5333
620 Lesher Pl, Lansing, MI 48912
For veterinary use only.

Polar Electro Inc. 1-800-227-1314
1111 Marcus Ave Ste M15, New Hyde Park, NY 11042
All Polar heart rate monitors are ECG accurate, wireless and water resistant to twenty meters. Every unit comes with the Polar lightweight, waterproof, 2 year maintenance free transmitter belt. Products available are: A-SERIES, M-SERIES, and S-SERIES.

Science-Electronics, Inc. 937-224-4444
521 Kiser St, Dayton, OH 45404

Thought Technology Ltd. 800-361-3651
2180 Belgrave Ave., Montreal, QUE H4A 2L8 Canada
CARDIOPRO, CARDIOPRO is a specialized biofeedback application that focuses on the physiology of the cardiovascular and repiratory systems and takes input from one EKG (electrocardiograph), two respiration, one temperature amd one BVP (blood volume pulse) sensor.

Welch Allyn Protocol Inc. 800-289-2500
8500 SW Creekside Pl, Beaverton, OR 97008

MONITOR, HEART RATE, R-WAVE (ECG) *(Cardiovascular) 74QZN*

Biosig Instruments, Inc. 800-463-5470
PO Box 860, Champlain, NY 12919
INSTA-PULSE Portable, patented fitness device, measures heart rate from the hands based on a beat to beat or 4 beat average. 5 models to choose from.

Elmed, Inc. 630-543-2792
60 W Fay Ave, Addison, IL 60101

Ge Medical Systems Information Technologies 800-643-6439
8200 W Tower Ave, Milwaukee, WI 53223
Multi-lead arrhythmia and ST-segment analysis unit; smart lead-fail pinpoints failed electrode and switches to alternate lead; history of up to 36 events; four-level customizable alarm structure.

Hokanson Inc., D.E. 800-999-8251
12840 NE 21st Pl, Bellevue, WA 98005
ANS2000 is an ECG monitor and respiration pacer that measures heart rate variability in response to respiration and postural maneuvers. This test is an indicator of cardiac autonomic neuropathy.

Instromedix, A Card Guard Co. 800-633-3361
10255 W Higgins Rd Ste 100, Rosemont, IL 60018

Lds Life Science (Formerly Gould Instrument Systems Inc.) 216-328-7000
5525 Cloverleaf Pkwy, Valley View, OH 44125

Mennen Medical Corp. 800-223-2201
2540 Metropolitan Dr, Trevose, PA 19053
ENVOY patient monitor.

MONITOR, HEMODIALYSIS UNIT CONDUCTIVITY
(Gastro/Urology) 78QZX

Mesa Laboratories, Inc. 800-992-6372
12100 W 6th Ave, Lakewood, CO 80228
METERS, for measuring temp./cond./pressure/pH/TDS/Resistivity. Western 90DX,NEO-2, pHoenix, NEO-STAT+, HYDRA instruments for the calibration and monitoring of hemodialysis equipment and dialysis water treatment systems.

MONITOR, HEMODIALYSIS UNIT CONDUCTIVITY *(cont'd)*

Transonic Systems Inc. 800-353-3569
34 Dutch Mill Rd, Warren Road Business Park, Ithaca, NY 14850
TRANSONIC Hemodialysis Monitor Measurement during patient dialysis of access recirculation, access flow, cardiac output, and blood line flow.

MONITOR, HEMODYNAMIC *(Anesthesiology) 73VJA*

Aga Linde Healthcare P.R. Inc. 787-622-7900
PO Box 363868, GPO Box 364727, San Juan, PR 00936
Anesth/Pul Med.

Buxco Research Systems 910-794-6980
219 Station Rd Ste 202, Wilmington, NC 28405

Cardiodynamics International Corp. 888-482-9449
21919 30th Dr SE, Bothell, WA 98021
The Bioz.com® from CardioDynamics is a noninvasive hemodynamic monitor utilizing clinically proven Impedance Cardiography (ICG) technology. The BioZ.com displays twelve hemodynamic parameters, including cardiac output, systemic vascular resistance and fluid status. BioZ® Impedance Cardiography (ICG) Module from CardioDynamics brings noninvasive hemodynamic monitoring to GE's Solar patient monitoring systems. The BioZ ICG Module allows rapid, accurate and continuous assessment of a patient's hemodynamic status, including cardiac output, systemic vascular resistance, and fluid status. When incorporated into initial clinical assessment, BioZ ICG may help to assess baseline status, identify appropriate therapeutic interventions, and distinguish those patients with early therapy response. The use of ICG may also help shorten length of stay, reduce overall hospital charges, and potentially improve patient outcomes.

Life Sensing Instrument Company, Inc. 800-624-2732
329 W Lincoln St, Tullahoma, TN 37388

Tecnomed International S.A. De C.V. 52-55-5519-7234
Andalucia 25, Alamos, Ciudad De Mexico, DF 03400 Mexico
BIOZ CARDIODYNAMICS and NICCOMO MEDIS, ICG (IMPEDANCE)non-invasive, hemodynamic monitoring systems.

MONITOR, IMPEDANCE PNEUMOGRAPH
(Anesthesiology) 73RBQ

Mennen Medical Corp. 800-223-2201
2540 Metropolitan Dr, Trevose, PA 19053
ENVOY patient monitor C51-104-000 or C51-112-000 provides ECG and impedance pneumonography for Envoy patient monitor.

U.F.I. 805-772-1203
545 Main St Ste C2, Morro Bay, CA 93442
$435.00 for Model RESPI; $525.00 for Model 2991.

MONITOR, INFUSION, GRAVITY FLOW *(General) 80FLN*

Argon Medical Devices Inc. 903-675-9321
1445 Flat Creek Rd, Athens, TX 75751
Pressure monitoring injection lines.

Bemis Mfg. Co. 920-467-5206
Hwy. Pp West, Sheboygan Falls, WI 53085
Sight chamber; burette chamber.

Kawasumi Laboratories America, Inc. 800-529-2786
4723 Oak Fair Blvd, Tampa, FL 33610
GRAVITY IV administration set - filter (0.22 micron). IV administration set and Y injection site. Needleless Y sites available.

Smith & Nephew Inc., Endoscopy Div. 978-749-1000
76 S Meridian Ave, Oklahoma City, OK 73107
Fluid level sensor.

MONITOR, INTRACRANIAL PRESSURE *(Cns/Neurology) 84RLW*

Integra Radionics 800-466-6814
22 Terry Ave, Burlington, MA 01803

MONITOR, INTRACRANIAL PRESSURE, CONTINUOUS
(Cns/Neurology) 84GWM

Flowtronics, Inc. 602-997-1364
10250 N 19th Ave Ste B, Phoenix, AZ 85021
Ventriculostomy catheter with ICP,Cerebral Blood Flow & Cortical Temperature continuous monitoring with CSF drain.

Integra Neurosciences 800-762-1574
5955 Pacific Center Blvd, San Diego, CA 92121
Device, intracranial pressure monitoring.

Integra Radionics 800-466-6814
22 Terry Ave, Burlington, MA 01803

Medtronic Neurosurgery 800-468-9710
125 Cremona Dr, Goleta, CA 93117
Sterile becker intracranial pressure system.

MONITOR, LINE ISOLATION *(Cardiovascular) 74DRI*

Bender, Inc. 800-356-4266
700 Fox Chase, Highlands Corp. Center, Coatesville, PA 19320
LIM2000 Monitors leakage on isolated power systems. Trip level 2 or 5 mA; various voltages.

Navilyst Medical 800-833-9973
100 Boston Scientific Way, Marlborough, MA 01752
Pressure monitoring line.

Post Glover Lifelink 800-287-4123
167 Gap Way, Erlanger, KY 41018
Monitors leakage in the equipment used in an operating room and identifies any power problems.

MONITOR, MEDICATION *(General) 80WKH*

American Medical Industries 605-428-5501
330 E 3rd St Ste 2, Dell Rapids, SD 57022
EZ-Store Electronic Pill Box/Timer and Clock. A pill box with two storage compartments plus a timer that tracks two medication times. Pocket-sized and easy to use.

MONITOR, MICROBIAL GROWTH *(Microbiology) 83JTA*

Bd Diagnostic Systems 800-675-0908
7 Loveton Cir, Sparks, MD 21152
BACTEC 9240 blood culture systems. A continuous monitoring, non-invasive device for the detection of microorganisms. Can hold and test up to 240 culture vials at one time. Media available: PLUS Aerobic/F, PLUS Anaerobic/F, PEDS PLUS/F & LYTIC/F.

Industrial Municipal Equipment, Inc. 410-795-0500
1430 Progress Way Ste 105, Eldersburg, MD 21784
Negative microbial urine screen.

New Brunswick Scientific Co., Inc. 800-631-5417
PO Box 4005, Edison, NJ 08818
Slit-to-agar microbial air samplers draw a precise volume of air onto a rotating 150-mm plate for subsequent incubation and analysis. For clean room environments, capable of sampling volume up to 5 cubic meters (5000 liters). In environments with more viable particles, can sample as little as 0.03 cubic meters (30 liters.)

Trek Diagnostic Systems, Inc. 608-8373788
210 Business Park Dr, Sun Prairie, WI 53590
Automated microbial detection system.

MONITOR, MUSCLE, DENTAL *(Dental And Oral) 76KZM*

Bio-Research Associates, Inc. 414-357-7525
9275 N 49th St Ste 150, Brown Deer, WI 53223
Electromyograph, 8 channel.

Electronic Waveform Laboratory, Inc. 800-874-9283
16168 Beach Blvd Ste 232, Huntington Beach, CA 92647

Myotronics-Noromed, Inc. 206-243-4214
5870 S 194th St, Kent, WA 98032
$765.00 for MS-100 single channel surface electromyograph scanner, battery operated, handheld.

Reflex Technologies, Inc. 305-892-0584
12565 Palm Rd Ste B, North Miami, FL 33181
Comfortron, m.a.n. stim, manstim.

MONITOR, NEONATAL *(Obstetrics/Gyn) 85TDE*

Bio-Med Devices, Inc. 800-224-6633
61 Soundview Rd, Guilford, CT 06437
Multifunction neonatal monitor for use with any ventillator. Monitors and displays PEAK, PEEP, MEAN pressure, PWI, RATE, I/E, I and E times, oxygen and temperature.

Colin Medical Instruments Corp. 800-829-6427
5850 Farinon Dr, San Antonio, TX 78249

Ivy Biomedical Systems, Inc. 800-247-4614
11 Business Park Dr, Branford, CT 06405
Model 700/701 Transport monitor adult and neonate.

Mennen Medical Corp. 800-223-2201
2540 Metropolitan Dr, Trevose, PA 19053
ENVOY patient monitor

Nihon Kohden America, Inc. 800-325-0283
90 Icon, Foothill Ranch, CA 92610

PerkinElmer 800-762-4000
940 Winter St, Waltham, MA 02451
DELFIA, AUTODELFIA: Neonatal screening assays for metabolic acylcarnitine, thyroid, hemoglobin, and other disorders. Also for AFP, UE3, HCG, and others.

MONITOR, NEONATAL, BLOOD PRESSURE, INVASIVE *(General) 80FLP*

Mennen Medical Corp. 800-223-2201
2540 Metropolitan Dr, Trevose, PA 19053
ENVOY patient monitor

Pace Tech, Inc. 800-722-3024
510 N Garden Ave, Clearwater, FL 33755

MONITOR, NEONATAL, HEART RATE *(General) 80FLO*

Ge Medical Systems Information Technologies 800-643-6439
8200 W Tower Ave, Milwaukee, WI 53223

Ivy Biomedical Systems, Inc. 800-247-4614
11 Business Park Dr, Branford, CT 06405
$2,200 for Model 301.

Mennen Medical Corp. 800-223-2201
2540 Metropolitan Dr, Trevose, PA 19053
ENVOY patient monitor

Respironics Georgia, Inc. 724-387-4559
175 Chastain Meadows Ct NW, Kennesaw, GA 30144
SMARTMONITOR Two models, both monitor pulse and respirator; alarms for brachycardia, tachycardia, and power failure.

MONITOR, NEONATAL, PHYSIOLOGICAL *(Obstetrics/Gyn) 85TDR*

Bio-Logic Systems Corp. 800-323-8326
1 Bio Logic Plz, Mundelein, IL 60060
ABAER, AUDX I and AuDX PRO - systems which perform automated infant hearing screening (ABAER requires notebook computer interface). AUDX I system (two line LCD display)provides DPOAE or TEOAE screening. AuDX Pro system provides DPOAE and TEOAE screening with a built in color display.

Ivy Biomedical Systems, Inc. 800-247-4614
11 Business Park Dr, Branford, CT 06405
$2,640 for Model 303A.

Mennen Medical Corp. 800-223-2201
2540 Metropolitan Dr, Trevose, PA 19053
ENVOY patient monitor

Nihon Kohden America, Inc. 800-325-0283
90 Icon, Foothill Ranch, CA 92610

MONITOR, ORTHOTIC/PROSTHETIC *(Physical Med) 89NHF*

Feels Good Footwear, Inc 203-740-8504
1 Whispering Way, Brookfld Ctr, CT 06804
Running,walking shoe.

MONITOR, OXYGEN *(General) 80SHT*

Aga Linde Healthcare P.R. Inc. 787-622-7900
PO Box 363868, GPO Box 364727, San Juan, PR 00936
General.

Enmet Corp. 734-761-1270
PO Box 979, Ann Arbor, MI 48106
Oxygen deficiency monitor.

Hamamatsu Photonic Systems 800-524-0504
360 Foothill Rd, Bridgewater, NJ 08807
Non-invasive monitoring of cerebral oxygenation using near-infrared light. NIRO 200 near-infrared oxygenation monitor.

Norco 800-657-6672
1125 W Amity Rd, Boise, ID 83705

Perimed, Inc. 877-374-3589
6785 Wallings Rd Ste 2C-2D, North Royalton, OH 44133
Measures oxygen in the skin and is widely used for assessment of non-healing wounds, hyperbaric oxygen treatment,and determination of microcirculation.

MONITOR, OXYGEN (VENTILATORY) W/WO ALARM *(Anesthesiology) 73BXC*

Aga Linde Healthcare P.R. Inc. 787-622-7900
PO Box 363868, GPO Box 364727, San Juan, PR 00936
Anesth/Pul Med.

Bio-Med Devices, Inc. 800-224-6633
61 Soundview Rd, Guilford, CT 06437
$395 for M-1 high/low pressure monitor, hand-held, battery operated,high/low alarm; $495 for M-2 oxygen/temperature monitor; hand-held, battery operated, high-low alarm; $1,400 for M-10 10-function ventilation monitor; hand-held, battery operated, monitoring PEAK, PEEP, mean airway, PWI, rate, I/E, inspiratory & expiratory times, oxygen and temperature, with automatic alarm settings.

MONITOR, OXYGEN (VENTILATORY) W/WO ALARM *(cont'd)*

Respironics Colorado 800-345-6443
12301 Grant St Unit 190, Thornton, CO 80241
$520.00 for remote alarm that monitors ventilator alarms and sounds alert at nurses' station or in other room in homecare setting.

Teledyne Analytical Instruments 888-789-8168
16830 Chestnut St, City Of Industry, CA 91748
MDL AX 300, MX 300

Vascular Technology Incorporated 800-550-0856
12 Murphy Dr, Nashua, NH 03062
VTI-200, oxygen analyzer. VTI-102, oxygen monitor.

MONITOR, OXYGEN, BRAIN *(Cns/Neurology) 84WYU*

Allegro Biodiesel Corporation 800-949-4762
6245 Bristol Pkwy Ste 263, Culver City, CA 90230
Neurotrend cerebral tissue-monitoring system measures p02, pC02, pH, and temperature.

MONITOR, OXYGEN, CUTAN. (NOT FOR INFANT OR UNDER GAS ANEST.) *(Anesthesiology) 73LPP*

Aga Linde Healthcare P.R. Inc. 787-622-7900
PO Box 363868, GPO Box 364727, San Juan, PR 00936
Anesth/Pul Med.

MONITOR, OXYGEN, CUTANEOUS *(Anesthesiology) 73KLK*

Draeger Medical Systems, Inc. 215-660-2626
16 Electronics Ave, Danvers, MA 01923
Monitor.

Respironics California, Inc. 724-387-4559
2271 Cosmos Ct, Carlsbad, CA 92011
Transcutaneous monitor.

Respironics Novametrix, Llc. 724-387-4559
5 Technology Dr, Wallingford, CT 06492
Transcutaneous monitor.

MONITOR, PATIENT POSITION, LIGHT BEAM *(Radiology) 90IWE*

Diacor, Inc. 800-342-2679
3191 Valley St Ste 100A, Salt Lake City, UT 84109
CENTRALITE patient positioning laser light, $1,650.00 to $3,300.00, complete family of HeNe and diode laser lights including infrared controlled motorized beam positioning.

Gammex Rmi 800-426-6391
PO Box 620327, Middleton, WI 53562

Lrl Logix 800-800-3650
1301 Justin Rd Ste 201, Lewisville, TX 75077
Monitor, patient position, light-beam.

Marconi Medical Systems 800-323-0550
595 Miner Rd, Cleveland, OH 44143

Medical Alignment Systems 801-733-6787
3656 Macintosh Ln, Salt Lake City, UT 84121
Patient positioning light.

Minrad, Inc. 716-855-1068
50 Cobham Dr, Orchard Park, NY 14127
Patient position indicator.

Nualine Laser 801-304-9678
1213 Twelve Pines Cir, Sandy, UT 84094
Red and green positioning lasers.

Standard Imaging, Inc. 608-831-0025
3120 Deming Way, Middleton, WI 53562
Positioning tool.

MONITOR, PENILE TUMESCENCE *(Gastro/Urology) 78LIL*

Behavioral Technology, Inc. 888-363-9017
24 M St, Salt Lake City, UT 84103
MONARCH 21 Penile Plethysmograph System.

Carolina Medical, Inc. 800-334-4531
157 Industrial Dr, King, NC 27021
$5,795.00 for AP102V VASCUMAP volume-calibrated air plethysmograph. Records volume changes in penile air cuff in cc's. $4,995 for AP102R VASCUMAP. Combines oscillometric BP results with waveforms for automatic vascular monitoring. With chart recorder. AP102V VASCUMAP volume-calibrated air plethysmograph for arterial and venous use. Weighs 16lb. Gives results in cc's.

D.M. Davis Inc. 201-833-0513
460 Warwick Ave, Teaneck, NJ 07666
penis gages, signal conditioners/adapters,calibrators

Timm Medical Technologies, Inc. 800-966-2796
6585 City West Pkwy, Eden Prairie, MN 55344
RIGISCAN.

MONITOR, PERINATAL *(Obstetrics/Gyn) 85HGM*

Airstrip Technologies, Lp 210-828-6131
11 Lynn Batts Ste 100, San Antonio, TX 78218
Pocket pc doctors remote data viewing software application.

Analogic Corporation 978-326-4000
8 Centennial Dr, Peabody, MA 01960

Cardinal Healthcare 209, Inc. 610-862-0800
5225 Verona Rd, Fitchburg, WI 53711
Test monitor.

E.Care Solutions, Inc. 912-897-6480
1345 Wilmington Island Rd, Savannah, GA 31410
Perinatal monitoring system accessory.

Ge Healthcare It 847-277-5000
540 W Northwest Hwy, Barrington, IL 60010
Various perinatal monitoring systems and accessories.

Hill-Rom Manufacturing, Inc. 800-445-3730
1225 Crescent Green Dr., Suite 200, Cary, NC 27511
The watchchild(tm) system.

Huntleigh Healthcare Llc. 800-223-1218
40 Christopher Way, Eatontown, NJ 07724
Fetal Assist - a handheld full specification antepartum fetal monitor with telemonitoring capability. Baby Dopplex 4000 - a compact and lightweight antepartum fetal monitor. Baby Dopplex 4002-Twins - a compact and lightweight antepartum twins fetal monitor that has a unique wide printout option making it possible to view both fetal heart rates as separate traces.

Lms Medical Systems Ltd. 514-488-3461
314-5252 Boul De Maisonneuve O, Montreal H4A 3S5 Canada
Calm system (computer assisted labor monitoring)

Spacelabs Medical Inc. 800-522-7212
5150 220th Ave SE, Issaquah, WA 98029
Fetal monitor.

MONITOR, PH *(Anesthesiology) 73RKP*

Analytical Measurements, Inc. 800-635-5580
100 Hoffman Pl, Hillside, NJ 07205
5 models - $685.00 to $1,000.00, solid state with strip chart recorder. BEST-1 Microprocessor based pH controller.

Brinkmann Instruments (Canada) Ltd. 800-263-8715
6670 Campobello Rd., Mississauga, ONT L5N 2L8 Canada

Narco Bio-Systems 800-433-5615
8508 Cross Park Dr, Austin, TX 78754
24 hour ambulatory pH monitoring 1-2 channels.

Sandhill Scientific, Inc. 800-468-4556
9150 Commerce Center Cir Ste 500, Highlands Ranch, CO 80129
Sleuth ambulatory impedance-pH monitoring system for assessing both acid and nonacid reflux. GERDCheck ambulatory acid reflux pH monitoring system.

Zinetics Medical, Inc. 800-648-4070
1050 E South Temple, Salt Lake City, UT 84102
PH monitor as well as gastric pH monitor system.

MONITOR, PHYSIOLOGICAL, ACUTE CARE
(Anesthesiology) 73RLA

Bio-Logic Systems Corp. 800-323-8326
1 Bio Logic Plz, Mundelein, IL 60060
BRAIN ATLAS,CEEGRAPH - microcomputer based systems which perform diagnostic monitoring of EEG.

Datascope Corp. 800-288-2121
14 Philips Pkwy, Montvale, NJ 07645
2000A monitor - Anesthesia monitors - OR/Recovery/Emergency Room. 2100 monitor; with recorder - Combination of non-invasive blood pressure, ECG and recording capability; ACCUTORR Central monitor; printer - Remote display from up to four bedside ACCUTORR monitors.

Mennen Medical Corp. 800-223-2201
2540 Metropolitan Dr, Trevose, PA 19053
ENVOY patient monitor Envoy, modular patient monitor 32 parameters capable, 24 individuals modules, ECG/resp/apnea/invasive/non-invasive BP's, cardiac output, etCO2, SpO2, 2 temp recording capabilities, data management.

Mortara Instrument, Inc. 800-231-7437
7865 N 86th St, Milwaukee, WI 53224
Monitor for myocardial infarct patients using 12-lead system.

Nihon Kohden America, Inc. 800-325-0283
90 Icon, Foothill Ranch, CA 92610

MONITOR, PHYSIOLOGICAL, ACUTE CARE *(cont'd)*

Physio-Control, Inc. 800-442-1142
11811 Willows Rd NE, Redmond, WA 98052
LIFEPAK 9 defibrillator/monitor.

Vitalog, Inc 650-366-8676
643 Bair Island Rd Ste 212, Redwood City, CA 94063
Monitor.

MONITOR, PHYSIOLOGICAL, CARDIAC CATHETERIZATION
(Cardiovascular) 74RLB

Mennen Medical Corp. 800-223-2201
2540 Metropolitan Dr, Trevose, PA 19053
HORIZON 9000 WS cath-lab information system.

Sorin Group Usa 800-289-5759
14401 W 65th Way, Arvada, CO 80004

MONITOR, PHYSIOLOGICAL, PATIENT *(Cardiovascular) 74MHX*

Cas Medical Systems, Inc. 800-227-4414
44 E Industrial Rd, Branford, CT 06405
Vital signs monitor measuring NIBP, SpO2, Temp, ECG, RR, EtCO2

Colin Medical Instruments Corp. 800-829-6427
5850 Farinon Dr, San Antonio, TX 78249
PILOT multi-parameter, configurable physiological monitor. NIPB, EGG(2), IBP(2), SpO2, ETCO2/N2, agent analysis, and continuous NIBP using arterial tonometry to provide beat-by-beat NIBP values and arterial waveform via totally noninvasive means.

Criticare Systems, Inc. 262-798-5361
20925 Crossroads Cir, Waukesha, WI 53186
Various models.

Draeger Medical Systems, Inc. 215-660-2626
16 Electronics Ave, Danvers, MA 01923
Multiple infinity systems.

Edwards Lifesciences Technology Sarl 949-250-2500
State Rd. 402 N.km 1.4, Anasco, PR 00610-1577
Monitor, physiological, patient(with arrhythmia detection or alarms).

Intellectual Property, Llc 608-798-0904
8030 Stagecoach Rd, Cross Plains, WI 53528
A non-contact monitor for respiratory and cardiac activity.

Mennen Medical Corp. 800-223-2201
2540 Metropolitan Dr, Trevose, PA 19053
ENVOY patient monitor allows access to clinical data management with patient monitoring functions through 'Quick Knob' on Envoy.

Nihon Kohden America, Inc. 800-325-0283
90 Icon, Foothill Ranch, CA 92610

Nkus Lab 949-474-9207
2446 Dupont Dr, Irvine, CA 92612
Various.

Spacelabs Healthcare 800-522-7025
5150 220th Ave SE, Issaquah, WA 98029
(WITH ARRHYTHMIA DETECTION OR ALARMS) - Ultraview Digital Telemetry, Ultraview SL Capnograph Module

Spacelabs Medical Inc. 800-522-7212
5150 220th Ave SE, Issaquah, WA 98029
Various models of physiological monitors.

Witt Biomedical Corporation 800-669-1328
305 North Dr, Melbourne, FL 32934
CALYSTO CENTRAL STATION Patient Care Monitor. Provides uninterrupted monitoring of all patients, up to eight-bed capacity per station. Two real-time waveforms per patient. ECG, NIBP, SPO2, resp. one body temperature, cardiac output; programmable user-defined alarms.

MONITOR, PHYSIOLOGICAL, PATIENT(WITHOUT ARRHYTHMIA DETECTION OR ALARMS) *(Cardiovascular) 74MWI*

Criticare Systems, Inc. 262-798-5361
20925 Crossroads Cir, Waukesha, WI 53186
8500 vital signs monitor.

Integriti Systems, Llc 206-652-4700
80 S Jackson St Apt 407, Seattle, WA 98104
Monitor, physiological, patient.

Invivo Corporation 425-487-7000
12601 Research Pkwy, Orlando, FL 32826
Mri patient monitoring system.

Stinger Industries 615-896-1652
1152 Park Ave, Murfreesboro, TN 37129
Vital signs monitor.

MONITOR, PHYSIOLOGICAL, PATIENT(WITHOUT ARRHYTHMIA DETECTION OR ALARMS) *(cont'd)*

Volcano Corporation 800-228-4728
3661 Valley Centre Dr Ste 200, San Diego, CA 92130
Pressure guide wire system.

Welch Allyn Protocol Inc. 800-289-2500
8500 SW Creekside Pl, Beaverton, OR 97008
Monitor, physiological, patient.

MONITOR, PHYSIOLOGICAL, STRESS EXERCISE
(Cardiovascular) 74RLC

Bio-Medical Instruments, Inc. 800-521-4640
2387 E 8 Mile Rd, Warren, MI 48091
Computer-physiological monitoring, software & interfacing.

Biomation 888-667-2324
335 Perth St., P.O. Box 156, Almonte, ON K0A 1A0 Canada
MEDAC System/3 Psychological Stress Assessment Equipment.

Capintec, Inc. 800-631-3826
6 Arrow Rd, Ramsey, NJ 07446

Colin Medical Instruments Corp. 800-829-6427
5850 Farinon Dr, San Antonio, TX 78249
STBP-780 noninvasive BP monitor for exercise stress testing. Interfaces with existing EKG monitors. Accurately provides NIBP/PR readings during exercise testing on treadmill or ergometers. Built-in printer.

Cybex International, Inc. 508-533-4300
10 Trotter Dr, Medway, MA 02053
Cardiovascular equipment.

Ge Medical Systems Information Technologies 800-643-6439
8200 W Tower Ave, Milwaukee, WI 53223

Nautilus, Inc. 360-859-2900
16400 SE Nautilus Dr, Vancouver, WA 98683
Full line of variable resistance strength training machines, including single station, multi-station and rehabilitation machines. These machines include four-bar linkage, range limiters and other safety-oriented features for safe and productive training.

New Life Systems, Inc. 954-972-4600
PO Box 8767, Coral Springs, FL 33075
All types with or without interpretation.

Nihon Kohden America, Inc. 800-325-0283
90 Icon, Foothill Ranch, CA 92610

Physio-Dyne Instrument Corporation 800-860-5930
PO Box 5025, Quogue, NY 11959
Exercising physiology testing equipment.

Suntech Medical, Inc. 800-421-8626
507 Airport Blvd Ste 117, Morrisville, NC 27560
The Tango exercise BP monitor is designed to automatically measure and display your patient's systolic and diastolic BP along with heart rate. It is specifically designed for use in treadmill, ergometer, and pharmacological stress-test environments. Tango is also ideal for use in research environments. Tango excels where other BP monitors have failed by making use of SunTech's proprietary Dimensional K-Sound Analysis (DKA). DKA was developed as a result of SunTech's pioneering work in 24-Hour ambulatory blood-pressure monitoring. It's this experience which provides SunTech's research and development team with invaluable insight into the relationship between the host of variables involved in determining blood pressure on a patient in motion. These variables include, but are not limited to, the patients ECG, K-sounds, overall body shape, foot-strike characteristics, arm movements, and age, along with treadmill and ergometer noise. With Tango's 'hands free' interface, BP readings can be initiated automatically by many stress ECG systems. Upon completion of the BP reading, the TANGO monitor automatically reports its results back to your stress ECG system for immediate display and printout, giving you the freedom to concentrate on your patient's performance instead of taking manual BP readings.

Thought Technology Ltd. 800-361-3651
2180 Belgrave Ave., Montreal, QUE H4A 2L8 Canada
$90.00 for GSR2 hand held unit and four stress management or fear of flying tapes and manual. $80.00 ea. for GSR2 and two tapes on the following behavioural management programs: SLEEP WELL; STOP SMOKING; WEIGHT CONTROL; TAKING TESTS WITH CONFIDENCE; PUBLIC SPEAKING; PAIN CONTROL; BREATHING FOR HEALTH; and JUST SAY KNOW. Visit www.mindgrowth.com

Tsi Medical Ltd. 800-661-7263
47 Athabascan Ave., Unit 105, Sherwood Park, AB T8A-4H3 Canada

MONITOR, PRESSURE, INTRACOMPARTMENTAL
(Orthopedics) 87LXC

Millennium Medical Technologies, Inc. 505-988-7595
460 Saint Michaels Dr Ste 901, Santa Fe, NM 87505
Compartment pressure monitor.

Stryker Puerto Rico, Ltd. 939-307-2500
Hwy. 3, Km. 131.2, Las Guasimas Ind. Park, Arroyo, PR 00714
Pressure monitor and various types of sterile and non-sterile accessories.

MONITOR, PRESSURE, INTRACRANIAL, IMPLANTABLE
(Cns/Neurology) 84LII

Innerspace, Inc. 877.HUM.BIRD
1622 Edinger Ave Ste C, Tustin, CA 92780
Hummingbird Parenchyma - ICP monitor

MONITOR, PRESSURE, INTRAUTERINE *(Obstetrics/Gyn) 85KXO*

American Catheter Corp. 800-345-6714
13047 S Highway 475, Ocala, FL 34480

MONITOR, PRESSURE, VENOUS, CENTRAL, POWERED
(Cardiovascular) 74FYN

Terumo Cardiovascular Systems, Corp 800-521-2818
6200 Jackson Rd, Ann Arbor, MI 48103

Welch Allyn Protocol Inc. 800-289-2500
8500 SW Creekside Pl, Beaverton, OR 97008

MONITOR, PULSE RATE *(Anesthesiology) 73BWS*

Bio-Medical Instruments, Inc. 800-521-4640
2387 E 8 Mile Rd, Warren, MI 48091
Pulse rate photoelectric, digital or meter, battery or line powered.

Colin Medical Instruments Corp. 800-829-6427
5850 Farinon Dr, San Antonio, TX 78249
PRESS-MATE Model 8800 SATP NiBP with continuous pulse-oximetry measurement. Incorporates deluxe rolling stand, accessories, electronic/tympanic temperature options. Includes new smart features and offers expanded memory and choice of printouts.

Datascope Corp. 800-288-2121
14 Philips Pkwy, Montvale, NJ 07645
Finger sensor, radial sensor for use with Datascope monitors.

Elmed, Inc. 630-543-2792
60 W Fay Ave, Addison, IL 60101

Fitness Motivation Institute Of America, Inc. 800-538-7790
26685 Sussex Hwy Ste A, Seaford, DE 19973
$129.95 for heart monitor.

Ge Medical Systems Information Technologies 800-558-5544
4502 Woodland Corporate Blvd, Tampa, FL 33614

Ge Medical Systems Information Technologies 800-643-6439
8200 W Tower Ave, Milwaukee, WI 53223

Her-Mar, Inc. 800-327-8209
8550 NW 30th Ter, Doral, FL 33122
$95.00 per unit (standard).

Industrial & Biomedical Sensors Corp. 781-891-4201
1377 Main St, Waltham, MA 02451
$380 and up for monitor that measures the heart/pulse rate.

Koaman International 909-983-4888
656 E D St, Ontario, CA 91764
Vital signs monitor.

Mennen Medical Corp. 800-223-2201
2540 Metropolitan Dr, Trevose, PA 19053
ENVOY patient monitor with SpO2 module.

New Life Systems, Inc. 954-972-4600
PO Box 8767, Coral Springs, FL 33075
All types.

Pace Tech, Inc. 800-722-3024
510 N Garden Ave, Clearwater, FL 33755
Pulse rate monitor, VITALMAX 800 & 500 series. $995 - 2,295.

Polar Electro Inc. 1-800-227-1314
1111 Marcus Ave Ste M15, New Hyde Park, NY 11042

U.F.I. 805-772-1203
545 Main St Ste C2, Morro Bay, CA 93442
$550 for Model SC2000/1 Simple Scope.

MONITOR, RADIATION *(Radiology) 90RNV*

Biodex Medical Systems, Inc. 800-224-6339
20 Ramsey Rd, Shirley, NY 11967

MONITOR, RADIATION *(cont'd)*

Capintec, Inc. 800-631-3826
6 Arrow Rd, Ramsey, NJ 07446
16 well units, multi detecting gamma counters with RIA data reduction and QC management.

Electronic Control Concepts 800-847-9729
160 Partition St, Saugerties, NY 12477
kVp Meter / Exposure Time Meter

Johnson & Associates Inc., Wm. B. 304-645-6568
200 AEI Dr., Lewisburg, WV 24902
$2,500 per unit, Model TR-5 tritium monitor, 50 uc/M3.

Landauer, Inc. 800-323-8830
2 Science Rd, Glenwood, IL 60425
Personnel radiation dosimeters to measure x-ray, beta, gamma radiation and neutrons. NVLAP accredited, full range of reports, ALARA aids; interactive computer system, dosimetry management PC software. CBT Radiation Safety Training and related services. Low-level gamma radiation dosimeter, down to 1/10 millirem. Comprehensive diagnostic evaluation backed by over 50 years experience.

Lnd, Inc. 516-678-6141
3230 Lawson Blvd, Oceanside, NY 11572

Ludlum Measurements, Inc. 800-622-0828
501 Oak St, Sweetwater, TX 79556
Full line, $320.00 to $1,475.00 per unit; survey meters; neutron, random flask and shielded well counters. Accessories such as survey meter dials and cables also available.

Marconi Medical Systems 800-323-0550
595 Miner Rd, Cleveland, OH 44143

Mirion Technologies 925-543-0800
3000 Executive Pkwy Ste 222, Bishop Ranch 8, San Ramon, CA 94583
Film badges, TLD badges, neutron badges, x-ray badges, personnel radiation monitoring badges, dosimeters.

Narda Safety Test Solutions 631-231-1700
435 Moreland Rd, Hauppauge, NY 11788
Radio-frequency monitor - Nardalert XT. Allows data logging of exposures to RF/microwave fields from 100 kHz to 100 GHz. Useful for exposed hospital personnel, and to rooftop workers where RF communications systems have been installed.

Owens Scientific Inc. 281-394-2311
23230 Sandsage Ln, Katy, TX 77494
For compliance and QA testing.

Radcal Corp. 800-423-7169
426 W Duarte Rd, Monrovia, CA 91016
All radiation dose monitors feature Radcal's patented current-to-frequency conversion allowing for a wide range. Ion Chambers for Radiography, Fluoroscopy, Mammography, CT, leakage, scatter, low and high level dose measurements. Dynalyzer for invasive kVp and mA/mAs measuremnts and Accu-kV for non-invasive kVp -

S.E. International, Inc. 800-293-5759
436 Farm Rd, PO Box 39, Summertown, TN 38483
8 models available from $279.00 to $685.00 for handheld ionizing radiation detectors.

Scanditronix - Wellhofer North America 901-386-2242
3150 Stage Post Dr Ste 110, Bartlett, TN 38133
Direct Patient Dosemeter, 3-channel electrometer system primarily intended for in vivo dosimetry priced from $3,800 to $4,500. Direct Patient Dosemeter, 12-channel electrometer with application software. Use for entrance/exit dose, risk organ monitoring, TBI measurements and intracavitary measurements for radiation therapy, and brachy therapy priced from $7,800 up to $10,000.

Trace Laboratories-East 410-584-9099
5 N Park Dr, Hunt Valley, MD 21030
Liquid scintillation for determining levels.

MONITOR, RESPIRATORY *(Surgery) 79FYZ*

Brytech Inc. 613-731-5800
600 Peter Morand Crescent, Suite 240, Ottawa, ONT K1G-5Z3 Canada
PAM

Commercial/Medical Electronics, Inc. 800-324-4844
1519 S Lewis Ave, Tulsa, OK 74104

Datascope Corp. 800-288-2121
14 Philips Pkwy, Montvale, NJ 07645
MULTINEX 4300, compact unit measures end-tidal CO2, inspired CO2, O2 and respiration rate with trend and diagnostics.

MONITOR, RESPIRATORY *(cont'd)*

Engler Engineering Corp. 800-445-8581
1099 E 47th St, Hialeah, FL 33013
SENTINEL - Veterinary Respiratory Monitor; 2 LED displays monitor time elapsed between each breath and number of breaths taken during the last sixty seconds.

Ge Industrial, Sensing 800-833-9438
1100 Technology Park Dr, Billerica, MA 01821

Ge Medical Systems Information Technologies 800-643-6439
8200 W Tower Ave, Milwaukee, WI 53223
The advantage multiplexed mass spectrometer system is capable of connecting up to 31 ICU/CCU or operating rooms. Measures and displays inspired and expired concentrations of O2, N2, N20, CO2, halothane, ethrane, suprane, and forane. The in-room display presents this data along with waveforms of all measured gases. Trend analysis of all stored parameters up to 16 hours. Remote observatory units may be connected with direct blood-gas input available. Hard-copy documentation for permanent record of patient data. CO2 mainstream and sidestream modules which measure and display inspired and expired CO2, CO2 waveforms, respiration rate, warmup time less than 45 seconds. Annual calibration required. SAM Module (multigas) infrared monitor, utilizes the near- and mid-band infrared analysis of anesthetic agents. Carbon dioxide, nitrous oxide, and oxygen paramagnetic. This module is an accessory for the Tramscope and Solar vital signs monitoring products. RAMS Quadrupole Mass Spectrometer, capable of simultaneous measuring of up to 10 gas channels within a dynamic range of 1-250 AMU. This unit is configurable and allows for use in many applications such as anethesia, stress testing, pulmonary function, hyperbaric studies, and research applications. The unit is software controlled and can be reprogrammed to measure new gases for different applications.

Mennen Medical Corp. 800-223-2201
2540 Metropolitan Dr, Trevose, PA 19053
ENVOY patient monitor with ECG/RESP module.

Servicios Paracliniclos S.A. 83-33-8400
Madero No. 3330 Pte., Monterrey N.L. 64020 Mexico

U.F.I. 805-772-1203
545 Main St Ste C2, Morro Bay, CA 93442
$550 for Model SC2000/1 Simple Scope.

MONITOR, RESPONSE, SKIN, GALVANIC *(Cns/Neurology) 84GZO*

Bio-Medical Instruments, Inc. 800-521-4640
2387 E 8 Mile Rd, Warren, MI 48091
Galvanic skin response, meter or digital, battery powered.

Galloway Technologies, Llc 801-766-3929
3736 Panarama Dr, Saratoga Spgs, UT 84045
Galvanic skin response device.

U.F.I. 805-772-1203
545 Main St Ste C2, Morro Bay, CA 93442
$625.00 for Model 2701.

MONITOR, SKIN RESISTANCE/SKIN TEMPERATURE, FOR INSULIN REACTIONS *(General) 80LMY*

Sensor Scientific, Inc. 800-524-1610
6 Kingsbridge Rd, Fairfield, NJ 07004
RTD, Platinum (Resistance Temperature Detector); standard and custom RTD elements for all biomedical applications; skin temperature, core body temperature, and hot wire flow measurement.

MONITOR, SPINE CURVATURE *(Physical Med) 89LZW*

JTECH Medical 800-985-8324
470 West Longdale Dr., Suite G, Salt Lake City, UT 84115

Lafayette Instrument Company 800-428-7545
PO Box 5729, 3700 Sagamore Pkwy,, Lafayette, IN 47903
Acumar Dual and Single Inclinometer

MONITOR, ST SEGMENT (WITH ALARM) *(General) 80MLD*

Draeger Medical Systems, Inc. 215-660-2626
16 Electronics Ave, Danvers, MA 01923
Multiple.

Welch Allyn Protocol Inc. 800-289-2500
8500 SW Creekside Pl, Beaverton, OR 97008
ST analysis.

MONITOR, TEMPERATURE (SELF-CONTAINED) *(General) 80KLL*

Biosynergy, Inc. 800-255-5274
1940 E Devon Ave, Elk Grove Village, IL 60007
FOODGARDE Multistage Irreversible Time/Temperature Monitor monitors the time/temperature history of food products throughout processing, shipping, warehousing and distribution.

MONITOR, TEMPERATURE (SELF-CONTAINED) *(cont'd)*

Cmt, Inc. 800-659-9140
PO Box 297, Hamilton, MA 01936

Colin Medical Instruments Corp. 800-829-6427
5850 Farinon Dr, San Antonio, TX 78249
PRESS-MATE Model 8800 FP, $3,445.00 to 3,895.00 with NIBP, PR, electronic temperature, deluxe rolling stand, accessories, optional printer, pulse-oximetry option. Includes new smart features and has expanded memory and choice of printouts.

Control Products Inc. 952-448-2217
1724 Lake Dr W, Chanhassen, MN 55317

Dickson Co 800-757-3747
930 S Westwood Ave, Addison, IL 60101
Chart Recorders and Data Loggers

Lake Shore Cryotronics, Inc. 614-891-2243
575 McCorkle Blvd, Westerville, OH 43082

Physitemp Instruments, Inc. 800-452-8510
154 Huron Ave, Clifton, NJ 07013
$610.00 per unit (standard w/o probe).

MONITOR, TEMPERATURE (WITH PROBE)

(Anesthesiology) 73BWX

Bio-Feedback Systems, Inc. 303-444-1411
2736 47th St, Boulder, CO 80301
2 models: $175 and $945 for biofeedback units.

Bio-Medical Instruments, Inc. 800-521-4640
2387 E 8 Mile Rd, Warren, MI 48091
Temperature monitor (with probe), digital or meter, battery or line powered.

Datascope Corp. 800-288-2121
14 Philips Pkwy, Montvale, NJ 07645
Rectal/esophageal probe for use with phys. monitor.

Dickson Co 800-757-3747
930 S Westwood Ave, Addison, IL 60101
K-Thermocouple data loggers, chart recorders and indicators

Everest Interscience, Inc. 800-422-4342
1891 N Oracle Rd, Tucson, AZ 85705
Non-contact non-invasive monitor without probe.

Ge Medical Systems Information Technologies 800-643-6439
8200 W Tower Ave, Milwaukee, WI 53223

Medtronic Perfusion Systems 800-328-3320
7611 Northland Dr N, Brooklyn Park, MN 55428
TM 147T temperature monitor with disposable temperature probes including Esophageal Stethoscope, Skin Surface, Myocardial Needle, Foley Catheter and Esophageal/Rectal/Nasopharyngeal temperature probes.

Mennen Medical Corp. 800-223-2201
2540 Metropolitan Dr, Trevose, PA 19053
ENVOY patient monitor with 2BP/2TEMP module.

Noral, Inc. 800-348-2345
23600 Mercantile Rd, Beachwood Commerce Park
Cleveland, OH 44122

Novamed, Llc 800-425-3535
4 Westchester Plz, Elmsford, NY 10523
NovaTemp Dual Display Temperature Monitor - Lightweight, portable and battery operated - ideal to monitor temperature simultaneously on two temperature sites. Use in conjunction with NovaTemp Skin Surface Temp Sensors.

Pace Tech, Inc. 800-722-3024
510 N Garden Ave, Clearwater, FL 33755
VITALMAX 800 & 500 series. $1,495 to $2295. Multiparameter monitor, LED readout optoins, NIBP, SpO2, respiration.

Pmt Corp. 800-626-5463
1500 Park Rd, Chanhassen, MN 55317

Psg Controls, Inc. 800-523-2558
1225 Tunnel Rd, Perkasie, PA 18944

Simpson Electric Co. 715-588-3311
520 Simpson Ave, PO Box 99, Lac Du Flambeau, WI 54538
$151.41 per unit (standard).

Terumo Cardiovascular Systems, Corp 800-521-2818
6200 Jackson Rd, Ann Arbor, MI 48103

MONITOR, TEMPERATURE, DIALYSIS *(Gastro/Urology) 78FLA*

Heatron, Inc. 913-651-4420
3000 Wilson Ave, Leavenworth, KS 66048
Dialysis heater.

MONITOR, TEMPERATURE, NEUROSURGERY, DIRECT CONTACT, POWERED *(Cns/Neurology) 84HCS*

Artronics 864-859-4755
464 Sweetbriar Way, Easley, SC 29640
Powered direct contact temperature measurement device.

Flowtronics, Inc. 602-997-1364
10250 N 19th Ave Ste B, Phoenix, AZ 85021
Priced from $6,450 to $21,500 for cerebral blood flow monitors.

Kale Research And Technology 864-574-4800
426 E Blackstock Rd, Spartanburg, SC 29301
Spinal differential tester and temperature differential scanner.

Titronics Research & Development Co. 800-705-2307
400 Stephans St, PO Box 470, Tiffin, IA 52340
Computer-aided paraspinal scanning system.

MONITOR, TEMPERATURE, SURGERY *(Surgery) 79FZA*

Dickson Co 800-757-3747
930 S Westwood Ave, Addison, IL 60101
Monitor room temperature

Ge Medical Systems Information Technologies 800-643-6439
8200 W Tower Ave, Milwaukee, WI 53223
Unit measuring two surface or internal temperatures and differences. Adjustable high and low alarm settings. Temperature surface or internal sensor accepted with five-year warranty.

Novamed, Llc 800-425-3535
4 Westchester Plz, Elmsford, NY 10523
NovaTemp 1400D Dual Display Temperature Monitor provides accurate measurement and display of two separate temperature sites. Portable and battery operated -- to provide an economical alternative to more expensive patient monitors without compromising accuracy and patient care. Ideal for any clinical application that necessitates continuous monitoring.

Pmt Corp. 800-626-5463
1500 Park Rd, Chanhassen, MN 55317

Sharn, Inc. 800-325-3671
4517 George Rd Ste 200, Tampa, FL 33634
CRYSTALINE II, CRYSTALINE and CRYSTALINE ST advanced liquid crystal technology displays free-moving gold line, indicates skin or body temperature, reads in both Fahrenheit and Celsius. Electronic probes, esophageal, general purpose, and skin.

Trademark Medical Llc 800-325-9044
449 Soverign Ct, St. Louis, MO 63011
Temperature monitor for anesthesia. (F deg.&C deg.)

MONITOR, TEST, HIV-1 *(Hematology) 81MTL*

Abbott Molecular, Inc. 847-937-6100
1300 E Touhy Ave, Des Plaines, IL 60018
Pcr hiv-1 assay.

Roche Molecular Systems, Inc. 925-730-8110
4300 Hacienda Dr, Pleasanton, CA 94588
Various hiv-1 monitor tests.

Zeptometrix Corporation 800-274-5487
872 Main St, Buffalo, NY 14202
HIV-1 IIIB, HIV-1 MN, HIV-1 BaL, CMV, HSV, Toxoplasma, EBV viral lysates.

MONITOR, TRANSCUTANEOUS, CARBON-DIOXIDE *(Anesthesiology) 73ULU*

Radiometer America, Inc. 800-736-0600
810 Sharon Dr, Westlake, OH 44145
TINA 50-sec response time, 0.1% accuracy.

MONITOR, TRANSCUTANEOUS, OXYGEN *(Anesthesiology) 73ULV*

Radiometer America, Inc. 800-736-0600
810 Sharon Dr, Westlake, OH 44145
TINA programmable unit with alarms, weighing 6 lb; recorder with event marker, 20-sec response time, 0.1% accuracy.

MONITOR, ULTRASONIC, NON-FETAL *(Radiology) 90JAF*

Agfa Corp. 800-581-2432
100 Challenger Rd, Ridgefield Park, NJ 07660

Cardinal Healthcare 209, Inc. 610-862-0800
5225 Verona Rd, Fitchburg, WI 53711
Monitor.

MONITOR, UTERINE CONTRACTION, EXTERNAL *(Obstetrics/Gyn) 85HFM*

Bio-Feedback Systems, Inc. 303-444-1411
2736 47th St, Boulder, CO 80301
Research Electrohysterograph. Cervix-based electrical signal sensing. IRB Approval required. Applications include drug discovery and general diagnosis for uterine dysfunctions such as endometriosis, pelvic pain, dysmenorrhea, etc.

Parker Hannifin Corporation. 805-658-2984
3007 Bunsen Ave Units K&L, Ventura, CA 93003
Toco.

MONITOR, VENTILATION *(Anesthesiology) 73SES*

Aga Linde Healthcare P.R. Inc. 787-622-7900
PO Box 363868, GPO Box 364727, San Juan, PR 00936
Anesth/Pul Med.

Covidien Lp 508-261-8000
15 Hampshire St, Mansfield, MA 02048
RESPIRADYNE II PLUS pulmonary function/ventilation monitor, ideal for bedside use, easy to carry, compact tray holds monitor and printer.

Sdi Diagnostics, Inc. 800-678-5782
10 Hampden Dr, South Easton, MA 02375
Various spirometers.

MONITOR, VENTILATORY FREQUENCY *(Anesthesiology) 73BZQ*

Bio-Med Devices, Inc. 800-224-6633
61 Soundview Rd, Guilford, CT 06437
10-function monitor for all ventilators with high-low alarms including PEEK, PEEP, MEAN, PWI, rate, O2, and temperature.

Cardinal Health 207, Inc. 610-862-0800
1100 Bird Center Dr, Palm Springs, CA 92262
Respiratory exhaled volume monitor.

Draeger Medical Systems, Inc. 215-660-2626
16 Electronics Ave, Danvers, MA 01923
Multiple infinity systems.

Dymedix Corporation 888-212-1100
5985 Rice Creek Pkwy Ste 201, Shoreview, MN 55126
Breathing/airflow sensors, snoring sensors, respiratory effort belts. Available in disposable and reusable.

Ge Medical Systems Information Technologies 800-643-6439
8200 W Tower Ave, Milwaukee, WI 53223
Mass spec.

Gereonics, Inc. 949-929-9319
25501 Aria Dr, Mission Viejo, CA 92692
Respiratory and limb movement sensors.

Grass Technologies, An Astro-Med, Inc. Product Gro 401-828-4002
53 Airport Park Drive, Rockland, MA 02370
Respiratory airflow sensor.

Invivo Corporation 425-487-7000
12601 Research Pkwy, Orlando, FL 32826
Respiration monitor.

Medtronic Neuromodulation 763-514-4000
710 Medtronic Pkwy, Minneapolis, MN 55432
Various types of breathing frequency monitors.

Non-Invasive Monitoring Systems, Inc. 305-575-4200
4400 Biscayne Blvd, Miami, FL 33137
Repitrace plus, respibands, respicentral.

Pace Tech, Inc. 800-722-3024
510 N Garden Ave, Clearwater, FL 33755
Breathing frequency, Class II. VITALMAX 500, VITALMAX 800 series, MINIPACK 911 series. $2295 to $4495.

Pro-Tech Services, Inc. 800-350-5511
4338 Harbour Pointe Blvd SW, Mukilteo, WA 98275
Periodic limb movement sensor (various configurations).

Rochester Electro Medical, Inc. 813-963-2933
4212 Cypress Gulch Dr, Lutz, FL 33559
Respiration monitors and sensors.

MONITOR, VIDEO, ENDOSCOPE *(General) 80TFB*

Ams Innovative Center-San Jose 800-356-7600
3070 Orchard Dr, San Jose, CA 95134

Cadmet, Inc. 800-543-7282
155 Planebrook Rd, P.O. Box 24, Malvern, PA 19355

MONITOR, VIDEO, ENDOSCOPE *(cont'd)*

Conrac, Inc. 626-480-0095
5124 Commerce Dr, Baldwin Park, CA 91706
$357 and up per unit, low to high resolution imaging monochrome monitors, 9in., 15in., 19in., Series 2600. $2,865 and up for 19in. high resolution color imaging monitor.

Elmed, Inc. 630-543-2792
60 W Fay Ave, Addison, IL 60101

Hitachi Kokusai Electric America, Ltd. 516-921-7200
150 Crossways Park Dr, Woodbury, NY 11797

JVC Americas Corp. 973-315-5000
1700 Valley Rd, Wayne, NJ 07470
High definition videotape monitor.

Karl Storz Endoscopy-America Inc. 800-421-0837
600 Corporate Pointe, Culver City, CA 90230

Mahe International Inc. 800-294-7946
468 Craighead St, Nashville, TN 37204

Olympus America, Inc. 800-645-8160
3500 Corporate Pkwy, PO Box 610, Center Valley, PA 18034

Richard Wolf Medical Instruments Corp. 800-323-9653
353 Corporate Woods Pkwy, Vernon Hills, IL 60061

Smith & Nephew, Inc., Endoscopy Division 800-343-8386
150 Minuteman Rd, Andover, MA 01810

Sony Electronics, Inc., Medical Systems Div. 800-686-7669
1 Sony Dr, Park Ridge, NJ 07656

Stryker Corp. 800-726-2725
2825 Airview Blvd, Portage, MI 49002

Stryker Endoscopy 800-435-0220
5900 Optical Ct, San Jose, CA 95138

Transamerican Technologies International 800-322-7373
2246 Camino Ramon, San Ramon, CA 94583
HDTV, high definition video system for microsurgery and endoscopic surgery.

Welch Allyn, Inc. 800-535-6663
4341 State Street Rd, Skaneateles Falls, NY 13153

MONITOR, X-RAY FILM PROCESSOR QUALITY CONTROL
(Radiology) 90SGL

Cone Instruments, Inc. 800-321-6964
5201 Naiman Pkwy, Solon, OH 44139
X-ray quality-assurance products; x-ray darkroom and processing accessories.

Marconi Medical Systems 800-323-0550
595 Miner Rd, Cleveland, OH 44143

St. John Companies 800-435-4242
25167 Anza Dr, PO Box 800460, Santa Clarita, CA 91355
Top name brands of x-ray quality control equipment at competitive prices to assure x-ray quality: sensitometers, densitometers, phantoms, etc.

White Mountain Imaging 603-648-2124
1617 Battle St, Webster, NH 03303
Processing accessories and supply.

X-Rite, Inc. 888-826-3044
4300 44th St SE, Grand Rapids, MI 49512
$675.00 & $875.00 for dual-color sensitometers for blue- or green-sensitive film; $1,850 & $2,650 for auto-reading densitometers with RS-232 interface.

MONITOR, X-RAY TUBE *(Radiology) 90VGH*

Capintec, Inc. 800-631-3826
6 Arrow Rd, Ramsey, NJ 07446

MONOCHROMATOR, FOR CLINICAL USE *(Chemistry) 75JRP*

Horiba Jobin Yvon Inc 866-JOBINYVON
3880 Park Ave, Edison, NJ 08820

Princeton Instruments - Acton 978-263-3584
15 Discovery Way, Acton, MA 01720
Monochromators and spectrographs with focal lengths from .150 meters to 2.0 meters.

Thermo Oriel 800-715-393
150 Long Beach Blvd, Stratford, CT 06615

MOTOR, DRILL, ELECTRIC *(Cns/Neurology) 84HBC*

Anspach Effort, Inc. 800-327-6887
4500 Riverside Dr, Palm Beach Gardens, FL 33410
eMax 2 Instrument System: high speed electric drill system for all facets of ENT and Neurosurgical surgery.

MOTOR, DRILL, ELECTRIC *(cont'd)*

Medtronic Powered Surgical Solutions 800-643-2773
4620 N Beach St, Haltom City, TX 76137
Electric high speed drill.

Wisap America 800-233-8448
8231 Melrose Dr, Lenexa, KS 66214

MOTOR, DRILL, PNEUMATIC *(Cns/Neurology) 84HBB*

Anspach Effort, Inc. 800-327-6887
4500 Riverside Dr, Palm Beach Gardens, FL 33410
XMax and microMax Instrument Systems: high speed pneumatic drill systems for all facets of surgery.

Brasseler Usa - Medical 805-650-5209
4837 McGrath St Ste J, Ventura, CA 93003
Surgical Instrument System

Medtronic Image-Guided Neurologics, Inc. 800-707-0933
2290 W Eau Gallie Blvd, Melbourne, FL 32935
Cranial drill.

Medtronic Powered Surgical Solutions 800-643-2773
4620 N Beach St, Haltom City, TX 76137
Various models of motors/drills.

Tava Surgical Instruments 805-650-5209
4837 McGrath St Ste J, Ventura, CA 93003
Surgical Instrument System.

MOTOR, SURGICAL INSTRUMENT, AC-POWERED
(Surgery) 79GEY

Abbott Vascular, Cardiac Therapies 800-227-9902
26531 Ynez Rd, Mailing P.O. Box 9018, Temecula, CA 92591
Sterile motor drive unit.

Aesthetic Technologies, Inc. 303-469-0965
14828 W 6th Ave Ste 9B, Golden, CO 80401
Dermabrasion.

Arthrex, Inc. 239-643-5553
1370 Creekside Blvd, Naples, FL 34108
Ar-8200s shaver system.

Biomet Microfixation Inc. 800-874-7711
1520 Tradeport Dr, Jacksonville, FL 32218
Battery powered screwdriver.

Biomet Sports Medicine 530-226-5800
6704 Lockheed Dr, Redding, CA 96002
Shaver, various sizes and speeds.

Bioplate, Inc. 310-815-2100
3643 Lenawee Ave, Los Angeles, CA 90016
Powered screwdriver.

Depuy Orthopaedics, Inc. 800-473-3789
700 Orthopaedic Dr, P.O. Box 988, Warsaw, IN 46582
Various type of motors (surgical instrument, ac-powered).

Depuy-Raynham, A Div. Of Depuy Orthopaedics 800-451-2006
325 Paramount Dr, Raynham, MA 02767
Various type of motors (surgical instrument, ac-powered).

E-Global Medical Equipment, L.L.C. 866-422-1845
2f 500 Lincoln St., Allston, MA 02134
Morcellator.

Focus Medical, Llc. 866-633-5273
23 Francis J Clarke Cir, Bethel, CT 06801
Microdermabrasion system.

Maximum Dental, Inc. 631-245-2176
600 Meadowlands Pkwy Ste 269, Secaucus, NJ 07094

Medisiss 866-866-7477
2747 SW 6th St, Redmond, OR 97756
Various ac powered surgical instruments,sterile.

Medtronic Powered Surgical Solutions 800-643-2773
4620 N Beach St, Haltom City, TX 76137
Electric high speed motor & various sterile & non sterile accessories.

Medtronic Sofamor Danek Instrument Manufacturing 901-396-3133
7375 Adrianne Pl, Bartlett, TN 38133
Various surgical drills.

Medtronic Sofamor Danek Usa, Inc. 901-396-3133
4340 Swinnea Rd, Memphis, TN 38118
Various surgical drills.

Pro-Dex, Inc. 800-562-6204
2361 McGaw Ave, Irvine, CA 92614
Various types of electric handpiece and irrigation systems.

MOTOR, SURGICAL INSTRUMENT, AC-POWERED *(cont'd)*

Promex Technologies, Llc 317-736-0128
3049 Hudson St, Franklin, IN 46131
Tissue morcellation system, surgical cutter.

Terumo Cardiovascular Systems, Corp 800-521-2818
6200 Jackson Rd, Ann Arbor, MI 48103

Warsaw Orthopedic, Inc. 901-396-3133
2500 Silveus Xing, Warsaw, IN 46582
Various surgical drills.

MOTOR, SURGICAL INSTRUMENT, DC-POWERED
(Surgery) 79SJM

Brailsford & Co., Inc. 603-588-2880
15 Elm Ave, Antrim, NH 03440
Mode T brushless DC motors.

MOTOR, SURGICAL INSTRUMENT, PNEUMATIC-POWERED
(Surgery) 79GET

Alexandria Research Technologies, Llc 952-949-2235
13755 1st Ave N Ste 100, Plymouth, MN 55441
Various types of sterile and non-sterile accessories/attachments for surgical in.

Clarus Medical, Llc. 763-525-8400
1000 Boone Ave N Ste 300, Minneapolis, MN 55427
Motor, surgical instrument, pneumatic powered.

Medisiss 866-866-7477
2747 SW 6th St, Redmond, OR 97756
Various pneumatic powered surgical instruments,sterile.

Medtronic Powered Surgical Solutions 800-643-2773
4620 N Beach St, Haltom City, TX 76137
Various models of motors.

Pretika Corporation, North America Market Headquarters 949-481-8818
16 Salermo, Laguna Niguel, CA 92677
Various types of oscillating,battery-operated brushes, massagers.

Symmetry Medical Usa, Inc. 574-267-8700
486 W 350 N, Warsaw, IN 46582
Surgical instrument motors and accessories-attachments.

MOUNT, EQUIPMENT *(General) 80WKM*

C.J.T. Enterprises, Inc. 714-751-6295
PO Box 10028, Costa Mesa, CA 92627
The Profiler-Lite; is durable, light weight and extemely adjustable. Easy to attach to round or non-round tubing the Profiler-Lite is the perfect swith mount and camera mount. ProLite; is great for carrying light weight AAC devices, cameras and tables. A pleasing blend of style, adjustability and strength the ProLite is an ideal mount.

Concepts International, Inc. 800-627-9729
224 E Main St, Summerton, SC 29148
Film bins. ABS wall mount holds four sizes of x-ray film.

Ergotron, Inc. 800-888-8458
1181 Trapp Rd, Saint Paul, MN 55121
Medical arm can be used in ICUs, ORs, ERs or patient rooms.

Gcx Corp. 800-228-2555
3875 Cypress Dr, Petaluma, CA 94954
POLYMOUNT Information Technology (IT) mounts: mounting solutions for IT component hardware including keyboards or other input devices, monitors, CPUs, and UPS units.

Golden Metal Products Co. 800-978-9058
50 Bushes Ln, Elmwood Park, NJ 07407
Chasses, enclosures and bracketry; sheet metal fabrication of chassis for hematology systems, scanners and laboratory equipment.

Intersurgical Inc. 315-451-2900
417 Electronics Pkwy, Liverpool, NY 13088
Catheter mounts and patient elbow connections. Micro mount.

Quality Rapid Service Mounts, Inc. 800-418-8342
8617 Eagle Point Blvd, Lake Elmo, MN 55042
ECG/EKG mounts.

Steelcraft, Inc. 800-225-7710
115 W Main St, Millbury, MA 01527

Ziamatic Corp. 800-711-FIRE
10 W College Ave, Yardley, PA 19067
QUIC STRAP mounting systems.

MOUNT, MONITOR (SUPPORT) *(General) 80RHM*

Da-Lite Screen Co., Inc. 800-622-3737
3100 N Detroit St, PO Box 137, Warsaw, IN 46582
Wall or ceiling mount, 13-31 in. diagonal.

MOUNT, MONITOR (SUPPORT) *(cont'd)*

Ergotron, Inc. 800-888-8458
1181 Trapp Rd, Saint Paul, MN 55121
Medical arm can be used in ICUs, ORs, ERs or patient rooms.

Gcx Corp. 800-228-2555
3875 Cypress Dr, Petaluma, CA 94954
POLYMOUNT wall mounting system; ceiling mounts; countertop mounts, floor-to-ceiling equipment support columns.

Independent Solutions, Inc. 847-498-0500
900 Skokie Blvd Ste 118, Northbrook, IL 60062
GCX Polymount Adjustable (up/down/swivel/tilt/pivot); surface wall mounted, or ceiling hung; seismic approved (OSHPOD); short or long arm; pivot block models available.

Medved Products, Inc. 651-482-8413
PO Box 120883, Saint Paul, MN 55112
Custom mobile roll stands for monitors and other equipment

Mennen Medical Corp. 800-223-2201
2540 Metropolitan Dr, Trevose, PA 19053

Phelan Manufacturing Corp. 800-328-2358
2523 Minnehaha Ave, Minneapolis, MN 55404
$767.00 for ceiling mounted monitor (support) mount.

Steelcraft, Inc. 800-225-7710
115 W Main St, Millbury, MA 01527

MOUNT, SURGICAL MICROSCOPE *(Surgery) 79UMJ*

Biomedics, Inc. 949-458-1998
23322 Peralta Dr Ste 11, Laguna Hills, CA 92653

Jedmed Instruments Co. 314-845-3770
5416 Jedmed Ct, Saint Louis, MO 63129

MOUNT, TELEVISION SET *(General) 80UMW*

Crest Healthcare Supply 800-328-8908
195 3rd St, Dassel, MN 55325
TV support devices and mounts.

Da-Lite Screen Co., Inc. 800-622-3737
3100 N Detroit St, PO Box 137, Warsaw, IN 46582
Wall or ceiling mount, 13-31 in. diagonal.

Gcx Corp. 800-228-2555
3875 Cypress Dr, Petaluma, CA 94954
Mounting solutions for hospital-grade televisions.

Independent Solutions, Inc. 847-498-0500
900 Skokie Blvd Ste 118, Northbrook, IL 60062
GCX Powermount (up/down/swivel/tilt), surface wall mounted, clean, modern, hygienic, unobtrusive, clear satin anod. alum, manual or portable motor operated.

MOUNT, X-RAY TUBE, DIAGNOSTIC *(Radiology) 90IYB*

Bay Shore Medical Equipment Corp. 631-586-1991
235 S Fehr Way, Bay Shore, NY 11706
Multiple.

Del Medical Systems 800-800-6006
11550 King St, Franklin Park, IL 60131
Ceiling tube mount.

Flow X-Ray Corporation 800-356-9729
100 W Industry Ct, Deer Park, NY 11729

Ge Medical Systems, Llc 262-548-2355
3000 N Grandview Blvd, W-417, Waukesha, WI 53188
Various types of tube supports and hangers.

Hologic, Inc. 800-343-9729
35 Crosby Dr, Bedford, MA 01730
OMNIFLEX TUBE CRANE

Phoxxor 251-408-0208
5600 Commerce Blvd E # A, Mobile, AL 36619
Super Stand 5000 tube stand.

Quantum Medical Imaging, Llc 631-567-5800
2002 Orville Dr N Ste B, Ronkonkoma, NY 11779
Various.

Wolf X-Ray Corporation 800-356-9729
100 W Industry Ct, Deer Park, NY 11729

MOUNTING MEDIA, OIL SOLUBLE *(Pathology) 88KEP*

Anatech, Ltd. 800-262-8324
1020 Harts Lake Rd, Battle Creek, MI 49037
REFRAX; 1 pint bottle

E K Industries, Inc. 877-EKI-CHEM
1403 Herkimer St, Joliet, IL 60432
Mounting media.

MOUNTING MEDIA, OIL SOLUBLE *(cont'd)*

Medical Chemical Corp. 800-424-9394
19430 Van Ness Ave, Torrance, CA 90501
$7.75 per 100ml.

Polysciences, Inc. 800-523-2575
400 Valley Rd, Warrington, PA 18976
100 ml - plastic mount.

Sci Gen, Inc. 310-324-6576
333 E Gardena Blvd, Gardena, CA 90248
FDA: Medical Device Manufacturing and packaging. Focus on Histology, Cytology, Analytical and General purpose Reagents, Chemistry, and Sterling and Disinfecting agents.

Statlab Medical Products, Inc. 800-442-3573
106 Hillside Dr, Lewisville, TX 75057
ACRYMOUNT M-1 mounting media and liquid coverslip.

MOUTH PROP *(Dental And Oral) 76UDZ*

Moyco Technologies, Inc. 800-331-8837
200 Commerce Dr, Montgomeryville, PA 18936

MOUTHGUARD *(Dental And Oral) 76MQC*

Abel Dental Lab 952-541-9622
2 W Main St, National City Bank Building, Uniontown, PA 15401
Occlusal splint.

Cooley & Cooley, Ltd. 800-215-4487
8550 Westland West Blvd, Houston, TX 77041
Athletic Sports Mouthguard- a boil and bite system for athletes of all ages to enjoy a custom fitted mouthguard by a dentist.

Dahlin Laboratory 952-541-9622
393 S Harlan St Ste 210, Lakewood, CO 80226
Occlusal splint.

Denplus Inc. 800-344-4424
205 - 1221 Labadie, Longueuil, QUE J4N 1E2 Canada

Dental Services Group Of Pittsburgh 952-541-9622
101 S 10th St, Pittsburgh, PA 15203
Occlusal splint.

Denticon International Inc. 952-541-9622
841 N Grand Ave Ste 13, Nogales, AZ 85621
Occlusal splint.

Dresch/Tolson Dental Lab 952-345-6300
4024 N Holland Sylvania Rd, Toledo, OH 43623
Occlusal splint.

General Dental Products, Inc. 888-367-6212
201 Ogden Ave, Ely, NV 89301
Tru-Pak (TM)

Hansen Dental Lab 952-541-9622
6700 Squibb Rd Ste 208, Mission, KS 66202
Occlusal splint.

Harrison & Cardillo Dental Lab 952-541-9622
3703 S 19th St, Tacoma, WA 98405
Occlusal splint.

Heumann & Associates Dental Lab 952-541-9622
520 SE 5th St, Topeka, KS 66607
Occlusal splint.

Ivoclar Vivadent, Inc. 800-533-6825
175 Pineview Dr, Amherst, NY 14228
SR IVOCAP ELASTOMER

Masel Co., Inc. 800-423-8227
2701 Bartram Rd, Bristol, PA 19007

Muth & Mumma Dental Lab 952-541-9622
6360 Flank Dr Ste 500, Harrisburg, PA 17112
Occlusal splint.

Pearce-Turk Dental Lab 952-541-9622
201 N Emporia St, Wichita, KS 67202
Occlusal splint.

Power Products, Inc.-Splintek 816-531-1900
3325 Wyoming St, Kansas City, MO 64111
Mouthguard.

Progressive Dental Services Lab 952-541-9622
21006 N 22nd St Ste B1, Phoenix, AZ 85024
Occlusal splint.

Research Information Svcs. 978-283-3030
1 Essex Ave, Gloucester, MA 01930
Ris.

Simon Dechatlet Labs 952-541-9622
4484 N Dixie Dr, Dayton, OH 45414
Occlusal splint.

MOUTHGUARD *(cont'd)*

Snorex, Inc. 800-276-6739
2813 Calvin Ct, Fremont, CA 94536
SNOR-X: tongue sleeve, mouth/teeth guard.

Sportsguard Laboratories, Inc. 330-673-6932
5960 Horning Rd Ste 100, Kent, OH 44240
Various mouthguards and various materials.

Standard Dental Lab 952-541-9622
431 Clark St, Clarksburg, WV 26301
Occlusal splint.

Stelray Plastic Products, Inc 203-735-2331
50 Westfield Ave, Ansonia, CT 06401
Dental protector.

Tincher/Butler Dental Labs 952-541-9622
525 1st Ave, South Charleston, WV 25303
Occlusal splint.

Trigroup Technologies, Ltd. 972-226-4600
200 Adell Blvd, Sunnyvale, TX 75182
Mouthguard.

Windl Dental Lab 952-541-9622
314 Maple Dr, New Castle, PA 16105
Occlusal splint.

MOUTHPIECE, BREATHING *(Anesthesiology) 73BYP*

A-M Systems, Inc. 800-426-1306
131 Business Park Loop, Sequim, WA 98382
12 types-disposable or reusable - Re-usable Thermoplastic rubber, Disposable paper mouthpieces

Amici, Inc. 610-948-7100
518 Vincent St, Spring City, PA 19475
TRU-FIT and SEAL-RITE mouthpieces (disposable) for nuclear medicine applications. Aerosol systems, corrugated tubing and interconnecting components. XENON administration system also available, along with KRYPTON administration systems.

Creative Health Products, Inc. 800-742-4478
5148 Saddle Ridge Rd, Plymouth, MI 48170
$45.00 per box of 1000 3/8' dia disposable mouthpieces, $35.00 per box of 500 1 1/8' dia disposable mouthpieces.

Custom Paper Tubes Inc. 216-362-2964
15900 Industrial Pkwy, Cleveland, OH 44135
Disposable mouthpiece (various sizes).

El-Fax Company, Inc. (Lung Gym) 610-896-6853
PO Box 407, 32 Llanfair Road,, Ardmore, PA 19003
Sani-cone.

Glenroe Technologies 800-237-4060
1912 44th Ave E, Bradenton, FL 34203
Orthodontic sportsguard mouthpiece.

Hans Rudolph, Inc. 816-363-5522
7200 Wyandotte St, Kansas City, MO 64114
Mouthpiece.

Intersurgical Inc. 315-451-2900
417 Electronics Pkwy, Liverpool, NY 13088

Kidsneb, Inc. 630-930-9412
310 N Villa Ave, Villa Park, IL 60181
Mouthpiece for aerosol therapy.

Normed 800-288-8200
PO Box 3644, Seattle, WA 98124
Mouth to mouth resuscitation shield.

Numask, Inc. 818-596-2100
6320 Canoga Ave Ste 1502, Woodland Hills, CA 91367
Anesthesia,resuscitation mask.

Opap, Inc. 831-458-5626
3523 Deanes Ln, Capitola, CA 95010
Intr-oral mouthpiece used with orally applied cpap or bilevel ventilation.

Primary Care Physician Platform Llc Dba Qrs Diagnostic 763-559-8492
14755 27th Ave N, Minneapolis, MN 55447

Respironics New Jersey, Inc. 800-804-3443
5 Woodhollow Rd, Parsippany, NJ 07054
$15.50 per box of 100pcs. ASSESS adult or pediatric disposable mouthpieces for ASSESS peak flow meter unit. $15.50 per box of 100 pcs. Disposable mouthpieces for use with PERSONAL BEST. $65.00 per box of 200 disposable Safety Mouthpieces with one way valve for ASSESS.

MOUTHPIECE, BREATHING *(cont'd)*

Respond Industries, Inc. 1-800-523-8999
9500 Woodend Rd, Edwardsville, KS 66111
Various styles of mouthpieces.

Sdi Diagnostics, Inc. 800-678-5782
10 Hampden Dr, South Easton, MA 02375
One-way cardboard Safe-T-Chek mouthpiece for expiratory testing; prevents patient from breathing in contaminants.

Seven Harvest Intl. Import & Export 765-456-3584
108 N Dixon Rd, Kokomo, IN 46901
Mouthpiece.

Smiths Medical Asd Inc. 800-258-5361
10 Bowman Dr, Keene, NH 03431
Various types of mouthpieces.

Smiths Medical Asd, Inc. 847-793-0135
330 Corporate Woods Pkwy, Vernon Hills, IL 60061
Mouthpiece.

Thayer Medical Corp. 520-790-5393
4575 S Palo Verde Rd Ste 337, Tucson, AZ 85714
Mouthpiece adapter.

Vacumed 800-235-3333
4538 Westinghouse St, Ventura, CA 93003
Cold-air breathing device (heat exchanger).

Vitalograph, Inc. 800-255-6626
13310 W 99th St, Lenexa, KS 66215
SAFETWAY safety mouthpiece to overcome concern about possibility of patient cross-infection during expiratory-only testing. Box of 200 $76.00.

MOUTHPIECE, SALIVA EJECTOR *(Dental And Oral) 76DYN*

Better Dental Products 402-934-4996
8540 I St, Omaha, NE 68127
Oral mouth prop.

Crosstex International, Inc. 516-482-9001
534 Vine Ave, Sharon, PA 16146

Dental Innovators, Inc. 877-921-3919
1642 N Mockingbird Pl, Orange, CA 92867

Glenroe Technologies 800-237-4060
1912 44th Ave E, Bradenton, FL 34203
Orthodontic saliva ejector.

H & H Co. 909-390-0373
4435 E Airport Dr Ste 108, Ontario, CA 91761
Mouth prop, suction tips, all types.

Hager Worldwide, Inc. 800-328-2335
13322 Byrd Dr, Odessa, FL 33556
BULLFROG (stainless steel), INVINCIBLE (titanium), MINI VAC (stainless steel), HYDRO VAC (aluminum), SERVICEABLE (aluminum/plastic).

Harry J. Bosworth Company 800-323-4352
7227 Hamlin Ave, Skokie, IL 60076
FLEXO - Saliva injectors.

Heraeus Kulzer, Inc., Dental Products Division 574-299-6662
4315 S Lafayette Blvd, South Bend, IN 46614
Oral evacuation mouthpieces.

Plasdent Corp. 909-620-0289
1290 Price Ave, Pomona, CA 91767
Surgical tips evacution tip, high volume.

Pulpdent Corp. 800-343-4342
80 Oakland St, Watertown, MA 02472
No common name listed.

Team Technologies, Inc. 423-587-2199
5949 Commerce Blvd, Morristown, TN 37814
Covered yankauer.

Tidi Products, Llc 920-751-4380
570 Enterprise Dr, Neenah, WI 54956
Saliva ejector.

Trigroup Technologies, Ltd. 972-226-4600
200 Adell Blvd, Sunnyvale, TX 75182
Intra oral device.

MULLER'S COLLOIDAL IRON *(Pathology) 88HZD*

American Mastertech Scientific, Inc. 209-368-4031
1330 Thurman St, Lodi, CA 95240
Multiple.

MULTI ANALYTE MIXTURE, CALIBRATOR *(Chemistry) 75JIX*

Alfa Wassermann, Inc. 800-220-4488
4 Henderson Dr, West Caldwell, NJ 07006

MULTI ANALYTE MIXTURE, CALIBRATOR *(cont'd)*

Bayer Healthcare, Llc 574-256-3430
430 S Beiger St, Mishawaka, IN 46544
Calibrator.

Beckman Coulter, Inc. 800-635-3497
740 W 83rd St, Hialeah, FL 33014
S-Cal hematology calibrator, DACAL chemistry calibrator.

Biocell Laboratories, Inc. 800-222-8382
2001 E University Dr, Rancho Dominguez, CA 90220
Lipid/APO A-1, APO-B, triglycerides, cholesterol, LDL, HDL.

Carolina Liquid Chemistries Corp. 800-471-7272
510 W Central Ave Ste C, Brea, CA 92821
Medical reagent calibrators.

Dade Behring, Inc. 800-948-3233
1717 Deerfield Rd, Deerfield, IL 60015

Fisher Diagnostics 877-722-4366
11515 Vanstory Dr Ste 125, Huntersville, NC 28078

Health Chem Diagnostics Llc 954-979-3845
3341 W McNab Rd, Pompano Beach, FL 33069
Calibrator, multi-analyte mixture.

Hemagen Diagnostics, Inc. 800-436-2436
9033 Red Branch Rd, Columbia, MD 21045
Various multi-analyte mixture calibrators.

Hycor Biomedical, Inc. 800-382-2527
7272 Chapman Ave, Garden Grove, CA 92841
Hematology calibrator.

Jas Diagnostics, Inc. 305-418-2320
7220 NW 58th St, Miami, FL 33166
Multi-analyte calibrator.

Maine Standards Company, Llc 800-377-9684
765 Roosevelt Trl Ste 9A, Windham, ME 04062
Various multi-analyte chemistry calibrators.

Nerl Diagnostics Llc. 401-824-2046
14 Almeida Ave, East Providence, RI 02914
Various multi-analyte mixture calibrators.

Synermed Intl., Inc. 317-896-1565
17408 Tiller Ct Ste 1900, Westfield, IN 46074
Clinical chemistry calibrator.

Thermo Fisher Scientific Inc. 781-622-1000
81 Wyman St, Waltham, MA 02451

Vital Diagnostics Inc. 714-672-3553
1075 W Lambert Rd Ste D, Brea, CA 92821
Various calibrators and calibration standards.

MYCOPLASMA SPP. DNA REAGENTS *(Microbiology) 83LQG*

Gen-Probe, Inc. 800-523-5001
10210 Genetic Center Dr, San Diego, CA 92121
GEN-PROBE® Mycoplasma Tissue Culture Non-Isotopic (MTC-NI) Rapid Detection System - DNA probe test for the detection of mycoplasma contamination in tissue culture. Not intended for diagnostic use.

Prodesse, Inc. 888-589-6974
W229N1870 Westwood Dr, Waukesha, WI 53186
Pneumoplex® - Multiplex PCR Reagents for simultaneous detection and differentiation of Mycoplasma pneumoniae, Legionella pneumophila, Legionella micdadei, Chlamydophila pneumoniae and Bordetella pertussis - Research Use Only.

Wescor, Inc. 800-453-2725
459 S Main St, Logan, UT 84321
Mycofast US has been designed for the detection, enumeration and identification of Ureaplasma urealyticum and Mycoplasma hominis in endocervical,urethral, urinary, gastric and sperm specimens.

MYELOPEROXIDASE, IMMUNOASSAY, SYSTEM, TEST *(Immunology) 82NTV*

Prognostix, Inc. 216-445-1380
10265 Carnegie Ave, Cleveland, OH 44106
Myeloperoxidase (mpo) test.

MYOGRAPH *(Physical Med) 89GWP*

Bio-Medical Instruments, Inc. 800-521-4640
2387 E 8 Mile Rd, Warren, MI 48091
Clinical scanner-electromyographic, digital, battery powered plus ambulatory electromyography unit.

MYOGRAPH *(cont'd)*

Biofeedback Instrument Corp. 212-222-5665
255 W 98th St Apt 3D, New York, NY 10025
Myotrac EMG ideal for PT work on all rehabilitation, Bruxism, Incontinence, $500. Myotrac2 EMG, dual channel, $1,600 w/computer option. EMG Retrainer - dual channel unit $795 Autogenic AT33 EMG biofeedback unit $850.

Biomation 888-667-2324
335 Perth St., P.O. Box 156, Almonte, ON K0A 1A0 Canada
MEGA Ambulatory muscle tester.

Neurodyne Medical Corp. 800-963-8633
186 Alewife Brook Pkwy, Cambridge, MA 02138
Neuromuscular System/3 offers two-, four-, and eight-channel computerized surface EMG instruments for relaxation training and muscular reeducation. NEUSCAN two-channel computerized surface EMG system features four- and eight-channel expansion capability.

Noraxon Usa, Inc. 800-364-8985
13430 N Scottsdale Rd Ste 104, Scottsdale, AZ 85254
Multiple choices of TeleMyo telemetric systems with a variety of channel choices; 4, 8, 12 and 16, with possibilities of up to 24 channels.

NAD REDUCTION/NADH OXIDATION, CPK OR ISOENZYMES
(Chemistry) 75CGS

Abbott Diagnostics Div. 626-440-0700
820 Mission St, South Pasadena, CA 91030
Various assay for dtection of creatine kinase.

Caldon Bioscience, Inc. 909-628-9944
2100 S Reservoir St, Pomona, CA 91766
Creatine kinase.

Carolina Liquid Chemistries Corp. 800-471-7272
510 W Central Ave Ste C, Brea, CA 92821
Ck.

Intersect Systems, Inc. 360-577-1062
1152 3rd Avenue, Suite D & E, Longview, WA 98632
Creatine phosphokinase/creatine kinase, Liquid Stable CK-NAC.

Jas Diagnostics, Inc. 305-418-2320
7220 NW 58th St, Miami, FL 33166
Cpk (creatine kinase).

Sterling Diagnostics, Inc. 800-637-2661
36645 Metro Ct, Sterling Heights, MI 48312
Cpk-uv reagent set.

Synermed Intl., Inc. 317-896-1565
17408 Tiller Ct Ste 1900, Westfield, IN 46074
Creatine kinase reagent kit.

Vital Diagnostics Inc. 714-672-3553
1075 W Lambert Rd Ste D, Brea, CA 92821
Various creatine kinase reagents.

NAD REDUCTION/NADH OXIDATION, LACTATE DEHYDROGENASE *(Chemistry) 75CFJ*

Abbott Diagnostics Div. 626-440-0700
820 Mission St, South Pasadena, CA 91030
Lactate dehydrogenase.

Beckman Coulter, Inc. 800-635-3497
740 W 83rd St, Hialeah, FL 33014
$0.11 per test.

Biomerieux Inc. 800-682-2666
100 Rodolphe St, Durham, NC 27712

Caldon Bioscience, Inc. 909-628-9944
2100 S Reservoir St, Pomona, CA 91766
Lactate dehydrogenase.

Caldon Biotech, Inc. 757-224-0177
2251 Rutherford Rd, Carlsbad, CA 92008
Ld.

Carolina Liquid Chemistries Corp. 800-471-7272
510 W Central Ave Ste C, Brea, CA 92821
Ld-l.

Genchem, Inc. 714-529-1616
510 W Central Ave Ste D, Brea, CA 92821
Ldh.

Health Chem Diagnostics Llc 954-979-3845
3341 W McNab Rd, Pompano Beach, FL 33069
Nad reduction/nadh oxidation, lactate dehydrogenase.

Jas Diagnostics, Inc. 305-418-2320
7220 NW 58th St, Miami, FL 33166
Ldh (lactate dehydrogerase).

NAD REDUCTION/NADH OXIDATION, LACTATE DEHYDROGENASE *(cont'd)*

Pointe Scientific, Inc. 800-445-9853
5449 Research Dr, Canton, MI 48188

Raichem, Division Of Hemagen Diagnostics, Inc. 800-438-6100
8225 Mercury Ct, San Diego, CA 92111

Sterling Diagnostics, Inc. 800-637-2661
36645 Metro Ct, Sterling Heights, MI 48312
Lactate dehydrogenase (uv-rate) reagent set.

Synermed Intl., Inc. 317-896-1565
17408 Tiller Ct Ste 1900, Westfield, IN 46074
Lactate dehydrogenase test system.

Teco Diagnostics 714-693-7788
1268 N Lakeview Ave, Anaheim, CA 92807
Lactate dehydrogenase.

Vital Diagnostics Inc. 714-672-3553
1075 W Lambert Rd Ste D, Brea, CA 92821
Various lactate dehydrogenase reagents.

NADH OXIDATION/NAD REDUCTION, AST/SGOT
(Chemistry) 75CIT

Abbott Diagnostics Div. 626-440-0700
820 Mission St, South Pasadena, CA 91030
Aspartate aminotransferase.

Bayer Healthcare Llc 914-524-2955
555 White Plains Rd Fl 5, Tarrytown, NY 10591
Test for sgot in plasma or serum.

Beckman Coulter, Inc. 800-635-3497
740 W 83rd St, Hialeah, FL 33014
$0.08 per test.

Biomerieux Inc. 800-682-2666
100 Rodolphe St, Durham, NC 27712

Caldon Bioscience, Inc. 909-628-9944
2100 S Reservoir St, Pomona, CA 91766
Ast/sgot.

Caldon Biotech, Inc. 757-224-0177
2251 Rutherford Rd, Carlsbad, CA 92008
Ast/sgot.

Carolina Liquid Chemistries Corp. 800-471-7272
510 W Central Ave Ste C, Brea, CA 92821
Ast.

Genchem, Inc. 714-529-1616
510 W Central Ave Ste D, Brea, CA 92821
Ast/sgot reagent.

Health Chem Diagnostics Llc 954-979-3845
3341 W McNab Rd, Pompano Beach, FL 33069
Nadh oxidation/nad reduction, ast/sgot.

Hemagen Diagnostics, Inc. 800-436-2436
9033 Red Branch Rd, Columbia, MD 21045
Various ast/sgot methods.

Jas Diagnostics, Inc. 305-418-2320
7220 NW 58th St, Miami, FL 33166
Ast (got).

Pointe Scientific, Inc. 800-445-9853
5449 Research Dr, Canton, MI 48188

Raichem, Division Of Hemagen Diagnostics, Inc. 800-438-6100
8225 Mercury Ct, San Diego, CA 92111

Sterling Diagnostics, Inc. 800-637-2661
36645 Metro Ct, Sterling Heights, MI 48312
Ast/sgot reagent set.

Synermed Intl., Inc. 317-896-1565
17408 Tiller Ct Ste 1900, Westfield, IN 46074
Ast/got reagent kit.

Teco Diagnostics 714-693-7788
1268 N Lakeview Ave, Anaheim, CA 92807
Ast/sgot liquid reagent-kinetic method.

Vital Diagnostics Inc. 714-672-3553
1075 W Lambert Rd Ste D, Brea, CA 92821
Various ast/sgot reagents.

NAIL, FIXATION, BONE *(Orthopedics) 87JDS*

Alphatec Spine, Inc. 760-494-6769
5818 El Camino Real, Carlsbad, CA 92008
Compression hip screw.

Depuy Ace, A Johnson & Johnson Company 800-473-3789
700 Orthopaedic Dr, Warsaw, IN 46582

NAIL, FIXATION, BONE *(cont'd)*

Depuy Orthopaedics, Inc. 800-473-3789
700 Orthopaedic Dr, P.O. Box 988, Warsaw, IN 46582
Various types of bone fixation nails.

Depuy Spine, Inc. 800-227-6633
325 Paramount Dr, Raynham, MA 02767
Bone nail.

Depuy-Raynham, A Div. Of Depuy Orthopaedics 800-451-2006
325 Paramount Dr, Raynham, MA 02767
Various types of bone fixation nails.

International Hospital Supply Co. 800-398-9450
6914 Canby Ave Ste 105, Reseda, CA 91335

Keller Engineering, Inc. 310-326-6291
3203 Kashiwa St, Torrance, CA 90505

Onyx Medical Corp. 901-323-6699
152 Collins St, Memphis, TN 38112

Paramedical Distributors 800-245-3278
2020 Grand Blvd, Kansas City, MO 64108

Stryker Spine 866-457-7463
2 Pearl Ct, Allendale, NJ 07401

Zimmer Holdings, Inc. 800-613-6131
1800 W Center St, PO Box 708, Warsaw, IN 46580

Zimmer Manufacturing B.V. 800-613-6131
Route 1, Km. 123.4, Bldg. 1, Turpeaux Industrial Park
Mercedita, PR 00715
Various types and sizes of sliding and non-sliding bone nails & nail/plate combi.

NAIL/BLADE/PLATE APPLIANCE *(Orthopedics) 87KWK*

Truform Orthotics & Prosthetics 800-888-0458
3960 Rosslyn Dr, Cincinnati, OH 45209

NAPHTHYL PHOSPHATE, ACID PHOSPHATASE
(Chemistry) 75CKB

Abbott Diagnostics Div. 626-440-0700
820 Mission St, South Pasadena, CA 91030
Acid phosphatase.

Jas Diagnostics, Inc. 305-418-2320
7220 NW 58th St, Miami, FL 33166
Acid phosphatase.

Teco Diagnostics 714-693-7788
1268 N Lakeview Ave, Anaheim, CA 92807
Acid phosphatase.

NASOPHARYNGOSCOPE (FLEXIBLE OR RIGID)
(Ear/Nose/Throat) 77EOB

Acclarent, Inc. 877-775-2789
1525B Obrien Dr, Menlo Park, CA 94025
Microendoscope.

Clinimed, Incorporated 877-CLINIMED
303 Markus Ct, Sandy Brae Industrial Park, Newark, DE 19713

Entellus Medical 866-620-7615
6705 Wedgwood Ct N, Maple Grove, MN 55311
Entellus Medical Flexible Endoscope

Gyrus Ent L.L.C., Sub. Of Gyrus Acmi, Inc. 508-804-2739
2925 Appling Rd, Bartlett, TN 38133
Various types and sizes of nasopharyngoscopes.

Henke Sass Wolf Of America, Inc. 508-671-9300
135 Schofield Ave, Dudley, MA 01571

J. Jamner Surgical Instruments, Inc 800-431-1123
9 Skyline Dr, Hawthorne, NY 10532

Jedmed Instruments Co. 314-845-3770
5416 Jedmed Ct, Saint Louis, MO 63129

Karl Storz Endoscopy-America Inc. 800-421-0837
600 Corporate Pointe, Culver City, CA 90230

Kelleher Medical, Inc. 804-378-9956
3049 St Marys Way, Powhatan, VA 23139

Mahe International Inc. 800-294-7946
468 Craighead St, Nashville, TN 37204

Minrad, Inc. 716-855-1068
50 Cobham Dr, Orchard Park, NY 14127
Sinuscope.

Olympus America, Inc. 800-645-8160
3500 Corporate Pkwy, PO Box 610, Center Valley, PA 18034

Optim Incorporated 800-225-7486
64 Technology Park Rd, Sturbridge, MA 01566

NASOPHARYNGOSCOPE (FLEXIBLE OR RIGID) *(cont'd)*

Pentax Medical Company 800-431-5880
102 Chestnut Ridge Rd, Montvale, NJ 07645
Various models of flexible naso-pharyngo-laryngoscopes, with distal tip diameters and channel sizes; fully immersible. Call for quote.

Pentax Southern Region Service Center 201-571-2300
8934 Kirby Dr, Houston, TX 77054
Nasopharyngoscope.

Pentax West Coast Service Center 800-431-5880
10410 Pioneer Blvd Ste 2, Santa Fe Springs, CA 90670
Pentax nasopharyngoscope.

Richard Wolf Medical Instruments Corp. 800-323-9653
353 Corporate Woods Pkwy, Vernon Hills, IL 60061

Rtc Inc.-Memcath Technologies Llc
1777 Oakdale Ave, West St Paul, MN 55118
Endoscope sheath.

Vision-Sciences, Inc. 800-874-9975
40 Ramland Rd S Ste 1, Orangeburg, NY 10962

Welch Allyn, Inc. 800-535-6663
4341 State Street Rd, Skaneateles Falls, NY 13153

NASOSCOPE *(Ear/Nose/Throat) 77RHS*

Aztec Medical Products, Inc. 800-223-3859
106 Ingram Rd, Williamsburg, VA 23188
Nasoflex. Nasopharyngyscope, flexible 3.8mm diameter, 300 mm working distance complete with optic cable and deluxe carrying case.

Cameron-Miller, Inc. 800-621-0142
5410 W Roosevelt Rd, Road #241, Chicago, IL 60644

Kelleher Medical, Inc. 804-378-9956
3049 St Marys Way, Powhatan, VA 23139

NEBULIZER, DIRECT PATIENT INTERFACE
(Anesthesiology) 73CAF

Airsep Corp. 800-874-0202
401 Creekside Dr, Amherst, NY 14228

Allied Healthcare Products, Inc. 800-444-3954
1720 Sublette Ave, Saint Louis, MO 63110

Amici, Inc. 610-948-7100
518 Vincent St, Spring City, PA 19475
AeroSol Radioaerosol System; Swirler Nebulizer; Swirler Aerosol System

Biodex Medical Systems, Inc. 800-224-6339
20 Ramsey Rd, Shirley, NY 11967

Catalent Pharma Solutions 866-720-3148
2200 Lake Shore Dr, Woodstock, IL 60098
Multiple

Contemporary Products, Inc. 800-424-2444
530 Riverside Industrial Pkwy, Portland, ME 04103
Heavy-duty 50psi compressor. Used for continuous aerosol therapy and for delivery of thicker medications. Also used for heated aerosol treatments with a J-bar attachment.

Destal Industries, Inc. 973-227-1830
201 Washington St, Columbus, IN 47201
Unit dose inhaler.

Dhd Healthcare Corporation 800-847-8000
PO Box 6, One Madison Street, Wampsville, NY 13163
ACE MDI holding chamber, acapella and acapella choice Vibratory PEP Devices, TheraPEP PEP System.

Forest Pharmaceutical, Inc. 212-421-7850
3721 Laclede Ave, Saint Louis, MO 63108
Aerosol holding chambers.

Futuremed America, Inc. 800-222-6780
15700 Devonshire St, Granada Hills, CA 91344
$150.00 to $250.00.

Holopack Intl. Corp. 803-806-3300
1 Technology Cir, Columbia, SC 29203
Various.

Intersurgical Inc. 315-451-2900
417 Electronics Pkwy, Liverpool, NY 13088
CIRRUS, MICROCIRRUS.

Kaz, Inc. 518-828-0450
1 Vapor Trl, Hudson, NY 12534
Various types of vaporizers.

Kentron Health Care, Inc. 615-384-0573
3604 Kelton Jackson Rd, P.o. Box 120, Springfield, TN 37172
Nebulizer.

NEBULIZER, DIRECT PATIENT INTERFACE *(cont'd)*

Medi/Nuclear Corp. 800-321-5981
4610 Littlejohn St, Baldwin Park, CA 91706
AERO/VENT lung aerosol unit. INSTA/VENT lung aerosol unit.

Medical Depot 516-998-4600
99 Seaview Blvd, Port Washington, NY 11050
Nebulizer.

Medical Industries America Inc. 800-759-3038
2636 289th Pl, Adel, IA 50003
AQUATOWER II, disposable nebulizer kit.

Meditrack Products, Llc 800-863-9633
433 Main St, Hudson, MA 01749
Dose counter for metered inhalation medication cannisters.

Monaghan Medical Corp. 800-833-9653
5 Latour Ave Ste 1600, P.O. Box 2805, Plattsburgh, NY 12901
AEROECLIPSE, breath activated aerosol delivery device w/disposalbe nebulizer.

Nspire Health, Inc 800-574-7374
1830 Lefthand Cir, Longmont, CO 80501
KoKo Dosimeter and KoKo DigiDoser for administration of nebulized medications in quantifiable methodology, specifically used for methacholine challenge testing.

Smiths Medical Asd Inc. 800-258-5361
10 Bowman Dr, Keene, NH 03431
Various types of nebulizers & accessories.

Smiths Medical Asd, Inc. 847-793-0135
330 Corporate Woods Pkwy, Vernon Hills, IL 60061
Various types of sterile nebulizers.

Superior Products, Inc. 216-651-9400
3786 Ridge Rd, Cleveland, OH 44144
Valved holding chamber.

Thayer Medical Corp. 520-790-5393
4575 S Palo Verde Rd Ste 337, Tucson, AZ 85714
Various.

The Respiratory Group 314-659-4311
4150 Carr Lane Ct, Saint Louis, MO 63119
Nebulizer.

Ventlab Corp. 336-753-5000
155 Boyce Dr, Mocksville, NC 27028
Spacer (mdi).

Weiler Engineering, Inc. 847-697-4900
1395 Gateway Dr, Elgin, IL 60124

Westmed, Inc. 800-975-7987
5580 S Nogales Hwy, Tucson, AZ 85706
Heart 8-hour continuous nebulizer, high flow (10-15 L/min.). High output (up to 50 mL/hour). IV Heart 4-hour continuous nebulizer high flow (10-15 L/min.). MiniHeart low flow (1-2 L/min.) continuous nebulizer ideal for ventilator use, up to 10 hours continuous nebulization. UniHeart low flow (2-4 L/min.) continuous nebulizer, up to 2 hours continuous, 10-cc reservoir. MiniHeart Hiflo (8L/min)1hour of continuous nebulization. VIXONE, high-output nebulizer.

NEBULIZER, HEATED *(Anesthesiology) 73RHT*

Dhd Healthcare Corporation 800-847-8000
PO Box 6, One Madison Street, Wampsville, NY 13163
Thera-Mist Air Entrainment Nebulizer; Thera-Mist Closed Dilution Nebulizer

Pegasus Research Corp. 877-632-0255
3505 Cadillac Ave Ste G5, Costa Mesa, CA 92626
For infant incubators and hand-held models.

NEBULIZER, MEDICINAL *(Ear/Nose/Throat) 77EPN*

A-M Systems, Inc. 800-426-1306
131 Business Park Loop, Sequim, WA 98382
$73.00 for case of 50.

Allied Healthcare Products, Inc. 800-444-3954
1720 Sublette Ave, Saint Louis, MO 63110

Bryan Corp. 800-343-7711
4 Plympton St, Woburn, MA 01801
Sclerosol Inrapleural Aerosol, for the treatment of Malignant Pleural Effusion (MPE). Sclerosol is aerosolized sterile talc.

Burton Medical Products, Inc. 800-444-9909
21100 Lassen St, Chatsworth, CA 91311

Dorel Design & Development Center 781-364-3542
25 Forbes Blvd, Foxboro, MA 02035

Intersurgical Inc. 315-451-2900
417 Electronics Pkwy, Liverpool, NY 13088

NEBULIZER, MEDICINAL *(cont'd)*

Invacare Corporation 800-333-6900
1 Invacare Way, Elyria, OH 44035
Sidestream reusable and disposable nebulizers with Venturi effect

Jayza Corp. 305-477-1136
7215 NW 41st St Ste A, Miami, FL 33166

Mada, Inc. 800-526-6370
625 Washington Ave, Carlstadt, NJ 07072

Meinhard Glass Products 303-277-9776
700 Corporate Cir Ste A, Golden, CO 80401
Nebulizer for use in inductively coupled plasma spectrometer. (Atomic Emmission and and Mass Spectrometer.)

Respironics Georgia, Inc. 724-387-4559
175 Chastain Meadows Ct NW, Kennesaw, GA 30144
INSPIRATION 929, 929K compressor-driven nebulizer aerosol therapy treatment with instructive coloring book and stickers for children.

Respironics New Jersey, Inc. 800-804-3443
5 Woodhollow Rd, Parsippany, NJ 07054
INSPIRATION 626, is a compressor driven nebulizer for medication delivery. Portable and lightweight, the 626 is easy to use and reliable for all ages.

Salter Labs 800-235-4203
100 Sycamore Rd, Arvin, CA 93203
NEBUTECH HDN-Disposable, hand-held nebulizer.

Thayer Medical Corp. 520-790-5393
4575 S Palo Verde Rd Ste 337, Tucson, AZ 85714
Metered dose actuator.

NEBULIZER, MEDICINAL, NON-VENTILATORY (ATOMIZER)
(Anesthesiology) 73CCQ

Afton Medical Llc 707-577-0685
3137 Swetzer Rd Ste C, Loomis, CA 95650
Aerosol delivery nebulizer.

Aradigm Corp. 510-265-9000
3929 Point Eden Way, Hayward, CA 94545
Smartmist respiratory management system.

Centurion Medical Products Corp. 517-545-1135
3310 S Main St, Salisbury, NC 28147

Emergency Medical Systems 214-704-7077
PO Box 111034, Carrollton, TX 75011
BVM/Ventilator assisted nebulizer kit.

Kentron Health Care, Inc. 615-384-0573
3604 Kelton Jackson Rd, P.o. Box 120, Springfield, TN 37172
Medicinal nebulizers.

Medical Depot 516-998-4600
99 Seaview Blvd, Port Washington, NY 11050
Nebulizer kit.

Nspire Health, Inc 800-574-7374
1830 Lefthand Cir, Longmont, CO 80501
KOKO Dosimeter automated, stand-alone dosimeter used to deliver reproducible, variable doses of an aerosol for challenge testing, diagnosis and therapy.

ReNu Medical Inc. 877-252-1110
9800 Evergreen Way, Everett, WA 98204
MULTIPLE MODELS; REPROCESSED NEBULIZER (ATOMIZER)

Respironics New Jersey, Inc. 800-804-3443
5 Woodhollow Rd, Parsippany, NJ 07054
OPTIHALER, Drug Delivery System for use with MDI $20.00., OptiChamber Valved Holding Chamber and OptiChamber with mask.

Tennessee Medical Equipment, Inc. 731-635-2119
4637 Highway 19 E, Ripley, TN 38063
Various.

Tri-State Hospital Supply Corp. 517-545-1135
3173 E 43rd St, Yuma, AZ 85365

NEBULIZER, NON-HEATED *(Anesthesiology) 73RHU*

A&H Products, Inc. 918-835-8081
PO Box 470686, Tulsa, OK 74147

Allied Healthcare Products, Inc. 800-444-3954
1720 Sublette Ave, Saint Louis, MO 63110
Electronic nebulizer.

Dedicated Distribution 800-325-8367
640 Miami Ave, Kansas City, KS 66105
AERO GEN.

NEBULIZER, NON-HEATED *(cont'd)*

Dhd Healthcare Corporation 800-847-8000
PO Box 6, One Madison Street, Wampsville, NY 13163
Thera-Mist Air Entrainment Nebulizer and Thera-Mist Closed Dilution Nebulizer

Intersurgical Inc. 315-451-2900
417 Electronics Pkwy, Liverpool, NY 13088
CIRRUS, MICRO CIRRUS.

Pari Respiratory Equipment, Inc. 800-327-8632
2943 Oak Lake Blvd, Midlothian, VA 23112
Aerosol system DURA-NEB 2000 compressor, portable, battery or AC/DC operation and LC JET + nebulizer. Particle size range 0.5-5 microns. PRONEB AC compressor also available with LC JET + nebulizer.

Vacumed 800-235-3333
4538 Westinghouse St, Ventura, CA 93003

NEBULIZER, ULTRASONIC *(Anesthesiology) 73RHV*

Allied Healthcare Products, Inc. 800-444-3954
1720 Sublette Ave, Saint Louis, MO 63110

Habley Medical Technology Corp. 800-729-1994
15721 Bernardo Heights Pkwy Ste B-30, San Diego, CA 92128
Breath-activated ultrasonic nebulizer for precise dose administration.

Lumiscope Company, Inc. 800-672-8293
1035 Centennial Ave, Piscataway, NJ 08854
Compact and portable

Medsonic U.S.A., Inc. 716-565-1700
8865 Sheridan Dr, Clarence, NY 14031
Ultrasonic COMPACT continuous cool or heated aerosol at 6.5cc/min.; ultrasonic SPIRAL battery-operated medication inhaler; and ultrasonic MINI MAX & MINI MAX II semi-portable medication inhaler.

Norco 800-657-6672
1125 W Amity Rd, Boise, ID 83705

Sunrise Medical 800-333-4000
7477 Dry Creek Pkwy, Longmont, CO 80503

NEEDLE, ACUPUNCTURE *(Anesthesiology) 73BWI*

Electro Therapeutic Devices Inc. 800-268-3834
570 Hood Rd., Ste. 14, Markham, ONT L3R 4G7 Canada
For intra muscular stimulation.

Kenshin Trading Corp. 800-766-1313
22353 S Western Ave Ste 201, Torrance, CA 90501
Wheelchair chains.

M.E.D. Servi-Systems Canada Ltd. 800-267-6868
8 Sweetnam Dr., Stittsville, ONT K2S 1G2 Canada

NEEDLE, ACUPUNCTURE, SINGLE USE *(General) 80MQX*

Helio Medical Supplies, Inc. 408-433-3355
606 Charcot Ave, San Jose, CA 95131
Sterile acupuncture needles.

Henry's Acupuncture Equipment 415-337-8290
241 Leland Ave, San Francisco, CA 94134
Acupuncture needle.

Kenshin Trading Corp. 800-766-1313
22353 S Western Ave Ste 201, Torrance, CA 90501
Acupuncture needle.

Seirin-America, Inc. 800-337-9338
230 Libbey Industrial Pkwy, Weymouth, MA 02189
SEIRIN needles.

NEEDLE, ANGIOGRAPHIC *(Cns/Neurology) 84HAQ*

Cadence Science Inc. 888-717-7677
1979 Marcus Ave Ste 215, New Hyde Park, NY 11042
14 types - all reusable.

Cook Inc. 800-457-4500
PO Box 489, Bloomington, IN 47402

Merit Medical Systems, Inc. 800-356-3748
1600 Merit Pkwy, South Jordan, UT 84095
Majestik Series Angiographic and Shielded Needles, Advance, SecureLoc

Tegra Medical Inc. 508-541-4200
9 Forge Pkwy, Franklin, MA 02038

NEEDLE, ASPIRATION AND INJECTION, DISPOSABLE *(Surgery) 79GAA*

B. Braun Medical, Inc. 610-596-2536
901 Marcon Blvd, Allentown, PA 18109

NEEDLE, ASPIRATION AND INJECTION, DISPOSABLE *(cont'd)*

Bd Medical - Diabetes Care 201-847-4298
1329 W US Highway 6 # &34, Holdrege, NE 68949
Biopsy, radiology, pharmacy, filter and other specialty needles.

Becton, Dickinson & Co. 308-872-6811
150 S 1st Ave, Broken Bow, NE 68822
Biopsy, radiology, pharmacy, filter and other specialty needles.

Becton, Dickinson & Co., (Bd) Preanalytical System 201-847-6280
1575 Airport Rd, Sumter, SC 29153
Various.

Bemis Mfg. Co. 920-467-5206
Hwy. Pp West, Sheboygan Falls, WI 53085
Needle recapping device.

Biocompatibles Inc. 877-783-5463
115 Hurley Rd Bldg 3, Oxford, CT 06478
Epidural needle.

Bioform Medical, Inc. 262-835-3323
4133 Courtney Rd Ste 10, Franksville, WI 53126
Various types of general surgery sterile injection needles.

Boston Scientific Corporation 508-652-5578
8600 NW 41st St, Doral, FL 33166

Busse Hospital Disposables, Inc. 631-435-4711
75 Arkay Dr, Hauppauge, NY 11788
Aspiration needle.

Churchill Medical Systems, Inc. 800-468-0585
935 Horsham Rd Ste M, Horsham, PA 19044
Kit, Disposable Procedure/General.

Collagen Matrix, Inc. 201-405-1477
509 Commerce St, Franklin Lakes, NJ 07417
Bone marrow harvest needles.

Cook Endoscopy 336-744-0157
4900 Bethania Station Rd # &, 5951 Grassy Creek Blvd. Winston Salem, NC 27105
Chiba needle, injection needle, lung biopsy needle.

Covidien Lp 508-261-8000
15 Hampshire St, Mansfield, MA 02048

Depuy Spine, Inc. 800-227-6633
325 Paramount Dr, Raynham, MA 02767
Needle, aspiration and injection, disposable.

Exelint International Co. 800-940-3935
5840 W Centinela Ave, Los Angeles, CA 90045

Havel's Inc. 800-638-4770
3726 Lonsdale St, Cincinnati, OH 45227

Hurricane Medical 941-751-0588
5315 Lena Rd, Bradenton, FL 34211
Disposable aspiration & injection needle.

Inrad 800-558-4647
4375 Donkers Ct SE, Kentwood, MI 49512
Senti-loc injectable breast localization wire.

Integra Lifesciences Corp. 609-275-0500
311 Enterprise Dr, Plainsboro, NJ 08536
Osteoject needle.

Ispg, Inc. 860-355-8511
517 Litchfield Rd, New Milford, CT 06776
Custom needles

Jorgensen Laboratories 970-669-2500
1450 Van Buren Ave, Loveland, CO 80538

Medical Device Technologies, Inc. (Md Tech) 800-338-0440
3600 SW 47th Ave, Gainesville, FL 32608
SELIS.

Medone Surgical, Inc. 941-359-3129
670 Tallevast Rd, Sarasota, FL 34243
Various.

Medtronic Spine Llc 877-690-5353
1221 Crossman Ave, Sunnyvale, CA 94089
Sterile needles (various types) with stylets.

Nanomed Devices, Inc. 518-862-0151
116 Kennewyck Cir, Slingerlands, NY 12159
Hand held disposable needles.

Norfolk Medical Products, Inc. 847-674-7075
7350 Ridgeway Ave, Skokie, IL 60076
Huber point needls - various gauges and lengths.

Novosci Corp. 281-363-4949
2828 N Crescentridge Dr, The Woodlands, TX 77381

NEEDLE, ASPIRATION AND INJECTION, DISPOSABLE *(cont'd)*

Osseon Therapeutics, Inc. 877-567-7366
2330 Circadian Way, Santa Rosa, CA 95407
OsseoFlex 1.0 Steerable Needle

Peregrine Surgical, Ltd. 215-348-0456
51 Britain Dr, Doylestown, PA 18901
Needle, aspiration and injection, disposable.

Pneumrx Inc 650-625-8910
530 Logue Ave, Mountain View, CA 94043
Sterile & non-sterile needle, aspiration & injection, disposable.

Princeton Medical Group, Inc. 800-875-0869
1189 Royal Links Dr, Mt Pleasant, SC 29466

Psi/Eye-Ko, Inc. 636-447-1010
804 Corporate Centre Dr, O Fallon, MO 63368
Retrobulbar, peribulbar needles.

Rhein Mfg., Inc. 314-997-1775
2269 Grissom Dr, Saint Louis, MO 63146
Endoscopic surgical instrument.

Rocket Medical Plc. 800-707-7625
150 Recreation Park Dr Ste 3, Hingham, MA 02043
Disposable VERRES needle.

Sterex Corp. 800-603-5045
4501 126th Ave N, Clearwater, FL 33762
Various sizes of sterile, disposable dental hypodermic needles.

Synthes (Usa) - Development Center 719-481-5300
1230 Wilson Dr, West Chester, PA 19380
Needle, aspiration and injection, disposable.

Tegra Medical Inc. 508-541-4200
9 Forge Pkwy, Franklin, MA 02038

Uroplasty, Inc. 952-426-6140
5420 Feltl Rd, Minnetonka, MN 55343

NEEDLE, ASPIRATION AND INJECTION, REUSABLE
(Surgery) 79GDM

Aesculap Implant Systems Inc. 1-800-234-9179
3773 Corporate Pkwy, Center Valley, PA 18034

Bausch & Lomb Surgical 636-255-5051
3365 Tree Court Ind Blvd, Saint Louis, MO 63122

Biomet Microfixation Inc. 800-874-7711
1520 Tradeport Dr, Jacksonville, FL 32218
Various types of needles.

Dermatologic Lab & Supply, Inc. 800-831-6273
608 13th Ave, Council Bluffs, IA 51501
No common name listed.

Havel's Inc. 800-638-4770
3726 Lonsdale St, Cincinnati, OH 45227

Integra Lifesciences Corp. 609-275-0500
311 Enterprise Dr, Plainsboro, NJ 08536
Osteoject needle.

Pneumrx Inc 650-625-8910
530 Logue Ave, Mountain View, CA 94043
Sterile & non-sterle needle, aspiration & injection, reusable.

Princeton Medical Group, Inc. 800-875-0869
1189 Royal Links Dr, Mt Pleasant, SC 29466
Needle Holder.

Psi/Eye-Ko, Inc. 636-447-1010
804 Corporate Centre Dr, O Fallon, MO 63368
Atkinson retrobulbar needle.

Ranfac Corp. 800-2RANFAC
30 Doherty Ave, Avon Industrial Park, Avon, MA 02322

Tegra Medical Inc. 508-541-4200
9 Forge Pkwy, Franklin, MA 02038
Biopsy aspiration needle.

NEEDLE, ASPIRATION, CYST, LAPAROSCOPIC *(Surgery) 79RIJ*

Ranfac Corp. 800-2RANFAC
30 Doherty Ave, Avon Industrial Park, Avon, MA 02322

Richard Wolf Medical Instruments Corp. 800-323-9653
353 Corporate Woods Pkwy, Vernon Hills, IL 60061

NEEDLE, ASSISTED REPRODUCTION *(Obstetrics/Gyn) 85MQE*

Cook Ob/Gyn 800-541-5591
1100 W Morgan St, Spencer, IN 47460

Genx International 888-GEN-XNOW
393 Soundview Rd, Guilford, CT 06437

NEEDLE, ASSISTED REPRODUCTION *(cont'd)*

Inntec, Inc. 608-444-4544
401 E Edgewater St, Portage, WI 53901
Assisted reproduction needle.

NEEDLE, BIOPSY, CARDIOVASCULAR *(Cardiovascular) 74DWO*

Argon Medical Devices Inc. 903-675-9321
1445 Flat Creek Rd, Athens, TX 75751
Cut biopsy needle.

Cadence Science Inc. 888-717-7677
1979 Marcus Ave Ste 215, New Hyde Park, NY 11042
22 types - all reusable.

Civco Medical Instruments Co., Inc. 319-656-4447
102 1st St S, Kalona, IA 52247
Disposable endocavity,ultrasound-disposable,ultrasound needle guide.

Covidien Lp 508-261-8000
15 Hampshire St, Mansfield, MA 02048

Integra Radionics 800-466-6814
22 Terry Ave, Burlington, MA 01803

Medtronic, Inc. 800-633-8766
710 Medtronic Pkwy, Minneapolis, MN 55432
BLOODPORTER, HILITER, THE POINT PRO, SAMPLE MASTER, SCABBARD, SURESTOP; needles and accessories.

Pneumrx Inc 650-625-8910
530 Logue Ave, Mountain View, CA 94043
Sterile & non-sterile needle, biopsy, cardiovascular.

Ranfac Corp. 800-2RANFAC
30 Doherty Ave, Avon Industrial Park, Avon, MA 02322
Various types in small gauges.

Tegra Medical Inc. 508-541-4200
9 Forge Pkwy, Franklin, MA 02038

Vita Needle Company 781-444-1780
919 Great Plain Ave, Needham, MA 02492
Reuseable, non-sterile manufacture to order, short and long runs. Gauges 3-34, ss 304 and ss 316.

NEEDLE, BIOPSY, MAMMARY *(Obstetrics/Gyn) 85WJD*

Anchor Products Company 800-323-5134
52 W Official Rd, Addison, IL 60101

Angiotech 800-424-6779
241 W Palatine Rd, Wheeling, IL 60090

Havel's Inc. 800-638-4770
3726 Lonsdale St, Cincinnati, OH 45227

Incisiontech 800-213-7809
9 Technology Dr, Staunton, VA 24401

Livingston Products, Inc. 800-822-2156
260 Holbrook Dr Unit A, Wheeling, IL 60090
Laser Positioner-Crosshair locator for breast biopsy

Mcdalt Medical Corp. 800-841-5774
2225 Prestonwood Dr Ste 100-A, Arlington, TX 76012
CT, ultrasound, MRI, and interventional radiology.'HS Medical', Inc.

Medical Device Technologies, Inc. (Md Tech) 800-338-0440
3600 SW 47th Ave, Gainesville, FL 32608
Hawkins breast localization needle. Homer Mammolok breast localization needle.

Milex Products, Inc. 800-621-1278
4311 N Normandy Ave, Chicago, IL 60634
$15.00 per unit with three-finger-control syringe.

Ranfac Corp. 800-2RANFAC
30 Doherty Ave, Avon Industrial Park, Avon, MA 02322
Breast and foreign-body instrument.

Tegra Medical Inc. 508-541-4200
9 Forge Pkwy, Franklin, MA 02038
Biopsy needle for soft tissue; also, biopsy aspiration needle.

NEEDLE, BLOOD COLLECTION *(General) 80RHY*

Bio-Plexus, Inc. 800-223-0010
129 Reservoir Rd, Vernon, CT 06066

Cadence Science Inc. 888-717-7677
1979 Marcus Ave Ste 215, New Hyde Park, NY 11042
Reusable only.

Covidien Lp 508-261-8000
15 Hampshire St, Mansfield, MA 02048

Dma Med-Chem Corporation 800-362-1833
49 Watermill Ln, Great Neck, NY 11021

NEEDLE, BLOOD COLLECTION *(cont'd)*

Fenwal Inc. 800-766-1077
3 Corporate Dr, Lake Zurich, IL 60047
Blood recipient sets, transfer sets, transfusion sets.

Garren Scientific, Inc. 800-342-3725
15916 Blythe St Unit A, Van Nuys, CA 91406

Habley Medical Technology Corp. 800-729-1994
15721 Bernardo Heights Pkwy Ste B-30, San Diego, CA 92128
Safety blood-collection devices.

International Technidyne Corp. 800-631-5945
23 Nevsky St, Edison, NJ 08820
Heel incision device. Disposable incision making device for infant heel blood sampling. Available for premature infants and toddlers as well.

Palco Labs, Inc. 800-346-4488
8030 Soquel Ave Ste 104, Santa Cruz, CA 95062
EZ-let sterile needles for obtaining capillary blood samples. EZ-LETS II sterile, single use, disposable needles for obtaining capillary blood samples.

Specialized Health Products International, Inc. 800-306-3360
585 W 500 S, Bountiful, UT 84010
Monoject Magellan Safety Blood Collection Needle includes a needle, barrel, and built-in safety device for clinician safety. This innovative and cost effective integral design ensures that a new barrel is used for each patient, significantly reducing the risk of crosscontamination from reused barrels and accidental needlestick injuries.

Terumo Medical Corp. 800-283-7866
2101 Cottontail Ln, Somerset, NJ 08873

NEEDLE, BLUNT *(General) 80RHZ*

B. Braun Oem Division, B. Braun Medical Inc. 866-8-BBRAUN
824 12th Ave, Bethlehem, PA 18018

Cadence Science Inc. 888-717-7677
1979 Marcus Ave Ste 215, New Hyde Park, NY 11042
Reusable only.

Covidien Lp 508-261-8000
15 Hampshire St, Mansfield, MA 02048

Hamilton Company 800-648-5950
4990 Energy Way, Reno, NV 89502

Medical Device Technologies, Inc. (Md Tech) 800-338-0440
3600 SW 47th Ave, Gainesville, FL 32608
HAWKINS.

Ranfac Corp. 800-2RANFAC
30 Doherty Ave, Avon Industrial Park, Avon, MA 02322

Tegra Medical Inc. 508-541-4200
9 Forge Pkwy, Franklin, MA 02038

The Electrode Store 360-829-0400
PO Box 188, Enumclaw, WA 98022

NEEDLE, BONE MARROW *(Surgery) 79SGU*

Cadence Science Inc. 888-717-7677
1979 Marcus Ave Ste 215, New Hyde Park, NY 11042
7 types.

Havel's Inc. 800-638-4770
3726 Lonsdale St, Cincinnati, OH 45227

Lee Medical Ltd. 800-826-2360
5500 Lincoln Dr Ste 100, Minneapolis, MN 55436
Disposable bone marrow needles for aspiration, transplant and biopsy.

Ranfac Corp. 800-2RANFAC
30 Doherty Ave, Avon Industrial Park, Avon, MA 02322
$22.00 for biopsy needles. Goldenberg Snarecoil disposable bone-marrow instrument.

Rocket Medical Plc. 800-707-7625
150 Recreation Park Dr Ste 3, Hingham, MA 02043

Tegra Medical Inc. 508-541-4200
9 Forge Pkwy, Franklin, MA 02038

NEEDLE, CARDIAC *(Cardiovascular) 74RIA*

Boston Scientific Corporation 800-225-2732
1 Boston Scientific Pl, Natick, MA 01760
Entry needles for cardiovascular procedures.

Cadence Science Inc. 888-717-7677
1979 Marcus Ave Ste 215, New Hyde Park, NY 11042
Reusable only.

NEEDLE, CARDIAC *(cont'd)*

Covidien Lp 508-261-8000
15 Hampshire St, Mansfield, MA 02048
CARDIOPOINT cardiac surgery needles and ROTOGRIP sternal closure needles.

Ethicon, Inc. 800-4-ETHICON
Route 22 West, Somerville, NJ 08876

Tegra Medical Inc. 508-541-4200
9 Forge Pkwy, Franklin, MA 02038

NEEDLE, CATHETER *(Surgery) 79GCB*

Abbott Diagnostics Intl, Biotechnology Ltd 787-846-3500
Road #2 KM. 58.0 , PO Box 278, Cruce Davila, Barceloneta, PR 00617
Various types of catheter sets (sterile).

Angiotech 800-424-6779
241 W Palatine Rd, Wheeling, IL 60090
Interventional drainage catheters for nephrostomy, biliary, and general abcess drainage.

Becton Dickinson Infusion Therapy Systems, Inc. 888-237-2762
9450 S State St, Sandy, UT 84070

Bioform Medical, Inc. 262-835-3323
4133 Courtney Rd Ste 10, Franksville, WI 53126
Connector.

Cadence Science Inc. 888-717-7677
1979 Marcus Ave Ste 215, New Hyde Park, NY 11042

Kelsar, S.A. 508-261-8000
Blvd. Insurgentes, Libriamento a La, Tijuana 22450 Mexico
Thoracentesis systems, procedure trays

Kentron Health Care, Inc. 615-384-0573
3604 Kelton Jackson Rd, P.o. Box 120, Springfield, TN 37172
Scalp vein set.

Orthovita, Inc. 610-640-1775
77 Great Valley Pkwy, Malvern, PA 19355
Introduction catheter.

Tfx Medical Oem 800-548-6600
50 Plantation Dr, Jaffrey, NH 03452

NEEDLE, CHOLANGIOGRAPHY *(Cardiovascular) 74RIB*

Cadence Science Inc. 888-717-7677
1979 Marcus Ave Ste 215, New Hyde Park, NY 11042

Karl Storz Endoscopy-America Inc. 800-421-0837
600 Corporate Pointe, Culver City, CA 90230

Mahe International Inc. 800-294-7946
468 Craighead St, Nashville, TN 37204

Tegra Medical Inc. 508-541-4200
9 Forge Pkwy, Franklin, MA 02038

NEEDLE, CONDUCTION, ANESTHESIA (W/WO INTRODUCER) *(Anesthesiology) 73BSP*

Alcon Manufacturing, Ltd. 817-551-6813
714 Columbia Ave, Sinking Spring, PA 19608
Various retrobulbar and peribulbar ophthalmic anesthesia needles.

Avid Medical 800-886-0584
9000 Westmont Dr, Stonehouse Commerce Park, Toano, VA 23168
POLYMEDIC pencil-point spinal needles, tapered; also, regular pencil-point spinals. REGANES epidural needles, disposable metal- or plastic-hubbed Tuohy, Hustead, and Crawford epidural needles; sterile/non-sterile, custom kits available.

Ballard Medical Products 770-587-7835
12050 Lone Peak Pkwy, Draper, UT 84020
Epidural and spinal needles.

Busse Hospital Disposables, Inc. 631-435-4711
75 Arkay Dr, Hauppauge, NY 11788
Anesthesia conduction needles.

Cadence Science Inc. 888-717-7677
1979 Marcus Ave Ste 215, New Hyde Park, NY 11042
Reusable only.

Covidien Lp 508-261-8000
15 Hampshire St, Mansfield, MA 02048

Demetech Corp. 888-324-2447
3530 NW 115th Ave, Doral, FL 33178
Dental needle.

Dyna Medical Corp. 800-268-1181
843 Wellington St., London, ONT N6A-3S6 Canada
Atraumatic special sprotte needle

Havel's Inc. 800-638-4770
3726 Lonsdale St, Cincinnati, OH 45227

NEEDLE, CONDUCTION, ANESTHESIA (W/WO INTRODUCER) *(cont'd)*

Life-Tech, Inc. 281-491-6600
4235 Greenbriar Dr, Stafford, TX 77477
ProBloc insulated hypodermic needles for nerve location and nerve block anesthesia. ProLong insulated hypodermic needle and catheter kit for continuous nerve block anesthesia.

Medtronic Spine Llc 877-690-5353
1221 Crossman Ave, Sunnyvale, CA 94089
Sterile functional anaesthesia discography catheter system.

Neo Medical Inc. 888-450-3334
42514 Albrae St, Fremont, CA 94538
Regional anesthesia needle-sterile.

Spectra Medical Devices, Inc. 978-657-0889
260H Fordham Rd, Wilmington, MA 01887
Spinal needles & Epidural needles, metal and plastic hubs

NEEDLE, CUTTING, BIPOLAR, ELECTROCAUTERIZATION *(Surgery) 79SJW*

Gyrus Medical, Inc. 800-852-9361
6655 Wedgwood Rd N Ste 105, Maple Grove, MN 55311

NEEDLE, DENTAL *(Dental And Oral) 76DZM*

B&E Medical Systems 503-233-4872
1006 NE 2nd Ave, Portland, OR 97232
Needle cap holder.

Cadco Dental Products 800-833-8267
600 E Hueneme Rd, Oxnard, CA 93033
28g long or short nondeflecting needles. $7.00 each for use with hydrocolloid syringe.

Clive Craig Co. 805-488-1122
600 E Hueneme Rd, Oxnard, CA 93033
Needle, dental, various.

Covidien Lp 508-261-8000
15 Hampshire St, Mansfield, MA 02048
Available in two styles: 400 plastic self-threading hub and 401 metal pre-threaded hub-double-ended; Gauges: 25, 27 and 30 ga. needles; 25 and 27 ga. short and long lengths; 30 ga. short and extra short.

Dshealthcare Inc. 201-871-1232
85 W Forest Ave, Englewood, NJ 07631
Dental injection needle.

Dux Dental 800-833-8267
600 E Hueneme Rd, Oxnard, CA 93033
$7.00 each for use with hydrocolloid syringe. 28g long or short non-deflecting needle.

Exelint International Co. 800-940-3935
5840 W Centinela Ave, Los Angeles, CA 90045
EXEL SUPERJECT Dental Needle

Inter-Med, Inc. 877-418-4782
2200 Northwestern Ave, Racine, WI 53404
Needle tip.

Lightspeed Technology, Inc. 210-495-4942
403 E Ramsey Rd Ste 205, San Antonio, TX 78216
Dental sealer needle.

Myco Medical 800-454-6926
158 Towerview Ct, Cary, NC 27513

Pac-Dent Intl., Inc. 909-839-0888
21078 Commerce Point Dr, Walnut, CA 91789
Bendable needle tips.

Pulpdent Corp. 800-343-4342
80 Oakland St, Watertown, MA 02472
No common name listed.

Rocket Medical Plc. 800-707-7625
150 Recreation Park Dr Ste 3, Hingham, MA 02043

Specialty Appliance Works, Inc. 800-522-4636
4905 Hammond Industrial Dr, Cumming, GA 30041

Tegra Medical Inc. 508-541-4200
9 Forge Pkwy, Franklin, MA 02038

Ultradent Products, Inc. 801-553-4586
505 W 10200 S, South Jordan, UT 84095
Needle, dental.

Vita Needle Company 781-444-1780
919 Great Plain Ave, Needham, MA 02492
Reuseable, non-sterile manufacture to order, short and long runs. Gauges 3-34, ss 304 and ss 316.

NEEDLE, DENTAL *(cont'd)*

Young Microbrush Llc 262-375-4011
1376 Cheyenne Ave, Grafton, WI 53024

NEEDLE, DIALYSIS *(Gastro/Urology) 78RIC*

Kawasumi Laboratories America, Inc. 800-529-2786
4723 Oak Fair Blvd, Tampa, FL 33610

Medisystems Corporation 800-369-6334
439 S Union St Fl 5, Lawrence, MA 01843

NEEDLE, EMERGENCY AIRWAY *(Anesthesiology) 73BWC*

Instrumentation Industries, Inc. 800-633-8577
2990 Industrial Blvd, Bethel Park, PA 15102

Smiths Medical Asd 800-424-8662
5700 W 23rd Ave, Gary, IN 46406
Pedia-Trake kit and Nutrake kit components.

NEEDLE, ENDOSCOPIC *(Gastro/Urology) 78FBK*

Ballard Medical Products 770-587-7835
12050 Lone Peak Pkwy, Draper, UT 84020
Injection needle catheter.

Bryan Corp. 800-343-7711
4 Plympton St, Woburn, MA 01801
5mm/33cm suction/irrigation with needle, Bruhat Manlles coagulating needle 5mm insulated.

Cook Urological, Inc. 800-457-4500
1100 W Morgan St, P.O. Box 227, Spencer, IN 47460

Greenwald Surgical Co., Inc. 219-962-1604
2688 Dekalb St, Gary, IN 46405
Orandi injection needle.

Gyrus Acmi, Inc. 508-804-2739
93 N Pleasant St, Norwalk, OH 44857
Endoscopes and accessories.

Hobbs Medical, Inc. 860-684-5875
8 Spring St, Stafford Springs, CT 06076
Injection needle.

Karl Storz Endoscopy-America Inc. 800-421-0837
600 Corporate Pointe, Culver City, CA 90230

Mahe International Inc. 800-294-7946
468 Craighead St, Nashville, TN 37204

Ranfac Corp. 800-2RANFAC
30 Doherty Ave, Avon Industrial Park, Avon, MA 02322

Reznik Instrument, Inc. 847-673-3444
7337 Lawndale Ave, Skokie, IL 60076
Accessories (probes, suction tubes, needles, and electrodes).

Richard Wolf Medical Instruments Corp. 800-323-9653
353 Corporate Woods Pkwy, Vernon Hills, IL 60061

Tegra Medical Inc. 508-541-4200
9 Forge Pkwy, Franklin, MA 02038

United States Endoscopy Group 800-769-8226
5976 Heisley Rd, Mentor, OH 44060
ARTICULATOR Injection Needle, Disposable 5 mm 14 guage needle with needle introducer.

NEEDLE, FILTER *(General) 80VCQ*

Globetec Nonwovens 410-287-2207
40 Industrial Rd, North East, MD 21901

NEEDLE, FISTULA *(Gastro/Urology) 78FIE*

B. Braun Medical Inc., Renal Therapies Div. 800-854-6851
824 12th Ave, Bethlehem, PA 18018

Baxter Healthcare Corporation, Renal 888-229-0001
1620 S Waukegan Rd, Waukegan, IL 60085
Arteriovenous fistula sets with ultra thin wall needle and clamp.

Cadence Science Inc. 888-717-7677
1979 Marcus Ave Ste 215, New Hyde Park, NY 11042

Diasol, Inc. 800-366-0546
13212 Raymer St, North Hollywood, CA 91605
Fistulok & Needlelok: Mounts over a fistula needle, and encloses needle at removal time, protecting the personnel. Same with Needlelok, but for syringe/needle combo. Diaset: Bloodlines for dialysis use.

Exelint International Co. 800-940-3935
5840 W Centinela Ave, Los Angeles, CA 90045
EXEL A.V. Fistula needle sets.

Kentron Health Care, Inc. 615-384-0573
3604 Kelton Jackson Rd, P.o. Box 120, Springfield, TN 37172
Arterio venous fistula needles.

NEEDLE, FISTULA *(cont'd)*

Nxstage Medical, Inc. 866-697-8243
439 S Union St Fl 5, Lawrence, MA 01843
Apheresis Needle, Hemodialysis Fistula Needle Set, Medisystems ButtonHole Needle Set

Terumo Medical Corporation 800-283-7866
950 Elkton Blvd, P.O.Box 605, Elkton, MD 21921
Av fistula needle set.

NEEDLE, GASTRO-UROLOGY *(Gastro/Urology) 78FHR*

Avid Medical 800-886-0584
9000 Westmont Dr, Stonehouse Commerce Park, Toano, VA 23168
Seed-implant needles. Needles for brachytherapy procedures.

Biocompatibles Inc. 877-783-5463
115 Hurley Rd Bldg 3, Oxford, CT 06478
Aspiration biopsy needles.

Biomet Microfixation Inc. 800-874-7711
1520 Tradeport Dr, Jacksonville, FL 32218
Various types of needles.

Boston Scientific Corporation 508-652-5578
780 Brookside Dr, Spencer, IN 47460

Covidien Lp 508-261-8000
15 Hampshire St, Mansfield, MA 02048

International Hospital Supply Co. 800-398-9450
6914 Canby Ave Ste 105, Reseda, CA 91335

NEEDLE, HYPODERMIC *(General) 80RIE*

Air-Tite Products Co., Inc. 800-231-7762
565 Central Dr Ste 101, Virginia Beach, VA 23454
Henke Sass Wolf, TSK, Terumo Excel, $55 per thousand sterile disposable, hypodermic, single lumen needles in various sizes 32G to 14G available.

Cadence Science Inc. 888-717-7677
1979 Marcus Ave Ste 215, New Hyde Park, NY 11042
Over 100 sizes - all reusable - from 13G to 27G, 1/4in. to 3-1/2in., 5 types of points .

Chagrin Safety Supply, Inc. 800-227-0468
8227 Washington St # 1, Chagrin Falls, OH 44023

Cotran Corp. 800-345-4449
574 Park Ave, PO Box 130, Portsmouth, RI 02871
Stainless steel and disposable.

Covidien Lp 508-261-8000
15 Hampshire St, Mansfield, MA 02048

Dma Med-Chem Corporation 800-362-1833
49 Watermill Ln, Great Neck, NY 11021

Engineers Express, Inc. 800-255-8823
7 Industrial Park Rd, Medway, MA 02053

Exelint International Co. 800-940-3935
5840 W Centinela Ave, Los Angeles, CA 90045
EXEL Hypodermic Needles

Md Works, Inc. 770-409-9639
1895 Beaver Ridge Cir Ste 410, Norcross, GA 30071
Safety needle system

Myco Medical 800-454-6926
158 Towerview Ct, Cary, NC 27513
Reusable and disposable.

Precision Medical Products, Inc. 717-335-3700
44 Denver Rd, PO Box 300, Denver, PA 17517

Ranfac Corp. 800-2RANFAC
30 Doherty Ave, Avon Industrial Park, Avon, MA 02322
Made to customer specs - from 6 to 33 Gauge, any length, and with 6 different point styles and 7 hub types.

Specialized Health Products International, Inc. 800-306-3360
585 W 500 S, Bountiful, UT 84010
Monoject Magellan Safety Syringe Needle has a built-in safety mechanism that reduces the risk of accidental needlestick injuries. It may be activated by a simple press of the finger, or other hard surface, such as a table.

Tegra Medical Inc. 508-541-4200
9 Forge Pkwy, Franklin, MA 02038

Vita Needle Company 781-444-1780
919 Great Plain Ave, Needham, MA 02492
Reuseable, non-sterile manufacture to order, short and long runs. Gauges 3-34, ss 304 and ss 316.

NEEDLE, HYPODERMIC, SINGLE LUMEN WITH SYRINGE *(General) 80FMI*

Argon Medical Devices Inc. 903-675-9321
1445 Flat Creek Rd, Athens, TX 75751
Various types and sizes of sterile needles.

Atrion Medical Products, Inc. 800-343-9334
1426 Curt Francis Rd NW, Arab, AL 35016
Sharps Isolation and Counting Devices. Devices to monitor contaminated sharps and facilitate safe transfer or disposal.

Avid Medical 800-886-0584
9000 Westmont Dr, Stonehouse Commerce Park, Toano, VA 23168
REGANES vascular-access Huber-point infusion needles for vascular-access ports.

B. Braun Medical, Inc. 610-596-2536
901 Marcon Blvd, Allentown, PA 18109

Bard Reynosa S.A. De C.V. 908-277-8000
Blvd. Montebello #1, Parque Industrial Colonial
Reynosa, Tamaulipas Mexico
Various

Bd Medical 760-631-6520
4665 North Ave, Oceanside, CA 92056
Various.

Bd Medical - Diabetes Care 201-847-4298
1329 W US Highway 6 # &34, Holdrege, NE 68949
Pen needle.

Becton Dickinson And Company 800-284-6845
1 Becton Dr, Franklin Lakes, NJ 07417

Busse Hospital Disposables, Inc. 631-435-4711
75 Arkay Dr, Hauppauge, NY 11788
Needle stick block.

Cytyc Surgical Products 800-442-9892
250 Campus Dr, Marlborough, MA 01752
Hypodermic single lumen needle.

Daniels Sharpsmart, Inc. 559-351-9593
4144 E Therese Ave, Fresno, CA 93725
Sharps container.

Engineers Express, Inc. 800-255-8823
7 Industrial Park Rd, Medway, MA 02053

Gettig Pharmaceutical Instrument Co., Div Of Gettig Technologies Inc. 814-422-8892
1 Streamside Pl. W., Spring Mills, PA 16875-0085
Gettig Guard Safety Needle. Hypodermic needle with engineered needlestick prevention features.

Griff Industries, Inc. 800-709-4743
19761 Bahama St, Northridge, CA 91324
Point-lok needle safety device.

Health Care Logistics, Inc. 800-848-1633
450 Town St, PO Box 25, Circleville, OH 43113
Various.

Icu Medical (Ut), Inc 949-366-2183
4455 Atherton Dr, Salt Lake City, UT 84123
Sterile needle for blood collection.

Icu Medical, Inc. 800-824-7890
951 Calle Amanecer, San Clemente, CA 92673
Sterile needle for blood collection.

Ingenious Technologies Corp. 941-966-0690
1109 Millpond Ct, Osprey, FL 34229
Needle recapper.

International Medication Systems, Ltd. 800-423-4136
1886 Santa Anita Ave, South El Monte, CA 91733
Safety needle.

Kentron Health Care, Inc. 615-384-0573
3604 Kelton Jackson Rd, P.o. Box 120, Springfield, TN 37172
Hypodermic needles.

Lexamed 419-693-5307
705 Front St, Northwood, OH 43605
Blunt cannula, various types sterile.

Marquette Medical, Inc. 410-987-2994
1114 Benfield Blvd Ste L, Millersville, MD 21108
Various sizes of sterile, disposable hollow lumen needles.

Medical Action Industries, Inc. 800-645-7042
25 Heywood Rd, Arden, NC 28704
Needles.

NEEDLE, HYPODERMIC, SINGLE LUMEN WITH SYRINGE *(cont'd)*

Midwest Medical Solutions, Llc 800-451-6244
1310 Michigan St, Gary, IN 46402
Sharps container.

Navilyst Medical 800-833-9973
100 Boston Scientific Way, Marlborough, MA 01752
Various types of sterile needles.

North Safety Products 401-943-4400
1101 B Calle Neutron, Parque Industrial Maran, Mexicali, B.c. Mexico
Needle

Nxstage Medical, Inc. 866-697-8243
439 S Union St Fl 5, Lawrence, MA 01843
Multiple

Procedure Products, Inc. 360-693-1832
6622 Oakridge Dr, Gladstone, OR 97027
Needle, cardiovascular.

Scs Corporation 630-797-7300
1901 Powis Rd, West Chicago, IL 60185
Mail-back Disposal sharps/medical waste systems.

Stericycle 847-367-5910
28161 N Keith Dr, Lake Forest, IL 60045
Biobox Funnel Top (Various Sizes), Biobox Trap Top (Various Sizes)

Sterilogic Waste Systems, Inc. 315-455-5600
6691 Pickard Dr, Syracuse, NY 13211
Reusable sharps disposal container-accessory to hypodermic needle.

Terumo Cardiovascular Systems (Tcvs) 800-283-7866
28 Howe St, Ashland, MA 01721
Hypodermic needle.

Terumo Medical Corporation 800-283-7866
950 Elkton Blvd, P.O.Box 605, Elkton, MD 21921
Various hypodermic needle and accessories.

Therapeutic Silicone Technologies, Inc. 212-606-0830
909 5th Ave, New York, NY 10021
Hypodermic needle (30g x 400') with metal hub and luer lok.

Thomas Medical Products, Inc. 866-446-3003
65 Great Valley Pkwy, Malvern, PA 19355
Introducer needle.

Vascular Solutions, Inc. 763-656-4300
5025 Cheshire Ln N, Plymouth, MN 55446
Sclerotherapy kit.

Vidacare Corp. 800-680-4911
4350 Lockhill Selma Rd Ste 150, Shavano Park, TX 78249
EZ-IO

Vita Needle Company 781-444-1780
919 Great Plain Ave, Needham, MA 02492
Reuseable, non-sterile manufacture to order, short and long runs. Gauges 3-34, ss 304 and ss 316.

NEEDLE, HYPODERMIC, SINGLE LUMEN, REPROCESSED *(General) 80NKK*

Retractable Technologies, Inc. 888-806-2626
511 Lobo Ln, PO Box 9, Little Elm, TX 75068
VanishPoint Blood Collection Tube H; VanishPoint Small Tube Adapter

Stericycle 847-367-5910
28161 N Keith Dr, Lake Forest, IL 60045
Biobox Traptop (Various Sizes)

NEEDLE, INSUFFLATION, LAPAROSCOPIC *(Surgery) 79RKN*

Aesculap Implant Systems Inc. 1-800-234-9179
3773 Corporate Pkwy, Center Valley, PA 18034

Ams Innovative Center-San Jose 800-356-7600
3070 Orchard Dr, San Jose, CA 95134

Boss Instruments, Ltd. 800-210-2677
395 Reas Ford Rd Ste 120, Earlysville, VA 22936

Elmed, Inc. 630-543-2792
60 W Fay Ave, Addison, IL 60101

Ethicon Endo-Surgery, Inc. 800-USE-ENDO
4545 Creek Rd, Cincinnati, OH 45242
ENDOPATH 120mm and 150mm, ultra Veress needle.

Genicon 800-936-1020
6869 Stapoint Ct Ste 114, Winter Park, FL 32792
Disposable Veress Needles in both 120mm and 150mm working lengths

NEEDLE, INSUFFLATION, LAPAROSCOPIC *(cont'd)*

Gibbons Surgical Corp. 800-959-1989
1112 Jensen Dr Ste 101, Virginia Beach, VA 23451

Mectra Labs, Inc. 800-323-3968
PO Box 350, Two Quality Way, Bloomfield, IN 47424
Single patient use 120mm and 150mm lengths

Ranfac Corp. 800-2RANFAC
30 Doherty Ave, Avon Industrial Park, Avon, MA 02322
12- and 15-cm lenghts, color indicator and audible click.

Richard Wolf Medical Instruments Corp. 800-323-9653
353 Corporate Woods Pkwy, Vernon Hills, IL 60061

Smith & Nephew, Inc., Endoscopy Division 800-343-8386
150 Minuteman Rd, Andover, MA 01810

Synectic Medical Product Development 203-877-8488
60 Commerce Park, Milford, CT 06460

Tegra Medical Inc. 508-541-4200
9 Forge Pkwy, Franklin, MA 02038

NEEDLE, INTRA-ARTERIAL *(Cardiovascular) 74RIF*

Cadence Science Inc. 888-717-7677
1979 Marcus Ave Ste 215, New Hyde Park, NY 11042
Reusable only.

Ranfac Corp. 800-2RANFAC
30 Doherty Ave, Avon Industrial Park, Avon, MA 02322

Tegra Medical Inc. 508-541-4200
9 Forge Pkwy, Franklin, MA 02038

NEEDLE, INTRAVENOUS *(General) 80RIG*

Amsino International, Inc. 800-MD-AMSINO
855 Towne Center Dr, Pomona, CA 91767

B. Braun Oem Division, B. Braun Medical Inc. 866-8-BBRAUN
824 12th Ave, Bethlehem, PA 18018

Baxa Corporation 800-567-2292
9540 S Maroon Circle, Suite 400, Englewood, CO 80112
Huber point, 16 and 19 g only.

Baxter Healthcare Corporporation, Alternate Care And Channel Team 888-229-0001
25212 W Il Route 120, Round Lake, IL 60073
Solution Sets, Secondary Medication Sets, Extension Sets, IV Filtration Sets, Buretrol Solution Sets, Blood Sets, Blood Recipient Sets, Infusion Sets.

Becton Dickinson Infusion Therapy Systems, Inc. 888-237-2762
9450 S State St, Sandy, UT 84070

Cadence Science Inc. 888-717-7677
1979 Marcus Ave Ste 215, New Hyde Park, NY 11042
90 sizes & types - all reusable.

Covidien Lp 508-261-8000
15 Hampshire St, Mansfield, MA 02048

Kawasumi Laboratories America, Inc. 800-529-2786
4723 Oak Fair Blvd, Tampa, FL 33610
Winged small vein infusicn sets, K-Shield safety and standard available

Tegra Medical Inc. 508-541-4200
9 Forge Pkwy, Franklin, MA 02038

Vygon Corp. 800-544-4907
2495 General Armistead Ave, Norristown, PA 19403

NEEDLE, ISOTOPE, GOLD, TITANIUM, PLATINUM *(Radiology) 90IWF*

Isotope Products Laboratories, Inc. 661-309-1010
24937 Avenue Tibbitts, Valencia, CA 91355

NEEDLE, KNIFE *(Surgery) 79RDG*

Becton Dickinson And Co. 866-906-8080
411 Waverley Oaks Rd, Waltham, MA 02452

Fortrad Eye Instruments Corp. 973-543-2371
8 Franklin Rd, Mendham, NJ 07945

Miltex Inc. 800-645-8000
589 Davies Dr, York, PA 17402

NEEDLE, OPHTHALMIC *(Ophthalmology) 86RID*

Akorn, Inc. 800-535-7155
2500 Millbrook Dr, Buffalo Grove, IL 60089
Disposable retrobulbar and peribulbar needles.

Cadence Science Inc. 888-717-7677
1979 Marcus Ave Ste 215, New Hyde Park, NY 11042
12 sizes reusable lacrimal needles.

NEEDLE, OPHTHALMIC *(cont'd)*

Ethicon, Inc. 800-4-ETHICON
Route 22 West, Somerville, NJ 08876

Incisiontech 800-213-7809
9 Technology Dr, Staunton, VA 24401

Jedmed Instruments Co. 314-845-3770
5416 Jedmed Ct, Saint Louis, MO 63129

Miltex Inc. 800-645-8000
589 Davies Dr, York, PA 17402

Oasis Medical, Inc. 800-528-9786
514 S Vermont Ave, Glendora, CA 91741
Air and fluid injection.

Ranfac Corp. 800-2RANFAC
30 Doherty Ave, Avon Industrial Park, Avon, MA 02322
Eight types - from $7.50 to $13.00 each.

Rhein Medical, Inc. 800-637-4346
5460 Beaumont Center Blvd Ste 500, Suite 500, Tampa, FL 33634
Retrobulbar and peribulbar, disposable and reusable.

Stephens Instruments, Inc. 800-354-7848
2500 Sandersville Rd, Lexington, KY 40511
$11.67 each.

Tegra Medical Inc. 508-541-4200
9 Forge Pkwy, Franklin, MA 02038

NEEDLE, OTHER *(General) 80RIL*

Ad-Tech Medical Instrument Corp. 800-776-1555
1901 William St, Racine, WI 53404
Disposable biopsy needle. High quality, low cost needle with luer fitting hubs.

Air-Tite Products Co., Inc. 800-231-7762
565 Central Dr Ste 101, Virginia Beach, VA 23454
Becton Dickinson & Terumo 18G to 27G winged infusion sets. Ultra thin wall needles. Color coded with kink resistant tubing. TSK brand hypodermic needles up to 32G. Sterile and disposable.

B. Braun Medical, Inc. 610-596-2536
901 Marcon Blvd, Allentown, PA 18109
Duplex System

Bagshaw Company, Inc., W.H. 800-343-7467
1 Pine Street Ext, PO Box 766, Nashua, NH 03060
Vaccination needles.

Baxa Corporation 800-567-2292
9540 S Maroon Circle, Suite 400, Englewood, CO 80112
Two-Fer Needles. Non-coring Huber-point needles that can operate as vented or non-vented for IV admixture reconstitution and withdrawal.

Churchill Medical Systems, Inc. 800-468-0585
935 Horsham Rd Ste M, Horsham, PA 19044
Non-coring needle. Needleless sets and accessories.

Colorado Serum Company 303-295-7527
4950 York St, PO Box 16428, Denver, CO 80216
Veterinary needles.

Covidien Lp 508-261-8000
15 Hampshire St, Mansfield, MA 02048

Dapco Industries 800-597-2726
241 Ethan Allen Hwy, Ridgefield, CT 06877
Ultrasonic hydrophone needle probes.

Dma Med-Chem Corporation 800-362-1833
49 Watermill Ln, Great Neck, NY 11021

Engineers Express, Inc. 800-255-8823
7 Industrial Park Rd, Medway, MA 02053

Exelint International Co. 800-940-3935
5840 W Centinela Ave, Los Angeles, CA 90045
Multi-drawing needles, port access Huber needles and sets, non-coring needles. EXEL Secure Touch Safety P.S.V. and A.V. sets.

Fenwal Inc. 800-766-1077
3 Corporate Dr, Lake Zurich, IL 60047
Ultra thinwall donor.

Gish Biomedical, Inc. 800-938-0531
22942 Arroyo Vis, Rancho Santa Margarita, CA 92688
Huber port access needle with extension tubing.

Gyrus Medical, Inc. 800-852-9361
6655 Wedgwood Rd N Ste 105, Maple Grove, MN 55311
BILAP electrosurgical single-wire bipolar needle electrode used for cutting in laparscopic procedures.

NEEDLE, OTHER *(cont'd)*

Halkey-Roberts Corp. 800-303-4384
2700 Halkey Roberts Pl N, Saint Petersburg, FL 33716
ROBERTSITE Swabable Needleless Valves

Harmac Medical Products, Inc. 716-897-4500
2201 Bailey Ave, Buffalo, NY 14211
Private-labeled Huber needle assemblies and extension sets. Available in 19, 20, and 22 gauge needles of various lengths, with or without injection site. Custom packaging and labeling available. Now offering Huber needle extension sets with DEHP-free, polyethylene-lined inner tubing.

Hart Enterprises, Inc. 616-887-0400
400 Apple Jack Ct, Sparta, MI 49345
Special application needles for guidewire introduction, FNA biopsy, and core biopsy.

Hospira Inc. 877-946-7747
275 N Field Dr, Lake Forest, IL 60045
Hospira Butterfly

Hospital Marketing Svcs. Company, Inc. 800-786-5094
162 Great Hill Rd./ Ind. Park, Naugatuck, CT 06770

Integral Design Inc. 781-740-2036
52 Burr Rd, Hingham, MA 02043

Ispg, Inc. 860-355-3511
517 Litchfield Rd, New Milford, CT 06776
Epidural and spinal needles, huber, chiba needles, custom cannulae.

Kawasumi Laboratories America, Inc. 800-529-2786
4723 Oak Fair Blvd, Tampa, FL 33610
Huber needle infusion sets, K-Shield safety and standard

Kck Industries 888-800-1967
14941 Calvert St, Van Nuys, CA 91411

Medi-Globe Corporation 800-966-1431
110 W Orion St Ste 136, Tempe, AZ 85283
Sclerotherapy needles; double lumina coaxial needles, G.I. ultrasonic aspiration and biopsy needles.

Medikmark Inc. 800-424-3520
3600 Burwood Dr, Waukegan, IL 60085
Specialty needles.

Mps Acacia 800-486-6677
785 Challenger St, Brea, CA 92821

Neogen Corporation 800-234-5333
620 Lesher Pl, Lansing, MI 48912
Disposable needles for veterinary use only.

Smiths Medical Asd 800-424-3662
5700 W 23rd Ave, Gary, IN 46406
TE puncture kit for Tracheosopaheal puncture. Needle, guidewire and 14Fr Silicone dilator.

Smiths Medical Asd, Inc. 800-433-5832
1265 Grey Fox Rd, Saint Paul, MN 55112
GRIPPER PLUS safety huber needles and PORT-A-CATH plastic hub needles for use with implantable vascular access systems.

Tegra Medical Inc. 508-541-4200
9 Forge Pkwy, Franklin, MA 02038
Epidural needle.

Telemed Systems Inc. 800-481-3718
8 Kane Industrial Dr, Hudson, MA 01749
Transbronchial needles.

Tfx Medical Oem 800-548-3600
50 Plantation Dr, Jaffrey, NH 03452

Vlv Associates, Inc. 973-428-2884
30C Ridgedale Ave, East Hanover, NJ 07936
Safety Huber Needle

Wisap America 800-233-8448
8231 Melrose Dr, Lenexa, KS 66214

NEEDLE, PHACOEMULSIFICATION, REPROCESSED
(Ophthalmology) 86NKX

Ascent Healthcare Solutions 480-763-5300
10232 S 51st St, Phoenix, AZ 85044
Phaco tip.

Medisiss 866-866-7477
2747 SW 6th St, Redmond, OR 97756
Various reprocessed phacoemulsification tips, sterile.

Sterilmed, Inc. 763-488-3400
11400 73rd Ave N Ste 100, Maple Grove, MN 55369
Phaco tips.

NEEDLE, PNEUMOPERITONEUM, SIMPLE
(Gastro/Urology) 78FHP

Elmed, Inc. 630-543-2792
60 W Fay Ave, Addison, IL 60101

Ethicon Endo-Surgery, Inc. 877-384-4266
3801 University Blvd SE, Albuquerque, NM 87106
Sterile veress needle.

Karl Storz Endoscopy-America Inc. 800-421-0837
600 Corporate Pointe, Culver City, CA 90230

Mahe International Inc. 800-294-7946
468 Craighead St, Nashville, TN 37204

Richard Wolf Medical Instruments Corp. 800-323-9653
353 Corporate Woods Pkwy, Vernon Hills, IL 60061

NEEDLE, PNEUMOPERITONEUM, SPRING LOADED
(Gastro/Urology) 78FHO

Apple Medical Corp. 508-357-2700
28 Lord Rd Ste 135, Marlborough, MA 01752
Laparoscopic insufflation needle.

Ethicon Endo-Surgery, Inc. 877-384-4266
3801 University Blvd SE, Albuquerque, NM 87106
Various sterile disposable pneumoperitoneum needles.

Gyrus Acmi, Inc. 508-804-2739
93 N Pleasant St, Norwalk, OH 44857
Veress needle.

Gyrus Acmi, Inc. 508-804-2739
300 Stillwater P.o.box 1971, Stamford, CT 06902
Veress needle.

Karl Storz Endoscopy-America Inc. 800-421-0837
600 Corporate Pointe, Culver City, CA 90230

Mahe International Inc. 800-294-7946
468 Craighead St, Nashville, TN 37204

Ranfac Corp. 800-2RANFAC
30 Doherty Ave, Avon Industrial Park, Avon, MA 02322

Ussc Puerto Rico, Inc. 203-845-1000
Building 911-67, Sabanetas Industrial Park, Ponce, PR 00731
Various sizes and types of pneumoperioneum needles.

NEEDLE, RADIOGRAPHIC *(Radiology) 90RIH*

Cadence Science Inc. 888-717-7677
1979 Marcus Ave Ste 215, New Hyde Park, NY 11042

Havel's Inc. 800-638-4770
3726 Lonsdale St, Cincinnati, OH 45227

Ranfac Corp. 800-2RANFAC
30 Doherty Ave, Avon Industrial Park, Avon, MA 02322
Ten types - from $24.00 to $60.00 each.

Spectra Medical Devices, Inc. 978-657-0889
260H Fordham Rd, Wilmington, MA 01887
guidewire introducer needles

Tegra Medical Inc. 508-541-4200
9 Forge Pkwy, Franklin, MA 02038

NEEDLE, SCALP *(Cns/Neurology) 84RII*

Exelint International Co. 800-940-3935
5840 W Centinela Ave, Los Angeles, CA 90045
Scalp Vein (Butterfly) Sets

Myco Medical 800-454-6926
158 Towerview Ct, Cary, NC 27513
Safety and standard winged infusion sets 19-26G. Epidural and spinal needles.

Vygon Corp. 800-544-4907
2495 General Armistead Ave, Norristown, PA 19403
Scalp vein needle.

NEEDLE, SPINAL, SHORT-TERM *(General) 80MIA*

Avid Medical 800-886-0584
9000 Westmont Dr, Stonehouse Commerce Park, Toano, VA 23168
REGANES disposable Quincke-point spinals and Whitacre-style pencil-point needles.

B. Braun Oem Division, B. Braun Medical Inc. 866-8-BBRAUN
824 12th Ave, Bethlehem, PA 18018

Biocompatibles Inc. 877-783-5463
115 Hurley Rd Bldg 3, Oxford, CT 06478
Spinal needle.

Cadence Science Inc. 888-717-7677
1979 Marcus Ave Ste 215, New Hyde Park, NY 11042
60 sizes - all reusable - 12G to 26G, 1-1/2in. to 7in., 3 point types.

NEEDLE, SPINAL, SHORT-TERM *(cont'd)*

Covidien Lp 508-261-8000
15 Hampshire St, Mansfield, MA 02048

Engineers Express, Inc. 800-255-8823
7 Industrial Park Rd, Medway, MA 02053

Exelint International Co. 800-940-3935
5840 W Centinela Ave, Los Angeles, CA 90045
EXEL Spinal Needles (Quinkee Bevel)

Hart Enterprises, Inc. 616-887-0400
400 Apple Jack Ct, Sparta, MI 49345
Disposable Quincke and atraumatic spinal needles.

Ispg, Inc. 860-355-8511
517 Litchfield Rd, New Milford, CT 06776

Kmedic 800-955-0559
190 Veterans Dr, Northvale, NJ 07647
Kerrison Punch, CLEANPUNCH new Kerrison spinal punch designed to be completely cleaned. Easily disassembles and reassembles - all parts remain connected. Patented.

Myco Medical 800-454-6926
158 Towerview Ct, Cary, NC 27513
Phoenix spinal, epidural, and biopsy needles.

Pain Products International 800-359-5756
4763 Hamilton Wolfe Rd # 210, San Antonio, TX 78229

Promex Technologies, Llc 317-736-0128
3049 Hudson St, Franklin, IN 46131
Spinal needle.

Ranfac Corp. 800-2RANFAC
30 Doherty Ave, Avon Industrial Park, Avon, MA 02322
Made to order RW or TW from 25 Ga. to 10 Ga., up to 12 L; reusable.

Smith & Nephew, Inc., Endoscopy Division 800-343-8386
130 Forbes Blvd, Mansfield, MA 02048

Spectra Medical Devices, Inc. 978-657-0889
260H Fordham Rd, Wilmington, MA 01887
custom manufactured spinals

Tegra Medical Inc. 508-541-4200
9 Forge Pkwy, Franklin, MA 02038

Vita Needle Company 781-444-1780
919 Great Plain Ave, Needham, MA 02492
Short runs, non-short-term. Reuseable, non-sterile manufacture to order, short and long runs. Gauges 3-34, ss 304 and ss 316.

Vygon Corp. 800-544-4907
2495 General Armistead Ave, Norristown, PA 19403
Epidural.

NEEDLE, SUTURE, DISPOSABLE *(Surgery) 79GAB*

Alcon Research, Ltd. 800-862-5266
6201 South Fwy, Fort Worth, TX 76134

Anchor Products Company 800-323-5134
52 W Official Rd, Addison, IL 60101
$240.00 per 144 (72/2 in).

Biomet Microfixation Inc. 800-874-7711
1520 Tradeport Dr, Jacksonville, FL 32218
Various types of needles.

Boston Scientific - Marina Bay Customer Fulfillment Center 617-689-6000
500 Commander Shea Blvd, Quincy, MA 02171
Various.

Boston Scientific Corporation 508-652-5578
8600 NW 41st St, Doral, FL 33166

Boston Scientific Corporation 508-652-5578
780 Brookside Dr, Spencer, IN 47460

Cincinnati Surgical Company 800-544-3100
11256 Cornell Park Dr, Cincinnati, OH 45242

Depuy Mitek, A Johnson & Johnson Company 800-451-2006
50 Scotland Blvd, Bridgewater, MA 02324
Eyed suturing needle.

Ethicon, Inc. 800-4-ETHICON
Route 22 West, Somerville, NJ 08876

Hospital Marketing Svcs. Company, Inc. 800-786-5094
162 Great Hill Rd./ Ind. Park, Naugatuck, CT 06770
HMS TORRINGTON - 100 (1 box) sterile, french spring eye.

Kelsar, S.A. 508-261-8000
Blvd. Insurgentes, Libriamento a La, Tijuana 22450 Mexico
Suturing, dental, fistula, gastro-urology, neurosurgical, opthalmic, tonsil

NEEDLE, SUTURE, DISPOSABLE *(cont'd)*

Lemaitre Vascular, Inc. 781-221-2266
63 2nd Ave, Burlington, MA 01803
GRICE SUTURE NEEDLE

Myco Medical 800-454-6926
158 Towerview Ct, Cary, NC 27513
Full line of absorbable and nonabsorbable sutures.

Roboz Surgical Instrument Co., Inc. 800-424-2984
PO Box 10710, Gaithersburg, MD 20898

Suturtek Incorporated
51 Middlesex St, North Chelmsford, MA 01863
Suture, needle.

NEEDLE, SUTURE, OPHTHALMIC *(Ophthalmology) 86HNM*

Escalon Trek Medical 800-433-8197
2440 S 179th St, New Berlin, WI 53146
Suturing needle.

Fischer Surgical Inc. 314-303-7753
1343 Pine Dr, Arnold, MO 63010
Various types of ophthalmic suturing needleholders.

Fortrad Eye Instruments Corp. 973-543-2371
8 Franklin Rd, Mendham, NJ 07945

Hai Laboratories, Inc. 781-862-9884
320 Massachusetts Ave, Lexington, MA 02420
Ophthalmic suturing needle - various types.

Harvey Precision Instruments 707-793-2600
217 Fairway Rd, Cape Haze, FL 33947
Various ophthalmic suturing needles and accessories.

Surgical Instrument Manufacturers, Inc. 800-521-2985
1650 Headland Dr, Fenton, MO 63026

NEEDLE, SUTURE, REUSABLE *(Surgery) 79GDL*

Anchor Products Company 800-323-5134
52 W Official Rd, Addison, IL 60101
$12.30 per 12 (1/2 in).

Cincinnati Surgical Company 800-544-3100
11256 Cornell Park Dr, Cincinnati, OH 45242

Havel's Inc. 800-638-4770
3726 Lonsdale St, Cincinnati, OH 45227

Hospital Marketing Svcs. Company, Inc. 800-786-5094
162 Great Hill Rd./ Ind. Park, Naugatuck, CT 06770
HMS TORRINGTON - french spring eye, and regular eye, 12 per package.

Miltex Inc. 800-645-8000
589 Davies Dr, York, PA 17402

NEISSERIA, DNA REAGENTS *(Microbiology) 83LSL*

Abbott Molecular, Inc. 847-937-6100
1300 E Touhy Ave, Des Plaines, IL 60018
Pcr ct-ng assay.

Qiagen Gaithersburg, Inc. 800-344-3631
1201 Clopper Rd, Gaithersburg, MD 20878
Reagents for the detection of neisseria gonorrheae (gc) dna.

Roche Molecular Systems, Inc. 925-730-8110
4300 Hacienda Dr, Pleasanton, CA 94588
Various neisseria gonorrhoea tests, gonorrhoea serological reagents.

NEPHELOMETER *(Chemistry) 75JQX*

Beckman Coulter, Inc. 800-742-2345
250 S Kraemer Blvd, PO Box 8000, Brea, CA 92821

Dade Behring, Inc. 800-948-3233
1717 Deerfield Rd, Deerfield, IL 60015
BN ProSpec; BN100 system; BNII system.

Lamotte Co. 800-344-3100
802 Washington Ave, PO Box 329, Chestertown, MD 21620
Digital, portable meter measures 0-20 and 0-200 NTU turbidity levels.

Orbeco Analytical Systems, Inc. 800-922-5242
185 Marine St, Farmingdale, NY 11735
$995.00 ea. digital EPA accepted 0-1000 ntu. in 3 ranges.

NEPHELOMETER, IMMUNOLOGY *(Immunology) 82JZW*

Beckman Coulter, Inc. 800-742-2345
250 S Kraemer Blvd, PO Box 8000, Brea, CA 92821

Diasorin Inc 800-328-1482
1951 Northwestern Ave S, PO Box 285, Stillwater, MN 55082

NEPHELOMETRIC INHIBITION IMMUNOASSAY, PHENOBARBITAL *(Toxicology) 91LFN*

Beckman Coulter, Inc. 800-635-3497
740 W 83rd St, Hialeah, FL 33014

NEPHELOMETRIC METHOD, IMMUNOGLOBULINS (G, A, M) *(Chemistry) 75CFN*

Beckman Coulter, Inc. 800-635-3497
740 W 83rd St, Hialeah, FL 33014
$0.90 per test.

Kamiya Biomedical Company 206-575-8068
12779 Gateway Dr S, Tukwila, WA 98168
Diagnostic immunoturbidimetric assay kits for IgG, IgA, IgM and calibrators. K-ASSAY High Sensitive CRP(2) & (3), all liquid reagents adaptable to automated chemistry analyzers for the measurement of low level C-reactive protein in serum.

Raichem, Division Of Hemagen Diagnostics, Inc. 800-438-6100
8225 Mercury Ct, San Diego, CA 92111
SPIA IgA, IgM, and IgG Reagent, Immunoturbidimetric Assay System.

NEPHELOMETRIC METHOD, LIPOPROTEINS *(Chemistry) 75JHQ*

Dade Behring, Inc. 800-948-3233
1717 Deerfield Rd, Deerfield, IL 60015

NEPHELOMETRIC, AMYLASE *(Chemistry) 75KHM*

Dade Behring, Inc. 800-948-3233
1717 Deerfield Rd, Deerfield, IL 60015

NEPHROSCOPE SET *(Gastro/Urology) 78FGA*

Karl Storz Endoscopy-America Inc. 800-421-0837
600 Corporate Pointe, Culver City, CA 90230

Mahe International Inc. 800-294-7946
468 Craighead St, Nashville, TN 37204

Pentax Southern Region Service Center 201-571-2300
8934 Kirby Dr, Houston, TX 77054
Nephroscope.

Pentax West Coast Service Center 800-431-5880
10410 Pioneer Blvd Ste 2, Santa Fe Springs, CA 90670
Pentax nephroscope.

NEPHROSCOPE, FLEXIBLE *(Gastro/Urology) 78RIM*

Olympus America, Inc. 800-645-8160
3500 Corporate Pkwy, PO Box 610, Center Valley, PA 18034

Pentax Medical Company 800-431-5880
102 Chestnut Ridge Rd, Montvale, NJ 07645
$16,170.00 for choledocho-nephro fiberscopes with distal tip diameter 4.8mm and channel size 2.2mm; fully immersible. $19,950.00 for choledocho-nephro video endoscope with monochrome CCD chip technology. Distal tip diameter of 5.3mm and channel size 2.0mm.

Richard Wolf Medical Instruments Corp. 800-323-9653
353 Corporate Woods Pkwy, Vernon Hills, IL 60061

NEPHROSCOPE, RIGID *(Gastro/Urology) 78RIN*

Karl Storz Endoscopy-America Inc. 800-421-0837
600 Corporate Pointe, Culver City, CA 90230

Mahe International Inc. 800-294-7946
468 Craighead St, Nashville, TN 37204

Richard Wolf Medical Instruments Corp. 800-323-9653
353 Corporate Woods Pkwy, Vernon Hills, IL 60061

NERVE, STIMULATOR, ELECTRICAL, PERCUTANEOUS (PENS) FOR PAIN RELIEF *(Cns/Neurology) 84NHI*

Biowave Corporation 203-855-8610
16 Knight St, Norwalk, CT 06851
Pens.

NEURAMININASE (SIALIDASE) *(Pathology) 88IBE*

Lonza Walkersville, Inc. 201-316-9200
8830 Biggs Ford Rd, Walkersville, MD 21793
Receptor-destroying enzyme (vibrio cholerae extract).

NINHYDRIN AND L-LEUCYL-L-ALANINE (FLUORIMETRIC) *(Chemistry) 75JNB*

Astoria-Pacific,Inc. 800-536-3111
PO Box 830, Clackamas, OR 97015
For measuring phenylalanine content in infant blood serum.

Neo-Genesis, A Division Of Natus 503-657-8000
15140 SE 82nd Dr Ste 270, Clackamas, OR 97015
Phenylalanine test system.

NINHYDRIN, NITROGEN (AMINO-NITROGEN) *(Chemistry) 75JMX*

Beckman Coulter, Inc. 800-742-2345
250 S Kraemer Blvd, PO Box 8000, Brea, CA 92821

NIPPER, MALLEUS *(Ear/Nose/Throat) 77JYR*

Aesculap Implant Systems Inc. 1-800-234-9179
3773 Corporate Pkwy, Center Valley, PA 18034

Bausch & Lomb Surgical 636-255-5051
3365 Tree Court Ind Blvd, Saint Louis, MO 63122

Biomet Microfixation Inc. 800-874-7711
1520 Tradeport Dr, Jacksonville, FL 32218
Nipper, malleus.

Toolmex Corporation 800-992-4766
1075 Worcester St, Natick, MA 01760

NIPPLE, FEEDING *(General) 80FNN*

Hi-Tech Rubber, Inc. 800-924-4832
3191 E La Palma Ave, Anaheim, CA 92806

Hospira 800-441-4100
268 E 4th St, Ashland, OH 44805
Bottle nipple.

Monroe Mfg., Inc. 318-338-3172
3030 Aurora Ave, 2nd Fl., Monroe, LA 71201
Los- mos-lol-mol pacifier with medium/large orthodontic silicone/ latex nipple.

NITROPHENYLPHOSPHATE, ALKALINE PHOSPHATASE OR ISOENZYMES *(Chemistry) 75CJE*

Abbott Diagnostics Div. 626-440-0700
820 Mission St, South Pasadena, CA 91030
Alkaline phosphatase.

Amresco Inc. 800-366-1313
30175 Solon Industrial Pkwy, Solon, OH 44139
Hitachi, technicon RA, SMAC and SMA systems.

Biomerieux Inc. 800-682-2666
100 Rodolphe St, Durham, NC 27712

Caldon Bioscience, Inc. 909-628-9944
2100 S Reservoir St, Pomona, CA 91766
Alkaline phosphatase.

Caldon Biotech, Inc. 757-224-0177
2251 Rutherford Rd, Carlsbad, CA 92008
Alkaline phosphatase.

Carolina Liquid Chemistries Corp. 800-471-7272
510 W Central Ave Ste C, Brea, CA 92821
Alp.

Genchem, Inc. 714-529-1616
510 W Central Ave Ste D, Brea, CA 92821
Alkaline phosphatase reagent.

Health Chem Diagnostics Llc 954-979-3845
3341 W McNab Rd, Pompano Beach, FL 33069
Nitrophenylphosphate, alkaline phosphatase or isoenzymes.

Hemagen Diagnostics, Inc. 800-436-2436
9033 Red Branch Rd, Columbia, MD 21045
Various alkaline phosphatase test methods.

Jas Diagnostics, Inc. 305-418-2320
7220 NW 58th St, Miami, FL 33166
Alkaline phosphatase.

Sterling Diagnostics, Inc. 800-637-2661
36645 Metro Ct, Sterling Heights, MI 48312
Alkaline phosphatase (rate) reagent set.

Synermed Intl., Inc. 317-896-1565
17408 Tiller Ct Ste 1900, Westfield, IN 46074
Alkaline phosphatase reagent kit.

Teco Diagnostics 714-693-7788
1268 N Lakeview Ave, Anaheim, CA 92807
Alkaline phosphatase, kinetic.

Vital Diagnostics Inc. 714-672-3553
1075 W Lambert Rd Ste D, Brea, CA 92821
Various alkaline phosphatase reagents.

NITROPRUSSIDE, KETONES (URINARY, NON-QUANTITATIVE) *(Chemistry) 75JIN*

Abbott Diagnostics Intl, Biotechnology Ltd 787-846-3500
Road #2 KM. 58.0 , PO Box 278, Cruce Davila, Barceloneta, PR 00617
Various: B ketone or glucose test strips and control solutions.

Arkray Factory Usa, Inc. 952-646-3168
5182 W 76th St, Minneapolis, MN 55439
Urine test strips.

NITROPRUSSIDE, KETONES (URINARY, NON-QUANTITATIVE) *(cont'd)*

Bayer Healthcare Llc 914-524-2955
555 White Plains Rd Fl 5, Tarrytown, NY 10591
Test for glucose & ketones in urine.

Bayer Healthcare, Llc 574-256-3430
430 S Beiger St, Mishawaka, IN 46544
Test for glucose & ketones in urine.

D-Tek Llc 215-245-5270
3580 Progress Dr Ste J3, Bensalem, PA 19020

Global Healthcheck, Inc. 949-757-0639
2417 34th St Unit 17, Santa Monica, CA 90405
Urine ketone test.

Lamotte Chemical Products Company 856-467-2000
802 Washington Ave, Chestertown, MD 21620
Urine ketone test.

Neo Pharm Inc. 714-226-0070
10532 Walker St Ste B, Cypress, CA 90630
Ketones (non-quantitative) test system.

Nipro Diagnostics, Inc. 1-800-342-7226
2400 NW 55th Ct, Fort Lauderdale, FL 33309
Test strips for ketones in urine.

Stanbio Life Sciences, Division Of Stanbio Laboratory 830-249-0772
25235 Leer Dr, Elkhart, IN 46514

Teco Diagnostics 714-693-7788
1268 N Lakeview Ave, Anaheim, CA 92807
Urine reagent strip-ik (urs-ik).

NITROSALICYLATE REDUCTION, AMYLASE *(Chemistry) 75CJD*

Teco Diagnostics 714-693-7788
1268 N Lakeview Ave, Anaheim, CA 92807
Same.

NITROUS ACID & NITROSONAPHTHOL, 5-HYDROXYINDOLE ACETIC ACID *(Chemistry) 75CDA*

Bio-Rad Laboratories Inc., Clinical Systems Div. 800-224-6723
4000 Alfred Nobel Dr, Hercules, CA 94547
5-hiaa by hplc.

NONABSORBABLE GAUZE, SURGICAL SPONGE, & WOUND DRESSING FOR EXTERNAL USE (WITH A DRUG) *(General) 80MXI*

Elamex S.A. De C.V. 52-16-164333
Av. Insurgentes 4145 lote., Cd. Jiarex, Chih Mexico
Various

NUCLEAR MAGNETIC RESONANCE EQUIPMENT, LABORATORY *(Chemistry) 75UGY*

Jeol Usa, Inc. 978-536-2270
11 Dearborn Rd, Peabody, MA 01960

Kontes Glass Co. 888-546-2531
1022 Spruce St, Vineland, NJ 08360

NUCLEAR MAGNETIC RESONANCE IMAGING SYSTEM *(Radiology) 90LNH*

Aurora Imaging Technology, Inc. 978-975-7530
39 High St, North Andover, MA 01845
Aurora.

Avotec, Inc. 800-272-2238
603 NW Buck Hendry Way, Stuart, FL 34994
Silent Scan-Hearing Protect

Chamco, Inc. 888-674-6683
798 Clearlake Rd, Cocoa, FL 32922
Various.

Diagnosoft, Inc. 650-320-9397
3461 Kenneth Dr, Palo Alto, CA 94303
Harp.

Engineering Services Kenneth C. Saltrick Inc. 330-425-9279
2200 E Enterprise Pkwy, Twinsburg, OH 44087
Mri internal cable assemblies accessory mri communication devices.

Fonar Corp. 888-NEEDMRI
110 Marcus Dr, Melville, NY 11747

Ge Magnets 847-277-5002
3001 W Radio Dr, Florence, SC 29501
Various models of magnetic resonance imaging systems.

Ge Medical Systems, Llc 262-312-7117
3200 N Grandview Blvd, Waukesha, WI 53188
Various models of magnetic resonance imaging systems.

NUCLEAR MAGNETIC RESONANCE IMAGING SYSTEM *(cont'd)*

Hitachi Medical Systems America, Inc. 800-800-3106
1959 Summit Commerce Park, Twinsburg, OH 44087
Hitachi Medical Systems America, Inc. is the leader in the advancement of Open Magnet Resonance imaging systems. Hitachi offers the AIRIS Elite, Altaire and AIRIS II MR systems. AIRIS Elite breaks through mid-field price/performance conventions with throughput and advanced capabilities previously considered high-field only. Features available on AIRIS Elite include Scaleable Dual Quad RF system, higher-orde active shim technology and higher-performance gradients, sequences such as RF FatSat, Single-Shot EPI-based Diffusion Weighted Imaging with ADC mapping, Balanced SARGE, Contrast Enhanced MRA and more. Altaire combines high-field performance with the patient comfort of Open MR, offering a no-compromise imaging platform. Altaire employs superconducting technology to generate a 0.7 Tesla field strength in a vertical orientation with extremely high homogeneity. Its high power, high slew rate gradients are competitive with those of traditional high-field sytems, and a variety of advanced imaging techniques can be applied with Altaire. The advanced RF system employs a quadrature transmitter design for exceptionally high uniformity. The multiple array receiver platform offers high uniform noise coverage, enhancing patient throughput and reducing study times. The computer system uses state-of-the-art technology featuring extremely fast processors with comprehensive multi-tasking capabilities. The AIRIS II premium performance Open MR system provides a 0.3T field strength and advanced permanent magnet technology for outstanding image quality. AIRIS II also offers superb imaging for a wide range of clinical applications and diagnostic procedures. Both products feature Hitachi's award-winning asymmetric two-post gantry design that provides easy patient access from all four sides in a non-claustrophobic environment for the ultimate in patient comfort.

I.Z.I. Medical Products, Inc. 800-231-1499
7020 Tudsbury Rd, Baltimore, MD 21244
Fat saturatuin and mri accessory device.

Icad Inc 603-882-5200
245 Main St Ste 620, White Plains, NY 10601
Medical imaging software.

Icad Inc. 866-280-2239
98 Spit Brook Rd Ste 100, Nashua, NH 03062
Specra/VividLook CADvue

Invivo 800-331-3220
12501 Research Pkwy, Orlando, FL 32826

Magna-Lab, Inc. 516-393-5874
6800 Jericho Tpke Ste 120W, Syosset, NY 11791
Magna-sl.

Magne Vu 760-929-8000
1916 Palomar Oaks Way Ste 150, Carlsbad, CA 92008
Magnetic resonance imaging system.

Marconi Medical Systems 800-323-0550
595 Miner Rd, Cleveland, OH 44143

Medtronic Image-Guided Neurologics, Inc. 800-707-0933
2290 W Eau Gallie Blvd, Melbourne, FL 32935
Equipment cover/drape.

Neurognostics, Inc. 414-727-7950
10437 W Innovation Dr Ste 309, Milwaukee, WI 53226
Functional magnetic resonance imaging.

Oni Medical Systems, Inc. 978-658-0020
301 Ballardvale St Ste 4, Wilmington, MA 01887
Orthopedic magnetic resonance imaging system

Penn Diagnostics 301-279-5958
14 Clemson Ct, Rockville, MD 20850
Medical imaging processing system.

Portal, Inc. 435-753-3598
1350 N 200 W Ste 6, Logan, UT 84341
Axial compression device.

Prism Clinical Imaging, Inc. 414-727-1930
851 S 70th St Ste 103, Milwaukee, WI 53214
Medical imaging software applications.

Resonance Innovations Llc 402-934-2650
10957 Lake Ridge Dr, Omaha, NE 68136
Multiple.

Resonance Technology, Inc. 818-882-1997
18121 Parthenia St, Northridge, CA 91325
Mri audio/video system.

Sherman Ophthalmic Supplies, Inc. 714-738-0209
428 S Brea Blvd Ste B, Brea, CA 92821
Anti-claustrophobia glasses, redirects patient's view to tv screen.

NUCLEAR MAGNETIC RESONANCE IMAGING SYSTEM *(cont'd)*

Spectron Corp. 425-827-9317
934 S Burlington Blvd # 603, Burlington, WA 98233

Sun Nuclear Corp. 321-259-6862
425 Pineda Ct Ste A, Melbourne, FL 32940
Various energy qed diode detectors:models 1112,1113,1114,1115,and 1116.

Toshiba America Medical Systems 800-421-1968
2441 Michelle Dr, Tustin, CA 92780
Models MRT-600, MRT-1501.

Usa Instruments, Inc. 330-562-1000
1515 Danner Dr, Aurora, OH 44202
Various types of magnetic resonance imaging coils.

NUCLEAR MAGNETIC RESONANCE SPECTROSCOPIC SYSTEM *(Radiology) 90LNI*

Ge Medical Systems, Llc 262-312-7117
3200 N Grandview Blvd, Waukesha, WI 53188
Various models of magnetic resonance spectroscopic systems.

NUCLEIC ACID AMPLIFICATION ASSAY SYSTEM, GROUP B STREPTOCOCCUS, DIRECT SPECIMEN TEST *(Microbiology) 83NJR*

Cepheid 408-400-8460
904 E Caribbean Dr, Sunnyvale, CA 94089
Nucleic acid amplification assay system.

NURSE CALL SYSTEM *(General) 80RIO*

Aiphone Corporation 425-455-0510
1700 130th Ave NE, Bellevue, WA 98005

Alpha Communications 800-666-4800
42 Central Dr, Farmingdale, NY 11735
Visual tone/light nurse-call system for hospitals and nursing homes

Callcare 800-345-9414
1370 Arcadia Rd, Lancaster, PA 17601
Nurse's annunciators, pillow speakers, nurse call cords, new and replacement patient stations.

Crest Healthcare Supply 800-328-8908
195 3rd St, Dassel, MN 55325
Desk/wall nurse call stations; incandescent lamp or push-button display. Pillow speakers. Locking nurse call buttons.

Curbell, Inc. Electronics 800-235-7500
7 Cobham Dr, Orchard Park, NY 14127
Replacement parts and accessories for pillow speaker. Bed controls and bed-repair services also available.

Dickey Engineering 603-763-5202
17 Autumn Ln, Newbury, NH 03255
$62.50 for nurse call sponge-switch, activated by slight patient movement. Size: 3 x 4.5 x 1.25in, weight: 3oz. With removable cloth cover.

Dukane Communication Systems 519-748-5352
461 Manitou Dr., Kitchener, ON N2C 1L5 Canada
Audio and visual nurse-call systems: StarCare; ProCare 1000, 2000, 2600, 6000.

Dwyer Precision Products, Inc. 800-422-3894
266 20th St N, Jacksonville Beach, FL 32250
Call cord devices - nurse call air activated. $30 and up for nurse call system using air bulb; $120 and up for BREATHCALL, air-puff activated nurse call system. These systems also include call cords.

Hospital Comm. & Electronics, Inc. 800-558-3957
7915 N 81st St, Milwaukee, WI 53223
$100.00 to $1,000.00 per bed, microprocessor based. $1500.00 to $2700.00 per bed, w/central computer, logging, RP interface. Centralized Nurse Call Linux platform to 'network' control units to one central database for report generation of all nurse call activity. Tone-Visual nurse call simple, straight forward low-cost tone-visual system for nursing homes, clinics, assisted living facilities.

Intercall Systems Inc. 516-294-4524
86 Denton Ave, Garden City Park, NY 11040
ULTRA 9000, a nurse call system featuring room-to-room communication.

Jeron Electronic Systems, Inc. 800-621-1903
1743 W Rosehill Dr # 55, Chicago, IL 60660
Touchscreen IP is Jeron's next generation master for Provider. It is a LAN-based master console that incorporates the power of the Ethernet. Advantages include increased number of masters per main, overall cost savings, reduced equipment requirements, assured reliability - LAN interruption has no effect on nurse call system operation, and virus immunity.

NURSE CALL SYSTEM *(cont'd)*

Kelkom Systems 800-985-3556
418 MacArthur Ave, Redwood City, CA 94063
Staff Vector light message communication system for combination doctor/nurse follower, room status, and emergency call.

Ledtronics 800-579-4875
23105 Kashiwa Ct, Torrance, CA 90505

Med Labs Inc. 800-968-2486
28 Vereda Cordillera, Goleta, CA 93117
E-Z CALL universal/quadriplegic nurse call switch- $74.00. PA-1 optional Portable Alarm, 9 VOLT battery powered- $49.90. The PA-1 can be used with E-Z CALL.

Pacific Electronics 800-281-7782
10200 US Highway 14, Woodstock, IL 60098
Repairs and replacement parts for X-L-COM systems,NC-9100 tone visual,NC-7 visual nurse call,emergency systems and door monitor systems.

Pioneer Medical Systems 800-234-0683
3408 Howell St Ste D, Duluth, GA 30096

Protex Central Inc. 800-274-0888
1239 N Minnesota Ave, PO Box 1467, Hastings, NE 68901
Service.

Rauland-Borg Corp. 800-752-7725
3450 Oakton St, Skokie, IL 60076
RESPONDER IV Nurse Call System for acute-care facilities. With more than 250 priorities, the system interfaces with wireless technology for anywhere communications. Customized for each facility. RESPONDER 4000 for long-term-care facilities integrates wireless technology such as wireless phones and pocket paging for anywhere communications.

Rf Technologies 800-669-9946
3125 N 126th St, Brookfield, WI 53005
Wireless communication call system notifies staff of need for assistance. Quick Response is an emergency call system. Sensatec home monitoring and fall prevention systems also available.

Senior Technologies 800-824-2996
PO Box 80238, 1620 N 20th Circle, Lincoln, NE 68501
Arial wireless communication system allows residents to signal for assistance from anywhere within the monitored areas of the facility. Portable pendants/staff pagers.

NYSTAGMOGRAPH *(Cns/Neurology) 84GWN*

Fall Prevention Technologies, Llc 937-434-5455
4601 Gateway Cir, Kettering, OH 45440
Videonystagmograph.

Gn Otometrics North America 800-289-2150
125 Commerce Dr, Schaumburg, IL 60173
Nystagmograph.

Intellinetx 877-370-0477
2301 W 205th St Ste 102, Torrance, CA 90501
Electronystagmograph system.

Western Systems Research, Inc. 626-578-7363
127 N Madison Ave Ste 24, Pasadena, CA 91101
Electronystagmography.

NYSTAGMOGRAPH, ENT *(Ear/Nose/Throat) 77ETO*

Md International, Inc. 305-669-9003
11300 NW 41st St, Doral, FL 33178

Tsi Medical Ltd. 800-661-7263
47 Athabascan Ave., Unit 105, Sherwood Park, AB T8A-4H3 Canada

OBSERVERSCOPE *(General) 80RIP*

Karl Storz Endoscopy-America Inc. 800-421-0837
600 Corporate Pointe, Culver City, CA 90230

Mahe International Inc. 800-294-7946
468 Craighead St, Nashville, TN 37204

Pentax Medical Company 800-431-5880
102 Chestnut Ridge Rd, Montvale, NJ 07645
FO-T3 lightweight and compact observerscope with right or left side positioning. Mounts directly to standard PENTAX eyepiece. Adapters are available for use with scopes from other manufacturers. Call for quote.

OBTURATOR, CEMENT *(Orthopedics) 87LZN*

Codman & Shurtleff, Inc 800-225-0460
325 Paramount Dr, Raynham, MA 02767

Depuy Orthopaedics, Inc. 800-473-3789
700 Orthopaedic Dr, P.O. Box 988, Warsaw, IN 46582
Various types of cement obturators.

OBTURATOR, CEMENT *(cont'd)*

Stryker Puerto Rico, Ltd. 939-307-2500
Hwy. 3, Km. 131.2, Las Guasimas Ind. Park, Arroyo, PR 00714
Obturator.

Warsaw Orthopedic, Inc. 901-396-3133
2500 Silveus Xing, Warsaw, IN 46582
Cement restrictor.

Zimmer Trabecular Metal Technology 800-613-6131
10 Pomeroy Rd, Parsippany, NJ 07054
Cement restrictor system.

OBTURATOR, CLEFT PALATE *(Ear/Nose/Throat) 77UCZ*

Bausch & Lomb Surgical 636-255-5051
3365 Tree Court Ind Blvd, Saint Louis, MO 63122

OBTURATOR, ENDOSCOPIC *(Gastro/Urology) 78FEC*

Aesculap Implant Systems Inc. 1-800-234-9179
3773 Corporate Pkwy, Center Valley, PA 18034

Bioteque America, Inc. 800-889-9008
340 E Maple Ave Ste 204A, Langhorne, PA 19047

Deknatel Snowden-Pencer 800-367-7874
5175 S Royal Atlanta Dr, Tucker, GA 30084
Hasson obturator available in 10/11mm and 12/13mm, with ability to convert existing cannulas to a Hasson-style cannula.

Ethicon Endo-Surgery, Inc. 800-USE-ENDO
4545 Creek Rd, Cincinnati, OH 45242

Frantz Medical Development Ltd. 440-255-1155
7740 Metric Dr, Mentor, OH 44060
Cap and connector assembly, bottle, endoscopic.

Gyrus Acmi, Inc. 508-804-2739
93 N Pleasant St, Norwalk, OH 44857
Obturator.

Gyrus Acmi, Inc. 508-804-2739
300 Stillwater P.o.box 1971, Stamford, CT 06902
Obturator.

Karl Storz Endoscopy-America Inc. 800-421-0837
600 Corporate Pointe, Culver City, CA 90230

Mahe International Inc. 800-294-7946
468 Craighead St, Nashville, TN 37204

Richard Wolf Medical Instruments Corp. 800-323-9653
353 Corporate Woods Pkwy, Vernon Hills, IL 60061

Smith & Nephew, Inc., Endoscopy Division 800-343-8386
150 Minuteman Rd, Andover, MA 01810

OCCLUDER, CARDIOVASCULAR *(Cardiovascular) 74WOZ*

Acro Associates 800-672-2276
1990 Olivera Rd Ste A, Concord, CA 94520
Solenoid and pneumatically-operated pinch valves for flexible, disposable tubing or tubesets.

Genesee Biomedical, Inc. 800-786-4890
1308 S Jason St, Denver, CO 80223
INTRA-ART Coronary Artery Occluders. Minimize hemorrhage from the anastomotic site.

In Vivo Metric 707-433-2949
PO Box 397, Healdsburg, CA 95448
Inflatable cuff for constriction and occlusion of blood vessel from 2 to 24 lumen diameter. Silicone made cuff includes tubing of 90cm (36in) and inflatable diaphragm inside to compress vessel when being inflated. (The device is only to be used for animal research at the present time - 1988.) Priced $56-$102.

Medtronic, Inc. 800-633-8766
710 Medtronic Pkwy, Minneapolis, MN 55432

OCCLUDER, CATHETER TIP *(Cardiovascular) 74DQT*

Cook Inc. 800-457-4500
PO Box 489, Bloomington, IN 47402

OCCLUDER, OPHTHALMIC *(Ophthalmology) 86HKE*

Gulden Ophthalmics 800-659-2250
225 Cadwalader Ave, Elkins Park, PA 19027

Landec Corp. 650-306-1650
3603 Haven Ave, Menlo Park, CA 94025
LANDEC PURT punctual for retention of tears.

Total Molding Services, Inc. 215-538-9613
354 East Broad St., Trumbauersville, PA 18970
Various Styles/Colors of Occuluder handles.

OCCLUDER, PATENT DUCTUS, ARTERIOSUS
(Cardiovascular) 74MAE

Aga Medical Corporation. 888-546-4407
5050 Nathan Ln N, Plymouth, MN 55442
AMPLATZER® Duct Occluder--The AMPLATZER Duct Occluder is a self-expandable device made from a Nitinol wire mesh. A retention skirt on the aortic side provides secure positioning in the ampulla of the ductus. As the occluder is implanted, it expands outward and the wires push against the wall of the ductus. Polyester fabric is sewn into the occluder with polyester thread. The fabric induces thrombosis that closes the communication.

OCCLUDER, UMBILICAL *(General) 80FOD*

Ac Healthcare Supply, Inc. 905-448-4706
11651 230th St, Cambria Heights, NY 11411
Umbilical clamp.

Cadco Dental Products 800-833-8267
600 E Hueneme Rd, Oxnard, CA 93033

Centurion Medical Products Corp. 517-545-1135
3310 S Main St, Salisbury, NC 28147

Dux Dental 800-833-8267
600 E Hueneme Rd, Oxnard, CA 93033

Kentron Health Care, Inc. 615-384-0573
3604 Kelton Jackson Rd, P.o. Box 120, Springfield, TN 37172
Umbilical clamp.

Prosec Protection Systems, Inc. 732-886-0990
1985 Swarthmore Ave Ste 7, Lakewood, NJ 08701
Umbilical clamps with transponder.

Tri-State Hospital Supply Corp. 517-545-1135
3173 E 43rd St, Yuma, AZ 85365

OCULAR PEG *(Ophthalmology) 86MQU*

Fci Ophthalmics 800-932-4202
64 Schoosett St, Pembroke, MA 02359
Motility peg for orbital spheres.

OFFICE EQUIPMENT *(General) 80VBG*

Atd-American Co. 800-523-2300
135 Greenwood Ave, Wyncote, PA 19095

Bevco Ergonomic Seating 800-864-2991
2246 W Bluemound Rd Ste A, Waukesha, WI 53186
Office chairs, BEVCO hat and coat racks (one inch 18 gauge steel construction, chrome finish available in 2 ft. through 6 ft. lengths), BEVCO hangers (sturdy metal hangers constructed with 3/16in. wire 17 1/4in. long--available in bright chrome, brass or epoxy finish--list $18.35/doz). Office and laboratory chairs and stools, quantity discounts available.

Budget Buddy Company, Inc. 800-208-3375
PO Box 590, Belton, MO 64012
Folding wall desk $129.95-265.95 each.

Easi File Corp. 800-800-5563
6 Wrigley, Irvine, CA 92618
EASI FILE Vertical steel filing systems for storage of documents such as MRIs, X-rays, etc. Documents are vertically suspended via a unique rod system, easily viewed and sorted, quick retrieval, space saving designs.

Franklin Miller Inc 800-932-0599
60 Okner Pkwy, Livingston, NJ 07039
TASKMASTER, material shredder and cutter.

Hessler Forms & Labels 800-346-1304
106 Susan Dr Ste 1, Elkins Park, PA 19027
Business forms, labels and supplies.

Kardex Systems, Inc. 800-234-3654
114 Westview Ave, Marietta, OH 45750
Shelving, vertical carousel filing devices, file folders, automated storage devices.

Medirecord Systems 800-561-9791
P.O. Box 6201 Station A, Saint John, NB E2L 4R6 Canada
Medical record storage systems and file carts.

Rem Systems 305-499-4800
625 E 10th Ave, Hialeah, FL 33010
Full line of open shelf filing, carts, cabinets, and professional seating.

Richards-Wilcox, Inc. 800-253-5668
600 S Lake St, Aurora, IL 60506
Mobile, static, and rotary shelving systems for books and medical files finished with powder coating, an alternative to water-borne paint finishes. New rotary file, Times-2 2-Tier has been introduced for under workstation applications.

OFFICE EQUIPMENT *(cont'd)*

Valley Craft 800-328-1480
2001 S Highway 61, Lake City, MN 55041

OFFICE PRODUCT *(General) 80VBM*

Anthro Corporation 800-325-3841
10450 SW Manhasset Dr, Tualatin, OR 97062
The FIT SYSTEM from Anthro combines elegance with absolute functionality for all your technology needs. Like all Anthro furniture, the SYSTEM pieces are modular and flexible--start with various sizes of work surfaces; connect pieces together; build up using your vertical space; set desk heights in 1' increments; add over 30 accessories; move your SYSTEM to where you need it; reconfigure it as your needs change; it will always 'fit' you and your hardware. Sizes come in 30', 36', 48', 60', 72' widths. Choose from surfaces that are standard desk, adjustable with a simple squeeze of a paddle, or recessed for your monitor. Metal components are silver in color. Work surfaces are available in butter, bluestone, fog, blanc, and wine colors. FIT comes with standard 3' casters, with 5' casters optional. And like all Anthro furniture, FIT SYSTEM pieces easily hold 150 lbs., and come with a Lifetime Warranty.

Atd-American Co. 800-523-2300
135 Greenwood Ave, Wyncote, PA 19095

Deflecto Corp. 800-428-4328
7035 E 86th St, Indianapolis, IN 46250
Oversized CONFIDENTIAL WALL POCKET is made from durable black plastic. Great for medical settings where keeping personal health records private is crucial. The break resistant Confidential Wall Pocket can be mounted to the wall or used on the desktop. Tilts out for easy viewing and retrieval. Holds letter, legal and A4 size doucments. Also accomodates hanging file folders and regular folders.

Healthstream, Inc. 800-521-0574
209 10th Ave S Ste 450, Nashville, TN 37203

Hessler Forms & Labels 800-346-1304
106 Susan Dr Ste 1, Elkins Park, PA 19027
Business forms, labels and supplies.

Kardex Systems, Inc. 800-234-3654
114 Westview Ave, Marietta, OH 45750
File folders, inventory cards, vertical carousel filing devices, file folders, book units, medical panels.

Medirecord Systems 800-561-9791
P.O. Box 6201 Station A, Saint John, NB E2L 4R6 Canada
Medical charts, chart dividers, chart binders, medical chart alert tabs, report pockets, x-ray mailing envelopes and jackets.

Pm Company 800-327-4359
1500 Kemper Meadow Dr, Cincinnati, OH 45240
Preventa Antimicrobial pens with built in AgION technology prevents the growth of bacteria. Lasts the life of the pen. Available in a variety of security counter, stick and retractable pens.

Richards-Wilcox, Inc. 800-253-5668
600 S Lake St, Aurora, IL 60506
Mobile, static, and rotary shelving systems for books and medical files finished with powder coating, an alternative to water-borne paint finishes.

Smead Manufacturing Co. 1-88-USE-SMEAD
600 Smead Blvd, Hastings, MN 55033
Color coded filing system.

Spectrum Laboratories, Inc. 800-634-3300
18617 S Broadwick St, Rancho Dominguez, CA 90220
Laboratory organizers.

Sprayway, Inc. 800-332-9000
484 S Vista Ave, Addison, IL 60101
Screen opener/adhesive/magnetic tape head cleaner-sprays.

St. John Companies 800-435-4242
25167 Anza Dr, PO Box 800460, Santa Clarita, CA 91355
Labels, envelopes and category jackets for the medical imaging field.

Veriad 800-423-4643
650 Columbia St, Brea, CA 92821
Office label aids.

OIL, IMMERSION *(Hematology) 81GLF*

Accu-Scope, Inc. 516-759-1000
7 Littleworth Ln, Sea Cliff, NY 11579

Cargille Laboratories 973-239-6633
55 Commerce Rd, Cedar Grove, NJ 07009
Type A (low viscosity) or Type B (high viscosity), $5.90 for 1 oz., $13.00 for 4 oz., $28.50 for 16 oz.

Edmund Industrial Optics 800-363-1992
101 E Gloucester Pike, Barrington, NJ 08007

OIL, IMMERSION *(cont'd)*

Polysciences, Inc. 800-523-2575
400 Valley Rd, Warrington, PA 18976

OMNICARDIOGRAPH (CARDIOINTEGRAPH)
(Cardiovascular) 74RIS

Ocg Technology, Inc. 914-576-8457
56 Harrison St, New Rochelle, NY 10801
Cardiointegraph, used for early detection of CAD in patients with normal resting ECGs. Leased.

ONCOMETER *(Microbiology) 83RIT*

Wescor, Inc. 800-453-2725
459 S Main St, Logan, UT 84321
Colloid osmometer model 4420 with flow-through sample and reference chambers, rapid response time, extended membrane life, whole-blood capability, 300-500 microliter sample size, 0-40 mmHg measurement range, $6,795.00 per unit.

ONCOMETER, LABORATORY *(Chemistry) 75UGZ*

Wescor, Inc. 800-453-2725
459 S Main St, Logan, UT 84321
Colloid osmometer model 4420 with flow-through sample and reference chambers, rapid response time, extended membrane life, whole-blood capacity, 300-500 microliter sample size, 0-40 mmHg measurement range, $6,795.00 per unit.

OPERATIVE DENTAL TREATMENT UNIT *(Dental And Oral) 76EIA*

A-Dec, Inc. 800-547-1883
2601 Crestview Dr, Newberg, OR 97132
Various models of dental operative units.

Air Techniques, Inc. 800-247-8324
1295 Walt Whitman Rd, Melville, NY 11747

Alliance H. Inc Dentech Equipment 360-988-7080
901 W Front St, Sumas, WA 98295
Over-the-patient, wall mount, cabinet mount, mobile carts. 5-year warranty. CAB810 right/left handed rear delivery center.

Arrow Industries Llc 701-886-7722
530 5th Street, Neche, ND 58265-4033
Self-contained portable dental unit.

Asi Medical, Inc. 303-766-3646
14550 E Easter Ave Ste 700, Centennial, CO 80112
Various dental delivery systems.

Beaverstate Dental, Inc. 800-237-2303
115 S Elliott Rd, Newberg, OR 97132

Bell Dental Products, Llc. 303-292-2137
3003 Arapahoe St Unit 101B, Denver, CO 80205
Portabell.

Boyd Industries, Inc.
12900 44th St N, Clearwater, FL 33762
Various dental operative units.

Cadent, Inc. 201-842-0800
640 Gotham Pkwy, Carlstadt, NJ 07072
Dental digital models.

Denmed Technologies, Inc. 866-433-6633
1531 W Orangewood Ave, Orange, CA 92868
Intraoral camera.

Dentalez Group 866-DTE-INFO
101 Lindenwood Dr Ste 225, Valleybrooke Corporate Center
Malvern, PA 19355

Dentalez Group, Stardental Division 717-291-1161
1816 Colonial Village Ln, Lancaster, PA 17601
Unit, operative dental.

Dentalez Of Alabama 251-937-6781
2500 S US Highway 31, Bay Minette, AL 36507
Unit, operative dental.

Dntlworks Equipment Corporation 800-847-0694
7300 S Tucson Way, Centennial, CO 80112
Self-contained carts with dedicated compressor and vacuum components; units for office use and mobile applications. Portable units for basic treatment and field use.

Electro-Optical Sciences, Inc. 800-729-8849
1 Bridge St Ste 15, Irvington, NY 10533
Difoti system.

OPERATIVE DENTAL TREATMENT UNIT *(cont'd)*

Engle Dental Systems, Inc. 503-359-9390
4115 24th Ave Ste A, Forest Grove, OR 97116
The company offers several different control units, each featuring air/water adjustment for each handpiece, asepsis design, and a host of other features. Additional options include automatic handpiece actuation and fiber-optic tubings.

Garrison Dental Solutions 616-842-2244
110 Dewitt Ln, Spring Lake, MI 49456
H2pro dental unit water line treatment.

Genesis Dental Technologies, Llc 715-778-5816
200 Main Street, Elmwood, WI 54740
Sterilizable water delivery system.

Health Science Products, Inc. 800-237-5794
1489 Hueytown Rd, Hueytown, AL 35023
DENTASSIST LIBERTY transthoracic dental delivery unit, chair mounted, standard features: 3+ handpiece controls, air-water and/or air-only syringe(s), high and low volume suction, integratable options not limited to and including electric handpieces, electrosurgery unit, piezo scaler, LED curing wand, endodontic instruments and handpieces and lighted handpiece tubings among others; various instruments usually work from one rheostat foot control when integrated into the dental unit.

Jeremy Ethan Industries, Inc. 954-772-9779
809 NW 57th St, Fort Lauderdale, FL 33309
Portable dental cart.

Kerr Corp. 714-516-7400
28200 Wick Rd, Romulus, MI 48174
Various accessories.

Mastercraft Dental Co. Of Texas 972-775-8757
880 Eastgate Rd, P.O. Box 882, Midlothian, TX 76065
Floor or chair mounted.

Midmark Corporation 800-643-6275
60 Vista Dr, P.O. Box 286, Versailles, OH 45380

Miltex Dental Technologies, Inc. 516-576-6022
589 Davies Dr, York, PA 17402
Various accessories to operative dental unit(aspirator tips).

Mobile Dental Equipment Corp.(M-Dec) 425-747-5424
13300 SE 30th St Ste 101, Bellevue, WA 98005
PORT-OP III, portable dental operatory $9618.00.

Mrlb Intl., Inc. 715-425-8180
2450 College Way, Fergus Falls, MN 56537
Dental water purification cartridge.

Obsidian Dental Inc. 541-617-0129
62915 NE 18th St Ste 4, Bend, OR 97701
Dental delivery unit.

Orametrix Inc. 493-024-3091
2350 Campbell Creek Blvd Ste 400, Richardson, TX 75082
Suresmile 3-d intraoral camera & accessories.

Pac-Dent Intl., Inc. 909-839-0888
21078 Commerce Point Dr, Walnut, CA 91789
Impression mixing tip.

Pelton & Crane 704-588-2126
11727 Fruehauf Dr, Charlotte, NC 28273
Dental delivery unit.

Proma, Inc. 310-327-0035
730 Kingshill Pl, Carson, CA 90746
Various.

Sota Precision Optics, Inc. 714-532-6100
1073 N Batavia St, Orange, CA 92867
Intraoral camera system and accessories.

Sterilex Corp. 800-511-1659
11409 Cronhill Dr Ste L, Owings Mills, MD 21117
Accessory to dental unit.

Sterisil, Inc. 719-481-0937
835 S Highway 105 Unit D, Palmer Lake, CO 80133
Dental operative unit and accessories.

Tidi Products, Llc 920-751-4380
570 Enterprise Dr, Neenah, WI 54956
Dental camera cover (accessory).

Twist2it, Inc. 877-PRO-PHYS
3930A 62nd St, Flushing, NY 11377
Dental surgical handpiece.

Vista Research Group, Llc 419-281-3927
1554 Township Road 805, Ashland, OH 44805
Vistaclear dental waterline treatment system.

OPERATIVE DENTAL TREATMENT UNIT *(cont'd)*

Young O/S Llc 800-325-1881
1663 Fenton Business Park Ct, Fenton, MO 63026
Various models of dental operative units.

OPHTHALMOSCOPE, AC-POWERED *(Ophthalmology) 86HLI*

Carl Zeiss Meditec, Inc. 800-722-6393
10805 Rancho Bernardo Rd Ste 210, San Diego, CA 92127
The GDx NFA is the essential technology to detect and track glaucoma so you can act confidently to preserve your patients' vision sooner. And now retinal nerve fiber layer imaging just got better with the GDX NFA with Custom Corneal Compensation. The GDx NFA features a new, updated normative database, providing you with even more confidence in every exam. The image reproducibility allows precise, accurate follow-up of change over time with a serial analysis printout that clearly shows specific areas of disease progression. And the GDx NFA is as easy to use as an autorefractor, takes less than a second for imagingóabout 3 minutes for a complete examóand does not require dilation. GDx NFA is reimburseable using CPT code 92135, with the proper diagnosis codes.

Hai Laboratories, Inc. 781-862-9884
320 Massachusetts Ave, Lexington, MA 02420
Clinical specular microscope.

Independent Solutions, Inc. 847-498-0500
900 Skokie Blvd Ste 118, Northbrook, IL 60062
Portable, wall mounted, rail mounted, or stand mounted.

Keeler Instruments Inc. 800-523-5620
456 Park Way, Broomall, PA 19008

Mira, Inc. 508-278-7877
414 Quaker Hwy, Uxbridge, MA 01569
S p ophthalmoscope.

North American Medical Products, Inc. 800-488-6267
6 British American Blvd Ste B, Latham, NY 12110
Fiberoptic lighting.

Optos, Inc. 441-383-8433
67 Forest St, Marlborough, MA 01752
Scanning laser ophthalmoscope.

Optovue, Inc. 866-344-8948
45531 Northport Loop W, Fremont, CA 94538
Ophthalmic instrument.

Propper Manufacturing Co., Inc. 800-832-4300
3604 Skillman Ave, Long Island City, NY 11101

Topcon Medical Systems, Inc. 800-223-1130
37 W Century Rd, Paramus, NJ 07652
Two models of indirect ophthalmoscopes: $950.00 and $1,350.00.

OPHTHALMOSCOPE, BATTERY-POWERED
(Ophthalmology) 86HLJ

Armstrong Medical Industries, Inc. 800-323-4220
575 Knightsbridge Pkwy, Lincolnshire, IL 60069

Carley Lamps 310-325-8474
1502 W 228th St, Torrance, CA 90501

Creative Health Products, Inc. 800-742-4478
5148 Saddle Ridge Rd, Plymouth, MI 48170
RIESTER Ri-Mini Ophthalmoscope; $139.00 for CHP. RIESTER Ri-Mini Ophthalmoscope/Otoscope Combination Kit $209.00

Edmund Industrial Optics 800-363-1992
101 E Gloucester Pike, Barrington, NJ 08007

Her-Mar, Inc. 800-327-8209
8550 NW 30th Ter, Doral, FL 33122
$100.00 each.

Independent Solutions, Inc. 847-498-0500
900 Skokie Blvd Ste 118, Northbrook, IL 60062
Portable, wall mounted, rail mounted, or stand mounted.

Jedmed Instruments Co. 314-845-3770
5416 Jedmed Ct, Saint Louis, MO 63129

Md International, Inc. 305-669-9003
11300 NW 41st St, Doral, FL 33178

Propper Manufacturing Co., Inc. 800-832-4300
3604 Skillman Ave, Long Island City, NY 11101

Welch Allyn, Inc. 800-535-6663
4341 State Street Rd, Skaneateles Falls, NY 13153

OPHTHALMOSCOPE, DIRECT *(Ophthalmology) 86RIV*

American Diagnostic Corporation (Adc) 800-232-2670
55 Commerce Dr, Hauppauge, NY 11788
Pocket and standard 2.5v opthalmoscope

OPHTHALMOSCOPE, DIRECT *(cont'd)*

Carl Zeiss Surgical, Inc. 800-442-4020
1 Zeiss Dr, Thornwood, NY 10594

Independent Solutions, Inc. 847-498-0500
900 Skokie Blvd Ste 118, Northbrook, IL 60062
Portable, wall mounted, rail mounted or stand mounted.

Keeler Instruments Inc. 800-523-5620
456 Park Way, Broomall, PA 19008
$375.00 3.5V rechargeable, professional ophthalmoscope with rechargeable handle.

Md International, Inc. 305-669-9003
11300 NW 41st St, Doral, FL 33178

Topcon Canada Inc. 800-361-3515
110 Provencher Ave., Boisbriand, QUE J7G-1N1 Canada

Welch Allyn, Inc. 800-535-6663
4341 State Street Rd, Skaneateles Falls, NY 13153

OPHTHALMOSCOPE, INDIRECT *(Ophthalmology) 86RIW*

Carl Zeiss Surgical, Inc. 800-442-4020
1 Zeiss Dr, Thornwood, NY 10594

Independent Solutions, Inc. 847-498-0500
900 Skokie Blvd Ste 118, Northbrook, IL 60062
Portable, wall mounted, rail mounted or stand mounted.

Keeler Instruments Inc. 800-523-5620
456 Park Way, Broomall, PA 19008
$1095 and up for Fison, ALL PUPIL, SPECTRA & VANTAGE ophthalmoscope.

Lumiscope Company, Inc. 800-672-8293
1035 Centennial Ave, Piscataway, NJ 08854

OPHTHALMOSCOPE, LASER *(Ophthalmology) 86WTA*

Iridex Corporation 800-388-4747
1212 Terra Bella Ave, Mountain View, CA 94043
TruFocus laser indirect ophthalmoscope with TruFocus optics. Lightweight, comfortable, with clear-viewing video attachment also available.

OPHTHALMOSCOPE, LASER, SCANNING
(Ophthalmology) 86MYC

Optos, Inc. 441-383-8433
67 Forest St, Marlborough, MA 01752
Scanning laser opthhalmoscope.

OPTICAL POSITION/MOVEMENT RECORDING SYSTEM
(Physical Med) 89LXJ

Bio-Research Associates, Inc. 414-357-7525
9275 N 49th St Ste 150, Brown Deer, WI 53223
Mandibular movement recorder.

Motion Analysis Corp.
3617 Westwind Blvd, Santa Rosa, CA 95403
Motion analysis system.

Vicon 303-799-8686
7388 S Revere Pkwy Ste 901, Centennial, CO 80112
Video motion measurement system.

ORAL ADMINISTRATION SET *(General) 80LEY*

Kelsar, S.A. 508-261-8000
Blvd. Insurgentes, Libriamento a La, Tijuana 22450 Mexico
Gravity & pump sets easy cap bag w/wo bag,y-site extension set containers

O&M Enterprise 847-258-4515
641 Chelmsford Ln, Elk Grove Village, IL 60007
ORAL ADMINISTRATION

ORANGE STICK *(General) 80RIY*

Amson Products 718-435-3728
1401 42nd St, Brooklyn, NY 11219
Emery boards and manicure sticks.

ORCHIDOMETER *(General) 80WXO*

Seritex Inc. 973-472-4200
1 Madison St, East Rutherford, NJ 07073

ORGAN PRESERVATION SYSTEM *(Gastro/Urology) 78RIZ*

Waters Medical Systems 800-426-9877
2112 15th St NW, Rochester, MN 55901
RM3.

ORTHODONTIC INSTRUMENT *(Dental And Oral) 76RJA*

Aoa 800-262-5221
13931 Spring St, P.O. Box 725, Sturtevant, WI 53177
Appliances.

ORTHODONTIC INSTRUMENT *(cont'd)*

D.C.A. (Dental Corporation Of America) 800-638-6684
889 S Matlack St, West Chester, PA 19382
Including mouth guards, tracing acetate, arch wire, and brackets.

G & H Wire Co. 800-526-1026
2165 Earlywood Dr, Franklin, IN 46131

George Tiemann & Co. 800-843-6266
25 Plant Ave, Hauppauge, NY 11788

Orthoband Company, Inc. 800-325-9973
3690 Highway M, Imperial, MO 63052

Orthodontic Supply & Equipment Co., Inc. 800-638-4003
7851 Airpark Rd Ste 202, Gaithersburg, MD 20879

Selane Products, Inc./Space Maintainers Lab. 800-423-3270
9129 Lurline Ave, Chatsworth, CA 91311
Orthodontic and pediatric laboratory therapy appliances.

Tp Orthodontics, Inc. 800-348-8856
100 Center Plz, La Porte, IN 46350
Straight Shooter Ligature Gun.

Yates & Bird And Motloid 800-662-5021
300 N Elizabeth St, Chicago, IL 60607
ORTHO WELDER is an orthodontic welder - combination machine - 3 functions in 1 : orthodontic welder, electric solderer, wire annealer.

3m Unitek 800-634-5300
2724 Peck Rd, Monrovia, CA 91016
Hand instruments.

ORTHOPEDIC IMPLANT MATERIAL *(Orthopedics) 87MOO*

Biomet Sports Medicine, Inc 800-348-9500
56 E Bell Dr, Warsaw, IN 46582
A full ine of arthroscopic implants to include titanium, stainless steel, resorbable, porcine, and allograft.

C.O.R.E. Tech, Inc. 574-267-5744
542 E 200 N, Warsaw, IN 46582

Implex Corp. 800-613-6131
1800 W Center St, Warsaw, IN 46580
Hedrocel Trabecular Metal.

Medical Carbon Research Institute, Llc - Mcri 512-339-8000
8200 Cameron Rd Ste A196, Austin, TX 78754
On-X carbon--pure pyrolytic carbon for bioprosthetics

ORTHOPEDIC MANUAL SURGICAL INSTRUMENT
(Orthopedics) 87LXH

Advanced Bio-Surfaces, Inc. 952-912-5400
5909 Baker Rd Ste 550, Minnetonka, MN 55345
Pusher.

Advanced Biomaterial Systems, Inc. 973-635-9040
100 Passaic Ave, Chatham, NJ 07928
Access needle.

Advanced Orthopaedic Solutions, Inc. 310-533-9966
386 Beech Ave Unit B6, Torrance, CA 90501
Various types of surgical instruments.

Advanced Spine Technology, Inc. 415-241-2400
457 Mariposa St, San Francisco, CA 94107
Double ended foraminal probe; posterior disc evacuator.

Aesculap Implant Systems, Inc. 610-984-9074
9999 Hamilton Blvd Bldg 8, Breinigsville, PA 18031
Orthosis manual surgical instrument.

Alexandria Research Technologies, Llc 952-949-2235
13755 1st Ave N Ste 100, Plymouth, MN 55441
Various types of non-sterile orthopedic manual surgical instruments.

Amedica Corporation 801-839-3500
1885 W 2100 S, Salt Lake City, UT 84119
Valeo CP Instruments; Valeo PS Instruments; Valo VBR Instruments

Arthrex California, Inc. 239-643-5553
20509 Earlgate St, Walnut, CA 91789
Orthopedic manual surgical instrument.

Arthrex Manufacturing 239-643-5553
1958 Trade Center Way, Naples, FL 34109
Probe,driver,mallet,scissors.

Arthrex, Inc. 239-643-5553
1370 Creekside Blvd, Naples, FL 34108
Various.

Arthrosurface, Inc. 508-520-3003
28 Forge Pkwy, Franklin, MA 02038
Orthopedic resurfacing instrument.

ORTHOPEDIC MANUAL SURGICAL INSTRUMENT *(cont'd)*

Ascent Healthcare Solutions 480-763-5300
10232 S 51st St, Phoenix, AZ 85044
Carpal tunnel blade.

Atlas Spine Inc. 561-741-1108
1555 Jupiter Park Dr Ste 4, Jupiter, FL 33458
Rongeurs, forceps, drill guide, plate holder, screw drivers,.

Beere Precision Medical Instruments, Kmedic, Telef 919-544-8000
5307 95th Ave, Kenosha, WI 53144
Orthopedic manual surgical instruments.

Biomet Microfixation Inc. 800-874-7711
1520 Tradeport Dr, Jacksonville, FL 32218
Various types of manual instruments.

Biomet Sports Medicine, Inc 800-348-9500
56 E Bell Dr, Warsaw, IN 46582
A full line of instrumentation and delivery systems for arthroscopic surgery.

Biomet, Inc. 574-267-6639
56 E Bell Dr, PO Box 587, Warsaw, IN 46582
Various instruments, cement gun inserter applicators, templates, gage sets.

Bolt Bethel, Llc 763-434-5900
23530 University Avenue Ext NW, PO Box 135, Bethel, MN 55005

Bonutti Research, Inc. 217-342-3412
2600 S Raney St, Effingham, IL 62401
Various.

Brasseler Usa - Komet Medical 800-535-6638
1 Brasseler Blvd, Savannah, GA 31419

Centinel Spine Inc. 952-885-0500
505 Park Ave Fl 14, New York, NY 10022

Conformis, Inc. 781-860-5111
2 4th Ave, Burlington, MA 01803
Alignment guide, cutting blocks/guides, drill.

De Good Dimensional Concepts, Inc. 574-834-5437
7815 N State Road 13, North Webster, IN 46555

Depuy Mitek, A Johnson & Johnson Company 800-451-2006
50 Scotland Blvd, Bridgewater, MA 02324
Various types of manual orthopedic surgical instruments.

Depuy Orthopaedics, Inc. 800-473-3789
700 Orthopaedic Dr, P.O. Box 988, Warsaw, IN 46582
Various types of manual surgical orthopedic instruments.

Depuy Spine, Inc. 800-227-6633
325 Paramount Dr, Raynham, MA 02767
Various types of orthopedic instruments (depth gauge, retractor).

Depuy-Raynham, A Div. Of Depuy Orthopaedics 800-451-2006
325 Paramount Dr, Raynham, MA 02767
Various types of manual surgical orthopedic instruments.

Derron Surgical Instruments, Inc. 888-374-3622
1055 Scherer Way, Osprey, FL 34229
Orthopedic manual surgical instrument.

DFine Inc. 866-963-3463
3047 Orchard Pkwy, San Jose, CA 95134
VertecoR Cement Staging Osteotome

DJO Inc. 800-336-6569
1430 Decision St, Vista, CA 92081

Gauthier Biomedical, Inc. 262-546-0010
1235 Dakota Dr Ste G, Grafton, WI 53024
Orthopedic manual surgical instrument.

Hiatt Metal Products 765-284-8351
720 W Willard St, Muncie, IN 47302
Ortopedic manual surgical instrument.

Holmed Corporation 508-238-3351
40 Norfolk Ave, South Easton, MA 02375

In'Tech Medical, Incorporated 757-224-0177
2851 Lamb Pl Ste 15, Memphis, TN 38118
Distractor/compressor/screwdriver/bender/probe/forcep.

Invuity, Inc. 760-744-4447
334 Via Vera Cruz Ste 255, San Marcos, CA 92078
Various types and sizes of ortho. man. surg. instruments.

Invuity, Inc. 415-655-2100
39 Stillman St, San Francisco, CA 94107

Jb Medical Development Inc. 813-645-2855
3000 NW 25th Ave Ste 10, Pompano Beach, FL 33069
Orthopedic manual surgical instrument.

ORTHOPEDIC MANUAL SURGICAL INSTRUMENT *(cont'd)*

K2m, Inc. 866-526-4171
751 Miller Dr SE Ste F1, Leesburg, VA 20175
Various orthopedic manual surgical instrumnets.

Mark Medical Manufacturing, Inc. 610-269-4420
530 Brandywine Ave, Downingtown, PA 19335
Stainless-streel pliers, needle nose, wire cutters, wire twisters, and pin cutters.

Medcon Llc 410-744-8367
1002 Frederick Rd, Catonsville, MD 21228
Quick-connect pin chucks.

Medical Device Concepts, Llc. 201-446-6691
4 Lawrence Way, Cedar Grove, NJ 07009
Various hip retractors.

Medical Innovators, Inc. 888-422-7717
9277 E Star Hill Ln, Lone Tree, CO 80124
Orthopedic manual surgical instruments.

Medisiss 866-866-7477
2747 SW 6th St, Redmond, OR 97756
Various orthopedic manual surgical instruments,sterile.

Medtronic Puerto Rico Operations Co.,Med Rel 763-514-4000
Road 909, Km. 0.4., Barrio Mariana, Humacao, PR 00792
Orthopedic manual surgical instrument.

Medtronic Sofamor Danek Instrument Manufacturing 901-396-3133
7375 Adrianne Pl, Bartlett, TN 38133
Orthopedic manual surgical instrument.

Medtronic Sofamor Danek Usa, Inc. 901-396-3133
4340 Swinnea Rd, Memphis, TN 38118
Orthopedic manual surgical instrument.

Medtronic Spine Llc 877-690-5353
1221 Crossman Ave, Sunnyvale, CA 94089
Curette.

Millstone Medical Outsourcing 508-679-8384
1565 N Main St Ste 408, Fall River, MA 02720
Multiple and various.

minSURG International, Inc. 727-466-4550
611 Druid Rd E, Suite 200, Clearwater, FL 33756

Musculoskeletal Transplant Foundation 800-433-6576
125 May St Ste 300, Edison Corp Ctr, Edison, NJ 08837
Allofix cortical bone pin insertion kit.

Nemcomed Fw Llc 419-542-7743
8727 Clinton Park Dr, Fort Wayne, IN 46825
Various types of manual surgical instruments.

Nuvasive, Inc. 800-475-9131
7475 Lusk Blvd, San Diego, CA 92121
Orthopedic manual surgical instruments.

Omni Life Science, Inc 800-448-6664
175 Paramount Dr Ste 302, Raynham, MA 02767
Various types of orthopedic instruments.

Opi, Inc. 260-248-4414
700 S Main St, Columbia City, IN 46725

Orthohelix Surgical Designs, Inc. 330-869-9582
1815 W Market St Ste 205, Akron, OH 44313
Instruments.

Orthovita, Inc. 610-640-1775
77 Great Valley Pkwy, Malvern, PA 19355
Funnel.

Paradigm Biodevices, Inc. 781-982-9950
800 Hingham St Ste 102N, Rockland, MA 02370
Orthopedic manual surgical instrument.

Performance Machine Technologies 661-294-8617
25141 Avenue Stanford, Valencia, CA 91355
Various types of orthopedic components.

Platinum Surgical Instruments, Inc. 262-798-8540
2325 Parklawn Dr Ste F, Waukesha, WI 53186
Various manual surgical instruments.

Precimed 260-244-6300
4532 E Park 30 Dr, Columbia City, IN 46725

Precision Medical Technologies 574-267-6385
2059 N Pound Dr W, Warsaw, IN 46582

Rkl Technologies, Inc. 951-738-8000
245 Citation Cir, Corona, CA 92880
Various orthopedic manual surgical instruments.

ORTHOPEDIC MANUAL SURGICAL INSTRUMENT *(cont'd)*

Salumedica, L.L.C. 404-589-1727
4451 Atlanta Rd SE Ste 138, Smyrna, GA 30080
Prosthesis pusher and guide.

Shukla Medical 732-474-1762
151 Old New Brunswick Rd, Piscataway, NJ 08854

Small Bone Innovations, Inc. 215-428-1791
1380 S Pennsylvania Ave, Morrisville, PA 19067
Orthopedic manual surgical instrument.

Spinal Elements, Inc. 760-607-0121
2744 Loker Ave W Ste 100, Carlsbad, CA 92010
Orthopedic manual surgical instruments.

Spinal Kinetics, Inc. 609-254-3999
595 N Pastoria Ave, Sunnyvale, CA 94085
Orthopedics manual surgical instruments.

Spine Smith Partners L.P. 512-206-0770
8140 N MO Pac Expy Bldg 120, Austin, TX 78759
Spinal intervertebral body sizers.

Spine Wave, Inc. 203-944-9494
2 Enterprise Dr Ste 302, Shelton, CT 06484
Various types of distractors.

Spineworks Medical Inc. 408-986-8950
1735 N 1st St Ste 245, San Jose, CA 95112

Sterilmed, Inc. 763-488-3400
11400 73rd Ave N Ste 100, Maple Grove, MN 55369
Knife blade.

Stryker Endoscopy 800-435-0220
5900 Optical Ct, San Jose, CA 95138

Stryker Puerto Rico, Ltd. 939-307-2500
Hwy. 3, Km. 131.2, Las Guasimas Ind. Park, Arroyo, PR 00714
Various types of sterile, disposable brushes and cement sculps.

Surgical Implant Generation Network (Sign) 509-371-1107
451 Hills St, Richland, WA 99354
Shield.

Symmetry Medical Usa, Inc 207-786-2775
111 N Clay St, Claypool, IN 46510
Various types of manual instruments.

Symmetry Medical Usa, Inc. 574-267-8700
486 W 350 N, Warsaw, IN 46582
Hip instruments, knee instruments, orthopedic instruments.

Symmetry Medical, Inc. 574-268-2252
3724 N State Road 15, Warsaw, IN 46582
MULTIPLE

Synthes San Diego 858-452-1266
6244 Ferris Sq Ste B, San Diego, CA 92121
Pedicle screw system accessories,instruments.

T & L Sharpening, Inc. 574-583-3868
PO Box 338, 2663 S. Freeman Rd., Monticello, IN 47960

Tmj Solution, Inc 805-650-3391
1793 Eastman Ave, Ventura, CA 93003
Various.

Trinity Orthopedics, Llc 858-792-1235
8817 Production Ave, San Diego, CA 92121

Ussc Puerto Rico, Inc. 203-845-1000
Building 911-67, Sabanetas Industrial Park, Ponce, PR 00731
Raylor instruments and accessories.

V--Operations Management Consulting, 317-570-5830
7350 E 86th St, Indianapolis, IN 46256

Von Zabern Surgical 951-734-7215
4121 Tigris Way, Riverside, CA 92503
Various orthopedic manual surgical instruments.

W.L. Gore & Associates,Inc 928-526-3030
1505 North Fourth St., Flagstaff, AZ 86004
Gore smoother crucial tool.

Warsaw Orthopedic, Inc. 901-396-3133
2500 Silveus Xing, Warsaw, IN 46582
Orthopedic manual surgical instrument.

West Coast Surgical Llc. 650-728-8095
141 California Ave Ste 101, Half Moon Bay, CA 94019
Drill guide,screwdriver,drill,bone tamp.

Zimmer Spine, Inc. 800-655-2614
7375 Bush Lake Rd, Minneapolis, MN 55439
Various laparoscopic spinal fusion instruments.

ORTHOPEDIC MANUAL SURGICAL INSTRUMENT *(cont'd)*

Zimmer Trabecular Metal Technology 800-613-6131
10 Pomeroy Rd, Parsippany, NJ 07054
Acetabular trial shell.

3d Medical Concepts, Llc 205-987-0935
1061 Morgan Park Rd, Pelham, AL 35124
Various orthopedic manual surgical instruments.

ORTHOSIS, ABDOMINAL *(Physical Med) 89KTD*

American Orthopedic Supply Co., Inc.
37017 State Highway 79, Cleveland, AL 35049
Abdominal binders.

Biomet, Inc. 574-267-6639
56 E Bell Dr, PO Box 587, Warsaw, IN 46582
Various types of abdominal supports.

Chase Ergonomics, Inc. 800-621-5436
PO Box 92497, Albuquerque, NM 87199
Various types and models of lumbo-sacral orthosis.

Dj Orthopedics De Mexico, S.A. De C.V. 690-727-1280
Blvd., Delagacion La Presa, Tijuana 22397 Mexico
Various

Dj Orthopedics De Mexico, S.A. De C.V. 690-727-1280
Ave. Venustiano Carranza 6802, Castillo, Tijuana 22100 Mexico
Various

Dynatronics Corp. Chattanooga Operations 801-568-7000
6607 Mountain View Rd, Ooltewah, TN 37363
Abdominal orthosis.

Marena Group, Inc. 770-822-6925
650 Progress Industrial Blvd, Lawrenceville, GA 30043
Marena post-operative compression garment.

Otto Bock Healthcare, Lp 763-489-5106
9420 Delegates Dr Ste 100, Orlando, FL 32837
Various types of abdominal orthosis/accessories.

Patterson Medical Supply, Inc. 262-387-8720
W68N158 Evergreen Blvd, Cedarburg, WI 53012
Various types.

Ps Products, Llc 215-661-9595
329 Bradford Ln, Lansdale, PA 19446
Penile support device, psd.

R & R Industries, Inc. 949-361-9238
1000 Calle Cordillera, San Clemente, CA 92673
Back support belt.

Spio Inc. 253-893-0390
25826 108th Ave SE, Kent, WA 98030
Abdominal support.

The Align-Right Pillow Co. Ltd. 800-331-0907
107 Merner Ave., Kitchener, ONTAR N2H 1X5 Canada
Sleeping pillows.

ORTHOSIS, CERVICAL *(Physical Med) 89IQK*

Air A Med, Inc. 239-936-5590
2049 Beacon Manor Dr, Fort Myers, FL 33907
Contour head immobilizer.

Ambu A/S 457-225-2210
6740 Baymeadow Dr, Glen Burnie, MD 21060
Cervical collars/extrication collars.

American Orthopedic Supply Co., Inc.
37017 State Highway 79, Cleveland, AL 35049
Soft cervical collar.

Aspen Medical Products 949-681-0200
6481 Oak Cyn, Irvine, CA 92618
Cervical collar.

Azmec, Inc. 877-862-9632
519 N Smith Ave Ste 110, Corona, CA 92880
Orthosis, cervical collars.

Becker Orthopedic Appliance Co. 248-588-7480
635 Executive Dr, Troy, MI 48083
Various cervical orthoses.

Best Orthopedic And Medical Services, Inc. 800-344-5279
2356B Springs Rd NE, Hickory, NC 28601

Biomet, Inc. 574-267-6639
56 E Bell Dr, PO Box 587, Warsaw, IN 46582
Various types of cervical collars.

Bird & Cronin, Inc. 651-683-1111
1200 Trapp Rd, Saint Paul, MN 55121
Cervical collar-soft.

ORTHOSIS, CERVICAL *(cont'd)*

Blackstone Medical, Inc. 888-298-5400
90 Brookdale Dr, Springfield, MA 01104

C.D. Denison Orthopaedic Appliance Corp. 410-235-9645
220 W 28th St, Baltimore, MD 21211
Cervical collar orthosis, $360.00 per unit (standard). Cervical-thoracic extension kit, $149.50 per unit (standard). Cervical-trachea front kit, $146.00 per unit (standard). Cervical extra small collar, $425.00 per unit. Torticollis kit, $819.30. Sheepskin cover kit, $237.50.

Caguas Orthopedic Center, Inc. 787-744-2325
FF4 Calle 11, Villa Del Rey, Caguas, PR 00727
Orthosis cervical.

Circular Traction Supply, Inc. 800-247-6535
7602 Talbert Ave Ste 9, Huntington Beach, CA 92648
Neck brace.

Core Products International, Inc. 800-365-3047
808 Prospect Ave, Osceola, WI 54020

Dj Orthopedics De Mexico, S.A. De C.V. 690-727-1280
Blvd., Delagacion La Presa, Tijuana 22397 Mexico
Various

Dj Orthopedics De Mexico, S.A. De C.V. 690-727-1280
Ave. Venustiano Carranza 6802, Castillo, Tijuana 22100 Mexico
Various

DJO Inc. 800-336-6569
1430 Decision St, Vista, CA 92081

Dr. Len's Medical Products Llc 678-908-8180
412 Atwood Rd, Erdenheim, PA 19038
Soft collar or soft brace.

Dynatronics Corp. Chattanooga Operations 801-568-7000
6607 Mountain View Rd, Ooltewah, TN 37363
Cervical orthosis.

E-Stat Plastics, Division Of Fram Trak Industries, 732-424-1600
205 Hallock Ave, Middlesex, NJ 08846
Cervical collar - neck brace.

Emergency Medical Supply, Inc. 502-543-2401
238 Salt Well Rd, P.o.. Box 99, Shepherdsville, KY 40165
Cervical collar.

Ferno-Washington, Inc. 800-733-3766
70 Weil Way, Wilmington, OH 45177

Florida Brace Corporation 800-327-0870
601 W Webster Ave, Winter Park, FL 32789

Florida Manufacturing Corp. 800-447-2372
501 Beville Rd, South Daytona, FL 32119

Freeman Manufacturing Company 800-253-2091
900 W Chicago Rd, PO Box J, Sturgis, MI 49091

Imak Products Corp. 619-291-9990
2515 Camino Del Rio S Ste 240, San Diego, CA 92108
Various.

Jerome Medical 800-257-8440
305 Harper Dr, Moorestown, NJ 08057
Extrication collar, rehabilitation collar, thoracic extension, and pediatric collar. Miami Occian Collar Back for patients at risk for occipital breakdown. Also Papoose Infant Spinal Immobilizer, for infants up to 3 months old.

Kenad Sg Medical, Inc. 800-825-0606
2692 Huntley Dr, Memphis, TN 38132
Cervical collar.

Kennex Development Inc 626-458-0598
533 S Atlantic Blvd Ste 301, Monterey Park, CA 91754
Various types of cervical orthosis.

Larkotex Company 800-972-3037
1002 Olive St, Texarkana, TX 75501

Medical Collar Covers, Inc. 606-836-2575
600 Greenup Ave Ste 101, Raceland, KY 41169
Cervical collar cover/liner; cervical brace cover/liner; neck brace cover/liner.

Medical Depot 516-998-4600
99 Seaview Blvd, Port Washington, NY 11050
Cervical collar.

Mizuho Osi 800-777-4674
30031 Ahern Ave, Union City, CA 94587

Optp 888-819-0121
3800 Annapolis Ln N Ste 165, PO Box 47009, Minneapolis, MN 55447
$17.45 for Original McKenzie Cervical Roll.

ORTHOSIS, CERVICAL *(cont'd)*

Orthotic & Prosthetic Lab, Inc. 314-968-8555
748 Marshall Ave, Webster Groves, MO 63119
O&p cervical orthosis.

Ossur Americas 800-257-8440
1414 Metropolitan Ave, West Deptford, NJ 08066
Miami J Cervical collar, Philadelphia Tracheotomy Collar, Atlas Collar

Ossur Americas 949-268-3155
742 Pancho Rd, Camarillo, CA 93012

Otto Bock Healthcare, Lp 763-489-5106
9420 Delegates Dr Ste 100, Orlando, FL 32837
Various types of cervical orthoses/accessories.

Patterson Medical Supply, Inc. 262-387-8720
W68N158 Evergreen Blvd, Cedarburg, WI 53012
Cervical pillow.

Pmt Corp. 800-626-5463
1500 Park Rd, Chanhassen, MN 55317

Rinz-L-O 248-548-3993
340 W Maplehurst St, Ferndale, MI 48220
Orthosis, cervical.

Scott Specialties, Inc. 785-527-5627
1827 Meadowlark Rd, Clay Center, KS 67432
Various types of cervical collars.

Scott Specialties, Inc. 785-527-5627
1820 E 7th St, Concordia, KS 66901

Scott Specialties, Inc./Cmo Inc./Ginny Inc. 800-255-7136
512 M St, Belleville, KS 66935

Symmetric Designs, Ltd. 800-537-1724
2059 North End Rd., Salt Spring Island, BC V8K 1C9 Canada
Civic collar

Tartan Orthopedics, Ltd. 888-287-1456
10651 Irma Dr Unit C, Northglenn, CO 80233
$5.90 per unit (standard).

The Saunders Group 800-445-9836
4250 Norex Dr, Chaska, MN 55318
Cervical roll.

Truform Orthotics & Prosthetics 800-888-0458
3960 Rosslyn Dr, Cincinnati, OH 45209

Vmg Medical, Inc. 540-337-1996
542 Walnut Hills Rd, Staunton, VA 24401
Cervical support cushion.

Warsaw Orthopedic, Inc. 901-396-3133
2500 Silveus Xing, Warsaw, IN 46582
Various types of cervical collars.

Zimmer Holdings, Inc. 800-613-6131
1800 W Center St, PO Box 708, Warsaw, IN 46580

ORTHOSIS, CERVICAL-THORACIC, RIGID *(Physical Med) 89IQF*

A&A Orthopedics, Incorporated 757-224-0177
12250 SW 129th Ct Bldg 1, Miami, FL 33186
Orthosis, cervical-thoracic, rigid.

Becker Orthopedic Appliance Co. 248-588-7480
635 Executive Dr, Troy, MI 48083
Various cervical-thoracic, rigid orthoses.

Biomet, Inc. 574-267-6639
56 E Bell Dr, PO Box 587, Warsaw, IN 46582
Various types of cervical braces.

Confortaire Inc 662-842-2966
2133 S Veterans Blvd, Tupelo, MS 38804
Cervical collar, foam collar, plastic collar.

Cranial Technologies, Inc. 480-505-1840
1395 W Auto Dr, Tempe, AZ 85284
Doc brand.

Depuy Ace, A Johnson & Johnson Company 800-473-3789
700 Orthopaedic Dr, Warsaw, IN 46582

Emergency Medical Supply, Inc. 502-543-2401
238 Salt Well Rd, P.o.. Box 99, Shepherdsville, KY 40165
Kendrick extrication device or ked, truncal orthosis.

Emergency Products And Research 305-304-6933
890 W Main St, Kent, OH 44240
Extrication device.

Florida Brace Corporation 800-327-0870
601 W Webster Ave, Winter Park, FL 32789

Freeman Manufacturing Company 800-253-2091
900 W Chicago Rd, PO Box J, Sturgis, MI 49091

ORTHOSIS, CERVICAL-THORACIC, RIGID *(cont'd)*

Goodwill Industries Of Central Indiana, Inc. 317-524-4270
1635 W Michigan St, Indianapolis, IN 46222
Long and short spineboard.

Innovative Choices, Inc. 315-482-2583
700 Progress Ave, Scarborough M1H 2Z7 Canada
Pillow (cervical)

Larkotex Company 800-972-3037
1002 Olive St, Texarkana, TX 75501

Spinal Solutions, Inc. 770-922-2434
1971 Old Covington Rd NE Ste 103, Conyers, GA 30013
Various types of orthoses.

Surgitech Inc. 760-477-8191
870 Rancheros Dr, San Marcos, CA 92069
Cervical-thoracic brace.

Tartan Orthopedics, Ltd. 888-287-1456
10651 Irma Dr Unit C, Northglenn, CO 80233
$30.00 per unit (standard).

The Saunders Group 800-445-9836
4250 Norex Dr, Chaska, MN 55318
Cervical roll.

Truform Orthotics & Prosthetics 800-888-0458
3960 Rosslyn Dr, Cincinnati, OH 45209

ORTHOSIS, CORRECTIVE SHOE *(Physical Med) 89KNP*

Alimed, Inc. 800-225-2610
297 High St, Dedham, MA 02026

Atlantic Footcare 401-765-3600
761 Great Rd, North Smithfield, RI 02896

Bird & Cronin, Inc. 651-683-1111
1200 Trapp Rd, Saint Paul, MN 55121
Foot orthotics.

Breg, Inc., An Orthofix Company 800-897-BREG
2611 Commerce Way, Vista, CA 92081
Orthotic.

Commerce Atlantic Corp. 626-448-3905
2239 Tyler Ave Ste B, South El Monte, CA 91733
Orthosis, corrective shoe.

Crocs, Inc. 801-455-8558
6328 Monarch Park Pl, Longmont, CO 80503
Depth shoe with molded insert.

Dr. Roth's Footcare Products, Llc. 800-486-0325
1012 Brioso Dr Ste 105, Costa Mesa, CA 92627
FABS (Foot Arch Band Support) is a one-size-fits-all foot device that provides relief to tired, achy feet, plantar fascitis, shin splints, flat foot disorders, heel-spur syndrome, many lesser known foot discomforts and lower back pain. FABS acts to improve the posture of the foot and is the only arch support that can be worn with sandals or even barefoot!

Footmaxx Holdings Inc. 800-779-3668
468 Queen St. E, Ste. 400, Toronto, ONT M5A-1T7 Canada
Footmaxx orthotic.

Magic Walk, Inc. 408-435-7380
2372 Qume Dr Ste E, San Jose, CA 95131
Diabetic shoe.

Md Orthopaedics 877-766-7384
604 N Parkway St, Wayland, IA 52654
Afo.

Medical Solutions Distribution Group 501-450-9063
535 Enterprise Ave, Conway, AR 72032
Multiple density inserts.

Nobile Consulting Usa Llc 866-500-7463
1555 Jupiter Park Dr Ste 11, Jupiter, FL 33458
Orthosis, corrective shoe.

Otto Bock Healthcare 763-489-5106
3820 Great Lakes Dr, Salt Lake City, UT 84120
Orthotics (various models).

Otto Bock Healthcare, Lp 763-489-5106
9420 Delegates Dr Ste 100, Orlando, FL 32837
Various types of shoe orthoses/accessories.

P. W. Minor 585-815-0659
3 Treadeasy Ave, Batavia, NY 14020
Extra depth, therapeutic, orthopedic footwear.

Painless Shoe Co. 818-734-7080
21500 Osborne St, Canoga Park, CA 91304

ORTHOSIS, CORRECTIVE SHOE *(cont'd)*

Patterson Medical Supply, Inc. 262-387-8720
W68N158 Evergreen Blvd, Cedarburg, WI 53012
Corrective shoe.

Pedors Shoes 800-750-6729
1349 Old 41 Hwy NW Ste 130, Marietta, GA 30060

Pine Tree Orthopedic Lab L.L.C. 207-524-2079
2120 Route 106, Leeds, ME 04263
Custom orthotic.

Prime Materials Corp. 877-755-1649
6 Treadeasy Ave, PO Box 71, Batavia, NY 14020
Pre-made foot orthosis.

Remington Products Company Llc 800-491-1571
961 Seville Rd, Wadsworth, OH 44281
Arch supports.

Schering-Plough Healthcare Products, Inc. 862-245-5115
4207 Michigan Avenue Rd NE, Cleveland, TN 37323
Various inserts.

Sorbothane, Inc. 800-838-3906
2144 State Route 59, Kent, OH 44240
SORBOTHANE insoles, sizes women 5-11, men 5 1/2-13
SORBOTHANE shock absorbing insoles sizes women 5-11, men 5 1/2 - 13

Spectra Industries Corp. 800-220-7050
322 W Oak Ln, Glenolden, PA 19036
Corrective foot orthosis.

Viscolas, Inc. 800-548-2694
8801 Consolidated Dr, Soddy Daisy, TN 37379
Various types.

ORTHOSIS, CRANIAL *(Cns/Neurology) 84MVA*

Becker Orthopedic Appliance Co. 248-588-7480
635 Executive Dr, Troy, MI 48083
Orthosis, cranial.

Center For Orthotic & Prosthetic Care 502-637-7717
1931 West St, New Albany, IN 47150
Cranial orthosis.

Children's Hospital 402-955-3857
8200 Dodge St, Omaha, NE 68114
Cranial orthosis.

Cranial Solutions 973-835-7929
602 Lincoln Ave, Pompton Lakes, NJ 07442
Cranial moulding helmet.

Cranial Technologies, Inc. 480-505-1840
1395 W Auto Dr, Tempe, AZ 85284
Cranial orthosis, helmet, molding helmet.

Danmar Products, Inc. 734-761-1990
221 Jackson Industrial Dr, Ann Arbor, MI 48103
Cranial helmet, cranial band or helmet.

Eastern Cranial Affiliates 703-807-5899
1600 Wilson Blvd Ste 200, Arlington, VA 22209
Cranial orthosis.

Gema, Inc. 773-878-2445
2434 W Peterson Ave, Chicago, IL 60659
Cranial orthosis.

Orthomerica Products, Inc. 800-446-6770
6333 N Orange Blossom Trl Ste 220, Orlando, FL 32810
STARband cranial-remodeling orthosis and Starlight designs. Used to treat positional plagiocephaly, brachycephaly, scaphocephaly, and other head-shape deformities in infants 3-18 months of age. Received FDA 510(k) clearance in 2000.

Orthotic & Prosthetic Lab, Inc. 314-968-8555
748 Marshall Ave, Webster Groves, MO 63119
O&p cranial molding helmet.

Orthotic Solutions, Llc. 703-849-9200
2802 Merrilee Dr Ste 100, Fairfax, VA 22031
Cranial orthosis.

Otto Bock Healthcare 763-489-5106
3820 Great Lakes Dr, Salt Lake City, UT 84120
Cranial helmet.

Personal Performance Medical Corp. 801-364-3100
50 S 900 E Ste 1, Salt Lake City, UT 84102
Plagiocephalic applied pressure orthosis.

Precision Prosthetics & Orthotics, Inc. 314-843-3339
11102 Lindbergh Business Ct, Saint Louis, MO 63123
Cranial orthosis.

ORTHOSIS, CRANIAL *(cont'd)*

Restorative Health Services 615-225-6090
800 NW Broad St Ste 126, Murfreesboro, TN 37129
Cranial helmet.

ORTHOSIS, FIXATION, CERVICAL INTERVERTEBRAL BODY, SPINAL *(Orthopedics) 87MAT*

Depuy Spine, Inc. 800-227-6633
325 Paramount Dr, Raynham, MA 02767
Cervical anterior plate.

Warsaw Orthopedic, Inc. 901-396-3133
2500 Silveus Xing, Warsaw, IN 46582
Cervical implant fixation device.

Zimmer Spine, Inc. 800-655-2614
7375 Bush Lake Rd, Minneapolis, MN 55439
Spinal fixation plates and screws.

ORTHOSIS, FIXATION, PEDICLE, SPINAL *(Orthopedics) 87MNI*

Abbott Spine, Inc. 847-937-6100
12708 Riata Vista Cir Ste B-100, Austin, TX 78727
Pedicle screw system.

Advanced Spine Technology, Inc. 415-241-2400
457 Mariposa St, San Francisco, CA 94107
Trifix system.

Aesculap Implant Systems, Inc. 610-984-9074
9999 Hamilton Blvd Bldg 8, Breinigsville, PA 18031
Pedicle screw spinal system.

Allez Spine, Llc 949-752-7885
2301 Dupont Dr Ste 510, Irvine, CA 92612
Spinal fixation system.

Alphatec Spine, Inc. 760-494-6769
5818 El Camino Real, Carlsbad, CA 92008
Pedicle screw system.

Amedica Corporation 801-839-3500
1885 W 2100 S, Salt Lake City, UT 84119
Valeo PS

Depuy Spine, Inc. 800-227-6633
325 Paramount Dr, Raynham, MA 02767
Pedicle screw.

Innovasis, Inc. 801-261-2236
614 E 3900 S, Salt Lake City, UT 84107
Rod and screw spinal instrumentation.

Jemo Spine, Llc 801-266-4811
6170 S 380 W Ste 200, Murray, UT 84107
Pedicle screw spinal system.

K2m, Inc. 866-526-4171
751 Miller Dr SE Ste F1, Leesburg, VA 20175
Spine fixation system.

Lanx Inc. 303-443-7500
390 Interlocken Cres, Broomfield, CO 80021

Micron Precision Engineering, Inc. 310-874-4963
939 Evening Shade Dr, San Pedro, CA 90731
Pedicle screw fixation.

Nuvasive, Inc. 800-475-9131
7475 Lusk Blvd, San Diego, CA 92121
Spinal implants.

Orthotec, Llc 800-557-2988
9595 Wilshire Blvd Ste 502, Beverly Hills, CA 90212
Various.

Paramount Surgicals, Inc. 956-541-1220
942 Wildrose Ln Ste B, Brownsville, TX 78520
Spine pedicle screw system.

Pisharodi Surgicals, Inc. 956-541-6725
3475 W Alton Gloor Blvd, Brownsville, TX 78520
Spine pedicle screw system.

Scient'X Usa, Inc. 407-571-2550
1015 Maitland Center Commons Blvd Ste 10, Maitland, FL 32751
Multiple.

Seaspine 760-727-8399
2302 La Mirada Dr, Vista, CA 92081
Pedicle screw spine system.

Spine Wave, Inc. 203-944-9494
2 Enterprise Dr Ste 302, Shelton, CT 06484
Pedicle screw system.

Spinecraft Llc 708-531-9700
2215 Enterprise Dr, Westchester, IL 60154
Spinal fixation system.

ORTHOSIS, FIXATION, PEDICLE, SPINAL *(cont'd)*

Synthes (Usa) 610-719-5000
35 Airport Rd, Horseheads, NY 14845
Various types and sizes of pedicle fixation orthoses.

Us Spine Inc. 561-367-7463
3600 Fau Blvd Ste 101, Boca Raton, FL 33431
Pedicle screw system.

V--Operations Management Consulting, 317-570-5830
7350 E 86th St, Indianapolis, IN 46256

Vertebron, Inc. 203-380-9340
400 Long Beach Blvd, Stratford, CT 06615
Pedicle screw system.

Vertiflex (Tm), Incorporated 1-866-268-6486
1351 Calle Avanzado, San Clemente, CA 92673
Pedicle screw system.

Zimmer Spine, Inc. 800-655-2614
7375 Bush Lake Rd, Minneapolis, MN 55439
Spinal pedicle fixation systems.

ORTHOSIS, FIXATION, SPINAL, SPONDYLOLISTHESIS
(Orthopedics) 87MNH

Abbott Spine, Inc. 847-937-6100
12708 Riata Vista Cir Ste B-100, Austin, TX 78727
Pedicle screw system.

Advanced Spine Technology, Inc. 415-241-2400
457 Mariposa St, San Francisco, CA 94107
Triplefix system.

Aesculap Implant Systems, Inc. 610-984-9074
9999 Hamilton Blvd Bldg 8, Breinigsville, PA 18031
Pedicle screw spinal system.

Allez Spine, Llc 949-752-7885
2301 Dupont Dr Ste 510, Irvine, CA 92612
Spinal fixation system.

Alphatec Spine, Inc. 760-494-6769
5818 El Camino Real, Carlsbad, CA 92008
Pedicle screw spinal system.

Applied Spine Technologies, Inc. 203-503-0280
300 George St Ste 511, New Haven, CT 06511

Depuy Spine, Inc. 800-227-6633
325 Paramount Dr, Raynham, MA 02767
Med pedicle screw.

Medtronic Sofamor Danek Usa, Inc. 901-396-3133
4340 Swinnea Rd, Memphis, TN 38118
Multi-axial screw.

Nuvasive, Inc. 800-475-9131
7475 Lusk Blvd, San Diego, CA 92121
Spinal implants.

Orthotec, Llc 800-557-2988
9595 Wilshire Blvd Ste 502, Beverly Hills, CA 90212
Various.

Spine Wave, Inc. 203-944-9494
2 Enterprise Dr Ste 302, Shelton, CT 06484
Pedicle screw system.

Spinecraft Llc 708-531-9700
2215 Enterprise Dr, Westchester, IL 60154
Spinal fixation system.

Synthes (Usa) 610-719-5000
35 Airport Rd, Horseheads, NY 14845
Various types and sizes of spondylolisthesis spinal fixation orthoses.

Synthes San Diego 858-452-1266
6244 Ferris Sq Ste B, San Diego, CA 92121
Pedicle screw fixation system.

Ultimate Spine, Llc. 562-598-1753
1220 N Barsten Way, Anaheim, CA 92806
Spinal fixation device.

Us Spine Inc. 561-367-7463
3600 Fau Blvd Ste 101, Boca Raton, FL 33431
Pedicle screw fixation system.

Vertiflex (Tm), Incorporated 1-866-268-6486
1351 Calle Avanzado, San Clemente, CA 92673
Pedicle screw system.

Warsaw Orthopedic, Inc. 901-396-3133
2500 Silveus Xing, Warsaw, IN 46582
Multi-axial screw.

ORTHOSIS, FIXATION, SPINAL, SPONDYLOLISTHESIS *(cont'd)*

Zimmer Spine, Inc. 800-655-2614
7375 Bush Lake Rd, Minneapolis, MN 55439
Spondyloisthesis spinal fixation system.

ORTHOSIS, FUSION, INTERVERTEBRAL, SPINAL
(Orthopedics) 87MAX

Depuy Spine, Inc. 800-227-6633
325 Paramount Dr, Raynham, MA 02767
Interbody fusion cage and posterior pedicle screw fixation system-sterile and no.

Medtronic Sofamor Danek Usa, Inc. 901-396-3133
4340 Swinnea Rd, Memphis, TN 38118
Spinal fusion device.

Micron Precision Engineering, Inc. 310-874-4963
939 Evening Shade Dr, San Pedro, CA 90731
Spinal intervertebral implant-fusion.

Ussc Puerto Rico, Inc. 203-845-1000
Building 911-67, Sabanetas Industrial Park, Ponce, PR 00731
Spinal fusion device.

Warsaw Orthopedic, Inc. 901-396-3133
2500 Silveus Xing, Warsaw, IN 46582
Spinal fusion device.

Zimmer Spine, Inc. 800-655-2614
7375 Bush Lake Rd, Minneapolis, MN 55439
Interbody fusion cage.

ORTHOSIS, LIMB BRACE *(Physical Med) 89IQI*

A&A Orthopedics, Incorporated 757-224-0177
12250 SW 129th Ct Bldg 1, Miami, FL 33186
Arm splints.

Accu-Med Technologies, Inc. 718-244-5330
150 Bud Mil Dr, Buffalo, NY 14206
Leg brace.

Accumed Systems, Inc. 734-930-0461
6109 Jackson Rd, Ann Arbor, MI 48103
Wrist positioning splint.

Acustep, Inc. 785-826-2500
2775 Arnold Ave Ste A, Salina, KS 67401
Various types of foot orthoses.

Agp-Medical, Llc. 860-416-0590
539 N Main St, Suffield, CT 06078
Limb orthosis vaso-wrap.

Aircast Llc 800-321-9549
1430 Decision St, Vista, CA 92081
AIRCAST walking brace.

Alimed, Inc. 800-225-2610
297 High St, Dedham, MA 02026

Anodyne Therapy, Llc 813-645-2855
13570 Wright Cir, Tampa, FL 33626
Limb brace.

Armor Sports Holdings, Llc 520-623-9800
2030 N Forbes Blvd Ste 106, Tucson, AZ 85745
The airarmor leg protection system, knee brace, prophylactic knee brace.

Arthron, Inc. 800-758-5633
PO Box 1627, 1605 Ash Grove Ct., Brentwood, TN 37024
Acromioclavicular pad or bridge.

Arthur Finnieston Clinic 305-817-1604
2480 W 82nd St Unit 8, Hialeah, FL 33016

Avry's Orthotic Facility, Inc. 330-746-5385
1441 Wick Ave, Youngstown, OH 44505
Knee-ankle-foot orthosis; ankle-foot orthosis.

Azmec, Inc. 877-862-9632
519 N Smith Ave Ste 110, Corona, CA 92880
Limb brace, knee splint.

B & H Orthopedic Lab., Inc. 314-647-1617
2510 Hampton Ave, Saint Louis, MO 63139
Plastic or metal-long leg brace, short leg brace, arm brace, wrist splint, hand.

Back Pain Relief Clinic, P.C. 574-271-9444
5507 Singer Ct, Granger, IN 46530
Wrist-hand-finger brace.

Becker Orthopedic Appliance Co. 248-588-7480
635 Executive Dr, Troy, MI 48083
Various limb orthoses and orthosis components.

ORTHOSIS, LIMB BRACE *(cont'd)*

Bellacure, Inc. 206-762-2070
6327 W Marginal Way SW Bldg 2, Seattle, WA 98106
Various limb braces examples knee braces,hip braces,elbow braces, etc.

Biomet, Inc. 574-267-6639
56 E Bell Dr, PO Box 587, Warsaw, IN 46582
Various types of general purpose braces.

Bird & Cronin, Inc. 651-683-1111
1200 Trapp Rd, Saint Paul, MN 55121
Orthopedic splints.

Blake Manufacturing, Inc. 813-935-1841
9241 Lazy Ln, Tampa, FL 33614
Ankle foot orthosis.

Bledsoe Brace Systems 888-253-3763
2601 Pinewood Dr, Grand Prairie, TX 75051

Bonutti Research, Inc. 217-342-3412
2600 S Raney St, Effingham, IL 62401
Various models.

Boston Billows, Inc. 603-598-1200
28 Charron Ave Ste 3, Nashua, NH 03063
Billowpillow.

Breg, Inc., An Orthofix Company 800-897-BREG
2611 Commerce Way, Vista, CA 92081
Knee supports.

Brennen Medical, Llc 651-429-7413
1290 Hammond Rd, Saint Paul, MN 55110
Lower leg positioning device.

Brown Medical Industries 800-843-4395
1300 Lundberg Dr W, Spirit Lake, IA 51360
FLEX 8 Elbow Extension Stabilizer prevents and reduces elbow pain by stabilizing elbow extension and rotation. SHIN ICE shin cold and compression sleeve provides therapeutic ice and compression treatment for patients with shin splints. STEADY STEP WALKER is a walking splint and ankle-foot fracture orthesis that can be converted to an ankle stirrup. SHIN SLEEVE compression neoprene sleeve to wear on lower leg. BIO-DYNAMIX complete line fo heel cushions, shoe inserts and compression supports. HERBST CRADLE multi-podus device for prevention and healing of ulcers on the heel and malleoli. Features heel suspension of an anti-rotation bar and prevent unwanted hip positioning.

C.D. Denison Orthopaedic Appliance Corp. 410-235-9645
220 W 28th St, Baltimore, MD 21211
Patella knee orthosis, $27.60 per unit. Dorsiflexion foot orthosis, $32.75 per unit. Shoulder/arm support orthosis $49.95 per unit; Denison-Duke Wyre shoulder vest orthosis, $99.75 per unit; Elastic leg rotation control orthosis,s,m: $156.10 per unit, lg: $163.25 per unit.

Caguas Orthopedic Center, Inc. 787-744-2325
FF4 Calle 11, Villa Del Rey, Caguas, PR 00727
Orthosis, limb brace.

Cascade Dafo, Inc. 360-384-1858
1360 Sunset Ave, Ferndale, WA 98248
Various types of ankle foot orthoses.

Cc Medical Devices, Inc. 913-269-8400
14131 S Mur Len Rd, Olathe, KS 66062
Carpal tunnel restorer.

Cosco 800-582-6853
1602 Lakeside Dr, Redding, CA 96001

D.A. Pearson Co. 860-651-9073
4 Tim Clark Cir, P.O. Box 51, Simsbury, CT 06070
Multi-Podus Type Ankle/Foot Orthosis

Debusk Orthopedic Casting (Doc) 865-362-2334
420 Straight Creek Rd Ste 1, New Tazewell, TN 37825
Various types of splinting material and walkers.

Dj Orthopedics De Mexico, S.A. De C.V. 690-727-1280
Blvd., Delagacion La Presa, Tijuana 22397 Mexico
Orthopedic softgoods

Dj Orthopedics De Mexico, S.A. De C.V. 690-727-1280
Ave. Venustiano Carranza 6802, Castillo, Tijuana 22100 Mexico
Orthopedic softgoods

DJO Inc. 800-336-6569
1430 Decision St, Vista, CA 92081
Various off-the-shelf and custom bracing and supports.

Dynatronics Corp. Chattanooga Operations 801-568-7000
6607 Mountain View Rd, Ooltewah, TN 37363
Limb brace orthosis.

ORTHOSIS, LIMB BRACE *(cont'd)*

Ebi Patient Care, Inc. 973-299-9300
1 Electro-biology Blvd., Guaynabo, PR 00657
Braces.

Eischco, Inc. 503-492-2232
1232 SE 282nd Ave, Gresham, OR 97080
A.e.r boot walkabout model.

Empi 651-415-9000
Clear Lake Industrial Park, Clear Lake, SD 57226
Active range of motion device.

Equip For Independence, Inc. 800-216-4881
333 Mamaroneck Ave Ste 383, White Plains, NY 10605
LIFT-A-LIMB, Unique lightweight and portable elevator/positioners. Upper Extremity Unit (1 1/2 lbs)and Lower Extremity Unit (3 lbs). Adjustable in height and angle. Ideal for prepping, procedures, recovery, wound care, casting or splint application, Ultrasound, Laser, treatment procedures and elevation with or without icing pre and or post trauma/surgery in the Emergency Room, Operating Room, Recovery Room, professional offices and home care. Stabilize, control edema and inhibit complications. Usage facilitates ROM and rehab progress.

Fallgard Llc 800-828-0702
631 Alexandria Dr, Naperville, IL 60565
Hip brace.

Ferno-Washington, Inc. 800-733-3766
70 Weil Way, Wilmington, OH 45177

Fillauer Companies, Inc. 800-251-6398
2710 Amnicola Hwy, Chattanooga, TN 37406

Foot Levelers, Inc. 540-345-0008
518 Pocahontas Ave NE, P.o. Box 12611, Roanoke, VA 24012
Arch support; cervical pillow.

Freeman Manufacturing Company 800-253-2091
900 W Chicago Rd, PO Box J, Sturgis, MI 49091
Tennis elbow splint; ankle, foot, knee, wrist & forearm orthoses.

Gelsmart Llc 973-884-8995
30 Leslie Ct Ste B-202, Whippany, NJ 07981
Various type of arch supports.

Hart Independent Mobility Corp. 905-403-8471
1323 Kelly Rd., Mississauga, ONT L5J 3V1 Canada
Hart walker

Hely And Weber 800-221-5465
1185 E Main St, Santa Paula, CA 93060
Patella stabilizer.

Hosmer Dorrance Corp. 408-379-5151
561 Division St, Campbell, CA 95008
Insert, tube.

Independent Brace, Inc. 863-647-5559
3633 Century Blvd Ste 1, Lakeland, FL 33811
Various.

J. T. Posey Co. 800-447-6739
5635 Peck Rd, Arcadia, CA 91006

Just Packaging Inc. 908-753-6700
450 Oak Tree Ave, South Plainfield, NJ 07080
Various types of limb orthoses.

Juzo 800-222-4999
PO Box 1088, 80 Chart Road, Cuyahoga Falls, OH 44223
Various.

Kintech Orthopaedics Ltd. 905-828-9921
2170 Dunwin Dr, Unit 7, Mississauga, ONT L5L-1C7 Canada
Buffalo knee brace

Kneebourne Therapeutic, Llc 317-776-2770
15299 Stony Creek Way, Noblesville, IN 46060
Active range of motion device.

Larkotex Company 800-972-3037
1002 Olive St, Texarkana, TX 75501

Leeder Group, Inc. 305-436-5030
8508 NW 66th St, Miami, FL 33166
Elbow splint.

Life-Like Prosthetics, Llc 310-320-5777
1319 W Carson St, Torrance, CA 90501

Maco Bag 315-226-1019
412 Van Buren St, Newark, NY 14513
Lymb brace.

ORTHOSIS, LIMB BRACE *(cont'd)*

Maramed Orthopedic Systems 800-327-5830
2480 W 82nd St, No. 8, Hialeah, FL 33016
MIAMI Fracture Brace System: Humerus, ulna, colles, tibia, femur and tibia.

Marken International, Inc. 800-564-9248
W231N2811 Roundy Cir E Ste 100, Pewaukee, WI 53072
Various.

Medefficiency, Inc. 303-321-7755
8620 Wolff Ct Ste 120, Westminster, CO 80031
Total contact cast.

Midwest Orthotic Services, Llc 574-233-3352
17530 Dugdale Dr, South Bend, IN 46635
Surestep smo.

Mizuho Osi 800-777-4674
30031 Ahern Ave, Union City, CA 94587

New Options, Inc. 214-638-6422
2545 Merrell Rd, Dallas, TX 75229
New options.

Normed 800-288-8200
PO Box 3644, Seattle, WA 98124
Various types & sizes of external limb braces.

Omni Life Science, Inc. 800-448-OMNI
1390 Decision St, Vista, CA 92081
V-Force ready-to-fit and custom knee brace for OA and ligament instability, with medial/lateral rotation control and suppport.

Ongoing Care Solutions, Inc. 800-375-0207
6545 44th St N Ste 4007, Pinellas Park, FL 33781
Various orthosis limb braces.

Ortho Innovations, Inc. 507-269-2895
121 23rd Ave SW, Rochester, MN 55902
Braces.

Orthotic & Prosthetic Lab, Inc. 314-968-8555
748 Marshall Ave, Webster Groves, MO 63119
O&p orthosis.

Orthotic Mobility Systems, Inc. 301-949-2444
10421 Metropolitan Ave, Kensington, MD 20895
Limb orthosis.

Orthotic Rehabilitation Products, Inc. 813-620-0035
7002 E Broadway Ave, Tampa, FL 33619
Hand splint.

Orthotics Choice Llc. 407-321-0454
451 E Airport Blvd, Sanford, FL 32773
Various types of limb braces/accessories.

Osborn Medical Corp. 800-535-5865
100 W Main St N, PO Box 324, Utica, MN 55979
Knee Immobilizer for Below Knee Amputation.

Ossur Americas 949-268-3155
742 Pancho Rd, Camarillo, CA 93012

Ots Corp. 800-221-4769
220 Merrimon Ave, Weaverville, NC 28787
Leg braces. STEPLOCK knee joints. INTERLOCK knee joints. INTEGRATED ANKLE orthotic ankle joints. ASAP II, multi fit flexion-contracture braces.

Otto Bock Healthcare, Lp 763-489-5106
9420 Delegates Dr Ste 100, Orlando, FL 32837
Various types of limb braces/accessories.

Painless Shoe Co. 818-734-7080
21500 Osborne St, Canoga Park, CA 91304

Pal Health Systems 800-223-2957
1805 Riverway Dr, Pekin, IL 61554
Custom ankle brace.

Patterson Medical Supply, Inc. 262-387-8720
W68N158 Evergreen Blvd, Cedarburg, WI 53012
Splinting material.

Pedifix, Inc. 800-424-5561
310 Guinea Rd, Brewster, NY 10509

Pfs Med, Inc. 541-349-9646
3295 Cross St, Eugene, OR 97402
Clam shell.

Plasco, Inc. 847-662-4400
Carretera Presta La Amistad, Km.19, Acuna, Coahila Mexico
Immobilizing extremity splint

ORTHOSIS, LIMB BRACE *(cont'd)*

Polygell Llc. 973-884-8995
30 Leslie Ct, Whippany, NJ 07981
Various type of arch supports.

R & R Industries, Inc. 949-361-9238
1000 Calle Cordillera, San Clemente, CA 92673
Wrist support,elastic.

Restorative Care Of America Inc 800-627-1595
12221 33rd St N, Saint Petersburg, FL 33716
Amputee Knee Orthosis, Prevents/corrects knee flexion contractures in the below the knee amputee. Features lower adjustable bi-valve shell.

Restorative Medical, Inc. 270-422-5454
332 Broadway St, Brandenburg, KY 40108
Various types hand splints, cervical collars, afos.

Royce Medical 800-521-0601
742 Pancho Rd, Camarillo, CA 93012

Saebo, Inc. 888-284-5433
2725 Water Ridge Pkwy Ste 320, Charlotte, NC 28217
Wrist hand finger orthosis.

Scott Orthotic Labs, Inc. 800-821-5795
1831 E Mulberry St, Fort Collins, CO 80524
Shoulder elbow wrist hand orthosis.

Shoney Scientific, Inc. 262-970-0170
West 223 North 720 Saratoga Drive,, Suite 120, Waukesha, WI 53186
Arm support.

Solaris, Inc. 414-918-9180
6737 W Washington St Ste 3260, West Allis, WI 53214
Ankle, knee, wrist, elbow padded support.

Spio Inc. 253-893-0390
25826 108th Ave SE, Kent, WA 98030
Hand splint, limb support.

Surgitech Inc. 760-477-8191
870 Rancheros Dr, San Marcos, CA 92069
Wrist brace.

Symmetric Designs, Ltd. 800-537-1724
2059 North End Rd., Salt Spring Island, BC V8K 1C9 Canada
Limb extension orthoses

The Saunders Group 800-445-9836
4250 Norex Dr, Chaska, MN 55318
Shoulder stabilizer.

Top Shelf Manufacturing, Llc 209-834-8185
1851 Paradise Rd Ste B, Tracy, CA 95304
Various types of limb orthosis.

Truform Orthotics & Prosthetics 800-888-0458
3960 Rosslyn Dr, Cincinnati, OH 45209

Ultraflex Systems, Inc. 610-906-1410
237 South St Ste 200, Pottstown, PA 19464
Various dynamic ankle splints.

Vantage Orthopedics 513-563-1690
41 Techview Dr, Cincinnati, OH 45215
Vantage.

Vision Quest Industries, Inc. 800-266-6969
18011 Mitchell S, Irvine, CA 92614
Brace, knee brace.

Vq Orthocare
1390 Decision St Ste A, Vista, CA 92081
Limb orthosis.

Warsaw Orthopedic, Inc. 901-396-3133
2500 Silveus Xing, Warsaw, IN 46582
Various types of hard and soft limb and joint splints (supports, braces).

Whitman Corp. 513-541-3223
1725 Powers St, Cincinnati, OH 45223
Drop foot support.

X-Strap Systems 914-968-3381
81 Pondfield Rd Ste 157, Bronxville, NY 10708
FOOT DROP AFO BRACE

Zhang Enterprises 972-238-8260
400 N Greenville Ave Ste 9, Richardson, TX 75081
Various types of limb devices.

Zimmer Holdings, Inc. 800-613-6131
1800 W Center St, PO Box 708, Warsaw, IN 46580

ORTHOSIS, LUMBAR *(Physical Med) 89IQE*

Accu-Med Technologies, Inc. 718-244-5330
150 Bud Mil Dr, Buffalo, NY 14206
Back brace.

Alimed, Inc. 800-225-2610
297 High St, Dedham, MA 02026
McKenzie lumbar rolls counteract poor posture and correct lordosis while seated.

Anodyne Therapy, Llc 813-645-2855
13570 Wright Cir, Tampa, FL 33626
Lumbar support.

Aspen Medical Products 949-681-0200
6481 Oak Cyn, Irvine, CA 92618
Cervical thoracic.

B & H Orthopedic Lab., Inc. 314-647-1617
2510 Hampton Ave, Saint Louis, MO 63139
Custom made plastic body jacket.

Bauerfeind Usa, Inc. 800-423-3405
55 Chastain Rd NW Ste 112, Kennesaw, GA 30144
LUMBOTRAIN low-back support with viscoelastic insert.

Becker Orthopedic Appliance Co. 248-588-7480
635 Executive Dr, Troy, MI 48083
Various orthosis, lumbar.

Breg, Inc., An Orthofix Company 800-897-BREG
2611 Commerce Way, Vista, CA 92081
Truncal orthosis, back support.

Chase Ergonomics, Inc. 800-621-5436
PO Box 92497, Albuquerque, NM 87199
Cadet. New products include the Decade Accupressure back support (48030 series), which provides clinically proven protection from over-contraction of back muscles during unexpected loading events (e.g., accidents).

Dj Orthopedics De Mexico, S.A. De C.V. 690-727-1280
Blvd., Delagacion La Presa, Tijuana 22397 Mexico
Sacro-lumbar supports

Dj Orthopedics De Mexico, S.A. De C.V. 690-727-1280
Ave. Venustiano Carranza 6802, Castillo, Tijuana 22100 Mexico
Sacro-lumbar supports

DJO Inc. 800-336-6569
1430 Decision St, Vista, CA 92081
Various off-the-shelf Lumbar supports and braces.

Dynatronics Corp. Chattanooga Operations 801-568-7000
6607 Mountain View Rd, Ooltewah, TN 37363
Lumbar orthosis.

Fillauer Companies, Inc. 800-251-6398
2710 Amnicola Hwy, Chattanooga, TN 37406

Frank Stubbs Co., Inc 800-223-1713
2100 Eastman Ave Ste B, Oxnard, CA 93030

Frederick Lee Inc 787-834-4880
191 Calle Balboa, PO Box 3287, Mayaguez, PR 00680

Freeman Manufacturing Company 800-253-2091
900 W Chicago Rd, PO Box J, Sturgis, MI 49091

Homedics Inc. 800-333-8282
3000 N Pontiac Trl, Commerce Township, MI 48390
Adjustable lumbar cushion and back support, and custom inflatable back supports and massagers, with or without heat.

Jobar Intl., Inc. 310-222-8682
21022 Figueroa St, Carson, CA 90745
Various.

Kenad Sg Medical, Inc. 800-825-0606
2692 Huntley Dr, Memphis, TN 38132
Lumbar support.

Kinetic Diversified Industries, Inc. 858-566-4850
7746 Arjons Dr, San Diego, CA 92126
Orthopedics.

Larkotex Company 800-972-3037
1002 Olive St, Texarkana, TX 75501

Mobility Transfer Systems 800-854-4687
PO Box 253, Medford, MA 02155
SAFEHIP, the hip protector helps prevent hip fracture. Designed to disperse the weight of a blow during a fall. Comfortable, everyday wear pants.

ORTHOSIS, LUMBAR *(cont'd)*

Optp 888-819-0121
3800 Annapolis Ln N Ste 165, PO Box 47009, Minneapolis, MN 55447
Original McKenzie Lumbar Roll, Original McKenzie D-Section Lumbar Roll, Original McKenzie Air Back Lumbar Roll, Original McKenzie Super Roll and Original McKenzie night roll.

Orthomerica Products, Inc. 800-446-6770
6333 N Orange Blossom Trl Ste 220, Orlando, FL 32810
NEWPORT 4 HIP SYSTEM - the next generation of post-operative hip management systems, designed and engineered to provide the most comfortable hip orthosis for patients. Innovative new options increase function and control. CALIFORNIA SOFT SPINAL SYSTEM - a lightweight modular, 'soft' spinal system based on an LSO with modular options for posterior, anterior, thoracic, and mediolateral control. Combines velcro and velcro-friendly materials with a series of modular plastic inserts to customize the orthosis.

Orthotic & Prosthetic Lab, Inc. 314-968-8555
748 Marshall Ave, Webster Groves, MO 63119
O&p lumbar orthosis.

Orthotics Choice Llc. 407-321-0454
451 E Airport Blvd, Sanford, FL 32773
Various types of lumbar braces/accessories.

Ossur Americas 949-268-3155
742 Pancho Rd, Camarillo, CA 93012

Otto Bock Healthcare, Lp 763-489-5106
9420 Delegates Dr Ste 100, Orlando, FL 32837
Various types of lumbar orthoses/accessories.

Posture Dynamics, Inc. 732-278-2081
415 Jarob Ct, Point Pleasant Boro, NJ 08742
Various.

R & R Industries, Inc. 949-361-9238
1000 Calle Cordillera, San Clemente, CA 92673
Lumbar back support belt.

Roloke Company 800-533-8212
127 W Hazel St, Inglewood, CA 90302

Rs Medical 800-683-0353
14001 S.E. First St., Vancouver, WA 98684
RS-LFS Lumbar Functional System; RS-LSO Spinal Orthosis

Spio Inc. 253-893-0390
25826 108th Ave SE, Kent, WA 98030
Lumbar support.

St. Francis Medical Technologies, Inc. 408-548-6500
1201 Marina Village Pkwy Ste 200, Alameda, CA 94501
X-stop.

Surgitech Inc. 760-477-8191
870 Rancheros Dr, San Marcos, CA 92069
Lumbar brace.

The Saunders Group 800-445-9836
4250 Norex Dr, Chaska, MN 55318
Sacroilaiac pad.

Tiburon Medical Enterprises 909-654-2333
915 Industrial Way, San Jacinto, CA 92582
Various.

Truform Orthotics & Prosthetics 800-888-0458
3960 Rosslyn Dr, Cincinnati, OH 45209

Tytex, Inc. 401-762-4100
601 Park East Dr, Highland Industrial Park, Woonsocket, RI 02895
Hip protector.

Yeswin Corp. 213-383-8066
3200 Wilshire Blvd, Ste 1140, Los Angeles, CA 90010
Back support.

ORTHOSIS, LUMBOSACRAL *(Physical Med) 89IPY*

A&A Orthopedics, Incorporated 757-224-0177
12250 SW 129th Ct Bldg 1, Miami, FL 33186
Orthosis, lumbo-sacral.

American Orthopedic Supply Co., Inc.
37017 State Highway 79, Cleveland, AL 35049
Lumbosacral corset.

Avry's Orthotic Facility, Inc. 330-746-5385
1441 Wick Ave, Youngstown, OH 44505
Lumbo-sacral orthosis.

Azmec, Inc. 877-862-9632
519 N Smith Ave Ste 110, Corona, CA 92880
Lumbo-sacral orthosis.

ORTHOSIS, LUMBOSACRAL *(cont'd)*

Back Pain Relief Clinic, P.C. 574-271-9444
5507 Singer Ct, Granger, IN 46530
Back brace.

Becker Orthopedic Appliance Co. 248-588-7480
635 Executive Dr, Troy, MI 48083
Various lumbo-sacral orthoses.

Bio Cybernetics Intl. 800-220-4224
1815 Wright St, La Verne, CA 91750
Back brace - mechanical.

Biomet, Inc. 574-267-6639
56 E Bell Dr, PO Box 587, Warsaw, IN 46582
Various types of lumbo-sacral supports.

Biorthex Inc. 877-246-7843
9001 L'Acadie Blvd., Ste. 802, Montreal, QUE H4N 3H5 Canada
Dynamic corrective brace for scoliosis treatment

Bird & Cronin, Inc. 651-683-1111
1200 Trapp Rd, Saint Paul, MN 55121
Lumbo sacral garment.

Caguas Orthopedic Center, Inc. 787-744-2325
FF4 Calle 11, Villa Del Rey, Caguas, PR 00727
Orthosis lumbar.

Chase Ergonomics, Inc. 800-621-5436
PO Box 92497, Albuquerque, NM 87199
Various models of back supports.

Core Products International, Inc. 800-365-3047
808 Prospect Ave, Osceola, WI 54020
CORFIT System 700 patented lumbosacral support system that uses proportional sizing to fit right the first time, fitting 95% of people with just 4 belts.

Corflex, Inc. 800-426-7353
669 E Industrial Park Dr, Manchester, NH 03109

Dj Orthopedics De Mexico, S.A. De C.V. 690-727-1280
Blvd., Delagacion La Presa, Tijuana 22397 Mexico
Industrial back support

Dj Orthopedics De Mexico, S.A. De C.V. 690-727-1280
Ave. Venustiano Carranza 6802, Castillo, Tijuana 22100 Mexico
Industrial back support

DJO Inc. 800-336-6569
1430 Decision St, Vista, CA 92081
Various off-the-shelf Lumbosacral supports and braces.

Dynatronics Corp. Chattanooga Operations 801-568-7000
6607 Mountain View Rd, Ooltewah, TN 37363
Lumbo-sacral orthosis.

Fla Orthopedics, Inc. 800-327-4110
2881 Corporate Way, Miramar, FL 33025

Foot Levelers, Inc. 540-345-0008
518 Pocahontas Ave NE, P.o. Box 12611, Roanoke, VA 24012
Postural back rest.

Frederick Lee Inc 787-834-4880
191 Calle Balboa, PO Box 3287, Mayaguez, PR 00680

Freeman Manufacturing Company 800-253-2091
900 W Chicago Rd, PO Box J, Sturgis, MI 49091
Trade names: Cinch-it, convertible-invertible, stressbelt and ultra beige.

Innovative Orthotics & Rehabilitation, Inc. 404-222-9998
13oo Dekalb Ave., Atlanta, GA 30006
Truncal orthosis.

Jeunique International, Inc. 800-628-7747
19501 E Walnut Dr S, City Of Industry, CA 91748
Jeunique natal support.

Judah Mfg. Corp. 800-618-9792
13657 Jupiter Rd Ste 100, Dallas, TX 75238
Lumbar sacral orthosis (back brace).

Kenad Sg Medical, Inc. 800-825-0606
2692 Huntley Dr, Memphis, TN 38132
Lumbo-sacral support.

Larkotex Company 800-972-3037
1002 Olive St, Texarkana, TX 75501

Life Back Enterprises, Inc. 727-641-9042
416 Admiral Cv, Tarpon Springs, FL 34689
Lumbo-sacral orthosis.

Mizuho Osi 800-777-4674
30031 Ahern Ave, Union City, CA 94587

ORTHOSIS, LUMBOSACRAL *(cont'd)*

Normed 800-288-8200
PO Box 3644, Seattle, WA 98124
Various types & sizes of back braces.

Ny Orthopedic Usa, Inc. 718-852-5330
63 Flushing Ave Unit 333, Brooklyn, NY 11205
Lumbo-sacral support.

Optec Specialties, Inc. 770-513-7380
975 Progress Cir, Lawrenceville, GA 30043
Various-orthosis, lumbo-sacral.

Orthotic & Prosthetic Lab, Inc. 314-968-8555
748 Marshall Ave, Webster Groves, MO 63119
O&p lumbo-sacral-orthoris.

Ossur Americas 949-268-3155
742 Pancho Rd, Camarillo, CA 93012

Otto Bock Healthcare, Lp 763-489-5106
9420 Delegates Dr Ste 100, Orlando, FL 32837
Various types of lumbo-sacral orthoses/accessories.

Pasman Medeq, Inc. 574-252-5690
3296 Cambridge Ct, Mishawaka, IN 46545
Back brace.

Patterson Medical Supply, Inc. 262-387-8720
W68N158 Evergreen Blvd, Cedarburg, WI 53012
Lumbo-sacral dual support.

Pmt Corp. 800-626-5463
1500 Park Rd, Chanhassen, MN 55317

Progressive Appliance Corp. 978-649-9334
9 Gloria Ave, Tyngsboro, MA 01879
Multiple.

Restorative Medical, Inc. 270-422-5454
332 Broadway St, Brandenburg, KY 40108
Safe spine.

Rolliture Corp. 650-652-5675
665 Clearfield Dr, Millbrae, CA 94030
Seat cushion.

Scott Specialties, Inc. 785-527-5627
1827 Meadowlark Rd, Clay Center, KS 67432
Various types of lumbo-sacral supports.

Scott Specialties, Inc. 785-527-5627
1820 E 7th St, Concordia, KS 66901

Scott Specialties, Inc./Cmo Inc./Ginny Inc. 800-255-7136
512 M St, Belleville, KS 66935

Spinal Solutions, Inc. 770-922-2434
1971 Old Covington Rd NE Ste 103, Conyers, GA 30013
Various types pf orthoses.

Spio Inc. 253-893-0390
25826 108th Ave SE, Kent, WA 98030
Lumbo-sacral support.

Stars 225-752-4912
6630 Exchequer Dr, Baton Rouge, LA 70809
Copes scoliosis brace.

Surgical Appliance Industries 800-888-0458
3960 Rosslyn Dr, Cincinnati, OH 45209

Tartan Orthopedics, Ltd. 888-287-1456
10651 Irma Dr Unit C, Northglenn, CO 80233
$20.50 per unit (standard); lace-up back support with Keystone pad; Dorsal lumbar support with custom moldable insert, $120.00/unit.

The Renaissance Co. 480-969-1731
708 S Drew St, Mesa, AZ 85210
Various.

The Saunders Group 800-445-9836
4250 Norex Dr, Chaska, MN 55318
Mutiple.

Top Shelf Manufacturing, Llc 209-834-8185
1851 Paradise Rd Ste B, Tracy, CA 95304
Industrial back brace.

Truform Orthotics & Prosthetics 800-888-0458
3960 Rosslyn Dr, Cincinnati, OH 45209

Trulife, Inc. 360-697-5656
26296 12 Trees Ln NW, Poulsbo, WA 98370
Various types of lumbo-sacral brace,spinal brace,hyperextension brace.

Vq Orthocare
1390 Decision St Ste A, Vista, CA 92081
Back braces.

ORTHOSIS, LUMBOSACRAL *(cont'd)*

Warsaw Orthopedic, Inc. 901-396-3133
2500 Silveus Xing, Warsaw, IN 46582
Various types of lumbo-sacral supports with and without pelvic traction.

Wilson Spinal Systems 863-294-6867
3532 Waterfield Pkwy, Lakeland, FL 33803
Spinal orthosis.

Xback Bracing Services, Inc. 610-404-4900
341A W Main St, Birdsboro, PA 19508

Zimmer Holdings, Inc. 800-613-6131
1800 W Center St, PO Box 708, Warsaw, IN 46580

ORTHOSIS, MOLDABLE, SUPPORTIVE, SKIN PROTECTIVE
(Physical Med) 89MNE

Larson Medical Products, Inc. 614-235-9100
2844 Banwick Rd, Columbus, OH 43232
Medical splinting material(molding sheets).

ORTHOSIS, OTHER *(Physical Med) 89RJB*

Aetrex Worldwide, Inc 800-526-2739
414 Alfred Ave, Teaneck, NJ 07666
LYNCO, ready-to-wear, off the shelf foot orthotic that provides immediate relief for a wide variety of foot problems. FOAMART, foot impression system and APEX foot imprinter, used to evaluate foot conditions and make custom foot orthotics.

Aircast Llc 800-321-9549
1430 Decision St, Vista, CA 92081
AIRCAST infrapatellar band.

Cfi Medical Solutions (Contour Fabricators, Inc.) 810-750-5300
14241 N Fenton Rd, Fenton, MI 48430

Contour Form Products 800-223-8808
38 Stewart Ave, PO Box 328, Greenville, PA 16125
$40.25 for elastic back-support binder with moldable insert CONTOUR FORM.

Corflex, Inc. 800-426-7353
669 E Industrial Park Dr, Manchester, NH 03109
POLY CAST vacuum-molded bracing for fracture management.

Cosco 800-582-6853
1602 Lakeside Dr, Redding, CA 96001

Dm Systems, Inc. 800-254-5438
1316 Sherman Ave, Evanston, IL 60201
CADLOW™ SHOULDER STABILIZER is the only shoulder product in existence that provides glenohumeral stability while maintaining an athlete's full range of motion. It helps prevent recurrent subluxations/dislocations without restriction. It also strengthens the shoulder by providing graduated, variable resistance that can be adjusted as an athlete's strength increases. Each customized Cadlow™ set includes: Compression shorts, harness, armband, and a full compliment of variable resistance tubing.

Freeman Manufacturing Company 800-253-2091
900 W Chicago Rd, PO Box J, Sturgis, MI 49091
Maternity supports, head halters, dorso-lumbar supports and rigid frame spinal braces.

Gait-Aid Inc. 800-677-1796
5468 Dundas St. W., Ste. 1000, Toronto, ONT M9B 6E3 Canada
GAIT-AID shoe inserts products for both walking/sport shoes and high heel fashion shoes give correct alignment for feet and lower limbs.

Hersco Ortho Labs 718-391-0416
3928 Crescent St, Long Island City, NY 11101
Foot orthotics and supplies. Custom made orthopedic shoes.

Knit-Rite, Inc. 800-821-3094
120 Osage Ave, Kansas City, KS 66105
Torso-interface, CAST-RITE. Elasticized, form fitting garment for under body casts, lumbosacral supports, braces & upper body orthoses.

Langer, Inc. 800-645-5520
450 Commack Rd, Deer Park, NY 11729
Foot orthosis.

Larkotex Company 800-972-3037
1002 Olive St, Texarkana, TX 75501

Maramed Orthopedic Systems 800-327-5830
2480 W 82nd St, No. 8, Hialeah, FL 33016
PLASTICAST: Adjustable cast system.

Mizuho Osi 800-777-4674
30031 Ahern Ave, Union City, CA 94587

ORTHOSIS, OTHER *(cont'd)*

Novacare Orthodics 800-272-2464
151 Hempstead Tpke, West Hempstead, NY 11552
Custom made braces.

Omni Life Science, Inc. 800-448-OMNI
1390 Decision St, Vista, CA 92081
Icon custom knee braces for ligament instability and O.A.

Ortho-Med, Inc. 800-547-5571
3208 SE 13th Ave, Portland, OR 97202
Neoprene braces.

Ortholine 800-243-3351
13 Chapel St, Norwalk, CT 06850
Neoprene knee, ankle and wrist supports.

Paramedical Distributors 800-245-3278
2020 Grand Blvd, Kansas City, MO 64108
For knees, ankles, arms, elbow, wrist, neck, and torso.

Professional's Choice Sports Medicine Products, Inc. 800-331-9421
2025 Gillespie Way Ste 106, El Cajon, CA 92020
One-size knee orthosis fitts any size right or left knee. Neoprene.

Tetra Medical Supply Corp. 800-621-4041
6364 W Gross Point Rd, Niles, IL 60714

Tri Hawk Corporation 866-874-4295
150 Highland Rd, Massena, NY 13662
ORTHOFIT.

Truform Orthotics & Prosthetics 800-888-0458
3960 Rosslyn Dr, Cincinnati, OH 45209

U.S. Orthotics, Inc. 800-825-5228
8605 Palm River Rd, Tampa, FL 33619
Spina Plastic Spinal Orthoses - Fiway Spinal Modular System.

Variety Ability Systems Inc. 800-891-4514
2 Kelvin Ave., Unit 3, Toronto, ONT M4C-5C8 Canada
Standing frame orthoses; also, three sizes of the Rochester parapodium, Toronto (Mark II) parapodium and Mark3 Stander/parapodium.

Zimmer Holdings, Inc. 800-613-6131
1800 W Center St, PO Box 708, Warsaw, IN 46580

ORTHOSIS, PNEUMATIC STRUCTURE, RIGID
(Physical Med) 89IPO

Ferno-Washington, Inc. 800-733-3766
70 Weil Way, Wilmington, OH 45177

ORTHOSIS, RIB FRACTURE, SOFT *(Physical Med) 89IPX*

A&A Orthopedics, Incorporated 757-224-0177
12250 SW 129th Ct Bldg 1, Miami, FL 33186
Orthosis, rib fracture, soft.

American Orthopedic Supply Co., Inc.
37017 State Highway 79, Cleveland, AL 35049
Rib belt.

Azmec, Inc. 877-862-9632
519 N Smith Ave Ste 110, Corona, CA 92880
Orthosis, rib fracture, soft.

Biomet, Inc. 574-267-6639
56 E Bell Dr, PO Box 587, Warsaw, IN 46582
Various types of rib belts.

Bird & Cronin, Inc. 651-683-1111
1200 Trapp Rd, Saint Paul, MN 55121
Rib belts.

Dale Medical Products, Inc. 800-343-3980
7 Cross St, Plainville, MA 02762
2 panel 6 in. Female #425 28-50', #427 46-60'; 2 panel 6' Male #525 28-50' #527 46-60'

Dj Orthopedics De Mexico, S.A. De C.V. 690-727-1280
Blvd., Delagacion La Presa, Tijuana 22397 Mexico
Rib belt

Dj Orthopedics De Mexico, S.A. De C.V. 690-727-1280
Ave. Venustiano Carranza 6802, Castillo, Tijuana 22100 Mexico
Rib belt

DJO Inc. 800-336-6569
1430 Decision St, Vista, CA 92081
Off-the-shelf rib belts in various sizes.

Dynatronics Corp. Chattanooga Operations 801-568-7000
6607 Mountain View Rd, Ooltewah, TN 37363
Soft rib fracture orthosis.

Fla Orthopedics, Inc. 800-327-4110
2881 Corporate Way, Miramar, FL 33025

ORTHOSIS, RIB FRACTURE, SOFT *(cont'd)*

Frederick Lee Inc 787-834-4880
191 Calle Balboa, PO Box 3287, Mayaguez, PR 00680

Freeman Manufacturing Company 800-253-2091
900 W Chicago Rd, PO Box J, Sturgis, MI 49091

Hospital Marketing Svcs. Company, Inc. 800-786-5094
162 Great Hill Rd./ Ind. Park, Naugatuck, CT 06770
HMS FLEXITONE soft rib fracture orthosis.

Kenad Sg Medical, Inc. 800-825-0606
2692 Huntley Dr, Memphis, TN 38132
Rib belt.

Larkotex Company 800-972-3037
1002 Olive St, Texarkana, TX 75501

Mizuho Osi 800-777-4674
30031 Ahern Ave, Union City, CA 94587

Ossur Americas 949-268-3155
742 Pancho Rd, Camarillo, CA 93012

Professional's Choice Sports Medicine Products, Inc. 800-331-9421
2025 Gillespie Way Ste 106, El Cajon, CA 92020
Support and compression for rib and abdominal area.

Scott Specialties, Inc. 785-527-5627
1827 Meadowlark Rd, Clay Center, KS 67432
Various types of rib orthosis.

Scott Specialties, Inc. 785-527-5627
1820 E 7th St, Concordia, KS 66901

Scott Specialties, Inc./Cmo Inc./Ginny Inc. 800-255-7136
512 M St, Belleville, KS 66935

Tartan Orthopedics, Ltd. 888-287-1456
10651 Irma Dr Unit C, Northglenn, CO 80233
$7.50 per unit (standard).

Truform Orthotics & Prosthetics 800-888-0458
3960 Rosslyn Dr, Cincinnati, OH 45209

Warsaw Orthopedic, Inc. 901-396-3133
2500 Silveus Xing, Warsaw, IN 46582
Various types of rib belts.

Zimmer Holdings, Inc. 800-613-6131
1800 W Center St, PO Box 708, Warsaw, IN 46580

ORTHOSIS, SACROILIAC, SOFT *(Physical Med) 89IPW*

American Orthopedic Supply Co., Inc.
37017 State Highway 79, Cleveland, AL 35049
Sacroiliac corset.

Biomet, Inc. 574-267-6639
56 E Bell Dr, PO Box 587, Warsaw, IN 46582
Various types of sacral supports.

DJO Inc. 800-336-6569
1430 Decision St, Vista, CA 92081
Sacro with pad tucks.

Dynatronics Corp. Chattanooga Operations 801-568-7000
6607 Mountain View Rd, Ooltewah, TN 37363
Soft sacroiliac orthosis.

Fla Orthopedics, Inc. 800-327-4110
2881 Corporate Way, Miramar, FL 33025

Frank Stubbs Co., Inc 800-223-1713
2100 Eastman Ave Ste B, Oxnard, CA 93030

Frederick Lee Inc 787-834-4880
191 Calle Balboa, PO Box 3287, Mayaguez, PR 00680

Freeman Manufacturing Company 800-253-2091
900 W Chicago Rd, PO Box J, Sturgis, MI 49091

Just Packaging Inc. 908-753-6700
450 Oak Tree Ave, South Plainfield, NJ 07080
Soft back supports.

Larkotex Company 800-972-3037
1002 Olive St, Texarkana, TX 75501

Optp 888-819-0121
3800 Annapolis Ln N Ste 165, PO Box 47009, Minneapolis, MN 55447
SI-LOC, sacroiliac belt.

Sam Medical Products 503-639-5474
4909 South Coast Hwy., #245, Newport, OR 97365
Pelvic sling, circumferential sacroiliac sling orthosis.

Scott Specialties, Inc. 785-527-5627
1827 Meadowlark Rd, Clay Center, KS 67432
Orthosis, sacroiliac, soft.

ORTHOSIS, SACROILIAC, SOFT *(cont'd)*

Scott Specialties, Inc. 785-527-5627
1820 E 7th St, Concordia, KS 66901

Scott Specialties, Inc./Cmo Inc./Ginny Inc. 800-255-7136
512 M St, Belleville, KS 66935

Surgical Appliance Industries 800-888-0458
3960 Rosslyn Dr, Cincinnati, OH 45209

Tartan Orthopedics, Ltd. 888-287-1456
10651 Irma Dr Unit C, Northglenn, CO 80233
$14.90 per unit (standard) & tartan form, sacro lumbar $45.00/unit.

Truform Orthotics & Prosthetics 800-888-0458
3960 Rosslyn Dr, Cincinnati, OH 45209

Zimmer Holdings, Inc. 800-613-6131
1800 W Center St, PO Box 708, Warsaw, IN 46580

ORTHOSIS, SPINAL PEDICLE FIXATION, FOR DEGENERATIVE DISC DISEASE *(Orthopedics) 87NKB*

Abbott Spine, Inc. 847-937-6100
12708 Riata Vista Cir Ste B-100, Austin, TX 78727
Pedicle screw system.

Allez Spine, Llc 949-752-7885
2301 Dupont Dr Ste 510, Irvine, CA 92612
Spinal fixation system.

Amedica Corporation 801-839-3500
1885 W 2100 S, Salt Lake City, UT 84119
Valeo PS

Applied Spine Technologies, Inc. 203-503-0280
300 George St Ste 511, New Haven, CT 06511
STABILIMAX BAR SPINAL FUSION SYSTEM

Medtronic Sofamor Danek Usa, Inc. 901-396-3133
4340 Swinnea Rd, Memphis, TN 38118
Metallic bone fixation device.

Vertiflex (Tm), Incorporated 1-866-268-6486
1351 Calle Avanzado, San Clemente, CA 92673
Pedicle screw system.

Warsaw Orthopedic, Inc. 901-396-3133
2500 Silveus Xing, Warsaw, IN 46582
Metallic bone fixation device.

Zimmer Spine, Inc. 800-655-2614
7375 Bush Lake Rd, Minneapolis, MN 55439
Pedicle screw system.

ORTHOSIS, SPINE, PLATE, LAMINOPLASTY, METAL *(Orthopedics) 87NQW*

Medtronic Puerto Rico Operations Co.,Med Rel 763-514-4000
Road 909, Km. 0.4., Barrio Mariana, Humacao, PR 00792
Orthosis, spine, plate, laminoplasty, metal.

Medtronic Sofamor Danek Usa, Inc. 901-396-3133
4340 Swinnea Rd, Memphis, TN 38118
Orthosis, spine, plate, laminoplasty, metal.

Warsaw Orthopedic, Inc. 901-396-3133
2500 Silveus Xing, Warsaw, IN 46582
Orthosis, spine, plate, laminoplasty, metal.

ORTHOSIS, THORACIC *(Physical Med) 89IPT*

American Orthopedic Supply Co., Inc.
37017 State Highway 79, Cleveland, AL 35049
Dorsolumbar corset.

Aspen Medical Products 949-681-0200
6481 Oak Cyn, Irvine, CA 92618
Tlso.

Avry's Orthotic Facility, Inc. 330-746-5385
1441 Wick Ave, Youngstown, OH 44505
Thoracic lumbo-sacral orthosis.

Becker Orthopedic Appliance Co. 248-588-7480
635 Executive Dr, Troy, MI 48083
Various thoracic orthoses.

Biomet, Inc. 574-267-6639
56 E Bell Dr, PO Box 587, Warsaw, IN 46582
Various types of thoracic orthoses.

Caguas Orthopedic Center, Inc. 787-744-2325
FF4 Calle 11, Villa Del Rey, Caguas, PR 00727
Orthosis thoracic.

Circular Traction Supply, Inc. 800-247-6535
7602 Talbert Ave Ste 9, Huntington Beach, CA 92648
Spinal brace.

ORTHOSIS, THORACIC *(cont'd)*

Fillauer Companies, Inc. 800-251-6398
2710 Amnicola Hwy, Chattanooga, TN 37406

Freeman Manufacturing Company 800-253-2091
900 W Chicago Rd, PO Box J, Sturgis, MI 49091
Dorso-lumbar supports and rigid frame spinal braces.

Hospital Marketing Svcs. Company, Inc. 800-786-5094
162 Great Hill Rd./ Ind. Park, Naugatuck, CT 06770

Just Packaging Inc. 908-753-6700
450 Oak Tree Ave, South Plainfield, NJ 07080
Spinal support.

Oakworks, Inc. 800-558-8850
923 E Wellspring Rd, New Freedom, PA 17349
Peri-surgical prone support, post surgical prone support, prone support.

Orthotic Rehabilitation Products, Inc. 813-620-0035
7002 E Broadway Ave, Tampa, FL 33619
Same.

Orthotics Choice Llc. 407-321-0454
451 E Airport Blvd, Sanford, FL 32773
Various types of thoracic braces/accessories.

Otto Bock Healthcare, Lp 763-489-5106
9420 Delegates Dr Ste 100, Orlando, FL 32837
Various types of thoracic orthoses/accessories.

Pectus Services 757-224-0177
549 Pompton Ave Ste 210, Cedar Grove, NJ 07009
Pectus carinatum brace.

Pmt Corp. 800-626-5463
1500 Park Rd, Chanhassen, MN 55317
Inflatable thoracic lumbosacral orthosis.

Prenatal Cradle, Inc. 800-383-3068
1818 S Bluegill Rd, Clare, MI 48617
Prenatal cradle, NEW Adjustable Prenatal Cradle, Prenatal Cradle Plus, Mini Cradle, V2 Supporter, Hip Brace, Hip Brace/V2 Combo., Natural Embrace Baby Carrier, Ambulatory Compression Support Panty Hose, and Tummy Honey Stretch Mark Solution Products.

Restorative Care Of America Inc 800-627-1595
12221 33rd St N, Saint Petersburg, FL 33716
A Knight Taylor type TLSO made of heat moldable Rydex. Features washable foam liner.

Spinal Solutions, Inc. 770-922-2434
1971 Old Covington Rd NE Ste 103, Conyers, GA 30013
Thoracic lumbo sacral orthosis, rigid spinal brace.

Spio Inc. 253-893-0390
25826 108th Ave SE, Kent, WA 98030
Trunk support.

The Bremer Group Co. 800-428-2304
11243-5 Saint Johns Industrial Pkwy S, Pkwy. South Jacksonville, FL 32246
Various.

The Saunders Group 800-445-9836
4250 Norex Dr, Chaska, MN 55318
Posture support.

Truform Orthotics & Prosthetics 800-888-0458
3960 Rosslyn Dr, Cincinnati, OH 45209

Warsaw Orthopedic, Inc. 901-396-3133
2500 Silveus Xing, Warsaw, IN 46582
Various types of abdominal binders.

Wilson Spinal Systems 863-294-6867
3532 Waterfield Pkwy, Lakeland, FL 33803
Spinal orthosis.

ORTHOSIS, TRUNCAL/LIMB *(Physical Med) 89MRI*

American Orthopedic Supply Co., Inc.
37017 State Highway 79, Cleveland, AL 35049
Body jacket.

Atlantic Rim Brace Mfg. Corp. 603-886-8130
25-29 Front St. Suite 5a, Nashua, NH 03064
Various types of rigid and semi-rigid atlantic rim t.l.s.o.'s and l.s.o.'s.

Becker Orthopedic Appliance Co. 248-588-7480
635 Executive Dr, Troy, MI 48083
Various truncal-orthosis, limb.

Benik Corp. 360-692-5601
11871 Silverdale Way NW Ste 107, Silverdale, WA 98383
Trunk support.

ORTHOSIS, TRUNCAL/LIMB *(cont'd)*

Bill Frank Productions Bf Bio-Supports Inc. 614-840-0091
665 Old Pond Ln, Powell, OH 43065
Bio-back.

Fallgard Llc 800-828-0702
631 Alexandria Dr, Naperville, IL 60565
Hip pads and pocketed underwear hip impact protector.

G & F Industries, Inc. 508-347-9132
Rt. 20 Box 515, Sturbridge, MA 01566
Cervical head immobilizer device.

Hendricks Orthotic Prosthetic Enterprises, Inc. 407-850-0411
6439 Milner Blvd Ste 6, Orlando, FL 32809
Orthosis, truncal/orthosis, limb.

Joerns Healthcare, Inc. 715-341-3600
1032 N Fourth St, Baldwyn, MS 38824
Cervical neck pillow.

Orthotic & Prosthetic Lab, Inc. 314-968-8555
748 Marshall Ave, Webster Groves, MO 63119
O&p body jacket.

Otto Bock Healthcare, Lp 763-489-5106
9420 Delegates Dr Ste 100, Orlando, FL 32837
Various types of limb orthoses/accessories.

Pelvic Binder, Inc. 877-451-3000
3982 Fm 2653 South, Cumby, TX 75433
Pelvic binder.

Spinal Solutions, Inc. 770-922-2434
1971 Old Covington Rd NE Ste 103, Conyers, GA 30013
Various types of orthoses.

Spio Inc. 253-893-0390
25826 108th Ave SE, Kent, WA 98030
Trunk support.

Trulife, Inc. 360-697-5656
26296 12 Trees Ln NW, Poulsbo, WA 98370
Spinal braces,body jackets,hyperextension braces.

Zhang Enterprises 972-238-8260
400 N Greenville Ave Ste 9, Richardson, TX 75081
Various types of truncal devices.

ORTHOTOLUIDINE, GLUCOSE *(Chemistry) 75CGE*

Health Care Logistics, Inc. 800-848-1633
450 Town St, PO Box 25, Circleville, OH 43113
Sterile diabetic test syringe.

Health Chem Diagnostics Llc 954-979-3845
3341 W McNab Rd, Pompano Beach, FL 33069
Orthotoluidine, glucose.

OSCILLOMETER *(Cardiovascular) 74DRZ*

Propper Manufacturing Co., Inc. 800-832-4300
3604 Skillman Ave, Long Island City, NY 11101

OSCILLOSCOPE *(General) 80RJC*

Leader Instruments Corp. 800-645-5104
6484 Commerce Dr, Cypress, CA 90630
Wide range of oscilloscopes and related equipment.

Lecroy Corp. 800-553-2769
700 Chestnut Ridge Rd, Chestnut Ridge, NY 10977
Digital-storage oscilloscopes.

Phipps & Bird, Inc. 800-955-7621
1519 Summit Ave, Richmond, VA 23230
Oscilloscope for student education (physiology experiments).

Soltec Corp. 800-423-2344
12977 Arroyo St, San Fernando, CA 91340

OSMIUM TETROXIDE *(Pathology) 88KEE*

Colonial Metals, Inc. 410-398-7200
505 Blue Ball Rd Bldg 20, Elkton, MD 21921
Osmium tetroxide.

Polysciences, Inc. 800-523-2575
400 Valley Rd, Warrington, PA 18976

Stevens Metallurgical Corp. 800-794-7887
239 E 79th St, New York, NY 10075
Chemical electron microscopy grade.

OSMOMETER *(Chemistry) 75JJM*

Advanced Instruments Inc. 800-225-4034
2 Technology Way, Norwood, MA 02062
Three models, freezing point; $6800.00 for ADVANCED micro-osmometer, Model 3300, sample size of 20 microliters and range of 0-2000 mOsm/Kg H-2-O; $7000.00 for Model 3D3, single sample automatic, 0-4000; $19,360.00 for Model 3900 multi-sample, 0-2000.

Precision Systems, Inc. 508-655-7010
16 Tech Cir, Natick, MA 01760
OSMETTE; 8 models freezing point, 0-3000, from $5887 (wider ranges available); semi- and fully automatic; available with computer/printer for autocalibration and data logging, samples as small as 10 microliters.

Spectron Corp. 425-827-9317
934 S Burlington Blvd # 603, Burlington, WA 98233
Reconditioned equipment.

Wescor, Inc. 800-453-2725
459 S Main St, Logan, UT 84321
$5,995.00 for the Model 5520 (Vapro), Vapor pressure osmometer with 10 microliter sample size, 0-3,200 mmol/kg measurement range; $6,295.00 for Model 5520XR for research applications, 0-3600 mmol/kg. measurement range.

OSTEOTOME (ORTHOPEDIC) *(Surgery) 79HWM*

Abbott Spine, Inc. 847-937-6100
12708 Riata Vista Cir Ste B-100, Austin, TX 78727
Osteotome.

Aesculap Implant Systems Inc. 1-800-234-9179
3773 Corporate Pkwy, Center Valley, PA 18034

Biomet Microfixation Inc. 800-874-7711
1520 Tradeport Dr, Jacksonville, FL 32218
Osteotome.

Biomet, Inc. 574-267-6639
56 E Bell Dr, PO Box 587, Warsaw, IN 46582
Various types of osteotomes.

Codman & Shurtleff, Inc 800-225-0460
325 Paramount Dr, Raynham, MA 02767

DJO Inc. 800-336-6569
1430 Decision St, Vista, CA 92081

E.A. Beck & Co. 949-645-4072
657 W 19th St Ste E, P O Box 10857, Costa Mesa, CA 92627
Osteotome.

Elmed, Inc. 630-543-2792
60 W Fay Ave, Addison, IL 60101

Holmed Corporation 508-238-3351
40 Norfolk Ave, South Easton, MA 02375

Integral Design Inc. 781-740-2036
52 Burr Rd, Hingham, MA 02043

Kirwan Surgical Products, Inc. 888-547-9267
180 Enterprise Dr, PO Box 427, Marshfield, MA 02050

Kmedic 800-955-0559
190 Veterans Dr, Northvale, NJ 07647

Medisiss 866-866-7477
2747 SW 6th St, Redmond, OR 97756
Various osteomes,sterile.

Medtronic Sofamor Danek Instrument Manufacturing 901-396-3133
7375 Adrianne Pl, Bartlett, TN 38133
Multiple (orthopedic osteotomes).

Medtronic Sofamor Danek Usa, Inc. 901-396-3133
4340 Swinnea Rd, Memphis, TN 38118
Multiple (orthopedic osteotomes).

Micro-Aire Surgical Instruments, Inc. 800-722-0822
1641 Edlich Dr, Charlottesville, VA 22911

Miltex Inc. 800-645-8000
589 Davies Dr, York, PA 17402

Modular Cutting Systems, Inc. 203-336-3526
650 Clinton Ave, Bridgeport, CT 06605
Assistive bed roll& hand osteotomes.

Pappas Surgical Instruments, Llc 508-429-1049
7 October Hill Rd, Holliston, MA 01746
Various types of osteotomes.

Richards Micro-Tool, Inc. 508-746-6900
250 Nicks Road,, Plymouth, MA 02360-2800

OSTEOTOME (ORTHOPEDIC) *(cont'd)*

Small Bone Innovations, Inc. 215-428-1791
1380 S Pennsylvania Ave, Morrisville, PA 19067
Manual surgical instrument for general use.

Stryker Spine 866-457-7463
2 Pearl Ct, Allendale, NJ 07401

Tuzik Boston 800-886-6363
104 Longwater Dr, Assinippi Park, Norwell, MA 02061

Warsaw Orthopedic, Inc. 901-396-3133
2500 Silveus Xing, Warsaw, IN 46582
Multiple (orthopedic osteotomes).

Zimmer Trabecular Metal Technology 800-613-6131
10 Pomeroy Rd, Parsippany, NJ 07054
Box osteotome.

OSTEOTOME, MANUAL (PLASTIC SURGERY) *(Surgery) 79GFI*

Abbott Spine, Inc. 847-937-6100
12708 Riata Vista Cir Ste B-100, Austin, TX 78727
Osteotome.

Bausch & Lomb Surgical 636-255-5051
3365 Tree Court Ind Blvd, Saint Louis, MO 63122

Cardinal Health, Snowden Pencer Products 847-689-8410
5175 S Royal Atlanta Dr, Tucker, GA 30084
Various styles of manual osteotomes.

Depuy Spine, Inc. 800-227-6633
325 Paramount Dr, Raynham, MA 02767
Osteotome.

George Tiemann & Co. 800-843-6266
25 Plant Ave, Hauppauge, NY 11788

H & H Co. 909-390-0373
4435 E Airport Dr Ste 108, Ontario, CA 91761
Ridge expansion osteotome, all types.

Lenox-Maclaren Surgical Corp. 720-890-9660
657 S Taylor Ave Ste A, Colorado Technology Center
Louisville, CO 80027
Osteotome, manual / all sizes.

Micrins Surgical Instruments, Inc. 800-833-3380
28438 N Ballard Dr, Lake Forest, IL 60045

Miltex Inc. 800-645-8000
589 Davies Dr, York, PA 17402

Precision Medical Manufacturing Corporation 866-633-4626
852 Seton Ct, Wheeling, IL 60090

Spine Wave, Inc. 203-944-9494
2 Enterprise Dr Ste 302, Shelton, CT 06484
Osteotome.

Symmetry Medical Usa, Inc. 574-267-8700
486 W 350 N, Warsaw, IN 46582
Flexible osteotome.

Tuzik Boston 800-886-6363
104 Longwater Dr, Assinippi Park, Norwell, MA 02061

Zimmer Holdings, Inc. 800-613-6131
1800 W Center St, PO Box 708, Warsaw, IN 46580

Zimmer Trabecular Metal Technology 800-613-6131
10 Pomeroy Rd, Parsippany, NJ 07054
Proxilock box osteotome-small.

OSTEOTOME, OTHER *(Surgery) 79RJE*

Micro-Aire Surgical Instruments, Inc. 800-722-0822
1641 Edlich Dr, Charlottesville, VA 22911
Osteotome for cranial bone graft harvesting.

Miltex Inc. 800-645-8000
589 Davies Dr, York, PA 17402

OSTEOTOME, ROTO WITH BLADE *(Dental And Oral) 76EGR*

Stryker Corp. 800-726-2725
2825 Airview Blvd, Portage, MI 49002

OSTOMY APPLIANCE (ILEOSTOMY, COLOSTOMY) *(Gastro/Urology) 78RJF*

Coloplast Manufacturing Us, Llc 800-533-0464
1840 W Oak Pkwy, Marietta, GA 30062
CONSEAL plug for continent stoma to provide periods of continence for voluntary control of evacuation.

Cook Urological, Inc. 800-457-4500
1100 W Morgan St, P.O. Box 227, Spencer, IN 47460

OSTOMY APPLIANCE (ILEOSTOMY, COLOSTOMY) *(cont'd)*

Invacare Supply Group, An Invacare Co. 800-225-4792
75 October Hill Rd, Holliston, MA 01746
Carry full lines of ostomy supplies from: Hollister, Convatec, Coloplast, Genairex, Bard & Cymed.

Ldb Medical, Inc. 800-243-2554
2909 Langford Rd Ste B500, Norcross, GA 30071
LAPIDES.

Marlen Manufacturing & Development Co. 216-292-7060
5150 Richmond Rd, Bedford, OH 44146
ULTRA one-piece/Ileostomy (Disposable with skin barrier); ULTRA one-piece/Urolstomy (Disposable with skin barrier). ULTRA two-piece/Urolstomy (Disposable with skin barrier).

Mentor Corp. 800-525-0245
201 Mentor Dr, Santa Barbara, CA 93111
Ostomy kits.

Metro Medical Supply Wholesale 800-768-2002
200 Cumberland Bnd, Nashville, TN 37228

Smith & Nephew, Inc. 800-876-1261
11775 Starkey Rd, Largo, FL 33773
FEATHER-LITE disposable and semi disposable pouches, 1 and 2-piece ostomy appliances.

Torbot Group, Inc. 800-545-4254
1367 Elmwood Ave, Cranston, RI 02910

OTOSCOPE *(Ear/Nose/Throat) 77ERA*

Aesculap Implant Systems Inc. 1-800-234-9179
3773 Corporate Pkwy, Center Valley, PA 18034

Alimed, Inc. 800-225-2610
297 High St, Dedham, MA 02026
Frant comes with three aural and one nasal specula. Friston comes with three specula and a spare lamp.

American Diagnostic Corporation (Adc) 800-232-2670
55 Commerce Dr, Hauppauge, NY 11788
Pocket and standard 2.5v Otoscopes

Armstrong Medical Industries, Inc. 800-323-4220
575 Knightsbridge Pkwy, Lincolnshire, IL 60069

Astralite Corporation 800-345-7703
PO Box 689, Somerset, CA 95684

Bio-Gate Usa, Inc. 714-670-2771
6800 Orangethorpe Ave Ste E, Buena Park, CA 90620
Otoscope.

Biomet Microfixation Inc. 800-874-7711
1520 Tradeport Dr, Jacksonville, FL 32218
Otoscope.

Boehm Surgical Instrument Corp. 716-436-6584
966 Chili Ave, Rochester, NY 14611
Otoscope.

Cameron-Miller, Inc. 800-621-0142
5410 W Roosevelt Rd, Road #241, Chicago, IL 60644

Carolina Biological Supply Co. 800-334-5551
2700 York Rd, Burlington, NC 27215

Clinimed, Incorporated 877-CLINIMED
303 Markus Ct, Sandy Brae Industrial Park, Newark, DE 19713

Creative Health Products, Inc. 800-742-4478
5148 Saddle Ridge Rd, Plymouth, MI 48170
RIESTER Ri-Mini Otoscope; $99.00 each for CHP. RIESTER Economy Otoscope $64.90 each for CHP. RIESTER Ri-Mini Otoscope/Ophthalmoscope Combination Kit $209.00 each for CHP.

Dorel Design & Development Center 781-364-3542
25 Forbes Blvd, Foxboro, MA 02035

Edmund Industrial Optics 800-363-1992
101 E Gloucester Pike, Barrington, NJ 08007

G & G Medical Products, Inc. 518-542-0395
6 White Fir Dr, Loudonville, NY 12211
Otoscope.

Global Endoscopy, Inc. 888-434-3398
914 Estes Ct, Schaumburg, IL 60193
Otoscope.

Gyrus Ent L.L.C., Sub. Of Gyrus Acmi, Inc. 508-804-2739
2925 Appling Rd, Bartlett, TN 38133
Multiple.

Hal-Hen Company, Inc. 800-242-5436
180 Atlantic Ave, Garden City Park, NY 11040
$150.00 per unit (standard).

OTOSCOPE *(cont'd)*

Health Ent., Inc. 508-695-0727
90 George Leven Dr, North Attleboro, MA 02760
Aculife optical scope.

Henke Sass Wolf Of America, Inc. 508-671-9300
135 Schofield Ave, Dudley, MA 01571

Her-Mar, Inc. 800-327-8209
8550 NW 30th Ter, Doral, FL 33122
$75.00 per unit (standard).

Jedmed Instruments Co. 314-845-3770
5416 Jedmed Ct, Saint Louis, MO 63129

Karl Storz Endoscopy-America Inc. 800-421-0837
600 Corporate Pointe, Culver City, CA 90230
Diagnostic and operative.

Kelleher Medical, Inc. 804-378-9956
3049 St Marys Way, Powhatan, VA 23139

Levine Health Products 800-426-6763
21101 NE 108th St, Redmond, WA 98053
Pocket size otoscope is suitable for professional and home use. Features include halogen bulb, 4 x magnification, large viewing area. The Ware otoscope is battery operated by two AA batteries which are included. This otoscope comes in an attractive box and includes two each pediatric and two adult specula.

Lumiscope Company, Inc. 800-672-8293
1035 Centennial Ave, Piscataway, NJ 08854

Mahe International Inc. 800-294-7946
468 Craighead St, Nashville, TN 37204

Md International, Inc. 305-669-9003
11300 NW 41st St, Doral, FL 33178

Medrx, Inc. 727-584-9600
1200 Starkey Rd Ste 105, Largo, FL 33771
Video otoscope.

Miltex Inc. 800-645-8000
589 Davies Dr, York, PA 17402

North American Medical Products, Inc. 800-488-6267
6 British American Blvd Ste B, Latham, NY 12110
$75.00 to $99.00 - Diagnostic set available with 2C cell batteries or with rechargable handles and recharger.

Notoco Llc. 707-786-4400
PO Box 300, 660 Berding St., Ferndale, CA 95536
Otoscope.

Panex Corp. 800-662-4499
12300 Highway A1A Alt Ste 103, Palm Beach Gardens, FL 33410
EARLIGHT, ear examination kit.

Pedia Pals, Llc 888-733-4272
965 Highway 169 N, Plymouth, MN 55441
Otoscope Elephant face attachment and matching specula in 2.5mm and 4.0mm.

Prestige Medical Corporation 800-762-3333
8600 Wilbur Ave, Northridge, CA 91324

Propper Manufacturing Co., Inc. 800-832-4300
3604 Skillman Ave, Long Island City, NY 11101

Richard Wolf Medical Instruments Corp. 800-323-9653
353 Corporate Woods Pkwy, Vernon Hills, IL 60061

Shippert Medical Technologies Corp. 800-888-8663
6248 S Troy Cir Ste A, Centennial, CO 80111
Welch Allyn.

Trans American Medical / Tamsco Instruments 708-430-7777
7633 W 100th Pl, Bridgeview, IL 60455
Economy otoscope.

Tsi Medical Ltd. 800-661-7263
47 Athabascan Ave., Unit 105, Sherwood Park, AB T8A-4H3 Canada

Welch Allyn, Inc. 800-535-6663
4341 State Street Rd, Skaneateles Falls, NY 13153

OVEN *(Chemistry) 75RJG*

Applied Test Systems, Inc. 800-441-0215
154 Eastbrook Ln, Butler, PA 16002
Lab-test ovens to specifications in a wide variety of sizes and temperatures.

Associated Environmental Systems 978-772-0022
31 Willow Rd, Ayer, MA 01432

Boekel Scientific 800-336-6929
855 Pennsylvania Blvd, Feasterville Trevose, PA 19053
Hybridization.

OVEN *(cont'd)*

Centorr Vacuum Industries 800-962-8631
55 Northeastern Blvd, Nashua, NH 03062
High temperature controlled atmosphere furnaces for induction, melting, brazing, sintering and crystal growth.

Cober Electronics, Inc. 203-855-8755
151 Woodward Ave, Norwalk, CT 06854
Laboratory microwave ovens. Microwave system for laboratory animal brain fixation.

Cole-Parmer Instrument Inc. 800-323-4340
625 E Bunker Ct, Vernon Hills, IL 60061

Elatec Technology Division 978-374-4040
252 Primrose St # 260, Haverhill, MA 01830
Vacuum.

Hotpack 800-523-3608
10940 Dutton Rd, Philadelphia, PA 19154

Jordi Associates, Flp 508-966-1301
4 Mill St, Bellingham, MA 02019

L&L Special Furnace Co., Inc. 888-808-3676
20 Kent Rd, Aston, PA 19014

Microwave Research & Applications, Inc. 866-953-1771
8685 Cherry Ln, Laurel, MD 20707
Laboratory microwave ovens features true variable power, temperature probes and power venting of the cavity. The ovens can operate in a time or temperature control mode. Applications for these ovens include cell fixation, drying of samples and the warming of medical and personal care products. Specializes in microwave applications research and development.

Paramedical Distributors 800-245-3278
2020 Grand Blvd, Kansas City, MO 64108

Precision Quincy Corp. 800-338-0079
1625 W Lake Shore Dr, Woodstock, IL 60098
Features include oversize insulation bats to prevent sagging, reinforced cabinet with stainless-steel interior, and Incoloy-sheathed heating elements.

Pro Scientific Inc. 800-584-3776
99 Willenbrock Rd, Oxford, CT 06478
Memmert ovens from 30-220 degrees Celsius are available in a range of capacities from 14-749l, with the choice of convection or air turbine. Available in 3 different controller classes; mechanical, electronic (RS232 computer interface) or process controller (RS232 computer interface and new chip card technology).

Thermal Product Solutions 800-216-7725
2121 Reach Rd, Williamsport, PA 17701
Laboratory oven and furnace.

Thermcraft, Inc 336-784-4800
3950 Overdale Rd, PO Box 12037, Winston Salem, NC 27107
LAB-TEMP, 300 F to 3000 F custom, benchtop, stainless steel ovens. Configured to your requirments.

Thermo Fisher Scientific Inc. 563-556-2241
2555 Kerper Blvd, Dubuque, IA 52001

Whip-Mix Corporation 800-626-5651
361 Farmington Ave, PO Box 17183, Louisville, KY 40209

OVEN, PARAFFIN *(Pathology) 88IDR*

Thermal Product Solutions 800-216-7725
2121 Reach Rd, Williamsport, PA 17701

OXIDASE TEST DEVICE FOR GONORRHEA *(Microbiology) 83LGA*

Akers Biosciences, Inc. 800-451-8378
201 Grove Rd, West Deptford, NJ 08086
HEALTHTEST.

Culture Kits, Inc. 888-680-6853
14 Prentice St, PO Box 748, Norwich, NY 13815

E-Y Laboratories, Inc. 800-821-0044
107 N Amphlett Blvd, San Mateo, CA 94401
Gonorrhoeae test.

OXIMETER, EAR *(Cardiovascular) 74DPZ*

Draeger Medical Systems, Inc. 215-660-2626
16 Electronics Ave, Danvers, MA 01923
Pulse oximeter.

Nonin Medical, Inc. 800-356-8874
13700 1st Ave N, Plymouth, MN 55441
Oximeters for neonatal through adult monitoring. Reusable and FLEXI-FORM disposable sensors.

Respironics California, Inc. 724-387-4559
2271 Cosmos Ct, Carlsbad, CA 92011
Bedside/handheld pulse oximeters.

OXIMETER, EAR *(cont'd)*

Respironics Novametrix, Llc. 724-387-4559
5 Technology Dr, Wallingford, CT 06492
Bedside/handheld pulse oximeters.

Smiths Medical Asd, Inc. 610-578-9600
9255 Customhouse Plz Ste N, San Diego, CA 92154
Blood saturation monitor and accessories.

OXIMETER, FINGER *(General) 80VFN*

Aiv, Inc. (Formerly American Iv) 800-990-2911
7485 Shipley Ave, Harmans, MD 21077
Specialized repair services on reusable adult pulse oximeter finger sensors. Adapter cables connecting finger sensors to leading patient monitors are also available.

Datrend Systems Inc. 800-667-6557
3531 Jacombs Road, Unit 1, Richmond, BC V6V 1Z8 Canada
Pulse Oximeter Sensor Tester: Sensitest

Epic Medical Equipment Services, Inc. 800-327-3742
1800 10th St Ste 300, Plano, TX 75074
FLEXI-SITE System (Y sensor) finger sensors for pulse oximeters.

Kentec Medical Inc. 800-825-5996
17871 Fitch, Irvine, CA 92614
Ameritus Pulse Oximeter Probes. Reusable and Disposable, in neonatal through adult configurations compatible with most OEM monitors.

M & I Medical Sales, Inc. 305-663-3444
4711 SW 72nd Ave, Miami, FL 33155

Nonin Medical, Inc. 800-356-8874
13700 1st Ave N, Plymouth, MN 55441
Oximeters for neonatal through adult monitoring. Also, ONYX finger pulse oximeter for spot check monitoring of adults and infants.

Omni Medical Supply Inc. 800-860-6664
4153 Pioneer Dr, Commerce Township, MI 48390

Respironics Colorado 800-345-6443
12301 Grant St Unit 190, Thornton, CO 80241
Spot check oximeter - hand held, battery powered, stored data for 99 patients $1,023.00

Respironics, Inc 800-345-6443
1010 Murry Ridge Ln, Murrysville, PA 15668
OXYPLETH provides continuous display of functional oxygen saturation and pulse rate. SPO2T is a hand-held pulse oximeter.

OXIMETER, INTRACARDIAC *(Cardiovascular) 74DQA*

Advanced Medical Instruments, Inc. 918-250-0566
3061 W Albany St, Broken Arrow, OK 74012
Pulse oximeter.

Beta Biomed Services, Inc. 800-315-7551
2804 Singleton St, Rowlett, TX 75088
Pulse oximeter sensor.

Biotek Instruments, Inc. 802-655-4040
100 Tigan St, Highland Park, Winooski, VT 05404
Pulse oximeter simulator.

Criticare Systems, Inc. 262-798-5361
20925 Crossroads Cir, Waukesha, WI 53186
Various models of 504 pulse oximeters.

Dai Shin Technologies, Inc. 262-347-0500
W238N1690 Rockwood Dr Ste 400, Waukesha, WI 53188
Various types of pulse oximeter sensors.

Dolphin Medical Inc. 310-978-0516
12525 Chadron Ave, Hawthorne, CA 90250
Pulse oximeters & sensors.

Draeger Medical Systems, Inc. 215-660-2626
16 Electronics Ave, Danvers, MA 01923
Pulse oximeter.

Fukuda Denshi Usa, Inc. 800-365-6668
17725 NE 65th St Ste C, Redmond, WA 98052
Various.

Ge Medical Systems Information Technologies 800-643-6439
8200 W Tower Ave, Milwaukee, WI 53223

Grass Technologies, An Astro-Med, Inc. Product Gro 401-828-4002
53 Airport Park Drive, Rockland, MA 02370
Oximeter.

Honeywell Hommed, Llc 888-353-5440
3400 Intertech Dr Ste 200, Brookfield, WI 53045
Monitor.

OXIMETER, INTRACARDIAC *(cont'd)*

Hospira, Inc. 877-946-7747
755 Jarvis Dr, Morgan Hill, CA 95037
$13,000 for intracardiac oximeter system.

International Technidyne Corporation 732-548-5700
8 Olsen Ave, Edison, NJ 08820
Co-oximeter.

Invivo Corporation 425-487-7000
12601 Research Pkwy, Orlando, FL 32826
Various types of pulse oximeters/monitors.

Ivy Biomedical Systems, Inc. 800-247-4614
11 Business Park Dr, Branford, CT 06405
Model 2000 Pulse Oximeter, noninvasive calculation of the functional oxygen saturation of arterial hemoglobin (spo2) using Masimo Set technology.

Jabil Global Services 502-240-1000
11201 Electron Dr, Louisville, KY 40299
Pulse oximeter.

Jostra Bentley, Inc. 302-454-9959
Rd. 402 N. Km 1.4, Industrial Park, Anasco, PR 00610-1577
Oxygen saturation meter.

Lifewatch Services, Inc. 877-774-9846
10255 W Higgins Rd Ste 100, O'hare International Center II
Rosemont, IL 60018
Oximeter.

Masimo Corp. 800-326-4890
40 Parker, Irvine, CA 92618
Pulse Oximeter. Pulse CO-Oximeter.

Mediaid Inc. 714-367-2848
17517 Fabrica Way Ste H, Cerritos, CA 90703
Reusable and disposable sensors.

Parker Hannifin Corporation. 805-658-2984
3007 Bunsen Ave Units K&L, Ventura, CA 93003
Protective probe cover, accessory to oximeter.

Respironics California, Inc. 724-387-4559
2271 Cosmos Ct, Carlsbad, CA 92011
Handheld pulse oximeter.

Respironics Novametrix, Llc. 724-387-4559
5 Technology Dr, Wallingford, CT 06492
Handheld pulse oximeter.

Spacelabs Medical Inc. 800-522-7212
5150 220th Ave SE, Issaquah, WA 98029
Pulse oximeter modules and accessories.

Syntech International 949-752-9642
17171 Daimler St, Irvine, CA 92614
Oximeter.

Waters Medical Systems, Llc 205-612-5221
2112 15th St NW, Rochester, MN 55901
Blood oximeter.

Welch Allyn Protocol Inc. 800-289-2500
8500 SW Creekside Pl, Beaverton, OR 97008
Oximeter

OXIMETER, PULSE *(General) 80WOR*

Aiv, Inc. (Formerly American Iv) 800-990-2911
7485 Shipley Ave, Harmans, MD 21077
Specialized repair services on reusable adult pulse oximeter finger sensors. Adapter cables connecting finger sensors to leading patient monitors are also available.

Armstrong Medical Industries, Inc. 800-323-4220
575 Knightsbridge Pkwy, Lincolnshire, IL 60069
Hand-held, accurate for neonate to adult.

Cardiac Science Corp. 800-777-1777
500 Burdick Pkwy, Deerfield, WI 53531
Burdick OXY 100 and 200

Clinical Dynamics Corp. 800-247-6427
10 Capital Dr, Wallingford, CT 06492
Pulse oximetry analyzer.

Commercial/Medical Electronics, Inc. 800-324-4844
1519 S Lewis Ave, Tulsa, OK 74104

Datascope Corp. 800-288-2121
14 Philips Pkwy, Montvale, NJ 07645
ACCUSAT pulse oximeter.

Datrend Systems Inc. 800-667-6557
3531 Jacombs Road, Unit 1, Richmond, BC V6V 1Z8 Canada
Pulse Oximeter Tester: Oxitest Plus 7

OXIMETER, PULSE *(cont'd)*

Devon Medical 800-571-3135
1100 1st Ave Ste 100, King Of Prussia, PA 19406
Devon Medical manufactures a complete line of Fingertip and Handheld Pulse Oximeters that provide spot-check measurements of oxygen saturation of arterial hemoglobin. Widely used in hospitals, home healthcare, community medical centers, and more. It can monitor pulse oxygen saturation and pulse rate through patient's finger. It is also widely used for sports, climbing, and avionics.

Dma Med-Chem Corporation 800-362-1833
49 Watermill Ln, Great Neck, NY 11021

Fluke Biomedical 800-648-7952
6920 Seaway Blvd, Everett, WA 98203
Index 2XL

General Biomedical Service, Inc. 800-558-9449
1900 25th St, Kenner, LA 70062
New & remanufactured respiratory equipment, ventilators, and pulse oximeters.

Invacare Corporation 800-333-6900
1 Invacare Way, Elyria, OH 44035
INVACARE Pulse Oximeter IrC700, measures SpO2 and pulse rate. Also, IRC750, measures SpO2, pulse rate, spot check, continues monitoring and sleep screening, print and download capability.

Lynn Medical 888-596-6633
764 Denison Ct, Bloomfield Hills, MI 48302
POCKET PULSE hand held oximeter.

M & I Medical Sales, Inc. 305-663-6444
4711 SW 72nd Ave, Miami, FL 33155

Medical Cables, Inc. 800-314-51111
1365 Logan Ave, Costa Mesa, CA 92626

Nihon Kohden America, Inc. 800-325-0283
90 Icon, Foothill Ranch, CA 92610

Nonin Medical, Inc. 800-356-8874
13700 1st Ave N, Plymouth, MN 55441
Hand-held pulse oximeters with optional real-time printer. Also with memory option for data management and documentation of screening and diagnostic studies using nVISION software.

Norco 800-657-6672
1125 W Amity Rd, Boise, ID 83705

Omni Medical Supply Inc. 800-860-6664
4153 Pioneer Dr, Commerce Township, MI 48390

Pace Tech, Inc. 800-722-3024
510 N Garden Ave, Clearwater, FL 33755
VITALMAX 520/510. MINIPACK 300 $1395 to $1495. LED readout, optional battery.

Qrs Diagnostic, Llc 800-465-8408
14755 27th Ave N, Plymouth, MN 55447
OxiCard PC Card Pulse Oximeter works with Windows CE, Windows 98/ME/2000/XP computers with PC Card slot; Spot check and records pulse rate and SPO2%.

Respironics Georgia, Inc. 724-387-4559
175 Chastain Meadows Ct NW, Kennesaw, GA 30144
920 hand-held pulse oximeter, 930 standard oximeter.

Respironics, Inc 800-345-6443
1010 Murry Ridge Ln, Murrysville, PA 15668
OXYPLETH provides continuous display of functional oxygen saturation and pulse rate. SPO2T is a hand-held pulse oximeter.

Sharn, Inc. 800-325-3671
4517 George Rd Ste 200, Tampa, FL 33634
Reusable finger clips, ear clips, and Y sensors. Soft-tip sensors for BCI, Datex, Marquette, Nellcor, and Ohmeda pulse oximeters.

Smiths Medical Pm, Inc. 800-558-2345
N7W22025 Johnson Dr, Waukesha, WI 53186
Model 3301 Hand-Held Pulse Oximeter is a portable monitor that noninvasively and continuously reports arterial oxygen saturation and pulse rate. Values for oxygen saturation, pulse rate and quantitative signal strength are displayed with large light emitting diodes. The BCI Digit Finger Oximeter combines monitor and sensor into one unit that provides fast reliable SpO2, pulse rate, and pulse strength measurements on patients from pediatric to adult. The BCI Fingerprint Hand-Held Pulse Oximeter is low-cost, easy-to-use and has an integrated printer, it provides fast, reliable spot checking and hard copy documentation of SpO2, and pulse rate for patients neonate to adult and Print options include real time or trend data documentation of up to 99 patients. The BCI Autocorr Pulse Oximeter with SAC Technology (serial autocorrelation) uses refined noise-reducing hardware and a unique patented software algorithm to look at pulse oximetry date in a new way, it is adaptable

to clinical, home, and sleep environments, has an internal rechargeable battery, remote alarm, function available, and real time or trend printout available when used with a computer or printer. The BCI MiniCorr Hand-Held Pulse Oximeter monitors SpO2, pulse rate and pulse strength. It is designed to provide fast, reliable measurements on challenging patients, the device rejects spontaneous motion and other artifacts, informs the operator of excess artifacts and improper sensor positioning, and processess low perfusion signals. Designed for spot checking or bedside monitoring, this portable unit is ideal in home care and clinical environments, as well as during sleep screening. The BCI 3303 is ideal for patient transport, bedside monitoring, sleep study screening, or home care. It has an easy-to-read LED display with adjustable brightness, separate patient and system tones for recognition of patient alarms or monitor alerts, one-touch direct function keys for easy no-menu operation, 24 hour memory feature with on-screen recall for up to 99 patients SpO2 and pulse rate readings, and an internal rechargeable NiMH battery. A protective rubber boot is included, a pole mount is available and the monitor is compatible with a personal computer or commercially available printer. The BCI FingerPrint Sleep Hand-Held Pulse oximeter with built-in Summary Printer is ideal for sleep screening studies in the sleep lab, clinical environment or home. The unit automatically enters Data Collection Mode after 10 minutes of continuous use, and utilizes minimal LED display when in this mode to lengthen the battery life. A summary of the saturation screening can be immediately printed from the integrated printer. It also provides fast, reliable spot-checking measurements of SpO2, pulse rate and pulse strength for use in clinical or hospital environments. It is compatible with the BCI Oximetry Data Management Program that is a Windows based, easy-to-use software, that rapidly downloads information collected during sleep screening, oxygen therapy validation, and/or related studies. To assist in the Clinicaian interpretation, it analyzes SpO2 data, and stores and prints Statistical, Desaturation and Graphic Reports.

Welch Allyn Protocol Inc. 800-289-2500
8500 SW Creekside Pl, Beaverton, OR 97008

World Medical Equipment, Inc. 800-827-3747
3915 152nd St NE, Marysville, WA 98271

Zoll Medical Corp. 800-348-9011
269 Mill Rd, Chelmsford, MA 01824
ZOLL R Series

OXIMETER, PULSE, FETAL *(Obstetrics/Gyn) 85MMA*

Ob Scientific, Inc. 262-532-8200
N112W18741 Mequon Rd, Germantown, WI 53022
Fetal pulse oximeter.

OXIMETER, REPROCESSED *(Anesthesiology) 73NLF*

Sterilmed, Inc. 763-488-3400
11400 73rd Ave N Ste 100, Maple Grove, MN 55369
Reprocessed pulse oximeter sensors.

OXIMETER, TISSUE SATURATION *(Cardiovascular) 74MUD*

Aiv, Inc. (Formerly American Iv) 800-990-2911
7485 Shipley Ave, Harmans, MD 21077
Specialized repair services on reusable adult pulse oximeter finger sensors. Adapter cables connecting finger sensors to leading patient monitors are also available.

Cas Medical Systems, Inc. 800-227-4414
44 E Industrial Rd, Branford, CT 06405
Absolute Cerebral Oximeter

Hutchinson Technology, Inc. 320-587-3797
40 W Highland Park Dr NE, Hutchinson, MN 55350
Tissue oximeter.

Hypermed, Inc 781-229-5900
41 2nd Ave, Burlington, MA 01803
Hyperspectral tissue saturation oximeter.

Somanetics Corp. 800-359-7662
2600 Troy Center Dr, Troy, MI 48084
INVOS(TM) Cerebral/Somatic Oximeter; provides noninvasive monitoring of blood oxygen saturation in the brain, body or both simultaneously. Clinicians may monitor up to four areas at once.

Spectros Corporation 650-851-4040
808 Portola Rd, Portola Valley, CA 94028
T-Stat, T-Stat 303

Vioptix, Inc. 510-360-7506
47224 Mission Falls Ct, Fremont, CA 94539
Tissue oximeter.

OXIMETER, TISSUE SATURATION, REPROCESSED
(Cardiovascular) 74NMD

ReNu Medical Inc. 877-252-1110
9800 Evergreen Way, Everett, WA 98204
Nellcor All Types

Sterilmed, Inc. 763-488-3400
11400 73rd Ave N Ste 100, Maple Grove, MN 55369
Pulse oxisensor.

OXIMETER, WHOLE BLOOD *(Hematology) 81GLY*

Gish Biomedical, Inc. 800-938-0531
22942 Arroyo Vis, Rancho Santa Margarita, CA 92688
Oxygen-saturation monitor.

Nova Biomedical 800-458-5813
200 Prospect St, Waltham, MA 02453
Models include the STAT PROFILE pHOx blood gas/ oximeter and STAT PROFILE Critical Care Xpress for the stat analysis of pH, PCO2, PO2, hematocrit, hemoglobin, and oxygen saturation (SO2%), with built-in, automatic liquid calibration and QC.

Opti Medical Systems Inc. 770-510-4444
235 Hembree Park Dr, Roswell, GA 30076
Automated blood gas/ electrolyte analyzer.

Osmetech, Inc. 800-373-6767
757 S Raymond Ave, Pasadena, CA 91105
Automated blood gas/ electrolyte analyzer.

Radiometer America, Inc. 800-736-0600
810 Sharon Dr, Westlake, OH 44145

Texas Photonics, Inc. 972-412-7111
3213 Main St, Rowlett, TX 75088

Waters Medical Systems 800-426-9877
2112 15th St NW, Rochester, MN 55901

Waters Medical Systems, Llc 205-612-5221
2112 15th St NW, Rochester, MN 55901
Blood oximeter.

OXYGEN *(Anesthesiology) 73WVK*

Aga Linde Healthcare P.R. Inc. 787-622-7900
PO Box 363868, GPO Box 364727, San Juan, PR 00936

Air Products And Chemicals, Inc. 800-654-4567
7201 Hamilton Blvd, Allentown, PA 18195
Regular or liquified oxygen.

C & C Oxygen Co. 423-867-2369
3615 Rossville Blvd, Chattanooga, TN 37407

Life Corporation 800-700-0202
1776 N Water St, Milwaukee, WI 53202
LIFE, OxygenPac Portable emergency oxygen units, clear cover and wall-mounted, off/on lever control, resuscitation mask with one-way valve for hygiene, 6lpm 90min. supply, refillable. Also available 6 & 12 lpm NORM & HIGH, 0-25 lpm variable, and demand-valve for 100% oxygen resuscitation. GSA Federal Supply Schedule.

Lifegas Llc 866-543-3427
1500 Indian Trail Lilburn Rd, Norcross, GA 30093
LifeGas supplies medical liquid and cylinder gases. Cylinder gases are supplied in lightweight aluminum cylinder for ease of transport and pharmaceutical appearance.

Norco 800-657-6672
1125 W Amity Rd, Boise, ID 83705

OXYGENATOR, CARDIOPULMONARY BYPASS
(Cardiovascular) 74DTZ

Cardiovention, Inc. 408-873-3400
19200 Stevens Creek Blvd Ste 200, Cupertino, CA 95014
Oxygenator.

Gish Biomedical, Inc. 800-938-0531
22942 Arroyo Vis, Rancho Santa Margarita, CA 92688
VISION.

Jostra Bentley, Inc. 302-454-9959
Rd. 402 N. Km 1.4, Industrial Park, Anasco, PR 00610-1577
Blood oxygenstor.

Medtronic Perfusion Systems 800-854-3570
7611 Northland Dr N, Brooklyn Park, MN 55428

Medtronic, Inc. 800-633-8766
710 Medtronic Pkwy, Minneapolis, MN 55432
MAXIMA, MAXIMA II, MINIMAX, MAXIMA PLUS, MINIMAX PLUS.

Novosci Corp. 281-363-4949
2828 N Crescentridge Dr, The Woodlands, TX 77381

Sorin Group Usa 800-289-5759
14401 W 65th Way, Arvada, CO 80004

OXYGENATOR, CARDIOPULMONARY BYPASS *(cont'd)*

Terumo Cardiovascular Systems (Tcvs) 800-283-7866
125 Blue Ball Rd, Elkton, MD 21921
Cardipulmonary bypass oxygenator.

Terumo Cardiovascular Systems (Tcvs) 800-283-7866
28 Howe St, Ashland, MA 01721
Oxygenator and accessories.

Terumo Cardiovascular Systems, Corp 800-521-2818
6200 Jackson Rd, Ann Arbor, MI 48103
Membrane oxygenator with integrated heat exchanger.

OXYGENATOR, EXTRACORPOREAL PERFUSION
(Anesthesiology) 73RJP

Sorin Group Usa 800-289-5759
14401 W 65th Way, Arvada, CO 80004

OXYGENATOR, INTRAVASCULAR *(Anesthesiology) 73MEV*

Novosci Corp. 281-363-4949
2828 N Crescentridge Dr, The Woodlands, TX 77381

OXYGENATOR, ORGAN PRESERVATION *(Surgery) 79UAA*

Sorin Group Usa 800-289-5759
14401 W 65th Way, Arvada, CO 80004

OXYHEMOGLOBIN/CARBOXYHEMOGLOBIN CURVE, CARBON-MONOXIDE *(Toxicology) 91JKS*

International Technidyne Corporation 732-548-5700
8 Olsen Ave, Edison, NJ 08820
Co-oximeter.

Masimo Corp. 800-326-4890
40 Parker, Irvine, CA 92618

Radiometer America, Inc. 800-736-0600
810 Sharon Dr, Westlake, OH 44145
OSM3.

PACEMAKER, CARDIAC, EXTERNAL TRANSCUTANEOUS (NON-INVASIVE) *(Cardiovascular) 74DRO*

Ballard Medical Products 770-587-7835
12050 Lone Peak Pkwy, Draper, UT 84020
Pacemaker, cardiac, external transcutaneous (non-invasive).

Heartbeat Medical Corp. 505-823-1990
8917 Adams St NE, Albuquerque, NM 87113
External pacemaker.

Invivo Corporation 425-487-7000
12601 Research Pkwy, Orlando, FL 32826
Various external cardiac monitors.

Physio-Control, Inc. 800-442-1142
11811 Willows Rd NE, Redmond, WA 98052
LIFEPAK 9P, 10: defibrillator/monitor/pacemaker. LIFEPAK 11 defibrillator/pacemaker (mates to LIFEPAK 11 diagnostic cardiac monitor)

Tz Medical Inc. 800-944-0187
7272 SW Durham Rd Ste 800, Portland, OR 97224
Defib/cardiovert/pace/monitoring electrode.

Welch Allyn Protocol, Inc. 800-462-0777
2 Corporate Dr Ste 110, Long Grove, IL 60047

Zoll Medical Corp. 800-348-9011
269 Mill Rd, Chelmsford, MA 01824
ZOLL R Series

PACEMAKER, HEART, EXTERNAL *(Cardiovascular) 74DTE*

Cardio Command, Inc. 800-231-6370
4920 W Cypress St Ste 110, Tampa, FL 33607
Transesophageal atrial pacing and recording catheter (TAP) and P-wave amplification using TAPSCOPE, esophageal stethoscope; TAPCATH Five-French catheter.

Galix Biomedical Instrumentation, Inc. 305-534-5905
2555 Collins Ave Ste C-5, Miami Beach, FL 33140
Transitory single-chamber external pacemaker model PaceStar, provides selection of rate, amplitude, sensitivity, refractory period, hysteresis, and width as programmable parameters. Three methods of tachycardia termination are available. Up to 75 seconds of intracavitary ECG signal and more than 1500 events can be stored and, through an optically isolated data-logging module, transmitted to a computer to register events such as parameter changes, alarms, tachycardia events, frequency trends, and more. Operates for a period of more than 20 days with 2 AA batteries and with a safety mechanism that enables the user to individually replace batteries; only one battery can be changed at a time.

PACEMAKER, HEART, EXTERNAL *(cont'd)*

Mcpherson Enterprises, Inc. 813-931-4201
3851 62nd Ave N Ste A, Pinellas Park, FL 33781
No common name listed.

Oscor, Inc. 800-726-7267
3816 Desoto Blvd, Palm Harbor, FL 34683
External, pulse-generator pacemaker.

Osypka Medical, Inc. 858-454-0021
7855 Ivanhoe Ave Ste 226, La Jolla, CA 92037
Temporary cardiac pacemaker.

Pace Medical, Inc. 781-890-5656
391 Totten Pond Rd, Waltham, MA 02451
5 models: single chamber and dual chamber temporary cardiac pacemakers. Pacing modes cover: AAI, AOO, AAT, VOO, VVI, VVT, DOO, DVI, DDI and DDD, depending on model selected. (Certain models with 450 or 800ppm high rate capability.).

Seecor, Inc. 972-288-3278
844 Dalworth Dr Ste 6, Mesquite, TX 75149
STAT-PACE II: Transesophageal cardiac pacer. STAT-PACE IIA: transesophageal cardiac pacer, OEM. Model 2A, transesophageal cardiac pacer, OEM.

St. Jude Medical Cardiac Rhythm Management Div. 800-777-2237
15900 Valley View Ct, Sylmar, CA 91342
Dual-chamber, multi-mode including DDD, DVI and DDI, multiprogrammable parameters with rapid atrial pacing to 800 ppm.

PACEMAKER, HEART, EXTERNAL, PROGRAMMABLE
(Cardiovascular) 74JOQ

Ep Medsystems, Inc. 609-753-8533
575 N Route 73 Bldg D, West Berlin, NJ 08091
Ep-4 clinical stimulator.

Galix Biomedical Instrumentation, Inc. 305-534-5905
2555 Collins Ave Ste C-5, Miami Beach, FL 33140
Multiprogrammable stimulator for transesophageal/intracardiac electrophysiological studies, for Brady and tachycardia support: up to 3 independent extra stimuli. Three methods of tachycardia termination are available, with manual and automatic extra stimulation as well as a built-in multiprogrammable pacemaker.

Hi-Tronics Designs, Inc. 973-347-4865
999 Willow Grove St, Hackettstown, NJ 07840
Contract manufacturing and design of ECG recorders, arrhythmia monitors, bonegrowth stimulators, PC based programming wands for implantable medical devices and clinical digital cardiovascular stimulators.

PACEMAKER, HEART, IMPLANTABLE, DUAL CHAMBER
(Cardiovascular) 74ULJ

St. Jude Medical Cardiac Rhythm Management Div. 800-777-2237
15900 Valley View Ct, Sylmar, CA 91342
Dual-chamber with programmed and measured telemetry, intracardiac electrograms, auto threshold tests, pace and sense event markers; dual chamber rate-modulated with activity sensor, programmed and measured telemetry, histograms, intracardiac electrograms, auto threshold tests, pace and sense event markers.

PACEMAKER, HEART, IMPLANTABLE, PROGRAMMABLE
(Cardiovascular) 74DXY

Arizona Device Manufacturing 763-505-0874
2350 W Medtronic Way, Tempe, AZ 85281
Implantable pulse generator.

Boston Scientific Corp. 612-582-7448
6645 185th Ave NE, Redmond, WA 98052
Pulse generator, SSS.

Cardiac Pacemakers, Inc. 800-227-3422
4100 Hamline Ave N, P.O. Box 64079, Saint Paul, MN 55112
Numerous models in unipolar or bipolar. Other programmable parameters and increments vary according to unit.

Ela Medical, Inc. 800-352-6466
2950 Xenium Ln N, Plymouth, MN 55441
Symphony DR is a multiprogrammable dual chamber, dual-sensor rate responsive pacemaker with autothreshold. features include DDD/AMC, rest rate, dynamic TARP, multimode switching, auto AV delay, PMT algorithm, automatic interpretation of data analysis, 6 minute stored EGM.

Medtronic Puerto Rico Operations Co., Juncos 763-514-4000
Road 31, Km. 24, Hm 4, Ceiba Norte Industrial Park, Juncos, PR 00777
Implantable pulse generator.

PACEMAKER, HEART, IMPLANTABLE, PROGRAMMABLE
(cont'd)

Medtronic Puerto Rico Operations Co.,Med Rel — 763-514-4000
Road 909, Km. 0.4., Barrio Mariana, Humacao, PR 00792
Implantable pulse generator.

St. Jude Medical Cardiac Rhythm Management Div. — 800-777-2237
15900 Valley View Ct, Sylmar, CA 91342
Single-chamber and dual-chamber with programmed and measured telemetry, intracardiac electrograms, auto threshold tests, pace and sense event markers; single-chamber and dual-chamber rate-modulated with activity sensor, programmed and measured telemetry, histograms, intracardiac electrograms, auto threshold tests, pace and sense event markers.

PACEMAKER, HEART, IMPLANTABLE, RATE RESPONSIVE
(Cardiovascular) 74WST

St. Jude Medical Cardiac Rhythm Management Div. — 800-777-2237
15900 Valley View Ct, Sylmar, CA 91342
Single-chamber and dual-chamber rate-modulated with activity sensor, programmed and measured telemetry, histograms, intracardiac electrograms, auto threshold tests, pace and sense event markers.

PACEMAKER, RESPIRATORY *(Surgery) 79RJT*

Ventlab Corporation — 800-593-4654
155 Boyce Dr, Mocksville, NC 27028
Hyperinflation bag syctems.

PACHOMETER *(Surgery) 79VDT*

Bausch & Lomb Surgical — 636-255-5051
3365 Tree Court Ind Blvd, Saint Louis, MO 63122

Carl Zeiss Meditec Inc. — 877-486-7473
5160 Hacienda Dr, Dublin, CA 94568
The Humphrey Ultrasound Pachometer (HUP) is recognized for its fast and accurate objective measurement capability. The HUP has been designed to measure corneal thickness with greater precision, employing unique digital signal processing algorithms. The solid tip probe is easy to use and virtually maintenance-free.

D.G.H. Technology, Inc. — 800-722-3883
110 Summit Dr Ste B, Exton, PA 19341
PACHETTE 2 DGH550 ultrasonic pachymeter, DGH5100e A-scan/pachymeter combination unit, DGH5000e A-Scan, Diamond Knives

Nidek Inc. — 800-223-9044
47651 Westinghouse Dr, Fremont, CA 94539
Model UP-1800 a-scan and pachymeter.

Sonomed, Inc. — 800-227-1285
1979 Marcus Ave Ste C105, New Hyde Park, NY 11042
$2500 for model 200p+.

PACIFIER *(General) 80WRP*

Children's Medical Ventures, Inc. — 800-345-6443
191 Wyngate Dr, Monroeville, PA 15146
WEE THUMBIE & SOOTHIE, premature to newborn size, vanilla scent optional.

Dma Med-Chem Corporation — 800-362-1833
49 Watermill Ln, Great Neck, NY 11021
WEE-THUMBIE

Gerber Products Co. — 800-430-0150
120 N Commercial St Fl 4, Neenah, WI 54956

Ulster Scientific, Inc. — 845-255-2200
83 S Putt Corners Rd, PO Box 819, New Paltz, NY 12561
KIDZ MED, liquid medicine delivery and decongestant pacifier.

PACK, COLD *(General) 80QLO*

Achilles Usa, Inc. — 425-353-7000
1407 80th St SW, Everett, WA 98203
Development of vinyls and plastics for the medical industry.

Alimed, Inc. — 800-225-2610
297 High St, Dedham, MA 02026

Battle Creek Equipment Co. — 800-253-0854
307 Jackson St W, Battle Creek, MI 49037
ICE IT Deluxe Wrap, non-toxic reusable pack remains pliable when frozen. Washable covers feature hook and loop closures with detachable elastic strap. $15.99 to $39.99.

Bruder Healthcare Company — 888-827-8337
3150 Engineering Pkwy, Alpharetta, GA 30004
Conforming, Soothing Cold Packs, Assorted Shapes and Sizes

PACK, COLD *(cont'd)*

Chattanooga Group — 800-592-7329
4717 Adams Rd, Hixson, TN 37343
COLPAC, SPORT=PAC, BOO-BOO PAC AND COOLBAND.

Contour Pak, Inc. — 800-926-2228
346 Rheem Blvd Ste 104, Moraga, CA 94556
A highly effective, easy-to-use cold-therapy product, the Pak offers a patented design that molds to any part of the body, with elastic straps with Velcro to hold it snugly in place. Soft and durable, the reusable Pak stays therapeutically cold for 30 to 40 minutes, remains flexible even right out of the freezer, and has eye-catching packaging draws consumers' attention. Cold therapy is one of the best and most commonly recommended treatments for the relief of pain and swelling associated with many injuries, post-surgical trauma, and numerous medical conditions. Cold helps to shrink blood vessels, reducing bleeding and associated swelling. It also helps prevent muscle spasm and relieves pain. The Pak is significantly easier and more comfortable to use than the alternatives: other products can be cumbersome, limited in how they can be applied, and often give the user ice burn. A second product, Ice on the Run, shares the same patented design as The Pak, yet offers users the flexibility of not having to store the product in a freezer. Ice on the Run simply requires users to fill it with crushed ice and slide the closure mechanism in place, making it ready to use.

Dura-Kold Corp. — 800-541-7199
3525 S Purdue St, Oklahoma City, OK 73179
Reusable compression ice wraps for in- and out-patient orthopedic surgical procedures and rehabilitation, providing up to 2 hours of cold compression.

Ebi, Llc — 800-526-2579
100 Interpace Pkwy, Parsippany, NJ 07054
TEMPTEK: Controlled cold therapy for post-operative pain and swelling. EBICE: Cold therapy.

Hospital Marketing Svcs. Company, Inc. — 800-786-5094
162 Great Hill Rd./ Ind. Park, Naugatuck, CT 06770
Case of 4 boxes (12 packs per box), 6in. x 10in., #6620, or PERI PLUS extra absorbent perineal cold pack for labor and delivery, cat. no. 6300, 24/case.

I-Rep, Inc. — 800-828-0852
508 Chaney St Ste B, Lake Elsinore, CA 92530

Icd, Inc. — 866-791-2503
PO Box 218, Imperial Beach, CA 91933
Ice packs for sports injuries.

Medi Inc — 800-225-8634
75 York Ave, P.O. Box 302, Randolph, MA 02368

Mine Safety Appliances Company — 866-MSA-1001
121 Gamma Dr, Pittsburgh, PA 15238

Pi Professional Therapy Products — 888-818-9632
PO Box 1067, Athens, TN 37371

Polar Products, Inc. — 800-763-8423
540 S Main St Ste 951, Akron, OH 44311
Our line of patented Soft Ice cold & hot packs are non-toxic and yet stay remarkably soft and flexible when frozen. We manufacture economical professional quality packs ranging in size from 3î x 8î to 11î x 23î

Pristech Products, Inc — 800-432-8722
6952 Fairgrounds Pkwy, PO Box 680728, San Antonio, TX 78238

Rockford Medical & Safety Co. — 800-435-9451
2420 Harrison Ave, PO Box 5646, Rockford, IL 61108

Tcp Reliable, Inc. — 888-TCP-3393
551 Raritan Center Pkwy, Edison, NJ 08837
TEMP-GARD, CRYOGEL, & INSULATING VIAL TRAYS.

Tetra Medical Supply Corp. — 800-621-4041
6364 W Gross Point Rd, Niles, IL 60714

Thermosafe Brands — 847-398-0110
3930 N Ventura Dr Ste 450, Arlington Heights, IL 60004
U-TEK Refrigerant Packs, INSUL-ICE reusable ice singles and mat.

Tyco Healthcare Group Lp — 800-445-5025
2 Ludlow Park Dr, Chicopee, MA 01022
KOOL GEL innovative cold therapy hydropad used at room, refrigerated of freezer temperature. Remains flexible and self-adhering.

PACK, COLD, CHEMICAL *(General) 80FRS*

Cramer Products, Inc. — 800-255-6621
153 W Warren St, Gardner, KS 66030
$9.29/12pcs. $10.15/16pcs.

PACK, COLD, CHEMICAL *(cont'd)*

Cryopak Industries, Inc. 800-667-2532
1055 Derwent Way, Delta, BC V3M 5R4 Canada
Cryopak× Instant Cold Pack is a First-Aid Cold Treatment, that provides temporary relief for minor swelling, sprains and strains.

Hospital Marketing Svcs. Company, Inc. 800-786-5094
162 Great Hill Rd./ Ind. Park, Naugatuck, CT 06770
24 pcs. #6627, case of 24 pcs. #6300 (perineal instant cold pack), case of 24 pcs. #6000-019 COMFORT COLD instant cold pack.

Morrison Medical 800-438-6677
3735 Paragon Dr, Columbus, OH 43228
Disposable Cold Packs

Mueller Sports Medicine 800-356-9522
1 Quench Dr, P.O. Box 99, Prairie Du Sac, WI 53578
Cold packs, stretch tape, and hinges.

Packaging Products Corp. 800-225-0484
198 Herman Melville Blvd, New Bedford, MA 02740
ARCTIC PACK and GLACIER GEL artifical refrigerant gel.

Tetra Medical Supply Corp. 800-621-4041
6364 W Gross Point Rd, Niles, IL 60714

PACK, CUSTOM/SPECIAL PROCEDURE *(General) 80WXF*

Akorn, Inc. 800-535-7155
2500 Millbrook Dr, Buffalo Grove, IL 60089
Ophthalmic.

Alcon Research, Ltd. 800-862-5266
6201 South Fwy, Fort Worth, TX 76134

Gdm Electronic And Medical 408-945-4100
2070 Ringwood Ave, San Jose, CA 95131

General Econopak, Inc. 888-871-8568
1725 N 6th St, Philadelphia, PA 19122
Sheets, drapes, covers, and packs custom made to order.

Johnson & Johnson Medical Division Of Ethicon, Inc. 800-423-4018
2500 E Arbrook Blvd, Arlington, TX 76014

Lee Medical International, Inc. 800-433-8950
612 Distributors Row, Harahan, LA 70123
Universal and custom-designed precaution packs for hospitals.

Mckesson General Medical 800-446-3008
8741 Landmark Rd, Richmond, VA 23228

Medical Techniques Usa 801-936-4501
125 N 400 W Ste C, North Salt Lake, UT 84054

Medistat Medical - Hallmark Sales Corporation 888-MED-ISTA
1601 Peach Leaf St, Houston, TX 77039
Manufacturer of kits including first aid, body fluid spills, burns, emergency, medical, surgical, obstetrical, exams, minor surgery, biopsy, convenience, procedure trays, disposable instruments, sterile kits. Owns manufacturing and validated sterilization facilities. Can make custom or special order kits. Refills, supplies.

Mentor Corp. 800-525-0245
201 Mentor Dr, Santa Barbara, CA 93111
Eighteen different trays for various urological procedures.

Windstone Medical Packaging, Inc. 800-637-7056
1602 4th Ave N, Billings, MT 59101

PACK, HOT OR COLD, DISPOSABLE *(Physical Med) 89IMD*

Aerosol And Liquid Packaging, Inc. 410-342-6100
715 S Haven St, Baltimore, MD 21224
Hot or cold disposable pack.

Be Well Usa, Inc. 229-890-1627
3195 7th St SE, Moultrie, GA 31788
Various types of disposable hot cold compression.

Beekley Corp. 860-583-4700
150 Dolphin Rd, Bristol, CT 06010
Self - adhesive cold pack.

Biomet, Inc. 574-267-6639
56 E Bell Dr, PO Box 587, Warsaw, IN 46582
Disposable heat pack.

Brain Tunnelgenix Technologies Corp. 203-922-0105
375 Mather St, Hamden, CT 06514
Brain Tunnelgenix Cold Pack; Thermalgenix Temperature Management

Certified Safety Manufacturing 800-854-7474
1400 Chestnut Ave, Kansas City, MO 64127
Certi-Cool Instant Cold Pack. Certi-Heat Instant Hot Pack.

PACK, HOT OR COLD, DISPOSABLE *(cont'd)*

D&M Soomekh International, Inc. 323-266-2500
1260 S Boyle Ave, Los Angeles, CA 90023
Hot or cold instant pack.

G&M Research Company, Inc. 603-645-6655
31 Hale Ave, Hooksett, NH 03106
Sports ice.

Healer Products, Llc 914-663-6300
427 Commerce Ln Ste 1, West Berlin, NJ 08091
Cold pack.

Heatmax, Inc. 800-533-7349
505 Hill Rd, Dalton, GA 30721
Hot or cold pack.

Hospital Marketing Svcs. Company, Inc. 800-786-5094
162 Great Hill Rd./ Ind. Park, Naugatuck, CT 06770
Case of 24 pcs. #6627 case of 16 pcs., 6in. x 10in., Cat. no # 6616.

Industrial Support Services, Inc. 217-223-6180
2600 N 42nd St, Quincy, IL 62305
Heating pad.

Kentron Health Care, Inc. 615-384-0573
3604 Kelton Jackson Rd, P.o. Box 120, Springfield, TN 37172
Instant cold compress.

Medco Supply Company 800-556-3326
500 Fillmore Ave, Tonawanda, NY 14150
Instant hot & cold, and reusable hot & cold.

Medi Inc 800-225-8634
75 York Ave, P.O. Box 302, Randolph, MA 02368

Medi-Temp Technology Intl., Llc 888-669-0600
1000 E Butler Ave Ste 104, Flagstaff, AZ 86001
Instant cold pack, disposable.

Medlogix, Inc. 804-530-2906
9405 Burge Ave, Richmond, VA 23237

Mycoal Products Corporation Of Usa 678-765-4000
475 Horizon Dr, Suwanee, GA 30024
Hand or body warmers.

Normed 800-288-8200
PO Box 3644, Seattle, WA 98124
Cold pack.

North Safety Products 401-943-4400
1101 B Calle Neutron, Parque Industrial Maran, Mexicali, B.c. Mexico
Instant cold pak

Norwood Promotional Products, Inc. 651-388-1298
5151 Moundview Dr, Red Wing, MN 55066
Chemical hot pack.

Ortho-Med, Inc. 800-547-5571
3208 SE 13th Ave, Portland, OR 97202

Pi-Ptp 888-818-9632
215 Rocky Mount Rd, PO Box 1067, Athens, TN 37303
Cold/hot pack.

Pristech Products, Inc 800-432-8722
6952 Fairgrounds Pkwy, PO Box 680728, San Antonio, TX 78238

Procter & Gamble Paper Product Co. 229-430-8260
512 Liberty Expy SE, Albany, GA 31705
Heatpack.

Rapid Deployment Products 877-433-7569
157 Railroad Dr, Ivyland, PA 18974
No impact activation, Zero % failure guarantee, long lasting cold below 32 degrees and hot exceeding 130 degrees. The best hot and cold pack on the market!

Respironics Missouri 978-659-4252
2039 Concourse Dr, Saint Louis, MO 63146
OMNI INFANT HEEL WARMERS disposable infant heel warmers activate temperature of 105 degrees Fahrenheit. OMNI INFANT TRANSPORT MATTRESS heats to 105 deg. Fahrenheit to prevent infant hypothermia during transport; disposable. OMNI MULTI-PURPOSE WARMER heats to 108 deg. Fahrenheit; disposable. OMNI COLD GEL PACK cold pack (reusable and single) with temperatures between 15 to 27 degrees.

Respond Industries, Inc. 1-800-523-8999
9500 Woodend Rd, Edwardsville, KS 66111
Various sizes of instant ice packs.

Rinz-L-O 248-548-3993
340 W Maplehurst St, Ferndale, MI 48220
Pack, hot or cold, non-chemical.

PACK, HOT OR COLD, DISPOSABLE *(cont'd)*

Sunbeam Products, Inc. 561-912-4100
2381 NW Executive Center Dr, Boca Raton, FL 33431
Air-activated heating pad.

Tellus Medical Products, Inc. 760-200-9772
77971 Wildcat Dr Ste C, Palm Desert, CA 92211
Disposable hot or cold packs.

Velcro Usa, Inc. 603-669-4880
406 Brown Ave, Manchester, NH 03103
Cold therapy wrap.

PACK, HOT OR COLD, REUSABLE *(Physical Med) 89IME*

Abare Ent., Inc. 478-994-5555
44 W Chambers St, Forsyth, GA 31029
Cold or ice packs of various shapes and sizes.

Aqua-Cel Corp. 888-254-HEAT
17137 Sparkleberry St, Fountain Valley, CA 92708
$5 for single pack, $29 for TMJ reusable and microwavable hot & cold water pack, $7 for post-surgical reusable cold gel pack.

Back Support Systems 800-669-2225
67684 San Andreas St, Desert Hot Springs, CA 92240
ICE N HEAT Magnetic hot/cold pack and microwavable/freezable hot/cold compress is available in six sizes.

Bagblocker, Inc 317-538-6732
2159 Dockside Dr, Greenwood, IN 46143
Cold pack.

Be Well Usa, Inc. 229-890-1627
3195 7th St SE, Moultrie, GA 31788
Various types of reusable hot and-or cold compresses.

Bionix Development Corp. 800-551-7096
5154 Enterprise Blvd, Toledo, OH 43612
Reusable heat pad.

Breg, Inc., An Orthofix Company 800-897-BREG
2611 Commerce Way, Vista, CA 92081
Cold pack.

Brown Medical Industries 800-843-4395
1300 Lundberg Dr W, Spirit Lake, IA 51360
POLAR ICE cold therapy supports that offer compressional cold, promoting faster recovery following sugery or injury. Specifically designed for body parts.

Bruder Healthcare Company 888-827-8337
3150 Engineering Pkwy, Alpharetta, GA 30004
Microwave Moist Heat Packs

Chattanooga Group 800-592-7329
4717 Adams Rd, Hixson, TN 37343
SENSAFLEX, THERMA-WRAP & FLEXI-PAC. Hot or cold therapy; goes from the freezer to the microwave.

Cherry Blossom Enterprises Inc. 864-972-2920
305 S Union Rd, Westminster, SC 29693
Hot or cold pack.

Coldstar International, Inc. 423-538-5551
677 Mountain View Dr, Piney Flats, TN 37686
Hot & cold gel packs.

Core Products International, Inc. 800-365-3047
808 Prospect Ave, Osceola, WI 54020
Hot/Cold Therapy that stays in place using an exclusive strapping system. Frost Free cover elminiates need for bulky, seperate cover. Headache Ice Pillo provides medically recommended cold therapy combined with the comfort of a fiber cervical-support pillow. Compact size makes it convient for traveling.

Corflex, Inc. 800-426-7353
669 E Industrial Park Dr, Manchester, NH 03109
CRYOTHERM cold/hot gel packs; cold/hot therapy.

Cramer Products, Inc. 800-255-6621
153 W Warren St, Gardner, KS 66030
FLEXI-COLD $11.88/12pcs. regular size, $7.78/12pcs. small size.

Creations Magiques C.M. Inc. 514-753-3892
3001 Rue Visitation, Saint-Charles-Borromee J6E 7Y8 Canada
Pack,reusable hot or cold

Cryopak Industries, Inc. 800-667-2532
1055 Derwent Way, Delta, BC V3M 5R4 Canada
ICE-PAK® HOT-PAK® can be used in coolers. Microwavable to keep food warm and also can be used as an ice pack. Microban® anti-microbial protection built into plastic to inhibit growth of common household bacteria, fungi, mold, mildew and odors.

PACK, HOT OR COLD, REUSABLE *(cont'd)*

DJO Inc. 800-336-6569
1430 Decision St, Vista, CA 92081
Reusable cold packs for the neck, shoulder, back, wrist, elbow, groin, knee, leg, arm, foot, ankle, vest, collar and dental uses in various sizes.

Dorel Design & Development Center 781-364-3542
25 Forbes Blvd, Foxboro, MA 02035

Dynatronics Corp. Chattanooga Operations 801-568-7000
6607 Mountain View Rd, Ooltewah, TN 37363
Reuseable hot or cold pack.

Flax Organics, Inc. 636-896-0668
1721 Brookline Dr, Saint Charles, MO 63303
Hot or cold pack, flaxseed incased in fabric, organic

Homedics Inc. 800-333-3282
3000 N Pontiac Trl, Commerce Township, MI 48390
Hot/Cold therapy devices.

Hospital Marketing Svcs. Company, Inc. 800-786-5094
162 Great Hill Rd./ Ind. Park, Naugatuck, CT 06770
Box of 10 pcs. #7714; 6'x10' box of 24 pcs. #7727.

I.B.S. (Ice Bag Support) 270-443-0443
1117 N 8th St Ste 201, Paducah, KY 42001
Ibs.

Ibc Int'L, Inc. 727-551-2087
100 4th Ave S Apt 412, Saint Petersburg, FL 33701
Body comforter.

Imtek Environmental Corp. 770-667-8621
PO Box 2066, Alpharetta, GA 30023
THERAPRO hot/cold therapy products - Therapro provides soothing heat or cold for extended periods of time. Use of Therapro reduces swelling, aches, hemorrhaging, muscle spasms & pain. For more info, go to www.temtro.com.

Invotec Intl. 800-998-8580
6833 Phillips Industrial Blvd, Jacksonville, FL 32256
Cold pack.

Jobar Intl., Inc. 310-222-8682
21022 Figueroa St, Carson, CA 90745
Various.

Kees Goebel Medical Specialties, Inc. 800-354-0445
9663 Glades Dr, Hamilton, OH 45011

Kentron Health Care, Inc. 615-384-0573
3604 Kelton Jackson Rd, P.o. Box 120, Springfield, TN 37172
Hot and cold pack.

Leesan Maquilas S.A. De C.V. 52-5-561-526
Enrique Dunant No., 12 Centro, Tlalnepantla,edo.de Mexico Cp Mexico
Soft cooling gel sheet

Lg Medical Technology, Llc 360-668-0803
22529 39th Ave SE, Bothell, WA 98021
Hot and cold gel pack.

Lohmann & Rauscher, Inc. 800-279-3863
6001 SW 6th Ave Ste 101, Topeka, KS 66615

Marlene C. Roche 519-658-4519
96 Grey Abbey Trail, Cambridge N3C 3G1 Canada
Pack, hot or cold, reuseable

Mastercraft Of Seattle 206-768-1297
300 S Bennett St, Seattle, WA 98108
Hot and cold gel pack.

Maternal Care, Inc. 678-770-4355
11585 Jones Bridge Rd Ste 420-216, Alpharetta, GA 30022
Pack, hot or cold, reusable cold pack.

Medi Inc 800-225-8634
75 York Ave, P.O. Box 302, Randolph, MA 02368

Medi-Temp Technology Intl., Llc 888-669-0600
1000 E Butler Ave Ste 104, Flagstaff, AZ 86001
Hot cold compress.

Naimco, Inc. 423-648-7730
4120 S Creek Rd, Chattanooga, TN 37406
Various reuseable cold packs.

Natural Wonders Ca Inc. 818-341-7007
21011 Itasca St Ste E, Chatsworth, CA 91311
Cold,hot pack.

Nature's Way Therapeutic Products, Inc. 604-921-2601
91021-1427 Bellevue Ave, West Vancouver V7T 1C3 Canada
Multirest

PACK, HOT OR COLD, REUSABLE *(cont'd)*

Nora-Dall 919-942-2592
111 Glosson Cir, Carrboro, NC 27510
Cooler offer/warmer upper.

Obus Forme Ltd. 888-225-7378
550 Hopewell Ave., Toronto, ON M6E 2S6 Canada

Omniqur, Inc. 626-336-9737
15342B Valley Blvd, City Of Industry, CA 91746
Cold pack.

Pan-American 404-966-4230
1480 Terrell Mill Rd SE Ste F, Suite 662, Marietta, GA 30067
Cold pack.

Patterson Medical Supply, Inc. 262-387-8720
W68N158 Evergreen Blvd, Cedarburg, WI 53012
Hot/cold packs.

Pelton Shepherd Industries 800-258-3423
812B W Luce St, Stockton, CA 95203
Dental pack 3 x 5 in. 3212 throat-perineal flex-gel pack 3 in. x 13 in. 3214 compact flex-gel pack 5 in. x 5 in. 3216 finger flex-gel pack 5 in. x 5 in. 3218 standard flex-gel pack 5 in. x 10 in. 3222 in. cryoflex-gel pack 4 in. x 10 in. w/ disposable linen cover 3224 in. standard solid-gel pack 5 in. x 10 in. freezes solid 3226 hot/cold therapy pack 4 in. x 10 in. w/disposable linen cover 3218 standard flex gel 5in. x 10 in. 3280 large flex-gel pack 10in. x 12 in.; #3282 extra large flex-gel pack 10 in. x 16 in.; #3286, cervical, ankle-elbow 5 x 18 in. POLAR ICE - Economy Line 6' x 6', 6' x 12', 10' x 15'.

Pi Professional Therapy Products 888-818-9632
PO Box 1067, Athens, TN 37371
SOFTOUCH hot and cold packs, CP reusuable cold packs.

Pi-Ptp 888-818-9632
215 Rocky Mount Rd, PO Box 1067, Athens, TN 37303
Cold pack.

Polar Products, Inc. 800-763-8423
540 S Main St Ste 951, Akron, OH 44311
Our line of patented Soft Ice cold & hot packs are non-toxic and yet stay remarkably soft and flexible when frozen. We manufacture economical professional quality packs ranging in size from 3î x 8î to 11î x 23î.

Precision Therapeutics, Inc. 800-544-0076
8400 E Prentice Ave Ste 700, Greenwood Village, CO 80111
$9.00 to $4.25 for SOFT PACK, hot or cold compress, reusable, various sizes; also available, from $2.19 for SOFT ICE, hot or cold compress, reusable, various sizes.

Pristech Products, Inc 800-432-8722
6952 Fairgrounds Pkwy, PO Box 680728, San Antonio, TX 78238

Protector Canada Inc. 800-268-6594
1111 Flint Rd., Unit 23, Toronto, ON M3J 3C7 Canada

Regency Product International 800-845-7931
4732 E 26th St, Vernon, CA 90058
ICE N HEAT available in 5 sizes.

Rockford Medical & Safety Co. 800-435-9451
2420 Harrison Ave, PO Box 5646, Rockford, IL 61108

Rtr Industries, Inc. 519-438-3691
700 York St, London N5W 2S8 Canada
Cold pack

Southwest Technologies, Inc. 800-247-9951
1746 E Levee St, North Kansas City, MO 64116
Gel packs with Velcro straps. 40 different shapes and sizes.

Sunbeam Products, Inc. 561-912-4100
2381 NW Executive Center Dr, Boca Raton, FL 33431
Cold pack.

Tetra Medical Supply Corp. 800-621-4041
6364 W Gross Point Rd, Niles, IL 60714

The 50 Degree Company 321-956-0050
315 Stan Dr, Melbourne, FL 32904
Hot and cold packs.

The Saunders Group 800-445-9836
4250 Norex Dr, Chaska, MN 55318
Hot and cold paks.

Thera-Tronics, Inc. 800-267-6211
623 Mamaroneck Ave, Mamaroneck, NY 10543
Paraffin and units.

Therapy Innovations Llc 541-550-7347
840 SE Woodland Blvd Ste 185, Bend, OR 97702
Hot pack.

Thermal Logic, Inc. 318-345-5603
204 Timber Ln, Monroe, LA 71203
Various.

Thermalcare Products Ltd. 416-231-2746
16 Great Oak Dr., Toronto, ONT m9a1m9 Canada
Various styles of hot/cold reusable packs

Thermionics Corp. 800-800-5728
1214 Bunn Ave Unit 5, Springfield, IL 62703
THERMPAQ is a hot/cold Clay-Based pack that goes from freezer to microwave. Maintains therapeutic temperature for 30 minutes. Available in 2 sizes: 6 x 12 in. general purpose; 9.5 x 16 in. for the back. Also, THERMIBEADS avail for Moist Heat, 2 sizes.

Vesture Corp. 614-864-6400
120 E Pritchard St, Asheboro, NC 27203
Cold pack that provide cold therapy for body surfaces.

Vsm Healthcare Products 330-673-8227
15547 Main Market Road, Parkman, OH 44080
Cold pack.

Wendell-Alan Ltd. 216-881-8299
1768 E 25th St, Cleveland, OH 44114
Various sizes of reusable cold packs.

Zimmer Orthopaedic Surgical Products 800-321-5533
PO Box 10, 200 West Ohio Ave., Dover, OH 44622

3m Company 651-733-4365
601 22nd Ave S, Brookings, SD 57006

PACK, HOT OR COLD, WATER CIRCULATING
(Physical Med) 89ILO

Adroit Medical Systems, Inc. 800-267-6077
1146 Carding Machine Rd, Loudon, TN 37774
Soft-Temp cold-therapy systems. Portable coolers (motorized ice chests) with foam insulated cold therapy pads. Used post-op and for sport medicine applications. Pads are available sterile and non-sterile.

Aqueduct Medical Incorporated 415-896-0134
665 3rd St Ste 20, San Francisco, CA 94107
Cold pad.

Breg, Inc., An Orthofix Company 800-897-BREG
2611 Commerce Way, Vista, CA 92081
Hot or cold pack.

Burke Medical, Llc 727-532-8333
2310 Tall Pines Dr Ste 210, Largo, FL 33771
Thermal therapy system.

Coolsystems, Inc. 510-868-5378
1201 Marina Village Pkwy Ste 200, Alameda, CA 94501
Cold therapy product.

Cryotherapy Pain Relief Products, Inc. 954-893-9059
3460 Laurel Oaks Ln, Hollywood, FL 33021
Cylindrical cold pack, plastic applicator.

Debusk Orthopedic Casting (Doc) 865-362-2334
420 Straight Creek Rd Ste 1, New Tazewell, TN 37825
Cold therapy units and blankets.

Discount Dme 714-630-9590
1265 N Grove St Ste A, Anaheim, CA 92806
Cold therapy.

DJO Inc. 800-336-6569
1430 Decision St, Vista, CA 92081
CRYOLOGIC II cold therapy system.

Ebi Patient Care, Inc. 973-299-9300
1 Electro-biology Blvd., Guaynabo, PR 00657
Thermal therapy devices.

Genesis Manufacturing, Inc. 317-485-7887
720 E Broadway St, Fortville, IN 46040
Contract Radio-Frequency (RF) Welding. From development to manufacturing and packaging.

Hospital Therapy Products, Inc. 630-766-7101
757 N Central Ave, Wood Dale, IL 60191
Vest-used under barrier gown-has ice to keep comfortable.

J. Pohler 305-757-7733
8740 SW 21st St, Davie, FL 33324
Cylinorical cold pac plastic.

Leemah Electronics, Inc. 415-394-1288
1088 Sansome St, --, San Francisco, CA 94111

PACK, HOT OR COLD, WATER CIRCULATING *(cont'd)*

Life Enhancement Technologies, Inc. 408-330-6940
807 Aldo Ave Ste 101, Santa Clara, CA 95054
Mark i cooling console.

Ossur Americas 949-268-3155
742 Pancho Rd, Camarillo, CA 93012

Ossur Americas, Inc 800-222-4284
19762 Pauling, Foothill Ranch, CA 92610
Sustained cold therapy is one of the most effective and soothing treatments for reducing post-op pain and swelling. Suited for hospital, home of portable use. A variety of cool pads designed to deliver cold therapy to hip, knee, ankle, shoulder, back, hand and foot.

Pain Management Technologies 216-776-1335
744 Merriman Rd, Akron, OH 44303
Hot water therapy device.

Polar Products, Inc. 800-763-8423
540 S Main St Ste 951, Akron, OH 44311
Designed especially for after surgery when serious pain relief is required. Our unit delivers localized cold therapy to the patient either in home or during their hospital stay. The unit uses a motorized pump to circulate cold water to the desired body area. The unit comes standard with a universal cold therapy wrap that fits many areas of the body including: Knees, Shoulder, Ankle, Elbow, Calf and Limbs

Pro Trainers' Choice Company 801-375-6600
PO Box 3953, 5803 Nw Newberry Hill Rd., Silverdale, WA 98383
Therapeutic cold therapy device.

Regency Product International 800-845-7931
4732 E 26th St, Vernon, CA 90058

S4 Tech Inc 703-467-9034
12900 Wood Crescent Cir, Herndon, VA 20171
Temperature controlled recirculating thermal treatment pad.

Sanker Intl., Inc. 817-645-8015
106 S Old Betsy Rd Ste A, Keene, TX 76059
Hydrot.

Thermotek Inc. 877-242-3232
1454 Halsey Way, Carrollton, TX 75007
Various.

Trulife, Inc. 360-697-5656
26296 12 Trees Ln NW, Poulsbo, WA 98370
Cold therapy system.

Zeltiq 925-474-2500
4698 Willow Rd, Pleasanton, CA 94588
Zeltiq System

PACK, HOT, CHEMICAL *(General) 80FRY*

Hospital Marketing Svcs. Company, Inc. 800-786-5094
162 Great Hill Rd./ Ind. Park, Naugatuck, CT 06770
Box of 24 pcs. #6630,4'x10' instant warm pack, box of 24 pcs. #6632.

I-Rep, Inc. 800-828-0852
508 Chaney St Ste B, Lake Elsinore, CA 92530

Pristech Products, Inc 800-432-8722
6952 Fairgrounds Pkwy, PO Box 680728, San Antonio, TX 78238

Tetra Medical Supply Corp. 800-621-4041
6364 W Gross Point Rd, Niles, IL 60714

PACK, MOIST HEAT *(Physical Med) 89IMA*

Be Well Usa, Inc. 229-890-1627
3195 7th St SE, Moultrie, GA 31788
Moist heat pack.

Bruder Healthcare Company 888-827-8337
3150 Engineering Pkwy, Alpharetta, GA 30004
Microwave Moist Heat Packs, Reusable

Chattanooga Group 800-592-7329
4717 Adams Rd, Hixson, TN 37343
HYDROCOLLATOR.

Creations Magiques C.M. Inc. 514-753-3892
3001 Rue Visitation, Saint-Charles-Borromee J6E 7Y8 Canada
Pack,heat,moist

Dedicated Distribution 800-325-8367
640 Miami Ave, Kansas City, KS 66105

Dynatronics Corp. Chattanooga Operations 801-568-7000
6607 Mountain View Rd, Ooltewah, TN 37363
Moist heat pack.

Hospital Marketing Svcs. Company, Inc. 800-786-5094
162 Great Hill Rd./ Ind. Park, Naugatuck, CT 06770
Case of 10 pcs., 4'. x 10', #7718; Case of 24 6'x10' no. 7727.

PACK, MOIST HEAT *(cont'd)*

Kennex Development Inc 626-458-0598
533 S Atlantic Blvd Ste 301, Monterey Park, CA 91754
Various types of moist heat pack.

Medical Supplies Corporation T/A.Roberts Manufacturing Co., 800-451-9951
4002 Dillon St, Baltimore, MD 21224
$672.00 for 12 medium moist heat therapy pads, 13' x 13'; $79.95 each. $440.00 for 12 small moist heat therapy pads, 7' x 11'; $62.95 each.

Naimco, Inc. 423-648-7730
4120 S Creek Rd, Chattanooga, TN 37406
Various moist heat packs.

Natural Wonders Ca Inc. 818-341-7007
21011 Itasca St Ste E, Chatsworth, CA 91311
Moist heat pack.

Obus Forme Ltd. 888-225-7378
550 Hopewell Ave., Toronto, ON M6E 2S6 Canada

Patterson Medical Supply, Inc. 262-387-8720
W68N158 Evergreen Blvd, Cedarburg, WI 53012
Hydrocollator moist heat packs.

Pelton Shepherd Industries 800-258-3423
812B W Luce St, Stockton, CA 95203
7 sizes HYDROTHERM mst heat packs and covers canvas & bentonite; #5100 standard size 10 x 12 in.; #5102 cervical (neck) size 6.5 x 21 in.; #5104 oversize 15 x 24 in.; #5106 half-size 5 x 12 in.; #5114 large size 10 x 18 in.; #5116 ex-large size 10 x 24in.; #5118 knee-shoulder size 10 x 20 in.; #5110 standard cover 18 x 26 in. (open); #5112 cervical (neck) cover 17 x 23 in. (open); 5113 (oversize) 49 x 18 1/2 in.

Polar Products, Inc. 800-763-8423
540 S Main St Ste 951, Akron, OH 44311
Thera-Temp Microwaveable Moist Heat Wraps: Professional quality moist heat wraps that use non-organic, no-odor therapeutic beads to collect moisture from humidity in the air. These beads will never break down or become rancid as wraps using barley or other organic fill can.

Relief Wrap Ltd. 519-442-5071
15a Oak Ave, Paris N3L 3C6 Canada
Natural heating pad

Roloke Company 800-533-8212
127 W Hazel St, Inglewood, CA 90302
THERMAPAD automatic.

Zhang Enterprises 972-238-8260
400 N Greenville Ave Ste 9, Richardson, TX 75081
Various types of heat packs.

PACK, STERILIZATION WRAPPER (BAG AND ACCESSORIES) *(Surgery) 79KCT*

Advanced Sterilization Products 800-595-0200
33 Technology Dr, Irvine, CA 92618

Andersen Products, Inc., 800-523-1276
3202 Caroline Dr, Health Science Park, Haw River, NC 27258
SEAL & PEEL packaging for ethylene-oxide-gas steriliztaion.

Atd-American Co. 800-523-2300
135 Greenwood Ave, Wyncote, PA 19095

Avent S.A. De C.V. 602-748-6900
Camino De Libramiento, Km. 1.5, Nogales, Sonora Mexico
Various types of sterile, surgical packs

Beacon Converters, Inc. 201-797-2600
Bldg. P-1 Andrea Blvd., Saddle Brook, NJ 07663-8208

Chagrin Safety Supply, Inc. 800-227-0468
8227 Washington St # 1, Chagrin Falls, OH 44023

Classone Orthodontics, Inc. 806-799-0608
5064 50th St, Lubbock, TX 79414
Various types of sterilization cassettes.

Coltene/Whaledent Inc. 330-916-8858
235 Ascot Pkwy, Cuyahoga Falls, OH 44223
Instrument cassette.

Dshealthcare Inc. 201-871-1232
85 W Forest Ave, Englewood, NJ 07631
Sterilization pouch.

Ethox International 800-521-1022
251 Seneca St, Buffalo, NY 14204
Instrument, suture holder.

PACK, STERILIZATION WRAPPER (BAG AND ACCESSORIES) *(cont'd)*

Griff Industries, Inc. 800-709-4743
19761 Bahama St, Northridge, CA 91324
Surgical instrument protector--sterilization wrap.

Gs Medical Packaging Inc. 800-489-7125
865 Rangeview Rd., Mississauga, ONT L5E 1H1 Canada
Sterilization packaging

Gyrus Acmi, Inc. 508-804-2739
93 N Pleasant St, Norwalk, OH 44857
Sterilization wrap containers, trays, cassettes & other accessories.

Health-Pak, Inc. 315-724-8370
2005 Beechgrove Pl, Utica, NY 13501
CSR wrap, non-woven.

Kerr Group 800-524-3577
1400 Holcomb Bridge Rd, Roswell, GA 30076
KIMBERLY-CLARK Sterilization Pouches and Tubing. Peel pouches and tubing.

Maquilas Teta-Kawi, S.A. De C.V. 413-593-6400
Carretera Internacional, Km 1969, Enpalme, Sonora Mexico
Various

Medical Action Industries, Inc. 800-645-7042
25 Heywood Rd, Arden, NC 28704
Sterilization pouches.

Promedica, Inc. 800-899-5278
114 Douglas Rd E, Oldsmar, FL 34677
Ultra System sterilization containers.

Propper Manufacturing Co., Inc. 800-832-4300
3604 Skillman Ave, Long Island City, NY 11101
Sterilization pouches and tubes.

Quality Products Of Montana 406-544-0305
4022 Timberlane St, Missoula, MT 59802
Sterilization pouch, re-bag.

The Sewing Source, Inc. 919-478-3900
802 E Nash St, Spring Hope, NC 27882
Wrapper, sterilization.

White Knight Healthcare 800-851-4431
Calle 16, Number 780, Agua Prieta, Sonora Mexico
Various types ofm sterile & nonsterile packs

Worldpak Flexible Packaging, Llc. 775-359-0733
300 E Parr Blvd, Reno, NV 89512
Sterilization wrap container trays,cassettes and other accessories.

PACK, SURGICAL (DRAPE) *(Surgery) 79RXP*

Atd-American Co. 800-523-2300
135 Greenwood Ave, Wyncote, PA 19095

Foothills Industries, Inc. 828-652-4088
300 Rockwell Dr, Marion, NC 28752

Johnson & Johnson Medical Division Of Ethicon, Inc. 800-423-4018
2500 E Arbrook Blvd, Arlington, TX 76014

Kerr Group 800-524-3577
1400 Holcomb Bridge Rd, Roswell, GA 30076

Medical Techniques Usa 801-936-4501
125 N 400 W Ste C, North Salt Lake, UT 84054

Novosci Corp. 281-363-4949
2828 N Crescentridge Dr, The Woodlands, TX 77381
Perfusion packs, basin packs, open heart drape packs, tubing kits, Mayo trays and nurse packs.

Precept Medical Products, Inc. 800-438-5827
PO Box 2400, 370 Airport Road/, Arden, NC 28704

PACKAGING EQUIPMENT *(General) 80VAG*

Apple Converting, Inc. 607-337-4474
65 Hale St, Norwich, NY 13815

Arjo Wiggins Medical, Inc. 843-388-8080
1301 Charleston Regional Pkwy # 500, Charleston, SC 29492
Sterilizable packaging papers and wrappers.

Ark Services Corporation 708-371-3674
6118 W 123rd St, Palos Heights, IL 60463
Solutions for problems and opportunities for packaging machinery manufacturers and users.

PACKAGING EQUIPMENT *(cont'd)*

Belco Packaging Systems, Inc. 800-833-1833
910 S Mountain Ave, Monrovia, CA 91016
We offer single- and dual-station tray sealers in four platen sizes, at four levels of process-control capabilities. Also constant heat bar/pouch sealers with two levels of process-control capabilities. Industrial shrink-packaging systems are High-Speed Automatic Horizontal Form, Fill and Seal (productivity capabilities from 50-120 packages per minute); Infinite Length Side Sealers (20-50 PPM); Automatic L-Bar sealers (20-40 PPM); Semi-Automatic and Manual L-Bar sealers (5-20 PPM); and a comprehensive line of Shrink Tunnels complement the entire offering of heat sealers.

Bio-Rad, Diagnostics Group 800-854-6737
9500 Jeronimo Rd, Irvine, CA 92618
Packaging for many quality control products, using PET plastic trays to replace the fiberboard boxes. The clear plastic allows inventory assessment at a glance and the tray makes storage more convenient.

Delta Industrial Services, Inc. 800-279-3358
11501 Eagle St NW, Minneapolis, MN 55448
Delta hot or cold seal packager. Offers many processing options. Excellent as stand-alone packager or in-line with Delta web converter.

Engineering & Research Assoc., Inc. (D.B.A. Sebra) 800-625-5550
100 N Tucson Blvd, Tucson, AZ 85716
Catheter forming & welding equipment.

Ima Nova 978-537-8534
7 New Lancaster Rd, Leominster, MA 01453

Inmark, Inc. 800-646-6275
675 Hartman Rd Ste 100, Austell, GA 30168
Complete line of infectious and diagnostic shipping (IDS) systems, fully certified packages that allow the shipment of infectious substances by all modes of transportation.

Kimble Glass, Inc. 888-546-2531
537 Crystal Ave, Vineland, NJ 08360

Master Bond, Inc. 201-343-8983
154 Hobart St, Hackensack, NJ 07601
Adhesives, sealants and Coatings.

Mts Medication Technologies 800-671-0508
2003 Gandy Blvd N Ste 800, Saint Petersburg, FL 33702
Pharmaceutical packaging equipment.

National Instrument Llc 866-258-1914
4119 Fordleigh Rd, Baltimore, MD 21215
Monobloc Liquid Filling Systems, Digifil Liquid Filling Systems, Molten Product Filling System, as well as Semi-Automatic Benchtop Filling Systems.

Oliver Medical 800-253-3893
445 6th St NW, Grand Rapids, MI 49504
Sterilizable medical device packaging material.

R. A. Jones & Co., Inc. 859-341-0400
2701 Crescent Springs Pike, Covington, KY 41017
Cartoners and pouch machines.

Uhlmann Packaging Systems, Inc. 973-402-8855
44 Indian Ln E, Towaco, NJ 07082
Blister packaging machinery for oral solid dose, liquids, vials, syringes, ampoules, etc.

Vonco Products, Inc. 800-323-9077
201 Park Ave, Lake Villa, IL 60046
Flexible packaging and containers.

Westlund Engineering, Inc. 727-572-4343
12400 44th St N, Clearwater, FL 33762
Horizontal form, fill and seal pouch-making and sealing machine with automatic product loading.

PACKAGING EQUIPMENT *(cont'd)*

Wrapade Packaging Systems, Llc. 888-815-8564
27 Law Dr, Suite B/C, Fairfield, NJ 07004
Horizontal and Vertical form/fill/seal machines for soft and hard thin-profile products in four-side-sealed or peel-seal pouches for sterilization. Pouch sizes to 12 in. wide, in any length. A Small Pouch Machine for powders, liquids, tablets, capsules, swabs, and any small parts in pouch sizes 2 x 2-in., up to 6 x 9-in. without the need for change parts. Options include both Digital & Flexographic In-Line Printing, Emboss Coding, Tear Notching for easy opening of the pouch, and Computerized Product Memory for changeovers. All models incorporate the latest in Servo-Drive Technology interfaced with an Operator Touch-Screen Panel, and validation & monitoring software (including Diagnostic Message Display indicating the current operating conditions of the machine). Newly available is the Model K Benchtop Heal Sealer, which is ideal for hermetically sealing filled pouches (up to 20/minute) and for laboratory testing of all types of heat-sealable laminated and coextruded packaging films and printing inks. For quality assurance testing, the Model K's Sealing Jaws can be fabricated with the same sealing pattern as the jaws on the automatic packaging machines to determine whether the packaging material meets the specifications. In cleanroom operation, the smooth outer surfaces of the equipment permits easy and effective cleaning, and all exhaust air is discharged to a common manifold for delivery outside the cleanroom.

PACKAGING MATERIAL *(General) 80VAI*

Amcor Flexibles, Inc. 608-249-0404
4101 Lien Rd, Madison, WI 53704
Barrier pouches for diagnostic products, burn dressings, casting tapes, wound care, liquids and products requiring high-barrier properties.

Angiosystems, Inc. 800-441-4256
7 Hopkins Pl., Ducktown, TN 37326

Beacon Converters, Inc. 201-797-2600
Bldg. P-1 Andrea Blvd., Saddle Brook, NJ 07663-8208
Materials designed to withstand sterilization processes and maintain sterility.

Brentwood Industries, Inc. 610-374-5109
610 Morgantown Rd, Reading, PA 19611
Custom thermoform packaging, with capability to 66-in. lengths. Complete design and in-house tooling capabilities.

Caton Connector Corp. 877-522-2866
26 Wapping Rd, Kingston, MA 02364

Colonial Carton Co. 919-553-4113
1000 Ccc Dr, Clayton, NC 27520
Folding cartons.

Cryopak Industries, Inc. 800-667-2532
1055 Derwent Way, Delta, BC V3M 5R4 Canada
Flexible Ice Blanket delivers superior thermal protection for the packing, handling, shipping and storage of temperature sensitive products.

Custom Bottle/Lerman Container 800-315-6681
10 Great Hill Rd, Naugatuck, CT 06770
Containers, packaging, packaging supplies.

Extra Packaging, Corp. 800-872-7548
631 Golden Harbour Dr, Boca Raton, FL 33432
Flexible packaging material. Military barrier packaging. Nylon bags for oven use. Produce bags to extend shelf life. Bags, pouches, rollstock, emergency water storage bags.

Facet Technologies, Llc 800-526-2387
112 Townpark Dr NW Ste 300, Kennesaw, GA 30144

Gdm Electronic And Medical 408-945-4100
2070 Ringwood Ave, San Jose, CA 95131

J. G. Finneran Associates, Inc. 800-552-3696
3600 Reilly Ct, Vineland, NJ 08360
Glass and plastic.

Lps Industries, Inc. 800-275-4577
10 Caesar Pl, Moonachie, NJ 07074
Flexible barrier packaging - rollstock and preformed pouches. A variety of laminates including foil. Non-printed also available.

Medical Action Industries, Inc 800-645-7042
500 Express Dr S, Brentwood, NY 11717
Heat and self-seal pouches and tubes for packaging sterile hospital materials.

PACKAGING MATERIAL *(cont'd)*

Multisorb Technologies, Inc. 800-445-9890
325 Harlem Rd, Buffalo, NY 14224
DESIMAX desiccant labels, adhesive backed, alleviate concerns about ingestion and potential co-mingling with products. Easily inserted, hte labels are designed to fit into new or existing packaging.

Oliver Medical 800-253-3893
445 6th St NW, Grand Rapids, MI 49504
Sterilizable medical device packaging material including Ovantex, a revolutionary sterile-grade packaging material and Osurance zone coated lids.

Pacon Manufacturing Corporation 732-357-8020
400 Pierce St # B, Somerset, NJ 08873
Heat seal and cohesive coated roll goods.

Perfecseal 877-828-7501
PO Box 2968, 3500 North Main St., Oshkosh, WI 54903
PERFECSEAL products are heat-seal-coated materials: PERFECRAFT heat-seal-coated paper and laminations; PERFECFLEX multiple-layer coex and laminated films; vacuum-metallized laminates; peel pouches; tubing; BREATHER BAG header-bag packaging; PERFECFORM custom-thermoformed trays and die-cut lids; pharmaceutical labels; eight-color flexo and rotogravure printing.

Silverstone Packaging, Inc.-Your One Stop Supplier 800-413-1108
1401 Lakeland Ave, Bohemia, NY 11716

Sps Medical Supply Corp. 800-722-1529
6789 W. Hennetta Road, Rush, NY 14543

Surgical Technologies, Inc. 800-777-9987
292 E Lafayette Frontage Rd, Saint Paul, MN 55107

Tegrant Corporation, Protexic Brands 800-289-9966
800 5th Ave, P.O. Box 448, New Brighton, PA 15066
Protective packaging for medical devices

Vonco Products, Inc. 800-323-9077
201 Park Ave, Lake Villa, IL 60046
Flexible packaging and containers.

West Pharmaceutical Services, Inc. 800-231-3000
101 Gordon Dr, Franklin Ctr, PA 19341

PACKAGING SYSTEM, UNIT-DOSE *(General) 80VDO*

Apothecary Products, Inc. 800-328-2742
11750 12th Ave S, Burnsville, MN 55337
Memory Pac. Hot and Cold Seal Cards and Blisters.

Dpt Laboratories, Ltd. 866-225-5378
4040 Broadway St Ste 401, San Antonio, TX 78209

Medi-Dose, Inc. 800-523-8966
70 Industrial Dr, Ivyland, PA 18974
Packaging system for both solid and liquid medications.

Medical Packaging Inc. 800-257-5282
470 Route 31 N, PO Box 500, Ringoes, NJ 08551
AUTOPAK-BPM and AUTOPAK-UDD Automatic Unit-Dose System with on-line computerized printing and automatic feed. Automatically fills a multi-dose seven-day blister compliance card. Unit-dose strip packaging machine for solid tablets and capsules; packaging supplies for unit-dose machines and unit-dose carts.

Mts Medication Technologies 800-671-0508
2003 Gandy Blvd N Ste 800, Saint Petersburg, FL 33702
Generic oral solid unit dose packaging.

Uhlmann Packaging Systems, Inc. 973-402-8855
44 Indian Ln E, Towaco, NJ 07082
Blister packaging machinery for oral solid dose, liquids, vials, syringes, ampoules, etc.

PACKAGING, STERILIZATION *(General) 80RVT*

Andersen Products, Inc., 800-523-1276
3202 Caroline Dr, Health Science Park, Haw River, NC 27258
SEAL & PEEL packaging for ethylene-oxide-gas sterilization.

Arjo Wiggins Medical, Inc. 843-388-8080
1301 Charleston Regional Pkwy # 500, Charleston, SC 29492

B. Braun Oem Division, B. Braun Medical Inc. 866-8-BBRAUN
824 12th Ave, Bethlehem, PA 18018

Beacon Converters, Inc. 201-797-2600
Bldg. P-1 Andrea Blvd., Saddle Brook, NJ 07663-8208
Packaging designed to withstand sterilization processes and maintain sterility of product it contains.

PACKAGING, STERILIZATION *(cont'd)*

Cadco Dental Products 800-833-8267
600 E Hueneme Rd, Oxnard, CA 93033
Priced $18.00 to $55.00 for PEELVUE, sterilizing pouches available in seven sizes, 200 to a box.

Crosstex International 800-223-2497
10 Ranick Rd, Hauppauge, NY 11788
Sterilization pouches.

Crosstex International Ltd., W. Region 800-707-2737
14059 Stage Rd, Santa Fe Springs, CA 90670
Sterilization pouches.

Crosstex International,Inc. 888-276-7783
10 Ranick Rd, Hauppauge, NY 11788
CROSSTEX Sterilization pouches, SANIROLLS, SANITUBES.

Dux Dental 800-833-8267
600 E Hueneme Rd, Oxnard, CA 93033
Priced $18.00 to $55.00 for PEEL VUE, sterilizing pouches available in seven sizes, 200 to a box.

Extra Packaging, Corp. 800-872-7548
631 Golden Harbour Dr, Boca Raton, FL 33432
FLEXSEAL, Sterilizable packaging. Header bags, Chevron pouches, paper bands, forming web, autocare bags.

Facet Technologies, Llc 800-526-2387
112 Townpark Dr NW Ste 300, Kennesaw, GA 30144

General Econopak, Inc. 888-871-8568
1725 N 6th St, Philadelphia, PA 19122
Sterilization wrappers, pouches, heat-seal and self-seal sterility maintenance bags. Self-seal and heat-seal absorbent tray liners. Sterilization tubing in 2- 3- 4- 6- and 12-in. sizes.

Greatbatch Medical 716-759-5600
3735 N Arlington Ave, Indianapolis, IN 46218
Poly-paper self sealing pouches.

Medical Action Industries, Inc 800-645-7042
500 Express Dr S, Brentwood, NY 11717
Heat and self-seal pouches and tubes for packaging sterile hospital materials.

Medical Sterile Products, Inc. 800-292-2887
Road 413 Km. 0.2 BO. Ensenada, Rincon, PR 00743

Medical Techniques Usa 801-936-4501
125 N 400 W Ste C, North Salt Lake, UT 84054

Medtech Group Inc., The 800-348-2759
6 Century Ln, South Plainfield, NJ 07080

Mydent International 800-275-0020
80 Suffolk Ct, Hauppauge, NY 11788
DEFEND self-seal pouch, paper/plastic, 6 convenient sizes, economy packaging, medical grade paper.

Oliver Medical 800-253-3893
445 6th St NW, Grand Rapids, MI 49504
Sterilizable medical device packaging material.

Pacon Manufacturing Corporation 732-357-8020
400 Pierce St # B, Somerset, NJ 08873

Precision Medical Products, Inc. 717-335-3700
44 Denver Rd, PO Box 300, Denver, PA 17517
As required to support component assembly services.

Propper Manufacturing Co., Inc. 800-832-4300
3604 Skillman Ave, Long Island City, NY 11101

Riley Medical, Inc. 800-245-3300
27 Wrights Lndg, Auburn, ME 04210

Scican Inc. 800-572-1211
701 Technology Dr, Canonsburg, PA 15317

Sps Medical Supply Corp. 800-722-1529
6789 W. Hennetta Road, Rush, NY 14543

Sts Duotek, Inc 800-836-4850
370 Summit Point Dr, Henrietta, NY 14467
ETO and steam sterilization, testing, packaging in form/fill/seal, pouching, tray and lidding. Cleanrooms.

Techlem Medical Systems Inc. 905-812-9727
4-6620 Kitimat Rd, Mississauga, ON L5N 2B8 Canada
Rolls and pouches.

Thermo Fisher Scientific Inc. 563-556-2241
2555 Kerper Blvd, Dubuque, IA 52001

Zimmer Holdings, Inc. 800-613-6131
1800 W Center St, PO Box 708, Warsaw, IN 46580

PACKER, GAUZE *(General) 80RJU*

Miltex Inc. 800-645-8000
589 Davies Dr, York, PA 17402

PACKING, SURGICAL *(Surgery) 79RXO*

Amd-Ritmed, Inc. 800-445-0340
295 Firetower Road, Tonawanda, NY 14150

Johnson & Johnson Medical Division Of Ethicon, Inc. 800-423-4018
2500 E Arbrook Blvd, Arlington, TX 76014

Shippert Medical Technologies Corp. 800-888-8663
6248 S Troy Cir Ste A, Centennial, CO 80111
A complete line of nasal, sinus, and ear packing. RHINO ROCKET nasal tampon with applicator is comprised of EXPANDACELL medical-grade sponge designed to give gentle but firm compression to the nasal mucosa. SLIK PAK, Slik Pack Laminated Non-stick Nasal/Sinus Pak, is a post-operative and epistaxis nasal/sinus pack surrounded by two slick polymer sacks with multiple offset slits allowing entry of blood into the pack, preventing contact between the mucosa and foam. PLUS PAK, Plus Pak Nasal Pack with Advantage Applicator, easy insertion, features a unique radiopaque marker for detection on x-ray.

Ultracell Medical Technologies, Inc. 877-SPO-NGE1
183 Providence New London Tpke, North Stonington, CT 06359
ULTRACELL Nasal packing. Many sizes and shapes of P.V.A. sponges are available for treating all anterior and posterior epistaxis, plus ideally used for nasal packing, sinus, turbinate and customizing. ULTRACELL Ear packing. Comes in various sizes to prevent stenosis of the ear canal following otic surgery, and acts as a supporting device to prevent movement of the graft after tympanoplasty.

PAD, ALCOHOL *(General) 80LKB*

Bd Medical - Diabetes Care 201-847-4298
1329 W US Highway 6 # &34, Holdrege, NE 68949
Isopropyl alcohol pad.

Beacon Promotions, Inc. 507-354-3900
2121 S Bridge St, New Ulm, MN 56073
Various types of alcohol pad and alcohol swab.

Chagrin Safety Supply, Inc. 800-227-0468
8227 Washington St # 1, Chagrin Falls, OH 44023

Dynarex Corp. 888-356-2739
10 Glenshaw St, Orangeburg, NY 10962
DYNAREX alcohol prep pads for antiseptic skin preparation prior to injection or venipuncture. Impregnated with 70% isopropyl alcohol.

El Paso Lighthouse For The Blind 915-532-4495
200 Washington St, El Paso, TX 79905
Alcohol pad.

K. W. Griffen Co. 203-846-1923
100 Pearl St, Norwalk, CT 06850
Alcohol pad.

Medi-Hut Co., Inc. 800-882-0139
1935 Swarthmore Ave, Lakewood, NJ 08701

O&M Enterprise 847-258-4515
641 Chelmsford Ln, Elk Grove Village, IL 60007
PAD ALCOHOL

Respond Industries, Inc. 1-800-523-8999
9500 Woodend Rd, Edwardsville, KS 66111
Alcohol pads.

Specialty Medical Supplies, Inc. 954-752-5603
3882 NW 124th Ave, Coral Springs, FL 33065

PAD, BREAST *(Obstetrics/Gyn) 85QEJ*

Almost U 800-626-6007
91 Market St Ste 23, Wappingers Falls, NY 12590
Post Mastectomy Bras - most comfortable cotton pocketed bras. Available in 6 styles.

Dumex Medical Surgical Products Ltd. 800-463-9613
104 Shorting Rd., Scarborough, ONT M1S 3S4 Canada
CONFIDENCE

Finebrand Co. 323-588-3228
3720 S Santa Fe Ave, Vernon, CA 90058
Surgical pads constructed out of natural latex; cosmetic (fashion) pads constructed out of natural latex and Poly-Kodel.

Medela, Inc. 800-435-8316
1101 Corporate Dr, McHenry, IL 60050
Disposable or washable in 100% cotton design.

Pharmaceutical Innovations, Inc. 973-242-2900
897 Frelinghuysen Ave, Newark, NJ 07114
ULTRA PHONICS FOCUS - Conforming Gel Pad. Is a solidified gel pad which is used to obtain near field imaging, or for scanning over bony prominent areas. Available in 2 sizes: 1.5cm x 9cm = $6.50 each & 2.5cm x 9cm = $7.00 each.

PAD, DEFIBRILLATOR PADDLE *(Cardiovascular) 74QOQ*

Armstrong Medical Industries, Inc. 800-323-4220
575 Knightsbridge Pkwy, Lincolnshire, IL 60069

Katecho, Inc. 515-244-1212
4020 Gannett Ave, Des Moines, IA 50321
Disposable defibrillator pads.

PAD, DENTURE, OTC *(Dental And Oral) 76EHR*

Durasol Corp. 978-388-2020
1 Oakland St, P.o. Box 35, Amesbury, MA 01913
Endslip denture adhesives.

PAD, DRESSING *(General) 80QQS*

Brady Corporation 800-541-1686
6555 W Good Hope Rd, PO Box 571, Milwaukee, WI 53223
Dressings manufactured to customer specifications. Specializing in complex, close tolerance laminating, die cutting, island placement and printing.

Covidien Lp 508-261-8000
15 Hampshire St, Mansfield, MA 02048
INTERSORB sterile dry dressings, gauze bandages help reduce granulation entrapment and conform to wound contours, dry burn vests, custom burn pads.

Delstar Technologies, Inc. 800-521-6713
601 Industrial Rd, Middletown, DE 19709
STRATEX Nonadherent, absorbent pads and rollstock.

Ferris Mfg Corp. 800-765-9636
16 W300 83rd St., Burr Ridge, IL 60527-5848
PolyMem Wound Care Dressings, The Pink Dressing. A unique patented formula in 28 sizes and configurations include, non-adhesives, Island Dressings, Strips, Cavity Fillers, Calcium Alginates, Super Thick and Silver dressings

Johnson & Johnson Medical Division Of Ethicon, Inc. 800-423-4018
2500 E Arbrook Blvd, Arlington, TX 76014

Mylan Technologies, Inc. 800-532-5226
110 Lake St, Saint Albans, VT 05478
MEDIFILM, series of USP Class VI extruded Hytrel co-polyester, urethane and Pebax high moisture vapor films, available with hypoallergenic acrylic or hydrocolloid adhesive systems, laminated to synergistic absorbent foams and available in either rolls or converted, packaged dressings.

Profex Medical Products 800-325-0196
2224 E Person Ave, Memphis, TN 38114
Padding, felt/cast.

PAD, ELECTRODE *(Cardiovascular) 74WWU*

Md International, Inc. 305-669-9003
11300 NW 41st St, Doral, FL 33178

Taylor Industries, Inc. 800-339-1361
2706 Industrial Dr, Jefferson City, MO 65109

PAD, EYE *(Ophthalmology) 86HMP*

Afassco, Inc. 800-441-6774
2244 Park Pl Ste C, Minden, NV 89423

American White Cross - Houston 609-514-4744
15200 North Fwy, Houston, TX 77090
Various sterile eye pads.

Centurion Medical Products Corp. 517-545-1135
3310 S Main St, Salisbury, NC 28147

Dumex Medical Surgical Products Ltd. 800-463-9613
104 Shorting Rd., Scarborough, ONT M1S 3S4 Canada
SURECARE

Healer Products, Llc 914-663-6300
427 Commerce Ln Ste 1, West Berlin, NJ 08091
Eye pad.

Kentron Health Care, Inc. 615-384-0573
3604 Kelton Jackson Rd, P.o. Box 120, Springfield, TN 37172
Various types of eye pads.

Mine Safety Appliances Company 866-MSA-1001
121 Gamma Dr, Pittsburgh, PA 15238

Niagara Pharmaceuticals Div. 905-690-6277
60 Innovation Dr., Flamborough, ONT L9H-7P3 Canada
HEALTH SAVER light shield pad (below the eye).

North Safety Products 401-943-4400
1101 B Calle Neutron, Parque Industrial Maran, Mexicali, B.c. Mexico
Pad, eye

Tailored Label Products, Inc. 800-727-1344
W165N5731 Ridgewood Dr, Menomonee Falls, WI 53051

PAD, EYE *(cont'd)*

Tri-State Hospital Supply Corp. 517-545-1135
3173 E 43rd St, Yuma, AZ 85365

PAD, HEATING, CIRCULATING FLUID *(General) 80QZS*

Gaymar Industries, Inc. 800-828-7341
10 Centre Dr, Orchard Park, NY 14127
T/PADS T-pumps and pads for localized heat therapy.

Genesis Manufacturing, Inc. 317-485-7887
720 E Broadway St, Fortville, IN 46040
Contract Radio-Frequency (RF) Welding. From development to manufacturing and packaging.

PAD, HEATING, ELECTRICAL *(Physical Med) 89FPG*

Bruder Healthcare Company 888-827-8337
3150 Engineering Pkwy, Alpharetta, GA 30004

Medical Supplies Corporation T/A.Roberts Manufacturing Co., 800-451-9951
4002 Dillon St, Baltimore, MD 21224
$756.00 for 12 standard moist heat therapy pads, 13' x 27'; $89.95 each

Questech International, Inc. 800-966-5367
3810 Gunn Hwy, Tampa, FL 33618
The Thermopulse Pain Relief System features an analgesic cream used in conjunction with a thermopulsing electronic heating pad that maximizes the effectiveness of the ingredients in the analgesic.

PAD, HEATING, POWERED *(Physical Med) 89IRT*

Disenos Termoelectricos Luyfel 16-17-0425
7424 Juarez Porvenir, Cd. Juarez Mexico
Heating pad

Dynatronics Corp. Chattanooga Operations 801-568-7000
6607 Mountain View Rd, Ooltewah, TN 37363
Powered heating pad.

Health Equipment Manufacturers, Inc. 269-962-6181
702 S Reed Rd, Fremont, IN 46737
Automatic moist heat pack.

Ir Therapies, Llc 602-595-3426
19827 N 20th Way, Phoenix, AZ 85024
Infrared heating pad.

Kaz Usa, Inc. 518-828-0450
4755 Southpoint Dr, Memphis, TN 38118
Various types of electric heating pads.

Kaz, Inc. 518-828-0450
1 Vapor Trl, Hudson, NY 12534
Various types of electric heating pads.

Medical Depot 516-998-4600
99 Seaview Blvd, Port Washington, NY 11050
Powered heating pad.

Naimco, Inc. 423-648-7730
4120 S Creek Rd, Chattanooga, TN 37406
Heating pad.

Questech International, Inc. 800-966-5367
3810 Gunn Hwy, Tampa, FL 33618
CLARITY, pulsed heating pad for the face and body. Also avalaible THERMOPULS pain-relief system which is combination of a 'heat activator' and anti-inflammatory cream with a pulsating heat wrap.

Suarez Corporation Industries 330-494-5504
7800 Whipple Avenue N.w., North Canton, OH 44720
Heating pad.

Sunbeam Products, Inc. 561-912-4100
2381 NW Executive Center Dr, Boca Raton, FL 33431
Heating pad.

Sunbeam Products, Inc. 601-671-2277
224 Russell Dr, Waynesboro, MS 39367

Tridien Medical 954-340-0500
4200 NW 120th Ave, Coral Springs, FL 33065

PAD, INCONTINENCE (UNDERPAD) *(General) 80RBU*

Allman Products 800-223-6889
21101 Itasca St, Chatsworth, CA 91311

American Associated Companies, Inc. 800-849-7060
120 Carnegie Pl Ste 202, Fayetteville, GA 30214

Arc Home Health Products 800-278-8595
PO Box 615, Oneonta, NY 13820

Atd-American Co. 800-523-2300
135 Greenwood Ave, Wyncote, PA 19095

PAD, INCONTINENCE (UNDERPAD) *(cont'd)*

Best Manufacturing Group Llc 800-843-3233
1633 Broadway Fl 18, New York, NY 10019
BEST reusable underpads, all sizes, Birdseye and Ibex.

Bio-Medic Health Services, Inc. 800-525-0072
5041B Benois Rd Bldg B, Roanoke, VA 24018

Calmoseptine, Inc. 800-800-3405
16602 Burke Ln, Huntington Beach, CA 92647

Central Paper Products Company 800-339-4065
PO Box 4480, Manchester, NH 03108

Duraline Medical Products, Inc. 800-654-3376
324 Werner St, P.O. Box 67, Leipsic, OH 45856

East Atlantic Trading/Triangle Healthcare Inc. 800-243-4635
76 National Rd, Edison, NJ 08817

Essential Medical Supply, Inc. 800-826-8423
6420 Hazeltine National Dr, Orlando, FL 32822
QUIK-SORB.

Feather-Soft Disposable Hospital Products, Inc. 303-470-0200
P.O. Box 360470, Highlands Ranch, CO 80163-0470

Freestyle Medical Supplies, Inc. 800-841-5330
336 Green Rd, Stoney Creek, ON L8E 2B2 Canada
FREESTYLE Liners - contoured, washable liners for added absorbency with FREESTLYE Maxi Briefs (all-in-one garments for incontinence). FREESTYLE Bed and Chair Pads - protect mattresses, bed linens and chairs from staining and moisture. Bed Pads available in three styles - measure up to 36in. x 36in. Chair Pad measures 20in. x 20in. Launder up to 350 times. Also flushable biodegradable liners for insertion into reusable or disposable diapers. FREESTYLE underpads for chair and bed. Protect all surfaces from moisture and staining. Three sizes, 20 x 20 in., 28 x 36 in., 36 x 36 in. Largest pad has turn handles to move person in care.

Genesis Manufacturing, Inc. 317-485-7887
720 E Broadway St, Fortville, IN 46040
Contract Radio-Frequency (RF) Welding. From development to manufacturing and packaging.

Geri-Care Products 201-440-0409
250 Moonachie Ave, Moonachie, NJ 07074
Reusable incontinence underpads

Hill-Rom Manufacturing, Inc. 800-638-2546
4349 Corporate Rd, Charleston, SC 29405

Hospital Specialty Company 800-321-9832
500 Memorial Dr, Nicholasville, KY 40356

Howard Medical Company 800-443-1444
1690 N Elston Ave, Chicago, IL 60642
$30/case (150/count) for disposable 23x36 size large pads.

Humanicare International, Inc. 800-631-5270
9 Elkins Rd, East Brunswick, NJ 08816
DIGNITY reusable pads for light leakage; contoured for comfort. Can be worn in DIGNITY, FREE and ACTIVES or in user's own underwear.

Hygienics Industries Div.Of Kleinert's, Inc. 800-498-7051
3968 194th Trl, Golden Beach, FL 33160

Ivry 305-448-9858
216 Catalonia Ave Ste 106, Coral Gables, FL 33134
Pads, disposable and reusable, for incontinence.

Jms Converters Inc Dba Sabee Products & Stanford Prof Prod 215-396-3302
67 Buck Rd Ste B7, Huntingdon Valley, PA 19006
Disposable underpads.

Kareco International, Inc. 800-8KA-RECO
299 Rte. 22 E., Green Brook, NJ 08812-1714

Ldb Medical, Inc. 800-243-2554
2909 Langford Rd Ste B500, Norcross, GA 30071

Lew Jan Textile 800-899-0531
366 Veterans Memorial Hwy Ste 4, Commack, NY 11725

Medline Industries, Inc. 800-633-5886
1 Medline Pl, Mundelein, IL 60060

Mip Inc. 800-361-4964
9100 Ray Lawson Blvd., Montreal, QC H1J-1K8 Canada
Chamonix pads, super-eidersoff pads.

Paperpak 800-428-8363
545 W Terrace Dr, San Dimas, CA 91773
DRI-SORB, TUCK IN, DRI-SHEET, STA SMOOTH, DRI-SORB, ULTIMA, AIR-DRI, SUPERSORB, DRI-SORB, EZ-SORB, TUFFSORB. Tuckables, Breathables.

PAD, INCONTINENCE (UNDERPAD) *(cont'd)*

Principle Business Enterprises, Inc. 800-467-3224
PO Box 129, Dunbridge, OH 43414
TRANQUILITY Peach Sheet under pads (bed pads) for heavy incontinence; TRIMSHIELD pads for light to moderate incontinence; High Capacity pads for moderate incontinence and TopLiners (diaper liner) for heavy incontinence. Original High Capacity Pads moderate incontinence protection for use with Tranquility Naturals- incontinence briefs.

R. Sabee Company 920-882-7350
1718 W 8th St, Appleton, WI 54914

Ross Disposable Products 800-649-6526
401 Traders Blvd E, Unit 10, Mississauga, ON L4Z 2H8 Canada

Salk Inc. 800-343-4497
119 Braintree St Ste 701, 4th Floor, Boston, MA 02134
Incontinence liner (disposable & reusable).

Standard Textile 800-999-0400
1 Knollcrest Dr, Cincinnati, OH 45237
ULTIMATE quilted reusable underpad. One-piece, quilted laminated underpad provides a non-bunching, non-curling pad with a textured non-slip barrier.

Standard Textile Co., Inc. 888-999-0400
PO Box 371805, Cincinnati, OH 45222

PAD, INSULATION, CARDIAC *(General) 80WRF*

Genesee Biomedical, Inc. 800-786-4890
1308 S Jason St, Denver, CO 80223
HEART-CHILL Cardiac and Phrenic Insulator. Superior thermal insulation conforming to the demands of cardiovascular anatomy.

PAD, MEDICATED *(General) 80RGM*

Birchwood Laboratories, Inc. 800-328-6156
7900 Fuller Rd, Eden Prairie, MN 55344
AER, witch hazel dressings, jars of witch hazel dressings (40pads/jar, 20 jars/case and 100pads/jar, 12 jars/case). AER Traveler witch hazel towlettes (5 1/2in. x 5in. 50/box)

C.B. Fleet Company Inc. 804-528-4000
PO Box 11349, 4615 Murray Place, Lynchburg, VA 24506
Pain relief, pre-moistened rectal/vaginal pads; 100 count: 6/case. Pre-moistened rectal/hemorrhoidal pads with Pramoxine HCl.

Covidien Lp 508-261-8000
15 Hampshire St, Mansfield, MA 02048
Sterile ointment non-adhering dressing, absorbent gauze, impregnated with scarlet red in a medicated blend of white petrolatum, lanolin and olive oil.

Mylan Technologies, Inc. 800-532-5226
110 Lake St, Saint Albans, VT 05478
Completely integrated source providing design, development, testing and manufacture of pharmaceutically active wound care dressings specializing in the MEDIFILM series of extruded, high moisture vapor permeable elastomeric films.

Purdue Frederick Company 800-877-5666
1 Stamford Forum, Stamford, CT 06901
Betadine gauze pads and swab aids.

Safetec Of America, Inc. 800-456-7077
887 Kensington Ave, Buffalo, NY 14215
Safetec Sting Relief is an antiseptic and pain reliever. Also works great prior to needle sticks! Packaging: individually-wrapped, pre-moistened 1' x 5' pads, or 2 oz. spray bottle.

Senecare Enterprises, Inc. 800-442-4577
350 Central Ave Ste A, Bohemia, NY 11716
Senepad Lotion Pad provides low-friction technology that protects skin against the effects of friction and shear. The pre-lubricated facing sheet moves with the patient, diminishing friction and shear damage. Breathable Lotion Pad designed for use with air loss specialty beds.

Xttrium Laboratories, Inc. 800-587-3721
415 W Pershing Rd, Chicago, IL 60609
PERIES medicated wipes: 40/jar or 100/jar sizes.

PAD, MEDICATED, ADHESIVE, NON-ELECTRIC *(General) 80MLX*

Ac Healthcare Supply, Inc. 905-448-4706
11651 230th St, Cambria Heights, NY 11411
Medicated adhesive pad, non-electric.

DJO Inc. 800-336-6569
1430 Decision St, Vista, CA 92081

PAD, MENSTRUAL, SCENTED *(Obstetrics/Gyn) 85HHL*

Gh Gunther Huettlin Manufacturing, Inc. 613-961-8860
101 Petrie Pl, Belleville K8N 4Z6 Canada
Pad, menstrual, scented

PAD, MENSTRUAL, SCENTED *(cont'd)*

Indelpa, S.A. De C.V. 609-983-8006
Carlos B. Zetina No. 22, Xalostoc Mexico
Obstetrical/femenine pads

J&J Healthcare Products Div Mcneil-Ppc, Inc 866-565-2229
199 Grandview Rd, Skillman, NJ 08558

PAD, MENSTRUAL, UNSCENTED *(Obstetrics/Gyn) 85HHD*

Al's Merchandise, Inc. 562-690-0139
3652 Norwich Pl, Rowland Heights, CA 91748
Personal hygiene topics.

Busse Hospital Disposables, Inc. 631-435-4711
75 Arkay Dr, Hauppauge, NY 11788
Obstetrical kit.

Centurion Medical Products Corp. 517-545-1135
3310 S Main St, Salisbury, NC 28147

Gh Gunther Huettlin Manufacturing, Inc. 613-961-8860
101 Petrie Pl, Belleville K8N 4Z6 Canada
Pad, menstrual, unscented

Health Care Products, Inc. 419-678-9620
410 Nisco St, Coldwater, OH 45828
Maxi pad.

Indelpa, S.A. De C.V. 609-983-8006
Carlos B. Zetina No. 22, Xalostoc Mexico
Feminine hygienic products

J&J Healthcare Products Div Mcneil-Ppc, Inc 866-565-2229
199 Grandview Rd, Skillman, NJ 08558

Keepers!, Inc. 503-546-5696
PO Box 12648, Portland, OR 97212
All cotton reusable menstrual pad.

Paper Converting Of America Corp. 718-385-9100
633 Marlborough Rd, Brooklyn, NY 11226
Sanitary napkins.

Paperpak 800-428-8363
545 W Terrace Dr, San Dimas, CA 91773
SECURELY YOURS OB pads and incontinent liners.

Tri-State Hospital Supply Corp. 517-545-1135
3173 E 43rd St, Yuma, AZ 85365

Tri-State Hospital Supply Corp. 800-248-4058
301 Catrell Dr, PO Box 170, Howell, MI 48843
LIBERTY OB maternity absorbant size pads and knit stretch briefs.

PAD, NEONATAL EYE *(General) 80FOK*

Genesis Medical Products, Inc. 508-876-1063
40 Farm Hill Rd, Wrentham, MA 02093
Phototherady eye protectors.

Health Care Logistics, Inc. 800-848-1633
450 Town St, PO Box 25, Circleville, OH 43113
Various sizes.

Ross Disposable Products 800-649-6526
401 Traders Blvd E, Unit 10, Mississauga, ON L4Z 2H8 Canada

Small Beginnings Inc. 760-949-7707
17525 Alder St Ste 28, Hesperia, CA 92345
Photo-therapy mask neonatal eye pad.

PAD, PRESSURE, AIR *(General) 80RLZ*

Genesis Manufacturing, Inc. 317-485-7887
720 E Broadway St, Fortville, IN 46040
Contract Radio-Frequency (RF) Welding. From development to manufacturing and packaging.

Hermell Products, Inc. 800-233-2342
9 Britton Dr, PO Box 7345, Bloomfield, CT 06002
Kodel Decubitus pad.

Tuffcare 800-367-6160
3999 E La Palma Ave, Anaheim, CA 92807

PAD, PRESSURE, ANIMAL SKIN *(General) 80RMA*

Maven Medical Manufacturing, Inc. 800-562-7326
2250 Lake Ave SE, Largo, FL 33771
Synthetic sheepskin pads and materials.

Scott Specialties, Inc./Cmo Inc./Ginny Inc. 800-255-7136
512 M St, Belleville, KS 66935

Select Medical Products, Inc. 800-276-7237
6531 47th St N, Pinellas Park, FL 33781
Premium Quilt and Cool Quilt patient kits for all model continuous passive motion devices. Kinetec, Breg, Danninger, Artromot, Chattanooga, Sutter, and Phoenix! Buy direct from the manufacturer and save up to 50% off dealer prices.

PAD, PRESSURE, ANIMAL SKIN *(cont'd)*

Sheepskin Ranch, Inc. 800-366-9950
3408 Indale Rd, Fort Worth, TX 76116
$20.00 for elbow or heel pad, $99.00 per skin, $110.00 for wheelchair seat cover, $55.00 for wheelchair seat pad, $35.00 for crutch pad kit, $75.00 for sheepskin slippers(pair), $32.00 for wheelchair armrest pads & $400.00 for full hospital bed size : all made of SOFSHEEP lamb or sheepskin. Full bed size, genuine sheepskin.

PAD, PRESSURE, FOAM (ELBOW, HEEL) *(General) 80RMB*

Aetrex Worldwide, Inc 800-526-2739
414 Alfred Ave, Teaneck, NJ 07666
ANTI-SHOX, heel cradles are designed to provide immediate relief for plantar fasciitis and other forms of heel pain. The cradles absorb shock and shear and protect the foot.

Albahealth Llc 800-262-2404
425 N Gateway Ave, Rockwood, TN 37854
Albahealth Heel & Elbow Protector

Alimed, Inc. 800-225-2610
297 High St, Dedham, MA 02026

Aplix, Inc. 704-588-1920
12300 Steele Creek Rd, Charlotte, NC 28273

Bauerfeind Usa, Inc. 800-423-3405
55 Chastain Rd NW Ste 112, Kennesaw, GA 30144
VISCOSPOT viscoelastic heel cushion for relief of heel pain, shock-absorbent. VISCOHEEL viscoelastic heel cushion for relief of heel pain and other applications, shock-absorbent.

Brown Medical Industries 800-843-4395
1300 Lundberg Dr W, Spirit Lake, IA 51360
HEEL HUGGER, which stablizes the heel inside a shoe.

Dm Systems, Inc. 800-254-5438
1316 Sherman Ave, Evanston, IL 60201
ELBOWLIFT® SUSPENSION PAD has been developed for the prevention of elbow discomfort and injuries. Made from soft foam with smooth surfaces, Elbowlift® has an adjustable, well-padded hook-and-loop strap that wraps around the outside to keep it in position. This is a one size fits all product that is easily washable.

Dynamic Systems, Inc. 828-683-3523
235 Sunlight Dr, Leicester, NC 28748

Hermell Products, Inc. 800-233-2342
9 Britton Dr, PO Box 7345, Bloomfield, CT 06002
Self-adhering foam pads.

J. T. Posey Co. 800-447-6739
5635 Peck Rd, Arcadia, CA 91006

Kees Goebel Medical Specialties, Inc. 800-354-0445
9663 Glades Dr, Hamilton, OH 45011

Mizuho Osi 800-777-4674
30031 Ahern Ave, Union City, CA 94587

National Medical Products 800-940-3262
9775 Mining Dr Ste 104, Jacksonville, FL 32257

Orthoband Company, Inc. 800-325-9973
3690 Highway M, Imperial, MO 63052

Paramedical Distributors 800-245-3278
2020 Grand Blvd, Kansas City, MO 64108

Profex Medical Products 800-325-0196
2224 E Person Ave, Memphis, TN 38114

Spenco Medical Corp. 254-772-6000
PO Box 2501, Waco, TX 76702
Padding products; for elbow and heel made from SILICORE® fibers.

Sunrise Medical 800-333-4000
7477 Dry Creek Pkwy, Longmont, CO 80503

Tartan Orthopedics, Ltd. 888-287-1456
10651 Irma Dr Unit C, Northglenn, CO 80233
$160.00 per 10 (med).

Tetra Medical Supply Corp. 800-621-4041
6364 W Gross Point Rd, Niles, IL 60714

Tex-Tenn Corp. 800-251-3027
108 Kwickway Ln # 118, PO Box 8219, Gray, TN 37615

Trademark Medical Llc 800-325-9044
449 Soverign Ct, St. Louis, MO 63011
Convoluted foam heel and elbow protectors.

Truform Orthotics & Prosthetics 800-888-0458
3960 Rosslyn Dr, Cincinnati, OH 45209

Zimmer Holdings, Inc. 800-613-6131
1800 W Center St, PO Box 708, Warsaw, IN 46580

PAD, PRESSURE, FOAM (ELBOW, HEEL) *(cont'd)*

Zimmer Orthopaedic Surgical Products 800-321-5533
PO Box 10, 200 West Ohio Ave., Dover, OH 44622
ULTRA-CARE.

PAD, PRESSURE, FOAM CONVOLUTED *(General) 80RMC*

Alex Orthopedic, Inc. 800-544-2539
PO Box 201442, Arlington, TX 76006

Allman Products 800-223-6889
21101 Itasca St, Chatsworth, CA 91311

American Health Systems 800-234-6655
PO Box 26688, Greenville, SC 29616
ULTRAFORM; Mattress Overlay with reduced heel section that provides pressures below 14 mmHg. Helps prevent ulcers in high risk patients. Can be effective in treatment of Stage 1 and 2 Pressure Ulcers. IST Surface Design has 576 individual cells to cradle the body and prevent skin breakdown.

Cfi Medical Solutions (Contour Fabricators, Inc.) 810-750-5300
14241 N Fenton Rd, Fenton, MI 48430

Dumex Medical Surgical Products Ltd. 800-463-9613
104 Shorting Rd., Scarborough, ONT M1S 3S4 Canada

Hermell Products, Inc. 800-233-2342
9 Britton Dr, PO Box 7345, Bloomfield, CT 06002
Convoluted mattress pad.

J. T. Posey Co. 800-447-6739
5635 Peck Rd, Arcadia, CA 91006

O&M Enterprise 847-258-4515
641 Chelmsford Ln, Elk Grove Village, IL 60007
PAD PRESSURE

Profex Medical Products 800-325-0196
2224 E Person Ave, Memphis, TN 38114

Span-America Medical Systems, Inc. 800-888-6752
70 Commerce Ctr, Greenville, SC 29615
GEOMATT therapeutic mattress pads.

Sunrise Medical 800-333-4000
7477 Dry Creek Pkwy, Longmont, CO 80503

Tuffcare 800-367-6160
3999 E La Palma Ave, Anaheim, CA 92807

Ufp Technologies, Inc. 630-543-2855
1235 W National Ave, Addison, IL 60101
Custom manufacturer of convoluted cushion pads, standard convoluted bed and wheelchair pads, impregnated foams for patches and bandages, filters & operating table pads.

Zimmer Holdings, Inc. 800-613-6131
1800 W Center St, PO Box 708, Warsaw, IN 46580

Zimmer Orthopaedic Surgical Products 800-321-5533
PO Box 10, 200 West Ohio Ave., Dover, OH 44622
ZIMFOAM.

PAD, PRESSURE, GEL *(General) 80RMD*

David Scott Company 800-804-0333
59 Fountain St, Framingham, MA 01702
BLUE DIAMOND gel pads & positioners, various gel (polymer/viscous) cushioning O. R. positions & pads, as well as long term care bed and chair (wheelchair) pads.

Genesis Manufacturing, Inc. 317-485-7887
720 E Broadway St, Fortville, IN 46040
Contract Radio-Frequency (RF) Welding. From development to manufacturing and packaging.

Innovative Health Care Products, Inc. 678-320-0009
6850 Peachtree Dunwoody Rd NE Apt 402, Atlanta, GA 30328
Double membrane Gel Pad

Paramedical Distributors 800-245-3278
2020 Grand Blvd, Kansas City, MO 64108
GELBO Heel Elbow and Ankle Gel Pads; Patented mineral oil-based gel pad reduces pressure that can cause bed sores or heel/elbow pain. Softens and moistens dry, cracked skin.

Spenco Medical Corp. 254-772-6000
PO Box 2501, Waco, TX 76702
Skin Care pads for pressure reduction.

Tuffcare 800-367-6160
3999 E La Palma Ave, Anaheim, CA 92807

Xodus Medical, Inc. 800-963-8776
702 Prominence Dr, Westmoreland Business & Research Park
New Kensington, PA 15068
Gel Positioning Products

PAD, PRESSURE, GEL, OPERATING TABLE *(General) 80WMD*

Alimed, Inc. 800-225-2610
297 High St, Dedham, MA 02026

Bryton Corp. 800-567-9500
4310 Guion Rd, Indianapolis, IN 46254

Covidien Lp 508-261-8000
15 Hampshire St, Mansfield, MA 02048
Burn pads and vests.

Gaymar Industries, Inc. 800-828-7341
10 Centre Dr, Orchard Park, NY 14127
Pad, Pressure, Gel, Operating Room Table; PUR-GEL O.R. POSITIONER; Cost effective positioning devices designed to prevent pressure ulcers and properly position patients.

Stryker Medical 800-869-0770
3800 E Centre Ave, Portage, MI 49002

PAD, PRESSURE, SOFT RUBBER *(General) 80RME*

Chamberlin Rubber Company, Inc. 585-427-7780
3333 Brighton Henrietta Town Line Rd, PO Box 22700
Rochester, NY 14623

Pedifix, Inc. 800-424-5561
310 Guinea Rd, Brewster, NY 10509
Palliative products.

PAD, PRESSURE, WATER CUSHION *(General) 80RMF*

Genesis Manufacturing, Inc. 317-485-7887
720 E Broadway St, Fortville, IN 46040
Contract Radio-Frequency (RF) Welding. From development to manufacturing and packaging.

Tetra Medical Supply Corp. 800-621-4041
6364 W Gross Point Rd, Niles, IL 60714

Waterloo Bedding Co. Ltd. 800-203-4293
141 Weber St. S, Waterloo, ONT N2J 2A9 Canada

PAD, VACUUM STABILIZED *(General) 80SEJ*

Olympic Medical Corp. 206-767-3500
5900 1st Ave S, Seattle, WA 98108
Various sizes.

PADDIE, COTTONOID *(Cns/Neurology) 84HBA*

Codman & Shurtleff, Inc 800-225-0460
325 Paramount Dr, Raynham, MA 02767

Degasa, S.A. De C.V. 525-5-483 31
Prolongacion Canal De, Miramontes #3775 Col. Ex-Hacienda San Juan Del. Tlalpan Mexico
Protec surgical compress (x-ray detectable); protec simple surgical compress

Ultracell Medical Technologies, Inc. 877-SPO-NGE1
183 Providence New London Tpke, North Stonington, CT 06359
ULTRACELL Neuro sponges. Products include paddies, strips, drains and other specialties.

PADDING, CAST/SPLINT *(General) 80WKI*

Alimed, Inc. 800-225-2610
297 High St, Dedham, MA 02026

Bioseal 800-441-7325
167 W Orangethorpe Ave, Placentia, CA 92870
Sterile, various styles.

Bsn Medical, Inc 800-552-1157
5825 Carnegie Blvd, Charlotte, NC 28209
Cotton, synthetic and rayon cast padding.

Chamberlin Rubber Company, Inc. 585-427-7780
3333 Brighton Henrietta Town Line Rd, PO Box 22700
Rochester, NY 14623

Darco International, Inc. 800-999-8866
810 Memorial Blvd, Huntington, WV 25701

Grand Rapids Foam Technologies 877-GET-GRFT
2788 Remico St SW, Wyoming, MI 49519

Select Medical Products, Inc. 800-276-7237
6531 47th St N, Pinellas Park, FL 33781
Quilted Padding.

Southwest Technologies, Inc. 800-247-9951
1746 E Levee St, North Kansas City, MO 64116
Gel for padding under casts/splints or other areas where pressure and friciton occur.

PADS, MENSTRUAL, SCENTED-DEODORIZED
(Obstetrics/Gyn) 85NRC

Gomez Packaging Corp. 973-569-9500
75 Wood St, Paterson, NJ 07524
Menstrual pads.

PAGE TURNER (HANDICAPPED) *(General) 80TFY*

Maddak Inc. 800-443-4926
661 State Route 23, Wayne, NJ 07470
ABLEWARE.

Touch Turner Company 888-811-1962
13621 103rd Ave NE, Arlington, WA 98223
Over 50 years of serving the disabled community with our automatic page turner. Our variety of switch options makes it possible for the machines to be used for people with limited abilities of varying degrees. Battery operated or AC option available. Works with books or magazines of varying sizes. The forward only model sells for,$940.00 and the forward/reverse,$1133.00, models available. Satisfaction guaranteed, with 1 year parts and labor. Call for free brochure or order a video for $7.00 on line at www.touchturner.com, or call our toll free number 1-888-811-1962.

PAGER, NON-RADIO *(General) 80TDN*

Dukane Communication Systems 519-748-5352
461 Manitou Dr., Kitchener, ON N2C 1L5 Canada

Instantel Inc. 800-267-9111
309 Legget Dr., Kanata, ON K2K 3A3 Canada
Nurse pager for alarm events involving wandering patients.

Kelkom Systems 800-985-3556
418 MacArthur Ave, Redwood City, CA 94063

Rauland-Borg Corp. 800-752-7725
3450 Oakton St, Skokie, IL 60076
Paging amplifiers, microphones, speakers etc.

Rf Technologies 800-669-9946
3125 N 126th St, Brookfield, WI 53005

Signalcom Systems, Inc. 650-692-1056
1499 Bayshore Hwy Ste 134, Burlingame, CA 94010
Computer-controlled personnel paging and message systems.

Talk-A-Phone Co. 773-539-1100
5013 N Kedzie Ave, Chicago, IL 60625

Visicomm Industries 866-221-3131
911A Milwaukee Ave, Burlington, WI 53105
Physician call system with three LEDs (green, red, amber); one cable, low voltage, site-to-site, any number per site.

PAGER, VISUAL *(General) 80VDJ*

Crest Healthcare Supply 800-328-8908
195 3rd St, Dassel, MN 55325

Signalcom Systems, Inc. 650-692-1056
1499 Bayshore Hwy Ste 134, Burlingame, CA 94010
Message communication system.

PANENDOSCOPE (GASTRODUODENOSCOPE)
(Gastro/Urology) 78FAK

Olympus America, Inc. 800-645-8160
3500 Corporate Pkwy, PO Box 610, Center Valley, PA 18034

PANT, INCONTINENCE *(General) 80RBV*

Arc Home Health Products 800-278-8595
PO Box 615, Oneonta, NY 13820

Coloplast Manufacturing Us, Llc 800-533-0464
1840 W Oak Pkwy, Marietta, GA 30062
CONVEEN washable, reusable stretch net pants holds Conveen Drip Collector and other absorbent pads or dressings in place.

Duraline Medical Products, Inc. 800-654-3376
324 Werner St, P.O. Box 67, Leipsic, OH 45856

Essential Medical Supply, Inc. 800-826-8423
6420 Hazeltine National Dr, Orlando, FL 32822
QUIK-SORB.

Freestyle Medical Supplies, Inc. 800-841-5330
336 Green Rd, Stoney Creek, ON L8E 2B2 Canada
Freestyle mini briefs for light to moderate urinary incontinence. Unisex design. Easily worn under cloting with adjustable belt and pull-on design. Available in 3 sizes, small, medium, large.

Geri-Care Products 201-440-0409
250 Moonachie Ave, Moonachie, NJ 07074
Reusable incontinence Briefs

PANT, INCONTINENCE *(cont'd)*

Humanicare International, Inc. 800-631-5270
9 Elkins Rd, East Brunswick, NJ 08816
FREE & ACTIVE, genderized pants, DIGNITY PLUS for men & women, DIGNITY unisex pant, four sizes and reusable $8.95-13.95; DIGNITY men's boxershorts $14.95

Hy-Tape International 800-248-0101
70 Jon Barrett Rd, Robin Hill Corporate Park, Patterson, NY 12563
SANIGARM Washable, reusable incontinence brief.

Hygienics Industries Div.Of Kleinert's, Inc. 800-498-7051
3968 194th Trl, Golden Beach, FL 33160
SAFE AND DRY Super and Ultra gel,disposable, absorbent liners and patented Safe And Dry water-resistant cotton pant system for men and women; Also are the Ashley Lee brand of beautiful lace/cotton briefs for women with light stress incontinence.Also, MATURE BASICS mens cotton brief with paented waterproof cotton front panel.Also SAFE And DRY waterproof matrress pads and cover product line.

Principle Business Enterprises, Inc. 800-467-3224
PO Box 129, Dunbridge, OH 43414
TRANQUILITY Washable pant for use with high capacity pads for moderate incontinence.

Salk Inc. 800-343-4497
119 Braintree St Ste 701, 4th Floor, Boston, MA 02134
PREMIER reusable panties and briefs. Adults.

PAPAIN *(Pathology) 88IBF*

Bd Diagnostic Systems 800-675-0908
7 Loveton Cir, Sparks, MD 21152

PAPER, ARTICULATION *(Dental And Oral) 76EFH*

Almore International, Inc. 503-643-6633
PO Box 25214, Portland, OR 97298
$13.95 to $39.95.

Ched Markay, Inc. 312-566-3307
1065 E High St, Mundelein, IL 60060
Holg mark:rite articulating paper.

George Taub Products & Fusion Co., Inc. 800-828-2634
277 New York Ave, Jersey City, NJ 07307
Bright Spot liquids offer an alternative to articulation paper. These articulating liquids either highlight or become indicators showing the premature marks with minimum contact pressure. Will give multiple marks from the same application. Apply on opposing surface to find the high contact spot. Before applying on stone models, best to seal stone with Stone Die Hardener. Available in white, brownish red, red, blue, pink and light green. Great for finding high contact spots on machined metal surfaces, as well.

Harry J. Bosworth Company 800-323-4352
7227 Hamlin Ave, Skokie, IL 60076

Heraeus Kulzer, Inc., Dental Products Division 574-299-6662
4315 S Lafayette Blvd, South Bend, IN 46614
Articulating paper.

Kerr Corp. 714-516-7400
28200 Wick Rd, Romulus, MI 48174
Occlusal clearance tabs.

Mds Products, Inc. 800-637-2330
22991 La Cadena Dr, Laguna Hills, CA 92653
Tru-Spot 1 Red or Black .00075 thin Articulating film. Tru-Spot 2 .0009 thin Red/Black Articulating Film.

Miltex Dental Technologies, Inc. 516-576-6022
589 Davies Dr, York, PA 17402
Articulating paper.

Moyco Technologies, Inc. 800-331-8837
200 Commerce Dr, Montgomeryville, PA 18936
$5.00 per 10 books.

Parkell, Inc. 800-243-7446
300 Executive Dr, Edgewood, NY 11717
ACCU-FILM I, ACCU-FILM II

Pascal Co., Inc. 425-602-3633
2929 Northup Way, Bellevue, WA 98004
Multiple articulation paper/articulation spray/multiple (dental).

Pulpdent Corp. 800-343-4342
80 Oakland St, Watertown, MA 02472
No common name listed.

Rite-Dent Manufacturing Corp. 305-693-8626
3750 E 10th Ct, Hialeah, FL 33013
Various types of articulating paper.

PAPER, ARTICULATION *(cont'd)*

Ultradent Products, Inc. 801-553-4586
505 W 10200 S, South Jordan, UT 84095
High sight indicator.

Vacalon Company, Inc. 614-577-1945
12960 Stonecreek Dr Ste C, Pickerington, OH 43147
Articulation spray.

PAPER, CHART, RECORD, MEDICAL *(General) 80QJP*

A-M Systems, Inc. 800-426-1306
131 Business Park Loop, Sequim, WA 98382
38 types for respirometers, spirometers, etc. of various manufacturers

Alimed, Inc. 800-225-2610
297 High St, Dedham, MA 02026

Astro-Med, Inc. 800-343-4039
600 E Greenwich Ave, West Warwick, RI 02893
Wide range of thermal chart paper and ink writing chart papers

Beckman Coulter, Inc. 800-742-2345
250 S Kraemer Blvd, PO Box 8000, Brea, CA 92821

Bibbero Systems, Inc. 800-242-2376
1300 N McDowell Blvd, Petaluma, CA 94954
Folders, dividers, forms, labels and custom printing. CMS forms & envelopes. Many products to assist in HIPAA compliance.

Deflecto Corp. 800-428-4328
7035 E 86th St, Indianapolis, IN 46250
CONFIDENTIAL WALL POCKET holds patient information, files and charts that need to be kept private. Convenient pocket tilts forward for easy retrieval. Made from opaque black plastic. TILT BIN STORAGE SYSTEMS are an excellent way to store medical supplies. Use for cotton balls, gauze, toothpaste, toothbrush, latex gloves and more. Interlocking design allows you to create a specific configuration to fit your need. STAND TALL LITERATURE HOLDERS are perfect for holding magazines and pamphlets in lobby areas. Available as wall unit, desktop, counter, and floor. MULTIPLE BUSINESS CARD HOLDERS. Great for offices with multiple individuals. SIGN HOLDERS are great for displaying important messages to patients and office administration.

Impac Medical Systems, Inc. 888-464-6722
100 W Evelyn Ave, Mountain View, CA 94041
eCHART electronic medical record (EMR) for radiation and medical oncology.

Marathon Equipment Company 800-269-7237
950 County HWY 9 S., Vernon, AL 35592
Pharmaceutical/Medical document shredder. Also shredded prescription vials and labels. www.RxShredder.com

Medical Accessories, Inc. 800-275-1624
92 Youngs Rd, Trenton, NJ 08619

Medical Tactile, Inc. 310-641-8228
5757 W Century Blvd Ste 600, Los Angeles, CA 90045
Electronic documentation for the Clinical Breast Examination

Medirecord Systems 800-561-9791
P.O. Box 6201 Station A, Saint John, NB E2L 4R6 Canada
Medical charts, file folders, indexes, file equipment, X-ray bags and inserts.

National Systems Co. 877-672-4278
31B Durward Pl., Waterloo N2J 3Z9 Canada
Patient charts, chart holders, indexes, racks, labels and tape.

Omni Medical Supply Inc. 800-860-6664
4153 Pioneer Dr, Commerce Township, MI 48390
Complete product line of single, dual, three channel papers. Also available is a comprehensive line of thernal video black & white and color papers.

Pace Tech, Inc. 800-722-3024
510 N Garden Ave, Clearwater, FL 33755

Paper Systems Inc. 800-950-8590
185 S Pioneer Blvd, Springboro, OH 45066

Print Media, Inc. 800-994-3318
9002 NW 105th Way, Medley, FL 33178
Recording paper/charts for ECG, EEG, fetal heart, ultrasound/imaging and all other medical instruments are manufactured to meet or exceed original equipment manufacturer's specifications. Each paper is designed to work with the recorder, producing clear, accurate tracings and clearly defined alphanumeric characters. Custom products, private labeling and drop shipments available.

Tyco Healthcare Group Lp 800-445-5025
2 Ludlow Park Dr, Chicopee, MA 01022
TAP Thermal Array printer papers; fetal heart chart papers.

PAPER, CHART, RECORD, MEDICAL *(cont'd)*

Vacumed 800-235-3333
4538 Westinghouse St, Ventura, CA 93003
For all spirometers.

PAPER, ION *(Toxicology) 91DMG*

Whatman Inc. 732-885-6529
800 Centennial Ave Bldg 1, Piscataway, NJ 08854

PAPER, PHOTOGRAPHIC *(General) 80WMJ*

National Graphic Supply 800-223-7130
226 N Allen St, Albany, NY 12206
Full line supplier of photographic supplies, equipment and electronics.

PAPER, RECORDING, DATA *(General) 80WUP*

Misc Inc. 800-524-1155
1889 Route 9 Ste 97, Toms River, NJ 08755
MISC Medical Data Recording Paper includes an extensive array of thermal, bond, electrosensitive and video printer paper. These generic products are guaranteed totally compatible to the diagnostic and laboratory instruments listed in the MISC catalog. Catalog, prices, and warranty sent upon request.

Omni Medical Supply Inc. 800-860-6664
4153 Pioneer Dr, Commerce Township, MI 48390

Paper Systems Inc. 800-950-8590
185 S Pioneer Blvd, Springboro, OH 45066

Print Media, Inc. 800-994-3318
9002 NW 105th Way, Medley, FL 33178
Recording paper/charts for ECG, EEG, fetal heart, ultrasound/imaging and all other medical instruments are manufactured to meet or exceed original equipment manufacturer's specifications. Each paper is designed to work with the recorder, producing clear, accurate tracings and clearly defined alphanumeric characters. Custom products, private labeling and drop shipments available.

Science-Electronics, Inc. 937-224-4444
521 Kiser St, Dayton, OH 45404
DATALOGGERS: recording instruments.

PAPER, RECORDING, ECG/EEG *(General) 80VLR*

Cardiocontrol, Inc. 973-340-8000
101425 Overseas Hwy, P.O. Box 615, Key Largo, FL 33037

Elmed, Inc. 630-543-2792
60 W Fay Ave, Addison, IL 60101

Ge Medical Systems Information Technologies 800-643-6439
8200 W Tower Ave, Milwaukee, WI 53223

Hillusa Corp. 305-594-7474
7215 NW 46th St, Miami, FL 33166

Lumiscope Company, Inc. 800-672-8293
1035 Centennial Ave, Piscataway, NJ 08854

Maguire Enterprises, Inc. 800-548-9686
10289 NW 46th St, Sunrise, FL 33351
Top quality chart paper, LP10, LP11, LP12, LP20, Zoll PD & M series (roll and Zfold) and most other chart papers.

Medirex Systems Ltd. 800-387-9848
P.O. Box 40 Station F, Toronto, ONT M4Y 2L4 Canada

Omni Medical Supply Inc. 800-860-6664
4153 Pioneer Dr, Commerce Township, MI 48390

Print Media, Inc. 800-994-3318
9002 NW 105th Way, Medley, FL 33178
Recording paper/charts for ECG, EEG, fetal heart, ultrasound/imaging and all other medical instruments are manufactured to meet or exceed original equipment manufacturer's specifications. Each paper is designed to work with the recorder, producing clear, accurate tracings and clearly defined alphanumeric characters. Custom products, private labeling and drop shipments available.

Quality Rapid Service Mounts, Inc. 800-418-8342
8617 Eagle Point Blvd, Lake Elmo, MN 55042

Tyco Healthcare Group Lp 800-445-5025
2 Ludlow Park Dr, Chicopee, MA 01022

PAPILLOTOME *(Surgery) 79RJX*

Cameron-Miller, Inc. 800-621-0142
5410 W Roosevelt Rd, Road #241, Chicago, IL 60644

Medi-Globe Corporation 800-966-1431
110 W Orion St Ste 136, Tempe, AZ 85283
Precut, standard, rotatable.

Telemed Systems Inc. 800-481-6718
8 Kane Industrial Dr, Hudson, MA 01749

PARAFFIN, ALL FORMULATIONS *(Pathology) 88KEO*

American Mastertech Scientific, Inc. 209-368-4031
1330 Thurman St, Lodi, CA 95240
Multiple.

Covidien Lp 508-261-8000
15 Hampshire St, Mansfield, MA 02048

Fisher Scientific Co., Llc. 201-703-3131
1 Reagent Ln, Fair Lawn, NJ 07410
Embedding parafin.

Grimm Scientific Ind., Inc. 800-223-5395
1403 Pike St, PO Box 2143, Marietta, OH 45750
PARALIN, $24.00 for 10 lb. and $16.00 for 6 lb., medical- grade paraffin refills.

Leica Biosystems - St. Louis, Llc 847-317-7209
12100A Prichard Farm Rd, Maryland Heights, MO 63043
Tissue embedding medium.

Polysciences, Inc. 800-523-2575
400 Valley Rd, Warrington, PA 18976
Peel - A - Way MicroCut paraffin, 3 meeting temperatures

Sci Gen, Inc. 310-324-6576
333 E Gardena Blvd, Gardena, CA 90248
FDA: Medical Device Manufacturing and packaging. Focus on Histology, Cytology, Analytical and General purpose Reagents, Chemistry, and Sterling and Disinfecting agents.

Ventana Medical Systems, Inc. 800-227-2155
1910 E Innovation Park Dr, Oro Valley, AZ 85755
Liquid cover slip.

PARAFORMALDEHYDE *(Pathology) 88KEF*

Polysciences, Inc. 800-523-2575
400 Valley Rd, Warrington, PA 18976

Sci Gen, Inc. 310-324-6576
333 E Gardena Blvd, Gardena, CA 90248
FDA: Medical Device Manufacturing and packaging. Focus on Histology, Cytology, Analytical and General purpose Reagents, Chemistry, and Sterling and Disinfecting agents.

PARAQUAT ASSAY *(Chemistry) 75LTD*

Celera Corporation 510-749-4219
884 Dubuque Ave, S San Fran, CA 94080
Reagent, general purpose.

PARTIAL THROMBOPLASTIN TIME *(Hematology) 81GGW*

Bio/Data Corp. 215-441-4000
155 Gibraltar Rd, Horsham, PA 19044
Aptt reagent.

Biomerieux Inc. 800-682-2666
100 Rodolphe St, Durham, NC 27712
Activated Auto APTT - platelin L, platelin LS for determination of APTT: used for monitoring heparin therapy, detect lupus inhibitors or factor deficiencies auto is lyophilized, Platelin L is liguid, Platelin LS is liguid with increased sensitivity to heparin.

Diagnostica Stago, Inc. 800-222-COAG
5 Century Dr, Parsippany, NJ 07054

Life Therapeutics Inc. 404-300-5000
780 Park North Blvd Ste 100, Clarkston, GA 30021
Factor v leiden test.

R2 Diagnostics, Inc. 574-288-4377
1801 Commerce Dr, South Bend, IN 46628
Aptt-activated partial thromboplastin time reagent.

PARTIAL THROMBOPLASTIN TIME, REAGENT, CONTROL *(Hematology) 81GIT*

Analytical Control Systems, Inc. 317-841-0458
9058 Technology Dr, Fishers, IN 46038
SPECTRA APTT Activated cephaloplastin reagent (activated partial thromboplastin time).

Biomerieux Inc. 800-682-2666
100 Rodolphe St, Durham, NC 27712

Dade Behring, Inc. 800-948-3233
1717 Deerfield Rd, Deerfield, IL 60015

Diagnostica Stago, Inc. 800-222-COAG
5 Century Dr, Parsippany, NJ 07054

Health Chem Diagnostics Llc 954-979-3845
3341 W McNab Rd, Pompano Beach, FL 33069
Reagent & control, partial thromboplastin time.

PASSER *(Orthopedics) 87HWQ*

Arthrex California, Inc. 239-643-5553
20509 Earlgate St, Walnut, CA 91789
Suture retriver/passer.

Depuy Mitek, A Johnson & Johnson Company 800-451-2006
50 Scotland Blvd, Bridgewater, MA 02324
Suture passer.

Mizuho Osi 800-777-4674
30031 Ahern Ave, Union City, CA 94587
Tendon passer.

Zimmer Holdings, Inc. 800-613-6131
1800 W Center St, PO Box 708, Warsaw, IN 46580

PASSER, WIRE, ORTHOPEDIC *(Orthopedics) 87HXI*

Biomet Microfixation Inc. 800-874-7711
1520 Tradeport Dr, Jacksonville, FL 32218
Various types of wire.

Biomet, Inc. 574-267-6639
56 E Bell Dr, PO Box 587, Warsaw, IN 46582
Various orthopedic wire passers.

Interventional Spine, Inc. 800-497-0484
13700 Alton Pkwy Ste 160, Irvine, CA 92618
Various types of passer wires.

Kmedic 800-955-0559
190 Veterans Dr, Northvale, NJ 07647

RTI Biologics Inc. 877-343-6832
11621 Research Cir, Alachua, FL 32615
Interference screw guidewire.

Rush-Berivon, Inc. 800-251-7874
1010 19th St, P.O. Box 1851, Meridian, MS 39301
$165.00ea - with 2, 3, or 5cm loops. $165.00 for slotted, orthopedic wire passer.

Spine Wave, Inc. 203-944-9494
2 Enterprise Dr Ste 302, Shelton, CT 06484
Various types of guide wires.

Stryker Spine 866-457-7463
2 Pearl Ct, Allendale, NJ 07401

Zimmer Holdings, Inc. 800-613-6131
1800 W Center St, PO Box 708, Warsaw, IN 46580

PATCH, EYE *(Ophthalmology) 86UET*

Precision Therapeutics, Inc. 800-544-0076
8400 E Prentice Ave Ste 700, Greenwood Village, CO 80111
$4.64 ea. for PRESSPATCH tapeless pressure pad with headband; $1.29 ea. for PRESSPATCH pads, sterile foam replacement pad for PRESSPATCH; $2.86 ea. for Tapeless Eye Shield, pinhole eye shield with headband; $0.60 ea. for eye shields - polyethylene with pinholes (unbreakable); and $.34 ea. for Comfort Cushion foam ring around eye shield.

PATCH, MYOCARDIAL *(Cardiovascular) 74UJO*

Bard Peripheral Vascular, Inc. 800-321-4254
1625 W 3rd St, Tempe, AZ 85281
Vascular patch for vascular repair, 50x100mm.

PATCH, PERICARDIAL *(Cardiovascular) 74MFX*

Medtronic Cardiovascular Surgery, The Heart Valve Div. 800-328-2518
1851 E Deere Ave, Santa Ana, CA 92705
Patch, cardiovascular.

Medtronic Heart Valves 800-227-3191
8299 Central Ave NE, Spring Lake Park, MN 55432
Patch cardiovascular.

W.L. Gore & Associates,Inc 928-526-3030
1505 North Fourth St., Flagstaff, AZ 86004
Surgical membrane.

PATCH, TRANSDERMAL *(General) 80WOL*

Brady Corporation 800-541-1686
6555 W Good Hope Rd, PO Box 571, Milwaukee, WI 53223
Custom transdermal patches manufactured to customer designs. Iontophoresis and drug delivery experience.

Brady Precision Converting, Llc 214-275-9595
1801 Big Town Blvd Ste 100, Mesquite, TX 75149
Component fabrication and packaging. Topical cosmeceutical patches.

PATCH, TRANSDERMAL *(cont'd)*

Mylan Technologies, Inc. 800-532-5226
110 Lake St, Saint Albans, VT 05478
Fully integrated and tested source providing custom design, product development, testing and GMP manufacture of transdermal therapeutic systems.

Smi 920-876-3361
Industrial Park, 544 Sohn Drive, Elkhart Lake, WI 53020

PATIENT ISOLATION CHAMBER *(General) 80LGM*

Gentex Corporation 570-282-8350
324 Main St, P.o. Box 315, Simpson, PA 18407
Patient transport isolation chamber.

Innovative Technology, Inc. 877-462-4415
2 New Pasture Rd, Newburyport, MA 01950
Environmental chambers for isolation, containment & safety. Inert atmospheres available, oxygen control down to (1 PPM.

PATIENT PERSONAL HYGIENE KIT *(Dental And Oral) 76NSB*

Centurion Medical Products Corp. 517-545-1135
3310 S Main St, Salisbury, NC 28147

Medline Industries Holdings, L.P. 847-837-2759
9303 Stoneview Dr, Dallas, TX 75237
Admit kit.

Medline Industries Holdings, L.P. 847-837-2759
7267 Schantz Rd, Allentown, PA 18106
Patient admission kit.

Tri-State Hospital Supply Corp. 517-545-1135
3173 E 43rd St, Yuma, AZ 85365

PATIENT TRANSFER UNIT *(General) 80RKB*

A.R.C. Distributors 800-296-8724
PO Box 599, Centreville, MD 21617
SLIPP patient moving device to make transfers easy for both healthcare worker and patient. Polyurethane bonded to nylon surface of sealed fluid that reduces normal friction to a minimum. INVACARE Class Transfer Benches have a durable anodized aluminum frame, reversible back, nine height adjustments, non-marring, non-slip rubber tips, shower curtain opening, and arm rail for support.

Airpal Patient Transfer Systems Inc. 800-633-4725
5456 Northwood Dr, Center Valley, PA 18034
AIRPAL lateral patient transfer system.

Alimed, Inc. 800-225-2610
297 High St, Dedham, MA 02026
Friction-free surface allows an easy slide on a bed or stretcher.

Allen Medical Systems, Inc. 800-433-5774
1 Post Office Sq, Acton, MA 01720
Roller-free roller board

Arjo Canada, Inc. 800-665-4831
1575 South Gateway Rd., Unit C, Mississauga, ONT L4W-5J1 Canada

Arjo, Inc. 800-323-1245
50 Gary Ave Ste A, Roselle, IL 60172

Armstrong Medical Industries, Inc. 800-323-4220
575 Knightsbridge Pkwy, Lincolnshire, IL 60069

Bio-Logics Products, Inc. 800-426-7577
PO Box 505, West Jordan, UT 84084
Room transfer system using permanent room jackets.

Eagle Health Supplies, Inc. 800-755-8999
535 W Walnut Ave, Orange, CA 92868
EAGLE GLIDE - 30' long made of lightweight aluminum for patient transfer.

Frank Scholz X-Ray Corp. 508-586-8308
244 Liberty St, Brockton, MA 02301
ROLL AID patient shifter, 25', 30' and 67' length patient transfer device. Moves patient from one surface to another without lifting, pulling or disruption and with very little effort.

Gendron, Inc. 800-537-2521
400 E Lugbill Rd, Archbold, OH 43502
PHASE CHAIR, combination stretcher/chair for transfer and transport of bariatric patients.

Hovertech International 800-471-2776
513 S Clewell St, Fountain Hill, PA 18015
HOVERMATT Patient Transfer Technology, a product used to assist lateral patient transfers using air as a lubricant to reduce friction.

PATIENT TRANSFER UNIT *(cont'd)*

Integrated Medical Systems, Inc. 562-498-1776
1984 Obispo Ave, Signal Hill, CA 90755
The FDA-cleared, patented, international award-winning web-enabled LSTAT system is an individualized portable Intensive Care Unit and surgical platform only 5 inches thick. Integrated within the LSTAT system are a ventilator, oxygen, suction, 3-channel fluid/drug infusion pump, physiological monitor, clinical blood analyzer, and an automatic external defibrillator. The patented information architecture supports the capture, storage, and transmission of continuous time-synchronized multi-device multi-parameter patient data to local and remote caregivers. This unique data capability saves time for the caregiver and improves care for the patient by offering a more complete view of the interplay between therapy and patient response. The architecture also enables web-based remote technical analysis and support of the devices aboard the LSTAT, as well as e-commerce applications for re-supply of disposable medical supplies.

Mxe, Inc. 800-252-1801
12107 Jefferson Blvd, Culver City, CA 90230
MXE's Stretchair offers the benefits of a chair, wheelchair, stretcher, transport unit, and a lateral transfer aid - all in one piece of equipment. Ergonomically designed to help reduce caregiver back injuries, the Stretchair is available for patients up to 800 lbs.

Rand-Scot Inc. 800-467-7967
401 Linden Center Dr, Fort Collins, CO 80524
Priced from $1,200 to $3,500; EASY PIVOT 'no sling' lift for home or institution usage.

Rifton Equipment 800-571-8198
PO Box 260, Rifton, NY 12471
The Rifton Support Station is a transfer convenience aid installed for patients to self-assist transfer from wheelchair to commode with stand-by assist.

Schueler & Company, Inc. 516-487-1500
PO Box 528, Stratford, CT 06615

Total Care 800-334-3802
PO Box 1661, Rockville, MD 20849
patient shifter(72'x22')with handgrips for easy transfer from bed to stretcher,o.r.,x-ray table,etc.

PATIENT TRANSFER UNIT, POWERED *(General) 80FRZ*

Air Movement Technologies, Inc. 800-317-9582
320 Gateway Park Dr, Syracuse, NY 13212
Air assisted patient transfer device.

Arjo, Inc. 800-323-1245
50 Gary Ave Ste A, Roselle, IL 60172

Horcher Lifting Systems, Inc. 800-582-8732
324 Cypress Rd, Ocala, FL 34472
DIANA Electric floor model with dual wheel casters and remote control unit. 24 volt battery powered. Improved safety features. RAISA Patient stand-up lift with adjustable knee pads and remote control. LEXA mobile floor model with patented motorized patient positioner.

Tr Group, Inc. 800-752-6900
903 Wedel Ln, Glenview, IL 60025
Shower trolley.

Vivax Medical Corp. 866-847-7890
89 Putter Ln, Torrington, CT 06790
The Vivax Mobility System is in the most advanced medical device for helping address the medical, rehabilitation, mobility and health care needs of mobility impaired persons .

PELVIMETER *(Obstetrics/Gyn) 85RKE*

Codman & Shurtleff, Inc 800-225-0460
325 Paramount Dr, Raynham, MA 02767

Miltex Inc. 800-645-8000
589 Davies Dr, York, PA 17402

Rocket Medical Plc. 800-707-7625
150 Recreation Park Dr Ste 3, Hingham, MA 02043

PELVIMETER, EXTERNAL *(Obstetrics/Gyn) 85HER*

Biomet Microfixation Inc. 800-874-7711
1520 Tradeport Dr, Jacksonville, FL 32218
Various types of pelvimeters.

Marconi Medical Systems 800-323-0550
595 Miner Rd, Cleveland, OH 44143

Rocket Medical Plc. 800-707-7625
150 Recreation Park Dr Ste 3, Hingham, MA 02043

PEN, MARKING, SURGICAL *(Ophthalmology) 86HRP*

Accu-Line Products, Inc. 800-363-7740
379 Iyannough Rd Rear Bldg, Hyannis, MA 02601
Universal points, ultrafine points and separate flexible plastic rulers and labels. Packaged sterile in various combinations.

Biomet, Inc. 574-267-6639
56 E Bell Dr, PO Box 587, Warsaw, IN 46582
Surgical marking pen.

Dri Mark Products, Inc. 516-484-6200
15 Harbor Park Dr, Port Washington, NY 11050
Surgical marker.

Hospital Marketing Svcs. Company, Inc. 800-786-5094
162 Great Hill Rd./ Ind. Park, Naugatuck, CT 06770
HMS SKIN SKRIBE skin marker - cat. no. 6650, 10/box, HMS TWIN TIP - fine and broad line, cat. no. 6650-T, 10/box.

Jaece Industries, Inc. 716-694-2811
908 Niagara Falls Blvd, North Tonawanda, NY 14120
IDENTI-MARKER - Lab marker marks on IDENTI-PLUGS, plastic, glass, metal, cold, or wet surfaces and alcohol-resistant surfaces. Ideal for general lab, hospital, or industrial use.

K. W. Griffen Co. 203-846-1923
100 Pearl St, Norwalk, CT 06850
Surgical marking pen.

Medical Action Industries, Inc. 800-645-7042
25 Heywood Rd, Arden, NC 28704
Surgical marking pen.

Olsen Medical 800-297-6344
3001 W Kentucky St, Louisville, KY 40211
Skin marking pens.

Quint Company 215-533-1988
3725 Castor Ave # 26, Philadelphia, PA 19124
Marking devices.

PENETROMETER *(Radiology) 90RKF*

Koehler Instrument Co., Inc. 800-878-9070
1595 Sycamore Ave, Bohemia, NY 11716
Digital penetrometer determines the consistency of solid to semi-solid materials. Microprocessor based.

PENLIGHT, BATTERY-POWERED *(Ophthalmology) 86HJP*

American Diagnostic Corporation (Adc) 800-232-2670
55 Commerce Dr, Hauppauge, NY 11788
Disposable and reusable diagnostic penlights

Armstrong Medical Industries, Inc. 800-323-4220
575 Knightsbridge Pkwy, Lincolnshire, IL 60069

Bovie Medical Corp. 800-537-2790
5115 Ulmerton Rd, Clearwater, FL 33760
8 models - AA or AAA batteries; slit beam, cobalt or regular models.

Pocket Nurse Enterprises, Inc. 800-225-1600
200 1st St, Ambridge, PA 15003

Schueler & Company, Inc. 516-487-1500
PO Box 528, Stratford, CT 06615

PEPTIDES *(Chemistry) 75UHC*

Bachem Bioscience, Inc. 800-634-3183
3700 Horizon Dr, King Of Prussia, PA 19406

Research Organics, Inc. 800-321-0570
4353 E 49th St, Cleveland, OH 44125

PERCUSSOR *(Cns/Neurology) 84GWZ*

Ballard Medical Products 770-587-7835
12050 Lone Peak Pkwy, Draper, UT 84020
Manual percussor.

Codman & Shurtleff, Inc 800-225-0460
325 Paramount Dr, Raynham, MA 02767

Demetech Corp. 888-324-2447
3530 NW 115th Ave, Doral, FL 33178
Percussion hammer.

Depuy-Raynham, A Div. Of Depuy Orthopaedics 800-451-2006
325 Paramount Dr, Raynham, MA 02767
Various.

Dhd Healthcare Corporation 800-847-8000
PO Box 6, One Madison Street, Wampsville, NY 13163
PALMCUPS.

General Pysiotherapy, Inc. 800-237-1832
13222 Lakefront Dr, Earth City, MO 63045
Postural drainage percussors

PERCUSSOR *(cont'd)*

Genesen Pan America, Inc. 714-799-1735
7245 Garden Grove Blvd Ste D, Garden Grove, CA 92841
Accutouch, acurepatch.

Kentron Health Care, Inc. 615-384-0573
3604 Kelton Jackson Rd, P.o. Box 120, Springfield, TN 37172
Percussion hammers.

Pedia Pals, Llc 888-733-4272
965 Highway 169 N, Plymouth, MN 55441
Reflex hammer in the shape of Jamaal the Giraffe. Same durometer, hardness and balance of a typical reflex hammer.

Sweat Chiropractic Clinic 770-457-4430
3274 Buckeye Rd, Atlanta, GA 30341
Same.

Tuzik Boston 800-886-6363
104 Longwater Dr, Assinippi Park, Norwell, MA 02061

PERCUSSOR, POWERED *(Anesthesiology) 73BYI*

Electromed, Inc. 952-758-9299
502 6th Ave NW, New Prague, MN 56071
SmartVest Airway Clearance System

Med Systems 800-345-9061
2631 Ariane Dr, San Diego, CA 92117
FLUID FLO 2500 PNEUMATIC CHEST PERCUSSOR. USED IN PHYSICAL THERAPY AND BRONCHIAL DRAINAGE WITH COPD, EMPHYSEMA OR CYSTIC FIBROSIS.

Respiratory Technologies, Inc. 651-379-8999
1380 Energy Ln Ste 113, Saint Paul, MN 55108
Powered percussor.

Thayer Medical Corp. 520-790-5393
4575 S Palo Verde Rd Ste 337, Tucson, AZ 85714
Mucus clearance device.

The Foredom Electric Co. 203-792-8622
16 Stony Hill Rd, Bethel, CT 06801
Various models of percussion vibrators.

PERFORATOR, AMNIOTIC MEMBRANE *(Obstetrics/Gyn) 85RKH*

Precision Dynamics Corp. 800-772-1122
13880 Del Sur St, San Fernando, CA 91340
SECURLINE AMP.

PERFORATOR, ANTRUM *(Ear/Nose/Throat) 77KAT*

Aesculap Implant Systems Inc. 1-800-234-9179
3773 Corporate Pkwy, Center Valley, PA 18034

Biomet Microfixation Inc. 800-874-7711
1520 Tradeport Dr, Jacksonville, FL 32218
Perforator, antrum.

Codman & Shurtleff, Inc 800-225-0460
325 Paramount Dr, Raynham, MA 02767

PERFORATOR, EAR *(Ear/Nose/Throat) 77QRT*

Roman Research, Inc. 800-451-5700
800 Franklin St, Hanson, MA 02341

PERFORATOR, EAR-LOBE *(Ear/Nose/Throat) 77JYS*

Concept Marketing, Inc. 252-247-5285
1000 Arendell St, Morehead City, NC 28557
Earpiercing instrument.

Inverness Corp. 201-794-3400
6 Hazel St, Attleboro, MA 02703
Inverness ear piercing system.

J. Hewitt Incorporated 800-543-9488
6 Faraday Ste B, Irvine, CA 92618
MEDISYSTEM medical instruments and sterile disposable products used for piercing ears; sold to the professional and consumer markets.

Miltex Inc. 800-645-8000
589 Davies Dr, York, PA 17402

Onyx Industries, Inc./Quadrtech 310-851-6161
521 W Rosecrans Ave, Gardena, CA 90248
Ear piercing.

Roman Research, Inc. 800-451-5700
800 Franklin St, Hanson, MA 02341
Allergy proof pierced and clip-on earrings.

PERFUSION APPARATUS *(Pathology) 88KJH*

Biovest International, Inc. 866-3BIOVEST
8500 Evergreen Blvd NW, Minneapolis, MN 55433
CELL-PHARM and ACUSYST computer controlled tissue culture systems for generation of mammalian cell secreted products. CELL-PHARM 2500 and ACUSYST MAXIMER cell culture systems produces 30 grams a month of bioproducts. ACUSYST-XCELL produces commercial quantities of bioproducts, up to a kilogram a year.

Medtronic, Inc. 800-633-8766
710 Medtronic Pkwy, Minneapolis, MN 55432

Novosci Corp. 281-363-4949
2828 N Crescentridge Dr, The Woodlands, TX 77381
Perfusion adapter sets.

Transonic Systems Inc. 800-353-3569
34 Dutch Mill Rd, Warren Road Business Park, Ithaca, NY 14850
TRANSONIC Bypass Flowmeter, Sterile tubing clamp-on flow sensors for use during CP bypass, ECMO, dialysis, CAVH, organ preservation, circulatory device.

PERFUSION SYSTEM, KIDNEY *(Gastro/Urology) 78KDN*

Organ Recovery Systems, Inc. 847-824-2600
2570 E Devon Ave, Des Plaines, IL 60018
Cold storage solution.

Preservation Solutions, Inc. 262-723-6715
980 Proctor Dr, Elkhorn, WI 53121
Kidney transport solution.

Smc Medical Manufacturing Division 715-247-3500
360 Reed St, Somerset, WI 54025
Perfusion pack.

Waters Medical Systems, Llc 205-612-5221
2112 15th St NW, Rochester, MN 55901
Organ preservation system.

PERFUSION UNIT *(General) 80FSB*

Terumo Cardiovascular Systems, Corp 800-521-2818
6200 Jackson Rd, Ann Arbor, MI 48103

PERIMETER, AC-POWERED *(Ophthalmology) 86HOO*

Mast/Keystone View 800-806-6569
2200 Dickerson Rd, Reno, NV 89503
measures lateral peripheral vision with push-button ease, fits all model TELEBINOCULARS with molded plastic viewing heads, uses 9-volt battery, weighs 2 5/8 lbs., $420.00.

Paradigm Medical Industries, Inc. 801-977-8970
2355 S 1070 W, Salt Lake City, UT 84119
Ac-powered perimeter.

PERIMETER, AUTOMATIC, AC-POWERED *(Ophthalmology) 86HPT*

Carl Zeiss Meditec Inc. 877-486-7473
5160 Hacienda Dr, Dublin, CA 94568
HUMPHREY FIELD ANALYZER II - The Humphrey Field Analyzer II's testing strategies, ergonomic design and very short testing times provide new levels of diagnostic information and patient acceptance. Compact size, faster testing, times made possible with FASTPAC, superior accuracy and STATPAC 2, the common language of perimetry, are hallmarks of the HFA II. Models: 720, 735, 740, 750.

Dicon, Inc. 800-426-0493
2355 S 1070 W, Salt Lake City, UT 84119
Autoperimeters LD 400, SST, TKS 5000 and FieldLink feature kinetic fixation, multiple/single stimulus, capability to display Humphrey fields, and full threshold exams.

Marco Ophthalmic, Inc. 800-874-5274
11825 Central Pkwy, Jacksonville, FL 32224
$7,995.00 for automatic perimeter. (List price)

Nidek, Inc. 510-226-5700
47651 Westinghouse Dr, Fremont, CA 94539
Perimeter.

Paradigm Medical Industries, Inc. 801-977-8970
2355 S 1070 W, Salt Lake City, UT 84119
Autoperimeter.

The Peristat Group, Inc. 714-928-8507
3721 Fillmore St, San Francisco, CA 94123
Virtual perimetry.

PERIMETER, MANUAL *(Ophthalmology) 86HON*

Accutome, Inc. 610-889-0200
3222 Phoenixville Pike, Malvern, PA 19355
Trephines.

PERIMETER, MANUAL *(cont'd)*

Marco Ophthalmic, Inc. 800-874-5274
11825 Central Pkwy, Jacksonville, FL 32224
$9,495.00 for manual marking model, Goldmann type. (List price)

Mast/Keystone View 800-806-6569
2200 Dickerson Rd, Reno, NV 89503
Telebinocular attachment for measuring lateral peripheral vision, easily mounted using 2 thumb screws, $135.00.

PERINEOMETER *(Obstetrics/Gyn) 85HIR*

American Imex 800-521-8286
16520 Aston, Irvine, CA 92606
PERITRON, a precision perineometer.

Colonial Medical Supply 800-634-9334
1350 E Flamingo Rd # 343, Las Vegas, NV 89119
Pelvic muscle trainer.

Deschutes Medical Products, Inc. 800-383-2588
1011 SW Emkay Dr Ste 104, Bend, OR 97702
MYSELF direct to the consumer pelvic floor exercise biofeedback device.

Kegelmaster Inc. 352-625-2156
4125 S Highway 314A, Ocklawaha, FL 32179
Perineometer.

Self Regulation Systems, Inc. 800-345-5642
8672 154th Ave NE Bldg F, Redmond, WA 98052
Vaginal and anal sensors for pelvic floor rehabilitation/continence therapy: SRS SenseRx Sensors, the quality standard; Eisman-Tries MEP Anal Sensor; Eisman-Tries IVS-2 Intravaginal Sensor.

The Prometheus Group 603-749-0733
1 Washington St Ste 303, Dover, NH 03820
Perineometer.

PERIODIC ACID *(Pathology) 88KKS*

American Mastertech Scientific, Inc. 209-368-4031
1330 Thurman St, Lodi, CA 95240
Multiple types of periodic acid.

Richard-Allan Scientific 269-544-5628
4481 Campus Dr, Kalamazoo, MI 49008
Pas.

PERIODONTAL INSTRUMENT *(Dental And Oral) 76RKJ*

Dentalez Group 866-DTE-INFO
101 Lindenwood Dr Ste 225, Valleybrooke Corporate Center
Malvern, PA 19355

Miltex Inc. 800-645-8000
589 Davies Dr, York, PA 17402

PERITONEAL DIALYSIS UNIT (CAPD) *(Gastro/Urology) 78RKL*

Baxter Healthcare Corporation, Renal 888-229-0001
1620 S Waukegan Rd, Waukegan, IL 60085
HOMECHOICE automated PD system

Janin Group, Inc. 800-323-5389
14A Stonehill Rd, Oswego, IL 60543
Y-TEC Catheter implantation kit, catheter implantation instruments.

PERITONEOSCOPE *(Gastro/Urology) 78GCG*

Innovasive Devices, Inc. 800-435-6001
734 Forest St, Marlborough, MA 01752

Karl Storz Endoscopy-America Inc. 800-421-0837
600 Corporate Pointe, Culver City, CA 90230

Mahe International Inc. 800-294-7946
468 Craighead St, Nashville, TN 37204

PESSARY, VAGINAL *(Obstetrics/Gyn) 85HHW*

Calmia Medical, Inc. 416-441-9009
7-15 Lesmill Rd, Toronto M3B 2T3 Canada
Vaginal pessary

Milex Products, Inc. 800-621-1278
4311 N Normandy Ave, Chicago, IL 60634
Prolapse kit, $50 to $32.00. Incontinence pessaries kit, $50 to $39.00 per unit.

Ob Specialties, Inc. 800-325-6644
1799 Northwood Ct, Oakland, CA 94611
Vaginal support system.

Premier Medical Products 888-PREMUSA
1710 Romano Dr, Plymouth Meeting, PA 19462
Ring, Donut, Gellhorn, Cube and Fitting Set.

R Medical Supply 800-882-7578
620 Valley Forge Rd Ste F, Hillsborough, NC 27278

PH PAPER, OBSTETRIC *(Obstetrics/Gyn) 85LNW*

Edmund Industrial Optics — 800-363-1992
101 E Gloucester Pike, Barrington, NJ 08007

Fil-Chem, Inc. — 919-788-0909
PO Box 90833, Raleigh, NC 27675
Not obstetric.

PH RATE MEASUREMENT, CARBON-DIOXIDE
(Chemistry) 75JFL

Abbott Point Of Care Inc. — 609-443-9300
104 Windsor Center Dr, East Windsor, NJ 08520
Total carbon dioxide.

Analytical Measurements, Inc. — 800-635-5580
100 Hoffman Pl, Hillside, NJ 07205
$850.00 per unit (standard).

Carolina Liquid Chemistries Corp. — 800-471-7272
510 W Central Ave Ste C, Brea, CA 92821
Co2 buffer.

Genchem, Inc. — 714-529-1616
510 W Central Ave Ste D, Brea, CA 92821
Co2 reagent.

Vital Diagnostics Inc. — 714-672-3553
1075 W Lambert Rd Ste D, Brea, CA 92821
Various total carbon dioxide reagents.

PHACOEMULSIFICATION SYSTEM *(Ophthalmology) 86WQT*

Alcon Research, Ltd. — 800-862-5266
6201 South Fwy, Fort Worth, TX 76134

Allergan — 800-366-6554
2525 Dupont Dr, Irvine, CA 92612
4 PLUS phacoemulsification unit with I/A, phaco, cautery and vitrectomy functions.

American Optisurgical Inc. — 800-576-1266
25501 Arctic Ocean Dr, Lake Forest, CA 92630
Phaco-compatible handpieces for Alcon Legacy, Ten Thousand, MacKool, Allergan Sovereign, Series 4, OMS, Millennium, SIStem and Odyssey. Phaco U/S tips, tubing (both reusable and disposable, sterile and non-sterile), T-fittings, tip wrenches, I/A handpieces, I/A tips, diathermy cables, pencil and forceps, vitrectomy cutters and sleeves, phacoemulsification systems for Optikon Pulsar, P4000. AOI Horizon phacoemulsification system, Mentor SIStem and Odyssey phacoemulsification system. QuickRinse automated instrument rinsing system and MK QuickRinse automated microsurgical instrument care system. Phaco handpiece refurbish and I/A handle and tip repairs. Service contracts.

Bausch & Lomb Surgical — 636-255-5051
3365 Tree Court Ind Blvd, Saint Louis, MO 63122

Biomedics, Inc. — 949-458-1998
23322 Peralta Dr Ste 11, Laguna Hills, CA 92653
also Vitrectomy Units. [Alcon & Storz]

Lake Region Manufacturing, Inc. — 952-448-5111
340 Lake Hazeltine Dr, Chaska, MN 55318
Phaco tips contract manufacturing.

Medical Technical Products — 949-551-4762
14980 Sand Canyon Ave Ste 200, Irvine, CA 92618

PHACOFRAGMENTATION UNIT *(Ophthalmology) 86HQC*

A.M.O. Puerto Rico Manufacturing, Inc — 714-247-8656
Rd. 402, Km. 4.2, Anasco, PR 00610
Various.

Accellent Inc. — 866-899-1392
100 Fordham Rd, Wilmington, MA 01887

Alcon Manufacturing, Ltd. — 817-551-6813
714 Columbia Ave, Sinking Spring, PA 19608
Various models of operating room instrumentation for ocular surgery.

Bausch & Lomb Surgical — 636-255-5051
3365 Tree Court Ind Blvd, Saint Louis, MO 63122

Benjamin Biomedical, Inc. — 727-343-5503
3125 Tyrone Blvd N, Saint Petersburg, FL 33710
Ultrasonic phaco handpiece.

Biomedics, Inc. — 949-458-1998
23322 Peralta Dr Ste 11, Laguna Hills, CA 92653

Circuit Tree Medical, Inc. — 626-303-7902
1911 Walker Ave, Monrovia, CA 91016
The wave phaco.

PHACOFRAGMENTATION UNIT *(cont'd)*

Customed, Inc. — 787-801-0101
Calle Igualdad #7, Fajardo, PR 00738
Cataract pack ojos inc. (sterile).

Fibra-Sonics, A Division Of Misonix, Inc. — 631-694-9555
1938 New Hwy, Farmingdale, NY 11735
Phaco fragmentation + vitreous aspiration device.

Imonti And Associates Inc., M. — 949-248-1058
25707 Compass Way, San Juan Capistrano, CA 92675
MASKET ERGO TIP Bent PHACO tip with bend outside of the eye high energy at low power, reduced bubbles, parallel to the iris. TIP WRENCH ALCON LEGACY for removal of Phaco Tip on Alcon Legacy Phaco Handpiece. PRO-TOOL Nose Cone Repair Tool on Dented Alcon Legacy Phaco Handpiece. PHACOFRAGMENTATION TIP The Conical highly polished bubble free phaco tip compatible with most systems. PHACOFRAGMENTATION TIP Conical 'Plus' the alternative phaco tip for the Alcon Legacy highly polished finish to reduce bubbles and friction.

Medical Cables, Inc. — 800-314-51111
1365 Logan Ave, Costa Mesa, CA 92626
Phaco Emulsification Handpiece, used in ophthalmology for cataract surgery.

Medical Technical Products — 949-551-4762
14980 Sand Canyon Ave Ste 200, Irvine, CA 92618

Microsurgical Technology, Inc. — 425-556-0544
PO Box 2679, Redmond, WA 98073
Phaco Tips and Dewey Radius Phaco Tips. Phaco tips for most phaco handpieces.

Microvision, Inc. — 603-474-5566
34 Folly Mill Rd, Seabrook, NH 03874
Phaco needle.

Milvella Limited — 952-746-[illegible]369
12100 Singletree Ln, Eden Prairie, MN 55344
Phacofragmentation unit.

Nidek, Inc. — 510-226-5700
47651 Westinghouse Dr, Fremont, CA 94539
Phacoemulsification system.

Paradigm Medical Industries, Inc. — 801-977-8970
2355 S 1070 W, Salt Lake City, UT 84119
Phaco system with various devices & accessories.

Solos Endoscopy — 800-388-6445
65 Sprague St # B, Boston/dedham Commerce Park, Boston, MA 02[illegible]36
Phacofragmentation system.

Staar Surgical Co. — 800-292-7902
1911 Walker Ave, Monrovia, CA 91016
Phaco XL Small Incision System

Visx Incorporated, A Subsidiary Of Amo Inc. — 714-247-8656
1328 Kifer Rd, Sunnyvale, CA 94086
Phacofragmentation unit.

PHANTOM, ANTHROPOMORPHIC, NUCLEAR *(Radiology) 90IYP*

Biodex Medical Systems, Inc. — 800-224-6339
20 Ramsey Rd, Shirley, NY 11967

Capintec, Inc. — 800-631-3826
6 Arrow Rd, Ramsey, NJ 07446

Marconi Medical Systems — 800-323-0550
595 Miner Rd, Cleveland, OH 44143

Radiology Support Devices — 800-221-0527
1904 E Dominguez St, Long Beach, CA 90810

PHANTOM, ANTHROPOMORPHIC, RADIOGRAPHIC
(Radiology) 90IXG

Action Products, Inc. — 800-228-7763
954 Sweeney Dr, Hagerstown, MD 21740
$480.10 per set (standard).

Capintec, Inc. — 800-631-3826
6 Arrow Rd, Ramsey, NJ 07446

Computerized Imaging Reference Systems, Inc. — 757-855-2765
2428 Almeda Ave Ste 212, Norfolk, VA 23513
Cirs.

Gammex Rmi — 800-426-6391
PO Box 620327, Middleton, WI 53562

Ge Medical Systems, Llc — 262-548-2355
3000 N Grandview Blvd, W-417, Waukesha, WI 53188
Cardiovascular phantom.

PHANTOM, ANTHROPOMORPHIC, RADIOGRAPHIC *(cont'd)*

Hologic, Inc. 800-343-9729
35 Crosby Dr, Bedford, MA 01730
(HIP); (SPINE); ANTHROPOMORPHIC PHANTOM (BLOCK)

Image Analysis, Inc. 800-548-4849
1380 Burkesville St, Columbia, KY 42728

Medtec 800-842-8688
1401 8th St SE, PO Box 320, Orange City, IA 51041
Water phantom.

Radiology Support Devices 800-221-0527
1904 E Dominguez St, Long Beach, CA 90810
Phantom, radiographic.

Sandstrom Trade & Technology, Inc. 800-699-0745
610 Niagara St., Welland, ONT L3C 1L8 Canada
LUCY high performance quality assurance phantom. Spherical acrylic phantom for multiple imaging modalitics, and stereotactic parameters verification for radiosurgery and radiation therapy. Also available, Multimodality radiographic markers.

Scanditronix - Wellhofer North America 901-386-2242
3150 Stage Post Dr Ste 110, Bartlett, TN 38133
WELLHOFER WATER PHANTOM radiation therapy beam data acquisition systems. Priced from $50,000 up to $175,000. SCANDITRONIX WATER PHANTOM radiation therapy beam data acquisition systems priced from $25,000 to $150,000.

Standard Imaging, Inc. 608-831-0025
3120 Deming Way, Middleton, WI 53562
Imaging phantom.

Supertech, Inc. 800-654-1054
PO Box 186, Elkhart, IN 46515
Anthropomorphic Teaching devices. Accurate and reproducible means of instructing radiologic technologic students.

The Phantom Laboratory, Inc. 800-525-1190
PO Box 511, Salem, NY 12865
Various types of anthropomorphic radiographic phantoms.

PHANTOM, COMPUTED AXIAL TOMOGRAPHY (CAT, CT)
(Radiology) 90VHB

Capintec, Inc. 800-631-3826
6 Arrow Rd, Ramsey, NJ 07446

Gammex Rmi 800-426-6391
PO Box 620327, Middleton, WI 53562
CT Phantom can be used for routine quality assurance tests.

Image Analysis, Inc. 800-548-4849
1380 Burkesville St, Columbia, KY 42728

Radcal Corp. 800-423-7169
426 W Duarte Rd, Monrovia, CA 91016
CT Phantoms - $795 for head; $1265 for body.

Ultra-Cal, Inc. 760-741-7207
3014 Laurashawn Ln, Escondido, CA 92026
5 models: $125 to $945.

PHANTOM, DENTAL, RADIOGRAPHIC *(Dental And Oral) 76VDR*

Cone Instruments, Inc. 800-321-6964
5201 Naiman Pkwy, Solon, OH 44139

PHANTOM, DIGITAL SUBTRACTION ANGIOGRAPHY (DSA)
(Radiology) 90WNE

Ultra-Cal, Inc. 760-741-7207
3014 Laurashawn Ln, Escondido, CA 92026
$1,400/unit.

PHANTOM, FLOOD SOURCE, NUCLEAR *(Radiology) 90IYQ*

Biodex Medical Systems, Inc. 800-224-6339
20 Ramsey Rd, Shirley, NY 11967

Capintec, Inc. 800-631-3826
6 Arrow Rd, Ramsey, NJ 07446

International Isotopes Inc. 800-699-3108
4137 Commerce Cir, Idaho Falls, ID 83401
Various types of flood sources, sheet sources, 6-57 phantoms.

Marconi Medical Systems 800-323-0550
595 Miner Rd, Cleveland, OH 44143

Qsa-Global Inc. 781-272-2000
40 North Ave, Burlington, MA 01803
Flood source.

Sanders Medical Products, Inc. 865-588-8998
520 Bearden Park Cir, Knoxville, TN 37919
Various.

PHANTOM, MAMMOGRAPHIC *(Radiology) 90VGI*

Gammex Rmi 800-426-6391
PO Box 620327, Middleton, WI 53562

Owens Scientific Inc. 281-394-2311
23230 Sandsage Ln, Katy, TX 77494

Radiology Support Devices 800-221-0527
1904 E Dominguez St, Long Beach, CA 90810

Supertech, Inc. 800-654-1054
PO Box 186, Elkhart, IN 46515
Mammographic Accreditation Phantom, Mammo QC Compliance Kit, Mammo Service Tech Kit, Biopsy Phantom, and more

PHANTOM, NMR/MRI *(Radiology) 90VKD*

Ultra-Cal, Inc. 760-741-7207
3014 Laurashawn Ln, Escondido, CA 92026
$1,895/unit.

PHANTOM, RADIOTHERAPY *(Radiology) 90VHI*

Capintec, Inc. 800-631-3826
6 Arrow Rd, Ramsey, NJ 07446

Radiology Support Devices 800-221-0527
1904 E Dominguez St, Long Beach, CA 90810

Supertech, Inc. 800-654-1054
PO Box 186, Elkhart, IN 46515
Teaching devices. Accurate and reproducible means of instructing radiologic technology students.

PHANTOM, ULTRASOUND *(Radiology) 90RKQ*

Ats Laboratories, Inc. 203-579-2700
404 Knowlton St, Bridgeport, CT 06608
Multipurpose tissue mimicking phantoms are recommended for most clinical QA programs to evaluate routine performance of any ultrasound diagnostic imaging system.

Cone Instruments, Inc. 800-321-6964
5201 Naiman Pkwy, Solon, OH 44139

Gammex Rmi 800-426-6391
PO Box 620327, Middleton, WI 53562
RMI 411 tissue-mimicking phantom is acoustically correct and provides all targets necessary for standard QC tests. Also available RMI 403, 404, 405, 408.

Ultra-Cal, Inc. 760-741-7207
3014 Laurashawn Ln, Escondido, CA 92026
8 models: $275-$995.

PHARYNGOSCOPE *(Ear/Nose/Throat) 77RKR*

Clinimed, Incorporated 877-CLINIMED
303 Markus Ct, Sandy Brae Industrial Park, Newark, DE 19713

Mahe International Inc. 800-294-7946
468 Craighead St, Nashville, TN 37204

PHENYLPHOSPHATE, ALKALINE PHOSPHATASE OR ISOENZYMES *(Chemistry) 75CKF*

Biomerieux Inc. 800-682-2666
100 Rodolphe St, Durham, NC 27712

Quidel Corp. 858-552-1100
2981 Copper Rd, Santa Clara, CA 95051
Alkphase-b assay kit.

PHLEBOGRAPH, IMPEDANCE *(Cardiovascular) 74DQB*

U.F.I. 805-772-1203
545 Main St Ste C2, Morro Bay, CA 93442
$6,250 to $10,250 for Model 2994 (1 to 4 channels).

PHONOCARDIOGRAPH *(Cardiovascular) 74DQC*

Biosignetics Corporation 603-303-0708
29 Downing Ct, Exeter, NH 03833
Various types of phonocardiographs.

Stethographics, Inc. 508-320-2841
1153 Centre St Ste 4381, Jamaica Plain, MA 02130
Phonocardiograph.

Zargis Medical Corp. 609-488-4608
1 Atlantic St, 1st Floo, Stamford, CT 06901
Various models of phonocardiograph.

PHOSPHATASE, ACID *(Hematology) 81JCI*

Beckman Coulter, Inc. 800-635-3497
740 W 83rd St, Hialeah, FL 33014
$0.17 per test.

Biomerieux Inc. 800-682-2666
100 Rodolphe St, Durham, NC 27712

PHOSPHATASE, ACID *(cont'd)*

Dade Behring, Inc. 800-948-3233
1717 Deerfield Rd, Deerfield, IL 60015

Genzyme Corp. 800-325-2436
160 Christian St, Oxford, CT 06478
Total and prostatic assay.

Raichem, Division Of Hemagen Diagnostics, Inc. 800-438-6100
8225 Mercury Ct, San Diego, CA 92111
Acid phosphatase reagent.

Sigma-Aldrich Manufacturing, Llc 314-286-6600
3500 Dekalb St, Saint Louis, MO 63118
Acid phosphatase, histochemical demonstration of #385.

PHOSPHATASE, ALKALINE *(Hematology) 81JCJ*

Beckman Coulter, Inc. 800-635-3497
740 W 83rd St, Hialeah, FL 33014
$0.11 per test.

Beckman Coulter, Inc. 800-742-2345
250 S Kraemer Blvd, PO Box 8000, Brea, CA 92821

Biomerieux Inc. 800-682-2666
100 Rodolphe St, Durham, NC 27712

Biozyme Laboratories International Ltd. 800-423-8199
9939 Hibert St Ste 101, San Diego, CA 92131

Dade Behring, Inc. 800-948-3233
1717 Deerfield Rd, Deerfield, IL 60015

Diasorin Inc 800-328-1482
1951 Northwestern Ave S, PO Box 285, Stillwater, MN 55082

Genzyme Corp. 800-325-2436
160 Christian St, Oxford, CT 06478
pNPP kinetic.

Raichem, Division Of Hemagen Diagnostics, Inc. 800-438-6100
8225 Mercury Ct, San Diego, CA 92111
Alkaline phosphatase reagent.

Stanbio Laboratory, Inc. 830-249-0772
1261 N Main St, Boerne, TX 78006
$63.50 for 15 x 15ml buffered substrate (powder) and diluent (1 x 250ml).

PHOSPHORIC-TUNGSTIC ACID (SPECTROPHOTOMETRIC), CHLORIDE *(Chemistry) 75CHG*

Intersect Systems, Inc. 360-577-1062
1152 3rd Avenue, Suite D & E, Longview, WA 98632
Non-mercuric chloride.

Synermed Intl., Inc. 317-896-1565
17408 Tiller Ct Ste 1900, Westfield, IN 46074
Chloride reagent kit.

PHOSPHORUS REAGENT (TEST SYSTEM) *(Chemistry) 75CEO*

Abbott Diagnostics Div. 626-440-0700
820 Mission St, South Pasadena, CA 91030
Phosphorus.

Beckman Coulter, Inc. 800-635-3497
740 W 83rd St, Hialeah, FL 33014
$0.05 per test.

Biomerieux Inc. 800-682-2666
100 Rodolphe St, Durham, NC 27712

Caldon Bioscience, Inc. 909-628-9944
2100 S Reservoir St, Pomona, CA 91766
Phosphorus reagent.

Caldon Biotech, Inc. 757-224-0177
2251 Rutherford Rd, Carlsbad, CA 92008
Phosphorus reagent.

Carolina Liquid Chemistries Corp. 800-471-7272
510 W Central Ave Ste C, Brea, CA 92821
Phos.

Diagnostic Specialties 732-549-4011
4 Leonard St, Metuchen, NJ 08840
$41.50 per unit (standard).

Genchem, Inc. 714-529-1616
510 W Central Ave Ste D, Brea, CA 92821
Phosphorus reagent.

Genzyme Corp. 800-325-2436
160 Christian St, Oxford, CT 06478
Phosphomolybdate, endpoint.

Health Chem Diagnostics Llc 954-979-3845
3341 W McNab Rd, Pompano Beach, FL 33069
Phosphomolybdate (colorimetric), inorganic phosphorus.

PHOSPHORUS REAGENT (TEST SYSTEM) *(cont'd)*

Jas Diagnostics, Inc. 305-418-2320
7220 NW 58th St, Miami, FL 33166
Phosphorus.

Medical Chemical Corp. 800-424-9394
19430 Van Ness Ave, Torrance, CA 90501
$22.50 per unit (standard).

Raichem, Division Of Hemagen Diagnostics, Inc. 800-438-6100
8225 Mercury Ct, San Diego, CA 92111
Inorganic phosphorus reagent.

Sandare Intl., Inc. 972-293-7440
910 Kck Way, Cedar Hill, TX 75104
Phosphorus nolybdate reagent.

Stanbio Laboratory, Inc. 830-249-0772
1261 N Main St, Boerne, TX 78006
$31.50 for 125 test kits with reagent and standard.

Sterling Diagnostics, Inc. 800-637-2661
36645 Metro Ct, Sterling Heights, MI 48312
Phosphorus reagent set.

Synermed Intl., Inc. 317-896-1565
17408 Tiller Ct Ste 1900, Westfield, IN 46074
Phosphorus reagent kit.

Teco Diagnostics 714-693-7788
1268 N Lakeview Ave, Anaheim, CA 92807
Phosphorus (inorganic) reagent.

Vital Diagnostics Inc. 714-672-3553
1075 W Lambert Rd Ste D, Brea, CA 92821
Various inorganic phosphorus reagents.

PHOSPHOTUNGSTATE REDUCTION, URIC ACID *(Chemistry) 75CDH*

Biomerieux Inc. 800-682-2666
100 Rodolphe St, Durham, NC 27712

Diagnostic Specialties 732-549-4011
4 Leonard St, Metuchen, NJ 08840
$45.50 per 1000ml.

Health Chem Diagnostics Llc 954-979-3845
3341 W McNab Rd, Pompano Beach, FL 33069
Acid, uric, phosphotungstate reduction.

Medical Chemical Corp. 800-424-9394
19430 Van Ness Ave, Torrance, CA 90501
$21.50 per unit.

PHOTOCOAGULATOR *(Ophthalmology) 86HQB*

Coherent, Inc. 800-527-3786
5100 Patrick Henry Dr, Santa Clara, CA 95054

Nidek, Inc. 510-226-5700
47651 Westinghouse Dr, Fremont, CA 94539
Ophthalmic photocoagulator.

Synergetics Usa, Inc. 800-600-0565
3845 Corporate Centre Dr, O Fallon, MO 63368
Various.

Transamerican Technologies International 800-322-7373
2246 Camino Ramon, San Ramon, CA 94583
ACCU-BEAM, Laser Block Beam Splitters. For use with a surgical laser and microscope to provide protection to the observer from laser radiation.

PHOTOFLUOROSCOPE (CARDIAC CATHETERIZATION) *(Radiology) 90RKW*

Precise Optics/Pme, Inc. 800-242-3604
239 S Fehr Way, Bay Shore, NY 11706

PHOTOKERATOSCOPE *(Ophthalmology) 86HJA*

Jedmed Instruments Co. 314-845-3770
5416 Jedmed Ct, Saint Louis, MO 63129

PHOTOMETER *(Chemistry) 75RKX*

Air Techniques International 410-363-9696
11403 Cronridge Dr, Owings Mills, MD 21117
Portable photometer #TDA-2G features an audible alarm, blue LED light source, 0.0001% sensitivity, internal reference for DOP, PAO and other aerosols, RS-232 port for data logging capability and is microprocessor controlled.

Analytical Spectral Devices, Inc. 303-444-6522
2555 55th St Ste A, Boulder, CO 80301

PHOTOMETER *(cont'd)*

Awareness Technology, Inc. 722-283-6540
1935 SW Martin Hwy, Palm City, FL 34990
$2,600 to $4,800 per non-dedicated photometer, depending on features of various models. $2,595 for STAT FAX 1904 preprogrammed for rate and endpoint assay analysis; $4,800 for Stat Fax 3300 with result storage ability; also, $95 for REDI-CHECK photometer QC kit. $1,000 for Mosquito aspiration flow-cell accessory.

Beckman Coulter, Inc. 800-742-2345
250 S Kraemer Blvd, PO Box 8000, Brea, CA 92821

Biomerieux Inc. 800-682-2666
100 Rodolphe St, Durham, NC 27712

Brain Power, Inc. 800-327-2250
4470 SW 74th Ave, Miami, FL 33155
Measures lens transmissions of UV and visible light. Digital display and 3 signal lights indicate danger, caution, and safe readings.

Continental Hydrodyne Systems, Inc. 800-543-9283
1025 Mary Laidley Dr, Covington, KY 41017
Filter photometer used with test reagents to analyze water samples. AQUAKING patented colorimeter used to analyze water samples for over 60 different substances.

Hyperion, Inc. 305-238-3020
14100 SW 136th St, Miami, FL 33186
$965.00-$9,000.00.

International Light Technologies, Inc. 978-818-6180
10 Technology Dr, Peabody, MA 01960
Our IL1700 Photometer with SHD033/Y/W has a measurement range 1.1(10-6) to 2.2(10+3) lux, or with the SED033/Y/W: 7.9(10-4) to 7.9(10+5) lux. We also offer the IL1400A or IL1400BL (with a back lit display) which measures 167 mlux to 583 klux when used with our SCL110 illuminance probe. Luminance, luminous flux and luminous intensity probes are also available as well as a full line of low cost hand held spectroradiometers which can not only measure illuminance, they can also measure luminance, chromaticity, corrected color temperature, dominant wavelength and purity.

Labsphere, Inc. 603-927-4266
231 Shaker St., North Sutton, NH 03260-9986
Handheld and benchtop photometers to measure the luminous flux output of fiber illuminators, small lamps and LED's.

Li-Cor, Inc. 800-645-4267
4647 Superior St, Lincoln, NE 68504
Radiometer photometers - instantaneous & integrated. Automated DNA analysis and sequencing. Proteomics. Genomics.

Orbeco Analytical Systems, Inc. 800-922-5242
185 Marine St, Farmingdale, NY 11735
The Analyst Model 975 MP-10, $895.00, is a 94 test portable water analyzer with data storage for 2000 test results, output printer or computer. Mini Analysts Series 942 include 34 specific test portable water analyzers. Direct reading digital display. One-touch operation. Chlorine $249.00, Lead or Cyanide $299.00, and all other 61 models, $259.00 each.

Photo Research, Inc. 818-341-5151
9731 Topanga Canyon Pl, Chatsworth, CA 91311
PRITCHARD $24,000.00 per unit (standard). PR 880

Spectronics Corporation 800-274-8888
956 Brush Hollow Rd, Westbury, NY 11590

Strategic Diagnostics Inc. 800-544-8881
111 Pendacar Dr., Newark, DE 19702
System prices starting at $15,931 for MICROTOX Model 500 toxicity test system; real time measurement of toxicity within 30 min.

PHOTOMETER, FLAME, GENERAL USE *(Toxicology) 91DMW*

Buck Scientific, Inc. 800-562-5566
58 Fort Point St, Norwalk, CT 06855

Myco Instrumentation Source, Inc. 425-228-4239
PO Box 354, Renton, WA 98057

Spectron Corp. 425-827-9317
934 S Burlington Blvd # 603, Burlington, WA 98233
Reconditioned equipment.

PHOTOMETER, FLAME, LITHIUM *(Chemistry) 75JIH*

Thermo Fisher Scientific Inc. 781-622-1000
81 Wyman St, Waltham, MA 02451

PHOTOMETER, FLAME, POTASSIUM *(Chemistry) 75JGM*

Thermo Fisher Scientific Inc. 781-622-1000
81 Wyman St, Waltham, MA 02451

PHOTOMETER, FLAME, SODIUM *(Chemistry) 75JGT*

Thermo Fisher Scientific Inc. 781-622-1000
81 Wyman St, Waltham, MA 02451

PHOTOMETER, REFLECTANCE *(Chemistry) 75VFU*

Analytical Spectral Devices, Inc. 303-444-6522
2555 55th St Ste A, Boulder, CO 80301

Labsphere, Inc. 603-927-4266
231 Shaker St., North Sutton, NH 03260-9986
Reflectance spectroscopy accessories for most leading analytical spectrophotometers. Also modular component systems for specialized reflectance and transmittance measurement.

PHOTOMETRIC METHOD, IRON (NON-HEME) *(Chemistry) 75JIY*

Caldon Bioscience, Inc. 909-628-9944
2100 S Reservoir St, Pomona, CA 91766
Iron reagent.

Caldon Biotech, Inc. 757-224-0177
2251 Rutherford Rd, Carlsbad, CA 92008
Iron reagent.

Genchem, Inc. 714-529-1616
510 W Central Ave Ste D, Brea, CA 92821
Iron reagent.

Sandare Intl., Inc. 972-293-7440
910 Kck Way, Cedar Hill, TX 75104
No common name listed.

Vital Diagnostics Inc. 714-672-3553
1075 W Lambert Rd Ste D, Brea, CA 92821
Various total iron reagents.

PHOTOMETRIC METHOD, MAGNESIUM *(Chemistry) 75JGJ*

Abbott Diagnostics Div. 626-440-0700
820 Mission St, South Pasadena, CA 91030
Multiple.

Caldon Bioscience, Inc. 909-628-9944
2100 S Reservoir St, Pomona, CA 91766
Magnesium.

Caldon Biotech, Inc. 757-224-0177
2251 Rutherford Rd, Carlsbad, CA 92008
Magnesium.

Carolina Liquid Chemistries Corp. 800-471-7272
510 W Central Ave Ste C, Brea, CA 92821
Mg.

Genchem, Inc. 714-529-1616
510 W Central Ave Ste D, Brea, CA 92821
Magnesium reagent.

Genzyme Corp. 800-325-2436
160 Christian St, Oxford, CT 06478
Xylidyl blue, endpoint.

Jas Diagnostics, Inc. 305-418-2320
7220 NW 58th St, Miami, FL 33166
Magnesium.

Raichem, Division Of Hemagen Diagnostics, Inc. 800-438-6100
8225 Mercury Ct, San Diego, CA 92111
Colorimetric magnesium reagent.

Sterling Diagnostics, Inc. 800-637-2661
36645 Metro Ct, Sterling Heights, MI 48312
Magnesium reagent set.

Synermed Intl., Inc. 317-896-1565
17408 Tiller Ct Ste 1900, Westfield, IN 46074
Magnesium reagent kit.

Teco Diagnostics 714-693-7788
1268 N Lakeview Ave, Anaheim, CA 92807
Magnesium.

Vital Diagnostics Inc. 714-672-3553
1075 W Lambert Rd Ste D, Brea, CA 92821
Various magnesium reagents.

PHOTOSTIMULATOR *(General) 80RKY*

Lkc Technologies, Inc. 800-638-7055
2 Professional Dr Ste 222, Gaithersburg, MD 20879
Standard-size, fully automatic Ganzfeld available as a stand-alone model capable of attaching to non-LKC systems or as integrated models attached to either a UTAS-E3000mf or an EPIC-4000. Kurbisfeld (Mini-Ganzfeld) stimulators for electroreturnography and electrooculography are available in stand-alone and integrated versions. Kurbisfeld avaialbe in two models. The LKC MGS-2 is a white-only flash model and the LKC CMGS-1 is a color Mini-Ganzfeld model.

PHOTOSTIMULATOR, AC-POWERED *(Ophthalmology) 86HLX*

Cadwell Laboratories 800-245-3001
909 N Kellogg St, Kennewick, WA 99336
Included with Easy II EEG system.

Cardinal Healthcare 209, Inc. 610-862-0800
5225 Verona Rd, Fitchburg, WI 53711
Visual stimulator.

Electro-Diagnostic Imaging, Inc. 650-367-9293
200F Twin Dolphin Dr, Redwood City, CA 94065
Electro retinography device.

PHOTOTHERAPY UNIT (BILIRUBIN LAMP) *(General) 80RKZ*

Bulbworks, Inc. 800-334-2852
80 N Dell Ave Unit 5, Kenvil, NJ 07847
Replacement Lamps For All Types Of Bilirubin Units

Burton Medical Products, Inc. 800-444-9909
21100 Lassen St, Chatsworth, CA 91311

Interlectric Corp. 800-722-2184
1401 Lexington Ave, Warren, PA 16365

Medela, Inc. 800-435-8316
1101 Corporate Dr, McHenry, IL 60050
BILIBED Phototherapy Unit - self-contained, can be used in hospital bassinet to encourage rooming-in of mother and baby as well as a home care unit. BILICOMBI - washable and disposable, used with BiliBed to keep infant secure and warm.

O&M Enterprise 847-258-4515
641 Chelmsford Ln, Elk Grove Village, IL 60007
PHOTOTHERAPY UNIT AND EYE-MASK

Olympic Medical Corp. 206-767-3500
5900 1st Ave S, Seattle, WA 98108
$1993.50 per unit (standard).

PHOTOTHERAPY UNIT, NEONATAL *(General) 80LBI*

International Hospital Supply Co. 800-398-9450
6914 Canby Ave Ste 105, Reseda, CA 91335

Lumitex, Inc. 800-969-5483
8443 Dow Cir, Strongsville, OH 44136
Phototherapy lamp.

Ohmeda Medical 800-345-2700
8880 Gorman Rd, Laurel, MD 20723
Fiberoptic device and halogen lamp for treating infant jaundice.

Physician Engineered Products, Inc. 800-622-6240
103 Smith St, Fryeburg, ME 04037
Bili light.

PHOTOTIMER, RADIOGRAPHIC MOBILE *(Radiology) 90VGG*

Advanced Instrument Development, Inc. 800-243-9729
2545 Curtiss St, Downers Grove, IL 60515
MOBIL-AID automatic exposure control system using exit-type ion chamber, available for numerous mobile/portable generators. EXPOS-AID automatic exposure control system for stationary generators, accepts MOBIL-AID AEC phototiming paddle - available in several configurations plus optional single-phase forced extinction unit. ROTOR-AID rotor controller, heavy-duty, high- and low-speed tube starter. Available for single (radiographic) or multiple tubes (radiographic and fluoroscopic).

Electronic Control Concepts 800-847-9729
160 Partition St, Saugerties, NY 12477
Exposure Time Meter / Pulse Counter

PHYSICIAN REGISTRY *(General) 80TDQ*

Crest Healthcare Supply 800-328-8908
195 3rd St, Dassel, MN 55325

Kelkom Systems 800-985-3556
418 MacArthur Ave, Redwood City, CA 94063
Staff Vector light message communication system for combination doctor/nurse follower, room status, and emergency call.

Signalcom Systems, Inc. 650-692-1056
1499 Bayshore Hwy Ste 134, Burlingame, CA 94010
Computer-controlled personnel registry system.

Stat-Chek Company 800-248-6618
PO Box 9636, Bend, OR 97708

Talk-A-Phone Co. 773-539-1100
5013 N Kedzie Ave, Chicago, IL 60625

Visicomm Industries 866-221-3131
911A Milwaukee Ave, Burlington, WI 53105
Green LED - doctor is in; steady red LED - message in voice-mail; blinking red - call operator; amber LED - call referral.

PICK, MASSAGING *(Dental And Oral) 76JET*

Abrasive Technology, Inc. 740-548-4100
8400 Green Meadows Dr N, Lewis Center, OH 43035
Toothpicks.

Dental Concepts Llc 800-592-6661
90 N Broadway, Irvington, NY 10533
Brushpicks.

Dentek Oral Care, Inc. 865-983-1300
307 Excellence Way, Maryville, TN 37801
Interdental stimulator.

Icon Llc 501-374-2929
8 Ten Tee Dr, Maumelle, AR 72113
Pick, massager.

Johnson & Johnson Consumer Products, Inc. 908-874-1402
185 Tabor Rd, Morris Plains, NJ 07950
Plaque remover.

L.A.K. Enterprises, Inc. 800-824-3112
423 Broadway Ste 501, Millbrae, CA 94030
Various massaging pick or tip for oral hygiene.

Marquis Dental Mfg. Co. 303-344-5222
15370 Smith Rd Unit H, Aurora, CO 80011
Perio-aid toothpick holder.

Sunstar Butler 800-J BUTLER
4635 W Foster Ave, Chicago, IL 60630

Ultradent Products, Inc. 801-553-4586
505 W 10200 S, South Jordan, UT 84095
Massaging pick or tip for oral hygiene.

Water Pik, Inc. 970-221-6129
1730 E Prospect Rd, Fort Collins, CO 80525
Flosser.

PICK, MICROSURGICAL EAR *(Ear/Nose/Throat) 77JYT*

Aesculap Implant Systems Inc. 1-800-234-9179
3773 Corporate Pkwy, Center Valley, PA 18034

Bausch & Lomb Surgical 636-255-5051
3365 Tree Court Ind Blvd, Saint Louis, MO 63122

Biomet Microfixation Inc. 800-874-7711
1520 Tradeport Dr, Jacksonville, FL 32218
Pick, microsurgical, ear.

George Tiemann & Co. 800-843-6266
25 Plant Ave, Hauppauge, NY 11788

Jedmed Instruments Co. 314-845-3770
5416 Jedmed Ct, Saint Louis, MO 63129

Nbn Products, L.L.C. 800-792-9795
1310 Amesbury Ave, Liberty, MO 64068
Pressure earrings, compression earrings.

PILLOW *(General) 80WLC*

Alimed, Inc. 800-225-2610
297 High St, Dedham, MA 02026
Elbow pillows help to reduce pressure and provide comfort. Snooze pillows keep one's head erect while sleeping in a seated position.

Atd-American Co. 800-523-2300
135 Greenwood Ave, Wyncote, PA 19095

Avid Products 888-575-AVID
72 Johnny Cake Hill Rd, Aquidneck Industrial Park, Middletown, RI 02842
AVID reusable and disposable pillows. Disposable pillows are made of flame retardant polyester. Reusable pillows are made of a patented fluid resistant material

Bean Products 800-726-8365
1500 S Western Ave Ste 4BN, Chicago, IL 60608
Sleeping Bean, therapeutic cylindrical shaped body pillows and positioning aids in three sizes. Relieves bones, joints, skin and tissue from the compression of gravity. Helps prevent bedsores. Improves circulation and spine alignment.

Body Therapeutics, Div. Of I-Rep, Inc. 800-530-3722
508 Chaney St Ste 13, Lake Elsinore, CA 92530

Care Line, Inc. 800-251-1157
2210 Lake Rd, Greenbrier, TN 37073
Disposable and reusable menus.

Comfort Care Products Corp. 803-321-0020
258 Industrial Park Rd, Newberry, SC 29108
NOVEX Pillow. Novex patented ticking which is antimicrobial, flame retardant and filled with Flexi-Lon 2000 Antimicrobial Polyester fiber fill. FLEXI- PRO's complete line of positioning pillows (items).

PILLOW *(cont'd)*

Corflex, Inc. 800-426-7353
669 E Industrial Park Dr, Manchester, NH 03109
MEDIC-AIR air-filled cushions that provide adjustable support for the body.

Crest Healthcare Supply 800-328-8908
195 3rd St, Dassel, MN 55325
Pillow speaker unit for calling a nurse.

Elginex Corporation 800-279-3762
270 Eisenhower Ln N Unit 4-A, Lombard, IL 60148
Lumbar roll and back support pillows.

Essential Medical Supply, Inc. 800-826-8423
6420 Hazeltine National Dr, Orlando, FL 32822
E-Z SLEEP.

Galaxy Medical Manufacturing Co. 800-876-4599
5411 Sheila St, Commerce, CA 90040

Herculite Products, Inc. 800-772-0036
PO Box 435, Emigsville, PA 17318

Hermell Products, Inc. 800-233-2342
9 Britton Dr, PO Box 7345, Bloomfield, CT 06002
Lumbar cushion (molded foam) pillow. VISCO ELASTIC PILLOW Shaped to U Pillow. New viscoelastic pillow continuosly self-adjusts to your body's shape, weight and temperature. Two lobe design lets you choose wide or narrow edge. ORTHOPEDIC PILLOW Softeze Orthopedic pillow Our uniquely contoured orthopedic pillow has a raised outer edge and a concave center to properly support your head and neck as you sleep. It was specially designed to keep your spine correctly alligned, reducing muscle tension so you awake relaxed and refreshed. Ideal for side or back sleeping.

Hos-Pillow Corp. 800-468-7874
1011 Campus Dr, Mundelein, IL 60060
$1.65 to $16.50 ea. for disposable, reusable, polyester, or feather pillow; also, anti-bacterial, self-deodorizing and fire-retardant.

Jms Converters Inc Dba Sabee Products & Stanford Prof Prod 215-396-3302
67 Buck Rd Ste B7, Huntingdon Valley, PA 19006
Disposable pillow covers.

Lohmann & Rauscher, Inc. 800-279-3863
6001 SW 6th Ave Ste 101, Topeka, KS 66615

Medic-Air, A Division Of Corflex, Inc. 800-426-7353
669 E Industrial Park Dr, Manchester, NH 03109
MEDIC-AIR air-filled cushions that provide adjustable support.

Morrison Medical 800-438-6677
3735 Paragon Dr, Columbus, OH 43228
Disposable or STAPH-CHEK.

Muffin Enterprises, Inc. 800-338-9041
2 Brenneman Cir Ste 2, Mechanicsburg, PA 17050
SIR KOFF-A-LOT (Heart and Lung)or TUMMY TEDDY (Abdominal/Bariatric)Teddy Bear Pillow provides support for post-operative patients with a personal touch. KOFF HEART (Heart and Lung) heart-shaped designed splint provides firm, even, and effective sternal support for recovering patients in order to minimize post-operative respiratory complications, while its pricing structure meets the healthcare industry's need for cost efficiency. Made in the USA. KOFF KUSHION (Heart/Lung) oval-shaped splint provides the same support as our Koff Heart splint, can be used as an educational tool, and is also very cost efficient. Made in the USA.

Obus Forme Ltd. 888-225-7378
550 Hopewell Ave., Toronto, ON M6E 2S6 Canada
NECK & NECK pillow; standard pillow available; back; pregnancy; and L shape pillows.

Roloke Company 800-533-8212
127 W Hazel St, Inglewood, CA 90302
Well-Pil-O neck pillow. Patented modification of Wal-Pil-O, plus memory foam wrapping.

PILLOW *(cont'd)*

Sleep Devices, Inc. 866-935-9166
506 W Cherry St, Kissimmee, FL 34741
The Sona Pillow is designed to help modify sleeping behavior in order to address sleep apnea and snoring. Most people with mild sleep apnea and snoring will experience excellent results with regular use of the Sona Pillow, and it is highly recommended that the Sona Pillow be used for a minimum of 20 days in order for the user to adjust their sleeping behavior, and thereby achieve positive results. The Sona Pillow allows the user to maintain sleep in the side position, using gravity to reduce or eliminate obstruction from the back of the throat. Two inclined surfaces create the shape of the Sona Pillow. One surface is the primary sleeping surface, and there is a flatter, lower surface. When a user places their head on the inclined surface of the Sona Pillow, facing downward, the user is in the proper position for the jaw to be pulled forward by gravity. When the jaw is kept from falling backwards, there is less likelihood of an obstruction in the back of the throat to cause sleep apnea and snoring. The Sona Pillow comes with a washable custom made pillow case that has an arm recess, or sling, sewn on either side of the lower part of the triangular surface. This sling can be used to help train the user to adjust to their improved sleeping position, and because the sling is sewn on both sides of the pillow case, the user can choose to sleep either on their left or right side, and still maintain their head in the proper inclined position on the pillow. The Sona Pillow should be fluffed periodically. This can be done by pressing on the nonstriped surface from the side. With regular usage, it is recommended that the Sona Pillow be replaced annually. Instructions for use of the Sona Pillow are included with the pillow. It also comes with a washable custom pillow case, and a convenient clear plastic travel bag. Additional cases are available through the manufacturer. The Sona Pillow is warranted against manufacturer's defects, and in the unlikely event of a defect, the pillow may be exchanged within 30 days of purchase.www.sonapillow.com

The Neurological Research And Development Group 800-327-6759
115 Rotary Dr, West Hazleton, PA 18202
Over 50 different healthcare pillows.

Thera-P-Cushion 800-567-9926
331 Bowes Rd., #2, Concord, ONT L4K-1J2 Canada

Waterloo Bedding Co. Ltd. 800-203-4293
141 Weber St. S, Waterloo, ONT N2J 2A9 Canada

PILLOW, CERVICAL *(Orthopedics) 87RLE*

Alex Orthopedic, Inc. 800-544-2539
PO Box 201442, Arlington, TX 76006

Allman Products 800-223-6889
21101 Itasca St, Chatsworth, CA 91311

Back Support Systems 800-669-2225
67684 San Andreas St, Desert Hot Springs, CA 92240
CONFOURM, with memory foam, therapeutic neck pillow comes in six sizes, each for $50.00. POLIAIRE hot and cold adjustable self inflating cervical pillow with density options.

Battle Creek Equipment Co. 800-253-0854
307 Jackson St W, Battle Creek, MI 49037
BATTLE CREEK, cervical pillows, $16.95 to $39.95 per unit (standard).

Body Therapeutics, Div. Of I-Rep, Inc. 800-530-3722
508 Chaney St Ste 13, Lake Elsinore, CA 92530

Core Products International, Inc. 800-365-3047
808 Prospect Ave, Osceola, WI 54020
Memory Plus Pillow foam cervical pillow that combines a memory foam top with a resilient foam base. Provides memory conforming benefits with therapeutic value of a foam base not found in other memory foam pillows.

Elginex Corporation 800-279-3762
270 Eisenhower Ln N Unit 4-A, Lombard, IL 60148

Essential Medical Supply, Inc. 800-826-8423
6420 Hazeltine National Dr, Orlando, FL 32822
ECLIPSE.

Herculite Products, Inc. 800-772-0036
PO Box 435, Emigsville, PA 17318

Hermell Products, Inc. 800-233-2342
9 Britton Dr, PO Box 7345, Bloomfield, CT 06002
Contour pillow.

Jobri Llc 800-432-2225
520 N Division St, Konawa, OK 74849
CERV-O-CURVE

PILLOW, CERVICAL *(cont'd)*

Lohmann & Rauscher, Inc. 800-279-3863
6001 SW 6th Ave Ste 101, Topeka, KS 66615

Mccarty's Sacro-Ease Llc 800-635-3557
3329 Industrial Ave S, Coeur D Alene, ID 83815
Peach cervical pillow.

Medi-Dyne Healthcare Products, L.L.C. 800-810-1740
1812 Industrial Blvd, Colleyville, TX 76034
Soothing relief from headache/sinus pain without gel packs or drugs.

Medic-Air, A Division Of Corflex, Inc. 800-426-7353
669 E Industrial Park Dr, Manchester, NH 03109
MEDIC-Air air-filled cervical pillow supports cervical structures while subjects sleep.

Ooltewah Manufacturing 800-251-6040x25
5722 Main St, P.O. Box 587, Ooltewah, TN 37363

Ppr Direct, Inc. 800-526-3668
74 20th St, Brooklyn, NY 11232

Regency Product International 800-845-7931
4732 E 26th St, Vernon, CA 90058
CHIRO PILLOW available in 5 styles.

Roloke 800-533-8212
127 W Hazel St, Inglewood, CA 90302
WELL-PIL-O, PATENTED. '4-IN-1' comfort and support.

Roloke Company 800-533-8212
127 W Hazel St, Inglewood, CA 90302
WAL-PIL-O. ABM multi-positional cervical collar: a five-position collar allows user's head and neck to rest in any of five chosen positions. More stable than other available collars. Also, WELL-PIL-O, which combines the WAL-PIL-O with ROLOFOAM memory foam wrapping and inserts for a softer feel.

Shamrock Medical, Inc. 503-233-5055
3620 SE Powell Blvd, Portland, OR 97202

Slawner Ltd., J. 514-731-3378
5713 Cote Des Neiges Rd., Montreal, QUE H3S 1Y7 Canada

Span-America Medical Systems, Inc. 800-888-6752
70 Commerce Ctr, Greenville, SC 29615
Dorso cervical pillows.

Tempur-Medical, Inc. 888-255-3302
1713 Jaggie Fox Way, Lexington, KY 40511
Tempur-Med Neck Pillow

Tetra Medical Supply Corp. 800-621-4041
6364 W Gross Point Rd, Niles, IL 60714

Zimmer Orthopaedic Surgical Products 800-321-5533
PO Box 10, 200 West Ohio Ave., Dover, OH 44622

PILLOW, CERVICAL(FOR MILD SLEEP APNEA)
(Ear/Nose/Throat) 77MYB

Florida Pillow Company 800-560-1631
1012 Sligh Blvd, Orlando, FL 32806
Apnea pillow.

Nasa Tech Memory Foam Sleep Systems 727-447-0957
8300 Ulmerton Rd Ste 100, Largo, FL 33771
Cervical pillow.

Perry Chemical & Mfg. Co., Inc. 800-592-6614
2335 S 30th St # 47909, PO Box 6419, Lafayette, IN 47909
Pillow positive.

PIN, FIXATION, SMOOTH *(Orthopedics) 87HTY*

Acumed Llc 503-627-9957
5885 NW Cornelius Pass Rd, Hillsboro, OR 97124
Fixation pin.

American Medical Specialties, Inc. 800-808-2877
10650 77th St., Suite 405, Largo, FL 33777
Full line of pins and wires.

Arthrex Manufacturing 239-643-5553
1958 Trade Center Way, Naples, FL 34109
K-wire, pin.

Arthrex, Inc. 239-643-5553
1370 Creekside Blvd, Naples, FL 34108
Fixation pin.

Biomet, Inc. 574-267-6639
56 E Bell Dr, PO Box 587, Warsaw, IN 46582
Fixation pin or rod.

Brasseler Usa - Komet Medical 800-535-6638
1 Brasseler Blvd, Savannah, GA 31419
K-WIRE, STEINMAN pins.

PIN, FIXATION, SMOOTH *(cont'd)*

Brasseler Usa - Medical 805-650-5209
4837 McGrath St Ste J, Ventura, CA 93003
Various.

Depuy Mitek, A Johnson & Johnson Company 800-451-2006
50 Scotland Blvd, Bridgewater, MA 02324
Cross pins.

Depuy Orthopaedics, Inc. 800-473-3789
700 Orthopaedic Dr, P.O. Box 988, Warsaw, IN 46582
Various types of smooth fixation pins.

Depuy-Raynham, A Div. Of Depuy Orthopaedics 800-451-2006
325 Paramount Dr, Raynham, MA 02767
Various types of smooth fixation pins.

Hand Innovations, Llc. 800-800-8188
6303 Blue Lagoon Dr Ste 100, Miami, FL 33126
Intramedullary fixation system for the hand.

International Hospital Supply Co. 800-398-9450
6914 Canby Ave Ste 105, Reseda, CA 91335

Jurgan Development & Mfg., Ltd. 608-231-1742
6018 S Highlands Ave, Madison, WI 53705
Jurgan pin balls.

Kmedic 800-955-0559
190 Veterans Dr, Northvale, NJ 07647

Onyx Medical Corp. 901-323-6699
152 Collins St, Memphis, TN 38112

Rush-Berivon, Inc. 800-251-7874
1010 19th St, P.O. Box 1851, Meridian, MS 39301
$49.00 to $154.00 each for full line, original Rush pin, Rush condyle. 1.6 to 8mm, length 3/4in to 21in.

Simpex Medical, Inc. 800-851-9753
401 E Prospect Ave, Mount Prospect, IL 60056

Small Bone Innovations, Inc. 215-428-1791
1380 S Pennsylvania Ave, Morrisville, PA 19067
Smooth or threaded metallic bone fixation fastener.

Stryker Spine 866-457-7463
2 Pearl Ct, Allendale, NJ 07401

Synthes (Usa) 610-719-5000
35 Airport Rd, Horseheads, NY 14845
Various types and sizes of smooth fixation pins.

Tava Surgical Instruments 805-650-5209
4837 McGrath St Ste J, Ventura, CA 93003
K-Wires & Steinman Pins

Tegra Medical Inc. 508-541-4200
9 Forge Pkwy, Franklin, MA 02038

Warsaw Orthopedic, Inc. 901-396-3133
2500 Silveus Xing, Warsaw, IN 46582
Various styles of steinmann pins and kirshner wires.

Westcon Orthopedics, Inc. 800-382-4975
4 Craig Rd, Neshanic Station, NJ 08853
Pin, capping device, external

Zimmer Holdings, Inc. 800-613-6131
1800 W Center St, PO Box 708, Warsaw, IN 46580

PIN, FIXATION, THREADED *(Orthopedics) 87JDW*

Acumed Llc 503-627-9957
5885 NW Cornelius Pass Rd, Hillsboro, OR 97124
External fixation devive with threaded threaded fixation pins.

Alphatec Spine, Inc. 760-494-6769
5818 El Camino Real, Carlsbad, CA 92008
Alphatec external fixation hybrid system.

American Medical Specialties, Inc. 800-808-2877
10650 77th St., Suite 405, Largo, FL 33777
Full line of pins and wires.

Biomet, Inc. 574-267-6639
56 E Bell Dr, PO Box 587, Warsaw, IN 46582
Various types of threaded pins.

Brasseler Usa - Komet Medical 800-535-6638
1 Brasseler Blvd, Savannah, GA 31419

Brasseler Usa - Medical 805-650-5209
4837 McGrath St Ste J, Ventura, CA 93003
Various

Depuy Ace, A Johnson & Johnson Company 800-473-3789
700 Orthopaedic Dr, Warsaw, IN 46582

Depuy Mitek, A Johnson & Johnson Company 800-451-2006
50 Scotland Blvd, Bridgewater, MA 02324
Cross pins.

PIN, FIXATION, THREADED *(cont'd)*

Depuy Orthopaedics, Inc. 800-473-3789
700 Orthopaedic Dr, P.O. Box 988, Warsaw, IN 46582
Various types of threaded fixation pins.

Depuy-Raynham, A Div. Of Depuy Orthopaedics 800-451-2006
325 Paramount Dr, Raynham, MA 02767
Various types of threaded fixation pins.

DJO Inc. 800-336-6569
1430 Decision St, Vista, CA 92081

Kmedic 800-955-0559
190 Veterans Dr, Northvale, NJ 07647

Microcision Llc 800-264-3811
5805 Keystone St, Philadelphia, PA 19135

New Business Development, Llc 678-852-5504
605 Industrial Ct, Woodstock, GA 30189
Distraction pin.

Onyx Medical Corp. 901-323-6699
152 Collins St, Memphis, TN 38112

Promex Technologies, Llc 317-736-0128
3049 Hudson St, Franklin, IN 46131
Kirshner wires (k-wire) & steinmann pins.

R&R Medical, Inc. 877-776-9972
2225 Park Place Dr., Slatington, PA 18080
Smooth or threaded metallic bone fixation.

Simpex Medical, Inc. 800-851-9753
401 E Prospect Ave, Mount Prospect, IL 60056

Stryker Spine 866-457-7463
2 Pearl Ct, Allendale, NJ 07401

Synthes (Usa) 610-719-5000
35 Airport Rd, Horseheads, NY 14845
Various types and sizes of smooth fixation pins.

Tava Surgical Instruments 805-650-5209
4837 McGrath St Ste J, Ventura, CA 93003
Various.

Tegra Medical Inc. 508-541-4200
9 Forge Pkwy, Franklin, MA 02038

Vilex, Inc. 800-872-4911
345 Old Curry Hollow Rd, Pittsburgh, PA 15236

Warsaw Orthopedic, Inc. 901-396-3133
2500 Silveus Xing, Warsaw, IN 46582
Various styles of threaded steinmann pins and kirshner wires.

Westcon Orthopedics, Inc. 800-382-4975
4 Craig Rd, Neshanic Station, NJ 08853
Pin, capping device, external.

Zimmer Holdings, Inc. 800-613-6131
1800 W Center St, PO Box 708, Warsaw, IN 46580

PIN, RETENTIVE AND SPLINTING *(Dental And Oral) 76EBL*

Aesculap Implant Systems Inc. 1-800-234-9179
3773 Corporate Pkwy, Center Valley, PA 18034

Coltene/Whaledent Inc. 330-916-8858
235 Ascot Pkwy, Cuyahoga Falls, OH 44223
Auxilliary retention pin.

Ellman International, Inc. 800-835-5355
3333 Royal Ave, Rockville Centre, NY 11572

Nanzee Dental Products 717-792-9795
2916 Robin Rd, York, PA 17404
Nanzee reinforcements.

Oratronics, Inc. 212-986-0050
405 Lexington Ave, New York, NY 10174
Single tooth replacement and bridge abutment kit.

Productivity Training Company 800-448-8855
360 Cochrane Cir # A, Morgan Hill, CA 95037
Cross Pin Model Pinning System.

3m Unitek 800-634-5300
2724 Peck Rd, Monrovia, CA 91016

PIN, SAFETY *(General) 80WMU*

Hospital Marketing Svcs. Company, Inc. 800-786-5094
162 Great Hill Rd./ Ind. Park, Naugatuck, CT 06770
HMS TORRINGTON - sterile, 1in., 1 1/2in., 2in., 2 pins per pack, 50 packs/box.

PIN, TRANSFER, SOLUTION *(General) 80WYV*

Baxa Corporation 800-567-2292
9540 S Maroon Circle, Suite 400, Englewood, CO 80112
Dispensing Pin. Vented pin with 0.2-micron filter for adding and withdrawing solutions from a vial. Tethered cap.

PINWHEEL *(Cns/Neurology) 84GWY*

Kmedic 800-955-0559
190 Veterans Dr, Northvale, NJ 07647

Riverbank Laboratories 630-232-2207
2613 Kaneville Ct, PO Box 110, Geneva, IL 60134

PIPETTE *(Chemistry) 75WKU*

Asi Instruments, Inc. 800-531-1105
12900 E 10 Mile Rd, Warren, MI 48089

Beckman Coulter, Inc. 800-742-2345
250 S Kraemer Blvd, PO Box 8000, Brea, CA 92821

Corning Inc., Science Products Division 800-492-1110
45 Nagog Park, Acton, MA 01720
CORNING transfer pipette, used for general transfer of fluids where a disposable alternative is required.

Engineers Express, Inc. 800-255-8823
7 Industrial Park Rd, Medway, MA 02053

Friedrich & Dimmock, Inc. 800-524-1131
2127 Wheaton Ave, PO Box 230, Millville, NJ 08332
Precision glass tubing and rods made to custom specifications for hospitals, laboratories and the laser industry; also HIV testing glassware.

Garren Scientific, Inc. 800-342-3725
15916 Blythe St Unit A, Van Nuys, CA 91406
Transfer pipettes, drug testing bottles, safety caps, chain of evidence bags.

Globe Scientific, Inc. 800-394-4562
610 Winters Ave, Paramus, NJ 07652
Complete range of Diamond Line high-precision, adjustable volume, fixed-volume, and multi-channel pipettors.

Image Molding, Inc. 800-525-1875
4525 Kingston St, Denver, CO 80239

Intersciences Inc. 800-661-6431
169 Idema Rd., Markham, ONT L3R 1A9 Canada
CLONEPETTE Digital Pipette

Mg Scientific, Inc. 800-343-8338
8500 107th St, Pleasant Prairie, WI 53158

Moyco Technologies, Inc. 800-331-8837
200 Commerce Dr, Montgomeryville, PA 18936
Plastic.

Nutech Molding Corporation 1-800-423-5278
PO Box 840, 2024 Broad St,, Pocomoke City, MD 21851

Parter Medical Products 800-666-8282
17015 Kingsview Ave, Carson, CA 90746
Transfer pipettes.

Tudor Scientific Glass Co., Inc. 800-336-4666
555 Edgefield Rd, Belvedere, SC 29841

Ware Medics Glass Works, Inc. 845-429-6950
PO Box 368, Garnerville, NY 10923
All types.

PIPETTE TIP *(Chemistry) 75TGI*

Accu-Glass Llc 800-325-4796
10765 Trenton Ave, Saint Louis, MO 63132
Soda lime glass.

Bd Diagnostic Systems 800-675-0908
7 Loveton Cir, Sparks, MD 21152

Beckman Coulter, Inc. 800-742-2345
250 S Kraemer Blvd, PO Box 8000, Brea, CA 92821

Bio Plas, Inc. 415-472-3777
4340 Redwood Hwy Ste A15, San Rafael, CA 94903
Disposable polypropylene pipettor tips, more than 25 different tips offered (free tips included with each pkg.).

Bio-Rad Laboratories, Life Science Group 800-424-6723
2000 Alfred Nobel Dr, Hercules, CA 94547

Biomedical Technologies, Inc. 781-344-9942
378 Page St, Stoughton, MA 02072

Biomerieux Inc. 800-682-2666
100 Rodolphe St, Durham, NC 27712

Brinkmann Instruments (Canada) Ltd. 800-263-8715
6670 Campobello Rd., Mississauga, ONT L5N 2L8 Canada

PIPETTE TIP *(cont'd)*

Cole-Parmer Instrument Inc. 800-323-4340
625 E Bunker Ct, Vernon Hills, IL 60061

Corning Inc., Science Products Division 800-492-1110
45 Nagog Park, Acton, MA 01720

Covidien Lp 508-261-8000
15 Hampshire St, Mansfield, MA 02048

Engineers Express, Inc. 800-255-8823
7 Industrial Park Rd, Medway, MA 02053

Globe Scientific, Inc. 800-394-4562
610 Winters Ave, Paramus, NJ 07652
Complete range for most pipettors.

Harvard Apparatus, Inc. 800-272-2775
84 October Hill Rd, Holliston, MA 01746
AmiKa PreTip C-18 sample preparation and purification tip. New non-clogging tip that is used to prepare samples prior to mass spec. Available in 3 sizes with different packing materials.

Helena Laboratories 409-842-3714
PO Box 752, Beaumont, TX 77704

Helena Plastics 800-227-1727
3700 Lakeville Hwy Ste 200, Petaluma, CA 94954

Intersciences Inc. 800-661-6431
169 Idema Rd., Markham, ONT L3R 1A9 Canada

Labcon North America 800-227-1466
3700 Lakeville Hwy Ste 200, Petaluma, CA 94954
Various types of pipette tips.

Mg Scientific, Inc. 800-343-8338
8500 107th St, Pleasant Prairie, WI 53158

Quality Scientific Plastics 800-426-9595
1260 Holm Rd, Petaluma, CA 94954
Filtered pipette tips.

Standard Instrumentation, Div. Preiser Scientific 800-624-8285
94 Oliver St, Saint Albans, WV 25177

Thermo Fisher Scientific 800-345-0206
22 Friars Dr, Hudson, NH 03051
INTEGRITY filter tips/amplification enhancers to prevent contamination.

Tricontinent 800-937-4738
12555 Loma Rica Dr, Grass Valley, CA 95945

Tudor Scientific Glass Co., Inc. 800-336-4666
555 Edgefield Rd, Belvedere, SC 29841

Ulster Scientific, Inc. 845-255-2200
83 S Putt Corners Rd, PO Box 819, New Paltz, NY 12561
V3 VERI-TIP: disposable for liquid handling in labs.

Usa Scientific, Inc. 800-522-8477
PO Box 3565, Ocala, FL 34478
Tip One Pipette Tip: Tips for a variety of manual and automated systems.

PIPETTE, DILUTING *(Hematology) 81GGY*

Bd Biosciences Discovery Labware 978-901-7431
1 Becton Cir, Durham, NC 27712
Pipette, diluting.

Biohit Inc. 800-922-0784
PO Box 308, 3535 Rte. 66, Bldg. 4, Neptune, NJ 07754

Cole-Parmer Instrument Inc. 800-323-4340
625 E Bunker Ct, Vernon Hills, IL 60061

Corning Inc., Science Products Division 800-492-1110
45 Nagog Park, Acton, MA 01720

Covidien Lp 508-261-8000
15 Hampshire St, Mansfield, MA 02048
Lancer liquid handling devices.

Dade Behring, Inc. 800-948-3233
1717 Deerfield Rd, Deerfield, IL 60015

Drummond Scientific Co. 800-523-7480
500 Park Way # 700, Broomall, PA 19008
Pipet-Aid Hood Mate.

Garren Scientific, Inc. 800-342-3725
15916 Blythe St Unit A, Van Nuys, CA 91406

Hamilton Company 800-648-5950
4990 Energy Way, Reno, NV 89502

Nalge Nunc International 800-625-4327
75 Panorama Creek Dr, Rochester, NY 14625
NALGENE autoclavable, unbreakable pipets from 1 to 10ml.

PIPETTE, MICRO *(Chemistry) 75JRC*

Accu-Glass Llc 800-325-4796
10765 Trenton Ave, Saint Louis, MO 63132

Act-Aeromed Copan Technologies Llc. 951-549-8793
85 Commerce St, Glastonbury, CT 06033
Transfer pipettes.

Asi Instruments, Inc. 800-531-1105
12900 E 10 Mile Rd, Warren, MI 48089

Bd Diagnostic Systems 800-675-0908
7 Loveton Cir, Sparks, MD 21152

Beckman Coulter, Inc. 800-742-2345
250 S Kraemer Blvd, PO Box 8000, Brea, CA 92821

Bio-Rad Laboratories, Life Science Group 800-424-6723
2000 Alfred Nobel Dr, Hercules, CA 94547

Brinkmann Instruments (Canada) Ltd. 800-263-8715
6670 Campobello Rd., Mississauga, ONT L5N 2L8 Canada

Carolina Biological Supply Co. 800-334-5551
2700 York Rd, Burlington, NC 27215

Copan Diagnostics, Inc. 800-216-4016
26055 Jefferson Ave, Murrieta, CA 92562
Transfer Pipettes

Corning Inc., Science Products Division 800-492-1110
45 Nagog Park, Acton, MA 01720

Covidien Lp 508-261-8000
15 Hampshire St, Mansfield, MA 02048

Dade Behring, Inc. 800-948-3233
1717 Deerfield Rd, Deerfield, IL 60015

Globe Scientific, Inc. 800-394-4562
610 Winters Ave, Paramus, NJ 07652
For dispensing precise micro volumes.

Hamilton Company 800-648-5950
4990 Energy Way, Reno, NV 89502

Helena Laboratories 409-842-3714
PO Box 752, Beaumont, TX 77704

Humagen Fertility Diagnostics, Inc. 800-937-3210
2400 Hunters Way, Charlottesville, VA 22911
Box of 10 micro pipettes for use in IVF labs.

Intersciences Inc. 800-661-6431
169 Idema Rd., Markham, ONT L3R 1A9 Canada

Kimble Glass, Inc. 888-546-2531
537 Crystal Ave, Vineland, NJ 08360

Kloehn Co., Ltd. 800-358-4342
10000 Banburry Cross Dr, Las Vegas, NV 89144

Kontes Glass Co. 888-546-2531
1022 Spruce St, Vineland, NJ 08360

Matrix Technologies Corporation 800-345-0206
12 Executive Dr, Hudson, NH 03051

Mg Scientific, Inc. 800-343-8338
8500 107th St, Pleasant Prairie, WI 53158

Samco Scientific Corporation 800-522-3359
1050 Arroyo St, San Fernando, CA 91340
Fine Tip Pipets available for Micro-pipetting

Sarstedt, Inc. 800-257-5101
PO Box 468, 1025, St. James Church Road, Newton, NC 28658

Tudor Scientific Glass Co., Inc. 800-336-4666
555 Edgefield Rd, Belvedere, SC 29841

Zander Medical Supplies, Inc. / Zander Ivf, Inc. 800-820-3029
755 8th Ct Ste 4, Vero Beach, FL 32962
IVF microinjection and holding pipettes, ICSI and biopsy pipettes, holding pipettes, spiked and non-spiked injection pipettes, 1.0 mm glass borosilicate/sterilize.

PIPETTE, PASTEUR *(Hematology) 81GJW*

Chase Scientific Glass, Inc. 412-490-8425
234 Cardiff Valley Rd, Rockwood, TN 37854
Various pasteur pipettes.

Dade Behring, Inc. 800-948-3233
1717 Deerfield Rd, Deerfield, IL 60015

Garren Scientific, Inc. 800-342-3725
15916 Blythe St Unit A, Van Nuys, CA 91406

Globe Scientific, Inc. 800-394-4562
610 Winters Ave, Paramus, NJ 07652
Range of transfer pipettes from 1.5 to 7 mL.

K-Sera, Inc. 661-775-5988
27525 Newhall Ranch Rd Ste 8, Valencia, CA 91355
Transfer pipettes, pasteur.

PIPETTE, PASTEUR *(cont'd)*

Kimble Chase Life Science And Research Products, Llc. 865-717-2635
234 Cardiff Valley Rd, Ozone, TN 37854

Samco Scientific Corporation 800-522-3359
1050 Arroyo St, San Fernando, CA 91340

PIPETTE, QUANTITATIVE, HEMATOLOGY *(Hematology) 81GJG*

Bd Biosciences Discovery Labware 978-901-7431
1 Becton Cir, Durham, NC 27712
Blood cell diluting pipets.

Brinkmann Instruments (Canada) Ltd. 800-263-8715
6670 Campobello Rd., Mississauga, ONT L5N 2L8 Canada

C & A Scientific Co. Inc. 703-330-1413
7241 Gabe Ct, Manassas, VA 20109
PREMIERE Plastic transfer pipet, non-sterile, 3.5mL and 1.0mL, graduated.

Corning Inc., Science Products Division 800-492-1110
45 Nagog Park, Acton, MA 01720

Globe Scientific, Inc. 800-394-4562
610 Winters Ave, Paramus, NJ 07652

Hema Diagnostic Systems, Llc 305-867-6123
1666 Kennedy Causeway, Suite 401, North Bay Village, FL 33141

Labcon North America 800-227-1466
3700 Lakeville Hwy Ste 200, Petaluma, CA 94954
Disposable transfer pipettes: graduated, standard, sedimentation and jumbo.

Spectra Medical Devices, Inc. 866-938-8649
4C Henshaw St, Woburn, MA 01801

PIPETTE, SAHLI *(Hematology) 81GGX*

Dade Behring, Inc. 800-948-3233
1717 Deerfield Rd, Deerfield, IL 60015

Propper Manufacturing Co., Inc. 800-832-4300
3604 Skillman Ave, Long Island City, NY 11101

PIPETTER *(Hematology) 81RLF*

Bd Diagnostic Systems 800-675-0908
7 Loveton Cir, Sparks, MD 21152

Beckman Coulter, Inc. 800-742-2345
250 S Kraemer Blvd, PO Box 8000, Brea, CA 92821

Biohit Inc. 800-922-0784
PO Box 308, 3535 Rte. 66, Bldg. 4, Neptune, NJ 07754
Biohit Pipetters liquid handling instruments for accurate and precise delivery of microvolume samples.

Brinkmann Instruments (Canada) Ltd. 800-263-8715
6670 Campobello Rd., Mississauga, ONT L5N 2L8 Canada

Cadence Science Inc. 888-717-7677
1979 Marcus Ave Ste 215, New Hyde Park, NY 11042
5 sizes (glass syringe).

Drummond Scientific Co. 800-523-7480
500 Park Way # 700, Broomall, PA 19008
Programmable Pipet-Aid Elite.

Hamilton Company 800-648-5950
4990 Energy Way, Reno, NV 89502

Intersciences Inc. 800-661-6431
169 Idema Rd., Markham, ONT L3R 1A9 Canada

Marconi Medical Systems 800-323-0550
595 Miner Rd, Cleveland, OH 44143

Mg Scientific, Inc. 800-343-8338
8500 107th St, Pleasant Prairie, WI 53158

Thermo Fisher Scientific 800-345-0206
22 Friars Dr, Hudson, NH 03051
CellMate II Cordless Pipettor, Single Channel Manual Pipettors, Multi Channel Manual Pipettors, Impact2 Electronic Pipettors, Impact2 Singel Channel Pipettors, Impact2 Shorty Pipettors, Impact2 Multichannel Pipettors, Impact2 EXP Pipettors, Impact2 Equalizer

Tricontinent 800-937-4738
12555 Loma Rica Dr, Grass Valley, CA 95945

Ulster Scientific, Inc. 845-255-2200
83 S Putt Corners Rd, PO Box 819, New Paltz, NY 12561
V3-PLUS: pipettes for liquid handling in labs.

PIPETTER *(cont'd)*

Zymark Corporation 508-435-9500
68 Elm St, Hopkinton, MA 01748
RAPID PLATE pipetting workstation pipets to and from 96 and 384 well microplates and deepwells and reservoirs for dilution simultiaspirate applications. $40,000.00. PRESTO microplate sealing workstation seals the tops of microplatesusing polyester, chemical resistant seals. $20,000.00. PRESTO Microplate Bar Code Labeling Workstation labels either portrait or landscape sides of microplate with a chemical resistant bar code label. $20,000.00. ALLEGRO ultra-high throughput screening system screens up to 100,000 assay points per day, using a modular, assembly line platform. TWISTER Universal Microplate handler loads microplates to and from industry standard microplate readers, washers and dispensers.

PIPETTING AND DILUTING SYSTEM, AUTOMATED *(Chemistry) 75JQW*

Abbott Diagnostics Div. 847-937-7988
1921 Hurd Dr, Irving, TX 75038
Various pipetting & wash systems.

Abbott Molecular, Inc. 847-937-6100
1300 E Touhy Ave, Des Plaines, IL 60018
Automated sample preparation system.

Awareness Technology, Inc. 722-283-6540
1935 SW Martin Hwy, Palm City, FL 34990
Completely automated analyzer for ELISA and Biochemistry analysis using standard microwells as the reaction cuvettes.

Bd Biosciences 408-954-6307
2350 Qume Dr, San Jose, CA 95131
Pipetting and diluting station.

Bd Biosciences Discovery Labware 978-901-7431
1 Becton Cir, Durham, NC 27712
Pipets and diluting systems.

Beckman Coulter, Inc. 800-526-3821
11800 SW 147th Ave, Miami, FL 33196
Pipetting and diluting system for clinical use.

Beckman Coulter, Inc. 800-742-2345
250 S Kraemer Blvd, PO Box 8000, Brea, CA 92821

Bio-Rad Laboratories, Inc. 425-881-8300
6565 185th Ave NE, Redmond, WA 98052
Pipettor/dilutor.

Biotek Instruments, Inc. 802-655-4040
100 Tigan St, Highland Park, Winooski, VT 05404
Various models of manual & auto. microplate washers.

Brinkmann Instruments (Canada) Ltd. 800-263-8715
6670 Campobello Rd., Mississauga, ONT L5N 2L8 Canada

Capitol Vial 334-887-8311
2039 McMillan St, Auburn, AL 36832
Urine aliquotor.

Carolina Liquid Chemistries Corp. 800-471-7272
510 W Central Ave Ste C, Brea, CA 92821
Wash concentrate reagent.

Covidien Lp 508-261-8000
15 Hampshire St, Mansfield, MA 02048

Dade Behring, Inc. 800-948-3233
1717 Deerfield Rd, Deerfield, IL 60015

Dynex Technologies, Inc. 800-288-2354
14340 Sullyfield Cir, Chantilly, VA 20151
Peristaltic pumps, various models.

Hamilton Company 800-648-5950
4990 Energy Way, Reno, NV 89502

Hycor Biomedical, Inc. 800-382-2527
7272 Chapman Ave, Garden Grove, CA 92841
Transfer pipet.

Hyperion, Inc. 305-238-3020
14100 SW 136th St, Miami, FL 33186
$16,500.00 Pipetting and diluting station for clinical use.

Matrix Technologies Corporation 800-345-0206
12 Executive Dr, Hudson, NH 03051

Myers-Stevens Group, Inc. 903-566-6696
2931 Vail Ave, Commerce, CA 90040
Plastic components for standardized urinalysis.

National Instrument Co., Inc. 800-526-1301
4119 Fordleigh Rd, Baltimore, MD 21215

PIPETTING AND DILUTING SYSTEM, AUTOMATED *(cont'd)*

Ortho-Clinical Diagnostics, Inc. 800-828-6316
513 Technology Blvd, Rochester, NY 14626
Sample handling system.

Perkinelmer Life And Analytical Sciences 800-323-5891
2200 Warrenville Rd, Downers Grove, IL 60515
Pipetting and dilution system for sample preparation.

Pharmacia & Upjohn Co. 212-573-1000
7000 Portage Rd, Kalamazoo, MI 49001
Acap system.

Pss Bio Instruments, Inc. 925-960-9182
6052 Industrial Way Ste H, Livermore, CA 94551
Pipetting and diluting system.

Qiagen Gaithersburg, Inc. 800-344-3631
1201 Clopper Rd, Gaithersburg, MD 20878
Pipettor, microplate handler, incubator.

Tomtec 877-866-8323
1000 Sherman Ave, Hamden, CT 06514
QUADRA 96 is an automated programmable 96 well pipetting system to automate microplate 96 well protocols. Transfer volumes from 1 microliter to 450 microliters. Units for sterile and non-sterile operations. QUADRA PLUS, automated, programmable, multifunctional dual head pipettor for volumes 0.5ml to 40ml with 4 bi-directional stackers.

Tri-Continent Scientific, Inc. 530-274-4240
12555 Loma Rica Dr # 2, Grass Valley, CA 95945
Automatic diluter/dispenser.

Zymark Corporation 508-435-9500
68 Elm St, Hopkinton, MA 01748
RAPID PLATE pipetting workstation pipets to and from 96 and 384 well microplates and deepwells and reservoirs for dilution simultiaspirate applications. $40,000.00. PRESTO microplate sealing workstation seals the tops of microplates using polyester, chemical-resistant seals. $20,000.00. PRESTO microplate bar-code labeling workstation labels either portrait or landscape sides of microplate with a chemical-resistant bar-code label. $20,000.00. ALLEGRO ultra-high-throughput screening system screens up to 100,000 assay points per day, using a modular, assembly-line platform. TWISTER universal microplate handler loads microplates to and from industry standard microplate readers, washers, and dispensers.

PLANCHET *(Chemistry) 75UHH*

Coy Laboratory Products, Inc. 734-475-2200
14500 Coy Dr, Grass Lake, MI 49240

PLASMA, COAGULASE, HUMAN/HORSE/RABBIT
(Microbiology) 83JTL

Bd Diagnostic Systems 800-675-0908
7 Loveton Cir, Sparks, MD 21152

Health Chem Diagnostics Llc 954-979-3845
3341 W McNab Rd, Pompano Beach, FL 33069
Plasma, coagulase, human, horse and rabbit.

R2 Diagnostics, Inc. 574-288-4377
1801 Commerce Dr, South Bend, IN 46628
Plasmacon & plasmaref.

PLASMA, CONTROL, FIBRINOGEN *(Hematology) 81GIL*

Bio/Data Corp. 215-441-4000
155 Gibraltar Rd, Horsham, PA 19044
Fibrinogen calibrator and control plasma.

Clinical Controls International 805-528-4039
1236 Los Osos Valley Rd Ste T, Los Osos, CA 93402
Various types of plasma fibrinogen control.

Fisher Diagnostics 877-722-4366
11515 Vanstory Dr Ste 125, Huntersville, NC 28078

Precision Biologic, Inc. 800-267-2796
900 Windmill Rd., Ste. 100, Dartmouth, NS B3B 1P7 Canada
CRYOCHECK LOW FIBRINOGEN CONTROL

Wortham Laboratories Inc 423-296-0090
6340 Bonny Oaks Dr, Chattanooga, TN 37416
Fibrinogen control plasma.

PLASMA, CONTROL, NORMAL *(Hematology) 81GIZ*

Bio/Data Corp. 215-441-4000
155 Gibraltar Rd, Horsham, PA 19044
Normal control plasma.

Dade Behring, Inc. 800-948-3233
1717 Deerfield Rd, Deerfield, IL 60015

PLASMA, CONTROL, NORMAL *(cont'd)*

Health Chem Diagnostics Llc 954-979-3845
3341 W McNab Rd, Pompano Beach, FL 33069
Plasma, control, normal.

Helena Laboratories 409-842-3714
PO Box 752, Beaumont, TX 77704

Precision Biologic, Inc. 800-267-2796
900 Windmill Rd., Ste. 100, Dartmouth, NS B3B 1P7 Canada
CRYOCHECK POOLED NORMAL PLASMA and CRYOCHECK REFERENCE CONTROL NORMAL

Wortham Laboratories Inc 423-296-0090
6340 Bonny Oaks Dr, Chattanooga, TN 37416
Normal coagulation control.

PLASMA, DEFICIENT, FACTOR, COAGULATION
(Hematology) 81GJT

Baxter International Inc 800-422-9837
1 Baxter Pkwy, Deerfield, IL 60015
RECOMBINATE Antihemophilic Factor, HEMOFIL M Antihemophilic Factor, PROPLEX T Factor IX Complex. Coagulation inhibitors, immuno globulin and plasma expanders.

Bio/Data Corp. 215-441-4000
155 Gibraltar Rd, Horsham, PA 19044
Various.

Biomerieux Inc. 800-682-2666
100 Rodolphe St, Durham, NC 27712
A series of factor deficient plasmas (V, VII, VIII, IX, X, XI, XII) for detection and quantification of a specific factor deficiency.

Dade Behring, Inc. 800-948-3233
1717 Deerfield Rd, Deerfield, IL 60015

Fisher Diagnostics 877-722-4366
11515 Vanstory Dr Ste 125, Huntersville, NC 28078

Health Chem Diagnostics Llc 954-979-3845
3341 W McNab Rd, Pompano Beach, FL 33069
Plasma, coagulation factor deficient.

Precision Biologic, Inc. 800-267-2796
900 Windmill Rd., Ste. 100, Dartmouth, NS B3B 1P7 Canada
CRYOCHECK FACTOR DEFICIENT PLASMAS - immunodepleted and certified to have less than 1% activity for the depleted factors, while all other factors are assayed within normal activity levels.

R2 Diagnostics, Inc. 574-288-4377
1801 Commerce Dr, South Bend, IN 46628
Various factor deficient plasmas.

PLATE, AGAR, OUCHTERLONY *(Immunology) 82JZP*

Helena Laboratories 409-842-3714
PO Box 752, Beaumont, TX 77704

PLATE, BASE, SHELLAC *(Dental And Oral) 76EEA*

Dentsply Canada, Ltd. 800-263-1437
161 Vinyl Ct., Woodbridge, ONT L4L 4A3 Canada

Miltex Dental Technologies, Inc. 516-576-6022
589 Davies Dr, York, PA 17402
Shellac baseplate.

PLATE, BONE, ORTHODONTIC *(Dental And Oral) 76JEY*

Ace Surgical Supply Co., Inc. 800-441-3100
1034 Pearl St, Brockton, MA 02301

Acumed Llc 503-627-9957
5885 NW Cornelius Pass Rd, Hillsboro, OR 97124
Bone plate.

Aesculap Implant Systems Inc. 1-800-234-9179
3773 Corporate Pkwy, Center Valley, PA 18034
Bone plates for orthopedic and cervical fixation.

Biomet Microfixation Inc. 800-874-7711
1520 Tradeport Dr, Jacksonville, FL 32218
Curette, biopsy, bronchoscope (rigid).

Biomet, Inc. 574-267-6639
56 E Bell Dr, PO Box 587, Warsaw, IN 46582
Various types of bone plates such as compression, regular, semi-tubular, narrow .

Bioplate, Inc. 310-815-2100
3643 Lenawee Ave, Los Angeles, CA 90016
Bone plates and bone screws.

Creative Medical Designs, Inc. 813-875-9999
13914 Shady Shores Dr, Tampa, FL 33613
Lnar bone plate.

PLATE, BONE, ORTHODONTIC *(cont'd)*

Interphase Implants, Inc. 248-442-1460
19928 Farmington Rd, Livonia, MI 48152
Transosseous implant.

Kls-Martin L.P. 800-625-1557
11239-1 St. John`s Industrial, Parkway South
Jacksonville, FL 32250
Normed bidirectional/multidirectional jaw distractor.

Kmedic 800-955-0559
190 Veterans Dr, Northvale, NJ 07647

Medtronic Puerto Rico Operations Co.,Med Rel 763-514-4000
Road 909, Km. 0.4., Barrio Mariana, Humacao, PR 00792
Multiple (bone plates).

Medtronic Sofamor Danek Usa, Inc. 901-396-3133
4340 Swinnea Rd, Memphis, TN 38118
Multiple (bone plates).

Osteogenics Biomedical, Inc. 806-796-1923
4620 71st St Bldg 78-79, Lubbock, TX 79424
Titanium ridge augmentation mesh.

Synthes (Usa) 610-719-5000
35 Airport Rd, Horseheads, NY 14845
Various types and sizes of dental bone plates.

Unicare Biomedical, Inc. 949-643-6707
22971 Triton Way Ste B, Laguna Hills, CA 92653
Cytoflex precision titanium mesh to ensure the three-dimensional reconstruction of alveolar bone defects and to facilitate augmentation with adequate fixation of the augmentation material.

Warsaw Orthopedic, Inc. 901-396-3133
2500 Silveus Xing, Warsaw, IN 46582
Multiple (bone plates).

Zimmer Holdings, Inc. 800-613-6131
1800 W Center St, PO Box 708, Warsaw, IN 46580

PLATE, BONE, SKULL (CRANIOPLASTY) *(Cns/Neurology) 84RLI*

Holmed Corporation 508-238-3351
40 Norfolk Ave, South Easton, MA 02375

Kinamed, Inc. 800-827-5775
820 Flynn Rd, Camarillo, CA 93012
NEUROPRO - Craniofacial plating system. Specialty plating system for craniotomies and cranioplasty.

PLATE, BONE, SKULL, PREFORMED, ALTERABLE
(Cns/Neurology) 84GWO

Biomet, Inc. 574-267-6639
56 E Bell Dr, PO Box 587, Warsaw, IN 46582
Various types of cranioplasty plates.

Medtronic Neurosurgery 800-468-9710
125 Cremona Dr, Goleta, CA 93117
Bone fixation appliance or surical mesh.

Synthes (Usa) - Development Center 719-481-5300
1230 Wilson Dr, West Chester, PA 19380
Various types and sizes of preformed alterable cranioplasty plates.

PLATE, BONE, SKULL, PREFORMED, NON-ALTERABLE
(Cns/Neurology) 84GXN

Biomet Microfixation Inc. 800-874-7711
1520 Tradeport Dr, Jacksonville, FL 32218
Hard tissue replacement-patient matched implant.

Biomet, Inc. 574-267-6639
56 E Bell Dr, PO Box 587, Warsaw, IN 46582
Hard tissue replacement, patient matched implant.

Bioplate, Inc. 310-815-2100
3643 Lenawee Ave, Los Angeles, CA 90016
Craniotomy fixation system.

Stryker Spine 866-457-7463
2 Pearl Ct, Allendale, NJ 07401

PLATE, COOLING *(Chemistry) 75UFU*

Lytron, Inc. 781-933-7300
55 Dragon Ct, Woburn, MA 01801
Several technologies standard and custom parts available.

PLATE, CULTURE *(Microbiology) 83WNW*

Bd Diagnostic Systems 800-675-0908
7 Loveton Cir, Sparks, MD 21152

Q.I. Medical, Inc. 800-837-8361
440 Lower Grass Valley Rd Ste C, Nevada City, CA 95959

Qiagen Gaithersburg, Inc. 800-344-3631
1201 Clopper Rd, Gaithersburg, MD 20878

PLATE, CULTURE *(cont'd)*

Simport Plastics Ltd. 450-464-1723
2588 Bernard-Pilon, Beloeil, QUE J3G 4S5 Canada

PLATE, FIXATION, BONE *(Orthopedics) 87HRS*

Abbott Spine, Inc. 847-937-6100
12708 Riata Vista Cir Ste B-100, Austin, TX 78727
Ubp system.

Acumed Llc 503-627-9957
5885 NW Cornelius Pass Rd, Hillsboro, OR 97124
Single,multiple component bone fixation appliance and accessories.

Acute Innovations Llc 503-627-9957
21421 NW Jacobson Rd Ste 700, Hillsboro, OR 97124
Plate, fixation, bone.

Alphatec Spine, Inc. 760-494-6769
5818 El Camino Real, Carlsbad, CA 92008
4.5 compression plates.

Arthrex, Inc. 239-643-5553
1370 Creekside Blvd, Naples, FL 34108
Bone plate.

Bio-Technology Usa, Inc. 305-512-3522
6175 NW 167th St Ste G8, Hialeah, FL 33015
Maxillofacial bone plate, fixation, bone.

Biomet Microfixation Inc. 800-874-7711
1520 Tradeport Dr, Jacksonville, FL 32218
Retrosternal strut.

Biomet, Inc. 574-267-6639
56 E Bell Dr, PO Box 587, Warsaw, IN 46582
Poly-l-lactic acid/polyglycolic acid plates.

Bioplate, Inc. 310-815-2100
3643 Lenawee Ave, Los Angeles, CA 90016
Bone plates and screws.

Centerpulse Orthopedics Inc. 877-768-7349
9900 Spectrum Dr, Austin, TX 78717
Natural-Knee HTO System.

Creative Medical Designs, Inc. 813-875-9999
13914 Shady Shores Dr, Tampa, FL 33613
Ulnar, kienbock, radial plates & osteotomy devices.

Depuy Ace, A Johnson & Johnson Company 800-473-3789
700 Orthopaedic Dr, Warsaw, IN 46582

Depuy Orthopaedics, Inc. 800-473-3789
700 Orthopaedic Dr, P.O. Box 988, Warsaw, IN 46582
Various types of bone fixation plates.

Depuy Spine, Inc. 800-227-6633
325 Paramount Dr, Raynham, MA 02767
Bone plates.

Elekta, Inc. 800-535-7355
4775 Peachtree Industrial Blvd, Building 300, Suite 300
Norcross, GA 30092
Fixation system.

Gyrus Ent L.L.C., Sub. Of Gyrus Acmi, Inc. 508-804-2739
2925 Appling Rd, Bartlett, TN 38133
Various types and sizes of bone fixation plates.

Hand Innovations, Llc. 800-800-8188
6303 Blue Lagoon Dr Ste 100, Miami, FL 33126
Distal volar radius fracture repair system (dvr).

Holmed Corporation 508-238-3351
40 Norfolk Ave, South Easton, MA 02375

Integra Lifesciences Of Ohio 800-654-2873
4900 Charlemar Dr Bldg A, Cincinnati, OH 45227
Various bone plates.

Keller Engineering, Inc. 310-326-6291
3203 Kashiwa St, Torrance, CA 90505

Kls-Martin L.P. 800-625-1557
11239-1 St. John`s Industrial, Parkway South
Jacksonville, FL 32250

Kmedic 800-955-0559
190 Veterans Dr, Northvale, NJ 07647

Onyx Medical Corp. 901-323-6699
152 Collins St, Memphis, TN 38112

Orthohelix Surgical Designs, Inc. 330-869-9582
1815 W Market St Ste 205, Akron, OH 44313
Orthopedic plates and screws.

Orthopedic Sciences, Inc 562-799-5550
3020 Old Ranch Pkwy Ste 325, Seal Beach, CA 90740
Bone plate.

PLATE, FIXATION, BONE *(cont'd)*

Pioneer Surgical Technology 800-557-9909
375 River Park Cir, Marquette, MI 49855

Small Bone Innovations, Inc. 215-428-1791
1380 S Pennsylvania Ave, Morrisville, PA 19067
Internal fixation system.

Spine Wave, Inc. 203-944-9494
2 Enterprise Dr Ste 302, Shelton, CT 06484
Wafer system.

Stryker Spine 866-457-7463
2 Pearl Ct, Allendale, NJ 07401

Synthes (Usa) 610-719-5000
35 Airport Rd, Horseheads, NY 14845
Various types and sizes of bone plates.

Synthes (Usa) - Brandywine Technical Center 800-523-0322
1301-1303 Goshen Pky., West Chester, PA 19380

Warsaw Orthopedic, Inc. 901-396-3133
2500 Silveus Xing, Warsaw, IN 46582
Bone plate devices.

Zimmer Holdings, Inc. 800-613-6131
1800 W Center St, PO Box 708, Warsaw, IN 46580

Zimmer Manufacturing B.V. 800-613-6131
Route 1, Km. 123.4, Bldg. 1, Turpeaux Industrial Park
Mercedita, PR 00715
Various types and sizes of bone plates.

Zimmer Trabecular Metal Technology 800-613-6131
10 Pomeroy Rd, Parsippany, NJ 07054
Porous metal rod.

PLATE, FIXATION, BONE, NON-SPINAL, METALLIC
(Orthopedics) 87NDF

Warsaw Orthopedic, Inc. 901-396-3133
2500 Silveus Xing, Warsaw, IN 46582
Axis, timesh, atlas.

Zimmer Manufacturing B.V. 800-613-6131
Route 1, Km. 123.4, Bldg. 1, Turpeaux Industrial Park
Mercedita, PR 00715
Various types and sizes of bone plates.

PLATE, HOT *(Chemistry) 75UGM*

Carver Inc. 260-563-7577
1569 Morris St, Wabash, IN 46992
Hot plates, hydraulic laboratory presses, laminating presses, manifolds plus various press accessories.

Cole-Parmer Instrument Inc. 800-323-4340
625 E Bunker Ct, Vernon Hills, IL 60061

Corning Inc., Science Products Division 800-492-1110
45 Nagog Park, Acton, MA 01720

Edmund Industrial Optics 800-363-1992
101 E Gloucester Pike, Barrington, NJ 08007

Ika-Works, Inc. 800-733-3037
2635 Northchase Pkwy SE, Wilmington, NC 28405

Kernco Instruments Co., Inc. 800-325-3875
420 Kenazo Ave., El Paso, TX 79928-7338
Digital, programmable hot plate/stirrers.

Omega Engineering, Inc. 800-848-4286
1 Omega Dr, Stamford, CT 06907
Featuring both analog- and microprocessor-based temp control either at plate surface by internal sensor or at the sample by probe.

Reheat Co., Inc. 800-373-4328
10 School St, Danvers, MA 01923
Custom hot plates and reaction blocks.

Thermo Fisher Scientific Inc. 563-556-2241
2555 Kerper Blvd, Dubuque, IA 52001

Troemner Llc 800-352-7705
201 Wolf Dr, PO Box 87, West Deptford, NJ 08086
$122.00 for model 501.

PLATE, PATIENT *(Gastro/Urology) 78FDB*

Cameron-Miller, Inc. 800-621-0142
5410 W Roosevelt Rd, Road #241, Chicago, IL 60644

PLATE, RADIAL IMMUNODIFFUSION *(Immunology) 82JZQ*

Binding Site, Inc., The 800-633-4484
5889 Oberlin Dr Ste 101, San Diego, CA 92121
Human serum proteins, complement components.

Helena Laboratories 409-842-3714
PO Box 752, Beaumont, TX 77704

PLATE, RADIAL IMMUNODIFFUSION *(cont'd)*

Immuno-Mycologics, Inc. 800-654-3639
PO Box 1151, Norman, OK 73070
Fungal immunodiffusion test systems for Histo, Blasto and cocci.

Invitrogen Corporation 800-955-6288
101 Lincoln Centre Dr, Foster City, CA 94404

Kent Laboratories, Inc. 360-398-8641
777 Jorgensen Pl, Bellingham, WA 98226
Full line of immunodiffusion plates.

Meridian Bioscience, Inc. 800-696-0739
3471 River Hills Dr, Cincinnati, OH 45244
$35.00 for 12 fungal plates.

Thermo Fisher Scientific (Rochester) 585-899-7600
75 Panorama Creek Dr, Panorama, NY 14625
Various.

PLATE, SILICA GEL, TLC *(Toxicology) 91DKS*

United Chemical Technologies, Inc. 800-385-3153
2731 Bartram Rd, Bristol, PA 19007
CLEAN SCREEN specialty-bonded organo-silica gels.

PLATFORM, FORCE-MEASURING *(Physical Med) 89KHX*

Advanced Mechanical Technology, Inc. (Amti) 800-422-AMTI
176 Waltham St, Watertown, MA 02472

Bertec Corporation 877-237-8320
6171 Huntley Rd Ste J, Columbus, OH 43229
Force measuring platforms of all sizes appropriate for a wide range of applications. Includes force plates for gait analysis, balance plates for balance screening and training, and force-measuring treadmills for complete analysis and rehabilitation of gait and balance.

Biodex Medical Systems, Inc. 800-224-6339
20 Ramsey Rd, Shirley, NY 11967

Electro Mechanical Products Inc. 772-286-8848
41 SE Kindred St, Stuart, FL 34994
Sway meter.

Fall Prevention Technologies, Llc 937-434-5455
4601 Gateway Cir, Kettering, OH 45440
Force-measuring platform.

Neurocom International, Inc. 503-653-2144
9570 SE Lawnfield Rd, Clackamas, OR 97015
Various models of force-measuring platform balance testers.

Podo Technology, Inc 678-990-1881
750 Hammond Dr NE Bldg 2, Suite 310, Atlanta, GA 30328
Various types of force measuring platform systems.

Three Rivers Holdings, Llc 480-833-1829
1826 W Broadway Rd Ste 43, Mesa, AZ 85202
Force measurement device.

Vestibular Technologies, Llc 307-637-5711
205 County Road 128a, Suite 200, Cheyenne, WY 82007-1831
Various models of force platforms.

PLEDGET AND INTRACARDIAC PATCH, PETP, PTFE, POLYPROPYLENE *(Cardiovascular) 74DXZ*

Bard Shannon Limited 908-277-8000
San Geronimo Industrial Park, Lot # 1, Road # 3, Km 79.7
Humacao, PR 00791
Fabrics,grafts,pledgets.

Bridger Biomed, Inc. 908-277-8000
2430 N 7th Ave, Bozeman, MT 59715
Cardiovascular patch.

Chase Medical, Lp 972-783-0644
1876 Firman Dr, Richardson, TX 75081
Cardiovascular patch kit (sterile).

Cryolife, Inc. 800-438-8285
1655 Roberts Blvd NW, Kennesaw, GA 30144
CryoPatch SG Pulm. Human Cardia

Ethicon, Llc. 908-218-2887
Rd. 183, Km. 8.3,, Industrial Area Hato, San Lorenzo, PR 00754
Sterile teflon pledgets.

Maquet Cardiovascular LLC 888-880-2874
45 Barbour Pond Dr, Wayne, NJ 07470
HEMASHIELD

Mast Biosurgery Usa Inc. 858-550-8050
6749 Top Gun St Ste 108, San Diego, CA 92121
Intracardiac patch or pledget.

Shelhigh, Inc. 908-206-8706
650 Liberty Ave, Union, NJ 07083
Patch.

PLEDGET AND INTRACARDIAC PATCH, PETP, PTFE, POLYPROPYLENE *(cont'd)*

Somanetics Corp. 800-359-7662
2600 Troy Center Dr, Troy, MI 48084
CorRestore(TM) System; Bovine pericardial patch system uniquely designed for cardiac repair and reconstruction and especially well-suited for Surgical Ventricular Restoration (SVR).

Synovis Life Technologies, Inc 800-255-4018
2575 University Ave W, Saint Paul, MN 55114
Peri-Guard Cardiovascular Patch; Supple Peri-Guard; Vascu-Guard

Tuzik Boston 800-886-6363
104 Longwater Dr, Assinippi Park, Norwell, MA 02061

W.L. Gore & Associates,Inc 928-526-3030
1505 North Fourth St., Flagstaff, AZ 86004
Cardiovascular patch.

Yama, Inc. 908-206-8706
650 Liberty Ave, Union, NJ 07083
Patch 'sterile'.

PLEDGET, DACRON, TEFLON, POLYPROPYLENE
(Cardiovascular) 74DSX

Covidien Lp 508-261-8000
15 Hampshire St, Mansfield, MA 02048
Teflon suture pledgets.

Ethicon, Inc. 800-4-ETHICON
Route 22 West, Somerville, NJ 08876
Available in 2 sizes, firm or soft teflon. Also available free standing in 2 sizes, prethreaded.

Tuzik Boston 800-886-6363
104 Longwater Dr, Assinippi Park, Norwell, MA 02061

PLETHYSMOGRAPH, IMPEDANCE *(Cardiovascular) 74DSB*

Behavioral Technology, Inc. 888-363-9017
24 M St, Salt Lake City, UT 84103
Barlow Gauge, Sensor, male arousal.

Cardiobeat.Com 480-419-3957
8070 E Morgan Trl Ste 210, Scottsdale, AZ 85258
Impedance cardiographic hemodynamic monitoring system.

Dermed Diagnostics, Inc. 630-668-4644
2S558 White Birch Ln, Wheaton, IL 60189
Impedance cardiograph.

Dimensional Dosing Systems, Inc. 724-933-7874
2465 Dogwood Dr, Wexford, PA 15090
Body composition analyzer.

Elmed, Inc. 630-543-2792
60 W Fay Ave, Addison, IL 60101

Hemo Sapiens, Inc. 928-202-4453
325 Lookout Dr, Sedona, AZ 86351
Non-invasive hemodynamic monitoring & management system.

Instrumentation For Medicine, Inc. 203-637-8377
31 MacArthur Dr, Old Greenwich, CT 06870
Hic 2000.

Nu Gyn, Inc 763-398-0108
1633 County Highway 10 Ste 15, Spring Lake Park, MN 55432
Penile impedence plethysmography.

Rjl Systems, Inc. 586-790-0200
33939 Harper Ave, Clinton Township, MI 48035
Orthosis, cervical.

U.F.I. 805-772-1203
545 Main St Ste C2, Morro Bay, CA 93442
$6,250 to $10,250 for Model 2994 (1 to 4 channels).

PLETHYSMOGRAPH, OCULAR *(Cns/Neurology) 84JXF*

Parks Medical Electronics, Inc. 503-649-7007
PO Box 5669, Aloha, OR 97006

PLETHYSMOGRAPH, PHOTO-ELECTRIC, PNEUMATIC OR HYDRAULIC *(Cardiovascular) 74JOM*

Aci Medical, Inc. 800-667-9451
1857 Diamond St, San Marcos, CA 92078
APG(R) Air Plethysmograph is a diagnostic device that provides answers to venous disease. It non-invasively measures absolute limb blood volume changes.

Behavioral Technology, Inc. 888-363-9017
24 M St, Salt Lake City, UT 84103
Geer Gauge, Sensor, female arousal.

Bio-Feedback Systems, Inc. 303-444-1411
2736 47th St, Boulder, CO 80301
$695 for penile plethysmograph (for impotence). Special order.

PLETHYSMOGRAPH, PHOTO-ELECTRIC, PNEUMATIC OR HYDRAULIC *(cont'd)*

Cardinal Healthcare 209, Inc. 610-862-0800
5225 Verona Rd, Fitchburg, WI 53711
Doppler system.

Elmed, Inc. 630-543-2792
60 W Fay Ave, Addison, IL 60101

Grass Technologies, An Astro-Med, Inc. Product Gro 401-828-4002
53 Airport Park Drive, Rockland, MA 02370
Protoelectric plethysmograph transducer.

Hokanson Inc., D.E. 800-999-8251
12840 NE 21st Pl, Bellevue, WA 98005
Photo and pneumo plethysmographs available for peripheral blood flow exams, including digit blood pressures and segmental pulse volume recordings. Stand-alone and integrated models available for clinical practice. The AI6 Arterial Inflow Blood Flow Measurement System is a new integrated strain gauge plethysmography system for measuring arterial inflow (venous occlusion plethysmography). It is fully computer automated, with customizable protocols.

Koven Technology, Inc. 800-521-8342
12125 Woodcrest Executive Dr Ste 320, Saint Louis, MO 63141
PGV-20 Plug-in module for Koven-Hadeco Dopplers PNEUMO, PPG, arterial & venous modes.

Neurodyne Medical Corp. 800-963-8633
186 Alewife Brook Pkwy, Cambridge, MA 02138
Medac System/3 includes photoelectric plethysmography for real-time monotoring of peripherial blood-flow changes and heart rate.

Osborn Medical Corp. 800-535-5865
100 W Main St N, PO Box 324, Utica, MN 55979
Air (option: Strain Gauge) Phlethysmography. For Detection of outflow obstruction, calf pump function, and valvular disorder in venous system. Inexpensive and ease of operation. Complete battery of tests completed in under 5 minutes. Comes with Stabilizing Chair.

U.F.I. 805-772-1203
545 Main St Ste C2, Morro Bay, CA 93442
$155.00 for Model 1020.

Unetixs Vascular, Inc. 800-486-3849
115 Airport St, North Kingstown, RI 02852

PLETHYSMOGRAPH, PRESSURE (BODY)
(Anesthesiology) 73CCM

Cardinal Health 207, Inc. 800-231-2466
22745 Savi Ranch Pkwy, Yorba Linda, CA 92887
Whole body, nonpressure.

Elmed, Inc. 630-543-2792
60 W Fay Ave, Addison, IL 60101

Hans Rudolph, Inc. 816-363-5522
7200 Wyandotte St, Kansas City, MO 64114
Mouthshutter valve.

Medical Graphics Corporation 800-950-5597
350 Oak Grove Pkwy, Saint Paul, MN 55127
Fully automated system 1085 flow and pressure body box with IBM compatible; performs diagnostic and administrative functions and disposable flow sensor. Determines lung volumes, airway machines, diffusion, bronchial provocation.

Morgan Scientific Inc. 800-525-5002
151 Essex St, Haverhill, MA 01832
Body Box 5510 - Instrument for the measurement of TGV, AWR, SGAW, Spirometry (Dynamic and Static), Lung Volumes (by plethysmography and/or nitrogen dilution), DLCO, Membrane Diffusion and Capillary Blood Volume, Bronchial Challenge and Respiratory Pressures. Interfaced to PC with ComPAS SQL Windows software (runs fully networked or stand-alone).

Nspire Health, Inc 800-574-7374
1830 Lefthand Cir, Longmont, CO 80501
OWL - Digital Body Plethysmography incorporates instant temperature equilibration, the new Autoflow electro/magnetic breathing valve with almost no resistance to inhalation of test gases, and the most stable software platform & SQL database in the business. Testing capabilities include spirometry, lung volumes, airways resistance and diffusion. Backed by the Talon warranty program, OWL gives you a grip on your budget with the lowest cost of operation.

Quadromed Inc. 800-363-0192
5776 Thimens Ave., St-Laurent, QUE H4R 2K9 Canada

PLETHYSMOGRAPH, PRESSURE (BODY) *(cont'd)*

Vasamed 800-695-2737
7615 Golden Triangle Dr Ste C, Eden Prairie, MN 55344
LASERDOPP waveform.

PLETHYSMOGRAPH, VOLUME *(Anesthesiology) 73JEH*

Cardinal Health 207, Inc. 610-862-0800
1100 Bird Center Dr, Palm Springs, CA 92262
Complete lung function system.

Eresearchtechnology Inc. 215-972-0420
1818 Market St Ste 1000, Philadelphia, PA 19103

Phipps & Bird, Inc. 800-955-7621
1519 Summit Ave, Richmond, VA 23230
Finger plethysmograph for student education.

Research Instrumentation Associates, Inc. 440-729-1649
8753 Mayfield Rd, Chesterland, OH 44026
Respiraton monitor.

Unetixs Vascular, Inc. 800-486-3849
115 Airport St, North Kingstown, RI 02852

PLIERS, CRIMP *(Gastro/Urology) 78FJY*

Biomet Microfixation Inc. 800-874-7711
1520 Tradeport Dr, Jacksonville, FL 32218
Various types of pliers.

PLIERS, OPERATIVE *(Dental And Oral) 76EJY*

Aesculap Implant Systems Inc. 1-800-234-9179
3773 Corporate Pkwy, Center Valley, PA 18034

Bendistal Pliers 636-230-9933
175 Lamp and Lantern Vlg, Chesterfield, MO 63017
Bendistal pliers: orthodontic pliers to bend and activate superelastic wires.

Dental Usa, Inc. 815-363-8003
5005 McCullom Lake Rd, McHenry, IL 60050
Plier.

Dentalez Group 866-DTE-INFO
101 Lindenwood Dr Ste 225, Valleybrooke Corporate Center
Malvern, PA 19355

Dentalez Group, Stardental Division 717-291-1161
1816 Colonial Village Ln, Lancaster, PA 17601
Carbide bur.

Hu-Friedy Manufacturing Co., Inc. 800-483-7433
3232 N Rockwell St, Chicago, IL 60618
$55.35 to $135.00 for 22 types of tissue pliers.

Kmedic 800-955-0559
190 Veterans Dr, Northvale, NJ 07647

Miltex Dental Technologies, Inc. 516-576-6022
589 Davies Dr, York, PA 17402
Various dental operative pliers.

Oratronics, Inc. 212-986-0050
405 Lexington Ave, New York, NY 10174
Titanium-tipped adjusting pliers.

Premier Dental Products Co. 888-670-6100
1710 Romano Dr, PO Box 4500, Plymouth Meeting, PA 19462

Pulpdent Corp. 800-343-4342
80 Oakland St, Watertown, MA 02472
Crimper/cutter pliers.

PLIERS, ORTHODONTIC *(Dental And Oral) 76JEX*

Aesculap Implant Systems Inc. 1-800-234-9179
3773 Corporate Pkwy, Center Valley, PA 18034

Align Technology, Inc. 408-470-1000
881 Martin Ave, Santa Clara, CA 95050
Plier,orthodontic.

Coltene/Whaledent Inc. 330-916-8858
235 Ascot Pkwy, Cuyahoga Falls, OH 44223
Plier.

Dental Usa, Inc. 815-363-8003
5005 McCullom Lake Rd, McHenry, IL 60050
Plier.

Dentronix, Inc. 800-523-5944
235 Ascot Pkwy, Cuyahoga Falls, OH 44223
$99.00 per unit (standard). Dentronix manufactures a complete line of hand-crafted, high quality pliers...available in high gloss and satin finishes.

E.A. Beck & Co. 949-645-4072
657 W 19th St Ste E, P O Box 10857, Costa Mesa, CA 92627
Pliers.

PLIERS, ORTHODONTIC *(cont'd)*

Emporium Specialties Co., Inc. 814-647-8661
10 Foster St, Austin, PA 16720

Forestadent Usa 314-878-5985
2315 Weldon Pkwy, Saint Louis, MO 63146
Dental hand instrument, orthodontic plier.

G & H Wire Co. 800-526-1026
2165 Earlywood Dr, Franklin, IN 46131

Glenroe Technologies 800-237-4060
1912 44th Ave E, Bradenton, FL 34203
Mathieu; separating pliers.

Hu-Friedy Manufacturing Co., Inc. 800-483-7433
3232 N Rockwell St, Chicago, IL 60618
$125.50 for 16 types of wire bending pliers.

Lancer Orthodontics, Inc. 760-304-2705
253 Pawnee St, San Marcos, CA 92078
Orthodontic pliers.

Masel Co., Inc. 800-423-8227
2701 Bartram Rd, Bristol, PA 19007

Miltex Dental Technologies, Inc. 516-576-6022
589 Davies Dr, York, PA 17402
Various orthodontic pliers.

National Precision Instruments 215-355-7525
1621 Loretta Ave Unit 4, Feasterville Trevose, PA 19053
Various types of orthodontic pliers.

Ortho Organizers, Inc. 760-448-8730
1822 Aston Ave, Carlsbad, CA 92008
Various types of orthodontic pliers.

Orthodental S.A. De C.V. 011-526-5611
Calle Industria Del Acero 18, Parque Industrial El Vigia
Mexicali 21397 Mexico
Various types of pliers

Orthodontic Design And Production, Inc. 760-734-3995
1370 Decision St Ste D, Vista, CA 92081
Various types of orthodontic pliers.

Orthopli Corp.
10061 Sandmeyer Ln, Philadelphia, PA 19116
Various styles.

Oscar, Inc. 317-849-2618
11793 Technology Ln, Fishers, IN 46038
Orthodontic plier.

Pyramid Orthodontics 800-752-3884
4328 Redwood Hwy Ste 100, San Rafael, CA 94903

Sds De Mexico, S.A. De C.V. 714-516-7484
Circuito Sur 31, Parque Industrial Nelson, Mexicali 21395 Mexico
Orthodontic pliers

Senitech Medical Instruments 760-918-1904
6351 Corte Del Abeto Ste A105, Carlsbad, CA 92011
Pliers.

Small Bone Innovations, Inc. 215-428-1791
1380 S Pennsylvania Ave, Morrisville, PA 19067
Dental hand instrument.

Toolmex Corporation 800-992-4766
1075 Worcester St, Natick, MA 01760
Orthodontics pliers, wire, ligature cutters.

Tp Orthodontics, Inc. 800-348-3856
100 Center Plz, La Porte, IN 46350

Ultradent Products, Inc. 801-553-4586
505 W 10200 S, South Jordan, UT 84095
Dental hand instrument.

World Class Technology Corporation 503-472-3320
1300 NE Alpha Dr, McMinnville, OR 97128
Plier, orthodontic.

PLIERS, SURGICAL *(Orthopedics) 87HTC*

Beere Precision Medical Instruments, Kmedic, Telef 919-544-3000
5307 95th Ave, Kenosha, WI 53144
Various types of surgical pliers.

Biomet Microfixation Inc. 800-874-7711
1520 Tradeport Dr, Jacksonville, FL 32218
Various types of pliers.

Biomet, Inc. 574-267-6639
56 E Bell Dr, PO Box 587, Warsaw, IN 46582
Various types of surgical pliers.

PLIERS, SURGICAL *(cont'd)*

Dental Usa, Inc. 815-363-8003
5005 McCullom Lake Rd, McHenry, IL 60050
Dental pliers.

Depuy Spine, Inc. 800-227-6633
325 Paramount Dr, Raynham, MA 02767
Spinal rod holder.

Elmed, Inc. 630-543-2792
60 W Fay Ave, Addison, IL 60101

H & H Co. 909-390-0373
4435 E Airport Dr Ste 108, Ontario, CA 91761
Suture pliers.

Holmed Corporation 508-238-3351
40 Norfolk Ave, South Easton, MA 02375

Key Surgical, Inc. 800-541-7995
8101 Wallace Rd Ste 100, Eden Prairie, MN 55344
Stainless steel pliers.

Kmedic 800-955-0559
190 Veterans Dr, Northvale, NJ 07647

Medtronic Sofamor Danek Instrument Manufacturing 901-396-3133
7375 Adrianne Pl, Bartlett, TN 38133
Multiple pliers, surgical.

Medtronic Sofamor Danek Usa, Inc. 901-396-3133
4340 Swinnea Rd, Memphis, TN 38118
Multiple pliers, surgical.

Prosurge Instruments, Inc. 866-832-7874
199 Laidlaw Ave, Jersey City, NJ 07306

Small Bone Innovations, Inc. 215-428-1791
1380 S Pennsylvania Ave, Morrisville, PA 19067
Pliers, surgical.

Standard Imaging, Inc. 608-831-0025
3120 Deming Way, Middleton, WI 53562
Vacuum powered tweezer, needle guide.

Symmetry Medical Usa, Inc. 574-267-8700
486 W 350 N, Warsaw, IN 46582
Manual surgical instrument for general use.

Trans American Medical / Tamsco Instruments 708-430-7777
7633 W 100th Pl, Bridgeview, IL 60455
Floor and medium grade surgical stainless steel.

Warsaw Orthopedic, Inc. 901-396-3133
2500 Silveus Xing, Warsaw, IN 46582
Multiple pliers, surgical.

Zimmer Holdings, Inc. 800-613-6131
1800 W Center St, PO Box 708, Warsaw, IN 46580

PLIERS, TUBE *(Gastro/Urology) 78FJO*

Biomet, Inc. 574-267-6639
56 E Bell Dr, PO Box 587, Warsaw, IN 46582
Various tube pliers.

PLINTH *(Physical Med) 89INT*

Colonial Scientific Ltd. 902-468-1811
201 Brownlow Ave., Unit 52, Dartmouth, NS B3B-1W2 Canada
Physiotherapy plinths-treatment tables, traction tables.

Dynatronics Corp. Chattanooga Operations 801-568-7000
6607 Mountain View Rd, Ooltewah, TN 37363
Plinth.

Hospital Therapy Products, Inc. 630-766-7101
757 N Central Ave, Wood Dale, IL 60191
Plinth.

Medi-Man Rehabilitation Products, Inc. 800-268-4256
6200A Tomken Rd., Mississauga, ONT L5T-1X7 Canada
COMFERTECH Massage therapy plinth.

Rite Time Corporation 800-266-2924
2950 E Dover St, Mesa, AZ 85213
Rite-Time surgery-recovery equipment.

PLUG, CATHETER *(Gastro/Urology) 78QHJ*

Addto, Inc. 773-278-0294
816 N Kostner Ave, Chicago, IL 60651
Catheter plug & cover.

Maddak Inc. 800-443-4926
661 State Route 23, Wayne, NJ 07470
ABLEWARE.

Smiths Medical Asd, Inc. 800-848-1757
6250 Shier Rings Rd, Dublin, OH 43016

PLUG, CATHETER *(cont'd)*

Woodhead L.P. 847-272-7990
3411 Woodhead Dr, Northbrook, IL 60062

PLUG, EAR *(Ear/Nose/Throat) 77QRU*

Apothecary Products, Inc. 800-328-2742
11750 12th Ave S, Burnsville, MN 55337
Ezy Care. Antimicrobial Ear plugs.

Doc's Proplugs, Inc. 800-521-2982
719 Swift St Ste 100, Santa Cruz, CA 95060
Vented to assist in equalization when scuba diving or free diving.

Hal-Hen Company, Inc. 800-242-5436
180 Atlantic Ave, Garden City Park, NY 11040
Complete line of ear plugs.

Harc Mercantile Ltd. 800-445-9968
1111 W Centre Ave, Portage, MI 49024

Medical Safety Systems Inc. 888-803-9303
230 White Pond Dr, Akron, OH 44313
Disposable.

Mid-States Laboratories, Inc. 800-247-3669
600 N Saint Francis St, Wichita, KS 67214
$22.00 per pair of EAR-DEFENDER sound plugs custom ear protection. Floatable, colored swim protection ear plugs (custom). Custom sound plugs with Hocks filter.

Norwood Promotional Products, Inc. 651-388-1298
5151 Moundview Dr, Red Wing, MN 55066

Oto-Med, Inc. 800-433-7703
1090 Empire Dr, Lake Havasu City, AZ 86404
OTOPlug ear protectors are designed to provide a superior seal and comfortable fit. Offered in six sizes.

Zee Medical, Inc. 800-841-8417
22 Corporate Park, Irvine, CA 92606

PLUG, OSTOMY *(Gastro/Urology) 78WHR*

Coloplast Manufacturing Us, Llc 800-533-0464
1840 W Oak Pkwy, Marietta, GA 30062
CONSEAL ostomy plug for continent stoma to provide periods of continence for voluntary control of evacuation.

PLUG, PUNCTUM *(Ophthalmology) 86LZU*

Eagle Vision, Inc. 800-222-7584
8500 Wolf Lake Dr Ste 110, Memphis, TN 38133
INSERT, DRY EYE. Short-term Temporary Punctal Canalicular Collagen Implant. 2 lengths, 3 diameters each. (Non-aesthetic use). DuraPlug, synthetic extended temporary punctal/canalicular insert, effective 60-180 days, made of PCL. PLUG, PUNCTUM. Tapered-shaft punctum plugs, five sizes and flow controller punctum valve, four sizes. FlexPlug, tapered shaft with ribbed shaft punctum plugs, ten sizes. SuperEagle, most advanced silicone plug available, 3 sizes. SuperFlex, the ultimate punctum plug, comes in 9 sizes.

Fci Ophthalmics 800-932-4202
64 Schoosett St, Pembroke, MA 02359

Lacrimedics, Inc. 360-376-7095
9 Hope Ln, Eastsound, WA 98245
Dissolvable lacrimal plug.

Oasis Medical, Inc. 800-528-9786
514 S Vermont Ave, Glendora, CA 91741
Intracanalicular Long-Term Hydrogel Plug, Silicone Plug, Collagen Plug, Extended Duration Intracanalicular Plug

Odyssey Medical, Inc. 901-383-7777
5828 Shelby Oaks Dr, Memphis, TN 38134
Various types of punctum plugs.

Technical Products, Inc. 800-226-8434
805 Marathon Pkwy Ste 150, Lawrenceville, GA 30046
Silicone rods from 1 to 7 mm, in 1-mm increments. Provided in 12-in. (30-cm) lengths.

PLUGGER, ROOT CANAL, ENDODONTIC *(Dental And Oral) 76EKR*

Aesculap Implant Systems Inc. 1-800-234-9179
3773 Corporate Pkwy, Center Valley, PA 18034

American Eagle Instruments, Inc. 406-549-7451
6575 Butler Creek Rd, Missoula, MT 59808
Various sizes & styles of endodontic instruments.

Arnold Tuber Industries 716-648-3363
97 Main St, Hamburg, NY 14075
Plugger, root canal, endodontic, dental hand instruments.

PLUGGER, ROOT CANAL, ENDODONTIC *(cont'd)*

Biomet Microfixation Inc. 800-874-7711
1520 Tradeport Dr, Jacksonville, FL 32218
Plugger, root canal, endodontic.

Coltene/Whaledent Inc. 330-916-8858
235 Ascot Pkwy, Cuyahoga Falls, OH 44223
Plugger.

Dental Usa, Inc. 815-363-8003
5005 McCullom Lake Rd, McHenry, IL 60050
Plugger.

Dentalez Group 866-DTE-INFO
101 Lindenwood Dr Ste 225, Valleybrooke Corporate Center
Malvern, PA 19355

Dentalez Group, Stardental Division 717-291-1161
1816 Colonial Village Ln, Lancaster, PA 17601
Explorer, operative.

E.A. Beck & Co. 949-645-4072
657 W 19th St Ste E, P O Box 10857, Costa Mesa, CA 92627
Plugger.

Hu-Friedy Manufacturing Co., Inc. 800-483-7433
3232 N Rockwell St, Chicago, IL 60618
$18.85 each, 26 types.

Js Dental Mfg., Inc. 800-284-3368
196 N Salem Rd, Ridgefield, CT 06877
Finger plugger.

Kerr Corp. 714-516-7400
28200 Wick Rd, Romulus, MI 48174
Endodontic plugger.

Lightspeed Technology, Inc. 210-495-4942
403 E Ramsey Rd Ste 205, San Antonio, TX 78216
Endodontic root canal obturator.

Micro-Dent Inc. 866-526-1166
379 Hollow Hill Rd, Wauconda, IL 60084
Plugger, root canal, endodontic.

Miltex Dental Technologies, Inc. 516-576-6022
589 Davies Dr, York, PA 17402
Various types of hand-operated endodontic pluggers.

Moyco Technologies, Inc. 800-331-8837
200 Commerce Dr, Montgomeryville, PA 18936

Premier Dental Products Co. 888-670-6100
1710 Romano Dr, PO Box 4500, Plymouth Meeting, PA 19462

Pulpdent Corp. 800-343-4342
80 Oakland St, Watertown, MA 02472
No common name listed.

San Diego Swiss Machining, Inc. 858-571-6636
9177 Aero Dr Ste A, San Diego, CA 92123
Endodontic post removal system.

Sci-Dent, Inc. 800-323-4145
210 Dowdle St Ste 2, Algonquin, IL 60102

PLUNGER-LIKE JOINT MANIPULATOR *(Physical Med) 89LXM*

Advanced Orthogonal Equipment, Incorporated 757-224-0177
2201 62nd Ave N, Saint Petersburg, FL 33702
Advanced orthogonal percussion adjusting instrument.

Alfred Ueda 307-789-2088
145 Upland Cir, Corte Madera, CA 94925
Hand held adjusting instrument.

Innovative Machinery Packaging And Converting Inc. 503-581-3239
PO Box 535, Salem, OR 97308
Manipulator/adjustor.

Miltex Dental Technologies, Inc. 516-576-6022
589 Davies Dr, York, PA 17402
Various integrators, chiropratic mallets & accessories.

Neuromechanical Innovations, Llc 480-785-8448
11011 S 48th St Ste 220, Phoenix, AZ 85044
Impluse-adjusting instrument, cbp adjusting instrument.

Sense Technology, Inc. 800-628-9416
4241 William Penn Hwy Fl 1, Murrysville, PA 15668
Computerized spinal assessment and treatment.

Sigma Instruments, Inc. 724-776-9500
506 Thomson Park Dr, Cranberry Township, PA 16066
Adjusting or joint mobilization instrument.

PNEUMOCYSTIS CARINII *(Microbiology) 83LYF*

Bio-Rad Laboratories, Inc. 425-881-8300
6565 185th Ave NE, Redmond, WA 98052
Direct fluorescence test for pneumocystis carinii.

Meridian Bioscience, Inc. 800-696-0739
3471 River Hills Dr, Cincinnati, OH 45244
A direct immunofluorescent procedure for the detection of Pneumocystis carinii cysts and trophozoites in respiratory tract specimens.

PNEUMOGRAPH *(Anesthesiology) 73RLL*

Phipps & Bird, Inc. 800-955-7621
1519 Summit Ave, Richmond, VA 23230
Pneumograph for student education.

PNEUMOPERITONEUM APPARATUS, AUTOMATIC *(Gastro/Urology) 78FDP*

Entracare, Llc 913-451-2234
11315 Strang Line Rd, Lenexa, KS 66215
Enteral pump and gravity feeding sets, non-sterile.

Karl Storz Endoscopy-America Inc. 800-421-0837
600 Corporate Pointe, Culver City, CA 90230

Mahe International Inc. 800-294-7946
468 Craighead St, Nashville, TN 37204

PNEUMOTACHOGRAPH *(Anesthesiology) 73RLM*

Lds Life Science (Formerly Gould Instrument Systems Inc.) 216-328-7000
5525 Cloverleaf Pkwy, Valley View, OH 44125

Morgan Scientific Inc. 800-525-5002
151 Essex St, Haverhill, MA 01832
ScreenStar Pneumotachograph. Instrument for the measurement of Spirometry (Dynamic and Static)and Bronchial Challenge. Interfaced to PC running ComPAS SQL Software (full network or stand-alone).

Quadromed Inc. 800-363-0192
5776 Thimens Ave., St-Laurent, QUE H4R 2K9 Canada

Vacumed 800-235-3333
4538 Westinghouse St, Ventura, CA 93003

PNEUMOTACHOMETER *(Anesthesiology) 73JAX*

Carlsbad International Export, Inc. 760-438-5323
1954 Kellogg Ave, Carlsbad, CA 92008
Pneumotach.

Hans Rudolph, Inc. 816-363-5522
7200 Wyandotte St, Kansas City, MO 64114
Rudolph linear pneumotachometer.

Sdi Diagnostics, Inc. 800-678-5782
10 Hampden Dr, South Easton, MA 02375
FLOSENSE disposable pneumotach; alternative to Puritan-Bennett FS-200 and 250. Also FLOSENSE II our new alternative to Puritan Bennett's FS II flow sensor!

POINT, ABRASIVE *(Dental And Oral) 76EHL*

Abrasive Technology, Inc. 740-548-4100
8400 Green Meadows Dr N, Lewis Center, OH 43035
Abrasive point.

Aesculap Implant Systems Inc. 1-800-234-9179
3773 Corporate Pkwy, Center Valley, PA 18034

Align Technology, Inc. 408-470-1000
881 Martin Ave, Santa Clara, CA 95050
Point,abrasive.

Buffalo Dental Mfg. Co., Inc. 516-496-7200
159 Lafayette Dr, Syosset, NY 11791
Abrasives.

Dedeco Intl., Inc. 845-887-4840
11617 Route 97, Long Eddy, NY 12760
Various types of abrasive points.

Den-Mat Holdings, Llc 805-922-8491
2727 Skyway Dr, Santa Maria, CA 93455
No common name listed.

Ivoclar Vivadent, Inc. 800-533-6825
175 Pineview Dr, Amherst, NY 14228

Nobel Biocare Usa, Llc 800-579-6515
22715/22725 Savi Ranch Parkway, Yorba Linda, CA 92887
Abrasive device & accessory.

Shofu Dental Corporation 800-827-4638
1225 Stone Dr, San Marcos, CA 92078
DURA-GREEN, SHOFU DURA-WHITE

POINT, ABRASIVE *(cont'd)*

Ultradent Products, Inc. 801-553-4586
505 W 10200 S, South Jordan, UT 84095
Abrasive points.

POINT, PAPER, ENDODONTIC *(Dental And Oral) 76EKN*

Coltene/Whaledent Inc. 330-916-8858
235 Ascot Pkwy, Cuyahoga Falls, OH 44223
Paper points.

Dentalez Group 866-DTE-INFO
101 Lindenwood Dr Ste 225, Valleybrooke Corporate Center
Malvern, PA 19355

Endodent, Inc. 626-359-5715
851 Meridian St, Duarte, CA 91010
Sterile cellpack absorbent points. Sterilized bulk pack absorbent points.

Miltex Dental Technologies, Inc. 516-576-6022
589 Davies Dr, York, PA 17402
Various endodontic paper points.

Moyco Technologies, Inc. 800-331-8837
200 Commerce Dr, Montgomeryville, PA 18936

Precise Dental Internacional S.A.C.V. 818-992-5333
925 Parque Cuzin Belenes Norte, Zapopan, Jalisoo Mexico
Sterile absorbent paper points

Pulpdent Corp. 800-343-4342
80 Oakland St, Watertown, MA 02472
No common name listed.

Rite-Dent Manufacturing Corp. 305-693-8626
3750 E 10th Ct, Hialeah, FL 33013
Various types of endodontic paper point.

United Dental Manufacturers, Inc. 918-878-0450
PO Box 700874, Tulsa, OK 74170
ISO-DIN 13965 Gutta-percha points.

United Dental Mfg., Inc. 717-845-7511
608 Rolling Hills Dr, Johnson City, TN 37604
Paper points.

POINT, SILVER, ENDODONTIC *(Dental And Oral) 76EKL*

Dentalez Group 866-DTE-INFO
101 Lindenwood Dr Ste 225, Valleybrooke Corporate Center
Malvern, PA 19355

Dentalez Group, Stardental Division 717-291-1161
1816 Colonial Village Ln, Lancaster, PA 17601
Explorer, operative.

Miltex Dental Technologies, Inc. 516-576-6022
589 Davies Dr, York, PA 17402
Various silver points.

Moyco Technologies, Inc. 800-331-8837
200 Commerce Dr, Montgomeryville, PA 18936

Pacific Implant, Inc. 707-764-5602
920 Rio Dell Ave, Rio Dell, CA 95562
Endodontic point.

Pulpdent Corp. 800-343-4342
80 Oakland St, Watertown, MA 02472
No common name listed.

United Dental Manufacturers, Inc. 918-878-0450
PO Box 700874, Tulsa, OK 74170
ISO-DIN 13965, also Gutta-percha point, ISO-DIN 13965.

United Dental Mfg., Inc. 717-845-7511
608 Rolling Hills Dr, Johnson City, TN 37604
Various.

POLARIMETER *(Chemistry) 75JQZ*

Glas-Col , Llc 800-452-7265
711 Hulman St, PO Box 2128, Terre Haute, IN 47802

Index Instruments U.S. Inc. 407-932-3688
3305 Commerce Blvd, Kissimmee, FL 34741
Polarimeters and accessories from simple instruments for routine analysis to the latest high accuracy 3000 series NIR near infrared system.

Jasco, Inc. 800-333-5272
8649 Commerce Dr, Easton, MD 21601

Olis: On-Line Instrument Systems, Inc. 800-852-3504
130 Conway Dr Ste A, Bogart, GA 30622
Spectropolarimeters.

POLARIMETER *(cont'd)*

Rudolph Research Analytical 973-584-1558
55 Newburgh Rd, Hackettstown, NJ 07840
The AUTOPOL series of automatic polarimeters. Also available, the AUTOPOL series of automatic saccharimeters.

POLYETHYLENE GLYCOL (CARBOWAX) *(Pathology) 88IER*

Polysciences, Inc. 800-523-2575
400 Valley Rd, Warrington, PA 18976

Sci Gen, Inc. 310-324-6576
333 E Gardena Blvd, Gardena, CA 90248
FDA: Medical Device Manufacturing and packaging. Focus on Histology, Cytology, Analytical and General purpose Reagents, Chemistry, and Sterling and Disinfecting agents.

POLYGRAPH *(General) 80RLN*

Galix Biomedical Instrumentation, Inc. 305-534-5905
2555 Collins Ave Ste C-5, Miami Beach, FL 33140
Galix Physio Stim: PC-based high-resolution electrophysiology system. Digital acquisition of 12 surface and 16 intracavitary ECG channels. 16 simultaneous channels on a split-screen display for real-time and stored ECG signal monitoring. This device provides data storage on recordable compact or optical disks. The most reliable and versatile built-in E.P. stimulator with up to 3 independent extra stimuli, with the stimulation channel selected by software.

Lds Life Science (Formerly Gould Instrument Systems Inc.) 216-328-7000
5525 Cloverleaf Pkwy, Valley View, OH 44125

POLYMER, ENT COMPOSITE SYNTHETIC PTFE WITH CARBON-FIBER *(Ear/Nose/Throat) 77ESF*

W.L. Gore & Associates,Inc 928-526-3030
1505 North Fourth St., Flagstaff, AZ 86004
Implantable material for augmenting tissue deficiencies.

POLYMER, ENT SYNTHETIC POLYAMIDE (MESH OR FOIL MATERIAL) *(Ear/Nose/Throat) 77KHJ*

Genzyme Corporation 617-252-7500
1125 Pleasantview Ter, Ridgefield, NJ 07657
Nasal-sinus and otologic dressing.

Gyrus Ent L.L.C., Sub. Of Gyrus Acmi, Inc. 508-804-2739
2925 Appling Rd, Bartlett, TN 38133
Vocom.

POLYMER, ENT SYNTHETIC, POROUS POLYETHYLENE *(Ear/Nose/Throat) 77JOF*

Tino, S.A. De C.V. 800-024-77-55
Hospital #631, Guadalajara, JALIS 44200 Mexico

POLYMER, ENT SYNTHETIC-PIFE, SILICON ELASTOMER *(Ear/Nose/Throat) 77ESH*

Pillar Surgical, Inc. 800-367-0445
PO Box 8141, La Jolla, CA 92038
Silastic silicone sheeting in various thicknesses, 6 x 8 x desired thickness (0.005 to 0.080 in.).

Technical Products, Inc. 800-226-8434
805 Marathon Pkwy Ste 150, Lawrenceville, GA 30046
Silicone tubing.

POLYMER, SYNTHETIC, OTHER *(General) 80WTJ*

Advansource Biomaterials Corp. 978-657-0075
229 Andover St, Wilmington, MA 01887
CHRONOFLEX AL ether-free, biodurable aliphatic thermoplastic polyurethane elastomers. CHRONOFLEX AR aromatic, solution-grade biodurable segmented polyurethane elastomers. CHRONO FLEX C ether free, biodurable aromatic thermoplastic polyurethane elastomer. CHRONOPRENE extremely soft, rubbery thermoplastic elastomer. CHRONOTHANE aromatic thermoplastic polyurethane elastomers. HYDROTHANE aliphatic, hydrophilic thermoplastic polyurethane elastomeric hydrogels. POLYBLEND aromatic, polyurethane hybrid elastoplastic mixtures. POLYWELD two-component reactive cast elastomer for potting/encapsulating.

Bangs Laboratories, Inc. 800-387-0672
9025 Technology Dr, Fishers, IN 46038
Uniform polymer particles (or microspheres) for medical diagnostic tests and immunoassays. Sizes 20nm - 650um. ProActive Protein Coated Microspheres, streptavidin, protein A, goat anti-mouse and other protein-coated microspheres, magnetic, polymeric, and silica.

Diamond Polymers, Inc. 888-437-4674
1353 Exeter Rd, Akron, OH 44306
SOFTFLEX alloys.

POLYMER, SYNTHETIC, OTHER *(cont'd)*

Filtrona Extrusion, Inc./Pexcor Medical Products Div. 800-755-7528
764 S Athol Rd, P.O. Box 659, Athol, MA 01331
Thermoplastic elastomer.

Kensey Nash Corporation 484-713-2100
735 Pennsylvania Dr, Exton, PA 19341
Contract research and development of absorbable polymer products with focus primarily on orthopedic applications.

Kent Elastomer Products, Inc. 800-331-4762
1500 Saint Clair Ave, PO Box 668, Kent, OH 44240
Thermoplastic elastomer.

Polymer Laboratories, Now A Part Of Varian, Inc. 800-767-3963
160 Old Farm Rd, Amherst Fields Research Park, Amherst, MA 01002
Polymers for drug therapy.

Polyzen, Inc. 919-319-9599
1041 Classic Rd, Apex, NC 27539
Polyurethane films. Polyurethane and silicone dip molding. Custom polymer forumulations.

Saint-Gobain Performance Plastics--Akron 800-798-1554
2664 Gilchrist Rd, Akron, OH 44305
PHARMED tubing provides unequaled flex life in peristaltic pump applications.

Saint-Gobain Performance Plastics/Clearwater 800-541-6880
4451 110th Ave N, Clearwater, FL 33762

Sonoco Crellin, Inc. 518-392-2000
87 Center St, Chatham, NY 12037
Wide range of press sizes and polymers available.

Sunlite Plastics, Inc. 262-253-0600
W194N11340 McCormick Dr, Germantown, WI 53022
Thermoplastic elastomer.

Waters Corp. 800-252-4752
34 Maple St, Milford, MA 01757

POLYVINYL METHYLETHER MALEIC ACID-CALCIUM-SODIUM DBL. SALT *(Dental And Oral) 76KOO*

Block Drug Co., Inc. 973-889-2578
2149 Harbor Ave., Memphis, TN 38113
Denture powder, cream, liquid, gel.

Dentek Oral Care, Inc. 865-983-1300
307 Excellence Way, Maryville, TN 37801
Secure denture adhesive.

Organics Corporation Of America 973-890-9002
55 W End Rd, Paterson, NJ 07512
Denture adhesive.

Perrigo New York, Inc. 269-686-2916
1700 Bathgate Ave, Bronx, NY 10457
Denture adhesive cream.

Procter & Gamble Co. 513-622-4851
6200 Bryan Park Rd, Browns Summit, NC 27214

POLYVINYL METHYLETHER MALEIC ACID/CARBOXYMETHYLCELLULOSE *(Dental And Oral) 76KOT*

Block Drug Co., Inc. 973-889-2578
2149 Harbor Ave., Memphis, TN 38113
Denture adhensive,powder, cream, liquid, gel.

Novocol, Inc. 303-665-7535
416 S Taylor Ave, Louisville, CO 80027
Denture adhesive.

Team Technologies, Inc. 423-587-2199
5949 Commerce Blvd, Morristown, TN 37814
Denture adhesive cream.

PORT & CATHETER, INFUSION, IMPLANTED, SUBCUT., INTRAPERIT. *(General) 80MDX*

Neo Medical Inc. 888-450-3334
42514 Albrae St, Fremont, CA 94538
Implantable vascular access portal.

PORT & CATHETER, INFUSION, IMPLANTED, SUBCUTANEOUS, INTRASPINAL *(General) 80MDV*

Bolt Bethel, Llc 763-434-5900
23530 University Avenue Ext NW, PO Box 135, Bethel, MN 55005

PORT, VASCULAR ACCESS *(Cardiovascular) 74THP*

Angiodynamics, Inc. 800-472-5221
1 Horizon Way, Manchester, GA 31816
TRIUMPH I, LIFEPORT, VORTEX, INFUSE-A-PORT, OMEGA-PORT, TITAN-PORT vascular access systems.

PORT, VASCULAR ACCESS *(cont'd)*

Arrow International, Inc. 800-523-8446
2400 Bernville Rd, Reading, PA 19605
A-PORT implantable vascular access port.

B. Braun Oem Division, B. Braun Medical Inc. 866-8-BBRAUN
824 12th Ave, Bethlehem, PA 18018

Cardio-Nef, S.A. De C.V. 01-800-024-0240
Rio Grijalva 186, Col. Mitras Norte, Monterrey, N.L. 64320 Mexico

Dma Med-Chem Corporation 800-362-1833
49 Watermill Ln, Great Neck, NY 11021
Ports and catheters.

Gish Biomedical, Inc. 800-938-0531
22942 Arroyo Vis, Rancho Santa Margarita, CA 92688
VASPORT lightweight venous and arterial port with high-density silicone septum. Port-access Huber needle with extension tubing.

Medi-Dose, Inc. 800-523-8966
70 Industrial Dr, Ivyland, PA 18974

Smiths Medical Asd, Inc. 800-433-5832
1265 Grey Fox Rd, Saint Paul, MN 55112
PORT-A-CATH implantable venous access systems. P.A.S.PORT ELITE implantable peripheral venous access system. ProPort plastic implantable venous access system.

Specialized Health Products International, Inc. 800-306-3360
585 W 500 S, Bountiful, UT 84010
The MiniLoc™ Safety Infusion Set uses an innovative, built-in safety mechanism to reduce the risk of accidental needlestick injuries by shielding the needle during port deaccess. MiniLoc™'s ultra-low profile, stability, easy-to-use design conforms to user technique. All standard sizes available, call 1-800-306-3360 for more information.

POSITIONER, SOCKET *(Orthopedics) 87KIL*

Alimed, Inc. 800-225-2610
297 High St, Dedham, MA 02026

Allen Medical Systems, Inc. 800-433-5774
1 Post Office Sq, Acton, MA 01720
Positioning device for shoulder

Allesee Orthodontic Appliances 714-516-7484
13931 Spring St, Sturtevant, WI 53177
Tongue positioner and excerciser,tongue positioner and exerciser palate.

Andronic Devices 800-563-7557
2335 Bayswater St., Vancouver, BC V6K-4B2 Canada

Tri-Medics, Inc. 401-490-5321
10 Pine Tree Ln, Lincoln, RI 02865
Positioner.

Voss Medical Products 210-650-3124
4235 Centergate St, San Antonio, TX 78217
Head rest.

Zimmer Trabecular Metal Technology 800-613-6131
10 Pomeroy Rd, Parsippany, NJ 07054
Retractors.

POSITIONER, SPINE, SURGICAL *(Orthopedics) 87WWB*

Alimed, Inc. 800-225-2610
297 High St, Dedham, MA 02026

Allen Medical Systems, Inc. 800-433-5774
1 Post Office Sq, Acton, MA 01720
Spinal suite of products to accommodate spine surgery in facility.

Imperial Surgical Ltd. 800-661-5432
581 Orly Ave., Dorval, ONT H9P-1G1 Canada
Priced $3500. scoliosis operating frame.

Lossing Orthopedic 800-328-5216
PO Box 6224, Minneapolis, MN 55406
LOSSING variable spine roll with interchangeable cores allows you to select comfort level - soft, medium or firm.

Northstar Medical. Inc, 800-457-3217
38 Buckingham Dr, Rogers, AR 72758
For shoulder.

POSITIONER, TOOTH, PREFORMED *(Dental And Oral) 76KMY*

Align Technology, Inc. 408-470-1000
881 Martin Ave, Santa Clara, CA 95050
Button kit.

Allesee Orthodontic Appliances 714-516-7484
13931 Spring St, Sturtevant, WI 53177
Positioners.

POSITIONER, TOOTH, PREFORMED *(cont'd)*

Allesee Orthodontic Appliances (Calexico) 714-516-7400
341 E 1st St, Calexico, CA 92231
Positioners.

Allesee Orthodontic Appliances, Inc. - Connecticut 949-255-8766
6 Niblick Rd, Enfield, CT 06082
Positioners.

Aurum Ceramic Dental Laboratories Llp 403-228-5199
1320 N Howard St, Spokane, WA 99201
Orthodontic appliance.

G & H Wire Co. 800-526-1026
2165 Earlywood Dr, Franklin, IN 46131

Glenroe Technologies 800-237-4060
1912 44th Ave E, Bradenton, FL 34203
Mouthguard.

Schueler & Company, Inc. 516-487-1500
PO Box 528, Stratford, CT 06615

Specialty Appliance Works, Inc. 800-522-4636
4905 Hammond Industrial Dr, Cumming, GA 30041

Tp Orthodontics, Inc. 800-348-8856
100 Center Plz, La Porte, IN 46350
Custom-made positioners.

POST, ROOT CANAL *(Dental And Oral) 76ELR*

Abrasive Technology, Inc. 740-548-4100
8400 Green Meadows Dr N, Lewis Center, OH 43035
Root canal posts.

Alceram Tech Inc 516-849-3666
57 2nd St, Ronkonkoma, NY 11779
Posts,manufactured out of FDA approved Ceramic Material.

Bisco, Inc. 847-534-6000
1100 W Irving Park Rd, Schaumburg, IL 60193
Post-various types.

Coltene/Whaledent Inc. 330-916-8858
235 Ascot Pkwy, Cuyahoga Falls, OH 44223
Endodontic post.

Den-Mat Holdings, Llc 805-922-8491
2727 Skyway Dr, Santa Maria, CA 93455
No common name listed.

Dentalez Group 866-DTE-INFO
101 Lindenwood Dr Ste 225, Valleybrooke Corporate Center
Malvern, PA 19355

Essential Dental Systems, Inc. 800-223-5394
89 Leuning St, South Hackensack, NJ 07606

Farpin, Inc. 801-262-8406
333 E 4500 S Apt 13, Murray, UT 84107
Root canal post.

Foremost Dental Llc. 201-894-5500
242 S Dean St, Englewood, NJ 07631
Root canal post.

Ivoclar Vivadent, Inc. 800-533-6825
175 Pineview Dr, Amherst, NY 14228
COSMOPOST, FRC POSTEC.

J. Morita Usa, Inc. 888-566-7482
9 Mason, Irvine, CA 92618
CF CARBON FIBER POST and GF GLASS FIBER POST: Both consist of strong fiber bundles embedded in a special composite material, which will chemically bond with the dental material used for cementation and core buildup. The braided plait form of the fiber bundles, in a multi-axial arrangement, gives the posts superior resistance to bending and torsion forces than fibers in a typical single-axial arrangement. Both posts have similar elasticity as dentin, enabling them to flex with the natural dentin. They dissipate occlusal stress rather than transmitting it as metal posts do. They are non-corrosive and biocompatible.

Metalor Technologies Usa 800-554-5504
255 John L Dietsch Blvd, PO Box 255, North Attleboro, MA 02763
Root canal post.

Miltex Dental Technologies, Inc. 516-576-6022
589 Davies Dr, York, PA 17402
Various root canal posts and post systems.

Moyco Technologies, Inc. 800-331-8837
200 Commerce Dr, Montgomeryville, PA 18936
Solid or hollow.

POST, ROOT CANAL *(cont'd)*

Oco Inc. 800-228-0477
600 Paisano St NE Ste A, Albuquerque, NM 87123
Root canal post.

Parkell, Inc. 800-243-7446
300 Executive Dr, Edgewood, NY 11717
CI Post - Glass composite, Stainless steel, or Burnout pattern

Pentron Clinical Technologies 203-265-7397
68-70 North Plains Industrial, Road, Wallingford, CT 06492
Post,root canal.

Pentron Laboratory Technologies 203-265-7397
53 N Plains Industrial Rd, Wallingford, CT 06492
Post, root canal.

Precision Dental Int, Inc. 818-992-1888
21361 Deering Ct, Canoga Park, CA 91304
Root canal post.

Promident Llc 845-634-3997
242 N Main St, New City, NY 10956

Sterngold 800-243-9942
23 Frank Mossberg Dr, PO Box 2967, Attleboro, MA 02703
ROTEX, HADER.

Ultradent Products, Inc. 801-553-4586
505 W 10200 S, South Jordan, UT 84095
Root canal post and drills.

Zenith Point Manufacturing 805-499-6808
3867 Old Conejo Rd, Newbury Park, CA 91320
Post.

POSTERIOR METAL/POLYMER SPINAL SYSTEM, FUSION *(Orthopedics) 87NQP*

Synthes San Diego 858-452-1266
6244 Ferris Sq Ste B, San Diego, CA 92121
Pedicle screw system.

POTASSIUM DICHROMATE, ALCOHOL *(Toxicology) 91DOJ*

Varian Inc 650-424-5078
25200 Commercentre Dr, Lake Forest, CA 92630
Alcohol test.

POTENTIATOR, BLOOD ANTIBODY *(Hematology) 81UJP*

Dade Behring, Inc. 800-948-3233
1717 Deerfield Rd, Deerfield, IL 60015

POTENTIOMETER *(Chemistry) 75UHJ*

Krohn-Hite Corporation 877-549-7781
15 Jonathan Dr Ste 4, Brockton, MA 02301
Standards of electricity. Calibrators, references, AC & DC voltage, current, and resistance.

POUCH, COLOSTOMY *(Gastro/Urology) 78EZQ*

Coloplast Manufacturing Us, Llc 800-533-0464
1840 W Oak Pkwy, Marietta, GA 30062
Transparent and opaque, one and two-piece pouches for colostomy with skin barrier.

Marlen Manufacturing & Development Co. 216-292-7060
5150 Richmond Rd, Bedford, OH 44146
Ileostomy, urostomy and colostomy appliances.

Spectrum Technology 513-471-8770
3120 Warsaw Ave, Cincinnati, OH 45205
Colostomy deodorant.

POUCH, TELEMETRY *(General) 80WME*

General Econopak, Inc. 888-871-8568
1725 N 6th St, Philadelphia, PA 19122

Neotech Products, Inc. 800-966-0500
27822 Fremont Ct, Valencia, CA 91355
TELE-TOTE, EZ TOTE, VERSA TOTE, CLIP TOTE, VALU-TOTE, & SOF-TOTE telemetry transmitter holders.

Rnd Signs 800-328-4009
7605 Equitable Dr, Eden Prairie, MN 55344
Disposable Holter monitor pouch without recorder.

POWDER, PORCELAIN *(Dental And Oral) 76EIH*

American Tooth Industries 800-235-4639
1200 Stellar Dr, Oxnard, CA 93033
JUSTI low-fusion porcelain.

Bisco, Inc. 847-534-6000
1100 W Irving Park Rd, Schaumburg, IL 60193
Porcelain powders - various types.

POWDER, PORCELAIN *(cont'd)*

Cdl Technologies Inc. 619-702-1806
645 Front St Unit 2007, San Diego, CA 92101
Dental frame material for dental prosthesis.

Ceragroup Industries Inc. 954-670-0208
6555 Powerline Rd Ste 211, Ft Lauderdale, FL 33309
Powder, porcelain.

Chameleon Dental Products, Inc. 913-281-5552
200 N 6th St, Kansas City, KS 66101
No common name listed.

D. Sign Dental Lab, Inc. 757-224-0177
690 W Fremont Ave Ste 9C, Sunnyvale, CA 94087
Porcelain powder.

Dds Services, Inc. 720-435-9052
15000 W 6th Ave Ste 150, Golden, CO 80401
Dental restorative material.

Den-Mat Holdings, Llc 805-922-8491
2727 Skyway Dr, Santa Maria, CA 93455
No common name listed.

Dentsply Canada, Ltd. 800-263-1437
161 Vinyl Ct., Woodbridge, ONT L4L 4A3 Canada

Foundation Milling Centre 716-579-3724
235 Aero Dr Ste 2, Buffalo, NY 14225
Porcelain powder.

Gc America, Inc. 708-597-0900
3737 W 127th St, Alsip, IL 60803
Porcelain stain kit.

Golden Triangle Dental Laboratory Inc. 972-910-9912
7475 Las Colinas Blvd Ste A, Irving, TX 75063
Crown/bridges, inlay/onlay.

Gresco Products, Inc. 800-527-3250
13391 Murphy Rd, P.o. Box 865, Stafford, TX 77477
Silane coupling agent.

Heraeus Kulzer, Inc. 800-431-1785
99 Business Park Dr, Armonk, NY 10504
For use with porcelain to metal dental alloys.

Ivoclar Vivadent, Inc. 800-533-6825
175 Pineview Dr, Amherst, NY 14228
IPS CLASSIC PORCELAIN, IPS d.SIGN, IPS ERIS, IPS EMPRESS.

Jensen Industries, Inc. 203-239-2090
50 Stillman Rd, North Haven, CT 06473
Pressible porcelain ingot,layering porcelain.

Js Dental Mfg., Inc. 800-284-3368
196 N Salem Rd, Ridgefield, CT 06877
Dental ceramic inlays.

Nobel Biocare Usa, Llc 800-579-6515
22715/22725 Savi Ranch Parkway, Yorba Linda, CA 92887
Procelain powder & related products.

Pentron Laboratory Technologies 203-265-7397
53 N Plains Industrial Rd, Wallingford, CT 06492
Stylepress.

Prismatik Dentalcraft, Inc. 949-440-2683
2181 Dupont Dr, Irvine, CA 92612
Dental porcelain.

Somerset Dental Products (Pentron Ceramics, Inc.) 800-496-9600
500 Memorial Dr, Somerset, NJ 08873
Porcelain powder.

Ultradent Products, Inc. 801-553-4586
505 W 10200 S, South Jordan, UT 84095
Etching gel barrier.

Vident 800-828-3839
3150 E Birch St, Brea, CA 92821
Vita In-Ceram YZ, Alumina and Spinell. VITA VM13 PFM Porcelain. VITA VM7 and VITA VM 9 All-Ceramic. Akzent stain kit.

POWDERS, ANTIMYCOBACTERIAL SUSCEPTIBILITY TEST
(Microbiology) 83MJA

Trek Diagnostic Systems, Inc. 608-8373788
210 Business Park Dr, Sun Prairie, WI 53590
Same.

POWER SUPPLY, ENDOSCOPIC, BATTERY-OPERATED
(General) 80QUD

Bovie Medical Corp. 800-537-2790
5115 Ulmerton Rd, Clearwater, FL 33760
Portable flexible shaft examination lights, 5 to 10 in.

Chiu Technical Corp. 631-544-0606
252 Indian Head Rd, Kings Park, NY 11754
$720.00 FO 150 - AC/DC.

Mahe International Inc. 800-294-7946
468 Craighead St, Nashville, TN 37204

Welch Allyn, Inc. 800-535-6663
4341 State Street Rd, Skaneateles Falls, NY 13153

POWER SUPPLY, ENDOSCOPIC, LINE-OPERATED
(General) 80QUE

Cameron-Miller, Inc. 800-621-0142
5410 W Roosevelt Rd, Road #241, Chicago, IL 60644

Welch Allyn, Inc. 800-535-6663
4341 State Street Rd, Skaneateles Falls, NY 13153

POWER SYSTEM, ISOLATED *(General) 80TCS*

Astralite Corporation 800-345-7703
PO Box 689, Somerset, CA 95684
ASTRALITE Shockproof Controller is a conveniently packaged auxiliary power source which converts line voltage to a variable low voltage output. Plugs directly into any grounded AC outlet.

Bender, Inc. 800-356-4266
700 Fox Chase, Highlands Corp. Center, Coatesville, PA 19320
IPP Isolated Power Systems for hospital operating rooms and ICUs.

Lake Shore Cryotronics, Inc. 614-891-2243
575 McCorkle Blvd, Westerville, OH 43082
Power supplies for superconducting magnets.

Maxwell Technologies Power Systems 877-511-4324
9244 Balboa Ave, San Diego, CA 92123
MEDI-GUARD 0.5- to 200-kVA power-line conditioners, UL544. All voltages and configurations for medical applications.

Mge Ups Sytems, Inc. 800-523-0142
1660 Scenic Ave, Costa Mesa, CA 92626
Total isolation, precise voltage regulation and power outage protection; systems in standard kVA ratings. 220VA-4500kVA.

Oneac Corporation 800-327-8801
27944 N Bradley Rd, Libertyville, IL 60048
75VA to 200kVA power conditioners; including low-leakage-current (UL2601 listed) versions for patient contact applications; isolation transformer based.

Powervar, Inc. 800-369-7179
1450 S Lakeside Dr, Waukegan, IL 60085
Laboratory power conditioners isolate sensitive laboratory equipment for increased reliability; medical power conditioners with low leakage current and safety agency listings, Global Power Interface is three phase power conditioners for higher power applications. All products are safety agency listed for both North America and international locations.

Rapid Power Technologies, Inc. 800-332-1111
18 Old Grays Bridge Rd, Brookfield, CT 06804
Isolation transformers with single and multiple shielding.

Woodhead L.P. 847-272-7990
3411 Woodhead Dr, Northbrook, IL 60062

POWER SYSTEMS, UNINTERRUPTIBLE (UPS) *(General) 80WMN*

Access Battery Inc. 800-654-9845
12104 W Carmen Ave, Division of Alpha Source, Inc.
Milwaukee, WI 53225
Full line sealed lead-acid UPS batteries.

Advanced Electronics Systems, Inc. 800-345-1280
2005 Lincoln Way E, Chambersburg, PA 17202

Advanced Instrument Development, Inc. 800-243-9729
2545 Curtiss St, Downers Grove, IL 60515
POWER-AID independent x-ray power source, supplies uninterruptible single- or three-phase power to operate a small x-ray generator such as a mammography unit. Available as 5 and 10 kVA units.

American Power Conversion 800-788-2208
132 Fairgrounds Rd, West Kingston, RI 02892
MATRIX-UPS midrange modular UPS protection.

Ametek Solidstate Controls 800-635-7300
875 Dearborn Dr, Columbus, OH 43085

PRINTER, IMAGE, VIDEO *(cont'd)*

Hitachi Kokusai Electric America, Ltd. 516-921-7200
150 Crossways Park Dr, Woodbury, NY 11797

Ideal Medical Source, Inc. 800-537-0739
2805 East. Oakland Blvd, Suite 352, Fort Lauderdale, FL 33306

Innervision Inc. 901-682-0417
6258 E Shady Grove Rd, Memphis, TN 38120

Karl Storz Endoscopy-America Inc. 800-421-0837
600 Corporate Pointe, Culver City, CA 90230

Lynn Medical 888-596-6633
764 Denison Ct, Bloomfield Hills, MI 48302

Mediflex Surgical Products 800-879-7575
250 Gibbs Rd, Islandia, NY 11749
Surgical grade, 5- by 7-in., image size, multi-image per page, publication-grade quality.

Meza Medical Equipment 888-308-7116
108 W Nakoma St, San Antonio, TX 78216

Pentax Medical Company 800-431-5880
102 Chestnut Ridge Rd, Montvale, NJ 07645
Several video printers in color or black and white and printer paper. Computer printers and accessories for use with PENTAX workstations are available. Call for quote.

Richard Wolf Medical Instruments Corp. 800-323-9653
353 Corporate Woods Pkwy, Vernon Hills, IL 60061

Smith & Nephew, Inc., Endoscopy Division 800-343-8386
150 Minuteman Rd, Andover, MA 01810

Sony Electronics, Inc., Medical Systems Div. 800-686-7669
1 Sony Dr, Park Ridge, NJ 07656
High resolution videographic printers.

Universal Ultrasound 800-842-0607
299 Adams St, Bedford Hills, NY 10507
Sony Medical, Mitsubishi.

PRINTER, RADIOGRAPHIC DUPLICATOR *(Radiology) 90RNW*

Bidwell Industrial Group, Inc., Blu-Ray Division 860-343-5353
2055 S Main St, Middletown, CT 06457
$1150 for MARK V duplicating printer (43 lb. wt.) - film returned in 6 sec.

Fujifilm Medical Systems Usa, Inc. 800-431-1850
419 West Ave, Stamford, CT 06902
Fuji Radiographic Duplicator

Marconi Medical Systems 800-323-0550
595 Miner Rd, Cleveland, OH 44143

Smith Companies Dental Products 800-336-3263
4368 Enterprise St, Fremont, CA 94538
PrintX Dental Film Printer. Makes diagnostic quality prints from #0-, 1- and 2-size dental x-rays. Stand-alone device, no computer is needed.

PRISM, ENDOSCOPIC *(Surgery) 79GCN*

Arw Optical Corp. 910-452-7373
6631 Amsterdam Way # B, Wilmington, NC 28405

PRISM, FRESNEL, OPHTHALMIC *(Ophthalmology) 86HKT*

Fresnel Prism & Lens Co. 952-496-0432
6824 Washington Ave S, Eden Prairie, MN 55344
Press-on prism.

3m Petaluma 707-765-3236
1331 Commerce St, Petaluma, CA 94954
Various styles and sizes of opthalmic press- on optics.

PRISM, ROTARY, OPHTHALMIC *(Ophthalmology) 86HKQ*

Astron International Inc. 239-435-0136
3410 Westview Dr, Naples, FL 34104
Prism, rotary, ophthalmic.

PROBE *(Orthopedics) 87HXB*

Accutome, Inc. 610-889-0200
3222 Phoenixville Pike, Malvern, PA 19355
Various opthalmic probes.

Allez Medical Applications, Inc. 714-641-2098
2141 S Standard Ave, Santa Ana, CA 92707
Various types of probes.

Arthrex California, Inc. 239-643-5553
20509 Earlgate St, Walnut, CA 91789
Probe.

Biomet, Inc. 574-267-6639
56 E Bell Dr, PO Box 587, Warsaw, IN 46582
Various.

PROBE *(cont'd)*

Civco Medical Instruments Co., Inc. 319-656-4447
102 1st St S, Kalona, IA 52247
Transesophageal probe sheath cover.

Dental Usa, Inc. 815-363-8003
5005 McCullom Lake Rd, McHenry, IL 60050
Dental probe.

Depuy Mitek, A Johnson & Johnson Company 800-451-2006
50 Scotland Blvd, Bridgewater, MA 02324
Various types of orthopedic probes.

Depuy Spine, Inc. 800-227-6633
325 Paramount Dr, Raynham, MA 02767
Orthopaedic probe.

Gyrus Medical, Inc. 800-852-9361
6655 Wedgwood Rd N Ste 105, Maple Grove, MN 55311
Laparoscope.

Innervision Inc. 901-682-0417
6258 E Shady Grove Rd, Memphis, TN 38120
Laparoscope.

Invuity, Inc. 760-744-4447
334 Via Vera Cruz Ste 255, San Marcos, CA 92078
Various types and sizes of probes.

Invuity, Inc. 415-655-2100
39 Stillman St, San Francisco, CA 94107

K2m, Inc. 866-526-4171
751 Miller Dr SE Ste F1, Leesburg, VA 20175
Feeler,probe.

Karl Storz Endoscopy-America Inc. 800-421-0837
600 Corporate Pointe, Culver City, CA 90230

Mectra Labs, Inc. 800-323-3968
PO Box 350, Two Quality Way, Bloomfield, IN 47424
Laparoscope.

Medtronic Puerto Rico Operations Co.,Med Rel 763-514-4000
Road 909, Km. 0.4., Barrio Mariana, Humacao, PR 00792
Various probes.

Micromanipulator Co., Inc., The 800-972-4032
1555 Forrest Way, Carson City, NV 89706
Products and accessories to aid in embyro recovery, grading, splitting, injection, micromanipulation and photomicrography.

Spine Wave, Inc. 203-944-9494
2 Enterprise Dr Ste 302, Shelton, CT 06484
Various types of probes.

Surgical Implant Generation Network (Sign) 509-371-1107
451 Hills St, Richland, WA 99354
Probe.

Symmetry Medical Usa, Inc. 574-267-8700
486 W 350 N, Warsaw, IN 46582
Orthopedic manual surgical instrument.

Symmetry Tnco 888-447-6661
15 Colebrook Blvd, Whitman, MA 02382

Wisap America 800-233-8448
8231 Melrose Dr, Lenexa, KS 66214

Zimmer Spine, Inc. 800-655-2614
7375 Bush Lake Rd, Minneapolis, MN 55439
Probe.

Zimmer Trabecular Metal Technology 800-613-6131
10 Pomeroy Rd, Parsippany, NJ 07054
Distal spacer sound.

Zinetics Medical, Inc. 800-648-4070
1050 E South Temple, Salt Lake City, UT 84102
PH probe.

PROBE, BLOOD FLOW, EXTRAVASCULAR
(Cardiovascular) 74DPT

Carolina Medical, Inc. 800-334-4531
157 Industrial Dr, King, NC 27021
Complete line of electromagnetic flow probes with lumens from 1 to 120mm circumference. Intra- and extra-corporeal types.

Genesee Biomedical, Inc. 800-786-4890
1308 S Jason St, Denver, CO 80223
INTRA-ART Coronary Artery Probes. Improves assessment and probing of the coronary arteries.

International Biophysics Corp. 512-326-3244
2101 E Saint Elmo Rd Ste 275, Austin, TX 78744
Floprobe.

PROBE, BLOOD FLOW, EXTRAVASCULAR *(cont'd)*

Numed, Inc. 315-328-4491
2880 Main St., Hopkinton, NY 12965
Intravascular catheter with transducer.

Terumo Cardiovascular Systems (Tcvs) 800-283-7866
28 Howe St, Ashland, MA 01721
Blood flow probe.

PROBE, COMMON DUCT *(Gastro/Urology) 78RMG*

Miltex Inc. 800-645-8000
589 Davies Dr, York, PA 17402

PROBE, DETECTOR, FLOW, BLOOD, LAPAROSCOPY, ULTRASONIC *(Surgery) 79RTA*

Intramedical Imaging Llc 800-519-3959
12340 Santa Monica Blvd Ste 227, Los Angeles, CA 90025
Gamma Radiation Detection Probe for sentinel nodes biopsy and detection of tumors using FDG

Neoprobe Corporation 800-793-0079
425 Metro Pl N Ste 300, Dublin, OH 43017
neo2000 gamma detection system including 14mm and laparoscopic probes

PROBE, ELECTROCAUTERIZATION, MULTI-USE *(Surgery) 79QEZ*

Ams Innovative Center-San Jose 800-356-7600
3070 Orchard Dr, San Jose, CA 95134

Gyrus Medical, Inc. 800-852-9361
6655 Wedgwood Rd N Ste 105, Maple Grove, MN 55311

Md International, Inc. 305-669-9003
11300 NW 41st St, Doral, FL 33178

Richard Wolf Medical Instruments Corp. 800-323-9653
353 Corporate Woods Pkwy, Vernon Hills, IL 60061

Synectic Medical Product Development 203-877-8488
60 Commerce Park, Milford, CT 06460

Vital Concepts, Inc. 800-984-2300
4334 Brockton Dr SE Ste F, Grand Rapids, MI 49512
Reusable, and disposable, J-hooks, L-hooks, spatulas, monopolar needle, knives in 5mm xia & 33 & 42 cm lengths. For use with Vita-Flow & Hydro-Pro Irrigation system.

PROBE, ELECTROCAUTERIZATION, SINGLE-USE *(Surgery) 79QHA*

Ams Innovative Center-San Jose 800-356-7600
3070 Orchard Dr, San Jose, CA 95134

Md International, Inc. 305-669-9003
11300 NW 41st St, Doral, FL 33178

Smith & Nephew, Inc., Endoscopy Division 800-343-8386
150 Minuteman Rd, Andover, MA 01810

Synectic Medical Product Development 203-877-8488
60 Commerce Park, Milford, CT 06460

PROBE, ELECTROSURGERY, ENDOSCOPY *(Surgery) 79SJC*

Angiodynamics, Inc. 510-771-0400
46421 Landing Pkwy, Fremont, CA 94538
The Starburst XLi is a state-of-the-art, minimally invasive RFA device designed to provide scalable, spherical ablations up to 7cm. Its real-time, multi-point temperature feedback system and unique micro-infusion technology ensures sustained target temperatures and enables the precise ablation of predictable volumes of tissue. The Starburst XLi not only reduces the time required to perform the procedure, in many cases, the patient can resume normal activity within days.

Clinical Innovations, Inc. 888-268-6222
747 W 4170 S, Murray, UT 84123
LATITUDE is a line of disposable motility catheters. LATITUDE incorporates the latest technology into single use esophageal motility and anorectal manometry catheters with every sensor circumferential.

Ethicon Endo-Surgery, Inc. 800-USE-ENDO
4545 Creek Rd, Cincinnati, OH 45242

Vital Concepts, Inc. 800-984-2300
4334 Brockton Dr SE Ste F, Grand Rapids, MI 49512
VITA-FLOW Irrigation and aspiration probe with tubing. Manual irrigation/aspiration trumpet valve with 28cm probe and tubing.

Xillix Technologies Corp. 800-665-2236
13775 Commerce Pkwy., Ste. 100, Richmond, BC V6V 2V4 Canada
Fluorescence endoscopy for improved cancer detection.

PROBE, FISTULA *(Gastro/Urology) 78RMI*

Miltex Inc. 800-645-8000
589 Davies Dr, York, PA 17402

PROBE, GASTROINTESTINAL *(Gastro/Urology) 78FGM*

Aesculap Implant Systems Inc. 1-800-234-9179
3773 Corporate Pkwy, Center Valley, PA 18034
Probe and director.

Biomet Microfixation Inc. 800-874-7711
1520 Tradeport Dr, Jacksonville, FL 32218
Various types of probes.

Gyrus Medical, Inc. 800-852-9361
6655 Wedgwood Rd N Ste 105, Maple Grove, MN 55311
Bipolar gastric coagulator; central lumen for irrigation.

Hansen Ophthalmic Development Lab 319-338-1285
745 Avalon Pl, Coralville, IA 52241
A grooved director modified the crawford stint.

Metabolic Solutions, Inc. 866-302-1998
460 Amherst St, Nashua, NH 03063
13c-octanoate gastric motility breath test.

Power Medical Interventions, Inc. 267-775-8154
2021 Cabot Blvd W, Langhorne, PA 19047
Rigid curve positioner.

Sandhill Scientific, Inc. 800-468-4556
9150 Commerce Center Cir Ste 500, Highlands Ranch, CO 80129
Combined impedance-manometry catheters for esophageal function testing(EFT). Both solid state and water perfused EFT models are available. ComforTEC Plus single use pH monitoring catheters. ComforTEC MII-pH impedance-pH monitoring catheters

Tuzik Boston 800-886-6363
104 Longwater Dr, Assinippi Park, Norwell, MA 02061

PROBE, LACRIMAL *(Ophthalmology) 86HNL*

Bausch & Lomb Surgical 636-255-5051
3365 Tree Court Ind Blvd, Saint Louis, MO 63122

Biomet Microfixation Inc. 800-874-7711
1520 Tradeport Dr, Jacksonville, FL 32218
Various types of probes.

Eagle Vision, Inc. 800-222-7584
8500 Wolf Lake Dr Ste 110, Memphis, TN 38133
Monocanalicular stent (2 sizes). Various probes, repair of lacerated canaliculi. Lacrimal intubation.

Eye Care And Cure 800-486-6169
4646 S Overland Dr, Tucson, AZ 85714
Lacrimal probe.

Fci Ophthalmics 800-932-4202
64 Schoosett St, Pembroke, MA 02359
Lacrimal intubation sets.

Fischer Surgical Inc. 314-303-7753
1343 Pine Dr, Arnold, MO 63010
Various types of lachrymal probes.

Fortrad Eye Instruments Corp. 973-543-2371
8 Franklin Rd, Mendham, NJ 07945

Gunther Weiss Scientific Glassblowing Co., Inc. 503-621-3463
14640 NW Rock Creek Rd, Portland, OR 97231
Jones tube.

Gyrus Ent L.L.C., Sub. Of Gyrus Acmi, Inc. 508-804-2739
2925 Appling Rd, Bartlett, TN 38133
Various.

Hurricane Medical 941-751-0588
5315 Lena Rd, Bradenton, FL 34211
Various.

Jedmed Instruments Co. 314-845-3770
5416 Jedmed Ct, Saint Louis, MO 63129
Crawford intubation set: stainless-steel probe with olive tips, wedged together by silicone tubing.

Katena Products, Inc. 800-225-1195
4 Stewart Ct, Denville, NJ 07834

Miltex Inc. 800-645-8000
589 Davies Dr, York, PA 17402

Princeton Medical Group, Inc. 800-875-0869
1189 Royal Links Dr, Mt Pleasant, SC 29466

Psi/Eye-Ko, Inc. 636-447-1010
804 Corporate Centre Dr, O Fallon, MO 63368
Various models of lachrymal probes.

PROBE, LACRIMAL *(cont'd)*

Stephens Instruments, Inc. 800-354-7848
2500 Sandersville Rd, Lexington, KY 40511
$18.00 per unit (standard).

Total Titanium, Inc. 618-473-2429
140 East Monroe St., Hecker, IL 62248
Various types of lacrimal probes.

PROBE, OPHTHALMIC *(Ophthalmology) 86RMH*

Alceram Tech Inc 516-849-3666
57 2nd St, Ronkonkoma, NY 11779
Specialty lenses to customer's design plus stock items.

Jedmed Instruments Co. 314-845-3770
5416 Jedmed Ct, Saint Louis, MO 63129

Stephens Instruments, Inc. 800-354-7848
2500 Sandersville Rd, Lexington, KY 40511
$15.00 per unit (standard).

PROBE, OTHER *(General) 80RMK*

Axiom Analytical, Inc. 949-757-9300
1451 Edinger Ave Ste A, Tustin, CA 92780
High performance immersion probes.

Bagshaw Company, Inc., W.H. 800-343-7467
1 Pine Street Ext, PO Box 766, Nashua, NH 03060
Neurologic, surgical probes (brain surgery).

Basi (Bioanalytical Systems, Inc.) 800-845-4246
2701 Kent Ave, West Lafayette, IN 47906
Microdialysis probe for monitoring analytes in the extracellular fluid of the body without removing liquid, and for introducing substances without injecting fluid. (Blood-vessel system copy). Probe consists of dialysing membrane (molecular cut-off is 30,000 daltons) with special design for brain, subdermal, bile duct, and I.V. use. For use with research animals only--not for humans.

Cardiofocus, Inc. 508-658-7200
500 Nickerson Rd Ste 500-200, Marlborough, MA 01752
Fiber-optic laser diffusing probes. Cylindrical, hemicylindrical, spherical, and micro lens. Fiber- optic catheters for spectroscopy.

Care Wise Medical Products Corp. 888-462-8725
15750 Vineyard Blvd Ste 160, Morgan Hill, CA 95037
Hand-held gamma probe.

Carl Zeiss Meditec Inc. 877-486-7473
5160 Hacienda Dr, Dublin, CA 94568
Ultrasonic Biometer has a solid probe that is equipped with a fixation light for easy alignment and precise axial length measurement for complete IOL calculations. A snap-in software module card interface allows the instrument to be updated with the latest IOL formulae and procedures. Help screens summarize operation procedures and simplify use.

Gammadirect Medical Division 847-267-5929
PO Box 383, Lake Forest, IL 60045
Micro-TC probe measures blood profusion, oxyegen synthesis and temperature at tissue in real time.

Ludlum Measurements, Inc. 800-622-0828
501 Oak St, Sweetwater, TX 79556
Proportional probes.

Medi-Globe Corporation 800-966-1431
110 W Orion St Ste 136, Tempe, AZ 85283
Bipolar coagulation probes.

Medrad, Inc. 800-633-7231
100 Global View Dr, Warrendale, PA 15086
MRINNERVU System with endorectal coils for the prostate, cervix and colon/rectum.

Medworks Instruments 800-323-9790
PO Box 581, Chatham, IL 62629
$2.00 per unit.Mall type.

Pelton Shepherd Industries 800-258-3423
812B W Luce St, Stockton, CA 95203
CRYOSTIM probe - ice massage for massage therapy and accupressure points. Each set (4002, 4012, 4036) includes two probes and one tube of conductor gel.

Princeton Medical Group, Inc. 800-875-0869
1189 Royal Links Dr, Mt Pleasant, SC 29466

Spaceage Control, Inc. 661-273-3000
38850 20th St E, Palmdale, CA 93550
miniature displacement sensor

PROBE, OTHER *(cont'd)*

United Electric Controls Co. 617-926-1000
180 Dexter Ave, P.O. Box 9143, Watertown, MA 02472
Thermocouples, R.T.D.'s, thermistors, thermowells, accessories, and transmilters

Vysis 800-553-7042
3100 Woodcreek Dr, Downers Grove, IL 60515
Fish for detecting Williams Syndrome.

PROBE, PERIODONTIC *(Dental And Oral) 76EIX*

Aesculap Implant Systems Inc. 1-800-234-9179
3773 Corporate Pkwy, Center Valley, PA 18034

Arnold Tuber Industries 716-648-3363
97 Main St, Hamburg, NY 14075
Probe, periodontic, dental hand instruments.

Coltene/Whaledent Inc. 330-916-8858
235 Ascot Pkwy, Cuyahoga Falls, OH 44223
Explorer.

Dental Usa, Inc. 815-363-8003
5005 McCullom Lake Rd, McHenry, IL 60050
Probe.

Dentalez Group 866-DTE-INFO
101 Lindenwood Dr Ste 225, Valleybrooke Corporate Center Malvern, PA 19355

Dentalez Group, Stardental Division 717-291-1161
1816 Colonial Village Ln, Lancaster, PA 17601
Unit, operative dental.

Florida Probe Corp. 352-372-1142
3700 NW 91st St Ste C100, Gainesville, FL 32606
Computerized periodontal probe.

H & H Co. 909-390-0373
4435 E Airport Dr Ste 108, Ontario, CA 91761
Probe, periodontic, all types.

Hu-Friedy Manufacturing Co., Inc. 800-483-7433
3232 N Rockwell St, Chicago, IL 60618
$17.45 to $29.80 each, 30 types.

Ivoclar Vivadent, Inc. 800-533-6825
175 Pineview Dr, Amherst, NY 14228

Marquis Dental Mfg. Co. 303-344-5222
15370 Smith Rd Unit H, Aurora, CO 80011
Probe.

Micro-Dent Inc. 866-526-1166
379 Hollow Hill Rd, Wauconda, IL 60084
Probe.

Miltex Dental Technologies, Inc. 516-576-6022
589 Davies Dr, York, PA 17402
Various periodontic probes.

Nordent Manufacturing, Inc. 800-966-7336
610 Bonnie Ln, Elk Grove Village, IL 60007
$17.50 each for color-coded units.

Pdt, Inc. 406-626-4153
12201 Moccasin Ct, Missoula, MT 59808
Various types of probes.

Premier Dental Products Co. 888-670-6100
1710 Romano Dr, PO Box 4500, Plymouth Meeting, PA 19462

Quden Inc. 450-243-6101
8 Maple, Cp 510, Knowlton J0E 1V0 Canada
Interoral perio probe

Sci-Dent, Inc. 800-323-4145
210 Dowdle St Ste 2, Algonquin, IL 60102

Stuart Allyn Co., Inc. 413-443-7306
17 Taconic Park Dr, Pittsfield, MA 01201
Periodontal probe.

Suter Dental Manufacturing Company, Inc. 800-368-8376
632 Cedar St, Chico, CA 95928

Wykle Research, Inc. 775-887-7500
2222 College Pkwy, Carson City, NV 89706
Periodontic probe.

Xinix Research, Inc. 603-433-9121
5 Pheasant Ln, Portsmouth, NH 03801
Periodontal probe.

PROBE, RADIOFREQUENCY LESION *(Cns/Neurology) 84GXI*

Bausch & Lomb Surgical 636-255-5051
3365 Tree Court Ind Blvd, Saint Louis, MO 63122

PROBE, RADIOFREQUENCY LESION *(cont'd)*

Neurotherm Inc. 978-777-3916
2 De Bush Ave, Middleton, MA 01949
Disposable rf cannula.

Oscor, Inc. 800-726-7267
3816 Desoto Blvd, Palm Harbor, FL 34683
RF catheter.

Trivirix International Inc. 320-982-8000
925 6th Ave NE, Milaca, MN 56353

PROBE, RECTAL, NON-POWERED *(Gastro/Urology) 78EXX*

Apple Medical Corp. 508-357-2700
28 Lord Rd Ste 135, Marlborough, MA 01752
Rectal probe.

Medrad Inc. 724-940-7940
625 Alpha Dr, Pittsburgh, PA 15238

Sandhill Scientific, Inc. 800-468-4556
9150 Commerce Center Cir Ste 500, Highlands Ranch, CO 80129
Anorectal manometry catheters in a comprehensive selection of both solid state and water perfused models.

Welch Allyn, Inc. 800-535-6663
4341 State Street Rd, Skaneateles Falls, NY 13153

PROBE, SINUS *(Ear/Nose/Throat) 77KAK*

Aesculap Implant Systems Inc. 1-800-234-9179
3773 Corporate Pkwy, Center Valley, PA 18034

Bausch & Lomb Surgical 636-255-5051
3365 Tree Court Ind Blvd, Saint Louis, MO 63122

Miltex Inc. 800-645-8000
589 Davies Dr, York, PA 17402

PROBE, SUCTION, IRRIGATOR/ASPIRATOR, LAPAROSCOPIC *(Surgery) 79QUQ*

Armm, Inc. 714-848-8190
17744 Sampson Ln, Huntington Beach, CA 92647
EndoSI suction/irrigation probes and wye sets for laparoscopic surgeries.

Atc Technologies, Inc. 781-939-0725
30B Upton Dr, Wilmington, MA 01887

Boss Instruments, Ltd. 800-210-2677
395 Reas Ford Rd Ste 120, Earlysville, VA 22936

Elmed, Inc. 630-543-2792
60 W Fay Ave, Addison, IL 60101

Ethicon Endo-Surgery, Inc. 800-USE-ENDO
4545 Creek Rd, Cincinnati, OH 45242

Mectra Labs, Inc. 800-323-3968
PO Box 350, Two Quality Way, Bloomfield, IN 47424
NIBBLER, 5mm (disposable) probe for tissue morcellation, sharp dissection and biopsy. Also, will function as suction/irrigator.

Mediflex Surgical Products 800-879-7575
250 Gibbs Rd, Islandia, NY 11749

Megadyne Medical Products, Inc. 800-747-6110
11506 S State St, Draper, UT 84020
ALL-IN-ONE, laparoscopic suction/irrigation/electrocautery hand control unit and electrodes.

Richard Wolf Medical Instruments Corp. 800-323-9653
353 Corporate Woods Pkwy, Vernon Hills, IL 60061

Rocket Medical Plc. 800-707-7625
150 Recreation Park Dr Ste 3, Hingham, MA 02043

Synectic Medical Product Development 203-877-8488
60 Commerce Park, Milford, CT 06460

Vital Concepts, Inc. 800-984-2300
4334 Brockton Dr SE Ste F, Grand Rapids, MI 49512
Hydro-Pro $ Vita-Flow, single use & reusable system for irrigation & aspiration during minimally invasive surgery.

PROBE, TEMPERATURE *(General) 80RMJ*

Berghof/America 800-544-5004
3773 NW 126th Ave Bldg 1, Coral Springs, FL 33065
Molded PTFE temperature probes can be used in any medium where there is chemical protection of both the medium and the probe.

Bsd Medical Corporation 801-972-5555
2188 W 2200 S, Salt Lake City, UT 84119
VITEK temperature probe.

Burling Instruments, Inc. 973-635-9481
16 River Rd, Chatham, NJ 07928
Temperature sensor.

PROBE, TEMPERATURE *(cont'd)*

Cas Medical Systems, Inc. 800-227-4414
44 E Industrial Rd, Branford, CT 06405
Neonatal skin-temperature sensor.

Cincinnati Sub-Zero Products, Inc., Medical Division 800-989-7373
12011 Mosteller Rd, Cincinnati, OH 45241
Reusable and single patient-use temperature probes available in rectal/esophageal (adult and infant) and skin surface versions.

Cornerstone Sensors, Inc. 800-955-1470
2128 Arnold Way Ste 4, Alpine, CA 91901

Dickson Co 800-757-3747
930 S Westwood Ave, Addison, IL 60101
Monitor temperatures from -300 to +2000F

Dma Med-Chem Corporation 800-362-1833
49 Watermill Ln, Great Neck, NY 11021

Kentec Medical Inc. 800-825-5996
17871 Fitch, Irvine, CA 92614
ACCUTEMP PROBE temperature probe, infant. Temperature probe for incubators and infant warmers.

Ludlow Technological Products 800-445-5025
2 Ludlow Park Dr, Chicopee, MA 01022
Pediatric and neonatal temperature probe covers.

Medtronic Perfusion Systems 800-328-3320
7611 Northland Dr N, Brooklyn Park, MN 55428

Mennen Medical Corp. 800-223-2201
2540 Metropolitan Dr, Trevose, PA 19053

Minco Products, Inc. 763-571-3121
7300 Commerce Ln NE, Minneapolis, MN 55432
Resistance temperature detectors, thermocouples and thermistors. Temperature pyrometer, platinum RTDs, thermocouples and thermistors; -200 to 200 degrees Celsius. Packaged in probe, ribbon and miniature configurations.

Noral, Inc. 800-348-2345
23600 Mercantile Rd, Beachwood Commerce Park
Cleveland, OH 44122

Oven Industries, Inc. 1-877-766-6836
207 Hempt Rd, Mechanicsburg, PA 17050

Physitemp Instruments, Inc. 800-452-8510
154 Huron Ave, Clifton, NJ 07013
$50.00 to $145.00 per unit.

Pmt Corp. 800-626-5463
1500 Park Rd, Chanhassen, MN 55317

Sensor Scientific, Inc. 800-524-1610
6 Kingsbridge Rd, Fairfield, NJ 07004
Thermistor-based temperature probes for all medical applications. Industry-standard 400 series, 700 series, and 10K other probes are available, in addition to custom designs.

U.F.I. 805-772-1203
545 Main St Ste C2, Morro Bay, CA 93442
$160.00 for Model 1070.

United Electric Controls Co. 617-926-1000
180 Dexter Ave, P.O. Box 9143, Watertown, MA 02472
Thermocouples, R.T.D.'s, thermistors, thermowells, accessories, and transmilters

PROBE, THERMODILUTION *(Cardiovascular) 74KRB*

Edwards Lifesciences Technology Sarl 949-250-2500
State Rd. 402 N.km 1.4, Anasco, PR 00610-1577
Co-set.

Icu Medical (Ut), Inc 949-366-2183
4455 Atherton Dr, Salt Lake City, UT 84123
Various types of thermodilution probes.

Mmj S.A. De C.V. 314-654-2000
716 Ponciano Arriaga, Cd. Juarez, Chih. Mexico
Myocardial sensor

PROBE, TRABECULOTOMY *(Ophthalmology) 86HNK*

Bausch & Lomb Surgical 636-255-5051
3365 Tree Court Ind Blvd, Saint Louis, MO 63122

Stephens Instruments, Inc. 800-354-7848
2500 Sandersville Rd, Lexington, KY 40511
$35.00 per unit (standard).

PROBE, ULTRASONIC *(Radiology) 90VCR*

Bard Access Systems, Inc. 800-545-0890
605 N 5600 W, Salt Lake City, UT 84116
$1,700 to $3,000 per ultrasound mechanical sector probe (8 models available).

Biomedix Inc. 877-854-0012
4215 White Bear Pkwy, Saint Paul, MN 55110
Doppler Untrasound Probes. Priced from $350 for pencil probes, available in 5mHz and 8 mHz.

Capistrano Labs, Inc. 949-492-0390
150 Calle Iglesia Ste B, San Clemente, CA 92672
Ultrasonic imagine probes, all types from $1750 to $4600.

Karl Storz Endoscopy-America Inc. 800-421-0837
600 Corporate Pointe, Culver City, CA 90230

Mahe International Inc. 800-294-7946
468 Craighead St, Nashville, TN 37204

Philips Medical Systems 949-450-0014
1590 Scenic Ave, Costa Mesa, CA 92626

Phillips Ultrasound 800-982-2011
22100 Bothell Everett Hwy, P.O. Box 3003, Bothell, WA 98021

Xma (X-Ray Marketing Associates, Inc.) 800-325-8880
1205 W Lakeview Ct, Windham Lakes Business Park
Romeoville, IL 60446

PROBE, UPTAKE, NUCLEAR *(Radiology) 90IZD*

Biodex Medical Systems, Inc. 800-224-6339
20 Ramsey Rd, Shirley, NY 11967
ATOMLAB 950 Thyroid Uptake System operates with powerful and intuitive Macintosh computer or Windows.

Capintec, Inc. 800-631-3826
6 Arrow Rd, Ramsey, NJ 07446
GAMMED II B Small, lightweight, hand-held probes with large direct readout with both digital and analog meters. This unit is able to read low or high energy radionuclide emitters.

Digirad Corp. 800-947-6134
13950 Stowe Dr, Poway, CA 92064
Various.

Intramedical Imaging Llc 800-519-3959
12340 Santa Monica Blvd Ste 227, Los Angeles, CA 90025
Intra-operative detection probes including Gamma probe for sentinel nodes, PET Probe for detetion of tumors using FDG, Beta Probe for detection of tumor margins and gamma probe for resection of Parathyroid adenoma.

Marconi Medical Systems 800-323-0550
595 Miner Rd, Cleveland, OH 44143

Neoprobe Corporation 800-793-0079
425 Metro Pl N Ste 300, Dublin, OH 43017
neo2000 Gamma Detection System; Neoprobe Portable Isotope Detector

Nortech Systems Incorporated 952-345-2244
1120 Wayzata Blvd E Ste 201, Wayzata, MN 55391

Parker Hannifin Corporation. 805-658-2984
3007 Bunsen Ave Units K&L, Ventura, CA 93003
Radiation detection probe.

Specialities Electronics Co., Inc. 609-267-5593
43 Washington St, Mount Holly, NJ 08060
Thyroid uptake system.

Sun Nuclear Corp. 321-259-6862
425 Pineda Ct Ste A, Melbourne, FL 32940
Atomlab thyroid uptakes: models 930 and 950.

PROCESSOR, CINE FILM *(Radiology) 90IXX*

Agfa Corporation 877-777-2432
PO Box 19048, 10 South Academy Street, Greenville, SC 29602

Fujifilm Medical Systems Usa, Inc. 800-431-1850
419 West Ave, Stamford, CT 06902

Simon & Company Inc., H.R. 800-638-9460
3515 Marmenco Ct, Baltimore, MD 21230

Ti-Ba Enterprises, Inc. 585-247-1212
25 Hytec Cir, Rochester, NY 14606
Ti-Ba sells ALL the Jamison and Vangurd processors, projectors and parts.

PROCESSOR, FROZEN BLOOD *(Hematology) 81KSW*

Haemonetics Corp. 781-848-7100
400 Wood Rd, P.O.Box 9114, Braintree, MA 02184
Centrifugal red cell washing system.

PROCESSOR, FROZEN BLOOD *(cont'd)*

Immucor, Inc. 800-829-2553
3130 Gateway Dr, PO Box 5625, Norcross, GA 30071
ROSYS PLATO High-Volume microplate processing system designed to provide processing of blood serology assays reader provides electronic interpretation. DYNEX DIAS PLUS, high volume microplate processing system. Reader provides electronic interpretation of blood serology assays.

PROCESSOR, RADIOGRAPHIC FILM, AUTOMATIC *(Radiology) 90IXW*

Afp Imaging Corp. 800-592-6666
250 Clearbrook Rd, Elmsford, NY 10523
$5,200 to $17,000 per unit; 8-17in. wide.

Agfa Corporation 877-777-2432
PO Box 19048, 10 South Academy Street, Greenville, SC 29602

Air Techniques, Inc. 800-247-8324
1295 Walt Whitman Rd, Melville, NY 11747
Peri-Pro; All-Pro 100 Plus; All-Pro 200; All-Pro 2010; AT2000XR

Alphatek 708-345-0500
2000 S 25th Ave, Broadview, IL 60155

Burkhart Roentgen Intl. Inc. 800-USA-XRAY
5201 8th Ave S, Gulfport, FL 33707
The new optimax and compact2. True 90 sec. processors.

Fischer Industries, Inc. 630-232-2803
2630 Kaneville Ct, Geneva, IL 60134
Various models of automatic x-ray film processors.

Fujifilm Medical Systems Usa, Inc. 800-431-1850
419 West Ave, Stamford, CT 06902
FPM 6000SP.

Ge Medical Systems, Llc 262-548-2355
3000 N Grandview Blvd, W-417, Waukesha, WI 53188
Multiple radiographic film processors.

Hale Imaging Systems, Inc. 800-321-4253
5314 Mill St, P.O. Box 184, Orient, OH 43146

Kodak Canada Inc., Health Imaging Division 800-295-5526
3500 Eglinton Ave. W., Toronto, ONT M6M 1V3 Canada

Marconi Medical Systems 800-323-0550
595 Miner Rd, Cleveland, OH 44143

Schueler & Company, Inc. 516-487-1500
PO Box 528, Stratford, CT 06615

Simon & Company Inc., H.R. 800-638-9460
3515 Marmenco Ct, Baltimore, MD 21230

Summit Industries, Inc. 800-729-9729
2901 W Lawrence Ave, Chicago, IL 60625

Tek Marketing, Inc. 215-364-4941
98 Railroad Dr, Warminster, PA 18974
X-ray film processor.

Ti-Ba Enterprises, Inc. 585-247-1212
25 Hytec Cir, Rochester, NY 14606
Ti-Ba sell new and remanufactured Kodak and Konica Minolta Medical X-ray film processors.

Xma (X-Ray Marketing Associates, Inc.) 800-325-8880
1205 W Lakeview Ct, Windham Lakes Business Park
Romeoville, IL 60446

PROCESSOR, RADIOGRAPHIC FILM, AUTOMATIC, DENTAL *(Dental And Oral) 76EGY*

Afp Imaging Corp. 800-592-6666
250 Clearbrook Rd, Elmsford, NY 10523
$5,200 to $17,000 per unit; 8-17in. wide.

J. Morita Usa, Inc. 888-566-7482
9 Mason, Irvine, CA 92618
FREEDOM Automatic Film Processor is a roller-less automatic film processor that processes all dental films dry-to-dry in 5 ¾ minutes. Using two reaction tanks the flow of work is smoother with less back up of undeveloped films. The Freedom processor has an optional 'quick view' feature that enables the clinician to read and measure endodontic files on an operatory monitor.

Schueler & Company, Inc. 516-487-1500
PO Box 528, Stratford, CT 06615

Simon & Company Inc., H.R. 800-638-9460
3515 Marmenco Ct, Baltimore, MD 21230

Smith Companies Dental Products 800-336-3263
4368 Enterprise St, Fremont, CA 94538
Replacement parts for Philips, Dent-X, and Air Techniques automatic dental radiographic x-ray film processors. Sold only through dental dealers.

PROCESSOR, RADIOGRAPHIC FILM, AUTOMATIC, DENTAL
(cont'd)

Star X-Ray Co., Inc. 800-374-2163
63 Ranick Dr S, Amityville, NY 11701

X-Ray Support Inc. 509-242-1011
3020 N Sullivan Rd Ste D, Spokane Valley, WA 99216
Dental x-ray automatic film processor.

PROCESSOR, RADIOGRAPHIC FILM, MANUAL
(Radiology) 90JAH

Schueler & Company, Inc. 516-487-1500
PO Box 528, Stratford, CT 06615

Whitehall Manufacturing 800-782-7706
15125 Proctor Ave, City Of Industry, CA 91746
2-gal., 3-gal., 5-gal. X-ray developing tank.

PROCESSOR, SLIDE, CYTOLOGY, AUTOMATED
(Pathology) 88MKQ

Cytyc Corporation 800-442-9892
445 Simarano Dr, Marlborough, MA 01752

Cytyc Surgical Products 800-442-9892
250 Campus Dr, Marlborough, MA 01752
Processor,cervical cytology slide, automated.

Monogen, Inc. 847-573-6700
3630 Burwood Dr, Waukegan, IL 60085
Cervical cytology, specimen collection and processing kit.

Tripath Imaging, Inc. 919-206-7140
780 Plantation Dr, Burlington, NC 27215
Cervical cytology preparation system.

PROCTOSCOPE *(Surgery) 79GCF*

Boehm Surgical Instrument Corp. 716-436-6584
966 Chili Ave, Rochester, NY 14611
Proctoscope.

Cameron-Miller, Inc. 800-621-0142
5410 W Roosevelt Rd, Road #241, Chicago, IL 60644

Codman & Shurtleff, Inc 800-225-0460
325 Paramount Dr, Raynham, MA 02767

Electro Surgical Instrument Co., Inc. 888-464-2784
37 Centennial St, Rochester, NY 14611
Various types, styles and sizes of fiberoptic lighted proctoscopes, sigmoidoscopes.

Karl Storz Endoscopy-America Inc. 800-421-0837
600 Corporate Pointe, Culver City, CA 90230

Mahe International Inc. 800-294-7946
468 Craighead St, Nashville, TN 37204

Md International, Inc. 305-669-9003
11300 NW 41st St, Doral, FL 33178

Miltex Inc. 800-645-8000
589 Davies Dr, York, PA 17402

Richard Wolf Medical Instruments Corp. 800-323-9653
353 Corporate Woods Pkwy, Vernon Hills, IL 60061

Welch Allyn, Inc. 800-535-6663
4341 State Street Rd, Skaneateles Falls, NY 13153

PROCTOSIGMOIDOSCOPE *(Gastro/Urology) 78RML*

Cameron-Miller, Inc. 800-621-0142
5410 W Roosevelt Rd, Road #241, Chicago, IL 60644

Md International, Inc. 305-669-9003
11300 NW 41st St, Doral, FL 33178

Welch Allyn, Inc. 800-535-6663
4341 State Street Rd, Skaneateles Falls, NY 13153

PRODUCTION EQUIPMENT *(General) 80VAP*

Ark Services Corporation 708-371-3674
6118 W 123rd St, Palos Heights, IL 60463
Testers to detect and measure leaks and flow rates. Tape and strip cutting equipment. Wide range of new custom equipment and improvements for existing machinery.

Arlington Machine & Tool Co. 973-276-1377
90 New Dutch Ln, Fairfield, NJ 07004

Athena Controls, Inc. 800-782-6776
5145 Campus Dr, Plymouth Meeting, PA 19462
Molding and process-control equipment. Thermocouples and temperature controllers.

PRODUCTION EQUIPMENT *(cont'd)*

Comco, Inc. 800-796-6626
2151 N Lincoln St, Burbank, CA 91504
Micro-abrasive blasting equipment for production of medical devices including deburring, cutting, cleaning, surface preparation, and material removal. Automated and manual systems.

Conoptics, Inc. 800-748-3349
19 Eagle Rd, Danbury, CT 06810
Laser system that encodes information onto a compact disk.

Delta Industrial Services, Inc. 800-279-3358
11501 Eagle St NW, Minneapolis, MN 55448
Delta Mod-Tech web-converting equipment. Features many process options including die cutting, laminating, placement, unwind/rewind, packaging, vision, printing, and more.

Drummond Scientific Co. 800-523-7480
500 Park Way # 700, Broomall, PA 19008
Tubing-processing equipment.

Eit, Inc. 703-478-0700
108 Carpenter Dr, Sterling, VA 20164
Adhesive-curing and process-control equipment.

Engineering & Research Assoc., Inc. (D.B.A. Sebra) 800-625-5550
100 N Tucson Blvd, Tucson, AZ 85716
Catheter manufacturing equipment, featuring fast, precise welding and shape forming on single- or multilumen catheters. Also medical bag manufacturing equipment, rollstock. Sterile connections for tubing. Safety seal cap welding.

Faustel 262-253-3333
W194N11301 McCormick Dr, Germantown, WI 53022
Customized equipment for coating and laminating basic rolls of paper, plastic films, and aluminum foil.

Hansco Technologies, Inc. 201-391-0700
17 Philips Pkwy, Montvale, NJ 07645
Machine tools for the production of surgical equipment components.

Littleford Day, Inc. 800-365-8555
PO Box 128, Florence, KY 41022
Various types of size reduction and mixing equipment.

Med-Rent, Inc. 800-233-7345
435 Bethany Rd, Burbank, CA 91504

National Instrument Llc 866-258-1914
4119 Fordleigh Rd, Baltimore, MD 21215
Filamatic's Fill/finish equipment includes liquid filling, tipping, plugging, capping and labeling. Capabilities include pre-capped/pre-sterlized tube filling equipment

Nypro Inc. 978-365-9721
101 Union St, Clinton, MA 01510
Assembly lines, automated systems, robotics, injection molds for medical device components and disposables.

Pedifix, Inc. 800-424-5561
310 Guinea Rd, Brewster, NY 10509
Vacuum press for orthotics molding.

Pva 518-371-2684
15 Solar Dr, Clifton Park, NY 12065
Adhesive-curing and automation equipment. PVA 3000, programmable adhesive dispensing system. PVA2000, selective conformal coating spray system for all chemistries. Programmable three-axis control eliminates masking and produces no overspray.

Sick, Inc. 800-325-7425
6900 W 110th St, Minneapolis, MN 55438
Material-handling and process-control equipment.

Tech Spray, L.P. 800-858-4043
1001 NW 1st Ave, Amarillo, TX 79107
Coatings and cleaners.

Thermo Fisher Scientific (Sales And Service) 800-227-8891
501 90th Ave NW, PROCESS INSTRUMENTS DIVISION Minneapolis, MN 55433
Checkweighers.

Ultra Tec Manufacturing, Inc. 877-542-0609
1025 E Chestnut Ave, Santa Ana, CA 92701
ULTRASLICE Precision Saw. Production saw machine for optical and structural medical components. MICROSLICE annular saw for the thinnest, lowest damage slices of fragile and/or expensive optical and crystal materials.

PROGRAMMER, PACEMAKER *(Cardiovascular) 74KRG*

Ela Medical, Inc. 800-352-6466
2950 Xenium Ln N, Plymouth, MN 55441
Orchestra Dedicated Programmer

PROGRAMMER, PACEMAKER *(cont'd)*

Trivirix International Inc. 320-982-8000
925 6th Ave NE, Milaca, MN 56353
Various types of non-sterile pulse generator controllers.

PROJECTOR, OPHTHALMIC *(Ophthalmology) 86HOS*

Accommodata Corporation 216-732-8888
20950 Edgecliff Dr, Euclid, OH 44123
Various types of computerized ophthalmic projectors.

Burton Co., R.H. 800-848-0410
3965 Brookham Dr, Grove City, OH 43123
BURTON 5000, chart projector. BURTON 6000 H halogen chart projector. BURTON CP-40, automatic chart projector.

M&S Technologies, Inc. / Marino 847-763-0500
5557 Howard St, Skokie, IL 60077

Marco Ophthalmic, Inc. 800-874-5274
11825 Central Pkwy, Jacksonville, FL 32224
$740.00 for chart projector; mounts available; $2,625.00 for automatic chart projector.

Reichert, Inc. 888-849-8955
3362 Walden Ave, Depew, NY 14043
AP250 auto projector is a remote-controlled, programmable, random-access, high-resolution ophthalmic projector. LongLife POC is a manual projector with an improved electro-optical system.

Topcon Medical Systems, Inc. 800-223-1130
37 W Century Rd, Paramus, NJ 07652
$990.00 for manual chart projector; $2,890.00 and $9,990.00 for automatic chart projectors.

Woodlyn, Inc. 800-331-7389
2920 Malmo Dr, Ophthalmic Instruments and Equipment
Arlington Heights, IL 60005
Model 31200. The Woodlyn Classic Projector features halogen illumination allowing cool operation and outlasting conventional incandescent lamps 20 to 1. Call for current prices.

PROJECTOR, X-RAY FILM *(Radiology) 90VGV*

Magnaplan Corp. 800-361-1192
1320 Rte. 9, Champlain, NY 12919-5007

Sony Electronics, Inc., Medical Systems Div. 800-686-7669
1 Sony Dr, Park Ridge, NJ 07656
Zoom, memory, and rotation features for cine video.

Ti-Ba Enterprises, Inc. 585-247-1212
25 Hytec Cir, Rochester, NY 14606
Ti-Ba sells ALL the Jamison and Vangurd processors, projectors and parts.

PROPHYLACTIC (CONDOM) *(General) 80FQT*

Barnett Intl. Corp. 704-587-0390
610 Greenway Industrial Dr, Charlotte, NC 28273

Polyzen, Inc. 919-319-9599
1041 Classic Rd, Apex, NC 27539
Custom male/female prophylactic device.

PROPHYLAXIS UNIT, ULTRASONIC, DENTAL *(Dental And Oral) 76DZY*

Danville Materials 800-827-7940
3420 Fostoria Way Ste A200, San Ramon, CA 94583
Air polishing dental prophylaxis unit.

Dentsply Canada, Ltd. 800-263-1437
161 Vinyl Ct., Woodbridge, ONT L4L 4A3 Canada

Engler Engineering Corp. 800-445-8581
1099 E 47th St, Hialeah, FL 33013
$865.00 POLI-X polisher. Variable speed polisher, 200 - 35,000 RPM's

Esma, Inc. 800-276-2466
450 Taft Dr, South Holland, IL 60473

PROPORTIONING APPARATUS *(Gastro/Urology) 78FKR*

Nxstage Medical, Inc. 866-697-8243
439 S Union St Fl 5, Lawrence, MA 01843
Proportioning system.

PROSTHESIS ALIGNMENT DEVICE *(Physical Med) 89IQO*

American Hand Prosthetics, Inc. 212-213-3700
73 Skillman Ave, Brooklyn, NY 11211
Upper & lower limb protheses.

Biomet, Inc. 574-267-6639
56 E Bell Dr, PO Box 587, Warsaw, IN 46582
Various.

PROSTHESIS ALIGNMENT DEVICE *(cont'd)*

Capro Solutions, Llc 518-456-1145
8 Corporate Cir., Karner Park, Albany, NY 12203
Dero prosthetic sock.

Hosmer Dorrance Corp. 408-379-5151
561 Division St, Campbell, CA 95008
Various.

Medical Industries Of America Llc. 203-254-8080
1735 Post Rd Ste 6, Fairfield, CT 06824
Supports a cast.

Simbex, Llc 603-448-2367
10 Water St Ste 410, Lebanon, NH 03766
Svgs-smart variable geometry socket accessory.

Solaris, Inc. 414-918-9180
6737 W Washington St Ste 3260, West Allis, WI 53214
Various types of padding.

Vq Orthocare
1390 Decision St Ste A, Vista, CA 92081
Prosthetic and orthotic accessory.

W.L. Gore & Associates,Inc 928-526-3030
1505 North Fourth St., Flagstaff, AZ 86004
Various types of cast liners.

PROSTHESIS IMPLANTATION INSTRUMENT, ORTHOPEDIC *(Orthopedics) 87RNB*

Holmed Corporation 508-238-3351
40 Norfolk Ave, South Easton, MA 02375

Micro-Aire Surgical Instruments, Inc. 800-722-0822
1641 Edlich Dr, Charlottesville, VA 22911

Nemcomed 800-255-4576
801 Industrial Dr, Hicksville, OH 43526

Stryker Spine 866-457-7463
2 Pearl Ct, Allendale, NJ 07401

Zimmer Holdings, Inc. 800-613-6131
1800 W Center St, PO Box 708, Warsaw, IN 46580

PROSTHESIS, ANKLE, NON-CONSTRAINED *(Orthopedics) 87KXC*

Endotec, Inc. 973-762-6100
2546 Hansrob Rd, Orlando, FL 32804
Buechel-pappas custom total ankle, bearing & talar component.

PROSTHESIS, ANKLE, SEMI-CONSTRAINED, METAL/POLYMER *(Orthopedics) 87HSN*

Depuy Orthopaedics, Inc. 800-473-3789
700 Orthopaedic Dr, P.O. Box 988, Warsaw, IN 46582
Various types.

S&B Biomedics, Inc. 972-288-3278
844 Dalworth Dr Ste 6, Mesquite, TX 75149
Also ceramic.

Stryker Spine 866-457-7463
2 Pearl Ct, Allendale, NJ 07401

Topez Orthopedics, Inc 303-865-5105
4820 63rd St Ste 104, Boulder, CO 80301
Ankle prosthesis.

Zimmer Holdings, Inc. 800-613-6131
1800 W Center St, PO Box 708, Warsaw, IN 46580

PROSTHESIS, ANKLE, TALAR COMPONENT *(Orthopedics) 87UBK*

Stryker Spine 866-457-7463
2 Pearl Ct, Allendale, NJ 07401

PROSTHESIS, ANKLE, TIBIAL COMPONENT *(Orthopedics) 87UBL*

Stryker Spine 866-457-7463
2 Pearl Ct, Allendale, NJ 07401

PROSTHESIS, ARM *(Orthopedics) 87RMN*

Arthur Finnieston Clinic 305-817-1604
2480 W 82nd St Unit 8, Hialeah, FL 33016
limbs.

Capital Prosthetic Manufacturing, Inc. 518-456-1145
8 Corporate Cir, Albany, NY 12203

Fillauer Companies, Inc. 800-251-6398
2710 Amnicola Hwy, Chattanooga, TN 37406

Motion Control, Inc. 888-696-2767
2401 S 1070 W Ste B, Salt Lake City, UT 84119
Utah Arm II above-elbow prosthesis, myoelectrically powered. Utah Pro Control below-elbow prosthesis, myoelectrically powered.

PROSTHESIS, ARM *(cont'd)*

Slawner Ltd., J. 514-731-3378
5713 Cote Des Neiges Rd., Montreal, QUE H3S 1Y7 Canada

Westcoast Brace & Limb 813-985-5000
5311 E Fletcher Ave, Temple Terrace, FL 33617

PROSTHESIS, ARTERIAL GRAFT, BOVINE CAROTID ARTERY *(Surgery) 79FZC*

Artegraft, Inc. 800-631-5264
220 N Center Dr, North Brunswick, NJ 08902
ARTEGRAFT collagen vascular grafts with natural advantages over synthetic. Indications for use include A-V access and peripheral bypass. Outside diameters from 6 to 8mm and lengths up to 52 cm.

PROSTHESIS, ARTERIAL GRAFT, SYNTHETIC, GREATER THAN 6MM *(Surgery) 79FZB*

Bard Peripheral Vascular, Inc. 800-321-4254
1625 W 3rd St, Tempe, AZ 85281
Regular, thin wall, straight or tapered IMPRA-FLEX grafts (PTFE).

Tuzik Boston 800-886-6363
104 Longwater Dr, Assinippi Park, Norwell, MA 02061

PROSTHESIS, ARTERIAL GRAFT, SYNTHETIC, LESS THAN 6MM *(Surgery) 79JCP*

Bard Peripheral Vascular, Inc. 800-321-4254
1625 W 3rd St, Tempe, AZ 85281
Regular, thin wall, straight or tapered IMPRA-FLEX grafts (PTFE).

Micrins Surgical Instruments, Inc. 800-833-3380
28438 N Ballard Dr, Lake Forest, IL 60045

Tuzik Boston 800-886-6363
104 Longwater Dr, Assinippi Park, Norwell, MA 02061

PROSTHESIS, BONE CERCLAGE *(Orthopedics) 87UCR*

Zimmer Holdings, Inc. 800-613-6131
1800 W Center St, PO Box 708, Warsaw, IN 46580

PROSTHESIS, BREAST, EXTERNAL *(Surgery) 79KCZ*

Airway Division Of Surgical Appliance Industries, Inc. 800-888-0458
3960 Rosslyn Dr, Cincinnati, OH 45209

Amoena 800-726-6362
1701 Barrett Lakes Blvd NW Ste 410, Kennesaw, GA 30144
Silicone & polyurethane.

B & B Lingerie Company, Inc. 800-262-2789
2417 Bank Dr Ste 201, Boise, ID 83705
BOSOM BUDDY All-fabric (contains no silicone or rubber), fully weighted, adjustable external breast prosthesis.

Coloplast Manufacturing Us, Llc 800-533-0464
1840 W Oak Pkwy, Marietta, GA 30062
Natural in appearance and feel, AMOENA, DISCRENE, AFFINITY, BALANCIA, CONTACT, LUXA, PREMA, and TRIA external silicon breast prostheses give women who have had mastectomy and lumpectomy surgeries a lifelike image and improved body alignment. Some forms fit in bra pockets and some attach directly to the chest wall. Supporting items include CoolPad pads that wick moisture away from the body; Skin Supports, Prep Pads, Back Pad, Skin Marker, Cream, Covers, Adhesive, Brush, Breast Form Wash, and ELEGANT CONTOURS mastectomy brassieres.

Finebrand Co. 323-588-3228
3720 S Santa Fe Ave, Vernon, CA 90058

Freeman Manufacturing Company 800-253-2091
900 W Chicago Rd, PO Box J, Sturgis, MI 49091
Temporary weighted breast forms and silicone breast forms.

La Charme Llc 718-816-1347
45 Main St Ste 309, Brooklyn, NY 11201
Breast prostheses, breast form.

Ladies First, Inc. 800-497-8285
PO Box 4400, Salem, OR 97302
Prosthetic Camisole

Medical Art Resources, Inc. 414-543-1002
10401 W Lincoln Ave Ste 105, West Allis, WI 53227
Custom breast prosthesis.

Nearly Me Technologies, Inc. 800-887-3370
3630 South I 35, Suite A, Waco, TX 76702-1475
Breast prosthesis.

Saville 1300, Inc. 888-824-9929
200 Culver Blvd Ste D, Playa Del Rey, CA 90293
Prosthesis, breast, external.

PROSTHESIS, BREAST, EXTERNAL *(cont'd)*

Truform Orthotics & Prosthetics 800-888-0458
3960 Rosslyn Dr, Cincinnati, OH 45209
Airway Division Post-Mastectomy products.

PROSTHESIS, BREAST, EXTERNAL, NO ADHESIVE *(Surgery) 79NOJ*

American Breast Care Lp 770-933-3444
2150 New Market Pkwy SE Ste 112, Marietta, GA 30067
Breast prosthesis breast form.

B & B Lingerie Co., Inc. 208-343-9696
2417 Bank Dr Ste 201, P.o. Box 5731, Boise, ID 83705
Breast prosthesis.

La Charme Llc 718-816-1347
45 Main St Ste 309, Brooklyn, NY 11201
Breast prostheses, breast form.

Soft Innovations, Inc. 909-678-3540
22300 Baxter Rd, Wildomar, CA 92595
Polymer breast prothesis.

PROSTHESIS, BREAST, INFLATABLE, INTERNAL *(Surgery) 79FWM*

Allergan 800-624-4261
71 S Los Carneros Rd, Goleta, CA 93117
Saline filled. Silicone gel filled breast implants.

Truform Orthotics & Prosthetics 800-888-0458
3960 Rosslyn Dr, Cincinnati, OH 45209
Airway Division Post-Mastectomy products.

Whalen Biomedical Incorporated 617-868-4433
11 Miller St, Somerville, MA 02143
An all silicone rubber, saline-filled prosthesis with microporous exterior surfaces to minimize fibrous tissue encapsulation.

PROSTHESIS, BREAST, NON-INFLATABLE, INTERNAL *(Surgery) 79FTR*

Adept-Med International, Inc. 800-222-8445
665 Pleasant Valley Rd, Diamond Springs, CA 95619
B.I.P. breast-implant protector assists in preventing implants from nicks and punctures.

Truform Orthotics & Prosthetics 800-888-0458
3960 Rosslyn Dr, Cincinnati, OH 45209
Airway Division Post-Mastectomy products.

PROSTHESIS, CARDIAC VALVE *(Cardiovascular) 74RMO*

ATS Medical, Inc. 800-399-1381
3905 Annapolis Ln N Ste 105, Minneapolis, MN 55447
ATS Simulus Annuloplasty Rings/Bands

Cryolife, Inc. 800-438-8285
1655 Roberts Blvd NW, Kennesaw, GA 30144
Storage and preservation (liquid nitrogen) of human tissue heart valves (pulmonary & aortic). Shipment of valves for implant within 24 hours.

Medical Carbon Research Institute, Llc - Mcri 512-339-8000
8200 Cameron Rd Ste A196, Austin, TX 78754
On-X bileaflet mechanical valve made with pure ON-X carbon.

Medicalcv, Inc. 800-328-2060
9725 S Robert Trl, Inver Grove Heights, MN 55077
OMNISCIENCE and OMNICARBON.

Medtronic, Inc. 800-633-8766
710 Medtronic Pkwy, Minneapolis, MN 55432
FREESTYLE, HANCOCK, MEDTRONIC HALL.

St. Jude Medical, Inc. 800-328-9634
1 Saint Jude Medical Dr, Saint Paul, MN 55117
Pryolytic carbon bileaflet prosthetic heart valves.

PROSTHESIS, CARDIAC VALVE, BIOLOGICAL *(Cardiovascular) 74DYE*

Cryolife, Inc. 800-438-8285
1655 Roberts Blvd NW, Kennesaw, GA 30144
Storage and preservation (liquid nitrogen) of human tissue heart valves (pulmonary & aortic). Shipment of valves for implant within 24 hours.

Edwards Lifesciences, Llc. 800-424-3278
1 Edwards Way, Irvine, CA 92614

Medtronic Cardiovascular Surgery, The Heart Valve Div. 800-328-2518
1851 E Deere Ave, Santa Ana, CA 92705
Various models & sizes of sterile mechanical & porcine bioprostheses & conduits.

PROSTHESIS, CARDIAC VALVE, BIOLOGICAL *(cont'd)*

Medtronic Heart Valves 800-227-3191
8299 Central Ave NE, Spring Lake Park, MN 55432
Various models.

St. Jude Medical, Inc. 800-328-9634
1 Saint Jude Medical Dr, Saint Paul, MN 55117
Porcine bioprosthetic heart valve.

PROSTHESIS, CHIN, INTERNAL *(Surgery) 79FWP*

Aesthetic And Reconstructive Technologies, Inc. 775-853-6800
3545 Airway Dr Ste 106, Reno, NV 89511
Silicone elastomer chin implant.

Allergan 800-624-4261
71 S Los Carneros Rd, Goleta, CA 93117

Allied Biomedical 800-276-1322
PO Box 392, Ventura, CA 93002

Hanson Medical, Inc. 800-771-2215
825 Riverside Ave Ste 2, Paso Robles, CA 93446
Chin implant - silicone.

Invotec Intl. 800-998-8580
6833 Phillips Industrial Blvd, Jacksonville, FL 32256
Chin implant.

Pillar Surgical, Inc. 800-367-0445
PO Box 8141, La Jolla, CA 92038
Various.

S Jackson Inc. 800-368-5225
PO Box 4487, Alexandria, VA 22303
SUPRAMESH $38.50 polyamide mentoplasty implant (3 sizes).

Spectrum Designs Medical, Inc. 800-239-6399
6387 Rose Ln Ste B, Carpinteria, CA 93013
Chin implants, sterile. Esigned to augment the chin area.

Surgical Technology Laboratories Inc. 803-462-1714
610 Clemson Rd, Columbia, SC 29229
Chin implant, straith, 5 different sizes.

PROSTHESIS, COCHLEAR *(Ear/Nose/Throat) 77UAI*

Advanced Bionics Corp. 800-678-2575
25129 Rye Canyon Loop, Santa Clarita, CA 91355
CLARION; cochlear implant designed to enable the deaf to hear; consists of implanted and external components, utilizes multiple sound-processing strategies.

Jedmed Instruments Co. 314-845-3770
5416 Jedmed Ct, Saint Louis, MO 63129

PROSTHESIS, CONDYLE, MANDIBULAR, TEMPORARY *(Dental And Oral) 76NEI*

Biomet Microfixation Inc. 800-874-7711
1520 Tradeport Dr, Jacksonville, FL 32218
Add-on condyle.

PROSTHESIS, DENTAL *(Dental And Oral) 76RMP*

Biogenic Dental Corp. 800-367-3322
PO Box 4119, 282-284 Genesee St., Utica, NY 13504

Dentsply Canada, Ltd. 800-263-1437
161 Vinyl Ct., Woodbridge, ONT L4L 4A3 Canada

Lifecore Biomedical, Inc. 952-368-4300
3515 Lyman Blvd, Chaska, MN 55318
PRIMA - dental implant system. STAGE-ONE - dental implant system. RENOVA - dental implant system. RESTORE close-tolerance dental-implant system.

Talon Acrylics, Inc. 888-433-2551
850 NE 102nd Ave, Portland, OR 97220
'TALON' and/or 'REVERE' Thermoplasic Acrylic Elastomer is used in fabrication of appliances for TMJ/D Splints, Night Guards, Repositioners, Sleep Apnea Anti-Snore Appliances, and Liners/Relines for Complete and Partial Dentures, Overdentures / Gaskets.

PROSTHESIS, DIAPHYSIS, CUSTOM *(Orthopedics) 87HWG*

Stryker Spine 866-457-7463
2 Pearl Ct, Allendale, NJ 07401

PROSTHESIS, EAR, INTERNAL *(Surgery) 79FZD*

Bausch & Lomb Surgical 636-255-5051
3365 Tree Court Ind Blvd, Saint Louis, MO 63122

Rocky Mountain Anaplastology, Inc. 303-973-8482
3405 S Yarrow St Unit C, Lakewood, CO 80227
Ear prosthesis [glue-on not implants].

PROSTHESIS, ELBOW, CONSTRAINED *(Orthopedics) 87JDC*

Biomet, Inc. 574-267-6639
56 E Bell Dr, PO Box 587, Warsaw, IN 46582
Various types of sterile & non-sterile elbow components.

Centerpulse Orthopedics Inc. 877-768-7349
9900 Spectrum Dr, Austin, TX 78717
GSB Elbow cemented contrained elbow.

Depuy Orthopaedics, Inc. 800-473-3789
700 Orthopaedic Dr, P.O. Box 988, Warsaw, IN 46582
Various types of elbow prostheses, constrained, cemented.

Zimmer Holdings, Inc. 800-613-6131
1800 W Center St, PO Box 708, Warsaw, IN 46580

PROSTHESIS, ELBOW, HEMI-, RADIAL, POLYMER *(Orthopedics) 87KWI*

Acumed Llc 503-627-9957
5885 NW Cornelius Pass Rd, Hillsboro, OR 97124
Prothesis, elbow joint radial head.

Ascension Orthopedics, Inc. 877-370-5001
8700 Cameron Rd, Austin, TX 78754
Ascension MRH

Biomet, Inc. 574-267-6639
56 E Bell Dr, PO Box 587, Warsaw, IN 46582
Various types of elbow prosthesis.

Depuy Orthopaedics, Inc. 800-473-3789
700 Orthopaedic Dr, P.O. Box 988, Warsaw, IN 46582
Various types of elbow prostheses, hemi-radial, polymer.

Small Bone Innovations, Inc. 215-428-1791
1380 S Pennsylvania Ave, Morrisville, PA 19067
Elbow joint radial (hemi-elbow) polymer prosthesis.

Zimmer Trabecular Metal Technology 800-613-6131
10 Pomeroy Rd, Parsippany, NJ 07054
Radial head replacement.

PROSTHESIS, ELBOW, NON-CONSTRAINED, UNIPOLAR *(Orthopedics) 87JDA*

Zimmer Holdings, Inc. 800-613-6131
1800 W Center St, PO Box 708, Warsaw, IN 46580

PROSTHESIS, ELBOW, SEMI-CONSTRAINED *(Orthopedics) 87JDB*

Biomet, Inc. 574-267-6639
56 E Bell Dr, PO Box 587, Warsaw, IN 46582
Various types of sterile and non-sterile total elbows.

Depuy Orthopaedics, Inc. 800-473-3789
700 Orthopaedic Dr, P.O. Box 988, Warsaw, IN 46582
Various types of semi-constrained, cemented, elbow prostheses.

Depuy-Raynham, A Div. Of Depuy Orthopaedics 800-451-2006
325 Paramount Dr, Raynham, MA 02767
Various types of semi-constrained, cemented, elbow prostheses.

Small Bone Innovations, Inc. 215-428-1791
1380 S Pennsylvania Ave, Morrisville, PA 19067
Elbow joint metal/polymer semi-constrained cemented prosthesis.

Stryker Spine 866-457-7463
2 Pearl Ct, Allendale, NJ 07401

Zimmer Holdings, Inc. 800-613-6131
1800 W Center St, PO Box 708, Warsaw, IN 46580

PROSTHESIS, ELBOW, TOTAL *(Orthopedics) 87UBM*

Biopro, Inc. 800-252-7707
2929 Lapeer Rd, Port Huron, MI 48060
The Townley total elbow system.

Variety Ability Systems Inc. 800-891-4514
2 Kelvin Ave., Unit 3, Toronto, ONT M4C-5C8 Canada
Electric elbows range of 2, for ages 3 to 8 & 8 to 12 years.

PROSTHESIS, ESOPHAGEAL *(Ear/Nose/Throat) 77ESW*

Boston Medical Products, Inc. 800-433-2674
117 Flanders Rd, Westborough, MA 01581
Montgomery esophageal tube (15mm o.d.), Montgomery salivary bypass tubes om sizes of 8mm, 10mm, 12mm, 14mm, 16mm, 18mm, and 20mm o.d.

Boston Scientific Corp. 800-323-6472
5905 Nathan Ln N, Minneapolis, MN 55442

Boston Scientific Corporation 800-225-2732
1 Boston Scientific Pl, Natick, MA 01760

PROSTHESIS, ESOPHAGEAL *(cont'd)*

Cook Endoscopy 336-744-0157
4900 Bethania Station Rd # &, 5951 Grassy Creek Blvd. Winston Salem, NC 27105
Esophageal prosthesis.

E. Benson Hood Laboratories, Inc. 800-942-5227
575 Washington St, Pembroke, MA 02359
Salivary bypass tubes: 8, 10, 12, 14, 16, 18, and 20mm O.D., esophageal stent.

Ev3 Inc. 800-716-6700
4600 Nathan Ln N, Plymouth, MN 55442
Esophageal prosthesis.

PROSTHESIS, ESOPHAGUS *(Surgery) 79JCQ*

E. Benson Hood Laboratories, Inc. 800-942-5227
575 Washington St, Pembroke, MA 02359
Esophageal tube with 15mm O.D.

Endochoice Inc. 888-682-3636
11810 Wills Rd Ste 100, Alpharetta, GA 30009
Bonastent Esophageal by Sewoon; Bonastent Esophageal design SST; Bonastent Esophageal mfg by Sewoon; EndoChoice Bonastent Esophageal

PROSTHESIS, EYE, INTERNAL (SPHERE) *(Surgery) 79FWO*

Custom Ocular Prosthetics 206-522-4222
10212 5th Ave NE Ste 210, Seattle, WA 98125
Artificial eye.

Richard Danz And Sons, Inc. 212-697-5722
104 E 40th St, New York, NY 10016
Custom artificial eye.

S Jackson Inc. 800-368-5225
PO Box 4487, Alexandria, VA 22303
SUPRAFOIL $35.50 for box of six sterile foil (nylon) pieces each 4 x 4 cm in various thicknesses from 0.05 to 2.0 mm.

Tomas L. Ortega 956-630-2887
San Borja 1361, Mexico City Mexico
Artificial eye

PROSTHESIS, EYELID *(Ophthalmology) 86RMQ*

Meddev Corporation 800-543-2789
730 N Pastoria Ave, Sunnyvale, CA 94085
GOLD EYELID IMPLANT are designed for the gravity assisted treatment of the functional defects of lagophthalmos resulting from facial paralysis. Available in a CONTOUR design spherically shaped to conform to the curvature of the globe. Seven standard sizes; ranging from 0.6 to 1.8 grams. Also available in the THINPROFILE® design. ThinProfile design incorporates many of the same proven features as the Contour design; however, it is significantly thinner. ThinProfile Eyelid Implants are only 0.6 mm thick, allowing for superior cosmesis and reduced migration and extrusion. Six standard sizes; ranging from 0.6 to 1.6 grams. Custom implants including platinum available upon request.

PROSTHESIS, FACIAL, MANDIBULAR IMPLANT
(Ear/Nose/Throat) 77JAZ

Biomet Microfixation Inc. 800-874-7711
1520 Tradeport Dr, Jacksonville, FL 32218
Various types of prothesis.

Biomet, Inc. 574-267-6639
56 E Bell Dr, PO Box 587, Warsaw, IN 46582
Hard tissue replacement (htr) granular.

Implantech Associates, Inc. 800-733-0833
6025 Nicolle St Ste B, Ventura, CA 93003
Flowers Mandibular Glove, MITTLEMAN Pre jowl chin, MITTLEMAN Prejowel.

Tmj Appliance 800 865-7246
130 Black Ferry Ct, Littleton, NC 27850
Intra-oral double mouthgard to end bruxing and repair temporomandibular-joint damage.

PROSTHESIS, FEMORAL *(Orthopedics) 87HSW*

Encore Medical Corporation 800-456-8696
9800 Metric Blvd, Austin, TX 78758
Total hip or knee replacements

Slawner Ltd., J. 514-731-3378
5713 Cote Des Neiges Rd., Montreal, QUE H3S 1Y7 Canada

Stryker Spine 866-457-7463
2 Pearl Ct, Allendale, NJ 07401

Zimmer Holdings, Inc. 800-613-6131
1800 W Center St, PO Box 708, Warsaw, IN 46580

PROSTHESIS, FEMORAL HEAD *(Orthopedics) 87UCE*

Kinamed, Inc. 800-827-5775
820 Flynn Rd, Camarillo, CA 93012
OPTION Total Hip System. CoCr cemented, Ti6Al4 press-fit, & revision stems. Low & full profile cups. CoCr & Ceramic femoral heads. Large ceramic femoral heads.

Signal Medical Corporation 800-246-6324
1000 Des Peres Rd Ste 140, Saint Louis, MO 63131
Ceramic, COCR

PROSTHESIS, FINGER *(Orthopedics) 87HSJ*

Touch Bionics 614-388-8075
3455 Mill Run Dr, Hilliard, OH 43026

Whalen Biomedical Incorporated 617-868-4433
11 Miller St, Somerville, MA 02143
A mechanical hinge joint for the proximal and distal interphalangeal positions designed to provide cosmetic as well as functional correction.

PROSTHESIS, FINGER, CONSTRAINED, METAL/POLYMER
(Orthopedics) 87KWG

Small Bone Innovations, Inc. 215-428-1791
1380 S Pennsylvania Ave, Morrisville, PA 19067
Finger joint metal/polymer constrained cemented prosthesis.

PROSTHESIS, FINGER, CONSTRAINED, POLYMER
(Orthopedics) 87KYJ

Ascension Orthopedics, Inc. 877-370-5001
8700 Cameron Rd, Austin, TX 78754
Ascension PIP

Depuy Orthopaedics, Inc. 800-473-3789
700 Orthopaedic Dr, P.O. Box 988, Warsaw, IN 46582
Mutiple.

Small Bone Innovations, Inc. 215-428-1791
1380 S Pennsylvania Ave, Morrisville, PA 19067
Finger joint polymer constrained prosthesis.

PROSTHESIS, FINGER, POLYMER *(Orthopedics) 87KWF*

Rocky Mountain Anaplastology, Inc. 303-973-8482
3405 S Yarrow St Unit C, Lakewood, CO 80227
Finger prosthesis [glue-on not implants].

PROSTHESIS, FINGER, TOTAL *(Orthopedics) 87UBQ*

Touch Bionics 614-388-8075
3455 Mill Run Dr, Hilliard, OH 43026

PROSTHESIS, FOOT *(Orthopedics) 87RMR*

College Park Industries, Inc. 800-728-7950
17505 Helro, Fraser, MI 48026
The TruStep® Foot is truly unique in its ability to mimic anatomical foot and ankle function. It helps restore confidence to patients by meeting or exceeding their daily ambulatory needs. The TruPer® Foot easily accommodates the ever-changing child. It is the first and only multi-axial, dynamic response foot made just for kids and is available in sizes 16 - 21 cm. The Venture Foot is the new solution for the active individual. It is a paragon of precise engineering that generates performance to suit the dynamic lifestyle without sacrificing comfort. It is the ultimate fusion of power and agility. The NEW Tribute Foot is the latest College Park innovation. It offers advanced simplicity and affordable mobility as a valuable solution for the dysvascular population. Combining College Park design principles, multi-axial and transverse rotation, with a full-length toe lever, the Tribute gives these individuals the mobility they need for the freedom they desire.

Kingsley Mfg. Co. 800-854-3479
1984 Placentia Ave, Costa Mesa, CA 92627

Life-Like Prosthetics, Llc 310-320-5777
1319 W Carson St, Torrance, CA 90501

Ohio Willow Wood Company 800-848-4930
15441 Scioto Darby Rd, Mount Sterling, OH 43143
CARBON COPY FEET - A complete line of 7 state-of-the-art prosthetic feet for every activity level and patient weight. PATHFINDER - Ohio Willow Wood's latest innovation, the PATHFINDER prosthetic foot is perfect for lower activity levels, as well as for amputees who are very active. The PATHFINDER's innovative triangular design results in optimal flexibility, stability, and comfort for the user.

Paramedical Distributors 800-245-3278
2020 Grand Blvd, Kansas City, MO 64108
Asstd. designs, brands, and products.

S&B Biomedics, Inc. 972-288-3278
844 Dalworth Dr Ste 6, Mesquite, TX 75149

PROSTHESIS, FOOT *(cont'd)*

Sgarlato Laboratories, Inc. 800-421-5303
2315 S Bascom Ave Ste 200, Campbell, CA 95008
LSI foot implant for indicated subtalar arthrosis.

Slawner Ltd., J. 514-731-3378
5713 Cote Des Neiges Rd., Montreal, QUE H3S 1Y7 Canada

PROSTHESIS, FOOT ARCH *(Orthopedics) 87UCN*

Langer, Inc. 800-645-5520
450 Commack Rd, Deer Park, NY 11729

PROSTHESIS, HAND *(Orthopedics) 87RMS*

Life-Like Prosthetics, Llc 310-320-5777
1319 W Carson St, Torrance, CA 90501

Motion Control, Inc. 888-696-2767
2401 S 1070 W Ste B, Salt Lake City, UT 84119
Motion Control Hand - electric hand prosthesis.

Touch Bionics 614-388-8075
3455 Mill Run Dr, Hilliard, OH 43026

Variety Ability Systems Inc. 800-891-4514
2 Kelvin Ave., Unit 3, Toronto, ONT M4C-5C8 Canada
Electric hands range of 4, for ages 3, 6, 9 & 11 years.

PROSTHESIS, HEART *(Cardiovascular) 74RMT*

Thoratec Corporation 800-456-1477
6101 Stoneridge Dr, Pleasanton, CA 94588
HEARTMATE left ventricle assist device with inner lining of biocompatible plastic FDA approval air-driven and electric.(IDE stage)

Whalen Biomedical Incorporated 617-868-4433
11 Miller St, Somerville, MA 02143

PROSTHESIS, HIP (METAL STEM/CERAMIC SELF-LOCKING BALL) *(Orthopedics) 87JDF*

Exactech, Inc. 800-392-2832
2320 NW 66th Ct, Gainesville, FL 32653
AcuMatch P-Series and Acumatch C-Series Total Hip System with CoCr or zirconia ceramic heads.

Precision Machine Products 860-399-5577
76 Westbrook Industrial Park, Westbrook, CT 06498

Signal Medical Corporation 800-246-6324
1000 Des Peres Rd Ste 140, Saint Louis, MO 63131
Quatroloc femoral stems.

PROSTHESIS, HIP, ACETABULAR COMPONENT, METAL, NON-CEMENTED *(Orthopedics) 87JDM*

Orchid Stealth Orthopedic Solutions 517-694-2300
1489 Cedar St, Holt, MI 48842

Stryker Spine 866-457-7463
2 Pearl Ct, Allendale, NJ 07401

Wright Medical Group, Inc. 800-238-7117
5677 Airline Rd, Arlington, TN 38002

PROSTHESIS, HIP, ACETABULAR MESH *(Orthopedics) 87JDJ*

Bio-Technology Usa, Inc. 305-512-3522
6175 NW 167th St Ste G8, Hialeah, FL 33015
Various types.

Depuy Orthopaedics, Inc. 800-473-3789
700 Orthopaedic Dr, P.O. Box 988, Warsaw, IN 46582
Prosthesis, hip, acetabular mesh (various types).

Stryker Spine 866-457-7463
2 Pearl Ct, Allendale, NJ 07401
Cobalt-chromium-molybdenum alloy.

Zimmer Holdings, Inc. 800-613-6131
1800 W Center St, PO Box 708, Warsaw, IN 46580

Zimmer Manufacturing B.V. 800-613-6131
Route 1, Km. 123.4, Bldg. 1, Turpeaux Industrial Park Mercedita, PR 00715
Acetabular reconstructive mesh.

PROSTHESIS, HIP, CEMENT RESTRICTOR *(Orthopedics) 87JDK*

Abbott Spine, Inc. 847-937-6100
12708 Riata Vista Cir Ste B-100, Austin, TX 78727
Cement restrictor.

Bio-Technology Usa, Inc. 305-512-3522
6175 NW 167th St Ste G8, Hialeah, FL 33015
Bio-technology spoac centralizer, hip.

Biomet, Inc. 574-267-6639
56 E Bell Dr, PO Box 587, Warsaw, IN 46582
Cement restrictor.

PROSTHESIS, HIP, CEMENT RESTRICTOR *(cont'd)*

Depuy Orthopaedics, Inc. 800-473-3789
700 Orthopaedic Dr, P.O. Box 988, Warsaw, IN 46582
Various types of hip prosthesis cement restrictors.

Depuy-Raynham, A Div. Of Depuy Orthopaedics 800-451-2006
325 Paramount Dr, Raynham, MA 02767
Prosthesis, hip, cement restrictor (various types).

Innovasis, Inc. 801-261-2236
614 E 3900 S, Salt Lake City, UT 84107
Cement restrictor implant system for use in orthopedic surgery.

Medtronic Sofamor Danek Usa, Inc. 901-396-3133
4340 Swinnea Rd, Memphis, TN 38118
Cement restrictor.

Nuvasive, Inc. 800-475-9131
7475 Lusk Blvd, San Diego, CA 92121
Cement restrictor.

Spinal Elements, Inc. 760-607-0121
2744 Loker Ave W Ste 100, Carlsbad, CA 92010
Various cement restrictors.

Stryker Puerto Rico, Ltd. 939-307-2500
Hwy. 3, Km. 131.2, Las Guasimas Ind. Park, Arroyo, PR 00714
Various types of sterile cement restrictors.

Stryker Spine 866-457-7463
2 Pearl Ct, Allendale, NJ 07401

Warsaw Orthopedic, Inc. 901-396-3133
2500 Silveus Xing, Warsaw, IN 46582
Cement restrictor.

Zimmer Holdings, Inc. 800-613-6131
1800 W Center St, PO Box 708, Warsaw, IN 46580

Zimmer Trabecular Metal Technology 800-613-6131
10 Pomeroy Rd, Parsippany, NJ 07054
Restrictor.

PROSTHESIS, HIP, CONSTRAINED, METAL *(Orthopedics) 87KXD*

Exactech, Inc. 800-392-2832
2320 NW 66th Ct, Gainesville, FL 32653
EXACTECH AcuMatch C-Series Cemented Total Hip System and EXACTECH AcuMatch A-Series Total Hip System.

PROSTHESIS, HIP, CONSTRAINED, METAL/POLYMER *(Orthopedics) 87KWZ*

Biomet, Inc. 574-267-6639
56 E Bell Dr, PO Box 587, Warsaw, IN 46582
Various types of hip prosthesis.

Depuy Orthopaedics, Inc. 800-473-3789
700 Orthopaedic Dr, P.O. Box 988, Warsaw, IN 46582
Various types.

Depuy-Raynham, A Div. Of Depuy Orthopaedics 800-451-2006
325 Paramount Dr, Raynham, MA 02767
Various types.

Endotec, Inc. 973-762-6100
2546 Hansrob Rd, Orlando, FL 32804
Buechel-pappas self-aligning acetabular component.

PROSTHESIS, HIP, FEMORAL COMPONENT, CEMENTED, METAL *(Orthopedics) 87JDG*

Bio-Technology Usa, Inc. 305-512-3522
6175 NW 167th St Ste G8, Hialeah, FL 33015
Bio-technology usa hip stem.

Biomet, Inc. 574-267-6639
56 E Bell Dr, PO Box 587, Warsaw, IN 46582
Various types of femoral total hip prosthesis.

Centerpulse Orthopedics Inc. 877-768-7349
9900 Spectrum Dr, Austin, TX 78717
FracSure System.

Depuy Orthopaedics, Inc. 800-473-3789
700 Orthopaedic Dr, P.O. Box 988, Warsaw, IN 46582
Various types of femoral hip prosthesis components.

Depuy-Raynham, A Div. Of Depuy Orthopaedics 800-451-2006
325 Paramount Dr, Raynham, MA 02767
Various types of femoral hip prosthesis components.

Endotec, Inc. 973-762-6100
2546 Hansrob Rd, Orlando, FL 32804
Buechel-pappas modular femoral stem.

Exactech, Inc. 800-392-2832
2320 NW 66th Ct, Gainesville, FL 32653
AcuMatch C-Series.

PROSTHESIS, HIP, FEMORAL COMPONENT, CEMENTED, METAL *(cont'd)*

Foster Manufacturing Corp. 262-633-7073
1652 Phillips Ave, Racine, WI 53403

Medtronic Sofamor Danek Usa, Inc. 901-396-3133
4340 Swinnea Rd, Memphis, TN 38118
Thompson.

Orchid Stealth Orthopedic Solutions 517-694-2300
1489 Cedar St, Holt, MI 48842

Stelkast Company 724-941-6368
200 Hidden Valley Rd, McMurray, PA 15317
Artificial hip replacement system.

Warsaw Orthopedic, Inc. 901-396-3133
2500 Silveus Xing, Warsaw, IN 46582
Thompson.

Zimmer Holdings, Inc. 800-613-6131
1800 W Center St, PO Box 708, Warsaw, IN 46580

Zimmer Manufacturing B.V. 800-613-6131
Route 1, Km. 123.4, Bldg. 1, Turpeaux Industrial Park
Mercedita, PR 00715
Hip joint femoral(hemi-hip) metallic cemented or uncemented prosthesis.

PROSTHESIS, HIP, FEMORAL, RESURFACING *(Orthopedics) 87KXA*

Arthrosurface, Inc. 508-520-3003
28 Forge Pkwy, Franklin, MA 02038
Femoral head resurfacing prosthesis.

Biomet, Inc. 574-267-6639
56 E Bell Dr, PO Box 587, Warsaw, IN 46582
Various resurfacing femoral hip components.

Biopro, Inc. 800-252-7707
2929 Lapeer Rd, Port Huron, MI 48060
Tara Hip hip femoral resurfacing.

Centerpulse Orthopedics Inc. 877-768-7349
9900 Spectrum Dr, Austin, TX 78717

PROSTHESIS, HIP, HEMI-, ACETABULAR, METAL *(Orthopedics) 87KWB*

Endotec, Inc. 973-762-6100
2546 Hansrob Rd, Orlando, FL 32804
Buechel-pappas acetabular bearing insert.

Zimmer Holdings, Inc. 800-613-6131
1800 W Center St, PO Box 708, Warsaw, IN 46580

PROSTHESIS, HIP, HEMI-, FEMORAL, METAL *(Orthopedics) 87KWL*

Depuy Orthopaedics, Inc. 800-473-3789
700 Orthopaedic Dr, P.O. Box 988, Warsaw, IN 46582
Various types of metal hemi-femoral hip prostheses.

PROSTHESIS, HIP, HEMI-, FEMORAL, METAL/POLYMER *(Orthopedics) 87KWY*

Bio-Technology Usa, Inc. 305-512-3522
6175 NW 167th St Ste G8, Hialeah, FL 33015
Biotechnology porous coated hip stem.

Biomet, Inc. 574-267-6639
56 E Bell Dr, PO Box 587, Warsaw, IN 46582
Various types of hip[prostheses.

Centerpulse Orthopedics Inc. 877-768-7349
9900 Spectrum Dr, Austin, TX 78717
Bipolar and unipolar endoprostheses.

Depuy Orthopaedics, Inc. 800-473-3789
700 Orthopaedic Dr, P.O. Box 988, Warsaw, IN 46582
Various types of cemented or uncemented metal/polymer, hemi-, femoral, hip prost.

Depuy-Raynham, A Div. Of Depuy Orthopaedics 800-451-2006
325 Paramount Dr, Raynham, MA 02767
Various types of cemented or uncemented metal/polymer, hemi-, femoral, hip prost.

Ortho Development Corp. 800-429-8339
12187 Business Park Dr, Draper, UT 84020
B2 Bipolar Cup. HEMISPHERE Modular Cup; cementless and cemented.

Stryker Spine 866-457-7463
2 Pearl Ct, Allendale, NJ 07401

Zimmer Holdings, Inc. 800-613-6131
1800 W Center St, PO Box 708, Warsaw, IN 46580

PROSTHESIS, HIP, HEMI-, FEMORAL, METAL/POLYMER *(cont'd)*

Zimmer Manufacturing B.V. 800-613-6131
Route 1, Km. 123.4, Bldg. 1, Turpeaux Industrial Park
Mercedita, PR 00715
Hip joint femoral (hemi-hip) metal/polymer cemented or cemented or uncemented pr.

Zimmer Trabecular Metal Technology 800-613-6131
10 Pomeroy Rd, Parsippany, NJ 07054
A-240 hep cemented hedrocel.

PROSTHESIS, HIP, SEMI-, UNCEMENTED, OSTEOPHILIC FINISH *(Orthopedics) 87MBL*

Biomet, Inc. 574-267-6639
56 E Bell Dr, PO Box 587, Warsaw, IN 46582
Various types of sterile hip components.

PROSTHESIS, HIP, SEMI-CONST., M/P, POR. UNCEM., CALC./PHOS. *(Orthopedics) 87MAZ*

Depuy Orthopaedics, Inc. 800-473-3789
700 Orthopaedic Dr, P.O. Box 988, Warsaw, IN 46582
Various sizes of sterile hip cups.

PROSTHESIS, HIP, SEMI-CONST., METAL/CERAMIC/CERAMIC, CEM. *(Orthopedics) 87LPF*

Bio-Technology Usa, Inc. 305-512-3522
6175 NW 167th St Ste G8, Hialeah, FL 33015
Bio-technology femoral head, hip, ceramic-zirconium.

Biomet, Inc. 574-267-6639
56 E Bell Dr, PO Box 587, Warsaw, IN 46582
Ceramic head component.

PROSTHESIS, HIP, SEMI-CONST., METAL/POLY., POROUS UNCEMENTED *(Orthopedics) 87LPH*

Biomet, Inc. 574-267-6639
56 E Bell Dr, PO Box 587, Warsaw, IN 46582
Various types of hip prosthesis.

Centerpulse Orthopedics Inc. 877-768-7349
9900 Spectrum Dr, Austin, TX 78717
APR Porous Hip System; Inbter-Op Acetabular System; Natural-Hip Porous Hip System and Inter-Op Durasul Acetabular insert system.

Depuy Orthopaedics, Inc. 800-473-3789
700 Orthopaedic Dr, P.O. Box 988, Warsaw, IN 46582
Various types.

Depuy-Raynham, A Div. Of Depuy Orthopaedics 800-451-2006
325 Paramount Dr, Raynham, MA 02767
Various types.

Global Medical Company 801-746-0208
3450 Highland Dr Ste 303, Salt Lake City, UT 84106
Prosthesis, hip, semi-constrained, metal polymer.

Implex Corp. 800-613-6131
1800 W Center St, Warsaw, IN 46580

Omni Life Science, Inc 800-448-6664
175 Paramount Dr Ste 302, Raynham, MA 02767
Hip prosthesis, uncemented.

Osteoimplant Technology, Inc. 410-785-0700
11201 Pepper Rd, Hunt Valley, MD 21031
OTI total hip systems consist of modular femoral components, acetabular components and acetabular screws for enhanced fixation. Standard femoral stems include ALFA porous and cemented, LSF porous and cemented. ALFA Acetabular System - porous coated, cluster screw, tri-spike or full dome options. 46mm to 64mm in 2mm increments. ALFA II and LSF II Modular Hip Systems - porous coated for press fit application. Modular neck configuration providing many combinations of neck length and off-set. Seven standard and small sizes, 3 neck lengths. R120 Modular Hip System - modular neck provides several combinations of neck lengths and off-set for cement fixation, seven standard sizes, three neck lengths.

Signal Medical Corp. 810-364-7070
400 Pyramid Dr, Marysville, MI 48040
Hip replacement system.

Stryker Howmedica Osteonics 201-831-5000
325 Corporate Dr, Mahwah, NJ 07430
Various types of hips.

Stryker Spine 866-457-7463
2 Pearl Ct, Allendale, NJ 07401

PROSTHESIS, HIP, SEMI-CONST., METAL/POLY., POROUS UNCEMENTED *(cont'd)*

Zimmer Manufacturing B.V. 800-613-6131
Route 1, Km. 123.4, Bldg. 1, Turpeaux Industrial Park
Mercedita, PR 00715
Biological ingrowth anatomic hip stem, femoral stems, acetabular cups.

Zimmer Trabecular Metal Technology 800-613-6131
10 Pomeroy Rd, Parsippany, NJ 07054
Sterile porous coated femoral hip stems.

PROSTHESIS, HIP, SEMI-CONST., UNCEM., NON-P., M/P, CA./PHOS. *(Orthopedics) 87MEH*

Biomet, Inc. 574-267-6639
56 E Bell Dr, PO Box 587, Warsaw, IN 46582
Bio-groove ha.

Centerpulse Orthopedics Inc. 877-768-7349
9900 Spectrum Dr, Austin, TX 78717
Precedent revision hip system with HA coating.

Depuy Orthopaedics, Inc. 800-473-3789
700 Orthopaedic Dr, P.O. Box 988, Warsaw, IN 46582
Various types of hip prostheses, (semi-constrained, uncemented, metal/polymer.

Depuy-Raynham, A Div. Of Depuy Orthopaedics 800-451-2006
325 Paramount Dr, Raynham, MA 02767
Various types of hip prostheses, (semi-constrained, uncemented, metal/polymer.

Exactech, Inc. 800-392-2832
2320 NW 66th Ct, Gainesville, FL 32653
EXACTECH BIPOLAR hip endoprosthesis.

Implex Corp. 800-613-6131
1800 W Center St, Warsaw, IN 46580

Osteoimplant Technology, Inc. 410-785-0700
11201 Pepper Rd, Hunt Valley, MD 21031
ALFA HA coated total hip system consists of ALFA modular femoral stems, ALFA modular acetabular components and an array of fixation screws.

Zimmer Trabecular Metal Technology 800-613-6131
10 Pomeroy Rd, Parsippany, NJ 07054
Sterile ha coated femoral hip stems and cups.

PROSTHESIS, HIP, SEMI-CONSTR., METAL/CERAMIC, CEMENTED/NC *(Orthopedics) 87LZO*

Biomet, Inc. 574-267-6639
56 E Bell Dr, PO Box 587, Warsaw, IN 46582
Various types of hip prosthesis and ceramic head.

Centerpulse Orthopedics Inc. 877-768-7349
9900 Spectrum Dr, Austin, TX 78717
APOLLO HIP SYSTEM; Natural Hip System -nonporous confemoral stem. APR II-T Non-porous femoral stem; Natural-Hip LD stem; MS-30 Hip Stem; Precedent revision hip stem; Alloclassic hip stem and Wagner revision hip stem.

Depuy Orthopaedics, Inc. 800-473-3789
700 Orthopaedic Dr, P.O. Box 988, Warsaw, IN 46582
Various types of hip prostheses, semi-constrained, metal/ceramic/polymer.

Depuy-Raynham, A Div. Of Depuy Orthopaedics 800-451-2006
325 Paramount Dr, Raynham, MA 02767
Various types of hip prostheses, semi-constrained, metal/ceramic/polymer.

Omni Life Science, Inc 800-448-6664
175 Paramount Dr Ste 302, Raynham, MA 02767
Ceramic femoral head.

Stelkast Company 724-941-6368
200 Hidden Valley Rd, McMurray, PA 15317
Artificial hip replacement components.

Stryker Spine 866-457-7463
2 Pearl Ct, Allendale, NJ 07401

Zimmer Trabecular Metal Technology 800-613-6131
10 Pomeroy Rd, Parsippany, NJ 07054
F-102 zirconia-implex ceramic head.

PROSTHESIS, HIP, SEMI-CONSTRAINED (CEMENTED ACETABULAR) *(Orthopedics) 87JDL*

Biomet, Inc. 574-267-6639
56 E Bell Dr, PO Box 587, Warsaw, IN 46582
Various types of sterile hip components.

PROSTHESIS, HIP, SEMI-CONSTRAINED (CEMENTED ACETABULAR) *(cont'd)*

Depuy Orthopaedics, Inc. 800-473-3789
700 Orthopaedic Dr, P.O. Box 988, Warsaw, IN 46582
Various types.

Depuy-Raynham, A Div. Of Depuy Orthopaedics 800-451-2006
325 Paramount Dr, Raynham, MA 02767
Various types.

Implex Corp. 800-613-6131
1800 W Center St, Warsaw, IN 46580

Stryker Spine 866-457-7463
2 Pearl Ct, Allendale, NJ 07401

Zimmer Trabecular Metal Technology 800-613-6131
10 Pomeroy Rd, Parsippany, NJ 07054
Acetabular cup system.

PROSTHESIS, HIP, SEMI-CONSTRAINED ACETABULAR *(Orthopedics) 87KWA*

Bio-Technology Usa, Inc. 305-512-3522
6175 NW 167th St Ste G8, Hialeah, FL 33015
Bio-technology porous coated acetabular cup hip.

Biomet, Inc. 574-267-6639
56 E Bell Dr, PO Box 587, Warsaw, IN 46582
Various types of hip prosthesis for sterile & non-sterile.

Centerpulse Orthopedics Inc. 877-768-7349
9900 Spectrum Dr, Austin, TX 78717
Metasul Acetabular system (metal-metal).

Depuy Orthopaedics, Inc. 800-473-3789
700 Orthopaedic Dr, P.O. Box 988, Warsaw, IN 46582
Various types of uncemented semi-constrained metal acetabular hip prosthesis com.

Depuy-Raynham, A Div. Of Depuy Orthopaedics 800-451-2006
325 Paramount Dr, Raynham, MA 02767
Various types of uncemented semi-constrained metal acetabular hip prosthesis com.

Hayes Medical, Inc. 800-240-0500
1115 Windfield Way Ste 100, El Dorado Hills, CA 95762
CONSENSUS HIP SYSTEM, CoCR, titanium, porous, non-porous, collared, non-collared or HA coated stems.

Stelkast Company 724-941-6368
200 Hidden Valley Rd, McMurray, PA 15317
Artificial hip replacement system.

PROSTHESIS, HIP, SEMI-CONSTRAINED, METAL/ CERAMIC/ CERAMIC/ METAL, CEMENTED OR UNCEMENTED *(Orthopedics) 87MRA*

Alceram Tech Inc 516-849-3666
57 2nd St, Ronkonkoma, NY 11779
Fermoral heads materials, Metals, Alumina, & Zirconia. Heads made for special requirements.

Biomet, Inc. 574-267-6639
56 E Bell Dr, PO Box 587, Warsaw, IN 46582
Hip prosthesis.

Depuy Orthopaedics, Inc. 800-473-3789
700 Orthopaedic Dr, P.O. Box 988, Warsaw, IN 46582
Various types of semi-constrained,metal ceramic,ceramic metal,cemented or unceme.

Tytex, Inc. 401-762-4100
601 Park East Dr, Highland Industrial Park, Woonsocket, RI 02895
Truncal orthosis.

PROSTHESIS, HIP, SEMI-CONSTRAINED, METAL/CERAMIC/POLYMER, CEMENTED OR NON-POROUS CEMENTED, OSTEOPHILIC FINISH *(Orthopedics) 87MAY*

Biomet, Inc. 574-267-6639
56 E Bell Dr, PO Box 587, Warsaw, IN 46582
Various types of sterile hip components.

Biopro, Inc. 800-252-7707
2929 Lapeer Rd, Port Huron, MI 48060
PSL Hip hip - metal/ceramic/PE.

Medtronic Sofamor Danek Usa, Inc. 901-396-3133
4340 Swinnea Rd, Memphis, TN 38118
Mueller.

Warsaw Orthopedic, Inc. 901-396-3133
2500 Silveus Xing, Warsaw, IN 46582
Mueller.

PROSTHESIS, HIP, SEMI-CONSTRAINED, METAL/POLYMER
(Orthopedics) 87JDI

Biomet, Inc. 574-267-6639
56 E Bell Dr, PO Box 587, Warsaw, IN 46582
Various types of hip, modular heads, andacetabular prosthesis.

Centerpulse Orthopedics Inc. 877-768-7349
9900 Spectrum Dr, Austin, TX 78717
Apollo hip system, All-poly acetabular cup, full and low profile all-poly cups and reinforced rings and cage.

Depuy Orthopaedics, Inc. 800-473-3789
700 Orthopaedic Dr, P.O. Box 988, Warsaw, IN 46582
Various types of semi-constrained, metal/polymer, cemented hip prostheses.

Depuy-Raynham, A Div. Of Depuy Orthopaedics 800-451-2006
325 Paramount Dr, Raynham, MA 02767
Various types of semi-constrained, metal/polymer, cemented hip prostheses.

Hayes Medical, Inc. 800-240-0500
1115 Windfield Way Ste 100, El Dorado Hills, CA 95762
Prosthesis, Hip, Total. Unisyn complete hip system; modular; porous acetabular components; bipolar mode.

Implex Corp. 800-613-6131
1800 W Center St, Warsaw, IN 46580

Macropore Biosurgery, Inc. 858-458-0900
6740 Top Gun St, San Diego, CA 92121
Cement restrictor.

Stelkast Company 724-941-6368
200 Hidden Valley Rd, McMurray, PA 15317
Artificial hip replacement components.

Stryker Howmedica Osteonics 201-831-5000
325 Corporate Dr, Mahwah, NJ 07430
Various types of hips.

Stryker Spine 866-457-7463
2 Pearl Ct, Allendale, NJ 07401

Warsaw Orthopedic, Inc. 901-396-3133
2500 Silveus Xing, Warsaw, IN 46582
Ultra high molecular weight polyethylene cup.

Zimmer Holdings, Inc. 800-613-6131
1800 W Center St, PO Box 708, Warsaw, IN 46580

Zimmer Manufacturing B.V. 800-613-6131
Route 1, Km. 123.4, Bldg. 1, Turpeaux Industrial Park
Mercedita, PR 00715
Various types and sizesof sterile acetabular cups and shells.

Zimmer Trabecular Metal Technology 800-613-6131
10 Pomeroy Rd, Parsippany, NJ 07054
Hep revision cup hedrocel.

PROSTHESIS, HIP, SEMI-CONSTRAINED, METAL/POLYMER, UNCEMENTED *(Orthopedics) 87LWJ*

Biomet, Inc. 574-267-6639
56 E Bell Dr, PO Box 587, Warsaw, IN 46582
Various types of hip prosthesis.

Depuy Orthopaedics, Inc. 800-473-3789
700 Orthopaedic Dr, P.O. Box 988, Warsaw, IN 46582
Various types of hip prostheses, semi-constrained, metal/polymer, uncemented.

Depuy-Raynham, A Div. Of Depuy Orthopaedics 800-451-2006
325 Paramount Dr, Raynham, MA 02767
Various types of hip prostheses, semi-constrained, metal/polymer, uncemented.

Stelkast Company 724-941-6368
200 Hidden Valley Rd, McMurray, PA 15317
Artificial hip replacement components.

Stryker Spine 866-457-7463
2 Pearl Ct, Allendale, NJ 07401

Zimmer Manufacturing B.V. 800-613-6131
Route 1, Km. 123.4, Bldg. 1, Turpeaux Industrial Park
Mercedita, PR 00715
Hip joint metal/polymer semi-constrained uncemented prosthesis.

Zimmer Trabecular Metal Technology 800-613-6131
10 Pomeroy Rd, Parsippany, NJ 07054
Implex hedrocel acetabular augment.

PROSTHESIS, INTERARTICULAR DISC (INTERPOSITIONAL IMPLANT) *(Dental And Oral) 76MPJ*

AxioMed Spine Corporation 216-587-5566
5350 Transportation Blvd Ste 18, Garfield Heights, OH 44125
Freedom Lumbar Disc

PROSTHESIS, JOINT, OTHER *(Orthopedics) 87RMV*

Mauch, Inc. 800-622-8742
3035 Dryden Rd, Moraine, OH 45439
$653.00 and $1043.00 per unit (standard). GAITMASTER lowprofile (for SNS, SNSJR, MICROLITE) aesthetic frame for above knee amputee. Prices are $670.00 and $855.00 and are availale in three sizes.

Osteoimplant Technology, Inc. 410-785-0700
11201 Pepper Rd, Hunt Valley, MD 21031
Including NEER II TYPE Shoulder, BIOMETRIC Total Hip System. Revision lengths and cemented stems available in all hip systems. ALFA Tri-spike porous coated acetabular arthroplasty cup with center drive with apical closure screw and 28 mm I.D. poly liners. Full dome and cluster styles.

Paramedical Distributors 800-245-3278
2020 Grand Blvd, Kansas City, MO 64108
Components.

Stryker Spine 866-457-7463
2 Pearl Ct, Allendale, NJ 07401

Zimmer Holdings, Inc. 800-613-6131
1800 W Center St, PO Box 708, Warsaw, IN 46580

PROSTHESIS, KNEE PATELLOFEMOROTIBIAL, PARTIAL, SEMI-CONSTRAINED, CEMENTED, POLYMER/METAL/POLYMER *(Orthopedics) 87NPJ*

Conformis, Inc. 781-860-5111
2 4th Ave, Burlington, MA 01803
Bicompartmental knee prosthesis.

PROSTHESIS, KNEE, FEMOROTIBIAL, CONSTRAINED, METAL
(Orthopedics) 87KRN

Implex Corp. 800-613-6131
1800 W Center St, Warsaw, IN 46580

PROSTHESIS, KNEE, FEMOROTIBIAL, CONSTRAINED, METAL/POLYMER *(Orthopedics) 87KRO*

Biomet, Inc. 574-267-6639
56 E Bell Dr, PO Box 587, Warsaw, IN 46582
Finn total knee.

Depuy Orthopaedics, Inc. 800-473-3789
700 Orthopaedic Dr, P.O. Box 988, Warsaw, IN 46582
Various types of cemented metal/polymer constrained femorotibial knee joint pros.

Depuy-Raynham, A Div. Of Depuy Orthopaedics 800-451-2006
325 Paramount Dr, Raynham, MA 02767
Various types of cemented metal/polymer constrained femorotibial knee joint pros.

Implex Corp. 800-613-6131
1800 W Center St, Warsaw, IN 46580

Stryker Spine 866-457-7463
2 Pearl Ct, Allendale, NJ 07401

Zimmer Holdings, Inc. 800-613-6131
1800 W Center St, PO Box 708, Warsaw, IN 46580

PROSTHESIS, KNEE, FEMOROTIBIAL, NON-CONSTRAINED
(Orthopedics) 87HSX

Biomet, Inc. 574-267-6639
56 E Bell Dr, PO Box 587, Warsaw, IN 46582
Stanmore total knee.

Conformis, Inc. 781-860-5111
2 4th Ave, Burlington, MA 01803
Unicondylar knee system.

Depuy Orthopaedics, Inc. 800-473-3789
700 Orthopaedic Dr, P.O. Box 988, Warsaw, IN 46582
Various types.

Depuy-Raynham, A Div. Of Depuy Orthopaedics 800-451-2006
325 Paramount Dr, Raynham, MA 02767
Various types.

Osteoimplant Technology, Inc. 410-785-0700
11201 Pepper Rd, Hunt Valley, MD 21031
OTI Condylar Knee System - standard total knee system available in five sizes.

Stelkast Company 724-941-6368
200 Hidden Valley Rd, McMurray, PA 15317
Unicondylar knee system.

Stryker Howmedica Osteonics 201-831-5000
325 Corporate Dr, Mahwah, NJ 07430
Various types of knees.

PROSTHESIS, KNEE, FEMOROTIBIAL, NON-CONSTRAINED *(cont'd)*

Stryker Spine 866-457-7463
2 Pearl Ct, Allendale, NJ 07401

Zimmer Holdings, Inc. 800-613-6131
1800 W Center St, PO Box 708, Warsaw, IN 46580

Zimmer Trabecular Metal Technology 800-613-6131
10 Pomeroy Rd, Parsippany, NJ 07054
Continuum knee system (cks).

PROSTHESIS, KNEE, FEMOROTIBIAL, NON-CONSTRAINED, METAL *(Orthopedics) 87KTX*

Osteoimplant Technology, Inc. 410-785-0700
11201 Pepper Rd, Hunt Valley, MD 21031
MJS tm Total Knee System - anatomic total knee system available in five sizes. Modular tibial plateau.

PROSTHESIS, KNEE, FEMOROTIBIAL, SEMI-CONSTRAINED *(Orthopedics) 87HRY*

Biomet, Inc. 574-267-6639
56 E Bell Dr, PO Box 587, Warsaw, IN 46582
Various types of knee prosthesis.

Centerpulse Orthopedics Inc. 877-768-7349
9900 Spectrum Dr, Austin, TX 78717
Natural-Knee Unicompartmental System, unicompartmental of the Natural-Knee system.

Depuy Orthopaedics, Inc. 800-473-3789
700 Orthopaedic Dr, P.O. Box 988, Warsaw, IN 46582
Various types of knee prostheses, semi-constrained, cemented, metal/polymer.

Depuy-Raynham, A Div. Of Depuy Orthopaedics 800-451-2006
325 Paramount Dr, Raynham, MA 02767
Various types of knee prostheses, semi-constrained, cemented, metal/polymer.

Stryker Howmedica Osteonics 201-831-5000
325 Corporate Dr, Mahwah, NJ 07430
Various types of knees.

Stryker Spine 866-457-7463
2 Pearl Ct, Allendale, NJ 07401

Zimmer Holdings, Inc. 800-613-6131
1800 W Center St, PO Box 708, Warsaw, IN 46580

Zimmer Manufacturing B.V. 800-613-6131
Route 1, Km. 123.4, Bldg. 1, Turpeaux Industrial Park
Mercedita, PR 00715
Various types and sizes of partially constrained total knee prostheses & accesso.

Zimmer Trabecular Metal Technology 800-613-6131
10 Pomeroy Rd, Parsippany, NJ 07054
Various sterile femoral knee, tibial knee and patella knee.

PROSTHESIS, KNEE, FEMOROTIBIAL, SEMI-CONSTRAINED, TRUNNION *(Orthopedics) 87LGE*

Stryker Spine 866-457-7463
2 Pearl Ct, Allendale, NJ 07401

PROSTHESIS, KNEE, HEMI-, FEMORAL *(Orthopedics) 87HSA*

Stryker Spine 866-457-7463
2 Pearl Ct, Allendale, NJ 07401

Usaeroteam 937-226-1900
1300 Grange Hall Rd, Dayton, OH 45430
Medical devices - implants - various types.

Wright Medical Group, Inc. 800-238-7117
5677 Airline Rd, Arlington, TN 38002

PROSTHESIS, KNEE, HEMI-, PATELLAR RESURFACING, UNCEMENTED *(Orthopedics) 87HTG*

Stryker Spine 866-457-7463
2 Pearl Ct, Allendale, NJ 07401

PROSTHESIS, KNEE, HEMI-, TIBIAL RESURFACING, UNCEMENTED *(Orthopedics) 87HSH*

Advanced Bio-Surfaces, Inc. 952-912-5400
5909 Baker Rd Ste 550, Minnetonka, MN 55345
Knee interpositional arthroplasty device.

Bio-Technology Usa, Inc. 305-512-3522
6175 NW 167th St Ste G8, Hialeah, FL 33015
Tibial knee.

Centerpulse Orthopedics Inc. 877-768-7349
9900 Spectrum Dr, Austin, TX 78717
Unispacer Knee System.

PROSTHESIS, KNEE, HEMI-, TIBIAL RESURFACING, UNCEMENTED *(cont'd)*

Conformis, Inc. 781-860-5111
2 4th Ave, Burlington, MA 01803
Various types of knee prosthesis, hemi-tibial.

Salumedica, L.L.C. 404-589-1727
4451 Atlanta Rd SE Ste 138, Smyrna, GA 30080
Interpositional spacer, fixed meniscus implant.

Stryker Spine 866-457-7463
2 Pearl Ct, Allendale, NJ 07401

PROSTHESIS, KNEE, HINGED (METAL-METAL) *(Orthopedics) 87HRZ*

Bolt Bethel, Llc 763-434-5900
23530 University Avenue Ext NW, PO Box 135, Bethel, MN 55005

Foster Manufacturing Corp. 262-633-7073
1652 Phillips Ave, Racine, WI 53403

Stryker Spine 866-457-7463
2 Pearl Ct, Allendale, NJ 07401

PROSTHESIS, KNEE, P/F, UNCONST., UNCEM., POR., CTD., P/M/P *(Orthopedics) 87MBD*

Bio-Technology Usa, Inc. 305-512-3522
6175 NW 167th St Ste G8, Hialeah, FL 33015
Patellar knee.

PROSTHESIS, KNEE, PATELLAR *(Orthopedics) 87UCD*

Encore Medical Corporation 800-456-8696
9800 Metric Blvd, Austin, TX 78758

Stryker Spine 866-457-7463
2 Pearl Ct, Allendale, NJ 07401

PROSTHESIS, KNEE, PATELLOFEMORAL, SEMI-CONSTRAINED *(Orthopedics) 87KRR*

Arthrosurface, Inc. 508-520-3003
28 Forge Pkwy, Franklin, MA 02038
Protello-femoral resurfacing prosthesis system.

Biomet, Inc. 574-267-6639
56 E Bell Dr, PO Box 587, Warsaw, IN 46582
Various types of knee prosthesis.

Centerpulse Orthopedics Inc. 877-768-7349
9900 Spectrum Dr, Austin, TX 78717
Natural-Knee Patellofemoral Joint.

Depuy Orthopaedics, Inc. 800-473-3789
700 Orthopaedic Dr, P.O. Box 988, Warsaw, IN 46582
Various types of knee prostheses, patello/femoral, semi-constrained, cemented.

Depuy-Raynham, A Div. Of Depuy Orthopaedics 800-451-2006
325 Paramount Dr, Raynham, MA 02767
Various types of knee prostheses, patello/femoral, semi-constrained, cemented.

Kinamed, Inc. 800-827-5775
820 Flynn Rd, Camarillo, CA 93012
KineMatch cemented PFR custom built to patient CT data.

Stryker Spine 866-457-7463
2 Pearl Ct, Allendale, NJ 07401

Wright Medical Group, Inc. 800-238-7117
5677 Airline Rd, Arlington, TN 38002

Zimmer Holdings, Inc. 800-613-6131
1800 W Center St, PO Box 708, Warsaw, IN 46580

PROSTHESIS, KNEE, PATELLOFEMOROTIBIAL, CONSTRAINED, METAL *(Orthopedics) 87KRP*

Exactech, Inc. 800-392-2832
2320 NW 66th Ct, Gainesville, FL 32653
Prous Coated Fined Tibial Tray Comp

Wright Medical Group, Inc. 800-238-7117
5677 Airline Rd, Arlington, TN 38002

PROSTHESIS, KNEE, PATELLOFEMOROTIBIAL, SEMI-CONSTRAINED *(Orthopedics) 87JWH*

Biomet, Inc. 574-267-6639
56 E Bell Dr, PO Box 587, Warsaw, IN 46582
Various types of knee prosthesis.

PROSTHESIS, KNEE, PATELLOFEMOROTIBIAL, SEMI-CONSTRAINED *(cont'd)*

Centerpulse Orthopedics Inc. 877-768-7349
9900 Spectrum Dr, Austin, TX 78717
NATURAL KNEE II porous and nonporous components; primary and revision with augmentation; all-poly and metal-backed patella components in four diameters and two thicknesses; varying thickness components for varying bone loss. PCL-saving and PCL-sacrificing options; anatomic component designs; all-poly tibial components. APOLLO TOTAL KNEE SYSTEM porous and nonporous femoral components; universal/total condylar femoral components; symmetric/universal tibial component; all-poly patella in four diameters and in three peg and one peg designs; PCL-saving and PCL-substituting designs. NATURAL KNEE Primary and Revision systems; ultracongruent and traditional posterior stabilized designs for PCL substitution; 10mm and 16mm distal femoral replacements; revision augmentation with femoral and tibial spacers and stems. Primary and Revision systems are interchangeable; Revision tibial baseplates with +4mm and +14mm thickness, porous and nonporous options. APOLLO TOTAL KNEE SYSTEM offers a total condylar (univeral) design for primary replacement with PCL-substituting designs.

Conformis, Inc. 781-860-5111
2 4th Ave, Burlington, MA 01803
Total knee prosthesis.

Depuy Orthopaedics, Inc. 800-473-3789
700 Orthopaedic Dr, P.O. Box 988, Warsaw, IN 46582
Various types of semi-constrained, cemented, polymer/metal/polymer, patellofemor.

Depuy-Raynham, A Div. Of Depuy Orthopaedics 800-451-2006
325 Paramount Dr, Raynham, MA 02767
Various types of semi-constrained, cemented, polymer/metal/polymer, patellofemor.

Endotec, Inc. 973-762-6100
2546 Hansrob Rd, Orlando, FL 32804
Knee system.

Omni Life Science, Inc 800-448-6664
175 Paramount Dr Ste 302, Raynham, MA 02767
Cemented total knee replacement

Stelkast Company 724-941-6368
200 Hidden Valley Rd, McMurray, PA 15317
Artificial knee replacement components.

Stryker Howmedica Osteonics 201-831-5000
325 Corporate Dr, Mahwah, NJ 07430
Various types of knees.

Stryker Spine 866-457-7463
2 Pearl Ct, Allendale, NJ 07401

Zimmer Holdings, Inc. 800-613-6131
1800 W Center St, PO Box 708, Warsaw, IN 46580

Zimmer Manufacturing B.V. 800-613-6131
Route 1, Km. 123.4, Bldg. 1, Turpeaux Industrial Park
Mercedita, PR 00715
Various plastic patellar surface replacements.

Zimmer Trabecular Metal Technology 800-613-6131
10 Pomeroy Rd, Parsippany, NJ 07054
Continuum knee system (cks).

PROSTHESIS, KNEE, PATELLOFEMOROTIBIAL, SEMI-CONSTRAINED, METAL/POLYMER, MOBILE BEARING *(Orthopedics) 87NJL*

Biomet, Inc. 574-267-6639
56 E Bell Dr, PO Box 587, Warsaw, IN 46582
Various types of knee prosthesis.

Depuy Orthopaedics, Inc. 800-473-3789
700 Orthopaedic Dr, P.O. Box 988, Warsaw, IN 46582
Various types of patellofemorotibial, semi-constrained, metal/polymer mobile bea.

Depuy-Raynham, A Div. Of Depuy Orthopaedics 800-451-2006
325 Paramount Dr, Raynham, MA 02767
Various types of patellofemorotibial, semi-constrained, metal/polymer mobile bea.

PROSTHESIS, KNEE, PATFEM., S-C., UHMWPE, PEGGED, UNC., P/M/P *(Orthopedics) 87MBV*

Biomet, Inc. 574-267-6639
56 E Bell Dr, PO Box 587, Warsaw, IN 46582
Various types of knee prosthesis.

PROSTHESIS, KNEE, PATFEM., S-C., UNC., POR., CTD., P/M/P *(Orthopedics) 87MBH*

Biomet, Inc. 574-267-6639
56 E Bell Dr, PO Box 587, Warsaw, IN 46582
Various types of knee components.

Depuy Orthopaedics, Inc. 800-473-3789
700 Orthopaedic Dr, P.O. Box 988, Warsaw, IN 46582
Various types.

Depuy-Raynham, A Div. Of Depuy Orthopaedics 800-451-2006
325 Paramount Dr, Raynham, MA 02767
Various types.

Zimmer Trabecular Metal Technology 800-613-6131
10 Pomeroy Rd, Parsippany, NJ 07054
Trabecular metal knee system augment.

PROSTHESIS, KNEE, TOTAL *(Orthopedics) 87UBR*

Biopro, Inc. 800-252-7707
2929 Lapeer Rd, Port Huron, MI 48060
The Biopro Uni-Compartmental knee. Total resurfacing, anatomically contoured knee.

Hayes Medical, Inc. 800-240-0500
1115 Windfield Way Ste 100, El Dorado Hills, CA 95762
CONSENSUS KNEE SYSTEM, complete knee system, porous and non-porous, posterior stabilized or PCL retaining, anatomic tibial components, CoCr/Ti femoral components.

Implex Corp. 800-613-6131
1800 W Center St, Warsaw, IN 46580

Kinamed, Inc. 800-827-5775
820 Flynn Rd, Camarillo, CA 93012
GEM Knee System total knee replacement system; cruciate sparing and posterior stabilized.

Orchid Stealth Orthopedic Solutions 517-694-2300
1489 Cedar St, Holt, MI 48842

Ortho Development Corp. 800-429-8339
12187 Business Park Dr, Draper, UT 84020
BALANCED KNEE System; Primary total knee, CR and PS options available.

Osteoimplant Technology, Inc. 410-785-0700
11201 Pepper Rd, Hunt Valley, MD 21031

Stryker Spine 866-457-7463
2 Pearl Ct, Allendale, NJ 07401

Wright Medical Group, Inc. 800-238-7117
5677 Airline Rd, Arlington, TN 38002

PROSTHESIS, LARYNGEAL (TAUB) *(Ear/Nose/Throat) 77EWL*

Bioform Medical, Inc. 262-835-3323
4133 Courtney Rd Ste 10, Franksville, WI 53126
Soft tissue bulking media.

Biomet Microfixation Inc. 800-874-7711
1520 Tradeport Dr, Jacksonville, FL 32218
Various types of prosthesis.

Boston Medical Products, Inc. 800-433-2674
117 Flanders Rd, Westborough, MA 01581
Montgomery small, medium, large adult and child size laryngeal stent. Also, Montgomery laryngeal keel, sizes 12mm, 14mm, and 16mm.

E. Benson Hood Laboratories, Inc. 800-942-5227
575 Washington St, Pembroke, MA 02359
Adult male, adult female, adolescent, and child size silicone laryngeal stents. Steg Stent for reconstruction after semi-laryngectomy. Laryngeal keel: 12mm, 14mm and 16mm, eliachar stent and inflatable stent.

Helix Medical, Inc. 800-266-4421
1110 Mark Ave, Carpinteria, CA 93013

PROSTHESIS, LARYNX *(Ear/Nose/Throat) 77FWN*

Bausch & Lomb Surgical 636-255-5051
3365 Tree Court Ind Blvd, Saint Louis, MO 63122

E. Benson Hood Laboratories, Inc. 800-942-5227
575 Washington St, Pembroke, MA 02359

Smiths Medical Asd 800-424-8662
5700 W 23rd Ave, Gary, IN 46406
Duckbill low resistance and ultra low resistance silicone voice prosthesis, 16Fr and 20Fr.

PROSTHESIS, LEG *(Orthopedics) 87RMX*

Capital Prosthetic Manufacturing, Inc. 518-456-1145
8 Corporate Cir, Albany, NY 12203

Fillauer Companies, Inc. 800-251-6398
2710 Amnicola Hwy, Chattanooga, TN 37406

PROSTHESIS, LEG *(cont'd)*

Ohio Willow Wood Company 800-848-4930
15441 Scioto Darby Rd, Mount Sterling, OH 43143
PATHFINDER, revolutionary prosthetic foot/ankle system that dramatically increases the comfort and performance of amputees ranging from moderately active to world-class athletics.

Slawner Ltd., J. 514-731-3378
5713 Cote Des Neiges Rd., Montreal, QUE H3S 1Y7 Canada

PROSTHESIS, LIGAMENT *(Orthopedics) 87HWF*

Cryolife, Inc. 800-438-8285
1655 Roberts Blvd NW, Kennesaw, GA 30144
Storage and preservation (liquid nitrogen) of human tissue ligaments. Shipment of tissue for implant within 24 hrs.

PROSTHESIS, MANDIBLE *(Surgery) 79JCR*

Tmj Implants, Inc. 800-825-4865
17301 W Colfax Ave Ste 135, Golden, CO 80401
Condylar Prosthesis.

PROSTHESIS, MANDIBULAR CONDYLE *(Dental And Oral) 76MPL*

Biomet Microfixation Inc. 800-874-7711
1520 Tradeport Dr, Jacksonville, FL 32218
Condyle implant.

PROSTHESIS, MAXILLOFACIAL *(Ear/Nose/Throat) 77LGK*

Medical Art Resources, Inc. 414-543-1002
10401 W Lincoln Ave Ste 105, West Allis, WI 53227
Custom external facial prosthesis.

PROSTHESIS, MEMBRANE *(Surgery) 79TDU*

Kensey Nash Corporation 484-713-2100
735 Pennsylvania Dr, Exton, PA 19341
EPI-GUIDE, bioresorbable OPLA periodontal matrix barrier is a bioresorbable polymer synthesized from D, D-L, L-lactic acid and is indicated for use as an adjunct to periodontal restorative surgeries in the treatment of periodontal defects.

PROSTHESIS, NAIL *(Surgery) 79MQZ*

Inro Medical Designs, Inc. 800-527-1093
PO Box 9, Desoto, TX 75123
Nail, nailsplint, temporary device to form a template for rejuvenating nail.

PROSTHESIS, NASAL, DORSAL *(Surgery) 79ESS*

Allergan 800-624-4261
71 S Los Carneros Rd, Goleta, CA 93117

Exmoor Plastics Inc. 317-244-1014
304 Gasoline Aly, Indianapolis, IN 46222
Sunderland nasal airway tubes and voice rehabilitation prostheses in various sizes.

Implantech Associates, Inc. 800-733-0833
6025 Nicolle St Ste B, Ventura, CA 93003
FLOWERS Dorsal Implant, BRINK Peripyriform, RIZZO Dorsal Implant, SHIRAKABE Nasal Implant.

PROSTHESIS, NIPPLE *(Obstetrics/Gyn) 85VLD*

Truform Orthotics & Prosthetics 800-888-0458
3960 Rosslyn Dr, Cincinnati, OH 45209
Airway Division Post-Mastectomy products.

PROSTHESIS, NOSE, INTERNAL *(Surgery) 79FZE*

Aesthetic And Reconstructive Technologies, Inc. 775-853-6800
3545 Airway Dr Ste 106, Reno, NV 89511
Silicone elastomer nasal implant.

Allied Biomedical 800-276-1322
PO Box 392, Ventura, CA 93002

Gyrus Ent L.L.C., Sub. Of Gyrus Acmi, Inc. 508-804-2739
2925 Appling Rd, Bartlett, TN 38133
Various.

Hanson Medical, Inc. 800-771-2215
825 Riverside Ave Ste 2, Paso Robles, CA 93446
Dorsal columella or dorsum.

Invotec Intl. 800-998-8580
6833 Phillips Industrial Blvd, Jacksonville, FL 32256
Nasel implant.

Pillar Surgical, Inc. 800-367-0445
PO Box 8141, La Jolla, CA 92038
Various.

Rocky Mountain Anaplastology, Inc. 303-973-8482
3405 S Yarrow St Unit C, Lakewood, CO 80227
Nose prosthesis (external).

PROSTHESIS, NOSE, INTERNAL *(cont'd)*

Spectrum Designs Medical, Inc. 800-239-6399
6387 Rose Ln Ste B, Carpinteria, CA 93013
Nasal implants, sterile. Designed to restore the nasal contour.

Surgical Technology Laboratories Inc. 803-462-1714
610 Clemson Rd, Columbia, SC 29229
15 different size straith nasal implant.

PROSTHESIS, ORBITAL RIM *(Ophthalmology) 86UBX*

Oculo Plastik Inc. 888-381-3292
200 Sauve West, Montreal, QUE H3L-1Y9 Canada
Acrylic socket and lid reconstruction prostheses, Putterman-Scott.

PROSTHESIS, OSSICULAR *(Ear/Nose/Throat) 77ETB*

Gyrus Ent L.L.C., Sub. Of Gyrus Acmi, Inc. 508-804-2739
2925 Appling Rd, Bartlett, TN 38133
Various types and sizes of partial ossicular replacements.

Jedmed Instruments Co. 314-845-3770
5416 Jedmed Ct, Saint Louis, MO 63129

Mednet Locator, Inc. 800-754-5070
7000 Shadow Oaks Dr, Memphis, TN 38125
Total and partial ossicular replacement prostheses.

PROSTHESIS, OSSICULAR (TOTAL), ABSORBABLE GELATIN MATERIAL *(Ear/Nose/Throat) 77LBO*

Jedmed Instruments Co. 314-845-3770
5416 Jedmed Ct, Saint Louis, MO 63129

PROSTHESIS, OSSICULAR, INCUS AND STAPES *(Ear/Nose/Throat) 77UBU*

Jedmed Instruments Co. 314-845-3770
5416 Jedmed Ct, Saint Louis, MO 63129

PROSTHESIS, OSSICULAR, POROUS POLYETHYLENE *(Ear/Nose/Throat) 77LBM*

Jedmed Instruments Co. 314-845-3770
5416 Jedmed Ct, Saint Louis, MO 63129

PROSTHESIS, OSSICULAR, TOTAL *(Ear/Nose/Throat) 77ETA*

Gyrus Ent L.L.C., Sub. Of Gyrus Acmi, Inc. 508-804-2739
2925 Appling Rd, Bartlett, TN 38133
Various types and sizes of total ossicular replacements.

PROSTHESIS, OSSICULAR, TOTAL, POROUS POLYETHYLENE *(Ear/Nose/Throat) 77LBN*

Jedmed Instruments Co. 314-845-3770
5416 Jedmed Ct, Saint Louis, MO 63129

PROSTHESIS, PENILE *(Gastro/Urology) 78FAE*

American Medical Systems, Inc. 800-328-3881
10700 Bren Rd W, Minnetonka, MN 55343
700 ULTREX and 700 ULTREX PLUS Penile Prostheses; AMS 700CX and AMS 700CXM Inflatable Penile Prostheses; and AMS MALLEABLE 650 and AMS MALLEABLE 600M Penile Prostheses.

Timm Medical Technologies, Inc. 800-966-2796
6585 City West Pkwy, Eden Prairie, MN 55344
DURA II.

PROSTHESIS, PENIS, INFLATABLE *(Surgery) 79JCW*

American Medical Systems, Inc. 800-328-3881
10700 Bren Rd W, Minnetonka, MN 55343
700 ULTREX and 700 ULTREX PLUS Penile Prostheses; AMS 700CX, AMS AMBICOR and AMS 700CXM Inflatable Penile Prostheses.

V.T.S.,Inc. 620-227-7434
1701 N 14th Ave, Dodge City, KS 67801
Various types of vacuum erection devices.

PROSTHESIS, PENIS, RIGID ROD, EXTERNAL *(Gastro/Urology) 78LKY*

Pos-T-Vac, Inc. 800-279-7434
1701 N 14th Ave, P.O. Box 1436, Dodge City, KS 67801
Battery-operated constriction erection device.

Repro-Med Systems, Inc. 845-469-2042
24 Carpenter Rd, Chester, NY 10918

V.T.S.,Inc. 620-227-7434
1701 N 14th Ave, Dodge City, KS 67801
Vt-1.

PROSTHESIS, PTFE/CARBON-FIBER *(Surgery) 79KDA*

Atrium Medical Corp. 800-528-7486
5 Wentworth Dr, Hudson, NH 03051
ATRIUM ADVANTA PTFE vascular prosthesis.

PROSTHESIS, RHINOPLASTY *(Surgery) 79ESR*

Allergan 800-624-4261
71 S Los Carneros Rd, Goleta, CA 93117

S Jackson Inc. 800-368-5225
PO Box 4487, Alexandria, VA 22303
$38.50 to 43.50 non-sterile SUPRAMESH mesh; implant (in 3 sizes).

PROSTHESIS, SENSORY *(Cns/Neurology) 84MHN*

Homedics Inc. 800-333-8282
3000 N Pontiac Trl, Commerce Township, MI 48390
Sensory therapy devices.

Spaceage Control, Inc. 661-273-3000
38850 20th St E, Palmdale, CA 93550
miniature displacement transducers

PROSTHESIS, SHOULDER *(Orthopedics) 87HSF*

Biopro, Inc. 800-252-7707
2929 Lapeer Rd, Port Huron, MI 48060
The Townley Modular shoulder. Porous coated; NFC; Cobalt chrome.

Exactech, Inc. 800-392-2832
2320 NW 66th Ct, Gainesville, FL 32653
Exactech Equinoxe Shoulder System

Stryker Spine 866-457-7463
2 Pearl Ct, Allendale, NJ 07401

Wright Medical Group, Inc. 800-238-7117
5677 Airline Rd, Arlington, TN 38002

Zimmer Holdings, Inc. 800-613-6131
1800 W Center St, PO Box 708, Warsaw, IN 46580

PROSTHESIS, SHOULDER, CONSTR., METAL/METAL OR POLYMER/CEM. *(Orthopedics) 87KWR*

Biomet, Inc. 574-267-6639
56 E Bell Dr, PO Box 587, Warsaw, IN 46582
Various types of sterile and non-sterile total shoulders.

PROSTHESIS, SHOULDER, HEMI-, GLENOID, METAL *(Orthopedics) 87KYM*

Encore Medical Corporation 800-456-8696
9800 Metric Blvd, Austin, TX 78758

Endotec, Inc. 973-762-6100
2546 Hansrob Rd, Orlando, FL 32804
Buechel-pappas glenoid fixation cup.

PROSTHESIS, SHOULDER, HEMI-, HUMERAL *(Orthopedics) 87HSD*

Acumed Llc 503-627-9957
5885 NW Cornelius Pass Rd, Hillsboro, OR 97124
Modular shoulder system.

Arthrex, Inc. 239-643-5553
1370 Creekside Blvd, Naples, FL 34108
Prosthesis,shoulder,hemi-,humeral,metallic uncemented.

Arthrosurface, Inc. 508-520-3003
28 Forge Pkwy, Franklin, MA 02038
Shoulder joint humeral (hemi-shoulder) metallic resurfacing prosthesis.

Ascension Orthopedics, Inc. 877-370-5001
8700 Cameron Rd, Austin, TX 78754
Ascension HRA

Biomet, Inc. 574-267-6639
56 E Bell Dr, PO Box 587, Warsaw, IN 46582
Various types of sterile and non-sterile shoulder prosthesis.

Depuy Orthopaedics, Inc. 800-473-3789
700 Orthopaedic Dr, P.O. Box 988, Warsaw, IN 46582
Various shoulder system components.

Endotec, Inc. 973-762-6100
2546 Hansrob Rd, Orlando, FL 32804
Buechel-pappas humeral stem.

Stryker Spine 866-457-7463
2 Pearl Ct, Allendale, NJ 07401

Zimmer Holdings, Inc. 800-613-6131
1800 W Center St, PO Box 708, Warsaw, IN 46580

PROSTHESIS, SHOULDER, HUMERAL, BIPOL., HEMI-, CONSTR., M/P *(Orthopedics) 87MJT*

Biomet, Inc. 574-267-6639
56 E Bell Dr, PO Box 587, Warsaw, IN 46582
Various types of shoulder prostheses.

PROSTHESIS, SHOULDER, METAL/POLYMER, UNCEMENTED *(Orthopedics) 87MBF*

Biomet, Inc. 574-267-6639
56 E Bell Dr, PO Box 587, Warsaw, IN 46582
Various types of sterile and non-sterile shoulder prosthesis.

Depuy Orthopaedics, Inc. 800-473-3789
700 Orthopaedic Dr, P.O. Box 988, Warsaw, IN 46582
Various types uncemented, metal-poly, semi-const. shoulder.

PROSTHESIS, SHOULDER, NON-CONSTRAINED, METAL/POLYMER CEM. *(Orthopedics) 87KWT*

Biomet, Inc. 574-267-6639
56 E Bell Dr, PO Box 587, Warsaw, IN 46582
Various types of sterile & non-sterile shoulder components.

Centerpulse Orthopedics Inc. 877-768-7349
9900 Spectrum Dr, Austin, TX 78717
The SELECT Shoulder system pegged and kelled all-poly glenoid components. Anatomical shoulder system all-poly glenoids.

Depuy Orthopaedics, Inc. 800-473-3789
700 Orthopaedic Dr, P.O. Box 988, Warsaw, IN 46582
Various types of shoulder prostheses, non-constrained, metal/polymer cemented.

Endotec, Inc. 973-762-6100
2546 Hansrob Rd, Orlando, FL 32804
Buechel-pappas glenoid bearing.

Stelkast Company 724-941-6368
200 Hidden Valley Rd, McMurray, PA 15317
Shoulder implant.

Zimmer Trabecular Metal Technology 800-613-6131
10 Pomeroy Rd, Parsippany, NJ 07054
Shoulder devices.

PROSTHESIS, SHOULDER, SEMI-CONSTRAINED, METAL/POLYMER CEM. *(Orthopedics) 87KWS*

Arthrex, Inc. 239-643-5553
1370 Creekside Blvd, Naples, FL 34108
Univers total shoulder,prosthesis,semi-contrained,metal/non-porous,cemented vari.

Biomet, Inc. 574-267-6639
56 E Bell Dr, PO Box 587, Warsaw, IN 46582
Bio-modular shoulder, bi-angular shoulder.

Centerpulse Orthopedics Inc. 877-768-7349
9900 Spectrum Dr, Austin, TX 78717
Select shoulder system and anatomical shoulder system; humeral stems and humeral heads (standard and offset).

Depuy Orthopaedics, Inc. 800-473-3789
700 Orthopaedic Dr, P.O. Box 988, Warsaw, IN 46582
Various types of shoulder prostheses, non-constrained, metal/polymer cemented.

Zimmer Trabecular Metal Technology 800-613-6131
10 Pomeroy Rd, Parsippany, NJ 07054
Shoulder devices.

PROSTHESIS, SOFT TISSUE *(Surgery) 79UCY*

Porex Surgical, Inc. 800-521-7321
15 Dart Rd, Newnan, GA 30265
MEDPOR porous polyethylene surgical implants for craniofacial reconstruction.

PROSTHESIS, SPINE, INTERVERTEBRAL DISC *(Orthopedics) 87MJO*

Depuy Spine, Inc. 800-227-6633
325 Paramount Dr, Raynham, MA 02767
Intervertebral disc prosthesis with related instrumentation.

Implex Corp. 800-613-6131
1800 W Center St, Warsaw, IN 46580

Ionics Medical Corp. 910-428-9726
248 Bird Haven Lane, Ether, NC 27247-0179
Vertically expandable, shock absorbing ALIF/nucleus replacement prosthesis, various sizes.

Medtronic Sofamor Danek Usa, Inc. 901-396-3133
4340 Swinnea Rd, Memphis, TN 38118
Intervertebral disc prosthesis.

Spinal Kinetics, Inc. 609-254-3999
595 N Pastoria Ave, Sunnyvale, CA 94085
Total artificial disc.

PROSTHESIS, SPINE, INTERVERTEBRAL DISC *(cont'd)*

Trimedyne, Inc. 800-733-5273
15091 Bake Pkwy, Irvine, CA 92618
Disc decompression devices. The Omni spinal introduction system and the Straightfire and Sidefire laser needles used with the Omnipulse holmium laser for performing cervical, thoracic, or lumbar percutaneous laser disc decompression/discectomy or endoscopic laser foraminoplasty.

Warsaw Orthopedic, Inc. 901-396-3133
2500 Silveus Xing, Warsaw, IN 46582
Intervertebral disc prosthesis.

PROSTHESIS, SUTURE, CERCLAGE *(Obstetrics/Gyn) 85HHY*

Ethicon, Inc. 800-4-ETHICON
Route 22 West, Somerville, NJ 08876
Available prethreaded on braided polyester suture material, 5mm tape.

Ethicon, Llc. 908-218-2887
Rd. 183, Km. 8.3,, Industrial Area Hato, San Lorenzo, PR 00754
Polyester fiber stripes.

PROSTHESIS, TENDON *(Surgery) 79FTP*

Cryolife, Inc. 800-438-8285
1655 Roberts Blvd NW, Kennesaw, GA 30144
Storage and preservation (liquid nitrogen) of human tissue tendons. Shipment of tissue for implant within 24 hrs.

PROSTHESIS, THIGH SOCKET, EXTERNAL COMPONENT *(Physical Med) 89ISS*

Caguas Orthopedic Center, Inc. 787-744-2325
FF4 Calle 11, Villa Del Rey, Caguas, PR 00727
Lower extremity prosthesis.

Genuine Care Rehab. Svc., Inc. 405-604-5907
2401 NW 23rd St Ste 17, Oklahoma City, OK 73107
Prosthetic sportswear garment.

Hosmer Dorrance Corp. 408-379-5151
561 Division St, Campbell, CA 95008
Various.

Ohio Willow Wood Company 800-848-4930
15441 Scioto Darby Rd, Mount Sterling, OH 43143
Structural components for ankle, foot, knee and thigh prostheses.

Orthotic & Prosthetic Lab, Inc. 314-968-8555
748 Marshall Ave, Webster Groves, MO 63119
O&p socket.

Trulife, Inc. 360-697-5656
26296 12 Trees Ln NW, Poulsbo, WA 98370
Socket liner.

PROSTHESIS, TIBIAL *(Orthopedics) 87RNA*

Encore Medical Corporation 800-456-8696
9800 Metric Blvd, Austin, TX 78758

Implex Corp. 800-613-6131
1800 W Center St, Warsaw, IN 46580

Slawner Ltd., J. 514-731-3378
5713 Cote Des Neiges Rd., Montreal, QUE H3S 1Y7 Canada

Zimmer Holdings, Inc. 800-613-6131
1800 W Center St, PO Box 708, Warsaw, IN 46580

PROSTHESIS, TOE *(Orthopedics) 87UCM*

Sgarlato Laboratories, Inc. 800-421-5303
2315 S Bascom Ave Ste 200, Campbell, CA 95008
Hammertoe implant for lesser digit; toe implant. Available in 3 sizes. GAIT toe implant for great toe, available in 3 sizes.

PROSTHESIS, TOE (METAPHAL.), JOINT, MET./POLY., SEMI-CONST. *(Orthopedics) 87LZJ*

Biomet, Inc. 574-267-6639
56 E Bell Dr, PO Box 587, Warsaw, IN 46582
Total toe.

PROSTHESIS, TOE, HEMI-, PHALANGEAL *(Orthopedics) 87KWD*

Arthrex, Inc. 239-643-5553
1370 Creekside Blvd, Naples, FL 34108
Prosthesis, toe, hemi-phalangeal.

Arthrosurface, Inc. 508-520-3003
28 Forge Pkwy, Franklin, MA 02038
Great toe resurfacing prosthesis.

Ascension Orthopedics, Inc. 877-370-5001
8700 Cameron Rd, Austin, TX 78754
Ascension CMC/TMT

PROSTHESIS, TOE, HEMI-, PHALANGEAL *(cont'd)*

Biopro, Inc. 800-252-7707
2929 Lapeer Rd, Port Huron, MI 48060
Great Toe toe hemi-phalangeal.

Small Bone Innovations, Inc. 215-428-1791
1380 S Pennsylvania Ave, Morrisville, PA 19067
Toe joint phalangeal (hemi-toe) polymer prosthesis.

Terray Corporation 613-623-3310
49 Jackson Lane, Pinegrove Industrial Pa
Arnprior, ON K7S-3 Canada
Trihedron System.

PROSTHESIS, TRACHEA *(Surgery) 79JCT*

Boston Medical Products, Inc. 800-433-2674
117 Flanders Rd, Westborough, MA 01581
Montgomery tracheal cannula system: short- and long-term, sizes 4, 6, 8 and 10, 6 lengths. Montgomery SAFE-T-TUBE set, o.d. sizes 6mm-16mm. Also available extra-long or with customizing kit. HMS system provides support as stent and offers inner cannula system for care and cleaning of tracheotomy during reconstruction.

Boston Scientific Corp. 800-323-6472
5905 Nathan Ln N, Minneapolis, MN 55442

Cook Endoscopy 336-744-0157
4900 Bethania Station Rd # &, 5951 Grassy Creek Blvd.
Winston Salem, NC 27105
Tracheal prothesis.

E. Benson Hood Laboratories, Inc. 800-942-5227
575 Washington St, Pembroke, MA 02359
T-Tubes with 4.5-16mm (standard), 5-18mm (long) 8-14mm (thoracic) outer diameters, T-Y Tubes with 10, 12, and 14mm OD. Tracheal stent with post. Ultra-smooth surface treatment.

Ev3 Inc. 800-716-6700
4600 Nathan Ln N, Plymouth, MN 55442
Tracheobronchial stent.

W.L. Gore & Associates,Inc 928-526-3030
1505 North Fourth St., Flagstaff, AZ 86004
Esopageal & tracheal endoprosthesis.

PROSTHESIS, TRACHEAL, EXPANDABLE, POLYMERIC *(Surgery) 79NYT*

W. L. Gore & Associates, Inc. 800-437-8181
PO Box 2400, Flagstaff, AZ 86003
Viabahn Endoprosthesis

PROSTHESIS, UPPER FEMORAL *(Orthopedics) 87JDD*

Biomet, Inc. 574-267-6639
56 E Bell Dr, PO Box 587, Warsaw, IN 46582
Various types of femoral hip prosthesis.

Stryker Spine 866-457-7463
2 Pearl Ct, Allendale, NJ 07401

Warsaw Orthopedic, Inc. 901-396-3133
2500 Silveus Xing, Warsaw, IN 46582
Thompson and moore type hip prostheses.

Zimmer Holdings, Inc. 800-613-6131
1800 W Center St, PO Box 708, Warsaw, IN 46580

PROSTHESIS, URETHRAL SPHINCTER *(Gastro/Urology) 78FAG*

American Medical Systems, Inc. 800-328-3881
10700 Bren Rd W, Minnetonka, MN 55343
AMS SPHINCTER 800 Urinary Prosthesis.

PROSTHESIS, VASCULAR GRAFT, LESS THAN 6MM DIAMETER *(Cardiovascular) 74DYF*

Angiotech Pharmaceuticals Inc., Vascular Graft Div 604-221-7676
23601 Ridge Route Dr Ste C, Laguna Hills, CA 92653
Vascular graft.

Bard Peripheral Vascular, Inc. 800-321-4254
1625 W 3rd St, Tempe, AZ 85281
Regular, thin wall, straight or tapered IMPRA-FLEX grafts (PTFE).

Bard Shannon Limited 908-277-8000
San Geronimo Industrial Park, Lot # 1, Road # 3, Km 79.7
Humacao, PR 00791
Fabrics,grafts,pledgets.

Corvita Corp. 305-599-3100
8210 NW 27th St, Doral, FL 33122
In clinical trials in U.S., Europe and Japan.

PROSTHESIS, VASCULAR GRAFT, LESS THAN 6MM DIAMETER *(cont'd)*

Cryolife, Inc. 800-438-8285
1655 Roberts Blvd NW, Kennesaw, GA 30144
Storage and preservation (liquid nitrogen) of human saphenous vein tissue. Shipment of vein for implant within 24 hrs.

Edwards Lifesciences, Llc. 800-424-3278
1 Edwards Way, Irvine, CA 92614
PTFE vascular graft.

Endovascular Instruments, Inc. 360-750-1150
2501 SE Columbia Way Ste 150, Vancouver, WA 98661

Maquet Cardiovascular LLC 888-880-2874
45 Barbour Pond Dr, Wayne, NJ 07470
Exxcel

Thoratec Corporation 800-456-1477
6101 Stoneridge Dr, Pleasanton, CA 94588

Tuzik Boston 800-886-6363
104 Longwater Dr, Assinippi Park, Norwell, MA 02061

W.L. Gore & Associates,Inc 928-526-3030
1505 North Fourth St., Flagstaff, AZ 86004
Sterile vascular graft.

PROSTHESIS, VASCULAR GRAFT, OF 6MM AND GREATER DIAMETER *(Cardiovascular) 74DSY*

Angiotech Pharmaceuticals Inc., Vascular Graft Div 604-221-7676
23601 Ridge Route Dr Ste C, Laguna Hills, CA 92653
Vascular graft.

Artegraft, Inc. 800-631-5264
220 N Center Dr, North Brunswick, NJ 08902
ARTEGRAFT. All collagen vascular grafts, available in 6, 7, and 8mm outside diameters and lengths up to 52cm.

Atrium Medical Corp. 800-528-7486
5 Wentworth Dr, Hudson, NH 03051
ATRIUM ADVANTA PTFE vascular grafts available in a wide range of sizes and configurations.

Bard Peripheral Vascular, Inc. 800-321-4254
1625 W 3rd St, Tempe, AZ 85281
Regular, thin wall, straight or tapered IMPRA-FLEX grafts (PTFE). VASCUTEK knitted and woven Dacron grafts.

Bard Shannon Limited 908-277-8000
San Geronimo Industrial Park, Lot # 1, Road # 3, Km 79.7
Humacao, PR 00791
Fabrics,grafts,pledgets.

Corvita Corp. 305-599-3100
8210 NW 27th St, Doral, FL 33122
In clinical trials in U.S., Commercialized in Europe, & Japan.

Cryolife, Inc. 800-438-8285
1655 Roberts Blvd NW, Kennesaw, GA 30144
Storage and preservation (liquid nitrogen) of human vascular graft tissue. Shipment of grafts for implant within 24 hrs.

Edwards Lifesciences, Llc. 800-424-3278
1 Edwards Way, Irvine, CA 92614
PTFE vascular graft.

Endovascular Instruments, Inc. 360-750-1150
2501 SE Columbia Way Ste 150, Vancouver, WA 98661

Maquet Cardiovascular LLC 888-880-2874
45 Barbour Pond Dr, Wayne, NJ 07470
HEMASHIELD

Thoratec Corporation 800-456-1477
6101 Stoneridge Dr, Pleasanton, CA 94588

Tuzik Boston 800-886-6363
104 Longwater Dr, Assinippi Park, Norwell, MA 02061

W.L. Gore & Associates,Inc 928-526-3030
1505 North Fourth St., Flagstaff, AZ 86004
Vascular graft.

PROSTHESIS, WRIST, 2 PART METAL-PLASTIC ARTICULATION *(Orthopedics) 87JWI*

Biomet, Inc. 574-267-6639
56 E Bell Dr, PO Box 587, Warsaw, IN 46582
Cfv wrist system.

PROSTHESIS, WRIST, 3 PART METAL-PLASTIC-METAL ARTICULATION *(Orthopedics) 87JWJ*

Biomet, Inc. 574-267-6639
56 E Bell Dr, PO Box 587, Warsaw, IN 46582
Various types of wrist prosthesis.

PROSTHESIS, WRIST, 3 PART METAL-PLASTIC-METAL ARTICULATION *(cont'd)*

Depuy Orthopaedics, Inc. 800-473-3789
700 Orthopaedic Dr, P.O. Box 988, Warsaw, IN 46582
Various wrist prostheses with sterile and non-sterile components.

Small Bone Innovations, Inc. 215-428-1791
1380 S Pennsylvania Ave, Morrisville, PA 19067
Wrist joint metal/polymer semi-constrained cemented prosthesis.

Stryker Spine 866-457-7463
2 Pearl Ct, Allendale, NJ 07401

PROSTHESIS, WRIST, CARPAL TRAPEZIUM *(Orthopedics) 87KYI*

Ascension Orthopedics, Inc. 877-370-5001
8700 Cameron Rd, Austin, TX 78754
Ascension PHS

Small Bone Innovations, Inc. 215-428-1791
1380 S Pennsylvania Ave, Morrisville, PA 19067
Wrist joint carpal trapezium polymer prosthesis.

Wright Medical Group, Inc. 800-238-7117
5677 Airline Rd, Arlington, TN 38002

PROSTHESIS, WRIST, HEMI-, ULNAR *(Orthopedics) 87KXE*

Aptis Medical, Llc. 502-899-9700
3602 Glenview Ave, Glenview, KY 40025
Distal ulna.

Small Bone Innovations, Inc. 215-428-1791
1380 S Pennsylvania Ave, Morrisville, PA 19067
Wrist joint ulnar (hemi-wrist) polymer prosthesis.

PROSTHESIS, WRIST, SEMI-CONSTRAINED *(Orthopedics) 87KWM*

Wright Medical Group, Inc. 800-238-7117
5677 Airline Rd, Arlington, TN 38002

PROSTHETIC DISC NUCLEUS DEVICE *(Orthopedics) 87MQO*

Raymedica, Llc 952-885-0500
9401 James Ave S Ste 120, Minneapolis, MN 55431
Same.

PROTAMINE SULPHATE *(Hematology) 81GFT*

International Technidyne Corp. 800-631-5945
23 Nevsky St, Edison, NJ 08820

Medtronic Blood Management 612-514-4000
18501 E Plaza Dr, Parker, CO 80134
Invitro diagnostic cartridges & controls.

PROTARGOL S *(Pathology) 88KKG*

Polysciences, Inc. 800-523-2575
400 Valley Rd, Warrington, PA 18976

PROTECTANT, SKIN *(Surgery) 79NEC*

Aspire Biotech, Inc. 719-522-9800
967 Elkton Dr, Colorado Springs, CO 80907
Various types of sterile and non-sterile liquid bandages.

Chemence Medical Products Inc. 770-664-6624
185 Bluegrass Valley Pkwy Ste 100, Alpharetta, GA 30005
Liquid occlusive wound bandage.

Chesson Laboratory Associates, Inc. 919-636-5773
603 Ellis Rd, Durham, NC 27703
Skin protectant.

Epien Medical, Inc. 651-653-3380
4225 White Bear Pkwy Ste 600, Saint Paul, MN 55110
Ulcer covering for pain relief.

Epikeia, Inc. 210-313-4600
500 Sandau Rd Ste 200, San Antonio, TX 78216
Liquid skin protectant.

Gel Concepts Llc. 973-884-8995
30 Leslie Ct, Whippany, NJ 07981
Natural hydrogel.

Maxpak, Llc 863-682-0123
2808 New Tampa Hwy, Lakeland, FL 33815
Liquid bandage.

Medspring Group, Inc. 801-295-9750
533 W 2600 S Ste 105, Bountiful, UT 84010
Liquid bandage.

PROTECTOR, DENTAL *(Anesthesiology) 73BRW*

Karwoski Dental 925-938-8977
418 Iron Hill St, Pleasant Hill, CA 94523
Lip protector.

Mainline Medical, Inc. 800-366-2084
3250 Peachtree Corners Cir Ste J, Norcross, GA 30092
Tooth protector.Adult size, protects patients teeth from tooth damage during intubation. Latex free.

Salmon Medical Innovations, Llc 301-279-2596
903 Willowleaf Way, Rockville, MD 20854
Dental protector.

Sunmed Healthcare 727-531-7266
12393 Belcher Rd S Ste 460, Largo, FL 33773

Superior Autocatheter Enterprises 800-243-1467
2137 Vermillion St Ste 250, Hastings, MN 55033
Teeth guard protector. Latex free product.

Ultradent Products, Inc. 801-553-4586
505 W 10200 S, South Jordan, UT 84095
Dental protector.

PROTECTOR, FINGER *(Orthopedics) 87QWH*

Alimed, Inc. 800-225-2610
297 High St, Dedham, MA 02026
Finger fracture splints have metal edges that have been buffed smooth.

Apothecary Products, Inc. 800-328-2742
11750 12th Ave S, Burnsville, MN 55337

Bsn Medical, Inc 800-552-1157
5825 Carnegie Blvd, Charlotte, NC 28209
STAX® FINGER SPLINTS are designed to support the distal joint of the finger in extension while permitting unrestricted movement of the proximal interphalangael joint.

Carex Health Brands 800-526-8051
921 E Amidon St, PO Box 2526, Sioux Falls, SD 57104
Finger splints.

Inland Specialties, Inc. 800-741-0022
7655 Matoaka Rd, Sarasota, FL 34243
Available in small, medium and large sizes.

Jurgan Development & Mfg. 800-587-4262
6018 S Highlands Ave, Madison, WI 53705
JURGAN PIN BALL system provides safe, dependable, easy to use protection from the hazards of all protruding pins and wires.

Mizuho Osi 800-777-4674
30031 Ahern Ave, Union City, CA 94587

Paramedical Distributors 800-245-3278
2020 Grand Blvd, Kansas City, MO 64108
Finger orthoses.

Unique Sports Products, Inc. 800-554-3707
840 McFarland Pkwy, Alpharetta, GA 30004
Finger Splints--used to hold finger in proper position. Made of aluminum with foam pad facing finger.

Zimmer Holdings, Inc. 800-613-6131
1800 W Center St, PO Box 708, Warsaw, IN 46580

PROTECTOR, HEARING (CIRCUMAURAL)
(Ear/Nose/Throat) 77EWE

Clark Company Inc., David 800-900-3434
360 Franklin St, Worcester, MA 01604

Gyrus Ent L.L.C., Sub. Of Gyrus Acmi, Inc. 508-804-2739
2925 Appling Rd, Bartlett, TN 38133
Shah aural dressing.

Natus Medical Inc. 800-255-3901
1501 Industrial Rd, San Carlos, CA 94070
MINIMUFFS neonatal noise attenuators provide a comfortable, easy-to-use solution for decreasing the noise levels to the newborn in the intensive care unit.

Niagara Pharmaceuticals Div. 905-690-6277
60 Innovation Dr., Flamborough, ONT L9H-7P3 Canada
EAR-MATE no. 228 plastic swim plugs (reversible, 3 pcs./case).

PROTECTOR, HEARING (INSERT) *(Ear/Nose/Throat) 77EWD*

Aearo Company 800-678-4163
5457 W 79th St, Indianapolis, IN 46268

Doc's Proplugs, Inc. 800-521-2982
719 Swift St Ste 100, Santa Cruz, CA 95060
Earplug, preformed protective. Protects the ear from high frequencies of music and light industry. Prevents swimmer's ear and surfer's ear (exostosis).

PROTECTOR, HEARING (INSERT) *(cont'd)*

Eckstein Brothers, Inc. 800-432-4913
2807 Oregon Ct Ste D5, Torrance, CA 90503
INFANT SCREENER. NOISE STIK model EB22 is a neonatal hearing screener with 60dB and 90db -white noise

Healer Products, Llc 914-663-6300
427 Commerce Ln Ste 1, West Berlin, NJ 08091
Ear plugs.

Hearing Components Inc. 800-872-8986
420 Hayward Ave N, Oakdale, MN 55128
ADHEAR stick-on wax guards and COMPLY canal tips. COMPLY soft wraps, adhesively bonded slow-recovery foam. A special foam tape to make earpierces active to match active ear canals. COMPLY snap tips, a novel instant fitting tip for earpieces. Includes user friendly delivery system of packaging.

Kerma Medical Products, Inc. 757-398-8400
400 Port Centre Pkwy, Portsmouth, VA 23704
Ear plugs.

Mckeon Products, Inc. 586-427-7560
25460 Guenther, Warren, MI 48091
Mack's pillow soft ear plugs.

Niagara Pharmaceuticals Div. 905-690-6277
60 Innovation Dr., Flamborough, ONT L9H-7P3 Canada
HEAR-SAVER no. 201 wax/cotton swim plugs; 6 pairs/case.

Santa Barbara Medco, Inc. 651-452-1977
1270 Eagan Industrial Rd, Eagan, MN 55121
Ear protector mold kit.

Sellstrom Manufacturing Co. 800-323-7402
1 Sellstrom Dr, Palatine, IL 60067
TONEDOWN NRR 2, TONEDOWN 200 NRR 26.

Westone Laboratories, Inc. 719-540-9333
2235 Executive Cir, Colorado Springs, CO 80906
Various models of hearing protectors.

Westone Laboratories, Inc. 719-540-9333
6287 American Ave, Portage, MI 49002

PROTECTOR, HEEL *(General) 80KIB*

Action Products, Inc. 800-228-7763
954 Sweeney Dr, Hagerstown, MD 21740
Heel cup protectors can be used in multiple modules to protect patients in any bony prominence area or other area vulnerable to high pressure during surgery or in the homecare market.

Alimed, Inc. 800-225-2610
297 High St, Dedham, MA 02026

Dm Systems, Inc. 800-254-5438
1316 Sherman Ave, Evanston, IL 60201
HEELIFT® and HEELIFT® SMOOTH SUSPENSION BOOTS aid in the prevention and treatment of heel pressure ulcers. They do so by suspending the heel in pressure-free space, while providing a comfortable, optimal healing environment for pressure ulcers. The only difference between the two boots is inside. The Original Heelift® Boot is made from soft convoluted foam for increased ventilation, while the New Heelift® Smooth Boot is made from soft smooth foam specifically designed for edematous legs.

Gaymar Industries, Inc. 800-828-7341
10 Centre Dr, Orchard Park, NY 14127
Sof-Care Heel Boot for prevention and treatment of pressure ulcers at the heels.

Hermell Products, Inc. 800-233-2342
9 Britton Dr, PO Box 7345, Bloomfield, CT 06002

Larkotex Company 800-972-3037
1002 Olive St, Texarkana, TX 75501

Senecare Enterprises, Inc. 800-442-4577
350 Central Ave Ste A, Bohemia, NY 11716
Lubricated heel protective.

Western Medical, Ltd. 800-628-8276
214 Carnegie Ctr Ste 100, Princeton, NJ 08540
Heel and elbow protectors.

PROTECTOR, MOUTH GUARD *(Dental And Oral) 76ELQ*

Certified Safety Manufacturing 800-854-7474
1400 Chestnut Ave, Kansas City, MO 64127
CPROTECTOR CPR, mouth-to-mouth barrier.

D.C.A. (Dental Corporation Of America) 800-638-6684
889 S Matlack St, West Chester, PA 19382
$39.75 for 12.

Masel Co., Inc. 800-423-8227
2701 Bartram Rd, Bristol, PA 19007

PROTECTOR, MOUTH GUARD *(cont'd)*

Medi/Nuclear Corp. 800-321-5981
4610 Littlejohn St, Baldwin Park, CA 91706
Safety shield mouthpiece, semi-rigid.

Orthodontic Supply & Equipment Co., Inc. 800-638-4003
7851 Airpark Rd Ste 202, Gaithersburg, MD 20879
Athletic mouth guard.

Ranir, Llc 616-698-8880
4701 E Paris Ave SE, Grand Rapids, MI 49512

Tp Orthodontics, Inc. 800-348-8856
100 Center Plz, La Porte, IN 46350
Varsity Guard, Free-N-Easy Mouthguard.

PROTECTOR, OSTOMY *(Gastro/Urology) 78EXE*

Bristol-Myers Squibb 732-227-7564
2400 W Lloyd Expy, Evansville, IN 47712
Skin barrier, absorber.

Hollister, Inc. 847-680-2849
366 Draft Ave, Stuarts Draft, VA 24477

Invacare Supply Group, An Invacare Co. 800-225-4792
75 October Hill Rd, Holliston, MA 01746
Carry full lines of ostomy systems from: Hollister, Convatec, Coloplast, Genairex, Bard & Cymed.

Mylan Technologies, Inc. 800-532-5226
110 Lake St, Saint Albans, VT 05478
Series of custom extruded polyolefin, Hytrel co-polyester, and urethane films optimized for comfort, conformability and security in ostomy barrier applications.

PROTECTOR, PUNCTURE, NEEDLE *(General) 80WUI*

Bio-Plexus, Inc. 800-223-0010
129 Reservoir Rd, Vernon, CT 06066

Medical Safety Systems Inc. 888-803-9303
230 White Pond Dr, Akron, OH 44313
Single handed needle recapper.

Micor, Inc. 412-487-1113
2855 Oxford Blvd, Allison Park, PA 15101
Guards, needle (LDPE, HDPE, PVC).

North American Medical Products, Inc. 800-488-6267
6 British American Blvd Ste B, Latham, NY 12110
SAFE-POINT Needle Cover System, for IM and IV use and blood gases, secondary sets to cover needle after use; fits all syringes. SAFETY NEEDLE which its all tube holders. SAFETY SHEATH covers needle after use.

PROTECTOR, SILICATE *(Dental And Oral) 76EFX*

Harry J. Bosworth Company 800-323-4352
7227 Hamlin Ave, Skokie, IL 60076

Lorvic Corp. 800-325-1881
13705 Shoreline Ct E, Earth City, MO 63045
Silicate lubricant.

PROTECTOR, SKIN PRESSURE *(General) 80FMP*

A&A Orthopedics, Incorporated 757-224-0177
12250 SW 129th Ct Bldg 1, Miami, FL 33186
Heel & elbow protectors.

Allen Medical Systems, Inc. 800-433-5774
1 Post Office Sq, Acton, MA 01720
Allen® offers a wide range of pressure management products

Amf Support Surfaces, Inc. 951-549-6800
1691 N Delilah St, Corona, CA 92879
Skin pressure protector.

Anatomic Concepts, Inc. 951-549-6800
1691 N Delilah St, Corona, CA 92879
Foam elbow and heel pads.

Aspen Medical Products 949-681-0200
6481 Oak Cyn, Irvine, CA 92618
Heel protection device.

Azmec, Inc. 877-862-9632
519 N Smith Ave Ste 110, Corona, CA 92880
Protector, skin pressure.

Biomedical Systems 800-877-6334
77 Progress Pkwy Bldg 1, Maryland Hts, MO 63043
Two products are available: a wheel-chair cushion and a heel protector.

Biomet, Inc. 574-267-6639
56 E Bell Dr, PO Box 587, Warsaw, IN 46582
Various types of protectors and pads.

PROTECTOR, SKIN PRESSURE *(cont'd)*

Bird & Cronin, Inc. 651-683-1111
1200 Trapp Rd, Saint Paul, MN 55121
Bed pad/heel/elbow protectors.

Brennen Medical, Llc 651-429-7413
1290 Hammond Rd, Saint Paul, MN 55110
Lower leg positioning device.

Carolina Narrow Fabric Co. 336-631-3000
1100 Patterson Ave, Winston Salem, NC 27101
Heel protector.

Cimex Medical Innovations, Llc 985-871-0802
72385 Industry Park Rd, Covington, LA 70435
Multiple.

Condex International, Inc. 310-618-8444
2441 W 205th St Ste C200E, Torrance, CA 90501
Skin pad.

Confortaire Inc 662-842-2966
2133 S Veterans Blvd, Tupelo, MS 38804
Protector, wedges, pillows.

Dj Orthopedics De Mexico, S.A. De C.V. 690-727-1280
Blvd., Delagacion La Presa, Tijuana 22397 Mexico
Heel, protector

Dj Orthopedics De Mexico, S.A. De C.V. 690-727-1280
Ave. Venustiano Carranza 6802, Castillo, Tijuana 22100 Mexico
Heel, protector

DJO Inc. 800-336-6569
1430 Decision St, Vista, CA 92081

Ethox International 800-521-1022
251 Seneca St, Buffalo, NY 14204
Skin pressure protector.

Frank Stubbs Co., Inc 800-223-1713
2100 Eastman Ave Ste B, Oxnard, CA 93030

Gelsmart Llc 973-884-8995
30 Leslie Ct Ste B-202, Whippany, NJ 07981
Skin protector pad.

Greenco Industries, Inc. 608-328-8311
1601 4th Ave W, Monroe, WI 53566
Various types of decubitus pads.

J. T. Posey Co. 800-447-6739
5635 Peck Rd, Arcadia, CA 91006

Joerns Healthcare, Inc. 715-341-3600
1032 N Fourth St, Baldwyn, MS 38824
Protector, wedges, pillows.

Kenad Sg Medical, Inc. 800-825-0606
2692 Huntley Dr, Memphis, TN 38132
Skin protector.

Kentron Health Care, Inc. 615-384-0573
3604 Kelton Jackson Rd, P.o. Box 120, Springfield, TN 37172
Protector, skin pressure.

Larkotex Company 800-972-3037
1002 Olive St, Texarkana, TX 75501

M.B.S. Fabricating & Coating, Inc. 704-871-1830
174 Crawford Rd Ste A, Po Box 249, Statesville, NC 28625
Heel, elbow protector.

Medical Action Industries, Inc. 800-645-7042
25 Heywood Rd, Arden, NC 28704
Comfort padding.

Mizuho Osi 800-777-4674
30031 Ahern Ave, Union City, CA 94587

Nearly Me Technologies, Inc. 800-887-3370
3630 South I 35, Suite A, Waco, TX 76702-1475
Silicone gel pads.

Neonatal, Infant, Pediatric, And Adult 305-267-8885
815 NW 57th Ave Ste 110, Miami, FL 33126
Skin pressure protectors.

Osborn Medical Corp. 800-535-5865
100 W Main St N, PO Box 324, Utica, MN 55979
Rooke boot/vascular system.

Ossur Americas 800-257-8440
1414 Metropolitan Ave, West Deptford, NJ 08066
Sorbatex Pads, IntuiTech Pads.

Patterson Medical Supply, Inc. 262-387-8720
W68N158 Evergreen Blvd, Cedarburg, WI 53012
Hapla stockinette; foam padding; countor foam polycushion.

PROTECTOR, SKIN PRESSURE *(cont'd)*

Polygell Llc. 973-884-8995
30 Leslie Ct, Whippany, NJ 07981
Skin protector pad.

Polymer Concepts, Inc. 877-820-3163
7561 Tyler Blvd Ste 8, Mentor, OH 44060
Various models of heel protector.

Premier Brands Of America, Inc. 914-667-6200
120 Pearl St, Mount Vernon, NY 10550
Various sizes and shapes of skin protector and cushions.

Primo, Inc. 770-486-7394
417 Dividend Dr Ste B, Peachtree City, GA 30269
Heel/elbow protectors,heel protectors relief products.

Royal Converting, Inc. 865-938-7828
1615 Highway 33 S, New Tazewell, TN 37825

Rx Textiles, Inc. 704-283-9787
3107 Chamber Dr, Monroe, NC 28110
Heel & elbow protector.

Scott Specialties, Inc. 785-527-5627
1827 Meadowlark Rd, Clay Center, KS 67432
Various types of skin pressure protectors.

Scott Specialties, Inc. 785-527-5627
1820 E 7th St, Concordia, KS 66901

Segufix Systems Ltd. 506-328-8636
110 Queen St., Woodstock, NB E7M-2M6 Canada

Senecare Enterprises, Inc. 800-442-4577
350 Central Ave Ste A, Bohemia, NY 11716
Senepad Lotion Pad provides low-friction technology that protects skin against the effects of friction and shear. The pre-lubricated facing sheet moves with the patient, diminishing friction and shear damage. Breathable Lotion Pad designed for use with air loss specialty beds.

Skil-Care Corp. 800-431-2972
29 Wells Ave, Yonkers, NY 10701

Snugfleece International Inc. 800-824-1177
2740 Pole Line Rd, Pocatello, ID 83201
Snugfleece wool mattress covers.

Sunrise Medical Hhg Inc 303-218-4505
2842 N Business Park Ave, Fresno, CA 93727

Thompson Medical Specialties 800-777-4949
3404 Library Ln, Saint Louis Park, MN 55426

Truform Orthotics & Prosthetics 800-888-0458
3960 Rosslyn Dr, Cincinnati, OH 45209

Viscolas, Inc. 800-548-2694
8801 Consolidated Dr, Soddy Daisy, TN 37379
Heel spur cushion.

Warsaw Orthopedic, Inc. 901-396-3133
2500 Silveus Xing, Warsaw, IN 46582
Various types of pads and heel and elbow protectors.

Wristies, Inc. 800-811-8290
650 Suffolk St # G-5, Lowell, MA 01854

Zimmer Holdings, Inc. 800-613-6131
1800 W Center St, PO Box 708, Warsaw, IN 46580

3m Company 651-733-4365
601 22nd Ave S, Brookings, SD 57006

PROTECTOR, SURGICAL INSTRUMENT *(Surgery) 79UEM*

Abbott Associates 203-878-2370
620 West Ave, Milford, CT 06461
Point Protectors, for instrument protection, PVC.

Fortrad Eye Instruments Corp. 973-543-2371
8 Franklin Rd, Mendham, NJ 07945

Key Surgical, Inc. 800-541-7995
8101 Wallace Rd Ste 100, Eden Prairie, MN 55344
Colored, clear, and tinted protectors for instruments including osteotomes, skin hooks, key elevators, chisels, and gouges. Clamp covers - silicone and fabric instrument covers reduce trauma while providing a positive grip.

Micromedics 800-624-5662
1270 Eagan Industrial Rd, Saint Paul, MN 55121
Instru-Safe systems keep surgical instruments organized in sets and protect the instruments during transportation, storage, and sterile processing...saving time in surgery and reducing instrument damage.

Scanlan International, Inc. 800-328-9458
1 Scanlan Plz, Saint Paul, MN 55107
TIP-GUARD instrument protectors.

PROTECTOR, SURGICAL INSTRUMENT *(cont'd)*

Sterion, Incorporated 800-328-7958
13828 Lincoln St NE, Ham Lake, MN 55304
Surgical instrument guards. Standard,vented,innervent, retractor, and weitlaner for all instruments including endoscopic, M.I.S., ENT, osteotomes.

PROTECTOR, TRANSDUCER, DIALYSIS *(Gastro/Urology) 78FIB*

Clinical Pharmacies, Inc. 800-669-6973
21622 Surveyor Cir # 8-C, Huntington Beach, CA 92646
Dialysis transducer filter (protector).

Millipore Corporation 800-MILLIPORE
80 Ashby Rd, Bedford, MA 01730
DUALEX transducer protector: prevents fluids from damaging transducer.

Molded Products Inc. 800-435-8957
1112 Chatburn Ave, Harlan, IA 51537
Protector, transducer, dialysis.

Terumo Cardiovascular Systems (Tcvs) 800-283-7866
28 Howe St, Ashland, MA 01721
Transducer protector.

PROTECTOR, WOUND, PLASTIC *(Gastro/Urology) 78EYF*

Biomet Microfixation Inc. 800-874-7711
1520 Tradeport Dr, Jacksonville, FL 32218
Marchac dura protector.

Genesis Manufacturing, Inc. 317-485-7887
720 E Broadway St, Fortville, IN 46040
Contract Radio-Frequency (RF) Welding. From development to manufacturing and packaging.

National Home Products Ltd. 416-661-2770
188 Limestone Crescent, Downsview, ONT M3J 2S4 Canada
Plastic adhesive bandage

PROTEINS, AMYLOID AND PRECURSOR *(Immunology) 82MME*

United Biotech, Inc. 650-961-2910
211 S Whisman Rd Ste E, Mountain View, CA 94041
ELISA detecting Protein S.

PROTHROMBIN TIME *(Hematology) 81GJS*

Abbott Point Of Care Inc. 609-443-9300
104 Windsor Center Dr, East Windsor, NJ 08520
Prothrombin tome test.

Bio/Data Corp. 215-441-4000
155 Gibraltar Rd, Horsham, PA 19044
Thromboplastin reagent.

Clinical Data Inc 800-937-5449
1 Gateway Ctr Ste 702, Newton, MA 02458
Fibron-1 optokinetic coagulation analyzer.

Dade Behring, Inc. 800-948-3233
1717 Deerfield Rd, Deerfield, IL 60015

Fisher Diagnostics 877-722-4366
11515 Vanstory Dr Ste 125, Huntersville, NC 28078

Helena Laboratories 409-842-3714
PO Box 752, Beaumont, TX 77704

Hemosense, Inc. 877-436-6444
651 River Oaks Pkwy, San Jose, CA 95134

International Technidyne Corp. 800-631-5945
23 Nevsky St, Edison, NJ 08820

International Technidyne Corporation 732-548-5700
8 Olsen Ave, Edison, NJ 08820
Pt test cuvette.

R2 Diagnostics, Inc. 574-288-4377
1801 Commerce Dr, South Bend, IN 46628
Pt-prothrombin time reagent.

Wortham Laboratories Inc 423-296-0090
6340 Bonny Oaks Dr, Chattanooga, TN 37416
Prothrombin time test.

PROTOPORPHYRIN ZINC METHOD, FLUOROMETRIC, LEAD *(Toxicology) 91DNX*

Aviv Biomedical, Inc. 732-370-1300
750 Vassar Ave, Lakewood, NJ 08701
Iron-deficiency screening.

PROTOPORPHYRIN, FLUOROMETRIC, LEAD
(Toxicology) 91DMK

Aviv Biomedical, Inc. 732-370-1300
750 Vassar Ave, Lakewood, NJ 08701
Lead-poisoning screening.

PROTRACTOR *(Orthopedics) 87HTH*

Arthrex, Inc. 239-643-5553
1370 Creekside Blvd, Naples, FL 34108
Protractor for clinical use.

Biomet, Inc. 574-267-6639
56 E Bell Dr, PO Box 587, Warsaw, IN 46582
Pocket protractor.

Medmetric Corp. 800-995-6066
7542 Trade St, San Diego, CA 92121
PCL Pro assists in the measurement of the disrupted PCL $810.00

Zimmer Holdings, Inc. 800-613-6131
1800 W Center St, PO Box 708, Warsaw, IN 46580

Zimmer Trabecular Metal Technology 800-613-6131
10 Pomeroy Rd, Parsippany, NJ 07054
Extramededullary tibial alignment guide.

PUBLIC ADDRESS SYSTEM *(General) 80TDL*

Signalcom Systems, Inc. 650-692-1056
1499 Bayshore Hwy Ste 134, Burlingame, CA 94010
Silent Message Indicator System.

PULSE GENERATOR, PACEMAKER, IMPLANTABLE, WITH CARDIAC RESYNCHRONIZATION *(Cardiovascular) 74NKE*

Medtronic, Inc. 800-633-8766
710 Medtronic Pkwy, Minneapolis, MN 55432
Multiple

PUMP, ABORTION UNIT, VACUUM *(Obstetrics/Gyn) 85HGF*

Rocket Medical Plc. 800-707-7625
150 Recreation Park Dr Ste 3, Hingham, MA 02043

PUMP, ABORTION, VACUUM, CENTRAL SYSTEM
(Obstetrics/Gyn) 85HHI

Allied Healthcare Products, Inc. 800-444-3954
1720 Sublette Ave, Saint Louis, MO 63110

PUMP, AIR, NON-MANUAL, ENDOSCOPIC
(Gastro/Urology) 78FEQ

Frantz Medical Development Ltd. 440-255-1155
7740 Metric Dr, Mentor, OH 44060
Endoscopy pumps and tubing sets.

Karl Storz Endoscopy-America Inc. 800-421-0837
600 Corporate Pointe, Culver City, CA 90230

Sensidyne, Inc. 800-451-9444
16333 Bay Vista Dr, Clearwater, FL 33760

PUMP, ALTERNATING PRESSURE PAD *(General) 80UBG*

American Bantex Corp. 800-633-4839
1815 Rollins Rd, Burlingame, CA 94010

Gaymar Industries, Inc. 800-828-7341
10 Centre Dr, Orchard Park, NY 14127
PILLO-PUMP, AIR FLO PLUS systems provide alternating pressure therapy for patients, with or without low air loss.

Huntleigh Healthcare Llc. 800-223-1218
40 Christopher Way, Eatontown, NJ 07724
$385.00 for ventilated ALPHACARE model, $285.00 for standard model and $198.00 for homecare model.

Nova Health Systems, Inc. 800-225-NOVA
1001 Broad St, Utica, NY 13501

Smith & Nephew, Inc. 800-876-1261
970 Lake Carillon Dr Ste 110, Saint Petersburg, FL 33716
NEGATIVE PRESSURE WOUND THERAPY POWERED SUCTION PUMP - Renasys -F Foam Dressing Kit, Renasys EZ, Modification to VersaTile 1 Wound V, Versatile 1 EZcare Wound Vacuum Sys, Versatil 1 Wound Vacuum System, BlueSky Vista Wound Vacuum System, Renasys Go Negative Pressure

Tuffcare 800-367-6160
3999 E La Palma Ave, Anaheim, CA 92807

PUMP, ASPIRATION, PORTABLE *(Anesthesiology) 73BTA*

Allied Healthcare Products, Inc. 800-444-3954
1720 Sublette Ave, Saint Louis, MO 63110

Ambu A/S 457-225-2210
6740 Baymeadow Dr, Glen Burnie, MD 21060
Suction pump/aspirator.

PUMP, ASPIRATION, PORTABLE *(cont'd)*

Ambu, Inc. 800-262-8462
6740 Baymeadow Dr, Glen Burnie, MD 21060
AMBU PPS compact for pharyngeal and tracheal suction.

Blue Sky Medical Group Incorporated 727-392-1261
5924 Balfour Ct Ste 102, Carlsbad, CA 92008
Wound vacuum.

Brailsford & Co., Inc. 603-588-2880
15 Elm Ave, Antrim, NH 03440
Miniature brushless DC diaphragm air pumps. No RFI filtering necessary. Can be mounted in any position.

Byron Medical 800-777-3434
602 W Rillito St, Tucson, AZ 85705
PSI-TEC.

Contemporary Products, Inc. 800-424-2444
530 Riverside Industrial Pkwy, Portland, ME 04103
Oilless aspirator model 6260, 6260A, or 6261. Heavy-duty aspirator that has adjustable vacuum ranges up to 22 in. of mercury (558 mm).

Covidien Lp 508-261-8000
15 Hampshire St, Mansfield, MA 02048

Encompas Unlimited, Inc. 800-825-7701
PO Box 516, Tallevast, FL 34270
$788 - $1150 for suction pump for all endoscopic applications, 2 sizes.

Fibra-Sonics, A Division Of Misonix, Inc. 631-694-9555
1938 New Hwy, Farmingdale, NY 11735
Aspirator, small or minute volume.

George Tiemann & Co. 800-843-6266
25 Plant Ave, Hauppauge, NY 11788

Gi Supply 800-451-5797
200 Grandview Ave, Camp Hill, PA 17011
Portable aspiration pump for paracentesis.

Health Care Logistics, Inc. 800-848-1633
450 Town St, PO Box 25, Circleville, OH 43113
Aspiration pump/portable suction unit.

Impact Instrumentation, Inc. 800-969-0750
27 Fairfield Pl, West Caldwell, NJ 07006
Models 305 and 305 GR, rechargeable battery-powered portable aspirators for oral, nasal, and tracheal suction. Vacuum from 0 to 550 mm Hg, free airflow exceeds 30 liters per minute. Diaphragm pump. Includes collection canister, rinse bottle, suction tips, Y-fitting catheters and tubing. Aeromedical versions available $575.00 to 675.00. Also available VAC-PACK and VAC-PAK GR, soft case, rechargeable battery-powered portable aspirators for oral, nasal, and tracheal suction. Vacuum from 0 to 550 mm Hg, free airflow exceeds 30 liters per minute. Diaphragm pump. Includes collection canister, rinse bottle, suction tips, Y-fitting catheters and tubing, $575.00 ot 675.00. Also available Models 320 and 320 GR ultra-lite series, rechargeable battery-powered portable aspirators for oral, nasal, and tracheal suction. Vacuum from 0 to 550 mm Hg, free airflow exceeds 30 liters per minute. Hard case, disposable collection canister. Diaphragm pump. Weighs approximately 5 lbs. Aeromedical versions available $540.00 to 715.00. Model 321 and 321 GR ultra-lite Series rechargeable battery-powered portable aspirators for oral, nasal, and tracheal suction. Vacuum from 0 to 550 mm Hg free airflow exceeds 30 liters per minute. Soft case, disposable collection canister, convertible carrying handle/shoulder strap. Diaphragm pump. Weighs approximately 5-lbs. Aeromedical versions available. $540.00to 815.00.

Industrial & Medical Design, Inc. 818-642-7501
4741 Deseret Dr, Woodland Hills, CA 91364
Flow and vacuum control modes. Low aspiration rate in stand-by automatically increases in presence of liquid and switches back to low rate when liquid extracted. No manual control during surgical procedure required.

Innovative Therapies, Inc. 866-484-6798
8 Metropolitan Ct Ste 2, Darnestown, MD 20878
Portable suction pump with sterile + non-sterile dressings.

Jedmed Instruments Co. 314-845-3770
5416 Jedmed Ct, Saint Louis, MO 63129

Medco Mfg. 281-379-3100
8319 Thora Ln Hngr A1, Spring, TX 77379
Aspirator.

PUMP, ASPIRATION, PORTABLE *(cont'd)*

Ohio Medical Corp. 800-662-5822
1111 Lakeside Dr, Gurnee, IL 60031
INSTAVAC II; tabletop aspirator for crash carts, scoping procedures, O.R. backup, clinics, etc.; high vacuum and flow. CARE-E-VAC tabletop AC powered economy aspirator for homecare and alternate care use; CARE-E-VAC AC, tabletop aspirator for crash cart or emergency, use AC and DC powered. TOTE-L-VAC DC powered aspirator for emergency or alternate care use.

Pentax Medical Company 800-431-5880
102 Chestnut Ridge Rd, Montvale, NJ 07645
Suction pumps with collection bottles. Suction pump accessories include cannisters, cannister lids, disposable bags, and cannister accessories. Call for quote.

Precision Medical, Inc. 800-272-7285
300 Held Dr, Northampton, PA 18067

Tennessee Medical Equipment, Inc. 731-635-2119
4637 Highway 19 E, Ripley, TN 38063
Various.

Thomas Products Division 920-457-4891
3524 Washington Ave, Sheboygan, WI 53081

Ussc Puerto Rico, Inc. 203-845-1000
Building 911-67, Sabanetas Industrial Park, Ponce, PR 00731
Aspiration pump.

Vital Concepts, Inc. 800-984-2300
4334 Brockton Dr SE Ste F, Grand Rapids, MI 49512
AC/DC powered irrigation and aspiration pumps for suction and irrigation during surgery. Capable of delivering up to 800Hg.

PUMP, BLOOD, CARDIOPULMONARY BYPASS, NON-ROLLER TYPE *(Cardiovascular) 74KFM*

Abiomed, Inc. 800-422-8666
22 Cherry Hill Dr, Danvers, MA 01923
Impella 2.5; MPC and Power Supply; Quick Set-up Kit

Cardiac Assist, Inc. 412-963-7770
240 Alpha Dr, Pittsburgh, PA 15238
Centrifugal blood pump.

Cardiovention, Inc. 408-873-3400
19200 Stevens Creek Blvd Ste 200, Cupertino, CA 95014
Nonroller-type blood pump.

International Biophysics Corp. 512-326-3244
2101 E Saint Elmo Rd Ste 275, Austin, TX 78744
Centrifugal blood pump.

Terumo Cardiovascular Systems (Tcvs) 800-283-7866
125 Blue Ball Rd, Elkton, MD 21921
Centrifugal pump.

Terumo Cardiovascular Systems (Tcvs) 800-283-7866
28 Howe St, Ashland, MA 01721
Centrifugal pump.

Terumo Cardiovascular Systems, Corp 800-521-2818
6200 Jackson Rd, Ann Arbor, MI 48103
Centrifugal pump system: disposable pump head, drive, monitor & mount accessories with ultrasonic flow meter.

PUMP, BLOOD, CARDIOPULMONARY BYPASS, ROLLER TYPE
(Cardiovascular) 74DWB

Medtronic, Inc. 800-633-8766
710 Medtronic Pkwy, Minneapolis, MN 55432
BIOPLUS.

Sorin Group Usa 800-289-5759
14401 W 65th Way, Arvada, CO 80004

Terumo Cardiovascular Systems, Corp 800-521-2818
6200 Jackson Rd, Ann Arbor, MI 48103

PUMP, BLOOD, EXTRA-LUMINAL *(Gastro/Urology) 78FIR*

Apheresis Technologies, Inc. 800-749-9284
PO Box 2081, Palm Harbor, FL 34682
Peristaltic plasma pump.

PUMP, BLOOD, HEMODIALYSIS UNIT *(Gastro/Urology) 78QZW*

Baxter Healthcare Corporation, Renal 888-229-0001
1620 S Waukegan Rd, Waukegan, IL 60085
BM11 blood pump and tubing.

Terumo Cardiovascular Systems, Corp 800-521-2818
6200 Jackson Rd, Ann Arbor, MI 48103

Whitehall Manufacturing 800-782-7706
15125 Proctor Ave, City Of Industry, CA 91746
Dialysis supply boxes.

PUMP, BREAST, NON-POWERED *(Obstetrics/Gyn) 85HGY*

Genesis Industries/Maternal Concepts 800-310-5817
130 S Public St, Elmwood, WI 54740
EVERT-IT nipple enhancer is used in assisting the correction of inverted or flattened nipples of the post-portum lactating mother by everting the nipple.

Genesis Instruments, Inc. 715-639-9209
200 Main St., Elmwood, WI 54740
Nipple everter.

Hospira 800-441-4100
268 E 4th St, Ashland, OH 44805

Medela, Inc. 800-435-8316
1101 Corporate Dr, McHenry, IL 60050
MANUALECTRIC - can be used as a manual unit and in connection with electric pump. HARMONY Manual Breastpump - single occasional-use pump.

PUMP, BREAST, POWERED *(Obstetrics/Gyn) 85HGX*

Allied Healthcare Products, Inc. 800-444-3954
1720 Sublette Ave, Saint Louis, MO 63110

Bailey Medical Engineering 805-528-5781
2216 Sunset Dr, Los Osos, CA 93402
Breast pump.

Gerber Products Co. 800-430-0150
120 N Commercial St Fl 4, Neenah, WI 54956

Limerick Incorporate 818-566-3060
2150 N Glenoaks Blvd, Burbank, CA 91504
Portable electric breast pump.

Medela, Inc. 800-435-8316
1101 Corporate Dr, McHenry, IL 60050
SYMPHONY w/2-Phase Expression Technology, a hospital grade double pump utilizing individual sterile and non-sterile kits. Model 015 CLASSIC with automatic operating mode, 110-240 mm Hg suction range, single patient reusable breast shields, weighs 21 lbs. Model 016S LACTINA ELECTRIC SELECT (7 lbs.) with rechargeable battery or vehicle use options and adjustable pumping speed. SINGLE DELUXE handheld unit with battery or manual or electric operation. PUMP IN STYLE provides double pumping professional performance in a discreet carrying/cooler bag. SWING provides single pumping, daily use.

Whittlestone, Inc. 877-608-6455
840 Eubanks Dr, Vacaville, CA 95688
Breast pump.

PUMP, COUNTERPULSATING, EXTERNAL
(Cardiovascular) 74DRN

Cardiomedics, Inc. 888-849-0200
18872 Bardeen Ave, Irvine, CA 92612
External Counterpulsation Device

Ecp Health, Inc. 817-881-4499
8416 Prairie Rose Ln, Fort Worth, TX 76123
External counter-pulsation device.

Nicore Equipment & Leasing, Inc. 813-901-0019
4897 W Waters Ave Ste J, Tampa, FL 33634
Counterpulastion device.

Vasomedical Inc. 800-455-3327
180 Linden Ave, Westbury, NY 11590

PUMP, DRUG ADMINISTRATION, CLOSED LOOP
(General) 80MQT

B. Braun Oem Division, B. Braun Medical Inc. 866-8-BBRAUN
824 12th Ave, Bethlehem, PA 18018

PUMP, EXTRACORPOREAL PERFUSION *(Cardiovascular) 74RNE*

Sorin Group Usa 800-289-5759
14401 W 65th Way, Arvada, CO 80004

Terumo Cardiovascular Systems, Corp 800-521-2818
6200 Jackson Rd, Ann Arbor, MI 48103
Pulsatile flow option.

PUMP, FOOD (ENTERAL FEEDING) *(General) 80RNF*

Abbott Laboratories 800-624-7677
1033 Kingsmill Pkwy, Columbus, OH 43229
Three models: FLEXIFLO III, computer controlled, flow rate of 1ml to 300ml/hr in 1-ml increments. Digital display of flow rate and volume/dose fed and to be fed. Alarms for occlusion/empty, low battery, cover open and dose complete, and with nurse call feature. COMPANION pump, lightweight, portable, volumetric pump with unique pump-set cassette; 300ml/hr in 1-ml increments, volume fed, easy to set up, no drop sensing. May be used in ambulatory mode without IV pole. QUANTUM pump, volumetric pump with cassette; 300ml/hr in 1ml increments, volume fed, close, no drop sensing, automatic set priming, protection against overdelivery. Optional two bag system clinically reduces tube clogging.

Cole-Parmer Instrument Inc. 800-323-4340
625 E Bunker Ct, Vernon Hills, IL 60061
For laboratory use only.

Covidien Lp 508-261-8000
15 Hampshire St, Mansfield, MA 02048
KANGAROO 22, KANGAROO 330 portable enteral feeding pumps, with handle, wide range of flow rates.

Frantz Medical Development Ltd. 440-255-1155
7740 Metric Dr, Mentor, OH 44060

Welcon, Inc. 800-877-0923
7409 Pebble Dr, Fort Worth, TX 76118
RATESAVER 3 enteral feeding pump is a rotary peristaltic device for use when accurate volumetric delivery of enteral tube feeding formulas is required. Provides set detection and set security features. PLAIN JANE Home Health Care enteral feeding pump is a rotary peristaltic device for use when accurate volumetric delivery of enteral feeding formula is required.

PUMP, INDUSTRIAL *(General) 80WSO*

Baxa Corporation 800-567-2292
9540 S Maroon Circle, Suite 400, Englewood, CO 80112
Rapid-Fill Automated Syringe Filler for sterile syringe batch filling, capping, and labeling.

Smiths Medical Asd, Inc. 800-848-1757
6250 Shier Rings Rd, Dublin, OH 43016
TRILOGY and KIDS large volume pumps.

PUMP, INFLATOR *(General) 80JOI*

Alimed, Inc. 800-225-2610
297 High St, Dedham, MA 02026

Brailsford & Co., Inc. 603-588-2880
15 Elm Ave, Antrim, NH 03440
Brushless D.C.

Essential Medical Supply, Inc. 800-826-8423
6420 Hazeltine National Dr, Orlando, FL 32822
ENDURANCE D9000, D8000.

Halkey-Roberts Corp. 800-303-4384
2700 Halkey Roberts Pl N, Saint Petersburg, FL 33716
Manually operated inflation and suction pumps, including blood-pressure pumps.

PUMP, INFUSION *(General) 80FRN*

Abbott Laboratories 800-223-2064
100 Abbott Park Rd, Abbott Park, IL 60064
Volumetric pump features selection dial that simplifies the user interface and a mode button for switching from primary to secondary fluid administration.

Acist Medical Systems, Inc. 888-667-6648
7905 Fuller Rd, Eden Prairie, MN 55344
Infusion pump.

Aiv, Inc. (Formerly American Iv) 800-990-2911
7485 Shipley Ave, Harmans, MD 21077
Specialized repair services for leading infusion pumps. AC Adapters, batteries, power cords and other service parts also available for sale.

Altron, Inc. 763-427-7735
6700 Bunker Lake Blvd NW, Ramsey, MN 55303
ENTERAL -

Arndorfer Medical Specialties 414-425-1661
5656 Grove Ter, Greendale, WI 53129
The pneumo-hydraulic capillary infusion system.

Arthrex, Inc. 239-643-5553
1370 Creekside Blvd, Naples, FL 34108
Arthroscopy pump and various types of tubing (sterile).

PUMP, INFUSION *(cont'd)*

Axiom Medical, Inc. 800-221-8569
19320 Van Ness Ave, Torrance, CA 90501
Multipurpose wound drain, multilumen drain allowing lavage and topical applications while continuing evacuation. Relocation/repositioning made easy. Multiple sizes.

B. Braun Oem Division, B. Braun Medical Inc. 866-8-BBRAUN
824 12th Ave, Bethlehem, PA 18018

Basi (Bioanalytical Systems, Inc.) 800-845-4246
2701 Kent Ave, West Lafayette, IN 47906
Syringe pump for microfilter/min perfusions. For use with research animals only-- not for for humans.

Baxa Corporation 800-567-2292
9540 S Maroon Circle, Suite 400, Englewood, CO 80112
MICRO FUSE, Dual Rate Infuser: 13-oz, portable, battery-operated syringe infuser with two selectable rates of flow. Custom infusers are available.; InFuse T10

Baxter Healthcare Corporation 847-473-6141
900 Corporate Grove Dr, Buffalo Grove, IL 60089
Various infusion pumps.

Baxter Healthcare Corporporation, Alternate Care And Channel Team 888-229-0001
25212 W Il Route 120, Round Lake, IL 60073
APII. INFUSO.R. INTERMATE system. INFUS.O.R.

Belmont Instrument Corp. 866-663-0212
780 Boston Rd, Billerica, MA 01821
Infusion pump with Warmer FMS 2000 fluid-management system for rapid infusion of warmed fluid, including blood products, up to 750 ml/min, with monitoring for air bubbles, line pressure, temperature, and volume infused.

Bionica, Inc. 916-643-2222
5112 Bailey Loop, McClellan, CA 95652
Ambulatory infusion pump.

Block Medical De Mexico S.A. De C.V. 949-206-2700
La Mesa Parque Industrial, Paseo Reforma S/n, Fracc. Tijuana, Bc Mexico
Infusion pump

Braemar, Inc. 800-328-2719
1285 Corporate Center Dr Ste 150, Eagan, MN 55121

Breg, Inc., An Orthofix Company 800-897-BREG
2611 Commerce Way, Vista, CA 92081
Multi-infusion.

Byron Medical 800-777-3434
602 W Rillito St, Tucson, AZ 85705
Infiltration system - automatic and syringe delivery. AUTOFUSE 10c multiple injection system. Also available, BIG BAG 3000 and PSI-TEC syringe pump.

Calibra Medical Inc. 650-298-4710
220 Saginaw Dr, Redwood City, CA 94063
Finesse Insulin Delivery System

Cmt, Inc. 800-659-9140
PO Box 297, Hamilton, MA 01936
Design and development of fluid management systems.

Curlin Medical, Inc. 714-893-2200
15751 Graham St, Huntington Beach, CA 92649
Infusion pump.

Delphi Medical Systems Colorado Corp. 248-813-6819
4300 Rd. 18, Longmont, CO 80504
Infusion pump and sterile iv administration sets.

Dma Med-Chem Corporation 800-362-1833
49 Watermill Ln, Great Neck, NY 11021

Ethox International 800-521-1022
251 Seneca St, Buffalo, NY 14204
Mechanical infusion pump.

Excelsior Medical Corp. 732-776-7525
1933 Heck Ave, Neptune, NJ 07753
Syringe pump.

Graymills Corp. 800-478-8673
3705 N Lincoln Ave, Chicago, IL 60613
Centrifuge and Diaphragm Pumps.

Haemonetics Corp. 781-848-7100
400 Wood Rd, P.O.Box 9114, Braintree, MA 02184
Blood warmer and pump.

PUMP, INFUSION *(cont'd)*

Harmac Medical Products, Inc. 716-897-4500
2201 Bailey Ave, Buffalo, NY 14211
OEM and private-labeled infusion bags and administration sets. Contract manufacturer of custom infusion disposables.

Harvard Apparatus, Inc. 800-272-2775
84 October Hill Rd, Holliston, MA 01746
Microprocessor controlled.

Hospira Inc. 877-946-7747
275 N Field Dr, Lake Forest, IL 60045
Multiple

Hospira, Inc. 877-946-7747
755 Jarvis Dr, Morgan Hill, CA 95037

Icu Medical (Ut), Inc 949-366-2183
4455 Atherton Dr, Salt Lake City, UT 84123
Various types of infusion pumps (non-sterile).

International Medication Systems, Ltd. 800-423-4136
1886 Santa Anita Ave, South El Monte, CA 91733
Sterile empty pca syringe.

Iradimed Corporation 407-677-8022
7457 Aloma Ave Ste 201, Winter Park, FL 32792
Infusion pump and accessories.

Kelsar, S.A. 508-261-8000
Blvd. Insurgentes, Libriamento a La, Tijuana 22450 Mexico
Enteral feeding pumps and accessories

Kmi Kolster Methods, Inc. 909-737-5476
3185 Palisades Dr, Corona, CA 92880
Infusion pump.

Medical Technology Products, Inc. 800-314-0210
2221 5th Ave Ste 16, Ronkonkoma, NY 11779
MTP 1001 $2,375 for general use peristaltic infusion pump.

Mediq/Prn 800-222-4776
1 Mediq Plaza, Pennsauken, NJ 08110

Medtronic Minimed 800-933-3322
18000 Devonshire St, Northridge, CA 91325

Mettler Electronics Corp. 800-854-9305
1333 S Claudina St, Anaheim, CA 92805
SILBERG TISSUE PREPARATION SYSTEM: consists of a peristaltic pump to infuse saline subcutaneously and disperse the saline into deeper tissues using ultrasound, $15,000.

Milestone Scientific Inc. 800-862-1125
45 Knightsbridge Rd, Piscataway, NJ 08854
COMPUFLO

Milestone Scientific Inc. 800-862-1125
220 S Orange Ave, Livingston, NJ 07039
COMPUFLO

Mtm Health Products Ltd. 800-263-8253
2349 Fairview St., Burlington, ONT L7R 2E3 Canada
IV-PUSH spring operated, constant pressure infusor with variable flow from 10ml per hour to 120ml per minute.

Mui Scientific 800-303-6611
145 Traders Blvd. E., Unit 34, Mississauga, ONT L4Z 3L3 Canada
Pneumohydraulic capillary infusion system for gastro-intestinal manometric studies. 8 Channel Electric US $4,050.00. 8 Channel Nitrogen US $3,450.00.

Omni Medical Supply Inc. 800-860-6664
4153 Pioneer Dr, Commerce Township, MI 48390
Rental of equipment.

Razel Scientific Instruments, Inc. 877-324-9914
PO Box 111, Saint Albans, VT 05478
$207.00 for pole mounted drug pump; $444.00 for ICU pump; also, oxytocin flow rate chart optional.

Sigma International, Llc. 800-356-3454
711 Park Ave, Medina, NY 14103
SIGMA 6000+, $2,995.00 volumetric pump, 0.1-999 ml/hr flow rate, linear peristaltic pump mechanism. Uses standard gravity IV sets. SIGMA 8000 Plus Infusion Pump - Linear peristaltic infusion pump utilizing standard gravity IV set. Set-based anti-free flow protection. 0.1 - 999 ml/hr flow rates, dose calculations and programs. Dual Channel available. EZ PUMP, Ambulatory Infusion Pump, six infusion modes in one device - PCA, Epidural, Continuous, Intermittent, Circadian and TPN. Simple to use. Flow rate range of .01 to 500 ml/hr. Light weight - only 10.2 oz. Dual channel available NOW. MULTI-DOSER, Syringe Delivery System, delivers multiple doses from a single 60cc BD or Monoject syringe. Most cost effective and time saving system for antibiotic drug delivery. No electronics. Simple to use in hospitals and homecare.

PUMP, INFUSION *(cont'd)*

Smisson-Cartledge Biomedical 1-866-944-9992
487 Cherry St, Third Street Tower, Macon, GA 31201
SMISSON-CARTLEDGE TIS-120; ThermaCor 1200; TIS-1200 Thermal Infusion System

Smith & Nephew Inc., Endoscopy Div. 978-749-1000
76 S Meridian Ave, Oklahoma City, OK 73107
Infusion pump and accessories.

Specialty Manufacturing Co., The 651-653-0599
5858 Centerville Rd, Saint Paul, MN 55127
Peristaltic.

Spectrum Laboratories, Inc. 800-634-3300
18617 S Broadwick St, Rancho Dominguez, CA 90220
Peristaltic pumps: routine lab use and chromatography applications.

Stryker Puerto Rico, Ltd. 939-307-2500
Hwy. 3, Km. 131.2, Las Guasimas Ind. Park, Arroyo, PR 00714
Infusion pump.

Terumo Cardiovascular Systems, Corp 800-521-2818
6200 Jackson Rd, Ann Arbor, MI 48103

Universal Medical Technologies 415-924-1133
15720 N Greenway Hayden Loop Ste 8, Scottsdale, AZ 85260
Ambulatory infusion pump.

Valeritas, Llc 508-845-1177
800 Boston Tpke, Shrewsbury, MA 01545
Infusion pump.

Walkmed Infusion Llc 303-420-9569
4080 Youngfield St, Wheat Ridge, CO 80033
Various models of infusion pumps.

Wells Johnson Co. 800-528-1597
8000 S Kolb Rd, Tucson, AZ 85756

3m Co. 888-364-3577
3M Center, Saint Paul, MN 55144

PUMP, INFUSION, AMBULATORY *(General) 80VEZ*

Abbott Laboratories 800-624-7677
1033 Kingsmill Pkwy, Columbus, OH 43229

Aiv, Inc. (Formerly American Iv) 800-990-2911
7485 Shipley Ave, Harmans, MD 21077
Specialized repair services for leading ambulatory infusion pumps.

Armstrong Medical Industries, Inc. 800-323-4220
575 Knightsbridge Pkwy, Lincolnshire, IL 60069

Baxter Healthcare Corporporation, Alternate Care And Channel Team 888-229-0001
25212 W Il Route 120, Round Lake, IL 60073
INTERMATE SYSTEM. PCA. INFUSOR.

Harmac Medical Products, Inc. 716-897-4500
2201 Bailey Ave, Buffalo, NY 14211
OEM and private-labeled infusion and medication bags and sets. Contract manufacturer of custom infusion disposables.

Hospira, Inc 877-946-7747
13520 Evening Creek Dr N Ste 200, San Diego, CA 92128
$3,495 for ambulatory TPNI pump provider one plus with taper functions, $3,495 for ambulatory PCA pump with remote bolus and lockbox. Also Multi-Therapy Ambulatory IV infusion Pump.

I-Flow Corporation 800-448-3569
20202 Windrow Dr, Lake Forest, CA 92630
VIVUS 4000 & VIVUS 4000/2 Infusion pumps, ambulatory multi-channel infusion systems.

Medical Technology Products, Inc. 800-314-0210
2221 5th Ave Ste 16, Ronkonkoma, NY 11779
MTP 1001 $2,375 for general use or transport peristaltic infusion pump.

Mps Acacia 800-486-6677
785 Challenger St, Brea, CA 92821

Smiths Medical Asd, Inc. 800-433-5832
1265 Grey Fox Rd, Saint Paul, MN 55112
CADD-LEGACY 1 ambulatory infusion pump for chemotherapy, CADD-LEGACY PLUS ambulatory infusion pump for antibiotic therapy, CADD-LEGACY PCA infusion ambulatory pump for pain management, and CADD-TPN ambulatory infusion system for nutritional therapy. CADD-PRIZM VIP (Variable Infusion Profile) multi-therapy pump for continuous, intermittent, PCA and TPN delivery.

Smiths Medical Asd, Inc. 800-848-1757
6250 Shier Rings Rd, Dublin, OH 43016
WALKMED PCA pumps.

PUMP, INFUSION, AMBULATORY *(cont'd)*

Sorenson Medical Product, Inc. 877-352-1888
1375 W 8040 S, West Jordan, UT 84088
The ambIT family of infusion products provides the healthcare profession with a low cost, therapy specific ambulatory infusion pumps. A New Standard In Pain Management The innovative ambIT PCA (Patient Controlled Analgesia) infusion pump provides a simple yet sophisticated solution for all types of post-operative local pain management as well as traditional IV delivery of PCA narcotics and regional nerve blocks. A New Standard In Local Pain Management The innovative ambIT Intermittent infusion pump provides a simple, sophisticated solution for intermittent dose infusions. All, with the same type of features and accuracy normally found on more expensive electronic ambulatory pumps. The innovative ambIT Continuous infusion pump provides a simple, sophisticated solution for continuous rate infusions. All, with the same type of features and accuracy normally found on more expensive electronic ambulatory pumps.

PUMP, INFUSION, ELASTOMERIC *(General) 80MEB*

Advanced Infusion, Inc. 909-305-9857
466 W Arrow Hwy Ste H, San Dimas, CA 91773
Elastomeric infusion pump.

Apex Medical Technologies, Inc. 800-345-3208
10064 Mesa Ridge Ct Ste 202, San Diego, CA 92121
Solace Post-Operative Pain Relief Infusion System

Baxter Healthcare Corporation, Medication Delivery 949-851-9066
17511 Armstrong Ave, Irvine, CA 92614
Infusor, elastomeric infusion pump.

Biomet, Inc. 574-267-6639
56 E Bell Dr, PO Box 587, Warsaw, IN 46582
Various types of infusion pumps.

Block Medical De Mexico S.A. De C.V. 949-206-2700
La Mesa Parque Industrial, Paseo Reforma S/n, Fracc. Tijuana, Bc Mexico
Various

Breg, Inc., An Orthofix Company 800-897-BREG
2611 Commerce Way, Vista, CA 92081
Pain care 2000.

Curlin Medical, Inc. 714-893-2200
15751 Graham St, Huntington Beach, CA 92649
Various models of infusion pumps.

Symbios Medical Products, Llc 317-225-4447
7301 Georgetown Rd Ste 150, Indianapolis, IN 46268
Disposable infusion pump kit.

Tandem Medical, Inc. 760-943-0100
535 Encinitas Blvd Ste 109, Encinitas, CA 92024
Innsion pump, various sterile disposables and non-sterile non-disposables.

Walkmed Infusion Llc 303-420-9569
4080 Youngfield St, Wheat Ridge, CO 80033
Disposable ambulatory infuser.

PUMP, INFUSION, IMPLANTABLE, GENERAL *(General) 80LKK*

Arrow International, Inc. 800-523-8446
2400 Bernville Rd, Reading, PA 19605

Dma Med-Chem Corporation 800-362-1833
49 Watermill Ln, Great Neck, NY 11021

Medtronic Neuromodulation 612-514-4000
800 53rd Ave NE, Minneapolis, MN 55421
Implantable infusion system.

Medtronic Puerto Rico Operations Co., Juncos 763-514-4000
Road 31, Km. 24, Hm 4, Ceiba Norte Industrial Park, Juncos, PR 00777
Implantable drug pump.

Medtronic, Inc. 800-633-8766
710 Medtronic Pkwy, Minneapolis, MN 55432
SYNCHROMED.

Proven Process Medical Devices, Inc. 508-261-0806
110 Forbes Blvd, Mansfield, MA 02048
Implantable programmable infusion pump.

Trivirix International Inc. 320-982-8000
925 6th Ave NE, Milaca, MN 56353
Implantable infusion system.

PUMP, INFUSION, IMPLANTABLE, NON-PROGRAMMABLE *(General) 80MDY*

Proven Process Medical Devices, Inc. 508-261-0806
110 Forbes Blvd, Mansfield, MA 02048
Implantable constant flow pump.

PUMP, INFUSION, LABORATORY *(Chemistry) 75UHO*

Cole-Parmer Instrument Inc. 800-323-4340
625 E Bunker Ct, Vernon Hills, IL 60061
Peristaltic pump confines fluid within the tubing to provide aseptic, noncontaminating pump chamber, chemical resistance, variable flow rates and more.

Harvard Apparatus, Inc. 800-272-2775
84 October Hill Rd, Holliston, MA 01746
For research use only. Also, computer interface pulse free pump.

Orion Research, Inc. 800-225-1480
166 Cummings Ctr, Beverly, MA 01915
SAGE 3 models of syringe pumps - $1,415 to $2,635 for 0.5-5.5cc/hr unit (NOT FOR HUMAN USE).

Razel Scientific Instruments, Inc. 877-324-9914
PO Box 111, Saint Albans, VT 05478
Model A-99.EM is $407. Model A-99.BHC, infusion-withdrawal with computer connection $466.

PUMP, INFUSION, OPHTHALMIC *(Ophthalmology) 86MRH*

Escalon Trek Medical 800-433-8197
2440 S 179th St, New Berlin, WI 53146
Continuous fluid/air exchange system, viscous fluid injection ad aspiration syst.

Iscience Interventional 650-421-2700
4055 Campbell Ave, Menlo Park, CA 94025
Viscoinjector.

PUMP, INFUSION, PATIENT CONTROLLED ANALGESIA (PCA) *(General) 80MEA*

Abbott Laboratories 800-223-2064
100 Abbott Park Rd, Abbott Park, IL 60064

Aiv, Inc. (Formerly American Iv) 800-990-2911
7485 Shipley Ave, Harmans, MD 21077
Specialized repair services for leading PCA pumps. AC Adapters available for sale as well.

Ardus Medical, Inc. 800-878-1388
11297 Grooms Rd, Cincinnati, OH 45242

Baxter Healthcare Corporation, Medication Delivery 949-851-9066
17511 Armstrong Ave, Irvine, CA 92614
Pca infusor, basal-bolus, pca infusor.

Integra Lifesciences Corp. 609-275-0500
311 Enterprise Dr, Plainsboro, NJ 08536
Verifuse.

Mps Acacia 800-486-6677
785 Challenger St, Brea, CA 92821

Smiths Medical Asd, Inc. 800-433-5832
1265 Grey Fox Rd, Saint Paul, MN 55112
CADD-LEGACY PCA ambulatory infusion pumps for management of acute, post-operative and chronic pain in the hospital or home setting. CADD-PRIZM VIP (Variable Infusion Profile) multi-therapy pump for continuous, intermittent, PCA and TPN delivery. CADD-PRIZM PCS II ambulatory infusion pump for continuous, clinician activated bolus infusion and patient activated dosing.

Walkmed Infusion Llc 303-420-9569
4080 Youngfield St, Wheat Ridge, CO 80033
Various models of PCA infusion pumps.

PUMP, INFUSION, SYRINGE *(General) 80RNG*

Aiv, Inc. (Formerly American Iv) 800-990-2911
7485 Shipley Ave, Harmans, MD 21077
Specialized repair services for leading syringe pumps. AC Adapters available for sale as well.

Basi (Bioanalytical Systems, Inc.) 800-845-4246
2701 Kent Ave, West Lafayette, IN 47906
Empis syringe drive.

Baxter Healthcare Corporporation, Alternate Care And Channel Team 888-229-0001
25212 W Il Route 120, Round Lake, IL 60073
MINI-INFUSER.

PUMP, INFUSION, SYRINGE *(cont'd)*

Cmt, Inc. 800-659-9140
PO Box 297, Hamilton, MA 01936
Dual 60cc syringe pump for endoscopic minimally invasive surgical procedures.

Harvard Apparatus, Inc. 800-272-2775
84 October Hill Rd, Holliston, MA 01746
3 models from $1,050 to $1,775 with AC synchronous motor, lead screw syringz driving mechanism; 0.19-281, 0.9-8.8, 0.1-99 cc/hr flow rate. $1,725 for model wth stepping motor, lead screw syringe driving mechanism; 0.1-99 cc/hr rate. For research use only. New units stepper motors, microprocessor controlled.

Marcal Medical, Inc. 800-628-9214
1114 Benfield Blvd Ste H, Millersville, MD 21108

Orion Research, Inc. 800-225-1480
166 Cummings Ctr, Beverly, MA 01915
SAGE 3 models of syringe pumps - $1,465 to $2,235 for 0.5-5.5cc/hr. unit (NOT FOR HUMAN USE).

Razel Scientific Instruments, Inc. 877-324-9914
PO Box 111, Saint Albans, VT 05478
MODEL A, $150 with AC synchronous motor and leadscrew syringe driving mechanism with a 0.6 - 72.4 cc/hr. flow rate. MODEL A-99, $370 with stepping motor and leadscrew driving mechanism with a 0.25 - 143 cc/hr. rate.

Smiths Medical Asd, Inc. 800-848-1757
6250 Shier Rings Rd, Dublin, OH 43016
2001, 2010, 2010i syringe pumps.

Tricontinent 800-937-4738
12555 Loma Rica Dr, Grass Valley, CA 95945
Syringe pumps range form standard, off-the-shelf products to highly customized designs to meet out-of-the-ordinary application requirements (standard, modified, and custom pumps). Services include concept development and design, testing and manufacturing, and return to testing for quality assurance and reliability.

PUMP, LABORATORY *(Chemistry) 75RNH*

Baxa Corporation 800-567-2292
9540 S Maroon Circle, Suite 400, Englewood, CO 80112
Exacta-Mix(TM) 2400 Compounder. Multi-source automated compounder for mixing IV solutions. Rapid-Fill(TM) Automated Syringe Filler. Fills, caps and labels sterile batch syringes automatically.

Beckman Coulter, Inc. 800-742-2345
250 S Kraemer Blvd, PO Box 8000, Brea, CA 92821

Blue White Industries, Inc. 714-893-8529
14931 Chestnut St, Westminster, CA 92683

Brinkmann Instruments (Canada) Ltd. 800-263-8715
6670 Campobello Rd., Mississauga, ONT L5N 2L8 Canada
Combination PTFE vacuum pump and controller for corrosive vapors. Contoller maintains a set pressure from 20 to 1200 mbar.

Cole-Parmer Instrument Inc. 800-323-4340
625 E Bunker Ct, Vernon Hills, IL 60061

Ems Pacific, Inc. 800-575-5093
4480 Enterprise St Ste D, Fremont, CA 94538
Pre-settable, adjustable shot range fluid-metering, dispensing pump with 99.7% accuracy and 99.9% repeatability; from 0.005 mL to 12.5 mL in different model of piston pumps; selections of pump models to handle variety of viscous fluid from 1,000 cps to 150,000 cps; pump cylinder and piston available in metal and non-metal wetted parts; selections of valve type: valve or valveless; in pneumatic or motorized configuration.

Encynova 303-465-4800
557 Burbank St Unit C, Broomfield, CO 80020
Achieve convenient and accurate dispensing and metering liquid in the lab, pilot plant, or any custom application with the Base Station and Satellite units. Use the built-in keypad to command fluid flow for simple procedures, or take advantage of the RS485 communication capability. The system can be controlled by a personal computer using LabVIEW or Visual Basic, or via a PLC using 8-bit ASCII commands. Up to four pumps can be commanded from the keypad of the Base Station unit.

Met-Pro Corporation 215-723-6751
160 Cassell Rd, P.O. Box 144, Harleysville, PA 19438
Small magnetic-drive pumps with sealless, horizontal compact pump that features leakproof design, run dry capability, polypropylene or Kynar, non-metalic construction, 206 pm.

Oerlikon Leybold Vacuum Usa Inc. 800-433-4021
5700 Mellon Rd, Export, PA 15632
Rough to ultra-high-vacuum pumps and pumping systems.

PUMP, LABORATORY *(cont'd)*

Thermo Savant 800-634-8886
100 Colin Dr, Holbrook, NY 11741
GELPUMP Oil-free vacuum pump for gel drying applications. No oil changes or maintenance required. VALUPUMP is rotary vane, oil-sealed vacuum pump for laboratory uses. Universal Vacuum Source combined vacuum pump and solvent recovery system for use with vacuum-dependent evaporation equipment. Built-in vacuum pump is oil-free/maintenance free.

Vindum Engineering, Inc. 925-275-0633
1 Woodview Ct, San Ramon, CA 94582
High-pressure, pulse-free metering pump.

PUMP, NEBULIZER, ELECTRIC *(Ear/Nose/Throat) 77JPW*

Allied Healthcare Products, Inc. 800-444-3954
1720 Sublette Ave, Saint Louis, MO 63110

Genadyne Biotechnologies, Inc. 516-487-8787
65 Watermill Ln, Great Neck, NY 11021
Foam air mattress.

Heyer America, Inc. 703-506-0040
1320 Old Chain Bridge Rd Ste 405, McLean, VA 22101
Nebulizer.

Lumiscope Company, Inc. 800-672-8293
1035 Centennial Ave, Piscataway, NJ 08854
Nebulizer compressor.

Precision Medical, Inc. 800-272-7285
300 Held Dr, Northampton, PA 18067

PUMP, NEBULIZER, MANUAL *(Ear/Nose/Throat) 77JPT*

Tsi Incorporated 800-874-2811
500 Cardigan Rd, Shoreview, MN 55126
Aerosol generator nebulizes a solution or liquid suspension. Mean droplet size is 0.3 micrometer with a geometric standard deviation of 1.8 to 2.0.

PUMP, SUCTION OPERATORY *(Dental And Oral) 76EBR*

A-Dec, Inc. 800-547-1883
2601 Crestview Dr, Newberg, OR 97132
Several styles of air, water and vacuum operated suction systems.

Allied Healthcare Products, Inc. 800-444-3954
1720 Sublette Ave, Saint Louis, MO 63110

Busse Hospital Disposables, Inc. 631-435-4711
75 Arkay Dr, Hauppauge, NY 11788
Various.

Dencraft 800-328-9729
PO Box 57, Moorestown, NJ 08057
A/R

Dentalez Group 866-DTE-INFO
101 Lindenwood Dr Ste 225, Valleybrooke Corporate Center Malvern, PA 19355

Koros Usa, Inc. 805-529-0825
610 Flinn Ave, Moorpark, CA 93021
Suction tube.

Maximum Dental, Inc. 631-245-2176
600 Meadowlands Pkwy Ste 269, Secaucus, NJ 07094

Milex Products, Inc. 800-621-1278
4311 N Normandy Ave, Chicago, IL 60634
$610.00 for endometrial suction pump.

Mycone Dental Supply Co. Inc. T/A Keystone Ind-Myerstown 717-866-7571
52 King St, Myerstown, PA 17067
Various.

Ramvac Dental Products Inc 800-572-6822
3100 1st Ave, Spearfish, SD 57783

Sds (Summit Dental Systems) 800-275-3368
3560 NW 53rd Ct, Fort Lauderdale, FL 33309

PUMP, VACUUM, CENTRAL *(Anesthesiology) 73SEI*

Air Dimensions, Inc. 800-650-3267
1371 W Newport Center Dr, Deerfield Beach, FL 33442
DIA VAC diaphragm pumps for gaseous sampling.

Allied Healthcare Products, Inc. 800-444-3954
1720 Sublette Ave, Saint Louis, MO 63110

Anko Products, Inc., Mityflex Div. 800-446-2656
3007 29th Ave E, Bradenton, FL 34208

Bei Technologies, Inc. 949-341-9500
170 Technology Dr, Irvine, CA 92618

Berkeley Medevices, Inc. 800-227-2388
1330 S 51st St, Richmond, CA 94804

PUMP, VACUUM, CENTRAL *(cont'd)*

Brailsford & Co., Inc. 603-588-2880
15 Elm Ave, Antrim, NH 03440
Brushless D.C.

Busch, Inc 800-872-7867
516 Viking Dr, Virginia Beach, VA 23452

Dansereau Health Products, Inc. 800-423-5657
250 E Harrison St, Corona, CA 92879
Dental central vacuum, DHP Precision 1001 - priced at $995.00, DHP Precision 2002 priced at $1,995.00.

Dentsply Canada, Ltd. 800-263-1437
161 Vinyl Ct., Woodbridge, ONT L4L 4A3 Canada

Emepe International, Inc. 813-994-9690
18108 Sugar Brooke Dr, Tampa, FL 33647
Large, for pipeline system. Also, smaller units for hospital aspiration in different kinds of applications (surgery, general, gastric, thoracic).

Enviro Guard, Inc. 800-438-1152
201 Shannon Oaks Cir Ste 115, Cary, NC 27511

Oerlikon Leybold Vacuum Usa Inc. 800-433-4021
5700 Mellon Rd, Export, PA 15632
Medical office, clinic, hospital, and lab applications.

Sterling Fluid Systems (Usa) 716-773-6450
303 Industrial Dr, Grand Island, NY 14072
Engineered medical/surgical vacuum systems.

Thomas Products Division 920-457-4891
3524 Washington Ave, Sheboygan, WI 53081

Ulvac Technologies, Inc. 800-998-5822
401 Griffin Brook Dr, Methuen, MA 01844
Sinku Kiko's DAM-010 dry vacuum pump features the ability to achieve low ultimate vacuum. The two-stage design reaches pressures as low as 3 Torr. The DAM-010 is compact, lightweight, and quiet, as well as being easy to use and maintain. Ideal for scientific, chemical and medical applications.

Varian Vacuum Products 800-882-7426
121 Hartwell Ave, Lexington, MA 02421

PUMP, VACUUM, ELECTRIC, SUCTION-TYPE ELECTRODE *(Orthopedics) 87MCJ*

Varian Vacuum Products 800-882-7426
121 Hartwell Ave, Lexington, MA 02421

PUMP, WITHDRAWAL/INFUSION *(Cardiovascular) 74DQI*

Biomet Sports Medicine 530-226-5800
6704 Lockheed Dr, Redding, CA 96002
Saline pump, orthopaedic.

Harvard Apparatus, Inc. 800-272-2775
84 October Hill Rd, Holliston, MA 01746
Programmable infusion/withdraw pump.

Karl Storz Endoscopy-America Inc. 800-421-0837
600 Corporate Pointe, Culver City, CA 90230

PUNCH, ADENOID *(Ear/Nose/Throat) 77KBS*

Aesculap Implant Systems Inc. 1-800-234-9179
3773 Corporate Pkwy, Center Valley, PA 18034

Bausch & Lomb Surgical 636-255-5051
3365 Tree Court Ind Blvd, Saint Louis, MO 63122

Biomet Microfixation Inc. 800-874-7711
1520 Tradeport Dr, Jacksonville, FL 32218
Various types of punches.

Tuzik Boston 800-886-6363
104 Longwater Dr, Assinippi Park, Norwell, MA 02061

PUNCH, ANTRUM *(Ear/Nose/Throat) 77KAW*

Aesculap Implant Systems Inc. 1-800-234-9179
3773 Corporate Pkwy, Center Valley, PA 18034

Bausch & Lomb Surgical 636-255-5051
3365 Tree Court Ind Blvd, Saint Louis, MO 63122

Biomet Microfixation Inc. 800-874-7711
1520 Tradeport Dr, Jacksonville, FL 32218
Various types of punches.

Symmetry Medical Usa, Inc. 574-267-8700
486 W 350 N, Warsaw, IN 46582
Ear, nose, and throat manual surgical instrument.

PUNCH, AORTIC *(Cardiovascular) 74RNI*

Codman & Shurtleff, Inc 800-225-0460
325 Paramount Dr, Raynham, MA 02767

PUNCH, AORTIC *(cont'd)*

Covidien Lp 508-261-8000
15 Hampshire St, Mansfield, MA 02048
CARDIOPUNCH disposable aortic punch.

Genesee Biomedical, Inc. 800-786-4890
1308 S Jason St, Denver, CO 80223

Scanlan International, Inc. 800-328-9458
1 Scanlan Plz, Saint Paul, MN 55107
Single use aorta/vein punch.

PUNCH, ATTIC *(Ear/Nose/Throat) 77JYX*

Aesculap Implant Systems Inc. 1-800-234-9179
3773 Corporate Pkwy, Center Valley, PA 18034

PUNCH, BIOPSY *(Gastro/Urology) 78FCI*

Aesculap Implant Systems Inc. 1-800-234-9179
3773 Corporate Pkwy, Center Valley, PA 18034

Cameron-Miller, Inc. 800-621-0142
5410 W Roosevelt Rd, Road #241, Chicago, IL 60644

Codman & Shurtleff, Inc 800-225-0460
325 Paramount Dr, Raynham, MA 02767

Elmed, Inc. 630-543-2792
60 W Fay Ave, Addison, IL 60101

Fray Products Corp. 800-288-6580
2495 Main St, Buffalo, NY 14214
BIOPUNCH Safety capped, sterile, seamless blade, sterility indicator, tamper evident pouch seal, hollow handle, color coded handle, pouch and dispenser box.

Karl Storz Endoscopy-America Inc. 800-421-0837
600 Corporate Pointe, Culver City, CA 90230

Kmedic 800-955-0559
190 Veterans Dr, Northvale, NJ 07647

Mahe International Inc. 800-294-7946
468 Craighead St, Nashville, TN 37204

Medgyn Products, Inc. 800-451-9667
328 Eisenhower Ln N, Lombard, IL 60148
Tischler biopsy punch, baby Tischler and Kevorkian biopsy punch. All German stainless.

Miltex Inc. 800-645-8000
589 Davies Dr, York, PA 17402
Disposable biopsy punches also available.

Premier Medical Products 888-PREMUSA
1710 Romano Dr, Plymouth Meeting, PA 19462
Uni-Punch method of obtaining dermal tissue samples for pathology. Electropolished carbon steel cutting tip available to provide sharp, precise incisions.

Princeton Medical Group, Inc. 800-875-0869
1189 Royal Links Dr, Mt Pleasant, SC 29466

Richard Wolf Medical Instruments Corp. 800-323-9653
353 Corporate Woods Pkwy, Vernon Hills, IL 60061

Rocket Medical Plc. 800-707-7625
150 Recreation Park Dr Ste 3, Hingham, MA 02043

Tuzik Boston 800-886-6363
104 Longwater Dr, Assinippi Park, Norwell, MA 02061

PUNCH, BIOPSY, SURGICAL *(Dental And Oral) 76EME*

Acuderm Inc. 800-327-0015
5370 NW 35th Ter Ste 106, Fort Lauderdale, FL 33309
Disposable skin biopsy punch.

Basic Dental Implant Systems, Inc. 505-884-1922
3321 Columbia Dr NE, Albuquerque, NM 87107
Tissue punch.

Elmed, Inc. 630-543-2792
60 W Fay Ave, Addison, IL 60101

George Tiemann & Co. 800-843-6266
25 Plant Ave, Hauppauge, NY 11788

H & H Co. 909-390-0373
4435 E Airport Dr Ste 108, Ontario, CA 91761
Dermal or circular punch.

International Hospital Supply Co. 800-398-9450
6914 Canby Ave Ste 105, Reseda, CA 91335

Kmedic 800-955-0559
190 Veterans Dr, Northvale, NJ 07647

Oratronics, Inc. 212-986-0050
405 Lexington Ave, New York, NY 10174
Tissue punch.

PUNCH, BIOPSY, SURGICAL *(cont'd)*
Shoney Scientific, Inc. 262-970-0170
West 223 North 720 Saratoga Drive,, Suite 120, Waukesha, WI 53186
Punch, biopsy, surgical.

Tuzik Boston 800-886-6363
104 Longwater Dr, Assinippi Park, Norwell, MA 02061

PUNCH, BONE *(Orthopedics) 87RNJ*
Codman & Shurtleff, Inc 800-225-0460
325 Paramount Dr, Raynham, MA 02767

Fehling Surgical Instruments 800-FEHLING
509 Broadstone Ln NW, Acworth, GA 30101

Stryker Spine 866-457-7463
2 Pearl Ct, Allendale, NJ 07401

Zimmer Holdings, Inc. 800-613-6131
1800 W Center St, PO Box 708, Warsaw, IN 46580

PUNCH, CATHETER *(Gastro/Urology) 78FEX*
Aesculap Implant Systems Inc. 1-800-234-9179
3773 Corporate Pkwy, Center Valley, PA 18034

Cook Urological, Inc. 800-457-4500
1100 W Morgan St, P.O. Box 227, Spencer, IN 47460

PUNCH, CORNEO-SCLERAL *(Ophthalmology) 86HNJ*
Barron Precision Instruments, L.L.C. 810-695-2080
8170 Embury Rd, Grand Blanc, MI 48439
Various types of sterile donor cornea punches.

Bausch & Lomb Surgical 636-255-5051
3365 Tree Court Ind Blvd, Saint Louis, MO 63122

Jedmed Instruments Co. 314-845-3770
5416 Jedmed Ct, Saint Louis, MO 63129

Katena Products, Inc. 800-225-1195
4 Stewart Ct, Denville, NJ 07834

Miltex Inc. 800-645-8000
589 Davies Dr, York, PA 17402

PUNCH, DENTAL, RUBBER DAM *(Dental And Oral) 76RNK*
Hager Worldwide, Inc. 800-328-2335
13322 Byrd Dr, Odessa, FL 33556
FIT.

Moyco Technologies, Inc. 800-331-8837
200 Commerce Dr, Montgomeryville, PA 18936

PUNCH, DERMAL *(Surgery) 79RNL*
Kmedic 800-955-0559
190 Veterans Dr, Northvale, NJ 07647

Princeton Medical Group, Inc. 800-875-0869
1189 Royal Links Dr, Mt Pleasant, SC 29466

PUNCH, ENT *(Ear/Nose/Throat) 77KTF*
Biomet Microfixation Inc. 800-874-7711
1520 Tradeport Dr, Jacksonville, FL 32218
Various types of punches.

Solos Endoscopy 800-388-6445
65 Sprague St # B, Boston/dedham Commerce Park, Boston, MA 02136
Punch,ent.

PUNCH, ETHMOID *(Ear/Nose/Throat) 77KAX*
Aesculap Implant Systems Inc. 1-800-234-9179
3773 Corporate Pkwy, Center Valley, PA 18034

Bausch & Lomb Surgical 636-255-5051
3365 Tree Court Ind Blvd, Saint Louis, MO 63122

PUNCH, FEMORAL NECK *(Orthopedics) 87HWP*
Biomet, Inc. 574-267-6639
56 E Bell Dr, PO Box 587, Warsaw, IN 46582
Moore hollow chisel.

Depuy Spine, Inc. 800-227-6633
325 Paramount Dr, Raynham, MA 02767
Bone screw extractor.

Fehling Surgical Instruments 800-FEHLING
509 Broadstone Ln NW, Acworth, GA 30101

Stryker Spine 866-457-7463
2 Pearl Ct, Allendale, NJ 07401

Warsaw Orthopedic, Inc. 901-396-3133
2500 Silveus Xing, Warsaw, IN 46582
Femoral neck punch.

Zimmer Holdings, Inc. 800-613-6131
1800 W Center St, PO Box 708, Warsaw, IN 46580

PUNCH, FEMORAL NECK *(cont'd)*
Zimmer Trabecular Metal Technology 800-613-6131
10 Pomeroy Rd, Parsippany, NJ 07054
Box osteotome.

PUNCH, GELFOAM *(Ear/Nose/Throat) 77JXZ*
Pharmacia & Upjohn Co. 212-573-1000
7000 Portage Rd, Kalamazoo, MI 49001
Various.

PUNCH, NASAL *(Ear/Nose/Throat) 77KAY*
Aesculap Implant Systems Inc. 1-800-234-9179
3773 Corporate Pkwy, Center Valley, PA 18034

Bausch & Lomb Surgical 636-255-5051
3365 Tree Court Ind Blvd, Saint Louis, MO 63122

Invotec Intl. 800-998-8580
6833 Phillips Industrial Blvd, Jacksonville, FL 32256
Nasal bropsy punch.

PUNCH, OTHER *(Surgery) 79RNO*
Symmetry Tnco 888-447-6661
15 Colebrook Blvd, Whitman, MA 02382
Endoscopic and arthroscopic punches.

Wisap America 800-233-8448
8231 Melrose Dr, Lenexa, KS 66214
Tissue Punch

PUNCH, SKULL *(Cns/Neurology) 84GXJ*
Biomet Microfixation Inc. 800-874-7711
1520 Tradeport Dr, Jacksonville, FL 32218
Various types of punches.

PUNCH, SURGICAL *(Surgery) 79LRY*
Acuderm Inc. 800-327-0015
5370 NW 35th Ter Ste 106, Fort Lauderdale, FL 33309
Elliptical excisional scalpel.

Arthrex California, Inc. 239-643-5553
20509 Earlgate St, Walnut, CA 91789
Punch.

Biomet Microfixation Inc. 800-874-7711
1520 Tradeport Dr, Jacksonville, FL 32218
Various types of punches.

Depuy Orthopaedics, Inc. 800-473-3789
700 Orthopaedic Dr, P.O. Box 988, Warsaw, IN 46582
Various punches.

Dermatologic Lab & Supply, Inc. 800-831-6273
608 13th Ave, Council Bluffs, IA 51501
Surgical punch.

DJO Inc. 800-336-6569
1430 Decision St, Vista, CA 92081

Fehling Surgical Instruments 800-FEHLING
509 Broadstone Ln NW, Acworth, GA 30101

Huot Instruments, Llc 262-373-1700
N50W13740 Overview Dr Ste A, Menomonee Falls, WI 53051
Dermal biopsy punch.

Kelsar, S.A. 508-261-8000
Blvd. Insurgentes, Libriamento a La, Tijuana 22450 Mexico
Aortic punch

Nobel Biocare Usa, Llc 800-579-6515
22715/22725 Savi Ranch Parkway, Yorba Linda, CA 92887
Surgical instrument.

Symmetry Medical Usa, Inc. 574-267-8700
486 W 350 N, Warsaw, IN 46582
Osteochondritis dessicans.

PUNCH, TONSIL *(Ear/Nose/Throat) 77KBT*
Aesculap Implant Systems Inc. 1-800-234-9179
3773 Corporate Pkwy, Center Valley, PA 18034

Bausch & Lomb Surgical 636-255-5051
3365 Tree Court Ind Blvd, Saint Louis, MO 63122

Biomet Microfixation Inc. 800-874-7711
1520 Tradeport Dr, Jacksonville, FL 32218
Various types of punches.

PUPILLOMETER *(Ophthalmology) 86TDV*
Burton Co., R.H. 800-848-0410
3965 Brookham Dr, Grove City, OH 43123
$375.00 for BURTON LLD P.D. meter with digital display.

PUPILLOMETER *(cont'd)*

Oasis Medical, Inc. 800-528-9786
514 S Vermont Ave, Glendora, CA 91741
Colvard Pupillometer with Reticle that provides measurement of vertical and horizontal corneal diameter.

PUPILLOMETER, AC-POWERED *(Ophthalmology) 86HLG*

Applied Science Laboratories 781-275-4000
175 Middlesex Tpke, Bedford, MA 01730
Priced from $8,000 to $17,000 for hand-held, portable binocular systems.

Indigo Micro Technologies, Inc. 815-874-3557
3220 Gunflint Trl, Rockford, IL 61109
Pupillometer.

Iritech, Inc. 703-787-7680
459 Herndon Pkwy Ste 21, Herndon, VA 20170
Drug screening system.

Neuroptics, Inc. 949-250-9792
1001 Avenida Pico Ste C495, San Clemente, CA 92673
Neuroptics pupillometer.

Pulse Medical Instruments, Inc. 301-816-9212
5951 Halpine Rd, Rockville, MD 20851
Fit 2000.

Topcon Medical Systems, Inc. 800-223-1130
37 W Century Rd, Paramus, NJ 07652
Digital PD meter: $590.00

PUPILLOMETER, MANUAL *(Ophthalmology) 86HLH*

Eye Care And Cure 800-486-6169
4646 S Overland Dr, Tucson, AZ 85714
Pupillometer.

Iritech, Inc. 703-787-7680
459 Herndon Pkwy Ste 21, Herndon, VA 20170
Pupillometer.

PURIFICATION FILTER, WATER, CHARCOAL *(Chemistry) 75SFX*

Cartwright Consulting Co. 952-854-4911
8324 16th Ave S, Minneapolis, MN 55425

Labconco Corp. 800-821-5525
8811 Prospect Ave, Kansas City, MO 64132
WaterPro PS Polishing Stations, RO Systems and Softener

Medro Systems, Inc. 972-542-8200
416 Industrial Blvd, McKinney, TX 75069
Carbon filters for removal of chlorine and chloramines.

PURIFICATION FILTER, WATER, PARTICULATE *(Chemistry) 75SFY*

G.E.M. Water Systems, Int'L., Llc 800-755-1707
6351 Orangethorpe Ave, Buena Park, CA 90620

Labconco Corp. 800-821-5525
8811 Prospect Ave, Kansas City, MO 64132
WaterPro Polishing Station, RO Systems and Softener

Leedal, Inc. 847-498-0111
3453 Commercial Ave, Northbrook, IL 60062

Medro Systems, Inc. 972-542-8200
416 Industrial Blvd, McKinney, TX 75069
Sand filters & softeners.

Millipore Corporation 800-MILLIPORE
80 Ashby Rd, Bedford, MA 01730
MILLIPAK.

Pall Corporation 800-521-1520
600 S Wagner Rd, Ann Arbor, MI 48103

Porvair Filtration Group Inc 803-327-5008
454 Anderson Rd S, BTC 514, Rock Hill, SC 29730

PURIFICATION SYSTEM, WATER *(Gastro/Urology) 78FIP*

Ameriwater 937-461-8833
1303 Stanley Ave, Dayton, OH 45404
Water treatment system.

Aqua Water Treatment, Inc. 850-939-9055
8195 E Bay Blvd, Navarre, FL 32566
Water purification system.

Better Water, Inc. 615-355-6063
698 Swan Dr, Smyrna, TN 37167
Water purification system for hemodialysis.

Bob J. Johnson & Associates 218-873-5555
16420 W Hardy Rd Ste 100, Houston, TX 77060
Activated carbon exchange tanks, water softener, deionizer exchange tanks, ca.

PURIFICATION SYSTEM, WATER *(cont'd)*

Bti Filtration 405-842-2517
7317 N Classen Blvd, Oklahoma City, OK 73116
Btro water purification system.

Dialysis Dimensions, Inc. 615-292-0333
2003 Blair Blvd, Nashville, TN 37212
Water treatment system for hemodialysis.

Dialysis Services, Inc. 615-384-4810
130 Elder Dr, Springfield, TN 37172
Water treatment system for hemodialysis.

Ge Ionics, Inc. 214-339-2135
4740 Bronze Way, Dallas, TX 75236
Various.

H20only Co. 800-338-4905
1101 Columbus Ave, Bay City, MI 48708
Water purification system.

Hydro Service & Supplies, Inc. 800-950-7426
PO Box 12197, Research Triangle Park, NC 27709
PICOTAP - faucets for ultrapure water.

Isopure Corp. 800-280-7873
141 Citizens Blvd, Simpsonville, KY 40067
Registered complete water purification system for multi-patient and single patient Reverse Osmosis Systems.

Lares Research 800-347-3289
295 Lockheed Ave, Chico, CA 95973
Sterile water delivery system

Mar Cor Purification 800-346-0365
4450 Township Line Road, Skippack, PA 19474-1429
Water-treatment system for kidney dialysis.

Medro Systems, Inc. 972-542-8200
416 Industrial Blvd, McKinney, TX 75069
Reverse osmosis water treatment equipment for kidney dialysis, 3-600 gal/hr. (11-2268 liters). Also pure water storage tanks and repressurization systems.

Millipore Corporation 800-MILLIPORE
80 Ashby Rd, Bedford, MA 01730
Milli-RO.

My Water House, Inc. 407-428-9377
3319 Bartlett Blvd, Orlando, FL 32811
Deionization systems with pre & post treatment and product water distribution co.

Neu-Ion, Inc. 410-944-5200
7200 Rutherford Rd Ste 100, Baltimore, MD 21244
Water purification system for dialysis.

Nxstage Medical, Inc. 866-697-8243
439 S Union St Fl 5, Lawrence, MA 01843
Water purification system.

Performance Water Systems, Llc 708-396-0136
13601 Kenton Ave, Crestwood, IL 60445
Water treatment system for hemodialysis.

Pure Water Solutions, Inc. 877-202-5871
520 Topeka Way Ste D, Castle Rock, CO 80109
Reverse osmosis central dialysis solution.

Pure Water, Inc. 864-375-0105
311 W Market St, Anderson, SC 29624
Water purification system for hemodialysis.

Purity Water Company Of San Antonio, Inc. 210-227-3601
1119 Paulsun St, San Antonio, TX 78219
ïDisinfection Systemsï Service Deionization Systems (SDI Systems)ï Reverse Osmosis Systemsï Water Softening Systemsï Ultra-Pure Water Systemsï Contract Regeneration Services, FDA Registered State-of-art Resin Regeneration Facility Resins Intended For Dialysis Applications

Serim Research Corp. 574-264-3440
3506 Reedy Dr, Elkhart, IN 46514
Test for low levels of chloramines and free chlorine in treated water.

Serv-A-Pure Company 800-338-4905
1101 Columbus Ave, Bay City, MI 48708
Water purification system.

Simply Clean Air & Water, Inc. 860-231-0687
28 Shepard Dr, Newington, CT 06111
Deionization system w/ pre & post treatment & water distribution components serv.

Sorb Technology, Inc. 405-682-1993
3631 SW 54th St, Oklahoma City, OK 73119
Ascorbic acid packet.

PURIFICATION SYSTEM, WATER *(cont'd)*

Steris Corporation 814-452-3100
2424 W 23rd St, Erie, PA 16506
Various sizes, components of water purification equipment.

Water & Power Technologies Of Texas, Inc. 801-974-5500
1501 Saint Andrews Rd, Po Box 21743, Columbia, SC 29210
Water purification system.

Water & Power Technologies, Inc. 817-640-1533
1217 Corporate Dr W, Arlington, TX 76006
FDA 510K Water Purification System.

PURIFICATION SYSTEM, WATER, DEIONIZATION
(Chemistry) 75SFZ

Hydro Service & Supplies, Inc. 800-950-7426
PO Box 12197, Research Triangle Park, NC 27709
PICOSYSTEM; Deionization: water purification systems. Water deionization and organic adsorption equipment.

Millipore Corporation 800-MILLIPORE
80 Ashby Rd, Bedford, MA 01730
MILLI-Q ultrapure water system.

Thermo Fisher Scientific Inc. 563-556-2241
2555 Kerper Blvd, Dubuque, IA 52001

PURIFICATION SYSTEM, WATER, REVERSE OSMOSIS
(Chemistry) 75SGA

Blue Spring Corp. 361-552-8898
45 Blue Spring Rd, Port Lavaca, TX 77979
RO Systems, Blue Spring; Reverse osmosis water purifiers for dialysis, central and acute.

G.E.M. Water Systems, Int'L., Llc 800-755-1707
6351 Orangethorpe Ave, Buena Park, CA 90620

Isopure Corp. 800-280-7873
141 Citizens Blvd, Simpsonville, KY 40067
MD 400 series reverse osmosis machine. Purified water for hemodialysis. Portable Reverse Osmosis Machine system which provides enough water for two systems available.

Medro Systems, Inc. 972-542-8200
416 Industrial Blvd, McKinney, TX 75069
Portable reverse osmosis water treatment equipment for kidney dialysis with an output of 3-600 gal./hour (11-2268 liter).

Millipore Corporation 800-MILLIPORE
80 Ashby Rd, Bedford, MA 01730
MILLI-RO system.

Rismed Oncology Systems 256-534-6993
2494 Washington St NW, Huntsville, AL 35811
RO water systems for 1 - 50 machine stations.

Thermo Fisher Scientific Inc. 563-556-2241
2555 Kerper Blvd, Dubuque, IA 52001

PURIFICATION SYSTEM, WATER, REVERSE OSMOSIS, REAGENT GRADE *(Chemistry) 75JRT*

G.E.M. Water Systems, Int'L., Llc 800-755-1707
6351 Orangethorpe Ave, Buena Park, CA 90620

Millipore Corporation 800-MILLIPORE
80 Ashby Rd, Bedford, MA 01730
MILLI-RO system.

PURIFICATION SYSTEM, WATER, ULTRAVIOLET
(Chemistry) 75SGB

Atlantic Ultraviolet Corp. 631-273-0500
375 Marcus Blvd, Hauppauge, NY 11788

Fuller Ultraviolet Corp. 815-469-3301
9416 Gulfstream Rd, Frankfort, IL 60423
$500.00 per unit (standard).

PURIFIER, AIR, ULTRAVIOLET *(General) 80FRA*

Abracair, Llc 502-445-9471
204 N 17th St, Louisville, KY 40203
Room air cleaner.

Atlantic Ultraviolet Corp. 631-273-0500
375 Marcus Blvd, Hauppauge, NY 11788
HYGEAIRE 3 models.

Calutech Corporation
6615 W 111th St, Worth, IL 60482
Purifier, air, ultraviolet, medical.

Clean Air Research & Environmental, Inc. 972-233-2777
13628 Beta Rd Ste B, Dallas, TX 75244
Rxair 3000.

PURIFIER, AIR, ULTRAVIOLET *(cont'd)*

Cloud 9 630-595-5000
777 N Edgewood Ave, Wood Dale, IL 60191

Innovative Health Care Products, Inc. 678-320-0009
6850 Peachtree Dunwoody Rd NE Apt 402, Atlanta, GA 30328
Medicair

Kesair Technologies, Llc 800-236-1846
3625 Kennesaw N Ind Pkwy NW, Kennesaw, GA 30144
Airocide TiO2 AiroCide kills airborne pathogens such as bacteria, mold, spores and viruses. AiroCides has two killing mechanisms 1) UV and 2) surface bound hydroxyl radicals. AiroCide is NOT a filter. AiroCide produces NO ozone. AiroCide has it own self-contained fan. AiroCide is a photocatalytic reactor (PCO). AiroCide oxidizes VOC's like ethylene gas into harmless CO2 and water vapor as well as many odors.

Lee Medical International, Inc. 800-433-8950
612 Distributors Row, Harahan, LA 70123
LEEZYME air freshener and odor eliminator.

Nbc Products, Inc. 952-226-1112
16873 Fish Point Rd SE, Prior Lake, MN 55372
Hospital grade air cleaner.

Peterson Air Purifiers, Llc 952-703-8962
9555 James Ave S Ste 220, Bloomington, MN 55431
Purifier, air, ultraviolet, medical.

Summit Hill Laboratories 800-922-0722
1 Sheila Dr, Tinton Falls, NJ 07724
MICRONAIRE and HEPANAIRE electrostatic precipitators.

Youngs, Inc. 800-523-5454
55 E Cherry Ln, Souderton, PA 18964

PURIFIER, WATER *(Chemistry) 75JRS*

A.J. Antunes & Co. 630-784-3469
180 Kehoe Blvd, Carol Stream, IL 60188
Various models of water filtration systems.

Barnstead International 412-490-8425
2555 Kerper Blvd, Dubuque, IA 52001
Various water purifiers.

Blue Spring Corp. 361-552-8898
45 Blue Spring Rd, Port Lavaca, TX 77979
RO Systems, Blue Spring; Reverse osmosis water purifiers for dialysis, central and acute.

Commonwealth H2o Services, Inc. 434-975-4426
325 Greenbrier Dr, Charlottesville, VA 22901
Deionization, various sizes, reverse osmosis, various sizes.

Consolidated Stills & Sterilizers 617-782-6072
76 Ashford St, Boston, MA 02134

Corning Inc., Science Products Division 800-492-1110
45 Nagog Park, Acton, MA 01720

Eagle Water Systems Of The Triangle 919-688-8558
2305 E Club Blvd, Durham, NC 27704
Deionzation-various sizes/reverse osmosis models.

Ecodyne Water Treatment, Inc. 800-228-9326
1270 Frontenac Rd, Naperville, IL 60563
Various types.

Millipore Corp. 781-533-2622
Prescott Rd., Jaffrey, NH 03452

Millipore Corporation 800-MILLIPORE
80 Ashby Rd, Bedford, MA 01730

Nerl Diagnostics Llc. 401-824-2046
14 Almeida Ave, East Providence, RI 02914
Reagent grade water.

Puretec Industrial Water 805-652-0552
3151 Sturgis Rd, Oxnard, CA 93030
Purified water.

Western Water Purifier Co. 800-55-WATER
PO Box 688, Woodland Hills, CA 91365
MULTIPURE, AMETEK, CUNO, EVERPURE, and OGDEN water filters; distribute standard and custom water-filtration equipment from California and Australia. Stock replacement cartridges and parts for most models. Water softeners -- small to commercial-sized units for the Australian and South Pacific market.

PUSHER, BAND, ORTHODONTIC *(Dental And Oral) 76ECS*

Biomet Microfixation Inc. 800-874-7711
1520 Tradeport Dr, Jacksonville, FL 32218
Pusher, band, orthodontic.

PUSHER, BAND, ORTHODONTIC *(cont'd)*

Coltene/Whaledent Inc. 330-916-8858
235 Ascot Pkwy, Cuyahoga Falls, OH 44223
Right angle handpiece: head, r.a. hdpce.

Dentronix, Inc. 800-523-5944
235 Ascot Pkwy, Cuyahoga Falls, OH 44223
$30.00 per unit (standard).

E.A. Beck & Co. 949-645-4072
657 W 19th St Ste E, P O Box 10857, Costa Mesa, CA 92627
Band pusher.

G & H Wire Co. 800-526-1026
2165 Earlywood Dr, Franklin, IN 46131

Glenroe Technologies 800-237-4060
1912 44th Ave E, Bradenton, FL 34203
Orthodontic elastic placer.

Hu-Friedy Manufacturing Co., Inc. 800-483-7433
3232 N Rockwell St, Chicago, IL 60618
$14.25 to $28.50 each, 4 types.

Lancer Orthodontics, Inc. 760-304-2705
253 Pawnee St, San Marcos, CA 92078
Pusher, band, orthodontic.

Masel Co., Inc. 800-423-8227
2701 Bartram Rd, Bristol, PA 19007

Orthodontic Design And Production, Inc. 760-734-3995
1370 Decision St Ste D, Vista, CA 92081
Type of orthodontic hand instrument.

Premier Dental Products Co. 888-670-6100
1710 Romano Dr, PO Box 4500, Plymouth Meeting, PA 19462

Pulpdent Corp. 800-343-4342
80 Oakland St, Watertown, MA 02472
No common name listed.

Sci-Dent, Inc. 800-323-4145
210 Dowdle St Ste 2, Algonquin, IL 60102

3m Unitek 800-634-5300
2724 Peck Rd, Monrovia, CA 91016

PUSHER, SOCKET *(Orthopedics) 87HXO*

Biomet, Inc. 574-267-6639
56 E Bell Dr, PO Box 587, Warsaw, IN 46582
Cup positioning and aiming device.

Depuy-Raynham, A Div. Of Depuy Orthopaedics 800-451-2006
325 Paramount Dr, Raynham, MA 02767
Various types of orthopedic socket pushers.

Medtronic Sofamor Danek Usa, Inc. 901-396-3133
4340 Swinnea Rd, Memphis, TN 38118
Socket.

Stryker Spine 866-457-7463
2 Pearl Ct, Allendale, NJ 07401

Warsaw Orthopedic, Inc. 901-396-3133
2500 Silveus Xing, Warsaw, IN 46582
Socket.

Zimmer Holdings, Inc. 800-613-6131
1800 W Center St, PO Box 708, Warsaw, IN 46580

Zimmer Trabecular Metal Technology 800-613-6131
10 Pomeroy Rd, Parsippany, NJ 07054
Retractor.

PYLON, POST SURGICAL *(Physical Med) 89ISM*

Ortho Innovations, Inc. 507-269-2895
121 23rd Ave SW, Rochester, MN 55902
Post surgical, dressing.

PYROMETER *(General) 80RNQ*

Capintec, Inc. 800-631-3826
6 Arrow Rd, Ramsey, NJ 07446

Cole-Parmer Instrument Inc. 800-323-4340
625 E Bunker Ct, Vernon Hills, IL 60061

Electronic Development Labs, Inc. 800-342-5335
244 Oakland Dr, Danville, VA 24540
Precision 1 deg. accuracy, 1 deg. repeatability, 1 deg. resolution. Portable digital RTD. Analog pyrometer, 1/2 percent reading accuracy, explosion proof (uses no batteries), pivot-jewel movement. Digital pyrometer, precision 1/10 percent accuracy, .1 deg. resolution, T.C. types k.j.e.t.n., R.F. shielded.

Mikron Infrared, Inc. 800-631-0176
16 Thornton Rd, Oakland, NJ 07436

PYROMETER *(cont'd)*

Noral, Inc. 800-348-2345
23600 Mercantile Rd, Beachwood Commerce Park
Cleveland, OH 44122
$199.00 per unit (standard).

Omega Engineering, Inc. 800-848-4286
1 Omega Dr, Stamford, CT 06907

Pyrometer Instrument Co. 800-468-7976
92 N Main St Bldg 18D, Windsor, NJ 08561
13 models - starting at $267.00, including optical pyrometer & infrared thermometers and laser pyrometer.

Simpson Electric Co. 715-588-3311
520 Simpson Ave, PO Box 99, Lac Du Flambeau, WI 54538
Models 29T & 3324, 3 1/2 in., 4 1/2 in., 4 in.x6 in. Panel mounted. $91.04-$153.12 per unit (standard).

QUALITATIVE CHEMICAL REACTIONS, URINARY CALCULI (STONE) *(Chemistry) 75JNQ*

Busse Hospital Disposables, Inc. 631-435-4711
75 Arkay Dr, Hauppauge, NY 11788
Calculi strainer.

Mission Pharmacal Co. 210-696-8400
10999 W Interstate 10 Ste 1000, San Antonio, TX 78230
STONE RISK Diagnostic profile for kidney stone disease: comprehensive 24-hour urinalysis test that measures all urinary risk factors and calculates relative supersaturation rate (RSR) for five stone classifications. A patented urine collection system and computerized graphic display reporting method are features unique to STONERISK Diagnostic Profile. CALCIBIND Diagnostics Assessment Urinalysis test is an abbreviated outpatient calcium fast and load test designed to classify hypercalciurias, important for appropriate dietary advice and use of adjunctive medications. URORISK Diagnostic Test Profile is our latest diagnostic test for kidney stone disease specifically designed for use in capitated managed care health plans. URORISK is a quantitative 24-hour urinalysis test that measures the major urinary risk factors responsible for stone formation. STONE COMP, Crystallographic Stone Analysis Test is our latest diagnostic test to precisely determine chemical components of urinary calculi.

Teco Diagnostics 714-693-7788
1268 N Lakeview Ave, Anaheim, CA 92807
Urinary calculi test strips.

QUANTITATION, ANTITHROMBIN III *(Hematology) 81JBQ*

Diagnostica Stago, Inc. 800-222-COAG
5 Century Dr, Parsippany, NJ 07054

Fisher Diagnostics 877-722-4366
11515 Vanstory Dr Ste 125, Huntersville, NC 28078

Millenia Diagnostics 619-957-6474
5909 Sea Lion Pl Ste D, Carlsbad, CA 92010
Rsv antigen detection.

Precision Biologic, Inc. 800-267-2796
900 Windmill Rd., Ste. 100, Dartmouth, NS B3B 1P7 Canada
CHROMOCHECK ANTITHROMBIN chromogenic assay kit.

Teco Diagnostics 714-693-7788
1268 N Lakeview Ave, Anaheim, CA 92807
Gamma-glutamyl transferase, kinetic or color.

QUANTITATION, HEMOGLOBIN, ABNORMAL *(Hematology) 81GKA*

Bio-Rad Laboratories Inc., Clinical Systems Div. 800-224-6723
4000 Alfred Nobel Dr, Hercules, CA 94547
Sickle cell program.

Helena Laboratories 409-842-3714
PO Box 752, Beaumont, TX 77704

PerkinElmer 800-762-4000
940 Winter St, Waltham, MA 02451
Total glycosolated hemoglobin assay and semi-automated GHb reader.

RACK, BEDPAN *(General) 80RNS*

American Specialties, Inc. 914-476-9000
441 Saw Mill River Rd, Yonkers, NY 10701

Imperial Surgical Ltd. 800-661-5432
581 Orly Ave., Dorval, ONT H9P-1G1 Canada
Various models available.

RACK, DRYING *(Chemistry) 75TDX*

DURHAM MANUFACTURING COMPANY 800-243-3774
201 Main St, Durham, CT 06422

RACK, DRYING *(cont'd)*

Nutech Molding Corporation 1-800-423-5278
PO Box 840, 2024 Broad St,, Pocomoke City, MD 21851

RACK, GLOVE, OPERATING ROOM *(Surgery) 79FSN*

Alimed, Inc. 800-225-2610
297 High St, Dedham, MA 02026

United Metal Fabricators, Inc. 800-638-5322
1316 Eisenhower Blvd, Johnstown, PA 15904
All stainless steel or enamel with stainless steel rack hooks.

RACK, INSTRUMENT, LAPAROSCOPY *(Surgery) 79SIO*

Belimed 800-457-4117
13840 SW 119th Ave, Miami, FL 33186
Instrument racks, laparoscopic/endoscopic racks and specialty racks.

RACK, MEDICAL CHART *(General) 80RGL*

First Healthcare Products 800-854-8304
6125 Lendell Dr, Sanborn, NY 14132
Mobile, floor and counter cabinet styles, revolving/carousel styles, flat and vertical storage. Standard and custom designs available.

Mayo Medical, S.A. De C.V. 800-715-3872
Edison 1141 Nte., Col. Talleres, Monterrey N.L. 64480 Mexico

Medi-Dose, Inc. 800-523-8966
70 Industrial Dr, Ivyland, PA 18974

Medirecord Systems 800-561-9791
P.O. Box 6201 Station A, Saint John, NB E2L 4R6 Canada

National Systems Co. 877-672-4278
31B Durward Pl., Waterloo N2J 3Z9 Canada
Patient charts, chart holders, indexes, racks etc.

Omnimed, Inc. (Beam Products) 800-257-2326
800 Glen Ave, Moorestown, NJ 08057

Peter Pepper Products, Inc. 800-496-0204
17929 S Susana Rd, PO Box 5769, Compton, CA 90221
For HIPAA.

RACK, SKIASCOPIC *(Ophthalmology) 86HMH*

Allegheny Plastics, Inc. 412-776-0100
1224 Freedom Rd, Cranberry Township, PA 16066
Corneal rust ring remover-eye spud.

RACK, SURGICAL INSTRUMENT *(Surgery) 79FSG*

Anchor Products Company 800-323-5134
52 W Official Rd, Addison, IL 60101
$12.20 each.

Codman & Shurtleff, Inc 800-225-0460
325 Paramount Dr, Raynham, MA 02767

Encompas Unlimited, Inc. 800-825-7701
PO Box 516, Tallevast, FL 34270
$99.00.

Intermetro Industries Corp. 800-441-2714
651 N Washington St, Wilkes Barre, PA 18705
STARSYS surgical-instrument cabinet.

Kmedic 800-955-0559
190 Veterans Dr, Northvale, NJ 07647

Lds Life Science (Formerly Gould Instrument Systems Inc.) 216-328-7000
5525 Cloverleaf Pkwy, Valley View, OH 44125

Mark Medical Manufacturing, Inc. 610-269-4420
530 Brandywine Ave, Downingtown, PA 19335
Quick-Rack, Weinstein, Sur-Lock and Stringers.

Micromedics 800-624-5662
1270 Eagan Industrial Rd, Saint Paul, MN 55121
Instru-Safe systems keep surgical instruments organized in sets and protect the instruments during transportation, storage, and sterile processing...saving time in surgery and reducing instrument damage.

Minnesota Bramstedt Surgical, Inc. 800-456-5052
1835 Energy Park Dr, Saint Paul, MN 55108

Phelan Manufacturing Corp. 800-328-2358
2523 Minnehaha Ave, Minneapolis, MN 55404
$17.00 per surgical instrument rack.

Precision Medical Manufacturing Corporation 866-633-4626
852 Seton Ct, Wheeling, IL 60090
Instrument Racks designed to stack forceps and scissors.They are cabinet space saver and allow to keep instruments securly organized.

RACK, SURGICAL INSTRUMENT *(cont'd)*

Rush-Berivon, Inc. 800-251-7874
1010 19th St, P.O. Box 1851, Meridian, MS 39301
$140.00 through $140.00 for orthopedic models for 1.6mm - 8mm pins.

Scanlan International, Inc. 800-328-9458
1 Scanlan Plz, Saint Paul, MN 55107

Stryker Corp. 800-726-2725
2825 Airview Blvd, Portage, MI 49002

Zimmer Holdings, Inc. 800-613-6131
1800 W Center St, PO Box 708, Warsaw, IN 46580

RACK, TEST TUBE *(Chemistry) 75RNT*

Beckman Coulter, Inc. 800-742-2345
250 S Kraemer Blvd, PO Box 8000, Brea, CA 92821

Berghof/America 800-544-5004
3773 NW 126th Ave Bldg 1, Coral Springs, FL 33065
Pure PTFE tube racks for use over temperature range +250 degrees C. Suitable for use in ovens and high temperature thermostats. Can be sterilized repeatedly.

Carolina Biological Supply Co. 800-334-5551
2700 York Rd, Burlington, NC 27215

Dade Behring, Inc. 800-948-3233
1717 Deerfield Rd, Deerfield, IL 60015

Dan Kar Corporation 800-942-5542
PO Box 279, 192 New Boston St C, Wilmington, MA 01887

Globe Scientific, Inc. 800-394-4562
610 Winters Ave, Paramus, NJ 07652
Complete range of test-tube racks.

Healthmark Industries 800-521-6224
22522 E 9 Mile Rd, Saint Clair Shores, MI 48080
$18.15 per unit (50-holes).

Image Molding, Inc. 800-525-1875
4525 Kingston St, Denver, CO 80239
Cardboard and acrylic.

Labcon North America 800-227-1466
3700 Lakeville Hwy Ste 200, Petaluma, CA 94954
Autoclavable, freezable, stackable rack for 24 test tubes.

Nalge Nunc International 800-625-4327
75 Panorama Creek Dr, Rochester, NY 14625
UNWIRE durable, non-corroding plastic racks for test tubes, microvials, collection tubes. Color-coded for easy identification and safety.

Nutech Molding Corporation 1-800-423-5278
PO Box 840, 2024 Broad St,, Pocomoke City, MD 21851

Post Medical, Inc. 800-876-8678
315 Bell Park Dr, Woodstock, GA 30188
Enamel coated wire test tube rack - 32 tube capacity.

Thermosafe Brands 847-398-0110
3930 N Ventura Dr Ste 450, Arlington Heights, IL 60004

Whitney Products, Inc. 800-338-4237
6153 W Mulford St Ste C, Niles, IL 60714
Test n, Toss disposable test tube rack holds up to 72 16 x 100-mm test tubes in a leak-resistant plastic shell. Stackable for storage incubator or refrigerator.

RADIAL IMMUNODIFFUSION, ALBUMIN *(Chemistry) 75CJQ*

Binding Site, Inc., The 800-633-4484
5889 Oberlin Dr Ste 101, San Diego, CA 92121
Immunoglobulin RID kits; CRP RID kit; complement component RID kits; and immunofixation kits.

Kent Laboratories, Inc. 360-398-8641
777 Jorgensen Pl, Bellingham, WA 98226
C-2 radial immunodiffusion.

RADIAL IMMUNODIFFUSION, LIPOPROTEINS *(Chemistry) 75JHP*

Binding Site, Inc., The 800-633-4484
5889 Oberlin Dr Ste 101, San Diego, CA 92121

RADIOASSAY, 17-HYDROXYCORTICOSTEROIDS *(Chemistry) 75JHE*

Bayer Healthcare Llc 914-524-2955
555 White Plains Rd Fl 5, Tarrytown, NY 10591
Test for occult blood in feces.

RADIOASSAY, ANGIOTENSIN CONVERTING ENZYME
(Chemistry) 75KQN

American Laboratory Products Co. 800-592-5726
26 Keewaydin Dr Ste G, Salem, NH 03079
Measure ACE in human serum, non-isotopic enzyme test also available.

Fujirebio Diagnostics, Inc. (Fdi) 877-861-7246
201 Great Valley Pkwy, Malvern, PA 19355
ACE Color Kit Colorimetric. $140.00 per kit (20 tests).

RADIOASSAY, INTRINSIC FACTOR BLOCKING ANTIBODY
(Chemistry) 75LIG

Abbott Diagnostics Intl, Biotechnology Ltd 787-846-3500
Road #2 KM. 58.0 , PO Box 278, Cruce Davila, Barceloneta, PR 00617
Enzyme assay to detect vitamin B12 in human serum or plasma.

RADIOASSAY, TRIIODOTHYRONINE UPTAKE
(Chemistry) 75KHQ

Calbiotech, Inc. 619-660-6162
10461 Austin Dr Ste G, Spring Valley, CA 91978
T-uptake elisa.

Health Chem Diagnostics Llc 954-979-3845
3341 W McNab Rd, Pompano Beach, FL 33069
Radioassay, triiodothyronine uptake.

Hemagen Diagnostics, Inc. 800-436-2436
9033 Red Branch Rd, Columbia, MD 21045
Various thyronine uptake methods.

Medicorp, Inc. 514-733-1900
5800 Royalmount, Montreal, QUE H4P 1K5 Canada

RADIOAUTOGRAPHIC EQUIPMENT *(Chemistry) 75UHP*

Electron Microscopy Sciences 800-523-5874
321 Morris Rd, Fort Washington, PA 19034

Polysciences, Inc. 800-523-2575
400 Valley Rd, Warrington, PA 18976
Ilford emulsions.

RADIOGRAPHIC PICTURE ARCHIVING/COMMUNICATION SYSTEM (PACS) *(Radiology) 90UMF*

Agfa Corp. 800-581-2432
100 Challenger Rd, Ridgefield Park, NJ 07660

AMD Technologies Inc. 800-423-3535
218 Bronwood Ave, Los Angeles, CA 90049
Catella voice-activated digital workstations: diagnostic and clinical review, digitizer stations, archives up to 95 TB, dictation and transcription, Web distribution. Call for literature or assistance and details.

Amicas, Inc. 800-490-8465
20 Guest St Ste 200, Brighton, MA 02135

Brit Systems Inc. 800-230-7227
1909 Hl Line Dr Ste A, Dallas, TX 75207

Dr Systems, Inc. 800-794-5955
10140 Mesa Rim Rd, San Diego, CA 92121
DR Systems PACS is an industry standards compliant workflow-efficiency system that includes: RIS Workstation for patient registration, scheduling, procedure ordering, document scanning, charge capture and management reports. Catapult Technologist Productivity Engine QC Workstation offers technologists with quick and easy to use tools to eliminate DICOM deficiencies and streamline other post processing tasks, providing the radiologists with read ready studies. Dominator Reading Station is the premier radiologist diagnostic tool with available DR Instant Reporter (dictation, reporting, and voice recognition), advanced 3D image processing and featuring DR Systems' exclusive patented auto-hanging protocol technology, automatically displays the radiologist's image format preferences. DR Central Server with a single, unified database stores all exams 'in-progress' and 'read' for the entire imaging enterprise. Communicator Web Server for instant report and image distribution over the Internet.

Elekta, Inc. 800-535-7355
4775 Peachtree Industrial Blvd, Building 300, Suite 300
Norcross, GA 30092
PRECISE NET, communications database to integrate the radiotherapy department with other hospital departments.

Emageon Inc 800-634-5151
900 Walnut Ridge Dr, Hartland, WI 53029
VERICIS for Cardiology - image and information management system for cardiovascular imaging modalities. Real-time digital study review from multiple networked review stations. Integrated physician reporting. Web viewing of images and reports.

RADIOGRAPHIC PICTURE ARCHIVING/COMMUNICATION SYSTEM (PACS) *(cont'd)*

Erad/Image Medical Corp. 864-234-7430
9 Pilgrim Rd Ste 312, Greenville, SC 29607
PracticeBuilder1i2i3™ is a web enabled Image Management System scalable from PACS to teleradiology

Image Systems Corporation 888-735-7373
6103 Blue Circle Dr, Minnetonka, MN 55343
Displays for medical imaging. LCD and CRT, color and greyscale, 9 in. to 24 in. Medical-grade, DICOM-compliant, NTSC to 5 megapixel, diagnostic and clinical. Legacy replacements.

Indec Systems, Inc. 408-986-1600
2210 Martin Ave, Santa Clara, CA 95050

International Radiographic, Inc. 404-405-7909
395 Grand Teton Cir, Fayetteville, GA 30215
PACS, CR, laser printers sales installation Service

Merge Healthcare 877-741-5369
6737 W Washington St Ste 2250, Milwaukee, WI 53214
Integrated RIS/PACS solution

Multi Imager Service, Inc 800-400-4549
13865 Magnolia Ave Bldg C, Chino, CA 91710
Founded in 1983, Multi Imager specializes in diagnostic-quality film imaging and digital imaging technologies, including film-based video imagers, wet-film-based laser imagers, dry-film imagers, digital acquisition/storage and transmission devices, computed radiography, PACS, and more. Multi Imager provides technical support and training, parts supply, and sales of new as well as refurbished equipment used with a broad range of modalities, including CT, MRI, ultrasound, nuclear medicine, and others.

Nai Tech Products 866-342-6629
12919 Earhart Ave, Auburn, CA 95602
MDR Network

Openmed Technologies Corporation 877-717-6215
256 W Cummings Park, Woburn, MA 01801
Complete, web-based, Clinical Image Management and Distribution System fully integrated into MEDITECH and Misys healthcare information systems

Skytron 800-759-8766
5085 Corporate Exchange Blvd SE, Grand Rapids, MI 49512
SkyVision advanced Video, Data and Communications Conrol System for the O.R. permits up to 6 monitors, PACS, GUI Touchscreen Control, optional Teleconferencing.

Sony Electronics, Inc., Medical Systems Div. 800-686-7669
1 Sony Dr, Park Ridge, NJ 07656
Medical image archive system designed to capture, archive, display, annotate and print incoming digital images from diagnostic scanners.

RADIOGRAPHIC UNIT, DIAGNOSTIC *(Radiology) 90KPR*

Advanced Instrument Development, Inc. 800-243-9729
2545 Curtiss St, Downers Grove, IL 60515
Rotor-AID rotor controller, high- and low-speed tube starter. Available for single (radiographic) or multiple tubes (radiographic and fluoroscopic).

Agfa Corporation 877-777-2432
PO Box 19048, 10 South Academy Street, Greenville, SC 29602

Americomp, Inc. 800-458-1782
2901 W Lawrence Ave, Chicago, IL 60625

Amrad 888-772-6723
2901 W Lawrence Ave, Chicago, IL 60625

Burkhart Roentgen Intl. Inc. 800-USA-XRAY
5201 8th Ave S, Gulfport, FL 33707
Portable and full sized units available with bucky and table plus accessories.

Calmaquip Engineering Corp. 305-592-4510
7240 NW 12th St, Miami, FL 33126

Faxitron X-Ray, Llc 888-465-9729
225 Larkin Dr Ste 1, Wheeling, IL 60090
The MX-20, the premium specimen x-ray system, provides unparalleled image resolution of breast specimens such as large-core needle biopsies. Specimens can be x-rayed, in the Film System, at up to 5x magnification. The versatility of the MX-20 is increased by adding digital camera options.

Ge Medical Systems, Llc 262-548-2355
3000 N Grandview Blvd, W-417, Waukesha, WI 53188
Various models of digital radiographic stationary x-ray systems.

Hale Imaging Systems, Inc. 800-321-4253
5314 Mill St, P.O. Box 184, Orient, OH 43146

RADIOGRAPHIC UNIT, DIAGNOSTIC *(cont'd)*

Hologic, Inc. 800-343-9729
35 Crosby Dr, Bedford, MA 01730
EPEX Direct-to-Digital Radiographic System, uses only one digital detector for the entire range of radiographic applications.

I.Z.I. Medical Products, Inc. 800-231-1499
7020 Tudsbury Rd, Baltimore, MD 21244
X-ray skin marker.

Jaco Medical Equipment Inc. 858-278-7743
4848 Ronson Ct Ste E, San Diego, CA 92111

Koch X-Ray Systems Inc 305-252-8770
10500 SW 184th Ter, Cutler Bay, FL 33157
X-ray equipment, Processors & Accessories, Service, Moving, Purchase of pre-owned x-ray

Kretchmer Corp., The 847-564-0323
3611 Commercial Ave, Northbrook, IL 60062

Marconi Medical Systems 800-323-0550
595 Miner Rd, Cleveland, OH 44143
Clinix Systems.

Mbi, Inc. 702-259-1999
1353 Arville St, Las Vegas, NV 89102
Bolin x-ray filter system.

Medimaging Tecnology, Inc. 800-244-9035
49 Herb Hill Rd, Glen Cove, NY 11542

Medlink Imaging, Inc. 800-456-7800
200 Clearbrook Rd, Elmsford, NY 10523

Minxray, Inc. 800-221-2245
3611 Commercial Ave, Northbrook, IL 60062

Owens Scientific Inc. 281-394-2311
23230 Sandsage Ln, Katy, TX 77494
Non-invasive x-ray test equipment.

Quantum Medical Imaging, Llc 631-567-5800
2002 Orville Dr N Ste B, Ronkonkoma, NY 11779
Radiographic x-ray system.

Raymax Medical Corp. 905-791-3020
20 Strathearn Ave, Unit 3, Brampton, ONT L6T 4P7 Canada
System '2100'-general radiographic unit

Sim Net, Inc. 804-752-2776
10471 Cobbs Rd, Glen Allen, VA 23059
X-ray machine.

Summit Industries, Inc. 800-729-9729
2901 W Lawrence Ave, Chicago, IL 60625
Radiographic equipment.

Toshiba America Medical Systems 800-421-1968
2441 Michelle Dr, Tustin, CA 92780
Stationary

Virtual Imaging, Inc. 954-428-6191
720 S Powerline Rd Ste E, Deerfield Bch, FL 33442
Stationary radiographic systems.

Xma (X-Ray Marketing Associates, Inc.) 800-325-8880
1205 W Lakeview Ct, Windham Lakes Business Park
Romeoville, IL 60446

RADIOGRAPHIC UNIT, DIAGNOSTIC, CHEST *(Radiology) 90QJT*

Control-X Medical, Inc. 800-777-9729
1755 Atlas St, Columbus, OH 43228

Del Medical Systems 800-800-6006
11550 King St, Franklin Park, IL 60131

Marconi Medical Systems 800-323-0550
595 Miner Rd, Cleveland, OH 44143

Medlink Imaging, Inc. 800-456-7800
200 Clearbrook Rd, Elmsford, NY 10523

RADIOGRAPHIC UNIT, DIAGNOSTIC, DENTAL (X-RAY)
(Dental And Oral) 76RNY

Alara Inc. 800-410-2525
47505 Seabridge Dr, Fremont, CA 94538

D & N Micro Products, Inc. 260-484-6414
2721 Corrinado Ct, Fort Wayne, IN 46808

Del Medical Systems 800-800-6006
11550 King St, Franklin Park, IL 60131

Dencraft 800-328-9729
PO Box 57, Moorestown, NJ 08057
X-Ray (interora) - panoramic.

Dntlworks Equipment Corporation 800-847-0694
7300 S Tucson Way, Centennial, CO 80112
Portable, digitally-capable x-ray unit with carrying cases.

RADIOGRAPHIC UNIT, DIAGNOSTIC, DENTAL (X-RAY) *(cont'd)*

Instrumentarium Imaging, Inc. 800-558-6120
300 W Edgerton Ave, Milwaukee, WI 53207

Mobile Dental Equipment Corp.(M-Dec) 425-747-5424
13300 SE 30th St Ste 101, Bellevue, WA 98005
PORT-XD, $5370.00 w/case & stand. PORT-XP, portable pediatric X-ray with several sizes of beam limiters and comes with orthoposer lead shield. PORT-XV, portable veterinary X-ray with several sizes of beam limiters.

Panoramic Corporation 800-654-2027
4321 Goshen Rd, Fort Wayne, IN 46818
Panoramic X-ray machines primarily used in dental offices and hospital trauma centers for taking non-invasive radiography of the oral cavity.

Planmeca U.S.A. Inc 630-529-2300
100 Gary Ave Ste A, Roselle, IL 60172
Panoramic X-Ray: film-based and digital panoramic and ceph imaging. EC Classic, Proline EC, Proline CC, ProMax.

Progeny Dental 888-924-3800
1407 Barclay Blvd, Buffalo Grove, IL 60089
JB-70 Dental Intraoral X-ray

Ti-Ba Enterprises, Inc. 585-247-1212
25 Hytec Cir, Rochester, NY 14606
Ti-Ba sells all the Kodak Dental Systems. The new Kodak 2100 and Kodak 2200 Intraoral X-ray Systems are now available.

York X-Ray And Orthopedic Supply, Inc. 800-334-6427
PO Box 326, 20 Hampton Rd.,, Lyman, SC 29365

RADIOGRAPHIC UNIT, DIAGNOSTIC, DENTAL, EXTRAORAL
(Dental And Oral) 76EHD

Aribex, Inc. 801-226-5522
744 S 400 E, Orem, UT 84097
Nomad dental x-ray system.

Cavitat Medical Technologies, Inc. 903-473-1710
118 S Texas St, PO Box 879, Emory, TX 75440
Cavitat ultrasonograph.

Dentalez Group 866-DTE-INFO
101 Lindenwood Dr Ste 225, Valleybrooke Corporate Center
Malvern, PA 19355

Dentalez Group, Stardental Division 717-291-1161
1816 Colonial Village Ln, Lancaster, PA 17601
Portable hdx intraoral x-ray system.

Dp Manufacture Corp. 305-640-9894
1460 NW 107th Ave Ste H, Doral, FL 33172
Bellini x-70.

Electronic Control Concepts 800-847-9729
160 Partition St, Saugerties, NY 12477
X-ray timer

Imaging Sciences International, Llc 215-997-5666
1910 N Penn Rd, Hatfield, PA 19440
Panoramic and tomographic x-ray machine.

Instrumentarium Imaging, Inc. 800-558-6120
300 W Edgerton Ave, Milwaukee, WI 53207

Practiceworks Systems, Llc. 800-944-6365
1765 the Exchange SE, Atlanta, GA 30339
Various types of extraoral source x-ray systems.

Progeny, Inc. 847-415-9800
675 Heathrow Dr, Lincolnshire, IL 60069
Dental x-ray system.

Tg Group 800-338-6236
10721 Keele St., P.O. Box 580, Maple, ONT L6A-1S5 Canada
X Genus AC/DC x-ray machine.

RADIOGRAPHIC UNIT, DIAGNOSTIC, FIXED (X-RAY)
(Radiology) 90RNZ

Control-X Medical, Inc. 800-777-9729
1755 Atlas St, Columbus, OH 43228

Del Medical Systems 800-800-6006
11550 King St, Franklin Park, IL 60131

Marconi Medical Systems 800-323-0550
595 Miner Rd, Cleveland, OH 44143

Shimadzu Medical Systems 800-228-1429
20101 S Vermont Ave, Torrance, CA 90502
4-way table Floating Top, 4-way Elevator Table, 4-way Elevator, tilt 90/15.

York X-Ray And Orthopedic Supply, Inc. 800-334-6427
PO Box 326, 20 Hampton Rd.,, Lyman, SC 29365

RADIOGRAPHIC UNIT, DIAGNOSTIC, HEAD *(Radiology) 90TEA*

Del Medical Systems 800-800-6006
11550 King St, Franklin Park, IL 60131

RADIOGRAPHIC UNIT, DIAGNOSTIC, INTRAORAL
(Dental And Oral) 76EAP

Certol International, Llc 303-799-9401
6120 E 58th Ave, Commerce City, CO 80022
Nonsterile,surface barrier.

Del Medical Systems 800-800-6006
11550 King St, Franklin Park, IL 60131

Dentalez Group, Stardental Division 717-291-1161
1816 Colonial Village Ln, Lancaster, PA 17601
X-ray machine, dental.

Ge Medical Systems, Llc 262-548-2355
3000 N Grandview Blvd, W-417, Waukesha, WI 53188
Dental x-ray system, various models.

Patterson Technology Center, Inc 800-475-5036
2202 Althoff Dr, Effingham, IL 62401
Clinical software used for record keeping and image review.

Planmeca U.S.A. Inc 630-529-2300
100 Gary Ave Ste A, Roselle, IL 60172
DIXI digital CCD sensor intraoral x-ray imaging system. PLANMECA INTRA DC generated intraoral x-ray.

The Gotzen Group, Inc. 905-607-1494
7-3505 Laird Rd, Mississauga L5L 5Y7 Canada
Image x system

RADIOGRAPHIC UNIT, DIAGNOSTIC, MAMMOGRAPHIC
(Radiology) 90IZH

American Mammographics, Inc. 423-624-9530
1302 Shawhan Ter, Chattanooga, TN 37411
Mammographic accessories, mammographic spot compression platforms & paddle; scre.

Ar Custom Medical Products, Ltd. 516-242-7501
19 W Industry Ct Ste A, Deer Park, NY 11729
Mammographic image receptor support device.

Bay Shore Medical Equipment Corp. 631-586-1991
235 S Fehr Way, Bay Shore, NY 11706
No common name listed.

Biocompatibles Inc. 877-783-5463
115 Hurley Rd Bldg 3, Oxford, CT 06478
Lorad needle guide.

Del Medical Systems 800-800-6006
11550 King St, Franklin Park, IL 60131

Frank Scholz X-Ray Corp. 508-586-8308
244 Liberty St, Brockton, MA 02301
$589.00 per unit (standard).

Ge Medical Systems, Llc 262-548-2355
3000 N Grandview Blvd, W-417, Waukesha, WI 53188
Mmx-2.

Health Care Exports, Inc. 800-847-0173
5701 NW 74th Ave, Miami, FL 33166
New and refurbished.

Instrumentarium Imaging, Inc. 800-558-6120
300 W Edgerton Ave, Milwaukee, WI 53207
$55,000 to $65,000 for ALPHA diagnostic mammography systems.

Linear Medical Corporation 303-962-5730
1130 W 124th Ave Ste 400, Westminster, CO 80234
Mammographic x-ray system.

Liv International Usa, Inc. 909-931-1719
2335 W Foothill Blvd, Suite 14 And 15, Upland, CA 91786
Liv(tm) breast self examination aid.

Lorad, A Hologic Company 800-321-4659
36 Apple Ridge Rd, Danbury, CT 06810
Elite system.

Marconi Medical Systems 800-323-0550
595 Miner Rd, Cleveland, OH 44143
Preference mammography system.

Mbf Sales, Llc 480-422-6742
7025 E Greenway Pkwy Ste 250, Scottsdale, AZ 85254
Breast self-exam pad.

Medical Coaches, Inc. 607-432-1333
399 County Highway 58, P.O. Box 129, Oneonta, NY 13820
Mobile mammography, multiphasic medical, general x-ray, and CT mobile coaches available.

RADIOGRAPHIC UNIT, DIAGNOSTIC, MAMMOGRAPHIC *(cont'd)*

Sante Feminine Limited 678-314-1649
1649 Sands Pl SE Ste C, Marietta, GA 30067
Mammographic accessory and or aid for breast self-examination.

Traxyz Medical, Inc. 781-249-6254
24 Lido Ln, Bedford, MA 01730
Traxyloc-1 system.

RADIOGRAPHIC UNIT, DIAGNOSTIC, MOBILE, EXPLOSION-SAFE *(Radiology) 90IZK*

Health Care Exports, Inc. 800-847-0173
5701 NW 74th Ave, Miami, FL 33166
Refurbished mobile x-ray units.

Marconi Medical Systems 800-323-0550
595 Miner Rd, Cleveland, OH 44143

RADIOGRAPHIC UNIT, DIAGNOSTIC, PHOTOFLUOROGRAPHIC
(Radiology) 90IZG

Advanced Spine Technology, Inc. 415-241-2400
457 Mariposa St, San Francisco, CA 94107
Radiographic discography kit.

RADIOGRAPHIC UNIT, DIAGNOSTIC, PORTABLE (X-RAY)
(Radiology) 90ROB

Marconi Medical Systems 800-323-0550
595 Miner Rd, Cleveland, OH 44143

RADIOGRAPHIC UNIT, DIAGNOSTIC, TOMOGRAPHIC
(Radiology) 90IZF

Del Medical Systems 800-800-6006
11550 King St, Franklin Park, IL 60131

Ge Medical Systems, Llc 262-548-2355
3000 N Grandview Blvd, W-417, Waukesha, WI 53188
Panoramic x-ray system.

Sim Net, Inc. 804-752-2776
10471 Cobbs Rd, Glen Allen, VA 23059
X-ray maching.

Tingle X-Ray Llc 349-162-3905
5481 Skyland Blvd E, Coaling, AL 35453
X-ray control with high voltage generator.

RADIOGRAPHIC UNIT, DIGITAL *(Radiology) 90TGL*

Afp Imaging Corp. 800-592-6666
250 Clearbrook Rd, Elmsford, NY 10523

Alara Inc. 800-410-2525
47505 Seabridge Dr, Fremont, CA 94538
Computed radiography system.

Altek Corp. 301-572-2555
12210 Plum Orchard Dr, Silver Spring, MD 20904
Digitizers for digital radiography; $3,550 for X-ray digitizing includes a backlit digitizer with .001 resolution.

Marconi Medical Systems 800-323-0550
595 Miner Rd, Cleveland, OH 44143

Precise Optics/Pme, Inc. 800-242-6604
239 S Fehr Way, Bay Shore, NY 11706

Stallion Technologies, Inc. 315-476-4330
1201 E Fayette St, Syracuse, NY 13210

Thales Components Corporation 973-812-9000
40G Commerce Way, PO Box 540, Totowa, NJ 07512
Pixium 4600 detector for digital capture of Radiographic Images

RADIOGRAPHIC UNIT, DIGITAL SUBTRACTION ANGIOGRAPHIC (DSA) *(Radiology) 90VLE*

Emergency Medical International 305-362-6050
6065 NW 167th St Ste B18, Hialeah, FL 33015
Add on unit for existing imaging system.

Ge Oec Medical Systems Inc. 800-874-7378
384 Wright Brothers Dr, Salt Lake City, UT 84116
SERIES 9600 Mobile Digital Imaging System with real-time DSA.

Indec Systems, Inc. 408-986-1600
2210 Martin Ave, Santa Clara, CA 95050

Infimed, Inc. 315-453-4545
121 Metropolitan Park Dr, Liverpool, NY 13088
Platinum One DSA and Platinum One RF provides advanced digital image acquisition, processing, review and DICOM communications for general RF, DSA & Urology applications. This innovative digital technolgoy is incredibly flexible and affordable and can be integrated into virtually any new, refurbished or exisiting fluoro or angio room.

RADIOGRAPHIC UNIT, DIGITAL SUBTRACTION ANGIOGRAPHIC (DSA) *(cont'd)*

Marconi Medical Systems — 800-323-0550
595 Miner Rd, Cleveland, OH 44143

Shimadzu Medical Systems — 800-228-1429
20101 S Vermont Ave, Torrance, CA 90502
Digital Subtraction Angiography; Digitex Alpha, Digitex Pro.

Stallion Technologies, Inc. — 315-476-4330
1201 E Fayette St, Syracuse, NY 13210

RADIOGRAPHIC/FLUOROSCOPIC UNIT, ANGIOGRAPHIC

(Radiology) 90IZI

Agfa Healthcare Corp. — 864-421-1815
1 Crosswind Dr, Westerly, RI 02891
Dicomview 'accessory to angiographic x-ray system'.

Chromodynamics — 732-730-1877
1195 Airport Rd, Lakewood, NJ 08701
HSi-300 Hyperspectral imaging System

Emergency Medical International — 305-362-6050
6065 NW 167th St Ste B18, Hialeah, FL 33015
Cathlab.

Medical Imaging Solutions, Inc. — 504-733-9729
800 Central Ave, Jefferson, LA 70121
Angiographic x-ray system.

Navilyst Medical — 800-833-9973
100 Boston Scientific Way, Marlborough, MA 01752
Various types of contrast management systems and accessories and contrast manage.

Optimed Technologies, Inc. — 973-575-9911
20 New Dutch Ln, Fairfield, NJ 07004
Central image library optical disk arching system.

Shimadzu Medical Systems — 800-228-1429
20101 S Vermont Ave, Torrance, CA 90502
Remote Radiographic/Fluoroscopic; RS 110.

Stallion Technologies, Inc. — 315-476-4330
1201 E Fayette St, Syracuse, NY 13210

Sterimed, Inc. — 770-387-0771
10 River Ct., Cartersville, GA 30120
Disposable fluoroscope and general equipment covers.

Toshiba America Medical Systems — 800-421-1968
2441 Michelle Dr, Tustin, CA 92780
Available models include 450D12A, 450D14A, 450D16A, 450D12A/PF, 450D14A/PF, 450D16A/PF, V1-UDP/100G-Infinix DP, V1-ASP/100G/3D-Infinix VC/3D, V1-ASP/100G-Infinix VC, V1-ABP/INF/3D-Infinix NB/3D, V1-ABP/INF-Infinix NB, V1-CSPC/100G-Infinix CC, V1-CBP/INF-Infinix CB, V1-CSPF/100G.

RADIOGRAPHIC/FLUOROSCOPIC UNIT, ANGIOGRAPHIC, DIGITAL *(Radiology) 90VHC*

Afp Imaging Corp. — 800-592-6666
250 Clearbrook Rd, Elmsford, NY 10523
Mobile image intensifier. C-Arm/rotating and stationary anode.

Infimed, Inc. — 315-453-4545
121 Metropolitan Park Dr, Liverpool, NY 13088
Platinum One DSA and Platinum One RF provides advanced digital image acquisition, processing, review and DICOM communications for general RF, DSA & Urology applications. This innovative digital technolgoy is incredibly flexible and affordable and can be integrated into virtually any new, refurbished or exisiting fluoro or angio room.

Stallion Technologies, Inc. — 315-476-4330
1201 E Fayette St, Syracuse, NY 13210

RADIOGRAPHIC/FLUOROSCOPIC UNIT, FIXED

(Radiology) 90QWR

Marconi Medical Systems — 800-323-0550
595 Miner Rd, Cleveland, OH 44143
Elite Systems and Clinix Systems.

Precise Optics/Pme, Inc. — 800-242-6604
239 S Fehr Way, Bay Shore, NY 11706

Stallion Technologies, Inc. — 315-476-4330
1201 E Fayette St, Syracuse, NY 13210

RADIOGRAPHIC/FLUOROSCOPIC UNIT, IMAGE-INTENSIFIED

(Radiology) 90JAA

Biomni Medical Systems, Inc. — 801-768-0166
160 S 1350 E, Lehi, UT 84043
CONTRAST-EASE Catheter Pacifier - Oral contrast media for radiological examination of the upper gastro-intestinal tract in infants and small children.

Brand X-Ray Co., Inc. — 630-543-5331
910 S Westwood Ave, Addison, IL 60101
Tube, x-ray.

Direx Systems Corp. — 339-502-6013
437 Turnpike St, Canton, MA 02021
Various models of fluoroscopic x-ray systems.

Dmx-Works, Inc. — 800-839-6757
4159 Corporate Ct Ste B, Palm Harbor, FL 34683
Various models of digital motion x-ray systems.

Ep Technologies, Inc. — 888-272-1001
2710 Orchard Pkwy, San Jose, CA 95134
Dc-coupled, isolated preamplifier.

Ge Medical Systems, Llc — 262-548-2355
3000 N Grandview Blvd, W-417, Waukesha, WI 53188
Mobile image intensifier unit.

Ge Oec Medical Systems — 978-552-5200
439 S Union St, Lawrence, MA 01843
Image guided surgical system.

Ge Oec Medical Systems Inc. — 800-874-7378
384 Wright Brothers Dr, Salt Lake City, UT 84116
SERIES 9600, COMPACT 7600, MINI-6600 and UROVIEW 2600 Mobile Digital Imaging Systems. Urology table with imaging.

I.Z.I. Medical Products, Inc. — 800-231-1499
7020 Tudsbury Rd, Baltimore, MD 21244
X-ray skin marker.

Image Diagnostics, Inc. — 978-422-8601
98 Pratts Junction Rd, Sterling, MA 01564
Arboards.

Lakeshore Technologies Inc. — 315-699-2975
7536 W Murray Dr, Cicero, NY 13039
Digital spot system.

Lifecare Imaging Intl., Ltd. — 815-477-1291
8411 Pyott Rd, Lake In The Hills, IL 60156
Mobilefluoroscopic c-arm.

Lixi, Inc. — 847-961-6666
11980 Oak Creek Pkwy, Huntley, IL 60142
Various models of lixiscope.

Medical Metrics, Inc. — 713-850-7500
4600 Post Oak Place Dr Ste 359, Houston, TX 77027
Kimax 1024.

Minrad, Inc. — 716-855-1068
50 Cobham Dr, Orchard Park, NY 14127
Remote control drape.

Omega Medical Imaging, Inc. — 407-323-9400
675 Hickman Cir, Sanford, FL 32771
C-arm and cantilevered table.

Precise Optics/Pme, Inc. — 800-242-6604
239 S Fehr Way, Bay Shore, NY 11706

Smith & Nephew Inc., Endoscopy Div. — 978-749-1000
76 S Meridian Ave, Oklahoma City, OK 73107
Discography system.

Stallion Technologies, Inc. — 315-476-4330
1201 E Fayette St, Syracuse, NY 13210

Tidi Products, Llc — 920-751-4380
570 Enterprise Dr, Neenah, WI 54956
Drape for image intensifier, fluoroscope.

Toshiba America Medical Systems — 800-421-1968
2441 Michelle Dr, Tustin, CA 92780
Tosrad Models CH/50, UH/50, UH/80, CPH/50, and UPH/50. Additional models include 450D12A, 450D14A, 450D16A, 450D12A/PF, 450D14A/PF, 450D16A/PF, EPS Plus, Ulti80X12A, Ulti80X12A/PF, Ulti80X16A, Ulti80X16A/PF, Ulti80X14A, Ulti80X14A/PF, XA-0420A--Ultimax/EPS Plus.

World Technologies, Inc. — 847-949-4948
708 Diamond Lake Rd Unit 6, Mundelein, IL 60060
Mobile c-arm.

RADIOGRAPHIC/FLUOROSCOPIC UNIT, MOBILE C-ARM *(Radiology) 90QWS*

Ge Oec Medical Systems Inc. 800-874-7378
384 Wright Brothers Dr, Salt Lake City, UT 84116
MINI-6600 mini C-Arm for use in extremity imaging.

Health Care Exports, Inc. 800-847-0173
5701 NW 74th Ave, Miami, FL 33166
Refurbished surgical image intensifiers/C-arms.

M & I Medical Sales, Inc. 305-663-6444
4711 SW 72nd Ave, Miami, FL 33155

Marconi Medical Systems 800-323-0550
595 Miner Rd, Cleveland, OH 44143
Orbitor-HF.

Shimadzu Medical Systems 800-228-1429
20101 S Vermont Ave, Torrance, CA 90502
3 models: 90/90, 90/45, 90/15, Remote 90/30, WHA-505, WHA-50N, UROMAX.

Stallion Technologies, Inc. 315-476-4330
1201 E Fayette St, Syracuse, NY 13210

Tower Medical System, Ltd. 631-699-3200
917 Lincoln Ave Ste 11, Holbrook, NY 11741
FCA 1000- Fixed Height C-Arm Table

Ziehm Imaging, Inc. 800-503-4952
4531 36th Street, Orlando, 32811 92501-1729
Ziehm Vision mobile C-arm; Ziehm Vista mobile C-arm; Ziehm 7000 mobile C-arm; Ziehm Compact mobile C-arm

RADIOGRAPHIC/FLUOROSCOPIC UNIT, NON-IMAGE-INTENSIFIED *(Radiology) 90JAB*

Stallion Technologies, Inc. 315-476-4330
1201 E Fayette St, Syracuse, NY 13210

RADIOGRAPHIC/FLUOROSCOPIC UNIT, SPECIAL PROCEDURE *(Radiology) 90THR*

Infimed, Inc. 315-453-4545
121 Metropolitan Park Dr, Liverpool, NY 13088
Platinum One DSA and Platinum One RF provides advanced digital image acquisition, processing, review and DICOM communications for general RF, DSA & Urology applications. This innovative digital technolgoy is incredibly flexible and affordable and can be integrated into virtually any new, refurbished or exisiting fluoro or angio room.

Precise Optics/Pme, Inc. 800-242-6604
239 S Fehr Way, Bay Shore, NY 11706

Shimadzu Medical Systems 800-228-1429
20101 S Vermont Ave, Torrance, CA 90502
5 models: angio, cardiac and neuro.

Stallion Technologies, Inc. 315-476-4330
1201 E Fayette St, Syracuse, NY 13210

RADIOIMMUNOASSAY, 17-HYDROXYPROGESTERONE *(Chemistry) 75JLX*

Beckman Coulter Inc. 800-231-7970
445 Medical Center Blvd, Webster, TX 77598
17alpha-OH Progesterone RIA and EIA

Bio-Analysis, Inc. 310-828-7423
1701 Berkeley St, Santa Monica, CA 90404
17-hydroxyprogesterone.

Neo-Genesis, A Division Of Natus 503-657-8000
15140 SE 82nd Dr Ste 270, Clackamas, OR 97015
Galactose test system.

Neometrics, A Division Of Natus 800-645-3616
150 Motor Pkwy Ste 203, Hauppauge, NY 11788
Neonatal Blood Spot 17P

RADIOIMMUNOASSAY, ACTH *(Chemistry) 75CKG*

American Laboratory Products Co. 800-592-5726
26 Keewaydin Dr Ste G, Salem, NH 03079
ELISA Adrenocorticotropic hormone. Quantitative ELISA to determine ACTH in plasma.

Beckman Coulter Inc. 800-231-7970
445 Medical Center Blvd, Webster, TX 77598
ACTH RIA

Celsis Laboratory Group 800-523-5227
165 Fieldcrest Ave, Edison, NJ 08837

Nichols Institute Diagnostics 949-940-7200
1311 Calle Batido, San Clemente, CA 92673
Multiple.

RADIOIMMUNOASSAY, ACTH *(cont'd)*

Scantibodies Laboratory, Inc. 619-258-9300
9336 Abraham Way, Santee, CA 92071
Acth irma.

RADIOIMMUNOASSAY, ALDOSTERONE *(Chemistry) 75CJM*

Beckman Coulter Inc. 800-231-7970
445 Medical Center Blvd, Webster, TX 77598
Aldosterone RIA

Diagnostics Biochem Canada Inc. 519-681-8731
1020 Hargrieve Rd., London, ONT N6E 1P5 Canada
$60.00 for 100 assay tubes.

Health Chem Diagnostics Llc 954-979-3845
3341 W McNab Rd, Pompano Beach, FL 33069
Radioimmunoassay, aldosterone.

RADIOIMMUNOASSAY, ANDROSTENEDIONE *(Chemistry) 75CIZ*

Beckman Coulter Inc. 800-231-7970
445 Medical Center Blvd, Webster, TX 77598
Androstenedione RIA and EIA

Diagnostics Biochem Canada Inc. 519-681-8731
1020 Hargrieve Rd., London, ONT N6E 1P5 Canada
$80.00 for 100 assay tubes, double antibody, liquid phase. $92.00 for 100 assay tubes, coated tubes, solid phase.

RADIOIMMUNOASSAY, ANGIOTENSIN I AND RENIN *(Chemistry) 75CIB*

American Laboratory Products Co. 800-592-5726
26 Keewaydin Dr Ste G, Salem, NH 03079
Quantitative angiotensin II to assist in diagnosis of hypertension of renal origin.

Beckman Coulter Inc. 800-231-7970
445 Medical Center Blvd, Webster, TX 77598
Renin IRMA

Health Chem Diagnostics Llc 954-979-3845
3341 W McNab Rd, Pompano Beach, FL 33069
Radioimmunoassay, angiotensin i and renin.

Nichols Institute Diagnostics 949-940-7200
1311 Calle Batido, San Clemente, CA 92673
Multiple.

RADIOIMMUNOASSAY, C PEPTIDES OF PROINSULIN *(Chemistry) 75JKD*

Beckman Coulter Inc. 800-231-7970
445 Medical Center Blvd, Webster, TX 77598
C-Peptide of Insulin RIA and ELISA

Diasorin Inc 800-328-1482
1951 Northwestern Ave S, PO Box 285, Stillwater, MN 55082

RADIOIMMUNOASSAY, CALCITONIN *(Chemistry) 75JKR*

Beckman Coulter Inc. 800-231-7970
445 Medical Center Blvd, Webster, TX 77598
Calcitonin RIA and Ultra-Sensitive Calcitonin RIA

Nichols Institute Diagnostics 949-940-7200
1311 Calle Batido, San Clemente, CA 92673
Multiple.

Scantibodies Laboratory, Inc. 619-258-9300
9336 Abraham Way, Santee, CA 92071
Calcitonin irma.

RADIOIMMUNOASSAY, CANNABINOID (S) *(Toxicology) 91LAT*

Psychemedics Corp. 800-628-8073
125 Nagog Park Ste 200, Acton, MA 01720

Psychmedics Corp. 978-206-8220
125 Nagog Park, Acton, MA 01720

RADIOIMMUNOASSAY, CHOLYGLYCINE, BILE ACIDS *(Chemistry) 75KWW*

Diazyme Laboratories 858-455-4761
12889 Gregg Ct, Poway, CA 92064
Total bile acids assay.

Genzyme Corp. 800-325-2436
160 Christian St, Oxford, CT 06478
Enzymatic, rate, 405/415 NM.

Teco Diagnostics 714-693-7788
1268 N Lakeview Ave, Anaheim, CA 92807
Bile acids reagent set.

RADIOIMMUNOASSAY, COCAINE METABOLITE
(Toxicology) 91KLN

Myers-Stevens Group, Inc. 903-566-6696
2931 Vail Ave, Commerce, CA 90040
Eia test for the detection of cocaine metabolites.

Psychemedics Corp. 800-628-8073
125 Nagog Park Ste 200, Acton, MA 01720

Psychmedics Corp. 978-206-8220
125 Nagog Park, Acton, MA 01720

RADIOIMMUNOASSAY, CORTISOL *(Chemistry) 75CGR*

Beckman Coulter Inc. 800-231-7970
445 Medical Center Blvd, Webster, TX 77598
Cortisol RIA and EIA and Cortisol (saliva) EIA

Bio-Rad Laboratories, Life Science Group 800-424-6723
2000 Alfred Nobel Dr, Hercules, CA 94547

Health Chem Diagnostics Llc 954-979-3845
3341 W McNab Rd, Pompano Beach, FL 33069
Radioimmunoassay, cortisol.

Immunospec Corporation 818-717-1840
9428 Eton Ave Ste O, Chatsworth, CA 91311
Cortisol.

Nichols Institute Diagnostics 949-940-7200
1311 Calle Batido, San Clemente, CA 92673
Multiple.

United Biotech, Inc. 650-961-2910
211 S Whisman Rd Ste E, Mountain View, CA 94041
ELISAs for detecting Human Steroid Hormones including: Cortisol, Product code: SH101; Estriol, Product code: SH202; Progesterone, Product code: SH301; Testosterone, Product code: SH401

RADIOIMMUNOASSAY, CYCLIC AMP *(Chemistry) 75CHO*

Biomedical Technologies, Inc. 781-344-9942
378 Page St, Stoughton, MA 02072
$295 per kit of 200 tubes.

Diasorin Inc 800-328-1482
1951 Northwestern Ave S, PO Box 285, Stillwater, MN 55082

RADIOIMMUNOASSAY, CYCLIC GMP *(Chemistry) 75CGT*

Biomedical Technologies, Inc. 781-344-9942
378 Page St, Stoughton, MA 02072
$295 per kit of 200 tubes.

Health Chem Diagnostics Llc 954-979-3845
3341 W McNab Rd, Pompano Beach, FL 33069
Radioimmunoassay, cyclic gmp.

RADIOIMMUNOASSAY, DEHYDROEPIANDROSTERONE (FREE AND SULFATE) *(Chemistry) 75JKC*

Beckman Coulter Inc. 800-231-7970
445 Medical Center Blvd, Webster, TX 77598
DHEA-S RIA, DHEA-S-7 RIA and EIA, DHEA-S-7 (saliva) RIA and EIA, DHEA RIA and EIA

Calbiotech, Inc. 619-660-6162
10461 Austin Dr Ste G, Spring Valley, CA 91978
Dhea-s elisa.

Immunalysis Corporation 909-482-0840
829 Towne Center Dr, Pomona, CA 91767
No common name listed.

Nichols Institute Diagnostics 949-940-7200
1311 Calle Batido, San Clemente, CA 92673
Dhea sulfate only test system.

RADIOIMMUNOASSAY, DESOXYCORTICOSTERONE
(Chemistry) 75JLE

Health Chem Diagnostics Llc 954-979-3845
3341 W McNab Rd, Pompano Beach, FL 33069
Radioimmunoassay, desoxycorticosterone.

RADIOIMMUNOASSAY, DIGITOXIN (3-H), RABBIT ANTIBODY, CHAR. *(Toxicology) 91DNW*

Health Chem Diagnostics Llc 954-979-3845
3341 W McNab Rd, Pompano Beach, FL 33069
Radioimmunoassay, digitoxin (3-h), rabbit antibody, charcoal sep.

RADIOIMMUNOASSAY, DIGOXIN *(Toxicology) 91DPI*

Monobind, Inc. 800-854-6265
100 N Pointe Dr, Lake Forest, CA 92630
$33.00/test kit of 100 Digoxin coated tubes.

RADIOIMMUNOASSAY, DIGOXIN (125-I), RABBIT, CHARCOAL
(Toxicology) 91DPB

Bio-Rad Laboratories, Life Science Group 800-424-6723
2000 Alfred Nobel Dr, Hercules, CA 94547

Dade Behring, Inc. 800-948-3233
1717 Deerfield Rd, Deerfield, IL 60015

RADIOIMMUNOASSAY, DIGOXIN (3-H), RABBIT, CHARCOAL
(Toxicology) 91DPD

Health Chem Diagnostics Llc 954-979-3845
3341 W McNab Rd, Pompano Beach, FL 33069
Radioimmunoassay, digoxin (3-h), rabbit antibody, charcoal sep.

RADIOIMMUNOASSAY, ESTRADIOL *(Chemistry) 75CHP*

Beckman Coulter Inc. 800-231-7970
445 Medical Center Blvd, Webster, TX 77598
Estradiol RIA and EIA, Ultra-Sensitive Estradiol RIA, 3rd Generation Estradiol RIA and EIA

Bio-Analysis, Inc. 310-828-7423
1701 Berkeley St, Santa Monica, CA 90404
Estradiol.

Biocheck, Inc. 650-573-1968
323 Vintage Park Dr, Foster City, CA 94404
Estradiol (e2) eia test kit.

Calbiotech, Inc. 619-660-6162
10461 Austin Dr Ste G, Spring Valley, CA 91978
Estrodiol immunoassy.

Diagnostics Biochem Canada Inc. 519-681-8731
1020 Hargrieve Rd., London, ONT N6E 1P5 Canada
$70.00 for 100 assay tubes, double antibody - liquid phase. $88.00 for 100 assay tubes, coated tubes - solid phase.

Diasorin Inc 800-328-1482
1951 Northwestern Ave S, PO Box 285, Stillwater, MN 55082

Terumo Medical Corporation 800-283-7866
950 Elkton Blvd, P.O.Box 605, Elkton, MD 21921
Same.

RADIOIMMUNOASSAY, ESTRIOL *(Chemistry) 75CGI*

Beckman Coulter Inc. 800-231-7970
445 Medical Center Blvd, Webster, TX 77598
Unconjugated Estriol RIA and EIA

Bio-Rad Laboratories, Life Science Group 800-424-6723
2000 Alfred Nobel Dr, Hercules, CA 94547

Calbiotech, Inc. 619-660-6162
10461 Austin Dr Ste G, Spring Valley, CA 91978
Estriol elisa.

Immunalysis Corporation 909-482-0840
829 Towne Center Dr, Pomona, CA 91767
Ria method to determine free estriol.

RADIOIMMUNOASSAY, ESTRONE *(Chemistry) 75CGF*

Beckman Coulter Inc. 800-231-7970
445 Medical Center Blvd, Webster, TX 77598
Estrone RIA and EIA, Estrone Sulfate RIA and EIA

Calbiotech, Inc. 619-660-6162
10461 Austin Dr Ste G, Spring Valley, CA 91978
Estron elisa.

Diagnostics Biochem Canada Inc. 519-681-8731
1020 Hargrieve Rd., London, ONT N6E 1P5 Canada
$70.00 for 100 assay tubes, double antibody, liquid phase. $88.00 for 100 assay tubes, coated tubes, solid phase.

Immuna Care Corp. 610-941-2167
13654 N 12th St Ste 3, Tampa, FL 33613
Eia kit for serum 16alpha-hydroxyestrone.

RADIOIMMUNOASSAY, FERRITIN *(Microbiology) 83JMG*

Abbott Diagnostics Intl, Biotechnology Ltd 787-846-3500
Road #2 KM. 58.0 , PO Box 278, Cruce Davila, Barceloneta, PR 00617
Ferritin.

Beckman Coulter Inc. 800-231-7970
445 Medical Center Blvd, Webster, TX 77598
Ferritin IRMA

Bio-Rad Laboratories, Life Science Group 800-424-6723
2000 Alfred Nobel Dr, Hercules, CA 94547

Biocheck, Inc. 650-573-1968
323 Vintage Park Dr, Foster City, CA 94404
Ferritin test kit.

RADIOIMMUNOASSAY, FERRITIN *(cont'd)*

Nichols Institute Diagnostics 949-940-7200
1311 Calle Batido, San Clemente, CA 92673
Multiple.

Ramco Laboratories, Inc. 281-313-1200
4100 Greenbriar Dr Ste 200, Stafford, TX 77477
Radioimmunoassay for quantifying the level of ferritin in human serum.

RADIOIMMUNOASSAY, FOLIC ACID *(Chemistry) 75CGN*

Bio-Rad Laboratories Inc., Clinical Systems Div. 800-224-6723
4000 Alfred Nobel Dr, Hercules, CA 94547
B12/folate-radioimmunoassay.

Bio-Rad Laboratories, Life Science Group 800-424-6723
2000 Alfred Nobel Dr, Hercules, CA 94547

Health Chem Diagnostics Llc 954-979-3845
3341 W McNab Rd, Pompano Beach, FL 33069
Acid, folic, radioimmunoassay.

RADIOIMMUNOASSAY, FOLLICLE STIMULATING HORMONE *(Chemistry) 75CGJ*

Abbott Diagnostics Intl, Biotechnology Ltd 787-846-3500
Road #2 KM. 58.0 , PO Box 278, Cruce Davila, Barceloneta, PR 00617
Follicle stimulating hormone.

Beckman Coulter Inc. 800-231-7970
445 Medical Center Blvd, Webster, TX 77598
FSH IRMA and ELISA

Bio-Medical Products Corp. 800-543-7427
10 Halstead Rd, Mendham, NJ 07945
FSH test.

Bio-Rad Laboratories, Life Science Group 800-424-6723
2000 Alfred Nobel Dr, Hercules, CA 94547

Biocheck, Inc. 650-573-1968
323 Vintage Park Dr, Foster City, CA 94404
Follicle-stimulating hormone eia test kit.

Calbiotech, Inc. 619-660-6162
10461 Austin Dr Ste G, Spring Valley, CA 91978
Follicle-stimulating hormone (fsh) elisa.

Celsis Laboratory Group 800-523-5227
165 Fieldcrest Ave, Edison, NJ 08837

Health Chem Diagnostics Llc 954-979-3845
3341 W McNab Rd, Pompano Beach, FL 33069
Radioimmunoassay, follicle-stimulating hormone.

Immunalysis Corporation 909-482-0840
829 Towne Center Dr, Pomona, CA 91767
No common name listed.

Immunospec Corporation 818-717-1840
9428 Eton Ave Ste O, Chatsworth, CA 91311
Fsh eia.

Innovacon, Inc. 858-535-2030
4106 Sorrento Valley Blvd, San Diego, CA 92121
Follicle-stimulating hormone test.

Inverness Medical Professional Diagnostics-San Die 858-535-2030
4106 Sorrento Valley Blvd, San Diego, CA 92121
Follicle-stimulating hormone test.

Medicorp, Inc. 514-733-1900
5800 Royalmount, Montreal, QUE H4P 1K5 Canada
FSH IRMA detection kit; also FSH ELISA.

Monobind, Inc. 800-854-6265
100 N Pointe Dr, Lake Forest, CA 92630
$62.50 per 100-test kit.

Nichols Institute Diagnostics 949-940-7200
1311 Calle Batido, San Clemente, CA 92673
Multiple.

Phamatech Inc. 858-643-5555
10151 Barnes Canyon Rd, San Diego, CA 92121
Fsh rapid test.

Solidphase, Inc. 207-797-0211
1039 Riverside St Ste 3, Portland, ME 04103
Radioimmunoassay for follicle stimulating hormone.

United Biotech, Inc. 650-961-2910
211 S Whisman Rd Ste E, Mountain View, CA 94041
ELISA for detecting FSH (Follicle Stimulating Hormone).

RADIOIMMUNOASSAY, FREE THYROXINE *(Chemistry) 75CEC*

Abbott Diagnostics Intl, Biotechnology Ltd 787-846-3500
Road #2 KM. 58.0 , PO Box 278, Cruce Davila, Barceloneta, PR 00617
Various.

Chemux Bioscience, Inc. 650-872-1800
50 S Linden Ave Ste 7, South San Francisco, CA 94080
Free thyroxine(t4) enzyme immunoassay kits.

Immunospec Corporation 818-717-1840
9428 Eton Ave Ste O, Chatsworth, CA 91311
Free t4 eia.

Nichols Institute Diagnostics 949-940-7200
1311 Calle Batido, San Clemente, CA 92673
Multiple.

Qualigen, Inc. 760-918-9165
2042 Corte Del Nogal, Carlsbad, CA 92011
Chemiluminescence assay for determination of free t4.

RADIOIMMUNOASSAY, GENTAMICIN (125-I), SECOND ANTIBODY *(Toxicology) 91DJB*

Bayer Healthcare, Llc 574-256-3430
430 S Beiger St, Mishawaka, IN 46544
Test for gentamicin in serum or plasma.

RADIOIMMUNOASSAY, HUMAN CHORIONIC GONADOTROPIN *(Chemistry) 75JHI*

Alfa Scientific Designs, Inc. 877-204-5071
13200 Gregg St, Poway, CA 92064
Various.

Ameditech, Inc. 858-535-1968
10340 Camino Santa Fe Ste F, San Diego, CA 92121
Human chorionic gonadotropin hcg test system.

Bayer Healthcare Llc 914-524-2955
555 White Plains Rd Fl 5, Tarrytown, NY 10591
Test for hcg in urine.

Biocheck, Inc. 650-573-1968
323 Vintage Park Dr, Foster City, CA 94404
Free beta-subunit of hcg eia test kit.

Genzyme Diagnostics 617-252-7500
6659 Top Gun St, San Diego, CA 92121
Pregnancy test.

Immunospec Corporation 818-717-1840
9428 Eton Ave Ste O, Chatsworth, CA 91311
Hcg.

Innovacon, Inc. 858-535-2030
4106 Sorrento Valley Blvd, San Diego, CA 92121
Hcg one step pregnancy test device, urine.

Inverness Medical Professional Diagnostics-San Die 858-535-2030
4106 Sorrento Valley Blvd, San Diego, CA 92121
Hcg one step pregnancy test device, urine.

Jas Diagnostics, Inc. 305-418-2320
7220 NW 58th St, Miami, FL 33166
Various combo pregnancy test.

Medicorp, Inc. 514-733-1900
5800 Royalmount, Montreal, QUE H4P 1K5 Canada
HCG IRMA detection kit; also HCG ELISA.

Monobind, Inc. 800-854-6265
100 N Pointe Dr, Lake Forest, CA 92630
$33.00/test kit of 100.

Myers-Stevens Group, Inc. 903-566-6696
2931 Vail Ave, Commerce, CA 90040
Quantitative hcg enzyme assay.

Nichols Institute Diagnostics 949-940-7200
1311 Calle Batido, San Clemente, CA 92673
Multiple.

Nubenco Ent., Inc. 800-633-1322
1 Kalisa Way Ste 207, Paramus, NJ 07652
Immunochromatographical test for the qualitative detection of hcg.

Phamatech Inc. 858-643-5555
10151 Barnes Canyon Rd, San Diego, CA 92121
Hcg rapid test.

Qualis Group Llc 515-243-3000
4600 Park Ave, Des Moines, IA 50321
Platform pregnancy test kit, midstream pregnancy test (1 test), (2 test).

RADIOIMMUNOASSAY, HUMAN CHORIONIC GONADOTROPIN
(cont'd)

Rapid Diagnostics, Div. Of Mp Biomedicals, Llc 800-888-7008
1429 Rollins Rd, Burlingame, CA 94010
HCG pregnancy test.

United Biotech, Inc. 650-961-2910
211 S Whisman Rd Ste E, Mountain View, CA 94041
ELISA for detecting hCG Pregnancy and hCG Quantitative.

W.H.P.M., Inc. 978-927-3808
9662 Telstar Ave, El Monte, CA 91731
Rapid pregnancy test.

RADIOIMMUNOASSAY, HUMAN GROWTH HORMONE
(Chemistry) 75CFL

Beckman Coulter Inc. 800-231-7970
445 Medical Center Blvd, Webster, TX 77598
Human GH IRMA and ELISA, Ultra-Sensitive Human GH ELISA, Immunofunctional Human GH ELISA; Human GHBP ELISA; IGF-I IRMA and ELISA (extraction and non-extraction methods available); Free IGF-I IRMA and ELISA; IGF-II IRMA and ELISA (extraction and non-extraction methods available); IGFBP-1, IGFBP-2, IGFBP-3, IGFBP-4, IGFBP-6 IRMAs and ELISAs; ALS ELISA

Biocheck, Inc. 650-573-1968
323 Vintage Park Dr, Foster City, CA 94404
Common growth hormone eia test kit.

Calbiotech, Inc. 619-660-6162
10461 Austin Dr Ste G, Spring Valley, CA 91978
Human growth hormone (hgh) elisa.

Medicorp, Inc. 514-733-1900
5800 Royalmount, Montreal, QUE H4P 1K5 Canada
GH IRMA detection kit; also GH ELISA.

Nichols Institute Diagnostics 949-940-7200
1311 Calle Batido, San Clemente, CA 92673
Multiple.

RADIOIMMUNOASSAY, IMMUNOGLOBULINS (D, E)
(Immunology) 82JHR

Biocheck, Inc. 650-573-1968
323 Vintage Park Dr, Foster City, CA 94404
Immunoglobulin e eia test kit.

RADIOIMMUNOASSAY, IMMUNOREACTIVE INSULIN
(Chemistry) 75CFP

Beckman Coulter Inc. 800-231-7970
445 Medical Center Blvd, Webster, TX 77598
Insulin RIA and ELISA

Health Chem Diagnostics Llc 954-979-3845
3341 W McNab Rd, Pompano Beach, FL 33069
Radioimmunoassay, immunoreactive insulin.

Ivd Technologies 714-549-5050
2002 S Grand Ave Ste A, Cowan Heights, CA 92705

Kronus, Inc. 800-822-6999
12554 W Bridger St Ste 108, Boise, ID 83713
Insulin antibody kit is an insulin antibody radioimmunoassay test kit for use in prediction and diagnosis of IDDM (Type 1).

Linco Research,Inc. 636-441-8400
6 Research Park Dr, Saint Charles, MO 63304
Insulin radioimmunoassay.

Medicorp, Inc. 514-733-1900
5800 Royalmount, Montreal, QUE H4P 1K5 Canada
Insulin IRMA detection kit.

RADIOIMMUNOASSAY, INFECTIOUS MONONUCLEOSIS
(Microbiology) 83THL

Lifesign 800-526-2125
71 Veronica Ave, Somerset, NJ 08873
UNISTEP-MONO.

RADIOIMMUNOASSAY, LUTEINIZING HORMONE
(Chemistry) 75CEP

Access Bio Incorporate 732-297-2222
2033 Rt. 130 Unit H, Monmouth Junction, NJ 08852
Ovulation test kit.

Alfa Scientific Designs, Inc. 877-204-5071
13200 Gregg St, Poway, CA 92064
Various.

RADIOIMMUNOASSAY, LUTEINIZING HORMONE *(cont'd)*

Ameritek Usa, Inc. 425-379-2580
125 130th St SE Ste 200, Everett, WA 98208
Lh test kit.

Beckman Coulter Inc. 800-231-7970
445 Medical Center Blvd, Webster, TX 77598
LH IRMA and ELISA

Biocheck, Inc. 650-573-1968
323 Vintage Park Dr, Foster City, CA 94404
Luteinizing hormone eia test kit.

Biotech Atlantic, Inc. 732-389-4789
Industrial Way W Bay F6, Eatontown, NJ 07724
Ovulation predictor.

Calbiotech, Inc. 619-660-6162
10461 Austin Dr Ste G, Spring Valley, CA 91978
Luteinizing hormone (lh) elisa.

Celsis Laboratory Group 800-523-5227
165 Fieldcrest Ave, Edison, NJ 08837

Chembio Diagnostic Systems, Inc. 631-924-1135
3661 Horseblock Rd, Medford, NY 11763
Immunochromotographic assay for visual detection of luteinizing hormone.

Germaine Laboratories, Inc. 210-692-4192
4139 Gardendale St Ste 101, San Antonio, TX 78229
Various types, ovulation test.

Immunalysis Corporation 909-482-0840
829 Towne Center Dr, Pomona, CA 91767
Ria method to determine luteinizing hormone in serum.

Innovacon, Inc. 858-535-2030
4106 Sorrento Valley Blvd, San Diego, CA 92121
Ovulation test.

Inverness Medical Professional Diagnostics-San Die 858-535-2030
4106 Sorrento Valley Blvd, San Diego, CA 92121
Ovulation test.

Jant Pharmacal Corp. 800-676-5565
16255 Ventura Blvd Ste 505, Encino, CA 91436
Various.

Medicorp, Inc. 514-733-1900
5800 Royalmount, Montreal, QUE H4P 1K5 Canada
LH IRMA detection kit; also LH ELISA

Monobind, Inc. 800-854-6265
100 N Pointe Dr, Lake Forest, CA 92630
$62.50 per 100-test kit.

Nichols Institute Diagnostics 949-940-7200
1311 Calle Batido, San Clemente, CA 92673
Multiple.

Phamatech Inc. 858-643-5555
10151 Barnes Canyon Rd, San Diego, CA 92121
Ovulation test.

Rapid Diagnostics, Div. Of Mp Biomedicals, Llc 800-888-7008
1429 Rollins Rd, Burlingame, CA 94010
LH test.

Scantibodies Laboratory, Inc. 619-258-9300
9336 Abraham Way, Santee, CA 92071
Various models of ovulation test kits.

Solidphase, Inc. 207-797-0211
1039 Riverside St Ste 3, Portland, ME 04103
Radioimmunoassay for luteinizing hormone.

St. Paul Biotech 714-903-1000
11555 Monarch St, Garden Grove, CA 92841
Ovulation test.

United Biotech, Inc. 650-961-2910
211 S Whisman Rd Ste E, Mountain View, CA 94041
ELISA for detecting LH (Luteinzing Hormone).

RADIOIMMUNOASSAY, MORPHINE (125-I), GOAT ANTIBODY
(Toxicology) 91DOE

Branan Medical Corp. 949-598-7166
140 Technology Dr Ste 400, Irvine, CA 92618
Immunochromatographical test for the qualitative determination of morphine 300.

RADIOIMMUNOASSAY, NETILMICIN (125-I) *(Toxicology) 91LCE*

Bayer Healthcare, Llc 574-256-3430
430 S Beiger St, Mishawaka, IN 46544
Test for netilmicin in serum or plasma.

RADIOIMMUNOASSAY, OTHER *(Chemistry) 75VKJ*

Amgen Inc. 206-265-7000
1201 Amgen Ct W, Seattle, WA 98119
$150 for c-peptide serum RIA kit, CAT #IMX108 IDDT; $160 for c-peptide urine RIA kit, CAT #IMX109 IDDT.

Biomedical Technologies, Inc. 781-344-9942
378 Page St, Stoughton, MA 02072
$310.00 per 100-tube human EGF RIA kit; $325.00 per 100 tubes for human osteocalcin RIA kit. $300 for 100 tubes of human EGF.

Biotecx Laboratories, Inc. 800-535-6286
15225 Gulf Hwy, #F106, Houston, TX 77034
Ty EIA Kit

Cidtech Research Inc. 519-621-3334
1200 Franklin Blvd, Cambridge, ON N1R 6T5 Canada
$230.00 to $350.00 for RIA melatonin antiserum; RIA 6-sulphatoxymelatonin antiserum; nerve growth factor antiserum; RIA metanephrine antiserum; all are for R&D purposes.

Diasorin Inc 800-328-1482
1951 Northwestern Ave S, PO Box 285, Stillwater, MN 55082

Drg International, Inc. 800-321-1167
1167 US Highway 22, Mountainside, NJ 07092

Kronus, Inc. 800-822-6999
12554 W Bridger St Ste 108, Boise, ID 83713
Voltage-Gated Calcium Channel (VGCC) antibody assay kit is a radioimmunoassay test kit for Lambert-Eaton Myasthenic Syndrome (LEMS).

Monobind, Inc. 800-854-6265
100 N Pointe Dr, Lake Forest, CA 92630
ELISA kits containing T3, T4, TSH, LH, FSH, PRL, h-CG, Digoxin, Anti-Tg, Anti-TPO, H-Pyroli, IgC, Igon V IgA

Nuclin Diagnostics, Inc. 847-498-5210
3322 Commercial Ave, Northbrook, IL 60062
Kits and supplies.

Princeton Biomeditech Corp. 732-274-1000
4242 US Highway 1, Monmouth Junction, NJ 08852
LifeSign CHF Nt-proBNP, rapid assay for detection of N-terminal pro-brain natriuretic peptide, indicator for congestive heart failure.

Ramco Laboratories, Inc. 281-313-1200
4100 Greenbriar Dr Ste 200, Stafford, TX 77477
Radioimmunoassay for the quantitation of erythropoietin in serum or plasma (EPO-RIA).

RADIOIMMUNOASSAY, PARATHYROID HORMONE *(Chemistry) 75CEW*

Beckman Coulter Inc. 800-231-7970
445 Medical Center Blvd, Webster, TX 77598
C-PTH RIA, MM-PTH RIA, Intact PTH IRMA and ELISA

Diasorin Inc 800-328-1482
1951 Northwestern Ave S, PO Box 285, Stillwater, MN 55082
PTHMM, N-TACT PTH IRMA (intact PTH I-84).

Nichols Institute Diagnostics 949-940-7200
1311 Calle Batido, San Clemente, CA 92673
Parathyroid hormone (1-84).

Scantibodies Laboratory, Inc. 619-258-9300
9336 Abraham Way, Santee, CA 92071
Pth irma kit.

RADIOIMMUNOASSAY, PHENCYCLIDINE *(Toxicology) 91LCL*

Immunalysis Corporation 909-482-0840
829 Towne Center Dr, Pomona, CA 91767
Ria method to determine phencyclidine in blood.

Psychemedics Corp. 800-628-8073
125 Nagog Park Ste 200, Acton, MA 01720

Psychmedics Corp. 978-206-8220
125 Nagog Park, Acton, MA 01720

RADIOIMMUNOASSAY, PLATELET FACTOR 4 *(Hematology) 81LCO*

Diagnostica Stago, Inc. 800-222-COAG
5 Century Dr, Parsippany, NJ 07054

Genetic Testing Institute 262-754-1000
20925 Crossroads Cir Ste 200, Waukesha, WI 53186
Platelet factor 4 assay.

RADIOIMMUNOASSAY, PROGESTERONE *(Chemistry) 75JLS*

Beckman Coulter Inc. 800-231-7970
445 Medical Center Blvd, Webster, TX 77598
Progesterone RIA and EIA

Bio-Analysis, Inc. 310-828-7423
1701 Berkeley St, Santa Monica, CA 90404
Progesterone.

Biocheck, Inc. 650-573-1968
323 Vintage Park Dr, Foster City, CA 94404
Progesterone eia test kit.

Calbiotech, Inc. 619-660-6162
10461 Austin Dr Ste G, Spring Valley, CA 91978
Progesterone elisa.

Health Chem Diagnostics Llc 954-979-3845
3341 W McNab Rd, Pompano Beach, FL 33069
Radioimmunoassay, progesterone.

Terumo Medical Corporation 800-283-7866
950 Elkton Blvd, P.O.Box 605, Elkton, MD 21921
Terumo sensibead eia progesterone kit.

RADIOIMMUNOASSAY, PROLACTIN (LACTOGEN) *(Chemistry) 75CFT*

Beckman Coulter Inc. 800-231-7970
445 Medical Center Blvd, Webster, TX 77598
Prolactin IRMA and ELISA

Bio-Medical Products Corp. 800-543-7427
10 Halstead Rd, Mendham, NJ 07945
Prolactin test.

Biocheck, Inc. 650-573-1968
323 Vintage Park Dr, Foster City, CA 94404
Prolactin eia test kit.

Calbiotech, Inc. 619-660-6162
10461 Austin Dr Ste G, Spring Valley, CA 91978
Probictin elisa.

Hope Laboratories 650-591-6271
409A Old County Rd, Belmont, CA 94002
Test kit for the quantitative measurement of prolactin in human serum.

Immunospec Corporation 818-717-1840
9428 Eton Ave Ste O, Chatsworth, CA 91311
Prolactin eia.

Medicorp, Inc. 514-733-1900
5800 Royalmount, Montreal, QUE H4P 1K5 Canada
PRL IRMA detection kit; also PRL ELISA.

Monobind, Inc. 800-854-6265
100 N Pointe Dr, Lake Forest, CA 92630
$80.00 per 100-test kit.

Nichols Institute Diagnostics 949-940-7200
1311 Calle Batido, San Clemente, CA 92673
Multiple.

United Biotech, Inc. 650-961-2910
211 S Whisman Rd Ste E, Mountain View, CA 94041
ELISA for detecting Prolactin.

RADIOIMMUNOASSAY, PROSTATE-SPECIFIC ANTIGEN (PSA) *(Immunology) 82MGY*

Beckman Coulter Inc. 800-231-7970
445 Medical Center Blvd, Webster, TX 77598
Total PSA IRMA and ELISA; Free PSA IRMA

United Biotech, Inc. 650-961-2910
211 S Whisman Rd Ste E, Mountain View, CA 94041
ELISA quantitative for detecting PSA (Prostatic Specific Antigen)

RADIOIMMUNOASSAY, T3 UPTAKE *(Chemistry) 75CDY*

Bio-Rad Laboratories, Life Science Group 800-424-6723
2000 Alfred Nobel Dr, Hercules, CA 94547

Monobind, Inc. 800-854-6265
100 N Pointe Dr, Lake Forest, CA 92630
$33.00 per 100-test kit.

RADIOIMMUNOASSAY, T4 *(Chemistry) 75UKB*

Bio-Rad Laboratories, Life Science Group 800-424-6723
2000 Alfred Nobel Dr, Hercules, CA 94547

Dade Behring, Inc. 800-948-3233
1717 Deerfield Rd, Deerfield, IL 60015

Monobind, Inc. 800-854-6265
100 N Pointe Dr, Lake Forest, CA 92630
$33.00/test kit of 100.

RADIOIMMUNOASSAY, TESTOSTERONES AND DIHYDROTESTOSTERONE *(Chemistry) 75CDZ*

Beckman Coulter Inc. 800-231-7970
445 Medical Center Blvd, Webster, TX 77598
Testosterone RIA and EIA; Free Testosterone RIA and EIA

Biocheck, Inc. 650-573-1968
323 Vintage Park Dr, Foster City, CA 94404
Testosterone eia test kit.

Diagnostics Biochem Canada Inc. 519-681-8731
1020 Hargrieve Rd., London, ONT N6E 1P5 Canada
$79.00 for 100 assay tubes, second antibody, liquid phase. $80.00 for 100 assay tubes, coated tubes, solid phase.

Diasorin Inc 800-328-1482
1951 Northwestern Ave S, PO Box 285, Stillwater, MN 55082

Health Chem Diagnostics Llc 954-979-3845
3341 W McNab Rd, Pompano Beach, FL 33069
Radioimmunoassay, testosterones and dihydrotestosterone.

Qualigen, Inc. 760-918-9165
2042 Corte Del Nogal, Carlsbad, CA 92011
Chemiluminescence assay for the determination of total testosterone.

RADIOIMMUNOASSAY, THYROID STIMULATING HORMONE
(Chemistry) 75JLW

Abbott Diagnostics Intl, Biotechnology Ltd 787-846-3500
Road #2 KM. 58.0 , PO Box 278, Cruce Davila, Barceloneta, PR 00617
Microparticle enzyme immunoassay for the quantitative measurement of thyroid sti.

Ameritek Usa, Inc. 425-379-2580
125 130th St SE Ste 200, Everett, WA 98208
Tsh test kit.

Beckman Coulter Inc. 800-231-7970
445 Medical Center Blvd, Webster, TX 77598
TSH IRMA and ELISA

Bio-Medical Products Corp. 800-543-7427
10 Halstead Rd, Mendham, NJ 07945
TSH test.qualatative and quantative test available.

Bio-Rad Laboratories, Life Science Group 800-424-6723
2000 Alfred Nobel Dr, Hercules, CA 94547

Biocheck, Inc. 650-573-1968
323 Vintage Park Dr, Foster City, CA 94404
Sensitive-tsh eia test kit.

Chemux Bioscience, Inc. 650-872-1800
50 S Linden Ave Ste 7, South San Francisco, CA 94080
Tsh enzyme immunoassay kits(eia kits).

Health Chem Diagnostics Llc 954-979-3845
3341 W McNab Rd, Pompano Beach, FL 33069
Radioimmunoassay, thyroid-stimulating hormone.

Immunospec Corporation 818-717-1840
9428 Eton Ave Ste O, Chatsworth, CA 91311
Tsh eia.

Medicorp, Inc. 514-733-1900
5800 Royalmount, Montreal, QUE H4P 1K5 Canada
TSH IRMA detection kit; also TSH ELISA.

Monobind, Inc. 800-854-6265
100 N Pointe Dr, Lake Forest, CA 92630
$50.00 per 100-test kit.

Myers-Stevens Group, Inc. 903-566-6696
2931 Vail Ave, Commerce, CA 90040
Eia test for the quantitation of tsh.

Neo-Genesis, A Division Of Natus 503-657-8000
15140 SE 82nd Dr Ste 270, Clackamas, OR 97015
Galactose test system.

Neometrics, A Division Of Natus 800-645-3616
150 Motor Pkwy Ste 203, Hauppauge, NY 11788
Neonatal blood spot TSH.

Nichols Institute Diagnostics 949-940-7200
1311 Calle Batido, San Clemente, CA 92673
Tsh reagent/kits.

Qualigen, Inc. 760-918-9165
2042 Corte Del Nogal, Carlsbad, CA 92011
Chemiluminescense assay for the determination of thyroid stimulating hormone.

Relia Diagnostic Systems, Llc 415-344-0844
1 Market St Ste 1475, Steuart Tower, San Francisco, CA 94105
Thyroid stimulation hormone test.

RADIOIMMUNOASSAY, THYROID STIMULATING HORMONE
(cont'd)

Repromedix Corp. 781-937-8893
86 Cummings Park, Woburn, MA 01801
Reprobead tsh enzyme immuno assay regent kit.

Scantibodies Laboratory, Inc. 619-258-9300
9336 Abraham Way, Santee, CA 92071
Tsh irma.

Teco Diagnostics 714-693-7788
1268 N Lakeview Ave, Anaheim, CA 92807
Thyroid stimulating hormone (tsh) eia set (bead assay).

United Biotech, Inc. 650-961-2910
211 S Whisman Rd Ste E, Mountain View, CA 94041
ELISA for detecting TSH (Thyroid Stimulating Hormone).

RADIOIMMUNOASSAY, THYROXINE BINDING GLOBULIN
(Chemistry) 75CEE

Neometrics, A Division Of Natus 800-645-3616
150 Motor Pkwy Ste 203, Hauppauge, NY 11788
Neonatal blood spot T4.

RADIOIMMUNOASSAY, TOTAL ESTROGEN, OTHER
(Chemistry) 75JMD

Immuna Care Corp. 610-941-2167
13654 N 12th St Ste 3, Tampa, FL 33613
Eia kit for urinary estrogen metabolites (2-hydroxyestrogen & 16a-hydroxyestrone.

RADIOIMMUNOASSAY, TOTAL THYROXINE *(Chemistry) 75CDX*

Beckman Coulter Inc. 800-231-7970
445 Medical Center Blvd, Webster, TX 77598
T4, Total RIA and EIA

Bio-Rad Laboratories, Life Science Group 800-424-6723
2000 Alfred Nobel Dr, Hercules, CA 94547

Diasorin Inc 800-328-1482
1951 Northwestern Ave S, PO Box 285, Stillwater, MN 55082

Monobind, Inc. 800-854-6265
100 N Pointe Dr, Lake Forest, CA 92630
$33.00 per 100-test kit Total Thyroxine coated tubes.

Neo-Genesis, A Division Of Natus 503-657-8000
15140 SE 82nd Dr Ste 270, Clackamas, OR 97015
Hcg test system.

Solidphase, Inc. 207-797-0211
1039 Riverside St Ste 3, Portland, ME 04103
Radioimmunoassay for total thyroxine (t4).

RADIOIMMUNOASSAY, TOTAL TRIIODOTHYRONINE
(Chemistry) 75CDP

Abbott Diagnostics Intl, Biotechnology Ltd 787-846-3500
Road #2 KM. 58.0 , PO Box 278, Cruce Davila, Barceloneta, PR 00617
Various.

Beckman Coulter Inc. 800-231-7970
445 Medical Center Blvd, Webster, TX 77598
T3, Total RIA and EIA

Bio-Rad Laboratories, Life Science Group 800-424-6723
2000 Alfred Nobel Dr, Hercules, CA 94547

Biocheck, Inc. 650-573-1968
323 Vintage Park Dr, Foster City, CA 94404
Total triiodothyronine eia test kit.

Calbiotech, Inc. 619-660-6162
10461 Austin Dr Ste G, Spring Valley, CA 91978
Triiodothyronine t3 elisa.

Chemux Bioscience, Inc. 650-872-1800
50 S Linden Ave Ste 7, South San Francisco, CA 94080
Total triiodothyronine (t3) enzyme immunoassay kits.

Health Chem Diagnostics Llc 954-979-3845
3341 W McNab Rd, Pompano Beach, FL 33069
Radioimmunoassay, total triiodothyronine.

Monobind, Inc. 800-854-6265
100 N Pointe Dr, Lake Forest, CA 92630
$33.00 per 100-test kit T3 coated tubes.

Nichols Institute Diagnostics 949-940-7200
1311 Calle Batido, San Clemente, CA 92673
Multiple.

Repromedix Corp. 781-937-8893
86 Cummings Park, Woburn, MA 01801
Reprobead t3 enyme immuno assay reagent kit.

RADIOIMMUNOASSAY, TRICYCLIC ANTIDEPRESSANT DRUGS
(Toxicology) 91LFG

American Bio Medica Corp. 800-227-1243
122 Smith Rd, Kinderhook, NY 12106
One step lateral flow immunoassay.

American Bio Medica Corp. 856-241-2320
603 Heron Dr Ste 3, Logan Township, NJ 08085
One step lateral flow immunoassay.

Germaine Laboratories, Inc. 210-692-4192
4139 Gardendale St Ste 101, San Antonio, TX 78229
Various types.

Innovacon, Inc. 858-535-2030
4106 Sorrento Valley Blvd, San Diego, CA 92121
Tricyclic antidepressants drug of abuse test.

Medtox Diagnostics, Inc. 800-334-1116
1640 Nova Ln, Burlington, NC 27215
Immunochromatographic assay for tricyclic antidepressants (tca).

QuantRx Biomedical Corp. 503-252-9565
5920 NE 112th Ave, Portland, OR 97220
ACCUSTEP DOA SINGLE AND

Ucp Biosciences, Inc. 408-392-0064
1445 Koll Cir Ste 111, San Jose, CA 95112
Tricyclic antidepressant test system.

Varian Inc 650-424-5078
25200 Commercentre Dr, Lake Forest, CA 92630
Drug testing device.

RADIOIMMUNOASSAY, VITAMIN B12 *(Chemistry) 75CDD*

Abbott Diagnostics Intl, Biotechnology Ltd 787-846-3500
Road #2 KM. 58.0 , PO Box 278, Cruce Davila, Barceloneta, PR 00617
Enzyme factor assay for determination of vitamin B12.

American Laboratory Products Co. 800-592-5726
26 Keewaydin Dr Ste G, Salem, NH 03079
Vitamin B6 REA (Pyridoxal -5 - Phosphate). Quantitative radioassay to determine the biologically active form of vitamin B6 in plasma.

Bio-Rad Laboratories, Life Science Group 800-424-6723
2000 Alfred Nobel Dr, Hercules, CA 94547

Health Chem Diagnostics Llc 954-979-3845
3341 W McNab Rd, Pompano Beach, FL 33069
Radioassay, vitamin b12.

RADIOMETER, LASER *(General) 80WRJ*

Coherent, Inc. 800-527-3786
5100 Patrick Henry Dr, Santa Clara, CA 95054

Gentec Electro-Optics Inc. 888-543-6832
445 St-Jean-Baptiste, Ste. 160, Quebec, QUE G2E-5N7 Canada
Laser Power and Energy Meters full line of detector heads and readouts for medical and surgical laser applications.

International Light Technologies, Inc. 978-818-6180
10 Technology Dr, Peabody, MA 01960
IL offers a full range of laser measurement systems for all types of applications including testing for photodynamic therapy. IL manufactures low cost, simple, accurate systems for measurement of low power continuous CW lasers (such as argone HeNE NdYAG) and laser diodes with a pulse greater than 5 microseconds.

Labsphere, Inc. 603-927-4266
231 Shaker St., North Sutton, NH 03260-9986
Laser power meters for lasers, laser diodes, and laser-driven fiber optics.

Laser Probe, Inc. 315-797-4492
23 Wells Ave, Utica, NY 13502

Ophir Optronics, Inc. 800-820-0814
260A Fordham Rd, Wilmington, MA 01887
Laser power/energy meters.

RADIOMETER, PHOTOTHERAPY *(General) 80ROE*

International Light Technologies, Inc. 978-818-6180
10 Technology Dr, Peabody, MA 01960
IL has a broad range of radiometers which can be used for phototherapy. By selecting either the IL1400 or IL1700 series radiometer and either/all of the UVA, UVB or Hyperbilirubinemia sensors, you can use one meter to make all of your phototherapy measurement. IL has also just released the new low cost specailist series radiometer IL74 for a low cost alternative for bilirubin testing.

Olympic Medical Corp. 206-767-3500
5900 1st Ave S, Seattle, WA 98108
$1,492.50 per unit (standard).

RADIOMETER, PHOTOTHERAPY *(cont'd)*

Photo Research, Inc. 818-341-5151
9731 Topanga Canyon Pl, Chatsworth, CA 91311
PR 705 SPECTRASCAN - SPECTRO RADIOMETER

Spectronics Corporation 800-274-8888
956 Brush Hollow Rd, Westbury, NY 11590
Ensures easy measurement of the complete ultraviolet range plus blue light. Designed for maximum usability, each radiometer offers a variety of features.

Thermo Oriel 800-715-393
150 Long Beach Blvd, Stratford, CT 06615

Uvp, Llc 800-452-6788
2066 W 11th St, Upland, CA 91786
UV Radiometer - for measurement of UV intensity.

RADIOMETER, ULTRAVIOLET *(General) 80VDS*

International Light Technologies, Inc. 978-818-6180
10 Technology Dr, Peabody, MA 01960
IL offers an extremely wide range of UV measurement systems including our new RPS200 and RPS900 hand held spectroradiometers and the IL52 radiometer. The IL52 performs continuous UV monotoring with filters and input optics custom designed to fit your application. The IL1400A or IL1400BL(Back lit LDC) Hand-held radiometer and our IL1700 research grade radiometer can be used with a large selection of off the shelf detectors, filters and optics for measuring UVA, UVB, UVC, phototherapy, photoresist, germicidal, actinic health hazard,Photostability/degredation, UV LED testing, solar UV, UV curing and general radiometric measurements. The RPS200 sepctroradioemter measures from 200-500 and the RPS900 measures from 200-1050 nm.

National Biological Corp. 800-338-5045
1532 Enterprise Pkwy, Twinsburg, OH 44087
UVA & UVB light meters.

Solar Light Co. 215-517-8700
100 E Glenside Ave, Glenside, PA 19038
UV radiometer

Spectronics Corporation 800-274-8888
956 Brush Hollow Rd, Westbury, NY 11590

RADIOMETRIC, FE59, IRON BINDING CAPACITY
(Chemistry) 75JQG

Stanbio Laboratory, Inc. 830-249-0772
1261 N Main St, Boerne, TX 78006
Iron and IBC test set.

RADIOTHERAPY TREATMENT PLANNING UNIT
(Radiology) 90ROG

Elekta, Inc. 800-535-7355
4775 Peachtree Industrial Blvd, Building 300, Suite 300
Norcross, GA 30092
Precise Treatment System, utilizes digital technology in linear accelerators and multi-leaf collimators.

Gammex Rmi 800-426-6391
PO Box 620327, Middleton, WI 53562

Indec Systems, Inc. 408-986-1600
2210 Martin Ave, Santa Clara, CA 95050

Rahd Oncology Products 800-844-0103
10762 Indian Head Industrial Blvd, Saint Louis, MO 63132
$65,000 to $247,000 for a RAHD Alpha 3D/PRO radiation therapy treatment planning system. Includes 3D Volumetric image fusion with a selection of 3D warp algorithims to merge functional and diagnostic images. Any DICOM image set for CT, MR, PET, SPECT and US.

RADIOTHERAPY UNIT, CHARGED-PARTICLE *(Radiology) 90LHN*

Bionix Development Corp. 800-551-7096
5154 Enterprise Blvd, Toledo, OH 43612
Various patient immobilization systems.

Computerized Medical Systems, Inc. 468-587-2550
1145 Corporate Lake Dr, Olivette, MO 63132
Radiation brachytherapy treatment planning system.

Hitachi America, Ltd., Power Systems Division 713-792-1804
1840 Old Spanish Trl, Houston, TX 77054
Proton beam therapy system.

Intraop Medical Corp. 408-636-1020
570 Del Rey Ave, Sunnyvale, CA 94085
Electron linear accelerator.

RADIOTHERAPY UNIT, CHARGED-PARTICLE *(cont'd)*

K&S Assoc., Inc. 615-883-9760
1926 Elm Tree Dr, Nashville, TN 37210
Dos software management program.

Lifeline Software, Inc. 903-894-9923
311 Hines Xing, Bullard, TX 75757
Radcalc.

Sicel Technologies, Inc. 919-465-2236
3800 Gateway Centre Blvd Ste 308, Morrisville, NC 27560
Radiation dosimeter.

Standard Imaging, Inc. 608-831-0025
3120 Deming Way, Middleton, WI 53562
Treatment planning computer program.

Varian Medical Systems, Oncology Systems 800 278-2747
911 Hansen Way, Bldg.3 M/S C-165, Palo Alto, CA 94304
Various types of radiation therapy systems.

RAIL, BATH *(General) 80TEB*

Alimed, Inc. 800-225-2610
297 High St, Dedham, MA 02026

American Specialties, Inc. 914-476-9000
441 Saw Mill River Rd, Yonkers, NY 10701

Bobrick Washroom Equipment, Inc. 818-764-1000
11611 Hart St, North Hollywood, CA 91605

Clarke Health Care Products, Inc. 888-347-4537
1003 International Dr, Oakdale, PA 15071
Handi-Grip portable grab bar uses suction pads to stick to most smooth surfaces, 3 sizes,telescoping length, easily installed and portable.

Elcoma Metal Fabricating Canada 705-526-9636
878 William St., P.O. Box 685, Midland, ONT L4R-4P4 Canada
Grab bars and other assistive devices. All colors, configurations, lengths and diameters.

Gendron, Inc. 800-537-2521
400 E Lugbill Rd, Archbold, OH 43502
$53.00 each.

Invacare Corporation 800-333-6900
1 Invacare Way, Elyria, OH 44035
INVACARE.

Maddak Inc. 800-443-4926
661 State Route 23, Wayne, NJ 07470
ABLEWARE.

RDL Supply 214-630-3965
11240 Gemini Ln, Dallas, TX 75229
ASI 1-1/2 in. diameter stainless steel bars for bathroom walls.

Sunrise Medical 800-333-4000
7477 Dry Creek Pkwy, Longmont, CO 80503

TFI Healthcare 800-526-0178
600 W Wythe St, Petersburg, VA 23803
Model #DME80/6 tub bar.

The C. D. Sparling Company 734-455-3121
498 Farmer St, Plymouth, MI 48170
Available in all standard sizes. Stainless-steel or decorative plastic with stainless-steel core. Shower seats also available. CHANNEL BACKER grab-bar and towel-bar fastening system for hollow-wall applications.

Tub Master Lc 800-833-0260
413 Virginia Dr, Orlando, FL 32803
ADA-Safety Grab Bars - Available in different textures, sizes, & colors.

Tuffcare 800-367-6160
3999 E La Palma Ave, Anaheim, CA 92807

Whitehall Manufacturing 800-782-7706
15125 Proctor Ave, City Of Industry, CA 91746
Standard and handicapped shower equipment.

Youngs, Inc. 800-523-5454
55 E Cherry Ln, Souderton, PA 18964
A.D.A compliant bathroom hardware.

RAIL, COMMODE *(General) 80TEC*

Alimed, Inc. 800-225-2610
297 High St, Dedham, MA 02026

American Specialties, Inc. 914-476-9000
441 Saw Mill River Rd, Yonkers, NY 10701

RAIL, COMMODE *(cont'd)*

Convaquip Industries, Inc. 800-637-8436
4834 Derrick Dr, PO Box 3417, Abilene, TX 79601
Bariatric Drop arm bedside commodes. Weight certified from 850 lb. to 1500 lbs., depending on item.

Sunrise Medical 800-333-4000
7477 Dry Creek Pkwy, Longmont, CO 80503

RAIL, WALL SIDE *(General) 80TED*

American Specialties, Inc. 914-476-9000
441 Saw Mill River Rd, Yonkers, NY 10701

Construction Specialties Inc. 800-233-8493
6696 Route. 405, Muncy, PA 17756

Handi-Ramp 800-876-7267
510 North Ave, Libertyville, IL 60048
Handrails are available stand alone or as a component on our ramp systems. We offer single- or double-bar construction and vertical pickets.

Independent Solutions, Inc. 847-498-0500
900 Skokie Blvd Ste 118, Northbrook, IL 60062

Inpro Corporation 800-222-5556
S80W18766 Apollo Dr, Muskego, WI 53150
InPro Corporation is your single source for all of your interior and exterior architectural products. With FOUR divisions; InPro IPC Door and Wall Protection Systems, InPro Signscape Signage and Wayfinding, InPro Clickeze Privacy Systems, and JointMaster Architectural Joint Systems, we have you covered from floor to ceiling.

Maddak Inc. 800-443-4926
661 State Route 23, Wayne, NJ 07470
ABLEWARE.

Pawling Corp., Architectural Prod. Div. 800-431-3456
32 Nelson Hill Rd, PO Box 200, Wassaic, NY 12592
Rail side rails; also bumper handrails.

RAILS, EQUIPMENT *(General) 80WRN*

Independent Solutions, Inc. 847-498-0500
900 Skokie Blvd Ste 118, Northbrook, IL 60062
Class 1, Fairfield, EASTERN & LifeSpan wall mounted, ambulance mounted, headwall mounted; over 10,000 accessories available; cart mounted, headwall mounted, boom mounted.

RAMP, WHEELCHAIR *(General) 80UKQ*

Alimed, Inc. 800-225-2610
297 High St, Dedham, MA 02026

Alumiramp, Inc. 800-800-3864
855 E Chicago Rd, Quincy, MI 49082
Mini Ramp Series telescopic channel ramps, folding curb ramps, threshold ramps. Modular aluminum ramp system for temporary or permanent installation; aluminum ramp kits that are modular in design and can be set up in most any configuration; portable curb and scooter ramps.

Electric Mobility Corporation 800-718-2082
591 Mantua Blvd, PO Box 450, Sewell, NJ 08080

Forward Motions, Inc. 877-364-8267
214 Valley St, Dayton, OH 45404

Handi-Ramp 800-876-7267
510 North Ave, Libertyville, IL 60048
Side- or rear-end-mountable van ramps with or w/o steps, portable suitcase/folding ramps, portable ramp tracks, platforms, threshold ramp, semi-permanent outdoor sectional ramp systems with handrails.

Handicap Unlimited, Inc. 888-371-0095
5640 Summer Ave Ste 3, Memphis, TN 38134

Handicaps, Inc. 800-782-4335
4335 S Santa Fe Dr, Englewood, CO 80110
Telescopic ramp, $500.00.

Homecare Products, Inc. 800-451-1903
1704 B St NW Ste 110, Auburn, WA 98001
EZ-ACCESS, portable ramps for wheelchairs and scooters, available in several different sizes and styles ranging from a 2 ft curb ramp to a 10 ft multi-purpose ramp. TRIFOLD RAMP, available in 5, 6, 7, 8 & 10 ft lengths. Unique 3-fold design provides compact storability. Made of aluminium, 700 lb. capacity with built-in carrying handle, 29' wide.

Kareco International, Inc. 800-8KA-RECO
299 Rte. 22 E., Green Brook, NJ 08812-1714
Portable aluminum ramps

RAMP, WHEELCHAIR *(cont'd)*

Rampmaster Division Of Thorweld 416-741-2501
174 Milvan Dr., Weston, ONT M9L 1Z9 Canada
Rampmaster portable wheelchair ramps & van wheelchair ramps.

Starr Industries/Portable Entry Systems 800-677-8377
87 Taylor St, Quincy, MI 49082
Portable wheelchair ramps, Permanent commercial and residential wheelchair ramps,

Stinson Manufacturing 800-932-2885
PO Box 3644, N. 414 Sycamore, Spokane, WA 99220
PRO-RAMP light-duty (1500-lb-capacity) aluminum ramps for wheelchair access.

Tuffcare 800-367-6160
3999 E La Palma Ave, Anaheim, CA 92807

RASP, BONE *(Orthopedics) 87HTR*

Abbott Spine, Inc. 847-937-6100
12708 Riata Vista Cir Ste B-100, Austin, TX 78727
Rasp.

Biomet Microfixation Inc. 800-874-7711
1520 Tradeport Dr, Jacksonville, FL 32218
Various types of rasps.

Biomet, Inc. 574-267-6639
56 E Bell Dr, PO Box 587, Warsaw, IN 46582
Various types of orthopedic rasps such as moore rasp, thompson rasp, and muller .

DJO Inc. 800-336-6569
1430 Decision St, Vista, CA 92081

Grace Manufacturing, Inc. 479-968-5455
614 Sr 247, Russellville, AR 72802

Integral Design Inc. 781-740-2036
52 Burr Rd, Hingham, MA 02043

Kirwan Surgical Products, Inc. 888-547-9267
180 Enterprise Dr, PO Box 427, Marshfield, MA 02050

Kmedic 800-955-0559
190 Veterans Dr, Northvale, NJ 07647

Medisiss 866-866-7477
2747 SW 6th St, Redmond, OR 97756
Various rasps,sterile.

Medtronic Sofamor Danek Instrument Manufacturing 901-396-3133
7375 Adrianne Pl, Bartlett, TN 38133
Various rasps.

Medtronic Sofamor Danek Usa, Inc. 901-396-3133
4340 Swinnea Rd, Memphis, TN 38118
Various rasps.

Pappas Surgical Instruments, Llc 508-429-1049
7 October Hill Rd, Holliston, MA 01746
Various types of rasps.

Pompano Precision Products, Inc. 954-946-6059
1100 SW 12th Ave, Pompano Beach, FL 33069

Spine Wave, Inc. 203-944-9494
2 Enterprise Dr Ste 302, Shelton, CT 06484
Bone rasp.

Stryker Spine 866-457-7463
2 Pearl Ct, Allendale, NJ 07401

Symmetry Medical Usa, Inc. 574-267-8700
486 W 350 N, Warsaw, IN 46582
Manual surgical instrument for general use.

Tuzik Boston 800-886-6363
104 Longwater Dr, Assinippi Park, Norwell, MA 02061

Vilex, Inc. 800-872-4911
345 Old Curry Hollow Rd, Pittsburgh, PA 15236
POWER RASP offers another option for precision bone rasping and sculpturing.

Warsaw Orthopedic, Inc. 901-396-3133
2500 Silveus Xing, Warsaw, IN 46582
Various rasps.

Zimmer Holdings, Inc. 800-613-6131
1800 W Center St, PO Box 708, Warsaw, IN 46580

Zimmer Spine, Inc. 800-655-2614
7375 Bush Lake Rd, Minneapolis, MN 55439
Rasp.

Zimmer Trabecular Metal Technology 800-613-6131
10 Pomeroy Rd, Parsippany, NJ 07054
Pf hip stem rasp assembly number 12.

RASP, EAR *(Ear/Nose/Throat) 77JYY*

Aesculap Implant Systems Inc. 1-800-234-9179
3773 Corporate Pkwy, Center Valley, PA 18034

Bausch & Lomb Surgical 636-255-5051
3365 Tree Court Ind Blvd, Saint Louis, MO 63122

Clinimed, Incorporated 877-CLINIMED
303 Markus Ct, Sandy Brae Industrial Park, Newark, DE 19713

Gyrus Ent L.L.C., Sub. Of Gyrus Acmi, Inc. 508-804-2739
2925 Appling Rd, Bartlett, TN 38133
Various types and sizes of ear rasps.

Princeton Medical Group, Inc. 800-875-0869
1189 Royal Links Dr, Mt Pleasant, SC 29466

RASP, FRONTAL-SINUS *(Ear/Nose/Throat) 77KAZ*

Aesculap Implant Systems Inc. 1-800-234-9179
3773 Corporate Pkwy, Center Valley, PA 18034

Bausch & Lomb Surgical 636-255-5051
3365 Tree Court Ind Blvd, Saint Louis, MO 63122

RASP, NASAL *(Ear/Nose/Throat) 77KBA*

Aesculap Implant Systems Inc. 1-800-234-9179
3773 Corporate Pkwy, Center Valley, PA 18034

Bausch & Lomb Surgical 636-255-5051
3365 Tree Court Ind Blvd, Saint Louis, MO 63122

Biomet Microfixation Inc. 800-874-7711
1520 Tradeport Dr, Jacksonville, FL 32218
Various types of rasps.

Clinimed, Incorporated 877-CLINIMED
303 Markus Ct, Sandy Brae Industrial Park, Newark, DE 19713

Codman & Shurtleff, Inc 800-225-0460
325 Paramount Dr, Raynham, MA 02767

Kmedic 800-955-0559
190 Veterans Dr, Northvale, NJ 07647

Miltex Inc. 800-645-8000
589 Davies Dr, York, PA 17402

Princeton Medical Group, Inc. 800-875-0869
1189 Royal Links Dr, Mt Pleasant, SC 29466

RASP, OTHER *(Surgery) 79ROI*

Kmedic 800-955-0559
190 Veterans Dr, Northvale, NJ 07647

Zimmer Holdings, Inc. 800-613-6131
1800 W Center St, PO Box 708, Warsaw, IN 46580

RASP, SURGICAL, GENERAL & PLASTIC SURGERY *(Surgery) 79GAC*

Aesculap Implant Systems Inc. 1-800-234-9179
3773 Corporate Pkwy, Center Valley, PA 18034

Ascent Healthcare Solutions 480-763-5300
10232 S 51st St, Phoenix, AZ 85044
Rasp.

Bausch & Lomb Surgical 636-255-5051
3365 Tree Court Ind Blvd, Saint Louis, MO 63122

Biomet Microfixation Inc. 800-874-7711
1520 Tradeport Dr, Jacksonville, FL 32218
Various types of rasps.

Biomet, Inc. 574-267-6639
56 E Bell Dr, PO Box 587, Warsaw, IN 46582
Various types of raspatory instruments.

Cardinal Health, Snowden Pencer Products 847-689-8410
5175 S Royal Atlanta Dr, Tucker, GA 30084
Various styles of general and plastic surgery rasps.

Grace Engineering Corp. 810-392-2181
34775 Potter St, Memphis, MI 48041
Bone rasp.

Grace Manufacturing, Inc. 479-968-5455
614 Sr 247, Russellville, AR 72802

Kmedic 800-955-0559
190 Veterans Dr, Northvale, NJ 07647

Maxilon Laboratories, Inc. 603-594-9300
105 State Route 101A Unit 8, Amherst, NH 03031
Various types of sterile and non-sterile bone grafting inst.

Miltex Inc. 800-645-8000
589 Davies Dr, York, PA 17402

Richard Wolf Medical Instruments Corp. 800-323-9653
353 Corporate Woods Pkwy, Vernon Hills, IL 60061

RASP, SURGICAL, GENERAL & PLASTIC SURGERY *(cont'd)*

Tuzik Boston 800-886-6363
104 Longwater Dr, Assinippi Park, Norwell, MA 02061

Vilex, Inc. 931-474-7550
111 Moffitt St, McMinnville, TN 37110

RASPATORY *(Surgery) 79ROH*

Codman & Shurtleff, Inc 800-225-0460
325 Paramount Dr, Raynham, MA 02767

Miltex Inc. 800-645-8000
589 Davies Dr, York, PA 17402

Zimmer Holdings, Inc. 800-613-6131
1800 W Center St, PO Box 708, Warsaw, IN 46580

REACHER (HANDICAPPED) *(General) 80TFZ*

Arcmate Mfg. Corp. 888-637-1926
637 S Vinewood St, Escondido, CA 92029
Available in standard, folding, locking & with light touch easy pull. 100% lifetime guarantee. Rainbow Reacher, new all plastic reacher, 16' only 3.7 oz. & the 26' is only 4/8 oz. E-Z REACHER w/SAF-T-LOK, this reacher has a patented SAF-T-LOK which enables one to release the handle while maintaining a secure grasp of the object. Great for overhead safety, lifting heavy objects, or people w/limited grip, strength. DRESS EZ, long handles shoehoe and S hook used by people with limited range of motion. Available in 24' and 30' with built up foam grip.

Cme Medical Equipment Corp. 908-561-0906
1130 Donemy Gln, Scotch Plains, NJ 07076
REHAB REACHER.

Geen Healthcare Inc. 800-565-4336
931 Progress Ave. Ste.13, Scarborough, ONT M1G 3V5 Canada

Maddak Inc. 800-443-4926
661 State Route 23, Wayne, NJ 07470
ABLEWARE.

Mailhawk Manufacturing Company 800-331-5070
5292 White House Pkwy, Hwy. 85-W, Warm Springs, GA 31830
$12.95 postpaid for 20 or 28' models and $14.95 postpaid for 42' model (quantity discounts). Long wooden handle with aluminum jaws covered with tapered vinyl for sensitive feel and pick up 28' model weighs 8ozs. Deduct $1.00ea. for order of 2 pcs. or more. Postage $4.50 per order. Quantity discounts available.

Mecanaids Co., Inc. 800-227-0877
21 Hampden Dr, South Easton, MA 02375
Handicapped dressing and reaching aids. Variety of daily living aids.

North Coast Medical, Inc. 800-821-9319
18305 Sutter Blvd, Morgan Hill, CA 95037

Paramedical Distributors 800-245-3278
2020 Grand Blvd, Kansas City, MO 64108

REACTION APPARATUS *(Microbiology) 83UHQ*

Berghof/America 800-544-5004
3773 NW 126th Ave Bldg 1, Coral Springs, FL 33065
Stainless steel, with fully encapsulated PTFE liners, sizes from 50ml to 1, 2, & 4 liters.

Parr Instrument Co. 800-872-7720
211 53rd St, Moline, IL 61265

Thermo Fisher Scientific Inc. 781-622-1000
81 Wyman St, Waltham, MA 02451
Reaction cuvettes for BM/Hitachi chemistry analyzers. ALKO now offers reaction cuvettes for use on Hitachi models 717, 747, 911 and 914.

READER, BAR CODE *(General) 80WMS*

Agr International, Inc. 724-482-2163
PO Box 149, 615 Whitestown Road, Butler, PA 16003
Vision or bar code inspection systems.

Data Hunter LLC 714-892-5461
5412 Bolsa Ave Ste G, Huntington Beach, CA 92649

Fluke Biomedical 800-648-7952
6920 Seaway Blvd, Everett, WA 98203

Howard Medical Company 800-443-1444
1690 N Elston Ave, Chicago, IL 60642
$2,500 Includes handheld reader with 35 key input, bar code and built in telephone modem.

Opticon, Inc. 800-636-0090
8 Olympic Dr, Orangeburg, NY 10962
Opticon offers a full family of both laser and CCD imaging readers that can be easily integrated into any product design. Opticon customizes readers to your meet your needs.

READER, BAR CODE *(cont'd)*

Sick, Inc. 800-325-7425
6900 W 110th St, Minneapolis, MN 55438
CLV 450 Bar Code Scanner. The new CLV 450 bar code scanner from SICK, Inc. is a very compact scanner with a long reading range. This model features dynamic focus control, which leads to high depth of field and expanded flexibility. This scanner is an excellent choice for demanding applications that require reading bar codes produced by ink jet printers, on corrugated surfaces and through shrink wrap. The CLV 450's SMART (SICK's Modular Advanced Recognition Technology) enables the scanner to read bar codes than can not be read by other scanners. The CLV 450 processes complete bar code images before decoding. This translates to a much higher percentage of successful reads, even with bar codes presented at high tilt angles or bar codes partially hidden from the scanner. The CLV 450 is especially suited to applications where space is at a premium because it is the smallest unit of its class. It has flash memory for easy updated via the software. Line and oscillating mirror versions are available. The dimensions are 3.5 x 2.4 x 1.4. The reading range for the CLV 450 is 8 to 63 in. The CLX 490 is the most compact, industrial omnidirectional scanner on the market. It incorporates automatic focus control, SMART technology, a high scan rate and package tracking into one unit. The CLX 490's SMART (SICK's Modular Advanced Recognition Technology) enables the scanner to read bar codes that could not be read by other scanners. The CLX 490 processes complete bar code images before decoding. This translates to a much higher percentage of successful reads, even with bar codes presented at high tilt angles or partially damaged bar codes. This scanner also allows small object spacing through its integrated tracking function. The CLX 490 is especially suited to applications where space is at a premium because it is the smallest unit of its class. The settings are stored in the memory plug for quick replacement if necessary. Optional internal heating is available. The scanner dimensions are 7x8x6 in. The reading range is 20 to 83 in. The scanning frequency is 1200 Hz for a complete x-pattern. The CLX 490 is ideal for conveyor widths up to 16 in (400 mm) and conveyor speeds up to 6.5 ft/sec (2 m/sec). The automatic focus control technology provides a large depth of field up to 32 in. The Windows based setup software 'CLV SETUP' provides an easy interface to optimize the performance of the scanner on-site.

READER, BAR, OPHTHALMIC *(Ophthalmology) 86HJY*

Ctp Coil Inc. 800-933-2645
1801 Howard St Ste D, Elk Grove Village, IL 60007
Various forms of hand, stand, and bar magnifiers.

READER, MICROPLATE *(General) 80WOD*

Awareness Technology, Inc. 722-283-6540
1935 SW Martin Hwy, Palm City, FL 34990
$3,000 to $5,000 for microtiter strip/plate reader; also, $4,895 for StatFax 3200, $3,950 for Stat Fax 2100, and $2,495 for StatFax 303 PLUS; $95 for QC DRI-DYE check strips for microplate and strip reader.

Biolog, Inc. 800-284-4949
21124 Cabot Blvd, Hayward, CA 94545
Semi-automatic reader for Biolog's MICROPLATE test kits.

Medtec, Inc. 919-241-1400
PO Box 16578, Chapel Hill, NC 27516
Validate your microplate via linearity checks using the Linear Validation Plate. Catalog Number MT03001.

Molecular Devices Corp. 800-635-5577
1311 Orleans Dr, Sunnyvale, CA 94089
VMAX, SOFTMAX, $3,500.00 to $12,000.00; kinetic microplate readers; SPECTRAMAX, uv/vis scanning microplate reader.

Tecan U.S., Inc. 800-338-3226
4022 Stirrup Creek Dr Ste 310, Durham, NC 27703
Sunrise.

Xiril 302-655-7035
91 Lukens Dr Ste A, New Castle, DE 19720
$6,500 for microplate reader.

READER, PRISM, OPHTHALMIC *(Ophthalmology) 86HJX*

Labtician Ophthalmics, Inc. 800-265-8391
2140 Winston Park Dr., Unit 6, Oakville, ONTAR L6H 5V5 Canada
Head-positioning glasses.

READER, RADIAL IMMUNODIFFUSION *(Microbiology) 83WJV*

Binding Site, Inc., The 800-633-4484
5889 Oberlin Dr Ste 101, San Diego, CA 92121
$1850.00 for electronic radial immunodiffusion reader (reads RID rings).

READER, SLIDE, CYTOLOGY, CERVICAL, AUTOMATED
(Pathology) 88MNM

Cytyc Surgical Products 800-442-9892
250 Campus Dr, Marlborough, MA 01752
Reader,cervical cytology slide, automated.

Tripath Imaging, Inc. 919-206-7140
8271 154th Ave NE, Redmond, WA 98052
Cervical cytology reader.

READER, ZONE, AUTOMATED *(Microbiology) 83KZK*

Giles Scientific, Inc. 800-603-9290
PO Box 4306, Santa Barbara, CA 93140
BIOMIC Vision automated antibiotic susceptibility and identification system for clinical bacteria and yeast testing; DIGICOUNTER microorganism-colony enumeration system; AUTOASSAY antibiotic potency/concentrations agar assay system. All systems use our color digital image analysis plate reader.

READING SYSTEM, CLOSED-CIRCUIT TELEVISION
(Ophthalmology) 86HJG

Assisted Access-Nfss, Inc. 800-950-9655
822 Preston Ct, Lake Villa, IL 60046
TV telecaption decoding equipment for the hearing impaired.

Innoventions, Inc. 800-854-6554
9593 Corsair Dr, Conifer, CO 80433
Electronic magnfier.

Insiphil (Us) Llc 408-616-8700
650 Vaqueros Ave Ste F, Sunnyvale, CA 94085
RAINDOW & ALADDIN image magnification system, using TV monitor to show enlargement of written material.

Magnisight, Inc. 800-753-4767
3631 N Stone Ave, Colorado Springs, CO 80907
Custom Focus - Sizes are available in 20', 17' & 14' models. It features auto focus, magnification up to 50 times depending on monitor size, variable brightness control, full-color or black & white camera models and easy-to-use manual focus override for unique focusing needs. Options available - Select-A-Color, Line Marking/ Windowing/ and Computer Compatiblility. MagniSight, Explorer Custom Focus, closed circuit television (CCTV) video magnifier: Magnisight,Exploer 20' Custom Focus CCTV Video Magnifier features auto focus, magnification up to 50 times, variable brightness control, full color or black & white camera models and easy-to-use manual focus override for unique focusing needs. Options available - Select-A-Color, Line Marking/Windowing and Computer Compatibility

Pasadena Scientific Industries 717-227-1220
5125 Pine View Dr, Glen Rock, PA 17327
Video print enlarger.

REAGENT, ACETYLCHOLINE CHLORIDE *(Toxicology) 91DLI*

Raichem, Division Of Hemagen Diagnostics, Inc. 800-438-6100
8225 Mercury Ct, San Diego, CA 92111

Sterling Diagnostics, Inc. 800-637-2661
36645 Metro Ct, Sterling Heights, MI 48312
Pseudocholinesterase (pche) reagent set.

REAGENT, ALBUMIN, COLORIMETRIC *(Chemistry) 75CJZ*

Amresco Inc. 800-366-1313
30175 Solon Industrial Pkwy, Solon, OH 44139
Hitachi, technicon RA, SMAC and SMA systems.

Beckman Coulter, Inc. 800-635-3497
740 W 83rd St, Hialeah, FL 33014
$0.045 per test.

Beckman Coulter, Inc. 800-742-2345
250 S Kraemer Blvd, PO Box 8000, Brea, CA 92821

Biomerieux Inc. 800-682-2666
100 Rodolphe St, Durham, NC 27712

Genzyme Corp. 800-325-2436
160 Christian St, Oxford, CT 06478
BCG, endpoint, acetate buffer.

Health Chem Diagnostics Llc 954-979-3845
3341 W McNab Rd, Pompano Beach, FL 33069
Acid, hydroxyazobenzene-benzoic, albumin.

Raichem, Division Of Hemagen Diagnostics, Inc. 800-438-6100
8225 Mercury Ct, San Diego, CA 92111

REAGENT, AMYLASE, COLORIMETRIC *(Chemistry) 75CJA*

Beckman Coulter, Inc. 800-635-3497
740 W 83rd St, Hialeah, FL 33014
$0.42 per test.

REAGENT, AMYLASE, COLORIMETRIC *(cont'd)*

Beckman Coulter, Inc. 800-742-2345
250 S Kraemer Blvd, PO Box 8000, Brea, CA 92821

Biomerieux Inc. 800-682-2666
100 Rodolphe St, Durham, NC 27712

Dade Behring, Inc. 800-948-3233
1717 Deerfield Rd, Deerfield, IL 60015

Raichem, Division Of Hemagen Diagnostics, Inc. 800-438-6100
8225 Mercury Ct, San Diego, CA 92111

Stanbio Laboratory, Inc. 830-249-0772
1261 N Main St, Boerne, TX 78006
$45.00 for 60 test kits containing buffered substrate (powder) and iodine reagent.

Sterling Diagnostics, Inc. 800-637-2661
36645 Metro Ct, Sterling Heights, MI 48312

REAGENT, ANALYZER, AMINO ACID *(Microbiology) 83UFK*

Beckman Coulter, Inc. 800-742-2345
250 S Kraemer Blvd, PO Box 8000, Brea, CA 92821

Bio-Rad Laboratories, Life Science Group 800-424-6723
2000 Alfred Nobel Dr, Hercules, CA 94547

REAGENT, ANTISTREPTOLYSIN-TITER/STREPTOLYSIN O
(Microbiology) 83GTQ

D-Tek Llc 215-245-5270
3580 Progress Dr Ste J3, Bensalem, PA 19020

Diagnostic Technology, Inc. 631-582-4949
175 Commerce Dr Ste L, Hauppauge, NY 11788
Latex slide test for the detection of antistreptolysin-o.

Jas Diagnostics, Inc. 305-418-2320
7220 NW 58th St, Miami, FL 33166
Antistreptolysin - titer/streptolysin o reagent microbiology.

Nerl Diagnostics Llc. 401-824-2046
14 Almeida Ave, East Providence, RI 02914
Aso latex kits.

REAGENT, BILIRUBIN (TOTAL OR DIRECT TEST SYSTEM)
(Chemistry) 75CIG

Abbott Diagnostics Div. 626-440-0700
820 Mission St, South Pasadena, CA 91030
Total bilirubin, direct bilirubin.

Advanced Instruments Inc. 800-225-4034
2 Technology Way, Norwood, MA 02062
Combined total and direct test kit.

Amresco Inc. 800-366-1313
30175 Solon Industrial Pkwy, Solon, OH 44139
RA, Hitachi systems.

Beckman Coulter, Inc. 800-635-3497
740 W 83rd St, Hialeah, FL 33014
$0.09 per test.

Beckman Coulter, Inc. 800-742-2345
250 S Kraemer Blvd, PO Box 8000, Brea, CA 92821

Biomerieux Inc. 800-682-2666
100 Rodolphe St, Durham, NC 27712

Caldon Bioscience, Inc. 909-628-9944
2100 S Reservoir St, Pomona, CA 91766
Bilirubin.

Caldon Biotech, Inc. 757-224-0177
2251 Rutherford Rd, Carlsbad, CA 92008
Bilirubin.

Carolina Liquid Chemistries Corp. 800-471-7272
510 W Central Ave Ste C, Brea, CA 92821
Bilirubin reagent.

Dade Behring, Inc. 800-948-3233
1717 Deerfield Rd, Deerfield, IL 60015

Diagnostic Specialties 732-549-4011
4 Leonard St, Metuchen, NJ 08840
$100.00 per unit (standard).

Elabsupply 714-446-8740
1001 Starbuck St Apt C306, Fullerton, CA 92833
Bilirubin Direct and Total clinical chemistry reagents in liquid format for Hitachi, Cobas Mira and Beckman Coulter CX series analyzers.

Genchem, Inc. 714-529-1616
510 W Central Ave Ste D, Brea, CA 92821
Total bilirubin reagent.

REAGENT, BILIRUBIN (TOTAL OR DIRECT TEST SYSTEM) *(cont'd)*

Genzyme Corp. 800-325-2436
160 Christian St, Oxford, CT 06478
DND, endpoint. Walters and gerarde, endpoint.

Globalemed Llc. 703-894-0710
1101 King St, Suites 370, 270, 170, Alexandria, VA 22314

Health Chem Diagnostics Llc 954-979-3845
3341 W McNab Rd, Pompano Beach, FL 33069
Diazo colorimetry, bilirubin.

Intersect Systems, Inc. 360-577-1062
1152 3rd Avenue, Suite D & E, Longview, WA 98632

Jas Diagnostics, Inc. 305-418-2320
7220 NW 58th St, Miami, FL 33166
Bilirubin (total & direct).

Sandare Intl., Inc. 972-293-7440
910 Kck Way, Cedar Hill, TX 75104
Diazo total and direct bilirubin methods.

Stanbio Laboratory, Inc. 830-249-0772
1261 N Main St, Boerne, TX 78006
$44.00 for 250ml reagent with oxidant and calibrator I (5ml/dl) and II (15mg/dl). $24.50 for 250ml direct bilirubin reagent.

Sterling Diagnostics, Inc. 800-637-2661
36645 Metro Ct, Sterling Heights, MI 48312
Total and direct bilirubin reagent set.

Synermed Intl., Inc. 317-896-1565
17408 Tiller Ct Ste 1900, Westfield, IN 46074
Direct bilirubin reagent kit, total bilirubin reagent kit.

Teco Diagnostics 714-693-7788
1268 N Lakeview Ave, Anaheim, CA 92807
Bilirubin, direct.

Vital Diagnostics Inc. 714-672-3553
1075 W Lambert Rd Ste D, Brea, CA 92821
Various total and direct bilirubin reagents.

REAGENT, BLOOD GAS/PH *(General) 80WRG*

Thermo Fisher Scientific Inc. 781-622-1000
81 Wyman St, Waltham, MA 02451

REAGENT, BLOOD UREA NITROGEN (BUN) *(Chemistry) 75UMB*

Amresco Inc. 800-366-1313
30175 Solon Industrial Pkwy, Solon, OH 44139
Bun reagent - conductivity rate/enzymatic.

Beckman Coulter, Inc. 800-635-3497
740 W 83rd St, Hialeah, FL 33014
$0.09 per test.

Beckman Coulter, Inc. 800-742-2345
250 S Kraemer Blvd, PO Box 8000, Brea, CA 92821

Biomerieux Inc. 800-682-2666
100 Rodolphe St, Durham, NC 27712

Genzyme Corp. 800-325-2436
160 Christian St, Oxford, CT 06478
Enzymatic rate.

Raichem, Division Of Hemagen Diagnostics, Inc. 800-438-6100
8225 Mercury Ct, San Diego, CA 92111

Stanbio Laboratory, Inc. 830-249-0772
1261 N Main St, Boerne, TX 78006
$80.00 for 250 urea nitrogen test sets with color reagent, acid reagent, and standards (25, 50 and 75mg/dl). $41.00 for 4 x 50ml enzymatic urea nitrogen test kits with enzyme and color reagent, and standard (25mg/dl). $42.00 for 20 x 6.5ml UV-rate urea nitrogen test kits with reagent and standard (30mg/dl).

REAGENT, BORRELIA, SEROLOGICAL *(Microbiology) 83LSR*

Bbi Diagnostics, A Division Of Seracare Life Scien 508-244-6428
375 West St, West Bridgewater, MA 02379
Various.

Chembio Diagnostic Systems, Inc. 631-924-1135
3661 Horseblock Rd, Medford, NY 11763
Lyme test.

Innominata dba GENBIO 800-288-4368
15222 Avenue of Science Ste A, San Diego, CA 92128
Immunowell borrelia (lyme) panel (igg & igm combined).

REAGENT, CALCIUM (TEST SYSTEM) *(Chemistry) 75JFO*

Amresco Inc. 800-366-1313
30175 Solon Industrial Pkwy, Solon, OH 44139
RA, Hitachi, SMA, SMAC.

Beckman Coulter, Inc. 800-635-3497
740 W 83rd St, Hialeah, FL 33014
$0.06 per test.

Beckman Coulter, Inc. 800-742-2345
250 S Kraemer Blvd, PO Box 8000, Brea, CA 92821

Biomerieux Inc. 800-682-2666
100 Rodolphe St, Durham, NC 27712

Elabsupply 714-446-8740
1001 Starbuck St Apt C306, Fullerton, CA 92833
Calcium clinical chemistry reagents in liquid format for use in Hitachi, Cobas Mira and Beckman Coulter CX series analyzers.

Genzyme Corp. 800-325-2436
160 Christian St, Oxford, CT 06478
Arsenzo III, endpoint.

Globalemed Llc. 703-894-0710
1101 King St, Suites 370, 270, 170, Alexandria, VA 22314

Raichem, Division Of Hemagen Diagnostics, Inc. 800-438-6100
8225 Mercury Ct, San Diego, CA 92111

Stanbio Laboratory, Inc. 830-249-0772
1261 N Main St, Boerne, TX 78006
$55.50 for 250 calcium test sets containing calcium color reagent, base reagent, standard I (10mg/dl) and II (15mg/dl).

REAGENT, CALIBRATION *(General) 80WRA*

Beckman Coulter, Inc. 800-635-3497
740 W 83rd St, Hialeah, FL 33014
The broad-based SYNCHRON reagents provide the ability to run DATs, TDMs, proteins, thyroids and general chemistries and elecrolytes all on one system.

Beckman Coulter, Inc. 800-742-2345
250 S Kraemer Blvd, PO Box 8000, Brea, CA 92821

Biocell Laboratories, Inc. 800-222-8382
2001 E University Dr, Rancho Dominguez, CA 90220
Multiple levels of bovine and human base calibrators.

Cliniqa Corporation 800-728-9558
774 N Twin Oaks Valley Rd Ste C, San Marcos, CA 92069
LINICAL instrument-specific human-serum-based, and liquid stable for calibration verification and linearity assessment. Kits include the major serum proteins for the Beckman Array, Behring BNA, and Olympus Au systems respectively.

Cytocolor, Inc. 800-776-6455
PO Box 401, Hinckley, OH 44233

Duke Scientific Corp. 800-334-3883
2463 Faber Pl, PO Box 50005, Palo Alto, CA 94303
Nanosphere size standards are calibrated in billionths of a meter. Used as standards for instrument calibration, quality control, filter checking, and biotechnology applications. Cyto-Cal--uniform-intensity calibration microspheres for flow cytometers.

Everest Interscience, Inc. 800-422-4342
1891 N Oracle Rd, Tucson, AZ 85705
High and low temperature calibration sources.

Laboratory Technologies, Inc. 800-542-1123
43 W 900 Rte. 64, Maple Park, IL 60151

Thermo Fisher Scientific Inc. 781-622-1000
81 Wyman St, Waltham, MA 02451

REAGENT, CHLORIDE (TEST SYSTEM) *(Chemistry) 75CHJ*

Beckman Coulter, Inc. 800-635-3497
740 W 83rd St, Hialeah, FL 33014
$0.07 per test.

Biomerieux Inc. 800-682-2666
100 Rodolphe St, Durham, NC 27712

Elabsupply 714-446-8740
1001 Starbuck St Apt C306, Fullerton, CA 92833
Clinical chemistry reagents for cloride in liquid format for use in Cobas Mira, Hitachi, and Beckman Coulter CX series analyzers.

Genzyme Corp. 800-325-2436
160 Christian St, Oxford, CT 06478
Iron thiocyanate, endpoint.

Health Chem Diagnostics Llc 954-979-3845
3341 W McNab Rd, Pompano Beach, FL 33069
Mercuric thiocyanate, colorimetry, chloride.

REAGENT, CHLORIDE (TEST SYSTEM) *(cont'd)*

Jas Diagnostics, Inc. 305-418-2320
7220 NW 58th St, Miami, FL 33166
Chloride.

Raichem, Division Of Hemagen Diagnostics, Inc. 800-438-6100
8225 Mercury Ct, San Diego, CA 92111

Sandare Intl., Inc. 972-293-7440
910 Kck Way, Cedar Hill, TX 75104
Thiocyanate chloride reagent.

Stanbio Laboratory, Inc. 830-249-0772
1261 N Main St, Boerne, TX 78006
$63.50 for 250 test kits containing color reagent, standard (100 mg/l), and blank.

Sterling Diagnostics, Inc. 800-637-2661
36645 Metro Ct, Sterling Heights, MI 48312
Chloride reagent set (colorimetric).

Teco Diagnostics 714-693-7788
1268 N Lakeview Ave, Anaheim, CA 92807
Chloride.

REAGENT, CHOLESTEROL (TOTAL TEST SYSTEM) *(Chemistry) 75CGO*

Amresco Inc. 800-366-1313
30175 Solon Industrial Pkwy, Solon, OH 44139
Direct HDL Cholesterol Reagent, Automatable R1-R2 reagent for the direct determination of HDL cholesterol.

Beckman Coulter, Inc. 800-635-3497
740 W 83rd St, Hialeah, FL 33014
$0.14 per test.

Beckman Coulter, Inc. 800-742-2345
250 S Kraemer Blvd, PO Box 8000, Brea, CA 92821

Bio-Medical Products Corp. 800-543-7427
10 Halstead Rd, Mendham, NJ 07945
Blood cholesterol screening and HDL test strips.

Genzyme Corp. 800-325-2436
160 Christian St, Oxford, CT 06478

Health Chem Diagnostics Llc 954-979-3845
3341 W McNab Rd, Pompano Beach, FL 33069
Lieberman-burchard/abell-kendall, colorimetric, cholesterol.

Helena Laboratories 409-842-3714
PO Box 752, Beaumont, TX 77704
REP Cholesterol Profile provides simultaneous, direct measurement of LDL and HDL.

Home Access Health Corp. 800-HIV-TEST
2401 Hassell Rd Ste 1510, Hoffman Estates, IL 60169
Home Access Instant Cholesterol Test allows a person to test their total cholesterol in 15 minutes without fasting.

Pointe Scientific, Inc. 800-445-9853
5449 Research Dr, Canton, MI 48188
Direct LDL cholesterol test kit. Auto cholesterol reagent is for the quantitative determination of high density lipoprotein cholesterol in human serum or plasma.

Raichem, Division Of Hemagen Diagnostics, Inc. 800-438-6100
8225 Mercury Ct, San Diego, CA 92111

Shared Systems, Inc. 888-474-2733
PO Box 211587, 3961 Columbia Rd, Augusta, GA 30917

Stanbio Laboratory, Inc. 830-249-0772
1261 N Main St, Boerne, TX 78006
$68.50 for 4 x 30ml, $177.00 for 500ml and $31.00 for 20ml, HDL precipitating reagent with standard.

REAGENT, CLOSTRIDIUM DIFFICILE TOXIN *(Microbiology) 83LLH*

Bd Diagnostic Systems 800-675-0908
7 Loveton Cir, Sparks, MD 21152

Bd Lee Laboratories 800-732-9150
1475 Athens Hwy, Grayson, GA 30017
C. diffile Toxin´A Antibody affinity purified antibodies to Clostridium Difficile Toxin A.

Biosite Incorporated 888-246-7483
9975 Summers Ridge Rd, San Diego, CA 92121
Enzymimmunoassay for detection of glutamate dehtdrogenase and toxin a.

Meridian Bioscience, Inc. 800-696-0739
3471 River Hills Dr, Cincinnati, OH 45244
Enzyme immunoassay for the detection of C. difficile common antigen in stool.

REAGENT, CLOSTRIDIUM DIFFICILE TOXIN *(cont'd)*

Oxoid, Inc. 800-567-8378
800 Proctor Ave, Ogdensburg, NY 13669

Prodesse, Inc. 888-589-6974
W229N1870 Westwood Dr, Waukesha, WI 53186
ProGastro Cd - PCR for toxigenic strains of Clostridium difficile - In Development

REAGENT, CREATININE (TEST SYSTEM) *(Chemistry) 75CGX*

Abbott Diagnostics Div. 626-440-0700
820 Mission St, South Pasadena, CA 91030
Creatinine.

Amresco Inc. 800-366-1313
30175 Solon Industrial Pkwy, Solon, OH 44139
Hitachi, technicon RA, SMAC and SMA systems picric acid method.

Bayer Healthcare Llc 914-524-2955
555 White Plains Rd Fl 5, Tarrytown, NY 10591
Test for creatinine.

Beckman Coulter, Inc. 800-635-3497
740 W 83rd St, Hialeah, FL 33014
$0.05 per test.

Beckman Coulter, Inc. 800-742-2345
250 S Kraemer Blvd, PO Box 8000, Brea, CA 92821

Biomerieux Inc. 800-682-2666
100 Rodolphe St, Durham, NC 27712

Caldon Bioscience, Inc. 909-628-9944
2100 S Reservoir St, Pomona, CA 91766
Creatinine.

Caldon Biotech, Inc. 757-224-0177
2251 Rutherford Rd, Carlsbad, CA 92008
Creatinine.

Carolina Liquid Chemistries Corp. 800-471-7272
510 W Central Ave Ste C, Brea, CA 92821
Creat.

Diagnostic Specialties 732-549-4011
4 Leonard St, Metuchen, NJ 08840
$44.00 per unit (standard).

Flexsite Diagnostics, Inc. 772-221-8893
3543 SW Corporate Pkwy, Palm City, FL 34990
Home sampling kit for self monitoring of urinary microalbumin.

Genchem, Inc. 714-529-1616
510 W Central Ave Ste D, Brea, CA 92821
Creatinine reagent.

Genzyme Corp. 800-325-2436
160 Christian St, Oxford, CT 06478
Jaffe, kinetic.

Health Chem Diagnostics Llc 954-979-3845
3341 W McNab Rd, Pompano Beach, FL 33069
Alkaline picrate, colorimetry, creatinine.

Intersect Systems, Inc. 360-577-1062
1152 3rd Avenue, Suite D & E, Longview, WA 98632
Alkaline picrate, colorimetry, creatine, Dual Vial Creatine.

Jas Diagnostics, Inc. 305-418-2320
7220 NW 58th St, Miami, FL 33166
Creatinine.

Raichem, Division Of Hemagen Diagnostics, Inc. 800-438-6100
8225 Mercury Ct, San Diego, CA 92111

Sita Associates 630-968-3727
720 Williamsburg Ct, Oak Brook, IL 60523
Rapid creatinine test kits for urine and serum/amniotic fluid.

Stanbio Laboratory, Inc. 830-249-0772
1261 N Main St, Boerne, TX 78006
$90.50 for 20 x 6.5ml Creatine Kinase/UV-Rate reagent, $49.00 for 100 creatinine test sets containing picric reagent, sodium hydroxide reagent, standards 2.5mg/dl and 5.0mg/dl. $51.50 for 250 direct creatinine test sets with 125ml ea. acid and base reagent and 5.0mg/dl standard.

Sterling Diagnostics, Inc. 800-637-2661
36645 Metro Ct, Sterling Heights, MI 48312
Creatinine reagent set.

Synermed Intl., Inc. 317-896-1565
17408 Tiller Ct Ste 1900, Westfield, IN 46074
Creatine reagent kit.

Teco Diagnostics 714-693-7788
1268 N Lakeview Ave, Anaheim, CA 92807
Creatinine.

REAGENT, CREATININE (TEST SYSTEM) *(cont'd)*

Vital Diagnostics Inc. 714-672-3553
1075 W Lambert Rd Ste D, Brea, CA 92821
Various creatinine reagents.

REAGENT, CYANOMETHEMOGLOBIN, WITH STANDARD
(Hematology) 81GJZ

Beckman Coulter, Inc. 800-635-3497
740 W 83rd St, Hialeah, FL 33014

Diagnostic Specialties 732-549-4011
4 Leonard St, Metuchen, NJ 08840
$32.00 per 1000ml.

Diagnostic Technology, Inc. 631-582-4949
175 Commerce Dr Ste L, Hauppauge, NY 11788
Cyanmethemoglobin reagent.

E K Industries, Inc. 877-EKI-CHEM
1403 Herkimer St, Joliet, IL 60432
Drabkin reagent.

Health Chem Diagnostics Llc 954-979-3845
3341 W McNab Rd, Pompano Beach, FL 33069
Cyanomethemoglobin reagent and standard solution.

Medical Chemical Corp. 800-424-9394
19430 Van Ness Ave, Torrance, CA 90501
$25.00 per unit.

Sandare Intl., Inc. 972-293-7440
910 Kck Way, Cedar Hill, TX 75104
Cyanhemoglobin standard.

Stanbio Laboratory, Inc. 830-249-0772
1261 N Main St, Boerne, TX 78006
$45.00 per pkg. (6 vials/pkg. = 6 x 2,000ml) of Drabkins cyanmethemoglobin powder, $53.00 for 3,800ml Drabkins liquid reagent. $41.00 for 6 x 15ml liquid standard (80 G/DL equivalent to 20 G/DL at 1:251 dilution).

Sterling Diagnostics, Inc. 800-637-2661
36645 Metro Ct, Sterling Heights, MI 48312

REAGENT, CYSTICERCOSIS *(Microbiology) 83MDJ*

Immunetics, Inc. 800-227-4765
27 Drydock Ave Ste 6, Boston, MA 02210
Cysticercosis Western Blot antibody detection kit.

Ivd Research, Inc. 760-929-7744
5909 Sea Lion Pl Ste D, Carlsbad, CA 92010
T.solium (cytirercosis) serum elisa.

United Biotech, Inc. 650-961-2910
211 S Whisman Rd Ste E, Mountain View, CA 94041
ELISA detecting Cysticercosis

REAGENT, DNA-PROBE, STREPTOCOCCAL
(Microbiology) 83MDK

Gen-Probe, Inc. 800-523-5001
10210 Genetic Center Dr, San Diego, CA 92121
AccuProbe Group A STREPTOCOCCUS Culture Identification Test - for the identification of Group A Streptococcus isolated from culture. AccuProbe Group B STREPTOCOCCUS Culture Identification Test - for the identification of Group B Streptococcus isolated from culture.

REAGENT, GENERAL PURPOSE *(Pathology) 88LDT*

Acuderm Inc. 800-327-0015
5370 NW 35th Ter Ste 106, Fort Lauderdale, FL 33309
Potassium hydroxide.

Alfa Wassermann, Inc. 800-220-4488
4 Henderson Dr, West Caldwell, NJ 07006
Liquid stable.

Alpha-Tec Systems, Inc. 800-221-6058
12019 NE 99th St Ste 1780, Vancouver, WA 98682
General purpose reagents & buffers.

Alt Bioscience,Llc 859-231-3061
235 Bolivar St, Lexington, KY 40508
Dilution of dtnb and coomassie brilliant blue.

Amresco Inc. 800-366-1313
30175 Solon Industrial Pkwy, Solon, OH 44139
Direct x-amylase quantitative kinetic determination of x-amylase activity in human serum and plasma by manual and automated procedures.

Asuragen, Inc. 877-777-1874
2150 Woodward St Ste 100, Austin, TX 78744
General purpose reagents.

REAGENT, GENERAL PURPOSE *(cont'd)*

Aviaradx, Inc. 877-886-6739
11025 Roselle St Ste 200, San Diego, CA 92121
General purpose reagents.

Bdh, Inc. 800-268-0310
350 Evans Ave., Toronto, ONT M8Z 1K5 Canada

Beckman Coulter, Inc. 714-871-4848
22900 W 8 Mile Rd, Southfield, MI 48033
Chemiluminescent detection reagents.

Bio-Rad Laboratories, Diagnostic Group 800-224-6723
524 Stone Rd Ste A, Benicia, CA 94510
Type i reagent grade water, isotonics solutions.

Bio-Synthesis, Inc 800-227-0627
612 E Main St, Lewisville, TX 75057
REAGENTS,SPECIFIC,ANALYTE

Biocare Medical, Llc 925-603-8003
4040 Pike Ln, Concord, CA 94520
Buffers, retrieval solutions and detection reagents.

Calbiotech, Inc. 619-660-6162
10461 Austin Dr Ste G, Spring Valley, CA 91978
Reagent, general purpose.

Celera Corporation 510-749-4219
884 Dubuque Ave, S San Fran, CA 94080
Reagent, general purpose.

Celera Corporation 510-749-4219
1401 Harbor Bay Pkwy, Alameda, CA 94502
Various types of general purpose reagents.

Cepheid 408-541-4191
904 E Caribbean Dr, Sunnyvale, CA 94089
SPECIFIC,ANALYTE

Cytocore, Inc. 312-379-4790
414 N Orleans St Ste 502, Chicago, IL 60654
Hpv buffer 1.

Cytyc Surgical Products 800-442-9892
250 Campus Dr, Marlborough, MA 01752
Fixative solution.

Diagnostic Biosystems 925-484-3350
1020 Serpentine Ln Ste 114, Pleasanton, CA 94566

E K Industries, Inc. 877-EKI-CHEM
1403 Herkimer St, Joliet, IL 60432
Picric acid solution.

eBioscience 888-999-1371
10255 Science Center Dr, San Diego, CA 92121
CD10 PE; CD14 PE; CD19 APC; CD19 PerCP-Cy5.5; CD20 FITC; CD3 eFluorTM 450; CD3 FITC; CD3 PerCP-Cy5.5; CD34 PE; CD38 PE; CD4 APC; CD4 eFluorTM 450; CD4 FITC; CD4 PE; CD45 PerCP-Cy5.5; CD7 FITC; CD8 APC; CD8 PE; HLA-DR PE; Ig lambda light chain PE; ZAP-70 PE

Edge Medical Imaging, Inc. 703-919-4732
6003 Woodlake Ln, Alexandria, VA 22315
General purpose reagent.

Exaxol Chemical Corp. 727-524-7732
14325 60th St N, Clearwater, FL 33760
Various.

Fertility Solutions, Inc. 800-959-7656
13000 Shaker Blvd, Cleveland, OH 44120
Sperm diluent.

Fisher Scientific Co., Llc. 201-703-3131
1 Reagent Ln, Fair Lawn, NJ 07410
Various histlogical reagents.

Gentra Systems, Inc. 763-543-0678
13355 10th Ave N Ste 120, Minneapolis, MN 55441
Various types of reagent, general purpose.

Horiba Abx 888-903-5001
34 Bunsen, Irvine, CA 92618
Liquid reagent used for general purposes in analyzer.

Iris Diagnostics 800-776-4747
9172 Eton Ave, Chatsworth, CA 91311
Reagent,general purpose.

Labchem, Inc. 412-826-5230
200 William Pitt Way, Pittsburgh, PA 15238
Multiple salt solutions.

Lgm International Inc. 410-472-9930
3030 Venture Ln Ste 106, Melbourne, FL 32934
Reagent, general purpose.

REAGENT, GENERAL PURPOSE *(cont'd)*

Micro Typing Systems, Inc. 908-218-8177
1295 SW 29th Ave, Pompano Beach, FL 33069
Wash solutions.

Nanogen, Inc. 877-626-6436
10398 Pacific Center Ct, San Diego, CA 92121
High and low salt buffer.

Nerl Diagnostics Llc. 401-824-2046
14 Almeida Ave, East Providence, RI 02914
Reagent, hematology general hematology reagents.

Nichols Institute Diagnostics 949-940-7200
1311 Calle Batido, San Clemente, CA 92673
Reagent controls.

Pochemco, Inc. 413-536-2900
724 Main St, Holyoke, MA 01040
Various types and strengths of general purpose reagents.

Promega Corp. 800-356-9526
2800 Woods Hollow Rd, Fitchburg, WI 53711

Qc Sciences 866-709-0523
4851 Lake Brook Dr, Glen Allen, VA 23060
Alcoholic agarose solution.

Qiagen Sciences, Inc. 301-944-7090
19300 Germantown Rd, Germantown, MD 20874
Various types of general purpose reagents.

R2 Diagnostics, Inc. 574-288-4377
1801 Commerce Dr, South Bend, IN 46628
Imidazole buffered saline.

Ricca Chemical Company Llc 888-467-4222
1841 Broad St, Pocomoke City, MD 21851
Various.

Ricca Chemical Company Llc 817-461-5601
1490 Lammers Pike, Batesville, IN 47006

Ricca Chemical Company, Llc 817-461-5601
448 W Fork Dr, Arlington, TX 76012
Various.

Richard-Allan Scientific 269-544-5628
4481 Campus Dr, Kalamazoo, MI 49008
General purpose reagents and buffers.

Sci Gen, Inc. 310-324-6576
333 E Gardena Blvd, Gardena, CA 90248
FDA: Medical Device Manufacturing and packaging. Focus on Histology, Cytology, Analytical and General purpose Reagents, Chemistry, and Sterling and Disinfecting agents.

Scientific Device Laboratory Inc. 847-803-9495
411 Jarvis Ave, Des Plaines, IL 60018
Snap n' digest, spiutolysin reagent.

Scytek Laboratories, Inc. 435-755-9848
205 S 600 W, Logan, UT 84321
Reagent, general purpose.

Sierra Molecular Inc. 209-536-0886
21109 Longeway Rd Ste C, Sonora, CA 95370
Nucleic acid preservative.

Statlab Medical Products, Inc. 800-442-3573
106 Hillside Dr, Lewisville, TX 75057
ANAPATH tap-water substitute.

Third Wave Technologies, Inc. 888-898-2357
502 S Rosa Rd, Madison, WI 53719
Cleavase enzyme & reagents.

Tripath Imaging, Inc. 919-206-7140
780 Plantation Dr, Burlington, NC 27215
Buffers, retreival solutions and detection reagents.

Vegamed, Inc. 787-807-0392
39 Calle Las Flores, Edificio Multifabril #5, Vega Baja, PR 00693
Detergent for hematology.

Ventana Medical Systems, Inc. 800-227-2155
1910 E Innovation Park Dr, Oro Valley, AZ 85755
Various general purpose reagents.

XDx Expression Diagnostics 415-287-2300
3260 Bayshore Blvd, Brisbane, CA 94005
PROCESSING PACK; ALLOMAP SAMPLE COLLECTION

Xtrana, Inc. 800-789-6534
590 Burbank St Unit 205, Broomfield, CO 80020
Xtra Amp.

REAGENT, GLOBULIN (TEST SYSTEM) *(Chemistry) 75JGE*

Irvine Scientific 800-437-5706
2511 Daimler St, Santa Ana, CA 92705
IMMUNOBEAD reagents provide fast and reproducible separation of primary antibody in immunoassays. Purified goat anti-rabbit (or anti-mouse) immunoglobulin antibody is covalently coupled to the Second Antibody IMMUNOBEAD. They exhibit low nonspecific binding and are insensitive to variations in sample protein concentration.

REAGENT, GLUCOSE (TEST SYSTEM) *(Chemistry) 75CGA*

Abbott Point Of Care Inc. 609-443-9300
104 Windsor Center Dr, East Windsor, NJ 08520
Various types of equipment and tests.

Access Bio Incorporate 732-297-2222
2033 Rt. 130 Unit H, Monmouth Junction, NJ 08852
Glucose test system.

Agamatrix 603-328-6000
10 Manor Pkwy, Salem, NH 03079
Blood glucose system.

Aimtronics Corp. 604-946-9666
100 Schneider Rd, Kanata K2K 1Y2 Canada
A)precision qid: 2)companion ii c)pen ii d) qid ii e)asteroid f)exac tec

Amresco Inc. 800-366-1313
30175 Solon Industrial Pkwy, Solon, OH 44139
Oxygen rate for Beckman systems.

Arkray Factory Usa, Inc. 952-646-3168
5182 W 76th St, Minneapolis, MN 55439
Blood glucose monitoring system.

Arkray Usa 800-818-8877
5198 W 76th St, Edina, MN 55439
Assure® Pro is specifically designed for multi-resident use in long-term care (LTC) facilities. This full-featured system offers qcProGuard™, the first of its kind, 24-hour reminder to conduct daily control solution testing as required in LTC settings. A íHypoî warning alerts users of low blood glucose readings and four programmable alarms can be used as test reminders. Assure Pro Test Strips are built using platinum technology and require a small blood sample size (1 μL). To test, simply insert the test strip in the convenient top-of-the-meter port. Results are displayed in 10 seconds on a large LCD and a backlight display (adjustable) assists for reading in low light conditions. A strip release button for strip disposal eliminates the need to touch a used strip, reducing the risk of exposure to infectious materials. For additional security, Assure Pro is designed with ProGrip™ to help secure a hold on the meter and reduce slipping on surfaces.

Bayer Healthcare Llc 914-524-2955
555 White Plains Rd Fl 5, Tarrytown, NY 10591
Blood clucose meter.

Bayer Healthcare, Llc 574-256-3430
430 S Beiger St, Mishawaka, IN 46544
Test for glucose in blood.

Beckman Coulter, Inc. 800-635-3497
740 W 83rd St, Hialeah, FL 33014
$0.08 per test.

Beckman Coulter, Inc. 800-742-2345
250 S Kraemer Blvd, PO Box 8000, Brea, CA 92821

Benchmark Winona 507-452-8932
6301 Bandel Rd NW, Rochester, MN 55901
Glucose test system.

Biomerieux Inc. 800-682-2666
100 Rodolphe St, Durham, NC 27712

Carolina Liquid Chemistries Corp. 800-471-7272
510 W Central Ave Ste C, Brea, CA 92821
Glucose reagent.

Chematics, Inc. 574-834-4080
Hwy. 13 South, North Webster, IN 46555
Solid phase determination of glucose, enzymatic glucose oxidase method.

Diagnostic Devices Inc. 704-285-6400
9300 Harris Corners Pkwy Ste 450, Charlotte, NC 28269
Glucose test system.

Firehouse Medical, Inc. 714-688-1575
1045 N Armando St Ste D, Anaheim, CA 92806
Blood glucose test device for emergency use.

Genchem, Inc. 714-529-1616
510 W Central Ave Ste D, Brea, CA 92821
Glucose oxidase reagent.

REAGENT, GLUCOSE (TEST SYSTEM) *(cont'd)*

Genzyme Corp. 800-325-2436
160 Christian St, Oxford, CT 06478
GOD-POD test system.

Gml, Inc. 651-486-3691
500 Oak Grove Pkwy, Saint Paul, MN 55127
Blood glucose test strips.

Harvey, R.J. Instrument Corp. 201-664-1380
123 Patterson St, Hillsdale, NJ 07642

Health Chem Diagnostics Llc 954-979-3845
3341 W McNab Rd, Pompano Beach, FL 33069
Glucose oxidase, glucose.

Health Hero Network, Inc. 650-779-9160
2000 Seaport Blvd Ste 400, Redwood City, CA 94063
Healthbuddy with device connect (glucose meter), buddy link, buddylink.

Jas Diagnostics, Inc. 305-418-2320
7220 NW 58th St, Miami, FL 33166
Glucose-oxidase.

Lifescan Llc. 408-263-9789
Rd. 308 Km 0.8, Pedernales Industrial Park, Cabo Rojo, PR 00623-5001
Reagent test strip for whole blood glucose determination.

Lifescan, Inc. 800-227-8862
1000 Gibraltar Dr, Milpitas, CA 95035
Reagent test strip for whole blood glucose determination.

Nipro Diagnostics, Inc. 1-800-342-7226
2400 NW 55th Ct, Fort Lauderdale, FL 33309
Blood glucose test system.

Nova Biomedical Corporation Diabetes Products 781-894-0800
205 Burlington Rd, Bedford, MA 01730
Glucose oxidase, glucose test system.

Opti Medical Systems Inc. 770-510-4444
235 Hembree Park Dr, Roswell, GA 30076
Automated blood gas/ electrolyte analyzer.

Osmetech, Inc. 800-373-6767
757 S Raymond Ave, Pasadena, CA 91105
Automated blood gas/ electrolyte analyzer.

Polymer Technology Systems, Inc. 317-870-5610
7736 Zionsville Rd, Indianapolis, IN 46268
Glucose monitoring system.

Quest Star Medical, Inc. 800-525-6718
10180 Viking Dr, Eden Prairie, MN 55344
Focus blood-glucose monitor and Focus test strips.

Raichem, Division Of Hemagen Diagnostics, Inc. 800-438-6100
8225 Mercury Ct, San Diego, CA 92111
Enzymatic reagent for determination of glucose at 500 nm.

Rockland Immunochemicals, Inc. 800-656-ROCK
PO Box 326, Gilbertsville, PA 19525
Glucose oxidase, anti-glucose oxidase.

Rose Technologies 425-637-2344
13400 NE 20th St Ste 32, Bellevue, WA 98005
Accessory to a blood glucose test system.

Sanmina-Sci Usa, Inc. 256-882-4800
13000 Memorial Pkwy SW, Huntsville, AL 35803
Glucose monitoring system.

Sterling Diagnostics, Inc. 800-637-2661
36645 Metro Ct, Sterling Heights, MI 48312
Glucose reagent set (trinder).

Synermed Intl., Inc. 317-896-1565
17408 Tiller Ct Ste 1900, Westfield, IN 46074
Glucose reagent kit.

Teco Diagnostics 714-693-7788
1268 N Lakeview Ave, Anaheim, CA 92807
Glucose reagent set.

Vital Diagnostics Inc. 714-672-3553
1075 W Lambert Rd Ste D, Brea, CA 92821
Various glucose reagents.

REAGENT, GUAIAC *(Hematology) 81GGG*

Aerscher Diagnostics 410-778-1144
353 High St, Chestertown, MD 21620
Hemaprompt-fecal occult blood kit, hemascreen seat coloncheck.

Beckman Coulter, Inc. Primary Care Diagnostics 714-961-3712
606 Elmwood Ave, Elmwood Court Three, Sharon Hill, PA 19079
Fecal occult blood test.

REAGENT, GUAIAC *(cont'd)*

Cambridge Diagnostic Products, Inc. 800-525-6262
6880 NW 17th Ave, Fort Lauderdale, FL 33309
Guaiac tablets and CAMCO Pak Guaiac.

REAGENT, IMMUNOASSAY, ACTIVATOR, C3, COMPLEMENT *(Immunology) 82KTP*

Quidel Corp. 858-552-1100
2981 Copper Rd, Santa Clara, CA 95051
Complement components, immunological test systems.

REAGENT, INOCULATOR CALIBRATION (LABORATORY) *(Microbiology) 83LIE*

Bangs Laboratories, Inc. 800-387-0672
9025 Technology Dr, Fishers, IN 46038
Standards for flow cytometry, fluorescent microspheres, calibration software.

REAGENT, IRON (TEST SYSTEM) *(Chemistry) 75CFM*

Abbott Diagnostics Div. 626-440-0700
820 Mission St, South Pasadena, CA 91030
Iron.

Amresco Inc. 800-366-1313
30175 Solon Industrial Pkwy, Solon, OH 44139
Hitachi systems.

Biomerieux Inc. 800-682-2666
100 Rodolphe St, Durham, NC 27712

Carolina Liquid Chemistries Corp. 800-471-7272
510 W Central Ave Ste C, Brea, CA 92821
Iron reagent.

Emd Chemicals Inc. 800-222-0342
480 S Democrat Rd, Gibbstown, NJ 08027

Genzyme Corp. 800-325-2436
160 Christian St, Oxford, CT 06478
FERENE Colorimetric iron & binding test, endpoint.

J&S Medical Associates 800-229-6000
35 Tripp St Ste 1, Framingham, MA 01702
$80.00 for 50-test kit of J & S iron saturating reagent.

Raichem, Division Of Hemagen Diagnostics, Inc. 800-438-6100
8225 Mercury Ct, San Diego, CA 92111

Stanbio Laboratory, Inc. 830-249-0772
1261 N Main St, Boerne, TX 78006
$92.50 for 110 iron & total iron binding capacity test kits with ferrozine color reagent, HA buffer, Tris buffer and iron standard, $131.50 for 220 test kits.

REAGENT, KINASE, PHOSPHATE, CREATINE *(Chemistry) 75JFX*

Amresco Inc. 800-366-1313
30175 Solon Industrial Pkwy, Solon, OH 44139
Hitachi, technicon RA, SMAC and SMA systems.

Beckman Coulter, Inc. 800-635-3497
740 W 83rd St, Hialeah, FL 33014
$0.12 per test.

Biomerieux Inc. 800-682-2666
100 Rodolphe St, Durham, NC 27712

Dade Behring, Inc. 800-948-3233
1717 Deerfield Rd, Deerfield, IL 60015

Elabsupply 714-446-8740
1001 Starbuck St Apt C306, Fullerton, CA 92833
Clinical chemistry reagents in liquid or powder format for use in Hitachi, Cobas Mira, and Beckman Coulter CX series analyzers.

Genzyme Corp. 800-325-2436
160 Christian St, Oxford, CT 06478
NAC activated, kinetic.

Globalemed Llc. 703-894-0710
1101 King St, Suites 370, 270, 170, Alexandria, VA 22314

Stanbio Laboratory, Inc. 830-249-0772
1261 N Main St, Boerne, TX 78006
$90.50 for 20 x 6.5ml Creatinine Kinase/UV-Rate reagent.

REAGENT, LEGIONELLA DETECTION *(Microbiology) 83UML*

Scimedx Corporation 800-221-5598
100 Ford Rd Ste 100-08, Denville, NJ 07834

REAGENT, LEISHMANII SEROLOGICAL *(Microbiology) 83LOO*

Inbios Intl., Inc. 866-INBIOS1
562 1st Ave S Ste 600, Seattle, WA 98104
Rapid test for the detection of visceral leishmaniasis.

REAGENT, LEISHMANII SEROLOGICAL *(cont'd)*

Ivd Research, Inc. 760-929-7744
5909 Sea Lion Pl Ste D, Carlsbad, CA 92010
Leishmania serum elisa.

United Biotech, Inc. 650-961-2910
211 S Whisman Rd Ste E, Mountain View, CA 94041
ELISA detecting Leishmania (IgM & IgM)

REAGENT, NAD-NADH, ALCOHOL ENZYME METHOD *(Toxicology) 91DML*

Abbott Diagnostics Div. 626-440-0700
820 Mission St, South Pasadena, CA 91030
Ethanol.

Biomerieux Inc. 800-682-2666
100 Rodolphe St, Durham, NC 27712

Raichem, Division Of Hemagen Diagnostics, Inc. 800-438-6100
8225 Mercury Ct, San Diego, CA 92111

Varian Inc 650-424-5078
25200 Commercentre Dr, Lake Forest, CA 92630
Alcohol test.

REAGENT, OCCULT BLOOD *(Hematology) 81KHE*

Ameritek Usa, Inc. 425-379-2580
125 130th St SE Ste 200, Everett, WA 98208
Occult blood test card.

Bayer Healthcare, Llc 574-256-3430
430 S Beiger St, Mishawaka, IN 46544
Test for occult blood in feces.

Beckman Coulter Primary Care Diagnostics 714-961-3712
1050 Page Mill Rd Bldg 2-B, Palo Alto, CA 94304
Test for fecal occult blood.

Beckman Coulter, Inc. Primary Care Diagnostics 714-961-3712
606 Elmwood Ave, Elmwood Court Three, Sharon Hill, PA 19079
Developer solutions for occult blood tests.

Bio-Medical Products Corp. 800-543-7427
10 Halstead Rd, Mendham, NJ 07945
Occult blood slide test kit. Fecal immunochromatographic 10 minute test.

Cambridge Diagnostic Products, Inc. 800-525-6262
6880 NW 17th Ave, Fort Lauderdale, FL 33309
Guaiac tablets and CAMCO Pak Guaiac.

Enterix Inc. 732-429-1899
236 Fernwood Ave, Edison, NJ 08837
Insure immunochemical fobt.

Immunostics, Inc. 800-722-7505
3505 Sunset Ave, Ocean, NJ 07712
HEMA SCREEN.

Innovacon, Inc. 858-535-2030
4106 Sorrento Valley Blvd, San Diego, CA 92121
Fecal occult blood test.

Inverness Medical Professional Diagnostics-San Die 858-535-2030
4106 Sorrento Valley Blvd, San Diego, CA 92121
Fecal occult blood test.

J&S Medical Associates 800-229-6000
35 Tripp St Ste 1, Framingham, MA 01702
ACCUCULT.

Propper Manufacturing Co., Inc. 800-832-4300
3604 Skillman Ave, Long Island City, NY 11101
SERACULT & SERACULT PLUS: Occult blood tests.

Teco Diagnostics 714-693-7788
1268 N Lakeview Ave, Anaheim, CA 92807
Rapid fecal occult blood card test.

W.H.P.M., Inc. 978-927-3808
9662 Telstar Ave, El Monte, CA 91731
Occult blood test.

REAGENT, OTHER *(General) 80WPW*

Analytical Control Systems, Inc. 317-841-0458
9058 Technology Dr, Fishers, IN 46038
SPECTRA APCT (activated plasma coagulation time). Available with 2 controls, Spectra APCT normal controls and Spectra APCT abnormal controls. Tests intrinsic system & PF3 release. Excellent stability. Able to screen for the Lupus Anticoagulant. Enhanced sensitivity to factors VIII, IX, X, XI, XII, Fitzgerald and Fletcher factors.

REAGENT, OTHER *(cont'd)*

Biokit Usa, Inc. 800-926-3353
101 Hartwell Ave, Lexington, MA 02421
QUANTEX RF, ASO CRP: Automated latex reagents.

Biolog, Inc. 800-284-4949
21124 Cabot Blvd, Hayward, CA 94545
GN MICROPLATE for biotyping & identifying aerobic gram-negative bacteria, GP MICROPLATE for biotyping and identifying aerobic gram-positive bacteria, ES MICROPLATE for biotyping E. Coli K12 and S. typhimurium LT2 strains.

Biomerieux Industry 800-634-7656
595 Anglum Rd, Hazelwood, MO 63042
Stains and reagents for microbiology and mycology.

Budenheim Usa, Inc 800-645-3044
245 Newtown Rd Ste 305, Plainview, NY 11803

Cholestech Corp. 800-733-0404
3347 Investment Blvd, Hayward, CA 94545
CHOLESTECH LDX and GDX Systems - CLIA Waived Lipid Profile, Glucose, ALT and HBA1C Test Results.

Crescent Chemical Co., Inc. 800-877-3225
2 Oval Dr, Islandia, NY 11749
HYDRANAL pyridine free reagents, buffers, atomic standards, ICP, environmental standards, Bis Benzimide, solvents and reagents.

Dominion Biologicals Ltd. 800-565-0653
5 Isnor Dr., Dartmouth, NS B3B 1M1 Canada
Red blood cell line.

Duke Scientific Corp. 800-334-3883
2463 Faber Pl, PO Box 50005, Palo Alto, CA 94303
Cyto-Plex--multiplex beads for flow-cytometry array analysis.

Electron Microscopy Sciences 800-523-5874
321 Morris Rd, Fort Washington, PA 19034
Chemicals for biological research.

Exocell, Inc. 800-234-3962
1880 John F Kennedy Blvd Ste 200, Philadelphia, PA 19103

Immunicon Corporation 215-830-0777
3401 Masons Mill Rd Ste 100, Huntingdon Valley, PA 19006
CellTracks kits use magnetic ferrofluid reagents for separating cells, viruses, bacteria, proteins, factors, and nucleic acids. Fluorescent reagents are used to differentiate and enumerate cells subsets. The CellSearch Circulating Tumor Cell Kit is to capture, count and characterize tumor cells in blood.

Inamco International Corp. 800-724-4003
801 Montrose Ave, South Plainfield, NJ 07080

Innovative Chemistry, Inc. 781-837-6709
PO Box 578, Marshfield, MA 02050
Enzyme reagents. Isoenzyme test kits for cell culture. Agarose gels.

Kamiya Biomedical Company 206-575-8068
12779 Gateway Dr S, Tukwila, WA 98168
Clinical chemistry, liquid-stable routine diagnostic reagents. Research assay kits for other serum proteins are available.

One Lambda, Inc. 800-822-8824
21001 Kittridge St, Canoga Park, CA 91303
HLA typing reagents; terasaki HLA-ABC/HLA-DR tissue typing trays; lambda monoclonal typing trays, traymates two-tray systems. HLA testing reagents; bult rabbit complement; controls; goat IgG anti-human kappa, mineral oil. HLA screening reagents; lambda cell trays.

Poly Scientific R&D Corp. 800-645-5825
70 Cleveland Ave, Bay Shore, NY 11706
Reagent assembly kit for histology. Alcohol reagent.

Polymer Laboratories, Now A Part Of Varian, Inc. 800-767-3963
160 Old Farm Rd, Amherst Fields Research Park, Amherst, MA 01002

Raichem, Division Of Hemagen Diagnostics, Inc. 800-438-6100
8225 Mercury Ct, San Diego, CA 92111
Fructosamine Reagent Test System.

Rockland Immunochemicals, Inc. 800-656-ROCK
PO Box 326, Gilbertsville, PA 19525
Purfied proteins.

Seradyn, Inc. 800-428-4072
7998 Georgetown Rd Ste 1000, Indianapolis, IN 46268
Cardiac risk assessment reagents/controls.

REAGENT, OTHER *(cont'd)*

Stanbio Laboratory, Inc. 830-249-0772
1261 N Main St, Boerne, TX 78006
$60.50 for 20 x 6.5ml LDH test kit (UV-rate). $38.00 for 4 x 30ml, $123.50 for 2 x 250ml magnesium test sets with reagent and standard. $92.50 for 50 potassium test kits with boron, sodium hydroxide, TCA precipitating reagent and postassium standard (4 meq/l).

Surgipath Medical Industries, Inc. 800-225-3035
PO Box 528, 5205 Route 12, Richmond, IL 60071

Surmodics, Inc. 866-SURMODX
9924 W 74th St, Eden Prairie, MN 55344
Surface modification reagents used to immobilize a wide variety of molecules to create unique performance-enhancing surfaces on medical devices. Customized reagent and processing formulations can provide increased lubricity, hemocompatibility, infection resistance, and/or drug elution.

Thermo Fisher Scientific Inc. 781-622-1000
81 Wyman St, Waltham, MA 02451

Vector Laboratories, Inc. 800-227-6666
30 Ingold Rd, Burlingame, CA 94010
$60.00 for 50 transfers biotinylated DNA molecular weight markers; $60.00 for 50 transfers biotinylated protein molecular weight markers. $60.00 for 50mg NEUROBIOTIN Tracer; $80.00 for 0.5mg PHOTOPROBE Biotin; $70.00 for 50mg Biotin (Long Arm) NHS, water soluble; $70.00 for 50mg Biotin (Long Arm) Hydrazide; and $45.00 for 7mL VECTABOND Tissue Secton Adhesive. $50.00 for 10ml VECTASHIELD mounting medium; $70.00 for peroxidase, alkaline, phosphate and glueose onidase substrate kits.

Wako Chemicals Usa, Inc. 877-714-1924
1600 Bellwood Rd, Richmond, VA 23237
Clinical chemistry reagents.

REAGENT, PLATELET AGGREGATION *(Hematology) 81GHR*

Bio/Data Corp. 215-441-4000
155 Gibraltar Rd, Horsham, PA 19044
Platelet aggregation reagents (collagen, epinephrine, ristocetin).

Chrono-Log Corp. 800-247-6665
2 W Park Rd, Havertown, PA 19083
ADP, Collagen, Ristocetin, Arachidonic Acid, Epinephrine and Ristocetin Cofactor Kits.

Dade Behring, Inc. 800-948-3233
1717 Deerfield Rd, Deerfield, IL 60015

Friedrich & Dimmock, Inc. 800-524-1131
2127 Wheaton Ave, PO Box 230, Millville, NJ 08332
Multi lumen glass & quartz micro capillary. Stock & custom bores (square,round, oval etc.) with or without locating flats to suit your high precision needs. Engineering assistance available from concept to protype to OEM requirements. Fax a print or drawing for fast service 856-327-4299.

Precision Biologic, Inc. 800-267-2796
900 Windmill Rd., Ste. 100, Dartmouth, NS B3B 1P7 Canada
CRYOCHECK Platelet Lysate

REAGENT, PROTEIN, TOTAL *(Chemistry) 75CEK*

Bayer Healthcare Llc 914-524-2955
555 White Plains Rd Fl 5, Tarrytown, NY 10591
Test for albumin in serum or plasma.

Beckman Coulter, Inc. 800-635-3497
740 W 83rd St, Hialeah, FL 33014
$0.035 per test.

Beckman Coulter, Inc. 800-742-2345
250 S Kraemer Blvd, PO Box 8000, Brea, CA 92821

Bio-Rad Laboratories, Life Science Group 800-424-6723
2000 Alfred Nobel Dr, Hercules, CA 94547

Biomerieux Inc. 800-682-2666
100 Rodolphe St, Durham, NC 27712

Caldon Bioscience, Inc. 909-628-9944
2100 S Reservoir St, Pomona, CA 91766
Total protein reagent.

Caldon Biotech, Inc. 757-224-0177
2251 Rutherford Rd, Carlsbad, CA 92008
Total protien reagent.

Carolina Liquid Chemistries Corp. 800-471-7272
510 W Central Ave Ste C, Brea, CA 92821
Mtp reagent.

Clin-Chem Mfg. Llc. 800-359-9691
2560 Business Pkwy Ste C, Minden, NV 89423
Protein reagent.

REAGENT, PROTEIN, TOTAL *(cont'd)*

Dade Behring, Inc. 800-948-3233
1717 Deerfield Rd, Deerfield, IL 60015

Genchem, Inc. 714-529-1616
510 W Central Ave Ste D, Brea, CA 92821
Total protein reagent.

Genzyme Corp. 800-325-2436
160 Christian St, Oxford, CT 06478
Total protein (micro) assay - pyrogallol, endpoint. Total protein assay - biuret, endpoint.

Health Chem Diagnostics Llc 954-979-3845
3341 W McNab Rd, Pompano Beach, FL 33069
Biuret (colorimetric), total protein.

Hemagen Diagnostics, Inc. 800-436-2436
9033 Red Branch Rd, Columbia, MD 21045
Various total protein (tp) methods.

Intersect Systems, Inc. 360-577-1062
1152 3rd Avenue, Suite D & E, Longview, WA 98632
Colorimetric, total protein, Urine/CSF microprotein.

Jas Diagnostics, Inc. 305-418-2320
7220 NW 58th St, Miami, FL 33166
Total protein.

Medical Chemical Corp. 800-424-9394
19430 Van Ness Ave, Torrance, CA 90501
$19.00 per unit (standard).

Peninsula Laboratories, Inc. 800-650-4442
305 Old County Rd, San Carlos, CA 94070
Synthetic peptides.

Quantimetrix Corporation 800-624-8380
2005 Manhattan Beach Blvd, Redondo Beach, CA 90278
QuanTest Red - Pyrogallol Red Reagent.

Raichem, Division Of Hemagen Diagnostics, Inc. 800-438-6100
8225 Mercury Ct, San Diego, CA 92111

Ricca Chemical Company, Llc 817-461-5601
448 W Fork Dr, Arlington, TX 76012
Various.

Sandare Intl., Inc. 972-293-7440
910 Kck Way, Cedar Hill, TX 75104
Total protein biuret method.

Stanbio Laboratory, Inc. 830-249-0772
1261 N Main St, Boerne, TX 78006
$34.50 for 500ml total protein reagent. $67.00 for total protein test set (CSF/urine) with TCA reagent and protein standard.

Synermed Intl., Inc. 317-896-1565
17408 Tiller Ct Ste 1900, Westfield, IN 46074
Total protein reagent kit.

Teco Diagnostics 714-693-7788
1268 N Lakeview Ave, Anaheim, CA 92807
Total protein reagent.

Vital Diagnostics Inc. 714-672-3553
1075 W Lambert Rd Ste D, Brea, CA 92821
Various total protein reagents.

REAGENT, QUALITY CONTROL *(General) 80WRB*

Analytical Control Systems, Inc. 317-841-0458
9058 Technology Dr, Fishers, IN 46038
SPAT (Slide platelet aggregation test). Reagent can screen for cogenital and for acquired platelet dysfunctions. Good correlation with the bleeding time test. Reagent very stable, quick and simple. PAA reagant can detect one dose of 81mg or 325mg aspirin & reopro use when used on an aggregometer.

Beckman Coulter, Inc. 800-742-2345
250 S Kraemer Blvd, PO Box 8000, Brea, CA 92821

Biochemical Diagnostics, Inc. 800-223-4835
180 Heartland Blvd, Edgewood, NY 11717
Urinary controls for toxicology proficiency.

Duke Scientific Corp. 800-334-3883
2463 Faber Pl, PO Box 50005, Palo Alto, CA 94303
Nanosphere size standards are calibrated in billionths of a meter. Used as standards for instrument calibration, quality control, filter checking, and biotechnology applications.

Quality Bioresources, Inc. 888-674-7224
1015 N Austin St, Seguin, TX 78155
OEM

REAGENT, RUSSEL VIPER VENOM *(Hematology) 81GIR*

American Diagnostica, Inc. 888-234-4435
500 West Ave, Stamford, CT 06902
DVV test reagent, lupue anticoagulent test kit.

Life Therapeutics Inc. 404-300-5000
780 Park North Blvd Ste 100, Clarkston, GA 30021
Simplified. drvvt for detection and confirmation of lupus.

Precision Biologic, Inc. 800-267-2796
900 Windmill Rd., Ste. 100, Dartmouth, NS B3B 1P7 Canada
CRYOCHECK LA CHECK screen reagent and CRYOCHECK LA SURE confirm reagent

REAGENT, SEROLOGICAL, DELTA, HEPATITIS
(Microbiology) 83LQI

United Biotech, Inc. 650-961-2910
211 S Whisman Rd Ste E, Mountain View, CA 94041
ELISA detecting HCV IgG

REAGENT, STREPTOLYSIN O/ANTISTREPTOLYSIN-TITER
(Microbiology) 83GTS

Arlington Scientific, Inc. Asi 800-654-0146
1840 N Technology Dr, Springville, UT 84663
ASO (Antitreptolysin O) kit; qualitative and semi-quantitative slide agglutination test for the determination of ASO in serum.

Bd Diagnostic Systems 800-675-0908
7 Loveton Cir, Sparks, MD 21152

Bd Lee Laboratories 800-732-9150
1475 Athens Hwy, Grayson, GA 30017
SLO Streptolysin O Reagent for latex applications.

J&S Medical Associates 800-229-6000
35 Tripp St Ste 1, Framingham, MA 01702
ACCUTEX qualitative and quantitative latex agglutination kits for RF, ASO, SLE, CRP, Mono and Staph.

Stanbio Laboratory, Inc. 830-249-0772
1261 N Main St, Boerne, TX 78006
$66.00 for 50 ASO tests with latex reagent, positive and negative control serum, NACL solution and six-cell slide.

Sterling Diagnostics, Inc. 800-637-2661
36645 Metro Ct, Sterling Heights, MI 48312

Wampole Laboratories 800-257-9525
2 Research Way, Princeton, NJ 08540
STREPTOZYNE Multiple enzyme/titers antistreptolysin.

REAGENT, TEST, CARBON MONOXIDE *(Toxicology) 91DKM*

Vitalograph, Inc. 800-255-6626
13310 W 99th St, Lenexa, KS 66215
Carbon monoxide monitor. $1,050.00

REAGENT, THROMBOPLASTIN, WITH CONTROL
(Hematology) 81GGO

Analytical Control Systems, Inc. 317-841-0458
9058 Technology Dr, Fishers, IN 46038
ULTRA-1 Factor VII insensitive. Ideal for assessing thrombotic risk as a coumadin patient is being stabilized. ISI of 1.0.

Dade Behring, Inc. 800-948-3233
1717 Deerfield Rd, Deerfield, IL 60015

Diagnostica Stago, Inc. 800-222-COAG
5 Century Dr, Parsippany, NJ 07054

Health Chem Diagnostics Llc 954-979-3845
3341 W McNab Rd, Pompano Beach, FL 33069
Reagent, thromboplastin and control.

REAGENT, VIRUS, GENERAL *(Pathology) 88UJH*

Akers Biosciences, Inc. 800-451-8378
201 Grove Rd, West Deptford, NJ 08086
The HEALTHTEST System, based on proprietary PIFA (Particle ImmunoFiltration Assay) technology; simple, two-step procedure requires no instrumentation or special training; results available in 3 minutes or less. All HEALTHTEST assays are self-contained, ready to use.

American Qualex, Inc. 800-772-1776
920 Calle Negocio Ste A, San Clemente, CA 92673

Dako North America, Inc 805-566-6655
6392 Via Real, Carpinteria, CA 93013

Prodesse, Inc. 888-589-6974
W229N1870 Westwood Dr, Waukesha, WI 53186
ProFlu+ Real Time PCR - Reagents for simultaneous detection and differentiation of Influenza A, Influenza B and RSV - Research Use Only - CE Mark pending - 510(k) pending

REAGENTS, SPECIFIC, ANALYTE *(Hematology) 81MVU*

Access Genetics 952-942-0671
7550 Market Place Dr, Eden Prairie, MN 55344
Various types of primer mix.

Asuragen, Inc. 877-777-1874
2150 Woodward St Ste 100, Austin, TX 78744
Various types of analytes.

Attostar Llc 952-920-6755
7600 W 27th St Ste 234, Saint Louis Park, MN 55426
Various types of starmaster mixes.

Autogenomics, Incorporated 760-477-2251
2890 Scott St, Vista, CA 92081
Analyte specific reagents(asr).

Bd Biosciences 408-954-6307
2350 Qume Dr, San Jose, CA 95131
Monoclonal antibodies.

Biocare Medical, Llc 925-603-3003
4040 Pike Ln, Concord, CA 94520
Analyte specific reagents.

Calbiotech, Inc. 619-660-6162
10461 Austin Dr Ste G, Spring Valley, CA 91978
Asr.

Celera Corporation 510-749-4219
884 Dubuque Ave, S San Fran, CA 94080
Reagent, specific analyte.

Celera Corporation 510-749-4219
1401 Harbor Bay Pkwy, Alameda, CA 94502
Various types of analyte specific reagents.

Cepheid 408-400-8460
904 E Caribbean Dr, Sunnyvale, CA 94089
Various types of analytes.

Cytocore, Inc. 312-379-4790
414 N Orleans St Ste 502, Chicago, IL 60654
Hpv mrna probe.

Diadexus, Inc. 650-246-6400
343 Oyster Point Blvd, South San Francisco, CA 94080
Diadexus analyte specific reagent.

Diagnostic Biosystems 925-484-3350
1020 Serpentine Ln Ste 114, Pleasanton, CA 94566

Diagnostic Hybrids, Inc. 740-589-3300
1055 E State St Ste 100, Athens, OH 45701
Vairous types of analytes.

Eragen Biosciences Inc. 608-662-9000
918 Deming Way Ste 201, Madison, WI 53717
Multiple

Eurogentec 858-793-2661
3347 Industrial Ct, San Diego, CA 92121
Various.

Gen Trak, Inc. 336-622-5266
121 W Swannanoa Ave, Liberty, NC 27298
Various.

Genetic Testing Institute 262-754-1000
20925 Crossroads Cir Ste 200, Waukesha, WI 53186
Various types of specific analyte reagents.

Invirion, Inc. 866-231-8378
2350 Pilgrim Hwy, Frankfort, MI 49635
Hiv probe cocktail.

Invivoscribe Technologies, Llc 858-623-8105
6330 Nancy Ridge Dr Ste 106, San Diego, CA 92121

Lab Vision Corp. 510-991-2800
47777 Warm Springs Blvd, Fremont, CA 94539
Various analyte specific reagents.

Nanogen Molecular Research Products Division 800-526-5544
21720 23rd Dr SE Ste 150, Bothell, WA 98021
Analyte specific reagents for detection.

Nanogen, Inc. 877-626-6436
10398 Pacific Center Ct, San Diego, CA 92121
Primer mixtures, probes, control dna for apo e, hfe, aspa, cftr factor v prothr.

Oligos Etc., Inc. 503-682-1814
9775 SW Commerce Cir Ste C6, Wilsonville, OR 97070
Oligonucleotides, various.

Pop Oligos, Llc 301-461-0457
9430 Key West Ave, Rockville, MD 20850
Oligonucleotides: nucleic acid chains.

REAGENTS, SPECIFIC, ANALYTE *(cont'd)*

Precision Biologic, Inc. 800-267-2796
900 Windmill Rd., Ste. 100, Dartmouth, NS B3B 1P7 Canada
CRYOCHECK HIT Antibodies

Qiagen Gaithersburg, Inc. 800-344-3631
1201 Clopper Rd, Gaithersburg, MD 20878
Nucleic acid probe for hpv.

Qiagen Sciences, Inc. 301-944-7090
19300 Germantown Rd, Germantown, MD 20874
Analyte specific reagent.

Roche Molecular Systems, Inc. 925-730-8110
4300 Hacienda Dr, Pleasanton, CA 94588
Various types of analytes.

Saladax Biomedical, Inc. 610-419-6731
116 Research Dr, Bethlehem, PA 18015
Busulfan antibody; busulfan hrp conjugate.

Scytek Laboratories, Inc. 435-755-9848
205 S 600 W, Logan, UT 84321
Analyte specific reagents.

Supertechs, Inc. 301-309-6695
9610 Medical Center Dr Ste 101, Rockville, MD 20850
Tdt antibodies.

Tepnel Lifecodes Corporation 203-328-9500
550 West Ave, Stamford, CT 06902
Various dna probes and primers for molecular hla typing.

Third Wave Technologies, Inc. 888-898-2357
502 S Rosa Rd, Madison, WI 53719
Invader assay oligonucleotides.

Trillium Diagnostics, Llc. 866-364-0028
915 Union St Ste 3, Bangor, ME 04401
Monoclonal Antibodies to CD163 MAC2-48, CD163 MAC2-158, CD163 R20, CD64 Clone 22, CD64 Clone 32.2, Fetal Hemoglobin (HbF), and human pan-Hemoglobin (PHb)

Tripath Imaging, Inc. 919-206-7140
780 Plantation Dr, Burlington, NC 27215
Various individual antibodies.

Ventana Medical Systems, Inc. 800-227-2155
1910 E Innovation Park Dr, Oro Valley, AZ 85755
Various.

REAMER *(Orthopedics) 87HTO*

Arthrex, Inc. 239-643-5553
1370 Creekside Blvd, Naples, FL 34108
Various sizes coring reamers and related items.

Ascent Healthcare Solutions 480-763-5300
10232 S 51st St, Phoenix, AZ 85044
Reamer.

Biomet, Inc. 574-267-6639
56 E Bell Dr, PO Box 587, Warsaw, IN 46582
Various types of reamers.

Case Medical, Inc. 888-227-2273
65 Railroad Ave, Ridgefield, NJ 07657
FINBLADE.

Depuy Mitek, A Johnson & Johnson Company 800-451-2006
50 Scotland Blvd, Bridgewater, MA 02324
Various orthopedic reamers.

Depuy Spine, Inc. 800-227-6633
325 Paramount Dr, Raynham, MA 02767
Various sizes of surgical orthopaedic reamers.

DJO Inc. 800-336-6569
1430 Decision St, Vista, CA 92081

Elite Medical Equipment 719-659-7926
5470 Kates Dr, Colorado Springs, CO 80919
Reamer.

Grace Manufacturing, Inc. 479-968-5455
614 Sr 247, Russellville, AR 72802
Orthopedic.

Holmed Corporation 508-238-3351
40 Norfolk Ave, South Easton, MA 02375

K2m, Inc. 866-526-4171
751 Miller Dr SE Ste F1, Leesburg, VA 20175
Reamer.

Medisiss 866-866-7477
2747 SW 6th St, Redmond, OR 97756
Various reamers,sterile.

REAMER *(cont'd)*

Medtronic Sofamor Danek Instrument Manufacturing 901-396-3133
7375 Adrianne Pl, Bartlett, TN 38133
Multiple (orthopedic reamers).

Medtronic Sofamor Danek Usa, Inc. 901-396-3133
4340 Swinnea Rd, Memphis, TN 38118
Multiple (orthopedic reamers).

minSURG International, Inc. 727-466-4550
611 Druid Rd E, Suite 200, Clearwater, FL 33756

Nobel Biocare Usa, Llc 800-579-6515
22715/22725 Savi Ranch Parkway, Yorba Linda, CA 92887
Surgical or prosthetic instrument.

Orthogenesis, Inc. 530-672-8560
4315 Product Dr # C, Cameron Park, CA 95682
Various sizes of acetabular cup reamers and associated handles.

Orthovita, Inc. 610-640-1775
77 Great Valley Pkwy, Malvern, PA 19355
Reamer.

Richards Micro-Tool, Inc. 508-746-6900
250 Nicks Road,, Plymouth, MA 02360-2800

Rush-Berivon, Inc. 800-251-7874
1010 19th St, P.O. Box 1851, Meridian, MS 39301
$123.00 each for 8 models - 1.6mm to 8mm dia., 3-1/2 to 10-3/8in length.

Stryker Corp. 800-726-2725
2825 Airview Blvd, Portage, MI 49002

Stryker Spine 866-457-7463
2 Pearl Ct, Allendale, NJ 07401

Surgical Implant Generation Network (Sign) 509-371-1107
451 Hills St, Richland, WA 99354
Reamer.

Synthes (Usa) 610-719-5000
35 Airport Rd, Horseheads, NY 14845
Various types and sizes of reamers.

Warsaw Orthopedic, Inc. 901-396-3133
2500 Silveus Xing, Warsaw, IN 46582
Multiple (orthopedic reamers).

Zimmer Holdings, Inc. 800-613-6131
1800 W Center St, PO Box 708, Warsaw, IN 46580
Retrograde, Trinkle fitting, 7-12mm.

Zimmer Spine, Inc. 800-655-2614
7375 Bush Lake Rd, Minneapolis, MN 55439
Reamer.

Zimmer Trabecular Metal Technology 800-613-6131
10 Pomeroy Rd, Parsippany, NJ 07054
Hip cylindrical reamer.

REAMER, PULP CANAL, ENDODONTIC *(Dental And Oral) 76EKP*

Acteon Inc. 800-289-6367
124 Gaither Dr Ste 140, Mount Laurel, NJ 08054

Aesculap Implant Systems Inc. 1-800-234-9179
3773 Corporate Pkwy, Center Valley, PA 18034

Dentalez Group 866-DTE-INFO
101 Lindenwood Dr Ste 225, Valleybrooke Corporate Center
Malvern, PA 19355

Ivoclar Vivadent, Inc. 800-533-6825
175 Pineview Dr, Amherst, NY 14228

Js Dental Mfg., Inc. 800-284-3368
196 N Salem Rd, Ridgefield, CT 06877
Reamer, engine reamer.

Kerr Corp. 714-516-7400
28200 Wick Rd, Romulus, MI 48174
Root canal reamer.

Lightspeed Technology, Inc. 210-495-4942
403 E Ramsey Rd Ste 205, San Antonio, TX 78216
Root canal reamer.

Medidenta International, Inc. 800-221-0750
3923 62nd St, PO Box 409, Woodside, NY 11377

Miltex Dental Technologies, Inc. 516-576-6022
589 Davies Dr, York, PA 17402
Hand-operated reamers and test reamers.

Moyco Technologies, Inc. 800-331-8837
200 Commerce Dr, Montgomeryville, PA 18936
Available in either metal or plastic.

REAMER, PULP CANAL, ENDODONTIC *(cont'd)*

Pulpdent Corp. 800-343-4342
80 Oakland St, Watertown, MA 02472
No common name listed.

United Dental Manufacturers, Inc. 918-878-0450
PO Box 700874, Tulsa, OK 74170
K-reamer.

United Dental Mfg., Inc. 717-845-7511
608 Rolling Hills Dr, Johnson City, TN 37604
Dental reamers.

Zenith Point Manufacturing 805-499-6808
3867 Old Conejo Rd, Newbury Park, CA 91320
Reamer.

REBREATHING SYSTEM, RADIONUCLIDE *(Radiology) 90IYT*

Amici, Inc. 610-948-7100
518 Vincent St, Spring City, PA 19475
Xenon Administration System; Krypton Administration System

Biodex Medical Systems, Inc. 800-224-6339
20 Ramsey Rd, Shirley, NY 11967
PULMONEX II Completely closed system for performing regional ventilator studies.

Diversified Diagnostic Products, Inc. 281-955-5323
11603 Windfern Rd, Houston, TX 77064
$13,100.00 : Xenon 133 or 127 and Xenon/CT administration equipment.

REBREATHING UNIT *(Anesthesiology) 73BYW*

Anecare Laboratories, Inc. 801-977-8877
3487 W 2100 S Ste 100, Salt Lake City, UT 84119
Rebreathing absorber.

Respironics California, Inc. 724-387-4559
2271 Cosmos Ct, Carlsbad, CA 92011
Non invasive cardiac output monitor.

Respironics Novametrix, Llc. 724-387-4559
5 Technology Dr, Wallingford, CT 06492
Non invasive cardiac output monitor.

RECEPTACLE, ELECTRICAL *(General) 80TEE*

Armstrong Medical Industries, Inc. 800-323-4220
575 Knightsbridge Pkwy, Lincolnshire, IL 60069
Hospital grade electrical outlet strip.

Crest Healthcare Supply 800-328-8908
195 3rd St, Dassel, MN 55325
Outlets and components.

Mercury Medical 800-237-6418
11300 49th St N, Clearwater, FL 33762
PowerBall, I. V. Pole mounted multi-outlet, UL approved.

Woodhead L.P. 847-272-7990
3411 Woodhead Dr, Northbrook, IL 60062
Hospital grade receptacles.

RECORDER, ANALOG/DIGITAL, OPHTHALMIC *(Ophthalmology) 86HMB*

Lkc Technologies, Inc. 800-638-7055
2 Professional Dr Ste 222, Gaithersburg, MD 20879

RECORDER, ATTENTION TASK PERFORMANCE *(Cns/Neurology) 84LQD*

Crist Instrument Co., Inc. 301-393-8615
111 W 1st St, Hagerstown, MD 21740
Recording Cylinders for cranial implantation, related devices for brain mapping and other neurological use. Electrodes for cell recordings.

Novavision, Inc. 561-558-2040
3651 Fau Blvd Ste 300, Boca Raton, FL 33431
Visual restoration therapy, therapy device, diagnostic device.

RECORDER, CHART, LABORATORY *(Chemistry) 75UHR*

Allen Datagraph Systems, Inc. 800-258-6360
56 Kendall Pond Rd, Derry, NH 03038
SERIES 4000 OEM strip-chart recorder modules feature a unique iron pen-motor design for accurate, lasting records of measurements as a function of time. SERIES 9000 compact thermal-array recorders offer simplicity and modularity for system flexibility in product design. OMNISCRIBE D-5000 stripchart recorders provide both inch and centimeter calibration on each instrument. One- or two-pen flatbed models are available.

Astro-Med, Inc. 800-343-4039
600 E Greenwich Ave, West Warwick, RI 02893
4- to 32-channel data acquisition chart recorders

RECORDER, CHART, LABORATORY *(cont'd)*

Beckman Coulter, Inc. 800-742-2345
250 S Kraemer Blvd, PO Box 8000, Brea, CA 92821

Bio-Rad Laboratories, Life Science Group 800-424-6723
2000 Alfred Nobel Dr, Hercules, CA 94547

Buck Scientific, Inc. 800-562-5566
58 Fort Point St, Norwalk, CT 06855
LC522-1 strip chart.

Charts-Inc. 800-882-9357
12977 Arroyo St, San Fernando, CA 91340
Recording charts & marking systems.

Climatronics Corp. 631-567-7300
140 Wilbur Pl, Bohemia, NY 11716

Cole-Parmer Instrument Inc. 800-323-4340
625 E Bunker Ct, Vernon Hills, IL 60061

Devar Inc. 800-566-6822
706 Bostwick Ave, Bridgeport, CT 06605
SMART CHART II compact process data logger featuring time extension recording and no computer configuration prior to use.

Dickson Co 800-757-3747
930 S Westwood Ave, Addison, IL 60101
Temperature or Temperature and Humidity chart recorders perfect for monitoring storage conditions, clean rooms, autoclaves, incubators, freezers, refrigerators and ovens.

Hokanson Inc., D.E. 800-999-8251
12840 NE 21st Pl, Bellevue, WA 98005
The MD6VR is a real-time thermal chart recorder compatible with MD6 Bidirectional Doppler, MD6RP Photo Plethysmograph and MD6PN Pneumo Plethysmograph.

iWorx Systems, Inc. 800-234-1757
1 Washington St Ste 404, Dover, NH 03820
Apple Macintosh based system for recording and analyzing ECG, EEG, EMG, blood pressure, pulse, etc.

Kipp & Zonen 631-589-2065
125 Wilbur Pl, Bohemia, NY 11716
Strip chart recorders.

Lds Life Science (Formerly Gould Instrument Systems Inc.) 216-328-7000
5525 Cloverleaf Pkwy, Valley View, OH 44125

Linseis, Inc. 800-732-6733
PO Box 666, Princeton Junction, NJ 08550
Strip chart and XY recorders.

Omega Engineering, Inc. 800-848-4286
1 Omega Dr, Stamford, CT 06907

Quintron Instrument Company 800-542-4448
3712 W Pierce St, Milwaukee, WI 53215
Single and dual pen-chart recorders, one or three spans from 1 mV to 1 volt F.S.

Rms Instruments 905-677-5533
6877-1 Goreway Dr., Mississauga, ONT L4V 1L9 Canada

Soltec Corp. 800-423-2344
12977 Arroyo St, San Fernando, CA 91340
Multichannel, 1-16 PENS. Flatbed and rackmount. Voltage, temperature, current inputs.

U.F.I. 805-772-1203
545 Main St Ste C2, Morro Bay, CA 93442

RECORDER, EVENT, IMPLANTABLE CARDIAC, (WITHOUT ARRHYTHMIA DETECTION) *(Cardiovascular) 74MXC*

Arizona Device Manufacturing 763-505-0874
2350 W Medtronic Way, Tempe, AZ 85281
Implantable cardiac monitor.

Medtronic Puerto Rico Operations Co., Juncos 763-514-4000
Road 31, Km. 24, Hm 4, Ceiba Norte Industrial Park, Juncos, PR 00777
Implantable cardiac monitor.

RECORDER, EXTERNAL, PRESSURE, AMPLIFIER & TRANSDUCER *(Gastro/Urology) 78FES*

Medtronic Neuromodulation 763-514-4000
710 Medtronic Pkwy, Minneapolis, MN 55432
Various types of external pressure, amplifier & transducer recorders.

RECORDER, LONG-TERM, BLOOD PRESSURE, PORTABLE *(Cardiovascular) 74ROK*

Instromedix, A Card Guard Co. 800-633-3361
10255 W Higgins Rd Ste 100, Rosemont, IL 60018
24-hour ambulatory blood-pressure recorder.

RECORDER, LONG-TERM, BLOOD PRESSURE, PORTABLE *(cont'd)*

Rozinn By Scottcare Corporation 800-243-9412
4791 W 150th St, Cleveland, OH 44135
Interfaces easily with Rozinn's state-of-the-art Holter scanning system, measures and records your patients' blood pressure at preset intervals; measurements can be carried out at a variety of preset intervals, stored, and printed with the RZ250, small, compact design, oscillometric measurement and large capacity memory stores data for 24 hours at 300 measurements per patient. Can be used as stand-alone system as well.

RECORDER, LONG-TERM, ECG *(Cardiovascular) 74ROL*

Biomedical Systems Corp. 800-877-6334
77 Progress Pkwy Bldg 1, Maryland Hts, MO 63043

Braemar, Inc. 800-328-2719
1285 Corporate Center Dr Ste 150, Eagan, MN 55121
ER300 ER310 ER320 portable event monitors, ER300 post event, ER310 1 channel looping, ER320 2 channel looping. Also available, ER710, ER720 portable event monitors with looping memory, programmable features, LCD display and R5232 data upload. ER710 is 1 channel, ER720 is 2 channel.

Ge Medical Systems Information Technologies 800-643-6439
8200 W Tower Ave, Milwaukee, WI 53223
Solid-state recorder acquires 24 hours of two-channel ECG data and analyzes it in real time. Tape recorder model can be used as either a two- or three-channel recorder for up to 48 hours recording.

Instromedix, A Card Guard Co. 800-633-3361
10255 W Higgins Rd Ste 100, Rosemont, IL 60018
Portable, with looping memory.

New Life Systems, Inc. 954-972-4600
PO Box 8767, Coral Springs, FL 33075
Tape or solid state.

Omni Medical Supply Inc. 800-860-6664
4153 Pioneer Dr, Commerce Township, MI 48390

Rozinn By Scottcare Corporation 800-243-9412
4791 W 150th St, Cleveland, OH 44135
The TTM for Windows Transtelephonic Cardiac Event Monitoring System includes Post Event & Looping Memory Recorders to satisfy all patient needs. They're very small and easily tolerated by elderly patients. The Software provides Physician, Patient, & Device tracking and includes complete reporting. Reports can be faxed, e-mailed, or mailed and can include full, ¾, and ⅓-size strips to conserve space.

U.F.I. 805-772-1203
545 Main St Ste C2, Morro Bay, CA 93442
$3,850 for model 3992.

RECORDER, LONG-TERM, ECG, PORTABLE (HOLTER MONITOR) *(Cardiovascular) 74ROM*

Aventric Technologies 800-228-3343
1551 E Lincoln Ave Ste 166, Madison Heights, MI 48071

Biomedical Systems Corp. 800-877-6334
77 Progress Pkwy Bldg 1, Maryland Hts, MO 63043
VX3 Digital Holter Recorder provides either 24 or 48 hours of continous 3-channel ECG recordings with an intuitive and simple user interface and LCD screen that guides the tech through patient hookup. DXP Digital Holter provides up to 48 hours of continous 3-channel ECG recording with a built-in LCD screen.

Braemar, Inc. 800-328-2719
1285 Corporate Center Dr Ste 150, Eagan, MN 55121
DL700 DL1250 Digital Holter monitor, flashcard technology, 24 hours of 2 or 3 channels with disclosure ECG data. Tape based Holter, Phillips cassette, 24 hours of 2 or 3 channel full disclosure ECG data. DXP1000 Digital Holter monitor, flash memory, 24-48 hours of 3 channel full disclosure ECG data, programmable features, pacemaker detection, LCD display and USB data upload.

Capintec, Inc. 800-631-3826
6 Arrow Rd, Ramsey, NJ 07446
Ambulatory measurement of ECG and LV function (ejection fraction), incorporating 2 channel ECG Holter monitor and miniature nuclear detector for measuring LV function.

Circadian Systems 800-669-7001
8099 Savage Way, Valley Springs, CA 95252
ACCU-SCANNER SUPRA--a computer-based system designed for the definitive diagnosis of complex cardiac cases and offers extensive arrhythmia classification, high accuracy and reproducibility; also, for chronic or transient cardiac problems, the ACCU-SCANNER SUPRA is a high precision in-office tool for assessing symptomatic or asymptomatic ischemia patients, post-coronary surgery, M.I. patients, and other complex cases.

RECORDER, LONG-TERM, ECG, PORTABLE (HOLTER MONITOR) *(cont'd)*

Ela Medical, Inc. 800-352-6466
2950 Xenium Ln N, Plymouth, MN 55441
Spiderview is a mulipurpose digital Holter recorder. It is small, compact adn easy to use. The user friendly Spiderview analysis software can be installed on your PC.

Galix Biomedical Instrumentation, Inc. 305-534-5905
2555 Collins Ave Ste C-5, Miami Beach, FL 33140
The GBI-3S is a 3-channel digital, 24/48 hour ambulatory ECG Holter recorder. This ultralight and ergonomic design records 3 channel of ECG data on a removable, reusable memory card. An interactive digital display indicates ECG output channel, recording mode, low-battery warning, etc. Has a security system that prevents recording over a nonprocessed memory card. Also offers short-term, very-high-resolution ECG data acquisition (1000 s/s) for further ventricular late potential analysis.

Ge Medical Systems Information Technologies 800-643-6439
8200 W Tower Ave, Milwaukee, WI 53223
Solid-state recorder acquires 24 hours of two-channel ECG data and analyzes it in real time. Tape recorder model can be used as either a two- or three-channel recorder for up to 48 hours recording.

Health Care Exports, Inc. 800-847-0173
5701 NW 74th Ave, Miami, FL 33166
Holter Plus III 3-channel holter system; user friendly, economical, very small.

Lynn Medical 888-596-6633
764 Denison Ct, Bloomfield Hills, MI 48302
LM-151 holter recorder.

Midmark Diagnostics Group 800-624-8950
3300 Fujita St, Torrance, CA 90505
The IQmark EZ Holter and IQmark Advanced Holter enables the physician to select the level of complexity they want to see in their Holter program. Both Holter systems provide 3-channel full disclosure capability. The EZ Holter can automatically scan, interpret and print the report so the physician only has to review and confirm. The Advanced Holter adds features that allow complete control over scanning, Template editing and other advanced report functions. The digital Holter RecorderCF displays the waveform during hook up, is lightweight, and has no moving parts.

Mortara Instrument, Inc. 800-231-7437
7865 N 86th St, Milwaukee, WI 53224
H-12, continuous Truis 12-lead Nolter data.

New Life Systems, Inc. 954-972-4600
PO Box 8767, Coral Springs, FL 33075
Computerized real-time, 24-hour Holter monitors.

Omni Medical Supply Inc. 800-860-6664
4153 Pioneer Dr, Commerce Township, MI 48390

Pulse Biomedical Inc. 610-666-5510
1305 Catfish Ln, Norristown, PA 19403
Holter Recorder

Q-Med, Inc. 732-544-5544
100 Metro Park S., 3rd Fl., South Amboy, NJ 08878
MONITOR ONE computerized ambulatory early warning system.

Rozinn By Scottcare Corporation 800-243-9412
4791 W 150th St, Cleveland, OH 44135
The RZ153+ Cardio ID+ is a Digital Holter Recorder of advanced design, capable of true 12-lead ECG studies and pacemaker detection. It uses removable CompactFlash Card Memory for NON-COMPRESSED storage of ECG data. The Model 151 series of two or three-channel cassette Holter monitors are versatile and compatible with virtually all scanning systems. Lightweight and yet rugged, the Energy-efficient design allows use of one 9V alkaline battery for up to 5 Holter recordings. Using rechargeable batteries allows for over 1,000 Holter recordings.

Tsi Medical Ltd. 800-661-7263
47 Athabascan Ave., Unit 105, Sherwood Park, AB T8A-4H3 Canada

U.F.I. 805-772-1203
545 Main St Ste C2, Morro Bay, CA 93442
$3850 for complete Ambulatory ECG Monitor System.

Vitalograph, Inc. 800-255-6626
13310 W 99th St, Lenexa, KS 66215
2110 Electronic PEV/FEV Diary for electronic peak flow meter. $350.00.

RECORDER, LONG-TERM, EEG *(Cns/Neurology) 84RON*

Cadwell Laboratories 800-245-3001
909 N Kellogg St, Kennewick, WA 99336
CADWELL EASY EEG (digital). Provides 24 or 32 channels. CADWELL CENTRAL EEG/EP/EMG is available with 24- or 32-channel EEG recording. Synchronous digital video/audio, spike detection and analysis, patient event button.

RECORDER, LONG-TERM, RESPIRATION *(Anesthesiology) 73VDC*

Konigsberg Instruments, Inc. 626-449-0016
2000 E Foothill Blvd, Pasadena, CA 91107
Implantable cardio/respiration system. Animal Research, Discovery Research, Safety Pharmacology, Special systems for Biocontainment Levels 2, 3 and 4.

U.F.I. 805-772-1203
545 Main St Ste C2, Morro Bay, CA 93442
$3850 for Biolog Model 3992.

RECORDER, LONG-TERM, TREND *(General) 80ROP*

Cardiac Science Corp. 800-777-1777
500 Burdick Pkwy, Deerfield, WI 53531
Model 92513 and 92510 Holter recorders

Eurotherm Inc. 703-443-0000
741F Miller Dr SE, Leesburg, VA 20175

Hillusa Corp. 305-594-7474
7215 NW 46th St, Miami, FL 33166
Holter EKG, three channel Holter system.

Lds Life Science (Formerly Gould Instrument Systems Inc.) 216-328-7000
5525 Cloverleaf Pkwy, Valley View, OH 44125

Md International, Inc. 305-669-9003
11300 NW 41st St, Doral, FL 33178

Respironics Georgia, Inc. 724-387-4559
175 Chastain Meadows Ct NW, Kennesaw, GA 30144
HDS.

Simpson Electric Co. 715-588-3311
520 Simpson Ave, PO Box 99, Lac Du Flambeau, WI 54538
Model 606. $1450.00 per unit (standard).

U.F.I. 805-772-1203
545 Main St Ste C2, Morro Bay, CA 93442
$3850 for Model 3992.

RECORDER, MAGNETIC TAPE/DISC *(Cardiovascular) 74DSH*

Braemar, Inc. 800-328-2719
1285 Corporate Center Dr Ste 150, Eagan, MN 55121
DL250 ECG tape transport with Phillips cassette. Two or three channels of data with 24 hour recording, designed for customer unique electronics, Halter applications.

Datrix 760-480-8874
340 State Pl, Escondido, CA 92029
Ecg cassette holter recorder.

Electro Medical Equipment Co., Inc. 800-423-2926
12015 Industriplex Blvd, Baton Rouge, LA 70809
Multiple.

Lifewatch Services, Inc. 877-774-9846
10255 W Higgins Rd Ste 100, O'hare International Center II Rosemont, IL 60018
Telephone, electrocardograph transmitter and record.

Memtec Corp. 603-893-8080
68 Stiles Rd Ste D, Salem, NH 03079
Holter recorder.

Northeast Monitoring, Inc. 866-346-5837
2 Clock Tower Pl Ste 555, Maynard, MA 01754
Digital Holter and Event Recorder

Rms Instruments 905-677-5533
6877-1 Goreway Dr., Mississauga, ONT L4V 1L9 Canada

Spacelabs Medical Inc. 800-522-7212
5150 220th Ave SE, Issaquah, WA 98029
Various magnetic tape/disk recorders.

RECORDER, PAPER CHART *(Cardiovascular) 74DSF*

Astro-Med, Inc. 800-343-4039
600 E Greenwich Ave, West Warwick, RI 02893
Wide range of thermal chart paper and ink writing chart papers

Beckman Coulter, Inc. 800-742-2345
250 S Kraemer Blvd, PO Box 8000, Brea, CA 92821

Cole-Parmer Instrument Inc. 800-323-4340
625 E Bunker Ct, Vernon Hills, IL 60061

RECORDER, PAPER CHART *(cont'd)*

Draeger Medical Systems, Inc. 215-660-2626
16 Electronics Ave, Danvers, MA 01923
Recorder.

Electro Medical Equipment Co., Inc. 800-423-2926
12015 Industriplex Blvd, Baton Rouge, LA 70809

Eurotherm Inc. 703-443-0000
741F Miller Dr SE, Leesburg, VA 20175

Ge Medical Systems Information Technologies 800-643-6439
8200 W Tower Ave, Milwaukee, WI 53223
Four-channel, direct digital thermal head printer for hard copy of real-time waveforms as well as stored information.

Grass Technologies, An Astro-Med, Inc. Product Gro 401-828-4002
53 Airport Park Drive, Rockland, MA 02370
Physiological recorder.

Gri Medical Products, Inc. 800-291-9425
4937 E Red Range Way, Cave Creek, AZ 85331
Chart recorder paper.

Invivo Corporation 425-487-7000
12601 Research Pkwy, Orlando, FL 32826
Patient parameter strip chart recorder.

Kipp & Zonen 631-589-2065
125 Wilbur Pl, Bohemia, NY 11716
Strip chart recorder.

Lds Life Science (Formerly Gould Instrument Systems Inc.) 216-328-7000
5525 Cloverleaf Pkwy, Valley View, OH 44125

Linseis, Inc. 800-732-6733
PO Box 666, Princeton Junction, NJ 08550

Mennen Medical Corp. 800-223-2201
2540 Metropolitan Dr, Trevose, PA 19053
Single- or dual-channel paper chart recorders, used with patient monitors or at central station.

Meylan Corporation 888-769-9667
543 Valley Rd, Upper Montclair, NJ 07043
$415.00 for single stylus, $510.00 for double, $550.00 for triple. 8, 12, and 24hr. charts available. With and without totalizers.

Nihon Kohden America, Inc. 800-325-0283
90 Icon, Foothill Ranch, CA 92610

Payton Scientific Inc. 716-876-1813
964 Kenmore Ave, Buffalo, NY 14216
$2,275.00 single, $2,850.00 2-pen linear per unit for use with hematology aggregometers.

Respironics Georgia, Inc. 724-387-4559
175 Chastain Meadows Ct NW, Kennesaw, GA 30144

Richard Wolf Medical Instruments Corp. 800-323-9653
353 Corporate Woods Pkwy, Vernon Hills, IL 60061

Soltec Corp. 800-423-2344
12977 Arroyo St, San Fernando, CA 91340
SOLTEC Model TA220-3608/1000 series digital oscillographic recorders with color display with touch screen control. 8 & 16 channels, modular signal conditioning. Portable, high speed chart and large high speed sample memory.

Taylor Industries, Inc. 800-339-1361
2706 Industrial Dr, Jefferson City, MO 65109

Tyco Healthcare Group Lp 800-445-5025
2 Ludlow Park Dr, Chicopee, MA 01022

United Electric Controls Co. 617-926-1000
180 Dexter Ave, P.O. Box 9143, Watertown, MA 02472

Welch Allyn Protocol Inc. 800-289-2500
8500 SW Creekside Pl, Beaverton, OR 97008
Printer option.

RECORDER, RADIOGRAPHIC VIDEO TAPE *(Radiology) 90ROQ*

Agfa Corp. 800-581-2432
100 Challenger Rd, Ridgefield Park, NJ 07660
SCOPIX compact laser imaging center.

National Video Services, Inc. 203-270-0677
18 Commerce Rd, Newtown, CT 06470

RECORDER, TRANSIENT *(General) 80ROR*

Rms Instruments 905-677-5533
6877-1 Goreway Dr., Mississauga, ONT L4V 1L9 Canada

RECORDER, VENTILATORY EFFORT *(Anesthesiology) 73MNR*

Cardinal Health 207, Inc. 610-862-0800
1100 Bird Center Dr, Palm Springs, CA 92262
Screening device for cardiac monitoring during sleep te.

Greatbatch Inc 716-759-5600
1771 E 30th St, Cleveland, OH 44114
Airflow sensors.

Individual Monitoring Systems, Inc. 410-296-7723
1055 Taylor Ave Ste 300, Baltimore, MD 21286
Apnea check.

Neurotronics, Inc. 352-372-9955
912 NE 2nd St Ste 5, Gainesville, FL 32601
Polysmith.

Pro-Tech Services, Inc. 800-350-5511
4338 Harbour Pointe Blvd SW, Mukilteo, WA 98275
Various.

Sector Medical Corp. 770-975-1384
320 Northpoint Pkwy SE Ste Q, Acworth, GA 30102
Aplab.

Sleep Solutions, Inc. 408-255-0808
2450 El Camino Real Ste 101, Palo Alto, CA 94306
Adult apnea recorder.

Snap Laboratories, L.L.C. 847-777-0000
5210 Capitol Dr, Wheeling, IL 60090
Apnaa/snoring screening and analysis device.

Watermark Medical LLC. 877-710-6999
1750 Clint Moore Rd Ste 101, Boca Raton, FL 33487

RECORDER, VIDEOTAPE/VIDEODISC *(General) 80TEF*

All-Tronics Medical Systems 800-ALL-TRON
3289 E 55th St, Cleveland, OH 44127
HRV 4000EM Video recorder: high resolution multi-scan enhanced SVHS unit.

Eigen 888-924-2020
13366 Grass Valley Ave, Grass Valley, CA 95945
Eigen's EigenNet™ is an acquisition, archive and review network for cardiac cath labs. EigenNet™ allows fast image access over the hospital intranet as well as the Internet with security authentication and encryption software to protect the data. It provides full motion viewing of patient images at Diagnostic Viewstations within the hospital as well as viewing of summary case data remotely using personal computers. Enterprise EigenNet: Departmental or hospital-wide/network that uses standard internet protocols. Cardio EigenNet: Provides cardiologists remote access within the hospital or off site. Echo EigenNet: The Echo EigenNet provides the connectivity to all echo systems in your hospital or practice, into one reading location or mobile laptop PC.

Intermed Video Technologies Inc. 203-270-0677
18 Commerce Rd, Newtown, CT 06470
Used in x-ray imaging procedures, also includes monitors.

JVC Americas Corp. 973-315-5000
1700 Valley Rd, Wayne, NJ 07470
HDTV Videocassette recorders and videocassette editing recorders.

Karl Storz Endoscopy-America Inc. 800-421-0837
600 Corporate Pointe, Culver City, CA 90230

Lg Electronics U.S.A., Inc. 800-884-1742
2000 Millbrook Dr, Lincolnshire, IL 60069

Mahe International Inc. 800-294-7946
468 Craighead St, Nashville, TN 37204

Perkins Electronics 877-923-4545
700 International Pkwy Ste 100, Richardson, TX 75081
The Perkins Electronics EZ PIC DICOM Video Acquisition and Recording Workstation enables easy capturing, reviewing, recording to DVD, and transferring of video sequences to PACS. Other products include scan conversion, video switching & distribution, and video isolation.

Richard Wolf Medical Instruments Corp. 800-323-9653
353 Corporate Woods Pkwy, Vernon Hills, IL 60061

Soltec Corp. 800-423-2344
12977 Arroyo St, San Fernando, CA 91340

Sony Electronics, Inc., Medical Systems Div. 800-686-7669
1 Sony Dr, Park Ridge, NJ 07656
8mm, 1/2 3/4 in. VTR's for medical applications. Also, still video recorder/player to capture, store and retrieve black and white or color images. One 2in.-floppy disk holds up to 50 images with no need for film processing.

RECORDER, X-RAY IMAGE *(Radiology) 90VFM*

Eigen 888-924-2020
13366 Grass Valley Ave, Grass Valley, CA 95945
Eigen Digital Fluoro Loop™ (DFL)and Digital Fluoro Store™ (DFS). For Cardiology and Radiology, the DFL provides superior fluoro looping and freeze frame capability. Adds the ability to send studies to DICOM archive. Archive interface option is available. The Eigen DFS provides Hold Last Image capability and can store 100+ images

Intermed Video Technologies Inc. 203-270-0677
18 Commerce Rd, Newtown, CT 06470
X-ray imaging recorders for cath labs and R&F rooms. Records and plays back 525 to 1249 line systems automatically.

Witt Biomedical Corporation 800-669-1328
305 North Dr, Melbourne, FL 32934
CALYSTO IMAGE IV, real time lossless digital image acquisition and archival network.Accessory to angiographic x-ray system.

RECOVERY EQUIPMENT, GAS *(General) 80WWT*

Andersen Products, Inc., 800-523-1276
3202 Caroline Dr, Health Science Park, Haw River, NC 27258
100% EO gas disposal system.

Nucon International, Inc. 800-992-5192
7000 Huntley Rd, Columbus, OH 43229
NUSORB, activated carbon, broad range of gas and liquid phase carbons for contaminant removal and recovery. Custom impregnated adsorbents available on request. MERSORB Hg Removal Adsorbent, custom adsorbent to remove Hg from gas phase, water or hydrocarbon liquids.

RECOVERY EQUIPMENT, WASTE HEAT *(General) 80VBL*

Burkhart Roentgen Intl. Inc. 800-USA-XRAY
5201 8th Ave S, Gulfport, FL 33707

RECOVERY EQUIPMENT, WATER *(General) 80VAQ*

Ars Enterprises 800-735-9277
12900 Lakeland Rd, Santa Fe Springs, CA 90670
Steam sterilizer water recirculation system.

Burkhart Roentgen Intl. Inc. 800-USA-XRAY
5201 8th Ave S, Gulfport, FL 33707
Mobile x-ray barriers.

Filtertek Inc. 800-248-2461
11411 Price Rd, Hebron, IL 60034
Filter elements (parts).

REDUCER, PRESSURE, INTRAOCULAR *(Ophthalmology) 86WNV*

Eyetech Ltd. 847-470-1777
9408 Normandy Ave, Morton Grove, IL 60053
Episcleral venomanometer for measuring episcleral vein pressure

Lebanon Corp., The 800-428-2310
1700 N Lebanon St, Lebanon, IN 46052
#2055 HONAN IOP Reducer with relief valve, #2050 HONAN model, single use bellows and headband.

REFRACTOMETER *(Chemistry) 75JRE*

Index Instruments U.S. Inc. 407-932-3688
3305 Commerce Blvd, Kissimmee, FL 34741
Refractometers and accessories. We have 3 generations of temperature control refractometers and our full line of TCR 15-30, CLR 12-70, GPR 12-70, GPR53X, GPRE anything from petroleum, plastics, waxes, to food and candies, beverages, contact lens.

Iris Sample Processing 800-782-8774
60 Glacier Dr, Westwood, MA 02090
Refractomer and accessories.

Kernco Instruments Co., Inc. 800-325-3875
420 Kenazo Ave., El Paso, TX 79928-7338
$195.00 to $495.00 for urine specific gravity clinical refractometers; five models available. Model DR-CLIN is $795.00 and features small sample requirement (0.4 mL), automatic temperature comp., stainless-steel plate for optical sample prism, use on sample temp. up to 100 degrees Celsius, and a two-year warranty.

Lw Scientific 800-726-7345
865 Marathon Pkwy, Lawrenceville, GA 30046
Tests specific gravity in urine or protein in serum.

Mettler-Toledo, Inc. 800-METTLER
1900 Polaris Pkwy, Columbus, OH 43240
REFRACTO, portable, digital refractometer. Accurate to 0.0001.

Nsg Precision Cells, Inc. 631-249-7474
195 Central Ave Ste G, Farmingdale, NY 11735
$139.00 per unit (standard).

REFRACTOMETER *(cont'd)*

Rudolph Research Analytical 973-584-1558
55 Newburgh Rd, Hackettstown, NJ 07840
The J-Series of automatic refractometers.

Vee Gee Scientific, Inc. 800-423-8842
13600 NE 126th Pl Ste A, Kirkland, WA 98034
Clinical.

REFRACTOMETER, OPHTHALMIC *(Ophthalmology) 86HKO*

Allergan 800-366-6554
2525 Dupont Dr, Irvine, CA 92612
BARRAQUER-KRUMREICH-SWINGER refractive set: non-freeze technique for keratomileusis and epikeratophakia. BKS-1000 refractive set allows partial removal of cornea and reshaping without freezing tissue.

Amo Manufacturing Usa, Llc 714-247-8656
510 Cottonwood Dr, Milpitas, CA 95035

Amo Wavefront Sciences Llc 714-247-8656
14820 Central Ave SE, Albuquerque, NM 87123
Autorefractor.

Brookfield Optical Systems 508-867-6675
218 Wigwam Rd, West Brookfield, MA 01585
Ophthalmic refractometer.

Canon Development Americas, Inc 949-932-3100
15955 Alton Pkwy, Irvine, CA 92618
R-F10 Full Auto Ref.

Marco Ophthalmic, Inc. 800-874-5274
11825 Central Pkwy, Jacksonville, FL 32224
$4,795.00 for unit. $15,750.00 for ARK 900 refractor/keratometer automatic combination system. (List prices)

Nidek Inc. 800-223-9044
47651 Westinghouse Dr, Fremont, CA 94539
Model AR-600/660, AR-800/860, ARK-700/760. Model OPD-Scan wavefront, autorefractor and topography unit.

Topcon Medical Systems, Inc. 800-223-1130
37 W Century Rd, Paramus, NJ 07652
Four models of auto refractometers: $8,990.00, $14,490,00, and $18,490.00 (with built-in topography system). Also, wavefront analyzer: $39,990; and patient-driven subjective refraction system: $39,990.00.

Tracey Technologies Corp. 281-445-1666
16720 Hedgecroft Dr Ste 208, Houston, TX 77060
Refractometer.

Visx Incorporated, A Subsidiary Of Amo Inc. 714-247-8656
1328 Kifer Rd, Sunnyvale, CA 94086
Refractometer,auto-refractor.

REFRACTOMETRIC, TOTAL PROTEIN *(Chemistry) 75JGR*

Kernco Instruments Co., Inc. 800-325-3875
420 Kenazo Ave., El Paso, TX 79928-7338

REFRACTOR, OPHTHALMIC *(Ophthalmology) 86HKN*

Burton Co., R.H. 800-848-0410
3965 Brookham Dr, Grove City, OH 43123
AUTOCROSS 7500-I, manual refractor with B-W illumination system to illuminate sphere, cylinder power and axis scales, $3550. 8AR-7 Auto refractor $6,995. 8ARK-8 Auto Refkeratometer $9,995. Autorefractor Burton Bar7 Autorefractor $6,995.00 newly developed measurement method allows for high speed, high precision and reliable refractive measurement by computing pherical, cylinder powers and axis for cylinder.

Carl Zeiss Meditec Inc. 877-486-7473
5160 Hacienda Dr, Dublin, CA 94568
HUMPHREY AUTOMATIC REFRACTOR/KERATOMETER The Humphrey Automatic Refractor/Keratometer (HARK) Model 599 is the first full-featured combination automatic refractor/keratometer. The HARK allows for immediate patient response on refraction results with visual acuities. The operator control panel can be positioned at either 90 degrees or 180 degrees to meet office space requirements. COMMUNICOM links the HARK to the Humphrey Lens Analyzer for quick and easy comparison of current and new prescriptions.

Marco Ophthalmic, Inc. 800-874-5274
11825 Central Pkwy, Jacksonville, FL 32224
3 models - $11,050.00 for objective model; $15,750.00 for objective/subjective model. (List prices)

Progressive Dental Supply/Progressive Orthodontics Seminars 800-443-3106
1701 E Edinger Ave Ste C1, Santa Ana, CA 92705
Photo lateral refractors and occlusal photo refractors.

REFRACTOR, OPHTHALMIC *(cont'd)*

Reichert, Inc. 888-849-8955
3362 Walden Ave, Depew, NY 14043
Reichert's Ultramatic RX Master Phoroptor - the first and always the best refracting instrument - continues to be the industry standard after nearly 80 years

Topcon Medical Systems, Inc. 800-223-1130
37 W Century Rd, Paramus, NJ 07652
Manual models: $5,490.00. Automated model: $18,990.00. Patient-driven subjective refraction system: $39,990.00.

Woodlyn, Inc. 800-331-7389
2920 Malmo Dr, Ophthalmic Instruments and Equipment
Arlington Heights, IL 60005
Model 61300 & 61301. The Woodlyn Refractor incorporates several outstanding features. Automatically synchronized cross cylinder axis, 'Better-one Better-two' knob, child guard, and anti-reflective coating on all lenses. Call for current prices.

REFRIGERANT, TOPICAL (VAPOCOOLANT) *(Physical Med) 89MLY*

Ari 770-227-8222
2523 South Mcdonough Rd., Orchard Hill, GA 30266
Cold spray.

Gebauer Company 800-321-9348
4444 E 153rd St, Cleveland, OH 44128
Fluori-Methane; Ethyl Chloride, fine and medium. Gebauer's Fluro-Ethyl, vapocoolant (skin refrigerant) intended to control the pain with minor surgical procedures, dermabrasion, injections, and the temporary relief of minor sports injuries. Pain-Ease Mist Spray, vapocoolant to control pain associated with injections, minor surgical procedures, and temporary relief of minor sports injuries. It delivers in a mist spray. Accu-Stream Stream Spray, vapocoolant to control pain associated with pre-injection, minor surgical procedures, minor sports injuries, spray & stretch technique, myofascial pain, and restricted motion.

Iki Mfg. Co, Inc. 608-884-3411
116 Swift St, Edgerton, WI 53534
Aerosol topical coolant.

REFRIGERATOR, BIOLOGICAL *(Microbiology) 83ROS*

Bally Refrigerated Boxes, Inc. 800-24-BALLY
135 Little Nine Rd, Morehead City, NC 28557

Biocold Environmental 636-349-0300
239 Seebold Spur, Fenton, MO 63026
Stability refrigerators for testing medical devices.

Hotpack 800-523-3608
10940 Dutton Rd, Philadelphia, PA 19154

Marvel Scientific 800-962-2521
233 Industrial Pkwy, PO Box 997, Richmond, IN 47374
6.1- to 29-cu-ft refrigeration models for pharmaceutical and medical-related applications; also available, utility, hazardous-location, and flammable-material models. MARVEL refrigerator 6ADA complies with height for American With Disabilities Act, autocycle defrost, all refrigerator.

Scientific Industries, Inc. 888-850-6208
70 Orville Dr, Bohemia, NY 11716

So-Low Environmental Equipment 513-772-9410
10310 Spartan Dr, Cincinnati, OH 45215

Taylor Wharton 800-898-2657
4075 Hamilton Blvd, Theodore, AL 36582
HC-Series, XT-Series, CRYOPAK Shipper, LD Series, K-Series, RS-Series. Large and small, Dewars, freezers, shippers, liquid cylinders.

Ts Scientific 800-258-2796
PO Box 198, Perkasie, PA 18944
Programmable controlled-rate freezer for cryopreservation of biological material using liquid nitrogen.

REFRIGERATOR, BLOOD BANK *(Hematology) 81ROT*

Bally Refrigerated Boxes, Inc. 800-24-BALLY
135 Little Nine Rd, Morehead City, NC 28557

Helmer, Inc. 800-743-5637
15425 Herriman Blvd, Noblesville, IN 46060
Blood Bank Refrigerators

Medi-Tech International, Inc. 305-593-9373
2924 NW 109th Ave, Doral, FL 33172
JEWETT.

REFRIGERATOR, EXPLOSION-PROOF *(Chemistry) 75ROU*

So-Low Environmental Equipment 513-772-9410
10310 Spartan Dr, Cincinnati, OH 45215
Freezer only.

REFRIGERATOR, FOODSERVICE *(General) 80UKW*

Electrolux Home Products - North America 877-435-3287
250 Bobby Jones Expy, PO Box 212378, Augusta, GA 30907
Refrigerators and freezers.

Hoshizaki America, Inc. 800-438-6087
618 Highway 74 S, Peachtree City, GA 30269
A full line of refrigerators, freezers, and dual-temperature reach-ins.

U-Line Corporation 800-779-2547
8900 N 55th St, PO Box 245040, Milwaukee, WI 53223
Also, other related products.

Victory Refrigeration, Inc. 800-523-5008
110 Woodcrest Rd, Cherry Hill, NJ 08003
Refrigerators and freezers.

REFRIGERATOR, LABORATORY *(General) 80WRM*

Follett Corp. 800-523-9361
801 Church Ln, Easton, PA 18040
Under-counter refrigerator with locking handle and external digital temperature display. Stainless steel interior/exterior. Available in 4.8 cu. Ft. capacity or 4.0 cu. Ft. capacity (ADA-compliant).

Harris Environmental Systems, Inc. 888-771-4200
11 Connector Rd, Andover, MA 01810
Custom refrigeration systems.

Helmer, Inc. 800-743-5637
15425 Herriman Blvd, Noblesville, IN 46060
Laboratory Refrigerators

Lytron, Inc. 781-933-7300
55 Dragon Ct, Woburn, MA 01801
200w to 54,000w water chiller for refrigerated cooling.

Medi-Tech International, Inc. 305-593-9373
2924 NW 109th Ave, Doral, FL 33172
JEWETT.

Powers Scientific, Inc. 800-998-0500
PO Box 268, Pipersville, PA 18947

So-Low Environmental Equipment 513-772-9410
10310 Spartan Dr, Cincinnati, OH 45215

REFRIGERATOR, MORGUE, WALK-IN *(Pathology) 88ROV*

Bally Refrigerated Boxes, Inc. 800-24-BALLY
135 Little Nine Rd, Morehead City, NC 28557

Environmental Growth Chambers 800-321-6854
510 Washington St, Chagrin Falls, OH 44022
Stainless Steel 4C Cold Rooms without drawers or morgue tables

Hotpack 800-523-3608
10940 Dutton Rd, Philadelphia, PA 19154

Medi-Tech International, Inc. 305-593-9373
2924 NW 109th Ave, Doral, FL 33172
JEWETT refrigerators and tables.

Scientek Medical Equipment 604-273-9094
11151 Bridgeport Rd., Richmond, BC V6X 1T3 Canada

REFRIGERATOR, PHARMACY *(General) 80WRL*

Helmer, Inc. 800-743-5637
15425 Herriman Blvd, Noblesville, IN 46060
Pharmacy Refrigerators

So-Low Environmental Equipment 513-772-9410
10310 Spartan Dr, Cincinnati, OH 45215

Springer-Penguin, Inc. 800-835-8500
PO Box 310, 11 Brookdale Place,, Mount Vernon, NY 10551
Compact, kept at nurses station; available with left or right hinged doors and/or built in cylinder locks.

REGULATOR, ANESTHESIA *(Anesthesiology) 73ROW*

Aga Linde Healthcare P.R. Inc. 787-622-7900
PO Box 363868, GPO Box 364727, San Juan, PR 00936
Anesth/Pul Med.

Air Liquide America Corporation, Cambridge Div. 800-638-1197
821 Chesapeake Dr, Cambridge, MD 21613
Low flow high purity regulators.

Farley Inc., W.T. 800-327-5397
931 Via Alondra, Camarillo, CA 93012

REGULATOR, INTAKE, OXYGEN *(Anesthesiology) 73QWO*

Lifegas Llc 866-543-3427
1500 Indian Trail Lilburn Rd, Norcross, GA 30093
MEDICYL-E-Lite (TM) Portable Medical Oxygen Delivery System. Integrated regulatory flowmeter and valve assembly in a single unit. The E-Lite eliminates the need for regulator set-up, ready to administer oxygen therapy. Manufactured in an FDA registered and ISO 9001 certified facility. This product has received FDA 510(k) clearance as MRI-Safe and MRI-Compatible for MRI systems up to 3.0T (Tesla).

Medsonic U.S.A., Inc. 716-565-1700
8865 Sheridan Dr, Clarence, NY 14031
OXYGEN CONSERVER Medi S O2 Nic Conserver. Oxygen flow conserves oxygen by providing non-inhalation and shutting off during exhalation.

REGULATOR, LINE VOLTAGE *(General) 80WMM*

Btx Tech 800-666-0996
5 Skyline Dr, Hawthorne, NY 10532

Megger Inc. (Formerly Avo International) 800-723-2861
2621 Van Buren Ave, Norristown, PA 19403
$2,625 for power disturbance analyzer.

Northern Technologies Inc. 509-927-0401
23123 E Mission Ave, Liberty Lake, WA 99019

Online Power, Inc. 800-227-8899
5701 Smithway St, Commerce, CA 90040

Rapid Power Technologies, Inc. 800-332-1111
18 Old Grays Bridge Rd, Brookfield, CT 06804
Voltage regulators and power conditioners with a variety of input/output specifications.

Welch Allyn, Inc. 800-535-6663
4341 State Street Rd, Skaneateles Falls, NY 13153

REGULATOR, OXYGEN, MECHANICAL *(General) 80FQE*

Aerodyne Controls, Inc., A Circor International Company 631-737-1900
30 Haynes Ct, Ronkonkoma, NY 11779

Allied Healthcare Products, Inc. 800-444-3954
1720 Sublette Ave, Saint Louis, MO 63110

Armstrong Medical Industries, Inc. 800-323-4220
575 Knightsbridge Pkwy, Lincolnshire, IL 60069

Chad Therapeutics, Inc. 800-423-8870
21622 Plummer St, Chatsworth, CA 91311
Oxygen conservation products available.

Contemporary Products, Inc. 800-424-2444
530 Riverside Industrial Pkwy, Portland, ME 04103

Dedicated Distribution 800-325-8367
640 Miami Ave, Kansas City, KS 66105
Pulse oximetry monitor.

Dixie Ems Supply 800-347-3494
385 Union Ave, Brooklyn, NY 11211
$108.00 per unit (standard).

Erie Medical 800-932-2293
10225 82nd Ave, Lakeview Corporate Park, Pleasant Prairie, WI 53158
Piston-design flowmeter style, Bourdon gauge style or dial-style regulators for hospital, homecare, or emergency use.

Farley Inc., W.T. 800-327-5397
931 Via Alondra, Camarillo, CA 93012
$90 for oxygen regulators, $65 for oxygen vacuum or air manifolds, $0.75 for oxgyen nut and nipple plastic piece.

Flotec, Inc. 800-401-1723
7625 W New York St, Indianapolis, IN 46214
Flotecs' 'Flopac' portable oxygen delivery system is a fully integrated and permanently valved Regulator / Cylinder combination. Flotec's legendary reputation for safety and durability continues with Flopac as we demonstrate once again the uncompromised value in providing the industry's only all-metal-constructed product line. Flopac is MRI Compatible and Safe when valved onto aluminum or composite cylinders.

Haskel International, Inc. 818-843-4000
100 E Graham Pl, Burbank, CA 91502
Model 53310 oxygen gas boosters for recharging medical oxygen bottles up to 2500 Ps.

Life Corporation 800-700-0202
1776 N Water St, Milwaukee, WI 53202
Complete line LIFE oxygen regulators, O-25 LPM with 12 flow settings and guage with rubber boot.

REGULATOR, OXYGEN, MECHANICAL *(cont'd)*

Lifegas Llc 866-543-3427
1500 Indian Trail Lilburn Rd, Norcross, GA 30093
Regulators: LifeGas supplies medical regulators for a variety of applications/gases including preset oxygen, nitrous oxide therapy, medical air and special applications including blood gas analysis and other medical equipment.

Marsh Bellofram 800-727-5646
8019 Ohio River Blvd., Newell, WV 26050
Precision flow regulators for aspirator, suction, and anesthesia.

U O Equipment Co. 800-231-6372
5863 W 34th St, Houston, TX 77092

Western Medica 800-783-7890
875 Bassett Rd, Westlake, OH 44145
Medical gas control equipment and respiratory systems including: regulators, oxygen conserving devices, oxygen transferring systems, cylinders, fittings/quick connects and flowmeters.

REGULATOR, PRESSURE, GAS CYLINDER
(Anesthesiology) 73CAN

Aerodyne Controls, Inc., A Circor International Company 631-737-1900
30 Haynes Ct, Ronkonkoma, NY 11779

Aga Linde Healthcare P.R. Inc. 787-622-7900
PO Box 363868, GPO Box 364727, San Juan, PR 00936
Anesth/Pul Med.

Air Products And Chemicals, Inc. 800-654-4567
7201 Hamilton Blvd, Allentown, PA 18195

Allied Healthcare Products, Inc. 800-444-3954
1720 Sublette Ave, Saint Louis, MO 63110

Ameriflo Corp. 866-573-1658
478 Gradle Dr, Carmel Industrial Park, Carmel, IN 46032
Regulator.

Amg, Llc 317-329-4000
4030 Guion Ln, Indianapolis, IN 46268
Regulator.

Bradley Alarm Systems 402-791-2388
28801 S 96th St, Firth, NE 68358
Pressure gas cylinder.

Cardinal Health 207, Inc. 610-862-0800
1100 Bird Center Dr, Palm Springs, CA 92262
Oxygen regulator.

Concoa 800-225-0473
1501 Harpers Rd, Virginia Beach, VA 23454
Flowmeter, non-sack-pressure compensated, Bourdon gauge.

Confluent Surgical,Inc 888-734-2583
101A 1st Ave, Waltham, MA 02451
Flow regulator.

Depuy Orthopaedics, Inc. 800-473-3789
700 Orthopaedic Dr, P.O. Box 988, Warsaw, IN 46582
Nitrogen regulatory.

Emepe International, Inc. 813-994-9690
18108 Sugar Brooke Dr, Tampa, FL 33647
Regulators for oxygen and other gases; pressure or flow outlet.

Flotec, Inc. 800-401-1723
7625 W New York St, Indianapolis, IN 46214
All CGA and international inlet and outlet connections available, unibody window design, 12 flow positions, flow ranges from 20 ml thru 60 lpm in all medical gases and gas blends.

Harris Products Group 800-241-0804
2345 Murphy Blvd, Gainesville, GA 30504
Harris Calorific.

Inovo, Inc. 239-643-6577
2975 Horseshoe Dr S Ste 600, Naples, FL 34104
Regulator, intake, oxygen.

Life Corporation 800-700-0202
1776 N Water St, Milwaukee, WI 53202
Complete line of LIFE oxygen regulators, 0 to 25 LPM with 12 flow settings and pressure gauges with rubber boot.

Mada, Inc. 800-526-6370
625 Washington Ave, Carlstadt, NJ 07072

Matrx 716-662-6650
145 Mid County Dr, Orchard Park, NY 14127
Gas regulator, o2-n20.

Matrx By Midmark 800-847-1000
145 Mid County Dr, Orchard Park, NY 14127

REGULATOR, PRESSURE, GAS CYLINDER *(cont'd)*

Medical Depot 516-998-4600
99 Seaview Blvd, Port Washington, NY 11050
Oxygen regulator.

Mg Industries 610-695-7628
1 Steel Rd E, U.S. Industrial Park, Morrisville, PA 19067
Patient lift.

Micro-Aire Surgical Instruments, Inc. 800-722-0822
1641 Edlich Dr, Charlottesville, VA 22911

Nichole Medical Equipment & Supply, Inc. 888-673-6335
2200 Michener St Ste 4, Philadelphia, PA 19115
Same.

Norco 800-657-6672
1125 W Amity Rd, Boise, ID 83705

O-Two Systems International Inc. 800-387-3405
7575 Kimbel St., Mississauga, ONT L5S 1C8 Canada

Ohmeda Medical 800-345-2700
8880 Gorman Rd, Laurel, MD 20723

Oxia U.S. Ltd. 262-369-1978
665 Industrial Ct Unit B, Hartland, WI 53029
Personal oxygen device, regulator.

Precision Medical, Inc. 800-272-7285
300 Held Dr, Northampton, PA 18067

Puritan Bennett Corp. 925-463-4371
2800 Airwest Blvd, Plainfield, IN 46168
Various.

Scott Specialty Gases 215-766-8861
6141 Easton Road Box 310, Plumsteadville, PA 18949
Pressure regulator.

Sherwood, Harsco Corp. 716-505-4831
2111 Liberty Dr, Niagara Falls, NY 14304
Grab and go, vipre (valve with integrated pressure regulator).

Southland Cryogenics, Inc. 800-872-2796
8350 Mosley Rd, Houston, TX 77075
Medical regulators for the controlled delivery of medical gases; variety of flow rates available.

Spiracle Technology 714-418-1091
16520 Harbor Blvd Ste D, Fountain Valley, CA 92708
Pressure regulator.

Stryker Corp. 800-726-2725
2825 Airview Blvd, Portage, MI 49002

Superior Products, Inc. 216-651-9400
3786 Ridge Rd, Cleveland, OH 44144
Medical gas regulator, compressed gas regulator.

Tennessee Medical Equipment, Inc. 731-635-2119
4637 Highway 19 E, Ripley, TN 38063
Various.

Tescom Corp. 800-447-9635
12616 Industrial Blvd NW, Elk River, MN 55330

The Respiratory Group 314-659-4311
4150 Carr Lane Ct, Saint Louis, MO 63119
20 & 50 psi regulators, fixed flow regulator, conserving regulator,flow selector.

Thermadyne Holdings, Corp. 940-381-1388
800 Henrietta Creek Rd, Roanoke, TX 76262
Medical regulators.

U O Equipment Co. 800-231-6372
5863 W 34th St, Houston, TX 77092

Western/Scott Fetzer Co. 440-871-2160
1354 Lear Industrial Pkwy, Avon, OH 44011
Pressure regulator, multiple.

Zimmer Holdings, Inc. 800-613-6131
1800 W Center St, PO Box 708, Warsaw, IN 46580

REGULATOR, SUCTION, SURGICAL *(General) 80CBB*

Boehringer Laboratories, Inc. 800-642-4945
500 E Washington St, Norristown, PA 19401
Boehringer offers both continuous and intermitting styles that can be easily sterilized. Ten-year warranty.

Datex-Ohmeda (Canada) 800-268-1472
1093 Meyerside Dr., Unit 2, Mississauga, ONT L5T-1J6 Canada

Emepe International, Inc. 813-994-9690
18108 Sugar Brooke Dr, Tampa, FL 33647
Regulator to attach to a wall or a ceiling gas outlet to suction patient fluids. Must be connected to a collecting bottle.

REGULATOR, SUCTION, THORACIC *(Anesthesiology) 73ROZ*

Allied Healthcare Products, Inc. 800-444-3954
1720 Sublette Ave, Saint Louis, MO 63110

Emepe International, Inc. 813-994-9690
18108 Sugar Brooke Dr, Tampa, FL 33647
Vacuum regulators (general, surgical, thoracic, gastric) and collection bottles. Accessories for suction.

Ohmeda Medical 800-345-2700
8880 Gorman Rd, Laurel, MD 20723
Intermittent suction unit.

REGULATOR, SUCTION, TRACHEAL (NASAL, ORAL) *(Ear/Nose/Throat) 77RPA*

Allied Healthcare Products, Inc. 800-444-3954
1720 Sublette Ave, Saint Louis, MO 63110

Datex-Ohmeda (Canada) 800-268-1472
1093 Meyerside Dr., Unit 2, Mississauga, ONT L5T-1J6 Canada

REGULATOR, TEMPERATURE *(Chemistry) 75JRR*

Aeroscout 706-867-0140
1300 Island Dr Ste 202, Redwood City, CA 94065

Burling Instruments, Inc. 973-635-9481
16 River Rd, Chatham, NJ 07928

Cmt, Inc. 800-659-9140
PO Box 297, Hamilton, MA 01936

Deltatrak, Inc. 800-962-6776
PO Box 398, Pleasanton, CA 94566
TEMPDOT time and temperature indicators - temperature labels that will provide accumulative temperature exposure time over specified temperature limit to indicate quality of product during transport.

Devar Inc. 800-566-6822
706 Bostwick Ave, Bridgeport, CT 06605

Kendro Laboratory Products 800-252-7100
308 Ridgefield Ct, Asheville, NC 28806

Omega Engineering, Inc. 800-848-4286
1 Omega Dr, Stamford, CT 06907

Thermo Fisher Scientific 877-843-7668
81 Wyman St, Waltham, MA 02451
Also, MRI recirculating coolers.

REGULATOR, THERMAL, CARDIOPULMONARY BYPASS *(Cardiovascular) 74DWJ*

Danbi, Inc. 310-398-0013
12099 W Washington Blvd Ste 304, Los Angeles, CA 90066
Hyperthermia unit with thermo couples/thermometry.

Icu Medical (Ut), Inc 949-366-2183
4455 Atherton Dr, Salt Lake City, UT 84123
Various.

Innercool Therapies, Inc.- A Delaware Corporation 858-713-5904
6740 Top Gun St, San Diego, CA 92121
Ccs catheters console & accessories.

Medisearch P.R., Inc. 787-864-0684
Machete Industrial Center, Guayama, PR 00784
Various.

Medivance, Inc. 303-926-1917
1172 W Century Dr Ste 240, Louisville, CO 80027
Hypo/hyperthermia system.

Merit Medical Systems, Inc. 801-253-1600
1111 S Velasco St, Angleton, TX 77515
Warmtouch patient warming system.

Mmj S.A. De C.V. 314-654-2000
716 Ponciano Arriaga, Cd. Juarez, Chih. Mexico
Warming system

North Safety Products 401-943-4400
1101 B Calle Neutron, Parque Industrial Maran, Mexicali, B.c. Mexico
Rescue blanket

Paragon Manufacturing Corp 425-438-0800
2615 W Casino Rd Ste 4C, Everett, WA 98204
Thermal regulating device.

Pi-Ptp 888-818-9632
215 Rocky Mount Rd, PO Box 1067, Athens, TN 37303
Warming blanket.

Smiths Medical Asd, Inc. 610-578-9600
9255 Customhouse Plz Ste N, San Diego, CA 92154
Warming blower, w/blanket.

REGULATOR, THERMAL, CARDIOPULMONARY BYPASS *(cont'd)*

Whitehall/A Division Of Acorn Engineering Co. 626-336-4561
15125 Proctor Ave, City Of Industry, CA 91746
Various models of water heating units.

REGULATOR, VACUUM *(General) 80KDP*

Aerodyne Controls, Inc., A Circor International Company 631-737-1900
30 Haynes Ct, Ronkonkoma, NY 11779

Composite Manufacturing, Inc. 949-361-7580
970 Calle Amanecer Ste B, San Clemente, CA 92673
Suction regulator.

Dornoch Medical Systems, Inc. 816-505-2226
4032 NW Riverside Dr, Riverside, MO 64150
Vacuum regulator.

Flotec, Inc. 800-401-1723
7625 W New York St, Indianapolis, IN 46214
Flotec's 'Suckrr' line of vacuum regulators has a planned introduction for the 4th quarter of 2006.

Handler Manufacturing Co. 800-274-2635
612 North Ave E, Westfield, NJ 07090
SANI-VAC, collect dust and debris from removal of nail and 'hard tissue' from foot.

Icu Medical (Ut), Inc 949-366-2183
4455 Atherton Dr, Salt Lake City, UT 84123
Various.

Maquet, Inc. 843-552-8652
7371 Spartan Blvd E, N Charleston, SC 29418
Various types of vacuum systems.

Medtek Devices, Inc. 716-835-7000
595 Commerce Dr, 155 Pineview Dr., Amherst, NY 14228
Smoke evacuator.

Ohmeda Medical 800-345-2700
8880 Gorman Rd, Laurel, MD 20723

Precision Medical, Inc. 800-272-7285
300 Held Dr, Northampton, PA 18067

Superior Products, Inc. 216-651-9400
3786 Ridge Rd, Cleveland, OH 44144
Vacuum regulator.

Terumo Cardiovascular Systems (Tcvs) 800-283-7866
28 Howe St, Ashland, MA 01721
Vacuum regulator.

Varian Vacuum Products 800-882-7426
121 Hartwell Ave, Lexington, MA 02421

RELINER, DENTURE, OTC *(Dental And Oral) 76EBP*

Holmes Dental Corp. 800-322-5577
50 S Penn St, Hatboro, PA 19040
STA-SOFT soft relining material.

REMINDER, MEDICATION *(Physical Med) 89NXQ*

Vocel 858-679-1919
13400 Sabre Springs Pkwy Ste 255, San Diego, CA 92128
Pill phone.

REMOVER, BLADE, SCALPEL *(General) 80WZH*

Cincinnati Surgical Company 800-544-3100
11256 Cornell Park Dr, Cincinnati, OH 45242

Medical Safety Systems Inc. 888-803-9303
230 White Pond Dr, Akron, OH 44313

Trademark Medical Llc 800-325-9044
449 Soverign Ct, St. Louis, MO 63011
BLADE-SAFE disposable surgical blade remover designed to prevent Sharps injury while removing surgical blades from scalpel handles. Can be used for blades up to size #20.

REMOVER, CLIP *(Surgery) 79QLA*

Mizuho America Inc. 800-699-2547
133 Brimbal Ave, Beverly, MA 01915
Aneurysm clip removers.

Okay Industries, Inc. 860-225-8707
200 Ellis St, P.O. Box 2470, New Britain, CT 06051

Roboz Surgical Instrument Co., Inc. 800-424-2984
PO Box 10710, Gaithersburg, MD 20898

REMOVER, CROWN *(Dental And Oral) 76EIS*

Almore International, Inc. 503-643-6633
PO Box 25214, Portland, OR 97298
$19.95 per unit (standard).

REMOVER, CROWN *(cont'd)*

American Eagle Instruments, Inc. 406-549-7451
6575 Butler Creek Rd, Missoula, MT 59808
Various types of crown removers.

Dental Usa, Inc. 815-363-8003
5005 McCullom Lake Rd, McHenry, IL 60050
Remover.

Dentalez Group 866-DTE-INFO
101 Lindenwood Dr Ste 225, Valleybrooke Corporate Center
Malvern, PA 19355

Gc America, Inc. 708-597-0900
3737 W 127th St, Alsip, IL 60803
Remover, crown.

H & H Co. 909-390-0373
4435 E Airport Dr Ste 108, Ontario, CA 91761
Remover, crown.

Hager Worldwide, Inc. 800-328-2335
13322 Byrd Dr, Odessa, FL 33556
CROWN CLICK & CROWN CLICK DELUXE.

Higa Manufacturing Ltd. 604-922-5261
Po Box 91160 Stn West Vancouver, West Vancouver V7V 3N6 Canada
No common name listed

J. Morita Usa, Inc. 888-566-7482
9 Mason, Irvine, CA 92618
ATD Automatic Crown and Bridge Remover by J. Morita USA is an automated device that has significantly advanced the technique of crown and bridge removal. This innovative system uses a specialized handpiece that can attach to either an electric or slow speed air driven handpiece motor with speeds between 5,000 rpm and 25,000 rpm. The ATD offers less stress on tooth structure by applying regular strokes and helps avoid and prevent damage to tooth, periodontium and the prosthesis. Both the intensity and frequency of the stroke force are adjustable. It is fully autoclavable and includes a wide range of hook and wire tips that are designed for removing any fixed prosthetic configuration. Available with connectors for either an E-type standard, Star Titan or Midwest Shorty Two-Speed.

Miltex Dental Technologies, Inc. 516-576-6022
589 Davies Dr, York, PA 17402
Miller-morrell type crown remover.

Pentron Laboratory Technologies 203-265-7397
53 N Plains Industrial Rd, Wallingford, CT 06492
Remover, crown.

Premier Dental Products Co. 888-670-6100
1710 Romano Dr, PO Box 4500, Plymouth Meeting, PA 19462

Pulpdent Corp. 800-343-4342
80 Oakland St, Watertown, MA 02472
Crown remover.

Salvin Dental Specialties, Inc. 800-535-6566
3450 Latrobe Dr, Charlotte, NC 28211
Various types of crown removers.

REMOVER, FOREIGN BODY, BRONCHOSCOPE (NON-RIGID) *(Anesthesiology) 73JEI*

Mahe International Inc. 800-294-7946
468 Craighead St, Nashville, TN 37204

Prosurge Instruments, Inc. 866-832-7874
199 Laidlaw Ave, Jersey City, NJ 07306

REMOVER, INTRAUTERINE DEVICE, CONTRACEPTIVE (HOOK TYPE) *(Obstetrics/Gyn) 85HHF*

Tuzik Boston 800-886-6363
104 Longwater Dr, Assinippi Park, Norwell, MA 02061

REMOVER, PARTICULATE *(Surgery) 79UMK*

The Evercare Company 800-435-6223
3440 Preston Ridge Rd Ste 650, Alpharetta, GA 30005
Adhesive lint remover (4 x 30) for picking up lint and foreign particles from surgical packs, wrappers and gowns.

REMOVER, STAPLE, SURGICAL *(Surgery) 79VLT*

Covidien Lp 508-261-8000
15 Hampshire St, Mansfield, MA 02048
APPOSE disposable skin staple remover.

Cypress Medical Products 800-334-3646
1202 S. Rte. 31, McHenry, IL 60050
Staple remover kits with staple remover, alcohol prep pad, 3x3 gauze sponge and PVP prep pad.

REMOVER, STAPLE, SURGICAL *(cont'd)*

Ethicon Endo-Surgery, Inc. 800-USE-ENDO
4545 Creek Rd, Cincinnati, OH 45242
PROXIMATE, squeeze handle or ring handle. ENDOPATH extractor, 5mm with handle or ratchet handle, reuseable.

Roboz Surgical Instrument Co., Inc. 800-424-2984
PO Box 10710, Gaithersburg, MD 20898

REMOVER, TISSUE *(Surgery) 79SHW*

Technical Products International, Inc. 800-729-4421
5918 Evergreen Blvd, Saint Louis, MO 63134
Flesh/fresh fixed tissue sectioning system.

REPROCESSING UNIT, DIALYZER *(Gastro/Urology) 78VHO*

Mesa Laboratories, Inc. 800-992-6372
12100 W 6th Ave, Lakewood, CO 80228
ECHO, for automated hemodialyzer reprocessing.

RESCUE EQUIPMENT *(General) 80WMZ*

Armstrong Medical Industries, Inc. 800-323-4220
575 Knightsbridge Pkwy, Lincolnshire, IL 60069

Bashaw Medical, Inc. 800-499-3857
4909 Mobile Hwy Ste B, Pensacola, FL 32506
EMS VEST & HARNESS & RESCUE VEST.

Dixie Ems Supply 800-347-3494
385 Union Ave, Brooklyn, NY 11211
A flame retardant vest with pouches to be used for emergency evacuation of infants.

Emergency Vehicles, Inc. 800-848-3652
705 13th St, Lake Park, FL 33403
Quick Attack vehicles. Rescue vehicles; haz-mat, rescue, specialty vehicles, command/communications vehicles, S.W.A.T. units, quick attack vehicles and brush trucks.

Ferno-Washington, Inc. 800-733-3766
70 Weil Way, Wilmington, OH 45177

Garaventa (Canada) Ltd. 800-663-6556
7505 - 134A St., Surrey, BC V3W-7B3 Canada
$2,195 for EVACU-TRAC emergency evacuation chair.

Iron Duck, A Div. Of Fleming Industries, Inc. 800-669-6900
20 Veterans Dr, Chicopee, MA 01022
Rope storage cases for rescue squads; storage units for turnout gear; nylon equipment bags; nylon mesh stretcher caddies.

Kinman Of Indianapolis, Inc. 800-444-8891
1401 Harding Ct Ste K, Indianapolis, IN 46217
Hydraulic rescue tool & ram. Also, hydraulic rescue tool-cutter and spreader combination tool, with 12 volt power unit, also hydraulic power ram and stroke multiplier. Also supplied, storage box and all accessories. Hose Reels with 100 feet of cable/hose assembly for Rescue Units.

Knox Company 800-552-5669
1601 W Deer Valley Rd, Phoenix, AZ 85027
Key vault for rapid entry by emergency response teams. Available in three sizes - both surface and recessed mounts. Available in door hanger model for temporary convalescing.

Life Corporation 800-700-0202
1776 N Water St, Milwaukee, WI 53202
LIFE Emergency oxygen units, regulators, masks, etc.

Rapid Deployment Products 877-433-7569
157 Railroad Dr, Ivyland, PA 18974
MP Carrier - High Density, Roto-Molded Polyethylene plastic, Seamless Design Floats over 300 lbs (with stabilizers attached), Haz-Mat Decon Tray with garden hose fittings for containment, Multiple units stack together for easy storage, Speed clip pins available, Foam filled for flotation and patient insulation, Bottom runner width fits ground ladder rails for ladder slide, Stabilizer floats are available, and must be used for water or ice rescue

Skedco, Inc. 503-639-2119
16420 SW 72nd Ave, PO Box 230487, Portland, OR 97224
SKED portable, backpack-type emergency stretcher rescue system for aerial, vertical and confined space rescue.

Ziamatic Corp. 800-711-FIRE
10 W College Ave, Yardley, PA 19067
QUIC BAR forceful entry tools. Also, gas cylinder brackets and mountaing devices and brackets.

RESECTOSCOPE *(Gastro/Urology) 78FJL*

Boehm Surgical Instrument Corp. 716-436-6584
966 Chili Ave, Rochester, NY 14611
Resectoscope.

RESECTOSCOPE *(cont'd)*

Conceptus, Inc. 650-962-4000
331 E Evelyn Ave, Mountain View, CA 94041

Gyrus Acmi, Inc. 508-804-2739
93 N Pleasant St, Norwalk, OH 44857
Resectoscope and accessories.

Karl Storz Endoscopy-America Inc. 800-421-0837
600 Corporate Pointe, Culver City, CA 90230
Gynecologic and urologic. Standard, continuous flow, rotating and fixed resectoscope sheaths in a range of sizes.

Mahe International Inc. 800-294-7946
468 Craighead St, Nashville, TN 37204

Olympus America, Inc. 800-645-8160
3500 Corporate Pkwy, PO Box 610, Center Valley, PA 18034

Princeton Medical Group, Inc. 800-875-0869
1189 Royal Links Dr, Mt Pleasant, SC 29466

Richard Wolf Medical Instruments Corp. 800-323-9653
353 Corporate Woods Pkwy, Vernon Hills, IL 60061

Superior Medical Limited 800-268-7944
520 Champagne Dr., Toronto, ONT M3J 2T9 Canada

RESECTOSCOPE WORKING ELEMENT *(Gastro/Urology) 78FDC*

Gyrus Acmi, Inc. 508-804-2739
93 N Pleasant St, Norwalk, OH 44857
Various sizes and kinds of resectoscope working elements.

Gyrus Acmi, Inc. 508-804-2739
300 Stillwater P.o.box 1971, Stamford, CT 06902
Various sizes and kinds of resectoscope working elements.

Karl Storz Endoscopy-America Inc. 800-421-0837
600 Corporate Pointe, Culver City, CA 90230
Spring action, and rack and pinion.

Mahe International Inc. 800-294-7946
468 Craighead St, Nashville, TN 37204

Richard Wolf Medical Instruments Corp. 800-323-9653
353 Corporate Woods Pkwy, Vernon Hills, IL 60061

RESERVOIR, BLOOD, CARDIOPULMONARY BYPASS *(Cardiovascular) 74DTN*

Circulatory Technology, Inc. 516-624-2424
21 Singworth St, Oyster Bay, NY 11771
The v-bag.

Gish Biomedical, Inc. 800-938-0531
22942 Arroyo Vis, Rancho Santa Margarita, CA 92688

Jostra Bentley, Inc. 302-454-9959
Rd. 402 N. Km 1.4, Industrial Park, Anasco, PR 00610-1577
Cardiotomy venous reservoirs.

Medtronic Blood Management 612-514-4000
18501 E Plaza Dr, Parker, CO 80134
Cardiotomy reservoir.

Medtronic Perfusion Systems 800-854-3570
7611 Northland Dr N, Brooklyn Park, MN 55428

Novosci Corp. 281-363-4949
2828 N Crescentridge Dr, The Woodlands, TX 77381

Sorin Group Usa 800-289-5759
14401 W 65th Way, Arvada, CO 80004

Terumo Cardiovascular Systems (Tcvs) 800-283-7866
125 Blue Ball Rd, Elkton, MD 21921
Reservoir.

Terumo Cardiovascular Systems (Tcvs) 800-283-7866
28 Howe St, Ashland, MA 01721
Reservoir.

Terumo Cardiovascular Systems, Corp 800-521-2818
6200 Jackson Rd, Ann Arbor, MI 48103
Large and regular volume, filtered and non-filtered, also available in custom tube pack.

Vitalcor, Inc. 800-874-8358
100 Chestnut Ave, Westmont, IL 60559
Blood-reservoir cardiopulmonary bypass.

RESERVOIR, HYDROCEPHALIC CATHETER *(Cns/Neurology) 84UCC*

Microcision Llc 800-264-3811
5805 Keystone St, Philadelphia, PA 19135

RESERVOIR, SPINAL FLUID *(Cns/Neurology) 84TEG*

Biocell Laboratories, Inc. 800-222-8382
2001 E University Dr, Rancho Dominguez, CA 90220
Normal and abnormal.

RESIN, ION-EXCHANGE *(Pathology) 88KEA*

Bachem Bioscience, Inc. 800-634-3183
3700 Horizon Dr, King Of Prussia, PA 19406

RESIN, OTHER *(General) 80WWC*

Hospitales Y Quirofanos S.A. Dec.V. 5-611-8244
Murillo No. 44 Col. Nonoalco, Deleg. B. Juarez, D.F. 03700 Mexico
Material.

Polymer Laboratories, Now A Part Of Varian, Inc. 800-767-3963
160 Old Farm Rd, Amherst Fields Research Park, Amherst, MA 01002
Resins for combinatorial chemistry.

RESIN, PLASTIC *(General) 80VAK*

Composiflex, Inc. 800-673-2544
8100 Hawthorne Dr, Erie, PA 16509
orthotic/orthopedic supports,available in flexible or rigid composite systems.

Dur-A-Flex, Inc. 800-253-3539
95 Goodwin St, East Hartford, CT 06108
Epoxies.

The Lifestyle Co. Inc. 800-622-0777
1800 State Route 34 Ste 401, Wall Township, NJ 07719
SGP telefocon A, SGP II telefocon B and SGP 3 unifocon A contact lens material; clear, blue or green 1/2in. blanks. SGP and SGP II only, grey or brown 1/2in. blanks.

RESIN, ROOT CANAL FILLING *(Dental And Oral) 76KIF*

Bisco, Inc. 847-534-6000
1100 W Irving Park Rd, Schaumburg, IL 60193
Calcium hydroxide/iodoform root canal treatment paste.

Coltene/Whaledent Inc. 330-916-8858
235 Ascot Pkwy, Cuyahoga Falls, OH 44223
Sealer.

Cooley & Cooley, Ltd. 800-215-4487
8550 Westland West Blvd, Houston, TX 77041
DOC'S BEST COPPER ANTIMICROBIAL PULP(ROOT) CANAL SEALER- A COPPER BASED PRODUCT TO BE PLACED WITH GUTTA PERCHA. THE INGREDIENTS WILL CONTINUOUSLY KILL STREP MUTANS, STAPH AUREUS AND LACTOBACILLUS PARACASEI. NO ABSORPTION REPORTED AS WITH CALCIUM HYDROXIDE.

Dentsply Canada, Ltd. 800-263-1437
161 Vinyl Ct., Woodbridge, ONT L4L 4A3 Canada

Kerr Corp. 714-516-7400
28200 Wick Rd, Romulus, MI 48174
Pulp canal sealer and liner.

Novocol, Inc. 303-665-7535
416 S Taylor Ave, Louisville, CO 80027
Granitec root canal cement.

Pentron Clinical Technologies 203-265-7397
68-70 North Plains Industrial, Road, Wallingford, CT 06492
Root canal filling resin.

Pentron Laboratory Technologies 203-265-7397
53 N Plains Industrial Rd, Wallingford, CT 06492
Root canal sealant.

Pulpdent Corp. 800-343-4342
80 Oakland St, Watertown, MA 02472
Root canal filling material.

Rite-Dent Manufacturing Corp. 305-693-8626
3750 E 10th Ct, Hialeah, FL 33013
Various types of root canal resin.

Ultradent Products, Inc. 801-553-4586
505 W 10200 S, South Jordan, UT 84095
Root canal sealant.

RESINOUS COMPOUND *(Dental And Oral) 76UDV*

American Diversified Dental Systems 800-637-2330
22991 La Cadena Dr, Laguna Hills, CA 92653
American DieRock Resin Die Stone, 10 & 40 lbs Boxes.

3m Espe Dental Products 949-863-1360
2111 McGaw Ave, Irvine, CA 92614
$35.85/refill for microfill anterior restorative.

RESINOUS COMPOUND, CRANIAL *(Cns/Neurology) 84UCK*

Codman & Shurtleff, Inc 800-225-0460
325 Paramount Dr, Raynham, MA 02767

RESINS, ION EXCHANGE, LIQUID CHROMATOGRAPHY *(Toxicology) 91DNH*

Bio-Rad Laboratories, Life Science Group 800-424-6723
2000 Alfred Nobel Dr, Hercules, CA 94547
$60-$100 for resins.

Polymer Laboratories, Now A Part Of Varian, Inc. 800-767-3963
160 Old Farm Rd, Amherst Fields Research Park, Amherst, MA 01002

Sterogene Bioseparations, Inc. 800-535-2284
5922 Farnsworth Ct, Carlsbad, CA 92008

RESORCIN FUCHSIN *(Pathology) 88HZR*

Rowley Biochemical Institute 978-739-4883
10 Electronics Ave, Danvers Industrial Park, Danvers, MA 01923

Ventana Medical Systems, Inc. 800-227-2155
1910 E Innovation Park Dr, Oro Valley, AZ 85755
Dye solution stain.

RESPIRATOR, SURGICAL, COMBINATION PRODUCT *(General) 80MSH*

Inovel Llc 866-546-6835
10111 Jefferson Blvd, Culver City, CA 90232
Particulate respirator and surgical mask.

RESPIRATORY SYNCYTIAL VIRUS, ANTIGEN, ANTIBODY, IFA *(Microbiology) 83LKT*

Bd Diagnostic Systems 800-675-0908
7 Loveton Cir, Sparks, MD 21152
Respiratory syncytial virus test kit.

Dako North America, Inc 805-566-6655
6392 Via Real, Carpinteria, CA 93013

Hemagen Diagnostics, Inc. 800-436-2436
9033 Red Branch Rd, Columbia, MD 21045
Rsv ifa.

Meridian Bioscience, Inc. 800-696-0739
3471 River Hills Dr, Cincinnati, OH 45244
Direct immunofluorescent procedure for the detection of varicella zoster virus in vesicle smears, biopsy specimens and cell culture.

Meridian Life Science, Inc. 800-327-6299
5171 Wilfong Rd, Memphis, TN 38134

RESTORATION, BASE METAL *() NSQ*

Edmonds Dental Prosthetics, Inc. 417-881-8572
2065 W Woodland St, Springfield, MO 65807

RESTORATION, NOBLE METAL *() NSJ*

Edmonds Dental Prosthetics, Inc. 417-881-8572
2065 W Woodland St, Springfield, MO 65807

RESTORATION, PORCELAIN-FUSED-TO-METAL *() NSO*

Edmonds Dental Prosthetics, Inc. 417-881-8572
2065 W Woodland St, Springfield, MO 65807

RESTRAINT *(Physical Med) 89KID*

Bashaw Medical, Inc. 800-499-3857
4909 Mobile Hwy Ste B, Pensacola, FL 32506
Restraint belts.

Body Tech 1 Nw 866-315-0640
10727 47th Pl W, Mukilteo, WA 98275
Restraint.

Community Products, Llc 845-658-7723
Platte Clove Rd., Elka Park, NY 12427

Greenco Industries, Inc. 608-328-8311
1601 4th Ave W, Monroe, WI 53566
Wrist restraint.

Sure-Lok, Inc. 866-787-3565
2501 Baglyos Cir, Bethlehem, PA 18020
Wheelchair tie-downs and occupant restraint systems

RESTRAINT, ANKLE/FOOT *(General) 80RPB*

Bryton Corp. 800-567-9500
4310 Guion Rd, Indianapolis, IN 46254
Disposable and reusable restraint straps for surgical procedures.

Dixie Ems Supply 800-347-3494
385 Union Ave, Brooklyn, NY 11211
$130.00 per 10 (16in).

Formedica Ltd. 800-361-9671
1481 Rue Begin, St Laurent, QUE H4R 1V8 Canada
$120.00 per 10 (16in).

RESTRAINT, ANKLE/FOOT *(cont'd)*

Humane Restraint Co Inc 800-356-7472
912 Bethel Cir, Waunakee, WI 53597
Various types of ankle/foot and other restraints.

J. T. Posey Co. 800-447-6739
5635 Peck Rd, Arcadia, CA 91006

Morrison Medical 800-438-6677
3735 Paragon Dr, Columbus, OH 43228
Disposable or reusable restraints.

Profex Medical Products 800-325-0196
2224 E Person Ave, Memphis, TN 38114

Segufix Systems Ltd. 506-328-8636
110 Queen St., Woodstock, NB E7M-2M6 Canada

Tartan Orthopedics, Ltd. 888-287-1456
10651 Irma Dr Unit C, Northglenn, CO 80233
$50.00 per 10 (16in).

Zimmer Holdings, Inc. 800-613-6131
1800 W Center St, PO Box 708, Warsaw, IN 46580

RESTRAINT, ARM *(General) 80RPC*

Bryton Corp. 800-567-9500
4310 Guion Rd, Indianapolis, IN 46254
Disposable and reusable restraint straps for surgical procedures.

Formedica Ltd. 800-361-9671
1481 Rue Begin, St Laurent, QUE H4R 1V8 Canada
$120.00 per 10 (med).

Frank Stubbs Co., Inc 800-223-1713
2100 Eastman Ave Ste B, Oxnard, CA 93030

J. T. Posey Co. 800-447-6739
5635 Peck Rd, Arcadia, CA 91006

Medline Industries, Inc. 800-633-5886
1 Medline Pl, Mundelein, IL 60060

Profex Medical Products 800-325-0196
2224 E Person Ave, Memphis, TN 38114

RESTRAINT, CRIB *(General) 80RPD*

Pedicraft, Inc. 800-223-7649
4134 Saint Augustine Rd, Jacksonville, FL 32207
PEDI-CRIB TOP; $1,160.00 per unit (standard); $228.00 per unit (standard) for Infant Reflux Wedge; $ 57.00 per unit (standard) for Infant Reflux Sling. Canopy Enclosed Bed: Mesh-enclosed bed with padded frame. $4,550 to $6,845 includes bed, enclosure, bed rails, mattress, sheets, bed skirt and casters.

RESTRAINT, PATIENT, CONDUCTIVE *(Anesthesiology) 73BRT*

Airway Management Inc. 214-369-0978
6116 N Central Expy Ste 605, Dallas, TX 75206
Thermoplastic immobilization materials.

Alimed, Inc. 800-225-2610
297 High St, Dedham, MA 02026

Bryton Corp. 800-567-9500
4310 Guion Rd, Indianapolis, IN 46254
Conductive restraint straps for surgical tables. Patient restraint straps for arm boards, leg holders & knee crutches.

Griff Industries, Inc. 800-709-4743
19761 Bahama St, Northridge, CA 91324
Disposable and reusable restraining straps.

J. T. Posey Co. 800-447-6739
5635 Peck Rd, Arcadia, CA 91006

Larson Medical Products, Inc. 614-235-9100
2844 Banwick Rd, Columbus, OH 43232
Thermoplastic immobilization material.

Mckesson General Medical 800-446-3008
8741 Landmark Rd, Richmond, VA 23228

Orthoband Company, Inc. 800-325-9973
3690 Highway M, Imperial, MO 63052

Primo, Inc. 770-486-7394
417 Dividend Dr Ste B, Peachtree City, GA 30269
Various.

Profex Medical Products 800-325-0196
2224 E Person Ave, Memphis, TN 38114

Ripp Restraints, Inc. 386-775-2812
1220 E Industrial Dr, Orange City, FL 32763
Patient restraints.

Span-America Medical Systems, Inc. 800-888-6752
70 Commerce Ctr, Greenville, SC 29615

RESTRAINT, PROTECTIVE (BODY) *(General) 80FMQ*

A&A Orthopedics, Incorporated 757-224-0177
12250 SW 129th Ct Bldg 1, Miami, FL 33186
Wrist & ankle restraints.

Alimed, Inc. 800-225-2610
297 High St, Dedham, MA 02026

Atd-American Co. 800-523-2300
135 Greenwood Ave, Wyncote, PA 19095

Barjan Mfg., Ltd. 631-420-5588
28 Baiting Place Rd, Farmingdale, NY 11735
No common name listed.

Bashaw Medical, Inc. 800-499-3857
4909 Mobile Hwy Ste B, Pensacola, FL 32506

Bennett Industries, Inc. 931-432-4011
1805 Burgess Falls Rd, Cookeville, TN 38506
Crib-top.

Biomet Microfixation Inc. 800-874-7711
1520 Tradeport Dr, Jacksonville, FL 32218
Restraint, protective.

Biomet, Inc. 574-267-6639
56 E Bell Dr, PO Box 587, Warsaw, IN 46582
Various types of restraints.

Bioplastics Co. 800-487-2358
34655 Mills Rd, North Ridgeville, OH 44039
Biothane security straps.

Bird & Cronin, Inc. 651-683-1111
1200 Trapp Rd, Saint Paul, MN 55121
Limb restraint.

Bryton Corp. 800-567-9500
4310 Guion Rd, Indianapolis, IN 46254
Restraint devices & straps for all types of operating room tables.

DJO Inc. 800-336-6569
1430 Decision St, Vista, CA 92081
Various waist, vest, bed, ankle, wrist and mitt restraints.

Emergency Products And Research 305-304-6933
890 W Main St, Kent, OH 44240
Straps.

Extended Care Air Therapy Systems, Inc. 740-697-0845
7165 Payne Rd, Roseville, OH 43777
Bed enclosure.

Formedica Ltd. 800-361-9671
1481 Rue Begin, St Laurent, QUE H4R 1V8 Canada
$160.00 per 10 (58in).

Ge Medical Systems, Llc 262-548-2355
3000 N Grandview Blvd, W-417, Waukesha, WI 53188
Head immobilizer strap set for ge ct/n.

Geriatric Products, Inc. 718-384-5700
72 Division Pl, Brooklyn, NY 11222
Protective restraint.

Gillen Industries 877-444-5536
1576 Bella Vista Cruz Drive, Suite 320, the villages, FL 32159
Restraint, protective.

Health Care Logistics, Inc. 800-848-1633
450 Town St, PO Box 25, Circleville, OH 43113
Pediatric arm and leg restraints/immobilizers.

Humane Restraint Co Inc 800-356-7472
912 Bethel Cir, Waunakee, WI 53597
Various types of body restraints including straight jackets.

J. T. Posey Co. 800-447-6739
5635 Peck Rd, Arcadia, CA 91006

Kenad Sg Medical, Inc. 800-825-0606
2692 Huntley Dr, Memphis, TN 38132
Various restraints,protective.

Kerr Group 800-524-3577
1400 Holcomb Bridge Rd, Roswell, GA 30076

Mcneil Healthcare, Inc. 203-932-6263
481 Elm St, West Haven, CT 06516
Conforming bandage,textured gauze roll,elastic gauze roll.

Morrison Medical 800-438-6677
3735 Paragon Dr, Columbus, OH 43228
For ambulance backboards, any size, style, webbing nylon, polypro and impervious.

Olympic Medical Corp. 206-767-3500
5900 1st Ave S, Seattle, WA 98108
$198.50 per unit.

RESTRAINT, PROTECTIVE (BODY) *(cont'd)*

Pedicraft, Inc. 800-223-7649
4134 Saint Augustine Rd, Jacksonville, FL 32207
STANG CIRC CHAIR, $345.00, positions infant for circumcision. Provides surgical access, prevents movement.

Primo, Inc. 770-486-7394
417 Dividend Dr Ste B, Peachtree City, GA 30269
Wrist restraint, vest restraint,or arm/table strap, gait belt.

Profex Medical Products 800-325-0196
2224 E Person Ave, Memphis, TN 38114
OR table restraint.

Segufix Systems Ltd. 506-328-8636
110 Queen St., Woodstock, NB E7M-2M6 Canada

Skil-Care Corp. 800-431-2972
29 Wells Ave, Yonkers, NY 10701

Sure-Lok, Inc. 866-787-3565
2501 Baglyos Cir, Bethlehem, PA 18020

Tartan Orthopedics, Ltd. 888-287-1456
10651 Irma Dr Unit C, Northglenn, CO 80233
$140.00 per 10 (58in).

Thompson Medical Specialties 800-777-4949
3404 Library Ln, Saint Louis Park, MN 55426
Positioning protective body.

Truform Orthotics & Prosthetics 800-888-0458
3960 Rosslyn Dr, Cincinnati, OH 45209

Vivax Medical Corp. 866-847-7890
89 Putter Ln, Torrington, CT 06790
The Soma Safe Enclosure (collapsible frame with a netted canopy which fits over most standard hospital beds) and the Soma Safe Enclosure Bed, which is an enclosed bed system secured with a netted canopy, provide a safe, patient friendly, easy to use, clinically proven and cost-effective alternative to caring for a patient that is subject to falling, wandering, confusion, delirium, aggression or seizures.

Zimmer Holdings, Inc. 800-613-6131
1800 W Center St, PO Box 708, Warsaw, IN 46580

RESTRAINT, VEST *(General) 80RPE*

Bdm Medical, Inc. 800-238-4655
518 Main St., Ashton, ID 83420-0515
Spider Strap for patients.

Formedica Ltd. 800-361-9671
1481 Rue Begin, St Laurent, QUE H4R 1V8 Canada
$160.00 per 10 (med).

J. T. Posey Co. 800-447-6739
5635 Peck Rd, Arcadia, CA 91006

Profex Medical Products 800-325-0196
2224 E Person Ave, Memphis, TN 38114

Schueler & Company, Inc. 516-487-1500
PO Box 528, Stratford, CT 06615

Zimmer Holdings, Inc. 800-613-6131
1800 W Center St, PO Box 708, Warsaw, IN 46580

RESTRAINT, WHEELCHAIR *(General) 80RPF*

Advanced Mobility Systems Corp. 800-661-6716
621 Justus Dr., Kingston, ONT K7M-4H5 Canada
A manual tilt-in-space wheelchair with manual recline. This wheelchair has a great range in seating and floor-to-seat height adjustment. The chair is built to order, meeting the client's specific seating and mobility requirements.

Alimed, Inc. 800-225-2610
297 High St, Dedham, MA 02026

Cfi Medical Solutions (Contour Fabricators, Inc.) 810-750-5300
14241 N Fenton Rd, Fenton, MI 48430

Complete Mobility Systems Inc. 800-788-7479
1915 County Road C W, Roseville, MN 55113
For drivers and passengers in wheelchairs.

Formedica Ltd. 800-361-9671
1481 Rue Begin, St Laurent, QUE H4R 1V8 Canada
$120.00 per 10 (med).

Geen Healthcare Inc. 800-565-4336
931 Progress Ave. Ste.13, Scarborough, ONT M1G 3V5 Canada

Handi-Ramp 800-876-7267
510 North Ave, Libertyville, IL 60048
Wall and floor clamps.

J. T. Posey Co. 800-447-6739
5635 Peck Rd, Arcadia, CA 91006

RESTRAINT, WHEELCHAIR *(cont'd)*

Profex Medical Products 800-325-0196
2224 E Person Ave, Memphis, TN 38114

Segufix Systems Ltd. 506-328-8636
110 Queen St., Woodstock, NB E7M-2M6 Canada

Total Care 800-334-3802
PO Box 1661, Rockville, MD 20849

Zimmer Holdings, Inc. 800-613-6131
1800 W Center St, PO Box 708, Warsaw, IN 46580

RESTRAINT, WRIST/HAND *(General) 80RPG*

Boehringer Laboratories, Inc. 800-642-4945
500 E Washington St, Norristown, PA 19401
Velcro/rubberized nylon restraint.

Dixie Ems Supply 800-347-3494
385 Union Ave, Brooklyn, NY 11211
$70.00 per 10 (11in).

Formedica Ltd. 800-361-9671
1481 Rue Begin, St Laurent, QUE H4R 1V8 Canada
$120.00 per 10 (11in).

Geen Healthcare Inc. 800-565-4336
931 Progress Ave. Ste.13, Scarborough, ONT M1G 3V5 Canada

Humane Restraint Co Inc 800-356-7472
912 Bethel Cir, Waunakee, WI 53597
Various types of wrist/hand and other restraints.

J. T. Posey Co. 800-447-6739
5635 Peck Rd, Arcadia, CA 91006

Morrison Medical 800-438-6677
3735 Paragon Dr, Columbus, OH 43228
Disposable or reusable restraints, all sizes.

North Coast Medical, Inc. 800-821-9319
18305 Sutter Blvd, Morgan Hill, CA 95037
Progress Functional Resting Splint.

Profex Medical Products 800-325-0196
2224 E Person Ave, Memphis, TN 38114

Segufix Systems Ltd. 506-328-8636
110 Queen St., Woodstock, NB E7M-2M6 Canada

Tartan Orthopedics, Ltd. 888-287-1456
10651 Irma Dr Unit C, Northglenn, CO 80233
$50.00 per 10 (11in); also available carpal tunnel, motion limiting device $79.50 / 10.

Zimmer Holdings, Inc. 800-613-6131
1800 W Center St, PO Box 708, Warsaw, IN 46580

RESUSCITATOR, CARDIAC, MECHANICAL, COMPRESSOR
(Anesthesiology) 73BTZ

Ams Innovative Center-San Jose 800-356-7600
3070 Orchard Dr, San Jose, CA 95134

Banyan International Corp. 800-351-4530
PO Box 1779, 2118 E. Interstate 20, Abilene, TX 79604
Stat Kit 900 - $965.00

Brunswick Laboratories 800-362-3482
50 Commerce Way, Norton, MA 02766
HLR emergency medical equipment.

Life Corporation 800-700-0202
1776 N Water St, Milwaukee, WI 53202
LIFE, OxygenPac Portable emergency oxygen units, clear cover and wall-mounted, off/on lever control, resuscitation mask with one-way valve for hygiene, 6lpm 90min. supply, refillable. Also available 6 & 12 lpm NORM & HIGH, 0-25 lpm variable, and demand-valve for 100% oxygen resuscitation. GSA Federal Supply Schedule.

RESUSCITATOR, CARDIOPULMONARY *(Cardiovascular) 74RPH*

Allied Healthcare Products, Inc. 800-444-3954
1720 Sublette Ave, Saint Louis, MO 63110

Cw Medical, Inc. 909-591-5220
5595 Daniels St Ste E, Chino, CA 91710
Resuscitator: a product used to restore respiration. Two great benefits of this device are the strap/holder and 1 piece mask. The strap/holder gives a tight grip, therefore the resuscitator doesn't fall out of ones hand during the process. The 1 piece mask is a feature to easily apply to the patient. The no cushion mask will give a direct effect to the patient for better respiration.

Dixie Ems Supply 800-347-3494
385 Union Ave, Brooklyn, NY 11211
$3,694.00 per unit (standard).

RESUSCITATOR, CARDIOPULMONARY *(cont'd)*

Michigan Instruments, Inc. 800-530-9939
4717 Talon Ct SE, Grand Rapids, MI 49512
THUMPER Mechanical CPR System performs cardiopulmonary resuscitation according to AHA guidelines.

Tagg Industries L.L.C. 800-548-3514
23210 Del Lago Dr, Laguna Hills, CA 92653
PTP and PTP II Mouth to mask resuscitation units.

U O Equipment Co. 800-231-6372
5863 W 34th St, Houston, TX 77092

RESUSCITATOR, EMERGENCY OXYGEN *(Dental And Oral) 76DZX*

Allied Healthcare Products, Inc. 800-444-3954
1720 Sublette Ave, Saint Louis, MO 63110

Ambu, Inc. 800-262-8462
6740 Baymeadow Dr, Glen Burnie, MD 21060

Banyan International Corp. 800-351-4530
PO Box 1779, 2118 E. Interstate 20, Abilene, TX 79604
$216.50 for Model 3000 emergency oxygen unit.

Dixie Ems Supply 800-347-3494
385 Union Ave, Brooklyn, NY 11211
$60.70 per unit (standard).

Emepe International, Inc. 813-994-9690
18108 Sugar Brooke Dr, Tampa, FL 33647
Manual resuscitators for CPR (adult, child, infant) and accessories (valves, gages, PEEP valves, etc.).

Erie Medical 800-932-2293
10225 82nd Ave, Lakeview Corporate Park, Pleasant Prairie, WI 53158
Disposable single-patient-use resuscitator with mask and oxygen inlet port.

Life Corporation 800-700-0202
1776 N Water St, Milwaukee, WI 53202
LIFE, OxygenPac Portable emergency oxygen units, clear cover and wall-mounted, off/on lever control, resuscitation mask with one-way valve for hygiene, 6lpm 90min. supply, refillable. Also available 6 & 12 lpm NORM & HIGH, 0-25 lpm variable, and demand-valve for 100% oxygen resuscitation. GSA Federal Supply Schedule.

Mada, Inc. 800-526-6370
625 Washington Ave, Carlstadt, NJ 07072

Matrx By Midmark 800-847-1000
145 Mid County Dr, Orchard Park, NY 14127

Southland Cryogenics, Inc. 800-872-2796
8350 Mosley Rd, Houston, TX 77075
Emergency Oxygen Kit, contains oxygen bottle, hand cart, regulator and canula mask.

U O Equipment Co. 800-231-6372
5863 W 34th St, Houston, TX 77092
Model 10700FC demand valve resuscitator with adjustable flow inhalator, portable. List price $675.00. Also available with aspirator.

RESUSCITATOR, EMERGENCY, PROTECTIVE, INFECTION
(Anesthesiology) 73WJE

Allied Healthcare Products, Inc. 800-444-3954
1720 Sublette Ave, Saint Louis, MO 63110

Ambu, Inc. 800-262-8462
6740 Baymeadow Dr, Glen Burnie, MD 21060
Single-patient-use resuscitators in adult and infant/child models.

Armstrong Medical Industries, Inc. 800-323-4220
575 Knightsbridge Pkwy, Lincolnshire, IL 60069

Life Corporation 800-700-0202
1776 N Water St, Milwaukee, WI 53202
LIFE, CPR Masks, LIFE CPR Shields, and Portable emergency oxygen units, clear cover and wall-mounted, off/on lever control, resuscitation mask with one-way valve for hygiene, 6lpm 90min. supply, refillable. Also available 6 & 12 lpm NORM & HIGH, 0-25 lpm variable, and demand-valve for 100% oxygen resuscitation. GSA Federal Supply Schedule.

Medical Safety Systems Inc. 888-803-9303
230 White Pond Dr, Akron, OH 44313

Mtm Health Products Ltd. 800-263-8253
2349 Fairview St., Burlington, ONT L7R 2E3 Canada
MTM MOUTH TO MASK one-way valve emergency resuscitator with adult and pediatric facemasks, with standard oxygen ports and head strap.

RESUSCITATOR, EMERGENCY, PROTECTIVE, INFECTION
(cont'd)

O-Two Systems International Inc. 800-387-3405
7575 Kimbel St., Mississauga, ONT L5S 1C8 Canada
Bio-Barrier bacterial/viral CPR Facesheild for mouth-to-mouth ressucitation; K960995. Revive Aid CPR Barrier with one-way valve and filter; K940927.

Quadromed Inc. 800-363-0192
5776 Thimens Ave., St-Laurent, QUE H4R 2K9 Canada

U O Equipment Co. 800-231-6372
5863 W 34th St, Houston, TX 77092

RESUSCITATOR, MANUAL, NON SELF-INFLATING
(Anesthesiology) 73NHK

Ventlab Corp. 336-753-5000
155 Boyce Dr, Mocksville, NC 27028
Hyperinflation system.

RESUSCITATOR, PULMONARY, GAS *(General) 80RPI*

Allied Healthcare Products, Inc. 800-444-3954
1720 Sublette Ave, Saint Louis, MO 63110

Erie Medical 800-932-2293
10225 82nd Ave, Lakeview Corporate Park, Pleasant Prairie, WI 53158
Same as 76DZX.

Life Corporation 800-700-0202
1776 N Water St, Milwaukee, WI 53202
LIFE, OxygenPac Portable emergency oxygen units, clear cover and wall-mounted, off/on lever control, resuscitation mask with one-way valve for hygiene, 6lpm 90min. supply, refillable. Also available 6 & 12 lpm NORM & HIGH, 0-25 lpm variable, and demand-valve for 100% oxygen resuscitation. GSA Federal Supply Schedule.

Mada, Inc. 800-526-6370
625 Washington Ave, Carlstadt, NJ 07072

Mercury Medical 800-237-6418
11300 49th St N, Clearwater, FL 33762

O-Two Systems International Inc. 800-387-3405
7575 Kimbel St., Mississauga, ONT L5S 1C8 Canada
CAREVENT range of pneumatically powered, automatic transport ventilators, and resuscitators. For emergency, toxic, environment rescue, and transport use; K991195.

Rockford Medical & Safety Co. 800-435-9451
2420 Harrison Ave, PO Box 5646, Rockford, IL 61108

U O Equipment Co. 800-231-6372
5863 W 34th St, Houston, TX 77092
Oxygen-powered resuscitators.

RESUSCITATOR, PULMONARY, MANUAL (DEMAND VALVE)
(General) 80FQB

Allied Healthcare Products, Inc. 800-444-3954
1720 Sublette Ave, Saint Louis, MO 63110

Ambu, Inc. 800-262-8462
6740 Baymeadow Dr, Glen Burnie, MD 21060
SPUR, AMBU Silicone $125 to $145, 300mL/min, pediatric, transparent with mask, 6oz; 13oz for adult model (MARK III), 1,300mL/min.

Anesthesia Associates, Inc. 760-744-6561
460 Enterprise St, San Marcos, CA 92078
Various styles and sizes available.

Armstrong Medical Industries, Inc. 800-323-4220
575 Knightsbridge Pkwy, Lincolnshire, IL 60069

Gammadirect Medical Division 847-267-5929
PO Box 383, Lake Forest, IL 60045
AukuVent CPR Kit for the clinical professional who does not do resuscitation on a regular basis. Economical and easy to use.

Life Corporation 800-700-0202
1776 N Water St, Milwaukee, WI 53202
LIFE, OxygenPac Portable emergency oxygen units, clear cover and wall-mounted, off/on lever control, resuscitation mask with one-way valve for hygiene, 6lpm 90min. supply, refillable. Also available 6 & 12 lpm NORM & HIGH, 0-25 lpm variable, and demand-valve for 100% oxygen resuscitation. GSA Federal Supply Schedule.

Mada, Inc. 800-526-6370
625 Washington Ave, Carlstadt, NJ 07072

Matrx By Midmark 800-847-1000
145 Mid County Dr, Orchard Park, NY 14127

Mercury Medical 800-237-6418
11300 49th St N, Clearwater, FL 33762
CPR BAG disposable resuscitators.

RESUSCITATOR, PULMONARY, MANUAL (DEMAND VALVE)
(cont'd)

O-Two Systems International Inc. 800-387-3405
7575 Kimbel St., Mississauga, ONT L5S 1C8 Canada
SMART BAG manual resuscitation bag/ valve mask device designed to reduce gatric insufflation and provide consistent ventilation. Flynn III resusitation bag, k832495.

Porter Instrument Division Parker Hannifin Corp 800-457-2001
245 Township Line Rd, Hatfield, PA 19440
$600 per unit for emergency oxygen positive pressure/demand flow resuscitation equipment.

U O Equipment Co. 800-231-6372
5863 W 34th St, Houston, TX 77092

Ventlab Corporation 800-593-4654
155 Boyce Dr, Mocksville, NC 27028

Vitalograph, Inc. 800-255-6626
13310 W 99th St, Lenexa, KS 66215

RETAINER, BANDAGE (ELASTIC NET) *(General) 80RPJ*

Albahealth Llc 800-262-2404
425 N Gateway Ave, Rockwood, TN 37854
XX-SPAN.

Delstar Technologies, Inc. 800-521-6713
601 Industrial Rd, Middletown, DE 19709
Naltex: Extruded netting for filter spacers and supports.

Hyginet Corp. Of America 800-245-1036
505 North Dr, I 79 North Industrial Park, Sewickley, PA 15143

Medi-Tech International Corp. 800-333-0109
26 Court St, Brooklyn, NY 11242
Open netted tubular elastic dressing retainer.

Western Medical, Ltd. 800-628-8276
214 Carnegie Ctr Ste 100, Princeton, NJ 08540
SURGILAST tubular elastic net, BANDNET tubular elastic net, SURGILAST latex-free tubular elastic net.

RETAINER, DENTAL *(Dental And Oral) 76RPK*

Hermanson Dental 800-328-9648
1055 Highway 36 E, Saint Paul, MN 55109

Miltex Inc. 800-645-8000
589 Davies Dr, York, PA 17402

Specialty Appliance Works, Inc. 800-522-4636
4905 Hammond Industrial Dr, Cumming, GA 30041
Hawley retainers.

RETAINER, MATRIX *(Dental And Oral) 76JEP*

C.E.J. Dental Products Inc. 949-493-2449
32332 Camino Capistrano Ste 101, San Juan Capistrano, CA 92675
Matrix retainer, multiple sizes and shapes.

Dencraft 800-328-9729
PO Box 57, Moorestown, NJ 08057

Dental Usa, Inc. 815-363-8003
5005 McCullom Lake Rd, McHenry, IL 60050
Retainer.

Dockum Research Lab 626-794-1821
844 E Mariposa St, Altadena, CA 91001
Wizard wedges.

E.A. Beck & Co. 949-645-4072
657 W 19th St Ste E, P O Box 10857, Costa Mesa, CA 92627
Retainer.

Garrison Dental Solutions 616-842-2244
110 Dewitt Ln, Spring Lake, MI 49456
Sectional matrix retainer system kit.

Guy Griffiths Orthodontic Lab (1984) Inc. 514-482-1267
4927 Rue Sherbrooke O, Westmount H3Z 1H2 Canada
Retainer

Hager Worldwide, Inc. 800-328-2335
13322 Byrd Dr, Odessa, FL 33556
TOFFLEMEIR.

Miltex Dental Technologies, Inc. 516-576-6022
589 Davies Dr, York, PA 17402
Tofflemire matrix retainers.

Moyco Technologies, Inc. 800-331-8837
200 Commerce Dr, Montgomeryville, PA 18936

Premier Dental Products Co. 888-670-6100
1710 Romano Dr, PO Box 4500, Plymouth Meeting, PA 19462

Pulpdent Corp. 800-343-4342
80 Oakland St, Watertown, MA 02472
Strip holder.

RETAINER, MATRIX *(cont'd)*

Ultradent Products, Inc. 801-553-4586
505 W 10200 S, South Jordan, UT 84095
Matrix retainer and band.

Water Pik, Inc. 970-221-6129
1730 E Prospect Rd, Fort Collins, CO 80525
Matrix retainers.

Wykle Research, Inc. 775-887-7500
2222 College Pkwy, Carson City, NV 89706
Wooden or interproximal wedge.

RETAINER, SCREW EXPANSION, ORTHODONTIC
(Dental And Oral) 76DYJ

Allesee Orthodontic Appliances 714-516-7484
13931 Spring St, Sturtevant, WI 53177
Orthodontic retainers / appliances.

Allesee Orthodontic Appliances (Calexico) 714-516-7400
341 E 1st St, Calexico, CA 92231
Orthodontic retainers-appliances.

Allesee Orthodontic Appliances, Inc. - Connecticut 949-255-8766
6 Niblick Rd, Enfield, CT 06082
Orthodontic retainers / appliances.

Aurum Ceramic Dental Laboratories Llp 403-228-5199
1320 N Howard St, Spokane, WA 99201
Orthodontic appliance.

Beloit Precision Incorporated 608-362-9085
1525 Office Park Ln, Beloit, WI 53511
Orthodontics.

Classone Orthodontics, Inc. 806-799-0608
5064 50th St, Lubbock, TX 79414
Various types of expansion screws.

Forestadent Usa 314-878-5985
2315 Weldon Pkwy, Saint Louis, MO 63146
Orthodontic expansion screw retainer.

G & H Wire Co. 800-526-1026
2165 Earlywood Dr, Franklin, IN 46131

K.O.L. Island Retainer, Llc. 808-871-8577
360 Papa Pl Ste 203, Kahului, HI 96732
Retainer.

Lancer Orthodontics, Inc. 760-304-2705
253 Pawnee St, San Marcos, CA 92078
Rapid palatal expander.

Nose Breathe 808-949-8876
2065 S King St Ste 304, Honolulu, HI 96826
Retainer.

Ortho Organizers, Inc. 760-448-8730
1822 Aston Ave, Carlsbad, CA 92008
Palatal expander.

Rideau Orthodontic Mfg., Ltd. 613-283-6841
69 Beckwith St N, Smiths Falls K7A 2B6 Canada
Multiple

Space Maintainers Lab 818-998-7460
9129 Lurline Ave, Chatsworth, CA 91311

Superscrew-Superspring Co. 800-494-7594
135 Stables Ct, Highwood, IL 60040
Palatal expander.

Tp Orthodontics, Inc. 800-348-8856
100 Center Plz, La Porte, IN 46350

3m Unitek 800-634-5300
2724 Peck Rd, Monrovia, CA 91016

RETAINER, SURGICAL *(Surgery) 79GCZ*

Abbott Spine, Inc. 847-937-6100
12708 Riata Vista Cir Ste B-100, Austin, TX 78727
Distractor.

Depuy Spine, Inc. 800-227-6633
325 Paramount Dr, Raynham, MA 02767
Spreader, distractor.

Frontier Devices 205-733-0901
153A Cahaba Valley Pkwy, Indian Spgs, AL 35124

Greer Medical, Inc. 805-962-5883
314 E Carrillo St Ste 1, Santa Barbara, CA 93101

K. W. Griffen Co. 203-846-1923
100 Pearl St, Norwalk, CT 06850
Cathetener retainer clip.

RETAINER, SURGICAL *(cont'd)*

Mectra Labs, Inc. 800-323-3968
PO Box 350, Two Quality Way, Bloomfield, IN 47424
Tissue sampler retainer. Specimen trap permits easy collection/retention of tissue specimens. Attaches to suction line of mectra devices.

RETAINER, VISCERAL *(Surgery) 79RPL*

Adept-Med International, Inc. 800-222-8445
665 Pleasant Valley Rd, Diamond Springs, CA 95619
The FISH. Available in 7 sizes, pediatric to ex-large. Retains the omentum and viscera during closure of abdominal cavity.

RETENTION DEVICE, SUTURE *(Surgery) 79KGS*

Angiodynamics, Inc. 518-795-1400
14 Plaza Drive, Latham, NY 12110
PERCHIK BUTTON

Arthrex, Inc. 239-643-5553
1370 Creekside Blvd, Naples, FL 34108
Suture.

Biomet, Inc. 574-267-6639
56 E Bell Dr, PO Box 587, Warsaw, IN 46582
Various types of suture buttons.

Boston Scientific Corporation 508-652-5578
780 Brookside Dr, Spencer, IN 47460

Covidien Lp 508-261-8000
15 Hampshire St, Mansfield, MA 02048
DERMALON CE-24 needles.

Ethicon Endo-Surgery, Inc. 877-384-4266
3801 University Blvd SE, Albuquerque, NM 87106
Sterile absorbable suture clips.

Ethicon, Llc. 908-218-2887
Rd. 183, Km. 8.3,, Industrial Area Hato, San Lorenzo, PR 00754
Sterile retention suture bridge.

RETINOL-BINDING PROTEIN, ANTIGEN, ANTISERUM, CONTROL *(Immunology) 82CZS*

Dako North America, Inc 805-566-6655
6392 Via Real, Carpinteria, CA 93013

RETINOSCOPE, AC-POWERED *(Ophthalmology) 86HKL*

Keeler Instruments Inc. 800-523-5620
456 Park Way, Broomall, PA 19008
$395 for professional combi retinoscope.

Md International, Inc. 305-669-9003
11300 NW 41st St, Doral, FL 33178

Welch Allyn, Inc. 800-535-6663
4341 State Street Rd, Skaneateles Falls, NY 13153

RETINOSCOPE, BATTERY-POWERED *(Ophthalmology) 86HKM*

Md International, Inc. 305-669-9003
11300 NW 41st St, Doral, FL 33178

Stereo Optical Co., Inc. 800-344-9500
3539 N Kenton Ave, Chicago, IL 60641

Vision Research Corp. 205-942-8011
211 Summit Pkwy Ste 105, Birmingham, AL 35209
Same.

Welch Allyn, Inc. 800-535-6663
4341 State Street Rd, Skaneateles Falls, NY 13153

RETRACTOR *(Orthopedics) 87HXM*

Boss Instruments, Ltd. 800-210-2677
395 Reas Ford Rd Ste 120, Earlysville, VA 22936
Ophthalmic, vascular/cardiovascular, ENT, plastic surgery; neurosurgical, spine (cervical and lumbar), orthopedic, micro surgery, general surgery.

Carl Heyer, Inc. 800-284-5550
1872 Bellmore Ave, North Bellmore, NY 11710

Cloward Instrument Corporation 808-734-3511
3787 Diamond Head Rd, Honolulu, HI 96816
CLOWARD Double hinge retractor.

Elmed, Inc. 630-543-2792
60 W Fay Ave, Addison, IL 60101

Fine Surgical Instrument, Inc. 800-851-5155
741 Peninsula Blvd, Hempstead, NY 11550

Genesee Biomedical, Inc. 800-786-4890
1308 S Jason St, Denver, CO 80223
HEART-LIFT Cardiac Retraction Sling. Provides easy access to the circumflex branch of the coronary artery.

RETRACTOR *(cont'd)*

George Tiemann & Co. 800-843-6266
25 Plant Ave, Hauppauge, NY 11788

International Hospital Supply Co. 800-398-9450
6914 Canby Ave Ste 105, Reseda, CA 91335

Kapp Surgical Instrument, Inc. 800-282-5277
4919 Warrensville Center Rd, Cleveland, OH 44128

Karl Storz Endoscopy-America Inc. 800-421-0837
600 Corporate Pointe, Culver City, CA 90230

Kmedic 800-955-0559
190 Veterans Dr, Northvale, NJ 07647

Mediflex Surgical Products 800-879-7575
250 Gibbs Rd, Islandia, NY 11749

Microsurgical Laboratories 713-723-6900
11333 Chimney Rock Rd Ste 120, Houston, TX 77035

Nemcomed 800-255-4576
801 Industrial Dr, Hicksville, OH 43526
MIS-TKA Technique Specific Retractor Set.

Omni-Tract Surgical, A Div. Of Minnesota Scientific, Inc. 800-367-8657
4849 White Bear Pkwy, Saint Paul, MN 55110
OmniAccess table-mounted retractor for total hip arthroplasty and revisions improves exposure and eliminates assistants.

Signal Medical Corporation 800-246-6324
1000 Des Peres Rd Ste 140, Saint Louis, MO 63131
Bent, anterior acetabular, posterior acetabular (left)with or without light cord brackets, and posterior acetabular (right) retractors with or without light cord brackets.

Stryker Corp. 800-726-2725
2825 Airview Blvd, Portage, MI 49002

Stryker Spine 866-457-7463
2 Pearl Ct, Allendale, NJ 07401

Tuzik Boston 800-886-6363
104 Longwater Dr, Assinippi Park, Norwell, MA 02061

Zimmer Holdings, Inc. 800-613-6131
1800 W Center St, PO Box 708, Warsaw, IN 46580

RETRACTOR, ABDOMINAL *(Surgery) 79RPM*

Codman & Shurtleff, Inc 800-225-0460
325 Paramount Dr, Raynham, MA 02767

Elmed, Inc. 630-543-2792
60 W Fay Ave, Addison, IL 60101

Mediflex Surgical Products 800-879-7575
250 Gibbs Rd, Islandia, NY 11749
Abdominal, variable-angle retractor ring; also, retractor ring; abdominal retractor type with holder/positioner. New Bookler Table Mounted Retractor Systems for many disciplines.

Miltex Inc. 800-645-8000
589 Davies Dr, York, PA 17402

Precision Medical Manufacturing Corporation 866-633-4626
852 Seton Ct, Wheeling, IL 60090
O'Sullivan -O'Connor Abdominal Retractor very strong constraction,locks automaticaly and unlocks easily. It opens to full ins. diameter of approx. 8-1/4 larger than any other O'Sullivan - O'Connor retractor on the market. Lateral swivel blades are permanently attached.

Richard Wolf Medical Instruments Corp. 800-323-9653
353 Corporate Woods Pkwy, Vernon Hills, IL 60061

Scanlan International, Inc. 800-328-9458
1 Scanlan Plz, Saint Paul, MN 55107

Thompson Surgical Instruments, Inc. 800-227-7543
10170 E Cherry Bend Rd, Traverse City, MI 49684
Table mounted system used for all procedures.

Zimmer Holdings, Inc. 800-613-6131
1800 W Center St, PO Box 708, Warsaw, IN 46580

RETRACTOR, ALL TYPES *(Dental And Oral) 76EIG*

American Eagle Instruments, Inc. 406-549-7451
6575 Butler Creek Rd, Missoula, MT 59808
Various types of retractors.

Arista Surgical Supply Co. Inc. 800-223-1984
297 High St, Dedham, MA 02026

Biomet Microfixation Inc. 800-874-7711
1520 Tradeport Dr, Jacksonville, FL 32218
Various types of retractors.

RETRACTOR, ALL TYPES *(cont'd)*

Classone Orthodontics, Inc. 806-799-0608
5064 50th St, Lubbock, TX 79414
Various types of retractors.

Dental Usa, Inc. 815-363-8003
5005 McCullom Lake Rd, McHenry, IL 60050
Dental retractors.

Dentsply Canada, Ltd. 800-263-1437
161 Vinyl Ct., Woodbridge, ONT L4L 4A3 Canada

G & H Wire Co. 800-526-1026
2165 Earlywood Dr, Franklin, IN 46131
Cheek Retractors

George Tiemann & Co. 800-843-6266
25 Plant Ave, Hauppauge, NY 11788

Glenroe Technologies 800-237-4060
1912 44th Ave E, Bradenton, FL 34203
Orthodontic photo retractors.

H & H Co. 909-390-0373
4435 E Airport Dr Ste 108, Ontario, CA 91761
Retractors all types.

Hager Worldwide, Inc. 800-328-2335
13322 Byrd Dr, Odessa, FL 33556
SPANDEX/MIRAHOLD (autoclavable) & LIP-EX (cold sterilizable).

Hu-Friedy Manufacturing Co., Inc. 800-483-7433
3232 N Rockwell St, Chicago, IL 60618
$90.00 to $122.00 for surgical units; others are $25.00 to $65.00; 66 types.

International Hospital Supply Co. 800-398-9450
6914 Canby Ave Ste 105, Reseda, CA 91335

J. Morita Usa, Inc. 888-566-7482
9 Mason, Irvine, CA 92618
FREE ACCESS II cheek and lip retractor offers convenient hands-free retraction and improved clinical performance. Its new transparent material makes it ideal for a variety of clinical situations and photography. Unique intraoral extensions retract powerful buccinator muscles, increasing visibility and access to the intraoral work area. Tensity can be adjusted for maximum patient comfort. It is safe for autoclave or dry heat sterilization, and is available in small and large sizes.

Kmedic 800-955-0559
190 Veterans Dr, Northvale, NJ 07647

Lenox-Maclaren Surgical Corp. 720-890-9660
657 S Taylor Ave Ste A, Colorado Technology Center Louisville, CO 80027
Retractor, all types.

Medcon Llc 410-744-8367
1002 Frederick Rd, Catonsville, MD 21228
Various hip retractors.

Miltex Inc. 800-645-8000
589 Davies Dr, York, PA 17402

Premier Dental Products Co. 888-670-6100
1710 Romano Dr, PO Box 4500, Plymouth Meeting, PA 19462

Salvin Dental Specialties, Inc. 800-535-6566
3450 Latrobe Dr, Charlotte, NC 28211
Various types of oral retractors.

Stryker Corp. 800-726-2725
2825 Airview Blvd, Portage, MI 49002

Symmetry Medical Usa, Inc. 574-267-8700
486 W 350 N, Warsaw, IN 46582
Dental hand instrument.

Trans American Medical / Tamsco Instruments 708-430-7777
7633 W 100th Pl, Bridgeview, IL 60455
Medium grade surgical stainless steel.

Tuzik Boston 800-886-6363
104 Longwater Dr, Assinippi Park, Norwell, MA 02061

Ultradent Products, Inc. 801-553-4586
505 W 10200 S, South Jordan, UT 84095
Bite block.

3m Unitek 800-634-5300
2724 Peck Rd, Monrovia, CA 91016

RETRACTOR, BLADDER *(Gastro/Urology) 78RPN*

Codman & Shurtleff, Inc 800-225-0460
325 Paramount Dr, Raynham, MA 02767

Elmed, Inc. 630-543-2792
60 W Fay Ave, Addison, IL 60101

RETRACTOR, BLADDER *(cont'd)*

Miltex Inc. 800-645-8000
589 Davies Dr, York, PA 17402

Richard Wolf Medical Instruments Corp. 800-323-9653
353 Corporate Woods Pkwy, Vernon Hills, IL 60061

Thompson Surgical Instruments, Inc. 800-227-7543
10170 E Cherry Bend Rd, Traverse City, MI 49684

RETRACTOR, BRAIN *(Cns/Neurology) 84RPO*

Codman & Shurtleff, Inc 800-225-0460
325 Paramount Dr, Raynham, MA 02767

Elmed, Inc. 630-543-2792
60 W Fay Ave, Addison, IL 60101

Fehling Surgical Instruments 800-FEHLING
509 Broadstone Ln NW, Acworth, GA 30101

Schaerer Mayfield Usa 800-755-6381
4900 Charlemar Dr, Cincinnati, OH 45227
BUDDE Halo Brain Retractor System featuring 360-degree Continutrac ring.

Zimmer Holdings, Inc. 800-613-6131
1800 W Center St, PO Box 708, Warsaw, IN 46580

RETRACTOR, BRAIN DECOMPRESSION *(Cns/Neurology) 84RPP*

Codman & Shurtleff, Inc 800-225-0460
325 Paramount Dr, Raynham, MA 02767

Zimmer Holdings, Inc. 800-613-6131
1800 W Center St, PO Box 708, Warsaw, IN 46580

RETRACTOR, CARDIAC *(Cardiovascular) 74RPQ*

Elmed, Inc. 630-543-2792
60 W Fay Ave, Addison, IL 60101

Genesee Biomedical, Inc. 800-786-4890
1308 S Jason St, Denver, CO 80223
GENESEE Sternal Retractors. Neonatal, pediatric, child and adult.

Kapp Surgical Instrument, Inc. 800-282-5277
4919 Warrensville Center Rd, Cleveland, OH 44128
COSGROVE mitral-valve retractors.

Scanlan International, Inc. 800-328-9458
1 Scanlan Plz, Saint Paul, MN 55107
CARDIOVASIVE retractor system for minimally invasive cardiothoracic surgery.

RETRACTOR, ENT (THORACIC) *(Ear/Nose/Throat) 77KAL*

Aesculap Implant Systems Inc. 1-800-234-9179
3773 Corporate Pkwy, Center Valley, PA 18034

Boss Instruments, Ltd. 800-210-2677
395 Reas Ford Rd Ste 120, Earlysville, VA 22936

Codman & Shurtleff, Inc 800-225-0460
325 Paramount Dr, Raynham, MA 02767

Elmed, Inc. 630-543-2792
60 W Fay Ave, Addison, IL 60101

Micro Medical Instruments 314-845-3663
123 Cliff Cave Rd, Saint Louis, MO 63129
Ophthalmic retractors.

Miltex Inc. 800-645-8000
589 Davies Dr, York, PA 17402

Princeton Medical Group, Inc. 800-875-0869
1189 Royal Links Dr, Mt Pleasant, SC 29466

RETRACTOR, FAN-TYPE, LAPAROSCOPY *(Surgery) 79RXS*

Automated Medical Products Corp. 800-832-4567
PO Box 2508, Edison, NJ 08818
ECCENTRIC Y; NATHANSON HOOK LIVER RETRACTOR; DBALY HOOKS; O'BRIEN INTRODUCER; O'BRIEN PLACER; O'BRIEN CLOSER; PEDIATRIC HOOK LIVER RETRACTORS.

Elmed, Inc. 630-543-2792
60 W Fay Ave, Addison, IL 60101

Md International, Inc. 305-669-9003
11300 NW 41st St, Doral, FL 33178

RETRACTOR, FIBEROPTIC *(Gastro/Urology) 78FDG*

Automated Medical Products Corp. 800-832-4567
PO Box 2508, Edison, NJ 08818

Bausch & Lomb Surgical 636-255-5051
3365 Tree Court Ind Blvd, Saint Louis, MO 63122

Biomet Microfixation Inc. 800-874-7711
1520 Tradeport Dr, Jacksonville, FL 32218
Various types of retractors.

RETRACTOR, FIBEROPTIC *(cont'd)*

Cardinal Health, Snowden Pencer Products 847-689-8410
5175 S Royal Atlanta Dr, Tucker, GA 30084
Various types of lighted retractors.

Codman & Shurtleff, Inc 800-225-0460
325 Paramount Dr, Raynham, MA 02767

Electro Surgical Instrument Co., Inc. 888-464-2784
37 Centennial St, Rochester, NY 14611
Various types and sizes of fiberoptic retractors.

Elmed, Inc. 630-543-2792
60 W Fay Ave, Addison, IL 60101

Invuity, Inc. 760-744-4447
334 Via Vera Cruz Ste 255, San Marcos, CA 92078
Illuminating cannula retractor,retractor blade illuminator.

Invuity, Inc. 415-655-2100
39 Stillman St, San Francisco, CA 94107

Kmi Kolster Methods, Inc. 909-737-5476
3185 Palisades Dr, Corona, CA 92880
Fiberoptic retractor.

Lumitex, Inc. 800-969-5483
8443 Dow Cir, Strongsville, OH 44136
LightMat Surgical Illuminator, with light attached to retractor to illuminate surgical site.

Marina Medical Instruments, Inc. 800-697-1119
955 Shotgun Rd, Sunrise, FL 33326
Various.

Sterilmed, Inc. 763-488-3400
11400 73rd Ave N Ste 100, Maple Grove, MN 55369
Fiberoptic retractor.

Stryker Corp. 800-726-2725
2825 Airview Blvd, Portage, MI 49002

Techman Int'L Corp. 508-248-2900
242 Sturbridge Rd, Charlton, MA 01507
Retractor.

RETRACTOR, LAMINECTOMY *(Surgery) 79RPS*

Codman & Shurtleff, Inc 800-225-0460
325 Paramount Dr, Raynham, MA 02767

Elmed, Inc. 630-543-2792
60 W Fay Ave, Addison, IL 60101

Fehling Surgical Instruments 800-FEHLING
509 Broadstone Ln NW, Acworth, GA 30101

International Hospital Supply Co. 800-398-9450
6914 Canby Ave Ste 105, Reseda, CA 91335

Miltex Inc. 800-645-8000
589 Davies Dr, York, PA 17402

Zimmer Holdings, Inc. 800-613-6131
1800 W Center St, PO Box 708, Warsaw, IN 46580

RETRACTOR, LAPAROSCOPY, OTHER *(Surgery) 79RZZ*

Automated Medical Products Corp. 800-832-4567
PO Box 2508, Edison, NJ 08818
IRON INTERN robotic retractor.

Ranfac Corp. 800-2RANFAC
30 Doherty Ave, Avon Industrial Park, Avon, MA 02322

RETRACTOR, MAMMARY *(Obstetrics/Gyn) 85WWA*

Scanlan International, Inc. 800-328-9458
1 Scanlan Plz, Saint Paul, MN 55107

RETRACTOR, MANUAL *(Cns/Neurology) 84GZW*

Applied Medical Technology, Inc. 800-869-7382
8000 Katherine Blvd, Brecksville, OH 44141

Automated Medical Products Corp. 800-832-4567
PO Box 2508, Edison, NJ 08818

Elmed, Inc. 630-543-2792
60 W Fay Ave, Addison, IL 60101

Fortrad Eye Instruments Corp. 973-543-2371
8 Franklin Rd, Mendham, NJ 07945
Hirschman 4.13 in./105mm, 9mm shaft. Kuglen 4.65 /118mm, 19mm shaft straight or angled 45deg. Sinskey lens hook, straight shank, Harris-Sinskey 4.53 in./115mm, shaft angled 45 degrees, Sinskey II hook angled 90deg. Tennant lens manipulating hook. Schepens Forked Orbital Retractor.

International Hospital Supply Co. 800-398-9450
6914 Canby Ave Ste 105, Reseda, CA 91335

RETRACTOR, MANUAL *(cont'd)*

Kls-Martin L.P. 800-625-1557
11239-1 St. John`s Industrial, Parkway South
Jacksonville, FL 32250
Soft tissue retractors.

Kmedic 800-955-0559
190 Veterans Dr, Northvale, NJ 07647

Precision Medical Manufacturing Corporation 866-633-4626
852 Seton Ct, Wheeling, IL 60090
Gardner wells Skull Traction Tongs an instrument to apply traction to the cervical spine. The thongs can be used on children and adults.

Toolmex Corporation 800-992-4766
1075 Worcester St, Natick, MA 01760

Tuzik Boston 800-886-6363
104 Longwater Dr, Assinippi Park, Norwell, MA 02061

Ussc Puerto Rico, Inc. 203-845-1000
Building 911-67, Sabanetas Industrial Park, Ponce, PR 00731
Manual retractors and accessories.

Zimmer Holdings, Inc. 800-613-6131
1800 W Center St, PO Box 708, Warsaw, IN 46580

RETRACTOR, MASTOID *(Ear/Nose/Throat) 77RPT*

Elmed, Inc. 630-543-2792
60 W Fay Ave, Addison, IL 60101

RETRACTOR, NON-SELF-RETAINING *(Gastro/Urology) 78FGN*

Aesculap Implant Systems Inc. 1-800-234-9179
3773 Corporate Pkwy, Center Valley, PA 18034

Greenwald Surgical Co., Inc. 219-962-1604
2688 Dekalb St, Gary, IN 46405
Retractor.

Tuzik Boston 800-886-6363
104 Longwater Dr, Assinippi Park, Norwell, MA 02061

RETRACTOR, OPHTHALMIC *(Ophthalmology) 86HNI*

B. Graczyk, Inc. 269-782-2100
27826 Burmax Park, Dowagiac, MI 49047
Various types of retractors.

Back-Mueller, Inc. 314-531-6640
2700 Clark Ave, Saint Louis, MO 63103
Various types of retractors.

Bausch & Lomb Surgical 636-255-5051
3365 Tree Court Ind Blvd, Saint Louis, MO 63122

Diamond Edge Co. 727-586-2927
928 W Bay Dr, Largo, FL 33770
Retractor.

Elmed, Inc. 630-543-2792
60 W Fay Ave, Addison, IL 60101

Escalon Trek Medical 800-433-8197
2440 S 179th St, New Berlin, WI 53146
Ophthalmic retractor.

Fci Ophthalmics 800-932-4202
64 Schoosett St, Pembroke, MA 02359
Iris retractors and Mackool capsular support system

Fortrad Eye Instruments Corp. 973-543-2371
8 Franklin Rd, Mendham, NJ 07945

George Tiemann & Co. 800-843-6266
25 Plant Ave, Hauppauge, NY 11788

Gulden Ophthalmics 800-659-2250
225 Cadwalader Ave, Elkins Park, PA 19027

Gyrus Ent L.L.C., Sub. Of Gyrus Acmi, Inc. 508-804-2739
2925 Appling Rd, Bartlett, TN 38133
Various.

International Hospital Supply Co. 800-398-9450
6914 Canby Ave Ste 105, Reseda, CA 91335

Jedmed Instruments Co. 314-845-3770
5416 Jedmed Ct, Saint Louis, MO 63129

Karl Storz Endoscopy-America Inc. 800-421-0837
600 Corporate Pointe, Culver City, CA 90230

Katena Products, Inc. 800-225-1195
4 Stewart Ct, Denville, NJ 07834

Miltex Inc. 800-645-8000
589 Davies Dr, York, PA 17402

Mira, Inc. 508-278-7877
414 Quaker Hwy, Uxbridge, MA 01569
Forked retractor.

RETRACTOR, OPHTHALMIC *(cont'd)*

Psi/Eye-Ko, Inc. 636-447-1010
804 Corporate Centre Dr, O Fallon, MO 63368
Various types and models of ophthalmic retractors.

Rhein Medical, Inc. 800-637-4346
5460 Beaumont Center Blvd Ste 500, Suite 500, Tampa, FL 33634

Rhein Mfg., Inc. 314-997-1775
2269 Grissom Dr, Saint Louis, MO 63146
General surgical instrument.

Stephens Instruments, Inc. 800-354-7848
2500 Sandersville Rd, Lexington, KY 40511
$18.00 each.

Total Titanium, Inc. 618-473-2429
140 East Monroe St., Hecker, IL 62248
Various types of ophthalmic retractors.

RETRACTOR, ORBITAL *(Surgery) 79RPU*

Bausch & Lomb Surgical 636-255-5051
3365 Tree Court Ind Blvd, Saint Louis, MO 63122

Elmed, Inc. 630-543-2792
60 W Fay Ave, Addison, IL 60101

RETRACTOR, OTHER *(Surgery) 79RPY*

Automated Medical Products Corp. 800-832-4567
PO Box 2508, Edison, NJ 08818
IRON INTERN Table-mounted retraction systems.

Elmed, Inc. 630-543-2792
60 W Fay Ave, Addison, IL 60101

Fortrad Eye Instruments Corp. 973-543-2371
8 Franklin Rd, Mendham, NJ 07945

Holmed Corporation 508-238-3351
40 Norfolk Ave, South Easton, MA 02375

Kapp Surgical Instrument, Inc. 800-282-5277
4919 Warrensville Center Rd, Cleveland, OH 44128
Total-knee-implant retractor.

Kmedic 800-955-0559
190 Veterans Dr, Northvale, NJ 07647

Lone Star Medical Products, Inc. 800-331-7427
11211 Cash Rd, Stafford, TX 77477
Cantilevered ring retractor, stainless steel, aluminum or disposable plastic. Uniquely designed to allow precise retraction from any angle along the ring without obstruction. Available in various geometric configurations.

Mediflex Surgical Products 800-879-7575
250 Gibbs Rd, Islandia, NY 11749
Nathanson Liver Retraction System (Endoscopic retractor).

Precision Medical Manufacturing Corporation 866-633-4626
852 Seton Ct, Wheeling, IL 60090
Burford Finochetto Rib retractor . Ahavy duty rib retractor of conventional Finochetto design.Locks automaticly in position. Powerfull laverage is provided and the handle folds flat out of the way when not in use.

Scanlan International, Inc. 800-328-9458
1 Scanlan Plz, Saint Paul, MN 55107
Pediatric retractors.

Thompson Surgical Instruments, Inc. 800-227-7543
10170 E Cherry Bend Rd, Traverse City, MI 49684
Table mounted retractor system for anterior and posterior approaches to spine surgery.

Zimmer Holdings, Inc. 800-613-6131
1800 W Center St, PO Box 708, Warsaw, IN 46580
Z-shaped, guides suture needle.

RETRACTOR, RECTAL *(Gastro/Urology) 78RPV*

Codman & Shurtleff, Inc 800-225-0460
325 Paramount Dr, Raynham, MA 02767

Elmed, Inc. 630-543-2792
60 W Fay Ave, Addison, IL 60101

Miltex Inc. 800-645-8000
589 Davies Dr, York, PA 17402

RETRACTOR, RIB *(Orthopedics) 87RPW*

Codman & Shurtleff, Inc 800-225-0460
325 Paramount Dr, Raynham, MA 02767

Elmed, Inc. 630-543-2792
60 W Fay Ave, Addison, IL 60101

Miltex Inc. 800-645-8000
589 Davies Dr, York, PA 17402

RETRACTOR, RIB *(cont'd)*

Scholten Surgical Instruments, Inc. 209-365-1393
170 Commerce St Ste 101, Lodi, CA 95240
Chest retractor for adult/pediatric purposes.

RETRACTOR, SELF-RETAINING *(Gastro/Urology) 78FFO*

Aesculap Implant Systems Inc. 1-800-234-9179
3773 Corporate Pkwy, Center Valley, PA 18034
Robotrac passive retraction system - OR table mounted pneumatic retraction system, prerobotic approach to surgical retraction.

Applied Medical Technology, Inc. 800-869-7382
8000 Katherine Blvd, Brecksville, OH 44141
TLC self-retaining retractor system.

Automated Medical Products Corp. 800-832-4567
PO Box 2508, Edison, NJ 08818
IRON INTERN.

Codman & Shurtleff, Inc 800-225-0460
325 Paramount Dr, Raynham, MA 02767

Elmed, Inc. 630-543-2792
60 W Fay Ave, Addison, IL 60101
RETRACT-ROBOT for self-retaining retraction for vascular, orthopedic, general, and gynecological surgery.

International Hospital Supply Co. 800-398-9450
6914 Canby Ave Ste 105, Reseda, CA 91335

Kagawa Shears.Com, Llc. 404-931-0258
3605 Swiftwater Park Dr, Suwanee, GA 30024

Kmedic 800-955-0559
190 Veterans Dr, Northvale, NJ 07647

Koros Usa, Inc. 805-529-0825
610 Flinn Ave, Moorpark, CA 93021
Laminectomy,self-retaining retractor.

Lone Star Medical Products, Inc. 800-331-7427
11211 Cash Rd, Stafford, TX 77477
The Lone Star Retractor System consists of two components, a cantilevered ring available in stainless steel, aluminum or plastic, and disposable elastic stays. The system is uniquely designed to allow precise retraction from any desired angle along the ring with excellent visualization. Rings are available in various geometric configurations and elastic stays are offered in various hook sizes to cover a broad range of surgery.

Omni-Tract Surgical, A Div. Of Minnesota Scientific, Inc. 800-367-8657
4849 White Bear Pkwy, Saint Paul, MN 55110
Omni-Tract Surgical Abdominal Retractor - surgical retractor for gastroenterology.

Schaerer Mayfield Usa 800-755-6381
4900 Charlemar Dr, Cincinnati, OH 45227
BUDDE Halo Brain Retractor and TEW Cranial/Spinal Retractor Systems.

Tuzik Boston 800-886-6363
104 Longwater Dr, Assinippi Park, Norwell, MA 02061

RETRACTOR, SELF-RETAINING, NEUROLOGY *(Cns/Neurology) 84GZT*

Abbott Spine, Inc. 847-937-6100
12708 Riata Vista Cir Ste B-100, Austin, TX 78727
Surgical retractor.

Biomet, Inc. 574-267-6639
56 E Bell Dr, PO Box 587, Warsaw, IN 46582
Various types of self retaining retractors.

Codman & Shurtleff, Inc 800-225-0460
325 Paramount Dr, Raynham, MA 02767

Compass International, Inc. 800-933-2143
1815 14th St NW, Rochester, MN 55901
Compass cylindrical retractor(s) for stereotactic neurosurgery.

Depuy Spine, Inc. 800-227-6633
325 Paramount Dr, Raynham, MA 02767
Retractor, self-retaining, for neurosurgery.

Elekta Inc. 800-535-7355
4775 Peachtree Industrial Blvd, Bldg. 300, Suite 300
Norcross, GA 30092

Elmed, Inc. 630-543-2792
60 W Fay Ave, Addison, IL 60101

Integra Lifesciences Of Ohio 800-654-2873
4900 Charlemar Dr Bldg A, Cincinnati, OH 45227
Various self retaining retractors.

International Hospital Supply Co. 800-398-9450
6914 Canby Ave Ste 105, Reseda, CA 91335

RETRACTOR, SELF-RETAINING, NEUROLOGY *(cont'd)*

Mediflex Surgical Products 800-879-7575
250 Gibbs Rd, Islandia, NY 11749

Northwest Stamping & Precision, Inc. 541-747-4269
86365 College View Rd, Eugene, OR 97405
leadframes for pulse oxymetry and other medical sensors

Schaerer Mayfield Usa 800-755-6381
4900 Charlemar Dr, Cincinnati, OH 45227
BUDDE Halo Brain Retractor and TEW Cranial/Spinal Retractor Systems.

Teleflex Medical 800-334-9751
2917 Weck Drive, Research Triangle Park, NC 27709
DURMAHOOK.

Thompson Surgical Instruments, Inc. 800-227-7543
10170 E Cherry Bend Rd, Traverse City, MI 49684

Zimmer Holdings, Inc. 800-613-6131
1800 W Center St, PO Box 708, Warsaw, IN 46580

RETRACTOR, SURGICAL *(Surgery) 79GAD*

Abbott Spine, Inc. 847-937-6100
12708 Riata Vista Cir Ste B-100, Austin, TX 78727
Retractor.

Aesculap Implant Systems Inc. 1-800-234-9179
3773 Corporate Pkwy, Center Valley, PA 18034

Alto Development Corp. 732-938-2266
5206 Asbury Rd, Wall Township, NJ 07727
Illuminated Hand Held Retractor

Atek Medical 800-253-1540
620 Watson St SW, Grand Rapids, MI 49504
Retractor adapter.

Atricure, Inc. 888.347.5403
6217 Centre Park Dr, West Chester, OH 45069
Retractor.

Automated Medical Products Corp. 800-832-4567
PO Box 2508, Edison, NJ 08818
IRON INTERN.

Axiom Medical, Inc. 800-221-8569
19320 Van Ness Ave, Torrance, CA 90501
Hook-type retractors of non-conductive plastic for use with electrosurgical knives and lasers to prevent arcing, reusable and sterilizable.

Bausch & Lomb Surgical 636-255-5051
3365 Tree Court Ind Blvd, Saint Louis, MO 63122

Biomet Microfixation Inc. 800-874-7711
1520 Tradeport Dr, Jacksonville, FL 32218
Various types of retractors.

Biomet, Inc. 574-267-6639
56 E Bell Dr, PO Box 587, Warsaw, IN 46582
Various types of manual retractors.

Cardinal Health, Snowden Pencer Products 847-689-8410
5175 S Royal Atlanta Dr, Tucker, GA 30084
Various styles of general plastic surgery surgical retractors.

Depuy Spine, Inc. 800-227-6633
325 Paramount Dr, Raynham, MA 02767
Retractor.

DJO Inc. 800-336-6569
1430 Decision St, Vista, CA 92081

E.A. Beck & Co. 949-645-4072
657 W 19th St Ste E, P O Box 10857, Costa Mesa, CA 92627
Retractor.

Elmed, Inc. 630-543-2792
60 W Fay Ave, Addison, IL 60101

Engineered Medical Solutions Co. Llc. 908-213-9001
85 Industrial Rd Bldg B, Phillipsburg, NJ 08865
Retractor.

Fehling Surgical Instruments 800-FEHLING
509 Broadstone Ln NW, Acworth, GA 30101

Gyrus Acmi, Inc. 508-804-2739
93 N Pleasant St, Norwalk, OH 44857
Retractor.

Innervision Inc. 901-682-0417
6258 E Shady Grove Rd, Memphis, TN 38120

Integra Neurosciences Pr 800-654-2873
Road 402 North, Km 1.2, Anasco, PR 00610
Silicone brain retractor.

RETRACTOR, SURGICAL *(cont'd)*

International Hospital Supply Co. 800-398-9450
6914 Canby Ave Ste 105, Reseda, CA 91335

Interventional Spine, Inc. 800-497-0484
13700 Alton Pkwy Ste 160, Irvine, CA 92618
Retractor.

Invuity, Inc. 760-744-4447
334 Via Vera Cruz Ste 255, San Marcos, CA 92078
Retractor.

Invuity, Inc. 415-655-2100
39 Stillman St, San Francisco, CA 94107

Kelsar, S.A. 508-261-8000
Blvd. Insurgentes, Libriamento a La, Tijuana 22450 Mexico
Retraction tape, polyester

Kmedic 800-955-0559
190 Veterans Dr, Northvale, NJ 07647

Marina Medical Instruments, Inc. 800-697-1119
955 Shotgun Rd, Sunrise, FL 33326
Various.

Mediflex Surgical Products 800-879-7575
250 Gibbs Rd, Islandia, NY 11749

Medisiss 866-866-7477
2747 SW 6th St, Redmond, OR 97756
Various retractors,sterile.

Medtronic Sofamor Danek Instrument Manufacturing 901-396-3133
7375 Adrianne Pl, Bartlett, TN 38133
Multiple retractors.

Medtronic Sofamor Danek Usa, Inc. 901-396-3133
4340 Swinnea Rd, Memphis, TN 38118
Multiple retractors.

Miltex Inc. 800-645-8000
589 Davies Dr, York, PA 17402

Northwest Stamping & Precision, Inc. 541-747-4269
86365 College View Rd, Eugene, OR 97405
bone screws, cervical plates

Omni-Tract Surgical, A Div. Of Minnesota Scientific, Inc. 800-367-8657
4849 White Bear Pkwy, Saint Paul, MN 55110
Omni-Tract Surgical MRI Fastsystem - surgical retractor for use in an MRI environment.

Oratronics, Inc. 212-986-0050
405 Lexington Ave, New York, NY 10174
Manual tissue retractor.

Orthovation, Llc 979-885-2012
2060 Highway 90 W, Sealy, TX 77474
Retractor.

Pemco, Inc. - Medical Div. 216-524-2990
5663 Brecksville Rd, Cleveland, OH 44131

Precision Medical Manufacturing Corporation 866-633-4626
852 Seton Ct, Wheeling, IL 60090
Balfour Retractors trigger positive controlled automatic retractor retaining design. Made of high quality stainless steel, large selections of sizes and changeable blades make the instrument adaptable and appropriate for pediatric, adult and obese patients. The fourth blade attachment doubles the incision exposure of Balfour Retractors. Variety of different retractors as Malleable, Kelly, Harrington, Gelpi Point Richardson, Deaver all available with bookwalter style handle.

Precision Products, Inc. 706-673-6900
681 N Varnell Rd, Tunnel Hill, GA 30755
Retractor.

Precision Surgical Intl., Inc. 800-776-8493
PO Box 726, Noblesville, IN 46061
Various styles and sizes of retractors.

Rocket Medical Plc. 800-707-7625
150 Recreation Park Dr Ste 3, Hingham, MA 02043

Scanlan International, Inc. 800-328-9458
1 Scanlan Plz, Saint Paul, MN 55107

Spine Smith Partners L.P. 512-206-0770
8140 N MO Pac Expy Bldg 120, Austin, TX 78759
Screw retractor.

Spine Wave, Inc. 203-944-9494
2 Enterprise Dr Ste 302, Shelton, CT 06484
Various types of nerve root retractors.

RETRACTOR, SURGICAL *(cont'd)*

Sterilmed, Inc. 763-488-3400
11400 73rd Ave N Ste 100, Maple Grove, MN 55369
Retractor.

Surgical Instrument Manufacturers, Inc. 800-521-2985
1650 Headland Dr, Fenton, MO 63026

Symmetry Medical Usa, Inc. 574-267-8700
486 W 350 N, Warsaw, IN 46582
Pcl retractor.

Teleflex Medical 800-334-9751
2917 Weck Drive, Research Triangle Park, NC 27709
DERMAHOOK elastic skin retractor.

Thompson Surgical Instruments, Inc. 800-227-7543
10170 E Cherry Bend Rd, Traverse City, MI 49684

Tuzik Boston 800-886-6363
104 Longwater Dr, Assinippi Park, Norwell, MA 02061

Vitalcor, Inc. 800-874-8358
100 Chestnut Ave, Westmont, IL 60559
Carpentier and IMA cardio-thoracic retractors.

Warsaw Orthopedic, Inc. 901-396-3133
2500 Silveus Xing, Warsaw, IN 46582
Multiple retractors.

Zimmer Spine, Inc. 800-655-2614
7375 Bush Lake Rd, Minneapolis, MN 55439
Retractor.

Zimmer Trabecular Metal Technology 800-613-6131
10 Pomeroy Rd, Parsippany, NJ 07054
Distractor.

RETRACTOR, VAGINAL *(Obstetrics/Gyn) 85HDL*

Aesculap Implant Systems Inc. 1-800-234-9179
3773 Corporate Pkwy, Center Valley, PA 18034

Automated Medical Products Corp. 800-832-4567
PO Box 2508, Edison, NJ 08818

Biomet Microfixation Inc. 800-874-7711
1520 Tradeport Dr, Jacksonville, FL 32218
Various types of retractors.

Boston Scientific Corporation 508-652-5578
780 Brookside Dr, Spencer, IN 47460

Centurion Medical Products Corp. 517-545-1135
3310 S Main St, Salisbury, NC 28147

Codman & Shurtleff, Inc 800-225-0460
325 Paramount Dr, Raynham, MA 02767

Coopersurgical, Inc. 800-243-2974
95 Corporate Dr, Trumbull, CT 06611

Elmed, Inc. 630-543-2792
60 W Fay Ave, Addison, IL 60101

George Tiemann & Co. 800-843-6266
25 Plant Ave, Hauppauge, NY 11788

Greatbatch Inc 716-759-5600
1771 E 30th St, Cleveland, OH 44114
Various types of vaginal retractors.

International Hospital Supply Co. 800-398-9450
6914 Canby Ave Ste 105, Reseda, CA 91335

Lone Star Medical Products, Inc. 800-331-7427
11211 Cash Rd, Stafford, TX 77477
The Lone Star Retractor System consists of two components, a cantilevered ring available in stainless steel, aluminum or plastic, and disposable elastic stays. The system is uniquely designed to allow precise retraction from any desired angle along the ring with excellent visualization. Rings are available in various geometric configurations and elastic stays are offered in various hook sizes for vaginal surgery.

Marina Medical Instruments, Inc. 800-697-1119
955 Shotgun Rd, Sunrise, FL 33326
Various.

Miltex Inc. 800-645-8000
589 Davies Dr, York, PA 17402

Precision Medical Manufacturing Corporation 866-633-4626
852 Seton Ct, Wheeling, IL 60090
The Guttmann Obstetrical retractor, self retaining, positive locking and ease of operation and strong stainless steel construction. Guttmann Vaginal Speculum positive self retaining and far greater exposure contured blades designed to fit pubic arch and to minimize pressure on soft tissue.

Premier Medical Products 888-PREMUSA
1710 Romano Dr, Plymouth Meeting, PA 19462

RETRACTOR, VAGINAL *(cont'd)*

Princeton Medical Group, Inc. 800-875-0869
1189 Royal Links Dr, Mt Pleasant, SC 29466

Thompson Surgical Instruments, Inc. 800-227-7543
10170 E Cherry Bend Rd, Traverse City, MI 49684

Tri-State Hospital Supply Corp. 517-545-1135
3173 E 43rd St, Yuma, AZ 85365

Tuzik Boston 800-886-6363
104 Longwater Dr, Assinippi Park, Norwell, MA 02061

RETRACTOR, VESSEL *(Cardiovascular) 74RPX*

Codman & Shurtleff, Inc 800-225-0460
325 Paramount Dr, Raynham, MA 02767

Elmed, Inc. 630-543-2792
60 W Fay Ave, Addison, IL 60101

Fehling Surgical Instruments 800-FEHLING
509 Broadstone Ln NW, Acworth, GA 30101

REVERSE GROUPING CELLS *(Hematology) 81UJT*

Dade Behring, Inc. 800-948-3233
1717 Deerfield Rd, Deerfield, IL 60015

REVERSE OSMOSIS MEMBRANE EQUIPMENT *(Chemistry) 75UHS*

Hydro Service & Supplies, Inc. 800-950-7426
PO Box 12197, Research Triangle Park, NC 27709
Ultrafiltration, reverse osmosis and point of use microbiological purity water purification equipment.

Isopure Corp. 800-280-7873
141 Citizens Blvd, Simpsonville, KY 40067
MD100 Portable Reverse Osmosis Machine produces enough water to supply two patients, 100% diversion-to-drain above a set-point, Intergrated HydroBLAST system.

Millipore Corporation 800-MILLIPORE
80 Ashby Rd, Bedford, MA 01730

Thermo Fisher Scientific Inc. 563-556-2241
2555 Kerper Blvd, Dubuque, IA 52001

RHEOENCEPHALOGRAPH *(Cns/Neurology) 84GZN*

U.F.I. 805-772-1203
545 Main St Ste C2, Morro Bay, CA 93442
$6,250 to $10,250 for Model 2994 (1 to 4 channels).

RHINOANEMOMETER (MEASUREMENT OF NASAL DECONGESTION) *(Anesthesiology) 73BXQ*

E. Benson Hood Laboratories, Inc. 800-942-5227
575 Washington St, Pembroke, MA 02359
ECCOVISION acoustic rhinometry system & acoustic pharyngometer system.

RHINOMANOMETER *(Anesthesiology) 73RQA*

E. Benson Hood Laboratories, Inc. 800-942-5227
575 Washington St, Pembroke, MA 02359
ECCOVISION acoustic rhinometry system & acoustic pharyngometer system.

RHINOSCOPE *(Ear/Nose/Throat) 77RQB*

Advanced Endoscopy Devices, Inc. 818-227-2720
22134 Sherman Way, Canoga Park, CA 91303
Endoscope for sinus surgery. Compatible with all manufacturer's instruments.

Clinimed, Incorporated 877-CLINIMED
303 Markus Ct, Sandy Brae Industrial Park, Newark, DE 19713

Karl Storz Endoscopy-America Inc. 800-421-0837
600 Corporate Pointe, Culver City, CA 90230
For adult and pediatric applications.

Kaypentax 800-289-5297
2 Bridgewater Ln, Lincoln Park, NJ 07035
Rhino-laryngeal stroboscope (RLS Model 9200) provides otolaryngologists, speech-language pathologists, and voice researchers with a system for viewing laryngeal anatomy and physiology; various options available.

Mahe International Inc. 800-294-7946
468 Craighead St, Nashville, TN 37204

Tsi Medical Ltd. 800-661-7263
47 Athabascan Ave., Unit 105, Sherwood Park, AB T8A-4H3 Canada

RICKETTSIA SEROLOGICAL REAGENTS, OTHER *(Microbiology) 83LSQ*

Access Bio Incorporate 732-297-2222
2033 Rt. 130 Unit H, Monmouth Junction, NJ 08852
Scrub typhus test.

Focus Diagnostics, Inc. 714-220-1900
10703 Progress Way, Cypress, CA 90630
Various.

Fuller Laboratories 714-525-7660
1135 E Truslow Ave, Fullerton, CA 92831
Spotted fever group rickettsia antibody, typhus group rickettsia antibody.

RING DRAPE RETENTION, INTERNAL (WOUND PROTECTOR) *(Surgery) 79KGW*

Apogee Medical, Llc 919-570-9605
90 Weathers Ct, Youngsville, NC 27596
Protractor retractor,protractor retractor with drape.

RING, ANNULOPLASTY *(Cardiovascular) 74KRH*

Medtronic Cardiovascular Surgery, The Heart Valve Div. 800-328-2518
1851 E Deere Ave, Santa Ana, CA 92705
Various models & sizes of annuloplasty rings.

Medtronic Heart Valves 800-227-3191
8299 Central Ave NE, Spring Lake Park, MN 55432
Various models.

Medtronic, Inc. 800-633-8766
710 Medtronic Pkwy, Minneapolis, MN 55432
SCULPTOR.

MiCardia Corporation 949-951-4888
30 Hughes Ste 206, Irvine, CA 92618

Shelhigh, Inc. 908-206-8706
650 Liberty Ave, Union, NJ 07083
Annuloplasty ring.

RING, CRIMP *(Gastro/Urology) 78FJX*

Aesculap Implant Systems Inc. 1-800-234-9179
3773 Corporate Pkwy, Center Valley, PA 18034

RING, DENTAL (CASTING) *(Dental And Oral) 76QOZ*

American Diversified Dental Systems 800-637-2330
22991 La Cadena Dr, Laguna Hills, CA 92653
Spiracast Ringless Casting System.

RING, ENDOCAPSULAR *(Ophthalmology) 86MRJ*

Fci Ophthalmics 800-932-4202
64 Schoosett St, Pembroke, MA 02359
Morcher capsular tension rings and Cionni rings

RING, LAPAROTOMY *(Gastro/Urology) 78FHI*

Precision Medical Manufacturing Corporation 866-633-4626
852 Seton Ct, Wheeling, IL 60090
Abdominal Ring Retractor available in 4'or 6' diameter. Four blades are included with ring. Two blades are solid and two are fenestrated. Used for minor abdominal surgery to provide good exposure. The instrument can be used in child surgery as well.

RING, OPHTHALMIC (FLIERINGA) *(Ophthalmology) 86HNH*

Accutome, Inc. 610-889-0200
3222 Phoenixville Pike, Malvern, PA 19355
Various.

B. Graczyk, Inc. 269-782-2100
27826 Burmax Park, Dowagiac, MI 49047
Various sizes of rings.

Bausch & Lomb Surgical 636-255-5051
3365 Tree Court Ind Blvd, Saint Louis, MO 63122

Katena Products, Inc. 800-225-1195
4 Stewart Ct, Denville, NJ 07834
Global fixation.

Micro Medical Instruments 314-845-3663
123 Cliff Cave Rd, Saint Louis, MO 63129
Ophthalmic rings.

Total Titanium, Inc. 618-473-2429
140 East Monroe St., Hecker, IL 62248
Various types of ophthalmic rings (flieringa).

RING, SUTURE *(Surgery) 79RXT*

Olympic Medical Corp. 206-767-3500
5900 1st Ave S, Seattle, WA 98108
$194.50 per unit (non-sterile).

RING, SYMBLEPHARON *(Ophthalmology) 86UBE*

Fci Ophthalmics 800-932-4202
64 Schoosett St, Pembroke, MA 02359
Small, medium and large symblepharon rings

Jardon Eye Prosthetics, Inc. 248-424-8560
15920 W 12 Mile Rd, Southfield, MI 48076

Oculo Plastik Inc. 888-381-3292
200 Sauve West, Montreal, QUE H3L-1Y9 Canada
PMMA, clear. Round: 20mm, 22.5mm, and 25mm. Elongated: 23mm, 25mm, and 27mm.

RING, TEETHING, FLUID-FILLED *(Dental And Oral) 76KKO*

Danara Intl. Ltd. 201-295-1448
8101 Tonnelle Ave, North Bergen, NJ 07047
Teething ring fluid filled.

Dorel Design & Development Center 781-364-3542
25 Forbes Blvd, Foxboro, MA 02035

Plastic And Metal Center, Inc. 949-770-8230
23162 La Cadena Dr, Laguna Hills, CA 92653

RING, TEETHING, NON-FLUID-FILLED *(Dental And Oral) 76MEF*

Ark Therapeutic Services, Inc. 803-438-9779
PO Box 340, 862 A Hwy. 1 South, Lugoff, SC 29078
Teething ring.

Monroe Mfg., Inc. 318-338-3172
3030 Aurora Ave, 2nd Fl., Monroe, LA 71201
Chewies.

Nose Breathe 808-949-8876
2065 S King St Ste 304, Honolulu, HI 96826
Baby pacifier.

Vibe 2000 805-377-2709
511 Higuera Dr, Oxnard, CA 93030
Teething ring.

ROD, COLOSTOMY *(Gastro/Urology) 78EZP*

Hollister, Inc. 847-680-2849
366 Draft Ave, Stuarts Draft, VA 24477

Kelsar, S.A. 508-261-8000
Blvd. Insurgentes, Libriamento a La, Tijuana 22450 Mexico
Colostomy rod

Marlen Manufacturing & Development Co. 216-292-7060
5150 Richmond Rd, Bedford, OH 44146
Surgeons' ostomy rod.

Tools For Surgery, Llc 631-444-4448
1339 Stony Brook Rd, Stony Brook, NY 11790
Colostomy rod.

ROD, FIXATION, INTRAMEDULLARY *(Orthopedics) 87HSB*

Acumed Llc 503-627-9957
5885 NW Cornelius Pass Rd, Hillsboro, OR 97124
Ulna, radius, fibula rod.

Advanced Orthopaedic Solutions, Inc. 310-533-9966
386 Beech Ave Unit B6, Torrance, CA 90501
Intramedullary femoral nail.

Alphatec Spine, Inc. 760-494-6769
5818 El Camino Real, Carlsbad, CA 92008
Alphatec intramedallary nail system.

Biomet Microfixation Inc. 800-874-7711
1520 Tradeport Dr, Jacksonville, FL 32218
Rod, fixation, intramedullary.

Biomet, Inc. 574-267-6639
56 E Bell Dr, PO Box 587, Warsaw, IN 46582
Various sterile & non-sterile intramdullary pins.

Biopro, Inc. 800-252-7707
2929 Lapeer Rd, Port Huron, MI 48060
Wujin #3 Intramedullary Nail System

Depuy Orthopaedics, Inc. 800-473-3789
700 Orthopaedic Dr, P.O. Box 988, Warsaw, IN 46582
Various.

Modular Cutting Systems, Inc. 203-336-3526
650 Clinton Ave, Bridgeport, CT 06605
Guidance system for placement of intramedullary rod.

Pioneer Surgical Technology 800-557-9909
375 River Park Cir, Marquette, MI 49855
STAYFUSE (Interdigital fusion system), two piece AV titanium, intramedullary implant for fixation of small bone fusions and fractures. Most commonly used for the correction of Hammertoe deformities.

ROD, FIXATION, INTRAMEDULLARY *(cont'd)*

Small Bone Innovations, Inc. 215-428-1791
1380 S Pennsylvania Ave, Morrisville, PA 19067
Intramedullary fixation rod.

Stryker Spine 866-457-7463
2 Pearl Ct, Allendale, NJ 07401

Surgical Implant Generation Network (Sign) 509-371-1107
451 Hills St, Richland, WA 99354
Various sizes of i.m. tibial nails.

Warsaw Orthopedic, Inc. 901-396-3133
2500 Silveus Xing, Warsaw, IN 46582
Various types of intramedullary rods.

Zimmer Holdings, Inc. 800-613-6131
1800 W Center St, PO Box 708, Warsaw, IN 46580

Zimmer Manufacturing B.V. 800-613-6131
Route 1, Km. 123.4, Bldg. 1, Turpeaux Industrial Park
Mercedita, PR 00715
Various types and sizes of intramedullary nails, pins, and sets containing vario.

ROD, FIXATION, INTRAMEDULLARY AND ACCESSORIES, METALLIC AND NON-COLLAPSIBLE *(Orthopedics) 87NDE*

Advanced Orthopaedic Solutions, Inc. 310-533-9966
386 Beech Ave Unit B6, Torrance, CA 90501
Intramedullary femoral nail.

Zimmer Manufacturing B.V. 800-613-6131
Route 1, Km. 123.4, Bldg. 1, Turpeaux Industrial Park
Mercedita, PR 00715
Various types and sizes of intramedullary nails, pins, and sets containing varis.

ROD, MEASURING EAR *(Ear/Nose/Throat) 77JYZ*

Aesculap Implant Systems Inc. 1-800-234-9179
3773 Corporate Pkwy, Center Valley, PA 18034

Non-Invasive Monitoring Systems, Inc. 305-575-4200
4400 Biscayne Blvd, Miami, FL 33137
Breathing monitors.

ROLLER, PATIENT *(General) 80RJZ*

Mizuho Osi 800-777-4674
30031 Ahern Ave, Union City, CA 94587

Wenzelite Rehab Supplies, Llc 800-706-9255
220 36th St, 99 Seaview Blvd, Brooklyn, NY 11232
Safety roller for pediatric use with forearm platforms, four wheels and automatic brakes. Also obese and extra tall models. Indoor/Outdoor models with large, all-terrain wheels and seat. All with Dial-A-Brake.

RONGEUR, DENTAL *(Dental And Oral) 76RQC*

Hu-Friedy Manufacturing Co., Inc. 800-483-7433
3232 N Rockwell St, Chicago, IL 60618
$195.00 to $332.00 each, 25 types.

Nordent Manufacturing, Inc. 800-966-7336
610 Bonnie Ln, Elk Grove Village, IL 60007
$200.00 per unit (standard).

RONGEUR, INTERVERTEBRAL DISK *(Orthopedics) 87RQD*

Princeton Medical Group, Inc. 800-875-0869
1189 Royal Links Dr, Mt Pleasant, SC 29466

RONGEUR, LACRIMAL SAC *(Ophthalmology) 86HNG*

Addition Technology, Inc. 847-297-8419
155 Moffett Park Dr Ste B-1, Sunnyvale, CA 94089

Bausch & Lomb Surgical 636-255-5051
3365 Tree Court Ind Blvd, Saint Louis, MO 63122

RONGEUR, MANUAL, NEUROSURGICAL *(Cns/Neurology) 84HAE*

Baxano, Inc. 408-514-2200
655 River Oaks Pkwy, San Jose, CA 95134
Microblade shaver and accessories, ultra low profile rongeur.

Biomet Microfixation Inc. 800-874-7711
1520 Tradeport Dr, Jacksonville, FL 32218
Various types of rongeurs.

Biomet, Inc. 574-267-6639
56 E Bell Dr, PO Box 587, Warsaw, IN 46582
Various types of rongeurs.

Codman & Shurtleff, Inc 800-225-0460
325 Paramount Dr, Raynham, MA 02767

Elmed, Inc. 630-543-2792
60 W Fay Ave, Addison, IL 60101

Fehling Surgical Instruments 800-FEHLING
509 Broadstone Ln NW, Acworth, GA 30101

RONGEUR, MANUAL, NEUROSURGICAL *(cont'd)*

Miltex Inc. 800-645-8000
589 Davies Dr, York, PA 17402

Schaerer Mayfield Usa 800-755-6381
4900 Charlemar Dr, Cincinnati, OH 45227
MAYFIELD black pearl rongeurs.

RONGEUR, MASTOID *(Ear/Nose/Throat) 77JZA*

Bausch & Lomb Surgical 636-255-5051
3365 Tree Court Ind Blvd, Saint Louis, MO 63122

Clinimed, Incorporated 877-CLINIMED
303 Markus Ct, Sandy Brae Industrial Park, Newark, DE 19713

RONGEUR, NASAL *(Ear/Nose/Throat) 77KBB*

Biomet Microfixation Inc. 800-874-7711
1520 Tradeport Dr, Jacksonville, FL 32218
Various types of rongeurs.

Clinimed, Incorporated 877-CLINIMED
303 Markus Ct, Sandy Brae Industrial Park, Newark, DE 19713

Princeton Medical Group, Inc. 800-875-0869
1189 Royal Links Dr, Mt Pleasant, SC 29466

RONGEUR, OTHER *(Surgery) 79RQE*

Centinel Spine Inc. 952-885-0500
505 Park Ave Fl 14, New York, NY 10022
Stalif C Rongeur

Elmed, Inc. 630-543-2792
60 W Fay Ave, Addison, IL 60101

Kmedic 800-955-0559
190 Veterans Dr, Northvale, NJ 07647

Roboz Surgical Instrument Co., Inc. 800-424-2984
PO Box 10710, Gaithersburg, MD 20898

RONGEUR, POWERED *(Cns/Neurology) 84HAD*

E-Z-Em, Inc. 516-333-8230
750 Summa Ave, Westbury, NY 11590
Guidewires for catheters, various types.

RONGEUR, RIB *(Orthopedics) 87HTX*

Abbott Spine, Inc. 847-937-6100
12708 Riata Vista Cir Ste B-100, Austin, TX 78727
Rongeur.

Ascent Healthcare Solutions 480-763-5300
10232 S 51st St, Phoenix, AZ 85044
Rongeur.

Biomet, Inc. 574-267-6639
56 E Bell Dr, PO Box 587, Warsaw, IN 46582
Various types of orthopedic rongeur.

Codman & Shurtleff, Inc 800-225-0460
325 Paramount Dr, Raynham, MA 02767

Dental Usa, Inc. 815-363-8003
5005 McCullom Lake Rd, McHenry, IL 60050
Dental rongeur.

Depuy Spine, Inc. 800-227-6633
325 Paramount Dr, Raynham, MA 02767
Various sizes and configurations of rongeurs.

Elmed, Inc. 630-543-2792
60 W Fay Ave, Addison, IL 60101

Invuity, Inc. 760-744-4447
334 Via Vera Cruz Ste 255, San Marcos, CA 92078
Various types and sizes of rongeurs.

Invuity, Inc. 415-655-2100
39 Stillman St, San Francisco, CA 94107

Kmedic 800-955-0559
190 Veterans Dr, Northvale, NJ 07647

Koros Usa, Inc. 805-529-0825
610 Flinn Ave, Moorpark, CA 93021
Disc ronguer.

M-P Mfg., Inc. 815-334-1112
13802 Washington St Ste B, Woodstock, IL 60098
Various types of rongeur, orthopedic manual surgical instrument.

Medtronic Sofamor Danek Instrument Manufacturing 901-396-3133
7375 Adrianne Pl, Bartlett, TN 38133
Various (rongeurs).

Medtronic Sofamor Danek Usa, Inc. 901-396-3133
4340 Swinnea Rd, Memphis, TN 38118
Various (rongeurs).

RONGEUR, RIB *(cont'd)*

Miltex Inc. 800-645-8000
589 Davies Dr, York, PA 17402

Scanlan International, Inc. 800-328-9458
1 Scanlan Plz, Saint Paul, MN 55107

Spine Wave, Inc. 203-944-9494
2 Enterprise Dr Ste 302, Shelton, CT 06484
Various types of pituitary rongeurs.

Symmetry Medical Usa, Inc. 574-267-8700
486 W 350 N, Warsaw, IN 46582
Orthopedic manual surgical instrument.

Ussc Puerto Rico, Inc. 203-845-1000
Building 911-67, Sabanetas Industrial Park, Ponce, PR 00731
Various.

Warsaw Orthopedic, Inc. 901-396-3133
2500 Silveus Xing, Warsaw, IN 46582
Various (rongeurs).

Zimmer Spine, Inc. 800-655-2614
7375 Bush Lake Rd, Minneapolis, MN 55439
Rongeur.

Zimmer Trabecular Metal Technology 800-613-6131
10 Pomeroy Rd, Parsippany, NJ 07054
Ronguer.

ROOM, ACOUSTICAL *(Ear/Nose/Throat) 77TAB*

Proudfoot Company, Inc. 800-445-0034
588 Pepper St, Monroe, CT 06468
NOISEMASTER and SOUNDBLOX acoustical rooms. Quilted sound screens, baffles, wall panels, pipe and duct lagging, pattented resonator absorbers, electronic sound masking systems.

ROTATOR, TRANSVERSE *(Physical Med) 89IQP*

Dade Behring, Inc. 800-948-3233
1717 Deerfield Rd, Deerfield, IL 60015

Lw Scientific 800-726-7345
865 Marathon Pkwy, Lawrenceville, GA 30046
Variable-speed rotator with tachometer and timer. Also available is a tube rocker that gently rocks 15 tubes at 24 cycles/minute.

Tillotson Rubber Co., Inc. 781-402-1731
59 Waters Ave, Everett, MA 02149
Glove, protective, radiographic.

ROWING UNIT *(Physical Med) 89RQF*

Alimed, Inc. 800-225-2610
297 High St, Dedham, MA 02026

Med-Fit Systems, Inc. 800-831-7665
3553 Rosa Way, Fallbrook, CA 92028

RUBELLA, OTHER ASSAYS *(Microbiology) 83LSD*

Arlington Scientific, Inc. Asi 800-654-0146
1840 N Technology Dr, Springville, UT 84663
The ASI Rubella Test is a rapid latex particle agglutination test for the qualitative and semiquantitative determination of rubella virus antibodies in serum. The test aids in the diagnosis of recent or active rubella infection and in the determination of immune status.

Hemagen Diagnostics, Inc. 800-436-2436
9033 Red Branch Rd, Columbia, MD 21045
Rubella ifa.

United Biotech, Inc. 650-961-2910
211 S Whisman Rd Ste E, Mountain View, CA 94041
ELISAs detecting: Rubella IgG, Rubella IgM

RULER, NEARPOINT (PUNCTOMETER) *(Ophthalmology) 86HLE*

Fortrad Eye Instruments Corp. 973-543-2371
8 Franklin Rd, Mendham, NJ 07945

Gulden Ophthalmics 800-659-2250
225 Cadwalader Ave, Elkins Park, PA 19027

SACCHAROGENIC, AMYLASE *(Chemistry) 75CIJ*

Caldon Bioscience, Inc. 909-628-9944
2100 S Reservoir St, Pomona, CA 91766
Amylase.

Caldon Biotech, Inc. 757-224-0177
2251 Rutherford Rd, Carlsbad, CA 92008
Amylase.

Genchem, Inc. 714-529-1616
510 W Central Ave Ste D, Brea, CA 92821
Amylase reagent.

SAFE, RADIONUCLIDE *(Radiology) 90JAS*

Biodex Medical Systems, Inc. 800-224-6339
20 Ramsey Rd, Shirley, NY 11967

Capintec, Inc. 800-631-3826
6 Arrow Rd, Ramsey, NJ 07446

SAFELIGHT, X-RAY *(Radiology) 90VGO*

Americomp, Inc. 800-458-1782
2901 W Lawrence Ave, Chicago, IL 60625

Bar-Ray Products, Inc. 800-359-6115
95 Monarch St, Littlestown, PA 17340

Bulbtronics, Inc. 800-624-2852
45 Banfi Plz N, Farmingdale, NY 11735

Bulbworks, Inc. 800-334-2852
80 N Dell Ave Unit 5, Kenvil, NJ 07847
Replacement Lamps For All Types Of X-Ray Safelights

Carr Corporation 800-952-2398
1547 11th St, Santa Monica, CA 90401

S&S Technology 281-815-1300
10625 Telge Rd, Houston, TX 77095

Schueler & Company, Inc. 516-487-1500
PO Box 528, Stratford, CT 06615

Star X-Ray Co., Inc. 800-374-2163
63 Ranick Dr S, Amityville, NY 11701
$ 92.25 fluorescent safelight.

Ti-Ba Enterprises, Inc. 585-247-1212
25 Hytec Cir, Rochester, NY 14606
Ti-Ba sell all saflights and filters by Kodak. Please call for pricing.

Xma (X-Ray Marketing Associates, Inc.) 800-325-8880
1205 W Lakeview Ct, Windham Lakes Business Park
Romeoville, IL 60446

SAFETY EQUIPMENT, LABORATORY *(Chemistry) 75RDT*

Argus-Hazco 800-332-0435
6501 Centerville Business Pkwy, Dayton, OH 45459
Personal protective equipment.

Aura Lens Products, Inc. 800-281-2872
51 8th St N, PO Box 763, St. Cloud,, Sauk Rapids, MN 56379
Safety shields.

Bedcolab Ltd. 800-461-6414
2305 Francis Hughes, Laval, QUE H7S 1N5 Canada

Biomerieux Industry 800-634-7656
595 Anglum Rd, Hazelwood, MO 63042
Laboratory equipment and supplies.

Dosimeter Division Of Arrow Tech Inc 800-322-8258
5 Eastmans Rd, Parsippany, NJ 07054
$995 per unit, a/v gamma alarm, 1 mR/hr to 100 R/hr range with adjustable alarm set point (low range,1 mR/h to 2 R/h also available). Remote probes optional.

Elvex Corporation 800-888-6582
13 Trowbridge Dr, Bethel, CT 06801

Justrite Manufacturing Co., L.L.C. 800-798-9250
2454 E Dempster St, Des Plaines, IL 60016
Justrite offers safety cans, cabinets, dispensing bottles, jackets, ChemCor™ lined corrosive cabinets, Stainless Steel Corrosive Cabinets, HPLC container and Biohazard waste cans for laboratory use.

Lab Safety Supply, Inc. 800-356-0783
401 S Wright Rd, Janesville, WI 53546

Olsen Medical 800-297-6344
3001 W Kentucky St, Louisville, KY 40211
Laser safety products.

Orthoband Company, Inc. 800-325-9973
3690 Highway M, Imperial, MO 63052

Safe-T-Rack Systems, Inc. 800-344-0619
4325 Dominguez Rd Ste A, Rocklin, CA 95677
Compressed gas cylinder restraint and storage system for interior or exterior use.

Sellstrom Manufacturing Co. 800-323-7402
1 Sellstrom Dr, Palatine, IL 60067
10-10 spill station with 1 liter spill pillows; 4 liter spill pillows available.

Troemner Llc 800-352-7705
201 Wolf Dr, PO Box 87, West Deptford, NJ 08086
Cylinder safety equipment.

SALIVA, ARTIFICIAL *(Dental And Oral) 76LFD*

Boehringer Ingelheim Roxane Inc.
1809 Wilson Rd, P.o. Box 16532, Columbus, OH 43228
Saliva substitute.

Catalent Pharma Solutions 866-720-3148
2200 Lake Shore Dr, Woodstock, IL 60098
Caphosol

Century Pharmaceuticals, Inc. 317-849-4210
10377 Hague Rd, Indianapolis, IN 46256
Moi-stir (mouth moistener).

Gebauer Company 800-321-9348
4444 E 153rd St, Cleveland, OH 44128
SALIVART, oral moisturizer.

Parnell Pharmaceuticals, Inc. 415-256-1800
1525 Francisco Blvd E Ste 15, San Rafael, CA 94901
Mouthkote.

Span Packaging Services Llc. 864-627-4155
4611A Dairy Dr, Greenville, SC 29607
Moi stir oral swab sticks.

SAMPLER, AIR *(General) 80QAI*

Air Techniques International 410-363-9696
11403 Cronridge Dr, Owings Mills, MD 21117
Air quality test and measurement equipment, respirator fit testing equipment.

Assay Technology Inc 800-833-1258
1252 Quarry Ln, Pleasanton, CA 94566
TraceAir Organic Vapor Monitor with prepaid analysis, five monitors per box.

Biotest Diagnostic Corp. 800-522-0090
400 Commons Way, Rockaway, NJ 07866
Microbiological air sampler.

Cds Analytical, Inc. 800-541-6593
465 Limestone Rd, Oxford, PA 19363

Esa, Inc. 800-959-5095
22 Alpha Rd, Chelmsford, MA 01824

Hamilton Company 800-648-5950
4990 Energy Way, Reno, NV 89502

Millipore Corporation 800-MILLIPORE
80 Ashby Rd, Bedford, MA 01730

New Brunswick Scientific Co., Inc. 800-631-5417
PO Box 4005, Edison, NJ 08818
Slit-to-agar microbial air samplers draw a precise volume of air onto a rotating 150-mm plate for subsequent incubation and analysis. For clean room environments, capable of sampling volume up to 5 cubic meters (5000 liters). In environments with more viable particles, can sample as little as 0.03 cubic meters (30 liters.)

Thermo Fisher Scientific 800-241-6898
500 Technology Ct SE, Smyrna, GA 30082
Microbial air sampler collects airborne bacteria; unit required to use pre-filled standard Petri dishes and a vacuum source. Sampler differentiates between respirable and non-respirable bacteria, and levels of airborne bacteria can be measured and maintained. Also available, vapor collectors, particulate samplers and SUMMA passivated canister for air toxics collection.

SAMPLER, AMNIOTIC FLUID (AMNIOCENTESIS TRAY) *(Obstetrics/Gyn) 85HIO*

Busse Hospital Disposables, Inc. 631-435-4711
75 Arkay Dr, Hauppauge, NY 11788
Amniocentesis tray.

Cook Ob/Gyn 800-541-5591
1100 W Morgan St, Spencer, IN 47460

Cytyc Corporation 888-773-8376
1240 Elko Dr, Sunnyvale, CA 94089
Specimen collection kit.

Cytyc Surgical Products 800-442-9892
250 Campus Dr, Marlborough, MA 01752
Specimen collection kit.

SAMPLER, BLOOD, FETAL *(Obstetrics/Gyn) 85HGW*

Kelsar, S.A. 508-261-8000
Blvd. Insurgentes, Libriamento a La, Tijuana 22450 Mexico
Fetal blood sampler

Richard Wolf Medical Instruments Corp. 800-323-9653
353 Corporate Woods Pkwy, Vernon Hills, IL 60061

SAMPLER, GAS *(Chemistry) 75QXY*

Draeger Safety, Inc. 800-922-5518
101 Technology Dr, Pittsburgh, PA 15275

Hamilton Company 800-648-5950
4990 Energy Way, Reno, NV 89502

Nasorcap Medical, Inc. 412-466-1412
1077 Huston Dr, West Mifflin, PA 15122
$5.00 per unit for NAZORCAP 9112 sampler. $6.00 per unit for NAZORCAP LD/9112. Disposable auxilliary products for capnographic respiratory monitoring during spontaneous natural-airway breathing with supplemented oxygen delivering capability. Volume discount pricing available. Both 9112 models are premium products with both oral and nasal CO2 sampling capability. NAZORCAP 9801 and 9802 models are nasal end tidal CO2 sampling and nasal/oral O2 delivery cannula products. These models are effective, low cost alternative with nasal CO2 sampling capability only and can be supplied in various lengths for additional cost saving considerations.

Praxair, Inc. 800-PRAXAIR
39 Old Ridgebury Rd, Danbury, CT 06810
Industrial.

Spectrex Corp. 800-822-3940
3580 Haven Ave, Redwood City, CA 94063
$299.00 for gas sampling pump.

SAMPLER, PARTICULATE *(General) 80WWH*

Thermo Fisher Scientific 800-241-6898
500 Technology Ct SE, Smyrna, GA 30082
Small, lightweight personal monitor for respirable TLVs.

SAND BAG *(Radiology) 90RQJ*

Alimed, Inc. 800-225-2610
297 High St, Dedham, MA 02026
Anti-magnetic sand filling will not interfere with MRI scans.

Cfi Medical Solutions (Contour Fabricators, Inc.) 810-750-5300
14241 N Fenton Rd, Fenton, MI 48430

Morrison Medical 800-438-6677
3735 Paragon Dr, Columbus, OH 43228
U.FILL & HANDY SANDY sand bags: 3, 5, 7, & 10lbs. Has handle with or without grommet.

Profex Medical Products 800-325-0196
2224 E Person Ave, Memphis, TN 38114

Rockford Medical & Safety Co. 800-435-9451
2420 Harrison Ave, PO Box 5646, Rockford, IL 61108

Xma (X-Ray Marketing Associates, Inc.) 800-325-8880
1205 W Lakeview Ct, Windham Lakes Business Park
Romeoville, IL 60446

SAND BAG, X-RAY *(Radiology) 90SGN*

Flow X-Ray Corporation 800-356-9729
100 W Industry Ct, Deer Park, NY 11729

Marconi Medical Systems 800-323-0550
595 Miner Rd, Cleveland, OH 44143
4000 pound sand bags.

Techno-Aide, Inc. 800-251-2629
7117 Centennial Blvd, Nashville, TN 37209

Wolf X-Ray Corporation 800-356-9729
100 W Industry Ct, Deer Park, NY 11729

Xma (X-Ray Marketing Associates, Inc.) 800-325-8880
1205 W Lakeview Ct, Windham Lakes Business Park
Romeoville, IL 60446

SANITIZER *(General) 80RQL*

Beaumont Products, Inc. 800-451-7096
1560 Big Shanty Dr NW, Kennesaw, GA 30144
Citrus II Instant Hand Sanitizing Lotion is a moisture-rich gel

Colonial Scientific Ltd. 902-468-1811
201 Brownlow Ave., Unit 52, Dartmouth, NS B3B-1W2 Canada
sterilizer

Crosstex International 800-223-2497
10 Ranick Rd, Hauppauge, NY 11788
SANITEX PLUS Surface spray disinfectant and cleaner.

Derma Sciences 609-514-4744
214 Carnegie Ctr Ste 300, Princeton, NJ 08540

SANITIZER *(cont'd)*

Gentell 800-840-9041
3600 Boundbrook Ave, Trevose, PA 19053
GENTELL INSTANT HAND SANITIZER is a cleansing and moisturizing solution designed to facilitate anti-bacterial hand washing without soap or water. It can also be used as an anti-bacterial supplement to regular hand-hygiene practices that kill 99.99% of bacteria. GENTELL INSTANT HAND SANITIZER is ethyl alcohol based and formulated with aloe and vitamins A & D. GENTELL INSTANT HAND SANITIZER is available in 4oz squeeze bottle, 8oz hand pump and 800mL Wall Dispenser Refill Bags.

Independent Solutions, Inc. 847-498-0500
900 Skokie Blvd Ste 118, Northbrook, IL 60062
SEMCO freestanding sanitizer.

Innovative Health Care Products, Inc. 678-320-0009
6850 Peachtree Dunwoody Rd NE Apt 402, Atlanta, GA 30328
NoRinse hand sanitizer.With or without alcohol.

Meritech, Inc. 800-932-7707
600 Corporate Cir Ste H, Golden, CO 80401

Nilodor, Inc. 800-443-4321
10966 Industrial Pkwy NW, Bolivar, OH 44612
Aerosol, wick, drop or pump-spray deodorizer.

No Rinse Laboratories, Llc. 800-223-9348
868 Pleasant Valley Dr, Springboro, OH 45066
No Rinse Hand Sanitizer, non-alcohol, antibacterial foaming formula with aloe vera. Approximately 125 applications per bottle.

Palmero Health Care 800-344-6424
120 Goodwin Pl, Stratford, CT 06615
Aerosol spray disinfectant deordorant spray.

Pl Medical Co., Llc. 800-874-0120
321 Ellis St, New Britain, CT 06051
Heavy metal and chemical recovery unit. This unit removes all metal, organic, and inorganic chemicals before discharging the spent x-ray developing chemicals into municipal drain. Full compliance with EPA waste water standards.

Professional Disposables International, Inc. 800-999-6423
2 Nice Pak Park, Orangeburg, NY 10962

Safetec Of America, Inc. 800-456-7077
887 Kensington Ave, Buffalo, NY 14215
ANTISEPTIC BIO-HAND CLEANER (a.b.h.c), waterless hand sanitizer, kills 99.99% of most germs in as little as 15 seconds! Contains 66.5% Ethyl Alcohol and aloe vera to add moisture to skin. Available in original Fresh or Citrus Scents. Packaging: 3 gram pouch, 1/2 oz. pouch, 2 oz. and 4 oz. flip-top bottles, 16 oz. and 64 oz. pump bottles, and 27.05 oz. bag for dispensers.

Unit Chemical Corp. 800-879-8648
7360 Commercial Way, Henderson, NV 89011
TIMSEN packets & Liquid TIMSEN.

Weiman Healthcare Solutions 800-837-8140
755 Tri State Pkwy, Gurnee, IL 60031
Cleaning products for the operating room.

Woodward Laboratories, Inc. 800-780-6999
125 Columbia Ste B, Aliso Viejo, CA 92656
HANDCLENS alcohol-free instant hand sanitizer. Kills 99.99% of disease-causing germs in 15 seconds without drying skin. Non-flammable, non-irritating, won't burn small cuts and abrasions, and persistence of activity exceeds FDA standards.

Xttrium Laboratories, Inc. 800-587-3721
415 W Pershing Rd, Chicago, IL 60609
ALCO-GEL instant hand sanitizer gel. Waterless hand sanitizer.

SAW, AUTOPSY *(Pathology) 88RQM*

Bsn Medical, Inc 800-552-1157
5825 Carnegie Blvd, Charlotte, NC 28209
M-PACT

SAW, BONE CUTTING *(Orthopedics) 87HSO*

Bestway Products Co. 310-329-0600
16602 S Broadway St, Gardena, CA 90248
Round single wire toothed saw blade (Gigli) for trauma, neuro, and orthopedic surgery.

Biomet, Inc. 574-267-6639
56 E Bell Dr, PO Box 587, Warsaw, IN 46582
Various types of sterile and non-sterile orthopedic saws.

Elmed, Inc. 630-543-2792
60 W Fay Ave, Addison, IL 60101

Kmedic 800-955-0559
190 Veterans Dr, Northvale, NJ 07647

SAW, BONE CUTTING *(cont'd)*

Stryker Corp. 800-726-2725
2825 Airview Blvd, Portage, MI 49002

Stryker Spine 866-457-7463
2 Pearl Ct, Allendale, NJ 07401

Tuzik Boston 800-886-6363
104 Longwater Dr, Assinippi Park, Norwell, MA 02061

Warsaw Orthopedic, Inc. 901-396-3133
2500 Silveus Xing, Warsaw, IN 46582
Various bone saws.

Zimmer Holdings, Inc. 800-613-6131
1800 W Center St, PO Box 708, Warsaw, IN 46580

SAW, BONE CUTTING, MICRO *(Orthopedics) 87VHR*

Aesculap Implant Systems Inc. 1-800-234-9179
3773 Corporate Pkwy, Center Valley, PA 18034
3 models available: Oscillating model with 4.8 in. length; 8 mm optional blade. SagiHal model with 4.8 in. length; optional 10, 15, 20 mm straight blades. Reciprocating model with 6.2 in. length; optional 5, 10, 30, 35 mm straight and 17, 22 mm curved blades.

Micro-Aire Surgical Instruments, Inc. 800-722-0822
1641 Edlich Dr, Charlottesville, VA 22911
$1,550 for sagittal and reciprocating models with 7" length; 0.7" diameter, 4.4 or 4.7 oz weight. $1,650 for oscillating model with 8.6 or 7.8" length; 4.8 oz weight. All with optional choice of Zimmer, Stryker, or 3M air hose connector.

Stryker Corp. 800-726-2725
2825 Airview Blvd, Portage, MI 49002

Vilex, Inc. 800-872-4911
345 Old Curry Hollow Rd, Pittsburgh, PA 15236

SAW, BONE, PNEUMATIC *(Orthopedics) 87RQN*

Micro-Aire Surgical Instruments, Inc. 800-722-0822
1641 Edlich Dr, Charlottesville, VA 22911

Stryker Corp. 800-726-2725
2825 Airview Blvd, Portage, MI 49002

Zimmer Holdings, Inc. 800-613-6131
1800 W Center St, PO Box 708, Warsaw, IN 46580
Also battery & electric. Sternum saw, small & large bone orthopedic saws.

SAW, ELECTRIC *(Cardiovascular) 74DWI*

Aesculap Implant Systems Inc. 1-800-234-9179
3773 Corporate Pkwy, Center Valley, PA 18034

Altair Instruments, Inc. 805-388-8503
330 Wood Rd Ste J, Camarillo, CA 93010

H&H Instruments
4950 Crescent Technical Ct, St Augustine, FL 32086
Hhi reciprocating saw.

Stryker Corp. 800-726-2725
2825 Airview Blvd, Portage, MI 49002

Terumo Cardiovascular Systems, Corp 800-521-2818
6200 Jackson Rd, Ann Arbor, MI 48103

Vilex, Inc. 931-474-7550
111 Moffitt St, McMinnville, TN 37110

SAW, LARYNGEAL *(Ear/Nose/Throat) 77JZZ*

Clinimed, Incorporated 877-CLINIMED
303 Markus Ct, Sandy Brae Industrial Park, Newark, DE 19713

SAW, MANUAL, AND ACCESSORIES *(Surgery) 79GDR*

Aesculap Implant Systems Inc. 1-800-234-9179
3773 Corporate Pkwy, Center Valley, PA 18034

Bestway Products Co. 310-329-0600
16602 S Broadway St, Gardena, CA 90248
Round single wire toothed saw blade (Gigli) for trauma, neuro, and orthopedic surgery.

Biomet Microfixation Inc. 800-874-7711
1520 Tradeport Dr, Jacksonville, FL 32218
Various types of saws.

Biomet, Inc. 574-267-6639
56 E Bell Dr, PO Box 587, Warsaw, IN 46582
Various types of saws.

Elmed, Inc. 630-543-2792
60 W Fay Ave, Addison, IL 60101

Miltex Inc. 800-645-8000
589 Davies Dr, York, PA 17402

Zimmer Holdings, Inc. 800-613-6131
1800 W Center St, PO Box 708, Warsaw, IN 46580

SAW, MANUAL, NEUROLOGICAL (WITH ACCESSORIES)
(Cns/Neurology) 84HAC

Bestway Products Co. 310-329-0600
16602 S Broadway St, Gardena, CA 90248
Round, single wire, toothed saw blade (Gigli) for trauma, neuro, and orthopedic surgery

SAW, NASAL *(Ear/Nose/Throat) 77KBC*

Acme Of Precision Surgical Co., Inc. 973-373-6797
485 21st St, Irvington, NJ 07111
Knight, nasal.

Aesculap Implant Systems Inc. 1-800-234-9179
3773 Corporate Pkwy, Center Valley, PA 18034

Bausch & Lomb Surgical 636-255-5051
3365 Tree Court Ind Blvd, Saint Louis, MO 63122

Biomet Microfixation Inc. 800-874-7711
1520 Tradeport Dr, Jacksonville, FL 32218
Various types of saws.

Clinimed, Incorporated 877-CLINIMED
303 Markus Ct, Sandy Brae Industrial Park, Newark, DE 19713

Tuzik Boston 800-886-6363
104 Longwater Dr, Assinippi Park, Norwell, MA 02061

SAW, OTHER *(Surgery) 79RQO*

Aesculap Implant Systems Inc. 1-800-234-9179
3773 Corporate Pkwy, Center Valley, PA 18034
Saw, bone, AC-powered.

Brasseler Usa - Komet Medical 800-535-6638
1 Brasseler Blvd, Savannah, GA 31419
Orthopedic small and large sawblades.

Kmedic 800-955-0559
190 Veterans Dr, Northvale, NJ 07647

Mizzy, Inc. Of National Keystone 800-333-3131
616 Hollywood Ave, Cherry Hill, NJ 08002
HYDRO AIR CARVER, fully pneumatic 300,000 rpm air turbine with or without spray. A versatile, compact unit with lightweight handpiece for precise shaping of high strength core ceramic materials. The Hydro-Air Carver consists of base unit with filter, pressure regulator, manometer, water container and spray regulators.

Motloid Company 800-662-5021
300 N Elizabeth St, Chicago, IL 60607
DI-CUT Model Saw automates the tedious and time-consuming chore of hand-sawing crowns and bridge models.

Stryker Corp. 800-726-2725
2825 Airview Blvd, Portage, MI 49002

Ultra Tec Manufacturing, Inc. 877-542-0609
1025 E Chestnut Ave, Santa Ana, CA 92701
ULTRASLICE Precision Saw. Production saw machine for optical and structural medical components. MICROSLICE annular saw for the thinnest, lowest damage slices of fragile and/or expensive optical and crystal materials.

SAW, PNEUMATICALLY POWERED *(Surgery) 79KFK*

Depuy Orthopaedics, Inc. 800-473-3789
700 Orthopaedic Dr, P.O. Box 988, Warsaw, IN 46582
Various types of pneumatically powered saws.

Depuy-Raynham, A Div. Of Depuy Orthopaedics 800-451-2006
325 Paramount Dr, Raynham, MA 02767
Various.

Medtronic Powered Surgical Solutions 800-643-2773
4620 N Beach St, Haltom City, TX 76137
Various models motors & various models of sterile & non sterile accessories.

SAW, POWERED, AND ACCESSORIES *(Cns/Neurology) 84HAB*

Arthrex, Inc. 239-643-5553
1370 Creekside Blvd, Naples, FL 34108
Various.

Ascent Healthcare Solutions 480-763-5300
10232 S 51st St, Phoenix, AZ 85044
Saw, powered, and accessories/saw blade.

Brasseler Usa - Medical 805-650-5209
4837 McGrath St Ste J, Ventura, CA 93003
Sterile sawblade.

Depuy Orthopaedics, Inc. 800-473-3789
700 Orthopaedic Dr, P.O. Box 988, Warsaw, IN 46582
Various types of powered saws and accessories.

SAW, POWERED, AND ACCESSORIES *(cont'd)*

Depuy-Raynham, A Div. Of Depuy Orthopaedics 800-451-2006
325 Paramount Dr, Raynham, MA 02767
Various types of powered saws and accessories.

Orrex Medical Technologies, Llp 940-458-7150
403 Acker St, Sanger, TX 76266
Surgical drill, surgical reamer, oscillating saw, reciprocating saw, sterbum saw.

Tava Surgical Instruments 805-650-5209
4837 McGrath St Ste J, Ventura, CA 93003
Sterile saw blade.

SAW, SURGICAL, ENT (ELECTRIC OR PNEUMATIC) *(Ear/Nose/Throat) 77EWQ*

Clinimed, Incorporated 877-CLINIMED
303 Markus Ct, Sandy Brae Industrial Park, Newark, DE 19713

Karl Storz Endoscopy-America Inc. 800-421-0837
600 Corporate Pointe, Culver City, CA 90230

SCALE, AUTOPSY *(Pathology) 88RQP*

Algen Scale Corp. 800-836-8445
68 Enter Ln, Islandia, NY 11749
Hanging type or tabletop; digital or mechanical.

SCALE, BED *(General) 80RQQ*

Apollo Research Corporation 800-418-1718
2300 Walden Ave Ste 200, Buffalo, NY 14225

Arjo, Inc. 800-323-1245
50 Gary Ave Ste A, Roselle, IL 60172

Asi Medical Equipment, Ltd. 800-527-0443
1735 N Interstate 35E, Carrollton, TX 75006
Bed with built-in weighing system.

Convaquip Industries, Inc. 800-637-8436
4834 Derrick Dr, PO Box 3417, Abilene, TX 79601
ConvaQuip offers Bariatric scales to stand on or roll a wheelchair on with capacities up to 1000 lbs.

Md International, Inc. 305-669-9003
11300 NW 41st St, Doral, FL 33178

Scale-Tronix, Inc. 800-873-2001
200 E Post Rd, White Plains, NY 10601
$3,650 for Model 2002 SlingScale 550/250 kg. with printer, weight recall, cordless. $3,250 for Model 2001 SlingScale 450lb./200kg.; $4,295. for under-bed scales. All scales are electronic with no need for calibration.

Sr Instruments, Inc. 800-654-6360
600 Young St, Tonawanda, NY 14150
Four models: 550 kg/1200 lb patient and bed load. 300 kg/660 lb patient weight, 0.1-kg res., 20-kg patient weight change 10-g res. Other types of scales and weighing modules available. OEM inquiries welcome.

SCALE, BLOOD *(Hematology) 81RQR*

Engineering & Research Assoc., Inc. (D.B.A. Sebra) 800-625-5550
100 N Tucson Blvd, Tucson, AZ 85716
SEBRA, blood weight monitor.

Highland Labs, Inc. 508-429-2918
42 Pope Rd # B, Holliston, MA 01746
Highland's Automatic Donor Scale Model #368, is precisely designed to clamp off the donor tubing when the desired blood volume has been collected. Designed, engineered and manufactured by Highland Laboratories, Inc.

SCALE, CHAIR *(General) 80RQS*

Algen Scale Corp. 800-836-8445
68 Enter Ln, Islandia, NY 11749
$580 for mechanical beam balance model with self-contained chair and scale unit. English/metric units; 350 lb/140 kg capacity. Mechanical beam is at eye level. Digital models also available.

Arjo, Inc. 800-323-1245
50 Gary Ave Ste A, Roselle, IL 60172

Md International, Inc. 305-669-9003
11300 NW 41st St, Doral, FL 33178

Pelstar Llc (Health O Meter Professional) 800-815-6615
7400 W 100th Pl, Bridgeview, IL 60455

SCALE, CHAIR *(cont'd)*

Scale-Tronix, Inc. 800-873-2001
200 E Post Rd, White Plains, NY 10601
$2,495 for permanently mounted upholstered chair, large rubber wheels, swing-away arms and foot-rest, reads in lbs. and kilos; $2,495. for under-chair scale for continuous weight monitoring of dialysis patients, fits all chairs.

Seca Corp. 800-542-7322
1352 Charwood Rd Ste E, Hanover, MD 21076
Three models self-contained chair and scale units with fold away arms, mechanical beam balance, digital with computer interface option, wheel brakes and collapsible seat scale for UPS shipment or storage.

Sr Instruments, Inc. 800-654-6360
600 Young St, Tonawanda, NY 14150
Dialysis chair platform Model 455, 200-kg patient weight, 0.1-kg res., 20-kg weight change, 10-g res. Other types of scales and weighing modules available. OEM inquiries welcome.

SCALE, CHAIR, TRANSFER *(General) 80WXD*

Porto-Lift Corp. 800-321-1454
PO Box 5, Higgins Lake, MI 48627
$1,266.00 for scale: electronic scale with digital display in pounds and kilograms; compact, 9-volt battery operation, no wires.

Rice Lake Weighing Systems 800-472-6703
230 W Coleman St, Rice Lake, WI 54868
Designed especially for people who need assistance, equipped with a large, flat platform to accommodate people in wheel chairs or seated during dialysis.

Stretchair Patient Transfer Systems, Inc, 800-237-1162
8110 Ulmerton Rd, Largo, FL 33771
T-TLC, transfer transport light chair, get patient out of bed with only one attendant. Goes vertical or horizontal; for use in home, nursing home or hospital.

SCALE, INFANT *(General) 80FRW*

Algen Scale Corp. 800-836-8445
68 Enter Ln, Islandia, NY 11749
Portable or stationary, mechanical, battery or AC operated.

Alimed, Inc. 800-225-2610
297 High St, Dedham, MA 02026

Befour, Inc. 800-367-7109
102 N Progress Dr, Saukville, WI 53080
Various types of patient scales.

Cardinal Scale Mfg. Co. 800-641-2008
203 E Daugherty St # 151, Webb City, MO 64870
Various neonatal/pediatric/adult scales.

Champion Mfg. Inc. 800-998-5018
2601 Industrial Pkwy, Elkhart, IN 46516
Scale.

Ims, Inc. 847-956-1940
600 Bonnie Ln, Elk Grove Village, IL 60007
Hanging scale, lift scale (various types).

Jabil Global Services 502-240-1000
11201 Electron Dr, Louisville, KY 40299
Scale display.

Kentec Medical Inc. 800-825-5996
17871 Fitch, Irvine, CA 92614
Diaper weighing scale for I&O monitoring in NICU, Nursery, L&D. 2000 gram capacity, 1 gram accuracy, full range tare, battery operated with removable weighing bowl.

Mastercare Patient Equipment, Inc. 800-798-5867
2071 14th Ave, PO Box 1435, Columbus, NE 68601
Patient scale.

Mayo Medical, S.A. De C.V. 800-715-3872
Edison 1141 Nte., Col. Talleres, Monterrey N.L. 64480 Mexico

Md International, Inc. 305-669-9003
11300 NW 41st St, Doral, FL 33178

Medela, Inc. 800-435-8316
1101 Corporate Dr, McHenry, IL 60050
BABYWEIGH scale - infant scale that also automatically calculates breastmilk intake. BABYCHECKER scale for infant through toddler weighing.

O&M Enterprise 847-258-4515
641 Chelmsford Ln, Elk Grove Village, IL 60007
SCALES INFANT

Ohmeda Medical 800-345-2700
8880 Gorman Rd, Laurel, MD 20723

SCALE, INFANT *(cont'd)*

Olympic Medical Corp. 206-767-3500
5900 1st Ave S, Seattle, WA 98108
$2989.50 for SMART SCALE Model 20; $2989.50 for SMART SCALE Model 42 (Intensive care); $3,641.50 for Model 25 (Roll-Around). WARM-SCALE $3,189.50 keeps baby warm during weighing. $3,249.75 for SMART SCALE Model 60.

Pelstar Llc (Health O Meter Professional) 800-815-6615
7400 W 100th Pl, Bridgeview, IL 60455
Pediatric, chair or portable scales.

Penner Manufacturing Inc 800-732-0717
102 Grant St, PO Box 523, Aurora, NE 68818
Various.

Rice Lake Weighing Systems 800-472-6703
230 W Coleman St, Rice Lake, WI 54868
Ideal for a hospital or clinic, this convenient model allows operators to compare the baby's current weight to a stored weight without looking up records. Precision weight measurements show on a large, easy to read LCD display.

Scale-Tronix, Inc. 800-873-2001
200 E Post Rd, White Plains, NY 10601
$1,895 for four electronic models with no need for calibration; battery and line-cord operated; 45 lb./20kg, pediatric capacity, 2/10oz., 5 & 1 gram accuracy; $2,395 for incubator Model #4002 for continuous monitoring of patient weight in incubator or warmer; $1,295 for diaper scale for measuring output; one gram accurate, portable and repeatable.

Schueler & Company, Inc. 516-487-1500
PO Box 528, Stratford, CT 06615

Seca Corp. 800-542-7322
1352 Charwood Rd Ste E, Hanover, MD 21076
Seven models of manual beam balance and digtal, portable with carry case options, with and without length measures and a/c and/or battery versions.

Sr Instruments, Inc. 800-654-6360
600 Young St, Tonawanda, NY 14150
Model 615 (20,000 weight readings) with 60-lb/27-kg range, lb/oz or kg/g readout, 1/4 oz, 10-g res. Battery operated. Other types of scales and weighing modules available. OEM inquiries welcome.

Tanita Corporation Of America, Inc. 877-682-6482
2625 S Clearbrook Dr, Arlington Heights, IL 60005
Digital baby scale

United Metal Fabricators, Inc. 800-638-5322
1316 Eisenhower Blvd, Johnstown, PA 15904

SCALE, LABORATORY *(Chemistry) 75RQT*

A&D Medical 800-726-7099
1756 Automation Pkwy, San Jose, CA 95131

Algen Scale Corp. 800-836-8445
68 Enter Ln, Islandia, NY 11749
Digital or mechanical analytical balances.

Alimed, Inc. 800-225-2610
297 High St, Dedham, MA 02026

Burkhart Roentgen Intl. Inc. 800-USA-XRAY
5201 8th Ave S, Gulfport, FL 33707
Radio-opaque measuring scales, x-ray caliper, cranial angulator.

Cole-Parmer Instrument Inc. 800-323-4340
625 E Bunker Ct, Vernon Hills, IL 60061

Edmund Industrial Optics 800-363-1992
101 E Gloucester Pike, Barrington, NJ 08007

Md International, Inc. 305-669-9003
11300 NW 41st St, Doral, FL 33178

Scientech, Inc. 303-444-1361
5649 Arapahoe Ave, Boulder, CO 80303
22 electronic models -$995 to $3,495 with capacities from 150 to 12000 g.

Sr Instruments, Inc. 800-654-6360
600 Young St, Tonawanda, NY 14150
200-gram x 0.1-gram scale.

Troemner Llc 800-352-7705
201 Wolf Dr, PO Box 87, West Deptford, NJ 08086
Precision calibration weights

SCALE, PLATFORM, WHEELCHAIR *(Physical Med) 89INF*

Algen Scale Corp. 800-836-8445
68 Enter Ln, Islandia, NY 11749
Digital or mechanical; portable or stationary. Wheel 'n Weigh.

SCALE, PLATFORM, WHEELCHAIR *(cont'd)*

Alimed, Inc. 800-225-2610
297 High St, Dedham, MA 02026

Befour, Inc. 800-367-7109
102 N Progress Dr, Saukville, WI 53080
Wheelchair scale.

Cardinal Scale Mfg. Co. 800-641-2008
203 E Daugherty St # 151, Webb City, MO 64870
Various digital wheelchair scales.

Fairbanks Scales, Inc. 800-451-4107
821 Locust St, Kansas City, MO 64106
Wheelchair scale.

Kistler Instrument Corp. 716-691-5100
75 John Glenn Dr, Amherst, NY 14228
$8150 for Model 9281B11, less electronics; 6-variable measure, piezoelectric; measures 3 orthogonal directions, point of force, and free moment.

Pelstar Llc (Health O Meter Professional) 800-815-6615
7400 W 100th Pl, Bridgeview, IL 60455

Richardson Products, Inc. 888-928-7297
9408 Gulfstream Rd, Frankfort, IL 60423
Wheelchair scale.

Scale-Tronix, Inc. 800-873-2001
200 E Post Rd, White Plains, NY 10601
$2,250 for Model 6002 ramp scale for weighing patients in wheelchairs; electronic cordless, reads in pounds and kilograms, 880lb. capacity; $2,750 for Model 6702, 880lb. capacity, rubber wheels, optional hand rail for standing patients; $4,550 for flush mounted floor scale, used for wheelchair, standing and stretcher patients, 800lb. capacity. And Bariatric Stand-On Scales. 1000 Lb. Capacity. Low profile platforms $1600 - $3000.

Sr Instruments, Inc. 800-654-6360
600 Young St, Tonawanda, NY 14150
Wheelchair scale Model 755, 1000 lb/450 kg range, 0.1-kg or 1-lb res., auto-tare. Handrails and height bar available; battery operation - 20,000 weight readings. Other types of scales and weighing modules available. OEM inquiries welcome.

SCALE, SPONGE, SURGICAL, ELECTRICALLY-POWERED
(General) 80MRL

Pondus Medical, Inc. 215-219-9152
5044 Davis Dr, Doylestown, PA 18902

SCALE, STAND-ON *(General) 80FRI*

Algen Scale Corp. 800-836-8445
68 Enter Ln, Islandia, NY 11749
Obesity scale (800 to 1,000 lb capacity); mailroom scale, physician scale and platform laundry scales. Scale, Medical Waste - Weighs and tracks hazardous medical waste bags for disposal or carting.

Alimed, Inc. 800-225-2610
297 High St, Dedham, MA 02026
Balance beam, step-on floor and electronic models.

Armstrong Medical Industries, Inc. 800-323-4220
575 Knightsbridge Pkwy, Lincolnshire, IL 60069

Atd-American Co. 800-523-2300
135 Greenwood Ave, Wyncote, PA 19095

Befour, Inc. 800-367-7109
102 N Progress Dr, Saukville, WI 53080
Various types of patient scales.

Cardinal Scale Mfg. Co. 800-641-2008
203 E Daugherty St # 151, Webb City, MO 64870
Various types of doctor office/hospital/patient scales.

Cardiocom LLC 888-243-8881
7980 Century Blvd, Chanhassen, MN 55317
Stand-on scale.

Chirotron, Inc. 206-364-1262
20126 Ballinger Way NE # 295, Shoreline, WA 98155
Chirotron, electronic body balance scale.

Creative Health Products, Inc. 800-742-4478
5148 Saddle Ridge Rd, Plymouth, MI 48170
Balance beam scales, DETECTO $204.00,HEALTH-O-METER $209.00, SECA $235.00. Strain Gauge Digital Floor Scales, A&D ENGINEERING $120.00 from CHP.

Demetech Corp. 888-324-2447
3530 NW 115th Ave, Doral, FL 33178
Dr's office patient scales (stand-on).

Express Manufacturing, Inc. 714-979-2228
3519 W Warner Ave, Santa Ana, CA 92704

SCALE, STAND-ON *(cont'd)*

Fairbanks Scales, Inc. 800-451-4107
821 Locust St, Kansas City, MO 64106
Health scale.

Health Hero Network, Inc. 650-779-9160
2000 Seaport Blvd Ste 400, Redwood City, CA 94063
Scale, stand on, patient.

Honeywell Hommed, Llc 888-353-5440
3400 Intertech Dr Ste 200, Brookfield, WI 53045
Scale.

Mayo Medical, S.A. De C.V. 800-715-3872
Edison 1141 Nte., Col. Talleres, Monterrey N.L. 64480 Mexico

Md International, Inc. 305-669-9003
11300 NW 41st St, Doral, FL 33178

O&M Enterprise 847-258-4515
641 Chelmsford Ln, Elk Grove Village, IL 60007
SCALES PHYSICIAN, TRANSFER

Pelstar Llc (Health O Meter Professional) 800-815-6615
7400 W 100th Pl, Bridgeview, IL 60455
New digital weighing scale. New 500# capacity beam scale

Rice Lake Weighing Systems 800-472-6703
230 W Coleman St, Rice Lake, WI 54868
The quintessential physician's scale, combines precision weighing with height measurement. With a focus on patient comfort this scale is equipped with a slip-resistant, heavy duty cast iron base that eliminates the need for a mat. Ideal for weight loss centers, clinics, and fitness clubs.

Scale-Tronix, Inc. 800-873-2001
200 E Post Rd, White Plains, NY 10601
$1,195 to $2,195 for 4 models of low platform stand-on scales; stable, mobile, repeatable electronic, no need for recalibration, battery and line cord operated; Model 5002: capacity, 1/10lb./100 gram accuracy; wrap-around hand rail $2,195.00 for physicians' stand-on scale, 19x15 platform 11/4 high, 800lb. capacity; $1,395 for portable stand-on scale, 400lb. capacity, designed for visiting nurse usage $1,195.

Schueler & Company, Inc. 516-487-1500
PO Box 528, Stratford, CT 06615

Seca Corp. 800-542-7322
1352 Charwood Rd Ste E, Hanover, MD 21076
Twenty one models of mechanical beam, digital, digital computer interface, dial spring, strain gauge, a/c and/or battery (alkaline, nicad, lithium), compact floor or upright and portable with carry bags.

Servicios Paraclinicios S.A. 83-33-8400
Madero No. 3330 Pte., Monterrey N.L. 64020 Mexico

Sr Instruments, Inc. 800-654-6360
600 Young St, Tonawanda, NY 14150
Stand-on scale Model 555, 1000 lb/450 kg range, 0.1-kg or 1-lb res., auto-tare, casting. Optional side rails and height bar available. Operates on D cell batteries. 20,000+ weight readings.

Sunbeam Products, Inc. 561-912-4100
2381 NW Executive Center Dr, Boca Raton, FL 33431
Scale.

System Sensor 630-377-6674
3825 Ohio Ave, Saint Charles, IL 60174

Tanita Corporation Of America, Inc. 877-682-6482
2625 S Clearbrook Dr, Arlington Heights, IL 60005
Patient scale

Vestibular Technologies, Llc 307-637-5711
205 County Road 128a, Suite 200, Cheyenne, WY 82007-1831
Various models of scales.

SCALE, SURGICAL SPONGE *(General) 80FQA*

Scale-Tronix, Inc. 800-873-2001
200 E Post Rd, White Plains, NY 10601
$1,295.00 for one gram accurate stainless steel tray.

SCALER, PERIODONTIC *(Dental And Oral) 76EMN*

Aesculap Implant Systems Inc. 1-800-234-9179
3773 Corporate Pkwy, Center Valley, PA 18034

Arnold Tuber Industries 716-648-3363
97 Main St, Hamburg, NY 14075
Scaler, periodontic, dental hand instruments.

Biomet Microfixation Inc. 800-874-7711
1520 Tradeport Dr, Jacksonville, FL 32218
Scaler.

SCALER, PERIODONTIC *(cont'd)*

Dental Usa, Inc. 815-363-8003
5005 McCullom Lake Rd, McHenry, IL 60050
Scaler.

Dentalez Group 866-DTE-INFO
101 Lindenwood Dr Ste 225, Valleybrooke Corporate Center
Malvern, PA 19355

Dentalez Group, Stardental Division 717-291-1161
1816 Colonial Village Ln, Lancaster, PA 17601
Rc cement non-staining.

Disposable Surgical Innovations 516-377-1497
958 Church St, Baldwin, NY 11510
Implant cleaner.

Dp Manufacture Corp. 305-640-9894
1460 NW 107th Ave Ste H, Doral, FL 33172
Periodontic scaler.

E.A. Beck & Co. 949-645-4072
657 W 19th St Ste E, P O Box 10857, Costa Mesa, CA 92627
Scaler.

H & H Co. 909-390-0373
4435 E Airport Dr Ste 108, Ontario, CA 91761
Scaler, periodontic.

Hartzell & Son, G. 800-950-2206
2372 Stanwell Cir, Concord, CA 94520

Hu-Friedy Manufacturing Co., Inc. 800-483-7433
3232 N Rockwell St, Chicago, IL 60618
$24.60 to $28.50 each, 160 types.

Lemoy International, Inc. 847-427-0840
95 King St, Elk Grove Village, IL 60007
AUTOTRAC Piezoelectric scaler for dentists/veterinarians 100% American made and made to order.

Maximum Dental, Inc. 631-245-2176
600 Meadowlands Pkwy Ste 269, Secaucus, NJ 07094

Micro-Dent Inc. 866-526-1166
379 Hollow Hill Rd, Wauconda, IL 60084
Scaler, periodontic.

Nobel Biocare Usa, Llc 800-579-6515
22715/22725 Savi Ranch Parkway, Yorba Linda, CA 92887
Prosthetic instrument.

Nordent Manufacturing, Inc. 800-966-7336
610 Bonnie Ln, Elk Grove Village, IL 60007
$19.00 each.

Pac-Dent Intl., Inc. 909-839-0888
21078 Commerce Point Dr, Walnut, CA 91789
Implant scaler.

Pdt, Inc. 406-626-4153
12201 Moccasin Ct, Missoula, MT 59808
Various.

Premier Dental Products Co. 888-670-6100
1710 Romano Dr, PO Box 4500, Plymouth Meeting, PA 19462

Pulpdent Corp. 800-343-4342
80 Oakland St, Watertown, MA 02472
No common name listed.

Sci-Dent, Inc. 800-323-4145
210 Dowdle St Ste 2, Algonquin, IL 60102

Small Bone Innovations, Inc. 215-428-1791
1380 S Pennsylvania Ave, Morrisville, PA 19067
Scaler, periodontic.

Suter Dental Manufacturing Company, Inc. 800-368-8376
632 Cedar St, Chico, CA 95928

Tpc Advanced Technology, Inc. 626-810-4337
18525 Gale Ave, City Of Industry, CA 91748
Advanced 750 Piezo Scaler--dental periodontal scaler.

Wykle Research, Inc. 775-887-7500
2222 College Pkwy, Carson City, NV 89706
Periodontic scaler.

SCALER, ROTARY *(Dental And Oral) 76ELB*

Aesculap Implant Systems Inc. 1-800-234-9179
3773 Corporate Pkwy, Center Valley, PA 18034

Dentalez Group 866-DTE-INFO
101 Lindenwood Dr Ste 225, Valleybrooke Corporate Center
Malvern, PA 19355

Ellman International, Inc. 800-835-5355
3333 Royal Ave, Rockville Centre, NY 11572

SCALER, ULTRASONIC *(Dental And Oral) 76ELC*

A-Dec, Inc. 800-547-1883
2601 Crestview Dr, Newberg, OR 97132
Ultrasonic scaler.

Acteon Inc. 800-289-6367
124 Gaither Dr Ste 140, Mount Laurel, NJ 08054
SUPRASSON, PMAX, P5 BOOSTER.

America Green Dent., Mfg. 323-265-7000
3432 E 14th St, Commerce, CA 90023
Dental ultrasonic scaler.

American Eagle Instruments, Inc. 406-549-7451
6575 Butler Creek Rd, Missoula, MT 59808
Types of ultrasonic dental scalers.

Coltene/Whaledent Inc. 330-916-8858
235 Ascot Pkwy, Cuyahoga Falls, OH 44223
Scaler.

D.B.I. America Corp. 813-909-9005
254 Crystal Grove Blvd, Lutz, FL 33548
Ultrasonic scaler.

Dentalez Group 866-DTE-INFO
101 Lindenwood Dr Ste 225, Valleybrooke Corporate Center
Malvern, PA 19355

Dentalez Group, Stardental Division 717-291-1161
1816 Colonial Village Ln, Lancaster, PA 17601
Explorer, operative.

Dentronix, Inc. 800-523-5944
235 Ascot Pkwy, Cuyahoga Falls, OH 44223
Biosonic Ultrasonic Scaler System, ultrasonic scaler designed for removal of adhesive during debonding procedures.

Engler Engineering Corp. 800-445-8581
1099 E 47th St, Hialeah, FL 33013
Ultrasonic scaler, $1655.00 SON-MATE-Ultrasonic scaler/polisher; SONUS V Ultrasonic Scaler- $785.00

Health Science Products, Inc. 800-237-5794
1489 Hueytown Rd, Hueytown, AL 35023
HSP ART PIEZO SCALER is a quiet and effective scaler with little required coolant water that can be built into the HSP unit or is available in a tabletop version.

Hu-Friedy Manufacturing Co., Inc. 800-483-7433
3232 N Rockwell St, Chicago, IL 60618
Ultrasonic inserts for ultrasonic sealing units, $94.00-$140.00.

Kinetic Instruments, Inc. 800-233-2346
17 Berkshire Blvd, Bethel, CT 06801
Vipersonic endo/scaler.

Mti Precision Products 732-905-7440
175 Oberlin Ave N, Lakewood, NJ 08701
Scaler, sonic.

Obtura Spartan 800-344-1321
13729 Shoreline Ct E, Earth City, MO 63045
Piezo electric ultrasonic.

Osada, Inc. 800-426-7232
8436 W 3rd St Ste 695, Los Angeles, CA 90048
ENAC.

Parkell, Inc. 800-243-7446
300 Executive Dr, Edgewood, NY 11717
TurboSENSOR ultrasonic scaler without tips, (features autoclavable handpiece sheath). TurboPIEZO scaler.

South East Instruments Corp. 352-332-0125
3706 NW 97th Blvd, Gainesville, FL 32606
Ultrasonic scaler.

Tpc Advanced Technology, Inc. 626-810-4337
18525 Gale Ave, City Of Industry, CA 91748
Ultrasonic scaler.

Ultrasonic Services, Inc. 713-665-4949
7126 Mullins Dr, Houston, TX 77081
Ultrasonic dental scaler.

Westside Packaging, Llc. 909-570-3508
1700 S Baker Ave Ste A, Ontario, CA 91761
Ultrasonic scaler insert.

Young Colorado, Llc. 800-325-1881
13705 Shoreline Ct E, Earth City, MO 63045
Ultrasonic cleaner for dental.

Young O/S Llc 800-325-1881
1663 Fenton Business Park Ct, Fenton, MO 63026
Ultrasonic scaler, various.

SCALES, DIALYSIS *(General) 80KOF*

Lee Medical International, Inc. 800-433-8950
612 Distributors Row, Harahan, LA 70123
Detecto scales.

SCALPEL, ONE-PIECE (KNIFE) *(Surgery) 79GDX*

Aesculap Implant Systems Inc. 1-800-234-9179
3773 Corporate Pkwy, Center Valley, PA 18034

American Safety Razor Co. 540-248-8000
1 Razor Blade Ln, Verona, VA 24482
Safety disposable scalpel.

Arista Surgical Supply Co. Inc. 800-223-1984
297 High St, Dedham, MA 02026

Arkray Factory Usa, Inc. 952-646-3168
5182 W 76th St, Minneapolis, MN 55439
Safety scalpel.

Bd Caribe, Ltd. 201-847-4298
Rd. 183, Km. 20.3, Las Piedras, PR 00771
Disposable scalpel.

C & A Scientific Co. Inc. 703-330-1413
7241 Gabe Ct, Manassas, VA 20109
PREMIERE Scalpel w/ plastic handle. Sterile, high carbon.

Cincinnati Surgical Company 800-544-3100
11256 Cornell Park Dr, Cincinnati, OH 45242
Disposable scalpels and mini-scalpels.

Controlled Molding, Inc. 724-253-3550
3043 Perry Hwy, Hadley, PA 16130
Scapel.

Depuy Mitek, A Johnson & Johnson Company 800-451-2006
50 Scotland Blvd, Bridgewater, MA 02324
Graft knives.

Globe Medical Tech, Inc. 713-365-9595
1766 W Sam Houston Pkwy N, Houston, TX 77043
Safety retractable scalpel, size #10, #11, #15.

Griff Industries, Inc. 800-709-4743
19761 Bahama St, Northridge, CA 91324
BladeGlove safety scalpel system in both disposable and reusable configurations

Habley Medical Technology Corp. 800-729-1994
15721 Bernardo Heights Pkwy Ste B-30, San Diego, CA 92128
Safety scalpels that do not need internal springs.

Havel's Inc. 800-638-4770
3726 Lonsdale St, Cincinnati, OH 45227

Healer Products, Llc 914-663-6300
427 Commerce Ln Ste 1, West Berlin, NJ 08091
Scalpel.

Health Care Logistics, Inc. 800-848-1633
450 Town St, PO Box 25, Circleville, OH 43113
Various sizes of sterile, disposable surgical scalpels.

Hospital Marketing Svcs. Company, Inc. 800-786-5094
162 Great Hill Rd./ Ind. Park, Naugatuck, CT 06770
HMS SURGIBLADE - sizes 10, 11, 12, 15, 20, 21, 22, 23. Cat. No 5510, 5511, 5512, 5515, 5520, 5521, 5522, 5523.

Lampac International Ltd. 636-797-3659
230 N Lake Dr, Hillsboro, MO 63050
Disposable, with stainless steel blade.

Medisiss 866-866-7477
2747 SW 6th St, Redmond, OR 97756
Various one piece scalpels,sterile.

Miltex Inc. 800-645-8000
589 Davies Dr, York, PA 17402

Myco Medical 800-454-6926
158 Towerview Ct, Cary, NC 27513
Full range of Safety and Non-safety Scalpels

Oratronics, Inc. 212-986-0050
405 Lexington Ave, New York, NY 10174
Scalpel handle.

Personna Medical/Div. Of American Safety Razor Co. 800-457-2222
1 Razor Blade Ln, Verona, VA 24482
PERSONNA PLUS Disposable Safety Scalpel has an innovative plastic sheath utilizing the PERSONNA PLUS surgical blades with microcoat. You never have to touch the blade, no loading or unloading. 5 blade sizes available. Also available, PERSONNA Safety Scalpel, 3 blade sizes, retractable blade shield; sterile, disposable scalpels.

SCALPEL, ONE-PIECE (KNIFE) *(cont'd)*

Propper Manufacturing Co., Inc. 800-832-4300
3604 Skillman Ave, Long Island City, NY 11101

Smith & Nephew, Inc., Endoscopy Division 800-343-8386
130 Forbes Blvd, Mansfield, MA 02048

Tran Pa-C, Inc. 321-276-5407
3348 Herringridge Dr, Orlando, FL 32812
Trans-catheter dissector.

SCALPEL, ULTRASONIC *(Surgery) 79SJE*

Incisiontech 800-213-7809
9 Technology Dr, Staunton, VA 24401

SCALPEL, ULTRASONIC, REPROCESSED *(Surgery) 79NLQ*

Medisiss 866-866-7477
2747 SW 6th St, Redmond, OR 97756
Various reprocessed ultrasonic instruments, sterile.

Sterilmed, Inc. 763-488-3400
11400 73rd Ave N Ste 100, Maple Grove, MN 55369
Harmonic scalpels.

SCANNER, BREAST, THERMOGRAPHIC, ULTRASONIC, COMPUTER-ASSTD. *(Obstetrics/Gyn) 85MGK*

Medical Tactile, Inc. 310-641-8228
5757 W Century Blvd Ste 600, Los Angeles, CA 90045
Electronic Palpation device for documenting the Clinical Breast Examination (CBE.

SCANNER, COLOR *(Dental And Oral) 76KZN*

Advanced American Biotechnology (Aab) 714-870-0290
1166 E Valencia Dr Unit 6C, Fullerton, CA 92831
Laser Densitometry Station: 0-4.2 OD linear range. Reflectance-transmission-UV fluorescence and white light. High speed; one lane per 2 secs, 2D in 12 minutes..1D, @d, DNA, RFLP software. Scanner attachment to scan 35x45cm x-ray film ...$14,500.

SCANNER, COMPUTED TOMOGRAPHY, CINE
(Radiology) 90WMF

M & I Medical Sales, Inc. 305-663-6444
4711 SW 72nd Ave, Miami, FL 33155

SCANNER, COMPUTED TOMOGRAPHY, X-RAY (CAT, CT)
(Cns/Neurology) 84JXD

Consumaquip Corporation 305-592-4510
7240 NW 12th St, Miami, FL 33126

Marconi Medical Systems 800-323-0550
595 Miner Rd, Cleveland, OH 44143
PQ and IQ Systems.

Myco Instrumentation Source, Inc. 425-228-4239
PO Box 354, Renton, WA 98057

Schaerer Mayfield Usa 800-755-6381
4900 Charlemar Dr, Cincinnati, OH 45227
Mayfield Mobilscan CT Portable CAT Scanner: Portable CT that can be used in a multitude of departments (OR, ICU, ER).

Spectron Corp. 425-827-9317
934 S Burlington Blvd # 603, Burlington, WA 98233
Reconditioned equipment.

SCANNER, COMPUTED TOMOGRAPHY, X-RAY, FULL BODY
(Radiology) 90THS

Atlas Medical Technologies 909-923-7887
1137 E Philadelphia St, Ontario, CA 91761
GE and Marconi (Picker) are our specialties; Multi slice, single slice and Big bore.

Calmaquip Engineering Corp. 305-592-4510
7240 NW 12th St, Miami, FL 33126

Hitachi Medical Systems America, Inc. 800-800-3106
1959 Summit Commerce Park, Twinsburg, OH 44087
Hitachi's CXR4 is a clinical application and performance-driven multi-slice CT featuring high quality imaging, efficient workflow, and Hitachi's tradition of high reliability. By combining the advantages of a high efficiency ceramic detector array with proprietary technologies for high pitch acquisitions, real-time reconstruction and display, large volume data transmission, and advanced clinical application software, Hitachi has created a multi-slice CT solution that is expansive in clinical applications, easy for the user to operate and comfortable for the patient.

King's Medical 330-653-3968
1894 Georgetown Rd, Hudson, OH 44236
Fee for service of fixed site and mobile CT scanners.

SCANNER, COMPUTED TOMOGRAPHY, X-RAY, FULL BODY
(cont'd)

Marconi Medical Systems 800-323-0550
595 Miner Rd, Cleveland, OH 44143

Radiographic Digital Imaging, Inc. 310-921-9559
20406 Earl St, Torrance, CA 90503

Shimadzu Medical Systems 800-228-1429
20101 S Vermont Ave, Torrance, CA 90502
3 Models: SCT-7000T Series, SCT-6800T Series, SCT-4800TZ Series.

SCANNER, COMPUTED TOMOGRAPHY, X-RAY, HEAD
(Radiology) 90TEI

Atlas Medical Technologies 909-923-7887
1137 E Philadelphia St, Ontario, CA 91761

Carl Zeiss Meditec Inc. 877-486-7473
5160 Hacienda Dr, Dublin, CA 94568
OPTICAL COHERENCE TOMOGRAPHY SCANNER - The Humphrey Optical Coherence Tomography (OCT) Scanner is a new diagnostic tool for cross-sectional imaging of the retina. The high-resolution images (15 um) show the living histology of the posterior pole with 10 times greater resolution than any other technique available. OCT reproducibly quantifies Retinal and Nerve Fiber Layer Thickness to better than 11 um. An OCT examination is non-contact, non-invasive and is performed simular to infrared slit-lamp ophthalmoscopy. OCT is an invaluable research tool and has demonstrated clinical efficacy for diagnosing macular holes and monitoring glaucoma and diabetic retinopathy.

Marconi Medical Systems 800-323-0550
595 Miner Rd, Cleveland, OH 44143

SCANNER, COMPUTED TOMOGRAPHY, X-RAY, SPECIAL PROCEDURE *(Radiology) 90JAK*

Aadco Medical, Inc. 800-225-9014
2279 VT Route 66, Randolph, VT 05060
Injector mount.

Analogic Corporation 978-326-4000
8 Centennial Dr, Peabody, MA 01960

Atlas Medical Technologies 909-923-7887
1137 E Philadelphia St, Ontario, CA 91761

Ge Medical Systems, Llc 262-548-2355
3000 N Grandview Blvd, W-417, Waukesha, WI 53188
Various models of ct systems.

Imaging Sciences International, Llc 215-997-5666
1910 N Penn Rd, Hatfield, PA 19440
Computed tomography x-ray system.

Imtec Imaging L.L.C. 800-226-3220
2401 N Commerce St, Ardmore, OK 73401
Cone beam computed tomography scanner.

Marconi Medical Systems 800-323-0550
595 Miner Rd, Cleveland, OH 44143

Medical Devices International 504-455-8311
3724 Severn Ave, Metairie, LA 70002
pre owned

Neurologica Corporation 978-564-8500
14 Electronics Ave, Danvers, MA 01923
Ct x-ray system.

Portal, Inc. 435-753-3598
1350 N 200 W Ste 6, Logan, UT 84341
Axial compression device.

Radiomed Corporation 866-649-0300
1 Industrial Way, Tyngsboro, MA 01879
Visicoil Linear Flexible tissue tracking marker.

Superdimension Inc. 763-210-4015
161 Cheshire Ln N Ste 100, Minneapolis, MN 55441
Bronchoscope.

Toshiba America Medical Systems 800-421-1968
2441 Michelle Dr, Tustin, CA 92780
Models TSX-101A/6D, TSX-101A/4D, TSX-021A/3D, TSX-021A/6D, TSX-021A/4D, TSX-021A/1D, TSX-021B/1F.

Varian Medical Systems Interay 800-468-3729
3235 Fortune Dr, North Charleston, SC 29418
Scanner tube housing assembly.

Viatronix, Inc. 631-444-9700
25 Health Sciences Dr Ste 203, Stony Brook, NY 11790
Image processing system.

SCANNER, COMPUTED TOMOGRAPHY, X-RAY, SPECIAL PROCEDURE *(cont'd)*

Xoran Technologies, Inc. 800-709-6726
309 N 1st St, Ann Arbor, MI 48103
Computed tomography (ct), cone-beam ct, volume ct.

SCANNER, EMISSION COMPUTED TOMOGRAPHY
(Radiology) 90KPS

Areeda Assoc., Ltd. 323-653-5515
1160 Glen Arbor Ave, Los Angeles, CA 90041
Image processing system.

Cardiovascular Imaging Technologies, Llc 816-531-2842
4320 Wornall Rd Ste 55, Kansas City, MO 64111
Display & processing nuclear computer syst. for gated spect & pet myocardial per.

Digirad Corp. 800-947-6134
13950 Stowe Dr, Poway, CA 92064
Gamma cameras and accessories.

Ge Medical Systems, Llc 262-548-2355
3000 N Grandview Blvd, W-417, Waukesha, WI 53188
Various models of pet systems.

Invia, Llc 734-205-1231
3025 Boardwalk St Ste 200, Ann Arbor, MI 48108
Software for nuclear medicine imaging systems.

Is2 Research Inc. 613-228-8755
3 6-20 Gurdwara Rd, Nepean K2E 8B3 Canada
Multiple

Medimage, Inc. 734-665-5400
6276 Jackson Rd Ste G, Ann Arbor, MI 48103
Galen, deltamanager, m-link.

Medx, Inc. 847-463-2020
3456 N Ridge Ave Ste 100, Arlington Heights, IL 60004
Emission computed tomography system.

Mie America, Inc. 847-981-6100
420 Bennett Rd, Elk Grove Village, IL 60007
Nuclear medicine computer for various gamma cameras.

Mimvista Corp. 216-896-9798
25200 Chagrin Blvd Ste 200, Cleveland, OH 44122
Mim.

Naviscan Inc. 858-587-3641
6865 Flanders Dr Ste B, San Diego, CA 92121
Pet scanner.

Nuclear Cardiology Systems, Inc. 303-541-0044
5660 Airport Blvd Ste 101, Boulder, CO 80301
Gamma camera.

Positron Corporation 800-766-2984
1304 Langham Creek Dr Ste 300, Houston, TX 77084
Attrius PET Scanner

Terarecon, Inc. 877-354-1100
2955 Campus Dr Ste 325, San Mateo, CA 94403
Gamma camera.

The Regents Of The University Of Michigan
3003 S State St Rm 1072, Ann Arbor, MI 48109
Software medical imaging systems.

Toshiba America Medical Systems 800-421-1968
2441 Michelle Dr, Tustin, CA 92780
T.CAM 1E, T.CAM2AP, T.CAM2E, T.CAM/CARDIO/V, T.CAM2E/D.

Transphoton Corporation 305-234-0836
14350 SW 142nd Ave, Miami, FL 33186
Gamma camera-spect gamma camera; emission computed tomography (ect) system.

Trionix Research Laboratory, Inc. 330-425-9055
8037 Bavaria Rd, Twinsburg, OH 44087
Nuclear medical imaging device.

Ugm Medical Systems, Inc. 425-487-7000
3611 Market St, Philadelphia, PA 19104
Emission computed tomography systems and accessories.

Verista Imaging Inc. 712-353-6225
201 S 4th St, Castana, IA 51010
Isocam gamma camera.

SCANNER, FLUORESCENT *(Radiology) 90JAO*

Marconi Medical Systems 800-323-0550
595 Miner Rd, Cleveland, OH 44143

SCANNER, LONG-TERM, ECG, RECORDING
(Cardiovascular) 74RQU

Braemar, Inc. 800-328-2719
1285 Corporate Center Dr Ste 150, Eagan, MN 55121
CD350 High speed Holter scanner, 3.5 in. form factor with optional interface electronics. SYS350, high speed Holter scanner subsystem.

Ge Medical Systems Information Technologies 800-643-6439
8200 W Tower Ave, Milwaukee, WI 53223
Several models available; accepts cassette tapes, reel tapes, and solid-state recordings. Fully automated analysis of Holter data, including pacemaker analysis provided. Options include batch processing, expanded on-line availability, and report transmissions and storage. CENTRA system offers optional resting ECG, exercise ECG, signal-averaged ECG, and pacemaker evaluation.

New Life Systems, Inc. 954-972-4600
PO Box 8767, Coral Springs, FL 33075
Holter scanners, cassettes or reel to reel.

Telescan Medical Systems 800-388-4324
26424 Table Meadow Rd, Auburn, CA 95602
Telescan offers a complete line of cardiac event recording transtelephonic monitoring devices and services. In addition to the 12 bed memory, ECG pager sized recorders are offered for chest or fingertip ECG recordings, and loop-memory recorders are available for pre-symptom event recording.

SCANNER, MAGNETIC RESONANCE (NMR/MRI)
(Radiology) 90JAM

Atlas Medical Technologies 909-923-7887
1137 E Philadelphia St, Ontario, CA 91761

Consumaquip Corporation 305-592-4510
7240 NW 12th St, Miami, FL 33126

Fonar Corp. 888-NEEDMRI
110 Marcus Dr, Melville, NY 11747
ULTIMATE low-cost MRI scanners (.3T resistive and .3T permanent magnet) with quiet, non-claustrophobic Open Gap and negligible fringe field for various body images. Stand-up scanner can accomodate a standing patient, allowing images of the spine and joints to be taken while the patient is bearing his or her full weight. Stand-Up MRI, allows patients to simply walk in and be scanned. This MRI allows all parts of the body to be imaged in the weight bearing state.

King's Medical 330-653-3968
1894 Georgetown Rd, Hudson, OH 44236
Lessors of fixed site and mobile interim MRI scanners. Fee for service, equity participation.

Magnevu 760-929-8000
2225 Faraday Ave Ste F, Carlsbad, CA 92008
MagneVu makes MRI available in settings where the use of traditional systems is not feasible due their high cost and complexity of operation. The MagneVu point-of-care scanner expands the use of MRI beyond the centralized imaging facility to front-line physicians and new clinical settings. Using breakthrough imaging techniques, Magnevu eliminates 90% of the cost, weight, and power consumption of traditional MRI. Current applications include rheumatology, orthopedics, and diabetic wound care.

Marconi Medical Systems 800-323-0550
595 Miner Rd, Cleveland, OH 44143
0.23T outlook, 0.5 asset, 1.0T vista and 1.5T edge.

Medical Devices International 504-455-8311
3724 Severn Ave, Metairie, LA 70002
3 to 5 years old

Numa, Inc. 603-883-1909
10 Northern Blvd Ste 12, Amherst, NH 03031
Image translation system.

SCANNER, NUCLEAR EMISSION COMPUTED TOMOGRAPHY (ECT) *(Radiology) 90THG*

Diagnostix Plus, Inc. 516-536-2670
100 N Village Ave Ste 33, Rockville Centre, NY 11570

Marconi Medical Systems 800-323-0550
595 Miner Rd, Cleveland, OH 44143
Prism Series.

SCANNER, NUCLEAR, RECTILINEAR *(Radiology) 90IYW*

Marconi Medical Systems 800-323-0550
595 Miner Rd, Cleveland, OH 44143

SCANNER, NUCLEAR, TOMOGRAPHIC *(Radiology) 90JWM*

Marconi Medical Systems 800-323-0550
595 Miner Rd, Cleveland, OH 44143

SCANNER, NUCLEAR, TOMOGRAPHIC *(cont'd)*

Numa, Inc. 603-883-1909
10 Northern Blvd Ste 12, Amherst, NH 03031
Nuclear medicine acquisition system.

Toshiba America Medical Systems 800-421-1968
2441 Michelle Dr, Tustin, CA 92780

Trionix Research Laboratory, Inc. 330-425-9055
8037 Bavaria Rd, Twinsburg, OH 44087
Monad.

SCANNER, POSITRON EMISSION TOMOGRAPHY (PET)
(Radiology) 90ULI

Atlas Medical Technologies 909-923-7887
1137 E Philadelphia St, Ontario, CA 91761

Diagnostix Plus, Inc. 516-536-2670
100 N Village Ave Ste 33, Rockville Centre, NY 11570

Hitachi Medical Systems America, Inc. 800-800-3106
1959 Summit Commerce Park, Twinsburg, OH 44087
Hitachi offers the Sceptre, a dedicated whole body system that features Lutetium Oxyorthosilicate (LSO) crystal technology. One-touch automatic protocols and an ergonomic gantry design for patient comfort allows fast, accurate patient positioning and improved workflow. Combining advanced technologies in 3D acquisition, iterative reconstruction and randoms and scatter corrections, Sceptre offers unparalleled diagnostic efficacy, operational efficiency and long-term economic value.

SCANNER, ULTRASONIC (PULSED DOPPLER)
(Radiology) 90IYN

Advanced Biosensor, Inc. 803-407-3044
400 Arbor Lake Dr Ste B450, Columbia, SC 29223
Peripheral vascular doppler.

Blatek, Inc. 814-231-2085
2820 E College Ave Ste F, State College, PA 16801

Boston Scientific-Neurovascular 510-440-7700
47900 Bayside Pkwy, Fremont, CA 94538
Ultrasonic pulsed doppler.

Cardinal Healthcare 209, Inc. 610-862-0800
5225 Verona Rd, Fitchburg, WI 53711
Doppler ultrasound.

Ep Medsystems, Inc. 609-753-8533
575 N Route 73 Bldg D, West Berlin, NJ 08091
Ultrasonic pulsed doppler imaging system.

Evolve Manufacturing Technologies Inc. 650-968-9292
960 Linda Vista Ave, Mountain View, CA 94043
Diagnostic ultrasound.

Ge Medical Systems Ultrasound And Primary Care Dia 608-826-7050
726 Heartland Trl, Madison, WI 53717
Ultrasonic imaging systems.

Ge Medical Systems, Llc 847-277-5002
4855 W Electric Ave, West Milwaukee, WI 53219
Various models of diagnostic doppler ultrasound systems.

Huntleigh Healthcare Llc. 800-223-1218
40 Christopher Way, Eatontown, NJ 07724

Imacor Llc. 516-393-0970
50 Charles Lindbergh Blvd Ste 200, Uniondale, NY 11553
ClariTEE probe; Zura system

Inceptio Medical Technologies, Lc 801-593-6300
532 N Kays Dr, Kaysville, UT 84037
Diagnostic pulsed doppler imaging system ,pulse echo imaging system.

Jaco Medical Equipment Inc. 858-278-7743
4848 Ronson Ct Ste E, San Diego, CA 92111

Nu Gyn, Inc 763-398-0108
1633 County Highway 10 Ste 15, Spring Lake Park, MN 55432
Bi-directional vascular doppler with spectral analysis.

Pentax Southern Region Service Center 201-571-2300
8934 Kirby Dr, Houston, TX 77054
Ultrasound endoscope.

Pentax West Coast Service Center 800-431-5880
10410 Pioneer Blvd Ste 2, Santa Fe Springs, CA 90670
Pentax ultrasound endoscope.

Phillips Ultrasound 800-982-2011
22100 Bothell Everett Hwy, P.O. Box 3003, Bothell, WA 98021

SCANNER, ULTRASONIC (PULSED DOPPLER) *(cont'd)*

Sonosite, Inc. 888-482-9449
21919 30th Dr SE, Bothell, WA 98021
iLook ultrasonic scanners are application-specific tools for visual medicine. Each unit weighs only 3 lb and gives healthcare providers a new dimension of visual information to improve routine care. Ultrasonic scanner SonoSite TITAN, the company's flagship product, is a full-featured high-resolution modular ultrasound system with advanced imaging technologies, a state-of-the-art operating system, and an intuitive interface for use in clinical environments. The SonoSite 180PLUS highly portable ultrasound system is a battery or AC power operated system weighing 5.4 lb (2.4 kg) with one transducer. It is an all digital, broadband ultrasound system. High-quality imaging is comparable to more-expensive cart-based systems. Pulsed wave Doppler, color power Doppler, M-Mode, tissue harmonic imaging, and PC direct connectivity are capabilities.

Terarecon, Inc. 877-354-1100
2955 Campus Dr Ste 325, San Mateo, CA 94403
General purpose ultrasound with doppler.

Toshiba America Medical Systems 800-421-1968
2441 Michelle Dr, Tustin, CA 92780
Models SSA-370A, SSA-550A, SSA-770R, SSA-325A, SSA-320A.

Universal Ultrasound 800-842-0607
299 Adams St, Bedford Hills, NY 10507
SHIMADZU ultrasound, MEDISON ultrasound, BIOSOUND ultrasound.

W. L. Gore And Associates, Inc. 888-914-4673
555 Paper Mill Rd Bldg 120, Newark, DE 19711
Imaging ultrasound system and transducers.

Zonare Medical Systems, Inc. 877-966-2731
420 Bernardo Ave, Mountain View, CA 94043
Diagnostic ultrasound.

SCANNER, ULTRASONIC (PULSED ECHO) *(Radiology) 90IYO*

Accutome Ultrasound, Inc. 610-889-0200
3222 Phoenixville Pike, Malvern, PA 19355
Various.

Accutome, Inc. 610-889-0200
3222 Phoenixville Pike, Malvern, PA 19355
Ophthalmic a-scan system.

Biosound Esaote, Inc. 800-428-4374
8000 Castleway Dr, Indianapolis, IN 46250
MyLab 30CV, MyLab 50, MEGAS ES, TECHNOS, TECHNOS MPX

Blatek, Inc. 814-231-2085
2820 E College Ave Ste F, State College, PA 16801

Boston Scientific-Neurovascular 510-440-7700
47900 Bayside Pkwy, Fremont, CA 94538
Ultrasound diagnostic imaging system.

Cardinal Healthcare 209, Inc. 610-862-0800
5225 Verona Rd, Fitchburg, WI 53711
System, ultrasound.

Civco Medical Instruments Co., Inc. 319-656-4447
102 1st St S, Kalona, IA 52247
Ultrasound probe cover-latex,poly.

Dicomit Dicom Information Technologies Corp. 905-477-3354
12-250 Cochrane Dr, Markham L3R 8E5 Canada
Mini pacs

Ellis Ophthalmic Technologies, Inc. 718-656-7390
147-39, 175 St.,, Suite #128, Jamaica, NY 11434
Ophthalmic a-scan.

Envisioneering Medical Technologies 314-429-7367
1982 Innerbelt Business Center Dr, Drive, Overland, MO 63114
Ultrasound system.

Fukuda Denshi Usa, Inc. 800-365-6668
17725 NE 65th St Ste C, Redmond, WA 98052
System, imaging, pulsed echo, ultrasonic.

Ge Medical Systems Ultrasound And Primary Care Dia 608-826-7050
726 Heartland Trl, Madison, WI 53717
Ultrasonic imaging systems.

Ge Medical Systems, Llc 847-277-5002
4855 W Electric Ave, West Milwaukee, WI 53219
Various models of diagnostic ultrasound systems.

Hillusa Corp. 305-594-7474
7215 NW 46th St, Miami, FL 33166

SCANNER, ULTRASONIC (PULSED ECHO) *(cont'd)*

Indiana Technology Development, Inc. 317-814-6194
4181 E 96th St Ste 200, Indianapolis, IN 46240
Automated ultrasound breast scanners.

Iscience Interventional 650-421-2700
4055 Campbell Ave, Menlo Park, CA 94025
Ophthalmic ultrasonic imaging system.

Kiltex Corp. 330-644-6746
2064 Killian Rd, Akron, OH 44312
Kiltex probe cover.

Medchannel Llc 617-314-9861
1241 Adams St Apt 110, Dorchester Center, MA 02124
Doppler bloodflowmeter.

Medge Platforms, Inc. 212-351-5029
100 Park Ave Rm 1600, New York, NY 10017
Sonocubic,3d ultrasound software,accessory to ultrasonic pulsed echo imaging sys.

Micro Medical Devices, Inc. 818-874-0000
23945 Calabasas Rd Ste 110, Calabasas, CA 91302
Ascan, pachymeter ultrasound for ophthalmic use.

Mobilsonic, Inc. 408-930-4197
560 Parrott St, San Jose, CA 95112
Diagnostic ultrasound system.

Nidek, Inc. 510-226-5700
47651 Westinghouse Dr, Fremont, CA 94539
Ultrasonic pulse echo imaging system.

Ophthalmic Technologies, Inc. 416-631-9123
12-37 Kodiak Cres, Downsview M3J 3E5 Canada
Ophthalmic a and b scan

Paradigm Medical Industries, Inc. 801-977-8970
2355 S 1070 W, Salt Lake City, UT 84119
Ultrasonic bio-microscope.

Philips Medical Systems 949-450-0014
1590 Scenic Ave, Costa Mesa, CA 92626

Phillips Ultrasound 800-982-2011
22100 Bothell Everett Hwy, P.O. Box 3003, Bothell, WA 98021

Ramsoft, Inc. 416-674-1347
37 Bankview Cir, Etobicoke M9W 6S6 Canada
Workstation for teleradiology, mini-pacs

Sante Feminine Limited 678-314-1649
1649 Sands Pl SE Ste C, Marietta, GA 30067
Mammographic access-aid- self exam-breast.

Scannex, Inc. 954-974-2000
5100 W Copans Rd Ste 1000, Margate, FL 33063
Scannex-sv; the hrl advanced imaging unit.

Sonogage, Inc. 216-464-1119
26650 Renaissance Pkwy, Cleveland, OH 44128
Ultrasonic pachometer.

Sonosite, Inc. 888-482-9449
21919 30th Dr SE, Bothell, WA 98021
SONOHEART PLUS Highly Portable Echocardiography battery or AC power operated system weighing 5.4 lbs. (2.4 kg) with one transducer. All digital, broadband ultrasound system. High-quality imaging comparable to more expensive cart-based systems. Directional color power Doppler assessment of blood flow. Pulsed wave Doppler, tissue harmonic imaging, ECG capability and PC direct connectivity.

Techniscan, Inc. 888-268-3030
1011 Murray Holladay Rd Ste 130, Salt Lake City, UT 84117
Ultrasound imaging system.

Teratech Corp. 781-270-4143
77-79 Terrace Hall Ave, Burlington, MA 01803
Diagnostic ultrasound imaging system.

Toshiba America Medical Systems 800-421-1968
2441 Michelle Dr, Tustin, CA 92780

U-System, Inc. 408-571-0777
110 Rose Orchard Way, San Jose, CA 95134
Ultrasound system.

Verathon Inc. 800-331-2313
21222 30th Dr SE Ste 120, Bothell, WA 98021
BLADDERSCAN hand-held, battery powered ultrasound device measures bladder volume. It is a non-invasive tool for determining post-void residuals, urinary retention or overdistention. Diagnostic catheterization is eliminated. BLADDERMANAGER is a hand-held, battery powered ultrasound device. Bladder volume is measured non-invasively. The BLADDERMANAGER is designed for individuals to use daily as part of their bladder management program. Individuals catheterize or void based on volume. A volume-dependent intermittent catheterization program minimizes the risk of UTI and reduces the incidence of overdistention, which may lead to hydronephrosis. The risks associated with time-dependent intermittent catheterization or timed voiding schedules are reduced.

Volcano Corporation 800-228-4728
3661 Valley Centre Dr Ste 200, San Diego, CA 92130
Intravascular ultrasound imaging system.

W. L. Gore And Associates, Inc. 888-914-4673
555 Paper Mill Rd Bldg 120, Newark, DE 19711
Ultrasound imaging system.

Zonare Medical Systems, Inc. 877-966-2731
420 Bernardo Ave, Mountain View, CA 94043
Diagnostic ultrasound.

3g Ultrasound, Inc. 201-825-3116
200 Williams Dr, Ramsey, NJ 07446
Ultrasound scanner with transducers.

SCANNER, ULTRASONIC, ABDOMINAL *(Radiology) 90RQV*

Biosound Esaote, Inc. 800-428-4374
8000 Castleway Dr, Indianapolis, IN 46250
MyLab 30CV, MyLab 25, MyLab 50, PICUS PRO, TECHNOS, TECHNOS MPX.

Blatek, Inc. 814-231-2085
2820 E College Ave Ste F, State College, PA 16801

Health Care Exports, Inc. 800-847-0173
5701 NW 74th Ave, Miami, FL 33166
New and refurbished.

Hillusa Corp. 305-594-7474
7215 NW 46th St, Miami, FL 33166

New Life Systems, Inc. 954-972-4600
PO Box 8767, Coral Springs, FL 33075
All types.

Philips Medical Systems 949-450-0014
1590 Scenic Ave, Costa Mesa, CA 92626

Phillips Ultrasound 800-982-2011
22100 Bothell Everett Hwy, P.O. Box 3003, Bothell, WA 98021

Shimadzu Medical Systems 800-228-1429
20101 S Vermont Ave, Torrance, CA 90502
4 Models: SDU-350XL , SDU-450XL, SDU-1200, SDU-2200.

SCANNER, ULTRASONIC, BREAST (MAMMOGRAPHIC)
(Obstetrics/Gyn) 85RQW

Imaging Diagnostic Systems, Inc. 800-992-9008
5307 NW 35th Ter, Ft Lauderdale, FL 33309
Imaging Diagnostic Systems, Inc., has developed the world's first patented laser based breast imaging system that utilizes state of the art laser technology and proprietary and patented algorithms to create three-dimensional cross sectional images of the breast. Our Computed Tomography Laser Breast Imaging System (CTLM®) is a non-invasive, painless examination that does not expose the patient to radiation or require breast compression.

SCANNER, ULTRASONIC, GENERAL PURPOSE
(Radiology) 90TEJ

Cone Instruments, Inc. 800-321-6964
5201 Naiman Pkwy, Solon, OH 44139

Health Care Exports, Inc. 800-847-0173
5701 NW 74th Ave, Miami, FL 33166
New and refurbished. Parts and Accessories

SCANNER, ULTRASONIC, GENERAL PURPOSE *(cont'd)*

Hitachi Medical Systems America, Inc. 800-800-3106
1959 Summit Commerce Park, Twinsburg, OH 44087
Hitachi Medical Systems America, Inc. offers a full line of diagnostic ultrasound systems designed to meet the clinical needs and price point of almost every customer in the diagnostic imaging community. Hitachi Ultrasound systems support an extensive array of general transducers as well as specialty probes such as laproscopic, endoscopic, fingertip and bi-plane probes, allowing our units to be tailored to meet the clinical requirements of even the most specialized customer. The systems and probes are engineered and manufactured by Hitachi, utilizing the resources and expertise of one of the world's largest electronics companies to assure that quality, efficiency and innovation are fully represented in every ultrasound unit.

Jaco Medical Equipment Inc. 858-278-7743
4848 Ronson Ct Ste E, San Diego, CA 92111

Medical Devices International 504-455-8311
3724 Severn Ave, Metairie, LA 70002
new systems all transducers

Philips Medical Systems 949-450-0014
1590 Scenic Ave, Costa Mesa, CA 92626
Diagnostic ultrasound medical systems. Famiy of products addressing high and medium performance pricing ranges P600 systems, SONO DIAGNOST 800.

Phillips Ultrasound 800-982-2011
22100 Bothell Everett Hwy, P.O. Box 3003, Bothell, WA 98021

Universal Ultrasound 800-842-0607
299 Adams St, Bedford Hills, NY 10507
SHIMADZU ultrasound: OB/GYN, urology, podiatric, and musculoskeletal scanning. , MEDISON ultrasound: MEDISON Sono Ace Pico and MySono-- OB/GYN, urology, podiatric, and musculoskeletal scanning. BIOSOUND ultrasound: MyLab, color-flow portable system used for abdominal, cardiac, and vascular applications.

SCANNER, ULTRASONIC, OBSTETRICAL/GYNECOLOGICAL *(Obstetrics/Gyn) 85HEM*

Cone Instruments, Inc. 800-321-6964
5201 Naiman Pkwy, Solon, OH 44139

Health Care Exports, Inc. 800-847-0173
5701 NW 74th Ave, Miami, FL 33166
New and refurbished.

Hillusa Corp. 305-594-7474
7215 NW 46th St, Miami, FL 33166

Jaco Medical Equipment Inc. 858-278-7743
4848 Ronson Ct Ste E, San Diego, CA 92111

Phillips Ultrasound 800-982-2011
22100 Bothell Everett Hwy, P.O. Box 3003, Bothell, WA 98021

Sdi Medical Consultants 619-267-1391
4190 Bonita Rd Ste 211, Bonita, CA 91902
Scanners ultrasound. 3D/4D and Color Doppler

Solomon Technology Labs 520-568-8007
22374 N Dietz Dr, Maricopa, AZ 85138
Ob/gyn computer software.

SCANNER, ULTRASONIC, OBSTETRICAL/GYNECOLOGICAL, MOBILE *(Obstetrics/Gyn) 85RQX*

Biosound Esaote, Inc. 800-428-4374
8000 Castleway Dr, Indianapolis, IN 46250
PICUS, PICUS PRO, AQUILA, TECHNOS, TECHNOS MPX.

Cone Instruments, Inc. 800-321-6964
5201 Naiman Pkwy, Solon, OH 44139

Hillusa Corp. 305-594-7474
7215 NW 46th St, Miami, FL 33166

Jaco Medical Equipment Inc. 858-278-7743
4848 Ronson Ct Ste E, San Diego, CA 92111

Main Line International, Inc. 800-397-9020
151 Ben Burton Cir, Coggins Park, Bogart, GA 30622

New Life Systems, Inc. 954-972-4600
PO Box 8767, Coral Springs, FL 33075
New or used scanners.

Philips Medical Systems 949-450-0014
1590 Scenic Ave, Costa Mesa, CA 92626

Phillips Ultrasound 800-982-2011
22100 Bothell Everett Hwy, P.O. Box 3003, Bothell, WA 98021

SCANNER, ULTRASONIC, OPHTHALMIC *(Radiology) 90HPR*

Blatek, Inc. 814-231-2085
2820 E College Ave Ste F, State College, PA 16801

D.G.H. Technology, Inc. 800-722-3883
110 Summit Dr Ste B, Exton, PA 19341
DGH3000Band DGH400B A-scan/pachymeter combination unit.

Nidek Inc. 800-223-9044
47651 Westinghouse Dr, Fremont, CA 94539
Model US-2500/2520 A/B Scan, Model US-2000 A-Scan.

Sonomed, Inc. 800-227-1285
1979 Marcus Ave Ste C105, New Hyde Park, NY 11042
Ophthalmic Ultrasound - $13,000 E/Z-scan B-scan system with color LCD and touch Screen interface // $16,500 A&B-scan version // $4,500 MICROSCAN 100A notebook size A+ Scan system // SONOMED 300 SERIES A-SCAN/PACHYMETER, 300AP - $8,000 // A-SCAN ONLY, 300A - $5000.00 // PACHYMETER ONLY - $3500.00 for corneal thickness measurement. Touch screen user interface. VuMax High Frequency ultrasound biomicroscope for anterior segment imaging using 35MHz or 50MHz transducers. U.S. Price $35,000.00

SCANNER, ULTRASONIC, OTHER *(Radiology) 90RQZ*

Bard Access Systems, Inc. 800-545-0890
605 N 5600 W, Salt Lake City, UT 84116
$10,000 - $15,000 for portable, battery operated ultrasound scanner (2 models); also, ultrasonic scanner for needle guidance in central venous line placement.

Biomedical Systems Corp. 800-877-6334
77 Progress Pkwy Bldg 1, Maryland Hts, MO 63043
Century Holter Scanning Systems, Versions C3000, C2000, and C1000. Plus the Century Review Station. Prodvides customized Holter reports from 24-48 hour Holter recordings with up to 12 leads. Options include QT Analysis, Enhanced ST, HRV, Data Export, and Multi-User networking.

Cone Instruments, Inc. 800-321-6964
5201 Naiman Pkwy, Solon, OH 44139
Urological ultrasonic scanner.

Ideal Medical Source, Inc. 800-537-0739
2805 East. Oakland Blvd, Suite 352, Fort Lauderdale, FL 33306

Jaco Medical Equipment Inc. 858-278-7743
4848 Ronson Ct Ste E, San Diego, CA 92111
New and used reconditioned scanners.

Linscan Ultrasound 800-533-7226
202 W 9th St Ste 301, PO Box 1217, Rolla, MO 65401
Intra-operative ultrasonic scanner, priced $35,000 - $60,000.

Medison America, Inc. 800-829-SONO
11075 Knott Ave Ste C, Cypress, CA 90630

Multigon Industries, Inc. 800-289-6858
1 Odell Plz, Yonkers, NY 10701

New Laser Science, Inc. 858-487-5880
PO Box 27210, San Diego, CA 92198

New Life Systems, Inc. 954-972-4600
PO Box 8767, Coral Springs, FL 33075
All types and frequencies.

Philips Medical Systems 949-450-0014
1590 Scenic Ave, Costa Mesa, CA 92626

Phillips Ultrasound 800-982-2011
22100 Bothell Everett Hwy, P.O. Box 3003, Bothell, WA 98021

Products Group International, Inc. 800-336-5299
447 Main St., Lyons, CO 80540

Shimadzu Medical Systems 800-228-1429
20101 S Vermont Ave, Torrance, CA 90502
OBGYN: SDU-1200, SDU-2200, SDU-450XL, SDU-350XL, Urology: SDU-1200, SDU-2200, SDU-450XL, SDU-350XL, MUSKULOSKELETAL: SDU-350XL, SDU-450XL, VET: SDU-350XL, SDU-450XL.

Universal Ultrasound 800-842-0607
299 Adams St, Bedford Hills, NY 10507
SHIMADZU --OB/GYN, infertility, abdominal, and rectal scanning. Medison SonoAce Pico, OB/GYN, Musculoskeletal. Mindray Musculoskeletal, Biosound MyLab Shared service, Abdominal, cardiac and Vascular

Verathon Inc. 800-331-2313
21222 30th Dr SE Ste 120, Bothell, WA 98021
BLADDERSCAN portable ultrasound instrument that measures bladder volume non-invasively. It provides immediate results, reducing patient trauma and discomfort. It also eliminates diagnostic catheterizations, minimizing the risk of urinary tract infections.

SCANNER, ULTRASONIC, PEDIATRIC *(Radiology) 90RQY*

Philips Medical Systems 949-450-0014
1590 Scenic Ave, Costa Mesa, CA 92626

Phillips Ultrasound 800-982-2011
22100 Bothell Everett Hwy, P.O. Box 3003, Bothell, WA 98021

Toshiba America Medical Systems 800-421-1968
2441 Michelle Dr, Tustin, CA 92780
SSA-270A, SSA-250A.

Verathon Inc. 800-331-2313
21222 30th Dr SE Ste 120, Bothell, WA 98021
BLADDERSCAN portable ultrasound scanner automatically calculates bladder volume. It is effective in measuring post-void residual volume as a determination of the bladder's emptying function. In pediatric urology, this is commonly done in the management of patients with myclodysplasia, dysfunctional voiding and urinary tract infections.

SCANNER, ULTRASONIC, SMALL PARTS *(Radiology) 90TEK*

Biosound Esaote, Inc. 800-428-4374
8000 Castleway Dr, Indianapolis, IN 46250
Aquila, PICUS PRO, TECHNOS, TECHNOS MPX

Cone Instruments, Inc. 800-321-6964
5201 Naiman Pkwy, Solon, OH 44139

Health Care Exports, Inc. 800-847-0173
5701 NW 74th Ave, Miami, FL 33166
New and refurbished.

New Life Systems, Inc. 954-972-4600
PO Box 8767, Coral Springs, FL 33075
New or used scanners.

Philips Medical Systems 949-450-0014
1590 Scenic Ave, Costa Mesa, CA 92626

Phillips Ultrasound 800-982-2011
22100 Bothell Everett Hwy, P.O. Box 3003, Bothell, WA 98021

Toshiba America Medical Systems 800-421-1968
2441 Michelle Dr, Tustin, CA 92780
SSA-270A, SSA-250A.

SCANNER, ULTRASONIC, SURGICAL *(Surgery) 79UMD*

Linscan Ultrasound 800-533-7226
202 W 9th St Ste 301, PO Box 1217, Rolla, MO 65401
Intra-operative ultrasound imaging, priced $35,000 - $60,000.

Universal Ultrasound 800-842-0607
299 Adams St, Bedford Hills, NY 10507

SCANNER, ULTRASONIC, VASCULAR *(Radiology) 90VCV*

Bard Access Systems, Inc. 800-545-0890
605 N 5600 W, Salt Lake City, UT 84116
Site-Rite II and Site-Rite III facilitates percutaneous vascular punctures and nerve blocks. Provides real-time viewing of the desired target vein or artery.

Biosound Esaote, Inc. 800-428-4374
8000 Castleway Dr, Indianapolis, IN 46250
MyLab 30CV, MyLab 25, MyLab 50, CARIS PLUS, MEGAS ES, TECHNOS, TECHNOS MPX

Health Care Exports, Inc. 800-847-0173
5701 NW 74th Ave, Miami, FL 33166
New and refurbished.

Multigon Industries, Inc. 800-289-6858
1 Odell Plz, Yonkers, NY 10701
Color vascular image.

New Life Systems, Inc. 954-972-4600
PO Box 8767, Coral Springs, FL 33075
B/W or color.

Philips Medical Systems 949-450-0014
1590 Scenic Ave, Costa Mesa, CA 92626

Phillips Ultrasound 800-982-2011
22100 Bothell Everett Hwy, P.O. Box 3003, Bothell, WA 98021

Unetixs Vascular, Inc. 800-486-3849
115 Airport St, North Kingstown, RI 02852
MULTILAB SERIES 2-LHS Advanced Vascular Diagnostic Lab Workstation features touch screen controls, dual calibrated P.V.R. and dual channel PPG 5R8 Maz Stereo Doppler. MULTILAB SERIES 2 (CP) is a portable version of MULTILAB SERIES 2-LHS. MULTILAB SERIES 2/IMG - First instrument capable of both physiological testing and ultrasound testing.

SCANNER, ULTRAVIOLET *(Chemistry) 75UHX*

Advanced American Biotechnology (Aab) 714-870-0290
1166 E Valencia Dr Unit 6C, Fullerton, CA 92831

SCANNER, ULTRAVIOLET *(cont'd)*

Camag Scientific, Inc. 800-334-3909
515 Cornelius Harnett Dr, Wilmington, NC 28401

SCAVENGER, GAS *(Anesthesiology) 73CBN*

Matrx 716-662-6650
145 Mid County Dr, Orchard Park, NY 14127
Gas scavenger.

Porter Instrument Division Parker Hannifin Corp 800-457-2001
245 Township Line Rd, Hatfield, PA 19440
$500 to $900 per unit. AVS-Automatic Vacuum Switch, AVS-5000 automatic vacuum switch used in conjunction with scavenging systems to control vacuum flow. Porter Scavenging System, a scavenging system used to deliver/remove analgesic gases usually used in dentistry.

SCAVENGER, GAS, ANESTHESIA UNIT *(Anesthesiology) 73QBA*

Aga Linde Healthcare P.R. Inc. 787-622-7900
PO Box 363868, GPO Box 364727, San Juan, PR 00936
Anesth/Pul Med.

Anesthesia Associates, Inc. 760-744-6561
460 Enterprise St, San Marcos, CA 92078
Various units, styles and systems. Inline, bagtail, adapter, self standing, and absorber output. Units generally adjustable from 0 to 60 cmH2O backpressure, all include checkvalves. Scavenger Vacuum Manifolds with dual safety check valves available to retrofit systems without existing scavenger capabilities.

Datex-Ohmeda (Canada) 800-268-1472
1093 Meyerside Dr., Unit 2, Mississauga, ONT L5T-1J6 Canada

SCISSORS WITH REMOVABLE TIPS, LAPAROSCOPY *(Surgery) 79SEP*

Ams Innovative Center-San Jose 800-356-7600
3070 Orchard Dr, San Jose, CA 95134

Smith & Nephew, Inc., Endoscopy Division 800-343-8386
150 Minuteman Rd, Andover, MA 01810

Synectic Medical Product Development 203-877-8488
60 Commerce Park, Milford, CT 06460

SCISSORS, BANDAGE/GAUZE/PLASTER *(General) 80RRB*

Afassco, Inc. 800-441-6774
2244 Park Pl Ste C, Minden, NV 89423

Alimed, Inc. 800-225-2610
297 High St, Dedham, MA 02026

Carl Heyer, Inc. 800-284-5550
1872 Bellmore Ave, North Bellmore, NY 11710

Clinimed, Incorporated 877-CLINIMED
303 Markus Ct, Sandy Brae Industrial Park, Newark, DE 19713

Codman & Shurtleff, Inc 800-225-0460
325 Paramount Dr, Raynham, MA 02767

Dixie Ems Supply 800-347-3494
385 Union Ave, Brooklyn, NY 11211
$4.50 per unit (5-1/2in).

Elmed, Inc. 630-543-2792
60 W Fay Ave, Addison, IL 60101

Fine Surgical Instrument, Inc. 800-851-5155
741 Peninsula Blvd, Hempstead, NY 11550

Kern Surgical Supply, Inc. 800-582-3939
2823 Gibson St, Bakersfield, CA 93308

Kmedic 800-955-0559
190 Veterans Dr, Northvale, NJ 07647
Cut thick layers of stockinette, bandages, drapes and pre-splinting material with ease. Available in two sizes and require minimal hand strength.

Kta, Instruments, Inc. 888-830-9KTA
3051 Brighton-Third St., 1st Fl., Brooklyn, NY 11235

Lydia's Professional Uniforms 800-942-3378
2547 3 Mile Rd NW Ste F, Grand Rapids, MI 49534

Medcare Technologies 800-388-6235
850 Saint Paul St, Rochester, NY 14605
Fin or punch tips, 7 1/2 in. and Mini 5 1/2 in. NSN 6515-00-935-7138 & 6505-01-030-4465.

Medworks Instruments 800-323-9790
PO Box 581, Chatham, IL 62629
$1.85 per unit (7-1/2in), autocalvable.

Miltex Inc. 800-645-8000
589 Davies Dr, York, PA 17402

Pocket Nurse Enterprises, Inc. 800-225-1600
200 1st St, Ambridge, PA 15003

SCISSORS, BANDAGE/GAUZE/PLASTER *(cont'd)*

Prestige Medical Corporation 800-762-3333
8600 Wilbur Ave, Northridge, CA 91324

Prosurge Instruments, Inc. 866-832-7874
199 Laidlaw Ave, Jersey City, NJ 07306

Rockford Medical & Safety Co. 800-435-9451
2420 Harrison Ave, PO Box 5646, Rockford, IL 61108

Scanlan International, Inc. 800-328-9458
1 Scanlan Plz, Saint Paul, MN 55107

Schueler & Company, Inc. 516-487-1500
PO Box 528, Stratford, CT 06615

Trans American Medical 800-626-9232
7633 W 100th Pl, Bridgeview, IL 60455
LISTER 5.5 and 7.5 in satin or polished. U.S. made.

Trans American Medical / Tamsco Instruments 708-430-7777
7633 W 100th Pl, Bridgeview, IL 60455
All types. Diagnostic.

Zimmer Holdings, Inc. 800-613-6131
1800 W Center St, PO Box 708, Warsaw, IN 46580

SCISSORS, CARDIOVASCULAR *(Cardiovascular) 74RRC*

Codman & Shurtleff, Inc 800-225-0460
325 Paramount Dr, Raynham, MA 02767

Deknatel Snowden-Pencer 800-367-7874
5175 S Royal Atlanta Dr, Tucker, GA 30084

Elmed, Inc. 630-543-2792
60 W Fay Ave, Addison, IL 60101

Fehling Surgical Instruments 800-FEHLING
509 Broadstone Ln NW, Acworth, GA 30101

J. Jamner Surgical Instruments, Inc 800-431-1123
9 Skyline Dr, Hawthorne, NY 10532

Miltex Inc. 800-645-8000
589 Davies Dr, York, PA 17402

Prosurge Instruments, Inc. 866-832-7874
199 Laidlaw Ave, Jersey City, NJ 07306

Scanlan International, Inc. 800-328-9458
1 Scanlan Plz, Saint Paul, MN 55107
ULTRA SHARP and SUPER CUT scissors.

SCISSORS, COLLAR AND CROWN *(Dental And Oral) 76EIR*

Acme Of Precision Surgical Co., Inc. 973-373-6797
485 21st St, Irvington, NJ 07111
Collar and crown scissors.

Buffalo Dental Mfg. Co., Inc. 516-496-7200
159 Lafayette Dr, Syosset, NY 11791
Scissors, collar and crown.

Coltene/Whaledent Inc. 330-916-8858
235 Ascot Pkwy, Cuyahoga Falls, OH 44223
Collar and crown scissors.

Dentronix, Inc. 800-523-5944
235 Ascot Pkwy, Cuyahoga Falls, OH 44223
$15.00 per unit (standard).

E.A. Beck & Co. 949-645-4072
657 W 19th St Ste E, P O Box 10857, Costa Mesa, CA 92627
Crown scissors.

Kmedic 800-955-0559
190 Veterans Dr, Northvale, NJ 07647

Miltex Dental Technologies, Inc. 516-576-6022
589 Davies Dr, York, PA 17402
Cutting (crown) scissors.

Premier Dental Products Co. 888-670-6100
1710 Romano Dr, PO Box 4500, Plymouth Meeting, PA 19462

Toolmex Corporation 800-992-4766
1075 Worcester St, Natick, MA 01760

Trans American Medical / Tamsco Instruments 708-430-7777
7633 W 100th Pl, Bridgeview, IL 60455
Floor grade surgical stainless steel.

SCISSORS, CORNEAL *(Ophthalmology) 86RRD*

Allergan 800-366-6554
2525 Dupont Dr, Irvine, CA 92612
BKS-1000 refractive set allows partial removal of cornea and reshaping without freezing tissue.

Codman & Shurtleff, Inc 800-225-0460
325 Paramount Dr, Raynham, MA 02767

Elmed, Inc. 630-543-2792
60 W Fay Ave, Addison, IL 60101

SCISSORS, CORNEAL *(cont'd)*

Fortrad Eye Instruments Corp. 973-543-2371
8 Franklin Rd, Mendham, NJ 07945

J. Jamner Surgical Instruments, Inc 800-431-1123
9 Skyline Dr, Hawthorne, NY 10532

Katena Products, Inc. 800-225-1195
4 Stewart Ct, Denville, NJ 07834

Miltex Inc. 800-645-8000
589 Davies Dr, York, PA 17402

Stephens Instruments, Inc. 800-354-7848
2500 Sandersville Rd, Lexington, KY 40511
$155.00 per unit (standard).

SCISSORS, CYSTOSCOPIC *(Gastro/Urology) 78KGD*

Gyrus Acmi, Inc. 508-804-2739
93 N Pleasant St, Norwalk, OH 44857
Various sizes and kinds of scissors.

Gyrus Acmi, Inc. 508-804-2739
300 Stillwater P.o.box 1971, Stamford, CT 06902
Various sizes and kinds of scissors.

Karl Storz Endoscopy-America Inc. 800-421-0837
600 Corporate Pointe, Culver City, CA 90230

Mahe International Inc. 800-294-7946
468 Craighead St, Nashville, TN 37204

Miltex Inc. 800-645-8000
589 Davies Dr, York, PA 17402

SCISSORS, DISPOSABLE *(General) 80JOK*

Acme Of Precision Surgical Co., Inc. 973-373-6797
485 21st St, Irvington, NJ 07111
Various types and sizes of medical scissors.

Bausch & Lomb Surgical 636-255-5051
3365 Tree Court Ind Blvd, Saint Louis, MO 63122

Biomet Microfixation Inc. 800-874-7711
1520 Tradeport Dr, Jacksonville, FL 32218
Various types of scissors.

Busse Hospital Disposables, Inc. 631-435-4711
75 Arkay Dr, Hauppauge, NY 11788
Various.

Centurion Medical Products Corp. 517-545-1135
3310 S Main St, Salisbury, NC 28147

Ethicon Endo-Surgery, Inc. 800-USE-ENDO
4545 Creek Rd, Cincinnati, OH 45242
ENDOPATH 5mm hook, micro, and curved, with unipolar cautery.

Healer Products, Llc 914-663-6300
427 Commerce Ln Ste 1, West Berlin, NJ 08091
Scissors.

Health Care Logistics, Inc. 800-848-1633
450 Town St, PO Box 25, Circleville, OH 43113
Various makes of scissors and shears.

K. W. Griffen Co. 203-846-1923
100 Pearl St, Norwalk, CT 06850
Scissors.

Kenyon Industries, Inc. 973-962-4844
235 Margaret King Ave, Ringwood, NJ 07456

Kmedic 800-955-0559
190 Veterans Dr, Northvale, NJ 07647

Lyons Tool And Die Company 800-422-9363
185 Research Pkwy, Meriden, CT 06450
Rapid prototyping. Production of medical devices in class 10,000 clean rooms. Medical knives and scissors. Precision metal stamping. Engineering services.

North Safety Products 401-943-4400
1101 B Calle Neutron, Parque Industrial Maran, Mexicali, B.c. Mexico
Scissors

Pulpdent Corp. 800-343-4342
80 Oakland St, Watertown, MA 02472
No common name listed.

Rocket Medical Plc. 800-707-7625
150 Recreation Park Dr Ste 3, Hingham, MA 02043

Std Med, Inc. 781-828-4400
75 Mill St, PO Box 420, Stoughton, MA 02072
Laparoscopic scissors.

Synectic Medical Product Development 203-877-8488
60 Commerce Park, Milford, CT 06460

SCISSORS, DISPOSABLE *(cont'd)*

Trans American Medical / Tamsco Instruments 708-430-7777
7633 W 100th Pl, Bridgeview, IL 60455
Floor grade surgical stainless steel.

Tri-State Hospital Supply Corp. 517-545-1135
3173 E 43rd St, Yuma, AZ 85365

Tuzik Boston 800-886-6363
104 Longwater Dr, Assinippi Park, Norwell, MA 02061

Vartex Instrument Corp. 718-486-5050
311 Wallabout St, Brooklyn, NY 11206
Various scissors.

Zimmer Holdings, Inc. 800-613-6131
1800 W Center St, PO Box 708, Warsaw, IN 46580

SCISSORS, EAR *(Ear/Nose/Throat) 77JZB*

Aesculap Implant Systems Inc. 1-800-234-9179
3773 Corporate Pkwy, Center Valley, PA 18034

Bausch & Lomb Surgical 636-255-5051
3365 Tree Court Ind Blvd, Saint Louis, MO 63122

Biomet Microfixation Inc. 800-874-7711
1520 Tradeport Dr, Jacksonville, FL 32218
Various types of scissors.

Clinimed, Incorporated 877-CLINIMED
303 Markus Ct, Sandy Brae Industrial Park, Newark, DE 19713

Deknatel Snowden-Pencer 800-367-7874
5175 S Royal Atlanta Dr, Tucker, GA 30084
Serrated scissors for reconstructive surgery.

Medone Surgical, Inc. 941-359-3129
670 Tallevast Rd, Sarasota, FL 34243
Various.

Prosurge Instruments, Inc. 866-832-7874
199 Laidlaw Ave, Jersey City, NJ 07306

Trans American Medical / Tamsco Instruments 708-430-7777
7633 W 100th Pl, Bridgeview, IL 60455
Floor grade surgical stainless steel.

Tuzik Boston 800-886-6363
104 Longwater Dr, Assinippi Park, Norwell, MA 02061

SCISSORS, ENUCLEATION *(Ophthalmology) 86RRE*

Elmed, Inc. 630-543-2792
60 W Fay Ave, Addison, IL 60101

Fortrad Eye Instruments Corp. 973-543-2371
8 Franklin Rd, Mendham, NJ 07945

J. Jamner Surgical Instruments, Inc 800-431-1123
9 Skyline Dr, Hawthorne, NY 10532

Katena Products, Inc. 800-225-1195
4 Stewart Ct, Denville, NJ 07834

Miltex Inc. 800-645-8000
589 Davies Dr, York, PA 17402

Stephens Instruments, Inc. 800-354-7848
2500 Sandersville Rd, Lexington, KY 40511
$35.00 per unit (standard).

SCISSORS, EPISIOTOMY *(Obstetrics/Gyn) 85HDK*

Acme Of Precision Surgical Co., Inc. 973-373-6797
485 21st St, Irvington, NJ 07111
Various types and sizes of episiotomy scissors.

Biomet Microfixation Inc. 800-874-7711
1520 Tradeport Dr, Jacksonville, FL 32218
Various types of scissors.

Kmedic 800-955-0559
190 Veterans Dr, Northvale, NJ 07647

Tuzik Boston 800-886-6363
104 Longwater Dr, Assinippi Park, Norwell, MA 02061

SCISSORS, GENERAL DISSECTING *(General) 80RRI*

Clinimed, Incorporated 877-CLINIMED
303 Markus Ct, Sandy Brae Industrial Park, Newark, DE 19713

Codman & Shurtleff, Inc 800-225-0460
325 Paramount Dr, Raynham, MA 02767

Deknatel Snowden-Pencer 800-367-7874
5175 S Royal Atlanta Dr, Tucker, GA 30084

Elmed, Inc. 630-543-2792
60 W Fay Ave, Addison, IL 60101

J. Jamner Surgical Instruments, Inc 800-431-1123
9 Skyline Dr, Hawthorne, NY 10532

SCISSORS, GENERAL DISSECTING *(cont'd)*

Lican Medical Products Ltd. 519-737-1142
5120 Halford Dr., Windsor, ON N9A 6J3 Canada

Medworks Instruments 800-323-9790
PO Box 581, Chatham, IL 62629
$1.90 per unit (standard).

Miltex Inc. 800-645-8000
589 Davies Dr, York, PA 17402

Nordent Manufacturing, Inc. 800-966-7336
610 Bonnie Ln, Elk Grove Village, IL 60007
$57.50 per unit (standard).

Princeton Medical Group, Inc. 800-875-0869
1189 Royal Links Dr, Mt Pleasant, SC 29466
TITANIUM & S/S INSTRUMENTS

Prosurge Instruments, Inc. 866-832-7874
199 Laidlaw Ave, Jersey City, NJ 07306

Zimmer Holdings, Inc. 800-613-6131
1800 W Center St, PO Box 708, Warsaw, IN 46580

SCISSORS, GYNECOLOGICAL *(Obstetrics/Gyn) 85RRJ*

Codman & Shurtleff, Inc 800-225-0460
325 Paramount Dr, Raynham, MA 02767

Deknatel Snowden-Pencer 800-367-7874
5175 S Royal Atlanta Dr, Tucker, GA 30084

Elmed, Inc. 630-543-2792
60 W Fay Ave, Addison, IL 60101

Miltex Inc. 800-645-8000
589 Davies Dr, York, PA 17402

Prosurge Instruments, Inc. 866-832-7874
199 Laidlaw Ave, Jersey City, NJ 07306

SCISSORS, IRIS *(Ophthalmology) 86RRF*

Akorn, Inc. 800-535-7155
2500 Millbrook Dr, Buffalo Grove, IL 60089
Titanium, 10mm blades, 4.5mm long, round handle with straight, curved, or angled tips plus diamond knives and other titanium instruments.

Deknatel Snowden-Pencer 800-367-7874
5175 S Royal Atlanta Dr, Tucker, GA 30084

Elmed, Inc. 630-543-2792
60 W Fay Ave, Addison, IL 60101

Fortrad Eye Instruments Corp. 973-543-2371
8 Franklin Rd, Mendham, NJ 07945

Howard Instruments, Inc. 205-553-4453
4749 Appletree Ln, Tuscaloosa, AL 35405

J. Jamner Surgical Instruments, Inc 800-431-1123
9 Skyline Dr, Hawthorne, NY 10532

Katena Products, Inc. 800-225-1195
4 Stewart Ct, Denville, NJ 07834

Kmedic 800-955-0559
190 Veterans Dr, Northvale, NJ 07647

Miltex Inc. 800-645-8000
589 Davies Dr, York, PA 17402

Nordent Manufacturing, Inc. 800-966-7336
610 Bonnie Ln, Elk Grove Village, IL 60007
$44.50 per unit (standard).

Princeton Medical Group, Inc. 800-875-0869
1189 Royal Links Dr, Mt Pleasant, SC 29466
TITANIUM & S/S INSTRUMENTS

Prosurge Instruments, Inc. 866-832-7874
199 Laidlaw Ave, Jersey City, NJ 07306

Rhein Medical, Inc. 800-637-4346
5460 Beaumont Center Blvd Ste 500, Suite 500, Tampa, FL 33634

Stephens Instruments, Inc. 800-354-7848
2500 Sandersville Rd, Lexington, KY 40511
$32.00 per unit (4-1/2in).

Trans American Medical 800-626-9232
7633 W 100th Pl, Bridgeview, IL 60455
4.5 in. straight and curved, satin or polished. U.S. made.

Trans American Medical / Tamsco Instruments 708-430-7777
7633 W 100th Pl, Bridgeview, IL 60455

Zimmer Holdings, Inc. 800-613-6131
1800 W Center St, PO Box 708, Warsaw, IN 46580

SCISSORS, LAPAROSCOPY *(Surgery) 79SAZ*

Aesculap Implant Systems Inc. 1-800-234-9179
3773 Corporate Pkwy, Center Valley, PA 18034

SCISSORS, LAPAROSCOPY *(cont'd)*

Genicon 800-936-1020
6869 Stapoint Ct Ste 114, Winter Park, FL 32792
Laparoscopic Scissors, both disposable and reusable, available in 33cm & 45cm working lengths and curved Metz., Straight and Hook styles.

Incisiontech 800-213-7809
9 Technology Dr, Staunton, VA 24401

Lyons Tool And Die Company 800-422-9363
185 Research Pkwy, Meriden, CT 06450
Rapid prototyping. Production of medical devices in class 10,000 clean rooms. Medical knives and scissors. Precision metal stamping. Engineering services.

Mediflex Surgical Products 800-879-7575
250 Gibbs Rd, Islandia, NY 11749

Okay Industries, Inc. 860-225-8707
200 Ellis St, P.O. Box 2470, New Britain, CT 06051

Putnam Precision Products 845-278-2141
3859 Danbury Rd, Brewster, NY 10509

Wisap America 800-233-8448
8231 Melrose Dr, Lenexa, KS 66214

SCISSORS, LAPAROSCOPY, BIPOLAR, ELECTROSURGICAL
(Surgery) 79SJL

Genicon 800-936-1020
6869 Stapoint Ct Ste 114, Winter Park, FL 32792
Bipolar scissors both reusable and disposable, available in 33cm & 45cm working lenghts.

Gyrus Medical, Inc. 800-852-9361
6655 Wedgwood Rd N Ste 105, Maple Grove, MN 55311

Okay Industries, Inc. 860-225-8707
200 Ellis St, P.O. Box 2470, New Britain, CT 06051

Princeton Medical Group, Inc. 800-875-0869
1189 Royal Links Dr, Mt Pleasant, SC 29466

SCISSORS, LAPAROSCOPY, ELECTROSURGICAL
(Surgery) 79WZE

Gyrus Medical, Inc. 800-852-9361
6655 Wedgwood Rd N Ste 105, Maple Grove, MN 55311
EVERSHEARS scissors, intended for laparoscopic and other MIS procedures. Available in straight or curved blade, 33- or 45-cm lengths for $95.00.

H.S. International Co., Inc. 800-811-0072
5040 Commercial Cir Ste A, Concord, CA 94520
Disposable and Reusable Laparoscopic Scissors, available in straight or curved blade in various lengths.

SCISSORS, LAPAROSCOPY, UNIPOLAR, ELECTROSURGICAL
(Surgery) 79SGV

Genicon 800-936-1020
6869 Stapoint Ct Ste 114, Winter Park, FL 32792
Reusable and Disposable products availalbe in 33cm and 45cm working lengths.

SCISSORS, NASAL *(Ear/Nose/Throat) 77KBD*

Acme Of Precision Surgical Co., Inc. 973-373-6797
485 21st St, Irvington, NJ 07111
Knight nasal scissors.

Aesculap Implant Systems Inc. 1-800-234-9179
3773 Corporate Pkwy, Center Valley, PA 18034

Bausch & Lomb Surgical 636-255-5051
3365 Tree Court Ind Blvd, Saint Louis, MO 63122

Biomet Microfixation Inc. 800-874-7711
1520 Tradeport Dr, Jacksonville, FL 32218
Various types of scissors.

Clinimed, Incorporated 877-CLINIMED
303 Markus Ct, Sandy Brae Industrial Park, Newark, DE 19713

Codman & Shurtleff, Inc 800-225-0460
325 Paramount Dr, Raynham, MA 02767

Deknatel Snowden-Pencer 800-367-7874
5175 S Royal Atlanta Dr, Tucker, GA 30084

Elmed, Inc. 630-543-2792
60 W Fay Ave, Addison, IL 60101

Invotec Intl. 800-998-8580
6833 Phillips Industrial Blvd, Jacksonville, FL 32256
Nasal scissors.

Jedmed Instruments Co. 314-845-3770
5416 Jedmed Ct, Saint Louis, MO 63129

SCISSORS, NASAL *(cont'd)*

Miltex Inc. 800-645-8000
589 Davies Dr, York, PA 17402

Prosurge Instruments, Inc. 866-832-7874
199 Laidlaw Ave, Jersey City, NJ 07306

Symmetry Medical Usa, Inc. 574-267-8700
486 W 350 N, Warsaw, IN 46582
Ear, nose, and throat manual surgical instrument.

Tuzik Boston 800-886-6363
104 Longwater Dr, Assinippi Park, Norwell, MA 02061

SCISSORS, NEUROSURGICAL (DURA) *(Cns/Neurology) 84RRK*

Codman & Shurtleff, Inc 800-225-0460
325 Paramount Dr, Raynham, MA 02767

Deknatel Snowden-Pencer 800-367-7874
5175 S Royal Atlanta Dr, Tucker, GA 30084

Elmed, Inc. 630-543-2792
60 W Fay Ave, Addison, IL 60101

Fehling Surgical Instruments 800-FEHLING
509 Broadstone Ln NW, Acworth, GA 30101

J. Jamner Surgical Instruments, Inc 800-431-1123
9 Skyline Dr, Hawthorne, NY 10532

Miltex Inc. 800-645-8000
589 Davies Dr, York, PA 17402

Prosurge Instruments, Inc. 866-832-7874
199 Laidlaw Ave, Jersey City, NJ 07306

Scanlan International, Inc. 800-328-9458
1 Scanlan Plz, Saint Paul, MN 55107

SCISSORS, OPHTHALMIC *(Ophthalmology) 86HNF*

Accutome, Inc. 610-889-0200
3222 Phoenixville Pike, Malvern, PA 19355
Scissors.

B. Graczyk, Inc. 269-782-2100
27826 Burmax Park, Dowagiac, MI 49047
Various types of scissors.

Bausch & Lomb Surgical 636-255-5051
3365 Tree Court Ind Blvd, Saint Louis, MO 63122

Berring Precision Blades Llc 352-383-8333
9236 Wildwood Ln, Robertsville, MO 63072
Ophthalmic scissors.

Boss Instruments, Ltd. 800-210-2677
395 Reas Ford Rd Ste 120, Earlysville, VA 22936
Ophthalmic; vascualr/cardiovascular; ENT, plastic surgery; neurosurgical, orthopedic, micro surgery, general surgery.

Codman & Shurtleff, Inc 800-225-0460
325 Paramount Dr, Raynham, MA 02767

Deknatel Snowden-Pencer 800-367-7874
5175 S Royal Atlanta Dr, Tucker, GA 30084

Demetech Corp. 888-324-2447
3530 NW 115th Ave, Doral, FL 33178
Ophthalmic scissors.

Diamond Edge Co. 727-586-2927
928 W Bay Dr, Largo, FL 33770
Scissors.

Dutch Ophthalmic Usa, Inc. 800-753-8824
10 Continental Dr Bldg 1, Exeter, NH 03833
Various models of scissors.

Elmed, Inc. 630-543-2792
60 W Fay Ave, Addison, IL 60101

Eye Care And Cure 800-486-6169
4646 S Overland Dr, Tucson, AZ 85714
Scissors.

Fischer Surgical Inc. 314-303-7753
1343 Pine Dr, Arnold, MO 63010
Various types of ophthalmic scissors.

Fortrad Eye Instruments Corp. 973-543-2371
8 Franklin Rd, Mendham, NJ 07945

George Tiemann & Co. 800-843-6266
25 Plant Ave, Hauppauge, NY 11788

Gyrus Ent L.L.C., Sub. Of Gyrus Acmi, Inc. 508-804-2739
2925 Appling Rd, Bartlett, TN 38133
Various.

H.S. International Co., Inc. 800-811-0072
5040 Commercial Cir Ste A, Concord, CA 94520
Pneumatic vertical/horizontal intraocular micro-scissors.

SCISSORS, OPHTHALMIC *(cont'd)*

Hai Laboratories, Inc. 781-862-9884
320 Massachusetts Ave, Lexington, MA 02420
Ophthalmic scissors - various types.

Harvey Precision Instruments 707-793-2600
217 Fairway Rd, Cape Haze, FL 33947
Straight, curved, blunt and angled eye scissors.

Jedmed Instruments Co. 314-845-3770
5416 Jedmed Ct, Saint Louis, MO 63129

Katena Products, Inc. 800-225-1195
4 Stewart Ct, Denville, NJ 07834
Capsulotomy scissors.

Kmedic 800-955-0559
190 Veterans Dr, Northvale, NJ 07647

Medone Surgical, Inc. 941-359-3129
670 Tallevast Rd, Sarasota, FL 34243
Various types of micro scissors.

Micrins Surgical Instruments, Inc. 800-833-3380
28438 N Ballard Dr, Lake Forest, IL 60045

Precision Surgical Intl., Inc. 800-776-8493
PO Box 726, Noblesville, IN 46061
Iris scissors.

Rhein Medical, Inc. 800-637-4346
5460 Beaumont Center Blvd Ste 500, Suite 500, Tampa, FL 33634
Titanium, vannas scissors, needleholders, lens manipulators, hooks, forceps and diamond knives.

Stephens Instruments, Inc. 800-354-7848
2500 Sandersville Rd, Lexington, KY 40511
$90.00 each.

Surgical Instrument Manufacturers, Inc. 800-521-2985
1650 Headland Dr, Fenton, MO 63026

Symmetry Medical Usa, Inc. 574-267-8700
486 W 350 N, Warsaw, IN 46582
Manual ophthalmic surgical instrument.

Synergetics Usa, Inc. 800-600-0565
3845 Corporate Centre Dr, O Fallon, MO 63368
Scissors.

Total Titanium, Inc. 618-473-2429
140 East Monroe St., Hecker, IL 62248
Various types of ophthalmic scissors.

Tuzik Boston 800-886-6363
104 Longwater Dr, Assinippi Park, Norwell, MA 02061

SCISSORS, ORTHOPEDIC *(Orthopedics) 87HRR*

Arthrex California, Inc. 239-643-5553
20509 Earlgate St, Walnut, CA 91789
Scissors.

Biomet Microfixation Inc. 800-874-7711
1520 Tradeport Dr, Jacksonville, FL 32218
Various types of scissors.

Biomet, Inc. 574-267-6639
56 E Bell Dr, PO Box 587, Warsaw, IN 46582
Various types of orthopedic scissors.

Deknatel Snowden-Pencer 800-367-7874
5175 S Royal Atlanta Dr, Tucker, GA 30084

Dental Usa, Inc. 815-363-8003
5005 McCullom Lake Rd, McHenry, IL 60050
Dental scissors.

DJO Inc. 800-336-6569
1430 Decision St, Vista, CA 92081

Elmed, Inc. 630-543-2792
60 W Fay Ave, Addison, IL 60101

George Tiemann & Co. 800-843-6266
25 Plant Ave, Hauppauge, NY 11788

J. Jamner Surgical Instruments, Inc 800-431-1123
9 Skyline Dr, Hawthorne, NY 10532

Karl Storz Endoscopy-America Inc. 800-421-0837
600 Corporate Pointe, Culver City, CA 90230
For arthroscopy use.

Kenad Sg Medical, Inc. 800-825-0606
2692 Huntley Dr, Memphis, TN 38132
Orthopedic scissors.

Kentron Health Care, Inc. 615-384-0573
3604 Kelton Jackson Rd, P.o. Box 120, Springfield, TN 37172
Bandage scissors.

SCISSORS, ORTHOPEDIC *(cont'd)*

Kmedic 800-955-0559
190 Veterans Dr, Northvale, NJ 07647

Mahe International Inc. 800-294-7946
468 Craighead St, Nashville, TN 37204

Medisiss 866-866-7477
2747 SW 6th St, Redmond, OR 97756
Various orthopedic surgical scissors,sterile.

Medtronic Sofamor Danek Instrument Manufacturing 901-396-3133
7375 Adrianne Pl, Bartlett, TN 38133
Multiple (scissors).

Medtronic Sofamor Danek Usa, Inc. 901-396-3133
4340 Swinnea Rd, Memphis, TN 38118
Multiple (scissors).

Patterson Medical Supply, Inc. 262-387-8720
W68N158 Evergreen Blvd, Cedarburg, WI 53012
Various types of sicissors and cast spreaders.

Princeton Medical Group, Inc. 800-875-0869
1189 Royal Links Dr, Mt Pleasant, SC 29466

Prosurge Instruments, Inc. 866-832-7874
199 Laidlaw Ave, Jersey City, NJ 07306

Scanlan International, Inc. 800-328-9458
1 Scanlan Plz, Saint Paul, MN 55107

Smith & Nephew, Inc., Endoscopy Division 800-343-8386
150 Minuteman Rd, Andover, MA 01810

Symmetry Tnco 888-447-6661
15 Colebrook Blvd, Whitman, MA 02382

Tuzik Boston 800-886-6363
104 Longwater Dr, Assinippi Park, Norwell, MA 02061

Warsaw Orthopedic, Inc. 901-396-3133
2500 Silveus Xing, Warsaw, IN 46582
Multiple (scissors).

Zimmer Holdings, Inc. 800-613-6131
1800 W Center St, PO Box 708, Warsaw, IN 46580

SCISSORS, PEDIATRIC *(General) 80RRL*

Deknatel Snowden-Pencer 800-367-7874
5175 S Royal Atlanta Dr, Tucker, GA 30084

Elmed, Inc. 630-543-2792
60 W Fay Ave, Addison, IL 60101

Miltex Inc. 800-645-8000
589 Davies Dr, York, PA 17402

Scanlan International, Inc. 800-328-9458
1 Scanlan Plz, Saint Paul, MN 55107

Southpaw Enterprises, Inc. 800-228-1698
PO Box 1047, Dayton, OH 45401
These innovative scissors provide guides for proper finger placement, aiding children in developing good habits early. The adjustable loop isolates the index finger allowing it to act as the ìguidingî finger. The specialized thumb hole promotes thumb flexion resulting in increased web space and allows greater leverage while cutting.

SCISSORS, PLASTIC SURGERY (DISSECTING) *(Surgery) 79RRM*

Adler Instrument Co. 866-382-3537
6191 Atlantic Blvd, Norcross, GA 30071

Arosurgical Instruments Corp. 800-776-1751
537 Newport Center Dr Ste 101, Newport Beach, CA 92660
AROSurpercut scissors for Plastic surgeons. We have a wide variety. go to www.arosurgical.com for complete listing.

Bausch & Lomb Surgical 636-255-5051
3365 Tree Court Ind Blvd, Saint Louis, MO 63122

Deknatel Snowden-Pencer 800-367-7874
5175 S Royal Atlanta Dr, Tucker, GA 30084

Elmed, Inc. 630-543-2792
60 W Fay Ave, Addison, IL 60101

Fehling Surgical Instruments 800-FEHLING
509 Broadstone Ln NW, Acworth, GA 30101

J. Jamner Surgical Instruments, Inc 800-431-1123
9 Skyline Dr, Hawthorne, NY 10532

Jedmed Instruments Co. 314-845-3770
5416 Jedmed Ct, Saint Louis, MO 63129

Micrins Surgical Instruments, Inc. 800-833-3380
28438 N Ballard Dr, Lake Forest, IL 60045
Stille, Supercut, micrins razor-edge scissors, plastic surgery.

SCISSORS, PLASTIC SURGERY (DISSECTING) *(cont'd)*

Miltex Inc. 800-645-8000
589 Davies Dr, York, PA 17402

Nordent Manufacturing, Inc. 800-966-7336
610 Bonnie Ln, Elk Grove Village, IL 60007
$57.50 per unit (5-1/2in).

Princeton Medical Group, Inc. 800-875-0869
1189 Royal Links Dr, Mt Pleasant, SC 29466
TITANIUM & S/S MICROSURGICAL INSTRUMENTS

Prosurge Instruments, Inc. 866-832-7874
199 Laidlaw Ave, Jersey City, NJ 07306

Rhein Medical, Inc. 800-637-4346
5460 Beaumont Center Blvd Ste 500, Suite 500, Tampa, FL 33634

Scanlan International, Inc. 800-328-9458
1 Scanlan Plz, Saint Paul, MN 55107

Trans American Medical / Tamsco Instruments 708-430-7777
7633 W 100th Pl, Bridgeview, IL 60455

SCISSORS, RECTAL *(Gastro/Urology) 78RRN*

Deknatel Snowden-Pencer 800-367-7874
5175 S Royal Atlanta Dr, Tucker, GA 30084

Elmed, Inc. 630-543-2792
60 W Fay Ave, Addison, IL 60101

Mark Medical Manufacturing, Inc. 610-269-4420
530 Brandywine Ave, Downingtown, PA 19335
Rectal surgical instruments.

Miltex Inc. 800-645-8000
589 Davies Dr, York, PA 17402

Prosurge Instruments, Inc. 866-832-7874
199 Laidlaw Ave, Jersey City, NJ 07306

SCISSORS, SURGICAL TISSUE, DENTAL (ORAL)
(Dental And Oral) 76EGN

Acme Of Precision Surgical Co., Inc. 973-373-6797
485 21st St, Irvington, NJ 07111
Various types and sizes of dental tissue scissors.

Aesculap Implant Systems Inc. 1-800-234-9179
3773 Corporate Pkwy, Center Valley, PA 18034

Biomet Microfixation Inc. 800-874-7711
1520 Tradeport Dr, Jacksonville, FL 32218
Various types of scissors.

Deknatel Snowden-Pencer 800-367-7874
5175 S Royal Atlanta Dr, Tucker, GA 30084

Dentalez Group, Stardental Division 717-291-1161
1816 Colonial Village Ln, Lancaster, PA 17601
Scissors, surgical tissue, dental.

E.A. Beck & Co. 949-645-4072
657 W 19th St Ste E, P O Box 10857, Costa Mesa, CA 92627
Tissue scissor.

H & H Co. 909-390-0373
4435 E Airport Dr Ste 108, Ontario, CA 91761
Scissors, surgical, dental.

Hartzell & Son, G. 800-950-2206
2372 Stanwell Cir, Concord, CA 94520

Hu-Friedy Manufacturing Co., Inc. 800-483-7433
3232 N Rockwell St, Chicago, IL 60618
$50.00 to $233.00 each, 59 types.

Kmedic 800-955-0559
190 Veterans Dr, Northvale, NJ 07647

Koros Usa, Inc. 805-529-0825
610 Flinn Ave, Moorpark, CA 93021
Reusable interchangeable shaft, endoscopic scissors or graspers with slide-on in.

Miltex Dental Technologies, Inc. 516-576-6022
589 Davies Dr, York, PA 17402
Various tissue and gum cutting scissors.

Miltex Inc. 800-645-8000
589 Davies Dr, York, PA 17402

Nordent Manufacturing, Inc. 800-966-7336
610 Bonnie Ln, Elk Grove Village, IL 60007
$49.50 per unit (5-1/2in).

Oratronics, Inc. 212-986-0050
405 Lexington Ave, New York, NY 10174
Tissue scissors.

Premier Dental Products Co. 888-670-6100
1710 Romano Dr, PO Box 4500, Plymouth Meeting, PA 19462

SCISSORS, SURGICAL TISSUE, DENTAL (ORAL) *(cont'd)*

Prosurge Instruments, Inc. 866-832-7874
199 Laidlaw Ave, Jersey City, NJ 07306

Salvin Dental Specialties, Inc. 800-535-6566
3450 Latrobe Dr, Charlotte, NC 28211
Various types of surgical dental scissors.

Symmetry Medical Usa, Inc. 574-267-8700
486 W 350 N, Warsaw, IN 46582
Dental hand instrument.

Toolmex Corporation 800-992-4766
1075 Worcester St, Natick, MA 01760

Trans American Medical / Tamsco Instruments 708-430-7777
7633 W 100th Pl, Bridgeview, IL 60455
Floor grade surgical stainless steel.

Tuzik Boston 800-886-6363
104 Longwater Dr, Assinippi Park, Norwell, MA 02061

SCISSORS, SUTURE *(Surgery) 79RRO*

Codman & Shurtleff, Inc 800-225-0460
325 Paramount Dr, Raynham, MA 02767

Deknatel Snowden-Pencer 800-367-7874
5175 S Royal Atlanta Dr, Tucker, GA 30084

Elmed, Inc. 630-543-2792
60 W Fay Ave, Addison, IL 60101

George Tiemann & Co. 800-843-6266
25 Plant Ave, Hauppauge, NY 11788

Hager Worldwide, Inc. 800-328-2335
13322 Byrd Dr, Odessa, FL 33556
ROBUSTA CUT.

Havel's Inc. 800-638-4770
3726 Lonsdale St, Cincinnati, OH 45227

Kmedic 800-955-0559
190 Veterans Dr, Northvale, NJ 07647

Miltex Inc. 800-645-8000
589 Davies Dr, York, PA 17402

Nordent Manufacturing, Inc. 800-966-7336
610 Bonnie Ln, Elk Grove Village, IL 60007
$49.50 per unit (standard).

Premier Medical Products 888-PREMUSA
1710 Romano Dr, Plymouth Meeting, PA 19462

Toolmex Corporation 800-992-4766
1075 Worcester St, Natick, MA 01760

Wexler Surgical Supplies 800-414-1076
11333 Chimney Rock Rd Ste 110, Houston, TX 77035

SCISSORS, TENOTOMY *(Ophthalmology) 86RRH*

Codman & Shurtleff, Inc 800-225-0460
325 Paramount Dr, Raynham, MA 02767

Elmed, Inc. 630-543-2792
60 W Fay Ave, Addison, IL 60101

Fortrad Eye Instruments Corp. 973-543-2371
8 Franklin Rd, Mendham, NJ 07945

Jedmed Instruments Co. 314-845-3770
5416 Jedmed Ct, Saint Louis, MO 63129

Katena Products, Inc. 800-225-1195
4 Stewart Ct, Denville, NJ 07834

Miltex Inc. 800-645-8000
589 Davies Dr, York, PA 17402

Prosurge Instruments, Inc. 866-832-7874
199 Laidlaw Ave, Jersey City, NJ 07306

Scanlan International, Inc. 800-328-9458
1 Scanlan Plz, Saint Paul, MN 55107

Stephens Instruments, Inc. 800-354-7848
2500 Sandersville Rd, Lexington, KY 40511
$32.00 each.

Zimmer Holdings, Inc. 800-613-6131
1800 W Center St, PO Box 708, Warsaw, IN 46580

SCISSORS, THORACIC *(Cardiovascular) 74RRP*

Boss Instruments, Ltd. 800-210-2677
395 Reas Ford Rd Ste 120, Earlysville, VA 22936

Codman & Shurtleff, Inc 800-225-0460
325 Paramount Dr, Raynham, MA 02767

Deknatel Snowden-Pencer 800-367-7874
5175 S Royal Atlanta Dr, Tucker, GA 30084

Elmed, Inc. 630-543-2792
60 W Fay Ave, Addison, IL 60101

SCISSORS, THORACIC *(cont'd)*

Karl Storz Endoscopy-America Inc. 800-421-0837
600 Corporate Pointe, Culver City, CA 90230

Miltex Inc. 800-645-8000
589 Davies Dr, York, PA 17402

Scanlan International, Inc. 800-328-9458
1 Scanlan Plz, Saint Paul, MN 55107

SCISSORS, UMBILICAL *(Obstetrics/Gyn) 85HDJ*

Gammadirect Medical Division 847-267-5929
PO Box 383, Lake Forest, IL 60045
Seal'n Snip disposable clamp and scissors, single action. 'Father friendly'.

Prosurge Instruments, Inc. 866-832-7874
199 Laidlaw Ave, Jersey City, NJ 07306

Thomas Medical Inc. 800-556-0349
5610 West 82 2nd Street, Indianpolis, IN 46278

Toolmex Corporation 800-992-4766
1075 Worcester St, Natick, MA 01760

Trans American Medical / Tamsco Instruments 708-430-7777
7633 W 100th Pl, Bridgeview, IL 60455
Floor grade surgical stainless steel.

Tuzik Boston 800-886-6363
104 Longwater Dr, Assinippi Park, Norwell, MA 02061

SCISSORS, WIRE CUTTING, ENT *(Ear/Nose/Throat) 77JYA*

Acme Of Precision Surgical Co., Inc. 973-373-6797
485 21st St, Irvington, NJ 07111
Wire cutting scissors.

Aesculap Implant Systems Inc. 1-800-234-9179
3773 Corporate Pkwy, Center Valley, PA 18034

Bausch & Lomb Surgical 636-255-5051
3365 Tree Court Ind Blvd, Saint Louis, MO 63122

Biomet Microfixation Inc. 800-874-7711
1520 Tradeport Dr, Jacksonville, FL 32218
Various types of scissors.

Bryan Corp. 800-343-7711
4 Plympton St, Woburn, MA 01801
Scissors, graspers, dissectors 90 and 45 degree, curved, straight biopsy and grasper forceps with and without suction, curette, suction tubes.

Clinimed, Incorporated 877-CLINIMED
303 Markus Ct, Sandy Brae Industrial Park, Newark, DE 19713

Deknatel Snowden-Pencer 800-367-7874
5175 S Royal Atlanta Dr, Tucker, GA 30084

Elmed, Inc. 630-543-2792
60 W Fay Ave, Addison, IL 60101

Gyrus Ent L.L.C., Sub. Of Gyrus Acmi, Inc. 508-804-2739
2925 Appling Rd, Bartlett, TN 38133
Various types and size of ent wire cutting scissors.

Kmedic 800-955-0559
190 Veterans Dr, Northvale, NJ 07647

Precision Surgical Intl., Inc. 800-776-8493
PO Box 726, Noblesville, IN 46061
Wire cutting scissors.

Prosurge Instruments, Inc. 866-832-7874
199 Laidlaw Ave, Jersey City, NJ 07306

Tuzik Boston 800-886-6363
104 Longwater Dr, Assinippi Park, Norwell, MA 02061

SCLERAL PLUG *(Ophthalmology) 86LXP*

Alcon Manufacturing, Ltd. 817-551-6813
714 Columbia Ave, Sinking Spring, PA 19608
Scleral plug.

SCLEROTOME *(Ophthalmology) 86RRQ*

Miltex Inc. 800-645-8000
589 Davies Dr, York, PA 17402

SCOOP, COMMON DUCT *(Gastro/Urology) 78RRR*

Aesculap Implant Systems Inc. 1-800-234-9179
3773 Corporate Pkwy, Center Valley, PA 18034

SCOOP, GALLSTONE *(Gastro/Urology) 78FHL*

Biomet Microfixation Inc. 800-874-7711
1520 Tradeport Dr, Jacksonville, FL 32218
Scoop.

Codman & Shurtleff, Inc 800-225-0460
325 Paramount Dr, Raynham, MA 02767

SCOOP, GALLSTONE *(cont'd)*

Miltex Inc. 800-645-8000
589 Davies Dr, York, PA 17402

SCOOTER (MOTORIZED 3-WHEELED VEHICLE)
(Physical Med) 89INI

Access Mobility, Inc. 800-336-1147
5240 Elmwood Ave, Indianapolis, IN 46203

Aceme Technologies Int'L. 916-549-2170
278 Howe Ave Apt B, Sacramento, CA 95825
Various.

Alan's Wheelchairs & Repairs 800-693-4344
109 S Harbor Blvd Ste B, Fullerton, CA 92832
Also available with 4 wheels.

Alc, Inc. 262-502-4665
N114W19049 Clinton Dr, Germantown, WI 53022
Scooter.

Amigo Mobility International 800-248-9131
6693 Dixie Hwy, Bridgeport, MI 48722
NEW Amigo Classic traveling aid with front-wheel drive! Amigo Rear Drive models include: Amigo RD, Amigo RT Express and RT Express Jr, Amigo HD450 and Amigo EXT350.

Bruno Independent Living Aids, Inc. 800-882-8183
1780 Executive Dr, Oconomowoc, WI 53066
Aluminum frame, 3 and 4 wheel, battery operated rear wheel drive REGAL scooter, tubular steel frame, 3-wheel, battery operated, front drive regal cub scooter. TYPHOON C3 SCOOTER, is an exceptionally portable high-performance scooter, attractively priced with everything you would expect in a higher-priced scooter. Typhoon has a 300 lb. weight capacity and has a travel speed up to 4.5 mph. Rear-wheel drive, impressive maneuverability in space-restrict areas, plus access to more areas in the house and wherever you choose to go. BRUNO TURNY, a low cost transportation solution. Easy installation: the Turny Component of the system easily installs quickly with no structural modification to the vehicle. This allows for easy removal to restore the vehicle to its original condition not compromising the resale value.

Complete Mobility Systems Inc. 800-788-7479
1915 County Road C W, Roseville, MN 55113
Electric scooters.

Eagle Parts & Products, Inc. 706-790-6687
1411 Marvin Griffin Rd, Augusta, GA 30906
3 wheel personal scooter.

Electric Mobility Corporation 800-718-2082
591 Mantua Blvd, PO Box 450, Sewell, NJ 08080

Golden Technologies, Inc. 800-624-6374
401 Bridge St, Old Forge, PA 18518
Golden Technologies offers four lines of personal scooters in three and four-wheel models: Buzzaround, Companion I, Companion II and Avenger, with weight capacities ranging from 250 to 500 pounds.

Handicap Unlimited, Inc. 888-371-0095
5640 Summer Ave Ste 3, Memphis, TN 38134

Hoveround Corporation 800-964-6837
2151 Whitfield Industrial Way, Sarasota, FL 34243
HOVEROUND TRANSPORTER SCOOTERS adult 3 & 4 wheeled power scooters.

Invacare Corporation 800-333-6900
1 Invacare Way, Elyria, OH 44035
Invacare Zoom 220 Highly Maneuverable Vehicle (HMV), Zoom 300 HMV, Zoom 400 HMV

Leisure-Lift, Inc. 800-255-0285
1800 Merriam Ln, Kansas City, KS 66106
3- and 4-wheeled battery-powered scooters.

Med-Lift & Mobility, Inc. 800-748-9438
310 S. Madison, Calhoun City, MS 38916
The CTM is a three wheel direct drive scooter.

Medical Depot 516-998-4600
99 Seaview Blvd, Port Washington, NY 11050
Motorized 3-wheeled vehicle.

Pride Mobility Products Corp. 800-800-8586
401 York Ave, Duryea, PA 18642
Various types of 3 and 4 wheel scooters.

Pride Mobility Products Corp. 800-800-8586
182 Susquehanna Ave, Exeter, PA 18643
Electric 3 wheel and 4 wheel.

Ranger All Season Corp. 800-225-3811
2002 Kingbird Ave, George, IA 51237

SCOOTER (MOTORIZED 3-WHEELED VEHICLE) *(cont'd)*

Tuffcare 800-367-6160
3999 E La Palma Ave, Anaheim, CA 92807

Wheelchair Sales And Service Co., Inc. 877-736-0376
315 Main St, West Springfield, MA 01089
Leisure Lift, Pride Mobility.

Wright-Way, Inc. 800-241-8839
175 E Interstate 30, Garland, TX 75043
The anchor is an assessory used to tie down an unoccupied scooter in a vehicle.

SCOPE, FIBEROPTIC INTUBATION *(Anesthesiology) 73VDU*

North American Medical Products, Inc. 800-488-6267
6 British American Blvd Ste B, Latham, NY 12110
PORT-O-SCOPE III- a portable, fiberoptic, flexible scope that is rechargeable battery operated for difficult intubations. Also light source-powered with adaptable cable connector to fit various light sources.

Pentax Medical Company 800-431-5880
102 Chestnut Ridge Rd, Montvale, NJ 07645
$8,085.00 to $8,925.00 for fully immersible ultra-slim intubation fiberscopes with various distal tip diameters (2.4mm to 5.1mm) and channel sizes (1.2mm to 2.6mm).

Vision-Sciences, Inc. 800-874-9975
40 Ramland Rd S Ste 1, Orangeburg, NY 10962

SCRAPER, CYTOLOGY (CERVICAL) *(Obstetrics/Gyn) 85RRS*

Puritan Medical Products Company Llc 800-321-2313
31 School St., Guilford, ME 04443-0149

Solon Manufacturing Co. 800-341-6640
338 Madison Ave Ste 7, Skowhegan, ME 04976
Finest white birch wood, smooth finish. Four styles available. Seven in. sterile or non-sterile.

Surgipath Medical Industries, Inc. 800-225-3035
PO Box 528, 5205 Route 12, Richmond, IL 60071

SCRAPER, SPECIMEN, SKIN *(Surgery) 79LXK*

Citmed 251-866-5519
18601 S Main St, Citronelle, AL 36522
Scraper, cytology (cervical), 7' ayre style.

SCRAPER, TONGUE *(Dental And Oral) 76LCN*

Amden Corp. 949-581-9988
2533 N Carson St, Carson City, NV 89706
Tongue scraper or tongue cleaner.

Beyond 21st Century Inc. 888-484-2587
13706 W 75th Pl, Lenexa, KS 66216
Breath Ace Breathfreshener. Tongue cleaner.

Biocurv Medical Instruments, Inc. 1-800-589-3043
245 Dryden Ct SW, Canton, OH 44706
Tongue sweeper.

Dental Resources 717-866-7571
52 King St, Myerstown, PA 17067
Tongue scraper.

Dentek Oral Care, Inc. 865-983-1300
307 Excellence Way, Maryville, TN 37801
Tongue scraper.

Inter-Med, Inc. 877-418-4782
2200 Northwestern Ave, Racine, WI 53404
Tongue brush/tongue scraper.

Oralgiene Usa, Inc. 800-933-6725
8460 Higuera St, Culver City, CA 90232
Etc. Tongue Cleaner vibrates and is battery powered to gentaly remove debris from tongue without causing a gag reflex.

Team Technologies, Inc. 423-587-2199
5949 Commerce Blvd, Morristown, TN 37814
Tongue, scraper.

Water Pik, Inc. 970-221-6129
1730 E Prospect Rd, Fort Collins, CO 80525
Tongue cleaner.

SCREEN, ANESTHESIA *(Anesthesiology) 73RRT*

Alimed, Inc. 800-225-2610
297 High St, Dedham, MA 02026
Winged screen featuring two extension arms to support sugical drapes.

Bryton Corp. 800-567-9500
4310 Guion Rd, Indianapolis, IN 46254

Medrecon, Inc. 877-526-4323
257 South Ave, Garwood, NJ 07027

SCREEN, ANESTHESIA *(cont'd)*

Phelan Manufacturing Corp. 800-328-2358
2523 Minnehaha Ave, Minneapolis, MN 55404
Anesthesia screens: $220 for pediatric size, $230 for standard size and $242 for tall size.

SCREEN, BEDSIDE *(General) 80RRU*

Armstrong Medical Industries, Inc. 800-323-4220
575 Knightsbridge Pkwy, Lincolnshire, IL 60069

Bruin Plastics Co. 800-556-7764
61 Joslin Rd, Glendale, RI 02826

Herculite Products, Inc. 800-772-0036
PO Box 435, Emigsville, PA 17318

Larkotex Company 800-972-3037
1002 Olive St, Texarkana, TX 75501

Mayo Medical, S.A. De C.V. 800-715-3872
Edison 1141 Nte., Col. Talleres, Monterrey N.L. 64480 Mexico
Single and triple, chrome structure with polyester curtain,

Omnimed, Inc. (Beam Products) 800-257-2326
800 Glen Ave, Moorestown, NJ 08057

Presco-Webber Corporation 336-722-1067
440 Cotton St, Winston Salem, NC 27101
Folding bed screens and room dividers.

SCREEN, INTENSIFYING, RADIOGRAPHIC *(Radiology) 90IXM*

Burkhart Roentgen Intl. Inc. 800-USA-XRAY
5201 8th Ave S, Gulfport, FL 33707
Calcium tungstate and rare earth screens available in all current formats.

Flow X-Ray Corporation 800-356-9729
100 W Industry Ct, Deer Park, NY 11729
Over 100 different types.

Marconi Medical Systems 800-323-0550
595 Miner Rd, Cleveland, OH 44143

Mci Optonix, Div. Of Usr Optonix Inc. 800-678-6649
253 E Washington Ave, Washington, NJ 07882

Pl Medical Co., Llc. 800-874-0120
321 Ellis St, New Britain, CT 06051

Soyee Products, Inc. 800-574-4743
459 Thompson Rd, Thompson, CT 06277
KIRAN intensifying screens.

Spectronics Corporation 800-274-8888
956 Brush Hollow Rd, Westbury, NY 11590
SPECTROLINE calcium tungstate and rare earth; all speeds and sizes.

Umi Intl. 888-511-8655
2 E Union Ave, PO Box 170, East Rutherford, NJ 07073

Wolf X-Ray Corporation 800-356-9729
100 W Industry Ct, Deer Park, NY 11729
Over 100 different types.

SCREEN, INTENSIFYING, RADIOGRAPHIC, DENTAL *(Dental And Oral) 76EAM*

Addent, Inc. 203-778-0200
43 Miry Brook Rd, Danbury, CT 06810
The Microlux DL is to be used in conjunction with a traditional visual and tactile examination. The exam is performed by a dentist or health care provider to increase identification, evaluation, and monitoring of oral mucosal abnormalities found on the soft tissues of the oral environment. After rinsing with the DL solution, irregular cells will take on a whitish hue which will contrast with the surrounding tissues making it more obvious to the examiner. The Microlux DL is used to help detect abnormal oral tissue. It is sold as a kit (the Microlux, the DL light guide, batteries plus 6 bottles of acetic acid solution). The light guide and solution can be purchased separately. Once the kit has been purchased, the refill bottles of acetic acid are all that is necessary to perform an exam. Cost of exam will be about $6.00 per patient!

Agfa Corporation 877-777-2432
PO Box 19048, 10 South Academy Street, Greenville, SC 29602

Cone Instruments, Inc. 800-321-6964
5201 Naiman Pkwy, Solon, OH 44139

Ge Medical Systems, Llc 262-548-2355
3000 N Grandview Blvd, W-417, Waukesha, WI 53188
Intensifying screens, in various sizes.

Kodak Canada Inc., Health Imaging Division 800-295-5526
3500 Eglinton Ave. W., Toronto, ONT M6M 1V3 Canada

Mci Optonix, Div. Of Usr Optonix Inc. 800-678-6649
253 E Washington Ave, Washington, NJ 07882

SCREEN, TANGENT, FELT (CAMPIMETER)
(Ophthalmology) 86HOL

A&A Orthopedics, Incorporated 757-224-0177
12250 SW 129th Ct Bldg 1, Miami, FL 33186
Orthopedic felt.

Richmond Products, Inc. 505-275-2406
4400 Silver Ave SE, Albuquerque, NM 87108
Hematocrit control.

SCREEN, TANGENT, TARGET *(Ophthalmology) 86HOJ*

Gulden Ophthalmics 800-659-2250
225 Cadwalader Ave, Elkins Park, PA 19027

Richmond Products, Inc. 505-275-2406
4400 Silver Ave SE, Albuquerque, NM 87108
Hematocrit control.

SCREW, CRANIOPLASTY PLATE *(Cns/Neurology) 84UAU*

Kls-Martin L.P. 800-625-1557
11239-1 St. John`s Industrial, Parkway South
Jacksonville, FL 32250

Zimmer Holdings, Inc. 800-613-6131
1800 W Center St, PO Box 708, Warsaw, IN 46580

SCREW, FIXATION, BONE *(Orthopedics) 87HWC*

Abbott Spine, Inc. 847-937-6100
12708 Riata Vista Cir Ste B-100, Austin, TX 78727
Ubp system.

Acumed Llc 503-627-9957
5885 NW Cornelius Pass Rd, Hillsboro, OR 97124
Bone fixation screw, acutrak, acutrail plus, extremity, fusion, mini acutrak.

Acute Innovations Llc 503-627-9957
21421 NW Jacobson Rd Ste 700, Hillsboro, OR 97124
Screw, fixation, bone.

Aesculap Implant Systems Inc. 1-800-234-9179
3773 Corporate Pkwy, Center Valley, PA 18034
Bone screws for orthopedic and cervical fixation.

Alphatec Spine, Inc. 760-494-6769
5818 El Camino Real, Carlsbad, CA 92008
Cannulated cancellous bone screw & cortical screws.

Arc Surgical Llc. 503-627-9957
21300 NW Jacobson Rd, Hillsboro, OR 97124
Smooth or threaded metallic bone fixation fastener.

Arthrex Manufacturing 239-643-5553
1958 Trade Center Way, Naples, FL 34109
Screw.

Arthrex, Inc. 239-643-5553
1370 Creekside Blvd, Naples, FL 34108
Various.

Ascension Orthopedics, Inc. 877-370-5001
8700 Cameron Rd, Austin, TX 78754
Cannulated Screw System

Bio-Technology Usa, Inc. 305-512-3522
6175 NW 167th St Ste G8, Hialeah, FL 33015
Maxillofacial screw fixation bone.

Biomet Microfixation Inc. 800-874-7711
1520 Tradeport Dr, Jacksonville, FL 32218
Various types of screws.

Biomet, Inc. 574-267-6639
56 E Bell Dr, PO Box 587, Warsaw, IN 46582
Poly-l-lactic acid/polyglycolic acid screws.

Coapt Systems, Inc. 650-461-7600
1820 Embarcadero Rd, Palo Alto, CA 94303
Chin lift device and installation tools.

Comco, Inc. 800-796-6626
2151 N Lincoln St, Burbank, CA 91504
Micro-abrasive blasting equipment for deburring, cleaning, and surface prep of bone screws and other implant devices.

Depuy Ace, A Johnson & Johnson Company 800-473-3789
700 Orthopaedic Dr, Warsaw, IN 46582

Depuy Mitek, A Johnson & Johnson Company 800-451-2006
50 Scotland Blvd, Bridgewater, MA 02324
Appliance for reconstruction of bone and soft tissue.

Depuy Orthopaedics, Inc. 800-473-3789
700 Orthopaedic Dr, P.O. Box 988, Warsaw, IN 46582
Various types of bone fixation screws.

SCREW, FIXATION, BONE *(cont'd)*

Depuy Spine, Inc. 800-227-6633
325 Paramount Dr, Raynham, MA 02767
Bone screw.

Depuy-Raynham, A Div. Of Depuy Orthopaedics 800-451-2006
325 Paramount Dr, Raynham, MA 02767
Various types of bone fixation screws.

DJO Inc. 800-336-6569
1430 Decision St, Vista, CA 92081

Doctors Research Group, Inc. 800-371-2535
574 Heritage Rd Ste 202, Southbury, CT 06488
Self-Drilling and Self-Tapping Screws with patented suture retention features

Endotec, Inc. 973-762-6100
2546 Hansrob Rd, Orlando, FL 32804
Buechel-pappas cancellous bone screw.

Gyrus Ent L.L.C., Sub. Of Gyrus Acmi, Inc. 508-804-2739
2925 Appling Rd, Bartlett, TN 38133
Various types and sizes of bone fixation screws.

Holmed Corporation 508-238-3351
40 Norfolk Ave, South Easton, MA 02375

Instratek, Inc. 281-890-8020
210 Spring Hill Dr Ste 130, Spring, TX 77386
Titanium cannulated bone-screw system.

Integra Lifesciences Of Ohio 800-654-2873
4900 Charlemar Dr Bldg A, Cincinnati, OH 45227
Various bone screws.

Internal Fixation Systems, Inc. 305-491-9133
10100 NW 116th Way Ste 18, Medley, FL 33178
Cannulated bone screw.

Interventional Spine, Inc. 800-497-0484
13700 Alton Pkwy Ste 160, Irvine, CA 92618
Compression anchor system.

Kls-Martin L.P. 800-625-1557
11239-1 St. John`s Industrial, Parkway South
Jacksonville, FL 32250

Kmedic 800-955-0559
190 Veterans Dr, Northvale, NJ 07647

Medtronic Sofamor Danek Usa, Inc. 901-396-3133
4340 Swinnea Rd, Memphis, TN 38118
Bone screw.

Microcision Llc 800-264-3811
5805 Keystone St, Philadelphia, PA 19135

Millennium Medical Technologies, Inc. 505-988-7595
460 Saint Michaels Dr Ste 901, Santa Fe, NM 87505
Bone screw.

Orthohelix Surgical Designs, Inc. 330-869-9582
1815 W Market St Ste 205, Akron, OH 44313
Cannulated screw.

Pioneer Surgical Technology 800-557-9909
375 River Park Cir, Marquette, MI 49855

RTI Biologics Inc. 877-343-6832
11621 Research Cir, Alachua, FL 32615
Interference screw.

Si-Bone Inc. 408-207-0700
550 S Winchester Blvd Ste 620, San Jose, CA 95128
SI-BONE

Signal Medical Corporation 800-246-6324
1000 Des Peres Rd Ste 140, Saint Louis, MO 63131
Cancellous Bone screws.

Simplicity Orthopedic Solutions, Llc 866-623-0033
77 Main St Ste 2, Andover, MA 01810
Various bone fasteners.

Small Bone Innovations, Inc. 215-428-1791
1380 S Pennsylvania Ave, Morrisville, PA 19067
Internal fixation system.

Smith & Nephew, Inc., Endoscopy Division 800-343-8386
150 Minuteman Rd, Andover, MA 01810
ENDOFIX Absorbable interference surgical fixation screw for bone-tendon-bone graft fixation in anterior cruciate ligament (ACL) surgery.

Stryker Spine 866-457-7463
2 Pearl Ct, Allendale, NJ 07401

SCREW, FIXATION, BONE *(cont'd)*

Supreme Screw Products, Inc. 718-293-6600
1368 Cromwell Ave, Bronx, NY 10452
Fixation devices (bone screws and other components).

Synthes (Usa) 610-719-5000
35 Airport Rd, Horseheads, NY 14845
Various types and sizes of bone fixation screws.

Synthes (Usa) - Brandywine Technical Center 800-523-0322
1301-1303 Goshen Pky., West Chester, PA 19380

Tornier Inc. 978-232-9997
100 Cummings Ctr Ste 444C, Beverly, MA 01915
Bone achor.

Ussc Puerto Rico, Inc. 203-845-1000
Building 911-67, Sabanetas Industrial Park, Ponce, PR 00731
Bone fixation.

Warsaw Orthopedic, Inc. 901-396-3133
2500 Silveus Xing, Warsaw, IN 46582
Bone screws-sterile and non-sterile.

Zimmer Holdings, Inc. 800-613-6131
1800 W Center St, PO Box 708, Warsaw, IN 46580
Also, compression hip screw.

Zimmer Manufacturing B.V. 800-613-6131
Route 1, Km. 123.4, Bldg. 1, Turpeaux Industrial Park
Mercedita, PR 00715
Various types and sizes of bones screws.

Zimmer Trabecular Metal Technology 800-613-6131
10 Pomeroy Rd, Parsippany, NJ 07054
Sterile cancellous bone screws and non-sterile instruments.

SCREW, FIXATION, BONE, NON-SPINAL, METALLIC
(Orthopedics) 87NDJ

Advanced Orthopaedic Solutions, Inc. 310-533-9966
386 Beech Ave Unit B6, Torrance, CA 90501
Bone screw.

Surgical Implant Generation Network (Sign) 509-371-1107
451 Hills St, Richland, WA 99354
Various sizes of cortical screws.

Warsaw Orthopedic, Inc. 901-396-3133
2500 Silveus Xing, Warsaw, IN 46582
Ucss, atlas.

Zimmer Manufacturing B.V. 800-613-6131
Route 1, Km. 123.4, Bldg. 1, Turpeaux Industrial Park
Mercedita, PR 00715
Various types and sizes of bone screws.

SCREW, FIXATION, INTRAOSSEOUS *(Dental And Oral) 76DZL*

Biomet Microfixation Inc. 800-874-7711
1520 Tradeport Dr, Jacksonville, FL 32218
Various types of screws.

Biomet, Inc. 574-267-6639
56 E Bell Dr, PO Box 587, Warsaw, IN 46582
Intraosseous fixation screw or wire.

Bioplate, Inc. 310-815-2100
3643 Lenawee Ave, Los Angeles, CA 90016
Screw, fixation, intraosseous.

Glenroe Technologies 800-237-4060
1912 44th Ave E, Bradenton, FL 34203
Ete coated nickel titanium wire.

Kmedic 800-955-0559
190 Veterans Dr, Northvale, NJ 07647

Renick Ent., Inc. 561-863-4183
1211 W 13th St, Riviera Beach, FL 33404
custom bone and attachment screws

Straumann Manufacturing, Inc. 978-747-2575
60 Minuteman Rd, Andover, MA 01810
Fixation screws and instruments.

SCREW, ORAL *(Ear/Nose/Throat) 77KBW*

Biomet Microfixation Inc. 800-874-7711
1520 Tradeport Dr, Jacksonville, FL 32218
Various types of screws.

E.A. Beck & Co. 949-645-4072
657 W 19th St Ste E, P O Box 10857, Costa Mesa, CA 92627
Wood screw.

SCREWDRIVER *(Orthopedics) 87HXX*

Abbott Spine, Inc. 847-937-6100
12708 Riata Vista Cir Ste B-100, Austin, TX 78727
Screwdriver.

Biomet Microfixation Inc. 800-874-7711
1520 Tradeport Dr, Jacksonville, FL 32218
Orthopedic screwdriver.

Biomet, Inc. 574-267-6639
56 E Bell Dr, PO Box 587, Warsaw, IN 46582
Various types of orthopedic screwdrivers.

Centinel Spine Inc. 952-885-0500
505 Park Ave Fl 14, New York, NY 10022
Stalif C 2.5 Universal Screwdriver

Depuy Mitek, A Johnson & Johnson Company 800-451-2006
50 Scotland Blvd, Bridgewater, MA 02324
Various orthopedic screwdrivers.

Depuy Spine, Inc. 800-227-6633
325 Paramount Dr, Raynham, MA 02767
Screwdriver, hexhead.

DJO Inc. 800-336-6569
1430 Decision St, Vista, CA 92081

Gauthier Biomedical, Inc. 262-546-0010
1235 Dakota Dr Ste G, Grafton, WI 53024
Screwdriver.

Holmed Corporation 508-238-3351
40 Norfolk Ave, South Easton, MA 02375

Interventional Spine, Inc. 800-497-0484
13700 Alton Pkwy Ste 160, Irvine, CA 92618
Various types of drivers.

K2m, Inc. 866-526-4171
751 Miller Dr SE Ste F1, Leesburg, VA 20175
Screw inserter, driver.

Kls-Martin L.P. 800-625-1557
11239-1 St. John`s Industrial, Parkway South
Jacksonville, FL 32250

Kmedic 800-955-0559
190 Veterans Dr, Northvale, NJ 07647

Medtronic Sofamor Danek Instrument Manufacturing 901-396-3133
7375 Adrianne Pl, Bartlett, TN 38133
Screwdriver, orthopedic.

Medtronic Sofamor Danek Usa, Inc. 901-396-3133
4340 Swinnea Rd, Memphis, TN 38118
Screwdriver, orthopedic.

Microcision Llc 800-264-3811
5805 Keystone St, Philadelphia, PA 19135

Nobel Biocare Usa, Llc 800-579-6515
22715/22725 Savi Ranch Parkway, Yorba Linda, CA 92887
Prosthetic instrument.

RTI Biologics Inc. 877-343-6832
11621 Research Cir, Alachua, FL 32615
Modular handle, screwdriver.

Salvin Dental Specialties, Inc. 800-535-6566
3450 Latrobe Dr, Charlotte, NC 28211
Various types of dental screwdrivers and accessories.

Small Bone Innovations, Inc. 215-428-1791
1380 S Pennsylvania Ave, Morrisville, PA 19067
Orthopedic manual surgical instrument.

Spine Wave, Inc. 203-944-9494
2 Enterprise Dr Ste 302, Shelton, CT 06484
Various types of screwdrivers.

Stryker Corp. 800-726-2725
2825 Airview Blvd, Portage, MI 49002

Stryker Spine 866-457-7463
2 Pearl Ct, Allendale, NJ 07401

Surgical Implant Generation Network (Sign) 509-371-1107
451 Hills St, Richland, WA 99354
Screw driver.

Vilex, Inc. 931-474-7550
111 Moffitt St, McMinnville, TN 37110

Warsaw Orthopedic, Inc. 901-396-3133
2500 Silveus Xing, Warsaw, IN 46582
Screwdriver, orthopedic.

Zimmer Holdings, Inc. 800-613-6131
1800 W Center St, PO Box 708, Warsaw, IN 46580

SCREWDRIVER *(cont'd)*

Zimmer Spine, Inc. 800-655-2614
7375 Bush Lake Rd, Minneapolis, MN 55439
Screwdriver.

Zimmer Trabecular Metal Technology 800-613-6131
10 Pomeroy Rd, Parsippany, NJ 07054
Acetabular screw driver.

SCREWDRIVER, SKULLPLATE *(Cns/Neurology) 84GXL*

Medtronic Image-Guided Neurologics, Inc. 800-707-0933
2290 W Eau Gallie Blvd, Melbourne, FL 32935
Screwdriver.

SCREWDRIVER, SURGICAL *(Surgery) 79LRZ*

Cardinal Health, Snowden Pencer Products 847-689-8410
5175 S Royal Atlanta Dr, Tucker, GA 30084
Manual surgical instrument.

Interphase Implants, Inc. 248-442-1460
19928 Farmington Rd, Livonia, MI 48152
Screwdriver.

Kls-Martin L.P. 800-625-1557
11239-1 St. John`s Industrial, Parkway South
Jacksonville, FL 32250

Microcision Llc 800-264-3811
5805 Keystone St, Philadelphia, PA 19135

Millennium Devices, Inc. 631-582-6424
250 Gibbs Rd, Islandia, NY 11749
Screw driver device.

SCRUB MACHINE, SURGICAL *(Surgery) 79RRX*

Medical Technologies Co. 800-280-3220
1728 W Park Center Dr Ste A, Fenton, MO 63026
Single, dual and triple surgical scrub stations.

Scientek Medical Equipment 604-273-9094
11151 Bridgeport Rd., Richmond, BC V6X 1T3 Canada
Stainless steel scrub sinks with knee or hip operated soap & water dispensers. Thermostatic water temperature controls. Optional infrared activated water & soap dispensing controls.

Sloan Valve Co. 800-9VA-LVE9
10500 Seymour Ave, Franklin Park, IL 60131
Electronic surgical scrub sink.

Whitehall Manufacturing 800-782-7706
15125 Proctor Ave, City Of Industry, CA 91746
Stainless steel surgical scrub sinks accommodate on or off-floor configurations in one-two-three station: all compact, durable and sanitary.

SEALANT, PIT AND FISSURE, AND CONDITIONER, RESIN *(Dental And Oral) 76EBC*

American Dental Products, Inc. 800-846-7120
603 Country Club Dr Ste B, Bensenville, IL 60106
Pit & fissure sealant.

Bisco, Inc. 847-534-6000
1100 W Irving Park Rd, Schaumburg, IL 60193
Sealant & conditioner-various types.

Block Drug Co., Inc. 973-889-2578
2149 Harbor Ave., Memphis, TN 38113
Dentinal sealant.

Cadco Dental Products 800-833-8267
600 E Hueneme Rd, Oxnard, CA 93033
Priced from $195.00 to $795.00 for five models of hydrocolloid conditioners.

Cao Group, Inc. 801-256-9282
4628 Skyhawk Dr, West Jordan, UT 84084
Pit and fissure sealant.

Den-Mat Holdings, Llc 805-922-8491
2727 Skyway Dr, Santa Maria, CA 93455
No common name listed.

Denali R&D Corporation 781-826-9190
134 Old Washington St, Hanover, MA 02339
Pit & fissure sealant and conditioner.

Dental Resources 717-866-7571
52 King St, Myerstown, PA 17067
Tissue sealant.

Dental Technologies, Inc. 847-677-5500
6901 N Hamlin Ave, Lincolnwood, IL 60712
Enamel bond system w/etchant.

SEALANT, PIT AND FISSURE, AND CONDITIONER, RESIN *(cont'd)*

Dux Dental 800-833-8267
600 E Hueneme Rd, Oxnard, CA 93033
Prices from $195.00 to $795.00 for five models of hydrocolloid conditioners.

Foremost Dental Llc. 201-894-5500
242 S Dean St, Englewood, NJ 07631
Toth etch agent.

Gresco Products, Inc. 800-527-3250
13391 Murphy Rd, P.o. Box 865, Stafford, TX 77477
Acid etching gel metal.

Ivoclar Vivadent, Inc. 800-533-6825
175 Pineview Dr, Amherst, NY 14228
HELIOSEAL F fluoride-releasing sealant in opaque shade. HELIOSEAL CLEAR CHROMA. Clear sealant with reversible color change.

Kerr Corp. 949-255-8766
1717 W Collins Ave, Orange, CA 92867
Pit and fissure sealant and conditioner.

Medental Intl. 760-727-5889
3008 Palm Hill Dr, Vista, CA 92084
Pit & fissure sealant & primers.

Novocol, Inc. 303-665-7535
416 S Taylor Ave, Louisville, CO 80027
Pit and fissure sealant.

Oratech, Llc 801-553-4493
475 W 10200 S, South Jordan, UT 84095
Pit and fissure sealant and conditioner.

Pentron Clinical Technologies 203-265-7397
68-70 North Plains Industrial, Road, Wallingford, CT 06492
Pit and fissure sealant.

Pentron Laboratory Technologies 203-265-7397
53 N Plains Industrial Rd, Wallingford, CT 06492
Pit and fissure sealant, c-22.

Protech Professional Products, Inc. 561-493-9818
2900 Commerce Park Dr Ste 10, Boynton Beach, FL 33426
Sealant.

Pulpdent Corp. 800-343-4342
80 Oakland St, Watertown, MA 02472
Fluoride-releasing pit and fissure sealant.

Rite-Dent Manufacturing Corp. 305-693-8626
3750 E 10th Ct, Hialeah, FL 33013
Various types of pit and fissure dental sealant.

Scientific Pharmaceuticals, Inc. 800-634-3047
3221 Producer Way, Pomona, CA 91768
$60.00 for 25-g kit with accessories.

Ultradent Products, Inc. 801-553-4586
505 W 10200 S, South Jordan, UT 84095
Pit and fissure sealant.

Zenith/Dmg Brand 800-662-6383
242 S Dean St, Division of Foremost Dental LLC, Englewood, NJ 07631

3m Espe Dental Products 949-863-1360
2111 McGaw Ave, Irvine, CA 92614
$140.50 per unit.

SEALANT, POLYMERIZING *(General) 80NBE*

Confluent Surgical,Inc 888-734-2583
101A 1st Ave, Waltham, MA 02451
Absorbable surgical sealant.

SEALER, PACKAGING *(General) 80TDK*

Baxter Healthcare Corporation Nutrition 888-229-0001
1 Baxter Pkwy, Deerfield, IL 60015
CLINTEC hand sealer and hand sealer clips.

Belco Packaging Systems, Inc. 800-833-1833
910 S Mountain Ave, Monrovia, CA 91016
Belco Packaging Systems, Inc. has manufactured heat-sealing equipment for since 1957, with 25 years dedicated to manufacturing medical device packaging machinery. As the industry demand for process control capabilities evolved, so has the product line.

SEALER, PACKAGING *(cont'd)*

Eraser Company, Inc. 800-724-0594
123 Oliva Dr, Mattydale, NY 13211
GLORING infrared heat tool for heat shrinking and tube forming. Suitable for cleanroom use. Used for sealing security seals of exit ports of I.V. bags and for shrinking tubing on probes, seals on catheters, and wire harnesses of medical equipment. Lightweight; can be used as a hand tool or bench mounted. With or without heat control.

Gdm Electronic And Medical 408-945-4100
2070 Ringwood Ave, San Jose, CA 95131

Mes, Inc. 800-423-2215
1968 E US Highway 90, Seguin, TX 78155
Impulse sealers in three sizes: Part#0108 for 8 inch, 0112 for 12 inch, and 1116 for 16 inch

National Instrument Co., Inc. 800-526-1301
4119 Fordleigh Rd, Baltimore, MD 21215

Saint-Gobain Performance Plastics--Akron 800-798-1554
2664 Gilchrist Rd, Akron, OH 44305
SEAL-VIEW laboratory sealing film for sealing glass, plastic or metal vessels and containers.

Trudell Medical Marketing Ltd. 800-265-5494
926 Leathorne St., London, ON N5Z-3M5 Canada

Westlund Engineering, Inc. 727-572-4343
12400 44th St N, Clearwater, FL 33762
Versatile benchtop sealer for trays, blisters, or pouches.

SECURITY EQUIPMENT/SUPPLIES *(General) 80VAY*

Argus-Hazco 800-332-0435
6501 Centerville Business Pkwy, Dayton, OH 45459
Laboratory supplies.

Assisted Access-Nfss, Inc. 800-950-9655
822 Preston Ct, Lake Villa, IL 60046
Fire and smoke alarm systems; visual alerting systems.

Atd-American Co. 800-523-2300
135 Greenwood Ave, Wyncote, PA 19095
Safety and protective security items such as metal detectors, security mirrors, etc.

Callcare 800-345-9414
1370 Arcadia Rd, Lancaster, PA 17601
Door and sign security systems and replacement parts.

Care Electronics, Inc. 303-444-2273
4700 Sterling Dr Ste D, Boulder, CO 80301
PATIENTCARE WANDERER Monitoring System monitors doorways and halls for attempts to exit. The system monitors 50 residents and identifies the wanderer attempting to exit. Adjustable sensitivity and long battery life transmitters are standard. PATIENTCARE 16/64 Wireless Monitoring System provides wireless nurse-call features, door monitoring, pendant 'help' buttons, and Deluxe Occupancy transmitters. System is fully supervised for reliability. WANDERCARE 100 Monitoring System monitors wanderers at home and notifies caregivers when the wanderer leaves the area. Long range tracking (up to one mile) is included. System can also notify others by phone and pager of the emergency.

Cmt, Inc. 800-659-9140
PO Box 297, Hamilton, MA 01936
HABITAT MONITOR is ideal for any controlled environment. The precision CLIMATE SECURITY SYSTEM is a thermo-hygrometric device with accuracies of + or - 2% Relative Humidity and = or - 1 degree Fahrenheit.

Construction Specialties Inc. 800-233-8493
6696 Route. 405, Muncy, PA 17756
PEDISYSTEMS, color matched entryway systems.

Crest Healthcare Supply 800-328-8908
195 3rd St, Dassel, MN 55325
Fire and smoke alarms; surveillance equipment; door alarms; tamper-proof security screw kit.

Healthmark Industries 800-521-6224
22522 E 9 Mile Rd, Saint Clair Shores, MI 48080
$13.60 to 29.00 per 100 tamper-evident locks for carts.

Idesco Corp. 800-336-1383
37 W 26th St, New York, NY 10010
Photo identification for hospital security.

J.M. Baragano Biomedical P.M. And Consulting, Inc. 787-722-4007
808 Ave Fernandez Juncos, San Juan, PR 00907
DYNAVISION/CONTROL SCREENING, security screening equipment for access control. X-ray screening, metal detectors, and controlled substance sniffers. TOPDATA Biometric Scanners.

SECURITY EQUIPMENT/SUPPLIES *(cont'd)*

Key-Bak 800-685-2403
4245 Pacific Privado, Ontario, CA 91761
Retractable key chain reels, key returns, and products for the key security industry. MINI-BAK ID combination badgeholder/retractor. TWIST FREE MINI-BAK and badge access control badgeholder/retractor is the best way to ensure your message is viewed every day. SUPER 48 KEY REEL extension unwinds directly from the reel in the same direction you pull. The Super 48 case has a wide slit along the front edge that lets the cable come straight off the reel tangentially. Unnecessary friction and wear are eliminated; spring action is 100% efficient; your KEY-BAK works easier; and its service life is enhanced.

Md International, Inc. 305-669-9003
11300 NW 41st St, Doral, FL 33178
Turnkey projects.

Metro Cad, Inc 612-302-8056
2277 49th Ave N, Minneapolis, MN 55430
ACTIVE RFID For local and remote Real Time locating of personel, patients, wheelchairs, equipment and samples. Simple and Cost Effective.

Minatronics Corp. 412-488-6435
1 Trimont Ln Apt 850C, Pittsburgh, PA 15211
Alarm system for 24-hour internal theft protection of computer and laboratory equipment. LIGHTGARD fiber optic system protects unit and internal circuit boards.

Rf Technologies 800-669-9946
3125 N 126th St, Brookfield, WI 53005
Electromagnetic door locks; Staff Alert panel annunciators; perimeter alarms. Also, infant and child security systems to prevent infant or child abductions from hospital nursery or pediatric wards. Infant/Child Security System (ICSS) 'Safe Place.' RF-based Wander Monitoring. 'PinPoint' asset management system to track and secure your most valuable assets.

Secure Care Products, Inc. 800-451-7917
39 Chenell Dr, Concord, NH 03301
ADVANTAGE 500 DE provides security for exits and meets safety code 101.

Shure Manufacturing Corp. 800-227-4873
1901 W Main St, Washington, MO 63090
SHURESAFE security thru-wall drawers for transferring prescriptions, etc.; SHURESAFE SHIELD safety enclosures and security systems for pharmacy usage.

Tork 914-664-3542
1 Grove St, Mount Vernon, NY 10550
Time Switches, Photocontrols, Facility Management Systems, signaling devices for hazardous warning for vehicles, buildings, dock-loading.

Uniflex Inc., Medical Packaging Division 800-223-0564
383 W John St, Hicksville, NY 11801
UNIVAULT Tamper evident patient valuable bags.

Valley Craft 800-328-1480
2001 S Highway 61, Lake City, MN 55041

Vicon Industries Inc. 800-645-9116
89 Arkay Dr, Hauppauge, NY 11788
Closed circuit television security systems, including digital video recorders and management systems.

SEED, ISOTOPE, GOLD, TITANIUM, PLATINUM
(Radiology) 90IWG

Alpha-Omega Services, Inc. 800-346-7894
9156 Rose St, Bellflower, CA 90706
Iridium-192 seeds for brachytherapy and endocurietherapy.

SEMINAL FLUID, ANTIGEN, ANTISERUM, CONTROL
(Immunology) 82DGB

Biomerieux Inc. 800-682-2666
100 Rodolphe St, Durham, NC 27712

SENSITIVITY TEST POWDER, ANTIMICROBIAL
(Microbiology) 83JTT

Roquette America 319-524-5757
1417 Exchange St, PO Box 6647, Keokuk, IA 52632
Surgical and examination dusting powder.

SENSITOMETER, RADIOGRAPHIC *(Radiology) 90VGP*

Owens Scientific Inc. 281-394-2311
23230 Sandsage Ln, Katy, TX 77494

Supertech, Inc. 800-654-1054
PO Box 186, Elkhart, IN 46515
Nuclear Associates and ESECO brands available.

SENSITOMETER, RADIOGRAPHIC *(cont'd)*

X-Rite, Inc. 888-826-3044
4300 44th St SE, Grand Rapids, MI 49512

SENSOR, BLOOD GAS, IN-LINE, CARDIOPULMONARY BYPASS
(Cardiovascular) 74DTY

International Biophysics Corp. 512-326-3244
2101 E Saint Elmo Rd Ste 275, Austin, TX 78744
Sensor, blood-gas, cardiopulmonary bypass.

Terumo Cardiovascular Systems (Tcvs) 800-283-7866
28 Howe St, Ashland, MA 01721
In-line blood gas monitor.

SENSOR, ELECTRO-OPTICAL(FOR CERVICAL CANCER)
(Obstetrics/Gyn) 85MWM

Medispectra Inc 781-372-2430
45 Hartwell Ave, Lexington, MA 02421
Optical detection system.

Spectrascience, Inc. 858-847-0200
11568 Sorrento Valley Rd Ste 11, San Diego, CA 92121
Luma(tm) Cervical Imaging System

SENSOR, GLUCOSE, INVASIVE *(General) 80MDS*

Dexcom, Inc. 858-200-0200
6340 Sequence Dr, San Diego, CA 92121
Continuous glucose sensor.

Medtronic Minimed 800-933-3322
18000 Devonshire St, Northridge, CA 91325
Cgms.

SENSOR, MOISTURE *(General) 80WSZ*

Cmt, Inc. 800-659-9140
PO Box 297, Hamilton, MA 01936

Edgetech 800-276-3729
19 Brigham St Unit 8, Marlborough, MA 01752
Model 1-C DewTrace Trace Moisture Analyzer. Also available, DPM-99 Dew Point Monitor which consists of the sensor, audible and visual alarms, and flow controller contained within a mountable enclosure.

Enviro Guard, Inc. 800-438-1152
201 Shannon Oaks Cir Ste 115, Cary, NC 27511

Wr Medical Electronics Co. 800-321-6387
123 2nd St N, Stillwater, MN 55082
Q-Sweat Quantitative Sweat Measurement System: diagnostic device precisely measures human sweat output in order to characterize the autonomic nervous system.

SENSOR, OPTICAL CONTOUR, PHYSICAL MEDICINE
(Physical Med) 89LDK

Medical Tactile, Inc. 310-641-8228
5757 W Century Blvd Ste 600, Los Angeles, CA 90045
Electronic documentation device for the clinical breast examination.

S&S Technology 281-815-1300
10625 Telge Rd, Houston, TX 77095

SENSOR, OXYGEN *(Anesthesiology) 73RSA*

Accu Scan Instruments, Inc. 800-822-1344
5098 Trabue Rd, Columbus, OH 43228
For laboratory animals; also measures CO2.

Cardinal Health 207, Inc. 800-231-2466
22745 Savi Ranch Pkwy, Yorba Linda, CA 92887
Non-invasive oxygen and carbon dioxide sensor.

Maxtec, Inc. 800-748-5355
6526 Cottonwood St, Salt Lake City, UT 84107
Replacement sensors for oxygen monitoring devices.

Quadromed Inc. 800-363-0192
5776 Thimens Ave., St-Laurent, QUE H4R 2K9 Canada

Sensidyne, Inc. 800-451-9444
16333 Bay Vista Dr, Clearwater, FL 33760
SensAid is the first system that combines the comfort and performance of a disposable SpO2 sensor with the economy and convenience of a disposable sensor.

Servomex 800-862-0200
525 Julie Rivers Dr Ste 185, Sugar Land, TX 77478
Paramagnetic O2 sensor. Non-depleting sensor, low power requirements, and high accuracy. SERVOMEX, Paracube, unique paramagnetic oxygen sensor for OEM applications.

SENSOR, OXYGEN *(cont'd)*

Sharn, Inc. 800-325-3671
4517 George Rd Ste 200, Tampa, FL 33634
Replacement sensors and long-life sensors for oxygen monitoring equipment.

Vascular Technology Incorporated 800-550-0856
12 Murphy Dr, Nashua, NH 03062
Polarographic or galvanic oxygen sensors and supplies.

SENSOR, PRESSURE, ANEURYSM, IMPLANTABLE
(Cardiovascular) 74NQH

CardioMEMS, Inc. 866-240-3335
387 Technology Cir NW Ste 500, Atlanta, GA 30313
ENDOSURE WIRELESS PRES, EndoSure s2, EndoSure

SEPARATION MEDIA *(Microbiology) 83TDG*

Bangs Laboratories, Inc. 800-387-0672
9025 Technology Dr, Fishers, IN 46038
Uniform silica particles for DNA separation and immunoassays. Sizes 0.15 to 7um.

SEPARATOR, BLOOD CELL, AUTOMATED *(Hematology) 81GKT*

Baxter Healthcare Corp., Renal Division 847-948-2000
7511 114th Ave, Largo, FL 33773
Various cell separators & sterile and non-sterile accessories.

Baxter Healthcare S.A. 847-948-2000
Rd. 721, Km. 0.3, Aibonito, PR 00609
Various cell separators and sterile and non-sterile accessories.

Biomerieux Inc. 800-682-2666
100 Rodolphe St, Durham, NC 27712

Caridianbct Inc. 800-525-2623
10810 W Collins Ave, Lakewood, CO 80215
COBE Spectra Apheresis System.

Fenwal Inc. 800-766-1077
3 Corporate Dr, Lake Zurich, IL 60047
CS-3000 Blood cell separator and apheresis kits.

Fenwal International, Inc. 847-550-7908
Camino Real Industrial Park,, Road #122
Ext Mans San German, PR 00683
Various cell separators & sterile/non-sterile accessories.

Fenwal International, Inc. 847-550-7908
Road 357, Km. 0.8, Maricao, PR 00606
Various cell separators & sterile & non-sterile accessories.

Haemonetics Corp. 800-225-5242
400 Wood Rd, P.O. Box 9114, Braintree, MA 02184
PCS2-wireless

Jostra Bentley, Inc. 302-454-9959
Rd. 402 N. Km 1.4, Industrial Park, Anasco, PR 00610-1577
Blood conservation, hemoconcentration systems.

SEPARATOR, BLOOD CELL/PLASMA, THERAPEUTIC
(Gastro/Urology) 78LKN

Accellent El Paso 915-771-9112
31 Butterfield Trail Blvd Ste C, El Paso, TX 79906
Spectratherm

Caridianbct Inc. 800-525-2623
10810 W Collins Ave, Lakewood, CO 80215
COBE Spectra Apheresis System.

Cytori Therapeutics, Inc. 877-470-8000
3020 Callan Rd, San Diego, CA 92121
Celution 800/CRS

SEPARATOR, DURAL *(Cns/Neurology) 84RSB*

Codman & Shurtleff, Inc 800-225-0460
325 Paramount Dr, Raynham, MA 02767

Miltex Inc. 800-645-8000
589 Davies Dr, York, PA 17402

Zimmer Holdings, Inc. 800-613-6131
1800 W Center St, PO Box 708, Warsaw, IN 46580

SEPARATOR, PROTEIN *(Chemistry) 75UHN*

Applied Biosystems 800-345-5724
850 Lincoln Centre Dr, Foster City, CA 94404
$36,000 for model 130A protein/peptide microbore separation system. $19,100 for model 150A protein/peptide separator. 3 systems for separation and purification of DNA, proteins and peptides.

Protein Sciences Corp. 800-488-7099
1000 Research Pkwy, Meriden, CT 06450
Custom protein expression. Purification for insect cells available.

SEPARATOR, PYLORUS *(Gastro/Urology) 78RSC*

Miltex Inc. 800-645-8000
589 Davies Dr, York, PA 17402

SEPARATOR, TOE *(Orthopedics) 87RSE*

Alimed, Inc. 800-225-2610
297 High St, Dedham, MA 02026

Pedifix, Inc. 800-424-5561
310 Guinea Rd, Brewster, NY 10509
Palliative products.

Slawner Ltd., J. 514-731-3378
5713 Cote Des Neiges Rd., Montreal, QUE H3S 1Y7 Canada

SERUM SEPARATION SYSTEM *(Hematology) 81UJN*

Biomerieux Inc. 800-682-2666
100 Rodolphe St, Durham, NC 27712
SURE-SEP device. Can be used to separate serum or plasma from red cells.

Covidien Lp 508-261-8000
15 Hampshire St, Mansfield, MA 02048

SERUM, ANIMAL *(Pathology) 88KIS*

Antibodies, Inc. 800-824-8540
PO Box 1560, Davis, CA 95617
Animal sera from various spp.

Biocell Laboratories, Inc. 800-222-8382
2001 E University Dr, Rancho Dominguez, CA 90220
Fetal bovine serum, rabbit, equine, goat, porcine, and fractions (albumin and gamma globulin).

Biologos, Inc. 800-246-4088
2235 Cornell Ave, Montgomery, IL 60538
Animal serum.

Biomerieux Industry 800-634-7656
595 Anglum Rd, Hazelwood, MO 63042
Animal blood products.

Central Biomedia, Inc. 800-448-0016
9900 Pflumm Rd Unit 61-63, Lenexa, KS 66215
Custom process animal serum.

Chisolm Biological Lab. 803-663-9618
PO Box 1289, Aiken, SC 29802
Animal serums, bloods, plasmas, albumin, and blood fractions Ex IgG, transfer factors.

Covance Laboratories ,Inc 800-742-8378
3301 Kinsman Blvd, Madison, WI 53704

Dako North America, Inc 805-566-6655
6392 Via Real, Carpinteria, CA 93013

Gemini Bio-Products, Inc. 916-273-5215
930 Riverside Pkwy, West Sacramento, CA 95605
Sera,animal and human.

Hyclone Laboratories, Inc. 435-792-8000
925 W 1800 S, Logan, UT 84321
Sera, animal and human (various types).

Immunostics, Inc. 800-722-7505
3505 Sunset Ave, Ocean, NJ 07712

Jr Scientific, Inc. 530-666-9868
1242 Commerce Ave Ste D, Woodland, CA 95776
Sera, animal and human.

Lampire Biological Laboratories, Inc. 215-795-2838
405 S Main St, Coopersburg, PA 18036
Sera, animal and human.

Lonza Walkersville, Inc. 201-316-9200
8830 Biggs Ford Rd, Walkersville, MD 21793
Animal and human sera.

Nova-Tech, Inc. 308-381-8841
1982 E Citation Way, Central Ne. Regional Airport
Grand Island, NE 68801
Animal and human sera.

Rockland Immunochemicals, Inc. 800-656-ROCK
PO Box 326, Gilbertsville, PA 19525

Safc Biosciences, Inc. 913-469-5580
13804 W 107th St, Lenexa, KS 66215

Seracare Life Sciences 800-676-1881
37 Birch St, Milford, MA 01757
Various.

The Metrix Co. 800-752-3148
4400 Chavenelle Rd, Dubuque, IA 52002
Centrifuged fetal calf and other animal serum.

SERUM, ANIMAL *(cont'd)*

Tissue Culture Biologicals 800-845-1445
19766 S Highway 99 Unit A, Suite 300, Tulare, CA 93274
Animal blood serums.

Vector Laboratories, Inc. 800-227-6666
30 Ingold Rd, Burlingame, CA 94010
$45.00 for 20 mL of normal goat, horse, rabbit, chicken or swine serum.

SERUM, BIOLOGICAL, GENERAL *(Toxicology) 91UHZ*

Antibodies, Inc. 800-824-8540
PO Box 1560, Davis, CA 95617
Sera, antisera, and labeled conjugates. Various purifications available. Monoclonal and polyclonal antibodies.

Bd Diagnostic Systems 800-675-0908
7 Loveton Cir, Sparks, MD 21152

Biocell Laboratories, Inc. 800-222-8382
2001 E University Dr, Rancho Dominguez, CA 90220
Tissue-culture sera.

Chisolm Biological Lab. 803-663-9618
PO Box 1289, Aiken, SC 29802
Animal serums, bloods, plasmas, albumin, and blood fractions Ex IgG, transfer factors.

Colorado Serum Company 303-295-7527
4950 York St, PO Box 16428, Denver, CO 80216
Animal blood products for tissue culture.

Dade Behring, Inc. 800-948-3233
1717 Deerfield Rd, Deerfield, IL 60015

Lampire Biological Laboratories 215-795-2838
PO Box 270, Pipersville, PA 18947
Calf, bovine, horse, lamb, and goat.

Rockland Immunochemicals, Inc. 800-656-ROCK
PO Box 326, Gilbertsville, PA 19525
Stopped sera and heat-treated sera, human and other animals.

The Metrix Co. 800-752-3148
4400 Chavenelle Rd, Dubuque, IA 52002

Vector Laboratories, Inc. 800-227-6666
30 Ingold Rd, Burlingame, CA 94010
Lectins & biotin/avidin reagents.

SERUM, CONTROL, DIGITOXIN, RIA *(Toxicology) 91DJK*

Biocell Laboratories, Inc. 800-222-8382
2001 E University Dr, Rancho Dominguez, CA 90220

SERUM, CONTROL, DIGOXIN, RIA *(Toxicology) 91DMP*

Health Chem Diagnostics Llc 954-979-3845
3341 W McNab Rd, Pompano Beach, FL 33069
Digoxin control serum, ria.

SERUM, HUMAN *(Pathology) 88KPC*

Biocell Laboratories, Inc. 800-222-8382
2001 E University Dr, Rancho Dominguez, CA 90220
Seranormal, analyte stripped, and fractions.

Interstate Blood Bank, Inc. 800-258-9557
5700 Pleasant View Rd, Memphis, TN 38134
Whole blood, red blood cells, source leukocytes (buffy coats), platelet concentrate, platelet rich or poor plasma, cryoprecipitate, cryo rich or poor fresh frozen plasma, serum from clotted whole blood; regular, modified, heparinized, liquid or tetanus-immune source plasma, diseased state plasma/serum, factor deficient plasma, specific antibody plasma/serum, recovered human plasma. All products prepared according to customer specifications.

Rockland Immunochemicals, Inc. 800-656-ROCK
PO Box 326, Gilbertsville, PA 19525

Seracare Life Sciences 800-676-1881
37 Birch St, Milford, MA 01757

SERUM, REACTIVE AND NON-SPECIFIC CONTROL, FTA-ABS TEST *(Microbiology) 83GMR*

Bd Diagnostic Systems 800-675-0908
7 Loveton Cir, Sparks, MD 21152

SERUM, SCREENING, BLOOD *(Hematology) 81UJU*

Biotest Diagnostic Corp. 800-522-0090
400 Commons Way, Rockaway, NJ 07866

Dade Behring, Inc. 800-948-3233
1717 Deerfield Rd, Deerfield, IL 60015

Kamiya Biomedical Company 206-575-8068
12779 Gateway Dr S, Tukwila, WA 98168
Research assay kits for other serum proteins.

SERUM, SCREENING, BLOOD *(cont'd)*

Ubi 631-273-2828
25 Davids Dr, Hauppauge, NY 11788
Enzyme immunoassay for the qualitative detection of antibodies to hepatitis C virus (HCV) in human serum of plasma of blood donors or individuals of known or unknown risk.

SERVICE, ARCHITECTURAL *(General) 80VAR*

Calmaquip Engineering Corp. 305-592-4510
7240 NW 12th St, Miami, FL 33126
Evaluation of existing facilities, space utilization, feasibility studies in conjunction with equipment requirements. Supervision of construction, interior design, furnishings and signage.

Cochran, Stephenson & Donkervoet, Inc. Architects 410-539-2080
323 W Camden St Ste 700, The Warehouse at Camden Yards Baltimore, MD 21201
Architectural interior design and planning for medical and lifecare projects.

Cromwell Architects Engineers 501-372-2900
101 S Spring St, Little Rock, AR 72201
Medical equipment planning.

Fkp Architects,Inc 713-621-2100
8 Greenway Plz Ste 300, Houston, TX 77046
Health planning and interior architecture. Medical and laboratory equipment planning.

Holabird & Root Llc 312-357-1771
140 S Dearborn St, Chicago, IL 60603
Architecture, engineering, and interior design. Renovations and constructions; provide ongoing services for healthcare/laboratory clients.

Identita Designers, Inc. 813-871-5511
4115 W Cypress St, Tampa, FL 33607
Designing of hospital sign systems, traffic analysis, functional planning, interior design, fire safety.

Page Southerland Page, Llp 512-472-6721
400 W Cesar Chavez St Ste 500, Austin, TX 78701

Smith Group 800-227-3008
225 Bush St Fl 11, San Francisco, CA 94104

SERVICE, ATTORNEY, PATENT *(General) 80WTQ*

Synectic Medical Product Development 203-877-8488
60 Commerce Park, Milford, CT 06460
Medical/surgical product development, consulting and trouble-shooting services available; experienced in mechanical engineering, industrial design, materials application, medical product manufacturing, tooling and Quality Control. Special consideration given to ergonomics and aesthetic factors; we bring together medical practitioners, industrial designers, engineers and marketing groups; our methods reduce time to market, develop and design product as well as enhancing productivity during and after the development process.

SERVICE, COMPUTER *(General) 80VBS*

Digital Dynamics, Inc. 800-765-1288
5 Victor Sq, Scotts Valley, CA 95066
Control computers for large EtO sterilization chambers.

Dynamic Energy Systems, Inc. 800-326-0314
1500 S Central Expy, McKinney, TX 75070
Computer and equipment consultants.

Legacy Integrators, Llc 800-272-5169
68 Forman St, Fair Haven, NJ 07704
Data Integration from bed side devices to charting system.

Pacifiq Systems Llc 949-442-2454
5015 Birch St, Newport Beach, CA 92660
Software implementation and validation of manufacturing and distribution systems for FDA-regulated companies.

Psyche Systems 800-345-1514
321 Fortune Blvd, Milford, MA 01757
Developing/marketing turnkey clinical, laboratory data processing systems (Digital Corp. hardware). Pathway - Anatomic pathology/cytology system for the small laboratory.

Qualityworx, Inc. 877-825-4379
11 Valley Rd, Kinnelon, NJ 07405
Custom solutions for software validation and GMP compliance. Specialized services include software testing assistance, turnkey test automation and GMP assessments through mock FDA audits of software development process.

SERVICE, CONSULTING *(General) 80VBN*

Applied Medical Systems, Inc. 617-577-1604
581 Boylston St Ste 500, Boston, MA 02116

Ark Services Corporation 708-371-3674
6118 W 123rd St, Palos Heights, IL 60463
PROEXPERTS.ORG - a place to find expert independent consultants.

Automated Imaging Association 800-994-6099
900 Victors Way, PO Box 3724, Ann Arbor, MI 48108
AIA is the world's largest trade association for the machine vision industry. Our members are suppliers, integrators and end users of imaging components in the medical and other manufacturing industries.

Bio-Reg Associates, Inc. 301-623-2500
11800 Baltimore Ave Ste 105, Beltsville, MD 20705
Bio-Reg Associates provide cost-effective regulatory, quality, clinical consulting services that consistently produce positive results for both domestic and international medical device, pharmaceutical, biotech and biologic firms. Bio-Reg's ultimate goal is to assist clients in getting their products to market and in keeping them there. Bio-Reg's core services include QSR/cGMP compliance, GMP/QSR audits, assisting with 483 and warning letters, consent decrees, and injunctions, quality system review and development, product, process, and software performance, validations, clinical study design, management and monitoring, preparation of regulatory applications and submissions, regulatory strategy development, regulatory training, FDA liaison, and electromechanical laboratory services.

Biomed Ink 720-493-5199
3411 Westhaven Pl, Littleton, CO 80126
labeling; package inserts; submissions; operating procedures; instruction for use; user manuals; online help; web-based training; books, articles, papers; beta testing and usability testing; desktop publishing and technical illustrations; document design and style guides; project management; research; single-source publishing.

Biosure, Inc. 800-345-2267
12301 Loma Rica Dr Unit G, Grass Valley, CA 95945

Breazeale & Associates, Inc. 770-447-4418
2909 Langford Rd Ste B500, Norcross, GA 30071
Development and implementation of worldwide strategies for start-ups, acquisitions, divestitures and for marketing, sales and distribution of a single product or an entire company.

Calmaquip Engineering Corp. 305-592-4510
7240 NW 12th St, Miami, FL 33126
Medical equipment contractor, supplier and consultant specializing in equipping hospitals on turnkey basis such as laboratory, sterilization, surgery, dental, diagnostic, anesthesia, pharmaceutical, and rooms equipment.

Capitol Management Consulting, Inc. 609-737-9963
30 Pleasant Valley Harbourton, Titusville, NJ 08560-2101
Business process improvement, information technology and regulatory compliance.

Ch Ellis Company Inc. 800-466-3351
2432 Southeastern Ave, Indianapolis, IN 46201

Clean Air Technology, Inc. 800 459 6320
41105 Capital Dr, Canton, MI 48187
Cleanroom consulting services, USP 797 consulting services for in-patient hospital pharmacy upgrades for compliance.

Cmt, Inc. 800-659-9140
PO Box 297, Hamilton, MA 01936
Research, design and development of diagnostic and therapeutic devices. 15+ years experience in the medical field applying mechanical and electrical engineering from technology assessment to production.

Concord Consulting Group, Inc. 978-369-8744
30 Monument Sq Ste 215, Concord, MA 01742
Management and marketing consulting for medical equipment manufacturers and hospitals with a particular focus on imaging equipment and applications.

Cuno Filter Systems 800-243-6894
400 Research Pkwy, Meriden, CT 06450
Broad line of solid support for biochemical development of diagnostic kits, for incorporation into filtration devices or for use as specialty porous substrates. Novel matrices for specialized applications generated by research and engineering groups.

D.J. Lacher Company, Inc. 516-931-0646
380 N Broadway, Jericho, NY 11753

Day & Zimmermann Validation Services 215-299-8000
1818 Market St, Philadelphia, PA 19103

SERVICE, CONSULTING *(cont'd)*

Design & Evaluation, Inc. 856-228-3800
1451B Chews Landing Rd, Laurel Springs, NJ 08021
The company offers electronic engineering analysis consulting services, specializing in worst-case circuit analysis (power supplies, analog, digital, RF circuits), worst-case part-variation databases, reliability engineering, failure modes and effects analysis, safety hazards analysis, and worst-case circuit-analysis training courses and handbooks.

Dma Med-Chem Corporation 800-362-1833
49 Watermill Ln, Great Neck, NY 11021

Dynamic Energy Systems, Inc. 800-326-0314
1500 S Central Expy, McKinney, TX 75070
Computer and equipment consultants.

Electronic Industries Alliance 703-907-7500
2500 Wilson Blvd, Arlington, VA 22201
National Trade Organization involved in the design and manufacture of electronic components, parts, systems and equipment for communications, industrial, government and consumer uses.

Enova Medical Technologies 866-773-0539
1839 Buerkle Rd, Saint Paul, MN 55110
Design and regulatory consulting.

Evans Group, Inc., The 973-616-1400
230 W Parkway Unit 7-1, Pompton Plains, NJ 07444
Professional Multi-Discipline Consulting Firm specializing in the Healthcare Industry. Each staff member has many years of experience in the Healthcare Industry most having served in Senior Level Management Positions of various disciplines for Fortune 500 companies. Expertise include Product Development, Manufacturing, and Validation of Production and Testing Processes.

Evergreen Research, Inc. 303-526-7402
433 Park Point Dr Ste 140, Golden, CO 80401

Fitzpatrick Management Resources 800-357-0509
9116 Fishers Pond Dr, Charlotte, NC 28277
Interim management for turnarounds and businesses in transition. Also, development of strategic plans and marketing strategies.

Grant Memorial Hospital/Petersburg, Wv 304-257-1026
Grant Memorial Drive, Petersburg, WV 26847
Advises buyers on where to find various hospital goods.

Hill-Rom Manufacturing, Inc. 800-638-2546
4349 Corporate Rd, Charleston, SC 29405

Imsi, Integrated Modular Systems Inc. 800-220-9729
2500 W Township Line Rd, PO Box 616, Havertown, PA 19083
We take a 'modular' approach to medical imaging technology and have helped numerous sites enter into the digital world.

Inc Research 866-462-7373
4700 Falls of Neuse Rd Ste 400, Raleigh, NC 27609
Manage global clinical trials for pharma, biotech and device companies developing drugs and/or devices in CNS, Oncology and pediatrics.

Independent Solutions, Inc. 847-498-0500
900 Skokie Blvd Ste 118, Northbrook, IL 60062
Headwall design, patient service console design, power column design.

Integral Design Inc. 781-740-2036
52 Burr Rd, Hingham, MA 02043
Medical and surgical product design and development.

John Cudia And Associates, Inc. 408-782-2628
18440 Technology Dr Ste 110, Morgan Hill, CA 95037
Representative for medical company.

John Goodman & Associates, Inc. 310-828 - 504
1734 Colorado Ave, Santa Monica, CA 90404
Cardiology business consulting.

King's Medical 330-653-3968
1894 Georgetown Rd, Hudson, OH 44236
Technical service, engineering consulting, financial services.

Koaman International 909-983-4888
656 E D St, Ontario, CA 91764
Disposable products from Asia (Far East).

Lenox Laser 800-494-6537
12530 Manor Rd, Glen Arm, MD 21057
Optical pinholes and slits, high-quality optical pinholes and slits for different optical applications (x-ray systems, confocal microscopy, high power systems, etc.). E-Blox 3D optical workstation for electro-optical systems. Microscopic hole drilling--drilling of microscopic holes in virtually any material.

SERVICE, CONSULTING *(cont'd)*

Lexicon Branding, Inc. 415-332-1811
30 Liberty Ship Way Ste 3360, Sausalito, CA 94965
Create medical and pharmaceutical tradenames. Visualink and Sounder.

Lyons Tool And Die Company 800-422-9363
185 Research Pkwy, Meriden, CT 06450
Rapid prototyping. Production of medical devices in class 10,000 clean rooms. Medical knives and scissors. Precision metal stamping. Engineering services.

Med-Con, Inc. 800-366-1366
PO Box 244, Antioch, IL 60002
Med-Gas Systems

Medi-Dyn, Inc. 800-776-6441
13111 E Briarwood Ave Ste 225, Englewood, CO 80112
Consulting & contract management service for housekeeping and laundry departments.

Medical Equipment Development, Inc. 520-743-7874
PO Box 85820, Tucson, AZ 85754
Consulting service to medical device manufacturers for quality assurance and FDA regulatory affairs including: 510(k), PMA, IDE, MDR, CGMP, quality systems, GLP, clinical studies design and monitoring, verification and validation procedures (hardware and software), reliability analysis, design control procedures and methods, ISO 9000 and CE Mark. Also, provides device evaluation and market analysis services.

Medical Marketing Services 800-927-0791
2322 Nazareth Rd, Kalamazoo, MI 49048
Assistance in developing overseas sales operations for U.S. medical device products; development of training programs for overseas medical distributors; selection and training of new distributors.

Medical Safety Systems Inc. 888-803-9303
230 White Pond Dr, Akron, OH 44313
In-office consultation service on the implementation of an OSHA compliance program.

Meta Health Technology Inc. 800-334-6840
330 7th Ave, New York, NY 10001
Data Processing consulting; implementation services.

Migliara/Kaplan Associates 410-581-8188
9 Park Center Ct, Owings Mills, MD 21117
Market research consulting service; ad testing, product positioning and pricing studies. A member of the NFO Research, Inc. group of companies.

Mylan Technologies, Inc. 800-532-5226
110 Lake St, Saint Albans, VT 05478
Design and production consultation on-site at production plant - experimental, pilot and final-stage production runs.

New Life Systems, Inc. 954-972-4600
PO Box 8767, Coral Springs, FL 33075
Broker of medical business sales mergers and acquisitions, medical investments, financing, leasing.

North American Science Associates, Inc. 866-666-9455
6750 Wales Rd, Northwood, OH 43619
Preclinical and clinical testing and consulting services.

Optimal Healthcare Products 800-364-8574
11444 W Olympic Blvd Ste 900, Los Angeles, CA 90064

Parexel International Corp. 781-487-9900
195 West St, Waltham, MA 02451
Medical device, pharmaceutical and biotechnology product development. Industry seminars offered.

Patient Instrumentation Corp. 610-799-4436
4117 Route 309, Schnecksville, PA 18078
Consulting service for medical gas systems, plus testing of the systems. Drawings of actual medical gas piping systems. PIC Medical Gas Tracking & Mapping; piping drawings of entire medical gas systems that have been on-site verified. Color coded.

Photovac Laser Corp., Inc. 614-875-3300
3513 Farm Bank Way, Grove City, OH 43123

Promatura Group, Llc 800-201-1483
19 County Road 168, Oxford, MS 38655
Market research and consulting group, provides services under two categories. Consumer Products and Services and Seniors Housing.

SERVICE, CONSULTING *(cont'd)*

Questech International, Inc. 800-966-5367
3810 Gunn Hwy, Tampa, FL 33618
Consulting service to aid in transfer of medical technology to consumer product marketplace; export consulting on U.S market for overseas manufacturers; import consulting on overseas manufacturers for U.S. distributors and product development consulting.

Revere Healthcare Ltd. 800-826-4900
10 Spring St, Cary, IL 60013

Rockland Technimed Limited Rtl 845-426-1136
3 Larissa Ct, Airmont, NY 10952
Strategic Planning for infrastructure development in evolving healthcare marketplace for delivery of services in healthcare facilities. Five-year technology plans and budgets, contract negotiations, specification writing, procurement, etc.

Rocky Mountain Helicopters 801-375-1124
800 S 3110 W, Provo, UT 84601
Medical aircraft transport training.

Rozynski & Associates 202-974-6222
2120 L St NW Ste 245, Washington, DC 20037

Sajan, Inc. 877-426-9505
625 Whitetail Blvd, River Falls, WI 54022
Sajan offers ISO-certified services fused with technology to offer a web-based solution that centrally manages and streamlines the entire content creation and translation workflow processes. GCMS is a hosted online offering so there is no buying, installing or learning additional applications or tools. Sajan integrates and simplifies what has been a disparate and hard-to-manage process within most companies. Sajan specializes in a wide range of services that include document translating, website localization, graphic design, globalization consulting, and software localization.

Scc Soft Computer 800-763-8352
5400 Tech Data Dr, Clearwater, FL 33760
SCC Soft Computer is a recognized leader in LIS development, installation and implementation for hospitals and independent laboratories, specializing in multi-site integration and consolidation. SCC supplies innovative technologies to meet the diverse needs and strictest demands of the Healthcare Industry by providing best-of-breed clinical information solutions to laboratories worldwide.

Science Applications International Corp. 800-430-7629
10260 Campus Point Dr, San Diego, CA 92121
Integrated solutions.

Surgical Implants, Inc. 941-366-1882
962 S. Tamiami Trail, Suite 203, Sarasota, FL 34236
Consultations regarding implants.

Surgical Technologies, Inc. 800-777-9987
292 E Lafayette Frontage Rd, Saint Paul, MN 55107
Consulting service for FDA-GMP related questions. Provides assistance to companies seeking CE mark for products and conducting clinical trials, authorized representative services and European/U.S. warehousing, office space, office support staff, logistic services and a training facility in Amsterdam.

Thermo Uscs 800-558-6377
120 Bishops Way Ste 100, Box 0951, Brookfield, WI 53005
Equipment maintenance management and cost reduction. Capital asset management services.

Virtec Enterprises, Llc 440-352-8970
11351 Prouty Rd, Painesville, OH 44077
Product development, mechanical, electronic products. FDA, UL, CE compliance. Contract manufacturing, offshore sourcing.

Vital Concepts, Inc. 800-984-2300
4334 Brockton Dr SE Ste F, Grand Rapids, MI 49512

SERVICE, DESIGN, IMPLANT, CUSTOM *(Orthopedics) 87WIV*

Holmed Corporation 508-238-3351
40 Norfolk Ave, South Easton, MA 02375

Innovation Genesis, Llc 617-234-0070
1 Canal Park, Cambridge, MA 02141
Technology and product strategy, design and development for medical device companies. Experience with devices ranging from home health care, diagnostics, imaging, surgical tools and procedures, and cardiology to advanced ER and OR systems.

Protein Sciences Corp. 800-488-7099
1000 Research Pkwy, Meriden, CT 06450
Gene Xpress, produce proteins in insect cells as a service to the pharmaceutical and biotech industry.

SERVICE, DEVICE COATING, PROTECTIVE *(General) 80SHG*

Implant Sciences Corp. 781-246-0700
107 Audubon Rd Ste 5, Wakefield, MA 01880
Ion implantation and coating services for the biomedical and dental industries, including surface modification by ion implantation, radiopaque coatings, antimicrobial coatings and graded-interface ceramic coatings.

Labsphere, Inc. 603-927-4266
231 Shaker St., North Sutton, NH 03260-9986
SPECTRAFLECT, DURAFLECT, INFRAGOLD, and INFRAGOLD-LF are four diffuse reflectance coatings that are offered for specific applications. Applications include flat panel displays, holographic imaging illuminator panels, integrating spheres, lamp housings, line illuminators, line scanners, optical components, remote sensing targets, and spectral diffuser panels.

Spire Corp. 800-510-4815
1 Patriots Park, Bedford, MA 01730

Surmodics, Inc. 866-SURMODX
9924 W 74th St, Eden Prairie, MN 55344
Surface modification technology used to immobilize a wide variety of molecules to create unique performance-enhancing surfaces on medical devices. Customized reagent and processing formulations can provide increased lubricity, hemocompatibility, infection resistance, and/or drug elution.

Tua Systems, Inc. 321-453-3200
3645 N Courtenay Pkwy, Merritt Island, FL 32953

Vergason Technology, Inc. 607-589-4429
166 State Route 224, Van Etten, NY 14889
VTI's coating services group has provided hard coatings and metalizing coatings since 1987. We utilize our patented Cat Arc® low temperature PVD methods and sputtering processes to supply a wide variety of quality coating solutions. VTI supplies strippable CrN coatings as well as TiN, TiAlN/AlTiN, TiB2, ZrN and TiCN for medical, decorative, aerospace & defense, electronic, machine tools, components and other applications.

SERVICE, ENGINEERING/DESIGN *(General) 80WND*

Aci Medical, Inc. 800-667-9451
1857 Diamond St, San Marcos, CA 92078
Electronic and plastic parts.

Adolfson & Peterson, Inc 612-544-1561
6701 W 23rd St, Minneapolis, MN 55426
Cleanroom design and building.

Advanced Polymers, Inc. 603-327-0600
29 Northwestern Dr, Salem, NH 03079
OEM design, development, and fabrication of angioplasty balloons and custom balloon catheters.

American Bio-Medical Service Corporation (Abmsc) 800-755-9055
631 W Covina Blvd, Sales,Service and Refurbishing Center
San Dimas, CA 91773
Reconditioned surgical equipment.

ARRK Product Development Group 800-735-2775
8880 Rehco Rd, San Diego, CA 92121
Complete rapid product development services include rapid prototyping, CAD/CAM and CNC machining, vacu-pressure moldings and castings, QuickCast and aluminum castings, fabrication and rapid tooling. Aluminum and steel injection.

Associated Design And Manufacturing Co. 800-837-8257
8245 Backlick Rd Ste K, Lorton, VA 22079

Atrion Medical Products, Inc. 800-343-9334
1426 Curt Francis Rd NW, Arab, AL 35016

Awareness Technology, Inc. 722-283-6540
1935 SW Martin Hwy, Palm City, FL 34990

Benchmark Electronics, Inc. 507-452-8932
4065 Theurer Blvd, Winona, MN 55987
Electronics design services, PCB layout, design for excellence (DFx), NPI, electronic prototypes, test development.

Brytech Inc. 613-731-5800
600 Peter Morand Crescent, Suite 240, Ottawa, ONT K1G-5Z3 Canada

Cadco Dental Products 800-833-8267
600 E Hueneme Rd, Oxnard, CA 93033
Innovative design, compact packaging and 11 standard sizes.

Certified Facilities Corp. 206-622-2508
208 Columbia St, Seattle, WA 98104
For cleanrooms.

SERVICE, ENGINEERING/DESIGN *(cont'd)*

Clean Air Technology, Inc. 800 459 6320
41105 Capital Dr, Canton, MI 48187
Cleanroom Design & Build services, AutoCAD construction drawings through to Professional Engineer P.E. review and seal for architectural, mechanical and/or electrical specialities for your state.

Cmt, Inc. 800-659-9140
PO Box 297, Hamilton, MA 01936
Research, design and development of diagnostic and therapeutic devices. 15+ years experience in the medical field applying mechanical and electrical engineering from technology assessment to production.

Colonial/Han-Dee Spring, Llc 860-589-3231
95 Valley St, PO Box 1079, Bristol, CT 06010
General engineering services, prototypes, and preproduction runs. Springs, stampings, wire forms and custom metal parts.

Concord Consulting Group, Inc. 978-369-8744
30 Monument Sq Ste 215, Concord, MA 01742
Product design and development.

Controltek, Inc. 360-896-9375
3905 NE 112th Ave, Vancouver, WA 98682
Electronic design.

Day & Zimmermann Validation Services 215-299-8000
1818 Market St, Philadelphia, PA 19103
Validation of construction technology, consultation, model simulation, and laboratory staff support.

Design & Evaluation, Inc. 856-228-3800
1451B Chews Landing Rd, Laurel Springs, NJ 08021
The company offers electronic engineering analysis consulting services, specializing in worst-case circuit analysis (power supplies, analog, digital, RF circuits), worst-case part-variation databases, reliability engineering, failure modes and effects analysis, safety hazards analysis, and worst-case circuit-analysis training courses and handbooks.

Drummond Scientific Co. 800-523-7480
500 Park Way # 700, Broomall, PA 19008

Dux Dental 800-833-8267
600 E Hueneme Rd, Oxnard, CA 93033
Innovative design, compact packaging and 11 standard sizes.

Electronic Industries Alliance 703-907-7500
2500 Wilson Blvd, Arlington, VA 22201
National Trade Organization involved in the design and manufacture of electronic components, parts, systems and equipment for communications, industrial, government and consumer uses.

Enpath Medical, Inc. 800-559-2613
2300 Berkshire Ln N, Minneapolis, MN 55441
Device development and manufacturing of catheters, introducers, implant tools, delivery systems, and leads and adapters for CRM, neuromodulation, and hearing restoration.

Evans Group, Inc., The 973-616-1400
230 W Parkway Unit 7-1, Pompton Plains, NJ 07444
Evaluation, Design and Fabrication of special Production and Testing Equipment. Automation of Production and Testing Processes. CAD services with AutoCad and Intergraph, CNC machining, and Machine/Model Shop.

Evergreen Research, Inc. 303-526-7402
433 Park Point Dr Ste 140, Golden, CO 80401

First Level Inc 717-266-2450
3109 Espresso Way, York, PA 17406

Florida Life Systems 727-321-9554
3446 5th Ave N, Saint Petersburg, FL 33713

Globe Medical Tech, Inc. 713-365-9595
1766 W Sam Houston Pkwy N, Houston, TX 77043
Provide turn key service for product design, development, prototype, FDA application, injection molding and clean room assembly / manufacturing.

Gw Plastics, Inc. 802-234-9941
239 Pleasant St, Bethel, VT 05032
In-house tooling and engineering of plastic components.

Habley Medical Technology Corp. 800-729-1994
15721 Bernardo Heights Pkwy Ste B-30, San Diego, CA 92128
Custom medical device design and engineering.

Harmac Medical Products, Inc. 716-897-4500
2201 Bailey Ave, Buffalo, NY 14211
Contract manufacturer of custom disposable plastic medical devices. Product design and development engineering services.

Hayes Medical, Inc. 800-240-0500
1115 Windfield Way Ste 100, El Dorado Hills, CA 95762

SERVICE, ENGINEERING/DESIGN *(cont'd)*

Heatron, Inc. 913-651-4420
3000 Wilson Ave, Leavenworth, KS 66048

Helix Medical, Inc. 800-266-4421
1110 Mark Ave, Carpinteria, CA 93013

Hi-Tronics Designs, Inc. 973-347-4865
999 Willow Grove St, Hackettstown, NJ 07840
Contract design and prototype for various external and implantable devices. Medical grade software development and qualification, custom integrated circuit design.

Innovation Genesis, Llc 617-234-0070
1 Canal Park, Cambridge, MA 02141
Technology and product strategy, design and development for medical device companies. Experience with devices ranging from home health care, diagnostics, imaging, surgical tools and procedures, and cardiology to advanced ER and OR systems.

Integral Design Inc. 781-740-2036
52 Burr Rd, Hingham, MA 02043
Medical and surgical product design and development including concept generation, engineering and industrial design and prototype development.

Ipax, Inc. 303-975-2444
2622 S Zuni St, Englewood, CO 80110
Interactive models.

J-Pac, Llc 603-692-9955
25 Centre Rd, Somersworth, NH 03878
J-PAC offers tooling and automation design and development services in conjunction with in-house packaging and manufacturing activities. Sterile, disposable package design and validation is a specialty, including the development and validation of all applicable fabrication processes.

Lacey Manufacturing Co. 203-336-0121
1146 Barnum Ave, PO Box 5156, Bridgeport, CT 06610

Ledtronics 800-579-4875
23105 Kashiwa Ct, Torrance, CA 90505
LEDs (light-emitting diodes), incandescent lamp replacement based LEDs, low-cost snap-in relampable panel-mount LEDs, high-intensity sunlight visible discrete, PCB circuit-board status indicators, and SMT LEDs.

Logic Product Development 612-672-9495
411 Washington Ave N Ste 101, Minneapolis, MN 55401
Logic provides a completely integrated product development process that helps clients get to market faster. Our services include Design and Strategy, Systems and Software Engineering, Mechanical Engineering, PCB Design and Layout, Electrical Engineering, and FPGA/DSP Design.

Lucomed Inc. 800-633-7877
45 Kulick Rd, Fairfield, NJ 07004

Luwa Lepco 713-461-1131
1750 Stebbins Dr, Houston, TX 77043
Cleanrooms; sterile facilities; complex process suppport systems. Ultra pure air systems.

Lyons Tool And Die Company 800-422-9363
185 Research Pkwy, Meriden, CT 06450
Rapid prototyping. Production of medical devices in class 10,000 clean rooms. Medical knives and scissors. Precision metal stamping. Engineering services.

Med Covers, Inc. 800-327-4571
500 W Goldsboro St, Kenly, NC 27542
Custom design and manufacturing of protective carrying cases and covers for medical and electronical equipment - patient containment systems, low loss air mattress, bolsters and comforters, non-stick sheets, oxygen cylinder bags, wheelchair and scooter accessories.

Medical Sterile Products, Inc. 800-292-2887
Road 413 Km. 0.2 BO. Ensenada, Rincon, PR 00743
Disposable and reusable surgical blades and knives.

Mediflex Surgical Products 800-879-7575
250 Gibbs Rd, Islandia, NY 11749

Medtech Group Inc., The 800-348-2759
6 Century Ln, South Plainfield, NJ 07080
Full design and engineering of disposable medical devices.

Micro-Aire Surgical Instruments, Inc. 800-722-0822
1641 Edlich Dr, Charlottesville, VA 22911
Development and prototyping to full OEM production of new products.

SERVICE, ENGINEERING/DESIGN *(cont'd)*

Mosaic Industries, Inc. 510-790-8222
5437 Central Ave Ste 1, Newark, CA 94560
QVGA Controller, a C-programmable computer with 1/4 VGA display and touchscreen-operated graphical interface. PANEL-TOUCH Controller, a C-programmable computer with 128x240 display and built-in graphical user interface. Wildcards - stackable I/O expansion modules. QED Board: I/O -rich, palm-sized microcontroller board. Precoded software libraries and keypad/display interface make it ideal for animating medical instruments.

Mylan Technologies, Inc. 800-532-5226
110 Lake St, Saint Albans, VT 05478
Design and production consultation on-site at production plant - experimental, pilot and final-stage production runs.

Navion Biomedical Corp. 781-341-8058
312 Tosca Dr, Stoughton, MA 02072

Page Southerland Page, Llp 512-472-6721
400 W Cesar Chavez St Ste 500, Austin, TX 78701

Pegasus Research Corp. 877-632-0255
3505 Cadillac Ave Ste G5, Costa Mesa, CA 92626
Contract design/engineering.

Penn United Technology, Inc. 724-352-1507
799 N Pike Rd, Cabot, PA 16023
Designing and building precision carbide dies, metal-stamping disposable components, prototyping, automatic assembly, CAD/CAM, and CNC machining and grinding.

Pgm 585-458-4300
1305 Emerson St, Rochester, NY 14606
Design, development, and running of unique manufacturing processes for critical components and assemblies.

Photovac Laser Corp., Inc. 614-875-3300
3513 Farm Bank Way, Grove City, OH 43123
Specializing in many types of lasers, tubes, fibers, optics design, prototyping, manufacturing, reprocessing and repair.

Plexus Corp 425-482-1300
20001 N Creek Pkwy, Bothell, WA 98011
Service organization to respond to issues facing today's competitive medical electronics industry, including providing design resources for new product development, enhancing existing products to provide logical extensions, supporting product manufacturing requirements, contributing expertise to non-electronic related companies, and entering into partnerships with start-up companies.

Plexus Corp. 877-733-5919
55 Jewelers Park Dr, PO Box 156, Neenah, WI 54956
Electronic product development.

Plitek, L.L.C 800-966-1250
69 Rawls Rd, Des Plaines, IL 60018
High-speed rotary die cutting, precision male and female die cutting, precision slitting, steel rule die cutting, prototyping, laminating and engineering design services.

Precision Medical Products, Inc. 717-335-3700
44 Denver Rd, PO Box 300, Denver, PA 17517

Precision Optics Corp. 800-447-2812
22 E Broadway, Gardner, MA 01440
Advanced lens design, optical system design, structural design and analysis, prototype production and evaluation, optics testing, and high-volume optical system manufacture.

Pulse Systems, Inc. 505-662-7599
422 Connie Ave, Los Alamos, NM 87544

Questech International, Inc. 800-966-5367
3810 Gunn Hwy, Tampa, FL 33618
Product engineering and technology assessment; product development consulting.

R&Da Co. 508-747-5803
37 Dwight Ave, Plymouth, MA 02360
Mechanical design & creation; cost reduction; total project eng'g; materials: composites; polymers.

Rocky Mountain Helicopters 801-375-1124
800 S 3110 W, Provo, UT 84601
Medical aircraft modifications/completions.

Scicon Technologies Corp. 888-295-8630
27525 Newhall Ranch Rd Ste 2, Valencia, CA 91355
Concurrent engineering and rapid prototype service bureau, using solid-modeling software to convert 2-D drawings into prototype parts.

SERVICE, ENGINEERING/DESIGN *(cont'd)*

Scientek Medical Equipment 604-273-9094
11151 Bridgeport Rd., Richmond, BC V6X 1T3 Canada
Autopsy suite planning and engineering services.

Smp Technology 408-778-4777
15940 Concord Cir, Morgan Hill, CA 95037
SMP designs and builds special OEM products, processes, and test equipment for the medical and pharmaceutical industries.

Sonoco Crellin, Inc. 518-392-2000
87 Center St, Chatham, NY 12037

Sparton Electronics Florida, Inc. 800-824-0682
5612 Johnson Lake Rd, De Leon Springs, FL 32130
Electro-mechanical product design of therapeutic, diagnostic, surgical, and laboratory equipment. Mechanical and electronic producibility enhancement and cost reduction. Microprocessor and embedded-software design and development.

Specialized Medical Devices, Llc 800-463-1874
300 Running Pump Rd, Lancaster, PA 17603
Design, development of precision components.

Spectralytics 800-543-0163
145 3rd St, PO Box L, Dassel, MN 55325
Full-service laser job shop featuring CO2, CO2 Tea, Excimer, and YAG laser processing in metals, plastics, and ceramics. Also, complete system integration.

Spin-Cast Plastics, Inc. 800-422-3625
3300 N Kenmore St, South Bend, IN 46628

Spire Corp. 800-510-4815
1 Patriots Park, Bedford, MA 01730
Surface treatments for improved resistance to wear, thrombo resistance and infection resistance. Surface coating services for improved biocompatibility.

Sr Instruments, Inc. 800-654-6360
600 Young St, Tonawanda, NY 14150

Sunrise Labs, Inc. 888-420-9600
5 Dartmouth Dr, Auburn, NH 03032
Contract product development, complete system design, analog and digital design, industrial and mechanical design, regulatory and FDA approvals, software development, user-interface design, embedded systems, 21 CFR Part 11.

Surgical Technologies, Inc. 800-777-9987
292 E Lafayette Frontage Rd, Saint Paul, MN 55107
Complete product development.

Synectic Medical Product Development 203-877-8488
60 Commerce Park, Milford, CT 06460
Medical/surgical product development, consulting, and trouble-shooting services available. Experienced in mechanical engineering, industrial design, materials application, medical product manufacturing, tooling, and quality control. Special consideration given to ergonomics and aesthetic factors. Additionally, we combine knowledge from medical practitioners, industrial designers, engineers, and marketing groups. Our methods reduce time to market, develop and design products, and enhance productivity during and after the development process.

Tcp Reliable, Inc. 888-TCP-3393
551 Raritan Center Pkwy, Edison, NJ 08837

Tmp Technologies, Inc. 716-895-6100
1200 Northland Ave, Buffalo, NY 14215
General.

Ufp Technologies, Inc. 630-543-2855
1235 W National Ave, Addison, IL 60101
Foam products. Gaskets, filters, pads, medical packaging components, totes, tote liners, impregnation services.

Westlund Engineering, Inc. 727-572-4343
12400 44th St N, Clearwater, FL 33762
Design and fabrication of custom machines, including cartoners and assembly and product-handling equipment.

SERVICE, EQUIPMENT LEASING *(General) 80WMP*

Americorp Financial, Inc. 800-233-1574
877 S Adams Rd, Birmingham, MI 48009
Innovative leasing and financing programs.

Angelus Medical & Optical Co., Inc. 310-769-6060
13007 S Western Ave, Gardena, CA 90249
Medical, ophthalmic, surgical & X-ray.

Bryton Corp. 800-567-9500
4310 Guion Rd, Indianapolis, IN 46254
Leasing of surgical tables, obstetrical tables, orthopedic tables & urology tables.

SERVICE, EQUIPMENT LEASING *(cont'd)*

Ge Capital 800-323-6217
3000 Lakeside Dr Ste 200N, Bannockburn, IL 60015

Leasing Innovations Incorporated 800-532-7388
437 S Highway 101 Ste 104, Solana Beach, CA 92075
Specializes in all types of medical equipment. Leasing to cities, states, towns, and other municipal agencies throughout the U.S. Leasing to Tribal Nationals through the U.S.

Mediq/Prn 800-222-4776
1 Mediq Plaza, Pennsauken, NJ 08110
IV infusion pump rentals. All major manufacturers available.

Medrecon, Inc. 877-526-4323
257 South Ave, Garwood, NJ 07027

Parimist Funding Corp. 800-645-6598
40 Commerce Pl, Hicksville, NY 11801
Lasers, imaging equipment (X-ray, ultrasound mammography, CT, PET, SPECT), analyzers (chemistry, blood, etc.), MR, processors, scopes, computers, ophthalmic equipment, isokinetic testing, EEG, EMG, brain mapping, microscopes, phaco/emulsification, monitors and sterilizers.

Sigmacon Health Products Corp. 800-898-7455
436 Limestone Cres, North York, ON M3J 2S4 Canada
Laser equipment and other medical devices.

Sterile Technologies, Inc. 518-793-7077
PO Box 4742, 63 Park Rd., Queensbury, NY 12804
Gas sterilizer and steam autoclave manufacturer. Sterilization process controls, facility temperature monitoring systems, sterilizer validation systems, environmental monitoring systems. Complete facility design and licensing.

Studebaker-Worthington Leasing Corp. 800-645-7242
100 Jericho Quadrangle, Jericho, NY 11753

World Medical Equipment, Inc. 800-827-3747
3915 152nd St NE, Marysville, WA 98271
Specialize in refurbished operating room tables, lights, autoclaves, anesthesia, monitors, and accessories.

2d Imaging, Inc. 800-449-1332
4745 E Wesley Dr, Anaheim, CA 92807
Sales and leasing and exchanges of all medical ultrasound euipment, servicing and sales of all ultrasound parts, supplies and accessories.

SERVICE, IMPORT/EXPORT *(General) 80WMQ*

American Medical Link, Inc. 908-359-9328
5 Homestead Road, Bldg. 5, Units 1 & 2, Hillsborough, NJ 08844

Applied Technologies International
70 Ovendon Square, Scarborough, ONT M13 2M5 Canada

Calmaquip Engineering Corp. 305-592-4510
7240 NW 12th St, Miami, FL 33126
Exporter of new medical equipment. Specializing in turnkey projects including building construction materials for new or remodeled hospitals and clinics.

Csi International, Inc. 303-795-8273
4301 S Federal Blvd Ste 116, Englewood, CO 80110

Dufort & Lavigne Ltee. 800-361-0655
2165 Parthenais Street, Montreal, QUE H2K 3T3 Canada

Dukal Corporation 800-243-0741
5 Plant Ave, Hauppauge, NY 11788

General Biomedical Service, Inc. 800-558-9449
1900 25th St, Kenner, LA 70062
New & remanufactured respiratory equipment, ventilators, and pulse oximeters.

Globe Medical Tech, Inc. 713-365-9595
1766 W Sam Houston Pkwy N, Houston, TX 77043
Manufacturer and worldwide exporter of IV administration sets, scalp vein sets, burettes, blood sets, syringes and needles, latex exam gloves, powder-free exam gloves, sterile surgical gloves, scalpels, etc.

Hillusa Corp. 305-594-7474
7215 NW 46th St, Miami, FL 33166

Inamco International Corp. 800-724-4003
801 Montrose Ave, South Plainfield, NJ 07080

Intermetra Corp. 305-889-1194
10100 NW 116th Way Ste 11, Medley, FL 33178
Exporter to South & Central America.

International Hospital Supply Co. 800-398-9450
6914 Canby Ave Ste 105, Reseda, CA 91335
Surgical, specialty, orthopedic, neuro, endoscopic, and dental instruments.

SERVICE, IMPORT/EXPORT *(cont'd)*

Ivry 305-448-9858
216 Catalonia Ave Ste 106, Coral Gables, FL 33134
Exporter of surgical, home healthcare products, and used medical equipment.

Kamiya Biomedical Company 206-575-8068
12779 Gateway Dr S, Tukwila, WA 98168
Import/export of research biochemicals.

Koaman International 909-983-4888
656 E D St, Ontario, CA 91764

Lampac International Ltd. 636-797-3659
230 N Lake Dr, Hillsboro, MO 63050

Life Medical Equipment 800-749-4646
7874 NW 64th St, Miami, FL 33166
Purchase and sell used equipment for labs and hospital clinics.

Metronix 813-972-1212
12421 N Florida Ave Ste D201, Tampa, FL 33612
Hospital turnkey project and Hospital Waste Management Systems.

New Life Systems, Inc. 954-972-4600
PO Box 8767, Coral Springs, FL 33075
Worldwide.

Pharaoh Trading Company 866-929-4913
9701 Brookpark Rd, Knollwood Plaza, Suite 241, Cleveland, OH 44129

Questech International, Inc. 800-966-5367
3810 Gunn Hwy, Tampa, FL 33618
Internet-international medical and healthcare network of manufacturers and distributors for faster worldwide design & distribution.

Repex Medical Products, Inc. 305-740-0133
5240 SW 64th Ave, Miami, FL 33155
Product Registration in Latin America, specially services providing product registration in Brazil. Business Development in Latin America, Europe and Arab countries.

Schneider International Ltd. 201-568-5166
600 Sylvan Ave, East Wing - First Floor, Englewood, NJ 07632

Sdi Medical Consultants 619-267-1391
4190 Bonita Rd Ste 211, Bonita, CA 91902
Ultrasound and imaging equipment sales. Service, leasing, trade-in, accessories and supplies.

Serrano International 760-773-5140
45175 Panorama Dr Ste G, Palm Desert, CA 92260
Importer/exporter of orthopedic implants and instruments, hospital equipment and supplies, hospital electric and manual beds, aneurism clips and burs.

Source Medical Corporation 888-871-5945
60 International Blvd., Toronto, ON M9W 6J2 Canada

South American Dental Export Corp. 305-512-4705
8205 W 20th Ave, Hialeah, FL 33014

Technical Marketing, Inc. 954-370-0855
1776 N Pine Island Rd Ste 306, Plantation, FL 33322
Distributions of generic pharmaceuticals manufactured in Ec. Intl. Accreditation 'BP.' Not for sale in USA.

Trans Med Usa, Inc. 978-670-6000
77 Alexander Rd Ste 9, Billerica, MA 01821

Xenotec Ltd. 949-640-4053
511 Hazel Dr, Corona Del Mar, CA 92625
Unique, innovative medical products from quality U.S.A. manufacturers.

SERVICE, LICENSING, DEVICE, MEDICAL *(General) 80WIE*

Bio-Reg Associates, Inc. 301-623-2500
11800 Baltimore Ave Ste 105, Beltsville, MD 20705
Bio-Reg Associates provide cost-effective regulatory, quality, clinical consulting services that consistently produce positive results for both domestic and international medical device, pharmaceutical, biotech and biologic firms. Bio-Reg's ultimate goal is to assist clients in getting their products to market and in keeping them there. Bio-Reg's core services include QSR/cGMP compliance, GMP/QSR audits, assisting with 483 and warning letters, consent decrees, and injunctions, quality system review and development, product, process, and software performance, validations, clinical study design, management and monitoring, preparation of regulatory applications and submissions, regulatory strategy development, regulatory training, FDA liaison, and electromechanical laboratory services.

SERVICE, LICENSING, DEVICE, MEDICAL *(cont'd)*

Biomed Ink 720-493-5199
3411 Westhaven Pl, Littleton, CO 80126
submissions; labeling; package inserts; operating procedures; instruction for use; user manuals; beta testing and usability testing; research; single-source publishing.

Explor Bioventures Llc 314-991-2004
21 Godwin Ln, Saint Louis, MO 63124
Global medical marketing and business development.

King's Medical 330-653-3968
1894 Georgetown Rd, Hudson, OH 44236
Radiologist practice assessment and management, outsourced radiology, fee for service - nuclear medicine, radiation therapy, and cardiac cath.

Met Laboratories, Inc. 800-638-6057
914 W Patapsco Ave, Baltimore, MD 21230
MET Laboratories is an accredited test and certification laboratory for medical devices for the global market. Met's accreditations include: NRTL (US), SCC (Canada), IECEE Scheme (over thirty countries), Brazil, other Latin American countries.

Orion Registrar Inc. 800-267-0861
47 Webster Way, Georgetown, ONT L7G 5J5 Canada

Rozynski & Associates 202-974-6222
2120 L St NW Ste 245, Washington, DC 20037

SERVICE, MAINTENANCE/REPAIR *(General) 80VBJ*

Adler Instrument Co. 866-382-3537
6191 Atlantic Blvd, Norcross, GA 30071
Surgical, microsurgical, and laparoscopic instruments repair. Scope repair.

Advanced Endoscopy Devices, Inc. 818-227-2720
22134 Sherman Way, Canoga Park, CA 91303
All makes and models of endoscopic instrument repair.

Aesculap Implant Systems Inc. 1-800-234-9179
3773 Corporate Pkwy, Center Valley, PA 18034

Air Techniques International 410-363-9696
11403 Cronridge Dr, Owings Mills, MD 21117
Calibration services for aerosol generators, photometers and respirator testers.

Aiv, Inc. (Formerly American Iv) 800-990-2911
7485 Shipley Ave, Harmans, MD 21077
Specialized repair services for leading infusion pumps, fetal transducers and pulse oximeter finger sensors. Service parts available for sale as well.

Alan's Wheelchairs & Repairs 800-693-4344
109 S Harbor Blvd Ste B, Fullerton, CA 92832

Appropriate Technical Resources, Inc. 800-827-5931
9157 Whiskey Bottom Rd, PO Box 460, Laurel, MD 20723

Assisted Access-Nfss, Inc. 800-950-9655
822 Preston Ct, Lake Villa, IL 60046
Repair service TTYs and visual alerting systems.

Atlas Medical Technologies 909-923-7887
1137 E Philadelphia St, Ontario, CA 91761
Atlas repairs and maintains CT and MR devices.

Aventric Technologies 800-228-3343
1551 E Lincoln Ave Ste 166, Madison Heights, MI 48071
Repair of long-term, portable Holter monitor, ECG recorders.

Bryan Corp. 800-343-7711
4 Plympton St, Woburn, MA 01801

Bryton Corp. 800-567-9500
4310 Guion Rd, Indianapolis, IN 46254
Complete remanufacturing of surgical and examination tables.

C.E. Tech 800-333-7477
800 Prudential Dr, Jacksonville, FL 32207
Repair of x-ray, biomedical and laboratory equipment.

California Medical Electronics 707-456-0990
2325 Perch Dr, Willits, CA 95490
Servicing of x-ray units.

Comeg Endoscopes, U.S.A. 800-248-5799
13790 E Rice Pl, Aurora, CO 80015
Arthroscopy, ENT, general surgery, gynecology, urology and video.

Cryofab, Inc. 800-426-2186
540 N Michigan Ave, Kenilworth, NJ 07033
Liquid-oxygen repair facility for respiratory equipment.

Dicon, Inc. 800-426-0493
2355 S 1070 W, Salt Lake City, UT 84119

SERVICE, MAINTENANCE/REPAIR *(cont'd)*

Elmed, Inc. 630-543-2792
60 W Fay Ave, Addison, IL 60101

Entech 800-451-0591
7300 W Detroit St, Chandler, AZ 85226
Biomedical, respiratory, anesthesia, metrology (test equipment calibration); medical imaging and telemetry-equipment repair.

Epic Medical Equipment Services, Inc. 800-327-3742
1800 10th St Ste 300, Plano, TX 75074
For all manufacturers of pulse oximeter sensors and cables, fetal monitoring transducers, respirometers and Holter recorders.

General Biomedical Service, Inc. 800-558-9449
1900 25th St, Kenner, LA 70062
Exporters of new, used and remanufactured medical equipment, specializing in ventilators and other respiratory equipment.

Hot Cell Services 800-562-2439
22626 85th Pl S, Kent, WA 98031

Image Technology, Inc. 877-WEI-MAGE
205 North Beckley, De Soto, TX 75115
Full service organization for all makes and models of MRI and CT. Specializing in Toshiba, General Electric, Philips, Picker, and Hitachi. Additionally, we provide telephone technical support for MRI technicians that have questions or comments on setup, protocols, or the general operation and maintenance of MRI systems. Deinstallations and installations.

J.M. Baragano Biomedical P.M. And Consulting, Inc. 787-722-4007
808 Ave Fernandez Juncos, San Juan, PR 00907
Preventative maintenance and repair of medical equipment. Installation, repair and preventive maintenance of security equipment.

Karl Storz Endoscopy-America Inc. 800-421-0837
600 Corporate Pointe, Culver City, CA 90230

Laser Solutions, Inc. 800-230-7705
44 Bullion Rd, Basking Ridge, NJ 07920
Medical laser service.

Latam Medical 1-877-989-4040
400 Belleville Ave, Bloomfield, NJ 07003

Life Medical Equipment 800-749-4646
7874 NW 64th St, Miami, FL 33166
Sale and repair of new and used medical equipment for operating room, cardiovacsular, endoscope, intensive care units (neonatal), respiratory and apnea monitors, neurology, radiology, laboratory equipment/accessories, rectives, analytic instruments, practice setup.

Mark Medical Manufacturing, Inc. 610-269-4420
530 Brandywine Ave, Downingtown, PA 19335
Surgical-instrument repair specializing in microsurgical repair, bipolar and monopolar forceps, Leep or Lete instruments recoatings. Ebonizing or laser recoatings.

Mass Medical Equipment Co., Inc. 781-246-3368
1 Melvin St Unit A, Wakefield, MA 01880
Refurbishing of medical, surgical, laboratory and diagnostic equipment.

Medi-Tek, Inc. 661-940-0030
4555 W Avenue G Ste 6, Lancaster, CA 93536

Medical Accessories, Inc. 800-275-1624
92 Youngs Rd, Trenton, NJ 08619
Repair service for Hewlett Packard, Corometrics, and other fetal monitoring ultrasonic transducers, tocotransducers and legplates.

Medical Cables, Inc. 800-314-51111
1365 Logan Ave, Costa Mesa, CA 92626

Medical Sales & Service Group 888-357-6520
10 Woodchester Dr, Acton, MA 01720
Repair and refurbishment of medical equipment.

Medical Technologies Co. 800-280-3220
1728 W Park Center Dr Ste A, Fenton, MO 63026
Surgical equipment: OR tables, lights, sterilizers, glassware washers and dryers.

Medivision Endoscopy 800-349-5367
1210 N Jefferson St, Anaheim, CA 92807
Independent service center specializing in rigid endoscope repairs and sales. Quality Control Department on premises. Provide customized maintenance reports to customers and distributors. Conduct technical training seminars and in-service programs.

Medrecon, Inc. 877-526-4323
257 South Ave, Garwood, NJ 07027
Operating room tables, all makes, models, onsite, p.m.

SERVICE, MAINTENANCE/REPAIR *(cont'd)*

Meena Medical Equipment, Inc. 888-225-2502
1904 Industrial Blvd Ste 105, Colleyville, TX 76034
Calibrate medical & laboratory equipment.

Mikron Digital Imaging, Inc. 800-925-3905
30425 8 Mile Rd, Livonia, MI 48152
X-ray service, specializing in Techicare DR-960.

Minnesota Bramstedt Surgical, Inc. 800-456-5052
1835 Energy Park Dr, Saint Paul, MN 55108
Surgical instruments: scissors, forceps (cracked box locks), retractors etc. Bone instruments: osteotomes, gouges, curettes, rongeurs (Kerrisons) etc. Needle holders: reinserted, milled & inserted, welded. Micro surgery instruments: ENT, micro and delicate. Cardiovascular instruments; titanium instruments. Arthroscopy instruments: punches, shavers, scissors etc. Cautery forceps (recoated, repaired, new cords); blood-pressure units (all types); rebuilt cast cutters (Stryker). Instrument recoating, color coding, modifying, and prototyping. Laser matte finish for all types of instruments.

Mobile Instrument Service And Repair, Inc. 800-722-3675
333 Water Ave, Bellefontaine, OH 43311
Sharpening and repair of all hand-held surgical instruments; laparoscopic instrument refurbishing; electrosurgical reinsulation; color coding and needleholder insert placement; repair and refurbishment of all makes and models of rigid and flexible endoscopes (minor and major repair) and power, pneumatic surgical equipment. Phacoemulsification equipment, diamond knife & cataract knife repair.

Mxe, Inc. 800-252-1801
12107 Jefferson Blvd, Culver City, CA 90230
X-ray cassette & ID camera repair.

Nashville Medical Electronics, Inc. 800-966-1001
319 Fesslers Ln Ste A, Nashville, TN 37210
Medical equipment maintenance service plus electrical safety maintenance programs in hospitals.

New Life Systems, Inc. 954-972-4600
PO Box 8767, Coral Springs, FL 33075
All types of medical equipment.

Nuell, Inc. 800-829-7694
PO Box 55, 312 East Van Buren St., Leesburg, IN 46538
Repair of powered surgical equipment.

Omega Medical Electronics Ltd. 910-763-9331
725 Wellington Ave, Wilmington, NC 28401
Reconditioning, Repair, Installation, Training and servicing of most brands of Clinical Laboratory Instrumentation.

Ortho-Cycle Co., Inc. 800-82-CYCLE
2026 Scott St, Hollywood, FL 33020
Refurbishing/recycling of orthodontic supplies.

Patient Instrumentation Corp. 610-799-4436
4117 Route 309, Schnecksville, PA 18078
Testing and certification of medical gas systems.

Photovac Laser Corp., Inc. 614-875-3300
3513 Farm Bank Way, Grove City, OH 43123
Specializing in many types of lasers, tubes, fibers, optics design, prototyping, manufacturing, reprocessing and repair.

Pro Science, Inc., Glass Shop Div. 800-267-1616
92 Railside Rd., Toronto, ONT M3A 1A3 Canada
Repair services for laboratory glassware.

R And L Hearing Services 800-444-8920
3005 Niagara Ln N Ste 2, Minneapolis, MN 55447
Hearing aid repair service.

Rocky Mountain Helicopters 801-375-1124
800 S 3110 W, Provo, UT 84601
Aircraft overhaul/repair.

Rozinn By Scottcare Corporation 800-243-9412
4791 W 150th St, Cleveland, OH 44135
Holter monitor repair specialists. Rozinn repairs all manufacturers' Cassette Holter Recorders on a flat fee plus parts basis.

Rsti (Radiological Service Training Institute) 800-229-7784
30745 Solon Rd, Solon, OH 44139
Training programs for the repair and maintenance of diagnostic imaging systems.

Rx Honing Machine Corporation 800-346-6464
1301 E 5th St, Mishawaka, IN 46544
RX Honing Machine Corp.'s laboratory sharpens surgical, hospital and dental instruments with a 48 hour turnaround. Also, retipping and refurbishing service. 1-800-346-6464.

Standard Supply Co. 800-453-7036
3424 S Main St, Salt Lake City, UT 84115
Battery packs serviced and repaired.

Starkey Florida 800-327-7939
2200 N Commerce Pkwy, Weston, FL 33326
Hearing aid repairs.

Sun Medical, Inc. 800-678-6633
2607 Aero Dr, Grand Prairie, TX 75052

Symmetry Tnco 888-447-6661
15 Colebrook Blvd, Whitman, MA 02382

Telsar Laboratories Inc 800-255-9938
1 Enviro Way Ste 100, Wood River, IL 62095
Maintenance and repair of laser equipment.

U.S. Technologies, Inc. 800-234-0862
1701 Pollitt Dr, Fair Lawn, NJ 07410
Equipment testing/repair. Intel Multibus, power supplies.

Zoetek Medical Sales & Service, Inc. 800-388-3223
668 Phillips Rd, Victor, NY 14564
Bio-medical equipment preventative maintenance and repair. Zoetek services hospitals, physicians offices, surgery centers, physical therapists, veterinarians, dentists, etc.

SERVICE, MODIFICATION, PRODUCT *(General) 80WWR*

Accellent Inc. 866-899-1392
100 Fordham Rd, Wilmington, MA 01887
Grinding service, precision grinding of microminiature wire products for the medical industry.

Cuno Filter Systems 800-243-6894
400 Research Pkwy, Meriden, CT 06450

Genesis Manufacturing, Inc. 317-485-7887
720 E Broadway St, Fortville, IN 46040
Contract Radio-Frequency (RF) Welding. From development to manufacturing and packaging.

Implant Sciences Corp. 781-246-0700
107 Audubon Rd Ste 5, Wakefield, MA 01880

Morris Latex Products, Inc. 405-872-3486
1101 E Maguire Rd, Noble, OK 73068
Custom latex dipped products.

Prime Solutions 510-490-2299
4261 Business Center Dr, Fremont, CA 94538
Laser marking, demarking and printing services as well as various cleaning processes for medical devices.

Rocky Mountain Helicopters 801-375-1124
800 S 3110 W, Provo, UT 84601
Medical aircraft modifications/completions.

Spire Corp. 800-510-4815
1 Patriots Park, Bedford, MA 01730
Surface modification technologies for use on metal, polymer, or ceramic substrates to impart improved wear, blood, and biological properties.

Zirc Company 800-328-3899
3918 State Highway 55 SE, Buffalo, MN 55313
Infection control products, Needle Capper - one-handed uncapping and recapping; Handi-Hopper - disposes of waste at chair side.

SERVICE, PARTS, REPAIR *(General) 80WTD*

Aetrex Worldwide, Inc 800-526-2739
414 Alfred Ave, Teaneck, NJ 07666
E-Z FIT, a broad range of products used in shoe fitting and repair including insoles, taps, heel grips and heel pads.

Aiv, Inc. (Formerly American Iv) 800-990-2911
7485 Shipley Ave, Harmans, MD 21077
AC Adapters, batteries, power cords and other service parts for leading infusion pumps available for sale.

Akorn, Inc. 800-535-7155
2500 Millbrook Dr, Buffalo Grove, IL 60089
Expert repair to microsurgical instruments and diamond knives.

American Autoclave Co. 800 421 5161
7819 Riverside Rd E, Sumner, WA 98390
Parts for sterilizers, autoclaves, OR tables.

Bryton Corp. 800-567-9500
4310 Guion Rd, Indianapolis, IN 46254
Manufacture parts for all makes and models of surgical, orthopedic, urological, obstetrical, and endoscopic tables.

Comeg Endoscopes, U.S.A. 800-248-5799
13790 E Rice Pl, Aurora, CO 80015

SERVICE, PARTS, REPAIR *(cont'd)*

Crest Healthcare Supply 800-328-8908
195 3rd St, Dassel, MN 55325
Nut and bolt set; electrical terminal/conductor set.

Ctronics 800-472-9909
6333 Pacific Ave, Stockton, CA 95207

Diestco Manufacturing Corp. 800-795-2392
PO Box 6504, Chico, CA 95927
Wheelchair Parts, replacement parts for wheelchairs. Various sizes and types of caster and bearings available. Various upholstery and replacement wheels and tires for wheelchairs. Wheelchair tubes, various tubes for wheelchair tires, pneumatic, flat-free and urethane.

East Penn Manufacturing 610-682-6361
Deka Road, Lyon Station, PA 19536-0147
Parts for powered wheelchairs, including batteries. 7/14/93.MC

Epic Medical Equipment Services, Inc. 800-327-3742
1800 10th St Ste 300, Plano, TX 75074
Repair of pulse oximeters, finger sensors and cables. Sale of finger sensors and cables.

General Biomedical Service, Inc. 800-558-9449
1900 25th St, Kenner, LA 70062
Exporters of new, used and remanufactured medical equipment, specializing in ventilators and other respiratory equipment.

Gould Discount Medical 800-876-6846
3901 Dutchmans Ln Ste 100, Louisville, KY 40207
Parts for powered wheelchairs.

Kapp Surgical Instrument, Inc. 800-282-5277
4919 Warrensville Center Rd, Cleveland, OH 44128
Instrument repairs.

Mark Medical Manufacturing, Inc. 610-269-4420
530 Brandywine Ave, Downingtown, PA 19335
Surgical-instrument repair specializing in microsurgical repair, bipolar and monopolar forceps, Leep or Lete instruments recoatings, ebonizing or laser recoatings.

Mxe, Inc. - X-Ray Cassette Repair 800-252-1801
12107 Jefferson Blvd, Culver City, CA 90230
X-Ray cassette and ID camera repair company.

Pyramid Medical Llc 800-764-1154
10940 Portal Dr, Los Alamitos, CA 90720
ULTRASOUND SYSTEM, PARTS, PROBES, REPAIR. Depot or on-site service for multi-vendors. Monitors repaired or replaced.

Remedpar 800-624-3994
101 Old Stone Bridge Rd, Goodlettsville, TN 37072

Replacement Parts Industries, Inc. 800-221-9723
20338 Corisco St, Chatsworth, CA 91311
Parts for repair of aspirators, autoclaves, blood gas analyzers, cast cutters, centrifuges, dental operatories, ECGs, examination tables, flame photometers, hydrocollators, spectrophotometers, sterilizers (bulk and table top), suction pumps, traction units, ventilators, incubators, and miscellaneous accessories; also, dental X-ray film processors, lamps and bulbs.

Rocky Mountain Helicopters 801-375-1124
800 S 3110 W, Provo, UT 84601
Aircraft overhaul/repair.

Vectron International 717-486-6060
100 Watts St, Mount Holly Springs, PA 17065
Electric Parts

Wheelchair Sales And Service Co., Inc. 877-736-0376
315 Main St, West Springfield, MA 01089
Services manual and powered wheelchairs, scooters, beds, chairs (seat lift), walking aids, and bathroom accessories.

World Medical Equipment, Inc. 800-827-3747
3915 152nd St NE, Marysville, WA 98271

SERVICE, PRINTING *(General) 80WYM*

Astro-Med, Inc. 800-343-4039
600 E Greenwich Ave, West Warwick, RI 02893
Contract services, supplies and materials.

Bibbero Systems, Inc. 800-242-2376
1300 N McDowell Blvd, Petaluma, CA 94954
Custom printing. Personalized stationery, envelopes, business cards, statements, super bills, prescription form blanks in single, duplicate, alterproof, and blanks for states requiring special security features.

Brady Corporation 800-541-1686
6555 W Good Hope Rd, PO Box 571, Milwaukee, WI 53223
Flexographic printing, performed in tandem with lamination/die cutting services. Up to six colors with four-color process capability.

SERVICE, PRINTING *(cont'd)*

Challenge Printing Company, The 800-654-1234
2 Bridewell Pl, Clifton, NJ 07014

Gdm Electronic And Medical 408-945-4100
2070 Ringwood Ave, San Jose, CA 95131

Medegen 800-520-7999
930 S Wanamaker Ave, Ontario, CA 91761

Pepin Manufacturing, Inc. 800-291-6505
1875 S Highway 61, Lake City, MN 55041
Flexo and screen.

Tailored Label Products, Inc. 800-727-1344
W165N5731 Ridgewood Dr, Menomonee Falls, WI 53051

Thermo Fisher Scientific - Checkweighing, Metal And X-Ray Detection 800-227-8891
501 90th Ave NW, Minneapolis, MN 55433
Contact coding systems for printing fixed text, graphics and variable information onto various substrates. TT53 IM Thermal Coder 300 DPI on-line contact coder for printing date codes, logos, graphics, bar codes and other information without the need for labor intensive type. TT53 IM Vacuum Carton Coder feeds cartons and flat, stackable material via a vacuum table for direct thermal transfer coding of bar codes, lot & date codes, graphics and other variable information.

Ultratec, Inc. 800-482-2424
450 Science Dr, Madison, WI 53711
SUPERPRINT 4425 and MINIPRINT 425 TTY Printing communication device. SUPERPRINT 4425 TTY deluxe printing, direct connect or acoustic use, E-Turbo, Turbo Code, auto answer, remote message retrieval, keyboard dialing. MINIPRINT 425 TTY basic printer with direct connect.

SERVICE, PUBLICATION ACQUISITION *(General) 80WNM*

Parexel International Corp. 781-487-9900
195 West St, Waltham, MA 02451
Publications include: US Regulatory Reporter, New Drug Development: A Regulatory Overview, Biologics Development: A Regulatory Overview, CANADA 1995: An International Regulatory and Strategy Report. New; Parexel's Pharmaceutical R&D Statistical Sourcebook 1996. Worldwide Pharmaceutical Regulation Series. Expediting Drug and Biologics Development.

SERVICE, REPAIR, ENDOSCOPIC *(General) 80QBN*

Advanced Endoscopy Devices, Inc. 818-227-2720
22134 Sherman Way, Canoga Park, CA 91303
A national independent repair company of rigid endoscopes and instruments. Any manufacturers. 50%-80% below manufacturer prices.

Aesculap Implant Systems Inc. 1-800-234-9179
3773 Corporate Pkwy, Center Valley, PA 18034

Comeg Endoscopes, U.S.A. 800-248-5799
13790 E Rice Pl, Aurora, CO 80015

Endoscopy Support Services, Inc. 800-349-3636
3 Fallsview Ln, Brewster, NY 10509

Hmb Endoscopy Products 800-659-5743
3746 SW 30th Ave, Fort Lauderdale, FL 33312
Repair of Flexible and Rigid Endoscopes as well as endoscopic accessories.

Matlock Endoscopic Repairs, Sales, And Service, Inc. 800-394-9822
4320 Kenilwood Dr Ste 107, Nashville, TN 37204

SERVICE, TISSUE BANK *(General) 80WXG*

Allosource 800-873-8330
6278 S Troy Cir, Centennial, CO 80111
Human Allograft

Lifenet Health 800-847-7831
1864 Concert Dr, Virginia Beach, VA 23453

SERVICE, USED EQUIPMENT *(General) 80WMO*

American Autoclave Co. 800 421 5161
7819 Riverside Rd E, Sumner, WA 98390
Remanufactured sterilizers.

Angelus Medical & Optical Co., Inc. 310-769-6060
13007 S Western Ave, Gardena, CA 90249
Buy/sell/trade/appraise all medical equipment.

Atlas Medical Technologies 909-923-7887
1137 E Philadelphia St, Ontario, CA 91761
Refurbishers of CT scanners.

SERVICE, USED EQUIPMENT *(cont'd)*

Bryton Corp. 800-567-9500
4310 Guion Rd, Indianapolis, IN 46254
Complete service as well as extensive scheduled maintenance programs for all types of surgical, orthopedic, urological, obstetrical, and major examination tables and surgical lights.

Cardio-Vascular Sales 888-287-8700
27111 Aliso Creek Rd Ste 130, Aliso Viejo, CA 92656
Retail dealer of preowned echocardiography, general ultrasound and stress echo equipment. Specializing in sales of reconditioned color and spectral Doppler ultrasound systems; serving cardiology, radiology, vascular surgery, neurology, anesthesiology and perinatology.

Cranford X-Ray Co. 800-285-8329
8106 Berwyn Dr, Houston, TX 77037
New and used x-ray and EKG equipment.

Ctronics 800-472-9909
6333 Pacific Ave, Stockton, CA 95207
CT and MRI scanners.

D.R.E., Inc. 800-462-8195
1800 Williamson Ct, Louisville, KY 40223
DRE operates within your budget by offering a wide range of new, used, and refurbished medical and surgical equipment. Brands such as Drager, Datex-Ohmeda, Nellcor, Valleylab, Sarns, Puritan Bennett, Amsco, Sechrist, Siemens, and more.

Davis Medical Electronics, Inc. 800-422-3547
2441 Cades Way Ste 200, Vista, CA 92081
Refurbished cardiac equipment.

General Biomedical Service, Inc. 800-558-9449
1900 25th St, Kenner, LA 70062
New & remanufactured respiratory equipment, ventilators, and pulse oximeters.

Gvs - New York 631-753-2100
46 Central Ave, Farmingdale, NY 11735
AMSCO surgery tables, defibrillators, autoclaves, pulse oximeters, stress and exam tables and more.

Health Care Exports, Inc. 800-847-0173
5701 NW 74th Ave, Miami, FL 33166
Exporter of new and refurbished ultrasound. Nuclear medicine, mammography, C-arms, x-ray, cardiology, surgical equipment to Latin America, the Caribbean, South Asia.

Ideal Medical Source, Inc. 800-537-0739
2805 East. Oakland Blvd, Suite 352, Fort Lauderdale, FL 33306

Instru-Med, Co. 404-252-6188
5775 Glenridge Dr NE, East Building Suite 360, Atlanta, GA 30328
Including dialysis and endoscopy equipment.

International Radiographic, Inc. 404-405-7909
395 Grand Teton Cir, Fayetteville, GA 30215
Radiation oncology products--Linear Accelerators and CT simulators. Used and reconditioned.

Ivry 305-448-9858
216 Catalonia Ave Ste 106, Coral Gables, FL 33134
Anesthesia and surgical tables, electrosurgical and imaging equipment, and diagnostic monitors.

J&S Medical Associates 800-229-6000
35 Tripp St Ste 1, Framingham, MA 01702
Remanufactured COULTER S & IV PLUS, I, II, and IV; also BECKMAN ASTRA, COULTER STKR, ROCHE MIRA, COULTER T 890, 660, 540.

John Cudia And Associates, Inc. 408-782-2628
18440 Technology Dr Ste 110, Morgan Hill, CA 95037

Laboratory Environment Support Systems, Inc. 800-621-6404
7755 E Evans Rd, Scottsdale, AZ 85260
Patented cuvette reprocessing service. Distributor of refurbished clinical analyzers, reagents, other consumables, and instrument service.

Labworld, Inc. 800-447-2428
471 Page St Ste 4, Stoughton, MA 02072

Leasing Innovations Incorporated 800-532-7388
437 S Highway 101 Ste 104, Solana Beach, CA 92075
Specializes in all types of medical equipment.

Lenox Laser 800-494-6537
12530 Manor Rd, Glen Arm, MD 21057
Laser systems including flow calibrated orifices, gas mixtures, optical apertures, and hole drilling service. Flow Calibrated Orifice, currently the most accurate gas flow system available.

SERVICE, USED EQUIPMENT *(cont'd)*

Life Medical Equipment 800-749-4646
7874 NW 64th St, Miami, FL 33166
Refurbish all types of used medical and laboratory equipment.

M.J.S. & Associates 727-934-5000
40347 US Highway 19 N, Tarpon Springs, FL 34689
Provider of refurbished and experienced surgical equimpment - video, endoscopic, laparoscopic, arthroscopic and instrumentation of varied specialties.

Mass Medical Equipment Co., Inc. 781-246-3368
1 Melvin St Unit A, Wakefield, MA 01880
Buy and sell medical and lab equipment.

Medi-Tek, Inc. 661-940-0030
4555 W Avenue G Ste 6, Lancaster, CA 93536

Medical Sales & Service Group 888-357-6520
10 Woodchester Dr, Acton, MA 01720

Medrecon, Inc. 877-526-4323
257 South Ave, Garwood, NJ 07027
Surgical tables, remanufactured.

Meza Medical Equipment 888-308-7116
108 W Nakoma St, San Antonio, TX 78216
Diagnostic ultrasound equipment and accessories.

Mfi Medical Equipment Inc 800-633-1558
7929 Silverton Ave Ste 610, San Diego, CA 92126
Listings of hospital equipment for resale.

Midwest Laser Products 815-462-9500
PO Box 262, Frankfort, IL 60423
Buys and sells used medical lasers.

Mit Service, Inc. 800-343-8828
1354 Swallow Dr Ste 104, El Cajon, CA 92020
Refurbished clinical laboratory instrumentation and spare parts.

Multi Imager Service, Inc 800-400-4549
13865 Magnolia Ave Bldg C, Chino, CA 91710
Founded in 1983, Multi Imager specializes in diagnostic-quality film imaging and digital imaging technologies, including film-based video imagers, wet-film-based laser imagers, dry-film imagers, digital acquisition/storage and transmission devices, computed radiography, PACS, and more. Multi Imager provides technical support and training, parts supply, and sales of new as well as refurbished equipment used with a broad range of modalities, including CT, MRI, ultrasound, nuclear medicine, and others.

Myco Instrumentation Source, Inc. 425-228-4239
PO Box 354, Renton, WA 98057

Mylin Medical Systems, Inc. 630-321-1450
11904 Heritage Dr, Burr Ridge, IL 60527
Sales: Used/Refurbished MRI, CT, X-ray,Nuclear Medicine, Ultrasound and Radiation Therapy systems.

Nashville Medical Electronics, Inc. 800-966-1001
319 Fesslers Ln Ste A, Nashville, TN 37210
All types of Medical Equipment available for purchase.

New Laser Science, Inc. 858-487-5880
PO Box 27210, San Diego, CA 92198

New Life Systems, Inc. 954-972-4600
PO Box 8767, Coral Springs, FL 33075
Laboratory, radiology, cardiology and pulmonary equipment.

Photovac Laser Corp., Inc. 614-875-3300
3513 Farm Bank Way, Grove City, OH 43123

Products Group International, Inc. 800-336-5299
447 Main St., Lyons, CO 80540
Wide selection of used ultrasound scanners, probes and accessories.

Progressive Medical International 800-764-0636
2460 Ash St, Vista, CA 92081
EMS supplies: Defibrillators and cardiac monitors from LifePak, HP, Zoll, Physio Control and Marquette. Infusion pumps from IVAC, Siemens, MTP and Baxter.

Pyramid Medical Llc 800-764-1154
10940 Portal Dr, Los Alamitos, CA 90720
Ultrasound equipment, parts, probes, monitors, cameras and accessories for multi-vendors. Including ACUSON, ATL, HP, DIASONICS, Siemens, Toshiba, Aloka and others. Reseller - ultrasound specialists for 25 years.

Remedpar 800-624-3994
101 Old Stone Bridge Rd, Goodlettsville, TN 37072
Remanufactured CT, MRI and X-ray systems.

SERVICE, USED EQUIPMENT *(cont'd)*

Rozinn By Scottcare Corporation 800-243-9412
4791 W 150th St, Cleveland, OH 44135
Holter equipment and supplies. We usually have used Holter Recorders for sale.

Second Exposure, Inc. 985-845-0933
PO Box 609, Madisonville, LA 70447
Used medical imaging systems; ie. MRI, CT, cardiac cath

Spectron Corp. 425-827-9317
934 S Burlington Blvd # 603, Burlington, WA 98233

Traco Medical Equipment 605-339-9339
3505 S Norton Ave, Sioux Falls, SD 57105
Specializing in laboratory equipment, exam tables, birthing beds and defibrillators.

Whittemore Enterprises, Inc. 800-999-2452
11149 Arrow Rte, Rancho Cucamonga, CA 91730
Flexible and rigid endoscopes and operating room equipment.

World Medical Equipment, Inc. 800-827-3747
3915 152nd St NE, Marysville, WA 98271
Specialize in refurbished operating room tables, lights, autoclaves, anesthesia, monitors, and accessories.

SERVICE, WASTE MANAGEMENT *(General) 80WUN*

American Autoclave Co. 800 421 5161
7819 Riverside Rd E, Sumner, WA 98390
Complete plant for processing biological waste.

Rmc Medical 800-332-0672
3019 Darnell Rd, Philadelphia, PA 19154
HAZMAT decontamination equipment.

Security Engineered Machinery 800-225-9293
5 Walkup Dr, Westborough, MA 01581

SET, ADMINISTRATION, INTRAVENOUS, NEEDLE-FREE *(General) 80WZG*

B. Braun Medical, Inc. 610-596-2536
901 Marcon Blvd, Allentown, PA 18109
INTRAVASCULAR ADMINISTRATION SET

B. Braun Oem Division, B. Braun Medical Inc. 866-8-BBRAUN
824 12th Ave, Bethlehem, PA 18018
SAFSITE and Ultrasite needle-free valves to replace injection sites and needles in intravenous therapy.

Baxter Healthcare Corporporation, Alternate Care And Channel Team 888-229-0001
25212 W Il Route 120, Round Lake, IL 60073
INTERLINK IV Access System.

Globe Medical Tech, Inc. 713-365-9595
1766 W Sam Houston Pkwy N, Houston, TX 77043
Syringes, small vein sets; blood sets, burettes also available.

Harmac Medical Products, Inc. 716-897-4500
2201 Bailey Ave, Buffalo, NY 14211
OEM and private-labeled custom infusion disposable bags and sets. Also extension sets (latex-free) and infusion components.

Hospira Inc. 877-946-7747
275 N Field Dr, Lake Forest, IL 60045
Multiple

Intravascular Incorporated 800-917-3234
3600 Burwood Dr, Waukegan, IL 60085
FloStar Needleless Connector - patented 'dual-valve' needle free connector for use on venous or arterial lines with luer lock or luer slip in intravenous therapy. Available stand alone or on extension sets.

Meridian Medical Technologies 800-638-8093
10240 Old Columbia Rd, Columbia, MD 21046
INTRAJECT disposable needle-free injector for self administration.

Vascular Solutions, Inc. 888-240-6001
6464 Sycamore Ct N, Maple Grove, MN 55369

SET, HOLDER, DIALYZER *(Gastro/Urology) 78FKI*

Molded Products Inc. 800-435-8957
1112 Chatburn Ave, Harlan, IA 51537
Dialyzer Holder for Tandem Dialysis

SETTER, BAND, ORTHODONTIC *(Dental And Oral) 76ECR*

G & H Wire Co. 800-526-1026
2165 Earlywood Dr, Franklin, IN 46131

Orthodontic Design And Production, Inc. 760-734-3995
1370 Decision St Ste D, Vista, CA 92081
Type of orthodontic hand instrument.

SETTER, BAND, ORTHODONTIC *(cont'd)*

Premier Dental Products Co. 888-670-6100
1710 Romano Dr, PO Box 4500, Plymouth Meeting, PA 19462

3m Unitek 800-634-5300
2724 Peck Rd, Monrovia, CA 91016

SGOT, COLORIMETRIC *(Chemistry) 75CIS*

Biomerieux Inc. 800-682-2666
100 Rodolphe St, Durham, NC 27712

Dade Behring, Inc. 800-948-3233
1717 Deerfield Rd, Deerfield, IL 60015

Diagnostic Specialties 732-549-4011
4 Leonard St, Metuchen, NJ 08840
$138.00 per unit (standard).

SGOT, ULTRAVIOLET *(Chemistry) 75CIQ*

Beckman Coulter, Inc. 800-635-3497
740 W 83rd St, Hialeah, FL 33014
$0.08 per test.

Beckman Coulter, Inc. 800-742-2345
250 S Kraemer Blvd, PO Box 8000, Brea, CA 92821

Biomerieux Inc. 800-682-2666
100 Rodolphe St, Durham, NC 27712

Genzyme Corp. 800-325-2436
160 Christian St, Oxford, CT 06478
Kinetic.

Health Chem Diagnostics Llc 954-979-3845
3341 W McNab Rd, Pompano Beach, FL 33069
Diazo, ast/sgot.

Sterling Diagnostics, Inc. 800-637-2661
36645 Metro Ct, Sterling Heights, MI 48312
Sgot reagent set.

Teco Diagnostics 714-693-7788
1268 N Lakeview Ave, Anaheim, CA 92807
Ast/sgot (color).

SGPT, COLORIMETRIC *(Chemistry) 75CKD*

Bio-Rad Laboratories, Inc. 425-881-8300
6565 185th Ave NE, Redmond, WA 98052
Various.

Biomerieux Inc. 800-682-2666
100 Rodolphe St, Durham, NC 27712

Dade Behring, Inc. 800-948-3233
1717 Deerfield Rd, Deerfield, IL 60015

Diagnostic Specialties 732-549-4011
4 Leonard St, Metuchen, NJ 08840
$138.00 per unit (standard).

Health Chem Diagnostics Llc 954-979-3845
3341 W McNab Rd, Pompano Beach, FL 33069
Hydrazone colorimetry, alt/sgpt.

Sterling Diagnostics, Inc. 800-637-2661
36645 Metro Ct, Sterling Heights, MI 48312
Sgpt reagent set.

Teco Diagnostics 714-693-7788
1268 N Lakeview Ave, Anaheim, CA 92807
Alt (sgpt) (color).

SGPT, ULTRAVIOLET *(Chemistry) 75CKA*

Abbott Diagnostics Div. 626-440-0700
820 Mission St, South Pasadena, CA 91030
Varioius assays for detection of sgpt (alt).

Bayer Healthcare Llc 914-524-2955
555 White Plains Rd Fl 5, Tarrytown, NY 10591
Test for sgpt in plasma or serum.

Beckman Coulter, Inc. 800-635-3497
740 W 83rd St, Hialeah, FL 33014
$0.08 per test.

Beckman Coulter, Inc. 800-742-2345
250 S Kraemer Blvd, PO Box 8000, Brea, CA 92821

Biomerieux Inc. 800-682-2666
100 Rodolphe St, Durham, NC 27712

Caldon Bioscience, Inc. 909-628-9944
2100 S Reservoir St, Pomona, CA 91766
Alt/sgpt.

Caldon Biotech, Inc. 757-224-0177
2251 Rutherford Rd, Carlsbad, CA 92008
Alt/sgpt.

SGPT, ULTRAVIOLET *(cont'd)*

Carolina Liquid Chemistries Corp. 800-471-7272
510 W Central Ave Ste C, Brea, CA 92821
Alt.

Genchem, Inc. 714-529-1616
510 W Central Ave Ste D, Brea, CA 92821
Alt/sgpt reagent.

Genzyme Corp. 800-325-2436
160 Christian St, Oxford, CT 06478
Kinetic.

Health Chem Diagnostics Llc 954-979-3845
3341 W McNab Rd, Pompano Beach, FL 33069
Nadh oxidation/nad reduction, alt/sgpt.

Hemagen Diagnostics, Inc. 800-436-2436
9033 Red Branch Rd, Columbia, MD 21045
Various alt/sgpt methods.

Jas Diagnostics, Inc. 305-418-2320
7220 NW 58th St, Miami, FL 33166
Alt (gpt).

Raichem, Division Of Hemagen Diagnostics, Inc. 800-438-6100
8225 Mercury Ct, San Diego, CA 92111
Alanine aminotransferase.

Sterling Diagnostics, Inc. 800-637-2661
36645 Metro Ct, Sterling Heights, MI 48312
Alt/sgpt reagent set.

Synermed Intl., Inc. 317-896-1565
17408 Tiller Ct Ste 1900, Westfield, IN 46074
Alt/gpt reagent kit.

Teco Diagnostics 714-693-7788
1268 N Lakeview Ave, Anaheim, CA 92807
Alt liquid reagent.

Vital Diagnostics Inc. 714-672-3553
1075 W Lambert Rd Ste D, Brea, CA 92821
Various alt/sgpt reagents.

SHAKER, WATERBATH *(Chemistry) 75VLS*

Eberbach Corp. 800-422-2558
505 S Maple Rd, Ann Arbor, MI 48103

Polyscience, Division Of Preston Industries Inc. 800-229-7569
6600 W Touhy Ave, Niles, IL 60714

Pro Scientific Inc. 800-584-3776
99 Willenbrock Rd, Oxford, CT 06478
Memmert water baths, from 10-100 degrees Celsius are available with an optional shaker unit for the 14L and 22l size. Standard features; high grade stainless steel, microprocessor PID control, integral self-diagnostics, digital timer, digital temperature display, overtemperature protection and corrosion proof large-area heating system on three sides of the working space ensuring optimum temperature uniformity.

Thermal Product Solutions 800-216-7725
2121 Reach Rd, Williamsport, PA 17701

Thermo Fisher Scientific 877-843-7668
81 Wyman St, Waltham, MA 02451

SHAKER/STIRRER *(Chemistry) 75JRQ*

Appropriate Technical Resources, Inc. 800-827-5931
9157 Whiskey Bottom Rd, PO Box 460, Laurel, MD 20723

Barnstead International 412-490-8425
2555 Kerper Blvd, Dubuque, IA 52001
Rotator.

Boekel Scientific 800-336-6929
855 Pennsylvania Blvd, Feasterville Trevose, PA 19053
Incubator.

Csc Scientific Co. 800-621-4778
2810 Old Lee Hwy, Fairfax, VA 22031
Sieve shaker with rheostat speed control, movable platform and adjustable sieve-holding rods. Holds up to 6 standard 8in. sieves and can adapt to 5in. sieves. Timer optional. MEINZER Meinzer II Sieve Shaker portable, compact sieve shaker, powered by electromagnetics - no moving parts so maintenance-free, built-in timer, affordable, accepts up to 10 FH 8' sieves.

Eberbach Corp. 800-422-2558
505 S Maple Rd, Ann Arbor, MI 48103
Reciprocating shaker and rotating (orbital) shaker.

Glas-Col , Llc 800-452-7265
711 Hulman St, PO Box 2128, Terre Haute, IN 47802
Various sizes for laboratory applications.

SHAKER/STIRRER *(cont'd)*

Haemonetics Corp. 800-225-5242
400 Wood Rd, P.O. Box 9114, Braintree, MA 02184

New Brunswick Scientific Co., Inc. 800-631-5417
PO Box 4005, Edison, NJ 08818
Over 30 biological shakers are offered for cell culture, hybridization, gel staining/destaining and more. Open-air 'platform' shakers, as well as environmentally-controlled models with optional incubation, refrigeration, photosynthetic lighting, and humidity control are offered. NBS shakers are designed for continuous day-in and day-out use, and are known to last for decades. Portable, benchtop, floor model, and space-saving stackable models are available, with a range of options.

Pro Scientific Inc. 800-584-3776
99 Willenbrock Rd, Oxford, CT 06478
The VSOS-4 Orbital Shaker provides orbital shaking motion for a variety of applications and can support up to 110 pounds. It has a digital readout for specific speed adjustments from 25-400 rpm and 60 minute timer with 'hold'. The VSR-50 Variable Speed Rocker is can support up to 30 pounds while limiting vibration and is equipped with a 60 minute timer with a 'hold' feature. The rocker is available with 12' x 14' or 16' x 20' tables with an adjustable table angle. The Variable Speed Rocker allows 5 to 100 rocking motions per minute.

Scientific Industries, Inc. 888-850-6208
70 Orville Dr, Bohemia, NY 11716

Thermo Fisher Scientific (Asheville) Llc 740-373-4763
Millcreek Rd., Marietta, OH 45750
Various models of shakers.

Thermo Fisher Scientific Inc. 563-556-2241
2555 Kerper Blvd, Dubuque, IA 52001

Troemner Llc 800-352-7705
201 Wolf Dr, PO Box 87, West Deptford, NJ 08086

SHARPENER, DENTAL *(Dental And Oral) 76RSF*

Hu-Friedy Manufacturing Co., Inc. 800-483-7433
3232 N Rockwell St, Chicago, IL 60618
$11.00-$78.00.

Moyco Technologies, Inc. 800-331-8837
200 Commerce Dr, Montgomeryville, PA 18936
$19.95 per unit (set of 6).

Rx Honing Machine Corporation 800-346-6464
1301 E 5th St, Mishawaka, IN 46544
RX Honing Machines: Sharpening sets: dental #90201 and periodontal #90602 include Rx sharpening machines and components for easily honing instruments. Video/manuals included.

Suter Dental Manufacturing Company, Inc. 800-368-8376
632 Cedar St, Chico, CA 95928

SHARPENER, INSTRUMENT, SURGICAL *(Surgery) 79WVB*

American Surgical Instrument Corp. 800-628-2879
26 Plaza Dr, Westmont, IL 60559
Diamond knive.

Prosurge Instruments, Inc. 866-832-7874
199 Laidlaw Ave, Jersey City, NJ 07306

Rx Honing Machine Corporation 800-346-6464
1301 E 5th St, Mishawaka, IN 46544
RX Honing Machines: Complete dermatology #90704, ophthalmology #91203, plastic/ent #92502, surgical #92701, laboratory #93002 and hospital #92801 sharpening sets from Rx Honing.

SHARPENER, KNIFE *(Surgery) 79RSG*

Rx Honing Machine Corporation 800-346-6464
1301 E 5th St, Mishawaka, IN 46544
RX Honing Machines: System II Sharpening Machine with surgical set #92701 or hospital set #92801 include all components for sharpening surgical knives.

Zimmer Holdings, Inc. 800-613-6131
1800 W Center St, PO Box 708, Warsaw, IN 46580

SHARPENER, MICROTOME BLADE *(Pathology) 88RSH*

Hacker Instruments And Industries Inc. 800-442-2537
1132 Kincaid Bridge Rd, PO Box 1176, Winnsboro, SC 29180
H/I-76 Microtome Knife Sharpener. Sharpens and reconditions microtome knives in minutes.

Hu-Friedy Manufacturing Co., Inc. 800-483-7433
3232 N Rockwell St, Chicago, IL 60618
$7.35 to $58.00 each, 17 types.

SHEATH, ENDOSCOPIC *(Gastro/Urology) 78FED*

Clarus Medical, Llc. 763-525-8400
1000 Boone Ave N Ste 300, Minneapolis, MN 55427
Sheath, access.

Comfort Products, Inc. 800-822-7500
705 Linton Ave, Croydon, PA 19021

Gyrus Acmi, Inc. 508-804-2739
93 N Pleasant St, Norwalk, OH 44857
Various sizes and kinds of sheaths for endoscopes.

Gyrus Acmi, Inc. 508-804-2739
300 Stillwater P.o.box 1971, Stamford, CT 06902
Various sizes and kinds of sheaths for endoscopes.

Karl Storz Endoscopy-America Inc. 800-421-0837
600 Corporate Pointe, Culver City, CA 90230

Mahe International Inc. 800-294-7946
468 Craighead St, Nashville, TN 37204

Polyzen, Inc. 919-319-9599
1041 Classic Rd, Apex, NC 27539

Richard Wolf Medical Instruments Corp. 800-323-9653
353 Corporate Woods Pkwy, Vernon Hills, IL 60061

Rtc Inc.-Memcath Technologies Llc
1777 Oakdale Ave, West St Paul, MN 55118
Endoscope sheath.

Spirus Medical, Inc. 781-297-7220
1063 Turnpike St, PO Box 258, Stoughton, MA 02072
Endoscopic overtube.

SHEET, BURN *(General) 80FPY*

Boyd Converting Co., Inc. 800-262-2242
PO Box 287, South Lee, MA 01260
Burn sheet.

Dixie Ems Supply 800-347-3494
385 Union Ave, Brooklyn, NY 11211
$47.75 per 10 (1ft x 1ft).

Healer Products, Llc 914-663-6300
427 Commerce Ln Ste 1, West Berlin, NJ 08091
Sheet, burn.

Kentron Health Care, Inc. 615-384-0573
3604 Kelton Jackson Rd, P.o. Box 120, Springfield, TN 37172
Burn sheet.

Milliken & Company 864-503-2844
920 Milliken Rd, Spartanburg, SC 29303

North Safety Products 401-943-4400
1101 B Calle Neutron, Parque Industrial Maran, Mexicali, B.c. Mexico
Burn sheet sterile

Respond Industries, Inc. 1-800-523-8999
9500 Woodend Rd, Edwardsville, KS 66111
Various sizes of pads and dressings.

Tidi Products, Llc 920-751-4380
570 Enterprise Dr, Neenah, WI 54956
Sheet, burn.

W. L. Gore & Associates, Inc. 800-437-8181
PO Box 2400, Flagstaff, AZ 86003
PROCEL BURN COVER

W.L. Gore & Associates,Inc 928-526-3030
1505 North Fourth St., Flagstaff, AZ 86004
Burn dressing.

Zimmer Holdings, Inc. 800-613-6131
1800 W Center St, PO Box 708, Warsaw, IN 46580

Zimmer Orthopaedic Surgical Products 800-321-5533
PO Box 10, 200 West Ohio Ave., Dover, OH 44622
ULTRA-CARE; Disposable.

SHEET, DRAPE *(Surgery) 79RSK*

Atd-American Co. 800-523-2300
135 Greenwood Ave, Wyncote, PA 19095

Foothills Industries, Inc. 828-652-4088
300 Rockwell Dr, Marion, NC 28752

Health-Pak, Inc. 315-724-8370
2005 Beechgrove Pl, Utica, NY 13501
Table covers, bed and stretcher sheets.

SHEET, DRAPE *(cont'd)*

Rockland Industries, Inc. 800-876-2566
1601 Edison Hwy, Baltimore, MD 21213
ROC LON TLC (Total Light Control) blackout lining system to combat sleep deprivation. Blackout drapery lining and drapery fabrics plus invisible magnetic closure provides ultimate in sleep-inducing darkness by making the bedroom light-tight, eliminating any gaps for outside light to peek through.

Ross Disposable Products 800-649-6526
401 Traders Blvd E, Unit 10, Mississauga, ON L4Z 2H8 Canada

SHEET, DRAPE, DISPOSABLE *(Surgery) 79RSL*

Atd-American Co. 800-523-2300
135 Greenwood Ave, Wyncote, PA 19095

Foothills Industries, Inc. 828-652-4088
300 Rockwell Dr, Marion, NC 28752

Graham Medical Products/Div. Of Little Rapids Corp 866-429-1408
2273 Larsen Rd, Green Bay, WI 54303
Full line of patient exam drapes. Various colors and materials, available in sleeve packaging. Stretch sheets.

Johnson & Johnson Medical Division Of Ethicon, Inc. 800-423-4018
2500 E Arbrook Blvd, Arlington, TX 76014

Kerr Group 800-524-3577
1400 Holcomb Bridge Rd, Roswell, GA 30076

Vital Concepts, Inc. 800-984-2300
4334 Brockton Dr SE Ste F, Grand Rapids, MI 49512

SHEET, EXAMINATION TABLE, DISPOSABLE *(General) 80RSM*

Atd-American Co. 800-523-2300
135 Greenwood Ave, Wyncote, PA 19095

Bibbero Systems, Inc. 800-242-2376
1300 N McDowell Blvd, Petaluma, CA 94954
Crepe & smooth finish exam table paper. Also Dri-Perf deluxe table paper. 2-ply & 3-ply disposable exam drape sheets and stretcher sheets.

Graham Medical Products/Div. Of Little Rapids Corp 866-429-1408
2273 Larsen Rd, Green Bay, WI 54303
Paper in crepe or smooth finish, white or prints, and POLYPERF.

Howard Medical Company 800-443-1444
1690 N Elston Ave, Chicago, IL 60642
$32.00 per case of 12 rolls exam paper, 18 2 300' smooth.

Jero Medical Equipment & Supplies, Inc. 800-457-0644
1701 W 13th St, Chicago, IL 60608

Jms Converters Inc Dba Sabee Products & Stanford Prof Prod 215-396-3302
67 Buck Rd Ste B7, Huntingdon Valley, PA 19006
Table paper - drape sheets.

SHEET, OPERATING ROOM *(Surgery) 79RSN*

Atd-American Co. 800-523-2300
135 Greenwood Ave, Wyncote, PA 19095

Best Manufacturing Group Llc 800-843-3233
1633 Broadway Fl 18, New York, NY 10019
Cotton and blends; barrier made to specs.

Johnson & Johnson Medical Division Of Ethicon, Inc. 800-423-4018
2500 E Arbrook Blvd, Arlington, TX 76014

Kerr Group 800-524-3577
1400 Holcomb Bridge Rd, Roswell, GA 30076

SHEET, OPERATING ROOM, DISPOSABLE *(Surgery) 79RSO*

Atd-American Co. 800-523-2300
135 Greenwood Ave, Wyncote, PA 19095

Johnson & Johnson Medical Division Of Ethicon, Inc. 800-423-4018
2500 E Arbrook Blvd, Arlington, TX 76014

SHEETING, EXAMINATION TABLE *(General) 80RSJ*

Atd-American Co. 800-523-2300
135 Greenwood Ave, Wyncote, PA 19095

General Econopak, Inc. 888-871-8568
1725 N 6th St, Philadelphia, PA 19122
Disposable, cut and folded (not roll stock).

SHEETING, EXAMINATION TABLE *(cont'd)*

Graham Medical Products/Div. Of Little Rapids Corp 866-429-1408
2273 Larsen Rd, Green Bay, WI 54303
Paper in crepe or smooth finish, white or prints, and POLYPERF.

Health-Pak, Inc. 315-724-8370
2005 Beechgrove Pl, Utica, NY 13501

Jms Converters Inc Dba Sabee Products & Stanford Prof Prod 215-396-3302
67 Buck Rd Ste B7, Huntingdon Valley, PA 19006
Exam table paper.

Kerr Group 800-524-3577
1400 Holcomb Bridge Rd, Roswell, GA 30076

Mckesson General Medical 800-446-3008
8741 Landmark Rd, Richmond, VA 23228

R. Sabee Company 920-882-7350
1718 W 8th St, Appleton, WI 54914

SHEETING, STRETCHER *(General) 80WKD*

Casco Manufacturing Solutions, Inc. 800-843-1339
3107 Spring Grove Ave, Cincinnati, OH 45225

General Econopak, Inc. 888-871-8568
1725 N 6th St, Philadelphia, PA 19122
Disposable, all sizes.

Precept Medical Products, Inc. 800-438-5827
PO Box 2400, 370 Airport Road/, Arden, NC 28704

Schueler & Company, Inc. 516-487-1500
PO Box 528, Stratford, CT 06615

SHELL, SCLERAL *(Ophthalmology) 86HQT*

Accutome Ultrasound, Inc. 610-889-0200
3222 Phoenixville Pike, Malvern, PA 19355
Scleral immersion shell.

Advanced Ocular Prosthetics Inc. 412-787-7277
1111 Oakdale Rd Ste 5, Oakdale, PA 15071
Scleral shell.

Austin Ocular Prosthetics Center, Llc 512-452-3100
711 W 38th St Ste G1A, Austin, TX 78705

Center For Ocular Reconstruction 301-652-9282
4833 Rugby Ave Fl 4, Bethesda, MD 20814

Erickson Labs Northwest 425-823-1861
12911 120th Ave NE Ste C10, Kirkland, WA 98034
Scleral shell.

Esi, Inc. 763-473-2533
2915 Everest Ln N, Plymouth, MN 55447
Scleral immersion shell.

Frank Tanaka, Ocularist, Inc. 813-978-1142
3000 E Fletcher Ave Ste 310, Tampa, FL 33613
Scleral shell.

Hansen Ophthalmic Development Lab 319-338-1285
745 Avalon Pl, Coralville, IA 52241
Echo shells used for echography.

Henthorn Ocular Prosthetics 316-688-5235
744 S Hillside St, Wichita, KS 67211
Shell, scleral.

John J. Kelley Associates Ltd. 215-567-1377
1528 Walnut St Ste 1801, Mid City East, PA 19102
Scleral protective shields (acrylic & teflon).

June R.R. Nichols, Ocularist Ltd. 847-803-5050
1767 E Oakton St, Des Plaines, IL 60018
Artificial eye.

Miller Artificial Eye Laboratory, Inc. 419-474-3939
3030 W Sylvania Ave Ste 13, Toledo, OH 43613
Scleral shell.

Randal Minor Ocular Prosthetics Inc. 813-949-2500
1628 Dale Mabry Hwy Ste 110, Lutz, FL 33548
Scleral cover shell.

Soper Brothers & Associates 713-521-1263
1213 Hermann Dr Ste 320, Houston, TX 77004
Scleral shell.

Southwest Artificial Eyes, Inc. 210-737-3937
PO Box 100636, San Antonio, TX 78201
Scleral shell.

Thompson Ocular Prosthetics, Inc. 210-223-3754
4118 McCullough Ave Ste 16, San Antonio, TX 78212
Scleral cover shell prosthesis.

SHELL, SCLERAL *(cont'd)*

Turntine Ocular Prosthetics, Inc 913-962-6299
6342 Long Ave Ste H, Lenexa, KS 66216
Scleral shell.

SHIELD RADIO FREQUENCY *(Radiology) 90TEM*

Data Hunter LLC 714-892-5461
5412 Bolsa Ave Ste G, Huntington Beach, CA 92649
Miniature radio frequency data link.

Intermark (Usa), Inc. 408-971-2055
1310 Tully Rd Ste 117, San Jose, CA 95122
Broad range of advanced and sophisticated EMI/RFI-shielding and ESD components, including ferrites, gaskets, jackets, and grounding parts.

SHIELD, BREAST *(Obstetrics/Gyn) 85RSQ*

Alimed, Inc. 800-225-2610
297 High St, Dedham, MA 02026

Bar-Ray Products, Inc. 800-359-6115
95 Monarch St, Littlestown, PA 17340

Medela, Inc. 800-435-8316
1101 Corporate Dr, McHenry, IL 60050

SHIELD, BUNION *(Orthopedics) 87RSR*

Aetna Foot Products/Div. Of Aetna Felt Corporation 800-390-3668
2401 W Emaus Ave, Allentown, PA 18103
SCOTT FOOT CARE.

Hermell Products, Inc. 800-233-2342
9 Britton Dr, PO Box 7345, Bloomfield, CT 06002
Bunion cushion.

Mark Medical 800-433-3668
1168 Aster Ave Ste C, Sunnyvale, CA 94086
BUNION SOCK cushions & protects painful bone protrusions. The product alleviates friction, pressure & shearing in casual and dress shoes.

Pedifix, Inc. 800-424-5561
310 Guinea Rd, Brewster, NY 10509
Palliative products and Hallus valgus splints.

Slawner Ltd., J. 514-731-3378
5713 Cote Des Neiges Rd., Montreal, QUE H3S 1Y7 Canada

SHIELD, CORNEAL *(Ophthalmology) 86WRV*

Oasis Medical, Inc. 800-528-9786
514 S Vermont Ave, Glendora, CA 91741
Collagen corneal shields. Under 12, 12-hour, 24-hour and 72-hour dissolution times.

Precision Therapeutics, Inc. 800-544-0076
8400 E Prentice Ave Ste 700, Greenwood Village, CO 80111

Southmedic Inc. 800-463-7146
50 Alliance Blvd., Barrie, ONT L4M-5K3 Canada
Universal Eye Shield. Plastic injection molded, available in adult and pediatric sizes.

Ultracell Medical Technologies, Inc. 877-SPO-NGE1
183 Providence New London Tpke, North Stonington, CT 06359
ULTRACELL P.V.A. Corneal Light Shield, LASIK shields and LASIK spears.

SHIELD, EYE, OPHTHALMIC *(Ophthalmology) 86HOY*

Abb Optical Of North America 954-733-2300
125 Enterprise Dr, Marshfield, MA 02050

Alimed, Inc. 800-225-2610
297 High St, Dedham, MA 02026

Alphaprotech, Inc. 229-242-1931
1287 W Fairway Dr, Nogales, AZ 85621

Anissa's Fun Patches 423-234-3404
PO Box 455, Chuckey, TN 37641
Ophthalmic eye shield. To be used primarily by children with lazy eye, or to conceal the eye after surgery, etc. for adults as well as children.

Astron International Inc. 239-435-0136
3410 Westview Dr, Naples, FL 34104
Shield, eye, ophthalmic (including sunlamp protective eye).

B. Graczyk, Inc. 269-782-2100
27826 Burmax Park, Dowagiac, MI 49047
Various types of shields.

Bausch & Lomb Surgical 636-255-5051
3365 Tree Court Ind Blvd, Saint Louis, MO 63122

SHIELD, EYE, OPHTHALMIC *(cont'd)*

Brady Precision Converting, Llc 214-275-9595
1801 Big Town Blvd Ste 100, Mesquite, TX 75149
Anti-fog coated shields for surgical and face masks.

Ctp Coil Inc. 800-933-2645
1801 Howard St Ste D, Elk Grove Village, IL 60007
Various types of safety shields and spectacle frame mounted occulars.

Eagle Laboratories 800-782-6534
10201 Trademark St Ste A, Rancho Cucamonga, CA 91730

Edge I-Wear Corp. 909-598-7679
1775 Curtiss Ct, La Verne, CA 91750
Edge i-wear corp.

Ferguson Production, Inc. 865-982-5552
2130 Industrial Dr, Conway, KS 67460

Fresnel Prism & Lens Co. 952-496-0432
6824 Washington Ave S, Eden Prairie, MN 55344
Ophthalmic eye shield.

General Scientific Safety Equipment Co. 800-523-0166
2553 E Somerset St Fl 1, Philadelphia, PA 19134

George Tiemann & Co. 800-843-6266
25 Plant Ave, Hauppauge, NY 11788

Greattec Vision S.A. De C.V.
Circuito De La Amistad #2700, Mexicali B.c. Mexico
Safety glasses

Gulden Ophthalmics 800-659-2250
225 Cadwalader Ave, Elkins Park, PA 19027

Hurricane Medical 941-751-0588
5315 Lena Rd, Bradenton, FL 34211
Eye shield, light shield.

J.E.M. Sales Ltd. 416-663-7313
6-110 Norfinch Dr, Toronto M3N 1X1 Canada
Eye mask

Jardon Eye Prosthetics, Inc. 248-424-8560
15920 W 12 Mile Rd, Southfield, MI 48076

Jedmed Instruments Co. 314-845-3770
5416 Jedmed Ct, Saint Louis, MO 63129

K Medical 800-478-5633
PO Box 5224, Fort Lauderdale, FL 33310

Lt Acquisition, Inc. 616-698-1830
4489 E Paris Ave SE, Grand Rapids, MI 49512
Tanning booth eyewear.

Maverick Technologies, Inc. 727-791-6151
1754 Grove Dr, Clearwater, FL 33759
Ablatable mask.

Medegen Medical Products, Llc 800-233-1987
209 Medegen Drive, Gallaway, TN 38036-0228
SAFE-CHOICE Disposable.

Medone Surgical, Inc. 941-359-3129
670 Tallevast Rd, Sarasota, FL 34243
Various.

Megadyne Medical Products, Inc. 800-747-6110
11506 S State St, Draper, UT 84020
E-Z CLEAN eye shield.

Neotech Products, Inc. 800-966-0500
27822 Fremont Ct, Valencia, CA 91355
NEOSHADES: Phototherapy Eye Shields. Cute phototherapy mask with sunglasses printed on one side. Fun for parents, patients and staff.

Niagara Pharmaceuticals Div. 905-690-6277
60 Innovation Dr., Flamborough, ONT L9H-7P3 Canada
HEALTH SAVER #134 (large concave), #234 (regular concave), #334 (large flat), or #434 (regular flat).

Perioptix, Inc. 949-366-3333
230 Market Pl, Escondido, CA 92029
Safety shields.

Pro-Optics, Inc. 800-323-3846
317 N Woodwork Ln, Palatine, IL 60067
$47.30 per box of 50 pcs. of PRO-SHIELDS.

Protech Leaded Eyewear 561-627-9769
4087 Burns Rd, Palm Beach Gardens, FL 33410
Radiation filtering glasses.

Richmond Products, Inc. 505-275-2406
4400 Silver Ave SE, Albuquerque, NM 87108
Hematocrit control.

SHIELD, EYE, OPHTHALMIC *(cont'd)*

Sharn, Inc. 800-325-3671
4517 George Rd Ste 200, Tampa, FL 33634

Sun-Med 800-433-2797
12393 Belcher Rd S Ste 450, Largo, FL 33773
Eye protector.

Total Molding Services, Inc. 215-538-9613
354 East Broad St., Trumbauersville, PA 18970
Pediatric & Adult Eye Shields.

Trident Medical Products 800-647-4448
1201 Summit Ave, Fort Worth, TX 76102
SAFE-EDGE malleable ophthalmic aluminum eyeshield and Universal Polycarbonate plastic eyeshield with U.V. additive.

U.V. Vision Corp. 480-948-5350
7755 E Gray Rd Ste 100, Scottsdale, AZ 85260

Ultracell Medical Technologies, Inc. 877-SPO-NGE1
183 Providence New London Tpke, North Stonington, CT 06359
ULTRACELL PVA corneal light shields and LASIK shields.

SHIELD, GONADAL *(Radiology) 90IWT*

Aadco Medical, Inc. 800-225-9014
2279 VT Route 66, Randolph, VT 05060
X-ray protective gonad shield.

Bar-Ray Products, Inc. 800-359-6115
95 Monarch St, Littlestown, PA 17340

Ge Medical Systems, Llc 262-548-2355
3000 N Grandview Blvd, W-417, Waukesha, WI 53188
Patient gonadal shield when doing chest radiography.

Marconi Medical Systems 800-323-0550
595 Miner Rd, Cleveland, OH 44143

Protech Leaded Eyewear 561-627-9769
4087 Burns Rd, Palm Beach Gardens, FL 33410
Radiation filtering gonad or ovarian shields.

S&S Technology 281-815-1300
10625 Telge Rd, Houston, TX 77095

Save The Gonads, Ltd. 513-385-8147
5710 Sheits Rd, Cincinnati, OH 45252
Infant gonadal sheild.

Shadow Shield 866-838-8400
313 Cross Rd, Alamo, CA 94507
X-ray shielding device.

Shielding International, Inc. 800-292-2247
PO Box Z, 2150 NW Andrews Drive, Madras, OR 97741
Full line of asst. gonadal and ovarian x-ray protective accessories.

Shielding Intl., Inc. 541-475-7211
2150 N.w. Andrews Dr., Madras, OR 97741
Various -gonadal shields.

Supertech, Inc. 800-654-1054
PO Box 186, Elkhart, IN 46515
Clear-Pb Adult and Pediatric Gonad Shields

SHIELD, HEAT, INFANT *(General) 80RSS*

Cas Medical Systems, Inc. 800-227-4414
44 E Industrial Rd, Branford, CT 06405
Temperature probe heat reflector.

Freedom Designs, Inc. 800-331-8551
2241 N Madera Rd, Simi Valley, CA 93065
INFANT KNIT CAP for newborns used for retainnig heat.

SHIELD, MAGNETIC FIELD *(Radiology) 90RSP*

Amuneal Manufacturing Corp. 800-755-9843
4737 Darrah St, Philadelphia, PA 19124
Magnetic shielding of medical instruments and facilities. Magnetically shielded rooms (MSR) for MRI installations. Magnetic site surveys and consulting.

Braden Shielding Systems 918-624-2888
9260 Broken Arrow Expy, Tulsa, OK 74145
Radio frequency; EMI shielding.

Intermark (Usa), Inc. 408-971-2055
1310 Tully Rd Ste 117, San Jose, CA 95122
EMI-shielding products. EMI ferrite suppressors, cable shielding materials, and grounding connectors.

Supertech, Inc. 800-654-1054
PO Box 186, Elkhart, IN 46515
Mobile MRI Shield

SHIELD, NIPPLE *(Obstetrics/Gyn) 85HFS*

Blaine Labs, Inc. 800-307-8818
11037 Lockport Pl, Santa Fe Springs, CA 90670
Nipple shield.

Medela, Inc. 800-435-8316
1101 Corporate Dr, McHenry, IL 60050
Odorless, silicone nipple shield to aid breastfeeding mothers with sore nipples.

Omron Healthcare, Inc. 847-680-6200
300 Lakeview Pkwy, Vernon Hills, IL 60061
Nipple, shield.

Ware Medics Glass Works, Inc. 845-429-6950
PO Box 368, Garnerville, NY 10923

SHIELD, OPHTHALMIC, RADIOLOGICAL *(Radiology) 90IWS*

Aadco Medical, Inc. 800-225-9014
2279 VT Route 66, Randolph, VT 05060
X-ray protective eye wear.

Aura Lens Products, Inc. 800-281-2872
51 8th St N, PO Box 763, St. Cloud,, Sauk Rapids, MN 56379
X-ray shielding eyeglasses, prescription and non-prescription.

Bar-Ray Products, Inc. 800-359-6115
95 Monarch St, Littlestown, PA 17340

Barrier Eyewear 561-317-5324
840 13th St Ste 31, Lake Park, FL 33403
Lead eyewear.

Burkhart Roentgen Intl. Inc. 800-USA-XRAY
5201 8th Ave S, Gulfport, FL 33707
Lead glass spectacles and goggles with or w/o prescription lenses as well as full wrap-around protection.

Flow X-Ray Corporation 800-356-9729
100 W Industry Ct, Deer Park, NY 11729
Radiation shielding eyeglasses (.75 mm lead equivalency).

K Medical 800-478-5633
PO Box 5224, Fort Lauderdale, FL 33310

Lt Acquisition, Inc. 616-698-1830
4489 E Paris Ave SE, Grand Rapids, MI 49512
Disposable protective eyewear.

Oberon Company ,Div Of The Paramount Corp. 800-322-3348
22 Logan St, PO Box 61008, New Bedford, MA 02740
Benchtop portable work shields provide protection from splash, flying particles and beta radiation up to 2 MeV.

Supertech, Inc. 800-654-1054
PO Box 186, Elkhart, IN 46515
X-ray protective eyeglasses.

Wolf X-Ray Corporation 800-356-9729
100 W Industry Ct, Deer Park, NY 11729
Radiation shielding eyeglasses (.75mm lead equivalency).

SHIELD, PROTECTIVE, PERSONNEL *(Radiology) 90KPY*

Aadco Medical, Inc. 800-225-9014
2279 VT Route 66, Randolph, VT 05060
X-ray protective wear.

Ak, Ltd. 503-669-0986
18412 NE Halsey St, Portland, OR 97230
Patented, acrylic benchtop shields, 12 in.x 12 in. x12 in. - 3/8 in. or 16 in.x 12 in.x 20 in. H - 3/8 in. Also, Coulter Shields with U Channel mounting to machinery, 6 in. x 4 in. x 6 or 8 in.x10x 4 1/4.

Angiosystems, Inc. 800-441-4256
7 Hopkins Pl., Ducktown, TN 37326

Apollo Corporation 800-247-5490
PO Box 219, Somerset, WI 54025
The SHIELD prevents splash-back while emptying or flushing containers of potentially infectious materials.

Bar-Ray Products, Inc. 800-359-6115
95 Monarch St, Littlestown, PA 17340

Biodex Medical Systems, Inc. 800-224-6339
20 Ramsey Rd, Shirley, NY 11967

Burkhart Roentgen Intl. Inc. 800-USA-XRAY
5201 8th Ave S, Gulfport, FL 33707
Personal protective gear - lead aprons, thyroid protectors, hats, gloves, glasses, patient aprons & gonad (M&F) protection.

F & L Medical Products Co. 724-845-7028
1129 Industrial Park Rd Ste 3, Vandergrift, PA 15690
Ct shields.

SHIELD, PROTECTIVE, PERSONNEL *(cont'd)*

Ge Medical Systems, Llc 262-548-2355
3000 N Grandview Blvd, W-417, Waukesha, WI 53188
Leaded x-ray protective screens two styles one mobile and one pivoted.

Global Healthcare 800-601-3880
1495 Hembree Rd Ste 700, Roswell, GA 30076
Full face shields.

Intec Industries, Inc. 205-251-5600
2024 12th Ave N, Birmingham, AL 35234

K Medical 800-478-5633
PO Box 5224, Fort Lauderdale, FL 33310

Lite Tech, Inc. 610-650-8690
975 Madison Ave, Norristown, PA 19403
Thyroid shields & half-aprons.

Molded Products Inc. 800-435-8957
1112 Chatburn Ave, Harlan, IA 51537
Safety visor w/shield.

Morgan Medesign, Inc. 888-799-4633
947 Piner Pl, Santa Rosa, CA 95403
SCATTER-BAN(R)Radiation Barrier offers clinically significant reductions in scatter-radiation (up to 99%) while allowing C-arm mobility around table. It is designed to use in conjunction with lead aprons. Compatible with most 20- to 22-in.-wide table tops. Protected by U.S. Patent.

Mwt Materials, Inc. 973-472-5161
90 Dayton Ave Ste 6, Passaic, NJ 07055
Mri isolation blanket.

North American Scientific, Inc. 818-734-8600
8300 Aurora Ave N, Seattle, WA 98103
Various shield protective personnel.

Oberon Company ,Div Of The Paramount Corp. 800-322-3348
22 Logan St, PO Box 61008, New Bedford, MA 02740
One piece light weight, disposable shield to meet Bloodborn Pathogon rule.

Oncology Automation, Inc. 337-998-6837
105 Water Oaks Dr, Lafayette, LA 70503
Intravascular brachytherapy beta shield.

Op-D-Op, Inc. 916-783-5741
8559 Washington Blvd, Roseville, CA 95678
Face shield with visor extending down over face.

Protech Leaded Eyewear 561-627-9769
4087 Burns Rd, Palm Beach Gardens, FL 33410
Radiation filtering shields.

Shielding International, Inc. 800-292-2247
PO Box Z, 2150 NW Andrews Drive, Madras, OR 97741
Half arons; demi aprons; VDT aprons and thyroid collars; full-line of protective eyewear.

Shielding Intl., Inc. 541-475-7211
2150 N.w. Andrews Dr., Madras, OR 97741
Lead vinyl blocker/sheeting.

Standard Imaging, Inc. 608-831-0025
3120 Deming Way, Middleton, WI 53562
Shields and protective apparatus.

Supertech, Inc. 800-654-1054
PO Box 186, Elkhart, IN 46515
Mobile and Modular Barriers made from leaded acrylic and opaque panels

Trademark Medical Llc 800-325-9044
449 Soverign Ct, St. Louis, MO 63011
Surgical patient arm shield. Provides safe ledge for surgeon to lean against during surgery.

Vascular Performance Products, Llc. 888-364-7004
6945 Southbelt Dr SE, Caledonia, MI 49316
Radiation protective tray.

Youngs, Inc. 800-523-5454
55 E Cherry Ln, Souderton, PA 18964

SHIELD, SYRINGE *(General) 80RST*

Alimed, Inc. 800-225-2610
297 High St, Dedham, MA 02026

Becton Dickinson Infusion Therapy Systems, Inc. 888-237-2762
9450 S State St, Sandy, UT 84070
Translucent needle shield to protect the healthcare worker and patient from needlestick injuries. Specially designed for small and compromised veins.

SHIELD, SYRINGE *(cont'd)*

Capintec, Inc. 800-631-3826
6 Arrow Rd, Ramsey, NJ 07446

Zerowet, Inc. 800-438-0938
PO Box 4375, Palos Verdes Peninsula, CA 90274
Syringe-mounted splash shield completely protects MD or RN from contaminated splash during wound irrigation. Eliminates use of needle. Meets OSHA regulations.

SHIELD, VIAL *(Radiology) 90IWW*

Aadco Medical, Inc. 800-225-9014
2279 VT Route 66, Randolph, VT 05060
X-ray protective shielding.

Biodex Medical Systems, Inc. 800-224-6339
20 Ramsey Rd, Shirley, NY 11967

Capintec, Inc. 800-631-3826
6 Arrow Rd, Ramsey, NJ 07446

SHIELD, WOUND, INJECTION SITE *(General) 80RSU*

Kawasumi Laboratories America, Inc. 800-529-2786
4723 Oak Fair Blvd, Tampa, FL 33610
Intermittent injection site.

SHIELD, X-RAY *(Radiology) 90RSW*

AMD Technologies Inc. 800-423-3535
218 Bronwood Ave, Los Angeles, CA 90049
Radiation protective garments.

Bar-Ray Products, Inc. 800-359-6115
95 Monarch St, Littlestown, PA 17340
X-ray accessories - all types.

Biodex Medical Systems, Inc. 800-224-6339
20 Ramsey Rd, Shirley, NY 11967
Fixed and mobile Radiation Shields for radiology, nuclear medicine and PET.

Burkhart Roentgen Intl. Inc. 800-USA-XRAY
5201 8th Ave S, Gulfport, FL 33707
Table to floor protection, replacement window skirts, windows with special cut-outs.

Carr Corporation 800-952-2398
1547 11th St, Santa Monica, CA 90401

Cbs Scientific Co., Inc. 800-243-4959
PO Box 856, Del Mar, CA 92014
Beta Radiation Shields.

Cone Instruments, Inc. 800-321-6964
5201 Naiman Pkwy, Solon, OH 44139

Dan Kar Corporation 800-942-5542
PO Box 279, 192 New Boston St C, Wilmington, MA 01887
Radiation protection supplies and shields.

Flow X-Ray Corporation 800-356-9729
100 W Industry Ct, Deer Park, NY 11729

Huestis Medical 800-972-9222
68 Buttonwood St, Bristol, RI 02809
STYRO-FORMER x-ray shield.

Itm Partners, Ltd. 210-651-9066
5925 Corridor Pkwy, Schertz, TX 78154
Blocking trays that allow only a specific area to be exposed to radiation.

Lead Enterprises Inc. 800-253-4249
3300 NW 29th St, Miami, FL 33142
Custom X-ray shields. Shields for sheet rock, gypsum board and drywalls.

Marconi Medical Systems 800-323-0550
595 Miner Rd, Cleveland, OH 44143

Medlink Imaging, Inc. 800-456-7800
200 Clearbrook Rd, Elmsford, NY 10523

Protech Leaded Eyewear 561-627-9769
4087 Burns Rd, Palm Beach Gardens, FL 33410
Radiation filtering shields.

S&S Technology 281-815-1300
10625 Telge Rd, Houston, TX 77095
X-ray booths, mobile protective screens, stationary screens, and hinged screens.

St. John Companies 800-435-4242
25167 Anza Dr, PO Box 800460, Santa Clarita, CA 91355
Full line of protective aprons. Technologically advanced materials used to provide maximum protection with lightest weight.

SHIELD, X-RAY *(cont'd)*

Ti-Ba Enterprises, Inc. 585-247-1212
25 Hytec Cir, Rochester, NY 14606
Ti-Ba is the North American distributor of MAVIG, GmbH. The leader in radiation protection and ceiling suspended monitor displays. Please call us for pricing.

Wehmer Corporation 800-323-0229
1151 N Main St, Lombard, IL 60148
$40.00 for lead cervical collar (dental).

Wolf X-Ray Corporation 800-356-9729
100 W Industry Ct, Deer Park, NY 11729

Xma (X-Ray Marketing Associates, Inc.) 800-325-8880
1205 W Lakeview Ct, Windham Lakes Business Park
Romeoville, IL 60446

SHIELD, X-RAY, BRICK *(Radiology) 90RSV*

Marconi Medical Systems 800-323-0550
595 Miner Rd, Cleveland, OH 44143

SHIELD, X-RAY, DOOR *(Radiology) 90TDY*

Lead Enterprises Inc. 800-253-4249
3300 NW 29th St, Miami, FL 33142
Sheet Rock/gypsum board/drywall.

SHIELD, X-RAY, LEAD-PLASTIC *(Radiology) 90WPD*

Bar-Ray Products, Inc. 800-359-6115
95 Monarch St, Littlestown, PA 17340

California Medical Electronics 707-456-0990
2325 Perch Dr, Willits, CA 95490

Owens Scientific Inc. 281-394-2311
23230 Sandsage Ln, Katy, TX 77494

Protech Leaded Eyewear 561-627-9769
4087 Burns Rd, Palm Beach Gardens, FL 33410
Radiation filtering shields.

Shielding International, Inc. 800-292-2247
PO Box Z, 2150 NW Andrews Drive, Madras, OR 97741
Clear Pb mobile x-ray barriers; portable and fixed shields.

SHIELD, X-RAY, LEADED *(Dental And Oral) 76EAK*

Aadco Medical, Inc. 800-225-9014
2279 VT Route 66, Randolph, VT 05060
X-ray protective overhead barrier.

Bard Brachytherapy, Inc 908-277-8000
295 E Lies Rd, Carol Stream, IL 60188
Leaded shield radiation shield.

Burlington Medical Supplies, Inc. 800-221-3466
3 Elmhurst St, PO Box 3194, Newport News, VA 23603

Lead Enterprises Inc. 800-253-4249
3300 NW 29th St, Miami, FL 33142
Lead shielding, lead building materials.

One Zone Devices 858-350-9284
3525 Del Mar Heights Rd # 366, San Diego, CA 92130
Radiation screen.

SHIELD, X-RAY, PORTABLE *(Radiology) 90TEN*

Bar-Ray Products, Inc. 800-359-6115
95 Monarch St, Littlestown, PA 17340

Burkhart Roentgen Intl. Inc. 800-USA-XRAY
5201 8th Ave S, Gulfport, FL 33707
Mobile barriers, curtains (soft lead), table to floor shields.

Md Works, Inc. 770-409-9639
1895 Beaver Ridge Cir Ste 410, Norcross, GA 30071
Lead free rdiation shipping container

Owens Scientific Inc. 281-394-2311
23230 Sandsage Ln, Katy, TX 77494

Protech Leaded Eyewear 561-627-9769
4087 Burns Rd, Palm Beach Gardens, FL 33410
Radiation filtering portable shields.

Pulse Medical Inc. 800-342-5973
4131 SW 47th Ave Ste 1404, Davie, FL 33314
Lead radiographic shields in all sizes, styles and colors. Shields can be custom designed for your needs.

SHIELD, X-RAY, THROAT *(Radiology) 90VGQ*

AMD Technologies Inc. 800-423-3535
218 Bronwood Ave, Los Angeles, CA 90049

Bar-Ray Products, Inc. 800-359-6115
95 Monarch St, Littlestown, PA 17340

SHIELD, X-RAY, THROAT *(cont'd)*

Burkhart Roentgen Intl. Inc. 800-USA-XRAY
5201 8th Ave S, Gulfport, FL 33707
Lens and thyroid protector: 1mm lead protection suspended from ceiling, wall or table. Mounted onto a feather-touch counter balanced arm for precise positioning and ease of movement.

SHIELD, X-RAY, TRANSPARENT *(Radiology) 90VLA*

Bar-Ray Products, Inc. 800-359-6115
95 Monarch St, Littlestown, PA 17340

Lead Enterprises Inc. 800-253-4249
3300 NW 29th St, Miami, FL 33142
Leaded glass and Leaded acrylic

Protech Leaded Eyewear 561-627-9769
4087 Burns Rd, Palm Beach Gardens, FL 33410
Radiation filtering transparent shields.

Supertech, Inc. 800-654-1054
PO Box 186, Elkhart, IN 46515
Mobile and Modular Barriers made from leaded acrylic and opaque panels

SHOE AND SHOE COVER, CONDUCTIVE *(Anesthesiology) 73BWP*

Alphaprotech, Inc. 229-242-1931
1287 W Fairway Dr, Nogales, AZ 85621

Chagrin Safety Supply, Inc. 800-227-0468
8227 Washington St # 1, Chagrin Falls, OH 44023

Global Healthcare 800-601-3880
1495 Hembree Rd Ste 700, Roswell, GA 30076
Non-skid and standard.

Grand Medical Products 800-521-2055
7222 Ertel Ln, Houston, TX 77040

Jero Medical Equipment & Supplies, Inc. 800-457-0644
1701 W 13th St, Chicago, IL 60608
Various.

Scientimed Corp. 510-763-5405
4109 Balfour Ave, Oakland, CA 94610
Conductive shoecovers.

SHOE, CAST *(Physical Med) 89IPG*

A&A Orthopedics, Incorporated 757-224-0177
12250 SW 129th Ct Bldg 1, Miami, FL 33186
Cast shoe, fracture walker.

Alimed, Inc. 800-225-2610
297 High St, Dedham, MA 02026

Biomet, Inc. 574-267-6639
56 E Bell Dr, PO Box 587, Warsaw, IN 46582
Various types of cast shoe.

Bird & Cronin, Inc. 651-683-1111
1200 Trapp Rd, Saint Paul, MN 55121
Post op shoe.

Corflex, Inc. 800-426-7353
669 E Industrial Park Dr, Manchester, NH 03109

Darco International, Inc. 800-999-8866
810 Memorial Blvd, Huntington, WV 25701
ORTHO WEDGE heal shoe; HEELWEDGE healing shoe.

DJO Inc. 800-336-6569
1430 Decision St, Vista, CA 92081
Assorted styles and sizes of off-the-shelf cast shoes.

Dm Systems, Inc. 800-254-5438
1316 Sherman Ave, Evanston, IL 60201
GAITKEEPER® CAST SHOE allows improved gait patterns, holding position throughout gait, and guaranteed durability for the lifetime of the cast. It also provides improved patient comfort by reducing impact loading of the injured leg. Five sizes are available (XS, S, M, L, XL) for one low price.

Etonic Worldwide Llc 781-419-3060
260 Charles St, Waltham, MA 02453
Etonic shoe.

Frank Stubbs Co., Inc 800-223-1713
2100 Eastman Ave Ste B, Oxnard, CA 93030

Freeman Manufacturing Company 800-253-2091
900 W Chicago Rd, PO Box J, Sturgis, MI 49091
Cast sandal, cast boot and post-op shoes.

Griswold Tool And Die, Inc. 517-741-7433
PO Box 86, 8500 M-60 East, Union City, MI 49094
Cast heels (for walking casts) various sizes.

SHOE, CAST *(cont'd)*

Jobri Llc 800-432-2225
520 N Division St, Konawa, OK 74849
MOR-LOC.

Kenad Sg Medical, Inc. 800-825-0606
2692 Huntley Dr, Memphis, TN 38132
Shoe cast.

Lord Custom Molded Shoes, Inc. 631-471-3090
1395 Lakeland Ave Ste 1, Bohemia, NY 11716
Shoes from cast.

Lunax Corp. 800-355-8629
6669 W Ridge Dr, Brighton, MI 48116
Lunax boot.

Maramed Orthopedic Systems 800-327-5830
2480 W 82nd St, No. 8, Hialeah, FL 33016

Ortholine 800-243-3351
13 Chapel St, Norwalk, CT 06850
Multiple sizes and types. Canvas, Vinyl, Open Toe, Closed Toe. Flat and Rocker styles

Ossur Americas 949-268-3155
742 Pancho Rd, Camarillo, CA 93012

Paramedical Distributors 800-245-3278
2020 Grand Blvd, Kansas City, MO 64108
Casting and post-op shoes, walking shoes.

Pedinol Pharmacal, Inc. 800-733-4665
30 Banfi Plz N, Farmingdale, NY 11735
PNS UNNA Boot (non-sterile).

Primo, Inc. 770-486-7394
417 Dividend Dr Ste B, Peachtree City, GA 30269
Cast shoe.

Scott Specialties, Inc. 785-527-5627
1827 Meadowlark Rd, Clay Center, KS 67432
Various types of cast shoes/boots.

Scott Specialties, Inc. 785-527-5627
1820 E 7th St, Concordia, KS 66901

Scott Specialties, Inc./Cmo Inc./Ginny Inc. 800-255-7136
512 M St, Belleville, KS 66935

Seattle Systems 360-697-5656
26296 12 Trees Ln NW Bldg 1, Poulsbo, WA 98370

Sroufe Healthcare Products Llc 888-894-4171
PO Box 347, 601 Sroufe St., Ligonier, IN 46767
Vinyl, canvas and other laminates.

Stryker Corp. 800-726-2725
2825 Airview Blvd, Portage, MI 49002

Tartan Orthopedics, Ltd. 888-287-1456
10651 Irma Dr Unit C, Northglenn, CO 80233
$100.00 per 10 (med).

Taylorcraft, Inc. 877-376-4756
313 Harbor Watch Dr., Chesapeake, VA 23320
Prosthetic retro-fit cast.

Tetra Medical Supply Corp. 800-621-4041
6364 W Gross Point Rd, Niles, IL 60714

Top Shelf Manufacturing, Llc 209-834-3185
1851 Paradise Rd Ste B, Tracy, CA 95304
Cast shoe.

Total Care 800-334-3802
PO Box 1661, Rockville, MD 20849
2 shoe models available - cast and post-op.

Warsaw Orthopedic, Inc. 901-396-3133
2500 Silveus Xing, Warsaw, IN 46582
Cast boot.

Zimmer Holdings, Inc. 800-613-6131
1800 W Center St, PO Box 708, Warsaw, IN 46580

Zimmer Orthopaedic Surgical Products 800-321-5533
PO Box 10, 200 West Ohio Ave., Dover, OH 44622

SHOE, OPERATING ROOM *(Surgery) 79FXW*

General Econopak, Inc. 888-871-8568
1725 N 6th St, Philadelphia, PA 19122
GEPCO disposable OR safety boots--waterproof, slip-resistant. OR slippers--non-skid, fluid-proof, universal size.

Hammill International 800-228-2129
PO Box 4968, Orange, CA 92863
MEDIPLOGS and PLOGS operating shoes. PLOGS 100% polyurethane honeycombed with air. MEDIPLOGS 100% polyurethane, washable, ventilated clog style shoes.

SHOE, OPERATING ROOM *(cont'd)*

Ortholine 800-243-3351
13 Chapel St, Norwalk, CT 06850
Post-operative rigid sole & hard rubber sole with 15 styles & types.

Primo, Inc. 770-486-7394
417 Dividend Dr Ste B, Peachtree City, GA 30269
Post op shoe, post surgical shoe.

SHOE, ORTHOPEDIC *(Orthopedics) 87TEO*

Alimed, Inc. 800-225-2610
297 High St, Dedham, MA 02026

Bsn Medical, Inc 800-552-1157
5825 Carnegie Blvd, Charlotte, NC 28209
Variety of orthopedic cast shoes available.

Friddle's Orthopedic Appliances, Inc. 800-528-9339
12306 Belton Honea Path Hwy, Honea Path, SC 29654
Devices, Orthopedic.

Ortho Active Appliances Ltd. 800-663-1254
103-250 Schoolhouse St., Coquitlam, BC V3K 6V7 Canada
Orthopedic and sports supports; orthotic sheet material.

Ortholine 800-243-3351
13 Chapel St, Norwalk, CT 06850
Aetrex Worldwide Foot Health Products

Pedors Shoes 800-750-6729
1349 Old 41 Hwy NW Ste 130, Marietta, GA 30060

Professional's Choice Sports Medicine Products, Inc. 800-331-9421
2025 Gillespie Way Ste 106, El Cajon, CA 92020

Slawner Ltd., J. 514-731-3378
5713 Cote Des Neiges Rd., Montreal, QUE H3S 1Y7 Canada

Tetra Medical Supply Corp. 800-621-4041
6364 W Gross Point Rd, Niles, IL 60714
Black nylon exterior, Velcro closure, strong heel counter.

Tru-Mold Shoes, Inc. 800-843-6653
42 Breckenridge St, Buffalo, NY 14213
Custom molded prescription footwear for individuals with diabetes, arthritis, post-polio and foot deformities.

SHOWER, EMERGENCY *(Chemistry) 75TEP*

Arjo, Inc. 800-323-1245
50 Gary Ave Ste A, Roselle, IL 60172
Stretcher-type mobile shower, functions both as patient stretcher and shower unit.

Hemco Corp. 816-796-2900
111 S Powell Rd, Independence, MO 64056
Emergency shower booth with pull rod activated overhead drench shower head and rear wall-mounted eye/face wash (also with additional spray nozzle heads built-in).

Lab Safety Supply, Inc. 800-356-0783
401 S Wright Rd, Janesville, WI 53546

SHUNT, ARTERIOVENOUS *(Gastro/Urology) 78RTB*

Angiodynamics, Inc. 800-472-5221
1 Horizon Way, Manchester, GA 31816
Full range of shunts and vessel tips including S-300 Series, Allen-Brown, pediatric, and ST-Series with integral tips.

Covidien Lp 508-261-8000
15 Hampshire St, Mansfield, MA 02048

SHUNT, CAROTID *(Cardiovascular) 74WWF*

Covidien Lp 508-261-8000
15 Hampshire St, Mansfield, MA 02048
VASCU-FLO silicone balloon carotid shunt.

Lemaitre Vascular, Inc. 781-221-2266
63 2nd Ave, Burlington, MA 01803
Maintains cerebral blood flow while reducing the risk of vessel lesions or trauma through clamping.

SHUNT, CENTRAL NERVE, WITH COMPONENT
(Cns/Neurology) 84JXG

Bioplate, Inc. 310-815-2100
3643 Lenawee Ave, Los Angeles, CA 90016
Shunt connector.

Codman & Shurtleff, Inc 800-225-0460
325 Paramount Dr, Raynham, MA 02767

Integra Neurosciences Pr 800-654-2873
Road 402 North, Km 1.2, Anasco, PR 00610
Various styles and shapes of shunts and components.

SHUNT, CENTRAL NERVE, WITH COMPONENT *(cont'd)*

Medtronic Neurosurgery 800-468-9710
125 Cremona Dr, Goleta, CA 93117
Flow and siphon control shunt assembly & associated components.

Neuro Diagnostic Devices 888-SHUNT-OK
3701 Market St Fl 3, Philadelphia, PA 19104
Thermal convection shunt analysis system.

Qualitel Corporation 425-423-8388
4608 150th Ave NE, Redmond, WA 98052
Shunt.

SHUNT, HYDROCEPHALIC *(Cns/Neurology) 84RTC*

Codman & Shurtleff, Inc 800-225-0460
325 Paramount Dr, Raynham, MA 02767

SHUNT, INTRAOCULAR *(Ophthalmology) 86WQB*

Tamcenan Corp. 800-950-0113
1703 S Minnesota Ave, Sioux Falls, SD 57105
Glaucoma pump shunt.

SHUNT, PORTOSYSTEMIC, ENDOPROSTHESIS
(Cardiovascular) 74MIR

W.L. Gore & Associates,Inc 928-526-3030
1505 North Fourth St., Flagstaff, AZ 86004
Tips endoprosthesis.

SIEVE, HEMATOLOGY *(Hematology) 81VCW*

Gilson Company, Inc. 800-444-1508
PO Box 200, Lewis Center, OH 43035

SIEVE, TISSUE *(Pathology) 88IDX*

Gilson Company, Inc. 800-444-1508
PO Box 200, Lewis Center, OH 43035

SIGMOIDOSCOPE, FLEXIBLE *(Gastro/Urology) 78FAM*

Olympus America, Inc. 800-645-8160
3500 Corporate Pkwy, PO Box 610, Center Valley, PA 18034

Pentax Medical Company 800-431-5880
102 Chestnut Ridge Rd, Montvale, NJ 07645
$5,775.00 for flexible sigmoido-fiberscope with insertion tube diameter, 11.5mm and channel diameter, 3.5mm. $16,275.00 to $16,800.00 for video sigmoidoscopes with CCD chip technology and insertion tube diameter, 12.8mm and channel size, 3.8mm to 4.2mm.

Pentax Southern Region Service Center 201-571-2300
8934 Kirby Dr, Houston, TX 77054
Sigmoidoscope.

Pentax West Coast Service Center 800-431-5880
10410 Pioneer Blvd Ste 2, Santa Fe Springs, CA 90670
Pentax sigmoidoscope.

Vision-Sciences, Inc. 800-874-9975
40 Ramland Rd S Ste 1, Orangeburg, NY 10962
ENDOSHEATH SYSTEM, disposable protective cover for proprietary sigmoidoscopic system.

Welch Allyn, Inc. 800-535-6663
4341 State Street Rd, Skaneateles Falls, NY 13153

SIGMOIDOSCOPE, RIGID, ELECTRICAL *(Gastro/Urology) 78FAN*

Boehm Surgical Instrument Corp. 716-436-6584
966 Chili Ave, Rochester, NY 14611
Sigmoidoscope.

Md International, Inc. 305-669-9003
11300 NW 41st St, Doral, FL 33178

Welch Allyn, Inc. 800-535-6663
4341 State Street Rd, Skaneateles Falls, NY 13153

SIGMOIDOSCOPE, RIGID, NON-ELECTRICAL
(Gastro/Urology) 78KDM

Cameron-Miller, Inc. 800-621-0142
5410 W Roosevelt Rd, Road #241, Chicago, IL 60644

Karl Storz Endoscopy-America Inc. 800-421-0837
600 Corporate Pointe, Culver City, CA 90230

Mahe International Inc. 800-294-7946
468 Craighead St, Nashville, TN 37204

Md International, Inc. 305-669-9003
11300 NW 41st St, Doral, FL 33178

Richard Wolf Medical Instruments Corp. 800-323-9653
353 Corporate Woods Pkwy, Vernon Hills, IL 60061

Welch Allyn, Inc. 800-535-6663
4341 State Street Rd, Skaneateles Falls, NY 13153

SIGN, HOSPITAL *(General) 80TEQ*

Arthur Blank & Co., Inc. 800-776-7333
225 Rivermoor St, Boston, MA 02132
Printed plastic signs.

Asi-Modulex 800-274-7732
3860 W Northwest Hwy Ste 350, Dallas, TX 75220
Architectural sign systems that direct the flow of visitors through a facility.

Atd-American Co. 800-523-2300
135 Greenwood Ave, Wyncote, PA 19095

Biodex Medical Systems, Inc. 800-224-6339
20 Ramsey Rd, Shirley, NY 11967

Brevis Corp. 800-383-3377
225 W 2855 S, Salt Lake City, UT 84115
Infection control hospital signs.

Champion America 800-521-7000
PO Box 3092, Branford, CT 06405
Full line of identification products: symbol-of-access signs ($8.95 to $58.75 ea), braille signs, OSHA signs, & badges, tags, & plaques.

Crest Healthcare Supply 800-328-8908
195 3rd St, Dassel, MN 55325
Signage, hospital/nursing home.

Identita Designers, Inc. 813-871-5511
4115 W Cypress St, Tampa, FL 33607
Designing of hospital sign systems; exterior and interior signs, patient room identification. Also, ADA code compliance signs, safety signage, OSHA signage and functional planning and signage design.

Idesco Corp. 800-336-1383
37 W 26th St, New York, NY 10010
Premade arch signs and make-your-own sign systems.

Intersign Corp. 800-322-8426
2156 Amnicola Hwy, Chattanooga, TN 37406
All kinds of signs.

Kroy, Llc 888-888-5769
3830 Kelley Ave, Cleveland, OH 44114

Lab Safety Supply, Inc. 800-356-0783
401 S Wright Rd, Janesville, WI 53546

Recognition Express 800-573-6444
502 Sunnyside Ave, Wheaton, IL 60187
Personalized name badges, permanently engraved.

Rockford Medical & Safety Co. 800-435-9451
2420 Harrison Ave, PO Box 5646, Rockford, IL 61108

SILASTIC ELASTOMER (ANGULAR DEFORMITY PREVENTION) *(Surgery) 79MBR*

Technical Products, Inc. 800-226-8434
805 Marathon Pkwy Ste 150, Lawrenceville, GA 30046
Available in nonreinforced and reinforced with polyester mesh, in sterile and nonsterile packaging. Various thicknesses and sheet sizes.

SILICONE SHEETING *(General) 80RTE*

Ace Hose & Rubber Company 888-223-4673
1333 S Jefferson St, Chicago, IL 60607

Allied Biomedical 800-276-1322
PO Box 392, Ventura, CA 93002
Long- and short-term implantable silicone sheeting: reinforced and nonreinforced, sterile.

Chamberlin Rubber Company, Inc. 585-427-7780
3333 Brighton Henrietta Town Line Rd, PO Box 22700
Rochester, NY 14623

Donell 800-324-7455
1801 Taylor Ave, Louisville, KY 40213
DURASIL-K silicone occlusive sheeting, treats hypertrophic scars and keloids. One sheet will last 12 months or more. Very cost effective, 6mm thick, soft and pliable. 88% success rate per studies. DURASIL-K durable silicone occlusive sheeting for treatment of hypertrophic scars and keloids. Thin, soft and pliable sheet will last 12 to 15 months. The most cost effective.

Specialty Manufacturing, Inc. 800-269-6204
2210 Midland Rd, Saginaw, MI 48603

SILICONE, LIQUID, INJECTABLE *(Surgery) 79KGM*

Therapeutic Silicone Technologies, Inc. 212-606-0830
909 5th Ave, New York, NY 10021
Sterile silicone oil for use as a prolonged retinal tamponade.

SILVER NITRATE *(Pathology) 88HZX*

Poly Scientific R&D Corp. 800-645-5825
70 Cleveland Ave, Bay Shore, NY 11706

Polysciences, Inc. 800-523-2575
400 Valley Rd, Warrington, PA 18976

Rocky Mountain Reagents,Inc. 303-762-0800
3207 W Hampden Ave, Englewood, CO 80110

SILVER RECOVERY EQUIPMENT *(Radiology) 90TER*

Hallmark Refining Corp. Inc. 360-428-5880
1016 Dale Ln, Mount Vernon, WA 98274

X-Rite, Inc. 888-826-3044
4300 44th St SE, Grand Rapids, MI 49512
$490.00 to $535.00 for manual systems - 2 models; $670.00 to $2,155.00 for automatic systems.

Xma (X-Ray Marketing Associates, Inc.) 800-325-8880
1205 W Lakeview Ct, Windham Lakes Business Park
Romeoville, IL 60446

SIMULATOR, ARRHYTHMIA *(Cardiovascular) 74RTF*

Fluke Biomedical 800-648-7952
6920 Seaway Blvd, Everett, WA 98203
Multiparameter simulator measuring arrhythmia, dual blood pressure, temperature & respiration, programmable via RS 232 line, line & battery powered. Also avail. with 1 more BP channel with automatic Swan-Ganz procedure.

Medical Plastics Laboratory, Inc. 800-433-5539
226 FM 116, Industrial Air Park, PO Box 38, Gatesville, TX 76528
Arrhythmia Scenario Trainer: Electronic trainer designed for independent use or to be integrated with MPL manikins, featuring the ability to interchange menus for training in arrhythmia interpretation. Features: Nine scenarios of up to nine steps each may be programmed into the trainer's memory; Arrhythmia interpretation with most 3-lead monitors is possible; Interchangeable menu features a total of 16 adult rhythms including Sinus Rhythm, Tachydysrhythmias, Bradydysrhythmias, Absent Collapse and Disorganized Rhythms. Additional menus available (adult & pediatric). Kit includes: Trainer, Menu, 9-Volt Battery, and Accessory Case.

Netech, Corp. 800-547-3557
110 Toledo St, Farmingdale, NY 11735
Several hand held patient simulators are offered. The MicroSim 400ARH simulates a 5 lead ECG with 10 arrhythmias while the MicroSim 400 simulates a 5 lead ECG with one invasive blood pressure and performance waveforms. The MiniSim 1000 is a comprehensive multiparameter simulator with full 12 lead ECG simulation, 45 arrhythmias, performance waveforms, 2 invasive blood preesures, respiration, and temperature. The model 1100 is a standalone Cardiac Output Simulator that simulates 32 curves and square waves. In addition there are specific Holter and EEG simulators. All simulators are powered by a single 9 Volt alkaline battery.

Pinnacle Technology Group, Inc. 800-345-5123
7076 Schnipke Dr, Ottawa Lake, MI 49267
TUTORS 15 models for arrhythmias, hemodynamics, and heart sounds, murmurs and breathing sounds. Recognition training. We carry the basic to the more advanced units.

SIMULATOR, BLOOD PRESSURE *(Cardiovascular) 74RTG*

Clinical Dynamics Corp. 800-247-6427
10 Capital Dr, Wallingford, CT 06492
SMARTARM NIBP simulator analyzer tests oscillometric and auscultatory monitors. Compact, lightweight unit includes digital manometer, hi-res graphic display, serial port, battery.

Fluke Biomedical 800-648-7952
6920 Seaway Blvd, Everett, WA 98203
Multiparameter simulator measuring arrhythmia, dual blood pressure, temperature & respiration, programmable via RS 232 line, line & battery powered. Also avail. with 1 more BP channel with automatic Swan-Ganz procedure.

Medical Plastics Laboratory, Inc. 800-433-5539
226 FM 116, Industrial Air Park, PO Box 38, Gatesville, TX 76528
Blood Pressure Training Arm: Lifelike, adult male arm with electronic trainer designed for training the procedure of NIBP measurement. Features: Palpable antecubital pulse; Blood Pressure Trainer with LCD guided operation; Systolic, diastolic, heart rate and auscultatory gap are programmable; Representation of both systolic and diastolic pressures; Indication of gauge reading as pressure is increased or decreased; Volume adjustable. Includes arm, blood pressure trainer, cuff, 9-volt battery and carry case.

SIMULATOR, BLOOD PRESSURE *(cont'd)*

Nasco 800-558-9595
901 Janesville Ave, PO Box 901, Fort Atkinson, WI 53538
$779.00 A blood-pressure training simulator.

Pocket Nurse Enterprises, Inc. 800-225-1600
200 1st St, Ambridge, PA 15003
variety of BP simulators

SIMULATOR, ECG *(Cardiovascular) 74RTH*

Armstrong Medical Industries, Inc. 800-323-4220
575 Knightsbridge Pkwy, Lincolnshire, IL 60069
Available in three models. TV interface and patient simulator available. Optional 12-lead ECG.

Fluke Biomedical 800-648-7952
6920 Seaway Blvd, Everett, WA 98203
Multiparameter simulator measuring arrhythmia, dual blood pressure, temperature & respiration, programmable via RS 232 line, line & battery powered. Also avail. with 1 more BP channel with automatic Swan-Ganz procedure and as pocket size unit with 12 lead/12 waveform output.

Nasco 800-558-9595
901 Janesville Ave, PO Box 901, Fort Atkinson, WI 53538
Interactive ECG simulator; arrythmia simulator with convent and pacing features.

Phipps & Bird, Inc. 800-955-7621
1519 Summit Ave, Richmond, VA 23230
Model 450A with 20-200 variable and 60 selectable rates. 9V battery with 20 hour operation time. Weighs 0.5 lb.

Respironics Georgia, Inc. 724-387-4559
175 Chastain Meadows Ct NW, Kennesaw, GA 30144

U.F.I. 805-772-1203
545 Main St Ste C2, Morro Bay, CA 93442
$170.00 for Model 1504.

SIMULATOR, EEG TEST SIGNAL *(Cns/Neurology) 84GWR*

U.F.I. 805-772-1203
545 Main St Ste C2, Morro Bay, CA 93442
$170 for Model 1504

SIMULATOR, HEART SOUND *(Cardiovascular) 74RTI*

Medical Plastics Laboratory, Inc. 800-433-5539
226 FM 116, Industrial Air Park, PO Box 38, Gatesville, TX 76528
Multi-Sounds Trainer Kits: Electronic trainer, designed for independent use or to be integrated with MPL manikins, featuring the ability to interchange sound menus for training in recognition of normal and abnormal heart, lung and bowel sounds. Sound volume is adjustable. External speaker features individual sound volume control. Recall button allows for alternation between two sounds. Total of nine menus available featuring adult, pediatric and infant sounds. Kit includes: Trainer, Menu, External Speaker, 9-Volt Batteries (2), and accessory case.

Nasco 800-558-9595
901 Janesville Ave, PO Box 901, Fort Atkinson, WI 53538
$2,370.00 LIFE/FORM Auscultation Trainer and SmartScope allows you to select by wirelss remore control a menu of heart and lung conditions.

Pocket Nurse Enterprises, Inc. 800-225-1600
200 1st St, Ambridge, PA 15003
variety of heart sound simulators

SIMULATOR, LUNG *(Anesthesiology) 73RTJ*

Dixie Ems Supply 800-347-3494
385 Union Ave, Brooklyn, NY 11211
$2,947.00 per unit (standard).

Ingmar Medical, Ltd. 800-583-9910
PO Box 10106, Pittsburgh, PA 15232
IngMar Medical offers several lung models, breathing simulators and test lungs for use in training, testing and R&D.

Michigan Instruments, Inc. 800-530-9939
4717 Talon Ct SE, Grand Rapids, MI 49512
TTL test lungs and PneuView ventilator testing and training systems are designed to simulate human pulmonary mechanics. Ideal for evaluating, testing, or demonstrating mechanical ventilation devices.

Pocket Nurse Enterprises, Inc. 800-225-1600
200 1st St, Ambridge, PA 15003

Radiology Support Devices 800-221-0527
1904 E Dominguez St, Long Beach, CA 90810

SIMULATOR, RADIOTHERAPY *(Radiology) 90RTL*

Atlas Medical Technologies 909-923-7887
1137 E Philadelphia St, Ontario, CA 91761

Huestis Medical 800-972-9222
68 Buttonwood St, Bristol, RI 02809
HUESTIS CASCADE radiotherapy simulator with fluoroscopic capabilities. Used to simulate radiation therapy treatment plan.

IZI Medical Products 800-231-1499
7020 Tudsbury Rd, Baltimore, MD 21244
IZ Port Skin Markers

Toshiba America Medical Systems 800-421-1968
2441 Michelle Dr, Tustin, CA 92780

Varian Medical Systems 800-544-4636
3100 Hansen Way, Palo Alto, CA 94304
Acuity X-ray system for treatment planning, simulation, and treatment plan verification, with exact simulation of Varian linear accelerators. This imager is also part of Varian's suite for image-guided brachytherapy.

SIMULATOR, RADIOTHERAPY, SPECIAL PURPOSE *(Radiology) 90KPQ*

Atlas Medical Technologies 909-923-7887
1137 E Philadelphia St, Ontario, CA 91761
Atlas is a leading CT simulator supplier. Connectivity is our specialty.

Best Nomos Corp. 800-70-NOMOS
1 Best Dr, Pittsburgh, PA 15202
PEACOCK system for dynamic conformal radiation therapy. CORVUS treatment planning system.

Computerized Medical Systems, Inc. 468-587-2550
1145 Corporate Lake Dr, Olivette, MO 63132
Contouring workstation.

Elekta, Inc. 800-535-7355
4775 Peachtree Industrial Blvd, Building 300, Suite 300
Norcross, GA 30092
Radiation therapy simulation systems. PRECISE SIM, treatment simulator.

I.Z.I. Medical Products, Inc. 800-231-1499
7020 Tudsbury Rd, Baltimore, MD 21244
Radiographic markers.

Medicalibration Physics Consultant Services, Inc. 209-524-6789
558 Van Dyken Way, Ripon, CA 95366
System, simulation, radiation therapy (various types).

Multidata Systems International Corp. 314-968-6880
9801 Manchester Rd, Saint Louis, MO 63119
Dss or rtp.

Prowess, Inc. 925-356-0360
1370 Ridgewood Dr Ste 20, Chico, CA 95973
Radiation therapy treatment planning system.

Rahd Ocology Products / Electronic Services Mart, Inc. 314-524-0103
500 Airport Rd, Saint Louis, MO 63135
Radiation therapy treatment plan simulation system.

Sim Net, Inc. 804-752-2776
10471 Cobbs Rd, Glen Allen, VA 23059
Radiation simulation device.

SIMULATOR, RESPIRATION *(Anesthesiology) 73RTK*

D.M. Davis Inc. 201-833-0513
460 Warwick Ave, Teaneck, NJ 07666
Stick-on adhesive piezo respiration sensors.

Fluke Biomedical 800-648-7952
6920 Seaway Blvd, Everett, WA 98203
Multiparameter simulator measuring arrhythmia, dual blood pressure, temperature & respiration, programmable via RS 232 line, line & battery powered. Also avail. with 1 more BP channel with automatic Swan-Ganz procedure.

Respironics Georgia, Inc. 724-387-4559
175 Chastain Meadows Ct NW, Kennesaw, GA 30144

SIMULTAN (INCLUDING CROSSED CYLINDER) *(Ophthalmology) 86HOR*

Eye Care And Cure 800-486-6169
4646 S Overland Dr, Tucson, AZ 85714
Cross cylinder.

SINGLE CHAMBER, SENSOR DRIVEN, IMPLANTABLE PULSE GENERATOR *(Cardiovascular) 74LWO*

Boston Scientific Corp. 612-582-7448
6645 185th Ave NE, Redmond, WA 98052
Pulse generator, DR, SR.

SINK, HOSPITAL *(General) 80TES*

Advance Tabco 800-645-3166
200 Heartland Blvd, Edgewood, NY 11717
Multi wash handsink.

American Specialties, Inc. 914-476-9000
441 Saw Mill River Rd, Yonkers, NY 10701

Blickman 800-247-5070
39 Robinson Rd, Lodi, NJ 07644
Stainless steel scrub sinks include Windsor model with 8' bowl and 22' scrub area. Infrared or knee-activated water. The 8000 Series sinks include wall or floor mounted units with infrared or knee-activated water. Optional knee-activated soap dispenser, scrub timer with display, storage shelf and in-wall chair carrier.

Colonial Scientific Ltd. 902-468-1811
201 Brownlow Ave., Unit 52, Dartmouth, NS B3B-1W2 Canada
Scrub sinks.

Concepts International, Inc. 800-627-9729
224 E Main St, Summerton, SC 29148
HYDROFLOW automatic faucets--hands-free, infrared activated; promotes infection control, water conservation.

Continental Metal Products Co., Inc. 800-221-4439
35 Olympia Ave, Woburn, MA 01801
Scrub sink, stainless steel.

Getinge Usa, Inc. 800-475-9040
1777 E Henrietta Rd, Rochester, NY 14623
GETINGE, scrub sinks.

Health Science Products, Inc. 800-237-5794
1489 Hueytown Rd, Hueytown, AL 35023
Sink cabinet with a mechanical hands-free knee-operated sanitary on/off water control system and faucet.

Highland Labs, Inc. 508-429-2918
42 Pope Rd # B, Holliston, MA 01746
Thigh operated water control valves and fluid dispensers.

Independent Solutions, Inc. 847-498-0500
900 Skokie Blvd Ste 118, Northbrook, IL 60062
AMERIMED plam or stainless steel or epoxy resin. Also ISI renal dialysis sink: stainless steel; flush wall mounted or headwall mounted; one-piece, funnel bottom.

Mayo Medical, S.A. De C.V. 800-715-3872
Edison 1141 Nte., Col. Talleres, Monterrey N.L. 64480 Mexico

Meritech, Inc. 800-932-7707
600 Corporate Cir Ste H, Golden, CO 80401
CLEANTECH 2000S, 4000S, and 400 automatic handwashing machines spray water and antibacterial solution on hands, cleaning them in 10 seconds. Units are activated by photo sensor to prevent contamination.

Sdi Medical Consultants 619-267-1391
4190 Bonita Rd Ste 211, Bonita, CA 91902
Scanner, ultrasonic, general purpose. 3D/4D Color Doppler.

Skytron 800-759-8766
5085 Corporate Exchange Blvd SE, Grand Rapids, MI 49512
Stainless scrub sinks with automatically dispensed pre-set water temperatures. Hands-free operation eliminates contact with both sink and the controls.

Unilab, Inc. 9058559093
2355 Royal Windsor Dr., Unit 3, Mississauga, ON L5M-5R5 Canada
Stainless steel sinks, faucets and gas taurets.

Whitehall Manufacturing 800-782-7706
15125 Proctor Ave, City Of Industry, CA 91746
Washware hospital sink to service up to eight people with easy access for wheelchair users.

SINK, LABORATORY *(Chemistry) 75TET*

Electra-Tec Inc. 800-225-3532
PO Box 17, Otsego, MI 49078

Kewaunee Scientific Corp. 704-873-7202
2700 W Front St, PO Box 1842, Statesville, NC 28677
Steel and resin.

Lab Fabricators Company 888-431-5444
1802 E 47th St, Cleveland, OH 44103
Sinks are available in a variety of materials in undercounter mount and grip rim mount styles. Sink cabinets and tables are also available.

SINK, LABORATORY *(cont'd)*

Nalge Nunc International 800-625-4327
75 Panorama Creek Dr, Rochester, NY 14625
NALGENE corrosion-resistant plastic sinks in several sizes and configurations.

Nutech Molding Corporation 1-800-423-5278
PO Box 840, 2024 Broad St,, Pocomoke City, MD 21851

Scientek Medical Equipment 604-273-9094
11151 Bridgeport Rd., Richmond, BC V6X 1T3 Canada
Dissection sinks, stainless steel, hydro aspirators (suction/flushing), hot & cold mixing valves, vacuum breakers, c/w overflows. Optional lever or knee operated drains.

Suburban Surgical Co., Inc. 800-323-7366
275 12th St, Wheeling, IL 60090
Stainless steel.

Terriss-Consolidated Industries 800-342-1611
807 Summerfield Ave, Asbury Park, NJ 07712
Stainless steel.

SIRIUS RED *(Pathology) 88HZY*

Poly Scientific R&D Corp. 800-645-5825
70 Cleveland Ave, Bay Shore, NY 11706

SIZER, DEVICE, ANASTOMOSIS *(Surgery) 79SIX*

Covidien Lp 508-261-8000
15 Hampshire St, Mansfield, MA 02048

SIZER, HEART VALVE PROSTHESIS *(Cardiovascular) 74DTI*

Ats Medical, Inc. 949-380-9333
20412 James Bay Cir, Lake Forest, CA 92630

ATS Medical, Inc. 800-399-1381
3905 Annapolis Ln N Ste 105, Minneapolis, MN 55447
3f Handle; 3f Sizers; Accessory Tray; Open Pivot Handles; Open Pivot Heart Valve Sizer; Simulus Handle; Simulus Sizers

Intuitive Surgical, Inc. 888-409-4774
1266 Kifer Rd, Sunnyvale, CA 94086
Prosthetic heart valve sizer.

Medtronic Cardiovascular Surgery, The Heart Valve Div. 800-328-2518
1851 E Deere Ave, Santa Ana, CA 92705
Sizer or obturator.

Medtronic Heart Valves 800-227-3191
8299 Central Ave NE, Spring Lake Park, MN 55432
Sizer or obturator.

SIZER, MAMMARY, BREAST IMPLANT VOLUME *(Surgery) 79MRD*

Specialty Surgical Products, Inc. 406-961-0102
1131 US Highway 93 N, Victor, MT 59875
Various.

SKID, BONE *(Orthopedics) 87HWO*

Biomet, Inc. 574-267-6639
56 E Bell Dr, PO Box 587, Warsaw, IN 46582
Various types of bone skids.

George Tiemann & Co. 800-843-6266
25 Plant Ave, Hauppauge, NY 11788

Integral Design Inc. 781-740-2036
52 Burr Rd, Hingham, MA 02043

Kirwan Surgical Products, Inc. 888-547-9267
180 Enterprise Dr, PO Box 427, Marshfield, MA 02050

Tuzik Boston 800-886-6363
104 Longwater Dr, Assinippi Park, Norwell, MA 02061

Warsaw Orthopedic, Inc. 901-396-3133
2500 Silveus Xing, Warsaw, IN 46582
Bone skid.

Zimmer Holdings, Inc. 800-613-6131
1800 W Center St, PO Box 708, Warsaw, IN 46580

SLEEP ASSESSMENT EQUIPMENT *(Cns/Neurology) 84LEL*

Bio-Logic Systems Corp. 800-323-8326
1 Bio Logic Plz, Mundelein, IL 60060
SLEEPSCAN, collects and analyzes data from the analog outputs of conventional polysomnograph. SLEEPSCAN TRAVELER, is a portable collector for home studies. Data is read on a SLEEPSCAN reader station.

SLEEP ASSESSMENT EQUIPMENT *(cont'd)*

Cadwell Laboratories 800-245-3001
909 N Kellogg St, Kennewick, WA 99336
CADWELL EASY II EEG and PSG for scoring sleep stages and marking events. Allows stages to be scored and events to be marked in a single pass. Provides dedicated on screen buttons for sleep stages and events. For sleep reports, the program produces printouts of staging activity and separate histograms that can be selected for each event. Auto-detect of heart rate, desaturation, respiratory & movement events. Q-video, Scorer to Scorer, Satellite view.

Cardinal Health 207, Inc. 800-231-2466
22745 Savi Ranch Pkwy, Yorba Linda, CA 92887
Automated polysomnograph and sleep diagnostic instrumentation.

Cardinal Healthcare 209, Inc. 610-862-0800
5225 Verona Rd, Fitchburg, WI 53711
Sleep assessment device for recording and scoring sleep and respiration data.

Koven Technology, Inc. 800-521-8342
12125 Woodcrest Executive Dr Ste 320, Saint Louis, MO 63141
B-SMART Patient response device for carotid endarterectomy under regional anesthesia.

Mini-Mitter Company, Inc. 800-685-2999
20300 Empire Ave Ste B3, Bend, OR 97701
ACTIWATCH and ACTIWATCH-L are wrist or ankle worn activity monitors for analyzing circadian rhythms and sleep parameters; assessing activity in any instance where quantifiable analysis of physical motion is desired. ACTIWATCH-SCORE combines the capabilities of ACTIWATCH with a built-in score pad that allows patients to subjectively assign and enter a score. The score pad can be used as a substitute or in addition to a patient diary.

Nihon Kohden America, Inc. 800-325-0283
90 Icon, Foothill Ranch, CA 92610
POLYSMITH Sleep Analysis Program for use in the diagnosis and study of sleep disorders. It provides comprehensive reporting for OSAS, UARS, GER, narcolepsy and Restless Leg Syndrome.

Respironics Georgia, Inc. 724-387-4559
175 Chastain Meadows Ct NW, Kennesaw, GA 30144
Systems for diagnostic evaluation. Also available, Tranquility Bilevel.

Sleepmed Incorporated 800-334-5085
200 Corporate Pl Ste 5-B, Peabody, MA 01960
The DigiTrace Home Sleep System is an 18 channel completely portable polysomnogram recorder. Continuous digital recording of all standard PSG channels including EEG, EOG, EMG, respiratory, airflow, SAO2, body position, snoring sensor.

Telediagnostic Systems 800-227-3224
2483 Old Middlefield Way Ste 202, Mountain View, CA 94043
Nightron: 32-channel Polysomnography System.

SLEEVE, COMPRESSIBLE LIMB *(Cardiovascular) 74JOW*

Aci Medical, Inc. 800-667-9451
1857 Diamond St, San Marcos, CA 92078
VenaPulse; ArtAssist; VenAssist

Alimed, Inc. 800-225-2610
297 High St, Dedham, MA 02026

Ascent Healthcare Solutions 480-763-5300
10232 S 51st St, Phoenix, AZ 85044
Compression sleeves.

Bio Compression Systems, Inc. 800-888-0908
120 W Commercial Ave, Moonachie, NJ 07074
Sequential Circulator

Chattanooga Group 800-592-7329
4717 Adams Rd, Hixson, TN 37343
PRESSION Compression Therapy.

Circulator Boot Corp. 610-240-9980
72 Pennsylvania Ave, Malvern, PA 19355

Compression Therapy Concepts, Inc. 800-993-9013
1750 Brielle Ave Ste B6, Ocean, NJ 07712
Deep vein thrombosis (DVT) system.

Healthcare Service And Supply 714-669-8803
10602 Mira Vista Dr, Santa Ana, CA 92705
Sleeve or garment for limb compression.

Huntleigh Healthcare Llc. 800-223-1218
40 Christopher Way, Eatontown, NJ 07724
$27.00 for SP101 single patient use, half-leg, $97.00 for L101 half-leg boot, $160.00 for L102 full-leg boot, $100.00 for S120 full-arm, $86.00 for S220 half-arm.

SLEEVE, COMPRESSIBLE LIMB *(cont'd)*

Kinetic Concepts, Inc. 800-275-4524
8023 Vantage Dr, San Antonio, TX 78230
Intermittent,external pneumatic comppression device.

Lohmann & Rauscher, Inc. 800-279-3863
6001 SW 6th Ave Ste 101, Topeka, KS 66615
epX Products

Medi Usa 800-633-6334
6481 Franz Warner Pkwy, Whitsett, NC 27377
Lymphedema sleeves.

Medisiss 866-866-7477
2747 SW 6th St, Redmond, OR 97756
Various compression limb sleeves, sterile.

Medmark Technologies, Llc 215-249-1540
724 H West Rt 313 Dublin Park, Perkasie, PA 18944
Compresion therapy pump, compresion pump.

ReNu Medical Inc. 877-252-1110
9800 Evergreen Way, Everett, WA 98204
ALP

Sterilmed, Inc. 763-488-3400
11400 73rd Ave N Ste 100, Maple Grove, MN 55369
Sleeve, limb, compressible.

Syntech International 949-752-9642
17171 Daimler St, Irvine, CA 92614
Leg pressure system.

University Of Utah Hospitals And Clinics 801-581-2742
50 N Medical Dr, Salt Lake City, UT 84132
Reprocessed compression sleeve device.

Wright Linear Pump, Inc. 800-631-9535
103B International Dr, Oakdale, PA 15071
pneumatic compression technology

SLEEVE, TROCAR *(Surgery) 79SHV*

Elmed, Inc. 630-543-2792
60 W Fay Ave, Addison, IL 60101

Ethicon Endo-Surgery, Inc. 800-USE-ENDO
4545 Creek Rd, Cincinnati, OH 45242
ENDOPATH, 5mm, 12mm, 10/11mm long; sleeve for ENDOPATH TS112.

Innervision Inc. 901-682-0417
6258 E Shady Grove Rd, Memphis, TN 38120

Karl Storz Endoscopy-America Inc. 800-421-0837
600 Corporate Pointe, Culver City, CA 90230

Laser, Inc. 800-367-5694
27831 Commercial Park Ln, Tomball, TX 77375
Reusable & self-sealing sleeves.

Mediflex Surgical Products 800-879-7575
250 Gibbs Rd, Islandia, NY 11749

Miltex Inc. 800-645-8000
589 Davies Dr, York, PA 17402

Putnam Precision Products 845-278-2141
3859 Danbury Rd, Brewster, NY 10509

SLIDE AND COVERSLIP *(Hematology) 81GJO*

Edmund Industrial Optics 800-363-1992
101 E Gloucester Pike, Barrington, NJ 08007

Image Molding, Inc. 800-525-1875
4525 Kingston St, Denver, CO 80239
Four test standardized acrylic slide with glass coverslip.

Jayza Corp. 305-477-1136
7215 NW 41st St Ste A, Miami, FL 33166

Sakura Finetek U.S.A., Inc. 800-725-8723
1750 W 214th St, Torrance, CA 90501
TISSUE-TEK $30,315 for automated coverslipper system.

Serum International Inc. 800-361-7726
4400 Autoroute Chomeoey, Laval, QUE H7R-6E9 Canada

SLIDE, CONTROL, QUALITY *(Microbiology) 83LJG*

Diagnostic Hybrids, Inc. 740-589-3300
1055 E State St Ste 100, Athens, OH 45701
Various qc slides.

Fertility Solutions, Inc. 800-959-7656
13000 Shaker Blvd, Cleveland, OH 44120
Sperm morphology smears-sperm viability smears.

SLIDE, CONTROL, QUALITY *(cont'd)*

Microbiologics, Inc. 800-599-BUGS
217 Osseo Ave N, Saint Cloud, MN 56303
KWIK-QC™ SLIDES & MICROBIOLOGY QUALITY CONTROL SLIDES

Scientific Device Laboratory Inc. 847-803-9495
411 Jarvis Ave, Des Plaines, IL 60018
Quality control slides.

SLIDE, MICROSCOPE *(Pathology) 88KEW*

American Mastertech Scientific, Inc. 209-368-4031
1330 Thurman St, Lodi, CA 95240
Microscope slides and coverslips.

C & A Scientific Co. Inc. 703-330-1413
7241 Gabe Ct, Manassas, VA 20109
PREMIERE Plain, single frost, double frost, & concavity. Color end frosted microscope slides available in white & 4 other colors. Charged slides.

Cytyc Surgical Products 800-442-9892
250 Campus Dr, Marlborough, MA 01752
Tissue processing equipment.

Edmund Industrial Optics 800-363-1992
101 E Gloucester Pike, Barrington, NJ 08007

Erie Scientific 603-431-8410
20 Post Rd, Portsmouth Park, Newington, NH 03801
Various slides.

Garren Scientific, Inc. 800-342-3725
15916 Blythe St Unit A, Van Nuys, CA 91406

Grace Bio-Labs, Inc. 541-318-1208
PO Box 228, Bend, OR 97709
Various types of microscope slides & tissue processing equipment.

Hycor Biomedical, Inc. 800-382-2527
7272 Chapman Ave, Garden Grove, CA 92841
Microscope slide.

Image Molding, Inc. 800-525-1875
4525 Kingston St, Denver, CO 80239
10 test and 4 test standardized acrylic slides hold a standardized volume and depth. Overflow wells prevent contact with sample and each well is segregated to prevent cross-contamination.

Immuno Concepts N.A. Ltd. 800-251-5115
9779 Business Park Dr, Sacramento, CA 95827

Iris Sample Processing 800-782-8774
60 Glacier Dr, Westwood, MA 02090
Tube with integrated microscope slide and cap.

Kreisers Inc. 800-843-7948
2200 W 46th St, Sioux Falls, SD 57105
Various types & sizes, plus laboratory accessories.

Medical Packaging Corporation 800-792-0600
941 Avenida Acaso, Camarillo, CA 93012
Printed microscope slides (any design or color).

Polysciences, Inc. 800-523-2575
400 Valley Rd, Warrington, PA 18976
Tissue Tack aminoalkylsilane coated slides and Poly-L-Lysine coated slides

Propper Manufacturing Co., Inc. 800-832-4300
3604 Skillman Ave, Long Island City, NY 11101

Rayson Co. Inc., W.R. 800-526-1526
720 S Dickerson St, Burgaw, NC 28425
Plastic microslides.

Spectra Medical Devices, Inc. 866-938-8649
4C Henshaw St, Woburn, MA 01801

Statlab Medical Products, Inc. 800-442-3573
106 Hillside Dr, Lewisville, TX 75057
ANAPATH, various sizes.

Surgipath Medical Industries, Inc. 800-225-3035
PO Box 528, 5205 Route 12, Richmond, IL 60071

Tripath Imaging, Inc. 919-206-7140
780 Plantation Dr, Burlington, NC 27215
Microscope slides.

Ware Medics Glass Works, Inc. 845-429-6950
PO Box 368, Garnerville, NY 10923

SLING, ARM *(Physical Med) 89ILI*

Alex Orthopedic, Inc. 800-544-2539
PO Box 201442, Arlington, TX 76006

Alimed, Inc. 800-225-2610
297 High St, Dedham, MA 02026

SLING, ARM *(cont'd)*

American Orthopedic Supply Co., Inc.
37017 State Highway 79, Cleveland, AL 35049
Arm sling.

Arthron, Inc. 800-758-5633
PO Box 1627, 1605 Ash Grove Ct., Brentwood, TN 37024
Arm sling.

Barjan Mfg., Ltd. 631-420-5588
28 Baiting Place Rd, Farmingdale, NY 11735
No common name listed.

Best Orthopedic And Medical Services, Inc. 800-344-5279
2356B Springs Rd NE, Hickory, NC 28601

Biomet, Inc. 574-267-6639
56 E Bell Dr, PO Box 587, Warsaw, IN 46582
Various types of arm sling.

Bird & Cronin, Inc. 651-683-1111
1200 Trapp Rd, Saint Paul, MN 55121
Arm sling.

Breg, Inc., An Orthofix Company 800-897-BREG
2611 Commerce Way, Vista, CA 92081
Arm sling.

Core Products International, Inc. 800-365-3047
808 Prospect Ave, Osceola, WI 54020

Corflex, Inc. 800-426-7353
669 E Industrial Park Dr, Manchester, NH 03109

Dj Orthopedics De Mexico, S.A. De C.V. 690-727-1280
Blvd., Delagacion La Presa, Tijuana 22397 Mexico
Orthopedic softgoods

Dj Orthopedics De Mexico, S.A. De C.V. 690-727-1280
Ave. Venustiano Carranza 6802, Castillo, Tijuana 22100 Mexico
Orthopedic softgoods

DJO Inc. 800-336-6569
1430 Decision St, Vista, CA 92081

Douglas & Harper Mfg. Co., Inc. 912-367-4149
1126 S Main St, Baxley, GA 31513
Arm slings.

Dynatronics Corp. Chattanooga Operations 801-568-7000
6607 Mountain View Rd, Ooltewah, TN 37363
Arm sling.

Faretec, Inc. 440-350-9510
1610 W Jackson St Unit 6, Concord Twp, OH 44077
Arm sling.

Formedica Ltd. 800-361-9671
1481 Rue Begin, St Laurent, QUE H4R 1V8 Canada
$45.00 per 10 (med).

Frank Stubbs Co., Inc 800-223-1713
2100 Eastman Ave Ste B, Oxnard, CA 93030

Freeman Manufacturing Company 800-253-2091
900 W Chicago Rd, PO Box J, Sturgis, MI 49091

Galveston Manufacturing Co., Inc. 800-634-3309
7810 FM 646 Rd S, Santa Fe, TX 77510
Gaveston cuff and collar sling.

Hermell Products, Inc. 800-233-2342
9 Britton Dr, PO Box 7345, Bloomfield, CT 06002

J. T. Posey Co. 800-447-6739
5635 Peck Rd, Arcadia, CA 91006

Jobri Llc 800-432-2225
520 N Division St, Konawa, OK 74849
MOR-LOC, E-Z FIT.

K W Griffen Company 800-424-5556
100 Pearl St, Norwalk, CT 06850

K. W. Griffen Co. 203-846-1923
100 Pearl St, Norwalk, CT 06850
Sling.

Kenad Sg Medical, Inc. 800-825-0606
2692 Huntley Dr, Memphis, TN 38132
Arm sling.

Kentron Health Care, Inc. 615-384-0573
3604 Kelton Jackson Rd, P.o. Box 120, Springfield, TN 37172
Arm sling.

Larkotex Company 800-972-3037
1002 Olive St, Texarkana, TX 75501

Maddak Inc. 800-443-4926
661 State Route 23, Wayne, NJ 07470
ABLEWARE.

SLING, ARM *(cont'd)*

Marcote, Llc 907-345-1377
1120 Huffman Rd, Anchorage, AK 99515
Slingshots.

North Safety Products 401-943-4400
1101 B Calle Neutron, Parque Industrial Maran, Mexicali, B.c. Mexico
Triangular bandage

Ny Orthopedic Usa, Inc. 718-852-5330
63 Flushing Ave Unit 333, Brooklyn, NY 11205
Sling, arm.

Ortholine 800-243-3351
13 Chapel St, Norwalk, CT 06850
Thirteen styles, pediatric sizes.

Ossur Americas 949-268-3155
742 Pancho Rd, Camarillo, CA 93012

Paramedical Distributors 800-245-3278
2020 Grand Blvd, Kansas City, MO 64108

Patterson Medical Supply, Inc. 262-387-8720
W68N158 Evergreen Blvd, Cedarburg, WI 53012
Hemi arm sling with cuff adaptor.

Primo, Inc. 770-486-7394
417 Dividend Dr Ste B, Peachtree City, GA 30269
Arm sling.

Rehabilitation Technical Components, Corp. 919-732-1705
3913 Devonwood Rd, Hillsborough, NC 27278
Arm sling.

Respond Industries, Inc. 1-800-523-8999
9500 Woodend Rd, Edwardsville, KS 66111
Various types of triangular bandages.

Scott Specialties, Inc. 785-527-5627
1827 Meadowlark Rd, Clay Center, KS 67432
Various types of arm slings.

Scott Specialties, Inc. 785-527-5627
1820 E 7th St, Concordia, KS 66901

Scott Specialties, Inc./Cmo Inc./Ginny Inc. 800-255-7136
512 M St, Belleville, KS 66935
12 different types.

Sroufe Healthcare Products Llc 888-894-4171
PO Box 347, 601 Sroufe St., Ligonier, IN 46767

Sunshine Co. 410-435-1771
415 Homeland Ave, Baltimore, MD 21212
Perfect comfort arm sling.

Tartan Orthopedics, Ltd. 888-287-1456
10651 Irma Dr Unit C, Northglenn, CO 80233
$29.50 per 10 (med).

Tetra Medical Supply Corp. 800-621-4041
6364 W Gross Point Rd, Niles, IL 60714

Tillotson Healthcare Corp. 888-335-7500
10 Glenshaw St, Orangeburg, NY 10962
TRI GUARD, non-sterile; 100% cotton muslin; natural color triangular bandage.

Top Shelf Manufacturing, Llc 209-834-8185
1851 Paradise Rd Ste B, Tracy, CA 95304
Various types of arm slings & shoulder immobilizers.

Truform Orthotics & Prosthetics 800-888-0458
3960 Rosslyn Dr, Cincinnati, OH 45209

U.S. Orthotics, Inc. 800-825-5228
8605 Palm River Rd, Tampa, FL 33619
Velcro closures or hook & catch.

Warsaw Orthopedic, Inc. 901-396-3133
2500 Silveus Xing, Warsaw, IN 46582
Various types arm slings and arm/shoulder immobilizers.

Zimmer Holdings, Inc. 800-613-6131
1800 W Center St, PO Box 708, Warsaw, IN 46580

Zimmer Orthopaedic Surgical Products 800-321-5533
PO Box 10, 200 West Ohio Ave., Dover, OH 44622

SLING, ARM, OVERHEAD SUPPORTED *(Physical Med) 89ILE*

A&A Orthopedics, Incorporated 757-224-0177
12250 SW 129th Ct Bldg 1, Miami, FL 33186
Cradle sling, pouch sling, sling.

Biomet, Inc. 574-267-6639
56 E Bell Dr, PO Box 587, Warsaw, IN 46582
Arm elevator.

SLING, ARM, OVERHEAD SUPPORTED *(cont'd)*

Dj Orthopedics De Mexico, S.A. De C.V. 690-727-1280
Blvd., Delagacion La Presa, Tijuana 22397 Mexico
Arm elevator sting

Dj Orthopedics De Mexico, S.A. De C.V. 690-727-1280
Ave. Venustiano Carranza 6802, Castillo, Tijuana 22100 Mexico
Arm elevator sting

DJO Inc. 800-336-6569
1430 Decision St, Vista, CA 92081

Frank Stubbs Co., Inc 800-223-1713
2100 Eastman Ave Ste B, Oxnard, CA 93030

Guitar Suspension Solutions 207-324-5717
183A Jagger Mill Rd, Sanford, ME 04073
Sound-attitude (tm) arm sling.

Maramed Orthopedic Systems 800-327-5830
2480 W 82nd St, No. 8, Hialeah, FL 33016
Wrist and hand holder.

Mizuho Osi 800-777-4674
30031 Ahern Ave, Union City, CA 94587

Tartan Orthopedics, Ltd. 888-287-1456
10651 Irma Dr Unit C, Northglenn, CO 80233
$49.50 per 10 (med).

Zimmer Holdings, Inc. 800-613-6131
1800 W Center St, PO Box 708, Warsaw, IN 46580

SLING, KNEE *(Orthopedics) 87RTU*

Mizuho Osi 800-777-4674
30031 Ahern Ave, Union City, CA 94587

Tartan Orthopedics, Ltd. 888-287-1456
10651 Irma Dr Unit C, Northglenn, CO 80233
$67.50 per 10 (med).

Tetra Medical Supply Corp. 800-621-4041
6364 W Gross Point Rd, Niles, IL 60714

Zimmer Holdings, Inc. 800-613-6131
1800 W Center St, PO Box 708, Warsaw, IN 46580

Zimmer Orthopaedic Surgical Products 800-321-5533
PO Box 10, 200 West Ohio Ave., Dover, OH 44622

SLING, LEG *(Orthopedics) 87RTV*

Paramedical Distributors 800-245-3278
2020 Grand Blvd, Kansas City, MO 64108

Tetra Medical Supply Corp. 800-621-4041
6364 W Gross Point Rd, Niles, IL 60714

Zimmer Holdings, Inc. 800-613-6131
1800 W Center St, PO Box 708, Warsaw, IN 46580

Zimmer Orthopaedic Surgical Products 800-321-5533
PO Box 10, 200 West Ohio Ave., Dover, OH 44622

SLING, OVERHEAD SUSPENSION, WHEELCHAIR *(Physical Med) 89INE*

Air Movement Technologies, Inc. 800-317-9582
320 Gateway Park Dr, Syracuse, NY 13212
Patient transfer device.

Koros Usa, Inc. 805-529-0825
610 Flinn Ave, Moorpark, CA 93021
Shoulder suspension device.

Medical Depot 516-998-4600
99 Seaview Blvd, Port Washington, NY 11050
Sling.

SLIPPERS *(General) 80RTW*

Albahealth Llc 800-262-2404
425 N Gateway Ave, Rockwood, TN 37854
TERRY-TREADS: Safety slippers. CARE-STEPS: Safety slippers.

Alert Care, Inc. 800-826-7444
591 Redwood Hwy Ste 5200, Mill Valley, CA 94941
WALK ALERT slippers. WALK ALERT are a distinct bright blue which easily indicates to caregivers throughout the facility those patients who have been screened to be high risk for falling. On the outside surface, Walk Alerts have a strong tread which enhances walking stability and reduces foot slippage. One size fits most patients with foot size from 4-13.

Geen Healthcare Inc. 800-565-4336
931 Progress Ave. Ste.13, Scarborough, ONT M1G 3V5 Canada

Lsl Industries, Inc. 888-225-5575
5535 N Wolcott Ave, Chicago, IL 60640

SLIPPERS *(cont'd)*

O&M Enterprise 847-258-4515
641 Chelmsford Ln, Elk Grove Village, IL 60007
SLIPPER

Principle Business Enterprises, Inc. 800-467-3224
PO Box 129, Dunbridge, OH 43414
PILLOW PAWS disposable slippers, footwear. MEDTREADS & TRED MATES custom imprinted slipper socks.

Salk Inc. 800-343-4497
119 Braintree St Ste 701, 4th Floor, Boston, MA 02134
Terrycloth.

Sroufe Healthcare Products Llc 888-894-4171
PO Box 347, 601 Sroufe St., Ligonier, IN 46767
Vinyl-canvas post-op shoes.

Zimmer Holdings, Inc. 800-613-6131
1800 W Center St, PO Box 708, Warsaw, IN 46580

SNARE, EAR *(Ear/Nose/Throat) 77JZD*

Aesculap Implant Systems Inc. 1-800-234-9179
3773 Corporate Pkwy, Center Valley, PA 18034

Bausch & Lomb Surgical 636-255-5051
3365 Tree Court Ind Blvd, Saint Louis, MO 63122

Biomet Microfixation Inc. 800-874-7711
1520 Tradeport Dr, Jacksonville, FL 32218
Various types of snares.

Clinimed, Incorporated 877-CLINIMED
303 Markus Ct, Sandy Brae Industrial Park, Newark, DE 19713

SNARE, ENDOSCOPIC *(Surgery) 79ULT*

Cameron-Miller, Inc. 800-621-0142
5410 W Roosevelt Rd, Road #241, Chicago, IL 60644

Elmed, Inc. 630-543-2792
60 W Fay Ave, Addison, IL 60101

Karl Storz Endoscopy-America Inc. 800-421-0837
600 Corporate Pointe, Culver City, CA 90230

Mahe International Inc. 800-294-7946
468 Craighead St, Nashville, TN 37204

Pentax Medical Company 800-431-5880
102 Chestnut Ridge Rd, Montvale, NJ 07645
Oval snares with or without handle. Call for quote.

Richard Wolf Medical Instruments Corp. 800-323-9653
353 Corporate Woods Pkwy, Vernon Hills, IL 60061

United States Endoscopy Group 800-769-8226
5976 Heisley Rd, Mentor, OH 44060
ROTATOR Rotatable polypectomy snare, Disposable and disposable retro fit, fits bard, olympus, & microvasive active cords. Oval & min. oval snare configuration, 230cm, 2.5mm sheath.

SNARE, ENUCLEATING *(Ophthalmology) 86HNE*

Bausch & Lomb Surgical 636-255-5051
3365 Tree Court Ind Blvd, Saint Louis, MO 63122

SNARE, FLEXIBLE *(Gastro/Urology) 78FDI*

Accellent El Paso 915-771-9112
31 Butterfield Trail Blvd Ste C, El Paso, TX 79906
Endoscopic snares

Annex Medical, Inc. 952-942-7576
6018 Blue Circle Dr, Minnetonka, MN 55343
3.0 or smaller, oval retrieval snare.

Boston Scientific Corporation 800-225-2732
1 Boston Scientific Pl, Natick, MA 01760

Cameron-Miller, Inc. 800-621-0142
5410 W Roosevelt Rd, Road #241, Chicago, IL 60644

Cook Endoscopy 336-744-0157
4900 Bethania Station Rd # &, 5951 Grassy Creek Blvd. Winston Salem, NC 27105
Snare, flexible snare, polypectomy devices.

SNARE, FLEXIBLE, REPROCESSED *(Gastro/Urology) 78NLT*

Sterilmed, Inc. 763-488-3400
11400 73rd Ave N Ste 100, Maple Grove, MN 55369
Polypectomy snare.

SNARE, NASAL *(Ear/Nose/Throat) 77KBE*

Aesculap Implant Systems Inc. 1-800-234-9179
3773 Corporate Pkwy, Center Valley, PA 18034

Bausch & Lomb Surgical 636-255-5051
3365 Tree Court Ind Blvd, Saint Louis, MO 63122

SNARE, NASAL *(cont'd)*

Biomet Microfixation Inc. 800-874-7711
1520 Tradeport Dr, Jacksonville, FL 32218
Various types of snares.

Cameron-Miller, Inc. 800-621-0142
5410 W Roosevelt Rd, Road #241, Chicago, IL 60644

SNARE, NON-ELECTRICAL *(Gastro/Urology) 78FGX*

Cook Endoscopy 336-744-0157
4900 Bethania Station Rd # &, 5951 Grassy Creek Blvd. Winston Salem, NC 27105
Cold snare.

SNARE, OTHER *(Surgery) 79RTZ*

Cameron-Miller, Inc. 800-621-0142
5410 W Roosevelt Rd, Road #241, Chicago, IL 60644

United States Endoscopy Group 800-769-8226
5976 Heisley Rd, Mentor, OH 44060
Laparoscopic disposable 5mm snare retractor/grasper; snare net for use in flexible endoscope to capture foreign bodies or polyps, 230 cm. 2.5 mm sheath.

SNARE, POLYP *(Surgery) 79RTY*

American Catheter Corp. 800-345-6714
13047 S Highway 475, Ocala, FL 34480

Cameron-Miller, Inc. 800-621-0142
5410 W Roosevelt Rd, Road #241, Chicago, IL 60644

Elmed, Inc. 630-543-2792
60 W Fay Ave, Addison, IL 60101

Gyrus Medical, Inc. 800-852-9361
6655 Wedgwood Rd N Ste 105, Maple Grove, MN 55311
BISNARE Polypectomy Snare: electrical, bipolar snare for gastropolypectomy; disposable, regular and mini-oval sizes.

Karl Storz Endoscopy-America Inc. 800-421-0837
600 Corporate Pointe, Culver City, CA 90230

Mahe International Inc. 800-294-7946
468 Craighead St, Nashville, TN 37204

Medi-Globe Corporation 800-966-1431
110 W Orion St Ste 136, Tempe, AZ 85283
Rotatable.

Miltex Inc. 800-645-8000
589 Davies Dr, York, PA 17402

SNARE, RIGID SELF-OPENING *(Gastro/Urology) 78FDJ*

Aesculap Implant Systems Inc. 1-800-234-9179
3773 Corporate Pkwy, Center Valley, PA 18034

Cameron-Miller, Inc. 800-621-0142
5410 W Roosevelt Rd, Road #241, Chicago, IL 60644

Cathguide, Division Of Scilogy Corp. 305-269-0500
9135 Fontainebleau Blvd Apt 5, Miami, FL 33172

SNARE, SURGICAL *(Surgery) 79GAE*

Beatty Marketing & Sales, Llc 425-895-1656
17371 NE 67th Ct Ste A12, Redmond, WA 98052
Snare, surgical.

Cameron-Miller, Inc. 800-621-0142
5410 W Roosevelt Rd, Road #241, Chicago, IL 60644

Electro Surgical Instrument Co., Inc. 888-464-2784
37 Centennial St, Rochester, NY 14611
Cautery snare in various sizes and wire loop types and various attachments.

Elmed, Inc. 630-543-2792
60 W Fay Ave, Addison, IL 60101

Medisiss 866-866-7477
2747 SW 6th St, Redmond, OR 97756
Various surgical snares,sterile.

SNARE, TONSIL *(Ear/Nose/Throat) 77KBZ*

Aesculap Implant Systems Inc. 1-800-234-9179
3773 Corporate Pkwy, Center Valley, PA 18034

Bausch & Lomb Surgical 636-255-5051
3365 Tree Court Ind Blvd, Saint Louis, MO 63122

Biomet Microfixation Inc. 800-874-7711
1520 Tradeport Dr, Jacksonville, FL 32218
Various types of snares.

Cameron-Miller, Inc. 800-621-0142
5410 W Roosevelt Rd, Road #241, Chicago, IL 60644

Elmed, Inc. 630-543-2792
60 W Fay Ave, Addison, IL 60101

SNARE, TONSIL (cont'd)

Miltex Inc. 800-645-8000
589 Davies Dr, York, PA 17402

Precision Medical Manufacturing Corporation 866-633-4626
852 Seton Ct, Wheeling, IL 60090
Designed to snare the tonsils slowly in stages without any backpressure to the hand uses cut formed wires.

SOAP (General) 80WPU

Alimed, Inc. 800-225-2610
297 High St, Dedham, MA 02026

AmSan 800-327-3528
1930 Energy Park Dr Ste 260, Saint Paul, MN 55108
Antimicrobial soaps.

Anatech, Ltd. 800-262-8324
1020 Harts Lake Rd, Battle Creek, MI 49037
Hand cleaners to remove hematoxylin, eosin, and Schiff stains from hands and clothing: Hematoxylin Hand Cleaner, Eosin Hand Cleaner, Schiff's Hand Cleaner

Cambridge Diagnostic Products, Inc. 800-525-6262
6880 NW 17th Ave, Fort Lauderdale, FL 33309
Erada-Stain [cream]. Erado-Sol [liquid]. E-Sol Foamy[Foam dispenser]. Stain Rx [liquid]

Carochem, Inc. 919-682-5121
744 E Markham Ave # 15699, Durham, NC 27701
Solution of castile soap.

Carrington Laboratories, Inc. 800-527-5216
2001 W Walnut Hill Ln, Irving, TX 75038
$8.00 for 8 oz. for perineal cleansing foam.

Carroll Co. 800-527-5722
2900 W Kingsley Rd, Garland, TX 75041
Hand microbial hand cleaners.

Cenorin 800-426-1042
6324 S 199th Pl Ste 107, Kent, WA 98032
Consumable products include Clean 505 biodegradable detergent, liquid/powder, preventive maintenance kits, cleaning kits, mesh bags, superfine and HEPA filters.

Chester Labs, Inc. 800-354-9709
1900 Section Rd, Cincinnati, OH 45237
Liquid soap.

Coloplast Manufacturing Us, Llc 800-533-0464
1840 W Oak Pkwy, Marietta, GA 30062
Gentle and thorough hand cleansers.

Deb Sbs, Inc. 704-263-4240
1100 Highway 27, Stanley, NC 28164
Green and UltraGreen antibacterial lotion soaps. SBS-71 lotion soap, SANITANE E-2 skin cleanser. AQUARESS hand and body shampoo and IMPRESS shower gel. AERO, foam soap dispenses antibacterial soap in economical and hygienically sealed format.

Global Dental Products 516-221-8844
PO Box 537, Bellmore, NY 11710
Urea based hand soap, without detergent. It will kill bacteria & moisturize the skin.

Gojo Industries, Inc 800-321-9647
1 Gojo Plz Ste 500, Akron, OH 44311
PROVON, PURELL, DERMAPRO.

Home Health 800-445-7137
2100 Smithtown Ave, Ronkonkoma, NY 11779
Shampoo.

Meritech, Inc. 800-932-7707
600 Corporate Cir Ste H, Golden, CO 80401
Cleansing products; products for hand sanitation.

New World Imports 800-329-1903
160 Athens Way, Nashville, TN 37228
FRESHSCENT deodorant soap, roll-on, alcohol-free antiperspirant deodorant, solid stick dedorants, baby powder, cornstarch powder, body powder and aerosol shaving cream. Soap dishes, shampoo packets and shower caps also available.

No Rinse Laboratories, Llc. 800-223-9348
868 Pleasant Valley Dr, Springboro, OH 45066
No-Rinse Shampoo, Body Bath, Body Wash personal cleansing products. No Rinse Bathing Wipes, 8 premoistened bathing cloths provide one complete bath. No Rinse Shampoo Cap-one piece cap, shampoo & condition hair with no water.

Orthodontic Supply & Equipment Co., Inc. 800-638-4003
7851 Airpark Rd Ste 202, Gaithersburg, MD 20879
Hand soaps.

SOAP (cont'd)

Palmero Health Care 800-344-6424
120 Goodwin Pl, Stratford, CT 06615
Cleansing products; hand sanitation.

Pharmaceutical Innovations, Inc. 973-242-2900
897 Frelinghuysen Ave, Newark, NJ 07114
Defoaming agent, $12.45 for 16 fl. oz. to $84.95 for gallon of D-FOAM, hydrotherapy additive.

Professional Disposables International, Inc. 800-999-6423
2 Nice Pak Park, Orangeburg, NY 10962
SANI-DEX Cleansing products; hand sanitation.

The Dial Corporation, A Henkel Company 480-754-3425
15501 N Dial Blvd, Scottsdale, AZ 85260

Ulmer Pharmacal Co. 800-848-5637
PO Box 408, 1614 Industry Ave., Park Rapids, MN 56470
LOBANA hand soap, liquid anti-microbial, $5.29 per 1000 ml.

SOCK, CAST TOE (Orthopedics) 87RUA

Darco International, Inc. 800-999-8866
810 Memorial Blvd, Huntington, WV 25701

Mark Medical 800-433-3668
1168 Aster Ave Ste C, Sunnyvale, CA 94086
HAMERTOE HOLDOWNS, single and double sleeves with metatarsal pad. The nylon, foam product alleviates corns and calluses as it straightens and cushions toes.

SOCK, FRACTURE (Orthopedics) 87RUB

Comfort Products, Inc. 800-822-7500
705 Linton Ave, Croydon, PA 19021
Prosthetic sock. All sizes and materials

Knit-Rite, Inc. 800-821-3094
120 Osage Ave, Kansas City, KS 66105
CAST-RITE fracture socks & arm sleeves for use under casts or braces, and torso shirt for use under upper body casts or braces.

Paramedical Distributors 800-245-3278
2020 Grand Blvd, Kansas City, MO 64108
Fracture socks, cast socks, AFO socks, etc.

Slawner Ltd., J. 514-731-3378
5713 Cote Des Neiges Rd., Montreal, QUE H3S 1Y7 Canada

Zimmer Holdings, Inc. 800-613-6131
1800 W Center St, PO Box 708, Warsaw, IN 46580

SOCK, NON-COMPRESSION (General) 80WVI

Paramedical Distributors 800-245-3278
2020 Grand Blvd, Kansas City, MO 64108
Seamless Diabetic Sock, true seamless diabetic socks in white, black, standard high length or shorties. TheraSock diabetic socks, a broad line of white, black, standard, shorties, single and double layered socks. THERASOCK Diabetic Socks; TheraSock, Custom System Plus, Wide Sock, Comfort System Lite, Care Sox Plus.

SOCK, PROTECTIVE, SKIN (General) 80WVH

Geen Healthcare Inc. 800-565-4336
931 Progress Ave. Ste.13, Scarborough, ONT M1G 3V5 Canada
GEEN DIABETESOX Pressure Free Socks for diabetes patients.

Knit-Rite, Inc. 800-821-3094
120 Osage Ave, Kansas City, KS 66105
THERASOCK and SMARTKNIT.

SOCK, STUMP COVER (General) 80RUC

Alimed, Inc. 800-225-2610
297 High St, Dedham, MA 02026

Comfort Products, Inc. 800-822-7500
705 Linton Ave, Croydon, PA 19021
Prosthetic Stump Shrinker - AK & BK in 3 lengths and 5 sizes. Comforgel Liner - prosthetic gel liner, AK & BK in 2 thicknesses and 3 lengths.

Freeman Manufacturing Company 800-253-2091
900 W Chicago Rd, PO Box J, Sturgis, MI 49091
Cast socks, stump socks, prosthetic sheath, stockinette and stump shrinker.

Knit-Rite, Inc. 800-821-3094
120 Osage Ave, Kansas City, KS 66105
Prosthetic sock and AMPU-TALC talcum powder for amputees.

SOFTWARE, BLOOD BANK (STAND-ALONE PRODUCTS) (Hematology) 81MMH

Abbott Diagnostics Div. 847-937-7988
1921 Hurd Dr, Irving, TX 75038
Various stand alone blood bank software products.

SOFTWARE, BLOOD BANK (STAND-ALONE PRODUCTS) (cont'd)

American National Red Cross Headquarters 202-303-5640
2025 E St NW, Washington, DC 20006
Blood banking software.

Blood Bank Computer Systems, Inc. 253-333-0046
1002 15th St SW Ste 120, Auburn, WA 98001
Bbcs.

Blood Trac Systems, Inc. 416-364-8441
300-49 Front St E, Toronto M5E 1B3 Canada
Bloodtrac

Bloodnetusa, Inc. 863-687-8925
3200 Lakeland Hills Blvd, Lakeland, FL 33805
Blood establishment software.

Cardinal Health 303, Inc. 571-521-8907
12120 Sunset Hills Rd Fl 3, Reston, VA 20190
Blood administration verification software.

Community Blood Center Of Greater K.C. 816-968-4025
4040 Main St, Kansas City, MO 64111
Cbc blood system.

Defense Blood Standard System (Dbss) 703-681-3901
5205 Leesburg Pike Ste 1000, Falls Church, VA 22041
Blood bank computer and software.

Digi-Trax Corp. 847-613-2100
650 Heathrow Dr, Lincolnshire, IL 60069
Donor-ID. Electronic blood donor record system. Hema Trax.LPS on-demand FDA compliance labeling for ISBT128

Edward Hines Va Hospital 708-786-5905
5th Ave & Roosevelt Rd., Hines, IL 60141
Various.

Healthcare Management Systems, Inc. 615-844-7320
3102 W End Ave Ste 400, Nashville, TN 37203
Blood transfusion software.

Healthcare-Id, Inc. 847-465-9047
1635 Barclay Blvd, Buffalo Grove, IL 60089
Donor-id 2.2.

Inreach Corporation 888-517-3224
2017 Cardinal Cir, Anderson, SC 29621
Winreach.

Korchek Technologies, Llc 203-452-8295
115 Technology Dr Unit B206, Trumbull, CT 06611
Carechek.

Medical Information Technology, Inc. (Meditech) 781-821-3000
Meditech Circle, Westwood, MA 02090

Mediware Dallas Service Center 913-307-1000
4545 Fuller Dr Ste 320, Irving, TX 75038
Lifetrak aka online care.

Medserv Biologicals, Llc 631-757-8401
1019 Fort Salonga Rd Ste 109, Northport, NY 11768
Pds3-computer software for plasmapheresis ctr.

Ortho-Clinical Diagnostics, Inc. 800-828-6316
513 Technology Blvd, Rochester, NY 14626
Laboratory qperations and management system.

Prescott Ideas, Llc 520-886-4399
8960 E Anna Pl, Tucson, AZ 85710
Blood bank software.

Roche Molecular Systems, Inc. 925-730-8110
4300 Hacienda Dr, Pleasanton, CA 94588
Blood pooling/data output management system software.

Rubin & Poor, Inc. 973-762-9009
155 Maplewood Ave Ste 5, Maplewood, NJ 07040
Configurable manual blot.

Scc Soft Computer 800-763-8352
5400 Tech Data Dr, Clearwater, FL 33760
SCC's centralized transfusion service management system combines high performance functionality with advanced features such as electronic crossmatch with embedded critical safety features.

Talisman Limited 703-242-4200
421 Church St NE Ste F, Vienna, VA 22180
Blood donor self interviewing computer software.

Wyndgate Technologies 800-996-3428
4925 Robert J Mathews Pkwy Ste 100, El Dorado Hills, CA 95762
Software to manage and track blood products from collection to transfusion.

SOLUTION, ANTIBACTERIAL CLEANER *(General) 80TGE*

Afassco, Inc. 800-441-6774
2244 Park Pl Ste C, Minden, NV 89423
Antimicrobial wipes, soap and surface cleaner.

AmSan 800-327-3528
1930 Energy Park Dr Ste 260, Saint Paul, MN 55108

Arjo, Inc. 800-323-1245
50 Gary Ave Ste A, Roselle, IL 60172
Equipment disinfectants, bath additive/skin conditioner, shampoo and complete line of skin care products.

Betco Corp. 800-462-3826
1001 Brown Ave, Toledo, OH 43607

Bio-Medical Products Corp. 800-543-7427
10 Halstead Rd, Mendham, NJ 07945
Foam cleaner. $48.50/box of 12; $3.25 ea.; SAFETY SOFT 3.2 oz. handy pocket-size can of antimicrobial hand degerming foam.

Brulin & Co. Inc. 800-776-7149
2920 Drive A.J. Brown Avenue, Indianapolis, IN 46205
Disinfectant used against HIV-1 (Human Immunodificiency Virus). Maxima is effective against Hepatitis B and HIV.

Canberra Corp. 419-841-6616
3610 N Holland Sylvania Rd, Toledo, OH 43615

Carrington Laboratories, Inc. 800-527-5216
2001 W Walnut Hill Ln, Irving, TX 75038
$14.30 for 5 oz. antifungal cream.

Carroll Co. 800-527-5722
2900 W Kingsley Rd, Garland, TX 75041

Chester Labs, Inc. 800-354-9709
1900 Section Rd, Cincinnati, OH 45237
Perineum wash for incontinent patients.

Crosstex International 800-223-2497
10 Ranick Rd, Hauppauge, NY 11788
Surface & Hand Cleaners

Crosstex International Ltd., W. Region 800-707-2737
14059 Stage Rd, Santa Fe Springs, CA 90670

Crosstex International,Inc. 888-276-7783
10 Ranick Rd, Hauppauge, NY 11788
SANITEX plus.

Essential Industries Inc. 800-551-9679
PO Box 12, 28391 Essential Road, Merton, WI 53056

Gentell 800-840-9041
3600 Boundbrook Ave, Trevose, PA 19053
GENTELL WOUND CLEANSER - pH-balanced, no-rinse cleanser that aids in the removal of wound contaminants and debris. 'Trigger SPray' adjusts from a fine mist to an irrigating stream delivering 8-10 PSI of force. GENTELL WOUND CLEANSER is available in 8oz and 16oz adjustable spray bottle.

Geritrex Corp. 800-736-3437
144 E Kingsbridge Rd, Mount Vernon, NY 10550
For whirlpool tubs.

Global Dental Products 516-221-8844
PO Box 537, Bellmore, NY 11710
TUBULICID RED. Smear layer remover, disinfectant, dentin wetting agent.

Gojo Industries, Inc 800-321-9647
1 Gojo Plz Ste 500, Akron, OH 44311
PROVON, PURELL, DERMAPRO

Graymills Corp. 800-478-8673
3705 N Lincoln Ave, Chicago, IL 60613
All sizes of solvent and heated detergent cleaning equipment.

Johnsondiversey, Inc. 262-631-4001
8310 16th St, P.O. Box 902, Sturtevant, WI 53177

Jvs Solutions 800-325-3303
1200 Switzer Ave, Saint Louis, MO 63147
Sanitizing Solution.

KIK Custom Products 800-479-6603
1 W Hegeler Ln, Danville, IL 61832

Laboratory Technologies, Inc. 800-542-1123
43 W 900 Rte. 64, Maple Park, IL 60151

Medical Chemical Corp. 800-424-9394
19430 Van Ness Ave, Torrance, CA 90501
SURGICIDE povidone-iodine solution - $4.00/16oz, $17.00/gal.

SOLUTION, ANTIBACTERIAL CLEANER *(cont'd)*

Mpm Medical, Inc. 800-232-5512
2301 Crown Ct, Irving, TX 75038
MPM Antiseptic Wound and Skin Cleanser is designed to be used on infected wounds. Effective against MRSA, VRE and many other gram-positive and -negative organisms such as pseudomonas, e. coli, staph and strep. Product is availabe in an 8 oz. and 4 oz. spray bottle.

Niagara Pharmaceuticals Div. 905-690-6277
60 Innovation Dr., Flamborough, ONT L9H-7P3 Canada
HEALTHSAVER disinfectant respirator disinfecting solution and pre-moistened towelette.

Pedinol Pharmacal, Inc. 800-733-4665
30 Banfi Plz N, Farmingdale, NY 11735
Castellani paint with or without color; Fungoid, Fungoid Solution, and Fungoid Tincture.

Pharmacal Research Labs. Inc. 800-243-5350
PO Box 369, Naugatuck, CT 06770
Laboratory animal care.

Safetec Of America, Inc. 800-456-7077
887 Kensington Ave, Buffalo, NY 14215
SANIZIDE PLUS and BIOZIDE help you comply with OSHA Bloodborne Pathogens Standard. Ready-to-use, broad spectrum, hospital grade, hard surface disinfectants/deodorizers. Both are EPA registered. SANIZIDE PLUS is tuberculocidal and virucidal -- kills HIV, HBV, and HCV! Dual quaternary ammonium compound is alcohol-free and non-flammable. Packaging: 2 oz., 16 oz., or 32 oz. Spray Bottles, or 1 gallon Refill. BIOZIDE is a tuberculocidal, virucidal, phenolic formula. Safe on surfaces that will not be harmed by alcohol. Packaging: Single-use Pouch with a heavy-duty dry 8' x 8' Wipe, in 2 oz., 4 oz. or 16 oz. Spray Bottles, or 1 gallon Refill.

Spartan Chemical Company, Inc. 800-537-8990
1110 Spartan Dr, Maumee, OH 43537
NABC One-step, non-acid disinfectant bathroom cleaner, staphylocidal, pseudomonicidal, salmonellacidal, virucidal kills HIV-1, Herpes Simplex type 2 and Influenza A2/Hong Kong viruses on hard inanimate nonporous environmental surfaces.

Stepan Co. 800-745-7837
22 W Frontage Rd, Northfield, IL 60093

The Hymed Group Corp. 610-865-9876
1890 Bucknell Dr, Bethlehem, PA 18015
PiercingCare is a first-aid antiseptic to help reduce bacterial contamination in wounds such as cuts, scrapes, and burns.

Tri-State Surgical Supply & Equipment 800-424-5227
409 Hoyt St, Brooklyn, NY 11231
Perineum wash lotion.

Urocare Products, Inc. 800-423-4441
2735 Melbourne Ave, Pomona, CA 91767
16 oz. bottle urinary appliance cleaner and deodorant.

West Penetone Corp 800-631-1652
700 Gotham Pkwy, Carlstadt, NJ 07072

Woodward Laboratories, Inc. 800-780-6999
125 Columbia Ste B, Aliso Viejo, CA 92656
THUROCLENS, a rapid-rinse cationic soap-free cleanser for regular hand-washing has broad-spectrum antimicrobial activity.

Xttrium Laboratories, Inc. 800-587-3721
415 W Pershing Rd, Chicago, IL 60609
DR. C.: Medicated creme for irritation and/or diaper rash.

Y.I. Ventures, Llc 314-344-0010
2260 Wendt St, Algonquin, IL 60102
DERMASEPTIC bactericidal hand-washing cleanser.

SOLUTION, ANTIMICROBIAL *(Microbiology) 83LOP*

Armstrong Medical Industries, Inc. 800-323-4220
575 Knightsbridge Pkwy, Lincolnshire, IL 60069
Hand washes.

Crosstex International,Inc. 888-276-7783
10 Ranick Rd, Hauppauge, NY 11788
SANISEPT, ALOE CARE soaps and lotions, SANICARE, BARRIER CREAM, SANICLENZ soap, Also, SANITYZE waterless moisturizing antimicrobial gel; kills up to 99% of bacteria in as little as five seconds; leaves hands safe, soft, protected, moisturized, and conditioned; requires no water, towels, or air dryers; latex compatible.

Omni Medical Supply Inc. 800-860-6664
4153 Pioneer Dr, Commerce Township, MI 48390

SOLUTION, ANTIMICROBIAL *(cont'd)*

Veridien Corp. 800-345-5444
7600 Bryan Dairy Rd Ste F, Largo, FL 33777
VIRAGUARD, antimicrobial hand gel, waterless antiseptic hand gel, kills 99.9% pathogenic organisms, emollient protects and moisturizes hands.

Woodward Laboratories, Inc. 800-780-6999
125 Columbia Ste B, Aliso Viejo, CA 92656
Mycocide NS Antimicrobial Nail Solution. Convenient, conservative, cost-effective, first line alternative. Antimicrobial formula penetrates to the nail matrix and promotes new healthy nail formation.

SOLUTION, BALANCED SALT *(Pathology) 88KIP*

Clinical Diagnostic Solutions, Inc. 954-791-1773
1800 NW 65th Ave, Plantation, FL 33313
Sheath reagent.

Diagnostic Hybrids, Inc. 740-589-3300
1055 E State St Ste 100, Athens, OH 45701
Hbss; balanced salt solution.

Lonza Walkersville, Inc. 201-316-9200
8830 Biggs Ford Rd, Walkersville, MD 21793
Balanced salt solutions.

Mediatech, Inc. 800-235-5476
13884 Park Center Rd, Herndon, VA 20171

Sigma-Aldrich Manufacturing, Llc. 913-469-5580
3506 S Broadway, Saint Louis, MO 63118
Various balanced salt soultions.

SOLUTION, CEMENT DISSOLVING *(Dental And Oral) 76KZP*

American Diversified Dental Systems 800-637-2330
22991 La Cadena Dr, Laguna Hills, CA 92653
ADDS-IT Tip Cleaner Kit.

Den-Mat Holdings, Llc 805-922-8491
2727 Skyway Dr, Santa Maria, CA 93455
Solvenex tm.

Mavidon Medical Products 800-654-0385
1820 2nd Ave N, Lake Worth, FL 33461
Collodion remover, acetone, body adhesive remover.

SOLUTION, COPPER SULFATE, FOR SPECIFIC GRAVITY TEST
(Hematology) 81KSL

Ricca Chemical Company Llc 888-467-4222
1841 Broad St, Pocomoke City, MD 21851
Various

Ricca Chemical Company Llc 817-461-5601
1490 Lammers Pike, Batesville, IN 47006

Ricca Chemical Company, Llc 817-461-5601
448 W Fork Dr, Arlington, TX 76012
Copper sulfate solutions.

Richard-Allan Scientific 269-544-5628
4481 Campus Dr, Kalamazoo, MI 49008
Copper sulfate solution.

SOLUTION, DIALYSIS *(Gastro/Urology) 78LLJ*

Baxter Healthcare Corporation, Renal 888-229-0001
1620 S Waukegan Rd, Waukegan, IL 60085
CAPD. DIANEAL low calcium. Electrolyte. Kidney preservation.

SOLUTION, FORMALIN/SODIUM ACETATE *(Pathology) 88IGB*

Alpha-Tec Systems, Inc. 800-221-6058
12019 NE 99th St Ste 1780, Vancouver, WA 98682
SAF fixative.

Hydrol Chemical Co. 610-622-3603
520 Commerce Dr, Yeadon, PA 19050
Solution, formalin-sodium acetate.

Meridian Bioscience, Inc. 800-696-0739
3471 River Hills Dr, Cincinnati, OH 45244
For the routine collection, transportation, preservation and examination of stool specimens for intestinal parasites.

Sci Gen, Inc. 310-324-6576
333 E Gardena Blvd, Gardena, CA 90248
FDA: Medical Device Manufacturing and packaging. Focus on Histology, Cytology, Analytical and General purpose Reagents, Chemistry, and Sterling and Disinfecting agents.

SOLUTION, INSTRUMENT CLEANER *(General) 80TGF*

Air Techniques, Inc. 800-247-8324
1295 Walt Whitman Rd, Melville, NY 11747
VACUSELTZER, granular evacuation system cleaner for dental vacuum system.

SOLUTION, INSTRUMENT CLEANER *(cont'd)*

Blue Wave Ultrasonics 800-373-0144
960 S Rolff St, Davenport, IA 52802
Concentrated detergent for medical ultrasonic cleaning.

Cambridge Diagnostic Products, Inc. 800-525-6262
6880 NW 17th Ave, Fort Lauderdale, FL 33309
Erado-Sol liquid stain remover - $13.00 for 16-oz, $19.00 for 32-oz., $52 .00 per gallon; E-Sol Foamy - $9.00 for 8 oz; 6-oz Erada-Stain cream stain remover for $9.60. Stain Rx $8.00 for 3.75 oz, $12 for 16 oz.

Carochem, Inc. 919-682-5121
744 E Markham Ave # 15699, Durham, NC 27701
Homogeneous blend for cleaning surgical instruments; enzymatic powder cleaner: enzymatic detergent blend for cleaning surgical instruments; enzymatic liquid cleaner: enzyme, detergent, stabilizer blend for cleaning surgical instruments.

Case Medical, Inc. 888-227-2273
65 Railroad Ave, Ridgefield, NJ 07657
Pentaprep pre soak, Pentazyme washer decontaminator low foam

Clinimed, Incorporated 877-CLINIMED
303 Markus Ct, Sandy Brae Industrial Park, Newark, DE 19713

Deknatel Snowden-Pencer 800-367-7874
5175 S Royal Atlanta Dr, Tucker, GA 30084
NUTRA-ZYME endoscopic instrument cleaner for use with ENDO-CLEAN unit. Formulation of enzymes, surfactants, digesters and antimicrobial agents for cleaning and disinfecting.

Haemo-Sol, Inc. 800-821-5676
7301 York Rd, Baltimore, MD 21204

L&R Manufacturing Co. 201-991-5330
577 Elm St, PO Box 607, Kearny, NJ 07032

Leander Health Technologies/Healthcare Division 800-635-8188
1525 Vivian Ct, Port Orchard, WA 98367
Keyston Vinyl Cleaner is specially formulated to clean leather and vinyl upholstery.

Md International, Inc. 305-669-9003
11300 NW 41st St, Doral, FL 33178

Mettler Electronics Corp. 800-854-9305
1333 S Claudina St, Anaheim, CA 92805
$103.00 for case of four 1-gal. containers.

Miltex Inc. 800-645-8000
589 Davies Dr, York, PA 17402
Surgical instrument cleaner and stain remover.

Parker Laboratories, Inc. 800-631-8888
286 Eldridge Rd, Fairfield, NJ 07004
TRANSEPTIC transducer, probe cleanser.

Thermo Fisher Scientific Inc. 781-622-1000
81 Wyman St, Waltham, MA 02451

Ultra Clean Systems, Inc. 877-935-6624
12700 Dupont Cir, Tampa, FL 33626
Ultra Clean Surgical Milk concentrated solution for lubricating surgical instruments.

Wave Form Systems, Inc. 800-332-8749
7737 SW Nimbus Ave, Beaverton, OR 97008
ANTI-FOG SOLUTION for endoscopes and cameras.

Xttrium Laboratories, Inc. 800-587-3721
415 W Pershing Rd, Chicago, IL 60609
BENZ-ALL: Germicidal concentrate/instrument disinfectant.

SOLUTION, INSTRUMENT, LAPAROSCOPIC, ANTI-FOG
(General) 80WYR

Richard Wolf Medical Instruments Corp. 800-323-9653
353 Corporate Woods Pkwy, Vernon Hills, IL 60061

Surgicorp, Inc. 727-934-5000
40347 US Highway 19 N Ste 121, Tarpon Springs, FL 34689
Alcohol-free anti-fog comes in 6cc or 30cc vials, or in pre-packaged sterile wipes.

Vital Concepts, Inc. 800-984-2300
4334 Brockton Dr SE Ste F, Grand Rapids, MI 49512
VCI Anit-Fog, alcohol area & alcohol based solution availiable in kits or presaturated sponges for reduction of fog formation on laparoscope.

SOLUTION, INTRAVENOUS *(General) 80TGA*

B. Braun Oem Division, B. Braun Medical Inc. 866-8-BBRAUN
824 12th Ave, Bethlehem, PA 18018

SOLUTION, INTRAVENOUS *(cont'd)*

Baxter Healthcare Corporation Nutrition 888-229-0001
1 Baxter Pkwy, Deerfield, IL 60015
Fat emulsion, dextrose injections, sterile water for injection, parenteral nutrition solutions.

Baxter Healthcare Corporation, Global Drug Delivery 888-229-0001
25212 W Il Route 120, Round Lake, IL 60073
Large and small volume parenterals, premix medications.

Baxter Healthcare Corporation, Medication Delivery 888-229-0001
25212 W Il Route 120, Round Lake, IL 60073

SOLUTION, ISOTONIC *(Hematology) 81JCE*

Health Care Logistics, Inc. 800-848-1633
450 Town St, PO Box 25, Circleville, OH 43113
Sterile buffered isotonic eyewash.

Nerl Diagnostics Llc. 401-824-2046
14 Almeida Ave, East Providence, RI 02914
Various.

Niagara Pharmaceuticals Div. 905-690-6277
60 Innovation Dr., Flamborough, ONT L9H-7P3 Canada
HEALTH SAVER saline buffered isotonic eye wash.

Pochemco, Inc. 413-536-2900
724 Main St, Holyoke, MA 01040
Sodium chloride.

Poly Scientific R&D Corp. 800-645-5825
70 Cleveland Ave, Bay Shore, NY 11706

Ricca Chemical Company Llc 817-461-5601
1490 Lammers Pike, Batesville, IN 47006

Ricca Chemical Company, Llc 817-461-5601
448 W Fork Dr, Arlington, TX 76012
Sodium chloride solution.

SOLUTION, NUTRITION, ENTERAL *(Gastro/Urology) 78WWM*

Novartis Nutrition 800-333-3785
1600 Utica Ave S Ste 600, PO Box 370, Minneapolis, MN 55416
Closed and open system packaging; full line of standard and disease specific formulas.

SOLUTION, NUTRITION, PARENTERAL *(Gastro/Urology) 78TGK*

Astellas Pharma Us, Inc. 800-888-7704
3 Parkway N, Deerfield, IL 60015
MURI-LUBE.

Baxter Healthcare Corporation Nutrition 888-229-0001
1 Baxter Pkwy, Deerfield, IL 60015
NOVAMINE, TRAVASOL, RENAMIN, AMINESS, BRANCHAMIN, INTRALIPID.

SOLUTION, OSTOMY, ODOR CONTROL *(Gastro/Urology) 78VKQ*

Beaumont Products, Inc. 800-451-7096
1560 Big Shanty Dr NW, Kennesaw, GA 30144
Citrus II Odor Eliminating Air Fragrance - The fresh, all natural way to eliminate tough odors on contact

Coloplast Manufacturing Us, Llc 800-533-0464
1840 W Oak Pkwy, Marietta, GA 30062
COLOPLAST liquid solution eliminates odors from ostomy appliances; rinses resusable appliances.

Gentell 800-840-9041
3600 Boundbrook Ave, Trevose, PA 19053
GENTELL EASE ODOR ELIMINATOR destroys biological and airborne odors; effective with malodorous wounds; contains light fragrance that dissipates within minutes. GENTELL EASE is available in 2oz spray bottle.

Hospitales Y Quirofanos S.A. Dec.V. 5-611-8244
Murillo No. 44 Col. Nonoalco, Deleg. B. Juarez, D.F. 03700 Mexico
Femenine deodorant spray for vaginal area.

Humanicare International, Inc. 800-631-5270
9 Elkins Rd, East Brunswick, NJ 08816
DIGNITY odor eliminator in 2- and 8-oz sprays.

Imtek Environmental Corp. 770-667-8621
PO Box 2066, Alpharetta, GA 30023
Smelleze Ostomy Bag Deodorizer absorbs, neutralizes and encapsulates pungent urine and fecal odors without masking them with fragrances. Smelleze Hospital Deodorizer Pouch, eliminates offensive odors from medicine, sick rooms, urine, feces, vomit, spills, perspiration, bacteria, mildew, etc. Safe, non-toxic & natural.

SOLUTION, OSTOMY, ODOR CONTROL *(cont'd)*

Innovative Health Care Products, Inc. 678-320-0009
6850 Peachtree Dunwoody Rd NE Apt 402, Atlanta, GA 30328
SUNZYME safely eliminates odor without masking(unscented), and is safe for the environment. Neutralizes all types of odors and can be used around people safely.It is also non-flammable, non-toxic and biodegradable. An all natural product formulated with enzymes.Good for surfaces and atmosphere.

Orange-Sol Medical Products, Inc. 800-877-7771
1400 N Fiesta Blvd Ste 100, Gilbert, AZ 85233

Smith & Nephew, Inc. 800-876-1261
11775 Starkey Rd, Largo, FL 33773
BANISH II ostomy appliance deodorant in liquid form and ODO-WAY deodorant in pill form.

Surco Products 800-556-0111
292 Alpha Dr, RIDC Industrial Park, Pittsburgh, PA 15238
Aerosol and dispensers.

SOLUTION, PATHOLOGY, CARNOY'S *(Pathology) 88IGM*

American Mastertech Scientific, Inc. 209-368-4031
1330 Thurman St, Lodi, CA 95240
Carnoy's solution.

E K Industries, Inc. 877-EKI-CHEM
1403 Herkimer St, Joliet, IL 60432
Carnoy's solution.

Hydrol Chemical Co. 610-622-3603
520 Commerce Dr, Yeadon, PA 19050
Solution, carnoy's.

Poly Scientific R&D Corp. 800-645-5825
70 Cleveland Ave, Bay Shore, NY 11706

Ricca Chemical Company Llc 817-461-5601
1490 Lammers Pike, Batesville, IN 47006

Ricca Chemical Company, Llc 817-461-5601
448 W Fork Dr, Arlington, TX 76012

SOLUTION, PATHOLOGY, DECALCIFIER, ACID CONTAINING
(Pathology) 88KDX

American Mastertech Scientific, Inc. 209-368-4031
1330 Thurman St, Lodi, CA 95240
Decalcifying solution.

E K Industries, Inc. 877-EKI-CHEM
1403 Herkimer St, Joliet, IL 60432
Decalcifying solution.

Fisher Scientific Co., Llc. 201-703-3131
1 Reagent Ln, Fair Lawn, NJ 07410
Decalcifying solution.

Hydrol Chemical Co. 610-622-3603
520 Commerce Dr, Yeadon, PA 19050
Solution, decalcifier, acid containing.

Poly Scientific R&D Corp. 800-645-5825
70 Cleveland Ave, Bay Shore, NY 11706

Ricca Chemical Company Llc 888-467-4222
1841 Broad St, Pocomoke City, MD 21851
Decalcifying Solution

Ricca Chemical Company Llc 817-461-5601
1490 Lammers Pike, Batesville, IN 47006

Ricca Chemical Company, Llc 817-461-5601
448 W Fork Dr, Arlington, TX 76012
Decalcifying solution.

Richard-Allan Scientific 269-544-5628
4481 Campus Dr, Kalamazoo, MI 49008
General purpose reagent.

Sci Gen, Inc. 310-324-6576
333 E Gardena Blvd, Gardena, CA 90248
FDA: Medical Device Manufacturing and packaging. Focus on Histology, Cytology, Analytical and General purpose Reagents, Chemistry, and Sterling and Disinfecting agents.

Spectra-Tint 585-546-8050
250 Cumberland St Ste 228, Rochester, NY 14605
Organic acid fixing decalcifier.

Statlab Medical Products, Inc. 800-442-3573
106 Hillside Dr, Lewisville, TX 75057
DECAL PLUS REDECAL rapid with fixative.

U S Biotex Corp. 606-652-4700
RR 1 Box 62, Webbville, KY 41180
Decalcifying solution.

SOLUTION, PATHOLOGY, FONTANNA SILVER
(Pathology) 88HYE

Poly Scientific R&D Corp. 800-645-5825
70 Cleveland Ave, Bay Shore, NY 11706

SOLUTION, PATHOLOGY, FORMALIN-ALCOHOL-ACETIC ACID
(Pathology) 88IGF

E K Industries, Inc. 877-EKI-CHEM
1403 Herkimer St, Joliet, IL 60432
Formalin-aceto-alcohol solution.

Hydrol Chemical Co. 610-622-3603
520 Commerce Dr, Yeadon, PA 19050
Solution, formalin-alcohol-acetic acid.

Labchem, Inc. 412-826-5230
200 William Pitt Way, Pittsburgh, PA 15238
Acid alcohol, multiple (lc10500, lc10520), various concentrations.

Poly Scientific R&D Corp. 800-645-5825
70 Cleveland Ave, Bay Shore, NY 11706

Ricca Chemical Company Llc 817-461-5601
1490 Lammers Pike, Batesville, IN 47006

Ricca Chemical Company, Llc 817-461-5601
448 W Fork Dr, Arlington, TX 76012
Formalin-aceto-alcohol solution (f-a-a mixture).

Rocky Mountain Reagents,Inc. 303-762-0800
3207 W Hampden Ave, Englewood, CO 80110

Sci Gen, Inc. 310-324-6576
333 E Gardena Blvd, Gardena, CA 90248
FDA: Medical Device Manufacturing and packaging. Focus on Histology, Cytology, Analytical and General purpose Reagents, Chemistry, and Sterling and Disinfecting agents.

Spectra-Tint 585-546-8050
250 Cumberland St Ste 228, Rochester, NY 14605
Forma-fix iii.

SOLUTION, PATHOLOGY, LUGOL'S *(Pathology) 88IAM*

Labchem, Inc. 412-826-5230
200 William Pitt Way, Pittsburgh, PA 15238
Iodine, lugols (lc15675).

Medical Chemical Corp. 800-424-9394
19430 Van Ness Ave, Torrance, CA 90501
$13.50 per 100ml.

Pochemco, Inc. 413-536-2900
724 Main St, Holyoke, MA 01040
Iodine, Lugol's.

Poly Scientific R&D Corp. 800-645-5825
70 Cleveland Ave, Bay Shore, NY 11706

Ricca Chemical Company Llc 817-461-5601
1490 Lammers Pike, Batesville, IN 47006

Ricca Chemical Company, Llc 817-461-5601
448 W Fork Dr, Arlington, TX 76012
Lugol's iodine.

Richard-Allan Scientific 269-544-5628
4481 Campus Dr, Kalamazoo, MI 49008
Solution, lugol's.

Rocky Mountain Reagents,Inc. 303-762-0800
3207 W Hampden Ave, Englewood, CO 80110

SOLUTION, PATHOLOGY, ORTH'S *(Pathology) 88IFN*

Ricca Chemical Company Llc 817-461-5601
1490 Lammers Pike, Batesville, IN 47006

Ricca Chemical Company, Llc 817-461-5601
448 W Fork Dr, Arlington, TX 76012
Orth's decolorizing fluid.

SOLUTION, PATHOLOGY, ZENKER'S *(Pathology) 88IFH*

American Mastertech Scientific, Inc. 209-368-4031
1330 Thurman St, Lodi, CA 95240
Zenker's solution.

E K Industries, Inc. 877-EKI-CHEM
1403 Herkimer St, Joliet, IL 60432
Zenker's solution.

Poly Scientific R&D Corp. 800-645-5825
70 Cleveland Ave, Bay Shore, NY 11706

Ricca Chemical Company Llc 817-461-5601
1490 Lammers Pike, Batesville, IN 47006

Ricca Chemical Company, Llc 817-461-5601
448 W Fork Dr, Arlington, TX 76012
Zenker's fixative solution.

SOLUTION, PATHOLOGY, ZENKER'S *(cont'd)*

Richard-Allan Scientific 269-544-5628
4481 Campus Dr, Kalamazoo, MI 49008
Zenker's solution.

SOLUTION, PATIENT PREPARATION *(General) 80TGG*

Crosstex International,Inc. 888-276-7783
10 Ranick Rd, Hauppauge, NY 11788
CROSSZYME EFFERZYME Ultrasonic solutions and tablets.

J. Hewitt Incorporated 800-543-9488
6 Faraday Ste B, Irvine, CA 92618
Pierced ear antiseptic.

Miller-Stephenson Chemical Company, Inc. 800-992-2424
George Washington Highway, Danbury, CT 06810-7378

Professional Disposables International, Inc. 800-999-6423
2 Nice Pak Park, Orangeburg, NY 10962
DUO-SWAB and IO-GONE Iodine preps and swabs.

Purdue Frederick Company 800-877-5666
1 Stamford Forum, Stamford, CT 06901
Betadine prep solution.

SOLUTION, PH BUFFER *(Chemistry) 75UHD*

Analytical Measurements, Inc. 800-635-5580
100 Hoffman Pl, Hillside, NJ 07205
$10.00 per pint.

Beckman Coulter, Inc. 800-742-2345
250 S Kraemer Blvd, PO Box 8000, Brea, CA 92821

Brinkmann Instruments (Canada) Ltd. 800-263-8715
6670 Campobello Rd., Mississauga, ONT L5N 2L8 Canada

Cole-Parmer Instrument Inc. 800-323-4340
625 E Bunker Ct, Vernon Hills, IL 60061

Crescent Chemical Co., Inc. 800-877-3225
2 Oval Dr, Islandia, NY 11749

Dade Behring, Inc. 800-948-3233
1717 Deerfield Rd, Deerfield, IL 60015

Extech Instruments Corp. 781-890-7440
285 Bear Hill Rd, Waltham, MA 02451

Myron L Company 760-438-2021
2450 Impala Dr, Carlsbad, CA 92010
Buffer solution

Orbeco Analytical Systems, Inc. 800-922-5242
185 Marine St, Farmingdale, NY 11735

Orion Research, Inc. 800-225-1480
166 Cummings Ctr, Beverly, MA 01915
ORION $9.50 per 475ml bottle.

Stanbio Laboratory, Inc. 830-249-0772
1261 N Main St, Boerne, TX 78006
$15.50 for 500ml, buffer solution.

Thermo Fisher Scientific Inc. 781-622-1000
81 Wyman St, Waltham, MA 02451

SOLUTION, SALINE(WOUND DRESSING) *(Surgery) 79MUG*

Ac Healthcare Supply, Inc. 905-448-4706
11651 230th St, Cambria Heights, NY 11411
Saline solution wound dressing.

Health Care Logistics, Inc. 800-848-1633
450 Town St, PO Box 25, Circleville, OH 43113
Sterile wound cleanser.

Oculus Innovative Sciences, Inc. 707-559-7191
1135 N McDowell Blvd, Petaluma, CA 94954
Wound dressing.

Revalesio Corporation 253-922-2600
5102 20th St E Ste 100, Fife, WA 98424
Sterile saline solution.

Winchester Laboratories Llc 630-377-7880
11 S 2nd Ave, Saint Charles, IL 60174
Various.

SOLUTION, SILVER CARBONATE *(Pathology) 88KKP*

Ventana Medical Systems, Inc. 800-227-2155
1910 E Innovation Park Dr, Oro Valley, AZ 85755
Chemical solution stain.

SOLUTION, STABILIZED ENZYME *(Hematology) 81KSK*

American Red Cross Diagnostic Manufacturing Divisi 202-303-5640
9319 Gaither Rd, Gaithersburg, MD 20877
Freeze dried bromelain.

SOLUTION, STERILIZING, COLD *(Dental And Oral) 76LFE*

Pascal Co., Inc. 425-602-3633
2929 Northup Way, Bellevue, WA 98004
Cold sterilizing solution.

SOLUTION, SURGICAL SCRUB *(General) 80TGD*

Covidien Lp 508-261-8000
15 Hampshire St, Mansfield, MA 02048

Medical Chemical Corp. 800-424-9394
19430 Van Ness Ave, Torrance, CA 90501
$16.95 per gal.

Purdue Frederick Company 800-877-5666
1 Stamford Forum, Stamford, CT 06901
Betadine solution.

Xttrium Laboratories, Inc. 800-587-3721
415 W Pershing Rd, Chicago, IL 60609
Chlorhexidine gluconate scrub solution for general skin cleaning.

SOLUTION-TEST, STANDARD-CONDUCTIVITY, DIALYSIS *(Gastro/Urology) 78FKH*

Alden Medical Llc 413-747-9717
360 Cold Spring Ave, West Springfield, MA 01089
Conductivity standard solutions.

H & S Technical Services, Inc. 480-517-4918
1833 W Main St Ste 119, Mesa, AZ 85201
Standard solution, conductivity for dialysis.

Myron L Company 760-438-2021
2450 Impala Dr, Carlsbad, CA 92010

SOLVENT *(Chemistry) 75UIB*

Elantec Med, Inc. 303-278-7672
85 S Union Blvd Ste M160, Lakewood, CO 80228
TAG OFF non-toxic adhesive remover for labels, tags, tape, etc. Cleaning products.

Honeywell Burdick & Jackson 800-368-0050
1953 Harvey St, Muskegon, MI 49442

Innovative Technology, Inc. 877-462-4415
2 New Pasture Rd, Newburyport, MA 01950
SPS 400, solvent purification system.

Reade Advanced Materials 401-433-7000
PO Box 15039, Riverside, RI 02915
Chromatography.

The Electrode Store 360-829-0400
PO Box 188, Enumclaw, WA 98022
For the removal of collodion and other adhesives.

Ulmer Pharmacal Co. 800-848-5637
PO Box 408, 1614 Industry Ave., Park Rapids, MN 56470
KLER-RO biodegradable blood solvent and multipurpose solvents, $8.16 per 1000 g.

Veltek Associates, Inc. 888-478-3745
15 Lee Blvd, Malvern, PA 19355
DECON-AHOL Sterile alcohol available in gallons, spays or wet and dry wipes.

Warner Graham Co., The 800-872-2300
160 Church Ln, Cockeysville, MD 21030

Yates & Bird And Motloid 800-662-5021
300 N Elizabeth St, Chicago, IL 60607
Wax solvent.

SOLVENT, ADHESIVE TAPE *(Surgery) 79KOX*

Elantec Med, Inc. 303-278-7672
85 S Union Blvd Ste M160, Lakewood, CO 80228
STR Surgical/sports tape remover is non-toxic, non-flammable and odorless.

Ferndale Laboratories, Inc. 248-548-0900
780 W 8 Mile Rd, Detroit, MI 48220
Detachol.

Ldb Medical, Inc. 800-243-2554
2909 Langford Rd Ste B500, Norcross, GA 30071
LAPIDES.

Mavidon Medical Products 800-654-0385
1820 2nd Ave N, Lake Worth, FL 33461
Adhesive remover.

Miller-Stephenson Chemical Company, Inc. 800-992-2424
George Washington Highway, Danbury, CT 06810-7378

Smith & Nephew, Inc. 800-876-1261
11775 Starkey Rd, Largo, FL 33773
UNI-SOLVE adhesive remover.

SOLVENT, ADHESIVE TAPE *(cont'd)*

Smith & Nephew, Inc. 800-876-1261
970 Lake Carillon Dr Ste 110, Saint Petersburg, FL 33716
UNISOLVE ADHESIVE REMOVER; REMOVE

Span Packaging Services Llc. 864-627-4155
4611A Dairy Dr, Greenville, SC 29607
Bard adhesive barrier film remover.

Sterion, Incorporated 800-328-7958
13828 Lincoln St NE, Ham Lake, MN 55304
Same day tape remover, solvent to remove identification tape.

Ulmer Pharmacal Co. 800-848-5637
PO Box 408, 1614 Industry Ave., Park Rapids, MN 56470
TA-POFF $21.16 per 1000 ml.

Veriad 800-423-4643
650 Columbia St, Brea, CA 92821
Label, tape and adhesive remover.

Weiman Healthcare Solutions 800-837-8140
755 Tri State Pkwy, Gurnee, IL 60031
Removes tape and adhesive from skin and surgical equipment.

3m Co. 888-364-3577
3M Center, Saint Paul, MN 55144
3M BRAND REMOVER LOTION; 3M WATER DDISPERSIBLE ADHESIVE TAPE

SOLVENT, SPECTROPHOTOMETER *(Chemistry) 75UIE*

Beckman Coulter, Inc. 800-742-2345
250 S Kraemer Blvd, PO Box 8000, Brea, CA 92821

Buck Scientific, Inc. 800-562-5566
58 Fort Point St, Norwalk, CT 06855

Honeywell Burdick & Jackson 800-368-0050
1953 Harvey St, Muskegon, MI 49442

SONOMETER, BONE *(Radiology) 90MUA*

Ge Medical Systems Ultrasound And Primary Care Dia 608-826-7050
726 Heartland Trl, Madison, WI 53717
Bone sonometer.

Hologic, Inc. 800-343-9729
35 Crosby Dr, Bedford, MA 01730

SORBENT, FTA-ABS TEST *(Microbiology) 83GMW*

Bd Diagnostic Systems 800-675-0908
7 Loveton Cir, Sparks, MD 21152

SORTER, CELL (SEPARATOR) *(Pathology) 88KEX*

Beckman Coulter, Inc. 800-635-3497
740 W 83rd St, Hialeah, FL 33014
$110,000 to $274,800 for flow cytometer (9 models).

Hamamatsu Corp. 800-524-0504
360 Foothill Rd, Bridgewater, NJ 08807

Immunicon Corporation 215-830-0777
3401 Masons Mill Rd Ste 100, Huntingdon Valley, PA 19006
The CellTracks AutoPrep System is a walk-away instrument designed for isolation of rare cells from whole blood using magnetic separation and enrichment.

SOUND, URETHRAL, METAL OR PLASTIC
(Gastro/Urology) 78FBX

Aesculap Implant Systems Inc. 1-800-234-9179
3773 Corporate Pkwy, Center Valley, PA 18034

Biomet Microfixation Inc. 800-874-7711
1520 Tradeport Dr, Jacksonville, FL 32218
Various types of sounds.

Candela Corp. 800-733-8550
530 Boston Post Rd, Wayland, MA 01778

Codman & Shurtleff, Inc 800-225-0460
325 Paramount Dr, Raynham, MA 02767

Greenwald Surgical Co., Inc. 219-962-1604
2688 Dekalb St, Gary, IN 46405
Various types of urethral sounds.

Miltex Inc. 800-645-8000
589 Davies Dr, York, PA 17402

Tuzik Boston 800-886-6363
104 Longwater Dr, Assinippi Park, Norwell, MA 02061

SOUND, UTERINE *(Obstetrics/Gyn) 85HHM*

Aesculap Implant Systems Inc. 1-800-234-9179
3773 Corporate Pkwy, Center Valley, PA 18034

SOUND, UTERINE *(cont'd)*

Biomet Microfixation Inc. 800-874-7711
1520 Tradeport Dr, Jacksonville, FL 32218
Various types of sound.

Clinical Innovations, Inc. 888-268-6222
747 W 4170 S, Murray, UT 84123
Disposable sound-dilator is molded plastic with centimeter graduation marks, one-step dilation, safety ends, and lubricious feel.

Codman & Shurtleff, Inc 800-225-0460
325 Paramount Dr, Raynham, MA 02767

Cook Ob/Gyn 800-541-5591
1100 W Morgan St, Spencer, IN 47460

Cytyc Surgical Products 800-442-9892
250 Campus Dr, Marlborough, MA 01752
Uterine sound.

George Tiemann & Co. 800-843-6266
25 Plant Ave, Hauppauge, NY 11788

Miltex Inc. 800-645-8000
589 Davies Dr, York, PA 17402

Premier Medical Products 888-PREMUSA
1710 Romano Dr, Plymouth Meeting, PA 19462

Princeton Medical Group, Inc. 800-875-0869
1189 Royal Links Dr, Mt Pleasant, SC 29466

Reznik Instrument, Inc. 847-673-3444
7337 Lawndale Ave, Skokie, IL 60076
Uterine manipulators.

Shoney Scientific, Inc. 262-970-0170
West 223 North 720 Saratoga Drive,, Suite 120, Waukesha, WI 53186
Uterine sound.

SOURCE, BRACHYTHERAPY, RADIONUCLIDE
(Radiology) 90KXK

Ati Medical, Inc. 858-946-2228
1 Palmer Sq E Ste 515, Princeton, NJ 08542
Isorod pd-103 implant brachytherapy source.

Bard Brachytherapy, Inc 908-277-8000
295 E Lies Rd, Carol Stream, IL 60188
Iodine seeds.

Best Medical International, Inc. 800-336-4970
7643 Fullerton Rd, Springfield, VA 22153
Iridium 192 in Nylon RIbbons, Gold 198 Seeds; different applicators (Fletcher-Suit-Delclos, Kumar, Hilaris-Nori, Burnett, Wang, etc.) Tubes, Buttons, Needles, Crimper; Calibrators and Survey Meters. Iodine 125 and Palladium-103. IODINE 125, Best Double Wall Iodine 125 for prostate & other brachytherapy treatments. PALLADIUM-103, Best Double Wall Palladium 103 Source for prostate and other brachytherapy treatments.

Cis-Us, Inc. 800-221-7554
10 Deangelo Dr, Bedford, MA 01730
Cs 137, Ir 191.

Cp Medical Corporation 800-950-2763
803 NE 25th Ave, Portland, OR 97232
Absorbable seeding spacers, bone-waxed needles, grids, carrier sleeve for use during brachytherapy procedures.

Cytyc Surgical Products 800-442-9892
250 Campus Dr, Marlborough, MA 01752
Source, brachytherapy, radionuclide.

Eckert & Ziegler Isotope Products 661-309-1034
24937 Avenue Tibbitts, Valencia, CA 91355
Various: cesium-137 tube sources, ruthenium eye applicators, ect.

International Brachytherapy, Inc. 770-582-0662
6000 Live Oak Pkwy Ste 107, Norcross, GA 30093
Brachytherapy source.

Isoaid, L.L.C. 727-815-3262
7824 Clark Moody Blvd, Port Richey, FL 34668
Radionuclide brachytherapy source.

Medi-Physics, Inc., Dba Ge Healthcare 800-633-4123
3350 N Ridge Ave, Arlington Heights, IL 60004
Iodine-125 seeds.

Mills Biopharmaceuticals, Llc 405-523-1868
120 NE 26th St, Oklahoma City, OK 73105
Mbi i-125 brachtherapy seed models 125sl, 125sh.

Qsa-Global Inc. 781-272-2000
40 North Ave, Burlington, MA 01803
Hdr source.

SOURCE, BRACHYTHERAPY, RADIONUCLIDE *(cont'd)*

Sun Nuclear Corp. 321-259-6862
425 Pineda Ct Ste A, Melbourne, FL 32940
Brachytherapy re-entrant chamber: model 1008.

Theragenics Corp. 770-271-0233
5203 Bristol Industrial Way, Buford, GA 30518
TheraStrand; In-STANT Stranding System; TheraLoad; TheraSleeve; TheraStrand; TheraSeed; I-Seed

SOURCE, CHEMILUMINESCENT LIGHT *(Obstetrics/Gyn) 85MPU*

Zila Technical, Inc. 602-266-6700
3418 S 48th St Ste 9, Phoenix, AZ 85040
Gynecologic laparoscope and accessories.

Zila, Inc. 800-228-5595
701 Centre Ave, Fort Collins, CO 80526
ViziLite Comprehensive Exam Tray; ViziLite Plus; ViziLite Single; ViziLite Supplemental Kit

SOURCE, HEAT, BLEACHING, TEETH, DENTAL
(Dental And Oral) 76EEG

Air Techniques, Inc. 800-247-8324
1295 Walt Whitman Rd, Melville, NY 11747
ARC light rapid curing and bleaching system.

Almore International, Inc. 503-643-6633
PO Box 25214, Portland, OR 97298
$240.00 to $280.00 for tooth bleaching instrument.

Beks Incorporated 630-480-0476
401 14th Ave NE Ste 2, Jasper, AL 35504
Teeth whitening system.

Bsml, Inc. 561-988-4098
7777 Glades Rd Ste 100, Boca Raton, FL 33434
One visit, one hour patented, light-activated teeth whitening. Distributed via company-owned whitening spas and Associated Center dentists. Line of aftercare maintenance products.

Cao Group, Inc. 801-256-9282
4628 Skyhawk Dr, West Jordan, UT 84084
Heat source for bleaching teeth.

Dp Manufacture Corp. 305-640-9894
1460 NW 107th Ave Ste H, Doral, FL 33172
Bleaching lights.

Lumalite, Inc. 800-400-2262
2830 Via Orange Way Ste B, Spring Valley, CA 91978
L.E.D. light source for bleaching teeth.

Miltex Dental Technologies, Inc. 516-576-6022
589 Davies Dr, York, PA 17402
Various.

Pac-Dent Intl., Inc. 909-839-0888
21078 Commerce Point Dr, Walnut, CA 91789
Ac powered device to apply to light to teeth after bleaching.

Shofu Dental Corporation 800-827-4638
1225 Stone Dr, San Marcos, CA 92078
NIVEOUS

Ultradent Products, Inc. 801-553-4586
505 W 10200 S, South Jordan, UT 84095
Accessory to laser for bleaching teeth.

Westside Packaging, Llc. 909-570-3508
1700 S Baker Ave Ste A, Ontario, CA 91761
Ac powered device applying light to teeth.

SOURCE, ISOTOPE, SEALED, GOLD, TITANIUM, PLATINUM
(Radiology) 90IWI

Medi-Physics, Inc., Dba Ge Healthcare 800-633-4123
3350 N Ridge Ave, Arlington Heights, IL 60004
Iodine-125 rapid strand.

Wilkinson Company, Inc. 208-777-8332
590 S Clearwater Loop Ste C, Post Falls, ID 83854

SOURCE, RADIOISOTOPE REFERENCE *(Chemistry) 75UIC*

Capintec, Inc. 800-631-3826
6 Arrow Rd, Ramsey, NJ 07446

Isotope Products Laboratories, Inc. 661-309-1010
24937 Avenue Tibbitts, Valencia, CA 91355

SOURCE, TELETHERAPY, RADIONUCLIDE *(Radiology) 90IWH*

Alpha-Omega Services, Inc. 800-346-7894
9156 Rose St, Bellflower, CA 90706
Radioactive source and treatment units (cobalt). Iridium seeds for interstitial implants, brachytherapy and endocurietherapy supplies and accessories.

SOURCE, TELETHERAPY, RADIONUCLIDE *(cont'd)*

Best Medical International, Inc. 800-336-4970
7643 Fullerton Rd, Springfield, VA 22153
All accessories for mold room, positioning devices, styrofoam, Bolus, low-melting alloy, trays, Aqua plast etc.

International Isotopes Inc. 800-699-3108
4137 Commerce Cir, Idaho Falls, ID 83401

Neutron Products Inc 800-424-8169
22301 Mount Ephraim Rd # 68, Dickerson, MD 20842
Cobalt-60 teletherapy sources for units manufactured by AECL/Theratronics/MDSNordon, Picker/AMS, TEM Instruments, Siemens, Toshiba and CIS-bio.

Neutron Products, Inc. 301-349-5001
22301 Mount Ephraim Rd, Dickerson, MD 20842

SOURCE, WIRE, RADIOACTIVE IRIDIUM *(Radiology) 90IWA*

Alpha-Omega Services, Inc. 800-346-7894
9156 Rose St, Bellflower, CA 90706
Seeds for interstitial implants & iridium/platinum isotope seeds. 10 curie iridium-192 sources for high dose remote afterloading.

Starmet Corporation 978-369-5410
2229 Main St, Concord, MA 01742

SPACER, CEMENT *(Orthopedics) 87LTO*

Depuy Orthopaedics, Inc. 800-473-3789
700 Orthopaedic Dr, P.O. Box 988, Warsaw, IN 46582
Various types of cement spacers.

Depuy-Raynham, A Div. Of Depuy Orthopaedics 800-451-2006
325 Paramount Dr, Raynham, MA 02767
Various types of cement spacers.

SPACER, TENDON *(Orthopedics) 87UBS*

Technical Products, Inc. 800-226-8434
805 Marathon Pkwy Ste 150, Lawrenceville, GA 30046
Silicone oval shapes; 24-cm lengths. See Web site for dimensions.

SPATULA, BRAIN *(Cns/Neurology) 84RUD*

Codman & Shurtleff, Inc 800-225-0460
325 Paramount Dr, Raynham, MA 02767

Miltex Inc. 800-645-8000
589 Davies Dr, York, PA 17402

Zimmer Holdings, Inc. 800-613-6131
1800 W Center St, PO Box 708, Warsaw, IN 46580

SPATULA, CEMENT *(Dental And Oral) 76RUE*

Hu-Friedy Manufacturing Co., Inc. 800-483-7433
3232 N Rockwell St, Chicago, IL 60618
$21.55 to $27.55.

Ivoclar Vivadent, Inc. 800-533-6825
175 Pineview Dr, Amherst, NY 14228

Miltex Inc. 800-645-8000
589 Davies Dr, York, PA 17402

Moyco Technologies, Inc. 800-331-8837
200 Commerce Dr, Montgomeryville, PA 18936

Wehmer Corporation 800-323-0229
1151 N Main St, Lombard, IL 60148
$650 for vacuum spatulator.

SPATULA, CERVICAL, CYTOLOGY *(Obstetrics/Gyn) 85HHT*

Amsino International, Inc. 800-MD-AMSINO
855 Towne Center Dr, Pomona, CA 91767
AMSINO Ayres style, white birch, 7 in. 500/BOX 10 BOX/CS. Item AS025.

C & A Scientific Co. Inc. 703-330-1413
7241 Gabe Ct, Manassas, VA 20109
PREMIERE Wood cervical scrapers in two styles.

Canadian Medical Brush, Inc. 905-405-1075
11-7686 Kimbel St, Mississauga L5S 1E9 Canada
Non sterile cytology brush cmb 1010

Centurion Medical Products Corp. 517-545-1135
3310 S Main St, Salisbury, NC 28147

Diamics, Inc. 415-883-0414
6 Hamilton Lndg Ste 200, Novato, CA 94949
Cercol cervical sample collector.

Kentron Health Care, Inc. 615-384-0573
3604 Kelton Jackson Rd, P.o. Box 120, Springfield, TN 37172
Wooden cervical scrapers.

Milex Products, Inc. 800-621-1278
4311 N Normandy Ave, Chicago, IL 60634
$0.20 each in quantities of 500.

SPATULA, CERVICAL, CYTOLOGY *(cont'd)*

Puritan Medical Products Company Llc 800-321-2313
31 School St., Guilford, ME 04443-0149

Qiagen Gaithersburg, Inc. 800-344-3631
1201 Clopper Rd, Gaithersburg, MD 20878
Cervical brush and specimen transport media (stm).

Solon Manufacturing Co. 800-341-6640
338 Madison Ave Ste 7, Skowhegan, ME 04976
7-in. sterile or non-sterile, smooth finish, white birch wood. Four styles available.

Statlab Medical Products, Inc. 800-442-3573
106 Hillside Dr, Lewisville, TX 75057
ANAPATH, wood and plastic.

Team Technologies, Inc. 423-587-2199
5949 Commerce Blvd, Morristown, TN 37814
Twisted wire brush.

Tri-State Hospital Supply Corp. 517-545-1135
3173 E 43rd St, Yuma, AZ 85365

Wallach Surgical Devices, Inc. 800-243-2463
235 Edison Rd, Orange, CT 06477
Full-spectrum Cervical Cell Collector.

SPATULA, MIDDLE EAR *(Ear/Nose/Throat) 77RUG*

Bausch & Lomb Surgical 636-255-5051
3365 Tree Court Ind Blvd, Saint Louis, MO 63122

Jedmed Instruments Co. 314-845-3770
5416 Jedmed Ct, Saint Louis, MO 63129

Miltex Inc. 800-645-8000
589 Davies Dr, York, PA 17402

SPATULA, OPHTHALMIC *(Ophthalmology) 86HND*

Accutome, Inc. 610-889-0200
3222 Phoenixville Pike, Malvern, PA 19355
Spatula.

Addition Technology, Inc. • 847-297-8419
155 Moffett Park Dr Ste B-1, Sunnyvale, CA 94089

Akorn, Inc. 800-535-7155
2500 Millbrook Dr, Buffalo Grove, IL 60089
Titanium lens spatula, Sinskey II, Kuglen and Lester plus diamond knives and other titanium instruments.

B. Graczyk, Inc. 269-782-2100
27826 Burmax Park, Dowagiac, MI 49047
Various types of spatulas sterile & non-sterile.

Back-Mueller, Inc. 314-531-6640
2700 Clark Ave, Saint Louis, MO 63103
Various types of spatulas.

Bausch & Lomb Surgical 636-255-5051
3365 Tree Court Ind Blvd, Saint Louis, MO 63122

Demetech Corp. 888-324-2447
3530 NW 115th Ave, Doral, FL 33178
Ophthalmic spatula.

Diamond Edge Co. 727-586-2927
928 W Bay Dr, Largo, FL 33770
Spatula.

Fischer Surgical Inc. 314-303-7753
1343 Pine Dr, Arnold, MO 63010
Various types of ophthalmic spatulas.

Fortrad Eye Instruments Corp. 973-543-2371
8 Franklin Rd, Mendham, NJ 07945

George Tiemann & Co. 800-843-6266
25 Plant Ave, Hauppauge, NY 11788

Hai Laboratories, Inc. 781-862-9884
320 Massachusetts Ave, Lexington, MA 02420
Ophthalmic spatula - various types.

Jedmed Instruments Co. 314-845-3770
5416 Jedmed Ct, Saint Louis, MO 63129

Katena Products, Inc. 800-225-1195
4 Stewart Ct, Denville, NJ 07834

Medone Surgical, Inc. 941-359-3129
670 Tallevast Rd, Sarasota, FL 34243
Various styles of spatulas.

Micro Medical Instruments 314-845-3663
123 Cliff Cave Rd, Saint Louis, MO 63129
Spatula, ophthalmic.

Microsurgical Technology, Inc. 425-556-0544
PO Box 2679, Redmond, WA 98073

SPATULA, OPHTHALMIC *(cont'd)*

Miltex Inc. 800-645-8000
589 Davies Dr, York, PA 17402

Psi/Eye-Ko, Inc. 636-447-1010
804 Corporate Centre Dr, O Fallon, MO 63368
Bechert roatotor; irrigrating vectis; simcole nucleus spatula.

Stephens Instruments, Inc. 800-354-7848
2500 Sandersville Rd, Lexington, KY 40511
$40.00 per unit (standard).

Surgical Instrument Manufacturers, Inc. 800-521-2985
1650 Headland Dr, Fenton, MO 63026

Total Titanium, Inc. 618-473-2429
140 East Monroe St., Hecker, IL 62248
Various types of ophthalmic spatulas.

SPATULA, OTHER *(Surgery) 79RUH*

Akorn, Inc. 800-535-7155
2500 Millbrook Dr, Buffalo Grove, IL 60089
Rothchild double-ended PRK Instrument. Spatula for removing epithelium on one end, 7mm optical zone marker on opposite end.

Carolina Biological Supply Co. 800-334-5551
2700 York Rd, Burlington, NC 27215

Fortrad Eye Instruments Corp. 973-543-2371
8 Franklin Rd, Mendham, NJ 07945

Miltex Inc. 800-645-8000
589 Davies Dr, York, PA 17402

Wehmer Corporation 800-323-0229
1151 N Main St, Lombard, IL 60148
Vacuum spatulator: to be used with dental plastic.

SPATULA, SURGICAL, GENERAL & PLASTIC SURGERY *(Surgery) 79GAF*

Aesculap Implant Systems Inc. 1-800-234-9179
3773 Corporate Pkwy, Center Valley, PA 18034

Bausch & Lomb Surgical 636-255-5051
3365 Tree Court Ind Blvd, Saint Louis, MO 63122

Biomet Microfixation Inc. 800-874-7711
1520 Tradeport Dr, Jacksonville, FL 32218
Spatula, surgical, general & plastic surgery.

Biomet, Inc. 574-267-6639
56 E Bell Dr, PO Box 587, Warsaw, IN 46582
Various types of spatula.

Dental Usa, Inc. 815-363-8003
5005 McCullom Lake Rd, McHenry, IL 60050
Dental spatula.

Jedmed Instruments Co. 314-845-3770
5416 Jedmed Ct, Saint Louis, MO 63129

Synthes (Usa) - Development Center 719-481-5300
1230 Wilson Dr, West Chester, PA 19380
Spatula, surgical.

Temrex Corp. 516-868-6221
112 Albany Ave, P.o. Box 182, Freeport, NY 11520
Various sizes + styles of spatulas.

Total Molding Services, Inc. 215-538-9613
354 East Broad St., Trumbauersville, PA 18970
Various Styles: Disk Spatula single Use Lap Cautery Probe.

Trans American Medical / Tamsco Instruments 708-430-7777
7633 W 100th Pl, Bridgeview, IL 60455

Tuzik Boston 800-886-6363
104 Longwater Dr, Assinippi Park, Norwell, MA 02061

Zimmer Holdings, Inc. 800-613-6131
1800 W Center St, PO Box 708, Warsaw, IN 46580

SPECTACLE MICROSCOPE, LOW-VISION *(Ophthalmology) 86HKC*

Bio-Optics, Inc. 503-493-8000
1525 NE 41st Ave, Portland, OR 97232
Specular Microscope Contact and noncontact clinical and eye bank specular microscopes for photographing & documenting ocular tissue.

Mastel Precision, Inc. 800-657-8057
2843 Samco Rd Unit A, Rapid City, SD 57702
Spectacle microscope, low-vision.

SPECTACLE, MAGNIFIER *(Ophthalmology) 86HOI*

Ctp Coil Inc. 800-933-2645
1801 Howard St Ste D, Elk Grove Village, IL 60007
Face mounted spectacle binoculars and hyperocular microscopic spectacles.

E-Z-Em, Inc. 516-333-8230
750 Summa Ave, Westbury, NY 11590
Amnicentesis needle.

Edmund Industrial Optics 800-363-1992
101 E Gloucester Pike, Barrington, NJ 08007

Edroy Products Co., Inc. 800-233-8803
245 N Midland Ave, PO Box 998, Nyack, NY 10960
OPTICAID clip-on, $21.10-23.10 per unit, 1.5, 1.75, 2.00, 2.25, 2.75, 3.5x (standard). OPTICAID SPRING-TOP, $26.45-28.10 per unit. 1.5, 1.75, 2.00, 2.25, 2.75, 3.5x.

Eschenbach Optik Of America, Inc. 800-487-5389
904 Ethan Allen Hwy, Ridgefield, CT 06877

Eye Care And Cure 800-486-6169
4646 S Overland Dr, Tucson, AZ 85714
Reading glasses.

Greattec Vision S.A. De C.V.
Circuito De La Amistad #2700, Mexicali B.c. Mexico
Spectacle, magnifying

Lehrer Brillenperfektion Werks, Inc. 818-407-1890
3908 N 5th St, North Las Vegas, NV 89032
Reading glasses.

Magnivision, Inc. 954-986-9000
3700 Commerce Pkwy, Miramar, FL 33025
Reading glasses - over the counter.

Marcolin Usa 888-627-2654
7543 E Tierra Buena Ln, Scottsdale, AZ 85260

Peter M. Tolliver 585-244-8788
42 Varinna Dr, Rochester, NY 14618
Low vision aid; to compensate for homoymous hemianopsia.

SPECTACLE, OPERATING (LOUPE), OPHTHALMIC *(Ophthalmology) 86HOH*

B. Graczyk, Inc. 269-782-2100
27826 Burmax Park, Dowagiac, MI 49047
Various styles of loupes.

Eschenbach Optik Of America, Inc. 800-487-5389
904 Ethan Allen Hwy, Ridgefield, CT 06877

Jedmed Instruments Co. 314-845-3770
5416 Jedmed Ct, Saint Louis, MO 63129

Laservision Usa 651-357-1800
595 Phalen Blvd, Saint Paul, MN 55130

SPECTROGRAPH, MASS *(Chemistry) 75UGU*

Headwall Photonics, Inc. 978-353-4100
601 River St, Fitchburg, MA 01420
Single or dual beam, designed for research or OEM.

Myco Instrumentation Source, Inc. 425-228-4239
PO Box 354, Renton, WA 98057

Spectron Corp. 425-827-9317
934 S Burlington Blvd # 603, Burlington, WA 98233
Reconditioned equipment.

Thermo - Industrial Hygiene Division 508-520-0430
27 Forge Pkwy, Franklin, MA 02038

Thermo Oriel 800-715-393
150 Long Beach Blvd, Stratford, CT 06615

Vacumed 800-235-3333
4538 Westinghouse St, Ventura, CA 93003
Supplies and accessories for mass spectroscopy.

SPECTROMETER, INFRARED *(Chemistry) 75WHI*

Analytical Spectral Devices, Inc. 303-444-6522
2555 55th St Ste A, Boulder, CO 80301

Bomem Inc. 800-858-FTIR
585 Charest Blvd. East, Suite 300, Quebec City, QUE G1K-9H4 Canada
Infrared spectrometer with .002cm resolution for QC applications. CHIRALIR- VDC spectrometer for chiral molecule analysis.

Guided Wave Inc. 916-939-4300
5190 Golden Foothill Pkwy, El Dorado Hills, CA 95762
NIR Spectroscopy- Process Analysis

SPECTROMETER, INFRARED *(cont'd)*

Labsphere, Inc. 603-927-4266
231 Shaker St., North Sutton, NH 03260-9986
Reflectance spectroscopy accessories for leading FTIR spectrometers permit accurate reflectance and transmittance measurement of scattering samples.

Olis: On-Line Instrument Systems, Inc. 800-852-3504
130 Conway Dr Ste A, Bogart, GA 30622
UV/VIS OLIS RSM (from $70,000) dual beam, rapid-scanning spectrometer for absorbance and fluorescence research; fully computerized.

Trace Laboratories-East 410-584-9099
5 N Park Dr, Hunt Valley, MD 21030

Waters Corp. 800-252-4752
34 Maple St, Milford, MA 01757

SPECTROMETER, NUCLEAR *(Chemistry) 75RUJ*

Canberra Industries 800-243-3955
800 Research Pkwy, Meriden, CT 06450

Ludlum Measurements, Inc. 800-622-0828
501 Oak St, Sweetwater, TX 79556
$4,250.00 for Model 42-5 neutron spectrometer.

SPECTROPHOTOMETER, ATOMIC ABSORPTION, GENERAL USE *(Toxicology) 91JXR*

Buck Scientific, Inc. 800-562-5566
58 Fort Point St, Norwalk, CT 06855
200--simple, sturdy, and one of the most sensitive available manual flames. 210--VGP built-in computer; 16-line LCD display; cookbook in memory and room for 90 to 100 more procedures; unique Graphie furnace; 2-background correction system.

SPECTROPHOTOMETER, FLUORESCENCE *(Chemistry) 75RUL*

Hitachi High Technologies America, Inc. 800-548-9001
3100 N 1st St, San Jose, CA 95134
Offering two models of fluorescence spectrophotometers, the F-2500 and F-7000 with a wide range of accessories.

Jasco, Inc. 800-333-5272
8649 Commerce Dr, Easton, MD 21601

Photon Technology International, Inc. 609-894-4420
300 Birmingham Road, Birmingham, NJ 08011-0272
TIMEMASTER, Fluorescence Lifetime Spectrometer, uses time-domain techniques to measure fluorescence lifetimes as low as 100 picoseconds. RATIO MASTER, dual wavelength spectrofluorometer for detection of calcium and other ions, using patented deltascan illuminator. IMAGEMASTER, quantitative ratio fluorescence imaging system for spatial detection of calcium and other ions in living cells.

Thermo Spectronic 800-654-9955
820 Linden Ave, Rochester, NY 14625
Fluorescence spectrofluorometer and lifetime spectrofluorometer; 3-kilobar high-pressure spectroscopy cell; epifluorescence microscope interface for T-OPTICS spectrofluorometer. Multiparameter cation-measuring spectrophotometer, multi-harmonic Fourier fluorometer.

SPECTROPHOTOMETER, INFRARED *(Chemistry) 75RUM*

Analytical Spectral Devices, Inc. 303-444-6522
2555 55th St Ste A, Boulder, CO 80301

Buck Scientific, Inc. 800-562-5566
58 Fort Point St, Norwalk, CT 06855
M500 Scanning. 4000 to 600 cm-1. Complete with software.

Harrick Scientific Products, Inc. 800-248-3847
141 Tomkins Avenue, Pleasantville, N 10570 United

Horiba Jobin Yvon Inc 866-JOBINYVON
3880 Park Ave, Edison, NJ 08820

Infrared Fiber Systems, Inc. 301-622-7131
2301 Broadbirch Dr Ste A, Silver Spring, MD 20904
Spectrophotometer, infrared.

Jasco, Inc. 800-333-5272
8649 Commerce Dr, Easton, MD 21601

Labsphere, Inc. 603-927-4266
231 Shaker St., North Sutton, NH 03260-9986
Reflectance spectroscopy accessories for leading FTIR spectrometers permit accurate reflectance and transmittance measurement of scattering samples.

SPECTROPHOTOMETER, U.V./VISIBLE *(Chemistry) 75RUO*

Beckman Coulter, Inc. 800-742-2345
250 S Kraemer Blvd, PO Box 8000, Brea, CA 92821

SPECTROPHOTOMETER, U.V./VISIBLE *(cont'd)*

Buck Scientific, Inc. 800-562-5566
58 Fort Point St, Norwalk, CT 06855
CECIL complete series of UV/basic to R&D grade.

Headwall Photonics, Inc. 978-353-4100
601 River St, Fitchburg, MA 01420
Spectrometer, UV - NIR; Holographic Diffraction Gratings.

Hitachi High Technologies America, Inc. 800-548-9001
3100 N 1st St, San Jose, CA 95134
Hitachi offers a wide range of UV-Visible Spectroscopy systems, from routine to research grade.

Intersciences Inc. 800-661-6431
169 Idema Rd., Markham, ONT L3R 1A9 Canada

Jasco, Inc. 800-333-5272
8649 Commerce Dr, Easton, MD 21601

Labsphere, Inc. 603-927-4266
231 Shaker St., North Sutton, NH 03260-9986
Reflectance spectroscopy accessories for most leading analytical spectrophotometers.

Medicos Laboratories, Inc. (Mdt) 800-724-4003
801 Montrose Ave, South Plainfield, NJ 07080

Mg Scientific, Inc. 800-343-8338
8500 107th St, Pleasant Prairie, WI 53158

Molecular Devices Corp. 800-635-5577
1311 Orleans Dr, Sunnyvale, CA 94089
SPECTRAMAX 340 and SPECTRAMAX 190, $12,000.00 to $25,000.00; are 96-well spectrophotometers.

Olis: On-Line Instrument Systems, Inc. 800-852-3504
130 Conway Dr Ste A, Bogart, GA 30622
UV/VIS/NIR OLIS 14 (from $35,000) dual beam, high resolution spectrophotometer with 180-2600nm spectral range; fully computerized operation.

Omega Engineering, Inc. 800-848-4286
1 Omega Dr, Stamford, CT 06907

Photon Technology International, Inc. 609-894-4420
300 Birmingham Road, Birmingham, NJ 08011-0272
QUANTAMASTER, steady-state fluorescence & phosphorescence spectrometer.

Princeton Instruments - Acton 978-263-3584
15 Discovery Way, Acton, MA 01720

Spectral Instruments, Inc. 520-884-8821
420 N Bonita Ave, Tucson, AZ 85745

Spectrex Corp. 800-822-3940
3580 Haven Ave, Redwood City, CA 94063
$7,500.00 for direct-reading spectroscope.

Spectron Corp. 425-827-9317
934 S Burlington Blvd # 603, Burlington, WA 98233

Terumo Medical Corp. 800-283-7866
2101 Cottontail Ln, Somerset, NJ 08873

Thermo Spectronic 800-654-9955
820 Linden Ave, Rochester, NY 14625
Dual-wavelength and diode-array spectrophotometers.

United Products & Instruments, Inc. 800-588-9776
182 Ridge Rd Ste E, Dayton, NJ 08810
Unico is proud to introduce the all new complete SpectroQuest line of UV-Visible spectrophotometers. All SpectroQuest spectrophotometers features high performance sealed optics mounted on a stable machined platform. The innovative optical layout and state of art monochromator with high grade blazed holographic grating ensure accuracy. Its integrated design assures long term stability and durability. The precisely aligned detector and quality deuterium and halogen lamps enhance

Waters Corp. 800-252-4752
34 Maple St, Milford, MA 01757

SPECTROPHOTOMETER, ULTRAVIOLET *(Chemistry) 75RUN*

Beckman Coulter, Inc. 800-742-2345
250 S Kraemer Blvd, PO Box 8000, Brea, CA 92821

Harrick Scientific Products, Inc. 800-248-3847
141 Tomkins Avenue, Pleasantville, N 10570 United

Horiba Jobin Yvon Inc 866-JOBINYVON
3880 Park Ave, Edison, NJ 08820

Jasco, Inc. 800-333-5272
8649 Commerce Dr, Easton, MD 21601
$7,800.00 per unit (standard).

SPECTROPHOTOMETER, VISIBLE *(Chemistry) 75RUP*

Analytical Spectral Devices, Inc. 303-444-6522
2555 55th St Ste A, Boulder, CO 80301

Beckman Coulter, Inc. 800-742-2345
250 S Kraemer Blvd, PO Box 8000, Brea, CA 92821

Horiba Jobin Yvon Inc 866-JOBINYVON
3880 Park Ave, Edison, NJ 08820

Hunter Associates Lab., Inc. 703-471-6870
11491 Sunset Hills Rd, Reston, VA 20190
These instruments measure the reflected or transmitted color of a wide range of pharmaceutical products. Use them to measure the reflected color of tablets, caplets, capsules and dip strips or to measure the color of clear liquids such as increasing yellowness with drug aging.

Jasco, Inc. 800-333-5272
8649 Commerce Dr, Easton, MD 21601

Optometrics Llc 978-772-1700
8 Nemco Way, Stony Brook Ind. Pk., Ayer, MA 01432
Clinical spectrophotometer with grating monochromator has built-in sipper with electrical temperature control of flowcell and printer. Performs 35 tests.

United Products & Instruments, Inc. 800-588-9776
182 Ridge Rd Ste E, Dayton, NJ 08810
UNICO has added a new reliable model to their economic line. The Model 1200 allows for Absorbance, Transmittance and Concentration modes, it also allows for automatic zeroing and blanking with a single button. Model 1200 features optional Window® based software for easy data collection for Microsoft Excel®. A tool-free and alignment

SPECTROPHOTOMETRIC, UROPORPHYRIN *(Chemistry) 75JQL*

Bio-Rad Laboratories Inc., Clinical Systems Div. 800-224-6723
4000 Alfred Nobel Dr, Hercules, CA 94547
Porphyrins test system.

SPECULUM, EAR *(Ear/Nose/Throat) 77EPY*

Aesculap Implant Systems Inc. 1-800-234-9179
3773 Corporate Pkwy, Center Valley, PA 18034
ENT.

Bausch & Lomb Surgical 636-255-5051
3365 Tree Court Ind Blvd, Saint Louis, MO 63122

Biomet Microfixation Inc. 800-874-7711
1520 Tradeport Dr, Jacksonville, FL 32218
Various types of speculums.

Bionix Development Corp. 800-551-7096
5154 Enterprise Blvd, Toledo, OH 43612
Bionix disposable nasal speculum.

Cameron-Miller, Inc. 800-621-0142
5410 W Roosevelt Rd, Road #241, Chicago, IL 60644

Centurion Medical Products Corp. 517-545-1135
3310 S Main St, Salisbury, NC 28147

Codman & Shurtleff, Inc 800-225-0460
325 Paramount Dr, Raynham, MA 02767

Elmed, Inc. 630-543-2792
60 W Fay Ave, Addison, IL 60101

Gyrus Ent L.L.C., Sub. Of Gyrus Acmi, Inc. 508-804-2739
2925 Appling Rd, Bartlett, TN 38133
Various types of ent speculum.

H & H Co. 909-390-0373
4435 E Airport Dr Ste 108, Ontario, CA 91761
Nasal speculum.

Jedmed Instruments Co. 314-845-3770
5416 Jedmed Ct, Saint Louis, MO 63129

Md International, Inc. 305-669-9003
11300 NW 41st St, Doral, FL 33178

Micrins Surgical Instruments, Inc. 800-833-3380
28438 N Ballard Dr, Lake Forest, IL 60045

Miltex Inc. 800-645-8000
589 Davies Dr, York, PA 17402

Princeton Medical Group, Inc. 800-875-0869
1189 Royal Links Dr, Mt Pleasant, SC 29466

Propper Manufacturing Co., Inc. 800-832-4300
3604 Skillman Ave, Long Island City, NY 11101

Prosurge Instruments, Inc. 866-832-7874
199 Laidlaw Ave, Jersey City, NJ 07306

Shoney Scientific, Inc. 262-970-0170
West 223 North 720 Saratoga Drive,, Suite 120, Waukesha, WI 53186
Nasal speculum.

SPECULUM, EAR *(cont'd)*

Speclinc 731-286-4211
361 Haynes Rd, Dyersburg, TN 38024
Otoscope speculum.

Trans American Medical / Tamsco Instruments 708-430-7777
7633 W 100th Pl, Bridgeview, IL 60455

Tri-State Hospital Supply Corp. 517-545-1135
3173 E 43rd St, Yuma, AZ 85365

Tuzik Boston 800-886-6363
104 Longwater Dr, Assinippi Park, Norwell, MA 02061

Welch Allyn, Inc. 800-535-6663
4341 State Street Rd, Skaneateles Falls, NY 13153

SPECULUM, ILLUMINATED *(Surgery) 79FXF*

Cameron-Miller, Inc. 800-621-0142
5410 W Roosevelt Rd, Road #241, Chicago, IL 60644

Electro Surgical Instrument Co., Inc. 888-464-2784
37 Centennial St, Rochester, NY 14611
Various types and sizes of fiberoptic lighted specula.

SPECULUM, NASAL *(Ear/Nose/Throat) 77RUR*

Bausch & Lomb Surgical 636-255-5051
3365 Tree Court Ind Blvd, Saint Louis, MO 63122

Codman & Shurtleff, Inc 800-225-0460
325 Paramount Dr, Raynham, MA 02767

Elmed, Inc. 630-543-2792
60 W Fay Ave, Addison, IL 60101

Jedmed Instruments Co. 314-845-3770
5416 Jedmed Ct, Saint Louis, MO 63129

Md International, Inc. 305-669-9003
11300 NW 41st St, Doral, FL 33178

Miltex Inc. 800-645-8000
589 Davies Dr, York, PA 17402

Propper Manufacturing Co., Inc. 800-832-4300
3604 Skillman Ave, Long Island City, NY 11101

Prosurge Instruments, Inc. 866-832-7874
199 Laidlaw Ave, Jersey City, NJ 07306

Trans American Medical / Tamsco Instruments 708-430-7777
7633 W 100th Pl, Bridgeview, IL 60455

Welch Allyn, Inc. 800-535-6663
4341 State Street Rd, Skaneateles Falls, NY 13153

SPECULUM, NON-ILLUMINATED *(Surgery) 79FXE*

Biomet Microfixation Inc. 800-874-7711
1520 Tradeport Dr, Jacksonville, FL 32218
Various types of speculums.

Cardinal Health, Snowden Pencer Products 847-689-8410
5175 S Royal Atlanta Dr, Tucker, GA 30084
Various types of speculums.

Kmi Kolster Methods, Inc. 909-737-5476
3185 Palisades Dr, Corona, CA 92880
Speculum.

Olsen Medical 800-297-6344
3001 W Kentucky St, Louisville, KY 40211
Graves Speculum with and without smoke tube. Open sided speculum.

SPECULUM, OPHTHALMIC *(Ophthalmology) 86HNC*

Accutome, Inc. 610-889-0200
3222 Phoenixville Pike, Malvern, PA 19355
Specula.

B. Graczyk, Inc. 269-782-2100
27826 Burmax Park, Dowagiac, MI 49047
Various types of sterile & non-sterile specula.

Bausch & Lomb Surgical 636-255-5051
3365 Tree Court Ind Blvd, Saint Louis, MO 63122

Diamond Edge Co. 727-586-2927
928 W Bay Dr, Largo, FL 33770
Lid specula.

Elmed, Inc. 630-543-2792
60 W Fay Ave, Addison, IL 60101

Envision Eyes, Llc 303-880-1031
5368 Wildcat Ct, Morrison, CO 80465
Sterile and non-sterile disposable speculum.

Eye Care And Cure 800-486-6169
4646 S Overland Dr, Tucson, AZ 85714
Speculum.

SPECULUM, OPHTHALMIC *(cont'd)*

Fischer Surgical Inc. 314-303-7753
1343 Pine Dr, Arnold, MO 63010
Various types of ophthalmic speculas.

Fortrad Eye Instruments Corp. 973-543-2371
8 Franklin Rd, Mendham, NJ 07945

Hai Laboratories, Inc. 781-862-9884
320 Massachusetts Ave, Lexington, MA 02420
Eye speculum - various types.

Harvey Precision Instruments 707-793-2600
217 Fairway Rd, Cape Haze, FL 33947
Wire, closed and adjustable eye specula and lid retractors.

Innovative Excimer Solutions, Inc. 416-410-1868
3340a Yonge St, Toronto M4N 2M4 Canada
Eye specula-barraquer

Jedmed Instruments Co. 314-845-3770
5416 Jedmed Ct, Saint Louis, MO 63129

Katena Products, Inc. 800-225-1195
4 Stewart Ct, Denville, NJ 07834

Miltex Inc. 800-645-8000
589 Davies Dr, York, PA 17402

Pedia Pals, Llc 888-733-4272
965 Highway 169 N, Plymouth, MN 55441
Opthalmoscope Mouse attachments, fits Welch Allyn opthalmoscopes.

Peregrine Surgical, Ltd. 215-348-0456
51 Britain Dr, Doylestown, PA 18901
Speculum, ophthalmic.

Princeton Medical Group, Inc. 800-875-0869
1189 Royal Links Dr, Mt Pleasant, SC 29466

Prosurge Instruments, Inc. 866-832-7874
199 Laidlaw Ave, Jersey City, NJ 07306

Psi/Eye-Ko, Inc. 636-447-1010
804 Corporate Centre Dr, O Fallon, MO 63368
Barraquer infant; barraquer spread blade; katz eye.

Stephens Instruments, Inc. 800-354-7848
2500 Sandersville Rd, Lexington, KY 40511
$15.00 each.

Surgical Instrument Manufacturers, Inc. 800-521-2985
1650 Headland Dr, Fenton, MO 63026

Total Titanium, Inc. 618-473-2429
140 East Monroe St., Hecker, IL 62248
Various types of ophthalmic specula.

SPECULUM, OTHER *(General) 80RUS*

Astralite Corporation 800-345-7703
PO Box 689, Somerset, CA 95684
GYN-A-LITE illuminator, speculum, vaginal clips to speculum, low-voltage, special bulb projects beam.

Elmed, Inc. 630-543-2792
60 W Fay Ave, Addison, IL 60101

Fortrad Eye Instruments Corp. 973-543-2371
8 Franklin Rd, Mendham, NJ 07945

Kmedic 800-955-0559
190 Veterans Dr, Northvale, NJ 07647

SPECULUM, RECTAL *(Gastro/Urology) 78FFQ*

Aesculap Implant Systems Inc. 1-800-234-9179
3773 Corporate Pkwy, Center Valley, PA 18034

Biomet Microfixation Inc. 800-874-7711
1520 Tradeport Dr, Jacksonville, FL 32218
Various types of speculums.

Clearwater Colon Hydrotherapy, Inc. 888-869-6191
3145 SW 74th Ter, Ocala, FL 34474
Speculum, rectal.

Codman & Shurtleff, Inc 800-225-0460
325 Paramount Dr, Raynham, MA 02767

Electro Surgical Instrument Co., Inc. 888-464-2784
37 Centennial St, Rochester, NY 14611
Various types, sizes and styles of lighted and unlighted rectal specula.

Elmed, Inc. 630-543-2792
60 W Fay Ave, Addison, IL 60101

Kmedic 800-955-0559
190 Veterans Dr, Northvale, NJ 07647

Miltex Inc. 800-645-8000
589 Davies Dr, York, PA 17402

SPECULUM, RECTAL *(cont'd)*

Monarch Molding Inc. 888-767-5116
120 Liberty St, Council Grove, KS 66846
$0.9975 each for rectal Disposo-Scope (9cm). Professional price.

Prosurge Instruments, Inc. 866-832-7874
199 Laidlaw Ave, Jersey City, NJ 07306

Tuzik Boston 800-886-6363
104 Longwater Dr, Assinippi Park, Norwell, MA 02061

Ultimate Concepts, Inc. 801-566-3241
5056 Crimson Patch Way, Riverton, UT 84096
Cleansing tip.

Welch Allyn, Inc. 800-535-6663
4341 State Street Rd, Skaneateles Falls, NY 13153

SPECULUM, VAGINAL, METAL *(Obstetrics/Gyn) 85HDF*

Biomet Microfixation Inc. 800-874-7711
1520 Tradeport Dr, Jacksonville, FL 32218
Various types of speculums.

Cameron-Miller, Inc. 800-621-0142
5410 W Roosevelt Rd, Road #241, Chicago, IL 60644

Centurion Medical Products Corp. 517-545-1135
3310 S Main St, Salisbury, NC 28147

Codman & Shurtleff, Inc 800-225-0460
325 Paramount Dr, Raynham, MA 02767

Coopersurgical, Inc. 800-243-2974
95 Corporate Dr, Trumbull, CT 06611
29 different sizes and models.

Dental Usa, Inc. 815-363-8003
5005 McCullom Lake Rd, McHenry, IL 60050
Speculum.

Elmed, Inc. 630-543-2792
60 W Fay Ave, Addison, IL 60101

Fine Surgical Instrument, Inc. 800-851-5155
741 Peninsula Blvd, Hempstead, NY 11550

Health Care Logistics, Inc. 800-848-1633
450 Town St, PO Box 25, Circleville, OH 43113
Various types of vaginal speculums.

Her-Mar, Inc. 800-327-8209
8550 NW 30th Ter, Doral, FL 33122
3 sizes. $10.00 each.

Kmedic 800-955-0559
190 Veterans Dr, Northvale, NJ 07647

Kta, Instruments, Inc. 888-830-9KTA
3051 Brighton-Third St., 1st Fl., Brooklyn, NY 11235

Marina Medical Instruments, Inc. 800-697-1119
955 Shotgun Rd, Sunrise, FL 33326
Various.

Md International, Inc. 305-669-9003
11300 NW 41st St, Doral, FL 33178

Medgyn Products, Inc. 800-451-9667
328 Eisenhower Ln N, Lombard, IL 60148
Graves, Pederson & various types. All German stainless.

Miltex Inc. 800-645-8000
589 Davies Dr, York, PA 17402

Precision Medical Manufacturing Corporation 866-633-4626
852 Seton Ct, Wheeling, IL 60090
Guttmann Vaginal Speculum Positive self-retaining contoured blades designed to fit pubic arch and to maximaze pressure on soft tissue.

Premier Medical Products 888-PREMUSA
1710 Romano Dr, Plymouth Meeting, PA 19462

Princeton Medical Group, Inc. 800-875-0869
1189 Royal Links Dr, Mt Pleasant, SC 29466

Prosurge Instruments, Inc. 866-832-7874
199 Laidlaw Ave, Jersey City, NJ 07306

R Medical Supply 800-882-7578
620 Valley Forge Rd Ste F, Hillsborough, NC 27278

Richard Wolf Medical Instruments Corp. 800-323-9653
353 Corporate Woods Pkwy, Vernon Hills, IL 60061

Rocket Medical Plc. 800-707-7625
150 Recreation Park Dr Ste 3, Hingham, MA 02043

Schueler & Company, Inc. 516-487-1500
PO Box 528, Stratford, CT 06615

Trans American Medical / Tamsco Instruments 708-430-7777
7633 W 100th Pl, Bridgeview, IL 60455
Medium grade surgical stainless steel.

SPECULUM, VAGINAL, METAL *(cont'd)*

Tri-State Hospital Supply Corp. 517-545-1135
3173 E 43rd St, Yuma, AZ 85365

Tuzik Boston 800-886-6363
104 Longwater Dr, Assinippi Park, Norwell, MA 02061

Welch Allyn, Inc. 800-535-6663
4341 State Street Rd, Skaneateles Falls, NY 13153

SPECULUM, VAGINAL, METAL, FIBEROPTIC
(Obstetrics/Gyn) 85HDG

Codman & Shurtleff, Inc 800-225-0460
325 Paramount Dr, Raynham, MA 02767

Prosurge Instruments, Inc. 866-832-7874
199 Laidlaw Ave, Jersey City, NJ 07306

SPECULUM, VAGINAL, NON-METAL *(Obstetrics/Gyn) 85HIB*

Ac Healthcare Supply, Inc. 905-448-4706
11651 230th St, Cambria Heights, NY 11411
Speculum, vaginal, nonmetal.

Advanced Medical Devices, Inc. 416-833-6681
15 Keele Street South Unit 2, Po Box 520, King City L7B 1A7 Canada
Speculum, vaginal, nonmetal

Amsino International, Inc. 800-MD-AMSINO
855 Towne Center Dr, Pomona, CA 91767
AMSINO available in small and medium 100/CS or 240/CS. Items AS031 and AS032.

Astralite Corporation 800-345-7703
PO Box 689, Somerset, CA 95684
Sterilizable - excellent for x-ray/oncology.

Cameron-Miller, Inc. 800-621-0142
5410 W Roosevelt Rd, Road #241, Chicago, IL 60644

Directmed, Inc. 516-656-3377
150 Pratt Oval, Glen Cove, NY 11542
HOSPITAL'S SPEC sterile/non-sterile vaginal specula available in three sizes.

Feminica Inc. 514-875-4422
3216 Rue Monsabre, Montreal H1N 2L5 Canada
Vaginal speculum non-metallic disposable

Femsuite, Llc 415-561-2565
220 Halleck St Ste 120B, San Francisco, CA 94129
Disposable vaginal speculum.

Global Healthcare 800-601-3880
1495 Hembree Rd Ste 700, Roswell, GA 30076
Small, medium and large disposables.

Intermed Group, Inc. 561-586-3667
3550 23rd Ave S Ste 1, Lake Worth, FL 33461
Vaginal speculum, non-metal.

Kentron Health Care, Inc. 615-384-0573
3604 Kelton Jackson Rd, P.o. Box 120, Springfield, TN 37172
Disposable vaginal speculum.

Marina Medical Instruments, Inc. 800-697-1119
955 Shotgun Rd, Sunrise, FL 33326
Plastic speculum.

Md International, Inc. 305-669-9003
11300 NW 41st St, Doral, FL 33178

Medline Industries, Inc. 800-633-5886
1 Medline Pl, Mundelein, IL 60060

Medline Manufacturing And Services Llc 847-837-2759
1 Medline Pl, Mundelein, IL 60060
Vaginal speculum.

Miami Medical Equipment & Supply Corp. 305-592-0111
2150 NW 93rd Ave, Doral, FL 33172

Monarch Molding Inc. 888-767-5116
120 Liberty St, Council Grove, KS 66846
$0.63 per unit (medium and small). Professional price.

Ob Specialties, Inc. 800-325-6644
1799 Northwood Ct, Oakland, CA 94611
4-way Speculum.

Prd, Inc. 317-241-1111
747 Washboard Rd, Springville, IN 47462
Disposable vaginal speculum.

Redyref A Division Of Dawnex Industries 800-628-3603
3861 11th St, Long Island City, NY 11101
Disposable plastic vaginal speculum.

SPECULUM, VAGINAL, NON-METAL *(cont'd)*

Solon Manufacturing Co. 800-341-6640
338 Madison Ave Ste 7, Skowhegan, ME 04976
Small, medium, and large; six position; smooth edged plastic resin; pre-lubricated; single use.

Southern Tier Plastics, Inc. 607-723-2601
PO Box 2015, 94 Industrial Park, Binghamton, NY 13902

Specialty Manufacturers, Medical Products Division 317-241-1111
2410 Executive Dr, Indianapolis, IN 46241
Disposable vaginal speculum.

Welch Allyn, Inc. 800-535-6663
4341 State Street Rd, Skaneateles Falls, NY 13153

SPECULUM, VAGINAL, NON-METAL, FIBEROPTIC
(Obstetrics/Gyn) 85HIC

Alliance Precision Plastics 585-426-2630
595 Trabold Rd, Rochester, NY 14624
Vaginal speculum.

Doctors Research Group, Inc. 800-371-2535
574 Heritage Rd Ste 202, Southbury, CT 06488
Inflatable Vaginal Speculum

SPEECH THERAPY UNIT (TRAINER) *(Ear/Nose/Throat) 77RUT*

Kaypentax 800-289-5297
2 Bridgewater Ln, Lincoln Park, NJ 07035
Visi-Pitch displays intensity and pitch of speech for analysis and therapy of speech disorders; requires IBM-compatible PC.

Phonic Ear, Inc. 800-227-0735
3880 Cypress Dr, Petaluma, CA 94954

SPEECH TRAINING AID, AC-POWERED *(Ear/Nose/Throat) 77LEZ*

Intelligent Hearing Systems, Corp. 800-447-9783
6860 SW 81st St, Miami, FL 33143
LIPP easy and efficient computerized transcription and analysis system, which provides remappable keyboard, phonetic symbol generation, dictionaries, data storage and printing.

SPHERE, OPHTHALMIC (IMPLANT) *(Ophthalmology) 86HPZ*

Evera Medical, Inc. 650-287-2884
353 Vintage Park Dr Ste F, Foster City, CA 94404
Sterile augmentation implant.

Gulden Ophthalmics 800-659-2250
225 Cadwalader Ave, Elkins Park, PA 19027

Jardon Eye Prosthetics, Inc. 248-424-8560
15920 W 12 Mile Rd, Southfield, MI 48076
Silicone/also veterinary eye implants.

John J. Kelley Associates Ltd. 215-567-1377
1528 Walnut St Ste 1801, Mid City East, PA 19102
'mull sphere implant' (non-sterile).

Oculo Plastik Inc. 888-381-3292
200 Sauve West, Montreal, QUE H3L-1Y9 Canada
Various ocular implants Includes the NEW-ALLEN, UNIVERSAL, SILICONE and PMMA-SPHERES.

W.L. Gore & Associates,Inc 928-526-3030
1505 North Fourth St., Flagstaff, AZ 86004
Eye sphere implant.

SPHYGMOMANOMETER, ANEROID (ARTERIAL PRESSURE)
(General) 80FLY

Alimed, Inc. 800-225-2610
297 High St, Dedham, MA 02026

American Diagnostic Corporation (Adc) 800-232-2670
55 Commerce Dr, Hauppauge, NY 11788
Pocket, palm, multicuff, clock aneroid sphygs, accessories and replacement parts

Carolina Biological Supply Co. 800-334-5551
2700 York Rd, Burlington, NC 27215

Cypress Medical Products 800-334-3646
1202 S. Rte. 31, McHenry, IL 60050
Available in 5 calibrated cuff sizes from infant to thigh. Both latex and latex-free versions. 10yr warranty on guage.

Dixie Ems Supply 800-347-3494
385 Union Ave, Brooklyn, NY 11211
$19.90 per unit (portable, 300mm).

Global Healthcare 800-601-3880
1495 Hembree Rd Ste 700, Roswell, GA 30076

SPHYGMOMANOMETER, ANEROID (ARTERIAL PRESSURE)
(cont'd)

Hokanson Inc., D.E. 800-999-8251
12840 NE 21st Pl, Bellevue, WA 98005
The S300 aneroid sphygmomanometer inflates up to 300 mmHg.

Invacare Supply Group, An Invacare Co. 800-225-4792
75 October Hill Rd, Holliston, MA 01746
Carry full lines of blood pressure monitors from: Omron, Invacare.

Lydia's Professional Uniforms 800-942-3378
2547 3 Mile Rd NW Ste F, Grand Rapids, MI 49534

Md International, Inc. 305-669-9003
11300 NW 41st St, Doral, FL 33178

Ortho-Med, Inc. 800-547-5571
3208 SE 13th Ave, Portland, OR 97202

Prestige Medical Corporation 800-762-3333
8600 Wilbur Ave, Northridge, CA 91324

Propper Manufacturing Co., Inc. 800-832-4300
3604 Skillman Ave, Long Island City, NY 11101

Protector Canada Inc. 800-268-6594
1111 Flint Rd., Unit 23, Toronto, ON M3J 3C7 Canada
ACCOSON sphygmomanometers.

Schueler & Company, Inc. 516-487-1500
PO Box 528, Stratford, CT 06615

Terumo Cardiovascular Systems, Corp 800-521-2818
6200 Jackson Rd, Ann Arbor, MI 48103

Trimline Medical Products Corp. 800-526-3538
34 Columbia Rd, Branchburg, NJ 08876
HADER aneroid gauge; pocket type gauge with carrying case and inflation systems, all latex-free. Also available, large face aneroids in wall, stand and desk models.

Tuzik Boston 800-886-6363
104 Longwater Dr, Assinippi Park, Norwell, MA 02061

Welch Allyn, Inc. 800-535-6663
4341 State Street Rd, Skaneateles Falls, NY 13153

SPHYGMOMANOMETER, ELECTRONIC (ARTERIAL PRESSURE) *(General) 80THH*

Lumiscope Company, Inc. 800-672-8293
1035 Centennial Ave, Piscataway, NJ 08854
$59.95 for standard unit; $79.95 for unit with audible/visual display, microphone; $199.95 for uP-based, digital display unit with auto zero, memory and recall.

Lydia's Professional Uniforms 800-942-3378
2547 3 Mile Rd NW Ste F, Grand Rapids, MI 49534

SPHYGMOMANOMETER, ELECTRONIC, AUTOMATIC
(General) 80UDM

American Diagnostic Corporation (Adc) 800-232-2670
55 Commerce Dr, Hauppauge, NY 11788
Arm and wrist based digital blood pressure monitors

Armstrong Medical Industries, Inc. 800-323-4220
575 Knightsbridge Pkwy, Lincolnshire, IL 60069

Bio-Medical Instruments, Inc. 800-521-4640
2387 E 8 Mile Rd, Warren, MI 48091

Carolina Biological Supply Co. 800-334-5551
2700 York Rd, Burlington, NC 27215

Cas Medical Systems, Inc. 800-227-4414
44 E Industrial Rd, Branford, CT 06405
Neonatal and adult non-invasive blood-pressure monitor. Also available with pulse oximetry and temperature options.

Datascope Corp. 800-288-2121
14 Philips Pkwy, Montvale, NJ 07645
ACCUTORR 1A non-invasive blood pressure monitor with printer - ACCUTORR 2A non-invasive blood pressure monitor without printer.

Her-Mar, Inc. 800-327-8209
8550 NW 30th Ter, Doral, FL 33122
$80 for standard unit.

Md International, Inc. 305-669-9003
11300 NW 41st St, Doral, FL 33178

Mennen Medical Corp. 800-223-2201
2540 Metropolitan Dr, Trevose, PA 19053

Propper Manufacturing Co., Inc. 800-832-4300
3604 Skillman Ave, Long Island City, NY 11101

SPHYGMOMANOMETER, ELECTRONIC, AUTOMATIC *(cont'd)*

Science Products 800-888-7400
1043 Lancaster Ave, Berwyn, PA 19312
$229.00 for Model #1597 Voice Modulator Omron 747IC Sphygmo, easy-to-use blood pressure and pulse monitor. Displays and announces, systolic/diastolic and pulse. Voice Modular for Omron 747IC Professional Digital Blood Pressure Monitor.

Welch Allyn, Inc. 800-535-6663
4341 State Street Rd, Skaneateles Falls, NY 13153

SPHYGMOMANOMETER, ELECTRONIC, MANUAL
(General) 80UDN

A&D Medical 800-726-7099
1756 Automation Pkwy, San Jose, CA 95131
$39.95 for Model UA-704 hand held manual inflate digital, $49.95 UA-705 fully featured manual inflate digital. $89.95 for Model UA 767 one-step autoinflation, jumbo display. $129.95 for Model UA-853AC Premium autoinflation, fuzzy logic. UA-787EJ Quick Response with Easy Fit Cuff feature; UA-767P One Step Plus Memory; UB-511 Wrist Ultra Compact; UB-328 Wrist Auto-Inflation, UB-512 Dual Memory Wrist.

American Bantex Corp. 800-633-4839
1815 Rollins Rd, Burlingame, CA 94010

American Diagnostic Corporation (Adc) 800-232-2670
55 Commerce Dr, Hauppauge, NY 11788
Arm manual inflate blood pressure monitors

Armstrong Medical Industries, Inc. 800-323-4220
575 Knightsbridge Pkwy, Lincolnshire, IL 60069

Carolina Biological Supply Co. 800-334-5551
2700 York Rd, Burlington, NC 27215

Crest Healthcare Supply 800-328-8908
195 3rd St, Dassel, MN 55325

Frontier Medical Products, Inc. 800-367-6828
140 S Park St, Port Washington, WI 53074

Her-Mar, Inc. 800-327-8209
8550 NW 30th Ter, Doral, FL 33122
$50.00 for standard unit.

Lumiscope Company, Inc. 800-672-8293
1035 Centennial Ave, Piscataway, NJ 08854

O&M Enterprise 847-258-4515
641 Chelmsford Ln, Elk Grove Village, IL 60007
SPHYGMOMANOMETER ELECTRONIC/MANUAL

Propper Manufacturing Co., Inc. 800-832-4300
3604 Skillman Ave, Long Island City, NY 11101

Rockford Medical & Safety Co. 800-435-9451
2420 Harrison Ave, PO Box 5646, Rockford, IL 61108

SPHYGMOMANOMETER, MERCURY (ARTERIAL PRESSURE)
(General) 80FLX

American Diagnostic Corporation (Adc) 800-232-2670
55 Commerce Dr, Hauppauge, NY 11788
desk, wall, and mobile mercury sphygs, accessories and replacement parts

Her-Mar, Inc. 800-327-8209
8550 NW 30th Ter, Doral, FL 33122
$70.00 for standard unit.

Md International, Inc. 305-669-9003
11300 NW 41st St, Doral, FL 33178

Phipps & Bird, Inc. 800-955-7621
1519 Summit Ave, Richmond, VA 23230
Blood pressure experimental kits for student education.

Propper Manufacturing Co., Inc. 800-832-4300
3604 Skillman Ave, Long Island City, NY 11101

Trimline Medical Products Corp. 800-526-3538
34 Columbia Rd, Branchburg, NJ 08876
TRIMLINE sphygmomanometers made of breakage-resistant, high impact polystyrene, available as wall, desk or stand models; also cuff containers and inflation systems, all latex-free.

Tuzik Boston 800-886-6363
104 Longwater Dr, Assinippi Park, Norwell, MA 02061

SPINAL CHANNELING INSTRUMENT, VERTEBROPLASTY
(Orthopedics) 87OCJ

Benvenue Medical, Inc. 408-454-9300
3052 Bunker Hill Ln Ste 120, Santa Clara, CA 95054
Benvenue VCF Osteo Coil System

Spineworks Medical Inc. 408-986-8950
1735 N 1st St Ste 245, San Jose, CA 95112

SPINNER, SLIDE, AUTOMATED *(Hematology) 81GKJ*

Beckman Coulter, Inc. 800-526-3821
11800 SW 147th Ave, Miami, FL 33196
Automated slide spinner.

Iris Sample Processing 800-782-8774
60 Glacier Dr, Westwood, MA 02090
Slide spinner and accessories.

Statspin, Inc. 800-782-8774
60 Glacier Dr, Westwood, MA 02090
DIFFSPIN 2 slide spinner prepares uniform monolayer of blood cells in less than 3 seconds.

SPIROMETER, DIAGNOSTIC (RESPIROMETER)
(Anesthesiology) 73BZG

A-M Systems, Inc. 800-426-1306
131 Business Park Loop, Sequim, WA 98382
New line of spirometers from SDI Diagnostics, and Schiller America.

Aesculap Implant Systems Inc. 1-800-234-9179
3773 Corporate Pkwy, Center Valley, PA 18034

Allied Healthcare Products, Inc. 800-444-3954
1720 Sublette Ave, Saint Louis, MO 63110

Anesthesia Associates, Inc. 760-744-6561
460 Enterprise St, San Marcos, CA 92078
Wide variety of styles and configurations of traditional Wright Respirometers, as well as an economical and rugged Digital Respirometer (PN 00-295). Pocket Spirometers and Peak Flow Meters also available.

Boehringer Laboratories, Inc. 800-642-4945
500 E Washington St, Norristown, PA 19401
FVC-guaranteed handheld spirometer that can be easily sterilized.

Cardiac Science Corp. 800-777-1777
500 Burdick Pkwy, Deerfield, WI 53531
Spirotouch and Sensaire. Spirocard.

Cdx Corporation 800-245-9949
1 Richmond Sq, Providence, RI 02906
Four models designed for basic and advanced testing. Portable fully functional spirometer with touch screen, onboard printer and multiple patient storage.

Commercial/Medical Electronics, Inc. 800-324-4844
1519 S Lewis Ave, Tulsa, OK 74104

Compleware Corp. 319-626-8888
2865 Stoner Ct, North Liberty, IA 52317
Diagnostic spirometer.

Compumed, Inc. 800-421-3395
5777 W Century Blvd Ste 360, Los Angeles, CA 90045
Spirometer.

Creative Biomedics, Inc. 949-366-2300
924 Calle Negocio Ste A, San Clemente, CA 92673
WinDX Spirometer

Creative Health Products, Inc. 800-742-4478
5148 Saddle Ridge Rd, Plymouth, MI 48170
SPIRO-PET $136.50.00 for CHP dry portable unit.

Eresearchtechnology Inc. 215-972-0420
1818 Market St Ste 1000, Philadelphia, PA 19103

Futuremed America, Inc. 800-222-6780
15700 Devonshire St, Granada Hills, CA 91344
For $1,590.00, SPIROVISION SV-1000 (SV-III) 3rd generation, PC based spirometer for easily converting a PC to a sophisticated but simple to use spirometer. DISCOVERY Portable spirometer, $1995.00, full spirometry capability, memory, full page printouts, PC interface.

Jones Medical Instrument Co. 800-323-7336
200 Windsor Dr, Oak Brook, IL 60523
$1,250 for PULMONAIRE 10 volume displacement system; bellows warranted for 5 years. Unit may be leased. Usable with all Jones processors. $1495 for full function handheld Satellite spirometer. Disposable transducer minimizes sterilization.

Medtronic Neuromodulation 763-514-4000
710 Medtronic Pkwy, Minneapolis, MN 55432
Various types of diagnostic spirometers.

Meza Medical Equipment 888-308-7116
108 W Nakoma St, San Antonio, TX 78216

SPIROMETER, DIAGNOSTIC (RESPIROMETER) *(cont'd)*

Midmark Diagnostics Group 800-624-8950
3300 Fujita St, Torrance, CA 90505
The IQmark Digital Spirometer has met or exceeded the requirements of the ATS. All standard spirometry measurements are available including FEV6, as recommended by the NLHEP. Standard features on this computer-based spirometer include full-loop, FVC, SVC, MVV, and pre/post BD tests; local or network database storage; trending software; and archive and e-mail capabilities. It is lightweight, weighing only 10 oz., and has no moving parts.

New Life Systems, Inc. 954-972-4600
PO Box 8767, Coral Springs, FL 33075
All types.

Norco 800-657-6672
1125 W Amity Rd, Boise, ID 83705

Nspire Health, Inc 800-574-7374
1830 Lefthand Cir, Longmont, CO 80501
KoKo Spirometer, KoKo Trek Spirometer and KoKo DigiDoser portable, computerized spirometer displays flow-volume loops side-by-side with volume time curve. Also a hand held office spirometer called KoKoMate.

Propper Manufacturing Co., Inc. 800-832-4300
3604 Skillman Ave, Long Island City, NY 11101

Respironics California, Inc. 724-387-4559
2271 Cosmos Ct, Carlsbad, CA 92011
Esprit ventilator with respiratory mechanics.

Vacumed 800-235-3333
4538 Westinghouse St, Ventura, CA 93003
4 models available.

Vitalograph, Inc. 800-255-6626
13310 W 99th St, Lenexa, KS 66215
COMPACT II, $2990.00

SPIROMETER, MONITORING (VOLUMETER)
(Anesthesiology) 73BZK

Cdx Corporation 800-245-9949
1 Richmond Sq, Providence, RI 02906
CDX offers a complete line of computerized spirometers.

Creative Health Products, Inc. 800-742-4478
5148 Saddle Ridge Rd, Plymouth, MI 48170
SPIRO-PET; $136.50 for CHP dry portable unit.

Datex-Ohmeda (Canada) 800-268-1472
1093 Meyerside Dr., Unit 2, Mississauga, ONT L5T-1J6 Canada

Dci Incorporated 913-982-5672
846 N Martway Ct, Olathe, KS 66061
Respiratory or ventiliatory monitor.

Draeger Medical Systems, Inc. 215-660-2626
16 Electronics Ave, Danvers, MA 01923
Spirometer.

Jones Medical Instrument Co. 800-323-7336
200 Windsor Dr, Oak Brook, IL 60523
Portable microcomputerized volumetric spirometer with automatic FVC and MVV. Pre- vs. post-comparisons, interpretation, and legal-size hard-copy graph. Also, hand-held spirometer, full function and portable, for bedside testing. $1,995.00.

Non-Invasive Monitoring Systems, Inc. 305-575-4200
4400 Biscayne Blvd, Miami, FL 33137
Respitrace.

Nspire Health, Inc 800-574-7374
1830 Lefthand Cir, Longmont, CO 80501
A full range of personal diary spirometers, including PiKo-1, KoKoPeak Pro and Accutrax, provide a simplified approach to monitoring FEV1 and PEFR in asthma and COPD patients at home.

Piko Healthcare Products, Inc. 888-737-5656
908 Main St, Louisville, CO 80027
The PiKo line of peak flow, FEV1, FEV6, and diary-information electronic monitoring spirometers. All products are electronic. (See BZK.)

Qrs Diagnostic, Llc 800-465-8408
14755 27th Ave N, Plymouth, MN 55447
SpiroCard PC Card Spirometer. Works with Windows CE, Windows 98/ME/2000/XP computers w/PC card slot FVC, MVV, SVC. SpirOxCard PC Card Spirometer/Pulse Oximeter. Works with Windows CE, Windows 98/ME/2000/XP computers w/PC card slot. Sensaire Pocket Spirometer, portable spirometer for the mobile practitioner; FVC, MVV, SVC, real-time graphs, full volume loop.

SPIROMETER, MONITORING (VOLUMETER) *(cont'd)*

Respironics California, Inc. 724-387-4559
2271 Cosmos Ct, Carlsbad, CA 92011
Spirometer, monitoring, w/wo alarm.

Respironics Novametrix, Llc. 724-387-4559
5 Technology Dr, Wallingford, CT 06492
Spirometer, monitoring, w/wo alarm.

Vitalograph, Inc. 800-255-6626
13310 W 99th St, Lenexa, KS 66215
2120 Recording spirometer. $1590.00

SPIROMETER, THERAPEUTIC (INCENTIVE)
(Anesthesiology) 73BWF

Ballard Medical Products 770-587-7835
12050 Lone Peak Pkwy, Draper, UT 84020
Spirometer, therapeutic (incentive).

Covidien Lp 508-261-8000
15 Hampshire St, Mansfield, MA 02048

Dhd Healthcare Corporation 800-847-8000
PO Box 6, One Madison Street, Wampsville, NY 13163
DHD COACH, COACH JR.are volumetric incentive spirometers, DHD CliniFLO is a flow based incentive spirometer. EzPAP, positive airway pressure therapy device.

El-Fax Company, Inc. (Lung Gym) 610-896-6853
PO Box 407, 32 Llanfair Road,, Ardmore, PA 19003
The Heart / Lung Gym.

Futuremed America, Inc. 800-222-6780
15700 Devonshire St, Granada Hills, CA 91344
SPIROBANK Multifunction Spirometer: Operates as handheld unit for asthma treatment or homecare, direct print on all printers, download to PC $950.00

Imetrikus, Inc. 760-804-8800
5875 Avenida Encinas, Carlsbad, CA 92008
Various models of spirometers.

Smiths Medical Asd Inc. 800-258-5361
10 Bowman Dr, Keene, NH 03431
Incentive spirometer.

Vitalograph, Inc. 800-255-6626
13310 W 99th St, Lenexa, KS 66215
AIM; $920.00 for aerosol inhalation device used to train patients to use metered dose inhalator correctly.

SPLINT, ABDUCTION, CONGENITAL HIP DISLOCATION
(Physical Med) 89IOZ

Alimed, Inc. 800-225-2610
297 High St, Dedham, MA 02026

Biomet, Inc. 574-267-6639
56 E Bell Dr, PO Box 587, Warsaw, IN 46582
Various types of abduction splints.

Bird & Cronin, Inc. 651-683-1111
1200 Trapp Rd, Saint Paul, MN 55121
Hip abduction splint.

Confortaire Inc 662-842-2966
2133 S Veterans Blvd, Tupelo, MS 38804
Hip abduction pillow.

Depuy Ace, A Johnson & Johnson Company 800-473-3789
700 Orthopaedic Dr, Warsaw, IN 46582

Dj Orthopedics De Mexico, S.A. De C.V. 690-727-1280
Blvd., Delagacion La Presa, Tijuana 22397 Mexico
Hip abduction kit

Dj Orthopedics De Mexico, S.A. De C.V. 690-727-1280
Ave. Venustiano Carranza 6802, Castillo, Tijuana 22100 Mexico
Hip abduction kit

Fillauer Companies, Inc. 800-251-6398
2710 Amnicola Hwy, Chattanooga, TN 37406

Larkotex Company 800-972-3037
1002 Olive St, Texarkana, TX 75501

Ortho Innovations, Inc. 507-269-2895
121 23rd Ave SW, Rochester, MN 55902
Braces.

Restorative Care Of America Inc 800-627-1595
12221 33rd St N, Saint Petersburg, FL 33716
Hip and knee abductor, provides abduction for scissoring or tight thigh adductors. Features static or reciprocating for bed bound or ambulatory patients. Adduction Bar provides adjustable abduction control. Nylon ball sockets duplicate the motion of hip joint. Breathable neoprene liner.

SPLINT, ABDUCTION, CONGENITAL HIP DISLOCATION *(cont'd)*

Tartan Orthopedics, Ltd. 888-287-1456
10651 Irma Dr Unit C, Northglenn, CO 80233
$50.00 per unit (med).

Truform Orthotics & Prosthetics 800-888-0458
3960 Rosslyn Dr, Cincinnati, OH 45209

Zimmer Holdings, Inc. 800-613-6131
1800 W Center St, PO Box 708, Warsaw, IN 46580

SPLINT, ABDUCTION, SHOULDER *(Orthopedics) 87WUU*

Alimed, Inc. 800-225-2610
297 High St, Dedham, MA 02026

Border Opportunity Saver Systems, Inc. 830-775-0992
10 Finegan Rd, Del Rio, TX 78840

Corflex, Inc. 800-426-7353
669 E Industrial Park Dr, Manchester, NH 03109
Ultra Shoulder Abduction Pillow with sling immobilizes shoulder and arm following separation, dislocation, or other shoulder injuries. Features V-lock strapping system to minimize roll and shifting from neutral position.

Depuy Mitek, Inc. 800-451-2006
325 Paramount Dr, Raynham, MA 02767

Professional's Choice Sports Medicine Products, Inc. 800-331-9421
2025 Gillespie Way Ste 106, El Cajon, CA 92020

Slawner Ltd., J. 514-731-3378
5713 Cote Des Neiges Rd., Montreal, QUE H3S 1Y7 Canada

Surgical Appliance Industries 800-888-0458
3960 Rosslyn Dr, Cincinnati, OH 45209

Wisap America 800-233-8448
8231 Melrose Dr, Lenexa, KS 66214

SPLINT, CLAVICLE *(Physical Med) 89IQJ*

A&A Orthopedics, Incorporated 757-224-0177
12250 SW 129th Ct Bldg 1, Miami, FL 33186
Splint, clavicle.

American Orthopedic Supply Co., Inc.
37017 State Highway 79, Cleveland, AL 35049
Clavicle splint.

Biomet, Inc. 574-267-6639
56 E Bell Dr, PO Box 587, Warsaw, IN 46582
Various types of clavical splints.

Bird & Cronin, Inc. 651-683-1111
1200 Trapp Rd, Saint Paul, MN 55121
Clavical brace.

Core Products International, Inc. 800-365-3047
808 Prospect Ave, Osceola, WI 54020

DJO Inc. 800-336-6569
1430 Decision St, Vista, CA 92081

Faretec, Inc. 440-350-9510
1610 W Jackson St Unit 6, Concord Twp, OH 44077
Arm sling.

Frank Stubbs Co., Inc 800-223-1713
2100 Eastman Ave Ste B, Oxnard, CA 93030

Freeman Manufacturing Company 800-253-2091
900 W Chicago Rd, PO Box J, Sturgis, MI 49091

Kenad Sg Medical, Inc. 800-825-0606
2692 Huntley Dr, Memphis, TN 38132
Clavical splint.

Larkotex Company 800-972-3037
1002 Olive St, Texarkana, TX 75501

Lots Corp. 520-730-6068
10977 E Tanque Verde Rd, Tucson, AZ 85749
Pcd 'pelvic compression device'.

Mizuho Osi 800-777-4674
30031 Ahern Ave, Union City, CA 94587

Ortholine 800-243-3351
13 Chapel St, Norwalk, CT 06850
Adult, heavy duty, and pediatric sizes.

Ossur Americas 949-268-3155
742 Pancho Rd, Camarillo, CA 93012

Pelvic Binder, Inc. 877-451-3000
3982 Fm 2653 South, Cumby, TX 75433
Pelvic binder.

SPLINT, CLAVICLE *(cont'd)*

Scott Specialties, Inc. 785-527-5627
1827 Meadowlark Rd, Clay Center, KS 67432
Various types of clavicle supports or splints.

Scott Specialties, Inc. 785-527-5627
1820 E 7th St, Concordia, KS 66901

Scott Specialties, Inc./Cmo Inc./Ginny Inc. 800-255-7136
512 M St, Belleville, KS 66935

Stryker Corp. 800-726-2725
2825 Airview Blvd, Portage, MI 49002

Surgical Appliance Industries 800-888-0458
3960 Rosslyn Dr, Cincinnati, OH 45209

Tartan Orthopedics, Ltd. 888-287-1456
10651 Irma Dr Unit C, Northglenn, CO 80233
$8.25 per unit (med).

Truform Orthotics & Prosthetics 800-888-0458
3960 Rosslyn Dr, Cincinnati, OH 45209

Warsaw Orthopedic, Inc. 901-396-3133
2500 Silveus Xing, Warsaw, IN 46582
Various types of clavical, acromioclavicular, and shoulder splints and braces.

Zimmer Holdings, Inc. 800-613-6131
1800 W Center St, PO Box 708, Warsaw, IN 46580

SPLINT, DENIS BROWN *(Physical Med) 89ITN*

Biomet, Inc. 574-267-6639
56 E Bell Dr, PO Box 587, Warsaw, IN 46582
Various types of clubfoot splints.

Fillauer Companies, Inc. 800-251-6398
2710 Amnicola Hwy, Chattanooga, TN 37406

Freeman Manufacturing Company 800-253-2091
900 W Chicago Rd, PO Box J, Sturgis, MI 49091

Larkotex Company 800-972-3037
1002 Olive St, Texarkana, TX 75501

Md Orthopaedics 877-766-7384
604 N Parkway St, Wayland, IA 52654
Foot, abduction rotation bar.

Zimmer Holdings, Inc. 800-613-6131
1800 W Center St, PO Box 708, Warsaw, IN 46580

SPLINT, ENDODONTIC STABILIZER *(Dental And Oral) 76ELS*

Dentalez Group 866-DTE-INFO
101 Lindenwood Dr Ste 225, Valleybrooke Corporate Center
Malvern, PA 19355

Glasspan, Inc. 610-363-2300
The Commons at Lincoln Center, 101 J.R. Thomas Drive
Exton, PA 19341
Flexible dental ceramic reinforcement device.

Oratronics, Inc. 212-986-0050
405 Lexington Ave, New York, NY 10174
Endodontic stabilization kit.

Pentron Clinical Technologies 203-265-7397
68-70 North Plains Industrial, Road, Wallingford, CT 06492
Splint,endodontic stabilizing.

Pentron Laboratory Technologies 203-265-7397
53 N Plains Industrial Rd, Wallingford, CT 06492
Splint, endodontic stabilizing.

Pulpdent Corp. 800-343-4342
80 Oakland St, Watertown, MA 02472
No common name listed.

SPLINT, EXTERMITY, NON-INFLATABLE, EXTERNAL, NON-STERILE *(Surgery) 79NOC*

Dr. Len's Medical Products Llc 678-908-8180
412 Atwood Rd, Erdenheim, PA 19038
Soft collar or soft brace.

Emergency Products And Research 305-304-6933
890 W Main St, Kent, OH 44240
Vaccum arm splint.

Healer Products, Llc 914-663-6300
427 Commerce Ln Ste 1, West Berlin, NJ 08091
Finger splint, wire splint.

Innovative Medical Products-Pjc,Llc 216-961-8735
3510 Chatham Ave, Cleveland, OH 44113
Aluminum splints, temporary splints.

Itec/Ems Llp 903-365-6390
400 All Star Dr, Winnsboro, TX 75494
Splint, various.

SPLINT, EXTERMITY, NON-INFLATABLE, EXTERNAL, NON-STERILE *(cont'd)*

Parker Athletic Products, Llc 704-370-0400
2401 Distribution St, Charlotte, NC 28203
Non-inflatable extremity splint.

SPLINT, EXTREMITY, INFLATABLE, EXTERNAL *(Surgery) 79FZF*

Afassco, Inc. 800-441-6774
2244 Park Pl Ste C, Minden, NV 89423

Alimed, Inc. 800-225-2610
297 High St, Dedham, MA 02026

Armstrong Medical Industries, Inc. 800-323-4220
575 Knightsbridge Pkwy, Lincolnshire, IL 60069

Dixie Ems Supply 800-347-3494
385 Union Ave, Brooklyn, NY 11211
$145.00 per 10 (1/2leg, med).

Normed 800-288-8200
PO Box 3644, Seattle, WA 98124
Inflatable air splint.

Schueler & Company, Inc. 516-487-1500
PO Box 528, Stratford, CT 06615
Schueler Air Splint. Perfect emergency first-aid treatment for common sprains, fractures and dislocations. Ready to use and orally inflates in seconds. More comfortable than traditional bandage/splint techniques. Can be completely washed and sterilized (by gas or cold solution). Can be deflated easily and reused. Helps prevent further damage to soft tissue and immobilizes and cushions injured limbs. Available in adult and children's sizes.

SPLINT, EXTREMITY, NON-INFLATABLE, EXTERNAL *(Surgery) 79FYH*

Anodyne Therapy, Llc 813-645-2855
13570 Wright Cir, Tampa, FL 33626
Extremity splint.

Bct Midwest, Inc. 785-856-1414
1220 Wagon Wheel Rd, Lawrence, KS 66049
Splint,synthetic,non-sterile.

Biomet, Inc. 574-267-6639
56 E Bell Dr, PO Box 587, Warsaw, IN 46582
Various types of splints.

Brown Medical Industries 800-843-4395
1300 Lundberg Dr W, Spirit Lake, IA 51360
N'ICE STRETCH Plantar Fasciitis Night Splint is a night splint designed to reduce heel and plantar fascia pain, used at night while sleeping.

Bsn Medical, Inc. 800-552-1157
100 Beiersdorf Drive, Rutherford College, NC 28671
Splint.

Carolina Narrow Fabric Co. 336-631-3000
1100 Patterson Ave, Winston Salem, NC 27101
Various.

Chase Ergonomics, Inc. 800-621-5436
PO Box 92497, Albuquerque, NM 87199
Splint wrist brace.

Cramer Products, Inc. 800-255-6621
153 W Warren St, Gardner, KS 66030
MARK I articulated adjustable emergency splint.

Depuy-Raynham, A Div. Of Depuy Orthopaedics 800-451-2006
325 Paramount Dr, Raynham, MA 02767
Various kinds of non-inflatable external extremity splints.

Dj Orthopedics De Mexico, S.A. De C.V. 690-727-1280
Blvd., Delagacion La Presa, Tijuana 22397 Mexico
Various

Dj Orthopedics De Mexico, S.A. De C.V. 690-727-1280
Ave. Venustiano Carranza 6802, Castillo, Tijuana 22100 Mexico
Various

DJO Inc. 800-336-6569
1430 Decision St, Vista, CA 92081
Patella, shin, foot, finger and leg splints in various sizes.

Dr. Len's Medical Products Llc 678-908-8180
412 Atwood Rd, Erdenheim, PA 19038
Soft collar or soft brace.

Freeman Manufacturing Company 800-253-2091
900 W Chicago Rd, PO Box J, Sturgis, MI 49091
Knee; wrist (canvas, thermo cast); humeral (thermo cast).

SPLINT, EXTREMITY, NON-INFLATABLE, EXTERNAL *(cont'd)*

Galveston Manufacturing Co., Inc. 800-634-3309
7810 FM 646 Rd S, Santa Fe, TX 77510
I-plus system humeral & ulnar fracture brace.

International Medication Systems, Ltd. 800-423-4136
1886 Santa Anita Ave, South El Monte, CA 91733
Finger splint.

Larson Medical Products, Inc. 614-235-9100
2844 Banwick Rd, Columbus, OH 43232
Various types of external splints for body extremities.

Millennium Devices, Inc. 631-582-6424
250 Gibbs Rd, Islandia, NY 11749
External fixator.

Minto R&D, Inc. 530-222-2373
20270 Charlanne Dr, Redding, CA 96002
$315 for single leg splint SAGER S-301, $352 for Bilateral INFANT SAGER INF-300, $436.00 for super bilateral leg splint SAGER S-304.

Neurotron Medical 609-896-3444
800 Silvia St, Ewing, NJ 08628
Support, wrist.

Normed 800-288-8200
PO Box 3644, Seattle, WA 98124
Wire splint.

North Coast Medical, Inc. 800-821-9319
18305 Sutter Blvd, Morgan Hill, CA 95037

Patterson Medical Supply, Inc. 262-387-8720
W68N158 Evergreen Blvd, Cedarburg, WI 53012
Various types of foot splints and supports.

Respond Industries, Inc. 1-800-523-8999
9500 Woodend Rd, Edwardsville, KS 66111
Splint wire 30.

Sam Medical Products 503-639-5474
4909 South Coast Hwy., #245, Newport, OR 97365
Universal malleable splint.

Select Medical Products, Inc. 800-276-7237
6531 47th St N, Pinellas Park, FL 33781
Patented, Adjustable Ankle/Foot Splint telescopes from Medium to XXLarge! Provides custom fit with an off-the-shelf device! Splints are also available in non-adjusting sizes, Small, Medium and Large. Both versions treat foot drop and rotation of the leg.

Sunmedica 530-229-1600
1661 Zachi Way, Redding, CA 96003
HIPGRIP Lateral positioning system. KNEEGRIP positioning device used to hold the knee in a flexed position during surgery. LEGGRIP secures the lower extremity for skin preparation prior to surgery. Works well with the patient in a lateral position. OTHRORAP compressive, supportive tapeless dressing used to secure a sterile dressing after breast/chest surgery.

Tartan Orthopedics, Ltd. 888-287-1456
10651 Irma Dr Unit C, Northglenn, CO 80233
$145.00 per 10 (1/2leg, med).

SPLINT, HAND, AND COMPONENT *(Physical Med) 89ILH*

A&A Orthopedics, Incorporated 757-224-0177
12250 SW 129th Ct Bldg 1, Miami, FL 33186
Wrist splint & wrist & forearm splint.

Air A Med, Inc. 239-936-5590
2049 Beacon Manor Dr, Fort Myers, FL 33907
Splints, hand and components.

Alimed, Inc. 800-225-2610
297 High St, Dedham, MA 02026

American Orthopedic Supply Co., Inc.
37017 State Highway 79, Cleveland, AL 35049
Wrist, hand, thumb, and splints.

Becker Orthopedic Appliance Co. 248-588-7480
635 Executive Dr, Troy, MI 48083
Various splints, hand orthoses and splints, hand orthotic components.

Benik Corp. 360-692-5601
11871 Silverdale Way NW Ste 107, Silverdale, WA 98383
Wrist support.

Biomet Microfixation Inc. 800-874-7711
1520 Tradeport Dr, Jacksonville, FL 32218
Splint, hand, and components.

Biomet, Inc. 574-267-6639
56 E Bell Dr, PO Box 587, Warsaw, IN 46582
Various types of finger & hand splints.

SPLINT, HAND, AND COMPONENT *(cont'd)*

Blake Manufacturing, Inc. 813-935-1841
9241 Lazy Ln, Tampa, FL 33614
Hand splint/orthosis.

Brown Medical Industries 800-843-4395
1300 Lundberg Dr W, Spirit Lake, IA 51360
PLASTALUME. Complete line of finger, hand, arm and leg splints.

Cosco 800-582-6853
1602 Lakeside Dr, Redding, CA 96001

Dalco International, Inc. 888-354-5515
8433 Glazebrook Ave, Richmond, VA 23228
Orthopedic hand and finger splints.

Daren Industries, Inc 574-534-3418
2452 Lincolnway E, Goshen, IN 46526
Universal splint, various types and styles of splints.

Dj Orthopedics De Mexico, S.A. De C.V. 690-727-1280
Blvd., Delagacion La Presa, Tijuana 22397 Mexico
Wrist management

Dj Orthopedics De Mexico, S.A. De C.V. 690-727-1280
Ave. Venustiano Carranza 6802, Castillo, Tijuana 22100 Mexico
Wrist management

DJO Inc. 800-336-6569
1430 Decision St, Vista, CA 92081
Various styles and sizes of hand and finger splints.

Faretec, Inc. 440-350-9510
1610 W Jackson St Unit 6, Concord Twp, OH 44077
Hand splint.

Formedica Ltd. 800-361-9671
1481 Rue Begin, St Laurent, QUE H4R 1V8 Canada
$20.00 per 10 hand splints.

Frank Stubbs Co., Inc 800-223-1713
2100 Eastman Ave Ste B, Oxnard, CA 93030

Freeman Manufacturing Company 800-253-2091
900 W Chicago Rd, PO Box J, Sturgis, MI 49091
Carpal tunnel and hand splint.

Galveston Manufacturing Co., Inc. 800-634-3309
7810 FM 646 Rd S, Santa Fe, TX 77510
Galveston metacarpel brace.

Hartmann-Conco Inc. 800-243-2294
481 Lakeshore Pkwy, Rock Hill, SC 29730
Alumafoam, Stax.

Health Ent., Inc. 508-695-0727
90 George Leven Dr, North Attleboro, MA 02760
Finger splint.

Imak Products Corp. 619-291-9990
2515 Camino Del Rio S Ste 240, San Diego, CA 92108
Various.

Inland Specialties, Inc. 800-741-0022
7655 Matoaka Rd, Sarasota, FL 34243
Frog style splints, Baseball splints and Spoon finger splints available in small, medium and large; Stax style splints (sizes 1 through 7); Padded finger strips in sizes .5 x 18in., .75 x 18in., 1 x 18in., .5 x 9in., .75 x 9in., and 1 x 9in.; Burnham thumb and finger splints also available.

Just Packaging Inc. 908-753-6700
450 Oak Tree Ave, South Plainfield, NJ 07080
Wrists splints.

Kenad Sg Medical, Inc. 800-825-0606
2692 Huntley Dr, Memphis, TN 38132
Hand splint.

Kennex Development Inc 626-458-0598
533 S Atlantic Blvd Ste 301, Monterey Park, CA 91754
Various types of wrist & hand splints.

Larkotex Company 800-972-3037
1002 Olive St, Texarkana, TX 75501

Larson Medical Products, Inc. 614-235-9100
2844 Banwick Rd, Columbus, OH 43232
Splint, hand splint.

Leeder Group, Inc. 305-436-5030
8508 NW 66th St, Miami, FL 33166
Hand splint.

LinkBio Corp. 800-932-0616
300 Round Hill Dr, Rockaway, NJ 07866
Finger splints.

SPLINT, HAND, AND COMPONENT *(cont'd)*

M.B.S. Fabricating & Coating, Inc. 704-871-1830
174 Crawford Rd Ste A, Po Box 249, Statesville, NC 28625
Various digital splints, splints kits, hand and leg splints.

Maramed Orthopedic Systems 800-327-5830
2480 W 82nd St, No. 8, Hialeah, FL 33016

Mckie Splints, Llc 888-477-5468
PO Box 16046, Duluth, MN 55816
McKie Thumb Splint. Hand Splint.

Mizuho Osi 800-777-4674
30031 Ahern Ave, Union City, CA 94587

Ortholine 800-243-3351
13 Chapel St, Norwalk, CT 06850
Universal, sized, canvas, padded foam, tricote, lacing wrist splints, thumb spikas aluminum finger splints. Pediatric sizes.

Orthotic & Prosthetic Lab, Inc. 314-968-8555
748 Marshall Ave, Webster Groves, MO 63119
O&p hand splint.

Ossur Americas 949-268-3155
742 Pancho Rd, Camarillo, CA 93012

Patterson Medical Supply, Inc. 262-387-8720
W68N158 Evergreen Blvd, Cedarburg, WI 53012
Various types of splints (wrist, dorsal, thumb, finger hand cone).

Rehabilitation Technical Components, Corp. 919-732-1705
3913 Devonwood Rd, Hillsborough, NC 27278
Hand orthosis.

Restorative Care Of America Inc 800-627-1595
12221 33rd St N, Saint Petersburg, FL 33716
Non component. Resting hand promotes functional alignment of the hand and wrist. Made of heat modable Kydex plastic. Foam liner included. Dorsal Resting Hand promotes functional alignment of the hand and wrist when spasticity is present. Reduces stimulation in the flexars of the hand. Made of heat moldable plastic, liner included. Resting Hand Burn Unit promotes functional alignment of the wrist and fingers in the burn patient. Closed cell foam liner repels fluids and resists bacteria. Splint made of heat moldable plastic for customization.

Richardson Products, Inc. 888-928-7297
9408 Gulfstream Rd, Frankfort, IL 60423
Hand splint devices and parts.

Sam Medical Products 503-639-5474
4909 South Coast Hwy., #245, Newport, OR 97365
Structural aluminum maleable splint.

Scott Specialties, Inc. 785-527-5627
1827 Meadowlark Rd, Clay Center, KS 67432
Various types of hand splints.

Scott Specialties, Inc. 785-527-5627
1820 E 7th St, Concordia, KS 66901

Scott Specialties, Inc./Cmo Inc./Ginny Inc. 800-255-7136
512 M St, Belleville, KS 66935

Silver Ring Splint Co. 434-971-4052
1140 E Market St, Charlottesville, VA 22902
Various types of finger splints.

Tiburon Medical Enterprises 909-654-2333
915 Industrial Way, San Jacinto, CA 92582
Various.

Top Shelf Manufacturing, Llc 209-834-8185
1851 Paradise Rd Ste B, Tracy, CA 95304
Various types of wrist & forearm supports.

Truform Orthotics & Prosthetics 800-888-0458
3960 Rosslyn Dr, Cincinnati, OH 45209

Ultraflex Systems, Inc. 610-906-1410
237 South St Ste 200, Pottstown, PA 19464
Various dynamic hand splints.

Warsaw Orthopedic, Inc. 901-396-3133
2500 Silveus Xing, Warsaw, IN 46582
Various types of wrist, hand and finger splints and soft good supports.

Wire Cloth Manufacturers Inc. 800-947-3626
110 Iron Mountain Rd, Randolph Industrial Park, Mine Hill, NJ 07803
Splint, hand, and components.

Zimmer Holdings, Inc. 800-613-6131
1800 W Center St, PO Box 708, Warsaw, IN 46580

Zimmer Orthopaedic Surgical Products 800-321-5533
PO Box 10, 200 West Ohio Ave., Dover, OH 44622

SPLINT, MOLDED, ALUMINUM *(Orthopedics) 87RUW*

Coopercare Lastrap Inc 416-741-9675
Highway H, Koopman Ln., Elkhorn, WI 53121

Corflex, Inc. 800-426-7353
669 E Industrial Park Dr, Manchester, NH 03109

Hartmann-Conco Inc. 800-243-2294
481 Lakeshore Pkwy, Rock Hill, SC 29730
Alumafoam.

Mizuho Osi 800-777-4674
30031 Ahern Ave, Union City, CA 94587

Nemcomed 800-255-4576
801 Industrial Dr, Hicksville, OH 43526
Full-line of splints: finger, hand, arm, leg, and customized splints.

Tetra Medical Supply Corp. 800-621-4041
6364 W Gross Point Rd, Niles, IL 60714

Truform Orthotics & Prosthetics 800-888-0458
3960 Rosslyn Dr, Cincinnati, OH 45209

Zimmer Holdings, Inc. 800-613-6131
1800 W Center St, PO Box 708, Warsaw, IN 46580

Zimmer Orthopaedic Surgical Products 800-321-5533
PO Box 10, 200 West Ohio Ave., Dover, OH 44622

SPLINT, MOLDED, PLASTIC *(Orthopedics) 87RUX*

Cfi Medical Solutions (Contour Fabricators, Inc.) 810-750-5300
14241 N Fenton Rd, Fenton, MI 48430

Larkotex Company 800-972-3037
1002 Olive St, Texarkana, TX 75501

Maramed Orthopedic Systems 800-327-5830
2480 W 82nd St, No. 8, Hialeah, FL 33016

Paramedical Distributors 800-245-3278
2020 Grand Blvd, Kansas City, MO 64108
Assorted adjustable wrist, hand, ankle, etc.

Pedifix, Inc. 800-424-5561
310 Guinea Rd, Brewster, NY 10509
Bunion splint.

Products International Co. 800-521-5123
2320 W Holly St, Phoenix, AZ 85009
The TABBAND PROTECTO-SPLINT is a simple, inexpensive finger splint and finger protector. Made of plastic, it's washable and may be x-rayed.

Restorative Care Of America Inc 800-627-1595
12221 33rd St N, Saint Petersburg, FL 33716
MULTI-PODUS System treats foot/ankle contractures, hip rotation, and heel pressure sores. Available in small, medium, large and x-large sizes.

Ross Disposable Products 800-649-6526
401 Traders Blvd E, Unit 10, Mississauga, ON L4Z 2H8 Canada

Slawner Ltd., J. 514-731-3378
5713 Cote Des Neiges Rd., Montreal, QUE H3S 1Y7 Canada

Total Care 800-334-3802
PO Box 1661, Rockville, MD 20849

Zimmer Holdings, Inc. 800-613-6131
1800 W Center St, PO Box 708, Warsaw, IN 46580

Zimmer Orthopaedic Surgical Products 800-321-5533
PO Box 10, 200 West Ohio Ave., Dover, OH 44622

SPLINT, NASAL *(Ear/Nose/Throat) 77EPP*

Andrew J. Diamond, M.D. 770-933-8214
551 Hackney Dr SE, Marietta, GA 30067
Customized external nasal splint.

Bausch & Lomb Surgical 636-255-5051
3365 Tree Court Ind Blvd, Saint Louis, MO 63122

Biomet, Inc. 574-267-6639
56 E Bell Dr, PO Box 587, Warsaw, IN 46582
Nasal splint.

E. Benson Hood Laboratories, Inc. 800-942-5227
575 Washington St, Pembroke, MA 02359
Doyle Shark nasal splint, post-sinus-surgery splint. Tellez splint, Eliacher nasal splint.

Exmoor Plastics Inc. 317-244-1014
304 Gasoline Aly, Indianapolis, IN 46222
Septal splints in many patterns and materials supplied sterile, priced from $5.00 each.

Gyrus Ent L.L.C., Sub. Of Gyrus Acmi, Inc. 508-804-2739
2925 Appling Rd, Bartlett, TN 38133
Various types and sizes of nasal splints.

SPLINT, NASAL *(cont'd)*

Hartmann-Conco Inc. 800-243-2294
481 Lakeshore Pkwy, Rock Hill, SC 29730
AlumaFoam.

Invotec Intl. 800-998-8580
6833 Phillips Industrial Blvd, Jacksonville, FL 32256
External nasal splints.

Larson Medical Products, Inc. 614-235-9100
2844 Banwick Rd, Columbus, OH 43232
Palatel stent.

Micromedics 800-624-5662
1270 Eagan Industrial Rd, Saint Paul, MN 55121
Micromedics' offers the most popular designs for temporary, postsurgical splinting. Our Breeze Nasal Airway, Doyle Spacer Splints, Bi-Valve Nasal Airway Splints are precision-made and hand assembled and finished for outstanding quality. Splints are available in a variety of sizes and thicknesses to meet your broad range of patient needs. The Denver Nasal Splint stablizies nasal bones and cartilage and reduces edema after nasal surgery or trauma.

Shippert Medical Technologies Corp. 800-888-8663
6248 S Troy Cir Ste A, Centennial, CO 80111
The Denver Splint is used after nasal surgery or trauma to reduce edema and stabilze bones. Complete line of adhesive nasal splinting.

Sientra, Inc 888-423-7600
11220 Grader St Ste 100, Dallas, TX 75238
Nasal splint.

Surgical Technology Laboratories Inc. 803-462-1714
610 Clemson Rd, Columbia, SC 29229
Various sizes nasal splints.

Zimmer Holdings, Inc. 800-613-6131
1800 W Center St, PO Box 708, Warsaw, IN 46580

SPLINT, OTHER *(Orthopedics) 87RVC*

Aegis Medical 203-838-9081
10 Wall St, Norwalk, CT 06850

Apothecary Products, Inc. 800-328-2742
11750 12th Ave S, Burnsville, MN 55337
Finger splints, including a new patented splint with velcro tape

Bashaw Medical, Inc. 800-499-3857
4909 Mobile Hwy Ste B, Pensacola, FL 32506
B-SPLINT FRACTURE KIT.

Better Hands Glove Products 800-242-2850
PO Box 21641, Concord, CA 94521
For prevention and treatment of wrist injuries, carpal tunnel syndrome, repetitive strain injury, and tendinitis. Claims for prevention and treatment have been cleared with the FDA

Cmo, Inc. 800-344-0011
PO Box 147, Barberton, OH 44203
Carpal-tunnel splint.

Corflex, Inc. 800-426-7353
669 E Industrial Park Dr, Manchester, NH 03109
Carpal-tunnel wrist splint. POLY CAST Plantar Fasciities Splints are ultrarigid, high-density black polyethylene plastic with grey terry foam lining (or all-padded version) to treat plantar fasciitis or achilles tendonitis disorders. POLY CAST Cubital Tunnel Splint is ultrarigid high-density black polyethylene plastic with soft grey terry lining to treat cubital tunnel syndrome.

Cosco 800-582-6853
1602 Lakeside Dr, Redding, CA 96001

Dalco International, Inc. 888-354-5515
8433 Glazebrook Ave, Richmond, VA 23228
Finger splints.

Formedica Ltd. 800-361-9671
1481 Rue Begin, St Laurent, QUE H4R 1V8 Canada
$7.00 per 10 (finger, med).

Geen Healthcare Inc. 800-565-4336
931 Progress Ave. Ste.13, Scarborough, ONT M1G 3V5 Canada
SPEEDSPLINT Multi-purpose speedsplint.

Health Enterprises 800-633-4243
90 George Leven Dr, North Attleboro, MA 02760
Finger splints.

Ita-Med Co. 888-9IT-AMED
310 Littlefield Ave, South San Francisco, CA 94080
Flexible splint that provides excellent immobilization in emergency situations. Easy to use, light, washable, and reusable.

SPLINT, OTHER *(cont'd)*

Langer, Inc. 800-645-5520
450 Commack Rd, Deer Park, NY 11729
Pediatric Anti-rotation Splint.

Lohmann & Rauscher, Inc. 800-279-3863
6001 SW 6th Ave Ste 101, Topeka, KS 66615

Morrison Medical 800-438-6677
3735 Paragon Dr, Columbus, OH 43228
Plain or padded cardboard splints, 12in., 18in., 24in. & 34in. Also plastic waterproof. Air Splints.

Ortholine 800-243-3351
13 Chapel St, Norwalk, CT 06850
Orthopedic soft bracing. Rib Belts, Abdominal Binders. Shoulder Immobilizers.

Precision Dynamics Corp. 800-772-1122
13880 Del Sur St, San Fernando, CA 91340

Protector Canada Inc. 800-268-6594
1111 Flint Rd., Unit 23, Toronto, ON M3J 3C7 Canada
Foam and metal type splints. Alco inflatable splints.

Reel R&D, Inc. 800-348-7335
9533 Sunnyside Ave, Ben Lomond, CA 95005
Traction/Immobilizer/Articulators - list price $459.95.

Restorative Care Of America Inc 800-627-1595
12221 33rd St N, Saint Petersburg, FL 33716
MULTI-PODUS System treats foot/ankle contractures, hip rotation and heel pressure sores. Phase II offers adjustable degree of angle for static stretch of the plantar flexors when serial casting is indicated.

Seaberg Company Inc., The 800-818-4726
4909 South Coast Hwy, Ste 245, Newport, OR 97365
Universal splint.

Slawner Ltd., J. 514-731-3378
5713 Cote Des Neiges Rd., Montreal, QUE H3S 1Y7 Canada

Tp Orthodontics, Inc. 800-348-8856
100 Center Plz, La Porte, IN 46350
Orthodontic dental splints.

Unisplint Corp. 770-271-0646
4485 Commerce Dr Ste 106, Buford, GA 30518
$55.00/pkg. (12 units/pkg.). $25.00 each for fracture kit.

Zimmer Orthopaedic Surgical Products 800-321-5533
PO Box 10, 200 West Ohio Ave., Dover, OH 44622
Molded others.

SPLINT, PADDED STAYS *(Orthopedics) 87RUY*

Border Opportunity Saver Systems, Inc. 830-775-0992
10 Finegan Rd, Del Rio, TX 78840

Cfi Medical Solutions (Contour Fabricators, Inc.) 810-750-5300
14241 N Fenton Rd, Fenton, MI 48430

Chamberlin Rubber Company, Inc. 585-427-7780
3333 Brighton Henrietta Town Line Rd, PO Box 22700
Rochester, NY 14623

Inland Specialties, Inc. 800-741-0022
7655 Matoaka Rd, Sarasota, FL 34243
Metal insert aluminum stays; split wrist cockup and palmar spoon stays.

Kees Goebel Medical Specialties, Inc. 800-354-0445
9663 Glades Dr, Hamilton, OH 45011

Mizuho Osi 800-777-4674
30031 Ahern Ave, Union City, CA 94587

Morrison Medical 800-438-6677
3735 Paragon Dr, Columbus, OH 43228
Disposable, economical or reusable, all sizes.

Tetra Medical Supply Corp. 800-621-4041
6364 W Gross Point Rd, Niles, IL 60714

Truform Orthotics & Prosthetics 800-888-0458
3960 Rosslyn Dr, Cincinnati, OH 45209

Zimmer Holdings, Inc. 800-613-6131
1800 W Center St, PO Box 708, Warsaw, IN 46580

Zimmer Orthopaedic Surgical Products 800-321-5533
PO Box 10, 200 West Ohio Ave., Dover, OH 44622

SPLINT, PNEUMATIC *(Orthopedics) 87RUZ*

Ferno-Washington, Inc. 800-733-3766
70 Weil Way, Wilmington, OH 45177

Medi Inc 800-225-8634
75 York Ave, P.O. Box 302, Randolph, MA 02368

SPLINT, PNEUMATIC *(cont'd)*

Mine Safety Appliances Company 866-MSA-1001
121 Gamma Dr, Pittsburgh, PA 15238

Precision Dynamics Corp. 800-772-1122
13880 Del Sur St, San Fernando, CA 91340

Rockford Medical & Safety Co. 800-435-9451
2420 Harrison Ave, PO Box 5646, Rockford, IL 61108

Sroufe Healthcare Products Llc 888-894-4171
PO Box 347, 601 Sroufe St., Ligonier, IN 46767
Laminated vinyl for compression and cold therapy.

SPLINT, SEPTAL, INTRANASAL *(Ear/Nose/Throat) 77LYA*

Applied Therapeutics, Inc. 877-682-2777
3104 Cherry Palm Dr Ste 220, Tampa, FL 33619
Sinu-Knit, a dissolvable sinus dressing for FESS, and other nasal dressings available in multiple sizes and configurations.

Arthrocare Corp. 800-797-6520
680 Vaqueros Ave, Sunnyvale, CA 94085
Nasal Dressing

Carbylan Biosurgery, Inc. 650-855-6777
3181 Porter Dr, Palo Alto, CA 94304
Sinus packing gel.

Evera Medical, Inc. 650-287-2884
353 Vintage Park Dr Ste F, Foster City, CA 94404
Intranasal splint.

Genzyme Corp. 617-252-7500
51 New York Ave. 1 Mountain Rd, 76-80 New York Avenue
Framingham, MA 01701
Nasal dressing and sinus stent.

Genzyme Corporation 617-252-7500
1125 Pleasantview Ter, Ridgefield, NJ 07657
Intranasal splint.

Gyrus Ent L.L.C., Sub. Of Gyrus Acmi, Inc. 508-804-2739
2925 Appling Rd, Bartlett, TN 38133
Various.

Jedmed Instruments Co. 314-845-3770
5416 Jedmed Ct, Saint Louis, MO 63129

Micromedics 800-624-5662
1270 Eagan Industrial Rd, Saint Paul, MN 55121
Middle Meatal Antrostomy Stent designed to be placed following functional endoscopic sinus surgery. Maintain patency of antrostomy and minimize adhesions between the middle turbinate and lateral nasal wall.

Ultracell Medical Technologies, Inc. 877-SPO-NGE1
183 Providence New London Tpke, North Stonington, CT 06359
Nasal splints are available in various sizes with or without airway.

SPLINT, TEMPORARY TRAINING *(Physical Med) 89IQM*

Alimed, Inc. 800-225-2610
297 High St, Dedham, MA 02026

Biomet, Inc. 574-267-6639
56 E Bell Dr, PO Box 587, Warsaw, IN 46582
Finger stall.

Bsn Medical, Inc 800-552-1157
5825 Carnegie Blvd, Charlotte, NC 28209
OCL® POLYLITE® SYNTHETIC SPLINTING SYSTEM has a polyester substrate that is fiberglass free, which means no sharp edges and more patient comfort. Easy to cut, easy to prepare; saves you time. Available in rolls or singles splints in a variety of sizes. OCL® SPLINT ROLL® -2 PLASTER SPLINTING SYSTEM'S foam and flannel covering. Easy application with no need for pre-padding. Available in rolls from 2- to 6-in. wide.

C.D. Denison Orthopaedic Appliance Corp. 410-235-9645
220 W 28th St, Baltimore, MD 21211
$222.90,s,m,l per unit standard; $282.10 combination unit.

Darco International, Inc. 800-999-8866
810 Memorial Blvd, Huntington, WV 25701
Darco Toe Alignment Splint

Gelsmart Llc 973-884-8995
30 Leslie Ct Ste B-202, Whippany, NJ 07981
Various type of toe regulators.

Glenroe Technologies 800-237-4060
1912 44th Ave E, Bradenton, FL 34203
Orthodontic sullivan bruxism splint.

National Dentex Corp 508-907-7800
2 Vision Dr Ste 3, Natick, MA 01760
Prosthetic and orthotic accessory.

SPLINT, TEMPORARY TRAINING *(cont'd)*

Pedifix, Inc. 800-424-5561
310 Guinea Rd, Brewster, NY 10509
Hammer-toe, bunion.

Polygell Llc. 973-884-8995
30 Leslie Ct, Whippany, NJ 07981
Various type of toe regulators.

Restorative Medical, Inc. 270-422-5454
332 Broadway St, Brandenburg, KY 40108
Various.

Stephan Wood Products, Inc. 989-348-5496
605 Huron St, Grayling, MI 49738
Splint wood.

Tmp Technologies, Inc. 716-895-6100
1200 Northland Ave, Buffalo, NY 14215

SPLINT, TRACTION *(Orthopedics) 87HSP*

A&A Orthopedics, Incorporated 757-224-0177
12250 SW 129th Ct Bldg 1, Miami, FL 33186
Buck's traction.

Armstrong Medical Industries, Inc. 800-323-4220
575 Knightsbridge Pkwy, Lincolnshire, IL 60069

Biomet, Inc. 574-267-6639
56 E Bell Dr, PO Box 587, Warsaw, IN 46582
Various types of traction splints.

Bird & Cronin, Inc. 651-683-1111
1200 Trapp Rd, Saint Paul, MN 55121
Bucks traction boot.

DJO Inc. 800-336-6569
1430 Decision St, Vista, CA 92081

Emergency Products And Research 305-304-6933
890 W Main St, Kent, OH 44240
Kendrick traction device.

Faretec, Inc. 440-350-9510
1610 W Jackson St Unit 6, Concord Twp, OH 44077
Traction leg splint.

Geen Healthcare Inc. 800-565-4336
931 Progress Ave. Ste.13, Scarborough, ONT M1G 3V5 Canada
SPEEDSPLINT Femoral traction speedsplint kit.

Lots Corp. 520-730-6068
10977 E Tanque Verde Rd, Tucson, AZ 85749
Iqs integrated quick splint.

Minto R&D, Inc. 530-222-2373
20270 Charlanne Dr, Redding, CA 96002
$352.00 model INF-300 infant SAGER bilateral splint, $289.00 model S-301 SAGER FORM III single splint, $436.00 model S-304 SAGER FORM III bilateral splint.

Mizuho Osi 800-777-4674
30031 Ahern Ave, Union City, CA 94587

Paramedical Distributors 800-245-3278
2020 Grand Blvd, Kansas City, MO 64108

Patterson Medical Supply, Inc. 262-387-8720
W68N158 Evergreen Blvd, Cedarburg, WI 53012
Head halter.

Reel R&D, Inc. 800-348-7335
9533 Sunnyside Ave, Ben Lomond, CA 95005
$239.00 list price.

Rk Froom & Co., Inc. 310-327-5125
903 Cunningham Ln S, Salem, OR 97302
Various models of splints.

Tetra Medical Supply Corp. 800-621-4041
6364 W Gross Point Rd, Niles, IL 60714

Truform Orthotics & Prosthetics 800-888-0458
3960 Rosslyn Dr, Cincinnati, OH 45209

Warsaw Orthopedic, Inc. 901-396-3133
2500 Silveus Xing, Warsaw, IN 46582
Aeroplane splint.

Zimmer Holdings, Inc. 800-613-6131
1800 W Center St, PO Box 708, Warsaw, IN 46580

Zimmer Orthopaedic Surgical Products 800-321-5533
PO Box 10, 200 West Ohio Ave., Dover, OH 44622

SPLINT, URETERAL *(Gastro/Urology) 78FAD*

Boston Scientific - Marina Bay Customer Fulfillment Center 617-689-6000
500 Commander Shea Blvd, Quincy, MA 02171
Ureteral stent.

C. R. Bard, Inc., Bard Urological Div. 888-367-2273
13183 Harland Dr NE, Covington, GA 30014

Hobbs Medical, Inc. 860-684-5875
8 Spring St, Stafford Springs, CT 06076
Ureteral stent sets.

SPLINT, VACUUM *(Orthopedics) 87RVA*

Cramer Products, Inc. 800-255-6621
153 W Warren St, Gardner, KS 66030
$269.28 for complete set of 3 splints, pump & bag. (sold as set and separately).

Hartwell Medical Corp. 800-633-5900
6352 Corte Del Abeto Ste J, Carlsbad, CA 92011
EVAC-U-SPLINT extremity set immobilizes injured areas without circumferential pressure. Ideal for fractures and dislocations. Used by paramedics and sports medicine personnel. Available in small, medium, and large sizes with compact manual vacuum pump. NEW FASPLINT provides the benefits of a vacuum splint in a semi-disposable product. If equipment loss or retrieval is an issue, then the FASPLINT is the product of choice. Hartwell Medical now offers both a durable and a semi-disposable vacuum splint to suit the needs of each customer.

Olympic Medical Corp. 206-767-3500
5900 1st Ave S, Seattle, WA 98108
Various sizes.

SPLINT, WIRE BOARD *(Orthopedics) 87RVB*

Schueler & Company, Inc. 516-487-1500
PO Box 528, Stratford, CT 06615

SPONGE, DISSECTOR *(Pathology) 88RVD*

Amd-Ritmed, Inc. 800-445-0340
295 Firetower Road, Tonawanda, NY 14150

Surgic Aid, Inc. 800-338-5213
37 Crystal Ave # 287, Derry, NH 03038

Ultracell Medical Technologies, Inc. 877-SPO-NGE1
183 Providence New London Tpke, North Stonington, CT 06359
ULTRACELL Dissector/tonsil. Various sizes of dissector sponges are available including microsponge for ENT surgery.

SPONGE, EXTERNAL *(Surgery) 79GER*

A Plus International, Inc 909-591-5168
5138 Eucalyptus Ave, Chino, CA 91710
Various sizes of lap sponges 100% cotton.

American Fiber & Finishing, Inc. 800-522-2438
PO Box 2488, Albemarle, NC 28002
Rymplecloth sponge, 100% cotton gauze.

American Silk Sutures, Inc. 781-592-7200
82 Sanderson Ave, Lynn, MA 01902
External sponge.

Aso Corporation 941-379-0300
300 Sarasota Center Blvd, Sarasota, FL 34240
Non-woven Pads, Non-Adherent Dressings

Aso Llc 941-379-0300
12120 Esther Lama Dr Ste 112, El Paso, TX 79936
Sterile pads.

First Aid Bandage Co., Inc. 888-813-8214
3 State Pier Rd, New London, CT 06320
Self-adhering gauze, muslin rolls, bandage rolls.

Johnson & Johnson Medical Division Of Ethicon, Inc. 800-423-4018
2500 E Arbrook Blvd, Arlington, TX 76014

Kerma Medical Products, Inc. 757-398-8400
400 Port Centre Pkwy, Portsmouth, VA 23704
Lap sponge, burn dressing pad.

Marel Corporation 203-934-8187
5 Saw Mill Rd, West Haven, CT 06516
Non-woven sponge, non-adherent sponge, combine PAS.

Mcneil Healthcare, Inc. 203-932-6263
481 Elm St, West Haven, CT 06516
Non woven sponge,non adherent sponge.

Omnia, Inc. 863-619-8100
3125 Drane Field Rd Ste 29, Lakeland, FL 33811
Various types and sizes of sterile and non sterile sponges.

SPONGE, EXTERNAL *(cont'd)*

Tillotson Healthcare Corp. 888-335-7500
10 Glenshaw St, Orangeburg, NY 10962
COTTON PLUS, non-sterile, high absorbent; USP Type VII gauze. Features a cotton fiber interior for extra absorbency and effective packing.

U-Ten Corporation 630-289-8058
1286 Humbracht Cir, Bartlett, IL 60103
Lap sponges.

Ultracell Medical Technologies, Inc. 877-SPO-NGE1
183 Providence New London Tpke, North Stonington, CT 06359
ULTRACELL Various P.V.A. sponges are available for external use.

SPONGE, EXTERNAL, NEUROLOGICAL *(Cns/Neurology) 84HAY*

American Silk Sutures, Inc. 781-592-7200
82 Sanderson Ave, Lynn, MA 01902
Sponge.

Lenzing Fibers Inc. 251-679-2811
12950 Highway 43 N, Axis, AL 36505
Topical wound dressing.

Surgic Aid, Inc. 800-338-5213
37 Crystal Ave # 287, Derry, NH 03038

Ultracell Medical Technologies, Inc. 877-SPO-NGE1
183 Providence New London Tpke, North Stonington, CT 06359

SPONGE, EXTERNAL, RUBBER *(Surgery) 79GEQ*

Chamberlin Rubber Company, Inc. 585-427-7780
3333 Brighton Henrietta Town Line Rd, PO Box 22700
Rochester, NY 14623

SPONGE, EXTERNAL, SYNTHETIC *(Surgery) 79GEP*

Axiom Medical, Inc. 800-221-8569
19320 Van Ness Ave, Torrance, CA 90501
For use at wound site. polyurethane

Tillotson Healthcare Corp. 888-335-7500
10 Glenshaw St, Orangeburg, NY 10962
COMFORT GUARD, sterile or non-sterile; highly absorbent 100% cotton gauze for IV and drain dressings. Cushioned IV and drain dressings are comprised of non-woven fabric with perforated openings. NEW WEAVE, sterile or non-sterile; quick wicking non-woven sponges & dressings.

Tmp Technologies, Inc. 716-895-6100
1200 Northland Ave, Buffalo, NY 14215
Surgical prep. Swabs.

Ultracell Medical Technologies, Inc. 877-SPO-NGE1
183 Providence New London Tpke, North Stonington, CT 06359

SPONGE, GAUZE *(Dental And Oral) 76EFQ*

A Plus International, Inc 909-591-5168
5138 Eucalyptus Ave, Chino, CA 91710
Various sizes of gauze sponge 100% cotton.

Adi Medical Division Of Asia Dynamics (Group) Inc. 877-647-7699
1565 S Shields Dr, Waukegan, IL 60085

Amd-Ritmed, Inc. 800-445-0340
295 Firetower Road, Tonawanda, NY 14150

American White Cross - Houston 609-514-4744
15200 North Fwy, Houston, TX 77090
Various.

Aso Llc 941-379-0300
12120 Esther Lama Dr Ste 112, El Paso, TX 79936
Sterile gauze roll.

Baldur Systems Corporation 800-736-4716
33235 Transit Ave, Union City, CA 94587
2x2 cotton-filled gauze sponges, non-sterile, 125-130 grams per pack, 200 pcs per pack, 25 packs per box, 4 boxes per carton.

Barnhardt Mfg. Co. 704-376-0380
1100 Hawthorne Ln, Charlotte, NC 28205
Various sizes of sterile and non-sterile gauze sponges.

Certified Safety Manufacturing 800-854-7474
1400 Chestnut Ave, Kansas City, MO 64127

Chagrin Safety Supply, Inc. 800-227-0468
8227 Washington St # 1, Chagrin Falls, OH 44023

Cypress Medical Products 800-334-3646
1202 S. Rte. 31, McHenry, IL 60050
Sterile or non-sterile gauze sponges, and cotton-filled dental sponges.

SPONGE, GAUZE *(cont'd)*

Dermapac, Inc. 203-924-7148
PO Box 852, Shelton, CT 06484
Procedural kits/packs. Custom kits.

Dukal Corporation 800-243-0741
5 Plant Ave, Hauppauge, NY 11788

Dumex Medical Surgical Products Ltd. 800-463-9613
104 Shorting Rd., Scarborough, ONT M1S 3S4 Canada
DUCARE Dumex Pak-Its plain guaze packing strips: for packing wounds.

Elastic Corporation Of America 704-328-5381
455 Highway 70, Columbiana, AL 35051
Gauze-various sizes.

Galia Textil S.A. De C.V. 246-1-6-066
Lote 3 Manzana 4, Parque Industrial, Tlaxcala Mexico
Sponge, gauze

General Econopak, Inc. 888-871-8568
1725 N 6th St, Philadelphia, PA 19122
100% cotton, all sizes, sterile.

Grand Medical Products 800-521-2055
7222 Ertel Ln, Houston, TX 77040

Johnson & Johnson Consumer Products, Inc. 800-526-3967
199 Grandview Rd, Skillman, NJ 08558

K. W. Griffen Co. 203-846-1923
100 Pearl St, Norwalk, CT 06850
Various types of gauze sponges and pads.

Kentron Health Care, Inc. 615-384-0573
3604 Kelton Jackson Rd, P.o. Box 120, Springfield, TN 37172
Gauze sponges.

Marel Corporation 203-934-8187
5 Saw Mill Rd, West Haven, CT 06516
Gauze sponge, filled sponge, fluff sponge, cut gauze, gauze bolt.

Mcneil Healthcare, Inc. 203-932-6263
481 Elm St, West Haven, CT 06516
Multiple.

Medspring Group, Inc. 801-295-9750
533 W 2600 S Ste 105, Bountiful, UT 84010
Gauze.

Mine Safety Appliances Company 866-MSA-1001
121 Gamma Dr, Pittsburgh, PA 15238

Normed 800-288-8200
PO Box 3644, Seattle, WA 98124
Various sterile/non-sterile absorbent gauze (external).

Omnia, Inc. 863-619-8100
3125 Drane Field Rd Ste 29, Lakeland, FL 33811
Dental and medical sponge.

Pac-Dent Intl., Inc. 909-839-0888
21078 Commerce Point Dr, Walnut, CA 91789
Gauze sponges.

Parker Anderson Llc 888-799-4289
5030 Paradise Rd Ste A214, Las Vegas, NV 89119
Hemostatic gauze (sterile) non absorbable for internal use.

Patterson Medical Supply, Inc. 262-387-8720
W68N158 Evergreen Blvd, Cedarburg, WI 53012
Gauze; gauze bandages;gauze sponges.

Pharaoh Trading Company 866-929-4913
9701 Brookpark Rd, Knollwood Plaza, Suite 241, Cleveland, OH 44129

Stryker Puerto Rico, Ltd. 939-307-2500
Hwy. 3, Km. 131.2, Las Guasimas Ind. Park, Arroyo, PR 00714
Various types of sterile,disposable femoral sponges.

Surgic Aid, Inc. 800-338-5213
37 Crystal Ave # 287, Derry, NH 03038

Tidi Products, Llc 920-751-4380
570 Enterprise Dr, Neenah, WI 54956
Non absorbent gauze sponge, various sizes and types, sterile and non-sterile.

SPONGE, GAUZE *(cont'd)*

Tillotson Healthcare Corp. 888-335-7500
10 Glenshaw St, Orangeburg, NY 10962
MULTI CARE SPONGE, non sterile; highly absorbent USP Type VII gauze sponge. COMFORT GUARD, sterile or non-sterile, highly absorbent 100% cotton gauze for tracheotomy dressings. Tracheotomy dressing feature pre-cut fenestrations that are sewn and cross-stiched. SUPER FLUFF SPONGE, sterile or non-sterile; highly absorbent USP Type VII gauze sponge. Features a diamond fold with diagonal measure and unique highly absorbent crinkle weave pattern. STERILE CARE SPONGE, sterile; highly absorbent USP Type VII gauze sponge. Feature excellent absorbency and fast wicking action. SURGI CARE SPONGE, sterile; highly absorbent USP Type VII gauze sponge. Feature finished and folded edges.

U-Ten Corporation 630-289-8058
1286 Humbracht Cir, Bartlett, IL 60103
Gauze sponge.

White Knight Healthcare 800-851-4431
Calle 16, Number 780, Agua Prieta, Sonora Mexico
Sponge, gauze

SPONGE, HEMOSTATIC, ABSORBABLE COLLAGEN
(Surgery) 79THO

Biocell Laboratories, Inc. 800-222-8382
2001 E University Dr, Rancho Dominguez, CA 90220
Modified collagen hemostat.

Johnson & Johnson Medical Division Of Ethicon, Inc. 800-423-4018
2500 E Arbrook Blvd, Arlington, TX 76014

SPONGE, INTERNAL *(Cns/Neurology) 84HAZ*

Carwild Corp. 860-442-4914
3 State Pier Rd, New London, CT 06320

Intl. Medsurg Connection, Inc. 847-619-9926
935 N Plum Grove Rd Ste V, Schaumburg, IL 60173
Laparotomy sponges.

Mcneil Healthcare, Inc. 203-932-6263
481 Elm St, West Haven, CT 06516
Neuro sponge.

Surgic Aid, Inc. 800-338-5213
37 Crystal Ave # 287, Derry, NH 03038

Tillotson Healthcare Corp. 888-335-7500
10 Glenshaw St, Orangeburg, NY 10962
VIEW GUARD, sterile x-ray detectable; USP Type VII gauze sponges. Features a built-in element for rapid sponge detection. TONSIL SPONGE, sterile, x-ray detectable; USP Type VII gauze sponges. Features a built-in element for rapid sponge detection.

Ultracell Medical Technologies, Inc. 877-SPO-NGE1
183 Providence New London Tpke, North Stonington, CT 06359
ULTRACELL P.V.A. surgical sponges of various sizes are available for internal use.

SPONGE, LAPAROTOMY *(Surgery) 79RVG*

Adi Medical Division Of Asia Dynamics (Group) Inc. 877-647-7699
1565 S Shields Dr, Waukegan, IL 60085

Amd-Ritmed, Inc. 800-445-0340
295 Firetower Road, Tonawanda, NY 14150

Dukal Corporation 800-243-0741
5 Plant Ave, Hauppauge, NY 11788

Dumex Medical Surgical Products Ltd. 800-463-9613
104 Shorting Rd., Scarborough, ONT M1S 3S4 Canada
DULAP

Grand Medical Products 800-521-2055
7222 Ertel Ln, Houston, TX 77040
Sterile and non-sterile.

SPONGE, NEURO *(Cns/Neurology) 84RVH*

Amd-Ritmed, Inc. 800-445-0340
295 Firetower Road, Tonawanda, NY 14150
X-ray or non-x-ray detectable, strung or unstrung, in strip or circular form.

Carwild Corp. 860-442-4914
3 State Pier Rd, New London, CT 06320

Dumex Medical Surgical Products Ltd. 800-463-9613
104 Shorting Rd., Scarborough, ONT M1S 3S4 Canada

Surgic Aid, Inc. 800-338-5213
37 Crystal Ave # 287, Derry, NH 03038

SPONGE, OPHTHALMIC *(Ophthalmology) 86HOZ*

Alcon Manufacturing, Ltd. 817-551-6813
714 Columbia Ave, Sinking Spring, PA 19608
Disposable ophthalmic sponges.

Amd-Ritmed, Inc. 800-445-0340
295 Firetower Road, Tonawanda, NY 14150
Eye spears: sterile, in peel pack of 10 pcs.

B. Graczyk, Inc. 269-782-2100
27826 Burmax Park, Dowagiac, MI 49047
Various sizes and shapes of sterile and non-sterile sponges.

Bausch & Lomb Surgical 636-255-5051
3365 Tree Court Ind Blvd, Saint Louis, MO 63122

Eagle Laboratories 800-782-6534
10201 Trademark St Ste A, Rancho Cucamonga, CA 91730

Hurricane Medical 941-751-0588
5315 Lena Rd, Bradenton, FL 34211
Various.

Jedmed Instruments Co. 314-845-3770
5416 Jedmed Ct, Saint Louis, MO 63129

Med-Logics, Inc. 949-582-3891
26061 Merit Cir Ste 102, Laguna Hills, CA 92653
Eye spear.

Ocusoft, Inc. 281-342-3350
PO Box 429, Richmond, TX 77406
Opthalmic sponge.

Solos Endoscopy 800-388-6445
65 Sprague St # B, Boston/dedham Commerce Park, Boston, MA 02136
Ophthalmic sponge.

Ultracell Medical Technologies, Inc. 877-SPO-NGE1
183 Providence New London Tpke, North Stonington, CT 06359
ULTRACELL Ophthalmic sponges. Various P.V.A. sponges are available. LASIK spears, LASIK drains, LASIK shields and LASIK wipes.

SPONGE, OTHER *(General) 80RVL*

Amd-Ritmed, Inc. 800-445-0340
295 Firetower Road, Tonawanda, NY 14150
Peanut/Cherry; x-ray detectable, in holder or strung on count card. Cylindrical: x-ray or non-x-ray detectable, end or center strung. Stick: sterile or non-sterile. Kittners: strung or non-strung, in holder or strung on count card. Needlets: double magnet, foam/magnet, foam strip/magnet. Tracheotomy, tonsil and nasal.

Cfi Medical Solutions (Contour Fabricators, Inc.) 810-750-5300
14241 N Fenton Rd, Fenton, MI 48430

Contec, Inc. 800-289-5762
525 Locust Grv, Spartanburg, SC 29303
VK Sponge incorporates the same high sorbency of polyester foam with the abrasion resistance of Polynit fabric. This sponge is designed for general cleaning adn wiping and ideal for use in the laboratory.

Custom Healthcare Systems, Inc. 804-421-5959
4205 Eubank Rd, Richmond, VA 23231

Cypress Medical Products 800-334-3646
1202 S. Rte. 31, McHenry, IL 60050
Non-sterile tracheostomy gauze sponges, 4x4 12-ply, sewn. Also, conforming stretch gauze, sterile or non-sterile.

Dukal Corporation 800-243-0741
5 Plant Ave, Hauppauge, NY 11788

Encompas Unlimited, Inc. 800-825-7701
PO Box 516, Tallevast, FL 34270
Disposable, endoscopic sponge. $1.04/sponge - for effective & safe endoscope cleaning.

Grand Medical Products 800-521-2055
7222 Ertel Ln, Houston, TX 77040

Kensey Nash Corporation 484-713-2100
735 Pennsylvania Dr, Exton, PA 19341
DRILAC, polylactic acid OPLA surgical dressing, surgical sponge for dental extraction wound management.

Mckesson General Medical 800-446-3008
8741 Landmark Rd, Richmond, VA 23228
Non-sterile sponges.

Medicom 800-361-2862
9404 Cote de Liesse, Lachine, QUE H8T 1A1 Canada
SAFEGAUZE Non-Woven Gauze Sponge. Non-sterile and sterile, 100% cotton.

SPONGE, OTHER *(cont'd)*

Multisorb Technologies, Inc. — 800-445-9890
325 Harlem Rd, Buffalo, NY 14224
DRIMOP, absorbs blood and urine.

Mydent International — 800-275-0020
80 Suffolk Ct, Hauppauge, NY 11788

Rogers Foam Corp. — 714-538-3033
808 W Nicolas Ave, Orange, CA 92868
Operating sponges, orthopedic.

Surgical Tools, Inc. — 800-774-2040
1106 Monroe St, Bedford, VA 24523

Ultracell Medical Technologies, Inc. — 877-SPO-NGE1
183 Providence New London Tpke, North Stonington, CT 06359
Ultracell epistaxis packing. Various sizes made of PVA sponge. Ultacell nasal packing with or without airway.

SPONGE, RAYON CELLULOSE *(General) 80RVI*

Global Healthcare — 800-601-3880
1495 Hembree Rd Ste 700, Roswell, GA 30076
Non Woven Sterile and Non Sterile Gauze Sponges

Katena Products, Inc. — 800-225-1195
4 Stewart Ct, Denville, NJ 07834
Sponge, hydro-cellulose.

Ultracell Medical Technologies, Inc. — 877-SPO-NGE1
183 Providence New London Tpke, North Stonington, CT 06359

SPONGE, SCRUB *(Surgery) 79RVJ*

Amd-Ritmed, Inc. — 800-445-0340
295 Firetower Road, Tonawanda, NY 14150

SPONGE, X-RAY DETECTABLE *(Surgery) 79RVK*

Codman & Shurtleff, Inc — 800-225-0460
325 Paramount Dr, Raynham, MA 02767

Surgic Aid, Inc. — 800-338-5213
37 Crystal Ave # 287, Derry, NH 03038

Ultracell Medical Technologies, Inc. — 877-SPO-NGE1
183 Providence New London Tpke, North Stonington, CT 06359

SPOON, EAR *(Ear/Nose/Throat) 77JZE*

Aesculap Implant Systems Inc. — 1-800-234-9179
3773 Corporate Pkwy, Center Valley, PA 18034

Bausch & Lomb Surgical — 636-255-5051
3365 Tree Court Ind Blvd, Saint Louis, MO 63122

SPOON, MEDICINE *(General) 80VLJ*

Amsino International, Inc. — 800-MD-AMSINO
855 Towne Center Dr, Pomona, CA 91767
AMSINO 3-in. white birch. Item AS024.

Apothecary Products, Inc. — 800-328-2742
11750 12th Ave S, Burnsville, MN 55337

Carex Health Brands — 800-526-8051
921 E Amidon St, PO Box 2526, Sioux Falls, SD 57104
Precisely calibrated in cc and tsp increments for dosages of up to two teaspoons (10 cc).

Health Enterprises — 800-633-4243
90 George Leven Dr, North Attleboro, MA 02760

Solon Manufacturing Co. — 800-341-6640
338 Madison Ave Ste 7, Skowhegan, ME 04976
3-, 3-5/8-, or 5-in. non-sterile wood medical spoons. Available in wrapped or non-wrapped.

SPOON, OPHTHALMIC *(Ophthalmology) 86HNB*

Accutome, Inc. — 610-889-0200
3222 Phoenixville Pike, Malvern, PA 19355
Spoons.

B. Graczyk, Inc. — 269-782-2100
27826 Burmax Park, Dowagiac, MI 49047
Various types of spoons.

Bausch & Lomb Surgical — 636-255-5051
3365 Tree Court Ind Blvd, Saint Louis, MO 63122

Hai Laboratories, Inc. — 781-862-9884
320 Massachusetts Ave, Lexington, MA 02420
Lens spoon - various types.

Katena Products, Inc. — 800-225-1195
4 Stewart Ct, Denville, NJ 07834

Stephens Instruments, Inc. — 800-354-7848
2500 Sandersville Rd, Lexington, KY 40511
$20.00 per unit (standard).

SPOT FILM DEVICE *(Radiology) 90IXL*

Ge Medical Systems, Llc — 262-548-2355
3000 N Grandview Blvd, W-417, Waukesha, WI 53188
Various types of spotfilm devices.

Marconi Medical Systems — 800-323-0550
595 Miner Rd, Cleveland, OH 44143

SPRAYER, THIN LAYER CHROMATOGRAPHY *(Chemistry) 75UIF*

Camag Scientific, Inc. — 800-334-3909
515 Cornelius Harnett Dr, Wilmington, NC 28401

Whatman Inc. — 732-885-6529
800 Centennial Ave Bldg 1, Piscataway, NJ 08854

SPREADER, BLADDER NECK *(Gastro/Urology) 78FHK*

Aesculap Implant Systems Inc. — 1-800-234-9179
3773 Corporate Pkwy, Center Valley, PA 18034

Island Biosurgical, Llc — 425-251-3455
18 Meadow Ln, Mercer Island, WA 98040
Mesh bolster for endopelvic fascia support. Suspension kit for correction of stress incontinence.

SPREADER, OTHER *(Surgery) 79RVQ*

Akorn, Inc. — 800-535-7155
2500 Millbrook Dr, Buffalo Grove, IL 60089
Ophthalmic incision spreader plus diamond knives and other titanium instruments.

Holmed Corporation — 508-238-3351
40 Norfolk Ave, South Easton, MA 02375

Inland Specialties, Inc. — 800-741-0022
7655 Matoaka Rd, Sarasota, FL 34243
Spreader block sizes 2in., 2.5in., and 3in.

Zimmer Holdings, Inc. — 800-613-6131
1800 W Center St, PO Box 708, Warsaw, IN 46580

SPREADER, PLASTER (CAST) *(Orthopedics) 87RVN*

Alimed, Inc. — 800-225-2610
297 High St, Dedham, MA 02026

Bsn Medical, Inc — 800-552-1157
5825 Carnegie Blvd, Charlotte, NC 28209
M-PACT CAST SPREADERS are made of solid stainless steel to resist corrosion and abrasive handling. Available in two models - Small Office Model and Large Hospital Model.

Codman & Shurtleff, Inc — 800-225-0460
325 Paramount Dr, Raynham, MA 02767

Kmedic — 800-955-0559
190 Veterans Dr, Northvale, NJ 07647

Miltex Inc. — 800-645-8000
589 Davies Dr, York, PA 17402

Ortho-Med, Inc. — 800-547-5571
3208 SE 13th Ave, Portland, OR 97202

Zimmer Holdings, Inc. — 800-613-6131
1800 W Center St, PO Box 708, Warsaw, IN 46580

Zimmer Orthopaedic Surgical Products — 800-321-5533
PO Box 10, 200 West Ohio Ave., Dover, OH 44622

SPREADER, PULP CANAL FILLING MATERIAL, ENDODONTIC *(Dental And Oral) 76EKK*

Acteon Inc. — 800-289-6367
124 Gaither Dr Ste 140, Mount Laurel, NJ 08054

Aesculap Implant Systems Inc. — 1-800-234-9179
3773 Corporate Pkwy, Center Valley, PA 18034

Coltene/Whaledent Inc. — 330-916-8858
235 Ascot Pkwy, Cuyahoga Falls, OH 44223
Spreader.

Dental Usa, Inc. — 815-363-8003
5005 McCullom Lake Rd, McHenry, IL 60050
Spreader.

Dentalez Group — 866-DTE-INFO
101 Lindenwood Dr Ste 225, Valleybrooke Corporate Center Malvern, PA 19355

Dentalez Group, Stardental Division — 717-291-1161
1816 Colonial Village Ln, Lancaster, PA 17601
Explorer, operative.

Hu-Friedy Manufacturing Co., Inc. — 800-483-7433
3232 N Rockwell St, Chicago, IL 60618
$12.15 to $12.65 each, 18 types.

Js Dental Mfg., Inc. — 800-284-3368
196 N Salem Rd, Ridgefield, CT 06877
Finger spreader.

SPREADER, PULP CANAL FILLING MATERIAL, ENDODONTIC *(cont'd)*

Kerr Corp. 714-516-7400
28200 Wick Rd, Romulus, MI 48174
Endodontic spreader.

Miltex Dental Technologies, Inc. 516-576-6022
589 Davies Dr, York, PA 17402
Various types of hand-operated endodontic spreaders.

Moyco Technologies, Inc. 800-331-8837
200 Commerce Dr, Montgomeryville, PA 18936

Premier Dental Products Co. 888-670-6100
1710 Romano Dr, PO Box 4500, Plymouth Meeting, PA 19462

Pulpdent Corp. 800-343-4342
80 Oakland St, Watertown, MA 02472
No common name listed.

San Diego Swiss Machining, Inc. 858-571-6636
9177 Aero Dr Ste A, San Diego, CA 92123
Ultrasonic tips.

Sci-Dent, Inc. 800-323-4145
210 Dowdle St Ste 2, Algonquin, IL 60102

SPREADER, RIB *(Orthopedics) 87RVO*

Fehling Surgical Instruments 800-FEHLING
509 Broadstone Ln NW, Acworth, GA 30101

Karl Storz Endoscopy-America Inc. 800-421-0837
600 Corporate Pointe, Culver City, CA 90230

Princeton Medical Group, Inc. 800-875-0869
1189 Royal Links Dr, Mt Pleasant, SC 29466

SPREADER, VEIN *(Cardiovascular) 74RVP*

Codman & Shurtleff, Inc 800-225-0460
325 Paramount Dr, Raynham, MA 02767

SPRING, ORTHODONTIC *(Dental And Oral) 76ECO*

Acme-Monaco Corp. 860-224-1349
75 Winchell Rd, New Britain, CT 06052
Springs and Wireforms

American Orthodontics Corp. 800-558-7687
1714 Cambridge Ave, Sheboygan, WI 53081

Barnhart Industries, Inc. 800-325-9973
3690 Highway M, Imperial, MO 63052
Traction springs.

Classone Orthodontics, Inc. 806-799-0608
5064 50th St, Lubbock, TX 79414
Various types of springs.

Forestadent Usa 314-878-5985
2315 Weldon Pkwy, Saint Louis, MO 63146
Orthodontic spring.

G & H Wire Co. 800-526-1026
2165 Earlywood Dr, Franklin, IN 46131
Both Nickel Titanium and Apollo Stainless Steel Open & Closed Springs

Highland Metals, Inc. 800-368-6484
419 Perrymont Ave, San Jose, CA 95125
Various.

Lancer Orthodontics, Inc. 760-304-2705
253 Pawnee St, San Marcos, CA 92078
Spring, orthodontic.

Ortho Organizers, Inc. 760-448-8730
1822 Aston Ave, Carlsbad, CA 92008
Various types of orthodontic springs.

Orthoband Company, Inc. 800-325-9973
3690 Highway M, Imperial, MO 63052

Orthodontic Design And Production, Inc. 760-734-3995
1370 Decision St Ste D, Vista, CA 92081
Types of separating and de-impaction springs.

Oscar, Inc. 317-849-2618
11793 Technology Ln, Fishers, IN 46038
Coil springs.

Pacific Coast Mfg., Inc. 425-485-8866
15604 163rd Ave NE, Woodinville, WA 98072
Support chair.

Ultimate Wireforms, Inc. 800-999-6484
200 Central St, Bristol, CT 06010
Nickel titanium and Stainless Steel springs in a variety of wire and lumen sizes.

SPRING, ORTHODONTIC *(cont'd)*

3m Unitek 800-634-5300
2724 Peck Rd, Monrovia, CA 91016

SPUD, OPHTHALMIC *(Ophthalmology) 86HNA*

B. Graczyk, Inc. 269-782-2100
27826 Burmax Park, Dowagiac, MI 49047
Various types of spuds.

Bausch & Lomb Surgical 636-255-5051
3365 Tree Court Ind Blvd, Saint Louis, MO 63122

Demetech Corp. 888-324-2447
3530 NW 115th Ave, Doral, FL 33178
Various manual ophthalmic spuds.

Eye Care And Cure 800-486-6169
4646 S Overland Dr, Tucson, AZ 85714
Spud.

Fischer Surgical Inc. 314-303-7753
1343 Pine Dr, Arnold, MO 63010
Various types of ophthalmic spuds.

Fortrad Eye Instruments Corp. 973-543-2371
8 Franklin Rd, Mendham, NJ 07945

Katena Products, Inc. 800-225-1195
4 Stewart Ct, Denville, NJ 07834

Stephens Instruments, Inc. 800-354-7848
2500 Sandersville Rd, Lexington, KY 40511
$35.00 each.

The Alger Company, Inc. 800-320-1043
320 Flightline Rd, Lago Vista, TX 78645
Corneal rust ring remover-eye spud.

STABILIZER, HEART, NON-COMPRESSION, REPROCESSED *(Cardiovascular) 74NQG*

Maquet Cardiovascular LLC 888-880-2874
45 Barbour Pond Dr, Wayne, NJ 07470

Sterilmed, Inc. 763-488-3400
11400 73rd Ave N Ste 100, Maple Grove, MN 55369
Heart stabilizer.

STABILIZER, VEIN *(General) 80LBJ*

Ac Healthcare Supply, Inc. 905-448-4706
11651 230th St, Cambria Heights, NY 11411
Scalp vein set.

Donell 800-324-7455
1801 Taylor Ave, Louisville, KY 40213
K-DERM Cream Vitamin K cream. Therapy to improve the appearance of bruises and purpura.

STAGE, MICROSCOPE *(Pathology) 88KEJ*

Accu-Scope, Inc. 516-759-1000
7 Littleworth Ln, Sea Cliff, NY 11579

Edmund Industrial Optics 800-363-1992
101 E Gloucester Pike, Barrington, NJ 08007
Microscope stages; various microscope accessories (objectives, eyepieces, stages, illuminators).

One Lambda, Inc. 800-822-8824
21001 Kittridge St, Canoga Park, CA 91303
LAMBDA SCAN PLUS II and LAMBDA SCAN PLUS II fluoro semi-automated stage HLA tray evaluation systems.

Physitemp Instruments, Inc. 800-452-8510
154 Huron Ave, Clifton, NJ 07013
Thermal microscope stage to accommodate a large tissue culture dish (up to 100 mm) and maintains specimen temperature between -20 and +100 degrees C.

Western Scientific Co., Inc. 877-489-3726
4104 24th St # 183, San Francisco, CA 94114

STAIN, ACID FUCHSIN *(Pathology) 88IDF*

American Mastertech Scientific, Inc. 209-368-4031
1330 Thurman St, Lodi, CA 95240
Multiple types of fuchsin acid.

Bd Diagnostic Systems 800-675-0908
7 Loveton Cir, Sparks, MD 21152

Biomerieux Inc. 800-682-2666
100 Rodolphe St, Durham, NC 27712

Poly Scientific R&D Corp. 800-645-5825
70 Cleveland Ave, Bay Shore, NY 11706

STAIN, ACRIDINE ORANGE *(Pathology) 88IDC*

Bd Diagnostic Systems 800-675-0908
7 Loveton Cir, Sparks, MD 21152

STAIN, ACRIDINE ORANGE *(cont'd)*

Pml Microbiologicals — 800-628-7014
27120 SW 95th Ave, Wilsonville, OR 97070

Polysciences, Inc. — 800-523-2575
400 Valley Rd, Warrington, PA 18976
C.I. 46005

STAIN, ALCIAN BLUE *(Pathology) 88IDA*

American Mastertech Scientific, Inc. — 209-368-4031
1330 Thurman St, Lodi, CA 95240
Multiple.

Anatech, Ltd. — 800-262-8324
1020 Harts Lake Rd, Battle Creek, MI 49037
Alcian Blue, certified by Biological Stain Commission, 25 gram bottle, powder.

Poly Scientific R&D Corp. — 800-645-5825
70 Cleveland Ave, Bay Shore, NY 11706

Rowley Biochemical Institute — 978-739-4883
10 Electronics Ave, Danvers Industrial Park, Danvers, MA 01923

Ventana Medical Systems, Inc. — 800-227-2155
1910 E Innovation Park Dr, Oro Valley, AZ 85755
Dye solution stain.

STAIN, ALDEHYDE FUCHSIN *(Pathology) 88IDB*

American Mastertech Scientific, Inc. — 209-368-4031
1330 Thurman St, Lodi, CA 95240
Multiple.

Pochemco, Inc. — 413-536-2900
724 Main St, Holyoke, MA 01040
Schiff's reagent.

STAIN, ALIZARIN RED *(Pathology) 88IDD*

American Mastertech Scientific, Inc. — 209-368-4031
1330 Thurman St, Lodi, CA 95240
Multiple.

Budenheim Usa, Inc — 800-645-3044
245 Newtown Rd Ste 305, Plainview, NY 11803

Rocky Mountain Reagents,Inc. — 303-762-0800
3207 W Hampden Ave, Englewood, CO 80110

STAIN, AMMONIACAL SILVER HYDROXIDE SILVER NITRATE *(Pathology) 88ICZ*

American Mastertech Scientific, Inc. — 209-368-4031
1330 Thurman St, Lodi, CA 95240
Multiple.

Poly Scientific R&D Corp. — 800-645-5825
70 Cleveland Ave, Bay Shore, NY 11706

Polysciences, Inc. — 800-523-2575
400 Valley Rd, Warrington, PA 18976

Ventana Medical Systems, Inc. — 800-227-2155
1910 E Innovation Park Dr, Oro Valley, AZ 85755
Ammoniacal silver nitrate.

STAIN, ANILINE BLUE *(Pathology) 88KFD*

A. J. P. Scientific, Inc. — 973-472-7200
82 Industrial St E, Clifton, NJ 07012
Aniline blue.

American Mastertech Scientific, Inc. — 209-368-4031
1330 Thurman St, Lodi, CA 95240
Multiple.

Poly Scientific R&D Corp. — 800-645-5825
70 Cleveland Ave, Bay Shore, NY 11706

Polysciences, Inc. — 800-523-2575
400 Valley Rd, Warrington, PA 18976
C.I. 42755, water soluble

Richard-Allan Scientific — 269-544-5628
4481 Campus Dr, Kalamazoo, MI 49008
Aniline blue stain.

Rocky Mountain Reagents,Inc. — 303-762-0800
3207 W Hampden Ave, Englewood, CO 80110

STAIN, AURAMINE O *(Pathology) 88KJK*

Alpha-Tec Systems, Inc. — 800-221-6058
12019 NE 99th St Ste 1780, Vancouver, WA 98682
Auramine O Stain

Bd Diagnostic Systems — 800-675-0908
7 Loveton Cir, Sparks, MD 21152

STAIN, AURAMINE O *(cont'd)*

Polysciences, Inc. — 800-523-2575
400 Valley Rd, Warrington, PA 18976
C.I.41000

STAIN, BIEBRICH SCARLET *(Pathology) 88ICN*

American Mastertech Scientific, Inc. — 209-368-4031
1330 Thurman St, Lodi, CA 95240
Multiple.

Poly Scientific R&D Corp. — 800-645-5825
70 Cleveland Ave, Bay Shore, NY 11706

Polysciences, Inc. — 800-523-2575
400 Valley Rd, Warrington, PA 18976
C.I. 26905

Richard-Allan Scientific — 269-544-5628
4481 Campus Dr, Kalamazoo, MI 49008
Biebrich scarlet.

STAIN, BIOLOGICAL, GENERAL *(Pathology) 88UIG*

Bd Diagnostic Systems — 800-675-0908
7 Loveton Cir, Sparks, MD 21152

Budenheim Usa, Inc — 800-645-3044
245 Newtown Rd Ste 305, Plainview, NY 11803

Carolina Biological Supply Co. — 800-334-5551
2700 York Rd, Burlington, NC 27215

Dade Behring, Inc. — 800-948-3233
1717 Deerfield Rd, Deerfield, IL 60015

Medical Chemical Corp. — 800-424-9394
19430 Van Ness Ave, Torrance, CA 90501

STAIN, BISMARCK BROWN Y *(Pathology) 88KJM*

American Mastertech Scientific, Inc. — 209-368-4031
1330 Thurman St, Lodi, CA 95240
Multiple.

STAIN, BRILLIANT CRESYL BLUE *(Pathology) 88KJN*

Ricca Chemical Company Llc — 817-461-5601
1490 Lammers Pike, Batesville, IN 47006

Ricca Chemical Company, Llc — 817-461-5601
448 W Fork Dr, Arlington, TX 76012
Brilliant crystal blue.

STAIN, BRILLIANT GREEN *(Pathology) 88KJO*

Bd Diagnostic Systems — 800-675-0908
7 Loveton Cir, Sparks, MD 21152

STAIN, BRILLIANT YELLOW *(Pathology) 88ICM*

Polysciences, Inc. — 800-523-2575
400 Valley Rd, Warrington, PA 18976
C.I. 24890, sodium salt

STAIN, CARBOL FUCHSIN *(Pathology) 88ICL*

A. J. P. Scientific, Inc. — 973-472-7200
82 Industrial St E, Clifton, NJ 07012
Carbol fuchsin.

Alpha-Tec Systems, Inc. — 800-221-6058
12019 NE 99th St Ste 1780, Vancouver, WA 98682
Carbol Fuchsin (Ziehl-Neelsen, Kinyoun).

American Mastertech Scientific, Inc. — 209-368-4031
1330 Thurman St, Lodi, CA 95240
Multiple.

Bd Diagnostic Systems — 800-675-0908
7 Loveton Cir, Sparks, MD 21152

E K Industries, Inc. — 877-EKI-CHEM
1403 Herkimer St, Joliet, IL 60432
Carbol-fuchsin, ziehi-neelsen.

Labchem, Inc. — 412-826-5230
200 William Pitt Way, Pittsburgh, PA 15238
Carbol fuchsin - kinyoun (lc12880).

Medical Chemical Corp. — 800-424-9394
19430 Van Ness Ave, Torrance, CA 90501
$11.00 per 100ml.

Poly Scientific R&D Corp. — 800-645-5825
70 Cleveland Ave, Bay Shore, NY 11706

Ricca Chemical Company Llc — 888-467-4222
1841 Broad St, Pocomoke City, MD 21851
Various.

Ricca Chemical Company Llc — 817-461-5601
1490 Lammers Pike, Batesville, IN 47006

STAIN, CARBOL FUCHSIN *(cont'd)*

Ricca Chemical Company, Llc 817-461-5601
448 W Fork Dr, Arlington, TX 76012
Various.

Richard-Allan Scientific 269-544-5628
4481 Campus Dr, Kalamazoo, MI 49008
Carbol fuchsin.

Rocky Mountain Reagents,Inc. 303-762-0800
3207 W Hampden Ave, Englewood, CO 80110

Ventana Medical Systems, Inc. 800-227-2155
1910 E Innovation Park Dr, Oro Valley, AZ 85755
Various dye stains.

STAIN, CARMINE *(Pathology) 88KJP*

American Mastertech Scientific, Inc. 209-368-4031
1330 Thurman St, Lodi, CA 95240
Multiple.

Polysciences, Inc. 800-523-2575
400 Valley Rd, Warrington, PA 18976
C.I. 75470

STAIN, CHEMICAL SOLUTION *(Pathology) 88LED*

Anatech, Ltd. 800-262-8324
1020 Harts Lake Rd, Battle Creek, MI 49037
Hp BLUE and Hp YELLOW, used to demonstrate Helicobacter in tissue sections

Bdh, Inc. 800-268-0310
350 Evans Ave., Toronto, ONT M8Z 1K5 Canada

Biogenex Laboratories 800-421-4149
4600 Norris Canyon Rd, San Ramon, CA 94583
HISTOGEN, STREPTAUIDEN; Immunohistology kits: peroxidase-antiperoxidase (PAP), avidin-biotin immunoperoxidase (AB); or indirect immunoperoxidase (IIP) methods.

Covance Research Products Inc. 800-223-0796
180 Rustcraft Rd Ste 140, Dedham, MA 02026
Immunohistology kits: peroxidase/anti-peroxidase (pap), avidin/biotin (abc), or streptavidin/biotin (HRP and alkaline phosphates labels) biotin free polymer detection (ACUITY), biotin free mouse-on-mouse detection (ACUITY MoM).

Fertility Solutions, Inc. 800-959-7656
13000 Shaker Blvd, Cleveland, OH 44120
Sperm viability stain.

Richard-Allan Scientific 269-544-5628
4481 Campus Dr, Kalamazoo, MI 49008
Various stains.

Scandinavian Formulas, Inc. 215-453-2507
140 E Church St, Sellersville, PA 18960
Lozenge.

STAIN, CHLORAZOL BLACK E *(Pathology) 88KJQ*

Polysciences, Inc. 800-523-2575
400 Valley Rd, Warrington, PA 18976
C.I. 30234

STAIN, CONGO RED *(Pathology) 88ICH*

A. J. P. Scientific, Inc. 973-472-7200
82 Industrial St E, Clifton, NJ 07012
Congo red.

American Mastertech Scientific, Inc. 209-368-4031
1330 Thurman St, Lodi, CA 95240
Multiple.

Poly Scientific R&D Corp. 800-645-5825
70 Cleveland Ave, Bay Shore, NY 11706

Richard-Allan Scientific 269-544-5628
4481 Campus Dr, Kalamazoo, MI 49008
Congo red.

Rocky Mountain Reagents,Inc. 303-762-0800
3207 W Hampden Ave, Englewood, CO 80110

Rowley Biochemical Institute 978-739-4883
10 Electronics Ave, Danvers Industrial Park, Danvers, MA 01923

Ventana Medical Systems, Inc. 800-227-2155
1910 E Innovation Park Dr, Oro Valley, AZ 85755
Congo red.

STAIN, CRESYL VIOLET ACETATE *(Pathology) 88ICG*

American Mastertech Scientific, Inc. 209-368-4031
1330 Thurman St, Lodi, CA 95240
Multiple.

STAIN, CRESYL VIOLET ACETATE *(cont'd)*

Imagepath Systems, Inc. 269-699-7182
23126 S Shore Dr, Edwardsburg, MI 49112
Cresyl violet acetate.

STAIN, CRYSTAL VIOLET, HISTOLOGY *(Pathology) 88ICF*

American Mastertech Scientific, Inc. 209-368-4031
1330 Thurman St, Lodi, CA 95240
Multiple.

Bd Diagnostic Systems 800-675-0908
7 Loveton Cir, Sparks, MD 21152

Fisher Healthcare 800-766-7000
9999 Veterans Memorial Dr, Houston, TX 77038
Histology Chemicals.

Hycor Biomedical, Inc. 800-382-2527
7272 Chapman Ave, Garden Grove, CA 92841
Urine stain.

Pochemco, Inc. 413-536-2900
724 Main St, Holyoke, MA 01040
Grain crystal violet.

Poly Scientific R&D Corp. 800-645-5825
70 Cleveland Ave, Bay Shore, NY 11706

Ricca Chemical Company Llc 888-467-4222
1841 Broad St, Pocomoke City, MD 21851
Various.

Ricca Chemical Company Llc 817-461-5601
1490 Lammers Pike, Batesville, IN 47006

Ricca Chemical Company, Llc 817-461-5601
448 W Fork Dr, Arlington, TX 76012
Various.

Richard-Allan Scientific 269-544-5628
4481 Campus Dr, Kalamazoo, MI 49008
Crystal violet.

Rocky Mountain Reagents,Inc. 303-762-0800
3207 W Hampden Ave, Englewood, CO 80110

Sci Gen, Inc. 310-324-6576
333 E Gardena Blvd, Gardena, CA 90248
FDA: Medical Device Manufacturing and packaging. Focus on Histology, Cytology, Analytical and General purpose Reagents, Chemistry, and Sterling and Disinfecting agents.

STAIN, DYE POWDER *(Pathology) 88LEF*

Fisher Scientific Co., Llc. 201-703-3131
1 Reagent Ln, Fair Lawn, NJ 07410
Various histological strains.

Richard-Allan Scientific 269-544-5628
4481 Campus Dr, Kalamazoo, MI 49008
Dye powders.

Sci Gen, Inc. 310-324-6576
333 E Gardena Blvd, Gardena, CA 90248
FDA: Medical Device Manufacturing and packaging. Focus on Histology, Cytology, Analytical and General purpose Reagents, Chemistry, and Sterling and Disinfecting agents.

STAIN, DYE SOLUTION *(Pathology) 88LEE*

American Mastertech Scientific, Inc. 209-368-4031
1330 Thurman St, Lodi, CA 95240
Various type of special stains.

Anatech, Ltd. 800-262-8324
1020 Harts Lake Rd, Battle Creek, MI 49037
Brazilin/Brazilliant (Red nuclear stain); Amyloid Red (demonstrates amyloid); EZ Mucicarmine (red mucus stain); EZ Green (green cytoplasmic stain)

Biosure, Inc. 800-345-2267
12301 Loma Rica Dr Unit G, Grass Valley, CA 95945
BioSure Propidium Iodide staining solution for staining cellular organelles. Two part staining reagent with a longer shelf life.

Invitrogen Corporation 800-955-6288
101 Lincoln Centre Dr, Foster City, CA 94404

Myers-Stevens Group, Inc. 903-566-6696
2931 Vail Ave, Commerce, CA 90040
Urine cell stain.

Ricca Chemical Company Llc 888-467-4222
1841 Broad St, Pocomoke City, MD 21851
Various

Ricca Chemical Company Llc 817-461-5601
1490 Lammers Pike, Batesville, IN 47006

STAIN, DYE SOLUTION *(cont'd)*

Ricca Chemical Company, Llc 817-461-5601
448 W Fork Dr, Arlington, TX 76012
Various.

Richard-Allan Scientific 269-544-5628
4481 Campus Dr, Kalamazoo, MI 49008
Various.

Trigon Technology, Inc. 269-699-7182
23126 S Shore Dr, Edwardsburg, MI 49112
Blue feulgen schiff reagent for feulgen stain procedure.

Tripath Imaging, Inc. 919-206-7140
780 Plantation Dr, Burlington, NC 27215
Hematoxylin stain.

Ventana Medical Systems, Inc. 800-227-2155
1910 E Innovation Park Dr, Oro Valley, AZ 85755
Dye solution stains.

STAIN, EOSIN B *(Pathology) 88ICC*

Sci Gen, Inc. 310-324-6576
333 E Gardena Blvd, Gardena, CA 90248
FDA: Medical Device Manufacturing and packaging. Focus on Histology, Cytology, Analytical and General purpose Reagents, Chemistry, and Sterling and Disinfecting agents.

STAIN, EOSIN Y *(Pathology) 88HYB*

American Mastertech Scientific, Inc. 209-368-4031
1330 Thurman St, Lodi, CA 95240
Multiple.

Anatech, Ltd. 800-262-8324
1020 Harts Lake Rd, Battle Creek, MI 49037
Alcoholic eosin stain

Fisher Scientific Co., Llc. 201-703-3131
1 Reagent Ln, Fair Lawn, NJ 07410
Eosin y solution (alcoholic eosin solution).

Labchem, Inc. 412-826-5230
200 William Pitt Way, Pittsburgh, PA 15238
Eosin y, 1% alcoholic (lc14030).

Medical Chemical Corp. 800-424-9394
19430 Van Ness Ave, Torrance, CA 90501
$9.00 per 100ml.

Pochemco, Inc. 413-536-2900
724 Main St, Holyoke, MA 01040
Stain, sosin Y.

Poly Scientific R&D Corp. 800-645-5825
70 Cleveland Ave, Bay Shore, NY 11706
1% Alcoholic or Agueos.

Ricca Chemical Company Llc 817-461-5601
1490 Lammers Pike, Batesville, IN 47006

Ricca Chemical Company, Llc 817-461-5601
448 W Fork Dr, Arlington, TX 76012
Various.

Richard-Allan Scientific 269-544-5628
4481 Campus Dr, Kalamazoo, MI 49008
Eosin-y.

Rocky Mountain Reagents,Inc. 303-762-0800
3207 W Hampden Ave, Englewood, CO 80110

Rowley Biochemical Institute 978-739-4883
10 Electronics Ave, Danvers Industrial Park, Danvers, MA 01923

Sci Gen, Inc. 310-324-6576
333 E Gardena Blvd, Gardena, CA 90248
FDA: Medical Device Manufacturing and packaging. Focus on Histology, Cytology, Analytical and General purpose Reagents, Chemistry, and Sterling and Disinfecting agents.

Scytek Laboratories, Inc. 435-755-9848
205 S 600 W, Logan, UT 84321
Eosin y.

Spectra-Tint 585-546-8050
250 Cumberland St Ste 228, Rochester, NY 14605
Alcoholic eosin histological counterstain.

STAIN, FAST GREEN *(Pathology) 88HYC*

American Mastertech Scientific, Inc. 209-368-4031
1330 Thurman St, Lodi, CA 95240
Multiple.

Richard-Allan Scientific 269-544-5628
4481 Campus Dr, Kalamazoo, MI 49008
Fast green stwin.

STAIN, FAST GREEN *(cont'd)*

Rocky Mountain Reagents,Inc. 303-762-0800
3207 W Hampden Ave, Englewood, CO 80110

STAIN, FETAL HEMOGLOBIN *(Hematology) 81GHQ*

A. J. P. Scientific, Inc. 973-472-7200
82 Industrial St E, Clifton, NJ 07012
Fetal hemoglobin stain.

Simmler, Inc. 800-325-0786
4564 N Square Dr, High Ridge, MO 63049
Priced at $202.00 for a 300 test kit and $133.00 for a 100 test kit, a screening test for the detection of erythrocytes containing fetal hemoglobin in maternal blood.

Sure-Tech Diagnostic Associates, Inc. 314-894-8933
11040 Lin Valle Dr Ste D, Saint Louis, MO 63123
Fetal hemoglobin staining procedure no. 101.

STAIN, GIEMSA *(Pathology) 88HYF*

A. J. P. Scientific, Inc. 973-472-7200
82 Industrial St E, Clifton, NJ 07012
Giemsa.

American Mastertech Scientific, Inc. 209-368-4031
1330 Thurman St, Lodi, CA 95240
Multiple.

E K Industries, Inc. 877-EKI-CHEM
1403 Herkimer St, Joliet, IL 60432
Giemsa stain.

Gam Rad, Inc. 540-646-5466
Star Rt. 608 (river Rd.), Chilhowie, VA 24319
Geisma stain.

Labchem, Inc. 412-826-5230
200 William Pitt Way, Pittsburgh, PA 15238
Giemsa stain (lc14840).

Lide Laboratories, Inc. 952-758-9760
401 4th Ave SW, New Prague, MN 56071
In vitro diagnostic hansel stain.

Medical Chemical Corp. 800-424-9394
19430 Van Ness Ave, Torrance, CA 90501
$14.00 per 100ml.

Pochemco, Inc. 413-536-2900
724 Main St, Holyoke, MA 01040
Giesma stain.

Ricca Chemical Company Llc 888-467-4222
1841 Broad St, Pocomoke City, MD 21851
Giemsa stain.

Ricca Chemical Company Llc 817-461-5601
1490 Lammers Pike, Batesville, IN 47006

Ricca Chemical Company, Llc 817-461-5601
448 W Fork Dr, Arlington, TX 76012
Giemsa stain.

Richard-Allan Scientific 269-544-5628
4481 Campus Dr, Kalamazoo, MI 49008
Giemsa stain.

Rowley Biochemical Institute 978-739-4883
10 Electronics Ave, Danvers Industrial Park, Danvers, MA 01923

Stanbio Laboratory, Inc. 830-249-0772
1261 N Main St, Boerne, TX 78006
$26.00 for 500ml, Miles stain.

Ventana Medical Systems, Inc. 800-227-2155
1910 E Innovation Park Dr, Oro Valley, AZ 85755
Giemsa stain.

STAIN, GIEMSA, HEMATOLOGY *(Hematology) 81GLP*

Cambridge Diagnostic Products, Inc. 800-525-6262
6880 NW 17th Ave, Fort Lauderdale, FL 33309
$60.00 for CAMCO Quik Stain II 32-oz Wright's-Giemsa stain.

Chemical Service Labs, Llc 214-691-3484
5543 Dyer St, Dallas, TX 75206
Giemsa #5, Giemsa Stain (Stock)

Medical Chemical Corp. 800-424-9394
19430 Van Ness Ave, Torrance, CA 90501
$14.00 per 100ml.

Poly Scientific R&D Corp. 800-645-5825
70 Cleveland Ave, Bay Shore, NY 11706

Polysciences, Inc. 800-523-2575
400 Valley Rd, Warrington, PA 18976
Certified Giemsa stain powder.

STAIN, GIEMSA, HEMATOLOGY *(cont'd)*

Rocky Mountain Reagents,Inc. 303-762-0800
3207 W Hampden Ave, Englewood, CO 80110

Volu-Sol, Inc. 801-974-9474
2100 South 5095 West, Salt Lake City, UT 84121

STAIN, GOLD CHLORIDE *(Pathology) 88HYH*

American Mastertech Scientific, Inc. 209-368-4031
1330 Thurman St, Lodi, CA 95240
Multiple.

Poly Scientific R&D Corp. 800-645-5825
70 Cleveland Ave, Bay Shore, NY 11706
Any size or dilution.

Ricca Chemical Company Llc 817-461-5601
1490 Lammers Pike, Batesville, IN 47006

Ricca Chemical Company, Llc 817-461-5601
448 W Fork Dr, Arlington, TX 76012
Gold chloride.

Richard-Allan Scientific 269-544-5628
4481 Campus Dr, Kalamazoo, MI 49008
Gold chloride.

STAIN, GRAMS IODINE *(Pathology) 88HYI*

A. J. P. Scientific, Inc. 973-472-7200
82 Industrial St E, Clifton, NJ 07012
Gram iodine.

American Mastertech Scientific, Inc. 209-368-4031
1330 Thurman St, Lodi, CA 95240
Multiple.

Bd Diagnostic Systems 800-675-0908
7 Loveton Cir, Sparks, MD 21152

E K Industries, Inc. 877-EKI-CHEM
1403 Herkimer St, Joliet, IL 60432
Gram iodine.

Labchem, Inc. 412-826-5230
200 William Pitt Way, Pittsburgh, PA 15238
Iodine d'antoni (lc15674).

Medical Chemical Corp. 800-424-9394
19430 Van Ness Ave, Torrance, CA 90501
$19.50 per 1000ml.

Pochemco, Inc. 413-536-2900
724 Main St, Holyoke, MA 01040
Stain gram iodine.

Poly Scientific R&D Corp. 800-645-5825
70 Cleveland Ave, Bay Shore, NY 11706
All grams stain.

Ricca Chemical Company Llc 817-461-5601
1490 Lammers Pike, Batesville, IN 47006

Ricca Chemical Company, Llc 817-461-5601
448 W Fork Dr, Arlington, TX 76012
Grams iodine.

Richard-Allan Scientific 269-544-5628
4481 Campus Dr, Kalamazoo, MI 49008
Iodine, grams.

Rocky Mountain Reagents,Inc. 303-762-0800
3207 W Hampden Ave, Englewood, CO 80110

STAIN, HEINZ BODY *(Hematology) 81GJJ*

A. J. P. Scientific, Inc. 973-472-7200
82 Industrial St E, Clifton, NJ 07012
Heinz body stain.

STAIN, HEMATOLOGY *(Pathology) 88KQC*

Cytocolor, Inc. 800-776-6455
PO Box 401, Hinckley, OH 44233
Hematology reagents, reagent kits and stains.

Image Molding, Inc. 800-525-1875
4525 Kingston St, Denver, CO 80239
Modified Sternheimer-Malbin supravital stain with no-spill delivery system.

Labchem, Inc. 412-826-5230
200 William Pitt Way, Pittsburgh, PA 15238
New methylene blue -n, for reticulocytes (lc17660).

Poly Scientific R&D Corp. 800-645-5825
70 Cleveland Ave, Bay Shore, NY 11706

Richard-Allan Scientific 269-544-5628
4481 Campus Dr, Kalamazoo, MI 49008
Hematology stain.

STAIN, HEMATOXYLIN *(Pathology) 88HYJ*

American Mastertech Scientific, Inc. 209-368-4031
1330 Thurman St, Lodi, CA 95240
Multiple.

Anatech, Ltd. 800-262-8324
1020 Harts Lake Rd, Battle Creek, MI 49037
Hematoxylin nuclear stains: Hematoxylin Extra (equivalent to Gill 3 hematoxylin), Hematoxylin Normal (equivalent to Gill 2 hematoxylin), Harris Hematoxylin

Biocare Medical, Llc 925-603-8003
4040 Pike Ln, Concord, CA 94520
Chromogens & counterstains.

Emd Chemicals Inc. 800-222-0342
480 S Democrat Rd, Gibbstown, NJ 08027
Gill's Formula I, Formula II, Formula III; of Harri's formula.

Poly Scientific R&D Corp. 800-645-5825
70 Cleveland Ave, Bay Shore, NY 11706
Harris, Gills I, II, III.

Polysciences, Inc. 800-523-2575
400 Valley Rd, Warrington, PA 18976
Gill's Hematoxylin #1, #2, #3

Ricca Chemical Company Llc 817-461-5601
1490 Lammers Pike, Batesville, IN 47006

Ricca Chemical Company, Llc 817-461-5601
448 W Fork Dr, Arlington, TX 76012
Various.

Richard-Allan Scientific 269-544-5628
4481 Campus Dr, Kalamazoo, MI 49008
Hematoxylin.

Sci Gen, Inc. 310-324-6576
333 E Gardena Blvd, Gardena, CA 90248
FDA: Medical Device Manufacturing and packaging. Focus on Histology, Cytology, Analytical and General purpose Reagents, Chemistry, and Sterling and Disinfecting agents.

Scytek Laboratories, Inc. 435-755-9848
205 S 600 W, Logan, UT 84321
Hematoxylin.

Statlab Medical Products, Inc. 800-442-3573
106 Hillside Dr, Lewisville, TX 75057
ANAPATH Harris and Gill stains.

Ventana Medical Systems, Inc. 800-227-2155
1910 E Innovation Park Dr, Oro Valley, AZ 85755
Hematoxylin.

STAIN, HEMATOXYLIN, HARRIS'S *(Pathology) 88HYK*

A. J. P. Scientific, Inc. 973-472-7200
82 Industrial St E, Clifton, NJ 07012
Hematoxylin harris's.

American Mastertech Scientific, Inc. 209-368-4031
1330 Thurman St, Lodi, CA 95240
Multiple.

E K Industries, Inc. 877-EKI-CHEM
1403 Herkimer St, Joliet, IL 60432
Harris hematoxylin stain.

Emd Chemicals Inc. 800-222-0342
480 S Democrat Rd, Gibbstown, NJ 08027
Mercury free.

Fisher Scientific Co., Llc. 201-703-3131
1 Reagent Ln, Fair Lawn, NJ 07410
Harris hematoxklin stain.

Medical Chemical Corp. 800-424-9394
19430 Van Ness Ave, Torrance, CA 90501
$16.50 per 500ml.

Polysciences, Inc. 800-523-2575
400 Valley Rd, Warrington, PA 18976

Ricca Chemical Company Llc 888-467-4222
1841 Broad St, Pocomoke City, MD 21851
Harris hematoxylin.

Ricca Chemical Company Llc 817-461-5601
1490 Lammers Pike, Batesville, IN 47006

Ricca Chemical Company, Llc 817-461-5601
448 W Fork Dr, Arlington, TX 76012
Harris hematoxylin.

Richard-Allan Scientific 269-544-5628
4481 Campus Dr, Kalamazoo, MI 49008
Modified harris hematoxylin.

STAIN, HEMATOXYLIN, HARRIS'S *(cont'd)*

Rowley Biochemical Institute 978-739-4883
10 Electronics Ave, Danvers Industrial Park, Danvers, MA 01923

STAIN, HEMATOXYLIN, MAYER'S *(Pathology) 88HYL*

A. J. P. Scientific, Inc. 973-472-7200
82 Industrial St E, Clifton, NJ 07012
Hematoxylin mayer's.

American Mastertech Scientific, Inc. 209-368-4031
1330 Thurman St, Lodi, CA 95240
Multiple.

Medical Chemical Corp. 800-424-9394
19430 Van Ness Ave, Torrance, CA 90501
$23.50 per 500ml.

Poly Scientific R&D Corp. 800-645-5825
70 Cleveland Ave, Bay Shore, NY 11706

Richard-Allan Scientific 269-544-5628
4481 Campus Dr, Kalamazoo, MI 49008
Modified mayer's.

Rowley Biochemical Institute 978-739-4883
10 Electronics Ave, Danvers Industrial Park, Danvers, MA 01923

Sci Gen, Inc. 310-324-6576
333 E Gardena Blvd, Gardena, CA 90248
FDA: Medical Device Manufacturing and packaging. Focus on Histology, Cytology, Analytical and General purpose Reagents, Chemistry, and Sterling and Disinfecting agents.

Scytek Laboratories, Inc. 435-755-9848
205 S 600 W, Logan, UT 84321
Hematoxylin,mayer's.

Ventana Medical Systems, Inc. 800-227-2155
1910 E Innovation Park Dr, Oro Valley, AZ 85755
Hematoxylin, mayer's.

STAIN, INDIGOCARMINE *(Pathology) 88KJT*

Polysciences, Inc. 800-523-2575
400 Valley Rd, Warrington, PA 18976
C.I. 73015

STAIN, IRON *(Pathology) 88GGH*

A. J. P. Scientific, Inc. 973-472-7200
82 Industrial St E, Clifton, NJ 07012
Iron stains.

American Mastertech Scientific, Inc. 209-368-4031
1330 Thurman St, Lodi, CA 95240
Multiple.

Richard-Allan Scientific 269-544-5628
4481 Campus Dr, Kalamazoo, MI 49008
Iron stains.

Rowley Biochemical Institute 978-739-4883
10 Electronics Ave, Danvers Industrial Park, Danvers, MA 01923

Ventana Medical Systems, Inc. 800-227-2155
1910 E Innovation Park Dr, Oro Valley, AZ 85755
Iron stain.

STAIN, JENNER STAIN *(Pathology) 88KJX*

American Mastertech Scientific, Inc. 209-368-4031
1330 Thurman St, Lodi, CA 95240
Multiple.

Richard-Allan Scientific 269-544-5628
4481 Campus Dr, Kalamazoo, MI 49008
Jenner stain.

STAIN, LIGHT GREEN *(Pathology) 88HYS*

American Mastertech Scientific, Inc. 209-368-4031
1330 Thurman St, Lodi, CA 95240
Multiple.

E K Industries, Inc. 877-EKI-CHEM
1403 Herkimer St, Joliet, IL 60432
Light green sf, 1%.

Poly Scientific R&D Corp. 800-645-5825
70 Cleveland Ave, Bay Shore, NY 11706
Any dilution.

Polysciences, Inc. 800-523-2575
400 Valley Rd, Warrington, PA 18976
SF yellowish, C.I. 42095

Richard-Allan Scientific 269-544-5628
4481 Campus Dr, Kalamazoo, MI 49008
Trend counter stain.

STAIN, LIGHT GREEN *(cont'd)*

Rocky Mountain Reagents,Inc. 303-762-0800
3207 W Hampden Ave, Englewood, CO 80110

Ventana Medical Systems, Inc. 800-227-2155
1910 E Innovation Park Dr, Oro Valley, AZ 85755
Light green.

STAIN, LUXOL FAST BLUE *(Pathology) 88HYT*

American Mastertech Scientific, Inc. 209-368-4031
1330 Thurman St, Lodi, CA 95240
Multiple.

Poly Scientific R&D Corp. 800-645-5825
70 Cleveland Ave, Bay Shore, NY 11706

Polysciences, Inc. 800-523-2575
400 Valley Rd, Warrington, PA 18976

STAIN, MALACHITE GREEN *(Pathology) 88KJY*

American Mastertech Scientific, Inc. 209-368-4031
1330 Thurman St, Lodi, CA 95240
Multiple.

Bd Diagnostic Systems 800-675-0908
7 Loveton Cir, Sparks, MD 21152

STAIN, MALLORY'S TRICHROME *(Pathology) 88HYW*

Poly Scientific R&D Corp. 800-645-5825
70 Cleveland Ave, Bay Shore, NY 11706

Richard-Allan Scientific 269-544-5628
4481 Campus Dr, Kalamazoo, MI 49008
Mallory's trichrome stain.

Ventana Medical Systems, Inc. 800-227-2155
1910 E Innovation Park Dr, Oro Valley, AZ 85755
Trichrome stain, mallory's.

STAIN, METANIL YELLOW *(Pathology) 88HYY*

American Mastertech Scientific, Inc. 209-368-4031
1330 Thurman St, Lodi, CA 95240
Multiple.

Poly Scientific R&D Corp. 800-645-5825
70 Cleveland Ave, Bay Shore, NY 11706

Polysciences, Inc. 800-523-2575
400 Valley Rd, Warrington, PA 18976
C.I. 13065

Ricca Chemical Company Llc 817-461-5601
1490 Lammers Pike, Batesville, IN 47006

Ricca Chemical Company, Llc 817-461-5601
448 W Fork Dr, Arlington, TX 76012
Metanil yellow stain.

STAIN, METHENAMINE SILVER *(Pathology) 88HYZ*

American Mastertech Scientific, Inc. 209-368-4031
1330 Thurman St, Lodi, CA 95240
Multiple.

Poly Scientific R&D Corp. 800-645-5825
70 Cleveland Ave, Bay Shore, NY 11706

Richard-Allan Scientific 269-544-5628
4481 Campus Dr, Kalamazoo, MI 49008
Various.

Ventana Medical Systems, Inc. 800-227-2155
1910 E Innovation Park Dr, Oro Valley, AZ 85755
Chemical solution stains.

STAIN, METHYL GREEN *(Pathology) 88HZA*

American Mastertech Scientific, Inc. 209-368-4031
1330 Thurman St, Lodi, CA 95240
Multiple.

Poly Scientific R&D Corp. 800-645-5825
70 Cleveland Ave, Bay Shore, NY 11706
Pyronin.

Polysciences, Inc. 800-523-2575
400 Valley Rd, Warrington, PA 18976
C.I. 42590

Richard-Allan Scientific 269-544-5628
4481 Campus Dr, Kalamazoo, MI 49008
Various methyl green stains.

Rocky Mountain Reagents,Inc. 303-762-0800
3207 W Hampden Ave, Englewood, CO 80110

Scytek Laboratories, Inc. 435-755-9848
205 S 600 W, Logan, UT 84321
Methyl green.

STAIN, METHYL GREEN *(cont'd)*

Ventana Medical Systems, Inc. 800-227-2155
1910 E Innovation Park Dr, Oro Valley, AZ 85755
Methyl green.

STAIN, METHYLENE BLUE *(Pathology) 88KFC*

A. J. P. Scientific, Inc. 973-472-7200
82 Industrial St E, Clifton, NJ 07012
New methylene blue stain.

American Mastertech Scientific, Inc. 209-368-4031
1330 Thurman St, Lodi, CA 95240
Multiple.

Bd Diagnostic Systems 800-675-0908
7 Loveton Cir, Sparks, MD 21152

E K Industries, Inc. 877-EKI-CHEM
1403 Herkimer St, Joliet, IL 60432
New methylene blue N.

Labchem, Inc. 412-826-5230
200 William Pitt Way, Pittsburgh, PA 15238
Methylene blue, loeffler (lc16960).

Poly Scientific R&D Corp. 800-645-5825
70 Cleveland Ave, Bay Shore, NY 11706

Ricca Chemical Company Llc 888-467-4222
1841 Broad St, Pocomoke City, MD 21851
Various.

Ricca Chemical Company Llc 817-461-5601
1490 Lammers Pike, Batesville, IN 47006

Ricca Chemical Company, Llc 817-461-5601
448 W Fork Dr, Arlington, TX 76012
Various.

Richard-Allan Scientific 269-544-5628
4481 Campus Dr, Kalamazoo, MI 49008
Methylene blue tissue stain.

Rocky Mountain Reagents,Inc. 303-762-0800
3207 W Hampden Ave, Englewood, CO 80110
Methylene Blue Terry's Polychrome.

Rowley Biochemical Institute 978-739-4883
10 Electronics Ave, Danvers Industrial Park, Danvers, MA 01923

STAIN, METHYLENE BLUE, NEW *(Hematology) 81GFR*

Medical Chemical Corp. 800-424-9394
19430 Van Ness Ave, Torrance, CA 90501
$13.50 per 100ml.

Poly Scientific R&D Corp. 800-645-5825
70 Cleveland Ave, Bay Shore, NY 11706

Rocky Mountain Reagents,Inc. 303-762-0800
3207 W Hampden Ave, Englewood, CO 80110
Methylene blue terry polychrome (path.).

STAIN, MICROBIOLOGICAL *(Microbiology) 83JTS*

Alpha-Tec Systems, Inc. 800-221-6058
12019 NE 99th St Ste 1780, Vancouver, WA 98682
Various microbiologic stains.

Anomeric, Inc. 225-268-3052
755 Delgado Dr, Baton Rouge, LA 70808
Various.

Astral Diagnostics, Inc. 856-224-0900
1224 Forest Pkwy, West Deptford, NJ 08066
Stains, microbiologic.

Bd Diagnostic Systems 800-675-0908
7 Loveton Cir, Sparks, MD 21152

Biomerieux Industry 800-634-7656
595 Anglum Rd, Hazelwood, MO 63042
Stains and reagents for microbiology and mycology.

E K Industries, Inc. 877-EKI-CHEM
1403 Herkimer St, Joliet, IL 60432
Sudan IV, herxhelmer fat stain.

Emd Chemicals Inc. 800-222-0342
480 S Democrat Rd, Gibbstown, NJ 08027
HARLECO gram stain set 4 x 500ml.

Iris Diagnostics 800-776-4747
9172 Eton Ave, Chatsworth, CA 91311
Urine stain.

Medical Chemical Corp. 800-424-9394
19430 Van Ness Ave, Torrance, CA 90501
$13.00 per set.

STAIN, MICROBIOLOGICAL *(cont'd)*

Meridian Bioscience, Inc. 800-696-0739
3471 River Hills Dr, Cincinnati, OH 45244
WHEATLEY'S TRICHROME STAIN and TRICHROME BLUE
Conventional trichrome stain for the examination of intestinal parasites.

Pml Microbiologicals 800-628-7014
27120 SW 95th Ave, Wilsonville, OR 97070

Pochemco, Inc. 413-536-2900
724 Main St, Holyoke, MA 01040
Lacto phenol-cotton blue.

Poly Scientific R&D Corp. 800-645-5825
70 Cleveland Ave, Bay Shore, NY 11706

Richard-Allan Scientific 269-544-5628
4481 Campus Dr, Kalamazoo, MI 49008
Various.

Rocky Mountain Reagents,Inc. 303-762-0800
3207 W Hampden Ave, Englewood, CO 80110

Rowley Biochemical Institute 978-739-4883
10 Electronics Ave, Danvers Industrial Park, Danvers, MA 01923

Surgipath Medical Industries, Inc. 800-225-3035
PO Box 528, 5205 Route 12, Richmond, IL 60071

Volu-Sol, Inc. 801-974-9474
2100 South 5095 West, Salt Lake City, UT 84121

STAIN, MUCICARMINE *(Pathology) 88HZC*

A. J. P. Scientific, Inc. 973-472-7200
82 Industrial St E, Clifton, NJ 07012
Mucicarmine.

American Mastertech Scientific, Inc. 209-368-4031
1330 Thurman St, Lodi, CA 95240
Multiple.

E K Industries, Inc. 877-EKI-CHEM
1403 Herkimer St, Joliet, IL 60432
Mayer's muci-carmine stain.

Poly Scientific R&D Corp. 800-645-5825
70 Cleveland Ave, Bay Shore, NY 11706

Richard-Allan Scientific 269-544-5628
4481 Campus Dr, Kalamazoo, MI 49008
Mucicarmine.

Rocky Mountain Reagents,Inc. 303-762-0800
3207 W Hampden Ave, Englewood, CO 80110

Rowley Biochemical Institute 978-739-4883
10 Electronics Ave, Danvers Industrial Park, Danvers, MA 01923

Ventana Medical Systems, Inc. 800-227-2155
1910 E Innovation Park Dr, Oro Valley, AZ 85755
Mucicarmine.

STAIN, NEUTRAL RED *(Pathology) 88KFE*

Polysciences, Inc. 800-523-2575
400 Valley Rd, Warrington, PA 18976
C.I. 50040

Rocky Mountain Reagents,Inc. 303-762-0800
3207 W Hampden Ave, Englewood, CO 80110

STAIN, NILE BLUE *(Pathology) 88HZE*

A. J. P. Scientific, Inc. 973-472-7200
82 Industrial St E, Clifton, NJ 07012
Nile blue.

STAIN, NUCLEAR FAST RED *(Pathology) 88HZF*

A. J. P. Scientific, Inc. 973-472-7200
82 Industrial St E, Clifton, NJ 07012
Nuclear fast red.

Poly Scientific R&D Corp. 800-645-5825
70 Cleveland Ave, Bay Shore, NY 11706

Richard-Allan Scientific 269-544-5628
4481 Campus Dr, Kalamazoo, MI 49008
Nuclear fast red stain.

Rowley Biochemical Institute 978-739-4883
10 Electronics Ave, Danvers Industrial Park, Danvers, MA 01923

Scytek Laboratories, Inc. 435-755-9848
205 S 600 W, Logan, UT 84321
Nuclear fast red.

Ventana Medical Systems, Inc. 800-227-2155
1910 E Innovation Park Dr, Oro Valley, AZ 85755
Nuclear fast red.

STAIN, OIL RED O *(Pathology) 88HZG*

Poly Scientific R&D Corp. 800-645-5825
70 Cleveland Ave, Bay Shore, NY 11706

Polysciences, Inc. 800-523-2575
400 Valley Rd, Warrington, PA 18976
C.I. 26125

Rocky Mountain Reagents,Inc. 303-762-0800
3207 W Hampden Ave, Englewood, CO 80110

STAIN, ORANGE G *(Pathology) 88HZH*

Bio-Scientific Specialty Products, Inc. 516-868-2553
197 N Main St # 99, P.o. Box 521, Freeport, NY 11520
Og-g papinicolau counterstain - modified.

E K Industries, Inc. 877-EKI-CHEM
1403 Herkimer St, Joliet, IL 60432
Orange G.

Polysciences, Inc. 800-523-2575
400 Valley Rd, Warrington, PA 18976
C.I. 16230.

STAIN, OTHER *(Pathology) 88WRC*

Bd Diagnostic Systems 800-675-0908
7 Loveton Cir, Sparks, MD 21152

Biomerieux Industry 800-634-7656
595 Anglum Rd, Hazelwood, MO 63042
Stains and reagents for mycology.

Cytocolor, Inc. 800-776-6455
PO Box 401, Hinckley, OH 44233
Bone marrow stain. Stain for fine needle aspirates. Stain for imprints. Cytology stain.

Helena Laboratories 409-842-3714
PO Box 752, Beaumont, TX 77704
Automated.

Medical Chemical Corp. 800-424-9394
19430 Van Ness Ave, Torrance, CA 90501

One Lambda, Inc. 800-822-8824
21001 Kittridge St, Canoga Park, CA 91303
STAIN-FIX stain and fixative. Fluoroquench stain/quench reagent.

Orbeco Analytical Systems, Inc. 800-922-5242
185 Marine St, Farmingdale, NY 11735

Poly Scientific R&D Corp. 800-645-5825
70 Cleveland Ave, Bay Shore, NY 11706
Gram's stains (all). Microwave stain kits, 8oz and 16oz. Halt use in water bath for better tissue adhesive. Solution lymph node. Stain kits for microwave procedures.

Polysciences, Inc. 800-523-2575
400 Valley Rd, Warrington, PA 18976
FungiFluor fungal identification stain; vital hydroethidine stain; acid-fast fluorescent stain kit, TB fluorostain kit, Micro Silver ammoniacal silver stain kit.

Surgipath Medical Industries, Inc. 800-225-3035
PO Box 528, 5205 Route 12, Richmond, IL 60071

Volu-Sol, Inc. 801-974-9474
2100 South 5095 West, Salt Lake City, UT 84121
Stain: Histology

STAIN, PAPANICOLAU *(Pathology) 88HZJ*

A. J. P. Scientific, Inc. 973-472-7200
82 Industrial St E, Clifton, NJ 07012
Papanicolaou stain.

American Mastertech Scientific, Inc. 209-368-4031
1330 Thurman St, Lodi, CA 95240
Papanicolaou stains.

Bio-Scientific Specialty Products, Inc. 516-868-2553
197 N Main St # 99, P.o. Box 521, Freeport, NY 11520
Various papanicolau stains.

Cytyc Surgical Products 800-442-9892
250 Campus Dr, Marlborough, MA 01752
Biological stain.

E K Industries, Inc. 877-EKI-CHEM
1403 Herkimer St, Joliet, IL 60432
Various types of papanicolaou stain.

Emd Chemicals Inc. 800-222-0342
480 S Democrat Rd, Gibbstown, NJ 08027
PAP-EA 36, PAP-EA 50, or PAP-EA 65; PAP-OG-6.

Fisher Scientific Co., Llc. 201-703-3131
1 Reagent Ln, Fair Lawn, NJ 07410
Pap stains.

STAIN, PAPANICOLAU *(cont'd)*

Medical Chemical Corp. 800-424-9394
19430 Van Ness Ave, Torrance, CA 90501
$12.50 per 500ml.

Poly Scientific R&D Corp. 800-645-5825
70 Cleveland Ave, Bay Shore, NY 11706
Microwave kits that include all solutions in one box that are necessary to do a Papanicolaou microwave procedure.

Polysciences, Inc. 800-523-2575
400 Valley Rd, Warrington, PA 18976

Ricca Chemical Company Llc 888-467-4222
1841 Broad St, Pocomoke City, MD 21851
Various.

Ricca Chemical Company Llc 817-461-5601
1490 Lammers Pike, Batesville, IN 47006

Ricca Chemical Company, Llc 817-461-5601
448 W Fork Dr, Arlington, TX 76012
Various.

Richard-Allan Scientific 269-544-5628
4481 Campus Dr, Kalamazoo, MI 49008
Papanicolau stain.

Statlab Medical Products, Inc. 800-442-3573
106 Hillside Dr, Lewisville, TX 75057
ANAPATH EA & OG stains.

STAIN, PERIODIC ACID SCHIFF (PAS) *(Pathology) 88HZK*

Polysciences, Inc. 800-523-2575
400 Valley Rd, Warrington, PA 18976

STAIN, PHLOXINE B *(Pathology) 88HZL*

Rocky Mountain Reagents,Inc. 303-762-0800
3207 W Hampden Ave, Englewood, CO 80110

Sci Gen, Inc. 310-324-6576
333 E Gardena Blvd, Gardena, CA 90248
FDA: Medical Device Manufacturing and packaging. Focus on Histology, Cytology, Analytical and General purpose Reagents, Chemistry, and Sterling and Disinfecting agents.

STAIN, PHOSPHOTUNGSTIC ACID HEMATOXYLIN *(Pathology) 88HZM*

A. J. P. Scientific, Inc. 973-472-7200
82 Industrial St E, Clifton, NJ 07012
Phosphoturgstic acid hematoxylin.

Poly Scientific R&D Corp. 800-645-5825
70 Cleveland Ave, Bay Shore, NY 11706

Rowley Biochemical Institute 978-739-4883
10 Electronics Ave, Danvers Industrial Park, Danvers, MA 01923

STAIN, PONCEAU *(Pathology) 88HZO*

Rocky Mountain Reagents,Inc. 303-762-0800
3207 W Hampden Ave, Englewood, CO 80110

STAIN, PONCEAU, HEMATOLOGY *(Hematology) 81GFL*

Dade Behring, Inc. 800-948-3233
1717 Deerfield Rd, Deerfield, IL 60015

Helena Laboratories 409-842-3714
PO Box 752, Beaumont, TX 77704

Rocky Mountain Reagents,Inc. 303-762-0800
3207 W Hampden Ave, Englewood, CO 80110

STAIN, PYRONIN *(Pathology) 88HZP*

Polysciences, Inc. 800-523-2575
400 Valley Rd, Warrington, PA 18976
C.I. 45005

Richard-Allan Scientific 269-544-5628
4481 Campus Dr, Kalamazoo, MI 49008
Various pyronin y stains.

STAIN, REAGENT, SCHIFF *(Pathology) 88HZT*

A. J. P. Scientific, Inc. 973-472-7200
82 Industrial St E, Clifton, NJ 07012
Schiff reagant (periodic acid schiff).

American Mastertech Scientific, Inc. 209-368-4031
1330 Thurman St, Lodi, CA 95240
Schiff's reagent.

E K Industries, Inc. 877-EKI-CHEM
1403 Herkimer St, Joliet, IL 60432
Schiff reagent.

Poly Scientific R&D Corp. 800-645-5825
70 Cleveland Ave, Bay Shore, NY 11706

STAIN, REAGENT, SCHIFF *(cont'd)*

Ricca Chemical Company Llc 817-461-5601
1490 Lammers Pike, Batesville, IN 47006

Richard-Allan Scientific 269-544-5628
4481 Campus Dr, Kalamazoo, MI 49008
Schiff reagent.

Rowley Biochemical Institute 978-739-4883
10 Electronics Ave, Danvers Industrial Park, Danvers, MA 01923

Ventana Medical Systems, Inc. 800-227-2155
1910 E Innovation Park Dr, Oro Valley, AZ 85755
Dye stain.

STAIN, RETICULOCYTE *(Hematology) 81GJH*

A. J. P. Scientific, Inc. 973-472-7200
82 Industrial St E, Clifton, NJ 07012
Stain, reticulocyte.

Bd Biosciences 408-954-6307
2350 Qume Dr, San Jose, CA 95131
Reticulocyte.

Becton Dickinson And Company 800-284-6845
1 Becton Dr, Franklin Lakes, NJ 07417
RETIC-COUNT; UNOPETTE

Clinical Diagnostic Solutions, Inc. 954-791-1773
1800 NW 65th Ave, Plantation, FL 33313
Stain, reticulocyte.

Medical Chemical Corp. 800-424-9394
19430 Van Ness Ave, Torrance, CA 90501
$13.00 per 100ml.

Pochemco, Inc. 413-536-2900
724 Main St, Holyoke, MA 01040
New methylene blue stain.

Ricca Chemical Company Llc 817-461-5601
1490 Lammers Pike, Batesville, IN 47006

Richard-Allan Scientific 269-544-5628
4481 Campus Dr, Kalamazoo, MI 49008
Reticulocyte stain.

Rocky Mountain Reagents,Inc. 303-762-0800
3207 W Hampden Ave, Englewood, CO 80110

STAIN, ROMANOWSKY *(Hematology) 81GJL*

Astral Diagnostics, Inc. 856-224-0900
1224 Forest Pkwy, West Deptford, NJ 08066
Romanowsky stains.

Rowley Biochemical Institute 978-739-4883
10 Electronics Ave, Danvers Industrial Park, Danvers, MA 01923

STAIN, SAFRANIN *(Pathology) 88HZS*

A. J. P. Scientific, Inc. 973-472-7200
82 Industrial St E, Clifton, NJ 07012
Safranin.

Bd Diagnostic Systems 800-675-0908
7 Loveton Cir, Sparks, MD 21152

E K Industries, Inc. 877-EKI-CHEM
1403 Herkimer St, Joliet, IL 60432
Safranin, safranin stain, 1%.

Labchem, Inc. 412-826-5230
200 William Pitt Way, Pittsburgh, PA 15238
Safranin, 1% alcoholic (lc22360).

Medical Chemical Corp. 800-424-9394
19430 Van Ness Ave, Torrance, CA 90501
$22.00 per 1000ml.

Pochemco, Inc. 413-536-2900
724 Main St, Holyoke, MA 01040
Stain safranin.

Poly Scientific R&D Corp. 800-645-5825
70 Cleveland Ave, Bay Shore, NY 11706

Polysciences, Inc. 800-523-2575
400 Valley Rd, Warrington, PA 18976
Certified.

Ricca Chemical Company Llc 888-467-4222
1841 Broad St, Pocomoke City, MD 21851
Various.

Ricca Chemical Company Llc 817-461-5601
1490 Lammers Pike, Batesville, IN 47006

Ricca Chemical Company, Llc 817-461-5601
448 W Fork Dr, Arlington, TX 76012
Various.

STAIN, SAFRANIN *(cont'd)*

Richard-Allan Scientific 269-544-5628
4481 Campus Dr, Kalamazoo, MI 49008
Safranin.

Rocky Mountain Reagents,Inc. 303-762-0800
3207 W Hampden Ave, Englewood, CO 80110

STAIN, SUDAN BLACK B *(Pathology) 88HZZ*

A. J. P. Scientific, Inc. 973-472-7200
82 Industrial St E, Clifton, NJ 07012
Sudan black b.

Poly Scientific R&D Corp. 800-645-5825
70 Cleveland Ave, Bay Shore, NY 11706

STAIN, TOLUIDINE BLUE *(Pathology) 88IAB*

A. J. P. Scientific, Inc. 973-472-7200
82 Industrial St E, Clifton, NJ 07012
Toluidine blue.

Medical Chemical Corp. 800-424-9394
19430 Van Ness Ave, Torrance, CA 90501
$12.00 per 100ml.

Polysciences, Inc. 800-523-2575
400 Valley Rd, Warrington, PA 18976
C.I. 52040 certfied and purified

Ricca Chemical Company Llc 817-461-5601
1490 Lammers Pike, Batesville, IN 47006

Ricca Chemical Company, Llc 817-461-5601
448 W Fork Dr, Arlington, TX 76012
Toluidine blue.

Rocky Mountain Reagents,Inc. 303-762-0800
3207 W Hampden Ave, Englewood, CO 80110

STAIN, TOLUIDINE BLUE, HEMATOLOGY *(Hematology) 81GIX*

Rocky Mountain Reagents,Inc. 303-762-0800
3207 W Hampden Ave, Englewood, CO 80110

STAIN, TRYPAN BLUE *(Pathology) 88LGY*

Polysciences, Inc. 800-523-2575
400 Valley Rd, Warrington, PA 18976
C.I. 23850

STAIN, VAN GIESON'S *(Pathology) 88IAC*

Poly Scientific R&D Corp. 800-645-5825
70 Cleveland Ave, Bay Shore, NY 11706

Richard-Allan Scientific 269-544-5628
4481 Campus Dr, Kalamazoo, MI 49008
Van gieson's stain.

Rowley Biochemical Institute 978-739-4883
10 Electronics Ave, Danvers Industrial Park, Danvers, MA 01923

STAIN, WEIGERT'S IRON HEMATOXYLIN *(Pathology) 88IAE*

A. J. P. Scientific, Inc. 973-472-7200
82 Industrial St E, Clifton, NJ 07012
Weighert's iron hematoxylin.

American Mastertech Scientific, Inc. 209-368-4031
1330 Thurman St, Lodi, CA 95240
Multiple.

Poly Scientific R&D Corp. 800-645-5825
70 Cleveland Ave, Bay Shore, NY 11706
Solutions A & B.

Richard-Allan Scientific 269-544-5628
4481 Campus Dr, Kalamazoo, MI 49008
Weigert's iron hematoxylin.

STAIN, WRIGHT'S *(Pathology) 88IAF*

A. J. P. Scientific, Inc. 973-472-7200
82 Industrial St E, Clifton, NJ 07012
Wright stain.

Bayer Healthcare, Llc 574-256-3430
430 S Beiger St, Mishawaka, IN 46544
Dye and clinical solution stains.

Bio-Scientific Specialty Products, Inc. 516-868-2553
197 N Main St # 99, P.o. Box 521, Freeport, NY 11520
Wright stain.

Cambridge Diagnostic Products, Inc. 800-525-6262
6880 NW 17th Ave, Fort Lauderdale, FL 33309
$60.00 for 32-oz CAMCO Quik Stain. $65.00 for 32-oz CAMCO Poly-Tet stain.

STAIN, WRIGHT'S *(cont'd)*

E K Industries, Inc. 877-EKI-CHEM
1403 Herkimer St, Joliet, IL 60432
Wright stain fixative & buffer.

Gam Rad, Inc. 540-646-5466
Star Rt. 608 (river Rd.), Chilhowie, VA 24319
Wright's stain.

Medical Chemical Corp. 800-424-9394
19430 Van Ness Ave, Torrance, CA 90501
$22.00 per 1000ml.

Pochemco, Inc. 413-536-2900
724 Main St, Holyoke, MA 01040
Wright stain.

Polysciences, Inc. 800-523-2575
400 Valley Rd, Warrington, PA 18976
Wright's stain, certified, Wright's Giensa solution.

Ricca Chemical Company Llc 888-467-4222
1841 Broad St, Pocomoke City, MD 21851
Various

Ricca Chemical Company Llc 817-461-5601
1490 Lammers Pike, Batesville, IN 47006

Ricca Chemical Company, Llc 817-461-5601
448 W Fork Dr, Arlington, TX 76012
Various.

Richard-Allan Scientific 269-544-5628
4481 Campus Dr, Kalamazoo, MI 49008
Wright stain.

Rocky Mountain Reagents,Inc. 303-762-0800
3207 W Hampden Ave, Englewood, CO 80110

Volu-Sol, Inc. 801-974-9474
2100 South 5095 West, Salt Lake City, UT 84121

STAIN, WRIGHT'S, HEMATOLOGY *(Hematology) 81GJK*

Beckman Coulter, Inc. 800-635-3497
740 W 83rd St, Hialeah, FL 33014
Stain packs and fixatives.

Cambridge Diagnostic Products, Inc. 800-525-6262
6880 NW 17th Ave, Fort Lauderdale, FL 33309
$60.00 for CAMCO Quik Stain II 32-oz Wright's-Giemsa stain. $65.00 for 32-oz CAMCO Poly-Tet stain.

Chemical Service Labs, Llc 214-691-3484
5543 Dyer St, Dallas, TX 75206
Q-Stain, a modified Wright's Stain

Dade Behring, Inc. 800-948-3233
1717 Deerfield Rd, Deerfield, IL 60015

Poly Scientific R&D Corp. 800-645-5825
70 Cleveland Ave, Bay Shore, NY 11706

Rocky Mountain Reagents,Inc. 303-762-0800
3207 W Hampden Ave, Englewood, CO 80110

Volu-Sol, Inc. 801-974-9474
2100 South 5095 West, Salt Lake City, UT 84121

STAINER, SLIDE, AUTOMATED *(Pathology) 88KPA*

Bayer Healthcare, Llc 574-256-3430
430 S Beiger St, Mishawaka, IN 46544
Hematologic slide stainer.

Beckman Coulter, Inc. 800-526-3821
11800 SW 147th Ave, Miami, FL 33196
Automated slide stainer.

Biocare Medical, Llc 925-603-8003
4040 Pike Ln, Concord, CA 94520
Automated slide stainer.

Dako Colorado, Inc. 454-485-9500
4850 Innovation Dr, Fort Collins, CO 80525
Slide stainer, automated.

Hacker Industries, Inc. 803-712-6100
1132 Kincaid Bridge Rd, Winnsboro, SC 29180
H/i automated stainer.

Hacker Instruments And Industries Inc. 800-442-2537
1132 Kincaid Bridge Rd, PO Box 1176, Winnsboro, SC 29180
Automatic slide staining machine; up to 1000 slides per hour; Continous loading. Extremely user friendly.Made in USA.

Lab Vision Corp. 510-991-2800
47777 Warm Springs Blvd, Fremont, CA 94539
Various.

STAINER, SLIDE, AUTOMATED *(cont'd)*

Leica Microsystems (Canada) Inc. 800-205-3422
400 - 111 Granton Drive, Richmond Hill, ONT L4B 1L5 Canada
LEICA

Medical Sales & Service Group 888-357-6520
10 Woodchester Dr, Acton, MA 01720

Medtec, Inc. 919-241-1400
PO Box 16578, Chapel Hill, NC 27516
Automated Western-blot processor.

Peripheral Dynamics Inc. 800-253-0253
5150 Campus Dr, Plymouth Meeting, PA 19462

Rushabh Instruments, Llc 215-491-0081
1750 Costner Dr Ste A, Warrington, PA 18976
Hematology slide stainer.

Tomtec 877-866-8323
1000 Sherman Ave, Hamden, CT 06514
Automated Grams stain equipment with staining basket holding 1 to 25 slides. No operator attendance required.

Tripath Imaging, Inc. 919-206-7140
780 Plantation Dr, Burlington, NC 27215
Automated slide stainers.

Ventana Medical Systems, Inc. 800-227-2155
1910 E Innovation Park Dr, Oro Valley, AZ 85755
Automated slide stainer & accessories.

Wescor, Inc. 800-453-2725
459 S Main St, Logan, UT 84321
$8,195.00 Model the model 7320 AEROSPRAY Gram Slide Stainer/Cytocentrifuge with 6 decolorizer settings for different thicknesses of smears for minimal stain consumption with clean cycle for minimal maintenance. $2,095.00 optional rotor allows cytocentrifugation. Model 7720 AEROSPRAY microbiology acid-fast bacteria slide stainer/cytocentrifuge. Automated acid-fast staining with no cross-contamination. The AFB stainer performs either carbol fuchsin or fluorescence staining, $8,195.00, an optional CytoPro rotor allows cytocentrifugation, $2,095.00.

STAINER, SLIDE, HEMATOLOGY *(Hematology) 81RTS*

Emd Chemicals Inc. 800-222-0342
480 S Democrat Rd, Gibbstown, NJ 08027
MIDAS III slide stainer for hematology and microbiology.

Hacker Instruments And Industries Inc. 800-442-2537
1132 Kincaid Bridge Rd, PO Box 1176, Winnsboro, SC 29180
Stainer, Slide, Hematology & Special Stain. 'INTERSTAIN-6' - Fully enclosed, automatic slide stainer for hematology and multiple special stain applications. Fully programmable with 6 stations and 25 steps per program.

Wescor, Inc. 800-453-2725
459 S Main St, Logan, UT 84321
$8,095.00 for the Model 7120 AEROSPRAY Hematology Slide Stainer/Cytocentrifuge with 7 stain intensities for peripheral smears and 3 stain intensities for bone marrow. Programmable for 2,4,6,12 slides in 3 minutes for minimal stain consumption with clean cycle for minimal maintenance. $2,095.00 optional rotor allows cytocentrifugation.

STAINER, SLIDE, HEMATOLOGY, AUTOMATED *(Hematology) 81GKD*

Horiba Abx 888-903-5001
34 Bunsen, Irvine, CA 92618

Sakura Finetek U.S.A., Inc. 800-725-8723
1750 W 214th St, Torrance, CA 90501
$23,950.00 for TISSUE-TEK DRS 2000 automatic slide stainer.

Wescor, Inc. 800-453-2725
459 S Main St, Logan, UT 84321
$ 8,295.00 for the model 7150 Aerospray Hematology Slide Stainer/Cytocentrifuge with 4 preprogrammed stain modes: Rapid Wright Giemsa, Wright Giemsa, May-grunwald Giemsa and a Custom Stain. Total programmability for user preferences, $ 2,095.00 for an optional rotor that allows cytocentrifugation.

STAINER, SLIDE, HISTOLOGY *(Microbiology) 83RTT*

Hacker Instruments And Industries Inc. 800-442-2537
1132 Kincaid Bridge Rd, PO Box 1176, Winnsboro, SC 29180
Automatic slide staining machine; up to 1000 slides per hour; made in USA.

Medical Sales & Service Group 888-357-6520
10 Woodchester Dr, Acton, MA 01720

STAINER, SLIDE, IMMERSION TYPE *(Pathology) 88KIO*

Barnstead International 412-490-8425
2555 Kerper Blvd, Dubuque, IA 52001
Various slide stainers.

Surgipath Medical Industries, Inc. 800-225-3035
PO Box 528, 5205 Route 12, Richmond, IL 60071

STAINER, TISSUE, AUTOMATED *(Pathology) 88KEY*

Abbott Molecular, Inc. 847-937-6100
1300 E Touhy Ave, Des Plaines, IL 60018
Slide processor and stainer.

Technical Products International, Inc. 800-729-4421
5918 Evergreen Blvd, Saint Louis, MO 63134
Universal slide stainer for histology and cytology. TST 33

Ted Pella, Inc. 800-237-3526
4595 Mountain Lakes Blvd, Redding, CA 96003
1 - Microwave tissue processor and accessories.

Ventana Medical Systems, Inc. 800-227-2155
1910 E Innovation Park Dr, Oro Valley, AZ 85755
Automated slide stainer.

STAND, BASIN *(General) 80QCQ*

Bedcolab Ltd. 800-461-6414
2305 Francis Hughes, Laval, QUE H7S 1N5 Canada

Blickman 800-247-5070
39 Robinson Rd, Lodi, NJ 07644
Basin stands have a single or double basin with your choice of supporting shelf or H-brace.

Pedigo Products 360-695-3500
4000 SE Columbia Way, Vancouver, WA 98661
Single or double basin, chrome or stainless steel.

Phelan Manufacturing Corp. 800-328-2358
2523 Minnehaha Ave, Minneapolis, MN 55404
$410.00 per double, adjustable basin holder.

Schueler & Company, Inc. 516-487-1500
PO Box 528, Stratford, CT 06615

STAND, CASTING *(Orthopedics) 87UES*

Innovative Medical Products, Inc. 800-467-4944
87 Spring Lane, Plainville Industrial Pk, Plainville, CT 06062
IMP Casting Stands, TURNSTILE casting stand, (folding). $495.00, (non-folding). IMP Cast Stand.

Kronner Medical 800-706-3533
1443 Upper Cleveland Rapids Rd, Roseburg, OR 97471
KRONNER foot casting stand.

Mizuho Osi 800-777-4674
30031 Ahern Ave, Union City, CA 94587

Ortho-Med, Inc. 800-547-5571
3208 SE 13th Ave, Portland, OR 97202

STAND, GAS CYLINDER *(Anesthesiology) 73QXX*

Air Products And Chemicals, Inc. 800-654-4567
7201 Hamilton Blvd, Allentown, PA 18195

Allied Healthcare Products, Inc. 800-444-3954
1720 Sublette Ave, Saint Louis, MO 63110

Farley Inc., W.T. 800-327-5397
931 Via Alondra, Camarillo, CA 93012
$98.00 for OXYSTAND oxygen six cylinder floor stand, Model ES106. OXYSTAND 12 cylinder floor stand, MODEL ES112, $108.00.

Life Corporation 800-700-0202
1776 N Water St, Milwaukee, WI 53202
LIFE, OxygenPac Portable emergency oxygen units, clear cover and wall-mounted, off/on lever control, resuscitation mask with one-way valve for hygiene, 6lpm 90min. supply, refillable. Also available 6 & 12 lpm NORM & HIGH, 0-25 lpm variable, and demand-valve for 100% oxygen resuscitation. GSA Federal Supply Schedule.

Praxair, Inc. 800-PRAXAIR
39 Old Ridgebury Rd, Danbury, CT 06810

STAND, INSTRUMENT, AC-POWERED, OPHTHALMIC
(Ophthalmology) 86HMF

Global Surgical Corp. 314-861-3388
3610 Tree Court Industrial Blvd, Saint Louis, MO 63122
System 1 instrument stand.

Ocular Instruments, North Facility 425-455-5200
5030 208th St SW Ste 1, Lynnwood, WA 98036
Opthalmic instrument stand.

STAND, INSTRUMENT, AC-POWERED, OPHTHALMIC *(cont'd)*

Phakosystems, Inc. 416-503-4200
14 Plastics Ave, Toronto M8Z 4B7 Canada
Irrigation/aspiration system c/w sterile tubing and handpieces

Topcon Medical Systems, Inc. 800-223-1130
37 W Century Rd, Paramus, NJ 07652
Two instrument stands: $4,490.00 and $5,490.00. Three models of instrument delivery/refraction systems - desk type (please call for current pricing).

Woodlyn, Inc. 800-331-7389
2920 Malmo Dr, Ophthalmic Instruments and Equipment
Arlington Heights, IL 60005
Model 01-2002-001. The Woodlyn Millennium Instrument Stand was designed to offer state-of-the-art functionality for the operator while conveniently accommodating patients. Wheel-chair accessible. Call for current prices.

STAND, INSTRUMENT, OPHTHALMIC *(Ophthalmology) 86HMG*

HAAG-STREIT USA, INC. 800-787-5426
3535 Kings Mills Rd, Mason, OH 45040
Floor Unit, $3995 (standard) for ophthalmic instrument floor unit. $450 for manual instrument table (opthalmic).

Jedmed Instruments Co. 314-845-3770
5416 Jedmed Ct, Saint Louis, MO 63129

Marco Ophthalmic, Inc. 800-874-5274
11825 Central Pkwy, Jacksonville, FL 32224
$4,220.00 for ophthalmic stand. (List price)

Pryor Products 800-854-2280
1819 Peacock Blvd, Oceanside, CA 92056
Custom medical device stands can be created for any new product. Custom and standard healthcare computer stands are also available for use with laptops, pen tablets and thin or thick PCs.

STAND, LAUNDRY HAMPER *(General) 80TCM*

Blickman 800-247-5070
39 Robinson Rd, Lodi, NJ 07644
Five models in chrome and two in stainless offer many options. Models 2010, 2118 and 2300 have lids and are chrome foot-operated units. Models 2301SS and 7772SS-LFP are stainless foot-operated lid models.

Hos-Pillow Corp. 800-468-7874
1011 Campus Dr, Mundelein, IL 60060
Laundry hamper bags, laundry hamper stands and laundry bags.

Medical Safety Systems Inc. 888-803-9303
230 White Pond Dr, Akron, OH 44313

Meese Orbitron Dunne Co. 800-829-3230
535 N Midland Ave, Saddle Brook, NJ 07663

R&B Wire Products, Inc. 800-634-0555
2902 W Garry Ave, Santa Ana, CA 92704
Stationary and portable; portable with footpedal; fits standard disposable poly bags (35 to 40 gallons) in wire and tubular construction.

Steele Canvas Basket Co., Inc. 800-541-8929
201 Williams St, Chelsea, MA 02150

STAND, OPERATING ROOM INSTRUMENT (MAYO)
(Surgery) 79FSH

Alimed, Inc. 800-225-2610
297 High St, Dedham, MA 02026

Blickman 800-247-5070
39 Robinson Rd, Lodi, NJ 07644
Six models in stainless and three in chrome. Tray sizes are 13-3/4' x 19-1/8' or 16' x 21'. Model 8771SS is a double post jumbo mayo stand with a 20' x 25' tray. Choose foot-operated, friction knob or thumb control height adjustment

Brandt Industries, Inc. 800-221-8031
4461 Bronx Blvd, Bronx, NY 10470
Mayo stands, instrument stands, and trays.

Brewer Company, The 888-873-9371
N88W13901 Main St, Menomonee Falls, WI 53051
#43460: Mayo Instrument Stand, 'U' Base, #43465: Mobile Instrument Stand, #11100: Mayo Instrument Stand, 'California Style' Base

Cameron-Miller, Inc. 800-621-0142
5410 W Roosevelt Rd, Road #241, Chicago, IL 60644

Codman & Shurtleff, Inc 800-225-0460
325 Paramount Dr, Raynham, MA 02767

Elmed, Inc. 630-543-2792
60 W Fay Ave, Addison, IL 60101

STAND, OPERATING ROOM INSTRUMENT (MAYO) *(cont'd)*

Galaxy Medical Manufacturing Co. 800-876-4599
5411 Sheila St, Commerce, CA 90040

Healthmark Industries 800-521-6224
22522 E 9 Mile Rd, Saint Clair Shores, MI 48080
Plastic Mayo trays.

International Hospital Supply Co. 800-398-9450
6914 Canby Ave Ste 105, Reseda, CA 91335

Jedmed Instruments Co. 314-845-3770
5416 Jedmed Ct, Saint Louis, MO 63129

Omnimed, Inc. (Beam Products) 800-257-2326
800 Glen Ave, Moorestown, NJ 08057
Power Lifter automated I.V. stand, battery operated I.V. stand designed to automatically lift heavy irrigation containers used during arthroscopic, cytoscopic and urologic procedures.

Pedigo Products 360-695-3500
4000 SE Columbia Way, Vancouver, WA 98661
Foot operated, stainless steel.

STAND/HOLDER, EQUIPMENT, LABORATORY *(Chemistry) 75WKC*

Diagnostic Instruments Inc. 586-731-6000
6540 Burroughs Ave, Sterling Heights, MI 48314
Microscope stand.

Howard Medical Company 800-443-1444
1690 N Elston Ave, Chicago, IL 60642
$5.45 for wire-formed glove-box holder.

Jaece Industries, Inc. 716-694-2811
908 Niagara Falls Blvd, North Tonawanda, NY 14120
Foam racks, securely fit for many tube sizes. Made of closed-cell foam, small racks feature 9-mm holes; large racks have 13-mm holes. Both racks have a capacity of 50 tubes.

Kapp Surgical Instrument, Inc. 800-282-5277
4919 Warrensville Center Rd, Cleveland, OH 44128
Strip Ts instrument holder.

Moyco Technologies, Inc. 800-331-8837
200 Commerce Dr, Montgomeryville, PA 18936
Endodontic instrument stand.

Rem Systems 305-499-4800
625 E 10th Ave, Hialeah, FL 33010
Slide-a-Shelf: New processor stand where bottom shelf slides out to allow for easy replacement of five-gallon jugs of processor fluids.

Snug Seat, Inc. 800-336-7684
12801 E Independence Blvd, PO Box 1739, Matthews, NC 28105
GIRAFFE nonlaboratory pediatric standing frame. Prone, supine, and upright stander in one unit. Accommodates children from 18 to 60 in. tall.

Thermo Fisher Scientific 800-345-0206
22 Friars Dr, Hudson, NH 03051
MEMOWELL LED lightbox aids in remembering where next to pipette.

Trademark Medical Llc 800-325-9044
449 Soverign Ct, St. Louis, MO 63011
O.R. POCKITS self sticking instrument holder keeps instruments neatly available for easy use or storage when necessary. Clear polyolefin.

STANDARD, AMINO ACID *(Chemistry) 75UIH*

Baxter Healthcare Corporation Nutrition 888-229-0001
1 Baxter Pkwy, Deerfield, IL 60015
NOVAMINE, TRAVASOL, RENAMIN, AMINESS, BRANCHAMIN, INTRALIPID.

Beckman Coulter, Inc. 800-742-2345
250 S Kraemer Blvd, PO Box 8000, Brea, CA 92821

Bio-Rad Laboratories, Life Science Group 800-424-6723
2000 Alfred Nobel Dr, Hercules, CA 94547

Hospira, Inc. 877-946-7747
8484 US 70 Bus Hwy W, Clayton, NC 27520

STANDARD, CARBOHYDRATE *(Chemistry) 75UII*

Accurate Chemical & Scientific Corp. 800-645-6264
300 Shames Dr, Westbury, NY 11590

Seikagaku America, Inc. 800-848-3248
124 Bernard St. Jean Dr., East Falmouth, MA 02536-4445

STANDARD, FIBRINOGEN *(Hematology) 81GFX*

Fisher Diagnostics 877-722-4366
11515 Vanstory Dr Ste 125, Huntersville, NC 28078

STANDARD, FIBRINOGEN *(cont'd)*

Precision Biologic, Inc. 800-267-2796
900 Windmill Rd., Ste. 100, Dartmouth, NS B3B 1P7 Canada
CRYOCHECK NORMAL REFERENCE PLASMA

STANDARD, LIPID *(Chemistry) 75UIJ*

Accurate Chemical & Scientific Corp. 800-645-6264
300 Shames Dr, Westbury, NY 11590

Avanti Polar Lipids, Inc. 800-227-0651
700 Industrial Park Dr, Alabaster, AL 35007
Phospholipids. Surfactants.

Biocell Laboratories, Inc. 800-222-8382
2001 E University Dr, Rancho Dominguez, CA 90220
Cholesterol, LDL, HDL, Apo A and Apo B, triglycerides.

Cliniqa Corporation 800-728-9558
774 N Twin Oaks Valley Rd Ste C, San Marcos, CA 92069

Creative Laboratory Products, Inc. 317-293-2991
6420 Guion Rd, Indianapolis, IN 46268

Dade Behring, Inc. 800-948-3233
1717 Deerfield Rd, Deerfield, IL 60015

Gilead Sciences 650-574-3000
333 Lakeside Dr, Foster City, CA 94404
Liposome products.

Hospira, Inc. 877-946-7747
8484 US 70 Bus Hwy W, Clayton, NC 27520
INTRALIPID.

Raichem, Division Of Hemagen Diagnostics, Inc. 800-438-6100
8225 Mercury Ct, San Diego, CA 92111
Elevated lipids control for use in calibrating kinetic triglycerides assays, evaluating ability of a reagent to hydrolyze triglycerides and as control for cholesterol assays.

Zeptometrix Corporation 800-274-5487
872 Main St, Buffalo, NY 14202
Oxi-Tek: TBARS assay used for screening and monitoring lipid peraxidation, a major indicator of oxidative stress.

STANDARD, ULTRAVIOLET REFERENCE *(Chemistry) 75UJC*

Beckman Coulter, Inc. 800-742-2345
250 S Kraemer Blvd, PO Box 8000, Brea, CA 92821

STANDARD/CONTROL, ALL TYPES *(Chemistry) 75UKC*

Advanced Instruments Inc. 800-225-4034
2 Technology Way, Norwood, MA 02062
Osmometer standards.

Beckman Coulter, Inc. 800-635-3497
740 W 83rd St, Hialeah, FL 33014

Beckman Coulter, Inc. 800-742-2345
250 S Kraemer Blvd, PO Box 8000, Brea, CA 92821

Bio-Rad, Diagnostics Group 800-854-6737
9500 Jeronimo Rd, Irvine, CA 92618
Spec. Controls: IA, TDM, tumor marker, hemoglobin, anemia, spinal fluid, chemistry, pediatric, toxicology, immunology, urine, blood gas, whole blood, isoenzyme, drug free serum and endocrine, hematology, cardiac marker, diabetes, alcohol, urine metals.

Biochemical Diagnostics, Inc. 800-223-4835
180 Heartland Blvd, Edgewood, NY 11717
Drug standard mixtures (DEA exempt).

Biomerieux Inc. 800-682-2666
100 Rodolphe St, Durham, NC 27712

Covidien Lp 508-261-8000
15 Hampshire St, Mansfield, MA 02048

Dade Behring, Inc. 800-948-3233
1717 Deerfield Rd, Deerfield, IL 60015

Diagnostica Stago, Inc. 800-222-COAG
5 Century Dr, Parsippany, NJ 07054

Frontier Scientific, Inc., 453-753-1901
PO Box 31, Logan, UT 84323

Labsphere, Inc. 603-927-4266
231 Shaker St., North Sutton, NH 03260-9986
Spectralon diffuse reflectance standards for calibration and validation of spectrophotometers and other reflectance measurement systems.

Precision Systems, Inc. 508-655-7010
16 Tech Cir, Natick, MA 01760
CON-TROL, reference standards for osmometers.

STANDARD/CONTROL, ALL TYPES *(cont'd)*

Raichem, Division Of Hemagen Diagnostics, Inc. 800-438-6100
8225 Mercury Ct, San Diego, CA 92111
Albumin-protein, calcium, calcium/phosphorus, chloride, cholesterol, creatinine, glucose, glycerol, phosphorus, bilirubin-free and conjugate, urea nitrogen, uric acid, carbon dioxide, uric acid standards.

Stanbio Laboratory, Inc. 830-249-0772
1261 N Main St, Boerne, TX 78006
$27.00 for 30ml albumin standard, $17.00 for 30ml calcium standard (10mg/dL), $22.00 for 30ml cholesterol standard (200mg/dL), $22.00 for 30ml HDL-cholesterol standard (50mg/dL), $22.00 for 30ml cratinine standard (5mg/dL), $17.00 for 30ml glucose standard (100mg/dL), $27.50 for 30ml phosphorus standard (10mg/dL), $27.50 for 30ml total protein standard (10mg/dL), $33.00 for 30ml triglyceride standard (200mg/dL), $27.50 for 30ml uric acid standard (8mg/dL).

Thermo Fisher Scientific Inc. 781-622-1000
81 Wyman St, Waltham, MA 02451
Standard and custom.

Wampole Laboratories 800-257-9525
2 Research Way, Princeton, NJ 08540

STANDARD/CONTROL, FIBRINOGEN DETERMINATION
(Hematology) 81GFK

Biomerieux Inc. 800-682-2666
100 Rodolphe St, Durham, NC 27712
VERIFY LFC, low-ibrinogen control, lyophilized.

Dade Behring, Inc. 800-948-3233
1717 Deerfield Rd, Deerfield, IL 60015

Helena Laboratories 409-842-3714
PO Box 752, Beaumont, TX 77704

Precision Biologic, Inc. 800-267-2796
900 Windmill Rd., Ste. 100, Dartmouth, NS B3B 1P7 Canada
CRYOCHECK NORMAL REFERENCE PLASMA

STANDARD/CONTROL, HEMOGLOBIN, NORMAL/ABNORMAL
(Hematology) 81GFS

Analytical Control Systems, Inc. 317-841-0458
9058 Technology Dr, Fishers, IN 46038
AFCS, AF, AS, AC, AD, AE, AFS, AFC, NAFSC, A2, A1C, Gal-1-Put, G-6-PDH, Hemoglobin Fractions (A2, AF, AC, & AS) and Total Hemoglobin controls available.

Beckman Coulter, Inc. 800-635-3497
740 W 83rd St, Hialeah, FL 33014
HB-5/10/20 G/DL, aqueous calibrator set.

Bio-Rad Laboratories, Diagnostic Group 800-224-6723
524 Stone Rd Ste A, Benicia, CA 94510
Hemoglobin calibrator.

Bionostics, Inc. 978-772-7070
7 Jackson Rd, Devens, MA 01434
Control for the instrumentationlaboratory 282 co-oximeter.

Bioresource Technology, Inc. 954-792-5222
11924 Miramar Pkwy, Flamingo Park Of Commerce, Miramar, FL 33025
Quality control, assayed materials.

Diagnostic Technology, Inc. 631-582-4949
175 Commerce Dr Ste L, Hauppauge, NY 11788
Count-a-part cyanmethemoglobin standard set.

Health Chem Diagnostics Llc 954-979-3845
3341 W McNab Rd, Pompano Beach, FL 33069
Standards and controls, hemoglobin, normal and abnormal.

Helena Laboratories 409-842-3714
PO Box 752, Beaumont, TX 77704

PerkinElmer 800-762-4000
940 Winter St, Waltham, MA 02451
For GHb test.

STAPLE, ABSORBABLE *(Orthopedics) 87MNU*

Arthrex, Inc. 239-643-5553
1370 Creekside Blvd, Naples, FL 34108
Staple.

STAPLE, FIXATION, BONE *(Orthopedics) 87JDR*

Acumed Llc 503-627-9957
5885 NW Cornelius Pass Rd, Hillsboro, OR 97124
Suture anchor.

Arthrex, Inc. 239-643-5553
1370 Creekside Blvd, Naples, FL 34108
Bone staple.

STAPLE, FIXATION, BONE *(cont'd)*

Biomedical Enterprises, Inc. 800-880-6528
14785 Omicron Dr Ste 205, San Antonio, TX 78245
OSStaple/OSSplate, shape memory nitinol staples and accessories for setting and warming the staples with the OSSforce to achieve fracture, osteotomy or arthrodesis compression.

Biomet, Inc. 574-267-6639
56 E Bell Dr, PO Box 587, Warsaw, IN 46582
Meniscal staple.

Depuy Mitek, A Johnson & Johnson Company 800-451-2006
50 Scotland Blvd, Bridgewater, MA 02324
Appliance for reconstruction of bone and soft tissue.

Depuy Orthopaedics, Inc. 800-473-3789
700 Orthopaedic Dr, P.O. Box 988, Warsaw, IN 46582
Various types of bone fixation staples.

Depuy-Raynham, A Div. Of Depuy Orthopaedics 800-451-2006
325 Paramount Dr, Raynham, MA 02767
Various types of bone fixation staples.

Holmed Corporation 508-238-3351
40 Norfolk Ave, South Easton, MA 02375

Innovasive Devices, Inc. 800-435-6001
734 Forest St, Marlborough, MA 01752

Intelifuse, Inc. 504-561-1100
1515 Poydras St Ste 1490, New Orleans, LA 70112
Staple, fixation, bone.

International Hospital Supply Co. 800-398-9450
6914 Canby Ave Ste 105, Reseda, CA 91335

Smith & Nephew, Inc., Endoscopy Division 800-343-8386
130 Forbes Blvd, Mansfield, MA 02048

Stryker Spine 866-457-7463
2 Pearl Ct, Allendale, NJ 07401

Tapco Medical, Inc. 818-225-5376
23981 Craftsman Rd, Calabasas, CA 91302
Fastlok

Ussc Puerto Rico, Inc. 203-845-1000
Building 911-67, Sabanetas Industrial Park, Ponce, PR 00731
Various.

V--Operations Management Consulting, 317-570-5830
7350 E 86th St, Indianapolis, IN 46256

Warsaw Orthopedic, Inc. 901-396-3133
2500 Silveus Xing, Warsaw, IN 46582
Staple.

Zimmer Holdings, Inc. 800-613-6131
1800 W Center St, PO Box 708, Warsaw, IN 46580

STAPLE, IMPLANTABLE *(Surgery) 79GDW*

Aesculap Implant Systems Inc. 1-800-234-9179
3773 Corporate Pkwy, Center Valley, PA 18034

Bard Shannon Limited 908-277-8000
San Geronimo Industrial Park, Lot # 1, Road # 3, Km 79.7
Humacao, PR 00791
Salute.

Biomet, Inc. 574-267-6639
56 E Bell Dr, PO Box 587, Warsaw, IN 46582
Clip for suturing apparatus.

Davol Inc., Sub. C.R. Bard, Inc. 800-556-6275
100 Crossings Blvd, Warwick, RI 02886
Stapling device and sterile stainless steel staple.

Devicor Medical Products Inc. 262-857-9300
10505 Corporate Dr Ste 207, Pleasant Prairie, WI 53158
MicroMARK II Tissue Marker MicroM

Edusa Corp. 651-733-4365
11751 Alameda Ave, Socorro, TX 79927
Surgical staples.

Ethicon Endo-Surgery, Inc. 877-384-4266
3801 University Blvd SE, Albuquerque, NM 87106
Various types of implantable staples and staplers.

Gyrus Ent L.L.C., Sub. Of Gyrus Acmi, Inc. 508-804-2739
2925 Appling Rd, Bartlett, TN 38133
Williams microclip.

Incisive Surgical, Inc. 877-246-7672
14405 21st Ave N Ste 130, Plymouth, MN 55447
INSORB (R) Absorbable Subcuticular Staple

Inrad 800-558-4647
4375 Donkers Ct SE, Kentwood, MI 49512
Clip / staple / tissue marker.

STAPLE, IMPLANTABLE *(cont'd)*

Medchannel Llc 617-314-9861
1241 Adams St Apt 110, Dorchester Center, MA 02124
Staple.

Okay Industries, Inc. 860-225-8707
200 Ellis St, P.O. Box 2470, New Britain, CT 06051

Power Medical Interventions, Inc. 267-775-8154
2021 Cabot Blvd W, Langhorne, PA 19047
Circular stapler.

Safestitch Medical Inc. 305-575-4145
4400 Biscayne Blvd Ste 760, Miami, FL 33137

Senorx, Inc. 949-362-4800
11 Columbia, Aliso Viejo, CA 92656
Biopsy site marker.

Tools For Surgery, Llc 631-444-4448
1339 Stony Brook Rd, Stony Brook, NY 11790
Hemorrhage occluder pin.

Ussc Puerto Rico, Inc. 203-845-1000
Building 911-67, Sabanetas Industrial Park, Ponce, PR 00731
Various sizes and types of sterile disposable staple cartridges.

Warsaw Orthopedic, Inc. 901-396-3133
2500 Silveus Xing, Warsaw, IN 46582
Staple.

STAPLE, IMPLANTABLE, REPROCESSED *(Surgery) 79NLL*

Sterilmed, Inc. 763-488-3400
11400 73rd Ave N Ste 100, Maple Grove, MN 55369
Reprocessed reloadable cutters & staplers.

STAPLE, REMOVABLE (SKIN) *(Surgery) 79GDT*

Design Standards Corp. 603-826-7744
Ceda Industrial Park, Charlestown, NH 03603
Removable (skin) staple extractor.

Edusa Corp. 651-733-4365
11751 Alameda Ave, Socorro, TX 79927
Various styles and sizes of removable skin staples.

Ethicon Endo-Surgery, Inc. 877-384-4266
3801 University Blvd SE, Albuquerque, NM 87106
Various of skin staples and staplers.

Kelsar, S.A. 508-261-8000
Blvd. Insurgentes, Libriamento a La, Tijuana 22450 Mexico
Staple removal

Teleflex Medical 800-334-9751
2917 Weck Drive, Research Triangle Park, NC 27709
VISISTAT.

STAPLER, LAPAROSCOPIC *(Surgery) 79WZO*

Ethicon Endo-Surgery, Inc. 800-USE-ENDO
4545 Creek Rd, Cincinnati, OH 45242
ENDOPATH EAS endoscopic articulating multifeed stapler.

Lyons Tool And Die Company 800-422-9363
185 Research Pkwy, Meriden, CT 06450
Rapid prototyping. Production of medical devices in class 10,000 clean rooms. Medical knives and scissors. Precision metal stamping. Engineering services.

Okay Industries, Inc. 860-225-8707
200 Ellis St, P.O. Box 2470, New Britain, CT 06051

Putnam Precision Products 845-278-2141
3859 Danbury Rd, Brewster, NY 10509

STAPLER, SURGICAL *(Surgery) 79GAG*

Avail Medical Products, Inc. 858-635-2206
1900 Carnegie Ave, --, Santa Ana, CA 92705

Covidien Lp 508-261-8000
15 Hampshire St, Mansfield, MA 02048
APPOSE unity, ULC & ULTRA stapler models.

Demetech Corp. 888-324-2447
3530 NW 115th Ave, Doral, FL 33178
Disposable skin stapler.

STAPLER, SURGICAL *(cont'd)*

Ethicon Endo-Surgery, Inc. 800-USE-ENDO
4545 Creek Rd, Cincinnati, OH 45242
PROXIMATE linear staplers (reload), titanium and linear staplers (reload) RL Plus, titanium: 30mm for TP30 and TL30, 60mm for TP60 and TPL60, 90mm for TL90; heavy wire: 30mm for TPH30 and TLH30, 60mm for TPH60 and TLH 60, 90mm for TPH 90 and TLH90; vascular 30mm for TPV30 and TLV30. Circular ILS stapler: 33mm dia, straight, detachable head, dark green; 21mm dia, light green anvil; 25mm dia, white anvil; 29mm dia, blue anvil; all with straight detachable heads, also available curved. Plus skin stapler, RH skin stapler and skin stapler III: 15, 25 and 35 stainless steel regular, 15, 25 and 35 stainless steel wide, also 55 wide for Plus skin stapler.

Gw Plastics, Inc. 802-234-9941
239 Pleasant St, Bethel, VT 05032

Ironwood Plastics, Inc. 906-932-5025
1235 Wall St, Ironwood, MI 49938
Surgical staple remover.

Kelsar, S.A. 508-261-8000
Blvd. Insurgentes, Libriamento a La, Tijuana 22450 Mexico
Skin stapler, ulc disposable, ultra unity, disposable, staples & remover

Lacey Manufacturing Co. 203-336-0121
1146 Barnum Ave, PO Box 5156, Bridgeport, CT 06610

Lyons Tool And Die Company 800-422-9363
185 Research Pkwy, Meriden, CT 06450
Rapid prototyping. Production of medical devices in class 10,000 clean rooms. Medical knives and scissors. Precision metal stamping. Engineering services.

Medisiss 866-866-7477
2747 SW 6th St, Redmond, OR 97756
Various surgical staplers,sterile.

Okay Industries, Inc. 860-225-8707
200 Ellis St, P.O. Box 2470, New Britain, CT 06051

Safestitch Medical Inc. 305-575-4145
4400 Biscayne Blvd Ste 760, Miami, FL 33137

Sterilmed, Inc. 763-488-3400
11400 73rd Ave N Ste 100, Maple Grove, MN 55369
Stapler.

Synectic Medical Product Development 203-877-8488
60 Commerce Park, Milford, CT 06460

Ussc Puerto Rico, Inc. 203-845-1000
Building 911-67, Sabanetas Industrial Park, Ponce, PR 00731
Multiple.

STARCH-DYE BOUND POLYMER, AMYLASE *(Chemistry) 75CIW*

Teco Diagnostics 714-693-7788
1268 N Lakeview Ave, Anaheim, CA 92807
Amylase.

STARTER, BONE SCREW *(Orthopedics) 87HWD*

Kls-Martin L.P. 800-625-1557
11239-1 St. John`s Industrial, Parkway South
Jacksonville, FL 32250

Surgical Implant Generation Network (Sign) 509-371-1107
451 Hills St, Richland, WA 99354
Punch.

W.L. Gore & Associates,Inc 928-526-3030
1505 North Fourth St., Flagstaff, AZ 86004
Bone screw.

Zimmer Trabecular Metal Technology 800-613-6131
10 Pomeroy Rd, Parsippany, NJ 07054
Drill bit starter tip.

STATION PIPETTING *(Chemistry) 75JRD*

Biodex Medical Systems, Inc. 800-224-6339
20 Ramsey Rd, Shirley, NY 11967
L-Block Shield & Dose Drawing Station, units combine to provide the ideal and safe workstation for drawing a dose of PET radionuclide into a syringe.

STATION, AUTOPSY *(Pathology) 88VFV*

Scientek Medical Equipment 604-273-9094
11151 Bridgeport Rd., Richmond, BC V6X 1T3 Canada
Grossing workstations formalin treatment hoods, wall mounted stations with sinks, air extraction, cart locks. AIDS morturary and autopsy tables, electric cadaver hoists, cadaver storage racking, etc.

STATION, NOURISHMENT *(General) 80UMU*

Continental Metal Products Co., Inc. 800-221-4439
35 Olympia Ave, Woburn, MA 01801
Nourishment and medicine centers.

Independent Solutions, Inc. 847-498-0500
900 Skokie Blvd Ste 118, Northbrook, IL 60062
CMP stainless steel, UL and NSF labeled.

Intermetro Industries Corp. 800-441-2714
651 N Washington St, Wilkes Barre, PA 18705
STARSYS nourishment room casework.

Piper Products, Inc. 800-492-3431
300 S 84th Ave, Wausau, WI 54401
Meal serving systems.

STATION, NURSING *(General) 80TBD*

Colonial Scientific Ltd. 902-468-1811
201 Brownlow Ave., Unit 52, Dartmouth, NS B3B-1W2 Canada

Independent Solutions, Inc. 847-498-0500
900 Skokie Blvd Ste 118, Northbrook, IL 60062
BWM wood or plastic laminate.

Intermetro Industries Corp. 800-441-2714
651 N Washington St, Wilkes Barre, PA 18705
STARSYS satellite nursing station.

Jamestown Metal Products 716-665-5313
178 Blackstone Ave, Jamestown, NY 14701

Life Sensing Instrument Company, Inc. 800-624-2732
329 W Lincoln St, Tullahoma, TN 37388

R.C. Smith Company 800-747-7648
14200 Southcross Dr W, Burnsville, MN 55306

STENT, CARDIOVASCULAR *(Cardiovascular) 74MAF*

Abbott Vascular, Cardiac Therapies 800-227-9902
3200 Lakeside Dr, Santa Clara, CA 95054
Sterile single use coronary stent.

Abbott Vascular, Cardiac Therapies 800-227-9902
26531 Ynez Rd, Mailing P.O. Box 9018, Temecula, CA 92591
Sterile single use coronary stent.

Advanced Bio Prosthetic Surfaces, Ltd 210-696-5300
4778 Research Dr, San Antonio, TX 78240
Sesame covered stent system.

Advanced Stent Technologies 508-650-8798
6900 Koll Center Pkwy Ste 415, Pleasanton, CA 94566
Various models of sterile coronary stent & delivery systems.

Atrium Medical Corp. 800-528-7486
5 Wentworth Dr, Hudson, NH 03051
Atrium Flyer Coronary Stent.

Avantec Vascular Corp. 408-329-5425
605 W California Ave, Sunnyvale, CA 94086
Coronary stent.

Biosensors International - Usa 949-553-8300
20280 SW Acacia St Ste 300, Newport Beach, CA 92660
Matrix™ Drug-Eluting Stent featuring Biolimus A-9 anti-restenotic compound (investigational device, not for sale); S-Stent Coronary Stent Delivery System (not available for sale in US).

Bolton Medical, Inc. 954-838-9699
799 International Pkwy, Sunrise, FL 33325
Stents-various types.

Boston Scientific - Marina Bay Customer Fulfillment Center 617-689-6000
500 Commander Shea Blvd, Quincy, MA 02171
Coronary stent.

Boston Scientific Corp. 800-323-6472
5905 Nathan Ln N, Minneapolis, MN 55442
WALLSTENT for peripheral use.

Cardio-Nef, S.A. De C.V. 01-800-024-0240
Rio Grijalva 186, Col. Mitras Norte, Monterrey, N.L. 64320 Mexico

Comco, Inc. 800-796-6626
2151 N Lincoln St, Burbank, CA 91504
Micro-abrasive blasting equipment for deburring, cleaning, and material removal on stents, pacemakers, cannula, IV components, and other medical devices.

Cook Inc. 800-457-4500
PO Box 489, Bloomington, IN 47402

Cordis Corporation 800-327-7714
14201 NW 60th Ave, Miami Lakes, FL 33014
Drug eluting stent.

STENT, CARDIOVASCULAR *(cont'd)*

Cordis Llc 877-338-4235
Road 362 Km 0.5, San German, PR 00683
Sterile stents.

Devax, Inc. 949-334-2333
20996 Bake Pkwy Ste 106, Lake Forest, CA 92630
Various modles of axxess stent system.

Drg International, Inc. 800-321-1167
1167 US Highway 22, Mountainside, NJ 07092

Insitu Technologies, Inc. 651-389-1017
5810 Blackshire Path, Inver Grove Heights, MN 55076
Coronary stent.

M & I Medical Sales, Inc. 305-663-6444
4711 SW 72nd Ave, Miami, FL 33155

Maxcor Inc 714-367-2847
17517 Fabrica Way Ste H, Artesia, CA 90703

Medtronic, Inc. 800-633-8766
710 Medtronic Pkwy, Minneapolis, MN 55432

Orbusneich Medical, Inc. 852-280-2228
5363 NW 35th Ave, Ft Lauderdale, FL 33309
Stent, stent delivery system.

Svelte Medical Systems Inc. 908-264-2194
675 Central Ave Ste 2, New Providence, NJ 07974

Thermopeutix Inc. 858-549-1760
9925 Businesspark Ave Ste B, San Diego, CA 92131
Intravascular stent with delivery system.

Tryton Medical, Inc. 919-226-1490
1000 Park Forty Plz Ste 325, Durham, NC 27713
Tryton Side Branch Stent System

STENT, COLONIC, METALIC, EXPANDABLE *(Gastro/Urology) 78MQR*

Cook Endoscopy 336-744-0157
4900 Bethania Station Rd # &, 5951 Grassy Creek Blvd. Winston Salem, NC 27105
Colon stent.

STENT, CORONARY, DRUG-ELUTING *(Cardiovascular) 74NIQ*

Cordis Llc 877-338-4235
Road 362 Km 0.5, San German, PR 00683
Sterile stents.

Elixir Medical Corporation 408-636-2000
870 Hermosa Ave, Sunnyvale, CA 94085
Coronary Stent System; Elixir Medical Novolimus-Eluting; with Durable Polyme

Icon Interventional Systems, Inc. 216-382-3119
1414 S Green Rd Ste 309, Cleveland, OH 44121
Various models of drug eluting coronary stents.

TriReme Medical Inc. 925-931-1300
7060 Koll Center Pkwy Ste 300, Pleasanton, CA 94566
Antares

STENT, INTRACRANIAL NEUROVASCULAR *(Cns/Neurology) 84NJE*

Abbott Vascular, Vascular Solutions 800-227-9902
26531 Ynez Rd, Temecula, CA 92591
Neurological stent.

Cordis Neurovascular, Inc. 800-327-7714
14201 NW 60th Ave, Miami Lakes, FL 33014
Intracranial stent.

STENT, METALLIC, EXPANDABLE *(Anesthesiology) 73MEW*

Cordis Endovascular 877-338-4235
7 Powderhorn Dr, Warren, NJ 07059

STENT, OTHER *(Obstetrics/Gyn) 85UAN*

Aci Medical, Inc. 800-667-9451
1857 Diamond St, San Marcos, CA 92078
UNNA-SLEEVE - peripheral vascular support device for chronic venous disease.

Boston Scientific Interventional Technologies 858-268-4488
3574 Ruffin Rd, San Diego, CA 92123
Stent, Coronary.

Bryan Corp. 800-343-7711
4 Plympton St, Woburn, MA 01801
Tracheobronchial Dumon style silicone stents in various sizes.

Telemed Systems Inc. 800-481-6718
8 Kane Industrial Dr, Hudson, MA 01749
Amsterdam stent available. Carr-Locke stent remover available.

STENT, SUPERFICIAL FEMORAL ARTERY *(Cardiovascular) 74NIP*

Abbott Vascular, Vascular Solutions 800-227-9902
26531 Ynez Rd, Temecula, CA 92591
Sterile peripheral stent.

Ev3 Inc. 800-716-6700
4600 Nathan Ln N, Plymouth, MN 55442
Femoropopliteal stent.

W.L. Gore & Associates,Inc 928-526-3030
1505 North Fourth St., Flagstaff, AZ 86004
Vascular endoprosthesis.

STENT, TRACHEAL *(Anesthesiology) 73WLI*

E. Benson Hood Laboratories, Inc. 800-942-5227
575 Washington St, Pembroke, MA 02359
Adult male, adult female, adolescent, and child size silicone stents; laryngeal keels, bronchial stents, custom diameters and lengths, Y stents; Eliacher laryngeal stent. Tracheal stent with post.

STENT, URETERAL *(Gastro/Urology) 78UAM*

American Medical Systems, Inc. 800-328-3881
10700 Bren Rd W, Minnetonka, MN 55343
UROLUME endourethral prosthesis.

C. R. Bard, Inc., Bard Urological Div. 888-367-2273
13183 Harland Dr NE, Covington, GA 30014

Cook Urological, Inc. 800-457-4500
1100 W Morgan St, P.O. Box 227, Spencer, IN 47460

Redi-Tech Medical Products,Llc 800-824-1793
529 Front St Ste 125, Berea, OH 44017

Saint-Gobain Performance Plastics/Clearwater 800-541-6880
4451 110th Ave N, Clearwater, FL 33762

STENT, VASCULAR *(Cardiovascular) 74WLQ*

Atrium Medical Corp. 800-528-7486
5 Wentworth Dr, Hudson, NH 03051
Atrium V-12 PTFE Perepheral Stent Graft.Atrium iCAST PTFE Covered Tracheal Bronchial Stent Graft

Cardio-Nef, S.A. De C.V. 01-800-024-0240
Rio Grijalva 186, Col. Mitras Norte, Monterrey, N.L. 64320 Mexico

Cordis Endovascular 877-338-4235
7 Powderhorn Dr, Warren, NJ 07059

Drg International, Inc. 800-321-1167
1167 US Highway 22, Mountainside, NJ 07092

Lemaitre Vascular, Inc. 781-221-2266
63 2nd Ave, Burlington, MA 01803
EndoFit's® unique design and construction offers a wide range of solutions for your abdominal and Thoracic endovascular graft needs.

STEREOSCOPE, AC-POWERED *(Ophthalmology) 86HJQ*

Mast/Keystone View 800-806-6569
2200 Dickerson Rd, Reno, NV 89503
Suited to home training applications, tests are available for fusion, retinal rivalry, scotomas, hemianopsia and diplopias, several models available.

Stereo Optical Co., Inc. 800-344-9500
3539 N Kenton Ave, Chicago, IL 60641

Topcon Medical Systems, Inc. 800-223-1130
37 W Century Rd, Paramus, NJ 07652
Screenoscope: $1,450.00.

Western Scientific Co., Inc. 800-48W-ESCO
2112 W Burbank Blvd, Burbank, CA 91506

STEREOTAXY EQUIPMENT *(Cns/Neurology) 84HAW*

Associated Design And Manufacturing Co. 800-837-8257
8245 Backlick Rd Ste K, Lorton, VA 22079
Stereotactic adapter for CAT-scan equipment.

Best Nomos Corp. 800-70-NOMOS
1 Best Dr, Pittsburgh, PA 15202

Biomet, Inc. 574-267-6639
56 E Bell Dr, PO Box 587, Warsaw, IN 46582
Various software navigation applications.

STEREOTAXY EQUIPMENT *(cont'd)*

Compass International, Inc. 800-933-2143
1815 14th St NW, Rochester, MN 55901
Compass Image-Guided Stereotactic System. Computer-assisted stereotactic neurosurgical hardware and software. Compass instruments for stereotactic neurosurgery including biopsy needle, forceps, coagulation probe, scissors, and sharp pins. COMPASS Framed Image-guided stereotatic surgery system, hardware and software for intra/extra-cranial procedures. Cygnus-PFS(Portable Frameless System) Image-Guided stereotactic surgery system. Hardware and software for intra/extra-cranial procedures.

Depuy Orthopaedics, Inc. 800-473-3789
700 Orthopaedic Dr, P.O. Box 988, Warsaw, IN 46582
Various types of stereotaxic instruments.

Depuy-Raynham, A Div. Of Depuy Orthopaedics 800-451-2006
325 Paramount Dr, Raynham, MA 02767
Various types of stereotaxic instruments.

Elekta, Inc. 800-535-7355
4775 Peachtree Industrial Blvd, Building 300, Suite 300
Norcross, GA 30092
Surgical treatment planning.

Fhc, Inc 800-326-2905
1201 Main St, Bowdoin, ME 04287
microTargeting® Drive and Platform System

I.Z.I. Medical Products, Inc. 800-231-1499
7020 Tudsbury Rd, Baltimore, MD 21244
Passive reflective marker.

Integra Radionics 800-466-6814
22 Terry Ave, Burlington, MA 01803

Mako Surgical Corp. 954-927-2044
2555 Davie Rd Ste 110, Plantation, FL 33317
Image guided surgery system.

Med-Surgical Services Inc. 408-617-2000
465 E Evelyn Ave, Sunnyvale, CA 94086
Cbyon surgical operating system.

Medtronic Image-Guided Neurologics, Inc. 800-707-0933
2290 W Eau Gallie Blvd, Melbourne, FL 32935
Microdrive and trajectory guide.

Medtronic Navigation, Inc. 888-580-8860
826 Coal Creek Cir, Louisville, CO 80027
Stereotactic device and accessories.

Ortho Development Corp. 800-429-8339
12187 Business Park Dr, Draper, UT 84020
Disposable biopsy probes. Stereotactic micro instrument CT/MRI, center of the arc system.

Orthosoft, Inc. 514-861-4074
75 Queen St., Ste. 3300, Montreal, QUE H3C-2N6 Canada
NAVITRACK computer assisted surgery system operates in real time using virtual 3D images. This offers a level ofprecision and safety that was previously unavailable for the implantation of prostheses.

Sandstrom Trade & Technology, Inc. 800-699-0745
610 Niagara St., Welland, ONT L3C 1L8 Canada
STEREOADAPTER patented, CT/MRI compatible, non-invasive localizer and head holder for neuro-imaging, stereotactic image-guided radiation therapy and neurosurgery. Full line of surgical and positioning accessories for multiple indications.

Schaerer Mayfield Usa 800-755-6381
4900 Charlemar Dr, Cincinnati, OH 45227
PELORUS stereotactic system. MAYFIELD/ACCISS Image Guided Surgery System.

Tipal Instruments Ltd. 514-484-9741
128 Prom Ronald, Montreal-Ouest H4X 1M8 Canada
No common name listed

Varian Medical Systems, Oncology Systems 800 278-2747
911 Hansen Way, Bldg.3 M/S C-165, Palo Alto, CA 94304
Various types of stereotaxic instruments.

Z-Kat, Inc. 954-927-2044
2903 Simms St, Hollywood, FL 33020
Various types of stereotaxic instruments.

STERILANT, MEDICAL DEVICE *(General) 80MED*

Alden Medical Llc 413-747-9717
360 Cold Spring Ave, West Springfield, MA 01089
Various sterilants for medical devices.

Andersen Products, Inc., 800-523-1276
3202 Caroline Dr, Health Science Park, Haw River, NC 27258
100% EO industrial sterilization systems.

STERILANT, MEDICAL DEVICE *(cont'd)*

Barnstead International 412-490-8425
2555 Kerper Blvd, Dubuque, IA 52001
Various liquid sterilants.

Certol International, Llc 303-799-9401
6120 E 58th Ave, Commerce City, CO 80022
Liquid chemical sterilant.

Cetylite Industries, Inc. 856-665-6111
9051 River Rd, Pennsauken, NJ 08110
Glutaraldehyde,liquid chemical sterilant/high-level disinfectant.

Dshealthcare Inc. 201-871-1232
85 W Forest Ave, Englewood, NJ 07631
Liquid chemical sterilant/high level disinfectant.

Lyne Laboratories, Inc. 508-583-8700
10 Burke Dr, Brockton, MA 02301
Peroxyacetic acid (dialyzer reprocessing concentrate).

Medsci, Inc. 336-274-3496
201 Pine St, Greensboro, NC 27401
Sterilant/high level disinfectant.

Pascal Co., Inc. 425-602-3633
2929 Northup Way, Bellevue, WA 98004
Glutaraldehyde solution.

Serim Research Corp. 574-264-3440
3506 Reedy Dr, Elkhart, IN 46514
Test for glutaraldehyde potency in specific 14-day activated dialdehyde solutios.

Smiths Medical Asd, Inc. 847-793-0135
330 Corporate Woods Pkwy, Vernon Hills, IL 60061
Germicide.

Sporicidin International 800-424-3733
121 Congressional Ln, Rockville, MD 20852
SPORICIDIN sterilizing and disinfecting solution is 100% effective with only 1% glutaraldehyde. It achieves high-level disinfection in only 20 minutes. FDA 510(k) cleared.

Young Colorado, Llc. 800-325-1881
13705 Shoreline Ct E, Earth City, MO 63045
Liquid chimical sterilants/high level disinfectants.

STERILIZATION INDICATOR *(Surgery) 79LRT*

North American Science Associates, Inc. 866-666-9455
6750 Wales Rd, Northwood, OH 43619
Chemical process indicator. Standard or custom product for steam, ethylene oxide, and radiation sterilization processes.

Princeton Medical Group, Inc. 800-875-0869
1189 Royal Links Dr, Mt Pleasant, SC 29466
INDICATORS, SECURITY SEALS & FILTERS

Ronpak, Inc. 732-968-8000
4301 New Brunswick Ave, South Plainfield, NJ 07080

Scican Inc. 800-572-1211
701 Technology Dr, Canonsburg, PA 15317

Tapco Medical, Inc. 818-225-5376
23981 Craftsman Rd, Calabasas, CA 91302

STERILIZATION PROCESS INDICATOR, BIOLOGICAL

(General) 80FRC

Andersen Products, Inc., 800-523-1276
3202 Caroline Dr, Health Science Park, Haw River, NC 27258
STERITEST biological indicators for use with ethylene-oxide sterilization.

Barnstead International 412-490-8425
2555 Kerper Blvd, Dubuque, IA 52001
Biological indicator.

Confirm Monitoring Systems, Inc. 303-699-3356
109 Inverness Dr E Ste F, Englewood, CO 80112
Biological indicator.

Getinge Usa, Inc. 800-475-9040
1777 E Henrietta Rd, Rochester, NY 14623
GETINGE

North American Science Associates, Inc. 866-666-9455
6750 Wales Rd, Northwood, OH 43619
Spore strips, discs, and suspensions for sterilization cycle validation. Available for ethylene oxide, dry heat, steam, and radiation sterilization.

Propper Manufacturing Co., Inc. 800-832-4300
3604 Skillman Ave, Long Island City, NY 11101

STERILIZATION PROCESS INDICATOR, BIOLOGICAL *(cont'd)*

Raven Biological Laboratories, Inc. 800-728-5702
8607 Park Dr, PO Box 27261, Omaha, NE 68127
Spore Strips, Suspensions, Prospore2 SCBI are available for EO, Steam, Dry Heat, Irradiation and/or Peroxide.

Sns Biosystems 805-925-1616
527B Oak St, Santa Maria, CA 93454
Biological indicator for chemical vapor, dry heat and steam sterilization process.

Sps Medical Supply Corp. 800-722-1529
6789 W. Hennetta Road, Rush, NY 14543

Sterilator Company, Inc. 585-968-2377
30 Water St, Cuba, NY 14727
Biological indicators and spore suspensions for ethylene oxide, steam, dry heat, and radiation sterilization processes.

Steris Biological Operations Facility 440-354-2600
9325 Pinecone Dr, Mentor, OH 44060
Biological indicator.

Sts Division Of Ethox International 800.836.4850
7500 W Henrietta Rd, Rush, NY 14543
Various types of sterilization biological indicators for the evaluation of moist.

Sts Duotek, Inc 800-836-4850
370 Summit Point Dr, Henrietta, NY 14467
Spore strips and suspensions for gas, steam, dry heat, and radiation sterilization.

Thermo Fisher Scientific Inc. 563-556-2241
2555 Kerper Blvd, Dubuque, IA 52001
SPOR-TEST biological sterilization process indicator.

STERILIZATION PROCESS INDICATOR, CHEMICAL

(General) 80RVU

Andersen Products, Inc., 800-523-1276
3202 Caroline Dr, Health Science Park, Haw River, NC 27258
DOSIMETER chemical integrator for use with ANDERSEN gas-sterilization systems.

Case Medical, Inc. 888-227-2273
65 Railroad Ave, Ridgefield, NJ 07657
sterilization container transport and storage

Getinge Usa, Inc. 800-475-9040
1777 E Henrietta Rd, Rochester, NY 14623
GETINGE

Kem Medical Products Corp. 800-553-0330
75 Price Pkwy, Farmingdale, NY 11735
KEMSURE sterilization indicators.

M&C Specialties Co. 800-441-6996
90 James Way, Southampton, PA 18966

Propper Manufacturing Co., Inc. 800-832-4300
3604 Skillman Ave, Long Island City, NY 11101

Sps Medical Supply Corp. 800-722-1529
6789 W. Hennetta Road, Rush, NY 14543

Sterion, Incorporated 800-328-7958
13828 Lincoln St NE, Ham Lake, MN 55304
SafeClean Instrument and Channel Cleaning Brushes used to clean surgical/medical instruments and endoscopic devices. Instrument ID tape

Thermo Fisher Scientific Inc. 563-556-2241
2555 Kerper Blvd, Dubuque, IA 52001

Thorn Smith Laboratories 231-882-7251
7755 Narrow Gauge Rd, Beulah, MI 49617
DIACK & DRYTOL; DIACK is $17.00 retail per box of 100 chemical sterilization monitors. DIACK monitors are used for a regular steam cycle (121 C). DRYTROL is $20.00 retail per box of 100 chemical sterilization monitors. DRYTROL monitors are used for a dry heat cycle.

Veriad 800-423-4643
650 Columbia St, Brea, CA 92821

STERILIZATION PROCESS INDICATOR, PHYSICAL/CHEMICAL

(General) 80JOJ

Advanced Sterilization Products 800-595-0200
33 Technology Dr, Irvine, CA 92618

Alden Medical Llc 413-747-9717
360 Cold Spring Ave, West Springfield, MA 01089
Various indicators.

Barnstead International 412-490-8425
2555 Kerper Blvd, Dubuque, IA 52001
Various physical/chemical sterilization indicators.

STERILIZATION PROCESS INDICATOR, PHYSICAL/CHEMICAL *(cont'd)*

Biosure, Inc. 800-345-2267
12301 Loma Rica Dr Unit G, Grass Valley, CA 95945
BIOSURE steam sterilization integrator. Validate the sterility of your autoclave without culturing spore strips or sending samples to a reference laboratory for sterility verification.

Dana Products, Inc. 847-455-2881
11457 Melrose Ave, Franklin Park, IL 60131
Sterilization indicator.

Hu-Friedy Manufacturing Co., Inc. 800-483-7433
3232 N Rockwell St, Chicago, IL 60618
$24.55 for 250 per box.

Indilab, Inc. 800-441-5000
10367 Franklin Ave, Franklin Park, IL 60131
Chemical indicator strips. Chemical indicator tapes

Industrias Tuk, S.A. De C.V. 8-313-7421-2
Antigua Carretera a Roma, Km 7 5¯, Apodaca 66632 Mexico
Indicator tape

Lorvic Corp. 800-325-1881
13705 Shoreline Ct E, Earth City, MO 63045
Autoclave indicator tape; process indicators.

Medical Action Industries, Inc 800-645-7042
500 Express Dr S, Brentwood, NY 11717
Bowie Dick test packs and other sterilization indicators.

Products For Medicine 800-333-3087
1201 E Ball Rd Ste H, Anaheim, CA 92805
Sterilization indicator on tamper-evident arrows.

Propper Manufacturing Co., Inc. 800-832-4300
3604 Skillman Ave, Long Island City, NY 11101

Serim Research Corp. 574-264-3440
3506 Reedy Dr, Elkhart, IN 46514
Test for potency of peracetic acid in dialllyzer reuse.

Steris Biological Operations Facility 440-354-2600
9325 Pinecone Dr, Mentor, OH 44060
Chemical indicator.

Steris Corporation 440-354-2600
6515 Hopkins Rd, Mentor, OH 44060
Air removal indicator for pre vacuum steam sterilizers.

Steritec Products, Inc. 303-660-4201
599 Topeka Way Ste 400, Castle Rock, CO 80109
Various types of process indicators.

Thorn Smith Laboratories 231-882-7251
7755 Narrow Gauge Rd, Beulah, MI 49617
VAC $17.00 per box of 100 physical/chemical sterilization monitors. VAC monitors are used for a flash steam cycle (134 C).

Willow Graphics, Inc. 631-454-6565
608 Oak St, Copiague, NY 11726
Chemical sterilizer indicators.

3m Espe Dental Products 949-863-1360
2111 McGaw Ave, Irvine, CA 92614
$8.85 to $13.25 for steam indicator tape.

STERILIZER, BOILING WATER *(Dental And Oral) 76ECG*

Dp Manufacture Corp. 305-640-9894
1460 NW 107th Ave Ste H, Doral, FL 33172
Autoclave.

Waterclave, L.L.C. 913-312-5860
6731 W 121st St, Overland Park, KS 66209
Waterclave.

STERILIZER, BULK, STEAM & ETHYLENE-OXIDE *(General) 80UDL*

Acteon Inc. 800-289-6367
124 Gaither Dr Ste 140, Mount Laurel, NJ 08054
VELA 160A Autoclave pressurized steam sterilizer for dental equipment and instruments.

Environmental Tectonics Corp. 215-355-9100
125 James Way, Southampton, PA 18966
Clean gas and steam sterilizers for pharmaceutical, medical waste, hospital, and laboratory applications; custom and standard models available; also animal care; cGMP, stainless steel; 3 cu. ft. to 3,000 cu. ft.

STERILIZER, CHEMICAL *(General) 80MLR*

Barnstead International 412-490-8425
2555 Kerper Blvd, Dubuque, IA 52001
Chemiclave.

STERILIZER, CHEMICAL *(cont'd)*

Chemisphere Corp. 314-644-1300
2101 Clifton Ave, Saint Louis, MO 63139

Eastman Medical Products Inc. 800-373-4410
2000 Powell St Ste 1540, Emeryville, CA 94608
EASTMAN ABSORBENT POLYMER--anionic polyacrylamide. Used to reduce or eliminate bacteria growth by depriving bacteria of nutrition.

Roger L. Goodman, D.D.S., P.C. 517-676-5200
200 Temple St, Mason, MI 48854
Alcohol solution for use in chemiclave sterilizers.

Steris Corporation 440-354-2600
6515 Hopkins Rd, Mentor, OH 44060
Liquid chemical sterilization system and accessories.

Xenotec Ltd. 949-640-4053
511 Hazel Dr, Corona Del Mar, CA 92625
Glutaraldehyde solution retains potency up to 28 days after activation. This same formulation is used safely in major hospitals throughout the world to sterilize or disinfect surgical instruments and implements.

STERILIZER, DRY HEAT *(General) 80KMH*

Coltene/Whaledent Inc. 330-916-8858
235 Ascot Pkwy, Cuyahoga Falls, OH 44223
Dry heat sterilizer.

Dencraft 800-328-9729
PO Box 57, Moorestown, NJ 08057
Wayne sterilizer.

Dentronix, Inc. 800-523-5944
235 Ascot Pkwy, Cuyahoga Falls, OH 44223
$2995.00 per unit (standard).

Pro Scientific Inc. 800-584-3776
99 Willenbrock Rd, Oxford, CT 06478
Memmert hot air sterilizers from 30-220 degrees Celsius are available in a range of capacities, from 14-749l, with the choice of convection or air turbine. These sterilizers are available in 3 different controller classes; mechanical, electronic (RS232 computer interface) or process controller (RS232 computer interface and new chip card technology).

Roboz Surgical Instrument Co., Inc. 800-424-2984
PO Box 10710, Gaithersburg, MD 20898
Germinator Glass Bead Sterilizer

Schueler & Company, Inc. 516-487-1500
PO Box 528, Stratford, CT 06615

STERILIZER, DRY HEAT, DENTAL *(Dental And Oral) 76ECF*

Cpac Equipment, Inc. 800-333-9729
2364 Leicester Road, Leicester, NY 14481-0175

Dentalez Group 866-DTE-INFO
101 Lindenwood Dr Ste 225, Valleybrooke Corporate Center
Malvern, PA 19355

Dentronix, Inc. 800-523-5944
235 Ascot Pkwy, Cuyahoga Falls, OH 44223
DDS 7000 Dry Heat Sterilizer features a Cool Down Cycle for safety, self-diagnostic system and comport for printing cycle data.

Her-Mar, Inc. 800-327-8209
8550 NW 30th Ter, Doral, FL 33122
$600.00 per unit (standard).

Kadan Co. Inc., D.A. 800-325-2326
1 Brigadoon Ln, Waxhaw, NC 28173

Mexicana De Equipos Dentales, S,A, 523-684-8110
Guillermo Baca 3738, Lomas De Polanco, Guadalajara 44960 Mexico
No common name listed

Murdock Laboratories, Inc. 800 439-2497
123 Primrose Rd, Burlingame, CA 94010

Pelton & Crane Co., 704-588-2126
11727 Fruehauf Dr, Charlotte, NC 28273

STERILIZER, ETHYLENE-OXIDE GAS *(General) 80FLF*

Aga Linde Healthcare P.R. Inc. 787-622-7900
PO Box 363868, GPO Box 364727, San Juan, PR 00936
General.

Andersen Products, Inc., 800-523-1276
3202 Caroline Dr, Health Science Park, Haw River, NC 27258
ANPROLENE, EOGAS, and STERIJET ANDERSEN sterilizers for healthcare and industrial use; 100% EO gas-diffusion technology.

Ars Enterprises 800-735-9277
12900 Lakeland Rd, Santa Fe Springs, CA 90670

STERILIZER, ETHYLENE-OXIDE GAS *(cont'd)*

Environmental Tectonics Corp. 215-355-9100
125 James Way, Southampton, PA 18966
Ethylene oxide gas sterilizers for medical device applications; sizes range from 1 unit to turnkey system.

H&W Technology, Llc. 585-218-0385
PO Box 20281, Rochester, NY 14602
The ILE20 resistometer for all ethylene oxide processes meets the requirements of ISO 11140 and AAMI ST44. And, new to the market, SteriCert (healthcare) and SteriMagic (industrial) ethylene oxide control systems are now available for blend (non-100%) ethylene oxide sterilizers and legacy controls replacements.

Mg Industries 610-695-7628
1 Steel Rd E, U.S. Industrial Park, Morrisville, PA 19067
Patient lift.

Sterigenics International, Inc. 800-472-4508
2015 Spring Rd Ste 650, Oak Brook, IL 60523
Custom contract ethylene oxide sterilization services at 17 locations in North America, Europe, and the Pacific Rim. Laboratory services include contract testing, contract research and product development using pilot EO and steam vessels. BIER vessel. Protocol and validation services.

Steris Corporation 814-452-3100
2424 W 23rd St, Erie, PA 16506
Eto sterilizer.

STERILIZER, ETHYLENE-OXIDE GAS, OPERATING ROOM *(Surgery) 79FSJ*

International Hospital Supply Co. 800-398-9450
6914 Canby Ave Ste 105, Reseda, CA 91335

STERILIZER, ETHYLENE-OXIDE, BULK *(General) 80UDJ*

Andersen Products, Inc., 800-523-1276
3202 Caroline Dr, Health Science Park, Haw River, NC 27258
STERIJET system industrial EO sterilization system; gas-diffusion process reduces gas consumption.

STERILIZER, ETHYLENE-OXIDE, TABLE TOP *(General) 80UDK*

Andersen Products, Inc., 800-523-1276
3202 Caroline Dr, Health Science Park, Haw River, NC 27258
ANPROLENE 100% EO unit-dose cartridge system employs gas-diffusion technology to reduce gas consumption.

STERILIZER, GLASS BEAD *(Dental And Oral) 76ECC*

Dentalez Group 866-DTE-INFO
101 Lindenwood Dr Ste 225, Valleybrooke Corporate Center
Malvern, PA 19355

Pulpdent Corp. 800-343-4342
80 Oakland St, Watertown, MA 02472
Glass bead sterilizer.

STERILIZER, LABORATORY *(Microbiology) 83UIM*

American Autoclave Co. 800 421 5161
7819 Riverside Rd E, Sumner, WA 98390

Brinkmann Instruments, Inc. 800-645-3050
PO Box 1019, Westbury, NY 11590

Buxton Medical Equipment Corp. 631-957-4500
1178 Route 109, Lindenhurst, NY 11757
All sizes available.

Consolidated Stills & Sterilizers 617-782-6072
76 Ashford St, Boston, MA 02134
Full line from $6,000 to $56,000 each.

Container Research Corp. 610-459-2160
PO Box 159, Hollow Hill Road, Glen Riddle, PA 19037
Specialized field-use sterilizer. Uses various fuels.

Covidien Lp 508-261-8000
15 Hampshire St, Mansfield, MA 02048

Eastman Medical Products Inc. 800-373-4410
2000 Powell St Ste 1540, Emeryville, CA 94608
MICRO-SORB--polymer added to laboratory fluids such as blood, urine. Turns fluids into solid state. For use in research laboratories or other areas where canisters containing fluids need neutralization.

Getinge Usa, Inc. 800-475-9040
1777 E Henrietta Rd, Rochester, NY 14623
GETINGE.

International Hospital Supply Co. 800-398-9450
6914 Canby Ave Ste 105, Reseda, CA 91335

Medi-Tech International, Inc. 305-593-9373
2924 NW 109th Ave, Doral, FL 33172
Market Forge.

STERILIZER, LABORATORY *(cont'd)*

New Brunswick Scientific Co., Inc. 800-631-5417
PO Box 4005, Edison, NJ 08818
Automated agar/media sterilizer, 1 to 10 L.

Thermo Fisher Scientific Inc. 563-556-2241
2555 Kerper Blvd, Dubuque, IA 52001

STERILIZER, LOOP, INOCULATING *(Microbiology) 83VLZ*

Coy Laboratory Products, Inc. 734-475-2200
14500 Coy Dr, Grass Lake, MI 49240

Fisher Healthcare 800-766-7000
9999 Veterans Memorial Dr, Houston, TX 77038

Sigma-Aldrich Corp. 800-521-8956
3050 Spruce St, Saint Louis, MO 63103

Vista Technology, Inc. 780-468-0020
8432 45th St. NW, Edmonton, ALB T6B-2N6 Canada
ISOLOOP, reusable streaking loop for automated petri dish streaking in the ISOPLATER.

STERILIZER, RADIATION *(General) 80RVX*

Neutron Products, Inc. 301-349-5001
22301 Mount Ephraim Rd, Dickerson, MD 20842
Gamma irradiator for research.

Sterigenics International, Inc. 800-472-4508
2015 Spring Rd Ste 650, Oak Brook, IL 60523
Sterigenics medical sterilization and analytical labs provides gamma, electron beam and X-ray sterilization and microorganism reduction services to the healthcare, labware, pharmaceutical, packaging and medical device industries. Headquartered in Oak Brook, IL, Sterigenics is ISO 9002 registered, EN46002 and EN552, with each of its certified facilities individually audited. Two facilities (Charlotte, NC and Corona, CA) offer ExCell services, the only company in the world able to deliver precise dose tolerences required by ANSI/AAMI/ISO 11137. Such precision is critical when a product's treatment specifications include a tight minimum and maximum dose range (i.e. 20-30 kGY).

STERILIZER, SOFT LENS, THERMAL, AC-POWERED *(Ophthalmology) 86HRD*

Atrion Medical Products, Inc. 800-343-9334
1426 Curt Francis Rd NW, Arab, AL 35016

Bausch & Lomb, Vision Care 800-553-5340
1400 Goodman St N, Rochester, NY 14609

STERILIZER, STEAM (AUTOCLAVE) *(General) 80FLE*

A-Dec, Inc. 800-547-1883
2601 Crestview Dr, Newberg, OR 97132
Autoclave or sterilizer.

Accutome, Inc. 610-889-0200
3222 Phoenixville Pike, Malvern, PA 19355
Stanley steam cleaning machine.

American Autoclave Co. 800 421 5161
7819 Riverside Rd E, Sumner, WA 98390

American Bio-Medical Service Corporation (Abmsc) 800-755-9055
631 W Covina Blvd, Sales,Service and Refurbishing Center
San Dimas, CA 91773

American Biomed Instruments, Inc. 718-235-8900
11 Wyona St, Brooklyn, NY 11207

Ars Enterprises 800-735-9277
12900 Lakeland Rd, Santa Fe Springs, CA 90670
General purpose (gravity) or pre-vacuum.

Barnstead International 412-490-8425
2555 Kerper Blvd, Dubuque, IA 52001
Steam sterilizer.

Better Containers Mfg. Co., Inc. 800-831-6049
530 Hyde Park Ave, Hillside, IL 60162
Metal autoclavable bags.

Brinkmann Instruments (Canada) Ltd. 800-263-8715
6670 Campobello Rd., Mississauga, ONT L5N 2L8 Canada
Four models

Buxton Medical Equipment Corp. 631-957-4500
1178 Route 109, Lindenhurst, NY 11757
All sizes available.

Cantylight 716-625-4227
6100 Donner Rd, Lockport, NY 14094

STERILIZER, STEAM (AUTOCLAVE) *(cont'd)*

Cd Nelson Manufacturing Co. 847-487-4870
26920 N Grace St, Wauconda, IL 60084
STEAMSHINE Steam-cleaning equipment JEWELSHINE Ultrasonics.

Chambermaid Products , Inc. 800-549-5356
12050 Suellen Cir, Wellington, FL 33414
Asepti-Clave. Fast with no electronics to fail. All cycle water is vented from unit after each operation. Eliminates the nasty job of cleaning the bio-mass from unit. Instruments are dry after sterilization cycle.

Consolidated Machine Corp. 617-782-6072
76 Ashford St, Boston, MA 02134
Sterilizer, autoclave.

Consolidated Stills & Sterilizers 617-782-6072
76 Ashford St, Boston, MA 02134
$6,000 to $56,000 per unit.

Crosstex International,Inc. 888-276-7783
10 Ranick Rd, Hauppauge, NY 11788
CROSSTEX.

Easter Services, Inc. 309-754-8303
3031 N Shore Dr, Moline, IL 61265
Steam sterilizers.

Elatec Technology Division 978-374-4040
252 Primrose St # 260, Haverhill, MA 01830
ETC manufactures vacuum equipment custom designed to specification.

Fluitron, Inc. 215-355-9970
30 Industrial Dr, Ivyland, PA 18974

Future Health Concept's, Inc. 407-322-3672
1211 E 30th St, Sanford, FL 32773
Sterilizer, steam.

Getinge Usa, Inc. 800-475-9040
1777 E Henrietta Rd, Rochester, NY 14623
GETINGE Steam Sterilizers provide superior sterility assurance, cycle flexibility, real-time information access and advanced operator control.

H&W Technology, Llc. 585-218-0385
PO Box 20281, Rochester, NY 14602
The state of the art in resistometers, the ILS-20, meets all requriements of ISO 11138 and 11140, and AAMI ST44-2002. It is also the basis for H & W's SteriMagic industrial steam controls, which use Allen-Bradley PLC's and a Windows user interface. SteriMagic is available to control new sterilizers or as a replacement for legacy controls.

Innovative Health Care Products, Inc. 678-320-0009
6850 Peachtree Dunwoody Rd NE Apt 402, Atlanta, GA 30328
Statim sterilizer. Fast,gentile with closed transport system.

Intersciences Inc. 800-661-6431
169 Idema Rd., Markham, ONT L3R 1A9 Canada

Kadan Co. Inc., D.A. 800-325-2326
1 Brigadoon Ln, Waxhaw, NC 28173

Kavo Dental Corp. 800-323-8029
340 East Route 22, Lake Zurich, IL 60047

Mcgill Airpressure Corp. 614-829-1200
1777 Refugee Rd, Columbus, OH 43207

Md International, Inc. 305-669-9003
11300 NW 41st St, Doral, FL 33178

Medical Sales & Service Group 888-357-6520
10 Woodchester Dr, Acton, MA 01720

Medicos Laboratories, Inc. (Mdt) 800-724-4003
801 Montrose Ave, South Plainfield, NJ 07080

Mg Scientific, Inc. 800-343-8338
8500 107th St, Pleasant Prairie, WI 53158

Midmark Corporation 800-643-6275
60 Vista Dr, P.O. Box 286, Versailles, OH 45380

Pelton & Crane 704-588-2126
11727 Fruehauf Dr, Charlotte, NC 28273
Sterilizer.

Pelton & Crane Co., 704-588-2126
11727 Fruehauf Dr, Charlotte, NC 28273
DELTA & MAGNA CLAVE

Primus Sterilizer Company, Llc. 620-793-7900
5520 10th St, Great Bend, KS 67530
Steam sterilizer.

STERILIZER, STEAM (AUTOCLAVE) *(cont'd)*

San-I-Pak,Pacific Inc. 800-875-7264
23535 S Bird Rd, Tracy, CA 95304
AUTO-CLAVE SAN-I-PAK, sterilizer and compactor system for biohazardous and non-hazardous hospital waste treatment and disposal. It is designed for small and large waste volume generators, will process 1000 lbs per hour (no AUTOCLAVE bags are required). Polypropylene bags used in infectious waste or instrument and steam sterlizers along with cart systems.

Schueler & Company, Inc. 516-487-1500
PO Box 528, Stratford, CT 06615

Scican 800-667-7733
1440 Don Mills Rd., Toronto, ON M3B 3P9 Canada
The Quantim 16 Autoclave--a gravity steam unit designed to process medical and dental instruments to achieve successful sterilization.

Scican Inc. 800-572-1211
701 Technology Dr, Canonsburg, PA 15317
STATIM 5000 - This steam cassette autoclave has an incredibly fast cycle time of 9 minutes. It is extremely gentle on instruments since it expels 98% of the air which causes oxidation in conventional autoclaves.

Sparco, Inc. 800-783-8309
2605 Oceanside Blvd Ste F, Oceanside, CA 92054
FLASH-GUARD - Flash Sterilization and Transport Container System - Designed for fast, safe, and reliable flash and transport of instruments from the autoclave/sterilizer to the point of use. - The only flash container to meet both 3- and 10-minute flash sterilization requirements. - Works in both gravity and pre-vac autoclaves. - Patented product is easy to use; offered since 1984; requires no valves or filters; low maintenance; no moving parts during sterilization.

Spectron Corp. 425-827-9317
934 S Burlington Blvd # 603, Burlington, WA 98233
Reconditioned equipment.

Spectrum Laboratories, Inc. 800-634-3300
18617 S Broadwick St, Rancho Dominguez, CA 90220
Systems for operating tangential flow membrane modules. Autoclavable and steam-sterilizable systems for tangential flow separations.

Standard Instrumentation, Div. Preiser Scientific 800-624-8285
94 Oliver St, Saint Albans, WV 25177

Sterile Resources, Inc. 800-317-6472
8117 Virginia Pine Ct, Richmond, VA 23237
Steam sterilizer.

Steris Corporation 814-452-3100
2424 W 23rd St, Erie, PA 16506
Various models of steam sterilizers.

Thermo Fisher Scientific Inc. 563-556-2241
2555 Kerper Blvd, Dubuque, IA 52001
HARVEY steam sterilizer, Model MC10.

Tuttnauer Usa Co. Ltd. 800-624-5836
25 Power Dr, Hauppauge, NY 11788
Horizontal autoclaves - custom made. Gravity, lab. All autoclaves have microprocessor controls. A.S.M.E. standard, UL. Gravity and pre-vacuum type standard equipment in hospital center supply, laboratory, research. biotechnology, and pharmaceutical industries, (various sizes).

Ubs Instruments Corporation 818-710-1195
7745 Alabama Ave Ste 7, Canoga Park, CA 91304
Tabletop steam sterilizer autoclaves with various chamber-size models.

Utech Products, Inc. 800-828-8324
135 Broadway, Schenectady, NY 12305

Ward's Natural Science Establishment, Inc. 800-962-2660
PO Box 92912, 5100 W. Henrietta Rd., Rochester, NY 14692

Wisconsin Aluminum Foundry Co., Inc. 920-682-8627
838 S 16th St, Manitowoc, WI 54220
ALL-AMERICAN Portable Pressure Steam Sterilizers; Model 1915X, 15 1/2qt. liquid capacity; Model 1925X, 25qt. liquid capacity; Model 1941X, 41 1/2qt. liquid capacity. ALL-AMERICAN Electric Pressure Steam Sterilizers; Model 25X- 120V; and Model 25X-240V, 25qt. liquid capacity. Model 50X-120 Volt and 50X-240 Volt Electric Pressure Steam Sterilizer, 25qt. liquid capacity, Model 75X-120V and 75X-240 Electric Pressure Steam Sterilizer, 41.5 qt. liquid capacity.

STERILIZER, STEAM (AUTOCLAVE) *(cont'd)*

World Medical Equipment, Inc. 800-827-3747
3915 152nd St NE, Marysville, WA 98271
Specialize in refurbished autoclaves such as AMSCO/Steris, and Castle/Getinge as well as OR tables, lights, anesthesia machines, monitors, and accessories.

STERILIZER, STEAM (AUTOCLAVE), DENTAL
(Dental And Oral) 76ECH

Alfa Medical Equipment 800-801-9934
59 Madison Ave, Hempstead, NY 11550

Dencraft 800-328-9729
PO Box 57, Moorestown, NJ 08057

Midmark Corporation 800-643-6275
60 Vista Dr, P.O. Box 286, Versailles, OH 45380

STERILIZER, STEAM (AUTOCLAVE), SURGICAL
(Surgery) 79FSI

American Autoclave Co. 800 421 5161
7819 Riverside Rd E, Sumner, WA 98390

Buxton Medical Equipment Corp. 631-957-4500
1178 Route 109, Lindenhurst, NY 11757
All sizes available.

Kadan Co. Inc., D.A. 800-325-2326
1 Brigadoon Ln, Waxhaw, NC 28173

Medical Technologies Co. 800-280-3220
1728 W Park Center Dr Ste A, Fenton, MO 63026

Pelton & Crane Co., 704-588-2126
11727 Fruehauf Dr, Charlotte, NC 28273
DELTA & MAGNA CLAVE

Whittemore Enterprises, Inc. 800-999-2452
11149 Arrow Rte, Rancho Cucamonga, CA 91730

STERILIZER, STEAM, BULK *(General) 80UCS*

Belimed 800-457-4117
13840 SW 119th Ave, Miami, FL 33186
All stainless steel, pure steam ready, sliding doors, computer interface availability, touch screen controls, no service room required and a wide range of available sizes.

Buxton Medical Equipment Corp. 631-957-4500
1178 Route 109, Lindenhurst, NY 11757
All sizes available.

Consolidated Stills & Sterilizers 617-782-6072
76 Ashford St, Boston, MA 02134
Models SR 24C, D & E with solid-state digital automatic controls or microcomputer controls with alphanumeric printer. Air removal by gravity only or vacuum/gravity combination. Circle chart recorder on digital and alpha numeric printer on micro.

Getinge Usa, Inc. 800-475-9040
1777 E Henrietta Rd, Rochester, NY 14623
GETINGE

STERILIZER, STEAM, TABLE TOP *(General) 80UCT*

Electro-Steam Generator Corp. 888-783-2624
1000 Bernard St, Alexandria, VA 22314
Steam generator.

Independent Solutions, Inc. 847-498-0500
900 Skokie Blvd Ste 118, Northbrook, IL 60062

Innovative Health Care Products, Inc. 678-320-0009
6850 Peachtree Dunwoody Rd NE Apt 402, Atlanta, GA 30328
Statim sterilizer. Fast, gentle with closed transport system.

Midmark Corporation 800-643-6275
60 Vista Dr, P.O. Box 286, Versailles, OH 45380

Scican 800-667-7733
1440 Don Mills Rd., Toronto, ON M3B 3P9 Canada
The StatIM Cassette Autoclave is a unique table-top steam sterilizer designed for the efficient, economical, and rapid steam sterilization of medical and dental devices in clinical settings.

Tuttnauer Usa Co. Ltd. 800-624-5836
25 Power Dr, Hauppauge, NY 11788
Table-top TUTTNAUER manual autoclave models available: 2340M(9' x 18'), 2540M(10' x 18'), Valueklave1730(7' x 13') & 3870M(15' x 30'). Manual KWIKLAVE: model 2540MK (220v). Fully Automatic Electronic models with air pump for closed door drying: EZ9(9' x 18'), EZ10(10' x 18') & 3870EA(15' x 30'). Fully Automatic KWIKLAVE: model EZ10k(220v).

Zoetek Medical Sales & Service, Inc. 800-388-6223
668 Phillips Rd, Victor, NY 14564
All Brand Name Manufacturer's, Midmark, Tuttnauer & Pelton Crane

STERILIZER, TONOMETER *(Ophthalmology) 86HKZ*

Eyetech Ltd. 847-470-1777
9408 Normandy Ave, Morton Grove, IL 60053
Sterilizer/cleaning container for Goldman Tonometer Prism

Gulden Ophthalmics 800-659-2250
225 Cadwalader Ave, Elkins Park, PA 19027

Numa Corp. 800-327-2212
2290 N CR 427 Ste 136, Longwood, FL 32750
Sterilization monitors.

STERILIZER, ULTRAVIOLET *(General) 80RVY*

Atlantic Ultraviolet Corp. 631-273-0500
375 Marcus Blvd, Hauppauge, NY 11788
MIGHTY-PURE.

Bhk, Inc. 909-983-2973
1480 N Claremont Blvd, Claremont, CA 91711

Fuller Ultraviolet Corp. 815-469-3301
9416 Gulfstream Rd, Frankfort, IL 60423
$400.00 per unit (standard).

Hanovia Specialty Lighting Llc 800-229-3666
825 Lehigh Ave, Union, NJ 07083
STERITRON $650.00 per unit (standard).

Uvp, Llc 800-452-6788
2066 W 11th St, Upland, CA 91786
Lamps, cabinets and crosslinkers emitting 254 mm shortwave UV.

Waldmann Lighting 800-634-0007
9 Century Dr, Wheeling, IL 60090

STERILIZER, VAPOR *(General) 80RVZ*

Advanced Sterilization Products 800-595-0200
33 Technology Dr, Irvine, CA 92618
STERRAD System uses peroxide gas plasma technology to sterilize metal, non-metal, and heat- and moisture-sensitive instruments without any toxic residues. The entire process takes about an hour. STERRAD 50 sterilization system uses hydrogen peroxide, gas plasma with a rapid dry, low temperature cycle, which safely sterilizes metal and nonmetal instruments; process takes about 45 minutes.

American Autoclave Co. 800 421 5161
7819 Riverside Rd E, Sumner, WA 98390

Consolidated Stills & Sterilizers 617-782-6072
76 Ashford St, Boston, MA 02134
$6,000 to $30,000 per unit (standard).

Environmental Tectonics Corp. 215-355-9100
125 James Way, Southampton, PA 18966

Thermo Fisher Scientific Inc. 563-556-2241
2555 Kerper Blvd, Dubuque, IA 52001
CHEMICLAVE vapor sterilizer.

STERILIZER/COMPACTOR *(General) 80WWY*

American Autoclave Co. 800 421 5161
7819 Riverside Rd E, Sumner, WA 98390

Hanovia Specialty Lighting Llc 800-229-3666
825 Lehigh Ave, Union, NJ 07083
LETHARY Mobile room sterilizer - sterilizes in 15 minutes or less. Air duct sterilizer provides sterile air from HVAC.

San-I-Pak,Pacific Inc. 800-875-7264
23535 S Bird Rd, Tracy, CA 95304
AUTO-CLAVE SAN-I-PAK, sterilizer and compactor system for biohazardous and non-hazardous hospital waste treatment and disposal. It is designed for small and large waste volume generators, will process 1000 lbs per hour (no AUTOCLAVE bags are required). Polypropylene bags used in infectious waste or instrument and steam sterlizers along with cart systems.

Tuttnauer Usa Co. Ltd. 800-624-5836
25 Power Dr, Hauppauge, NY 11788
TUTTNAUER medical waste sterilizer, specialized high vacuum autoclaves just for the treatment of regulated medical waste, (various sizes).

Zirc Company 800-328-3899
3918 State Highway 55 SE, Buffalo, MN 55313
Accessories: cassettes, bur-blocks, instrument mats.

STERILIZER/WASHER, ENDOSCOPE *(General) 80THI*

Custom Ultrasonics, Inc. 215-364-1477
144 Railroad Dr, Hartsville, PA 18974
System 83 automated systems for processing endoscopic instruments and accessories; Pre-processing sink designed for endoscopic instruments and accessories.

STERILIZER/WASHER, ENDOSCOPE *(cont'd)*

Deknatel Snowden-Pencer 800-367-7874
5175 S Royal Atlanta Dr, Tucker, GA 30084
ENDO-CLEAN portable unit plugs into standard electrical outlets. Microprocessor controlled to deliver metered amounts of cleaning solution and lubricant to the instruments.

Encompas Unlimited, Inc. 800-825-7701
PO Box 516, Tallevast, FL 34270
$138.50 for #SS-40 soaking system for all endoscopes. $99.00 for safe soak pan for all flexible submersible scopes.

STEROTAXIC UNIT *(Cns/Neurology) 84RVR*

Integra Radionics 800-466-6814
22 Terry Ave, Burlington, MA 01803

STETHOSCOPE, AMPLIFIED *(General) 80VKO*

Armstrong Medical Industries, Inc. 800-323-4220
575 Knightsbridge Pkwy, Lincolnshire, IL 60069

Dixie Ems Supply 800-347-3494
385 Union Ave, Brooklyn, NY 11211
POT BELLY.

Lydia's Professional Uniforms 800-942-3378
2547 3 Mile Rd NW Ste F, Grand Rapids, MI 49534

Md International, Inc. 305-669-9003
11300 NW 41st St, Doral, FL 33178

Ultrascope 800-677-2673
2401 Distribution St, Charlotte, NC 28203
All models w/o batteries or moving parts, and filter external noises while amplifying heart/lung sounds. $89.95 for ULTRA SCOPE for hearing impaired: 30% thicker PVC tubing than MAXI-SCOPE, internal spring, clear head; has no batteries or moving parts. ULTRA-T teaching scope $99.95. ULTRA-TOT is pediate model $89.95 and neonatal scope is ULTRA-MINI at $89.95. ULTRA-CLASSIC for severe hearing impaired at $99.95.

Welch Allyn, Inc. 800-535-6663
4341 State Street Rd, Skaneateles Falls, NY 13153

STETHOSCOPE, DIRECT (ACOUSTIC), ULTRASONIC *(Surgery) 79FXD*

Doctors Research Group, Inc. 800-371-2535
574 Heritage Rd Ste 202, Southbury, CT 06488
Cardiology scopes

Md International, Inc. 305-669-9003
11300 NW 41st St, Doral, FL 33178

STETHOSCOPE, ELECTRONIC (AUSCULTOSCOPE) *(Cardiovascular) 74DQD*

A&D Medical 800-726-7099
1756 Automation Pkwy, San Jose, CA 95131
Single head, dual head, Sprague Rappaport type in a variety of colors.

American Telecare, Inc. 800-323-6667
15159 Technology Dr, Eden Prairie, MN 55344

Argon Medical Devices Inc. 903-675-9321
1445 Flat Creek Rd, Athens, TX 75751
Cvp catheterization kit/tray.

Bio-Research Associates, Inc. 414-357-7525
9275 N 49th St Ste 150, Brown Deer, WI 53223
Joint vibration recorder for joint sounds.

Biomet Microfixation Inc. 800-874-7711
1520 Tradeport Dr, Jacksonville, FL 32218
Electronic stethoscope.

Cardinal Healthcare 209, Inc. 610-862-0800
5225 Verona Rd, Fitchburg, WI 53711
Stethoscope.

Edmund Industrial Optics 800-363-1992
101 E Gloucester Pike, Barrington, NJ 08007

Hal-Hen Company, Inc. 800-242-5436
180 Atlantic Ave, Garden City Park, NY 11040
$350.00 per unit for medical doctors and nurses.

Heartsounds Corp. 416-383-1520
314-801 York Mills Rd, Don Mills M3B 1X7 Canada
Analyst digital stethoscope

Her-Mar, Inc. 800-327-8209
8550 NW 30th Ter, Doral, FL 33122
$225.00 per unit (standard).

Inovise Medical, Inc. 503-431-3800
10565 SW Nimbus Ave Ste 100, Portland, OR 97223
Ecg sensor w/ heartsound microphone.

STETHOSCOPE, ELECTRONIC (AUSCULTOSCOPE) *(cont'd)*

Lumiscope Company, Inc. 800-672-8293
1035 Centennial Ave, Piscataway, NJ 08854

Medtronic Blood Management 612-514-4000
18501 E Plaza Dr, Parker, CO 80134
Stethoscope amplifier.

Rnk Products, Inc. 612-414-0289
12700 Diamond Dr, Burnsville, MN 55337
Electronic stethoscope.

Tuzik Boston 800-886-6363
104 Longwater Dr, Assinippi Park, Norwell, MA 02061

Zargis Medical Corp. 609-488-4608
1 Atlantic St, 1st Floo, Stamford, CT 06901
Various models of electronic stethoscopes.

3m Co. 888-364-3577
3M Center, Saint Paul, MN 55144
3M Littmann Stethoscope

STETHOSCOPE, ELECTRONIC-AMPLIFIED *(Surgery) 79FXC*

Novamed, Llc 800-425-3535
4 Westchester Plz, Elmsford, NY 10523
LifeSound Telemetric Heart and Breath Sound System enhances monitoring by improving sound clarity and fidelty while simplifying continuous monitoring of patients. Its telemetric capabilty provides unrestricted mobility -- LifeSound is connected to the patient via microphonic sensors that couple directly to the patient or to any standard precordial chest piece or esophageal stethoscope. Highly regarded for clinical applications including pediatric monitoring, in teaching institutions, by oral/maxillo and plastic surgeons.

Starkey Laboratories, Inc. 800-328-8602
6700 Washington Ave S, Eden Prairie, MN 55344
$289.50 for unit with volume & tone control switches.

STETHOSCOPE, ESOPHAGEAL *(Anesthesiology) 73BZW*

Covidien Lp 508-261-8000
15 Hampshire St, Mansfield, MA 02048

Ge Industrial, Sensing 800-833-9438
1100 Technology Park Dr, Billerica, MA 01821

Kentron Health Care, Inc. 615-384-0573
3604 Kelton Jackson Rd, P.o. Box 120, Springfield, TN 37172
Disposable esophageal stethoscope.

Novamed, Llc 800-425-3535
4 Westchester Plz, Elmsford, NY 10523
To monitor heart /breath sounds and temperature with 400 and 700 Series Thermistor. Available sizes 9FR, 12FR, 18FR and 24FR. Packaged in boxes of 40 pcs/ cases of 160.

Sun-Med 800-433-2797
12393 Belcher Rd S Ste 450, Largo, FL 33773

STETHOSCOPE, ESOPHAGEAL, WITH ELECTRICAL CONDUCTORS *(Anesthesiology) 73BZT*

Cardio Command, Inc. 800-231-6370
4920 W Cypress St Ste 110, Tampa, FL 33607
TAPSCOPE stethoscope. Transesophageal atrial pacing (TAP), P-wave amplification and temperature monitoring with an esophageal stethoscope.

Mmj S.A. De C.V. 314-654-2000
716 Ponciano Arriaga, Cd. Juarez, Chih. Mexico
Mon-a-therm esophageal stethoscope with temperature sensor

Sharn, Inc. 800-325-3671
4517 George Rd Ste 200, Tampa, FL 33634

Shore Medical, Inc. 714-628-9785
1050 N Batavia St Ste C, Orange, CA 92867
Various.

STETHOSCOPE, FETAL *(Obstetrics/Gyn) 85HGN*

Allen Medical Instruments Corp. 949-646-3215
177 Riverside Ave Ste F602, Newport Beach, CA 92663
$101.00 for Series #10 fetal stethoscope.

Md International, Inc. 305-669-9003
11300 NW 41st St, Doral, FL 33178

Tuzik Boston 800-886-6363
104 Longwater Dr, Assinippi Park, Norwell, MA 02061

STETHOSCOPE, MANUAL *(Cardiovascular) 74LDE*

A&D Medical 800-726-7099
1756 Automation Pkwy, San Jose, CA 95131
Stethoscope

A.M.G. Medical, Inc. 888-396-1213
8505 Dalton Rd., Montreal, QUE H4T-IV5 Canada

STETHOSCOPE, MANUAL *(cont'd)*

American Diagnostic Corporation (Adc) 800-232-2670
55 Commerce Dr, Hauppauge, NY 11788
Institutional and professional stethoscopes and accessories.

Bhs International, Inc. 410-721-5055
2431 Crofton Ln Ste 9, Crofton, MD 21114

Carolina Biological Supply Co. 800-334-5551
2700 York Rd, Burlington, NC 27215

Centurion Medical Products Corp. 517-545-1135
3310 S Main St, Salisbury, NC 28147

Creative Health Products, Inc. 800-742-4478
5148 Saddle Ridge Rd, Plymouth, MI 48170
Large selection of major brand name stethoscopes from AMERICAN DIAGNOSTIC, PHILIPS MEDICAL, LITMANN, MABIS, TYCOS at CHP discounted prices.

Cypress Medical Products 800-334-3646
1202 S. Rte. 31, McHenry, IL 60050
Single head, dual head and Sprague Rappaport types. Tubing length 22'. Available in a variety of colors.

Demetech Corp. 888-324-2447
3530 NW 115th Ave, Doral, FL 33178
Stethoscope.

Global Healthcare 800-601-3880
1495 Hembree Rd Ste 700, Roswell, GA 30076

Healer Products, Llc 914-663-6300
427 Commerce Ln Ste 1, West Berlin, NJ 08091
Stethoscope, manual.

Jayza Corp. 305-477-1136
7215 NW 41st St Ste A, Miami, FL 33166

Kck Industries 888-800-1967
14941 Calvert St, Van Nuys, CA 91411

Kentron Health Care, Inc. 615-384-0573
3604 Kelton Jackson Rd, P.o. Box 120, Springfield, TN 37172
Stethoscopes.

Kerma Medical Products, Inc. 757-398-8400
400 Port Centre Pkwy, Portsmouth, VA 23704
Stethoscope.

Lydia's Professional Uniforms 800-942-3378
2547 3 Mile Rd NW Ste F, Grand Rapids, MI 49534

Max Bloom, M.D. 401-785-9671
111 Roger Williams Cir, Cranston, RI 02905
The Bloom Stethoscope.

Md International, Inc. 305-669-9003
11300 NW 41st St, Doral, FL 33178

North Safety Products 401-943-4400
1101 B Calle Neutron, Parque Industrial Maran, Mexicali, B.c. Mexico
Stethoscope

Pedia Pals, Llc 888-733-4272
965 Highway 169 N, Plymouth, MN 55441
Stethoscope cover accessories in smiling animal shapes, dino's, dalmatians, lions and tigers.

ReNu Medical Inc. 877-252-1110
9800 Evergreen Way, Everett, WA 98204
MULTIPLE MODELS; REPROCESSED STETHOSCOPE MANUAL

Schueler & Company, Inc. 516-487-1500
PO Box 528, Stratford, CT 06615

Stethocap, Inc. 866-691-4181
3401 Wellington Ct Unit 115, Rolling Mdws, IL 60008

Tri-State Hospital Supply Corp. 517-545-1135
3173 E 43rd St, Yuma, AZ 85365

Ultrascope 800-677-2673
2401 Distribution St, Charlotte, NC 28203
$39.95 for MAXI-SCOPE. All models w/o batteries or moving parts, and filter external noises while amplifying heart/lung sounds. $89.95 for ULTRA SCOPE for hearing impaired: 30% thicker PVC tubing than MAXI-SCOPE, internal spring, clear head; has no batteries or moving parts.

Welch Allyn, Inc. 800-535-6663
4341 State Street Rd, Skaneateles Falls, NY 13153

3m Company 651-733-4365
601 22nd Ave S, Brookings, SD 57006

STETHOSCOPE, MECHANICAL *(General) 80FLT*

Allen Medical Instruments Corp. 949-646-3215
177 Riverside Ave Ste F602, Newport Beach, CA 92663
Manual equipment. $180.00 - $190.00 for Gemini twin channel cardiology model. $155.00 for Solitaire, twin channel, no-bell Gemini series. $165.00 for Series 12, single, $185.00 for Series 5A, $101.00 for series 10 fetal. GEMINI-P twin channel pediatric stethoscope. GEMINI-L twin channel lightweight. $120.00 for new mark 10 cardiology rotary switch model.

Armstrong Medical Industries, Inc. 800-323-4220
575 Knightsbridge Pkwy, Lincolnshire, IL 60069

Crest Healthcare Supply 800-328-8908
195 3rd St, Dassel, MN 55325

Dixie Ems Supply 800-347-3494
385 Union Ave, Brooklyn, NY 11211
$80.00 per 10 (standard).

Her-Mar, Inc. 800-327-8209
8550 NW 30th Ter, Doral, FL 33122
$9.00 for std unit.

Lumiscope Company, Inc. 800-672-8293
1035 Centennial Ave, Piscataway, NJ 08854
Dual, nurse, neonatal, pediatric, adult.

Md International, Inc. 305-669-9003
11300 NW 41st St, Doral, FL 33178

Medworks Instruments 800-323-9790
PO Box 581, Chatham, IL 62629
$28.00 Definer stainless steel adult dual, $6.50 Wing Ace lightweight adult dual.

Miltex Inc. 800-645-8000
589 Davies Dr, York, PA 17402

Pocket Nurse Enterprises, Inc. 800-225-1600
200 1st St, Ambridge, PA 15003

Prestige Medical Corporation 800-762-3333
8600 Wilbur Ave, Northridge, CA 91324

Sun-Med 800-433-2797
12393 Belcher Rd S Ste 450, Largo, FL 33773
SOFTEAR Disposable Monascope uses transmission of sound through a system dependent on a complete seal in the system. Earpiece utilizes a foam ear piece that contours into the ear canal allowing for enhanced sound transmission.

Trimline Medical Products Corp. 800-526-3538
34 Columbia Rd, Branchburg, NJ 08876
Full line of cardiology, traditional and disposable stethoscopes

Ultrascope 800-677-2673
2401 Distribution St, Charlotte, NC 28203
$39.95 for MAXI-SCOPE. All models w/o batteries or moving parts, and filter external noises while amplifying heart/lung sounds. $89.95 for ULTRA SCOPE for hearing impaired: 30% thicker PVC tubing than MAXI-SCOPE, internal spring, clear head; has no batteries or moving parts.

Welch Allyn, Inc. 800-535-6663
4341 State Street Rd, Skaneateles Falls, NY 13153

STICK, URINALYSIS TEST *(Chemistry) 75UKD*

Bio-Rad Laboratories, Life Science Group 800-424-6723
2000 Alfred Nobel Dr, Hercules, CA 94547

Chagrin Safety Supply, Inc. 800-227-0468
8227 Washington St # 1, Chagrin Falls, OH 44023

Covidien Lp 508-261-8000
15 Hampshire St, Mansfield, MA 02048

STILL, SOLVENT RECOVERY *(Chemistry) 75UIA*

B/R Instrument Corp. 800-922-9206
9119 Centreville Rd, Easton, MD 21601
Models 9300 & 9400, PROCYCLER, high purity solvent recycling systems; automatic recycling of organic solvents like xylene, xylene substitutes and alcohol for reuse in histology and cytology laboratories.

Brinkmann Instruments (Canada) Ltd. 800-263-8715
6670 Campobello Rd., Mississauga, ONT L5N 2L8 Canada

Kimble Glass, Inc. 888-546-2531
537 Crystal Ave, Vineland, NJ 08360
KONTES.

Kontes Glass Co. 888-546-2531
1022 Spruce St, Vineland, NJ 08360

STILL, WATER *(Chemistry) 75UIN*

Colonial Scientific Ltd. 902-468-1811
201 Brownlow Ave., Unit 52, Dartmouth, NS B3B-1W2 Canada
Stills.

Kontes Glass Co. 888-546-2531
1022 Spruce St, Vineland, NJ 08360

Thermo Fisher Scientific Inc. 563-556-2241
2555 Kerper Blvd, Dubuque, IA 52001

STIMULATOR, ACUPUNCTURE *(Anesthesiology) 73UKR*

Biomedical Life Systems, Inc. 800-726-8367
2448 Cades Way, Vista, CA 92081

STIMULATOR, ARTHRITIS, NON-INVASIVE *(Physical Med) 89MKC*

Cbs Medical Technologies Inc. 514-582-9098
225 Chemin des Grands Ducs, Piedmont, QUE J0R 1K0 Canada

STIMULATOR, AUDIO *(Cns/Neurology) 84RWB*

Crist Instrument Co., Inc. 301-393-8615
111 W 1st St, Hagerstown, MD 21740
Provides audio signals that originate equidistant from the center of a subject's head. 360-degree rotation.

STIMULATOR, AUDITORY, EVOKED RESPONSE *(Cns/Neurology) 84GWJ*

Cadwell Laboratories 800-245-3001
909 N Kellogg St, Kennewick, WA 99336
Optional headphones available with SIERRA II.

Cardinal Healthcare 209, Inc. 610-862-0800
5225 Verona Rd, Fitchburg, WI 53711
Auditory evoked response system.

Gn Otometrics North America 800-289-2150
125 Commerce Dr, Schaumburg, IL 60173
Evoked response auditory stimulator.

Grass Technologies, An Astro-Med, Inc. Product Gro 401-828-4002
53 Airport Park Drive, Rockland, MA 02370
Auditory evoked response stimulator.

Sonamed Corp. 781-889-6499
1250 Main St, Waltham, MA 02451
Clarity system.

STIMULATOR, CALORIC AIR *(Ear/Nose/Throat) 77KHH*

Gn Otometrics North America 800-289-2150
125 Commerce Dr, Schaumburg, IL 60173
Air caloric stimulator.

Jedmed Instruments Co. 314-845-3770
5416 Jedmed Ct, Saint Louis, MO 63129

Tsi Medical Ltd. 800-661-7263
47 Athabascan Ave., Unit 105, Sherwood Park, AB T8A-4H3 Canada

STIMULATOR, CALORIC WATER *(Ear/Nose/Throat) 77ETP*

Gn Otometrics North America 800-289-2150
125 Commerce Dr, Schaumburg, IL 60173
Water caloric stimulator.

Jedmed Instruments Co. 314-845-3770
5416 Jedmed Ct, Saint Louis, MO 63129

Tsi Medical Ltd. 800-661-7263
47 Athabascan Ave., Unit 105, Sherwood Park, AB T8A-4H3 Canada

STIMULATOR, CEREBELLAR, FULL IMPLANT (PAIN RELIEF) *(Cns/Neurology) 84LGW*

Boston Scientific Neuromodulation Corporation 508-652-5578
25155 Rye Canyon Loop, Valencia, CA 91355
Spinal cord stimulator.

Medtronic Puerto Rico Operations Co., Juncos 763-514-4000
Road 31, Km. 24, Hm 4, Ceiba Norte Industrial Park, Juncos, PR 00777
Various types of sterile and non-sterile spinal cord stimulation systems.

Medtronic Puerto Rico Operations Co., Villalba 763-514-4000
PO Box 6001, Rd. 149, Km. 56.3, Villalba, PR 00766
Various types of sterile and non-sterile spinal cord stimulation systems.

STIMULATOR, CEREBRAL, IMPLANTABLE *(Cns/Neurology) 84GZA*

Avery Biomedical Devices, Inc. 631-864-1600
61 Mall Dr, Commack, NY 11725
Cerebellar stimulator.

STIMULATOR, COLLECTION, SPERM, ELECTRICAL *(Gastro/Urology) 78LNL*

G & S Instrument Co. 972-723-0856
6851 Montgomery Rd, Midlothian, TX 76065
Electroejaculator system.

Irvine Scientific 800-437-5706
2511 Daimler St, Santa Ana, CA 92705
Model IS-300 centrifuge is designed for sperm processing and is preset to operate at 300 x g, which eliminates overheating and overcompensation of the sperm; up to six 15-ml tubes can be accommodated at one time. ISOLATE Sperm Separation Medium is a new, superior medium for separation of the motile fraction of sperm from its surrounding seminal fluids by density centrifugation.

STIMULATOR, CRANIAL ELECTROTHERAPY *(Cns/Neurology) 84JXK*

Biomedical Life Systems, Inc. 800-726-8367
2448 Cades Way, Vista, CA 92081

Chattanooga Group 800-592-7329
4717 Adams Rd, Hixson, TN 37343
Non-cranial. INTELECT stimulators.

Electromedical Products International, Inc. 800-367-7246
2201 Garrett Morris Pkwy, Mineral Wells, TX 76067
$495.00 ALPHA-STIM SCS (Stress-Control System). For relief from anxiety, depression, insomnia, and stress-related disorders. Ideal for home use.

Neurotone Systems, Inc. 972-271-1978
510 Nesbit Dr, Garland, TX 75041
Ces.

STIMULATOR, CRANIAL ELECTROTHERAPY (SITUATIONAL ANXIETY) *(Cns/Neurology) 84GZG*

Electromedical Products International, Inc. 800-367-7246
2201 Garrett Morris Pkwy, Mineral Wells, TX 76067
$895.00 for ALPHA-STIM 100 combined cranial electrotherapy and microcurrent stimulator (for acute, chronic and postoperative pain plus anxiety, depression, and insomnia). For clinical and home use.

STIMULATOR, CRANIAL, MAGNETIC PULSE (FOR PSYCHOTHERAPY) *(Cns/Neurology) 84MRT*

Aldagen, Inc 919-484-2571
2810 Meridian Pkwy Ste 148, Durham, NC 27713
Stem/progenitor cell enumeration kit.

STIMULATOR, DIAPHRAGMATIC/PHRENIC NERVE, IMPLANTABLE *(Cns/Neurology) 84GZE*

Avery Biomedical Devices, Inc. 631-864-1600
61 Mall Dr, Commack, NY 11725
Breathing pacemaker system.

Synapse Biomedical Inc. 440-774-2488
300 Artino St, Oberlin, OH 44074
NeuRx Diaphragm Pacing System(TM); NeuRx DPS(TM

STIMULATOR, DORSAL COLUMN *(Cns/Neurology) 84RWD*

Ebi, Llc 800-526-2579
100 Interpace Pkwy, Parsippany, NJ 07054
Spinal fusion stimulator.

STIMULATOR, ELECTRICAL, EVOKED RESPONSE *(Cns/Neurology) 84GWF*

Ad-Tech Medical Instrument Corp. 800-776-1555
1901 William St, Racine, WI 53404
Spinal Electrode for motor evoked potential monitoring during spinal surgery.

Cadwell Laboratories 800-245-3001
909 N Kellogg St, Kennewick, WA 99336
Included with SIERRA II.

Cardinal Healthcare 209, Inc. 610-862-0800
5225 Verona Rd, Fitchburg, WI 53711
Electrical evoked response.

Cybex International, Inc. 800-667-6544
10 Trotter Dr, Medway, MA 02053
$3,795 for KINESTIM electrotherapy system.

Integra Radionics 800-466-6814
22 Terry Ave, Burlington, MA 01803

Medtronic Sofamor Danek Usa, Inc. 901-396-3133
4340 Swinnea Rd, Memphis, TN 38118
Monopolar stimulating instrumentation.

STIMULATOR, ELECTRICAL, EVOKED RESPONSE *(cont'd)*

Nuvasive, Inc. 800-475-9131
7475 Lusk Blvd, San Diego, CA 92121
Electromyography, emg monitor/stimulator and accessory electrodes.

STIMULATOR, ELECTRICAL, FOR INCONTINENCE
(Gastro/Urology) 78EZW

Athena Feminine Technologies, Inc 866-308-4436
179 Moraga Way, Orinda, CA 94563
The Athena Pelvic Muscle Trainer is a cordless product that is inserted like a tampon and is controlled by a remote control. The PMT automatically stimulates the pelvic floor muscles to do Kegel exercises. It has a 15-minute cycle and then shuts off automatically. The intensity of the contractions is easily controlled. Clinical studies prove that the Athena PMT is safe and effective. The Athena Pelvic Muscle Trainer is FDA approved and Medicare reimbursable. It will be available by prescription.

Dedicated Distribution 800-325-8367
640 Miami Ave, Kansas City, KS 66105
MINNOVA pelvic floor stimulator for incontinence.

Empi, Inc. 800-328-2536
599 Cardigan Rd, Saint Paul, MN 55126
INNOVA home therapy system for incontinence. Intervaginal electric stimulation strengthens lax pelvic floor muscles and controls uninhibited detrusor contractions.

Medtronic Puerto Rico Operations Co., Juncos 763-514-4000
Road 31, Km. 24, Hm 4, Ceiba Norte Industrial Park, Juncos, PR 00777
Sacral nerve stimulator for voiding dysfunction.

STIMULATOR, ELECTRICAL, IMPLANTED (PARKINSONIAN TREMOR) *(Cns/Neurology) 84MHY*

Medtronic Neuromodulation 612-514-4000
800 53rd Ave NE, Minneapolis, MN 55421
Deep brain stimulator for tremor suppression.

Medtronic Puerto Rico Operations Co., Villalba 763-514-4000
PO Box 6001, Rd. 149, Km. 56.3, Villalba, PR 00766
Deep brain stimulator for tremor supression.

Medtronic Puerto Rico Operations Co.,Med Rel 763-514-4000
Road 909, Km. 0.4., Barrio Mariana, Humacao, PR 00792
Deep brain stimulator for tremor supression.

Trivirix International Inc. 320-982-8000
925 6th Ave NE, Milaca, MN 56353
Deep brain stimulator for tremor suppression.

STIMULATOR, ELECTRICAL, MUSCLE *(Physical Med) 89MPH*

Athena Feminine Technologies, Inc 866-308-4436
179 Moraga Way, Orinda, CA 94563
The Athena Pelvic Muscle Trainer is a cordless product that is inserted like a tampon and is controlled by a remote control. The PMT automatically stimulates the pelvic floor muscles to do Kegel exercises. It has a 15-minute cycle and then shuts off automatically. The intensity of the contractions is easily controlled. Clinical studies prove that the Athena PMT is safe and effective. The Athena Pelvic Muscle Trainer is FDA approved and Medicare reimbursable. It will be available by prescription.

Erp Group Professional Products Ltd. 800-361-3537
3232 Autoroute Laval W., Laval, QC H7T 2H6 Canada
Dynatronics electrotherapy products.

Jace Systems 800-800-4276
2 Pin Oak Ln Ste 200, Cherry Hill, NJ 08003
The JACE Tri-Stim provides three modalities in a single portable device. HVPC- decreases skin resistance for deeper therapy penetration. A/C:ASYM- a balanced universal muscle stimulation waveform. A/C:SYMM- a balanced waveform to enhance patient comfort for the stimulation of larger muscle groups.

Mylon-Tech Health Technologies Inc. 613-728-1667
301 Moodie Dr., Ste. 205, Ottawa, ON K2H 9C4 Canada
Many EMS devices in all price ranges.

STIMULATOR, ELECTRO-ANALGESIC *(Cns/Neurology) 84UFF*

Activator Methods International, Ltd 800-598-0224
2950 N 7th St Ste 200, Phoenix, AZ 85014
Activator Adjusting Instrument, chiropractic.

STIMULATOR, ELECTRO-ANALGESIC *(cont'd)*

Biofreeze Performance Health, Inc. 800-246-3733
1245 Home Ave, Akron, OH 44310
BIOFREEZE 'Cold Therapy' topical analgesic pain-relieving gel, convenient roll-on and new no-touch natural spray. Cool, non-greasy, vanishing scent. Biofreeze contains ILEX, a natural herb extract, which helps provide a deeper, faster, longer lasting pain relief than most conventional cooling gels. Biofreeze is not sold in retail stores. Biofreeze is available in 16 oz spray bottle, 16 oz., 32 oz, and gallon gel pump bottles and Gravity Dispenser Box filled with 100 5-g single use application packets for clinical use. The 4-oz gel tubes, spray bottle and 3-oz. roll-ons are perfect for use at home.

Biomedical Life Systems, Inc. 800-726-8367
2448 Cades Way, Vista, CA 92081

Rs Medical 800-683-0353
14001 S.E. First St., Vancouver, WA 98684
Vertis Percutaneous Neuromodulation Therapy (PNT) minimally invasive electrical stimulator system. Indicated for symptomatic relief and management of chronic or intractable cervical or lumbar pain. Physician-prescribed, in-office treatment.

STIMULATOR, ELECTRO/ACUPUNCTURE
(Anesthesiology) 73BWK

Ack Laboratories, Inc. 908-707-9244
540 Stony Brook Dr, Bridgewater, NJ 08807
Acupuncture stimulator.

Biomedical Life Systems, Inc. 800-726-8367
2448 Cades Way, Vista, CA 92081

STIMULATOR, EXTERNAL, NEUROMUSCULAR, FUNCTIONAL
(Physical Med) 89IPP

Biomedical Life Systems, Inc. 800-726-8367
2448 Cades Way, Vista, CA 92081

Bloomex International, Inc. 201-703-9799
295 Molnar Dr, Elmwood Park, NJ 07407
Multiple outlets neuromuscular stimulators. Programmable electrotherapy for treatment of pathological conditions, rehabilitation, and sports medicine needs.

Elmed, Inc. 630-543-2792
60 W Fay Ave, Addison, IL 60101

Mylon-Tech Health Technologies Inc. 613-728-1667
301 Moodie Dr., Ste. 205, Ottawa, ON K2H 9C4 Canada
Many NMES units to choose from.

Tetra Medical Supply Corp. 800-621-4041
6364 W Gross Point Rd, Niles, IL 60714
Portable digital units in carrying case.

STIMULATOR, GROWTH, BONE, NON-INVASIVE
(Orthopedics) 87LOF

Capstone Therapeutics 800-937-5520
1275 W Washington St, Tempe, AZ 85281
ORTHOLOGIC 1000

STIMULATOR, INCONTINENCE (NON-IMPLANTABLE), ELECTRICAL *(Gastro/Urology) 78KPI*

Avazzia, Inc. 214-575-2820
13154 Coit Rd Ste 200, Dallas, TX 75240
Incontinence probe.

Biomation 888-667-2324
335 Perth St., P.O. Box 156, Almonte, ON K0A 1A0 Canada
ELPHA II 3000 2-channel muscle stimulator. FemiScan biofeedback system. Femetone and ETS-190 Trophic Stimulator. Aquaflex weighted vaginal cone.

Empi, Inc. 800-328-2536
599 Cardigan Rd, Saint Paul, MN 55126

The Prometheus Group 603-749-0733
1 Washington St Ste 303, Dover, NH 03820
Pelvic floor training system.

STIMULATOR, INTESTINAL *(Gastro/Urology) 78LNQ*

Medtronic Puerto Rico Operations Co., Juncos 763-514-4000
Road 31, Km. 24, Hm 4, Ceiba Norte Industrial Park, Juncos, PR 00777
Stimulator, intestinal.

STIMULATOR, INTRACEREBRAL/SUBCORTICAL, IMPLANTABLE *(Cns/Neurology) 84GYZ*

Avery Biomedical Devices, Inc. 631-864-1600
61 Mall Dr, Commack, NY 11725
Electrical brain stimulator (e.b.s.) sterotatic.

STIMULATOR, MECHANICAL, EVOKED RESPONSE
(Cns/Neurology) 84GZP

4-D Neuroimaging 858-453-6300
9727 Pacific Heights Blvd, San Diego, CA 92121
Stimulator, mechanical, evoked response.

STIMULATOR, MUSCLE, DIAGNOSTIC *(Physical Med) 89ISB*

Alimed, Inc. 800-225-2610
297 High St, Dedham, MA 02026

Elmed, Inc. 630-543-2792
60 W Fay Ave, Addison, IL 60101
STIMULETTE.

Motion Control, Inc. 888-696-2767
2401 S 1070 W Ste B, Salt Lake City, UT 84119
Myolab II Electromyographic device to stimulate muscles for prosthetic use.

Rochester Electro Medical, Inc. 813-963-2933
4212 Cypress Gulch Dr, Lutz, FL 33559
Stimulator probes and stimulation needles.

STIMULATOR, MUSCLE, ELECTRICAL-POWERED (EMS)
(Physical Med) 89IPF

American Imex 800-521-8286
16520 Aston, Irvine, CA 92606
R-STIM - dual channel, reciprocal mode, adjustable parameters. R-STIM II-Dual channel, reciprocal & synchronous modes, adjustable parameters.

Amrex Electrotherapy Equipment 800-221-9069
641 E Walnut St, Carson, CA 90746
SYNCHROPULSE model HV752. Z-STIM IF150 interferential therapy. MS 322 low volt AC stimulator. MS324A Dual channel LV AC stimulator. Z-STIM IF 250 interferential therapy/Russian stimulator MS324AB dual channel LVAC stimulator AC or battery operable. LVG325A Low Voltage Galvanic.

Arizona Dme--Durable Medical Equipment, Inc. 888-665-2568
PO Box 15413, Scottsdale, AZ 85267
Galvanic stimulators, CPMS, Bracing C Custum, Post-op., etc.

Armstrong Industries, Inc. 972-547-1400
1801 W Louisiana St, McKinney, TX 75069
High volt galvani stimulator.

Athena Feminine Technologies, Inc 866-308-4436
179 Moraga Way, Orinda, CA 94563
The Athena Pelvic Muscle Trainer is a cordless product that is inserted like a tampon and is controlled by a remote control. The PMT automatically stimulates the pelvic floor muscles to do Kegel exercises. It has a 15-minute cycle and then shuts off automatically. The intensity of the contractions is easily controlled. Clinical studies prove that the Athena PMT is safe and effective. The Athena Pelvic Muscle Trainer is FDA approved and Medicare reimbursable. It will be available by prescription.

Biomedical Life Systems, Inc. 800-726-8367
2448 Cades Way, Vista, CA 92081

Bloomex International, Inc. 201-703-9799
295 Molnar Dr, Elmwood Park, NJ 07407
Battery powered $500.00 & up.

Care Rehab And Orthopaedic Products, Inc. 703-448-9644
3930 Horseshoe Bend Rd, Keysville, VA 23947
Powered muscle stimulator.

Chattanooga Group 800-592-7329
4717 Adams Rd, Hixson, TN 37343
INTELECT stimulators.

Comfort Technologies, Inc. 800-321-7846
381 Mountain Blvd, Watchung, NJ 07069
Digital Muscle Stimulator with LCD display, treatment timer, patient-compliance timer, and many other features.

Compex Technologies, Inc. 866-676-6489
1811 Old Highway 8 NW, New Brighton, MN 55112
NEUROMUSCULAR III (NMIII) dual channel NMS. GVII high-voltage galvanic stimulator. IFII portable, wearable interferential stimulator.

Control Solutions, Inc. 630-806-7062
2229 Diehl Rd, Aurora, IL 60502
CS3102 High Voltage Galvanic Stimulator

Discount Dme 714-630-9590
1265 N Grove St Ste A, Anaheim, CA 92806
Electrical stimulation.

Electro Therapeutic Devices Inc. 800-268-3834
570 Hood Rd., Ste. 14, Markham, ONT L3R 4G7 Canada

STIMULATOR, MUSCLE, ELECTRICAL-POWERED (EMS) *(cont'd)*

Electro-Med Health Industries 800-232-3644
PO Box 610484, Miami, FL 33261
EGS 100SL high voltage pulsed galvanic stimulator. Multiple frequency muscle stimulator VERSASTIM 380. EGXtra (EGS Model EGS4000) portable high voltage pulsed galvanic stimulator. EGXtra (Model EGS4000) high-voltage pulsed galvanic stimulator, portable two-channel, operates on one 9-volt battery, multiple switching rates, timer, independent intensity controls, visible indicators, compliance mechanism, two-second rise time, belt clip, approx. seven oz.

Electrotherapy Systems, Inc. 503-779-7039
476 Winding Ct SE, Salem, OR 97302
Neuromuscular electrical stimulator,electrical muscle stimulator.

Elmed, Inc. 630-543-2792
60 W Fay Ave, Addison, IL 60101
STIMULETTE.

Empi 651-415-9000
Clear Lake Industrial Park, Clear Lake, SD 57226
Stimulator, muscle, powered.

Excel Tech. Ltd. 905-829-5300
2568 Bristol Cir, Oakville L6H 5S1 Canada
Various

I-Rep, Inc. 800-828-0852
508 Chaney St Ste B, Lake Elsinore, CA 92530
Electrotherapy equipment for under $2,500.

Integrated Biomedical Corp. 702-450-1005
5030 S Decatur Blvd Ste E, Las Vegas, NV 89118
Various models of microcurrent muscle stimulators.

Kesner C.R. 630-232-8118
2520 Kaneville Ct, Geneva, IL 60134
Also available: combination units - muscle stimulator and therapeutic ultrasound, electrically powered.

Lsi Intl., Inc. 913-894-4493
11529 W 79th St, Lenexa, KS 66214
System ii.

Md International, Inc. 305-669-9003
11300 NW 41st St, Doral, FL 33178

Med Labs Inc. 800-968-2486
28 Vereda Cordillera, Goleta, CA 93117
Neuromuscular Stimulators: EMS-1C battery powered, Interrupted DC (Galvanic) output- $192.50. EMS-2C battery-powered, Interrupted DC and Pulsed (Faradic) output- $210.00.

Mednet Services, Inc. 612-788-6228
2855 Anthony Ln S Ste B10, Minneapolis, MN 55418
Neuromuscular stimulator.

Mettler Electronics Corp. 800-854-9305
1333 S Claudina St, Anaheim, CA 92805
*SYS*STIM neuromuscular stimulators, four models available, including interferential, medium frequency, pulsed and D.C. outputs, from $550.00 to $2,895.00.*

Multiplex Stimulator Ltd. 800-663-8576
2-1750 McLean Ave., Port Coquitlam, BC V3C 1M9 Canada

Myo/Kinetic Systems, Inc. 414-255-1005
North 84 West 13562 Leon Rd., Menomonee Falls, WI 53051
Therapeutic stimulator.

Neurocare, Inc. 877-571-3599
6252 Skyline Rd S, Salem, OR 97306
Electronic neuromuscular stimulator.

Newwave Medical Llc 888-513-9283
1239 Durham Rd, Whitewright, TX 75491
High voltage pulsed galvanic stimulator hupgs.

Physiodynamics, Inc. 303-713-0605
7200 E Dry Creek Rd Ste A202, Centennial, CO 80112
Therastim.

Rich-Mar Corporation 800-762-4665
PO Box 879, 15499 E 590 Rd, Inola, OK 74036
Full line of electro-simulators including multi-waveform devices, inferential, high volt, biphoric, and low volt waveforms for all therapy needs.

Rs Medical 800-683-0353
14001 S.E. First St., Vancouver, WA 98684
RS-2i Interferential Stimulator; RS-2m Muscle Stimulator

Soken Products, Inc. 972-939-8072
1906 Robin Meadow Dr, Carrollton, TX 75007
No common name listed.

STIMULATOR, MUSCLE, ELECTRICAL-POWERED (EMS) *(cont'd)*

Taylor Industries, Inc. 800-339-1361
2706 Industrial Dr, Jefferson City, MO 65109

Thera-Tronics, Inc. 800-267-6211
623 Mamaroneck Ave, Mamaroneck, NY 10543

Therapeutic Alliances, Inc. 937-879-0734
333 N Broad St, Fairborn, OH 45324
Powered muscle stimulator.

Universal Technology Systems, Inc. 904-778-8614
5150 Timuquana Rd Ste 4, Jacksonville, FL 32210
Pulse galvanic stimulator.

Vision Quest Industries, Inc. 800-266-6969
18011 Mitchell S, Irvine, CA 92614
Neuromuscular stimulation.

Zynex Inc. 800-495-6670
9990 Park Meadows Dr, Lone Tree, CO 80124
NeuroMove NM900, E-Wave, IF8000

STIMULATOR, MUSCLE, LOW INTENSITY *(Physical Med) 89LBF*

Comfort Technologies, Inc. 800-321-7846
381 Mountain Blvd, Watchung, NJ 07069
Digital TENS Stimulator with LCD display, treatment timer, patient compliance timer and many other features.

Dedicated Distribution 800-325-8367
640 Miami Ave, Kansas City, KS 66105

Nikomed U.S.A., Inc. 800-355-6456
2000 Pioneer Rd, Huntingdon Valley, PA 19006
Flip Tens, Tens Unit. Stimulator, nerve, transeutaneous, for pain relief. Prima Tens, Tens Unit. Stimulator, nerve, transcutaneous for pain relief.

Rpi Of Atlanta 800-554-1501
120 Interstate North Pkwy SE Ste 424, Atlanta, GA 30339
INTRACELL. Non-motorized soft tissue manipulator for treatment of muscular pain or stiffness.

Taylor Industries, Inc. 800-339-1361
2706 Industrial Dr, Jefferson City, MO 65109

STIMULATOR, MUSCLE, POWERED, INVASIVE
(Physical Med) 89MBN

Taylor Industries, Inc. 800-339-1361
2706 Industrial Dr, Jefferson City, MO 65109

STIMULATOR, MUSCLE, VAGINAL *(Obstetrics/Gyn) 85HII*

Athena Feminine Technologies, Inc 866-308-4436
179 Moraga Way, Orinda, CA 94563
The Athena Pelvic Muscle Trainer is a cordless product that is inserted like a tampon and is controlled by a remote control. The PMT automatically stimulates the pelvic floor muscles to do Kegel exercises. It has a 15-minute cycle and then shuts off automatically. The intensity of the contractions is easily controlled. Clinical studies prove that the Athena PMT is safe and effective. The Athena Pelvic Muscle Trainer is FDA approved and Medicare reimbursable. It will be available by prescription.

Mylon-Tech Health Technologies Inc. 613-728-1667
301 Moodie Dr., Ste. 205, Ottawa, ON K2H 9C4 Canada
EMG and EMS units for treatment of urge and stress incontinence.

STIMULATOR, NERVE LOCATING *(Cns/Neurology) 84UFH*

Bovie Medical Corp. 800-537-2790
5115 Ulmerton Rd, Clearwater, FL 33760

Dma Med-Chem Corporation 800-362-1833
49 Watermill Ln, Great Neck, NY 11021

Neuro Technology, Inc. 800-638-7689
164 Firefly Ln, Kerrville, TX 78028

Singer Medical Products, Inc. 800-222-2572
790 Maple Ln, Bensenville, IL 60106
AXOSTIM hand-held single use device for use during surgery.

STIMULATOR, NERVE LOCATING, FACIAL
(Cns/Neurology) 84UFI

Bovie Medical Corp. 800-537-2790
5115 Ulmerton Rd, Clearwater, FL 33760

STIMULATOR, NERVE, AC-POWERED *(Anesthesiology) 73BXM*

Cadwell Laboratories 800-245-3001
909 N Kellogg St, Kennewick, WA 99336
CADWELL MES-10 painless nerve stimulation system.

STIMULATOR, NERVE, AC-POWERED *(cont'd)*

Grass Technologies, An Astro-Med, Inc. Product Gro 401-828-4002
53 Airport Park Drive, Rockland, MA 02370
General purpose stimulator.

Nuvasive, Inc. 800-475-9131
7475 Lusk Blvd, San Diego, CA 92121
Electromyography (emg) monitor/stimulator & accessory electrodes.

STIMULATOR, NERVE, ANESTHESIA *(Anesthesiology) 73KOI*

Biomedical Life Systems, Inc. 800-726-8367
2448 Cades Way, Vista, CA 92081

Draeger Medical Systems, Inc. 215-660-2626
16 Electronics Ave, Danvers, MA 01923
Electric peripheral nerve stimulator.

Mercury Medical 800-237-6418
11300 49th St N, Clearwater, FL 33762

Neuro Technology, Inc. 800-638-7689
164 Firefly Ln, Kerrville, TX 78028

Sunmed Healthcare 727-531-7266
12393 Belcher Rd S Ste 460, Largo, FL 33773

STIMULATOR, NERVE, BATTERY-POWERED
(Anesthesiology) 73BXN

Biomedical Life Systems, Inc. 800-726-8367
2448 Cades Way, Vista, CA 92081

Canadian Medical Products, Ltd. 800-267-0572
850 Tapscott Rd., Unit 21, Scarborough, ONT M1X-1N4 Canada

Life-Tech, Inc. 281-491-6600
4235 Greenbriar Dr, Stafford, TX 77477

Neo Medical Inc. 888-450-3334
42514 Albrae St, Fremont, CA 94538
Nerve stimulator.

Neuro Technology, Inc. 800-638-7689
164 Firefly Ln, Kerrville, TX 78028

St. Jude Medical Neuromodulation Division 800-727-7846
6901 Preston Rd, Plano, TX 75024
Spinal cord stimulation systems for the treatment of chronic pain.

STIMULATOR, NERVE, ENT *(Ear/Nose/Throat) 77ETN*

Baxano, Inc. 408-514-2200
655 River Oaks Pkwy, San Jose, CA 95134
Neural Localization Probe; NeuroCheck Device

Blue Torch Medical Technologies 508-231-1080
200 Homer Ave, Center, Ashland, MA 01721
Nerve stimulator.

Cardinal Healthcare 209, Inc. 610-862-0800
5225 Verona Rd, Fitchburg, WI 53711
Nerve stimulator.

Grass Technologies, An Astro-Med, Inc. Product Gro 401-828-4002
53 Airport Park Drive, Rockland, MA 02370
General purpose stimulus isolator.

Gyrus Ent L.L.C., Sub. Of Gyrus Acmi, Inc. 508-804-2739
2925 Appling Rd, Bartlett, TN 38133
Various.

Medtronic Sofamor Danek Usa, Inc. 901-396-3133
4340 Swinnea Rd, Memphis, TN 38118
Monopolar stimulating instrumentation.

Ndi Medical, Inc. 216-378-9106
22901 Millcreek Blvd Ste 110, Cleveland, OH 44122
Surgical nerve stimulator-locator.

Neo Medical Inc. 888-450-3334
42514 Albrae St, Fremont, CA 94538
Nerve location device.

Nuvasive, Inc. 800-475-9131
7475 Lusk Blvd, San Diego, CA 92121
Electromyography, emg monitor/stimulator and accessory electrodes.

Paragon Medsystems, Llc. 858-613-1200
15920 Bernardo Center Dr, San Diego, CA 92127
Emg monitor/stimulator.

Rhythmlink International, LLC 866-633-3754
1140 First St. South, Columbia, SC 29209
MSP

STIMULATOR, NERVE, ENT *(cont'd)*

Singer Medical Products Inc., Md Systems Div. 630-860-6500
3800 Buckner St, El Paso, TX 79925
Disposable nerve stimulator.

Wr Medical Electronics Co. 800-321-6387
123 2nd St N, Stillwater, MN 55082
$869 to $6,850 for 3 different models: Hilger, Silverstein, and Brackmann facial-nerve monitors and stimulators.

STIMULATOR, NERVE, TRANSCUTANEOUS (PAIN RELIEF, TENS) *(Cns/Neurology) 84GZJ*

Alivio Corporation 231-275-1345
20429 Honor Hwy, Interlochen, MI 49643
Stimulator, nerve, transcutaneous for pain relief.

Allvetsusa:Attn:Us-It.Net 954-560-4257
500 S Australian Ave Ste 510, West Palm Beach, FL 33401
Computer neural stimulator, integrity.

American Imex 800-521-8286
16520 Aston, Irvine, CA 92606
ULTIMA microampere current. PREMIER TENS, USA made according to GMP, ANSI/AAMI, and ISO 9001 & ISO 9002; fully adjustable, extremely high quality and tolerances. EASY TENS, basic device with high/low/burst. AI-86 A-TENS, fully adjustable, cost effective. SDII Program, SD MODE III, BIOTENS, & IF-400 INTERFERENTIAL. MICROCARE II- Microcurrent device, dual channel.

Amrex Electrotherapy Equipment 800-221-9069
641 E Walnut St, Carson, CA 90746
SPECTRUM Micro 1000. Z-STIM 100 TENS, Advanteq 2000 two-channel, multi-feature TENS device.

Arizona Dme--Durable Medical Equipment, Inc. 888-665-2568
PO Box 15413, Scottsdale, AZ 85267

Armstrong Industries, Inc. 972-547-1400
1801 W Louisiana St, McKinney, TX 75069
Tens.

Arthrowave Medical Technologies, Llc 410-472-0360
53 Loveton Cir Ste 207, Glencoe, MD 21152
Tens (transcutaneous electrical nerve stimulator).

Avazzia, Inc. 214-575-2820
13154 Coit Rd Ste 200, Dallas, TX 75240
Transcutaneous electrical nerve stimulation (tens).

Avery Biomedical Devices, Inc. 631-864-1600
61 Mall Dr, Commack, NY 11725
Tns system.

Bbg, Inc. 757-366-9211
1708 S Park Ct, Chesapeake, VA 23320
Dr liberson's micropulsei.

Bio-Research Associates, Inc. 414-357-7525
9275 N 49th St Ste 150, Brown Deer, WI 53223
Tens transcutaneous electrical nerve stimulator.

Biofeedback Instrument Corp. 212-222-5665
255 W 98th St Apt 3D, New York, NY 10025
$850.00 per Alphastim (.5hz-100hz)clincial dual channel micro-current TENS, Acutron: clinical diagnostic units-Microcurrent TENS; 1500 - $5995.

Biomedical Life Systems, Inc. 800-726-8367
2448 Cades Way, Vista, CA 92081

Biowave Corporation 203-855-8610
16 Knight St, Norwalk, CT 06851
Tens.

Bloomex International, Inc. 201-703-9799
295 Molnar Dr, Elmwood Park, NJ 07407

Canadian Medical Products, Ltd. 800-267-0572
850 Tapscott Rd., Unit 21, Scarborough, ONT M1X-1N4 Canada

Care Rehab And Orthopaedic Products, Inc. 703-448-9644
3930 Horseshoe Bend Rd, Keysville, VA 23947
Stimulator, nerve, transcutaneous, for pain relief.

Comfort Technologies, Inc. 800-321-7846
381 Mountain Blvd, Watchung, NJ 07069
Single mode, dual channel stimulator - comtech, three mode, full function stimulator - comfort - stim.

Compex Technologies, Inc. 866-676-6489
1811 Old Highway 8 NW, New Brighton, MN 55112
Broad line of reusable and disposable, wearable TENS systems. Made in U.S.A.

STIMULATOR, NERVE, TRANSCUTANEOUS (PAIN RELIEF, TENS) *(cont'd)*

Dermawave, Llc 561-784-0599
15693 83rd Ln N, Loxahatchee, FL 33470
Transcutaneous electrical nerve/muscle stimulator for pain relief & accesories.

Digi-Com Electronics 805-522-6223
5327 Jacuzzi St, Richmond, CA 94804
Transcutaneous electrical nerve stimulator.

Dynatronics Corp. 800-874-6251
7030 Park Centre Dr, Salt Lake City, UT 84121

Dynawave Research Inc. 800-732-7877
Broadway W Prof Centre, 412-2150 Broadway W
Vancouver V6K 4 Canada
Micro current therapy,a.k.a. micro tens

Electro Medica Office 705-878-5894
33 Williams St. North, Lindsay, ONT K9V-3Z9 Canada
$180 for EMOTENS transcutaneous nerve stimulator.

Electro Medical Inc. 918-663-0297
9736 E 55th Pl, Tulsa, OK 74146
Transcutaneous electrical nerve stimulation.

Electro Surface Technologies, Inc. 760-431-8306
2280 Faraday Ave, Carlsbad, CA 92008
Dial away pain, tens device.

Electro Therapeutic Devices Inc. 800-268-3834
570 Hood Rd., Ste. 14, Markham, ONT L3R 4G7 Canada

Electro-Tech Products Inc. 909-592-1434
2001 E Gladstone St Ste A, Glendora, CA 91740
Microcurrent.

Electromedical Products International, Inc. 800-367-7246
2201 Garrett Morris Pkwy, Mineral Wells, TX 76067
$395.00 for ALPHA-STIM PPM (Personal Pain Manager) microcurrent stimulator for acute, chronic, and postoperative pain. Ideal for home use.

Electronic Waveform Laboratory, Inc. 800-874-9283
16168 Beach Blvd Ste 232, Huntington Beach, CA 92647
H-WAVE Muscular And Neurological Stimulator (MANS).

Elmed, Inc. 630-543-2792
60 W Fay Ave, Addison, IL 60101
NEUROPROBE.

Empi 651-415-9000
Clear Lake Industrial Park, Clear Lake, SD 57226
Stimulator, nerve, transcutaneous, for pain relief.

Empi, Inc. 800-328-2536
599 Cardigan Rd, Saint Paul, MN 55126
EPIX XL & ECLIPSE+ TENS systems.

Eprt Technologies, Inc. 805-522-6223
2139 Tapo St Ste 228, Simi Valley, CA 93063
Tens.

Eumedic Incorporated
1369 Forest Park Cir Ste 100, Lafayette, CO 80026
Transcutaneous nerve stimulation device.

Excel Tech. Ltd. 905-829-5300
2568 Bristol Cir, Oakville L6H 5S1 Canada
Various

Genadyne Biotechnologies, Inc. 516-487-8787
65 Watermill Ln, Great Neck, NY 11021
Gentens.

Grand Technology, Inc. 562-316-7869
PO Box 4746, 12145 Mora Drive, Unit 1, Cerritos, CA 90703
Tens.

Hako-Med Usa, Inc. 888-913-7900
1024 Puuwai St, Honolulu, HI 96819
Electrical stimulator.

Healthonics, Inc. 770-955-2006
903 Main St S, New Ellenton, SC 29809
Tens device.

Inovar, Inc. 435-792-4949
1073 W 1700 N, Logan, UT 84321
Nerve stimulator.

Integrated Biomedical Corp. 702-450-1005
5030 S Decatur Blvd Ste E, Las Vegas, NV 89118
Various models of micro-current neural stimulators.

International Plastics, Llc 262-781-2270
4965 N. Campbell Dr., Menomonee Falls, WI 53051
Tens device.

STIMULATOR, NERVE, TRANSCUTANEOUS (PAIN RELIEF, TENS) *(cont'd)*

Invacare Supply Group, An Invacare Co. 800-225-4792
75 October Hill Rd, Holliston, MA 01746
Carry full lines of TENS units from: Invacare, Biomedical Life Systems, & Rehabilicare.

Lsi Intl., Inc. 913-894-4493
11529 W 79th St, Lenexa, KS 66214
Transcutaneous nerve stimulator.

Lumiscope Company, Inc. 800-672-8293
1035 Centennial Ave, Piscataway, NJ 08854

M.E.D. Servi-Systems Canada Ltd. 800-267-6868
8 Sweetnam Dr., Stittsville, ONT K2S 1G2 Canada

Medi-Man Rehabilitation Products, Inc. 800-268-4256
6200A Tomken Rd., Mississauga, ONT L5T-1X7 Canada
MEDI-STIM multi-modality unit, including interferrential, micro current, high volt, Russian stim and ultrasound.

Mednet Services, Inc. 612-788-6228
2855 Anthony Ln S Ste B10, Minneapolis, MN 55418
Tens unit.

Micro Current Technology, Inc. 206-778-5717
2244 1st Ave S, Seattle, WA 98134
Stimulator, nerve, transcutaneous.

Microstim Technology, Inc. 772-283-0408
1849 SW Crane Creek Ave, Palm City, FL 34990
Tens nerve stimulator.

Multiplex Stimulator Ltd. 800-663-8576
2-1750 McLean Ave., Port Coquitlam, BC V3C 1M9 Canada

Mylon-Tech Health Technologies Inc. 613-728-1667
301 Moodie Dr., Ste. 205, Ottawa, ON K2H 9C4 Canada
Wide variety of TENS and EMS devices.

Myo/Kinetic Systems, Inc. 414-255-1005
North 84 West 13562 Leon Rd., Menomonee Falls, WI 53051
Tens.

Myotronics-Noromed, Inc. 206-243-4214
5870 S 194th St, Kent, WA 98032
$595.00 per unit, BNS-40 home treatment TENS and $1,445.00 for J-4 Myo-Monitor Stimulator unit.

Naimco, Inc. 423-648-7730
4120 S Creek Rd, Chattanooga, TN 37406
Transcutaneous electronic nerve stimulator, tens.

Neuro Resource Group, Inc. 972-665-1810
1100 Jupiter Rd Ste 190, Plano, TX 75074
Interactive neurostimulation device.

Neurotone Systems, Inc. 972-271-1978
510 Nesbit Dr, Garland, TX 75041
Transcutaneous nerve stimulation (tns).

Neurowave Medical Technologies 312-334-2505
200 E Randolph St, Suite 2200, Chicago, IL 60601
Multiple

Precision Microcurrent, Inc. 503-443-6100
705 S.springbrook Rd., Bld.a-135, Newberg, OR 97132
Microcurrent stimulator.

R & D Medical Products, Inc. 949-472-9346
20492 Crescent Bay Dr Ste 106, Lake Forest, CA 92630
TENS electrode.

Reflex Technologies, Inc. 305-892-0584
12565 Palm Rd Ste B, North Miami, FL 33181
Comfortron, m.a.n. stim, manstim.

Selective Med Components, Inc. 740-397-7838
564 Harcourt Rd, Mount Vernon, OH 43050
Reusable tens & nmes electrodes.

The Synaptic Corp. 800-685-7246
3176 S Peoria St Ste 100, Aurora, CO 80014
Tens.

Thera-Tronics, Inc. 800-267-6211
623 Mamaroneck Ave, Mamaroneck, NY 10543

Vision Quest Industries, Inc. 800-266-6969
18011 Mitchell S, Irvine, CA 92614
Transcutaneous electrical nerve stimulator.

Z Technologies, Llc 404-248-0159
2615 Woodacres Rd NE, Atlanta, GA 30345
Electrical Nerve Stimulator

STIMULATOR, NERVE, TRANSCUTANEOUS (PAIN RELIEF, TENS) *(cont'd)*

Zimmer Medizinsystems 800-327-3576
25 Mauchly Ste 300, Irvine, CA 92618
Dual channel, low and high rate, burst mode compact size, coaxial lead wires, 9V battery system.

Zynex Inc. 800-495-6670
9990 Park Meadows Dr, Lone Tree, CO 80124
TruWave

STIMULATOR, NEUROLOGICAL *(Surgery) 79FXA*

Bak Electronics, Inc. 800-894-6000
PO Box 623, Mount Airy, MD 21771

Biomedical Life Systems, Inc. 800-726-8367
2448 Cades Way, Vista, CA 92081

Elmed, Inc. 630-543-2792
60 W Fay Ave, Addison, IL 60101

Integra Radionics 800-466-6814
22 Terry Ave, Burlington, MA 01803

Md International, Inc. 305-669-9003
11300 NW 41st St, Doral, FL 33178

Nihon Kohden America, Inc. 800-325-0283
90 Icon, Foothill Ranch, CA 92610

Tegra Medical Inc. 508-541-4200
9 Forge Pkwy, Franklin, MA 02038

STIMULATOR, NEUROMUSCULAR, EXTERNAL FUNCTIONAL *(Cns/Neurology) 84GZI*

Alivio Corporation 231-275-1345
20429 Honor Hwy, Interlochen, MI 49643
Neuromuscular electrical stimulator.

American Imex 800-521-8286
16520 Aston, Irvine, CA 92606
High Volt Pulsed Galvanic Stimulator. PGS 3000 patient/practitioner friendly. Comfortable hidden controls for practitioner selection.

Bausch & Lomb Surgical 636-255-5051
3365 Tree Court Ind Blvd, Saint Louis, MO 63122

Biomedical Life Systems, Inc. 800-726-8367
2448 Cades Way, Vista, CA 92081

Chattanooga Group 800-592-7329
4717 Adams Rd, Hixson, TN 37343
INTELECT stimulators.

Comfort Technologies, Inc. 800-321-7846
381 Mountain Blvd, Watchung, NJ 07069
MYOTECH full-featured muscle stimulator.

Compex Technologies, Inc. 866-676-6489
1811 Old Highway 8 NW, New Brighton, MN 55112
NEUROMUSCULAR III (NMIII) dual channel NMS. GVII high-voltage galvanic stimulator. IFII portable, wearable interferential stimulator.

Dmedicus, Llc. 469-698-9939
842 Canterbury Dr, Rockwall, TX 75032
Neuromuscular stimulation device.

Elmed, Inc. 630-543-2792
60 W Fay Ave, Addison, IL 60101

Empi 651-415-9000
Clear Lake Industrial Park, Clear Lake, SD 57226
Stimulator, neuromuscular, external functional.

Empi, Inc. 800-328-2536
599 Cardigan Rd, Saint Paul, MN 55126
FOCUS

Humantronic, Inc 866-340-1648
1103 Leeland Heights Blvd E, Lehigh Acres, FL 33936
Intravesical Electro Stimulation Catheter

Kimball Electronics Tampa 813-814-8114
13750 Reptron Blvd, Tampa, FL 33626
Functional external neuromuscular stimulator.

R.J. Lindquist Co. 213-382-1268
2419 James M Wood Blvd, Los Angeles, CA 90006
Various models of chronowave electro-stimulator.

Reflex Technologies, Inc. 305-892-0584
12565 Palm Rd Ste B, North Miami, FL 33181
Comfortron, m.a.n. stim, manstim.

Rs Medical 800-683-0353
14001 S.E. First St., Vancouver, WA 98684
Relieving pain and improving function with a line of physician-prescribed RS-brand electrotherapy stimulators for home use.

STIMULATOR, NEUROMUSCULAR, EXTERNAL FUNCTIONAL
(cont'd)

Sterne Equipment Co., Ltd. 905-457-2524
7 Research Rd., Brampton, ONT L6W 1P4 Canada
Neurotrain

Vision Quest Industries, Inc. 800-266-6969
18011 Mitchell S, Irvine, CA 92614
Neuromuscular stimulator.

STIMULATOR, NEUROMUSCULAR, FUNCTIONAL WALKING, NON-INVASIVE *(Physical Med) 89MKD*

Sterne Equipment Co., Ltd. 905-457-2524
7 Research Rd., Brampton, ONT L6W 1P4 Canada
Same

Taylor Industries, Inc. 800-339-1361
2706 Industrial Dr, Jefferson City, MO 65109

STIMULATOR, OSTEOGENESIS, ELECTRIC, INVASIVE
(Orthopedics) 87HTM

Ebi, Llc 800-526-2579
100 Interpace Pkwy, Parsippany, NJ 07054
OSTEOGEN monitorable, with constant direct current field, 20 mA output. Power source: one lithium iodine battery with 32-35 week battery life, 10g weight. SpF-4 four lead constant direct current implantable bone growth stimulator for the enhancement of spinal fusions. SpF: Spinal fusion stimulator fully implantable with telemetry, delivers direct current to fusion site for six monthg. SpF-2 & SpF-4.

STIMULATOR, OSTEOGENESIS, ELECTRIC, NON-INVASIVE
(Orthopedics) 87WNT

Autogenesis, Inc. 410-665-2017
8700 Old Harford Rd, Baltimore, MD 21234
AUTOMATOR computerized, motor-driven, can be fitted to most manufacturers' circular fixators. The AUTOMATOR then distracts the fixation rings according to the physician's exact prescription. Research indicates the frequent distractions in small increments can promote superior new bone and soft tissue regeneration.

Biolectron, Inc. 800-524-0677
25 Commerce Dr, Allendale, NJ 07401
ORTHOPAK, portable, lightweight, battery-powered, non-invasive. SPINALPAK FUSION STIMULATOR, portable, lightweight, battery-powered, non-invasive stimulator that provides effective treatment for Lumbar Fusions.

Ebi, Llc 800-526-2579
100 Interpace Pkwy, Parsippany, NJ 07054
Portable EBI Bone Healing System Model 1200, with flx flexible treatment coils.

Orthofix Inc. 800-535-4492
1720 Bray Central Dr, McKinney, TX 75069
Physio-Stim bone growth stimulator with control module, U-shaped transducer coil, and battery. Spinal-Stim Pemf spinal-fusion system for surgical adjunct procedures and pseudoarthroses.

Slawner Ltd., J. 514-731-3378
5713 Cote Des Neiges Rd., Montreal, QUE H3S 1Y7 Canada

STIMULATOR, PERIPHERAL NERVE, BLOCKADE MONITOR
(Anesthesiology) 73UFG

Anesthesia Associates, Inc. 760-744-6561
460 Enterprise St, San Marcos, CA 92078
Battery operated, portable units. Available in both Compact (PN 00-100) and Full Size (PN 00-105) styles with many usefull features. Fully FDA Compliant and sold with ball electode set. Various alligator clip, snap button and extension sets (all compliant) available as well.

Life-Tech, Inc. 281-491-6600
4235 Greenbriar Dr, Stafford, TX 77477
Ministim, EZStim and Maxistim

STIMULATOR, PERIPHERAL NERVE, BLOCKADE MONITOR
(cont'd)

Neuro Technology, Inc. 800-638-7689
164 Firefly Ln, Kerrville, TX 78028
$495 for DIGISTIM II digital peripheral nerve stimulator; includes 1 pair of 6-ft leads with alligator clips and universal mounting bracket. $375 for DIGISTIM III with 1 pair of leads as DIGISTIM II. $120 for MICRO STIM, $20-$40/accessories (leads, needles, bracket, etc). $140 for MICROSTIM PLUS with belt clip, variable output, numbered dial, ball electrodes, leadwires, double-burst stimulation mode. $540 for DIGISTIM 2 PLUS with double-burst stimulation mode, IV pole mount, automatic power shutdown after 20 minutes nonuse, adjustable audio output, low current range for regional blocks, liquid crystal display of current delivered and battery voltage. $445 for DIGISTIM 3 PLUS with double-burst stimulation mode, automatic power shutdown after 20 minutes nonuse, adjustable audio output, low current range for regional blocks, liquid crystal display of current delivered and battery voltage.

Sunmed Healthcare 727-531-7266
12393 Belcher Rd S Ste 460, Largo, FL 33773

STIMULATOR, PERIPHERAL NERVE, IMPLANTABLE (PAIN RELIEF) *(Cns/Neurology) 84GZF*

Avery Biomedical Devices, Inc. 631-864-1600
61 Mall Dr, Commack, NY 11725
Peripheral nerve stimulator.

Medtronic Neuromodulation 612-514-4000
800 53rd Ave NE, Minneapolis, MN 55421
Various.

Medtronic Puerto Rico Operations Co., Villalba 763-514-4000
PO Box 6001, Rd. 149, Km. 56.3, Villalba, PR 00766
Various types of sterile and non-sterile peripheral nerve stimulation systems.

Medtronic Puerto Rico Operations Co.,Med Rel 763-514-4000
Road 909, Km. 0.4., Barrio Mariana, Humacao, PR 00792
Various types of sterile and non-sterile peripheral nerve stimulation systems.

Trivirix International Inc. 320-982-8000
925 6th Ave NE, Milaca, MN 56353
Various.

STIMULATOR, PHOTIC, EVOKED RESPONSE
(Cns/Neurology) 84GWE

Cadwell Laboratories 800-245-3001
909 N Kellogg St, Kennewick, WA 99336
3' LED Flash optional.

Cardinal Healthcare 209, Inc. 610-862-0800
5225 Verona Rd, Fitchburg, WI 53711
Evoked response.

Grass Technologies, An Astro-Med, Inc. Product Gro 401-828-4002
53 Airport Park Drive, Rockland, MA 02370
Photo stimulator.

Lkc Technologies, Inc. 800-638-7055
2 Professional Dr Ste 222, Gaithersburg, MD 20879
See photostimulator.

STIMULATOR, SACRAL NERVE, IMPLANTED
(Cns/Neurology) 84MQQ

Medtronic Neuromodulation 612-514-4000
800 53rd Ave NE, Minneapolis, MN 55421
Sacral nerve stimulator for voiding dysfunction.

Trivirix International Inc. 320-982-8000
925 6th Ave NE, Milaca, MN 56353
Sacral nerve stimulator for voiding dysfunction.

STIMULATOR, SCOLIOSIS, NEUROMUSCULAR, FUNCTIONAL
(Orthopedics) 87LWB

Encore Medical Corporation 800-456-8696
9800 Metric Blvd, Austin, TX 78758
Clincial and home rehabilitional electrotheraphy devices, including electrical stimulation, NMES, TENS, clinical ultrasound, laser technologies

Stars 225-752-4912
6630 Exchequer Dr, Baton Rouge, LA 70809
Copes scopliosis brace.

STIMULATOR, SPINAL CORD, IMPLANTABLE (PAIN RELIEF)
(Cns/Neurology) 84GZB

Avery Biomedical Devices, Inc. 631-864-1600
61 Mall Dr, Commack, NY 11725
Spinal cord stimulator.

Medtronic Neuromodulation 612-514-4000
800 53rd Ave NE, Minneapolis, MN 55421
Various.

Medtronic Puerto Rico Operations Co., Juncos 763-514-4000
Road 31, Km. 24, Hm 4, Ceiba Norte Industrial Park, Juncos, PR 00777
Various types of sterile and non-sterile spinal cord stimulation systems.

Medtronic Puerto Rico Operations Co., Villalba 763-514-4000
PO Box 6001, Rd. 149, Km. 56.3, Villalba, PR 00766
Various types of sterile and non-sterile spinal cord stimulation systems.

Medtronic Puerto Rico Operations Co.,Med Rel 763-514-4000
Road 909, Km. 0.4., Barrio Mariana, Humacao, PR 00792
Various types of sterile and non-sterile spinal cord stimulation systems.

Medtronic, Inc. 800-633-8766
710 Medtronic Pkwy, Minneapolis, MN 55432
ITREL, ITREL EZ, ITREL 3, ITREL II, PISCES, PISCES-QUAD, PISCES-QUAD PLUS, PISCES QUINTA, PISCES-SELECTRX, PISCES-SIGMA, SYMMIX, X-TREL.

Trivirix International Inc. 320-982-8000
925 6th Ave NE, Milaca, MN 56353
Various.

STIMULATOR, SPINAL CORD, IMPLANTABLE, BLADDER EVACUATOR *(Cns/Neurology) 84GZD*

Avery Biomedical Devices, Inc. 631-864-1600
61 Mall Dr, Commack, NY 11725
Micturition stimulator.

STIMULATOR, TRANSCUTANEOUS ELECTRICAL, FOR COSMETIC USE *(Cns/Neurology) 84NFO*

Care Rehab And Orthopaedic Products, Inc. 703-448-9644
3930 Horseshoe Bend Rd, Keysville, VA 23947
Transcutaneous electrical nerve stimulator.

Facemaster Of Beverly Hills, Inc. 818-222-2461
23961 Craftsman Rd Ste I, Calabasas, CA 91302
Facial toning system.

Salton, Inc. 202-408-9213
1955 W Field Ct, Lake Forest, IL 60045
Facial toning system.

STIMULATOR, ULTRASOUND, MUSCLE *(Physical Med) 89IMG*

Amrex Electrotherapy Equipment 800-221-9069
641 E Walnut St, Carson, CA 90746
SYNCHROSONIC combination US/50. SYNCHROSONIC COMBINATION US/54. SYNCHROSONIC combination US/752. SYNCHROSONIC combination U/HVG50.

Chattanooga Group 800-592-7329
4717 Adams Rd, Hixson, TN 37343
INTELECT ultrasound.

Dermawave, Llc 561-784-0599
15693 83rd Ln N, Loxahatchee, FL 33470
Ultrasound & muscle stimulators & powered muscle stimulators & accessories.

Dynatronics Corp. 800-874-6251
7030 Park Centre Dr, Salt Lake City, UT 84121

Elmed, Inc. 630-543-2792
60 W Fay Ave, Addison, IL 60101

Excel Tech. Ltd. 905-829-5300
2568 Bristol Cir, Oakville L6H 5S1 Canada
Various

Hill Laboratories Co. 877-445-5020
3 N Bacton Hill Rd, PO Box 2028, Frazer, PA 19355
HF27 Hands-Free Therapeutic Ultrasound delivers ultrasound and muscle stimulation without movement of the soundhead during treatment. Additionally, a special gel pad eliminates residue on the patient and contours to any curvature of the body.

Md International, Inc. 305-669-9003
11300 NW 41st St, Doral, FL 33178

STIMULATOR, ULTRASOUND, MUSCLE *(cont'd)*

Medelco Ltd. 800-268-7927
55 Queens Plate Dr., Unit 9, Toronto, ONT M9W 6P2 Canada
OMNISOUND 3000, therapeutic ultrasound for physical therapy. Applications inlude soft tissue repair and pain management for rehabilitation. OMNISTIM 500 and VECTORDYNE, electrical stimulators providing Interferential Current for use in physical therapy. Applications inlude soft tissue repair and pain management for rehabilitation.

Medi-Man Rehabilitation Products, Inc. 800-268-4256
6200A Tomken Rd., Mississauga, ONT L5T-1X7 Canada
MEDI-SOUND therapeutic ultrasound with 1 and 3 Mhz. Self-calibrating sound heads. In compact and clinical.

Mettler Electronics Corp. 800-854-9305
1333 S Claudina St, Anaheim, CA 92805
Semicator Plus 930, 940, 994 and 992 is two to four channel combination device with six stimulation waveforms and 1 and 3 MHz ultrosound. Price range from $2,895.00 to $4,250.00

R.J. Lindquist Co. 213-382-1268
2419 James M Wood Blvd, Los Angeles, CA 90006
Various models of chronosonic ultrasound stimulators.

Rich-Mar Corporation 800-762-4665
PO Box 879, 15499 E 590 Rd, Inola, OK 74036
Combination US and stim devices available - AUTOSOUND 7.6 HANDS-FREE ULTRASOUND/STIM COMBO $3499, THERATOUCH 7.7 $4799.00 and THERAMINI 3P $3869.00 (portable), THERAMINI 3C $3649.00).

Zimmer Medizinsystems 800-327-3576
25 Mauchly Ste 300, Irvine, CA 92618
SONO 3 reverberation free, lightweight head, coupling control through output independent analog, combination option.

STIMULATOR, VAGUS NERVE, EPILEPSY, IMPLANTED
(Cns/Neurology) 84MBY

Cyberonics, Inc. 800-332-1375
100 Cyberonics Blvd, The Cyberonics Building, Houston, TX 77058
NeuroCybernetic Prosthesis (NCP) pacemaker-like, signal generator implant and vagus nerve lead.

STIMULATOR, VAGUS NERVE, IMPLANTED, TREMOR
(Cns/Neurology) 84MUV

Maine Biotechnology Services, Inc. 207-797-5454
1037 Forest Ave # R, Portland, ME 04103
Analyte specific reagent, multiple.

STIMULATOR, WOUND HEALING *(Physical Med) 89WIN*

Capstone Therapeutics 800-937-5520
1275 W Washington St, Tempe, AZ 85281
ORTHOLOGIC 1000: Designed to stimulate and accelerate the repair of bone fractures that have failed to heal normally.

Certified Safety Manufacturing 800-854-7474
1400 Chestnut Ave, Kansas City, MO 64127
CERTI-BURN, burn cream, spray.

Covidien Lp 508-261-8000
15 Hampshire St, Mansfield, MA 02048
THERMAZENE cream, 1%, is a soft, water dispersible cream containing silver sulfadiazine in micronized form for topical application.

Genzyme Corp. 800-232-7546
64 Sidney St, Cambridge, MA 02139
Wound healing product.

Kck Industries 888-800-1967
14941 Calvert St, Van Nuys, CA 91411

STIRRER *(Chemistry) 75RWG*

Alfa Aesar, A Johnson Matthey Company 800-343-0660
26 Parkridge Rd, Ward Hill, MA 01835

Beckman Coulter, Inc. 800-742-2345
250 S Kraemer Blvd, PO Box 8000, Brea, CA 92821

Berghof/America 800-544-5004
3773 NW 126th Ave Bldg 1, Coral Springs, FL 33065
PTFE shaft stirrers and PTFE magnetic stirring bars available in a variety of shapes and sizes. Propeller stirrers and movable stirrer blades also available.

Caframo Ltd. 800-567-3556
RR#2 Airport Rd., Wiarton, ONT N0H 2T0 Canada
Hi-torque variable speed models. Stirrer accessories: clamps, stand, impellers.

Carolina Biological Supply Co. 800-334-5551
2700 York Rd, Burlington, NC 27215

STIRRER *(cont'd)*

Cole-Parmer Instrument Inc. 800-323-4340
625 E Bunker Ct, Vernon Hills, IL 60061

Eberbach Corp. 800-422-2558
505 S Maple Rd, Ann Arbor, MI 48103

Edmund Industrial Optics 800-363-1992
101 E Gloucester Pike, Barrington, NJ 08007

Fts Systems 800-824-0400
PO Box 158, 3538 Main Street,, Stone Ridge, NY 12484

Glas-Col , Llc 800-452-7265
711 Hulman St, PO Box 2128, Terre Haute, IN 47802

Ika-Works, Inc. 800-733-3037
2635 Northchase Pkwy SE, Wilmington, NC 28405
Magnetic stirrers ranging from basic systems to programmable, microprocessor controlled computer interfacing systems.

Kernco Instruments Co., Inc. 800-325-3875
420 Kenazo Ave., El Paso, TX 79928-7338
Digital, programmable hot plate/stirrers.

Kontes Glass Co. 888-546-2531
1022 Spruce St, Vineland, NJ 08360

Lightnin Mixers 888-MIX-BEST
135 Mount Read Blvd, Rochester, NY 14611
INLINER mixers, LIGHTNIN mixers and agitators, MIXCO agitators. LAB MASTER small mixers pc-controlled mixers that record and display 8 processing parameters. LIGHTNIN BIOMIXERS pc-controlled mixers for use with closed vessels in aseptic applications. Record and display 8 processing parameters. Up to 32 mixers can be controlled by a single computer for scale-up or pilot processes.

Nalge Nunc International 800-625-4327
75 Panorama Creek Dr, Rochester, NY 14625
NALGENE magnetic stirrer for use with 10- and 20-L NALGENE carboys. Chemical resistant, high-purity PVDF shaft with TFE stir bar.

Nutech Molding Corporation 1-800-423-5278
PO Box 840, 2024 Broad St,, Pocomoke City, MD 21851

Phipps & Bird, Inc. 800-955-7621
1519 Summit Ave, Richmond, VA 23230
FLOC testing four or six paddle stirrers.

Scientific Industries, Inc. 888-850-6208
70 Orville Dr, Bohemia, NY 11716

Sienco, Inc. 800-432-1624
7985 Vance Dr Ste 104, Arvada, CO 80003
Ion/stir, portable battery operated mechanical stirrer for ion-specific and pH electrodes. No stir bars needed. $249.00 for battery powered, portable ion electrode unit, which does not heat the sample. Runs up to a month on a single, heavy-duty D size battery.

Thermo Fisher Scientific Inc. 563-556-2241
2555 Kerper Blvd, Dubuque, IA 52001

Troemner Llc 800-352-7705
201 Wolf Dr, PO Box 87, West Deptford, NJ 08086
$142.00 for Model 500.

STIRRUP *(Gastro/Urology) 78EYD*

Allen Medical Systems, Inc. 800-433-5774
1 Post Office Sq, Acton, MA 01720
Yellofin Stirrups, legholders for ob/gyn, urology, colorectal, and general surgery

Bryton Corp. 800-567-9500
4310 Guion Rd, Indianapolis, IN 46254
Wide range of leg support devices to accommodate all types of surgical procedures.

Health Supply Company Inc., The 770-452-0090
2902 Marlin Cir, Atlanta, GA 30341
Multisurgical procedure stirrups for general surgery (including low anterior and A/P resections), GU/Cysto procedures (including radical prostatectomy, cystectomy, TUR's, insertion of penile prosthesis), GYN procedures (including D & C, laser surgery, laparoscopy, A&P repair and vaginal hysterectomy, labor and delivery with proper adaptor for birthing bed or table). Set of two includes reusable Nelson decubitus pads and in-service. TKO Telescoping Stirrups.

Medrecon, Inc. 877-526-4323
257 South Ave, Garwood, NJ 07027

Northeast Medical Systems Corp. 856-910-8111
901 Beechwood Ave, Cherry Hill, NJ 08002
Pneumatic leg stirrups, single-control to adjust height, 360-degree rotation. Pediatric stirrups for urology tables.

STIRRUP *(cont'd)*

Phelan Manufacturing Corp. 800-328-2358
2523 Minnehaha Ave, Minneapolis, MN 55404
$1,165.00 for a pair of stirrups.

Profex Medical Products 800-325-0196
2224 E Person Ave, Memphis, TN 38114

Repro-Med Systems, Inc. 845-469-2042
24 Carpenter Rd, Chester, NY 10918

Rms Medical Products 800-624-9600
24 Carpenter Rd, Chester, NY 10918
GYNELOOP stirrups.

Rycor Medical, Inc. 800-227-9267
2053 Atwater Dr, North Port, FL 34288
Greenfield/Wan infant stirrups support small infants' feet and legs for urological and general surgery.

United Metal Fabricators, Inc. 800-638-5322
1316 Eisenhower Blvd, Johnstown, PA 15904
Vinyl clad unit.

STIRRUP, EXTERNAL BRACE COMPONENT
(Physical Med) 89ITC

Becker Orthopedic Appliance Co. 248-588-7480
635 Executive Dr, Troy, MI 48083
Various stirrup orthoses and orthosis components.

Brown Medical Industries 800-843-4395
1300 Lundberg Dr W, Spirit Lake, IA 51360
PRO GEL conforms to contour of maaeoli for comfort and support. Gel can be refrigerated for cold therapy.

Dj Orthopedics De Mexico, S.A. De C.V. 690-727-1280
Blvd., Delagacion La Presa, Tijuana 22397 Mexico
Ankle brace

Dj Orthopedics De Mexico, S.A. De C.V. 690-727-1280
Ave. Venustiano Carranza 6802, Castillo, Tijuana 22100 Mexico
Ankle brace

Inverse Technology Corp. 800-222-5778
1000 W O St Ste B, Lincoln, NE 68528
Various models of protonics.

Leeder Group, Inc. 305-436-5030
8508 NW 66th St, Miami, FL 33166
Sewho.

Mansfield Orthotic & Prosthetic Center, Inc. 419-522-4171
240 Marion Ave, Mansfield, OH 44903
External orthotic ankle joint.

Scott Orthotic Labs, Inc. 800-821-5795
1831 E Mulberry St, Fort Collins, CO 80524
Ankle joint for external ankle foot orthotic.

STOCKINETTE *(Orthopedics) 87RWH*

Albahealth Llc 800-262-2404
425 N Gateway Ave, Rockwood, TN 37854
ALBAHEALTH Sterile.

Bioseal 800-441-7325
167 W Orangethorpe Ave, Placentia, CA 92870
Sterile bias & tubular in various sizes.

Brecon Knitting Mills, Inc. 800-841-2821
PO Box 478, Talladega, AL 35161
Cotton, polyester blend.

Comfort Products, Inc. 800-822-7500
705 Linton Ave, Croydon, PA 19021
Nylon, cotton, aralon, spectralon - all sizes.

Custom Healthcare Systems, Inc. 804-421-5959
4205 Eubank Rd, Richmond, VA 23231

Dermapac, Inc. 203-924-7148
PO Box 852, Shelton, CT 06484
Procedural kits/packs. Custom kits.

Hermell Products, Inc. 800-233-2342
9 Britton Dr, PO Box 7345, Bloomfield, CT 06002

Johnson & Johnson Medical Division Of Ethicon, Inc. 800-423-4018
2500 E Arbrook Blvd, Arlington, TX 76014

Kerr Group 800-524-3577
1400 Holcomb Bridge Rd, Roswell, GA 30076

Knit-Rite, Inc. 800-821-3094
120 Osage Ave, Kansas City, KS 66105
COMPRESSOGRIP tubular stockinette.

STOCKINETTE *(cont'd)*

Lohmann & Rauscher, Inc. 800-279-3863
6001 SW 6th Ave Ste 101, Topeka, KS 66615

Maramed Orthopedic Systems 800-327-5830
2480 W 82nd St, No. 8, Hialeah, FL 33016

O&M Enterprise 847-258-4515
641 Chelmsford Ln, Elk Grove Village, IL 60007
STOKINETTE

Paramedical Distributors 800-245-3278
2020 Grand Blvd, Kansas City, MO 64108
Cosmetic stockings, Therafirm compression hose.

Qmd Medical 800-665-9950
9800 Clark St., Montreal, QUE H3L 2R3 Canada
Tubular Stockinette

Slawner Ltd., J. 514-731-3378
5713 Cote Des Neiges Rd., Montreal, QUE H3S 1Y7 Canada

Tetra Medical Supply Corp. 800-621-4041
6364 W Gross Point Rd, Niles, IL 60714

STOCKINETTE, CAST *(Orthopedics) 87QHB*

Albahealth Llc 800-262-2404
425 N Gateway Ave, Rockwood, TN 37854
COPLEX.

Brecon Knitting Mills, Inc. 800-841-2821
PO Box 478, Talladega, AL 35161

Bsn Medical, Inc 800-552-1157
5825 Carnegie Blvd, Charlotte, NC 28209
M-PACT® STOCKINETTE is available in cotton or synthetic. Designed to provide maximum patient comfort with plaster of synthetic casting material.

Comfort Products, Inc. 800-822-7500
705 Linton Ave, Croydon, PA 19021
Casting socks available in AK and BK.

Freeman Manufacturing Company 800-253-2091
900 W Chicago Rd, PO Box J, Sturgis, MI 49091

Kingsley Mfg. Co. 800-854-3479
1984 Placentia Ave, Costa Mesa, CA 92627

Paramedical Distributors 800-245-3278
2020 Grand Blvd, Kansas City, MO 64108
Compressiongrip compression stockinette, casting stockinette.

Zimmer Orthopaedic Surgical Products 800-321-5533
PO Box 10, 200 West Ohio Ave., Dover, OH 44622

STOCKING, ELASTIC *(General) 80FQL*

Beocare Inc., Hudson 353-643-9400
1905 International Blvd, Hudson, NC 28638
Antimicrobial, antifungal compression stocking.

Bio-Concepts, Inc. 202-772-5333
2424 E University Dr, Phoenix, AZ 85034
Elastic stocking.

Biomet, Inc. 574-267-6639
56 E Bell Dr, PO Box 587, Warsaw, IN 46582
Stockinette.

Bsn-Jobst 704-554-9933
5825 Carnegie Blvd, Charlotte, NC 28209
Elastic stocking.

Crocs, Inc. 801-455-8558
6328 Monarch Park Pl, Longmont, CO 80503
Diabetic stockings various sizes.

Delfi Medical Innovations Inc. 800-933-3022
Suite 106, 1099 West 8th Avenue, Vancouver, BC V6H 1C3 Canada
Various.

Dr. Len's Medical Products Llc 678-908-8180
412 Atwood Rd, Erdenheim, PA 19038
Support stockings.

Frank Stubbs Co., Inc 800-223-1713
2100 Eastman Ave Ste B, Oxnard, CA 93030
Neoprene support.

Gottfried Medical, Inc. 419-474-2973
4105 W Alexis Rd, Toledo, OH 43623
Made-to-measure surgical elastic supports.

Ita-Med Co. 888-9IT-AMED
310 Littlefield Ave, South San Francisco, CA 94080
GABRIALLA--complete range of pantyhose, thigh highs, knee highs, and men's socks available in several colors, many sizes, and five levels of compression.

STOCKING, ELASTIC *(cont'd)*

Juzo 800-222-4999
PO Box 1088, 80 Chart Road, Cuyahoga Falls, OH 44223
Various.

Kayser-Roth Corp. 336-547-4603
3707 W 5th St, Lumberton, NC 28358
Compression hosiery.

Kerma Medical Products, Inc. 757-398-8400
400 Port Centre Pkwy, Portsmouth, VA 23704
Compression bandage.

Medi Usa 800-633-6334
6481 Franz Warner Pkwy, Whitsett, NC 27377
A complete line of medical compression stockings for the treatment of all stages of venous disease.

Redwood Sportswear Ltd. 920-898-1919
1828 Park Ave, New Holstein, WI 53061

Renfro Corporation 336-719-8345
661 Linville Rd, Mount Airy, NC 27030
Various types of socks with cupron yarn.

Sigvaris Inc. 800-322-7744
1119 Highway 74 S, Peachtree City, GA 30269
SIGVARIS® medical compression stockings offer patients the most effective compression therapy available for treatment of veno-lymphatic disorders. Manufactured to strict specifications, stockings are offered in various fabrics, colors, and compression ranges.

Solaris, Inc. 414-918-9180
6737 W Washington St Ste 3260, West Allis, WI 53214
Edema garment.

The Kendrick Co., Inc.
6139 Germantown Ave, Philadelphia, PA 19144
Kenlastic accordion stitch.

Venosan North America, Inc. 800-432-5347
300 Industrial Park Ave, PO Box 1067, Asheboro, NC 27205
VENOSAN Full line of therapeutic, medical compression stockings. Men's and ladies' streetwear support stockings and socks. All styles and sizes with four compression classes of seamless stockings and armsleeves.

Web-Tex, Inc. 888-633-2723
5445 De Gaspe Ave., Ste. 702, Montreal, QC H2T 3B2 Canada

STOCKING, ELASTIC, PHYSICAL MEDICINE
(Physical Med) 89ILG

Biacare Corporation 616-931-1267
140 W Washington Ave Ste 100, Zeeland, MI 49464
Elastic stockinette.

Compression Design 616-931-1267
140 W Washington Ave Ste 200, Zeeland, MI 49464
Stocking, elastic.

Freeman Manufacturing Company 800-253-2091
900 W Chicago Rd, PO Box J, Sturgis, MI 49091
Therapeutic compression stockings in 4 compression classes.

Venosan North America, Inc. 800-432-5347
300 Industrial Park Ave, PO Box 1067, Asheboro, NC 27205
VENOSAN Full line of therapeutic, medical compression stockings. All styles and sizes with 4 compression classes of seamless stockings and armsleeves. Swiss and American made products.

STOCKING, SUPPORT (ANTI-EMBOLIC) *(General) 80DWL*

Albahealth Llc 800-262-2404
425 N Gateway Ave, Rockwood, TN 37854
C.A.R.E.; LIFE-SPAN, P.A.S., PULSTAR.

Barton-Carey Medical Products, Inc. 419-887-1285
460 5th St, Jellico, TN 37762
Stocking, medical support.

Bauerfeind Usa, Inc. 800-423-3405
55 Chastain Rd NW Ste 112, Kennesaw, GA 30144
Venotrain Hosiery Collection--stylish and effective, gradient-compression hosiery. Available in a variety of consumer preferred styles, colors and finishes.

Bsn-Jobst 704-554-9933
5825 Carnegie Blvd, Charlotte, NC 28209
Support stockings.

Dedicated Distribution 800-325-8367
640 Miami Ave, Kansas City, KS 66105
Support and T.E.D. hosiery

STOCKING, SUPPORT (ANTI-EMBOLIC) *(cont'd)*

DJO Inc. 800-336-6569
1430 Decision St, Vista, CA 92081
Anti-embolism stockings and supports.

Dumex Medical Surgical Products Ltd. 800-463-9613
104 Shorting Rd., Scarborough, ONT M1S 3S4 Canada
Venimax Compression hosiery: medical support stocking

Elastic Therapy, Inc. 800-849-2497
718 Industrial Park Ave, P.O. Box 4068, Asheboro, NC 27205
Men's and women's firm compression graduated support stockings; medical and surgical compression stockings. Prescription fit.

Freeman Manufacturing Company 800-253-2091
900 W Chicago Rd, PO Box J, Sturgis, MI 49091

Hermell Products, Inc. 800-233-2342
9 Britton Dr, PO Box 7345, Bloomfield, CT 06002
Tubular orthopedic stockinette.

Incappe, Inc. 601-638-2345
9 Ashland Ave, Brandon, MS 39047
Hydroboot.

Ivry 305-448-9858
216 Catalonia Ave Ste 106, Coral Gables, FL 33134

Kayser-Roth Corp. 336-547-4603
3707 W 5th St, Lumberton, NC 28358
No nonsense renew !.

Medi Mfg., Inc. 336-449-4440
6481 Franz Warner Pkwy, Whitsett, NC 27377
Compression stocking.

Paramedical Distributors 800-245-3278
2020 Grand Blvd, Kansas City, MO 64108
Full line of men's and women's Therafirm compression hose, socks, and pantyhose.

Tetra Medical Supply Corp. 800-621-4041
6364 W Gross Point Rd, Niles, IL 60714

Therafirm, A Knit Rite Company 800-562-2701
120 Osage Ave, Kansas City, KS 66105
Women's support and maternity support stockings and pantyhose, 15-25 mm Hg compression. Also, men's medium support socks and regular firm weight socks. Stocking support hi-compression 20-30 & 30-40 mm Hg uni-sex knee high, thigh high, panty hose, open & closed toe waist high (w/belt) one-leg. (Anti-Embolic) Hospital type thromboembolic deterrent, knee-high, thigh-high, inspection toe.

Truform Orthotics & Prosthetics 800-888-0458
3960 Rosslyn Dr, Cincinnati, OH 45209
Truform Brand Gradient Support Stockings, anti-embolism stockings and diabetic footcare stockings.

Wells Hosiery Mills, Inc. 336-633-4881
1758 S Fayetteville St, Asheboro, NC 27205
Various sizes and styles and anti embolism stockings.

Zimmer Holdings, Inc. 800-613-6131
1800 W Center St, PO Box 708, Warsaw, IN 46580

STOOL, ANESTHETIST'S *(Anesthesiology) 73BRX*

Armstrong Medical Industries, Inc. 800-323-4220
575 Knightsbridge Pkwy, Lincolnshire, IL 60069

Biofit Engineered Products 800-597-0246
PO Box 109, Waterville, OH 43566
18 models of conductive stools.

Blickman 800-247-5070
39 Robinson Rd, Lodi, NJ 07644
Clifton stainless steel stool is height adjustable from 19'-31'. Seat comes with your choice of recessed vinyl insert or padding. Circular heel rest and flared legs sit on rubber tips or 2' casters.

Cameron-Miller, Inc. 800-621-0142
5410 W Roosevelt Rd, Road #241, Chicago, IL 60644

Camtec 410-228-1156
1959 Church Creek Rd, Cambridge, MD 21613
Stool anesthesia.

Galaxy Medical Manufacturing Co. 800-876-4599
5411 Sheila St, Commerce, CA 90040

Imperial Surgical Ltd. 800-661-5432
581 Orly Ave., Dorval, ONT H9P-1G1 Canada
Various models available.

Lic Care 800-323-5232
2935A Northeast Pkwy, Atlanta, GA 30360

STOOL, BEDSIDE *(General) 80RWJ*

Brewer Company, The 888-873-9371
N88W13901 Main St, Menomonee Falls, WI 53051

STOOL, BEDSIDE *(cont'd)*

Galaxy Medical Manufacturing Co. 800-876-4599
5411 Sheila St, Commerce, CA 90040
Bedside and step stools.

HAAG-STREIT USA, INC. 800-787-5426
3535 Kings Mills Rd, Mason, OH 45040

Lic Care 800-323-5232
2935A Northeast Pkwy, Atlanta, GA 30360

Ppr Direct, Inc. 800-526-3668
74 20th St, Brooklyn, NY 11232
Rolling 3-legged stool.

STOOL, DENTAL *(Dental And Oral) 76RWK*

Dansereau Health Products, Inc. 800-423-5657
250 E Harrison St, Corona, CA 92879
America Value Line Combo: Dentist & Assistant Seating $425.00 (both)

Dentalez Group 866-DTE-INFO
101 Lindenwood Dr Ste 225, Valleybrooke Corporate Center
Malvern, PA 19355

Dentsply Canada, Ltd. 800-263-1437
161 Vinyl Ct., Woodbridge, ONT L4L 4A3 Canada

Forest Dental Products Inc 800-423-3535
6200 NE Campus Ct, Hillsboro, OR 97124

Galaxy Medical Manufacturing Co. 800-876-4599
5411 Sheila St, Commerce, CA 90040

Health Science Products, Inc. 800-237-5794
1489 Hueytown Rd, Hueytown, AL 35023
Ergonomically designed dental, doctor and assistant stools for proper support and maximum comfort.

Midmark Corporation 800-643-6275
60 Vista Dr, P.O. Box 286, Versailles, OH 45380

Pelton & Crane Co., 704-588-2126
11727 Fruehauf Dr, Charlotte, NC 28273
SPIRIT 2000

Planmeca U.S.A. Inc 630-529-2300
100 Gary Ave Ste A, Roselle, IL 60172
PLANMECA Stools

Royal Dental Manufacturing, Inc. 425-743-0988
12414 Highway 99, Everett, WA 98204
$510.00 for operator Model RO2; $640.00 for Ergonomic Operator Model RO4/RO44; $570.00 for assistant Model RA2/RA24;$670.00 Domain 2110 Ergonomic Operator Stool. $600.00 Domain 2120 Assistant Stool; $840.00 Domain 2130 Operator Stool; $940.00 Domain 2140 Assistant Stool.

Sds (Summit Dental Systems) 800-275-3368
3560 NW 53rd Ct, Fort Lauderdale, FL 33309

United Metal Fabricators, Inc. 800-638-5322
1316 Eisenhower Blvd, Johnstown, PA 15904

STOOL, EXERCISE *(Physical Med) 89RWL*

Brandt Industries, Inc. 800-221-8031
4461 Bronx Blvd, Bronx, NY 10470
Treatment stools, skates.

Hausmann Industries, Inc. 888-428-7626
130 Union St, Northvale, NJ 07647
$152.00 per unit (standard).

STOOL, OPERATING ROOM, ADJUSTABLE *(Surgery) 79FZM*

Advantage Medical Systems, Inc. 800-810-1262
2876 S Wheeling Way, Aurora, CO 80014
Surgical stool.

Allergan 800-366-6554
2525 Dupont Dr, Irvine, CA 92612
Electric, hydraulic or manually adjustable stools.

Biofit Engineered Products 800-597-0246
PO Box 109, Waterville, OH 43566
34 models.

Blickman 800-247-5070
39 Robinson Rd, Lodi, NJ 07644
Adjustable and pneumatic stools including foot-operated models sit on a five leg 24' diameter cast aluminum base with Wall Savers to protect against scuffmarks and provide a foot grip. Travel on 2' twin wheel hooded casters.Choose from 32 colors. Optional backrest and foot ring.

Brandt Industries, Inc. 800-221-8031
4461 Bronx Blvd, Bronx, NY 10470
Various models

STOOL, OPERATING ROOM, ADJUSTABLE *(cont'd)*

Dexta Corporation 800-733-3982
962 Kaiser Rd, Napa, CA 94558
$600 for foot-operated unit.

Galaxy Medical Manufacturing Co. 800-876-4599
5411 Sheila St, Commerce, CA 90040

HAAG-STREIT USA, INC. 800-787-5426
3535 Kings Mills Rd, Mason, OH 45040
$775.00 for hydraulic stool for micro and laser surgery and $165 and $247 for pneumatic stool.

Hill-Rom, Inc. 812-934-7777
4115 Dorchester Rd Unit 600, North Charleston, SC 29405
Stool.

Imperial Surgical Ltd. 800-661-5432
581 Orly Ave., Dorval, ONT H9P-1G1 Canada
$490 per unit.

Jedmed Instruments Co. 314-845-3770
5416 Jedmed Ct, Saint Louis, MO 63129
Hydraulic with pneumatic foot; hand-operated unit also available.

Keeler Instruments Inc. 800-523-5620
456 Park Way, Broomall, PA 19008
$1,495.00 per unit.

Medical Technology Industries, Inc. 800-924-4655
3555 W 1500 S, Salt Lake City, UT 84104
Exam and surgery stools.

Midmark Corporation 800-643-6275
60 Vista Dr, P.O. Box 286, Versailles, OH 45380

Mobile Dental Equipment Corp.(M-Dec) 425-747-5424
13300 SE 30th St Ste 101, Bellevue, WA 98005
Portable operator's stool. $560.00.

Pedigo Products 360-695-3500
4000 SE Columbia Way, Vancouver, WA 98661
Various styles, chrome or stainless steel.

Stryker Medical 800-869-0770
3800 E Centre Ave, Portage, MI 49002

Surge Medical Solutions, Llc. 616-977-2516
3710 Sysco Ct SE, Grand Rapids, MI 49512
Stool, operating-room.

United Metal Fabricators, Inc. 800-638-5322
1316 Eisenhower Blvd, Johnstown, PA 15904
Air spring or threaded stem height adjustments. 4 or 5 leg base with optional foot ring and back rest. Height adjustable by screw stem or automatic gas spring.

Winco, Inc. 800-237-3377
5516 SW 1st Ln, Ocala, FL 34474
Chairs.

STOPCOCK *(General) 80FMG*

Ac Healthcare Supply, Inc. 905-448-4706
11651 230th St, Cambria Heights, NY 11411
Plastic disposable non-sterile stop cock.

B. Braun Medical, Inc. 610-596-2536
901 Marcon Blvd, Allentown, PA 18109
OTHER; DISCOFIX

B. Braun Oem Division, B. Braun Medical Inc. 866-8-BBRAUN
824 12th Ave, Bethlehem, PA 18018

B. Braun Of Puerto Rico, Inc. 610-691-5400
215.7 Insular Rd., Sabana Grande, PR 00637
Iv set stopcock.

Baxter Healthcare Corporporation, Alternate Care And Channel Team 888-229-0001
25212 W Il Route 120, Round Lake, IL 60073

Baxter Healthcare S.A. 847-948-2000
Rd. 721, Km. 0.3, Aibonito, PR 00609
Various stopcocks.

Berghof/America 800-544-5004
3773 NW 126th Ave Bldg 1, Coral Springs, FL 33065
PTFs, various types & sizes

Cadence Science Inc. 888-717-7677
1979 Marcus Ave Ste 215, New Hyde Park, NY 11042
Metal stopcocks in 30 sizes.

Churchill Medical Systems, Inc. 800-468-0585
935 Horsham Rd Ste M, Horsham, PA 19044

Cook Inc. 800-457-4500
PO Box 489, Bloomington, IN 47402

STOPCOCK *(cont'd)*

Covidien Lp 508-261-8000
15 Hampshire St, Mansfield, MA 02048

David Scott Company 800-804-0333
59 Fountain St, Framingham, MA 01702

Directmed, Inc. 516-656-3377
150 Pratt Oval, Glen Cove, NY 11542

Edwards Lifesciences Technology Sarl 949-250-2500
State Rd. 402 N.km 1.4, Anasco, PR 00610-1577
Stopcock, i.v. set.

Elcam Medical, Inc. 800-530-2441
2 University Plz Ste 620, Hackensack, NJ 07601

Engineers Express, Inc. 800-255-8823
7 Industrial Park Rd, Medway, MA 02053

Ernst Flow Industries 800-992-2843
116 Main St, Farmingdale, NJ 07727

Farmatap S.A. De C.V.
117 Alfonso Esparza Oteo, Mexico Df 01020 Mexico
No common name listed

Hospira Inc. 877-946-7747
275 N Field Dr, Lake Forest, IL 60045
MULTIPLE

Hospira, Inc. 877-946-7747
755 Jarvis Dr, Morgan Hill, CA 95037
INTRALOCK disposable stopcock.

Icu Medical (Ut), Inc 949-366-2183
4455 Atherton Dr, Salt Lake City, UT 84123
Intravascular administrtion set.

Icu Medical, Inc. 800-824-7890
951 Calle Amanecer, San Clemente, CA 92673
Intravascular administration set.

Interpore Cross International 800-722-4489
181 Technology Dr, Irvine, CA 92618
Ultraconcentrator manifold with extension set. Graft delivery syringe. Disposable system for intraoperative collection of autologous growth factors.

Kentron Health Care, Inc. 615-384-0573
3604 Kelton Jackson Rd, P.o. Box 120, Springfield, TN 37172
Stopcocks and iv sets.

Kontes Glass Co. 888-546-2531
1022 Spruce St, Vineland, NJ 08360

Merit Medical Systems, Inc. 801-253-1600
1111 S Velasco St, Angleton, TX 77515
Various types of stopcocks with luer lock adapters.

Mps Acacia 800-486-6677
785 Challenger St, Brea, CA 92821

Novosci Corp. 281-363-4949
2828 N Crescentridge Dr, The Woodlands, TX 77381

S4j Manufacturing Services, Inc. 888-S4J-LUER
2685 NE 9th Ave, Cape Coral, FL 33909

Smiths Medical Asd, Inc. 800-848-1757
6250 Shier Rings Rd, Dublin, OH 43016
HYPERAL stopcock, extension sets and T-connector.

Sorin Group Usa 800-289-5759
14401 W 65th Way, Arvada, CO 80004

Terumo Medical Corporation 800-283-7866
950 Elkton Blvd, P.O.Box 605, Elkton, MD 21921
Three way stopcock.

Vygon Corp. 800-544-4907
2495 General Armistead Ave, Norristown, PA 19403
Disposable stopcocks.

STOPPER *(General) 80WNN*

Berghof/America 800-544-5004
3773 NW 126th Ave Bldg 1, Coral Springs, FL 33065
PTFE Type S for glass joints, type F for flask lengths. Solid and hollow PTFE stoppers also available for test tubes.

Csi International, Inc. 303-795-8273
4301 S Federal Blvd Ste 116, Englewood, CO 80110
Stopper needle.

Hospira 800-441-4100
268 E 4th St, Ashland, OH 44805
Drug vial stoppers.

Jaece Industries, Inc. 716-694-2811
908 Niagara Falls Blvd, North Tonawanda, NY 14120
IDENTI-PLUGS, foam stoppers, diameter: 6 - 75 mm.

STOPPER *(cont'd)*

Plasticoid Co., The 410-398-2800
249 W High St, Elkton, MD 21921

RamÇ-Hart, Inc. 973-448-0305
95 Allen St, PO Box 400, Netcong, NJ 07857
Syringe stoppering system, auto-device to vacuum and stopper syringes.

Simport Plastics Ltd. 450-464-1723
2588 Bernard-Pilon, Beloeil, QUE J3G 4S5 Canada

Ware Medics Glass Works, Inc. 845-429-6950
PO Box 368, Garnerville, NY 10923

West Pharmaceutical Services, Inc. 800-231-3000
101 Gordon Dr, Franklin Ctr, PA 19341
Pharmaceutical serum and lyophilization stoppers.

STORAGE DEVICE, FLUOROSCOPIC IMAGE *(Radiology) 90VGY*

Imsi, Integrated Modular Systems Inc. 800-220-9729
2500 W Township Line Rd, PO Box 616, Havertown, PA 19083
i2ARM DICOM ARCHIVE. Any DICOM image may be archived and viewed with TeleRad and PACS. Extremely Cost Effective.

Stallion Technologies, Inc. 315-476-4330
1201 E Fayette St, Syracuse, NY 13210

STORAGE UNIT, X-RAY FILM *(Radiology) 90UAB*

Alimed, Inc. 800-225-2610
297 High St, Dedham, MA 02026

AMD Technologies Inc. 800-423-3535
218 Bronwood Ave, Los Angeles, CA 90049

Bar-Ray Products, Inc. 800-359-6115
95 Monarch St, Littlestown, PA 17340

Budget Buddy Company, Inc. 800-208-3375
PO Box 590, Belton, MO 64012

Carr Corporation 800-952-2398
1547 11th St, Santa Monica, CA 90401

Cone Instruments, Inc. 800-321-6964
5201 Naiman Pkwy, Solon, OH 44139

Flow X-Ray Corporation 800-356-9729
100 W Industry Ct, Deer Park, NY 11729

Hale Imaging Systems, Inc. 800-321-4253
5314 Mill St, P.O. Box 184, Orient, OH 43146
FILE 14, bankers' box style x-ray film storage box that holds up to 300 14x17 films in envelopes.

Imsi, Integrated Modular Systems Inc. 800-220-9729
2500 W Township Line Rd, PO Box 616, Havertown, PA 19083
Digitize and Store. Fast, Easy and Cost Effecitive. Viewing systems also available. DICOM Archive and Digitizer complete for under $30K.

Marconi Medical Systems 800-323-0550
595 Miner Rd, Cleveland, OH 44143

Mcdalt Medical Corp. 800-841-5774
2225 Prestonwood Dr Ste 100-A, Arlington, TX 76012
Medical Design System, 'MASS', complete line of Custom Storage Cabinets for Cath Labs, Radiology, ENDO, Surgery.

Medirecord Systems 800-561-9791
P.O. Box 6201 Station A, Saint John, NB E2L 4R6 Canada
X-ray bags and inserts, x-ray mobile work center and records file equipment.

Negafile Systems 800-523-5474
1560 Industry Rd, Hatfield, PA 19440

Rem Systems 305-499-4800
625 E 10th Ave, Hialeah, FL 33010
BSR Archival 15 inch shelve model and 18 inch shelve model.

S&S Technology 281-815-1300
10625 Telge Rd, Houston, TX 77095
Open steel shelving; vertifiles with or without doors.

Schueler & Company, Inc. 516-487-1500
PO Box 528, Stratford, CT 06615

Smead Manufacturing Co. 1-88-USE-SMEAD
600 Smead Blvd, Hastings, MN 55033
X-ray color coded envelopes.

Spacesaver Corporation 800-492-3434
1450 Janesville Ave, Fort Atkinson, WI 53538
PHARMASTOR, high density mobile storage systems.

Stackbin Corporation 800-333-1603
29 Powder Hill Rd, Lincoln, RI 02865
Stackfiles for storage of medical records or x-rays; combination units also available.

STORAGE UNIT, X-RAY FILM *(cont'd)*

Wolf X-Ray Corporation 800-356-9729
100 W Industry Ct, Deer Park, NY 11729

STRAP, CLAVICLE *(Orthopedics) 87RWP*

Alimed, Inc. 800-225-2610
297 High St, Dedham, MA 02026

Corflex, Inc. 800-426-7353
669 E Industrial Park Dr, Manchester, NH 03109

Formedica Ltd. 800-361-9671
1481 Rue Begin, St Laurent, QUE H4R 1V8 Canada
$7.00 per unit (med).

Mizuho Osi 800-777-4674
30031 Ahern Ave, Union City, CA 94587

Paramedical Distributors 800-245-3278
2020 Grand Blvd, Kansas City, MO 64108

Zimmer Holdings, Inc. 800-613-6131
1800 W Center St, PO Box 708, Warsaw, IN 46580

STRAP, ELECTRODE *(General) 80QSN*

Elmed, Inc. 630-543-2792
60 W Fay Ave, Addison, IL 60101

STRAP, HEAD, GAS MASK *(Anesthesiology) 73BTK*

Ac Healthcare Supply, Inc. 905-448-4706
11651 230th St, Cambria Heights, NY 11411
Gas mask head strap.

Advanced Circulatory Systems, Inc. 952-947-9590
7615 Golden Triangle Dr Ste A, Eden Prairie, MN 55344
Gas mask head strap.

Corpak Medsystems, Inc. 800-323-6305
100 Chaddick Dr, Wheeling, IL 60090
Head strap.

Eastmed Enterprises, Inc. 856-797-0131
11 Brandywine Dr, Marlton, NJ 08053
Various types of head harnesses.

Sharn, Inc. 800-325-3671
4517 George Rd Ste 200, Tampa, FL 33634

Smiths Medical Asd Inc. 800-258-5361
10 Bowman Dr, Keene, NH 03431
Various sizes of gas mask head strapes.

Sunmed Healthcare 727-531-7266
12393 Belcher Rd S Ste 460, Largo, FL 33773

The Saunders Group 800-445-9836
4250 Norex Dr, Chaska, MN 55318
Various sizes and uses.

STRAP, RESTRAINING *(General) 80RWQ*

Alimed, Inc. 800-225-2610
297 High St, Dedham, MA 02026

Aplix, Inc. 704-588-1920
12300 Steele Creek Rd, Charlotte, NC 28273
Hooks & loops.

Armstrong Medical Industries, Inc. 800-323-4220
575 Knightsbridge Pkwy, Lincolnshire, IL 60069

Bryton Corp. 800-567-9500
4310 Guion Rd, Indianapolis, IN 46254
Wide variety of restraint straps for surgical, orthopedic, urological and obstetrical tables. Restraint straps available in cotton, nylon, and electrically conductive rubber.

Fpp, Inc. 352-622-4595
6800 SW 66th St, Ocala, FL 34476
Disposable and reusable armboard straps.

Mizuho Osi 800-777-4674
30031 Ahern Ave, Union City, CA 94587
Patient positioning straps for OR tables.

Morrison Medical 800-438-6677
3735 Paragon Dr, Columbus, OH 43228
BEST STRAP strapping restraint system for ambulance cot. One complete system for total restraint in one. Also available Stretcher Straps Miscellanous which is an impervious webbing material (universal precaution) that is available in any style of many assorted buckles and end styles that are now available in a material that can be disinfected.

North Coast Medical, Inc. 800-821-9319
18305 Sutter Blvd, Morgan Hill, CA 95037
Comfort Cool Thumb CMC Restoration Splint.

STRAP, RESTRAINING *(cont'd)*

Ooltewah Manufacturing 800-251-6040x25
5722 Main St, P.O. Box 587, Ooltewah, TN 37363

Optp 888-819-0121
3800 Annapolis Ln N Ste 165, PO Box 47009, Minneapolis, MN 55447
$132.30 for set of 3 pcs. of POSITEX mobilization straps.

Profex Medical Products 800-325-0196
2224 E Person Ave, Memphis, TN 38114

Rapid Deployment Products 877-433-7569
157 Railroad Dr, Ivyland, PA 18974

Xodus Medical, Inc. 800-963-8776
702 Prominence Dr, Westmoreland Business & Research Park
New Kensington, PA 15068
O.R. Positioning Straps

STRAP, TRACHEOSTOMY TUBE *(Anesthesiology) 73VDM*

Dhd Healthcare Corporation 800-847-8000
PO Box 6, One Madison Street, Wampsville, NY 13163
DHD Tracheostomy Straps

Marpac Inc. 800-334-6413
8436 Washington Pl NE, Albuquerque, NM 87113
Marpac Tracheostomy collars comfortably secure tracheostomy tubes. Composed of a latex free, soft, breathable neckband and easy Velco adjustment tabs. One piece, 'Perfect Fit' collars come in boxes of 25 or 100. Two piece, 'One Size Fits All' collars come in boxes of 10 or 100.

STREPTOLYSIN O *(Pathology) 88IBA*

Bd Diagnostic Systems 800-675-0908
7 Loveton Cir, Sparks, MD 21152

Biomerieux Inc. 800-682-2666
100 Rodolphe St, Durham, NC 27712

Sa Scientific, Inc. 800-272-2710
4919 Golden Quail, San Antonio, TX 78240
Latex slide test.

STRETCHER, BASKET, PORTABLE *(General) 80VLO*

Armstrong Medical Industries, Inc. 800-323-4220
575 Knightsbridge Pkwy, Lincolnshire, IL 60069

Ferno-Washington, Inc. 800-733-3766
70 Weil Way, Wilmington, OH 45177

STRETCHER, COLLAPSIBLE *(General) 80WKO*

Armstrong Medical Industries, Inc. 800-323-4220
575 Knightsbridge Pkwy, Lincolnshire, IL 60069

International Hospital Supply Co. 800-398-9450
6914 Canby Ave Ste 105, Reseda, CA 91335

Protector Canada Inc. 800-268-6594
1111 Flint Rd., Unit 23, Toronto, ON M3J 3C7 Canada
Folding stretchers made of aluminum.

STRETCHER, EMERGENCY, OTHER *(General) 80WIG*

Armstrong Medical Industries, Inc. 800-323-4220
575 Knightsbridge Pkwy, Lincolnshire, IL 60069

Ferno-Washington, Inc. 800-733-3766
70 Weil Way, Wilmington, OH 45177

Florida Life Systems 727-321-9554
3446 5th Ave N, Saint Petersburg, FL 33713
Stretchers.

Iron Duck, A Div. Of Fleming Industries, Inc. 800-669-6900
20 Veterans Dr, Chicopee, MA 01022
Stretcher straps.

Mayo Medical, S.A. De C.V. 800-715-3872
Edison 1141 Nte., Col. Talleres, Monterrey N.L. 64480 Mexico

Nk Medical Products Inc. 800-274-2742
10123 Main St, PO Box 627, Clarence, NY 14031
Trauma/ICU transfer stretcher.

Rapid Deployment Products 877-433-7569
157 Railroad Dr, Ivyland, PA 18974
Pro-Lite Pedi-Lite pediatric spineboard - No rods, runners or rails, 100% X-Ray Translucent, Foam filled for flotation & patient insulation, Concave design for perfect patient centering & less deflection/warpage, Carrying case, head blocks, straps, and C-Collar included in PEDI-LITE Kit.

Schueler & Company, Inc. 516-487-1500
PO Box 528, Stratford, CT 06615

Skedco, Inc. 503-639-2119
16420 SW 72nd Ave, PO Box 230487, Portland, OR 97224
SKED portable, backpack-type emergency stretcher for aerial, vertical, water and confined space rescue.

STRETCHER, HAND-CARRIED *(General) 80FPP*

Access Now Llc 800-351-8375
1337 Burns Ave, Iowa City, IA 52240
Transfer sling to move people with disabilities and injuries from one location to another.

Amelife Llc 302-476-2631
702 N West St Ste 101, Wilmington, DE 19801

Anatomic Concepts, Inc. 951-549-6800
1691 N Delilah St, Corona, CA 92879
Stretcher pad.

Arizona Industries For The Blind 602-269-5131
3013 W Lincoln St Dept Economicsecurity, Phoenix, AZ 85009
Folding rigid pole aluminum litter (NSN#6530-01-380-7309) for the transport of injured patients and during emergency resonse situations. Designed for use by the military, emergency responders, homeland security response

Armstrong Medical Industries, Inc. 800-323-4220
575 Knightsbridge Pkwy, Lincolnshire, IL 60069

Bruin Plastics Co. 800-556-7764
61 Joslin Rd, Glendale, RI 02826

Chair Care-Mobile Cot, Inc. 803-564-3698
6241 Wagener Rd, Wagener, SC 29164
Stretcher, hand carried.

Descent Control Systems, Inc. 801-304-9299
8100 S 1300 W Ste D, West Jordan, UT 84088
Stair chair.

Dixie Ems Supply 800-347-3494
385 Union Ave, Brooklyn, NY 11211
$950.00 per 10 (med).

E-Z Sales & Manufacturing Inc. 310-324-5980
1432 W 166th St, Gardena, CA 90247
Stretcher.

Emergency Products And Research 305-304-6933
890 W Main St, Kent, OH 44240
Spineboard.

Farley Inc., W.T. 800-327-5397
931 Via Alondra, Camarillo, CA 93012
Adapts gurneys for easier transport and to hold ancillary equipment; $160 for aluminum oxygen manifold sytems, $50 for aluminum IV pole, $100 for oxygen cylinder holder for gurney.

Ferno-Washington, Inc. 800-733-3766
70 Weil Way, Wilmington, OH 45177

Formed Plastics, Inc. 516-334-2300
207 Stonehinge Ln, Carle Place, NY 11514
Spineboard.

General Scientific Safety Equipment Co. 800-523-0166
2553 E Somerset St Fl 1, Philadelphia, PA 19134

Henley Board, Inc. 301-831-6662
213 Crabb Ave, Rockville, MD 20850
Spine board, backboard, spinal immob.device.

Junkin Safety Appliance Co., Inc. 502-775-8303
3121 Millers Ln, Louisville, KY 40216
Strecher.

Kentron Health Care, Inc. 615-384-0573
3604 Kelton Jackson Rd, P.o. Box 120, Springfield, TN 37172
Hand carried stretcher.

Lifesaving Systems Corp. 813-645-2748
220 Elsberry Rd, Apollo Beach, FL 33572
Rescue litter.

Mayo Medical, S.A. De C.V. 800-715-3872
Edison 1141 Nte., Col. Talleres, Monterrey N.L. 64480 Mexico

Medex Para-Medical Equipment Inc. 450-581-3966
275 Boul Pierre-Legardeur, Le Gardeur J5Z 3A7 Canada
Stretcher (hand-carried)

Meza Medical Equipment 888-308-7116
108 W Nakoma St, San Antonio, TX 78216

Mine Safety Appliances Company 866-MSA-1001
121 Gamma Dr, Pittsburgh, PA 15238

Minto R&D, Inc. 530-222-2373
20270 Charlanne Dr, Redding, CA 96002
$340.00 model B-101 breakaway flat, $472.00 model B-104 maxi breakaway flat.

Patient Transfer Systems, Inc. 800-633-4725
5456 Northwood Dr, Center Valley, PA 18034
Patient transfer unit.

STRETCHER, HAND-CARRIED *(cont'd)*

Rapid Deployment Products 877-433-7569
157 Railroad Dr, Ivyland, PA 18974
Seamless design prevents fluids from entering and eliminates cross-contamination, With the unique design, two boards can be stored together in less than 4' of space, Foot section is angled slightly downward to assist rescuer in auto extrication, Compatible with all head immobilization devices, 100% guarantee of workmanship, Available with or without speed clip pins. Three styles to choose from.

Reeves Emergency Management Systems, Llc. 301-698-1596
1704 W 7th St, Frederick, MD 21702
Stretcher or litter.

Rockford Medical & Safety Co. 800-435-9451
2420 Harrison Ave, PO Box 5646, Rockford, IL 61108

Simulaids, Inc. 800-431-4310
16 Simulaids Dr, PO Box 1289, Saugerties, NY 12477
Flexible soft stretcher for stair chair or ladder.

Skedco, Inc. 503-639-2119
16420 SW 72nd Ave, PO Box 230487, Portland, OR 97224
SKED portable, backpack-type emergency stretcher rescue system for water, aerial, vertical and confined space rescue. Mass casualty/HAZ-MAT decontaminable SKED (HMD) stretcher for evacuation of patients from contaminated areas and mass-casualty evacuation of mass casualties.

Spectrum Products Usa 800-338-7581
3701 W Roanoke Ave, Phoenix, AZ 85009
Kwik strap.

Surge Medical Solutions, Llc. 616-977-2516
3710 Sysco Ct SE, Grand Rapids, MI 49512
Stretcher.

Symphony Medical Products 877-470-9995
6320 NW 84th Ave, Miami, FL 33166
Hand carrier stretcher.

Weevac, W. Murphy Enterprises, Inc. 613-584-9473
12 La Salle Dr., P.O. Box 1306, Deep River, ONT K0J 1P0 Canada
Portable rescue stretcher

STRETCHER, HYDRAULIC *(General) 80TEW*

A.R.C. Distributors 800-296-8724
PO Box 599, Centreville, MD 21617
GENDRON EASY ACCESS Hydraulic stretcher, Trendelenburg/Reverse. Extra wide mattress, tuck away side rails, Fowler assisted backrest. Trendelenburg/Reverse has self-storing IV pole and oxygen cylinder holder, dual side mount foot pedal, full length side rails and corner bumper, all surface casters. Series 2100 Hydraulic Elevate and Trendelenburg; Series 1200 Hydraulic Trendelenburg; Series 700 Hydraulic Trendelenburg/Pediatric.

Arjo, Inc. 800-323-1245
50 Gary Ave Ste A, Roselle, IL 60172

Hill-Rom Holdings, Inc. 800-445-3730
1069 State Road 46 E, Batesville, IN 47006

Lic Care 800-323-5232
2935A Northeast Pkwy, Atlanta, GA 30360
Fixed or variable height.

Schueler & Company, Inc. 516-487-1500
PO Box 528, Stratford, CT 06615

Stryker Medical 800-869-0770
3800 E Centre Ave, Portage, MI 49002

STRETCHER, ORTHOPEDIC *(Orthopedics) 87TEX*

Assisted Access-Nfss, Inc. 800-950-9655
822 Preston Ct, Lake Villa, IL 60046

Ferno-Washington, Inc. 800-733-3766
70 Weil Way, Wilmington, OH 45177

Hartwell Medical Corp. 800-633-5900
6352 Corte Del Abeto Ste J, Carlsbad, CA 92011
The COMBICARRIER is a split litter and a spineboard. Molded polyethylene with foam filling provides unique full-body immobilization that minimizes patient movement during application. Used for those with back, hip, and pelvis injuries, as well as for other trauma victims.

STRETCHER, PATIENT RESTRAINT *(General) 80NZD*

Amelife Llc 302-476-2631
702 N West St Ste 101, Wilmington, DE 19801

STRETCHER, RADIOGRAPHIC *(Radiology) 90TEY*

Composiflex, Inc. 800-673-2544
8100 Hawthorne Dr, Erie, PA 16509
Low absorption, carbon fiber radiographic stretcher tops.

Stryker Medical 800-869-0770
3800 E Centre Ave, Portage, MI 49002

Vermont Composites, Inc. 802-442-9964
25 Performance Dr, Bennington, VT 05201
Low absorption carbon stretcher.

STRETCHER, TRANSFER *(Surgery) 79FSL*

A.R.C. Distributors 800-296-8724
PO Box 599, Centreville, MD 21617
GENDRON, Prone Stretcher Cart self propelled stretcher with pad. GENDRON Series 600 stretcher folding transfer and emergency. Series1100 heavy duty transfer and emergency. Series 1000 general transfer and transport.

Armstrong Medical Industries, Inc. 800-323-4220
575 Knightsbridge Pkwy, Lincolnshire, IL 60069

Birkova Products 888-567-4502
809 4th St, Gothenburg, NE 69138
Stretchers, replacement stretcher mattresses or pads, transfer devices, and more.

Calmaquip Engineering Corp. 305-592-4510
7240 NW 12th St, Miami, FL 33126

David Scott Company 800-804-0333
59 Fountain St, Framingham, MA 01702
Patient slider allows easy transfer from one surface to another bed, stretcher, x-ray, or table.

Gendron, Inc. 800-537-2521
400 E Lugbill Rd, Archbold, OH 43502
$684.00 per unit (standard).

Hill-Rom Holdings, Inc. 800-445-3730
1069 State Road 46 E, Batesville, IN 47006

Ibiom Instruments Ltd. 450-678-5468
6640 Barry St., Brossard, QUE J4Z 1T8 Canada
ECHOFLEX. Ergonomic stretcher for ultrasound.

Imperial Surgical Ltd. 800-661-5432
581 Orly Ave., Dorval, ONT H9P-1G1 Canada
$1300 per unit.

International Hospital Supply Co. 800-398-9450
6914 Canby Ave Ste 105, Reseda, CA 91335

Lic Care 800-323-5232
2935A Northeast Pkwy, Atlanta, GA 30360

Md International, Inc. 305-669-9003
11300 NW 41st St, Doral, FL 33178

Nk Medical Products Inc. 800-274-2742
10123 Main St, PO Box 627, Clarence, NY 14031

Pedigo Products 360-695-3500
4000 SE Columbia Way, Vancouver, WA 98661
Fixed height, various accessories available.

Rockford Medical & Safety Co. 800-435-9451
2420 Harrison Ave, PO Box 5646, Rockford, IL 61108

Schueler & Company, Inc. 516-487-1500
PO Box 528, Stratford, CT 06615

Servicios Paraclinicos S.A. 83-33-8400
Madero No. 3330 Pte., Monterrey N.L. 64020 Mexico

Stryker Medical 800-869-0770
3800 E Centre Ave, Portage, MI 49002

Wy'East Medical Corp. 503-657-3101
16700 SE 120th Ave, PO Box 1625, Clackamas, OR 97015
TOTALIFT-250 Transfer Stretcher.

STRETCHER, WHEELED (MOBILE) *(General) 80FPO*

Alimed, Inc. 800-225-2610
297 High St, Dedham, MA 02026

Amelife Llc 302-476-2631
702 N West St Ste 101, Wilmington, DE 19801

Arjo, Inc. 800-323-1245
50 Gary Ave Ste A, Roselle, IL 60172

Armstrong Medical Industries, Inc. 800-323-4220
575 Knightsbridge Pkwy, Lincolnshire, IL 60069

Atlantic Medco, Inc. 800-203-8444
166 Bloomfield Ave, Verona, NJ 07044
$800.00 to $1,500.00.

STRETCHER, WHEELED (MOBILE) *(cont'd)*

Bay Shore Medical Equipment Corp. 631-586-1991
235 S Fehr Way, Bay Shore, NY 11706
Multiple.

Biodex Medical Systems, Inc. 800-224-6339
20 Ramsey Rd, Shirley, NY 11967
Non-magnetic for dedicated MRI use.

Cameron-Miller, Inc. 800-621-0142
5410 W Roosevelt Rd, Road #241, Chicago, IL 60644

Camtec 410-228-1156
1959 Church Creek Rd, Cambridge, MD 21613
Transportation stretcher.

Care Products Inc. 757-224-0177
10701 N Ware Rd, McAllen, TX 78504
Shower/transport gurney.

Chair Care-Mobile Cot, Inc. 803-564-3698
6241 Wagener Rd, Wagener, SC 29164
Stretcher, wheeled ambulance.

Descent Control Systems, Inc. 801-304-9299
8100 S 1300 W Ste D, West Jordan, UT 84088
Stretcher track device.

Dixie Ems Supply 800-347-3494
385 Union Ave, Brooklyn, NY 11211
$580.00 per unit (standard).

Duralife, Inc. 800-443-5433
195 Phillips Park Dr, Williamsport, PA 17702

Emergencia 2000, Inc. 757-224-0177
8160 NW 66th St, Miami, FL 33166
Medical devices: stretcher.

Ferno-Washington, Inc. 800-733-3766
70 Weil Way, Wilmington, OH 45177

Future Health Concept's, Inc. 407-322-3672
1211 E 30th St, Sanford, FL 32773
Stretcher.

Gendron, Inc. 800-537-2521
400 E Lugbill Rd, Archbold, OH 43502
From $656 to $2,432 for 12 models. Hydraulic, fixed height, mechanical, hand crank height control and Trendelenburg control. Folding, vertical drop, or swing away side rails. Weight from 90 to 325 lbs.

General Scientific Safety Equipment Co. 800-523-0166
2553 E Somerset St Fl 1, Philadelphia, PA 19134

HAAG-STREIT USA, INC. 800-787-5426
3535 Kings Mills Rd, Mason, OH 45040
$4,495 for surgical stretcher.

Harbor Metalcrafters, Inc./Medpro 631-242-2428
208 S Fehr Way, Bay Shore, NY 11706
Patient transport 'cot'.

Healthline Medical Products, Inc. 407-656-0704
1065 E Story Rd, Oakland, FL 34787

Hill-Rom, Inc. 812-934-7777
4115 Dorchester Rd Unit 600, North Charleston, SC 29405
Various.

Innovative Products Unlimited, Inc. 800-833-2826
2120 Industrial Dr, Niles, MI 49120
$1,030 per shower gurney.

Khl, Inc. 206-915-2115
18300 NE 146th Way, Woodinville, WA 98072
Mri stretcher.

Mac Medical 618-476-3550
820 S Mulberry St, Millstadt, IL 62260
Stretcher.

Mayo Medical, S.A. De C.V. 800-715-3872
Edison 1141 Nte., Col. Talleres, Monterrey N.L. 64480 Mexico

Md International, Inc. 305-669-9003
11300 NW 41st St, Doral, FL 33178
Mobile, mechanical, powered.

Medi-Tech International, Inc. 305-593-9373
2924 NW 109th Ave, Doral, FL 33172
GENDRON

Mjm International Corporation 956-781-5000
2003 N Veterans Blvd Ste 10, San Juan, TX 78589
Various models of shower gurneys.

STRETCHER, WHEELED (MOBILE) *(cont'd)*

Schaerer Mayfield Usa 800-755-6381
4900 Charlemar Dr, Cincinnati, OH 45227
900 Stretcher.

Schueler & Company, Inc. 516-487-1500
PO Box 528, Stratford, CT 06615

Stryker Medical 800-869-0770
3800 E Centre Ave, Portage, MI 49002

Symphony Medical Products 877-470-9995
6320 NW 84th Ave, Miami, FL 33166
Wheeled stretcher.

STRETCHER, WHEELED, MECHANICAL *(Physical Med) 89INJ*

Armstrong Medical Industries, Inc. 800-323-4220
575 Knightsbridge Pkwy, Lincolnshire, IL 60069

Ferno-Washington, Inc. 800-733-3766
70 Weil Way, Wilmington, OH 45177

Gendron, Inc. 800-537-2521
400 E Lugbill Rd, Archbold, OH 43502
$804.00 per unit (standard).

Imperial Surgical Ltd. 800-661-5432
581 Orly Ave., Dorval, ONT H9P-1G1 Canada
$2000 per unit.

Medi-Man Rehabilitation Products, Inc. 800-268-4256
6200A Tomken Rd., Mississauga, ONT L5T-1X7 Canada
NOMAD

Stryker Medical 800-869-0770
3800 E Centre Ave, Portage, MI 49002

United Metal Fabricators, Inc. 800-638-5322
1316 Eisenhower Blvd, Johnstown, PA 15904
Chrome plated side rails; double hook IV pole; 10 casters 2 in. with brake and swivel lock; six position head rest raises to full chair position. Optional stretcher cushion.

STRETCHER, WHEELED, POWERED *(Physical Med) 89INK*

Gator Custom Mobility, Inc. 352-373-9673
501 NE 23rd Ave, Gainesville, FL 32609
Powered wheeled stretcher, powered wheeled gurney.

Symphony Medical Products 877-470-9995
6320 NW 84th Ave, Miami, FL 33166
Wheeled powered stretcher.

STRIP, ADHESIVE *(Surgery) 79FPX*

A.M.G. Medical, Inc. 888-396-1213
8505 Dalton Rd., Montreal, QUE H4T-IV5 Canada

Almore International, Inc. 503-643-6633
PO Box 25214, Portland, OR 97298
Magnetic boxing strips. $15.95.

American Safety Razor Co. 540-248-8000
1 Razor Blade Ln, Verona, VA 24482
Adhesive skin closure strip.

Aso Corporation 941-379-0300
300 Sarasota Center Blvd, Sarasota, FL 34240
Butterfly closure device.

Aso Llc 941-379-0300
12120 Esther Lama Dr Ste 112, El Paso, TX 79936
Multiple.

Chamberlin Rubber Company, Inc. 585-427-7780
3333 Brighton Henrietta Town Line Rd, PO Box 22700
Rochester, NY 14623

Csi Holdings 615-452-9633
170 Commerce Way, Gallatin, TN 37066

Customs Hospital Products, Inc 800-426-2780
6336 SE 107th Ave, Portland, OR 97266
Montgomery straps-non-sterile.

Elementis Specialties 800-866-6800
329 Wyckoff Mills Rd, Hightstown, NJ 08520
DOUBLE-BUBBLE adhesive, job-sized maintenance and repair adhesive. Also called EPOWELD 2156A/EPOCURE 118B. ECLIPSE 203 UV-cure medical adhesive is a single-component polyurethane/acrylate adhesive designed for use between tight-fitting parts or for bonding flexible plastics to themselves or to rigid assemblies.

Ethicon, Inc. 800-4-ETHICON
Route 22 West, Somerville, NJ 08876
PROXI-STRIP skin closures in 6 sizes: 1/8in.x3in., 1/4in.x3in., 1/4in.x1.1/2in., 1/4in.x4in.x1/2in., 4in., 1in.x3in., packaged in 50-unit dispenser boxes.

STRIP, ADHESIVE *(cont'd)*

Healer Products, Llc 914-663-6300
427 Commerce Ln Ste 1, West Berlin, NJ 08091
Adhesive strips.

Johnson & Johnson Medical Division Of Ethicon, Inc. 800-423-4018
2500 E Arbrook Blvd, Arlington, TX 76014

Kapp Surgical Instrument, Inc. 800-282-5277
4919 Warrensville Center Rd, Cleveland, OH 44128
STRIP T adhesive strip to hold instruments and tubing in place.

M&C Specialties Co. 800-441-6996
90 James Way, Southampton, PA 18966

Maxpak, Llc 863-682-0123
2808 New Tampa Hwy, Lakeland, FL 33815
Wound closure strips.

Normed 800-288-8200
PO Box 3644, Seattle, WA 98124
Various types of adhesive strip skin closures.

Rockford Medical & Safety Co. 800-435-9451
2420 Harrison Ave, PO Box 5646, Rockford, IL 61108

Scapa Medical 310-419-0567
540 N Oak St, Inglewood, CA 90302

Smith & Nephew, Inc. 800-876-1261
11775 Starkey Rd, Largo, FL 33773
PRE-CUT adhesive support. HYPAFIX dressing retention sheet.

Tailored Label Products, Inc. 800-727-1344
W165N5731 Ridgewood Dr, Menomonee Falls, WI 53051

The Evercare Company 800-435-6223
3440 Preston Ridge Rd Ste 650, Alpharetta, GA 30005
4 x 30 refills for adhesive lint remover.

STRIP, CRANIOSYNOSTOSIS, PREFORMED
(Cns/Neurology) 84GXO

Elekta, Inc. 800-535-7355
4775 Peachtree Industrial Blvd, Building 300, Suite 300
Norcross, GA 30092
Lesion Neuro generator and accessories.

Integra Neurosciences Pr 800-654-2873
Road 402 North, Km 1.2, Anasco, PR 00610
U-channel silicone elastomer stripping.

STRIP, FLUORESCEIN *(Ophthalmology) 86KYC*

Accutome, Inc. 610-889-0200
3222 Phoenixville Pike, Malvern, PA 19355
Test strips.

Holles Laboratories, Inc. 800-356-4015
30 Forest Notch, Cohasset, MA 02025
Large molecular weight fluorescent solution for soft contact lens fitting and BUT testing.

STRIP, HAMA IGG, ELISA, IN VITRO TEST SYSTEM
(Immunology) 82MLH

Calbiotech, Inc. 619-660-6162
10461 Austin Dr Ste G, Spring Valley, CA 91978
Invitro diagnostic kits.

Immunomedics, Inc. 973-605-8200
300 the American Rd, Morris Plains, NJ 07950
ELISA assay for the detection and semi-quantification of human anti-mouse antibody

United Biotech, Inc. 650-961-2910
211 S Whisman Rd Ste E, Mountain View, CA 94041
ELISA for HAMA (Human Anti-mouse Antibody).

Zeptometrix Corporation 800-274-5487
872 Main St, Buffalo, NY 14202
Mouse IgG, Antigen ELISA; these are for research use only, not for in vitro diagnostic use! IMMUNO-TEK mouse IgG EIA kit is a rapid easy to use enzyme linked immunosorbent assay designed for the measurement of mouse IgG in cell culture supernatants, ascites or other biological fluid. Useful in monitoring the production and purification of mouse monoclonal antibodies. Results in less than two hours. IMMUNO-TEK ELISA construction system is an easy to use kit that enables scientists to rapidly prepare high-quality ELISA assays. Comparable quality to that of the world's leading immunodiagnostic companies. All components may be ordered individually to meet special needs and further optimize their ELISA assays.

STRIP, INDICATOR, PH, DIALYSATE *(Gastro/Urology) 78MNV*

Serim Research Corp. 574-264-3440
3506 Reedy Dr, Elkhart, IN 46514
Test for hydrogen ion concentration in bicarbonate buffer.

STRIP, POLISHING AGENT *(Dental And Oral) 76EHM*

Abrasive Technology, Inc. 740-548-4100
8400 Green Meadows Dr N, Lewis Center, OH 43035
Various types of abrasive strips.

Align Technology, Inc. 408-470-1000
881 Martin Ave, Santa Clara, CA 95050
Strip,polishing agent.

Almore International, Inc. 503-643-6633
PO Box 25214, Portland, OR 97298
$18.75 for polishing & finishing strips.

G & H Wire Co. 800-526-1026
2165 Earlywood Dr, Franklin, IN 46131

Gc America, Inc. 708-597-0900
3737 W 127th St, Alsip, IL 60803
Polishing strips.

Miltex Dental Technologies, Inc. 516-576-6022
589 Davies Dr, York, PA 17402
Various intra-oral abrasive strips.

Moyco Technologies, Inc. 800-331-8837
200 Commerce Dr, Montgomeryville, PA 18936
$14.95 per 150 strips.

Rite-Dent Manufacturing Corp. 305-693-8626
3750 E 10th Ct, Hialeah, FL 33013
Various types of polishing strip.

Ultradent Products, Inc. 801-553-4586
505 W 10200 S, South Jordan, UT 84095
Abrasive devices and accessories.

Water Pik, Inc. 970-221-6129
1730 E Prospect Rd, Fort Collins, CO 80525
Stainless steel polishing strip.

3m Espe Dental Products 949-863-1360
2111 McGaw Ave, Irvine, CA 92614
$16.35 per unit.

STRIP, SCHIRMER *(Ophthalmology) 86KYD*

Eagle Vision, Inc. 800-222-7584
8500 Wolf Lake Dr Ste 110, Memphis, TN 38133
COLOR BAR Schirmer Tear Test.

Nomax, Inc. 314-961-2500
40 N Rock Hill Rd, Saint Louis, MO 63119
Tear testing strips.

STRIP, TEST *(Chemistry) 75WTX*

Acon Laboratories, Inc. 858-535-2030
10125 Mesa Rim Rd, San Diego, CA 92121
Urinalysis Reagent Strips

Akers Biosciences, Inc. 800-451-8378
201 Grove Rd, West Deptford, NJ 08086

Bio-Medical Products Corp. 800-543-7427
10 Halstead Rd, Mendham, NJ 07945
One step screening diagnostic tests for UTI, PSA, Hepatitis, HIV, glucose, pregnancy, urinalysis, and narcotics for use by doctors, offices, and clinics.

Chagrin Safety Supply, Inc. 800-227-0468
8227 Washington St # 1, Chagrin Falls, OH 44023

Current Technologies Inc 800-456-4022
PO Box 21, Crawfordsville, IN 47933
BLEACH-RITE test strips to determine efficacy of bleach solutions for disinfection.

Fil-Chem, Inc. 919-788-0909
PO Box 90833, Raleigh, NC 27675
Iondetect Strips for the determination of various ions such as iron, copper, zinc, cyanide aluminum and peroxide water hardness, potassium, chloride, and many others.

Lamotte Co. 800-344-3100
802 Washington Ave, PO Box 329, Chestertown, MD 21620
Water Test Strips; for chlorine, chlorine dioxide, peroxide, q.a.c., iodine, pH, etc.

Lifescan, Inc. 800-227-8862
1000 Gibraltar Dr, Milpitas, CA 95035
ONE TOUCH test strips and GLUCOSCAN test strips.

Schueler & Company, Inc. 516-487-1500
PO Box 528, Stratford, CT 06615

STRIP, TEST *(cont'd)*

Smi 920-876-3361
Industrial Park, 544 Sohn Drive, Elkhart Lake, WI 53020
Diagnostic strips.

Xenotec Ltd. 949-640-4053
511 Hazel Dr, Corona Del Mar, CA 92625
Visual blood and meter glucose test for in vitro diagnostic use.

STRIP, TEST, REAGENT, RESIDUALS FOR DIALYSATE, DISINFECTANT *(Gastro/Urology) 78MSY*

Germaine Laboratories, Inc. 210-692-4192
4139 Gardendale St Ste 101, San Antonio, TX 78229
Various types.

Integrated Biomedical Technology, Inc. 574-264-0025
2931 Moose Trl, Elkhart, IN 46514
Glutaraldehyde test strips.

Rpc 800-647-3873
PO Box 35849, Tucson, AZ 85740
Micro-X Peroxide Residual Test Strips; Micro-X Peracetic Acid Potency Strips.

STRIPPER, ARTERY, INTRALUMINAL *(Cardiovascular) 74DWX*

Lemaitre Vascular, Inc. 781-221-2266
63 2nd Ave, Burlington, MA 01803
Schubart Periscope

STRIPPER, DONOR TUBE *(Hematology) 81RWS*

Fenwal Inc. 800-766-1077
3 Corporate Dr, Lake Zurich, IL 60047

Melco Engineering Corp. 888-635-2688
PO Box 8907, Calabasas, CA 91372
Melco Donor Tube Stripper model TS-2.

STRIPPER, OTHER *(Surgery) 79RWU*

Eraser Company, Inc. 800-724-0594
123 Oliva Dr, Mattydale, NY 13211
Magnet wire strippers (fiberglass and wire wheel) used to remove insulation and enamel from magnet wire. Also offered are coaxial cable strippers for use in the manufacture of cable connectors in medical devices.

STRIPPER, SURGICAL *(Orthopedics) 87HRT*

Biomet Microfixation Inc. 800-874-7711
1520 Tradeport Dr, Jacksonville, FL 32218
Various types of strippers.

Biomet, Inc. 574-267-6639
56 E Bell Dr, PO Box 587, Warsaw, IN 46582
Bunnell tendon stripper.

Depuy-Raynham, A Div. Of Depuy Orthopaedics 800-451-2006
325 Paramount Dr, Raynham, MA 02767
Various.

King Tool, Inc. 800-587-9445
5350 Love Ln, Bozeman, MT 59718
Tendon strippers.

Warsaw Orthopedic, Inc. 901-396-3133
2500 Silveus Xing, Warsaw, IN 46582
Tendon stripper.

Zimmer Holdings, Inc. 800-613-6131
1800 W Center St, PO Box 708, Warsaw, IN 46580

STRIPPER, TENDON *(Surgery) 79RWT*

Codman & Shurtleff, Inc 800-225-0460
325 Paramount Dr, Raynham, MA 02767

LinkBio Corp. 800-932-0616
300 Round Hill Dr, Rockaway, NJ 07866

Miltex Inc. 800-645-8000
589 Davies Dr, York, PA 17402

Princeton Medical Group, Inc. 800-875-0869
1189 Royal Links Dr, Mt Pleasant, SC 29466

Zimmer Holdings, Inc. 800-613-6131
1800 W Center St, PO Box 708, Warsaw, IN 46580

STRIPPER, VEIN, DISPOSABLE *(Surgery) 79GAJ*

Codman & Shurtleff, Inc 800-225-0460
325 Paramount Dr, Raynham, MA 02767

Depuy-Raynham, A Div. Of Depuy Orthopaedics 800-451-2006
325 Paramount Dr, Raynham, MA 02767
Codman disposable vein stripper.

STRIPPER, VEIN, EXTERNAL *(Cardiovascular) 74DWQ*

Aesculap Implant Systems Inc. 1-800-234-9179
3773 Corporate Pkwy, Center Valley, PA 18034

Lemaitre Vascular, Inc. 781-221-2266
63 2nd Ave, Burlington, MA 01803
The InvisiGrip® Vein Stripper provides a less traumatic alternative to standard vein strippers for removal of the saphenous vein. This technique reduces the likelihood of injury to adjacent structures. The additional benefit of the InvisiGrip device is that the vein can be removed with just one incision versus traditional two-incision procedures.

Tuzik Boston 800-886-6363
104 Longwater Dr, Assinippi Park, Norwell, MA 02061

STRIPPER, VEIN, REUSABLE *(Surgery) 79GAI*

Aesculap Implant Systems Inc. 1-800-234-9179
3773 Corporate Pkwy, Center Valley, PA 18034

Bausch & Lomb Surgical 636-255-5051
3365 Tree Court Ind Blvd, Saint Louis, MO 63122

Biomet Microfixation Inc. 800-874-7711
1520 Tradeport Dr, Jacksonville, FL 32218
Various types of strippers.

Codman & Shurtleff, Inc 800-225-0460
325 Paramount Dr, Raynham, MA 02767

Miltex Inc. 800-645-8000
589 Davies Dr, York, PA 17402

Richard Wolf Medical Instruments Corp. 800-323-9653
353 Corporate Woods Pkwy, Vernon Hills, IL 60061

Venosan North America, Inc. 800-432-5347
300 Industrial Park Ave, PO Box 1067, Asheboro, NC 27205
VENOSAN vein strippers by Wright, Fischer & Oesch. Phlebectomy re-usable hooks by Ramelet, Oesch, Muller, & Tretbar.

STROLLER, ADAPTIVE *(Physical Med) 89LBE*

Convaid Inc. 888-266-8243
PO Box 4209, Rolling Hills Estates, CA 90274
METRO, a low price basic lightweight, compact-folding Stroller line. Removable, reinforced fabric seat has a built-in Pelvic Stabilizer and is washable. Available in 12,14,16 and 18 inch seat widths. Crash tested.

Reha Partner Inc. 866-282-4558
530 Means St NW Ste 120, Atlanta, GA 30318
The Merlino Stroller system is easily foldable and comes with adjustable comfortable seating. It has 3 different front wheel options. (Jogger, swivel or fixed wheels). The Merlino stroller Seat features tilt in space and backrest reclining.

Wenzelite Rehab Supplies, Llc 800-706-9255
220 36th St, 99 Seaview Blvd, Brooklyn, NY 11232
The lightweight TRAVELER stroller base features front swivel wheels and oversized rear wheels. It accommodates the MSS Tilt & Recline seating system and will fold with the seating system in place.

STYLET, CATHETER *(Cardiovascular) 74DRB*

Acme-Monaco Corp. 860-224-1349
75 Winchell Rd, New Britain, CT 06052
Catheter wire stylets.

Diablo Sales & Marketing, Inc. 925-648-1611
PO Box 3219, Danville, CA 94526
Custom design and manufacturing of catheters and specialty guidewires. Guiding catheters; stent delivery and drug delivery systems.

Fort Wayne Metals Research Prod. Corp. 260-747-4154
9609 Ardmore Ave, Fort Wayne, IN 46809
Various grades, properties and shapes of precision wire.

Maquet Puerto Rico Inc. 408-635-3900
No. 12, Rd. #698, Dorado, PR 00646
Various models of stylets.

Navion Biomedical Corp. 781-341-8058
312 Tosca Dr, Stoughton, MA 02072
MAPCATH disposable stylet with sensor in its tip; replaces stylet in any standard catheter.

Ranfac Corp. 800-2RANFAC
30 Doherty Ave, Avon Industrial Park, Avon, MA 02322

Sanderson-Macleod, Inc. 866-522-3481
1199 S Main St, P.O. Box 50, Palmer, MA 01069

St. Jude Medical Atrial Fibrillation (Endocardial Solutions) 800-374-8038
1350 Energy Ln Ste 110, Saint Paul, MN 55108
Catheter stylet.

STYLET, CATHETER *(cont'd)*

Vygon Corp. 800-544-4907
2495 General Armistead Ave, Norristown, PA 19403

Wytech Industries, Inc. 732-396-3900
960 E Hazelwood Ave, Rahway, NJ 07065

STYLET, CATHETER, GASTRO-UROLOGY
(Gastro/Urology) 78EZB

Angiodynamics, Inc. 800-472-5221
1 Horizon Way, Manchester, GA 31816
Tunneling stylets in multiple lumen catheter kits.

Boston Scientific Corporation 508-652-5578
8600 NW 41st St, Doral, FL 33166

Boston Scientific Corporation 508-652-5578
780 Brookside Dr, Spencer, IN 47460

Greenwald Surgical Co., Inc. 219-962-1604
2688 Dekalb St, Gary, IN 46405
Various types of catheter stylets.

STYLET, NEEDLE *(General) 80RWX*

Cadence Science Inc. 888-717-7677
1979 Marcus Ave Ste 215, New Hyde Park, NY 11042

Spectra Medical Devices, Inc. 978-657-0889
260H Fordham Rd, Wilmington, MA 01887
Specialty needles

Tegra Medical Inc. 508-541-4200
9 Forge Pkwy, Franklin, MA 02038

Vygon Corp. 800-544-4907
2495 General Armistead Ave, Norristown, PA 19403

Wytech Industries, Inc. 732-396-3900
960 E Hazelwood Ave, Rahway, NJ 07065

STYLET, SURGICAL *(Surgery) 79GAH*

Aesculap Implant Systems Inc. 1-800-234-9179
3773 Corporate Pkwy, Center Valley, PA 18034
General and plastic surgery.

Bausch & Lomb Surgical 636-255-5051
3365 Tree Court Ind Blvd, Saint Louis, MO 63122

Biomet Microfixation Inc. 800-874-7711
1520 Tradeport Dr, Jacksonville, FL 32218
Stylet, surgical, general & plastic surgery.

Olsen Medical 800-297-6344
3001 W Kentucky St, Louisville, KY 40211
Stylet for irrigating forceps.

Orthovita, Inc. 610-640-1775
77 Great Valley Pkwy, Malvern, PA 19355
Needle stylet.

Osseon Therapeutics, Inc. 877-567-7366
2330 Circadian Way, Santa Rosa, CA 95407
OsseoFlex 1.0 Steerable Needle

Synthes (Usa) - Development Center 719-481-5300
1230 Wilson Dr, West Chester, PA 19380
Various stylets.

Wytech Industries, Inc. 732-396-3900
960 E Hazelwood Ave, Rahway, NJ 07065

STYLET, TRACHEAL TUBE *(Anesthesiology) 73BSR*

Aesculap Implant Systems Inc. 1-800-234-9179
3773 Corporate Pkwy, Center Valley, PA 18034

Anesthesia Associates, Inc. 760-744-6561
460 Enterprise St, San Marcos, CA 92078
Available in various adult and pediatric sizes, fabricated from malleable copper or stainless steel.

Armstrong Medical Industries, Inc. 800-323-4220
575 Knightsbridge Pkwy, Lincolnshire, IL 60069

Bovie Medical Corp. 800-537-2790
5115 Ulmerton Rd, Clearwater, FL 33760
Lighted.

Ccr Medical, Inc. 888-883-7331
967 43rd Ave NE, Saint Petersburg, FL 33703
Sytlet, introducer, flexible.

Cookgas Llc 314-781-5700
1167 Hillside Dr, Saint Louis, MO 63117
Tracheal tube stylet.

Eastmed Enterprises, Inc. 856-797-0131
11 Brandywine Dr, Marlton, NJ 08053
Various sizes of stylet.

STYLET, TRACHEAL TUBE *(cont'd)*

Green Field Medical Sourcing, Inc. 512-894-3002
14141 W Highway 290 Ste 410, Austin, TX 78737
Et tube introducer.

Gyrus Acmi, Inc. 508-804-2739
93 N Pleasant St, Norwalk, OH 44857
Various stylets.

Gyrus Acmi, Inc. 508-804-2739
300 Stillwater P.o.box 1971, Stamford, CT 06902
Various stylets.

Health Care Logistics, Inc. 800-848-1633
450 Town St, PO Box 25, Circleville, OH 43113
Intubation stylette.

Innovative Medical Devices, Inc. 516-766-3800
3571 Hargale Ct, Oceanside, NY 11572
Stylet, tracheal tube.

Innovative Medical Visions, Inc. 516-766-3800
3571 Hargale Ct, Oceanside, NY 11572
Stylet, tracheal tube.

Kentron Health Care, Inc. 615-384-0573
3604 Kelton Jackson Rd, P.o. Box 120, Springfield, TN 37172
Endotracheal tube stylets.

Mercury Medical 800-237-6418
11300 49th St N, Clearwater, FL 33762

Parker Medical 303-799-1990
7275 S Revere Pkwy Ste 804, Centennial, CO 80112
Endotracheal tube stylet with one-hand operation, requiring no pre-bending;easy thumb action allows curvature to be remotely adjusted during intubation.

Primary Medical Co., Inc. 727-520-1920
6541 44th St N Ste 6003, Pinellas Park, FL 33781
Various models non-sterile stylet.

Sharn, Inc. 800-325-3671
4517 George Rd Ste 200, Tampa, FL 33634

Shore Medical, Inc. 714-628-9785
1050 N Batavia St Ste C, Orange, CA 92867
Various.

Sun-Med 800-433-2797
12393 Belcher Rd S Ste 450, Largo, FL 33773

Sunmed Healthcare 727-531-7266
12393 Belcher Rd S Ste 460, Largo, FL 33773

STYLET, URETERAL *(Gastro/Urology) 78EYA*

Aesculap Implant Systems Inc. 1-800-234-9179
3773 Corporate Pkwy, Center Valley, PA 18034

SUBSTANCE, GROUPING, BLOOD (NON-HUMAN ORIGIN)
(Hematology) 81KSX

Genetic Testing Institute 262-754-1000
20925 Crossroads Cir Ste 200, Waukesha, WI 53186
Elution kit for rapid elution of antibodies from intact red blood cells.

SUCKER, CARDIOTOMY RETURN, CARDIOPULMONARY BYPASS *(Cardiovascular) 74DTS*

Atek Medical 800-253-1540
620 Watson St SW, Grand Rapids, MI 49504
Suction tube, sump.

California Medical Laboratories, Inc. 714-556-7365
1570 Sunland Ln, Costa Mesa, CA 92626

Edwards Lifesciences Research Medical 949-250-2500
6864 Cottonwood St, Midvale, UT 84047
Cardiac sucker.

International Biophysics Corp. 512-326-3244
2101 E Saint Elmo Rd Ste 275, Austin, TX 78744
Suction wand.

Jostra Bentley, Inc. 302-454-9959
Rd. 402 N. Km 1.4, Industrial Park, Anasco, PR 00610-1577
Disposable sucker.

Medtronic Blood Management 612-514-4000
18501 E Plaza Dr, Parker, CO 80134
Cardiopulmonary.

Terumo Cardiovascular Systems (Tcvs) 800-283-7866
28 Howe St, Ashland, MA 01721
Suckers.

Terumo Cardiovascular Systems, Corp 800-521-2818
6200 Jackson Rd, Ann Arbor, MI 48103

SUCTION APPARATUS, OPERATING ROOM, WALL VACUUM-POWERED *(Surgery) 79GCX*

Amelife Llc 302-476-2631
702 N West St Ste 101, Wilmington, DE 19801

Armstrong Medical Industries, Inc. 800-323-4220
575 Knightsbridge Pkwy, Lincolnshire, IL 60069

Bass Medical, Inc 800-214-9084
2539 John Hawkins Pkwy Ste 101, Birmingham, AL 35244
Fluid collection & removal system.

Biodrain Medical, Inc. 952-475-1989
699 Minnetonka Highlands Ln, Orono, MN 55356
Fluid collection device.

Brasseler Usa - Medical 805-650-5209
4837 McGrath St Ste J, Ventura, CA 93003
Suction.

Cascade Life Solutions, Llc 616-977-2505
3710 Sysco Ct SE, Grand Rapids, MI 49512
Sucker.

Chase Medical, Lp 972-783-0644
1876 Firman Dr, Richardson, TX 75081
Various models of suckers (sterile/non sterile).

Colby Manufacturing Corp. 800-969-3718
1016 Branagan Dr, Tullytown, PA 19007
WATERBUG Quiet Floor Suction Device efficiently suctions irrigants, blood and body fluids from the floor to ensure that the operating room is clean and safe.

Elite Medical Products, Inc. 661-273-6518
38606 Roma Ct, Palmdale, CA 93550
Meconium aspirator.

Gyrus Acmi, Inc. 508-804-2739
93 N Pleasant St, Norwalk, OH 44857
Apparatus, suction, operating-room, wall vacuum powered.

Icu Medical (Ut), Inc 949-366-2183
4455 Atherton Dr, Salt Lake City, UT 84123
Various.

International Hospital Supply Co. 800-398-9450
6914 Canby Ave Ste 105, Reseda, CA 91335

Maquet, Inc. 843-552-8652
7371 Spartan Blvd E, N Charleston, SC 29418
Various models of vacuum-powered body fluid suction apparatus.

Novosci Corp. 281-363-4949
2828 N Crescentridge Dr, The Woodlands, TX 77381
Suction systems.

Ohmeda Medical 800-345-2700
8880 Gorman Rd, Laurel, MD 20723
Ohmeda Thoracic and Continuous Suction Regulator and Ohmeda Surgical Free Flow Regulator.

Oto-Med, Inc. 800-433-7703
1090 Empire Dr, Lake Havasu City, AZ 86404
OTOMED Suction Tubing, Soft, lighweight silicone type end tubing with suction controls. Sterile, disposable, latex free

Steris Corporation 440-354-2600
6515 Hopkins Rd, Mentor, OH 44060
Blood fluid collection/disposal system.

Stryker Puerto Rico, Ltd. 939-307-2500
Hwy. 3, Km. 131.2, Las Guasimas Ind. Park, Arroyo, PR 00714
Suction irrigator.

Surge Medical Solutions, Llc. 616-977-2516
3710 Sysco Ct SE, Grand Rapids, MI 49512
Sucker.

Tava Surgical Instruments 805-650-5209
4837 McGrath St Ste J, Ventura, CA 93003
Suction.

Terumo Cardiovascular Systems (Tcvs) 800-283-7866
28 Howe St, Ashland, MA 01721
Fluid collection devices.

SUCTION APPARATUS, SINGLE PATIENT, PORTABLE, NON-POWERED *(Surgery) 79GCY*

Ambu A/S 457-225-2210
6740 Baymeadow Dr, Glen Burnie, MD 21060
Manual suction pump.

Aspen Surgical 800-328-7958
6945 Southbelt Dr SE, Caledonia, MI 49316
S-Vac Silicone and S-Vac PVC Bulb Evacuators.

SUCTION APPARATUS, SINGLE PATIENT, PORTABLE, NON-POWERED *(cont'd)*

Biomet, Inc. 574-267-6639
56 E Bell Dr, PO Box 587, Warsaw, IN 46582
Sterile reqi-vacette.

Byron Medical 800-777-3434
602 W Rillito St, Tucson, AZ 85705
Canisters & canister liners for collection systems.

Covidien Lp 508-261-8000
15 Hampshire St, Mansfield, MA 02048

Depuy Orthopaedics, Inc. 800-473-3789
700 Orthopaedic Dr, P.O. Box 988, Warsaw, IN 46582
Various types of suctions.

Dornoch Medical Systems, Inc. 816-505-2226
4032 NW Riverside Dr, Riverside, MO 64150
Suction canister.

E-Global Medical Equipment, L.L.C. 866-422-1845
2f 500 Lincoln St., Allston, MA 02134
Suction irrigation unit.

Edwards Lifesciences Technology Sarl 949-250-2500
State Rd. 402 N.km 1.4, Anasco, PR 00610-1577
Various.

Engineered Medical Solutions Co. Llc. 908-213-9001
85 Industrial Rd Bldg B, Phillipsburg, NJ 08865
Suction.

Erie Medical 800-932-2293
10225 82nd Ave, Lakeview Corporate Park, Pleasant Prairie, WI 53158
SUPER-VAC 110-V suction unit, AC powered, with single-patient-use disposable 1200-cc canister. Supplied with bacteria filter to prevent contamination.

K W Griffen Company 800-424-5556
100 Pearl St, Norwalk, CT 06850

Mada, Inc. 800-526-6370
625 Washington Ave, Carlstadt, NJ 07072

Medical Industries America Inc. 800-759-3038
2636 289th Pl, Adel, IA 50003
VACUMAX aspirator used for suctioning the upper airway.

R & D Medical Products, Inc. 949-472-9346
20492 Crescent Bay Dr Ste 106, Lake Forest, CA 92630
Closed wound suction drainage system holder.

Spine Smith Partners L.P. 512-206-0770
8140 N MO Pac Expy Bldg 120, Austin, TX 78759
Single use only sucker tip.

Std Med, Inc. 781-828-4400
75 Mill St, PO Box 420, Stoughton, MA 02072
Suction irrigation unit.

Stryker Puerto Rico, Ltd. 939-307-2500
Hwy. 3, Km. 131.2, Las Guasimas Ind. Park, Arroyo, PR 00714
Closed wound suction device with various sterile and nonsterile accessories.

Uresil, Llc 800-538-7374
5418 Touhy Ave, Skokie, IL 60077
TRU-CLOSE suction drainage reservoirs.

Zimmer Orthopaedic Surgical Products 800-321-5533
PO Box 10, 200 West Ohio Ave., Dover, OH 44622
PULSAVAC PLUS wound debridement system, provides suction and irrigation to clean and debride traumatic and chronic wounds.

SUCTION APPARATUS, WARD USE, PORTABLE, AC-POWERED *(Surgery) 79JCX*

Allied Healthcare Products, Inc. 800-444-3954
1720 Sublette Ave, Saint Louis, MO 63110

Aspen Surgical 800-328-7958
6945 Southbelt Dr SE, Caledonia, MI 49316
VariDyne portable vacuum controller.

Avail Medical Products, Inc. 858-635-2206
1225 N. 28th Avenue, Suite 500, Dallas, TX 75261
Vacuum assisted wound care dressing.

Boehringer Labs, Inc 888-390-4325
500 E Washington St Ste 2A, Black Horse, PA 19401
Negative pressure wound therapy system.

Contemporary Products, Inc. 800-424-2444
530 Riverside Industrial Pkwy, Portland, ME 04103

Depuy Orthopaedics, Inc. 800-473-3789
700 Orthopaedic Dr, P.O. Box 988, Warsaw, IN 46582
Various types of portable ac-powered suction apparatus.

SUCTION APPARATUS, WARD USE, PORTABLE, AC-POWERED *(cont'd)*

Dntlworks Equipment Corporation 800-847-0694
7300 S Tucson Way, Centennial, CO 80112
PROSEAL I AND PROSEAL II. Portable hygiene units with powerful, quiet suction pump. Small, quiet compressor pressurizes water reservoir and powers air/water syringe. PROSEAL II adds electric slowspeed prophy handpiece.

Erie Medical 800-932-2293
10225 82nd Ave, Lakeview Corporate Park, Pleasant Prairie, WI 53158
PORT-A-VAC 12-V-DC, battery operated, portable suction unit for emergency use. Also operates from vehicle cigarette-lighter outlet.

Impact Instrumentation, Inc. 800-969-0750
27 Fairfield Pl, West Caldwell, NJ 07006
Model 306 Programmable Intermittent Suction System, AC-DC rechargeable battery-powered aspirator for oral, nasal, and tracheal and post-operative gastrointestinal drainage suction. Drainage settings programmable to 144 different combinations. Vacuum from 0 to 600 mm HG and free airflow to 8 liters per minute for gastrointestinal suction. Rotary vane pump. $ 1310.00 to 1710.00. Also available, Model 308 and 308 GR, AC-DC rechargeable battery-powered portable aspirators for oral, nasal, and tracheal suction. Vacuum from 0 to 550 mm Hg, free airflow, exceeds 30 liters per minute. Diaphragm pump. Includes collection canister, rinse bottle, suction tips, Y-fitting catheters and tubing. Aeromedical versions available. $610.00 to 829.00. Also available, Model 326 ultra-lite Series, Programmable Intermittent Suction System, AC-DC-rechargeable battery-powered aspirator for oral, nasal, tracheal and post-operative gastrointestinal drainage suction. Drainage settings are programmable to 144 different combinations. Vacuum from 0 to 550 mm Hg and free airflow exceeding 30 liters per minute for ONT suction. Vacuum from 0 to 200 mm HG and free airflow to 8 liters per minute for gastrointestinal suction. Diaphragm pump. Includes aeromedical certification, DC-DC converter and 115/230 VAC, 50/60 Hz power supply. $ 1705.00. Also available, Impact/Sorensen Model 1120 General Purpose, AC-powered portable aspirator for oral, nasal, and tracheal suction. Vacuum from 0 to 550 mm HG, free airflow exceeds 30 liters per minute. Diaphragm pump. Available 32 oz or 64 collection canisters. $910.00 to 1035.00. Also available, Impact Sorensen Model 2110 General Purpose, AC-powered aspirator for oral, nasal, and tracheal suction. Cart-mounted. Vacuum from 0 to 550 mm Hg. Diaphragm pump. Available 32-, 64-, or 128-oz collection canisters. $1150.00 to 1270.00. Also available, Impact/Sorensen Model 2120 General Purpose, AC-powered, aspirator for oral, nasal, and tracheal suction. Cart-mounted version of Model 1120. Vacuum from 0 to 550 mm Hg, free airflow exceeds 30 liters per minute. Diaphragm pump. Includes 64 oz collection canister. $1330.00 to 1450.00. Also available, Impact/Sorensen Model 2135 General Purpose, AC-powered aspirator for oral, nasal, and tracheal suction. Cart-mounted. Vacuum from 0 to 550 mm Hg. Rotary vane pump. Available with 64 oz or 128 oz collection canisters. $1575.00 to 1700.00. Also available Impact/Sorensen Model 2492 Thoracic Drainage Unit, AC-powered for removal of air and fluids from the pleural cavity. Cart-mounted. Vacuum 0 to 58 cm H2O, high, airflow. Available with two, 128 oz collection canisters, $1325.00. Also available, Impact/Sorensen Model 2590 Low-Volume Thermotic Drainage, AC-powered aspirator for mild intermittent suction. Cart-mounted. Vacuum 90 or 120 mm Hg. Available with 128 oz collection canisters. $1415.00. Also available Impact/Sorensen Model 2591 Low Volume Thermotic Drainage, AC-powered aspirator for mild continuous or intermittent suction. Cart-mounted. Vacuum 30 to 180 mm Hg. Available with 128 oz collection canisters. $2035.00. Also available Impact/Sorensen Model 16666 Uterine portable aspiratotor for vacuum cutterage procedures. Vacuum to 29-in. Hg, high airflow. Double diaphragm pump. Available with two, 32 oz collection canisters. $2050.00 to 2120.00.

J. H. Emerson Co. 800-252-1414
22 Cottage Park Ave, Cambridge, MA 02140
Various models of suction pumps for pleural or gastric suction.

Kinetic Concepts, Inc. 800-275-4524
8023 Vantage Dr, San Antonio, TX 78230
Vacuum therapy unit.

Kmi Kolster Methods, Inc. 909-737-5476
3185 Palisades Dr, Corona, CA 92880
General aspirator.

Medical Device Resource Corporation 800-633-8423
23392 Connecticut St, Hayward, CA 94545

Neomedix Corp. 949-258-8355
15042 Parkway Loop Ste A, Tustin, CA 92780
Suction pump.

SUCTION APPARATUS, WARD USE, PORTABLE, AC-POWERED *(cont'd)*

Ohio Medical Corp. 800-662-5822
1111 Lakeside Dr, Gurnee, IL 60031
MOBLVAC III portable suction; provides constant or intermittent suction, quiet operation, high flow and vacuum.

Penumbra, Inc. 510-618-3223
1351 Harbor Bay Pkwy, Alameda, CA 94502
Aspiration pump.

Ubs Instruments Corporation 818-710-1195
7745 Alabama Ave Ste 7, Canoga Park, CA 91304
Suction Pump is a portable, general purpose suction pump with non-breakable containers. It is AC-powered with single/dual containers.

SUDAN III *(Pathology) 88KKJ*

E K Industries, Inc. 877-EKI-CHEM
1403 Herkimer St, Joliet, IL 60432

Ricca Chemical Company Llc 817-461-5601
1490 Lammers Pike, Batesville, IN 47006

Ricca Chemical Company, Llc 817-461-5601
448 W Fork Dr, Arlington, TX 76012
Sudan iii.

SUDAN IV *(Pathology) 88KKK*

Argon Medical Devices Inc. 903-675-9321
1445 Flat Creek Rd, Athens, TX 75751
Equipment covers & drapes.

E K Industries, Inc. 877-EKI-CHEM
1403 Herkimer St, Joliet, IL 60432

The Sewing Source, Inc. 919-478-3900
802 E Nash St, Spring Hope, NC 27882
Drape, surgical.

SUIT, PNEUMATIC COUNTERPRESSURE (ANTI-SHOCK) *(Cardiovascular) 74RLJ*

Allied Healthcare Products, Inc. 800-444-3954
1720 Sublette Ave, Saint Louis, MO 63110

Armstrong Medical Industries, Inc. 800-323-4220
575 Knightsbridge Pkwy, Lincolnshire, IL 60069

Clark Company Inc., David 800-900-3434
360 Franklin St, Worcester, MA 01604
Adult, pediatric or toddler sizes of Medical Anti-Shock Trousers (MAST), with max. 54in. or 30in. waist, and max. 74in. or 46in. to 58in. height. Fabric or transparent models. Machine wash, drip dry. 5lb. to 9 lb. weight. Pressure monitoring assembly available.

David Clark Company, Inc. 800-900-3434
360 Franklin St, Worcester, MA 01604
Medical anti-shock trouser

Rockford Medical & Safety Co. 800-435-9451
2420 Harrison Ave, PO Box 5646, Rockford, IL 61108

SUIT, SCRUB, DISPOSABLE *(Surgery) 79RRY*

Dna Products, Llc 800-535-3189
PO Box 306, New York, NY 10032
Unisex disposable head-to-ankle coverall made of soft polypropylene laminated for waterproofing. Lightweight, yet durable and roomy. Comes loaded with styling features such as a hooded top, white nylon zipper front with covered placket, and elasticized waist, sleeve cuff, and ankle openings. Front chest patch pocket easily holds id badge or pens. Rear seat patch pocket is perfect for storing a wallet or other small items. Intended to be worn once and discarded; available in 5 sizes (S-XXL); 1 white individually wrapped coverall per package; $2.55/package ($2.35/package for non-laminated coverall); 40 packages per carton (single size).

General Econopak, Inc. 888-871-8568
1725 N 6th St, Philadelphia, PA 19122
GEPCO.

Health-Pak, Inc. 315-724-8370
2005 Beechgrove Pl, Utica, NY 13501
Disposable non-woven scrub shirts and scrub pants.

Johnson & Johnson Medical Division Of Ethicon, Inc. 800-423-4018
2500 E Arbrook Blvd, Arlington, TX 76014

Kappler Protective Apparel & Fabrics 800-600-4019
115 Grimes Dr, Guntersville, AL 35976

Kerr Group 800-524-3577
1400 Holcomb Bridge Rd, Roswell, GA 30076

SUIT, SCRUB, DISPOSABLE *(cont'd)*

Mylan Technologies, Inc. 800-532-5226
110 Lake St, Saint Albans, VT 05478
High moisture vapor permeable yet biologically occlusive extrusion laminates of non-woven fabrics and the MEDIFILM series of USP Class VI elastomeric films in bulk rolls.

New York Hospital Disposables, Inc. 718-384-1620
101 Richardson St, Brooklyn, NY 11211
New York Hospital Disposables, Inc., Lab coat. Komlon Lab coat with pockets & elastic wrist.

Pfb Inter-Apparel Corp. 800-828-7629
1930 Harrison St Ste 304, Hollywood, FL 33020

SUIT, SCRUB, REUSABLE *(Surgery) 79RRZ*

Angelica Image Apparel 800-222-3112
700 Rosedale Ave, Saint Louis, MO 63112

Best Manufacturing Group Llc 800-843-3233
1633 Broadway Fl 18, New York, NY 10019
BEST, blended, reversible, color-coded.

Medline Industries, Inc. 800-633-5886
1 Medline Pl, Mundelein, IL 60060

SUIT, SURGICAL *(Surgery) 79FXO*

Angelica Image Apparel 800-222-3112
700 Rosedale Ave, Saint Louis, MO 63112

Avent S.A. De C.V. 770-587-8393
Carretera Intl., Salida Norte, Magdalena, Sonora Mexico
Hospital coverall

Dowling Textiles 770-957-3981
615 Macon Rd, McDonough, GA 30253
Various types of operating and scrub suits.

General Econopak, Inc. 888-871-8568
1725 N 6th St, Philadelphia, PA 19122
GEPCO disposable coveralls, jump suits, and OR entrance suits (with or without hood and shoe covers attached).

Pfb Inter-Apparel Corp. 800-828-7629
1930 Harrison St Ste 304, Hollywood, FL 33020

Sloan Corp. 402-597-5700
13316 A St, Omaha, NE 68144
Jumpsuit.

The Sewing Source, Inc. 919-478-3900
802 E Nash St, Spring Hope, NC 27882
Suit, scrub.

Tronex Healthcare Industries 800-833-1181
2 Cranberry Rd, One Tronex Centre, Parsippany, NJ 07054
Polypropylene spunbonded for breathability and cool, comfortable fit. Full coverage, fluid resistant. Styles also available with fluid impervious PE coating, hoods and booties, elastic or open cuffs and ankles. All have zippered fronts. Neatly packaged.

White Knight Healthcare 800-851-4431
Calle 16, Number 780, Agua Prieta, Sonora Mexico
Suit, surgical

SULFOPHOSPHOVANILLIN, COLORIMETRY, TOTAL LIPIDS
(Chemistry) 75CFD

Dade Behring, Inc. 800-948-3233
1717 Deerfield Rd, Deerfield, IL 60015

Medical Chemical Corp. 800-424-9394
19430 Van Ness Ave, Torrance, CA 90501
$22.00 per 120-test kit.

SUNGLASSES (INCLUDING PHOTOSENSITIVE)
(Ophthalmology) 86HQY

Aearo Canada Ltd. 617-371-4200
7115 Tomken Rd, Mississauga L5S 1R7 Canada
Spectacle frame, protective eyewear and faceshield

Aim International, Inc. 858-618-2799
16955 Via Del Campo Ste 260, San Diego, CA 92127
Sunglasses.

Alpha Optics, Llc. 212-431-9190
5408 46th St, Maspeth, NY 11378
Various.

Ao Eyewear, Inc. 508-764-3214
529 Ashland Ave Ste 3, P.o. Box 1064, Southbridge, MA 01550
Sunglasses.

Atlantic Optical Co., Inc. 800-423-5175
20801 Nordhoff St, Chatsworth, CA 91311

SUNGLASSES (INCLUDING PHOTOSENSITIVE) *(cont'd)*

Bayz Sunwear 410-939-2200
920 Revolution St, Havre De Grace, MD 21078
Bayz sunwear.

Cold River Unlimited, Inc. 662-286-3558
2070A S Tate St, Corinth, MS 38834
Eyewear / sunglasses.

Ctp Coil Inc. 800-933-2645
1801 Howard St Ste D, Elk Grove Village, IL 60007
Various clip-on sunglasses.

Dillon Optics 480-948-8009
8009 E Dillons Way, Scottsdale, AZ 85260
Sunglass lenses.

Dioptics Medical Products, Inc. 800-959-9040
125 Venture Ln, San Luis Obispo, CA 93401
SOLARSHIELD & SOLARETTES Sunglasses. SOLARSHIELD sunglasses for post-operative use in cataract and refractive surgery. SOLARETTES are disposable sunglasses for post-mydriatic use. SOLARSHIELD ULTRA contemporary frame and lens sunglasses that fit comfortably over prescription sunglasses. Sunglasses provide 40% more UV protection than ordinary sunglasses. Styles feature side lenses and top and lower shields. SOLARCOMFORT total protection sunglasses in a wear-alone style. Sunglasses feature side lenses and top and lower shields that provide 40% more UV blockage than ordinary sunglasses.

Eschenbach Optik Of America, Inc. 800-487-5389
904 Ethan Allen Hwy, Ridgefield, CT 06877

Euro-Frames, Inc. 800-422-2773
2985 Glendale Blvd, Los Angeles, CA 90039
CLUB L.A.

European Eyewear Corp. 941-322-6771
630 Myakka Rd, Sarasota, FL 34240
Sunglasses, ski goggles.

Eye Care And Cure 800-486-6169
4646 S Overland Dr, Tucson, AZ 85714
Sunglasses (non-prescription).

Eyes Of The World, Inc. 516-889-5800
4217 Austin Blvd, Island Park, NY 11558

Fine & Particular Ey 914-834-4358
2001 Palmer Ave Ste 103, Larchmont, NY 10538

Gladiator Sports 703-878-9434
3499 Cowes Mews, Woodbridge, VA 22193

Greattec Vision S.A. De C.V.
Circuito De La Amistad #2700, Mexicali B.c. Mexico
Sunglasses (non-prescription including photosensitive)

Hasbro, Inc. 401-431-8697
1027 Newport Ave, Pawtucket, RI 02861
Goggles.

Jay-Y Enterprise Co. 909-469-4898
632 New York Dr, Pomona, CA 91768

Jkruz Inc. 410-444-2944
7315 Harford Rd, Baltimore, MD 21234
Sunglasses.

Kerma Medical Products, Inc. 757-398-8400
400 Port Centre Pkwy, Portsmouth, VA 23704
Protective eyewear.

Klinger Eye Shields, Inc. 800-848-1244
1108A Singleton Dr, Selma, AL 36703
Eye shields, post-mydriatic.

Lehrer Brillenperfektion Werks, Inc. 818-407-1890
3908 N 5th St, North Las Vegas, NV 89032
Sunglasses.

Marcolin Usa 888-627-2654
7543 E Tierra Buena Ln, Scottsdale, AZ 85260
Ophthalmic frames & sunglasses.

Nike, Inc. 800-344-6453
1 SW Bowerman Dr, Beaverton, OR 97005
Nike.

Noir Manufacturing 800-521-9746
10125 Colonial Industrial Dr, South Lyon, MI 48178

Nomax, Inc. 314-961-2500
40 N Rock Hill Rd, Saint Louis, MO 63119
Amcon slip in mydriatic sunglasses.

SUNGLASSES (INCLUDING PHOTOSENSITIVE) *(cont'd)*

Norwood Promotional Products, Inc. 651-388-1298
5151 Moundview Dr, Red Wing, MN 55066
Sunglasses.

Oakley, Inc. 800-431-1439
1 Icon, Foothill Ranch, CA 92610
Sunglasses.

Ockiobel, Inc. 305-261-6144
777 NW 72nd Ave Ste 2K20, Miami, FL 33126
Sunglasses.

Opsales, Inc.
4217 Austin Blvd, Island Park, NY 11558
Clip-on/flip-up sunglasses.

Optical Ventures, Inc. 626-915-1533
150 N Grand Ave Ste 203, West Covina, CA 91791
Sunglass lenses.

Opticote Inc. 847-678-8900
10455 Seymour Ave, Franklin Park, IL 60131
Sunglasses.

Palco Marketing, Inc. 763-559-5539
8575 Monticello Ln N, Maple Grove, MN 55369
Protective eyewear.

Panoptx, Inc. 925-484-0292
1252 Quarry Ln Ste A, Pleasanton, CA 94566

Prairie Products, Inc. 717-292-1089
4660 Raycom Rd, Industrial Park, Dover, PA 17315
Sunglasses.

Randolph Engineering, Inc. 781-961-6070
26 Thomas Patten Dr, Randolph, MA 02368
Sunglasses (non prescription).

Revolution Eyewear, Inc. 310-777-8399
997 Flower Glen St, Simi Valley, CA 93065
Sunglasses, clip-on sunglasses.

Rochester Optical Mfg. Company 585-254-0022
1260 Lyell Ave, Rochester, NY 14606

Rollens Professional Products, Inc. 303-840-2238
16610 Amberstone Way, Parker, CO 80134
Rollens post-mydriatic sunglass.

Schott Glass Technologies, Inc. 570-457-7485
400 York Ave, Duryea, PA 18642

Smith Sports Optics, Inc. 208-726-4477
PO Box 2999, 280 Northwood Way, Ketchum, ID 83340
Sunglasses (non-prescription including photosensitive).

Spectrum Optical 323-931-4349
6154 W 6th St, Los Angeles, CA 90048
Sun wear, sunglasses.

Sunglass International Llc 888-478-6764
71 Cypress St, Warwick, RI 02888
Sunglasses.

Take One Llc 602-997-2888
10807 N Cave Creek Rd, Phoenix, AZ 85020
Sunglasses.

The Orvis Co., Inc. 802-362-3622
178 Conservation Way, Arlington, VT 05250

Transitions Optical, Inc. 727-545-0400
9251 Belcher Rd, Pinellas Park, FL 33782
Multiple transitions lenses.

U.S. Vision Optical, Inc. 856-228-1000
5 Harmon Dr, Blackwood, NJ 08012
Sunglasses.

United Syntek Corp. 888-665-2326
3557 Denver Dr, Denver, NC 28037
Sunglasses.

Wilson Optical Laboratories, Inc. 866-216-6225
190 Alpha Park, Cleveland, OH 44143
Non-prescription sunglasses - various styles.

Wilson Sporting Goods Co. 773-714-6400
8750 W Bryn Mawr Ave, Chicago, IL 60631
Sunglasses for Fury racquet pack.

Wink Lens Technologies 415-332-6694
200 Gate 5 Rd Ste 201, Sausalito, CA 94965
Sunglass lens.

Zyloware Corporation 800-765-3700
1136 46th Rd, Long Island City, NY 11101
UV protected, optical quality.

SUPPLEMENTARY NITROGLYCERIN CONTAINER
(General) 80LLC

Apothecary Products, Inc. 800-328-2742
11750 12th Ave S, Burnsville, MN 55337
EZY-DOSE, Adult Lock Weekly Pill Reminder, 7 cavity pill reminder with an easy to use lock bar to prevent spills.

SUPPLIES, BLOOD BANK *(Hematology) 81KSS*

Alpha Scientific Corp. 800-242-5989
287 Great Valley Pkwy, Malvern, PA 19355
Seg-safe segment processor.

Baxter Healthcare Corp., Renal Division 847-948-2000
7511 114th Ave, Largo, FL 33773
Various sterile and non-sterile blood bank supplies.

Biomet, Inc. 574-267-6639
56 E Bell Dr, PO Box 587, Warsaw, IN 46582
Various types of platelet separation kits.

Controlled Chemicals, Inc. 734-769-5940
317 S Division St Ste 9, Ann Arbor, MI 48104
Thermal exposure indicator.

Fenwal Inc. 800-766-1077
3 Corporate Dr, Lake Zurich, IL 60047
Blood sets, blood bags.

Icu Medical, Inc. 800-824-7890
951 Calle Amanecer, San Clemente, CA 92673
Needle protector.

Interstate Blood Bank, Inc. 800-258-9557
5700 Pleasant View Rd, Memphis, TN 38134
Whole blood, red blood cells, source leukocytes (buffy coats), platelet concentrate, platelet rich or poor plasma, cryoprecipitate, cryo rich or poor fresh frozen plasma, serum from clotted whole blood; regular, modified, heparinized, liquid or tetanus-immune source plasma, diseased state plasma/serum, factor deficient plasma, specific antibody plasma/serum, recovered human plasma. All products prepared according to customer specifications.

Micro Typing Systems, Inc. 908-218-8177
1295 SW 29th Ave, Pompano Beach, FL 33069
Dispensers, test tube racks, pipettors, incubators.

Nerl Diagnostics Llc. 401-824-2046
14 Almeida Ave, East Providence, RI 02914
Blood bank saline.

Ortho-Clinical Diagnostics, Inc. 800-828-6316
513 Technology Blvd, Rochester, NY 14626
Blood bank test kit.

Terumo Cardiovascular Systems (Tcvs) 800-283-7866
125 Blue Ball Rd, Elkton, MD 21921
Phlebotomy needle cap holder.

Terumo Cardiovascular Systems (Tcvs) 800-283-7866
28 Howe St, Ashland, MA 01721
Blood banking accessories.

SUPPORT, ABDOMINAL *(Physical Med) 89RXB*

Airway Division Of Surgical Appliance Industries, Inc. 800-888-0458
3960 Rosslyn Dr, Cincinnati, OH 45209
MY TIME Maternity girdle.

Alimed, Inc. 800-225-2610
297 High St, Dedham, MA 02026

Cmo, Inc. 800-344-0011
PO Box 147, Barberton, OH 44203
SUPPORT PLUS obesity support provides abdominal plus lumbar support for greatly oversized men and women.

Dale Medical Products, Inc. 800-343-3980
7 Cross St, Plainville, MA 02762
2 panel 6' wide: 28-50'; 3 panel 9' wide: #410 30-45', #411 46-62', #418 60-75' 4 panel 12' wide: #810 30-45', #811 46-62', #818 60-75', #819 72-84', #820 82-94' 5 panel 15 in. wide: #920 82-94 in.

Formedica Ltd. 800-361-9671
1481 Rue Begin, St Laurent, QUE H4R 1V8 Canada
$120.00 per 10 (10in, med).

Freeman Manufacturing Company 800-253-2091
900 W Chicago Rd, PO Box J, Sturgis, MI 49091

Hospital Marketing Svcs. Company, Inc. 800-786-5094
162 Great Hill Rd./ Ind. Park, Naugatuck, CT 06770
HMS FLEXITONE abdominal support no.7350.

Larkotex Company 800-972-3037
1002 Olive St, Texarkana, TX 75501

SUPPORT, ABDOMINAL *(cont'd)*

Lohmann & Rauscher, Inc. 800-279-3863
6001 SW 6th Ave Ste 101, Topeka, KS 66615

Medical Accessories, Inc. 800-275-1624
92 Youngs Rd, Trenton, NJ 08619

Paramedical Distributors 800-245-3278
2020 Grand Blvd, Kansas City, MO 64108
Asstd. designs available.

Scott Specialties, Inc./Cmo Inc./Ginny Inc. 800-255-7136
512 M St, Belleville, KS 66935

Shumsky Therapeutic Products 888-333-3677
811 E 4th St, Dayton, OH 45402
Heart shaped post-op pillows, lung post-op pillows, organ transplant pillows, abdominal post-op pillows and new mother/baby breast feeding, bottle feeding and support pillows.

Tetra Medical Supply Corp. 800-621-4041
6364 W Gross Point Rd, Niles, IL 60714

Total Care 800-334-3802
PO Box 1661, Rockville, MD 20849

Truform Orthotics & Prosthetics 800-888-0458
3960 Rosslyn Dr, Cincinnati, OH 45209

Variety Ability Systems Inc. 800-891-4514
2 Kelvin Ave., Unit 3, Toronto, ONT M4C-5C8 Canada
Flip2Sit™ offers two unique seats in one product. On one side, it provides a stable posture for table height activities. Flip the seat over and it becomes a floor-level positioning aide for playing!

Worldwide Products Heat Packs 800-554-6340
7031 N Via De Paesia, Scottsdale, AZ 85258
Non-electric, push button, self activating, reusable and portable heat pack. Low back therapy kit also includes Flex Ice Pack and Neo-Belt.

Zimmer Holdings, Inc. 800-613-6131
1800 W Center St, PO Box 708, Warsaw, IN 46580

SUPPORT, ANKLE *(Orthopedics) 87RXC*

Aircast Llc 800-321-9549
1430 Decision St, Vista, CA 92081
AIR-STIRRUP ankle brace.

Alex Orthopedic, Inc. 800-544-2539
PO Box 201442, Arlington, TX 76006

Alimed, Inc. 800-225-2610
297 High St, Dedham, MA 02026

Bauerfeind Usa, Inc. 800-423-3405
55 Chastain Rd NW Ste 112, Kennesaw, GA 30144
MALLEOTRAIN ankle support with viscoelastic insert; equal compression throughout.

Best Orthopedic And Medical Services, Inc. 800-344-5279
2356B Springs Rd NE, Hickory, NC 28601

Border Opportunity Saver Systems, Inc. 830-775-0992
10 Finegan Rd, Del Rio, TX 78840

Cho-Pat 800-221-1601
Mt. Holly Industrial Commons, Lippincott Lane, Unit 6, Mt. Holly, NJ 08060
Cho-Pat Achilles Tendon Strap, Cho-Pat Ankle Support

Core Products International, Inc. 800-365-3047
808 Prospect Ave, Osceola, WI 54020
Deluxe Ankle Support, patented lacing system features offset eyelets and vinyl side supports to help position heel and stabilize ankle. Removable straps for additional support.

Cropper Medical, Inc./Bio Skin 800-541-2455
240 E Hersey St Ste 2, Ashland, OR 97520
Bioskin Ankle brace and Trilok Ankle support system with foot strap.

Evs Sports Protection 800-229-4EVS
2146 E Gladwick St, Rancho Dominguez, CA 90220

Fla Orthopedics, Inc. 800-327-4110
2881 Corporate Way, Miramar, FL 33025
GEL BAND Ankle Trainer Brace; Ankle support for chronically weak and lax ankles. Reduces ankle instability and aids in rehabilitation.

Formedica Ltd. 800-361-9671
1481 Rue Begin, St Laurent, QUE H4R 1V8 Canada
$30.00 per 10 (med).

Frank Stubbs Co., Inc 800-223-1713
2100 Eastman Ave Ste B, Oxnard, CA 93030

Freeman Manufacturing Company 800-253-2091
900 W Chicago Rd, PO Box J, Sturgis, MI 49091

Hermell Products, Inc. 800-233-2342
9 Britton Dr, PO Box 7345, Bloomfield, CT 06002

SUPPORT, ANKLE *(cont'd)*

Hospital Marketing Svcs. Company, Inc. 800-786-5094
162 Great Hill Rd./ Ind. Park, Naugatuck, CT 06770
HMS FLEXITONE - trauma wraps, #7614.

I-Rep, Inc. 800-828-0852
508 Chaney St Ste B, Lake Elsinore, CA 92530

Kern Surgical Supply, Inc. 800-582-3939
2823 Gibson St, Bakersfield, CA 93308

Larkotex Company 800-972-3037
1002 Olive St, Texarkana, TX 75501

Lohmann & Rauscher, Inc. 800-279-3863
6001 SW 6th Ave Ste 101, Topeka, KS 66615

Longdon Corp. Division Of Scythes, Inc., The 800-268-1737
128 Sterling Rd., Toronto, ONT M6R-2B7 Canada

Maramed Orthopedic Systems 800-327-5830
2480 W 82nd St, No. 8, Hialeah, FL 33016

Mark Medical 800-433-3668
1168 Aster Ave Ste C, Sunnyvale, CA 94086
ANKLE BRAVE, Feather Sock, a mini ankle support that can be worn under street clothing with the Feather Step orthotic for a complete support solution.

Mizuho Osi 800-777-4674
30031 Ahern Ave, Union City, CA 94587

Omni Life Science, Inc. 800-448-OMNI
1390 Decision St, Vista, CA 92081
ISO8 Quickloc and Sport ankle supports and Focus stirrup-style ankle brace.

Ossur Americas, Inc 800-222-4284
19762 Pauling, Foothill Ranch, CA 92610
Support for mild to moderate ankle strains and sprains. Skin friendly, greptec reduces slippage, low profile, comfortable fit with any shoe, v-stirrup straps for medical lateral stability to reduce inversion/eversion.

Paramedical Distributors 800-245-3278
2020 Grand Blvd, Kansas City, MO 64108
Asstd. designs available, AFOs, walkers, braces.

Pedifix, Inc. 800-424-5561
310 Guinea Rd, Brewster, NY 10509
Elastic ankle braces.

Pro Orthopedic Devices, Inc. 800-523-5611
2884 E Ganley Rd, Tucson, AZ 85706
PRO Neoprene rubber joint sleeves and supports.

Professional's Choice Sports Medicine Products, Inc. 800-331-9421
2025 Gillespie Way Ste 106, El Cajon, CA 92020
Sock with dual straps simulating athletic taping procedure. Also, shin splints that provide compression support to tendons without restricting flexibility or motion; 3 sizes.

Protectair Inc. 800-235-7932
59 Eisenhower Ln S, Lombard, IL 60148

Royce Medical 800-521-0601
742 Pancho Rd, Camarillo, CA 93012
Orthopaedic supports and braces. Wrist splints, ankle braces, short leg walking casts, back supports, knee immobilizers and knee supports.

Scott Specialties, Inc./Cmo Inc./Ginny Inc. 800-255-7136
512 M St, Belleville, KS 66935

Serum International Inc. 800-361-7726
4400 Autoroute Chomeoey, Laval, QUE H7R-6E9 Canada

Spenco Medical Corp. 254-772-6000
PO Box 2501, Waco, TX 76702
FIBERFLEX™ elastic support.

Surgical Appliance Industries 800-888-0458
3960 Rosslyn Dr, Cincinnati, OH 45209

Tartan Orthopedics, Ltd. 888-287-1456
10651 Irma Dr Unit C, Northglenn, CO 80233
$30.00 per 10 (med), $16.95 for active ankle support, Neoprene ankle support, Neoprene fig. 8 ankle wrap.

Tetra Medical Supply Corp. 800-621-4041
6364 W Gross Point Rd, Niles, IL 60714

Total Care 800-334-3802
PO Box 1661, Rockville, MD 20849

U.S. Orthotics, Inc. 800-825-5228
8605 Palm River Rd, Tampa, FL 33619
Vinyl and neoprene.

SUPPORT, ANKLE *(cont'd)*

Zimmer Holdings, Inc. 800-613-6131
1800 W Center St, PO Box 708, Warsaw, IN 46580

SUPPORT, ARCH *(Physical Med) 89RXD*

Alimed, Inc. 800-225-2610
297 High St, Dedham, MA 02026

Baron Medical Supply 888-702-2766
709 Grand St, Brooklyn, NY 11211
Custom molded arches and custom molded shoes.

Langer, Inc. 800-645-5520
450 Commack Rd, Deer Park, NY 11729

Paramedical Distributors 800-245-3278
2020 Grand Blvd, Kansas City, MO 64108
Asstd. styles, materials, and sizes available.

Pedifix, Inc. 800-424-5561
310 Guinea Rd, Brewster, NY 10509
Orthotics, preforms, arch binder.

Pro Orthopedic Devices, Inc. 800-523-5611
2884 E Ganley Rd, Tucson, AZ 85706
PRO Neoprene rubber joint sleeves and supports.

Spenco Medical Corp. 254-772-6000
PO Box 2501, Waco, TX 76702
SPENCO® 3/4 length arch cushion, full length cushion.

Tri Hawk Corporation 866-874-4295
150 Highland Rd, Massena, NY 13662
ORTHOFIT series 9000 and 9001 pre-fabricated orthotics.

SUPPORT, ARM *(Physical Med) 89IOY*

Aircast Llc 800-321-9549
1430 Decision St, Vista, CA 92081
AIRCAST pneumatic armband.

Alimed, Inc. 800-225-2610
297 High St, Dedham, MA 02026

American Orthopedic Supply Co., Inc.
37017 State Highway 79, Cleveland, AL 35049
Humeral fracture.

Back Support Systems 800-669-2225
67684 San Andreas St, Desert Hot Springs, CA 92240
THE HUG T is used to prop or position the arm for side sleeping used for rotator cuff recovery.

Biomet, Inc. 574-267-6639
56 E Bell Dr, PO Box 587, Warsaw, IN 46582
Various types of immobilizers/supports.

Bryton Corp. 800-567-9500
4310 Guion Rd, Indianapolis, IN 46254
Arm supports for surgical tables.

C.G. Laboratories, Inc. 817-279-1945
1410 Southtown Dr, Granbury, TX 76048

Chase Ergonomics, Inc. 800-621-5436
PO Box 92497, Albuquerque, NM 87199
Slip-on wrist support.

Cho-Pat 800-221-1601
Mt. Holly Industrial Commons, Lippincott Lane, Unit 6, Mt. Holly, NJ 08060
Cho-Pat Upper Arm Strap, Cho-Pat Bicep/Triceps Cuff.

Dj Orthopedics De Mexico, S.A. De C.V. 690-727-1280
Blvd., Delagacion La Presa, Tijuana 22397 Mexico
Arm support

Dj Orthopedics De Mexico, S.A. De C.V. 690-727-1280
Ave. Venustiano Carranza 6802, Castillo, Tijuana 22100 Mexico
Arm support

DJO Inc. 800-336-6569
1430 Decision St, Vista, CA 92081
Various styles and sizes of off-the-shelf arm supports.

Dynatronics Corp. Chattanooga Operations 801-568-7000
6607 Mountain View Rd, Ooltewah, TN 37363
Arm support.

Fla Orthopedics, Inc. 800-327-4110
2881 Corporate Way, Miramar, FL 33025

Formedica Ltd. 800-361-9671
1481 Rue Begin, St Laurent, QUE H4R 1V8 Canada
$30.00 per 10 (med).

Freeman Manufacturing Company 800-253-2091
900 W Chicago Rd, PO Box J, Sturgis, MI 49091
Thermo cast (plastic).

SUPPORT, ARM *(cont'd)*

Health Care Logistics, Inc. 800-848-1633
450 Town St, PO Box 25, Circleville, OH 43113
Various sizes and types of arm supports.

Hospital Marketing Svcs. Company, Inc. 800-786-5094
162 Great Hill Rd./ Ind. Park, Naugatuck, CT 06770
HMS FLEXITONE - trauma wraps, #7618.

Jaeco Orthopedic Specialties, Inc. 501-623-5944
214 Drexel St, Hot Springs, AR 71901

Jobri Llc 800-432-2225
520 N Division St, Konawa, OK 74849
MOR-LOC.

Larkotex Company 800-972-3037
1002 Olive St, Texarkana, TX 75501

Maramed Orthopedic Systems 800-327-5830
2480 W 82nd St, No. 8, Hialeah, FL 33016

Mcconnell Orthopedic Mfg. Co. 513-573-0085
1324 East Interstate 30 Bldg. B, Floyd, TX 75401
No common name listed.

Medi Usa 800-633-6334
6481 Franz Warner Pkwy, Whitsett, NC 27377
Epicompylitis support.

Medrecon, Inc. 877-526-4323
257 South Ave, Garwood, NJ 07027

Mizuho Osi 800-777-4674
30031 Ahern Ave, Union City, CA 94587

Orthotic & Prosthetic Lab, Inc. 314-968-8555
748 Marshall Ave, Webster Groves, MO 63119
O&p arm support.

Ossur Americas 949-268-3155
742 Pancho Rd, Camarillo, CA 93012

Paramedical Distributors 800-245-3278
2020 Grand Blvd, Kansas City, MO 64108

Patterson Medical Supply, Inc. 262-387-8720
W68N158 Evergreen Blvd, Cedarburg, WI 53012
Various types of arm supports.

Phelan Manufacturing Corp. 800-328-2358
2523 Minnehaha Ave, Minneapolis, MN 55404
$74.00 - $75.00 for arm guards, L-shaped or curved.

Pre Pak Products, Inc. 800-544-7257
4055 Oceanside Blvd Ste L, Oceanside, CA 92056
SHOULDER EASE, $65.00 each for arm support with arm resting angles of 45 degree abduction, 25 degree horizontal abduction and neutral rotation.

Pro Orthopedic Devices, Inc. 800-523-5611
2884 E Ganley Rd, Tucson, AZ 85706
PRO Neoprene rubber joint sleeves and supports.

R & R Industries, Inc. 949-361-9238
1000 Calle Cordillera, San Clemente, CA 92673
Forearm guard,elbow support.

Restorative Medical, Inc. 270-422-5454
332 Broadway St, Brandenburg, KY 40108
Safe elbow separator.

Serola Biomechanics, Inc. 815-636-2780
5281 Zenith Pkwy, Loves Park, IL 61111

Tartan Orthopedics, Ltd. 888-287-1456
10651 Irma Dr Unit C, Northglenn, CO 80233
$30.00 per 10 (med).

Terumo Cardiovascular Systems, Corp 800-521-2818
6200 Jackson Rd, Ann Arbor, MI 48103

Tetra Medical Supply Corp. 800-621-4041
6364 W Gross Point Rd, Niles, IL 60714

Total Care 800-334-3802
PO Box 1661, Rockville, MD 20849

Unique Sports Products, Inc. 800-554-3707
840 McFarland Pkwy, Alpharetta, GA 30004
For tennis elbow: Air-Cell tennis elbow support; wrist support. Also, Wrist Pad--a patented ergonomic wrist pad that provides support and helps prevent carpal tunnel syndrome. Cotton wristband with foam insert.

Vq Orthocare
1390 Decision St Ste A, Vista, CA 92081
Limb orthosis.

SUPPORT, ARM *(cont'd)*

Wisap America 800-233-8448
8231 Melrose Dr, Lenexa, KS 66214
Flexible arm.

Xback Bracing Services, Inc. 610-404-4900
341A W Main St, Birdsboro, PA 19508

Zimmer Holdings, Inc. 800-613-6131
1800 W Center St, PO Box 708, Warsaw, IN 46580

SUPPORT, BACK *(Orthopedics) 87RXE*

Alex Orthopedic, Inc. 800-544-2539
PO Box 201442, Arlington, TX 76006

Alimed, Inc. 800-225-2610
297 High St, Dedham, MA 02026

Allman Products 800-223-6889
21101 Itasca St, Chatsworth, CA 91311
Lumbar support cushions and rolls.

Back Support Systems 800-669-2225
67684 San Andreas St, Desert Hot Springs, CA 92240
THE CURVE is a therapeutic cushion that relieves lower-back discomfort due to tension, fatigue and stress. CONFOURM lumbar pad with straps that conform to almost any lumbar position for maximum comfort and support. Also available, THE KNEE T is a side sleeping positioning device to support the back. BACK T thoracic and lumbar car support system allows support while driving. With its adjustable positions, it fits most people.

Ball Dynamics International, Llc 800-752-2255
14215 Mead St, Longmont, CO 80504

Bauerfeind Usa, Inc. 800-423-3405
55 Chastain Rd NW Ste 112, Kennesaw, GA 30144
LUMBOTRAIN low-back support with viscoelastic insert.

Body Therapeutics, Div. Of I-Rep, Inc. 800-530-3722
508 Chaney St Ste 13, Lake Elsinore, CA 92530

Border Opportunity Saver Systems, Inc. 830-775-0992
10 Finegan Rd, Del Rio, TX 78840

Cmo, Inc. 800-344-0011
PO Box 147, Barberton, OH 44203
MOTHER-TO-BE maternity support features 8-in.-wide elastic support for lumbar area, optional moldable insert; belly pad supports baby and increases circulation.

Contour Form Products 800-223-8808
38 Stewart Ave, PO Box 328, Greenville, PA 16125
$40.25 for elastic binder CONTOUR FORM with moldable insert. POWER CINCH industrial back support, Model 400, 9' high, constructed of 2 layers of vented elastic, 4 steel stays with detachable suspenders.

Coopercare Lastrap Inc 416-741-9675
Highway H, Koopman Ln., Elkhorn, WI 53121

Corflex, Inc. 800-426-7353
669 E Industrial Park Dr, Manchester, NH 03109
Moldable and lumbosacral supports; industrial and neoprene back supports.

Cropper Medical, Inc./Bio Skin 800-541-2455
240 E Hersey St Ste 2, Ashland, OR 97520
Bioskin double back support system with lombar pads.

Darco International, Inc. 800-999-8866
810 Memorial Blvd, Huntington, WV 25701

Ehob, Inc. 800-899-5553
250 N Belmont Ave, Indianapolis, IN 46222
Versatile ASTRO-BACK lumbar support worn around the lower back to prevent soft tissue distortion and to massage the back muscles.

Ergodyne 800-225-8238
1021 Bandana Blvd E Ste 220, Saint Paul, MN 55108

Fla Orthopedics, Inc. 800-327-4110
2881 Corporate Way, Miramar, FL 33025

Formedica Ltd. 800-361-9671
1481 Rue Begin, St Laurent, QUE H4R 1V8 Canada
$25.00 per unit (med).

Frank Stubbs Co., Inc 800-223-1713
2100 Eastman Ave Ste B, Oxnard, CA 93030
Industrial back support.

Freeman Manufacturing Company 800-253-2091
900 W Chicago Rd, PO Box J, Sturgis, MI 49091

Home-Aid-Healthcare, Inc. 888-297-9109
PO Box 801764, Santa Clarita, CA 91380
ECONOWEAR, neoprene industrial back supports.

SUPPORT, BACK *(cont'd)*

Hospital Marketing Svcs. Company, Inc. 800-786-5094
162 Great Hill Rd./ Ind. Park, Naugatuck, CT 06770
HMS FLEXITONE - trauma wraps, #7606.

Invacare Corporation 800-333-6900
1 Invacare Way, Elyria, OH 44035
ULti-Mate Air/Ulti-Mate air pneumatic, Personal Back10/Personal Back10 Plus, LoBack, UniBack10, DualFlex10.

Jobri Llc 800-432-2225
520 N Division St, Konawa, OK 74849
MOR-LOC, E-Z FIT, JOBRI,

Kern Surgical Supply, Inc. 800-582-3939
2823 Gibson St, Bakersfield, CA 93308

Lab Safety Supply, Inc. 800-356-0783
401 S Wright Rd, Janesville, WI 53546

Larkotex Company 800-972-3037
1002 Olive St, Texarkana, TX 75501

Leander Health Technologies/Healthcare Division 800-635-8188
1525 Vivian Ct, Port Orchard, WA 98367
An inter-trochanteric support device which will allow healing of Sacral/ilium ligamentous structure.

Lohmann & Rauscher, Inc. 800-279-3863
6001 SW 6th Ave Ste 101, Topeka, KS 66615

Mccarty's Sacro-Ease Llc 800-635-3557
3329 Industrial Ave S, Coeur D Alene, ID 83815
SACRO-EASE - Orthopedic back supports.

Medic-Air, A Division Of Corflex, Inc. 800-426-7353
669 E Industrial Park Dr, Manchester, NH 03109
MEDIC-AIR air-filled cushions that provide adjustable support for the back.

Medical Safety Systems Inc. 888-803-9303
230 White Pond Dr, Akron, OH 44313

Nada-Concepts 800-722-2587
2448 Larpenteur Ave W, Saint Paul, MN 55113
Orthopedic back supports. Acti-Vest, clothing vest with a built in back support in it.

Obus Forme Ltd. 888-225-7378
550 Hopewell Ave., Toronto, ON M6E 2S6 Canada
$56 for THE SEAT (buttock rest); also, support roll available.

Ok-1 Manufacturing Co., Inc. 800-654-9873
709 S Veterans Dr, PO Box 736, Altus, OK 73521
Back support belts, wrist supports, other personal ergonomic products including: gloves, antivibration gloves and knee pads.

Ooltewah Manufacturing 800-251-6040x25
5722 Main St, P.O. Box 587, Ooltewah, TN 37363
Therapeutic weight belt to correct spinal curvature.

Ortho Active Appliances Ltd. 800-663-1254
103-250 Schoolhouse St., Coquitlam, BC V3K 6V7 Canada
We have a wide range of back supports, competitively prices.

Ortholine 800-243-3351
13 Chapel St, Norwalk, CT 06850
L/S Supports, Industrial Back Supports, CMO Supports w/Moldable Inserts

Ossur Americas, Inc 800-222-4284
19762 Pauling, Foothill Ranch, CA 92610
Powertex Back support provides warmth, compression adn support for mild to moderate back sprains and strains.

Paramedical Distributors 800-245-3278
2020 Grand Blvd, Kansas City, MO 64108
Asstd. orthoses available.

Ppr Direct, Inc. 800-526-3668
74 20th St, Brooklyn, NY 11232

Pro Orthopedic Devices, Inc. 800-523-5611
2884 E Ganley Rd, Tucson, AZ 85706
PRO Neoprene rubber joint sleeves and supports.

Professional's Choice Sports Medicine Products, Inc. 800-331-9421
2025 Gillespie Way Ste 106, El Cajon, CA 92020
Lumbo-sacral back supports; one size fits all. Neoprene.

Roloke Company 800-533-8212
127 W Hazel St, Inglewood, CA 90302
LUVS YA BACK Pelvic Spinal Posture Seat. BACK ME spinal posture aid for lumbar and thoracic support, adjustable. GOOD 'N BED adjustable body positioner multi-adjustable wedge. CURVE SNUGGER lumbar support. BOTTOMS UP pelvic spinal posture seat cushion.

SUPPORT, BACK *(cont'd)*

Royce Medical 800-521-0601
742 Pancho Rd, Camarillo, CA 93012
Orthopaedic supports and braces. Wrist splints, ankle braces, short leg walking casts, back supports, knee immobilizers and knee supports.

Scott Specialties, Inc./Cmo Inc./Ginny Inc. 800-255-7136
512 M St, Belleville, KS 66935

Shamrock Medical, Inc. 503-233-5055
3620 SE Powell Blvd, Portland, OR 97202

Slawner Ltd., J. 514-731-3378
5713 Cote Des Neiges Rd., Montreal, QUE H3S 1Y7 Canada

Surgical Appliance Industries 800-888-0458
3960 Rosslyn Dr, Cincinnati, OH 45209

Tetra Medical Supply Corp. 800-621-4041
6364 W Gross Point Rd, Niles, IL 60714

Truform Orthotics & Prosthetics 800-888-0458
3960 Rosslyn Dr, Cincinnati, OH 45209

U.S. Orthotics, Inc. 800-825-5228
8605 Palm River Rd, Tampa, FL 33619
Metal, plastic, canvas, elastic, and neoprene.

Valeo, Inc. 800-634-2704
W248N5499 Executive Dr, Sussex, WI 53089
Belt, for prevention and rehabilitation of lower back strain and fatigue. Keeps back stable during all types of activity. Cam buckle/torque ring, high-tech tightening and locking device.

Zimmer Holdings, Inc. 800-613-6131
1800 W Center St, PO Box 708, Warsaw, IN 46580

Zimmer Orthopaedic Surgical Products 800-321-5533
PO Box 10, 200 West Ohio Ave., Dover, OH 44622

SUPPORT, BREATHING TUBE *(Anesthesiology) 73JAY*

Allied Healthcare Products, Inc. 800-444-3954
1720 Sublette Ave, Saint Louis, MO 63110

Hans Rudolph, Inc. 816-363-5522
7200 Wyandotte St, Kansas City, MO 64114
Various types of breathing valves supports.

Hawaii Medical, Llc 781-826-5565
750 Corporate Park Dr, Pembroke, MA 02359

Health Care Logistics, Inc. 800-848-1633
450 Town St, PO Box 25, Circleville, OH 43113
Tube support.

Instrumentation Industries, Inc. 800-633-8577
2990 Industrial Blvd, Bethel Park, PA 15102
Safety straps, flex arms, brackets.

Intersurgical Inc. 315-451-2900
417 Electronics Pkwy, Liverpool, NY 13088
KNUCKLEHEAD, tubing holder for 10, 15 and 22 mm breathing circuits.

Kinetic Concepts, Inc. 800-275-4524
8023 Vantage Dr, San Antonio, TX 78230
Endo collar.

Mercury Medical 800-237-6418
11300 49th St N, Clearwater, FL 33762

Nova Health Systems, Inc. 800-225-NOVA
1001 Broad St, Utica, NY 13501
HALO.

Precision Medical, Inc. 800-272-7285
300 Held Dr, Northampton, PA 18067

Primary Medical Co., Inc. 727-520-1920
6541 44th St N Ste 6003, Pinellas Park, FL 33781
Support breathing tube, various profiles.

Sunmed Healthcare 727-531-7266
12393 Belcher Rd S Ste 460, Largo, FL 33773

Vartec Solutions, Inc. 330-655-7930
7570 Foxdale Cir, Hudson, OH 44236
Support, breathing tube.

SUPPORT, CLAVICLE *(Orthopedics) 87RXG*

Formedica Ltd. 800-361-9671
1481 Rue Begin, St Laurent, QUE H4R 1V8 Canada
$7.00 per unit (med).

Freeman Manufacturing Company 800-253-2091
900 W Chicago Rd, PO Box J, Sturgis, MI 49091

Larkotex Company 800-972-3037
1002 Olive St, Texarkana, TX 75501

SUPPORT, CLAVICLE *(cont'd)*

Ossur Americas, Inc 800-222-4284
19762 Pauling, Foothill Ranch, CA 92610
Shoulder suppport garment to address many shoulder and posture conditions due to weaken muscle groups.

Paramedical Distributors 800-245-3278
2020 Grand Blvd, Kansas City, MO 64108

Scott Specialties, Inc./Cmo Inc./Ginny Inc. 800-255-7136
512 M St, Belleville, KS 66935

Tartan Orthopedics, Ltd. 888-287-1456
10651 Irma Dr Unit C, Northglenn, CO 80233
$5.25 per unit (med).

Tetra Medical Supply Corp. 800-621-4041
6364 W Gross Point Rd, Niles, IL 60714

Zimmer Holdings, Inc. 800-613-6131
1800 W Center St, PO Box 708, Warsaw, IN 46580

SUPPORT, COLUMN, GLC *(Toxicology) 91DJA*

Chromatography Sciences Co. (Csc) 800-668-4752
5750 Vanden Abeele, St-Laurent, QUE H4S 1R9 Canada
COLUMN LC (CSC-TRIBUTE), column for aqueous condition for very polar compounds (Equivalent to Aqua, YMC-AQÖ)

SUPPORT, ELBOW *(Orthopedics) 87RXF*

Alimed, Inc. 800-225-2610
297 High St, Dedham, MA 02026

Bauerfeind Usa, Inc. 800-423-3405
55 Chastain Rd NW Ste 112, Kennesaw, GA 30144
EPITRAIN elbow support with viscoelastic insert; equal compression throughout.

Cho-Pat 800-221-1601
Mt. Holly Industrial Commons, Lippincott Lane, Unit 6, Mt. Holly, NJ 08060
Cho-Pat Forearm (Tennis Elbow) Strap, Cho-Pat Elbow Compression Cuff.

Coopercare Lastrap Inc 416-741-9675
Highway H, Koopman Ln., Elkhorn, WI 53121

Cropper Medical, Inc./Bio Skin 800-541-2455
240 E Hersey St Ste 2, Ashland, OR 97520
Bioskin Elbow Skin support brace.

Equip For Independence, Inc. 800-216-4881
333 Mamaroneck Ave Ste 383, White Plains, NY 10605

Evs Sports Protection 800-229-4EVS
2146 E Gladwick St, Rancho Dominguez, CA 90220

Freeman Manufacturing Company 800-253-2091
900 W Chicago Rd, PO Box J, Sturgis, MI 49091

Hermell Products, Inc. 800-233-2342
9 Britton Dr, PO Box 7345, Bloomfield, CT 06002

Home-Aid-Healthcare, Inc. 888-297-9109
PO Box 801764, Santa Clarita, CA 91380
ECONOWEAR, neoprene elbow supports.

Larkotex Company 800-972-3037
1002 Olive St, Texarkana, TX 75501

Lohmann & Rauscher, Inc. 800-279-3863
6001 SW 6th Ave Ste 101, Topeka, KS 66615

Longdon Corp. Division Of Scythes, Inc., The 800-268-1737
128 Sterling Rd., Toronto, ONT M6R-2B7 Canada

Mizuho Osi 800-777-4674
30031 Ahern Ave, Union City, CA 94587

Paramedical Distributors 800-245-3278
2020 Grand Blvd, Kansas City, MO 64108

Pro Orthopedic Devices, Inc. 800-523-5611
2884 E Ganley Rd, Tucson, AZ 85706
PRO Neoprene rubber joint sleeves and supports.

Professional's Choice Sports Medicine Products, Inc. 800-331-9421
2025 Gillespie Way Ste 106, El Cajon, CA 92020

Restorative Care Of America Inc 800-627-1595
12221 33rd St N, Saint Petersburg, FL 33716
RESPOND ROM elbow provides flexion/extension stop settings and static lock pin. Heat moldable Kydex construction. Foam liner included. Gradually increases joint extension with static lock settings. Universal Arm Brace - bilateral hinges provide flexion/extension elbow control from 0 to 120 degrees. Adjustable length hinge arms. Strains, sprains, elbow surgery, stable fractures.

Scott Specialties, Inc./Cmo Inc./Ginny Inc. 800-255-7136
512 M St, Belleville, KS 66935

SUPPORT, ELBOW *(cont'd)*

Serum International Inc. 800-361-7726
4400 Autoroute Chomeoey, Laval, QUE H7R-6E9 Canada

Swb Elbow Brace, Ltd. 760-564-9853
56059 Winged Foot, La Quinta, CA 92253
Brace designed to limit extension of the elbow joint; allow joint to heal as activity continues; support the elbow joint laterally and be worn during activity.

Tetra Medical Supply Corp. 800-621-4041
6364 W Gross Point Rd, Niles, IL 60714

Total Care 800-334-3802
PO Box 1661, Rockville, MD 20849

U.S. Orthotics, Inc. 800-825-5228
8605 Palm River Rd, Tampa, FL 33619
Neoprene sleeves.

Zimmer Holdings, Inc. 800-613-6131
1800 W Center St, PO Box 708, Warsaw, IN 46580

SUPPORT, FOOT *(Orthopedics) 87RXH*

Aetrex Worldwide, Inc 800-526-2739
414 Alfred Ave, Teaneck, NJ 07666
ANTI-SHOX, foot supports absorb shock and treat the discomfort of heel pain, arch strain and ball of foot ailments. AMBULATOR, footwear specially designed to protect and comfort the diabetic and arthritic foot.

Alimed, Inc. 800-225-2610
297 High St, Dedham, MA 02026

Cropper Medical, Inc./Bio Skin 800-541-2455
240 E Hersey St Ste 2, Ashland, OR 97520
Bioskin Trilok and Bioskin Ankle brace support systems.

Dr. Roth's Footcare Products, Llc. 800-486-0325
1012 Brioso Dr Ste 105, Costa Mesa, CA 92627
TABS (Toe Arch Band Support) is a revolutionary, one-size-fits-all, front-of-the-foot orthotic device that provides relief to tired achy feet, stone bruise, metatarceligia, capsulitis, and many lesser known front-of-the-foot discomforts. TABS act to improve front-of-the-foot posture by stabilizing the metatarsal arch. The metatarsal arch is a long-ignored area of foot architecture that is a source of foot discomfort for a considerable percentage of the population. TABS is the first metatarsal-arch support ever designed to quickly and effectively bring relief to the area under the ball of the foot. In so doing, TABS provide a potential alternative to surgical correction or life-long discomfort.o act to improve the posture of the foot. Better foot posture will help increase endurance, decrease the likelihood of the pulling or tearing of a muscle, as well as, providing the foot with better balance and stability. TABS help to improve overall foot performance by assisting the foot to work more efficiently, with less fatigue, and with a decreased chance for injury. Due to its unique design, TABS is the only arch support that can be worn with sandals or even barefoot! Originally developed for dancers and athletes, TABS is a unique combination of compression banding technology and pressure offloading effect, which together help to alleviate foot discomfort quickly.

Equip For Independence, Inc. 800-216-4881
333 Mamaroneck Ave Ste 383, White Plains, NY 10605

Freeman Manufacturing Company 800-253-2091
900 W Chicago Rd, PO Box J, Sturgis, MI 49091

J. T. Posey Co. 800-447-6739
5635 Peck Rd, Arcadia, CA 91006

Kronner Medical 800-706-3533
1443 Upper Cleveland Rapids Rd, Roseburg, OR 97471
KRONNER foot stand.

Langer, Inc. 800-645-5520
450 Commack Rd, Deer Park, NY 11729

Larkotex Company 800-972-3037
1002 Olive St, Texarkana, TX 75501

Northeast Medical Systems Corp. 856-910-8111
901 Beechwood Ave, Cherry Hill, NJ 08002

Omni Life Science, Inc. 800-448-OMNI
1390 Decision St, Vista, CA 92081
Ultra Gait and Ultra Gait 2 Walker post-surgery and fracture orthosis and support.

SUPPORT, FOOT *(cont'd)*

Ossur Americas, Inc 800-222-4284
19762 Pauling, Foothill Ranch, CA 92610
Dynamic ankle-foot orthosis provides dynamic support for drop foot or similar complaints for which support of dorsiflexion is desirable. Simple to fit, provides visible improvement in patients gait. Ergonomic ankle strap and plastic inlay fits between the tongue and laces of patients shoe for an innovative patient friedly way to address drop foot.

Paramedical Distributors 800-245-3278
2020 Grand Blvd, Kansas City, MO 64108
Asstd. supports available.

Pedifix, Inc. 800-424-5561
310 Guinea Rd, Brewster, NY 10509
Arch binder, diabetic and ambulatory shoes.

Pro Orthopedic Devices, Inc. 800-523-5611
2884 E Ganley Rd, Tucson, AZ 85706
PRO Neoprene rubber joint sleeves and supports.

Restorative Care Of America Inc 800-627-1595
12221 33rd St N, Saint Petersburg, FL 33716
MULTI-PODUS System treats foot/ankle contractures, hip rotation, and heel pressure sores. Phase II offers adjustable degree of angle for static stretch of the plantar flexors when serial casting is indicated.

Serum International Inc. 800-361-7726
4400 Autoroute Chomeoey, Laval, QUE H7R-6E9 Canada

Spenco Medical Corp. 254-772-6000
PO Box 2501, Waco, TX 76702
Orthotic arch support, 3/4 length and full length.

Tetra Medical Supply Corp. 800-621-4041
6364 W Gross Point Rd, Niles, IL 60714

Western Medical, Ltd. 800-628-8276
214 Carnegie Ctr Ste 100, Princeton, NJ 08540
Heel protector.

Zimmer Holdings, Inc. 800-613-6131
1800 W Center St, PO Box 708, Warsaw, IN 46580

SUPPORT, HAND *(Orthopedics) 87RXI*

Alimed, Inc. 800-225-2610
297 High St, Dedham, MA 02026

Coopercare Lastrap Inc 416-741-9675
Highway H, Koopman Ln., Elkhorn, WI 53121

Cropper Medical, Inc./Bio Skin 800-541-2455
240 E Hersey St Ste 2, Ashland, OR 97520
Bioskin thumb spica, DP2 and DP3 wrist braces.

Equip For Independence, Inc. 800-216-4881
333 Mamaroneck Ave Ste 383, White Plains, NY 10605

Ergodyne 800-225-8238
1021 Bandana Blvd E Ste 220, Saint Paul, MN 55108

Formedica Ltd. 800-361-9671
1481 Rue Begin, St Laurent, QUE H4R 1V8 Canada
$80.00 per 10 (med).

Freeman Manufacturing Company 800-253-2091
900 W Chicago Rd, PO Box J, Sturgis, MI 49091

Hermell Products, Inc. 800-233-2342
9 Britton Dr, PO Box 7345, Bloomfield, CT 06002

Jaeco Orthopedic Specialties, Inc. 501-623-5944
214 Drexel St, Hot Springs, AR 71901
Wrist driven wrist hand orthosis. Functional hand orthosis for c5-6 and c6-7 Quad RA, PC, for the use of residual muscles to create prehension.

Larkotex Company 800-972-3037
1002 Olive St, Texarkana, TX 75501

Ossur Americas, Inc 800-222-4284
19762 Pauling, Foothill Ranch, CA 92610
Wrist brace and wrist bankd provides compression and support for mild to moderate wrist strains and sprains.

Paramedical Distributors 800-245-3278
2020 Grand Blvd, Kansas City, MO 64108
Wrist/hand splints, fabric supports, moldable supports, etc.

Pro Orthopedic Devices, Inc. 800-523-5611
2884 E Ganley Rd, Tucson, AZ 85706
PRO Neoprene rubber joint sleeves and supports.

Slawner Ltd., J. 514-731-3378
5713 Cote Des Neiges Rd., Montreal, QUE H3S 1Y7 Canada

Surgical Appliance Industries 800-888-0458
3960 Rosslyn Dr, Cincinnati, OH 45209

SUPPORT, HAND *(cont'd)*

Tetra Medical Supply Corp. 800-621-4041
6364 W Gross Point Rd, Niles, IL 60714

Zimmer Holdings, Inc. 800-613-6131
1800 W Center St, PO Box 708, Warsaw, IN 46580

SUPPORT, HEAD AND TRUNK, WHEELCHAIR
(Physical Med) 89IMS

Alimed, Inc. 800-225-2610
297 High St, Dedham, MA 02026

Alternative Products 904-378-9081
5351 Ramona Blvd Ste 7, Jacksonville, FL 32205
Back support.

Anodyne Therapy, Llc 813-645-2855
13570 Wright Cir, Tampa, FL 33626
Lumbar support.

Blue Earth, Inc. 518-237-5585
31 Ontario St, 2nd Floor - Front, Cohoes, NY 12047
Trunk support, head rest.

Body Tech 1 Nw 866-315-0640
10727 47th Pl W, Mukilteo, WA 98275
Support, head and trunk, wheelchair.

Daher Mfg., Inc. 204-663-3299
Mazenod Rd, Winnipeg R2J 4H2 Canada
Various

Danmar Products, Inc. 734-761-1990
221 Jackson Industrial Dr, Ann Arbor, MI 48103
Chest support.

Innovative Concepts 800-676-5030
300 N State St, Girard, OH 44420
Headrests and mounting hardware. Also, custom seats, backs, pads and various seating and positioning hardware.

Intarsia Ltd. 203-355-1357
14 Martha Ln, Gaylordsville, CT 06755
Various wheelchair supports (solid, drop, back; armrest; headrest).

Keyes Manufacturing & Supply Llc. 316-284-2200
2015 West 1st, Newton, KS 67114
Add-on reclining backrest with optional mechanical lumbar support for wheelchair.

Miller's Adaptive Technologies 800-837-4544
2023 Romig Rd, Akron, OH 44320
Two-step Super Soft Headrest;fits the contours of head and neck. Dynamic Headrest Interface-allows responsive movement to occur-fitted with a gas spring.

Numotech, Inc. 818-772-1579
9420 Reseda Blvd Ste 504, Northridge, CA 91324
Wheelchair accessory.

Patterson Medical Supply, Inc. 262-387-8720
W68N158 Evergreen Blvd, Cedarburg, WI 53012
Occipital release board.

Sunrise Medical Hhg Inc 303-218-4505
7128 Ambassador Rd, Baltimore, MD 21244
Various sizes and shapes of positioning supports.

Sunrise Medical Hhg Inc 303-218-4505
2010 E Spruce Cir, Olathe, KS 66062
Wheelchair belt.

Sunrise Medical Hhg Inc 303-218-4505
6724 Preston Ave # 1, Livermore, CA 94551

Sunrise Medical Hhg Inc 303-218-4505
2615 W Casino Rd # 2B, Everett, WA 98204

Sunrise Medical Hhg Inc 303-218-4505
2842 N Business Park Ave, Fresno, CA 93727

Symmetric Designs, Ltd. 800-537-1724
2059 North End Rd., Salt Spring Island, BC V8K 1C9 Canada
Mantis headrest

Therafin Corporation 800-843-7234
19747 Wolf Rd, Mokena, IL 60448
Various head and trunk positioning products.

Thompson Medical Specialties 800-777-4949
3404 Library Ln, Saint Louis Park, MN 55426

SUPPORT, HEAD, SURGICAL, ENT *(Ear/Nose/Throat) 77EPW*

Genesis Medical Products, Inc. 508-876-1063
40 Farm Hill Rd, Wrentham, MA 02093
Various.

SUPPORT, HEAD, SURGICAL, ENT *(cont'd)*

Gyrus Ent L.L.C., Sub. Of Gyrus Acmi, Inc. 508-804-2739
2925 Appling Rd, Bartlett, TN 38133
Various.

Morris Designs, Inc. 757-463-9400
2212 Commerce Pkwy, Virginia Beach, VA 23454
Chin strap.

Oto-Med, Inc. 800-433-7703
1090 Empire Dr, Lake Havasu City, AZ 86404
Surgical Dressings: Glasscock Ear Dressing (Adult & Pediatric sizes), Head and Neck Pressure Dressing, Tierney Otoplasty Dressing, Postauricular Bandage and Eye Protector.

Span-America Medical Systems, Inc. 800-888-6752
70 Commerce Ctr, Greenville, SC 29615
Adult head support, head cradle, O.R. table pillow.

SUPPORT, HERNIA *(Gastro/Urology) 78EXN*

Apparel Med 425-359-6510
4902 112th St SE, Everett, WA 98208
Ostomy belt with peristomal hernia support and leakage support.

DJO Inc. 800-336-6569
1430 Decision St, Vista, CA 92081
Various sizes of groin supports.

Frederick Lee Inc 787-834-4880
191 Calle Balboa, PO Box 3287, Mayaguez, PR 00680

Freeman Manufacturing Company 800-253-2091
900 W Chicago Rd, PO Box J, Sturgis, MI 49091

I.M.K. Distributors, Inc. 800-878-5552
19 W 34th St Rm 915, New York, NY 10001

Ita-Med Co. 888-9IT-AMED
310 Littlefield Ave, South San Francisco, CA 94080
Double-sided, with removable foam inserts.

Larkotex Company 800-972-3037
1002 Olive St, Texarkana, TX 75501

Truform Orthotics & Prosthetics 800-888-0458
3960 Rosslyn Dr, Cincinnati, OH 45209

SUPPORT, HOT/COLD PACK *(Physical Med) 89UEC*

Back Support Systems 800-669-2225
67684 San Andreas St, Desert Hot Springs, CA 92240
ICE N HEAT hot/cold packs are $2.00 each and come in 15 sizes.

Bean Products 800-726-8365
1500 S Western Ave Ste 4BN, Chicago, IL 60608
Back burner, Largest leakproof hot/cold wrap for lower back area. Increase circulation, performance, reduce injuries. Fastens securely. Neck wrap, unbleached cotton covered leakproof hot/cold gel designed for neck area. Microwavable, freezable, solid glycerin based hydrogel. Headache wrap, unbleached cotton covered thermal gel designed for hot/cold therapy. Secures in position for freedom of movement. Solid leakproof glycerin based hydrogel.

Bruder Healthcare Company 888-827-8337
3150 Engineering Pkwy, Alpharetta, GA 30004
Moist Heat/Soothing Cold Therapy Wrap

Hospital Marketing Svcs. Company, Inc. 800-786-5094
162 Great Hill Rd./ Ind. Park, Naugatuck, CT 06770
TEMP-WRAP - 30in. elastic support with hot/cold pack, 6in. wide, #7626, 12 each; 4in. wide, #7624, 12 each.

Lohmann & Rauscher, Inc. 800-279-3863
6001 SW 6th Ave Ste 101, Topeka, KS 66615

Regency Product International 800-845-7931
4732 E 26th St, Vernon, CA 90058
Available in 2 sizes.

Tetra Medical Supply Corp. 800-621-4041
6364 W Gross Point Rd, Niles, IL 60714
New, Kanga-Wrap binder with pocket for hot or cold pack. Originally designed as pressure binder following abdominal surgery.

SUPPORT, KNEE *(Physical Med) 89RXJ*

Aircast Llc 800-321-9549
1430 Decision St, Vista, CA 92081
AIRCAST patellar brace.

Alex Orthopedic, Inc. 800-544-2539
PO Box 201442, Arlington, TX 76006

Alimed, Inc. 800-225-2610
297 High St, Dedham, MA 02026

SUPPORT, KNEE *(cont'd)*

Bauerfeind Usa, Inc. 800-423-3405
55 Chastain Rd NW Ste 112, Kennesaw, GA 30144
GENUTRAIN knee support with viscoelastic insert; equal compression throughout.

Bryton Corp. 800-567-9500
4310 Guion Rd, Indianapolis, IN 46254
Knee supports for surgical table & examination tables.

Cho-Pat 800-221-1601
Mt. Holly Industrial Commons, Lippincott Lane, Unit 6, Mt. Holly, NJ 08060
Cho-Pat Dual Action Knee Strap, Cho-Pat's Original Knee Strap, Cho-Pat Counter-Force Knee Wrap, Cho-Pat Patellar Stabilizer, Cho-Pat Dynamic Knee Compression Sleeve

Core Products International, Inc. 800-365-3047
808 Prospect Ave, Osceola, WI 54020
Performance Wrap Knee Support, best unhinged knee support available. Unique, 4-way tensioning system for custom fit and circumferential compression wraparound design.

Ergodyne 800-225-8238
1021 Bandana Blvd E Ste 220, Saint Paul, MN 55108
PROFLEX knee pads, for kneeling on hard, slippery, or abrasive surfaces.

Evs Sports Protection 800-229-4EVS
2146 E Gladwick St, Rancho Dominguez, CA 90220

Fla Orthopedics, Inc. 800-327-4110
2881 Corporate Way, Miramar, FL 33025

Formedica Ltd. 800-361-9671
1481 Rue Begin, St Laurent, QUE H4R 1V8 Canada
$70.00 per 10 (med).

Frank Stubbs Co., Inc 800-223-1713
2100 Eastman Ave Ste B, Oxnard, CA 93030

Freeman Manufacturing Company 800-253-2091
900 W Chicago Rd, PO Box J, Sturgis, MI 49091
Trade names; airprene & palumbo.

Hermell Products, Inc. 800-233-2342
9 Britton Dr, PO Box 7345, Bloomfield, CT 06002

Home-Aid-Healthcare, Inc. 888-297-9109
PO Box 801764, Santa Clarita, CA 91380
ECONOWEAR, neoprene knee supports.

Hospital Marketing Svcs. Company, Inc. 800-786-5094
162 Great Hill Rd./ Ind. Park, Naugatuck, CT 06770
FLEXITONE - trauma wraps, #7602-7618.

Kern Surgical Supply, Inc. 800-582-3939
2823 Gibson St, Bakersfield, CA 93308

Larkotex Company 800-972-3037
1002 Olive St, Texarkana, TX 75501

Lohmann & Rauscher, Inc. 800-279-3863
6001 SW 6th Ave Ste 101, Topeka, KS 66615

Longdon Corp. Division Of Scythes, Inc., The 800-268-1737
128 Sterling Rd., Toronto, ONT M6R-2B7 Canada

Lossing Orthopedic 800-328-5216
PO Box 6224, Minneapolis, MN 55406
Knee crescent.

Mizuho Osi 800-777-4674
30031 Ahern Ave, Union City, CA 94587

Omni Life Science, Inc. 800-448-OMNI
1390 Decision St, Vista, CA 92081
CoolLite and CompLite post-surgery adjustable braces for rigid support.

Paramedical Distributors 800-245-3278
2020 Grand Blvd, Kansas City, MO 64108
Asstd. knee supports, orthoses--both hard-hinged and fabric.

Pro Orthopedic Devices, Inc. 800-523-5611
2884 E Ganley Rd, Tucson, AZ 85706
PRO Neoprene rubber joint sleeves and supports.

Professional's Choice Sports Medicine Products, Inc. 800-331-9421
2025 Gillespie Way Ste 106, El Cajon, CA 92020
Several styles available; includes flexible stays,patella pulls, post-arthroscopic stabilizer brace, and more.

SUPPORT, KNEE *(cont'd)*

Restorative Care Of America Inc 800-627-1595
12221 33rd St N, Saint Petersburg, FL 33716
RESPOND ROM knee provides flexion/extension stop settings and static lock pin. Heat moldable Kydex construction. Foam liner included. Gradually increases joint extension with static lock settings. Flex Cuff Knee provides rehabilitation for knee injuries and contracture. Wrap around foam lines with flexion/extension stop bilateral hinges. Universal Leg Brace - multiaxial hinge provides infinite degree of flexion/extension settings. 7 degree tibial offset. Adjustable length hinge arms. Strains, sprains, stable fractures, and total knee replacements. Postoperative Pin Knee Brace - drop pin hinge control flexion/extension in 7'2 degrees following ACL, PCL, MCL, and LCL surgeries. Available in long or short lengths. Long length can be converted into short length with breakaway capabilities.

Royce Medical 800-521-0601
742 Pancho Rd, Camarillo, CA 93012
Orthopaedic supports and braces. Wrist splints, ankle braces, short leg walking casts, back supports, knee immobilizers and knee supports.

Scott Specialties, Inc./Cmo Inc./Ginny Inc. 800-255-7136
512 M St, Belleville, KS 66935

Signal Medical Corporation 800-246-6324
1000 Des Peres Rd Ste 140, Saint Louis, MO 63131
Silent knee assistant, including femoral belt, tibial belt, PCL retractor, and lateral retractors (set of two).

Surgical Appliance Industries 800-888-0458
3960 Rosslyn Dr, Cincinnati, OH 45209

Tetra Medical Supply Corp. 800-621-4041
6364 W Gross Point Rd, Niles, IL 60714

Truform Orthotics & Prosthetics 800-888-0458
3960 Rosslyn Dr, Cincinnati, OH 45209

U.S. Orthotics, Inc. 800-825-5228
8605 Palm River Rd, Tampa, FL 33619
Neoprene, pull-on sleeves, hinges, spirals, patella buttress, wraparound.

Valeo, Inc. 800-634-2704
W248N5499 Executive Dr, Sussex, WI 53089

Zimmer Holdings, Inc. 800-613-6131
1800 W Center St, PO Box 708, Warsaw, IN 46580

Zimmer Orthopaedic Surgical Products 800-321-5533
PO Box 10, 200 West Ohio Ave., Dover, OH 44622

SUPPORT, LEG *(Physical Med) 89RXK*

Aircast Llc 800-321-9549
1430 Decision St, Vista, CA 92081
AIR-STIRRUP leg brace.

Alimed, Inc. 800-225-2610
297 High St, Dedham, MA 02026

Bryton Corp. 800-567-9500
4310 Guion Rd, Indianapolis, IN 46254
Stirrups & leg holders for surgical tables.

Cho-Pat 800-221-1601
Mt. Holly Industrial Commons, Lippincott Lane, Unit 6, Mt. Holly, NJ 08060
Cho-Pat Shin Splint Compression Sleeve, Cho-Pat ITB (Iliotibial Band) Strap

Comfort Care Products Corp. 803-321-0020
258 Industrial Park Rd, Newberry, SC 29108
Leg positioners elevate the leg while helping to prevent pressure ulcer formation at the heels and foot drop. There are three cotton/poly straps with tension release locks to assist in holding the leg in place.

Formedica Ltd. 800-361-9671
1481 Rue Begin, St Laurent, QUE H4R 1V8 Canada
$200.00 per 10 (med).

Freeman Manufacturing Company 800-253-2091
900 W Chicago Rd, PO Box J, Sturgis, MI 49091

Hermell Products, Inc. 800-233-2342
9 Britton Dr, PO Box 7345, Bloomfield, CT 06002
Calf/shin support.

Jobri Llc 800-432-2225
520 N Division St, Konawa, OK 74849
MOR-LOC, E-Z FIT.

Larkotex Company 800-972-3037
1002 Olive St, Texarkana, TX 75501

Maramed Orthopedic Systems 800-327-5830
2480 W 82nd St, No. 8, Hialeah, FL 33016

SUPPORT, LEG *(cont'd)*

Paramedical Distributors 800-245-3278
2020 Grand Blvd, Kansas City, MO 64108
Asstd. designs available.

Pro Orthopedic Devices, Inc. 800-523-5611
2884 E Ganley Rd, Tucson, AZ 85706
PRO Neoprene rubber joint sleeves and supports.

Royce Medical 800-521-0601
742 Pancho Rd, Camarillo, CA 93012
Orthopaedic supports and braces. Wrist splints, ankle braces, short leg walking casts, back supports, knee immobilizers and knee supports.

Scott Specialties, Inc./Cmo Inc./Ginny Inc. 800-255-7136
512 M St, Belleville, KS 66935

Tetra Medical Supply Corp. 800-621-4041
6364 W Gross Point Rd, Niles, IL 60714

Total Care 800-334-3802
PO Box 1661, Rockville, MD 20849

Zimmer Holdings, Inc. 800-613-6131
1800 W Center St, PO Box 708, Warsaw, IN 46580

Zimmer Orthopaedic Surgical Products 800-321-5533
PO Box 10, 200 West Ohio Ave., Dover, OH 44622

SUPPORT, PATIENT POSITION *(Anesthesiology) 73CCX*

Alimed, Inc. 800-225-2610
297 High St, Dedham, MA 02026
Nursing home positioners. PROTECTA-COAT available in variety of shapes and sizes with liquid-resistant, non-slip coating.

Ambu A/S 457-225-2210
6740 Baymeadow Dr, Glen Burnie, MD 21060
Head immobilizer.

Anna-Dote, Inc. 800-346-6132
40 Pullam Dr, West Middlesex, PA 16159
ANNA-DOTE positioning support fits over the backrest of either a wheelchair or geriatric chair, providing an extended, padded backrest to aid in sitting upright.

Biomet, Inc. 574-267-6639
56 E Bell Dr, PO Box 587, Warsaw, IN 46582
Various types of patient position supports.

Bone Foam 612-338-1400
700 10th Ave S, Minneapolis, MN 55415
Surgical patient stabilization blocks.

Bryton Corp. 800-567-9500
4310 Guion Rd, Indianapolis, IN 46254
Patient positioning systems for surgical procedures.

Burkhart Roentgen Intl. Inc. 800-USA-XRAY
5201 8th Ave S, Gulfport, FL 33707
Comfortable patient positioning aids & table pads for all types of tables.

Cloward Instrument Corporation 808-734-3511
3787 Diamond Head Rd, Honolulu, HI 96816
CLOWARD Surgical saddle.

Confortaire Inc 662-842-2966
2133 S Veterans Blvd, Tupelo, MS 38804
Various types of positioning wedges, pillows and rings.

Creative Foam Medical Systems 800-446-4644
405 Industrial Dr, Bremen, IN 46506
Various types of coated foam support & patient positioning pads.

Crosley Medical Products, Inc. 631-595-2547
60 S 2nd St Ste E, Deer Park, NY 11729

Dupaco, Inc. 800-546-4550
4144 Avenida De La Plata, Oceanside, CA 92056
Proneview Protective Helmet System.

Dynamic Systems, Inc. 828-683-3523
235 Sunlight Dr, Leicester, NC 28748

Ebi, Llc 800-526-2579
100 Interpace Pkwy, Parsippany, NJ 07054
AOA Soft Goods, Line of braces and supports.

Encompas Unlimited, Inc. 800-825-7701
PO Box 516, Tallevast, FL 34270
MZ-28 Endo Wedge: Designed to keep your patient firmly on their side.

Frank Scholz X-Ray Corp. 508-586-8308
244 Liberty St, Brockton, MA 02301
$320.00 per unit (standard).

SUPPORT, PATIENT POSITION *(cont'd)*

Freedom Designs, Inc. 800-331-8551
2241 N Madera Rd, Simi Valley, CA 93065
Seating/positioning systems.

Global Medical Foam, Inc. 419-529-9354
124 Plymouth St Ste A, Lexington, OH 44904
Various.

Health Care Logistics, Inc. 800-848-1633
450 Town St, PO Box 25, Circleville, OH 43113
Patient arm shield support.

Innovative Medical Products, Inc. 800-467-4944
87 Spring Lane, Plainville Industrial Pk, Plainville, CT 06062
IMP Universal Lateral Positioner for patient stability during hip arthroplasty; allows for surgeon's point of reference to be reproduced exactly for revision surgery. Disposable foam pads also available to help prevent pressure sores. IMP Universal Knee Positioner - used for total knee arthroplasty, ACL repair, IMP Knee Position Triangle. Equalizer: Surgical guide used during total hip arthoplasty to prevent leg length discrepancy. DeMayo Hip Positioner, Ducharme FX Alignment Device. Tibial Distractor: Used for tibial fractures requiring intramedullary nail. An adjustable height triangle with distraction of the ankle to align fracture. De Mayo Hip Positioner: For stable lateral decubiter positioning of the patient for THA and revision surgeries. Especially useful in positioning the obese patient.

Jerome Medical 800-257-8440
305 Harper Dr, Moorestown, NJ 08057
AirWay PAD (Pediatric Alignment Device)- A Broselow-Luten color coded device to quickly raise the thorax of a pediatric patient to the appropriate height to maintain an open airway and c-spine alignment.

Kaye Products, Inc. 919-732-6444
535 Dimmocks Mill Rd, Hillsborough, NC 27278
Prone positioner, supine positioner and vertical stander for children; also, prone stander for adults and children.

Lossing Orthopedic 800-328-5216
PO Box 6224, Minneapolis, MN 55406
LOSSING BASICTRAC provides lumbar positional distraction with no weights, water bags or pulleys; patient's own weight, combined with positioning, does the work. Several models available.

Mccarty's Sacro-Ease Llc 800-635-3557
3329 Industrial Ave S, Coeur D Alene, ID 83815

Mcconnell Orthopedic Mfg. Co. 513-573-0085
1324 East Interstate 30 Bldg. B, Floyd, TX 75401
No common name listed.

Medical Positioning, Inc. 800-593-3246
1717 Washington St, Kansas City, MO 64108
SAFETWEDGE non-skid positional cushion for patient head elevation and positioning. Available in 4 sizes and shapes or customized.

Mizuho Osi 800-777-4674
30031 Ahern Ave, Union City, CA 94587
Inflatable bolster, lateral positioner, Collins device.

National Medical Products 800-940-6262
9775 Mining Dr Ste 104, Jacksonville, FL 32257
POSI BLOCK positioning wedges: for body positioning, foot positioning block, foot drop blocks. Pediatric line available. Hip abduction blocks. Elbow and Heel protectors.

O.R. Comfort, Llc 973-239-1950
28 Appleton Rd, Glen Ridge, NJ 07028
Adjustable and inflatable surgical support pillow.

Oakworks, Inc. 800-558-8850
923 E Wellspring Rd, New Freedom, PA 17349
Post-vitrectomy face-down prone support positioner.

Optp 888-819-0121
3800 Annapolis Ln N Ste 165, PO Box 47009, Minneapolis, MN 55447
POSITEX Personal Wedge and POSITEX Professional positioning wedges.

Oxy-Sure Company, Llc 866-476-3800
13930 W 2nd Ave, Orofino, ID 83544
The Oxy-Sure 'Buddy' is a support device for stabilizing the position of a nasal cannula and minimizing the development of friction sores.

Prime Engineering 800-827-8263
4202 W Sierra Madre Ave, Fresno, CA 93722
Granstand III: Child to adult growth capable modular standing system and transfer device client height from 3' to 6'5'.

Profex Medical Products 800-325-0196
2224 E Person Ave, Memphis, TN 38114
Foam positioning pads; laminectomy positioners.

SUPPORT, PATIENT POSITION *(cont'd)*

Rinz-L-O 248-548-3993
340 W Maplehurst St, Ferndale, MI 48220
Support, patient position.

Royal Converting, Inc. 865-938-7828
1615 Highway 33 S, New Tazewell, TN 37825

Smithers Medical Products, Inc. 330-497-0690
4850 Hossler Dr NW, North Canton, OH 44720
Various sizes and types of patient immobilization. CT, MRI, PET, Therapeutic Radiology.

Span-America Medical Systems, Inc. 800-888-6752
70 Commerce Ctr, Greenville, SC 29615
SPAN+AIDS Patient positioners & body aligners and abduction pillows.

Telos Medical Equipment (Austin & Assoc., Inc.) 800-934-3029
1109 Sturbridge Rd, Fallston, MD 21047
TELOS O.R. supports maintain most all operative positions. Bi-directional pivoting with 360 degrees rotation. Attaches to any O.R. table.

The Saunders Group 800-445-9836
4250 Norex Dr, Chaska, MN 55318
Support, patient position.

Universal Service Associates, Inc. 800-601-1916
500 Ellis Ave, Darby, PA 19023
Laminectomy and surgery support.

SUPPORT, PATIENT POSITION, RADIOGRAPHIC *(Radiology) 90RNX*

Alimed, Inc. 800-225-2610
297 High St, Dedham, MA 02026
PROTECTA-COAT vinyl coated, multi-purpose positioners. Ideal for radiology with liquid-resistant, non-slip coating. Infant/small child positioners also available.

Biopro, Inc. 800-252-7707
2929 Lapeer Rd, Port Huron, MI 48060
Fix-Ray Device

Burlington Medical Supplies, Inc. 800-221-3466
3 Elmhurst St, PO Box 3194, Newport News, VA 23603
Positioning sponge (radiology).

Cfi Medical Solutions (Contour Fabricators, Inc.) 810-750-5300
14241 N Fenton Rd, Fenton, MI 48430

Composiflex, Inc. 800-673-2544
8100 Hawthorne Dr, Erie, PA 16509
Low absorption, high strength carbon fiber patient support systems.

Flow X-Ray Corporation 800-356-9729
100 W Industry Ct, Deer Park, NY 11729
Wolfoam nonabsorbant foam blocks.

Frank Scholz X-Ray Corp. 508-586-8308
244 Liberty St, Brockton, MA 02301
$489.50 for head holder with vacuum suction mounting; fixation/positioning device.

Gammex Rmi 800-426-6391
PO Box 620327, Middleton, WI 53562

Hokanson Inc., D.E. 800-999-8251
12840 NE 21st Pl, Bellevue, WA 98005
Patient positioning aids for plethysmographic studies. We offer a 5-piece foam block set for forearm studies and an 8-piece set for forearm and limb studies.

Infab Corp. 805-987-5255
3651 Via Pescador, Camarillo, CA 93012
Standard and custom shapes available in standard foam, super foam and temper foam.

Marconi Medical Systems 800-323-0550
595 Miner Rd, Cleveland, OH 44143

Modern Way Immobilizers, Inc. 866-694-7444
PO Box 660, 100 Johnson St, Clifton, TN 38425
Pigg-O-Stat infant immobilizer and positioner. Moder Way infant and child foot immobilizer and positioner.

Mtd, Inc. 908-362-6807
24 Slabtown Creek Rd, Hardwick, NJ 07825

Profex Medical Products 800-325-0196
2224 E Person Ave, Memphis, TN 38114

S&S Technology 281-815-1300
10625 Telge Rd, Houston, TX 77095

Techno-Aide, Inc. 800-251-2629
7117 Centennial Blvd, Nashville, TN 37209

SUPPORT, PATIENT POSITION, RADIOGRAPHIC *(cont'd)*

Vermont Composites, Inc. 802-442-9964
25 Performance Dr, Bennington, VT 05201
Low absorption carbon supports.

Wolf X-Ray Corporation 800-356-9729
100 W Industry Ct, Deer Park, NY 11729
Wolfoam nonabsorbant foam blocks.

Xma (X-Ray Marketing Associates, Inc.) 800-325-8880
1205 W Lakeview Ct, Windham Lakes Business Park
Romeoville, IL 60446

Zimmer Holdings, Inc. 800-613-6131
1800 W Center St, PO Box 708, Warsaw, IN 46580

SUPPORT, SCROTAL *(Gastro/Urology) 78EXO*

Truform Orthotics & Prosthetics 800-888-0458
3960 Rosslyn Dr, Cincinnati, OH 45209

SUPPORT, SCROTAL, THERAPEUTIC *(General) 80FQJ*

Truform Orthotics & Prosthetics 800-888-0458
3960 Rosslyn Dr, Cincinnati, OH 45209

SUPPORT, THIGH *(Physical Med) 89RXL*

Hermell Products, Inc. 800-233-2342
9 Britton Dr, PO Box 7345, Bloomfield, CT 06002

Hospital Marketing Svcs. Company, Inc. 800-786-5094
162 Great Hill Rd./ Ind. Park, Naugatuck, CT 06770

I-Rep, Inc. 800-828-0852
508 Chaney St Ste B, Lake Elsinore, CA 92530

Lohmann & Rauscher, Inc. 800-279-3863
6001 SW 6th Ave Ste 101, Topeka, KS 66615

Pro Orthopedic Devices, Inc. 800-523-5611
2884 E Ganley Rd, Tucson, AZ 85706
PRO Neoprene rubber joint sleeves and supports.

Professional's Choice Sports Medicine Products, Inc. 800-331-9421
2025 Gillespie Way Ste 106, El Cajon, CA 92020
Assists in management of groin pulls and strains.

Tetra Medical Supply Corp. 800-621-4041
6364 W Gross Point Rd, Niles, IL 60714

U.S. Orthotics, Inc. 800-825-5228
8605 Palm River Rd, Tampa, FL 33619
Also, calf support.

SUPPORT, TUBE, TEST *(Chemistry) 75WID*

Bio Plas, Inc. 415-472-3777
4340 Redwood Hwy Ste A15, San Rafael, CA 94903
Polyester foam test tube supports (floats in water bath).

Nutech Molding Corporation 1-800-423-5278
PO Box 840, 2024 Broad St,, Pocomoke City, MD 21851

SUPPORT, WRIST *(Physical Med) 89RXM*

Alex Orthopedic, Inc. 800-544-2539
PO Box 201442, Arlington, TX 76006

Alimed, Inc. 800-225-2610
297 High St, Dedham, MA 02026

Bauerfeind Usa, Inc. 800-423-3405
55 Chastain Rd NW Ste 112, Kennesaw, GA 30144
MANUTRAIN wrist support with viscoelastic insert.

Best Orthopedic And Medical Services, Inc. 800-344-5279
2356B Springs Rd NE, Hickory, NC 28601

Cho-Pat 800-221-1601
Mt. Holly Industrial Commons, Lippincott Lane, Unit 6, Mt. Holly, NJ 08060
Cho-Pat Wrist Support.

Contour Form Products 800-223-8808
38 Stewart Ave, PO Box 328, Greenville, PA 16125
WRIST BUDDIE, model 116-M or 116-L, for carpel tunnel support, 8' length, 4 flexible steel stays, vented elastic with 4' wrap around strap. Can be worn on either hand.

Ergodyne 800-225-8238
1021 Bandana Blvd E Ste 220, Saint Paul, MN 55108

Evs Sports Protection 800-229-4EVS
2146 E Gladwick St, Rancho Dominguez, CA 90220

Fla Orthopedics, Inc. 800-327-4110
2881 Corporate Way, Miramar, FL 33025
WORK ABOUT CARPAL MATE, CARPAL MATE Wrist Support; helps prevent and provide symptomatic relief of carpal tunnel syndrome

SUPPORT, WRIST *(cont'd)*

Formedica Ltd. 800-361-9671
1481 Rue Begin, St Laurent, QUE H4R 1V8 Canada
$80.00 per 10 (med).

Frank Stubbs Co., Inc 800-223-1713
2100 Eastman Ave Ste B, Oxnard, CA 93030

Freeman Manufacturing Company 800-253-2091
900 W Chicago Rd, PO Box J, Sturgis, MI 49091
Cock-up Wrist Splints, therapeutic wrist aid.

Hermell Products, Inc. 800-233-2342
9 Britton Dr, PO Box 7345, Bloomfield, CT 06002

Home-Aid-Healthcare, Inc. 888-297-9109
PO Box 801764, Santa Clarita, CA 91380
ECONOWEAR, neoprene wrist supports.

Hospital Marketing Svcs. Company, Inc. 800-786-5094
162 Great Hill Rd./ Ind. Park, Naugatuck, CT 06770

I-Rep, Inc. 800-828-0852
508 Chaney St Ste B, Lake Elsinore, CA 92530

Kinetikos Medical, Inc. 800-546-3845
6005 Hidden Valley Rd Ste 180, Carlsbad, CA 92011
SPIDER, 3-dimensional, stainless-steel plate indicated for 4-corner fusion in the wrist. Mini-Spider Limited Wrist Fusion Plate for STT and other limited fusions of the wrist.

Larkotex Company 800-972-3037
1002 Olive St, Texarkana, TX 75501

Lohmann & Rauscher, Inc. 800-279-3863
6001 SW 6th Ave Ste 101, Topeka, KS 66615

Longdon Corp. Division Of Scythes, Inc., The 800-268-1737
128 Sterling Rd., Toronto, ONT M6R-2B7 Canada

Maramed Orthopedic Systems 800-327-5830
2480 W 82nd St, No. 8, Hialeah, FL 33016

Medical Safety Systems Inc. 888-803-9303
230 White Pond Dr, Akron, OH 44313

Optp 888-819-0121
3800 Annapolis Ln N Ste 165, PO Box 47009, Minneapolis, MN 55447
Wrist Restore, increases the willingness of the patient to obtain and use treatment for an unstable wrist.

Paramedical Distributors 800-245-3278
2020 Grand Blvd, Kansas City, MO 64108
Asstd. wrist/hand supports and orthoses.

Pro Orthopedic Devices, Inc. 800-523-5611
2884 E Ganley Rd, Tucson, AZ 85706
PRO Neoprene rubber joint sleeves and supports.

Professional's Choice Sports Medicine Products, Inc. 800-331-9421
2025 Gillespie Way Ste 106, El Cajon, CA 92020
MAGIC WRIST; both left and right wrist; one size fits all. Neoprene.

Restorative Care Of America Inc 800-627-1595
12221 33rd St N, Saint Petersburg, FL 33716
Dorsal Carpal Tunnel Splint. Limits wrist flexion and extension during repetitive hand motion. Made of moldable Rydex material; foam liner included. New products include a Neoprene wrist-extension splint that limits wrist flexion and extension and features both palmar and dorsal stays; and a Neoprene universal thumb/wrist support with bendable metal stay that places the thumb in a position of function and limits extreme joint motion.

Royce Medical 800-521-0601
742 Pancho Rd, Camarillo, CA 93012
Orthopaedic supports and braces. Wrist splints, ankle braces, short leg walking casts, back supports, knee immobilizers and knee supports.

Scott Specialties, Inc./Cmo Inc./Ginny Inc. 800-255-7136
512 M St, Belleville, KS 66935

Sroufe Healthcare Products Llc 888-894-4171
PO Box 347, 601 Sroufe St., Ligonier, IN 46767
Canvas,vinyl and elastic wrist splints.

Star Medical Systems 800-626-3006
8301 Torresdale Ave Ste 13, Philadelphia, PA 19136

Surgical Appliance Industries 800-888-0458
3960 Rosslyn Dr, Cincinnati, OH 45209

Tetra Medical Supply Corp. 800-621-4041
6364 W Gross Point Rd, Niles, IL 60714

Therafirm, A Knit Rite Company 800-562-2701
120 Osage Ave, Kansas City, KS 66105
For relief from carpal tunnel syndrome.

SUPPORT, WRIST *(cont'd)*

Valeo, Inc. 800-634-2704
W248N5499 Executive Dr, Sussex, WI 53089

Zimmer Holdings, Inc. 800-613-6131
1800 W Center St, PO Box 708, Warsaw, IN 46580

SURGICAL BENCH VISE *(Surgery) 79LSA*

Biomet Microfixation Inc. 800-874-7711
1520 Tradeport Dr, Jacksonville, FL 32218
Vise, bench, surgical.

Bioquest 480-350-9944
2211 W 1st St Ste 106, Tempe, AZ 85281
Bone vise.

SURGICAL DEVICE, FOR ABLATION OF CARDIAC TISSUE
(Surgery) 79OCL

ATS Medical, Inc. 800-399-1381
3905 Annapolis Ln N Ste 105, Minneapolis, MN 55447
SURGIFROST PROBES; ATS MEDICAL CRYOABLATION SYSTEM SUR; CryoCath Frostbyte Clamp & Console; CryoCath Surgifrost 10cm Probe; CryoMaze Surgical Ablation System

Healthtronics Inc. 888-252-6575
9825 Spectrum Dr Bldg B, Austin, TX 78717

Minnetronix Inc. 888-301-1025
1635 Energy Park Dr, Saint Paul, MN 55108
EPICOR MEDICAL ABLATION SYSTEMS

nContact Surgical, Inc. 919-466-9810
1001 Aviation Pkwy Ste 400, Morrisville, NC 27560
nContact Guided Coagulation System; VisiTrax, Numeris Tethered Coagulation System, Numeris Guided Coagulation System

SURGICAL INSTRUMENT, CARDIOVASCULAR
(Cardiovascular) 74DWS

Abbott Vascular Inc. 800-227-9902
400 Saginaw Dr, Redwood City, CA 94063
Suture trimmer.

Accumed Systems, Inc. 734-930-0461
6109 Jackson Rd, Ann Arbor, MI 48103
Accugage vessel caliper.

Adler Instrument Co. 866-382-3537
6191 Atlantic Blvd, Norcross, GA 30071

Ascent Healthcare Solutions 480-763-5300
10232 S 51st St, Phoenix, AZ 85044
Tissue stabilizer.

Atek Medical 800-253-1540
620 Watson St SW, Grand Rapids, MI 49504
Tissue stabilizer.

Atrion Medical Products, Inc. 800-343-9334
1426 Curt Francis Rd NW, Arab, AL 35016
CLEANCUT(tm),OneTwo(tm) aortic punches. Also available, autogenous tissue collector used to collect autogenous bone for use in orthopedic and dental reconstrucion procedures.

ATS Medical, Inc. 800-399-1381
3905 Annapolis Ln N Ste 105, Minneapolis, MN 55447
ATS SurgiFrost probe for surgical cryoablation

Bard Peripheral Vascular, Inc. 800-321-4254
1625 W 3rd St, Tempe, AZ 85281
Kelley-Wick tunneler for vascular graft placement.

Bolt Bethel, Llc 763-434-5900
23530 University Avenue Ext NW, PO Box 135, Bethel, MN 55005

Boss Instruments, Ltd. 800-210-2677
395 Reas Ford Rd Ste 120, Earlysville, VA 22936

Boston Scientific Corp. 408-935-3400
150 Baytech Dr, San Jose, CA 95134
Access stabilizer.

Cardica, Inc. 888-544-7194
900 Saginaw Dr, Redwood City, CA 94063
Gauge.

Cascade Life Solutions, Llc 616-977-2505
3710 Sysco Ct SE, Grand Rapids, MI 49512
Cardiovascular accessories.

Chase Medical, Lp 972-783-0644
1876 Firman Dr, Richardson, TX 75081
Various models of clips, suture stay, retractor, basket sizer steril/non sterile.

Codman & Shurtleff, Inc 800-225-0460
325 Paramount Dr, Raynham, MA 02767

SURGICAL INSTRUMENT, CARDIOVASCULAR *(cont'd)*

Daily Medical Products, Inc. 800-550-1553
4620 Goldenrod Ln N, Plymouth, MN 55442

Drg International, Inc. 800-321-1167
1167 US Highway 22, Mountainside, NJ 07092

Edwards Lifesciences Research Medical 949-250-2500
6864 Cottonwood St, Midvale, UT 84047
Aortic sizer.

Elmed, Inc. 630-543-2792
60 W Fay Ave, Addison, IL 60101

Ethicon, Inc. 800-4-ETHICON
Route 22 West, Somerville, NJ 08876

Fehling Surgical Instruments 800-FEHLING
509 Broadstone Ln NW, Acworth, GA 30101

International Biophysics Corp. 512-326-3244
2101 E Saint Elmo Rd Ste 275, Austin, TX 78744
Identification instrument.

International Hospital Supply Co. 800-398-9450
6914 Canby Ave Ste 105, Reseda, CA 91335

J. Jamner Surgical Instruments, Inc 800-431-1123
9 Skyline Dr, Hawthorne, NY 10532

Kelsar, S.A. 508-261-8000
Blvd. Insurgentes, Libriamento a La, Tijuana 22450 Mexico
Aortic punch instrument

Kmedic 800-955-0559
190 Veterans Dr, Northvale, NJ 07647

Maquet Cardiovascular LLC 888-880-2874
45 Barbour Pond Dr, Wayne, NJ 07470

Maquet Puerto Rico Inc. 408-635-3900
No. 12, Rd. #698, Dorado, PR 00646
Cardiac off pump surgical stabilizer.

Mark Medical Manufacturing, Inc. 610-269-4420
530 Brandywine Ave, Downingtown, PA 19335
Endoscopic instruments.

Medisiss 866-866-7477
2747 SW 6th St, Redmond, OR 97756
Various cardiovascular surgical instruments,sterile.

Medtronic Cardiovascular Surgery, The Heart Valve Div. 800-328-2518
1851 E Deere Ave, Santa Ana, CA 92705
Various sizes and models of surgical instruments.

Medtronic Heart Valves 800-227-3191
8299 Central Ave NE, Spring Lake Park, MN 55432
Various sizes.

Navilyst Medical 800-833-9973
100 Boston Scientific Way, Marlborough, MA 01752
Introducer needle.

Precision Medical Manufacturing Corporation 866-633-4626
852 Seton Ct, Wheeling, IL 60090

Scanlan International, Inc. 800-328-9458
1 Scanlan Plz, Saint Paul, MN 55107
Diamond dust and titanium instrumentation.

Surge Medical Solutions, Llc. 616-977-2516
3710 Sysco Ct SE, Grand Rapids, MI 49512
Cardiovascular accessories.

Surgical Instrument Manufacturers, Inc. 800-521-2985
1650 Headland Dr, Fenton, MO 63026

Teleflex Medical 800-334-9751
2917 Weck Drive, Research Triangle Park, NC 27709

Terumo Cardiovascular Systems (Tcvs) 800-283-7866
28 Howe St, Ashland, MA 01721
Aspirator needle.

Thomas Medical Products, Inc. 866-446-3003
65 Great Valley Pkwy, Malvern, PA 19355
Pacing lead clamping system/tearaway intro. score propagating device.

Tuzik Boston 800-886-6363
104 Longwater Dr, Assinippi Park, Norwell, MA 02061

W. L. Gore & Associates, Inc. 800-437-8181
PO Box 2400, Flagstaff, AZ 86003
GORE HEMOSTATIC VALVE OPENER

W.L. Gore & Associates,Inc 928-526-3030
1505 North Fourth St., Flagstaff, AZ 86004
Reusable surgical instruments.

SURGICAL INSTRUMENT, DISPOSABLE *(Surgery) 79KDC*

Acra Cut, Inc. 978-263-0250
989 Main St, Acton, MA 01720
Distraction screw or pins.

Alcon Manufacturing, Ltd. 817-551-6813
714 Columbia Ave, Sinking Spring, PA 19608
Various disposable surgical instruments.

Ascent Healthcare Solutions 480-763-5300
10232 S 51st St, Phoenix, AZ 85044
Disposable surgical instruments.

Bd Caribe, Ltd. 201-847-4298
Rd. 183, Km. 20.3, Las Piedras, PR 00771
Disposable scalpel.

Bolt Bethel, Llc 763-434-5900
23530 University Avenue Ext NW, PO Box 135, Bethel, MN 55005

Busse Hospital Disposables, Inc. 631-435-4711
75 Arkay Dr, Hauppauge, NY 11788
Various types of sterile non-sterile disposable instruments.

Centurion Medical Products Corp. 517-545-1135
3310 S Main St, Salisbury, NC 28147

Chase Medical, Lp 972-783-0644
1876 Firman Dr, Richardson, TX 75081
Sucker.

Clinical Pharmacies, Inc. 800-669-6973
21622 Surveyor Cir # 8-C, Huntington Beach, CA 92646
Plastic tube occluding forceps.

Cornerstone Surgical, Llc 503-680-7281
10175 SW Barbur Blvd Ste 214-B, Portland, OR 97219
Distraction screw or pins.

David Scott Company 800-804-0333
59 Fountain St, Framingham, MA 01702

Eagle Laboratories 800-782-6534
10201 Trademark St Ste A, Rancho Cucamonga, CA 91730
Disposable blades and knives for microsurgery.

Esco Medical Instruments, Inc. 800-970-3726
21 William Penn Dr, Stony Brook, NY 11790
Sterile and disposable biopsy forceps.

Ese Acquisition Llc. 609-716-0600
666 Plainsboro Rd Ste 1271, Plainsboro, NJ 08536
Bone marrow biopsy and aspiration needle.

Ethicon Endo-Surgery, Inc. 800-USE-ENDO
4545 Creek Rd, Cincinnati, OH 45242
ENDOPATH curved scissors, hook and micro, short with unipolar cautery, and dissector (straight also), 5mm rotating; extractor/ratchet, 5mm, rotating, claw; grasper/ratchet and tooth graser, 5mm rotating with ratchet.

Genicon 800-936-1020
6869 Stapoint Ct Ste 114, Winter Park, FL 32792
Mono Polar and Bi Polar Disposable Laparoscopic Instrumentation

Her-Mar, Inc. 800-327-8209
8550 NW 30th Ter, Doral, FL 33122
Scissors, forceps, needle holders, handles, etc. Dissecting sets.

Hospira Inc. 877-946-7747
275 N Field Dr, Lake Forest, IL 60045
Multiple

Hydrocision, Inc. 888-747-7470
22 Linnell Cir Ste 102, Billerica, MA 01821
Hydrosurgical system for soft-tissue management, including traumatic and chronic wound debridement.

International Hospital Supply Co. 800-398-9450
6914 Canby Ave Ste 105, Reseda, CA 91335
Disposable scalpels.

Invacare Supply Group, An Invacare Co. 800-225-4792
75 October Hill Rd, Holliston, MA 01746

Koros Usa, Inc. 805-529-0825
610 Flinn Ave, Moorpark, CA 93021
Instrument, surgical, disposable.

Magnum Medical 800-336-9710
3265 N Nevada St, Chandler, AZ 85225
Single use plastic instruments.

Mckesson General Medical 800-446-3008
8741 Landmark Rd, Richmond, VA 23228

Medical Action Industries, Inc. 800-645-7042
25 Heywood Rd, Arden, NC 28704
Disposable instruments.

SURGICAL INSTRUMENT, DISPOSABLE *(cont'd)*

Olsen Medical 800-297-6344
3001 W Kentucky St, Louisville, KY 40211
Full line of Bipolar and Monopolar Forceps, & Monopolar Electrodes.

Putnam Precision Products 845-278-2141
3859 Danbury Rd, Brewster, NY 10509

Quality Aspirators 800-858-2121
1419 Godwin Ln, Duncanville, TX 75116
SCREEN VAC disposable high volume aspirator. Prevents grabbing of patient's tongue, cheek and soft tissue.

Ross Disposable Products 800-649-6526
401 Traders Blvd E, Unit 10, Mississauga, ON L4Z 2H8 Canada

Specialty Surgical Instrumentation, Inc. 800-251-3000
200 River Hills Dr, Nashville, TN 37210

Sterling Multi-Products, Inc. 815-537-2381
326 W 5th St, Prophetstown, IL 61277
Various disposable metal thumb forceps and suture removal scissors.

Surgical Safety Products, Inc. 800-953-7889
2018 Oak Ter Ste 400, Sarasota, FL 34231
Surgical assist device. Suturemate is designed for use by surgeons or surgical assistants during the suturing process. It has been clinically proven to reduce suture needlesticks and glove performations by all specialties.

Techstyles Manufacturing Division 800-826-4490
16415 Addison Rd Ste 660, Addison, TX 75001
Sterile and non-sterile disposable hypothermia prevention blankets and accessories.

Terumo Cardiovascular Systems (Tcvs) 800-283-7866
28 Howe St, Ashland, MA 01721
Pediatric sucker.

Tri-State Hospital Supply Corp. 517-545-1135
3173 E 43rd St, Yuma, AZ 85365

Tri-State Hospital Supply Corp. 800-248-4058
301 Catrell Dr, PO Box 170, Howell, MI 48843

Troy Manufacturing Co. 440-834-8262
17090 Rapids Rd, PO Box 448, Burton, OH 44021

SURGICAL INSTRUMENT, G-U, MANUAL *(Gastro/Urology) 78KOA*

Boston Scientific Corporation 508-652-5578
8600 NW 41st St, Doral, FL 33166

Boston Scientific Corporation 508-652-5578
780 Brookside Dr, Spencer, IN 47460

C. R. Bard, Inc., Bard Urological Div. 888-367-2273
13183 Harland Dr NE, Covington, GA 30014

Greenwald Surgical Co., Inc. 219-962-1604
2688 Dekalb St, Gary, IN 46405
Urethral/vesicourethral.

Gyrus Acmi, Inc. 508-804-2739
93 N Pleasant St, Norwalk, OH 44857
Surgical instruments, g-u, manual (and accessories).

Laprostop, Llc 858-705-3838
1845 Newport Avenue, San Diego, CA 92107
Surgical instrument accessory.

Lone Star Medical Products, Inc. 800-331-7427
11211 Cash Rd, Stafford, TX 77477
DILAMEZINSERT, a stainless steel surgical instrument utilizing disposable insert, which facilitates dilation, measurement and insertion of the penile prosthesis. Available in both the sharp tip (DMI) or blunt tip (DMI-B). Inguinal Reservoir Inserter (IRI), a stainless steel instrument consisting of two components: a carrier and inserter. They are used to facilitate implantaion and protection of reservoir during placement into prevesical space. Closing Tool (P-3), a stainless steel penile prosthesis protector used to prevent inadvertent puncture of penile prosthesis while closing incision.

Omnitech Systems, Inc. 866-266-9490
450 Campbell St Ste 2, Valparaiso, IN 46385
Stone dislodgers/graspers. Helical/flat-wire and custom shape-memory alloys.

Tools For Surgery, Llc 631-444-4448
1339 Stony Brook Rd, Stony Brook, NY 11790
Stapler sizers.

Tulip Medical Products 800-325-6526
PO Box 7368, San Diego, CA 92167
TULIP brand syringe instrumentation for soft tissue surgery.

U.S. Women Institute 714-546-3898
11160 Warner Ave Ste 117, Fountain Valley, CA 92708
Burch-sling device(BLADDER SAVER DEVICE).

SURGICAL INSTRUMENT, G-U, MANUAL *(cont'd)*

Urology-Tech Llc 806-798-0214
4710 FM 1585, Lubbock, TX 79424
Deep dorjal vein higator.

Uroplasty, Inc. 952-426-6140
5420 Feltl Rd, Minnetonka, MN 55343

SURGICAL INSTRUMENT, MANUAL (GENERAL USE)

(Surgery) 79MDW

Acuderm Inc. 800-327-0015
5370 NW 35th Ter Ste 106, Fort Lauderdale, FL 33309
Disposable comedone extractor.

Aesculap Implant Systems Inc. 1-800-234-9179
3773 Corporate Pkwy, Center Valley, PA 18034

Automated Medical Products Corp. 800-832-4567
PO Box 2508, Edison, NJ 08818
Articulating dissector.

Codman & Shurtleff, Inc 800-225-0460
325 Paramount Dr, Raynham, MA 02767

Deknatel Snowden-Pencer 800-367-7874
5175 S Royal Atlanta Dr, Tucker, GA 30084

Derron Surgical Instruments, Inc. 888-374-3622
1055 Scherer Way, Osprey, FL 34229
Instrument; manual, surgical, general use.

El Mar, Inc. 860-729-7232
43 Cody St, West Hartford, CT 06110
Tweezers with pinpoint precision.

Fehling Surgical Instruments 800-FEHLING
509 Broadstone Ln NW, Acworth, GA 30101

Her-Mar, Inc. 800-327-8209
8550 NW 30th Ter, Doral, FL 33122

Keeler Instruments Inc. 800-523-5620
456 Park Way, Broomall, PA 19008

Kls-Martin L.P. 800-625-1557
11239-1 St. John`s Industrial, Parkway South
Jacksonville, FL 32250

Kmedic 800-955-0559
190 Veterans Dr, Northvale, NJ 07647

Prosurge Instruments, Inc. 866-832-7874
199 Laidlaw Ave, Jersey City, NJ 07306
Wide range of scissors, including Lister bandage, operating, Kelly, Mayo, stitch, Littaur, and wire cutting.

Protectair Inc. 800-235-7932
59 Eisenhower Ln S, Lombard, IL 60148

Rx Honing Machine Corporation 800-346-6464
1301 E 5th St, Mishawaka, IN 46544
RX Honing Machines: Surgical instrument sharpening manual with over 150 pictures and diagrams giving detailed steps in the sharpening of surgical instruments with Rx Machine Set components.

Savoy Medical Supply 631-234-7003
745 Calebs Path, Hauppauge, NY 11788

Scanlan International, Inc. 800-328-9458
1 Scanlan Plz, Saint Paul, MN 55107

Troy Manufacturing Co. 440-834-8262
17090 Rapids Rd, PO Box 448, Burton, OH 44021

SURGICAL INSTRUMENT, NON-POWERED, NEUROSURGICAL

(Cns/Neurology) 84HAO

Abbott Spine, Inc. 847-937-6100
12708 Riata Vista Cir Ste B-100, Austin, TX 78727
Handle.

Acra Cut, Inc. 978-263-0250
989 Main St, Acton, MA 01720
Dura separotors.

Advanced Biomaterial Systems, Inc. 973-635-9040
100 Passaic Ave, Chatham, NJ 07928
Immedica.

Aztec Medical Products, Inc. 800-223-3859
106 Ingram Rd, Williamsburg, VA 23188
Surgical instruments.

Becton Dickinson And Co. 866-906-8080
411 Waverley Oaks Rd, Waltham, MA 02452

Biomet Microfixation Inc. 800-874-7711
1520 Tradeport Dr, Jacksonville, FL 32218
Non-powered surgical instrument.

SURGICAL INSTRUMENT, NON-POWERED, NEUROSURGICAL *(cont'd)*

Bioplate, Inc. 310-815-2100
3643 Lenawee Ave, Los Angeles, CA 90016
Non powered neurosurgical instrument.

Boss Instruments, Ltd. 800-210-2677
395 Reas Ford Rd Ste 120, Earlysville, VA 22936

Cynthia Flores Castrejon 52-5-780-36-97
Plazuela #24, Mz 12, Lt 8 Casa, 3 Plazas De Aragon
Nezahualcoyotl, EDO. 57139 Mexico
Various.

Depuy Spine, Inc. 800-227-6633
325 Paramount Dr, Raynham, MA 02767
Instrument handle, multiple use.

Depuy-Raynham, A Div. Of Depuy Orthopaedics 800-451-2006
325 Paramount Dr, Raynham, MA 02767
Instrument.

Elmed, Inc. 630-543-2792
60 W Fay Ave, Addison, IL 60101

Fischer Surgical Inc. 314-303-7753
1343 Pine Dr, Arnold, MO 63010
Various types of non-powered surgical instruments.

Integral Design Inc. 781-740-2036
52 Burr Rd, Hingham, MA 02043

Invacare Supply Group, An Invacare Co. 800-225-4792
75 October Hill Rd, Holliston, MA 01746

King Tool, Inc. 800-587-9445
5350 Love Ln, Bozeman, MT 59718
Instrument for removal of foreign objects from eye (battery powered).

Kirwan Surgical Products, Inc. 888-547-9267
180 Enterprise Dr, PO Box 427, Marshfield, MA 02050
Disposable neurosurgical dissecting needle.

Kmedic 800-955-0559
190 Veterans Dr, Northvale, NJ 07647

West Coast Surgical Llc. 650-728-8095
141 California Ave Ste 101, Half Moon Bay, CA 94019
Spreader-distractor.

SURGICAL INSTRUMENT, OBSTETRIC/GYNECOLOGIC *(Obstetrics/Gyn) 85KNA*

Adler Instrument Co. 866-382-3537
6191 Atlantic Blvd, Norcross, GA 30071

Apple Medical Corp. 508-357-2700
28 Lord Rd Ste 135, Marlborough, MA 01752
Various hand-held ob/gyn surgical instruments.

Centurion Medical Products Corp. 517-545-1135
3310 S Main St, Salisbury, NC 28147

Confluent Surgical,Inc 888-734-2583
101A 1st Ave, Waltham, MA 02451
Absorbable intrauterine stent.

Health Care Logistics, Inc. 800-848-1633
450 Town St, PO Box 25, Circleville, OH 43113
Umbilical cord clamp and cutter.

Omnitech Systems, Inc. 866-266-9490
450 Campbell St Ste 2, Valparaiso, IN 46385
Hysteroscopic resectoscope electrodes. Patented tips for endometrial ablation.

Princeton Medical Group, Inc. 800-875-0869
1189 Royal Links Dr, Mt Pleasant, SC 29466

Sterilis Inc. 714-437-9801
17092 Newhope St, Fountain Valley, CA 92708
Speculum, vaginal.

Tri-State Hospital Supply Corp. 517-545-1135
3173 E 43rd St, Yuma, AZ 85365

SURGICAL INSTRUMENT, OBSTETRIC/GYNECOLOGIC, GENERAL *(Obstetrics/Gyn) 85KOH*

Apple Medical Corp. 508-357-2700
28 Lord Rd Ste 135, Marlborough, MA 01752
Vaginal probe.

Cameron-Miller, Inc. 800-621-0142
5410 W Roosevelt Rd, Road #241, Chicago, IL 60644

Derron Surgical Instruments, Inc. 888-374-3622
1055 Scherer Way, Osprey, FL 34229
Instrument; manual, general obstetric-gynecologic.

SURGICAL INSTRUMENT, OBSTETRIC/GYNECOLOGIC, GENERAL *(cont'd)*

Greystone Of Lincoln, Inc. 401-333-0444
7 Wellington Rd, Lincoln, RI 02865
Endoscopic housing and metal tubes.

International Hospital Supply Co. 800-398-9450
6914 Canby Ave Ste 105, Reseda, CA 91335

Laprostop, Llc 858-705-3838
1845 Newport Avenue, San Diego, CA 92107
Trocar accessory.

Mark Medical Manufacturing, Inc. 610-269-4420
530 Brandywine Ave, Downingtown, PA 19335
Custom-made suction tubes, Leep or Lete instrument, custom manufacturer.

Purfybr, Inc. 800-947-9227
9384 Calumet Ave, Munster, IN 46321
Various types of sterile & non-sterile cytology brushes.

Rocket Medical Plc. 800-707-7625
150 Recreation Park Dr Ste 3, Hingham, MA 02043

Schueler & Company, Inc. 516-487-1500
PO Box 528, Stratford, CT 06615

SURGICAL INSTRUMENT, ORTHOPEDIC, AC-POWERED MOTOR *(Orthopedics) 87HWE*

Accellent Inc. 866-899-1392
100 Fordham Rd, Wilmington, MA 01887

Arthrex, Inc. 239-643-5553
1370 Creekside Blvd, Naples, FL 34108
Various.

Biomet Sports Medicine 530-226-5800
6704 Lockheed Dr, Redding, CA 96002
Micro power sugical system.

Biomet, Inc. 574-267-6639
56 E Bell Dr, PO Box 587, Warsaw, IN 46582
Various tyeps of electrical powered surgical instruments.

Brasseler Usa - Medical 805-650-5209
4837 McGrath St Ste J, Ventura, CA 93003
Surgical Instrument System.

Cloward Instrument Corporation 808-734-3511
3787 Diamond Head Rd, Honolulu, HI 96816
CLOWARD Posterior lumbar interbody fusion kit.

Depuy Orthopaedics, Inc. 800-473-3789
700 Orthopaedic Dr, P.O. Box 988, Warsaw, IN 46582
Various types of surgical instrument accessories/attachments, ac-powered.

Hydrocision, Inc. 888-747-7470
22 Linnell Cir Ste 102, Billerica, MA 01821
Arthroscopic hydrosurgery system for soft-tissue management and bone burring.

Kapp Surgical Instrument, Inc. 800-282-5277
4919 Warrensville Center Rd, Cleveland, OH 44128

Kinamed, Inc. 800-827-5775
820 Flynn Rd, Camarillo, CA 93012
NaviPro image free hip navigation system.

Kmedic 800-955-0559
190 Veterans Dr, Northvale, NJ 07647

LinkBio Corp. 800-932-0616
300 Round Hill Dr, Rockaway, NJ 07866
Instruments for surgery of the hand and foot.

Medtronic Sofamor Danek Instrument Manufacturing 901-396-3133
7375 Adrianne Pl, Bartlett, TN 38133
Various surgical burs.

Medtronic Sofamor Danek Usa, Inc. 901-396-3133
4340 Swinnea Rd, Memphis, TN 38118
Various surgical burs.

Micro-Aire Surgical Instruments, Inc. 800-722-0822
1641 Edlich Dr, Charlottesville, VA 22911

Microaire Surgical Instruments, Llc 434-975-8000
1641 Edlich Dr, Charlottesville, VA 22911

Modular Cutting Systems, Inc. 203-336-3526
650 Clinton Ave, Bridgeport, CT 06605
Hip core & bone grafting system.

SURGICAL INSTRUMENT, ORTHOPEDIC, AC-POWERED MOTOR *(cont'd)*

Ortho Development Corp. 800-429-8339
12187 Business Park Dr, Draper, UT 84020
Orion-I EMF System; used in general surgical purposes in coagulation, cutting & ablation of soft tissues.

Rx Honing Machine Corporation 800-346-6464
1301 E 5th St, Mishawaka, IN 46544
RX Honing Machines: Surgical #92701 or hospital #92801 sharpening sets include components, video and manual for orthopedic instrument sharpening.

Small Bone Innovations, Inc. 215-428-1791
1380 S Pennsylvania Ave, Morrisville, PA 19067
Surgical instrument and accessories/attachments.

Stryker Endoscopy 800-435-0220
5900 Optical Ct, San Jose, CA 95138

Symmetry Medical Usa, Inc. 574-267-8700
486 W 350 N, Warsaw, IN 46582
Reamers.

Tava Surgical Instruments 805-650-5209
4837 McGrath St Ste J, Ventura, CA 93003
Surgical Instrument System.

Thompson Surgical Instruments, Inc. 800-227-7543
10170 E Cherry Bend Rd, Traverse City, MI 49684

Vilex, Inc. 931-474-7550
111 Moffitt St, McMinnville, TN 37110

Warsaw Orthopedic, Inc. 901-396-3133
2500 Silveus Xing, Warsaw, IN 46582
Various surgical burs.

Zimmer Spine, Inc. 800-655-2614
7375 Bush Lake Rd, Minneapolis, MN 55439
Various.

Zimmer Trabecular Metal Technology 800-613-6131
10 Pomeroy Rd, Parsippany, NJ 07054
Oscillating saw blade.

SURGICAL INSTRUMENT, ORTHOPEDIC, BATTERY-POWERED *(Surgery) 79KIJ*

Acumed Llc 503-627-9957
5885 NW Cornelius Pass Rd, Hillsboro, OR 97124
Bone graft insruments.

Arthrex, Inc. 239-643-5553
1370 Creekside Blvd, Naples, FL 34108
Graft harvesting kit.

Medtronic Powered Surgical Solutions 800-643-2773
4620 N Beach St, Haltom City, TX 76137
Electric high speed motor & various sterile & non sterile accessories.

Putnam Precision Products 845-278-2141
3859 Danbury Rd, Brewster, NY 10509

S & S Orthopedic Ltd. 336-626-5167
701 Westmont Dr, Asheboro, NC 27205
Wire driver.

Smith & Nephew Inc., Endoscopy Div. 978-749-1000
76 S Meridian Ave, Oklahoma City, OK 73107
Powered hand instruments.

Smith & Nephew, Inc., Endoscopy Division 800-343-8386
150 Minuteman Rd, Andover, MA 01810

Symmetry Medical Usa, Inc. 574-267-8700
486 W 350 N, Warsaw, IN 46582
Reamers.

SURGICAL INSTRUMENT, RADIAL KERATOTOMY *(Ophthalmology) 86VKE*

Akorn, Inc. 800-535-7155
2500 Millbrook Dr, Buffalo Grove, IL 60089
Grene/Kenyon corneal marker, optical zone markers, plus diamond knives and titanium instruments.

Boss Instruments, Ltd. 800-210-2677
395 Reas Ford Rd Ste 120, Earlysville, VA 22936

H.S. International Co., Inc. 800-811-0072
5040 Commercial Cir Ste A, Concord, CA 94520
H.S.International has built a well-known reputation in the manufacture of wide range of ophthalmic instruments: Vitrectomy Cutters, Intraocular Micro-Scissors, Infusion Sleeves, Bi-Manual Irrigation and Aspiration, Titanium I/A, Phaco needles, etc. and provide a complete line of support and services, including repair.

SURGICAL INSTRUMENT, RADIAL KERATOTOMY *(cont'd)*

Incisiontech 800-213-7809
9 Technology Dr, Staunton, VA 24401

Kmi Surgical Ltd. 800-528-2900
110 Hopewell Rd, Laird Professional Building, Downingtown, PA 19335

SURGICAL INSTRUMENT, SONIC *(Orthopedics) 87JDX*

Biomet Sports Medicine 530-226-5800
6704 Lockheed Dr, Redding, CA 96002
Sonic, orthopedic surgical instrument system.

Biomet, Inc. 574-267-6639
56 E Bell Dr, PO Box 587, Warsaw, IN 46582
Various types of ultrasonic bone cutting instruments.

SURGICAL INSTRUMENT, ULTRASONIC *(Surgery) 79LFL*

Ethicon Endo-Surgery, Inc. 877-384-4266
3801 University Blvd SE, Albuquerque, NM 87106
Various types of ultrasonic surgical instruments & convience kits.

Fibra-Sonics, A Division Of Misonix, Inc. 631-694-9555
1938 New Hwy, Farmingdale, NY 11735
Ultrasonic surgical aspirator.

Misonix, Inc. 800-694-9612
1938 New Hwy, Farmingdale, NY 11735
The SonicOne is an innovative, ultrasonic wound care system that offers tissue specific debridement and cleansing for effective removal of devitalized tissue and fibrin deposits while sparing viable cellular structures. The SonicOne establishes a new standard in advanced wound care and ensures progress towards patient healing.

Sound Surgical Technologies Llc 888-471-4777
357 McCaslin Blvd Ste 100, Louisville, CO 80027
VASER® System for body sculpting. Using patented pulsed ultrasonic energy and small groove-tipped probes, the VASER System effectively emulsifies fat cells while leaving connective tissue, nerves and vessels largely intact.

SURGICAL, RAZOR *(Surgery) 79LWK*

American Safety Razor Co. 540-248-8000
1 Razor Blade Ln, Verona, VA 24482
Various types of surgical/medical prep razors.

Amson Products 718-435-3728
1401 42nd St, Brooklyn, NY 11219
Disposable.

Centurion Medical Products Corp. 517-545-1135
3310 S Main St, Salisbury, NC 28147

Derma-Safe Company 973-839-6383
32 Juniper Rd, Wayne, NJ 07470
DERMA-SAFE surgical prep razors: small straight type; double edge wet shave; single edge dry shave; wet and dry shave kits.

Encore Plastics Corporation 419-626-8000
725 Water St, Cambridge, OH 43725
Razor surgical.

Omni Medical Supply Inc. 800-860-6664
4153 Pioneer Dr, Commerce Township, MI 48390

Personna Medical/Div. Of American Safety Razor Co. 800-457-2222
1 Razor Blade Ln, Verona, VA 24482
PERSONNA DERMAGARD Safety Prep Razor is a heavyweight safety prep razor, with combs to lift and separate. Personna Medical's uniquely wrapped blade provides protection from nicks and cuts. If you have considered alternative methods for prepping because of concerns about nicks, cuts, and potential infection, this product may offer the protection you require. It takes shave preping to a new, higher level...Added safety - because the blade never touches the skin! PERSONNA Premium Double Edge Prep Razor is a heavyweight double edge prep razor with combs to lift and separate hair, manufactured with Personna Medical's high-quality COMFORT-COATED stainless steel blades, providing smooth, clean shaves.

Tri-State Hospital Supply Corp. 517-545-1135
3173 E 43rd St, Yuma, AZ 85365

Wahl Clipper Corp. 815-548-8342
2900 Locust St, Sterling, IL 61081
Surgical clipper.

SUSCEPTIBILITY TEST PANELS, ANTIMICROBIAL *(Microbiology) 83LTT*

Trek Diagnostic Systems 800-871-8909
982 Keynote Cir Ste 6, Cleveland, OH 44131

SUSPENSION SYSTEM, CELL CULTURE *(Pathology) 88KJF*

Biovest International, Inc. 866-3BIOVEST
8500 Evergreen Blvd NW, Minneapolis, MN 55433
RESCU-PRIMER Research Scale Cell Culture Kit is a disposable, single use perfusion cell culture kit which is ideal for producing research qualities of biologic protein and antibodies.

New Brunswick Scientific Co., Inc. 800-631-5417
PO Box 4005, Edison, NJ 08818
NBS offers a range of stirred tank fermentors and bioreactors, 1 to 1,500 L, for growth of virtually any bacterial, animal, mammalian, plant or insect cell. All are offered with numerous options, ranging from specialized impellers to a unique packed-bed for producing high-yields of secreted products.

North American Science Associates, Inc. 866-666-9455
6750 Wales Rd, Northwood, OH 43619
Growth-promotion test suspensions for qualifying culture media; available for a wide variety of organisms.

Thermo Fisher Scientific (Rochester) 585-899-7600
75 Panorama Creek Dr, Panorama, NY 14625
System, suspension, cell culture.

Thermo Fisher Scientific - Fairport 585-899-7600
236 Perinton Pkwy, Fairport, NY 14450
Various cell culture suspension systems.

SUTURE APPARATUS, STOMACH AND INTESTINAL
(Gastro/Urology) 78FHM

Medisiss 866-866-7477
2747 SW 6th St, Redmond, OR 97756
Various stomach and intestinal suturing apparatus,sterile.

Pare Surgical, Inc. 303-689-0187
7332 S Alton Way Ste H, Centennial, CO 80112
gi-Stitch for suturing in the gi track with a 2.8mm suturing device and pre-tied knot through the operating channel of a standard gastroscope,

SUTURE, ABSORBABLE *(Surgery) 79GAK*

Covidien Lp 508-261-8000
15 Hampshire St, Mansfield, MA 02048
DEXON S, DEXON II, MAXON chromic catgut.

Cp Medical Corporation 800-950-2763
803 NE 25th Ave, Portland, OR 97232
VISORB, MONO DOX, MONOSWIFT synthetic absorbable surgical sutures; polyglycolic acid, poly-glycolide-e-caprolactone, and polydioxanone sutures.

Ethicon Endo-Surgery, Inc. 877-384-4266
3801 University Blvd SE, Albuquerque, NM 87106
Sterile and nonsterile gut sutures.

Gramsmed, Llc 800-366-1976
2225 Dakota Dr, Grafton, WI 53024
Suture. Gramsorb (braided) or Monograms (monofilament) surgical suture, coated.

Havel's Inc. 800-638-4770
3726 Lonsdale St, Cincinnati, OH 45227

Myco Medical 800-454-6926
158 Towerview Ct, Cary, NC 27513
AILEE brand, synthetic and natural.

Surgical Specialties Corporation 800-523-3332
100 Dennis Dr, Reading, PA 19606
Suture absorbable catgut chromic and plain, with and without needles.

SUTURE, ABSORBABLE, NATURAL *(Surgery) 79GAL*

Cp Medical Corporation 800-950-2763
803 NE 25th Ave, Portland, OR 97232
Plain and Chromic Catgut, collagen suture.

Demetech Corp. 888-324-2447
3530 NW 115th Ave, Doral, FL 33178
Surgical suture catgut.

Ethicon, Llc. 908-218-2887
Rd. 183, Km. 8.3,, Industrial Area Hato, San Lorenzo, PR 00754
Absorbable suture.

Gramsmed, Llc 800-366-1976
2225 Dakota Dr, Grafton, WI 53024
Grams absorbable surgical suture, plain and chromic.

Grupo Manufacturero Rio Grande, S.A. De C.V. 878-237-70
Privada Aldama #113, Piedras Negras, Coah. Mexico
Natural suture

Hu-Friedy Manufacturing Co., Inc. 800-483-7433
3232 N Rockwell St, Chicago, IL 60618

SUTURE, ABSORBABLE, NATURAL *(cont'd)*

Kelsar, S.A. 508-261-8000
Blvd. Insurgentes, Libriamento a La, Tijuana 22450 Mexico
Plain catgut, surgical w/wo needle

Suturtek Incorporated
51 Middlesex St, North Chelmsford, MA 01863
Suture.

Ussc Puerto Rico, Inc. 203-845-1000
Building 911-67, Sabanetas Industrial Park, Ponce, PR 00731
Multiple.

SUTURE, ABSORBABLE, OPHTHALMIC *(Ophthalmology) 86HMO*

Covidien Lp 508-261-8000
15 Hampshire St, Mansfield, MA 02048
DEXON S, DEXON II, chromic, mild chromic catgut.

Kelsar, S.A. 508-261-8000
Blvd. Insurgentes, Libriamento a La, Tijuana 22450 Mexico
Catgut, chromic sutures

Surgical Instrument Manufacturers, Inc. 800-521-2985
1650 Headland Dr, Fenton, MO 63026

SUTURE, ABSORBABLE, SYNTHETIC *(Surgery) 79GAN*

Biomet, Inc. 574-267-6639
56 E Bell Dr, PO Box 587, Warsaw, IN 46582
Anchor, suture anchor.

Ethicon Endo-Surgery, Inc. 877-384-4266
3801 University Blvd SE, Albuquerque, NM 87106
Sterile synthetic, absorbable sutures.

Gramsmed, Llc 800-366-1976
2225 Dakota Dr, Grafton, WI 53024
Monograms snthetic absorbable surgical suture, monofilament suture.

Surgical Specialties Corporation 800-523-3332
100 Dennis Dr, Reading, PA 19606
PCL monofilament synthetic absorbable suture.

Ussc Puerto Rico, Inc. 203-845-1000
Building 911-67, Sabanetas Industrial Park, Ponce, PR 00731
Multiple.

SUTURE, ABSORBABLE, SYNTHETIC, POLYGLYCOLIC ACID
(Surgery) 79GAM

Accutome, Inc. 610-889-0200
3222 Phoenixville Pike, Malvern, PA 19355
Pga absorbable sutures.

Alcon Manufacturing, Ltd. 817-551-6813
714 Columbia Ave, Sinking Spring, PA 19608
Various types of sterile opthalmic sutures.

Coapt Systems, Inc. 650-461-7600
1820 Embarcadero Rd, Palo Alto, CA 94303
Midface lift device and installation tools.

Covidien Lp 508-261-8000
15 Hampshire St, Mansfield, MA 02048
DEXON S or DEXON II.

Demetech Corp. 888-324-2447
3530 NW 115th Ave, Doral, FL 33178
Suture, absorbable, polyglycolic acid.

Depuy Mitek, A Johnson & Johnson Company 800-451-2006
50 Scotland Blvd, Bridgewater, MA 02324
Suture anchors.

Ethicon Endo-Surgery, Inc. 877-384-4266
3801 University Blvd SE, Albuquerque, NM 87106
Sterile synthetic absorbable sutures.

Gramsmed, Llc 800-366-1976
2225 Dakota Dr, Grafton, WI 53024
Suture. Gramsorb synthetic absorbable polyglycolic-acid surgical suture, coated.

Hu-Friedy Manufacturing Co., Inc. 800-483-7433
3232 N Rockwell St, Chicago, IL 60618

Kelsar, S.A. 508-261-8000
Blvd. Insurgentes, Libriamento a La, Tijuana 22450 Mexico
Polyglycolic acid sutures w/wo coating, braided, synthetic

Kollsut Scientific Corporation 630-290-5746
3286 N 29th Ct, Hollywood, FL 33020
Absorbable surgical suture, synthetic (polyglycolic acid).

SUTURE, ABSORBABLE, SYNTHETIC, POLYGLYCOLIC ACID *(cont'd)*

Lsi Solutions Inc. 585-869-6641
7796 Victor Mendon Rd, Victor, NY 14564
Various sizes and lengths of absorbable syn. polyglycolic acid surgical suture.

SUTURE, CARDIOVASCULAR *(Cardiovascular) 74DTH*

Covidien Lp 508-261-8000
15 Hampshire St, Mansfield, MA 02048
MAXON CV polybutester, TICRON silicone treated braided polyester and SURGILENE polypropylene sutures.

Kelsar, S.A. 508-261-8000
Blvd. Insurgentes, Libriamento a La, Tijuana 22450 Mexico
Polyglyconate monofilament absorbable suture

SUTURE, CATGUT *(Surgery) 79RXV*

Covidien Lp 508-261-8000
15 Hampshire St, Mansfield, MA 02048
Plain/mild chromic catgut.

Ethicon, Inc. 800-4-ETHICON
Route 22 West, Somerville, NJ 08876
Plain and chromic surgical gut reverse cutting, micropoint reverse cutting, and straight cutting sutures.

Gramsmed, Llc 800-366-1976
2225 Dakota Dr, Grafton, WI 53024
Grams absorbable gut suture, plain and chromic.

Victor Surgical Gut Manufacturing Co. 630-654-9520
PO Box 208, Hinsdale, IL 60522
Non-sterile catgut string for sutures.

SUTURE, COTTON *(Surgery) 79RXW*

Covidien Lp 508-261-8000
15 Hampshire St, Mansfield, MA 02048

SUTURE, DENTAL *(Dental And Oral) 76DZG*

Biomet Microfixation Inc. 800-874-7711
1520 Tradeport Dr, Jacksonville, FL 32218
Suture, dental.

Demetech Corp. 888-324-2447
3530 NW 115th Ave, Doral, FL 33178
Dental suture.

Myco Medical 800-454-6926
158 Towerview Ct, Cary, NC 27513
AILEE brand, synthetic and natural.

SUTURE, LAPAROSCOPY *(Surgery) 79SGX*

Covidien Lp 508-261-8000
15 Hampshire St, Mansfield, MA 02048

Delco Wire Winding Company 610-296-0350
59 Street Rd, Newtown Square, PA 19073

Ethicon, Inc. 800-4-ETHICON
Route 22 West, Somerville, NJ 08876

Fort Wayne Metals Research Prod. Corp. 260-747-4154
9609 Ardmore Ave, Fort Wayne, IN 46809
Various grades, properties and shapes of precision wire.

Zimmer Holdings, Inc. 800-613-6131
1800 W Center St, PO Box 708, Warsaw, IN 46580

SUTURE, MULTIFILAMENT STEEL *(Surgery) 79RXY*

Covidien Lp 508-261-8000
15 Hampshire St, Mansfield, MA 02048
FLEXON suture.

Ethicon, Inc. 800-4-ETHICON
Route 22 West, Somerville, NJ 08876

Fort Wayne Metals Research Prod. Corp. 260-747-4154
9609 Ardmore Ave, Fort Wayne, IN 46809
Various grades, properties and shapes of precision wire.

SUTURE, NON-ABSORBABLE *(Surgery) 79GAO*

Arosurgical Instruments Corp. 800-776-1751
537 Newport Center Dr Ste 101, Newport Beach, CA 92660
AROSuture/MICROsuture; sizes 8-0 to 11-0, 140 to 70 micron needles, taper point and met point, 13.5cm suture length. CALL FOR FREE SAMPLES.

Covidien Lp 508-261-8000
15 Hampshire St, Mansfield, MA 02048

Cp Medical Corporation 800-950-2763
803 NE 25th Ave, Portland, OR 97232
Silk, nylon, and polyester sutures.

SUTURE, NON-ABSORBABLE *(cont'd)*

Ethicon, Inc. 800-4-ETHICON
Route 22 West, Somerville, NJ 08876

Hu-Friedy Manufacturing Co., Inc. 800-483-7433
3232 N Rockwell St, Chicago, IL 60618

Kelsar, S.A. 508-261-8000
Blvd. Insurgentes, Libriamento a La, Tijuana 22450 Mexico
Monofilament, polybutester & cotton sutures

Micrins Surgical Instruments, Inc. 800-833-3380
28438 N Ballard Dr, Lake Forest, IL 60045
Micrins microsuture, blackmono nylon.

Surgical Specialties Corporation 800-523-3332
100 Dennis Dr, Reading, PA 19606
Suture non-absorbable, cotton, with and without needles.

SUTURE, NON-ABSORBABLE, OPHTHALMIC *(Ophthalmology) 86HMN*

Alcon Manufacturing, Ltd. 817-551-6813
714 Columbia Ave, Sinking Spring, PA 19608
Various types of sterile opthalmic sutures.

Covidien Lp 508-261-8000
15 Hampshire St, Mansfield, MA 02048
DERMALON, silk, NOVAFIL sutures.

Kelsar, S.A. 508-261-8000
Blvd. Insurgentes, Libriamento a La, Tijuana 22450 Mexico
Nylon sutures

SUTURE, NON-ABSORBABLE, SILK *(Surgery) 79GAP*

Accutome, Inc. 610-889-0200
3222 Phoenixville Pike, Malvern, PA 19355
Silk sutures.

Alcon Manufacturing, Ltd. 817-551-6813
714 Columbia Ave, Sinking Spring, PA 19608
Various types of sterile opthalmic sutures.

Arthrex, Inc. 239-643-5553
1370 Creekside Blvd, Naples, FL 34108
Nonabsorbable silk suture.

Covidien Lp 508-261-8000
15 Hampshire St, Mansfield, MA 02048
Silk suture.

Demetech Corp. 888-324-2447
3530 NW 115th Ave, Doral, FL 33178
Surgical suture, nonabsorbable silk.

Ethicon Endo-Surgery, Inc. 877-384-4266
3801 University Blvd SE, Albuquerque, NM 87106
Sterile and nonsterile silk sutures.

Ethicon, Inc. 800-4-ETHICON
Route 22 West, Somerville, NJ 08876

Ethicon, Llc. 908-218-2887
Rd. 183, Km. 8.3,, Industrial Area Hato, San Lorenzo, PR 00754
Sterile and non-sterile silk sutures.

Gramsmed, Llc 800-366-1976
2225 Dakota Dr, Grafton, WI 53024
Surgical suture, braided and coated.

Havel's Inc. 800-638-4770
3726 Lonsdale St, Cincinnati, OH 45227

Hu-Friedy Manufacturing Co., Inc. 800-483-7433
3232 N Rockwell St, Chicago, IL 60618

Kelsar, S.A. 508-261-8000
Blvd. Insurgentes, Libriamento a La, Tijuana 22450 Mexico
Silk suture

Kollsut Scientific Corporation 630-290-5746
3286 N 29th Ct, Hollywood, FL 33020
Nonabsorbable surgical suture usp (black braided).

Surgical Specialties Corporation 800-523-3332
100 Dennis Dr, Reading, PA 19606
Suture non-absorbable, silk, with and without needles.

Ussc Puerto Rico, Inc. 203-845-1000
Building 911-67, Sabanetas Industrial Park, Ponce, PR 00731
Multiple.

SUTURE, NON-ABSORBABLE, STEEL, MONOFILAMENT & MULTIFILAMENT *(Surgery) 79GAQ*

Biomet, Inc. 574-267-6639
56 E Bell Dr, PO Box 587, Warsaw, IN 46582
Suture wire.

SUTURE, NON-ABSORBABLE, STEEL, MONOFILAMENT & MULTIFILAMENT *(cont'd)*

Covidien Lp 508-261-8000
15 Hampshire St, Mansfield, MA 02048
FLEXON stainless, multi-strand steel and monofilament stainless steel sutures.

Davol Inc., Sub. C.R. Bard, Inc. 800-556-6275
100 Crossings Blvd, Warwick, RI 02886
Stainless steel suture and suturing device.

Delco Wire Winding Company 610-296-0350
59 Street Rd, Newtown Square, PA 19073

Ethicon, Inc. 800-4-ETHICON
Route 22 West, Somerville, NJ 08876

Fort Wayne Metals Research Prod. Corp. 260-747-4154
9609 Ardmore Ave, Fort Wayne, IN 46809
Various grades, properties and shapes of precision wire.

Gramsmed, Llc 800-366-1976
2225 Dakota Dr, Grafton, WI 53024
Suture. Surgical steel monofilament or multifilament.

Kelsar, S.A. 508-261-8000
Blvd. Insurgentes, Libriamento a La, Tijuana 22450 Mexico
Monofilament polybutester surgical suture w/wo coating

Ortheon Medical, Llc. 866-836-6349
777 W Swan St, Columbus, OH 43212
Stainless steel suture for tendon repair kit.

Pioneer Surgical Technology 800-557-9909
375 River Park Cir, Marquette, MI 49855
Songer Sternal Cable System. Multifilament cable system used for the fixation of the sternum after a midline sternotomy.

Surgical Specialties Corporation 800-523-3332
100 Dennis Dr, Reading, PA 19606
Suture non-absorbable, steel, monofilament and multifilament, w/wo needle.

Suturtek Incorporated
51 Middlesex St, North Chelmsford, MA 01863
Suturing device.

Ussc Puerto Rico, Inc. 203-845-1000
Building 911-67, Sabanetas Industrial Park, Ponce, PR 00731
Various.

Zimmer Holdings, Inc. 800-613-6131
1800 W Center St, PO Box 708, Warsaw, IN 46580

SUTURE, NON-ABSORBABLE, SYNTHETIC, POLYAMIDE
(Surgery) 79GAR

Accutome, Inc. 610-889-0200
3222 Phoenixville Pike, Malvern, PA 19355
Nylon sutures.

Alcon Manufacturing, Ltd. 817-551-6813
714 Columbia Ave, Sinking Spring, PA 19608
Various types of sterile opthalmic sutures.

Alcon Research, Ltd. 800-862-5266
6201 South Fwy, Fort Worth, TX 76134

Boston Scientific Corp. 408-935-3400
150 Baytech Dr, San Jose, CA 95134
Suture.

Covidien Lp 508-261-8000
15 Hampshire St, Mansfield, MA 02048
SURGILON braided nylon; DERMALON monofilament nylon.

Demetech Corp. 888-324-2447
3530 NW 115th Ave, Doral, FL 33178
Surgical nylon suture.

Ethicon Endo-Surgery, Inc. 877-384-4266
3801 University Blvd SE, Albuquerque, NM 87106
Sterile nylon sutures.

Ethicon, Inc. 800-4-ETHICON
Route 22 West, Somerville, NJ 08876

Ethicon, Llc. 908-218-2887
Rd. 183, Km. 8.3,, Industrial Area Hato, San Lorenzo, PR 00754
Sterile nylon sutures.

Gramsmed, Llc 800-366-1976
2225 Dakota Dr, Grafton, WI 53024
Suture. Monofilament and braided surgical nylon.

Kelsar, S.A. 508-261-8000
Blvd. Insurgentes, Libriamento a La, Tijuana 22450 Mexico
Nylon surgical suture

SUTURE, NON-ABSORBABLE, SYNTHETIC, POLYAMIDE *(cont'd)*

Kollsut Scientific Corporation 630-290-5746
3286 N 29th Ct, Hollywood, FL 33020
Nonabsorbable surgical suture usp, monofilament polyamide.

S Jackson Inc. 800-368-5225
PO Box 4487, Alexandria, VA 22303
SUPRAMID available in 8 sizes with full range of needle types - priced from $20.75 to $149.50 per dozen.

Surgical Specialties Corporation 800-523-3332
100 Dennis Dr, Reading, PA 19606
Suture non-absorbable, synthetic, polyamide, with and without needles.

Ussc Puerto Rico, Inc. 203-845-1000
Building 911-67, Sabanetas Industrial Park, Ponce, PR 00731
Various.

SUTURE, NON-ABSORBABLE, SYNTHETIC, POLYESTER
(Surgery) 79GAS

Alcon Manufacturing, Ltd. 817-551-6813
714 Columbia Ave, Sinking Spring, PA 19608
Various types of sterile opthalmic sutures.

Alcon Research, Ltd. 800-862-5266
6201 South Fwy, Fort Worth, TX 76134

Arthrex, Inc. 239-643-5553
1370 Creekside Blvd, Naples, FL 34108
Suture.

Biomet, Inc. 574-267-6639
56 E Bell Dr, PO Box 587, Warsaw, IN 46582
Suture anchor.

Boston Scientific Corp. 408-935-3400
150 Baytech Dr, San Jose, CA 95134
Suture.

Covidien Lp 508-261-8000
15 Hampshire St, Mansfield, MA 02048
TI.CRON silicone treated, braided polyester fiber and DACRON braided polyester fiber sutures.

Depuy Mitek, A Johnson & Johnson Company 800-451-2006
50 Scotland Blvd, Bridgewater, MA 02324
Suture, nonabsorbable, synthetic, polyester.

Ethicon Endo-Surgery, Inc. 877-384-4266
3801 University Blvd SE, Albuquerque, NM 87106
Sterile polyester sutures.

Ethicon, Inc. 800-4-ETHICON
Route 22 West, Somerville, NJ 08876

Ethicon, Llc. 908-218-2887
Rd. 183, Km. 8.3,, Industrial Area Hato, San Lorenzo, PR 00754
Sterile polyester sutures.

Gramsmed, Llc 800-366-1976
2225 Dakota Dr, Grafton, WI 53024
Suture. Braided silicone coated, waxed coated, or uncoated.

Gudebrod, Inc. 877-249-2211
274 Shoemaker Rd, Pottstown, PA 19464

Hu-Friedy Manufacturing Co., Inc. 800-483-7433
3232 N Rockwell St, Chicago, IL 60618

Kelsar, S.A. 508-261-8000
Blvd. Insurgentes, Libriamento a La, Tijuana 22450 Mexico
Polyester sutures

Lsi Solutions Inc. 585-869-6641
7796 Victor Mendon Rd, Victor, NY 14564
Various sizes and lengths of nonabsorbable synthetic polyester surgical suture.

Regen Biologics, Inc. 415-562-0800
411 Hackensack Ave, Hackensack, NJ 07601
Suture with needle.

Surgical Specialties Corporation 800-523-3332
100 Dennis Dr, Reading, PA 19606
Suture non-absorbable synthetic polyester with and without needles.

Welco-Cgi Gas Technologies 440-234-1075
145 Shimersville Rd, Bethlehem, PA 18015
Gas mixtures, medical.

SUTURE, NON-ABSORBABLE, SYNTHETIC, POLYETHYLENE
(Surgery) 79GAT

Accutome, Inc. 610-889-0200
3222 Phoenixville Pike, Malvern, PA 19355
Polyester sutures.

SUTURE, NON-ABSORBABLE, SYNTHETIC, POLYETHYLENE
(cont'd)

Anulex Technologies, Inc 877-326-8539
5600 Rowland Rd Ste 280, Minnetonka, MN 55343
Surgical suture.

Arthrex, Inc. 239-643-5553
1370 Creekside Blvd, Naples, FL 34108
Suture.

Biomet, Inc. 574-267-6639
56 E Bell Dr, PO Box 587, Warsaw, IN 46582
Various types of nonabsorbable suture.

Covidien Lp 508-261-8000
15 Hampshire St, Mansfield, MA 02048

Cp Medical Corporation 800-950-2763
803 NE 25th Ave, Portland, OR 97232
Monofilament polypropylene, polyethylene and stainless steel sutures.

Demetech Corp. 888-324-2447
3530 NW 115th Ave, Doral, FL 33178
Surgical suture nonabsorbable polyethylene.

Ethicon Endo-Surgery, Inc. 877-384-4266
3801 University Blvd SE, Albuquerque, NM 87106
Suture knot-tying instrument and reloads.

Kollsut Scientific Corporation 630-290-5746
3286 N 29th Ct, Hollywood, FL 33020
Nonabsorbable surgical suture usp, coated & braided polyester.

Lsi Solutions Inc. 585-869-6641
7796 Victor Mendon Rd, Victor, NY 14564
Suture, nonabsorbable, synthetic, polyethylene.

Musculoskeletal Transplant Foundation 800-433-6576
125 May St Ste 300, Edison Corp Ctr, Edison, NJ 08837
Bone anchor.

Sutura, Inc. 714-437-9801
17080 Newhope St, Fountain Valley, CA 92708
Sterile suturing device.

Tornier Inc. 978-232-9997
100 Cummings Ctr Ste 444C, Beverly, MA 01915
Polyester suture.

Usgi Medical 949-369-3890
1140 Calle Cordillera, San Clemente, CA 92673
Sterile suture.

Ussc Puerto Rico, Inc. 203-845-1000
Building 911-67, Sabanetas Industrial Park, Ponce, PR 00731
Various.

SUTURE, NON-ABSORBABLE, SYNTHETIC, POLYPROPYLENE
(Surgery) 79GAW

Abbott Vascular Inc. 800-227-9902
400 Saginaw Dr, Redwood City, CA 94063
Perclose vascular suture device.

Alcon Manufacturing, Ltd. 817-551-6813
714 Columbia Ave, Sinking Spring, PA 19608
Various types of sterile ophthalmic sutures.

Demetech Corp. 888-324-2447
3530 NW 115th Ave, Doral, FL 33178
Surgical suture nonabsorbable polypropylene.

Ethicon, Inc. 800-4-ETHICON
Route 22 West, Somerville, NJ 08876

Ethicon, Llc. 908-218-2887
Rd. 183, Km. 8.3,, Industrial Area Hato, San Lorenzo, PR 00754
Sterile polypropylene suture.

Gramsmed, Llc 800-366-1976
2225 Dakota Dr, Grafton, WI 53024
Suture. Surgical monofilament polypropylene.

Hu-Friedy Manufacturing Co., Inc. 800-483-7433
3232 N Rockwell St, Chicago, IL 60618

Kelsar, S.A. 508-261-8000
Blvd. Insurgentes, Libriamento a La, Tijuana 22450 Mexico
Polypropylene suture

Kmi Kolster Methods, Inc. 909-737-5476
3185 Palisades Dr, Corona, CA 92880
Featherlift silhouette suture.

Kollsut Scientific Corporation 630-290-5746
3286 N 29th Ct, Hollywood, FL 33020
Nonabsorbable surgical suture usp, monofilament polypropylene.

SUTURE, NON-ABSORBABLE, SYNTHETIC, POLYPROPYLENE
(cont'd)

Lsi Solutions Inc. 585-869-6641
7796 Victor Mendon Rd, Victor, NY 14564
Various sizes & lengths of nonabsorbable syn. polypropylene surgical suture.

Surgical Specialties Corporation 800-523-3332
100 Dennis Dr, Reading, PA 19606
Suture non-absorbable, synthetic, polypropylene, with and without needles.

Tornier Inc. 978-232-9997
100 Cummings Ctr Ste 444C, Beverly, MA 01915
Suture applicator.

Ussc Puerto Rico, Inc. 203-845-1000
Building 911-67, Sabanetas Industrial Park, Ponce, PR 00731
Various.

W.L. Gore & Associates,Inc 302-738-4880
345 Inverness Dr S, Bldg. A, Ste. 120, Englewood, CO 80112
Suture.

SUTURE, OTHER *(Surgery) 79RYF*

Aegis Medical 203-838-9081
10 Wall St, Norwalk, CT 06850
Disposable sutures.

Alto Development Corp. 732-938-2266
5206 Asbury Rd, Wall Township, NJ 07727
Sternum sutures, 18in. long with different needle options.

Arista Surgical Supply Co. Inc. 800-223-1984
297 High St, Dedham, MA 02026
Dressings, surgical.

Arosurgical Instruments Corp. 800-776-1751
537 Newport Center Dr Ste 101, Newport Beach, CA 92660
AROSuture/COSMETIC Suture; sizes 3-0 to 6-0 black and blue nylon monofilament

Cincinnati Surgical Company 800-544-3100
11256 Cornell Park Dr, Cincinnati, OH 45242
Non-sterile suture.

Covidien Lp 508-261-8000
15 Hampshire St, Mansfield, MA 02048
MAXON polyglyconate suture.

Ethicon, Inc. 800-4-ETHICON
Route 22 West, Somerville, NJ 08876
Monocryl (poliglecaprone 25) sutures, coated vicryl (polyglactin 910) sutures, and PDS II (polydioxanone) sutures.

Jorgensen Laboratories 970-669-2500
1450 Van Buren Ave, Loveland, CO 80538

Key Surgical, Inc. 800-541-7995
8101 Wallace Rd Ste 100, Eden Prairie, MN 55344
Vinyl covers for mosquito hemostats to assist in grasping and tagging suture.

Lfi, Inc-Laser Fare, Inc. 401-231-4400
1 Industrial Dr S, Lan-Rex Industrial Pk., Smithfield, RI 02917

SUTURE, POLYPROPYLENE MONOFILAMENT *(Surgery) 79RYC*

Covidien Lp 508-261-8000
15 Hampshire St, Mansfield, MA 02048
SURGILENE monofilament polypropylene sutures.

Ethicon, Inc. 800-4-ETHICON
Route 22 West, Somerville, NJ 08876
PROLENE polypropylene sutures.

Innovative Med Inc. 877-779-9492
4 Autry Ste B, Irvine, CA 92618
threads

SUTURE, SILK *(Surgery) 79RYD*

Alcon Research, Ltd. 800-862-5266
6201 South Fwy, Fort Worth, TX 76134

Covidien Lp 508-261-8000
15 Hampshire St, Mansfield, MA 02048

Ethicon, Inc. 800-4-ETHICON
Route 22 West, Somerville, NJ 08876
PERMA-HAND silk sutures.

George Tiemann & Co. 800-843-6266
25 Plant Ave, Hauppauge, NY 11788

SUTURE, STAINLESS STEEL *(Surgery) 79RYE*

Covidien Lp 508-261-8000
15 Hampshire St, Mansfield, MA 02048
FLEXON.

SUTURE, STAINLESS STEEL *(cont'd)*

Delco Wire Winding Company — 610-296-0350
59 Street Rd, Newtown Square, PA 19073

Ethicon, Inc. — 800-4-ETHICON
Route 22 West, Somerville, NJ 08876
Surgical stainless steel sutures.

Fort Wayne Metals Research Prod. Corp. — 260-747-4154
9609 Ardmore Ave, Fort Wayne, IN 46809
Various grades, properties and shapes of precision wire.

Rahns Specialty Metals — 800-523-1777
70 Rahns Rd Rte 113, Collegeville, PA 19426
Strips of stainless steel.

SUTURE, SURGICAL, ABSORBABLE, POLYDIOXANONE *(Surgery) 79NEW*

Lsi Solutions Inc. — 585-869-6641
7796 Victor Mendon Rd, Victor, NY 14564
Various sizes & lengths of absorbable syn. polydioxanone surgical suture.

SUTURE, SURGICAL, NONABSORBABLE, EXPANDED, POLYTETRAFLOUROETHYLENE *(Surgery) 79NBY*

Osteogenics Biomedical, Inc. — 806-796-1923
4620 71st St Bldg 78-79, Lubbock, TX 79424
M-ptfe monofilament suture.

SWABS, ALCOHOL *(General) 80TGC*

A.M.G. Medical, Inc. — 888-396-1213
8505 Dalton Rd., Montreal, QUE H4T-IV5 Canada

Afassco, Inc. — 800-441-6774
2244 Park Pl Ste C, Minden, NV 89423

Mckesson General Medical — 800-446-3008
8741 Landmark Rd, Richmond, VA 23228

Miami Medical Equipment & Supply Corp. — 305-592-0111
2150 NW 93rd Ave, Doral, FL 33172

Omni Medical Supply Inc. — 800-860-6664
4153 Pioneer Dr, Commerce Township, MI 48390

Powell Products, Inc. — 800-840-9205
4940 Northpark Dr, Colorado Springs, CO 80918
Alcohol saturated foam swabs

Professional Disposables International, Inc. — 800-999-6423
2 Nice Pak Park, Orangeburg, NY 10962

Veltek Associates, Inc. — 888-478-3745
15 Lee Blvd, Malvern, PA 19355

SWABS, ANTISEPTIC *(General) 80RYG*

Afassco, Inc. — 800-441-6774
2244 Park Pl Ste C, Minden, NV 89423
Triple-action cut cleaners.

Chagrin Safety Supply, Inc. — 800-227-0468
8227 Washington St # 1, Chagrin Falls, OH 44023

Norpak Manufacturing Inc. — 905-427-0960
85 Chambers Dr., Unit 4, Ajax, ONT L1Z-1E2 Canada
Pad Plus povidone-iodine No-Touch infection control applicator for replacement of prep pads and swab sticks. Alcohol preps are available in medium and large sizes, both non-sterile and sterile. Institutional boxes of 200 and retail boxes of 100.

O&M Enterprise — 847-258-4515
641 Chelmsford Ln, Elk Grove Village, IL 60007
SWABS/PAD ANTISEPTIC

Powell Products, Inc. — 800-840-9205
4940 Northpark Dr, Colorado Springs, CO 80918
Antiseptic saturated foam swabs

Purdue Frederick Company — 800-877-5666
1 Stamford Forum, Stamford, CT 06901
Betadine swabsticks

Puritan Medical Products Company Llc — 800-321-2313
31 School St., Guilford, ME 04443-0149

SWABS, COTTON *(General) 80RYH*

Amd-Ritmed, Inc. — 800-445-0340
295 Firetower Road, Tonawanda, NY 14150

Birchwood Laboratories, Inc. — 800-328-6156
7900 Fuller Rd, Eden Prairie, MN 55344
SCOPETTES, Rayon.

Chagrin Safety Supply, Inc. — 800-227-0468
8227 Washington St # 1, Chagrin Falls, OH 44023

SWABS, COTTON *(cont'd)*

Clean Esd Products, Inc. — 510-257-5080
48340 Milmont Dr, Fremont, CA 94538
Six-inch cotton swabs.

Crosswell International Corporation — 305-648-0777
101 Madeira Ave, Coral Gables, FL 33134

Medical Packaging Corporation — 800-792-0600
941 Avenida Acaso, Camarillo, CA 93012
Dacron, rayon, calcium alginate, or cotton on wooden, plastic, stainless steel or aluminum shafts, sterile and non-sterile swabs. 100/pkg. and 1000/case. Custom swabs available upon request. Special scoring available.

Omnical, Inc. — 818-837-7531
557 Jessie St, San Fernando, CA 91340
Sealed polyester tips.

Pedinol Pharmacal, Inc. — 800-733-4665
30 Banfi Plz N, Farmingdale, NY 11735
Dispos-A-Swab.

Puritan Medical Products Company Llc — 800-321-2313
31 School St., Guilford, ME 04443-0149
Sterile cotton, rayon and polyester swabs.

Sentinel Consumer Products, Inc. — 440-974-8144
7750 Tyler Blvd, Mentor, OH 44060
Cotton swabs, cosmetic rounds and squares, cotton balls, footcare and fluffs.

Solon Manufacturing Co. — 800-341-6640
338 Madison Ave Ste 7, Skowhegan, ME 04976
3- and 6-in. sterile and non-sterile with plastic or wood shafts.

SWABS, ORAL CARE *(General) 80VLI*

Powell Products, Inc. — 800-840-9205
4940 Northpark Dr, Colorado Springs, CO 80918
Swabs for dental applications

Puritan Medical Products Company Llc — 800-321-2313
31 School St., Guilford, ME 04443-0149

SWABS, SPECIMEN COLLECTION *(General) 80RYI*

Bd Diagnostic Systems — 800-675-0908
7 Loveton Cir, Sparks, MD 21152

Birchwood Laboratories, Inc. — 800-328-6156
7900 Fuller Rd, Eden Prairie, MN 55344
SCOPETTES- Case with 500 16in. proctosigmoidoscopy swabs, case with 500 8in. OB/GYN swabs, case of 300 8in. rayon tip sterile swabs (50pkgs/6ea).

Medical Packaging Corporation — 800-792-0600
941 Avenida Acaso, Camarillo, CA 93012
Nucleic Acid Transport (NAT): A universal transport system for the collection of male and female urogenital swabs for the detection of c. trachomatis and n. gonorrhoeae DNA or RNA. This transport has been validated on the following asays: Abbott LCX, BD Probetec ET, Roche Cobas Amplicor, Gin Robe, Pace 2.

Porex Corporation — 800-241-0195
500 Bohannon Rd, Fairburn, GA 30213
POREX SQ-EASY diagnostic prefilter with swabs.

Powell Products, Inc. — 800-840-9205
4940 Northpark Dr, Colorado Springs, CO 80918
Synthetic swabs available for specimen collection.

Puritan Medical Products Company Llc — 800-321-2313
31 School St., Guilford, ME 04443-0149
Cotton, rayon, polyester and calcium alginate. CALGISWAB completely dissolves in bodily fluids when fibers detach during collection, allowing safer collection from open wounds, nasal passages and other sensitive regions without the risk of irritation or infection. TRANSETTES for transporting specimens to laboratories.

Schleicher & Schuell, Inc. — 800-245-4024
10 Optical Ave, PO Box 2012, Keene, NH 03431
ISOCODE blood/saliva collection device for preparing DNA template for PCR.

Starplex Scientific Inc. — 800-665-0954
50A Steinway Blvd., Etobicoke, ONT M9W 6Y3 Canada
STARSWABS Microbiology transport swabs with advanced designed biohazard cap. Available in a variety of formats and media.

SYNCHRONIZER, ECG/RESPIRATOR, RADIOGRAPHIC *(Radiology) 90IXO*

Medrecon, Inc. — 877-526-4323
257 South Ave, Garwood, NJ 07027
X-ray tops to fit all types of surgical tables.

SYNCHRONIZER, ECG/RESPIRATOR, RADIOGRAPHIC *(cont'd)*

Varian Medical Systems, Oncology Systems 800 278-2747
911 Hansen Way, Bldg.3 M/S C-165, Palo Alto, CA 94304
Respiratory gating.

SYNCHRONIZER, ELECTROCARDIOGRAPH, NUCLEAR *(Radiology) 90IYY*

Marconi Medical Systems 800-323-0550
595 Miner Rd, Cleveland, OH 44143

SYNCHRONIZER, NUCLEAR CAMERA *(Radiology) 90RYJ*

Diagnostix Plus, Inc. 516-536-2670
100 N Village Ave Ste 33, Rockville Centre, NY 11570
Radionuclide camera upgrades, specializing in Elscint,Sopha,SMV,Picker,Siemens,Toshiba and General Electric.

Marconi Medical Systems 800-323-0550
595 Miner Rd, Cleveland, OH 44143

SYNCHROTRON, MEDICAL *(Radiology) 90IWM*

Optivus Proton Therapy, Inc 888-PROTONS
PO Box 608, Loma Linda, CA 92354
Proton beam therapy system.

SYNOPTOPHORE *(Ophthalmology) 86WNQ*

Welch Allyn, Inc. 800-535-6663
4341 State Street Rd, Skaneateles Falls, NY 13153

SYNTHESIZER, DNA *(Chemistry) 75WJI*

Applied Biosystems 800-345-5724
850 Lincoln Centre Dr, Foster City, CA 94404
$46,750 for 1-column 380-B DNA synthesizer (upgradeable), $23,900 for 1-column model 381A (not upgradeable), $54,450 for 3-column model 380-B DNA synthesizer.

Beckman Coulter, Inc. 800-742-2345
250 S Kraemer Blvd, PO Box 8000, Brea, CA 92821

SYNTHESIZER, PEPTIDE & PROTEIN *(Chemistry) 75UIP*

Applied Biosystems 800-345-5724
850 Lincoln Centre Dr, Foster City, CA 94404
$88,000 for 1 vessel model 430A, $96,000 for 3 vessel model 430A peptide synthesizer. $21,700 for model 151A synthetic peptide purification system. $57,500 for model 431A peptide synthesizer.

Waters Corp. 800-252-4752
34 Maple St, Milford, MA 01757
Protein and peptide purification.

SYNTHESIZER, POLYNUCLEOTIDE *(Chemistry) 75UIQ*

Applied Biosystems 800-345-5724
850 Lincoln Centre Dr, Foster City, CA 94404
$46,750 for 1-column 380-B DNA synthesizer (upgradeable), $23,900 for 1-column model 381A (not upgradeable), $54,450 for 3-column model 380-B DNA synthesizer.

Beckman Coulter, Inc. 800-742-2345
250 S Kraemer Blvd, PO Box 8000, Brea, CA 92821

SYRINGE UNIT, AIR AND/OR WATER *(Dental And Oral) 76ECB*

Alltec Integrated Manufacturing,Inc. 805-595-3500
4330 Old Santa Fe Rd, San Luis Obispo, CA 93401
Hand held air,water suction.

Beaverstate Dental, Inc. 800-237-2303
115 S Elliott Rd, Newberg, OR 97132

Busse Hospital Disposables, Inc. 631-435-4711
75 Arkay Dr, Hauppauge, NY 11788
Various.

Dentalez Group 866-DTE-INFO
101 Lindenwood Dr Ste 225, Valleybrooke Corporate Center Malvern, PA 19355

Dentalez Group, Stardental Division 717-291-1161
1816 Colonial Village Ln, Lancaster, PA 17601
X-ray machine, dental.

Dentsply Canada, Ltd. 800-263-1437
161 Vinyl Ct., Woodbridge, ONT L4L 4A3 Canada

Dp Manufacture Corp. 305-640-9894
1460 NW 107th Ave Ste H, Doral, FL 33172
Tri way syringe.

Forest Dental Products Inc 800-423-3535
6200 NE Campus Ct, Hillsboro, OR 97124

Inter-Med, Inc. 877-418-4782
2200 Northwestern Ave, Racine, WI 53404
Air/water syringe plastic cover.

SYRINGE UNIT, AIR AND/OR WATER *(cont'd)*

L.L. Dental 541-822-3839
91780 Mill Creek Rd, Blue River, OR 97413
4-way syringe.

Midmark Corporation 800-643-6275
60 Vista Dr, P.O. Box 286, Versailles, OH 45380

Miltex Dental Technologies, Inc. 516-576-6022
589 Davies Dr, York, PA 17402
Various water and air bulb syringes.

Pac-Dent Intl., Inc. 909-839-0888
21078 Commerce Point Dr, Walnut, CA 91789
Three way- tip.

Sds (Summit Dental Systems) 800-275-3368
3560 NW 53rd Ct, Fort Lauderdale, FL 33309

Shoney Scientific, Inc. 262-970-0170
West 223 North 720 Saratoga Drive,, Suite 120, Waukesha, WI 53186
10cc syringe.

Ultradent Products, Inc. 801-553-4586
505 W 10200 S, South Jordan, UT 84095
Accessory to air/water syringe unit.

Westar Medical Products, Inc. 425-290-3945
4470 Chennault Beach Rd Ste 2, Mukilteo, WA 98275
Air/water syringe.

3m Unitek 800-634-5300
2724 Peck Rd, Monrovia, CA 91016

SYRINGE, ANESTHESIA *(Anesthesiology) 73RYM*

Cadence Science Inc. 888-717-7677
1979 Marcus Ave Ste 215, New Hyde Park, NY 11042
Reusable only.

Covidien Lp 508-261-8000
15 Hampshire St, Mansfield, MA 02048

Ispg, Inc. 860-355-8511
517 Litchfield Rd, New Milford, CT 06776
Glass syringes

Spectra Medical Devices, Inc. 978-657-0889
260H Fordham Rd, Wilmington, MA 01887

SYRINGE, ANGIOGRAPHIC *(Cns/Neurology) 84RYN*

Cadence Science Inc. 888-717-7677
1979 Marcus Ave Ste 215, New Hyde Park, NY 11042

Coeur, Inc 800-296-5893
704 Cadet Ct, Lebanon, TN 37087
Syringes for cardiological and radiological applications.

Cook Inc. 800-457-4500
PO Box 489, Bloomington, IN 47402

Medrad, Inc. 800-633-7231
100 Global View Dr, Warrendale, PA 15086
Disposable syringes, disposable syringes for angiography 60, 100, 130, 150, 200 and 260 ml.

SYRINGE, ANGIOPLASTY *(Cardiovascular) 74WTW*

Cardio-Nef, S.A. De C.V. 01-800-024-0240
Rio Grijalva 186, Col. Mitras Norte, Monterrey, N.L. 64320 Mexico

Coeur, Inc 800-296-5893
704 Cadet Ct, Lebanon, TN 37087
Disposable syringe used in conjunction with a power injection machine.

Medical Techniques Usa 801-936-4501
125 N 400 W Ste C, North Salt Lake, UT 84054

Total Molding Services, Inc. 215-538-9613
354 East Broad St., Trumbauersville, PA 18970
10cc Luer Lock & Luer Slip Cardiovascular Syringe.

SYRINGE, ANTISTICK *(General) 80MEG*

Arkray Factory Usa, Inc. 952-646-3168
5182 W 76th St, Minneapolis, MN 55439
Safety syringe.

Covidien Lp 508-261-8000
15 Hampshire St, Mansfield, MA 02048

Inter-Med, Inc. 877-418-4782
2200 Northwestern Ave, Racine, WI 53404
Safety Syringe

Magnum Plastics, Inc. 303-828-3156
425 Bonnell Ave, Erie, CO 80516
Safety syringe.

SYRINGE, ANTISTICK *(cont'd)*

Medical Action Industries, Inc. 800-645-7042
25 Heywood Rd, Arden, NC 28704
Syringe.

Medisystems Corporation 800-369-6334
439 S Union St Fl 5, Lawrence, MA 01843
Anti-stick needles.

Retractable Technologies, Inc. 888-806-2626
511 Lobo Ln, PO Box 9, Little Elm, TX 75068
VanishPoint syringe

Safecare Corporation 225-753-4664
6352 Quin Dr Apt A, Baton Rouge, LA 70817
Covertip.

Safepro Usa Inc. 904-880-1958
11497 Columbia Park Dr W, West Suite 9, Jacksonville, FL 32258
Hypodermic syringe.

Safety 1st Medical, Inc. 800-997-2331
1740 E Garry Ave Ste 109, Santa Ana, CA 92705
SAFE-1 disposable safety syringe and anti-needlesticks.

Safety Syringe Corporation Of America, Inc. 415-454-8054
58 Oakdale Ave, San Rafael, CA 94901
Syringe safety for injury prevention. Auto-Lock for IM injections ANGIO-LOCK IV

Safety Syringes, Inc. 760-918-9908
2875 Loker Ave E, Carlsbad, CA 92010
Ultrasafe dental injection system.

Sterion, Incorporated 800-328-7958
13828 Lincoln St NE, Ham Lake, MN 55304
One-handed syringe handling system to extract cap and to re-cap.

U.S. Medical Instruments, Inc. 619-661-5500
1490 Air Wing Rd, San Diego, CA 92154
Piston syringe.

Unilife Medical Solutions 1-800-324-7674
633 Lowther Rd, Lewisberry, PA 17339
Unitract

Univec, Inc. 410-347-9959
4810 Seton Dr, Baltimore, MD 21215
Hypodermic syringe with sharps protection.

SYRINGE, BALLOON INFLATION *(Cardiovascular) 74MAV*

Abbott Vascular, Cardiac Therapies 800-227-9902
26531 Ynez Rd, Mailing P.O. Box 9018, Temecula, CA 92591
Sterile low pressure inflation device.

Argon Medical Devices Inc. 903-675-9321
1445 Flat Creek Rd, Athens, TX 75751
Catheter inflation device.

Cardio-Nef, S.A. De C.V. 01-800-024-0240
Rio Grijalva 186, Col. Mitras Norte, Monterrey, N.L. 64320 Mexico

Cook Endoscopy 336-744-0157
4900 Bethania Station Rd # &, 5951 Grassy Creek Blvd. Winston Salem, NC 27105
Balloon inflation device.

Excel Medical Products, Llc 810-714-4775
3145 Copper Ave, Fenton, MI 48430
The Excel Angyo® Life Kit for balloon dilation procedures consists of a 25 ATM inflation device with luminescent gauge, 3-way stopcock, guidewire insertion tool, torque device and the Excel-9 large bore hemostasis y-connector valve.

Medtronic Spine Llc 877-690-5353
1221 Crossman Ave, Sunnyvale, CA 94089
Various types of sterile inflation syrings.

Medtronic Vascular 707-525-0111
3576 Unocal Pl, Santa Rosa, CA 95403

Merit Medical Systems, Inc. 801-253-1600
1111 S Velasco St, Angleton, TX 77515
Angioplasty balloon inflation device.

Merit Medical Systems, Inc. 800-356-3748
1600 Merit Pkwy, South Jordan, UT 84095
INTELLISYSTEM Inflation Device and Monitor; MONARCH and BASIX Inflation Devices.

Navilyst Medical 800-833-9973
100 Boston Scientific Way, Marlborough, MA 01752
Inflation devices and inflation device kits.

SYRINGE, BULB *(General) 80RYU*

Cadence Science Inc. 888-717-7677
1979 Marcus Ave Ste 215, New Hyde Park, NY 11042
Reusable only.

Colorado Serum Company 303-295-7527
4950 York St, PO Box 16428, Denver, CO 80216
Veterinary syringes.

Covidien Lp 508-261-8000
15 Hampshire St, Mansfield, MA 02048

Global Healthcare 800-601-3880
1495 Hembree Rd Ste 700, Roswell, GA 30076
Bulb, Flat top, and Thumb ring syringes

Lsl Industries, Inc. 888-225-5575
5535 N Wolcott Ave, Chicago, IL 60640
$27.50 for 50 sterile single 60ml bulb syringes with tip protector.

Medical Plastic Devices (Mpd), Inc. 866-633-9835
161 Oneida Dr., Pointe Claire, QUE H9R 1A9 Canada

Spectrum Laboratories, Inc. 800-634-3300
18617 S Broadwick St, Rancho Dominguez, CA 90220
Gas/Liquid syringes for chromatography, 5ul to 100 ml; fixed and removable needles.

Vygon Corp. 800-544-4907
2495 General Armistead Ave, Norristown, PA 19403

SYRINGE, BULB, AIR OR WATER *(Dental And Oral) 76DYY*

Covidien Lp 508-261-8000
15 Hampshire St, Mansfield, MA 02048

Hospira 800-441-4100
268 E 4th St, Ashland, OH 44805
Vinyl and rubber bulbs.

Moyco Technologies, Inc. 800-331-8837
200 Commerce Dr, Montgomeryville, PA 18936
$19.00 per unit (standard).

SYRINGE, CALIBRATION TESTING, SPIROMETER *(Anesthesiology) 73WTC*

A-M Systems, Inc. 800-426-1306
131 Business Park Loop, Sequim, WA 98382
Volume Calibration Syringe, Aluminum and Acrylic (Adjustable, 2,3, or 4L) - $240.75 Aluminum 3L to $347.75 Acryllic 3L

Cardiac Science Corp. 800-777-1777
500 Burdick Pkwy, Deerfield, WI 53531
3.00 L. calibration syringe for spirometers. All aluminum, guaranteed +/- 1% accuracy, traceable to NBS.

Vitalograph, Inc. 800-255-6626
13310 W 99th St, Lenexa, KS 66215
$270.00, 1-L precision syringe, integral valves.

SYRINGE, CARTRIDGE *(Dental And Oral) 76EJI*

Arnold Tuber Industries 716-648-3363
97 Main St, Hamburg, NY 14075
Cartridge syringe.

Centrix, Inc. 800-235-5862
770 River Rd, Shelton, CT 06484

Milestone Scientific Inc. 800-862-1125
45 Knightsbridge Rd, Piscataway, NJ 08854
Cartridge syringe.

Milestone Scientific Inc. 800-862-1125
220 S Orange Ave, Livingston, NJ 07039
COMPUDENT STA, The Wand, wand plus, handpiece; safety wand disposable, computer controlled anesthetic ; delivery system; Wand Plus, CompuDent

Miltex Dental Technologies, Inc. 516-576-6022
589 Davies Dr, York, PA 17402
Cartridge syringe.

Moyco Technologies, Inc. 800-331-8837
200 Commerce Dr, Montgomeryville, PA 18936

Sterex Corp. 800-603-5045
4501 126th Ave N, Clearwater, FL 33762
2 Ml aspirating syringe.

Ultradent Products, Inc. 801-553-4586
505 W 10200 S, South Jordan, UT 84095
Impulse sealer.

Vetter Pharma-Turm, Inc. 215-321-6930
1790 Yardley Langhorne Rd, Heston Hall/Carriage House, Suite 203 Yardley, PA 19067

SYRINGE, CATHETER *(General) 80RYO*

Cadence Science Inc. 888-717-7677
1979 Marcus Ave Ste 215, New Hyde Park, NY 11042
Reusable only.

Covidien Lp 508-261-8000
15 Hampshire St, Mansfield, MA 02048

Medi Inc 800-225-8634
75 York Ave, P.O. Box 302, Randolph, MA 02368

Welcon, Inc. 800-877-0923
7409 Pebble Dr, Fort Worth, TX 76118

SYRINGE, DENTAL *(Dental And Oral) 76RYP*

Air-Tite Products Co., Inc. 800-231-7762
565 Central Dr Ste 101, Virginia Beach, VA 23454
Henke Sass Wolf Henke-Ject intralignmental syringes. Hypo aspirating syringes.

Centrix, Inc. 800-235-5862
770 River Rd, Shelton, CT 06484
Impression material syringes.

Covidien Lp 508-261-8000
15 Hampshire St, Mansfield, MA 02048

Dental Components, Inc. 503-538-8343
305 N Springbrook Rd, Newberg, OR 97132

Dentalez Group 866-DTE-INFO
101 Lindenwood Dr Ste 225, Valleybrooke Corporate Center
Malvern, PA 19355

Dentsply Canada, Ltd. 800-263-1437
161 Vinyl Ct., Woodbridge, ONT L4L 4A3 Canada

Millstone Medical Outsourcing 508-679-8384
1565 N Main St Ste 408, Fall River, MA 02720
Multiple and various.

Miltex Inc. 800-645-8000
589 Davies Dr, York, PA 17402
Dental aspirating syringes.

SYRINGE, DRUG, LUER-LOCK *(Dental And Oral) 76DZF*

Air-Tite Products Co., Inc. 800-231-7762
565 Central Dr Ste 101, Virginia Beach, VA 23454
NORM-JECT, SOFT-JECT, Excel,Air-Tite & Terumo; 3cc luer lock disposable, sterile syringes with needles in various sizes. 1cc thru 60cc also available.

Cadence Science Inc. 888-717-7677
1979 Marcus Ave Ste 215, New Hyde Park, NY 11042

Engineers Express, Inc. 800-255-8823
7 Industrial Park Rd, Medway, MA 02053

SYRINGE, EAR *(Ear/Nose/Throat) 77KCP*

Aesculap Implant Systems Inc. 1-800-234-9179
3773 Corporate Pkwy, Center Valley, PA 18034
ENT.

Bausch & Lomb Surgical 636-255-5051
3365 Tree Court Ind Blvd, Saint Louis, MO 63122

Biomet Microfixation Inc. 800-874-7711
1520 Tradeport Dr, Jacksonville, FL 32218
Various types of syringes.

Bionix Development Corp. 800-551-7096
5154 Enterprise Blvd, Toledo, OH 43612
Single use irrigation tip.

Cadence Science Inc. 888-717-7677
1979 Marcus Ave Ste 215, New Hyde Park, NY 11042
3 sizes (reusable).

Dental Usa, Inc. 815-363-8003
5005 McCullom Lake Rd, McHenry, IL 60050
Dental syringe.

Dorel Design & Development Center 781-364-3542
25 Forbes Blvd, Foxboro, MA 02035

Ear-Clear, Inc. 866-290-4260
1920 Brunns Rd Lot 29, Sebring, FL 33872
Ear irrigation syringe.

Jedmed Instruments Co. 314-845-3770
5416 Jedmed Ct, Saint Louis, MO 63129

Lsl Industries, Inc. 888-225-5575
5535 N Wolcott Ave, Chicago, IL 60640
1, 2, and 3oz. ear ulcer syringe. $28.00 to $31.50.

Medi Inc 800-225-8634
75 York Ave, P.O. Box 302, Randolph, MA 02368

SYRINGE, EAR *(cont'd)*

Medline Industries, Inc. 800-633-5886
1 Medline Pl, Mundelein, IL 60060

Medline Manufacturing And Services Llc 847-837-2759
1 Medline Pl, Mundelein, IL 60060
Ear ulcer syringes.

Miltex Inc. 800-645-8000
589 Davies Dr, York, PA 17402

SYRINGE, HYPODERMIC *(General) 80RYQ*

British Marketing Enterprises, Inc. 800-358-8220
1825 Bush St, San Francisco, CA 94109

Cadence Science Inc. 888-717-7677
1979 Marcus Ave Ste 215, New Hyde Park, NY 11042
40 types - all reusable glass - from 1cc to 250ml; lock tip, metal tip, glass tip, or eccentric tip - list price for 10cc lock tip.

Chagrin Safety Supply, Inc. 800-227-0468
8227 Washington St # 1, Chagrin Falls, OH 44023

Cotran Corp. 800-345-4449
574 Park Ave, PO Box 130, Portsmouth, RI 02871

Covidien Lp 508-261-8000
15 Hampshire St, Mansfield, MA 02048

Exelint International Co. 800-940-3935
5840 W Centinela Ave, Los Angeles, CA 90045
1cc up to 60cc Syringes in L-Lock, L-Slip and Catheter Tips

Gettig Pharmaceutical Instrument Co., Div Of Gettig Technologies Inc. 814-422-8892
1 Streamside Pl. W., Spring Mills, PA 16875-0085

Globe Medical Tech, Inc. 713-365-9595
1766 W Sam Houston Pkwy N, Houston, TX 77043
Available in sizes 1 cc through 60 cc.

Gw Plastics, Inc. 802-234-9941
239 Pleasant St, Bethel, VT 05032

Ispg, Inc. 860-355-8511
517 Litchfield Rd, New Milford, CT 06776
Glass syringes.

Jorgensen Laboratories 970-669-2500
1450 Van Buren Ave, Loveland, CO 80538
Disposable syringes and needles.

Learning Curve Brands Inc. THE FIRST YEARS 800-225-0382
100 Technology Center Dr Ste 2A, Stoughton, MA 02072

Lockett Medical Corp. 401-421-6599
3 Richmond Sq, Providence, RI 02906
Glass syringes for epidural and reusable use.

Meridian Medical Technologies 800-638-8093
10240 Old Columbia Rd, Columbia, MD 21046
Pre-filled disposable.

Myco Medical 800-454-6926
158 Towerview Ct, Cary, NC 27513
Disposable and reusable syringes and needles; also, insulin syringes.

Xenotec Ltd. 949-640-4053
511 Hazel Dr, Corona Del Mar, CA 92625
Safe-1 Safety Syringe designed to give healthcare providers maximum protection with minimum inconvenience. The product has advantages over all other safety syringes.

SYRINGE, INSULIN *(General) 80RYR*

A.M.G. Medical, Inc. 888-396-1213
8505 Dalton Rd., Montreal, QUE H4T-IV5 Canada

Aimsco, Delta Hi-Tech, Inc. 800-378-0909
3762 Secord St, Salt Lake City, UT 84115
AIMSCO Insulin syringes 28, 29 and 30 gauge 1cc, 1/2cc and 3/10cc. 31 gauge Insulin syringe 1/2cc & 3/10cc.

Cadence Science Inc. 888-717-7677
1979 Marcus Ave Ste 215, New Hyde Park, NY 11042
12 types (reusable).

Chagrin Safety Supply, Inc. 800-227-0468
8227 Washington St # 1, Chagrin Falls, OH 44023

Covidien Lp 508-261-8000
15 Hampshire St, Mansfield, MA 02048
MONOJECT ULTRA-COMFORT insulin syringes.

Exelint International Co. 800-940-3935
5840 W Centinela Ave, Los Angeles, CA 90045
1/2cc & 1cc, 29G x 1/2'. 1/2cc & 1cc, 28G x 1/2'.

Lockett Medical Corp. 401-421-6599
3 Richmond Sq, Providence, RI 02906
Disposable and reusable.

SYRINGE, INSULIN *(cont'd)*

Medi-Hut Co., Inc. 800-882-0139
1935 Swarthmore Ave, Lakewood, NJ 08701

Microplastics, Inc. 630-513-2900
406 38th Ave, Saint Charles, IL 60174

Owen Mumford Usa, Inc. 800-421-6936
1755 W Oak Commons Ct Ste A, Marietta, GA 30062

Palco Labs, Inc. 800-346-4488
8030 Soquel Ave Ste 104, Santa Cruz, CA 95062
INSUL-EZE, insulin syringe loading device with magnifier. INSUL-TOTE Insulated all-weather carry tote for insulin meter, strips and syringes, and COLD POUCH insulated tote for carrying medication while in infusion pump. INSUL-CAP, insulin bottle caps, makes one-handed loading of syringes easier.

Terumo Medical Corp. 800-283-7866
2101 Cottontail Ln, Somerset, NJ 08873

Ulti Med, Inc. 877-858-4633
287 6th St E Ste 380, Saint Paul, MN 55101
UltiCare syringes come in all popular sizes and capacities. 28gauge 1cc and 1/2cc; 29gauge 1cc, 1/2cc and 3/10cc; and 30gauge 1cc, 1/2cc, and 3/10cc. The 28g and 29g needles are the standard 1/2inch needles and the 30g needles are the 'shorts' or 5/16 inch.

SYRINGE, IRRIGATING *(General) 80KYZ*

Alcon Manufacturing, Ltd. 817-551-6813
714 Columbia Ave, Sinking Spring, PA 19608
Sterile ophthalmic syringe.

Amsino International, Inc. 800-MD-AMSINO
855 Towne Center Dr, Pomona, CA 91767
AMSINO available in thumb-control ring or flat-top style, individually wrapped or bulk, or in I.V. pole bag non-sterile. Items AS012, AS018, AS016, AS112, AS118, and AS116.

B. Braun Medical, Inc. 610-596-2536
901 Marcon Blvd, Allentown, PA 18109

Ballard Medical Products 770-587-7835
12050 Lone Peak Pkwy, Draper, UT 84020
Syringe device,gastric lavage kit,.

Biomet, Inc. 574-267-6639
56 E Bell Dr, PO Box 587, Warsaw, IN 46582
Various types of non-dental syringes.

Bionix Development Corp. 800-551-7096
5154 Enterprise Blvd, Toledo, OH 43612
Splash shield accessory for irrigating syringe.

Busse Hospital Disposables, Inc. 631-435-4711
75 Arkay Dr, Hauppauge, NY 11788
Irrigation splash guard.

Byron Medical 800-777-3434
602 W Rillito St, Tucson, AZ 85705
Percutaneous stik -2cc reusable injection sysringe. LAMIS-reusable infiltration multiple port needles.

Centurion Medical Products Corp. 517-545-1135
3310 S Main St, Salisbury, NC 28147

Cytori Therapeutics, Inc. 877-470-8000
3020 Callan Rd, San Diego, CA 92121
Celbrush

Ear-Clear, Inc. 866-290-4260
1920 Brunns Rd Lot 29, Sebring, FL 33872
Infant earwax removal syringe, 3 year olds and over.

Ethox International 800-521-1022
251 Seneca St, Buffalo, NY 14204
Irrigation guard.

Genesis Biosystems, Inc. 888-577-7335
1500 Eagle Ct, Lewisville, TX 75057
Various tissue harvest and wash syringes.

Hasbro, Inc. 401-431-8697
1027 Newport Ave, Pawtucket, RI 02861
Ear syringe.

Health Care Logistics, Inc. 800-848-1633
450 Town St, PO Box 25, Circleville, OH 43113
Sterile disposable and reusable irrigating.

Health Ent., Inc. 508-695-0727
90 George Leven Dr, North Attleboro, MA 02760
Irrigating syringe.

Intl. Medsurg Connection, Inc. 847-619-9926
935 N Plum Grove Rd Ste V, Schaumburg, IL 60173
Bulb syringe.

SYRINGE, IRRIGATING *(cont'd)*

Kelsar, S.A. 508-261-8000
Blvd. Insurgentes, Libriamento a La, Tijuana 22450 Mexico
Bulb irrigation syringe, piston irrigation syringe (various)

Kentron Health Care, Inc. 615-384-0573
3604 Kelton Jackson Rd, P.o. Box 120, Springfield, TN 37172
Irrigation syringe.

Lsl Industries, Inc. 888-225-5575
5535 N Wolcott Ave, Chicago, IL 60640
$27.50 for case of 50.

Medline Manufacturing And Services Llc 847-837-2759
1 Medline Pl, Mundelein, IL 60060
Bulb syringe for feeding,irrigating.

Pedia Pals, Llc 888-733-4272
965 Highway 169 N, Plymouth, MN 55441
Elephant shaped pinnk and blue Ear/nasal syringe.

Terumo Cardiovascular Systems (Tcvs) 800-283-7866
28 Howe St, Ashland, MA 01721
Irrigating syringe.

Tri-State Hospital Supply Corp. 517-545-1135
3173 E 43rd St, Yuma, AZ 85365

Trinity Sterile, Inc. 410-860-5123
201 Kiley Dr, Salisbury, MD 21801

Ultracell Medical Technologies, Inc. 877-SPO-NGE1
183 Providence New London Tpke, North Stonington, CT 06359
Syringe, irrigating. Silicone irrigating bulbs are available for ophthalmic surgery. A 22cc blue autoclavable bulb is standard industry wide.

Wolfe Tory Medical, Inc. 801-281-3000
79 W 4500 S Ste 18, Salt Lake City, UT 84107
Wound irrigation syringe.

SYRINGE, IRRIGATING, DENTAL *(Dental And Oral) 76EIB*

Aesculap Implant Systems Inc. 1-800-234-9179
3773 Corporate Pkwy, Center Valley, PA 18034

Cadence Science Inc. 888-717-7677
1979 Marcus Ave Ste 215, New Hyde Park, NY 11042
6 sizes (reusable) 1/2 to 4 oz.

Centurion Medical Products Corp. 517-545-1135
3310 S Main St, Salisbury, NC 28147

Covidien Lp 508-261-8000
15 Hampshire St, Mansfield, MA 02048

Dentalez Group 866-DTE-INFO
101 Lindenwood Dr Ste 225, Valleybrooke Corporate Center
Malvern, PA 19355

Hu-Friedy Manufacturing Co., Inc. 800-483-7433
3232 N Rockwell St, Chicago, IL 60618
$131.75 for AQUA-FIX syringe; $14.65 for syringe tip.

Medi Inc 800-225-8634
75 York Ave, P.O. Box 302, Randolph, MA 02368

Tri-State Hospital Supply Corp. 517-545-1135
3173 E 43rd St, Yuma, AZ 85365

SYRINGE, IRRIGATING, STERILE *(General) 80KYY*

Amsino International, Inc. 800-MD-AMSINO
855 Towne Center Dr, Pomona, CA 91767
AMSINO available in thumb-control ring or flat-top style, sterile 50/CS. Items AS015 and AS115.

C. R. Bard, Inc., Bard Urological Div. 888-367-2273
13183 Harland Dr NE, Covington, GA 30014

SYRINGE, LABORATORY *(Chemistry) 75UIR*

Air-Tite Products Co., Inc. 800-231-7762
565 Central Dr Ste 101, Virginia Beach, VA 23454
Henke-Sass Wolf NORM-JECT syringes. 1cc all-plastic syringe for genetic research (non-cytotoxic). 1cc thru 50cc available. No rubber or silicone, with luer lock and luer slip.

Cadence Science Inc. 888-717-7677
1979 Marcus Ave Ste 215, New Hyde Park, NY 11042

Engineers Express, Inc. 800-255-8823
7 Industrial Park Rd, Medway, MA 02053

Hamilton Company 800-648-5950
4990 Energy Way, Reno, NV 89502
Chromatography and dual-gauge syringes for autosamplers.

Harvard Apparatus, Inc. 800-272-2775
84 October Hill Rd, Holliston, MA 01746

SYRINGE, LABORATORY *(cont'd)*

Spectra Medical Devices, Inc. 866-938-8649
4C Henshaw St, Woburn, MA 01801
Specializing in chromatography syringes.

SYRINGE, OPHTHALMIC *(Ophthalmology) 86HKA*

Bausch & Lomb Surgical 636-255-5051
3365 Tree Court Ind Blvd, Saint Louis, MO 63122

Labtician Ophthalmics, Inc. 800-265-8391
2140 Winston Park Dr., Unit 6, Oakville, ONTAR L6H 5V5 Canada
LSO™ QuickSet Silicone OIl injection system

SYRINGE, OTHER *(General) 80WVE*

Atlas Medical Resources (Amr) Corp. 800-267-1880
190 Colonnade Rd, Ste. 202, Ottawa, ON K2E 7J5 Canada
Non-reusable.

B. Braun Oem Division, B. Braun Medical Inc. 866-8-BBRAUN
824 12th Ave, Bethlehem, PA 18018

Baxter Healthcare Corporation, Baxter Biopharma Solutions 800-353-0887
927 S. Curry Pike Drive, Bloomington, IN 47402
CLEAR SHOT

Chagrin Safety Supply, Inc. 800-227-0468
8227 Washington St # 1, Chagrin Falls, OH 44023

Dma Med-Chem Corporation 800-362-1833
49 Watermill Ln, Great Neck, NY 11021
With/without needle.

Engineers Express, Inc. 800-255-8823
7 Industrial Park Rd, Medway, MA 02053

Exelint International Co. 800-940-3935
5840 W Centinela Ave, Los Angeles, CA 90045
Exel Secure Touch Safety Syringes.

Globe Medical Tech, Inc. 713-365-9595
1766 W Sam Houston Pkwy N, Houston, TX 77043
Safety Retractable Syringe

Greer Laboratories, Inc. 800-419-7302
639 Nuway Cir, PO Box 800, Lenoir, NC 28645
OPTIMIX mixing syringe.

Habley Medical Technology Corp. 800-729-1994
15721 Bernardo Heights Pkwy Ste B-30, San Diego, CA 92128
Safety-syringe needle.

Hamilton Company 800-648-5950
4990 Energy Way, Reno, NV 89502
Digital syringes.

Ipas 919-967-7052
PO Box 5027, Chapel Hill, NC 27514
Uterine manual vacuum aspiration syringe.

Ispg, Inc. 860-355-8511
517 Litchfield Rd, New Milford, CT 06776
Glass syringes.

Kloehn Co., Ltd. 800-358-4342
10000 Banburry Cross Dr, Las Vegas, NV 89144
Micro syringes (O.E.M.).

Lee Medical Ltd. 800-826-2360
5500 Lincoln Dr Ste 100, Minneapolis, MN 55436
LEE SYRINGE, a disposable syringe for fine needle aspiration biopsy.

Medi-Dose, Inc. 800-523-8966
70 Industrial Dr, Ivyland, PA 18974
Geriatric feeding appliance.

Medi-Hut Co., Inc. 800-882-0139
1935 Swarthmore Ave, Lakewood, NJ 08701
Safety syringe.

Medtech Group Inc., The 800-348-2759
6 Century Ln, South Plainfield, NJ 07080
Disposable-plastic, water-filled/gel-filled sterile syringes.

Neogen Corporation 800-234-5333
620 Lesher Pl, Lansing, MI 48912
Disposable syringes for veterinary use only.

Procedure Products, Inc. 360-693-1832
6622 Oakridge Dr, Gladstone, OR 97027
Color-coded syringes used in radiology/cardiac cath procedures.

Retractable Technologies, Inc. 888-806-2626
511 Lobo Ln, PO Box 9, Little Elm, TX 75068
VanishPoint Syringe and Blood Collection Tube Holder. Automatic retraction is passively activated by users while needle is still in patient's arm. Protects users from contaminated needles.

SYRINGE, OTHER *(cont'd)*

Safety 1st Medical, Inc. 800-997-2331
1740 E Garry Ave Ste 109, Santa Ana, CA 92705
SAFE-1 disposable safety syringe and anti-needlesticks.

Specialized Health Products International, Inc. 800-306-3360
585 W 500 S, Bountiful, UT 84010
LuproLoc is a safety device attached to TAP Pharmaceutical's Lupron Depot®. LuproLoc is activated by a simple press of the finger, or by pressing the device on a hard surface, such as a table. LuproLoc reduces the risk of accidental needlestick injuries by shielding the needle after use.

Spectra Medical Devices, Inc. 978-657-0889
260H Fordham Rd, Wilmington, MA 01887
Glass syringes with or without metal tips, bulk, non-sterile

Spectra Medical Devices, Inc. 866-938-8649
4C Henshaw St, Woburn, MA 01801
Plastic and glass syringes.

Total Molding Services, Inc. 215-538-9613
354 East Broad St., Trumbauersville, PA 18970
10 & 20cc plungers for 10 & 20 cc syringe barrels. 10 & 20cc Barrel Type Syringes.

Tulip Medical Products 800-325-6526
PO Box 7368, San Diego, CA 92167
Tulip brand syringe instrumentation for soft tissue surgery.

Ware Medics Glass Works, Inc. 845-429-6950
PO Box 368, Garnerville, NY 10923
Asepto syringes.

SYRINGE, PERIODONTIC, ENDODONTIC *(Dental And Oral) 76EIC*

Aesculap Implant Systems Inc. 1-800-234-9179
3773 Corporate Pkwy, Center Valley, PA 18034

Biolase Technology, Inc. 888-424-6527
4 Cromwell, Irvine, CA 92618

Biomet Microfixation Inc. 800-874-7711
1520 Tradeport Dr, Jacksonville, FL 32218
Various types of syringes.

Centrix, Inc. 800-235-5862
770 River Rd, Shelton, CT 06484

Covidien Lp 508-261-8000
15 Hampshire St, Mansfield, MA 02048
Sterile needle/syringe combination with special notched needle for endo irrigation.

Denbur, Inc. 630-969-6865
433 Plaza Dr Ste 4, Westmont, IL 60559
Irrigating tip.

Inter-Med, Inc. 877-418-4782
2200 Northwestern Ave, Racine, WI 53404
Syringe.

Js Dental Mfg., Inc. 800-284-3368
196 N Salem Rd, Ridgefield, CT 06877
Pipettes.

Miltex Dental Technologies, Inc. 516-576-6022
589 Davies Dr, York, PA 17402
Various luer and aspirating syringes.

Moyco Technologies, Inc. 800-331-8837
200 Commerce Dr, Montgomeryville, PA 18936

Pac-Dent Intl., Inc. 909-839-0888
21078 Commerce Point Dr, Walnut, CA 91789
Syringe.

Special Products, Inc. 800-538-6836
2540 Greenwood Dr, Kissimmee, FL 34744
Endodontic syringe.

Ultradent Products, Inc. 801-553-4586
505 W 10200 S, South Jordan, UT 84095
Syringe.

SYRINGE, PISTON *(General) 80FMF*

Advance Medical Designs, Inc. 800-221-3679
1241 Atlanta Industrial Dr, Marietta, GA 30066
Control Syringes

Air-Tite Products Co., Inc. 800-231-7762
565 Central Dr Ste 101, Virginia Beach, VA 23454
Henke-Sass Wolf Complete line of SOFT-JECT syringes available. AIR-TITE, insulin syringe, new line of .5ml, 1ml, 3ml, 5ml, and 10ml syringes, including insulin priced at economical levels. Offers high quality and low cost. Also Terumo,Excel,BD.

SYRINGE, PISTON *(cont'd)*

Alcon Manufacturing, Ltd. 817-551-6813
714 Columbia Ave, Sinking Spring, PA 19608
Sterile ophthalmic syringe.

Am2 Pat Inc. 919-552-9689
455 W Depot St, Angier, NC 27501
Normal saline flush.

Argon Medical Devices Inc. 903-675-9321
1445 Flat Creek Rd, Athens, TX 75751
Control syringe.

Arthrex Manufacturing 239-643-5553
1958 Trade Center Way, Naples, FL 34109
Aspirate kit.

Arthrex, Inc. 239-643-5553
1370 Creekside Blvd, Naples, FL 34108
Arthrex orthokin family syringes.

B. Braun Medical Inc., Renal Therapies Div. 800-854-6851
824 12th Ave, Bethlehem, PA 18018

B. Braun Medical, Inc. 610-596-2536
901 Marcon Blvd, Allentown, PA 18109
VARIOUS PISTON SYRINGES AND CAPS

Baxter Healthcare Corporation, Medication Delivery 949-851-9066
17511 Armstrong Ave, Irvine, CA 92614
Accessory grip.

Bd Medical - Diabetes Care 201-847-4298
1329 W US Highway 6 # &34, Holdrege, NE 68949
Various sizes of hypodermic, insulin, lor syringe and insulin pens.

Becton, Dickinson & Co. 308-872-6811
150 S 1st Ave, Broken Bow, NE 68822
Various sizes of hypodermic, insulin, lor syringes and insulin pens.

Biocompatibles Inc. 877-783-5463
115 Hurley Rd Bldg 3, Oxford, CT 06478
Loss of resistance syringe.

Biomet, Inc. 574-267-6639
56 E Bell Dr, PO Box 587, Warsaw, IN 46582
Various types of piston syringes.

Busse Hospital Disposables, Inc. 631-435-4711
75 Arkay Dr, Hauppauge, NY 11788
Vad access tray.

C. R. Bard, Inc., Bard Urological Div. 888-367-2273
13183 Harland Dr NE, Covington, GA 30014

Cardinal Health 303,Inc. 858-458-7830
1515 Ivac Way, Creedmoor, NC 27522
Various type of piston syringes.

Coeur, Inc 800-296-5893
704 Cadet Ct, Lebanon, TN 37087
Disposable control syringe.

Confluent Surgical,Inc 888-734-2583
101A 1st Ave, Waltham, MA 02451
Dual liquid applicator.

Covidien Lp 508-261-8000
15 Hampshire St, Mansfield, MA 02048
50cc and 60cc enteral feeding and irrigation syringes.

Daxor Corporation 865-425-0555
107 Meco Ln, Oak Ridge, TN 37830
Piston syringe.

Depuy Spine, Inc. 800-227-6633
325 Paramount Dr, Raynham, MA 02767
Syring, piston.

Eli Lilly And Co. 317-276-4000
Lilly Corporate Ctr, Drop Code 2622, Indianapolis, IN 46285
Insulin pen injector various.

Engineers Express, Inc. 800-255-8823
7 Industrial Park Rd, Medway, MA 02053

Ev3 Neurovascular 800-716-6700
9775 Toledo Way, Irvine, CA 92618
Sterile syringe.

Genchem, Inc. 714-529-1616
510 W Central Ave Ste D, Brea, CA 92821
Glucose reagent.

Haemacure Corp. 888-721-8076
2001 University Pkwy Ste 430, Sarasota, FL 34243 Canada
Sterile surgical applicator system.

SYRINGE, PISTON *(cont'd)*

Harvest Technologies, Corp. 508-732-7500
40 Grissom Rd Ste 100, Plymouth, MA 02360
Graft delivery system,dual liquid applicator.

Health Care Logistics, Inc. 800-848-1633
450 Town St, PO Box 25, Circleville, OH 43113
Sterile 'piston type' irrigation syringe and accessories.

Hospira Inc. 877-946-7747
275 N Field Dr, Lake Forest, IL 60045
HOSPIRA CARPUJECT HOLDER

Hosuk America Co. 303-750-3829
1583 S Tucson St, Aurora, CO 80012
Various.

Icu Medical (Ut), Inc 949-366-2183
4455 Atherton Dr, Salt Lake City, UT 84123
Vial access spike.

Icu Medical, Inc. 800-824-7890
951 Calle Amanecer, San Clemente, CA 92673
Vial access spike.

Indigo Orb, Inc. 949-784-0303
2454 Alton Pkwy, Irvine, CA 92606
Loss of resistance syringe.

Integra Lifesciences Corp. 609-275-0500
311 Enterprise Dr, Plainsboro, NJ 08536
Syringe.

Integra Lifesciences Corp. 801-886-9505
3395 W 1820 S, Salt Lake City, UT 84104
Piston syringe.

Interpore Cross International 800-722-4489
181 Technology Dr, Irvine, CA 92618
Ultraconcentrator manifold with extension set. Graft delivery syringe. Disposable system for intraoperative collection of autologous growth factors.

Ispg, Inc. 860-355-8511
517 Litchfield Rd, New Milford, CT 06776
Glass syringes.

K & W Medical Specialties, Inc. 215-675-4653
115 Pritchard Hollow Rd, Westfield, PA 16950
Ear plugs/ear molds.

Kelsar, S.A. 508-261-8000
Blvd. Insurgentes, Libriamento a La, Tijuana 22450 Mexico
Syringes, syringe tip caps, accessories (various)

Kentron Health Care, Inc. 615-384-0573
3604 Kelton Jackson Rd, P.o. Box 120, Springfield, TN 37172
Syringe.

Lsl Industries, Inc. 888-225-5575
5535 N Wolcott Ave, Chicago, IL 60640

Medical Techniques Usa 801-936-4501
125 N 400 W Ste C, North Salt Lake, UT 84054

Medline Manufacturing And Services Llc 847-837-2759
1 Medline Pl, Mundelein, IL 60060
Piston syringes.

Medtronic Minimed 800-933-3322
18000 Devonshire St, Northridge, CA 91325
MMT103 drug reservoir.

Medtronic Sofamor Danek Usa, Inc. 901-396-3133
4340 Swinnea Rd, Memphis, TN 38118
General purpose centrifuge.

Merit Medical Systems, Inc. 800-356-3748
1600 Merit Pkwy, South Jordan, UT 84095
CCS Control Syringe MEDALLION Series Syringes. VAKLOK syringes.

Milestone Scientific Inc. 800-862-1125
45 Knightsbridge Rd, Piscataway, NJ 08854
Piston syringe.

Milestone Scientific Inc. 800-862-1125
220 S Orange Ave, Livingston, NJ 07039
The Wand, computer controlled anesthetic ; delivery system; Wand Plus, CompuMed

Minrad, Inc. 716-855-1068
50 Cobham Dr, Orchard Park, NY 14127
Sterile syringe.

North Safety Products 401-943-4400
1101 B Calle Neutron, Parque Industrial Maran, Mexicali, B.c. Mexico
Syringe

SYRINGE, PISTON *(cont'd)*

Orthovita, Inc. 610-640-1775
77 Great Valley Pkwy, Malvern, PA 19355
Piston syringe.

Precision Medical Devices, Inc. 717-795-9480
5020 Ritter Rd Ste 211, Mechanicsburg, PA 17055
Bone cement syringe.

Retractable Technologies, Inc. 888-806-2626
511 Lobo Ln, PO Box 9, Little Elm, TX 75068
Patient Safe syringe

Safecare Corporation 225-753-4664
6352 Quin Dr Apt A, Baton Rouge, LA 70817
Covertip.

Safegard Medical Products, Inc. 800-389-7173
52 Dragon Ct, Woburn, MA 01801
Manual retraction safety syringes of various sizes.

Safety 1st Medical, Inc. 800-997-2331
1740 E Garry Ave Ste 109, Santa Ana, CA 92705

Safety Syringes, Inc. 760-918-9908
2875 Loker Ave E, Carlsbad, CA 92010
Various.

Shinamerica, Inc. 651-291-7909
710 Fourth St., Desmet, SD 57231
Various types of sterile syringes.

Squareone Medical, Inc. 805-987-2457
1640 Pierside Ln, Camarillo, CA 93010
Sq-1.

Stryker Puerto Rico, Ltd. 939-307-2500
Hwy. 3, Km. 131.2, Las Guasimas Ind. Park, Arroyo, PR 00714
Discography syringe.

Synthes (Usa) - Development Center 719-481-5300
1230 Wilson Dr, West Chester, PA 19380
Syringe.

Terumo Cardiovascular Systems (Tcvs) 800-283-7866
28 Howe St, Ashland, MA 01721
Syringe.

Terumo Medical Corporation 800-283-7866
950 Elkton Blvd, P.O.Box 605, Elkton, MD 21921
Hypodermic syringe and needle.

Therapeutic Silicone Technologies, Inc. 212-606-0830
909 5th Ave, New York, NY 10021
Automated injection syringe/aspiration system.

Thermogenesis Corp. 800-783-8357
2711 Citrus Rd, Rancho Cordova, CA 95742
Multiple

Univec, Inc. 410-347-9959
4810 Seton Dr, Baltimore, MD 21215
Hypodermic syring with sharps protection.

Vascular Solutions, Inc. 888-240-6001
6464 Sycamore Ct N, Maple Grove, MN 55369
Auto-Fill Syringe Kit

Vascular Solutions, Inc. 763-656-4300
5025 Cheshire Ln N, Plymouth, MN 55446
Lidocaine delivery system.

Warsaw Orthopedic, Inc. 901-396-3133
2500 Silveus Xing, Warsaw, IN 46582
General purpose centrifuge.

SYRINGE, RESTORATIVE AND IMPRESSION MATERIAL
(Dental And Oral) 76EID

Aesculap Implant Systems Inc. 1-800-234-9179
3773 Corporate Pkwy, Center Valley, PA 18034

Cadco Dental Products 800-833-8267
600 E Hueneme Rd, Oxnard, CA 93033
$24.00 for hydrocolloid syringe.

Centrix, Inc. 800-235-5862
770 River Rd, Shelton, CT 06484

Dux Dental 800-833-8267
600 E Hueneme Rd, Oxnard, CA 93033
$24.00 for hydrocolloid syringe.

Harry J. Bosworth Company 800-323-4352
7227 Hamlin Ave, Skokie, IL 60076
SUPERSIL, RE'CORD, ULTRATRIM.

Inter-Med, Inc. 877-418-4782
2200 Northwestern Ave, Racine, WI 53404
Impression syringe; disposable impression syringe.

SYRINGE, RESTORATIVE AND IMPRESSION MATERIAL *(cont'd)*

Kerr Corp. 714-516-7400
28200 Wick Rd, Romulus, MI 48174
Impression material syringe.

Pac-Dent Intl., Inc. 909-839-0888
21078 Commerce Point Dr, Walnut, CA 91789
Hp mixing tips, mixing tips for penta machine, cartridge mixing gun.

Plasdent Corp. 909-620-0289
1290 Price Ave, Pomona, CA 91767
Plastic impression syringes.

Plastodent 718-792-3554
2881 Middletown Rd, Bronx, NY 10461

Shofu Dental Corporation 800-827-4638
1225 Stone Dr, San Marcos, CA 92078
BEAUTIFIL, FL-BOND, SOLIDEX

Ultradent Products, Inc. 801-553-4586
505 W 10200 S, South Jordan, UT 84095
Syringe.

3m Unitek 800-634-5300
2724 Peck Rd, Monrovia, CA 91016

SYRINGE, TUBERCULIN *(General) 80RYT*

Cadence Science Inc. 888-717-7677
1979 Marcus Ave Ste 215, New Hyde Park, NY 11042
14 types (reusable).

Chagrin Safety Supply, Inc. 800-227-0468
8227 Washington St # 1, Chagrin Falls, OH 44023

Covidien Lp 508-261-8000
15 Hampshire St, Mansfield, MA 02048

Exelint International Co. 800-940-3935
5840 W Centinela Ave, Los Angeles, CA 90045
EXEL 1cc TB Syringe Zero Dead Syringe.

SYSTEM, ABLATION, ULTRASOUND AND ACCESSORIES
(Surgery) 79NTB

Minnetronix Inc. 888-301-1025
1635 Energy Park Dr, Saint Paul, MN 55108
EPICOR MEDICAL ABLATION SYSTEMS

SYSTEM, ALBATION, MICROWAVE AND ACCESSORIES
(Surgery) 79NEY

Boston Scientific Corp. 408-935-3400
150 Baytech Dr, San Jose, CA 95134
Microwave generator, flex 10, flex 4.

Maquet Puerto Rico Inc. 408-635-3900
No. 12, Rd. #698, Dorado, PR 00646
Ablation system.

SYSTEM, ANALYSIS, HEARING-AID *(Ear/Nose/Throat) 77EWM*

Fecom Corporation 800-292-3362
12 Stults Rd Ste 103, Dayton, NJ 08810
Digital Key-chain battery tester with LCD indicator for hearing aid batteries and household battery tester that tester sizes D, C, AA, AAA, 9 volt, and Lithium all in one unit

Frye Electronics, Inc. 800-547-8209
9826 SW Tigard St, Tigard, OR 97223
FONIX FP35 Hearing Aid Analyzer. The basic price is $3995. Options can be added bringing the cost to $5600 or more. Also available: the FONIX 40-D hearing aid analyzer: $5,250.00 per unit (standard). and the new top of the line FONIX 7000 Hearing Aid Test System. Several computer programs: WinCHAP, Press and GO, and FONIX NOAH 3 Module can be used with these instruments and our audiometer. Look on our web site for details and pricing. www.frye.com.

Starkey Laboratories, Inc. 800-328-8602
6700 Washington Ave S, Eden Prairie, MN 55344
$6,950 for HAL-P hearing aid laboratory with printer, not requiring sound-proof test box.

SYSTEM, APPLIANCE, FIXATION, SPINAL PEDICLE SCREW
(Orthopedics) 87MCV

Bio-Technology Usa, Inc. 305-512-3522
6175 NW 167th St Ste G8, Hialeah, FL 33015
Screw pedicular system, fixation.

Millstone Medical Outsourcing 508-679-8384
1565 N Main St Ste 408, Fall River, MA 02720
Multiple and various.

SYSTEM, APPLIANCE, FIXATION, SPINAL PEDICLE SCREW *(cont'd)*

Ortho Development Corp. 800-429-8339
12187 Business Park Dr, Draper, UT 84020
CONTOUR Spine System; Pedicle Screw fixation for lumbar spinal fusion. ENVISION Anterior Cervical Plate; one-step locking mechanism, self-drilling screws, large graft window. IBS Allograft; Interbody spacer with C-TLIF procedure, one-piece femoral cortical bone, precision-milled.

Orthopedic Sciences, Inc 562-799-5550
3020 Old Ranch Pkwy Ste 325, Seal Beach, CA 90740
Pedicle screw fixation system.

SYSTEM, AUTOMATED SCANNING MICROSCOPE AND IMAGE ANALYSIS FOR FLUORESCENCE IN SITU HYBRIDIZATION (FISH) ASSAYS *(Immunology) 82NTH*

Abbott Molecular, Inc. 847-937-6100
1300 E Touhy Ave, Des Plaines, IL 60018
Automated fluorescence in situ hybridization (fish) enumeration systems.

SYSTEM, AUTOMATED, MICROBIOLOGICAL *(Microbiology) 83QCC*

Gen-Probe, Inc. 800-523-5001
10210 Genetic Center Dr, San Diego, CA 92121
MultiPROBE 204 Robotic Liquid Handling System With Bar Code Reader - a fully automated sample and reagent pipetting system for use with GEN-PROBE assays. TECAN GENEIS RSP 100/4 System - an automated sample and reagent pipetting system for use with GEN-PROBE assays.TECAN GENESIS RSP 150/8 System - an automated sample and reagent pipetting system for use with GEN-PROBE assays. MultiPROBE 104/204 Robotic Liquid Handling System - a fully automated sample and reagent pipetting system for use with GEN-PROBE assays.

Medical Sales & Service Group 888-357-6520
10 Woodchester Dr, Acton, MA 01720

Thermo Spectra-Tech 800-243-9186
2 Research Dr, PO Box 869, Shelton, CT 06484
IRUS infrared microanalysis system combines optical microscopy and infrared spectroscopy along with dedicated IRUS microanalysis Windows-based software. The system allows the user to determine the chemical and molecular properties of a wide variety of organic and inorganic materials.

Trek Diagnostic Systems 800-871-8909
982 Keynote Cir Ste 6, Cleveland, OH 44131

Vista Technology, Inc. 780-468-0020
8432 45th St. NW, Edmonton, ALB T6B-2N6 Canada
ISOPLATER Automatic Petri Dish Streaking System. Automatically loads, streakes, and stacks up to 180 petri dishes per hour, thereby improving results, increasing safety, standardizing processes, and generating substantial cost savings by automating a repetitive, laborious 100-year-old manual procedure.

SYSTEM, BLOOD CULTURING *(Microbiology) 83MDB*

Bd Diagnostic Systems 800-675-0908
7 Loveton Cir, Sparks, MD 21152

Biomerieux Inc. 800-682-2666
100 Rodolphe St, Durham, NC 27712
BACT/ALERT: microbial blood culture detection system fully automated for detection of bacteria and fungi in blood cultures, available in 240 or 120 bottle capacity. BACT/ALERT 3D is a fully automated system for detecting the growth of microorganisms in blood and other body fluids and is FDA cleared for mycobacteria.

North American Medical Products, Inc. 800-488-6267
6 British American Blvd Ste B, Latham, NY 12110
SAFE-POINT VAC- System which provides vacutainer holder and blood collection needle with safety cover, pre-assembled.

Oxoid, Inc. 800-567-8378
800 Proctor Ave, Ogdensburg, NY 13669
One-bottle system.

Trek Diagnostic Systems 800-871-8909
982 Keynote Cir Ste 6, Cleveland, OH 44131

SYSTEM, CAMERA, 3-DIMENSIONAL *(Surgery) 79SGZ*

Integra Luxtec, Inc. 800-325-8966
99 Hartwell St, West Boylston, MA 01583
Microlux.

Olympus America, Inc. 800-645-8160
3500 Corporate Pkwy, PO Box 610, Center Valley, PA 18034

Richard Wolf Medical Instruments Corp. 800-323-9653
353 Corporate Woods Pkwy, Vernon Hills, IL 60061

SYSTEM, CANCER TREATMENT, HYPERTHERMIA, RF/MICROWAVE *(Radiology) 90LOC*

Bsd Medical Corporation 801-972-5555
2188 W 2200 S, Salt Lake City, UT 84119
Generates electromagnetic radiation for tumor heat treatment.

Celsion Corporation 800-262-0394
10220 Old Columbia Rd Ste L, Columbia, MD 21046
APA 1000 - Adaptive Phased Array System. For the treatment and management of surface and subsurface tumors in conjunction with radiation therapy.

Labthermics Technologies 217-351-7722
701 Devonshire Dr, Champaign, IL 61820
INTERTHERM 100 RF interstitial unit.

SYSTEM, CATHETER CONTROL, REPROCESSED *(Cardiovascular) 74NKR*

Ascent Healthcare Solutions 480-763-5300
10232 S 51st St, Phoenix, AZ 85044
Electrophysiology catheters, reprocessed.

SYSTEM, CODING, COLOR, INSTRUMENT *(Dental And Oral) 76UDU*

Key Surgical, Inc. 800-541-7995
8101 Wallace Rd Ste 100, Eden Prairie, MN 55344
Instrument identification tape in 1/8-, 1/4-, and 3/8-inch widths.

Mark Medical Manufacturing, Inc. 610-269-4420
530 Brandywine Ave, Downingtown, PA 19335
25 colors, surgical instruments fused with nylon coatings.

Scanlan International, Inc. 800-328-9458
1 Scanlan Plz, Saint Paul, MN 55107
SURG-I-BAND color coding.

SYSTEM, COMMUNICATION, IMAGE, DIGITAL *(Radiology) 90LMD*

Access Genetics 952-942-0671
7550 Market Place Dr, Eden Prairie, MN 55344
Web-enhanced telemedicine portal software.

Agfa Corporation 877-777-2432
PO Box 19048, 10 South Academy Street, Greenville, SC 29602
IMPAX, digital image management software. ADC, computer radiology.

Agfa Healthcare Corp. 864-421-1815
580 Gotham Pkwy, Carlstadt, NJ 07072
Gateway,hub,router,interface.

Agfa Healthcare Corp. 864-421-1815
1 Crosswind Dr, Westerly, RI 02891
Xa capture system.

Amicas, Inc. 800-490-8465
20 Guest St Ste 200, Brighton, MA 02135
Image communication device.

Barco, Inc 678-475-8137
3059 Premiere Pkwy, Duluth, GA 30097
Workstation,image workstation, and others.

Black Diamond Video, Inc. 215-348-3896
1151 Harbor Bay Pkwy Ste 208, Alameda, CA 94502
Dvi converter.

Canon U.S.A., Inc. 949-932-3100
15975 Alton Pkwy, Irvine, CA 92618
Various models.

Cardea Technology Inc. 617-627-9399
249 Elm St Ste NO1, Somerville, MA 02144
Radiological digital image communications system.

Carestream Health, Inc. 888-777-2072
150 Verona St, Rochester, NY 14608
Various types of digital image communication devices & accessories.

Compressus Inc. 202-742-4307
101 Constitution Ave NW Ste 800, Washington, DC 20001
Medical imaging software system.

Computer Programs And Systems, Inc. 251-639-8100
6600 Wall St, Mobile, AL 36695
Medical image communciations device.

Computerized Medical Systems, Inc. 468-587-2550
1145 Corporate Lake Dr, Olivette, MO 63132
Contouring workstation.

Compview Medical Llc 503-641-8439
10035 SW Arctic Dr, Beaverton, OR 97005
Medical imaging communication device.

SYSTEM, COMMUNICATION, IMAGE, DIGITAL *(cont'd)*

Dejarnette Research Systems 410-583-0680
401 Washington Ave Ste 1010, Towson, MD 21204
Protocol communications gateway.

Desacc, Inc. 866-638-0936
0844 SW Curry St, Portland, OR 97239
Medical imaging software.

Ebm Technologies Usa, Llc 808-945-3100
641 Keeaumoku St Ste 5, Honolulu, HI 96814

Empiric Systems, Llc 866-367-4742
3800 Paramount Pkwy Ste 130, Morrisville, NC 27560
Various medical imagecommunications and simple display functions used in conjunc.

Erad/Image Medical Corp. 864-234-7430
9 Pilgrim Rd Ste 312, Greenville, SC 29607
Medical image communication device.

Everybyte, Llc 805-279-3228
3940 Verde Vista Dr, Thousand Oaks, CA 91360
Everybyte image management system.

Ge Healthcare It 847-277-5000
540 W Northwest Hwy, Barrington, IL 60010
Medical image communications device.

Gencosoft Llc. 714-625-8972
17042 Pinehurst Ln Apt B, Huntington Beach, CA 92647
Autopacs.

Genesis Digital Imaging, Inc. 888-436-3444
12921 W Washington Blvd, Los Angeles, CA 90066

Heart Imaging Technologies, Llc 919-384-5044
5003 Southpark Dr Ste 140, Durham, NC 27713
Image management system.

Hipgraphics, Inc. 410-821-7040
100 West Rd Ste 302, Towson, MD 21204
3d ct/mr post-processing workstation.

Hopkins Imaging 951-302-8416
34721 El Mirador Corte, Temecula, CA 92592
Digital imaging systems.

Imco Technologies 800-300-7734
N27W23957 Paul Rd Ste 101, Pewaukee, WI 53072
IMCO-PACS consists of IMCO-view, IMCO-store, IMCO-web, IMCO-link, IMCO-Ortho for the viewing and storing of DICOM images.

Imsi, Integrated Modular Systems Inc. 800-220-9729
2500 W Township Line Rd, PO Box 616, Havertown, PA 19083
DICOM Archive and Viewing. Full functionality complete for under $100K. Over 600 installs worldwide.

Invoke Imaging, Inc. 630-271-8111
1250 Palmer St, Downers Grove, IL 60516
Various medical image communications devices.

Medical Data Technologies, Inc. 866-643-7424
1421 Oakfield Dr, Brandon, FL 33511
Direct rad.

Medical Metrx Solutions
12 Commerce Ave, West Lebanon, NH 03784
Medical image communications devices.

Medimaging Tecnology, Inc. 800-244-9035
49 Herb Hill Rd, Glen Cove, NY 11542

Medstrat, Inc. 630-960-8700
1901 Butterfield Rd Ste 600, Downers Grove, IL 60515
Medstrat data server.

Medweb 800-863-3932
667 Folsom St, San Francisco, CA 94107
Picture archiving & communications system (PACS), teleradiology, and telemedicine.

Merlin Engineering Works, Inc. 800-227-1980
1888 Embarcadero Rd, Palo Alto, CA 94303
ME-959 UNISCAN digital scan converter. ME-509 DownScan LT provides video scan conversion from 1023-1125/30 (1249/25) to 525/30 (625/30) for standard video. ME-511 DownscanLX provides video scan conversion, SVGA progressive scan signals to 525-625 line standard video.

National Electronic Attachment, Inc. 800-782-5150
4588 Winters Chapel Rd Ste 200, Atlanta, GA 30360
Fast attach.

Naviscan Inc. 858-587-3641
6865 Flanders Dr Ste B, San Diego, CA 92121
Image server, image viewer.

SYSTEM, COMMUNICATION, IMAGE, DIGITAL *(cont'd)*

Openmed Technologies Corporation 877-717-6215
256 W Cummings Park, Woburn, MA 01801
OpenMed Viewer, web-based clinical review workstation for clinician consults via the Internet

Pacsgear, Inc. 925-846-9600
7020 Koll Center Pkwy Ste 100, Pleasanton, CA 94566
Software utility package to interface pc to image digitizer.

Phillips Ultrasound 800-982-2011
22100 Bothell Everett Hwy, P.O. Box 3003, Bothell, WA 98021

Plexar Associates, Inc. 216-932-2069
3722 Meadowbrook Blvd, University Heights, OH 44118
DP-1 bridge. DICOM protocol converter for use with legacy laser imagers.

Polycom Inc. 925-924-6000
100 Minuteman Rd, Andover, MA 01810
Video conferencing system.

Provation Medical, Inc. 612-313-1564
800 Washington Ave N Ste 400, Minneapolis, MN 55401
Medical procedure documentation and coding compliance software.

Rahd Ocology Products / Electronic Services Mart, Inc. 314-524-0103
500 Airport Rd, Saint Louis, MO 63135
Picture archwing communications system.

Ramsoft, Inc. 416-674-1347
37 Bankview Cir, Etobicoke M9W 6S6 Canada
Pacs

Scimage, Inc. 866-724-6243
4916 El Camino Real Ste 200, Los Altos, CA 94022
PACS and Telemedicine System

Segami Corporation 410-381-2311
8325 Guilford Rd Ste B, Columbia, MD 21046
Juniper radiology information system.

Stair Systems, Inc. 336-852-9122
3723 W Market St Ste A, Greensboro, NC 27403
Various types of digital image communications devices.

Stryker Communications Corp. 866-726-3705
1410 Lakeside Pkwy, Flower Mound, TX 75028
Medical Video/Audio Routing System

Stryker Imaging 888-795-4624
1410 Lakeside Pkwy Ste 600, Flower Mound, TX 75028
Digital image communications system.

Sunquest Information Systems, Inc 520-570-2347
250 S Williams Blvd, Tucson, AZ 85711

Terarecon, Inc. 877-354-1100
2955 Campus Dr Ste 325, San Mateo, CA 94403
Lmd viewing station.

Thinking Systems Corporation 727-217-0909
750 94th Ave N Ste 211, Saint Petersburg, FL 33702
Image-review software.

Toshiba America Medical Systems 800-421-1968
2441 Michelle Dr, Tustin, CA 92780

Varian Medical Systems, Oncology Systems 800 278-2747
911 Hansen Way, Bldg.3 M/S C-165, Palo Alto, CA 94304
Various types of image communication device.

Visual Med, Inc.
11110 Westlake Dr, Charlotte, NC 28273
Image acquisition and transfer software.

Worldcare, Inc. 617-374-9001
1 Cambridge Ctr Ste 5, Cambridge, MA 02142
Pacs equipment, pacs components.

SYSTEM, CONCENTRATION, HEMATOPOIETIC STEM CELL
(Hematology) 81MZJ

Dendreon Corp. 866-477-6782
3005 1st Ave, Seattle, WA 98121
Buoyant densith solution 60 (bds60).

SYSTEM, COOLING, LASER *(Surgery) 79WOH*

Aec, Inc. 847-273-7700
1100 E Woodfield Rd Ste 588, Schaumburg, IL 60173
Chillers and heat transfer equipment.

Biomedics, Inc. 949-458-1998
23322 Peralta Dr Ste 11, Laguna Hills, CA 92653

SYSTEM, COOLING, LASER *(cont'd)*

Telsar Laboratories Inc 800-255-9938
1 Enviro Way Ste 100, Wood River, IL 62095
DermaChiller 4 skin cooling device for dermatology/plastic surgery.

SYSTEM, CRYOSURGICAL, LIQUID NITROGEN, FOR GASTROENTEROLOGY *(Gastro/Urology) 78NEJ*

Csa Medical, Inc. 443-921-8053
1101 E 33rd St, Third Floor, Ste. E305, Baltimore, MD 21218
Cryo-ablator.

SYSTEM, CYSTIC FIBROSIS TRANSMEMBRANE CONDUCTANCE REGULATOR, GENE MUTATION DETECTION *(Immunology) 82NUA*

Celera Corporation 510-749-4219
1401 Harbor Bay Pkwy, Alameda, CA 94502
Cf genotyping assay.

SYSTEM, DELIVERY, DRUG, NON-INVASIVE *(General) 80WOI*

Advansource Biomaterials Corp. 978-657-0075
229 Andover St, Wilmington, MA 01887

Antares Pharma, Inc. 800-328-3074
250 Phillips Blvd, Princeton Crossroads Corporate Center
Ewing, NJ 08618
VISION(R) Needle-Free Injection System for administration of insulin and growth hormone

Boston Scientific Corporation 800-225-2732
1 Boston Scientific Pl, Natick, MA 01760
Coronary iontophoresis drug delivery system for treating and/or preventing angioplasty associated complications.

General Medical Co. 800-432-5362
1935 Armacost Ave, Los Angeles, CA 90025
LECTRO PATCH Iontophoretic device - both long term and short term delivery. Patented safety features prevent skin injury.

Iomed, Inc. 800-621-3347
2441 S 3850 W Ste A, Salt Lake City, UT 84120
PHORESOR iontophoretic, painless drug delivery unit.

Mps Acacia 800-486-6677
785 Challenger St, Brea, CA 92821

Sgarlato Laboratories, Inc. 800-421-5303
2315 S Bascom Ave Ste 200, Campbell, CA 95008
PainFree Pump. Ambulatory, non-narcotic drug delivery system for pain control. Spring loaded & flow regulated device that delivers a continuous flow of pain medication directly to surgical site to help releive postoperative pain. Patient goes home with device.

Vivus, Inc. 650-934-5200
1172 Castro St, Mountain View, CA 94040
MUSE non-injectable delivery system for alprostadil. Is indicated for the treatment of erectile dysfunction. MUSE is a non-injectable, transurethral drug delivery system consisting of a prefilled plastic applicator containing a urethral suppository of alprostadil.

SYSTEM, DELIVERY, DRUG, OCULAR *(Ophthalmology) 86WVM*

Command Medical Products, Inc. 386-672-8116
15 Signal Ave, Ormond Beach, FL 32174
Huber winged infusion sets; microbore winged infusion sets for drug delivery.

Eagle Vision, Inc. 800-222-7584
8500 Wolf Lake Dr Ste 110, Memphis, TN 38133
Glaucoma drainage devices with and without valves; low profile; large surface area; supplied with cannula

SYSTEM, DELIVERY, DRUG, UNIT-DOSE *(General) 80SGR*

Akro-Mils, Inc. 800-253-2467
1293 S Main St, Akron, OH 44301

Arrow International, Inc. 800-523-8446
2400 Bernville Rd, Reading, PA 19605
Model M-3000 implantable drug delivery pump.

Artromick International, Inc. 800-848-6462
4800 Hilton Corporate Dr, Columbus, OH 43232

Baxa Corporation 800-567-2292
9540 S Maroon Circle, Suite 400, Englewood, CO 80112
KWIK-VIAL, unit dose containers.

Best Nomos Corp. 800-70-NOMOS
1 Best Dr, Pittsburgh, PA 15202
PEREGRINE Dose Calculation System.

Forest Dental Products Inc 800-423-3535
6200 NE Campus Ct, Hillsboro, OR 97124

Gw Plastics, Inc. 802-234-9941
239 Pleasant St, Bethel, VT 05032

SYSTEM, DELIVERY, DRUG, UNIT-DOSE *(cont'd)*

I-Flow Corporation 800-448-3569
20202 Windrow Dr, Lake Forest, CA 92630
PAINBUSTER, Continuous Infusion System, infusing local anesthetics directly into wound site. ON-Q, Continuous Infusion System, infusing local anesthetics directly into an inoperative site for postoperative pain management. PARAGON Low cost ambulatory IV system for chemotherapy and pain medications. SIDEKICK low cost ambulatory IV system for antibiotics.

Iomed, Inc. 800-621-3347
2441 S 3850 W Ste A, Salt Lake City, UT 84120
PHORESOR iontophoretic drug delivery system.

Mdrna, Inc. 425-908-3600
3830 Monte Villa Pkwy, Bothell, WA 98021
Nasal insulin delivery unit in development.

Mps Acacia 800-486-6677
785 Challenger St, Brea, CA 92821

Pro Med Pharmacies, Inc. 806-379-7311
3615 SW 45th Ave, Amarillo, TX 79109
Unit dose bronchodilator medications shipped directly to patient home of which PRO-MED assumes responsibility for billing any insurances involved.

Ventlab Corporation 800-593-4654
155 Boyce Dr, Mocksville, NC 27028
BREATHERITE spacer/holding chamber for MDI.

Westmed, Inc. 800-975-7987
5580 S Nogales Hwy, Tucson, AZ 85706
CIRCULAIRE aerosol drug-delivery system; straight drug and shorter, more-efficient therapy.

SYSTEM, DETECTION, BACTERIAL, FOR PLATELET TRANSFUSION PRODUCTS *(Immunology) 82MZC*

Medsep Corp., A Subsidiary Of Pall Corp. 516-484-5400
1630 W Industrial Park St, Covina, CA 91722
Bacterial detection system.

SYSTEM, DETERMINATION, FIBRINOGEN *(Hematology) 81KQJ*

Dade Behring, Inc. 800-948-3233
1717 Deerfield Rd, Deerfield, IL 60015

Diasorin Inc 800-328-1482
1951 Northwestern Ave S, PO Box 285, Stillwater, MN 55082

Fisher Diagnostics 877-722-4366
11515 Vanstory Dr Ste 125, Huntersville, NC 28078

Helena Laboratories 409-842-3714
PO Box 752, Beaumont, TX 77704

International Technidyne Corp. 800-631-5945
23 Nevsky St, Edison, NJ 08820

International Technidyne Corporation 732-548-5700
8 Olsen Ave, Edison, NJ 08820
Fibrinogen test and quality control reagents.

Wortham Laboratories Inc 423-296-0090
6340 Bonny Oaks Dr, Chattanooga, TN 37416
Fibrinogen control plasma.

SYSTEM, DRUG DISPENSING, PHARMACY, AUTOMATED *(General) 80SHI*

Life Care Technologies, Inc. 800-671-0580
4710 Eisenhower Blvd Ste A10, Tampa, FL 33634
MEDSERV & E-MAR automated dispensing & electronic mar.

SYSTEM, ELECTROGASTROGRAPHY(EGG) *(Gastro/Urology) 78MYE*

Medtronic Neuromodulation 763-514-4000
710 Medtronic Pkwy, Minneapolis, MN 55432
Various types of electrogastrography (egg) systems.

SYSTEM, EVACUATION, SMOKE, LASER *(Surgery) 79VCN*

Applied Medical Technology, Inc. 800-869-7382
8000 Katherine Blvd, Brecksville, OH 44141
SAF-T-VAC smoke evacuation for Bovie.

Biomedics, Inc. 949-458-1998
23322 Peralta Dr Ste 11, Laguna Hills, CA 92653

Buffalo Filter, A Division Of Medtek Devices Inc. 800-343-2324
595 Commerce Dr, Amherst, NY 14228
Porta PLUMESAFE 603 Smoke Evacuation System, PLUMESAFE Whisper 602 smoke evacuation system, VIROSAFE 12 and VIROSAFE 6 replacement filters for our PLUMESAFE Systems. PLUMESAFE Whisper Turbo Smoke Evacuation system, powerful Turbo button for extra suction on plume generated from Erbium:YAG laser procedures.

SYSTEM, EVACUATION, SMOKE, LASER *(cont'd)*

Cameron-Miller, Inc. 800-621-0142
5410 W Roosevelt Rd, Road #241, Chicago, IL 60644

Coopersurgical, Inc. 800-243-2974
95 Corporate Dr, Trumbull, CT 06611
$995.00 electrosurgical.

Ellman International, Inc. 800-835-5355
3333 Royal Ave, Rockville Centre, NY 11572

Fumex Inc. 800-432-7550
1150 Cobb International Pl NW Ste D, Kennesaw, GA 30152

Geiger Medical Technologies 800-320-9612
608 13th Ave, Council Bluffs, IA 51501
Geiger Smoke Evacuation System

Megadyne Medical Products, Inc. 800-747-6110
11506 S State St, Draper, UT 84020
The MEGA VAC smoke evacuation system can be used for evacuating both laser and electrosurgical plume.

Niche Medical, Inc. 800-633-1055
55 Access Rd, Warwick, RI 02886
SmartVac Smoke Evacuation System is ultra quiet, powerful, user friendly with a low cost per procedure. It safely collects hazardous surgical smoke/plume direct from the operative site.

Novosci Corp. 281-363-4949
2828 N Crescentridge Dr, The Woodlands, TX 77381
35 CFM Unit MINI or 55 CFM Unit (PLUME-INATOR)-mini with wheels, tabletop or cabinet. All disposables available.

Premier Medical Products 888-PREMUSA
1710 Romano Dr, Plymouth Meeting, PA 19462

Skytron 800-759-8766
5085 Corporate Exchange Blvd SE, Grand Rapids, MI 49512
SkyVac Smoke Evacuation successfully removes surgical smoke via built in system in Skyboom controlled automatically by surgeon with no footprint.

Sun Medical, Inc. 800-678-6633
2607 Aero Dr, Grand Prairie, TX 75052
SFE-200, smoke and fluid evacuation system; a closed circuit smoke evacuator system designed specifically for laparoscopic surgery with no loss of pneumoperitoneum.

Surgical Tools, Inc. 800-774-2040
1106 Monroe St, Bedford, VA 24523

Surgicorp, Inc. 727-934-5000
40347 US Highway 19 N Ste 121, Tarpon Springs, FL 34689
STACKHOUSE, smoke filtration systems and disposables.

Valleylab 800-255-8522
5920 Longbow Dr, Boulder, CO 80301
OPTIMUMM™ smoke evacuation system; smoke evacuation pencil attachment.

Wallach Surgical Devices, Inc. 800-243-2463
235 Edison Rd, Orange, CT 06477
BioVac Smoke Evacuator is a simple-to-operate electrical device designed to remove smoke particulate (smoke plume) generated as a by-product of certain electrosurgery, electrocautery, or laser surgery procedures.

SYSTEM, EXTRACTION, CEMENT REMOVAL
(Orthopedics) 87LZV

Biomet, Inc. 574-267-6639
56 E Bell Dr, PO Box 587, Warsaw, IN 46582
Ultrasonic surgical equipment.

Micro-Aire Surgical Instruments, Inc. 800-722-0822
1641 Edlich Dr, Charlottesville, VA 22911

SYSTEM, FACET SCREW SPINAL DEVICE *(Orthopedics) 87MRW*

Interventional Spine, Inc. 800-497-0484
13700 Alton Pkwy Ste 160, Irvine, CA 92618
Facet screw.

Nuvasive, Inc. 800-475-9131
7475 Lusk Blvd, San Diego, CA 92121
Facet screw.

Trans1 Incorporated 910-332-1700
411 Landmark Dr, Wilmington, NC 28412
Facet screw spinal device.

SYSTEM, GONADOTROPIN, CHORIONIC, HUMAN (NON-RIA)
(Chemistry) 75JZM

Beckman Coulter Inc. 800-231-7970
445 Medical Center Blvd, Webster, TX 77598
Intact hCG IRMA and ELISA; Free Beta hCG ELISA

SYSTEM, HEMODIALYSIS, ACCESS RECIRCULATION MONITORING *(Gastro/Urology) 78MQS*

Baxter Healthcare Corp., Renal Division 847-948-2000
7511 114th Ave, Largo, FL 33773
System, hemodialysis, access recirculation monitoring.

SYSTEM, HEMODIALYSIS, REMOTE ACCESSORIES
(Gastro/Urology) 78MON

Vasc-Alert, Inc. 765-775-2525
3000 Kent Ave, West Lafayette, IN 47906
Hemodialysis access site patency monitoring software.

SYSTEM, HYPERTHERMIA, RF/MICROWAVE (BENIGN PROSTATIC HYPERPLASIA), THERMOTHERAPY
(Gastro/Urology) 78MEQ

Celsion Corporation 800-262-0394
10220 Old Columbia Rd Ste L, Columbia, MD 21046
Celsion's Prolieve Thermodilation System for the Treatment of enlarged Prostates (BPH). The Prolieve system is a non-surgical dual modality thermotherapy and dilation single treatment system which could be used as an alternate to drug therapy (e.g., Finasteride(Proscar®)).

Focus Surgery, Inc. 317-541-1580
3940 Pendleton Way, Indianapolis, IN 46226
The Sonablate 500 is an integrated image-guided ultrasound therapy device using High Intensity Focused Ultrasound (HIFU) for the minimally invasive treatment of Localized Prostate Cancer (PCa) and Benign Prostatic Hyperplasia (BPH).

L&L Special Furnace Co., Inc. 888-808-3676
20 Kent Rd, Aston, PA 19014

Sanmina-Sci Usa, Inc. 256-882-4800
13000 Memorial Pkwy SW, Huntsville, AL 35803
Transurethral microwave thermotherapy (tumt) device.

Urologix, Inc. 800-475-1403
14405 21st Ave N, Minneapolis, MN 55447
TARGIS System treats patients with BPH. It has non-surgical high energy design.

SYSTEM, HYPOTHERMIA, INTRAVENOUS, COOLING
(Cns/Neurology) 84NCX

Alsius Corp. 949-453-0150
15770 Laguna Canyon Rd Ste 150, Irvine, CA 92618
Icy(single, triple lumen),cool line, fortius catheters,coolgard system.

Thermopeutix Inc. 858-549-1760
9925 Businesspark Ave Ste B, San Diego, CA 92131
Thermal regulating system.

SYSTEM, IDENTIFICATION, HEPATITIS B ANTIGEN
(Hematology) 81KSJ

Acon Laboratories, Inc. 858-535-2030
10125 Mesa Rim Rd, San Diego, CA 92121

Akers Biosciences, Inc. 800-451-8378
201 Grove Rd, West Deptford, NJ 08086
HEALTHTEST. Also Hepatitis C.

Bio-Medical Products Corp. 800-543-7427
10 Halstead Rd, Mendham, NJ 07945
Test with strip; $5.00 each. 15 minute test immunochromatographic serum test.

Dako North America, Inc 805-566-6655
6392 Via Real, Carpinteria, CA 93013

Diasorin Inc 800-328-1482
1951 Northwestern Ave S, PO Box 285, Stillwater, MN 55082
ETI-MAK PLUS for the detection of Hepatitis B surface Antigen. ETI-AB-AUK PLUS for the detection of antibodies to Hepatitis B surface Antigen.

Virotech International, Inc. 301-924-8000
12 Meem Ave Ste C, Gaithersburg, MD 20877
Hbsag.

SYSTEM, IDENTIFICATION, LENS, CONTACT
(Ophthalmology) 86LOH

Softchrome, Inc. 925-743-1285
2551 San Ramon Valley Blvd Ste 101, San Ramon, CA 94583
Tint System for soft contact lenses with FDA marketing certification. Tint torics, bi-focal, disposable & high +/- lenses.

SYSTEM, IMAGE MANAGEMENT, OPHTHALMIC
(Ophthalmology) 86NFJ

Cambridge Research & Instrumentation (CRi) 800-383-7924
35B Cabot Rd, Woburn, MA 01801
Pannoramic SCAN, Pannoramic MIDI, Pannoramic DESK

SYSTEM, IMAGING, ESOPHAGEAL, WIRELESS, CAPSULE
(Gastro/Urology) 78NSI

Given Imaging Inc. 770-662-0870
3950 Shackleford Rd Ste 500, Duluth, GA 30096
Given diagnostic system with pillcome eso capsule.

SYSTEM, IMAGING, FLUORESCENCE *(Ear/Nose/Throat) 77MRK*

Cambridge Research & Instrumentation (CRi) 800-383-7924
35B Cabot Rd, Woburn, MA 01801
Vectra

SYSTEM, IMAGING, GASTROINTESTINAL, WIRELESS, CAPSULE *(Gastro/Urology) 78NEZ*

Given Imaging Inc. 770-662-0870
3950 Shackleford Rd Ste 500, Duluth, GA 30096
Ingestible capsule system.

SYSTEM, IMAGING, LAPAROSCOPY, ULTRASONIC
(Radiology) 90SIK

Sonosite, Inc. 888-482-9449
21919 30th Dr SE, Bothell, WA 98021

SYSTEM, IMAGING, OPTICAL COHERENCE TOMOGRAPHY (OCT) *(Radiology) 90NQQ*

Imalux Corporation 216-502-0755
11000 Cedar Ave Ste 250, Cleveland, OH 44106
Oct imaging system.

LightLab Imaging Inc. 978-399-1000
1 Technology Park Dr, Westford, MA 01886
C7XR; M2x OCT Imaging System

SYSTEM, IMMUNOMAGNETIC, CIRCULATING CANCER CELL, ENUMERATION *(Immunology) 82NQI*

Veridex, Llc 877-837-4339
1001 US Highway Route 202 N., Raritan, NJ 08869
System immunomagnetic, circulating cancer cell, enumeration.

SYSTEM, IMPLANT, TOOTH *(Dental And Oral) 76LTE*

Productivity Training Company 800-448-8855
360 Cochrane Cir # A, Morgan Hill, CA 95037
Ball Bearing Bite Recorder System.

Tatum Surgical 888-360-5550
14010 Roosevelt Blvd Ste 705, Clearwater, FL 33762
Dental implant system and Dental Surgical instruments

SYSTEM, INFUSION, ADMINISTRATION, DRUG, IMPLANTABLE
(General) 80TGT

Alaris Medical Systems, Inc 800-854-7128
10221 Wateridge Cir, San Diego, CA 92121
Pre-filled IV drug administration container.

Basi (Bioanalytical Systems, Inc.) 800-845-4246
2701 Kent Ave, West Lafayette, IN 47906
Drug purity and characterization.

Encynova 303-465-4800
557 Burbank St Unit C, Broomfield, CO 80020
Encynova's pump modules are ideal for medical device system integration. Wetted parts made of ceramic, Pyrex™, Teflon™, PEEK and 316L SS are very chemically-compatible. With no valves to clog, and clean-in-place capabilities, the Travcyl™ system is ideal for chemical processing, reactor feed, pharmaceutical manufacturing, chemical and custom automation applications. A variety of models are available to help you achieve exceptional accuracy for metering or dispensing fluid.

Exelint International Co. 800-940-3935
5840 W Centinela Ave, Los Angeles, CA 90045
EXEL Huber Infusion sets (Conventional & Safety)

Kawasumi Laboratories America, Inc. 800-529-2786
4723 Oak Fair Blvd, Tampa, FL 33610
Winged small-vein infusion sets, safety and standard

SYSTEM, INFUSION, ENZYME, THROMBOLYTIC
(Cardiovascular) 74WYC

Cook Inc. 800-457-4500
PO Box 489, Bloomington, IN 47402

SYSTEM, LASER ASSISTED HATCHING *(Obstetrics/Gyn) 85MRX*

Hamilton Thorne Biosciences 978-921-2050
181 Elliott St, 100 Cummings Center-suite 465e, Beverly, MA 01915
Laser for laser assisted hatching.

SYSTEM, LASER, EXCIMER, OPHTHALMIC
(Ophthalmology) 86LZS

International Hospital Supply Co. 800-398-9450
6914 Canby Ave Ste 105, Reseda, CA 91335

Lasersight Technologies, Inc. 630-530-9700
6848 Stapoint Ct, Winter Park, FL 32792
Ophthalmic medical laser system.

Nidek Inc. 800-223-9044
47651 Westinghouse Dr, Fremont, CA 94539
Nidek EC-5000 excimer laser system for corneal surgery (PRK).

Nidek, Inc. 510-226-5700
47651 Westinghouse Dr, Fremont, CA 94539
Excimer laser system.

Princeton Instruments - Acton 978-263-3584
15 Discovery Way, Acton, MA 01720
Excimer laser optics.

Visx Incorporated, A Subsidiary Of Amo Inc. 714-247-8656
1328 Kifer Rd, Sunnyvale, CA 94086
Excimer laser systems(various models).

SYSTEM, LASER, FIBER OPTIC, PHOTODYNAMIC THERAPY
(Surgery) 79MVG

Cook Endoscopy 336-744-0157
4900 Bethania Station Rd # &, 5951 Grassy Creek Blvd.
Winston Salem, NC 27105
Photodynamic therapy balloon.

SYSTEM, LASER, PHOTODYNAMIC THERAPY *(Surgery) 79MVF*

Dusa Pharmaceuticals, Inc. 978-657-7500
25 Upton Dr, Wilmington, MA 01887
Photodynamic therapy illuminator.

Ra Medical Systems, Inc. 760-804-1648
2270 Camino Vida Roble Ste L, Carlsbad, CA 92011
Pharos ex-308 excimer laser.

SYSTEM, LASER, TRANSMYOCARDIAL REVASCULARIZATION
(Cardiovascular) 74MNO

Cardiogenesis Corp. 800-238-2205
11 Musick, Irvine, CA 92618
Holmium laser system, fiberoptic delivery system, handpiece. - Pearl 5.0 Handpiece Delivery System; Solargen2100s Ho:YAG Laser System; Sologrip III Handpiece Delivery Sys; TMR2000 Ho:YAG Laser System

Plc Systems Inc. 508-541-8800
10 Forge Pkwy, Franklin, MA 02038

SYSTEM, MARKING, FILM, RADIOGRAPHIC *(Radiology) 90JAC*

Agfa Corporation 877-777-2432
PO Box 19048, 10 South Academy Street, Greenville, SC 29602

Americomp, Inc. 800-458-1782
2901 W Lawrence Ave, Chicago, IL 60625

Burkhart Roentgen Intl. Inc. 800-USA-XRAY
5201 8th Ave S, Gulfport, FL 33707

Civco Medical Instruments Co., Inc. 319-656-4447
102 1st St S, Kalona, IA 52247
Skin marking device.

Coherent, Inc. 800-527-3786
5100 Patrick Henry Dr, Santa Clara, CA 95054

Cone Instruments, Inc. 800-321-6964
5201 Naiman Pkwy, Solon, OH 44139

Flow X-Ray Corporation 800-356-9729
100 W Industry Ct, Deer Park, NY 11729

Ge Medical Systems, Llc 262-548-2355
3000 N Grandview Blvd, W-417, Waukesha, WI 53188
Lead letters, numbers, patient i.d. labels & data processing card.

I.Z.I. Medical Products, Inc. 800-231-1499
7020 Tudsbury Rd, Baltimore, MD 21244
Non-invasive radiographic skin markers, non-sterile.

Livingston Products, Inc. 800-822-2156
260 Holbrook Dr Unit A, Wheeling, IL 60090
Film id system various models.

Lorad, A Hologic Company 800-321-4659
36 Apple Ridge Rd, Danbury, CT 06810
Various types of film i.d. systems.

Marconi Medical Systems 800-323-0550
595 Miner Rd, Cleveland, OH 44143

SYSTEM, MARKING, FILM, RADIOGRAPHIC *(cont'd)*

Pulse Medical Inc. 800-342-5973
4131 SW 47th Ave Ste 1404, Davie, FL 33314
X-Ray Film ID Printer, automatic, battery operated.

Solstice Corp. 207-874-7922
68 Marginal Way Fl 4, Portland, ME 04101
Various sizes film marking ring pads.

Southern Illinois X-Ray Markers 618-253-7375
513 E Locust St, Harrisburg, IL 62946
X-ray markers.

Wolf X-Ray Corporation 800-356-9729
100 W Industry Ct, Deer Park, NY 11729

SYSTEM, MARKING, LASER *(General) 80WXP*

Champion America 800-521-7000
PO Box 3092, Branford, CT 06405

Coherent, Inc. 800-527-3786
5100 Patrick Henry Dr, Santa Clara, CA 95054

Lfi, Inc-Laser Fare, Inc. 401-231-4400
1 Industrial Dr S, Lan-Rex Industrial Pk., Smithfield, RI 02917

Metron Optics, Inc. 858-755-4477
PO Box 690, 813 Academy Drive, Solana Beach, CA 92075
Marking systems: pens, syringes, non-toxic inks.

Multi Imager Service, Inc 800-400-4549
13865 Magnolia Ave Bldg C, Chino, CA 91710
AGFA-Kodak-Imation-3M-Sterling-DuPont Laser imagers. Buy, sell, service, trade, lease. Also Dry Laser Imagers and Printers.

SYSTEM, NETWORK AND COMMUNICATION, PHYSIOLOGICAL MONITORS *(Cardiovascular) 74MSX*

Draeger Medical Systems, Inc. 215-660-2626
16 Electronics Ave, Danvers, MA 01923
Multiple infinity systems.

Emageon Inc 800-634-5151
900 Walnut Ridge Dr, Hartland, WI 53029
VERICIS PhysioLog - physiologic monitoring and data collection system for the cardiac cath lab.

Imsi, Integrated Modular Systems Inc. 800-220-9729
2500 W Township Line Rd, PO Box 616, Havertown, PA 19083
RADIN Cariolology. Cardio Imaging Systems Software. Viewing, Manipulating, Archiving, Tools, Diagnosis, Re-view, etc. Cost Effective Licensing.

Masimo Corp. 800-326-4890
40 Parker, Irvine, CA 92618

Optimed Technologies, Inc. 973-575-9911
20 New Dutch Ln, Fairfield, NJ 07004
PACS system for Cardiology (Cath, Echo, Nuclear, Fast CT, MRI etc.). Automated report generation and distribution. WEB access to patient data.

Spacelabs Healthcare 800-522-7025
5150 220th Ave SE, Issaquah, WA 98029
Ultraview Waveform Pager System

Spacelabs Medical Inc. 800-522-7212
5150 220th Ave SE, Issaquah, WA 98029
Waveform pager.

Visicu, Inc. 410-276-1960
217 E Redwood St Ste 1900, Baltimore, MD 21202
Network & communication system.

SYSTEM, NON-COHERENT LIGHT, PHOTODYNAMIC THERAPY *(Surgery) 79MYH*

Dusa Pharmaceuticals, Inc. 978-657-7500
25 Upton Dr, Wilmington, MA 01887
Blue light photodynamic therapy illuminator.

SYSTEM, NUCLEIC ACID AMPLIFICATION TEST, DNA, METHICILLIN RESISTANT STAPHYLOCOCCUS AUREUS, DIRECT SPECIMEN *(Microbiology) 83NQX*

Cepheid 408-400-8460
904 E Caribbean Dr, Sunnyvale, CA 94089
Nucleic acid amplification system.

SYSTEM, NUCLEIC ACID AMPLIFICATION, MYCOBACTERIUM TUBERCULOSIS COMPLEX *(Microbiology) 83MWA*

Chembio Diagnostic Systems, Inc. 631-924-1135
3661 Horseblock Rd, Medford, NY 11763
Immunochromatographic assay for the visual detection of tb antibodies.

SYSTEM, NUCLEIC ACID AMPLIFICATION, MYCOBACTERIUM TUBERCULOSIS COMPLEX *(cont'd)*

Roche Molecular Systems, Inc. 925-730-8110
4300 Hacienda Dr, Pleasanton, CA 94588
Mycobacterium tuburculosis test.

SYSTEM, OPTICAL IMPRESSION, COMPUTER ASSISTED DESIGN AND MANUFACTURING (CAD/CAM) OF DENTAL RESTORATIONS *(Dental And Oral) 76NOF*

Brontes Technologies 781-541-5200
10 Maguire Rd Ste 310, Lexington, MA 02421
Cad/cam for dental restorations.

D4d Technologies, Llc 972-234-3880
630 International Pkwy Ste 150, Richardson, TX 75081
Optical impression system for dental cad/cam.

Nobel Biocare Usa, Llc 800-579-6515
22715/22725 Savi Ranch Parkway, Yorba Linda, CA 92887
Scanners.

Sculptec Dental Design Inc. 801-942-1874
6841 S 1300 E, Cottonwood Heights, UT 84121

SensAble Technologies, Inc. 781-937-8315
15 Constitution Way, Woburn, MA 01801
Free Form; SensAble Dental Lab System

3d Systems Corporation 803-326-3900
333 Three D Systems Cir, Rock Hill, SC 29730
Dental cad/cam system.

SYSTEM, ORIENTATION, IDENTIFICATION, SPECIMEN/TISSUE *(Pathology) 88MJI*

Beekley Corp. 860-583-4700
150 Dolphin Rd, Bristol, CT 06010
Specimen margin markers.

International Plastics, Llc 262-781-2270
4965 N. Campbell Dr., Menomonee Falls, WI 53051
Sterile specimen marker for pathological analysis.

SYSTEM, OXYGEN, AQUEOUS *(Cardiovascular) 74MWG*

Therox, Inc. 949-757-1999
17500 Cartwright Rd Ste 100, Irvine, CA 92614
Ao system and ao cartridge.

SYSTEM, PACING, ANTI-TACHYCARDIA *(Cardiovascular) 74LPD*

Medtronic, Inc. 800-633-8766
710 Medtronic Pkwy, Minneapolis, MN 55432

SYSTEM, PACING, TEMPORARY, ACUTE, INTERNAL ATRIAL DEFIBRILLATION *(Cardiovascular) 74MTE*

Ep Medsystems, Inc. 609-753-8533
575 N Route 73 Bldg D, West Berlin, NJ 08091
Acute temporary pacing system.

SYSTEM, PERITONEAL DIALYSIS, AUTOMATIC *(Gastro/Urology) 78FKX*

Baxter Healthcare Corp., Renal Division 847-948-2000
7511 114th Ave, Largo, FL 33773
Various automatic dialysis cycler systems.

Baxter Healthcare Corporation, Renal 888-229-0001
1620 S Waukegan Rd, Waukegan, IL 60085
HOMECHOICE PRO automated PD system

Baxter Healthcare S.A. 847-948-2000
Rd. 721, Km. 0.3, Aibonito, PR 00609
Various automatic dialysis cycler systems.

Erika De Reynosa, S.A. De C.V. 781-402-9068
Brecha E99 Sur; Parque, Industrial Reynos, Bldg. Ii
Cd, Reynosa, Tamps Mexico
Various

Haemonetics Corp. 781-848-7100
400 Wood Rd, P.O.Box 9114, Braintree, MA 02184
Sterile docking device.

Medionics International Inc. 800-463-6087
114 Anderson Ave., Markham, ONT L6E 1A5 Canada
Medionics International Inc. manufactures peritoneal dialysis cyclers and other accessories including PD catheters. 'Easy Care' is a revolutionary CAPD system designed to cut monthly operating costs by almost 50%. It weighs only 3 kgs and can also be used to perform CCPD, NIPD, one or two middle of the night exchanges or to initiate early incremental dialysis.

SYSTEM, PERITONEAL DIALYSIS, AUTOMATIC *(cont'd)*

Spectrum Laboratories, Inc. 800-634-3300
18617 S Broadwick St, Rancho Dominguez, CA 90220
DISPODIALYZER ready-to-use dialysis devices with cap and weight for 0.5ml, 1ml, 2ml and 5ml capacities. Easy-to-use, Float-A-Lyzer and Micro Dispodialyzer dialysis device for dialyzing sample volumes 10ul to 10ml.

Terumo Medical Corporation 800-283-7866
950 Elkton Blvd, P.O.Box 605, Elkton, MD 21921
Sterile tubing welder.

SYSTEM, PIPELINE, GAS *(General) 80WOE*

Aga Linde Healthcare P.R. Inc. 787-622-7900
PO Box 363868, GPO Box 364727, San Juan, PR 00936
General.

Dynacon, Inc. 573-594-3813
4924 Pike 451, Curryville, MO 63339
Piping systems for medical gases, regulators, manifolds, outlets, flowmeters, humidifiers, nebulizers, glass bottles for suction, compressors and pumps.

Emepe International, Inc. 813-994-9690
18108 Sugar Brooke Dr, Tampa, FL 33647
Outlet stations, zone valves, area alarms, manifolds, air compressors and dryers, vacuum pumps.

Enviro Guard, Inc. 800-438-1152
201 Shannon Oaks Cir Ste 115, Cary, NC 27511

Independent Solutions, Inc. 847-498-0500
900 Skokie Blvd Ste 118, Northbrook, IL 60062
Tri-Tech medical gas pipeline (distribution) systems. Air, oxygen, vacuum, nitrogen, nitrous oxide, carbon dioxide, evacuation (scavenger) outlets, alarms, valves, pumps, and compressors.

Reimers Systems, Inc. 877-734-6377
8210 Cinder Bed Rd Ste D, Lorton, VA 22079
Gas selection panels.

SYSTEM, PLANNING, RADIATION THERAPY TREATMENT
(Radiology) 90MUJ

.Decimal, Inc. 407-330-3300
121 Central Park Pl, Sanford, FL 32771
Radiation treatment planning system.

American Radiosurgery, Inc. 858-451-6173
16776 Bernardo Center Dr Ste 203, San Diego, CA 92128
Treatment planning system.

Computerized Medical Systems, Inc. 468-587-2550
1145 Corporate Lake Dr, Olivette, MO 63132
Radiation treatment planning system.

Permedics, Inc. 909-478-5000
1475 Victoria Ct, San Bernardino, CA 92408
Odyssey Treatment Planning software - 3D radiaton therapy treatment planning system supporting protons, electrons, and photons. Has sterotactic and whole body planning capabilities.

Prowess, Inc. 925-356-0360
1370 Ridgewood Dr Ste 20, Chico, CA 95973
Radiation therapy treatment planning system.

Varian Medical Systems 800-544-4636
3100 Hansen Way, Palo Alto, CA 94304
Eclipse treatment planning system for conventional radiotherapy, intensity-modulated radiotherapy (IMRT), image-guided radiotherapy (IGRT), brachytherapy, and proton radiotherapy.

Varian Medical Systems Brachytheraphy 888.666.7847
700 Harris St Ste 109, Charlottesville, VA 22903
Radiation therapy planning systems.

Varian Medical Systems, Oncology Systems 800 278-2747
911 Hansen Way, Bldg.3 M/S C-165, Palo Alto, CA 94304
Radiation therapy planning systems.

SYSTEM, RECORDING, DATA, ANESTHESIOLOGY
(Anesthesiology) 73WQI

Rms Instruments 905-677-5533
6877-1 Goreway Dr., Mississauga, ONT L4V 1L9 Canada
Chart recorder, data logger, magnetic tape recorder, transient recorder.

SYSTEM, RETROPERFUSION, ARTERY, CORONARY
(Cardiovascular) 74LPE

Abbott Vascular, Cardiac Therapies 800-227-9902
26531 Ynez Rd, Mailing P.O. Box 9018, Temecula, CA 92591
Perfusion catheter.

SYSTEM, RETROPERFUSION, ARTERY, CORONARY *(cont'd)*

Biomet Microfixation Inc. 800-874-7711
1520 Tradeport Dr, Jacksonville, FL 32218
System, coronary, artery, retroperfusion.

SYSTEM, ROBOT *(General) 80WTV*

Beckman Coulter, Inc. 800-742-2345
250 S Kraemer Blvd, PO Box 8000, Brea, CA 92821

Hamilton Company 800-648-5950
4990 Energy Way, Reno, NV 89502
Robotic and microwell plate sample preparation systems.

Phytron, Inc. 800-96P-HYTR
600 Blair Park Rd Ste 220, Williston, VT 05495
PAROS-HEXAPOD parallel robot operating system for micromanipulation in the medical industry.

Soltec Corp. 800-423-2344
12977 Arroyo St, San Fernando, CA 91340
ROBOTEST I Driving robot.

Tecan U.S., Inc. 800-338-3226
4022 Stirrup Creek Dr Ste 310, Durham, NC 27703
Sample processors.

Xiril 302-655-7035
91 Lukens Dr Ste A, New Castle, DE 19720

SYSTEM, SKIN CLOSURE *(Surgery) 79MKY*

Boehringer Labs, Inc 888-390-4325
500 E Washington St Ste 2A, Black Horse, PA 19401
Sterile wound closure device.

Medical Action Industries, Inc. 800-645-7042
25 Heywood Rd, Arden, NC 28704
Skin closures.

Medist International 901-380-9411
9160 Highway 64 Ste 12, Lakeland, TN 38002
Tissue extender.

SYSTEM, SUCTION, LIPOPLASTY *(Surgery) 79MUU*

Biosculpture Technology, Inc. 212-977-5400
40 Central Park S Ste 16E, New York, NY 10019
Surgical aspiration and lipoplasty device.

Cytori Therapeutics, Inc. 877-470-8000
3020 Callan Rd, San Diego, CA 92121
Suction lipoplasty system.

Kmi Kolster Methods, Inc. 909-737-5476
3185 Palisades Dr, Corona, CA 92880
Surgical aspiratoin & lipoplasty.

Macropore Biosurgery, Inc. 858-458-0900
6740 Top Gun St, San Diego, CA 92121
Cannister.

Misonix, Inc. 800-694-9612
1938 New Hwy, Farmingdale, NY 11735
LySonix 3000 Ultrasonic Surgical System

SYSTEM, SURGICAL, COMPUTER CONTROLLED INSTRUMENT
(Surgery) 79NAY

Intuitive Surgical, Inc. 888-409-4774
1266 Kifer Rd, Sunnyvale, CA 94086
Multiple.

Ortho-Clinical Diagnostics, Inc. 800-828-6316
513 Technology Blvd, Rochester, NY 14626
Laboratory date management system.

SYSTEM, TEST, AMINO ACIDS, FREE CARNITINES AND ACYLCARNITINES TANDEM MASS SPECTROMETRY
(Chemistry) 75NQL

PerkinElmer 800-762-4000
940 Winter St, Waltham, MA 02451
NEOGRAM AMINO ACIDS AND ACY; NEOGRAM AMINO ACIDS AND ACYLCARNI

SYSTEM, TEST, ANTIBODIES, B2 - GLYCOPROTEIN I (B2 - GPI)
(Immunology) 82MSV

Corgenix Medical Corporation 800-729-5661
11575 Main St, Broomfield, CO 80020
Multiple

Theratest Laboratories, Inc. 800-441-0771
1111 N Main St, Lombard, IL 60148
Beta 2 gp1 antibody ELISA test, screening, isotypes: IgM, IgG, IgA

SYSTEM, TEST, ANTICARDIOLIPIN, IMMUNOLOGICAL
(Immunology) 82MID

Corgenix Medical Corporation 800-729-5661
11575 Main St, Broomfield, CO 80020
Multiple

Immuno Concepts N.A. Ltd. 800-251-5115
9779 Business Park Dr, Sacramento, CA 95827

Innominata dba GENBIO 800-288-4368
15222 Avenue of Science Ste A, San Diego, CA 92128
Various.

Quest Intl., Inc. 305-592-6991
8127 NW 29th St, Doral, FL 33122
Anti-cardiolipin igg serological reagents.

Theratest Laboratories, Inc. 800-441-0771
1111 N Main St, Lombard, IL 60148
Enzyme immunoassay for cardiolipin antibodies (aCL), screening and isotypes.

SYSTEM, TEST, BLOOD GLUCOSE, OVER-THE-COUNTER
(Chemistry) 75NBW

Abbott Diabetes Care Inc. 510-749-5400
1360 S Loop Rd, Alameda, CA 94502
Glucose blood test system.

Access Bio Incorporate 732-297-2222
2033 Rt. 130 Unit H, Monmouth Junction, NJ 08852
Glucose test system.

Akers Biosciences, Inc. 800-451-8378
201 Grove Rd, West Deptford, NJ 08086
Rapid test measures glucose levels using urine (first test) or blood (second test).

Arkray Factory Usa, Inc. 952-646-3168
5182 W 76th St, Minneapolis, MN 55439
Blood glucose monitoring system.

Arkray Usa 800-818-8877
5198 W 76th St, Edina, MN 55439
GLUCOCARD X-METER BLOOD GLUCOSE METER AD STRIPS 0.3 μL samples size, 5 second test time, self coding. POCKETCHEM EZ BLOOD GLUCOSE METER AND STRIPS 10 second test time, 1 μL sample size, downloading capabilities, code chip calibration. ADVANCE MICRO-DRAW BLOOD GLUCOSE MONITORING SYSTEM WITH MICRO-DRAW TEST STRIPS-Results in 15 seoncds. Requires 1.5μL blood sample. Simple two step test. 14-day & 30-day averaging. GLUCOBALANCE SOFTWARE SYSTEM-electronic log book eliminates the need to record test results by hand. Useful in tracking the number of tests performed daily and recognizing trends.

Bayer Healthcare Llc 914-524-2955
555 White Plains Rd Fl 5, Tarrytown, NY 10591
Test for blood glucose.

Benchmark Winona 507-452-8932
6301 Bandel Rd NW, Rochester, MN 55901
Glucose test system.

Cardiocom LLC 888-243-8881
7980 Century Blvd, Chanhassen, MN 55317
Blood glucose measurement device.

Diagnostic Devices Inc. 704-285-6400
9300 Harris Corners Pkwy Ste 450, Charlotte, NC 28269
Glucose test system.

Lifescan Llc. 408-263-9789
Rd. 308 Km 0.8, Pedernales Industrial Park, Cabo Rojo, PR 00623-5001
Reagent test strip for whole blood glucose determination.

Lifescan, Inc. 800-227-8862
1000 Gibraltar Dr, Milpitas, CA 95035
Reagent test strip for whole blood glucose determination.

Medtronic Minimed 800-933-3322
18000 Devonshire St, Northridge, CA 91325
Glucose meter.

Nipro Diagnostics, Inc. 1-800-342-7226
2400 NW 55th Ct, Fort Lauderdale, FL 33309
Over the counter blood glucose testing system.

Nova Biomedical Corporation Diabetes Products 781-894-0800
205 Burlington Rd, Bedford, MA 01730
Blood glucose test system.

Polymer Technology Systems, Inc. 317-870-5610
7736 Zionsville Rd, Indianapolis, IN 46268
Bioscanner beyond glucose test system.

SYSTEM, TEST, BLOOD GLUCOSE, OVER-THE-COUNTER
(cont'd)

Sanmina-Sci Usa, Inc. 256-882-4800
13000 Memorial Pkwy SW, Huntsville, AL 35803
Glucose monitoring system.

St. Paul Biotech 714-903-1000
11555 Monarch St, Garden Grove, CA 92841
Blood glucose test.

SYSTEM, TEST, BREATH NITRIC OXIDE *(Chemistry) 75MXA*

Aerocrine, Inc. 468-629-0780
562 Central Ave, New Providence, NJ 07974
Nitric oxide monitoring system.

SYSTEM, TEST, DRUGS OF ABUSE *(Chemistry) 75MGX*

Acon Laboratories, Inc. 858-535-2030
10125 Mesa Rim Rd, San Diego, CA 92121
AMP, BAR, BZO, COC, MDMA, MET, MOP, MTD, OPI, PCP, TCA, THC, and multidrug tests.

Akers Biosciences, Inc. 800-451-8378
201 Grove Rd, West Deptford, NJ 08086
VISUALINE, Rapid drug-abuse test that can test for 1-10 drugs, same as the lab, FDA approved.

Alcopro 800-227-9890
2547 Sutherland Ave, Knoxville, TN 37919

Ameritek Usa, Inc. 425-379-2580
125 130th St SE Ste 200, Everett, WA 98208
Multi drug test kit.

Bio-Medical Products Corp. 800-543-7427
10 Halstead Rd, Mendham, NJ 07945
Cocaine drug abuse urine screening test strip. Also for benzodiazepine, PCP, amphetamine, methadone, barbiturate, cannabinoid, opiates, methamphetamine. These are 5 minute tests. Panels of 6 drugs.

Biochemical Diagnostics, Inc. 800-223-4835
180 Heartland Blvd, Edgewood, NY 11717
Thin layer chromatography (semi-automated) test.

Biosite Incorporated 888-246-7483
9975 Summers Ridge Rd, San Diego, CA 92121
Visul immunoassay for detection of drugs of abuse in urine.

Drg International, Inc. 800-321-1167
1167 US Highway 22, Mountainside, NJ 07092

J&S Medical Associates 800-229-6000
35 Tripp St Ste 1, Framingham, MA 01702
SENTRY urine control for all SAMSHA recommended analytes.

Jant Pharmacal Corp. 800-676-5565
16255 Ventura Blvd Ste 505, Encino, CA 91436
Tests to detect tobacco, alcohol, and various drugs of abuse.

Lifesign 800-526-2125
71 Veronica Ave, Somerset, NJ 08873
STATUS-DS one-stop immunoassay for drugs of abuse.

Metronix 813-972-1212
12421 N Florida Ave Ste D201, Tampa, FL 33612
ACCU-DOA-CHEK MET/THC One-Step Dual Screen Test Kit is a drug screening kit for marijuana and methamphetamine.

Orasure Technologies, Inc. 800-869-3538
220 E 1st St, Bethlehem, PA 18015
Intercept oral fluid drug test. QED saliva alcohol test.

Pan Probe Biotech, Inc. 858-689-9936
7396 Trade St, San Diego, CA 92121
Determination of cocaine in human urine.

Princeton Biomeditech Corp. 732-274-1000
4242 US Highway 1, Monmouth Junction, NJ 08852
AccuSign one-step, 5-minute urine tests for cocaine (COC), marijuana/ cannabis (THC), opiates (OPI), methamphetamine/ ecstasy (MET/XTC), amphetamine (AMP), phencyclidine (PCP), barbiturates (BAR), benzodiazepines (BZO), methadone (MTD), tricyclic antidepressants (TCA); 2-, 3-, 4-, 5-, 8-, and 10-in-1 drug panels; saliva alcohol.

Sirchie Finger Print Laboratories 800-356-7311
100 Hunter Pl, Youngsville, NC 27596

Syntron Bioresearch, Inc. 800-854-6226
2774 Loker Ave W, Carlsbad, CA 92010

Utak Laboratories, Inc. 800-235-3442
25020 Avenue Tibbitts, Valencia, CA 91355
UTAK Whole Blood Drugs of Abuse contains benzoylecgonine, cocaine, cocaethylene, d-amphetamine, d-methamphetamine, morphine, codeine and hydrocodone.

SYSTEM, TEST, HER-2/NEU, IHC *(Pathology) 88MVC*

Ventana Medical Systems, Inc. 800-227-2155
1910 E Innovation Park Dr, Oro Valley, AZ 85755
Her-2/new ihc test system.

SYSTEM, TEST, IMMUNOLOGICAL, ANTIGEN, TUMOR *(Immunology) 82MOI*

United Biotech, Inc. 650-961-2910
211 S Whisman Rd Ste E, Mountain View, CA 94041
ELISA for detecting Cancer Marker for: CEA (Carcinoembryonic Antigen), Free PSA (free Prostate Specific Antigen), Free Beta hCG (free Beta subunit (beta-hCG), NSE (Neuron Specific Enolase), CA-153 (Mucin Breast Cancer)

SYSTEM, TEST, LIPOPROTEIN(A) *(Chemistry) 75MSM*

Abbott Diagnostics Div. 626-440-0700
820 Mission St, South Pasadena, CA 91030
Various.

SYSTEM, TEST, LOW-DENSITY, LIPOPROTEIN *(Chemistry) 75MRR*

Polymer Technology Systems, Inc. 317-870-5610
7736 Zionsville Rd, Indianapolis, IN 46268
Low density lipoprotein cholesterol test strips.

Teco Diagnostics 714-693-7788
1268 N Lakeview Ave, Anaheim, CA 92807
Direct ldl cholesterol reagent.

Vital Diagnostics Inc. 714-672-3553
1075 W Lambert Rd Ste D, Brea, CA 92821
Various ldl-cholesterol reagents.

SYSTEM, TEST, SODIUM, ENZYMATIC METHOD *(Chemistry) 75MZU*

Diazyme Laboratories 858-455-4761
12889 Gregg Ct, Poway, CA 92064
Sodium enzymatic assay.

SYSTEM, TEST, THYROGLOBULIN *(Immunology) 82MSW*

Nichols Institute Diagnostics 949-940-7200
1311 Calle Batido, San Clemente, CA 92673
Tg.

SYSTEM, TEST, TOPIRAMATEE *(Toxicology) 91MSL*

Opus Diagnostics, Inc. 877-944-1777
1 Parker Plz, Fort Lee, NJ 07024
Innofluor toparimate reagent set.

SYSTEM, TEST, TUMOR MARKER, FOR DETECTION OF BLADDER CANCER *(Immunology) 82NAH*

United Biotech, Inc. 650-961-2910
211 S Whisman Rd Ste E, Mountain View, CA 94041
ELISA for detecting CA-242 (Pancreatic & Gastro-Intestinal Cancer - P&GC)

SYSTEM, TEST, VITAMIN D *(Chemistry) 75MRG*

Nichols Institute Diagnostics 949-940-7200
1311 Calle Batido, San Clemente, CA 92673
25-oh vit d.

SYSTEM, THERMOGRAPHIC, LIQUID CRYSTAL *(Obstetrics/Gyn) 85LHM*

E-Z-Em, Inc. 516-333-8230
750 Summa Ave, Westbury, NY 11590
Liquid crystal thermography device.

Liquid Crystal Resources, L.L.C. 800-527-1419
1820 Pickwick Ln, Glenview, IL 60026

SYSTEM, TRANSPORT, IN-HOUSE *(General) 80WIH*

A.R.C. Distributors 800-296-8724
PO Box 599, Centreville, MD 21617
POLECAT I.V. transport system for wheelchair and stretcher patients. POLECAT facilitates moving patients using infusion pumps mounted on portable (wheeled) IV poles. Forms a single unit for improved safety and productivity. FAST, SAFE AND EASY!! PREVENTS INJURIES TO PATIENT & TRANSPORTERS TOO!!!!!!

Healthmark Industries 800-521-6224
22522 E 9 Mile Rd, Saint Clair Shores, MI 48080
$30 to $220 for instrument retrieval systems. Meets OSHA guidelines for safe handling of contaminated reusable instruments.

SYSTEM, TRANSPORT, IN-HOUSE *(cont'd)*

Hygiene Specialties, Inc./Andermac, Inc. 800-824-0214
2626 Live Oak Blvd, Yuba City, CA 95991
The Anderlift System lifts, transports, showers and weighs patients up to 500 lbs. The Bariatic Unit will handle patients up to 800 lbs. All systems have radio translucent sheets and legs wide enough to fit over OR tables, gurneys and x-ray tables.

Inclinator Co. Of America 800-343-9007
601 Gibson Blvd, Harrisburg, PA 17104
HOMEWAITER '75 dumbwaiter.

SYSTEM, TREATMENT, AORTIC ANEURYSM, ENDOVASCULAR GRAFT *(Cardiovascular) 74MIH*

Aptus Endosystems Inc. 877-292-7887
777 N Pastoria Ave, Sunnyvale, CA 94085
Aptus AAA EndoGraft and Del. Sys.; Aptus EndoStapling System; Aptus Endovascular AAA Repair System

Corvita Corp. 305-599-3100
8210 NW 27th St, Doral, FL 33122
Under development.

Endologix, Inc. 800-983-2284
11 Studebaker, Irvine, CA 92618

W. L. Gore & Associates, Inc. 800-437-8181
PO Box 2400, Flagstaff, AZ 86003
Aaa bifurcated endoprosthesis.

W.L. Gore & Associates,Inc 928-526-3030
1505 North Fourth St., Flagstaff, AZ 86004
Aaa bifurcated endoprosthesis.

SYSTEM, URINE DRAINAGE, CLOSED, FOR NON-INDWELLING CATHETER, NON-STERILE *(Gastro/Urology) 78NNZ*

Arcus Medical Llc 704-332-3424
2327 Distribution St, Charlotte, NC 28203
Male incontinence management system.

SYSTEM, VOCAL CORD MEDIALIZATION *(Ear/Nose/Throat) 77MIX*

Bioform Medical, Inc. 262-835-3323
4133 Courtney Rd Ste 10, Franksville, WI 53126
Vocal chord medialization system.

Gyrus Ent L.L.C., Sub. Of Gyrus Acmi, Inc. 508-804-2739
2925 Appling Rd, Bartlett, TN 38133
Vocom implant.

Uroplasty, Inc. 952-426-6140
5420 Feltl Rd, Minnetonka, MN 55343

W.L. Gore & Associates,Inc 928-526-3030
1505 North Fourth St., Flagstaff, AZ 86004
Thyroplasty implant.

SYSTEM, WATER, REPRODUCTION, ASSISTED, AND PURIFICATION *(Obstetrics/Gyn) 85MTW*

Conception Technologies 858-824-0888
6835 Flanders Dr Ste 500, San Diego, CA 92121
Water for tissue culture.

Plomeria Especializada De Baja California, S.A. De 626-336-4561
Calle Maquiladoras No. 322, Seccion Dorada
Nueva Tijuana, Baja California Mexico
Various models of water heating units

Sage In-Vitro Fertilization Inc. 203-601-5200
1979 Locust St, Pasadena, CA 91107
Water for tissue culture.

Whitehall/A Division Of Acorn Engineering Co. 626-336-4561
15125 Proctor Ave, City Of Industry, CA 91746
Various models of water heating units.

SYSTEM, X-RAY, EXTRAORAL SOURCE, DIGITAL *(Radiology) 90MUH*

Camsight Co., Inc. 323-259-1900
3380 N San Fernando Rd, Glassell, CA 90065
Extraoral source x-ray system.

Cyber Medical Imaging, Inc. 310-859-3802
3054 Franklin Canyon Dr, Beverly Hills, CA 90210
Digital x-ray system.

Imaging Sciences International, Llc 215-997-5666
1910 N Penn Rd, Hatfield, PA 19440
Cone beam volumetric tomography, a digital x-ray device.

Practiceworks Systems, Llc. 800-944-6365
1765 the Exchange SE, Atlanta, GA 30339
Dental intraoral x-ray and video camera.

SYSTEM, X-RAY, EXTRAORAL SOURCE, DIGITAL *(cont'd)*

Progeny, Inc. 847-415-9800
675 Heathrow Dr, Lincolnshire, IL 60069
Extraoral source x-ray system.

Suni Medical Imaging, Inc. 408-227-6698
6840 Via Del Oro, San Jose, CA 95119
Digital x-ray system.

SYSTEM, X-RAY, MOBILE *(Radiology) 90IZL*

Del Medical Systems 800-800-6006
11550 King St, Franklin Park, IL 60131

Dynacon, Inc. 573-594-3813
4924 Pike 451, Curryville, MO 63339
Portable x-ray units

Ge Medical Systems Ultrasound And Primary Care Dia 608-826-7050
726 Heartland Trl, Madison, WI 53717
Mobile orthopedic c-arm.

Ge Medical Systems, Llc 262-548-2355
3000 N Grandview Blvd, W-417, Waukesha, WI 53188
Various types of mobile x-ray units.

Imaging Sciences International, Llc 215-997-5666
1910 N Penn Rd, Hatfield, PA 19440
Mobile x-ray machine.

Imaging3, Inc. 800-900-9729
3200 W Valhalla Dr, Burbank, CA 91505
Mobile x-ray system 'c-arm'.

Imsi, Integrated Modular Systems Inc. 800-220-9729
2500 W Township Line Rd, PO Box 616, Havertown, PA 19083
Mobile Unit Viewing Sytem. Web-Based. Need only internet connectivity for fast downloads and diagnostic viewing by remote radiologists. Very cost effective.

Innovative Medical Products, Inc. 800-467-4944
87 Spring Lane, Plainville Industrial Pk, Plainville, CT 06062
IMP Porta-View portable x-ray view box allows surgeons to view films & scans at surgical site without leaving sterile field and/or readjustments of magnifying lenses or loupes.

Lorad, A Hologic Company 800-321-4659
36 Apple Ridge Rd, Danbury, CT 06810
Various types of mobile x-ray units.

Marconi Medical Systems 800-323-0550
595 Miner Rd, Cleveland, OH 44143

Medtronic Navigation, Inc. (Littleton) 720-890-3325
300 Foster St, Harwood Station, Littleton, MA 01460
Mobile x-ray system.

Minrad, Inc. 716-855-1068
50 Cobham Dr, Orchard Park, NY 14127
Sterile drape.

Orthoscan, Inc. 480-503-8010
8212 E Evans Rd, Scottsdale, AZ 85260
Mini c-arm.

Precise Optics/Pme, Inc. 800-242-6604
239 S Fehr Way, Bay Shore, NY 11706

Remote Technologies, Inc. 800-733-9729
PO Box 1185, Greenwich, CT 06836
Cordless exposure switch (accessory for mobile x-ray unit).

Shimadzu Medical Systems 800-228-1429
20101 S Vermont Ave, Torrance, CA 90502
Mobile X-Ray; MU 125M, MU-125P, MUX-100H

Source-Ray, Inc. 631-244-8200
167 Keyland Ct, Bohemia, NY 11716
Portable X-Ray Systems.

Sterne Equipment Co., Ltd. 905-457-2524
7 Research Rd., Brampton, ONT L6W 1P4 Canada
Same

Tidi Products, Llc 920-751-4380
570 Enterprise Dr, Neenah, WI 54956
Drape for mobile x-ray unit.

Toshiba America Medical Systems 800-421-1968
2441 Michelle Dr, Tustin, CA 92780

Trac Electronics 919-876-8088
1100 W Chatham St, Cary, NC 27511
Orthotrac coaxial laser.

Trex Enterprises Corp. 858-646-5500
427 Ala Makani St, Kahului, HI 96732
Various models of x-ray systems.

SYSTEM, X-RAY, MOBILE *(cont'd)*

Virtual Imaging, Inc. 954-428-6191
720 S Powerline Rd Ste E, Deerfield Bch, FL 33442
Mobile radiographic x-ray systems.

X-Cel X-Ray Corporation 800-441-2470
4220 Waller St, Crystal Lake, IL 60012
$10,900 each for podiatric unit, regular extremity unit, dedicated hand

Xi Tec, Inc. 800-243-0084
4 New Park Rd, East Windsor, CT 06088
XISCAN MINI C-ARM $19,500 to 49,500 for XISCAN 1000, a portable fluoroscopic imaging system.

York X-Ray And Orthopedic Supply, Inc. 800-334-6427
PO Box 326, 20 Hampton Rd.,, Lyman, SC 29365

SYSTEM/DEVICE, PHARMACY COMPOUNDING *(General) 80NEP*

Baxter Healthcare Corp., Renal Division 847-948-2000
7511 114th Ave, Largo, FL 33773
System/device, pharmacy compounding.

Winland Electronics Inc. 507-625-7231
1950 Excel Dr, Mankato, MN 56001
Auto compounder.

TABLE, ANESTHETIST'S *(Anesthesiology) 73BWN*

Blickman 800-247-5070
39 Robinson Rd, Lodi, NJ 07644
Stainless steel table with your choice of 1- to 4-drawers, guard rails on three or four sides, travels on two-inch ballbearing swivel casters.

Civco Medical Instruments Co., Inc. 319-656-4447
102 1st St S, Kalona, IA 52247
Positioning system accessories.

Depuy Orthopaedics, Inc. 800-473-3789
700 Orthopaedic Dr, P.O. Box 988, Warsaw, IN 46582
Hand surgery table.

Tekquest Industries 800-327-7175
4200 Saint Johns Pkwy, Sanford, FL 32771
Surgical immobilizer.

Wellan Medical, Inc. 603-676-8601
10 Water St, Lebanon, NH 03766
Positioning system.

TABLE, AUTOPSY *(Pathology) 88RYV*

Imperial Surgical Ltd. 800-661-5432
581 Orly Ave., Dorval, ONT H9P-1G1 Canada
From $1,800-$8,900 for 5 models varying in size from 34 x 76 x 30" to 36 x 91 x 28". Optional removable headrest; table end or table center sink drain location & stainless steel removable instrument tray.

Medi-Tech International, Inc. 305-593-9373
2924 NW 109th Ave, Doral, FL 33172
JEWETT.

National Nonwovens 800-333-3469
PO Box 150, Easthampton, MA 01027
Autopsy table pads. Absorbs blood and washing fluids during autopsies.

Pacific Research Laboratories, Inc. 206-463-5551
10221 SW 188th St, PO Box 409, Vashon, WA 98070
Cadaver holders & trays for use at training sessions. Available for rent or purchase.

Scientek Medical Equipment 604-273-9094
11151 Bridgeport Rd., Richmond, BC V6X 1T3 Canada
Incl. sink, table spray, hydro aspirator, sump drain, vacuum breakers.

TABLE, BLOOD DONOR *(Hematology) 81RYW*

Arlington Scientific, Inc. Asi 800-654-0146
1840 N Technology Dr, Springville, UT 84663
ASI stationary lounges useful for drawing, apheresis and other applications. Horizon, Hampton and Space Saver. ASI Portable Donor Lounge.

Mayo Medical, S.A. De C.V. 800-715-3872
Edison 1141 Nte., Col. Talleres, Monterrey N.L. 64480 Mexico

Profex Medical Products 800-325-0196
2224 E Person Ave, Memphis, TN 38114

Schueler & Company, Inc. 516-487-1500
PO Box 528, Stratford, CT 06615

TABLE, CYSTOMETRIC, ELECTRIC *(Gastro/Urology) 78MMZ*

Direx Systems Corp. 339-502-6013
437 Turnpike St, Canton, MA 02021
Urological table.

TABLE, CYSTOMETRIC, NON-ELECTRICAL
(Gastro/Urology) 78KQS

Bryton Corp. 800-567-9500
4310 Guion Rd, Indianapolis, IN 46254
Tables for all types of urological and endoscopic procedures.

Medrecon, Inc. 877-526-4323
257 South Ave, Garwood, NJ 07027
Remanufactured units - 2 yr warranty.

TABLE, EXAMINATION/TREATMENT *(General) 80RYX*

Alimed, Inc. 800-225-2610
297 High St, Dedham, MA 02026

American Biomed Instruments, Inc. 718-235-8900
11 Wyona St, Brooklyn, NY 11207

Atd-American Co. 800-523-2300
135 Greenwood Ave, Wyncote, PA 19095

Atlantic Medco, Inc. 800-203-8444
166 Bloomfield Ave, Verona, NJ 07044
$500 to $3000.

Brandt Industries, Inc. 800-221-8031
4461 Bronx Blvd, Bronx, NY 10470
Hydraulic and non-hydraulic.

Brewer Company, The 888-873-9371
N88W13901 Main St, Menomonee Falls, WI 53051
Brewer Access Exam Table; Brewer Basic Exam Table

Bryton Corp. 800-567-9500
4310 Guion Rd, Indianapolis, IN 46254

Cardon Rehabilitation Products Inc 800-944-7868
908 Niagara Falls Blvd, Wurlitzer Industrial Park
North Tonawanda, NY 14120

Chattanooga Group 800-592-7329
4717 Adams Rd, Hixson, TN 37343
ADAPTA & TRITON Several styles with 1-5 sectioned tops, treatment, mobilization, and traction.

Custom Comfort Medtek 800-749-0933
3939 Forsyth Rd Ste A, Winter Park, FL 32792
The classic series of exam tables features heavy-duty steel legs and a baked-on epoxy finish. The contemporary series features warm wood design laminated with our Wilson Art platinum Formica. Both series come with a padded, medical-grade, seamless vinyl top in a choice of eighteen colors.

Elekta, Inc. 800-535-7355
4775 Peachtree Industrial Blvd, Building 300, Suite 300
Norcross, GA 30092
Precise Table Treatment, for linear accelerator.

Elmed, Inc. 630-543-2792
60 W Fay Ave, Addison, IL 60101

Enochs Examining Room Furniture, Inc. 800-428-2305
PO Box 50559, Indianapolis, IN 46250
$1,642.00 per unit (standard); $1,980.00 per pediatric table.

Fleetwood Group, Incorporated 800-257-6390
PO Box 1259, Holland, MI 49422
Padded treatment table with H bracing and adjustable backrest.

Florida Life Systems 727-321-9554
3446 5th Ave N, Saint Petersburg, FL 33713

Galaxy Medical Manufacturing Co. 800-876-4599
5411 Sheila St, Commerce, CA 90040
Adjustment table.

Good Sports 412-731-3032
1701 Monongahela Ave, Pittsburgh, PA 15218
Bailey Manufacturing.

Hausmann Industries, Inc. 888-428-7626
130 Union St, Northvale, NJ 07647
24 wooden models - $276 to $865 each.

Hill Laboratories Co. 877-445-5020
3 N Bacton Hill Rd, PO Box 2028, Frazer, PA 19355
Hill Laboratories custom manufactures over 20 elevation tables for every facet of the medical industry. Tables can be viewed at www.hilllabs.com.

I-Rep, Inc. 800-828-0852
508 Chaney St Ste B, Lake Elsinore, CA 92530

Imperial Surgical Ltd. 800-661-5432
581 Orly Ave., Dorval, ONT H9P-1G1 Canada
Various models available.

Jedmed Instruments Co. 314-845-3770
5416 Jedmed Ct, Saint Louis, MO 63129

TABLE, EXAMINATION/TREATMENT *(cont'd)*

Kadan Co. Inc., D.A. 800-325-2326
1 Brigadoon Ln, Waxhaw, NC 28173

Living Earth Crafts 800-358-8292
3210 Executive Rdg, Vista, CA 92081
Treatment tables: portable, hydraulic and electric models from $339.00 to $1,895.00. 5-year warranty, custom models available.

Mayo Medical, S.A. De C.V. 800-715-3872
Edison 1141 Nte., Col. Talleres, Monterrey N.L. 64480 Mexico

Md International, Inc. 305-669-9003
11300 NW 41st St, Doral, FL 33178

Medical Positioning, Inc. 800-593-3246
1717 Washington St, Kansas City, MO 64108
ECHO BED examination table for echocardigraphy and stress echo. Patented drop section allows full left lateral imaging. Also available with second drop section to facilitate right handed scanning. STRESS ECHO & ECHO BED examination bed for echocardiography and stress echo. Both products feature one hand release drop section to improve apical images. Pedal ergometer has eddy current brake resistance and application specific microprocessor controller designed for one button operation of ideal protocol.

Medrecon, Inc. 877-526-4323
257 South Ave, Garwood, NJ 07027
Remanufactured units - 2 yr warranty.

Midmark Corporation 800-643-6275
60 Vista Dr, P.O. Box 286, Versailles, OH 45380

Nk Medical Products Inc. 800-274-2742
10123 Main St, PO Box 627, Clarence, NY 14031
Specialty pediatric exam table designed in child-friendly themes.

Olympic Medical Corp. 206-767-3500
5900 1st Ave S, Seattle, WA 98108
$1844.50 each.

Pedia Pals, Llc 888-733-4272
965 Highway 169 N, Plymouth, MN 55441
Smiling animal shape ZooPals exam tables. 8 different animal shapes made of durable fiberglass construction.

Profex Medical Products 800-325-0196
2224 E Person Ave, Memphis, TN 38114
Standard examination/treatment and portable tables.

Pulley-Kellam Co., Inc. 260-356-6326
245 Erie St, Huntington, IN 46750
General use manual examination table with storage.

Recreation Equipment Unlimited, Inc. 412-731-3000
PO Box 4700, Pittsburgh, PA 15206
Bailey Manufacturing exam tables, therapeutic equipment, recovery.

S&W By Hausmann 888-428-7626
130 Union St, Northvale, NJ 07647
Hi-lo mat table.

Schueler & Company, Inc. 516-487-1500
PO Box 528, Stratford, CT 06615

Servicios Paraclinicios S.A. 83-33-8400
Madero No. 3330 Pte., Monterrey N.L. 64020 Mexico

Stille-Sonesta, Inc. 800-665-1614
1610 S Interstate 35E Ste 203, Carrollton, TX 75006

Suburban Surgical Co., Inc. 800-323-7366
275 12th St, Wheeling, IL 60090
For veterinary use only: stainless steel top, base tubular or cabinet.

Superior Medical Limited 800-268-7944
520 Champagne Dr., Toronto, ONT M3J 2T9 Canada

Tower Medical System, Ltd. 631-699-3200
917 Lincoln Ave Ste 11, Holbrook, NY 11741
MD250-2 Multi-Purpose Ultrasound Table. Exam Table.

Tri W-G Group 800-437-8011
215 12th Ave NE, PO Box 905, Valley City, ND 58072
Non-powered examination/treatment table. Powered examination/treatment table.

United Metal Fabricators, Inc. 800-638-5322
1316 Eisenhower Blvd, Johnstown, PA 15904
Vacuum formed vinyl upholstered top, all metal cabinet, adjustable length and width stirrups, enameled, color coordinated, power or manually adjustable. Two function (hi-lo and back) Model 5070 and 4 function (height, Trendelenburg, back and leg rest) Model 5000; also, pediatric examination table with integrated beam scale or digital electronic scale and measuring rule.

TABLE, INSTRUMENT, SURGICAL *(Surgery) 79FZN*

Alimed, Inc. 800-225-2610
297 High St, Dedham, MA 02026

Blickman 800-247-5070
39 Robinson Rd, Lodi, NJ 07644
Shelf or H-brace adjustable models.

Bryton Corp. 800-567-9500
4310 Guion Rd, Indianapolis, IN 46254

Eagle Mhc 800-637-5100
100 Industrial Blvd, Clayton, DE 19938
Stainless steel instrument tables provide an all-stainless work system for use as back tables in O.R. suite or as mobile work station for any department.

Elmed, Inc. 630-543-2792
60 W Fay Ave, Addison, IL 60101

Imperial Surgical Ltd. 800-661-5432
581 Orly Ave., Dorval, ONT H9P-1G1 Canada
Various models.

Mayo Medical, S.A. De C.V. 800-715-3872
Edison 1141 Nte., Col. Talleres, Monterrey N.L. 64480 Mexico

Pedigo Products 360-695-3500
4000 SE Columbia Way, Vancouver, WA 98661
Stainless steel, various sizes.

Phelan Manufacturing Corp. 800-328-2358
2523 Minnehaha Ave, Minneapolis, MN 55404
$5,550.00 for neurosurgical instrument table; also, $1,516.00 for straddle instrument table.

Schaerer Mayfield Usa 800-755-6381
4900 Charlemar Dr, Cincinnati, OH 45227
MAYFIELD overhead instrument.

Scientek Medical Equipment 604-273-9094
11151 Bridgeport Rd., Richmond, BC V6X 1T3 Canada

Steris Corporation 800-884-9550
5960 Heisley Rd, Mentor, OH 44060

United Metal Fabricators, Inc. 800-638-5322
1316 Eisenhower Blvd, Johnstown, PA 15904
All stainless steel or enameled with shelf or brace, with casters or rubber tips, various sizes.

TABLE, MECHANICAL *(Physical Med) 89INW*

Community Products, Llc 845-658-7723
2032 Route 213, Rifton, NY 12471
Prone stander, supine board.

Dynatronics Corp. Chattanooga Operations 801-568-7000
6607 Mountain View Rd, Ooltewah, TN 37363
Mechanical table.

Galaxy Medical Manufacturing Co. 800-876-4599
5411 Sheila St, Commerce, CA 90040
Massage table.

Grant Chiropractic, Llc 770-719-1917
155 Bradford Sq Ste C, Fayetteville, GA 30215
Stationary traction table.

Hamilton Mfg. Co. 888-871-5600
128 Berkeley Cir, Summerville, SC 29483
Table, mechanical.

Innovative Healthcare Products, Llc 231-755-0277
3120 S Getty St, Muskegon, MI 49444
Hydro massage unit.

Jwp & Associates, Inc. 636-536-5055
15259 Kingsman Cir, Chesterfield, MO 63017
Chiropractil stationary adjusting table.

Kyro Mfg. Co. 817-336-1319
2601 Weisenberger St, Fort Worth, TX 76107
Chiropractic adjusting tables.

Leander Health Technologies/Healthcare Division 800-635-8188
1525 Vivian Ct, Port Orchard, WA 98367
Motorized chiropractic table, Leander 900 Series, a Z series CPM, multi-purpose table. Also Leander Lite manual flexion chiropractic distraction table.

Living Earth Crafts 800-358-8292
3210 Executive Rdg, Vista, CA 92081
Treatment tables: portable, hydraulic and electric models from $339.00 to $1,895.00. 5-year warranty, custom models available.

Medical Depot 516-998-4600
99 Seaview Blvd, Port Washington, NY 11050
Mechanical table.

TABLE, MECHANICAL *(cont'd)*

Medtec 800-842-8688
1401 8th St SE, PO Box 320, Orange City, IA 51041
Transfer table.

N-K Products Company, Div. Of I-Rep,Inc. 800-462-6509
508 Chaney St Ste B, Lake Elsinore, CA 92530
Entry level priced three and five section hi-lo tables with outstanding stability and features.

Oakworks, Inc. 800-558-8850
923 E Wellspring Rd, New Freedom, PA 17349
Multiple brands of tables used in physical medicine.

Patterson Medical Supply, Inc. 262-387-8720
W68N158 Evergreen Blvd, Cedarburg, WI 53012
Ropox ergotables; economy treatment tables.

Pedia Pals, Llc 888-733-4272
965 Highway 169 N, Plymouth, MN 55441
Pediatric Exam Tables in the shape of animals. Smiling durable fiberglass tables that are a great distraction for kids. Matching wall decals available.

Pulley-Kellam Co., Inc. 260-356-6326
245 Erie St, Huntington, IN 46750
Treatment/examination table with padded surface.

Real Ideas Rehabilitation Div. Inc. 604-820-8916
34142 York Ave, Mission V2V 6Y5 Canada
Mechanical table

Schaerer Mayfield Usa 800-755-6381
4900 Charlemar Dr, Cincinnati, OH 45227
547 Surgical Lounge Stretcher, 540/545 Stretcher, 550/555 Stretcher, 511/516 Stretcher.

Simple Slant 828-245-8962
1218 Spooky Hollow Rd, Marion, NC 28752
Home stretch spinal system.

Stand-Rite Manufacturing Co. 562-782-6346
16655 Grand Ave, Bellflower, CA 90706
Standing frame.

Thera-Tronics, Inc. 800-267-6211
623 Mamaroneck Ave, Mamaroneck, NY 10543
Massage tables and vibrators.

Tumble Forms, Inc. 262-387-8720
1013 Barker Rd, Dolgeville, NY 13329
Standing frame.

U.S. Table, Inc. 847-741-3650
158 N Edison Ave, Elgin, IL 60123
Flex-8000.

TABLE, NUCLEAR MEDICINE *(Radiology) 90VHE*

Composiflex, Inc. 800-673-2544
8100 Hawthorne Dr, Erie, PA 16509
Low absorption, high strength carbon fiber nuclear imaging table tops.

Owens Scientific Inc. 281-394-2311
23230 Sandsage Ln, Katy, TX 77494

Vermont Composites, Inc. 802-442-9964
25 Performance Dr, Bennington, VT 05201
Low absorption carbon tops.

TABLE, OBSTETRICAL *(Obstetrics/Gyn) 85KNC*

Bryton Corp. 800-567-9500
4310 Guion Rd, Indianapolis, IN 46254
Obstetrical tables for C-section and natural childbirth deliveries.

Enochs Examining Room Furniture, Inc. 800-428-2305
PO Box 50559, Indianapolis, IN 46250
$2,057.00 per unit (standard).

Galaxy Medical Manufacturing Co. 800-876-4599
5411 Sheila St, Commerce, CA 90040
Gynecological table.

Hill-Rom Holdings, Inc. 800-445-3730
1069 State Road 46 E, Batesville, IN 47006

Mayo Medical, S.A. De C.V. 800-715-3872
Edison 1141 Nte., Col. Talleres, Monterrey N.L. 64480 Mexico

Medrecon, Inc. 877-526-4323
257 South Ave, Garwood, NJ 07027
Remanufactured units - 2 yr warranty.

Smith & Nephew Inc. 800-463-7439
2100 52nd Ave., Lachine, QUE H8T 2Y5 Canada

Sri Surgical 813-891-9550
6801 Longe St, Stockton, CA 95206
Delivery blanket.

TABLE, OBSTETRICAL, AC-POWERED *(Obstetrics/Gyn) 85HDD*

Bryton Corp. 800-567-9500
4310 Guion Rd, Indianapolis, IN 46254
Obstetrical tables for C-section & natural childbirth deliveries.

Enochs Examining Room Furniture, Inc. 800-428-2305
PO Box 50559, Indianapolis, IN 46250
$6,216.00 per unit (standard).

Hill-Rom, Inc. 812-934-7777
4115 Dorchester Rd Unit 600, North Charleston, SC 29405
Birthing beds (various).

Lic Care 800-323-5232
2935A Northeast Pkwy, Atlanta, GA 30360

Md International, Inc. 305-669-9003
11300 NW 41st St, Doral, FL 33178

Medrecon, Inc. 877-526-4323
257 South Ave, Garwood, NJ 07027

Midmark Corporation 800-643-6275
60 Vista Dr, P.O. Box 286, Versailles, OH 45380

Penner Manufacturing Inc 800-732-0717
102 Grant St, PO Box 523, Aurora, NE 68818
Birthing chairs.

Pulley-Kellam Co., Inc. 260-356-6326
245 Erie St, Huntington, IN 46750
Powered High-low exam table.

TABLE, OBSTETRICAL, MANUAL *(Obstetrics/Gyn) 85HHP*

Bryton Corp. 800-567-9500
4310 Guion Rd, Indianapolis, IN 46254
Obstetrical tables for natural childbirth and C-section deliveries.

Elmed, Inc. 630-543-2792
60 W Fay Ave, Addison, IL 60101

Kadan Co. Inc., D.A. 800-325-2326
1 Brigadoon Ln, Waxhaw, NC 28173

Lic Care 800-323-5232
2935A Northeast Pkwy, Atlanta, GA 30360

Maquet, Inc. 843-552-8652
7371 Spartan Blvd E, N Charleston, SC 29418
Various obstetrical tables manual.

Medrecon, Inc. 877-526-4323
257 South Ave, Garwood, NJ 07027
Remanufactured - 2 yr. warranty.

Pulley-Kellam Co., Inc. 260-356-6326
245 Erie St, Huntington, IN 46750
Exam table with storage, warmer and pelvic tilt.

Stryker Medical 800-869-0770
3800 E Centre Ave, Portage, MI 49002

United Metal Fabricators, Inc. 800-638-5322
1316 Eisenhower Blvd, Johnstown, PA 15904

TABLE, OPERATING ROOM, AC-POWERED *(Surgery) 79FQO*

Advantage Medical Systems, Inc. 800-810-1262
2876 S Wheeling Way, Aurora, CO 80014
Advantage Smart Table: Only major general surgery table with lower ideal height range for less-invasive procedures and higher range for open procedures. Allows laparoscopic surgeons to operate at correct height (less fatigue) without lifts (less dangerous).

Ams Innovative Center-San Jose 800-356-7600
3070 Orchard Dr, San Jose, CA 95134

Bryton Corp. 800-567-9500
4310 Guion Rd, Indianapolis, IN 46254
Complete range of electrically controlled operating tables for all types of surgical procedures.

Getinge Usa, Inc. 800-475-9040
1777 E Henrietta Rd, Rochester, NY 14623
MAQUET

Kma Remarketing Corp. 814-371-5242
302 Aspen Way, Dubois, PA 15801
Electric operating room table.

Maquet, Inc. 843-552-8652
7371 Spartan Blvd E, N Charleston, SC 29418
Various surgical tables, powered.

Md International, Inc. 305-669-9003
11300 NW 41st St, Doral, FL 33178

Medrecon, Inc. 877-526-4323
257 South Ave, Garwood, NJ 07027
Remanufactured - 2 yr. warranty.

TABLE, OPERATING ROOM, AC-POWERED *(cont'd)*

Smith & Nephew Inc. 800-463-7439
2100 52nd Ave., Lachine, QUE H8T 2Y5 Canada

Tekna Solutions, Inc. 269-978-3500
3400 Tech Cir, Kalamazoo, MI 49008
Operation room accessories.

Voss Medical Products 210-650-3124
4235 Centergate St, San Antonio, TX 78217
Leg positioner.

TABLE, OPERATING ROOM, MECHANICAL *(Surgery) 79FWX*

Amelife Llc 302-476-2631
702 N West St Ste 101, Wilmington, DE 19801

American Bio-Medical Service Corporation (Abmsc) 800-755-9055
631 W Covina Blvd, Sales,Service and Refurbishing Center
San Dimas, CA 91773

Bryton Corp. 800-567-9500
4310 Guion Rd, Indianapolis, IN 46254
Complete range of operating tables for all types of surgical procedures.

Kma Remarketing Corp. 814-371-5242
302 Aspen Way, Dubois, PA 15801
Manual operating room table.

Medical Technologies Co. 800-280-3220
1728 W Park Center Dr Ste A, Fenton, MO 63026
Surgical tables, O.B. tables, C-section tables, ortho/fracture tables.

Medrecon, Inc. 877-526-4323
257 South Ave, Garwood, NJ 07027
Remanufactured units - 2 yr warranty.

Pedigo Products 360-695-3500
4000 SE Columbia Way, Vancouver, WA 98661
Over operating table.

TABLE, OPERATING ROOM, PNEUMATIC *(Surgery) 79FWW*

Medrecon, Inc. 877-526-4323
257 South Ave, Garwood, NJ 07027
Remanufactured - 2 yr. warranty.

TABLE, OPHTHALMIC, INSTRUMENT, MANUAL *(Ophthalmology) 86HRK*

Allergan 800-366-6554
2525 Dupont Dr, Irvine, CA 92612
From $15 to $500 for over 800 hand-held surgical intruments.

Benjamin Biomedical, Inc. 727-343-5503
3125 Tyrone Blvd N, Saint Petersburg, FL 33710
Instruments.

HAAG-STREIT USA, INC. 800-787-5426
3535 Kings Mills Rd, Mason, OH 45040

Marco Ophthalmic, Inc. 800-874-5274
11825 Central Pkwy, Jacksonville, FL 32224
$405.00 for unit. (List price)

Ocular Instruments, Inc. 800-888-6616
2255 116th Ave NE, Bellevue, WA 98004

TABLE, OPHTHALMIC, INSTRUMENT, POWERED *(Ophthalmology) 86HRJ*

Allergan 800-366-6554
2525 Dupont Dr, Irvine, CA 92612
$610 per unit.

Benjamin Biomedical, Inc. 727-343-5503
3125 Tyrone Blvd N, Saint Petersburg, FL 33710
Instrument.

Cline Products Inc. 941-776-0230
11446 Savannah Lakes Dr, Parrish, FL 34219
Motorized instrument table.

HAAG-STREIT USA, INC. 800-787-5426
3535 Kings Mills Rd, Mason, OH 45040

Marco Ophthalmic, Inc. 800-874-5274
11825 Central Pkwy, Jacksonville, FL 32224
$1,245.00 for unit. (List price)

Ocular Instruments, Inc. 800-888-6616
2255 116th Ave NE, Bellevue, WA 98004

Topcon Medical Systems, Inc. 800-223-1130
37 W Century Rd, Paramus, NJ 07652
Three models of instrument tables: $990.00, $1,590.00, and $1,990.00 each.

TABLE, OPHTHALMIC, INSTRUMENT, POWERED *(cont'd)*

Woodlyn, Inc. 800-331-7389
2920 Malmo Dr, Ophthalmic Instruments and Equipment
Arlington Heights, IL 60005
Model 67600. The Woodlyn Motorized Instrument Table features sturdy construction and quiet operation. Call for current prices.

TABLE, OTHER *(General) 80RZB*

Atd-American Co. 800-523-2300
135 Greenwood Ave, Wyncote, PA 19095
Folding tables, conference room tables, cafeteria tables, table trucks to store your tables.

Back Solution, The 800-326-2724
6281 S Park Ave, Tucson, AZ 85706

Biodex Medical Systems, Inc. 800-224-6339
20 Ramsey Rd, Shirley, NY 11967
Echocardiography and ultrasound table.

Brandt Industries, Inc. 800-221-8031
4461 Bronx Blvd, Bronx, NY 10470
Massage, treatment.

Can-Dan Rehatec Ltd. 9056487522
3-1378 Sandhill Dr., Ancaster, ONT L9G-4V5 Canada
Electric Height-Adjustable Change Table for use in Orthopedic washroom, Treatment Centre, Schools. Infinitely variable in height. Different sizes avaiable. Models: Wall Mount or Mobile.

Cardon Rehabilitation Products Inc 800-944-7868
908 Niagara Falls Blvd, Wurlitzer Industrial Park
North Tonawanda, NY 14120
Gerontic rehabilitation tables.

Carolina Biological Supply Co. 800-334-5551
2700 York Rd, Burlington, NC 27215

Colonial Scientific Ltd. 902-468-1811
201 Brownlow Ave., Unit 52, Dartmouth, NS B3B-1W2 Canada
General and stainless steel.

Contamination Control Products 877-553-2676
1 3rd Ave # 578, Neptune, NJ 07753
Stainless steel tables & carts.

Crest Healthcare Supply 800-328-8908
195 3rd St, Dassel, MN 55325
Overbed and utility tables.

Da-Lite Screen Co., Inc. 800-622-3737
3100 N Detroit St, PO Box 137, Warsaw, IN 46582
Computer tables.

Elmed, Inc. 630-543-2792
60 W Fay Ave, Addison, IL 60101

Falcon Products, Inc. 800-873-3252
10650 Gateway Blvd, Saint Louis, MO 63132
Folding and flip top tables.

Fleetwood Group, Incorporated 800-257-6390
PO Box 1259, Holland, MI 49422
$1,180 to $2,010 42in. x 60in. adjustable, hydraulic table, manual operation. $520 for fixed height wheelchair table, height: 32in., width: 42in., length: 60in.

Galaxy Medical Manufacturing Co. 800-876-4599
5411 Sheila St, Commerce, CA 90040
Portable-chiropractic, portable-massage, and adjustment tables.

Getinge Usa, Inc. 800-475-9040
1777 E Henrietta Rd, Rochester, NY 14623
MAQUET, surgical table.

Hausmann Industries, Inc. 888-428-7626
130 Union St, Northvale, NJ 07647
$1,175.00 per unit.

Hemco Corp. 816-796-2900
111 S Powell Rd, Independence, MO 64056

Intermetro Industries Corp. 800-441-2714
651 N Washington St, Wilkes Barre, PA 18705
Stainless-steel reprocessing tables. Instrument-prep tables.

Kadan Co. Inc., D.A. 800-325-2326
1 Brigadoon Ln, Waxhaw, NC 28173

La Calhene 320-358-4713
1325 S Field Ave, PO Box 567, Rush City, MN 55069
Cleanroom tables.

Living Earth Crafts 800-358-8292
3210 Executive Rdg, Vista, CA 92081
Treatment tables: portable, hydraulic and electric models from $339.00 to $1,895.00. 5-year warranty, custom models available. SERENITY is a hydraulic lifting table.

TABLE, OTHER *(cont'd)*

Lm Air Technology, Inc. 866-381-8200
1467 Pinewood St, Cleanroom & Lab Equipment - Mfger
Rahway, NJ 07065
Stainless steel, Polypropylene & laminated.

Medical Positioning, Inc. 800-593-3246
1717 Washington St, Kansas City, MO 64108
Echo Positioning System for echo, stress echo and peripheral vascular exams. Controller allows height adjustment, Trendelenburg and reverse Trendelenburg plus lateral tilt positioning. DBI TABLE, table has drop sections enabling closer proximity for decubitus stereotactic core breast biopsies. Allows efficient, low cost use of a stereotactic add-on to a mammography machine. VASSCAN TABLE, Comes with a foot board and the ability to place the patient in a 30 degree reverse Trendelenburg position, this increases venous pooling resulting in easier & more accurate peripheral ultrasound/Doppler studies.ULTRASSCAN TABLE, comes with leg supports, footboard to support patient in 35 degree reverse Trendelenburg position, -15 degree Trendelenburg, and with/without pelvic cutout and fluid containment system, removable foot drop section for OB/GYN studies.

Mizuho Osi 800-777-4674
30031 Ahern Ave, Union City, CA 94587
OSI Orthopedic fracture and radiolucent tables. Orthopedic TraumaTable, Jackson Spinal Surgery Table, JST-2000, Modular Table System, Endourology Table.

N-K Products Company, Div. Of I-Rep,Inc. 800-462-6509
508 Chaney St Ste B, Lake Elsinore, CA 92530
The ORIGINAL NK-330 hamstring and quad exercise table.

Noa Medical Industries 800-633-6068
801 Terry Ln, Washington, MO 63090

Peter Pepper Products, Inc. 800-496-0204
17929 S Susana Rd, PO Box 5769, Compton, CA 90221
Desks.

Plymold 800-533-0480
615 Centennial Dr, Kenyon, MN 55946
Nursing home table, with an advanced hygienic, seamless, molded polyurethane edge which has color clear through for wearabiltiy.

Radix Corp. 204-697-2349
#2-572 South Fifth St., Pembina, ND 58271
NORDIC feeding and game tables (wheelchair accessible), children's furniture.

Scientek Medical Equipment 604-273-9094
11151 Bridgeport Rd., Richmond, BC V6X 1T3 Canada
Including: Anatomy table.

Stille-Sonesta, Inc. 800-665-1614
1610 S Interstate 35E Ste 203, Carrollton, TX 75006

Thera-Tronics, Inc. 800-267-6211
623 Mamaroneck Ave, Mamaroneck, NY 10543
Chiropractic, physical therapy and fluid therapy tables.

Thompson Contract Inc. 631-589-7337
41 Keyland Ct, Bohemia, NY 11716
Cafeteria, office and conference tables.

Tri W-G Group 800-437-8011
215 12th Ave NE, PO Box 905, Valley City, ND 58072
Fixed-height tilt table; and fixed-height mat table and hi-lo mat table.

World Dryer Corp. 800-323-0701
5700 McDermott Dr, Berkeley, IL 60163
WORLD DRYER Drybaby changing station.

TABLE, OVERBED *(General) 80RYY*

A.R.C. Distributors 800-296-8724
PO Box 599, Centreville, MD 21617
INVACARE Auto Touch Overbed Table, Tilt-top Overbed Table.

Alimed, Inc. 800-225-2610
297 High St, Dedham, MA 02026

Basic American Medical Products 800-849-6664
2935A Northeast Pkwy, Atlanta, GA 30360

Basic American Metal Products 800-365-2338
336 Trowbridge Dr, PO Box 907, Fond Du Lac, WI 54937

Brandt Industries, Inc. 800-221-8031
4461 Bronx Blvd, Bronx, NY 10470

Brewer Company, The 888-873-9371
N88W13901 Main St, Menomonee Falls, WI 53051
#11600: Gray Laminate- 'H' Base, #11610: Walnute Laminate- 'H' Base, #11620 Walnute Laminate- 'U' Base, #11630 - Gray Laminate- 'U' Base, #11640: Low Overbed Table- Walnute Laminate- 'H' Base

TABLE, OVERBED *(cont'd)*

Hard Manufacturing Co. 800-873-4273
230 Grider St, Buffalo, NY 14215
$123 for Model 711C overbed table; $295 for Model 4853 auto-rise with vanity.

Hill-Rom Holdings, Inc. 800-445-3730
1069 State Road 46 E, Batesville, IN 47006

M.C. Healthcare Products, Inc. 800-268-8671
4658 Ontario St., Beamsville, ONT L0R 1B4 Canada
Spring Assist Lifting. Moulded marine edge top or laminate top.

Mayo Medical, S.A. De C.V. 800-715-3872
Edison 1141 Nte., Col. Talleres, Monterrey N.L. 64480 Mexico

Nk Medical Products Inc. 800-274-2742
10123 Main St, PO Box 627, Clarence, NY 14031

Noa Medical Industries 800-633-6068
801 Terry Ln, Washington, MO 63090
$88.00 to $93.00 for automatic lift overbed table, solid construction.

Rockaway Chairs 800-256-6601
111 Alexander Rd Apt 11, West Monroe, LA 71291

Sunrise Medical 800-333-4000
7477 Dry Creek Pkwy, Longmont, CO 80503

Tuffcare 800-367-6160
3999 E La Palma Ave, Anaheim, CA 92807

TABLE, PHYSICAL MEDICINE, POWERED *(Physical Med) 89INQ*

Aggressive Solutions, Inc. 972-242-2164
1735 N Interstate 35E, Carrollton, TX 75006
Tilt table.

Armedica Mfg. Corp. 479-996-2612
212 Bell Rd, Greenwood, AR 72936
Physical therapy table.

Clinton Industries, Inc 717-848-3519
1140 Edison St, York, PA 17403
Various powered tables.

Country Medical Equipment 302-845-2462
3758 Williamsville Rd, Houston, DE 19954
Adjustable exam/treatment table.

Dynatronics Corp. Chattanooga Operations 801-568-7000
6607 Mountain View Rd, Ooltewah, TN 37363
Powered table.

Elekta, Inc. 800-535-7355
4775 Peachtree Industrial Blvd, Building 300, Suite 300
Norcross, GA 30092
Powered therapy table.

Enochs Examining Room Furniture, Inc. 800-428-2305
PO Box 50559, Indianapolis, IN 46250
$8,595.00 per unit (standard).

Hamilton Mfg. Co. 888-871-5600
128 Berkeley Cir, Summerville, SC 29483
Table, powered.

Hausmann Industries, Inc. 888-428-7626
130 Union St, Northvale, NJ 07647
$181 or $495 - 2 models.

Hcmi, Inc. 773-588-2444
2146 E Pythian St, Springfield, MO 65802
Hylo adjusting table.

Hill Laboratories Co. 877-445-5020
3 N Bacton Hill Rd, PO Box 2028, Frazer, PA 19355
Hill Air Flex. Designed predominately for chiropractors, this elevation table allows for the use of drops, flexion, distraction, elevation/dual drop/tilting cervical headpiece, rotation, and lateral movement, along with many other options.

I-Rep, Inc. 800-828-0852
508 Chaney St Ste B, Lake Elsinore, CA 92530
$1,600-$4,000 each for Hi-Lo powered physical medicine tables.

Jwp & Associates, Inc. 636-536-5055
15259 Kingsman Cir, Chesterfield, MO 63017
Electric flexion adjusting table.

Living Earth Crafts 800-358-8292
3210 Executive Rdg, Vista, CA 92081
Treatment tables: portable, hydraulic and electric models from $339.00 to $1,895.00. 5-year warranty, custom models available.

Med-Fit Systems, Inc. 800-831-7665
3553 Rosa Way, Fallbrook, CA 92028

TABLE, PHYSICAL MEDICINE, POWERED *(cont'd)*

Medi-Man Rehabilitation Products, Inc. 800-268-4256
6200A Tomken Rd., Mississauga, ONT L5T-1X7 Canada
MEDI-PLINTH, MINI-MATT. Electrically operated hi-low 3 and 5 sections treatment tables with a 90 degree drop of the head section.

Midmark Corporation 800-643-6275
60 Vista Dr, P.O. Box 286, Versailles, OH 45380

Synergistic Concepts, Ltd. 419-448-4868
1660 W Market St Ste D, Tiffin, OH 44883
Chiropractic table.

Track Corporation 616-850-9444
17024 Taft Rd, Spring Lake, MI 49456
Chiropractic adjusting table.

Tri W-G Group 800-437-8011
215 12th Ave NE, PO Box 905, Valley City, ND 58072
Motorized Hi-Lo mat tables and treatment tables.

U.S. Table, Inc. 847-741-3650
158 N Edison Ave, Elgin, IL 60123
Elevator table.

United Metal Fabricators, Inc. 800-638-5322
1316 Eisenhower Blvd, Johnstown, PA 15904
Ob/Gyn and proctologic.

Winco, Inc. 800-237-3377
5516 SW 1st Ln, Ocala, FL 34474
Lift table.

TABLE, PHYSICAL THERAPY *(Physical Med) 89JFB*

Activeaid, Inc. 800-533-5330
101 Activeaid Rd, Redwood Falls, MN 56283

Armedica Mfg. Corp. 479-996-2612
212 Bell Rd, Greenwood, AR 72936
Physical therapy tables.

Battle Creek Equipment Co. 800-253-0854
307 Jackson St W, Battle Creek, MI 49037
BATTLE CREEK, portable tables and permanent tables. $299.00 to $479.00/unit (standard).

Cardon Rehabilitation Products Inc 800-944-7868
908 Niagara Falls Blvd, Wurlitzer Industrial Park
North Tonawanda, NY 14120
Manual orthopedic tables.

Erp Group Professional Products Ltd. 800-361-3537
3232 Autoroute Laval W., Laval, QC H7T 2H6 Canada
Akron treatment tables.

Galaxy Medical Manufacturing Co. 800-876-4599
5411 Sheila St, Commerce, CA 90040

Hausmann Industries, Inc. 888-428-7626
130 Union St, Northvale, NJ 07647
2 models - $1,845 (manual) or $3,098 (electric).

Hayday Irrit-Easers 416-434-1400
883 Derry Crt, Oshawa L1J 6X8 Canada
No common name listed

Hcmi, Inc. 773-588-2444
2146 E Pythian St, Springfield, MO 65802
Intersegmental traction table.

Hill Laboratories Co. 877-445-5020
3 N Bacton Hill Rd, PO Box 2028, Frazer, PA 19355
Hill Physical Therapy Tables. Hill Laboratories custom manufactures many elevation tables for physical therapists, offering an enormous selection of options for each table.

I-Rep, Inc. 800-828-0852
508 Chaney St Ste B, Lake Elsinore, CA 92530
$300 to $15,000 each for benches, exercise tables and other equipment.

International Therapeutic Machines 877-848-2835
425 Lombard St, Thousand Oaks, CA 91360
Vivatek & p.t. machine.

Jwp & Associates, Inc. 636-536-5055
15259 Kingsman Cir, Chesterfield, MO 63017
Intersegmental roller table.

Kadan Co. Inc., D.A. 800-325-2326
1 Brigadoon Ln, Waxhaw, NC 28173

Living Earth Crafts 800-358-8292
3210 Executive Rdg, Vista, CA 92081
Treatment tables: portable, hydraulic and electric models from $339.00 to $1,895.00. 5-year warranty, custom models available.

TABLE, PHYSICAL THERAPY *(cont'd)*

Major Lab. Manufacturing 800-598-2621
4408 N Sewell Ave, Oklahoma City, OK 73118
$251.00 each.

Mylon-Tech Health Technologies Inc. 613-728-1667
301 Moodie Dr., Ste. 205, Ottawa, ON K2H 9C4 Canada

Noram Solutions 800-387-7103
PO Box 543, Lewiston, NY 14092
Multi-flex Hi-Lo physical therapy table.

Omni Medical Supply Inc. 800-860-6664
4153 Pioneer Dr, Commerce Township, MI 48390

Prime Engineering 800-827-8263
4202 W Sierra Madre Ave, Fresno, CA 93722
Granstand III: Pediactric to adult modular standing system and transfer device grows with the client from 3' to 6'5'. Symmetry Adult and Symmetry Youth solid seat standing system with full body support options.

Profex Medical Products 800-325-0196
2224 E Person Ave, Memphis, TN 38114

S&W By Hausmann 888-428-7626
130 Union St, Northvale, NJ 07647
Hi-lo mat table.

Tjn Manufacturing,Inc. 563-322-2162
416 N Perry St, Davenport, IA 52801
Chiropractic table.

Tri W-G Group 800-437-8011
215 12th Ave NE, PO Box 905, Valley City, ND 58072
Treatment, mat and tilt tables, bariatric tables.

U.S. Table, Inc. 847-741-3650
158 N Edison Ave, Elgin, IL 60123
Elevation physical therapy table.

TABLE, RADIOGRAPHIC *(Radiology) 90KXJ*

Americomp, Inc. 800-458-1782
2901 W Lawrence Ave, Chicago, IL 60625
Elevator table.

Amrad 888-772-6723
2901 W Lawrence Ave, Chicago, IL 60625

Composiflex, Inc. 800-673-2544
8100 Hawthorne Dr, Erie, PA 16509
Low absorption, high strength carbon fiber table tops.

Computron Medical Corp. 847-952-8800
1697 W Imperial Ct, Mount Prospect, IL 60056
Various models of c-arm x-ray tables.

Del Medical Systems 800-800-6006
11550 King St, Franklin Park, IL 60131
4-way float table, fixed height or elevator table.

Grady Research, Inc. 978-772-3303
323 W Main St, Ayer, MA 01432
Angiographic table.

Hologic, Inc. 800-343-9729
35 Crosby Dr, Bedford, MA 01730
INTEGRATED RADIOGRAPHY TABLE

Medtec 800-842-8688
1401 8th St SE, PO Box 320, Orange City, IA 51041
Couch top and table indexing system.

Medx, Inc. 847-463-2020
3456 N Ridge Ave Ste 100, Arlington Heights, IL 60004
Radiologic table.

Mizuho Osi 800-777-4674
30031 Ahern Ave, Union City, CA 94587
OSI imaging table. VACS tables, URO VACS tables and US imaging tables.

Quatro Composites 858-513-4300
13250 Gregg St Ste A1, Poway, CA 92064

Stille-Sonesta, Inc. 800-665-1614
1610 S Interstate 35E Ste 203, Carrollton, TX 75006

Surgical Tables Incorporated 888-737-5044
2 De Bush Ave Bldg 2, Middleton, MA 01949
Max 0, max 1, max 2, max 3, max 4, max 5.

Xma (X-Ray Marketing Associates, Inc.) 800-325-8880
1205 W Lakeview Ct, Windham Lakes Business Park
Romeoville, IL 60446

TABLE, RADIOGRAPHIC, NON-TILTING, POWERED

(Radiology) 90IZZ

Altek Corp. 301-572-2555
12210 Plum Orchard Dr, Silver Spring, MD 20904

Bay Shore Medical Equipment Corp. 631-586-1991
235 S Fehr Way, Bay Shore, NY 11706
Multiple.

Composiflex, Inc. 800-673-2544
8100 Hawthorne Dr, Erie, PA 16509
Low absorption, high strength carbon fiber table tops.

Control-X Medical, Inc. 800-777-9729
1755 Atlas St, Columbus, OH 43228

Quantum Medical Imaging, Llc 631-567-5800
2002 Orville Dr N Ste B, Ronkonkoma, NY 11779
Radiologic table.

Raymax Medical Corp. 905-791-3020
20 Strathearn Ave, Unit 3, Brampton, ONT L6T 4P7 Canada
Alpha-4-way float table

Toshiba America Medical Systems 800-421-1968
2441 Michelle Dr, Tustin, CA 92780
Tosrad Models CH/50, UH/50, UH/80, CPH/50, and UPH/50.

Vermont Composites, Inc. 802-442-9964
25 Performance Dr, Bennington, VT 05201
Low absorption carbon tops.

Virtual Imaging, Inc. 954-428-6191
720 S Powerline Rd Ste E, Deerfield Bch, FL 33442
Radiographic elevating table.

Xma (X-Ray Marketing Associates, Inc.) 800-325-8880
1205 W Lakeview Ct, Windham Lakes Business Park
Romeoville, IL 60446

York X-Ray And Orthopedic Supply, Inc. 800-334-6427
PO Box 326, 20 Hampton Rd.,, Lyman, SC 29365

TABLE, RADIOGRAPHIC, STATIONARY TOP *(Radiology) 90IXQ*

Altek Corp. 301-572-2555
12210 Plum Orchard Dr, Silver Spring, MD 20904

Anholt Technologies, Inc. 610-268-2758
440 Church Rd, Avondale, PA 19311
Table, radiographic, stationary.

Bryton Corp. 800-567-9500
4310 Guion Rd, Indianapolis, IN 46254
Complete range of radiographic imaging tables for all types of imaging procedures.

Composiflex, Inc. 800-673-2544
8100 Hawthorne Dr, Erie, PA 16509
Low absorption, high strength carbon fiber table tops.

Composites Horizons, Inc. 626-331-0861
1471 W Industrial Park St, Covina, CA 91722
Radiolucent composite table tops for x-ray, CT & nuclear medicine, and geography.

Control-X Medical, Inc. 800-777-9729
1755 Atlas St, Columbus, OH 43228

Del Medical Systems 800-800-6006
11550 King St, Franklin Park, IL 60131

Image Diagnostics, Inc. 978-422-8601
98 Pratts Junction Rd, Sterling, MA 01564
General purpose fluoroscopic table w/ stationary top.

Marconi Medical Systems 800-323-0550
595 Miner Rd, Cleveland, OH 44143

Mizuho Osi 800-777-4674
30031 Ahern Ave, Union City, CA 94587
Chemonucleolysis orthopedic table.

Quantum Medical Imaging, Llc 631-567-5800
2002 Orville Dr N Ste B, Ronkonkoma, NY 11779
Radiologic table.

Tingle X-Ray Llc 349-162-8905
5481 Skyland Blvd E, Coaling, AL 35453
Flat bucky table.

Vermont Composites, Inc. 802-442-9964
25 Performance Dr, Bennington, VT 05201
Low absorption carbon tops.

Xma (X-Ray Marketing Associates, Inc.) 800-325-8880
1205 W Lakeview Ct, Windham Lakes Business Park
Romeoville, IL 60446

York X-Ray And Orthopedic Supply, Inc. 800-334-6427
PO Box 326, 20 Hampton Rd.,, Lyman, SC 29365

TABLE, RADIOGRAPHIC, TILTING *(Radiology) 90IXR*

Altek Corp. 301-572-2555
12210 Plum Orchard Dr, Silver Spring, MD 20904

Arcoma North America, Inc. 464-707-0690
23151 Alcalde Dr Ste C8, Laguna Hills, CA 92653
X-ray table.

Asi Medical Equipment, Ltd. 800-527-0443
1735 N Interstate 35E, Carrollton, TX 75006
600T TILT TABLE is a radiolucent bed with articulating litter. Tilts from -15 to 82 degrees for head up tilt table testing, syncope evaluation, electrophysiology studies, controlled gradual rehab for orthopedic recovery and other weight bearing exersises.

Biodex Medical Systems, Inc. 800-224-6339
20 Ramsey Rd, Shirley, NY 11967
Surgical C-Arm Tables.

Composiflex, Inc. 800-673-2544
8100 Hawthorne Dr, Erie, PA 16509
Low absorption, high strength carbon fiber table tops.

Control-X Medical, Inc. 800-777-9729
1755 Atlas St, Columbus, OH 43228

Ge Medical Systems, Llc 262-548-2355
3000 N Grandview Blvd, W-417, Waukesha, WI 53188
Various types of patient handling devices.

Image Diagnostics, Inc. 978-422-8601
98 Pratts Junction Rd, Sterling, MA 01564
Fluoroscopic examination table.

Marconi Medical Systems 800-323-0550
595 Miner Rd, Cleveland, OH 44143

Medical Positioning, Inc. 800-593-3246
1717 Washington St, Kansas City, MO 64108
Non-invasive procedure room exam surface to facilitate syncope studies and all EP procedures.

Medstone International, Inc. 949-367-1238
229 Arnold Mill Rd Ste 200, Woodstock, GA 30188
Mobile radiologic table.

Morgan Medesign, Inc. 888-799-4633
947 Piner Pl, Santa Rosa, CA 95403
Morgan Medesign, Inc.'s custom-built fluoroscopy tables are utilized by leading pain management specialists throughout the U.S. Their features and motions contribute to patient and operator safety, procedure efficiency, minimal radiation exposure, and maximum C-Arm capabilities.

Nurad Medical Solutions Llc 949-737-7523
396 Cliffwood Park St, Brea, CA 92821
Mobile radiologic table.

Oakworks, Inc. 800-558-8850
923 E Wellspring Rd, New Freedom, PA 17349
Carbon Fiber Fluoroscopy Tables with Trendelenberg.

Perfection Enterprises 818-764-3447
7250 Hinds Ave, North Hollywood, CA 91605
Patient table.

Shimadzu Medical Systems 800-228-1429
20101 S Vermont Ave, Torrance, CA 90502
- 90/15 tilt.

Stille-Sonesta, Inc. 800-665-1614
1610 S Interstate 35E Ste 203, Carrollton, TX 75006

Stryker Medical 800-869-0770
3800 E Centre Ave, Portage, MI 49002

Toshiba America Medical Systems 800-421-1968
2441 Michelle Dr, Tustin, CA 92780
Models 450D12A, 450D14A, 450D16A, 450D12A/PF, 450D14A/PF, 450D16A/PF.

Tower Medical System, Ltd. 631-699-3200
917 Lincoln Ave Ste 11, Holbrook, NY 11741
MCA-1500- Fixed Height Motorized C-Arm Table. Chair, positioning, electric, table, tilting.

Vermont Composites, Inc. 802-442-9964
25 Performance Dr, Bennington, VT 05201
Low absorption carbon tops.

York X-Ray And Orthopedic Supply, Inc. 800-334-6427
PO Box 326, 20 Hampton Rd.,, Lyman, SC 29365

TABLE, SLIDE WARMING *(Pathology) 88IEG*

Abbott Molecular, Inc. 847-937-6100
1300 E Touhy Ave, Des Plaines, IL 60018
Slide warming table.

TABLE, SLIDE WARMING *(cont'd)*

Surgipath Medical Industries, Inc. 800-225-3035
PO Box 528, 5205 Route 12, Richmond, IL 60071

TABLE, SURGICAL WITH ORTHOPEDIC ACCESSORIES, AC-POWERED *(Surgery) 79JEA*

Bryton Corp. 800-567-9500
4310 Guion Rd, Indianapolis, IN 46254
Complete range of operating tables for all types of surgical procedures.

Composiflex, Inc. 800-673-2544
8100 Hawthorne Dr, Erie, PA 16509
Low x-ray absorption, high strength carbon fiber surgical table tops.

Frank Scholz X-Ray Corp. 508-586-8308
244 Liberty St, Brockton, MA 02301
$941.00 for Model 1564-X, radiotranslucent extension for C-arm work on surgical table, surgical table accessory.

Getinge Usa, Inc. 800-475-9040
1777 E Henrietta Rd, Rochester, NY 14623
MAQUET

Medrecon, Inc. 877-526-4323
257 South Ave, Garwood, NJ 07027

Nuvo, Inc. 814-899-4220
5368 Kuhl Rd., Corry, PA 16407
Surgical tables.

Valley Technology, Inc. 541-434-9180
1025 Conger St Ste 2, Eugene, OR 97402
Epidural positioning device.

TABLE, SURGICAL, ELECTRICAL *(Surgery) 79GDC*

Amelife Llc 302-476-2631
702 N West St Ste 101, Wilmington, DE 19801

Biomedics, Inc. 949-458-1998
23322 Peralta Dr Ste 11, Laguna Hills, CA 92653

Bryton Corp. 800-567-9500
4310 Guion Rd, Indianapolis, IN 46254
Complete range of electrically controlled operating tables for all types of surgical procedures.

Calmaquip Engineering Corp. 305-592-4510
7240 NW 12th St, Miami, FL 33126

Composiflex, Inc. 800-673-2544
8100 Hawthorne Dr, Erie, PA 16509
Low x-ray absorption, high strength carbon fiber surgical table tops.

Dexta Corporation 800-733-3982
962 Kaiser Rd, Napa, CA 94558
$5,995 for multi-purpose table unit.

Florida Life Systems 727-321-9554
3446 5th Ave N, Saint Petersburg, FL 33713

Getinge Usa, Inc. 800-475-9040
1777 E Henrietta Rd, Rochester, NY 14623
MAQUET

Kma Remarketing Corp. 814-371-5242
302 Aspen Way, Dubois, PA 15801
Electric operating room table.

Medrecon, Inc. 877-526-4323
257 South Ave, Garwood, NJ 07027
Remanufactured units - 2 yr warranty.

Medtronic Sofamor Danek Instrument Manufacturing 901-396-3133
7375 Adrianne Pl, Bartlett, TN 38133
Various sizes of surgical pillows.

Medtronic Sofamor Danek Usa, Inc. 901-396-3133
4340 Swinnea Rd, Memphis, TN 38118
Various sizes of surgical pillows.

Morgan Medesign, Inc. 888-799-4633
947 Piner Pl, Santa Rosa, CA 95403
Manufacturers of portable multi-purpose (MP) fluoroscopy procedure tables. The MP Series accommodates the positioning and radiographic needs of multiple specialists with astonishing versatility.

Schaerer Mayfield Usa 800-755-6381
4900 Charlemar Dr, Cincinnati, OH 45227
7300 Surgery table/surgery table for urology, orthopedics, gynecology. 7100 Surgery table/surgery table for general surgery.

TABLE, SURGICAL, ELECTRICAL *(cont'd)*

Skytron 800-759-8766
5085 Corporate Exchange Blvd SE, Grand Rapids, MI 49512
Nine models with full positioning capability. Tabletop rotates 180 (dgr)to 210 (dgr)-in 3 models. Optional raised tabletop is suitable for radiographic use, accepts standard X-ray cassettes up to 14" x 17". Specialty C-arm and microsurgery vascular and pain-management tables with multi-directional top slide.

Stille-Sonesta, Inc. 800-665-1614
1610 S Interstate 35E Ste 203, Carrollton, TX 75006

Surgical Table Services Company 330-253-7766
526 S Main St Ste 701E, Akron, OH 44311
Surgical table.

Warsaw Orthopedic, Inc. 901-396-3133
2500 Silveus Xing, Warsaw, IN 46582
Various sizes of surgical pillows.

World Medical Equipment, Inc. 800-827-3747
3915 152nd St NE, Marysville, WA 98271
Specialize in refurbished OR tables such as AMSCO/Steris, Skytron, Shampaine and Chick as well as lights, autoclaves, anesthesia machines, monitors, and accessories.

TABLE, SURGICAL, HYDRAULIC *(Surgery) 79FWY*

Berchtold Corp. 800-243-5135
1950 Hanahan Rd, Charleston, SC 29406
OPERON SL.

Brandt Industries, Inc. 800-221-8031
4461 Bronx Blvd, Bronx, NY 10470
Occupational therapy, hydraulic tables.

Bryton Corp. 800-567-9500
4310 Guion Rd, Indianapolis, IN 46254
Complete range of hydraulic operating tables for all types of surgical procedures.

Kma Remarketing Corp. 814-371-5242
302 Aspen Way, Dubois, PA 15801
Manual operating room table.

Medrecon, Inc. 877-526-4323
257 South Ave, Garwood, NJ 07027
Remanufactured units - 2 yr warranty.

Skytron 800-759-8766
5085 Corporate Exchange Blvd SE, Grand Rapids, MI 49512
Three Top Slide Models available. Model 3600B UltraSlide, 1000 lbs. Lift 800 lbs. articulation, 23 inches of top slide, removable back and leg sections., 24' low table height. Model 3501EZSlide Surgical Table, 700 lbs. Lift and 600 lb. articulation with 21 inches of top slide. Full function surgical table with removable leg section and durable pendant control. Model 3003 Impulse 4 way Top Slide Imaging Table with 83 inch carbon fiber top, 65 inch imaging window, 500 lb. capacity, optional sterile joy stick control for top slide, reverse and auto centering button. Features include 4 way slide, height adjustment, tilt, Trendelenburg, reverse Trendelenburg. Durable, back lit pendant control.

TABLE, SURGICAL, MANUAL *(General) 80FSE*

Arizona Industries For The Blind 602-269-5131
3013 W Lincoln St Dept Economicsecurity, Phoenix, AZ 85009
Portable Field Operating Table (NSN#6530-01-321-5592) Used by medical personel for emergency surgical procedures in field conditions. Designed for military, emergency responders, homeland security response

Bryton Corp. 800-567-9500
4310 Guion Rd, Indianapolis, IN 46254
Complete range of operating tables for all surgical procedures.

Composiflex, Inc. 800-673-2544
8100 Hawthorne Dr, Erie, PA 16509
Low x-ray absorption, high strength carbon fiber surgical table tops.

Elmed, Inc. 630-543-2792
60 W Fay Ave, Addison, IL 60101

International Hospital Supply Co. 800-398-9450
6914 Canby Ave Ste 105, Reseda, CA 91335

Kma Remarketing Corp. 814-371-5242
302 Aspen Way, Dubois, PA 15801
Manual operating room table.

Medrecon, Inc. 877-526-4323
257 South Ave, Garwood, NJ 07027
Remanufactured units - 2 yr warranty.

TABLE, SURGICAL, MANUAL *(cont'd)*

Mizuho Osi 800-777-4674
30031 Ahern Ave, Union City, CA 94587
OSI Spinal surgery frame and hand surgery tables. Andrews Spinal Surgery Table, SST-3000.

Rycor Medical, Inc. 800-227-9267
2053 Atwater Dr, North Port, FL 34288
Hand surgical table.

Schuerch Corp. 617-773-0927
48 Oval Rd, Quincy, MA 02170
Various.

Stryker Medical 800-869-0770
3800 E Centre Ave, Portage, MI 49002
TRIO: Mobile Surgery Platform.

Suburban Surgical Co., Inc. 800-323-7366
275 12th St, Wheeling, IL 60090
For veterinary use only: stainless steel top & hydraulic base. Available heated.

Supertech, Inc. 800-654-1054
PO Box 186, Elkhart, IN 46515
Biodex Surgery Tables: Surgery, G-arm brachytherapy

U.S. Table, Inc. 847-741-3650
158 N Edison Ave, Elgin, IL 60123
Bmk-stationary.

United Metal Fabricators, Inc. 800-638-5322
1316 Eisenhower Blvd, Johnstown, PA 15904
All stainless steel or enameled with stainless steel top. Optional vinyl covered pad, shoulder support and knee crutches. Anesthes brakes.

World Medical Equipment, Inc. 800-827-3747
3915 152nd St NE, Marysville, WA 98271
Specialize in refurbished OR tables such as AMSCO/Steris, Skytron, Shampaine and Chick as well as lights, autoclaves, anesthesia machines, monitors, and accessories.

TABLE, SURGICAL, ORTHOPEDIC *(Orthopedics) 87JEB*

Bryton Corp. 800-567-9500
4310 Guion Rd, Indianapolis, IN 46254
Orthopedic table for all types of surgical orthopedic procedures.

Citow Cervical Visualizer Company 646-460-2984
712 S Milwaukee Ave, Libertyville, IL 60048

Composiflex, Inc. 800-673-2544
8100 Hawthorne Dr, Erie, PA 16509
Low x-ray absorption, high strength carbon fiber surgical table tops.

Elmed, Inc. 630-543-2792
60 W Fay Ave, Addison, IL 60101

Frank Scholz X-Ray Corp. 508-586-8308
244 Liberty St, Brockton, MA 02301
$685.00 per unit (standard). Also available standard CLARK socket and combination CLARK socket fixation devices for standard orthopedic and surgical table side rails.

General Hospital Supply Corp. 704-225-9500
2844 Gray Fox Rd, Monroe, NC 28110
Knee positioner.

Hugh's Company 972-672-5092
4930 Mill Creek Rd, Dallas, TX 75244
Tilt table.

Md International, Inc. 305-669-9003
11300 NW 41st St, Doral, FL 33178

Medrecon, Inc. 877-526-4323
257 South Ave, Garwood, NJ 07027
Remanufactured units - 2 yr warranty.

Mizuho Osi 800-777-4674
30031 Ahern Ave, Union City, CA 94587
Ovation table. PROfx Table

Quatro Composites 858-513-4300
13250 Gregg St Ste A1, Poway, CA 92064

Schaerer Mayfield Usa 800-755-6381
4900 Charlemar Dr, Cincinnati, OH 45227
CHICK CLT Orthopedic and Surgical Operating Table. CHICK IOT Imagable Orthopedic Table. CHICK 703 Orthopedic & Surgical Operating Table.

Stryker Medical 800-869-0770
3800 E Centre Ave, Portage, MI 49002

TABLE, SURGICAL, ORTHOPEDIC *(cont'd)*

Telos Medical Equipment (Austin & Assoc., Inc.) 800-934-3029
1109 Sturbridge Rd, Fallston, MD 21047
TELOS O.R. table extension for orthopedic surgery of the hip, pelvis, and lower extremities.

White Surgical, Inc. 901-758-8768
1644 Dogwood Creek Rd, Germantown, TN 38139
Hip and knee positioner.

World Medical Equipment, Inc. 800-827-3747
3915 152nd St NE, Marysville, WA 98271
Specialize in refurbished OR tables such as AMSCO/Steris, OEC, OSI, and Chick as well as lights, autoclaves, anesthesia machines, monitors, and accessories.

TABLE, TRACTION *(Orthopedics) 87RYZ*

Alimed, Inc. 800-225-2610
297 High St, Dedham, MA 02026

Cardon Rehabilitation Products Inc 800-944-7868
908 Niagara Falls Blvd, Wurlitzer Industrial Park
North Tonawanda, NY 14120

Chattanooga Group 800-592-7329
4717 Adams Rd, Hixson, TN 37343
Triton or TX traction tables.

Hill Laboratories Co. 877-445-5020
3 N Bacton Hill Rd, PO Box 2028, Frazer, PA 19355
The Hill Anatomotor has been used successfully for over 50 years. The Anatomotor implements deep muscle therapy with cervical, arm, pelvic, lumbar, and arm-shoulder traction. This versatile table can also be used for passive motion and exercise.

Ossur Americas, Inc 800-222-4284
19762 Pauling, Foothill Ranch, CA 92610
Light weight, sterile traction hand surgery table, radiolucent material to allow x-ray in traction with C-arm.

TABLE, ULTRASOUND *(General) 80WNI*

Aesthetic Technologies, Inc. 303-469-0965
14828 W 6th Ave Ste 9B, Golden, CO 80401
Parisian Peel 'Elite' external ultrasound device, which uses a specially designed facial wand through which ultrasonic waves drive topical antioxidants into the skin, increasing absorption and retention.

Cone Instruments, Inc. 800-321-6964
5201 Naiman Pkwy, Solon, OH 44139

Mxe, Inc. 800-252-1801
12107 Jefferson Blvd, Culver City, CA 90230
Three adjustable sections, motorized hydraulic lift from 27' to 37' height. Stirrups and IV pole are optional.

Northeast Medical Systems Corp. 856-910-8111
901 Beechwood Ave, Cherry Hill, NJ 08002
Four-function motor-driven table with elevation, lateral tilt, Trendelenburg and Fowler.

Stille-Sonesta, Inc. 800-665-1614
1610 S Interstate 35E Ste 203, Carrollton, TX 75006

Supertech, Inc. 800-654-1054
PO Box 186, Elkhart, IN 46515
Biodex Ultrasound Tables: Foot controls, adjustable height, Trendelenberg, reverse Trendelenberg.

TABLE, UROLOGICAL (CYSTOLOGICAL) *(Gastro/Urology) 78RZA*

Bryton Corp. 800-567-9500
4310 Guion Rd, Indianapolis, IN 46254
Urological tables for performing all types of urology procedures.

Elmed, Inc. 630-543-2792
60 W Fay Ave, Addison, IL 60101

Life-Tech, Inc. 281-491-6600
4235 Greenbriar Dr, Stafford, TX 77477
Radiolucent examination tables

Md International, Inc. 305-669-9003
11300 NW 41st St, Doral, FL 33178

Medrecon, Inc. 877-526-4323
257 South Ave, Garwood, NJ 07027
Remanufactured - 2 yr. warranty.

Stille-Sonesta, Inc. 800-665-1614
1610 S Interstate 35E Ste 203, Carrollton, TX 75006

TABLE, UROLOGICAL, NON-ELECTRICAL
(Gastro/Urology) 78EYH

Biodex Medical Systems, Inc. 800-224-6339
20 Ramsey Rd, Shirley, NY 11967
Urology C-Arm Table. Portable, fluoroscopic and radiographic urological C-arm table.

Bryton Corp. 800-567-9500
4310 Guion Rd, Indianapolis, IN 46254
Urological tables for performing all types of urology procedures.

Medrecon, Inc. 877-526-4323
257 South Ave, Garwood, NJ 07027

TABLE, UROLOGICAL, RADIOGRAPHIC *(Gastro/Urology) 78UEE*

Altek Corp. 301-572-2555
12210 Plum Orchard Dr, Silver Spring, MD 20904

Bryton Corp. 800-567-9500
4310 Guion Rd, Indianapolis, IN 46254
Urological tables for performing all types of urological procedures.

Composiflex, Inc. 800-673-2544
8100 Hawthorne Dr, Erie, PA 16509
Low x-ray absorption, high strength carbon fiber urological table tops.

Medrecon, Inc. 877-526-4323
257 South Ave, Garwood, NJ 07027
Remanufactured - 2 yr. warranty.

Stille-Sonesta, Inc. 800-665-1614
1610 S Interstate 35E Ste 203, Carrollton, TX 75006

Vermont Composites, Inc. 802-442-9964
25 Performance Dr, Bennington, VT 05201
Low absorption carbon tops.

TACHOMETER *(General) 80UKT*

Cole-Parmer Instrument Inc. 800-323-4340
625 E Bunker Ct, Vernon Hills, IL 60061

Extech Instruments Corp. 781-890-7440
285 Bear Hill Rd, Waltham, MA 02451
Priced from $229.00 for combination tachometer which measures with or without contact.

Kernco Instruments Co., Inc. 800-325-3875
420 Kenazo Ave., El Paso, TX 79928-7338
Photo, non-contact tachometer: measures RPM speeds on digital centrifuges, up to 99,999 RPM.

Meylan Corporation 888-769-9667
543 Valley Rd, Upper Montclair, NJ 07043
2 digital models - $300.00 (contact) or $355.00 (non-contact).

TACK, SACCULOTOMY (CODY) *(Ear/Nose/Throat) 77ESX*

Gyrus Ent L.L.C., Sub. Of Gyrus Acmi, Inc. 508-804-2739
2925 Appling Rd, Bartlett, TN 38133
Various.

TACTILE HEARING-AID *(Ear/Nose/Throat) 77LRA*

Audiological Engineering Corp. 800-283-4601
9 Preston Rd, Somerville, MA 02143
TACTAID 7 - $2,955, seven-channel device - primarily used in speech training & structured teaching situations. LTD (mini-tactilator) - $975, two-channel device, general purpose, specifically designed for speech reading.

Insiphil (Us) Llc 408-616-8700
650 Vaqueros Ave Ste F, Sunnyvale, CA 94085

TAG, DEVICE STATUS *(General) 80QPG*

Bio-Logics Products, Inc. 800-426-7577
PO Box 505, West Jordan, UT 84084
Label printer makes labels from patient's tag in ID band.

Idesco Corp. 800-336-1383
37 W 26th St, New York, NY 10010

Key Surgical, Inc. 800-541-7995
8101 Wallace Rd Ste 100, Eden Prairie, MN 55344
Repair/code tags - sterilizable, tamper-proof, locking tags for coding in/out dates on trays. Tags for identifying instruments that are damaged and need repair. Twelve colors, two sizes available.

Medical Safety Systems Inc. 888-803-9303
230 White Pond Dr, Akron, OH 44313
Hazardous materials label kit; infection control labels and waterproof hazardous materials labels.

National Systems Co. 877-672-4278
31B Durward Pl., Waterloo N2J 3Z9 Canada
Alert flags for physicians, nurses, etc.

TAG, DEVICE STATUS *(cont'd)*

Tailored Label Products, Inc. 800-727-1344
W165N5731 Ridgewood Dr, Menomonee Falls, WI 53051

TAMP *(Orthopedics) 87HXG*

Abbott Spine, Inc. 847-937-6100
12708 Riata Vista Cir Ste B-100, Austin, TX 78727
Tamp.

Biomet, Inc. 574-267-6639
56 E Bell Dr, PO Box 587, Warsaw, IN 46582
Various types of orthopedic wire tamps.

Depuy Spine, Inc. 800-227-6633
325 Paramount Dr, Raynham, MA 02767
Impactor.

K2m, Inc. 866-526-4171
751 Miller Dr SE Ste F1, Leesburg, VA 20175
Tamp.

Medtronic Sofamor Danek Instrument Manufacturing 901-396-3133
7375 Adrianne Pl, Bartlett, TN 38133
Multple tamps.

Medtronic Sofamor Danek Usa, Inc. 901-396-3133
4340 Swinnea Rd, Memphis, TN 38118
Multple tamps.

Medtronic Spine Llc 877-690-5353
1221 Crossman Ave, Sunnyvale, CA 94089
Various types of sterile, inflatable bone tamps.

Osseon Therapeutics, Inc. 877-567-7366
2330 Circadian Way, Santa Rosa, CA 95407

Spine Wave, Inc. 203-944-9494
2 Enterprise Dr Ste 302, Shelton, CT 06484
Various types of tamps.

Symmetry Medical Usa, Inc. 574-267-8700
486 W 350 N, Warsaw, IN 46582
Bone tamp.

Warsaw Orthopedic, Inc. 901-396-3133
2500 Silveus Xing, Warsaw, IN 46582
Multple tamps.

Zimmer Holdings, Inc. 800-613-6131
1800 W Center St, PO Box 708, Warsaw, IN 46580

Zimmer Spine, Inc. 800-655-2614
7375 Bush Lake Rd, Minneapolis, MN 55439
Tamp.

Zimmer Trabecular Metal Technology 800-613-6131
10 Pomeroy Rd, Parsippany, NJ 07054
Acetabular, restrictor trial-tamp.

TAMPON, MENSTRUAL, SCENTED *(Obstetrics/Gyn) 85HIL*

Gomez Packaging Corp. 973-569-9500
75 Wood St, Paterson, NJ 07524
Scented or scented deodorized menstrual tampons.

J&J Healthcare Products Div Mcneil-Ppc, Inc 866-565-2229
199 Grandview Rd, Skillman, NJ 08558

Tambrands Manufacturing, Inc. 513-634-2466
2879 Hotel Rd, Auburn, ME 04210
Tampon, scented.

TAMPON, MENSTRUAL, UNSCENTED *(Obstetrics/Gyn) 85HEB*

C & D Industries, Inc. 413-534-6144
28 Appleton St, Holyoke, MA 01040
Tampax tampons.

Health Care Products, Inc. 419-678-9620
410 Nisco St, Coldwater, OH 45828
Tampon.

J&J Healthcare Products Div Mcneil-Ppc, Inc 866-565-2229
199 Grandview Rd, Skillman, NJ 08558
O.b. tampons.

Organic Essentials 800-765-6491
822 Baldridge St, Odonnell, TX 79351
Organic essentials.

Qpsi Mass, Llc 413-789-6500
609 Silver St, Agawam, MA 01001
Tampons.

QuantRx Biomedical Corp. 503-252-9565
5920 NE 112th Ave, Portland, OR 97220
INSYNC MINIFORM

TAMPON, MENSTRUAL, UNSCENTED *(cont'd)*

Tambrands Manufacturing, Inc. 513-634-2466
2879 Hotel Rd, Auburn, ME 04210
Menstrual tampon-vatrious absorbencies & applicator types.

TANK, DEVELOPING, TLC *(Toxicology) 91DKK*

Carr Corporation 800-952-2398
1547 11th St, Santa Monica, CA 90401

Schueler & Company, Inc. 516-487-1500
PO Box 528, Stratford, CT 06615

TANK, FULL BODY (BATH) *(General) 80RZD*

Arjo, Inc. 800-323-1245
50 Gary Ave Ste A, Roselle, IL 60172
Rectangular and butterfly-shaped tanks with or without patient lifts and disinfection system.

Burch Manufacturing Co., Inc. 515-573-4136
618 1st Ave N, Fort Dodge, IA 50501
One type of Kolaps-A-Tank is a Decontamination Booth comes vertial or horizon. Another type of Kolaps-A-Tank is FDA approved for storing drinking water.Kolaps-A-Tank portable water container, seven different sizes.

Contemporary Products, Inc. 800-424-2444
530 Riverside Industrial Pkwy, Portland, ME 04103
WAVE CONSERVER - a pulse demand unit, programmed to deliver bolus of oxygen at the peak inspiratory moment.

Ferno-Washington, Inc. 800-733-3766
70 Weil Way, Wilmington, OH 45177

Galaxy Aquatics, Inc. 713-464-0303
1075 W Sam Houston Pkwy N Ste 210, Houston, TX 77043
All-tile therapy pools and spas for hospitals and therapy clinics.

Samadhi Tank Co. 888-755-7700
PO Box 2119, Nevada City, CA 95959

Whitehall Manufacturing 800-782-7706
15125 Proctor Ave, City Of Industry, CA 91746
Total immersion body tanks in rectangular 260 or 300 gallons or Hubbard Tanks in 268 or 325 gallons. Ideal usage burn victims or a patient requiring rehabilitative hydrotherapy.

TANK, HOLDING, DIALYSIS *(Gastro/Urology) 78FIN*

Ameriwater 937-461-8833
1303 Stanley Ave, Dayton, OH 45404
Hemodialysis system and accessories.

Better Water, Inc. 615-355-6063
698 Swan Dr, Smyrna, TN 37167
Sodium bicarbonate mixing/delivery system & concentrate delivery system.

Civco Medical Instruments Co., Inc. 319-656-4447
102 1st St S, Kalona, IA 52247
Various types of ultrasound transducer holders.

Dialysis Dimensions, Inc. 615-292-0333
2003 Blair Blvd, Nashville, TN 37212
Bicarbonate mixing/delivery system.

G.E.M. Water Systems, Int'L., Llc 800-755-1707
6351 Orangethorpe Ave, Buena Park, CA 90620
Carbon tanks; dialysis mixing tank, sodium-carbonate with water.

Medical Solutions International, Inc. 757-224-0177
5646 Merriam Dr, Merriam, KS 66203
Bicarb mixing system for dialysis.

Pure Water, Inc. 864-375-0105
311 W Market St, Anderson, SC 29624
Various types of acidified storage & distribution system.

Whitehall Manufacturing 800-782-7706
15125 Proctor Ave, City Of Industry, CA 91746
Dialysis supply & waste boxes.

TAP, BONE *(Orthopedics) 87HWX*

Abbott Spine, Inc. 847-937-6100
12708 Riata Vista Cir Ste B-100, Austin, TX 78727
Tap.

Ascent Healthcare Solutions 480-763-5300
10232 S 51st St, Phoenix, AZ 85044
Tap.

Biomet Microfixation Inc. 800-874-7711
1520 Tradeport Dr, Jacksonville, FL 32218
Tap, bone.

Biomet, Inc. 574-267-6639
56 E Bell Dr, PO Box 587, Warsaw, IN 46582
Various types of bone screw taps.

TAP, BONE *(cont'd)*

Bioplate, Inc. 310-815-2100
3643 Lenawee Ave, Los Angeles, CA 90016
Tap, bone.

Depuy Mitek, A Johnson & Johnson Company 800-451-2006
50 Scotland Blvd, Bridgewater, MA 02324
Various bone taps.

Depuy Spine, Inc. 800-227-6633
325 Paramount Dr, Raynham, MA 02767
Bone tap.

DJO Inc. 800-336-6569
1430 Decision St, Vista, CA 92081

Grace Engineering Corp. 810-392-2181
34775 Potter St, Memphis, MI 48041
Bone tap.

Holmed Corporation 508-238-3351
40 Norfolk Ave, South Easton, MA 02375

Interventional Spine, Inc. 800-497-0484
13700 Alton Pkwy Ste 160, Irvine, CA 92618
Tap.

K2m, Inc. 866-526-4171
751 Miller Dr SE Ste F1, Leesburg, VA 20175
Tap.

Kmedic 800-955-0559
190 Veterans Dr, Northvale, NJ 07647

Lenox-Maclaren Surgical Corp. 720-890-9660
657 S Taylor Ave Ste A, Colorado Technology Center
Louisville, CO 80027
Tap, bone.

Medisiss 866-866-7477
2747 SW 6th St, Redmond, OR 97756
Various bone taps,sterile.

Onyx Medical Corp. 901-323-6699
152 Collins St, Memphis, TN 38112

RTI Biologics Inc. 877-343-6832
11621 Research Cir, Alachua, FL 32615
Ht tap, st tap.

Spine Wave, Inc. 203-944-9494
2 Enterprise Dr Ste 302, Shelton, CT 06484
Tap.

Sterilmed, Inc. 763-488-3400
11400 73rd Ave N Ste 100, Maple Grove, MN 55369
Bone tap.

Stryker Spine 866-457-7463
2 Pearl Ct, Allendale, NJ 07401

Synthes (Usa) 610-719-5000
35 Airport Rd, Horseheads, NY 14845
Various types and sizes of bone taps.

Tsugami / Rem Sales Inc. 860-687-3400
910 Day Hill Rd, Windsor, CT 06095
Specialized machinery for the production of taps, bone screws, fixation devices, and inplants.

Warsaw Orthopedic, Inc. 901-396-3133
2500 Silveus Xing, Warsaw, IN 46582
Bone tap.

Zimmer Holdings, Inc. 800-613-6131
1800 W Center St, PO Box 708, Warsaw, IN 46580

Zimmer Spine, Inc. 800-655-2614
7375 Bush Lake Rd, Minneapolis, MN 55439
Bone tap.

TAPE, ADHESIVE *(General) 80RZE*

Arlon Engineered Coated Products 800-232-7181
6110 Rittiman Rd, San Antonio, TX 78218
Skin contact.

Brady Precision Converting, Llc 214-275-9595
1801 Big Town Blvd Ste 100, Mesquite, TX 75149
Skin contact adhesive tapes.

Covidien Lp 508-261-8000
15 Hampshire St, Mansfield, MA 02048
EXPANDOVER elastic adhesive tape stretches evenly, unique elasticity, patient-friendly adhesive removal, exclusive design and construction, can be torn by hand.

Csi Holdings 615-452-9633
170 Commerce Way, Gallatin, TN 37066

TAPE, ADHESIVE *(cont'd)*

Delstar Technologies, Inc. 800-521-6713
601 Industrial Rd, Middletown, DE 19709
DEL PORE medical, porous polymer tape for adhering dressings & bandages.

Dukal Corporation 800-243-0741
5 Plant Ave, Hauppauge, NY 11788
Short rolls available.

Hartmann-Conco Inc. 800-243-2294
481 Lakeshore Pkwy, Rock Hill, SC 29730
AC-Tape latex-free all-cotton elastic adhesive tape that delivers unmatched strength and security. Pro's Choice latex-free athletic tape with superior tensile strength and firm support.

IZI Medical Products 800-231-1499
7020 Tudsbury Rd, Baltimore, MD 21244
Soft Strip

Johnson & Johnson Medical Division Of Ethicon, Inc. 800-423-4018
2500 E Arbrook Blvd, Arlington, TX 76014

Kck Industries 888-800-1967
14941 Calvert St, Van Nuys, CA 91411

Key Surgical, Inc. 800-541-7995
8101 Wallace Rd Ste 100, Eden Prairie, MN 55344
Instrument identification tape in 1/8-, 1/4-, and 3/8-in. widths.

M&C Specialties Co. 800-441-6996
90 James Way, Southampton, PA 18966

Medi Inc 800-225-8634
75 York Ave, P.O. Box 302, Randolph, MA 02368
Trainers tape. Athletic tape, athletic training supplies.

Pacon Manufacturing Corporation 732-357-8020
400 Pierce St # B, Somerset, NJ 08873
Surgical drape tape.

Pepin Manufacturing, Inc. 800-291-6505
1875 S Highway 61, Lake City, MN 55041
Precision slitting and rewinding of tape for all applications. Specializing in narrow widths.

Silverstone Packaging, Inc.-Your One Stop Supplier 800-413-1108
1401 Lakeland Ave, Bohemia, NY 11716

Smi 920-876-3361
Industrial Park, 544 Sohn Drive, Elkhart Lake, WI 53020

Sterion, Incorporated 800-328-7958
13828 Lincoln St NE, Ham Lake, MN 55304
ColorTrack Instrument Marking Tape--sheet and roll. Strips and solids in 70 color combinations. XtraGentle Surgical Tape coated with Gel-X pressure sensitive adhesive recommended for patients with friable or sensitive skin. STERION Surgical Tape Strips available in paper, elastic, transparent plastic or silk. Convenient to carry in pocket. DuoPlas HP&GP Double Adhesive Surgical Tape developed for medical uses such as configuring drapes, pouching, or securement of small devices to material.

Tailored Label Products, Inc. 800-727-1344
W165N5731 Ridgewood Dr, Menomonee Falls, WI 53051

Timemed Labeling Systems, Inc. 800-323-4840
144 Tower Dr, Burr Ridge, IL 60527
Assorted pressure sensitive tape and labeling systems.

TAPE, ADHESIVE, HYPOALLERGENIC *(General) 80RZF*

Brady Precision Converting, Llc 214-275-9595
1801 Big Town Blvd Ste 100, Mesquite, TX 75149
Adhesive tapes with FDA approved skin contact adhesives. Tapes can be made with very gentle relase to very aggressive adhesion.

Csi Holdings 615-452-9633
170 Commerce Way, Gallatin, TN 37066

Dumex Medical Surgical Products Ltd. 800-463-9613
104 Shorting Rd., Scarborough, ONT M1S 3S4 Canada

Global Healthcare 800-601-3880
1495 Hembree Rd Ste 700, Roswell, GA 30076
Impervious Clear, Paper, Silk, Transparent semi-permeable, and Zinc Oxide tapes.

H.B. Fuller Company 800-328-9673
1200 Willow Lake Blvd, PO Box 64683, Saint Paul, MN 55110
Packaging/converting latex-free adhesives for skin and medical tapes.

Johnson & Johnson Medical Division Of Ethicon, Inc. 800-423-4018
2500 E Arbrook Blvd, Arlington, TX 76014

TAPE, ADHESIVE, HYPOALLERGENIC *(cont'd)*

M&C Specialties Co. 800-441-6996
90 James Way, Southampton, PA 18966

Tailored Label Products, Inc. 800-727-1344
W165N5731 Ridgewood Dr, Menomonee Falls, WI 53051

Taylor Industries, Inc. 800-339-1361
2706 Industrial Dr, Jefferson City, MO 65109

TAPE, ADHESIVE, WATERPROOF *(General) 80RZG*

Hy-Tape International 800-248-0101
70 Jon Barrett Rd, Robin Hill Corporate Park, Patterson, NY 12563
HY-TAPE Adhesive tape with zinc oxide base that is soothing to delicate skin. Water resistant, washable and can be applied to wet or oily skin. Latex free.

Johnson & Johnson Consumer Products, Inc. 800-526-3967
199 Grandview Rd, Skillman, NJ 08558

Johnson & Johnson Medical Division Of Ethicon, Inc. 800-423-4018
2500 E Arbrook Blvd, Arlington, TX 76014

M&C Specialties Co. 800-441-6996
90 James Way, Southampton, PA 18966

Tailored Label Products, Inc. 800-727-1344
W165N5731 Ridgewood Dr, Menomonee Falls, WI 53051

Urocare Products, Inc. 800-423-4441
2735 Melbourne Ave, Pomona, CA 91767
URO-BOND, medical adhesive and CONSTAY tape.

TAPE, COTTON *(General) 80RZH*

Hartmann-Conco Inc. 800-243-2294
481 Lakeshore Pkwy, Rock Hill, SC 29730
AC-Tape latex-free all cotton elastic adhesive tape that delivers unmatched strength and security.

Valley Products Co. 800-451-8874
PO Box 187, York New Salem, PA 17371
Twill tapes, braided cords/ropes and printed cloth labels.

TAPE, GAUZE, ADHESIVE *(General) 80WMH*

Chagrin Safety Supply, Inc. 800-227-0468
8227 Washington St # 1, Chagrin Falls, OH 44023

Covidien Lp 508-261-8000
15 Hampshire St, Mansfield, MA 02048
EXPANDOVER is a patented, high strength, elastic adhesive tape. It is highly breathable, can be torn by hand, and allows for controlled compression.

Cypress Medical Products 800-334-3646
1202 S. Rte. 31, McHenry, IL 60050
Available in 1/2', 1' and 2' widths in paper, cloth and transparent. Hypoallergenic. Air and moisture permeable.

Johnson & Johnson Medical Division Of Ethicon, Inc. 800-423-4018
2500 E Arbrook Blvd, Arlington, TX 76014

M&C Specialties Co. 800-441-6996
90 James Way, Southampton, PA 18966

Mylan Technologies, Inc. 800-532-5226
110 Lake St, Saint Albans, VT 05478
MEDIDERM, high moisture vapor permeable yet biologically occlusive laminates.

Pedinol Pharmacal, Inc. 800-733-4665
30 Banfi Plz N, Farmingdale, NY 11735

Smith & Nephew, Inc. 800-876-1261
11775 Starkey Rd, Largo, FL 33773
HYPAFIX dressing retention sheet.

TAPE, MEASURING, RULER AND CALIPER *(Surgery) 79FTY*

Advanced Concept Innovations Llc 863-577-8055
4100 Frontage Rd S, Lakeland, FL 33815

Aesculap Implant Systems Inc. 1-800-234-9179
3773 Corporate Pkwy, Center Valley, PA 18034

Bausch & Lomb Surgical 636-255-5051
3365 Tree Court Ind Blvd, Saint Louis, MO 63122

Biomet Microfixation Inc. 800-874-7711
1520 Tradeport Dr, Jacksonville, FL 32218
Tape, measuring, rulers and calipers.

Biomet, Inc. 574-267-6639
56 E Bell Dr, PO Box 587, Warsaw, IN 46582
Various types of measuring devices.

TAPE, MEASURING, RULER AND CALIPER *(cont'd)*

Cardinal Health, Snowden Pencer Products 847-689-8410
5175 S Royal Atlanta Dr, Tucker, GA 30084
Various types of measuring instruments for surgery.

Cardiovascular Systems, Inc. 877-CSI-0360
651 Campus Dr, Saint Paul, MN 55112
ViperTrack

Creative Health Products, Inc. 800-742-4478
5148 Saddle Ridge Rd, Plymouth, MI 48170
$21.95 for CHP unit, Gulick type tension calibrated measuring tape.

Diamond Edge Co. 727-586-2927
928 W Bay Dr, Largo, FL 33770
Blade extension measuring reticle.

Ethicon, Inc. 800-4-ETHICON
Route 22 West, Somerville, NJ 08876

Ge Medical Systems, Llc 262-548-2355
3000 N Grandview Blvd, W-417, Waukesha, WI 53188
X-ray caliper.

Hansen Ophthalmic Development Lab 319-338-1285
745 Avalon Pl, Coralville, IA 52241
Curved ruler for measurement along the surface of the globe.

Integra Neurosciences Pr 800-654-2873
Road 402 North, Km 1.2, Anasco, PR 00610
Line level, rulers.

Miltex Dental Technologies, Inc. 516-576-6022
589 Davies Dr, York, PA 17402
Rulers.

Novel Products, Inc. 800-323-5143
PO Box 408, Rockton, IL 61072
Medical tensioning tape measure.

Pac-Dent Intl., Inc. 909-839-0888
21078 Commerce Point Dr, Walnut, CA 91789
Endodontic ruler.

S&S Technology 281-815-1300
10625 Telge Rd, Houston, TX 77095

Spinus, Llc 603-758-1444
8 Merrill Industrial Dr, Hampton, NH 03842
Radiopaque anterior spine center locator.

Symmetry Medical Usa, Inc. 574-267-8700
486 W 350 N, Warsaw, IN 46582
Caliper.

Vq Orthocare
1390 Decision St Ste A, Vista, CA 92081
Measuring tape.

Warsaw Orthopedic, Inc. 901-396-3133
2500 Silveus Xing, Warsaw, IN 46582
Ruler.

Zimmer Holdings, Inc. 800-613-6131
1800 W Center St, PO Box 708, Warsaw, IN 46580

Zimmer Spine, Inc. 800-655-2614
7375 Bush Lake Rd, Minneapolis, MN 55439
Tape, measuring, rulers and calipers.

TAPE, ORTHOPEDIC *(Orthopedics) 87HXT*

Arrowhead Athletics 800-225-1516
220 Andover St, PO Box 4264, Andover, MA 01810
Athletic and therapeutic tapes.

Debusk Orthopedic Casting (Doc) 865-362-2334
420 Straight Creek Rd Ste 1, New Tazewell, TN 37825
Fiberglass casting tape.

Dumex Medical Surgical Products Ltd. 800-463-9613
104 Shorting Rd., Scarborough, ONT M1S 3S4 Canada

Medist International 901-380-9411
9160 Highway 64 Ste 12, Lakeland, TN 38002
Tendon spacer.

Modern Aids, Inc. 847-437-8600
201 Bond St, Elk Grove Village, IL 60007
Gauztape.

Ossur Americas 949-268-3155
742 Pancho Rd, Camarillo, CA 93012

Patterson Medical Supply, Inc. 262-387-8720
W68N158 Evergreen Blvd, Cedarburg, WI 53012
Various sizes of orthopedic tape.

Valley Products Co. 800-451-8874
PO Box 187, York New Salem, PA 17371
Orthopedic elastic tapes and webbings.

TAPE, TELEVISION & VIDEO, ENDOSCOPIC
(Gastro/Urology) 78FET

Cardinal Health, Snowden Pencer Products 847-689-8410
5175 S Royal Atlanta Dr, Tucker, GA 30084
Surgical cameras,cables.

Karl Storz Endoscopy-America Inc. 800-421-0837
600 Corporate Pointe, Culver City, CA 90230

Minrad, Inc. 716-855-1068
50 Cobham Dr, Orchard Park, NY 14127
Color television camera.

Olympus America, Inc. 800-645-8160
3500 Corporate Pkwy, PO Box 610, Center Valley, PA 18034

Print Media, Inc. 800-994-3318
9002 NW 105th Way, Medley, FL 33178
Full Line of brand name audio, video and digital recording media available.

Richard Wolf Medical Instruments Corp. 800-323-9653
353 Corporate Woods Pkwy, Vernon Hills, IL 60061

Smith & Nephew, Inc., Endoscopy Division 800-343-8386
150 Minuteman Rd, Andover, MA 01810

Sony Electronics, Inc., Medical Systems Div. 800-686-7669
1 Sony Dr, Park Ridge, NJ 07656

Stryker Endoscopy 800-435-0220
5900 Optical Ct, San Jose, CA 95138

TAPE, UMBILICAL *(General) 80RZI*

Covidien Lp 508-261-8000
15 Hampshire St, Mansfield, MA 02048
Two strands, 1/8in. round x 30in. tape sizes.

Ethicon, Inc. 800-4-ETHICON
Route 22 West, Somerville, NJ 08876

Gudebrod, Inc. 877-249-2211
274 Shoemaker Rd, Pottstown, PA 19464
1/2in., 3/8in., 1/4in. & 1/8in. braided polyester.

TARGET, FUSION/STEREOSCOPIC *(Ophthalmology) 86HLP*

Mast/Keystone View 800-806-6569
2200 Dickerson Rd, Reno, NV 89503
Keystone view makes several fusion test target cards that can be used with the stereoscope instruments or the TELEBINOCULAR.

Stereo Optical Co., Inc. 800-344-9500
3539 N Kenton Ave, Chicago, IL 60641

Vision Assessment Corp. 847-239-5889
2675 Coyle Ave, Elk Grove Village, IL 60007
Stereo depth perception test.

TARTRATE INHIBITED, ACID PHOSPHATASE (PROSTATIC)
(Chemistry) 75JFH

Beckman Coulter, Inc. 800-635-3497
740 W 83rd St, Hialeah, FL 33014
$0.17 per test.

TEACHING ATTACHMENT, ENDOSCOPIC *(Gastro/Urology) 78FEA*

Jedmed Instruments Co. 314-845-3770
5416 Jedmed Ct, Saint Louis, MO 63129

Karl Storz Endoscopy-America Inc. 800-421-0837
600 Corporate Pointe, Culver City, CA 90230

Mahe International Inc. 800-294-7946
468 Craighead St, Nashville, TN 37204

Pentax Medical Company 800-431-5880
102 Chestnut Ridge Rd, Montvale, NJ 07645
$5,775.00 for assistant's observerscope, lightweight and compact. Photography possible through eyepiece. Adapters available for use with endoscopes from other manufacturers.

Pentax Southern Region Service Center 201-571-2300
8934 Kirby Dr, Houston, TX 77054
Observeroscope.

Pentax West Coast Service Center 800-431-5880
10410 Pioneer Blvd Ste 2, Santa Fe Springs, CA 90670
Pentax observeroscope.

Richard Wolf Medical Instruments Corp. 800-323-9653
353 Corporate Woods Pkwy, Vernon Hills, IL 60061

TEETH, ARTIFICIAL, BACKING AND FACING
(Dental And Oral) 76ELK

American Tooth Industries 800-235-4639
1200 Stellar Dr, Oxnard, CA 93033
JUSTI IMPERIAL acrylic teeth and plastic blended facings.

TEETH, ARTIFICIAL, BACKING AND FACING *(cont'd)*

Astron Dental Corporation 847-726-8787
815 Oakwood Rd Ste G, Lake Zurich, IL 60047
Vinyl teeth.

Dentsply Canada, Ltd. 800-263-1437
161 Vinyl Ct., Woodbridge, ONT L4L 4A3 Canada

Intergrated Dental Solutions, Inc. 858-643-1143
6195 Cornerstone Ct E Ste 108, San Diego, CA 92121
Gold coping,crown & bridge.

Ivoclar Vivadent, Inc. 800-533-6825
175 Pineview Dr, Amherst, NY 14228

Lactona Corporation 215-692-9000
1669 School Rd, P.o. Box 428, Hatfield, PA 19440

Tds U-Best Dental Technology 714-666-2288
2941 E Miraloma Ave Ste 6, Anaheim, CA 92806
Coping, crown, inlay, onlay, veneer.

TEETH, ARTIFICIAL, POSTERIOR WITH METAL INSERT
(Dental And Oral) 76ELJ

Advanced Aesthetic Solutions 757-224-0177
631 B/c Keeaumoku St., Honolulu, HI 96814

Aurum Ceramic Dental Laboratories Llp 403-228-5199
1320 N Howard St, Spokane, WA 99201
Dental prosthesis.

Dentsply Canada, Ltd. 800-263-1437
161 Vinyl Ct., Woodbridge, ONT L4L 4A3 Canada

Intergrated Dental Solutions, Inc. 858-643-1143
6195 Cornerstone Ct E Ste 108, San Diego, CA 92121
Pfm,crown & bridge.

Ivory Dental Laboratory 323-663-6422
4205 Santa Monica Blvd, Los Angeles, CA 90029
Fabricated porcelain tooth with metal insert.

Kainos Dental Laboratory 925-943-2332
1844 San Miguel Dr Ste 308B, Walnut Creek, CA 94596
Types of artifical teeth.

Orchid Dental Studio, Inc 469-619-2368
1101 E Plano Pkwy Ste J, Plano, TX 75074
Crowns and bridges / dental.

Scodenco, Inc. 918-627-6795
7405 E 31st Pl, Tulsa, OK 74145
O-so dental attachment.

TEETH, PORCELAIN *(Dental And Oral) 76ELL*

A Plus Dental Lab 215-996-4177
1700 Horizon Dr, --suite 104, Chalfont, PA 18914
Porcelain teeth.

American Dental Designs Inc. 215-643-3232
1116 Horsham Rd, North Wales, PA 19454
Full ceramic crown, pfm.

Aurident, Inc. 714-523-5544
610 S State College Blvd, Fullerton, CA 92831
Various porcelain names.

Cardent International, Inc. 866-764-6832
1568 NW 89th Ct, Doral, FL 33172

Carter Dental Lab, Llc 870-673-1568
301 S Grand Ave, Stuttgart, AR 72160
Porcelain crown.

Dentsply Canada, Ltd. 800-263-1437
161 Vinyl Ct., Woodbridge, ONT L4L 4A3 Canada

Eurotech Dental Laboratory, Inc. 307-234-6808
301 N McKinley St, Casper, WY 82601
Porcelain crowns, bridges, gold crowns.

Global Dentech Inc. 215-654-1237
1116 Horsham Rd, North Wales, PA 19454
Crown, pfm, bridges, veneer and denture.

Golden Empire Dental Lab Corp. 661-327-1888
929 21st St, Bakersfield, CA 93301
False teeth, bridges.

Hennessy Dental Laboratory 800-694-6862
3709 Interstate Park Rd S, Riviera Beach, FL 33404
EMPRESS II - All ceramic, full porcelain restorations.

Hermanson Dental 800-328-9648
1055 Highway 36 E, Saint Paul, MN 55109

TEETH, PORCELAIN *(cont'd)*

Ivoclar Vivadent, Inc. 800-533-6825
175 Pineview Dr, Amherst, NY 14228
VIVOPERL PE Offer precisely crafted construction. Each tooth features an intricate series of layers skillfully applied to achieve the subtleties of natural luminescense and esthetics.

Mason Dental Midwest, Inc. 734-525-1070
12752 Stark Rd, Livonia, MI 48150
Crown and bridge/partials and dentures.

Nobel Biocare Procera Llc. 714-282-5074
800 Corporate Dr, Mahwah, NJ 07430
Procera crowns.

Nobel Biocare Procera, Inc. 201-828-9268
800 Corporate Dr, Mahwah, NJ 07430
Procera.

Nobel Biocare Usa, Llc 800-579-6515
22715/22725 Savi Ranch Parkway, Yorba Linda, CA 92887
Crowns and copings.

Pentron Laboratory Technologies 203-265-7397
53 N Plains Industrial Rd, Wallingford, CT 06492
Porcelaintooth.

Read Dental Lab 337-496-3706
1508 Ford St, Lake Charles, LA 70601
Porcelain teeth, crowns, bridges.

Univac Dental Company 800-523-2559
113 Park Dr, PO Box 447, Montgomeryville, PA 18936
Porcelain Teeth

3m Espe Dental Products 949-863-1360
2111 McGaw Ave, Irvine, CA 92614
$89.95 for porcelain repair refill.

TELEMETRY UNIT, PHYSIOLOGICAL, ECG

(Cardiovascular) 74RZJ

Biotelemetrics, Inc. 561-394-0315
6520 Contempo Ln, Boca Raton, FL 33433
Implantable; $495.00 FM model CFM-8, single channel, DC to 7,000-Hz bandwidth; 87-145 MHz, tunable, 0.7 gm, implantable; also for external measurements. Also for measuring ECGs, EEGs, and EMGs externally compatible with most transducers and sensors.

Ge Medical Systems Information Technologies 800-643-6439
8200 W Tower Ave, Milwaukee, WI 53223
Includes multi-lead arrhythmia analysis; Einthoven lead scheme displays any 4 of the standard frontal plane leads of the 12-lead ECG, dual-diversity antenna reception, programmable receivers; 1-, 8- and 24-hour trends, lead-fail out-of-range indicator, low battery indicator, remote graph start, and alarm-off buttons. Select mode for either lead transmitted, QRS tones, and adjustable gain.

Konigsberg Instruments, Inc. 626-449-0016
2000 E Foothill Blvd, Pasadena, CA 91107
Medical Research, Discovery Research, Safety Pharmacology, Special systems for Biocontainment Levels 2, 3 and 4.

Life Sensing Instrument Company, Inc. 800-624-2732
329 W Lincoln St, Tullahoma, TN 37388

Maguire Enterprises, Inc. 800-548-9686
10289 NW 46th St, Sunrise, FL 33351
ECG modulator unit to convert defibrillator output into telephone or radio transmittable signals.

Mcdalt Medical Corp. 800-841-5774
2225 Prestonwood Dr Ste 100-A, Arlington, TX 76012
Health Monitoring Service, Cardiac Loop ECG Event Monitoring, Dual Holter/Ambulatory ABP, Telemetry @ Home HEARTLINK II, Sub-Maximal Stress Testing.

New Life Systems, Inc. 954-972-4600
PO Box 8767, Coral Springs, FL 33075
All types.

Nihon Kohden America, Inc. 800-325-0283
90 Icon, Foothill Ranch, CA 92610

Rozinn By Scottcare Corporation 800-243-9412
4791 W 150th St, Cleveland, OH 44135
TeleRehab™ Advantage a powerful and affordable telemetry monitoring system designed for cardiopulmonary rehabilitation. ScottCare has a flexible Advantage solution for you.

Vitalcom, Inc. 800-888-0077
15222 Del Amo Ave, Tustin, CA 92780

TELEMETRY UNIT, PHYSIOLOGICAL, EEG

(Cns/Neurology) 84RZK

Konigsberg Instruments, Inc. 626-449-0016
2000 E Foothill Blvd, Pasadena, CA 91107
Medical Research, Discovery Research, Safety Pharmacology, Special systems for Biocontainment Levels 2, 3 and 4.

Nihon Kohden America, Inc. 800-325-0283
90 Icon, Foothill Ranch, CA 92610

TELEMETRY UNIT, PHYSIOLOGICAL, EMG *(Physical Med) 89RZL*

Konigsberg Instruments, Inc. 626-449-0016
2000 E Foothill Blvd, Pasadena, CA 91107
Gait Analysis, Fnictional Assessment, Biomechanics, Medical Research, Discovery Research, Safety Pharmacology

TELEMETRY UNIT, PHYSIOLOGICAL, EOG

(Cns/Neurology) 84RZM

Konigsberg Instruments, Inc. 626-449-0016
2000 E Foothill Blvd, Pasadena, CA 91107
Medical Research, Discovery Research, Safety Pharmacology

TELEMETRY UNIT, PHYSIOLOGICAL, MULTIPLE CHANNEL

(General) 80TEZ

Ge Medical Systems Information Technologies 800-643-6439
8200 W Tower Ave, Milwaukee, WI 53223
Holter aquisition unit for telemetry allowing 2-lead Holter data to be recorded directly from the Series 7700 telemetry system, which transmits dual leads. Each acquisition unit allows 6 Holter modules to be used simultaneously. Up to two Holter acquisition units can be connected in series to allow a maximum of 12 patients for simultaneous Holter monitoring; single-patient remote receiver monitor, AC or battery powered, with QRS tones, high and low heart rate alarms, 4-second ECG display, HR trends. Telemetry Central Station, provides centralized monitoring for telemetry as well as bedside monitors. The display provides waveform as well as key vital-sign data in digital form for up to eight patients per central station. User-friendly interactive controls allow access of individual patient information for review and print, including graphic trends, tabular vital signs, arrhythmia history events, unit defaults, and all limits. Also Telemetry Antenna System, omni-directional, diversity type; the multi-field antenna is similar to that used in cellular telecommunications. A more stable and accurate signal from each monitored patient is attained by the reduction in signal fade or dropout.

Konigsberg Instruments, Inc. 626-449-0016
2000 E Foothill Blvd, Pasadena, CA 91107
Medical Research, Discovery Research, Safety Pharmacology, Special systems for Biocontainment Levels 2, 3 and 4.

Nihon Kohden America, Inc. 800-325-0283
90 Icon, Foothill Ranch, CA 92610

Vitalcom, Inc. 800-888-0077
15222 Del Amo Ave, Tustin, CA 92780

TELEMETRY UNIT, PHYSIOLOGICAL, NEUROLOGICAL

(Cns/Neurology) 84GYE

Cardinal Healthcare 209, Inc. 610-862-0800
5225 Verona Rd, Fitchburg, WI 53711
Multichannel biotelemetry system.

Criticare Systems, Inc. 262-798-5361
20925 Crossroads Cir, Waukesha, WI 53186
Various models of central monitor.

Ge Medical Systems Information Technologies 800-643-6439
8200 W Tower Ave, Milwaukee, WI 53223

Konigsberg Instruments, Inc. 626-449-0016
2000 E Foothill Blvd, Pasadena, CA 91107
Medical Research, Discovery Research, Safety Pharmacology, Special systems for Biocontainment Levels 2, 3 and 4.

TELEMETRY UNIT, PHYSIOLOGICAL, PRESSURE

(General) 80RZN

Ekeg Electronics Co. Ltd. 604-857-0828
PO Box 46199, Stn. D, Vancouver, BC V6J 5G5 Canada
$1,950 for multi-channel FM/FM unit, compatible with standard transducers.

Konigsberg Instruments, Inc. 626-449-0016
2000 E Foothill Blvd, Pasadena, CA 91107
Medical Research, Discovery Research, Safety Pharmacology, Special systems for Biocontainment Levels 2, 3 and 4.

TELEMETRY UNIT, PHYSIOLOGICAL, TEMPERATURE *(General) 80RZO*

Barrows Company 707-987-0460
18701 Glenwood Rd, Hidden Valley Lake, CA 95467
$120 - Model T implantable transmitter. Measures Temperature and Activity in laboratory animals.

Konigsberg Instruments, Inc. 626-449-0016
2000 E Foothill Blvd, Pasadena, CA 91107
Medical Research, Discovery Research, Safety Pharmacology, Special systems for Biocontainment Levels 2, 3 and 4.

TELEPHONE EQUIPMENT *(General) 80VAT*

Assisted Access-Nfss, Inc. 800-950-9655
822 Preston Ct, Lake Villa, IL 60046
Various equipment and devices for the hearing impaired, including TTY systems and telephone amplifiers; fax signallers. Repair services for these products also available.

Crest Healthcare Supply 800-328-8908
195 3rd St, Dassel, MN 55325
Dispensable phone.

Hitec Group Intl. 800-288-8303
8160 S Madison St, Burr Ridge, IL 60527
Telephone equipment for aiding the deaf.

R. D. Equipment, Inc. 508-362-7498
230 Percival Dr, West Barnstable, MA 02668
EZ Phone Holder.

Ring Communications, Inc. 516-585-7464
57 Trade Zone Dr, Ronkonkoma, NY 11779

Spectralink Corporation 800-676-5465
5755 Central Ave, Boulder, CO 80301
SpectraLink's NetLink Wireless Telephones provide healthcare staff with lightweight wireless handsets that make and receive telephone calls anywhere in the facility with no service charges or usage fees. In addition, these handsets seamlessly integrate with many third-party messaging applications such as nurse call systems and other patient monitoriing systems. NetLink wireless telephones are an IEEE 802.11 standards-based wireless LAN (WLAN) telephone system that provides high-quality mobile voice communications throughout the workplace using voice-over IP (VOIP) technology.

Talk-A-Phone Co. 773-539-1100
5013 N Kedzie Ave, Chicago, IL 60625
ADA compliant hands-free emergency phones.

Ultratec, Inc. 800-482-2424
450 Science Dr, Madison, WI 53711
PUBLIC TTY ST and PUBLIC TTY telephones for the deaf.

TELEPHONE, HANDICAPPED USE *(Physical Med) 89UME*

Assisted Access-Nfss, Inc. 800-950-9655
822 Preston Ct, Lake Villa, IL 60046
Various equipment and devices for the hearing impaired, including TTY systems and telephone amplifiers.

Assistive Technology, Inc. 800-793-9227
333 Elm St Ste 115, Dedham, MA 02026

Harc Mercantile Ltd. 800-445-9968
1111 W Centre Ave, Portage, MI 49024

Insiphil (Us) Llc 408-616-8700
650 Vaqueros Ave Ste F, Sunnyvale, CA 94085

Krown Manufacturing, Inc. 800-366-9950
3408 Indale Rd, Fort Worth, TX 76116
Portaview Junior (PV2JR), priced from $239.00 for basic TDD and comes with a 1 year warranty; Portaview Senior (PV20SR), Priced from $279.00 with direct connect keyboard dialing and printer port for auto answer, comes with 1 year warranty; Portaview Plus (PV20T), Priced from $339.00 with more memory, built in directory, electronic voice and remote message retrieval, comes with 1 year warranty; Portaview Plus A (PV20TA), Priced from $389.00 with ASCII to communicate with a modem, comes with 1 year warranty. All units have batteries plus AC adapter and 20 character display. PortaPrinter 2000 (PP2000), priced from $378.00 with built-in 24-character printer with upper and lower case printing, 3 sizes of print available, and electronic voice and TTY call alert, with 1 year warranty; PortaPrinter (PP2000D), priced from $409.00 with direct connect keyboard dialing, call program screen, and auto answer with fixed message, with 1 year warranty; MemoryPrinter 2000D (MP2000D), priced from $499.00 with direct connect and built-in 24 character printer, 32k memory, auto answer with programmable message, built-in clock and calendar, built-in help menu and more, available with ASCII code, with 1 year warranty; MemoryPrinter 2000Dx (MP2000DX), priced from $549.00 with additional built-in strobe to indicate incoming calls and available with ASCII cade, 1 year warranty; PayPhone TDD (PAYTDD), priced from $649.00 with 3 year warranty. The best on the market for pay phones. Spill resistant keyboard, stainless steel without accoustic couplers, and vandal proof. PVCO is used for persons who are deaf or late-deafened that can speak well. This device allows them to talk on the phone and read the responses via the state relay services.

Ultratec, Inc. 800-482-2424
450 Science Dr, Madison, WI 53711
UNIPHONE 1140 combination telephone with volume control and voice-carry-over capabilities. Also includes 8k memory, backlight, built-in flasher, and programmable auto answer. UNIPHONE 1000 combination telephone with volume control and voice-carry-over capabilities. CRYSTAL TONE Amplified Telephone, designed for individuals with mild to moderate hearing loss. Offers up to 35dB gain. A unique CRYSTAL TONE which lets users filter and enhance the incoming sound and adjust sound quality, frequency range, and pitch to their optimal hearing level. Also CRYSTAL TONE PLUS Amplified Telephone, designed for people who have difficulty hearing on the telephone, offers up to 50dB gain plus a built in speakerphone for hands-free use, 10 speed dial numbers, outgoing volume amplification, 3.5mm audio jack connection and more.

Weitbrecht Communications, Inc. 800-233-9130
926 Colorado Ave, Santa Monica, CA 90401
TTYs and amplified phones for the deaf or hard of hearing

TELESCOPE, HAND-HELD, LOW-VISION *(Ophthalmology) 86HKB*

Heine Usa Ltd. 800-367-4872
1 Washington St Ste 555, Dover, NH 03820

TELESCOPE, LARYNGEAL-BRONCHIAL *(Ear/Nose/Throat) 77ENZ*

Heine Usa Ltd. 800-367-4872
1 Washington St Ste 555, Dover, NH 03820

Jedmed Instruments Co. 314-845-3770
5416 Jedmed Ct, Saint Louis, MO 63129

Karl Storz Endoscopy-America Inc. 800-421-0837
600 Corporate Pointe, Culver City, CA 90230

Princeton Medical Group, Inc. 800-875-0869
1189 Royal Links Dr, Mt Pleasant, SC 29466

TELESCOPE, RIGID, ENDOSCOPIC *(Gastro/Urology) 78FBP*

Gyrus Acmi, Inc. 508-804-2739
93 N Pleasant St, Norwalk, OH 44857
Various sizes and kinds of rigid endoscopic telepscopes.

Gyrus Acmi, Inc. 508-804-2739
300 Stillwater P.o.box 1971, Stamford, CT 06902
Various sizes and kinds of rigid endoscopic telepscopes.

Karl Storz Endoscopy-America Inc. 800-421-0837
600 Corporate Pointe, Culver City, CA 90230

Mahe International Inc. 800-294-7946
468 Craighead St, Nashville, TN 37204

Md International, Inc. 305-669-9003
11300 NW 41st St, Doral, FL 33178

Olympus America, Inc. 800-645-8160
3500 Corporate Pkwy, PO Box 610, Center Valley, PA 18034

Richard Wolf Medical Instruments Corp. 800-323-9653
353 Corporate Woods Pkwy, Vernon Hills, IL 60061

TELESCOPE, SPECTACLE, LOW-VISION *(Ophthalmology) 86HKK*

Ctp Coil Inc. 800-933-2645
1801 Howard St Ste D, Elk Grove Village, IL 60007
Face mounted spectacle binoculars, jewelers loures and monocular clip-on flip-ups.

Eschenbach Optik Of America, Inc. 800-487-5389
904 Ethan Allen Hwy, Ridgefield, CT 06877

Sds-Surgical Acuity 888-822-8489
3225 Deming Way Ste 120, Middleton, WI 53562
Class II Galilean Dimension-3 and Hi Res EyeLites surgical flip-up and fixed, wide field loupes; and EyeMax Hi Res Class III and IV Prismatic flip-up and fixed, high magnification, wide field loupes. Superior Visualization Systems - EyeMax, EyeLites, Dimension-3 - Loupes that offer high resolution and wide fields for optimum operating comfort and visualization. Available in five magnification levels in both Prismatic and Galilean designs, and in either flip-up (front-lens mounted) or fixed (through-the-lens mounted). All systems are fully customized to meet the specific needs of the surgeon.

Zoom Focus Eyewear, Llc 818-785-7773
7065 Hayvenhurst Ave Ste 2, Lake Balboa, CA 91406

TELETHERAPY SYSTEM, RADIONUCLIDE *(Radiology) 90IWB*

American Radiosurgery, Inc. 858-451-6173
16776 Bernardo Center Dr Ste 203, San Diego, CA 92128
Tele gamma system, gammaknife.

Elekta, Inc. 800-535-7355
4775 Peachtree Industrial Blvd, Building 300, Suite 300
Norcross, GA 30092
Radionuclide radiation therapy system.

Neutron Products Inc 800-424-8169
22301 Mount Ephraim Rd # 68, Dickerson, MD 20842
Various types of cobalt-60 teletherapy units.

Neutron Products, Inc. 301-349-5001
22301 Mount Ephraim Rd, Dickerson, MD 20842

Patterson Medical Supply, Inc. 262-387-8720
W68N158 Evergreen Blvd, Cedarburg, WI 53012
Radiotherapy positioning device.

Sun Nuclear Corp. 321-259-6862
425 Pineda Ct Ste A, Melbourne, FL 32940
Various energy isorad diode detectors:models 1160,1161,1162,1163, and 11164.

TELETHERMOGRAPHIC SYSTEM *(Radiology) 90IYM*

American Thermal Instruments, Inc. 937-429-2114
2400 E River Rd, Moraine, OH 45439
Ati breast & body health system.

TELETHERMOGRAPHIC SYSTEM (ADJUNCTIVE USE)
(Radiology) 90LHQ

Advanced Biophotonics Inc. 631-244-8244
125 Wilbur Pl Ste 120, Bohemia, NY 11716
Infrared imaging system.

Compix Incorporated 503-639-8496
15824 Upper Boones Ferry Rd, Lake Oswego, OR 97035
Thermographic camera.

Infrared Sciences Corp. 516-482-9001
213 Hallock Rd Ste 5, Stony Brook, NY 11790
Adjunctive telethermographic system.

Meditherm Inc. 503-639-8496
400 Front St Ste 8, Beaufort, NC 28516
Thermographic camera.

TELEVISION MONITOR, MICROSCOPE *(General) 80TFC*

Accu-Scope, Inc. 516-759-1000
7 Littleworth Ln, Sea Cliff, NY 11579

JVC Americas Corp. 973-315-5000
1700 Valley Rd, Wayne, NJ 07470
Microscope monitor/recorder.

Leica Microsystems (Canada) Inc. 800-205-3422
400 - 111 Granton Drive, Richmond Hill, ONT L4B 1L5 Canada

Mccrone Microscopes & Accessories 800-622-8122
850 Pasquinelli Dr, Westmont, IL 60559
LINKAM heating and freezing microscope stages, freeze drying stages, DSC, shearing, cryo, FTIR, and peltier stages.

Micromanipulator Co., Inc., The 800-972-4032
1555 Forrest Way, Carson City, NV 89706
Products and accessories to aid in embryo recovery, grading, splitting, injection, micromanipulation and photomicrography.

TELEVISION MONITOR, MICROSCOPE *(cont'd)*

Sony Electronics, Inc., Medical Systems Div. 800-686-7669
1 Sony Dr, Park Ridge, NJ 07656
Wide range of monitors for medical applications.

Stryker Corp. 800-726-2725
2825 Airview Blvd, Portage, MI 49002

Stryker Endoscopy 800-435-0220
5900 Optical Ct, San Jose, CA 95138

Western Scientific Co., Inc. 877-489-3726
4104 24th St # 183, San Francisco, CA 94114
Complete line of video and digital imaging systems.

TELEVISION MONITOR, OPERATING ROOM *(General) 80TFD*

Berchtold Corp. 800-243-5135
1950 Hanahan Rd, Charleston, SC 29406
CHROMOVISION closed-circuit television.

Burton Medical Products, Inc. 800-444-9909
21100 Lassen St, Chatsworth, CA 91311
Available is XenaLux operating room satellite.

Jedmed Instruments Co. 314-845-3770
5416 Jedmed Ct, Saint Louis, MO 63129

Sony Electronics, Inc., Medical Systems Div. 800-686-7669
1 Sony Dr, Park Ridge, NJ 07656
High resolution monochrome and color monitors for surgery, lab, and more applications.

Stryker Corp. 800-726-2725
2825 Airview Blvd, Portage, MI 49002

Stryker Endoscopy 800-435-0220
5900 Optical Ct, San Jose, CA 95138

Wisap America 800-233-8448
8231 Melrose Dr, Lenexa, KS 66214

TELEVISION SYSTEM, SLOW SCAN *(Radiology) 90UEY*

Emed Technologies 866-363-3669
76 Blanchard Rd, Burlington, MA 01803

Sony Electronics, Inc., Medical Systems Div. 800-686-7669
1 Sony Dr, Park Ridge, NJ 07656

TELEVISION, PATIENT ROOM *(General) 80TFA*

Avid Products 888-575-AVID
72 Johnny Cake Hill Rd, Aquidneck Industrial Park, Middletown, RI 02842
AVID electronic television headset for hospital patient use; plastic headsets for communication between patient and MRI technician, assists during diagnostic or magnetic-resonance imaging.

HCI 800-783-8105
113 Commerce Dr, Loveland, OH 45140
Standard or personal patient and staff TV receivers, computer control services, patient and staff education, movie and satellite entertainment and educational programming. Special TV systems for critical care and dialysis applications. New products include the Bedmate 9-in. patient television system and the Ivod patient/staff digital education entertainment and information system.

Lg Electronics U.S.A., Inc. 800-884-1742
2000 Millbrook Dr, Lincolnshire, IL 60069
20 inch Healthview Series patient room television with closed caption, FM radio and intelligent pillow speaker interface.

TEMPERATURE STRIP, FOREHEAD, LIQUID CRYSTAL
(General) 80KPD

Biosynergy, Inc. 800-255-5274
1940 E Devon Ave, Elk Grove Village, IL 60007
TEMPTREND, a surface thermometer that measures temperature of urine samples/drug testing. TEMPTREND II, is a reversible forehead thermometer that measures core body temperature. LABTEMP is a disposable laboratory surface thermometer.

Carex Health Brands 800-526-8051
921 E Amidon St, PO Box 2526, Sioux Falls, SD 57104
Gives precise reading in only 15 seconds, and is reuseable without sterilizing.

Color Change Corp. 630-289-0900
1545 Burgundy Pkwy, Streamwood, IL 60107
E-Z temp I+ is available in Fahrenheit (9404M) or Celsius (3540M) scales. E-Z Temp II (8406M) reads in both Fahrenheit and Celsius scales. There are 100 forehead thermometers per box.

Dorel Design & Development Center 781-364-3542
25 Forbes Blvd, Foxboro, MA 02035

Healer Products, Llc 914-663-6300
427 Commerce Ln Ste 1, West Berlin, NJ 08091
Thermometer strips.

TEMPERATURE STRIP, FOREHEAD, LIQUID CRYSTAL *(cont'd)*

Lcr-Hallcrest--Florida 847-998-8580
6705 Parke East Blvd Unit A, Tampa, FL 33610
Strip, temperature, forehead, liquid crystal.

Liquid Crystal Resources, L.L.C. 800-527-1419
1820 Pickwick Ln, Glenview, IL 60026
Liquid crystal thermometers available as disposable or reusable. For use as anesthesiology thermometers, forehead skin thermometers, urine test thermometers.

Respironics Missouri 978-659-4252
2039 Concourse Dr, Saint Louis, MO 63146
OMNI ACCU-BAR 1 degree increment monitor with both Fahrenheit and celsius, and the only insta-read models available. OMNI SPECTRUM 1 degree incremental monitor with both farenheit and celsius.

Sharn, Inc. 800-325-3671
4517 George Rd Ste 200, Tampa, FL 33634
CRYSTALINE II, and CRYSTALINE ST liquid crystal technology indicates skin or body temperature, reads in both Fahrenheit and Celsius. TEMPALERT II, forehead temperature strip displays continuous temperature changes, reads both Fahrenheit and Celsius. NUMITEMP, forehead fever indicator for use on children provides a check of temperature in just a few seconds and is not invasive.

Thermo Products, Llc 303-796-8234
7767 S Valentia St, Centennial, CO 80112

Trademark Medical Llc 800-325-9044
449 Soverign Ct, St. Louis, MO 63011
REDI-TEMP temperature monitor for anesthesia.

TEMPLATE *(Orthopedics) 87HWT*

Abbott Spine, Inc. 847-937-6100
12708 Riata Vista Cir Ste B-100, Austin, TX 78727
Template.

Best Medical International, Inc. 800-336-4970
7643 Fullerton Rd, Springfield, VA 22153
Applicator; Syed-Neblett GYN I, II & III, Templates & Kits, Prostate, Urethral, Rectal Template & Kits; Disposable Prostate, Rectal & GYN Templates.

Biomet, Inc. 574-267-6639
56 E Bell Dr, PO Box 587, Warsaw, IN 46582
Deyerle femoral template.

Bioquest 480-350-9944
2211 W 1st St Ste 106, Tempe, AZ 85281
Fmoral neck cut guide.

Centinel Spine Inc. 952-885-0500
505 Park Ave Fl 14, New York, NY 10022
STALIF C Sizing Trial, var. sizes

Demetech Corp. 888-324-2447
3530 NW 115th Ave, Doral, FL 33178
Anatomical models.

Depuy Spine, Inc. 800-227-6633
325 Paramount Dr, Raynham, MA 02767
Template.

K2m, Inc. 866-526-4171
751 Miller Dr SE Ste F1, Leesburg, VA 20175
Template.

Kls-Martin L.P. 800-625-1557
11239-1 St. John`s Industrial, Parkway South
Jacksonville, FL 32250

Medical Modeling Inc 303-273-5344
17301 W Colfax Ave Ste 300, Golden, CO 80401
Anatomical models.

Medtronic Sofamor Danek Instrument Manufacturing 901-396-3133
7375 Adrianne Pl, Bartlett, TN 38133
Template.

Medtronic Sofamor Danek Usa, Inc. 901-396-3133
4340 Swinnea Rd, Memphis, TN 38118
Template.

Otismed Corporation 888-684-7633
1600 Harbor Bay Pkwy, Alameda, CA 94502
Multiple types of templates.

Protomed 303-422-2207
1329 W 121st Ave, Westminster, CO 80234
Anatomical models.

TEMPLATE *(cont'd)*

Small Bone Innovations, Inc. 215-428-1791
1380 S Pennsylvania Ave, Morrisville, PA 19067
Template.

Spine Wave, Inc. 203-944-9494
2 Enterprise Dr Ste 302, Shelton, CT 06484
Template.

Stryker Spine 866-457-7463
2 Pearl Ct, Allendale, NJ 07401

Summit Business Products, Inc. 260-244-1820
995 E Business 30, Columbia City, IN 46725

Surgical Implant Generation Network (Sign) 509-371-1107
451 Hills St, Richland, WA 99354
Jig.

Warsaw Orthopedic, Inc. 901-396-3133
2500 Silveus Xing, Warsaw, IN 46582
Template.

Zimmer Holdings, Inc. 800-613-6131
1800 W Center St, PO Box 708, Warsaw, IN 46580

Zimmer Manufacturing B.V. 800-613-6131
Route 1, Km. 123.4, Bldg. 1, Turpeaux Industrial Park
Mercedita, PR 00715
Various types of templates and gauge sets.

Zimmer Spine, Inc. 800-655-2614
7375 Bush Lake Rd, Minneapolis, MN 55439
Template.

Zimmer Trabecular Metal Technology 800-613-6131
10 Pomeroy Rd, Parsippany, NJ 07054
Drill template.

TEMPLATE, FEMORAL ANGLE CUTTING *(Orthopedics) 87HWS*

Zimmer Holdings, Inc. 800-613-6131
1800 W Center St, PO Box 708, Warsaw, IN 46580

TENACULUM, OTHER (FORCEPS) *(Surgery) 79RZQ*

Cardiovascular Research, Inc. 813-832-6222
4810 W Gandy Blvd, Tampa, FL 33611
Non-skid vascular surgical forceps.

Fortrad Eye Instruments Corp. 973-543-2371
8 Franklin Rd, Mendham, NJ 07945

Prosurge Instruments, Inc. 866-832-7874
199 Laidlaw Ave, Jersey City, NJ 07306

TENACULUM, THYROID *(Gastro/Urology) 78RZP*

Elmed, Inc. 630-543-2792
60 W Fay Ave, Addison, IL 60101

TENACULUM, UTERINE *(Obstetrics/Gyn) 85HDC*

Coopersurgical, Inc. 800-243-2974
95 Corporate Dr, Trumbull, CT 06611

Elmed, Inc. 630-543-2792
60 W Fay Ave, Addison, IL 60101

George Tiemann & Co. 800-843-6266
25 Plant Ave, Hauppauge, NY 11788

Karl Storz Endoscopy-America Inc. 800-421-0837
600 Corporate Pointe, Culver City, CA 90230

Marina Medical Instruments, Inc. 800-697-1119
955 Shotgun Rd, Sunrise, FL 33326
Various.

Premier Medical Products 888-PREMUSA
1710 Romano Dr, Plymouth Meeting, PA 19462

Princeton Medical Group, Inc. 800-875-0869
1189 Royal Links Dr, Mt Pleasant, SC 29466

Richard Wolf Medical Instruments Corp. 800-323-9653
353 Corporate Woods Pkwy, Vernon Hills, IL 60061

Thomas Medical Inc. 800-556-0349
5610 West 82 2nd Street, Indianpolis, IN 46278

Tuzik Boston 800-886-6363
104 Longwater Dr, Assinippi Park, Norwell, MA 02061

TENT, MIST *(General) 80RZS*

Allied Healthcare Products, Inc. 800-444-3954
1720 Sublette Ave, Saint Louis, MO 63110

Sunnydale Industries, Inc. 800-346-3515
6859 Audrain Road 9139, Centralia, MO 65240
$4.50 to $11.00 per unit.

TENT, OXYGEN (CANOPY) *(Anesthesiology) 73BYL*

Allied Healthcare Products, Inc. 800-444-3954
1720 Sublette Ave, Saint Louis, MO 63110

Nova Health Systems, Inc. 800-225-NOVA
1001 Broad St, Utica, NY 13501
BABYPORT.

Ohmeda Medical 800-345-2700
8880 Gorman Rd, Laurel, MD 20723

Sea-Long Medical Systems, Inc. 502-969-4949
1983 S Park Rd, Louisville, KY 40219
Oxygen tent.

Sunnydale Industries, Inc. 800-346-3515
6859 Audrain Road 9139, Centralia, MO 65240
$4.50 to $11.00 per unit.

TENT, OXYGEN, ELECTRIC *(Anesthesiology) 73BYK*

Allied Healthcare Products, Inc. 800-444-3954
1720 Sublette Ave, Saint Louis, MO 63110

Ohmeda Medical 800-345-2700
8880 Gorman Rd, Laurel, MD 20723

TENT, PEDIATRIC AEROSOL *(General) 80FNC*

Mes, Inc. 800-423-2215
1968 E US Highway 90, Seguin, TX 78155
Part#0236, Ohio Pediatric Canopy; also we have self-supporting Dispos-O-Tents in 4 sizes

Peace Medical, Inc. 973-672-2120
50 S Center St Ste 11, Orange, NJ 07050
Hoods.

Sunnydale Industries, Inc. 800-346-3515
6859 Audrain Road 9139, Centralia, MO 65240
Self-supporting, transparent cube for aerosol/oxygen therapy. Available in 7, 10, 12, 18, and 24 inch models.

TEST PATTERN, RADIOGRAPHIC *(Radiology) 90IXF*

Cortechs Labs, Inc. 858-459-9702
1020 Prospect St Ste 304, La Jolla, CA 92037
3d distortion phantom.

Ge Medical Systems, Llc 262-548-2355
3000 N Grandview Blvd, W-417, Waukesha, WI 53188
Penetrometers, test patterns, step wedges.

Owens Scientific Inc. 281-394-2311
23230 Sandsage Ln, Katy, TX 77494

Supertech, Inc. 800-654-1054
PO Box 186, Elkhart, IN 46515
Wide Selection of Test Patterns available

The Phantom Laboratory, Inc. 800-525-1190
PO Box 511, Salem, NY 12865
Various types of radiographic test-pattern devices.

TEST PATTERN/PHANTOM, RADIONUCLIDE *(Radiology) 90JAR*

Capintec, Inc. 800-631-3826
6 Arrow Rd, Ramsey, NJ 07446

Eckert & Ziegler Isotope Products 661-309-1034
24937 Avenue Tibbitts, Valencia, CA 91355
Various types of phantom or test-pattern sources with multiplenuclides.

TEST SYSTEM, ANTIMICROBIAL SUSCEPTIBILITY, AUTOMATED *(Microbiology) 83LON*

Trek Diagnostic Systems 800-871-8909
982 Keynote Cir Ste 6, Cleveland, OH 44131

TEST SYSTEM, ANTINEUTROPHIL CYTOPLASMIC ANTIBODIES (ANCA) *(Immunology) 82MOB*

Global Focus (G.F.M.D. Ltd.) 800-527-2320
2280 Springlake Rd Ste 106, Dallas, TX 75234

Hemagen Diagnostics, Inc. 800-436-2436
9033 Red Branch Rd, Columbia, MD 21045
Ifa.

Immuno Concepts N.A. Ltd. 800-251-5115
9779 Business Park Dr, Sacramento, CA 95827

Zeus Scientific, Inc. 800-286-2111
PO Box 38, Raritan, NJ 08869
MPO (pANCA); ANCA Screen; PR-3 (cANCA) 96 tests ELISA IgG only.

TEST SYSTEM, NICOTINE, COTININE, METABOLITES *(Toxicology) 91MRS*

Acon Laboratories, Inc. 858-535-2030
10125 Mesa Rim Rd, San Diego, CA 92121

Ameritek Usa, Inc. 425-379-2580
125 130th St SE Ste 200, Everett, WA 98208
Cotinine test kit.

Ucp Biosciences, Inc. 408-392-0064
1445 Koll Cir Ste 111, San Jose, CA 95112
Cotinine test system.

TEST, AGAR PLATE *(Microbiology) 83UJZ*

Bd Diagnostic Systems 800-675-0908
7 Loveton Cir, Sparks, MD 21152

New Brunswick Scientific Co., Inc. 800-631-5417
PO Box 4005, Edison, NJ 08818
MP-1000 (PourMatic) Automated agar plate filler and stacker, pours and stacks up to 320 high-quality plates in 20 minutes. Requires just 20 in. of bench space. Optional bi-plate dispensing kit, foot switch, and printer available. Can be coupled with NBS AS-10 automated agar sterilizer for a complete and compact automated agar-sterilization and plate-filling station.

Pml Microbiologicals 800-628-7014
27120 SW 95th Ave, Wilsonville, OR 97070

Simport Plastics Ltd. 450-464-1723
2588 Bernard-Pilon, Beloeil, QUE J3G 4S5 Canada

TEST, AGAR TUBE *(Microbiology) 83UKA*

Bd Diagnostic Systems 800-675-0908
7 Loveton Cir, Sparks, MD 21152
350 different prepared media.

Pml Microbiologicals 800-628-7014
27120 SW 95th Ave, Wilsonville, OR 97070

Raven Biological Laboratories, Inc. 800-728-5702
8607 Park Dr, PO Box 27261, Omaha, NE 68127
Soybean Casein Digest Broth specially formulated for us with our spore products. Dermatophyte Test Media, Mycobiotic Agar, Sabaraud Dextrose Agar, and Biggy agar for fungal isolation and ID are also available.

TEST, ALBUMIN COBALT BINDING *(Chemistry) 75NJV*

Ischemia Technologies, Inc. 720-540-0200
4600 W 60th Ave, Arvada, CO 80003
Albumin cobalt binding test.

TEST, ALLERGY *(Immunology) 82VKL*

Alerchek, Inc. 877-282-9542
203 Anderson St, Portland, ME 04101
Flip screen allergy tests for 400 different allergens in serum or plasma. Total Human IgE quantitative test for the level of human IgE in serum or plasma.

Biomerica, Inc. 800-854-3002
17571 Von Karman Ave, Irvine, CA 92614
#7190 90 Foods IgG kit ELISA,

Dexall Biomedical Labs, Inc. 301-840-1884
18904 Bonanza Way, Gaithersburg, MD 20879
*Allerg*E-EIA test kit for total serum IgE. Allerg*Ens-EIA test kit for allergen-specific IgE. LabDex ASR-spectrophotometer strip reader. LabDex APR-spectrophotometer plate reader. Visual*Ens immunochromatographic assay.*

Dms Laboratories, Inc. 800-567-4367
2 Darts Mill Rd, Flemington, NJ 08822
ALLERZYME Identifier Kit. Rapid presumptive evaluation for the presence of clinically significant levels of allergen-specific IgE in canine serum. Visual determination of test results in 15 minutes. 10 patient kit includes perennial and seasonal multi-allergen results within each evaluation.

Greer Laboratories, Inc. 800-419-7302
639 Nuway Cir, PO Box 800, Lenoir, NC 28645
GREERPICK allergy skin testing system with self-loading allergy test device for immediate hypersensitivity. Allergenic extracts and related supplies are also available.

Lincoln Diagnostics, Inc. 800-537-1336
PO Box 1128, Decatur, IL 62525
Skin testing devices for allergies.

TEST, ALPHA-FETOPROTEIN *(Pathology) 88UMR*

Bio-Medical Products Corp. 800-543-7427
10 Halstead Rd, Mendham, NJ 07945
Alpha-fetoprotein (AFP) screening strip test in serum.

TEST, ALPHA-FETOPROTEIN *(cont'd)*

Dako North America, Inc — 805-566-6655
6392 Via Real, Carpinteria, CA 93013

TEST, ANTIBIOTIC SUSCEPTIBILITY *(Microbiology) 83UJX*

Biomerieux Industry — 800-634-7656
595 Anglum Rd, Hazelwood, MO 63042
Antibiotic differentiation and susceptibility disks.

Celsis Laboratory Group — 800-523-5227
165 Fieldcrest Ave, Edison, NJ 08837

Giles Scientific, Inc. — 800-603-9290
PO Box 4306, Santa Barbara, CA 93140
BIOMIC Vision automated color-digital image analysis plate reader system with US-NCCLS recommended methods and materials for bacteria and yeast species identification and antibiotic susceptibility testing.

TEST, ANTIBODY, ACQUIRED IMMUNE DEFICIENCY SYNDROME (AIDS) *(Hematology) 81VJE*

Acon Laboratories, Inc. — 858-535-2030
10125 Mesa Rim Rd, San Diego, CA 92121

Akers Biosciences, Inc. — 800-451-8378
201 Grove Rd, West Deptford, NJ 08086
HEALTHTEST HIV 1 and 2 serum and whole blood based.

Bio-Medical Products Corp. — 800-543-7427
10 Halstead Rd, Mendham, NJ 07945
HIV I and II test kit screening test kit. Blood serum Immunochromatographic 10 minute test.

Biomerieux Inc. — 800-682-2666
100 Rodolphe St, Durham, NC 27712
VIRONOSTIKA HIV screening test kits. Also available is NASBA HIV-1 quatitative detection test. Quantitative determination of HIV-1 RNA levels in plasma/serum and other biological fluids.

Biorad Laboratories — 800-2BI-ORAD
1000 Alfred Nobel Dr, Hercules, CA 94547

Calypte Biomedical Corporation — 877-CALYPTE
16290 SW Upper Boones Ferry Rd, Portland, OR 97224
SENTINEL HIV-1 urine microwell-based EIA for antibodies to HIV-1 in urine.

Crosswell International Corporation — 305-648-0777
101 Madeira Ave, Coral Gables, FL 33134

Hema Diagnostic Systems, Llc — 305-867-6123
1666 Kennedy Causeway, Suite 401, North Bay Village, FL 33141
Rapid 1-2-3 hema whole blood test, strip form or in the new rapid 1-2-3 hema housing.

Home Access Health Corp. — 800-HIV-TEST
2401 Hassell Rd Ste 1510, Hoffman Estates, IL 60169
Anonymous home HIV-1 test. Development in sales telemedicine products.

Inamco International Corp. — 800-724-4003
801 Montrose Ave, South Plainfield, NJ 07080
MEDICOS.

Ubi — 631-273-2828
25 Davids Dr, Hauppauge, NY 11788
Enzyme immunoassy for the qualitative detection of antibodies to Human Immunodeficiency Virus Type 1 (HIV-1) in human serum or plasma of blood donors or individuals at unknown risk.

Zeptometrix Corporation — 800-274-5487
872 Main St, Buffalo, NY 14202
CELLKINES (Trade Name): TCGF, Recombinant IL-2, RETRO-TEK HTLV-1 ELISA kit, RETRO-TEK antibody probe to AIDS virus, RETRO-TEK, MONOBODY anti-p19 to HTLV-1 core protein. All tests for research use only.

TEST, ANTIGEN (CA125), TUMOR-ASSOCIATED, OVARIAN, EPITHELIAL *(Immunology) 82LTK*

Biocheck, Inc. — 650-573-1968
323 Vintage Park Dr, Foster City, CA 94404
Ovarian cancer antigen ca 125 eia test kit.

Fujirebio Diagnostics, Inc. (Fdi) — 877-861-7246
201 Great Valley Pkwy, Malvern, PA 19355
In vitro device for the quantitative measurement of OC-125-reative determinants associated with a high-molecular-weight glycoprotein in serum of women with primary epithelial ovarian cancer, excluding those with cancer of low malignant potential. The FDI CA 125II RIA is indicated for use as an aid in the detection of residual ovarian carcinoma in patients who have undergone first-line therapy and would be considered for diagnostic second-look procedures.

TEST, ANTIGEN (CA125), TUMOR-ASSOCIATED, OVARIAN, EPITHELIAL *(cont'd)*

United Biotech, Inc. — 650-961-2910
211 S Whisman Rd Ste E, Mountain View, CA 94041
ELISA for Cancer Marker for CA-125 (Epithelial Ovarian Cancer - EOC).

TEST, ANTIMICROBIAL SUSCEPTIBILITY *(Microbiology) 83JWY*

Bd Diagnostic Systems — 800-675-0908
7 Loveton Cir, Sparks, MD 21152

Dade Behring, Inc. — 800-948-3233
1717 Deerfield Rd, Deerfield, IL 60015
MicroSCAN microbiology systems.

Trek Diagnostic Systems — 800-871-8909
982 Keynote Cir Ste 6, Cleveland, OH 44131

TEST, ANTITHROMBIN III, TWO STAGE CLOTTING TIME *(Hematology) 81JPE*

Health Chem Diagnostics Llc — 954-979-3845
3341 W McNab Rd, Pompano Beach, FL 33069
Antithrombin iii, two stage clotting time assay.

R2 Diagnostics, Inc. — 574-288-4377
1801 Commerce Dr, South Bend, IN 46628
Thrombotek at.

TEST, B LYMPHOCYTE MARKER *(Hematology) 81LJD*

Binding Site, Inc., The — 800-633-4484
5889 Oberlin Dr Ste 101, San Diego, CA 92121
Cell surface markers including CD23.

Gen Trak, Inc. — 336-622-5266
121 W Swannanoa Ave, Liberty, NC 27298
Various configurations of hla dr phenotyping trays.

TEST, BACILLUS SUBTILIS MICROBIOLOGY, TOBRAMYCIN *(Toxicology) 91DID*

Beckman Coulter, Inc. — 800-742-2345
250 S Kraemer Blvd, PO Box 8000, Brea, CA 92821

TEST, BACTERIA CHARACTERIZATION *(General) 80WWZ*

Bd Diagnostic Systems — 800-675-0908
7 Loveton Cir, Sparks, MD 21152

Biolog, Inc. — 800-284-4949
21124 Cabot Blvd, Hayward, CA 94545
ES MICROPLATE for biotyping E. Coli K12 and S. Typhimurium LT2 strands; MT MICROPLATE for studying the metabolic properties of a given bacterium.

Syntron Bioresearch, Inc. — 800-854-6226
2774 Loker Ave W, Carlsbad, CA 92010
Streptococcus A test.

TEST, BACTERIAL DIAGNOSTIC *(Microbiology) 83VLF*

Bd Diagnostic Systems — 800-675-0908
7 Loveton Cir, Sparks, MD 21152

Biolog, Inc. — 800-284-4949
21124 Cabot Blvd, Hayward, CA 94545
Biolog, Inc. provides innovative cell analysis tools which solve challenges facing pharmaceutical and biotechnology industries. Biolog's Phenotype MicroArray and OmniLog PM System are used in drug discovery to determine gene function, optimize drug targets, and assess cellular toxicology, Biolog also provides tools for identification/characterization of microbes ranging from bacteria to fungi.

Biomerieux Inc. — 800-682-2666
100 Rodolphe St, Durham, NC 27712

Culture Kits, Inc. — 888-680-6853
14 Prentice St, PO Box 748, Norwich, NY 13815

TEST, BACTERIAL DIAGNOSTIC *(cont'd)*

Gen-Probe, Inc. 800-523-5001
10210 Genetic Center Dr, San Diego, CA 92121
AccuProbe MYCOBACTERIUM AVIUM Complex Culture Identification Test for identification of Mycobacterium aviumi complex isolated from culture. AccuProbe MYCOBACTERIUM AVIUM Culture Identification Test - for identification of Mycobacterium aviumi isolated from culture.AccuProbe MYCOBACTERIUM GORDONAE Culture Identification Test - for identification of Mycobacterium gordonae isolated from culture. AccuProbe MYCOBACTERIUM INTRACELLULARE Culture Identification Test - for identification of Mycobacterium intracellulare isolated from culture. AccuProbe MYCOBACTERIUM KANSASII Culture Identification Test - for identification of Mycobacterium kansasii isolated from culture. AccuProbe MYCOBACTERIUM TUBERCULOSIS Complex Culture Identification Test - for identification of Mycobacterium tuberculosis complex isolated from culture. AMPLIFIED MYCOBACTERIUM TUBERCULOSIS Direct (MTD) Test - direct target-amplified nucleic acid probe test for the in virto diagnostic detection of Mycobacterium tuberculosis complex rRNA in ascid-fact bacilli (AFB) smear positive and negative concentrated sediments from sputum, bronchial specimens, or tracheal aspirates.

Meridian Bioscience, Inc. 800-696-0739
3471 River Hills Dr, Cincinnati, OH 45244
24 immunodiffusion teichoic acid antibody tests.

Princeton Biomeditech Corp. 732-274-1000
4242 US Highway 1, Monmouth Junction, NJ 08852
BioSign H. pylori IgM/IgG/IgA total antibody test for ulcer-causing bacteria, from whole blood, serum, or plasma; results in 5 minutes.

Remel Atlanta, Div. Of Remel, Inc. 800-255-6730
2797 Peterson Pl, Norcross, GA 30071
RAPID SYSTEMS Rapid bacterial identification kits; oxichrome and staphylochrome reagents.

Shared Systems, Inc. 888-474-2733
PO Box 211587, 3961 Columbia Rd, Augusta, GA 30917
E. coli latex agglutination test kit.

Techlab, Inc. 800-832-4522
2001 Kraft Dr, Blacksburg, VA 24060
TOX-A TEST, a monoclonal antibody-based ELISA for the rapid and specific detection of toxin A in stool specimens. TOX-B TEST, a highly sensitive tissue culture assay for toxin B in stools. TOX A/B TEST, for detecting both toxins in stools and gives results in 1-hour, offers increased sensitivity and has no indeterminate zone. LEUKO-TEST, a latex test for the detection of elevated levels of fecal lactoferrin, a marker protein for fecal leukocytes. It quickly distinguishes non-inflammatory diarrheas from those that are inflammatory and more serious. E.HISTOLYTICA TEST, a monoclonal antibody-based ELISA for rapid detection of E. histolytica and the only ELISA that specifically detects E. histolytica. GIARDIA TEST, a monoclonal antibody-based ELISA with a variable incubation period for testing a few specimens or for batch processing. CRYPTOSPORIDIUM TEST, a highly specific, monoclonal antibody-based ELISA.

Ubi 631-273-2828
25 Davids Dr, Hauppauge, NY 11788
Test kit for detection of antibody to Severe Acute Respiratory Syndrome (SARS) coronavirus

United Biotech, Inc. 650-961-2910
211 S Whisman Rd Ste E, Mountain View, CA 94041
ELISAs detecting: Chagas, Cysticercosis, Leishmania

TEST, BETA 2 - MICROGLOBULIN *(Immunology) 82JZG*

Binding Site, Inc., The 800-633-4484
5889 Oberlin Dr Ste 101, San Diego, CA 92121
B2 microglobulin RID kit.

Biocheck, Inc. 650-573-1968
323 Vintage Park Dr, Foster City, CA 94404
Beta-2 microglobulin eia test kit.

United Biotech, Inc. 650-961-2910
211 S Whisman Rd Ste E, Mountain View, CA 94041
ELISA quantitative test for Beta-2-Microglobulin.

TEST, C-REACTIVE PROTEIN *(Immunology) 82DCN*

Abbott Diagnostics Div. 626-440-0700
820 Mission St, South Pasadena, CA 91030
C-reactive protein.

Access Bio Incorporate 732-297-2222
2033 Rt. 130 Unit H, Monmouth Junction, NJ 08852
C-reactive protein test.

TEST, C-REACTIVE PROTEIN *(cont'd)*

Arlington Scientific, Inc. Asi 800-654-0146
1840 N Technology Dr, Springville, UT 84663
The ASI CRP latex reagent qualitatively and semiquantitatively detects C-reactive protein (CRP) in human serum. The test is based on the immunologic agglutination reaction between CRP antigen and the corresponding antibody coated on the surface of the biologically inert latex particles. The CRP latex reagent provides a sensitivity of 6 mg/L.

Bio-Medical Products Corp. 800-543-7427
10 Halstead Rd, Mendham, NJ 07945
Test with latex slide. Also, hsCRP 5 minute test.

Biocheck, Inc. 650-573-1968
323 Vintage Park Dr, Foster City, CA 94404
High sensitive c-reactive protein eia test kit.

Biomerieux Inc. 800-682-2666
100 Rodolphe St, Durham, NC 27712

Dexall Biomedical Labs, Inc. 301-840-1884
18904 Bonanza Way, Gaithersburg, MD 20879
*Auro*Dex CRP immunogold card test for determination of C Reactive Protein in whole blood or serum/plasma.*

Diagnostic Technology, Inc. 631-582-4949
175 Commerce Dr Ste L, Hauppauge, NY 11788
Latex slide test for the detection of c-reative protein.

Diasorin Inc 800-328-1482
1951 Northwestern Ave S, PO Box 285, Stillwater, MN 55082
C-peptide radioimmunoassay test.

Immunostics, Inc. 800-722-7505
3505 Sunset Ave, Ocean, NJ 07712

J&S Medical Associates 800-229-6000
35 Tripp St Ste 1, Framingham, MA 01702
ACCUTEX qualitative and quantitative latex agglutination kits for RF, ASO, SLE, CRP, Mono and Staph.

Kent Laboratories, Inc. 360-398-8641
777 Jorgensen Pl, Bellingham, WA 98226
Radial immunodiffusion kit.

Pulse Scientific, Inc. 800-363-7907
5100 S. Service Rd., Unit 18, Burlington, ONT L7L-6A5 Canada
CRP Latex Test, latex agglutination test to detect C-reactive Protein.

Raichem, Division Of Hemagen Diagnostics, Inc. 800-438-6100
8225 Mercury Ct, San Diego, CA 92111
RAICHEM SPIA C-Reactive protein reagent and immunoturbidimetric assay system.

Sa Scientific, Inc. 800-272-2710
4919 Golden Quail, San Antonio, TX 78240
Latex slide test.

Stanbio Laboratory, Inc. 830-249-0772
1261 N Main St, Boerne, TX 78006
$38.00 for 50 CRP test kits with latex reagent, positive and negative control serum, glycine-saline buffer and six-cell.

Sterling Diagnostics, Inc. 800-637-2661
36645 Metro Ct, Sterling Heights, MI 48312

Teco Diagnostics 714-693-7788
1268 N Lakeview Ave, Anaheim, CA 92807
C-reactive protein (crp); a latex slide test.

United Biotech, Inc. 650-961-2910
211 S Whisman Rd Ste E, Mountain View, CA 94041
ELISA for detecting CRP (C-Reactive Protein)

Wampole Laboratories 800-257-9525
2 Research Way, Princeton, NJ 08540
IMMUNEX CRP Latex agglutination test.

TEST, C-REACTIVE PROTEIN, FITC *(Immunology) 82DCK*

Abbott Diagnostics Intl, Biotechnology Ltd 787-846-3500
Road #2 KM. 58.0 , PO Box 278, Cruce Davila, Barceloneta, PR 00617
Various assays for detection of C-reactive protein.

Biomerieux Inc. 800-682-2666
100 Rodolphe St, Durham, NC 27712

Carolina Liquid Chemistries Corp. 800-471-7272
510 W Central Ave Ste C, Brea, CA 92821
Crp reagent kit.

Jas Diagnostics, Inc. 305-418-2320
7220 NW 58th St, Miami, FL 33166
C-reactive protein hs.

TEST, C-REACTIVE PROTEIN, FITC *(cont'd)*

Kamiya Biomedical Company 206-575-8068
12779 Gateway Dr S, Tukwila, WA 98168
Diagnostic immunoturbidimetric assay kit for CRP including calibrator.

Nerl Diagnostics Llc. 401-824-2046
14 Almeida Ave, East Providence, RI 02914
Crp latex kits.

Raichem, Division Of Hemagen Diagnostics, Inc. 800-438-6100
8225 Mercury Ct, San Diego, CA 92111
RAICHEM CRP High Sensitivity Reagent

Vital Diagnostics Inc. 714-672-3553
1075 W Lambert Rd Ste D, Brea, CA 92821
C-reactive protein reagent.

TEST, CANCER DETECTION, DNA-PROBE *(Immunology) 82VJL*

Affymetrix, Inc. 888-DNA-CHIP
3420 Central Expy, Santa Clara, CA 95051

Vysis 800-553-7042
3100 Woodcreek Dr, Downers Grove, IL 60515

TEST, CANCER DETECTION, MONOCLONAL ANTIBODY
(Immunology) 82VJD

Biogenex Laboratories 800-421-4149
4600 Norris Canyon Rd, San Ramon, CA 94583
Antibodies for tumor-associated cell surface antigens including adenoCA, breast CA, lung CA, melanoma, pancreatic, and prostate CA.

Covance Research Products Inc. 800-223-0796
180 Rustcraft Rd Ste 140, Dedham, MA 02026
Tests for tumor-associated antigens in/on tissue, cells, body fluids.

Dako North America, Inc 805-566-6655
6392 Via Real, Carpinteria, CA 93013

Invitrogen Corporation 800-955-6288
101 Lincoln Centre Dr, Foster City, CA 94404

TEST, CANCER DETECTION, OTHER *(Hematology) 81VIA*

American Diagnostica, Inc. 888-234-4435
500 West Ave, Stamford, CT 06902
IMUBIND; Colon cancer prognosis. ICA & ELISA

Biomerica, Inc. 800-854-3002
17571 Von Karman Ave, Irvine, CA 92614
#1052 double Ab Alpha-Subunit RIA, T-markers controls serum with 13 tumor associated antigens incl. CEA, PTH, ferritin, gastrin & more, lyophilized 4x2ml vials per box, high & low. TRI-LEVEL with over 40 constituents, lyophilized 6x5ml vials per box. Thyroglobulin RIA #1042.

Dako North America, Inc 805-566-6655
6392 Via Real, Carpinteria, CA 93013

Elabsupply 714-446-8740
1001 Starbuck St Apt C306, Fullerton, CA 92833
Hemosure One-Step IFOB (Immuncological Fecal Occult Blood Test) for Initial colorectal cancer screening.

Exact Sciences, Inc. 866-333-9228
441 Charmany Dr, Madison, WI 53719
Colorectal screening. PRE GEN-26 non-invasive screen for colorectal cancer in individuals with hereditary non-polypesis colorectal cancer.

Immunomedics, Inc. 973-605-8200
300 the American Rd, Morris Plains, NJ 07950
Radiolabeled monoclonal antibody.

Neoprobe Corporation 800-793-0079
425 Metro Pl N Ste 300, Dublin, OH 43017
Radioimmunoguided surgery (RIGS) technology. neo2000 portable radioisotope detector.

Princeton Biomeditech Corp. 732-274-1000
4242 US Highway 1, Monmouth Junction, NJ 08852
Rapid one-step PSA test for prostate cancer marker.

TEST, CERVICAL MUCOUS PENETRATION *(Pathology) 88LIY*

Embryotech Laboratories, Inc. 800-673-7500
323 Andover St, Wilmington, MA 01887

TEST, CYSTIC FIBROSIS *(Chemistry) 75VIP*

Polychrome Medical 763-585-9328
2700 Freeway Blvd Ste 750, Brooklyn Center, MN 55430
Diagnostic test for Cystic Fibrosis.

TEST, DIRECT AGGLUTINATION, TOXOPLASMA GONDII
(Microbiology) 83LLA

Bio-Medical Products Corp. 800-543-7427
10 Halstead Rd, Mendham, NJ 07945
Test with latex slide. Blood serum membrane slide 10 minute immunochromatographic test.

Immunostics, Inc. 800-722-7505
3505 Sunset Ave, Ocean, NJ 07712

Polymer Laboratories, Now A Part Of Varian, Inc. 800-767-3963
160 Old Farm Rd, Amherst Fields Research Park, Amherst, MA 01002
PL-Latex is an established range of products, specifically designed and manufactured by Polymer Laboratories, for use as supports in immunodiagnostic assays. Also for use in membrane migration, capture assays or turbidimetric and nephelometric.

TEST, DISEASE, LYME *(Immunology) 82WVP*

Akers Biosciences, Inc. 800-451-8378
201 Grove Rd, West Deptford, NJ 08086
HEALTHTEST.

Diamedix Corp. 800-327-4565
2140 N Miami Ave, Miami, FL 33127
EIA assay for detection of antibodies to B. burgdorferi: IgM Catalog #720-510; IgG/IgM Catalog# 720-390

Immunetics, Inc. 800-227-4765
27 Drydock Ave Ste 6, Boston, MA 02210
Lyme disease Western blot antibody detection kit.

Princeton Biomeditech Corp. 732-274-1000
4242 US Highway 1, Monmouth Junction, NJ 08852
BioSign Lyme disease B. burgdorferi IgG antibody test.

Wampole Laboratories 800-257-9525
2 Research Way, Princeton, NJ 08540
ELISA kit.

Zeus Scientific, Inc. 800-286-2111
PO Box 38, Raritan, NJ 08869
96 tests ELISA IgG/M, IgM only and IgG only.

TEST, DNA-PROBE, OTHER *(Microbiology) 83WNY*

Aushon Biosystems, Inc. 978-436-6400
43 Manning Rd, Billerica, MA 01821
2470 Arrayer

Bd Diagnostic Systems 800-675-0908
7 Loveton Cir, Sparks, MD 21152
DNA probe test for vaginitis/vaginosis Affirm Vpill Microbial Indentification System. DNA Probe test for the rapid indentification of gardnerella vaginalis, trichomonas vaginalis and cardia spp. Directly from vaginal specimens.

Biogenex Laboratories 800-421-4149
4600 Norris Canyon Rd, San Ramon, CA 94583
In Situ hybridization detection systems for DNA and mRNA. In Situ hybridization kits for kappa and lambda mRNA, EBV, HPV.

Bioreliance 800-553-5372
14920 Broschart Rd, Rockville, MD 20850
Genetic Toxicology Testing.

Biotecx Laboratories, Inc. 800-535-6286
15225 Gulf Hwy, #F106, Houston, TX 77034
DNA isolation and DNA single tube test, Bioplaz plasmid DNA; also, RNA isolation and UltraSpec RNA.

Enzo Biochem, Inc. 212-583-0100
527 Madison Ave, New York, NY 10022
BIOPROBES for HSV I & II, Epstein-Barr virus, hepatitis B, cytomegalovirus, adenovirus, human papilloma virus, JC virus, BK virus, mycoplasma pneumoniae, chlamydia trachomatis, hepatitis A, campylobacter jejuni, oncogenes, herpes simplex virus. BIOPAP Human Papillomavirus DNA Typing Assay for cervical smears. PATHO GENE DNA probe assay kits for adenoviras, cytomegalovisus, Epstein-Barr virus, Herpes Simplex virus, Chlamydia trachomatis, Human Papilloma virus. Microplate hybridization assay for HIV, Mycobacterium, tuberculosis complex (MTB).

Immunetics, Inc. 800-227-4765
27 Drydock Ave Ste 6, Boston, MA 02210
Checkerboard DNA Hybridization System used in dot blot DNA application.

Immuno Concepts N.A. Ltd. 800-251-5115
9779 Business Park Dr, Sacramento, CA 95827
DNA antibody test systems or antigen control.

TEST, DNA-PROBE, OTHER *(cont'd)*

Jbm Service Limited 800-663-2280
1405 Menu Road, Westbank, BC V4T-2R9 Canada
SENSITEST PROBE TESTER tests oximeter probes with 2 line LCD. OXITEST PLUS and OXITEST PLUS7 oximeter simulator tests pulse oximetry of all makes via a 75 item menu by simulating SpO2 and pulse ampliture.

Promega Corp. 800-356-9526
2800 Woods Hollow Rd, Fitchburg, WI 53711
RNA/DNA probes.

Qiagen Gaithersburg, Inc. 800-344-3631
1201 Clopper Rd, Gaithersburg, MD 20878
Hybrid Capture HPV DNA assay.

Scimedx Corporation 800-221-5598
100 Ford Rd Ste 100-08, Denville, NJ 07834
Immunofluorescent indirect anti-DNA antibody.

TEST, DONOR, CMV *(Immunology) 82MZE*

Virotech International, Inc. 301-924-8000
12 Meem Ave Ste C, Gaithersburg, MD 20877
Cmv.

TEST, EQUIPMENT, STERILIZATION *(General) 80WLS*

Agion Technologies Inc. 781-224-7100
60 Audubon Rd, Wakefield, MA 01880
Agion's naturally-safe silver based antimicrobial combines the natural protection of ionic silver with a patented delivery system. It is tolerant of the high temperatures used in manufacturing operations and has been proven effective in independent laboratory testing against a broad spectrum of bacteria.

Air Techniques International 410-363-9696
11403 Cronridge Dr, Owings Mills, MD 21117
HEPA filter test equipment for cleanrooms, biosafety cabinets and laminar-flow workstations; Respirator test equipment and respirator fit test equipment for QNFT.

Andersen Products, Inc., 800-523-1276
3202 Caroline Dr, Health Science Park, Haw River, NC 27258
Various test equipment for use with ethylene-oxide sterilization.

Cadco Dental Products 800-833-8267
600 E Hueneme Rd, Oxnard, CA 93033

Dux Dental 800-833-8267
600 E Hueneme Rd, Oxnard, CA 93033

Hach Company / Environmental Test Systems 800-548-4381
23575 County Road 106, PO Box 4659, Elkhart, IN 46514
SteriChek Medical Test Strips measure peroxide, residual chlorine, total chloramines, peracetic acid, bicarb pH and hardness in water. Hach also offers SteriChek DPD test kits and refills.

Johnson & Johnson Medical Division Of Ethicon, Inc. 800-423-4018
2500 E Arbrook Blvd, Arlington, TX 76014

Scican Inc. 800-572-1211
701 Technology Dr, Canonsburg, PA 15317

Sterile Technologies, Inc. 518-793-7077
PO Box 4742, 63 Park Rd., Queensbury, NY 12804
Ethylene oxide sterilizer, steam autoclave, tabletop autoclave manufacturer, temperature/relative humidity monitoring systems. Environmental monitoring systems.

Surgical Technologies, Inc. 800-777-9987
292 E Lafayette Frontage Rd, Saint Paul, MN 55107

TEST, ERYTHROPOIETIN *(Hematology) 81GGT*

Beckman Coulter Inc. 800-231-7970
445 Medical Center Blvd, Webster, TX 77598
EPO RIA

Diasorin Inc 800-328-1482
1951 Northwestern Ave S, PO Box 285, Stillwater, MN 55082
EPO-TRAC erythropoietin RIA kit.

Nichols Institute Diagnostics 949-940-7200
1311 Calle Batido, San Clemente, CA 92673
Epo.

TEST, ETHYL ALCOHOL *(Toxicology) 91DMJ*

Acon Laboratories, Inc. 858-535-2030
10125 Mesa Rim Rd, San Diego, CA 92121
Alcohol Saliva Test Strips

Chematics, Inc. 574-834-4080
Hwy. 13 South, North Webster, IN 46555
Solid phase determination of ethyl alcohol.

TEST, ETHYL ALCOHOL *(cont'd)*

Draeger Safety, Inc. 800-922-5518
101 Technology Dr, Pittsburgh, PA 15275

Genzyme Corp. 800-325-2436
160 Christian St, Oxford, CT 06478
Kinetic rate. Alcohol dehydrogenase, endpoint.

Intoximeters, Inc. 800-451-8639
8110 Lackland Rd, Saint Louis, MO 63114

Medical & Clinical Consortium (Mcc) 877-622-8378
13740 Nelson Ave, City Of Industry, CA 91746
MCC Saliva Alcohol Test, is intended for the rapid semi-quantitative determination of ethyl alcohol level in human saliva.

Poly Scientific R&D Corp. 800-645-5825
70 Cleveland Ave, Bay Shore, NY 11706
95%.

TEST, EUGLOBULIN LYSIS *(Hematology) 81JBO*

Dade Behring, Inc. 800-948-3233
1717 Deerfield Rd, Deerfield, IL 60015

TEST, FACTOR II G20210A MUTATIONS, GENOMIC DNA PCR *(Hematology) 81NPR*

Autogenomics, Incorporated 760-477-2251
2890 Scott St, Vista, CA 92081
Test,factor ii g20210a mutations,genomic dna pcr.

TEST, FACTOR V LEIDEN MUTATIONS, GENOMIC DNA PCR *(Hematology) 81NPQ*

Autogenomics, Incorporated 760-477-2251
2890 Scott St, Vista, CA 92081
Test,factor v leiden mutations,genomic dna pcr.

TEST, FERTILITY MONITORING *(Obstetrics/Gyn) 85VJM*

Acon Laboratories, Inc. 858-535-2030
10125 Mesa Rim Rd, San Diego, CA 92121

Bio-Medical Products Corp. 800-543-7427
10 Halstead Rd, Mendham, NJ 07945
LH urine ovulation test. $15.00 for LH one-step ovulation test slide (6 per package) - two minute test.

Crosswell International Corporation 305-648-0777
101 Madeira Ave, Coral Gables, FL 33134

Drg International, Inc. 800-321-1167
1167 US Highway 22, Mountainside, NJ 07092
Ovulation test, one step (BEE-SURE).

Embryotech Laboratories, Inc. 800-673-7500
323 Andover St, Wilmington, MA 01887

Inverness Medical Inc. 732-308-3000
569 Halls Mill Rd, Freehold, NJ 07728
Ovulation predictor test.

Jant Pharmacal Corp. 800-676-5565
16255 Ventura Blvd Ste 505, Encino, CA 91436
LH Ovulation Test to detect the increase of luteinizing hormone (LH) and predict ovulation.

Princeton Biomeditech Corp. 732-274-1000
4242 US Highway 1, Monmouth Junction, NJ 08852
OvuSign LH, one-step ovulation predictor kit.

Syntron Bioresearch, Inc. 800-854-6226
2774 Loker Ave W, Carlsbad, CA 92010
Ovulation test.

Zetek, Inc. 800-367-2837
876 Ventura St, Aurora, CO 80011

TEST, FETAL HEMOGLOBIN *(Hematology) 81KQI*

Ortho-Clinical Diagnostics, Inc. 800-828-6316
513 Technology Blvd, Rochester, NY 14626
Screening kit, fetal blood cell tast.

TEST, FIBRINOGEN *(Hematology) 81GIS*

Bio/Data Corp. 215-441-4000
155 Gibraltar Rd, Horsham, PA 19044
Fibrinogen assay.

Biomerieux Inc. 800-682-2666
100 Rodolphe St, Durham, NC 27712
Fibriquik kit or components for quantitative fibrinogen determination.

Diasorin Inc 800-328-1482
1951 Northwestern Ave S, PO Box 285, Stillwater, MN 55082

Fisher Diagnostics 877-722-4366
11515 Vanstory Dr Ste 125, Huntersville, NC 28078
Thrombin time reagent & venom time reagent.

TEST, FIBRINOGEN *(cont'd)*

Kent Laboratories, Inc. 360-398-8641
777 Jorgensen Pl, Bellingham, WA 98226
2 ml antiserum.

R2 Diagnostics, Inc. 574-288-4377
1801 Commerce Dr, South Bend, IN 46628
Fibrinogen kit.

TEST, FOLLICLE STIMULATING HORMONE (FSH), OVER THE COUNTER *(Toxicology) 91NGA*

QuantRx Biomedical Corp. 503-252-9565
5920 NE 112th Ave, Portland, OR 97220

St. Paul Biotech 714-903-1000
11555 Monarch St, Garden Grove, CA 92841
Menopause test.

TEST, GLYCOSYLATED HEMOGLOBIN ASSAY *(Hematology) 81LCP*

Bayer Healthcare, Llc 574-256-3430
510 Oakmead Pkwy, Sunnyvale, CA 94085
Hba1c or a1c.

Bayer Healthcare, Llc 574-256-3430
430 S Beiger St, Mishawaka, IN 46544
Assay, glycosylated hemoglobin.

Bio-Rad Laboratories Inc., Clinical Systems Div. 800-224-6723
4000 Alfred Nobel Dr, Hercules, CA 94547
Hemoglobin a1c program.

Biorad Laboratories 800-2BI-ORAD
1000 Alfred Nobel Dr, Hercules, CA 94547

Carolina Liquid Chemistries Corp. 800-471-7272
510 W Central Ave Ste C, Brea, CA 92821
Glycohemoglobin reagent.

Diabetes Technologies, Inc. 229-227-1245
184 Big Star Dr, Thomasville, GA 31757
A1 c test.

Diazyme Laboratories 858-455-4761
12889 Gregg Ct, Poway, CA 92064
Glycated serum protein enzymatic assay.

Flexsite Diagnostics, Inc. 772-221-8893
3543 SW Corporate Pkwy, Palm City, FL 34990
Various.

Jas Diagnostics, Inc. 305-418-2320
7220 NW 58th St, Miami, FL 33166
Fructosamine.

Nerl Diagnostics Llc. 401-824-2046
14 Almeida Ave, East Providence, RI 02914
Glycohemoglobin test kit.

PerkinElmer 800-762-4000
940 Winter St, Waltham, MA 02451

Pointe Scientific, Inc. 800-445-9853
5449 Research Dr, Canton, MI 48188
Direct measurement HbA1c. Single channel immunoassay. No pretreatment, on board lyse parameters available.

Primus Diagnostics 800-377-4752
4231 E 75th Ter, Kansas City, MO 64132
PDQ--Glycohemoglobin analyzer system featuring an interference-free boronate affinity assay, a 2-minute throughput and a small footprint designed for the clinic and small to medium lab. Available in two models -- the direct injection PDQ Standalone or the automated PDQ Plus.

Sandare Intl., Inc. 972-293-7440
910 Kck Way, Cedar Hill, TX 75104
No common name listed.

Stanbio Laboratory, Inc. 830-249-0772
1261 N Main St, Boerne, TX 78006
$126.00 for glycohemoglobin (HbA1) test sets with ion-exchange resin, lysing reagent, standard, control and serum separators. $41.50 for 2 x 1ml glycohemoglobin control set with normal and abnormal control (1ml ea.). $52.50 for 2 x 1ml glycohemglobin standard.

Teco Diagnostics 714-693-7788
1268 N Lakeview Ave, Anaheim, CA 92807
Hemoglobin a1c reagent set.

Vital Diagnostics Inc. 714-672-3553
1075 W Lambert Rd Ste D, Brea, CA 92821
Hemoglobin a1c reagent kit.

TEST, HEMOGLOBIN BART'S *(Hematology) 81LGL*

Bio-Rad Laboratories Inc., Clinical Systems Div. 800-224-6723
4000 Alfred Nobel Dr, Hercules, CA 94547
Hemoglobin testing program.

PerkinElmer 800-762-4000
940 Winter St, Waltham, MA 02451
Alpha thalassemia screen.

TEST, HEPARIN (CLOTTING TIME) *(Hematology) 81KFF*

Celsis Laboratory Group 800-523-5227
165 Fieldcrest Ave, Edison, NJ 08837

Diagnostica Stago, Inc. 800-222-COAG
5 Century Dr, Parsippany, NJ 07054

Fisher Diagnostics 877-722-4366
11515 Vanstory Dr Ste 125, Huntersville, NC 28078

Haemachem, Inc. 314-644-3277
2335 S Hanley Rd, Saint Louis, MO 63144
Heparin assay.

Helena Laboratories 409-842-3714
PO Box 752, Beaumont, TX 77704

Heptest Laboratories, Inc. 314-962-3527
1431 Hanley Industrial Ct, Saint Louis, MO 63144
Heparin assay.

International Technidyne Corp. 800-631-5945
23 Nevsky St, Edison, NJ 08820

International Technidyne Corporation 732-548-5700
8 Olsen Ave, Edison, NJ 08820
Heparin response test, various.

TEST, HEPATITIS A (ANTIBODY AND IGM ANTIBODY) *(Microbiology) 83LOL*

Diasorin Inc 800-328-1482
1951 Northwestern Ave S, PO Box 285, Stillwater, MN 55082
ETI-AB-HAVK PLUS for the detection of Total Antibodies to Hepatitis A Virus. ETI-HA-IgMK PLUS for the detection of IgM Antibodies to Hepatitis A Virus.

Inamco International Corp. 800-724-4003
801 Montrose Ave, South Plainfield, NJ 07080
MEDICOS.

United Biotech, Inc. 650-961-2910
211 S Whisman Rd Ste E, Mountain View, CA 94041
ELISA detecting HbsAg (Hepatitis B Surface Antigen)

TEST, HIV DETECTION *(Immunology) 82MZF*

Bio-Medical Products Corp. 800-543-7427
10 Halstead Rd, Mendham, NJ 07945

Chembio Diagnostic Systems, Inc. 631-924-1135
3661 Horseblock Rd, Medford, NY 11763
Rapid test for detection of antibodies to hiv-1 and hiv-2.

Globalemed Llc. 703-894-0710
1101 King St, Suites 370, 270, 170, Alexandria, VA 22314

Maxim Biomedical Incorporated 301-251-0800
1500 E Gude Dr Ste A, Rockville, MD 20850
Hiv-1 urine eia.

United Biotech, Inc. 650-961-2910
211 S Whisman Rd Ste E, Mountain View, CA 94041
Antigens: HIV p24 Core Protein, Recombinant HIV p24-env (I) Protein, Recombinant HIV p24-env core (I) Protein, Recombinant HIV p24-env (II) Protein, Recombinant HIV p24-env Type O CNS, Recombinant HIV p17 Polypeptide, Recombinant HIV p66 Reverse Transciptase Polypeptide, HIV 17-24 Fusion Protein

Virotech International, Inc. 301-924-8000
12 Meem Ave Ste C, Gaithersburg, MD 20877
Hiv.

TEST, HUMAN CHORIONIC GONADOTROPIN *(Immunology) 82JZN*

Bio-Medical Products Corp. 800-543-7427
10 Halstead Rd, Mendham, NJ 07945
$125.00 for HCG one-step urine/serum pregnancy test slide (50 tests per package) - two minute test.

Celsis Laboratory Group 800-523-5227
165 Fieldcrest Ave, Edison, NJ 08837

Dako North America, Inc 805-566-6655
6392 Via Real, Carpinteria, CA 93013

Globalemed Llc. 703-894-0710
1101 King St, Suites 370, 270, 170, Alexandria, VA 22314

TEST, HUMAN CHORIONIC GONADOTROPIN *(cont'd)*

Immunostics, Inc. 800-722-7505
3505 Sunset Ave, Ocean, NJ 07712

Inverness Medical Inc. 732-308-3000
569 Halls Mill Rd, Freehold, NJ 07728
INVERNESS MEDICAL.

J&S Medical Associates 800-229-6000
35 Tripp St Ste 1, Framingham, MA 01702
ACCUTEX.

Sa Scientific, Inc. 800-272-2710
4919 Golden Quail, San Antonio, TX 78240
Latex slide test.

Stanbio Laboratory, Inc. 830-249-0772
1261 N Main St, Boerne, TX 78006
QUPID HCG Pregnancy test kit - 50 test or 25 test. One step for urine samples only. 5 minute test.

TEST, HUMAN CHORIONIC GONADOTROPIN, SERUM
(Immunology) 82DHA

Ameritek Usa, Inc. 425-379-2580
125 130th St SE Ste 200, Everett, WA 98208
Hcg 2 iu/ml test kit.

Azog, Inc. 908-213-2900
1011 US Highway 22, Alpha, NJ 08865
Various types of immunochromatographic test for urine pregnancy (hcg).

Bremancos Diagnostics Inc. 800-830-2593
6800 Kitimat Rd., Unit 2, Mississauga, ONT L5N-5M1 Canada

Chembio Diagnostic Systems, Inc. 631-924-1135
3661 Horseblock Rd, Medford, NY 11763
Various.

Diagnostic Technology, Inc. 631-582-4949
175 Commerce Dr Ste L, Hauppauge, NY 11788
Latex slide test for pregnancy.

Germaine Laboratories, Inc. 210-692-4192
4139 Gardendale St Ste 101, San Antonio, TX 78229
Various.

Globalemed Llc. 703-894-0710
1101 King St, Suites 370, 270, 170, Alexandria, VA 22314

Health Chem Diagnostics Llc 954-979-3845
3341 W McNab Rd, Pompano Beach, FL 33069
System, test, human chorionic gonadotropin.

Immunostics, Inc. 800-722-7505
3505 Sunset Ave, Ocean, NJ 07712

Jant Pharmacal Corp. 800-676-5565
16255 Ventura Blvd Ste 505, Encino, CA 91436
Solid phase immunochromatographic assay/detection of hcg.

Pan Probe Biotech, Inc. 858-689-9936
7396 Trade St, San Diego, CA 92121
Determination of hcg in human urine.

Sun Biomedical Laboratories, Inc. 888-440-8388
604 Vpr Center, 1001 Lower Landing Road, Blackwood, NJ 08012
Pregnancy urine test kit (dipstrip).

Teco Diagnostics 714-693-7788
1268 N Lakeview Ave, Anaheim, CA 92807
One-step pregnancy test.

Unotech Diagnostics, Inc. 510-352-3070
2235 Polvorosa Dr Ste 220, San Leandro, CA 94577
Hcg test.

Victorch Meditek, Inc. 858-530-9191
7313 Carroll Rd Ste A-B, San Diego, CA 92121
Hcg urine rapid test.

TEST, HUMAN PLACENTAL LACTOGEN *(Immunology) 82DHT*

Dako North America, Inc 805-566-6655
6392 Via Real, Carpinteria, CA 93013

TEST, IMMUNITY, CELL-MEDIATED, MYCOBACTERIUM TUBERCULOSIS *(Microbiology) 83NCD*

Bremancos Diagnostics Inc. 800-830-2593
6800 Kitimat Rd., Unit 2, Mississauga, ONT L5N-5M1 Canada
Dengue IgG/IgM, Strep A test

Scantibodies Laboratory, Inc. 619-258-9300
9336 Abraham Way, Santee, CA 92071
Mycobacteium tuberculosis,cell mediated immune response eia test.

TEST, INFECTIOUS MONONUCLEOSIS *(Immunology) 82KTN*

Acon Laboratories, Inc. 858-535-2030
10125 Mesa Rim Rd, San Diego, CA 92121

Akers Biosciences, Inc. 800-451-8378
201 Grove Rd, West Deptford, NJ 08086
HEALTHTEST.

Ameritek Usa, Inc. 425-379-2580
125 130th St SE Ste 200, Everett, WA 98208
Im test kit.

Bio-Medical Products Corp. 800-543-7427
10 Halstead Rd, Mendham, NJ 07945
$145.00 for mono one-step IgM test slide (30 per package).

Diagnostic Technology, Inc. 631-582-4949
175 Commerce Dr Ste L, Hauppauge, NY 11788
Rapid slide test for detection of heterophile antibodies associated with infecti.

Elabsupply 714-446-8740
1001 Starbuck St Apt C306, Fullerton, CA 92833
Teco Diagnostics Serology Infectious Monoucleosis Seriology Test in 50 and 100 test packages.

Genzyme Diagnostics 617-252-7500
6659 Top Gun St, San Diego, CA 92121
Mono test.

Germaine Laboratories, Inc. 210-692-4192
4139 Gardendale St Ste 101, San Antonio, TX 78229
Infectious mononucleosis immunological test system.

Hemagen Diagnostics, Inc. 800-436-2436
9033 Red Branch Rd, Columbia, MD 21045
Ebv-vca ifa.

Immunostics, Inc. 800-722-7505
3505 Sunset Ave, Ocean, NJ 07712

Innovacon, Inc. 858-535-2030
4106 Sorrento Valley Blvd, San Diego, CA 92121
Infectious mononucleosis immunological test.

Inverness Medical Professional Diagnostics-San Die 858-535-2030
4106 Sorrento Valley Blvd, San Diego, CA 92121
Infectious mononucleosis immun. test.

J&S Medical Associates 800-229-6000
35 Tripp St Ste 1, Framingham, MA 01702
ACCUTEX qualitative and quantitative latex agglutination kits for RF, ASO, SLE, CRP, Mono and Staph.

Jant Pharmacal Corp. 800-676-5565
16255 Ventura Blvd Ste 505, Encino, CA 91436
Accutest infectious mononucleosis WB test is a rapid visual test used for detection of IgM antibodies to infectious mononucleosis.

Meridian Bioscience, Inc. 800-696-0739
3471 River Hills Dr, Cincinnati, OH 45244
A qualitative and semiquantitative differential slide test for the heterophile antibody of infectious mononucleosis.

Nerl Diagnostics Llc. 401-824-2046
14 Almeida Ave, East Providence, RI 02914
Infectious mononucleosis assay.

Princeton Biomeditech Corp. 732-274-1000
4242 US Highway 1, Monmouth Junction, NJ 08852
BioSign Mono infectious mononucleosis test; detects IM heterophile antibody (IgM) from whole blood, serum, or plasma; results in 8 minutes.

Pulse Scientific, Inc. 800-363-7907
5100 S. Service Rd., Unit 18, Burlington, ONT L7L-6A5 Canada

Sa Scientific, Inc. 800-272-2710
4919 Golden Quail, San Antonio, TX 78240
Latex slide test.

Seradyn, Inc. 800-428-4072
7998 Georgetown Rd Ste 1000, Indianapolis, IN 46268
Color change red-cell agglutination. Also available, COLOR Q. Seradyn Color Q Mono. Rapid IgM test for the qualitative detection of infectious mononucleosis.

Wampole Laboratories 800-257-9525
2 Research Way, Princeton, NJ 08540
MONO-TEST, MONO-PLUS and MONO-LATEX Red cell or latex agglutination type.

TEST, INFLUENZA *(Microbiology) 83VIG*

Princeton Biomeditech Corp. 732-274-1000
4242 US Highway 1, Monmouth Junction, NJ 08852
BioSign Influenza A&B, rapid antigen test from a swab.

TEST, INFLUENZA *(cont'd)*

Prodesse, Inc. 888-589-6974
W229N1870 Westwood Dr, Waukesha, WI 53186
Hexaplex® Plus - Multiplex PCR Reagents for simultaneous detection and differentiation of Influenza A, Influenza B, Parainfluenza 1, 2 and 3, RSV and human metapneumovirus - Research Use Only and CE Marked.

Thermo Biostar, Inc. 800-637-3717
331 S 104th St, Louisville, CO 80027
The only rapid (15 minute) test for the detection of Influenza A & B viral antigen.

TEST, LEUKOCYTE TYPING *(Hematology) 81LGO*

Akers Biosciences, Inc. 800-451-8378
201 Grove Rd, West Deptford, NJ 08086
HEALTHTEST rapid blood typing.

Genetic Testing Institute 262-754-1000
20925 Crossroads Cir Ste 200, Waukesha, WI 53186
Hla abc tissue typing tray.

One Lambda, Inc. 800-822-8824
21001 Kittridge St, Canoga Park, CA 91303

Trans-Type Of Maryland, Inc. 301-695-7087
108 Byte Dr Ste 101, Frederick, MD 21702
Various types of lymphocyte phenotyping trays.

TEST, LUTEINIZING HORMONE (LH), OVER THE COUNTER
(Chemistry) 75NGE

Fertility Tech. Inc 702-233-2601
9405 Darwell Dr, Las Vegas, NV 89117
Luteinizing hormone test system.

Scantibodies Laboratory, Inc. 619-258-9300
9336 Abraham Way, Santee, CA 92071
Ovulation tests kits.

Sci International Inc. 301-696-8879
5902 Enterprise Ct, Frederick, MD 21703
In vitro ovulation test.

TEST, METHAMPHETAMINE, OVER THE COUNTER
(Toxicology) 91NGG

St. Paul Biotech 714-903-1000
11555 Monarch St, Garden Grove, CA 92841
Methamphetamine test.

TEST, MYOCARDIAL INFARCTION (HEART ATTACK)
(Chemistry) 75VIQ

Princeton Biomeditech Corp. 732-274-1000
4242 US Highway 1, Monmouth Junction, NJ 08852
LifeSign MI, rapid cardiac markers for heart attack; Troponin I, CK-MB, and myoglobin cardiac-marker panel tests.

TEST, NATRIURETIC PEPTIDE *(Chemistry) 75NBC*

Abbott Point Of Care Inc. 609-443-9300
104 Windsor Center Dr, East Windsor, NJ 08520
B-type natriuretic peptide.

Biosite Incorporated 888-246-7483
9975 Summers Ridge Rd, San Diego, CA 92121
B-type natriuretic peptide test system.

TEST, NEURAL TUBE DEFECT, ALPHA-FETOPROTEIN (AFP)
(Immunology) 82LOK

Abbott Diagnostics Intl, Biotechnology Ltd 787-846-3500
Road #2 KM. 58.0 , PO Box 278, Cruce Davila, Barceloneta, PR 00617
Alpha-fetoprotein.

TEST, NUCLEAR ANTIGEN, EPSTEIN-BARR VIRUS
(Microbiology) 83LLM

Focus Diagnostics, Inc. 714-220-1900
10703 Progress Way, Cypress, CA 90630
Multiple ebv serological reagents.

Innominata dba GENBIO 800-288-4368
15222 Avenue of Science Ste A, San Diego, CA 92128
Immunowell ebv ebna igg test.

Zeus Scientific, Inc. 800-286-2111
PO Box 38, Raritan, NJ 08869
100 EBV-NA IFA antibody test systems. EBNA 96 tests ELISA IgG. EBV-EA 96 tests ELISA IgG only.

TEST, PLATELET ANTIBODY *(Hematology) 81MYP*

Genetic Testing Institute 262-754-1000
20925 Crossroads Cir Ste 200, Waukesha, WI 53186
Antigen capture elisa for the detection of antibodies to platelet-specific antig.

TEST, PROSTATE SPECIFIC ANTIGEN, FREE, (NONCOMPLEXED) TO DISTINGUISH PROSTATE CANCER FROM BENIGN CONDITIONS *(Immunology) 82MTG*

Ameritek Usa, Inc. 425-379-2580
125 130th St SE Ste 200, Everett, WA 98208
Psa test kit.

Globalemed Llc. 703-894-0710
1101 King St, Suites 370, 270, 170, Alexandria, VA 22314

Qualigen, Inc. 760-918-9165
2042 Corte Del Nogal, Carlsbad, CA 92011
Chemi iminescence assay for the determination of free prostate specific antigen.

TEST, QUALITATIVE AND QUANTITATIVE FACTOR DEFICIENCY
(Hematology) 81GGP

Binding Site, Inc., The 800-633-4484
5889 Oberlin Dr Ste 101, San Diego, CA 92121

Bio/Data Corp. 215-441-4000
155 Gibraltar Rd, Horsham, PA 19044
Factor test.

Biosite Incorporated 888-246-7483
9975 Summers Ridge Rd, San Diego, CA 92121
Protein c test.

Chrono-Log Corp. 800-247-6665
2 W Park Rd, Havertown, PA 19083
RISTOCETIN Cofactor Assay Kit. For use in the quantitative determination of Factor VIII Ristocetin cofactor activity in citrated plasma.

Dade Behring, Inc. 800-948-3233
1717 Deerfield Rd, Deerfield, IL 60015

Diagnostica Stago, Inc. 800-222-COAG
5 Century Dr, Parsippany, NJ 07054

Genetic Testing Institute 262-754-1000
20925 Crossroads Cir Ste 200, Waukesha, WI 53186
Factor viii inhibitor assay.

Haemachem, Inc. 314-644-3277
2335 S Hanley Rd, Saint Louis, MO 63144
Activated factor x.

Heptest Laboratories, Inc. 314-962-3527
1431 Hanley Industrial Ct, Saint Louis, MO 63144
Factor xa_ bovine.

International Technidyne Corporation 732-548-5700
8 Olsen Ave, Edison, NJ 08820
Factor vi test and quality control reagent.

R2 Diagnostics, Inc. 574-288-4377
1801 Commerce Dr, South Bend, IN 46628
Thrombotek pc, ps & resistin.

Ramco Laboratories, Inc. 281-313-1200
4100 Greenbriar Dr Ste 200, Stafford, TX 77477
VFE is an enzyme immunoassay for measuring the level of VWF antigen in human plasma.

TEST, QUALITATIVE, FOR HLA, NON-DIAGNOSTIC
(Hematology) 81MZI

Genetic Testing Institute 262-754-1000
20925 Crossroads Cir Ste 200, Waukesha, WI 53186
Antibody monitoring system hla class i and class ii (ams1, ams1+2).

Tepnel Lifecodes Corporation 203-328-9500
550 West Ave, Stamford, CT 06902
Luminex 100 lficodes hla sso,screening assay for the detection of igg antibodies.

TEST, RADIO-ALLERGEN ABSORBENT (RAST)
(Immunology) 82DHB

Arlington Scientific, Inc. Asi 800-654-0146
1840 N Technology Dr, Springville, UT 84663
IVT RAST tracer unit intended for the semi-quantitative determination of allergen-specific IgE in serum.

Hitachi Chemical Diagnostics, Inc. 650-961-5501
630 Clyde Ct, Mountain View, CA 94043
Mast cla allergy systems.

TEST, RADIO-ALLERGEN ABSORBENT (RAST) *(cont'd)*

Hycor Biomedical, Inc. 800-382-2527
7272 Chapman Ave, Garden Grove, CA 92841
Various.

TEST, RADIORECEPTOR *(Chemistry) 75VKI*

Biomedical Technologies, Inc. 781-344-9942
378 Page St, Stoughton, MA 02072

Kronus, Inc. 800-822-6999
12554 W Bridger St Ste 108, Boise, ID 83713
TSH receptor Ab radioreceptor tests for Graves' disease diagnosis. Acetylcholine receptor Ab radioreceptor tests for myasthenia gravis diagnosis.

TEST, RADIORECEPTOR, NEUROLEPTIC DRUGS *(Toxicology) 91LPX*

Biomedical Technologies, Inc. 781-344-9942
378 Page St, Stoughton, MA 02072

TEST, REAGENT, BIOCHEMICAL, NEISSERIA GONORRHOEAE *(Microbiology) 83LTS*

Alpha Biosciences, Inc. 877-825-7428
3651 Clipper Mill Rd, Baltimore, MD 21211
GC agar, GC agar base, GC medium base.

Gen-Probe, Inc. 800-523-5001
10210 Genetic Center Dr, San Diego, CA 92121
PACE 2 Neisseria Gonorrhoeae Probe Competition Assay - supplemental test to verify non-specific signal in endocervical and male urethral swab specimens that test positive in the PACE 2 System assays for Neisseria gonorrhoeae. PACE 2 System for Neisseria Gonorrhoeae - for direct detection of Neisseria gonorrhoeae from endocervical and male urethral swab specimens.

TEST, RECEPTOR, INTERLEUKIN, SERUM *(Immunology) 82WPH*

Invitrogen Corporation 800-955-6288
101 Lincoln Centre Dr, Foster City, CA 94404

TEST, RHEUMATOID FACTOR *(Immunology) 82DHR*

Abbott Diagnostics Div. 626-440-0700
820 Mission St, South Pasadena, CA 91030
Rheumatoid factor.

Advanced Diagnostics, Inc. (Adi) 800-724-4003
801 Montrose Ave, South Plainfield, NJ 07080

Akers Biosciences, Inc. 800-451-8378
201 Grove Rd, West Deptford, NJ 08086
HEALTHTEST.

Ameritek Usa, Inc. 425-379-2580
125 130th St SE Ste 200, Everett, WA 98208
Rf test kit.

Arlington Scientific, Inc. Asi 800-654-0146
1840 N Technology Dr, Springville, UT 84663
RA (Rheumatoid Arthritis) kit, qualitative and quantitative slide agglutination test for the determination of rheumatoid factor (RF) in serum.

Bd Diagnostic Systems 800-675-0908
7 Loveton Cir, Sparks, MD 21152

Beckman Coulter, Inc. 800-742-2345
250 S Kraemer Blvd, PO Box 8000, Brea, CA 92821

Bio-Medical Products Corp. 800-543-7427
10 Halstead Rd, Mendham, NJ 07945
Test with latex slide.

Biomerieux Inc. 800-682-2666
100 Rodolphe St, Durham, NC 27712

Carolina Liquid Chemistries Corp. 800-471-7272
510 W Central Ave Ste C, Brea, CA 92821
Rheumatoid factor reagent.

Diagnostic Technology, Inc. 631-582-4949
175 Commerce Dr Ste L, Hauppauge, NY 11788
Latex slide test for rheumatoid factors.

Diamedix Corp. 800-327-4565
2140 N Miami Ave, Miami, FL 33127
Is-Rheumatoid Factor catalog #720-710.

Hycor Biomedical, Inc. 800-382-2527
7272 Chapman Ave, Garden Grove, CA 92841
Rf autoimmune kit.

Immunospec Corporation 818-717-1840
9428 Eton Ave Ste O, Chatsworth, CA 91311
Rf igm.

TEST, RHEUMATOID FACTOR *(cont'd)*

Immunostics, Inc. 800-722-7505
3505 Sunset Ave, Ocean, NJ 07712

J&S Medical Associates 800-229-6000
35 Tripp St Ste 1, Framingham, MA 01702
ACCUTEX qualitative and quantitative latex agglutination kits for RF, ASO, SLE, CRP, Mono and Staph.

Jas Diagnostics, Inc. 305-418-2320
7220 NW 58th St, Miami, FL 33166
Rheumatiid factor (rf).

Micro Detect, Inc. 714-832-8234
2852 Walnut Ave Ste H1, Tustin, CA 92780
Mdi-rf-test.

Nerl Diagnostics Llc. 401-824-2046
14 Almeida Ave, East Providence, RI 02914
Rf latex kits.

Pulse Scientific, Inc. 800-363-7907
5100 S. Service Rd., Unit 18, Burlington, ONT L7L-6A5 Canada
RF Latex Test, Latex Agglutination Test to detect Rheumatoid Factor (RF) as an aid to diagnosis Rheumatoid Arthritis.

Sa Scientific, Inc. 800-272-2710
4919 Golden Quail, San Antonio, TX 78240
Latex slide test.

Seradyn, Inc. 800-428-4072
7998 Georgetown Rd Ste 1000, Indianapolis, IN 46268
EIA screening and confirmatory diagnostic tests for connective-tissue and rheumatoid disease.

St. Paul Biotech 714-903-1000
11555 Monarch St, Garden Grove, CA 92841
Rheumatoid factor test.

Stanbio Laboratory, Inc. 830-249-0772
1261 N Main St, Boerne, TX 78006
$30.00 for 50 rheumathoid arthritis test kits with RA-latex reagent, positive and negative control serum, glycine-saline buffer and six-cell slide.

Sterling Diagnostics, Inc. 800-637-2661
36645 Metro Ct, Sterling Heights, MI 48312

Teco Diagnostics 714-693-7788
1268 N Lakeview Ave, Anaheim, CA 92807
Rheumatoid factor (rf) reagent: a latex slide test.

Theratest Laboratories, Inc. 800-441-0771
1111 N Main St, Lombard, IL 60148
Enzyme immunoassay for rheumatoid factor, IgM, IgG, IgA isotypes.

United Biotech, Inc. 650-961-2910
211 S Whisman Rd Ste E, Mountain View, CA 94041
ELISA for detecting RF IgM (Rheumatoid Factor)

Wampole Laboratories 800-257-9525
2 Research Way, Princeton, NJ 08540
RHEUMATEX Red Cell or latex agglutination.

Zeus Scientific, Inc. 800-286-2111
PO Box 38, Raritan, NJ 08869
Rheumatoid Factor 96 tests ELISA IgM only.

TEST, ROTAVIRUS *(Microbiology) 83WJX*

Lifesign 800-526-2125
71 Veronica Ave, Somerset, NJ 08873
DIARLEX tests. $120.00 per kit of 20 dual tests for Rotavirus and Adenovirus.

Meridian Bioscience, Inc. 800-696-0739
3471 River Hills Dr, Cincinnati, OH 45244
Latex agglutination test for rotavirus antigen in stool. Also culture confirmation latex agglutination test for Campylobacter jejuni, coli, laridis (50 tests).

Sa Scientific, Inc. 800-272-2710
4919 Golden Quail, San Antonio, TX 78240

Wampole Laboratories 800-257-9525
2 Research Way, Princeton, NJ 08540
Direct antigen detection from stool sample.

TEST, SICKLE CELL *(Hematology) 81GHM*

Biomerieux Inc. 800-682-2666
100 Rodolphe St, Durham, NC 27712
SICKLEQUIK for distinguishing both hetero and homozygous.

Chembio Diagnostic Systems, Inc. 631-924-1135
3661 Horseblock Rd, Medford, NY 11763
Sickle-stat hemoglobin s screening kit (qualitative).

TEST, SICKLE CELL *(cont'd)*

Creative Laboratory Products, Inc. 317-293-2991
6420 Guion Rd, Indianapolis, IN 46268

Dade Behring, Inc. 800-948-3233
1717 Deerfield Rd, Deerfield, IL 60015

Fisher Diagnostics 877-722-4366
11515 Vanstory Dr Ste 125, Huntersville, NC 28078

Michclone Associates, Inc. 248-583-1150
1197 Rochester Rd Ste L, Troy, MI 48083
Sickel cell solubility test.

Ortho-Clinical Diagnostics, Inc. 800-828-6316
513 Technology Blvd, Rochester, NY 14626
Tube test for hemoglobin s.

Sa Scientific, Inc. 800-272-2710
4919 Golden Quail, San Antonio, TX 78240

Sterling Diagnostics, Inc. 800-637-2661
36645 Metro Ct, Sterling Heights, MI 48312
Sickle cell reagent set.

TEST, SPECTACLE DISSOCIATION, BATTERY-POWERED (LANCASTER) *(Ophthalmology) 86HLO*

Gulden Ophthalmics 800-659-2250
225 Cadwalader Ave, Elkins Park, PA 19027

TEST, SYPHILIS (RPR OR VDRL) *(Microbiology) 83UMO*

Akers Biosciences, Inc. 800-451-8378
201 Grove Rd, West Deptford, NJ 08086
HEALTHTEST.

Arlington Scientific, Inc. Asi 800-654-0146
1840 N Technology Dr, Springville, UT 84663
Qualitative and semi-quantitative non-treponemal flocculation card test for the determination of reagin antibodies in serum.

Bd Diagnostic Systems 800-675-0908
7 Loveton Cir, Sparks, MD 21152
5ml VDRL cardiolpin antigen.

Biomerieux Inc. 800-682-2666
100 Rodolphe St, Durham, NC 27712
Reagin automated ELISA for syphillis screening. VISUWELL syphillis antibody automated assay for the detection of Ab to T. Pallidum.

Fujirebio Diagnostics, Inc. (Fdi) 877-861-7246
201 Great Valley Pkwy, Malvern, PA 19355
Confirmatory SERODIA TP-PA.

Hema Diagnostic Systems, Llc 305-867-6123
1666 Kennedy Causeway, Suite 401, North Bay Village, FL 33141
Rapid 1-2-3 hema syphilis whole blood test. Available in strip format or in the new rapid 1-2-3 hema housing.

Immunostics, Inc. 800-722-7505
3505 Sunset Ave, Ocean, NJ 07712

J&S Medical Associates 800-229-6000
35 Tripp St Ste 1, Framingham, MA 01702
ACCUTEX.

Sa Scientific, Inc. 800-272-2710
4919 Golden Quail, San Antonio, TX 78240

Stanbio Laboratory, Inc. 830-249-0772
1261 N Main St, Boerne, TX 78006
$34.00 for 100, $99.00 for 500 Rapid Plasma Reagent test kits with antigen suspension, positive and negative controls, dispensing bottle, needle tip, pipette/stirrers and disposable test cards.

United Biotech, Inc. 650-961-2910
211 S Whisman Rd Ste E, Mountain View, CA 94041
ELISA for detecting Syphilis IgG

Wampole Laboratories 800-257-9525
2 Research Way, Princeton, NJ 08540
WAMPOLE carbon particle RPR kit.

TEST, SYPHILIS, TREPONEMAL *(Hematology) 81MTN*

Ameritek Usa, Inc. 425-379-2580
125 130th St SE Ste 200, Everett, WA 98208
Syphilis test kit.

St. Paul Biotech 714-903-1000
11555 Monarch St, Garden Grove, CA 92841
Syphilis test.

TEST, SYSTEM, IMMUNOASSAY, LIPOPROTEIN-ASSOCIATED PHOSPHOLIPASE A2 *(Immunology) 82NOE*

Diadexus, Inc. 650-246-6400
343 Oyster Point Blvd, South San Francisco, CA 94080
Lp-pla2 test.

TEST, SYSTEM, POTASSIUM, ENZYMATIC METHOD

(Chemistry) 75MZV

Diazyme Laboratories 858-455-4761
12889 Gregg Ct, Poway, CA 92064
Potassium enzymatic assay.

TEST, SYSTEMIC LUPUS ERYTHEMATOSUS

(Immunology) 82DHC

Arlington Scientific, Inc. Asi 800-654-0146
1840 N Technology Dr, Springville, UT 84663
Deoxyribonucleoprotein (DNP) is the antigen to which most SLE (Systemic Lupus Erythematosus) autoantibodies are directed. Stabilized latex particles coated with DNP will agglutinate when mixed with serum from SLE patients. This makes the latex test a useful qualitative and semiquantitative screening test for SLE.

Bio-Medical Products Corp. 800-543-7427
10 Halstead Rd, Mendham, NJ 07945
Test with latex slide.

Corgenix Medical Corporation 800-729-5661
11575 Main St, Broomfield, CO 80020
Multiple

Corgenix, Inc. 800-729-5661
12061 Tejon St, Westminster, CO 80234
Enzyme-linked immunosorbent assay (ELISA) for the determination of anti-cardiolipin or anti-phosphotidylserine antibodies in human serum or plasma.

Immunostics, Inc. 800-722-7505
3505 Sunset Ave, Ocean, NJ 07712

J&S Medical Associates 800-229-6000
35 Tripp St Ste 1, Framingham, MA 01702
ACCUTEX qualitative and quantitative latex agglutination kits for RF, ASO, SLE, CRP, Mono and Staph.

Nerl Diagnostics Llc. 401-824-2046
14 Almeida Ave, East Providence, RI 02914
Sle latex kits.

R2 Diagnostics, Inc. 574-288-4377
1801 Commerce Dr, South Bend, IN 46628
Lupotek detectin, correctin.

Sa Scientific, Inc. 800-272-2710
4919 Golden Quail, San Antonio, TX 78240
Latex slide test.

Sterling Diagnostics, Inc. 800-637-2661
36645 Metro Ct, Sterling Heights, MI 48312

TEST, TETRAHYDROCANNABINOL *(Toxicology) 91DKE*

Ameritek Usa, Inc. 425-379-2580
125 130th St SE Ste 200, Everett, WA 98208
Thc test kit.

Biochemical Diagnostics, Inc. 800-223-4835
180 Heartland Blvd, Edgewood, NY 11717

Dyna-Tek, Inc. 913-438-6363
8369 Nieman Rd, Lenexa, KS 66214
Drug detection system.

Germaine Laboratories, Inc. 210-692-4192
4139 Gardendale St Ste 101, San Antonio, TX 78229
Thc marijuana.

Globalemed Llc. 703-894-0710
1101 King St, Suites 370, 270, 170, Alexandria, VA 22314

Immunalysis Corporation 909-482-0840
829 Towne Center Dr, Pomona, CA 91767
No common name listed.

Medtox Diagnostics Inc. 800-334-1116
1238 Anthony Rd, Burlington, NC 27215
EZ-SCREEN competitive enzyme immunoassay screening test for cannabinoids and metabolites.

Medtox Diagnostics, Inc. 800-334-1116
1640 Nova Ln, Burlington, NC 27215
Immunochromatographic assay for cannabinoids (thc).

Varian Inc 650-424-5078
25200 Commercentre Dr, Lake Forest, CA 92630
Test, substance/drug abuse cannabinoid;solid-phase extraction device.

W.H.P.M., Inc. 978-927-3808
9662 Telstar Ave, El Monte, CA 91731
Drug of abuse screening.

TEST, THROMBIN TIME *(Hematology) 81GJA*

Bio/Data Corp. 215-441-4000
155 Gibraltar Rd, Horsham, PA 19044
Thrombin clotting time.

Biomerieux Inc. 800-682-2666
100 Rodolphe St, Durham, NC 27712
THROMBOQUICK thrombin-time reagent.

Haemachem, Inc. 314-644-3277
2335 S Hanley Rd, Saint Louis, MO 63144
Thrombin.

Heptest Laboratories, Inc. 314-962-3527
1431 Hanley Industrial Ct, Saint Louis, MO 63144
Bovine thrombin.

International Technidyne Corp. 800-631-5945
23 Nevsky St, Edison, NJ 08820

International Technidyne Corporation 732-548-5700
8 Olsen Ave, Edison, NJ 08820
Thrombin test.

R2 Diagnostics, Inc. 574-288-4377
1801 Commerce Dr, South Bend, IN 46628
Multiple.

TEST, THROMBOPLASTIN GENERATION *(Hematology) 81GKQ*

Biomerieux Inc. 800-682-2666
100 Rodolphe St, Durham, NC 27712

TEST, THYROID AUTOANTIBODY *(Immunology) 82JZO*

American Laboratory Products Co. 800-592-5726
26 Keewaydin Dr Ste G, Salem, NH 03079
Quantitative anti-TG and anti-TPO with ready to use reagents in ELISA formats.

Bio-Rad Laboratories, Life Science Group 800-424-6723
2000 Alfred Nobel Dr, Hercules, CA 94547

Diagnostic Hybrids, Inc. 740-589-3300
1055 E State St Ste 100, Athens, OH 45701
Analyte specific reagents for defecting thyroid stimulating auto antibodies.

Globalemed Llc. 703-894-0710
1101 King St, Suites 370, 270, 170, Alexandria, VA 22314

Innominata dba GENBIO 800-288-4368
15222 Avenue of Science Ste A, San Diego, CA 92128
Immunodot thyroid auroimmunity panel.

Kronus, Inc. 800-822-6999
12554 W Bridger St Ste 108, Boise, ID 83713
TSH receptor Ab radioreceptor tests for Graves' disease. Thryoid peroxidase (TPO) Ab direct or thyroglobulin Ab direct RIA and EIA tests for Hashimoto's disease.

Nichols Institute Diagnostics 949-940-7200
1311 Calle Batido, San Clemente, CA 92673
Multiple.

Quest Intl., Inc. 305-592-6991
8127 NW 29th St, Doral, FL 33122
Thyroid autoantibody serological reagents.

Scimedx Corporation 800-221-5598
100 Ford Rd Ste 100-08, Denville, NJ 07834

Specialities Electronics Co., Inc. 609-267-5593
43 Washington St, Mount Holly, NJ 08060
Thyroid diagnostic counting system.

United Biotech, Inc. 650-961-2910
211 S Whisman Rd Ste E, Mountain View, CA 94041
ELISA quantitative for detecting Total T3 (Triiodothyronine)

TEST, UREA (BREATH OR BLOOD) *(Microbiology) 83MSQ*

Ameritek Usa, Inc. 425-379-2580
125 130th St SE Ste 200, Everett, WA 98208
H.pylori-uresa test kit.

Metabolic Solutions, Inc. 866-302-1998
460 Amherst St, Nashua, NH 03063
13c urea breath test to measure active H. pylori infection.

TEST, URINE LEUKOCYTE *(Hematology) 81LJX*

Arkray Factory Usa, Inc. 952-646-3168
5182 W 76th St, Minneapolis, MN 55439
Urine test strips.

Bayer Healthcare Llc 914-524-2955
555 White Plains Rd Fl 5, Tarrytown, NY 10591
Various tests.

TEST, URINE LEUKOCYTE *(cont'd)*

Bayer Healthcare, Llc 574-256-3430
430 S Beiger St, Mishawaka, IN 46544
Multiple.

Serim Research Corp. 574-264-3440
3506 Reedy Dr, Elkhart, IN 46514
Test for the presumptive identification of leukocytes in peritoneal dialysate.

Teco Diagnostics 714-693-7788
1268 N Lakeview Ave, Anaheim, CA 92807
Various.

TEST, VAGINAL, BACTERIAL SIALIDASE *(Chemistry) 75MXB*

Gryphus Diagnostics, L.L.C. 865-251-0101
2200 Sutherland Ave Ste H101, Knoxville, TN 37919
Bvblue.

TESTER, ALIGNMENT, LASER BEAM *(General) 80WZF*

Coherent, Inc. 800-527-3786
5100 Patrick Henry Dr, Santa Clara, CA 95054

TESTER, AUDITORY IMPEDANCE *(Ear/Nose/Throat) 77ETY*

Cardinal Healthcare 209, Inc. 610-862-0800
5225 Verona Rd, Fitchburg, WI 53711
Impedance meter, abr screener.

Fecom Corporation 800-292-3362
12 Stults Rd Ste 103, Dayton, NJ 08810
Digital Key-chain battery tester with LCD indicator for hearing aid batteries and household battery tester that tester sizes D, C, AA, AAA, 9 volt, and Lithium all in one unit

Intelligent Hearing Systems, Corp. 800-447-9783
6860 SW 81st St, Miami, FL 33143
SMART SCREENER automated newborn hearing screener, using evoked potentials. IVRA automated behavioral hearing evaluation.

Maico Diagnostics 888-941-4201
7625 Golden Triangle Dr, Eden Prairie, MN 55344
Tympanometers series for children (RACE CAR and Quik TYMP) as well as adult screening and diagnosis.

Md International, Inc. 305-669-9003
11300 NW 41st St, Doral, FL 33178

Micro Audiometrics Corp. 800-729-9509
655 Keller Rd, Murphy, NC 28906
$1,695.00 for EARSCAN Impedance. $100.00 for acoustic reflex option.

Neurocom International, Inc. 503-653-2144
9570 SE Lawnfield Rd, Clackamas, OR 97015
Pressure test accessory for equitest.

Singer Medical Products Inc., Md Systems Div. 630-860-6500
3800 Buckner St, El Paso, TX 79925
Screening audiometer & impedance analyzer.

Singer Medical Products, Inc. 800-222-2572
790 Maple Ln, Bensenville, IL 60106
$2,495 for portable impedance tester & audiometer MD-1, $1,995 for portable impedance tester MD-2, $3,195 for desk-top impedance tester & audiometer with printer model MD-3, $395 for MD-P printer for MD-1 or MD-2, $725 for portable audiometer MD-4, $1,095 for portable audiometer with printer.

Starkey Laboratories, Inc. 800-328-8602
6700 Washington Ave S, Eden Prairie, MN 55344
$249.50 for bone cross headband.

TESTER, COLOR VISION *(Ophthalmology) 86HIT*

Good-Lite Co. 800-362-3860
865 Muirfield Dr, Bartlett, IL 60133
OPTEC 2000 is a vision tester machine.

Gulden Ophthalmics 800-659-2250
225 Cadwalader Ave, Elkins Park, PA 19027

Lkc Technologies, Inc. 800-638-7055
2 Professional Dr Ste 222, Gaithersburg, MD 20879
Available as an Anomaloscope quadrant tester model AQT-10.

Mast/Keystone View 800-806-6569
2200 Dickerson Rd, Reno, NV 89503
TELEBINOCULAR, VS II; both instruments are used in conjunction with Dvorine Color Tests providing accurate information about the patients' color perception as well as far point, near point, depth perception and acuity. DVS II Driver Vision Screener. Specifically for DMV's, industrial drivers or any application where driver vision must be evaluated.

TESTER, COLOR VISION *(cont'd)*

National Optronics 434-295-9126
100 Avon St, Charlottesville, VA 22902
Vision tester.

Richmond Products, Inc. 505-275-2406
4400 Silver Ave SE, Albuquerque, NM 87108
Hematocrit control.

Titmus Optical Inc. 800-446-1802
690 Hp Way, 3811 CorPOrate Drive, Chester, VA 23836
3 base models for general use. $1,600.00-$2,100.00 for vision screening instrument (children or adults).

Vision Assessment Corp. 847-239-5889
2675 Coyle Ave, Elk Grove Village, IL 60007
Color test book.

TESTER, CONDUCTIVITY, FLOOR AND EQUIPMENT
(General) 80RZW

Anderson, W.E., Div. Dwyer Instruments, Inc. 800-872-9141
102 Highway 212, Michigan City, IN 46361
Measures conductivity on direct reading. Color-coded scale with range 0-5 megohm.

Sticht Inc., Herman H. 800-221-3203
45 Main St, Brooklyn, NY 11201
$585.00 for model F-7 conductivity test kit; includes carrying case, MEGOHMER, pair of 5-lb electrodes, 2-1/2in rubber discs, set of heavy duty test leads, supply of foil and heavy duty rubber bands; 18-lb wt.

TESTER, CONDUCTIVITY, SHOE AND GOWN *(General) 80RZX*

Anderson, W.E., Div. Dwyer Instruments, Inc. 800-872-9141
102 Highway 212, Michigan City, IN 46361
Shoe tester for electrostatic dissipating (ESD) footwear. Includes direct reading scale plus dual LED go/no go indicators.

TESTER, DEFIBRILLATOR *(Cardiovascular) 74DRL*

Biotek Instruments, Inc. 802-655-4040
100 Tigan St, Highland Park, Winooski, VT 05404
Defibrillator analyzer.

Fluke Biomedical 800-648-7952
6920 Seaway Blvd, Everett, WA 98203
2 output testers, 1 energy meter, & 1 waveform analyzer.

Netech, Corp. 800-547-6557
110 Toledo St, Farmingdale, NY 11735
Defibrillator Testers: DELTA 1000 tests monophasic and biphasic defibrillators. DELTA 1500 tests any AED. DELTA 2000 tests any defibrillators and any AEDs. DELTA 3000 tests any defibrillator and all external pacemakers including both transcutaneous and transvenous models. DELTA 3000A tests any defibrillator and transcutaneous pacemakers. Both the DELTA 3000 and DELTA 3000A include a 12 lead ECG/arrhythmia/performance waveform simulator.

Solid State Sonics & Electronics, Inc. 785-232-0497
4137 NW Lower Silver Lake Rd, Topeka, KS 66618
$295.00 for the FLASHER. Model DF-100 sterilizable defibrillator tester for the operating room, tests 5 to 50 joules, for use with internal defibrillators.

Welch Allyn Protocol, Inc. 800-462-0777
2 Corporate Dr Ste 110, Long Grove, IL 60047
$795 for MRL defibrillator tester model DT2000-A.

TESTER, ELECTROCARDIOGRAPH CABLE
(Cardiovascular) 74QSI

U.F.I. 805-772-1203
545 Main St Ste C2, Morro Bay, CA 93442
$385 for Model 1089.

TESTER, ELECTRODE *(General) 80RZY*

Elmed, Inc. 630-543-2792
60 W Fay Ave, Addison, IL 60101

U.F.I. 805-772-1203
545 Main St Ste C2, Morro Bay, CA 93442
$385 for Model 1089.

TESTER, ELECTRODE, SURFACE, ELECTROCARDIOGRAPH
(Cardiovascular) 74KRC

Echo Therapeutics, Inc. 508-553-8850
10 Forge Pkwy, Franklin, MA 02038
Impedance diagnostics (idx) system.

TESTER, ELECTRODE, SURFACE, ELECTROCARDIOGRAPH
(cont'd)

Lechnologies Research, Inc.. 866-321-2342
N64W24801 Main St Ste 107, Sussex, WI 53089
Electrode impedance tester checks the integrity of the electrode contacts for stress, Holter, and event-monitor hook-ups.

U.F.I. 805-772-1203
545 Main St Ste C2, Morro Bay, CA 93442
$385 for Model 1089.

TESTER, ELECTRODE/LEAD, ELECTROENCEPHALOGRAPH
(Cns/Neurology) 84GYA

Cadwell Laboratories 800-245-3001
909 N Kellogg St, Kennewick, WA 99336

Grass Technologies, An Astro-Med, Inc. Product Gro 401-828-4002
53 Airport Park Drive, Rockland, MA 02370
Lead tester.

Rochester Electro Medical, Inc. 813-963-2933
4212 Cypress Gulch Dr, Lutz, FL 33559
Impedance meter.

U.F.I. 805-772-1203
545 Main St Ste C2, Morro Bay, CA 93442
$385 for Model 1089.

TESTER, GROUND FAULT CIRCUIT INTERRUPTER
(General) 80QYV

Fluke Biomedical 800-648-7952
6920 Seaway Blvd, Everett, WA 98203

TESTER, GROUNDING SYSTEM *(General) 80QYY*

Megger Inc. (Formerly Avo International) 800-723-2861
2621 Van Buren Ave, Norristown, PA 19403
$466.00 per unit; also, tool/appliance tester.

TESTER, INFUSION PUMP *(General) 80AZZ*

Datrend Systems Inc. 800-667-6557
3531 Jacombs Road, Unit 1, Richmond, BC V6V 1Z8 Canada
Automated Infusion Device Analyzer: Infutest 2000 and Infutest Solo

Fluke Biomedical 800-648-7952
6920 Seaway Blvd, Everett, WA 98203
Micro-based unit with volumetric chambers & drop rate section to measure 6 parameters.

TESTER, ISOLATED POWER SYSTEM *(General) 80SAA*

Bender, Inc. 800-356-4266
700 Fox Chase, Highlands Corp. Center, Coatesville, PA 19320
LT3000, LT 2000; Isolated Power Test Kits; Tests isolated power systems for compliance with NFPA 99.

Fluke Biomedical 800-648-7952
6920 Seaway Blvd, Everett, WA 98203
2 models for use with electrical safety analyzers.

TESTER, PACEMAKER ELECTRODE FUNCTION
(Cardiovascular) 74DTA

Netech, Corp. 800-547-6557
110 Toledo St, Farmingdale, NY 11735
EXPMT 900 tests all functions of any external pacemaker. EXPMT 2000 with larger display and added features provides quick comprehensive testing of all external pacemakers.

TESTER, PULP *(Dental And Oral) 76EAT*

Coltene/Whaledent Inc. 330-916-8858
235 Ascot Pkwy, Cuyahoga Falls, OH 44223
Thermal pulp tester.

Ellman International, Inc. 800-835-5355
3333 Royal Ave, Rockville Centre, NY 11572

Hu-Friedy Manufacturing Co., Inc. 800-483-7433
3232 N Rockwell St, Chicago, IL 60618

Miltex Dental Technologies, Inc. 516-576-6022
589 Davies Dr, York, PA 17402
Pulp tester.

Moyco Technologies, Inc. 800-331-8837
200 Commerce Dr, Montgomeryville, PA 18936
MARK V.

Parkell, Inc. 800-243-7446
300 Executive Dr, Edgewood, NY 11717
Portable 'Gentle Pulse' analog or 'Digitest' digital electronic pulp vitality testers.

TESTER, PULP *(cont'd)*

Pelton & Crane Co., 704-588-2126
11727 Fruehauf Dr, Charlotte, NC 28273

Pulpdent Corp. 800-343-4342
80 Oakland St, Watertown, MA 02472
No common name listed.

TESTER, RADIOLOGY *(Radiology) 90LHO*

Bionix Development Corp. 800-551-7096
5154 Enterprise Blvd, Toledo, OH 43612
Bionix laser alignment cube.

Clinical Microsystems Intl. 703-920-4345
620 22nd St S, Arlington, VA 22202
Radiation dose display meter.

Computerized Medical Systems, Inc. 468-587-2550
1145 Corporate Lake Dr, Olivette, MO 63132
Dosimetry system.

Dome Imaging Systems, Inc. 866-752-6271
400 5th Ave, Waltham, MA 02451
Radiologic quality assurance instrument.

Electronic Systems Engineering Company 918-225-1266
730 E Eseco Rd, Cushing, OK 74023
X-ray film densitometer/sensitometer.

Integrated Medical Technologies 518-368-2400
157 First St., Troy, NY 12180
Radiologic phantom.

Modus Medical Devices Inc. 519-438-2409
17 Masonville Cres, London N5X 3T1 Canada
Quality assurance phantoms

Multidata Systems International Corp. 314-968-6880
9801 Manchester Rd, Saint Louis, MO 63119
Multidose.

Prowess, Inc. 925-356-0360
1370 Ridgewood Dr Ste 20, Chico, CA 95973
Qa tool.

Ramsoft, Inc. 416-674-1347
37 Bankview Cir, Etobicoke M9W 6S6 Canada
Ultrasound qa software

Scanditronix - Wellhofer North America 901-386-2242
3150 Stage Post Dr Ste 110, Bartlett, TN 38133
WELLHOFER WATERPHANTOM radiographic quality assurance instrument. Radiation therapy beam data acquisition systems priced from $50,000 up to $175,000. SCANDITRONIX Linear Detector Array for dynamic field dosimetry in water and air. For daily quality assurance, real time profile measurements, calculation of wedge angle. Priced from $14,000 up to $30,000.

Standard Imaging, Inc. 608-831-0025
3120 Deming Way, Middleton, WI 53562
Brachytherapy source counter and check tool.

Sun Nuclear Corp. 321-259-6862
425 Pineda Ct Ste A, Melbourne, FL 32940
Various beam analyzers and ion chambers:models 1003,1007,1090,1091,1092 and 1170.

Washington University School Of Medicine 314-362-8525
4921 Parkview Pl, Saint Louis, MO 63110
Motion phantom for radiology.

TESTER, RADIOLOGY QUALITY ASSURANCE *(Radiology) 90TDZ*

AMD Technologies Inc. 800-423-3535
218 Bronwood Ave, Los Angeles, CA 90049

Berkeley Nucleonics Corp. 800-234-7858
2955 Kerner Blvd, San Rafael, CA 94901

Capintec, Inc. 800-631-3826
6 Arrow Rd, Ramsey, NJ 07446

Marconi Medical Systems 800-323-0550
595 Miner Rd, Cleveland, OH 44143

Radcal Corp. 800-423-7169
426 W Duarte Rd, Monrovia, CA 91016
$1095.00 for test stand assembly for use with Radcal radiation monitors.

Rti Electronics, Inc. 800-222-7537
1275 Bloomfield Ave, Building 5, Unit 29A, Fairfield, NJ 07004
Barracuda, PMX I

Supertech, Inc. 800-654-1054
PO Box 186, Elkhart, IN 46515
X-ray exposure meter, densitometer, sensitometer.

TESTER, RADIOLOGY QUALITY ASSURANCE *(cont'd)*

Unisyn Medical Technologies. 877-386-3246
1150 Catamount Dr, Golden, CO 80403
Nickel, FirstCall

TESTER, RECEPTACLE, ELECTRICAL *(General) 80SAB*

Woodhead L.P. 847-272-7990
3411 Woodhead Dr, Northbrook, IL 60062

TESTER, RECEPTACLE, MECHANICAL *(General) 80SAC*

Woodhead L.P. 847-272-7990
3411 Woodhead Dr, Northbrook, IL 60062

TETRABROMO-M-CRESOLSULFONPHTHALEIN, ALBUMIN *(Chemistry) 75CJG*

Biomerieux Inc. 800-682-2666
100 Rodolphe St, Durham, NC 27712

TETRABROMOPHENOLPHTHALEIN, ALBUMIN *(Chemistry) 75CJF*

Health Chem Diagnostics Llc 954-979-3845
3341 W McNab Rd, Pompano Beach, FL 33069
Tetrabromophenolphthalein, albumin.

TETRAPHENYL BORATE, COLORIMETRY, POTASSIUM *(Chemistry) 75CEJ*

Diagnostic Specialties 732-549-4011
4 Leonard St, Metuchen, NJ 08840
Light scattering reagent.

Sterling Diagnostics, Inc. 800-637-2661
36645 Metro Ct, Sterling Heights, MI 48312
Potassium reagent set.

Teco Diagnostics 714-693-7788
1268 N Lakeview Ave, Anaheim, CA 92807
Potassium reagent set.

TETRAZOLIUM INT DYE-DIAPHORASE, LACTATE DEHYDROGENASE *(Chemistry) 75CFH*

Bayer Healthcare Llc 914-524-2955
555 White Plains Rd Fl 5, Tarrytown, NY 10591
Test for lactate dehydrogenase in plasma or serum.

Diagnostic Specialties 732-549-4011
4 Leonard St, Metuchen, NJ 08840
$34.50 per 1000ml.

Health Chem Diagnostics Llc 954-979-3845
3341 W McNab Rd, Pompano Beach, FL 33069
Tetrazolium int dye-diaphorase, lactate dehydrogenase.

Teco Diagnostics 714-693-7788
1268 N Lakeview Ave, Anaheim, CA 92807
Ldh-l (color).

THERAPEUTIC DEEP HEAT VITRECTOMY *(Ophthalmology) 86MLZ*

Peregrine Surgical, Ltd. 215-348-0456
51 Britain Dr, Doylestown, PA 18901
Vitreous cutter (guillotine style - pneumatic) ophthalmic surgery.

Visioncare Devices, Inc. 530-243-5047
1246 Redwood Blvd, Redding, CA 96003
Various types of vitrectomy cutters.

THERAPEUTIC X-RAY SYSTEM *(Radiology) 90JAD*

Bionix Development Corp. 800-551-7096
5154 Enterprise Blvd, Toledo, OH 43612
Various patient immobilization systems.

Diacor, Inc. 800-342-2679
3191 Valley St Ste 100A, Salt Lake City, UT 84109
$3,190.00 for MAMMORX Breast Treatment System, Model MBS-1 for simulation and reproducible setup, slant board, allows elevation for better positioning. (Optional slant board to be used with the breast board).

Elekta, Inc. 800-535-7355
4775 Peachtree Industrial Blvd, Building 300, Suite 300
Norcross, GA 30092

Topex, Inc 203-748-5918
10 Precision Rd, Danbury, CT 06810
X-ray systems.

Tri-Star Medical, Inc. 708-645-1107
14227 Winchester Ct, Orland Park, IL 60467
Various.

X-Cel X-Ray Corporation 800-441-2470
4220 Waller St, Crystal Lake, IL 60012
$23,300 for Grenz Ray radiotherapy unit.

THERAPEUTIC X-RAY SYSTEM *(cont'd)*

Xoft, Inc. 408-419-2300
345 Potrero Ave, Sunnyvale, CA 94085
X-ray radiation therapy system.

THERMISTOR *(General) 80SAF*

Brooklyn Thermometer Co., Inc. 800-241-6316
90 Verdi St, Farmingdale, NY 11735
Complete line of laboratory thermometers, precision thermometers with 1/100 degree accuracy, thermocouple/thermistor digital thermometers (NBS calibration).

Cole-Parmer Instrument Inc. 800-323-4340
625 E Bunker Ct, Vernon Hills, IL 60061

Cornerstone Sensors, Inc. 800-955-1470
2128 Arnold Way Ste 4, Alpine, CA 91901
Precision NTC thermistors.

Ge Industrial, Sensing 800-833-9438
1100 Technology Park Dr, Billerica, MA 01821
Negative and positive coefficient NTC thermistor temperature sensors for medical applications.

Minco Products, Inc. 763-571-3121
7300 Commerce Ln NE, Minneapolis, MN 55432
THERMAL-TAB, miniature surface sensors.

Noral, Inc. 800-348-2345
23600 Mercantile Rd, Beachwood Commerce Park
Cleveland, OH 44122

Omega Engineering, Inc. 800-848-4286
1 Omega Dr, Stamford, CT 06907

Sensor Scientific, Inc. 800-524-1610
6 Kingsbridge Rd, Fairfield, NJ 07004
Disposable and non-disposable temperature sensors for all medical applications: esophageal (400 and 700 Series), oral, skin, rectal and neonatal.

THERMOFORMING, EXTRUSION, CUSTOM *(General) 80WYK*

Command Medical Products, Inc. 386-672-8116
15 Signal Ave, Ormond Beach, FL 32174
Bubble tubing, taper tubing, straight tubing, paratubing and multi-lumen tubing and coextrusion. In-line printing on tubing available.

Ima Nova 978-537-8534
7 New Lancaster Rd, Leominster, MA 01453

J-Pac, Llc 603-692-9955
25 Centre Rd, Somersworth, NH 03878
J-PAC designs and manufactures custom thermoformed trays for the sterile, disposable medical device marketplace. Trays are formed in Class 100,000 cleanrooms. Package design services are offered and all forming tools are manufactured in-house. J-PAC works with hard-to-form materials, like polycarbonate and CPET. PETG and polystyrene are a specialty.

Surgical Technologies, Inc. 800-777-9987
292 E Lafayette Frontage Rd, Saint Paul, MN 55107

Tray-Pak Corporation 888-926-1777
PO Box 14804, Tuckerton Road & Reading Crest Avenue
Reading, PA 19612

THERMOGRAPHIC DEVICE, INFRARED *(Obstetrics/Gyn) 85SAG*

Dorex, Inc. 714-639-0700
954 N Lemon St, Orange, CA 92867

Everest Interscience, Inc. 800-422-4342
1891 N Oracle Rd, Tucson, AZ 85705
Infrared temperature transducers.

Linear Laboratories Corporation 800-536-0262
42025 Osgood Rd, Fremont, CA 94539

Mikron Infrared, Inc. 800-631-0176
16 Thornton Rd, Oakland, NJ 07436

THERMOGRAPHIC DEVICE, LIQUID CRYSTAL, ADJUNCTIVE
(Radiology) 90KXZ

Exergen Corp. 800-422-3006
400 Pleasant St, Watertown, MA 02472
Decade iii r.

THERMOGRAPHIC DEVICE, LIQUID CRYSTAL, NON-POWERED
(Radiology) 90KYA

Scantek Medical, Inc. 973-527-7100
1705 US Highway 46 Ste 5, Ledgewood, NJ 07852
Breast differential temperature sensor.

THERMOGRAVIMETRIC ANALYSIS EQUIPMENT
(Chemistry) 75UIS

Mettler-Toledo, Inc. 800-METTLER
1900 Polaris Pkwy, Columbus, OH 43240

Netzsch Instruments, Inc. 800-688-6738
37 North Ave, Burlington, MA 01803
Advanced TGA and TGA/DSC Equipment

THERMOMETER, CHEMICAL COLOR CHANGE *(General) 80FQZ*

American Thermal Instruments, Inc. 937-429-2114
2400 E River Rd, Moraine, OH 45439
Ati forehead thermometer.

General Scientific Safety Equipment Co. 800-523-0166
2553 E Somerset St Fl 1, Philadelphia, PA 19134

Lake Saint Louis Research Products, Inc. 816-373-8899
3624 NW Blue Jacket Dr, Lees Summit, MO 64064
Digital fever detector.

Lcr-Hallcrest--Florida 847-998-8580
6705 Parke East Blvd Unit A, Tampa, FL 33610
Various models of liquid crystal thermometers.

Liquid Crystal Resources, L.L.C. 800-527-1419
1820 Pickwick Ln, Glenview, IL 60026
Liquid crystal thermometers available as disposable or reusable. For use as anesthesiology thermometers, forehead skin thermometers, urine skin thermometers.

Medical Indicators, Inc. 609-737-1600
1589 Reed Rd, Pennington, NJ 08534
NEXTEMP STANDARD. Single-use clinical thermometer. Accurate, economical, non-toxic, long shelf life, store in virtually any environment without damage.

Respironics Missouri 978-659-4252
2039 Concourse Dr, Saint Louis, MO 63146
OMNI ACCU-BAR 1 degree increment monitor with both Fahrenheit and celsius and the only INSTA-READ models available.

Terumo Cardiovascular Systems, Corp 800-521-2818
6200 Jackson Rd, Ann Arbor, MI 48103

Trademark Medical Llc 800-325-9044
449 Soverign Ct, St. Louis, MO 63011
STAT-TEMP reg. model & for STAT-TEMP wide range model for hyper and hypothermia imbibing thermalsense backing

THERMOMETER, ELECTRONIC *(General) 80SAK*

A&D Medical 800-726-7099
1756 Automation Pkwy, San Jose, CA 95131
DT-703 - Digital Thermometer; DT-704 - Flex-tip; DT-705 - Jumbo Display; UT-202 - Ear Thermometer.

Alimed, Inc. 800-225-2610
297 High St, Dedham, MA 02026

American Bantex Corp. 800-633-4839
1815 Rollins Rd, Burlingame, CA 94010
Digital clinical thermometer.

American Diagnostic Corporation (Adc) 800-232-2670
55 Commerce Dr, Hauppauge, NY 11788
Stick digital thermometers, dual scale, oral, rectal or axillary use. Digital Hypthermia & Tympanic, Water resistant with memory.

Azonix Corporation 800-967-5558
900 Middlesex Tpke Bldg 6, Billerica, MA 01821

Biosynergy, Inc. 800-255-5274
1940 E Devon Ave, Elk Grove Village, IL 60007
STAFREEZ Non-electronic. Irreversible Freeze-Thaw thermometer for frozen material to detect thawing.

Brain Tunnelgenix Technologies Corp. 203-922-0105
375 Mather St, Hamden, CT 06514
Abreu BTT 700 System; BTT 700 System

Clinimed, Incorporated 877-CLINIMED
303 Markus Ct, Sandy Brae Industrial Park, Newark, DE 19713

Covidien Lp 508-261-8000
15 Hampshire St, Mansfield, MA 02048
FILAC F-1010, F-1500, F-2000 electronic thermometers, light-weight, fast, accurate temperature readings.

Deltatrak, Inc. 800-962-6776
PO Box 398, Pleasanton, CA 94566
FLASHLINK DATALOGGER records environmental conditions (temperature, humidity) and interfaces with PC to create numerical and graphical reports.

Everest Interscience, Inc. 800-422-4342
1891 N Oracle Rd, Tucson, AZ 85705

THERMOMETER, ELECTRONIC *(cont'd)*

Extech Instruments Corp. 781-890-7440
285 Bear Hill Rd, Waltham, MA 02451
Priced from $79.00 for minithermometers with single or dual input, Type K.

Faichney Medical Co. 800-548-0817
433 Scenic Dr Ste 103, Saint Peters, MO 63376
A complete line of Electronic Digital Fever thermometers. Fahrenheit, Celsius and Dual scales; oral, universal and baby/rectal types; rigid and flexible probe styles; consumer and commercial packaging.

Ge Industrial, Sensing 800-833-9438
1100 Technology Park Dr, Billerica, MA 01821

Lampac International Ltd. 636-797-3659
230 N Lake Dr, Hillsboro, MO 63050
Digital. Available in Fahrenheit and centigrade.

Linseis, Inc. 800-732-6733
PO Box 666, Princeton Junction, NJ 08550

LumaSense Technologies Inc. 408-727-1600
3301 Leonard Ct, Santa Clara, CA 95054
LumaSense Technologies FocalPoint; Luxtron Model 3100; Luxtron Model 3101; Luxtron Model 3102; Luxtron Model 3300

Lumiscope Company, Inc. 800-672-8293
1035 Centennial Ave, Piscataway, NJ 08854

Md International, Inc. 305-669-9003
11300 NW 41st St, Doral, FL 33178

Mikron Infrared, Inc. 805-644-9544
3033 Scott Blvd, Santa Clara, CA 95054

Pharaoh Trading Company 866-929-4913
9701 Brookpark Rd, Knollwood Plaza, Suite 241, Cleveland, OH 44129

Physitemp Instruments, Inc. 800-452-8510
154 Huron Ave, Clifton, NJ 07013

Prestige Medical Corporation 800-762-3333
8600 Wilbur Ave, Northridge, CA 91324

SanoMedics Development Corp. 305-433-7814
80 SW 8th St Ste 2180, Miami, FL 33130
Clinical

Sensor Scientific, Inc. 800-524-1610
6 Kingsbridge Rd, Fairfield, NJ 07004
Solid state thermistor thermometers are available for all popular monitor styles.

Simpson Electric Co. 715-588-3311
520 Simpson Ave, PO Box 99, Lac Du Flambeau, WI 54538
Model 383 $226.60 per unit (standard).

Uei 800-547-5740
8030 SW Mimbus, Beaverton, OR 97008

THERMOMETER, ELECTRONIC, CONTINUOUS *(General) 80FLL*

Bio-Feedback Systems, Inc. 303-444-1411
2736 47th St, Boulder, CO 80301
2 models: $175 and $945 for biofeedback units.

Cardinal Health 303,Inc. 858-458-7830
1515 Ivac Way, Creedmoor, NC 27522
Electronic thermometers and accessories.

Covidien Lp 508-261-8000
15 Hampshire St, Mansfield, MA 02048

Danbi, Inc. 310-398-0013
12099 W Washington Blvd Ste 304, Los Angeles, CA 90066
Tissue implantable thermocouple microprobe.

Diabetica Solutions, Inc. 210-692-1114
12665 Silicon Dr, San Antonio, TX 78249
Skin surface thermometer.

Draeger Medical Systems, Inc. 215-660-2626
16 Electronics Ave, Danvers, MA 01923
Multiple infinity systems.

Edmund Industrial Optics 800-363-1992
101 E Gloucester Pike, Barrington, NJ 08007

Entracare, Llc 913-451-2234
11315 Strang Line Rd, Lenexa, KS 66215
Thermometer, electronic.

Everest Interscience, Inc. 800-422-4342
1891 N Oracle Rd, Tucson, AZ 85705

Exergen Corp. 800-422-3006
400 Pleasant St, Watertown, MA 02472
Various models of infrared thermometer.

Ge Industrial, Sensing 800-833-9438
1100 Technology Park Dr, Billerica, MA 01821

THERMOMETER, ELECTRONIC, CONTINUOUS *(cont'd)*

Global One Medical, Inc. 561-842-7727
3707 Interstate Park Rd S, Riviera Beach, FL 33404
Probe cover: disposable probe cover; thermometer sheath.

Hq, Inc. 941-721-7588
210 9th Street Dr W # 208-210, Palmetto, FL 34221
Same.

Invivo Corporation 425-487-7000
12601 Research Pkwy, Orlando, FL 32826
Temperature monitor.

Jayza Corp. 305-477-1136
7215 NW 41st St Ste A, Miami, FL 33166

Kelsar, S.A. 508-261-8000
Blvd. Insurgentes, Libriamento a La, Tijuana 22450 Mexico
Electronic, digital thermometers and accessories

Kentron Health Care, Inc. 615-384-0573
3604 Kelton Jackson Rd, P.o. Box 120, Springfield, TN 37172
Electronic thermometer.

Kerma Medical Products, Inc. 757-398-8400
400 Port Centre Pkwy, Portsmouth, VA 23704
Thermometer.

Labthermics Technologies 217-351-7722
701 Devonshire Dr, Champaign, IL 61820
Fiberoptic, 8-channel model LT-300 and LT-100 16-channel thermocouple thermometry system.

Linseis, Inc. 800-732-6733
PO Box 666, Princeton Junction, NJ 08550

Md International, Inc. 305-669-9003
11300 NW 41st St, Doral, FL 33178

Medical Indicators, Inc. 609-737-1600
1589 Reed Rd, Pennington, NJ 08534
TRAXIT is a continuous-reading wearable thermometer. Applies under arm with a gentle medical tape backing. Accurate temperatures readings are provided for 48 hours. Apply and then read body temperature at any time.

Medport, Llc 978-927-3808
23 Acorn St, Providence, RI 02903
Electronic thermometer.

Medtronic Blood Management 612-514-4000
18501 E Plaza Dr, Parker, CO 80134
Various models of electronic thermometers.

Mmj S.A. De C.V. 314-654-2000
716 Ponciano Arriaga, Cd. Juarez, Chih. Mexico
Thermometer, temperature sensor

Noral, Inc. 800-348-2345
23600 Mercantile Rd, Beachwood Commerce Park
Cleveland, OH 44122
$199.00 per unit (standard).

Norwood Promotional Products, Inc. 651-388-1298
5151 Moundview Dr, Red Wing, MN 55066
Electronic thermometer.

O&M Enterprise 847-258-4515
641 Chelmsford Ln, Elk Grove Village, IL 60007
THERMOMETER ELECTRONIC

Physitemp Instruments, Inc. 800-452-8510
154 Huron Ave, Clifton, NJ 07013
$400 to $2,700 for 5 models with LCD display in 0.5 or 1" height. 25 to 45 or -10 to 60deg.C. Oral, rectal, skin, esophageal, implantable probe types. Benchtop, cabinet, column clamp or rack mounted. Weight from 3 to 50 lbs. $6,500 for NTE-2 temperature threshold measurement device. $2,995 and up for single channel temperature monitoring system for hyperthermia.

Prizm Medical, Inc. 770-622-0933
PO Box 40, Oakwood, GA 30566
Thermometer, skin.

Psg Controls, Inc. 800-523-2558
1225 Tunnel Rd, Perkasie, PA 18944

Questech International, Inc. 800-966-5367
3810 Gunn Hwy, Tampa, FL 33618
WEE CARE/THERMOMOMMY, digital thermometer pacifier for children 1 to 4 years old.

Rochester Electro Medical, Inc. 813-963-2933
4212 Cypress Gulch Dr, Lutz, FL 33559
Thermistor thermometer.

THERMOMETER, ELECTRONIC, CONTINUOUS *(cont'd)*

Shore Medical, Inc. 714-628-9785
1050 N Batavia St Ste C, Orange, CA 92867
Various.

Smiths Medical Asd, Inc. 610-578-9600
9255 Customhouse Plz Ste N, San Diego, CA 92154
Temperature sensor cover,airway temperature probe.

Telefelx Medical 919-544-8000
900 W University Dr, Arlington Heights, IL 60004
Temperature monitor.

Temp-Tronix 800-223-8367
7350 Trade St Ste B, San Diego, CA 92121
Accessories for clinical electronic thermometer.

Terumo Cardiovascular Systems (Tcvs) 800-283-7866
28 Howe St, Ashland, MA 01721
Temperature probe.

Terumo Cardiovascular Systems, Corp 800-521-2818
6200 Jackson Rd, Ann Arbor, MI 48103

Tidi Products, Llc 920-751-4380
570 Enterprise Dr, Neenah, WI 54956
Thermometer sheath for digital or mercury thermometers (non-rigid, disposable).

Welch Allyn, Inc. 800-535-6663
4341 State Street Rd, Skaneateles Falls, NY 13153
SURETEMP thermometer, electronic clinical thermometer.

Whitehall/A Division Of Acorn Engineering Co. 626-336-4561
15125 Proctor Ave, City Of Industry, CA 91746
Various models of water heating units.

THERMOMETER, FLUID COLUMN *(Surgery) 79FWS*

Francis L. Freas Glass Works, Inc. 610-828-0430
148 E 9th Ave, Conshohocken, PA 19428

THERMOMETER, INFRARED *(General) 80SAL*

Armstrong Medical Industries, Inc. 800-323-4220
575 Knightsbridge Pkwy, Lincolnshire, IL 60069

Deltatrak, Inc. 800-962-6776
PO Box 398, Pleasanton, CA 94566

Everest Interscience, Inc. 800-422-4342
1891 N Oracle Rd, Tucson, AZ 85705
MEDI-THERM: battery-operated portable unit measures precise skin temperature to confirm pain, pinpoint injection sites, and monitor organ temperature in surgery.

Linseis, Inc. 800-732-6733
PO Box 666, Princeton Junction, NJ 08550

Mikron Infrared, Inc. 800-631-0176
16 Thornton Rd, Oakland, NJ 07436

Unetixs Vascular, Inc. 800-486-3849
115 Airport St, North Kingstown, RI 02852

Vespo Marketing Assoc., Inc. 800-49-VESPO
9 Dogwood Dr, P.O. Box 60, Bloomingburg, NY 12721

THERMOMETER, LABORATORY *(Chemistry) 75UIT*

Brooklyn Thermometer Co., Inc. 800-241-6316
90 Verdi St, Farmingdale, NY 11735
Complete line of laboratory thermometers, precision thermometers with 1/100 degree accuracy, thermocouple/thermistor digital thermometers (NBS calibration).

Capintec, Inc. 800-631-3826
6 Arrow Rd, Ramsey, NJ 07446

Cole-Parmer Instrument Inc. 800-323-4340
625 E Bunker Ct, Vernon Hills, IL 60061

Linseis, Inc. 800-732-6733
PO Box 666, Princeton Junction, NJ 08550

Marsh Bellofram 800-727-5646
8019 Ohio River Blvd., Newell, WV 26050
Dial thermometers and pressure gauges, including low-pressure diaphragm gauge.

Minco Products, Inc. 763-571-3121
7300 Commerce Ln NE, Minneapolis, MN 55432
Flex-circuits and flex-coils, resistance thermometers.

Noshok, Inc. 440-243-0888
1010 W Bagley Rd, Berea, OH 44017
Bimetallic and remote types, 2 through 5 inch diameters. Minus 100 degrees Fahrenheit to plus-1,200 degrees. Various materials.

Omega Engineering, Inc. 800-848-4286
1 Omega Dr, Stamford, CT 06907

THERMOMETER, LABORATORY *(cont'd)*

Physitemp Instruments, Inc. 800-452-8510
154 Huron Ave, Clifton, NJ 07013
$495.00 for standard unit (also cryometer).

Pyrometer Instrument Co. 800-468-7976
92 N Main St Bldg 18D, Windsor, NJ 08561
13 models - starting at $267.00, including optical pyrometer & infrared thermometers and laser pyrometer.

Rdf Corp. 800-445-8367
23 Elm Ave, Hudson, NH 03051
Foil heaters and sensors, probe and surface temperature sensors.

Soltec Corp. 800-423-2344
12977 Arroyo St, San Fernando, CA 91340

Testo, Inc. 800-227-0729
40 White Lake Rd, Sparta, NJ 07871

Uei 800-547-5740
8030 SW Mimbus, Beaverton, OR 97008

THERMOMETER, LABORATORY, RECORDING *(General) 80VLX*

Everest Interscience, Inc. 800-422-4342
1891 N Oracle Rd, Tucson, AZ 85705
Infrared thermometer, record via software on PC.

Linseis, Inc. 800-732-6733
PO Box 666, Princeton Junction, NJ 08550

Mini-Mitter Company, Inc. 800-685-2999
20300 Empire Ave Ste B3, Bend, OR 97701

Omega Engineering, Inc. 800-848-4286
1 Omega Dr, Stamford, CT 06907

Rdf Corp. 800-445-8367
23 Elm Ave, Hudson, NH 03051
Surface Platinum RTD - Low cost, sealed platinum RTD . The IEC 751 sensor is refractory, sealed for 0.05 C stability. Toughness is provided by leads welded within the sealed RTD. Moisture resistance for condensing environments, shallow immersion or sterilization is provided by Kapton/Teflon lamination that completely encapsulates the assembly and lead entrance. Platinum RTD capsules have insulated lead wires welded and anchored internally. Assures reliable rugged embedment, insertion or probe assembly. Miniature flexible platinum RTD designed to easily conform on complex surfaces for accurate response in milliseconds. Sealed Metal Platinum RTD capsules are sealed in stainless steel. These capsules can outperform traditional RTD assemblies in a lower cost configuration. Void free construction.

Uei 800-547-5740
8030 SW Mimbus, Beaverton, OR 97008

THERMOMETER, LIQUID CRYSTALS *(Surgery) 79FWR*

Biosynergy, Inc. 800-255-5274
1940 E Devon Ave, Elk Grove Village, IL 60007
HEMOTEMP II Liquid crystals thermometer; blood bag thermometers that are reversible/irreversible, disposable and measure core temperature of blood bag. HEMOTEMP liquid crystal thermometer; blood bag thermometers that are reversible, disposable and measure core temperature of blood bag.

David Scott Company 800-804-0333
59 Fountain St, Framingham, MA 01702

Doxtech, Llc. 503-641-1865
10025 SW Allen Blvd, Beaverton, OR 97005
Adhesive back for monitoring urine temps/drug testing.

Learning Curve Brands Inc. THE FIRST YEARS 800-225-0382
100 Technology Center Dr Ste 2A, Stoughton, MA 02072

Liquid Crystal Resources, L.L.C. 800-527-1419
1820 Pickwick Ln, Glenview, IL 60026
Forehead skin thermometers; urine test thermometers; anesthesiology thermometers.

Medical Indicators, Inc. 609-737-1600
1589 Reed Rd, Pennington, NJ 08534
NEXTEMP ULTRA. An improvement on our standard model which provides a full 1 minute of signal retention time. ULTRA maintains all of the excellent characteristics of NEXTEMP, including clinical accuracy, non-toxic, long shelf life, can store in most any environment without damaging the product, disposable and economical. Please call for a free trial pack.

Novamed, Llc 800-425-3535
4 Westchester Plz, Elmsford, NY 10523
Latex-Free Liquid Crystal Forehead Temperature Monitoring with enhanced readability and safety tested hypoallergenic adhesive (for even the most sensitive skin). Utilized from pre-op through recovery and beyond, provides continuous, uninterrupted temperature readings with clinically proven accuracy.

THERMOMETER, LIQUID CRYSTALS *(cont'd)*

Respironics Missouri 978-659-4252
2039 Concourse Dr, Saint Louis, MO 63146
OMNI ACCU-BAR 1 degree increment monitor with both Fahrenheit and celsius, and the only INSTA-READ models available. OMNI SPECTRUM 1 degree increment monitor with both Farenheit and Celsius.

Sharn, Inc. 800-325-3671
4517 George Rd Ste 200, Tampa, FL 33634
CRYSTALINE II, CRYSTALINE and CRYSTALINE ST advanced liquid crystal technology displays free-moving gold line, indicates skin or body temperature, reads in both Fahrenheit and Celsius.

Trademark Medical Llc 800-325-9044
449 Soverign Ct, St. Louis, MO 63011
KWIK-SKAN liquid crystal temperature monitoring Fahrenheit & Celcius.

THERMOMETER, MERCURY *(General) 80FLK*

Amsino International, Inc. 800-MD-AMSINO
855 Towne Center Dr, Pomona, CA 91767
AMSINO clinical thermometers, mercury/clinical, oral or rectal, triangular tab tops. Color coded, yellow back. Meets ASTM E667 standards.

Armstrong Medical Industries, Inc. 800-323-4220
575 Knightsbridge Pkwy, Lincolnshire, IL 60069

C & A Scientific Co. Inc. 703-330-1413
7241 Gabe Ct, Manassas, VA 20109
PREMIERE oral & rectal in fahrenheit or celsius.

Global Healthcare 800-601-3880
1495 Hembree Rd Ste 700, Roswell, GA 30076

Global One Medical, Inc. 561-842-7727
3707 Interstate Park Rd S, Riviera Beach, FL 33404
Glass thermometer cover: glass thermometer sheath.

Healer Products, Llc 914-663-6300
427 Commerce Ln Ste 1, West Berlin, NJ 08091
Thermometer.

Jayza Corp. 305-477-1136
7215 NW 41st St Ste A, Miami, FL 33166

Kentron Health Care, Inc. 615-384-0573
3604 Kelton Jackson Rd, P.o. Box 120, Springfield, TN 37172
Clinical thermometer.

Lampac International Ltd. 636-797-3659
230 N Lake Dr, Hillsboro, MO 63050
Available in Fahrenheit and centigrade, oral, rectal,flat, enclosed scale and basal.

Learning Curve Brands Inc. THE FIRST YEARS 800-225-0382
100 Technology Center Dr Ste 2A, Stoughton, MA 02072

Medline Industries, Inc. 800-633-5886
1 Medline Pl, Mundelein, IL 60060

Medline Manufacturing And Services Llc 847-837-2759
1 Medline Pl, Mundelein, IL 60060
Thermomether.

Norwood Promotional Products, Inc. 651-388-1298
5151 Moundview Dr, Red Wing, MN 55066
Thermometer.

S.M.B. Ceksuys Co., Inc. 631-447-1198
PO Box 204, Plainview, NY 11803
$29.88/dozen, Celsius and Fahrenheit scales.

Smiths Medical Asd, Inc. 847-793-0135
330 Corporate Woods Pkwy, Vernon Hills, IL 60061
Disposable thermometers.

Ware Medics Glass Works, Inc. 845-429-6950
PO Box 368, Garnerville, NY 10923

THERMOMETER, TYMPANIC *(Ear/Nose/Throat) 77WXS*

Armstrong Medical Industries, Inc. 800-323-4220
575 Knightsbridge Pkwy, Lincolnshire, IL 60069

Covidien Lp 508-261-8000
15 Hampshire St, Mansfield, MA 02048
FIRSTTEMP GENIUS tympanic thermometer, takes an accurate, non-invasive temperature from the ear's tympanic membrane in under two seconds.

THIN LAYER CHROMATOGRAPHY, BENZOYLECGNONINE
(Toxicology) 91DOM

Jant Pharmacal Corp. 800-676-5565
16255 Ventura Blvd Ste 505, Encino, CA 91436
Test to detect benzoylecgonine in human urine.

THIN LAYER CHROMATOGRAPHY, COCAINE
(Toxicology) 91DMN

Ucp Biosciences, Inc. 408-392-0064
1445 Koll Cir Ste 111, San Jose, CA 95112
Cocaine test system.

THIN LAYER CHROMATOGRAPHY, METAMPHETAMINE
(Toxicology) 91DJC

Acro Biotech Llc. 909-466-6892
9500 7th St Ste M, Rancho Cucamonga, CA 91730
Point of care rapid test.

American Bio Medica Corp. 856-241-2320
603 Heron Dr Ste 3, Logan Township, NJ 08085
Methamphetamine test system.

Branan Medical Corp. 949-598-7166
140 Technology Dr Ste 400, Irvine, CA 92618
Immunochromatographical test for the qualitative determination of methamphetamin.

Express Diagnostics Int'L, Inc. 507-526-3951
1550 Industrial Dr, Blue Earth, MN 56013
Drugs of abuse screening test.

Medtox Diagnostics, Inc. 800-334-1116
1640 Nova Ln, Burlington, NC 27215
Immunochromatographic assay for methamphetamine and mdma (mamp-mdma).

Nano-Ditech Corporation 609-409-0700
7 Clarke Dr, Cranbury, NJ 08512
Thin layer chromatography, metamphetamine.

Psychemedics Corp. 800-628-8073
125 Nagog Park Ste 200, Acton, MA 01720

Psychmedics Corp. 978-206-8220
125 Nagog Park, Acton, MA 01720

QuantRx Biomedical Corp. 503-252-9565
5920 NE 112th Ave, Portland, OR 97220
ACCUSTEP DOA SINGLE AND

Rapid Diagnostics, Div. Of Mp Biomedicals, Llc 800-888-7008
1429 Rollins Rd, Burlingame, CA 94010
Various.

St. Paul Biotech 714-903-1000
11555 Monarch St, Garden Grove, CA 92841
Mdma, ecstasy, xtc test.

Ucp Biosciences, Inc. 408-392-0064
1445 Koll Cir Ste 111, San Jose, CA 95112
Methamphetamine test system.

W.H.P.M., Inc. 978-927-3808
9662 Telstar Ave, El Monte, CA 91731
Drug of abuse screening.

THIN LAYER CHROMATOGRAPHY, MORPHINE
(Toxicology) 91DNK

QuantRx Biomedical Corp. 503-252-9565
5920 NE 112th Ave, Portland, OR 97220
ACCUSTEP DOA SINGLE AND

THIN LAYER CHROMATOGRAPHY, OPIATES *(Toxicology) 91LAI*

Varian Inc 650-424-5078
25200 Commercentre Dr, Lake Forest, CA 92630
Chromatographic system, tlc, opiates.

THORACOSCOPE *(Cardiovascular) 74SAM*

Deknatel Snowden-Pencer 800-367-7874
5175 S Royal Atlanta Dr, Tucker, GA 30084

Gibbons Surgical Corp. 800-959-1989
1112 Jensen Dr Ste 101, Virginia Beach, VA 23451
Thoroscopic instruments.

Karl Storz Endoscopy-America Inc. 800-421-0837
600 Corporate Pointe, Culver City, CA 90230
Rod-lens optics; range of available sizes.

Mahe International Inc. 800-294-7946
468 Craighead St, Nashville, TN 37204

Md International, Inc. 305-669-9003
11300 NW 41st St, Doral, FL 33178

Olympus America, Inc. 800-645-8160
3500 Corporate Pkwy, PO Box 610, Center Valley, PA 18034
OES thoracoscope system.

Richard Wolf Medical Instruments Corp. 800-323-9653
353 Corporate Woods Pkwy, Vernon Hills, IL 60061

THORACOSCOPE *(cont'd)*

Welch Allyn, Inc. 800-535-6663
4341 State Street Rd, Skaneateles Falls, NY 13153

THREAD, STABILITY, TROCAR *(Surgery) 79SID*

Ethicon Endo-Surgery, Inc. 800-USE-ENDO
4545 Creek Rd, Cincinnati, OH 45242
ENDOPATH, 10/11mm, 7/8mm, 5mm, and 10/12mm, adjustable.

THROMBOPLASTIN, ACTIVATED PARTIAL *(Hematology) 81GFO*

Analytical Control Systems, Inc. 317-841-0458
9058 Technology Dr, Fishers, IN 46038
THROMBEX Thromboplastin with excellent sensitivity to II, V, VII & X. ISI is near 2.0.

Bio/Data Corp. 215-441-4000
155 Gibraltar Rd, Horsham, PA 19044
Platelet extract and aptt reagents.

Diagnostica Stago, Inc. 800-222-COAG
5 Century Dr, Parsippany, NJ 07054

Fisher Diagnostics 877-722-4366
11515 Vanstory Dr Ste 125, Huntersville, NC 28078

Health Chem Diagnostics Llc 954-979-3845
3341 W McNab Rd, Pompano Beach, FL 33069
Activated partial thromboplastin.

International Technidyne Corp. 800-631-5945
23 Nevsky St, Edison, NJ 08820

International Technidyne Corporation 732-548-5700
8 Olsen Ave, Edison, NJ 08820
Aptt (activated partial thromboplastin) test.

R2 Diagnostics, Inc. 574-288-4377
1801 Commerce Dr, South Bend, IN 46628
Phospholin rsa.

Wortham Laboratories Inc 423-296-0090
6340 Bonny Oaks Dr, Chattanooga, TN 37416
Activated partial thromboplastin time.

THYMOLPHTHALEIN MONOPHOSPHATE, ACID PHOSPHATASE *(Chemistry) 75CKE*

Health Chem Diagnostics Llc 954-979-3845
3341 W McNab Rd, Pompano Beach, FL 33069
Acid phosphatase, thymolphthale inmonophosphate.

Sandare Intl., Inc. 972-293-7440
910 Kck Way, Cedar Hill, TX 75104
No common name listed.

Teco Diagnostics 714-693-7788
1268 N Lakeview Ave, Anaheim, CA 92807
Acid phosphatase color.

THYMOLPHTHALEIN MONOPHOSPHATE, ALKALINE PHOSPHATASE *(Chemistry) 75CIO*

Diagnostic Specialties 732-549-4011
4 Leonard St, Metuchen, NJ 08840
$53.00 per 1000ml.

Health Chem Diagnostics Llc 954-979-3845
3341 W McNab Rd, Pompano Beach, FL 33069
Thymolphthalein monophosphate, alkaline phosphatase or isoenzymes.

Sandare Intl., Inc. 972-293-7440
910 Kck Way, Cedar Hill, TX 75104
No common name listed.

Sterling Diagnostics, Inc. 800-637-2661
36645 Metro Ct, Sterling Heights, MI 48312

Teco Diagnostics 714-693-7788
1268 N Lakeview Ave, Anaheim, CA 92807
Alkaline phosphatase.

THYROGLOBULIN, ANTIGEN, ANTISERUM, CONTROL *(Immunology) 82DDC*

Nichols Institute Diagnostics 949-940-7200
1311 Calle Batido, San Clemente, CA 92673
Tg.

Quest Intl., Inc. 305-592-6991
8127 NW 29th St, Doral, FL 33122
Thyroid autoantibody serological reagents.

United Biotech, Inc. 650-961-2910
211 S Whisman Rd Ste E, Mountain View, CA 94041
ELISA quantitative detecting Total T4 (Total Thyroxine - T4)

THYROGLOBULIN, ANTIGEN, ANTISERUM, CONTROL *(cont'd)*

Wampole Laboratories 800-257-9525
2 Research Way, Princeton, NJ 08540
Autoimmune disease elisa kit.

THYROGLOBULIN, FITC, ANTIGEN, ANTISERUM, CONTROL *(Immunology) 82DDJ*

Hemagen Diagnostics, Inc. 800-436-2436
9033 Red Branch Rd, Columbia, MD 21045
Ifa.

THYROID FUNCTION UNIT *(Chemistry) 75SAO*

Kronus, Inc. 800-822-6999
12554 W Bridger St Ste 108, Boise, ID 83713
OPTI QUANT Thyroglobulin IRMA Kit for detection of residual thyroid tissue secretion after thyroidectomy and/or radioiodine ablation therapy and confirmation of thyroid abnormalities.

Monobind, Inc. 800-854-6265
100 N Pointe Dr, Lake Forest, CA 92630

THYROID UPTAKE SYSTEM *(Radiology) 90VGR*

Capintec, Inc. 800-631-3826
6 Arrow Rd, Ramsey, NJ 07446

Microgenics Corporation 800-232-3342
46360 Fremont Blvd, Fremont, CA 94538
Non-radiolabeled thyroid uptake enzyme immunoassay.

Owens Scientific Inc. 281-394-2311
23230 Sandsage Ln, Katy, TX 77494

TIE GUN, DIALYSIS *(Gastro/Urology) 78FKF*

Alimed, Inc. 800-225-2610
297 High St, Dedham, MA 02026

Sorin Group Usa 800-289-5759
14401 W 65th Way, Arvada, CO 80004

TIMECLOCK *(General) 80VBA*

Crest Healthcare Supply 800-328-8908
195 3rd St, Dassel, MN 55325
Institutional battery or quartz clocks.

Spirig Advanced Technologies, Inc. 413-788-6191
144 Oakland St, Springfield, MA 01108
Count-down feature.

TIMER, APGAR *(General) 80LHB*

Medela, Inc. 800-435-8316
1101 Corporate Dr, McHenry, IL 60050
Battery operated liquid crystal display in minutes and seconds, acoustical signal after 1, 5, and 10 minutes, recording of birth time.

TIMER, CLOT, AUTOMATED *(Hematology) 81GKN*

Covidien Lp 508-261-8000
15 Hampshire St, Mansfield, MA 02048

International Technidyne Corp. 800-631-5945
23 Nevsky St, Edison, NJ 08820

International Technidyne Corporation 732-548-5700
8 Olsen Ave, Edison, NJ 08820
Clot timer.

TIMER, COAGULATION *(Hematology) 81JBT*

Bio/Data Corp. 215-441-4000
155 Gibraltar Rd, Horsham, PA 19044
Coagulation analyzer (kinetic) thrombokinetogram, tkg.

Covidien Lp 508-261-8000
15 Hampshire St, Mansfield, MA 02048

Dade Behring, Inc. 800-948-3233
1717 Deerfield Rd, Deerfield, IL 60015

International Technidyne Corp. 800-631-5945
23 Nevsky St, Edison, NJ 08820
2 models - $3,000 for whole blood coagulation timer, $3,500 for dual-well version.

TIMER, COAGULATION, AUTOMATED *(Hematology) 81SAQ*

Medical Sales & Service Group 888-357-6520
10 Woodchester Dr, Acton, MA 01720

TIMER, DIAGNOSTIC USE *(General) 80LHA*

Novel Products, Inc. 800-323-5143
PO Box 408, Rockton, IL 61072

TIMER, FLOW *(Anesthesiology) 73QWN*

Allied Healthcare Products, Inc. 800-444-3954
1720 Sublette Ave, Saint Louis, MO 63110
Oxygen flow timer.

TIMER, GENERAL LABORATORY *(Hematology) 81JBS*

Beckman Coulter, Inc. 800-526-3821
11800 SW 147th Ave, Miami, FL 33196
General purpose laboratory equipment labeled or promoted for a specific medical.

Beckman Coulter, Inc. 800-635-3497
740 W 83rd St, Hialeah, FL 33014
$275 for multi-timer replacing multiple timers for concurrent procedures.

Chrontrol Corporation 800-854-1999
PO Box 19537, San Diego, CA 92159
$289.00 per unit (standard): 8 or 16 digital inputs, 2 or 4 independent circuits, 20 or 40 operational programs. Chrontrol XT Table Top Timer XT-4, XT-2, XT-4.5, XT-2.5. $350.00 per unit (standard): 8 digital inputs, 2 or 4 independent circuits, 20 or 40 operational programs.

Coloplast Manufacturing Us, Llc 612-302-4992
1185 Willow Lake Blvd, Vadnais Heights, MN 55110
Clock/timer.

Dade Behring, Inc. 800-948-3233
1717 Deerfield Rd, Deerfield, IL 60015

Edmund Industrial Optics 800-363-1992
101 E Gloucester Pike, Barrington, NJ 08007

Eric Armin Inc. 800-272-0272
118 Bauer Dr, PO Box 7046, Oakland, NJ 07436
Countdown timers, general laboratory stopwatches, time study boards. Watches for pulse check, blood-pressure monitoring. Calculators with 256K memory, B.O.S.S./scientific programables/parts and peripherals. Printing stopwatch (with a printer), made by Seiko.

Meylan Corporation 888-769-9667
543 Valley Rd, Upper Montclair, NJ 07043
7 models of timers ($60.00 to $450.00), & 32 models of stopwatches ($60.00 to $226.00). $420.00 to $900.00 for digital time study boards.

TIMER, PHOTOTHERAPY *(General) 80SAR*

Olympic Medical Corp. 206-767-3500
5900 1st Ave S, Seattle, WA 98108
$319.50 each.

TIMER, RADIOGRAPHIC *(Radiology) 90SAS*

Advanced Instrument Development, Inc. 800-243-9729
2545 Curtiss St, Downers Grove, IL 60515
Automatic exposure controls and ionization chambers for AEC.

Chrontrol Corporation 800-854-1999
PO Box 19537, San Diego, CA 92159
$289.00 per unit (standard): 8 or 16 digital inputs, 2 or 4 independent circuits, 20 or 40 operational programs.

Dimco Gray Co. 800-876-8353
900 Dimco Way, Centerville, OH 45458
Prices starting at $92.65 ea.

Flow X-Ray Corporation 800-356-9729
100 W Industry Ct, Deer Park, NY 11729
3 models, 3 to 6 lb. Each.

Marconi Medical Systems 800-323-0550
595 Miner Rd, Cleveland, OH 44143

Wolf X-Ray Corporation 800-356-9729
100 W Industry Ct, Deer Park, NY 11729
3 models, 3 to 6 lb. each.

TIMER, SCRUB STATION *(Surgery) 79VLW*

Getinge Usa, Inc. 800-475-9040
1777 E Henrietta Rd, Rochester, NY 14623
GETINGE, scrub station.

TIP, ENEMA *(General) 80QUH*

Alimed, Inc. 800-225-2610
297 High St, Dedham, MA 02026

Hospira 800-441-4100
268 E 4th St, Ashland, OH 44805
Douche and enema tips.

Marconi Medical Systems 800-323-0550
595 Miner Rd, Cleveland, OH 44143

TIP, RUBBER, ORAL-HYGIENE *(Dental And Oral) 76JEW*

Arjo Canada, Inc. 800-665-4831
1575 South Gateway Rd., Unit C, Mississauga, ONT L4W-5J1 Canada

TIP, RUBBER, ORAL-HYGIENE *(cont'd)*

Denticator International, Inc. 800-325-1881
13705 Shoreline Ct E, Earth City, MO 63045
$75.00 per box of 166.

Powell Products, Inc. 800-840-9205
4940 Northpark Dr, Colorado Springs, CO 80918
Interdental brush.

TIP, SUCTION *(Anesthesiology) 73BSQ*

Aesculap Implant Systems Inc. 1-800-234-9179
3773 Corporate Pkwy, Center Valley, PA 18034
Rigid.

Cameron-Miller, Inc. 800-621-0142
5410 W Roosevelt Rd, Road #241, Chicago, IL 60644

Covidien Lp 508-261-8000
15 Hampshire St, Mansfield, MA 02048

Medi Inc 800-225-8634
75 York Ave, P.O. Box 302, Randolph, MA 02368

Medline Industries, Inc. 800-633-5886
1 Medline Pl, Mundelein, IL 60060

Miltex Inc. 800-645-8000
589 Davies Dr, York, PA 17402

Novosci Corp. 281-363-4949
2828 N Crescentridge Dr, The Woodlands, TX 77381

Pelton & Crane Co., 704-588-2126
11727 Fruehauf Dr, Charlotte, NC 28273

Stryker Corp. 800-726-2725
2825 Airview Blvd, Portage, MI 49002

Tuzik Boston 800-886-6363
104 Longwater Dr, Assinippi Park, Norwell, MA 02061

Vital Concepts, Inc. 800-984-2300
4334 Brockton Dr SE Ste F, Grand Rapids, MI 49512

Welch Allyn, Inc. 800-535-6663
4341 State Street Rd, Skaneateles Falls, NY 13153

TIP, SUCTION TUBE (YANKAUER, POOLE, ETC.) *(Surgery) 79ULE*

Advanced Medical Innovations, Inc. 888-367-2641
9410 De Soto Ave Ste J, Chatsworth, CA 91311
SAF-T-GRIP, disposable one-handed holder for the suction catheter or Yankauer that attaches to the rail of the OR table. Eliminates the contamination of the Catheter/Yankauer when it is placed under the pillow or matress in the operating room. There is also an OR version that adheres to the drapes and secures the electosurgical cord and suction tubing from falling and getting contaminated.

Alto Development Corp. 732-938-2266
5206 Asbury Rd, Wall Township, NJ 07727
Electrosurgical suction tubes.

Anspach Effort, Inc. 800-327-6887
4500 Riverside Dr, Palm Beach Gardens, FL 33410
KAM super sucker with large tapered bore and gradually increasing inner diameter to prevent bottleneck. Three sizes: 15 in., 10.5 in. (both straight) and 10.5 in. curved with flare tip.

Cameron-Miller, Inc. 800-621-0142
5410 W Roosevelt Rd, Road #241, Chicago, IL 60644

Codman & Shurtleff, Inc 800-225-0460
325 Paramount Dr, Raynham, MA 02767

Covidien Lp 508-261-8000
15 Hampshire St, Mansfield, MA 02048

Cpac Equipment, Inc. 800-333-9729
2364 Leicester Road, Leicester, NY 14481-0175

Global Healthcare 800-601-3880
1495 Hembree Rd Ste 700, Roswell, GA 30076
Yankauer suction tip with, and without Suction tubing. Tubing in 3/16', 1/4' various lengths.

Jedmed Instruments Co. 314-845-3770
5416 Jedmed Ct, Saint Louis, MO 63129

Medovations, Inc. 800-558-6408
102 E Keefe Ave, Milwaukee, WI 53212
Yankauer, flexible.

Miltex Inc. 800-645-8000
589 Davies Dr, York, PA 17402

Moldpro, Inc. 603-721-6286
36 Denman Thompson Hwy, Swanzey, NH 03446
Yankauers (bulk, non-sterile)

Novosci Corp. 281-363-4949
2828 N Crescentridge Dr, The Woodlands, TX 77381

TIP, SUCTION TUBE (YANKAUER, POOLE, ETC.) *(cont'd)*

Pelton & Crane Co., 704-588-2126
11727 Fruehauf Dr, Charlotte, NC 28273

Pmt Corp. 800-626-5463
1500 Park Rd, Chanhassen, MN 55317

Stryker Corp. 800-726-2725
2825 Airview Blvd, Portage, MI 49002

Welch Allyn, Inc. 800-535-6663
4341 State Street Rd, Skaneateles Falls, NY 13153

TIP, SUCTION, ELECTROSURGICAL *(Surgery) 79RWZ*

Alto Development Corp. 732-938-2266
5206 Asbury Rd, Wall Township, NJ 07727
Electrosurgical suction tubes.

Cameron-Miller, Inc. 800-621-0142
5410 W Roosevelt Rd, Road #241, Chicago, IL 60644

Jedmed Instruments Co. 314-845-3770
5416 Jedmed Ct, Saint Louis, MO 63129

Surgical Laser Technologies, Inc. 800-366-4758
147 Keystone Dr, Montgomeryville, PA 18936

TIP, SUCTION, FIBEROPTIC ILLUMINATED
(Anesthesiology) 73RXA

Cameron-Miller, Inc. 800-621-0142
5410 W Roosevelt Rd, Road #241, Chicago, IL 60644

Codman & Shurtleff, Inc 800-225-0460
325 Paramount Dr, Raynham, MA 02767

Quality Aspirators 800-858-2121
1419 Godwin Ln, Duncanville, TX 75116

TIP, VESSEL *(Gastro/Urology) 78FKW*

Lifemed Of California 800-543-3633
1216 S Allec St, Anaheim, CA 92805

TIPS AND PADS, CANE, CRUTCH AND WALKER
(Physical Med) 89INP

A&A Orthopedics, Incorporated 757-224-0177
12250 SW 129th Ct Bldg 1, Miami, FL 33186
Cane & crutch tips, etc..

Alimed, Inc. 800-225-2610
297 High St, Dedham, MA 02026

Arizona Dme--Durable Medical Equipment, Inc. 888-665-2568
PO Box 15413, Scottsdale, AZ 85267
All DME.

Assisted Access-Nfss, Inc. 800-950-9655
822 Preston Ct, Lake Villa, IL 60046

Biomet, Inc. 574-267-6639
56 E Bell Dr, PO Box 587, Warsaw, IN 46582
Various types of tips for canes, crutches, and walkers.

Bower, Inc. 205-884-7918
830 Pine Harbor Rd, Pell City, AL 35128
Safe arms safe legs.

DJO Inc. 800-336-6569
1430 Decision St, Vista, CA 92081

Gendron, Inc. 800-537-2521
400 E Lugbill Rd, Archbold, OH 43502
$4.50 per pair.

Global Franchise Consultants, Inc. 330-848-1956
3656 Durham Dr, Norton, OH 44203
Gimme-A-Lift or The Lift. A personal Lift aid.

Invacare Corporation 800-333-6900
1 Invacare Way, Elyria, OH 44035
INVACARE, WalkLite.

Keen Mobility Company 503-285-9090
6500 NE Halsey St Ste B, Portland, OR 97213

Larkotex Company 800-972-3037
1002 Olive St, Texarkana, TX 75501

Medical Depot 516-998-4600
99 Seaview Blvd, Port Washington, NY 11050
Tips, pads, cane, crutch and walker.

Medline Industries, Inc. 800-633-5886
1 Medline Pl, Mundelein, IL 60060

Paramedical Distributors 800-245-3278
2020 Grand Blvd, Kansas City, MO 64108

Patterson Medical Supply, Inc. 262-387-8720
W68N158 Evergreen Blvd, Cedarburg, WI 53012
Walker splint; care covers for crutches.

TIPS AND PADS, CANE, CRUTCH AND WALKER *(cont'd)*

Perfect Care 718-805-7800
8927 126th St, Richmond Hill, NY 11418
Tips and pads, cane, crutch and walker.

Pharmaceutical Innovations, Inc. 973-242-2900
897 Frelinghuysen Ave, Newark, NJ 07114
LEAN ON ME, $16.95 each, cane and crutch tip available 3/4 in., 7/8 in., and 1 in. sizes.

Productos Rubbermaid, Sociedad Anonima De Capital 540-542-8363
Kmi-Ote, Carretera Cadereyta-Allende
Cadereyta Jimenez 67450 Mexico
Various

Profex Medical Products 800-325-0196
2224 E Person Ave, Memphis, TN 38114

Richardson Products, Inc. 888-928-7297
9408 Gulfstream Rd, Frankfort, IL 60423
Walker pad.

Roll A Bout Corp. 302-335-5057
3240 Barratts Chapel Rd, Frederica, DE 19946
Wheel walker.

Wenzelite Rehab Supplies, Llc 800-706-9255
220 36th St, 99 Seaview Blvd, Brooklyn, NY 11232
MARVEL, Free Stander, pediatric vertical stander with four points support at the floor, pelvic and trunk level. OUT/STANDER, multi positioning stander, pediatric stander allows prone, supine and pediatric positioning. Standard accessories include tray, headrest, lateral supports, kneepads and hip and trunk support.

Xtol Products Co. 814-255-2298
522 Goucher St, Johnstown, PA 15905
Crutch ice tips.

Youngs, Inc. 800-523-5454
55 E Cherry Ln, Souderton, PA 18964

TISSUE CULTURE APPARATUS *(Microbiology) 83SAU*

Biologos, Inc. 800-246-4088
2235 Cornell Ave, Montgomery, IL 60538
Tissue culture.

Cadence Science Inc. 888-717-7677
1979 Marcus Ave Ste 215, New Hyde Park, NY 11042

Cbs Scientific Co., Inc. 800-243-4959
PO Box 856, Del Mar, CA 92014

Corning Inc., Science Products Division 800-492-1110
45 Nagog Park, Acton, MA 01720

Eberbach Corp. 800-422-2558
505 S Maple Rd, Ann Arbor, MI 48103

Irvine Scientific 800-437-5706
2511 Daimler St, Santa Ana, CA 92705
Tissue culture media & sera, and Chang medium for the culture of amniotic fluid cells.Serum free media and animal component free media.

Kontes Glass Co. 888-546-2531
1022 Spruce St, Vineland, NJ 08360

Labconco Corp. 800-821-5525
8811 Prospect Ave, Kansas City, MO 64132
Purifier Tissue Enclosure provides a non-ventilated, circulation-free work area designed to reduce cross-contamination during culture manipulation of non-hazardous samples.

Millipore Corporation 800-MILLIPORE
80 Ashby Rd, Bedford, MA 01730
STERICUP media filtration system.

Nalge Nunc International 800-625-4327
75 Panorama Creek Dr, Rochester, NY 14625
NALGENE sterile, disposable filtration apparatus for sterilization of media buffers and additives.

New Brunswick Scientific Co., Inc. 800-631-5417
PO Box 4005, Edison, NJ 08818
Test tube roller for growing mini-preps, tissue and bacterial culture by roller method. Available with four interchangeable drums to accommodate various-sized test tubes (13- to 30-mm in diameter). Two models provide choice of rotating speeds: 6 - 56 rpm or 0.20 - 3.5 rpm.

Nuaire, Inc. 800-328-3352
2100 Fernbrook Ln N, Plymouth, MN 55447

Scientific Industries, Inc. 888-850-6208
70 Orville Dr, Bohemia, NY 11716

TISSUE CULTURE APPARATUS *(cont'd)*
Thermo Fisher Scientific Inc. 563-556-2241
2555 Kerper Blvd, Dubuque, IA 52001
Virtis, An Sp Industries Company 800-431-8232
815 Route 208, Gardiner, NY 12525
Omni-Culture and Omni-Culture Plus fermenters.

TISSUE EMBEDDING EQUIPMENT/REAGENT *(Pathology) 88SAV*
Bio Plas, Inc. 415-472-3777
4340 Redwood Hwy Ste A15, San Rafael, CA 94903
Histological processing/embedding cassettes and capsules, histological biopsy pads.
Eberbach Corp. 800-422-2558
505 S Maple Rd, Ann Arbor, MI 48103
Kimble Glass, Inc. 888-546-2531
537 Crystal Ave, Vineland, NJ 08360
KONTES.
Leica Microsystems (Canada) Inc. 800-205-3422
400 - 111 Granton Drive, Richmond Hill, ONT L4B 1L5 Canada
LEICA
Polysciences, Inc. 800-523-2575
400 Valley Rd, Warrington, PA 18976
Full line of tissue embedding kits and reagents
Sakura Finetek U.S.A., Inc. 800-725-8723
1750 W 214th St, Torrance, CA 90501
TISSUE-TEK embedding console system. $8,995 for the system. TISSUE-TEK AutoTEC to embed automatically at a rate of 120 blocks per hour using the novel Paraform Sectionable Cassette System.
Surgipath Medical Industries, Inc. 800-225-3035
PO Box 528, 5205 Route 12, Richmond, IL 60071

TISSUE GRAFT OF 6MM AND GREATER *(Cardiovascular) 74LXA*
Artegraft, Inc. 800-631-5264
220 N Center Dr, North Brunswick, NJ 08902
ARTEGRAFT 100% collagen vascular grafts, available in 6, 7 and 8 mm O.D. and 15 to 52cm lengths. Indications include A-V access and peripheral bypass distal to the aorta.

TISSUE PROCESSOR (INFILTRATOR) *(Pathology) 88SAW*
Exakt Technologies, Inc. 800-866-7172
7002 Broadway Ext, Oklahoma City, OK 73116
For dehydrating and infiltrating undecalcified hard tissue.

TISSUE PROCESSOR, AUTOMATED *(Pathology) 88IEO*
Boeckeler Instruments, Inc. 800-552-2262
4650 S Butterfield Dr, Tucson, AZ 85714
EMP-5160 automated tissue processor - RMC Products line
Hacker Industries, Inc. 803-712-6100
1132 Kincaid Bridge Rd, Winnsboro, SC 29180
H/i flex 3000 tissue processor.
Hacker Instruments And Industries Inc. 800-442-2537
1132 Kincaid Bridge Rd, PO Box 1176, Winnsboro, SC 29180
Rapid HistoProcessing Systems. Automated, menu driven programs reduce all tissue processing to less than 3 hours. Biopsies in 20 minutes. Programs and modules for processing, rapid fixation, decalcification, histochemical staining, high temperature proceedures and gross hardening.
Leica Microsystems (Canada) Inc. 800-205-3422
400 - 111 Granton Drive, Richmond Hill, ONT L4B 1L5 Canada
LEICA
Leica Microsystems Inc. 800-248-0123
2345 Waukegan Rd, Bannockburn, IL 60015
ASP300 TISSUE PROCESSOR- convenient and versatile with protection of specimens and safe operation.
Medical Sales & Service Group 888-357-6520
10 Woodchester Dr, Acton, MA 01720
Myco Instrumentation Source, Inc. 425-228-4239
PO Box 354, Renton, WA 98057
Sakura Finetek U.S.A., Inc. 800-725-8723
1750 W 214th St, Torrance, CA 90501
$42,995 for TISSUE-TEK V.I.P. 5 System. Tissue-Tek Xpress rapid tissue processor processes 120 specimens per hour.
Spectron Corp. 425-827-9317
934 S Burlington Blvd # 603, Burlington, WA 98233
Reconditioned equipment.
Ted Pella, Inc. 800-237-3526
4595 Mountain Lakes Blvd, Redding, CA 96003
Microwave tissue and accessories.

TISSUE PROCESSOR, AUTOMATED *(cont'd)*
Tripath Imaging, Inc. 919-206-7140
780 Plantation Dr, Burlington, NC 27215
Automated tissue processor.

TISSUE, CORNEAL *(Ophthalmology) 86WQU*
Allergan 800-366-6554
2525 Dupont Dr, Irvine, CA 92612
KERATO-LENS and KERATO-PATCH processed corneal tissue epikeratophakia procedures.
Oasis Medical, Inc. 800-528-9786
514 S Vermont Ave, Glendora, CA 91741
Acelagraft Amniotic Membrane Allografts

TISSUE, TOILET *(General) 80VBE*
Washington Trade International, Inc. 800-327-3379
2633 Willamette Dr NE, Lacey, WA 98516
Just about ANY disposible that you need we can get for you.

TITRATOR *(Chemistry) 75SAX*
Analyticon Instruments Corp. 973-379-6771
99 Morris Ave, P.O. Box 92, Springfield, NJ 07081
Brinkmann Instruments (Canada) Ltd. 800-263-8715
6670 Campobello Rd., Mississauga, ONT L5N 2L8 Canada
Metrohm titration workstations with end point seeking and set point titration modes, method storage and software for data handling.
Brinkmann Instruments, Inc. 800-645-3050
PO Box 1019, Westbury, NY 11590
Mettler-Toledo, Inc. 800-METTLER
1900 Polaris Pkwy, Columbus, OH 43240
Many versatile, expandable automatic titrators available. Menu-driven systems with multiple burette operation.

TITRIMETRIC PHENOL RED, CARBON-DIOXIDE
(Chemistry) 75CHR
Medical Chemical Corp. 800-424-9394
19430 Van Ness Ave, Torrance, CA 90501
$15.00 per unit.

TITRIMETRIC WITH EDTA AND INDICATOR, CALCIUM
(Chemistry) 75CHW
Rocky Mountain Reagents,Inc. 303-762-0800
3207 W Hampden Ave, Englewood, CO 80110

TOMOGRAPHY, OPTICAL COHERENCE *(Ophthalmology) 86OBO*
Optovue, Inc. 866-344-8948
45531 Northport Loop W, Fremont, CA 94538
iVue; iVue 100

TONGS, SKULL *(Cns/Neurology) 84SBB*
Codman & Shurtleff, Inc 800-225-0460
325 Paramount Dr, Raynham, MA 02767
Miltex Inc. 800-645-8000
589 Davies Dr, York, PA 17402
Zimmer Holdings, Inc. 800-613-6131
1800 W Center St, PO Box 708, Warsaw, IN 46580

TONGS, SKULL, TRACTION *(Cns/Neurology) 84HAX*
Alphatec Spine, Inc. 760-494-6769
5818 El Camino Real, Carlsbad, CA 92008
Tong.
Biomet, Inc. 574-267-6639
56 E Bell Dr, PO Box 587, Warsaw, IN 46582
Various types of cranial tongs for skezeial traciton.
Codman & Shurtleff, Inc 800-225-0460
325 Paramount Dr, Raynham, MA 02767
Ossur Americas 800-257-8440
1414 Metropolitan Ave, West Deptford, NJ 08066
JTongs, ReSolve Halo
Zimmer Holdings, Inc. 800-613-6131
1800 W Center St, PO Box 708, Warsaw, IN 46580

TONOGRAPH *(Ophthalmology) 86HPK*
Konigsberg Instruments, Inc. 626-449-0016
2000 E Foothill Blvd, Pasadena, CA 91107
Chronically implantable Intra Optic Pressure Sensor and telemetry system. Medical Research, Discovery Research, Safety Pharmacology,

TONOMETER (CALIBRATION AND Q.C. OF BLOOD GAS INSTRUMENTS) *(Chemistry) 75LCH*

Bionostics, Inc. 978-772-7070
7 Jackson Rd, Devens, MA 01434
Blood gas tonometer.

Linear Tonometers, Inc. 800-786-2163
PO Box 322, Commack, NY 11725
Tonometer provides three widely spaced levels of blood gas controls. All control production is totally automatic and is instantly available at all times. There are no lot-to-lot test-value changes as are found in commercial controls. The stability of the system picks up blood-gas-analyzer problems and drifts earlier than ampuled controls. There is no room air contamination to shift control test values, and the system requires no routine maintenance. CO-OX controls are available for a wide selection of analyzers. System supports most commonly tested electrolyte analytes. The KGT Tonometer has been in wide use for twenty years.

Rna Medical, A Division Of Bionostics, Inc. 800-533-6162
7 Jackson Rd, Devens, MA 01434

Spec Connection Intl Inc. 813-618-0400
34310 State Road 54, Zephyrhills, FL 33543
Clinical blood gas.

TONOMETER, AC-POWERED *(Ophthalmology) 86HKX*

Bausch & Lomb Surgical 636-255-5051
3365 Tree Court Ind Blvd, Saint Louis, MO 63122

Canon Development Americas, Inc 949-932-3100
15955 Alton Pkwy, Irvine, CA 92618
TX-F non-contact air puff tonometer. Also available, TX-F non-contact tonometer world's first full auto-alignment tonometer.

Falck Medical Corporation 860-536-5162
35 Washington St Ste 2, Mystic, CT 06355
Tonometer.

Paradigm Medical Industries, Inc. 801-977-8970
2355 S 1070 W, Salt Lake City, UT 84119
Tonometer and accessories.

Reichert, Inc. 888-849-8955
3362 Walden Ave, Depew, NY 14043
AT555 auto non-contact tonometer, automatically measures inter-occular eye pressure. PT100, the world's first and only truly portable, cordless NCT

Topcon Medical Systems, Inc. 800-223-1130
37 W Century Rd, Paramus, NJ 07652
Noncontact tonometer: $9,490.00.

TONOMETER, MANUAL *(Ophthalmology) 86HKY*

Burton Co., R.H. 800-848-0410
3965 Brookham Dr, Grove City, OH 43123
Goldman type fits slit lamps 825, 830, 850, 2000 and Haag-Streit style slit lamps, $925.00.

Eyetech Ltd. 847-470-1777
9408 Normandy Ave, Morton Grove, IL 60053
Tonometry practice eye for use with Goldman Tonometer, Tonopen

Fortrad Eye Instruments Corp. 973-543-2371
8 Franklin Rd, Mendham, NJ 07945

Gulden Ophthalmics 800-659-2250
225 Cadwalader Ave, Elkins Park, PA 19027

Keeler Instruments Inc. 800-523-5620
456 Park Way, Broomall, PA 19008
$4,995 Pulsair EasyEye - Non Contact Tonometer. Clinically proven to be as accurate as Goldmann.

Kmedic 800-955-0559
190 Veterans Dr, Northvale, NJ 07647

Miltex Inc. 800-645-8000
589 Davies Dr, York, PA 17402
Hand-held.

Tra & Accessories 909-305-1944
449 W Allen Ave Ste 107, San Dimas, CA 91773
Tip covers for the tono pen.

TONSILLECTOME *(Ear/Nose/Throat) 77KCA*

Aesculap Implant Systems Inc. 1-800-234-9179
3773 Corporate Pkwy, Center Valley, PA 18034

Bausch & Lomb Surgical 636-255-5051
3365 Tree Court Ind Blvd, Saint Louis, MO 63122

Mahe International Inc. 800-294-7946
468 Craighead St, Nashville, TN 37204

TOOTH BONDING AGENT, RESIN RESTORATION *(Dental And Oral) 76KLE*

Addent, Inc. 203-778-0200
43 Miry Brook Rd, Danbury, CT 06810
The Calset Composite Warmer now has three temperature settings of 98×F (37×C), 130×F (54×C), and 155×F (68×C). The reason for the change in temperatures is to accommodate the newest tray which will be heated to body temperature. The temperature of 130×F remains the same as the previous unit for warming composite. The new 155×F temperature will give the doctor additional working time, due to composite cooling, before and after placement. Warming composite substantially reduces microleakage, shortens curing time and increases the depth of cure.

American Dental Products, Inc. 800-846-7120
603 Country Club Dr Ste B, Bensenville, IL 60106
Hg-35 desensitizer with fluoride.

Beutlich Lp, Pharmaceuticals 800-238-8542
1541 S Shields Dr, Waukegan, IL 60085
Hurriseal R Dentin Desensitizer

Biomat Sciences, Inc. 866-4-BIOMAT
7210A Corporate Ct, Frederick, MD 21703
Tooth bonding system.

Bisco, Inc. 847-534-6000
1100 W Irving Park Rd, Schaumburg, IL 60193
Dentin bonding systems.

Coltene/Whaledent Inc. 330-916-8858
235 Ascot Pkwy, Cuyahoga Falls, OH 44223
Dentin/enamel bonding system.

Deepak Products, Inc. 305-482-9669
5220 NW 72nd Ave Ste 15, Miami, FL 33166
Bonding system, etch gel.

Den-Mat Holdings, Llc 805-922-8491
2727 Skyway Dr, Santa Maria, CA 93455
Dry bond.

Dent Zar, Inc. 800-444-1241
6362 Hollywood Blvd Ste 214, Los Angeles, CA 90028
Bonding agents.

Drm Research Laboratories, Inc. 203-488-5555
29 Business Park Dr, Branford, CT 06405
Dental adhesive.

Gc America, Inc. 708-597-0900
3737 W 127th St, Alsip, IL 60803
Light-cured surface sealant.

Ivoclar Vivadent, Inc. 800-533-6825
175 Pineview Dr, Amherst, NY 14228
Excite, Syntac, Adhese.

J. Morita Usa, Inc. 888-566-7482
9 Mason, Irvine, CA 92618
ONE-UP BOND F is a self-etching, light-cured, and fluoride releasing bonding agent. One-Up Bond F contains a unique color chromatic agent which gives the clinician visual confirmation of polymerization by color change. One-Up Bond F contains the patented MAC-10 adhesive monomer offering strong adhesion to enamel and dentin.

Kerr Corp. 714-516-7400
28200 Wick Rd, Romulus, MI 48174
Tooth bonding resin agent.

Kerr Corp. 949-255-8766
1717 W Collins Ave, Orange, CA 92867
Multiple.

Lorvic Corp. 800-325-1881
13705 Shoreline Ct E, Earth City, MO 63045
Etching-gel, tooth conditioner.

Motloid Company 800-662-5021
300 N Elizabeth St, Chicago, IL 60607
COMPO-T Composite restoration material.

Novocol, Inc. 303-665-7535
416 S Taylor Ave, Louisville, CO 80027
Dentin bonding systems, enamel bonding systems.

Pac-Dent Intl., Inc. 909-839-0888
21078 Commerce Point Dr, Walnut, CA 91789
Dental bonding agent.

Parkell, Inc. 800-243-7446
300 Executive Dr, Edgewood, NY 11717
AMALGAMBOND dentin bonding agent that bonds composite or amalgam to tooth structure. Brush&Bond and Touch&Bond self-etching bonding agents.

TOOTH BONDING AGENT, RESIN RESTORATION *(cont'd)*

Pentron Clinical Technologies 203-265-7397
68-70 North Plains Industrial, Road, Wallingford, CT 06492
Resin tooth bonding agent.

Pentron Laboratory Technologies 203-265-7397
53 N Plains Industrial Rd, Wallingford, CT 06492
Dentin conditioning and adhesive sytem.

Pulpdent Corp. 800-343-4342
80 Oakland St, Watertown, MA 02472
Various.

Rite-Dent Manufacturing Corp. 305-693-8626
3750 E 10th Ct, Hialeah, FL 33013
Various types of enamel bonding.

Temrex Corp. 516-868-6221
112 Albany Ave, P.o. Box 182, Freeport, NY 11520
Resin veneer.

Ultradent Products, Inc. 801-553-4586
505 W 10200 S, South Jordan, UT 84095
Bonding resin.

Wykle Research, Inc. 775-887-7500
2222 College Pkwy, Carson City, NV 89706
Bonding agent.

TOOTHBRUSH, IONIC, BATTERY-POWERED
(Dental And Oral) 76MMD

Ranir, Llc 616-698-8880
4701 E Paris Ave SE, Grand Rapids, MI 49512

TOOTHBRUSH, MANUAL *(Dental And Oral) 76EFW*

Amden Corp. 949-581-9988
2533 N Carson St, Carson City, NV 89706
Toothbrush.

Amson Products 718-435-3728
1401 42nd St, Brooklyn, NY 11219
42 tufts.

Atd-American Co. 800-523-2300
135 Greenwood Ave, Wyncote, PA 19095

Ballard Medical Products 770-587-7835
12050 Lone Peak Pkwy, Draper, UT 84020
Toothbrush.

Block Drug Co., Inc. 973-889-2578
2149 Harbor Ave., Memphis, TN 38113
Toothbrush.

Bonita Dental Lab 239-495-3368
10915 Bonita Beach Rd SE Ste 1152, Bonita Springs, FL 34135
Toothbrush.

Bretton Square Industries 800-360-6126
812 E Jolly Rd Ste 216, Lansing, MI 48910
ADA Acceptable. Available in traditional colors or the new designer colors. Custom imprinting available.

Buffalo Dental Mfg. Co., Inc. 516-496-7200
159 Lafayette Dr, Syosset, NY 11791
Dental brushes.

Cal Hush Llc 505-763-0770
108 Calle De Oro, Clovis, NM 88101
Toothbrush wash.

Centurion Medical Products Corp. 517-545-1135
3310 S Main St, Salisbury, NC 28147

Classone Orthodontics, Inc. 806-799-0608
5064 50th St, Lubbock, TX 79414
Various types of toothbrushes.

Colgate Juncos, Inc. 212-310-2000
Rd #31 No 100, Juncos, PR 00777
Toothbrushes.

Collis Curve, Inc. 800-298-4818
6110 California Rd, Brownsville, TX 78521
COLLIS-CURVE Outer bristles are curved and straddle teeth, center bristle is short. ADA approved for assisted brushing technique. Brushes all surfaces.

Del Pharmaceuticals, Inc. 516-844-2020
1830 Carver Dr, Rocky Point, NC 28457
Toothbrush.

Dentek Oral Care, Inc. 865-983-1300
307 Excellence Way, Maryville, TN 37801
Tongue brush; Interdental brush

TOOTHBRUSH, MANUAL *(cont'd)*

Donovan Industries 800-334-4404
13401 McCormick Dr, Tampa, FL 33626
Nylon and polyester toothbrushes, fluoroide toothpastes and gels.

Dorel Design & Development Center 781-364-3542
25 Forbes Blvd, Foxboro, MA 02035

E-Z Floss 760-325-1888
PO Box 2292, Palm Springs, CA 92263
Swab tip & interdental brush.

Ethicare 954-742-3599
2190 NW 74th Ave, Sunrise, FL 33313
Plaq-ataq 1.

Floss & Go, Inc. 310-394-6700
1112 Montana Ave Ste D, Santa Monica, CA 90403
Toothbrush.

Gmz Associates, Ltd. 800-581-5088
86 Cain Dr, Brentwood, NY 11717
Toothbrush.

Hager Worldwide, Inc. 800-328-2335
13322 Byrd Dr, Odessa, FL 33556
HAPPY MORNING (disposable w/paste), HAPPY MORNING DELUXE, HAPPY MORNING 'SUPER SOFT', HAPPY MORNING TRAVELER, INFANT TOOTHBRUSH, JUNIOR BRUSH, MEGA BRUSH, MEGA BRUSH C, PARO ULTRA LITE.

Hasbro, Inc. 401-431-8697
1027 Newport Ave, Pawtucket, RI 02861
Toothbrushes with sound feature.

Hygo Plastic, Inc. 414-375-4011
1376 Cheyenne Ave, Grafton, WI 53024
Microbrush.

Inter-Med, Inc. 877-418-4782
2200 Northwestern Ave, Racine, WI 53404
Disposable brush applicator.

J&J Healthcare Products Div Mcneil-Ppc, Inc 866-565-2229
199 Grandview Rd, Skillman, NJ 08558

Kenyon Industries, Inc. 973-962-4844
235 Margaret King Ave, Ringwood, NJ 07456

L.A.K. Enterprises, Inc. 800-824-3112
423 Broadway Ste 501, Millbrae, CA 94030
Various types of manual tooth brushes.

Lactona Corporation 215-692-9000
1669 School Rd, P.o. Box 428, Hatfield, PA 19440

Lancer Orthodontics, Inc. 760-304-2705
253 Pawnee St, San Marcos, CA 92078
Toothbrush, manual.

Loops, L.L.C. 360-366-3009
PO Box 2936, Ferndale, WA 98248
Manual toothbrush.

Nagl Manufacturing Co. 423-587-2199
3626 Martha St, Omaha, NE 68105
Manual toothbrush.

New World Imports 800-329-1903
160 Athens Way, Nashville, TN 37228
Disposable toothbrushes, toothbrush holders and toothpaste.

Norwood Promotional Products, Inc. 651-388-1298
5151 Moundview Dr, Red Wing, MN 55066
Toothbrush.

Novamin Technology Inc. 386-418-1551
13859 Progress Blvd Ste 600, Alachua, FL 32615
Toothbrush.

Nysarc, Columbia County Chapter, Inc. 518-672-4451
PO Box 2, Mellenville, NY 12544
Griptight.

Oraceutical Llc 413-528-5070
815 Pleasant St, Lee, MA 01238
Toothbrush.

Oral Health Products, Inc. 918-622-9412
6847 E 40th St, Tulsa, OK 74145
Poh manual toothbrushes.

Oralbotic Research, Inc. 760-743-5160
701 S Andreasen Dr Ste C, Escondido, CA 92029
Manual toothbrush.

Orthodontic Supply & Equipment Co., Inc. 800-638-4003
7851 Airpark Rd Ste 202, Gaithersburg, MD 20879

TOOTHBRUSH, MANUAL *(cont'd)*

Patterson Medical Supply, Inc. 262-387-8720
W68N158 Evergreen Blvd, Cedarburg, WI 53012
Rolyan built-up & oral stimulation trainer set (toothbrush).

Peak Enterprises Inc 941-373-0046
635 S Orange Ave Ste 8, Sarasota, FL 34236
Tongue brush.

Quden Inc. 450-243-6101
8 Maple, Cp 510, Knowlton J0E 1V0 Canada
Various

Radius Corp. 800-626-6223
207 Railroad St, Kutztown, PA 19530
Radius.

Ranir, Llc 616-698-8880
4701 E Paris Ave SE, Grand Rapids, MI 49512
Dental travel kits also available.

Robell Research, Inc. 212-755-6577
635 Madison Ave, New York, NY 10022
Toothbrush.

Ross Disposable Products 800-649-6526
401 Traders Blvd E, Unit 10, Mississauga, ON L4Z 2H8 Canada
With and without dentifrice. Childs sizes also available.

Ruthal Industries Ltd. 800-445-6640
1 Industrial Ave., Mahwah, NJ 07430-2113

Schueler & Company, Inc. 516-487-1500
PO Box 528, Stratford, CT 06615

Staino, Llc 845-887-5746
11617 State Route 97, Long Eddy, NY 12760
Types of interdental brushes.

Sunstar Butler 800-J BUTLER
4635 W Foster Ave, Chicago, IL 60630

Team Technologies, Inc. 423-587-2199
5949 Commerce Blvd, Morristown, TN 37814
Various types of manual toothbrushes.

Tri-State Hospital Supply Corp. 517-545-1135
3173 E 43rd St, Yuma, AZ 85365

Ultradent Products, Inc. 801-553-4586
505 W 10200 S, South Jordan, UT 84095
Manual toothbrush.

Venturi, Inc. 231-929-7732
2299 Traversefield Dr, Traverse City, MI 49686
Disposable toothbrush with paste.

Via! For Travel 800-339-0628
22885 Savi Ranch Pkwy Ste C, Yorba Linda, CA 92887
Toothbrush, manual.

TOOTHBRUSH, POWERED *(Dental And Oral) 76JEQ*

Air Force, Inc. 616-399-8511
933 Butternut Dr, Holland, MI 49424
Dental cleaner and air powered oral irrigator.

Amden Corp. 949-581-9988
2533 N Carson St, Carson City, NV 89706
Electric toothbrush.

Conair Corp. 203-351-9000
150 Milford Rd, East Windsor, NJ 08520
Electric toothbrush (battery operated).

Del Pharmaceuticals, Inc. 516-844-2020
1830 Carver Dr, Rocky Point, NC 28457
Toothbrush.

Dentek Oral Care, Inc. 865-983-1300
307 Excellence Way, Maryville, TN 37801
Electric brush.

Homedics Inc. 800-333-8282
3000 N Pontiac Trl, Commerce Township, MI 48390

Oralbotic Research, Inc. 760-743-5160
701 S Andreasen Dr Ste C, Escondido, CA 92029
Hydrabrush & powered toothbrush.

Oralgiene Usa, Inc. 800-933-6725
8460 Higuera St, Culver City, CA 90232
ORALGIENE '60 second' TIME MACHINE TOOTHBRUSH, makes kids want to brush. Power toothbrush targeted at ages 3 years upward. It is clinically proven to brush faster and better than other manual/power toothbrushes. ORALGIENE, electric tongue cleaner gently and effectively removes bacteria from the tongue surface without causing a gag reflex.

TOOTHBRUSH, POWERED *(cont'd)*

Ranir, Llc 616-698-8880
4701 E Paris Ave SE, Grand Rapids, MI 49512

Salton, Inc. 202-408-9213
1955 W Field Ct, Lake Forest, IL 60045
Various types of toothbrushes and flossser.

Sunbeam Products, Inc. 561-912-4100
2381 NW Executive Center Dr, Boca Raton, FL 33431
Rechargeable toothbrush.

Sunstar Butler 800-J BUTLER
4635 W Foster Ave, Chicago, IL 60630

The Gillette Company 617-421-7000
800 Boylston St, Prudential Tower Bldg. Fl.45, Boston, MA 02199
Electric powered toothbrush.

Toothtickler Enterprises, Inc. 651-429-5187
5222 Bald Eagle Blvd E, White Bear Lake, MN 55110
Electric toothbrusssh.

Trademark Medical Llc 800-325-9044
449 Soverign Ct, St. Louis, MO 63011
PLAK-VAC oral evacuator brush to be attached to suction unit for eliminating food particles in patient's mouth. It is a suction toothbrush.

Ultreo 877-485-8736
9461 Willows Rd NE Ste 101, Redmond, WA 98052
Electric toothbrush.

United Laboratories And Manufacturing, Llc 703-787-9600
45000 Underwood Ln Ste F, Sterling, VA 20166
Powered toothbrush.

Wahl Clipper Corp. 815-548-8342
2900 Locust St, Sterling, IL 61081
Electric toothbrush.

Water Pik, Inc. 970-221-6129
1730 E Prospect Rd, Fort Collins, CO 80525
Powered toothbrush, electric toothbrush.

TOPOGRAPHER, CORNEAL *(Ophthalmology) 86MMQ*

Dicon, Inc. 800-426-0493
2355 S 1070 W, Salt Lake City, UT 84119
CT 200 features auto-alignment, auto-focus and a contact lens module. The topographer features a Bull's Eye keratoconus detection program.

Paradigm Medical Industries, Inc. 801-977-8970
2355 S 1070 W, Salt Lake City, UT 84119
Corneal topographer, ct.

Reichert, Inc. 888-849-8955
3362 Walden Ave, Depew, NY 14043
CTS Corneal Topography System has the most 'user friendly' software of any topography system.

Topcon Medical Systems, Inc. 800-223-1130
37 W Century Rd, Paramus, NJ 07652
KR-8000PA auto refractor with corneal topography: $18,490.00. KR-9000PW wavefront analyzer with corneal topography: $39,990.00. Color mapping software: $600.00.

TOURNIQUET *(General) 80SBD*

Adi Medical Division Of Asia Dynamics (Group) Inc. 877-647-7699
1565 S Shields Dr, Waukegan, IL 60085

Alimed, Inc. 800-225-2610
297 High St, Dedham, MA 02026

American Diagnostic Corporation (Adc) 800-232-2670
55 Commerce Dr, Hauppauge, NY 11788
Hook and loop adhesive tourniquet

Armstrong Medical Industries, Inc. 800-323-4220
575 Knightsbridge Pkwy, Lincolnshire, IL 60069

Clinimed, Incorporated 877-CLINIMED
303 Markus Ct, Sandy Brae Industrial Park, Newark, DE 19713

Kent Elastomer Products, Inc. 800-331-4762
1500 Saint Clair Ave, PO Box 668, Kent, OH 44240
FREE-BAND, latex free tourniquet band.

Medipoint, Inc. 800-445-0525
72 E 2nd St, Mineola, NY 11501
Tubular latex tourniquets that are tubular instead of flat.

Mine Safety Appliances Company 866-MSA-1001
121 Gamma Dr, Pittsburgh, PA 15238

TOURNIQUET *(cont'd)*

ReNu Medical Inc. 877-252-1110
9800 Evergreen Way, Everett, WA 98204
Tourniquet,Pneumatic; Zimmer

Schueler & Company, Inc. 516-487-1500
PO Box 528, Stratford, CT 06615

Zimmer Holdings, Inc. 800-613-6131
1800 W Center St, PO Box 708, Warsaw, IN 46580

TOURNIQUET, AIR PRESSURE *(Orthopedics) 87HTA*

Medtronic Perfusion Systems 800-328-3320
7611 Northland Dr N, Brooklyn Park, MN 55428
TCPM II tourniquet monitor has built-in features of internal pressure pump and air reservoir as well as AC/DC power capabilities.

Zimmer Holdings, Inc. 800-613-6131
1800 W Center St, PO Box 708, Warsaw, IN 46580

TOURNIQUET, AUTOMATIC ROTATING *(Cardiovascular) 74DRP*

Zimmer Holdings, Inc. 800-613-6131
1800 W Center St, PO Box 708, Warsaw, IN 46580

TOURNIQUET, NON-PNEUMATIC, SURGICAL *(Surgery) 79GAX*

Ac Healthcare Supply, Inc. 905-448-4706
11651 230th St, Cambria Heights, NY 11411
Nonpneumatic tourniquet.

Accumed Systems, Inc. 734-930-0461
6109 Jackson Rd, Ann Arbor, MI 48103
Hemostasis band.

Adi Medical Division Of Asia Dynamics (Group) Inc. 877-647-7699
1565 S Shields Dr, Waukegan, IL 60085

Becton Dickinson And Company 800-284-6845
1 Becton Dr, Franklin Lakes, NJ 07417
VACUTAINER BRAND BLOOD

Biomet Microfixation Inc. 800-874-7711
1520 Tradeport Dr, Jacksonville, FL 32218
Various types of tourniquets.

Blind & Vision Rehabilitation Services Of Pittsburgh 412-325-7504
1204 Western Ave Bldg 4, Pittsburgh, PA 15233
Dvi converter.

Canvas Specialties, Inc. 210-662-6412
5923 Distribution, San Antonio, TX 78218
Tourniquet, nonpneumatic#general and plastic surgery.

Centurion Medical Products Corp. 517-545-1135
3310 S Main St, Salisbury, NC 28147

Codman & Shurtleff, Inc 800-225-0460
325 Paramount Dr, Raynham, MA 02767

Donovan Industries 800-334-4404
13401 McCormick Dr, Tampa, FL 33626
Both latex and non-latex versions.

Formedica Ltd. 800-361-9671
1481 Rue Begin, St Laurent, QUE H4R 1V8 Canada
$2.00 per unit (standard).

Fulflex Of Vermont, Inc. 802-257-5256
32 Justin Holden Dr, Brattleboro, VT 05301
Non-sterile synthetic tourniquet.

H & H Associates, Inc. 757-224-0177
4173 G.w. Memorial Highway, Ordinary, VA 23131
Tourniquet.

Healer Products, Llc 914-663-6300
427 Commerce Ln Ste 1, West Berlin, NJ 08091
Tourniquet.

Health Care Logistics, Inc. 800-848-1633
450 Town St, PO Box 25, Circleville, OH 43113
Manual tourniquet.

Hydro-Med Products, Inc. 214-350-5100
3400 Royalty Row, Irving, TX 75062
Tourniquet, nonpneumatic.

Innovate Medical, L.L.C. 423-854-9694
225 White Top Rd. Ext., Bluff City, TN 37618
Tourniquet (rubber).

K. W. Griffen Co. 203-846-1923
100 Pearl St, Norwalk, CT 06850
Blood tourniquet.

TOURNIQUET, NON-PNEUMATIC, SURGICAL *(cont'd)*

Kelsar, S.A. 508-261-8000
Blvd. Insurgentes, Libriamento a La, Tijuana 22450 Mexico
Sentinel loops, silicone vascular tape

Kent Elastomer Products, Inc 330-628-1802
3890 Mogadore Industrial Pkwy, Mogadore, OH 44260
Non-latex tourniquet.

Kentron Health Care, Inc. 615-384-0573
3604 Kelton Jackson Rd, P.o. Box 120, Springfield, TN 37172
Tourniquets.

Medical Action Industries, Inc. 800-645-7042
25 Heywood Rd, Arden, NC 28704
Tourniquet.

Medline Manufacturing And Services Llc 847-837-2759
1 Medline Pl, Mundelein, IL 60060
Tourniquet.

Molded Products Inc. 800-435-8957
1112 Chatburn Ave, Harlan, IA 51537
Tourniquet.

Normed 800-288-8200
PO Box 3644, Seattle, WA 98124
Buckle tourniquet for first aid kits.

North Safety Products 401-943-4400
1101 B Calle Neutron, Parque Industrial Maran, Mexicali, B.c. Mexico
Tourniquet

Ohk Medical Devices Inc. 908-566-5745
715 South Ave E, Cranford, NJ 07016

Patriot Products 909-988-6578
12460 Park Ave, Chino, CA 91710
Tourniquet.

Propper Manufacturing Co., Inc. 800-832-4300
3604 Skillman Ave, Long Island City, NY 11101

Q-Teknologies, Inc. 321-631-3915
391 Brookcrest Cir, Rockledge, FL 32955
Tourniquet.

Richard-Allan Scientific 269-544-5628
4481 Campus Dr, Kalamazoo, MI 49008
Tourniquet.

The Hygenic Corp. 800-321-2135
1245 Home Ave, Akron, OH 44310
Various sizes of tourniquet straps.

Tri-State Hospital Supply Corp. 517-545-1135
3173 E 43rd St, Yuma, AZ 85365

TOURNIQUET, PNEUMATIC *(Surgery) 79KCY*

Ac Healthcare Supply, Inc. 905-448-4706
11651 230th St, Cambria Heights, NY 11411
Pneumatic tourniquet.

Ascent Healthcare Solutions 480-763-5300
10232 S 51st St, Phoenix, AZ 85044
Touriquet, pneumatic.

Biomet Microfixation Inc. 800-874-7711
1520 Tradeport Dr, Jacksonville, FL 32218
Various types of tourniquets.

Delfi Medical Innovations Inc. 800-933-3022
Suite 106, 1099 West 8th Avenue, Vancouver, BC V6H 1C3 Canada
Various.

Depuy Orthopaedics, Inc. 800-473-3789
700 Orthopaedic Dr, P.O. Box 988, Warsaw, IN 46582
Various types of pneumatic tourniquets.

Geen Healthcare Inc. 800-565-4336
931 Progress Ave. Ste.13, Scarborough, ONT M1G 3V5 Canada

Health Care Logistics, Inc. 800-848-1633
450 Town St, PO Box 25, Circleville, OH 43113
Inflatable tourniquet cuff.

Medisiss 866-866-7477
2747 SW 6th St, Redmond, OR 97756
Various pneumatic tourniquet cuffs,sterile.

Medtronic Blood Management 612-514-4000
18501 E Plaza Dr, Parker, CO 80134
Pneumatic tourniquet.

Patterson Medical Supply, Inc. 262-387-8720
W68N158 Evergreen Blvd, Cedarburg, WI 53012
Tourniquet, pneumatic.

Schueler & Company, Inc. 516-487-1500
PO Box 528, Stratford, CT 06615

TOURNIQUET, PNEUMATIC *(cont'd)*

Sterilmed, Inc. 763-488-3400
11400 73rd Ave N Ste 100, Maple Grove, MN 55369
Tourniquet cuff.

Zimmer Holdings, Inc. 800-613-6131
1800 W Center St, PO Box 708, Warsaw, IN 46580

TOWEL, SURGICAL *(Surgery) 79SBE*

Adi Medical Division Of Asia Dynamics (Group) Inc. 877-647-7699
1565 S Shields Dr, Waukegan, IL 60085

Amd-Ritmed, Inc. 800-445-0340
295 Firetower Road, Tonawanda, NY 14150

Atd-American Co. 800-523-2300
135 Greenwood Ave, Wyncote, PA 19095

Best Manufacturing Group Llc 800-843-3233
1633 Broadway Fl 18, New York, NY 10019
Imports and domestic, colors and various sizes.

Dukal Corporation 800-243-0741
5 Plant Ave, Hauppauge, NY 11788

Grand Medical Products 800-521-2055
7222 Ertel Ln, Houston, TX 77040
Sterile and non-sterile.

Jms Converters Inc Dba Sabee Products & Stanford Prof Prod 215-396-3302
67 Buck Rd Ste B7, Huntingdon Valley, PA 19006

Kerr Group 800-524-3577
1400 Holcomb Bridge Rd, Roswell, GA 30076

Medline Industries, Inc. 800-633-5886
1 Medline Pl, Mundelein, IL 60060

Pacon Manufacturing Corporation 732-357-8020
400 Pierce St # B, Somerset, NJ 08873

R. Sabee Company 920-882-7350
1718 W 8th St, Appleton, WI 54914

Riegel Consumer Products Div. 800-845-2232
PO Box E, 51 Riegel Road, Johnston, SC 29832
FDA certified Class I,100% Cotton absorbent towel features special low-lint weave, hemmed sides and is vat dyed. Colors include jade green, misty green and ceil blue. Toweling in bolt form is also available. Also available as X-Ray detectable

Viscot Medical, Llc 800-221-0658
32 West St, PO Box 351, East Hanover, NJ 07936
Available in tissue or tissue/poly plies.

TOWEL/TOWELETTE, PAPER *(General) 80WNF*

Alimed, Inc. 800-225-2610
297 High St, Dedham, MA 02026

Atd-American Co. 800-523-2300
135 Greenwood Ave, Wyncote, PA 19095
Absorbent paper towel for lab use.

Caltech Industries, Inc. 800-234-7700
2420 Schuette Rd, Midland, MI 48642
CALTECH disposable hospital cleaning towels with bleach provide cleaning of non-porous surfaces in healthcare facilities, laboratories, physician and dental offices. Fast Acting two minutes efficacy - in singles portable towels or 60 count soft pack.

Central Paper Products Company 800-339-4065
PO Box 4480, Manchester, NH 03108

Chester Labs, Inc. 800-354-9709
1900 Section Rd, Cincinnati, OH 45237
APRILFRESH WIPES. Personal Cleansing Washcloths. Premoistened with a gentle cleansing lotion. Contains Aloe and Lanolin to soften and soothe skin. Alcohol Free. Clamshell Tub, Soft Pack with Lid and Resealable Packs.

Cone Instruments, Inc. 800-321-6964
5201 Naiman Pkwy, Solon, OH 44139
Pre-moistened cleansing wipes.

Crosstex International 800-223-2497
10 Ranick Rd, Hauppauge, NY 11788
SANITEX PLUS disposable wipes.

Crosstex International Ltd., W. Region 800-707-2737
14059 Stage Rd, Santa Fe Springs, CA 90670
Sanitabs disposable.

Crosstex International,Inc. 888-276-7783
10 Ranick Rd, Hauppauge, NY 11788
CROSSTEX.

TOWEL/TOWELETTE, PAPER *(cont'd)*

General Econopak, Inc. 888-871-8568
1725 N 6th St, Philadelphia, PA 19122
GEPCO disposable bath/shower and hand towels, all sizes.

Global Concepts, Ltd. 818-363-7195
19464 Eagle Ridge Ln, Northridge, CA 91326
FRESH CLEANSE, antibacterial moist towlettes and antibacterial topical skin wipes.

Jms Converters Inc Dba Sabee Products & Stanford Prof Prod 215-396-3302
67 Buck Rd Ste B7, Huntingdon Valley, PA 19006
Disposable Professional Towels & Drapes

Palmero Health Care 800-344-6424
120 Goodwin Pl, Stratford, CT 06615
DISCIDE ULTRA disinfecting towelettes, hospital level.

Professional Disposables International, Inc. 800-999-6423
2 Nice Pak Park, Orangeburg, NY 10962
NICE CLEAN, NICE 'N CLEAN, HYGEA, and SANI-DEX Antiseptic towelettes and incontinent wipes and PCMX based antimicrobial handwipes.

Royal Paper Products, Inc. 800-666-6655
PO Box 151, Coatesville, PA 19320
Placemats and coasters made of paper. Napkin Bands paper napkin bands to go around napkins holding silverware.

Safetec Of America, Inc. 800-456-7077
887 Kensington Ave, Buffalo, NY 14215
Personal Antimicrobial Wipes by Safetec (p.a.w.s.) remove soil from hands and kill 99.99% of most germs in as little as 15 seconds. 5 x 8-in towelettes are formulated with PCMX and SD Alcohol, plus aloe vera to help moisturize the skin. Packaged as individually-wrapped, pre-moistened towelettes, or in pull-out, 50-count, and 160-count dispenser tubs. Available in original Fresh or Citrus Scents. BIOZIDE is a ready-to-use, broad-spectrum, hospital-grade, hard-surface disinfectant/deodorizer. BIOZIDE is a tuberculocidal, virucidal, phenolic formula. Safe on surfaces that will not be harmed by alcohol. EPA registered and helps you comply with OSHA Bloodborne Pathogens Standard. Packaging: single-use pouch with a heavy-duty, dry 8 x 8-in. wipe.

Silverstone Packaging, Inc.-Your One Stop Supplier 800-413-1108
1401 Lakeland Ave, Bohemia, NY 11716

Veridien Corp. 800-345-5444
7600 Bryan Dairy Rd Ste F, Largo, FL 33777
Antimicrobial towelette in canisters or sachets.

TRABECULOTOME *(Ophthalmology) 86HMZ*

Neomedix Corp. 949-258-8355
15042 Parkway Loop Ste A, Tustin, CA 92780
Glaucoma trabulotomy devices.

TRACING UNIT, ARCH *(Orthopedics) 87VDE*

Slawner Ltd., J. 514-731-3378
5713 Cote Des Neiges Rd., Montreal, QUE H3S 1Y7 Canada

TRACK AND CARRIER, CUBICLE CURTAIN *(General) 80SBK*

Covoc Corp. 800-725-3266
1194 E Valencia Dr, Fullerton, CA 92831
Cubicle curtain track and carriers; shower curtain tracks and carriers; shower curtain poles and rings.

Crest Healthcare Supply 800-328-8908
195 3rd St, Dassel, MN 55325
Cubicle track and hardware.

General Cubicle Co. 800-869-4606
49 Meeker Ave, Cranford, NJ 07016
Cubicle curtains, track, track carriers, hardware, IV tracks and carriage systems

Imperial Fastener Co., Inc. 954-782-7130
1400 SW 8th St, Pompano Beach, FL 33069
Tracks - custom made as to type, size, shape etc.

Independent Solutions, Inc. 847-498-0500
900 Skokie Blvd Ste 118, Northbrook, IL 60062
ARNCO flush or surface celing mounted or suspended clear anodized aluminum or white enamel finish.

Makita Usa Inc. - Drapery Opener Div. 800-462-5482
14930 Northam St, La Mirada, CA 90638
Motorized drapery opener system. Automatic Drapery Opening System - motorized drapery opener system.

Salsbury Industries 800-640-4341
1010 E 62nd St, Los Angeles, CA 90001

TRACK AND CARRIER, CUBICLE CURTAIN *(cont'd)*

Webb Manufacturing Co. 800-932-2634
1241 Carpenter St, Philadelphia, PA 19147

TRACK AND CARRIER, INTRAVENOUS *(General) 80SBL*

Covoc Corp. 800-725-3266
1194 E Valencia Dr, Fullerton, CA 92831
Ceiling mount I.V. Track, I.V. carriers, and I.V. trees (bottle hangers).

Imperial Fastener Co., Inc. 954-782-7130
1400 SW 8th St, Pompano Beach, FL 33069

Independent Solutions, Inc. 847-498-0500
900 Skokie Blvd Ste 118, Northbrook, IL 60062
ARNCO flush or surface ceiling mounted, clear satin anodized or white enamel finish; conductive or non-conductive twist-lock carriers, adjustable or fixed bottleholders.

Medical Skyhook Company 801-262-1471
PO Box 17213, Salt Lake City, UT 84117
Track for intravenous hanger.

Pryor Products 800-854-2280
1819 Peacock Blvd, Oceanside, CA 92056
A wide variety of ceiling mounted IV hangers are available.

Salsbury Industries 800-640-4341
1010 E 62nd St, Los Angeles, CA 90001

TRACTION UNIT, HIP, NON-POWERED, NON-PENETRATING

(Orthopedics) 87HSR

Biomet, Inc. 574-267-6639
56 E Bell Dr, PO Box 587, Warsaw, IN 46582
Various types of non-powered, non-penetrating hip traction units.

Depuy Ace, A Johnson & Johnson Company 800-473-3789
700 Orthopaedic Dr, Warsaw, IN 46582

Truform Orthotics & Prosthetics 800-888-0458
3960 Rosslyn Dr, Cincinnati, OH 45209

TRACTION UNIT, NON-POWERED *(Orthopedics) 87HST*

A&A Orthopedics, Incorporated 757-224-0177
12250 SW 129th Ct Bldg 1, Miami, FL 33186
Accessories, frame, cord, etcc...

A.M.G. Medical, Inc. 888-396-1213
8505 Dalton Rd., Montreal, QUE H4T-IV5 Canada

Arc Surgical Llc. 503-627-9957
21300 NW Jacobson Rd, Hillsboro, OR 97124
Apparatus, traction, non-powered.

Arthrex Manufacturing 239-643-5553
1958 Trade Center Way, Naples, FL 34109
Traction device.

Arthrex, Inc. 239-643-5553
1370 Creekside Blvd, Naples, FL 34108
Shoulder holder.

Back Bubble 858-481-8715
621 Seabright Ln, Solana Beach, CA 92075
A non-powered orthopedic traction apparatus.

Back Support Systems 800-669-2225
67684 San Andreas St, Desert Hot Springs, CA 92240
THE ANGLE lumbar traction unit is priced from $34.95 and comes in two sizes. THE CURVE lumbar traction unit is priced at $119.95.

Bagrad 904-272-6369
84 Sleepy Hollow Rd, Middleburg, FL 32068
Pelvic traction unit.

Biomet, Inc. 574-267-6639
56 E Bell Dr, PO Box 587, Warsaw, IN 46582
Various types of traction (cart, reame, cord, weight) accessories.

Bird & Cronin, Inc. 651-683-1111
1200 Trapp Rd, Saint Paul, MN 55121
Various traction kits and accessories.

Breg, Inc., An Orthofix Company 800-897-BREG
2611 Commerce Way, Vista, CA 92081
Arm traction device.

Core Products International, Inc. 800-365-3047
808 Prospect Ave, Osceola, WI 54020

Depuy Mitek, Inc. 800-451-2006
325 Paramount Dr, Raynham, MA 02767
Cervical traction devices.

Depuy Orthopaedics, Inc. 800-473-3789
700 Orthopaedic Dr, P.O. Box 988, Warsaw, IN 46582
Various types of non-powered tration apparatus.

TRACTION UNIT, NON-POWERED *(cont'd)*

Dj Orthopedics De Mexico, S.A. De C.V. 690-727-1280
Blvd., Delagacion La Presa, Tijuana 22397 Mexico
Traction accessories

Dj Orthopedics De Mexico, S.A. De C.V. 690-727-1280
Ave. Venustiano Carranza 6802, Castillo, Tijuana 22100 Mexico
Traction accessories

Dynatronics Corp. Chattanooga Operations 801-568-7000
6607 Mountain View Rd, Ooltewah, TN 37363
Overdoor traction set.

Elite Medical Equipment 719-659-7926
5470 Kates Dr, Colorado Springs, CO 80919
Hand wheel.

Endorphin Corporation 800-940-9844
6901 90th Ave, Pinellas Park, FL 33782
Vertican Traction System is a non-powered traction device for treating back pain in both the lumbar region and the cervical region. It can utilize focused traction to treat spondylolisthesis, retrolisthesis and other problems associated with the lumbar spine.

Faretec, Inc. 440-350-9510
1610 W Jackson St Unit 6, Concord Twp, OH 44077
Traction weights.

Gilliam Enterprises, Llc 866-655-0517
5830 Briercliff Rd, Knoxville, TN 37918
Apparatus, traction, non-powered.

Glacier Cross, Inc. 800-388-4828
1694 Whalebone Dr, Kalispell, MT 59901
PRONEX is a patient controlled pneumatic cervical traction device. HOMESTRETCH is a patient controlled pneumatic lumbar traction device.

Hill-Rom, Inc. 812-934-7777
4115 Dorchester Rd Unit 600, North Charleston, SC 29405
Adaptors.

Ihn, Inc. 517-706-0060
4572 Ottawa Dr Ste 105, Okemos, MI 48864
Knee extension device.

Kenshin Trading Corp. 800-766-1313
22353 S Western Ave Ste 201, Torrance, CA 90501
Apparatus, traction, non-powered.

Lohmann & Rauscher, Inc. 800-279-3863
6001 SW 6th Ave Ste 101, Topeka, KS 66615

Lossing Orthopedic 800-328-5216
PO Box 6224, Minneapolis, MN 55406
Clinical cervical unit, lumbar clinical unit.

Lumiscope Company, Inc. 800-672-8293
1035 Centennial Ave, Piscataway, NJ 08854
Cervical traction sets.

Malcomtech International 510-293-0580
26200 Industrial Blvd, Hayward, CA 94545
Traction equipment.

Medical Depot 516-998-4600
99 Seaview Blvd, Port Washington, NY 11050
Carts, frames, weight, cords.

Mictron, Inc. 941-371-6659
6050 Porter Way, Sarasota, FL 34232
Leg holder with integrated tourniquet.

Midwest Health Care Consultants Inc. 231-354-7482
154 Southern Shores Dr, Brooklyn, MI 49230
Arch attachment, shrp traction attachment.

Physical Research Company 508-410-1928
451 Worcester Rd, Charlton, MA 01507
$249 for SPINALAID (3'x2'x7') back traction system, $145 for cervical & thoracic bench.

Posture Pro, Inc. 714-847-8607
18584 Main St, Huntington Beach, CA 92648

Preeminent, Llc 925-979-9090
1440 Maria Ln Ste 250, Walnut Creek, CA 94596
Ruch carpal tunnel glove.

Pro-Zooics Research Associates 650-322-2455
711 Central Ave, Menlo Park, CA 94025
Traction apparatus.

Promedica, Inc. 800-899-5278
114 Douglas Rd E, Oldsmar, FL 34677
Shoulder suspension system.

TRACTION UNIT, NON-POWERED *(cont'd)*

Rs Medical 800-683-0353
14001 S.E. First St., Vancouver, WA 98684
Pronex

Serola Biomechanics, Inc. 815-636-2780
5281 Zenith Pkwy, Loves Park, IL 61111

Shamrock Medical, Inc. 503-233-5055
3620 SE Powell Blvd, Portland, OR 97202
Lumbar and supine cervical traction system for home or clinical use.

Smith & Nephew Inc., Endoscopy Div. 978-749-1000
76 S Meridian Ave, Oklahoma City, OK 73107
Hip distraction system,hardware.

Spinal Designs Intl. 701-265-4927
708 Division Ave S., Cavalier, ND 58220
Lumbar rehabilitation system.

Spinal Traction Products, Llc. 636-947-9086
5 Lake Forest Ct E, Saint Charles, MO 63301
Ambulatory.

Synthes (Usa) 610-719-5000
35 Airport Rd, Horseheads, NY 14845
Various types and sizes of non-powered traction components.

The Pettibon System 888-774-6258
2118 Jackson Hwy, Chehalis, WA 98532
Cervical traction.

The Saunders Group 800-445-9836
4250 Norex Dr, Chaska, MN 55318
Cervical traction device.

Top Shelf Manufacturing, Llc 209-834-8185
1851 Paradise Rd Ste B, Tracy, CA 95304
Knee extension board.

Total Motion Restoration, Llc 678-910-0156
9990 Devonshire St, Douglasville, GA 30135
Orthopedic traction device.

Truform Orthotics & Prosthetics 800-888-0458
3960 Rosslyn Dr, Cincinnati, OH 45209

Tubular Fabricators Industry, Inc. 804-733-4000
600 W Wythe St, Petersburg, VA 23803
Traction stand.

Vmg Medical, Inc. 540-337-1996
542 Walnut Hills Rd, Staunton, VA 24401
Traction device.

Warsaw Orthopedic, Inc. 901-396-3133
2500 Silveus Xing, Warsaw, IN 46582
Various types of weights, cord, frames, and other traction acc.

TRACTION UNIT, POWERED, MOBILE *(Orthopedics) 87SBN*

Alimed, Inc. 800-225-2610
297 High St, Dedham, MA 02026

I-Rep, Inc. 800-828-0852
508 Chaney St Ste B, Lake Elsinore, CA 92530
Digital portable intermittant traction unit, capable of up to 200 lbs. traction force.

TRACTION UNIT, STATIC, BED *(Orthopedics) 87SBO*

Alimed, Inc. 800-225-2610
297 High St, Dedham, MA 02026

Florida Manufacturing Corp. 800-447-2372
501 Beville Rd, South Daytona, FL 32119

Freeman Manufacturing Company 800-253-2091
900 W Chicago Rd, PO Box J, Sturgis, MI 49091

Paramedical Distributors 800-245-3278
2020 Grand Blvd, Kansas City, MO 64108

Tetra Medical Supply Corp. 800-621-4041
6364 W Gross Point Rd, Niles, IL 60714

Truform Orthotics & Prosthetics 800-888-0458
3960 Rosslyn Dr, Cincinnati, OH 45209

Zimmer Holdings, Inc. 800-613-6131
1800 W Center St, PO Box 708, Warsaw, IN 46580

TRACTION UNIT, STATIC, CHAIR *(Orthopedics) 87SBP*

Freeman Manufacturing Company 800-253-2091
900 W Chicago Rd, PO Box J, Sturgis, MI 49091
Over-door and bed traction units.

Paramedical Distributors 800-245-3278
2020 Grand Blvd, Kansas City, MO 64108

Zimmer Holdings, Inc. 800-613-6131
1800 W Center St, PO Box 708, Warsaw, IN 46580

TRACTION UNIT, STATIC, OTHER *(Orthopedics) 87SBQ*

Florida Manufacturing Corp. 800-447-2372
501 Beville Rd, South Daytona, FL 32119

Mizuho Osi 800-777-4674
30031 Ahern Ave, Union City, CA 94587

Paramedical Distributors 800-245-3278
2020 Grand Blvd, Kansas City, MO 64108

Thera-Tronics, Inc. 800-267-6211
623 Mamaroneck Ave, Mamaroneck, NY 10543
Traction tables & units.

Truform Orthotics & Prosthetics 800-888-0458
3960 Rosslyn Dr, Cincinnati, OH 45209

Ultron Systems, Inc. 805-529-1485
5105 Maureen Ln, Moorpark, CA 93021
Ionizing Air Pencil. Neutralizes static on small parts and devices. Pencil sized for fine point-of-use applications.

Zimmer Orthopaedic Surgical Products 800-321-5533
PO Box 10, 200 West Ohio Ave., Dover, OH 44622
ZIMCODE.

TRAINER, AUDITORY *(Ear/Nose/Throat) 77SBR*

Armstrong Medical Industries, Inc. 800-323-4220
575 Knightsbridge Pkwy, Lincolnshire, IL 60069
Ear diagnostic trainer.

Phonic Ear, Inc. 800-227-0735
3880 Cypress Dr, Petaluma, CA 94954
SOLARIS sleek and durable binaural hearing system includes two hearing aids and fits mild to profound hearing losses. With the system's 40 built-in channels, students simply dial to the appropriate frequency - no crystals are needed. Moreover, its detented fitter controls can be set separately for each ear with repeatable precision.

Telex Communications, Inc.-Hearing Instrument Grp. 800-328-8212
1200 Portland Avenue S, Burnsville, MN 55357
CLASSMATE & SELECT, personal FM sound systems for the hard of hearing and sound field amplification systems for classrooms.

TRAINER, LAPAROSCOPY *(Surgery) 79SHA*

Ethicon Endo-Surgery, Inc. 800-USE-ENDO
4545 Creek Rd, Cincinnati, OH 45242

Richard Wolf Medical Instruments Corp. 800-323-9653
353 Corporate Woods Pkwy, Vernon Hills, IL 60061

TRAINING AID *(Orthopedics) 87UFE*

Armstrong Medical Industries, Inc. 800-323-4220
575 Knightsbridge Pkwy, Lincolnshire, IL 60069
Early defibrillation training system, complete with RHYTHMSIM, manikin, and TV interface. Compatible with all defibrillators.

Burkhart Roentgen Intl. Inc. 800-USA-XRAY
5201 8th Ave S, Gulfport, FL 33707

Clarke Health Care Products, Inc. 888-347-4537
1003 International Dr, Oakdale, PA 15071
DST Dynamic Stair Trainer, electronically adjust the height of the stairs from flat plane to 6.5' height in 1cm increments. Use as stair trainer or parallel bars. Patient can set stairs to individual needs. Display shows progress to prepare patient charts.

Ibiom Instruments Ltd. 450-678-5468
6640 Barry St., Brossard, QUE J4Z 1T8 Canada
Video teaching system.

Immersion Medical 800-929-4709
55 W Watkins Mill Rd, Gaithersburg, MD 20878
CATHSIM Intravenous Training System, medical simulator for training intravenous procedures. Includes the 'Accutouch' tactile feedback device, a robotic device that simulates the feel of the actual procedure. Also, preop endoscopy simulator for practicing endoscopic procedures.

Kilgore International, Inc. 800-892-9999
36 W Pearl St, Coldwater, MI 49036

Medikmark Inc. 800-424-8520
3600 Burwood Dr, Waukegan, IL 60085
OSHA compliance kits.

TRAINING AID *(cont'd)*

Medsim-Eagle Simulation Inc. 607-779-6000
151 Court St, Binghamton, NY 13901
Medical Training Simulator, a full-body, computer controlled patient mannequin with lifelike qualities. The simulation software models cardiovascular and pulmonary functions, metabolic effects and drug reactions-simulating the mannequin, anesthesia machine and monitors to provide information. The simulator realistically simulates the look, feel, symptoms and responses of a human patient in an O.R./E.R./C.C. or I.C.U. environment.

Microscopy/Microscopy Education 413-746-6931
125 Paridon St Ste 102, Springfield, MA 01118
MME provides customized on-site training in all areas of microscopy and sample preparation; image analysis. Book 'Optimizing Light Microscopy for Biological and Clinical Laboratories' a new microscopy text which is great for classes or learning on your own. It is also a wonderful reference for any laboratory or library, containing nearly 200 pp. of helpful tips, quick experiments and new ideas for getting the best from a microscope. Over 100 simple diagrams and illustrative photos.

N-K Products Company, Div. Of I-Rep,Inc. 800-462-6509
508 Chaney St Ste B, Lake Elsinore, CA 92530
Stairs.

Nasco 800-558-9595
4825 Stoddard Rd, PO Box 3837, Modesto, CA 95356

Optp 888-819-0121
3800 Annapolis Ln N Ste 165, PO Box 47009, Minneapolis, MN 55447
$10.00 each for Treat Your Own Back and Treat Your Own Neck patient education books.

Ossur Americas, Inc 800-222-4284
19762 Pauling, Foothill Ranch, CA 92610
Bodylines progressive elastic resistance technology. Resistance system represents the latest advance in closed chain rehab and exercise. Designed for use in clinic, home or office settings. Effective for both rehab and conditioning.

Pacific Research Laboratories, Inc. 206-463-5551
10221 SW 188th St, PO Box 409, Vashon, WA 98070
Training aids include deformed foot bones, bony pathologies, vertebral column, arthroscopy models plus psychomotor skills kit.

Rsti (Radiological Service Training Institute) 800-229-7784
30745 Solon Rd, Solon, OH 44139
Radiology service training.

Rx Honing Machine Corporation 800-346-6464
1301 E 5th St, Mishawaka, IN 46544
Detailed instrument sharpening manuals with over 150 pictures and diagrams of surgical instruments being sharpened with the Rx System II Sharpening Machine.

Veritech Corporation 413-525-3368
168 Denslow Rd, East Longmeadow, MA 01028
6-part interactive video disc education program, includes Anatomy of the Hip, Spine and Knee (3-D anatomy with human anatomy examples), two part sales course, x-ray analysis and templating of hip and knee; runs on Learning Exchange.

TRAINING AID, ARRHYTHMIA RECOGNITION *(Cardiovascular) 74VCZ*

Armstrong Medical Industries, Inc. 800-323-4220
575 Knightsbridge Pkwy, Lincolnshire, IL 60069
RHYTHMSIM display arrhythmia and BP on TV for large classroom settings.

Health & Radiological Seminars, Inc. 800-969-4774
550 Highland St Ste 100, Frederick, MD 21701
Nuclear Cardiology Course. 200 Hour, didactic training course for nuclear cardiologist licensure.

TRAINING MANIKIN, CPR (RESUSCITATION) *(General) 80SBS*

Ambu, Inc. 800-262-8462
6740 Baymeadow Dr, Glen Burnie, MD 21060
AMBUMAN unit.

Armstrong Medical Industries, Inc. 800-323-4220
575 Knightsbridge Pkwy, Lincolnshire, IL 60069
ACTAR D-FIB adult CPR manikin with CPR teaching features and AED training features. Actar AED Trainer and Little Joe economical CPR manikin.

Dixie Ems Supply 800-347-3494
385 Union Ave, Brooklyn, NY 11211
$290.00 per unit (standard).

Nasco 800-558-9595
4825 Stoddard Rd, PO Box 3837, Modesto, CA 95356

TRAINING MANIKIN, CPR (RESUSCITATION) *(cont'd)*

Pocket Nurse Enterprises, Inc. 800-225-1600
200 1st St, Ambridge, PA 15003
Variety of CPR manikins

Rockford Medical & Safety Co. 800-435-9451
2420 Harrison Ave, PO Box 5646, Rockford, IL 61108

Simulaids, Inc. 800-431-4310
16 Simulaids Dr, PO Box 1289, Saugerties, NY 12477
Regular & choking models: CPR TIMMY, CPR KIM, CPR KEVIN, CPR KYLE, BRAD, SANI MAN, SANI BABY and the new JT BRAD.

TRAINING MANIKIN, INTRAVENOUS ARM *(General) 80TFF*

Armstrong Medical Industries, Inc. 800-323-4220
575 Knightsbridge Pkwy, Lincolnshire, IL 60069

Medical Plastics Laboratory, Inc. 800-433-5539
226 FM 116, Industrial Air Park, PO Box 38, Gatesville, TX 76528
Multi-Venous IV Training Arms: Male & Female available. Features: Venipuncture possible in the antecubital fossa or dorsum of the hand; Rotation at the deltoid for easier access during peripheral IV line insertion and removal; Accessible veins include median, basilic and cephalic; Palpable veins enable site selection and preparation; Infusible veins allow peripheral therapy with IV bolus or push injection method; Intermittent Infusion Device insertion or conversion of existing IV line is possible; Peripheral IV line maintenance, including assessment and rotation of site and dressing, solution and tubing change; Replaceable skin and vein system ensure longevity of model; May articulate to adult MPL manikins. Kits include: Replacement skin and Multi-Vein system, blood concentrate, blood bag w/tubing & connector, clamp and hook, syringes (5), lubricant and carry case. Pediatric Multi-Venous Arm, Standard IV Arm & Hand, Foam IV Arm, Elbow & Hand also available.

Nasco 800-558-9595
901 Janesville Ave, PO Box 901, Fort Atkinson, WI 53538
$450.00 per unit (standard).

Nasco 800-558-9595
4825 Stoddard Rd, PO Box 3837, Modesto, CA 95356

Pocket Nurse Enterprises, Inc. 800-225-1600
200 1st St, Ambridge, PA 15003
variety of IV training arms

Rockford Medical & Safety Co. 800-435-9451
2420 Harrison Ave, PO Box 5646, Rockford, IL 61108

Simulaids, Inc. 800-431-4310
16 Simulaids Dr, PO Box 1289, Saugerties, NY 12477
Arm & hand models, ALS Adult Trainer, ALS Pediatric Trainer, STAT, PDA STAT, patient simulators.

TRAINING MANIKIN, OTHER *(General) 80SBT*

Ambu, Inc. 800-262-8462
6740 Baymeadow Dr, Glen Burnie, MD 21060
AMBU MECACODE Intubation trainer, BLS master. AMBU cardiac care.

Armstrong Medical Industries, Inc. 800-323-4220
575 Knightsbridge Pkwy, Lincolnshire, IL 60069
OB training manikins, ear syringing models and patient care manikins, basic and advanced; X-ray positioning manikin.

Mammatech Corp. 800-626-2273
930 NW 8th Ave, Gainesville, FL 32601
$125.00 for training models for breast lump detection.

Medical Plastics Laboratory, Inc. 800-433-5539
226 FM 116, Industrial Air Park, PO Box 38, Gatesville, TX 76528
The Laerdal SimMan Universal Patient Simulator: Extremely realistic, yet affordable and portable, the SimMan simulator was specifically designed to meet the scenario-based training needs of nursing, anesthesia, ACLS, ATLS and difficult airway management. The Laerdal AirMan Difficult Airway Simulator (torso) offers the capability of presenting a multitude of difficult airway situations with the touch of a button and was specifically designed to meet the scenario-based training needs of difficult airway management for healthcare providers. A full line of full body manikins and torso models: Male, Female, Pediatric & Infant Patient Care Manikins (Complete Care Doll); Birthing Simulators; Sounds Auscultation Torso; NG Tube & Trach Care Torso; Urinary Catheterization Models; Vascular Access Simulators; Neonatal Task Trainers; Adult & Pediatric ACLS manikins (MegaCode); Airway Management Trainers; Femoral Access Models; Neonatal Resuscitation Baby; First Aid, CPR, Extrication & Immobilization Manikins; Choking Charlie; Weighted Rescue Manikins (Tuff Kelly).

TRAINING MANIKIN, OTHER *(cont'd)*

Medsim-Eagle Simulation Inc. 607-779-6000
151 Court St, Binghamton, NY 13901
Medical Training Simulator, a full-body, computer controlled patient mannequin with lifelike qualities. The simulation software models cardiovascular and pulmonary functions, metabolic effects and drug reactions-simulating the mannequin, anesthesia machine and monitors to provide information. The simulator realistically simulates the look, feel, symptoms and responses of a human patient in an O.R./E.R./C.C. or I.C.U. environment.

Nasco 800-558-9595
901 Janesville Ave, PO Box 901, Fort Atkinson, WI 53538
$995.00 for Intraosseous Infusion Simulator to aid in the training of adult sternal intraosseous infusion with the F.A.S.T. 1 Training System

Pocket Nurse Enterprises, Inc. 800-225-1600
200 1st St, Ambridge, PA 15003
Variety of Manikins and Simulators for education

Rockford Medical & Safety Co. 800-435-9451
2420 Harrison Ave, PO Box 5646, Rockford, IL 61108

Simulaids, Inc. 800-431-4310
16 Simulaids Dr, PO Box 1289, Saugerties, NY 12477
Male catheterization, breast self examination, rescue, gynecological and tension pneumothorax procedure training manikins.

TRAINING MANIKIN, WOUND MOULAGE *(General) 80TFO*

Armstrong Medical Industries, Inc. 800-323-4220
575 Knightsbridge Pkwy, Lincolnshire, IL 60069

Dixie Ems Supply 800-347-3494
385 Union Ave, Brooklyn, NY 11211
$65.00 per unit (standard).

Medical Plastics Laboratory, Inc. 800-433-5539
226 FM 116, Industrial Air Park, PO Box 38, Gatesville, TX 76528
The Ultimate Hurt manikin features three interchangeable heads for teaching airway management and the assessment of facial and cranial trauma, plus a set of interchangeable wound modules. The First Aid/CPR Training full body manikin combines CPR capabilities with wound modules for simulating first aid scenarios. The BTLS Victim Injury Set contains over 30 wound lay-ons with Velcro design, blood splats and simulated blood for use on either humans or manikins to simulate injuries required in 12 scenarios from the BTLS Instructor's Manual. The Trauma Make-Up Kit contains materials for moulaging realistic trauma on both humans and manikins. Interchangeable Wound Module Sets, Bleeding Control Limb Modules, and Wound Care & Assessment Modules are availble for use with MPL manikins or as stand-alone models.

Pocket Nurse Enterprises, Inc. 800-225-1600
200 1st St, Ambridge, PA 15003
variety of wound moulage packages

Simulaids, Inc. 800-431-4310
16 Simulaids Dr, PO Box 1289, Saugerties, NY 12477
Wound moulage training manikin for burns, punctures, lacerations, fractures & foreign body protrusions.

TRANSDUCER, BLOOD FLOW, INVASIVE *(Anesthesiology) 73BXG*

Flowtronics, Inc. 602-997-1364
10250 N 19th Ave Ste B, Phoenix, AZ 85021
$350.00 and up for each cerebral blood flow sensor, thermal diffusion method.

Hospira, Inc. 877-946-7747
755 Jarvis Dr, Morgan Hill, CA 95037

TRANSDUCER, BLOOD PRESSURE *(General) 80SBW*

Apollo Research Corporation 800-418-1718
2300 Walden Ave Ste 200, Buffalo, NY 14225
Pressure Pulse Sensor is a piezoelectric pressure sensor (22-mm diameter) with built-in signed conditioning microelectronics.

B. Braun Oem Division, B. Braun Medical Inc. 866-8-BBRAUN
824 12th Ave, Bethlehem, PA 18018

Biosensors International - Usa 949-553-8300
20280 SW Acacia St Ste 300, Newport Beach, CA 92660
BIOTRANS II, a new high-tech next-generation disposable/reusable transducer system for effective continuous blood-pressure measurement.

Datascope Corp. 800-288-2121
14 Philips Pkwy, Montvale, NJ 07645
3 models.

David Scott Company 800-804-0333
59 Fountain St, Framingham, MA 01702
Transducer, disposable.

TRANSDUCER, BLOOD PRESSURE *(cont'd)*

Hospira, Inc. 877-946-7747
755 Jarvis Dr, Morgan Hill, CA 95037
$25 for disposable TRANSPAC transducer with monitoring kit.

Konigsberg Instruments, Inc. 626-449-0016
2000 E Foothill Blvd, Pasadena, CA 91107
Custom devices for OEM and research requirements.

Millar Instruments, Inc. 800.669.2343
6001 Gulf Fwy Ste A, Houston, TX 77023
Pressure wave form for pulse pressure measurement.

Sensym Ict 800-573-6796
1804 McCarthy Blvd, Milpitas, CA 95035
$38.00 for 0-300mm Hg Blood pressure sensor. Disposable and general purpose pressure sensors.

Smiths Medical Asd, Inc. 800-848-1757
6250 Shier Rings Rd, Dublin, OH 43016
Multi-use and disposable types.

U.F.I. 805-772-1203
545 Main St Ste C2, Morro Bay, CA 93442
$205 for Model 1050.

TRANSDUCER, BLOOD PRESSURE, CATHETER TIP
(Cardiovascular) 74DXO

Edwards Lifesciences, Llc. 800-424-3278
1 Edwards Way, Irvine, CA 92614

Escalon Trek Medical 800-433-8197
2440 S 179th St, New Berlin, WI 53146
Doppler vascular access device.

Millar Instruments, Inc. 800.669.2343
6001 Gulf Fwy Ste A, Houston, TX 77023
Direct measurement of physiological pressures (sizes 2F-8F). Also with fluid-velocity sensor.

Volcano Corporation 800-228-4728
3661 Valley Centre Dr Ste 200, San Diego, CA 92130
Pressure guide wire.

TRANSDUCER, BLOOD PRESSURE, EXTRAVASCULAR
(Cardiovascular) 74DRS

Argon Medical Devices Inc. 903-675-9321
1445 Flat Creek Rd, Athens, TX 75751
Various.

Biotek Instruments, Inc. 802-655-4040
100 Tigan St, Highland Park, Winooski, VT 05404
Vacuum, pressure & temperature circuit testers.

Edwards Lifesciences Technology Sarl 949-250-2500
State Rd. 402 N.km 1.4, Anasco, PR 00610-1577
Disposable pressure dome.

Edwards Lifesciences, Llc. 800-424-3278
1 Edwards Way, Irvine, CA 92614

Grass Technologies, An Astro-Med, Inc. Product Gro 401-828-4002
53 Airport Park Drive, Rockland, MA 02370
Blood pressure transducer.

Harvard Apparatus, Inc. 800-272-2775
84 October Hill Rd, Holliston, MA 01746
Model 72-4496 physiological blood pressure transducer.

Icu Medical (Ut), Inc 949-366-2183
4455 Atherton Dr, Salt Lake City, UT 84123
Various.

Jetcor, Inc. 206-243-2230
15001 8th Ave SW Ste 16, Burien, WA 98166
Transducer, blood-pressure extravascular.

Merit Medical Systems, Inc. 800-356-3748
1600 Merit Pkwy, South Jordan, UT 84095
Meritrans Physiologic Transducers.

Millar Instruments, Inc. 800.669.2343
6001 Gulf Fwy Ste A, Houston, TX 77023

Navilyst Medical 800-833-9973
100 Boston Scientific Way, Marlborough, MA 01752
Various types of blood pressure transducers and disposable blood pressure kits.

Sorin Group Usa 800-289-5759
14401 W 65th Way, Arvada, CO 80004

Terumo Cardiovascular Systems (Tcvs) 800-283-7866
28 Howe St, Ashland, MA 01721
Transducer.

TRANSDUCER, FLOW, CATHETER TIP *(Cardiovascular) 74WLT*

Dynamics Research Corp. 800-522-4321
60 Frontage Rd, Andover, MA 01810

Millar Instruments, Inc. 800.669.2343
6001 Gulf Fwy Ste A, Houston, TX 77023

TRANSDUCER, FORCE *(General) 80SBV*

Apollo Research Corporation 800-418-1718
2300 Walden Ave Ste 200, Buffalo, NY 14225
Triaxial Force Sensor (three-axis) and Uniaxial Force Sensor (single-axis) piezoelectric force sensors with built-in signal-conditioning microelectronics.

Himmelstein & Co., S. 800-632-7873
2490 Pembroke Ave, Hoffman Estates, IL 60169
Pancake style load cells

Hoggan Health Industries, Inc. 800-678-7888
8020 S 1300 W, West Jordan, UT 84088
MICROFET3 handheld electronic force gauge transducer for muscle testing and inclinometer for range of motion testing in one compact device. MICROFET2 handheld electronic transducer for muscle testing. Software available for both.

Nasco 800-558-9595
901 Janesville Ave, PO Box 901, Fort Atkinson, WI 53538
CPaRlene manikins and torsos. BASIC BUDDY/BABY BUDDY manikins (CPR). CPR Prompt manikins. CPR Prompt Audio Rescue and Practice Aid that talks individuals through every step of CPR in real time.

U.F.I. 805-772-1203
545 Main St Ste C2, Morro Bay, CA 93442
$335 for standard unit (Model 1030).

TRANSDUCER, GAS PRESSURE, DIFFERENTIAL *(Anesthesiology) 73BYR*

Grass Technologies, An Astro-Med, Inc. Product Gro 401-828-4002
53 Airport Park Drive, Rockland, MA 02370
Plethesmograph transducer.

TRANSDUCER, HEART SOUND *(Cardiovascular) 74JOO*

Grass Technologies, An Astro-Med, Inc. Product Gro 401-828-4002
53 Airport Park Drive, Rockland, MA 02370
Stethoscope microphone.

TRANSDUCER, MINIATURE PRESSURE *(Physical Med) 89IKE*

Apollo Research Corporation 800-418-1718
2300 Walden Ave Ste 200, Buffalo, NY 14225
Acoustic Contact Sensor is a small (13-mm) piezoelectric pressure sensor with built-in microelectronic voltage amplifiers.

Asi Medical Equipment, Ltd. 800-527-0443
1735 N Interstate 35E, Carrollton, TX 75006
IPC 200 is a portable interface pressure measuring device which is battery powered.

Bio-Logic Systems Corp. 800-323-8326
1 Bio Logic Plz, Mundelein, IL 60060
SLEEPSCAN AF, airflow pressure transducer. Works on the basis of pressure not temperature so it can detect shallow breathing where temperature related transducers remain substantially unchanged.

Cleveland Medical Devices, Inc. 877-253-8363
4415 Euclid Ave, Cleveland, OH 44103
PRESSORE Monitor. Hand-held digital instrument measures wrapping pressure for bandages and pressure between body and support surfaces. Also, PRESSORE Reminder a pressure relief reminder, audible or vibratory, for wheelchair users

Diagnostic Support Usa Inc. 305-532-1586
1900 Sunset Harbour Dr., Suite 1902, Miami Beach, FL 33139
Baropodometer.

Dynatronics Corp. 800-874-6251
7030 Park Centre Dr, Salt Lake City, UT 84121

Global Services Group 757-220-8282
350 McLaws Cir Ste 2, Williamsburg, VA 23185

Medtronic Blood Management 612-514-4000
18501 E Plaza Dr, Parker, CO 80134
Transducer.

Millar Instruments, Inc. 800.669.2343
6001 Gulf Fwy Ste A, Houston, TX 77023

TRANSDUCER, PRESSURE, INTRAUTERINE *(Obstetrics/Gyn) 85HFN*

Aiv, Inc. (Formerly American Iv) 800-990-2911
7485 Shipley Ave, Harmans, MD 21077
Specialized repair services on fetal transducers.

Argon Medical Devices Inc. 903-675-9321
1445 Flat Creek Rd, Athens, TX 75751
Intrauterine pressure monitor kit.

Clinical Innovations, Inc. 888-268-6222
747 W 4170 S, Murray, UT 84123
Koala intrauterine pressure system.

TRANSDUCER, STETHOSCOPE *(Anesthesiology) 73BZS*

Ccr Medical, Inc. 888-883-7331
967 43rd Ave NE, Saint Petersburg, FL 33703
Stethoscope, chestpiece, various size.

Greystone Of Lincoln, Inc. 401-333-0444
7 Wellington Rd, Lincoln, RI 02865
Stethoscope diaphram housing.

Primary Medical Co., Inc. 727-520-1920
6541 44th St N Ste 6003, Pinellas Park, FL 33781
Various models non-sterile stethoscope.

Sun-Med 800-433-2797
12393 Belcher Rd S Ste 450, Largo, FL 33773

U.F.I. 805-772-1203
545 Main St Ste C2, Morro Bay, CA 93442
$160 for Model 1010C.

TRANSDUCER, TREMOR *(Cns/Neurology) 84GYD*

Grass Technologies, An Astro-Med, Inc. Product Gro 401-828-4002
53 Airport Park Drive, Rockland, MA 02370
Tremor transducer.

U.F.I. 805-772-1203
545 Main St Ste C2, Morro Bay, CA 93442
$170 for Model 1110.

TRANSDUCER, ULTRASONIC *(Cardiovascular) 74JOP*

Blatek, Inc. 814-231-2085
2820 E College Ave Ste F, State College, PA 16801

Cardinal Healthcare 209, Inc. 610-862-0800
5225 Verona Rd, Fitchburg, WI 53711
Vascular recorder.

Channel Industries, Inc. 805-967-0171
839 Ward Dr, Santa Barbara, CA 93111

Cone Instruments, Inc. 800-321-6964
5201 Naiman Pkwy, Solon, OH 44139

Dapco Industries 800-597-2726
241 Ethan Allen Hwy, Ridgefield, CT 06877
Ultrasonic doppler

Ellis Ophthalmic Technologies, Inc. 718-656-7390
147-39, 175 St.,, Suite #128, Jamaica, NY 11434
Ultrasound a scan probe/transducer.

Elmed, Inc. 630-543-2792
60 W Fay Ave, Addison, IL 60101

Ge Inspection Technologies, Lp 717-447-1278
50 Industrial Park Rd, Lewistown, PA 17044

Hokanson Inc., D.E. 800-999-8251
12840 NE 21st Pl, Bellevue, WA 98005
Extra or replacement Doppler transducers compatible with Hokanson Dopplers.

Huntleigh Healthcare Llc. 800-223-1218
40 Christopher Way, Eatontown, NJ 07724

Ideal Medical Source, Inc. 800-537-0739
2805 East. Oakland Blvd, Suite 352, Fort Lauderdale, FL 33306

Integra Radionics 800-466-6814
22 Terry Ave, Burlington, MA 01803

Main Line International, Inc. 800-397-9020
151 Ben Burton Cir, Coggins Park, Bogart, GA 30622

Medical Accessories, Inc. 800-275-1624
92 Youngs Rd, Trenton, NJ 08619
New ultrasonic transducers, tocotransducers and leg plates compatible with Corometrics and Hewlett-Packard fetal monitors.

Philips Medical Systems 949-450-0014
1590 Scenic Ave, Costa Mesa, CA 92626

Phillips Ultrasound 800-982-2011
22100 Bothell Everett Hwy, P.O. Box 3003, Bothell, WA 98021

TRANSDUCER, ULTRASONIC *(cont'd)*

Products Group International, Inc. 800-336-5299
447 Main St., Lyons, CO 80540

Shimadzu Medical Systems 800-228-1429
20101 S Vermont Ave, Torrance, CA 90502
TRUEVISION, ENDFIREPLUS.

Volcano Corporation 800-228-4728
3661 Valley Centre Dr Ste 200, San Diego, CA 92130
No common name listed.

2d Imaging, Inc. 800-449-1332
4745 E Wesley Dr, Anaheim, CA 92807

TRANSDUCER, ULTRASONIC, DIAGNOSTIC *(Radiology) 90ITX*

Blatek, Inc. 814-231-2085
2820 E College Ave Ste F, State College, PA 16801

Boston Scientific Corporation 800-225-2732
1 Boston Scientific Pl, Natick, MA 01760

Boston Scientific-Neurovascular 510-440-7700
47900 Bayside Pkwy, Fremont, CA 94538
Diagnostic ultrasound transducer.

Cardinal Healthcare 209, Inc. 610-862-0800
5225 Verona Rd, Fitchburg, WI 53711
Transducer 2,4,8mhz pulsed & continuous wave.

Civco Medical Instruments Co., Inc. 319-656-4447
102 1st St S, Kalona, IA 52247
Polyisoprene cover,stand-off,brachystepper,brachystepper template,brachystand su.

Consumaquip Corporation 305-592-4510
7240 NW 12th St, Miami, FL 33126

Cook Vascular, Incorporated 800-457-4500
1186 Montgomery Ln, Vandergrift, PA 15690
COOK-SWARTZ Doppler Flow Probe and Monitor System - Implantable cuff with probe used during and following microvascular surgical procedures to help determine the presence of blood flow to transplanted tissue flaps.

Fukuda Denshi Usa, Inc. 800-365-6668
17725 NE 65th St Ste C, Redmond, WA 98052
Transducer, ultrasonic, diagnostic.

Ge Inspection Technologies, Lp 717-447-1278
50 Industrial Park Rd, Lewistown, PA 17044

Ge Medical Systems, Llc 847-277-5002
4855 W Electric Ave, West Milwaukee, WI 53219
Varous models of diagnostic ultrasound transducers.

Ge Parallel Design, Inc. 262-544-3894
365 S 52nd St, Tempe, AZ 85281
Various models of diagnostic ultrasonic transducers.

Healthtronics Inc. 888-252-6575
9825 Spectrum Dr Bldg B, Austin, TX 78717

Imacor Llc. 516-393-0970
50 Charles Lindbergh Blvd Ste 200, Uniondale, NY 11553
ImaCor Zura Imaging System; ImaCor Zura TEE system; Zura

Koven Technology, Inc. 800-521-8342
12125 Woodcrest Executive Dr Ste 320, Saint Louis, MO 63141
Surgical Doppler probes for blood flow sound or velocity detection.

Md International, Inc. 305-669-9003
11300 NW 41st St, Doral, FL 33178

Medtronic Vascular 707-525-0111
3576 Unocal Pl, Santa Rosa, CA 95403
Pioneer.

Noshok, Inc. 440-243-0888
1010 W Bagley Rd, Berea, OH 44017
Ultrastable thin film and Hall effect technologies produces plus or minus .25% and plus or minus .5% accuracies, three year warranty. Pressure Switch. Electronic pressure switches in normally open and normally closed configurations with PNP and NPN outputs.

Pentax Southern Region Service Center 201-571-2300
8934 Kirby Dr, Houston, TX 77054
Ultrasound endoscope.

Pentax West Coast Service Center 800-431-5880
10410 Pioneer Blvd Ste 2, Santa Fe Springs, CA 90670
Pentax ultrasound endoscope.

Phillips Ultrasound 800-982-2011
22100 Bothell Everett Hwy, P.O. Box 3003, Bothell, WA 98021

Protek Medical Products, Inc. 319-545-7100
4125 Westcor Ct, Coralville, IA 52241
Various.

TRANSDUCER, ULTRASONIC, DIAGNOSTIC *(cont'd)*

Sheathing Technologies, Inc. 408-782-2720
18431 Technology Dr, Morgan Hill, CA 95037
Ultrasound probe cover.

The Newman Group, Llc 847-283-9177
42 Sherwood Ter Ste 2, Lake Bluff, IL 60044
Diagnostic ultrasonic transducer.

Toshiba America Medical Systems 800-421-1968
2441 Michelle Dr, Tustin, CA 92780
Models include the following: PC-19M, PC-50V, PEM-508SC, PEF-510MB, PEF-704LA, PLF-308P, PLM-503AT, PLM-703AT, PLM-805AT, PLM-1202S, PLM-1204AT, PSM-20CT, PSM-25AT, PSM-37AT, PSM-37CT, PSM-50AT, PSM-70AT, PVF-381MT, PVF-575AT, PVF-620ST, PVF-738H, PVF-738F, PVF-745V, PVM-375AT, PVM-651VT, PVM-662AT, PVM-740RT, PLG-805S, PVG-366M, PVG-601V, PVG-681S, PVG-720S, PVG-381M, PLG-506M, PLG-308P, PVG-600S, PC-20M, PLT-704AT, PLT-805AT, PLT-1204AT, PLT-1204AX, PST-20CT, PST-25AT, PST-37CT, PST-65AT, PVT-375AT, PVT-661VT.

Volcano Corporation 800-228-4728
3661 Valley Centre Dr Ste 200, San Diego, CA 92130
Ultrasound transducer.

W. L. Gore And Associates, Inc. 888-914-4673
555 Paper Mill Rd Bldg 120, Newark, DE 19711
Ultrasound imaging transducer.

Zonare Medical Systems, Inc. 877-966-2731
420 Bernardo Ave, Mountain View, CA 94043
Diagnostic ultrasound.

TRANSDUCER, ULTRASONIC, INTRAVAGINAL
(Obstetrics/Gyn) 85WOP

Aiv, Inc. (Formerly American Iv) 800-990-2911
7485 Shipley Ave, Harmans, MD 21077
Specialized repair services on fetal transducers.

Blatek, Inc. 814-231-2085
2820 E College Ave Ste F, State College, PA 16801

Consumaquip Corporation 305-592-4510
7240 NW 12th St, Miami, FL 33126

TRANSDUCER, ULTRASONIC, OBSTETRICAL
(Obstetrics/Gyn) 85HGL

Aiv, Inc. (Formerly American Iv) 800-990-2911
7485 Shipley Ave, Harmans, MD 21077
Specialized repair services on fetal transducers.

Blatek, Inc. 814-231-2085
2820 E College Ave Ste F, State College, PA 16801

Epic Medical Equipment Services, Inc. 800-327-3742
1800 10th St Ste 300, Plano, TX 75074
Sale and repair of all fetal transducers.

Kentec Medical Inc. 800-825-5996
17871 Fitch, Irvine, CA 92614
Ameritus Toco and Ultrasonic transducer replacements for most GE Corometrics and Phillips fetal monitors.

Medical Accessories, Inc. 800-275-1624
92 Youngs Rd, Trenton, NJ 08619
New ultrasonic transducers, tocotransducers and leg plates compatible with Corometrics and Hewlett-Packard fetal monitors.

Philips Medical Systems 949-450-0014
1590 Scenic Ave, Costa Mesa, CA 92626

Phillips Ultrasound 800-982-2011
22100 Bothell Everett Hwy, P.O. Box 3003, Bothell, WA 98021

TRANSFER AID *(Physical Med) 89IKX*

Alimed, Inc. 800-225-2610
297 High St, Dedham, MA 02026

Arjo, Inc. 800-323-1245
50 Gary Ave Ste A, Roselle, IL 60172
Floor-mount lift chair attached next to bathtub allowing independent access to bathtub.

Barjan Mfg., Ltd. 631-420-5588
28 Baiting Place Rd, Farmingdale, NY 11735
No common name listed.

Biogrip, Inc. 916-483-2686
3904 New York Ave, Fair Oaks, CA 95628
Hand grips.

Costonde Products Llc 810-743-1167
419 Tennyson Ave, Flint, MI 48507
Toilet transfer board.

TRANSFER AID *(cont'd)*

David Scott Company 800-804-0333
59 Fountain St, Framingham, MA 01702

George J. Kamilar 516-665-7167
240 Windsor Ave, Brightwaters, NY 11718
Easy over, over easy.

Hillmor Products 734-721-3485
39292 Montana Dr, Romulus, MI 48174
Extend a hand.

Hospira, Inc. 877-946-7747
Hwy. 301 North, Rocky Mount, NC 27801
Various types.

Icu Medical (Ut), Inc 949-366-2183
4455 Atherton Dr, Salt Lake City, UT 84123
Various types of transfer aids.

International Medication Systems, Ltd. 800-423-4136
1886 Santa Anita Ave, South El Monte, CA 91733
Various types of closed, aseptic fluid transfer devices.

Leeder Group, Inc. 305-436-5030
8508 NW 66th St, Miami, FL 33166
Seat lifting devices.

Liftvest U.S.A, Llc 800-300-5671
35 W 83rd St, New York, NY 10024
PonchoVest: a stylish denim poncho with webbing harness that slips over head for easy transfers. See Liftvest.

Lytron, Inc. 781-933-7300
55 Dragon Ct, Woburn, MA 01801
Heat transfer system.

Mizuho Osi 800-777-4674
30031 Ahern Ave, Union City, CA 94587

Mobility Inc. 858-456-8121
5726 La Jolla Blvd Ste 104, La Jolla, CA 92037
Toilet seat, hydraulic.

Needle Aid, Ltd. 902-895-8015
23 Lower Truro Rd, Truro B2N 5A9 Canada
Needle aid device

Noram Seating, Inc. 866-236-7328
18 Market St, Union City, PA 16438
Liftchairs, bed handles and rails.

Patterson Medical Supply, Inc. 262-387-8720
W68N158 Evergreen Blvd, Cedarburg, WI 53012
Transfer aid, daily activity assist device.

Perfect Care 718-805-7800
8927 126th St, Richmond Hill, NY 11418
Aid, transfer, bath seat.

Rapid Deployment Products 877-433-7569
157 Railroad Dr, Ivyland, PA 18974
Pro-Lite patient slide is great for hospitals, nursing homes, morticians, X-Ray departments or EMS crews for bed to stretcher transfers. The PRO-SLIDE has the most hand holes (12) available on the market for quick grip.

Richardson Products, Inc. 888-928-7297
9408 Gulfstream Rd, Frankfort, IL 60423
Transfer device.

Rifton Equipment 800-571-8198
PO Box 260, Rifton, NY 12471
With zero-lifting, a single caregiver can transfer adult clients from their wheelchair to an upright standing or mobility device. Additionally, by lifting entirely from above the waist, the Rifton SoloLift offers convenience and dignity for toileting.

Solo Step, Inc. 866-453-9442
7421 W Luke Dr, Sioux Falls, SD 57106
Rehabilitation.

Therafin Corporation 800-843-7234
19747 Wolf Rd, Mokena, IL 60448
Various types of transfer boards.

Therapeutic Dimensions, Inc. 509-323-9275
319 W Hastings Rd, Po Box 28307, Spokane, WA 99218
Orthopedic leg support scooter.

Tubular Fabricators Industry, Inc. 804-733-4000
600 W Wythe St, Petersburg, VA 23803
Various models of transfer bench.

We Care Design's, L.L.C. 504-624-8282
428 Bill Dr, Mandeville, LA 70448
Transfer aide.

TRANSFER AID *(cont'd)*

Xtol Products Co. 814-255-2298
522 Goucher St, Johnstown, PA 15905
Drug eluting stent and delivery system.

TRANSFER DEVICE, PATIENT, MANUAL *(General) 80FMR*

Air Movement Technologies, Inc. 800-317-9582
320 Gateway Park Dr, Syracuse, NY 13212
Air assisted patient transfer device.

Alimed, Inc. 800-225-2610
297 High St, Dedham, MA 02026

Arjo, Inc. 800-323-1245
50 Gary Ave Ste A, Roselle, IL 60172

Armstrong Medical Industries, Inc. 800-323-4220
575 Knightsbridge Pkwy, Lincolnshire, IL 60069

Bams Manufacturing Co., Inc. 847-647-6990
6273 W Howard St, Niles, IL 60714
Manual patient transfer device.

Bionix Development Corp. 800-551-7096
5154 Enterprise Blvd, Toledo, OH 43612
Bionix patient mover.

Bird & Cronin, Inc. 651-683-1111
1200 Trapp Rd, Saint Paul, MN 55121
Transfer board.

Cameron-Miller, Inc. 800-621-0142
5410 W Roosevelt Rd, Road #241, Chicago, IL 60644

Camtec 410-228-1156
1959 Church Creek Rd, Cambridge, MD 21613
Bassinets cadtec.

Clever Solutions, Inc. 800-743-6165
10163 Faetano Ln, Milan, MI 48160
Easy Does It Bath Transfer System - Rotating, Sliding, and Foldable transfer system.

Dick Medical Supply, Llc 614-444-2300
630 Marion Rd, Columbus, OH 43207
Stretcher strap.

Dixie Ems Supply 800-347-3494
385 Union Ave, Brooklyn, NY 11211
$129.95 for SMOOTH MOVER patient mover.

Duralife, Inc. 800-443-5433
195 Phillips Park Dr, Williamsport, PA 17702
Wheeled shower bed/transport.

Eclectic Grey Mater Designs 801-296-0741
279 E 650 N, Bountiful, UT 84010
Patient transfer board, slicker board.

Ergodyne 800-225-8238
1021 Bandana Blvd E Ste 220, Saint Paul, MN 55108
Ergodyne(R) On3(R) Transfer Surface. Designed for patient lateral transfer and repositioning, the On3(R) Transfer Surface eliminates the need for vertical lifting and saves on people power. Reduces associated back injury costs, increases productivity, and improves patient dignity. It's simply the most economical way to perform comfortable patient transfers. We apply a special heat-sealed wax treatment to a rugged 140 denier nylon material. The slick result reduces friction and makes transfers smoother. Rugged polyester webbing handles are stitched to last. Includes tote/storage bag. Available in two sizes: 27 x 66 in. (69 x 168 cm) black handles; 32 x 72 in. (81 x 183 cm) gray handles.

Evacu Technologies Inc. 905-372-0322
2-20 Strathy Rd, Cobourg K9A 5J7 Canada
Evacu-sled,evacuation device for patients

Gendron, Inc. 800-537-2521
400 E Lugbill Rd, Archbold, OH 43502
EASY GLIDE Bath Transfer designed to assist transferring obese patient for bathing or showering. 700 pound weight capacity.

Gymstandy Llc 503-684-4990
9055 SW Mountain View Ln, Tigard, OR 97224
Manual transfer device.

Hospira, Inc. 877-946-7747
1776 Centennial Dr, McPherson, KS 67460
Syringe holder.

Intarsia Ltd. 203-355-1357
14 Martha Ln, Gaylordsville, CT 06755
Transfer board.

Itec/Ems Llp 903-365-6390
400 All Star Dr, Winnsboro, TX 75494
Stretcher, patient transfer device.

TRANSFER DEVICE, PATIENT, MANUAL *(cont'd)*

Liftvest U.S.A, Llc 800-300-5671
35 W 83rd St, New York, NY 10024
Stylish denim vest with webbing harness permits manual transfer with safety and eliminates caregiver back injuries. Does away with armpit lift.

Maine Anti-Gravity Systems, Inc. 207-775-3800
98 Gray St, Portland, ME 04102
Ipps.

Mastercare Patient Equipment, Inc. 800-798-5867
2071 14th Ave, PO Box 1435, Columbus, NE 68601
Manual patient transfer device.

Medex Para-Medical Equipment Inc. 450-581-3966
275 Boul Pierre-Legardeur, Le Gardeur J5Z 3A7 Canada
Dorso-lite

Medical Associates Network 818-500-7711
801 N Brand Blvd Ste 690, Glendale, CA 91203
Needleless ampoule transfer device method to extract fluids from ampoules wihtout risk of injury plus integral disposal housing.

Mizuho Osi 800-777-4674
30031 Ahern Ave, Union City, CA 94587
TRANSTRACK & HALF TRACK.

Mjm International Corporation 956-781-5000
2003 N Veterans Blvd Ste 10, San Juan, TX 78589
Various models of transfer benches.

Parsons A.D.L. Inc. 800-263-1281
R.R. #2, 1986 Sideroad 15, Tottenham, ONT L0G 1W0 Canada
Transfer discs, both soft and ridgid for floor and seated use, glide sheets, E - Z Turn stand and turn device, patient lifting slings (manual lift), gait belts

Patient Transfer Systems, Inc. 800-633-4725
5456 Northwood Dr, Center Valley, PA 18034
Patient transfer unit.

Perfect Care 718-805-7800
8927 126th St, Richmond Hill, NY 11418
Transfer bench.

Profex Medical Products 800-325-0196
2224 E Person Ave, Memphis, TN 38114

Reeves Emergency Management Systems, Llc. 301-698-1596
1704 W 7th St, Frederick, MD 21702
Spineboard and sleeve.

Regal Medi-Spa Co., Inc. 905-477-7689
166 Torbay Rd, Markham L3R 1G6 Canada
Patient transporter

Schuerch Corp. 617-773-0927
48 Oval Rd, Quincy, MA 02170
Patient transfer device.

Stryker Medical 800-869-0770
3800 E Centre Ave, Portage, MI 49002

Sunrise Medical 800-333-4000
7477 Dry Creek Pkwy, Longmont, CO 80503

Sunrise Medical Hhg Inc 303-218-4505
7128 Ambassador Rd, Baltimore, MD 21244
Various sizes and styles of transfer board.

Symphony Medical Products 877-470-9995
6320 NW 84th Ave, Miami, FL 33166
Manual transfer stretcher.

Total Innovative Manufacturing 616-738-8299
12688 New Holland St, Holland, MI 49424
Device, transfer, patient, manual.

Tr Group, Inc. 800-752-6900
903 Wedel Ln, Glenview, IL 60025
Shower trolley.

Tuffcare 800-367-6160
3999 E La Palma Ave, Anaheim, CA 92807

Wright Products, Inc. 800-356-6911
1909 S Taylorville Rd Ste 100, Decatur, IL 62521
SLIPP.

Wy'East Medical Corp. 503-657-3101
16700 SE 120th Ave, PO Box 1625, Clackamas, OR 97015
TOTALIFT-II, transfer chair. TOTALLIFT-MPL, powerful manual patient lift transfer system. TOTALIFT-PPL, portable, patient vertical lift for home use.

TRANSFER UNIT, BLOOD *(Hematology) 81KSB*

B. Braun Of Puerto Rico, Inc. 610-691-5400
215.7 Insular Rd., Sabana Grande, PR 00637
Blood/plasma transfer set.

Baxter Healthcare S.A. 847-948-2000
Rd. 721, Km. 0.3, Aibonito, PR 00609
Transfer sets.

Charter Medical, Ltd. 336-768-6447
3948 Westpoint Blvd Ste A, Winston Salem, NC 27103
Transfer set.

Fenwal Inc. 800-766-1077
3 Corporate Dr, Lake Zurich, IL 60047
Pack unit.

Kawasumi Laboratories America, Inc. 800-529-2786
4723 Oak Fair Blvd, Tampa, FL 33610
Tubing and blood bag for therapeutic phlebotomy.

Medi Inc 800-225-8634
75 York Ave, P.O. Box 302, Randolph, MA 02368

Medsep Corp., A Subsidiary Of Pall Corp. 516-484-5400
1630 W Industrial Park St, Covina, CA 91722
Sterile, disposable harness for automated plasma collection system.

Terumo Cardiovascular Systems (Tcvs) 800-283-7866
28 Howe St, Ashland, MA 01721
Fluid delivery set.

The Metrix Co. 800-752-3148
4400 Chavenelle Rd, Dubuque, IA 52002
Custom contract manufacturer.

TRANSFER UNIT, IV FLUID *(General) 80LHI*

Accellent El Paso 915-771-9112
31 Butterfield Trail Blvd Ste C, El Paso, TX 79906
Fluid transfer sets and spikes.

Avail Medical Products 858-635-2206
5950 Nancy Ridge Dr Ste 500, San Diego, CA 92121
Transfer set.

B. Braun Oem Division, B. Braun Medical Inc. 866-8-BBRAUN
824 12th Ave, Bethlehem, PA 18018

B. Braun Of Puerto Rico, Inc. 610-691-5400
215.7 Insular Rd., Sabana Grande, PR 00637
Various dispensing pins/connectors and fluid transfer sets.

Baxa Corporation 800-567-2292
9540 S Maroon Circle, Suite 400, Englewood, CO 80112
Exacta-Mix 600 Universal Pump - six-source compounder and pharmacy pump for automated compounding and multi-source solution mixing. One system for accurate fluid delivery and base-solution compounding. REPEATER PUMP - peristaltic pump for accurate fluid transfer procedures. Automates routine filling procedures in the pharmacy. Exacta-Mix 2400 Compounder - twenty-four source compounder for automated mixing of macro and micro volume ingredients.

Baxter Healthcare Corporation Nutrition 888-229-0001
1 Baxter Pkwy, Deerfield, IL 60015
Solution transfer sets.

Baxter Healthcare Corporporation, Alternate Care And Channel Team 888-229-0001
25212 W Il Route 120, Round Lake, IL 60073
Solution transfer sets.

Baxter Healthcare S.A. 847-948-2000
Rd. 721, Km. 0.3, Aibonito, PR 00609
Chemotherapy dispensing pin.

Benlan Inc. 905-829-5004
2760 Brighton Rd., Oakville, ONT L6H 5T4 Canada

Cardinal Health 303,Inc. 858-458-7830
1515 Ivac Way, Creedmoor, NC 27522
Single dose dispensing pin.

Churchill Medical Systems, Inc. 800-468-0585
935 Horsham Rd Ste M, Horsham, PA 19044

Directmed, Inc. 516-656-3377
150 Pratt Oval, Glen Cove, NY 11542

Ethox International 800-521-1022
251 Seneca St, Buffalo, NY 14204
Emergency infusion.

Excelsior Medical Corp. 732-776-7525
1933 Heck Ave, Neptune, NJ 07753
Dispensing pump tubing.

TRANSFER UNIT, IV FLUID *(cont'd)*

Health Care Logistics, Inc. 800-848-1633
450 Town St, PO Box 25, Circleville, OH 43113
Various.

Hospira Inc. 877-946-7747
275 N Field Dr, Lake Forest, IL 60045
Multiple

Inrad 800-558-4647
4375 Donkers Ct SE, Kentwood, MI 49512
I.v. decanter-flexible.

Kawasumi Laboratories America, Inc. 800-529-2786
4723 Oak Fair Blvd, Tampa, FL 33610
Tubing set for therapeutic phlebotomy.

Lifemed Of California 800-543-3633
1216 S Allec St, Anaheim, CA 92805
INSTAFIL, Transfer unit, high flow or gravity.

Medikmark Inc. 800-424-8520
3600 Burwood Dr, Waukegan, IL 60085
I.V. extension sets.

Mps Acacia 800-486-6677
785 Challenger St, Brea, CA 92821

Smiths Medical Asd, Inc. 800-848-1757
6250 Shier Rings Rd, Dublin, OH 43016

Venetec International., Inc. 888-685-0565
12555 High Bluff Dr Ste 100, San Diego, CA 92130
I.V. safety connector.

West Pharmaceutical Services, Inc. 610-594-3105
6453 US Highway 15, Montgomery, PA 17752
Fluid transfer set.

TRANSFORMER, ENDOSCOPE *(Surgery) 79GCW*

Electro Surgical Instrument Co., Inc. 888-464-2784
37 Centennial St, Rochester, NY 14611
Transformer.

Rapid Power Technologies, Inc. 800-332-1111
18 Old Grays Bridge Rd, Brookfield, CT 06804
Isolation Transformers.

TRANSILLUMINATOR, AC-POWERED, OPHTHALMIC
(Ophthalmology) 86HJM

Electro Surgical Instrument Co., Inc. 888-464-2784
37 Centennial St, Rochester, NY 14611
Various types, styles and sizes transilluminators.

Keeler Instruments Inc. 800-523-5620
456 Park Way, Broomall, PA 19008
$175.00 per unit.

Mira, Inc. 508-278-7877
414 Quaker Hwy, Uxbridge, MA 01569
Fiber optic light source.

Synergetics Usa, Inc. 800-600-0565
3845 Corporate Centre Dr, O Fallon, MO 63368
Various.

Translite 281-240-3111
8410 Highway 90A, Sugar Land, TX 77478
Skin examination microscope.

TRANSILLUMINATOR, AC-POWERED, OTHER
(Ophthalmology) 86ETJ

Chiu Technical Corp. 631-544-0606
252 Indian Head Rd, Kings Park, NY 11754
$446.00 for transilluminator of the neonate.

Md International, Inc. 305-669-9003
11300 NW 41st St, Doral, FL 33178

Richard Wolf Medical Instruments Corp. 800-323-9653
353 Corporate Woods Pkwy, Vernon Hills, IL 60061

Uvp, Llc 800-452-6788
2066 W 11th St, Upland, CA 91786
2UV and 3UV single intensity, dual intensity, or white/UV, also multiple ultraviolet wavelength units and white light models. Also available are high-performance UV transilluminators, 25-watt tubes for high power and UV intensity.

Welch Allyn, Inc. 800-535-6663
4341 State Street Rd, Skaneateles Falls, NY 13153

TRANSILLUMINATOR, BATTERY-POWERED
(Ophthalmology) 86HJN

Lumitex, Inc. 800-969-5483
8443 Dow Cir, Strongsville, OH 44136
Transilluminator.

Md International, Inc. 305-669-9003
11300 NW 41st St, Doral, FL 33178

Olympic Medical Corp. 206-767-3500
5900 1st Ave S, Seattle, WA 98108
$985.50 for hand-held transilluminator; allows patients to locate veins for home IV treatment.

Richard Wolf Medical Instruments Corp. 800-323-9653
353 Corporate Woods Pkwy, Vernon Hills, IL 60061

Sylvan Fiberoptics 800-628-3836
PO Box 501, Irwin, PA 15642
Fiberoptic battery-powered transilluminator.

Venoscope, Llc 337-234-8993
1018 Harding St Ste 104, Lafayette, LA 70503

Venoscope, Llc 800-284-7655
1018 Harding St Ste 104, Lafayette, LA 70503

Welch Allyn, Inc. 800-535-6663
4341 State Street Rd, Skaneateles Falls, NY 13153

TRANSILLUMINATOR, FIBER OPTIC *(Ear/Nose/Throat) 77MQW*

Jedmed Instruments Co. 314-845-3770
5416 Jedmed Ct, Saint Louis, MO 63129

TRANSILLUMINATOR, LABORATORY *(Chemistry) 75UIW*

Camag Scientific, Inc. 800-334-3909
515 Cornelius Harnett Dr, Wilmington, NC 28401

Ultra-Lum, Inc. 800-809-6559
1480 N Claremont Blvd, Claremont, CA 91711
Electronic Transilluminators.

TRANSMITTER, IMAGE & DATA, RADIOGRAPHIC
(Radiology) 90WOG

All-Tronics Medical Systems 800-ALL-TRON
3289 E 55th St, Cleveland, OH 44127
LB5 Film-to-video converter for use in conjunction with teleradiography transceiver.

Avotec, Inc. 800-272-2238
603 NW Buck Hendry Way, Stuart, FL 34994
SILENT SCAN MRI Audio System with Real Friend Companion Headset, Silver Screen Movie Projector System with Real Friend Visual System, SILENT VISION functional MRI Fiber Optic Visual System, Silent Vision LCD Projector Visual System, and REAL EYE Imaging System.

Dr Systems, Inc. 800-794-5955
10140 Mesa Rim Rd, San Diego, CA 92121
DR Systems' industry standards compliant workflow-efficiency system includes: RIS Workstation for patient registration, scheduling, procedure ordering, document scanning, charge capture and management reports. Catapult Technologist Productivity Engine QC Workstation offers technologists with quick and easy to use tools to eliminate DICOM deficiencies and streamline other post processing tasks, providing the radiologists with read ready studies. Dominator Reading Station is the premier radiologist diagnostic tool with available DR Instant Reporter (dictation, reporting, and voice recognition), advanced 3D image processing and featuring DR Systems' exclusive patented auto-hanging protocol technology, automatically displays the radiologist's image format preferences. DR Central Server with a single, unified database stores all exams 'in-progress' and 'read' for the entire imaging enterprise. Communicator Web Server for instant report and image distribution over the Internet.

Emed Technologies 866-363-3669
76 Blanchard Rd, Burlington, MA 01803

Gammasonics 800-253-0145
170 Dutcher St, Hopedale, MA 01747
PACS

Images-On-Call 214-902-8337
10290 Monroe Dr Ste 202, Dallas, TX 75229
Teleradiology systems to transmit images from radiology to doctors at home or hospital. Image distribution networks to distribute radiographic images to multiple locations throughout hospital.

Radiographic Digital Imaging, Inc. 310-921-9559
20406 Earl St, Torrance, CA 90503

TRANSMITTER/RECEIVER SYSTEM, ECG, TELEPHONE MULTI-CHANNEL *(Cardiovascular) 74QRY*

Commercial/Medical Electronics, Inc. 800-324-4844
1519 S Lewis Ave, Tulsa, OK 74104

Eresearchtechnology Inc. 215-972-0420
1818 Market St Ste 1000, Philadelphia, PA 19103

Ge Medical Systems Information Technologies 800-643-6439
8200 W Tower Ave, Milwaukee, WI 53223

Med-Com Systems Corp. 800-324-3283
1519 S Lewis Ave, Tulsa, OK 74104
Receiving and/or transmission of 3-channel ECG via telephone, Marquette, FAA and HIP compatible. Multi-channel transceiver for remote ICU monitoring also available.

Mortara Instrument, Inc. 800-231-7437
7865 N 86th St, Milwaukee, WI 53224
3-4 channels with interpretation, battery powered.

TRANSMITTER/RECEIVER SYSTEM, ECG, TELEPHONE SINGLE-CHANNEL *(Cardiovascular) 74QRZ*

Braemar, Inc. 800-328-2719
1285 Corporate Center Dr Ste 150, Eagan, MN 55121
EVENT MANAGER is a software/hardware kit that allows a standard Pentium PC to be used as an event receiving station. Transtelephonic and RS232 ECG transmission. ECG VIEWER is a software package that can receive ECG data via serial port from ER710 and ER720 event monitors.

Commercial/Medical Electronics, Inc. 800-324-4844
1519 S Lewis Ave, Tulsa, OK 74104
Analog transmitters and receivers with 2-way a/v signaling, 12-lead ECG strip transmitter.

Ge Medical Systems Information Technologies 800-643-6439
8200 W Tower Ave, Milwaukee, WI 53223
Transmitting ECG carts.

Instromedix, A Card Guard Co. 800-633-3361
10255 W Higgins Rd Ste 100, Rosemont, IL 60018
System for pacemakers.

Integrated Medical Devices, Inc. 888-486-6900
549 Electronics Pkwy, Liverpool, NY 13088
Transtelephonic Pacemaker Transmitter

Med-Com Systems Corp. 800-324-3283
1519 S Lewis Ave, Tulsa, OK 74104
12 lead single channel ECG telephone transmitters and receivers.

Mednet Healthcare Technologies, Inc. 800-606-5511
100 Ludlow Dr, Ewing, NJ 08638
CARDIOSTATION Pacemaker, ICD and cardiac event monitoring system 'Focusing on Follow-Up'

Meridian Medical Technologies 800-638-8093
10240 Old Columbia Rd, Columbia, MD 21046
CARDIOBEERER pocket size transmitter for cardiac risk management (plus service).

TRANSMITTER/RECEIVER SYSTEM, FETAL MONITOR, TELEPHONE *(General) 80VFH*

Commercial/Medical Electronics, Inc. 800-324-4844
1519 S Lewis Ave, Tulsa, OK 74104
Manual or semi-automatic, 2 or 3 channel.

TRANSMITTER/RECEIVER SYSTEM, PHYSIOLOGICAL, RADIOFREQUENCY *(Cardiovascular) 74DRG*

Barrows Company 707-987-0460
18701 Glenwood Rd, Hidden Valley Lake, CA 95467
$400 - Model RDT Receiver/Demodulator receives and demodulates Temperature and Activity data. To be used with Model T implantable transmitters.

Bl Healthcare, Inc. 508-543-4150
33 Commercial St Ste 3, Foxboro, MA 02035
Telehealth system.

Confidant International, Llc 919-806-4323
2530 Meridian Pkwy Ste 300, Durham, NC 27713
Data reporting and feedback system.

Criticare Systems, Inc. 262-798-5361
20925 Crossroads Cir, Waukesha, WI 53186
Mpt 24 and vital view 24.

Draeger Medical Systems, Inc. 215-660-2626
16 Electronics Ave, Danvers, MA 01923
Various models of telemetry systems.

eCardio Diagnostics 888-747-1442
1717 N Sam Houston Pkwy W, Houston, TX 77038
eVolution

TRANSMITTER/RECEIVER SYSTEM, PHYSIOLOGICAL, RADIOFREQUENCY *(cont'd)*

Fukuda Denshi Usa, Inc. 800-365-6668
17725 NE 65th St Ste C, Redmond, WA 98052
Transmitters and receivers, physiological signal, radiofrequency.

Ge Medical Systems Information Technologies 800-643-6439
8200 W Tower Ave, Milwaukee, WI 53223

Honeywell Hommed, Llc 888-353-5440
3400 Intertech Dr Ste 200, Brookfield, WI 53045
Monitor.

Intel Corp. Digital Health Group 916-356-8080
1900 Prairie City Rd, FM7-197, Folsom, CA 95630
INTEL HEALTH GUIDE, MODEL: PHS6000

Jabil Global Services 502-240-1000
11201 Electron Dr, Louisville, KY 40299
Physiological signal transmitter and receiver.

Kimball Electronics Tampa 813-814-8114
13750 Reptron Blvd, Tampa, FL 33626
Wireless ecg system.

Konigsberg Instruments, Inc. 626-449-0016
2000 E Foothill Blvd, Pasadena, CA 91107
Medical Research, Discovery Research, Safety Pharmacology, Special systems for Biocontainment Levels 2, 3 and 4.

Lifesync Corporation 866-324-3888
1 E Broward Blvd Ste 1701, Fort Lauderdale, FL 33301
Wireless ecg system.

Millar Instruments, Inc. 800.669.2343
6001 Gulf Fwy Ste A, Houston, TX 77023

Nihon Kohden America, Inc. 800-325-0283
90 Icon, Foothill Ranch, CA 92610

Spacelabs Medical Inc. 800-522-7212
5150 220th Ave SE, Issaquah, WA 98029
Various telemetry transmitters and receivers.

Televital, Inc. 408-441-1199
1172 Murphy Ave # 229, San Jose, CA 95131
Physiological transmitter and receiver.

Welch Allyn Protocol Inc. 800-289-2500
8500 SW Creekside Pl, Beaverton, OR 97008
Telemetry.

TRANSMITTER/RECEIVER SYSTEM, PHYSIOLOGICAL, TELEPHONE *(Cardiovascular) 74DXH*

Advanced Monitored Caregiving 201-727-1703
111 John St Rm 250, New York, NY 10038
Telephone patient monitoring system.

Commercial/Medical Electronics, Inc. 800-324-4844
1519 S Lewis Ave, Tulsa, OK 74104
Remote monitoring for ICU/CCU applications, 6-channel.

Compumed, Inc. 800-421-3395
5777 W Century Blvd Ste 360, Los Angeles, CA 90045
Computer assisted, electrocardiographic equipment.

Covance Cardiac Safety Services, Inc. 215-282-5588
9390 Gateway Dr, Reno, NV 89521
Transmitting electrocardiograph.

Cybernet Systems Corp. 734-668-2567
727 Airport Blvd, Ann Arbor, MI 48108
Various types of medical data transmitters and receivers.

Ep Medsystems, Inc. 609-753-8533
575 N Route 73 Bldg D, West Berlin, NJ 08091
Teletrace iii ecg receiver, transtelephonic ecg receiver.

Instromedix, A Card Guard Co. 800-633-3361
10255 W Higgins Rd Ste 100, Rosemont, IL 60018

Integrated Medical Devices, Inc. 888-486-6900
549 Electronics Pkwy, Liverpool, NY 13088
PC Based Transelephonic Cardiac Event Receiving Software

Lifewatch Services, Inc. 877-774-9846
10255 W Higgins Rd Ste 100, O'hare International Center II
Rosemont, IL 60018
Medical phone system.

Medicomp, Inc. 800-23-HEART
7845 Ellis Rd, Melbourne, FL 32904
CardioPAL event monitor that features both post-activation mode and looping mode. CardioPAL AI event monitor that also features auto trigger capabilities based on rate, rhythm and morphology.

TRANSMITTER/RECEIVER SYSTEM, PHYSIOLOGICAL, TELEPHONE *(cont'd)*

Medtronic Inc, Paceart — 763-514-4000
4265 Lexington Ave N, Arden Hills, MN 55126
Electrocardiograph transmitters and receivers.

Millar Instruments, Inc. — 800.669.2343
6001 Gulf Fwy Ste A, Houston, TX 77023

Mortara Instrument, Inc. — 800-231-7437
7865 N 86th St, Milwaukee, WI 53224
3-4 channels with interpretation, battery powered.

Pinmed, Inc — 412-687-6964
245 Melwood Ave Apt 501, Pittsburgh, PA 15213
Electrocardiographic systems.

Pori & Rowe Assoc., Inc. — 650-359-5175
1825 Palmetto Ave, Pacifica, CA 94044
E.e.g. transmitter and receiver.

Ppi-Time Zero Inc. — 973-278-6500
262 Buffalo Ave, Paterson, NJ 07503
Vital signs recorder and transmitter.

Trivirix International Inc. — 320-982-8000
925 6th Ave NE, Milaca, MN 56353
Various types of ecg telephone transmitters & receivers.

Tz Medical Inc. — 800-944-0187
7272 SW Durham Rd Ste 800, Portland, OR 97224
Telephone electrocardiograph transmitter.

Universal Medical, Inc. — 800-606-5511
101 Ludlow Dr, Ewing, NJ 08638
Transtelephonic cardiac monitoring station.

7n Gabriela Naydenov;, Inc. — 973-278-0866
503 E 40th St, Paterson, NJ 07504
Event recorder 'heart access plus'.

TRANSMITTER/RECEIVER SYSTEM, PULMONARY MONITOR, TELEPHONE *(General) 80VFI*

Commercial/Medical Electronics, Inc. — 800-324-4844
1519 S Lewis Ave, Tulsa, OK 74104

Ge Medical Systems Information Technologies — 800-643-6439
8200 W Tower Ave, Milwaukee, WI 53223
The Telemetry Transmitter is compact, lightweight, and programmable to frequency on site. The transmitter may be either single channel or multi channel. Both varieties are equipped to indicate battery status, electrode failure, and alarm pause status. Each is powered by two inexpensive AA batteries. Also, Telemetry Receiver Cabinet which houses up to sixteen receivers that are multi-channel and tuned to frequency at the time of admission. All arrhythmia processing is accomplished at the receiver tower via software. Software upgrading is accomplished via floppy disk drive without interrupting patient monitoring.

TRANSMITTER/RECEIVER, EEG, TELEPHONE *(Cns/Neurology) 84QSC*

Telediagnostic Systems — 800-227-3224
2483 Old Middlefield Way Ste 202, Mountain View, CA 94043
$7,000 per receiver (10-channel) $7,500 per transmitter (10-channel). $12,000 per receiver (24-channel). $12,500 per transmitter (24-channel). DT-24, DR-24: Transmitter and receiver for 24-channel digital EEG transmission over standard telephone line (POTS).

Telemedx Corp. — 800-231-1009
2550 S Sam Houston Pkwy W, Houston, TX 77047
Digital or analog equipment available. Secure FTP site for processing patient data.

TRANSMITTER/RECEIVER, PHYSIOLOGICAL SIGNAL, INFRARED *(Cardiovascular) 74MFL*

Eurotherm Inc. — 703-443-0000
741F Miller Dr SE, Leesburg, VA 20175

TRANSPORT SYSTEM, AEROBIC *(Microbiology) 83JTW*

Bd Diagnostic Systems — 800-675-0908
7 Loveton Cir, Sparks, MD 21152

Globe Scientific, Inc. — 800-394-4562
610 Winters Ave, Paramus, NJ 07652
O-P TECT OVA and parasite transport kit. Vials with spoon containing PVA and formalin.

Pml Microbiologicals — 800-628-7014
27120 SW 95th Ave, Wilsonville, OR 97070

Sierra Molecular Inc. — 209-536-0886
21109 Longeway Rd Ste C, Sonora, CA 95370
Urine collection & transport system.

TRANSPORT SYSTEM, ANAEROBIC *(Microbiology) 83JTX*

Bd Diagnostic Systems — 800-675-0908
7 Loveton Cir, Sparks, MD 21152

Becton, Dickinson & Co. — 308-872-6811
150 S 1st Ave, Broken Bow, NE 68822
Various sterile anaerobic transport systems.

Fitzco, Inc. — 952-471-1185
4300 Shoreline Dr, Spring Park, MN 55384
Fitapak urine transport system.

Pml Microbiologicals — 800-628-7014
27120 SW 95th Ave, Wilsonville, OR 97070

Spec Connection Intl Inc. — 813-618-0400
34310 State Road 54, Zephyrhills, FL 33543
Anaerobic blend artificial atmosphere.

Welco-Cgi Gas Technologies — 440-234-1075
145 Shimersville Rd, Bethlehem, PA 18015
Anaerobic gas mixture.

TRANSPORT, PATIENT, POWERED *(Physical Med) 89ILK*

Aero Medical Products Co., Inc. — 262-677-0535
4514 Maple Rd, West Bend, WI 53095
Transport, patient, powered.

Arjo, Inc. — 800-323-1245
50 Gary Ave Ste A, Roselle, IL 60172

Summit Lifts, Inc. — 866-378-6648
18505 E 163rd St, Lake Winnebago, MO 64034
Stairway lift.

TRAP, BUBBLE *(Cardiovascular) 74SBY*

Terumo Cardiovascular Systems, Corp — 800-521-2818
6200 Jackson Rd, Ann Arbor, MI 48103

TRAP, MUCUS *(Anesthesiology) 73SBZ*

Axcan Pharma Inc. — 800-950-8085
22 Inverness Center Pkwy, Birmingham, AL 35242

Covidien Lp — 508-261-8000
15 Hampshire St, Mansfield, MA 02048

Tri-State Hospital Supply Corp. — 800-248-4058
301 Catrell Dr, PO Box 170, Howell, MI 48843
Suction specimen trap with barrier filter located inside trap designed to prevent accidental flow of material through exit port.

Vygon Corp. — 800-544-4907
2495 General Armistead Ave, Norristown, PA 19403
With and without filter.

TRAP, STERILE SPECIMEN *(Anesthesiology) 73BYZ*

Busse Hospital Disposables, Inc. — 631-435-4711
75 Arkay Dr, Hauppauge, NY 11788
Various sterile speciman traps.

Covidien Lp — 508-261-8000
15 Hampshire St, Mansfield, MA 02048

Kelsar, S.A. — 508-261-8000
Blvd. Insurgentes, Libriamento a La, Tijuana 22450 Mexico
Various

Ludwig Medical, Inc. — 217-342-6570
1010 N Parkview St, P.o. Box 207, Effingham, IL 62401
Lukens tube.

M D Technologies, Inc. — 800-201-3060
PO Box 60, Galena, IL 61036
Environ-Mate PT20 disposable, non-sterile single specimen/polyp collector.

Medical Action Industries, Inc. — 800-645-7042
25 Heywood Rd, Arden, NC 28704
Trap, specimen.

Medline Manufacturing And Services Llc — 847-837-2759
1 Medline Pl, Mundelein, IL 60060
Trap,sterile specimen.

Terumo Cardiovascular Systems (Tcvs) — 800-283-7866
28 Howe St, Ashland, MA 01721
Mucus trap.

TRAY, BLOOD COLLECTION *(Hematology) 81GJE*

Dade Behring, Inc. — 800-948-3233
1717 Deerfield Rd, Deerfield, IL 60015

Daxor Corporation — 865-425-0555
107 Meco Ln, Oak Ridge, TN 37830
Various collections of released parts, bagged for convenience.

TRAY, BLOOD COLLECTION *(cont'd)*

Health Chem Diagnostics Llc 954-979-3845
3341 W McNab Rd, Pompano Beach, FL 33069
Tray, blood collection.

Healthmark Industries 800-521-6224
22522 E 9 Mile Rd, Saint Clair Shores, MI 48080

Kelsar, S.A. 508-261-8000
Blvd. Insurgentes, Libriamento a La, Tijuana 22450 Mexico
Various types and sizes of blood collection systems and needles

Merit Medical Systems Inc. 804-416-1030
12701 Kingston Ave, Chesterfield, VA 23837

Pioneer Center For Human Services 815-344-1230
4001 W Dayton St, McHenry, IL 60050
Well reaction trays.

TRAY, CIRCUMCISION, REUSABLE *(Obstetrics/Gyn) 85QKH*

Tri-State Hospital Supply Corp. 800-248-4058
301 Catrell Dr, PO Box 170, Howell, MI 48843
Disposable instruments, all components for procedure included.

TRAY, CUSTOM/SPECIAL PROCEDURE *(General) 80WNH*

Allergan 800-366-6554
2525 Dupont Dr, Irvine, CA 92612
Disposable packs for vitrectomy I/A and phacoemulsification. Balanced salt solution in 500cc and 30cc bottles.

American Medical Devices, Inc. 800-788-9876
287 S Stoddard Ave, San Bernardino, CA 92401
Custom medical kits and trays: wound closure, delivery, dressing change, IV administration, umbilical, circumcision, skin care, cataract, angiography, pelvic exam, etc.

Angiosystems, Inc. 800-441-4256
7 Hopkins Pl., Ducktown, TN 37326
Standard PTCA and art. packs. Standard and custom cardiac catheter packs.

Armstrong Medical Industries, Inc. 800-323-4220
575 Knightsbridge Pkwy, Lincolnshire, IL 60069

Benlan Inc. 905-829-5004
2760 Brighton Rd., Oakville, ONT L6H 5T4 Canada
Anesthesia, dressing, foley, orathral, irrigations and suture removal trays.

Biotest Diagnostic Corp. 800-522-0090
400 Commons Way, Rockaway, NJ 07866
HLA ABC trays, HLA DR trays, and HLA sera.

Bound Tree Medical, Llc 800-533-0523
5200 Rings Rd Ste A, Dublin, OH 43017
Emergency obstetrics, infection control and complete airway management kits (CAM kit). Nasal intubation and immobilization kit.

Cadco Dental Products 800-833-8267
600 E Hueneme Rd, Oxnard, CA 93033
Unit dose fluoride treatment trays, 1.23% APF, FLUREZE pre-impregnated, available in small, medium or large sizes; also, BANDETTES, disposable single dose prophylactic paste.

Cypress Medical Products 800-334-3646
1202 S. Rte. 31, McHenry, IL 60050
Stock and custom kits available. Stock kits include tracheostomy care, urological care, suture and skin staple removal, IV start and laceration. Private label kits available.

Cytosol Ophthalmics, Inc. 800-234-5166
PO Box 1408, 1325 William White Place, NE, Lenoir, NC 28645
Ophthalmic disposables and sterile irrigation solutions (cataract extraction procedures).

David Scott Company 800-804-0333
59 Fountain St, Framingham, MA 01702
Radiology special procedure trays.

Dux Dental 800-833-8267
600 E Hueneme Rd, Oxnard, CA 93033
Unit dose fluoride treatment trays, 1.23% APF, FLUREZE pre-impregnated, available in small, medium, or large; also BANDETTES, disposable single dose prophylactic paste.

General Dental Products, Inc. 888-367-6212
201 Ogden Ave, Ely, NV 89301
TRU-TRAY (TM)

Greatbatch Medical 716-759-5600
3735 N Arlington Ave, Indianapolis, IN 46218
Reusable aluminum, stainless steel and plastic trays.

International Hospital Supply Co. 800-398-9450
6914 Canby Ave Ste 105, Reseda, CA 91335

TRAY, CUSTOM/SPECIAL PROCEDURE *(cont'd)*

Johnson & Johnson Medical Division Of Ethicon, Inc. 800-423-4018
2500 E Arbrook Blvd, Arlington, TX 76014

Lsl Industries, Inc. 888-225-5575
5535 N Wolcott Ave, Chicago, IL 60640
$32.95 for 20 sterile Foley catheterization trays without catheter (for 5cc balloon catheters) containing: 1 package of 3 povidone iodine saturated swabs, 10cc prefilled syringe, 2 gloves, lubricating jelly, waterproof drape, fenestrated drape, specimen container with lid & label, 1100ml tray. $35.50 for same but for 30cc balloon catheters. Premium wrapped trays also available.

Medical Design Concepts, Inc. 951-296-2600
41980 Winchester Rd, Temecula, CA 92590

Medical Techniques Usa 801-936-4501
125 N 400 W Ste C, North Salt Lake, UT 84054

Medikmark Inc. 800-424-8520
3600 Burwood Dr, Waukegan, IL 60085

Medistat Medical - Hallmark Sales Corporation 888-MED-ISTA
1601 Peach Leaf St, Houston, TX 77039
Manufacturer of kits including first aid, body fluid spills, burns, emergency, medical, surgical, obstetrical, exams, minor surgery, biopsy, convenience, procedure trays, disposable instruments, sterile kits. Owns manufacturing and validated sterilization facilities. Can make custom or special order kits. Refills, supplies.

Meditron Inc D.B.A. Medcare Usa 800-243-2442
3435 Montee Gagnon, Terrebonne, QUEBE J6Y-1J4 Canada
For usage in hospitals, nursing home or home health care.

Mentor Corp. 800-525-0245
201 Mentor Dr, Santa Barbara, CA 93111
Procedure trays, catheter injection trays and accessories.

Merit Medical Systems Inc. 804-416-1030
12701 Kingston Ave, Chesterfield, VA 23837

Packaging Plus Llc 714-522-5400
14450 Industry Cir, La Mirada, CA 90638
Thermoformed custom trays to 64 in. long.

Packaging Plus, Inc. 763-566-8808
6840 Shingle Creek Pkwy, Minneapolis, MN 55430
Custom shipping trays and blisters. Sterilizable medical grade plastics.

Pain Products International 800-359-5756
4763 Hamilton Wolfe Rd # 210, San Antonio, TX 78229
Pain management trays.

Post Medical, Inc. 800-876-8678
315 Bell Park Dr, Woodstock, GA 30188
Laboratory trays. Two styles: one features an open top with closable drawer, the other features a closed system with lid for transporting specimens. Lid can be locked.

Precision Medical Products, Inc. 717-335-3700
44 Denver Rd, PO Box 300, Denver, PA 17517

Primesource Healthcare, Inc. 888-842-6999
3708 E Columbia St Ste 100, Tucson, AZ 85714

Riley Medical, Inc. 800-245-3300
27 Wrights Lndg, Auburn, ME 04210
Custom sterilization trays.

Shippert Medical Technologies Corp. 800-888-8663
6248 S Troy Cir Ste A, Centennial, CO 80111
Busse Laceration, Busse Sharp Debridement, Busse Facial Wound Closure, Busse Primary Dressing Change.

Vital Concepts, Inc. 800-984-2300
4334 Brockton Dr SE Ste F, Grand Rapids, MI 49512

Windstone Medical Packaging, Inc. 800-637-7056
1602 4th Ave N, Billings, MT 59101

TRAY, FLUORIDE *(Dental And Oral) 76UDW*

Harry J. Bosworth Company 800-323-4352
7227 Hamlin Ave, Skokie, IL 60076

Plastodent 718-792-3554
2881 Middletown Rd, Bronx, NY 10461
Sodium floride solutions.

TRAY, FLUORIDE, DISPOSABLE *(Dental And Oral) 76KMT*

Archtek, Inc. 303-763-8916
12105 W Cedar Dr, Lakewood, CO 80228
Customizable bleaching tray.

Chameleon Dental Products, Inc. 913-281-5552
200 N 6th St, Kansas City, KS 66101
Fluoride luting composite kit.

TRAY, FLUORIDE, DISPOSABLE *(cont'd)*

Deepak Products, Inc. 305-482-9669
5220 NW 72nd Ave Ste 15, Miami, FL 33166
Disposable fluoride trays.

Dental Resources 717-866-7571
52 King St, Myerstown, PA 17067
Fluoride trays.

Inman Orthodontic Laboratories, Inc. 954-340-8477
9381 W Sample Rd, Coral Springs, FL 33065
Dental tray.

Inter-Med, Inc. 877-418-4782
2200 Northwestern Ave, Racine, WI 53404
Disposable fluoride tray.

Kerr Corp. 714-516-7400
28200 Wick Rd, Romulus, MI 48174
Fluoride tray.

Lorvic Corp. 800-325-1881
13705 Shoreline Ct E, Earth City, MO 63045
Disposable wax and foam trays.

Ohlendorf Company 314-533-3440
2840 Clark Ave, Saint Louis, MO 63103
Dental tray.

Perio Protect Llc 202-672-5430
3929 Bayless Ave, Saint Louis, MO 63125
Dental tray.

Young Colorado, Llc. 800-325-1881
13705 Shoreline Ct E, Earth City, MO 63045
Disposable fluoride tray.

TRAY, FOODSERVICE *(General) 80TFH*

LIFTnWALK LP 972-837-4615
PO Box 742855, Dallas, TX 75374
BUDDY SAFETY ROLLER TRAY (BSR SEAT), snap on tray with cup indent.

Tray-Pak Corporation 888-926-1777
PO Box 14804, Tuckerton Road & Reading Crest Avenue
Reading, PA 19612
Custom thermoformed trays and clamshells and bowls with lids.

TRAY, IMPRESSION *(Dental And Oral) 76EHY*

Align Technology, Inc. 408-470-1000
881 Martin Ave, Santa Clara, CA 95050
Tray,impression,preformed.

Alltec Integrated Manufacturing,Inc. 805-595-3500
4330 Old Santa Fe Rd, San Luis Obispo, CA 93401
Dental tray.

Alrand, Inc./Boca Dental Supply, Inc. 800-5004908
3401 N Federal Hwy Ste 203, Boca Raton, FL 33431
Various types.

Aluwax Dental Products Co. 616-895-4385
5260 Edgewater Dr, Allendale, MI 49401

American Tooth Industries 800-235-4639
1200 Stellar Dr, Oxnard, CA 93033
POZZI.

Arnold Tuber Industries 716-648-3363
97 Main St, Hamburg, NY 14075
Preformed impression trays.

Blue Sky Bio, Llc 847-548-8499
888 E Belvidere Rd Ste 212, Grayslake, IL 60030
Impression tray.

Cadco Dental Products 800-833-8267
600 E Hueneme Rd, Oxnard, CA 93033
20 types of water-cooled trays, $16.00 for standard units; also, $9.50 each for autoclavable impression trays, alignate type, all sizes, uppers and lowers.

Ceragroup Industries Inc. 954-670-0208
6555 Powerline Rd Ste 211, Ft Lauderdale, FL 33309
Tray, impression, preformed.

Citizens Development Center 214-637-2911
8800 Ambassador Row, Dallas, TX 75247
Whitening kits.

Coltene/Whaledent Inc. 330-916-8858
235 Ascot Pkwy, Cuyahoga Falls, OH 44223
Impression tray.

TRAY, IMPRESSION *(cont'd)*

Cooley & Cooley, Ltd. 800-215-4487
8550 Westland West Blvd, Houston, TX 77041
ELFIT- a mouth tray softened in very hot water, placed in mouth; patient sucks air & water from around tray to mold to dentitives. Uses: nightguard to prevent grinding teeth; bleaching tray to bleach teeth with whitening gel; disposable impression tray.

D.C.A. (Dental Corporation Of America) 800-638-6684
889 S Matlack St, West Chester, PA 19382
METAL TRAYS $8.75 each.

Denplus Inc. 800-344-4424
205 - 1221 Labadie, Longueuil, QUE J4N 1E2 Canada

Dental Technologies, Inc. 847-677-5500
6901 N Hamlin Ave, Lincolnwood, IL 60712
Disposable impression trays.

Dental Usa, Inc. 815-363-8003
5005 McCullom Lake Rd, McHenry, IL 60050
Dental impression tray.

Dux Dental 800-833-8267
600 E Hueneme Rd, Oxnard, CA 93033
20 types of water-cooled trays, $16.00 for standard units; also, $9.50 each for autoclavable impression trays, alignate type, all sizes, uppers and lowers.

G & H Wire Co. 800-526-1026
2165 Earlywood Dr, Franklin, IN 46131
Disposable impression tray.

Hager Worldwide, Inc. 800-328-2335
13322 Byrd Dr, Odessa, FL 33556
ALGILOCK (stainless steel), MIRATRAY (plastic), MINITRAY (plastic quadrant tray), MIRATRAY PLUS (autoclavable/plastic).

Harry J. Bosworth Company 800-323-4352
7227 Hamlin Ave, Skokie, IL 60076
Stainless steel impression trays, TRAY-AWAYS disposable trays, BIG BITE bite registration trays.

Inter-Med, Inc. 877-418-4782
2200 Northwestern Ave, Racine, WI 53404
Impression tray.

Jardon Eye Prosthetics, Inc. 248-424-8560
15920 W 12 Mile Rd, Southfield, MI 48076
Ophthalmic impression tray.

Lancer Orthodontics, Inc. 760-304-2705
253 Pawnee St, San Marcos, CA 92078
Tray, impression.

Miltex Dental Technologies, Inc. 516-576-6022
589 Davies Dr, York, PA 17402
Various crown and bridge trays.

Moyco Technologies, Inc. 800-331-8837
200 Commerce Dr, Montgomeryville, PA 18936

Ortho Organizers, Inc. 760-448-8730
1822 Aston Ave, Carlsbad, CA 92008
Impression trays.

Orthopli Corp.
10061 Sandmeyer Ln, Philadelphia, PA 19116
Various styles.

Oscar, Inc. 317-849-2618
11793 Technology Ln, Fishers, IN 46038
Disposable impression trays.

Pac-Dent Intl., Inc. 909-839-0888
21078 Commerce Point Dr, Walnut, CA 91789
Dental impression tray.

Pentron Clinical Technologies 203-265-7397
68-70 North Plains Industrial, Road, Wallingford, CT 06492
Preformed impression tray.

Pulpdent Corp. 800-343-4342
80 Oakland St, Watertown, MA 02472
Disposable impression tray.

Reliance Dental Mfg., Co. 708-597-6694
5805 W 117th Pl, Alsip, IL 60803
Trays, perforated impression.

Rite-Dent Manufacturing Corp. 305-693-8626
3750 E 10th Ct, Hialeah, FL 33013
Various types of preformed impression trays.

Superior Dental & Test 800-528-7297
1501 SE Village Green Dr, Port St Lucie, FL 34952

TRAY, IMPRESSION *(cont'd)*

Symmetry Medical Usa, Inc. 574-267-8700
486 W 350 N, Warsaw, IN 46582
Preformed impression tray.

Temrex Corp. 516-868-6221
112 Albany Ave, P.o. Box 182, Freeport, NY 11520
Bite relator for regular & large rite bite trays.

Texstar Technology Inc. 806-748-1184
2306 120th St Unit D, Lubbock, TX 79423
Preformed dental impression tray.

Tp Orthodontics, Inc. 800-348-8856
100 Center Plz, La Porte, IN 46350
Extend-O, Norm-O, Solay Disposable trays.

Ultradent Products, Inc. 801-553-4586
505 W 10200 S, South Jordan, UT 84095
Impression tray.

Water Pik, Inc. 970-221-6129
1730 E Prospect Rd, Fort Collins, CO 80525
Dental impression tray.

Westside Packaging, Llc. 909-570-3508
1700 S Baker Ave Ste A, Ontario, CA 91761
Dental impression trays.

Yates & Bird And Motloid 800-662-5021
300 N Elizabeth St, Chicago, IL 60607

3m Unitek 800-634-5300
2724 Peck Rd, Monrovia, CA 91016

TRAY, IMPRESSION, FOOT *(Orthopedics) 87WPM*

Freeman Manufacturing Company 800-253-2091
900 W Chicago Rd, PO Box J, Sturgis, MI 49091

Precision Dynamics Corp. 800-772-1122
13880 Del Sur St, San Fernando, CA 91340
KLEEN-PRINT, QUICK-PRINT, PERMA-PRINT Newborn footprinter.

TRAY, MEDICINE *(General) 80SCA*

Covidien Lp 508-261-8000
15 Hampshire St, Mansfield, MA 02048

Healthmark Industries 800-521-6224
22522 E 9 Mile Rd, Saint Clair Shores, MI 48080
$389.50 per 10 (med). Also, autoclavable soaking trays.

Homak Manufacturing Company Inc. 800-874-6625
1605 Old Route 18 Ste 4-36, Wampum, PA 16157

Lewis Bins+ 877-97L-EWIS
PO Box 389, Oconomowoc, WI 53066
Full line of plastic bins & trays.

Maddak Inc. 800-443-4926
661 State Route 23, Wayne, NJ 07470
ABLEWARE.

Orbis Corporation 800-890-7292
1055 Corporate Center Dr, PO Box 389, Oconomowoc, WI 53066
Full line of plastic bins & trays.

Surgical Tools, Inc. 800-774-2040
1106 Monroe St, Bedford, VA 24523

Youngs, Inc. 800-523-5454
55 E Cherry Ln, Souderton, PA 18964

TRAY, MICRO (MIC PLATE) *(Microbiology) 83ULL*

Polar Plastic Ltd. 514-331-0207
4210 Thimens Blvd., St. Laurent, QUE H4R 2B9 Canada
POLAR RX. Bi-plates, tri-plates and quad-plates.

TRAY, START/STOP (INCLUDING CONTENTS), DIALYSIS *(Gastro/Urology) 78FKG*

Aoss Medical Supply, Inc. 318-325-8290
4971 Central Ave, Monroe, LA 71203
Convenience kit.

Argon Medical Devices Inc. 903-675-9321
1445 Flat Creek Rd, Athens, TX 75751
Dual lumen catheter, kit & tray.

Erika De Reynosa, S.A. De C.V. 781-402-9068
Brecha E99 Sur; Parque, Industrial Reynos, Bldg. Ii Cd, Reynosa, Tamps Mexico
Peritoneal dialysis on/off tray (sterile)

Lee Medical International, Inc. 800-433-8950
612 Distributors Row, Harahan, LA 70123

Megamed Corporation 305-665-6876
7432 SW 48th St, Miami, FL 33155

TRAY, START/STOP (INCLUDING CONTENTS), DIALYSIS *(cont'd)*

Merit Medical Systems Inc. 804-416-1030
12701 Kingston Ave, Chesterfield, VA 23837

TRAY, STERILIZATION, INSTRUMENT *(Surgery) 79SIC*

Advanced Medical Innovations, Inc. 888-367-2641
9410 De Soto Ave Ste J, Chatsworth, CA 91311
IN-STRINGER, L-shaped, keeps the instruments in the open position during sterilization. Works together with the instrument rack. Saves a lot of time in stringing instruments in a standard stringer.

Advantis Medical 888-625-4497
2121 Southtech Dr Ste 600, Greenwood, IN 46143
Stainless steel and aluminum sterilization trays, cassettes and case/tray systems for orthopedic and surgical instruments and reusable medical devices.

Alimed, Inc. 800-225-2610
297 High St, Dedham, MA 02026
Clear plastic trays cool down in 60 seconds after flash sterilization. Clear plastic scope trays include custom-made silicone strips to secure scopes for sterilization.

American Surgical Instrument Corp. 800-628-2879
26 Plaza Dr, Westmont, IL 60559

Micromedics 800-624-5662
1270 Eagan Industrial Rd, Saint Paul, MN 55121
Sterilization trays for rigid endoscopes, endoscopic video cameras, and laparoscopic procedures.

Miltex Inc. 800-645-8000
589 Davies Dr, York, PA 17402

Moyco Technologies, Inc. 800-331-8837
200 Commerce Dr, Montgomeryville, PA 18936

Packaging Plus, Inc. 763-566-8808
6840 Shingle Creek Pkwy, Minneapolis, MN 55430
ROTA-PLUS, STRAIGHT PACK handling trays. Multiple-length catheter tubing and wire trays and covers. PETG plastic. ROTA-PLUS, COIL PACK 18 x 18 x 2 PETG trays and covers for coiled tubing and wires for catheters.

Princeton Medical Group, Inc. 800-875-0869
1189 Royal Links Dr, Mt Pleasant, SC 29466
MICROSURGICAL & GENERAL INSTRUMENT STERILIZATION CONTAINERS & LAPAROSCOPIC BRIDGE INSERTS

Riley Medical, Inc. 800-245-3300
27 Wrights Lndg, Auburn, ME 04210
MULTIPAK instrument processing, handling, and sterilization tray stsem.

TRAY, SURGICAL *(Surgery) 79LRP*

Advance Tabco 800-645-3166
200 Heartland Blvd, Edgewood, NY 11717
Mobile tray unit.

Armm, Inc. 714-848-8190
17744 Sampson Ln, Huntington Beach, CA 92647
Custom through contract services.

B. Braun Medical, Inc. 610-596-2536
901 Marcon Blvd, Allentown, PA 18109

Biomet Microfixation Inc. 800-874-7711
1520 Tradeport Dr, Jacksonville, FL 32218
Container (tray).

Centurion Medical Products Corp. 517-545-1135
3310 S Main St, Salisbury, NC 28147

Cpt Med, Inc. 770-242-1165
195 Commerce Ctr # A, Greenville, SC 29615
Various styles of surgical trays.

Cytyc Surgical Products 800-442-9892
250 Campus Dr, Marlborough, MA 01752
Tray, minor surgical procedures.

E-Z-Em, Inc. 516-333-8230
750 Summa Ave, Westbury, NY 11590
Procedure tray.

Elamex S.A. De C.V. 52-16-164333
Av. Insurgentes 4145 lote., Cd. Jiarex, Chih Mexico
37270-lf latex or prep tray

General Hospital Supply Corp. 704-225-9500
2844 Gray Fox Rd, Monroe, NC 28110
Sterilization tray corner guard.

Mckesson General Medical 800-446-3008
8741 Landmark Rd, Richmond, VA 23228

Medical Techniques Usa 801-936-4501
125 N 400 W Ste C, North Salt Lake, UT 84054

TRAY, SURGICAL *(cont'd)*

Merit Medical Systems Inc. 804-416-1030
12701 Kingston Ave, Chesterfield, VA 23837

Micrins Surgical Instruments, Inc. 800-833-3380
28438 N Ballard Dr, Lake Forest, IL 60045

Micromedics 800-624-5662
1270 Eagan Industrial Rd, Saint Paul, MN 55121
Instru-Safe systems keep surgical instruments organized in sets and protect the instruments during transportation, storage, and sterile processing...saving time in surgery and reducing instrument damage.

Prosurge Instruments, Inc. 866-832-7874
199 Laidlaw Ave, Jersey City, NJ 07306

Qfc Plastics, Inc. 817-649-7400
728 111th St, Arlington, TX 76011
Surgical instrument tray.

Quantum Medical Concepts, Llc. 503-708-0702
3518 SE 21st Ave, Portland, OR 97202
Sterilization tray, autoclave tray, surgical instrument tray.

Riley Medical, Inc. 800-245-3300
27 Wrights Lndg, Auburn, ME 04210

Rogers Foam Corporation 859-497-0702
120 Clarence Dr, Woodland Industrial Park, Mt Sterling, KY 40353
Various foam containers and accessories.

Salumedica, L.L.C. 404-589-1727
4451 Atlanta Rd SE Ste 138, Smyrna, GA 30080
Tray.

Salvin Dental Specialties, Inc. 800-535-6566
3450 Latrobe Dr, Charlotte, NC 28211
Various types of surgical trays and cassettes.

Savoy Medical Supply 631-234-7003
745 Calebs Path, Hauppauge, NY 11788

Small Bone Innovations, Inc. 215-428-1791
1380 S Pennsylvania Ave, Morrisville, PA 19067
Tray, surgical.

Symmetry Medical, Inc. - Polyvac 207-786-2775
253 Abby Rd, Manchester, NH 03103
Surgical trays.

Tri-State Hospital Supply Corp. 517-545-1135
3173 E 43rd St, Yuma, AZ 85365

Zirc Company 800-328-3899
3918 State Highway 55 SE, Buffalo, MN 55313
Set-up trays, cabinet trays, procedure tubs.

TRAY, SURGICAL INSTRUMENT *(Surgery) 79FSM*

Abbott Spine, Inc. 847-937-6100
12708 Riata Vista Cir Ste B-100, Austin, TX 78727
Instrument tray.

Accutome, Inc. 610-889-0200
3222 Phoenixville Pike, Malvern, PA 19355
Trays.

Aesculap Implant Systems Inc. 1-800-234-9179
3773 Corporate Pkwy, Center Valley, PA 18034

Alcon Research, Ltd. 800-862-5266
6201 South Fwy, Fort Worth, TX 76134

Apple Medical Corp. 508-357-2700
28 Lord Rd Ste 135, Marlborough, MA 01752
Instrument organizer.

Arthrex, Inc. 239-643-5553
1370 Creekside Blvd, Naples, FL 34108
Various.

B. Graczyk, Inc. 269-782-2100
27826 Burmax Park, Dowagiac, MI 49047
Various types of trays.

Bausch & Lomb Surgical 636-255-5051
3365 Tree Court Ind Blvd, Saint Louis, MO 63122

Biomet Microfixation Inc. 800-874-7711
1520 Tradeport Dr, Jacksonville, FL 32218
Tray, surgical, instrument.

Biomet, Inc. 574-267-6639
56 E Bell Dr, PO Box 587, Warsaw, IN 46582
Various types of instrument trays.

Brandt Industries, Inc. 800-221-8031
4461 Bronx Blvd, Bronx, NY 10470
Mayo stands.

TRAY, SURGICAL INSTRUMENT *(cont'd)*

Busse Hospital Disposables, Inc. 631-435-4711
75 Arkay Dr, Hauppauge, NY 11788
Sterile-general purpose instrument trays,wound closure trays,minor laceration tr.

Cadco Dental Products 800-833-8267
600 E Hueneme Rd, Oxnard, CA 93033

Centinel Spine Inc. 952-885-0500
505 Park Ave Fl 14, New York, NY 10022
STALIF C Instrument case system

Codman & Shurtleff, Inc 800-225-0460
325 Paramount Dr, Raynham, MA 02767

Davol Inc., Sub. C.R. Bard, Inc. 800-556-6275
100 Crossings Blvd, Warwick, RI 02886
Sterilization tray.

Demetech Corp. 888-324-2447
3530 NW 115th Ave, Doral, FL 33178
Instrument stand.

Dencraft 800-328-9729
PO Box 57, Moorestown, NJ 08057

Dental Usa, Inc. 815-363-8003
5005 McCullom Lake Rd, McHenry, IL 60050
Dental instrument tray.

Depuy Mitek, A Johnson & Johnson Company 800-451-2006
50 Scotland Blvd, Bridgewater, MA 02324
Sterilization tray.

Depuy Spine, Inc. 800-227-6633
325 Paramount Dr, Raynham, MA 02767
Instrument tray.

Depuy-Raynham, A Div. Of Depuy Orthopaedics 800-451-2006
325 Paramount Dr, Raynham, MA 02767
Multiple surgical instrument trays.

Diamond Edge Co. 727-586-2927
928 W Bay Dr, Largo, FL 33770
Sterilization tray.

DJO Inc. 800-336-6569
1430 Decision St, Vista, CA 92081

Dux Dental 800-833-8267
600 E Hueneme Rd, Oxnard, CA 93033

Eagle Vision, Inc. 800-222-7584
8500 Wolf Lake Dr Ste 110, Memphis, TN 38133

Elamex S.A. De C.V. 52-16-164333
Av. Insurgentes 4145 lote., Cd. Jiarex, Chih Mexico
Various

Eriem Surgical 800-833-3380
28438 N Ballard Dr, Lake Forest, IL 60045

General Hospital Supply Corp. 704-225-9500
2844 Gray Fox Rd, Monroe, NC 28110
Corner protector for surgical instrument and tray and wrap.

Gregstrom Corp. 781-935-6600
64 Holton St, Woburn, MA 01801
Soaking tray.

Gyrus Ent L.L.C., Sub. Of Gyrus Acmi, Inc. 508-804-2739
2925 Appling Rd, Bartlett, TN 38133
Various.

Hager Worldwide, Inc. 800-328-2335
13322 Byrd Dr, Odessa, FL 33556
STERIRACK.

Healthmark Industries 800-521-6224
22522 E 9 Mile Rd, Saint Clair Shores, MI 48080
$167.00 per 20 Mayo trays (9pc), $20ea. per autoclavable tray, $35ea. per soaking tray.

Integra Lifesciences Of Ohio 800-654-2873
4900 Charlemar Dr Bldg A, Cincinnati, OH 45227
Instrument tables.

Invuity, Inc. 760-744-4447
334 Via Vera Cruz Ste 255, San Marcos, CA 92078
Sterilization trays.

Invuity, Inc. 415-655-2100
39 Stillman St, San Francisco, CA 94107

Jedmed Instruments Co. 314-845-3770
5416 Jedmed Ct, Saint Louis, MO 63129

Karl Storz Endoscopy-America Inc. 800-421-0837
600 Corporate Pointe, Culver City, CA 90230
Variety of tray styles for KARL STORZ instruments and scopes.

TRAY, SURGICAL INSTRUMENT *(cont'd)*

Kelsar, S.A. 508-261-8000
Blvd. Insurgentes, Libriamento a La, Tijuana 22450 Mexico
Paracentesis procedure needle & tray

Kls-Martin L.P. 800-625-1557
11239-1 St. John`s Industrial, Parkway South
Jacksonville, FL 32250
Sterilizing tray (without contents).

Lenox-Maclaren Surgical Corp. 720-890-9660
657 S Taylor Ave Ste A, Colorado Technology Center
Louisville, CO 80027
Tray, surgical, instrument.

Mahe International Inc. 800-294-7946
468 Craighead St, Nashville, TN 37204

Mark Medical Manufacturing, Inc. 610-269-4420
530 Brandywine Ave, Downingtown, PA 19335

Mckesson General Medical 800-446-3008
8741 Landmark Rd, Richmond, VA 23228

Medegen Medical Products, Llc 800-233-1987
209 Medegen Drive, Gallaway, TN 38036-0228
MED ASSIST Stainless steel.

Medical Techniques Usa 801-936-4501
125 N 400 W Ste C, North Salt Lake, UT 84054

Medikmark Inc. 800-424-8520
3600 Burwood Dr, Waukegan, IL 60085

Medistat Medical - Hallmark Sales Corporation 888-MED-ISTA
1601 Peach Leaf St, Houston, TX 77039
Manufacturer of kits including first aid, body fluid spills, burns, emergency, medical, surgical, obstetrical, exams, minor surgery, biopsy, convenience, procedure trays, disposable instruments, sterile kits. Owns manufacturing and validated sterilization facilities. Can make custom or special order kits. Refills, supplies.

Medtronic Sofamor Danek Instrument Manufacturing 901-396-3133
7375 Adrianne Pl, Bartlett, TN 38133
Case/tray.

Medtronic Sofamor Danek Usa, Inc. 901-396-3133
4340 Swinnea Rd, Memphis, TN 38118
Case/tray.

Micrins Surgical Instruments, Inc. 800-833-3380
28438 N Ballard Dr, Lake Forest, IL 60045

Minnesota Bramstedt Surgical, Inc. 800-456-5052
1835 Energy Park Dr, Saint Paul, MN 55108
Sterilizable instrument tray for The Woodpecker - a total hip broaching device.

Nobel Biocare Usa, Llc 800-579-6515
22715/22725 Savi Ranch Parkway, Yorba Linda, CA 92887
Surgical instrument.

Northeast Medical Systems Corp. 856-910-8111
901 Beechwood Ave, Cherry Hill, NJ 08002

Pac-Dent Intl., Inc. 909-839-0888
21078 Commerce Point Dr, Walnut, CA 91789
Plastic tray.

Palmero Health Care 800-344-6424
120 Goodwin Pl, Stratford, CT 06615

Polar Ware Co. 800-237-3655
2806 N 15th St, Sheboygan, WI 53083
Stainless steel - many sizes available. Solid or perforated design available.

Princeton Medical Group, Inc. 800-875-0869
1189 Royal Links Dr, Mt Pleasant, SC 29466

RTI Biologics Inc. 877-343-6832
11621 Research Cir, Alachua, FL 32615
Interference screw system instrument tray.

Scientek Medical Equipment 604-273-9094
11151 Bridgeport Rd., Richmond, BC V6X 1T3 Canada

Silverglide Surgical Technologies 303-444-1970
5398 Manhattan Cir Ste 120, Boulder, CO 80303
Surgical instrument tray.

Small Bone Innovations, Inc. 215-428-1791
1380 S Pennsylvania Ave, Morrisville, PA 19067
Surgical tray.

Spine Wave, Inc. 203-944-9494
2 Enterprise Dr Ste 302, Shelton, CT 06484
Various instrument cases.

TRAY, SURGICAL INSTRUMENT *(cont'd)*

Sri Surgical 813-891-9550
6801 Longe St, Stockton, CA 95206
Surgical instrument tray various.

Sri Surgical 813-891-9550
7086 Industrial Row Dr, Mason, OH 45040

Sri Surgical 813-891-9550
1416 Dogwood Way, Mebane, NC 27302

Sri Surgical 813-891-9550
2595 Custer Rd Ste B, Salt Lake City, UT 84104

Sri Surgical 813-891-9550
6675 Business Pkwy Ste A, Elkridge, MD 21075

Sri Surgical 813-891-9550
12950 Executive Dr, Sugar Land, TX 77478

Sri Surgical 813-891-9550
6024 Century Oaks Dr, Chattanooga, TN 37416

Sri Surgical 813-891-9550
1441 Patton Pl Ste 139, Carrollton, TX 75007

Sri Surgical 813-891-9550
2240 E Artesia Blvd, Long Beach, CA 90805

Sri Surgical Express Inc. 813-891-9550
4501 Acline Dr E Ste 170, Tampa, FL 33605

Stryker Spine 866-457-7463
2 Pearl Ct, Allendale, NJ 07401

Suturtek Incorporated
51 Middlesex St, North Chelmsford, MA 01863
Sterilization tray.

Symmetry Medical, Inc. - Polyvac 207-786-2775
253 Abby Rd, Manchester, NH 03103
Tray, surgical instruments.

Synovis Micro Companies Alliance, Inc. 651-603-3700
439 Industrial Ln, Birmingham, AL 35211
Surgical instrument tray, container.

Teleflex Medical 800-334-9751
2917 Weck Drive, Research Triangle Park, NC 27709

Trinity Sterile, Inc. 410-860-5123
201 Kiley Dr, Salisbury, MD 21801

Tuzik Boston 800-886-6363
104 Longwater Dr, Assinippi Park, Norwell, MA 02061

Warsaw Orthopedic, Inc. 901-396-3133
2500 Silveus Xing, Warsaw, IN 46582
Case/tray.

West Coast Surgical Llc. 650-728-8095
141 California Ave Ste 101, Half Moon Bay, CA 94019
Tray,surgical,instrument.

Zimmer Holdings, Inc. 800-613-6131
1800 W Center St, PO Box 708, Warsaw, IN 46580

Zimmer Manufacturing B.V. 800-613-6131
Route 1, Km. 123.4, Bldg. 1, Turpeaux Industrial Park
Mercedita, PR 00715
Various instrument trays.

Zimmer Spine, Inc. 800-655-2614
7375 Bush Lake Rd, Minneapolis, MN 55439
Surgical instrument tray.

Zimmer Trabecular Metal Technology 800-613-6131
10 Pomeroy Rd, Parsippany, NJ 07054
Proximal tibial prep tray case top tray.

TRAY, WALKER *(General) 80UEL*

Helping Hand Trays 303-781-4019
4351 S Galapago St, Englewood, CO 80110
Food trays for walkers.

Invacare Corporation 800-333-6900
1 Invacare Way, Elyria, OH 44035
INVACARE.

Plastic And Metal Center, Inc. 949-770-8230
23162 La Cadena Dr, Laguna Hills, CA 92653

Sunrise Medical 800-333-4000
7477 Dry Creek Pkwy, Longmont, CO 80503

TRAY, WHEELCHAIR *(Physical Med) 89IMX*

Alimed, Inc. 800-225-2610
297 High St, Dedham, MA 02026

Broda Enterprises Inc. 800-668-0637
385 Phillip St., Waterloo, ONT N2L 5R8 Canada
BRODA SEATING.

TRAY, WHEELCHAIR *(cont'd)*

Diestco Manufacturing Corp. 800-795-2392
PO Box 6504, Chico, CA 95927
MEGATRAY, polycarbonate wheelchair tray and MINITRAY flip up tray for scooters and MIGHTY TRAY wheelchair tray.

Falcon Products, Inc. 800-873-3252
10650 Gateway Blvd, Saint Louis, MO 63132
Woop leg, wheelchair height tables.

Flaghouse, Inc. 800-793-7900
601 US Highway 46 W, Hasbrouck Heights, NJ 07604

Innovative Concepts 800-676-5030
300 N State St, Girard, OH 44420
3/8' or 1/4' polycarbonate, blank or complete w/stomach cutout, edges on three sides and adjustable toggle clamps; small, medium, large and x-large sizes, custom sizes available.

Intarsia Ltd. 203-355-1357
14 Martha Ln, Gaylordsville, CT 06755
Tray, anterior, upper extremity support surface.

Kayjae Mfg. Co. Inc. 888-452-9523
PO Box 95, Rte. 198 at Chapel Creek Road, Cobbs Creek, VA 23035
This product can be easily used under the legs of a person sitting in a wheelchair. The base comes in different sizes to fit comfortably, and the center supports extend upward with a table-top attached. The adjustability ranges from level for eating to slanted for reading. It is constructed of lightweight birch veneer with a durable finish. Weighs less than five lbs. and folds flat for portability.

Maddak Inc. 800-443-4926
661 State Route 23, Wayne, NJ 07470
ABLEWARE.

Medical Depot 516-998-4600
99 Seaview Blvd, Port Washington, NY 11050
Board.

Parsons A.D.L. Inc. 800-263-1281
R.R. #2, 1986 Sideroad 15, Tottenham, ONT L0G 1W0 Canada
Molded plastic trays in both transparent and solid beige colours, flat trays in Lexan and wood, padded trays, full size trays and half lap trays, velcro and mechanical mounting systems

Patterson Medical Supply, Inc. 262-387-8720
W68N158 Evergreen Blvd, Cedarburg, WI 53012
Wheelchair lap trays.

Profex Medical Products 800-325-0196
2224 E Person Ave, Memphis, TN 38114

Richardson Products, Inc. 888-928-7297
9408 Gulfstream Rd, Frankfort, IL 60423
Wheelchair tray.

Sunrise Medical Hhg Inc 303-218-4505
7128 Ambassador Rd, Baltimore, MD 21244
Various sizes of wheelchair trays.

Sunrise Medical Hhg Inc 303-218-4505
2010 E Spruce Cir, Olathe, KS 66062
Wheelchair lapboard.

Sunrise Medical Hhg Inc 303-218-4505
6724 Preston Ave # 1, Livermore, CA 94551

Sunrise Medical Hhg Inc 303-218-4505
2615 W Casino Rd # 2B, Everett, WA 98204

Sunrise Medical Hhg Inc 303-218-4505
2842 N Business Park Ave, Fresno, CA 93727

Therafin Corporation 800-843-7234
19747 Wolf Rd, Mokena, IL 60448
Various types of wheelchair trays.

Trayco 512-341-3709
1101 Pecan St W, Pflugerville, TX 78660
Wheelchair accessories.

Tuffcare 800-367-6160
3999 E La Palma Ave, Anaheim, CA 92807

TREADMILL, MECHANICAL *(Physical Med) 89IOG*

Accu Scan Instruments, Inc. 800-822-1344
5098 Trabue Rd, Columbus, OH 43228
Electromechanical treadmills for laboratory animals.

Battle Creek Equipment Co. 800-253-0854
307 Jackson St W, Battle Creek, MI 49037
HEALTH WALKER, $469.00 to $499.00 per unit (standard).

TREADMILL, MECHANICAL *(cont'd)*

Bertec Corporation 877-237-8320
6171 Huntley Rd Ste J, Columbus, OH 43229
6-component force-measurement treadmill to measure forces and moments associated with each foot. Appropriate for gait analysis and rehabilitation of individuals with locomotor problems.

Eagle Sports Chairs 800-932-9380
2351 Parkwood Rd, Snellville, GA 30039
PRO-ROLLER treadmill exerciser for wheelchair, $499.00.

Elmed, Inc. 630-543-2792
60 W Fay Ave, Addison, IL 60101

New Life Systems, Inc. 954-972-4600
PO Box 8767, Coral Springs, FL 33075
Electrical only.

TREADMILL, POWERED *(Physical Med) 89IOL*

Alimed, Inc. 800-225-2610
297 High St, Dedham, MA 02026

Battle Creek Equipment Co. 800-253-0854
307 Jackson St W, Battle Creek, MI 49037
WALKABOUT, $999.95.

Biodex Medical Systems, Inc. 800-224-6339
20 Ramsey Rd, Shirley, NY 11967
RTM Up to 15 degrees incline/decline, forward and reverse for retro walking or running. Competitively priced.

Cardiac Science Corp. 800-777-1777
500 Burdick Pkwy, Deerfield, WI 53531
TM 55, TM 65.

Cardinal Health 207, Inc. 800-231-2466
22745 Savi Ranch Pkwy, Yorba Linda, CA 92887

Dedicated Distribution 800-325-8367
640 Miami Ave, Kansas City, KS 66105

Full Vision, Inc. 316-283-3344
3017 Full Vision Dr, Newton, KS 67114
Medical treadmill.

Ge Medical Systems Information Technologies 800-643-6439
8200 W Tower Ave, Milwaukee, WI 53223
Model 2000 with high, medium, and low speed range and 1 to 25% grade elevation. Steel-frame, polyester-tread, 1/4-hp elevation motor, 2-hp drive motor. Remote controller, analog meter display speed and elevation; 0-mph startup.

Hoggan Health Industries, Inc. 800-678-7888
8020 S 1300 W, West Jordan, UT 84088
SPRINT RUNNER, motorless manual treadmill with electronic displays.

Innoventor, Inc. 314-785-0900
3600 Rider Trl S, Earth City, MO 63045

Landice, Inc. 800-LANDICE
111 Canfield Ave, Randolph, NJ 07869
Zero starting speed; Actual 0.1 to 12.0 mph speed range; Ultra high-torque drive; 400-pound user weight capacity with the L7 Model; 500-pound user weight capacity with the L8 Model; 15% grade electric elevation; Variable elevation over-speed protection; 20 x 58 four-ply treadbelt; Low 5 3/4 step-up height; Extended parallel medical handrails; Patient-attachable safety lanyard; Size: 32 x 77.

Life Fitness 800-735-3867
10601 Belmont Ave, Franklin Park, IL 60131

Md International, Inc. 305-669-9003
11300 NW 41st St, Doral, FL 33178

Med-Fit Systems, Inc. 800-831-7665
3553 Rosa Way, Fallbrook, CA 92028

Mortara Instrument, Inc. 800-231-7437
7865 N 86th St, Milwaukee, WI 53224
Heavy duty treadmill with 1.5 to 10 mph (0.1 mph increments), 0 to 22 percent grade elevation (0.5 percent increments), and 18 in. x 56 in. walking surface.

New Life Systems, Inc. 954-972-4600
PO Box 8767, Coral Springs, FL 33075
Electrical.

Robertson Harness
261 W Cypress Dr # A, Henderson, NV 89015
Treadmill.

Simbex, Llc 603-448-2367
10 Water St Ste 410, Lebanon, NH 03766
Activestep treadmill.

TREADMILL, POWERED *(cont'd)*

Thera-Tronics, Inc. 800-267-6211
623 Mamaroneck Ave, Mamaroneck, NY 10543
All types of exercise equipment; upper cycle, elliptical, biofeedback (EMG), and balance system.

True Fitness 800-426-6570
865 Hoff Rd, St Peters, MO 63366
Heavy-duty, 23 in. x 63 in. training surface, 12-mph max speed, standard 13% incline. Displays time, distance, speed, grade, pace, calories, and mets. Heart-rate control system allows input of target hour, max speed, max time, and max grade. Control both speed and grade and keeps users heart-rate within 3 beats of selected target. TRUE 750 HRC is a heavy-duty, heart-rate-controlled commercial treadmill. TRUE 350 HRC is a residential, heart-rate-controlled treadmill.

Vacumed 800-235-3333
4538 Westinghouse St, Ventura, CA 93003

Woodway Usa, Inc. 262-548-6235
West 229 North 591 Foster Ct., Waukesha, WI 53186
Various types.

TREPHINE, BONE *(Orthopedics) 87HWK*

Ascent Healthcare Solutions 480-763-5300
10232 S 51st St, Phoenix, AZ 85044
Trephine.

Biomet, Inc. 574-267-6639
56 E Bell Dr, PO Box 587, Warsaw, IN 46582
Blackburn trephine.

Depuy Spine, Inc. 800-227-6633
325 Paramount Dr, Raynham, MA 02767
Trephinea.

DJO Inc. 800-336-6569
1430 Decision St, Vista, CA 92081
Various orthopedic trephines and accessories.

Kmedic 800-955-0559
190 Veterans Dr, Northvale, NJ 07647

Medical Innovations International Inc. 507-289-0761
6256 34th Ave NW, Rochester, MN 55901
Rochester Bone Biopsy Trephine™ and dowel graft trephine.

Medtronic Sofamor Danek Usa, Inc. 901-396-3133
4340 Swinnea Rd, Memphis, TN 38118
Holder, needle.

Orthopedic Sciences, Inc 562-799-5550
3020 Old Ranch Pkwy Ste 325, Seal Beach, CA 90740
Trephine.

Salvin Dental Specialties, Inc. 800-535-6566
3450 Latrobe Dr, Charlotte, NC 28211
Trephine drills.

Stryker Corp. 800-726-2725
2825 Airview Blvd, Portage, MI 49002

Symmetry Medical Usa, Inc. 574-267-8700
486 W 350 N, Warsaw, IN 46582
Trephine.

Warsaw Orthopedic, Inc. 901-396-3133
2500 Silveus Xing, Warsaw, IN 46582
Holder, needle.

Zimmer Holdings, Inc. 800-613-6131
1800 W Center St, PO Box 708, Warsaw, IN 46580

TREPHINE, MANUAL, OPHTHALMIC (CORNEAL) *(Ophthalmology) 86HRH*

Back-Mueller, Inc. 314-531-6640
2700 Clark Ave, Saint Louis, MO 63103
Various sizes of trephine blades.

Barron Precision Instruments, L.L.C. 810-695-2080
8170 Embury Rd, Grand Blanc, MI 48439
Various types of sterile manual opthalmic trephines.

Bausch & Lomb Surgical 636-255-5051
3365 Tree Court Ind Blvd, Saint Louis, MO 63122

Glaukos Corp. 949-367-9600
26051 Merit Cir Ste 103, Laguna Hills, CA 92653
Various type of sterile & non-sterile manual ophthalmic trephines.

Hai Laboratories, Inc. 781-862-9884
320 Massachusetts Ave, Lexington, MA 02420
Trephine - various types.

Jedmed Instruments Co. 314-845-3770
5416 Jedmed Ct, Saint Louis, MO 63129

TREPHINE, MANUAL, OPHTHALMIC (CORNEAL) *(cont'd)*

Jim's Instrument Mfg., Inc. 319-351-3429
1910 S Gilbert St, Iowa City, IA 52240
Ophthalmic trephine manual.

Katena Products, Inc. 800-225-1195
4 Stewart Ct, Denville, NJ 07834
Also disposable.

Miltex Inc. 800-645-8000
589 Davies Dr, York, PA 17402

Ultracell Medical Technologies, Inc. 877-SPO-NGE1
183 Providence New London Tpke, North Stonington, CT 06359

TREPHINE, SINUS *(Ear/Nose/Throat) 77KBF*

H & H Co. 909-390-0373
4435 E Airport Dr Ste 108, Ontario, CA 91761
Trephines, sinus.

TREPHINE, SKULL *(Cns/Neurology) 84SCB*

Codman & Shurtleff, Inc 800-225-0460
325 Paramount Dr, Raynham, MA 02767

Miltex Inc. 800-645-8000
589 Davies Dr, York, PA 17402

TRICALCIUM PHOSPHATE GRANULES FOR DENTAL BONE REPAIR *(Dental And Oral) 76LPK*

Gfs Chemicals, Inc. 800-858-9682
867 McKinley Ave, Columbus, OH 43222
Beta-tricalcium phosphate.

Steiner Laboratories 808-371-2700
590 Farrington Hwy, #1010 Suite 7, Kapolei, HI 96707
Socket graft.

Ultradent Products, Inc. 801-553-4586
505 W 10200 S, South Jordan, UT 84095
Bone grafting material.

TROCAR, ABDOMINAL *(Gastro/Urology) 78SCC*

Ams Innovative Center-San Jose 800-356-7600
3070 Orchard Dr, San Jose, CA 95134

Elmed, Inc. 630-543-2792
60 W Fay Ave, Addison, IL 60101

Karl Storz Endoscopy-America Inc. 800-421-0837
600 Corporate Pointe, Culver City, CA 90230
Reusable, multifunction trocars in a range of styles and sizes,

Mahe International Inc. 800-294-7946
468 Craighead St, Nashville, TN 37204

Richard Wolf Medical Instruments Corp. 800-323-9653
353 Corporate Woods Pkwy, Vernon Hills, IL 60061

Smith & Nephew, Inc., Endoscopy Division 800-343-8386
150 Minuteman Rd, Andover, MA 01810

Synectic Medical Product Development 203-877-8488
60 Commerce Park, Milford, CT 06460

Troy Manufacturing Co. 440-834-8262
17090 Rapids Rd, PO Box 448, Burton, OH 44021

TROCAR, AMNIOTIC *(Obstetrics/Gyn) 85SCD*

Codman & Shurtleff, Inc 800-225-0460
325 Paramount Dr, Raynham, MA 02767

Mahe International Inc. 800-294-7946
468 Craighead St, Nashville, TN 37204

Richard Wolf Medical Instruments Corp. 800-323-9653
353 Corporate Woods Pkwy, Vernon Hills, IL 60061

TROCAR, ANTRUM *(Ear/Nose/Throat) 77SCE*

Karl Storz Endoscopy-America Inc. 800-421-0837
600 Corporate Pointe, Culver City, CA 90230

Mahe International Inc. 800-294-7946
468 Craighead St, Nashville, TN 37204

Miltex Inc. 800-645-8000
589 Davies Dr, York, PA 17402

Richard Wolf Medical Instruments Corp. 800-323-9653
353 Corporate Woods Pkwy, Vernon Hills, IL 60061

TROCAR, CARDIOVASCULAR *(Cardiovascular) 74DRC*

Angiodynamics, Inc. 518-795-1400
14 Plaza Drive, Latham, NY 12110

Biocompatibles Inc. 877-783-5463
115 Hurley Rd Bldg 3, Oxford, CT 06478
Angiographic needles.

TROCAR, CARDIOVASCULAR *(cont'd)*

Depuy Orthopaedics, Inc. 800-473-3789
700 Orthopaedic Dr, P.O. Box 988, Warsaw, IN 46582
Various types of trocars.

Depuy-Raynham, A Div. Of Depuy Orthopaedics 800-451-2006
325 Paramount Dr, Raynham, MA 02767
Various types of trocars.

Diablo Sales & Marketing, Inc. 925-648-1611
PO Box 3219, Danville, CA 94526
Custom design and manufacturing of catheters and specialty guidewires. Guiding catheters; stent delivery and drug delivery systems.

E-Z-Em, Inc. 516-333-8230
750 Summa Ave, Westbury, NY 11590
Sterile angiographic needle.

Karl Storz Endoscopy-America Inc. 800-421-0837
600 Corporate Pointe, Culver City, CA 90230

Kelsar, S.A. 508-261-8000
Blvd. Insurgentes, Libriamento a La, Tijuana 22450 Mexico
Trocar, safety trocar, thoracostomy trays/kits (various)

Medtronic Blood Management 612-514-4000
18501 E Plaza Dr, Parker, CO 80134
Trocar.

Medtronic Cardiovascular Surgery, The Heart Valve Div. 800-328-2518
1851 E Deere Ave, Santa Ana, CA 92705
Various sizes of trocar blades & handles.

Medtronic Heart Valves 800-227-3191
8299 Central Ave NE, Spring Lake Park, MN 55432
Various sizes.

Medtronic Vascular 707-525-0111
3576 Unocal Pl, Santa Rosa, CA 95403
Transseptal needle

Merit Medical Systems, Inc. 801-253-1600
1111 S Velasco St, Angleton, TX 77515
Various sizes of sterile angiographic needles.

Miltex Inc. 800-645-8000
589 Davies Dr, York, PA 17402

Princeton Medical Group, Inc. 800-875-0869
1189 Royal Links Dr, Mt Pleasant, SC 29466

Surgistar Inc. 800-995-7086
2310 La Mirada Dr, Vista, CA 92081
Trocars.

Thomas Medical Products, Inc. 866-446-3003
65 Great Valley Pkwy, Malvern, PA 19355
Transseptal needle.

Troy Manufacturing Co. • 440-834-8262
17090 Rapids Rd, PO Box 448, Burton, OH 44021

TROCAR, ENT *(Ear/Nose/Throat) 77KTE*

Aesculap Implant Systems Inc. 1-800-234-9179
3773 Corporate Pkwy, Center Valley, PA 18034

Biomet Microfixation Inc. 800-874-7711
1520 Tradeport Dr, Jacksonville, FL 32218
Various types of trocars.

Surgistar Inc. 800-995-7086
2310 La Mirada Dr, Vista, CA 92081
Trocars.

Troy Manufacturing Co. 440-834-8262
17090 Rapids Rd, PO Box 448, Burton, OH 44021

TROCAR, GALLBLADDER *(Gastro/Urology) 78SCF*

Arrow International, Inc. 800-523-8446
2400 Bernville Rd, Reading, PA 19605

Codman & Shurtleff, Inc 800-225-0460
325 Paramount Dr, Raynham, MA 02767

Elmed, Inc. 630-543-2792
60 W Fay Ave, Addison, IL 60101

Richard Wolf Medical Instruments Corp. 800-323-9653
353 Corporate Woods Pkwy, Vernon Hills, IL 60061

Smith & Nephew, Inc., Endoscopy Division 800-343-8386
150 Minuteman Rd, Andover, MA 01810

TROCAR, GASTRO-UROLOGY *(Gastro/Urology) 78FBQ*

Aesculap Implant Systems Inc. 1-800-234-9179
3773 Corporate Pkwy, Center Valley, PA 18034

TROCAR, GASTRO-UROLOGY *(cont'd)*

Biomet Microfixation Inc. 800-874-7711
1520 Tradeport Dr, Jacksonville, FL 32218
Various types of trocars.

Gibbons Surgical Corp. 800-959-1989
1112 Jensen Dr Ste 101, Virginia Beach, VA 23451

Princeton Medical Group, Inc. 800-875-0869
1189 Royal Links Dr, Mt Pleasant, SC 29466

Richard Wolf Medical Instruments Corp. 800-323-9653
353 Corporate Woods Pkwy, Vernon Hills, IL 60061

Smith & Nephew, Inc., Endoscopy Division 800-343-8386
150 Minuteman Rd, Andover, MA 01810

Surgistar Inc. 800-995-7086
2310 La Mirada Dr, Vista, CA 92081
Trocars.

Synectic Medical Product Development 203-877-8488
60 Commerce Park, Milford, CT 06460

Troy Manufacturing Co. 440-834-8262
17090 Rapids Rd, PO Box 448, Burton, OH 44021

TROCAR, LAPAROSCOPIC *(Surgery) 79WYQ*

David Scott Company 800-804-0333
59 Fountain St, Framingham, MA 01702

Deknatel Snowden-Pencer 800-367-7874
5175 S Royal Atlanta Dr, Tucker, GA 30084
DIAMOND-POINT disposable trocars. Color coded to insure easy identification of sizes.

Dma Med-Chem Corporation 800-362-1833
49 Watermill Ln, Great Neck, NY 11021

Ethicon Endo-Surgery, Inc. 800-USE-ENDO
4545 Creek Rd, Cincinnati, OH 45242

Frantz Medical Development Ltd. 440-255-1155
7740 Metric Dr, Mentor, OH 44060
Disposable device.

Genicon 800-936-1020
6869 Stapoint Ct Ste 114, Winter Park, FL 32792
Laparoscopic Trocar and Cannula Systems including: Disposable and Reusable products configured as Pyramidal, Shielded, Open & Bladeless Tip Styles

Mediflex Surgical Products 800-879-7575
250 Gibbs Rd, Islandia, NY 11749

Princeton Medical Group, Inc. 800-875-0869
1189 Royal Links Dr, Mt Pleasant, SC 29466

Putnam Precision Products 845-278-2141
3859 Danbury Rd, Brewster, NY 10509

Stryker Endoscopy 800-435-0220
5900 Optical Ct, San Jose, CA 95138

Taut, Inc. 800-231-8288
2571 Kaneville Ct, Geneva, IL 60134
ADAPt PORTS dilate through tissue without cutting blades. The unique action of the asymmetrical tip stretches and divides fascial fibers, and avoids bladed injury. BALLOON OPEN ACCESS PORT, a unique latex-free balloon fully inflated with 10cc of saline. Foamseal locking plug secures & seals at the incision site. Balloon anchor provides an excellent seal for general, gynecological & bariatric surgery. OPEN ACCESS PORT has a Softseal elliptical plug designed for an excellent fit with the Hasson incision. Soft silicone plug construction, not rigid plastic or metal. Unique ADAPt floating seal and rotary valve. Latex Free

Tegra Medical Inc. 508-541-4200
9 Forge Pkwy, Franklin, MA 02038

Troy Manufacturing Co. 440-834-8262
17090 Rapids Rd, PO Box 448, Burton, OH 44021

Vital Concepts, Inc. 800-984-2300
4334 Brockton Dr SE Ste F, Grand Rapids, MI 49512
Trocars & cannulas, disposable & reusable trocars, reusable sleeves and accessories.

TROCAR, LARYNGEAL *(Ear/Nose/Throat) 77KAB*

Aesculap Implant Systems Inc. 1-800-234-9179
3773 Corporate Pkwy, Center Valley, PA 18034

Bausch & Lomb Surgical 636-255-5051
3365 Tree Court Ind Blvd, Saint Louis, MO 63122

Cadence Science Inc. 888-717-7677
1979 Marcus Ave Ste 215, New Hyde Park, NY 11042

Elmed, Inc. 630-543-2792
60 W Fay Ave, Addison, IL 60101

TROCAR, LARYNGEAL *(cont'd)*

Karl Storz Endoscopy-America Inc. 800-421-0837
600 Corporate Pointe, Culver City, CA 90230

Mahe International Inc. 800-294-7946
468 Craighead St, Nashville, TN 37204

ReNu Medical Inc. 877-252-1110
9800 Evergreen Way, Everett, WA 98204
OXYGEN NON-REBREATHING; REPROCESSED MASK

Richard Wolf Medical Instruments Corp. 800-323-9653
353 Corporate Woods Pkwy, Vernon Hills, IL 60061

Surgistar Inc. 800-995-7086
2310 La Mirada Dr, Vista, CA 92081
Trocars.

TROCAR, OTHER *(General) 80SCH*

Cadence Science Inc. 888-717-7677
1979 Marcus Ave Ste 215, New Hyde Park, NY 11042

Diablo Sales & Marketing, Inc. 925-648-1611
PO Box 3219, Danville, CA 94526
Custom design and manufacturing of catheters and specialty guidewires. Guiding catheters; stent delivery and drug delivery systems.

Incisiontech 800-213-7809
9 Technology Dr, Staunton, VA 24401

Karl Storz Endoscopy-America Inc. 800-421-0837
600 Corporate Pointe, Culver City, CA 90230

Medovations, Inc. 800-558-6408
102 E Keefe Ave, Milwaukee, WI 53212

Richard Wolf Medical Instruments Corp. 800-323-9653
353 Corporate Woods Pkwy, Vernon Hills, IL 60061

Spectra Medical Devices, Inc. 978-657-0889
260H Fordham Rd, Wilmington, MA 01887
trocars and tunnellers, custom manufactured

Surgistar Inc. 800-995-7086
2310 La Mirada Dr, Vista, CA 92081
Surgistar laparoscopic trocars and sleeves: Laparoscopic trocars and cannulas; a system of trocars and cannulas for laparoscopic incisions.

Tegra Medical Inc. 508-541-4200
9 Forge Pkwy, Franklin, MA 02038

Troy Manufacturing Co. 440-834-8262
17090 Rapids Rd, PO Box 448, Burton, OH 44021

Wisap America 800-233-8448
8231 Melrose Dr, Lenexa, KS 66214

Wytech Industries, Inc. 732-396-3900
960 E Hazelwood Ave, Rahway, NJ 07065

TROCAR, SHORT *(Surgery) 79SHB*

Ethicon Endo-Surgery, Inc. 800-USE-ENDO
4545 Creek Rd, Cincinnati, OH 45242

Putnam Precision Products 845-278-2141
3859 Danbury Rd, Brewster, NY 10509

Richard Wolf Medical Instruments Corp. 800-323-9653
353 Corporate Woods Pkwy, Vernon Hills, IL 60061

Tegra Medical Inc. 508-541-4200
9 Forge Pkwy, Franklin, MA 02038

TROCAR, SINUS *(Ear/Nose/Throat) 77KBG*

Aesculap Implant Systems Inc. 1-800-234-9179
3773 Corporate Pkwy, Center Valley, PA 18034

Jedmed Instruments Co. 314-845-3770
5416 Jedmed Ct, Saint Louis, MO 63129

Karl Storz Endoscopy-America Inc. 800-421-0837
600 Corporate Pointe, Culver City, CA 90230

Mahe International Inc. 800-294-7946
468 Craighead St, Nashville, TN 37204

Surgistar Inc. 800-995-7086
2310 La Mirada Dr, Vista, CA 92081
Trocars.

TROCAR, SURGICAL *(Surgery) 79SHU*

Ethicon Endo-Surgery, Inc. 800-USE-ENDO
4545 Creek Rd, Cincinnati, OH 45242
ENDOPATH: TRI-STAR, 10/11mm and 10/12mm, 100mm; 10/11mm blunt tip; thoracic, 10/12, 33mm, 18mm. Also with specimen cannula, 33mm and reducer.

TROCAR, THORACIC *(Cardiovascular) 74SCG*

Atrium Medical Corp. 800-528-7486
5 Wentworth Dr, Hudson, NH 03051

Axiom Medical, Inc. 800-221-8569
19320 Van Ness Ave, Torrance, CA 90501
Wide variety of sizes, straight, right angle, PVC

Diablo Sales & Marketing, Inc. 925-648-1611
PO Box 3219, Danville, CA 94526
Custom design and manufacturing of catheters and specialty guidewires. Guiding catheters; stent delivery and drug delivery systems.

Ethicon Endo-Surgery, Inc. 800-USE-ENDO
4545 Creek Rd, Cincinnati, OH 45242
FLEXIPATH thoracic trocar, available in 7mm, 15mm, and 20mm sizes.

Mahe International Inc. 800-294-7946
468 Craighead St, Nashville, TN 37204

Medovations, Inc. 800-558-6408
102 E Keefe Ave, Milwaukee, WI 53212

Miltex Inc. 800-645-8000
589 Davies Dr, York, PA 17402

Richard Wolf Medical Instruments Corp. 800-323-9653
353 Corporate Woods Pkwy, Vernon Hills, IL 60061

TROCAR, TRACHEAL *(Ear/Nose/Throat) 77KCI*

Aesculap Implant Systems Inc. 1-800-234-9179
3773 Corporate Pkwy, Center Valley, PA 18034

Miltex Inc. 800-645-8000
589 Davies Dr, York, PA 17402

Surgistar Inc. 800-995-7086
2310 La Mirada Dr, Vista, CA 92081
Trocars.

TROUSERS, ANTI-SHOCK *(Anesthesiology) 73LHX*

Allied Healthcare Products, Inc. 800-444-3954
1720 Sublette Ave, Saint Louis, MO 63110

Armstrong Medical Industries, Inc. 800-323-4220
575 Knightsbridge Pkwy, Lincolnshire, IL 60069

David Clark Company, Inc. 800-900-3434
360 Franklin St, Worcester, MA 01604
Medical anti-shock trouser

TRUSS, HERNIA (BELT) *(Gastro/Urology) 78SCI*

Freeman Manufacturing Company 800-253-2091
900 W Chicago Rd, PO Box J, Sturgis, MI 49091

Larkotex Company 800-972-3037
1002 Olive St, Texarkana, TX 75501

Lumiscope Company, Inc. 800-672-8293
1035 Centennial Ave, Piscataway, NJ 08854

Surgical Appliance Industries 800-888-0458
3960 Rosslyn Dr, Cincinnati, OH 45209

Truform Orthotics & Prosthetics 800-888-0458
3960 Rosslyn Dr, Cincinnati, OH 45209

TRUSS, UMBILICAL *(Gastro/Urology) 78EXM*

Ethicon Endo-Surgery, Inc. 877-384-4266
3801 University Blvd SE, Albuquerque, NM 87106
Various types of sterile and nonsterile umbilical tapes.

Ethicon, Inc. 800-4-ETHICON
Route 22 West, Somerville, NJ 08876

Larkotex Company 800-972-3037
1002 Olive St, Texarkana, TX 75501

The Kendrick Co., Inc.
6139 Germantown Ave, Philadelphia, PA 19144
Truss, umbilical.

Truform Orthotics & Prosthetics 800-888-0458
3960 Rosslyn Dr, Cincinnati, OH 45209

TRYPSIN *(Pathology) 88IBG*

Safc Biosciences, Inc. 913-469-5580
320 Swamp Bridge Rd, Denver, PA 17517
Trypsin.

Safc Biosciences, Inc. 913-469-5580
13804 W 107th St, Lenexa, KS 66215

Scytek Laboratories, Inc. 435-755-9848
205 S 600 W, Logan, UT 84321
Trypsin, stabilized solution.

TRYPSIN *(cont'd)*

Ventana Medical Systems, Inc. 800-227-2155
1910 E Innovation Park Dr, Oro Valley, AZ 85755
Enzyme.

TRYPTOPHAN MEASUREMENT (COLORIMETRIC), GLOBULIN *(Chemistry) 75JGC*

Health Chem Diagnostics Llc 954-979-3845
3341 W McNab Rd, Pompano Beach, FL 33069
Tryptophan measurement (colorimetric), globulin.

TUBAL OCCLUSIVE DEVICE *(Obstetrics/Gyn) 85KNH*

Bausch & Lomb Surgical 636-255-5051
3365 Tree Court Ind Blvd, Saint Louis, MO 63122

Coloplast Manufacturing Us, Llc 800-533-0464
1840 W Oak Pkwy, Marietta, GA 30062
Absorbent pocket designed for male dribbling or light bladder control. Adheres to underwear.

Richard Wolf Medical Instruments Corp. 800-323-9653
353 Corporate Woods Pkwy, Vernon Hills, IL 60061

TUBE, ASPIRATING, FLEXIBLE, CONNECTING *(Anesthesiology) 73BYY*

A-M Systems, Inc. 800-426-1306
131 Business Park Loop, Sequim, WA 98382
5 types (smooth interior, some autoclavable, pasteurizable, and or cold sterilizable)

Allied Healthcare Products, Inc. 800-444-3954
1720 Sublette Ave, Saint Louis, MO 63110

Ballard Medical Products 770-587-7835
12050 Lone Peak Pkwy, Draper, UT 84020
Aspiration catheter.

Benlan Inc. 905-829-5004
2760 Brighton Rd., Oakville, ONT L6H 5T4 Canada

Breg, Inc., An Orthofix Company 800-897-BREG
2611 Commerce Way, Vista, CA 92081
Disposable joint aspiration/injection kit.

Busse Hospital Disposables, Inc. 631-435-4711
75 Arkay Dr, Hauppauge, NY 11788
Various sizes of sterile aspirating tubing & handle.

Centurion Medical Products Corp. 517-545-1135
3310 S Main St, Salisbury, NC 28147

H2or, Inc. 918-744-4267
1638 S Main St, Tulsa, OK 74119
Floor aspirator.

Kelsar, S.A. 508-261-8000
Blvd. Insurgentes, Libriamento a La, Tijuana 22450 Mexico
Tubing connectors, conductive & non-conductive (various)

Medline Manufacturing And Services Llc 847-837-2759
1 Medline Pl, Mundelein, IL 60060
Connecting tubing.

Mercury Medical 800-237-6418
11300 49th St N, Clearwater, FL 33762

Princeton Medical Group, Inc. 800-875-0869
1189 Royal Links Dr, Mt Pleasant, SC 29466

Rd Medical Mfg. Inc. 787-716-6363
Road 183, Km 21.6, Las Piedras Industrial Park, Las Piedras, PR 00771
Various types of suction tubes.

Smiths Medical Asd, Inc. 610-578-9600
9255 Customhouse Plz Ste N, San Diego, CA 92154
Airway intubation set with accessories (sterile and non-sterile).

Tri-State Hospital Supply Corp. 517-545-1135
3173 E 43rd St, Yuma, AZ 85365

Wells Johnson Co. 800-528-1597
8000 S Kolb Rd, Tucson, AZ 85756

TUBE, ASPIRATING, RIGID BRONCHOSCOPE ASPIRATING *(Ear/Nose/Throat) 77KTR*

Ballard Medical Products 770-587-7835
12050 Lone Peak Pkwy, Draper, UT 84020
Bronchoscope (flexible or rigid) and accessories.

Kelsar, S.A. 508-261-8000
Blvd. Insurgentes, Libriamento a La, Tijuana 22450 Mexico
Aspirating tube

TUBE, AUTOCLAVING *(General) 80SCL*

A-M Systems, Inc. 800-426-1306
131 Business Park Loop, Sequim, WA 98382
Standard sizes; custom sizes available; wire reinforced tubing, Hytrel.

TUBE, BLOOD COLLECTION *(Chemistry) 75SCN*

Accu-Glass Llc 800-325-4796
10765 Trenton Ave, Saint Louis, MO 63132
Precision glass tubing for blood collection applications.

Becton Dickinson And Company 800-284-6845
1 Becton Dr, Franklin Lakes, NJ 07417
PBBCS with Preattached Holder; Push Button Blood Collection Set

Covidien Lp 508-261-8000
15 Hampshire St, Mansfield, MA 02048

Dade Behring, Inc. 800-948-3233
1717 Deerfield Rd, Deerfield, IL 60015

Drummond Scientific Co. 800-523-7480
500 Park Way # 700, Broomall, PA 19008

Exelint International Co. 800-940-3935
5840 W Centinela Ave, Los Angeles, CA 90045
EXEL Vacuum Blood Collection Tubes.

Filtrona Extrusion, Inc./Pexcor Medical Products Div. 800-755-7528
764 S Athol Rd, P.O. Box 659, Athol, MA 01331

Sunlite Plastics, Inc. 262-253-0600
W194N11340 McCormick Dr, Germantown, WI 53022

Terumo Medical Corp. 800-283-7866
2101 Cottontail Ln, Somerset, NJ 08873

TUBE, BLOOD MICROCOLLECTION *(Chemistry) 75SCM*

Accu-Glass Llc 800-325-4796
10765 Trenton Ave, Saint Louis, MO 63132

Covidien Lp 508-261-8000
15 Hampshire St, Mansfield, MA 02048
$8.55 per 100 (3cc).

Dade Behring, Inc. 800-948-3233
1717 Deerfield Rd, Deerfield, IL 60015

Drummond Scientific Co. 800-523-7480
500 Park Way # 700, Broomall, PA 19008

Ram Scientific, Inc. 800-535-6734
PO Box 348, Yonkers, NY 10703
100% plastic SAFE-T-FILL(R) Blood Gas Capillary Tube for clinical and reference applications. Prepared with either balanced heparin or sodium heparin.

TUBE, BRONCHIAL (W/WO CONNECTOR) *(Anesthesiology) 73BTS*

Avalon Laboratories, Inc. 866-938-6613
2610 Homestead Pl, Rancho Dominguez, CA 90220

Boehm Surgical Instrument Corp. 716-436-6584
966 Chili Ave, Rochester, NY 14611
Tube,bronchial (20/connector).

E. Benson Hood Laboratories, Inc. 800-942-5227
575 Washington St, Pembroke, MA 02359
T-Y tracheobronchial tubes in 3 sizes, Y-Tubes in multiple sizes, T-Y tube, bronchial stents with posts. Y-Tubes with posts with Ultra-smooth.

Richard Wolf Medical Instruments Corp. 800-323-9653
353 Corporate Woods Pkwy, Vernon Hills, IL 60061

TUBE, BRONCHOSCOPE, ASPIRATING *(Anesthesiology) 73JEM*

Covidien Lp 508-261-8000
15 Hampshire St, Mansfield, MA 02048
LUKI tubes.

TUBE, CAPILLARY *(Chemistry) 75SCO*

Accu-Glass Llc 800-325-4796
10765 Trenton Ave, Saint Louis, MO 63132

Covidien Lp 508-261-8000
15 Hampshire St, Mansfield, MA 02048

Dade Behring, Inc. 800-948-3233
1717 Deerfield Rd, Deerfield, IL 60015

Drummond Scientific Co. 800-523-7480
500 Park Way # 700, Broomall, PA 19008

Engineers Express, Inc. 800-255-8823
7 Industrial Park Rd, Medway, MA 02053

Jayza Corp. 305-477-1136
7215 NW 41st St Ste A, Miami, FL 33166

TUBE, CAPILLARY *(cont'd)*

Mckesson General Medical 800-446-3008
8741 Landmark Rd, Richmond, VA 23228

Radiometer America, Inc. 800-736-0600
810 Sharon Dr, Westlake, OH 44145
CLINITUBES.

Spectra Medical Devices, Inc. 866-938-8649
4C Henshaw St, Woburn, MA 01801

TUBE, CAPILLARY BLOOD COLLECTION *(Hematology) 81GIO*

Abbott Point Of Care Inc. 609-443-9300
104 Windsor Center Dr, East Windsor, NJ 08520
Capillary dispensers.

Accu-Glass Llc 800-325-4796
10765 Trenton Ave, Saint Louis, MO 63132

Becton Dickinson And Company 800-284-6845
1 Becton Dr, Franklin Lakes, NJ 07417
BACTO-CAPILLARY TUBES; MULTIPLE; PLASTIC CLAD MICRO HEMATOCRIT TUBES

Bio-Rad Laboratories, Diagnostic Group 800-224-6723
524 Stone Rd Ste A, Benicia, CA 94510
Microcapillary collection device.

Bionostics, Inc. 978-772-7070
7 Jackson Rd, Devens, MA 01434
Capillary blood collection tubes.

Chase Scientific Glass, Inc. 412-490-8425
234 Cardiff Valley Rd, Rockwood, TN 37854
Multiple.

Covidien Lp 508-261-8000
15 Hampshire St, Mansfield, MA 02048

Dade Behring, Inc. 800-948-3233
1717 Deerfield Rd, Deerfield, IL 60015

Health Care Logistics, Inc. 800-848-1633
450 Town St, PO Box 25, Circleville, OH 43113
Blood/vials.

Innovative Medical Technologies, Inc. 866-560-1820
15059 Cedar St, Leawood, KS 66224
Innovac Quick-Draw capillary whole blood collection system. Consists of disposable Quick-Draw collector and Innovac battery-powered vacuum device. Makes capillary collection quick, clean, and easy. Automatically mixes sample during collection, reducing microclot potential. Newborn screening samples are made nearly fool proof with new sample application technique.

Iris Sample Processing 800-782-8774
60 Glacier Dr, Westwood, MA 02090
Capillary blood collector.

Jayza Corp. 305-477-1136
7215 NW 41st St Ste A, Miami, FL 33166

Kimble Chase Life Science And Research Products, Llc. 865-717-2635
234 Cardiff Valley Rd, Ozone, TN 37854

Kimble Glass, Inc. 888-546-2531
537 Crystal Ave, Vineland, NJ 08360
KIMBLE.

Omni Medical Supply Inc. 800-860-6664
4153 Pioneer Dr, Commerce Township, MI 48390

Propper Manufacturing Co., Inc. 800-832-4300
3604 Skillman Ave, Long Island City, NY 11101

Ram Scientific, Inc. 800-535-6734
PO Box 348, Yonkers, NY 10703
100% plastic SAFE-T-FILL(R) Capillary Blood Collection device for hematology and chemistry applications. Prepared with EDTA, lithium heparin, sodium fluoride, sodium citrate, and plain. Also available with serum gel separator.

Rpc 800-647-3873
PO Box 35849, Tucson, AZ 85740
Port caps for reprocessed hemodialyzers.

Safe-Tec Clinical Products, Inc. 800-356-6033
142 Railroad Dr, Ivyland, PA 18974
MICROSAFE is a one-piece plastic tube used to collect and dispense whole blood from a fingerstick. This device fills automatically by capillary action while the air vent regulates the present volume. The sample is easily expelled by squeezing the unfilled portion of the tube, then discarded. No bulbs, dispensers, or other mechanical devices needed.

TUBE, CAPILLARY BLOOD COLLECTION *(cont'd)*

Separation Technology Inc 800-777-6668
1096 Rainer Dr, Altamonte Springs, FL 32714
ClearCRIT 100%-plastic microhematocrit tubes eliminate the risk of disease transmitted by blood via broken glass. The heparinized tubes are available in standard 75-mm length, 0.5- and 1.1-mm inside diameter. ClearCRIT self-sealing, Mylar plastic-coated hematocrit tubes require no sealing clay. Available in 75-mm length, 1.1mm inside diameter. Heparinized.

Statspin, Inc. 800-782-8774
60 Glacier Dr, Westwood, MA 02090
STATSAMPLER capillary tube collection system with volume of 100 uL or 200 uL; separation with gel in a micro-tube, or with EDTA for hematology.

TUBE, CEMENT VENTILATION *(Orthopedics) 87KII*

Biomet, Inc. 574-267-6639
56 E Bell Dr, PO Box 587, Warsaw, IN 46582
Vent tubing.

TUBE, CENTRIFUGE *(Chemistry) 75SCP*

Beckman Coulter, Inc. 800-742-2345
250 S Kraemer Blvd, PO Box 8000, Brea, CA 92821

Berghof/America 800-544-5004
3773 NW 126th Ave Bldg 1, Coral Springs, FL 33065
PTFE conical bottom tubes with or without rims, and round bottom tubes.

Bio Plas, Inc. 415-472-3777
4340 Redwood Hwy Ste A15, San Rafael, CA 94903
15ml styrene centrifuge tubes, and microcentrifuge tubes in 5 sizes with color coding and tight fitting closures. Screw cap, snap cap and flat top microcentrifuge tubes. G-TUBES microgentrifuge tubes available in 0.6ml, 1.5ml, and 2.0ml, at over 30,000 x g without cap locks.

Brinkmann Instruments (Canada) Ltd. 800-263-8715
6670 Campobello Rd., Mississauga, ONT L5N 2L8 Canada

Covidien Lp 508-261-8000
15 Hampshire St, Mansfield, MA 02048

Drummond Scientific Co. 800-523-7480
500 Park Way # 700, Broomall, PA 19008

Garren Scientific, Inc. 800-342-3725
15916 Blythe St Unit A, Van Nuys, CA 91406
Centrifuge tubes 15mL/50mL.

Globe Scientific, Inc. 800-394-4562
610 Winters Ave, Paramus, NJ 07652
Microcentrifuge tubes in 12-, 15-, 30- and 50-ml sizes.

Image Molding, Inc. 800-525-1875
4525 Kingston St, Denver, CO 80239
Disposable polysturene tubes graduated to 12mL designed to retain a standardized 0.4mL of sediment when decanted.

Jaece Industries, Inc. 716-694-2811
908 Niagara Falls Blvd, North Tonawanda, NY 14120
Racks and floating tube--these are polyfoam racks for PCR, microtubes, and centrifuge.

Labcon North America 800-227-1466
3700 Lakeville Hwy Ste 200, Petaluma, CA 94954
50ml and 15ml with screw cap and disposable micro-centrifuge tubes (0.25ml, 0.4ml, 0.5ml & 1.5ml). SUPERCLEAR micro centrifuge micro volume tubes.

Midwest Scientific 800-227-9997
280 Vance Rd, Valley Park, MO 63088
$29.00 per 1,000 1.5-mL, flattop, RNASE-free, freeze- and boil-safe microcentrifuge tubes.

Nalge Nunc International 800-625-4327
75 Panorama Creek Dr, Rochester, NY 14625
NALGENE conical-bottom, round-bottom and Oak Ridge style tubes. Round-, conical-, and flat-bottom bottles. A variety of sizes and materials. Sealing caps available for handling biohazardous samples.

Novosci Corp. 281-363-4949
2828 N Crescentridge Dr, The Woodlands, TX 77381

Quality Scientific Plastics 800-426-9595
1260 Holm Rd, Petaluma, CA 94954

Simport Plastics Ltd. 450-464-1723
2588 Bernard-Pilon, Beloeil, QUE J3G 4S5 Canada

Surgipath Medical Industries, Inc. 800-225-3035
PO Box 528, 5205 Route 12, Richmond, IL 60071

TUBE, CENTRIFUGE *(cont'd)*

United Products & Instruments, Inc. 800-588-9776
182 Ridge Rd Ste E, Dayton, NJ 08810
The PowerSpin M24 spins 1000 - 3400 RPM, to insure a lean and complete separation of cellular components yielding superior serum or plasma specimen. The all digital push

Usa Scientific, Inc. 800-522-8477
PO Box 3565, Ocala, FL 34478
Seal-Rite.

Ware Medics Glass Works, Inc. 845-429-6950
PO Box 368, Garnerville, NY 10923

TUBE, CONNECTING *(General) 80SCR*

Allied Healthcare Products, Inc. 800-444-3954
1720 Sublette Ave, Saint Louis, MO 63110

Benlan Inc. 905-829-5004
2760 Brighton Rd., Oakville, ONT L6H 5T4 Canada
Proprietory and custom, disposable and bulk assembled.

Coeur Inc., Sheboygan 800-874-4240
3411 Behrens Pkwy, Sheboygan, WI 53081

Covidien Lp 508-261-8000
15 Hampshire St, Mansfield, MA 02048

Filtrona Extrusion, Inc./Pexcor Medical Products Div. 800-755-7528
764 S Athol Rd, P.O. Box 659, Athol, MA 01331

Hospira Inc. 877-946-7747
275 N Field Dr, Lake Forest, IL 60045
THORACENTESIS SET

Medi Inc 800-225-8634
75 York Ave, P.O. Box 302, Randolph, MA 02368

Trademark Medical Llc 800-325-9044
449 Soverign Ct, St. Louis, MO 63011
Adjustable tube holder to prevent accidental disconnects.

TUBE, CULTURE *(Microbiology) 83SCS*

Bio-Medical Products Corp. 800-543-7427
10 Halstead Rd, Mendham, NJ 07945
Urine. Screw-cap, 12ml clear, sturdy, plastic tube.

Carolina Biological Supply Co. 800-334-5551
2700 York Rd, Burlington, NC 27215

Covidien Lp 508-261-8000
15 Hampshire St, Mansfield, MA 02048

Garren Scientific, Inc. 800-342-3725
15916 Blythe St Unit A, Van Nuys, CA 91406
All sizes glass and plastic.

Gen-Probe, Inc. 800-523-5001
10210 Genetic Center Dr, San Diego, CA 92121
DTS 1600 System - generates up to 1600 results in 8 hours; includes the primary equipment and ancillary items to operate the APTIMA Combo 2 Assay. DTS 400 System - generates up to 400 results in 8 hours; includes the primary equipment and ancillary items to operate the APTIMA Combo 2 Assay. DTS 800 System - generates up to 800 results in 8 hours; includes the primary equipment and ancillary items to operate the APTIMA Combo 2 Assay.

Globe Scientific, Inc. 800-394-4562
610 Winters Ave, Paramus, NJ 07652
Sterile and non-sterile.

Kimble Glass, Inc. 888-546-2531
537 Crystal Ave, Vineland, NJ 08360

Labcon North America 800-227-1466
3700 Lakeville Hwy Ste 200, Petaluma, CA 94954
10 x 75, 12 x 75, 13 x 100, 17 x 100.

Mckesson General Medical 800-446-3008
8741 Landmark Rd, Richmond, VA 23228

Micro-Bio-Logics.Inc 800-599-2847
217 Osseo Ave N, Saint Cloud, MN 56303

Quality Scientific Plastics 800-426-9595
1260 Holm Rd, Petaluma, CA 94954

Simport Plastics Ltd. 450-464-1723
2588 Bernard-Pilon, Beloeil, QUE J3G 4S5 Canada

Usa Scientific, Inc. 800-522-8477
PO Box 3565, Ocala, FL 34478

Ware Medics Glass Works, Inc. 845-429-6950
PO Box 368, Garnerville, NY 10923

TUBE, DECOMPRESSION *(General) 80SCT*

Cook Inc. 800-457-4500
PO Box 489, Bloomington, IN 47402

TUBE, DECOMPRESSION *(cont'd)*

Medovations, Inc. 800-558-6408
102 E Keefe Ave, Milwaukee, WI 53212

TUBE, DIALYSATE *(Gastro/Urology) 78FID*

Apheresis Technologies, Inc. 800-749-9284
PO Box 2081, Palm Harbor, FL 34682
Plasma exchange tubeset.

Lucomed Inc. 800-633-7877
45 Kulick Rd, Fairfield, NJ 07004
Hemodialysis blood tubing.

TUBE, DOUBLE LUMEN FOR INTESTINAL DECOMPRESSION
(Gastro/Urology) 78FEG

Andersen Products, Inc., 800-523-1276
3202 Caroline Dr, Health Science Park, Haw River, NC 27258
ANDERSEN.

Cook Endoscopy 336-744-0157
4900 Bethania Station Rd # &, 5951 Grassy Creek Blvd. Winston Salem, NC 27105
Colonic irrigation and aspiration catheter, gastrointestinal tube.

Cook Inc. 800-457-4500
PO Box 489, Bloomington, IN 47402

Covidien Lp 508-261-8000
15 Hampshire St, Mansfield, MA 02048

Filtrona Extrusion, Inc./Pexcor Medical Products Div. 800-755-7528
764 S Athol Rd, P.O. Box 659, Athol, MA 01331

Medovations, Inc. 800-558-6408
102 E Keefe Ave, Milwaukee, WI 53212

Neo Medical Inc. 888-450-3334
42514 Albrae St, Fremont, CA 94538
Gastro intestinal decompression tube.

Sunlite Plastics, Inc. 262-253-0600
W194N11340 McCormick Dr, Germantown, WI 53022

Terumo Cardiovascular Systems (Tcvs) 800-283-7866
28 Howe St, Ashland, MA 01721
Decompression / intubation tube.

TUBE, DRAINAGE *(Gastro/Urology) 78FFA*

Andersen Products, Inc., 800-523-1276
3202 Caroline Dr, Health Science Park, Haw River, NC 27258
ANDERSEN nasogastric tube with or without stylet, double-lumen, radio-opaque with anti-reflux filter.

Armm, Inc. 714-848-8190
17744 Sampson Ln, Huntington Beach, CA 92647
Thoracic, mediastinal, and closed wound drains.

Bentec Medical, Inc. 757-224-0177
1380 E Beamer St, Woodland, CA 95776
Suprapubic urological catheter.

Bipore, Inc. 201-767-1993
31 Industrial Pkwy, Northvale, NJ 07647

Boston Scientific Corporation 800-225-2732
1 Boston Scientific Pl, Natick, MA 01760

Cook Urological, Inc. 800-457-4500
1100 W Morgan St, P.O. Box 227, Spencer, IN 47460

Covidien Lp 508-261-8000
15 Hampshire St, Mansfield, MA 02048

Filtrona Extrusion, Inc./Pexcor Medical Products Div. 800-755-7528
764 S Athol Rd, P.O. Box 659, Athol, MA 01331

Geneva Medical Inc. 630-232-2507
2571 Kaneville Ct, Geneva, IL 60134
Sterile penrose type drain.

Gish Biomedical, Inc. 800-938-0531
22942 Arroyo Vis, Rancho Santa Margarita, CA 92688
Pleural drainage kit (chest-tube placement).

Icu Medical (Ut), Inc 949-366-2183
4455 Atherton Dr, Salt Lake City, UT 84123
Various sizes.

Ldb Medical, Inc. 800-243-2554
2909 Langford Rd Ste B500, Norcross, GA 30071

Medovations, Inc. 800-558-6408
102 E Keefe Ave, Milwaukee, WI 53212

Neo Medical Inc. 888-450-3334
42514 Albrae St, Fremont, CA 94538
Needle, intravenous sre intravadcular.

TUBE, DRAINAGE *(cont'd)*

Saint-Gobain Performance Plastics/Clearwater 800-541-6880
4451 110th Ave N, Clearwater, FL 33762
C-FLEX, non-latex, penrose drains.

Stryker Puerto Rico, Ltd. 939-307-2500
Hwy. 3, Km. 131.2, Las Guasimas Ind. Park, Arroyo, PR 00714
Evacuation tubes.

Sunlite Plastics, Inc. 262-253-0600
W194N11340 McCormick Dr, Germantown, WI 53022

Taut, Inc. 800-231-8288
2571 Kaneville Ct, Geneva, IL 60134
Suprapubic - see drain, penrose.

Urocare Products, Inc. 800-423-4441
2735 Melbourne Ave, Pomona, CA 91767
60in., 9/32in. lumen vinyl drainage tube. Also, extension tube with connector.

Zimmer Holdings, Inc. 800-613-6131
1800 W Center St, PO Box 708, Warsaw, IN 46580

Zimmer Orthopaedic Surgical Products 800-321-5533
PO Box 10, 200 West Ohio Ave., Dover, OH 44622
HEMOVAC.

TUBE, EAR SUCTION *(Ear/Nose/Throat) 77JZF*

Aesculap Implant Systems Inc. 1-800-234-9179
3773 Corporate Pkwy, Center Valley, PA 18034

Bausch & Lomb Surgical 636-255-5051
3365 Tree Court Ind Blvd, Saint Louis, MO 63122

Biomet Microfixation Inc. 800-874-7711
1520 Tradeport Dr, Jacksonville, FL 32218
Various types ear suction tubes.

Exmoor Plastics Inc. 317-244-1014
304 Gasoline Aly, Indianapolis, IN 46222
EXMOOR Tympanocentesis kit, procedure pack for infection typing (middle ear fluid).

Gyrus Ent L.L.C., Sub. Of Gyrus Acmi, Inc. 508-804-2739
2925 Appling Rd, Bartlett, TN 38133
Various types and sizes of ear suction tubes.

Spinus, Llc 603-758-1444
8 Merrill Industrial Dr, Hampton, NH 03842
Aspirator.

Surgical Instrument Manufacturers, Inc. 800-521-2985
1650 Headland Dr, Fenton, MO 63026

Symmetry Medical Usa, Inc. 574-267-8700
486 W 350 N, Warsaw, IN 46582
Ear, nose, and throat manual surgical instrument.

Tuzik Boston 800-886-6363
104 Longwater Dr, Assinippi Park, Norwell, MA 02061

TUBE, ENEMA *(Gastro/Urology) 78SCU*

Benlan Inc. 905-829-5004
2760 Brighton Rd., Oakville, ONT L6H 5T4 Canada

Cardiomed Supplies Inc. 800-387-9757
5 Gormley Industrial Ave., P.O. Box 575
Gormley, ONT L0H 1 Canada
Shandling enema catheter.

Filtrona Extrusion, Inc./Pexcor Medical Products Div. 800-755-7528
764 S Athol Rd, P.O. Box 659, Athol, MA 01331

Sunlite Plastics, Inc. 262-253-0600
W194N11340 McCormick Dr, Germantown, WI 53022

TUBE, ESOPHAGEAL, BLAKEMORE *(Gastro/Urology) 78SCV*

Brunswick Laboratories 800-362-3482
50 Commerce Way, Norton, MA 02766
EOA, EGTA - Esophageal Obturator Airway and Esophageal Gastric Tube Airway: Adjunct airway tubes to be used in an emergency environment.

TUBE, ESOPHAGEAL, REPLOGLE *(Gastro/Urology) 78SCW*

Covidien Lp 508-261-8000
15 Hampshire St, Mansfield, MA 02048

TUBE, ESOPHAGEAL, SENGSTAKEN *(Gastro/Urology) 78SCX*

E. Benson Hood Laboratories, Inc. 800-942-5227
575 Washington St, Pembroke, MA 02359

TUBE, FEEDING *(General) 80FPD*

Abbott Laboratories 800-624-7677
1033 Kingsmill Pkwy, Columbus, OH 43229
8Fr 36in. with stylet, 8Fr 45in., 8Fr 45in. with stylet, 12Fr 36in., 12Fr 45in. with stylet, 10Fr 45in. with stylet, 14Fr 36in., 16Fr 36in., enteral feeding tube. Balloon G-tubes (14Fr, 16Fr, 18Fr, 20Fr, 22Fr, 24Fr, and 26Fr); PEG kits (over-the-guidewire, introducer, versa-PEG); low-profile G-tubes (STOMATE in 18Fr and 22Fr sizes); J-tubes; and suction feeding tubes.

Accellent El Paso 915-771-9112
31 Butterfield Trail Blvd Ste C, El Paso, TX 79906
Line of external feeding sets and containers.

Benlan Inc. 905-829-5004
2760 Brighton Rd., Oakville, ONT L6H 5T4 Canada
Bulk assembled.

Biosearch Medical Products, Inc. 908-722-5000
35 Industrial Pkwy, Branchburg, NJ 08876
Biofeedback device.

Covidien Lp 508-261-8000
15 Hampshire St, Mansfield, MA 02048
ENDO-TUBE wire guided enteral feeding tube designed for precision placement in the small bowel using either endoscopy or fluoroscopy. Sold with guidewire and transfer cannula.

Entracare, Llc 913-451-2234
11315 Strang Line Rd, Lenexa, KS 66215
Enteral feeding tubes.

Ethox International 800-521-1022
251 Seneca St, Buffalo, NY 14204
Tube, feeding.

Farmatap S.A. De C.V.
117 Alfonso Esparza Oteo, Mexico Df 01020 Mexico
Alipso 1500 (system of forced feeding by tube)

Filtrona Extrusion, Inc./Pexcor Medical Products Div. 800-755-7528
764 S Athol Rd, P.O. Box 659, Athol, MA 01331

Health Care Logistics, Inc. 800-848-1633
450 Town St, PO Box 25, Circleville, OH 43113
Accessory to feeding tube/non-sterile.

Kelsar, S.A. 508-261-8000
Blvd. Insurgentes, Libriamento a La, Tijuana 22450 Mexico
Feeding tubes and sets

Manufacturing & Research, Inc.(Dba Mri Medical) 520-882-7794
4700 S Overland Dr, Tucson, AZ 85714
12Fr - 28Fr, silicone, (bi-funnel and tri-funnel); also, silicone, low profile, (balloon).

Moss Tubes, Inc. 800-827-0470
749 Columbia Tpke, East Greenbush, NY 12061
Transgastral.

Neo Medical Inc. 888-450-3334
42514 Albrae St, Fremont, CA 94538
Sterile jejunostomy feeding tube kit.

Novartis Nutrition 800-333-3785
1600 Utica Ave S Ste 600, PO Box 370, Minneapolis, MN 55416
J feeding tubes, nasogastric tubes, balloon replacement gastrostomy tube. Designed for quick and easy placement.

Sunlite Plastics, Inc. 262-253-0600
W194N11340 McCormick Dr, Germantown, WI 53022

Vital Concepts, Inc. 800-984-2300
4334 Brockton Dr SE Ste F, Grand Rapids, MI 49512
Adult and pediatric TPN connectors for feeding machines with one-way check valves and injection sites.

Vygon Corp. 800-544-4907
2495 General Armistead Ave, Norristown, PA 19403

Work, Inc. 800-898-0301
3 Arlington St, Quincy, MA 02171
ENTERAL FEEDING BAG WITH HANGER & TUBE ATTACHMENTS

Zinetics Medical, Inc. 800-648-4070
1050 E South Temple, Salt Lake City, UT 84102
Enteral feeding tube with pH level electrode/sensor at the tip; also, feeding tube.

TUBE, GASTRO-ENTEROSTOMY *(Gastro/Urology) 78KGC*

Abbott Laboratories 800-624-7677
1033 Kingsmill Pkwy, Columbus, OH 43229

Ballard Medical Products 770-587-7835
12050 Lone Peak Pkwy, Draper, UT 84020
Arious types of feeding tubes.

TUBE, GASTRO-ENTEROSTOMY *(cont'd)*

Bard Shannon Limited 908-277-8000
San Geronimo Industrial Park, Lot # 1, Road # 3, Km 79.7
Humacao, PR 00791
Feeding line.

Boston Scientific Corporation 508-652-5578
780 Brookside Dr, Spencer, IN 47460

Cook Endoscopy 336-744-0157
4900 Bethania Station Rd # &, 5951 Grassy Creek Blvd.
Winston Salem, NC 27105
Various sterile gastrostomy kits.

E K Industries, Inc. 877-EKI-CHEM
1403 Herkimer St, Joliet, IL 60432
Gomorl's trichrome stain.

Ethox International 800-521-1022
251 Seneca St, Buffalo, NY 14204
Tube, gastrostomy.

Manufacturing & Research, Inc.(Dba Mri Medical) 520-882-7794
4700 S Overland Dr, Tucson, AZ 85714
12-28Fr., silicone.

Moss Tubes, Inc. 800-827-0470
749 Columbia Tpke, East Greenbush, NY 12061

Southside Biotechnology 440-974-4074
8780 Tyler Blvd, Mentor, OH 44060
14,20,24 and 28-fr. silicone mushroom-head P.E.G. catheters.

TUBE, GASTROINTESTINAL *(Gastro/Urology) 78KNT*

Abbott Laboratories 800-624-7677
1033 Kingsmill Pkwy, Columbus, OH 43229
Basic and other gastrostomy kits with various sizes (14Fr, 16Fr, 18Fr, 20Fr, 22Fr, 24Fr, 26Fr). STOMATE low-profile gastrostomy devices in 18Fr and 22Fr sizes. Laparoscopic G-tube in 18 Fr size.

Andersen Products, Inc., 800-523-1276
3202 Caroline Dr, Health Science Park, Haw River, NC 27258
ANDERSEN long-weighted intestinal tube does not require mercury.

Applied Medical Technology, Inc. 800-869-7382
8000 Katherine Blvd, Brecksville, OH 44141
Percutaneous endoscopic gastrostomy, low-profile feeding devices; feeding accessories. New products include the Monarch G-Tube, a non-balloon gastrostomy tube for percutaneous placement/balloon replacement.

Autovage 412-653-5888
1631 Citation Dr, South Park, PA 15129
Gastric lavage kit.

B. Braun Of Puerto Rico, Inc. 610-691-5400
215.7 Insular Rd., Sabana Grande, PR 00637
Gavage administration set.

Ballard Medical Products 770-587-7835
12050 Lone Peak Pkwy, Draper, UT 84020
Enternal feeding tubes and accessories.

Bard Shannon Limited 908-277-8000
San Geronimo Industrial Park, Lot # 1, Road # 3, Km 79.7
Humacao, PR 00791
Feeding line.

Biosearch Medical Products, Inc. 908-722-5000
35 Industrial Pkwy, Branchburg, NJ 08876
Needle catheter jejunostomy kit.

Boston Scientific Corporation 508-652-5578
780 Brookside Dr, Spencer, IN 47460

Cook Endoscopy 336-744-0157
4900 Bethania Station Rd # &, 5951 Grassy Creek Blvd.
Winston Salem, NC 27105
Various gastroiontestinal tamponade cuffs, balloons, tubes.

Cook Inc. 800-457-4500
PO Box 489, Bloomington, IN 47402

Corpak Medsystems, Inc. 800-323-6305
100 Chaddick Dr, Wheeling, IL 60090
Tubes, gastrointestinal (and accessories).

Ethox International 800-521-1022
251 Seneca St, Buffalo, NY 14204
Gastrointestinal tube and accessories.

Icu Medical (Ut), Inc 949-366-2183
4455 Atherton Dr, Salt Lake City, UT 84123
Gastric valve-gastric lavage kit.

Icu Medical, Inc. 800-824-7890
951 Calle Amanecer, San Clemente, CA 92673
Gastric valve/gastric lavage kit.

TUBE, GASTROINTESTINAL *(cont'd)*

Medevices, Inc. 847-548-8499
888 E Belvidere Rd Ste 212, Grayslake, IL 60030
Dual lumen operational indicator.

Medovations, Inc. 800-558-6408
102 E Keefe Ave, Milwaukee, WI 53212

Navion Biomedical Corp. 781-341-8058
312 Tosca Dr, Stoughton, MA 02072
Bionavigation System feeding tube and catheter locating system. Sensor stylet and handheld electronic instrument used for tracking feeding tubes and central catheters during placement.

Neo Medical Inc. 888-450-3334
42514 Albrae St, Fremont, CA 94538
Gastro-j-cath gastrojejunal tube.

Neo-Care Arrow International 800-640-6428
5714 Epsilon, San Antonio, TX 78249
Neonatal.

Novartis Nutrition 800-333-3785
1600 Utica Ave S Ste 600, PO Box 370, Minneapolis, MN 55416
Stay-Put nasojejunal tubes.

Utah Medical Products, Inc. 800-533-4984
7043 Cottonwood St, Midvale, UT 84047
NUTRI-CATH neonatal silicone feeding tube for nasogastric or orogastric enteral feedings, in multiple sizes & lengths.

Vygon Corp. 800-544-4907
2495 General Armistead Ave, Norristown, PA 19403

TUBE, GASTROINTESTINAL DECOMPRESSION, BAKER JEJUNOSTOMY *(Gastro/Urology) 78VHP*

Abbott Laboratories 800-624-7677
1033 Kingsmill Pkwy, Columbus, OH 43229

Manufacturing & Research, Inc.(Dba Mri Medical) 520-882-7794
4700 S Overland Dr, Tucson, AZ 85714
Silicone.

TUBE, GASTROINTESTINAL DECOMPRESSION, CANTOR *(Gastro/Urology) 78SDB*

Andersen Products, Inc., 800-523-1276
3202 Caroline Dr, Health Science Park, Haw River, NC 27258
ANDERSEN tungsten-weighted intestinal tube does not require mercury.

TUBE, GASTROINTESTINAL DECOMPRESSION, MILLER-ABBOTT *(Gastro/Urology) 78SDD*

Andersen Products, Inc., 800-523-1276
3202 Caroline Dr, Health Science Park, Haw River, NC 27258
ANDERSEN.

TUBE, IMAGE AMPLIFIER, X-RAY *(Radiology) 90IZE*

Flow X-Ray Corporation 800-356-9729
100 W Industry Ct, Deer Park, NY 11729
DIGITAL X-Ray machine

Precise Optics/Pme, Inc. 800-242-6604
239 S Fehr Way, Bay Shore, NY 11706

Spellman High Voltage Electronics Corp. 631-630-3000
475 Wireless Blvd, Hauppauge, NY 11788

Thales Components Corporation 973-812-9000
40G Commerce Way, PO Box 540, Totowa, NJ 07512
X-ray image amplifier tube, tetrode power grid tubes, raditation therapy microwave tubes, charged coupled devices, solid state x-ray detectors.

Varian Medical Systems X-Ray Products 800-432-4422
1678 Pioneer Rd, Salt Lake City, UT 84104

TUBE, LARYNGECTOMY *(Ear/Nose/Throat) 77KAC*

Bausch & Lomb Surgical 636-255-5051
3365 Tree Court Ind Blvd, Saint Louis, MO 63122

Bentec Medical, Inc. 757-224-0177
1380 E Beamer St, Woodland, CA 95776
Laryngectomy tube.

E. Benson Hood Laboratories, Inc. 800-942-5227
575 Washington St, Pembroke, MA 02359
T-tubes, full size (27 sizes) range available.

TUBE, LEVINE *(General) 80FRQ*

Benlan Inc. 905-829-5004
2760 Brighton Rd., Oakville, ONT L6H 5T4 Canada

Covidien Lp 508-261-8000
15 Hampshire St, Mansfield, MA 02048

TUBE, LEVINE *(cont'd)*

Medline Manufacturing And Services Llc 847-837-2759
1 Medline Pl, Mundelein, IL 60060
Levine tubes, various.

Mmj S.A. De C.V. 314-654-2000
716 Ponciano Arriaga, Cd. Juarez, Chih. Mexico
Various

TUBE, MYRINGOTOMY *(Ear/Nose/Throat) 77SDE*

Exmoor Plastics Inc. 317-244-1014
304 Gasoline Aly, Indianapolis, IN 46222
Various patterns supplied sterile, priced from $3.60 each.

Micromedics 800-624-5662
1270 Eagan Industrial Rd, Saint Paul, MN 55121
Dozens of designs, six different materials, and convenient packaging choices.

Oto-Med, Inc. 800-433-7703
1090 Empire Dr, Lake Havasu City, AZ 86404
Sheehy Collar Button, Teflon

Saint-Gobain Performance Plastics/Clearwater 800-541-6880
4451 110th Ave N, Clearwater, FL 33762

Shippert Medical Technologies Corp. 800-888-8663
6248 S Troy Cir Ste A, Centennial, CO 80111
Full line of Ear Ventilation Tubes.

TUBE, NASOGASTRIC *(Anesthesiology) 73BSS*

Abbott Laboratories 800-624-7677
1033 Kingsmill Pkwy, Columbus, OH 43229
8Fr 36in. with stylet, 8Fr 45in., 8Fr 45in. with stylet, 12Fr 36in., 12Fr 45in. with stylet, 10Fr 45in. with stylet, and 14Fr 36in. enteral feeding tube. 12Fr and 16Fr 36in. clear with radiopaque strip feeding tubes. Pediatric nasogastric tubes also available - 5Fr and 8Fr, 17in., PVC tubes.

Andersen Products, Inc., 800-523-1276
3202 Caroline Dr, Health Science Park, Haw River, NC 27258
ANDERSEN nasogastric tube with or without stylet, double-lumen, radio-opaque with anti-reflux filter.

Benlan Inc. 905-829-5004
2760 Brighton Rd., Oakville, ONT L6H 5T4 Canada

Biosearch Medical Products, Inc. 908-722-5000
35 Industrial Pkwy, Branchburg, NJ 08876
Enteral feeding tube or nasogastric feeding tube.

Boston Medical Products, Inc. 800-433-2674
117 Flanders Rd, Westborough, MA 01581
Pharyngeal salivary bypass tube, for major oropharyngeal, laryngeal and esophageal resections in patients at high risk for development of postoperative fistula.

Covidien Lp 508-261-8000
15 Hampshire St, Mansfield, MA 02048

Kelsar, S.A. 508-261-8000
Blvd. Insurgentes, Libriamento a La, Tijuana 22450 Mexico
Silicone salem sump tubes w/wo arv

Manufacturing & Research, Inc.(Dba Mri Medical) 520-882-7794
4700 S Overland Dr, Tucson, AZ 85714
Nasal silicone gastrostomy and other 12-28Fr. silicone gastrostomy tubes.

Mormac Tube Guard Co. 800-445-2868
PO Box 40, Main St., North Loup, NE 68859
MORMAC Tube Guard tube holder for 8, 10, 14 and 18 Fr. single lumen and 18 Fr. double lumen nasogastric tubes.

Novartis Nutrition 800-333-3785
1600 Utica Ave S Ste 600, PO Box 370, Minneapolis, MN 55416

Omni Medical Supply Inc. 800-860-6664
4153 Pioneer Dr, Commerce Township, MI 48390

Trademark Medical Llc 800-325-9044
449 Soverign Ct, St. Louis, MO 63011
ANTI-REFLUX VALVE preventing reflux occuring from double lumen N/G tubes. Also anti-reflux valve for nasogastric sump tubes to prevent spills. Also available anti reflux valve for use with nasogastric tubes.

TUBE, NEPHROSTOMY *(Gastro/Urology) 78SDF*

Cook Urological, Inc. 800-457-4500
1100 W Morgan St, P.O. Box 227, Spencer, IN 47460

TUBE, ORTHODONTIC *(Dental And Oral) 76DZD*

American Orthodontics Corp. 800-558-7687
1714 Cambridge Ave, Sheboygan, WI 53081

TUBE, ORTHODONTIC *(cont'd)*

Classone Orthodontics, Inc. 806-799-0608
5064 50th St, Lubbock, TX 79414
Various types of tubing.

Forestadent Usa 314-878-5985
2315 Weldon Pkwy, Saint Louis, MO 63146
Orthodontic tube.

G & H Wire Co. 800-526-1026
2165 Earlywood Dr, Franklin, IN 46131
Weldable and bondable buccal tubes

Lancer Orthodontics, Inc. 760-304-2705
253 Pawnee St, San Marcos, CA 92078
Various sizes and styles of orthodontic tubes.

Ortho Organizers, Inc. 760-448-8730
1822 Aston Ave, Carlsbad, CA 92008
Various types of orthodontic buccal tubes.

Orthodontic Design And Production, Inc. 760-734-3995
1370 Decision St Ste D, Vista, CA 92081
Various types of orthodontic tubes.

Oscar, Inc. 317-849-2618
11793 Technology Ln, Fishers, IN 46038
Buccal tubes-various sizes.

Strite Industries Ltd. 800-267-7333
298 Shepherd Ave., Cambridge, ON N3C 1V1 Canada
$3.95 for single metal buccal tubes; $4.55 for double metal buccal tube.

Tp Orthodontics, Inc. 800-348-8856
100 Center Plz, La Porte, IN 46350
Molar.

3m Unitek 800-634-5300
2724 Peck Rd, Monrovia, CA 91016

TUBE, PUMP, CARDIOPULMONARY BYPASS *(Cardiovascular) 74DWE*

Cardiomed Supplies Inc. 800-387-9757
5 Gormley Industrial Ave., P.O. Box 575
Gormley, ONT L0H 1 Canada
CORD CARE device to facilitate placement of endotracheal tube

Gish Biomedical, Inc. 800-938-0531
22942 Arroyo Vis, Rancho Santa Margarita, CA 92688
Custom tube packs for extracorporeal, ECMO perfusion and bypass procedures.

Jostra Bentley, Inc. 302-454-9959
Rd. 402 N. Km 1.4, Industrial Park, Anasco, PR 00610-1577
Surgical grade tubing.

Medtronic Blood Management 612-514-4000
18501 E Plaza Dr, Parker, CO 80134
Tubing.

Medtronic Perfusion Systems 800-854-3570
7611 Northland Dr N, Brooklyn Park, MN 55428

Novosci Corp. 281-363-4949
2828 N Crescentridge Dr, The Woodlands, TX 77381

Sorin Group Usa 800-289-5759
14401 W 65th Way, Arvada, CO 80004

Terumo Cardiovascular Systems (Tcvs) 800-283-7866
125 Blue Ball Rd, Elkton, MD 21921
Pump tubing.

Terumo Cardiovascular Systems (Tcvs) 800-283-7866
28 Howe St, Ashland, MA 01721
Pump tubing.

Terumo Cardiovascular Systems, Corp 800-521-2818
6200 Jackson Rd, Ann Arbor, MI 48103

TUBE, RECTAL *(Gastro/Urology) 78SDH*

Benlan Inc. 905-829-5004
2760 Brighton Rd., Oakville, ONT L6H 5T4 Canada
Bulk assembled.

Manufacturing & Research, Inc.(Dba Mri Medical) 520-882-7794
4700 S Overland Dr, Tucson, AZ 85714
Custom silicone balloon catheters.

TUBE, SEDIMENTATION RATE *(Hematology) 81GHC*

Becton Dickinson And Company 800-284-6845
1 Becton Dr, Franklin Lakes, NJ 07417
Multiple

TUBE, SEDIMENTATION RATE *(cont'd)*

Chase Scientific Glass, Inc. 412-490-8425
234 Cardiff Valley Rd, Rockwood, TN 37854
Multiple.

Dade Behring, Inc. 800-948-3233
1717 Deerfield Rd, Deerfield, IL 60015

Globe Scientific, Inc. 800-394-4562
610 Winters Ave, Paramus, NJ 07652
SEDIGREN and SEDI-RATE sedimentation-rate vials for Westergren procedure.

Kimble Chase Life Science And Research Products, Llc. 865-717-2635
234 Cardiff Valley Rd, Ozone, TN 37854

Serum International Inc. 800-361-7726
4400 Autoroute Chomeoey, Laval, QUE H7R-6E9 Canada

Ware Medics Glass Works, Inc. 845-429-6950
PO Box 368, Garnerville, NY 10923

TUBE, SHUNT, ENDOLYMPHATIC *(Ear/Nose/Throat) 77ESZ*

E. Benson Hood Laboratories, Inc. 800-942-5227
575 Washington St, Pembroke, MA 02359
Huang/Gibson inner ear shunt.

TUBE, SHUNT, ENDOLYMPHATIC, WITH VALVE
(Ear/Nose/Throat) 77KLZ

E. Benson Hood Laboratories, Inc. 800-942-5227
575 Washington St, Pembroke, MA 02359
Arenberg inner ear valve shunt.

TUBE, SINGLE LUMEN, W MERCURY WT BALLOON
(Gastro/Urology) 78FEF

Covidien Lp 508-261-8000
15 Hampshire St, Mansfield, MA 02048

TUBE, SMOKE REMOVAL, ENDOSCOPIC *(Gastro/Urology) 78FCZ*

Maquet, Inc. 843-552-8652
7371 Spartan Blvd E, N Charleston, SC 29418
Various types of tubing for smoke removal.

Megadyne Medical Products, Inc. 800-747-6110
11506 S State St, Draper, UT 84020
The unique MEGA VAC Plus smoke evacuator can effectively remove smoke from the abdominal cavity without deflating the pneumoperitoneum.

Richard Wolf Medical Instruments Corp. 800-323-9653
353 Corporate Woods Pkwy, Vernon Hills, IL 60061

TUBE, STOMACH EVACUATOR (GASTRIC LAVAGE)
(Gastro/Urology) 78SDI

Benlan Inc. 905-829-5004
2760 Brighton Rd., Oakville, ONT L6H 5T4 Canada
Bulk assembled.

Vygon Corp. 800-544-4907
2495 General Armistead Ave, Norristown, PA 19403

TUBE, SUCTION *(General) 80WNO*

Armm, Inc. 714-848-8190
17744 Sampson Ln, Huntington Beach, CA 92647
Plastic / PVC.

Benlan Inc. 905-829-5004
2760 Brighton Rd., Oakville, ONT L6H 5T4 Canada

Filtrona Extrusion, Inc./Pexcor Medical Products Div. 800-755-7528
764 S Athol Rd, P.O. Box 659, Athol, MA 01331

Hager Worldwide, Inc. 800-328-2335
13322 Byrd Dr, Odessa, FL 33556
CLEAN FLEX (HVE, SE, air/water syringe tubing).

Medovations, Inc. 800-558-6408
102 E Keefe Ave, Milwaukee, WI 53212

Sunrise Medical 800-333-4000
7477 Dry Creek Pkwy, Longmont, CO 80503

Vital Concepts, Inc. 800-984-2300
4334 Brockton Dr SE Ste F, Grand Rapids, MI 49512
Bifurcated, trifurcated, quadfurcated irrigation tubing.

Vygon Corp. 800-544-4907
2495 General Armistead Ave, Norristown, PA 19403

TUBE, TEST *(Chemistry) 75RZV*

Aidlab, Inc. 416-410-5377
60 5th Street., Toronto, ONT M2N-6N1 Canada
AIDLAB; test tube and culture. Borosilicate glass round or flat bottom screw thread tubes for culture media. O.D. range - 13-25 mm, length 65mm to 150mm.

Berghof/America 800-544-5004
3773 NW 126th Ave Bldg 1, Coral Springs, FL 33065
PTFE test tubes with round bottom available with standard joints for stoppers, or PFA test tubes available with screw cap. Graduated cylinders also available.

Bio-Rad Laboratories, Life Science Group 800-424-6723
2000 Alfred Nobel Dr, Hercules, CA 94547
Micro test tubes for PCR featuring uniform walls for even heat transfer. Tubes fit thermal cyclers and are autoclavable up to 120 degrees C.

Carolina Biological Supply Co. 800-334-5551
2700 York Rd, Burlington, NC 27215

Edmund Industrial Optics 800-363-1992
101 E Gloucester Pike, Barrington, NJ 08007

Elabsupply 714-446-8740
1001 Starbuck St Apt C306, Fullerton, CA 92833
LABAID Test Tubes made from clear polypropylene or transparent poystrene. Round bottom, ideal for numerous testing applications. Available in plug cap for tight sealing, snap cap for easy handling, or no cap for simple testing.

Globe Scientific, Inc. 800-394-4562
610 Winters Ave, Paramus, NJ 07652
Complete range from 11 x 70 mm to 50 x 120 mm.

Kimble Glass, Inc. 888-546-2531
537 Crystal Ave, Vineland, NJ 08360
KIMAX.

Midwest Scientific 800-227-9997
280 Vance Rd, Valley Park, MO 63088
50-mL tubes - 50BS bulk, 50RS racked, sterile, graduated, caps; 15-mL tubes - 15BS bulk, 15RS racked, sterile, graduated, caps.

Quality Scientific Plastics 800-426-9595
1260 Holm Rd, Petaluma, CA 94954

Quartz Scientific, Inc. 800-229-2186
819 East St, Fairport Harbor, OH 44077

Simport Plastics Ltd. 450-464-1723
2588 Bernard-Pilon, Beloeil, QUE J3G 4S5 Canada

TUBE, THORPE, UNCOMPENSATED *(Anesthesiology) 73BYM*

Ingen Technologies, Inc. 757-224-0177
35193 Avenue A Apt C, Yucaipa, CA 92399
Flow meter.

TUBE, TISSUE CULTURE *(Pathology) 88KJG*

Chase Scientific Glass, Inc. 412-490-8425
234 Cardiff Valley Rd, Rockwood, TN 37854
Various tissue culture tubes.

Kimble Chase Life Science And Research Products, Llc. 865-717-2635
234 Cardiff Valley Rd, Ozone, TN 37854

TUBE, TONSIL SUCTION *(Ear/Nose/Throat) 77KCB*

Aesculap Implant Systems Inc. 1-800-234-9179
3773 Corporate Pkwy, Center Valley, PA 18034

Bausch & Lomb Surgical 636-255-5051
3365 Tree Court Ind Blvd, Saint Louis, MO 63122

Biomet Microfixation Inc. 800-874-7711
1520 Tradeport Dr, Jacksonville, FL 32218
Various types of tubes, tonsil suction.

E.A. Beck & Co. 949-645-4072
657 W 19th St Ste E, P O Box 10857, Costa Mesa, CA 92627
Suction tip; yankauer.

George Tiemann & Co. 800-843-6266
25 Plant Ave, Hauppauge, NY 11788

Medline Industries, Inc. 800-633-5886
1 Medline Pl, Mundelein, IL 60060

Novosci Corp. 281-363-4949
2828 N Crescentridge Dr, The Woodlands, TX 77381

Spinus, Llc 603-758-1444
8 Merrill Industrial Dr, Hampton, NH 03842
Multi-function suction instrument.

TUBE, TONSIL SUCTION *(cont'd)*

Symmetry Medical Usa, Inc. 574-267-8700
486 W 350 N, Warsaw, IN 46582
Ear, nose, and throat manual surgical instrument.

Tuzik Boston 800-886-6363
104 Longwater Dr, Assinippi Park, Norwell, MA 02061

TUBE, TRACHEAL (ENDOTRACHEAL) *(Anesthesiology) 73BTR*

Aesculap Implant Systems Inc. 1-800-234-9179
3773 Corporate Pkwy, Center Valley, PA 18034

Ambu A/S 457-225-2210
6740 Baymeadow Dr, Glen Burnie, MD 21060
Tubechek.

Arcadia Medical Corporation 847-330-4447
1450 American Ln Ste 1400, Schaumburg, IL 60173
100% Silicone Wire Reinforced Endotracheal Tubes in Cuffless or Air Cuff Models. Complete range of Pediatric and Adult sizes.

Avalon Laboratories, Inc. 866-938-6613
2610 Homestead Pl, Rancho Dominguez, CA 90220

Ballard Medical Products 770-587-7835
12050 Lone Peak Pkwy, Draper, UT 84020
Trans-tracheal catheter.

Cardiomed Supplies Inc. 800-387-9757
5 Gormley Industrial Ave., P.O. Box 575
Gormley, ONT L0H 1 Canada
Tube to provide ventilation during difficult intubatior/extubation.

Codman & Shurtleff, Inc 800-225-0460
325 Paramount Dr, Raynham, MA 02767

Covidien Lp 508-261-8000
15 Hampshire St, Mansfield, MA 02048

Dixie Ems Supply 800-347-3494
385 Union Ave, Brooklyn, NY 11211
$16.90 per 10 (Murphy, 6mm).

Dma Med-Chem Corporation 800-362-1833
49 Watermill Ln, Great Neck, NY 11021

Filtrona Extrusion, Inc./Pexcor Medical Products Div. 800-755-7528
764 S Athol Rd, P.O. Box 659, Athol, MA 01331

Gyrus Acmi, Inc. 508-804-2739
93 N Pleasant St, Norwalk, OH 44857
Intubation catheter.

Gyrus Acmi, Inc. 508-804-2739
300 Stillwater P.o.box 1971, Stamford, CT 06902
Intubation catheter.

Invotec Intl. 800-998-8580
6833 Phillips Industrial Blvd, Jacksonville, FL 32256
Tracheal T-tube.

Kentron Health Care, Inc. 615-384-0573
3604 Kelton Jackson Rd, P.o. Box 120, Springfield, TN 37172
Endotracheal tubes.

Lampac International Ltd. 636-797-3659
230 N Lake Dr, Hillsboro, MO 63050
Available cuffed and uncuffed.

Medline Industries, Inc. 800-633-5886
1 Medline Pl, Mundelein, IL 60060

Miltex Inc. 800-645-8000
589 Davies Dr, York, PA 17402

Parker Medical 303-799-1990
7275 S Revere Pkwy Ste 804, Centennial, CO 80112
The endotracheal tube's patented, soft, and flexible tip facilitates intubation by improving tip visibility, resulting in easier insertion and gentle skiing down tracheal walls.

Pulmonx 650-934-2604
1047 Elwell Ct, Palo Alto, CA 94303
Sterile tracheal tube//bronchoscope & fiberoptic lightsource & video display.

Rose Technologies Company 616-233-3000
1440 Front Ave NW, Grand Rapids, MI 49504

Smiths Medical Asd 800-424-8662
5700 W 23rd Ave, Gary, IN 46406
FOME-CUF, AIRE-CUF & TTS; Silicone with and without wire reinforced shafts; adult and pediatric. Also available for CO2 laser surgery with silicone jacketed armature with FOME-CUF.

Smiths Medical Asd, Inc. 610-578-9600
9255 Customhouse Plz Ste N, San Diego, CA 92154
Airwat intubation set with accessories (sterile & non-sterile).

TUBE, TRACHEAL (ENDOTRACHEAL) *(cont'd)*

Sun-Med 800-433-2797
12393 Belcher Rd S Ste 450, Largo, FL 33773
The Endotracheal Tube Introducer is Sterile & Disposable. The Disposable Bougie is Manufactured from Low Density Polyethylene & Provides Proper Stiffness for Ease of Insertion.

Unomedical, Inc. 800-634-6003
5701 S Ware Rd Ste 1, McAllen, TX 78503

Utah Medical Products, Inc. 800-533-4984
7043 Cottonwood St, Midvale, UT 84047
PALA-NATE, silicone molded to fit neonates upper mouth designed to protect against palatal grooves.

Vygon Corp. 800-544-4907
2495 General Armistead Ave, Norristown, PA 19403

Wolfe Tory Medical, Inc. 801-281-3000
79 W 4500 S Ste 18, Salt Lake City, UT 84107
Esophageal detector device.

TUBE, TRACHEAL/BRONCHIAL, DIFFERENTIAL VENTILATION *(Anesthesiology) 73CBI*

Passy-Muir Inc. 800-634-5397
4521 Campus Dr, Irvine, CA 92612
Passy-Muir™ closed-position 'no leak' Tracheostomy & Ventilator Swallowing and Speaking valves (PMVs.) The only swallowing & speaking valves that are interchangeable for use on or off the ventilator (with the exception of the PMV™ 2020 for metal trach tubes.) Independent research has shown that the closed position PMV improves swallowing, reduces aspiration, facilitates secretion management, and reduces weaning and decannulation time. Reimbursable by Medicare, Medicaid, MediCal, and CCS.

Smiths Medical Asd 800-424-8662
5700 W 23rd Ave, Gary, IN 46406

Vitaid Ltd. 800-267-9301
300 International Dr, Williamsville, NY 14221
TCB Univent Bronchial Blocking Tube. 'Uni-Blocker' bronchial blocker. 'SilBroncho' all silicone rubber double lumen tubes

TUBE, TRACHEOSTOMY (BREATHING TUBE), ENT *(Ear/Nose/Throat) 77EQK*

Bausch & Lomb Surgical 636-255-5051
3365 Tree Court Ind Blvd, Saint Louis, MO 63122

Boston Medical Products, Inc. 800-433-2674
117 Flanders Rd, Westborough, MA 01581
Montgomery silicone tracheal cannula system. TRACOE TRACHEOSTOMY long-term tube product line. 6 models, sizes from pediatric to large adult.

Catalent Pharma Solutions 866-720-3148
2200 Lake Shore Dr, Woodstock, IL 60098
Multiple

Covidien Lp 508-261-8000
15 Hampshire St, Mansfield, MA 02048

Dixie Ems Supply 800-347-3494
385 Union Ave, Brooklyn, NY 11211
$169.50 per 10 (8mm, 32fr).

E. Benson Hood Laboratories, Inc. 800-942-5227
575 Washington St, Pembroke, MA 02359
Stoma stent system.

Passy-Muir Inc. 800-634-5397
4521 Campus Dr, Irvine, CA 92612
Passy-Muir™ closed-position 'no leak' Tracheostomy & Ventilator Swallowing and Speaking valves (PMVs.) The only swallowing & speaking valves that are interchangeable for use on or off the ventilator (with the exception of the PMV™ 2020 for metal trach tubes.) Independent research has shown that the closed position PMV improves swallowing, reduces aspiration, facilitates secretion management, and reduces weaning and decannulation time. Reimbursable by Medicare, Medicaid, MediCal, and CCS.

Smiths Medical Asd 800-424-8662
5700 W 23rd Ave, Gary, IN 46406
AIRE-CUF, FOME-CUF & TTS Silicone fixed and adjustable neck flange; Adult and pediatric.

TUBE, TRACHEOSTOMY (W/WO CONNECTOR) *(Anesthesiology) 73BTO*

Arcadia Medical Corporation 847-330-4447
1450 American Ln Ste 1400, Schaumburg, IL 60173
100% Silicone Wire Reinforced Tracheostomy Tubes in Pediatric, Neonatal, Adult and Adjustable sytles. Available in cuffless, air cuff or foam cuff models. Custom Tracheostomy Tubes are also available.

TUBE, TRACHEOSTOMY (W/WO CONNECTOR) *(cont'd)*

Biomet Microfixation Inc. 800-874-7711
1520 Tradeport Dr, Jacksonville, FL 32218
Tracheostomy tube.

Busse Hospital Disposables, Inc. 631-435-4711
75 Arkay Dr, Hauppauge, NY 11788
Sterile trach care kit(s).

Crandall Medical Devices 949-369-9954
2209 Via Gavilan, San Clemente, CA 92673
Product engineering

Intl. Medical, Inc. 952-890-6547
14470 W Burnsville Pkwy, Burnsville, MN 55306
Double swivel connectors.

Passy-Muir Inc. 800-634-5397
4521 Campus Dr, Irvine, CA 92612
Passy-Muir™ closed-position 'no leak' Tracheostomy & Ventilator Swallowing and Speaking valves (PMVs.) The only swallowing & speaking valves that are interchangeable for use on or off the ventilator (with the exception of the PMV™ 2020 for metal trach tubes.) Independent research has shown that the closed position PMV improves swallowing, reduces aspiration, facilitates secretion management, and reduces weaning and decannulation time. Reimbursable by Medicare, Medicaid, MediCal, and CCS.

Respironics California, Inc. 724-387-4559
2271 Cosmos Ct, Carlsbad, CA 92011
Tube,tracheostomy.

Smiths Medical Asd 800-424-8662
5700 W 23rd Ave, Gary, IN 46406
AIRE-CUF, FOME-CUF & TTS Silicone fixed and adjustable neck flange; Adult and pediatric.

TUBE, TRANSFER *(General) 80SDJ*

Ace Surgical Supply Co., Inc. 800-441-3100
1034 Pearl St, Brockton, MA 02301

Bd Diagnostic Systems 800-675-0908
7 Loveton Cir, Sparks, MD 21152

Bio-Medical Products Corp. 800-543-7427
10 Halstead Rd, Mendham, NJ 07945
URI-TUBE plastic vacuum tube containing a preservative for C & S specimens. Urinalysis and urine culture transport tube. Closed system.

Dade Behring, Inc. 800-948-3233
1717 Deerfield Rd, Deerfield, IL 60015

Filtrona Extrusion, Inc./Pexcor Medical Products Div. 800-755-7528
764 S Athol Rd, P.O. Box 659, Athol, MA 01331

Globe Scientific, Inc. 800-394-4562
610 Winters Ave, Paramus, NJ 07652
Transfer pipettes.

Simport Plastics Ltd. 450-464-1723
2588 Bernard-Pilon, Beloeil, QUE J3G 4S5 Canada

TUBE, TYMPANOSTOMY *(Ear/Nose/Throat) 77ETD*

Bausch & Lomb Surgical 636-255-5051
3365 Tree Court Ind Blvd, Saint Louis, MO 63122

Gyrus Ent L.L.C., Sub. Of Gyrus Acmi, Inc. 508-804-2739
2925 Appling Rd, Bartlett, TN 38133
Various types and sizes of tympanostomy tubes.

Invotec Intl. 800-998-8580
6833 Phillips Industrial Blvd, Jacksonville, FL 32256

Micromedics 800-624-5662
1270 Eagan Industrial Rd, Saint Paul, MN 55121
Dozens of designs, six different materials, and convenient packaging choices.

Santa Barbara Medco, Inc. 651-452-1977
1270 Eagan Industrial Rd, Eagan, MN 55121
Ventilation tubes.

TUBE, VACUUM SAMPLE, WITH ANTICOAGULANT
(Hematology) 81GIM

Artefactos De Vidrio S.A. De C.V.
Canela, Granjas Mexico 346, Ciudad De Mexico 08400 Mexico
Various types of sterile and blood collection vacuum tubes with or

Covidien Lp 508-261-8000
15 Hampshire St, Mansfield, MA 02048

Greiner Bio-One North America, Inc. 410-592-2060
4238 Capital Dr, Monroe, NC 28110
Various types & sizes, sterile blood collection tubes w/ anticoagulant.

TUBE, VACUUM SAMPLE, WITH ANTICOAGULANT *(cont'd)*

International Technidyne Corp. 800-631-5945
23 Nevsky St, Edison, NJ 08820

Varian Sample Preparation Products 800-421-2825
24201 Frampton Ave, Harbor City, CA 90710
Liquid extraction tubes, sample preparation, also vacuum manifolds, sample preparation.

TUBE, X-RAY *(Radiology) 90VHF*

Afp Imaging Corp. 800-592-6666
250 Clearbrook Rd, Elmsford, NY 10523

Americomp, Inc. 800-458-1782
2901 W Lawrence Ave, Chicago, IL 60625
X-ray tube and stand.

Atlas Medical Technologies 909-923-7887
1137 E Philadelphia St, Ontario, CA 91761
CT and X-Ray tubes for most applications, installed.

Inmark Corporation 800-899-7947
4 Byington Pl, Norwalk, CT 06850
Diagnostic and CT tube assemblies for all medical applications.

M & I Medical Sales, Inc. 305-663-6444
4711 SW 72nd Ave, Miami, FL 33155

Marconi Medical Systems 800-323-0550
595 Miner Rd, Cleveland, OH 44143

Mikron Digital Imaging, Inc. 800-925-3905
30425 8 Mile Rd, Livonia, MI 48152
Service and installation.

Narragansett Imaging 401-767-4462
51 Industrial Dr, North Smithfield, RI 02896
X-ray camera tube.

Trace Laboratories-East 410-584-9099
5 N Park Dr, Hunt Valley, MD 21030
Feinfocus Cougar Series Real-Time X-Ray System

Varian Medical Systems 800-544-4636
3100 Hansen Way, Palo Alto, CA 94304
Varian Medical Systems makes X-ray tubes for CT scanners, mammography, and other medical imaging systems.

Varian Medical Systems X-Ray Products 800-432-4422
1678 Pioneer Rd, Salt Lake City, UT 84104

Xma (X-Ray Marketing Associates, Inc.) 800-325-8880
1205 W Lakeview Ct, Windham Lakes Business Park
Romeoville, IL 60446

TUBING, BRAIDED *(General) 80SDK*

Chamberlin Rubber Company, Inc. 585-427-7780
3333 Brighton Henrietta Town Line Rd, PO Box 22700
Rochester, NY 14623

Diablo Sales & Marketing, Inc. 925-648-1611
PO Box 3219, Danville, CA 94526
Custom design and manufacturing of catheters and specialty guidewires. Guiding catheters; stent delivery and drug delivery systems.

Filtrona Extrusion, Inc./Pexcor Medical Products Div. 800-755-7528
764 S Athol Rd, P.O. Box 659, Athol, MA 01331

Mercury Medical 800-237-6418
11300 49th St N, Clearwater, FL 33762

Tfx Medical Oem 800-548-6600
50 Plantation Dr, Jaffrey, NH 03452

TUBING, CONDUCTIVE *(General) 80SDL*

Anesthesia Associates, Inc. 760-744-6561
460 Enterprise St, San Marcos, CA 92078
Various types, lengths and styles of tubing available. Materials include polyester, EPDM, teflon, neoprene, and chrome plated brass. Many different end fitting available from silicone, delrin, stainless steel, chrome plated brass, teflon and neoprene.

Coeur Inc., Sheboygan 800-874-4240
3411 Behrens Pkwy, Sheboygan, WI 53081

Covidien Lp 508-261-8000
15 Hampshire St, Mansfield, MA 02048

Filtrona Extrusion, Inc./Pexcor Medical Products Div. 800-755-7528
764 S Athol Rd, P.O. Box 659, Athol, MA 01331

Medi Inc 800-225-8634
75 York Ave, P.O. Box 302, Randolph, MA 02368

Mercury Medical 800-237-6418
11300 49th St N, Clearwater, FL 33762

TUBING, CONDUCTIVE *(cont'd)*

Tfx Medical Oem 800-548-6600
50 Plantation Dr, Jaffrey, NH 03452

TUBING, CONNECTING *(General) 80WSP*

A-M Systems, Inc. 800-426-1306
131 Business Park Loop, Sequim, WA 98382
20 types (smooth interior) from $6.00 to $30.00 per tube.

Benlan Inc. 905-829-5004
2760 Brighton Rd., Oakville, ONT L6H 5T4 Canada

Carolina Biological Supply Co. 800-334-5551
2700 York Rd, Burlington, NC 27215

Engineers Express, Inc. 800-255-8823
7 Industrial Park Rd, Medway, MA 02053

Exelint International Co. 800-940-3935
5840 W Centinela Ave, Los Angeles, CA 90045
EXEL Luer Adapter and L-Holder

Filtrona Extrusion, Inc./Pexcor Medical Products Div. 800-755-7528
764 S Athol Rd, P.O. Box 659, Athol, MA 01331

Medegen 800-520-7999
930 S Wanamaker Ave, Ontario, CA 91761
Intravenous luer connectors, male and female luer-lock adaptors, caps and hubs.

Medovations, Inc. 800-558-6408
102 E Keefe Ave, Milwaukee, WI 53212
Surgical and 5-in-1 connectors.

Mps Acacia 800-486-6677
785 Challenger St, Brea, CA 92821

Novosci Corp. 281-363-4949
2828 N Crescentridge Dr, The Woodlands, TX 77381

Ormantine Usa Ltd. 321-676-7003
1740 Convair St SE, Palm Bay, FL 32909
Laboratory tubing.

Sunlite Plastics, Inc. 262-253-0600
W194N11340 McCormick Dr, Germantown, WI 53022

Vital Concepts, Inc. 800-984-2300
4334 Brockton Dr SE Ste F, Grand Rapids, MI 49512
Adult and pediatric TPN connectors with one way check valves and injection sites.

Vygon Corp. 800-544-4907
2495 General Armistead Ave, Norristown, PA 19403

TUBING, CORRUGATED *(General) 80SDM*

A-M Systems, Inc. 800-426-1306
131 Business Park Loop, Sequim, WA 98382
5 types (smooth interior, some autoclavable)

Intersurgical Inc. 315-451-2900
417 Electronics Pkwy, Liverpool, NY 13088

Mercury Medical 800-237-6418
11300 49th St N, Clearwater, FL 33762

Niche Medical, Inc. 800-633-1055
55 Access Rd, Warwick, RI 02886
Full line of corrugated and PVC tubing for use with smoke evacuation systems.

TUBING, DIALYSATE (AND CONNECTOR) *(Gastro/Urology) 78KQQ*

Molded Products Inc. 800-435-8957
1112 Chatburn Ave, Harlan, IA 51537
Dialysate Lines, Female Hansen Connectors, and Male Hansen Connectors

TUBING, FLEXIBLE, MEDICAL GAS, LOW-PRESSURE *(Anesthesiology) 73BYX*

A-M Systems, Inc. 800-426-1306
131 Business Park Loop, Sequim, WA 98382

Afton Medical Llc 707-577-0685
3137 Swetzer Rd Ste C, Loomis, CA 95650
Oxygen supply tube.

Allied Healthcare Products, Inc. 800-444-3954
1720 Sublette Ave, Saint Louis, MO 63110

Armm, Inc. 714-848-8190
17744 Sampson Ln, Huntington Beach, CA 92647

Busse Hospital Disposables, Inc. 631-435-4711
75 Arkay Dr, Hauppauge, NY 11788
Connectors, various.

TUBING, FLEXIBLE, MEDICAL GAS, LOW-PRESSURE *(cont'd)*

Coeur Inc., Sheboygan 800-874-4240
3411 Behrens Pkwy, Sheboygan, WI 53081

Corpak Medsystems, Inc. 800-323-6305
100 Chaddick Dr, Wheeling, IL 60090
Various respiratory accessories.

Covidien Lp 508-261-8000
15 Hampshire St, Mansfield, MA 02048

Datascope Corp., Cardiac Assist Division 201-307-5400
1300 MacArthur Blvd, Mahwah, NJ 07430
Pressure tubing.

Datex-Ohmeda Inc. 608-221-1551
3030 Ohmeda Dr, Madison, WI 53718
Breathing tube.

East Coast Surgical Inc. 717-361-0400
64 Pheasant Ct, Elizabethtown, PA 17022
Filtered insufflation tubing.

Filtrona Extrusion, Inc./Pexcor Medical Products Div. 800-755-7528
764 S Athol Rd, P.O. Box 659, Athol, MA 01331

Hans Rudolph, Inc. 816-363-5522
7200 Wyandotte St, Kansas City, MO 64114
Various tubing, stopcocks, directional control valves and connectors.

Instrumentation Industries, Inc. 800-633-8577
2990 Industrial Blvd, Bethel Park, PA 15102
Tubing (reusable). Reusable ventilator tubing for breathing circuit.

Intersurgical Inc. 315-451-2900
417 Electronics Pkwy, Liverpool, NY 13088

Kentron Health Care, Inc. 615-384-0573
3604 Kelton Jackson Rd, P.o. Box 120, Springfield, TN 37172
Oxygen tubing.

Life Corporation 800-700-0202
1776 N Water St, Milwaukee, WI 53202
LIFE oxygen tubing.

Medi Inc 800-225-8634
75 York Ave, P.O. Box 302, Randolph, MA 02368

Mercury Medical 800-237-6418
11300 49th St N, Clearwater, FL 33762

Perma Pure Llc 800-337-3762
8 Executive Dr, Toms River, NJ 08755
Soft PE sampling line used for CO2 sampling.

Quadromed Inc. 800-363-0192
5776 Thimens Ave., St-Laurent, QUE H4R 2K9 Canada

Salter Labs 800-235-4203
100 Sycamore Rd, Arvin, CA 93203

Shore Medical, Inc. 714-628-9785
1050 N Batavia St Ste C, Orange, CA 92867
Various.

Smiths Medical Asd Inc. 800-258-5361
10 Bowman Dr, Keene, NH 03431
Various types of tubing.

Superior Products, Inc. 216-651-9400
3786 Ridge Rd, Cleveland, OH 44144
Various types.

Terumo Cardiovascular Systems, Corp 800-521-2818
6200 Jackson Rd, Ann Arbor, MI 48103

Tfx Medical Oem 800-548-6600
50 Plantation Dr, Jaffrey, NH 03452

Ventlab Corp. 336-753-5000
155 Boyce Dr, Mocksville, NC 27028
Tubing, flexible, medical gas, low pressure.

TUBING, FLUID DELIVERY *(General) 80FPK*

Apothecary Products, Inc. 800-328-2742
11750 12th Ave S, Burnsville, MN 55337

B. Braun Oem Division, B. Braun Medical Inc. 866-8-BBRAUN
824 12th Ave, Bethlehem, PA 18018

Baxa Corporation 800-567-2292
9540 S Maroon Circle, Suite 400, Englewood, CO 80112
Liquid delivery systems and oral liquid tube sets.

Baxter Healthcare Corporporation, Alternate Care And Channel Team 888-229-0001
25212 W Il Route 120, Round Lake, IL 60073
MICRO-VOLUME Infusion Sets, Solution Sets, Extension Sets, IV Filtration Sets.

TUBING, FLUID DELIVERY *(cont'd)*

Benlan Inc. 905-829-5004
2760 Brighton Rd., Oakville, ONT L6H 5T4 Canada
Medical tubing for fluid delivery.

Codan Us Corporation 800-33-CODAN
3511 W Sunflower Ave, Santa Ana, CA 92704
Filtration sets.

Edwards Lifesciences Technology Sarl 949-250-2500
State Rd. 402 N.km 1.4, Anasco, PR 00610-1577
Tubing, fluid delivery.

Filtrona Extrusion, Inc./Pexcor Medical Products Div. 800-755-7528
764 S Athol Rd, P.O. Box 659, Athol, MA 01331

Health Care Logistics, Inc. 800-848-1633
450 Town St, PO Box 25, Circleville, OH 43113
Various accessories for fluid delivery tubing.

Hospira Inc. 877-946-7747
275 N Field Dr, Lake Forest, IL 60045
Multiple

Hurricane Medical 941-751-0588
5315 Lena Rd, Bradenton, FL 34211
Tubing, extension set.

Icu Medical (Ut), Inc 949-366-2183
4455 Atherton Dr, Salt Lake City, UT 84123
Various types of arterial pressure tubing.

Integra Lifesciences Corp. 609-275-0500
311 Enterprise Dr, Plainsboro, NJ 08536
Fluid transfer set.

Marquette Medical, Inc. 410-987-2994
1114 Benfield Blvd Ste L, Millersville, MD 21108
I.V. extension sets.

Merit Medical Systems, Inc. 800-356-3748
1600 Merit Pkwy, South Jordan, UT 84095
High-pressure tubing with SHERLOCK connectors.

Monogen, Inc. 847-573-6700
3630 Burwood Dr, Waukegan, IL 60085
Cytostraw.

Mps Acacia 800-486-6677
785 Challenger St, Brea, CA 92821

Nalge Nunc International 800-625-4327
75 Panorama Creek Dr, Rochester, NY 14625
NALGENE clear PVC, low-density polyethylene, polyproplylene, FEP, PFA, PVDF, PUR and platinum-cured silicone available.

Norfolk Medical Products, Inc. 847-674-7075
7350 Ridgeway Ave, Skokie, IL 60076
Drug delivery catheter system i.v.

Saint-Gobain Performance Plastics--Akron 800-798-1554
2664 Gilchrist Rd, Akron, OH 44305
TYGON tubing represents a broad range of materials and formulations to meet specific application requirements.

Spectra Medical Devices, Inc. 866-938-8649
4C Henshaw St, Woburn, MA 01801

Stryker Puerto Rico, Ltd. 939-307-2500
Hwy. 3, Km. 131.2, Las Guasimas Ind. Park, Arroyo, PR 00714
Irrigation tubing.

Sunlite Plastics, Inc. 262-253-0600
W194N11340 McCormick Dr, Germantown, WI 53022
Funneled, co-extrusion, multi-lumen, striped, radiopaque, coiled and cut-to-length. PVC, polyetheylene, nylon and other thermoplastics. Custom and standard tubing.

Tfx Medical Oem 800-548-6600
50 Plantation Dr, Jaffrey, NH 03452

The Metrix Co. 800-752-3148
4400 Chavenelle Rd, Dubuque, IA 52002
Custom contract manufacturer.

Thomas Medical Products, Inc. 866-446-3003
65 Great Valley Pkwy, Malvern, PA 19355
Tubing set.

Tss Hudson
19 Brent Dr, Hudson, MA 01749
Silicone rubber tubing & molded components.

TUBING, HYPODERMIC *(General) 80WHK*

Ispg, Inc. 860-355-8511
517 Litchfield Rd, New Milford, CT 06776
Stainless steel tubing.

TUBING, HYPODERMIC *(cont'd)*

Spectra Medical Devices, Inc. 866-938-8649
4C Henshaw St, Woburn, MA 01801
Full line of 304 and 316 stainless steel hypo tubing. Short lead time and attractive pricing.

Tegra Medical Inc. 508-541-4200
9 Forge Pkwy, Franklin, MA 02038

TUBING, IRRIGATION *(Surgery) 79SIT*

Armm, Inc. 714-848-8190
17744 Sampson Ln, Huntington Beach, CA 92647
High flow, non-toxic.

Benlan Inc. 905-829-5004
2760 Brighton Rd., Oakville, ONT L6H 5T4 Canada

Covidien Lp 508-261-8000
15 Hampshire St, Mansfield, MA 02048

Filtrona Extrusion, Inc./Pexcor Medical Products Div. 800-755-7528
764 S Athol Rd, P.O. Box 659, Athol, MA 01331

Surgin Surgical Instrumentation, Inc. (Surgin Inc.) 714-832-6300
37 Shield, Irvine, CA 92618

Valley Forge Scientific Corp. 610-666-7500
136 Green Tree Road, Suite 100, Oaks, PA 19456
Bipolar cord/irriigation tubing set, Coextruded with irrigation tubing set attached for bipolar electrosurgical procedures.

TUBING, LATEX *(General) 80SDN*

Ace Hose & Rubber Company 888-223-4673
1333 S Jefferson St, Chicago, IL 60607

Carolina Biological Supply Co. 800-334-5551
2700 York Rd, Burlington, NC 27215

Kent Elastomer Products, Inc. 800-331-4762
1500 Saint Clair Ave, PO Box 668, Kent, OH 44240

TUBING, MULTI-LUMEN *(General) 80WPT*

Axiom Medical, Inc. 800-221-8569
19320 Van Ness Ave, Torrance, CA 90501
Multilumen extrusions, wide variety of sizes, with or without radiopaque markings.

B. Braun Oem Division, B. Braun Medical Inc. 866-8-BBRAUN
824 12th Ave, Bethlehem, PA 18018

Diablo Sales & Marketing, Inc. 925-648-1611
PO Box 3219, Danville, CA 94526
Custom design and manufacturing of catheters and specialty guidewires. Guiding catheters; stent delivery and drug delivery systems.

Filtrona Extrusion, Inc./Pexcor Medical Products Div. 800-755-7528
764 S Athol Rd, P.O. Box 659, Athol, MA 01331

Sunlite Plastics, Inc. 262-253-0600
W194N11340 McCormick Dr, Germantown, WI 53022
PVC, polyethylene, polyurethane, Hytrel and other thermoplastics.

Tfx Medical Oem 800-548-6600
50 Plantation Dr, Jaffrey, NH 03452

Vygon Corp. 800-544-4907
2495 General Armistead Ave, Norristown, PA 19403

TUBING, NON-CONDUCTIVE *(General) 80SDO*

Benlan Inc. 905-829-5004
2760 Brighton Rd., Oakville, ONT L6H 5T4 Canada

Coeur Inc., Sheboygan 800-874-4240
3411 Behrens Pkwy, Sheboygan, WI 53081

Covidien Lp 508-261-8000
15 Hampshire St, Mansfield, MA 02048

Filtrona Extrusion, Inc./Pexcor Medical Products Div. 800-755-7528
764 S Athol Rd, P.O. Box 659, Athol, MA 01331

Medi Inc 800-225-8634
75 York Ave, P.O. Box 302, Randolph, MA 02368

Saint-Gobain Performance Plastics--Akron 800-798-1554
2664 Gilchrist Rd, Akron, OH 44305
Fluoropolymer, co-extrusion & radiopaque tubing.

Sunlite Plastics, Inc. 262-253-0600
W194N11340 McCormick Dr, Germantown, WI 53022
PVC compounding, funneled, co-extrusion, multi-lumen, striped, radiopaque, coiled, cut-to-length, custom and standard tubing. PVC and polyethylene.

TUBING, NON-CONDUCTIVE *(cont'd)*

Tfx Medical Oem 800-548-6600
50 Plantation Dr, Jaffrey, NH 03452

TUBING, NON-INVASIVE *(Surgery) 79GAZ*

Allied Healthcare Products, Inc. 800-444-3954
1720 Sublette Ave, Saint Louis, MO 63110

Amerivac Usa Inc. 908-486-5200
1207 Pennsylvania Ave, Linden, NJ 07036
Various, noninvasive suction tubing.

Artcraft Packaging Corp. 314-488-5566
212 Lions Estates Dr, Jonesburg, MO 63351
Canister manifold tubing.

Buffalo Filter, A Division Of Medtek Devices Inc. 800-343-2324
595 Commerce Dr, Amherst, NY 14228
VT HOSE

Byron Medical 800-777-3434
602 W Rillito St, Tucson, AZ 85705
Liposuction disposable tubing, infiltration tubing.

Covidien Lp 508-261-8000
15 Hampshire St, Mansfield, MA 02048

Filtrona Extrusion, Inc./Pexcor Medical Products Div. 800-755-7528
764 S Athol Rd, P.O. Box 659, Athol, MA 01331

Globalmed Inc. 613-394-9844
155 N. Murray St., Trenton, ONT K8V-5R5 Canada
Extruded corrugated and collapsible medical tubing.

Gyrus Acmi, Inc. 508-804-2739
93 N Pleasant St, Norwalk, OH 44857
Various sterile and non-sterile.

Gyrus Acmi, Inc. 508-804-2739
300 Stillwater P.o.box 1971, Stamford, CT 06902
Various sterile and non-sterile.

Gyrus Ent L.L.C., Sub. Of Gyrus Acmi, Inc. 508-804-2739
2925 Appling Rd, Bartlett, TN 38133
Various.

Icu Medical (Ut), Inc 949-366-2183
4455 Atherton Dr, Salt Lake City, UT 84123
Various.

Icu Medical, Inc. 800-824-7890
951 Calle Amanecer, San Clemente, CA 92673
Non-invasive tubing.

Invivo Corporation 425-487-7000
12601 Research Pkwy, Orlando, FL 32826
Co2 sample line.

Kentron Health Care, Inc. 615-384-0573
3604 Kelton Jackson Rd, P.o. Box 120, Springfield, TN 37172
Suction tubes.

Medical Action Industries, Inc. 800-645-7042
25 Heywood Rd, Arden, NC 28704
Clear connective tubing.

Medtek Devices, Inc. 716-835-7000
595 Commerce Dr, 155 Pineview Dr., Amherst, NY 14228
Vacuum hose.

Medtronic Blood Management 612-514-4000
18501 E Plaza Dr, Parker, CO 80134
Blood management set-disposable.

Mps Acacia 800-486-6677
785 Challenger St, Brea, CA 92821

North American Latex Corp. 812-268-6608
49 Industrial Park Dr, Sullivan, IN 47882
Tubing for urinal bag connection, latex.

Peregrine Surgical, Ltd. 215-348-0456
51 Britain Dr, Doylestown, PA 18901
Tubing lining for delivery of viscoelastic fluid.

Solos Endoscopy 800-388-6445
65 Sprague St # B, Boston/dedham Commerce Park, Boston, MA 02136
Vacuum-powered body fluid suction apparatus.

Specialty Medical Products Co. 801-295-6023
3063 S Davis Blvd, Bountiful, UT 84010
Perforated soaking tube.

Stryker Puerto Rico, Ltd. 939-307-2500
Hwy. 3, Km. 131.2, Las Guasimas Ind. Park, Arroyo, PR 00714
Handpiece and tubing set.

TUBING, NON-INVASIVE *(cont'd)*

Sunlite Plastics, Inc. 262-253-0600
W194N11340 McCormick Dr, Germantown, WI 53022
PVC compounding, funneled, co-extrusion, paratubing, multi-lumen, striped, radiopaque, coiled, cut-to-length, custom and standard tubing. PVC, polyethylene, polyurethane, nylon and other thermoplastics.

Surgin Surgical Instrumentation, Inc. (Surgin Inc.) 714-832-6300
37 Shield, Irvine, CA 92618
Phaco kit.

Terumo Cardiovascular Systems (Tcvs) 800-283-7866
28 Howe St, Ashland, MA 01721
Tubing.

The Hygenic Corp. 800-321-2135
1245 Home Ave, Akron, OH 44310
Various sizes of surgical latex tubing and rubber tubing.

TUBING, NYLON *(General) 80SDP*

Filtrona Extrusion, Inc./Pexcor Medical Products Div. 800-755-7528
764 S Athol Rd, P.O. Box 659, Athol, MA 01331

Tfx Medical Oem 800-548-6600
50 Plantation Dr, Jaffrey, NH 03452

TUBING, OTHER *(General) 80WWE*

A-M Systems, Inc. 800-426-1306
131 Business Park Loop, Sequim, WA 98382

Accu-Glass Llc 800-325-4796
10765 Trenton Ave, Saint Louis, MO 63132
Glass: tubing, rods & other forms; precision glass products for flow restrictors, flush devices, percise flow control, connectors & liquid measuring products.

Advanced Polymers, Inc. 603-327-0600
29 Northwestern Dr, Salem, NH 03079
Fabrication of ultra-thin-walled, high strength tubing and heat-shrink tubing. Single- and multi-lumen tubing.

Armm, Inc. 714-848-8190
17744 Sampson Ln, Huntington Beach, CA 92647
SuperFlow filtered insufflation tubing.

Atc Technologies, Inc. 781-939-0725
30B Upton Dr, Wilmington, MA 01887
Fluid transfer systems.

Axiom Medical, Inc. 800-221-8569
19320 Van Ness Ave, Torrance, CA 90501
Wide variety of diameters, single and multi-lumen, for insufflation/fluid transfer, systems, liposuction. various profiles.

Benlan Inc. 905-829-5004
2760 Brighton Rd., Oakville, ONT L6H 5T4 Canada
Tipping and piercing of tubing.

Carolina Biological Supply Co. 800-334-5551
2700 York Rd, Burlington, NC 27215

Drummond Scientific Co. 800-523-7480
500 Park Way # 700, Broomall, PA 19008
Plasticrit - Plastic hematocrit tubes, with or without heparin, 75mm length.

Equilibrated Bio Systems, Inc. 800-327-9490
22 Lawrence Ave Ste LL2, Smithtown, NY 11787
Zee Frame ventilation tubing management device.

Eraser Company, Inc. 800-724-0594
123 Oliva Dr, Mattydale, NY 13211
WC601 Series Rotary Tubing Cutter is an automatic cutter for medical tubing of all types up to 1-1/8-in. OD. Used in manufacture of disposable medical products and medical equipment. Rotary blade action cuts tubing with square flat ends and no crushing.

Fenwal Inc. 800-766-1077
3 Corporate Dr, Lake Zurich, IL 60047
Blood recipient sets, plasma transfer sets, specialty blood component transfusion sets.

Filtrona Extrusion, Inc./Pexcor Medical Products Div. 800-755-7528
764 S Athol Rd, P.O. Box 659, Athol, MA 01331

Ispg, Inc. 860-355-8511
517 Litchfield Rd, New Milford, CT 06776
Stainless steel tubing.

Kawasumi Laboratories America, Inc. 800-529-2786
4723 Oak Fair Blvd, Tampa, FL 33610
Secondary IV sets for piggy backing.

TUBING, OTHER *(cont'd)*

Kent Elastomer Products, Inc. 800-331-4762
1500 Saint Clair Ave, PO Box 668, Kent, OH 44240
Thermoplastic elastomers.

Laborie Medical Technologies Inc. 888-522-6743
6415 Northwest Dr., Units 7-14, Mississauga, ONT L4V-1X1 Canada
Laborie Urodynamic measurement tubing. Model 101T tubing available at $104.00 for 25. 576T tubing available for other manufacturers' systems except Browne. Call for quotation/pricing for volume purchase.

Lifemed Of California 800-543-3633
1216 S Allec St, Anaheim, CA 92805
Lifemed custom and specialized tubing.

Medovations, Inc. 800-558-6408
102 E Keefe Ave, Milwaukee, WI 53212
Universal funnel tubes.

Micro-Vac, Inc. 800-729-1020
5905 E 5th St, Tucson, AZ 85711
Patented antistatic vacuum tubing for cleanroom use.

Mydent International 800-275-0020
80 Suffolk Ct, Hauppauge, NY 11788
DEFEND Sterilization tubing. 16 25 mm thickness, 2, 3, 4, & 6 in. wide.

Neotech Products, Inc. 800-966-0500
27822 Fremont Ct, Valencia, CA 91355
NEOHOLD:Cannula/Tubing Holder secures cannula and tubing to patient with skin friendly hydrocolloid.

Northgate Technologies Inc. 800-348-0424
600 Church Rd, Elgin, IL 60123
High flow, disposable, insufflation, tubing for laparoscopic procedures.

Pre Pak Products, Inc. 800-544-7257
4055 Oceanside Blvd Ste L, Oceanside, CA 92056
EXER-BAND PAKS, come complete with one stretch tube with handle(s), one web door-strap and an exercise instruction book. Available in 5 resistance levels in both bilateral and unilateral configurations. Prices range from $9.50 to $11.50 based on resistance level and quantity purchased. EXER-BAND OPEN STOCK, products are also sold separately.

Saint-Gobain Performance Plastics--Akron 800-798-1554
2664 Gilchrist Rd, Akron, OH 44305
TYGON 2075 plasticizer-free, virtually no extractables and exceptionally low absorption. TYGON LR-40 latex-free alternative. CHEMFLUOR 367 features surface smoothness and clarity superior to other fluoropolymer tubings.Tygon S-95-E non-DEHP formulation with exceptional pump life.

Saint-Gobain Performance Plastics/Clearwater 800-541-6880
4451 110th Ave N, Clearwater, FL 33762
C-FLEX Flexible tubing, alternative to latex, puc and silicone.

Smiths Medical Asd 800-424-8662
5700 W 23rd Ave, Gary, IN 46406
Silicone, custom to OEM spec.

Spectra Medical Devices, Inc. 866-938-8649
4C Henshaw St, Woburn, MA 01801
Full line of 304 and 316 stainless steel hypo tubing. Short lead time and attractive pricing.

Sunlite Plastics, Inc. 262-253-0600
W194N11340 McCormick Dr, Germantown, WI 53022

Tegra Medical Inc. 508-541-4200
9 Forge Pkwy, Franklin, MA 02038

Tfx Medical Oem 800-548-6600
50 Plantation Dr, Jaffrey, NH 03452

Vital Concepts, Inc. 800-984-2300
4334 Brockton Dr SE Ste F, Grand Rapids, MI 49512
Insufflation tubing, .1 micron hydrophobic filter, sterile/non-sterile tubing in a variety of configurations.

Wells Johnson Co. 800-528-1597
8000 S Kolb Rd, Tucson, AZ 85756

Wisap America 800-233-8448
8231 Melrose Dr, Lenexa, KS 66214

Young Innovations, Inc. 800-325-1881
13705 Shoreline Ct E, Earth City, MO 63045
NYCLAVE reusable clear tubing for sterilization of instruments.

TUBING, OXYGEN CONNECTING *(General) 80VHQ*

Benlan Inc. 905-829-5004
2760 Brighton Rd., Oakville, ONT L6H 5T4 Canada

TUBING, OXYGEN CONNECTING *(cont'd)*

Chad Therapeutics, Inc. 800-423-8870
21622 Plummer St, Chatsworth, CA 91311

Coeur Inc., Sheboygan 800-874-4240
3411 Behrens Pkwy, Sheboygan, WI 53081

Covidien Lp 508-261-8000
15 Hampshire St, Mansfield, MA 02048

Dedicated Distribution 800-325-8367
640 Miami Ave, Kansas City, KS 66105

Filtrona Extrusion, Inc./Pexcor Medical Products Div. 800-755-7528
764 S Athol Rd, P.O. Box 659, Athol, MA 01331

Intersurgical Inc. 315-451-2900
417 Electronics Pkwy, Liverpool, NY 13088

Life Corporation 800-700-0202
1776 N Water St, Milwaukee, WI 53202
LIFE oxygen tubing.

Mada, Inc. 800-526-6370
625 Washington Ave, Carlstadt, NJ 07072

Medline Industries, Inc. 800-633-5886
1 Medline Pl, Mundelein, IL 60060

Medovations, Inc. 800-558-6408
102 E Keefe Ave, Milwaukee, WI 53212

Rockford Medical & Safety Co. 800-435-9451
2420 Harrison Ave, PO Box 5646, Rockford, IL 61108

Salter Labs 800-235-4203
100 Sycamore Rd, Arvin, CA 93203

Spectra Medical Devices, Inc. 866-938-8649
4C Henshaw St, Woburn, MA 01801

Sunrise Medical 800-333-4000
7477 Dry Creek Pkwy, Longmont, CO 80503

Vygon Corp. 800-544-4907
2495 General Armistead Ave, Norristown, PA 19403

TUBING, PLASTIC *(General) 80VKN*

Armm, Inc. 714-848-8190
17744 Sampson Ln, Huntington Beach, CA 92647

Benlan Inc. 905-829-5004
2760 Brighton Rd., Oakville, ONT L6H 5T4 Canada

Carolina Biological Supply Co. 800-334-5551
2700 York Rd, Burlington, NC 27215

Filtrona Extrusion, Inc./Pexcor Medical Products Div. 800-755-7528
764 S Athol Rd, P.O. Box 659, Athol, MA 01331

Intersurgical Inc. 315-451-2900
417 Electronics Pkwy, Liverpool, NY 13088

Ipax, Inc. 303-975-2444
2622 S Zuni St, Englewood, CO 80110

Kent Elastomer Products, Inc. 800-331-4762
1500 Saint Clair Ave, PO Box 668, Kent, OH 44240

Medovations, Inc. 800-558-6408
102 E Keefe Ave, Milwaukee, WI 53212

Novosci Corp. 281-363-4949
2828 N Crescentridge Dr, The Woodlands, TX 77381

Saint-Gobain Performance Plastics--Akron 800-798-1554
2664 Gilchrist Rd, Akron, OH 44305
TYGON S-50-HL flexible plastic tubing used in heart/lung surgical packs, compatible with blood and tissue. TYGON R-3603 laboratory tubing.

Saint-Gobain Performance Plastics/Clearwater 800-541-6880
4451 110th Ave N, Clearwater, FL 33762
C-FLEX, thermoplastic elastomer, custom and STD formulations 5A to 95A hardness, radiopaque.

Spectra Medical Devices, Inc. 866-938-8649
4C Henshaw St, Woburn, MA 01801

Sunlite Plastics, Inc. 262-253-0600
W194N11340 McCormick Dr, Germantown, WI 53022
PVC compounding, funneled, co-extrusion, paratubing, multi-lumen, striped, radiopaque, coiled, cut-to-length, custom and standard tubing. PVC, polyethylene, polyurethane, nylon and other thermoplastics.

Tfx Medical Oem 800-548-6600
50 Plantation Dr, Jaffrey, NH 03452

Vindum Engineering, Inc. 925-275-0633
1 Woodview Ct, San Ramon, CA 94582
Teflon and nylon.

TUBING, POLYETHYLENE *(General) 80SDQ*

Benlan Inc. 905-829-5004
2760 Brighton Rd., Oakville, ONT L6H 5T4 Canada
Thermoplastic medical tubing.

Coeur Inc., Sheboygan 800-874-4240
3411 Behrens Pkwy, Sheboygan, WI 53081

Coeur, Inc 800-296-5893
704 Cadet Ct, Lebanon, TN 37087
Curved fill tube for delivery of contrast media.

Cole-Parmer Instrument Inc. 800-323-4340
625 E Bunker Ct, Vernon Hills, IL 60061

Covidien Lp 508-261-8000
15 Hampshire St, Mansfield, MA 02048

Diablo Sales & Marketing, Inc. 925-648-1611
PO Box 3219, Danville, CA 94526
Custom design and manufacturing of catheters and specialty guidewires. Guiding catheters; stent delivery and drug delivery systems.

Filtrona Extrusion, Inc./Pexcor Medical Products Div. 800-755-7528
764 S Athol Rd, P.O. Box 659, Athol, MA 01331

Nalge Nunc International 800-625-4327
75 Panorama Creek Dr, Rochester, NY 14625
NALGENE 1/8 x 1/4 x 1/16 in. to 2 x 2 1/4 x 1/8 in. sizes.

Saint-Gobain Performance Plastics--Akron 800-798-1554
2664 Gilchrist Rd, Akron, OH 44305
Laboratory tubing.

Spectra Medical Devices, Inc. 866-938-8649
4C Henshaw St, Woburn, MA 01801

Sunlite Plastics, Inc. 262-253-0600
W194N11340 McCormick Dr, Germantown, WI 53022
Co-extrusion, multi-lumen, striped, radiopaque, coiled, cut-to-length, custom and standard polyethylene tubing.

Tfx Medical Oem 800-548-6600
50 Plantation Dr, Jaffrey, NH 03452

TUBING, POLYPROPYLENE *(General) 80WPS*

Benlan Inc. 905-829-5004
2760 Brighton Rd., Oakville, ONT L6H 5T4 Canada

Chamberlin Rubber Company, Inc. 585-427-7780
3333 Brighton Henrietta Town Line Rd, PO Box 22700
Rochester, NY 14623

Filtrona Extrusion, Inc./Pexcor Medical Products Div. 800-755-7528
764 S Athol Rd, P.O. Box 659, Athol, MA 01331

Spectra Medical Devices, Inc. 866-938-8649
4C Henshaw St, Woburn, MA 01801

Sunlite Plastics, Inc. 262-253-0600
W194N11340 McCormick Dr, Germantown, WI 53022
Co-extrusion, multi-lumen, striped, radiopaque, profiles, coiled, cut-to-length, custom or standard.

Tfx Medical Oem 800-548-6600
50 Plantation Dr, Jaffrey, NH 03452

TUBING, POLYTETRAFLUOROETHYLENE *(General) 80WTH*

Berghof/America 800-544-5004
3773 NW 126th Ave Bldg 1, Coral Springs, FL 33065
Fluoropolymer and PTFE tubing.

Tfx Medical Oem 800-548-6600
50 Plantation Dr, Jaffrey, NH 03452

TUBING, POLYVINYL CHLORIDE *(General) 80SDR*

Ace Hose & Rubber Company 888-223-4673
1333 S Jefferson St, Chicago, IL 60607

Armm, Inc. 714-848-8190
17744 Sampson Ln, Huntington Beach, CA 92647

Benlan Inc. 905-829-5004
2760 Brighton Rd., Oakville, ONT L6H 5T4 Canada

Coeur Inc., Sheboygan 800-874-4240
3411 Behrens Pkwy, Sheboygan, WI 53081

Coeur, Inc 800-296-5893
704 Cadet Ct, Lebanon, TN 37087
Syringe connector tubing.

Command Medical Products, Inc. 386-672-8116
15 Signal Ave, Ormond Beach, FL 32174

Covidien Lp 508-261-8000
15 Hampshire St, Mansfield, MA 02048

TUBING, POLYVINYL CHLORIDE *(cont'd)*

Csi Holdings 615-452-9633
170 Commerce Way, Gallatin, TN 37066

Filtrona Extrusion, Inc./Pexcor Medical Products Div. 800-755-7528
764 S Athol Rd, P.O. Box 659, Athol, MA 01331

Hospira 800-441-4100
268 E 4th St, Ashland, OH 44805
Dimensions 0.100-in. ID x 0.138 in. and 0.120-in. ID x 0.170 in.

Kent Elastomer Products, Inc. 800-331-4762
1500 Saint Clair Ave, PO Box 668, Kent, OH 44240

Lucomed Inc. 800-633-7877
45 Kulick Rd, Fairfield, NJ 07004

Nalge Nunc International 800-625-4327
75 Panorama Creek Dr, Rochester, NY 14625
1/16 x 1/8 x 1/32 in. to 2 x 2 1/2 x 1/4 in. sizes. Braided from 3/16 x 3/8 x 3/32 in. to 2 x 2 1/2 x 1/4 in.

Saint-Gobain Performance Plastics--Akron 800-798-1554
2664 Gilchrist Rd, Akron, OH 44305
Laboratory tubing.

Spectra Medical Devices, Inc. 866-938-8649
4C Henshaw St, Woburn, MA 01801
PVC extension sets.

Sunlite Plastics, Inc. 262-253-0600
W194N11340 McCormick Dr, Germantown, WI 53022
PVC compounding, funneled, co-extrusion, paratubing, multi-lumen, striped, radiopaque, coiled, cut-to-length, custom and standard tubing.

TUBING, RADIOPAQUE *(General) 80WNG*

Andersen Products, Inc., 800-523-1276
3202 Caroline Dr, Health Science Park, Haw River, NC 27258

Benlan Inc. 905-829-5004
2760 Brighton Rd., Oakville, ONT L6H 5T4 Canada

Diablo Sales & Marketing, Inc. 925-648-1611
PO Box 3219, Danville, CA 94526
Custom design and manufacturing of catheters and specialty guidewires. Guiding catheters; stent delivery and drug delivery systems.

Filtrona Extrusion, Inc./Pexcor Medical Products Div. 800-755-7528
764 S Athol Rd, P.O. Box 659, Athol, MA 01331

Polyzen, Inc. 919-319-9599
1041 Classic Rd, Apex, NC 27539
Radiopaque specialty compounds.

Spectra Medical Devices, Inc. 866-938-8649
4C Henshaw St, Woburn, MA 01801

Sunlite Plastics, Inc. 262-253-0600
W194N11340 McCormick Dr, Germantown, WI 53022
PVC compounding, funneled, co-extrusion, paratubing, multi-lumen, striped, coiled, cut-to-length. PVC and polyurethane.

Tfx Medical Oem 800-548-6600
50 Plantation Dr, Jaffrey, NH 03452

TUBING, REPLACEMENT, PHACOFRAGMENTATION UNIT *(Ophthalmology) 86MSR*

Accellent Inc. 866-899-1392
100 Fordham Rd, Wilmington, MA 01887

Hurricane Medical 941-751-0588
5315 Lena Rd, Bradenton, FL 34211
Tubing extension set.

TUBING, SILICONE *(General) 80SDS*

Ace Hose & Rubber Company 888-223-4673
1333 S Jefferson St, Chicago, IL 60607

Allied Biomedical 800-276-1322
PO Box 392, Ventura, CA 93002
Long Term Implantable and Healthcare Grade Silicone Tubing. 50' coils.

Armm, Inc. 714-848-8190
17744 Sampson Ln, Huntington Beach, CA 92647
Nontoxic, class VI.

Axiom Medical, Inc. 800-221-8569
19320 Van Ness Ave, Torrance, CA 90501
Penrose, ribbed and plain, wide range of flat and round tubing sizes. Various profiles, multi and single lumen.

TUBING, SILICONE *(cont'd)*

Chamberlin Rubber Company, Inc. — 585-427-7780
3333 Brighton Henrietta Town Line Rd, PO Box 22700
Rochester, NY 14623

Cole-Parmer Instrument Inc. — 800-323-4340
625 E Bunker Ct, Vernon Hills, IL 60061
Peroxide-cured and platinum-cured biocompatible tubing.

Covidien Lp — 508-261-8000
15 Hampshire St, Mansfield, MA 02048

Degania Silicone, Inc. — 401-333-8199
1226 Mendon Rd, Cumberland, RI 02864
Standard and custom sizes. Cut to various lengths. Numerous colors and printing capabilities available.

Diablo Sales & Marketing, Inc. — 925-648-1611
PO Box 3219, Danville, CA 94526
Custom design and manufacturing of catheters and specialty guidewires. Guiding catheters; stent delivery and drug delivery systems.

Helix Medical, Inc. — 800-266-4421
1110 Mark Ave, Carpinteria, CA 93013
Extruded, medical grade silicone tubing.

Hi-Tech Rubber, Inc. — 800-924-4832
3191 E La Palma Ave, Anaheim, CA 92806

Howard Instruments, Inc. — 205-553-4453
4749 Appletree Ln, Tuscaloosa, AL 35405

Johnson & Johnson Medical Division Of Ethicon, Inc. — 800-423-4018
2500 E Arbrook Blvd, Arlington, TX 76014

Rose Technologies Company — 616-233-3000
1440 Front Ave NW, Grand Rapids, MI 49504

Saint-Gobain Performance Plastics--Akron — 800-798-1554
2664 Gilchrist Rd, Akron, OH 44305
TYGON 3350 silicone and custom extrusions, profiles, multi-lumen tubing, molded parts and sheeting.

Smiths Medical Asd — 800-424-8662
5700 W 23rd Ave, Gary, IN 46406
Airway lines, buck or cut to length.

Specialty Manufacturing, Inc. — 800-269-6204
2210 Midland Rd, Saginaw, MI 48603

Spectra Medical Devices, Inc. — 866-938-8649
4C Henshaw St, Woburn, MA 01801

Vygon Corp. — 800-544-4907
2495 General Armistead Ave, Norristown, PA 19403

Zimmer Orthopaedic Surgical Products — 800-321-5533
PO Box 10, 200 West Ohio Ave., Dover, OH 44622
HEMOVAC.

TUBING, URETHANE *(General) 80VKF*

Coeur Inc., Sheboygan — 800-874-4240
3411 Behrens Pkwy, Sheboygan, WI 53081

Coeur, Inc — 800-296-5893
704 Cadet Ct, Lebanon, TN 37087
Syringe connector tubing.

Diablo Sales & Marketing, Inc. — 925-648-1611
PO Box 3219, Danville, CA 94526
Custom design and manufacturing of catheters and specialty guidewires. Guiding catheters; stent delivery and drug delivery systems.

Filtrona Extrusion, Inc./Pexcor Medical Products Div. — 800-755-7528
764 S Athol Rd, P.O. Box 659, Athol, MA 01331

Saint-Gobain Performance Plastics--Akron — 800-798-1554
2664 Gilchrist Rd, Akron, OH 44305
TYGOTHANE tubing for polyurethane applications requiring consistently tight dimensional tolerances.

Spectra Medical Devices, Inc. — 866-938-8649
4C Henshaw St, Woburn, MA 01801

Sunlite Plastics, Inc. — 262-253-0600
W194N11340 McCormick Dr, Germantown, WI 53022
Custom tubing: co-extrusion, multi-lumen, funneled, striped, radiopaque, coiled, cut-to-length.

Vygon Corp. — 800-544-4907
2495 General Armistead Ave, Norristown, PA 19403

TUBING, VENTILATOR *(Anesthesiology) 73BZO*

A-M Systems, Inc. — 800-426-1306
131 Business Park Loop, Sequim, WA 98382

TUBING, VENTILATOR *(cont'd)*

Globalmed Inc. — 613-394-9844
155 N. Murray St., Trenton, ONT K8V-5R5 Canada
Blue and natural corrugated tubing coils with dispenser box.

Intersurgical Inc. — 315-451-2900
417 Electronics Pkwy, Liverpool, NY 13088

Quadromed Inc. — 800-363-0192
5776 Thimens Ave., St-Laurent, QUE H4R 2K9 Canada

Smiths Medical Asd Inc. — 800-258-5361
10 Bowman Dr, Keene, NH 03431
Various types and lengths of ventilator tubing.

Smiths Medical Asd, Inc. — 847-793-0135
330 Corporate Woods Pkwy, Vernon Hills, IL 60061
Volume ventilator ste, ventilator circuit with manifold ventilator set.

Tiara Medical Systems, Inc. — 610-862-0800
4153 166th St, Oak Forest, IL 60452
Various types and lengths of cpap tubing.

Vacumed — 800-235-3333
4538 Westinghouse St, Ventura, CA 93003

TUBING, VINYL *(General) 80SDT*

Armm, Inc. — 714-848-8190
17744 Sampson Ln, Huntington Beach, CA 92647

Benlan Inc. — 905-829-5004
2760 Brighton Rd., Oakville, ONT L6H 5T4 Canada

Cole-Parmer Instrument Inc. — 800-323-4340
625 E Bunker Ct, Vernon Hills, IL 60061

Crown Mats — 800-628-5463
2100 Commerce Dr, Fremont, OH 43420
Vinyl products.

Filtrona Extrusion, Inc./Pexcor Medical Products Div. — 800-755-7528
764 S Athol Rd, P.O. Box 659, Athol, MA 01331

Kent Elastomer Products, Inc. — 800-331-4762
1500 Saint Clair Ave, PO Box 668, Kent, OH 44240

Maddak Inc. — 800-443-4926
661 State Route 23, Wayne, NJ 07470
ABLEWARE.

Saint-Gobain Performance Plastics--Akron — 800-798-1554
2664 Gilchrist Rd, Akron, OH 44305
Ethyl vinyl acetate tubing.

Spectra Medical Devices, Inc. — 866-938-8649
4C Henshaw St, Woburn, MA 01801

Sunlite Plastics, Inc. — 262-253-0600
W194N11340 McCormick Dr, Germantown, WI 53022
PVC compounding, funneled, co-extrusion, paratubing, multi-lumen, striped, radiopaque, coiled, cut-to-length, custom and standard tubing.

TUCKER, LIGATURE, ORTHODONTIC *(Dental And Oral) 76ECP*

American Orthodontics Corp. — 800-558-7687
1714 Cambridge Ave, Sheboygan, WI 53081
Orthodontic instruments.

Biomet Microfixation Inc. — 800-874-7711
1520 Tradeport Dr, Jacksonville, FL 32218
Various types of ligature.

Coltene/Whaledent Inc. — 330-916-8858
235 Ascot Pkwy, Cuyahoga Falls, OH 44223
Director.

G & H Wire Co. — 800-526-1026
2165 Earlywood Dr, Franklin, IN 46131
Various types of orthodontic hand instruments.

Glenroe Technologies — 800-237-4060
1912 44th Ave E, Bradenton, FL 34203
Orthodontic lingual instrument.

Hu-Friedy Manufacturing Co., Inc. — 800-483-7433
3232 N Rockwell St, Chicago, IL 60618

Ortho Organizers, Inc. — 760-448-8730
1822 Aston Ave, Carlsbad, CA 92008
Elastic attacher, elastic engager.

Ortho-Med Intl., Inc. — 760-357-5040
357A W 2nd St, Calexico, CA 92231
Various.

Orthodontic Design And Production, Inc. — 760-734-3995
1370 Decision St Ste D, Vista, CA 92081
Types of ligature tucking/tying instruments.

TUCKER, LIGATURE, ORTHODONTIC *(cont'd)*

Sci-Dent, Inc. 800-323-4145
210 Dowdle St Ste 2, Algonquin, IL 60102

Strite Industries Ltd. 800-267-7333
298 Shepherd Ave., Cambridge, ON N3C 1V1 Canada
$24.00 for ligature director.

3m Unitek 800-634-5300
2724 Peck Rd, Monrovia, CA 91016

TUNNELER, SURGICAL *(Surgery) 79WVC*

Bard Peripheral Vascular, Inc. 800-321-4254
1625 W 3rd St, Tempe, AZ 85281

Tegra Medical Inc. 508-541-4200
9 Forge Pkwy, Franklin, MA 02038

TURBIDIMETRIC METHOD, LIPOPROTEINS *(Chemistry) 75JHN*

Bacton Assay Systems, Inc. 760-471-4538
772 N Twin Oaks Valley Rd Ste A, San Marcos, CA 92069
Apolipoprotein al reagent.

Eucardio Laboratory, Inc. 760-632-1824
2216 Silver Peak Pl, Encinitas, CA 92024
Apo ai & b reagent.

TURBIDIMETRIC METHOD, PROTEIN OR ALBUMIN (URINARY) *(Chemistry) 75JIQ*

Abbott Diagnostics Div. 626-440-0700
820 Mission St, South Pasadena, CA 91030
Microalbumin.

Accumin Diagnostics, Inc. 212-659-0711
750 Lexington Ave Fl 20, New York, NY 10022
Microalbumin assay.

Cargille Laboratories 973-239-6633
55 Commerce Rd, Cedar Grove, NJ 07009
Albumin standards, $195.00 for 6 mL, $240.00 for 10 mL. Set of 8 standards.

Jas Diagnostics, Inc. 305-418-2320
7220 NW 58th St, Miami, FL 33166
Microalbumin.

Labchem, Inc. 412-826-5230
200 William Pitt Way, Pittsburgh, PA 15238
Sulfosalicylic acid, multiple solutions, various concentrations.

Ricca Chemical Company Llc 888-467-4222
1841 Broad St, Pocomoke City, MD 21851
Various.

Ricca Chemical Company Llc 817-461-5601
1490 Lammers Pike, Batesville, IN 47006

Ricca Chemical Company, Llc 817-461-5601
448 W Fork Dr, Arlington, TX 76012
Various.

Rocky Mountain Reagents,Inc. 303-762-0800
3207 W Hampden Ave, Englewood, CO 80110

TURBIDIMETRIC, TOTAL PROTEIN *(Chemistry) 75JGQ*

Abbott Diagnostics Div. 626-440-0700
820 Mission St, South Pasadena, CA 91030
Urine/csf protein.

Jas Diagnostics, Inc. 305-418-2320
7220 NW 58th St, Miami, FL 33166
Microprotein.

TWEEZERS *(General) 80SDU*

Afassco, Inc. 800-441-6774
2244 Park Pl Ste C, Minden, NV 89423

Carl Heyer, Inc. 800-284-5550
1872 Bellmore Ave, North Bellmore, NY 11710

Edmund Industrial Optics 800-363-1992
101 E Gloucester Pike, Barrington, NJ 08007

Miltex Inc. 800-645-8000
589 Davies Dr, York, PA 17402

Polysciences, Inc. 800-523-2575
400 Valley Rd, Warrington, PA 18976
Magnetic and non-magnetic types, medium and extra-fine pointed, curved, reverse action, Dumant and Peer.

TWISTER, BRACE SETTING *(Physical Med) 89ITO*

Becker Orthopedic Appliance Co. 248-588-7480
635 Executive Dr, Troy, MI 48083
Various twister, brace setting orthoses and orthosis comp.

TWISTER, BRACE SETTING *(cont'd)*

Burke Medical, Llc 727-532-8333
2310 Tall Pines Dr Ste 210, Largo, FL 33771
Knee brace.

TWISTER, WIRE *(Orthopedics) 87HXS*

Abbott Spine, Inc. 847-937-6100
12708 Riata Vista Cir Ste B-100, Austin, TX 78727
Wire twister.

Biomet Microfixation Inc. 800-874-7711
1520 Tradeport Dr, Jacksonville, FL 32218
Various types of wire.

Biomet, Inc. 574-267-6639
56 E Bell Dr, PO Box 587, Warsaw, IN 46582
Various types of wire twisters.

Deknatel Snowden-Pencer 800-367-7874
5175 S Royal Atlanta Dr, Tucker, GA 30084

Kls-Martin L.P. 800-625-1557
11239-1 St. John`s Industrial, Parkway South
Jacksonville, FL 32250
Wire twisting forceps.

Kmedic 800-955-0559
190 Veterans Dr, Northvale, NJ 07647

Lenox-Maclaren Surgical Corp. 720-890-9660
657 S Taylor Ave Ste A, Colorado Technology Center
Louisville, CO 80027
Probe.

Rgi Medical Manufacturing Inc. 352-378-3633
2321 NW 66th Ct Ste W4, Gainesville, FL 32653
Guidewire, stylet, braided stylet.

Steeger Usa, Llc 800-554-2082
2353 Highway 292, Inman, SC 29349
Fine wire braiders with 3-144 carriers with intelligent control. Suitable for catheters and medical devices. Also, make braiding equipment.

Tuzik Boston 800-886-6363
104 Longwater Dr, Assinippi Park, Norwell, MA 02061

Zimmer Holdings, Inc. 800-613-6131
1800 W Center St, PO Box 708, Warsaw, IN 46580

TYMPANOSCOPE *(Ear/Nose/Throat) 77JOG*

Tsi Medical Ltd. 800-661-7263
47 Athabascan Ave., Unit 105, Sherwood Park, AB T8A-4H3 Canada

U.V. METHOD, CPK ISOENZYMES *(Chemistry) 75JHW*

Abbott Diagnostics Intl, Biotechnology Ltd 787-846-3500
Road #2 KM. 58.0 , PO Box 278, Cruce Davila, Barceloneta, PR 00617
Assay for detection of creatine kinase.

Beckman Coulter, Inc. 800-635-3497
740 W 83rd St, Hialeah, FL 33014
$0.95 per test.

Codman & Shurtleff, Inc 800-225-0460
325 Paramount Dr, Raynham, MA 02767

Dade Behring, Inc. 800-948-3233
1717 Deerfield Rd, Deerfield, IL 60015

Health Chem Diagnostics Llc 954-979-3845
3341 W McNab Rd, Pompano Beach, FL 33069
U.v. method, cpk isoenzymes.

Raichem, Division Of Hemagen Diagnostics, Inc. 800-438-6100
8225 Mercury Ct, San Diego, CA 92111
CK-MB Reagent Test System.

U.V. SPECTROMETRY, THEOPHYLLINE *(Toxicology) 91LCY*

Hemagen Diagnostics, Inc. 800-436-2436
9033 Red Branch Rd, Columbia, MD 21045
Analyst theophylline.

ULTRACENTRIFUGE *(Chemistry) 75SDV*

Beckman Coulter, Inc. 800-742-2345
250 S Kraemer Blvd, PO Box 8000, Brea, CA 92821

Kendro Laboratory Products 800-252-7100
308 Ridgefield Ct, Asheville, NC 28806

ULTRAFILTRATION EQUIPMENT *(Chemistry) 75UIZ*

Ag Industries 800-875-3138
3637 Scarlet Oak Blvd, Saint Louis, MO 63122
Healthcare Filters.

Cartwright Consulting Co. 952-854-4911
8324 16th Ave S, Minneapolis, MN 55425

ULTRAFILTRATION EQUIPMENT *(cont'd)*

Hydro Service & Supplies, Inc. 800-950-7426
PO Box 12197, Research Triangle Park, NC 27709
Ultrafiltration, reverse osmosis, point of use microbiological purity water purification and polishing equipment.

Isopure Corp. 800-280-7873
141 Citizens Blvd, Simpsonville, KY 40067
MD600 Series 10,000 MWCO membranes with AAMI standard deionization exchange tank connections, automatic dual alternating distribution pumps.

Millipore Corporation 800-MILLIPORE
80 Ashby Rd, Bedford, MA 01730

Pall Corporation 800-521-1520
600 S Wagner Rd, Ann Arbor, MI 48103

Spectrum Laboratories, Inc. 800-634-3300
18617 S Broadwick St, Rancho Dominguez, CA 90220
Ultrafiltration systems: stirred cells, tangential flow cells for pressured filtration; also, ultrafiltration membranes.

ULTRASOUND, HYPERTHERMIA, CANCER TREATMENT *(Radiology) 90LSY*

Best Nomos Corp. 800-70-NOMOS
1 Best Dr, Pittsburgh, PA 15202
BAT Ultrasound localization system that provides quick localization of prostate and other organs that move from day to day.

Labthermics Technologies 217-351-7722
701 Devonshire Dr, Champaign, IL 61820
Multifrequency ultrasound hyperthermia cancer therapy system.

ULTRASOUND, INFUSION, SYSTEM *(Cardiovascular) 74NUI*

Ekos Corp. 888-400-3567
11911 N Creek Pkwy S, Bothell, WA 98011
Ultrasound infusion catheter system for diagnostic infusion.

ULTRASOUND, SKIN PERMEATION *(Surgery) 79NRJ*

Echo Therapeutics, Inc. 508-553-8850
10 Forge Pkwy, Franklin, MA 02038
Ultrasonic skin permeation system and procedure tray.

UNIT, ANESTHESIA, DENTAL, ELECTRIC *(Dental And Oral) 76LWM*

Midmark Corporation 800-643-6275
60 Vista Dr, P.O. Box 286, Versailles, OH 45380

Reflex Technologies, Inc. 305-892-0584
12565 Palm Rd Ste B, North Miami, FL 33181
Comfortron, m.a.n. stim, manstim.

UNIT, CONTROL, BED, PATIENT, POWERED *(General) 80WPL*

Colonial Scientific Ltd. 902-468-1811
201 Brownlow Ave., Unit 52, Dartmouth, NS B3B-1W2 Canada
Critical care beds

Crest Healthcare Supply 800-328-8908
195 3rd St, Dassel, MN 55325
Bed control conversion kits; bed control holders.

Linak U.S. Inc. 502-253-5595
2200 Stanley Gault Pkwy, Louisville, KY 40223

Sunrise Medical 800-333-4000
7477 Dry Creek Pkwy, Longmont, CO 80503

UNIT, COOLING, CARDIAC *(Cardiovascular) 74WIU*

Cardiomed Supplies Inc. 800-387-9757
5 Gormley Industrial Ave., P.O. Box 575
Gormley, ONT L0H 1 Canada
Heart and kidney cooling jackets.

Wallach Surgical Devices, Inc. 800-243-2463
235 Edison Rd, Orange, CT 06477
$13,475 for non-AC-powered cryocardiac unit.

UNIT, ELECTROSURGICAL, ENDOSCOPIC (WITH OR WITHOUT ACCESSORIES), REPROCESSED *(Gastro/Urology) 78NLR*

Apollo Endosurgery, Inc. 877-ENDO-130
7000 Bee Caves Rd Ste 350, Austin, TX 78746
Electrocautery Dilation Balloon

Sterilmed, Inc. 763-488-3400
11400 73rd Ave N Ste 100, Maple Grove, MN 55369
Sphinctertomes.

UNIT, EVALUATION, HEIGHT, LIFT *(Orthopedics) 87REX*

Linak U.S. Inc. 502-253-5595
2200 Stanley Gault Pkwy, Louisville, KY 40223
DESKLIFT, electrical height adjustment of desks and workstations. Ergonomics.

UNIT, EVALUATION, HEIGHT, LIFT *(cont'd)*

Porto-Lift Corp. 800-321-1454
PO Box 5, Higgins Lake, MI 48627

Spectrum Aquatics 406-542-9781
7100 Spectrum Ln, Missoula, MT 59808
Swim Lift.

UNIT, EXAMINING/TREATMENT, ENT *(Ear/Nose/Throat) 77ETF*

Global Surgical Corp. 314-861-3388
3610 Tree Court Industrial Blvd, Saint Louis, MO 63122
Maxi cabinets.

Gn Otometrics North America 800-289-2150
125 Commerce Dr, Schaumburg, IL 60173
E.n.g. table.

HAAG-STREIT USA, INC. 800-787-5426
3535 Kings Mills Rd, Mason, OH 45040
$2,495, $3,195 and $3,595 for manual ENT chairs; $4,395, $4,985 for motorized ENT chairs.

Jedmed Instruments Co. 314-845-3770
5416 Jedmed Ct, Saint Louis, MO 63129

Kelleher Medical, Inc. 804-378-9956
3049 St Marys Way, Powhatan, VA 23139

Khl, Inc. 206-915-2115
18300 NE 146th Way, Woodinville, WA 98072
8450 cardiac stress, lateral tilting, ultrasound exam table.

Stryker Medical 800-869-0770
3800 E Centre Ave, Portage, MI 49002

Tsi Medical Ltd. 800-661-7263
47 Athabascan Ave., Unit 105, Sherwood Park, AB T8A-4H3 Canada

Winco, Inc. 800-237-3377
5516 SW 1st Ln, Ocala, FL 34474
Chairs.

UNIT, FILTER, MEMBRANE *(Chemistry) 75JRL*

Byron Medical 800-777-3434
602 W Rillito St, Tucson, AZ 85705
.3 micron, 99.97% DOP Rating.

Corning Inc., Science Products Division 800-492-1110
45 Nagog Park, Acton, MA 01720

Filtertek Inc. 800-248-2461
11411 Price Rd, Hebron, IL 60034
Filter elements (parts).

Ge Infrastructure Water & Process Technologies 877-522-7867
5951 Clearwater Dr, Minnetonka, MN 55343

Hurricane Medical 941-751-0588
5315 Lena Rd, Bradenton, FL 34211
Unit, filter, membrane.

Inter-Med, Inc. 877-418-4782
2200 Northwestern Ave, Racine, WI 53404
Aqueous solutions filter component.

Medi-Dose, Inc. 800-523-8966
70 Industrial Dr, Ivyland, PA 18974

Met-Pro Corporation 215-723-6751
160 Cassell Rd, P.O. Box 144, Harleysville, PA 19438
Miniature filter systems.

Millipore Corp. 781-533-2622
Prescott Rd., Jaffrey, NH 03452

Millipore Corporation 800-MILLIPORE
80 Ashby Rd, Bedford, MA 01730

Monogen, Inc. 847-573-6700
3630 Burwood Dr, Waukegan, IL 60085
Filter membrane & plug, monoprep, filters and plugs standard, ultra clean.

Nalge Nunc International 800-625-4327
75 Panorama Creek Dr, Rochester, NY 14625
NALGENE sterile units from 115 to 1000ml. Polyethersulfone surfactant-free cellulose acetate, cellulose nitrate and nylon membranes available.

Schleicher & Schuell, Inc. 800-245-4024
10 Optical Ave, PO Box 2012, Keene, NH 03431

Spectrum Laboratories, Inc. 800-634-3300
18617 S Broadwick St, Rancho Dominguez, CA 90220
Tubular dialysis membranes. Available membranes: cellulose ester (CE), regenerated cellulose (RC), and polyvinylidene difleronde (PVDF).

UNIT, FILTER, MEMBRANE *(cont'd)*

Superior Products, Inc. 216-651-9400
3786 Ridge Rd, Cleveland, OH 44144
Filter.

Western Water Purifier Co. 800-55-WATER
PO Box 688, Woodland Hills, CA 91365
Solid carbon block filters and prefilters; both rated for removal of Giardia and Crypto. Plus, replacement filter cartridges for most major brands.

UNIT, IMAGING, THERMAL *(Radiology) 90WTF*

Agfa Corporation 877-777-2432
PO Box 19048, 10 South Academy Street, Greenville, SC 29602
DRYSTAR, dry and solid inkjet imaging. SCOPIX, laser imaging.

Boeckeler Instruments, Inc. 800-552-2262
4650 S Butterfield Dr, Tucson, AZ 85714
VIA: Video measuring and marking devices: allows measurements and annotation of video images without altering the image; IMG-100 image contrast controller increases contrast of video images for optional viewing or anlysis, shading and color inversion controls featured.

Cytogen Corp. 800-833-3533
600 College Rd E Ste 3100, Princeton, NJ 08540
PROSTA SCINT for prostate cancer imaging and tumor targeted radio immuno scintigraphy.

Dorex, Inc. 714-639-0700
954 N Lemon St, Orange, CA 92867

Multigon Industries, Inc. 800-289-6858
1 Odell Plz, Yonkers, NY 10701
Duplex imaging unit.

Print Media, Inc. 800-994-3318
9002 NW 105th Way, Medley, FL 33178
Black & White Video Imaging Rolls are produced to meet or exceed origial equipment manufacturer's specifications. Color Video Image Print Sets are specifically manufactured to provide optimal and indistinguishable image quality, with no printer adjustment required.

Sony Electronics, Inc., Medical Systems Div. 800-686-7669
1 Sony Dr, Park Ridge, NJ 07656
High resolution monochrome and color thermal videographic printers.

UNIT, MEASURING, POTENTIAL, EVOKED, AUDITORY
(Ear/Nose/Throat) 77EWN

Fecom Corporation 800-292-3362
12 Stults Rd Ste 103, Dayton, NJ 08810
Digital Key-chain battery tester with LCD indicator for hearing aid batteries and household battery tester that tester sizes D, C, AA, AAA, 9 volt, and Lithium all in one unit

Gn Otometrics 800-289-2150
125 Commerce Dr, Schaumburg, IL 60173
Auditory evoked potential. CHARTR EP, $18,900 per unit.

UNIT, MICROWAVE, TRANSURETHRAL *(Gastro/Urology) 78WYF*

Energy Beam Sciences, Inc. 800-992-9037
29 Kripes Rd Ste B, East Granby, CT 06026
Non-transurethral. 2 models. Laboratory microwave processor; vented, safety-interlocked for fixation, dehydration and embedding of histological specimens. Immunohistochemistry microwave; vented, safety-interlocked fiber-optically controlled for the incubation of histological specimens with immunizations.

UNIT, OPERATIVE DENTAL, ACCESSORIES
(Dental And Oral) 76NRD

Air Techniques, Inc. 800-247-8324
1295 Walt Whitman Rd, Melville, NY 11747
Vistacam Omni and Omni IC, SLC

Kavo Dental Manufacturing Inc 202-828-0850
901 W Oakton St, Des Plaines, IL 60018
Various models of dental operative units and accessories.

Winders Dental Equipment 206-772-1522
10624 Crestwood Dr S, Seattle, WA 98178
Dental air and vacuum systems.

UNIT, PAD, HEATING, PORTABLE *(Physical Med) 89WWS*

Achilles Usa, Inc. 425-353-7000
1407 80th St SW, Everett, WA 98203

Creative Health Products, Inc. 800-742-4478
5148 Saddle Ridge Rd, Plymouth, MI 48170
BATTLE CREEK THERMOPHORE HEATING PADS, moist deep heat: 14' X 25' $59.50, 14' x 14' $47.20, 4' x 17' $36.75 from CHP.

UNIT, SANITATION/STERILIZATION, TOOTHBRUSH, ULTRAVIOLET *(Dental And Oral) 76MCF*

Cooley & Cooley, Ltd. 800-215-4487
8550 Westland West Blvd, Houston, TX 77041
STERIL MED DENTAL UNIT WATERLINE CARTRIDGE SYSTEM-COPPER AND SILVER IONS CONTINUOUSLY SANITIZE THE WATERLINES FOR 365 DAYS WITH NO PURGING OR MAINTENANCE.

Health Ent., Inc. 508-695-0727
90 George Leven Dr, North Attleboro, MA 02760
Toothbrush sanitizer.

Murdock Laboratories, Inc. 800 439-2497
123 Primrose Rd, Burlingame, CA 94010
Ultraviolet toothbrush sanitizer.

Sutura, Inc. 714-437-9801
17080 Newhope St, Fountain Valley, CA 92708
Sterile knot pusher.

UNIT, THERAPY, BEHAVIOR *(General) 80QDG*

Accu Scan Instruments, Inc. 800-822-1344
5098 Trabue Rd, Columbus, OH 43228
Study behavior and test anxiety in small animals.

UNIT, THERAPY, CURRENT, INTERFERENTIAL
(Cns/Neurology) 84LIH

Biomedical Life Systems, Inc. 800-726-8367
2448 Cades Way, Vista, CA 92081

Care Rehab And Orthopaedic Products, Inc. 703-448-9644
3930 Horseshoe Bend Rd, Keysville, VA 23947
Interferential current therapy.

Chattanooga Group 800-592-7329
4717 Adams Rd, Hixson, TN 37343
INTELECT ultrasound, stimulators, and combo unit.

Control Solutions, Inc. 630-806-7062
2229 Diehl Rd, Aurora, IL 60502
Cs3101 interferential stimulator.

Dermawave, Llc 561-784-0599
15693 83rd Ln N, Loxahatchee, FL 33470
Interferential current therapy for pain relief & accessories.

Dynatronics Corp. 800-874-6251
7030 Park Centre Dr, Salt Lake City, UT 84121
Newly available is the DYNATRON SOLARIS Series, featuring optional infrared therapy, ultrasound, and combination 7 stims: interferential and premodulated with target feature; Russian stimulation; biphasic stimulation; microcurrent; direct current; multifrequency ultrasound with three frequencies and differently sized soundheads (Diadynamic can be added). DYNATRON 950--5 channels with ultrasound; DYNATRON 708--3 channels with ultrasound; DYNATRON 708--3 channels with ultrasound; DYNATRON 706--5 channels; DYNATRON 705--3 channels. DYNATRON 950 combination ultrasound/interferential unit. Interferential, premodulated, Russian stimulation, biphasic stimulation, microcurrent, multifrequency ultrasound with three frequencies and different sized sound. DYNATRON 550 is a 2 channel electrotherapy unit. Interfernetial, premodulated, Russian stimulation, biophasic stimulation, microcurrent, includes TARGET feature to target pain. And, DYNATRON 650 is a 4-channel electrotherapy unit. Includes inferential, premodulated, Russian stimulation, biophasic stimulation, microcurrent, and high voltage. Includes TARGET feature to target pain.

Electrostim Medical Services, Inc. 800-588-8383
3504 Cragmont Dr Ste 100, Tampa, FL 33619
Interferential stimulator.

Mednet Services, Inc. 612-788-6228
2855 Anthony Ln S Ste B10, Minneapolis, MN 55418
Interferential stimulator.

Multiplex Stimulator Ltd. 800-663-8576
2-1750 McLean Ave., Port Coquitlam, BC V3C 1M9 Canada

Newwave Medical Llc 888-513-9283
1239 Durham Rd, Whitewright, TX 75491
Smartwave IF 2000

Rs Medical 800-683-0353
14001 S.E. First St., Vancouver, WA 98684
RS-4i Sequential Stimulator

Spectrum Assembly Inc. 760-752-7008
970 Los Vallecitos Blvd Ste 140, San Marcos, CA 92069
Interferential current therapy.

UNIT, THERAPY, CURRENT, INTERFERENTIAL *(cont'd)*

Surgitech Inc. 760-477-8191
870 Rancheros Dr, San Marcos, CA 92069
Interferential current therapy.

Zynex Inc. 800-495-6670
9990 Park Meadows Dr, Lone Tree, CO 80124
IF8000

UNIT, THERAPY, TINNITUS *(Ear/Nose/Throat) 77SAT*

Adm Tronics Unlimited, Inc. 201-767-6040
224 Pegasus Ave, Northvale, NJ 07647
AUREX-3, electromedical device for the control and treatment of tinnitus.

Doc's Proplugs, Inc. 800-521-2982
719 Swift St Ste 100, Santa Cruz, CA 95060
Doc's Promold with Doc's Protune adapter holds earbud of cassette player in the ear to deliver white sound to relieve tinnitus.

Hal-Hen Company, Inc. 800-242-5436
180 Atlantic Ave, Garden City Park, NY 11040
$155.00 per unit for tinnitus sufferers.

Starkey Florida 800-327-7939
2200 N Commerce Pkwy, Weston, FL 33326

Starkey Laboratories, Inc. 800-328-8602
6700 Washington Ave S, Eden Prairie, MN 55344
$2,950 for tinnitus research audiometer with master and subject consoles.

UNIT, ULTRAVIOLET SANITATION/STERILIZATION (FOR TOOTHBRUSHES), NON-STERILE *(Dental And Oral) 76NOB*

Synergy Usa 786-222-1710
13899 Biscayne Blvd Ste 101, North Miami Beach, FL 33181

UNLOADER, CART *(General) 80WVS*

Mcclure Industries, Inc. 800-752-2821
9051 SE 55th Ave, Portland, OR 97206
Electric cart unloading equipment.

URANYL ACETATE/ZINC ACETATE, SODIUM *(Chemistry) 75CEI*

Teco Diagnostics 714-693-7788
1268 N Lakeview Ave, Anaheim, CA 92807
Sodium reagent set.

UREASE AND GLUTAMIC DEHYDROGENASE, UREA NITROGEN
(Chemistry) 75CDQ

Abbott Diagnostics Div. 626-440-0700
820 Mission St, South Pasadena, CA 91030
Urea nitrogen.

Amresco Inc. 800-366-1313
30175 Solon Industrial Pkwy, Solon, OH 44139

Biozyme Laboratories International Ltd. 800-423-8199
9939 Hibert St Ste 101, San Diego, CA 92131

Caldon Bioscience, Inc. 909-628-9944
2100 S Reservoir St, Pomona, CA 91766
Urease and glutamic dehydrogenase, urea nitrogen, clinical chemistry.

Caldon Biotech, Inc. 757-224-0177
2251 Rutherford Rd, Carlsbad, CA 92008
Bun.

Carolina Liquid Chemistries Corp. 800-471-7272
510 W Central Ave Ste C, Brea, CA 92821
Bun.

Genchem, Inc. 714-529-1616
510 W Central Ave Ste D, Brea, CA 92821
Bun reagent.

Hemagen Diagnostics, Inc. 800-436-2436
9033 Red Branch Rd, Columbia, MD 21045
Various urea nitrogen methods.

Jas Diagnostics, Inc. 305-418-2320
7220 NW 58th St, Miami, FL 33166
Urea nitrogen.

Pointe Scientific, Inc. 800-445-9853
5449 Research Dr, Canton, MI 48188

Raichem, Division Of Hemagen Diagnostics, Inc. 800-438-6100
8225 Mercury Ct, San Diego, CA 92111

Sterling Diagnostics, Inc. 800-637-2661
36645 Metro Ct, Sterling Heights, MI 48312

UREASE AND GLUTAMIC DEHYDROGENASE, UREA NITROGEN *(cont'd)*

Synermed Intl., Inc. 317-896-1565
17408 Tiller Ct Ste 1900, Westfield, IN 46074
Urea nitrogen reagent kit.

Teco Diagnostics 714-693-7788
1268 N Lakeview Ave, Anaheim, CA 92807
Cx3 reagent set for synchron cx system, bun, kinetic.

Vital Diagnostics Inc. 714-672-3553
1075 W Lambert Rd Ste D, Brea, CA 92821
Various urea/urea nitrogen reagents.

UREASE, PHOTOMETRIC, UREA NITROGEN *(Chemistry) 75CDN*

Bayer Healthcare Llc 914-524-2955
555 White Plains Rd Fl 5, Tarrytown, NY 10591
Test for urea nitrogen in whole blood.

Bayer Healthcare, Llc 574-256-3430
430 S Beiger St, Mishawaka, IN 46544
Test for urea nitrogen in whole blood.

Beckman Coulter, Inc. 800-635-3497
740 W 83rd St, Hialeah, FL 33014
$0.09 per test.

Dexall Biomedical Labs, Inc. 301-840-1884
18904 Bonanza Way, Gaithersburg, MD 20879
*Auro*Dex H-pylori MultiTest includes a single lateral flow strip for simultaneous determination of H-pylori IgA, IgG and IgM antibodies in serum/plasma.*

Health Chem Diagnostics Llc 954-979-3845
3341 W McNab Rd, Pompano Beach, FL 33069
Urease, photometric, urea nitrogen.

Teco Diagnostics 714-693-7788
1268 N Lakeview Ave, Anaheim, CA 92807
(bun0urea nitrogen (color).

URETEROSCOPE *(Gastro/Urology) 78FGB*

Cortek Endoscopy, Inc. 847-526-2266
260 Jamie Ln Ste D, Wauconda, IL 60084
Gastroenterology.

Global Endoscopy, Inc. 888-434-3398
914 Estes Ct, Schaumburg, IL 60193
Ureteroscope.

Gyrus Acmi, Inc. 508-804-2739
93 N Pleasant St, Norwalk, OH 44857
Ureteroscope and accessories.

Gyrus Acmi, Inc. 508-804-2739
300 Stillwater P.o.box 1971, Stamford, CT 06902
Ureteroscope and accessories.

Karl Storz Endoscopy-America Inc. 800-421-0837
600 Corporate Pointe, Culver City, CA 90230
New-generation semi-rigid ureteroscopes with straight and angles eyepieces; large, bright image.

Mahe International Inc. 800-294-7946
468 Craighead St, Nashville, TN 37204

Olympus America, Inc. 800-645-8160
3500 Corporate Pkwy, PO Box 610, Center Valley, PA 18034

Pentax Medical Company 800-431-5880
102 Chestnut Ridge Rd, Montvale, NJ 07645
$14,490.00 for fiber ureteroscopes with distal tip diameters, 3.0mm to 4.1mm and channel diameters, 1.2mm to 1.8mm; fully immersible.

Pentax Southern Region Service Center 201-571-2300
8934 Kirby Dr, Houston, TX 77054
Ureteroscope.

Pentax West Coast Service Center 800-431-5880
10410 Pioneer Blvd Ste 2, Santa Fe Springs, CA 90670
Pentax ureteroscope.

Richard Wolf Medical Instruments Corp. 800-323-9653
353 Corporate Woods Pkwy, Vernon Hills, IL 60061

Technology Delivery Systems, Inc. 866-629-4359
340 E Parker Blvd, Suite 240, Baton Rouge, LA 70808
Sterile, disposable ureteroscope.

URETEROTOME *(Gastro/Urology) 78SEA*

Karl Storz Endoscopy-America Inc. 800-421-0837
600 Corporate Pointe, Culver City, CA 90230

Mahe International Inc. 800-294-7946
468 Craighead St, Nashville, TN 37204

Olympus America, Inc. 800-645-8160
3500 Corporate Pkwy, PO Box 610, Center Valley, PA 18034

URETEROTOME *(cont'd)*
Richard Wolf Medical Instruments Corp. 800-323-9653
353 Corporate Woods Pkwy, Vernon Hills, IL 60061

URETHROMETER *(Gastro/Urology) 78FBR*
Richard Wolf Medical Instruments Corp. 800-323-9653
353 Corporate Woods Pkwy, Vernon Hills, IL 60061

URETHROSCOPE *(Gastro/Urology) 78FGC*
Gyrus Acmi, Inc. 508-804-2739
93 N Pleasant St, Norwalk, OH 44857
Various urethroscopes.
Gyrus Acmi, Inc. 508-804-2739
300 Stillwater P.o.box 1971, Stamford, CT 06902
Various urethroscopes.
Karl Storz Endoscopy-America Inc. 800-421-0837
600 Corporate Pointe, Culver City, CA 90230
Mahe International Inc. 800-294-7946
468 Craighead St, Nashville, TN 37204
Richard Wolf Medical Instruments Corp. 800-323-9653
353 Corporate Woods Pkwy, Vernon Hills, IL 60061

URETHROTOME *(Gastro/Urology) 78EZO*
Greenwald Surgical Co., Inc. 219-962-1604
2688 Dekalb St, Gary, IN 46405
Cold kinves for visual urethrotomes.
Gyrus Acmi, Inc. 508-804-2739
93 N Pleasant St, Norwalk, OH 44857
Various urthrotomes.
Gyrus Acmi, Inc. 508-804-2739
300 Stillwater P.o.box 1971, Stamford, CT 06902
Various urthrotomes.
Karl Storz Endoscopy-America Inc. 800-421-0837
600 Corporate Pointe, Culver City, CA 90230
Optical urethrotome and working element set.
Mahe International Inc. 800-294-7946
468 Craighead St, Nashville, TN 37204
Richard Wolf Medical Instruments Corp. 800-323-9653
353 Corporate Woods Pkwy, Vernon Hills, IL 60061

URICASE (COLORIMETRIC), URIC ACID *(Chemistry) 75KNK*
Amresco Inc. 800-366-1313
30175 Solon Industrial Pkwy, Solon, OH 44139
RA, Hitachi, SMA, SMAC.
Caldon Bioscience, Inc. 909-628-9944
2100 S Reservoir St, Pomona, CA 91766
Uric acid reagent.
Caldon Biotech, Inc. 757-224-0177
2251 Rutherford Rd, Carlsbad, CA 92008
Uric acid reagent.
Carolina Liquid Chemistries Corp. 800-471-7272
510 W Central Ave Ste C, Brea, CA 92821
Uric acid or ua.
Genchem, Inc. 714-529-1616
510 W Central Ave Ste D, Brea, CA 92821
Uric acid reagent.
Genzyme Corp. 800-325-2436
160 Christian St, Oxford, CT 06478
Enzymatic, endpoint.
Jas Diagnostics, Inc. 305-418-2320
7220 NW 58th St, Miami, FL 33166
Uric acid.
Raichem, Division Of Hemagen Diagnostics, Inc. 800-438-6100
8225 Mercury Ct, San Diego, CA 92111
Stanbio Laboratory, Inc. 830-249-0772
1261 N Main St, Boerne, TX 78006
$52.50 for 4 x 30ml set with liquid reagent & standard (8mg/dl) and $142.00 for 2 x 250ml.
Synermed Intl., Inc. 317-896-1565
17408 Tiller Ct Ste 1900, Westfield, IN 46074
Uric acid reagent kit.
Teco Diagnostics 714-693-7788
1268 N Lakeview Ave, Anaheim, CA 92807
Uric acid.
Vital Diagnostics Inc. 714-672-3553
1075 W Lambert Rd Ste D, Brea, CA 92821
Various uric acid reagents.

URICASE (COULOMETRIC), URIC ACID *(Chemistry) 75JHB*
Beckman Coulter, Inc. 800-635-3497
740 W 83rd St, Hialeah, FL 33014
$0.09 per test.
Beckman Coulter, Inc. 800-742-2345
250 S Kraemer Blvd, PO Box 8000, Brea, CA 92821
Hemagen Diagnostics, Inc. 800-436-2436
9033 Red Branch Rd, Columbia, MD 21045
Various uric acid methods.

URICASE (OXYGEN RATE), URIC ACID *(Chemistry) 75JHC*
Health Chem Diagnostics Llc 954-979-3845
3341 W McNab Rd, Pompano Beach, FL 33069
Acid, uric, uricase (oxygen rate).

URICASE (U.V.), URIC ACID *(Chemistry) 75CDO*
Abbott Diagnostics Div. 626-440-0700
820 Mission St, South Pasadena, CA 91030
Uric acid.
Health Chem Diagnostics Llc 954-979-3845
3341 W McNab Rd, Pompano Beach, FL 33069
Acid, uric, uricase (u.v.).

URINAL *(General) 80FNP*
Centurion Medical Products Corp. 517-545-1135
3310 S Main St, Salisbury, NC 28147
Dornoch Medical Systems, Inc. 816-505-2226
4032 NW Riverside Dr, Riverside, MO 64150
Suction canister.
E-Z-Em, Inc. 516-333-8230
750 Summa Ave, Westbury, NY 11590
Urine collection device.
Jones-Zylon Company 800-848-8160
305 N Center St, West Lafayette, OH 43845
Male and female specifications; autoclavable and disposable.
Lsl Industries, Inc. 888-225-5575
5535 N Wolcott Ave, Chicago, IL 60640
$18.00 for 50 pcs.
Med-Assist Technology, Inc. 801-296-6848
2441 S 1560 W, Woods Cross, UT 84087
Various models of urinary collection system.
Medegen Medical Products, Llc 800-233-1987
209 Medegen Drive, Gallaway, TN 38036-0228
ROOM-MATES Disposable and reusable.
Medline Industries, Inc. 800-633-5886
1 Medline Pl, Mundelein, IL 60060
Mobility Transfer Systems 800-854-4687
PO Box 253, Medford, MA 02155
Spillproof URSEC urinal.
Polar Ware Co. 800-237-3655
2806 N 15th St, Sheboygan, WI 53083
Stainless steel, reusable plastic, single-patient plastic.
Prosurge Instruments, Inc. 866-832-7874
199 Laidlaw Ave, Jersey City, NJ 07306
Reach Global Industries, Inc. (Reachgood) 888-518-8389
8 Corporate Park Ste 300, Irvine, CA 92606
Urinals.
Sunrise Medical 800-333-4000
7477 Dry Creek Pkwy, Longmont, CO 80503
Tri-State Hospital Supply Corp. 517-545-1135
3173 E 43rd St, Yuma, AZ 85365
Truform Orthotics & Prosthetics 800-888-0458
3960 Rosslyn Dr, Cincinnati, OH 45209
Urocare Products, Inc. 800-423-4441
2735 Melbourne Ave, Pomona, CA 91767
Male urinal kit. Three sizes available: large, standard and small.
Viscot Medical, Llc 800-221-0658
32 West St, PO Box 351, East Hanover, NJ 07936
Clear, graduated MILLIE female and VISCOT male urinals.

URINARY HOMOCYSTINE (NON-QUANTITATIVE) TEST SYSTEM *(Chemistry) 75LPS*
Bio-Rad Laboratories Inc., Clinical Systems Div. 800-224-6723
4000 Alfred Nobel Dr, Hercules, CA 94547
Homocysteine by hplc.
Carolina Liquid Chemistries Corp. 800-471-7272
510 W Central Ave Ste C, Brea, CA 92821
Homocysteine reagent.

URINARY HOMOCYSTINE (NON-QUANTITATIVE) TEST SYSTEM *(cont'd)*

Catch Incorporated 425-402-8960
11822 N Creek Pkwy N Ste 107, Bothell, WA 98011
Homocysteine reagent.

Diazyme Laboratories 858-455-4761
12889 Gregg Ct, Poway, CA 92064
Homocysteine microtiter plate assay.

Intersect Systems, Inc. 360-577-1062
1152 3rd Avenue, Suite D & E, Longview, WA 98632
Homocysteine reagents for routine chemistry analyzers-- FDA cleared--excellent correlation to IMX and HPCC

Jas Diagnostics, Inc. 305-418-2320
7220 NW 58th St, Miami, FL 33166
Homocysteine enzimatic assay kit.

URINOMETER, ELECTRICAL *(Gastro/Urology) 78EXS*

Iris Diagnostics 800-776-4747
9172 Eton Ave, Chatsworth, CA 91311
Specific gravity meter.

URINOMETER, NON-ELECTRICAL *(Gastro/Urology) 78EXT*

Francis L. Freas Glass Works, Inc. 610-828-0430
148 E 9th Ave, Conshohocken, PA 19428

Kelsar, S.A. 508-261-8000
Blvd. Insurgentes, Libriamento a La, Tijuana 22450 Mexico
Measurit urine meter with drainage bag

Profex Medical Products 800-325-0196
2224 E Person Ave, Memphis, TN 38114

Ware Medics Glass Works, Inc. 845-429-6950
PO Box 368, Garnerville, NY 10923

URODYNAMIC MEASUREMENT SYSTEM *(Gastro/Urology) 78SEF*

Laborie Medical Technologies Inc. 888-522-6743
6415 Northwest Dr., Units 7-14, Mississauga, ONT L4V-1X1 Canada
Windows Based software systems designed for ease of use and world-wide serviceability. Systems priced from $11,400.00 to 100,000.00 depending on user's requirements. Total video capability offered. Portable systems offered as well as on-line service and service contracts.

Life-Tech, Inc. 281-491-6600
4235 Greenbriar Dr, Stafford, TX 77477
Urolab Spectrum self contained table-top instrument. Urolab Novus, Urolab Opus, Urolab Janus and Urolab Maximus expandable, PC based urodynamic systems with interfaced Galen lower urinary tract charting system and database.

Richard Wolf Medical Instruments Corp. 800-323-9653
353 Corporate Woods Pkwy, Vernon Hills, IL 60061

Timm Medical Technologies, Inc. 800-966-2796
6585 City West Pkwy, Eden Prairie, MN 55344
Equipment.

UROFLOWMETER *(Gastro/Urology) 78EXY*

C. R. Bard, Inc., Bard Urological Div. 888-367-2273
13183 Harland Dr NE, Covington, GA 30014

Laborie Medical Technologies Inc. 888-522-6743
6415 Northwest Dr., Units 7-14, Mississauga, ONT L4V-1X1 Canada
Priced below $3000.00, this flow unit is compact and portable. Windows software upgrade package available to link to a PC.

Life-Tech, Inc. 281-491-6600
4235 Greenbriar Dr, Stafford, TX 77477
Microflo microprocessor controlled uroflowmeter with nomograms.

Medtronic Neuromodulation 763-514-4000
710 Medtronic Pkwy, Minneapolis, MN 55432
Uroflowmeter.

Myo/Kinetic Systems, Inc. 414-255-1005
North 84 West 13562 Leon Rd., Menomonee Falls, WI 53051
Urodynamic equipment.

Reach Global Industries, Inc. (Reachgood) 888-518-8389
8 Corporate Park Ste 300, Irvine, CA 92606
Various.

Richard Wolf Medical Instruments Corp. 800-323-9653
353 Corporate Woods Pkwy, Vernon Hills, IL 60061

The Prometheus Group 603-749-0733
1 Washington St Ste 303, Dover, NH 03820
Biofeedback uroflowmeter.

UROLOGICAL IRRIGATION SYSTEM *(Gastro/Urology) 78LJH*

B. Braun Of Puerto Rico, Inc. 610-691-5400
215.7 Insular Rd., Sabana Grande, PR 00637
Irrigation sets and accessories.

Baxter Healthcare S.A. 847-948-2000
Rd. 721, Km. 0.3, Aibonito, PR 00609
Irrigation sets.

Benlan Inc. 905-829-5004
2760 Brighton Rd., Oakville, ONT L6H 5T4 Canada

Insight Biodesign Llc 775-250-0267
1065 Waverly Dr, Reno, NV 89519
Simple cystometrogram kit.

Karl Storz Endoscopy-America Inc. 800-421-0837
600 Corporate Pointe, Culver City, CA 90230

Lsl Industries, Inc. 888-225-5575
5535 N Wolcott Ave, Chicago, IL 60640
$13.00 per case of 50 disposable 8oz. irrigation bottles.

Medi Inc 800-225-8634
75 York Ave, P.O. Box 302, Randolph, MA 02368

Nexus Medical, Llc 913-451-2234
11315 Strang Line Rd, Lenexa, KS 66215
Irrigation set.

Northgate Technologies Inc. 800-348-0424
600 Church Rd, Elgin, IL 60123
The Flo-Assist tubing set and Flo-Assistant mechanical pump for hands free usage allows for routine, uninterrupted high flow gravity fed fluid delivery for cystoscopy and ureteroscopy with a bolus flow of 40cc on demand.

UTENSIL, FOOD *(Physical Med) 89ILC*

Abbas' Grace 603-624-9559
52 Meadow Ln, Manchester, NH 03109
J.a.m. straw.

Adlib, Inc. 714-895-9529
5142 Bolsa Ave Ste 106, Huntington Beach, CA 92649
Protracting implement holder mouthstick.

Ellkar Corporation 727-442-8231
1137 Sunnydale Dr, Clearwater, FL 33755
Spoon, fork.

Equipment Shop, Inc. 800-525-7681
PO Box 33, Bedford, MA 01730
Feeding spoons in two sizes: Maroon Spoon/small (package of 10 spoons, $7.50) and Maroon Spoon/large (package of 10 spoons, $8.60). Flexible cut cups sold in packages of 5: 1oz., $7.40; 2oz., $8.25; 7oz., $10.60. Also Chewy Tubes and Ark grabbers for oral therapy

Evergreen Health Inc. 877-742-3555
401 Audubon St, Adair, IA 50002
Sip-tip.

Inglis Foundation 215-581-0725
2600 Belmont Ave, Phila, PA 19131
Water bottle.

Maddak Inc. 800-443-4926
661 State Route 23, Wayne, NJ 07470

Mealtime Partners, Inc. 817-237-9991
1137 Southeast Pkwy, Azle, TX 76020
Assistive dining device.

Paramedical Distributors 800-245-3278
2020 Grand Blvd, Kansas City, MO 64108

Parsons A.D.L. Inc. 800-263-1281
R.R. #2, 1986 Sideroad 15, Tottenham, ONT L0G 1W0 Canada
Adapted cutlery to solve a wide range of challenges, cups, plates and other dining aids.

Patterson Medical Supply, Inc. 262-387-8720
W68N158 Evergreen Blvd, Cedarburg, WI 53012
Eating utensil,daily activity assist device.

Rice Research, Inc. 847-869-0621
2001 Sherman Ave Apt 506, Evanston, IL 60201
WONDER-FLO VACUUM CUP for patient self-feeding of liquids without spilling. Monsanto nylon, capacity 8oz., liquid content 240cc.

Richardson Products, Inc. 888-928-7297
9408 Gulfstream Rd, Frankfort, IL 60423
Eating utensils and kitchen aids.

Therafin Corporation 800-843-7234
19747 Wolf Rd, Mokena, IL 60448
Various types of eating aids.

UTENSIL, FOOD *(cont'd)*

Transatlantic Engineering 818-716-0663
21637 Dumetz Rd, Woodland Hills, CA 91364
High quality material. Sleek design.

UTENSIL, HANDICAPPED AID *(Physical Med) 89IKW*

Adlib, Inc. 714-895-9529
5142 Bolsa Ave Ste 106, Huntington Beach, CA 92649
Portable door knob turner.

Alimed, Inc. 800-225-2610
297 High St, Dedham, MA 02026

American Printing House For The Blind, Inc. 800-223-1839
PO Box 6085, Louisville, KY 40206
Quick Braille Kit with slate, stylus, and fanfold paper (#1-00086-00); 4-track cassette player/recorder with rechargeable batteries (#1-07085-00); GrandStand portable reading stand (#1-03205-00); Metric/inch ruler with raised lines (#1-03100-00); Variable intensity lamp (#1-08940-00); Beginners Abacus (#1-03180-00).

Assisted Access-Nfss, Inc. 800-950-9655
822 Preston Ct, Lake Villa, IL 60046
Doorbells, clocks, bed vibrators, crying baby signaling equipment, audio link systems for theaters and auditoriums and other living aids for the deaf.

Cme Medical Equipment Corp. 908-561-0906
1130 Donemy Gln, Scotch Plains, NJ 07076
Aids for daily living.

Dynatronics Corp. Chattanooga Operations 801-568-7000
6607 Mountain View Rd, Ooltewah, TN 37363
Homemaking utensil.

Forward Motions, Inc. 877-364-8267
214 Valley St, Dayton, OH 45404

Handi-Cap Aids Company 800-689-0511
730 W Hefner Rd, Oklahoma City, OK 73114
Handicapped aids and customized products for the individual handicapped, including adaptive driving aids for drivers and passengers. Hand controls, steering devices, high-tech driving systems, specialized autmotive seating, lifting devices, and more.

Maddak Inc. 800-443-4926
661 State Route 23, Wayne, NJ 07470

Mecanaids Co., Inc. 800-227-0877
21 Hampden Dr, South Easton, MA 02375
Handicapped dressing and reaching aids. Variety of daily living aids. Hip Kits.

Multi Marketing & Manufacturing, Inc. 303-794-5955
PO Box 1070, 5401 Prince Street, Littleton, CO 80160
UN-SKRU $8.95 plus $3.00 s/h screw top opener for 1/2in to 5in size tops; to be mounted underneath the cabinet; available in white and brown to match kitchen and workshop cabinets.

Noram Seating, Inc. 866-236-7328
18 Market St, Union City, PA 16438
Foot protecter.

Patterson Medical Supply, Inc. 262-387-8720
W68N158 Evergreen Blvd, Cedarburg, WI 53012
Homemaking aid, daily activity assist device.

Richardson Products, Inc. 888-928-7297
9408 Gulfstream Rd, Frankfort, IL 60423
Household aids.

Therafin Corporation 800-843-7234
19747 Wolf Rd, Mokena, IL 60448
Various types of paring boards.

Uneek Concepts, Llc 888-686-7988
6435 Alloway Ct, Springfield, VA 22152
Half bed rails for home beds.

VACUUM, CAST CUTTER *(Orthopedics) 87QGY*

Bsn Medical, Inc 800-552-1157
5825 Carnegie Blvd, Charlotte, NC 28209
AMERICAN ORTHOPEDIC™ MOBILE VACUUM'S remote on/off switch give the ability to use the vacuum alone or with the saw. The disposable filter cartridge traps more dust particles without clogging and is easy and safe to replace. Powerful enough to pick up fine particles. Also available AMERICAN ORTHOPAEDIC™ PORTABLE VACUUM - convenient storage within the self-contained unit. Versatile- attaches easily to most cast cutters.

Stryker Corp. 800-726-2725
2825 Airview Blvd, Portage, MI 49002

VAGINOSCOPE *(Obstetrics/Gyn) 85SEL*

Karl Storz Endoscopy-America Inc. 800-421-0837
600 Corporate Pointe, Culver City, CA 90230

Mahe International Inc. 800-294-7946
468 Craighead St, Nashville, TN 37204

Monarch Molding Inc. 888-767-5116
120 Liberty St, Council Grove, KS 66846

Richard Wolf Medical Instruments Corp. 800-323-9653
353 Corporate Woods Pkwy, Vernon Hills, IL 60061

VALVE, BREATHING *(Anesthesiology) 73WHT*

Dey, L.P. 800-755-5560
2751 Napa Valley Corporate Dr, Napa, CA 94558
EASIVENT valved holding chamber is the only valved holding chamber designed to hold the complete MDI kit inside. Masks are available in small, medium, and large. EasiVent improves medication delivery and simplifies patient training with a one-way valve, universal port, instructions printed on the unit, and built-in coaching signal.

Intersurgical Inc. 315-451-2900
417 Electronics Pkwy, Liverpool, NY 13088

Life Corporation 800-700-0202
1776 N Water St, Milwaukee, WI 53202
One-way valve on LIFE CPR Masks and Shields.

Passy-Muir Inc. 800-634-5397
4521 Campus Dr, Irvine, CA 92612
Passy-Muir™ closed-position 'no leak' Tracheostomy & Ventilator Swallowing and Speaking valves (PMVs.) The only swallowing & speaking valves that are interchangeable for use on or off the ventilator (with the exception of the PMV™ 2020 for metal trach tubes.) Independent research has shown that the closed position PMV improves swallowing, reduces aspiration, facilitates secretion management, and reduces weaning and decannulation time. Reimbursable by Medicare, Medicaid, MediCal, and CCS.

Spiration Inc. 866-497-1700
6675 185th Ave NE, Redmond, WA 98052
IBV Valve System One-Way Air-Leak Valve

VALVE, CATHETER FLUSH *(Cardiovascular) 74QHH*

Hospira, Inc. 877-946-7747
755 Jarvis Dr, Morgan Hill, CA 95037

Smiths Medical Asd, Inc. 800-848-1757
6250 Shier Rings Rd, Dublin, OH 43016
Catheter flush and hemostasis Y valves.

VALVE, CATHETER FLUSH, CONTINUOUS *(Cardiovascular) 74QHI*

Becton Dickinson Infusion Therapy Systems, Inc. 888-237-2762
9450 S State St, Sandy, UT 84070

Hospira, Inc. 877-946-7747
755 Jarvis Dr, Morgan Hill, CA 95037

Smiths Medical Asd, Inc. 800-848-1757
6250 Shier Rings Rd, Dublin, OH 43016

VALVE, CPB CHECK, RETROGRADE, IN-LINE *(Anesthesiology) 73MJJ*

Alliant Healthcare Products 269-629-0300
8850 M89, Richland, MI 49083
Vent valve.

Terumo Cardiovascular Systems (Tcvs) 800-283-7866
28 Howe St, Ashland, MA 01721
Retrograde flow valve.

VALVE, EAR *(Ear/Nose/Throat) 77SEM*

E. Benson Hood Laboratories, Inc. 800-942-5227
575 Washington St, Pembroke, MA 02359
Inner ear valve.

VALVE, HEART, MECHANICAL *(Cardiovascular) 74LWQ*

ATS Medical, Inc. 800-399-1381
3905 Annapolis Ln N Ste 105, Minneapolis, MN 55447
ATS Open Pivot Mechanical Heart Valve

Cryolife, Inc. 800-438-8285
1655 Roberts Blvd NW, Kennesaw, GA 30144
Cryolife-Ross stentless porcine heart valve.

Edwards Lifesciences, Llc. 800-424-3278
1 Edwards Way, Irvine, CA 92614

Medtronic, Inc. 800-633-8766
710 Medtronic Pkwy, Minneapolis, MN 55432

VALVE, HEART, MECHANICAL *(cont'd)*

Plastic And Metal Center, Inc. 949-770-8230
23162 La Cadena Dr, Laguna Hills, CA 92653

St. Jude Medical, Inc. 800-328-9634
1 Saint Jude Medical Dr, Saint Paul, MN 55117

VALVE, HEART, TISSUE *(Cardiovascular) 74LWR*

Alabama Tissue Center, Inc. 205-934-4314
1900 University Blvd, 855 Tinsley Harrison Tower
Birmingham, AL 35233
Heart valve, tissue.

Ats Medical, Inc. 949-380-9333
20412 James Bay Cir, Lake Forest, CA 92630

Bio Breeders, Inc. 617-926-5278
116 Temperton Parkway, Watertown, MA 02472

Cryolife, Inc. 800-438-8285
1655 Roberts Blvd NW, Kennesaw, GA 30144

Edwards Lifesciences, Llc. 800-424-3278
1 Edwards Way, Irvine, CA 92614

Medtronic Cardiovascular Surgery, The Heart Valve Div. 800-328-2518
1851 E Deere Ave, Santa Ana, CA 92705
Various models and sizes of porcine bioprostheses and conduits.

RTI Biologics Inc. 877-343-6832
11621 Research Cir, Alachua, FL 32615
Aortic valve; pulmonic valve.

VALVE, LABORATORY *(Chemistry) 75WYH*

Acro Associates 800-672-2276
1990 Olivera Rd Ste A, Concord, CA 94520
Solenoid and pneumatically-operated pinch valves for flexible, disposable tubing or tubesets.

VALVE, NON-REBREATHING *(Anesthesiology) 73CBP*

Aerodyne Controls, Inc., A Circor International Company 631-737-1900
30 Haynes Ct, Ronkonkoma, NY 11779

Ambu A/S 457-225-2210
6740 Baymeadow Dr, Glen Burnie, MD 21060
E valve.

Cft, Inc./Life Mask 800-331-8844
14602 N Cave Creek Rd Ste B, Phoenix, AZ 85022
One way valve, non-rebreathing.

Corpak Medsystems, Inc. 800-323-6305
100 Chaddick Dr, Wheeling, IL 60090
Transport circuit.

Dhd Healthcare Corporation 800-847-8000
PO Box 6, One Madison Street, Wampsville, NY 13163
NIFTEE.

Eastmed Enterprises, Inc. 856-797-0131
11 Brandywine Dr, Marlton, NJ 08053
Guedel and Berman airways.

Hans Rudolph, Inc. 816-363-5522
7200 Wyandotte St, Kansas City, MO 64114
Rudolph respiratory valves and masks.

Instrumentation Industries, Inc. 800-633-8577
2990 Industrial Blvd, Bethel Park, PA 15102
Non-rebreathing T.

Intersurgical Inc. 315-451-2900
417 Electronics Pkwy, Liverpool, NY 13088
One-way exhalation valve that directs breathing flow to the patient and vents exhaled gases into the atmosphere.

Life Corporation 800-700-0202
1776 N Water St, Milwaukee, WI 53202
One-way valve on LIFE CPR Masks and Shields.

Nano Mask Inc. 888-656-3697
175 Cassia Way Ste A115, Henderson, NV 89014
RespAide - CPR assistance mask and valve

Passy-Muir Inc. 800-634-5397
4521 Campus Dr, Irvine, CA 92612
Passy-Muir™ closed-position 'no leak' Tracheostomy & Ventilator Swallowing and Speaking valves (PMVs.) The only swallowing & speaking valves that are interchangeable for use on or off the ventilator (with the exception of the PMV™ 2020 for metal trach tubes.) Independent research has shown that the closed position PMV improves swallowing, reduces aspiration, facilitates secretion management, and reduces weaning and decannulation time. Reimbursable by Medicare, Medicaid, MediCal, and CCS.

VALVE, NON-REBREATHING *(cont'd)*

Plasco, Inc. 847-662-4400
Carretera Presta La Amistad, Km.19, Acuna, Coahila Mexico
Exhaled air pulmonary resuscitator

Rondex Products, Inc. 815-226-0452
PO Box 1829, Rockford, IL 61110
CPR valve used with resuscitation mask for CPR.

Smiths Medical Asd Inc. 800-258-5361
10 Bowman Dr, Keene, NH 03431
Disposable resuscitation bag valve.

Spiracle Technology 714-418-1091
16520 Harbor Blvd Ste D, Fountain Valley, CA 92708
Resuscitation bag refill valve.

Tagg Industries L.L.C. 800-548-3514
23210 Del Lago Dr, Laguna Hills, CA 92653
PTP rebreathing air valve with oxygen mask.

U O Equipment Co. 800-231-6372
5863 W 34th St, Houston, TX 77092

Work 'N Leisure Products, Inc. 508-634-0939
455 Fortune Blvd, Milford, MA 01757
Cpr resuscitator.

VALVE, OPHTHALMIC *(Ophthalmology) 86SEN*

E. Benson Hood Laboratories, Inc. 800-942-5227
575 Washington St, Pembroke, MA 02359
Krupin eye valve in 4 sizes, with Ultra-smooth.

VALVE, OTHER *(Chemistry) 75UJD*

Aerodyne Controls, Inc., A Circor International Company 631-737-1900
30 Haynes Ct, Ronkonkoma, NY 11779
Pneumatic, solenoid, pressure, regulator, check and relief; miniature; plastic, brass and stainless steel; specialty and general purpose models available for most liquids and gases.

B. Braun Oem Division, B. Braun Medical Inc. 866-8-BBRAUN
824 12th Ave, Bethlehem, PA 18018

Bei Technologies, Inc. 949-341-9500
170 Technology Dr, Irvine, CA 92618
Pressure-vacuum.

Bicron Electronics 800-624-2766
50 Barlow St, Canaan, CT 06018
Solenoid.

Cte Chem Tec Equipment Co. 800-222-2177
234 SW 12th Ave, Deerfield Beach, FL 33442
Excess Flow Valves

Directmed, Inc. 516-656-3377
150 Pratt Oval, Glen Cove, NY 11542

Engineers Express, Inc. 800-255-8823
7 Industrial Park Rd, Medway, MA 02053

Filtertek Inc. 800-248-2461
11411 Price Rd, Hebron, IL 60034

Halkey-Roberts Corp. 800-303-4384
2700 Halkey Roberts Pl N, Saint Petersburg, FL 33716

Industrial Specialities Manufacturing, Inc. 800-781-8487
2741 W Oxford Ave Unit 6, Englewood, CO 80110
Check valve for air & liquid.

Kloehn Co., Ltd. 800-358-4342
10000 Banburry Cross Dr, Las Vegas, NV 89144
O.E.M. solenoid valves.

Kontes Glass Co. 888-546-2531
1022 Spruce St, Vineland, NJ 08360

Nalge Nunc International 800-625-4327
75 Panorama Creek Dr, Rochester, NY 14625
NALGENE liquid/gas check valves; needle-type valve; 2- and 3- way stopcock; assorted sanitary adapters.

Noshok, Inc. 440-243-0888
1010 W Bagley Rd, Berea, OH 44017
Precision needle valves. 6000 psi and 10,000 psi, carbon steel and 316 stainless steel construction. Soft and hard seat. All configurations.

Self Regulation Systems, Inc. 800-345-5642
8672 154th Ave NE Bldg F, Redmond, WA 98052
IN-FLOW intraurethral device with remote controlled valve-pump mechanism for female bladder drainage.

Specialty Manufacturing Co., The 651-653-0599
5858 Centerville Rd, Saint Paul, MN 55127
Flow-control.

VALVE, OTHER *(cont'd)*

Spectra Medical Devices, Inc. 866-938-8649
4C Henshaw St, Woburn, MA 01801
Stopcocks.

Vernay Laboratories, Inc. 800-666-5227
120 E South College St, Yellow Springs, OH 45387

Vital Concepts, Inc. 800-984-2300
4334 Brockton Dr SE Ste F, Grand Rapids, MI 49512
Hydro Pro & Virta Flow, Irrigation & aspiration valve system; high flow disposable trumpet system w/disposable or reusable probes including I/A electrode probes.

VALVE, POSITIVE END EXPIRATORY PRESSURE (PEEP)
(Anesthesiology) 73SEO

Ambu, Inc. 800-262-8462
6740 Baymeadow Dr, Glen Burnie, MD 21060
AMBU RMT-PEEP valves.

Armstrong Medical Industries, Inc. 800-323-4220
575 Knightsbridge Pkwy, Lincolnshire, IL 60069

Boehringer Laboratories, Inc. 800-642-4945
500 E Washington St, Norristown, PA 19401
2.5-, 5-, 10-, and 15-cm H2O units available. Peep valves designed to be used in CPAP and ventilator circuits, as well as in anesthesia systems.

Mercury Medical 800-237-6418
11300 49th St N, Clearwater, FL 33762
Single patient use peep valve.

Quadromed Inc. 800-363-0192
5776 Thimens Ave., St-Laurent, QUE H4R 2K9 Canada

VALVE, PRESSURE RELIEF, CARDIOPULMONARY BYPASS
(Cardiovascular) 74MNJ

Circulatory Technology, Inc. 516-624-2424
21 Singworth St, Oyster Bay, NY 11771
Pressure relief valve.

Terumo Cardiovascular Systems (Tcvs) 800-283-7866
28 Howe St, Ashland, MA 01721
Pressure relief valve.

VALVE, PROSTHESIS *(Physical Med) 89ISP*

E. Benson Hood Laboratories, Inc. 800-942-5227
575 Washington St, Pembroke, MA 02359
PANJE, Voicemaster & Grongingen.

Hosmer Dorrance Corp. 408-379-5151
561 Division St, Campbell, CA 95008
Various.

Orthotic & Prosthetic Lab, Inc. 314-968-8555
748 Marshall Ave, Webster Groves, MO 63119
O&p valve prosthesis.

Passy-Muir Inc. 800-634-5397
4521 Campus Dr, Irvine, CA 92612
Passy-Muir™ closed-position 'no leak' Tracheostomy & Ventilator Swallowing and Speaking valves (PMVs.) The only swallowing & speaking valves that are interchangeable for use on or off the ventilator (with the exception of the PMV™ 2020 for metal trach tubes.) Independent research has shown that the closed position PMV improves swallowing, reduces aspiration, facilitates secretion management, and reduces weaning and decannulation time. Reimbursable by Medicare, Medicaid, MediCal, and CCS.

VALVE, SPEAKING, TRACHEAL *(Ear/Nose/Throat) 77WRO*

Boston Medical Products, Inc. 800-433-2674
117 Flanders Rd, Westborough, MA 01581
Montgomery silicone speaking valves, for all Montgomery cannulas, adult Safe-T-Tubes, and standard tracheotomy tubes. Including a speaking valve for ventilator dependent patients.

E. Benson Hood Laboratories, Inc. 800-942-5227
575 Washington St, Pembroke, MA 02359
Speaking valve fits Stoma Stent System and 15mm connector.

Passy-Muir Inc. 800-634-5397
4521 Campus Dr, Irvine, CA 92612
Passy-Muir™ closed-position 'no leak' Tracheostomy & Ventilator Swallowing and Speaking valves (PMVs.) The only swallowing & speaking valves that are interchangeable for use on or off the ventilator (with the exception of the PMV™ 2020 for metal trach tubes.) Independent research has shown that the closed position PMV improves swallowing, reduces aspiration, facilitates secretion management, and reduces weaning and decannulation time. Reimbursable by Medicare, Medicaid, MediCal, and CCS.

VALVE, SPEAKING, TRACHEAL *(cont'd)*

Smiths Medical Asd 800-424-8662
5700 W 23rd Ave, Gary, IN 46406
Spring activated for laryngectomees to achieve hands-free voice when used with voice prosthesis.

Technical Products, Inc. 800-226-8434
805 Marathon Pkwy Ste 150, Lawrenceville, GA 30046
One-piece, integrated speech valve in the tracheal cannula. Improves phonation and airflow availability.

VALVE, SWITCHING (PLOSS) *(Anesthesiology) 73JFE*

Precision Medical, Inc. 800-272-7285
300 Held Dr, Northampton, PA 18067
Instant flow valve.

VALVULOTOME *(Cardiovascular) 74MGZ*

Biomet Microfixation Inc. 800-874-7711
1520 Tradeport Dr, Jacksonville, FL 32218
Valvulotome.

Edwards Lifesciences, Llc. 800-424-3278
1 Edwards Way, Irvine, CA 92614

Lemaitre Vascular, Inc. 781-221-2266
63 2nd Ave, Burlington, MA 01803
LEMAITRE Expandable Valvulotome, disposable self-sizing, self-centering valve cutter. Disposable and reusable valve cutters available in 7 sizes.

Scanlan International, Inc. 800-328-9458
1 Scanlan Plz, Saint Paul, MN 55107

Uresil, Llc 800-538-7374
5418 Touhy Ave, Skokie, IL 60077
For in situ bypass procedures.

VAPOR PRESSURE, OSMOLALITY OF SERUM & URINE
(Chemistry) 75JNA

Arkray Factory Usa, Inc. 952-646-3168
5182 W 76th St, Minneapolis, MN 55439
Urine test strips.

VAPORIZER *(General) 80SEQ*

Clover Medical Equipment Services, Inc. 800-550-4111
117 Albert Dr, Lancaster, NY 14086
Cleaning, repair, and calibration of Ohio, Cyprane, Ohmeda, and Drager vaporizers. Sales of remanufactured vaporizers. Vaporizer conversions.

Electro-Steam Generator Corp. 888-783-2624
1000 Bernard St, Alexandria, VA 22314
LITTLE GIANT electric steam generators.

P-Ryton Corp. 800-221-9840
504 50th Ave, Long Island City, NY 11101
SKIN DYNAMICS Console system and aroma vapor machines. Console system is a facial machine consisting of: a vapor brush, vac/spray, sanitizer(optional high frequency or galvanic current instead of sanitizer) with clamp(X3 Diopter). Aroma vapor is a facial steamer with aroma adapter.

Southmedic Inc. 800-463-7146
50 Alliance Blvd., Barrie, ONT L4M-5K3 Canada
Trolley bars (vaporizer accessory); anti-spill adaptor, which is used to fill funnel for vaporizer without spillage; funnel adaptor used to convert Funnel Fill vaporizer to key indexed vaporizer.

VAPORIZER, ANESTHESIA, NON-HEATED
(Anesthesiology) 73CAD

Aga Linde Healthcare P.R. Inc. 787-622-7900
PO Box 363868, GPO Box 364727, San Juan, PR 00936
Anesth/Pul Med.

Anesthetic Vaporizer Services 716-759-8490
10185 Main St, Clarence, NY 14031
Anesthetic vaporizer.

Clover Medical Equipment Services, Inc. 800-550-4111
117 Albert Dr, Lancaster, NY 14086

Datex-Ohmeda (Canada) 800-268-1472
1093 Meyerside Dr., Unit 2, Mississauga, ONT L5T-1J6 Canada

Datex-Ohmeda Inc. 608-221-1551
3030 Ohmeda Dr, Madison, WI 53718
Vaporizer.

Datex-Ohmeda, Inc. (Madison) 800-345-2700
3030 Ohmeda Dr, Madison, WI 53718

Health Care Logistics, Inc. 800-848-1633
450 Town St, PO Box 25, Circleville, OH 43113
Various types of vaporizer fillers.

VAPORIZER, ANESTHESIA, NON-HEATED *(cont'd)*

Sharn, Inc. 800-325-3671
4517 George Rd Ste 200, Tampa, FL 33634
VAPOFIL key fills without vapor lock; ANTI-SPIL adapter reduces spills.

Southmedic Inc. 800-463-7146
50 Alliance Blvd., Barrie, ONT L4M-5K3 Canada
ANAESLOCK HVA-003 anesthetic vaporizer lock; locks all but selected vaporizer in off position and shows vaporizer in use, made of aluminum. ANESLOCK ADAPTOR for use with CYPRANE vaporizer. PEN LEVEL unit for levelling transducers and catheters.

VARNISH *(Dental And Oral) 76EMC*

Cadco Dental Products 800-833-8267
600 E Hueneme Rd, Oxnard, CA 93033
$6.50 for 1/2 oz. Copa-seal cavity varnish.

Cooley & Cooley, Ltd. 800-215-4487
8550 Westland West Blvd, Houston, TX 77041
COPALITE dental cavity varnish is the number one selling dental varnish since 1933. Toxicology lab tests report no toxicity or mutagenicity. Innovative blend of resins and solvents penetrate deep into infected dental tubules to reach deep biofilm infestation. Decreases tooth sensitivity caused by mechanical, chemical or temperature factors.

Dux Dental 800-833-8267
600 E Hueneme Rd, Oxnard, CA 93033
$6.00 for 1/2 oz. Copa-seal cavity varnish.

Harry J. Bosworth Company 800-323-4352
7227 Hamlin Ave, Skokie, IL 60076
COPALINER, cavity varnish and sealant.

Scientific Pharmaceuticals, Inc. 800-634-3047
3221 Producer Way, Pomona, CA 91768
$15.00 for 15 cc.

Sterngold 800-243-9942
23 Frank Mossberg Dr, PO Box 2967, Attleboro, MA 02703
Stern Vantage Varnish LC - SternVantage Varnish LC is a light cure one-component surface coating material based on acrylates and cures without a smear layer caused by oxygen inhibition. It has been developed especially for cases where the surface of acrylate materials after polymerization exhibits an undesired or intolerable smear layer, where increased surface hardness is desirable or where the oral environment must be protected from elution of monomers out of freshly polymerized materials. Treatment of polymerized composite surfaces, custom trays or temporary crowns and bridges with Varnish LC yields a hard, high gloss, solvent and stain resistant, ultra dry finish with a smooth surface. Plaque formation and deposition of tartar is minimized. Varnish LC is cured with a common dental halogen light unit or in an UV or stroboscopic light unit.

Zila, Inc. 800-228-5595
701 Centre Ave, Fort Collins, CO 80526
ProDenRx

VARNISH, CAVITY *(Dental And Oral) 76LBH*

Cetylite Industries, Inc. 856-665-6111
9051 River Rd, Pennsauken, NJ 08110
Cavity varnish.

Chx Technologies, Inc. 416-233-3737
105-4800 Dundas St W, Toronto M9A 1B1 Canada
Cavity varnish

Dent Zar, Inc. 800-444-1241
6362 Hollywood Blvd Ste 214, Los Angeles, CA 90028
Cavity varnish.

Dental Resources 717-866-7571
52 King St, Myerstown, PA 17067
Cavity varnish.

Dentsply Canada, Ltd. 800-263-1437
161 Vinyl Ct., Woodbridge, ONT L4L 4A3 Canada

Dshealthcare Inc. 201-871-1232
85 W Forest Ave, Englewood, NJ 07631
Cavity varnish.

Gc America, Inc. 708-597-0900
3737 W 127th St, Alsip, IL 60803
Varnish.

Ivoclar Vivadent, Inc. 800-533-6825
175 Pineview Dr, Amherst, NY 14228
FLUOR PROTECTOR

VARNISH, CAVITY *(cont'd)*

Kerr Corp. 949-255-8766
1717 W Collins Ave, Orange, CA 92867
Vavity varnish.

Medental Intl. 760-727-5889
3008 Palm Hill Dr, Vista, CA 92084
Various.

Medical Products Laboratories, Inc. 215-677-2700
9990 Global Rd, Philadelphia, PA 19115
5% sodium fluoride varnish.

Novamin Technology Inc. 386-418-1551
13859 Progress Blvd Ste 600, Alachua, FL 32615
Inorganic apatite-forming tooth root conditioner and dentin tubule occluder.

Pascal Co., Inc. 425-602-3633
2929 Northup Way, Bellevue, WA 98004
Cavity varnish.

Pentron Clinical Technologies 203-265-7397
68-70 North Plains Industrial, Road, Wallingford, CT 06492
Varnish,cavity.

Rite-Dent Manufacturing Corp. 305-693-8626
3750 E 10th Ct, Hialeah, FL 33013
Various types of copal varnish.

Scientific Pharmaceuticals, Inc. 800-634-3047
3221 Producer Way, Pomona, CA 91768

Ultradent Products, Inc. 801-553-4586
505 W 10200 S, South Jordan, UT 84095
Disinfecting solution.

Water Pik, Inc. 970-221-6129
1730 E Prospect Rd, Fort Collins, CO 80525
Cavity varnish.

Westside Packaging, Llc. 909-570-3508
1700 S Baker Ave Ste A, Ontario, CA 91761
Compound to coat a tooth cavity.

Wykle Research, Inc. 775-887-7500
2222 College Pkwy, Carson City, NV 89706
Cavity varnish.

VASCULAR ACCESS GRAFT *(Gastro/Urology) 78LTH*

Artegraft, Inc. 800-631-5264
220 N Center Dr, North Brunswick, NJ 08902
ARTEGRAFT. The 100% collagen vascular graft and natural alternative to synthetic grafts. Proven long-term patency and surgical compliancy.

B. Braun Oem Division, B. Braun Medical Inc. 866-8-BBRAUN
824 12th Ave, Bethlehem, PA 18018

Bard Peripheral Vascular, Inc. 800-321-4254
1625 W 3rd St, Tempe, AZ 85281

Cook Inc. 800-457-4500
PO Box 489, Bloomington, IN 47402

Corvita Corp. 305-599-3100
8210 NW 27th St, Doral, FL 33122
Blood access for hemodialysis.

VECTORCARDIOGRAPH *(Cardiovascular) 74DYC*

Elmed, Inc. 630-543-2792
60 W Fay Ave, Addison, IL 60101

VEHICLE, HANDICAPPED *(Physical Med) 89WHH*

Champion Bus Inc. 800-776-4943
331 Graham Rd, Imlay City, MI 48444

Collins Bus Corporation 800-354-9802
415 W 6th Ave, P.O. Box 2946, South Hutchinson, KS 67505

Complete Mobility Systems Inc. 800-788-7479
1915 County Road C W, Roseville, MN 55113
Vehicles equipped for individuals and commercial applications - transporting ambulatory and wheelchair bound passengers. ADA certified.

Forward Motions, Inc. 877-364-8267
214 Valley St, Dayton, OH 45404
Vans (full size/mini) for use by people with disabilities (personal and commercial). Also, with equipment lifts to transport medical equipment less than 800 lbs.

Goshen Coach Div. Warrick Industries, Inc. 800-326-2062
25161 Leer Dr, Elkhart, IN 46514
GOSHEN COACH para-transit, has maximum headroom and wide aisles for easy access to seats and wheelchairs.

VEHICLE, HANDICAPPED *(cont'd)*

Hds Specialty Vehicles 866-826-6176
16290 Kenrick Loop, Lakeville, MN 55044
Converted van models for the handicapped, with or without raised roof. Also, ADA-approved transport vehicle with certified roll-bar system. Manufacturers of the DuraTran ADA Paratransit Van.

Kaye Products, Inc. 919-732-6444
535 Dimmocks Mill Rd, Hillsborough, NC 27278
Scoot-About, 4 swivel wheeled seat with hand rail. Adjustable height for children, 2 1/2 to adult. For mobile sitting.

Leisure-Lift, Inc. 800-255-0285
1800 Merriam Ln, Kansas City, KS 66106

Wright-Way, Inc. 800-241-8839
175 E Interstate 30, Garland, TX 75043
Conversion of vans for handicapped use.

VEHICLE/EQUIPMENT, RECREATIONAL (HANDICAPPED)
(General) 80SHN

Trace Laboratories-East 410-584-9099
5 N Park Dr, Hunt Valley, MD 21030
Bicycle.

Wright-Way, Inc. 800-241-8839
175 E Interstate 30, Garland, TX 75043
Products and services for the disabled senior citizens, injury and rehab markets. Also offer a free after-therapy catalog.

VENA CAVA BALLOON OCCLUDER *(Cardiovascular) 74LWT*

Docxs Biomedical Products And Accessories 707-462-2351
564 S Dora St Ste A-1, Ukiah, CA 95482
Implantable, 100% Silicone Rubber Vascular Occluders, Hepatic Shunts and Aritficial Uretheral Spincters for animal research and Veterinary use

VENEER, DENTAL *(Dental And Oral) 76VDX*

Scientific Pharmaceuticals, Inc. 800-634-3047
3221 Producer Way, Pomona, CA 91768
$150.00 for 15-g kit with accessories.

VENTILATOR, ANESTHESIA UNIT *(Anesthesiology) 73QBB*

Aga Linde Healthcare P.R. Inc. 787-622-7900
PO Box 363868, GPO Box 364727, San Juan, PR 00936
Anesth/Pul Med.

Datex-Ohmeda (Canada) 800-268-1472
1093 Meyerside Dr., Unit 2, Mississauga, ONT L5T-1J6 Canada

Ge Medical Systems Information Technologies 800-643-6439
8200 W Tower Ave, Milwaukee, WI 53223

Mallard Medical, Inc. 530-226-0727
20268 Skypark Dr, Redding, CA 96002

VENTILATOR, CONTINUOUS (RESPIRATOR)
(Anesthesiology) 73CBK

Airon Corporation 888-448-1238
751 North Dr Ste 6, Melbourne, FL 32934
Pneuton transport ventilator.

American Biomed Instruments, Inc. 718-235-8900
11 Wyona St, Brooklyn, NY 11207

Cardinal Health 207, Inc. 610-862-0800
1100 Bird Center Dr, Palm Springs, CA 92262
Seris 2000.

Cardiopulmonary Corp. 203-877-1999
200 Cascade Blvd, Milford, CT 06460
Venturi.

Datex-Ohmeda Inc. 608-221-1551
3030 Ohmeda Dr, Madison, WI 53718
Various continuous ventilators.

Draeger Medical Systems, Inc. 215-660-2626
16 Electronics Ave, Danvers, MA 01923
Various ventilators.

Draeger Safety, Inc. 800-922-5518
101 Technology Dr, Pittsburgh, PA 15275

Emergency Medical International 305-362-6050
6065 NW 167th St Ste B18, Hialeah, FL 33015
The Inspiration Ventilator.The Critical Care Ventilator that provides suppport for your infant through adult patients.Our innovative Ethernet interface and optional mini-webserver revolutionize patient monitoring.

VENTILATOR, CONTINUOUS (RESPIRATOR) *(cont'd)*

General Biomedical Service, Inc. 800-558-9449
1900 25th St, Kenner, LA 70062
New & remanufactured respiratory equipment, ventilators, and pulse oximeters.

Hamilton Medical, Inc. 800-426-6331
4990 Energy Way, Reno, NV 89502
GALILEO, VEOLAR & AMADEUS microprocessor-based adult/pediatric ventilators.

Health Chem Diagnostics Llc 954-979-3845
3341 W McNab Rd, Pompano Beach, FL 33069
Ventilator, continuous (respirator).

Impact Instrumentation, Inc. 800-969-0750
27 Fairfield Pl, West Caldwell, NJ 07006
Model 706, Uni-Vent Series, Automatic Resuscitator/Volume Ventilators. For emergency ventilation of non-breathing patients. Includes fixed rate/inspiratory time settings, adjustable volume. AC-DC-rechargeable battery-powered. $1525.00to $1546.00. Also available, Model 754 Eagle, Uni-Vent Portable Ventilator-Compressor-Air/Oxygen Mixer. Self-contained critical care ventilation system with AC-DC rechargeable battery operation. Multiple operating modes, graphics display, internal PEEP, automatic altitude compensation, internal backup ventilator and alarms. Includes aeromedical certification, autosensing universal power supply, hoses and ventilator circuit. $8995.00. Also available 750, Uni-Vent Portable Ventilator. Critical care, AC-DC rechargeable battery powered portable ventilator. Multiple operating modes, displays and alarms. Includes aeromedical certification, 115/230 VAC, 50/60 Hz power supply, hoses, ventilator circuit and patient valve. $5395.00

Lab Safety Supply, Inc. 800-356-0783
401 S Wright Rd, Janesville, WI 53546
Respirators.

Mine Safety Appliances Company 866-MSA-1001
121 Gamma Dr, Pittsburgh, PA 15238

Oceanic Medical Products, Inc. 913-874-2000
8005 Shannon Industrial Park, Ln., Atchison, KS 66002
Respiratory ventilator.

Pace Tech, Inc. 800-722-3024
510 N Garden Ave, Clearwater, FL 33755

Respironics California, Inc. 724-387-4559
2271 Cosmos Ct, Carlsbad, CA 92011
Respirator.

Sechrist Industries, Inc. 800-732-4747
4225 E La Palma Ave, Anaheim, CA 92807

Versamed Medical Systems, Inc. 800-475-9239
2 Blue Hill Plz, Pearl River, NY 10965
Ventilator.

883495 Ontario, Inc. 613-384-9550
2-759 Progress Ave, Kingston K7M 6N6 Canada
Bear cub infant ventilator

VENTILATOR, CONTINUOUS (RESPIRATOR), ACCESSORY
(Anesthesiology) 73MOD

Innovision Medical Technologies, Llc 410-694-9450
1302 Concourse Dr Ste 302, Linthicum, MD 21090
Software to view medical device data.

Sleepnet Corporation 800-742-3646
5 Merrill Industrial Dr, Hampton, NH 03842
IQ non-invasive nasal mask (non-US only)

Welch Allyn Protocol Inc. 800-289-2500
8500 SW Creekside Pl, Beaverton, OR 97008
Accessory to continuous ventilator (respirator).

VENTILATOR, CONTINUOUS, NON-LIFE SUPPORTING
(Anesthesiology) 73MNS

Respironics California, Inc. 724-387-4559
2271 Cosmos Ct, Carlsbad, CA 92011
Ventilator system.

VENTILATOR, EMERGENCY, MANUAL (RESUSCITATOR)
(Anesthesiology) 73BTM

Allied Healthcare Products, Inc. 800-444-3954
1720 Sublette Ave, Saint Louis, MO 63110

Ambu A/S 457-225-2210
6740 Baymeadow Dr, Glen Burnie, MD 21060
Resuscitators, various models.

VENTILATOR, EMERGENCY, MANUAL (RESUSCITATOR) *(cont'd)*

Ambu, Inc. 800-262-8462
6740 Baymeadow Dr, Glen Burnie, MD 21060
Mark 111 Resuscitator, Ambu Baby Resuscitator, Ambu Silicone Resuscitator, Ambu Spur; various models and Rescue Key.

Caligor 800-472-4346
846 Pelham Pkwy, Pelham, NY 10803

Corpak Medsystems, Inc. 800-323-6305
100 Chaddick Dr, Wheeling, IL 60090
Various.

Eastmed Enterprises, Inc. 856-797-0131
11 Brandywine Dr, Marlton, NJ 08053
Various types of head harnesses.

Engineered Medical Systems 317-246-5500
2055 Executive Dr, Indianapolis, IN 46241
Various models of manual resuscitators and accessories.

Health Care Logistics, Inc. 800-848-1633
450 Town St, PO Box 25, Circleville, OH 43113
Disposable resuscitators.

Kentron Health Care, Inc. 615-384-0573
3604 Kelton Jackson Rd, P.o. Box 120, Springfield, TN 37172
Manual resuscitator.

Life Corporation 800-700-0202
1776 N Water St, Milwaukee, WI 53202
LIFE, CPR Masks and Shield and LIFE Bags/Mask/Resuscitators Portable emergency oxygen units, clear cover and wall-mounted, off/on lever control, resuscitation mask with one-way valve for hygiene, 6lpm 90min. supply, refillable. Also available 6 & 12 lpm NORM & HIGH, 0-25 lpm variable, and demand-valve for 100% oxygen resuscitation. GSA Federal Supply Schedule.

Mada, Inc. 800-526-6370
625 Washington Ave, Carlstadt, NJ 07072

Matrx 716-662-6650
145 Mid County Dr, Orchard Park, NY 14127
Bag/valve/mask resuscitator.

Mtm Health Products Ltd. 800-263-8253
2349 Fairview St., Burlington, ONT L7R 2E3 Canada
Disposable MTM MOUTH TO MASK one-way valve emergency resuscitator with adult and pediatric facemasks, with standard oxygen ports and head strap.

Oemedic International, Inc. 886-2-22903959
No. 162, Atlantic Street, Pomona, CA 91768
Manual resuscitator.

Plasco, Inc. 847-662-4400
Carretera Presta La Amistad, Km.19, Acuna, Coahila Mexico
Exhale air pulmonary resuscitator

Smiths Medical Asd Inc. 800-258-5361
10 Bowman Dr, Keene, NH 03431
Manual resuscitator.

Ventlab Corp. 336-753-5000
155 Boyce Dr, Mocksville, NC 27028
Manual resuscitator.

Work 'N Leisure Products, Inc. 508-634-0939
455 Fortune Blvd, Milford, MA 01757
Resuscitator mask.

VENTILATOR, EMERGENCY, POWERED (RESUSCITATOR)
(Anesthesiology) 73BTL

Airon Corporation 888-448-1238
751 North Dr Ste 6, Melbourne, FL 32934
MACS CPAP System

Allied Healthcare Products, Inc. 800-444-3954
1720 Sublette Ave, Saint Louis, MO 63110

Ambu A/S 457-225-2210
6740 Baymeadow Dr, Glen Burnie, MD 21060
Ambu matic automatic resuscitator.

Bio-Med Devices, Inc. 800-224-6633
61 Soundview Rd, Guilford, CT 06437
$4500 for adult ICU/transport and $5300 for MRI model IC-2A volume ventilator, assist control/control, 8 1/2lbs., gas operated, SIMV, PEEP, CPAP, manual, calibrated controls: for adult and pediatric use. $2400 for P-7 adult transport volume ventilator, assist control/control, 6lbs., gas operated. $7000 for CV4 electronic transport volume ventilator/infant through adults. Functions include pressure support, 20-hour battery, 12 alarms, 8lbs. $3300 for MVP-10, 4lb. neonatal unit for ICU/transport. Gas-operated volume or pressure limited, calibrated controls, IMV, PEEP, CPAP blender. $3800 for MRI verison.

VENTILATOR, EMERGENCY, POWERED (RESUSCITATOR) *(cont'd)*

Gammadirect Medical Division 847-267-5929
PO Box 383, Lake Forest, IL 60045
Beta Vent Emergency and Transport ventilator kits. MRI compatible. Adult, pediatric and neonate.

Hartwell Medical Corp. 800-633-5900
6352 Corte Del Abeto Ste J, Carlsbad, CA 92011
The SUREVENT is a single-patient-use, oxygen-powered emergency transport ventilator for use by emergency-care personnel and paramedics. Provides smooth, consistent ventilations. Weighs 4 oz. Compact size ideal for disaster-preparedness personnel. New SUREVENT MCI Kit is a self-contained product that can accommodate up to 7 patients running off of an oxygen manifold. Can hold up to 10 SUREVENTs. Ideal for disaster cache.

Instrumentation Industries, Inc. 800-633-8577
2990 Industrial Blvd, Bethel Park, PA 15102
Manuel jet ventilator.

Life Corporation 800-700-0202
1776 N Water St, Milwaukee, WI 53202
LIFE OxygenPac and LIFE O2 SoftPac portable emergency oxygen units, clear cover and wall-mounted, off/on lever control, resuscitation mask with one-way valve for hygiene, 6lpm 90min. supply, refillable. Also available 6 & 12 lpm NORM & HIGH, 0-25 lpm variable, and demand-valve for 100% oxygen resuscitation. GSA Federal Supply Schedule.

Mada, Inc. 800-526-6370
625 Washington Ave, Carlstadt, NJ 07072

Matrx 716-662-6650
145 Mid County Dr, Orchard Park, NY 14127
Portable oxygen resuscitator.

Oxygen Therapy Institute 989-752-9891
106 W Johnson St, Saginaw, MI 48604
Portable oxygen inhalator.

Spiracle Technology 714-418-1091
16520 Harbor Blvd Ste D, Fountain Valley, CA 92708
Demand value resusciator.

U O Equipment Co. 800-231-6372
5863 W 34th St, Houston, TX 77092

Vortran Medical Technology 800-434-4034
21 Golden Land Ct, Sacramento, CA 95834
VORTRAN Automatic Resuscitator (VAR) is an inexpensive, hands-free, fully automatic resuscitator - ideal for on the scene, in transport and mass casualty incidents.

VENTILATOR, EXTERNAL BODY, NEGATIVE PRESSURE, (CUIRASS) *(Anesthesiology) 73BYT*

Porta-Lung Inc. 303-288-7575
7854 Logan St, Denver, CO 80229
PORTA-LUNG sealed pressure chamber in which the patient's body below the neck is enclosed within a pressurized cylinder. The patient's head remains outside the chamber.

Respironics Colorado 800-345-6443
12301 Grant St Unit 190, Thornton, CO 80241
$8,600.00 for NEV-100 ventilator, positive & negative pressure, best suited for CHEST SHELL or PULMO-WRAP, 120 VAC & 12 VDC, 35lbs. $640.00 for chest shell, standard with straps, used with negative pressure ventilators, 31 standard sizes and custom fits available, 10lbs. $596.00 for pulmo-wrap used with negative pressure ventilators, incl. garment back plate & grid. $826.00 for NU-MO suit used with ventilator equipment (negative pressure).

VENTILATOR, HIGH-FREQUENCY *(Anesthesiology) 73LSZ*

Bunnell Incorporated 800-800-4358
436 Lawndale Dr, Salt Lake City, UT 84115
High frequency jet ventilator for infants.

VENTILATOR, NEONATAL RESPIRATOR *(General) 80FQC*

Allied Healthcare Products, Inc. 800-444-3954
1720 Sublette Ave, Saint Louis, MO 63110

Bio-Med Devices, Inc. 800-224-6633
61 Soundview Rd, Guilford, CT 06437
$3,800 for MVP-10 4lb unit for ICU, anesthesia, transport & MRI gas operated, calibrated controls, volume or pressure limited IMV, CPAP, PEEP, Blender; $3,800 for MRI unit.

General Biomedical Service, Inc. 800-558-9449
1900 25th St, Kenner, LA 70062
New & remanufactured respiratory equipment, ventilators, and pulse oximeters.

VENTILATOR, NON-CONTINUOUS (RESPIRATOR)
(Anesthesiology) 73BZD

Aeiomed, Inc. 612-455-0550
1313 5th St SE Ste 205, Minneapolis, MN 55414
Cpap mask.

Bergquist Torrington Company 860-489-0489
89 Commercial Blvd, Torrington, CT 06790
Continuous positive airway pressure (cpap) device.

Cardinal Health 207, Inc. 610-862-0800
1100 Bird Center Dr, Palm Springs, CA 92262
Various models of ventilators, non-continuous.

Circadiance LLC 1-888-825-9640
1060 Corporate Ln, Export, PA 15632
Sleepweaver Soft Cloth CPAP Mask

Commercial/Medical Electronics, Inc. 800-324-4844
1519 S Lewis Ave, Tulsa, OK 74104

Hans Rudolph, Inc. 816-363-5522
7200 Wyandotte St, Kansas City, MO 64114
Face mask.

Henry G. Dietz Co., Inc. 718-726-7270
1426 28th Ave, Long Island City, NY 11102
Supplying intermittent flow of oxygen for inhalation therapy.

J. H. Emerson Co. 800-252-1414
22 Cottage Park Ave, Cambridge, MA 02140
Device, positive pressure breathing, intermittent.

Medical Electronic Devices, Inc. 310-618-0306
2807 Oregon Ct Ste D6, Torrance, CA 90503
Oxygen conserver.

Medical Industries America Inc. 800-759-3038
2636 289th Pl, Adel, IA 50003
REMREST, priced from $350.00; nasal C.P.A.P. system, to administer continuous positive airway pressure via nasal mask.

Mergenet Medical Inc. 888-925-2526
6601 Lyons Rd Ste B1-B4, Coconut Creek, FL 33073
Multiple

Millennia Technology, Inc. 724-274-7741
1105 Pittsburgh St, Cheswick, PA 15024
Respironics bipap remote control unit.

O-Two Systems International Inc. 800-387-3405
7575 Kimbel St., Mississauga, ONT L5S 1C8 Canada
Pocket Ventilator mouth to mask ventilator k841429.

Oceanic Medical Products, Inc. 913-874-2000
8005 Shannon Industrial Park, Ln., Atchison, KS 66002
Respiratory ventilator.

Resmed Inc. 800-424-0737
9001 Spectrum Center Blvd, San Diego, CA 92123
S8 Res Traxx

Stevenson Industries, Inc. 310-459-9393
881 Alma Real Dr Ste 310, Pacific Palisades, CA 90272
Cpap pro.

Thermadyne Holdings, Corp. 940-381-1388
800 Henrietta Creek Rd, Roanoke, TX 76262
02 on demand oxygen conserver.

Tiara Medical Systems, Inc. 610-862-0800
4153 166th St, Oak Forest, IL 60452
Nasal cpap mask.

Ventlab Corp. 336-753-5000
155 Boyce Dr, Mocksville, NC 27028
Nasal cpap cannula.

Viasys Sleep Systems, Llc. 847-689-8410
9305 Eton Ave, Chatsworth, CA 91311
Noncontinuous ventilator, cpap.

VENTILATOR, OTHER *(Anesthesiology) 73SEX*

Aearo Company 800-678-4163
5457 W 79th St, Indianapolis, IN 46268
Personal respirator (TB).

Avon-Isi 888-ISI-SAFE
922 Hurricane Shoals Rd NE, Lawrenceville, GA 30043
Self-contained breathing equipment with air tank.

Caddy Corporation 856-467-4222
509 Sharptown Road, Bridgeport, NJ 08014-0345

Controlair, Inc. 800-216-3636
8 Columbia Dr, Amherst, NH 03031
Gas regulators for use in ventilators.

VENTILATOR, OTHER *(cont'd)*

Farley Inc., W.T. 800-327-5397
931 Via Alondra, Camarillo, CA 93012
$264.00 for ventilator mounting arm with backplate.

General Biomedical Service, Inc. 800-558-9449
1900 25th St, Kenner, LA 70062
Exporters of new, used and remanufactured medical equipment, specializing in ventilators and other respiratory equipment.

Hamilton Medical, Inc. 800-426-6331
4990 Energy Way, Reno, NV 89502

Life Corporation 800-700-0202
1776 N Water St, Milwaukee, WI 53202
Portable emergency oxygen units, clear cover and wall-mounted, off/on lever control, resuscitation mask with one-way valve for hygiene, 6lpm 90min. supply, refillable. Also available 6 & 12 lpm NORM & HIGH, 0-25 lpm variable, and demand-valve for 100% oxygen resuscitation. GSA Federal Supply Schedule.

M & I Medical Sales, Inc. 305-663-6444
4711 SW 72nd Ave, Miami, FL 33155

Mada, Inc. 800-526-6370
625 Washington Ave, Carlstadt, NJ 07072

Monaghan Medical Corp. 800-833-9653
5 Latour Ave Ste 1600, P.O. Box 2805, Plattsburgh, NY 12901
AEROVENT aerosol holding chamber lets you deliver aerosol medications directly to the patient without compromising the integrity of the ventilator circuit. AEROCHAMBER valved holding chamber, AEROCHAMBER VHC with mask and AEROCHAMBER MV provide mechanical ventilation for intubated patients.

Newport Medical Instruments, Inc. 800-451-3111
1620 Sunflower Ave, Costa Mesa, CA 92626
The Newport HT50 Ventilator offers a patented, self-contained gas delivery system, long lasting internal battery, full mode selection (including pressure support) - all in a small, durable, easy to use package. The HT50 is ideal for homecare, transport or emergency settings.

Repex Medical Products, Inc. 305-740-0133
5240 SW 64th Ave, Miami, FL 33155
Intensive care & Transport ventilators; Adult, Pediatric & Neonate.

Respironics Colorado 800-345-6443
12301 Grant St Unit 190, Thornton, CO 80241
$6,400.00 for rocking bed ventilator, non-invasive ventilatory assist through diaphragmatic mobility, side rails available, 120 VAC, 300lbs. $440.00 for exsufflation belt with bladder; non-invasive ventilatory assist through intermittent abdominal pressure, 3 sizes, 2lbs.

Respironics Georgia, Inc. 724-387-4559
175 Chastain Meadows Ct NW, Kennesaw, GA 30144
QUANTUM PSV pressure support ventilator provides non-continuous, non-invasive support for airway management and ventilation.

VENTILATOR, PRESSURE CYCLED (IPPB MACHINE)
(Anesthesiology) 73SEU

A&H Products, Inc. 918-835-8081
PO Box 470686, Tulsa, OK 74147
Flow assist ventilators with nebulizer accessory.

General Biomedical Service, Inc. 800-558-9449
1900 25th St, Kenner, LA 70062
Exporters of new, used and remanufactured medical equipment, specializing in ventilators and other respiratory equipment.

Richard Wolf Medical Instruments Corp. 800-323-9653
353 Corporate Woods Pkwy, Vernon Hills, IL 60061

Smiths Medical Asd 800-424-8662
5700 W 23rd Ave, Gary, IN 46406
Jet ventilation device. Connector, tubing, regulator (factory set), trigger and wer fitments.

VENTILATOR, TIME CYCLED (IRON LUNG)
(Anesthesiology) 73SEV

Respironics Colorado 800-345-6443
12301 Grant St Unit 190, Thornton, CO 80241
$15,400.00 for non-invasive ventilatory support through negative pressure, 120 VAC.

VENTILATOR, VOLUME (CRITICAL CARE)
(Anesthesiology) 73SEW

Ambu, Inc. 800-262-8462
6740 Baymeadow Dr, Glen Burnie, MD 21060
Pneumatically powered transport ventilators with single circuit-volume constant and time-cycled and flow variable.

VENTILATOR, VOLUME (CRITICAL CARE) *(cont'd)*

Bio-Med Devices, Inc. 800-224-6633
61 Soundview Rd, Guilford, CT 06437
$7000 to $10,000 (depending on options) for CV-4 (CROSSVENT 4) volume ventilator, microprocessor based/intensive care and transport/infant through adult. Touch screen controls. All functions, including: built in PEEP, SIMV, pressure support, continuous flow, lung mechanics, 15 hour battery, 12 hi-lo alarms including exhaled tidal volume, 8 pounds. C -3 (CROSSVENT 3)Transport Volume Ventilator, $6,000-7,000 microprocessor based/pediatric through adult/transport. $4500 for adult ICU transport and $5300 MRI Model IC-2A volume ventilator, assist control/control, 8 1/2lbs weight, gas operated, SIMV, PEEP, CPAP manual, calibrated controls; for adult and pediatric use.

General Biomedical Service, Inc. 800-558-9449
1900 25th St, Kenner, LA 70062
New & remanufactured respiratory equipment, ventilators, and pulse oximeters.

Hamilton Medical, Inc. 800-426-6331
4990 Energy Way, Reno, NV 89502
GALILEO, VEOLAR & AMADEUS microprocessor-based adult/pediatric ventilators.

Impact Instrumentation, Inc. 800-969-0750
27 Fairfield Pl, West Caldwell, NJ 07006
Model 73X from Impact is a self-contained portable ventilator developed specifically for transport and mass casualty care. Impact's design team recognized that limited oxygen supplies would deplete during a mass casualty incident and need for an alternative gas source was imperative. The iXi can be used with external oxygen but more importantly it is operable via its own internal compressor using filtered ambient air. The iXi automatically switches to compressor operation should oxygen supplies become exhausted and simultaneously triggers an alarm. Interfaces with industry-standard HEPA or chemical/biologic filters, includes a digital airway pressure display, alarms suite, airway pressure limiting, continuous operation from external power

Mallard Medical, Inc. 530-226-0727
20268 Skypark Dr, Redding, CA 96002
Large and Small Animal Anesthesia Ventilator System

Newport Medical Instruments, Inc. 800-451-3111
1620 Sunflower Ave, Costa Mesa, CA 92626
The Newport e360 is a critical care ventilator that makes sophisticated technology simple to use. The e360 can easily transition from invasive to non-invasive ventilation for adult, pediatric or infant patients. It includes comprehensive mode selections, with graphics and extensive monitoring built into a single compact package.

Repex Medical Products, Inc. 305-740-0133
5240 SW 64th Ave, Miami, FL 33155

Respironics Colorado 800-345-6443
12301 Grant St Unit 190, Thornton, CO 80241
$9,600.00 for PLV-100 microprocessor controlled portable volume cycled ventilator, incl. control, assist/control & SIMV modes, visual displays, alarm & feedback system. 120VAC, 12VDC & internal battery, 28 lbs. $11,400.00 for volume ventilator PLV-102 with oxygen control dial allowing to set rate of oxygen, with no oxygen-waste feature plus same features as PLV-100.

Tkb International 714-429-8800
1620 Sunflower Ave, Costa Mesa, CA 92626

VIAL, HEMATOLOGY *(General) 80WPJ*

Globe Scientific, Inc. 800-394-4562
610 Winters Ave, Paramus, NJ 07652
FLEXIVIAL hematology cups for most cell counters.

Labcon North America 800-227-1466
3700 Lakeville Hwy Ste 200, Petaluma, CA 94954
Vials for automated hematology equipment (blood cell count).

Simport Plastics Ltd. 450-464-1723
2588 Bernard-Pilon, Beloeil, QUE J3G 4S5 Canada

VIAL, LIQUID SCINTILLATION COUNTING *(Chemistry) 75UJF*

Globe Scientific, Inc. 800-394-4562
610 Winters Ave, Paramus, NJ 07652
Disposable, high-density polyethylene vials are offered in three convenient sizes, provide consistently low background counts and good light transmission, and are suitable for low-activity counting.

Kimble Glass, Inc. 888-546-2531
537 Crystal Ave, Vineland, NJ 08360
KIMBLE.

Mg Scientific, Inc. 800-343-8338
8500 107th St, Pleasant Prairie, WI 53158

VIAL, LIQUID SCINTILLATION COUNTING *(cont'd)*

Sigma-Aldrich Corp. 800-521-8956
3050 Spruce St, Saint Louis, MO 63103

Simport Plastics Ltd. 450-464-1723
2588 Bernard-Pilon, Beloeil, QUE J3G 4S5 Canada

Standard Instrumentation, Div. Preiser Scientific 800-624-8285
94 Oliver St, Saint Albans, WV 25177

VIAL, MEDICATION *(General) 80TFK*

Apothecary Products, Inc. 800-328-2742
11750 12th Ave S, Burnsville, MN 55337

VIAL, OTHER *(General) 80WWJ*

Aidlab, Inc. 416-410-5377
60 5th Street., Toronto, ONT M2N-6N1 Canada
INTERGLASS serum vials. Type I borosilicate amber and clear vials, sizes 2 to 40ml. AIDPAK screw thread vials. Type 1 borosilicate amber and clear screw thread vials for sampling or packaging, sizes 2ml to 45ml.

Berghof/America 800-544-5004
3773 NW 126th Ave Bldg 1, Coral Springs, FL 33065
PFA vials and septum vials available with or without plastic trays.

Biohit Inc. 800-922-0784
PO Box 308, 3535 Rte. 66, Bldg. 4, Neptune, NJ 07754
VANGARD CRYOS Cryogenic storage vials.

Crosstex International 800-223-2497
10 Ranick Rd, Hauppauge, NY 11788
Plastic drinking cups.

Crosstex International Ltd., W. Region 800-707-2737
14059 Stage Rd, Santa Fe Springs, CA 90670
Plastic drinking cups.

Crosstex International,Inc. 888-276-7783
10 Ranick Rd, Hauppauge, NY 11788
CROSSTEX Plastic drinking cups.

Hollister-Stier Laboratories, Llc 800-992-1120
3525 N Regal St, Spokane, WA 99207
Sterile empty vials

J. G. Finneran Associates, Inc. 800-552-3696
3600 Reilly Ct, Vineland, NJ 08360
Versa Vial series. A clear vial measuring 2 ml.

Medical Associates Network 818-500-7711
801 N Brand Blvd Ste 690, Glendale, CA 91203
Needleless vial transfer device method to reconstitute lyophilized medications with needleless method.

Millipore Corporation 877-246-2247
290 Concord Rd, Billerica, MA 01821
Humidifier bag for respiratory therapy and irrigation fluid containers.

VIBRATION THRESHOLD MEASUREMENT DEVICE
(Cns/Neurology) 84LLN

Diabetica Solutions, Inc. 210-692-1114
12665 Silicon Dr, San Antonio, TX 78249
Vibration threshold measurement device.

Neuro-Diagnostic Assoc. 949-497-1207
2514 Temple Hills Dr, Laguna Beach, CA 92651
Current perception threshold device.

Physitemp Instruments, Inc. 800-452-8510
154 Huron Ave, Clifton, NJ 07013
$2,950 for VIBRATION II.

Wr Medical Electronics Co. 800-321-6387
123 2nd St N, Stillwater, MN 55082
$22,000 CASE IV computer-aided sensory evaluator for peripheral sensory nervous-system characterization.

VIBRATOR, BATTERY-POWERED *(Physical Med) 89IPE*

Alimed, Inc. 800-225-2610
297 High St, Dedham, MA 02026

VIBRATOR, THERAPEUTIC *(Physical Med) 89IRO*

Dnms Institute, Llc 210-561-7881
6421 Mondean St, San Antonio, TX 78240
Theratapper.

Dynatronics Corp. Chattanooga Operations 801-568-7000
6607 Mountain View Rd, Ooltewah, TN 37363
Battery powered, hand held vibrator.

Excel Tech. Ltd. 905-829-5300
2568 Bristol Cir, Oakville L6H 5S1 Canada
Electrical muscle stimulator

VIBRATOR, THERAPEUTIC *(cont'd)*

Global Sport Technology, Inc — 719-574-0584
4745 Signal Rock Rd, Colorado Springs, CO 80922
Vibration training or treatment.

Hasbro, Inc. — 401-431-8697
1027 Newport Ave, Pawtucket, RI 02861
30811 gentle vibes.

Healthsonix Inc. — 949-417-8880
14252 Culver Dr Ste 107, Irvine, CA 92604
Therapeutic vibrator.

Innovative Machinery Packaging And Converting Inc. — 503-581-3239
PO Box 535, Salem, OR 97308
Vibrator.

Medecon — 954-742-6300
10001 NW 50th St Ste W2, Sunrise, FL 33351
Vibrator, therapeutic.

Photoclear, Inc. — 888-789-3784
8819 Hoskins Rd, Freeport, TX 77541

Pretika Corporation, North America Market Headquarters — 949-481-8818
16 Salermo, Laguna Niguel, CA 92677
Facial massager.

VIDEOFLUOROSCOPIC UNIT *(Radiology) 90WJC*

York X-Ray And Orthopedic Supply, Inc. — 800-334-6427
PO Box 326, 20 Hampton Rd.,, Lyman, SC 29365

VIEW BOX, BLOOD GROUPING *(Hematology) 81KSY*

Micro Typing Systems, Inc. — 908-218-8177
1295 SW 29th Ave, Pompano Beach, FL 33069
Reader or viewing device.

VIEWER, RADIOGRAPHIC FILM, MOTORIZED
(Radiology) 90WUY

Broadwest Corp. — 800-232-2948
304 Elati St, Denver, CO 80223
Broadwest's Rolloscope M and ML® series automatic multiviewers features the unique One Touch System, which saves radiologists a substantial amount of time in the reading process. More specifically, one button on the Rolloscope® automatically dims the light, advances the film, masks to each frame's film configuration and brightens in about one second per frame. It also has the highest luminance level, though that feature is automatically dimmed and masked, and can be used as a roaming spot. The reliability of the Rolloscope is a proven feature and the transport belt has an exceptionally long life of 10 years or more. The Rolloscope M® holds the largest capacity of films in all three sizes, including both mammo sizes plus 14î X 17î film, such as MRI's or ultrasounds. The Rolloscope ML® features all the benefits of the Rolloscope M® with an additional capacity of 33% more films and 4 across of 14' x 17' film. Both the Rolloscope M and ML® also provide complete shutter control within each frame with four toggle switches for individual movement, as well as a roam function with a single joystick.

S&S Technology — 281-815-1300
10625 Telge Rd, Houston, TX 77095
Over 20 models to choose from, including mamography sizes. Capacity from 48-800 films plus large selection of quality illuminators. Send for free catalog.

Schueler & Company, Inc. — 516-487-1500
PO Box 528, Stratford, CT 06615

Xma (X-Ray Marketing Associates, Inc.) — 800-325-8880
1205 W Lakeview Ct, Windham Lakes Business Park
Romeoville, IL 60446

VIEWER/ANALYZER, 35MM ANGIO *(Radiology) 90SGP*

Advanced American Biotechnology (Aab) — 714-870-0290
1166 E Valencia Dr Unit 6C, Fullerton, CA 92831
Image anaylzer 11/6/98 LF.

VIEWER/MAGNIFIER *(Hematology) 81GLO*

Caprock Developments Inc. — 800-222-0325
475 Speedwell Ave, PO Box 95, Morris Plains, NJ 07950

Concepts International, Inc. — 800-627-9729
224 E Main St, Summerton, SC 29148
Clip-on magnifiers.

VIEWER/MAGNIFIER *(cont'd)*

Edroy Products Co., Inc. — 800-233-8803
245 N Midland Ave, PO Box 998, Nyack, NY 10960
STEREOPTIC MAGNIFIER $153.65 for U-66, $185.10 for U-68, $287.05 for U-66-2, $350.60 for U-68-2 single or double lens with lens powers from 2.75x to 5.5x for technical or other benchwork with halogen lamp, $66.00.

Eschenbach Optik Of America, Inc. — 800-487-5389
904 Ethan Allen Hwy, Ridgefield, CT 06877
Magnification aids.

Image Marketing Corp. — 800-466-7032
1636 N 24th St, PO Box 30935, Mesa, AZ 85213
CRYSTAL VIEW magnifier. For viewing all types of films and x-rays. Prefocused, hands-free viewing. 4 sizes, 2in., 2.5in., 3.5in and 4.5'. 4 times magnifier, gather light. POP UP POCKET MAGNIFIER a 4x push button actuated magnifier with built-in LED illumination.

Optelec U.S., Inc. — 800-828-1056
3030 Enterprise Ct Ste C, Vista, CA 92081
Video Magnifier - Spectrum Series - color magnification systems that enlarge text and graphics to a size that is easy to read. Come with 20' or 14' viewing screen. 20/20 Series - black and white magnification systems that enlarge text and pictures to a size that is easy to read. Come with 20' or 14' viewing screens.

Roldan Products Corp. — 866-922-6800
448 Sovereign Ct, Ballwin, MO 63011
$145 per unit (standard) for magnifier light.

VISCOELASTIC SURGICAL AID *(Ophthalmology) 86LZP*

Allergan — 800-366-6554
2525 Dupont Dr, Irvine, CA 92612

Cytosol Ophthalmics, Inc. — 800-234-5166
PO Box 1408, 1325 William White Place, NE, Lenoir, NC 28645
Shellgel, 1.2% concentration of sodium hyaluronate packaged in an 0.8-mL sterile syringe. 27G cannula included.

Eyekon Medical, Inc — 800-633-9248
2451 Enterprise Rd, Clearwater, FL 33763
HPMC - EyeCoat 4,000 cps and EyeCoat Plus 40,000 cps. Sodium Hyaluronate - EyeCoat SH

Eyekon Medical, Inc. — 800-633-9248
2451 Enterprise Rd, Clearwater, FL 33763

La Labs — 805-562-9889
7334 Hollister Ave Ste H, Goleta, CA 93117
Viscoelastic gel.

Staar Surgical Co. — 626-3037-902
27121 Aliso Creek Rd, Suite #100,105, 110 & 115
Aliso Viejo, CA 92656
Viscoeleatic.

VISCOMETER *(Chemistry) 75UJI*

Brinkmann Instruments, Inc. — 800-645-3050
PO Box 1019, Westbury, NY 11590

Cannon Instrument Co. — 800-676-6232
PO Box 16, State College, PA 16804
CANNON-FENSKE ROUTINE, priced at $77.50 per unit.

Cargille Laboratories — 973-239-6633
55 Commerce Rd, Cedar Grove, NJ 07009
ASTM time-test viscosity tubes, $42.00 for two dozen; Class G, 10.65 viscosity tubes, $37.50 for two dozen; Class V, 10.75 viscosity tubes, $34.00 for two dozen.

Koehler Instrument Co., Inc. — 800-878-9070
1595 Sycamore Ave, Bohemia, NY 11716
New constant-temperature-bath series with advanced temperature-control circuitry and integrated timing features for convenient, accurate glass capillary viscometry determinations. Microprocessor PID circuitry assures precise, reliable temperature control within ASTM-specified tolerances throughout the operating range of the bath.

Norcross Corp. — 617-969-7020
255 Newtonville Ave, Newton, MA 02458

Pac — 281-580-0339
300 Bammel Westfield Rd, Houston, TX 77090

Petrolab Company — 518-783-5133
874 Albany Shaker Rd, Latham, NY 12110

Polymer Laboratories, Now A Part Of Varian, Inc. — 800-767-3963
160 Old Farm Rd, Amherst Fields Research Park, Amherst, MA 01002
PL-BV 400RT room temperature viscometer and PL-BV 400HT high temperature viscometer.

Standard Instrumentation, Div. Preiser Scientific — 800-624-8285
94 Oliver St, Saint Albans, WV 25177

VISCOMETER *(cont'd)*

Tudor Scientific Glass Co., Inc. 800-336-4666
555 Edgefield Rd, Belvedere, SC 29841

VISCOMETER, MUCUS, CERVICAL *(Obstetrics/Gyn) 85LHZ*

Biosense Corporation 215-348-2977
450 East St, Doylestown, PA 18901
Viscometer for cervical mucus.

Boston Rheology, L.L.C. 617-912-1020
20 Whitney Dr, Chestnut Hill Medical Center, Sherborn, MA 01770
Rheometric measurement of human, animal, and industrial fluids.

VISCOMETER, PLASMA *(Chemistry) 75JJL*

Rheologics, Inc. 610-524-5427
15 E Uwchlan Ave Ste 414, Exton, PA 19341
Blood viscometer.

VISE, OSSICULAR FINGER *(Ear/Nose/Throat) 77JYB*

Gyrus Ent L.L.C., Sub. Of Gyrus Acmi, Inc. 508-804-2739
2925 Appling Rd, Bartlett, TN 38133
Various.

VISION AID, BRAILLE *(General) 80WMV*

American Printing House For The Blind, Inc. 800-223-1839
PO Box 6085, Louisville, KY 40206
Quick Braille Kit with slate, stylus, and perforated fanfold paper for brailling (#1-00086-00); 4-track cassette player/recorder with rechargeable batteries (#1-07085-00); braille paper (#1-04540-00); GrandStand portable reading stand (#1-03205-00); Metric/inch ruler with raised lines (#1-03100-00); Variable intensity lamp (#1-08940-00); ColorTest II (#1-03951-00), a portable hand-held device that reads color. Excellent for blind and color blind individuals. Calendars, cookbooks, dictionaries, recreational reading in braille and large print.

Duxbury Systems, Inc. 978-692-3000
270 Littleton Rd Ste 6, Westford, MA 01886
Duxbury System's DBT is the standard for braille translator word-processing software. DBT has versions for Windows XP, Windows 98, Windows 95, Windows NT, Windows 3.1, Macintosh, DOS, and UNIX. This simple-looking software does the hard work of translating and formatting your print document into braille. Handles over 30 braille languages and braille math. Also integrates wtih Braille Music Translator and handles braille graphics.

Enabling Technologies Company 800-777-DOTS
1601 NE Braille Pl, Jensen Beach, FL 34957
BRAILLE EXPRESS 150 interpoint embosser with a speed of 150 cps, $14,995; BRAILLE BOOKMAKER interpoint embosser with a speed of 80 cps, $7,995.00; ROMEO BRAILLE PRINTER, Model RB-25, personal braille printer with a speed of 25 cps, $2195.00; The TRANSEND LT enables user to produce braille and print on the same page available with choice of 3 braille printer. The JULIET INTERPOINT EMBOSSER MODELS, JULIET CLASSIC, JULIET PRO, and JULIET PRO 60, ranging from $3795.00-$4095.00; ROMEO BRAILLE PRINTER, MODEL PRO 50 - personal Braille printer with extra features, 50 cps, $2895; KGS BRAILLE LABELER - Small desktop unit makes clear, self-stick labels in Braille without Braille knowledge, $995; ROMEO ATTACHE - small transportable Braille Embosser. 16 pounds with 15 cps $1,895; ROMEO ATTACHE PRO - small transportable Braille Emboser with tractor and single sheet feed, ET speaks, 16 pounds with 15 cps $1,995.

Humanware 800-722-3393
175 Mason Cir, Concord, CA 94520
The BrailleNote PK is the worlds smallest Braille and speech personal digital assistant. This 18-cell model combines a crisp, high definition Braille display with clear responsive speech output. Features: bluetooth technology, WiFI connectibity, Internet Explorer v6. enhanced KeySoft media player. Every BrailleNote (with high definite Braille display and speech output) and VoiceNote (with speech output only) has the same powerful, user-friendly functions, including: word processor; e-mail; daily planner; book reader; medial player and activesync. The BrailleNote mPower the newest generation of mobile information management technology offers even more functionality with speed, memory and connectivity options.

VISION AID, ELECTRONIC, AC-POWERED
(Ophthalmology) 86HPF

Eschenbach Optik Of America, Inc. 800-487-5389
904 Ethan Allen Hwy, Ridgefield, CT 06877

Guerilla Technologies Inc. 772-283-0500
5029 SE Horseshoe Point Rd, Stuart, FL 34997
Stand-alone ocr.

VISION AID, ELECTRONIC, AC-POWERED *(cont'd)*

Optelec U.S., Inc. 800-828-1056
3030 Enterprise Ct Ste C, Vista, CA 92081
Low vision reading aid with camera and monitor connected to typewriter. Display can be chosen to appear in positive or negative form.

VISION AID, ELECTRONIC, BATTERY-POWERED
(Ophthalmology) 86HPG

B.E. Meyers & Co., Inc. 800-327-5648
14540 NE 91st St, Redmond, WA 98052
Hand-held passive infrared night-vision device.

Brytech Inc. 613-731-5800
600 Peter Morand Crescent, Suite 240, Ottawa, ONT K1G-5Z3 Canada
NOTE TELLER, identifies all U.S. bank notes for the blind and visually impaired. Announces in English or Spanish.

Purdy Electronics Corp. 408-523-8201
720 Palomar Ave, Sunnyvale, CA 94085
AND Optoelectronics high & ultra bright LED's.

VISION AID, IMAGE INTENSIFICATION, BATTERY-POWERED
(Ophthalmology) 86HOT

American Printing House For The Blind, Inc. 800-223-1839
PO Box 6085, Louisville, KY 40206
Magni-Cam (#1-03920-00) Hooks up to an ordinary television set to produce highly magnified images of text or pictures that are scanned with its hand-held camera. Also comes in a color model, and a more basic version. PocketViewer (#1-07560-00) is a portable hand-held battery operated magnifier with its own 4-inch black and white screen. It is lightweight and fits into a coat pocket or purse.

Ctp Coil Inc. 800-933-2645
1801 Howard St Ste D, Elk Grove Village, IL 60007
Various illuminated hand and stand magnifiers requiring battery powered source.

Eschenbach Optik Of America, Inc. 800-487-5389
904 Ethan Allen Hwy, Ridgefield, CT 06877
Illumination aids.

Insiphil (Us) Llc 408-616-8700
650 Vaqueros Ave Ste F, Sunnyvale, CA 94085

Itt Night Vision 800-448-8678
7635 Plantation Rd, Roanoke, VA 24019

Keeler Instruments Inc. 800-523-5620
456 Park Way, Broomall, PA 19008
$97 to $277 for illuminated magnifier 8x-20x.

VISION AID, OPTICAL, AC-POWERED *(Ophthalmology) 86HPI*

Ctp Coil Inc. 800-933-2645
1801 Howard St Ste D, Elk Grove Village, IL 60007
Various illuminated stand magnifiers requiring A.C. power source.

E.W. Pike & Company 908-352-0630
501 Pennsylvania Ave # 517, Elizabeth, NJ 07201

Eschenbach Optik Of America, Inc. 800-487-5389
904 Ethan Allen Hwy, Ridgefield, CT 06877

VISION AID, OPTICAL, BATTERY-POWERED
(Ophthalmology) 86HPE

Ctp Coil Inc. 800-933-2645
1801 Howard St Ste D, Elk Grove Village, IL 60007
Various hand and stand format magnifiers with battery powered illumination source.

Depuy-Raynham, A Div. Of Depuy Orthopaedics 800-451-2006
325 Paramount Dr, Raynham, MA 02767
Optical hand-piece.

Eschenbach Optik Of America, Inc. 800-487-5389
904 Ethan Allen Hwy, Ridgefield, CT 06877

Freedom Scientific Blv Group, Llc. 727-803-8000
11800 31st Ct N, Saint Petersburg, FL 33716
Various models of cctvs.

VISION AID, ULTRASONIC *(Ophthalmology) 86WOM*

Brytech Inc. 613-731-5800
600 Peter Morand Crescent, Suite 240, Ottawa, ONT K1G-5Z3 Canada
$1000 retail for SENSORY 6 with control unit, glasses with detectors, head phones, power supply, power charger and user manual in booklet and tape form. The device measures the distance between objects and user indicating the distance by using lower or higher pitched tones which are audible via the head phones. Specs.: 1-6 ft. short range, 1-12ft. long range. Detection pattern: 25 horizontal, 15 vertical. Frequency transmission: 50kHz, Audio: 150-3kHz, Weight: 0.71 lbs.

VOLTMETER *(Chemistry) 75SFD*

Iet Labs, Inc. 800-899-8438
534 Main St, Westbury, NY 11590
Product name: ECG Simulators: LIM/GFI testers, isolation transformers. Leakage current tester. Safety analyzer.

Leader Instruments Corp. 800-645-5104
6484 Commerce Dr, Cypress, CA 90630
Single and dual channel AC millivoltmeters.

Omega Engineering, Inc. 800-848-4286
1 Omega Dr, Stamford, CT 06907

Simpson Electric Co. 715-588-3311
520 Simpson Ave, PO Box 99, Lac Du Flambeau, WI 54538
Analog AC (Model 376) or DC (Model 377-2). $128.73 per unit (standard). Also, volt/OHM meter, Model 260 series.$161.18-$286.65.

Soltec Corp. 800-423-2344
12977 Arroyo St, San Fernando, CA 91340

VOLUMETER *(Chemistry) 75UJK*

Alimed, Inc. 800-225-2610
297 High St, Dedham, MA 02026
Foot, hand, and arm sets provide an objective measurement of changes in edema.

WALKER, MECHANICAL *(Physical Med) 89ITJ*

A.R.C. Distributors 800-296-8724
PO Box 599, Centreville, MD 21617
INVACARE adjustable, lightweight, easy to use with and without wheels, baskets, pouches and trays.

Able Walker, Ltd. 604-576-8488
16-2350 Beta Ave, Burnaby V5C 5M8 Canada
Assistive walking device

Access Mobility, Inc. 800-336-1147
5240 Elmwood Ave, Indianapolis, IN 46203

Allman Products 800-223-6889
21101 Itasca St, Chatsworth, CA 91311

American Innovations, Inc. 800-223-3913
123 N Main St, Dublin, PA 18917
The AMBULMATE Walker is the industry's first all-resin folding walker, featuring two-tiered handgrips (assists standing/sitting), built-in rubber mesh pockets, 6-in. semi-pneumatic wheels with rear ball glides, accessory adapters, and more. Available in four stylish colors.

Arjo, Inc. 800-323-1245
50 Gary Ave Ste A, Roselle, IL 60172
Lift walker equipment allows patients to be lifted from a sitting to a standing position for ambulation training. The unit includes suspension straps, hand grips, and safety belt.

Bio-Medic Health Services, Inc. 800-525-0072
5041B Benois Rd Bldg B, Roanoke, VA 24018

Biomet, Inc. 574-267-6639
56 E Bell Dr, PO Box 587, Warsaw, IN 46582
Various types of walkers.

Care Products Inc. 757-224-0177
10701 N Ware Rd, McAllen, TX 78504
Various daily assist devices.

Clarke Health Care Products, Inc. 888-347-4537
1003 International Dr, Oakdale, PA 15071
DOLOMITE Walkers--Legacy, Symphony, Maxi+ four-wheeled folding walkers with seats. Oxygen-tank holder with one-handed brake, cane holder, tray, tall handles. Alpha forearm-support walker with seat. Melody, cableless brake system uses stainless steel rods to accuate brake, available in 3 sizes.

Community Products, Llc 845-658-7723
2032 Route 213, Rifton, NY 12471
Walker.

WALKER, MECHANICAL *(cont'd)*

Convaquip Industries, Inc. 800-637-8436
4834 Derrick Dr, PO Box 3417, Abilene, TX 79601
Non-mechanical. Bariatric; weight certified to 850lb. Rigid, adjustable in height.

Demetech Corp. 888-324-2447
3530 NW 115th Ave, Doral, FL 33178
Mechanical walker.

Dolomite Home Care Products, Inc. 888-687-2390
50 Shields Crt, Markham, ONT L3R 9T5 Canada
Various model

Duralife, Inc. 800-443-5433
195 Phillips Park Dr, Williamsport, PA 17702

Dynatronics Corp. Chattanooga Operations 801-568-7000
6607 Mountain View Rd, Ooltewah, TN 37363
Various adjustable walkers.

Eagle Health Supplies, Inc. 800-755-8999
535 W Walnut Ave, Orange, CA 92868
EAGLE Rehab Walker, Gait training, aluminum made light weight with adjustable seat height and 4 wheels (4') caster. Also, Heavy Duty Rollator, 4 wheel H/D rollator. Weight capacity 310 lbs, locking brake.

Elyria Plastic Products 440-322-8577
710 Taylor St, Elyria, OH 44035
Walker, mechanical.

Enduro Medical Technology, Inc. 860-289-2299
310 Nutmeg Rd S Unit C5, South Windsor, CT 06074
S.A.M. Secure Ambulation Module- Robotic walker developed under NASA license, gait training and standing therapy - can handle patients up to 1000 pounds.

Essential Medical Supply, Inc. 800-826-8423
6420 Hazeltine National Dr, Orlando, FL 32822
ENDURANCE, FEATHERLIGHT, ROLL EASY, BLAZER, EXCALIBUR.

Farley Inc., W.T. 800-327-5397
931 Via Alondra, Camarillo, CA 93012
Combination walker and oxygen carrier provides a steady base for patient support while the dual cylinder holder allows users more freedom of movement.

Flaghouse, Inc. 800-793-7900
601 US Highway 46 W, Hasbrouck Heights, NJ 07604

G. Hirsch And Co., Inc. 650-692-8770
870 Mahler Rd, Burlingame, CA 94010
Various models of mechanical walkers.

Gendron, Inc. 800-537-2521
400 E Lugbill Rd, Archbold, OH 43502
$70.00 per unit (standard).

Gunnell, Inc. 800-551-0055
8440 State Rd, Millington, MI 48746

Handicap Unlimited, Inc. 888-371-0095
5640 Summer Ave Ste 3, Memphis, TN 38134

Hart Independent Mobility Corp. 905-403-8471
1323 Kelly Rd., Mississauga, ONT L5J 3V1 Canada
Hart walker

Hartford Walking Systems Inc. 315-735-1659
22 Pearl St, New Hartford, NY 13413
Ergonomically designed walking system.

Healthline Medical Products, Inc. 407-656-0704
1065 E Story Rd, Oakland, FL 34787

In-Step Mobility 847-676-1275
8027 Monticello Ave, Skokie, IL 60076
U-step walker.

Innovative Products Unlimited, Inc. 800-833-2826
2120 Industrial Dr, Niles, MI 49120
$300 each.

Invacare Canada 800-668-5324
5970 Chedworth Way, Mississauga, ONT L5R 3T9 Canada

Karman Healthcare, Inc. 800-805-2762
19255 San Jose Ave, City Of Industry, CA 91748
KARMAN 3 wheels/4 wheels rollators.

Kaye Products, Inc. 919-732-6444
535 Dimmocks Mill Rd, Hillsborough, NC 27278
Posture Control walker for adults and children.

Keen Mobility Company 503-285-9090
6500 NE Halsey St Ste B, Portland, OR 97213

WALKER, MECHANICAL *(cont'd)*

Kern Surgical Supply, Inc. 800-582-3939
2823 Gibson St, Bakersfield, CA 93308

LIFTnWALK LP 972-837-4615
PO Box 742855, Dallas, TX 75374
$599 for BUDDY SAFETY ROLLER variable resistance walker with heavy duty multi-braking system. BUDDY SAFETY ROLLER walker for stroke.

Medical Depot 516-998-4600
99 Seaview Blvd, Port Washington, NY 11050
Walker, mechanical.

Merry Walker Corp. 847-837-9580
21350 Sylvan Dr S Unit 9, Mundelein, IL 60060
MERRY WALKER foldable, ambulation device, available in all-steel or PVC construction, new sleek design, padded wipeable seat, offered in four sizes. Pediatric available; home care models in four sizes. MERRY WALKER PEDIATRIC allows disabled children walking capabilities by surrounding them with a framework and seat while walking. All-steel frame, folding, bottom-weighted, non-tipping. MERRY WALKER HOMECARE walker/chair combination allowing users to be completely surrounded by framework with seat to rest on, foldable, washable, non-tipping. 23-in. wide; allows wheelchair users to walk independently without fear of falling. MERRY CART, steel frame, lightweight, narrow in width, cart with three railings to hold nine snap-closed bins. Bins are fully washable and removable. Perfect for therapy or hostess cart, economical. MERRY WALKER INSTITUTIONAL, similiar to the new homecare unit but larger in width. A steel framework and lightweight walker/chair combination allows users to rest on a seat when fatigued. Foldable, washable, non-tipping, and restraint-free. The whole device surrounds the individual as he or she walks, preventing falls. MERRY WALKER MOTIVATOR allows end-user to move about using lower legs and also strengthens upper body. Height-adjustable, cushioned seat will assist in 'motivating' frail elderly to get up and walk after restoring muscle tone to upper and lower body. MERRY TRAVELER, recommended for use by persons who need only minimal assistance in walking, such as during rehabilition of knee or hip after surgery. Foldable and washable. MERRY STAND BY ME wheelchair stander allows a person in a wheelchair to stand up and practice sitting and standing in a rigid framework. MERRY WALKER BARIATRIC permits those weighing up to 500 lb to exercise and walk.

Metro Medical Supply Wholesale 800-768-2002
200 Cumberland Bnd, Nashville, TN 37228

Mjm International Corporation 956-781-5000
2003 N Veterans Blvd Ste 10, San Juan, TX 78589
Walker.

Mobility Research 480-829-1727
444 W Geneva Dr, Tempe, AZ 85282

Northeastern Biomechanical Manufacturing Corp. 716-692-9585
81 Penarrow Dr, Tonawanda, NY 14150
Adjustable sling walker.

Paramedical Distributors 800-245-3278
2020 Grand Blvd, Kansas City, MO 64108

Parsons A.D.L. Inc. 800-263-1281
R.R. #2, 1986 Sideroad 15, Tottenham, ONT L0G 1W0 Canada
Walkers & accessories.

Patterson Medical Supply, Inc. 262-387-8720
W68N158 Evergreen Blvd, Cedarburg, WI 53012
Walker.

Perfect Care 718-805-7800
8927 126th St, Richmond Hill, NY 11418
Walker.

Portacare Llc 509-928-0650
13023 E Tall Tree Rd, Spokane Valley, WA 99216
Ez-walker & accessories.

Productos Rubbermaid, Sociedad Anonima De Capital 540-542-8363
Kmi-Ote, Carretera Cadereyta-Allende
Cadereyta Jimenez 67450 Mexico
Various

Pryor Products 800-854-2280
1819 Peacock Blvd, Oceanside, CA 92056
Several products are available for patient support/walker applications, including the Walk N Roller folding walker.

Rehabilitation Center For Children Inc. 204-452-4311
633 Wellington Cres, Winnipeg R3M 0A8 Canada
Pommel walker

WALKER, MECHANICAL *(cont'd)*

Rifton Equipment 800-571-8198
PO Box 260, Rifton, NY 12471
Gait trainers. Pediatric to adult, 3 sizes. Adjustable prompts fully support very involved child while walking; prompts are removed as skills improve.

Roll A Bout Corp. 302-335-5057
3240 Barratts Chapel Rd, Frederica, DE 19946
Roll-a-bout 4 wheel walker.

Scott Orthotic Labs, Inc. 800-821-5795
1831 E Mulberry St, Fort Collins, CO 80524
Walker.

Sroufe Healthcare Products Llc 888-894-4171
PO Box 347, 601 Sroufe St., Ligonier, IN 46767
CHEVRON II short leg walker.

TFI Healthcare 800-526-0178
600 W Wythe St, Petersburg, VA 23803
Model #DME17/2 double button folding model; also, extra wide Model #2138/1 maximum weight 500 lbs.

The Anthros Medical Group 785-544-6592
807 E Spring St, Highland, KS 66035
Various daily assist devices.

Therafin Corporation 800-843-7234
19747 Wolf Rd, Mokena, IL 60448
Various walkers.

Tr Group, Inc. 800-752-6900
903 Wedel Ln, Glenview, IL 60025
Rolling walker.

Triaid, Inc. 301-759-3525
637 N Centre St, Cumberland, MD 21502
Arrow walker.

Truform Orthotics & Prosthetics 800-888-0458
3960 Rosslyn Dr, Cincinnati, OH 45209

Tuffcare 800-367-6160
3999 E La Palma Ave, Anaheim, CA 92807

Walkerworks 800-667-4111
4580 Hickmore St., Montreal, QUE H4T 1K2 Canada
Walker

Wenzelite Rehab Supplies, Llc 800-706-9255
220 36th St, 99 Seaview Blvd, Brooklyn, NY 11232
Four-wheel, automatic brakes. Safety roller permits disabled to stand or sit unassisted.

Wheelchair Sales And Service Co., Inc. 877-736-0376
315 Main St, West Springfield, MA 01089
Lumex; API; Invacare; Summit.

White Cap Ent. 781-925-3705
133 Beach Ave, Hull, MA 02045
Buddy.

WALLPAPER, ANTIBACTERIAL *(General) 80TFM*

Construction Specialties Inc. 800-233-8493
6696 Route. 405, Muncy, PA 17756

WARMER, ANESTHESIA TUBE *(Dental And Oral) 76EFC*

Addent, Inc. 203-778-0200
43 Miry Brook Rd, Danbury, CT 06810
A new tray for the Calset is now available. The tray is for warming anesthetic carpules to body temperature. The tray holds 3 carpules. When the anesthetic is warmed to body temperature, it benefits the patient by being more comfortable.

Premier Dental Products Co. 888-670-6100
1710 Romano Dr, PO Box 4500, Plymouth Meeting, PA 19462

WARMER, BEDPAN *(General) 80SFE*

Independent Solutions, Inc. 847-498-0500
900 Skokie Blvd Ste 118, Northbrook, IL 60062
Blickman stainless steel electric; UL listed.

WARMER, BLANKET *(General) 80SFF*

Alimed, Inc. 800-225-2610
297 High St, Dedham, MA 02026

Blickman 800-247-5070
39 Robinson Rd, Lodi, NJ 07644
Models 7921MG and 7921MS (single door) and 7924MG and 7924MS (double door) are 30 in. wide and 74.5 in. tall. Models SW30MG and SW30MS are 30 in. wide and 60 in. high. All units feature an open and adjustable shelf design for flexibility and expanded use, easy-to-use controls for setting internal temperaturwe, and glass or stainless-steel doors.

WARMER, BLANKET *(cont'd)*

Cincinnati Sub-Zero Products, Inc., Medical Division — 800-989-7373
12011 Mosteller Rd, Cincinnati, OH 45241

Colonial Scientific Ltd. — 902-468-1811
201 Brownlow Ave., Unit 52, Dartmouth, NS B3B-1W2 Canada

Genesis Manufacturing, Inc. — 317-485-7887
720 E Broadway St, Fortville, IN 46040
Contract Radio-Frequency (RF) Welding. From development to manufacturing and packaging.

Independent Solutions, Inc. — 847-498-0500
900 Skokie Blvd Ste 118, Northbrook, IL 60062
Blickman stainless steel electric or steam; one or two compartments; one or both compartments heated. U.L. listed. Pass through models available.

Scientek Medical Equipment — 604-273-9094
11151 Bridgeport Rd., Richmond, BC V6X 1T3 Canada
Mechanically convected electric or steam heat, thermostatic temperature control, dial thermometer, stainless steel constr.

Smiths Medical Asd, Inc. — 800-553-8351
160 Weymouth St, Rockland, MA 02370
SNUGGLEWARM Convective Warmer & Blankets, Convective blower/warmer & blankets.

WARMER, BLOOD AND PLASMA *(Hematology) 81KZL*

Arrow International, Inc. — 800-523-8446
2400 Bernville Rd, Reading, PA 19605

Cytotherm — 800-747-9699
110 Sewell Ave, Trenton, NJ 08610
CYTOTHERM frozen-plasma-thawing equipment. Tabletop units. Dry Thawing models CT-DR and CT-D4. Wet Thawing models CT-4T and CT-4S.

Nortech Systems Incorporated — 952-345-2244
1120 Wayzata Blvd E Ste 201, Wayzata, MN 55391
DEVICE, WARMING. BLOOD AND PLASMA

Smiths Medical Asd, Inc. — 800-553-8351
160 Weymouth St, Rockland, MA 02370

Thermo Fisher Scientific (Asheville) Llc — 740-373-4763
Millcreek Rd., Marietta, OH 45750
Various models of thawing devices.

Thermogenesis Corp. — 800-783-8357
2711 Citrus Rd, Rancho Cordova, CA 95742
THERMOGENESIS, Blood component thawer. Available in 3 sizes.

WARMER, BLOOD, COIL *(Hematology) 81SFG*

Filtrona Extrusion, Inc./Pexcor Medical Products Div. — 800-755-7528
764 S Athol Rd, P.O. Box 659, Athol, MA 01331

WARMER, BLOOD, NON-ELECTROMAGNETIC RADIATION *(Anesthesiology) 73BSB*

Adroit Medical Systems, Inc. — 800-267-6077
1146 Carding Machine Rd, Loudon, TN 37774
Fluido blood and fluid warmer. IV and trauma sets. Flow 15-800 ml/min. Temp range 30C-39C.

B. Braun Of Puerto Rico, Inc. — 610-691-5400
215.7 Insular Rd., Sabana Grande, PR 00637
Blood warming coil.

Belmont Instrument Corp. — 866-663-0212
780 Boston Rd, Billerica, MA 01821
Belmont buddy is a low cost in-line blood and fluid warmer for routine use during surgery with advanced features, including close-to-the-patient warming without a water bath, very large microporous membrane for venting air from crystalloid, and No Flow/Empty Set alarm.

Estill Medical Technologies, Inc. — 877-354-0286
4144 N Central Expy Ste 260, Dallas, TX 75204
Sterile fluid path, in-line blood/fluid warmer.

Mmj S.A. De C.V. — 314-654-2000
716 Ponciano Arriaga, Cd. Juarez, Chih. Mexico
Fluid warmer, heat exchanger

Thermo Fisher Scientific (Asheville) Llc — 740-373-4763
Millcreek Rd., Marietta, OH 45750
Various modles of blood thawing baths.

WARMER, BLOOD, WATER BATH *(Hematology) 81VLV*

Smiths Medical Asd, Inc. — 800-553-8351
160 Weymouth St, Rockland, MA 02370
IV fluid/blood warmers. System 1025; using counter-current (not static) technology; HOTLINE warmer for routine surgery fluid warmer.

WARMER, DIALYSATE, PERITONEAL *(Gastro/Urology) 78MLW*

Thermasolutions, Inc. — 651-209-3900
1889 Buerkle Rd, Saint Paul, MN 55110
Thermal infusion fluid warmer.

WARMER, ENDOSCOPE *(Surgery) 79SHE*

Elmed, Inc. — 630-543-2792
60 W Fay Ave, Addison, IL 60101

Richard Wolf Medical Instruments Corp. — 800-323-9653
353 Corporate Woods Pkwy, Vernon Hills, IL 60061

Wisap America — 800-233-8448
8231 Melrose Dr, Lenexa, KS 66214

WARMER, GEL *(General) 80WLV*

Coopersurgical, Inc. — 800-243-2974
95 Corporate Dr, Trumbull, CT 06611

Cryopak Industries, Inc. — 800-667-2532
1055 Derwent Way, Delta, BC V3M 5R4 Canada
Simply Cozy microwaves in minutes for hours of warm, cozy comfort. Portable, soothing therapy; flexible for hot and cold therapy. Flannel cover is machine washable.

Genesis Manufacturing, Inc. — 317-485-7887
720 E Broadway St, Fortville, IN 46040
Contract Radio-Frequency (RF) Welding. From development to manufacturing and packaging.

Ideal Products — 800-321-5490
1287 County Road 623, Broseley, MO 63932
Priced from $79.00, ultrasound gel warmer, stainless-steel device available in 14 diferent models, 2-year warranty.

Parker Laboratories, Inc. — 800-631-8888
286 Eldridge Rd, Fairfield, NJ 07004
THERMASONIC, ultrasound gel warmer unit.

R Medical Supply — 800-882-7578
620 Valley Forge Rd Ste F, Hillsborough, NC 27278

WARMER, INFUSION FLUID, THERMAL *(General) 80LGZ*

Accellent El Paso — 915-771-9112
31 Butterfield Trail Blvd Ste C, El Paso, TX 79906
Fluid warming sets

Arizant Healthcare Inc. — 800-733-7775
10393 W 70th St, Eden Prairie, MN 55344
BAIR HUGGER 241 fluid warming system. RANGER blood/fluid warming system designed to meet flow rates from KVO to 30,000 ml/hr.

C.F. Electronics, Inc. — 307-742-5200
2052 N 3rd St, Laramie, WY 82072
IV Fluid Warmer, Portable

Futuremed America, Inc. — 800-222-6780
15700 Devonshire St, Granada Hills, CA 91344
ANIMEC Fluid Warmers: Device for warming I.V. fluid and blood for flow rates of 0-150 cc per minute. ASTOTHERM Blood Warmer for O.R: Device using standard tubing for warming blood in operating rooms.

Gaymar Industries, Inc. — 800-828-7341
10 Centre Dr, Orchard Park, NY 14127
MediTemp blood/fluid warming system, uses dry heat plate warming technology.

Mcdalt Medical Corp. — 800-841-5774
2225 Prestonwood Dr Ste 100-A, Arlington, TX 76012
Thermal Angel.

Mfg One, Llc — 703-437-9838
3900 Skyhawk Dr, Chantilly, VA 20151
Heat stack, various models.

Nxstage Medical, Inc. — 866-697-8243
439 S Union St Fl 5, Lawrence, MA 01843
Fluid warming system and accessories.

Smiths Medical Asd, Inc. — 800-553-8351
160 Weymouth St, Rockland, MA 02370
IV fluid/blood warmers. System 1025; using counter-current (not static) technology; HOTLINE warmer for routine surgery fluid warmer.

WARMER, INFUSION FLUID, THERMAL *(cont'd)*

Thermogenesis Corp. 800-783-8357
2711 Citrus Rd, Rancho Cordova, CA 95742
BIOARCHIVE System, automated liquid nitrogen storage system with integrated controlled rate freezer modules.

WARMER, IRRIGATION SOLUTION *(General) 80LHC*

Inter-Med, Inc. 877-418-4782
2200 Northwestern Ave, Racine, WI 53404
Solution warmer.

Mfg One, Llc 703-437-9838
3900 Skyhawk Dr, Chantilly, VA 20151
Surgical solution warmer.

Smiths Medical Asd, Inc. 800-553-8351
160 Weymouth St, Rockland, MA 02370
Normothermic Irrigating System 1129 with power pole for high-flow irrigating.

WARMER, RADIANT, ADULT *(General) 80SFJ*

Aragona Medical, Inc. 201-664-8822
184 Rivervale Rd, Rivervale, NJ 07675
Thermal Ceiling: Mobile and Ceiling Mounted. Requires no disposables.

WARMER, RADIANT, INFANT *(General) 80FMT*

Aragona Medical, Inc. 201-664-8822
184 Rivervale Rd, Rivervale, NJ 07675
Thermal Ceiling: mobile unit and baby warmer with light. Requires no disposables.

Hill-Rom Holdings, Inc. 800-445-3730
1069 State Road 46 E, Batesville, IN 47006

International Hospital Supply Co. 800-398-9450
6914 Canby Ave Ste 105, Reseda, CA 91335

J. H. Emerson Co. 800-252-1414
22 Cottage Park Ave, Cambridge, MA 02140
Various types of infant radiant warmers.

Ohmeda Medical 800-345-2700
8880 Gorman Rd, Laurel, MD 20723
Ohio Infant Warming System for use in hospital neonatal intensive care units.

Promotora Biomedica Internacional, S.A. De C.V. 42157770
San Francisco 1, Ste. 2, San Miguel de Allende, Gto. 26033 Mexico

WARMER, SOLUTION *(Chemistry) 75SFL*

Independent Solutions, Inc. 847-498-0500
900 Skokie Blvd Ste 118, Northbrook, IL 60062
Blickman stainless steel electric, one or two compartment; one or both compartments heated. U.L. listed. Pass through models available.

Phipps & Bird, Inc. 800-955-7621
1519 Summit Ave, Richmond, VA 23230
Portable dialysate warmer. A self-contained warming pouch for dialysate solution used in C.A.P.D. procedures. 120V and 12V.

Scientek Medical Equipment 604-273-9094
11151 Bridgeport Rd., Richmond, BC V6X 1T3 Canada
Mechanically convected electric or steam heat, thermostatic temperature control, dial thermometer, stainless steel constr.

WASHER, CART *(General) 80SFN*

Belimed 800-457-4117
13840 SW 119th Ave, Miami, FL 33186
Manual and automated versions available, can be installed with and without a pit, short drying times and most economical to use.

Buxton Medical Equipment Corp. 631-957-4500
1178 Route 109, Lindenhurst, NY 11757
All sizes available.

Damas Corp. 609-695-9121
1977 N Olden Avenue Ext Ste 289, Ewing, NJ 08618

Getinge Usa, Inc. 800-475-9040
1777 E Henrietta Rd, Rochester, NY 14623
GETINGE.

Independent Solutions, Inc. 847-498-0500
900 Skokie Blvd Ste 118, Northbrook, IL 60062
Girton.

Mcclure Industries, Inc. 800-752-2821
9051 SE 55th Ave, Portland, OR 97206
Automatic wash systems, conveyors, ejectors.

WASHER, CART *(cont'd)*

Meese Orbitron Dunne Co. 800-829-3230
535 N Midland Ave, Saddle Brook, NJ 07663
CART HANDLER automated system to service laundry or hospital hand carts and trucks. Up to 240 carts per hour may be washed, sanitized and dried.

Scientek Medical Equipment 604-273-9094
11151 Bridgeport Rd., Richmond, BC V6X 1T3 Canada

WASHER, CELL (FROZEN BLOOD PROCESSOR)
(Hematology) 81SFO

Caridianbct Inc. 800-525-2623
10810 W Collins Ave, Lakewood, CO 80215
COBE 2991 Cell Processor.

Dade Behring, Inc. 800-948-3233
1717 Deerfield Rd, Deerfield, IL 60015

WASHER, CLEANER, AUTOMATED, ENDOSCOPE
(Gastro/Urology) 78NVE

Langford Ic Systems, Inc. 520-745-6201
310 S Williams Blvd Ste 270, Tucson, AZ 85711
Device cleaner.

WASHER, LABWARE *(Chemistry) 75SFP*

American Autoclave Co. 800 421 5161
7819 Riverside Rd E, Sumner, WA 98390
Various sizes.

Buxton Medical Equipment Corp. 631-957-4500
1178 Route 109, Lindenhurst, NY 11757
All sizes available.

Damas Corp. 609-695-9121
1977 N Olden Avenue Ext Ste 289, Ewing, NJ 08618

Getinge Usa, Inc. 800-475-9040
1777 E Henrietta Rd, Rochester, NY 14623
GETINGE.

Hotpack 800-523-3608
10940 Dutton Rd, Philadelphia, PA 19154
$2,500 to $25,000 for free-standing, bench, or undercounter, five models with jet spray washer; tank size varies from 17x13x13" to 23x25x40". Electric water heater type; also, steam heated models available.

Labconco Corp. 800-821-5525
8811 Prospect Ave, Kansas City, MO 64132
STEAMSCRUBBER, FLASKSCRUBBER, and new Vantage Series Glassware Washers; Three models: mobile, undercounter, freestanding; high heat models available, optional viewing window (standard on Vantage), a variety of basket inserts to accommodate BOD bottles, petrie dishes, culture tubes, etc.

Lancer Usa, Inc. 800-332-1855
140 State Road 419, Winter Springs, FL 32708
32 models available of glassware washers from $10,000 to $115,000. Washers are equipped with self-diagnostic fault finding and program to 40 different wash cycles.

Medical Technologies Co. 800-280-3220
1728 W Park Center Dr Ste A, Fenton, MO 63026

Scientek Medical Equipment 604-273-9094
11151 Bridgeport Rd., Richmond, BC V6X 1T3 Canada

WASHER, LAUNDRY *(General) 80TFN*

Bausch & Stroebel Machine Company, Inc. 866-512-2637
112 Nod Rd Ste 17, Clinton, CT 06413

Consumaquip Corporation 305-592-4510
7240 NW 12th St, Miami, FL 33126

Dexter Apache Holdings, Inc. 800-524-2954
2211 W Grimes Ave, Fairfield, IA 52556
DEXTER.

Electrolux Home Products - North America 877-435-3287
250 Bobby Jones Expy, PO Box 212378, Augusta, GA 30907

Harco Co., Ltd. 905-890-1220
395 Brunel Rd., Mississauga, ONT L4Z 1Z5 Canada

Hoyt Corp. 800-343-9411
251 Forge Rd, Westport, MA 02790
Laundry and drapery washers and dryers. PETRO-MISER petroleum recovery tumbler, PETRO-WASH petroleum washer, distillation equipment.

WASHER, LAUNDRY *(cont'd)*

Huebsch Sales 800-553-5120
PO Box 990, Shepard Street, Ripon, WI 54971
Huebsch, solid-mount washer-extractors in 20lb, 30lb, 40lb, 60lb, and 80lb capacities. Huebsch, soft-mount washer-extractors in 18lb, 25lb, 35lb, 55lb, 75lb, 100lb, 135lb, & 165lb capacities.

Ipso Usa, Inc. 800-872-4776
PO Box 990, Shepard Street, Ripon, WI 54971
IPSO, D'HOOGE, LAUNDERCENTER - Heavy duty washers, 18 lbs through 125 lbs. Stainless steel cabinet, tub and basket, Hygienic version in 50 and 125 lbs. IPSO commercial dryers 20 lbs. to 190 lbs.

Pellerin Milnor Corp. 800-469-8780
PO Box 400, Kenner, LA 70063
Laundry washer-extractors, 35- to 750-lb capacity, continuous-batch washers, dryers, and materials-handling systems.

Wascomat Laundry Equipment 800-645-2204
461 Doughty Blvd, Inwood, NY 11096
WASCOMAT, Washer extractors, from 10 lb. capacity to 250 lb. capacities.

WASHER, MICROPLATE *(General) 80WLU*

Awareness Technology, Inc. 722-283-6540
1935 SW Martin Hwy, Palm City, FL 34990
Automatic, single-plate washer, microprocessor controlled, $3,495. STAT WASH, $725, semi-automatic microwell washer; handheld, with push-button controls.

Hyperion, Inc. 305-238-3020
14100 SW 136th St, Miami, FL 33186
Autoclavable microplate washer with Teflon coated tubes and individual aspirate and dispense tubes. MICROWASHER 4 PLUS, automated, programmable microplate washer stores 50 custom protocols; 8-way manifold standard; 12-way manifold optional.

Tecan U.S., Inc. 800-338-3226
4022 Stirrup Creek Dr Ste 310, Durham, NC 27703
96 PW, Columbus, PW 384.

Tricontinent 800-937-4738
12555 Loma Rica Dr, Grass Valley, CA 95945

Xiril 302-655-7035
91 Lukens Dr Ste A, New Castle, DE 19720
$4,000 for microplate washer.

WASHER, PIPETTE *(Chemistry) 75SFQ*

Boekel Scientific 800-336-6929
855 Pennsylvania Blvd, Feasterville Trevose, PA 19053

Buxton Medical Equipment Corp. 631-957-4500
1178 Route 109, Lindenhurst, NY 11757
All sizes available.

Getinge Usa, Inc. 800-475-9040
1777 E Henrietta Rd, Rochester, NY 14623
GETINGE.

Nalge Nunc International 800-625-4327
75 Panorama Creek Dr, Rochester, NY 14625
NALGENE one-piece leakproof washer/rinser for pipets up to 24in. long. Operates at a wide range of cycling speeds.

Scientek Medical Equipment 604-273-9094
11151 Bridgeport Rd., Richmond, BC V6X 1T3 Canada

Standard Instrumentation, Div. Preiser Scientific 800-624-8285
94 Oliver St, Saint Albans, WV 25177

WASHER, RECEPTACLE, WASTE, BODY *(General) 80FLH*

Cdx Corporation 800-245-9949
1 Richmond Sq, Providence, RI 02906
BIOSPONSE Blood/Biohazard Clean-up Kit: A compact, easy-to-use spill kit to contain and clean up blood and other bodily fluid spills.

Centurion Medical Products Corp. 517-545-1135
3310 S Main St, Salisbury, NC 28147

Dornoch Medical Systems, Inc. 816-505-2226
4032 NW Riverside Dr, Riverside, MO 64150
Suction canister washer.

Gentell 800-840-9041
3600 Boundbrook Ave, Trevose, PA 19053
GENTELL LIQUID CLEAN is a soothing, antimicrobial skin cleanser in a convenient non-aerosol dispenser. Rinse free skin cleanser cleans, moisturizes and conditions the area to which it is applied. GENTELL LIQUID CLEAN contains aloe vera gel and a proven broad spectrum antimicrobial with a persistent bactericidal effect against micoorganisms that cause skin breakdown and odor. GENTELL LIQUID CLEAN is available in an 8oz spray bottle.

WASHER, RECEPTACLE, WASTE, BODY *(cont'd)*

Multisorb Technologies, Inc. 800-445-9890
325 Harlem Rd, Buffalo, NY 14224
SANISORB, used in E/R and O/R for bodily waste.

Promethean Medical Technologies, Inc. 763-259-0559
105 Old Highway #8, Suite 1, New Brighton, MN 55112
Disposable fluid control island.

Tri-State Hospital Supply Corp. 517-545-1135
3173 E 43rd St, Yuma, AZ 85365

WASHER, RESPIRATORY/ANESTHESIA EQUIPMENT *(General) 80WPY*

Custom Ultrasonics, Inc. 215-364-1477
144 Railroad Dr, Hartsville, PA 18974
SYSTEM 80 automated systems for reprocessing, disinfecting/sterilizing/pasteurizing reusable anesthesia/respiratory therapy equipment.

WASHER, UTENSIL *(General) 80SFR*

Buxton Medical Equipment Corp. 631-957-4500
1178 Route 109, Lindenhurst, NY 11757
Tunnel type washers, glassware washers and dryers, instrument washers.

Getinge Usa, Inc. 800-475-9040
1777 E Henrietta Rd, Rochester, NY 14623
GETINGE.

Independent Solutions, Inc. 847-498-0500
900 Skokie Blvd Ste 118, Northbrook, IL 60062
Girton.

Scientek Medical Equipment 604-273-9094
11151 Bridgeport Rd., Richmond, BC V6X 1T3 Canada
Also available: cage and rack washer.

WASHER/DISINFECTOR *(General) 80WWK*

Abbott Associates 203-878-2370
620 West Ave, Milford, CT 06461
Medical device disinfector, soap pads.

Belimed 800-457-4117
13840 SW 119th Ave, Miami, FL 33186
Washer/Disinfector with large chamber size, glass doors, short cycle times with lowest operational costs and a wide variety of available racks.

Capital Controls, MicroChem 215-997-4000
3000 Advance Ln, Colmar, PA 18915
Disinfecting equipment and instrumentation.

Dentronix, Inc. 800-523-5944
235 Ascot Pkwy, Cuyahoga Falls, OH 44223
Ultrasonic Cleaning Solution MP-US Plus cleaner concentrate, no rinse formula, highly concentrated general-purpose solution. Contains no phosphates, and is formulated with a rust inhibitor. $49.50/box of 4 8-oz. bottles

Getinge Usa, Inc. 800-475-9040
1777 E Henrietta Rd, Rochester, NY 14623
GETINGE Washer/Disinfectors deliver a powerful combination of cleaning and moist thermal heat disinfection in a compact, space-saving design.

Lancer Usa, Inc. 800-332-1855
140 State Road 419, Winter Springs, FL 32708
32 models available of glassware washers from $10,000 to $115,000. Washers are equipped with self-diagnostic fault finding and program to 40 different wash cycles.

Miele Professional Products Group 800-843-7231
9 Independence Way, Princeton, NJ 08540
Hot water disinfection (95 degrees C/203 degrees F for 10 minutes)of surgical/digital instruments with simultaneous cleaning. Washer disinfector for dental instruments.

Scican 800-667-7733
1440 Don Mills Rd., Toronto, ON M3B 3P9 Canada
Hydrim C51w Washer--a high-speed instrument washer designed to prepare soiled medical and dental instruments for sterilization.

Skytron 800-759-8766
5085 Corporate Exchange Blvd SE, Grand Rapids, MI 49512
I Series Washer-Disinfectors including I3 Under the Counter and I5 Series Stand Alone and Pass Through.

Spartan Chemical Company, Inc. 800-537-8990
1110 Spartan Dr, Maumee, OH 43537

PRODUCT DIRECTORY

WASHER/DISINFECTOR *(cont'd)*

Unit Chemical Corp. 800-879-8648
7360 Commercial Way, Henderson, NV 89011
Pre-measured dry disinfectant packets with 200 ppm with no rinse HIV claim.

WASHER/STERILIZER *(General) 80SFM*

Almore International, Inc. 503-643-6633
PO Box 25214, Portland, OR 97298
STERITUBE Sterilization Instrument. $21.95 per unit.

American Autoclave Co. 800 421 5161
7819 Riverside Rd E, Sumner, WA 98390

Brulin & Co. Inc. 800-776-7149
2920 Drive A.J. Brown Avenue, Indianapolis, IN 46205
Parts Cleaner/Process Cleaner: water-based process detergent for immersion, ultrasonic cleaning, and spray wash cleaning.

Buxton Medical Equipment Corp. 631-957-4500
1178 Route 109, Lindenhurst, NY 11757
All sizes available.

Cadco Dental Products 800-833-8267
600 E Hueneme Rd, Oxnard, CA 93033
$12.50 for STERICAGE, sterilizing pouches.

Consolidated Stills & Sterilizers 617-782-6072
76 Ashford St, Boston, MA 02134
From $21,770 for model with 16 x 16 x 26" chamber. Single or double manual doors. Jet spray washer. Cabinet enclosed or recessed in wall installation. Microcomputer controls with CRT display. Circular chart recorder or alphanumeric printer.

Dux Dental 800-833-8267
600 E Hueneme Rd, Oxnard, CA 93033
$12.50 for STERICAGE, sterilizing cassettes.

Environmental Tectonics Corp. 215-355-9100
125 James Way, Southampton, PA 18966
Sterilizer for medical/infectious waste.

Harrick Scientific Products, Inc. 800-248-3847
141 Tomkins Avenue, Pleasantville, N 10570 United
Cleaner and sterilizer.

Innovative Health Care Products, Inc. 678-320-0009
6850 Peachtree Dunwoody Rd NE Apt 402, Atlanta, GA 30328
Statim/Hydrim combo

Medco Equipment, Inc. 800-717-3626
105 Old Highway 8 NW Ste 3, New Brighton, MN 55112
Washing machine for wheelchair, walker, cart, chair.

Medi-Tech International, Inc. 305-593-9373
2924 NW 109th Ave, Doral, FL 33172
PRIMUS STERILIZERS

Spartan Chemical Company, Inc. 800-537-8990
1110 Spartan Dr, Maumee, OH 43537
TB-CIDE PLUS: Phenolic-based cleaner. Disinfectant kills TB and HIV-1 (AIDS Virus) on inanimate surfaces. 10% blood serum/1000 ppm water hardness. HEPACIDE QUAT: ready to use EPA registered disinfectant with Hepatitis B claims.

Steris Corporation 800-884-9550
5960 Heisley Rd, Mentor, OH 44060
Surface disinfectant.

WASTE DISPOSAL UNIT, SHARPS *(General) 80SFS*

Amd-Ritmed, Inc. 800-445-0340
295 Firetower Road, Tonawanda, NY 14150
Sharps count and disposal cases.

American Surgical Instrument Corp. 800-628-2879
26 Plaza Dr, Westmont, IL 60559
Disposable knife.

Armstrong Medical Industries, Inc. 800-323-4220
575 Knightsbridge Pkwy, Lincolnshire, IL 60069

Bemis Mfg. Co. 800-558-7651
300 Mill St, Sheboygan Falls, WI 53085
Sharps containers in all sizes from 1 Qt. to 11 gallons. Includes a 5 Qt. and 3 Gal. locking wall cabinet.

Covidien Lp 508-261-8000
15 Hampshire St, Mansfield, MA 02048

Johnson & Johnson Medical Division Of Ethicon, Inc. 800-423-4018
2500 E Arbrook Blvd, Arlington, TX 76014

Lampac International Ltd. 636-797-3659
230 N Lake Dr, Hillsboro, MO 63050
Chimney top horizontal entry and chemotherapy models.

WASTE DISPOSAL UNIT, SHARPS *(cont'd)*

Medical Safety Systems Inc. 888-803-9303
230 White Pond Dr, Akron, OH 44313

Post Medical, Inc. 800-876-8678
315 Bell Park Dr, Woodstock, GA 30188
In-room sharps disposal Leak Tight Locking Top containers and laboratory sharps disposable containers. Also, phlebotomy sharps disposable container for laboratory personnel for automatically unwinding blood collection needles. Leak Tight Locking Top sharps disposal containers for home health, nursing homes, POL, etc.

Sharps Compliance Corp. 713-432-0300
9220 Kirby Dr Ste 500, Houston, TX 77054
Sharps Disposal By Mail Systems, manufactured by Sharps Compliance, Inc., represent the first complete disposal system pioneered for simplified management of used needles, syringes, and other small-quantity medical waste. Sharps Disposal By Mail Systems is the ideal disposal solution for small-quantity medical waste generators, businesses, and individual patients who are self-injectors of drug therapies. The Sharps Disposal By Mail System comprises a sharps container, a government-approved return by mail system, and instructions for use. When the drug therapy is concluded, or when the sharps container is full, the patient or generator of the medical waste returns the sharps container to its original packaging. The original packaging is a postage pre-paid return box, which is returned to Sharps via the U.S. Postal Service (USPS). Upon receipt via the USPS, Sharps documents the receipt, weight, and destruction of each sharps container and its contents of used syringes. The safe disposal of used needles and other sharps is a critical public health safety issue.

Simport Plastics Ltd. 450-464-1723
2588 Bernard-Pilon, Beloeil, QUE J3G 4S5 Canada
BIODISPOSER.

WASTE DISPOSAL UNIT, SURGICAL INSTRUMENT (SHARPS)

(Surgery) 79KDB

Advanced Medical Innovations, Inc. 888-367-2641
9410 De Soto Ave Ste J, Chatsworth, CA 91311
SAF-T-SHELL, sharps collection containers for disposal of used syringes & other sharps.

Bemis Mfg. Co. 800-558-7651
300 Mill St, Sheboygan Falls, WI 53085
Large Volume Sharps Containers in 8 & 11 gallon sizes for use in Operating Rooms.

Covidien Lp 508-261-8000
15 Hampshire St, Mansfield, MA 02048

Hospital Marketing Svcs. Company, Inc. 800-786-5094
162 Great Hill Rd./ Ind. Park, Naugatuck, CT 06770
DISPOS-A-SHARP waste disposal unit (sharps, needles, suture needles, surgeon's blades).

Medical Safety Systems Inc. 888-803-9303
230 White Pond Dr, Akron, OH 44313

Schiffmayer Plastics Corporation 847-658-8140
1201 Armstrong St, Algonquin, IL 60102
Various types of instrument, disposal, surgical, (sharps).

WASTE DISPOSAL UNIT, SYRINGE *(General) 80SFT*

American Autoclave Co. 800 421 5161
7819 Riverside Rd E, Sumner, WA 98390

Bemis Mfg. Co. 800-558-7651
300 Mill St, Sheboygan Falls, WI 53085
Sharps disposal containers in all sizes from 1 Qt. to 11 Gal. including our new 5 Qt. and 3 Gal. locking wall cabinets.

Bio-Plexus, Inc. 800-223-0010
129 Reservoir Rd, Vernon, CT 06066

Covidien Lp 508-261-8000
15 Hampshire St, Mansfield, MA 02048

Post Medical, Inc. 800-876-8678
315 Bell Park Dr, Woodstock, GA 30188
New patented, safely transportable insulin needle disposal unit, the VOYAGER, which destroys insulin needles and syringe barrels in one easy step. New VOYAGER unit will accept most pen needles for disposal as well.

Security Engineered Machinery 800-225-9293
5 Walkup Dr, Westborough, MA 01581
SEM Security Disintegrator waste-disposal unit, syringe.

WASTE RECEPTACLE, CONTAMINATED *(General) 80SFU*

American Autoclave Co. 800 421 5161
7819 Riverside Rd E, Sumner, WA 98390

WASTE RECEPTACLE, CONTAMINATED *(cont'd)*

Cdx Corporation 800-245-9949
1 Richmond Sq, Providence, RI 02906
BIOPAIL Blood/Biohazard Cleanup Kit: A large, easy-to-use spill cleanup kit to contain large spills and dispose of sharps and hazardous waste.

Enpac Corp. 800-936-7229
34355 Melinz Pkwy, Eastlake, OH 44095
20 gallon containers.

Lee Medical International, Inc. 800-433-8950
612 Distributors Row, Harahan, LA 70123
Sharps containers.

M & M Industries 800-331-5305
316 Corporate Pl, Chattanooga, TN 37419
LIFE LATCH medical waste containers available in variety of sizes.Plastic containers for biohazard and chemo-therapy waste, UN certified for solids and liquids. Easy-to-seal screw-top covers with child-resistant and tamper evident features.

Precision Quincy Corp. 800-338-0079
1625 W Lake Shore Dr, Woodstock, IL 60098
HAZ-BIN portable containment shelter for safer storage of hazardous materials. Sizes up to 1,400 sq ft.

Wes-Pak, Inc. 1-800-493-7725
11610 Vimy Ridge Rd, Alexander, AR 72002
MED-PAK slotless, solid bottom, corrugated container - lined with cross-laminated polyethylene liner knocks down flat for transportation as well as for storage. Available in five sizes: 10, 18, 24, 30, and 40 gallons. PATH PACK unlined solid bottom, collapsible containers can help you reduce product handling and minimize packaging waste.

Whitney Products, Inc. 800-338-4237
6153 W Mulford St Ste C, Niles, IL 60714
TERMINAL BENCH-TOPKEEPER; heavy paperboard carton with plastic lining available in 2 sizes to collect biohazard waste. TERMINAL SAFE-KEEPER; paperboard container hangs up at workbench and collects biohazard waste. TERMINAL PIPET KEEPER; paperboard container holds up to 14' pipets with plastic lining to prevent leaks and soak through of liquids. SAFETY TOSS Biohazard Disposal Container is a solid cardboard container lined with biohazard bag. Available as floor model or bench top model. With RECLOSE-A/REMOVE-A-LID.

Youngs, Inc. 800-523-5454
55 E Cherry Ln, Souderton, PA 18964

WASTE RECEPTACLE, GENERAL PURPOSE *(General) 80UKO*

Atd-American Co. 800-523-2300
135 Greenwood Ave, Wyncote, PA 19095

Bennett Manufacturing Co., Inc. 800-345-2142
13315 Railroad St, Alden, NY 14004
Step-on receptacles and fire-safe receptacles.

Bobrick Washroom Equipment, Inc. 818-764-1000
11611 Hart St, North Hollywood, CA 91605

Brewer Company, The 888-873-9371
N88W13901 Main St, Menomonee Falls, WI 53051
#35266: Step On Metal Waste Can

Chem-Tainer Industries, Inc. 800-ASK-CHEM
361 Neptune Ave, West Babylon, NY 11704

Continental Manufacturing Co. 800-325-1051
13330 Lakefront Dr, Earth City, MO 63045
Step-on painted or stainless steel in 5-, 8-, 12-, and 24-gallon capacity. Also available, tilt trucks, 1/2 and one cubic yard standard and heavy-duty industrial plastic.

DURHAM MANUFACTURING COMPANY 800-243-3774
201 Main St, Durham, CT 06422

Eagle Manufacturing 304-737-3171
2400 Charles St, Wellsburg, WV 26070
High-density polyethylene disposal safety cans are supplied in 3- and 5-gallon sizes. Disposal cans provide an intermediate station for temporary storage of liquid waste.

Enochs Examining Room Furniture, Inc. 800-428-2305
PO Box 50559, Indianapolis, IN 46250
$357.00 per unit (standard).

Freund Container 800-363-9822
4200 Commerce Ct Ste 206, Corporate Center II, Lisle, IL 60532

Hygolet Usa 800-494-6538
349 SE 2nd Ave, Deerfield Beach, FL 33441
WALLBOX Sanitary napkin metal receptacle. Wall mounts with drop-down botton for the sanitary removal of the plastic bag. Accessories available.

WASTE RECEPTACLE, GENERAL PURPOSE *(cont'd)*

Justrite Manufacturing Co., L.L.C. 800-798-9250
2454 E Dempster St, Des Plaines, IL 60016
Smokers Cease-fire® Waste receptacles are specially contoured to direct smoke and gas from any fire inside the container, back into the combustion area, cutting off the air supply and extinguishing glames in seconds. Available in five different colors.

Marathon Equipment Company 800-269-7237
950 County HWY 9 S., Vernon, AL 35592
Industrial-sized stationary and self-contained compactors. Industrial and stockroom-sized balers.

O&M Enterprise 847-258-4515
641 Chelmsford Ln, Elk Grove Village, IL 60007
WASTER RECEPTACLE

Peter Pepper Products, Inc. 800-496-0204
17929 S Susana Rd, PO Box 5769, Compton, CA 90221

Protectoseal Co. 800-323-2268
225 Foster Ave, Bensenville, IL 60106
Safety containers for flammable and hazardous liquids.

Safco Products Company 800-328-3020
9300 Research Center Rd W, Minneapolis, MN 55428
Stainless steel waste receptacles, waste baskets & step on cans. SMOKE DOME - covered ash/trash receptacle. TROPHY COLLECTION - plastic indoor/outdoor receptacles.

Spin-Cast Plastics, Inc. 800-422-3625
3300 N Kenmore St, South Bend, IN 46628

United Metal Fabricators, Inc. 800-638-5322
1316 Eisenhower Blvd, Johnstown, PA 15904
Vinyl clad steel in woodgrain pattern or enamel to match suite color.

United Receptacle 800-233-0314
1400 Laurel Blvd, Pottsville, PA 17901
Defenders Series step cans, both powder coated and #304 non magnetic stainless steel, COllect A Cubes for HIPAA Compliance, indoor/outdoor fire-safe waste receptacles and related accessories; also available, smoking urns and planters.

Whitney Products, Inc. 800-338-4237
6153 W Mulford St Ste C, Niles, IL 60714
TERMINAL Broken Glass Benchtop Keeper. Available as floor model. Sturdy cardboard container for non-biohazard broken glass with clear plastic bag and RECLOSE-A/REMOVE-A-LID. Collects non-contaminated broken glass to protect the employee.

WASTE RECEPTACLE, KICK BUCKET *(General) 80RDD*

Alimed, Inc. 800-225-2610
297 High St, Dedham, MA 02026

Armstrong Medical Industries, Inc. 800-323-4220
575 Knightsbridge Pkwy, Lincolnshire, IL 60069

Blickman 800-247-5070
39 Robinson Rd, Lodi, NJ 07644
Blickman offers two model kickbuckets, 1900SS (flat bumper) and 7766SS (encircling bumper) and one sponge receptacle-model 8766SS. Both kickbuckets support a 12-1/2qt. pail and travel on 2' swivel casters.

Brandt Industries, Inc. 800-221-8031
4461 Bronx Blvd, Bronx, NY 10470

Mayo Medical, S.A. De C.V. 800-715-3872
Edison 1141 Nte., Col. Talleres, Monterrey N.L. 64480 Mexico

Medegen Medical Products, Llc 800-233-1987
209 Medegen Drive, Gallaway, TN 38036-0228
MED-ASSIST Stainless steel.

Medical Safety Systems Inc. 888-803-9303
230 White Pond Dr, Akron, OH 44313

Pedigo Products 360-695-3500
4000 SE Columbia Way, Vancouver, WA 98661
Stainless steel.

WASTE RECEPTACLE, RADIOACTIVE *(Radiology) 90SFV*

Dan Kar Corporation 800-942-5542
PO Box 279, 192 New Boston St C, Wilmington, MA 01887

WATER, DISTILLED (IRRIGATION) *(Gastro/Urology) 78TGB*

Baxter Healthcare Corporation, Global Drug Delivery 888-229-0001
25212 W Il Route 120, Round Lake, IL 60073
Sterile.

Welcon, Inc. 800-877-0923
7409 Pebble Dr, Fort Worth, TX 76118

WATER, THERAPY, RESPIRATORY *(Microbiology) 83WKT*

Aqua Products Company, Inc. 800-849-4264
14301 C R Koon Hwy, Newberry, SC 29108
Electric Water Heaters blow-molded polybutylene tank is impervious to rust and corrosion. Available in 30, 40, 50, 75, 85 and 105 gallon models. Energy efficient and insulated with Envirofoam insulation which is free ozone depletin CFC's and HCFC's. For more information call 1-800-849-4264

Atlantic Medical Specialties 888-487-5568
3620 Horizon Dr, King Of Prussia, PA 19406

Dey, L.P. 800-755-5560
2751 Napa Valley Corporate Dr, Napa, CA 94558
0.45%, 0.9%, 3% and 10% sodium chloride solutions for inhalation therapy. Cromolyn sodium, albuterol sulfate, and USP purified water also available. Ipratropium bromide inhalation solution; 0.02%, 2.5 mL. Metaproterenol inhalation solution; 0.4%, 2.5 mL; 0.6%, 2.5 mL. Branded products include AccuNeb (albuterol sulfate) 0.63 mg and 1.25 mg* Inhalation Solution(*Potency expressed as albuterol, equivalent to 0.75 mg and 1.5 mg albuterol sulfate), DuoNeb (ipratropium 0.5mg/albuterol sulfate 3.0mg*) Inhalation Solution *Equivalent to 2.5 mg albuterol base, and EpiPen epinephrine Auto-injectors.*

Promotora Biomedica Internacional, S.A. De C.V. 42157770
San Francisco 1, Ste. 2, San Miguel de Allende, Gto. 26033 Mexico

WAX, BONE *(Surgery) 79MTJ*

Ceremed, Inc. 310-815-2125
3643 Lenawee Ave, Los Angeles, CA 90016
Bone wax.

Ethicon, Inc. 800-4-ETHICON
Route 22 West, Somerville, NJ 08876

Ethicon, Llc. 908-218-2887
Rd. 183, Km. 8.3,, Industrial Area Hato, San Lorenzo, PR 00754
Bone wax.

Musculoskeletal Transplant Foundation 800-433-6576
125 May St Ste 300, Edison Corp Ctr, Edison, NJ 08837
Bone wax.

Surgical Specialties Corporation 800-523-3332
100 Dennis Dr, Reading, PA 19606
Bone wax.

WAX, DENTAL *(Dental And Oral) 76EGD*

Almore International, Inc. 503-643-6633
PO Box 25214, Portland, OR 97298
$8.00 to $25.00 per lb.

Aluwax Dental Products Co. 616-895-4385
5260 Edgewater Dr, Allendale, MI 49401
ALUWAX $10.55 to $15.00 per box; registration and impression material. 7 different styles available.

American Diversified Dental Systems 800-637-2330
22991 La Cadena Dr, Laguna Hills, CA 92653
Production Dipwax & Rapid Wax By James Pitre, Granulated 6 & 16 oz Bottles.

Astron Dental Corporation 847-726-8787
815 Oakwood Rd Ste G, Lake Zurich, IL 60047
Dental waxes.

Classone Orthodontics, Inc. 806-799-0608
5064 50th St, Lubbock, TX 79414
Various types of dental wax.

Coltene/Whaledent Inc. 330-916-8858
235 Ascot Pkwy, Cuyahoga Falls, OH 44223
Wax.

Corning Wax 631-738-0041
1744 Julia Goldbach Ave, Ronkonkoma, NY 11779
Wax, dental, intraoral, various types.

Denplus Inc. 800-344-4424
205 - 1221 Labadie, Longueuil, QUE J4N 1E2 Canada

Dentek Oral Care, Inc. 865-983-1300
307 Excellence Way, Maryville, TN 37801
Brace wax.

Dentsply Canada, Ltd. 800-263-1437
161 Vinyl Ct., Woodbridge, ONT L4L 4A3 Canada

G & H Wire Co. 800-526-1026
2165 Earlywood Dr, Franklin, IN 46131

General Dental Products, Inc. 888-367-6212
201 Ogden Ave, Ely, NV 89301

WAX, DENTAL *(cont'd)*

Glenroe Technologies 800-237-4060
1912 44th Ave E, Bradenton, FL 34203
Orthodontic silicone felief wax.

Harry J. Bosworth Company 800-323-4352
7227 Hamlin Ave, Skokie, IL 60076
Tacky wax, occlusal plane wax.

Heraeus Kulzer, Inc. 800-431-1785
99 Business Park Dr, Armonk, NY 10504
Various dental waxes for laboratory use.

Heraeus Kulzer, Inc., Dental Products Division 574-299-6662
4315 S Lafayette Blvd, South Bend, IN 46614
Various types of dental waxes.

Kay See Dental Mfg. Co. 816-842-2817
124 Missouri Ave, Kansas City, MO 64106
Hydro-cast (various).

Kerr Corp. 714-516-7400
28200 Wick Rd, Romulus, MI 48174
Dental wax.

Kindt Collins Co. 800-321-3170
12651 Elmwood Ave, Cleveland, OH 44111
INTRAORAL - MULTIPLE

Lancer Orthodontics, Inc. 760-304-2705
253 Pawnee St, San Marcos, CA 92078
Relief wax.

Memphis Dental Mfg. Co., Inc. 901-526-6328
402 S 2nd St, Memphis, TN 38103
Bite wax.

Miltex Dental Technologies, Inc. 516-576-6022
589 Davies Dr, York, PA 17402
Various intra-oral dental waves.

Mizzy, Inc. Of National Keystone 800-333-3131
616 Hollywood Ave, Cherry Hill, NJ 08002
Try Allcezon Base Plate, Byte Ryte or our Special Formula waxes for all your dental impression needs.

Motloid Company 800-662-5021
300 N Elizabeth St, Chicago, IL 60607
Waxes: sticky, dipping, red-refined, bite rims, baseplate, casting, etc.

Moyco Technologies, Inc. 800-331-8837
200 Commerce Dr, Montgomeryville, PA 18936
$36.00 per unit.

Ortho Organizers, Inc. 760-448-8730
1822 Aston Ave, Carlsbad, CA 92008
Relief wax.

Pemaco, Inc. 314-231-3399
2030 S 3rd St, Saint Louis, MO 63104
Dental wax.

The Hygenic Corp. 800-321-2135
1245 Home Ave, Akron, OH 44310
Original & renewal handpiece tubings and accessories for.

Whip-Mix Corporation 800-626-5651
361 Farmington Ave, PO Box 17183, Louisville, KY 40209

Yates & Bird And Motloid 800-662-5021
300 N Elizabeth St, Chicago, IL 60607
Features Digital Wax Pot. It is a precise temperature-controlled wax pot that quickly reaches and maintains desired temperature to make perfect copings every time.

WEARABLE, DEFIBRILLATOR, AUTOMATIC, EXTERNAL *(Cardiovascular) 74MVK*

Zoll Lifecor Corporation 800-543-3267
121 Freeport Rd, Blawnox, PA 15238
Wearable cardioverter defibrillator.

WEDGES *(Dental And Oral) 76UMQ*

Almore International, Inc. 503-643-6633
PO Box 25214, Portland, OR 97298
$14.75 for 500 plastic wedges.

WEIGHT, IV POLE *(General) 80WTM*

Evergreen Research, Inc. 303-526-7402
433 Park Point Dr Ste 140, Golden, CO 80401
OEM precision scale with 6-kg and 2-gm capacity used for hanging loads such as I.V. solution bags or bottles, various models available.

Northeast Medical Systems Corp. 856-910-8111
901 Beechwood Ave, Cherry Hill, NJ 08002
For urology, cardiac and electrophysiology tables.

WEIGHT, IV POLE *(cont'd)*

Tuffcare 800-367-6160
3999 E La Palma Ave, Anaheim, CA 92807

WEIGHTS, EYELID, EXTERNAL *(Ophthalmology) 86MML*

Jedmed Instruments Co. 314-845-3770
5416 Jedmed Ct, Saint Louis, MO 63129

Labtician Ophthalmics, Inc. 800-265-8391
2140 Winston Park Dr., Unit 6, Oakville, ONTAR L6H 5V5 Canada
Labtician Lid Load™ gold eyelid weights.

Meddev Corporation 800-543-2789
730 N Pastoria Ave, Sunnyvale, CA 94085
EYECLOSE EXTERNAL EYELID WEIGHTS are taped to the outside of the eyelid for the gravity assisted treatment of the functional defects of lagophthalmos resulting from temporary or permanent facial paralysis.

WELL, AMALGAM *(Dental And Oral) 76VLM*

Hager Worldwide, Inc. 800-328-2335
13322 Byrd Dr, Odessa, FL 33556
Stainless steel.

Hu-Friedy Manufacturing Co., Inc. 800-483-7433
3232 N Rockwell St, Chicago, IL 60618
$22.35 for amalgam well.

Miltex Inc. 800-645-8000
589 Davies Dr, York, PA 17402

Moyco Technologies, Inc. 800-331-8837
200 Commerce Dr, Montgomeryville, PA 18936

WHEEL, POLISHING AGENT *(Dental And Oral) 76EJQ*

Align Technology, Inc. 408-470-1000
881 Martin Ave, Santa Clara, CA 95050
Wheel,polishing agent.

Almore International, Inc. 503-643-6633
PO Box 25214, Portland, OR 97298
$29.95 for disposable buffing wheel kit.

Axis Dental 800-355-5063
800 W Sandy Lake Rd Ste 100, Coppell, TX 75019

Dentsply Canada, Ltd. 800-263-1437
161 Vinyl Ct., Woodbridge, ONT L4L 4A3 Canada

Grobet File Co. 800-847-4188
1912 Whitney Rd, Cheyenne, WY 82007
Polishing felts.

Handler Manufacturing Co. 800-274-2635
612 North Ave E, Westfield, NJ 07090

Heraeus Kulzer, Inc., Dental Products Division 574-299-6662
4315 S Lafayette Blvd, South Bend, IN 46614
Polishing wheels.

Ivoclar Vivadent, Inc. 800-533-6825
175 Pineview Dr, Amherst, NY 14228
WILLIAMS Diamond Polishing Paste System. Fast, easy to use, multi-purpose system that provides a highly glazed more natural looking finish for porcelain jackets, veneers, inlays and denture teeth without additional firing.

Productivity Training Company 800-448-8855
360 Cochrane Cir # A, Morgan Hill, CA 95037
Also includes finishing stones and burs.

Reliable Buff Co., Inc. 800-338-2833
226 N Bivens Rd, Monroe, NC 28110
Muslin buff - size range 3/4' through 6'

Shofu Dental Corporation 800-827-4638
1225 Stone Dr, San Marcos, CA 92078
DURA-GREEN WHEELS, CHIPLESS WHEELS, CUT-OFF DISKS, SPRUCUT WHEELS

Ultradent Products, Inc. 801-553-4586
505 W 10200 S, South Jordan, UT 84095
Polishing brush.

Wehmer Corporation 800-323-0229
1151 N Main St, Lombard, IL 60148
$1,125 for dual wheel trimmer. Also single wheel trimmer.

WHEELCHAIR, MANUAL *(Physical Med) 89IOR*

A.R.C. Distributors 800-296-8724
PO Box 599, Centreville, MD 21617
E&J,EVERMED,GENDRON,INVACARE,MEDLINE,THERADYNE, TUFFCARE MANUFACTURERS. E&J = Vista, Metro. GENDRON = Tracker Series, Travel About,Tracker Youth, Tracker Transport, Regency XL - 450lb. 600lb 700lb 750lb 850lb. weight capacities. INVACARE = Tracer EX2, Transport Chairs, Tracer SX5, Tracer SX5 Recliner,9000 Series Wheelchairs, 9000 Topaz-700lb capacity, Tracer IV 350lb & 450lb capacities, 9000 Jymni-Pediatric wheelchair or recliner, 125-lb capacity. MEDLINE = Excell Series-2000, narrow, extra-wide, 350- and 450-lb capacities; Shuttle 600-lb capacity, Recliner, Transport. THERADYNE = Envoy Transport, Maxium, Maxium LBW, Venture, Venture Wide, Venture Recliner, and Venture Plus, 800-lb capacity. Large variety of sizes and models with accessories and options.

Access Mobility, Inc. 800-336-1147
5240 Elmwood Ave, Indianapolis, IN 46203

Aero Innovative Research, Inc. 316-755-3477
500 W Clay St, Valley Center, KS 67147
Mechanical wheelchair.

Alan's Wheelchairs & Repairs 800-693-4344
109 S Harbor Blvd Ste B, Fullerton, CA 92832

Alex Orthopedic, Inc. 800-544-2539
PO Box 201442, Arlington, TX 76006
Standard wheelchair.

American Bantex Corp. 800-633-4839
1815 Rollins Rd, Burlingame, CA 94010

American Biomed Instruments, Inc. 718-235-8900
11 Wyona St, Brooklyn, NY 11207

American Track Roadsters, Inc. 303-986-9300
3535 S Kipling St Unit A, Lakewood, CO 80235
Various models of manual wheelchairs.

Arizona Dme--Durable Medical Equipment, Inc. 888-665-2568
PO Box 15413, Scottsdale, AZ 85267
All DME.

Armstrong Medical Industries, Inc. 800-323-4220
575 Knightsbridge Pkwy, Lincolnshire, IL 60069

Basic American Medical Products 800-849-6664
2935A Northeast Pkwy, Atlanta, GA 30360

Bio-Medic Health Services, Inc. 800-525-0072
5041B Benois Rd Bldg B, Roanoke, VA 24018

Broda Enterprises Inc. 800-668-0637
385 Phillip St., Waterloo, ONT N2L 5R8 Canada
BRODA SEATING Fully reclining wheelchair, semi-reclining wheelchair, tilt-in space wheelchair.

Camtec 410-228-1156
1959 Church Creek Rd, Cambridge, MD 21613
Converta litter.

Convaid Inc. 888-266-8243
PO Box 4209, Rolling Hills Estates, CA 90274
EZ RIDER, a lightweight, compact-folding positioning wheelchair with upright seating for children and teenagers with upper body control. It's adjustable and offers a wide range of positioning options. Available in 10', 12', 14', 16', 18' seat widths. Crash tested. CRUISER, a lightweight, compact-folding, positioning mobility base with a fixed 30 degree tilt, and offering a wide range of adjustments and positioning adaptations. Four sizes from infants to teenagers. Crash tested. SAFARI-TILT, a unique compact-folding tilt-in-space chair. It's a lightweight adjustable positioning wheelchair with an adjustable tilt from 5 degrees-45 degrees, and offering a wide range of adjustments and positioning adaptations. Available in 12', 14',16' and 18' seat sizes. The frame only offers an excellent base for sophisticated seating inserts by others. Crash tested. SCOUT, compact-foldng all terrain wheelchair with upright seating for children and adults with upper body control. Available in 12in, 14in, 16in, and 18in.

Demetech Corp. 888-324-2447
3530 NW 115th Ave, Doral, FL 33178
Mechanical wheelchair.

Eagle Sports Chairs 800-932-9380
2351 Parkwood Rd, Snellville, GA 30039
HURRICANE & TORNADO, SCREAMING EAGLE and SOARING EAGLE racers; $1,200.00 to $1,800.00 for basketball, tennis, track and road-racing sports wheelchairs.

Enduro Wheelchair Co. 860-289-2299
310 Nutmeg Rd S Unit C5, South Windsor, CT 06074
Various types of custom tilt-in-space mechanical wheelchairs, including forward tilt and side tilt.

WHEELCHAIR, MANUAL *(cont'd)*

Essential Medical Supply, Inc. 800-826-8423
6420 Hazeltine National Dr, Orlando, FL 32822
Roll Easy standard and color transport chairs and Roll Easy Plus lightweight aluminum transport chairs. Two models, both with folding backs; 30% lighter than standard transports. One model with 12-in. rear wheel and hand brakes. Endurance Heavy Duty transport chair comes in 20- and 22-in. seat widths and supports users weighing up to 400 lb.

Evermed Corp. 714-777-9997
4999 E La Palma Ave, Anaheim, CA 92807
Wheelchair.

Fortress Scientifique Du Quebec Ltee. 418-847-5225
2160 Rue De Celles, Quebec G2C 1X8 Canada
Various mechanical wheelchairs,varying in shape,size and features

Freedom Designs, Inc. 800-331-8551
2241 N Madera Rd, Simi Valley, CA 93065
SPECTRUM & SOLUTION pediatric folding wheelchairs. SOLUTION allows tilt-in-space and recline feature.

G. Hirsch And Co., Inc. 650-692-8770
870 Mahler Rd, Burlingame, CA 94010
Various.

Gendron, Inc. 800-537-2521
400 E Lugbill Rd, Archbold, OH 43502
ACTI-LITE $676.00-1,500.00 Lightweight, adjustable frame wheelchairs for active users. $344.00 per unit (standard). Also standard duty lightweight wheelchair; 35 lbs., $531.00.

Good Sports 412-731-3032
1701 Monongahela Ave, Pittsburgh, PA 15218
Everest and Jennings wheelchairs.

Great Lakes Innovation Inc 248-680-8671
1103 Winthrop Dr, Troy, MI 48083
Innolife size adjustable wheelchair.

Handicap Unlimited, Inc. 888-371-0095
5640 Summer Ave Ste 3, Memphis, TN 38134

Hannah's Miracle Shoe, Inc. 801-329-9802
11237 Aubrey Meadow Cir, South Jordan, UT 84095
Wheelchair wheel cover.

Icca, A Division Of Internet Services Corporation 800-624-5940
1300 Altura Rd, Fort Mill, SC 29708
Durable Medical Equipment: Rollators, Transport Chairs, Canes, and Bathroom accessories.

International Hospital Supply Co. 800-398-9450
6914 Canby Ave Ste 105, Reseda, CA 91335

Invacare Canada 800-668-5324
5970 Chedworth Way, Mississauga, ONT L5R 3T9 Canada

Invacare Corporation 800-333-6900
1 Invacare Way, Elyria, OH 44035
INVACARE, Top End, IVC, Tracer Transport, Tracer EX2, Tracer SX5, 9000 SL, 9000 XT, 9000 Topaz, 9000 XDT, Tracer IV, 900.

Invacare Top End 800-532-8677
4501 63rd Cir N, Pinellas Park, FL 33781
Manual wheelchair.

Invamex S.A. De C.V. 440-329-6595
Carretera Reynosa-Matamros,, Km#1, Reynosa Tamaulipas Mexico
Various

J&J Engineering Llc 503-626-7812
11791 SW Crater Loop, Beaverton, OR 97008
The 'Quantum Runner' is a new and innovative lever propelled wheelchair. It provides forward propulsion with the push and pull of its lever. This ergonomically correct positioning allows the user to sit in the upright position and change gears depending on the power needed. The chair will normally be used in an 'automatic' mode where the 4-speed gears change according to the speed of the wheel. In addition, the propulsion system can be disabled completely and the chair used in the conventional wheel-push manual method. Disc brakes are provided for safety and quick turning. The combination of these attributes gives the user freedom to go places that would not otherwise be possible with a conventional chair such as dirt paths, grass, carpet, hills etc.

Jason Marine Enterprises, Inc. 954-346-5240
5494 NW 22nd Ave, Ft Lauderdale, FL 33309
Same.

Joerns Healthcare, Inc. 715-341-3600
1032 N Fourth St, Baldwyn, MS 38824
Manual wheelchair.

WHEELCHAIR, MANUAL *(cont'd)*

Kareco International, Inc. 800-8KA-RECO
299 Rte. 22 E., Green Brook, NJ 08812-1714
Manual wheelchair styles include standards, lightweights, heavy-duty wides, recliners, hemis's, and travel chairs. Suggested retail prices range from $250.00 - $1,050.

Karman Healthcare, Inc. 800-805-2762
19255 San Jose Ave, City Of Industry, CA 91748
Specialized in mobility products including lightweight aluminum, steel Standard, recliner, walkers, rollators, power wheelchairs and scooters, and other healthcare products.

Kern Surgical Supply, Inc. 800-582-3939
2823 Gibson St, Bakersfield, CA 93308

L.P.A. Medical, Inc. 888-845-6447
460 Desrochers, Ste. 150D, Vanier, QUEBE G1M 1C2 Canada
OPTIMUM Posturo-Pedic positioning chair, Series 1600.

Lakeview Center, Inc. 850-595-1330
1221 W Lakeview Ave, Pensacola, FL 32501
Mechanical wheelchairs.

Maple Leaf Wheelchair Mfg., Inc. 905-602-0566
12/13-1655 Sismet Rd, Mississauga L4W 1Z4 Canada
Various types of wheelchairs (manual)

Marken International, Inc. 800-564-9248
W231N2811 Roundy Cir E Ste 100, Pewaukee, WI 53072
Mechanical wheelchair.

Medical Depot 516-998-4600
99 Seaview Blvd, Port Washington, NY 11050
Wheelchir, mechanical.

Medisol U.S.A., Inc. 626-350-6662
9713 Factorial Way, South El Monte, CA 91733
Medisol customized wheel chairs.

Metro Medical Supply Wholesale 800-768-2002
200 Cumberland Bnd, Nashville, TN 37228

Nova Health Products, Llc 843-673-0702
1138 Annelle Dr, Florence, SC 29505
Standard weight and/or light weight manual wheelchairs.

Ocelco, Inc. 800-328-5343
1111 Industrial Park Rd SW, Brainerd, MN 56401

Palmer Industries 800-847-1304
PO Box 5707, Endicott, NY 13763
PALMER $1595.00 3 speed 3 wheeled handcycle.

Pdg Product Design Group, Inc. 888-858-4422
Unit 102, 366 East Kent Ave. South, Vancouver, BC V5X 4N6 Canada
Bentley manual-tilt wheelchair; Eclipse extra-wide manual wheelchair; Stellar manual-tilt wheelchair.

Portacare Llc 509-928-0650
13023 E Tall Tree Rd, Spokane Valley, WA 99216
Sideslider wheelchair.

Product Design Group 888-858-4422
366 East Kent Ave. South, Unit 102, Vancouver, BC V5X-4N6 Canada
Bentley Manual Tilt Wheelchair; Eclipse Extra Wide Manual Wheelchair; Stellar Manual Tilt Wheelchair.

Recreation Equipment Unlimited, Inc. 412-731-3000
PO Box 4700, Pittsburgh, PA 15206
Everest and Jennings wheelchairs.

Rehab Innovations, Inc. 402-445-4335
8727 Ames Ave, Omaha, NE 68134
The ue ranger.

Respiratory Science Industries Ltd 516-561-6161
1325 M St, Elmont, NY 11003
Repair of wheelchairs.

Snug Seat, Inc. 800-336-7684
12801 E Independence Blvd, PO Box 1739, Matthews, NC 28105
The ETAC STING, a lightweight, ergonomically designed wheelchair, provides children with more mobility than do comparable chairs. The adjustable seating system also allows for a number of accessories to position any child.

Specmat Technologies Inc. 011-441-5687
215 Dunavant Dr, Rockford, TN 37853
Various types of wheelchairs.

Stryker Medical 800-869-0770
3800 E Centre Ave, Portage, MI 49002

The Universal Handicycle Wheelchair 604-595-8632
2214 Belmont Ave, Victoria V8R 3Z8 Canada
Universal handicycle wheelchair

WHEELCHAIR, MANUAL *(cont'd)*

Theradyne Products Division 800-328-4014
395 Ervin Industrial Dr, Jordan, MN 55352

Tisport, Llc 800-545-2266
1426 E 3rd Ave, Kennewick, WA 99337
Rigid manual wheelchair.

Tuffcare 800-367-6160
3999 E La Palma Ave, Anaheim, CA 92807

Turbo Wheelchair Co., Inc. 843-322-0486
45 Laurel Bay Rd, Suite 3 & 15, Beaufort, SC 29906
Manual wheelchair.

Wheelchair Sales And Service Co., Inc. 877-736-0376
315 Main St, West Springfield, MA 01089
Invacare: Everest & Jennings.

Wheelchairs Of Kansas 800-537-6454
204 W 2nd St, Ellis, KS 67637
BCW Wheelchair and BCW ADVANTAGE are heavy-duty wide wheelchairs. BCW Wheelchair can be ordered with up to 1000 lb weight capacity with customized specifications. The ADVANTAGE holds 850 lbs.and customized seat width to 34 in. Both chairs have stainless steel construction and have expectional warranties.

Youngs, Inc. 800-523-5454
55 E Cherry Ln, Souderton, PA 18964

WHEELCHAIR, POWERED *(Physical Med) 89ITI*

A.R.C. Distributors 800-296-8724
PO Box 599, Centreville, MD 21617
INVACARE, E & J Action, Quest, Metro Series powered wheelchairs. Large variety of sizes and models with all accessories and options. Also available, Youth Mobile and Action Series. Wheelchairs of Kansas, Overlander, battery operated, 750lb limit.

Access Mobility, Inc. 800-336-1147
5240 Elmwood Ave, Indianapolis, IN 46203

Alan's Wheelchairs & Repairs 800-693-4344
109 S Harbor Blvd Ste B, Fullerton, CA 92832
Six-wheeled, power wheelchair that combines high performance with elegant style.

American Biomed Instruments, Inc. 718-235-8900
11 Wyona St, Brooklyn, NY 11207

Applied Resources Corp. 973-575-0650
1275 Bloomfield Ave, Fairfield, NJ 07004
Rtd robotic arm.

Chief Power Chair, Llc 520-722-5265
8051 E Lakeside Pkwy Ste 113, Tucson, AZ 85730
Power wheelchair.

Eagle Health Supplies, Inc. 800-755-8999
535 W Walnut Ave, Orange, CA 92868
EAGLE 2 in 1 Commode Wheelchair - Wheelchair has commode built in so that patient does not need to leave chair in order to use the commode.

Eagle Parts & Products, Inc. 706-790-6687
1411 Marvin Griffin Rd, Augusta, GA 30906
Wheel power (electric) wheelchair.

Electric Mobility Corporation 800-718-2082
591 Mantua Blvd, PO Box 450, Sewell, NJ 08080

Enhanced Mobility Solutions
6910 Dixie Ave, Inver Grove Heights, MN 55076
Powered wheelchair.

Evermed Corp. 714-777-9997
4999 E La Palma Ave, Anaheim, CA 92807
Powered wheelchair.

Fortress Scientifique Du Quebec Ltee. 418-847-5225
2160 Rue De Celles, Quebec G2C 1X8 Canada
Various powered wheelchairs varying in shape,size and features

Golden Technologies, Inc. 800-624-6374
401 Bridge St, Old Forge, PA 18518
Golden Technologies offers four different power wheelchairs: The Alero, The Golden Compass, The Alante and The Alante HD. Weight capacities range from 250 to 425 pounds.

Gould Discount Medical 800-876-6846
3901 Dutchmans Ln Ste 100, Louisville, KY 40207

Handicap Unlimited, Inc. 888-371-0095
5640 Summer Ave Ste 3, Memphis, TN 38134

Hoveround Corporation 800-964-6837
2151 Whitfield Industrial Way, Sarasota, FL 34243
MPV4, TEKNIQUE FWD, TEKNIQUE XHD, TEKNIQUE GT and TEKNIQUE RWD.

WHEELCHAIR, POWERED *(cont'd)*

Invacare Canada 800-668-5324
5970 Chedworth Way, Mississauga, ONT L5R 3T9 Canada

Invacare Corporation 800-333-6900
1 Invacare Way, Elyria, OH 44035
INVACARE Pronto M51, M71, M71 jr, M91, M94; Storm Series Arrow, Ranger X and Torque SP; TDX3, TDX4, TDX5; MKIV and MK5 electronics

Jason Marine Enterprises, Inc. 954-346-5240
5494 NW 22nd Ave, Ft Lauderdale, FL 33309
Same.

Joerns Healthcare, Inc. 715-341-3600
1032 N Fourth St, Baldwyn, MS 38824
Powered wheelchair.

Leisure-Lift, Inc. 800-255-0285
1800 Merriam Ln, Kansas City, KS 66106
Scout power wheelchair.

Medical Depot 516-998-4600
99 Seaview Blvd, Port Washington, NY 11050
Powered wheelchair.

Mobilife, Llc 262-646-5433
78 Enterprise Rd Unit D, Delafield, WI 53018
Powered wheelchair.

Motion Concepts 905-695-0134
84 Citation Dr., Concord, ONTAR L4K 3C1 Canada
Power tilt/recline system.

Movingpeople.Net Canada, Inc. 416-739-8333
500 Norfinch Dr, Downsview M3N 1Y4 Canada
Various powered wheelchairs varying in shape, size and features

Ocelco, Inc. 800-328-5343
1111 Industrial Park Rd SW, Brainerd, MN 56401

Palmer Industries 800-847-1304
PO Box 5707, Endicott, NY 13763
$3,700.00 for 3-wheel outdoor wheelchair.

Permobil, Inc. 800-736-0925
6961 Eastgate Blvd, Lebanon, TN 37090
CHAIRMAN Seating system helps maintain skin integrity and reduces the need for help in changing positions. For both adults and children with different power options: recline, tilt, stand, elevate and seat-to-floor.

Pride Mobility Products Corp. 800-800-8586
182 Susquehanna Ave, Exeter, PA 18643

Rivertrail Mobility 501-745-6790
369 Factory Rd, Clinton, AR 72031
Powered wheelchair.

Steven Motor Chair Co. 530-637-5915
20580 Placer Hills Rd, Colfax, CA 95713
Wheel chair.

Teftec Corp. 210-477-0330
12450 Network Blvd, San Antonio, TX 78249
Powered wheelchair.

Theradyne Products Division 800-328-4014
395 Ervin Industrial Dr, Jordan, MN 55352

Trac About, Inc. 800-458-8616
PO Box 502, 1801 SE 9th St., Newton, KS 67114
TracAbout, IRV2000 indoor/outdoor all terrain power chair with tracks.

Tuffcare 800-367-6160
3999 E La Palma Ave, Anaheim, CA 92807

Wheelchair Carrier, Inc. 800-541-3213
203 Matzinger Rd, Toledo, OH 43612
The Roamer Riding Chair, this one-of-a-kind mobility chair weighs only 35 pounds without the battery, folds for compact storage, and will travel 3-6 hours per battery charge.

Wheelchair Sales And Service Co., Inc. 877-736-0376
315 Main St, West Springfield, MA 01089
Invacare, Everest & Jennings, Pride Mobility.

WHEELCHAIR, POWERED *(cont'd)*

Wheelchairs Of Kansas 800-537-6454
204 W 2nd St, Ellis, KS 67637
BCW POWERCHAIR & OVERLANDER/PEV: BCW Powerchair is a traditional powerchair for bariatric individuals for up to 600 lbs., custom built to individuals' specs with stainless steel construction, two 4-pole motors, widths to 26 in., 5-year frame warranty. OVERLANDER/PEV comes in 750 lb. capacity with heavy-duty contruction and widths to 28 in, it meets the mobility needs of the individual with rugged tires, a durable steel frame for strength and power, tested to meet ANSI/RESNA standards, suspension is adjustable allowing for fine-tuning of the individual rider, gear belt drive system and 4-ply tires virtually create an all terrain powerchiar.

21st Century Scientific, Inc. 800-448-3680
4915 N Industrial Way, Coeur D Alene, ID 83815
Power wheelchair.

WHEELCHAIR, SPECIAL GRADE *(Physical Med) 89IQC*

A.R.C. Distributors 800-296-8724
PO Box 599, Centreville, MD 21617
Theradyne, Medline, Wheelchairs of Kansas, Convaquip, Invacare, Gendron Tracer IV, Regency XL manual wheelchairs specifically designed to accommodate special requirements of the bariatric patient. Weight capacities from 350 to 700 lbs. with many accessories and options available. Heavy duty and extra wide. Transcart wheelchair and cart. Because of its size, it discourages theft; anti-fold wheelchair, cart ultramodern design. Wheelchair for patient, cart for belongings. Weight limit 500 lbs. Also available, Stretchair series stretcher to wheelchair, wheelchair to stretcher. Many models available with all accessories. Weight capacity 250 to 800 lbs.

Colours Wheelchair 800-892-8998
860 E Parkridge Ave, Corona, CA 92879
Custom and Ultlalightweigh wheelchairs including; Suspension wheelchairs, 14 lb. wheelchair, sports and pediatric models. Some of the coolest chairs on the planet.

Eagle Sports Chairs 800-932-9380
2351 Parkwood Rd, Snellville, GA 30039

Gendron, Inc. 800-537-2521
400 E Lugbill Rd, Archbold, OH 43502
$394.00 per unit (standard).

Gunnell, Inc. 800-551-0055
8440 State Rd, Millington, MI 48746

Invacare Top End Sports And Recreation Products 800-532-8677
4501 63rd Cir N, Pinellas Park, FL 33781
Terminator custom built wheelchairs used for sports or everyday use. Includes basketball, tennis and quad rugby. Also available, Terminator SS, Terminator Titanium: custom built lightweight wheelchair, with front and rear suspension to give user a very comfortable ride. Invacare Top End Excelerator XLT Pro handcycle.

Leisure-Lift, Inc. 800-255-0285
1800 Merriam Ln, Kansas City, KS 66106
Powered wheelchairs.

Metro Rehab Services 708-361-7060
11551 S Ridgeland Ave, Alsip, IL 60803

Palmer Industries 800-847-1304
PO Box 5707, Endicott, NY 13763
$4,300.00 for large 3-wheel outdoor wheelchair.

Per4max Medical, Llc 972-641-6773
2550 114th St Ste 190, Grand Prairie, TX 75050
Shockwave.

Permobil, Inc. 800-736-0925
6961 Eastgate Blvd, Lebanon, TN 37090
CHAIRMAN ENTRA, front wheeled drive power wheelchair, alternative drive capable. CHAIRMAN 2K, suspension frame power wheelchair - modular seating system. Front wheel drive with alternative drive capabilities.

Primo, Inc. 770-486-7394
417 Dividend Dr Ste B, Peachtree City, GA 30269
Cervical collar.

Stretchair Patient Transfer Systems, Inc, 800-237-1162
8110 Ulmerton Rd, Largo, FL 33771
STRETCHAIR, converts from wheelchair to stretcher in a single movement, able to accommodate patients weighing up to 800lbs

Triaid, Inc. 301-759-3525
637 N Centre St, Cumberland, MD 21502
Dodgem.

WHEELCHAIR, SPECIAL GRADE *(cont'd)*

Wheelchairs Of Kansas 800-537-6454
204 W 2nd St, Ellis, KS 67637
BCW RECLINER is designed to give the bariatric client a variety of options for positioning and comfort. It is a manual wheelchair constructed with a durable, heavy-duty steel frame, signature double x-brace and powered 45 degree reclining back. It is equipped with a 12 volt battery and user-friendly recharging system.

WHEELCHAIR, STAIR CLIMBING *(Physical Med) 89IMK*

Garaventa (Canada) Ltd. 800-663-6556
7505 - 134A St., Surrey, BC V3W-7B3 Canada
$6,295 for STAIR-TRAC portable wheelchair stair climbing device.

WHEELCHAIR, STANDUP *(Physical Med) 89IPL*

American Emergency Vehicles 800-374-9749
165 American Way, Jefferson, NC 28640
Interfleet wheelchair and transport units.

Davismade, Inc. 866-742-0581
2511 Davison Rd, Flint, MI 48506
STANDING DANI mobile prone wheeled stander.

Levo Usa 888-538-6872
7105 Northland Ter N, Brooklyn Park, Minneapolis, MN 55428

Nestor Machine Co Inc 818-707-1678
5537 Fairview Pl, Agoura Hills, CA 91301
Stand up wheelchair.

Stand-Rite Manufacturing Co. 562-782-6346
16655 Grand Ave, Bellflower, CA 90706
Standing frame, stand aid.

Theradyne Products Division 800-328-4014
395 Ervin Industrial Dr, Jordan, MN 55352

WHOLE BLOOD HEMOGLOBIN DETERMINATION
(Hematology) 81KHG

American Diagnostica, Inc. 888-234-4435
500 West Ave, Stamford, CT 06902
ADIAFLO, flow cytometry whole blood assay kits and monoclonal antibodies.

Teco Diagnostics 714-693-7788
1268 N Lakeview Ave, Anaheim, CA 92807
Hemoglobin.

WHOLE HUMAN PLASMA, ANTIGEN, ANTISERUM, CONTROL
(Immunology) 82DGQ

Bio-Heme 801-277-9392
3710 Ceres Dr, Salt Lake City, UT 84124
Supplier of bulk, disease-state plasma for diagnostic tests.

Biocell Laboratories, Inc. 800-222-8382
2001 E University Dr, Rancho Dominguez, CA 90220

Cell Science Systems, Ltd. Corp. 954-426-2304
1239 E Newport Center Dr Ste 101, Deerfield Beach, FL 33442
White blood cell size and number test kit.

Cortex Biochem, Inc. 800-888-7713
1933 Davis St Ste 321, San Leandro, CA 94577
Primary antibodies for infectious disease, signal enhancement.

Dako North America, Inc 805-566-6655
6392 Via Real, Carpinteria, CA 93013

Fertility Solutions, Inc. 800-959-7656
13000 Shaker Blvd, Cleveland, OH 44120
Antisperm antibody test.

Fitzgerald Industries International, Inc. 800-370-2222
34 Junction Square Dr, Concord, MA 01742

Health Chem Diagnostics Llc 954-979-3845
3341 W McNab Rd, Pompano Beach, FL 33069
Whole blood plasma, antigen, antiserum, control.

Valley Biomedical Products/Ser., Inc. 540-868-0800
121 Industrial Dr, Winchester, VA 22602
Dental curing light.

WICK, EAR *(Ear/Nose/Throat) 77KCN*

Eagle Laboratories 800-782-6534
10201 Trademark St Ste A, Rancho Cucamonga, CA 91730

First Aid Bandage Co., Inc. 888-813-8214
3 State Pier Rd, New London, CT 06320
Ivalon PVA earwicks

Gyrus Ent L.L.C., Sub. Of Gyrus Acmi, Inc. 508-804-2739
2925 Appling Rd, Bartlett, TN 38133
Various types and sizes of ear wicks.

WICK, EAR *(cont'd)*

Micromedics 800-624-5662
1270 Eagan Industrial Rd, Saint Paul, MN 55121
MicroWick for treatment of inner ear disease; MicroWick ET for treatment of chronic eustacian tube dysfunction

Oto-Med, Inc. 800-433-7703
1090 Empire Dr, Lake Havasu City, AZ 86404
Improved faster wicking with controlled expansion. Unique fine open pore structure. 9mm dia.x15mm. Biocompatible

Ultracell Medical Technologies, Inc. 877-SPO-NGE1
183 Providence New London Tpke, North Stonington, CT 06359
ULTRACELL Ear wick; various sizes of ear wick for treating otitis external plus packing the ear canal where other conditions require packing and medication. Available from 7mm to 15mm diameter.

WIPE, INSTRUMENT *(General) 80WPO*

Brain Power, Inc. 800-327-2250
4470 SW 74th Ave, Miami, FL 33155
Kimwipes--$2.25/box of 270, $99.95/case with 60 boxes--highly-creped, bleached-fiber laboratory wipes.

Caig Laboratories, Inc. 800-224-4123
12200 Thatcher Ct, Poway, CA 92064
DeoxIT Gold Wipes for contact and connector conditioning and protecting for electric or battery operated equipment.

Eagle Laboratories 800-782-6534
10201 Trademark St Ste A, Rancho Cucamonga, CA 91730

Globetec Nonwovens 410-287-2207
40 Industrial Rd, North East, MD 21901
Nonwoven substrate for disposable patient wipes. We can provide wipe substrates including Rayon, Tencel, polyester, and polypropylene fibers.

Medela, Inc. 800-435-8316
1101 Corporate Dr, McHenry, IL 60050
QUICK CLEAN WIPES - general cleaning wipes for breastpumps. QUICK CLEAN MICRO-STEAM BAGS - quick sanitizing system for breastpump components.

Palmero Health Care 800-344-6424
120 Goodwin Pl, Stratford, CT 06615
DISCIDE ULTRA disinfecting towelettes. Kills HIV, Herpes and Adenovirus in one minute. Foil packets and canisters.

Ultracell Medical Technologies, Inc. 877-SPO-NGE1
183 Providence New London Tpke, North Stonington, CT 06359
ULTRACELL Instrument wipe. A P.V.A. sponge wipe is used to wipe off delicate surgical instruments. P.V.A. material contains no lint and when moist will not snag in box locks. LASIK wipe.

WIRE, BONE *(Orthopedics) 87UBT*

Fort Wayne Metals Research Prod. Corp. 260-747-4154
9609 Ardmore Ave, Fort Wayne, IN 46809
Various grades, properties and shapes of precision wire, including strands and cables.

Kls-Martin L.P. 800-625-1557
11239-1 St. John`s Industrial, Parkway South
Jacksonville, FL 32250
MARTIN implant tantalum wire made of pure nonalloyed tantalum metal. Optimal deformation, break-proof, bio- compatible.

Kmedic 800-955-0559
190 Veterans Dr, Northvale, NJ 07647
.028 through .062 and Steinmann pins 5/64in. through 3/16in., diamond and trocar styles.

Onyx Medical Corp. 901-323-6699
152 Collins St, Memphis, TN 38112

Simpex Medical, Inc. 800-851-9753
401 E Prospect Ave, Mount Prospect, IL 60056

Stryker Spine 866-457-7463
2 Pearl Ct, Allendale, NJ 07401

Wytech Industries, Inc. 732-396-3900
960 E Hazelwood Ave, Rahway, NJ 07065
Also instrument wire.

WIRE, FIXATION, INTRAOSSEOUS *(Dental And Oral) 76DZK*

Biomet Microfixation Inc. 800-874-7711
1520 Tradeport Dr, Jacksonville, FL 32218
Wire, fixation, intraosseous.

DJO Inc. 800-336-6569
1430 Decision St, Vista, CA 92081
Various suture wires.

WIRE, FIXATION, INTRAOSSEOUS *(cont'd)*

Ideatrics, Inc. 303-417-6353
4845 Pearl East Cir Ste 101, Boulder, CO 80301
Intraosseous fixation wire.

Kmedic 800-955-0559
190 Veterans Dr, Northvale, NJ 07647

Synthes (Usa) 610-719-5000
35 Airport Rd, Horseheads, NY 14845
Various types of sizes of intraosseous fixation wires.

Zimmer Holdings, Inc. 800-613-6131
1800 W Center St, PO Box 708, Warsaw, IN 46580

WIRE, LIGATURE *(Surgery) 79SGE*

Delco Wire Winding Company 610-296-0350
59 Street Rd, Newtown Square, PA 19073

Fort Wayne Metals Research Prod. Corp. 260-747-4154
9609 Ardmore Ave, Fort Wayne, IN 46809
Various grades, properties and shapes of precision wire.

Miltex Inc. 800-645-8000
589 Davies Dr, York, PA 17402

Westcon Orthopedics, Inc. 800-382-4975
4 Craig Rd, Neshanic Station, NJ 08853
Wire, capping device, internal and external.

Wytech Industries, Inc. 732-396-3900
960 E Hazelwood Ave, Rahway, NJ 07065

Zimmer Holdings, Inc. 800-613-6131
1800 W Center St, PO Box 708, Warsaw, IN 46580

WIRE, ORTHODONTIC *(Dental And Oral) 76DZC*

Ace Surgical Supply Co., Inc. 800-441-3100
1034 Pearl St, Brockton, MA 02301

Acme-Monaco Corp. 860-224-1349
75 Winchell Rd, New Britain, CT 06052

Aesculap Implant Systems Inc. 1-800-234-9179
3773 Corporate Pkwy, Center Valley, PA 18034

American Orthodontics Corp. 800-558-7687
1714 Cambridge Ave, Sheboygan, WI 53081

Atlanta Orthodontics 800-535-7166
1247 Zonolite Rd NE, Atlanta, GA 30306
$3.95 per one ART AUXILIARY wire for anterior root torquing. $4.50 per one ACTION ARCHWIRE, a compound curve, 2 loop, stainless archwire.

Biomet Microfixation Inc. 800-874-7711
1520 Tradeport Dr, Jacksonville, FL 32218
Various types of wire.

Cablestrand Corp. 562-595-4527
2660 Signal Pkwy, Signal Hill, CA 90755
Orthodontic arch wire.

Classone Orthodontics, Inc. 806-799-0608
5064 50th St, Lubbock, TX 79414
Various types of wire.

D.C.A. (Dental Corporation Of America) 800-638-6684
889 S Matlack St, West Chester, PA 19382

Forestadent Usa 314-878-5985
2315 Weldon Pkwy, Saint Louis, MO 63146
Orthodontic wire.

Fort Wayne Metals Research Prod. Corp. 260-747-4154
9609 Ardmore Ave, Fort Wayne, IN 46809
Various grades, properties and shapes of precision wire, including turkshead forms.

G & H Wire Co. 800-526-1026
2165 Earlywood Dr, Franklin, IN 46131
Orthodontic arch wire.

Glenroe Technologies 800-237-4060
1912 44th Ave E, Bradenton, FL 34203
Various orthodontic wires.

Gold'N Braces, Inc. 800-785-1970
2595 Tampa Rd Ste 1, Palm Harbor, FL 34684
Gold-plated orthodontic wires.

Highland Metals, Inc. 800-368-6484
419 Perrymont Ave, San Jose, CA 95125
Various.

Kmedic 800-955-0559
190 Veterans Dr, Northvale, NJ 07647

Lancer Orthodontics, Inc. 760-304-2705
253 Pawnee St, San Marcos, CA 92078
Various sizes, finishes and types of orthodontic wire.

WIRE, ORTHODONTIC *(cont'd)*

Lee Pharmaceuticals 626-442-3141
1434 Santa Anita Ave, El Monte, CA 91733
Orthodontic wire.

Masel Co., Inc. 800-423-8227
2701 Bartram Rd, Bristol, PA 19007

Models Plus 800-522-4044
PO Box 600, 605 Grayton Road, Kingsford Heights, IN 46346

Ormco Corp. 800-672-5068
1332 S Lone Hill Ave, Glendora, CA 91740

Ortho Organizers, Inc. 760-448-8730
1822 Aston Ave, Carlsbad, CA 92008
Various types, shapes and sizes of orthodontic wire.

Ortho-Tain, Inc.
Carr 861 # KM5.0, Pinas, Toa Alta, PR 00953
Orthodontic accessory - bumper.

Orthodontic Design And Production, Inc. 760-734-3995
1370 Decision St Ste D, Vista, CA 92081
Various types of orthodontic wire.

Orthodontic Supply & Equipment Co., Inc. 800-638-4003
7851 Airpark Rd Ste 202, Gaithersburg, MD 20879

Oscar, Inc. 317-849-2618
11793 Technology Ln, Fishers, IN 46038
Orthodontic wire.

Prosurge Instruments, Inc. 866-832-7874
199 Laidlaw Ave, Jersey City, NJ 07306

Pyramid Orthodontics 800-752-8884
4328 Redwood Hwy Ste 100, San Rafael, CA 94903

Tp Orthodontics, Inc. 800-348-8856
100 Center Plz, La Porte, IN 46350
Reflex Nickel Titanium, TiMolium, Bow-Flex Preformed archwire.

Ultimate Wireforms, Inc. 800-999-6484
200 Central St, Bristol, CT 06010
Highest quality Nickel titanium, stainless steel, and our own BIII-CNA® wire are used to manufacture archwires and straights in a wide variety of shapes, sizes, and forces.

Ultradent Products, Inc. 801-553-4586
505 W 10200 S, South Jordan, UT 84095
Orthodontic appliance and accessories.

Wytech Industries, Inc. 732-396-3900
960 E Hazelwood Ave, Rahway, NJ 07065

3m Unitek 800-634-5300
2724 Peck Rd, Monrovia, CA 91016

WIRE, SURGICAL *(Orthopedics) 87LRN*

Kls-Martin L.P. 800-625-1557
11239-1 St. John`s Industrial, Parkway South
Jacksonville, FL 32250
MARTIN IMPLANT tantalum wire made of pure nonalloyed tantalum metal. Optimal deformation, break-proof, bio- compatible.

Kmedic 800-955-0559
190 Veterans Dr, Northvale, NJ 07647
Wire Cutter with safety inserts. K-Wire cutter with silicon inserts prevents pieces of cut wire from flying across the O.R.

Koros Usa, Inc. 805-529-0825
610 Flinn Ave, Moorpark, CA 93021
Sternatomy suture.

Synthes (Usa) 610-719-5000
35 Airport Rd, Horseheads, NY 14845
Various types and sizes of surgical wires.

Vilex, Inc. 800-872-4911
345 Old Curry Hollow Rd, Pittsburgh, PA 15236

Warsaw Orthopedic, Inc. 901-396-3133
2500 Silveus Xing, Warsaw, IN 46582
Surgical cable.

WOUND CLEANER, ULTRASOUND *(Surgery) 79NRB*

Celleration, Inc. 952-224-8700
10250 Valley View Rd Ste 137, Eden Prairie, MN 55344
Ultrasonic wound debrider.

WRAP, STERILIZATION *(General) 80FRG*

Abbott Associates 203-878-2370
620 West Ave, Milford, CT 06461
Tyvek lids and pouches, printed & unprinted.

WRAP, STERILIZATION *(cont'd)*

Aesculap Implant Systems Inc. 1-800-234-9179
3773 Corporate Pkwy, Center Valley, PA 18034
STERILCONTAINER system for holding, transporting, storing, and sterilizing surgical instruments.

Ahlstrom Windsor Locks Llc 860-654-8300
2 Elm St, Windsor Locks, CT 06096

Andersen Products, Inc., 800-523-1276
3202 Caroline Dr, Health Science Park, Haw River, NC 27258

Atd-American Co. 800-523-2300
135 Greenwood Ave, Wyncote, PA 19095

Boyd Converting Co., Inc. 800-262-2242
PO Box 287, South Lee, MA 01260
Sterilization wrap.

Busse Hospital Disposables, Inc. 631-435-4711
75 Arkay Dr, Hauppauge, NY 11788
Csr wrap.

Case Medical, Inc. 888-227-2273
65 Railroad Ave, Ridgefield, NJ 07657
MEDITRAY-STERITITE sealed container. The STERITITE product line is a reusable rigid sterilization container system intended to be used for the sterilization of surgical instruments.

Clive Craig Co. 805-488-1122
600 E Hueneme Rd, Oxnard, CA 93033
Sterilization pouch.

Coltene/Whaledent Inc. 330-916-8858
235 Ascot Pkwy, Cuyahoga Falls, OH 44223
Instrument cassette.

Conflex 800-225-4296
6637 N Sidney Pl, Milwaukee, WI 53209
Shrink packaging for form, fill and seal.

Deuteronomy Management Services,Inc. 850-897-3321
1439 Live Oak St Ste A, Niceville, FL 32578
Various.

Dowling Textiles 770-957-3981
615 Macon Rd, McDonough, GA 30253
Sterilization wrap.

East Texas Lighthouse For The Blind 903-595-3444
500 N Bois D Arc Ave, Tyler, TX 75702
No common name listed.

General Hospital Supply Corp. 704-225-9500
2844 Gray Fox Rd, Monroe, NC 28110
Sterilization wrap.

Global Healthcare 800-601-3880
1495 Hembree Rd Ste 700, Roswell, GA 30076
SMS Sterilization Wraps in various sizes

Health-Pak, Inc. 315-724-8370
2005 Beechgrove Pl, Utica, NY 13501

Hpk Industries Llc 315-724-0196
1208 Broad St, Utica, NY 13501
Csr wrap various types for sizes.

Hu-Friedy Manufacturing Co., Inc. 800-483-7433
3232 N Rockwell St, Chicago, IL 60618
$99.50 to $159.50 per case, 4 sizes.

Icd, Inc. 866-791-2503
PO Box 218, Imperial Beach, CA 91933
Neoprene wraps.

Jms Converters Inc Dba Sabee Products & Stanford Prof Prod 215-396-3302
67 Buck Rd Ste B7, Huntingdon Valley, PA 19006

Kerr Group 800-524-3577
1400 Holcomb Bridge Rd, Roswell, GA 30076

Kleen Laundry & Drycleaning Services, Inc. 603-448-1134
1 Foundry St, Lebanon, NH 03766
Sterile wrapper.

Lorvic Corp. 800-325-1881
13705 Shoreline Ct E, Earth City, MO 63045
Nylon tubing.

M & Q Packaging Corp. 877-726-7287
Earl Street, Schuylkill Haven, PA 17972
Nylon sterilization tubing and bags.

Medical Action Industries, Inc. 800-645-7042
25 Heywood Rd, Arden, NC 28704
Overwrap.

WRAP, STERILIZATION *(cont'd)*

Medline Industries, Inc. 800-633-5886
1 Medline Pl, Mundelein, IL 60060

Medtronic Navigation, Inc. 888-580-8860
826 Coal Creek Cir, Louisville, CO 80027
Sterilization wrap.

Mydent International 800-275-0020
80 Suffolk Ct, Hauppauge, NY 11788
DEFEND Blue tinted transparent film assists in detecting any tears caused by instruments. Indicator arrows change color when sterilization is complete.

Pacon Manufacturing Corporation 732-357-8020
400 Pierce St # B, Somerset, NJ 08873

Pelton Shepherd Industries 800-258-3423
812B W Luce St, Stockton, CA 95203
Reusable compression wrap for 5 x 10 ice pack.

Products For Medicine 800-333-3087
1201 E Ball Rd Ste H, Anaheim, CA 92805
Disposable sterilization wrap.

Propper Manufacturing Co., Inc. 800-832-4300
3604 Skillman Ave, Long Island City, NY 11101

Quality Products Of Montana 406-544-0305
4022 Timberlane St, Missoula, MT 59802
Reusable sterilization pouch.

Sri Surgical 813-891-9550
6801 Longe St, Stockton, CA 95206
Sterilization wrap, sterile and non-sterile.

Standard Textile Co., Inc. 888-999-0400
PO Box 371805, Cincinnati, OH 45222
Wrappers.

Steris Corporation 440-354-2600
6515 Hopkins Rd, Mentor, OH 44060
Sterilization container system.

Terumo Cardiovascular Systems (Tcvs) 800-283-7866
28 Howe St, Ashland, MA 01721
Sterile wrap.

The Hygenic Corp. 800-321-2135
1245 Home Ave, Akron, OH 44310
Various.

Tidi Products, Llc 920-751-4380
570 Enterprise Dr, Neenah, WI 54956
Sterilization wrap, csr wrap.

Zimmer Holdings, Inc. 800-613-6131
1800 W Center St, PO Box 708, Warsaw, IN 46580

Zoetek Medical Sales & Service, Inc. 800-388-6223
668 Phillips Rd, Victor, NY 14564
Complete line of all medical consumables for hospitals, OB/GYN, Vet, ENT and private offices.

WRAPPER, SURGICAL INSTRUMENT (STERILE)
(General) 80SGG

Angelica Image Apparel 800-222-3112
700 Rosedale Ave, Saint Louis, MO 63112

Atd-American Co. 800-523-2300
135 Greenwood Ave, Wyncote, PA 19095

Best Manufacturing Group Llc 800-843-3233
1633 Broadway Fl 18, New York, NY 10019
Cotton, blended barrier, 99% polyester, 1% carbon filament.

Chagrin Safety Supply, Inc. 800-227-0468
8227 Washington St # 1, Chagrin Falls, OH 44023

General Econopak, Inc. 888-871-8568
1725 N 6th St, Philadelphia, PA 19122
GEPCO.

Standard Textile 800-999-0400
1 Knollcrest Dr, Cincinnati, OH 45237

Viscot Medical, Llc 800-221-0658
32 West St, PO Box 351, East Hanover, NJ 07936
2 levels of quality in CSR wrap; 15 sizes (10x10 to 60x72).

WRENCH *(Orthopedics) 87HXC*

Abbott Spine, Inc. 847-937-6100
12708 Riata Vista Cir Ste B-100, Austin, TX 78727
Wrench.

Biomet Microfixation Inc. 800-874-7711
1520 Tradeport Dr, Jacksonville, FL 32218
Wrench.

WRENCH *(cont'd)*

Biomet, Inc. 574-267-6639
56 E Bell Dr, PO Box 587, Warsaw, IN 46582
Various types of orthopedic wrenches.

Depuy Spine, Inc. 800-227-6633
325 Paramount Dr, Raynham, MA 02767
Orthopaedic wrench.

DJO Inc. 800-336-6569
1430 Decision St, Vista, CA 92081

Emporium Specialties Co., Inc. 814-647-8661
10 Foster St, Austin, PA 16720
ES Tools stainless steel wrenches.

Feiter's Inc 414-355-7575
8700 W Port Ave, Milwaukee, WI 53224
Wrench.

Holmed Corporation 508-238-3351
40 Norfolk Ave, South Easton, MA 02375

K2m, Inc. 866-526-4171
751 Miller Dr SE Ste F1, Leesburg, VA 20175
Wrench.

Medtronic Sofamor Danek Instrument Manufacturing 901-396-3133
7375 Adrianne Pl, Bartlett, TN 38133
Various types of orthopedic wrenches.

Medtronic Sofamor Danek Usa, Inc. 901-396-3133
4340 Swinnea Rd, Memphis, TN 38118
Various types of orthopedic wrenches.

Nobel Biocare Usa, Llc 800-579-6515
22715/22725 Savi Ranch Parkway, Yorba Linda, CA 92887
Surgical or prosthetic instrument.

Seven Harvest Intl. Import & Export 765-456-3584
108 N Dixon Rd, Kokomo, IN 46901
Cylinder wrench.

Spine Wave, Inc. 203-944-9494
2 Enterprise Dr Ste 302, Shelton, CT 06484
Wrench.

Stryker Spine 866-457-7463
2 Pearl Ct, Allendale, NJ 07401

Symmetry Medical Usa, Inc. 574-267-8700
486 W 350 N, Warsaw, IN 46582
Orthopedic manual surgical instrument.

Warsaw Orthopedic, Inc. 901-396-3133
2500 Silveus Xing, Warsaw, IN 46582
Various types of orthopedic wrenches.

Zimmer Holdings, Inc. 800-613-6131
1800 W Center St, PO Box 708, Warsaw, IN 46580

Zimmer Spine, Inc. 800-655-2614
7375 Bush Lake Rd, Minneapolis, MN 55439
Wrench.

Zimmer Trabecular Metal Technology 800-613-6131
10 Pomeroy Rd, Parsippany, NJ 07054
Cross bar handle.

WRIST, EXTERNAL LIMB COMPONENT, POWERED
(Physical Med) 89KGH

Jace Systems 800-800-4276
2 Pin Oak Ln Ste 200, Cherry Hill, NJ 08003
The JACE Wrist is a portable anatomical CPM allowing for 135 degrees of total motion for flexion/extension and radial/ulnar deviation. With Features including a Warm-up mode- gently and gradually progresses to the full range of programmed motion, and Dynamic Tension mode- converts CPM to low-load prolonged stress to the tissues while reading tissue resistance and automatically adjusting range of motion.

WRISTLET, PATIENT RETURN *(Gastro/Urology) 78FDL*

Cameron-Miller, Inc. 800-621-0142
5410 W Roosevelt Rd, Road #241, Chicago, IL 60644

Secure Care Products, Inc. 800-451-7917
39 Chenell Dr, Concord, NH 03301
Wandering patient electronic monitoring system.

X-RAY, TOMOGRAPHY, COMPUTED, DENTAL
(Radiology) 90OAS

Veran Medical Technologies, Inc. 314-659-8500
5743 W Park Ave, Saint Louis, MO 63110
IG4

XENON SYSTEM *(Anesthesiology) 73SGH*

Medi/Nuclear Corp. 800-321-5981
4610 Littlejohn St, Baldwin Park, CA 91706
Xenon/Master integrated delivery trapping system.

YOKE, MEDICAL GAS *(Anesthesiology) 73CAM*

Matrx 716-662-6650
145 Mid County Dr, Orchard Park, NY 14127
Yoke blocks.

Matrx By Midmark 800-847-1000
145 Mid County Dr, Orchard Park, NY 14127

Richard Wolf Medical Instruments Corp. 800-323-9653
353 Corporate Woods Pkwy, Vernon Hills, IL 60061

Superior Products, Inc. 216-651-9400
3786 Ridge Rd, Cleveland, OH 44144
Various types.

ZINC OXIDE EUGENOL *(Dental And Oral) 76EMB*

Cadco Dental Products 800-833-8267
600 E Hueneme Rd, Oxnard, CA 93033
$11.00 for ZONE impression paste kit.

Dentek Oral Care, Inc. 865-983-1300
307 Excellence Way, Maryville, TN 37801
DenTek Temparin Filling Material; DenTek Thin Set Cap & Crown Cement

Dshealthcare Inc. 201-871-1232
85 W Forest Ave, Englewood, NJ 07631
Various root canal sealers-periodontal packs.

Dux Dental 800-833-8267
600 E Hueneme Rd, Oxnard, CA 93033
$11.00 for ZONE impression paste kit.

Kerr Corp. 714-516-7400
28200 Wick Rd, Romulus, MI 48174
Dental cement.

Miltex Dental Technologies, Inc. 516-576-6022
589 Davies Dr, York, PA 17402
Zinc oxide for use in dental cements.

Moyco Technologies, Inc. 800-331-8837
200 Commerce Dr, Montgomeryville, PA 18936

Nanomaterials, Inc. 401-433-7022
9 Preston Dr, Barrington, RI 02806
A nanoparticle-sized zince oxide with a spherical morphology. Residual impurity levels meet USP standards for cosmetic formulations. CAS # 1314-13-2

Novocol, Inc. 303-665-7535
416 S Taylor Ave, Louisville, CO 80027
Temporary cement.

Oratech, Llc 801-553-4493
475 W 10200 S, South Jordan, UT 84095
Dental cement (zoe).

Plastodent 718-792-3554
2881 Middletown Rd, Bronx, NY 10461

Pulpdent Corp. 800-343-4342
80 Oakland St, Watertown, MA 02472
Eugenol.

Rite-Dent Manufacturing Corp. 305-693-8626
3750 E 10th Ct, Hialeah, FL 33013
Various types of eugenol USP.

Temrex Corp. 516-868-6221
112 Albany Ave, P.o. Box 182, Freeport, NY 11520
Zinc oxide eugenol with ca (oh 2) temporary cement.

Ultradent Products, Inc. 801-553-4586
505 W 10200 S, South Jordan, UT 84095
Dental cement.

1-NITROSO-2-NAPHTHOL (FLUOROMETRIC), FREE TYROSINE
(Chemistry) 75CDR

Astoria-Pacific,Inc. 800-536-3111
PO Box 830, Clackamas, OR 97015
For measuring free tyrosine in blood serum.

11-DEHYDRO THROMBOXANE B2 KIT, URINARY
(Hematology) 81OBW

Corgenix Medical Corporation 800-729-5661
11575 Main St, Broomfield, CO 80020
11dhTxB2 Test Kit; ASPIRINWORKS TEST KIT

2, 4-DINITROPHENYLHYDRAZINE, LACTATE DEHYDROGENASE
(Chemistry) 75CER

Amresco Inc. 800-366-1313
30175 Solon Industrial Pkwy, Solon, OH 44139
Hitachi, technicon RA, SMAC and SMA systems.

Beckman Coulter, Inc. 800-742-2345
250 S Kraemer Blvd, PO Box 8000, Brea, CA 92821

Dade Behring, Inc. 800-948-3233
1717 Deerfield Rd, Deerfield, IL 60015

Genzyme Corp. 800-325-2436
160 Christian St, Oxford, CT 06478
Pyruvate, kinetic.

Helena Laboratories 409-842-3714
PO Box 752, Beaumont, TX 77704

Raichem, Division Of Hemagen Diagnostics, Inc. 800-438-6100
8225 Mercury Ct, San Diego, CA 92111
LDH (L-P and P-L) lactate dehydrogenase.

2ND ANTIBODY (SPECIES SPECIFIC ANTI-ANIMAL GAMMA GLOBULIN) *(Immunology) 82KTS*

Antibodies, Inc. 800-824-8540
PO Box 1560, Davis, CA 95617
Custom and catalog second antibodies from various antigens and host spp.

Binding Site, Inc., The 800-633-4484
5889 Oberlin Dr Ste 101, San Diego, CA 92121

Biocell Laboratories, Inc. 800-222-8382
2001 E University Dr, Rancho Dominguez, CA 90220

Cortex Biochem, Inc. 800-888-7713
1933 Davis St Ste 321, San Leandro, CA 94577
Magnetic particles; 2nd antibodies-magnetic particles; magnetic separators.

Dako North America, Inc 805-566-6655
6392 Via Real, Carpinteria, CA 93013

Invitrogen Corporation 800-955-6288
101 Lincoln Centre Dr, Foster City, CA 94404

Polysciences, Inc. 800-523-2575
400 Valley Rd, Warrington, PA 18976

Qed Bioscience, Inc. 800-929-2114
10919 Technology Pl Ste C, San Diego, CA 92127
Affinity-purified secondary antibodies either unconjugated or conjugated to horseradish peroxidase, alkaline phosphatase, FITC, or biotin.

Quality Bioresources, Inc. 888-674-7224
1015 N Austin St, Seguin, TX 78155
Liquid or lyophilized.

Grey House Publishing 2011 Title List

Visit **www.greyhouse.com** for Product Information, Table of Contents and Sample Pages

General Reference

American Environmental Leaders: From Colonial Times to the Present
An African Biographical Dictionary
Encyclopedia of African-American Writing
Encyclopedia of American Industries
Encyclopedia of Emerging Industries
Encyclopedia of Global Industries
Encyclopedia of Gun Control & Gun Rights
Encyclopedia of Invasions & Conquests
Encyclopedia of Prisoners of War & Internment
Encyclopedia of Religion & Law in America
Encyclopedia of Rural America
Encyclopedia of the United States Cabinet, 1789-2010
Encyclopedia of Warrior Peoples & Fighting Groups
Environmental Resource Handbook
From Suffrage to the Senate: America's Political Women
Global Terror & Political Risk Assessment
Historical Dictionary of War Journalism
Human Rights in the United States
Nations of the World
Political Corruption in America
Speakers of the House of Representatives, 1789-2009
The Environmental Debate: A Documentary History
The Evolution Wars: A Guide to the Debates
The Religious Right: A Reference Handbook
The Value of a Dollar: 1860-2009
The Value of a Dollar: Colonial Era
University & College Museums, Galleries & Related Facilities
Weather America
World Cultural Leaders of the 20th & 21st Centuries
Working Americans 1880-1999 Vol. I: The Working Class
Working Americans 1880-1999 Vol. II: The Middle Class
Working Americans 1880-1999 Vol. III: The Upper Class
Working Americans 1880-1999 Vol. IV: Their Children
Working Americans 1880-2003 Vol. V: At War
Working Americans 1880-2005 Vol. VI: Women at Work
Working Americans 1880-2006 Vol. VII: Social Movements
Working Americans 1880-2007 Vol. VIII: Immigrants
Working Americans 1770-1869 Vol. IX: Revol. War to the Civil War
Working Americans 1880-2009 Vol. X: Sports & Recreation
Working Americans 1880-2010 Vol. XI: Entrepreneurs & Inventors

Bowker's Books In Print® Titles

Books In Print®
Books In Print® Supplement
American Book Publishing Record® Annual
American Book Publishing Record® Monthly
Books Out Loud™
Bowker's Complete Video Directory™
Children's Books In Print®
Complete Directory of Large Print Books & Serials™
El-Hi Textbooks & Serials In Print®
Forthcoming Books®
Law Books & Serials In Print™
Medical & Health Care Books In Print™
Publishers, Distributors & Wholesalers of the US™
Subject Guide to Books In Print®
Subject Guide to Children's Books In Print®

Business Information

Directory of Business Information Resources
Directory of Mail Order Catalogs
Directory of Venture Capital & Private Equity Firms
Food & Beverage Market Place
Grey House Homeland Security Directory
Grey House Performing Arts Directory
Hudson's Washington News Media Contacts Directory
New York State Directory
Sports Market Place Directory
The Rauch Guides – Industry Market Research Reports

Statistics & Demographics

America's Top-Rated Cities
America's Top-Rated Small Towns & Cities
America's Top-Rated Smaller Cities
Comparative Guide to American Suburbs
Comparative Guide to Health in America
Profiles of... Series – State Handbooks

Health Information

Comparative Guide to American Hospitals
Comparative Guide to Health in America
Complete Directory for Pediatric Disorders
Complete Directory for People with Chronic Illness
Complete Directory for People with Disabilities
Complete Mental Health Directory
Directory of Health Care Group Purchasing Organizations
Directory of Hospital Personnel
HMO/PPO Directory
Medical Device Register
Older Americans Information Directory

Education Information

Charter School Movement
Comparative Guide to American Elementary & Secondary Schools
Complete Learning Disabilities Directory
Educators Resource Directory
Special Education

TheStreet.com Ratings Guides

TheStreet.com Ratings Consumer Box Set
TheStreet.com Ratings Guide to Bank Fees & Service Charges
TheStreet.com Ratings Guide to Banks & Thrifts
TheStreet.com Ratings Guide to Bond & Money Market Mutual Funds
TheStreet.com Ratings Guide to Common Stocks
TheStreet.com Ratings Guide to Credit Unions
TheStreet.com Ratings Guide to Exchange-Traded Funds
TheStreet.com Ratings Guide to Health Insurers
TheStreet.com Ratings Guide to Life & Annuity Insurers
TheStreet.com Ratings Guide to Property & Casualty Insurers
TheStreet.com Ratings Guide to Stock Mutual Funds
TheStreet.com Ratings Ultimate Guided Tour of Stock Investing

Canadian General Reference

Associations Canada
Canadian Almanac & Directory
Canadian Environmental Resource Guide
Canadian Parliamentary Guide
Financial Services Canada
History of Canada
Libraries Canada